MAYO CLINIC
PRACTICE OF CARDIOLOGY

MAYO CLINIC PRACTICE OF CARDIOLOGY

EMILIO R. GIULIANI, M.D.
Chair, Division of Cardiovascular Diseases,
Mayo Clinic Scottsdale, Scottsdale, Arizona;
Professor of Medicine, Mayo Medical School;
Rochester, Minnesota

BERNARD J. GERSH, M.B.,Ch.B., D.Phil.
Chief, Division of Cardiology,
W. Proctor Harvey Teaching Professor of Cardiology,
Georgetown University Medical Center, Washington, D.C.
(Formerly, Consultant, Division of Cardiovascular Diseases and Internal Medicine,
Mayo Clinic and Mayo Foundation;
Professor of Medicine, Mayo Medical School)

MICHAEL D. McGOON, M.D.
Consultant, Division of Cardiovascular Diseases and Internal Medicine,
Mayo Clinic and Mayo Foundation;
Associate Professor of Medicine, Mayo Medical School;
Rochester, Minnesota

DAVID L. HAYES, M.D.
Consultant, Division of Cardiovascular Diseases and Internal Medicine,
Mayo Clinic and Mayo Foundation;
Professor of Medicine, Mayo Medical School;
Rochester, Minnesota

HARTZELL V. SCHAFF, M.D.
Consultant, Section of Cardiovascular Surgery,
Mayo Clinic and Mayo Foundation;
Professor of Surgery, Mayo Medical School;
Rochester, Minnesota

THIRD EDITION

Mosby

St. Louis Baltimore Boston Carlsbad Chicago Naples New York Philadelphia Portland
London Madrid Mexico City Singapore Sydney Tokyo Toronto Wiesbaden

Mosby
Dedicated to Publishing Excellence

A Times Mirror
Company

Publisher: Anne Patterson
Acquisition Editor: Laura DeYoung
Project Manager: Patricia Tannian
Book Design Manager: Gail Morey Hudson
Cover Designer: Gail Morey Hudson
Manufacturing Supervisor: David Graybill

THIRD EDITION

Printed in the United States of America
Composition by Graphic World, Inc.
Printing/binding by Courier Corporation

Mosby–Year Book, Inc.
11830 Westline Industrial Drive
St. Louis, Missouri 63146

Library of Congress Cataloging in Publication Data

Mayo Clinic practice of cardiology / [edited by] Emilio R. Giuliani
... [et al.]. – 3rd ed.
p. cm.
Rev. ed. of: Cardiology. 2nd ed. c1991.
Includes bibliographical references and index.
ISBN 0-8151-4040-1 (hardcover)
1. Heart–Diseases. 2. Cardiology. I. Giuliani, Emilio R.
(Emilio Romolo, 1927- . II. Mayo Clinic. III. Cardiology.
[DNLM: 1. Heart Diseases. WG 200 M473 1996]
RC681.C179 1996
616.1′2–dc20
DNLM/DLC
for Library of Congress 95-36794
CIP

95 96 97 98 99 / 9 8 7 6 5 4 3 2 1

This book is dedicated to
our families

Contributing editors

RICK A. NISHIMURA, M.D.
Consultant, Division of Cardiovascular Diseases and Internal Medicine,
Mayo Clinic and Mayo Foundation;
Professor of Medicine, Mayo Medical School;
Rochester, Minnesota

DAVID R. HOLMES, Jr., M.D.
Consultant, Division of Cardiovascular Diseases and Internal Medicine,
Mayo Clinic and Mayo Foundation;
Professor of Medicine, Mayo Medical School;
Rochester, Minnesota

Contributors

Charles F. Abboud, M.D.
Consultant, Division of Endocrinology, Metabolism, and Internal Medicine, Mayo Clinic and Mayo Foundation; Associate Professor of Medicine, Mayo Medical School; Rochester, Minnesota

Martin D. Abel, M.D.
Consultant, Department of Anesthesiology, Mayo Clinic and Mayo Foundation; Associate Professor of Anesthesiology, Mayo Medical School; Rochester, Minnesota

Thomas G. Allison, Ph.D.
Consultant, Division of Cardiovascular Diseases and Internal Medicine, Mayo Clinic and Mayo Foundation; Assistant Professor of Medicine, Mayo Medical School; Rochester, Minnesota

William T. Bardsley, M.D.
Consultant, Division of Cardiovascular Diseases and Internal Medicine, Mayo Clinic and Mayo Foundation; Assistant Professor of Medicine, Mayo Medical School; Rochester, Minnesota

Malcolm R. Bell, M.B.,B.S.
Consultant, Division of Cardiovascular Diseases and Internal Medicine, Mayo Clinic and Mayo Foundation; Associate Professor of Medicine, Mayo Medical School; Rochester, Minnesota

Peter B. Berger, M.D.
Consultant, Division of Cardiovascular Diseases and Internal Medicine, Mayo Clinic and Mayo Foundation; Assistant Professor of Medicine, Mayo Medical School; Rochester, Minnesota

Joseph L. Blackshear, M.D.
Consultant, Division of Cardiovascular Diseases, Mayo Clinic Jacksonville, Jacksonville, Florida; Associate Professor of Medicine, Mayo Medical School; Rochester, Minnesota

Robert O. Brandenburg, M.D.
Emeritus Member, Division of Cardiovascular Diseases and Internal Medicine, Mayo Clinic and Mayo Foundation; Emeritus Professor of Medicine, Mayo Medical School; Rochester, Minnesota

Jerome F. Breen, M.D.
Consultant, Department of Diagnostic Radiology, Mayo Clinic and Mayo Foundation; Assistant Professor of Radiology, Mayo Medical School; Rochester, Minnesota

Mahlon K. Burbank, M.D.
Consultant, Division of Cardiovascular Diseases and Internal Medicine, Mayo Clinic and Mayo Foundation; Assistant Professor of Medicine, Mayo Medical School; Rochester, Minnesota

John C. Burnett, Jr., M.D.
Consultant, Division of Cardiovascular Diseases and Internal Medicine, and Consultant, Department of Physiology and Biophysics, Mayo Clinic and Mayo Foundation; Professor of Medicine and of Physiology, Mayo Medical School; Rochester, Minnesota

Mark J. Callahan, M.D.
Consultant, Division of Cardiovascular Diseases and Internal Medicine, Mayo Clinic and Mayo Foundation; Assistant Professor of Medicine, Mayo Medical School; Rochester, Minnesota

James H. Chesebro, M.D.
Associate Director, Cardiovascular Institute; Professor of Medicine, Mount Sinai Medical Center; New York, New York (Formerly, Consultant, Division of Cardiovascular Diseases and Internal Medicine, Mayo Clinic and Mayo Foundation; Professor of Medicine, Mayo Medical School)

Ian P. Clements, M.D.
Consultant, Division of Cardiovascular Diseases and Internal Medicine, Mayo Clinic and Mayo Foundation; Assistant Professor of Medicine, Mayo Medical School; Rochester, Minnesota

Roger L. Click, M.D., Ph.D.

Consultant, Division of Cardiovascular Diseases and Internal Medicine, Mayo Clinic and Mayo Foundation; Assistant Professor of Medicine, Mayo Medical School; Rochester, Minnesota

Gordon K. Danielson, M.D.

Consultant, Section of Cardiovascular Surgery, Mayo Clinic and Mayo Foundation; Professor of Surgery, Mayo Medical School; Rochester, Minnesota

David J. Driscoll, M.D.

Head, Section of Pediatric Cardiology, Mayo Clinic and Mayo Foundation; Professor of Pediatrics, Mayo Medical School; Rochester, Minnesota

Brooks S. Edwards, M.D.

Consultant, Division of Cardiovascular Diseases and Internal Medicine, Mayo Clinic and Mayo Foundation; Associate Professor of Medicine, Mayo Medical School; Rochester, Minnesota

William D. Edwards, M.D.

Consultant, Division of Anatomic Pathology, Mayo Clinic and Mayo Foundation; Professor of Pathology, Mayo Medical School; Rochester, Minnesota

Maurice Enriquez-Sarano, M.D.

Consultant, Division of Cardiovascular Diseases and Internal Medicine, Mayo Clinic and Mayo Foundation; Assistant Professor of Medicine, Mayo Medical School; Rochester, Minnesota

Titus C. Evans, Jr., M.D., Ph.D.

Consultant, Division of Cardiovascular Diseases and Internal Medicine, Mayo Clinic and Mayo Foundation; Associate Professor of Medicine, Mayo Medical School; Rochester, Minnesota

William P. Fay, M.D.

Assistant Professor of Internal Medicine, Department of Internal Medicine, University of Michigan Medical Center, Ann Arbor, Michigan

Robert H. Feldt, M.D.

Consultant, Section of Pediatric Cardiology, Mayo Clinic and Mayo Foundation; Professor of Pediatrics, Mayo Medical School; Rochester, Minnesota

Lee A. Forstrom, M.D., Ph.D.

Consultant, Department of Diagnostic Radiology, Mayo Clinic and Mayo Foundation; Assistant Professor of Radiology, Mayo Medical School; Rochester, Minnesota

William K. Freeman, M.D.

Cardiology Consultant, Diagnostic and Interventional Cardiology Consultants, Sacramento, California (Formerly, Consultant, Division of Cardiovascular Diseases and Internal Medicine, Mayo Clinic and Mayo Foundation; Assistant Professor of Medicine, Mayo Medical School)

Valentin Fuster, M.D.

Arthur M. & Hilda A. Master Professor of Medicine, The Mount Sinai School of Medicine; Director, Cardiovascular Institute, The Mount Sinai Medical Center; New York, New York (Formerly, Consultant, Division of Cardiovascular Diseases and Internal Medicine, Mayo Clinic and Mayo Foundation)

Kirk N. Garratt, M.D.

Consultant, Division of Cardiovascular Diseases and Internal Medicine, Mayo Clinic and Mayo Foundation; Assistant Professor of Medicine, Mayo Medical School; Rochester, Minnesota

Gerald T. Gau, M.D.

Consultant, Division of Cardiovascular Diseases and Internal Medicine, Mayo Clinic and Mayo Foundation; Associate Professor of Medicine, Mayo Medical School; Rochester Minnesota

Raymond J. Gibbons, M.D.

Consultant, Division of Cardiovascular Diseases and Internal Medicine, Mayo Clinic and Mayo Foundation; Professor of Medicine, Mayo Medical School; Rochester, Minnesota

Donald J. Hagler, M.D.

Consultant, Section of Pediatric Cardiology, Mayo Clinic and Mayo Foundation; Professor of Pediatrics, Mayo Medical School; Rochester, Minnesota

Stephen C. Hammill, M.D.

Consultant, Division of Cardiovascular Diseases and Internal Medicine, Mayo Clinic and Mayo Foundation; Professor of Medicine, Mayo Medical School; Rochester, Minnesota

Sharonne N. Hayes, M.D.

Consultant, Division of Cardiovascular Diseases and Internal Medicine, Mayo Clinic and Mayo Foundation; Assistant Professor of Medicine, Mayo Medical School; Rochester, Minnesota

Stuart T. Higano, M.D.

Consultant, Division of Cardiovascular Diseases and Internal Medicine, Mayo Clinic and Mayo Foundation; Assistant Professor of Medicine, Mayo Medical School; Rochester, Minnesota

Donald L. Johnston, M.D.

Consultant, Division of Cardiovascular Diseases, Mayo Clinic and Mayo Foundation; Associate Professor of Medicine, Mayo Medical School; Rochester, Minnesota

Paul R. Julsrud, M.D.

Consultant, Department of Diagnostic Radiology, Mayo Clinic and Mayo Foundation; Associate Professor of Radiology, Mayo Medical School; Rochester, Minnesota

Barry L. Karon, M.D.

Consultant, Division of Cardiovascular Diseases and Internal Medicine, Mayo Clinic and Mayo Foundation; Instructor in Medicine, Mayo Medical School; Rochester, Minnesota

Stephen L. Kopecky, M.D.

Consultant, Division of Cardiovascular Diseases and Internal Medicine, Mayo Clinic and Mayo Foundation; Assistant Professor of Medicine, Mayo Medical School; Rochester, Minnesota

Thomas E. Kottke, M.D.

Consultant, Division of Cardiovascular Diseases and Internal Medicine, Mayo Clinic and Mayo Foundation; Professor of Medicine, Mayo Medical School; Rochester, Minnesota

J.T. Lie, M.D.

Professor and Director, Divison of Anatomic Pathology, University of California Davis Medical Center, Sacramento, California (Formerly, Consultant, Division of Anatomic Pathology and Division of Cardiovascular Diseases and Internal Medicine, Mayo Clinic and Mayo Foundation; former Professor of Pathology, Mayo Medical School)

John J. Lynch, M.D.

Consultant, Division of Cardiovascular Diseases, Mayo Clinic Scottsdale, Scottsdale, Arizona; Assistant Professor of Medicine, Mayo Medical School; Rochester, Minnesota

Douglas D. Mair, M.D.

Consultant, Section of Pediatric Cardiology, and Consultant, Division of Cardiovascular Diseases and Internal Medicine, Mayo Clinic and Mayo Foundation; Professor of Pediatrics and Associate Professor of Medicine, Mayo Medical School; Rochester, Minnesota

Sylvia A. Mamby, M.D.

Consultant, Division of Cardiovascular Diseases, Mayo Clinic Scottsdale, Scottsdale, Arizona; Assistant Professor of Medicine, Mayo Medical School; Rochester, Minnesota

Harold T. Mankin, M.D.

Emeritus Member, Division of Cardiovascular Diseases and Internal Medicine, Mayo Clinic and Mayo Foundation; Emeritus Assistant Professor of Medicine, Mayo Medical School; Rochester, Minnesota

Craig N. Mattson, R.Ph., M.S., M.B.A.

Pharmacist, Mayo Clinic and Mayo Foundation, Rochester, Minnesota

Dwight C. McGoon, M.D.

Emeritus Member, Division of Cardiovascular Diseases and Internal Medicine, Mayo Clinic and Mayo Foundation; Emeritus Professor of Medicine, Mayo Medical School; Rochester, Minnesota

Christopher G. A. McGregor, M.D.

Consultant, Section of Cardiovascular Surgery, Mayo Clinic and Mayo Foundation; Professor of Surgery, Mayo Medical School; Rochester, Minnesota

Virginia V. Michels, M.D.

Chair, Department of Medical Genetics, Mayo Clinic and Mayo Foundation; Professor of Medical Genetics, Mayo Medical School; Rochester, Minnesota

Fletcher A. Miller, Jr., M.D.

Consultant, Division of Cardiovascular Diseases and Internal Medicine, Mayo Clinic and Mayo Foundation; Associate Professor of Medicine, Mayo Medical School; Rochester, Minnesota

Todd D. Miller, M.D.

Consultant, Division of Cardiovascular Diseases and Internal Medicine, Mayo Clinic and Mayo Foundation; Associate Professor of Medicine, Mayo Medical School; Rochester, Minnesota

Wayne L. Miller, M.D.

Consultant, Division of Cardiovascular Diseases and Internal Medicine, Mayo Clinic and Mayo Foundation; Assistant Professor of Medicine, Mayo Medical School; Rochester, Minnesota

Michael B. Mock, M.D.

Consultant, Division of Cardiovascular Diseases and Internal Medicine, Mayo Clinic and Mayo Foundation; Professor of Medicine, Mayo Medical School; Rochester, Minnesota

James P. Morgan, M.D., Ph.D.

Beth Israel Hospital, Boston, Massachusetts (Formerly, Senior Clinical Fellow, Division of Cardiovascular Diseases and Internal Medicine, Mayo Clinic and Mayo Foundation)

Pamela B. Morris, M.D.

Consultant, Division of Cardiovascular Diseases and Internal Medicine, Mayo Clinic and Mayo Foundation; Assistant Professor of Medicine, Mayo Medical School; Rochester, Minnesota

Charles J. Mullany, M.B.,B.S.
Consultant, Section of Cardiovascular Surgery, Mayo Clinic and Mayo Foundation; Associate Professor of Surgery, Mayo Medical School; Rochester, Minnesota

Tu T. Nguyen, M.D.
Consultant, Division of Endocrinology, Metabolism, and Internal Medicine, Mayo Clinic and Mayo Foundation; Assistant Professor of Medicine, Mayo Medical School; Rochester, Minnesota

Barbara A. Nichols, R.N., R.D.C.S.
Supervisor, Division of Cardiovascular Diseases and Internal Medicine, Mayo Clinic and Mayo Foundation; Rochester, Minnesota

Michael K. O'Connor, Ph.D.
Consultant, Department of Diagnostic Radiology, Mayo Clinic and Mayo Foundation; Associate Professor of Radiologic Physics, Mayo Medical School; Rochester, Minnesota

Jae K. Oh, M.D.
Consultant, Division of Cardiovascular Diseases and Internal Medicine, Mayo Clinic and Mayo Foundation; Associate Professor of Medicine, Mayo Medical School; Rochester, Minnesota

Byron A. Olney, M.D.
Consultant, Division of Cardiovascular Diseases and Internal Medicine, Mayo Clinic and Mayo Foundation; Assistant Professor of Medicine, Mayo Medical School; Rochester, Minnesota

Lyle J. Olson, M.D.
Consultant, Division of Cardiovascular Diseases and Internal Medicine, Mayo Clinic and Mayo Foundation; Assistant Professor of Medicine, Mayo Medical School; Rochester, Minnesota

Michael J. Osborn, M.D.
Consultant, Division of Cardiovascular Diseases and Internal Medicine, Mayo Clinic and Mayo Foundation; Assistant Professor of Medicine, Mayo Medical School; Rochester, Minnesota

Douglas L. Packer, M.D.
Consultant, Division of Cardiovascular Diseases and Internal Medicine, Mayo Clinic and Mayo Foundation; Associate Professor of Medicine, Mayo Medical School; Rochester, Minnesota

Patricia A. Pellikka, M.D.
Consultant, Division of Cardiovascular Diseases and Internal Medicine, Mayo Clinic and Mayo Foundation; Assistant Professor of Medicine, Mayo Medical School; Rochester, Minnesota

Francisco J. Puga, M.D.
Chair, Division of Thoracic and Cardiovascular Surgery, Mayo Clinic and Mayo Foundation; Professor of Surgery, Mayo Medical School; Rochester, Minnesota

Margaret M. Redfield, M.D.
Consultant, Division of Cardiovascular Diseases and Internal Medicine, Mayo Clinic and Mayo Foundation; Assistant Professor of Medicine, Mayo Medical School; Rochester, Minnesota

Guy S. Reeder, M.D.
Consultant, Division of Cardiovascular Diseases and Internal Medicine, Mayo Clinic and Mayo Foundation; Professor of Medicine, Mayo Medical School; Rochester, Minnesota

Richard J. Rodeheffer, M.D.
Consultant, Division of Cardiovascular Diseases and Internal Medicine, Mayo Clinic and Mayo Foundation; Associate Professor of Medicine, Mayo Medical School; Rochester, Minnesota

Thom W. Rooke, M.D.
Consultant, Division of Cardiovascular Diseases and Internal Medicine, Mayo Clinic and Mayo Foundation; Associate Professor of Medicine, Mayo Medical School; Rochester, Minnesota

Edward C. Rosenow III, M.D., M.S.
Consultant, Division of Thoracic Diseases and Internal Medicine, Mayo Clinic and Mayo Foundation; Professor of Medicine, Mayo Medical School; Rochester, Minnesota

John A. Rumberger, Ph.D., M.D.
Consultant, Division of Cardiovascular Diseases and Internal Medicine, Mayo Clinic and Mayo Foundation; Associate Professor of Medicine, Mayo Medical School; Rochester, Minnesota

Jay H. Ryu, M.D.
Consultant, Division of Thoracic Diseases and Internal Medicine, Mayo Clinic and Mayo Foundation; Associate Professor of Medicine, Mayo Medical School; Rochester, Minnesota

Robert E. Safford, M.D., Ph.D.
Chair, Division of Cardiovascular Diseases, Mayo Clinic Jacksonville, Jacksonville, Florida; Associate Professor of Medicine, Mayo Medical School; Rochester, Minnesota

Thomas T. Schattenberg, M.D.
Consultant, Division of Cardiovascular Diseases and Internal Medicine, Mayo Clinic and Mayo Foundation; Associate Professor of Medicine, Mayo Medical School; Rochester, Minnesota

John P. Scott, M.D.

Consultant, Division of Thoracic Diseases and Internal Medicine, Mayo Clinic and Mayo Foundation; Associate Professor of Medicine, Mayo Medical School; Rochester, Minnesota

James B. Seward, M.D.

Consultant, Division of Cardiovascular Diseases and Internal Medicine, and Consultant, Section of Pediatric Cardiology, Mayo Clinic and Mayo Foundation; Professor of Medicine and of Pediatrics, Mayo Medical School; Rochester, Minnesota

Patrick F. Sheedy, M.D.

Consultant, Department of Diagnostic Radiology, Mayo Clinic and Mayo Foundation; Professor of Radiology, Mayo Medical School; Rochester, Minnesota

Win-Kuang Shen, M.D.

Consultant, Division of Cardiovascular Diseases and Internal Medicine, Mayo Clinic and Mayo Foundation; Associate Professor of Medicine, Mayo Medical School; Rochester, Minnesota

Sheldon G. Sheps, M.D.

Chair, Division of Hypertension and Internal Medicine, Mayo Clinic and Mayo Foundation; Professor of Medicine, Mayo Medical School; Rochester, Minnesota

Clarence Shub, M.D.

Consultant, Division of Cardiovascular Diseases and Internal Medicine, Mayo Clinic and Mayo Foundation; Professor of Medicine, Mayo Medical School; Rochester, Minnesota

J. Christopher Sill, M.B.,B.S.

Consultant, Department of Anesthesiology, Mayo Clinic and Mayo Foundation; Associate Professor of Anesthesiology, Mayo Medical School; Rochester, Minnesota

Hugh C. Smith, M.D.

Consultant, Division of Cardiovascular Diseases and Internal Medicine, Mayo Clinic and Mayo Foundation; Professor of Medicine, Mayo Medical School; Rochester, Minnesota

Peter C. Spittell, M.D.

Consultant, Division of Cardiovascular Diseases and Internal Medicine, Mayo Clinic and Mayo Foundation; Assistant Professor of Medicine, Mayo Medical School; Rochester, Minnesota

Ray W. Squires, Ph.D.

Director, Cardiovascular Health Clinic, Mayo Clinic and Mayo Foundation; Associate Professor of Medicine, Mayo Medical School; Rochester, Minnesota

Anthony W. Stanson, M.D.

Consultant, Department of Diagnostic Radiology, Mayo Clinic and Mayo Foundation; Associate Professor of Radiology, Mayo Medical School; Rochester, Minnesota

Robert G. Tancredi, M.D.

Consultant, Division of Cardiovascular Diseases, Mayo Clinic Scottsdale, Scottsdale, Arizona; Associate Professor of Medicine, Mayo Medical School; Rochester, Minnesota

Eric G. Tangalos, M.D.

Consultant, Division of Community Internal Medicine, Mayo Clinic and Mayo Foundation; Associate Professor of Medicine, Mayo Medical School; Rochester, Minnesota

Juergen E. Thomas, M.D.

Emeritus Member, Department of Neurology, Mayo Clinic and Mayo Foundation; Emeritus Professor of Neurology, Mayo Medical School; Rochester, Minnesota

Carole A. Warnes, M.D.

Consultant, Division of Cardiovascular Diseases and Internal Medicine, Mayo Clinic and Mayo Foundation; Associate Professor of Medicine, Mayo Medical School; Rochester, Minnesota

William H. Weidman, M.D.

Emeritus Member, Section of Pediatric Cardiology, Mayo Clinic and Mayo Foundation; Emeritus Professor of Pediatrics, Mayo Medical School; Rochester, Minnesota

Arnold M. Weissler, M.D.

Consultant, Division of Cardiovascular Diseases and Internal Medicine, Mayo Clinic and Mayo Foundation; Professor of Medicine, Mayo Medical School; Rochester, Minnesota

Roger D. White, M.D.

Consultant, Division of Cardiovascular and Thoracic Anesthesia, Mayo Clinic and Mayo Foundation; Professor of Anesthesiology, Mayo Medical School; Rochester, Minnesota

Douglas L. Wood, M.D.

Consultant, Division of Cardiovascular Diseases and Internal Medicine, Mayo Clinic and Mayo Foundation; Associate Professor of Medicine, Mayo Medical School; Rochester, Minnesota

Prince K. Zachariah, M.D., Ph.D.

Chair, Division of Hypertension/Nephrology, Mayo Clinic Jacksonville, Jacksonville, Florida; Professor of Medicine and Assistant Professor of Pharmacology, Mayo Medical School; Rochester, Minnesota

Foreword

WE hold this book today and wonder about its impact on the future of Cardiology in much the same way a voyager planning an expedition into wild, uncharted country prepares for that experience. That voyager must provide for protection from the elements, for regular sustenance, and for a reasonable amount of comfort. His potential for success will be enhanced by having even partial maps of the region and knowledge of its hazards, of its beauty spots, of its history, and of the experiences of travelers who have preceded him.

Foremost, however, the voyager must have a keen desire for exploration and a curiosity about the hidden. The desire will offset the inevitable hardships; the curiosity will allow openness to new, perhaps as yet undescribed, phenomena and thus permit better delineation and understanding of what others have observed earlier.

Not the least of the requirements for the successful and rewarding experience is that the voyager share with those who have gone before and with those who will follow, share not only in the excitement of witnessing phenomena but also in understanding their meaning. With such sharing, even the novice is not a complete novice. Without such sharing, a swelling apparent at the top of a Norway pine, for example, is an unexplained swelling. With sharing, even the novice may recognize that it is a bald eagle perched on the tree. And recognizing and watching, he may prove to himself that it is so even as the bird flies away from its perch. Without sharing, all waters may look alike. With sharing, the novice may know ahead of time about shallow, rocky bottoms and avoid their potential hazards.

The voyager who has prepared adequately and who maintains a keen awareness comes back having achieved personal fulfillment and having become a source of valuable information and help to others who someday will travel the same area. In a manner, any student in Medicine, the Cardiologist included, is a voyager into country that is only partially charted. This book may be considered a comprehensive guide for the Cardiology voyager. Among those who will use it as a guide, experience in Cardiology will be of the greatest possible diversity; these voyagers will range from the novice to the highly experienced physician. Despite this broad array of experience, this book will have knowledge new to each. No voyager, however experienced, will have seen every element of the terrain.

This book is a handbook, comprehensive and detailed, designed to invite, excite, and guide the Cardiologist. Its foundation is the extensive experience of its many authors, experience that collectively is as broad as the entire field of medicine. The many areas of interest among the authors might have led, without proper coordination, to many unintegrated chapters. But that has been avoided by the close teamwork and interdigitation of ideas among members of the Staff of the Mayo Clinic.

The result of this teamwork is even more positive: a collection of facts and concepts that are coordinated beautifully, presented clearly, and illustrated elegantly. Of biblical type, it holds both facts and implications for deductions, so that it is both a source of illumination and a stimulus of thought.

To those who make use of it in the future, this book will supply facts about phenomena, will show how seemingly subtle phenomena can be woven into diagnoses, and will describe what can be done to help the patient affected by cardiac disease. The book will do more. Its approach is such as to magnify curiosity, and this is one of the elements of its greatness because it is only through curiosity that the unknown of today will be revealed tomorrow.

Jesse E. Edwards, M.D.

Senior Consultant,
Registry of Cardiovascular Diseases,
United Hospital,
St. Paul, Minnesota;
Professor of Pathology,
University of Minnesota,
Minneapolis, Minnesota

Preface

THE purpose of this book, *Mayo Clinic Practice of Cardiology*, is to share with our readers the experience of one institution's integrated clinical approach to the management of patients with cardiac disorders. To achieve this goal in the third edition, we have changed our format for presenting the basic science portion of the book. In previous editions, basic mechanisms were presented in separate chapters at the beginning of the textbook. In this edition, pertinent aspects of basic physiology and pathophysiology are incorporated in each chapter.

We have shortened most chapters, limited references to those we believe most relevant, and added more illustrations, graphs, and tables. The primary purpose of these changes was to condense the material into one volume. By achieving this, we believe that the book will be more user-friendly for physicians responsible for the care of patients with cardiac disorders.

Significant revisions have been made in nearly every chapter and major revisions in most chapters. New chapters have been added to incorporate the progress in cardiology since the previous edition.

An undertaking of this magnitude requires the combined effort of many individuals, and we the editors are indebted to all those who contributed to this edition. First, we wish to express gratitude to our authors, each of whom made important contributions. They all have been most gracious in accepting criticism and revising their chapters to meet the goals of this project.

A special thank you is extended to John L. Prickman, Editor; Roberta Schwartz, Supervisor; Sharon Wadleigh, Lead Editorial Assistant and Coordinator; Mary Schwager, Lead Proofreader; Jen Schlotthauer, Office Assistant; and all their colleagues in the Section of Publications at the Mayo Clinic. Their contribution to this book is enormous.

It has been a singular pleasure to work with Laura DeYoung, Acquisitions Editor, and her associates at Mosby. Their enthusiasm, interest, and commitment were vital and are sincerely appreciated.

With this third edition, I will join the other original editors, Drs. Robert O. Brandenburg, Valentin Fuster, and Dwight C. McGoon, in passing on the responsibility for succeeding editions. In doing so, I am convinced that the "ship" we give the editors of the fourth edition is sound and traveling the proper course. I have full confidence that these editors and the editors to follow will continue with the same philosophical perspective embodied in the first three editions.

Emilio R. Giuliani, M.D.

Contents

Mayo Clinic
Practice of Cardiology

PART I *Diagnostic and Therapeutic Modalities*

CHAPTER

1

The history

Arnold M. Weissler, M.D.

MEDICINE is an art based on scientific knowledge and principles and practiced for the benefit of ailing human beings. Cardiology is a branch of that art, devoted to the care of those with disorders of the heart and circulation. In practicing his* art, the cardiologist has three primary goals: to discover what is wrong, to know how to ameliorate it, and to render care and bring comfort to his patient. In meeting these goals, he directs the breadth of his knowledge, judgment, and skills in cardiovascular medicine to the individual needs of the patients who seek his aid. Nowhere in the disciplined approach to the evaluation of the patient is there a more opportune occasion to approach such individualization than that provided during the taking of the cardiovascular history. Through the history, the consultant acquires a base of information from which he will plan and implement the initial evaluation and treatment of his patient. At the same time, he establishes a blending of human trust and confidence between physician and patient, which is the setting for his third goal, care of the patient.

In our contemporary era of advancing science and technology, of constraints on time and resources, and of economic preoccupation, some have attempted to relegate the history to vicarious practices such as interviews by a physician's assistant or nurse-clinician, use of computer questionnaires, or working of simple checklists. In the view of the author, this is a singularly regrettable and indeed regressive practice. When one considers the unprecedented scientific and technologic advances of recent decades, the uncertainties in diagnosis and treatment that nevertheless continue to exist, and the breadth of knowledge and acuity that cardiovascular practice demands, the responsibility for eliciting the history directly from the patient rests today, all the more, on the shoulders of the most expert member of the health care team, the physician. This view is supported in studies documenting the critical position of the cardiovascular history in the hierarchy of diagnostic procedures[1,2] and the clear diagnostic superiority of the physician's history over that acquired by nonphysicians or self-administered questionnaires.[3]

Previous volumes of this textbook have presented a detailed review of the basic mechanisms for the cardinal cardiovascular symptoms. In this chapter, these discussions are not reiterated. Rather, the focus is on the process of history-taking, with emphasis on the skills that are fundamental to its success as a precursor to diagnosis, therapy, and patient care.

THE PSYCHOLOGIC ENVIRONMENT OF THE HISTORY

Much remains beyond the realm of scientific scrutiny in the contemporary practice of cardiology. This is most evident when one reflects on the interaction between patient and consultant during their initial meeting. The reasons for the need of a specialist range widely: a worrisome symptom; a constellation of abnormalities; an unresolved observation; inquiry related to a previously detected disorder; interpretation of a laboratory abnormality, risk factor, or family trait; and, commonly, advice on therapeutic options. In virtually all these circumstances, the patient seeks counsel about a disorder that, with few exceptions, is regarded as potentially life-limiting or disabling. The expert view of the cardiologist is hence sought in an atmosphere of anxiety and apprehension, often shrouded in misconception and modified by an incomplete understanding of the disorder that afflicts the cardiac patient. How the consultant should behave in this emotionally charged atmosphere is not easily taught or learned; the response has not been subjected to critical evaluation and has no firm scientific basis. Nevertheless, the appropriateness of the physician's reactions during this initial meeting remains at the foundation of all that can be accomplished in diagnosis, treatment, and care for the patient.

*Throughout this chapter, "he" and "his" refer to both genders.

The early moments of the meeting with the patient should be directed toward creating a welcome and placid environment conducive to easing the patient's emotional and physical distress. If medical exigencies are absent, the consultant should cordially introduce himself to the patient and greet members of the family. It is proper for the consultant to describe his professional role and to succinctly outline the processes that will take place. Much can be learned at the outset if the patient is given the opportunity to describe his life situation, occupation, and family relationships even before he is asked about the current clinical symptoms. Such expressions ensure that the physician's interests go well beyond illness alone.

THE DIAGNOSTIC SYNTHESIS

The pursuit of the patient's symptom complex must follow an organized and logical pattern of inquiry. The patient should be asked to describe major disabling symptoms, not only his chief complaint but also all symptoms that have a bearing on the current state of his well-being. The patient should be allowed a nondirected interval in which to convey his feelings and reactions. With these first words, the consultant's cerebral computer begins to generate a differential diagnosis. On this basis, the consultant chooses several pathways of inquiry to clarify the diagnosis. These include the *chronologic*, which takes diagnostic advantage of nature's timetables of disease; the *descriptive*, for clarification of character and severity of symptoms; and the *associative*, in which the relationships of the symptoms to underlying disease mechanisms, past events, and related illness are pursued. In the course of these inquiries, the consultant searches for diagnostic insights stemming from the observations of other physicians, the consequences of previous episodes of the illness, and the patient's response to therapeutic interventions. The differential diagnostic approach leads to a branching search for entities and relationships that can explain the underlying disease mechanism. These include inquiries about familial, genetic, and risk factors; occupational exposure; remote illness; potential iatrogenic disorders; psychogenic influences; and, when appropriate, the patient's personal habits, including diet, exercise, sexual behavior, and exposure to tobacco, alcohol, illicit drugs, stimulants, and depressants. Throughout this line of inquiry, the consultant assesses the patient's emotional state and its influence on the character and intensity of the patient's symptoms. As the history progresses, the consultant must reassure the patient and explain that a detailed inquiry is essential for clarification of the nature and cause of his malady.

In the course of the interview, the consultant should observe the patient's physical reactions and gestures. The subliminal language of body movement often reveals details of diagnostic significance; the common fist clenching of angina pectoris is but one of many bodily reactions that amplify the character of the symptom and its cause. Of recurring value to the author are such gestures as the gripping movement of pleuritic pain, the sighing respiration of emotional distress, the pointing finger of fleeting noncardiac chest pain, and the chest patting defining regular or irregular cardiac rhythm.

As the interview progresses, the consultant focuses on questions related to physiologic, psychologic, and pathologic aspects of the patient's symptoms. Questions that regularly arise are as follows: Do the patient's symptoms truly reflect disease? Are they a deviation from the norm? Do they result from exaggerated normal responses? By this process, the consultant arrives at one or more leading hypotheses to explain the underlying mechanism of the patient's symptom complex.

SOURCES OF INFORMATION

Although the patient remains the essential figure in the acquiring of data, additional sources include letters and notes from the referral physician; telephone communication; office, hospital, and emergency room records; and laboratory reports. It is prudent to review the material that is received before the patient's appointment and to be well informed of its content before beginning the interview. Other valuable sources of information are the patient's spouse and immediate relatives. Their commentary serves to amplify the existing base of knowledge and provides a focus on the living relationships in which the patient functions.

It is important to recognize that the patient may well have information he would prefer to reserve for private and personal communication. Accordingly, it is advisable to politely dismiss members of the patient's family to allow for a personal and confidential exchange. At times, the social dynamics of the family group preempt a favorable flow of information. Under such circumstances, it is appropriate to dismiss family members early. Not infrequently, members of the family, particularly the patient's spouse, prefer a confidential meeting with the consultant to relate their personal concerns, to offer details that otherwise might prove embarrassing to the patient, or to augment information the patient may have failed to retain. The consultant, with due diplomacy, should encourage such exchanges.

THE HISTORY AS PREPARATION FOR LABORATORY STUDIES, TREATMENT, AND PROGNOSIS

Having gained enough information to advance a firm hypothesis on the cause of the patient's illness, the consultant now turns to a line of inquiry related to the need for diagnostic testing. In considering the array of available laboratory procedures, their merits, limitations, and hazards, and the frequent need for patient participation, the consultant must consider such matters as the patient's tolerance to the test procedure, his exercise capacity, the potential for adverse responses to the stress of the test or to pharmacologic testing agents, the influence of comorbid disease on test results, and the relative diagnostic predictive value of the proposed tests.

The plan of one's laboratory evaluation is often influenced by the findings reported by the referring physician. Questions often raised include the following:

Do tests previously performed need repetition? Were the tests performed at appropriate standards and with adequate pretest preparation? Are the results consistent with the overall clinical presentation? Were relevant tests deleted?

The history generally provides information pertinent to the patient's current and previous therapy. Of particular interest in considering future therapeutic options are the effectiveness of current medications and previous interventions, the occurrence of possible adverse reactions to previous therapeutic maneuvers, and the influence of noncardiovascular drugs and drug interactions on the patient's status.

The consultant's thoughts must in addition lean toward an evaluation of the intensity of the patient's disease and estimates of its short- and long-term prognoses. The information acquired through the history provides a framework for evaluating the status of the patient's disease, its stability, and the level of cardiovascular compensation. These data permit assessment of the presence and severity of ventricular dysfunction, myocardial ischemia, and cardiac arrhythmia and of the effectiveness of previous therapy, thus providing a basis for initial projection of the patient's clinical risk.

THE CONSULTANT'S BEHAVIOR

The contemporary medical history does not constitute a mere collection of patient complaints. Rather, it provides a broad-based information bank from which the full spectrum of clinical thinking emerges. As clinical experience grows, so does the consultant's effectiveness in history-taking. Indeed, in eliciting the history, the experienced specialist performs much like an accomplished musician who can interpret a wide breadth of musical scores with immediate virtuosity and interpretive sensitivity.

The taking of the history should for the most part remain a continuous and uninterrupted process. For the experienced consultant, the intense processing of the history flows in a seemingly extemporaneous pattern. Of course, pauses for brief note-taking and review of the information forwarded by the primary physician are expected. The consultant should explain such pauses and inform the patient when there is a need to interrupt the history or to leave the office temporarily for review of films or graphic data. In the course of the interview, the patient often recollects previously unmentioned events or symptoms. He should be encouraged to elaborate on these thoughts when they come to mind.

A common pattern of behavior among patients is their attempt to offer a personal diagnosis. This does not reflect a desire to display their own knowledge of medicine. Rather, it is a maneuver, for the most part, to stimulate discussion on the cause of their symptoms. The contemporary patient is commonly aware that the outcome of his illness is intrinsically related to the severity of the underlying disease mechanism. The introduction of the patient's theory provides an opportunity for the consultant to discuss the patient's feelings, to offer reassurance that medicine has much to offer, and to reinforce the value of a thorough cardiovascular examination. Allowing the patient to explain his views without adverse criticism affords reassurance that his physician is interested and tolerant. Such discussion does much to solidify the patient's confidence in his consultant.

During the interview, the consultant must maintain composure and professional equanimity. Despite the volume of information to be gathered, the interview must be conducted unhurriedly. Not uncommonly, the patient's responses are vague and indefinite – a circumstance that can prove frustrating to the consultant. Despite such an impediment, the consultant must remain sympathetic and supportive. He should always speak directly to the patient in language that is understandable and unambiguous. The interview should be flexible and unmechanical, allowing for diversion in direction and attention as dictated by the patient's emotional and physical states. Although the patient's responses should not be biased by leading questions and direct suggestion, it is not inappropriate to guide the patient's thinking and to help in describing the characteristics of his symptoms. Rarely can patients project precise recollection of the time, place, and circumstances of their symptoms. Memory failure in patients is common in the emotional atmosphere of an intense interview and may be accentuated by disease and aging. The consultant should expect imperfect recall of events and details and must work with the patient in establishing a meaningful portrayal of the progression of his illness.

A common trend in contemporary subspecialty practice, including cardiovascular medicine, is a progressive narrowing of clinical perspective among consultants. The cardiologist should never consider himself one who confines his inquiry solely to the analysis of the cardiovascular problem. The exclusion of the thinking of the general internist and the failure to keep abreast of advances in noncardiovascular subspecialties narrow the cardiologist's perspective and have an eroding influence on his clinical effectiveness. Failure to appreciate the ever-expanding breadth of clinical knowledge in other subspecialties eventually relegates the practice of the cardiologist to that of a technical colleague who is called on merely to purvey or perform laboratory procedures.

RECORDING THE HISTORY

Having gathered pertinent information from all available sources, the consultant reaches the point at which he is prepared to dictate or write the information that he has gathered through the history-taking process. Some consultants prefer to move directly to the physical examination at this juncture, and others take time to record the history forthwith. Whatever the approach, the consultant must be aware of the singular value of a well-inscribed synthesis of the patient's historical data. Although the patient's information base may have been acquired somewhat haphazardly, the inscribed medical history should conform to sound medical reasoning, constituting a critical rearrangement and analysis of the information derived from the history. Composed in logical and succinct descriptive paragraphs, the summary of the history will remain an intellectual biopsy of the patient's cardiovascular problem, a reliable and efficient source of clinical information to which the consultant and colleagues can refer in the future. When the history is written by hand, the consultant must recognize the essential need for legibility. In his written or transcribed summary, he should avoid cryptic, uninterpretable abbreviations, locally adopted acronyms, and medical jargon. One rarely encounters anything more frustrating than a medical report describing a critical illness in undecipherable script. The typewritten history remains an invaluable asset, particularly so in our era of rapid transtelephonic fax communication. To facilitate such transfer of patient information, the consultant's dictated history should be composed in concise, organized, and logical language.

It is to be recognized that pertinent historical information is often derived after the formal process of history-taking is completed. Findings uncovered during the physical examination and by laboratory studies often prompt new inquiry. This information should be incorporated in an addendum to the history. If it is a telling observation, it should be highlighted for emphasis.

Table 1-1 Etiology of cardiovascular disease
A basic classification

1. Coronary artery disease
2. Hypertensive heart disease
3. Valvular heart disease
4. Myocardial disease and myocarditis
5. Pulmonary hypertension
6. Pulmonary embolic disease
7. Congenital heart disease
8. Arrhythmia and conduction abnormalities
9. Pericardial disease
10. Infective endocarditis
11. Cardiac tumors
12. Cardiac trauma
13. Endocrinopathic heart disease
14. Rheumatic and connective tissue disease
15. Neuromyopathic cardiac disease
16. Drug-induced cardiac dysfunction
17. Diseases of the aorta
18. Cerebrovascular disease
19. Peripheral arterial disease
20. Cardiovascular disease related to noncardiac and systemic disease

SUMMARIZING THE HISTORY

After completing the history and before proceeding to the formal physical examination, the prudent physician summarizes the impressions gleaned from the information gathered during the history. A valuable exercise is to attempt an organized assessment of the historical database according to the following categories: (1) the patient's primary problems; (2) differential diagnosis; (3) anatomic abnormalities; (4) physiologic abnormalities, including assessment of systolic and diastolic dysfunction and arrhythmia; (5) cardiovascular status with respect to compensation and stability; (6) past and current therapy; (7) prognosis; and (8) unanswered questions. With such an outline in mind, the consultant approaches the ensuing physical examination and laboratory evaluation with a well-conceived differential diagnosis and an appreciation for areas of his clinical uncertainty. At this juncture, the consultant is advised to consider, from memory, a comprehensive list of the basic causes of cardiovascular disease. Such a disciplined approach uncovers pathways of diagnostic consideration that may otherwise have been left unexplored. Table 1-1 presents such a listing of 20 basic etiologic categories of cardiovascular disease that may exist as independent or combined disorders.

The major progress in the basic sciences of the early and middle decades of this century together with the emergence of cellular and molecular biology in more recent years has promoted a remarkable new technology in cardiovascular medicine. The promise of this technology to bring definitive and certain diagnosis and treatment, however, has not been realized. Rather, our current era is characterized by a plurality of improved diagnostic and therapeutic options, few of which yield decisive answers. As a consequence, the care of the patient in this era of new but incomplete technology requires more considered guidance and personalized attention than ever. The key step in preparing for such care resides in that uniquely important exercise, the clinical history. The practice of history-taking remains today a vital skill to be learned and perfected by every consultant in cardiovascular medicine.

REFERENCES

1. Hampton JR, Harrison MJG, Mitchell JRA, et al: Relative contributions of history-taking, physical examination, and laboratory investigation to diagnosis and management of medical outpatients. *Br Med J* 2:486-489, 1975

2. Sandler G: The importance of the history in the medical clinic and the cost of unnecessary tests. *Am Heart J* 100:928-931, 1980

3. Hickam DH, Sox HC Jr, Sox CH: Systematic bias in recording the history in patients with chest pain. *J Chronic Dis* 38:91-100, 1985

CHAPTER

2

Physical examination

Titus C. Evans, Jr., M.D., Ph.D., Emilio R. Giuliani, M.D., Robert G. Tancredi, M.D., and Robert O. Brandenburg, M.D.

GENERAL APPEARANCE

The role of the physical examination varies widely in the diagnosis and management of patients with cardiovascular disease.

The technologic developments of the past decade have lessened the time and attention devoted to the physical examination. This is understandable but unfortunate because in many instances the two different approaches complement each other. In many cases an accurate physical assessment leads to a more intelligent and selective use of additional studies. In others it avoids errors, sometimes major, when decisions are based solely on laboratory results. Palpation, in particular, seems to be a declining skill. Almost two decades ago, it was found that 81% of patients who had the left ventricular impulse limited to one intercostal space had normal left ventricular volumes; in contrast, almost the same percentage of those whose left ventricular impulse was palpated in two or more intercostal spaces had cardiac enlargement. In addition, it was noted that a sustained left ventricular impulse correctly indicated an increased left ventricular mass in 88% of patients, whereas when the apical impulse was confined to early systole, the left ventricular mass was normal in 78%.[1] Subsequent workers confirmed that an apical impulse diameter of at least 3 cm predicted left ventricular enlargement.[2] This degree of accuracy in detection of left ventricular hypertrophy and left ventricular mass may not be attained by conventional electrocardiographic and roentgenographic criteria.[3,4]

An integral part of a clinician's diagnostic acumen and expertise in management of patients is the ability to interweave the facts in the history and the findings on the physical examination. A clinician who does a careful and complete physical examination of the patient is always alert for noncardiovascular abnormalities as well as cardiovascular abnormalities, particularly correctable or treatable ones. He or she knows when to exercise the patient and listen again and when to use the effect of respiration, Valsalva maneuver, positional changes, or amyl nitrite.

Another important aspect is awareness of the many common illnesses that may affect the symptoms of stable cardiac conditions – e.g., the gradual worsening of angina in the elderly patient, due not to progression of the coronary disease but to anemia secondary to carcinoma of the ascending colon. Similarly, fever, hyperthyroidism, or personal stresses may cause exacerbations of mild stable cardiac symptoms.

Traditionally, the history of the patient's illnesses is taken before the physical examination is begun, but, in practice, the examination actually begins with the introduction of the patient and usual handshake. These few seconds allow the physician to identify sex, approximate age, size, body build, and personal hygiene and to obtain a glimpse of the personality involved. The demeanor is of particular importance – anxiety, depression, anger, hostility. The comments the patient makes about his or her other physicians may be of significance.

During the first few moments of getting acquainted, one can evaluate the severity and acuteness of the problem. At a glance, one becomes aware of pallor, sweating, tremor, pain, evidence of weight loss, abnormal skin pigmentation, elevated jugular venous pulsation, or abnormal carotid arterial pulsation. Hence, before the systematic physical examination begins, a great amount of useful information has been obtained.

Head

Cardiovascular abnormalities frequently have an associated facial component (Fig 2-1). There is a malar flush and slight cyanosis associated with mitral stenosis with severe pulmonary hypertension; a different type of malar butterfly erythema occurs in the occasional patient with systemic lupus erythematosus (Fig 2-2). The leathery, atrophic, immobile skin of scleroderma (Fig 2-3) particularly affects the mouth, giving the classic "pinched" look. In myxedema there is puffy, dry skin with periorbital edema, large tongue, and sparse eyebrows laterally. A round face with "hidden ears" may be seen in severe stenosis of the pulmonary valve and Cushing's syndrome.

A host of anomalies are associated with alterations in

We acknowledge and thank Dr. James A. Shaver (Professor of Medicine and Director of Division of Cardiology, School of Medicine, University of Pittsburgh, PA) who furnished many excellent illustrations used in this chapter.

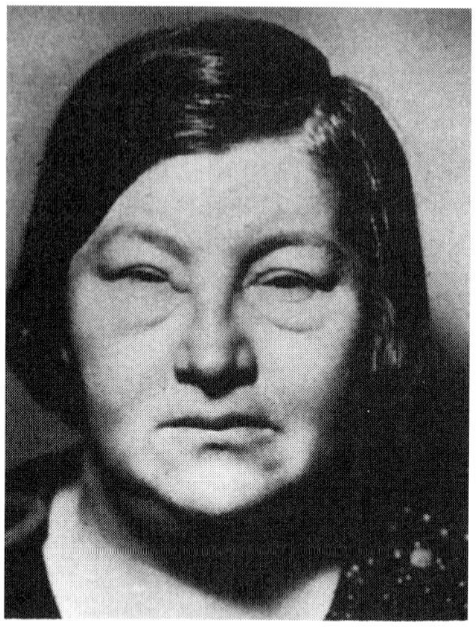

Fig 2-1 Patient with myxedema. (Courtesy of Charles F. Abboud, M.D.)

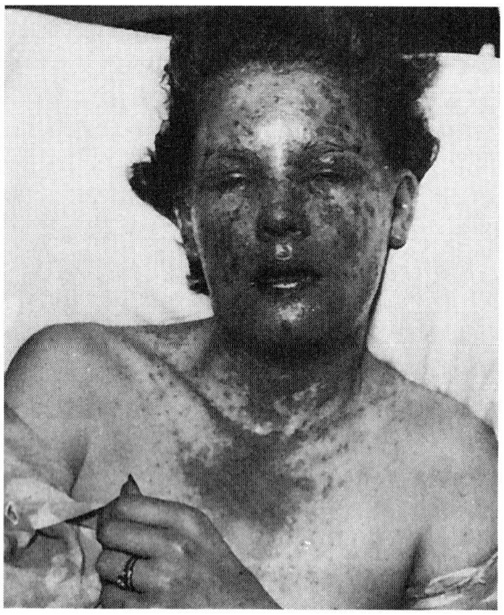

Fig 2-2 Facial rash in patient with systemic lupus erythematosus.

facial anatomy. The more common of these are: Down's syndrome, with small nose and eyes, epicanthal folds, and large tongue, which is often associated with atrioventricular (AV) canal defects or other defects of septation; Noonan's syndrome, with hypertelorism (wide-set eyes) and pulmonic stenosis; Turner's syndrome, with short webbed neck, epicanthal folds, hypertelorism, low-set ears (Fig 2-4), and coarctation of the aorta; the nonfamilial type of supravalvular aortic stenosis with elfin-like features, hypertelorism, a wide mouth with large lips, full cheeks, and large, low-set ears; and the long, narrow face with arched palate of Marfan's syndrome (Fig 2-5).

The muscular dystrophies are also associated with facial alterations. In myotonia dystrophica, there is a dull masklike expression, receding hairline, ptosis, and atrophy of the temporal and sternocleidomastoid muscles (Fig 2-6).

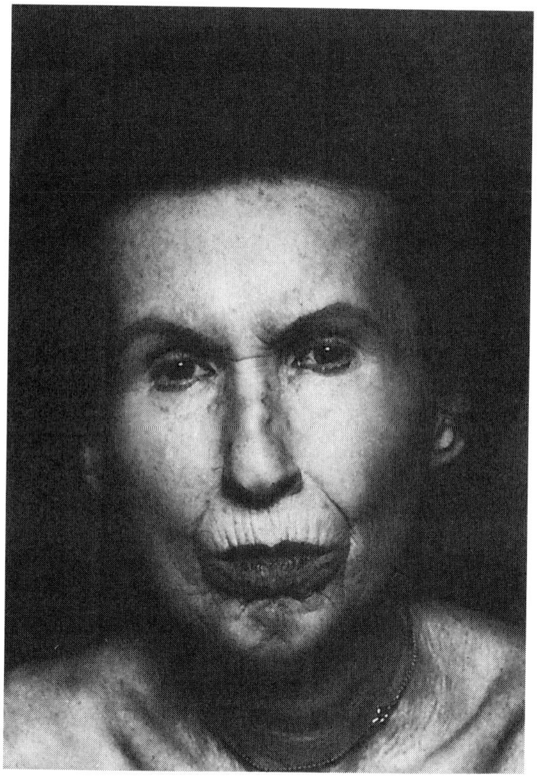

Fig 2-3 Appearance in scleroderma.

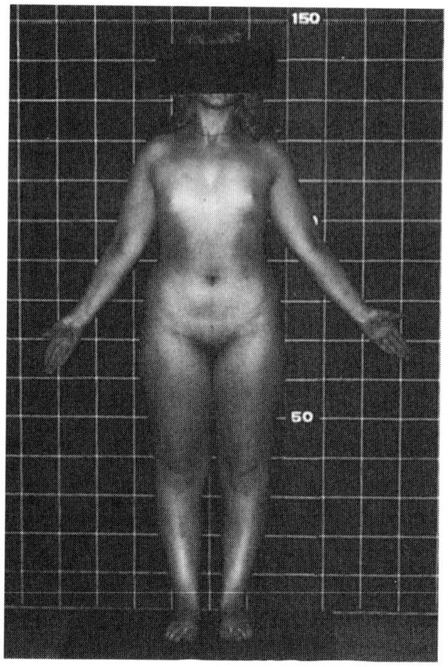

Fig 2-4 Turner's syndrome. (Courtesy of H. Gordon, M.D.)

Eyes. The appearance of the retinal vessels allows detection of hypertension, hemorrhages secondary to vasculitis, infective endocarditis (Fig 2-7), and retinal occlusions due to emboli (calcific and atheromatous from

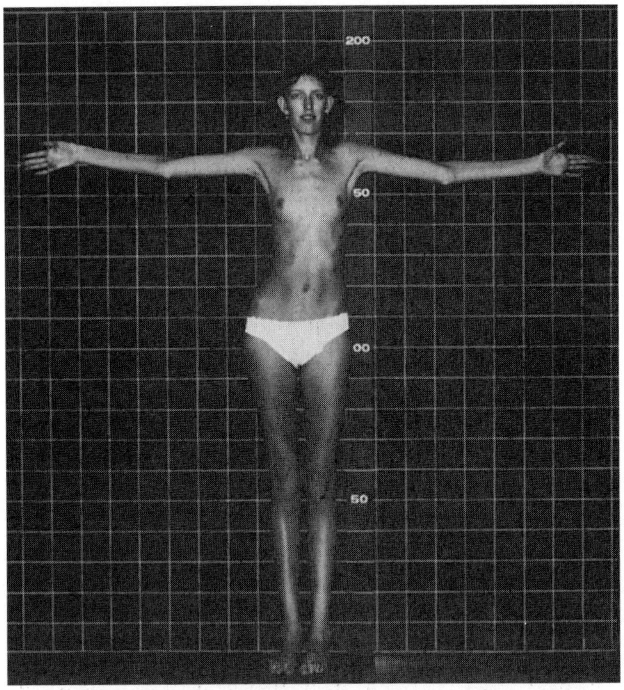

Fig 2-5 Marfan's syndrome.

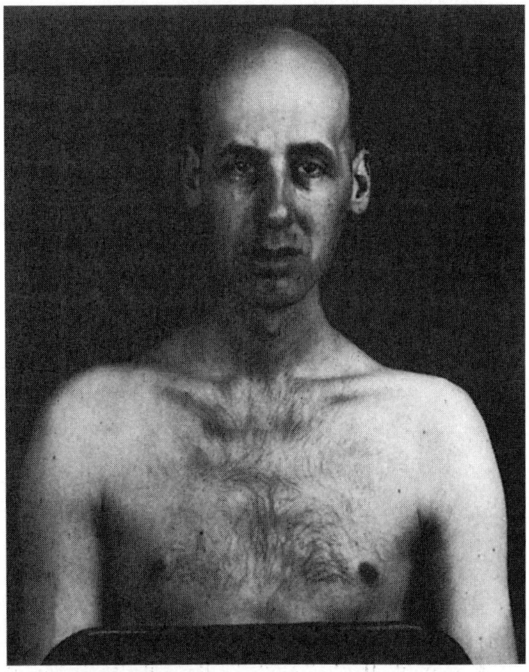

Fig 2-6 Patient with myotonia dystrophica.

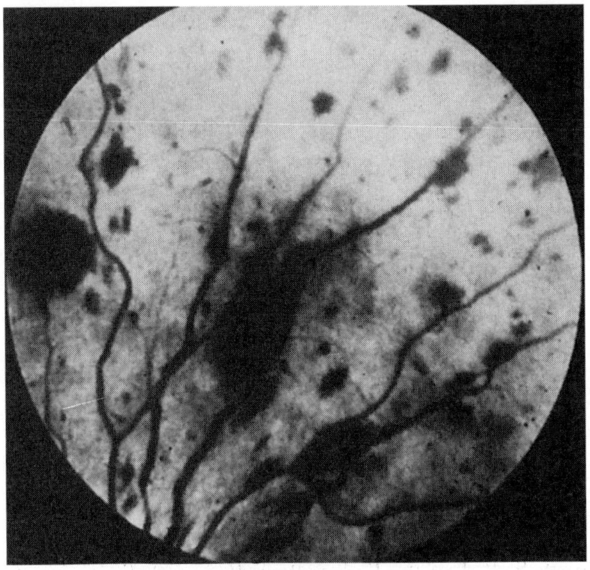

Fig 2-7 Appearance of optic fundus in infective endocarditis.

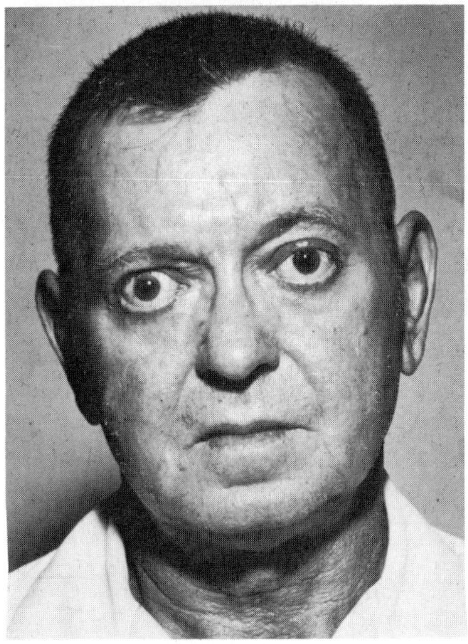

Fig 2-8 Exophthalmos in Graves' disease. (Courtesy of Charles Abboud, M.D.)

the aorta and carotid arteries; thrombi and myxomas from the left atrium). Papilledema may occur with hypoxia (cor pulmonale) and in malignant hypertension.

Exophthalmos with stare may occur with Graves' disease and chronic congestive heart failure (Fig 2-8). External ophthalmoplegia and ptosis occur in the ocular muscular dystrophy described by Kearns and Sayre[5] with myocardial disease and complete heart block. Conjunctivae may reveal the pallor of anemia and the subjunctional hemorrhages and petechiae of infective endocarditis (Fig 2-9). The iris may be tremulous due to poor support in Marfan's disease, and iritis may occur in sarcoidosis and rheumatoid disease, both with cardiac manifestations. Blue sclera may be present in osteogenesis imperfecta, Marfan's syndrome, and the Ehlers-Danlos syndrome, which may be associated with thoracic aortic dilatation,

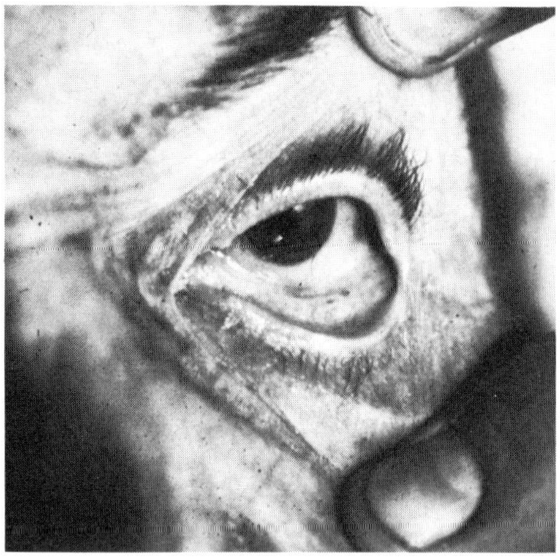

Fig 2-9 Conjunctival petechiae in patient with documented infective endocarditis.

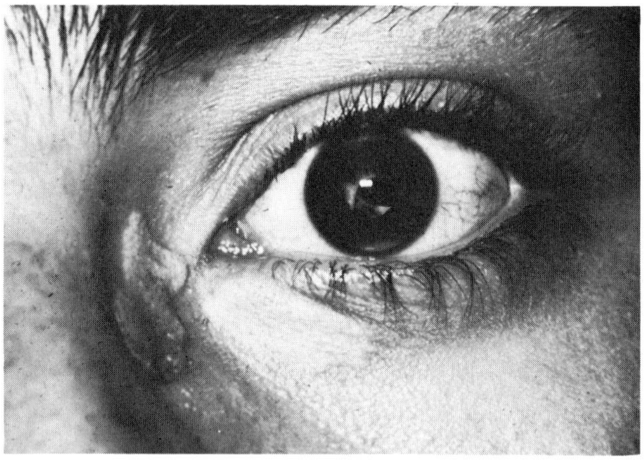

Fig 2-10 Xanthelasma in patient with premature atherosclerosis. (Courtesy of T.T. Schattenberg, M.D.)

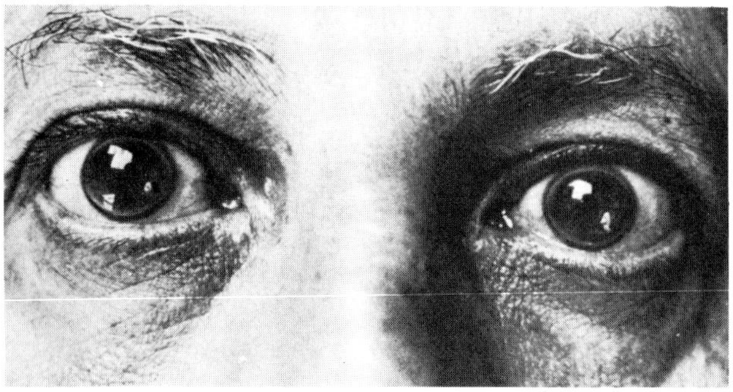

Fig 2-11 Arcus senilis.

aortic valve incompetence, aortic dissection, and mitral valve prolapse.

Cataracts occur in a multitude of conditions with a cardiac component and are of little diagnostic aid. The Argyll Robertson pupil—an irregular pupil that is small

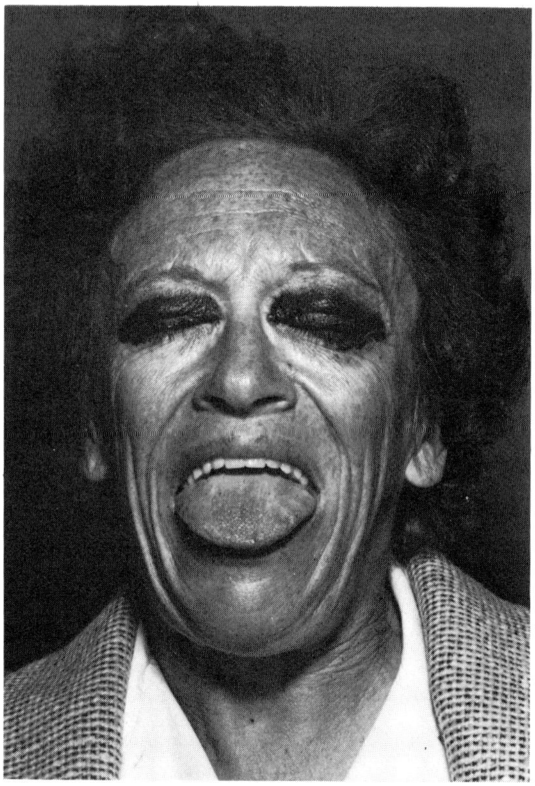

Fig 2-12 Macroglossia and periorbital purpura in amyloidosis.

and unequal to the opposite pupil, fails to respond to light, and does not dilate properly—is seldom seen now. It is diagnostic of central nervous system syphilis which may be associated with aortic disease (aneurysm, aortic valve incompetence, and coronary ostial stenosis). Xanthelasma (yellowish fatty deposits on or below the eyelids) may be associated with premature atherosclerosis, especially in men under age 40 years (Fig 2-10). There is a similar association for arcus senilis in the young (Fig 2-11).

Mouth. An enlarged tongue may occur in systemic amyloidosis (Fig 2-12), Down's syndrome, hypothyroidism, and Hurler's syndrome. The buccal mucosa may show petechiae in infective endocarditis. A high-arched palate is characteristic of Marfan's and Turner's syndromes. Cleft palate and lip are associated with an increased incidence of congenital heart disease. Central cyanosis (intracardiac or intrapulmonary right-to-left shunts) will be manifested by cyanosis of the oral mucosa.

Skin

The skin exhibits a multitude of abnormalities of diagnostic value. Irregular and lumpy tumors between and over the knuckles and in the Achilles tendon are xanthomas that also are associated with premature atherosclerosis. The velvety hyperelastic skin of the Ehlers-Danlos syndrome may be associated with aortic dissection or rupture and mitral valve prolapse. Bronze or

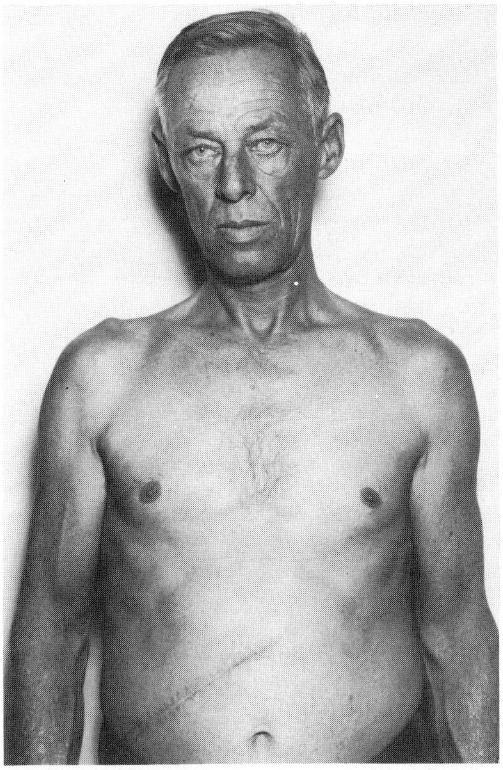

Fig 2-13 Hemochromatosis. (Courtesy of J. Kiely, M.D.)

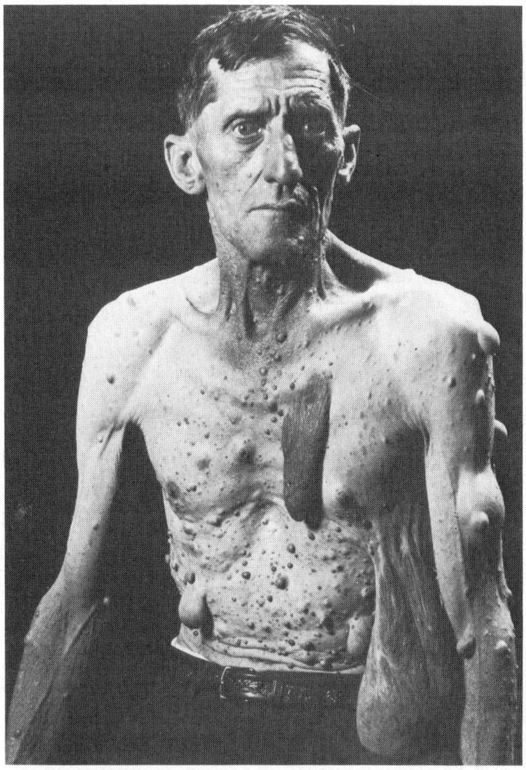

Fig 2-14 Subcutaneous neurofibromas suggest the possibility of pheochromocytoma.

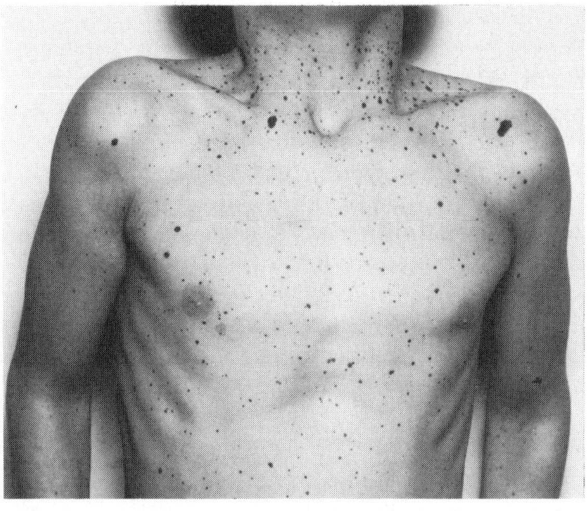

Fig 2-15 Lentigines. Diagnosis by clinical examination and histologic studies. Patient had associated hypertrophic cardiomyopathy.

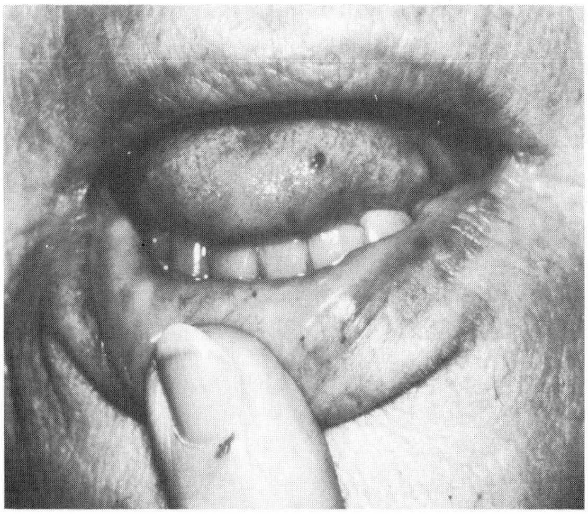

Fig 2-16 Lesions of tongue and lips in hereditary telangiectasis.

gray coloration of the skin and loss of axillary and pubic hair are characteristic of hemochromatosis (Fig 2-13), which is associated with myocardial involvement and congestive heart failure.

Argyria, a slate-gray skin color due to deposition of silver, must be distinguished from cyanosis due to an intracardiac right-to-left shunt. Subcutaneous neurofibromas with café-au-lait spots (Fig 2-14) and hypertension suggest the possibility of renal artery stenosis or pheochromocytoma. Lentiginosis (Fig 2-15), characterized by freckle-like lesions not affected by sunlight, is associated with hypertrophic cardiomyopathy. Erythema marginatum, the rapidly changing skin lesions of acute rheumatic fever, may be associated with subcutaneous nodules over the extensor surface of the elbows or, less often, over the spinal column. Subcutaneous nodules over the elbows are also seen in advanced rheumatoid arthritis with pericardial involvement. Hereditary telangiectasia of the skin may resemble the spider nevi of liver disease; it is often accompanied by lesions of the tongue and lips (Fig 2-16), pulmonary arteriovenous fistulas causing cyanosis, and gastrointestinal lesions causing bleeding. Punctate purplish angiokeratomas on the trunk and lip occur with Fabry's disease, which is associated with deposits of lipid and glycogen in blood vessels and in the myocardium, causing arrhythmias, myocardial infarction, mitral incompetence, and congestive failure.

Thorax

Alterations in thoracic anatomy should immediately raise the possibility of congenital heart disease, particularly in younger patients, and may lead to abnormal respiration with resultant hypoxia, vasoconstriction, and obstruction to pulmonary flow. Cor pulmonale from increased pulmonary vascular resistance may develop from kyphoscoliosis, ankylosing spondylitis, or spinal cord disease or as a sequela to poliomyelitis, chronic lung disease, or pneumonectomy.

The straight back syndrome with and without pectus excavatum may lead to the false diagnosis of cardiomegaly by compressing or flattening the heart or displacing it to the left. A pulmonary outflow murmur and minor right ventricular conduction delay on the electrocardiogram (ECG) may be present with this syndrome or with pectus excavatum, leading to the erroneous diagnosis of atrial septal defect. However, the straight back syndrome is associated with an increased incidence of congenital heart disease, especially atrial septal defect. Scoliosis is often present with cyanotic congenital heart disease. Mitral valve prolapse has an increased incidence in all of the above – i.e., straight back syndrome, pectus excavatum, and scoliosis. Localized bulges of the anterior thorax may be seen with certain diseases: a bulge of the upper left sternal area with atrial septal defect, and of the lower left sternal area with ventricular septal defect. A bulge with pulsations over the upper right sternum may be present with an aneurysm of the ascending aorta, and a bulge with pulsations over the left upper anterior chest may be noted with an aneurysm of the upper descending thoracic aorta. Tortuous intercostal arteries with increased pulsations are present on the lateral and posterior aspects of the chest wall with coarctation of the aorta.

Abdomen

Examination of the abdomen should include careful auscultation for renal artery bruits in the presence of hypertension and renal artery fistula and palpation of the abdominal aorta for evidence of dilatation and aneurysm. A friction rub over the liver suggests gonococcal endocarditis. The kidneys may be enlarged and palpable if hypertension or renal failure is due to polycystic disease.

Splenomegaly is frequent in chronic long-standing congestive heart failure from any cause but especially with chronic constrictive pericarditis. Palpable splenomegaly is infrequent in infective endocarditis; when present, it may be painful. Splenic infarcts also may be painful.

Liver congestion secondary to cardiac failure is often associated with right upper quadrant and epigastric fullness and discomfort. With severe, acute onset, it may simulate gallbladder colic. When the congestion is chronic, the liver becomes firm to palpation, and tenderness and discomfort wane. Even then, however, percussion over the liver usually causes discomfort. Systolic pulsation of the liver is associated with tricuspid valve incompetence.

In the presence of ascites, the jugular venous pressure should be carefully examined. If normal, the heart is excluded as the cause, and other causes should be sought such as cirrhosis or ovarian tumor.

Extremities

The extremities, particularly the hands, are associated with many congenital and acquired cardiac diseases. Cyanosis and clubbing (Fig 2-17) of the fingers and toes are characteristic of right-to-left shunting in congenital heart disease as well as in pulmonary arteriovenous fistulas. Clubbing also may occur with infective endocarditis, carcinoma of the lung, emphysema, sarcoidosis, regional enteritis, or biliary cirrhosis.

Differential cyanosis has interesting diagnostic implications. Cyanosis more marked in the fingers than the toes suggests transposition of the great vessels with interruption of the aortic arch or preductal coarctation with pulmonary hypertension and a reversed shunt through a ductus arteriosus. If cyanosis and clubbing of the toes are associated with pink fingernails of the right hand and slight cyanosis in the left, a reversing patent ductus arteriosus due to severe pulmonary hypertension is suggested.

Alterations in the shape and number of fingers are often associated with congenital heart disease. The Holt-Oram syndrome is characterized by a "fingerized" thumb in the same plane as the rest of the fingers and short forearms with limited pronation and supination. Atrial septal defect is the usual associated cardiac lesion. Atrial and ventricular septal defects are associated with polydactyly and dystrophic nails in the Ellis–van Creveld syndrome. Arachnodactyly is characteristic of Marfan's syndrome

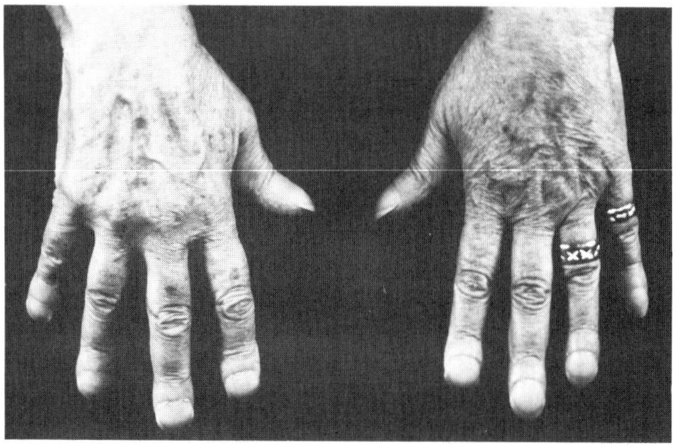

Fig 2-17 Clubbing of fingers. (Courtesy of Edward Rosenow, M.D.)

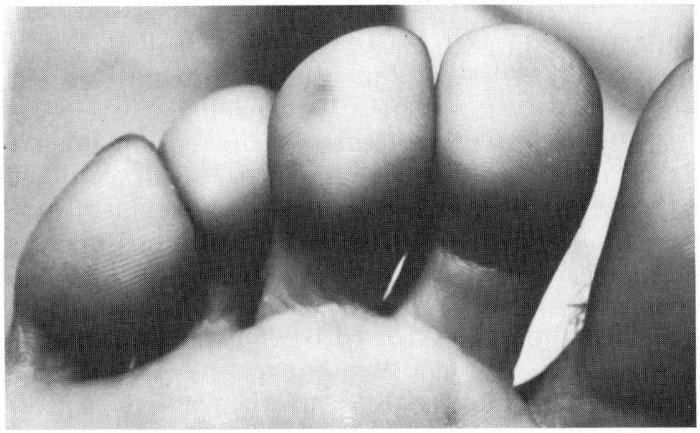

Fig 2-18 Osler's nodes in patient with proven infective endocarditis.

(see Fig 2-5). In addition, when the fist is clenched over the thumb, the thumb will extend well beyond the ulnar side of the hand. The Laurence-Moon-Biedl syndrome is also associated with polydactyly and various cardiac lesions, but mental retardation and retinitis pigmentosa usually also are present.

After myocardial infarction, cerebral infarction, or arterial occlusion, the shoulder-hand syndrome may develop, producing a shiny, swollen, stiff, painful, semi-immobile hand. Sickle cell disease may also be associated with painful swollen hands (and feet); the associated cardiovascular lesions are pulmonary vascular thrombosis and high-output cardiac failure. Visible pulsation of the nail beds is evidence of significant aortic runoff, as in aortic valve incompetence or ruptured sinus of Valsalva. Splinter hemorrhages of the nails occur in many conditions and in normal persons. Occasionally, they are helpful in leading to the diagnosis of infective endocarditis. The Janeway lesions, areas of localized vasculitis on the palms or soles, are nontender and hemorrhagic; they may be helpful in diagnosing infectious endocarditis. Osler's nodes (Fig 2-18), tender, reddish, raised nodules of the distal finger and toe pads, occur occasionally in patients with infective endocarditis.

INSPECTION AND PALPATION: NORMAL AND ABNORMAL PULSATIONS OF THE VEINS, ARTERIES, AND HEART

Analysis of cardiovascular pulsations is extremely important. Enough information is often available in the various waveforms to suggest the correct cardiovascular diagnosis or to confirm it, thereby rendering such analysis valuable to both patient management and cost control. It requires more effort and understanding than most other areas of physical diagnosis.

In this section, divided into four areas of discussion—General, Jugular Venous Pulsations, Carotid Arterial Pulsations, and Chest Wall and Apex Pulsations—the approach is geared to the evaluation of the patient at the bedside rather than in the laboratory. In reviewing the conclusions of other authors, it is apparent that differences of opinion still exist about the causes of some physical findings and the relative importance and merit of various examination techniques.

General

Encouragement. The interpretation of the motions of cardiovascular structures is an essential part of a complete cardiac examination. Observation of pulsations often yields the diagnosis quickly and makes the subsequent auscultation much more certain, expeditious, and satisfying to the physician.

Pulsations in the chest and neck may be rapid or slow and tall or short. Location, timing with respect to the cardiac cycle, and extent of normalcy or abnormality also are features to be determined for each pulse or waveform. Because events are repetitive over several cardiac cycles, take advantage of repeated observations to compare the results of different maneuvers. Only a few seconds are usually required to evaluate each pulse.

The jugular venous pressure and pulse waveforms are influenced by the right atrium and right ventricle; the carotid arterial pulse and the cardiac apex impulse are influenced by the left atrium and the left ventricle. The jugular venous pulse, the carotid arterial pulse, and the cardiac apex pulse are the three most important areas of interest.

Caution. The cardiologist must expect to encounter, from time to time, a patient who is difficult to examine or who presents findings that are subtle or confusing. Patients with obese or short necks, with various degrees of pericardial constriction, with restriction of diastolic heart filling, or with low jugular venous pressure may be especially difficult to evaluate. Pulsations and motions are sometimes small in amplitude and hard to assess. Arrhythmias or extrasystoles can create uncertainty if not recognized in advance. Even normal patients are sometimes difficult to evaluate.

Before examining for the venous levels and varius pulse waves in the neck and chest, remember to optimize the patient's body position and respiration. Take full advantage of the effects of gravity, hydraulic pressure, and pneumatic pressure to alter vascular and cardiac blood volumes and thereby maximize the information present for observation.

General sequence of evaluation. The patient's history is the starting point for planning modifications in the usual sequence of steps in the physical examination. The symptoms usually indicate the general areas of cardiovascular disease. Findings on examination reveal where new emphasis is needed. If the examination of the cardiovascular system is being combined with a general examination of the entire body, then various areas of the body may be examined in a somewhat different, more opportune, sequence in order to avoid repetition, excessive time, and additional unnecessary changes in body position by the patient. The approach presented herein is a typical simplified scheme.

Consider the patient's feelings; start with the peripheral examination. Allowing the patient a short period in which to become at ease with the examination setting will often result in better rapport and less total time being required for the examination. Placing a gown across the front of the patient's chest and a sheet across the abdomen and lap will reassure the patient and provide warmth and comfort. Some patients exhibit tachycardia or hypertension due to natural anxiety if the examiner proceeds too rapidly to examine the neck, chest, or abdomen. To reduce such apprehension, one might begin the examination with an evaluation of the various pulses in the peripheral limbs and measurement of the systemic arterial blood pressure in the right and left brachial arteries before proceeding to evaluate the neck, chest, abdomen, and femoral pulses.

Blood pressure should be measured in both arms. It is important to note any significant difference between the two sides of the body, abnormalities of systolic or diastolic pressure, widened pulse pressure, paradoxic pulse, pulsus alternans, bigeminy, or other arrhythmias.

If the brachial artery blood pressure sounds are difficult to hear due to obesity, emptying the capillaries and veins of the arm will often augment the Korotkoff sounds significantly. Position the uninflated cuff, pump it up only until it remains in place, elevate the patient's arm for about 5 seconds (the patient may close and open the fist once or twice) to allow time for venous and capillary emptying, pump up the cuff above systolic pressure, lower the patient's arm, apply the stethoscope to the brachial artery, and listen as the cuff is gradually deflated in the usual manner.

Central cardiovascular examination. After examination of the peripheral arteries, the pulsations of the veins and arteries of the neck may be examined, followed by those of the chest and heart. The motions of the liver, abdominal aorta, and femoral arteries are checked last. This sequence allows the patient to start the examination in the sitting position and to change to the supine position only once. Subsequent use of the left semilateral decubitus position, sit-ups, leg lifts, prompt squatting, and prompt standing may be needed in individual cases. The examiner should always be prepared to repeat a step or to search further to confirm an initial impression. Combination of steps in the usual examination procedure is encouraged wherever expedient. For instance, palpation and auscultation of carotid pulses during suspended respiration immediately following the hyperventilation for auscultation of the lungs will allow the patient to cooperate for a longer time. Also, palpation of the liver for size, pulsations, and hepatojugular reflux, the abdominal examination for ascites, the abdominal aortic palpation and auscultation, and the femoral artery palpation and auscultation may be done in close sequence at the end of the cardiac examination.

Inspection, palpation, auscultation, and percussion. In the analysis of the various pulsations of the veins, arteries, and structures of the chest and abdomen, the experienced clinician alternates frequently between visual inspection and palpation. In some instances, these two techniques are combined for greater advantage, as in observing the motion of the palpating fingers or hand or in watching the stethoscope for rocking or inward and outward motion when applied to the apex during auscultation.[6]

Auscultation is often heavily influenced by the results of the preceding inspection and palpation.

Percussion of the heart may reveal the cardiac borders of an enlarged heart. Usually, better clues to cardiac enlargement are found by inspection and palpation. Determination of pleural effusions and of liver size are certainly bona fide uses for extracardiac percussion.

Inspection means observing with the eyes, appreciating the significance of various findings, and identifying them as representing normal or abnormal cardiovascular function. Normally it precedes the other methods of examination and usually begins at a distance of a few feet from the patient so that large areas may be scanned in a short time. Inspection generally reveals body features, pulsations, and fluid accumulations; these findings influence subsequent observations and interpretations. Waveforms that merit special attention may be apparent in the neck, chest, or abdomen. As the examiner moves closer to the patient, the visual field is narrowed and one tends to limit attention to a small area of the body. Several areas should be scanned in sequence. If such orderly inspection is omitted or deferred until after palpation or auscultation, a great opportunity will be lost.

Palpation, the "laying on of hands," follows inspection. It can be used to detect a fine body tremor in thyrotoxicosis, rapid vibrations (thrills), coarse vibrations (carotid shudders), outward lifts from the aortic arch, pulmonary artery, right ventricle, or left ventricle, arterial pulsations, forceful venous waves, pericardial knocks, intense valve closure impulses, tumor plops, the general level of cardiac activity, and other cardiovascular impulses. Precise localization of these areas is often best achieved by palpation and then reinspection. Certain abnormal findings—such as the forceful beating of the left ventricle in hypertrophic cardiomyopathy, the forceful aortic valve closure shock when the ascending aorta has been replaced with a graft or conduit, and the forceful pulmonary valve closure impulse in pulmonary hypertension—may yield nearly instant diagnosis.

By the time inspection and palpation have been completed, the cardiologist often has an excellent idea of the general, if not specific, cardiac diagnosis and can predict the approximate results of subsequent auscultation. Discrepancies between findings on inspection and palpation and findings on auscultation will then be greatly minimized. When they occur, repeat examination need be directed only to the involved regions of the body. Thus, all such modalities of examination are complementary.

Accurate determination of systole and diastole. The task of determining and timing systole and diastole when examining the veins, arteries, and chest wall motions sometimes can be troublesome. Difficulties may arise when waveforms are small, heart tones are faint, heart rate is rapid, heart rhythm is irregular, or several cardiac-related events occur in rapid sequence. It is not uncommon to confuse the diastolic murmurs of aortic insufficiency in bacterial endocarditis or of mitral stenosis with systolic murmurs because of a hyperdynamic apex or an increased heart rate. Uncertainty about the exact timing of the cardiac cycle will destroy even the best efforts to identify and to characterize the various pulsations.

Fortunately, a relatively straightforward method exists for identifying both systole and diastole. It should be used after the determination of the jugular venous pressure and before the evaluation of the venous, arterial, and chest pulsations.

To identify systole and diastole, listen to the first and second heart sounds while holding the diaphragm of the stethoscope against the left anterior chest wall with one hand. At the same time, gently palpate one common carotid artery below the bulb with the fingers of the other hand. Using the outward systolic carotid pulse as a reference, identify the first heart sound as preceding this rise and the second heart sound as following this rise. Accordingly, systole and diastole are accurately demarcated by these heart sounds and distinguished by the carotid pulse.

Unless otherwise stated, the terms "systole" and "diastole" refer to ventricular events and not to atrial events.

Timing of venous, arterial, and chest pulsations. Of these three types of pulsations, venous waves are the most difficult to understand. To time venous waveforms, palpate the left common carotid arterial upstroke and watch the venous pulsations in the opposite internal jugular vein over several cardiac cycles. Establish which are systolic events and which are diastolic events. Note when each wave appears in the cardiac cycle. Generally, one can then determine fairly easily if the major venous deflection in systole is an upright v wave which is nearly synchronous with the carotid pulse or slightly delayed (v wave of tricuspid insufficiency vs. normal v wave, respectively), or if it is a downward y descent immediately following the end of systole. Once this has been positively identified, it is no longer necessary to continue to listen to the heart sounds.

Timing of the carotid and chest pulsations is more direct but should also involve carotid pulse palpation along with auscultation of the first and second heart sounds.

How to detect vibrations (thrills). Small, rapidly alternating waveforms, such as vibrations (thrills), may be palpated with the heel of the palm of the hand placed with light to moderate pressure against the chest or with the tips of the fingers placed gently against the skin over the subclavian, carotid, or other superficial arteries. By first feeling over a wide area of the chest with the palm held flat, one can determine where the intensity of the vibrations is greatest. One then moves the heel of the hand or the fingers to this area for more precise localization. Subsequent auscultation should include this location. A palpable thrill is nearly always accompanied by an audible murmur or bruit and implies a jet of blood whose force, velocity, or flow is great.

The location of a thrill on the skin is downstream from the location of its production. This is why thrills of aortic valve stenosis are over the right upper sternum or lower carotid arteries, thrills of ventricular septal defects are over the middle and lower sternal region, and thrills of mitral insufficiency are over the left anterior chest (as in flail posterior leaflet), left posterior chest (as in flail anterior leaflet), or left anterolateral chest. Similarly, thrills over arteries are somewhat downstream of the area of stenosis or arteriovenous connection.

The causes of thrills will be discussed in the carotid artery section for arterial lesions and in the chest section for cardiac lesions.

Large, visible, or palpable waveforms. Large, relatively slow waveforms may be observed with the eye or palpated with the hand or fingers. Venous pulses and the height of the jugular venous column are observed with the eye. In cases of significant pressure waves, they may also be palpated in the internal jugular vein and in the liver (large, early forceful v wave of significant tricuspid insufficiency or rapid y descent and rapid rebound of constrictive pericarditis).

Arterial pulses are evaluated by palpation and, in the case of the carotid artery, also by observation. Watch the motion of the examining fingers by sighting lengthwise along them. In many cases of a tardus and parvus pulse, this visual observation of the gently palpating fingers is easier to appreciate and to quantitate than is subjective tactile palpation alone.

Chest wall motions in response to cardiac events are often easily appreciated by both visual examination and palpation. Pay special attention to the aortic, pulmonary, right ventricular, and left ventricular areas. Palpate these areas and other areas of visible pulsation with the patient in the sitting, supine, and left semilateral decubitus positions. In searching for the best sites for auscultation it is helpful first to locate such visible and palpable pulsations in order to save time and avoid missing important physical signs. At times, it can be easier for the examiner to see the third or fourth heart sounds with the eyes or to palpate them with the palm of the hand as ventricular filling waves than it is to hear them with the stethoscope.

Overactive cardiovascular motions. In patients with overactive hearts and vascular pulsations due to anemia, thyrotoxicosis, drugs, volume overload (aortic or mitral insufficiency), or hypertrophic cardiomyopathy, there may be an area of visible precordial or vessel motion that is forceful, rapid, large in area, or large in amplitude. In patients with significant mitral insufficiency, a rapid heart rate, and an abnormal ventricular gallop sound at the apex (abnormal third heart sound, palpable rapid-filling wave), the skin of the chest wall or left breast may jiggle with the cardiac cycle. This is due to the increased volumes of blood in the left atrium and left ventricle that undergo rapid, alternate changes in direction of motion, causing the heart to move at rates and amplitudes sufficient to approximate a natural resonance frequency of the external chest wall structures. This is a helpful finding, even if the murmur or third heart sound is faint or if the rapid-filling wave is not distinct.

Conclusions. Analysis of vibrations and pulsations created by movement of the blood and of the walls of the veins, arteries, and heart can reveal a wealth of information about the status of a patient and the extent of disease. It frequently is possible to arrive at the correct diagnosis from these motions, even before auscultation is performed. The following three sections deal with individual systems in which such an analysis can be put to good use.

Jugular venous pulsations

The jugular venous examination is logically performed before the carotid arterial, chest, and cardiac apex examinations because it reveals information about right heart events, primarily relating to inflow of blood to the chest. The other modalities reveal details about left heart events related to outflow of blood from the chest. It is helpful to determine the jugular venous pressure before looking for individual venous waveforms because optimal positioning of the patient depends on recognition of the top of the venous column of blood. The jugular venous pressure is one of the most important clues to body fluid volume and to right heart failure. Peripheral leg edema or abdominal ascites associated with normal or low jugular venous pressure implies a noncardiac cause; a high pressure in the jugular veins implies a cardiac or pericardial cause.

Jugular venous pressure, waves, and associated volume changes. The inflow of blood from the peripheral veins to the central venous system is nonpulsatile and relatively constant, whereas the outflow through the right heart is cyclic and intermittent. The motions of the right heart and its valves and the breathing muscles produce momentary changes in direction of flow, in velocity of flow, and in pressure and volume of blood within the superior vena cava and jugular venous system. Because these vessels are large in diameter and very flexible, the lowest regions will be distended by blood, and the highest regions will be collapsed. The level of transition will change throughout the cardiac cycle, and the diameter of the veins just below this level will vary accordingly. The waveforms created in the top of the venous column of blood and in the walls of the jugular veins can be analyzed to yield valuable information about cardiac function. The upper level relates to the jugular venous pressure; the motions are called, collectively, the "jugular venous pulse."

A situation analogous to the jugular venous system would be a faucet running water into a partially filled sink in which the drain stopper is being opened and closed repeatedly. The level of water in the sink is dependent upon the rate of water entering from the tap, the amount of water already present, and the position of the stopper in the drain. The water level rises when the drain is plugged, falls rapidly when the stopper is removed, falls slowly when the drain is partially plugged, and shows a surface shock wave if the stopper is suddenly plunged into or pulled out of the drain opening.

The jugular venous pressure is determined by the volume of blood and the height to which it rises in the jugular veins above the right atrium. It is a measure of right heart filling pressure and compensation. Given a relatively steady state of right heart function over a period of several cardiac cycles, the volumes of blood entering and leaving the jugular venous system must be equal, regardless of whether the jugular venous pressure is high, normal, or low. Thus, the jugular venous pressure does not reveal cardiac output. In summary, the jugular venous pressure indicates right heart filling pressure, and the individual waveforms in the jugular venous pulse relate to respiratory and right heart events.

Examination position and lighting. The patient should sit comfortably with arms in the lap, legs down, and face forward. The top of the venous column of blood and the venous waves can best be visualized by having the patient sit on the side of the bed or examination table facing daylight from a window. A fixed light in front of the patient or a hand-held light is a good substitute. A ceiling light or a light positioned beside the patient is less desirable. If possible, stand in front of or beside the patient in the office or sit beside the patient on the hospital bed when examining the right and left jugular venous systems.

Reference levels and units of jugular venous pressure. The concept of jugular venous pressure is simple but potentially confusing due to terminology. The level of the right atrium is defined as the zero reference level for the purpose of measuring the jugular venous pressure, regardless of whether the patient is sitting upright, partially reclining, or supine. Because blood has mass and exerts a downward force (its weight) due to gravity, the pressure in the right atrium at any instant is determined by the jugular venous pressure level, which is the true vertical height of blood above the right atrium. The local pressure is greatest at the bottom of the column in the right atrium and gradually decreases to zero at the top of the venous column in the neck, where the difference between the distended and collapsed portions of the jugular venous system can be observed. The physician must be careful not to confuse the number assigned to the jugular venous pressure level and the actual venous pressure at that venous location. In summary, the value of the jugular venous pressure relates to the filling pressure of the right atrium and is measured by the height of the venous column of blood (described in cm H_2O) in a true vertical direction above the right atrium.

With the patient sitting upright, legs down and hands in lap, and with the right atrium as the zero reference level, a venous blood column level at the clavicles represents about 10 cm H_2O. The normal jugular venous pressure is about or slightly less than this value. A level less than 5 cm H_2O suggests dehydration, diuresis, or blood loss. A column up to the level of the angle of the jaw signifies a jugular venous pressure of about 20 cm H_2O (10 cm H_2O above normal) and a column up to the earlobe, about 22 cm H_2O (12 cm H_2O above normal).

When the patient reclines, the normal jugular venous pressure may cause the jugular veins to distend well into the upper neck or lower head, often contributing to nocturnal nasal stuffiness and head congestion. If the patient has a congested liver or distended varicose veins, then the jugular venous column of blood may rise disproportionately more than usual in the neck on partial or full reclining, making estimation of the exact jugular venous pressure more speculative. One must be aware that such a congested liver can act as a venous reservoir in right-sided congestive heart failure, reducing the increase in jugular venous pressure level when the patient sits up and augmenting the increase when the patient reclines. This combination is a helpful clue to combined right heart failure and liver congestion.

The jugular venous pressure is the only cardiovascular measurement determined at the bedside that is reported as cm H_2O. Cardiac catheterization and peripheral blood pressure data are measured in mm Hg. The different unit systems must not be confused, even though both are used in describing jugular venous and right heart pressure.

How to measure jugular venous pressure level. Gentle compression of the internal or external jugular venous system low in the neck with the side of a thin ballpoint pen for a few seconds is a safe procedure for measuring the venous pressure level and waveforms. The trachea and sternocleidomastoid muscle prevent the pen from indenting the neck significantly in the region of the lower common carotid artery, which is deeper in the neck. Obviously, if carotid occlusive disease is suspected or if the carotid arteries are tortuous or superficial, compression of neck veins should be done very cautiously.

To determine the jugular venous level, watch the area of skin overlying the carotid sheath which contains the internal jugular vein. This vein runs from near the sternoclavicular joint to beneath the angle of the jaw. In most patients the right jugular veins are closer and more directly connected to the superior vena cava than are the left jugular veins. Thus, they are usually, but not always, less affected by mechanical compression within the chest and neck which might dampen the waveforms or falsely elevate the top of the jugular venous column of blood.[6]

Place the side of a ballpoint pen (with the point retracted) gently against the lower portion of one carotid sheath just above the clavicle in a transverse (usually horizontal) manner to compress the neck veins slightly. This causes the veins above to distend. Remove the pen and observe the level to which the column of blood falls. This lowest level is usually the jugular venous pressure level. A few trials and repositionings of the pen may be needed. Under certain circumstances, such as compression of the jugular venous system by the clavicle, additional testing may reveal that the true jugular venous pressure level is lower than indicated. Accordingly, certain criteria for identifying the correct level are helpful.

Check both right and left internal jugular venous system levels. The lower of the two pressure levels is used. Because the internal jugular veins are quite distensible and typically may expand enough to move a 3-cm-wide area of neck skin, they usually are easily detected. The external jugular veins are more superficial, are smaller in diameter, run more parallel to the long axis of the neck, and may be more lateral or anterior than the internal jugular veins. They have valves at their lower ends, which may distort backward transmission of venous waveforms and pressures, so they are utilized mainly when the internal jugular veins are not readily visible. They are satisfactory for measurement of the jugular venous pressure level but not for jugular venous pulse waveforms.

With gentle external compression of the venous system high in the neck, the return of blood from the head is reduced, and the more central venous blood column, especially in the external jugular veins (sometimes falsely elevated by compression in the subclavicular region), may then fall. The jugular venous pressure level is also at least as low as this second lowest level. By comparing the lowest levels of the venous columns after release of low neck venous compression and during high neck venous compression, one can determine the natural level of the jugular venous column.

If there are large waves present in the venous system due to heart contraction or sudden changes in cardiac filling, the most reliable reading of the passive venous pressure in the right atrium is usually the average level in the internal jugular vein at those times in the cardiac cycle other than when a large positive or negative wave is occurring.

Effects of body position on jugular venous pressure level. Measurements of venous pressure use the right atrium as the zero reference point. They are evaluated in a vertical direction with respect to gravity and not according to the particular alignment of the chest and neck. The jugular venous column height represents the right atrial pressure when the patient sits upright with the legs dependent.

For best observation, it is necessary to lower the head and torso of a sitting patient when the peak of the jugular venous column and the jugular venous pulse waves are below the middle and lower anterolateral neck region. Conversely, it is necessary to raise the head and torso when the peak of the jugular venous column and the jugular venous pulse waves are above this region. When using this tilt method for jugular venous pressure measurements, the angles from the vertical must be estimated carefully; one must still consider the true vertical difference in height between the right atrium and the top of the venous column of blood.

As the patient reclines, two phenomena occur that affect venous volumes. When the patient becomes more horizontal, the diameter of neck vein distention increases at each venous location in the lower neck as blood extends farther cephalad, but the top of the venous column of blood may spread out over a few centimeters of the upper neck, appearing as a thin ellipse, and may be obscure. The venous waveforms and respiratory variations in jugular venous level aid in detecting this level. Also, when the patient reclines, inflow of blood from a congested liver may increase lower neck vein distention, elevating the actual venous pressure spuriously but also greatly aiding in recognition of elevated right atrial pressure and enhancing the regurgitant v wave (also called cv wave or r wave) of tricuspid insufficiency.

Respiratory effects on jugular venous pressure. During active inspiration, the intrathoracic pressure is decreased, so the inflow of blood from the peripheral and central veins to the right heart is augmented, and the amount of blood in the superior vena cava and the internal jugular vein is diminished. The average level, excluding waveforms, of the blood column in the internal jugular vein indicating the venous pressure in the right atrium decreases throughout inspiration and becomes lowest at the end of active inspiration.[6] Once inspiration stops, there is an increase in intrathoracic pressure; this also occurs during the Valsalva maneuver. One must not confuse the important jugular venous events that occur during active inspiration with those that occur after the end of inspiration or during held inspiration.

Conversely, during active exhalation, the intrathoracic pressure is increased, so blood from the jugular venous system cannot drain as easily into the right atrium. Hence, the average level of blood standing in the internal jugular vein increases. The jugular venous pressure and the right atrial pressure increase according to the rise in height of this blood column.

Kussmaul's sign: true paradoxic increase in jugular venous pressure during inspiration. During inspiration the diaphragm descends and carries with it the inferior portion of the pericardium, causing elongation of the pericardial sac. The normally compliant pericardium and myocardium can easily adapt to this elongated shape, in part by stretching, so the pressures within the pericardial space and within the heart chambers are essentially unaffected. The normal slight drop in jugular venous pressure level still occurs.

With constriction of the pericardium due to scarring and thickening, the ability of the right atrium to distend and fill with blood from the superior vena cava and jugular veins during ventricular systole is inhibited. The right ventricular distensibility and filling during diastole are also limited. The latter conditions occur as well in restrictive heart disease. The net effect is an increased jugular venous pressure level which is in part compensatory.

During active inspiration, elongation of a noncompliant pericardial sac or of a noncompliant heart within it decreases the maximum potential volume within the pericardial space and heart chambers, because a spherical shape contains the largest volume for a fixed surface area of pericardium or myocardium. Fast (cine) computed tomographic scanning of the heart in held inspiration in patients with constrictive pericarditis often demonstrates an elongated, banana-shaped pericardial contour (personal observation of T.C.E.). With this limited volume in the heart chambers during inspiration, there is decreased filling of the right heart, and the jugular venous pressure increases instead of decreases – Kussmaul's sign.[7,8] This is a true paradoxic situation and is different from the arterial paradoxic pulse, which is an exaggerated normal decrease in pressure. Occasionally, hyperexpansion of the lungs, when the diaphragm is already lower than normal in the thorax, or a mediastinal tumor mass, can impede right atrial filling and produce similar changes. It is not uncommon to see the height of "a" and v waves increase somewhat with inspiration in this setting and at times in normal patients when they are supine.[6] One must be careful to recognize if a rapid x or a rapid y descent in constrictive or restrictive disease is the dominant wave when the jugular venous pressure increases during inspiration. Observe the neck veins during the middle and late phases of active inspiration, when the greatest changes occur, and not after the end of inspiration, because an unintentional Valsalva maneuver can mimic Kussmaul's sign.

O'Rourke[9] noted that Kussmaul's sign may be positive in severe right ventricular failure. The large right atrium and ventricle, more spherical than usual, are operating with high filling pressures and may develop increased internal pressure when the diaphragm descends and distorts their optimal shapes. Kussmaul's sign may be present temporarily after acute right ventricular infarction.[10] Kussmaul's sign is uncommon in obstructive or asthmatic lung disease; the jugular venous pressure may show an excessive inspiratory decrease and expiratory increase due to the extreme pressure effects of the respiratory muscles.[8]

Rapid manipulation of venous volumes when venous pressure is markedly increased. When the jugular venous pressure is too high (generally, more than 22 cm H_2O) to allow for visualization of the top of the venous column of blood or waveforms, as in severe, chronic constrictive pericarditis or obstruction of the superior vena cava, one may be able to lower the top of the jugular venous column and reduce the jugular venous distention for a few seconds to permit better observation. If the patient is able to do so, ask him or her to stand on the floor and then squat. The venous return from the lower extremities will increase, and the jugular venous pressure will rise temporarily. Support the patient so that he or she does not fall over and have the patient raise his or her arms over the head to drain venous blood from the upper limbs toward the heart. After a few seconds, have the patient stand up quickly and immediately lower the arms. This will reverse the process, allowing blood in the venous system to fill up the arm veins and the lower extremity veins more fully and decreasing the venous return to the right heart. This often results in a temporary drop in the internal jugular venous pressure and the corresponding level of the jugular venous column. During this period of a few seconds, one may locate the top of the jugular venous column of blood in order to evaluate the venous waveforms. Note whether a rapid x or y descent is present or whether there are no venous waves at all (chronic constrictive pericarditis or superior vena caval obstruction, respectively). In all cases of extremely high jugular venous pressure, one should search for collateral veins over the upper chest.[7]

Although sometimes associated with very high jugular venous pressure, severe tricuspid insufficiency produces bounding jugular venous v waves which mimic the bounding carotid arterial pulse contour of valvular aortic insufficiency. Obliteration of the more cranial v wave by compression of the lower jugular venous column with the side of a ballpoint pen identifies the pulse as venous and not arterial in origin. One must never compress the carotid artery or displace it during such testing.

Hepatojugular reflux. The hepatojugular reflux (i.e., reverse flow; distention of the jugular veins induced by pressure over the liver) is an excellent method for demonstrating liver congestion due to increased venous pressure in this organ. Place the patient in a semisupine position (the upright position may be appropriate in some cases) to bring the upper portion of the venous column of blood into the lower internal jugular venous system, easily observed just above the clavicle. Use moderate palpation with continued, steady, posterior pressure on the right upper abdominal quadrant portion of the liver for several seconds. This forces some of the extrahepatic venous and inferior vena caval blood to flow upward in the inferior vena cava and right atrium and to reflux into the superior vena cava and internal jugular veins. Avoid pressing on the abdominal aorta, because no reflux will occur. It is also important that the patient breathe normally and avoid straining or performing an inadvertent Valsalva maneuver, which would impede right atrial filling and lead to a false interpretation of the jugular venous pressure increase.[8,11]

A positive hepatojugular reflux is an increase in the jugular venous pressure level of a few centimeters; if the patient is semirecumbent, this may extend several centimeters up the neck. It usually occurs in less than 5 to 10 seconds in patients with significant hepatic congestion due to increased inferior vena caval (and therefore increased superior vena caval and jugular venous) pressure. If more than 30 seconds of compression is required, the rise is usually minimal, and the reliability and value are questionable. On release of the compression of the liver, the jugular venous pressure level should decrease promptly and reach the original level in a few seconds. Because the initial jugular venous pressure level does not have to be markedly elevated for the hepatojugular reflux to be positive, this test is sometimes helpful in patients treated with diuretics.

A liver that is large because of venous congestion and that can be partially compressed to create a positive hepatojugular reflux thus can be differentiated from hepatomegaly due to certain other causes. The hepatojugular reflux will be positive in conditions of liver congestion of cardiac origin such as right heart congestive failure, constrictive pericarditis, cardiac tamponade, right atrial myxoma, tricuspid stenosis, and tricuspid insufficiency associated with increased right heart filling pressure. A partially obstructing inferior vena caval thrombus or tumor between the liver and the right heart might yield a positive hepatojugular reflux. The hepatojugular reflux will not be positive in cases of superior vena caval obstruction, inferior vena caval obstruction below the level of the hepatic veins, left heart congestive failure, hypoalbuminemia, cirrhosis of the liver, or other causes of hepatomegaly, ascites, or lower limb edema. Just before or just after the test for the hepatojugular reflux is a convenient time to observe the liver and palpate it gently to check for abnormally tall v waves or deep y descents.

Some cardiologists find no special advantage to palpation over the liver rather than over the remainder of the abdomen. They believe that the increase in jugular venous pressure indicates the right ventricle's inability to adapt to increased venous return. Here the increased venous return probably comes from several abdominal organs and not just from the liver. This would better be termed the "abdominojugular reflux."[8] Ewy[12] has shown that a positive abdominojugular test (abrupt drop in jugular venous pressure of 4 cm after release of 10 seconds of firm midabdominal pressure) is sometimes correlated with a pulmonary arterial wedge pressure of 15 mm Hg or greater.

Ascites and the jugular venous pressure. Ascites associated with chronic constrictive pericarditis may not correlate with the apparent elevation in the average jugular venous pressure; it may be inconsequential or disproportionately massive. It is usually well tolerated by the patient.

Hepatosplenomegaly and the jugular venous pressure. Chronic elevation of the jugular venous pressure often results in progressive hepatomegaly and splenomegaly. The hepatomegaly is usually dominant, so the liver is superior to the spleen as an organ for palpation of the regurgitant v wave in tricuspid insufficiency. Both hepatic and splenic enlargement may become permanent after several years of chronic jugular venous pressure elevation.

The peripheral venous examination: pressures and pulsations. Upper limb veins usually collapse promptly when the veins being observed are elevated above the jugular venous pressure level in the neck; hand and antecubital veins are the most readily observed. If the veins do not collapse, then reduced central venous drainage due to external compression within the subclavian area (usually benign), superior vena caval obstruction, or true elevation of the central venous pressure may exist. The central venous waveforms are absent because of the venous valves. Observation of limb veins is an additional way to determine the status of central venous drainage and to estimate the central venous pressure level when the jugular veins are difficult to observe or when the jugular venous pressure level is uncertain. In most patients, however, routine examination of the upper limb veins in detail is not necessary.

Distended upper limb veins have no major significance when they are below the jugular venous pressure level, nor do constricted hand veins in a cool environment, but they are a source of anxiety for some patients.

Abnormal tortuosity or distention of superficial thoracic or longitudinally oriented thoracoabdominal veins implies that they are being used as accessory pathways for central venous return, as in inferior vena caval obstruction. The practice of trying to strip blood in each direction to determine the direction of flow (caudad in superior vena caval obstruction and craniad in inferior vena caval obstruction) is well known[6] but is often of doubtful value. The blood is usually pressurized on each side of the stripped venous segment, and flow velocity on release may be equal despite valves or else may be spuriously unequal because of valves. Similarly, waveforms in these veins are of little use due to valves, distance from the heart, and small size with respect to the jugular veins. The presence of increased jugular venous pressure is a valuable adjunctive test of superior vena caval obstruction; the increase is not present in inferior vena caval obstruction.

Veins of the lower extremities may show the large pulsatile systolic v wave of significant tricuspid insufficiency if they have incompetent venous valves. In this high degree of tricuspid insufficiency, one would also expect to find increased jugular venous pressure, an enlarged and pulsatile liver, and possibly some ascites. Palpate such pulsating foot or leg veins and a nearby artery on the same foot simultaneously to check for an arteriovenous malformation or fistula. In tricuspid insufficiency, the venous v wave should be more delayed than the arterial pulse peak, whereas the abnormal venous pulsation in an arteriovenous malformation or fistula should involve only a single limb.

Sequence of the jugular venous waves. In normal sinus rhythm the sequence of jugular venous waves is "a," x, c, x′, v, y, and h.[6,7,9,11] The waves correspond to the rising

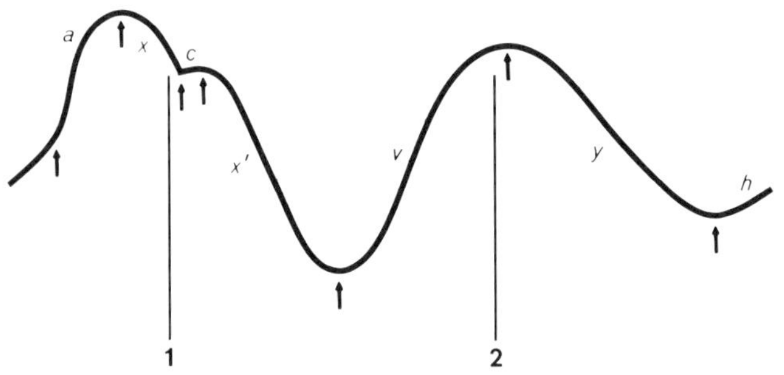

Fig 2-19 Jugular venous pulse. *Arrows* indicate junctions between the named waves. The upward "a" wave is due to right atrial contraction. The downward x descent is due to right atrial relaxation. The brief upward c wave is caused by cephalad motion of the tricuspid valve during its closure. The downward x′ descent is a continuation of the original x descent after tricuspid valve closure. The normal upward v wave is a passive wave due to continued right atrial filling. The downward y descent is caused by tricuspid valve opening. The rising h wave is a shallow upward deflection due to continued inflow of blood to the jugular venous system during diastole. The numbers represent the first and second heart sounds. The first heart sound slightly precedes the c wave, and the second heart sound slightly precedes the end of the v wave.

or falling phases and begin or end with the peaks and valleys (Fig 2-19). The waves usually do not have sharp demarcations between them, so the sequence of waves must be observed over several cycles and correlated with the onset and ending of both ventricular systole and diastole in order to make proper identification. Without this appreciation for the total cardiac cycle, the individual rises and falls are sometimes too subtle to appreciate fully. Although convention varies in the literature, we will use lower-case letters for jugular venous waves and capital letters for carotid and chest impulses.

Jugular venous pulse waves in sequence of occurrence in sinus rhythm

"a" WAVE. The positive jugular venous wave due to blood that is forced backward into the jugular veins from right atrial systole. It precedes ventricular systole in sinus rhythm.

x DESCENT. The negative jugular venous wave after the "a" wave, due to more rapid filling of the partly emptied right atrium. The total wave ends in the x point or x trough.

c WAVE. The small positive jugular venous wave due to upward (craniad) closure of the tricuspid valve and the ensuing brief retrograde fluid shock wave in the jugular veins. It is seen within the total x descent. It may be absent or very small.

x′ DESCENT. The portion of the total x descent after the c wave.

v WAVE. The positive jugular venous wave after the x descent, due to continued filling of the right atrium when the blood begins to back up in the jugular veins while the tricuspid valve is closed during ventricular systole. It is a passive wave and is not due to right ventricular systole itself unless there is tricuspid insufficiency.

cv OR r WAVE. The v wave of tricuspid insufficiency. It is earlier, taller, and more forceful than the normal passive v wave.

y DESCENT. The negative jugular venous wave after the v wave. It begins with opening of the tricuspid valve as the right atrial blood and the jugular venous column of blood above it fall into the partly emptied right ventricle.

h WAVE. The slowly rising baseline between the end of the y descent and the next "a" or c wave. It is due to continued passive atrial filling in ventricular diastole.

"a" wave: the visible right atrial kick. The rising jugular venous "a" (atrial) wave is due to right atrial contraction. Because there is no valve between the right atrium, the superior vena cava, and the internal jugular vein, the active contraction of the right atrium due to electrical stimulation must use the weight of the column of venous blood above it as a buttress to force extra blood into the nearly filled right ventricle. Ventricular systole must soon follow to close the tricuspid valve and thereby capture this extra volume of blood or much of it will reflux back into the right atrium and have little continued right ventricular stretching effect or contribution to right ventricular stroke volume. If ventricular systole is delayed (as in first-degree heart block and in some beats of second-degree heart block) or asynchronous (as in AV dissociation or third-degree heart block), the advantages of the atrial kick are reduced or lost.

The normal rapid right atrial contraction distributes extra atrial blood forward into the right ventricle. The temporary rise in the jugular venous column of blood and the associated dilation of the jugular veins represent the corresponding reaction, a brief reflux pulse named the "a" wave. In normal sinus rhythm the right atrial contraction occurs in late ventricular diastole when the right atrium has been nearly filled with blood and the incoming venous blood has risen passively in the internal jugular veins to a relatively high level (the basic jugular venous pressure level), so the "a" wave normally is the highest positive jugular venous wave.[7]

"a" waves in late diastole: normal sinus rhythm. Normal sinus rhythm can be confirmed by detecting "a" waves just before the onset of right ventricular systole. This pattern excludes atrial fibrillation.

Large "a" waves: pressure and volume changes in sinus rhythm. Restriction of diastolic filling of the right ventricle due to right ventricular hypertrophy and loss of compliance (primary or secondary pulmonary hypertension, pulmonary embolism, pulmonary stenosis, hypertrophic cardiomyopathy, or infiltrative cardiomyopathy) or tricuspid obstruction (stenosis, myxoma, or atresia) leads to hypertrophy of the right atrium. There is greater than normal intra-atrial pressure during contraction and thus more jugular venous reflux, causing a large "a" wave.[6,7,11] Tetralogy of Fallot is not characterized by an increased "a" wave[7,8] because the large ventricular septal defect allows decompression of the right ventricle.

Increased blood volume in the right atrium (atrial septal defect, partial anomalous pulmonary venous connection, or tricuspid insufficiency) also results in a large "a" wave. In the case of an atrial septal defect, the "a" wave and the subsequent large, peaked v wave may

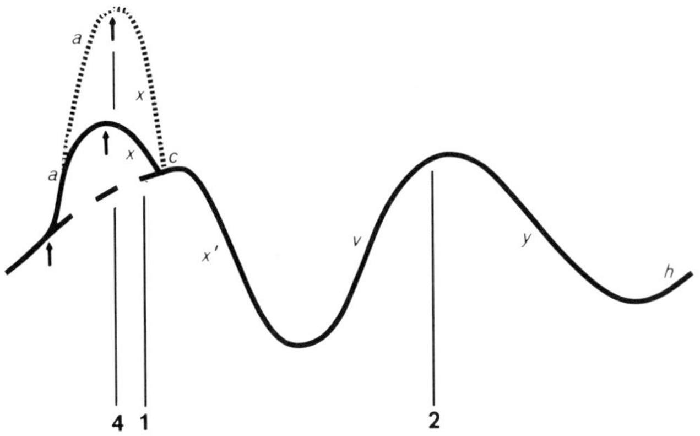

Fig 2-20 Jugular venous pulse. The normal contour is shown by the *solid line.* The "a" wave is absent in atrial fibrillation *(dashed line).* The "a" wave becomes large or giant when the right atrium contracts against a greater-than-normal volume of blood, a noncompliant or hypertrophied right ventricle, or a closing or closed tricuspid valve *(dotted line). Arrows* indicate the beginning and end of the "a" wave. The numbers represent the first, second, and fourth heart sounds. The fourth heart sound coincides with the peak of the large or giant "a" wave.

together resemble a sawtooth pattern that is due to accentuation of the heights of both waves from the increased right atrial blood return; the double venous waves for each single carotid pulse wave may be quite striking.

Giant "a" waves: rhythm changes. Giant "a" waves (cannon "a" waves) yield valuable clues to certain cardiac rhythms (Fig 2-20). When the right atrium contracts and the tricuspid valve is either closing or is already closed due to increased ventricular systolic pressure, the atrial blood cannot enter the tricuspid valve and right ventricle. The "a" wave in the jugular veins can be driven quite high by the extra regurgitant blood. It is easily visualized as a very large, quick "a" wave and actually may be palpated with the fingers. It is important to time such giant "a" waves with every carotid pulse by palpation of the opposite carotid artery over a series of cardiac cycles.

Determine if the giant "a" waves occur with every carotid cycle (very short P-R interval,[11] marked first-degree heart block, junctional rhythm, or regular retrograde rhythm), with occasional cycles but near the regular time (late-coupled ventricular premature beats), with only occasional cycles while the "a" wave rate is greater than the carotid pulse rate (third-degree heart block), with only occasional cycles while the "a" wave rate is less than the carotid pulse rate (AV dissociation, ventricular tachycardia, or ventricular demand pacemaker rhythm), or during single premature beats (atrial or junctional premature beats).[6,7,11] Second-degree heart block with 2:1 conduction sometimes may be manifested by alternating "a" wave amplitudes at twice the carotid pulse rate, but the tallest "a" waves are not always giant.[11]

Small or absent "a" waves may mean rapid or disorganized atrial activity. In atrial flutter, the frequent small "a" waves are called f (flutter) waves. They sometimes may be seen in the right internal jugular vein if the top of the venous column can be adjusted, by body positioning, to appear just above the clavicle. In atrial fibrillation, the atrial waves are absent (see Fig 2-20). Do not assume, however, that absent, obscure, or low-volume "a" waves automatically mean an abnormal cardiac rhythm. Many normal patients in normal sinus rhythm may have low-amplitude venous waves ("a," v, or both). Right atrial injury after cardiopulmonary bypass may[13] or may not[14] depress the "a" wave amplitude.

Timing of "a" waves. The jugular pulse recording apparatus can record the timing, amplitude, and rhythm of the "a" waves. They are delayed slightly due to hydraulic lag in the neck veins to about the same extent that the right-sided fourth heart sound of right ventricular distention is delayed by hydraulic and mechanical lags. Hence, the jugular "a" wave and the right-sided fourth heart sound are essentially simultaneous events.[7]

The x descent, the c wave, and the x′ descent: atrial filling as ventricular contraction begins. With right atrial relaxation after the "a" wave, the jugular venous column of blood can drop into the atrium easily due to the decline in active and passive tension in the atrial walls, the low volume of blood remaining in the atrium, the increased potential filling capacity of the collapsed atrial chamber, and the low atrial pressure resulting from these factors. The downward motion of the top of the jugular venous column immediately after the "a" wave is called the x descent. The x descent begins in late diastole. It is a passive wave and is not due to contraction of a cardiac chamber. It is most easily recognized in sinus rhythm as the downward wave in the jugular veins just before the carotid arterial upstroke.

During early right ventricular systole the tricuspid valve closes and sends a small rising hydraulic shock wave, called the c wave, up the jugular venous system as the downward motion of the column of blood is temporarily disturbed. This c wave is not due to transmission of movement of either the carotid arterial wall or the carotid arterial blood. Although it is an active wave due to contraction of the right ventricle and tricuspid valve motion, it usually is too small to be recognized in most patients. A technically poor jugular venous pulse recording may include the carotid pulse upstroke phase by mistake and this artifact may simulate a jugular venous pulse c wave.

Sometimes the portion of the total x descent in right ventricular diastole before tricuspid valve closure is called the x descent and that portion after the c wave in right ventricular systole is called the x′ descent. One important feature of this subclassification is to alert the observer to the possibility of seeing multiple waveforms in some individuals. Most cardiologists lump the x and x′ waves together simply as the x descent.[6,7]

Ventricular premature beats produce c waves (also called early v waves) as part of the y descent or pre-"a" wave phase if they are early-coupled or giant "a" waves if they are late-coupled. In atrial fibrillation, the "a" waves are absent and the c waves may be more easily recognized if they are present.

The slope of the total x descent may be enhanced (rapid x descent) in constrictive pericarditis or cardiac tamponade in which the jugular venous pressure is elevated as a compensatory mechanism to augment right heart filling.[6,7] The total x descent may be greater than the subsequent y descent in a few patients with constrictive pericarditis, active pericarditis,[11] or cardiac tamponade. Conversely, injury to the right atrium after cannulation for cardiopulmonary bypass may reduce the amplitude of the total x descent.[13]

Blood that enters the jugular venous system and the venae cavae during ventricular systole is used to fill the right atrium. As the entry of blood into the right atrium slows due to chamber distention and increasing pressure, the flow from the jugular veins also subsides and the x descent ends with a smooth transition to a brief horizontal slope. Normally, the end of the total x descent, the x point, has the greatest negative value of all the venous waves.

The v wave: usually passive, sometimes active. The normal upward v wave in the jugular venous system occurs as a passive event. Blood enters the jugular venous system at a relatively constant rate and is used in ventricular systole to fill the right atrium (x′ descent). However, as the atrium becomes distended, its rate of filling declines continually and the excess blood must back up into the superior vena cava and the jugular venous system during the remainder of systole. The x′ descent in the jugular veins is thus ended and followed, in about midsystole, by a smooth transition to a subsequent rising wave called the v wave. The v wave continues to rise until the end of ventricular systole. The increasing venous pressure aids in the completion of passive right atrial filling. With the end of systole and the opening of the tricuspid valve, the jugular venous column of blood drops successively into the superior vena cava, the right atrium, the tricuspid valve opening, and the right ventricle. The start of this fall signals the end of the v wave.

A large, sharp-peaked v wave appears in atrial septal defect or partial anomalous pulmonary venous connection due to increased right atrial blood entry.[7]

An abnormally large v wave occurs if the tricuspid valve is incompetent. It is an active regurgitant wave due to right ventricular contraction (ventricularization of the venous pulse wave).[11] The rise begins early in systole, the rate of rise is rapid, and the peak is higher than normal; it follows the c wave more closely and shortens the duration and amplitude of the x′ descent. It is also called a cv wave or r (regurgitant) wave by some authors.[6,11] It lasts most of systole and has a smooth peak (Fig 2-21).

The forcefulness and size of this abnormal v wave in the internal jugular vein or in the pulsatile liver yield important clues to the severity of tricuspid insufficiency. Severe tricuspid insufficiency may create giant v waves that move the skin over the entire visible course of the internal jugular vein and the earlobes, even with the patient sitting. One may use the side of a ballpoint pen to compress the lower internal jugular vein and attenuate or block the v wave above it, thereby distinguishing it from the bounding carotid pulse of aortic insufficiency. Slight extra force may be necessary to accomplish this compression, because of the strength of the regurgitant v wave.

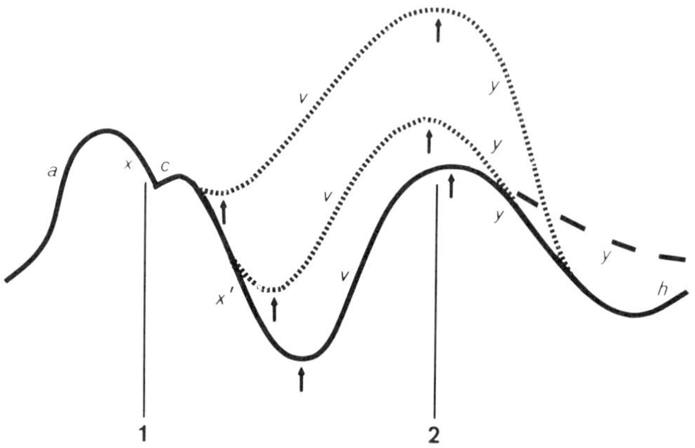

Fig 2-21 Jugular venous pulse. The normal contour is shown by the *solid line.* The v wave begins earlier and its peak is taller than normal in tricuspid insufficiency. The *upper dotted line* represents severe tricuspid insufficiency; the *lower dotted line* represents mild tricuspid insufficiency. *Arrows* indicate the beginning and end of the v wave. This regurgitant v wave is also termed a cv or r wave (see text). The early onset of the v wave in tricuspid insufficiency encroaches upon the x′ descent, shortening this latter wave's duration and amplitude. The peak of the regurgitant v wave may rise above the peak of the normal "a" wave. The downslope of the regurgitant v wave, the y descent, is correspondingly increased but has no functional significance by itself. The y descent in tricuspid stenosis is shallow *(dashed line).* The numbers represent the first and second heart sounds.

The compression must be done cautiously and for only one or two cardiac cycles to minimize carotid compression.

In atrial fibrillation the v wave is the only major positive wave; the "a" wave is absent.

In complete heart block, the v waves are less frequent but may be taller than normal. When "a" and v waves occur together in this type of heart block, the resulting venous wave may become a giant wave.

If the v wave is not easily recognized, then the patient's head and chest position should be changed gradually, either up or down, until the top of the jugular venous column is in the lower neck where the relative motions of the jugular venous system are the easiest to see. If the patient has a low jugular venous pressure due to dehydration, use of diuretics, or blood loss, the v wave may be small and difficult to recognize unless the patient is placed in the reclining position. In tricuspid insufficiency, an increased amplitude of the v wave in the reclining position may be the only major physical clue to this lesion because there may be no murmur or right ventricular lift. An abnormally large v wave or a v wave that increases greatly in the supine position should always be sought in associated mitral valve disease, right ventricular failure, increased jugular venous pressure, or hepatomegaly, and especially before planning cardiac surgery or liver biopsy.

In the presence of constrictive pericarditis the v wave may appear to be increased in amplitude although the y descent following it, deeper and more rapid than usual, in reality is the dominant wave. Restrictive heart disease causes similar but somewhat delayed v and y descent waves. The overlap in timing ranges of these waves makes it difficult to differentiate constriction from restriction by bedside venous wave measurements.

The hepatic v wave in tricuspid insufficiency. The regurgitant v wave of tricuspid insufficiency observed and palpated in the liver is a smoothly rising impulse throughout much of systole. Its upstroke and overall contour are less abrupt than those of the abdominal aorta or an abdominal aortic aneurysm. Such a liver is usually enlarged enough to be easily palpated below the right costal margin. By lightly palpating in the right upper abdominal quadrant and avoiding the midline, one generally can be sure the pulsations are hepatic in origin. It is also good practice to observe the palpating hand visually to estimate the pulse volume and contour.

If the v wave pulsations in the liver are disproportionately more forceful than those in the jugular vein in systole, one should suspect a rare condition such as an arteriovenous malformation in the liver (hereditary hemorrhagic telangiectasia), a localized hepatic artery aneurysm, or transmitted pulsations from an unusually positioned abdominal aortic aneurysm. Auscultation of the region would be especially appropriate in these circumstances.

The y descent: a measure of tricuspid valve flow. With cessation of right ventricular systole and opening of the tricuspid valve, the blood in the right atrium and in the jugular veins above it drops into the relatively empty, collapsed right ventricle; the associated falling jugular venous wave is called the y descent.

If the maximal effective opening of the tricuspid valve is relatively small due to tricuspid stenosis or a right atrial myxoma, the rate of tricuspid flow is limited and the slope of the y descent is abnormally shallow (see Fig 2-21). This is a difficult feature to appreciate, and there are relatively few such patients to provide experience. In the presence of rheumatic mitral or aortic valvular disease or of tricuspid insufficiency, one must examine the y descent for just such slowing. Failure to correct associated organic tricuspid stenosis at the time of operation on other valves can lead to a poor surgical result. A great deal of time should be spent examining normal and rheumatic heart disease patients so that the subtle slowing of the y descent will be recognized when it is present. Pulmonary valve stenosis with marked right ventricular hypertrophy and reduced compliance also may produce a slow "y" descent,[6,7,11] and the y descent may become diminished or even disappear when cardiac tamponade is present.[15]

In tricuspid insufficiency or in atrial septal defect, in which the tricuspid flow in diastole is increased, the slightly increased size of the y descent is simply the backslope of a larger-than-normal v wave.[7]

Constrictive pericarditis often causes an elevated jugular venous pressure with a rapid and deep y descent followed by a sudden, rapid rebound to the higher-than-normal resting jugular venous pressure level, termed the h plateau (Fig 2-22). The pattern of the jugular venous pulse recording resembles a square root sign.[7,16] It is only in the early diastolic filling phase of the right ventricle during the y descent that the abnormally high pressures within the right ventricle, right atrium, and jugular venous system are temporarily decreased as the pericardial sac is depressurized and partially collapsed around the contracted right ventricle. Due to the high jugular venous pressure level, the rate of filling is rapid, accounting for the steepness of the y descent. The right ventricle quickly fills to the maximal capacity permitted by the reexpanded, nonstretchable, pericardial sac, and then the filling ceases abruptly. The higher-than-normal pressure in all the right-sided cardiac structures is restored rapidly. Accordingly, the rapid y descent ends abruptly with a rapidly rising wave to the high jugular venous pressure level again. Recognizing that the dominant wave is a rapid y descent and not a tall v wave takes practice; one often can see this best from a distance of 2 or 3 feet from the neck. Do not fail to look for this feature during the initial inspection of the jugular veins; the diagnosis of constrictive pericarditis is easiest when made early during the physical examination.

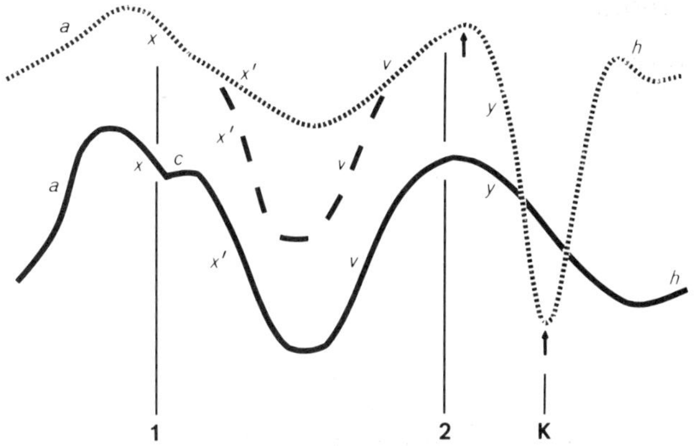

Fig 2-22 Jugular venous pulse. The normal contour is shown by the *solid line.* The upper contour *(dotted line)* represents the usual shape of the jugular venous pulse tracing in constrictive pericarditis. The *dashed line* indicates a variation in this curve. The steepness of the x′ descent may be increased, with the corresponding v wave being somewhat increased in its own slope. The opening of the tricuspid valve *(first arrow)* allows rapid right ventricular filling, resulting in a more rapid and steeper-than-usual y descent. It ends with the distention of the right ventricle and pericardium being abruptly halted by the inability of the pericardium to stretch once it has adopted its most efficient and maximal size *(second arrow).* The pericardial knock *(K)* is heard at this time. The jugular venous pressure then rebounds rapidly, with the h wave having a very steep slope until it attains the high jugular venous pressure associated with constrictive pericarditis. The shape of the rapid y descent and rapid h rebound wave followed by the h plateau resembles a mathematical square root sign. The numbers represent the first and second heart sounds.

Braunwald[6] stated that Kussmaul's sign is more characteristic of constriction than of tamponade, whereas

Table 2-1 Diagnostic significance of visible and palpable jugular venous pulse waves

Diagnosis	Jugular venous pressure	Jugular venous waves
Superior vena caval obstruction	Very high	No waves
Constrictive pericarditis	High to very high, Kussmaul's sign positive	Rapid x or y descent, h plateau
Pericardial tamponade	High	Rapid x or y descent (uncommon)
Restrictive cardiomyopathy	High	Rapid y descent
Right heart failure	High	Normal to increased v wave
Right atrial myxoma	Normal to slightly elevated	Increased "a" wave, shallow x or y descent
Tricuspid stenosis	Normal to slightly elevated	Increased "a" wave, shallow y descent
Tricuspid insufficiency	Normal to elevated	Reduced x descent, early and increased v wave (cv or r wave)
Atrial septal defect	Normal	Increased "a" wave, increased and peaked v wave
Partial anomalous pulmonary venous connection	Normal	Increased "a" and v waves
Ebstein's anomaly of tricuspid valve	Normal	Large "a" or v wave
Normal sinus rhythm	...	Regular, normal waves
Atrial fibrillation	...	Absent "a" wave
Atrial flutter	...	Flutter waves
First-degree block (marked)	...	Increased "a" wave
Second-degree block	...	Regular "a" wave, variation in size
Third-degree block	...	Infrequent giant "a" wave
AV dissociation, ventricular tachycardia	...	Infrequent giant "a" wave
Pacemaker rhythm (ventricular)	...	Infrequent giant "a" wave
Junctional rhythm	...	Regular giant "a" waves
Atrial premature contractions	...	Irregular, extra "a" waves
Ventricular premature contractions	...	Irregular, extra v waves or giant "a" waves
Junctional premature contractions	...	Irregular, extra giant "a" waves
Hypertrophic cardiomyopathy	...	Increased "a" wave
Pulmonary valve stenosis	...	Increased "a" wave
Pulmonary hypertension	...	Increased "a" wave
Low venous volume	Low	Decreased waves
Noncardiac peripheral edema	Normal	Normal waves
Right heart ischemia	Normal to elevated	Increased "a" wave

Spodick[17] emphasized that it is not a feature of tamponade. Kussmaul's sign, discussed above, should always be sought whenever the venous pressure is elevated or the jugular venous pulse demonstrates prominent negative waves. A prominent y descent with a rapid rebound to an h plateau is seen in some patients with restrictive heart disease or with severe right heart failure with high right ventricular end-diastolic and jugular venous pressures.[11] Conversely, a deep y descent without an ensuing rapid rebound to an h plateau is of no major significance.

The h plateau (wave): passive filling in late diastole. The h plateau in constrictive pericarditis is a manifestation of the increased jugular venous pressure. In normal patients, sometimes a distinct late diastolic h wave of low amplitude can be identified, especially if the sinus rate is slow.[16]

Possible diagnoses. Diagnoses that may be suggested on the basis of examination of the jugular venous pressure and waveforms include superior vena caval obstruction, constrictive pericarditis, pericardial tamponade, restrictive cardiomyopathy, right heart failure, right atrial myxoma, tricuspid valve stenosis, tricuspid valve insufficiency, atrial septal defect, partial anomalous pulmonary venous connection, Ebstein's anomaly, normal sinus rhythm, atrial fibrillation, atrial flutter, first-degree heart block, second-degree heart block, complete heart block, AV dissociation, pacemaker rhythm, junctional rhythm, atrial premature beats, ventricular premature beats, junctional premature beats, hypertrophic cardiomyopathy, pulmonary valve stenosis, pulmonary hypertension, dehydration, peripheral edema of noncardiac cause associated with low jugular venous pressure, and right heart ischemia (Table 2-1). The large number of possible diagnoses indicates the importance of studying the jugular venous pressure and waveforms in the assessment of the cardiac patient.

Conclusions. Evaluation of the jugular venous pressure is one of the first steps in cardiac physical diagnosis. The jugular venous pressure and waves are abnormal or characteristic in a large number of cardiovascular conditions. Right heart events are readily evaluated by this important diagnostic modality.

Carotid arterial pulsations

Carotid arterial pulse volume and contour. Valuable information about the characteristics of the left ventricle, its output, and its outflow tract can be obtained by analysis of the pulse volume and contour of the carotid artery in the neck. Such evaluation of the carotid pulse volume and contour is an important part of the total cardiac examination and should not be omitted or performed with only casual interest. Unless the patient is very obese, has a short neck, or is confined to the supine position in bed, it is nearly always possible to inspect and palpate the carotid pulse. The carotid pulse contour is often easier to analyze than either the jugular venous pulse waves or the motions of the cardiac apex. Time spent in analysis of the carotid contour is time well spent and will often reward the examiner with enough information to confirm or to exclude certain cardiac diagnoses with a high degree of confidence.

Why the carotid is the best artery to use for wave recognition. The carotid artery yields the best pulse contour of all of the easily palpable arteries for evaluation of the status of the left heart. Each carotid artery is relatively large and simple to locate. The upper portion of the common carotid artery just below the midneck is the best location for inspection and palpation.

The carotid artery is close to the aorta and left ventricle, so the pattern of distention of the artery by blood passing through it retains the primary pulse volume and waveform contours generated by the left ventricle, aortic valve, and proximal aorta. As blood travels farther from the heart, however, the elastic and volume properties of the more peripheral arteries distort the amplitude and contour of the original wave to make it relatively taller, shorter in duration, smoother in contour, more symmetric in the rising and falling phases, and single rather than multiple in its peak.[6-9] This smoothing and narrowing effect on the arterial pulse wave as it travels away from the heart is similar to the modification of a square wave telegraph signal into a smooth curve which declines in amplitude as it travels along an electric wire without reamplification. The arterial properties are somewhat analogous to the space and time constants of a wire, a nerve cell, or a skeletal muscle cell. Thus, the characteristic slopes, notches, peaks, and oscillations in the carotid arterial pulse contour frequently are reduced or absent distally in certain cardiac diseases.

Nevertheless, marked aortic valve stenosis or marked aortic valve insufficiency may produce pulses with sufficient abnormality of contour to be preserved and recognized peripherally as well as more centrally (tardus and parvus pulse in aortic stenosis, and a bounding pulse in aortic insufficiency).

Examining the carotid artery: position the patient properly and avoid reduction in cerebral blood flow during palpation. The carotid artery may contain significant atheromas, especially at its bifurcation and in the lower internal carotid artery in the middle of the neck. It is extremely important to know its course and to avoid compression or distortion during palpation or auscultation. If the patient has symptoms or signs of decreased cerebral perfusion, it is wise to defer palpation and auscultation of the carotid artery until one has enough experience to be sure of not compressing or distorting the carotid arterial system.

The carotid artery usually is easy to locate in both sides of the neck. Have the patient sit upright on the examining table or bed, facing daylight from a window or light from a lamp in front of the neck. Place one hand behind the patient's upper neck or lower head and apply gentle forward pressure. The patient will automatically resist this motion by contracting the posterior neck muscles and relaxing the anterior neck muscles. These relaxed anterior muscles will allow easier palpation of the carotid arteries. Some observers prefer to palpate the carotid arteries with the patient in the supine position and the head supported on a pillow (see "An alternative method").

Where to palpate: the upper common carotid artery. Place the tips of the second, third, and fourth fingers of the second hand (or any adjacent two of these three, depending on your own finger lengths) gently against the skin of the lower anterior neck over the upper common carotid artery between the sternocleidomastoid muscle and the trachea. Using multiple fingertips minimizes neck pressure in a given location and reduces the danger of compression while maintaining adequate tactile sensation. The thumb, which is stronger, should not be used.

The common carotid artery becomes more superficial in the neck as it proceeds toward the head, so the upper portion of the common carotid artery is the region most easily palpated. It is just below the carotid bulb, which is in the middle of the neck between the clavicle and the angle of the jaw. Most carotid atheromatous disease of hemodynamic importance is above this level in the upper bulb and adjacent lower internal carotid region. Although large lesions also can involve the upper common carotid artery and the lower carotid bulb in some patients, the lumens of the common carotid artery and bulb are generally large in this region, and the chance for inadvertent compression with distortion or occlusion of the carotid system is relatively slight.

Look at your fingers, not elsewhere; inspection is important. The examining fingers should palpate the upper common carotid artery very softly so that carotid arterial wall motions are transmitted directly to these fingers. Vibrations (shudders and thrills) associated with murmurs and bruits and arterial waveforms thus may be both felt through the fingers' tactile sensation and observed by careful sighting along the fingers with the eye. The visual perception capabilities are better than the tactile sensations for most waves, because the mind is more accustomed to analyzing and remembering motion that is visualized against a stationary background than motion that is felt. Features such as rate of rise, amplitude of total displacement, waveforms, and variations in timing or amplitude from one cycle to the next are readily appreciated in this manner. One must not palpate both carotid arteries at the same time; each should be examined independently.

Internal carotid artery and external carotid artery; beware. The internal carotid artery usually is a direct and linear continuation of the common carotid artery and bulb, whereas the external carotid artery arises at an acute angle from the main axis of the common carotid artery and bulb. Both are smaller in diameter than the common carotid artery. There can be marked branching asymmetry in the direction of the carotid bifurcation and in the orientation of the internal and external carotid arteries, both from patient to patient and between the two sides in a given patient. As a general rule the external carotid artery is slightly more anterior in the neck but more medial to the internal carotid artery at and just above the bifurcation and therefore is not easily palpated. The internal carotid artery, fortunately, is usually lateral in position and is more easily palpated above the carotid bulb. The external carotid artery crosses over the internal carotid artery in the upper lateral neck to assume its named external position. Tortuosity or atherosclerosis may distort the usual orientations and positions of these two arteries.

Because the primary location for significant atherosclerosis in the carotid system is in the upper carotid bulb and the entrance to the internal carotid artery, and because additional lesions may be found just above this in the proximal internal carotid artery, it is extremely important to avoid strong palpation of the lower internal carotid artery above the bulb. Adhere to the rules of gentle palpation and observation of surface motion without any compression, displacement, or bending of the bulb or the internal carotid artery. In addition, avoid rapid changes in contact pressure in this region because the carotid sinus mechanism may be stimulated inadvertently; reflex vasovagal orthostatism or bradycardia with syncope may result.

The internal carotid artery should be palpated and observed only briefly, and even then mainly for the purpose of determining the pulse volume in comparison to volumes in the opposite internal carotid artery and both common carotid arteries. A thrill due to carotid atherosclerosis should be noted if present. Distinguishing between an internal and an external carotid source may be difficult. Both atherosclerosis and tortuosity may cause carotid bruits,[8] but thrills are chiefly due to atherosclerotic narrowing and hence are more specific. One can also determine the location and course of the internal carotid artery during palpation, for the purpose of subsequent auscultation.

The internal carotid artery is not palpated primarily for evaluation of the pulse contour and subtleties such as slope, anacrotic notch, and shudder. These features should be sought in the common carotid artery below the bulb.

An alternative method. Another excellent method for examination of the carotid artery is to have the patient recline with the head and thorax slightly elevated on a pillow. This technique also relaxes the anterior neck muscles and allows for relatively easy palpation of the carotid artery. In obese patients or patients with a short neck in whom carotid exposure is difficult, one might try both the vertical and the horizontal method of positioning the patient if either alone is not satisfactory. The advantage of the horizontal position is that it reduces the chance of cerebral hypotension.

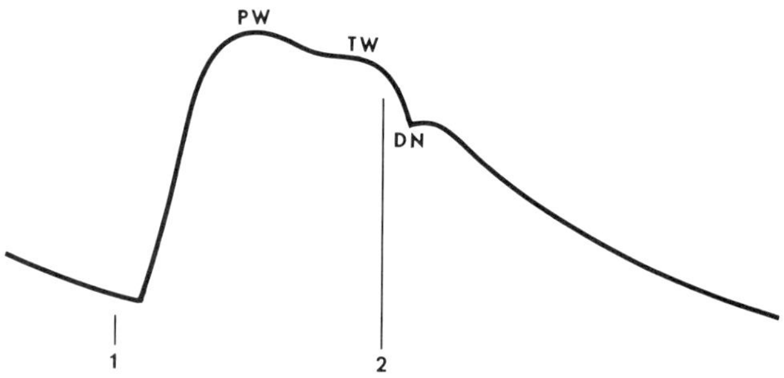

Fig 2-23 Carotid arterial pulse. The normal contour is shown for a single cardiac cycle. The rising percussion wave *(PW)* and subsequent tidal wave *(TW)* are systolic events. Aortic valve closure produces the dicrotic notch *(DN)*, or incisura. The gradual declining diastolic wave that follows has no specific name. The numbers represent the first and second heart sounds. Note that both the upstroke of the percussion wave and the dicrotic notch follow the respective heart sounds by a short time interval.

One must *never* produce cerebral hypotension by carotid compression of any sort, regardless of the patient's position.

Features of the carotid arterial pulse. The carotid system shows one major positive rise for each ventricular systole with relatively minor perturbations called "notches" or "shudders" and larger alterations called "waves." The slopes of the waves, their relative amplitudes, and the effects of pulse rate and cardiac output must be considered in determining if a given feature of the carotid pulse is normal or abnormal. Outward carotid wall expansion is plotted as an upward wave and inward retraction, as a downward wave on the carotid pulse tracing (Fig 2-23).

Terms used with carotid arterial pulse waves. Letter and word descriptions are used to identify features of the carotid pulse contour. Several Greek and Latin terms are retained and are listed below with their English explanations in parentheses.[18] Terms for the events are listed in order of occurrence after the onset of left ventricular systole.[6-9]

(1) Onset of upstroke, no designating term; (2) upstroke or rising phase, anacrotic (*Gr,* up or again beating) limb; (3) anacrotic notch, AN; (4) shudder, no abbreviation; (5) peak, also called the percussion wave, P; (6) initial systolic decline, no designating term; (7) second peak or tidal wave, T, due to reflected energy from the aorta (sometimes T is earlier than normal and peaked, resulting in P and T appearing together as a bifid [*L,* split in two] pulse or pulsus bisferiens [*L,* twice-beating pulse]; in hypertrophic cardiomyopathy, T may be delayed and round, a secondary wave, SW); (8) dicrotic (*Gr,* double beating) notch, DN, also called the incisura (*L,* notch) in early diastole, I; (9) dicrotic pulse or wave, DW, a large diastolic wave following aortic valve closure in significant left

ventricular disease and increased peripheral arterial resistance; (10) descending or runoff phase.

Additional pulsus (*L,* pulse) terms are used in connection with the overall carotid pulse contour. In valvular aortic stenosis, parvus (*L,* small) refers to the reduced peak amplitude and tardus (*L,* slow rising) to the shallower-than-usual upslope of the systolic portion of the carotid pulse. Alternans (*L,* alternating) indicates successive tall and short pulse amplitudes or pressures, and bigeminus (*L,* bigeminy—i.e., twice + twin) means paired beats occurring in sequence.

Sequence of the carotid arterial waves. The carotid arterial waves occur in the order given above. Not all of these features are present in any one carotid pulse. Unlike the jugular venous pulse waves or the apex impulse waves, in the carotid arterial waves the sequence is constant for a single beat regardless of the cardiac rhythm. The carotid pulse usually is physically stronger and more easily palpated than either the jugular venous pulse or the cardiac apex pulse. This makes it the easiest to locate, but the modifications that need to be detected are sometimes much smaller in relative amplitude. Observing the fingers or using a small wooden dowel as a magnifying lever to increase the motions are important diagnostic aids to overcome this deficiency.

The onset and ending of systole and the onset and ending of diastole may be determined with precision in the same manner as for the jugular venous pulse. By using the first and second heart sounds as the reference marks, these two periods are easily separable, with the carotid pulse rise identifying systole. The timing and distinction of a tidal wave and a dicrotic wave depend upon this identification method.

The carotid arterial upstroke: cardiac output and obstruction. The entire carotid arterial pulse may be conveniently divided into the upstroke, peak, and downstroke (runoff) phases. The upstroke phase is usually the most important of the three for aiding proper cardiac diagnosis.

Before left ventricular systole, the diastolic blood pressure and the rate of decline in pressure in the carotid arteries are minimal. The carotid pulse contour is a smooth, shallow, decreasing wave. Upon this relatively tranquil background, the next left ventricular stroke volume is expelled into the aorta and carotid arteries, suddenly producing a rapidly rising systolic wave of pressure and distention of each carotid artery. If present, the aortic ejection sound occurs with this initial upstroke.[7] The slope of outward carotid wall motion quickly reaches a maximum and then decreases toward zero, gradually at first and then with increasing rapidity. The total ascent curve usually has an S-shaped contour, reaching a peak when aortic ejection is also at a maximum. This initial rise is called the anacrotic limb of the percussion wave.[7,9] Certain features of the ascending portion of the percussion wave have diagnostic value (Fig 2-24).

First, the maximum rate of rise indicates whether or not there is outflow obstruction (discrete subvalvular, valvular, or supravalvular aortic stenosis), because the fixed maximum area of the narrowest portion of the left ventricular outflow tract or aortic root limits the peak volume of flow per unit of time. This produces various degrees of parvus

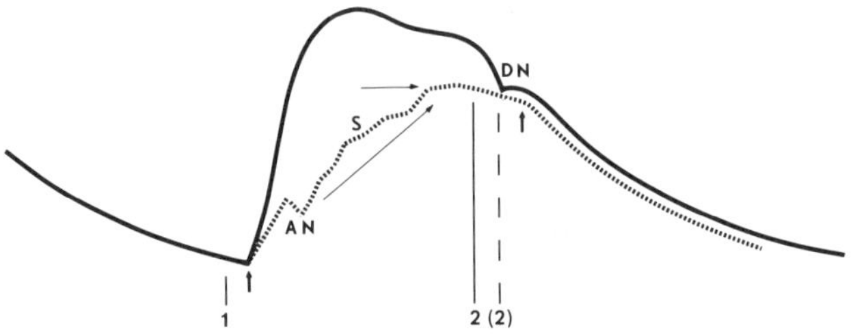

Fig 2-24 Carotid arterial pulse. The normal contour is shown by the solid line. The *dotted line* shows a typical contour of calcific aortic valve stenosis. The initial upstroke contains an anacrotic notch *(AN),* after which there is an irregular contour to the continuation of the rising percussion wave. The irregularity is sometimes easily palpable as a shudder *(S).* The average rising slope *(long, thin arrow)* is more shallow (tardus) than the normal percussion wave slope. The maximum of the pulse amplitude *(short, thin arrow)* is less (parvus) than normal. *Vertical arrows* indicate the beginning and end of the systolic portion of this carotid pulse contour. Note that the left ventricular ejection time is prolonged. The numbers represent the first and second heart sounds. The second heart sound is delayed in valvular aortic stenosis; the corresponding dicrotic notch *(DN)* may be obscure.

(small total amplitude of the peak) and tardus (shallow average and maximal slopes) of the upstroke phase of the pulse. Supravalvular aortic stenosis often involves preferential flow of blood to the right subclavian and carotid systems with resulting higher pulse volume and blood pressure than in the left-side arteries.[6-9]

Second, the left ventricular ejection time in aortic stenosis is increased but the heart rate is not increased at rest, two features that help the left ventricle to maintain its output and to compensate for the outlet obstruction.

Third, a small downward indentation, the anacrotic notch, sometimes appears on or just after the middle of the upstroke (anacrotic) wave.[9] With increasing severity of valvular aortic stenosis, the anacrotic notch occurs earlier and may be accentuated.[7] Use of a small wooden dowel against the surface of the common carotid artery as a magnifying lever permits the anacrotic notch to be seen more easily. Similarly, watching the motion of the palpating fingers also often will reveal the anacrotic notch. This notch is most easily recognized in aortic stenosis because the carotid upstroke is more gradual and lasts longer than usual.

Fourth, the upstroke phase after the anacrotic notch in valvular aortic stenosis may have a series of palpable, rough vibrations, called a carotid shudder.[7] Such a shudder is more coarse than a thrill over the carotid artery or over the base of the chest but is basically the same manifestation—systolic vibrations relating to a jet of blood through a narrowed opening. It is most intense in the lowest portion of the common carotid artery just above the clavicle. Unless accompanied by a parvus or tardus pulse, however, a carotid shudder or thrill may mean a stenotic atherosclerotic lesion in this carotid artery or in the adjacent subclavian artery near its origin.

Rating the damped carotid arterial upstroke. The normal carotid arterial pulse volume is used as a reference against which other carotid arterial pulses may be compared. Obviously, because many patients have abnormal carotid arterial pulses on both sides of the neck, the reference must be to the average expected normal pulse for such a patient based on age, body habitus, and heart rate.

Normal slope and amplitude would be designated 100%. Many cardiologists use a scale of 0 (pulse absent) to 4 (normal), each unit representing an increment of 25% of normal. A pulse graded 2 is 50% of normal; 2+ is greater than 50% but less than 62.5% of normal; and 3- is greater than 62.5% but less than 75% of normal. Carotid atherosclerosis or arteritis, aortic stenosis, low-output left ventricular failure, and systemic hypotension are conditions in which reduced pulse volume may occur.

Rankings of parvus and tardus features of carotid pulse upstrokes proceed in the opposite direction from the estimations of normality because these two descriptive terms automatically indicate abnormality. A pulse that is parvus 2 and tardus 3 is 50% of normal in height and only 25% of normal in rapidity of rise. This would imply severe aortic stenosis.

Beware of the normal-appearing carotid arterial pulse in the older patient. Because of the normal loss of elastic properties in the arterial walls and the tendency for kyphosis, aortic arch tortuosity, and carotid arterial tortuosity to occur with aging, the normal carotid pulse acquires a sharper rate of rise but is more limited in its ultimate peak amplitude. The net effect is to produce a higher systolic blood pressure and a shock-wave type of carotid upstroke in some older patients.[6] This is the same age group in which aortic stenosis is increasingly common. Unfortunately, this change in carotid arterial wall properties may mask the expected slowing and dampening of the carotid arterial upstroke wave in aortic stenosis. A basal thrill, a low pitch or rough quality of the ejection murmur, a sustained and forceful left ventricular lift, or a history of angina, syncope, or decreasing tolerance on exertion must be sought and considered carefully in such cases. Echocardiography or cardiac catheterization may be needed to complete the evaluation.

The carotid arterial upstroke that is more rapid than usual. Aortic insufficiency is the prototype cause of the bounding carotid arterial upstroke pulse (Fig 2-25). Extra blood is ejected in systole to compensate for the subsequent diastolic regurgitant volume of blood; the cardiac rate is increased. The rate of rise and the peak amplitude of the arterial pulse are both increased. The contour up to the peak is usually smooth, but a systolic thrill may be palpable due to the ejection of extra blood at increased velocity, even if little or no associated aortic stenosis is present.[8,16] The twin peak waves sometimes present will be discussed later.

If the runoff of blood into a peripheral artery or vein is rapid due to low peripheral resistance, then the upstroke pulse wave also will be more rapid and taller than usual. Truncus arteriosus (with or without quadricuspid insufficiency), bacterial endocarditis, patent ductus arteriosus, peripheral arteriovenous malformation or shunt, fever,

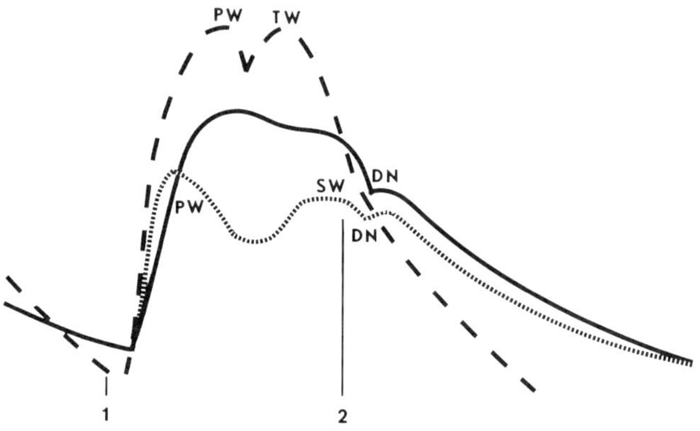

Fig 2-25 Carotid arterial pulse. The normal contour is shown by the *solid line.* The difference between a bifid *(dashed line)* and a bisferiens *(dotted line)* pulse is often confusing, and they sometimes may appear to be similar in contour. The bifid contour in aortic insufficiency involves the percussion wave *(PW)* and tidal wave *(TW)* occurring close together with a small cleft between them *(dashed line).* The upstroke is rapid during the percussion wave and the downslope of the tidal wave is also increased in its slope. The dicrotic notch *(DN)* may be obscure, although a decrease in diastolic slope may then occur. The remainder of the runoff phase in diastole is also steeper than normal. Systole is slightly prolonged but diastole is shortened. The diastolic pressure is lower than normal. In hypertrophic cardiomyopathy, a "spike-and-dome" contour of the bisferiens pulse may appear *(dotted line).* The percussion wave is rapid in its upslope but halts abruptly and then declines in midsystole. During late systole, there is a secondary wave *(SW)* that may be easily palpable. Neither a bifid nor a bisferiens pulse has the same tardus and parvus upslope characteristics of the pulse in aortic stenosis (compare Fig 2-24). The numbers represent the first and second heart sounds.

sepsis, beriberi, anemia, thyrotoxicosis, anxiety, catecholamine excess, and arrhythmias may cause such increased carotid arterial upstroke pulses.[6-9] Occlusion of the artery supplying an arteriovenous shunt will effectively increase peripheral arterial resistance, reduce the pulse rate (Nicoladoni-Branham sign) through a reflex mechanism, and reduce the pulse amplitude.[19]

The rapid carotid arterial upstroke in hypertrophic cardiomyopathy: a special case. Ordinarily, one might expect an obstructive process in the subaortic valvular outflow tract of the left ventricle such as hypertrophic cardiomyopathy to reduce the upstroke phase of the carotid arterial pulse. This it does do, but not initially. With the onset of left ventricular ejection, the anterior mitral leaflet is not yet close to the thick subaortic portion of the interventricular septum, so the muscular left ventricle initially propels blood into the aortic root and carotid arteries with vigor. The upstroke wave in the carotid arterial wall is rapid in rise and essentially normal in amplitude.

The sum of kinetic and potential energies in the outflow

tract must decrease as blood leaves the energy source, the left ventricle. Because the rapid passage of blood past the mitral valve and interventricular septal wall represents increased kinetic energy of the ejected blood, the associated potential energy, manifested as laterally directed pressure, must be decreased correspondingly (Venturi effect). The reduced lateral blood pressure draws the anterior mitral leaflet toward the thick interventricular septum, progressively and rapidly accentuating these features and resulting in sudden, marked left ventricular outlet obstruction. The carotid arterial upstroke ceases abruptly and prematurely.

The carotid arterial peak: single and double systolic bumps. The carotid pulse wave usually has a single peak, the percussion wave. Sometimes a second pulse, the tidal wave, is present before the end of systole.[6-8] In aortic stenosis the peak is usually single, low in total amplitude, blunt, and delayed, and the duration of systole is prolonged to compensate for the limited flow at a given instant (see Fig 2-24).

In aortic insufficiency, the peak usually is sharp due to the rapid rate of upstroke and rapid central runoff, but sometimes in aortic insufficiency or in combined aortic stenosis and insufficiency there are two sharp peaks (percussion and tidal waves) close together in time and separated by a small cleft, creating a bifid or split pulse (see Fig 2-25). The finger observation and dowel lever amplification methods for detecting the double peaks work very well. The bifid pulse, if present, serves to identify the pulse as that of aortic insufficiency and helps to exclude overactive pulses of hormonal or metabolic causes. The ejection time is prolonged due to the increased systolic stroke volume; the heart rate may be increased. None of the pulse characteristics can be quantitated and correlated with the severity of aortic insufficiency to the same extent as the parvus and tardus features of aortic stenosis, but a rapidly rising, bifid-peaked, rapidly falling pulse does suggest significant aortic insufficiency. If the two systolic peaks are both prominent and separated by a major cleft, the term pulsus bisferiens (twice-beating pulse) may be used.[6-9]

In hypertrophic cardiomyopathy the carotid arterial upstroke is steep, the percussion peak is early and abrupt, and the systolic portion of the curve immediately after the peak shows a shallow decline, a plateau, or a second flattened or rounded peak that may undulate. After the onset of the first peak, the outflow obstruction at the mitral valve-interventricular septal level may decline a bit or vary temporarily about an average value. This depends on several factors such as stroke volume, velocity of ejected blood, area of outflow tract remaining, peripheral runoff of arterial blood, completion of ventricular emptying, extent of left ventricular cavity obliteration, and heart rate. The peak or peaks begin early but the blood is still being forcefully ejected for a while longer. Thus, the pulse remains partially elevated around the initial peak value for much of the duration of systole, in comparison to normal pulses. The second pulse is variable and probably represents a combination of a continued percussion wave and a tidal wave. The rapid rise, sudden moderation, and prolonged hang-up pattern of the peaks is unique for this condition (see Fig 2-25). It may be accentuated by the use of amyl nitrite. The bisferiens pulse sometimes appears as a "spike-and-dome."[7-9,16]

The tidal wave in otherwise normal patients becomes relatively more prominent with aging or hypertension, in part due to higher velocity of the reflected pulse waves.[7,9]

The carotid arterial pulse waves in mitral stenosis and mitral insufficiency are relatively normal in rate of rise and show a smooth, rounded, single-peak contour. The ejection time is shortened due to reduced forward ejection of blood.[6,7] The entire systolic pulse contour is smoother in mitral insufficiency than in other conditions because the increased left atrial volume, regurgitation, and distensibility help moderate and filter abrupt changes in carotid flow and pressure.

The carotid arterial runoff phase. In most cardiac conditions, analysis of the runoff phase is of less diagnostic importance than analysis of either the rising phase or the peak. However, there is merit in evaluating the declining portion of the carotid pulse in aortic insufficiency; the steepness of its initial slope is in proportion to the incompetency of the aortic valve. The dicrotic notch follows the end of left ventricular systole and the closure of the aortic valve by a constant time interval. It is seen on the upper portion of the downslope of the carotid arterial pulse as a small negative indentation.[7] In aortic insufficiency, the dicrotic notch may be low on the downslope phase and small in amplitude or absent; the slope of the runoff phase is altered little from before to after the dicrotic notch.[8] Because the aortic valve fails to halt aortic reflux into the left ventricle, the aorta has both distal and proximal retrograde runoff, and the diastolic pressure and arterial pulse volumes may drop to relatively low values before the next systolic upstroke. The increased cardiac rate, bounding upstroke, brief peak or twin peaks, and increased runoff without a normal dicrotic notch or major slope change are characteristic of significant aortic insufficiency (see Fig 2-25).

Aortic stenosis may accompany aortic insufficiency or exist by itself. The thickened aortic valve may not permit rapid initial reflux of aortic root blood, rapid closure of the remainder of the valve orifice, or abrupt termination of the reversed aortic root flow as does a normal aortic valve. Hence, the dicrotic notch is flattened or not very impressive (see Fig 2-24).

In mitral insufficiency the dicrotic notch is sometimes well preserved and must not be confused with the earlier second peak in the systolic phase of hypertrophic cardiomyopathy. Use of the aortic second sound as a reference will help identify the dicrotic notch properly. Such a prominent dicrotic notch is also labeled the incisura because it looks like a tooth mark on a graph of the pulse contour.

An unusual type of carotid arterial downslope is the dicrotic (double-beating) pulse in which there is a single, relatively smooth percussion wave in systole, a significant late systolic collapse to a low dicrotic notch, and then a rebound in diastole of a major second pulse wave, the dicrotic wave (Fig 2-26). Common causes are conditions leading to left ventricular failure with systemic hypotension, such as congestive cardiomyopathy, coronary athero-

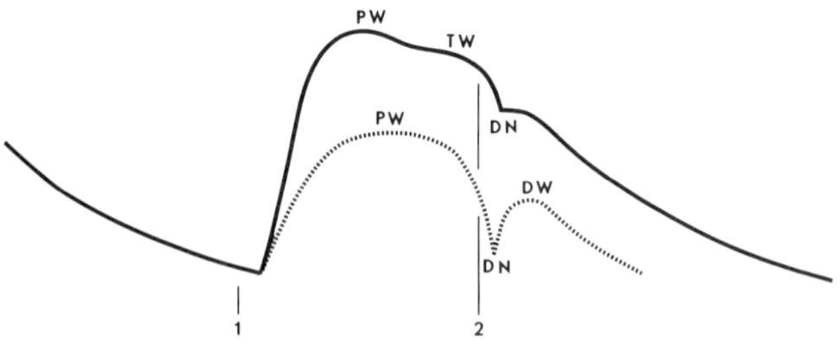

Fig 2-26 Carotid arterial pulse. The normal contour is shown by the *solid line.* A special type of carotid pulse contour occurs in very sick patients with reduced cardiac output *(dotted line).* The percussion wave *(PW)* is lower than normal in amplitude and its contour is smoother than usual. The dicrotic notch *(DN)* occurs at a much lower pressure than normal. Following the dicrotic notch is a second wave occurring entirely in diastole, the dicrotic wave *(DW).* The numbers represent the first and second heart sounds. *TW,* tidal wave.

sclerosis, myocardial infarction, and hypertensive heart disease. It may appear in the morbid patient receiving intensive drug therapy for cardiovascular support. Fever, youth, constrictive or tamponadal pericardial disease, low peripheral arterial resistance, and high peripheral arterial resistance have been associated with a prominent dicrotic wave.[6-9,16]

Carotid pulse features of left ventricular failure. A failing left ventricle may produce certain arterial signs. These include reduced amplitude of the carotid arterial pulse (palpable as a weak or mushy rise without the usual force), reduced arterial systolic pressure, low dicrotic notch with large following dicrotic wave, and pulsus alternans (every other cardiac cycle has a lower systolic blood pressure and pulse amplitude).[8] The cardiac rhythm should be regular to make a diagnosis of pulsus alternans.

Effects of premature heartbeats on the carotid pulse contour. Ventricular premature beats or supraventricular premature beats usually are associated with a reduced carotid pulse volume. The amount of relative prematurity influences the extent of the decrease. The following normally conducted beat, the postextrasystolic beat, is often amplified due to the increased stroke volume. In hypertrophic cardiomyopathy, however, it is decreased instead because of the increased outflow obstruction associated with the heart's attempt to eject the extra blood at increased velocity.[6-8] In ventricular bigeminy the carotid pulse shows pulsus bigeminus (paired large and small pulses) or else a 2:1 pulse deficit.[8]

Paradoxic pulse: a nonparadoxic sign. Pulsus paradoxus (paradoxic pulse) refers to a greater-than-normal decrease in systolic blood pressure during the active phase of inspiration. In constrictive pericarditis or restrictive heart disease, and especially in pericardial tamponade, this fall may exceed 10 mm Hg. It occurs in the normal direction and thus is not truly paradoxic, just excessive. Lesser degrees of exaggerated systolic pressure decrease during inspiration may occur in chronic obstructive pulmonary disease and asthma, when the diaphragm is lower than normal during respiration.[8]

The peripheral cardiovascular examination: arteries and their pulsations. A slow-rising (tardus) pulse of normal or low (parvus) volume in the peripheral limb arteries occasionally may be found in valvular aortic stenosis or combined valvular aortic stenosis and insufficiency. Although the carotid arteries are superior for purposes of pulse waveform analysis, one should not fail to recognize such dampened peripheral pulses when they are present.

A bounding, rapidly rising and collapsing, peripheral arterial pulse implies valvular aortic insufficiency or rapid runoff of arterial blood. A delayed peak in a femoral pulse, compared with the ipsilateral radial pulse, suggests coarctation of the aorta distal to the corresponding subclavian artery. Atherosclerosis, on the other hand, tends to reduce the amplitude of the distal pulses without producing significant delay, presumably due to the more distal location of partial obstruction and the smaller capacity of the arteries beyond the stenotic area.[7]

Thrills from arterial lesions. Thrills over arteries may be associated with stenotic regions (atherosclerosis or coarctation of the aorta), kinked arteries (carotid, innominate, or subclavian), dilated intercostal arteries (coarctation of the aorta), or arteriovenous fistulas. Check both the lower common carotid and carotid bulb (bifurcation) regions. An innominate artery thrill (and bruit), especially before middle age, usually is innocent. Subclavian thrills may indicate stenosis or distortion due to atherosclerosis or a cervical rib. Abdominal or peripheral arterial thrills (e.g., femoral or popliteal) usually indicate atherosclerosis or an arteriovenous fistula. Fibromuscular dysplasia may produce a thrill, although such disease in the carotid artery is frequently in the lower intracranial region, which is not accessible to palpation.

Possible diagnoses. Diagnoses that may be suspected on the basis of the carotid pulse characteristics include aortic stenosis, aortic insufficiency, combined aortic stenosis and insufficiency, hypertrophic cardiomyopathy, left ventricular failure, constrictive pericarditis, pericardial tamponade, and atherosclerosis of the carotid arteries (Table 2-2). Certain other cardiovascular and systemic diseases alter the carotid pulse volume and contour in ways that permit the observer to place them in general categories. Examples include: excess cardiac stimulation from catecholamines, hormones, or drugs; high cardiac output from anemia, fever, or peripheral arteriovenous shunt; and low cardiac output from hypovolemia or cardiac failure.

Conclusions. Palpation of the carotid pulse with simultaneous observation of the motion of the fingers can yield extremely valuable information about several cardiovascular diseases. Although caution must be used in this examination, good technique will permit study of nearly every patient without the risk of inadvertent compression of the carotid artery being examined. In patients with valvular aortic stenosis, the carotid pulse evaluation is often the single most important step in the clinical estimation of the seriousness of this disorder. The carotid pulse examination is a valuable adjunct to the other portions of the cardiac physical examination and should be considered a routine part of a complete cardiac workup.

Table 2-2 Diagnostic significance of visible and palpable carotid arterial pulse waves

Diagnosis	Carotid arterial pulse
Aortic stenosis	Early anacrotic notch, shudder, tardus and parvus rise, prolonged duration
Aortic insufficiency	Rapid rise, bifid peak, prolonged duration, reduced dicrotic notch, rapid runoff
Aortic stenosis and insufficiency	Bifid or bisferiens pulse
Hypertrophic cardiomyopathy	Rapid rise, early abrupt peak, plateau or gentle second hump (bisferiens pulse)
Mitral stenosis	Smooth contour, normal or reduced amplitude and duration
Mitral insufficiency	Smooth contour, normal or reduced amplitude and duration
Left ventricular ischemia	Low amplitude
Left ventricular failure	Low amplitude, pulsus alternans
Constrictive pericarditis	Reduced amplitude, paradoxic pulse
Pericardial tamponade	Reduced amplitude, paradoxic pulse
Coarctation of aorta	Increased force, femoral delay or damping
Atherosclerosis	Reduced amplitude, thrill
Peripheral arteriovenous fistula	Rapid rise and runoff
Anemia, fever, sepsis, thyrotoxicosis	Increased pulse amplitude and rate

Chest wall and apex pulsations

Lifts, thrills, and waveforms. "Lift" is a term used to indicate a systolic rise in the skin over a cardiovascular structure in the chest. "Thrill" is used for a palpable vibration in the skin over a jet of blood in a cardiovascular structure. Waveforms are features of systolic and diastolic skin pulsations transmitted from cardiovascular structures. Certain important areas of the chest should be checked visually for lifts and pulsations and then palpated for thrills, lifts, and pulsations. Various features of these motions will be discussed in detail.

Specific areas for examination. Several areas of the thorax are useful for examination of chest wall impulses and motions. These regions should be inspected visually and then palpated. The aortic area, pulmonary area, right ventricular area, and left ventricular area (apex) are the most important and are usually studied in this sequence. Additional areas for observation include the epigastric (subxiphoid) area, the right and left subclavian arterial areas, the sternoclavicular area, the left upper anterior chest area, the left subaxillary area, the posterior thorax, and any other regions of the chest wall that may be opportune.

Thrills caused by cardiac lesions. Typical thrills due to cardiac lesions include the following cases.

1. Apical systolic thrill of mitral insufficiency, often to the left of the midclavicular line or near the anterior or midaxillary lines.
2. Anterior left chest systolic thrill of mitral insufficiency due to posterior mitral leaflet prolapse or to flail posterior mitral leaflet (Merendino's sign).
3. Posterior left chest systolic thrill, between the left scapula and spinal column, of mitral insufficiency due to anterior mitral leaflet prolapse or to flail anterior mitral leaflet (Giuliani's sign).[20]
4. Basal systolic thrill or common carotid arterial shudder of aortic stenosis (subvalvular, valvular, or supravalvular, nearly always with significant hemodynamic gradient), slightly delayed after the onset of the left ventricular apical lift. A thrill is unusual in hypertrophic cardiomyopathy over either the base or apex, even though both aortic outflow tract obstruction and mitral regurgitation may exist.
5. Left lower to midsternal border (or adjacent left parasternal area) systolic thrill of a ventricular septal defect with left-to-right jet of blood.[21] Early, mid, or late systolic timing, if present, may be helpful in its recognition because most other systolic thrills from the heart are more holosystolic.
6. Tricuspid area systolic thrill of tricuspid insufficiency. This is uncommon, even if the murmur is loud. With right atrial and right ventricular enlargement, the right ventricle may be displaced to the left, so the observer must shift mentally the expected locations for the thrill and auscultatory findings.
7. Apical diastolic thrill of rapid flow through an incompetent mitral valve due to the extra volume of blood in diastole and the closer approximation of the enlarged left ventricle to the left chest wall.[21]
8. Apical diastolic thrill of severe mitral stenosis.[21]
9. Left or right sternal border diastolic thrill of aortic insufficiency. A more rightward location suggests aortic root enlargement or aneurysm.
10. Pulmonary systolic thrill of pulmonary valve stenosis, localized to the area of the systolic murmur.[21]

The aortic area. Located in the second intercostal space just to the right of the sternum, the aortic area is the region where skin motions due to the aortic valve and the ascending thoracic aortic arch can be most easily inspected and palpated. Although the aortic valve is located within the center of the heart, the jet of blood that enters the ascending aorta from it may have a profound influence on the chest wall motions in the aortic area several centimeters above it. Palpation usually is much more helpful than inspection.

In a patient with aortic stenosis or with a normal aortic prosthetic valve with slight functional stenosis, there may exist a palpable systolic thrill in the aortic area on the chest wall. The thrill also may be palpated in the supraclavicular regions (subclavian arteries) or carotid arteries (carotid shudder).

The thrill may be most easily palpated when the patient is sitting. One should also palpate over the aortic area when the patient is supine on the examining table or bed. Once the best area is located, lighter tactile pressure in this area may be more satisfactory. Heavier pressure on palpation is needed for higher-frequency or lower-amplitude thrills. Such a thrill indicates relatively fixed valvular aortic stenosis or a rare supravalvular or subvalvular web. Its intensity does not correlate well with the amount of stenosis, although its presence does confirm a narrowed outflow tract.

The aortic area systolic lift is normally quite low in amplitude and often may be undetectable. Yet, palpation here should not be omitted. In valvular aortic stenosis the left ventricular apical lift may be palpated as a strong rising phase over the left ventricular area (cardiac apex) significantly in advance of the parvus (reduced) or tardus (delayed) lift over the aortic area. The timing and rates of rise of each of these two lifts are helpful in confirming the presence of aortic outflow obstruction from a stenotic aortic valve or fixed web. A prompt initial upstroke in the aortic area, on the other hand, is more characteristic of hypertrophic cardiomyopathy. By using two hands to palpate the left ventricular and aortic areas simultaneously, one may be able to detect these alterations in timing and thus differentiate significant aortic valvular stenosis from hypertrophic cardiomyopathy.

Patients with aortic valve sclerosis without stenosis have a normal aortic area lift and no delay with respect to the left ventricular area lift. A left ventricular aneurysm from a previous myocardial infarction or mitral insufficiency does not yield a major delay in the aortic area lift.

With aortic insufficiency or with a hyperdynamic heart due to low systemic arterial resistance, the rates of rise and collapse of the aortic area lift may be increased and thus helpful in estimating the amount of aortic regurgitation or peripheral arterial runoff.

When the ascending aorta or part of the aortic arch has been replaced by an inelastic conduit—whether or not there is an aortic valve prosthesis or the aortic valve is diseased—the aortic closure shock may be very forceful and quite characteristic on palpation. The aortic valve closure impulse is accentuated in systemic arterial hypertension and decreased in aortic stenosis and aortic insufficiency. It may be increased when the patient has an aortic ball-and-cage prosthesis.

Increase in the systolic expansion of an ascending aortic arch aneurysm against the aortic area may yield a low-amplitude, widely distributed lift that is smooth in its contour.

Displacement of a tortuous aortic arch cephalad due to thoracic kyphosis may produce an increase in the aortic arch lift as well as buckled subclavian and carotid arteries. These should not be mistaken for aneurysms.

The pulmonary (pulmonic) area. The pulmonary area is on the left side of the sternum at the same or a slightly lower level (second or third intercostal space) on the anterior chest wall. It should be inspected and then palpated, in the sitting patient, with the palm of the hand pressed firmly against the skin while the palm of the opposite hand provides an opposite and equal counterpressure on the back of the thorax. The supine patient position usually is even better for inspection and palpation than the sitting position.

Increased pulmonary artery pressure occurs in primary and secondary pulmonary hypertension, certain congenital or postoperative congenital cardiac conditions, and those left heart diseases that increase pulmonary venous pressure (left atrial myxoma, mitral stenosis, mitral insufficiency, left ventricular failure, and advanced aortic stenosis). Pulmonary hypertension may be detected on palpation by the presence of an increased and sustained pulmonary area lift, a palpable pulmonary valve closure impulse over the pulmonary area, or both.[6,21] The pulmonary valve closure impulse is decreased in pulmonary stenosis and in tetralogy of Fallot. A systolic thrill without a lift may be palpable over the pulmonary area in pulmonary valve stenosis.

Pulmonary artery volume overload, as in atrial septal defect, partial AV canal defect, partial anomalous pulmonary venous connection, and ventricular septal defect, may yield a pulmonary area lift that is larger and slightly more rapid but less sustained than in pulmonary hypertension.[21]

In the case of an increased lift over either or both sides of the upper parasternal region it is a good idea to palpate the aortic and pulmonary areas alternately to determine which side of the sternum demonstrates the greatest lift and which has the greatest associated semilunar valvular closure sensation. This may aid in the differentiation of aortic and pulmonary hypertension or excess flow, aortic and pulmonary valve disease, and left and right ventricular disease. Because the pulmonary artery is closer to the sternum than is the aortic arch, a small amount of pulmonary arterial hypertension produces a greater pulmonary area lift than does the same relative amount of systemic hypertension for the aortic area lift.

The right ventricular area. The right ventricular area, sometimes called the "left parasternal or tricuspid area," is a variable region over the central and left lower sternum and adjacent left parasternal area. In obese patients it is somewhat higher on the sternum, about one-third of the way from the xiphoid process to the manubrium. In thin patients or those with chronic obstructive pulmonary disease it is lower, just above the xiphoid process. In palpating this area, one should avoid pressure on the xiphoid process itself because it often is tender and it may be fractured by excess pressure. Although the right ventricular area may be palpated with the patient in the sitting position, it has been personal experience (T.C.E.) that the supine position is best. Begin by inspecting and then palpating with the palm over this area to locate the point of maximal lift of the lower sternum.

A systolic thrill in or just above the lower left sternal area is characteristic of a ventricular septal defect with an anteriorly directed jet of blood. Rarely, tricuspid valve regurgitation may produce a localized thrill in this region. A diastolic thrill may be palpated in significant aortic insufficiency.

Pulmonary hypertension (primary or secondary), cor pulmonale, pulmonary valve stenosis, mitral valve stenosis, and mitral valve insufficiency may be associated with a sustained right ventricular precordial lift due to right ventricular hypertrophy.[6,7,21] A late right ventricular lift also may occur with marked mitral valve insufficiency, but without pulmonary hypertension or right ventricular hypertrophy, due to systolic expansion of the left atrium pushing the right ventricle anteriorly. Right ventricular enlargement may displace the associated lift farther to the left than usual.

Conditions leading to volume overload of the right ventricle, such as atrial septal defect, partial anomalous pulmonary venous connection, ventricular septal defect, and tricuspid valve insufficiency, may produce a less forceful, somewhat more rapid and brief right ventricular lift.[21] Differentiation between pressure and volume overload conditions should not be attempted on the basis of the quality of the right ventricular lift alone, however. Tricuspid atresia with a small right ventricle and tetralogy of Fallot are not associated with a significant right ventricular lift.

The left ventricular area (apex). The left ventricular area, also known as the mitral area or cardiac apex, is the last of the four major regions of interest in the chest for evaluation of cardiac pulsations. The study of its complex motions has been given the title "apexcardiography." The cardiac apical impulse, also called "beat," "lift," or "thrust," is due to motion of the left ventricular wall in contact with the left anterior chest wall. It results from contraction of the left atrium and left ventricle and from passive expansion of the left ventricle. The apex beat actually represents contributions of motion from the entire left ventricle and not just its true apex. It is typically found in about the fifth or sixth left intercostal space at or just medial to the midclavicular line.[7,21]

The apex impulse may be displaced from the expected position or may be difficult to locate in some patients. Knowledge of body build and of possible diagnoses will aid in searching for the apex in the most likely locations. It may be higher in reclining or obese patients, lower in sitting or thin patients, or more lateral in some patients with marked pectus excavatum or with left ventricular enlargement, hypertrophy, dyskinesis, or aneurysm. Because of the potential variability of location from patient to patient and in different body orientations, the extra seconds spent locating the best area for examination are quite important for future results. The apex may not be detectable in some normal patients. It also may be obscure in other patients because of overexpansion of the lungs, kyphoscoliosis, large or small chest sizes, obesity, or weakness of the impulse.[21]

By using frontal or tangential light, observe the left anterior and lateral chest wall for the apex impulse in the fourth to eighth intercostal spaces, concentrating first on the fifth and sixth interspaces. One first should have a good idea of the pulse rate from the carotid or radial pulse or from the blood pressure measurement. Observe several cardiac cycles once the apparent apex is located visually to prevent inadvertent fixation of attention on a spurious adjacent location that also shows some pulsation. Next, palpate the apical region with the palm, note the exact location of the maximal outward systolic motion, and shift the palm accordingly if indicated. The normal apex impulse is usually less than 3 cm in diameter. Aneurysms, dyskinetic zones, and enlargement of the left ventricle may yield larger apical impulses.[21]

Body position is important; be sure to check more than one position. Although the left semilateral decubitus position empirically would seem to be the best of the three main positions to permit gravity to press the left ventricular apex against the left anterior chest wall, in contrast to the upright and supine positions, this is not always the case. Some patients with left ventricular hypertrophy or enlargement paradoxically may provide the best apical impulse for examination while sitting or supine. Thus, it is good practice to check, in sequence, all three positions by visual inspection and manual palpation. Study the patient during exhalation as well as during normal breathing before choosing the best body orientation and chest wall location for the definitive apex waveform evaluations. Remember, failure to find the best apical impulse makes the subsequent testing difficult or futile.

Terms used with chest and cardiac apex pulse waves. The terms relating to chest and apical impulses are taken mainly from apexcardiography. Outward skin motion is plotted on the apexcardiogram as an upward wave; inward skin motion is plotted as a downward wave.[7,21,22] The terms are listed here in order of occurrence in normal sinus rhythm (Fig 2-27).

A WAVE. The slight outward motion of the skin over the left ventricle (upward apexcardiogram wave) in late diastole as the left atrial contraction distends the left ventricle prior to systole in normal sinus rhythm. It is synchronous with the left ventricular fourth heart sound. The declining inward phase of this wave has no name.[7]

C POINT. The abrupt onset of the outward motion of the skin over the left ventricle (upward rise in the apexcardiogram wave) at the onset of left ventricular systole (start of isovolumetric contraction). The remainder of the outward motion (upward slope) is large but has no name. The left ventricle rotates and uses the chest wall as a buttress in the early part of systole, producing the apex motion.[6]

E POINT. The peak of the outward systolic motion of the skin over the left ventricle (upward apexcardiogram peak) as ejection of blood into the aorta decreases the left ventricular volume and allows the contracting myocardium to begin to pull away from the chest wall. Following the E point is an initial rapid inward motion (downward apexcardiogram wave) and then a less-rapid inward motion (still downward apexcardiogram wave but with a reduced slope) as ventricular contraction is maintained.

As systole ends, the left ventricle relaxes, the inward motion of the skin rapidly accelerates, and the apexcardiogram shows a large descending wave. There is no name for this large negative wave which spans both the end of systole and the beginning of diastole.

A small artifact due to aortic valve closure may be transmitted through the left ventricle and its blood and is recorded on the apexcardiogram as a brief upward spike on the steep portion of this major negative wave. It closely follows the aortic closure sound and is the counterpart of the dicrotic notch of the carotid arterial pulse wave.[7]

O POINT. The abrupt reversal, in early diastole, from inward to outward motion of the skin over the left ventricle (negative trough on the apexcardiogram) as the mitral valve opens and blood begins to flow into the left

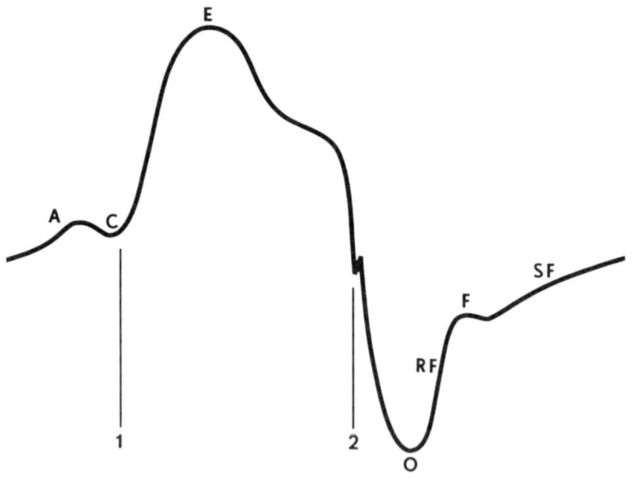

Fig 2-27 Apex pulse (apexcardiogram). The normal apex pulse has several waves. The A wave is caused by outward expansion of the skin beneath the left ventricle due to left atrial contraction. A brief retraction occurs before left ventricular contraction begins *(C)*. The rapid upward slope indicates outward motion of the skin over the left ventricle prior to the time of approximate maximal ejection of blood from the left ventricle *(E)*. After this most-outward excursion point there is an increasing decline in the slope (there is a temporary shoulder in this decline just before the end of systole). When systole ends, there is a more rapid inward retraction of the apex pulse, interrupted only by a small artifact that corresponds to the dicrotic notch in the carotid arterial pulse contour. The numbers represent the first and second heart sounds. Note that the C point is virtually synchronous with the first heart sound and that the artifact on the downslope of the curve is also nearly synchronous with the second heart sound. The apex pulse then retracts further until the mitral valve opening occurs (O point) and then it expands again. An initial rapid-filling *(RF)* wave is noted until the ventricle becomes unfolded, at which time the rapid-filling slope moderates *(F)*. A slow-filling *(SF)* wave follows this as the ventricle becomes distended with additional blood and stretching of myocardial fibers in diastole is necessary.

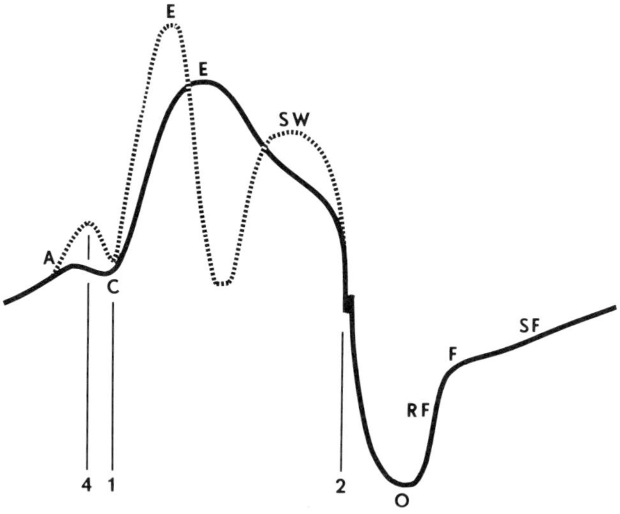

Fig 2-28 Apex pulse (apexcardiogram). The normal contour is shown by the *solid line*. A larger-than-normal set of waves occurs in hypertrophic cardiomyopathy *(dotted line)*. The A wave is increased in amplitude and is often easily palpable. It corresponds to the fourth heart sound *(4)* from the left ventricle. The rate of rise of the apex impulse is rapid and the impulse is large and very forceful (C to E slope). At the E point, which occurs early, there is a sudden moderation and withdrawal of the apex impulse until midsystole, when there may occur a large secondary wave *(SW)*. These systolic ventricular waves may also be palpable, yielding a bifid or trifid apical impulse. Other letters and numbers are explained in Fig 2-27 legend.

ventricle. It is synchronous with the opening snap in mitral valve stenosis.

RF WAVE. The rapid outward motion early in diastole of the skin over the left ventricle (upward apexcardiogram wave) due to swift inflow of blood from the left atrium to the left ventricle, called the rapid-filling wave.

F POINT. The outward peak (upward apexcardiogram peak) in diastole of the rapid-filling wave as the rate of left ventricular filling suddenly diminishes due to achievement of a more spherical chamber shape and the onset of left ventricular stretching. It is synchronous with the left ventricular third heart sound or pericardial knock. Other explanations have also been published.[23,24]

SF WAVE. The outward motion of the skin over the left ventricle (upward wave on the apexcardiogram) as left ventricular filling continues in mid and late diastole at a slower pace, called the slow-filling wave.

STASIS. The flattened horizontal ending of the slow-filling wave in late diastole.

Modifications of the apex impulse in cardiac disease. When the apex impulse can be visualized and palpated or recorded with accuracy, one can determine a great deal of information about the left atrium and left ventricle. A given normal feature of one of the series of waves may by itself be sufficient to exclude certain cardiac abnormalities. A particular abnormal feature may be adequate to confirm a certain cardiac diagnosis.

The normal A wave is usually less than 15% of the total apexcardiogram amplitude. A larger-than-normal apical A wave prior to systole is evidence of decreased left ventricular compliance, often due to ischemia or hypertrophy (Fig 2-28). Classic examples include coronary atherosclerosis, acute myocardial infarction, systemic arterial hypertension, aortic stenosis (subvalvular, valvular, or supravalvular), and hypertrophic cardiomyopathy.[7,16] Most such diseases involve pressure load increases on the left ventricle or on the residual contractile myocardium. The A wave of hypertrophic cardiomyopathy may be very forceful and part of the overall trifid apex impulse.[6,7] Occasionally, the A wave of aortic insufficiency also is large.[7]

A short P-R interval causes the A wave to merge with the closely following systolic upstroke wave, masking the separate identity of the A wave. Mitral valve stenosis or an obstructing left atrial myxoma produces small A waves.

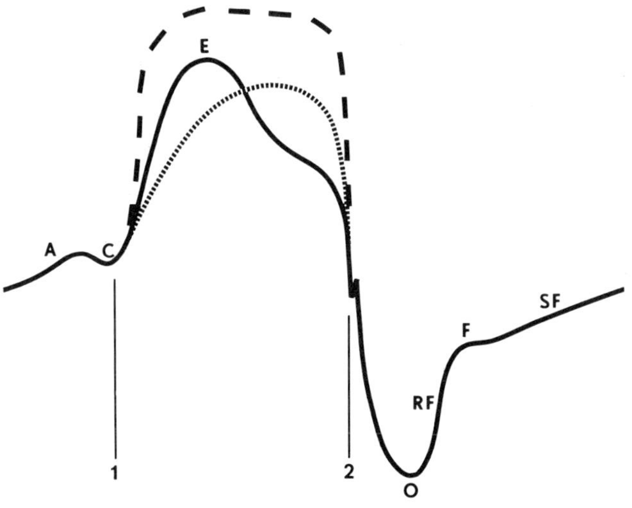

Fig 2-29 Apex pulse (apexcardiogram). The normal contour is shown by the *solid line.* In left ventricular hypertrophy due to aortic stenosis the upstroke of the apex impulse is strong, steady, and continuous, reaching a peak that is relatively sustained in late systole *(dotted line).* With a left ventricular aneurysm, there is marked dyskinesis of the apex impulse and the contour is a smooth, sustained impulse that may extend over a large area corresponding to the ventricular aneurysm *(dashed line).* Letters and numbers are explained in Fig 2-27 legend.

Conversely, a large A wave excludes significant mitral valve stenosis.[7]

Because most normal individuals have A waves that are difficult to detect, only large, easily visible or palpable A waves should be considered definitely abnormal; undetectable or small-amplitude A waves are not necessarily abnormal.

The apical tap (here used to mean a light, rapid blow) of an intensive mitral valve closure impulse at the onset of systole may help identify mitral valve stenosis and, occasionally, mitral valve insufficiency.[6,21]

The upstroke phase and the E point of the apexcardiogram are variable enough in slope, amplitude, and duration from patient to patient to make this early systolic portion of the apex impulse of somewhat less value than the later systolic phase for clinical interpretation.

The portion of the apex impulse after the E point during the last half of systole has considerable diagnostic merit and should be studied carefully in cases of suspected left ventricular disease. In aortic valve stenosis the last portion of this wave is sustained with a strong outward apical thrust or lift in the form of a plateau that easily and smoothly raises the palpating hand (Fig 2-29). The total amplitude may not always be much increased, but the persistent late systolic quality and longer duration of the apex impulse are abnormal.[7,16] The carotid upstroke lags behind the apical outward thrust in significant aortic valve stenosis.[25]

In hypertrophic cardiomyopathy the apex impulse may be bifid during systole and have a very strong force, as though the heart is a muscular fist that is clenching and unclenching or punching within the chest. Coupled with the large A wave, the combination of waves may be trifid and easily recognizable as characteristic of this disorder.[6,7] The term systolic wave (SW) has been applied to the large, second, extra mid to late systolic wave in hypertrophic cardiomyopathy (see Fig 2-28).

In aortic insufficiency, the large, brief, initial outward thrust is not sustained and declines rapidly and smoothly in late systole.[6,7,16]

A left ventricular dyskinetic area of an aneurysm may be palpated as a fairly large region, of several square centimeters, which rises smoothly early in systole and then remains expanded as a single wave during the remainder of systole; it is not as forceful as in the two forms of left ventricular outflow obstruction just discussed.[7] The location on the chest wall corresponds approximately to the position of the Q wave scar or the T wave ischemia on the ECG, so this often provides a good example of the displaced cardiac apex (see Fig 2-29). The important qualities in these systolic lifts are the timing and the overall shape. Precise recording of the onset, peaks, and duration of waves is rarely needed if the examining physician takes time to look and then to feel carefully at the bedside.

It has been reported that the peak systolic wave in a patient with a midsystolic click of mitral valve prolapse may retract in systole.[7,16,26] This may produce a bifid apex impulse. Most patients lack a significant apex impulse in mitral valve prolapse, so one should not spend inordinate time searching for these findings.

Mitral insufficiency may produce an apical systolic thrill or lift.

Abnormalities of diastolic apexcardiographic events relate to diseases of the mitral and aortic valves (Fig 2-30). The cessation of the diastolic decline at the O point is due to the opening of the mitral valve. In mitral valve stenosis the opening snap is heard at this moment. It may be palpable. The echocardiogram has been found to be more precise than the apex impulse for timing of the mitral valve opening.[16] After the O point the normal rapid-filling, outward-moving wave is limited to a more shallow slope as the narrowed mitral opening restricts this first phase of left ventricular filling. The normal transition through the peak of the rapid-filling wave (F point) to the slow-filling wave is also gradual or indistinct. Essentially, the O point is followed by a protracted slow-filling wave, during which there usually is neither a palpable rapid-filling peak nor an audible third heart sound. If an opening snap is present it always precedes whatever rapid-filling wave and peak may be present. A diastolic thrill may be noted on palpation of the apex in severe mitral valve stenosis. Aortic valve stenosis in adults may be associated with a long, slow-filling wave.[7]

In patients with mitral or aortic valve insufficiency, the rapid-filling wave and its peak are accentuated as extra blood enters the left ventricle in early diastole. The peak of the rapid-filling wave is simultaneous with the third heart sound. An experienced cardiologist often can palpate an increased rapid-filling wave and its peak even though the third heart sound has not yet become loud enough to hear. The rapid-filling wave usually peaks with the greatest amplitudes in cases of left ventricular

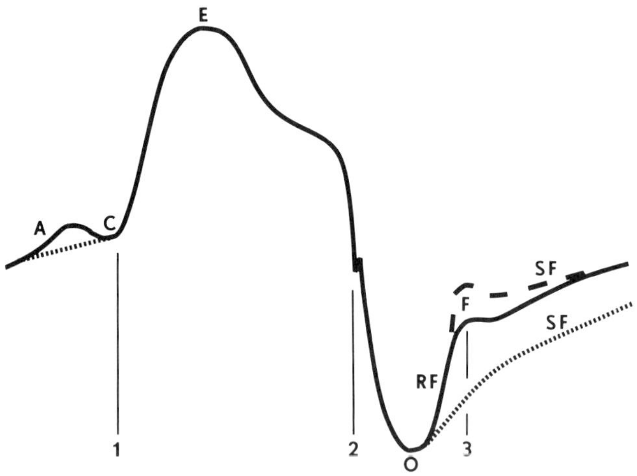

Fig 2-30 Apex pulse (apexcardiogram). The normal contour is shown by the *solid line.* In atrial fibrillation, there is no A wave *(dotted line below the A wave).* In mitral valve disease, the diastolic portion of the apex pulse waves is important. In mitral valve insufficiency, the rapid-filling *(RF)* wave is steep and tall and the F point is more readily palpable than normal. It corresponds to the third heart sound *(3).* The slow-filling *(SF)* wave is more shallow in slope than the previous rapid-filling wave *(dashed line).* In mitral stenosis the rapid-filling wave is drastically reduced, and the F point is often absent. There is usually a more moderate slow-filling wave which follows the O point and replaces the rapid-filling wave *(dotted line).* The opening snap of the mitral valve occurs at about the O point. Points and other numbers are explained in Fig 2-27 legend.

enlargement due to volume overload. Examples include chronic mitral insufficiency, chronic significant left ventricular failure with dilatation, congestive (dilated) cardiomyopathy, aortic valve insufficiency, and subacute or chronic aortic or mitral valve endocarditis with dilatation of the volume-overloaded left ventricle. Hyperthyroidism, anemia, and peripheral arteriovenous connection may be associated with increased rapid-filling waves also. An occasional patient with advanced hypertrophic cardiomyopathy also has an increased rapid-filling wave.[7]

Patients with combined mitral valve stenosis and insufficiency or patients with a previous mitral valve commissurotomy may show a hybrid pattern between the O point and the slow-filling wave in which there is an F point. Some of these patients produce an early diastolic sound that requires phonocardiographic recording for interpretation.

The O point (opening snap) in normal patients varies from 30 to 120 msec after the aortic closure sound, whereas the F point (third heart sound) is usually 100 to 200 msec after the aortic closure sound. Neither the hand nor the ear is as accurate as a phonocardiogram in timing the O point and the F point.[7]

In constrictive pericarditis the knock is produced when rapid left and right ventricular and pericardial expansions are suddenly halted. It occurs slightly earlier than the peak of the usual rapid-filling wave. On palpation the knock may be a shock-like impulse widely distributed over an area larger than the apparent cardiac apex, even in the sitting position.

In left ventricular failure with a compensatory increase in heart rate, the peaks of the rapid-filling wave and the following A wave may occur close to each other or merge into a large, palpable apical wave. This is the physical displacement equivalent of sequential third and fourth heart sounds and of a summation gallop. The word "gallop" takes its name from the sound of a horse galloping and implies that the heart rate is rapid enough to warrant this palpable and auditory metaphor.[7]

Other thoracic areas. Pulsations in other thoracic areas sometimes provide valuable information about cardiovascular diseases. These will be discussed next.

EPIGASTRIC (SUBXIPHOID) AREA. After palpation of the right ventricular area over the sternum while the patient is supine, one should reach under the xiphoid process and try to palpate the bottom portion of the right ventricle in the epigastric region. An enlarged or hypertrophied right ventricle is often easily palpated in this area and produces a downward thrust toward the abdomen, in contrast to the anterior pulsation of the abdominal aorta.

SUBCLAVIAN ARTERIAL AREAS. The right and left subclavian arteries should be palpated for thrills and for the volume of the pulse, especially if a subclavian bruit is noted, a carotid bruit or thrill exists, an upper limb pulse is reduced, an upper limb shows distal embolic infarction, or the aortic or pulmonic areas have a thrill, murmur, or aneurysmal lift. Two common mistakes are assigning a murmur, bruit, or thrill to the wrong cause or location and failing to detect such physical signs because of lack of complete palpation. Inspection of the subclavian arteries may reveal a region of tortuosity. Palpation can confirm this and exclude an aneurysm if the arterial diameter is determined gently between two fingers. An innominate or proximal right subclavian bruit or thrill occasionally is discovered in a healthy young or middle-aged adult and is almost always harmless.

STERNOCLAVICULAR AREA. The suprasternal notch may contain systolic pulsations from a buckled innominate, subclavian, or carotid artery and occasionally from a thoracic aortic aneurysm. Visible pulsations here should be palpated and then traced to the appropriate arterial structure.

LEFT UPPER ANTERIOR CHEST AREA. A large aneurysm of the upper descending thoracic aorta may produce a lift in the left upper anterior chest in the sitting or supine position. When the patient is rolled to the left semilateral decubitus position, it may become less palpable in the original area and more palpable in the subaxillary space in the midaxillary line. Two-dimensional echocardiography may be helpful in distinguishing this type of lift from that of a high lateral or anterior left ventricular aneurysm.

LEFT SUBAXILLARY AREA. A high lateral or anterolateral left ventricular aneurysm may be palpable in the left subaxillary area far from the usual cardiac apical location. The left semilateral decubitus position usually is the best for this purpose.

POSTERIOR THORAX. Thrills of mitral valve insufficiency (anterior leaflet prolapse or flail anterior leaflet) at times may be palpable over the posterior left thorax or between

Table 2-3 Diagnostic significance of visible and palpable chest wall pulsations

Diagnosis	Area	Chest wall pulse
Supravalvular aortic stenosis	Aortic (high)	Systolic thrill
	Apex	Increased lift
Valvular aortic stenosis	Aortic	Systolic thrill
	Apex	Increased lift
Subvalvular aortic stenosis	Aortic (low)	Systolic thrill
	Apex	Increased lift
Aortic insufficiency	Aortic	Increased lift
	Left parasternal	Diastolic thrill
	Apex	Brief lift
Hypertrophic cardiomyopathy	Apex	Large A wave, forceful trifid impulse
Aortic valve prosthesis	Aortic	Increased aortic valve closure impulse
Aortic arch conduit	Aortic	Forceful aortic valve closure impulse
Systemic hypertension	Aortic	Increased aortic valve closure impulse
Pulmonary hypertension	Pulmonary	Increased pulmonary valve closure impulse
Pulmonary valve stenosis	Pulmonary	Systolic thrill
	Right ventricular	Increased lift
Atrial septal defect	Pulmonary	Brief lift
	Right ventricular	Brief lift
Partial anomalous pulmonary venous connection	Pulmonary	Brief lift
	Right ventricular	Brief lift
Ventricular septal defect	Left parasternal	Systolic thrill
	Right ventricular	Brief lift
Tricuspid insufficiency	Right ventricular	Brief lift
Left atrial myxoma	Left ventricular	Forceful plop
Mitral valve stenosis	Pulmonary	Increased lift
	Right ventricular	Increased lift
	Apex	Increased mitral valve closure impulse, diastolic thrill
Mitral valve insufficiency	Pulmonary	Increased lift
	Right ventricular	Increased lift
	Apex	Increased mitral valve closure impulse, systolic thrill
Prolapsed or flail anterior mitral leaflet	Posterior left thorax	Systolic thrill
Prolapsed or flail posterior mitral leaflet	Apex and left parasternal	Systolic thrill
Left ventricular dyskinesis	Apex	Increased A wave, systolic expansion
Left ventricular aneurysm	Apex (may be displaced to left)	Increased A wave, large systolic expansion
Left ventricular failure or volume overload; severe aortic or mitral valve insufficiency	Apex	Rapid filling wave or summation gallop (RF wave merges with A wave)
Constrictive pericarditis	Right or left ventricular	Forceful knock impulse
Coarctation of aorta	Anterior or posterior left thorax	Systolic thrill
	Aortic	Increased aortic valve closure impulse

the scapulae. Thrills of arterial origin (coarctation of the aorta) may be detected by palpation over the posterior thorax.

Possible diagnoses. Diagnoses that may be suggested on the basis of examination of the cardiac apex and other chest wall impulses include supravalvular, valvular, and subvalvular aortic stenosis, aortic valve insufficiency, hypertrophic cardiomyopathy, aortic valve prosthesis, aortic arch conduit, systemic hypertension, pulmonary hypertension, pulmonary valve stenosis, atrial septal defect, partial anomalous pulmonary venous connection, ventricular septal defect, tricuspid insufficiency, left atrial myxoma, mitral valve stenosis, mitral valve insufficiency, prolapsed or flail anterior or posterior mitral leaflets, left ventricular dyskinesis, left ventricular aneurysm, left ventricular failure or volume overload, constrictive pericarditis, and coarctation of the aorta (Table 2-3).

Conclusions. Searching for chest wall vibrations and pulsations is important. Both normal findings and abnormalities are important clues to the nature of the cardiovascular diagnosis. Those who rely on auscultation alone are omitting one of the most valuable parts of the cardiac physical diagnosis. Although every patient need not be scrutinized with exhaustive efforts, the best cardiologists always spend whatever time is warranted in inspection and palpation of the chest wall motions. There are no substitutes for interest, compulsiveness, and thoroughness.

AUSCULTATION: HEART SOUNDS

Heart sounds are due to sudden acceleration and deceleration of columns of blood that set up vibrations in the entire system; that is, the entire heart is put into motion, producing sound.[27-33] The intracardiac valves are essential components in abruptly halting the movement of these blood columns.

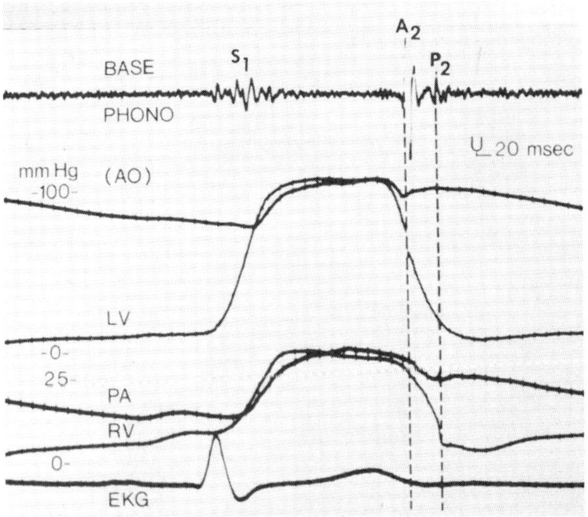

Fig 2-31 The cardiac cycle as depicted by high-fidelity catheter-tip micromanometers in the right *(RV)* and left *(LV)* ventricles, aorta *(AO)*, and pulmonary artery *(PA)*. S_1 occurs shortly after increase in LV pressure. A_2 is coincident with the incisura of the central aortic pressure, and P_2 is coincident with the incisura of the pulmonary artery pressure. (Courtesy of James A. Shaver, M.D., with modification.)

First heart sound

Normal. The first heart sound consists of four components. The first component is low in frequency; it usually is inaudible but can be recorded in most normal subjects. This is followed by two high-frequency, easily audible sounds. Finally, a series of inaudible but recordable low-frequency vibrations follow. The genesis of the first heart sound remains controversial.[34-37]

The first sound occurs at the time of or shortly after the pressure begins to increase in the left ventricle (Fig 2-31). Hemodynamic studies have shown that the pressure in the left ventricle exceeds atrial pressure for 10 to 15 msec before the onset of the first heart sound.[28] The first heart sound is generated at the time of closure of the AV valves;[34,35] phonoechocardiographic studies have confirmed this association in normal subjects.[27,33,35-38]

The initial low-frequency component of the first heart sound probably represents vibrations caused by contraction of the left ventricle and deceleration of antegrade blood flow across the mitral valve.[39]

The first high-frequency component coincides with the closure of the mitral valve, and the second coincides with the closure of the tricuspid valve. The interval between the high-frequency components of the first heart sound (i.e., the interval between mitral and tricuspid valve closures) in a normal subject varies between 20 and 30 msec.[40] The two high-frequency components can be heard in most normal subjects.[41] Ventricular contraction probably accounts for the low-frequency vibrations preceding the first major component of the first heart sound and those following the second high-frequency component.

The first heart sound can be heard best by using the diaphragm of the stethoscope at the apex in order to appreciate its high-frequency components.[42]

Wide splitting of first heart sound. Abnormal splitting of the first heart sound occurs when there is delayed or prolonged contraction of the right ventricle due to abnormalities in electrical activation or mechanical performance. Disorders of electrical activation include right bundle-branch block,[43] left ventricular ectopic beats, left-sided preexcitation,[43] and artificial epicardial pacemakers triggering initial left ventricular contraction.[44,45]

A typical mechanical cause of wide splitting of the first heart sound is Ebstein's anomaly. In this condition, phonoechocardiographic studies have demonstrated that the second high-frequency component of the first heart sound coincides with tricuspid valve closure and that the increased splitting is due to mechanical delay of this valve closure.[46] In severe mitral valve stenosis, mitral valve closure and its resultant sound are delayed.[47] Unmasking of the tricuspid valve component of the first sound is enhanced in pulmonary hypertension, which increases the intensity of this sound.[48]

Sounds that may be confused with wide splitting of the first heart sound include prominent atrial gallops and systolic ejection sounds. Differential characteristics of these sounds will be reviewed below.

Intensity of first heart sound. The intensity of the first heart sound depends on three factors: (1) distance of the heart from the chest wall, (2) sequence of electrical activation of the heart, and (3) mechanical function of the heart. The last two factors determine the position of the AV valve at the onset of systole[49-51] (Fig 2-32). The state of the myocardium determines the rate of rise of intraventricular pressure[43,52-55] and therefore the velocity of closure of the AV valve. The extent of disease of the mitral apparatus determines the ability of the valve to close.[56]

Increased intensity of the first heart sound may be caused by increased flow from a preventricular left-to-right shunt.[57,58] The second high-frequency component

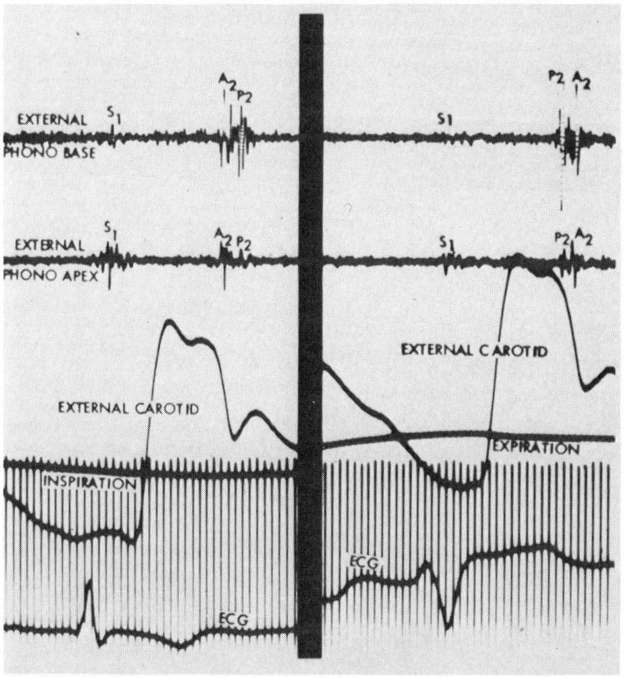

Fig 2-32 Variation in the intensity of the first heart sound in a patient whose intraventricular conduction changes from the normal pattern *(left side)* to left bundle-branch block *(right side)*. There is a marked decrease in the intensity of the first heart sound and paradoxic splitting of the second heart sound. (From Thompson ME, Shaver JA, Leon DF, et al: Pathodynamics of the first heart sound. In *Physiologic Principles of Heart Sounds and Murmurs* [American Heart Association Monograph No 46]. Edited by DF Leon, JA Shaver. New York, American Heart Association, 1975, pp 8-18. By permission.)

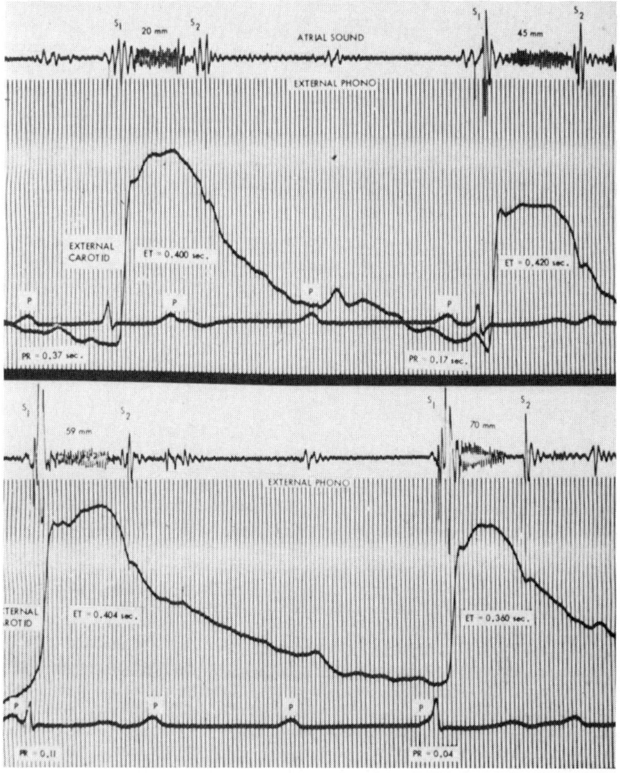

Fig 2-33 Simultaneous apexphonocardiogram, external carotid pulse tracing, and ECG in patient with complete heart block. Note variation in intensity of the first heart sound with the P-R interval. *ET,* ejection time. (From Thompson ME, Shaver JA, Leon DF, et al: Pathodynamics of the first heart sound. In *Physiologic Principles of Heart Sounds and Murmurs* [American Heart Association Monograph No 46]. Edited by DF Leon, JA Shaver. New York, American Heart Association, 1975, pp 8-18. By permission.)

usually is increased in atrial septal defect.[57] The loudness of the first sound is increased in patients with tachycardia and hyperthyroidism, due to increased contractility of the myocardium. In mitral valve stenosis, the first heart sound is accentuated, usually the first high-frequency component, due to delay in mitral valve closure (reversed splitting of S_1).[48]

Decreased intensity of the first sound most commonly is due to poor conduction of sound through the chest and chest wall, as may be noted in patients who are obese or who have chronic obstructive lung disease, constrictive pericarditis, or pericardial effusions. The first heart sound is also decreased when there is first-degree AV block because the effect of atrial systole in extending the valve leaflets is nearly lost as a result of the prolonged delay prior to ventricular contraction. A soft delayed first heart sound is often found in left bundle-branch block.[59,60] The most likely explanation is that left bundle-branch block is frequently associated with impaired ventricular contraction due to myocardial disease. The first sound is also diminished in patients with impaired ventricular function from any cause, with aortic valve insufficiency, or with a heavily calcified, nonpliable mitral valve.

Variations in intensity of the components of the first heart sound occur with phasic respiration in the normal patient.[61] These variations are further influenced in patients with atrial fibrillation because of varying ventricular filling periods and therefore different positions of the AV valves at the end of diastole.[62,63] In complete heart block, there is also variability in the intensity of the first heart sound, depending on the timing of atrial contraction and, therefore, of the AV valve positions at the end of diastole (short P-R interval = loud S_1)[64] (Fig 2-33). By the same mechanism, in ventricular tachycardia with AV dissociation the intensity of the first heart sound is variable.

Second heart sound

Normal. The second heart sound consists of two high-frequency components. The first component (A_2) coincides with aortic valve closure and the second (P_2), with pulmonary valve closure (Fig 2-34).

The asynchronous contraction of the right and left ventricles contributes somewhat to the separation of the

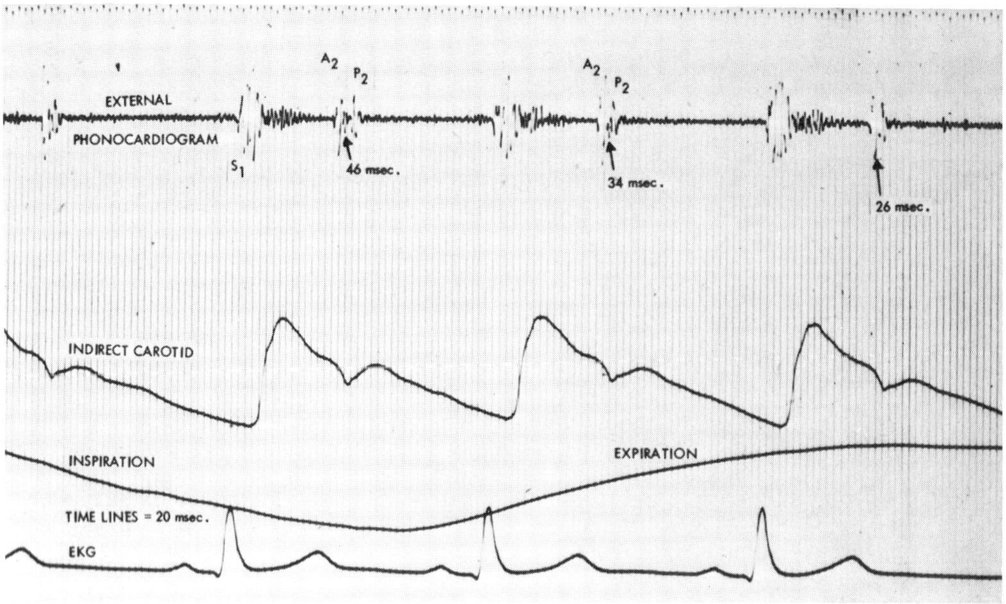

Fig 2-34 Patient with a functional systolic murmur. Note normal physiologic splitting of the second heart sound. (Courtesy of James A. Shaver, M.D.)

aortic and pulmonary valve closure components; however, the most important determining factor is the relative impedance of the pulmonary and systemic vascular beds.[65-67] Identification of these two sounds is best achieved with the diaphragm placed at the second interspace to the left of the sternum. In the newborn, the second heart sound is single. With the decrease in pulmonary vascular resistance that occurs in the first few days of life, the two components separate during inspiration. Normally, at end-expiration, the interval between these two sounds varies from 10 to 20 msec[68] (see Fig 2-34). With augmentation of right ventricular filling during inspiration, the two sounds separate by 50 to 90 msec. Because the relationship is influenced by body position, evaluation of S_2 must be done with the patient in the sitting position during normal respiration. Although the mechanism for this normal splitting has been considered to be prolongation of right ventricular ejection compared to left ventricular ejection, the relationships between the two sounds are the result of a complex interplay between altered venous return to the right and left heart and changes in impedance that occur in the pulmonary vasculature during a normal respiratory cycle.[66,69] Rarely, normal subjects will show wide splitting of the first heart sound and persistent splitting of the second heart sound.

Careful analysis of the relationship of these two components of the second heart sound and their relative intensities provides important clinical clues. It allows appreciation of the relative duration of left and right ventricular systoles (which may be important in acquired heart disease). It may lead one to suspect congenital heart disease such as atrial septal defects,[57] and it may suggest the presence or absence of pulmonary hypertension,[57] and its severity.

Normally, the aortic valve component of the second heart sound is much louder than P_2 and therefore can be heard over the entire precordium. The pulmonary component is heard best in the second intercostal space to the left of the sternum and is poorly transmitted. For this reason, a normal pulmonary valve closure sound is rarely heard at the right upper parasternal area or at the cardiac apex.

The timing of the second heart sound clinically and phonocardiographically coincides with the closure of the semilunar valves—the first component with aortic valve closure[42,70,71] and the second component with pulmonary valve closure[70,72] (see Fig 2-31). Hemodynamic studies, however, demonstrate that closure of each valve precedes its respective sound by 12 msec.[69,72,73]

Electrical as well as mechanical events will influence the relationship of the two components of the second heart sound as well as the intensity of these sounds.

Intensity of second heart sound. The intensity of the aortic valve component is increased in patients with systemic hypertension or coarctation of the aorta or when the aorta is closer to the chest wall as in dilatation of the ascending aorta and transposition of the great arteries. It is diminished when cusps become immobile as in calcific aortic valve disease.

The pulmonary valve component of the second heart sound is increased in intensity in pulmonary hypertension from any cause[74,75] (Fig 2-35). This finding remains valid as a clinical sign of pulmonary hypertension whether or not right ventricular failure occurs.[76] The intensity of this sound is decreased in either valvular or infundibular pulmonary stenosis.

Persistent splitting of second heart sound. Persistent expiratory splitting of more than 30 msec is abnormal. Various electrical and mechanical abnormalities will

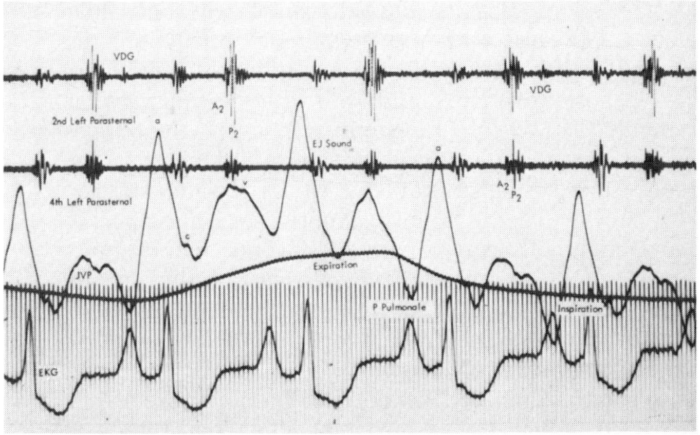

Fig 2-35 Patient with primary pulmonary hypertension. "P" pulmonale is seen on the ECG; prominent A waves are present. Note narrow splitting with an increased intensity of the pulmonary valve component of S_2. *EJ,* ejection; *JVP,* jugular venous pressure; *VDG,* ventricular diastolic gallop. (Courtesy of James A. Shaver, M.D.)

cause this abnormal wide splitting of the second heart sound (Table 2-4).

Complete right bundle-branch block delays right ventricular activation, which delays right ventricular mechanical systole, which results in later-than-normal pulmonary valve closure[43] (Fig 2-36). Normal respiratory variation, however, is usually present, and the cause of the abnormal splitting can be identified as right bundle-branch block by the presence of abnormal splitting of the first heart sound due to delayed tricuspid valve closure.

Other electrical causes of persistent splitting of the second sound are left ventricular pacing, premature contractions originating in the left ventricle, and, in some patients, left ventricular preexcitation.

Atrial septal defect is an important mechanical cause of persistent splitting of the second heart sound. Inspiratory increase in right ventricular volume was considered in the past to be the sole cause of inspiratory splitting of the second sound.[40,57,61] More recent observations indicate that it is not only the volume increase in the ventricle but also the altered impedance in the pulmonary vascular bed that delays the pulmonary valve closure sound.[65] Atrial septal defect (secundum) is characterized by a wide, persistent, relatively fixed split of the second sound during the entire respiratory cycle (Fig 2-37). If pulmonary vascular resistance is low, the wide split is due to the delayed pulmonary component of the second sound (evidenced by the pulmonary artery incisura moving away from the right ventricular pressure pulse).[65] The "fixed" split is attributed to right and left ventricular ejection times remaining constant. Inspiration increases systemic venous return to the right ventricle, but the left-to-right shunt also decreases and left ventricular filling is maintained. Pulmonary vascular impedance is already low and does not decrease further with inspiration, and, hence, there is no further inspiratory delay in the pulmonary valve component of the second sound.[64]

Table 2-4 Abnormal splitting of second heart sound

- Persistent splitting
  - Electrical delay of pulmonary component
    - Right bundle-branch block
    - Left ventricular ectopic beats
    - Preexcitation (left ventricular tract)
    - Left ventricular pacemaker
  - Mechanical delay of pulmonary component
    - Pulmonary valve stenosis
    - Subvalvular pulmonary obstruction
    - Large pulmonary embolus
    - Right ventricular dysfunction
  - Decrease in pulmonary vascular impedance
    - Dilatation of pulmonary artery
    - Atrial septal defect
    - After surgical repair of atrial septal defect
  - Early aortic component
    - Mitral regurgitation
    - Ventricular septal defect
    - Preexcitation (left ventricular tract)
- Paradoxic splitting
  - Electrical delay of aortic component
    - Left bundle-branch block
    - Right ventricular ectopic beats
    - Right ventricular pacemaker
    - Coronary heart disease
  - Mechanical delay of aortic component
    - Aortic valve stenosis
    - Hypertrophic cardiomyopathy
    - Coronary heart disease
    - Patent ductus arteriosus
    - Aortic regurgitation
  - Early closure of pulmonary valve
    - Tricuspid regurgitation

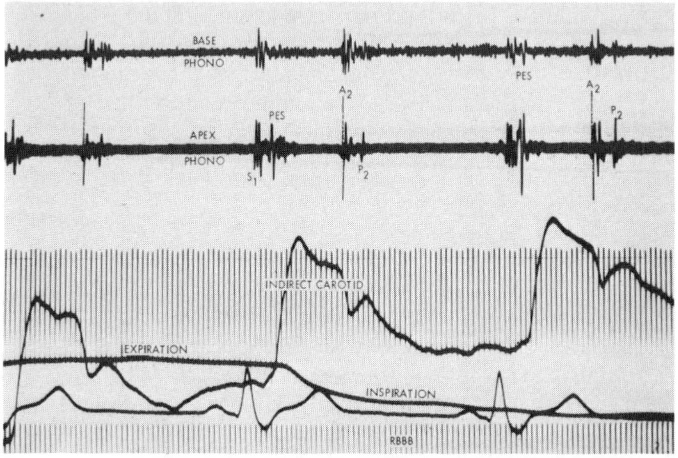

Fig 2-36 Wide splitting of second heart sound in patient with complete right bundle-branch block *(RBBB). PES,* pulmonary ejection sound. (Courtesy of James A. Shaver, M.D.)

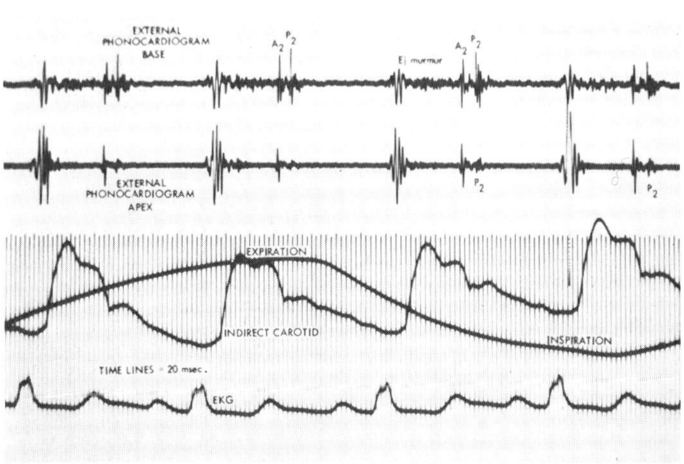

Fig 2-37 Wide splitting of second heart sound in patient with a large atrial septal defect. Note also the short systolic ejection *(Ej)* murmur. (Courtesy of James A. Shaver, M.D.)

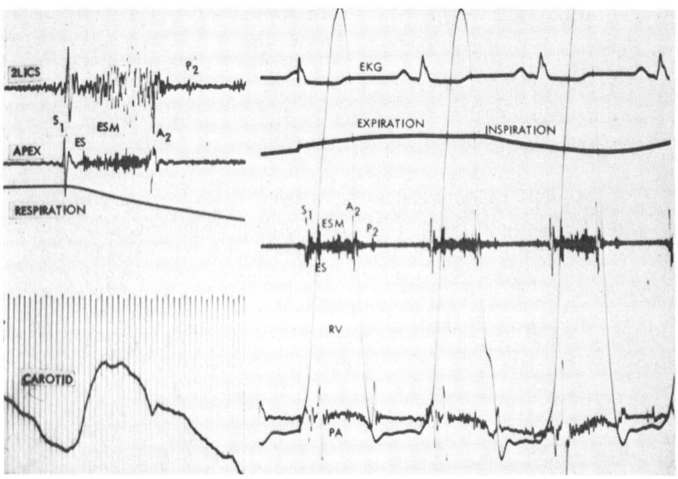

Fig 2-38 Patient with severe pulmonary valve stenosis, wide splitting of the second heart sound, and a late-peaking systolic murmur. *Right,* simultaneous pressure recordings showing a peak right ventricular pressure of 170 mm Hg. *ES,* ejection sound; *ESM,* ejection systolic murmur; *PA,* pulmonary artery; *2LICS,* second left intercostal space. (Courtesy of James A. Shaver, M.D.)

After repair, the normal relationship of the two components of the second sound usually occurs early.[57] However, in some cases, persistent splitting of the second sound persists in the absence of complete right bundle-branch block. Right ventricular dysfunction, along with persistent changes in the pulmonary vasculature, explains this finding in some patients.[65] In pulmonary valve stenosis with intact ventricular septum, the cause of delay in the pulmonary valve component of the second heart sound is also mechanical[77] (Fig 2-38). In this condition, the pulmonary valve component is very soft and can be heard best in the second intercostal space along the left sternal border.[78] Because the duration of right ventricular ejection increases with the degree of obstruction, the interval of the splitting during expiration in pulmonary valve stenosis correlates quite well with the transvalvular gradient.[78] However, if the stenosis is severe, the pulmonary valve component may not be heard and therefore the second sound is single and due to aortic valve closure. With subvalvular pulmonary stenosis, separation of the second sound also may persist. Right ventricular dysfunction at times may produce persistent splitting of the second sound.

In constrictive pericarditis, there may be less variation in the relationships of the two components of the second heart sound compared to normal, but they are rarely "fixed." Although right ventricular filling, and therefore stroke volume, is fixed, the aortic valve component of the second sound occurs earlier with inspiration because of the inspiratory decrease in left ventricular filling that occurs in constrictive pericarditis.[79]

Persistent or wide splitting of the second heart sound occurs in severe mitral valve insufficiency[80] and in ventricular septal defect.[81] In both there is retrograde ejection of left ventricular blood into a low-pressure chamber which results in an abnormally short left ventricular ejection time and thus early aortic valve closure. The respiratory variation is preserved and readily heard.

Paradoxic splitting of second heart sound. Paradoxic splitting of the second sound (i.e., pulmonary valve component precedes aortic valve component) may be caused by electrical or mechanical abnormalities (see Table 2-4).

Delay in aortic valve closure sufficient to allow the pulmonary valve component of the second sound to precede the aortic valve component results in reverse splitting of the second heart sound. When this occurs, the two sounds come closer together and at times fuse during inspiration; in expiration, the sounds separate.[82]

The most common cause of paradoxic splitting of the second heart sound is left bundle-branch block (see Fig 2-32). Delayed activation of the left ventricle also occurs with right ventricular ectopic beats, right endocardial pacemakers, and some cases of right ventricular preexcitation.

With obstruction to the left ventricular outflow, paradoxic splitting can be heard (Fig 2-39). This includes both aortic valve stenosis and hypertrophic cardiomyopathy. In aortic valve stenosis, it is most obvious in the congenital variety because the aortic valve closure sound remains preserved, in contrast to calcific aortic bicuspid or rheumatic disease in which the aortic valve closure sound is decreased in intensity or absent. In both aortic valve stenosis and hypertrophic cardiomyopathy, paradoxic splitting of the second heart sound implies hemodynamically significant obstruction.

Paradoxic splitting of the second heart sound may be observed during episodes of "ischemic cardiac pain."[83] Prolongation of left ventricular ejection time due to hypertension may produce paradoxic splitting of the second heart sound.[84] Reversed splitting of the second heart sound due to tricuspid regurgitation has been reported.[85]

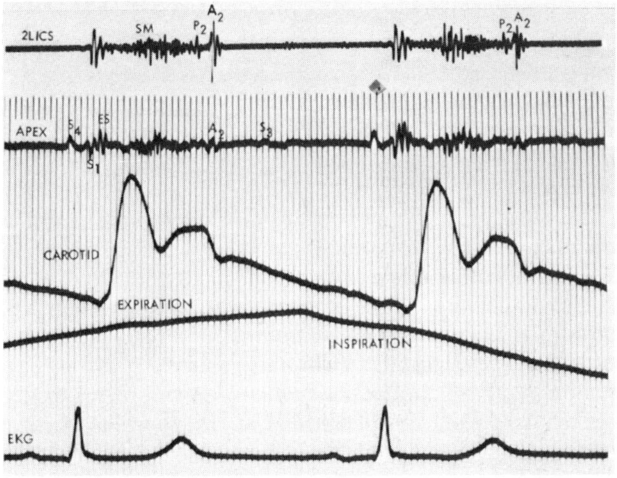

Fig 2-39 Classic carotid pulse of hypertrophic cardiomyopathy with paradoxic splitting of the second heart sound, crescendo-decrescendo murmur, and atrial and ventricular gallop. Note delayed A_2. *ES,* ejection sound; *SM,* systolic murmur; *2LICS,* second left intercostal space. (From Shaver JA: Current uses of phonocardiography in clinical practice. *Cardiol Update,* 1981, pp 327-378. By permission of Elsevier Science Publishing Company.)

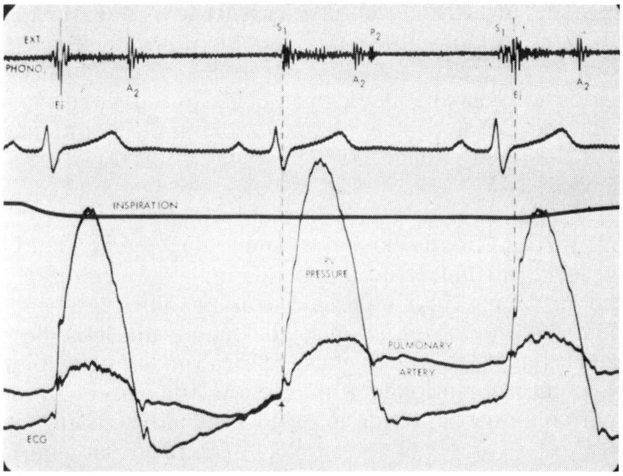

Fig 2-40 Mechanism responsible for variation in intensity of a right-sided ejection sound with respiration. With inspiration, there is an increase in venous return, equalizing the diastolic pressure in the pulmonary artery and right ventricle and resulting in early opening of the pulmonary valve in diastole. Therefore, during isometric contraction there is no doming of the valve and no opening sound. In the next cycle, there is a diastolic gradient at the time of isometric contraction associated with doming of the valve and a loud pulmonary valve ejection sound. *Ej,* ejection. (Courtesy of James A. Shaver, M.D.)

Single second heart sound. A single audible second sound occurs as a result of synchronous closure of both semilunar valves or decreased intensity or absence of one component. The most common cause of decreased intensity of the pulmonary valve component is the increased anteroposterior chest dimension seen in older adults.[66] In patients with severe pulmonary valve stenosis, a single second heart sound is due to poor transmission of a soft pulmonary valve component. Other conditions associated with an "audible" single second heart sound (aortic) are tetralogy of Fallot and transposition of the great arteries. In all of these, two components of the second sound are present; however, the pulmonary valve component is inaudible.

A single second sound due to synchrony of the two components throughout the respiratory cycle is seen normally at birth and in patients with Eisenmenger's disease. It implies identical impedance and capacitance in the pulmonary and systemic circulations.[65] In truncus arteriosus the single second sound (not invariably present) is the result of the presence of only one semilunar valve.

Ejection sounds

An ejection sound (click) follows the first heart sound and is produced at the time of ejection of blood from a ventricle into a great artery. The sound is brief and of high frequency; it is best heard with the diaphragm of the stethoscope. With rare exceptions, the presence of an ejection click implies underlying cardiovascular disease. The sound may be caused by vibration of the aortic or pulmonary valve as it reaches its maximal level of ascent into the great artery, or it may result from sudden distention of the aorta or pulmonary artery.

Pulmonary ejection sounds. Pulmonary ejection sounds (Fig 2-40) are heard best in the second and third left interspaces along the sternum and occur earlier than aortic ejection sounds. They are heard poorly along the lower left sternal border and apex. The sounds fluctuate in intensity with respiration, diminishing or disappearing with inspiration and increasing in intensity with expiration. The change in intensity is considered to be related to the position of the valve at the beginning of right ventricular contraction.[86] During inspiration there is augmentation of right ventricular filling that results in displacement of the mobile pulmonary valve to a more open position before systole.

Pulmonary ejection sounds are heard in congenital pulmonary valve stenosis,[86] idiopathic dilatation of the pulmonary artery,[87] and pulmonary hypertension.[88,89] These sounds are not present in patients with supravalvular or muscular subvalvular obstruction.

The recognition of an ejection sound occurring in the right side of the heart is useful in distinguishing pulmonary valve stenosis from infundibular pulmonary stenosis and for distinguishing pulmonary valve stenosis from atrial septal defect. All of these conditions have in common a systolic ejection murmur and persistent splitting of the second heart sound, but a pulmonary ejection sound is usually present in mild to moderate pulmonary valve stenosis and is less common in atrial septal defect and infundibular pulmonary stenosis.

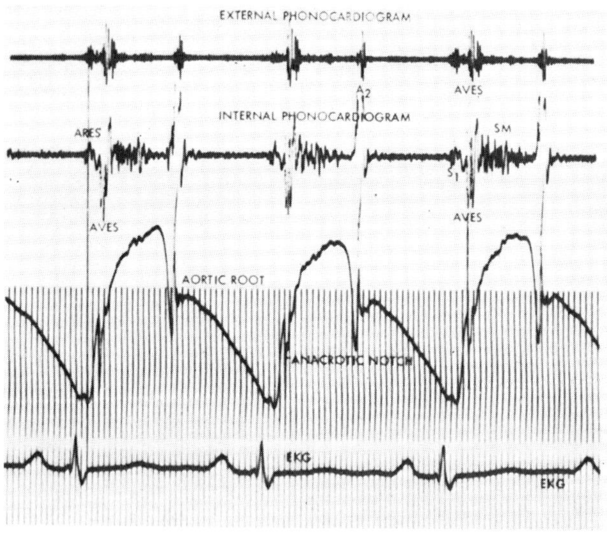

Fig 2-41 Patient with mild aortic valve stenosis and a prominent ejection sound *(AVES)* introducing a short ejection murmur *(SM),* ending well before a well-preserved aortic closure sound. The aortic ejection sound *(ARES)* coincides with the anacrotic notch on the high-fidelity catheter in the central aorta. (From Whittaker AV, Shaver JA, Gray S III, et al: Sound-pressure correlates of the aortic ejection sound: an intracardiac sound study. *Circulation* 39:475-486, 1969. By permission of American Heart Association.)

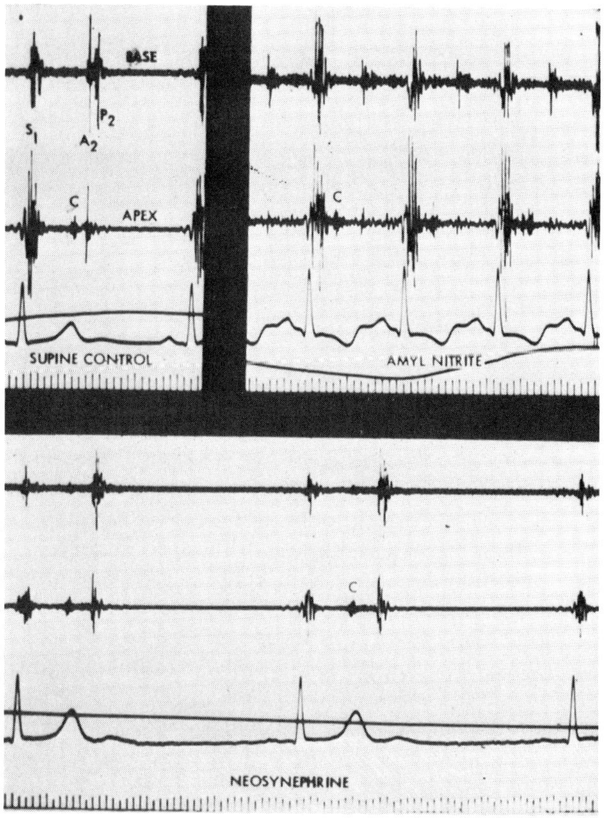

Fig 2-42 Effect of amyl nitrite and phenylephrine (Neo-Synephrine) on movement of the click *(C).* With amyl nitrite, the click moves toward the first heart sound; with phenylephrine, the click moves back toward the second heart sound. (Courtesy of James A. Shaver, M.D.)

Aortic ejection sounds. Aortic ejection sounds are heard best at the base but are widely transmitted over the entire precordium. They do not vary in intensity with respiration, in contrast to pulmonary ejection sounds (Fig 2-41).

The aortic ejection sound is frequently present in patients with aortic valve disease (both stenosis and insufficiency) with dilatation of the aortic root due to hypertension, aneurysm of the ascending aorta, and coarctation of the aorta.[90,91] This sound is rarely present in supravalvular or subaortic muscular obstruction.

Of practical diagnostic importance are the following facts: (1) The presence of this sound indicates mobility of the aortic cusp(s) in patients with aortic valve stenosis; therefore, an ejection sound is not heard when the valve becomes immobile in patients with significant calcific aortic valve stenosis. (2) In the absence of other auscultatory findings, an aortic ejection sound may be the first clue to the presence of bicuspid aortic valve; in fact, an aortic ejection sound may precede the appearance of a murmur or significant aortic valve obstruction by many years. (3) If an aortic ejection sound is present in a patient with coarctation, bicuspid aortic valve is usually present.

Nonejection systolic sounds

In the past, sounds occurring in the middle or later part of systole were thought to be pericardial or extracardiac in origin.[61,92] However, whether single or multiple and whether associated with a late systolic murmur or not, nearly all of these sounds are now known to be due to abnormalities in structure of the mitral valve apparatus.[93-96]

Nonejection systolic sounds are heard best along the lower left sternal border and toward the apex. They are poorly heard at the base of the heart. Like ejection sounds, the midsystolic sounds are very crisp, high-frequency sounds (Figs 2-42 and 2-43). They should not be confused with the first or second heart sound or ejection sounds. On occasion, a late systolic sound may be misinterpreted as the second heart sound and the late systolic murmur, as a diastolic murmur.

The systolic sound occurs when the prolapsed mitral leaflet reaches its maximal excursion and there is sudden deceleration of intracardiac columns of blood. Multiple sounds may result from multiple redundant valve scallops that are prolapsing into the left atrium at different times. Patients with systolic sounds due to mitral valve prolapse may develop late systolic murmurs and holosystolic murmurs. When only a click is heard, a diagnosis of mitral valve prolapse cannot be made with certainty because midsystolic sounds may arise from various intracardiac and extracardiac mechanisms. Pneumothorax has been well documented as a cause of nonejection sounds. Midsystolic sounds have also been reported with idio-

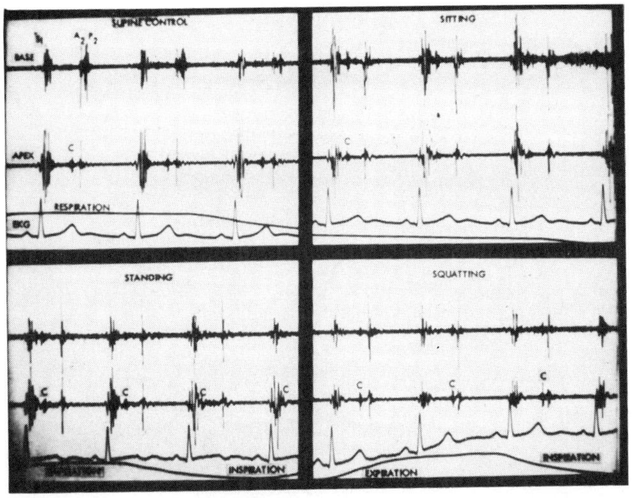

Fig 2-43 Effect of change in posture on the click *(C).* In the sitting patient, the click moves toward the first heart sound; in the standing patient, it moves toward the first heart sound. When the patient squats, it moves toward the second heart sound. (From Shaver JA: Current uses of phonocardiography in clinical practice. *Cardiol Update,* 1981, pp 327-378. By permission of Elsevier Science Publishing Company.)

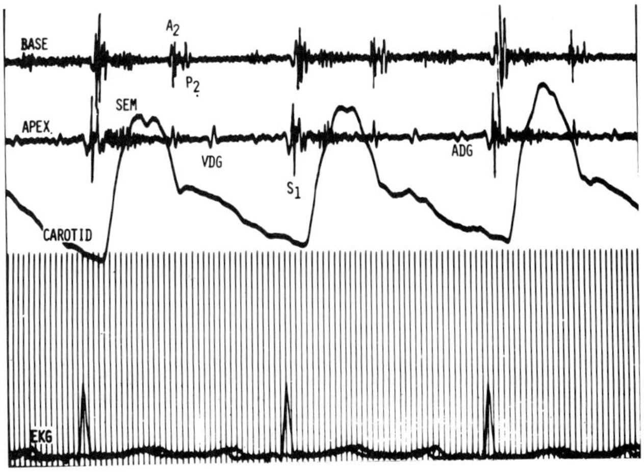

Fig 2-44 Functional systolic ejection murmur *(SEM)* of high-output state of thyrotoxicosis. Note both atrial and ventricular filling sounds. *ADG,* atrial diastolic gallop; *VDG,* ventricular diastolic gallop. (From Shaver JA: Innocent murmurs. *Hosp Med* 14:8-35, April 1978. By permission of Hospital Publications.)

pathic left ventricular subannular aneurysm, with epicardial pacing, and after cardiac surgery. Finally, Barlow and Bosman[94] described five patients with mitral stenosis and fibrous chordae. Systolic sounds have developed after mitral valvotomy. In the majority of instances, however, midsystolic clicks are part of the spectrum of the mitral valve prolapse syndrome.[97]

The timing of the click and murmur in systole is influenced by left ventricular volume during systole, and in each patient there is a point of critical volume during systole at which prolapse will occur. Various bedside maneuvers that influence ventricular volume will influence timing and intensity of both the click and the murmur (see Figs 2-42 and 2-43). Interventions that result in decreased left ventricular volume during systole produce earlier prolapse associated with an earlier onset of the click and the systolic murmur. Maneuvers that increase left ventricular volume, on the other hand, will delay the systolic click or murmur and, on occasion, may even prevent prolapse and thus obliterate the murmur and click. Bedside maneuvers that can be used to decrease left ventricular volume include sitting, standing, and the Valsalva maneuver (phase II or straining phase). The maneuvers resulting in a larger left ventricular volume include prompt squatting, isometrics, and elevation of legs from the recumbent position.

Pharmacologic agents are also helpful in identifying the nonejection sounds as mitral in origin. Vasodilators, such as amyl nitrite, produce a significant decrease in systemic vascular resistance with subsequently increased stroke volume, decreased regurgitation fraction, and decreased ventricular volume; thus, the click and murmur occur earlier in systole. On the other hand, vasopressors, such as phenylephrine, increase the systemic blood pressure and delay the nonejection sounds and murmur.

Third heart sound

Third heart sounds result from vibrations that occur in early diastole. Two main factors are responsible for most abnormal third heart sounds: abnormal ventricular compliance as in ventricular failure, and an increase in the rate and volume of AV flow during the passive filling stage of the cardiac cycle.[66,98,99] The sound is often heard in normal children and adolescents. It also may be heard in the normal young adult and may be a typical finding in high-output states such as thyrotoxicosis and pregnancy (Fig 2-44). In pathologic states, as in volume overload (examples are mitral regurgitation and aortic regurgitation), the third heart sound is associated with an increase in ventricular volume but not necessarily in diastolic pressure. Normal filling of a ventricle whose function is impaired results in a relative volume overload (i.e., restrictive cardiomyopathy), often accompanied by an increase in diastolic pressure, and is the likely explanation of the ventricular filling sound in patients with latent or overt left ventricular dysfunction. The ventricular filling sound from the left ventricle is heard best at the apex.

Nearly all normal subjects under the age of 40 have a recordable heart sound.[100]

Although a third heart sound is an important clinical sign, clinicians often cannot agree reliably about whether or not it is present.[101]

The third heart sound of right ventricular origin is heard best along the lower sternal borders and over the xiphoid. It is often present in patients with cor pulmonale. In some instances it is heard in the epigastrium and at times beneath the right lower rib cage. A right-sided third sound also implies underlying cardiac disease – specifically, impaired right ventricular function. It is distinguished from a left ventricular third sound not only by its location but also by its augmentation during inspiration. The explanation for the genesis of the right-sided third sound is similar to that of a left-sided third sound.

Fourth heart sound

The fourth heart sound results from atrial contraction and occurs before the onset of ventricular activation. In the normal heart, the atrial contribution to ventricular filling is of minor importance and, hence, fourth sounds are less commonly heard[102-106] (see Fig 2-44). Physiologic fourth heart sounds occur in patients with hyperthyroidism,[107] anemia, or peripheral arteriovenous fistulas. In this clinical setting, the sound is associated with increased ventricular filling volume as part of an increased blood volume and is not secondary to abnormal ventricular compliance.[102] The fourth heart sound of left-sided origin is best heard inside the cardiac apex or just at the apex when the patient is lying in the left lateral position. The right-sided fourth heart sound is best heard along the left sternal border and xiphoid and, like most events in the right side, is augmented with inspiration.

Left-sided fourth heart sounds are heard in patients with decreased left ventricular compliance.[108] Examples include left ventricular hypertrophy due to hypertension, aortic valve stenosis,[109] hypertrophic cardiomyopathy, and primary and secondary myocardial disease.[110] Common to all patients is a left ventricle with decreased compliance and a rapid change in intraventricular pressure due to atrial systole and late diastolic distention of the ventricle. The presence or absence of the fourth heart sound is quantitatively related to the left atrial filling fraction and appears to predict atrial filling fraction greater than or equal to or less than 35% reasonably well.[111] A fourth heart sound arising in the right heart is heard in pulmonary hypertension, pulmonary valve stenosis, and hypertrophic cardiomyopathy,[77,112] conditions producing decreased right ventricular compliance.

An audible fourth heart sound does provide evidence for cardiac disease, and increasing examiner experience renders this finding fairly specific.[113]

In patients with sinus tachycardia, at times it is difficult to separate the two diastolic sounds because they tend to coalesce and become a single loud sound (summation gallop). When the heart rate is slowed by use of carotid sinus massage, the two sounds separate and are clearly identified. It is important to identify the filling sounds properly; the fourth heart sound is associated with a better prognosis than the third heart sound.[107]

Third and fourth sounds often are intermittent and may be accentuated with exercise or by an increase in blood pressure, such as attained by simple isometric hand exercise. These sounds are of such low frequency that often they are better felt than heard. For this reason, close inspection of the apical impulse helps to confirm the presence of ventricular as well as atrial filling sounds.

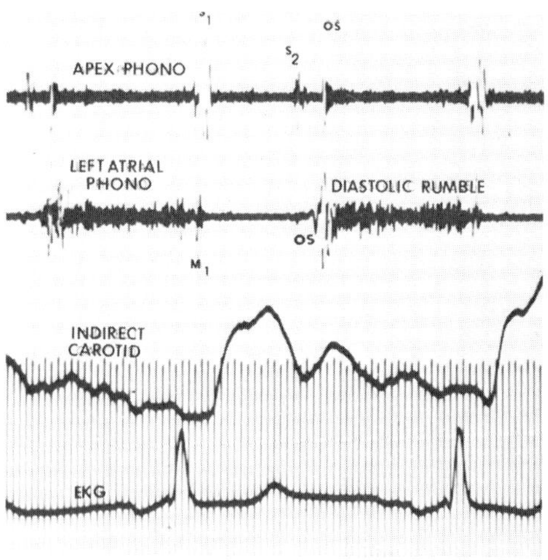

Fig 2-45 Patient with pure mitral valve stenosis with a loud first heart sound and a loud opening snap *(OS)* initiating a diastolic rumble. (Courtesy of James A. Shaver, M.D.)

Opening snaps

The opening snap of mitral valve stenosis occurs 30 to 120 msec after the aortic valve component of the second heart sound (Fig 2-45). It is a brief, high-pitched sound with wide radiation. It is caused by the "tambourine effect" of a valve with fused commissures snapping into the ventricle rather than opening to allow free flow of blood. It is best heard at the point of maximal apical impulse; it also is heard easily along the left sternal border with the patient in the recumbent position. The opening snap in patients with mitral valve stenosis implies pliability of the mitral leaflet, particularly the anterior leaflet.[114,115] In addition to the implication of disease of the mitral valve, almost always rheumatic, the relationship of this sound to the aortic valve component of the second sound is helpful in assessing the severity of the mitral valve stenosis[116] (Fig 2-46). At any given heart rate and blood pressure, in a patient with mitral valve stenosis the more severe the stenosis, the higher the left atrial pressure, and therefore the shorter the time interval between aortic valve closure and opening snap. Exceptions are older patients and patients with systemic hypertension, in whom severe mitral valve stenosis can occur without a short interval because left ventricular systolic pressure takes longer to fall below left atrial pressure.[66] With some experience, intervals as short as 20 msec can be appreciated at the bedside.

The opening snap of the mitral valve may be difficult to differentiate from other sounds. The most frequent problem involves separation of the opening snap from the pulmonary valve component of the second heart sound, particularly when pulmonary hypertension is a consequence of severe mitral valve stenosis. There are two helpful findings. First, when an early diastolic sound is heard in the right second parasternal interspace ("aortic area"), it almost invariably represents a mitral valve

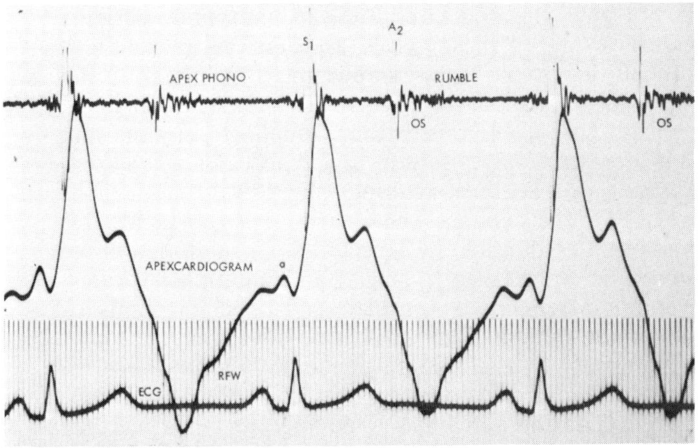

Fig 2-46 Apexcardiogram in patient with very mild mitral valve stenosis. Note the late opening snap *(OS),* the short early rumble, and the persistence of an "a kick" on the apexcardiogram, all favoring mild stenosis. *RFW,* rapid-filling wave. (From Shaver JA: Current uses of phonocardiography in clinical practice. *Cardiol Update,* 1978, pp 327-378. By permission of Elsevier Science Publishing Company.)

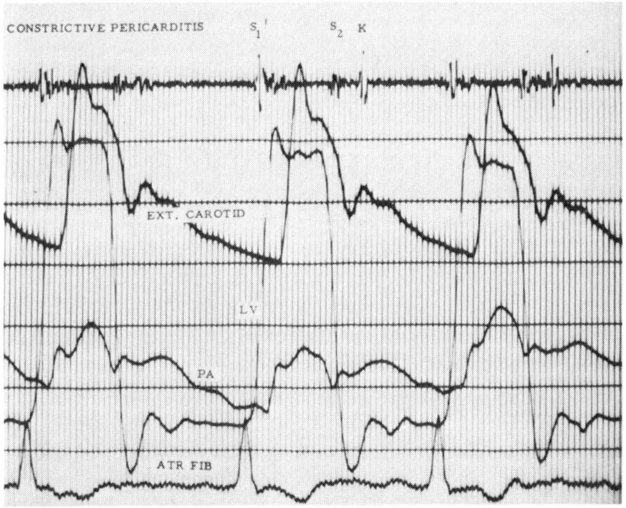

Fig 2-47 Pericardial knock *(K)* in patient with constrictive pericarditis. Note the "square root sign" on the left ventricular pressure tracing and the lack of variation in the peak pressure of the left ventricle *(LV)* with varying cycle length. The end-diastolic pressure in the left ventricle is the same in all cycles. *ATR FIB,* atrial fibrillation; *PA,* pulmonary artery. (From Shaver JA: Current uses of phonocardiography in clinical practice. *Cardiol Update,* 1978, pp 327-378. By permission of Elsevier Science Publishing Company.)

opening snap (personal observation). It is rare to hear a pulmonary valve component, even in the presence of pulmonary hypertension, a third heart sound, or a pericardial knock in this area. Second, with careful auscultation at the second left interspace during the entire respiratory phase, three heart sounds can be identified. With inspiration, the second heart sound separates into aortic and pulmonary components and can be identified. If an opening snap is present, this third high-frequency component is readily heard. This then distinguishes the opening snap from the pulmonary valve component of the second heart sound. This may be an important observation in patients who have an atrial septal defect. These patients may be considered to have mitral valve stenosis because the pulmonary valve closure component is misinterpreted as a mitral valve opening snap. A sound with acoustic characteristics similar to those of the opening snap is heard in some patients with left atrial myxoma. The sound occurs when the tumor moves into the left ventricle in early diastole.

The opening snap of the tricuspid valve is seldom appreciated on auscultation and for this reason is of little clinical help in the diagnosis of tricuspid valve stenosis. Because rheumatic tricuspid valve stenosis is rarely, if ever, an isolated lesion, the clinical findings usually are dominated by the findings of mitral valve stenosis or mitral and aortic valve disease. The diagnosis of associated tricuspid valve stenosis is based on other clinical findings.

Although mitral and tricuspid valve opening snaps usually imply diseased valves, they can occur with normal AV valves when an increased diastolic flow across the valve produces an increased velocity of opening. Mitral valve opening snaps have been reported in mitral valve regurgitation, ventricular septal defect, patent ductus arteriosus, and high-degree AV block.[117] A tricuspid valve opening snap may be heard in atrial septal defect with a large left-to-right shunt.

Pericardial knock

Corrigan first reported the early diastolic sound of constrictive pericarditis,[118] and it first was recognized by Potain[119] as a valuable sign in the diagnosis of pericardial constriction. This high-frequency sound occurs between 90 and 120 msec after aortic closure (Fig 2-47). The cause of this sound is considered to be the sudden cessation of ventricular filling. In patients with a ventricular filling sound, the decrease in ventricular compliance interferes with ventricular filling; in patients with constrictive pericarditis, the pericardium acts as a constricting force, preventing normal ventricular diastolic expansion. This sound occurs later than an opening snap and earlier than the ventricular filling sound. Identification of this sound in noncalcific constrictive pericarditis is particularly important.[120] The most common misinterpretation is confusing this sound with the opening snap of mitral valve stenosis. In mitral valve stenosis there are, in addition, the auscultatory apical diastolic rumble, pulmonary lift, and right ventricular lift when the mitral valve stenosis is severe and of long standing. The opening snap does not vary with the respiratory cycle. In the majority of patients with constrictive pericarditis and a pericardial knock, there is an alteration of the intensity of the pericardial knock with inspiration. The inspiratory phase of respiration augments the pericardial knock, whereas it has no influence on the intensity of the opening snap of mitral valve stenosis. Rarely, early diastolic sounds (pseudoknock sounds) produced by noncardiac disease have been reported.[121]

SOUNDS PRODUCED BY PACEMAKERS, CATHETERS, AND ARTIFICIAL VALVES

Cardiac pacing occasionally produces a sound that occurs synchronously with the pacing impulse. This sound occurs in presystole and is related to either skeletal muscle or diaphragmatic contraction rather than being cardiac in origin. This extracardiac sound rarely, if ever, causes diagnostic problems. Systolic sounds induced by intracardiac catheters have been reported.[122] The sound is thought to be due to the slapping of the catheter against the right ventricular septum during systole.[123]

There are four basic types of artificial valves in current use: ball cage, floating or tilting disk, bileaflet valves, and biologic valves. Each of these valves has had numerous modifications during development. Each valve makes distinctive valve sounds. Unfortunately, most physicians do not have the opportunity to examine many patients who have one of these valves, and, for this reason, it is difficult for a physician to become familiar with the characteristics of the sounds made by the various artificial devices. The problem is further complicated by the fact that multiple valves often are placed in a patient. Furthermore, at times, multiple valves of different types are used in the same patient. Despite these obstacles, it is possible to identify, by auscultation, malfunction of prosthetic valves, both single and multiple. Clinical evaluation remains a sensitive and specific means of identifying patients with prosthetic valve dysfunction.[124]

Noninvasive assessment, including phonoechocardiography, two-dimensional echocardiography, and Doppler echocardiography, has gradually replaced cardiac catheterization for quantitative assessment of prosthetic valve function. It is now possible with the development of pulsed, continuous-wave, and color-flow Doppler echocardiography to characterize prosthetic valve function precisely and noninvasively. Flow characteristics of normal[125] (Tables 2-5 and 2-6) and abnormal prosthetic heart valves have been reported by many investiga-

Table 2-5 Normal values for prosthesis in the mitral position*

Prosthesis	Number of patients	Mitral valve area (cm^2)	Mean gradient (mm Hg)	Regurgitant valves (5)
Mechanical				
Starr-Edwards	43	2.01 ± 0.49	4.6 ± 2.4	36
St. Jude	156	2.88 ± 0.64	3.5 ± 1.3	30
Björk-Shiley	128	2.44 ± 0.62	2.9 ± 1.6	16
Lillehei-Kaster	9	NI	3.35	NI
Beall	16	NI	6.0 ± 2.0	NI
Tissue				
Ionescu-Shiley	29	2.36 ± 0.75	3.3 ± 1.2	NI
Carpentier-Edwards	75	2.45 ± 0.74	6.5 ± 2.1	NI
Hancock	114	1.71 ± 0.41	4.3 ± 2.1	20

NI, not included.
*Pooled data adapted from Reisner SA, Meltzer RS: Normal values of prosthetic valve Doppler echocardiographic parameters: a review. *J Am Soc Echocardiography* 1:201-210, 1988.

Table 2-6 Normal values for prosthesis in the aortic position*

Prosthesis	Number of patients	Peak gradient (mm Hg)	Mean gradient (mm Hg)	Regurgitant valves (%)
Mechanical				
St. Jude	70	25.5 ± 5.1	12.5 ± 6.3	51
Björk-Shiley	102	23.8 ± 8.8	14.3 ± 5.2	22
Starr-Edwards	56	38.6 ± 11.7	24.0 ± 4.0	52
Tissue				
Carpentier-Edwards	143	23.2 ± 8.7	14.4 ± 5.7	20
Hancock	91	23.0 ± 6.7	11.0 ± 2.3	27
Ionescu-Shiley	32	24.7 ± 7.6	14.0 ± 4.3	NI

NI, not included.
*Pooled data adapted from Reisner SA, Meltzer RS: Normal values of prosthetic valve Doppler echocardiographic parameters: a review. *J Am Soc Echocardiography* 1:201-210, 1988.

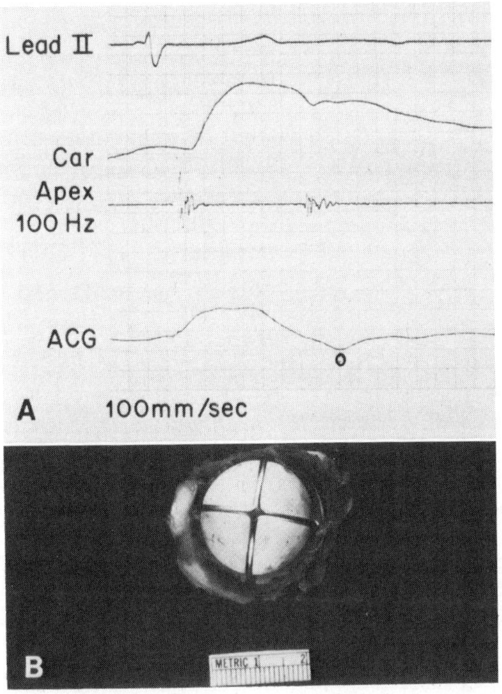

Fig 2-48 **A,** phonocardiogram from patient with Starr-Edwards mitral ball-valve prosthesis. Note absence of opening click at O point on apexcardiogram. *Car,* carotid; *ACG,* apexcardiogram. **B,** swollen, discolored poppet that was found to be fixed in open position at time of operation. (From Brandenburg RO, Fuster V, Giuliani ER, et al: Postoperative follow-up of the cardiac surgical patient. *Cardiovasc Clin* 10 No 3:231-240, 1980. By permission of FA Davis Company.)

tors.[126-128] A working knowledge of the normal characteristics of each prosthetic valve in each of the four locations within the heart is essential in identifying the abnormally functioning prosthetic valve. Color-flow Doppler echocardiography is useful in identifying the site of origin and severity of regurgitation. Transesophageal color-flow Doppler echocardiography is most useful in the evaluation of mitral prostheses.[129,130]

Mitral valves

Ball-cage prostheses. The intensity of the closure sound(s) varies depending on multiple factors (discussed later under "Mitral valve stenosis"). The opening sound may be single or multiple, but usually there are two distinct components. The second component is attributed to bouncing of the ball against the struts. Generally, the mechanical valves produce high-frequency, crisp, loud sounds that are readily audible. The intensity varies with the model used. The interval between aortic valve closure and the opening sound normally varies between 80 and 120 msec. If the opening click is absent (Fig 2-48) or if the interval is less than 70 msec (Fig 2-49) or varies more than 20 msec in patients with normal sinus rhythm, malfunction of the prosthesis is the most likely explanation. In patients

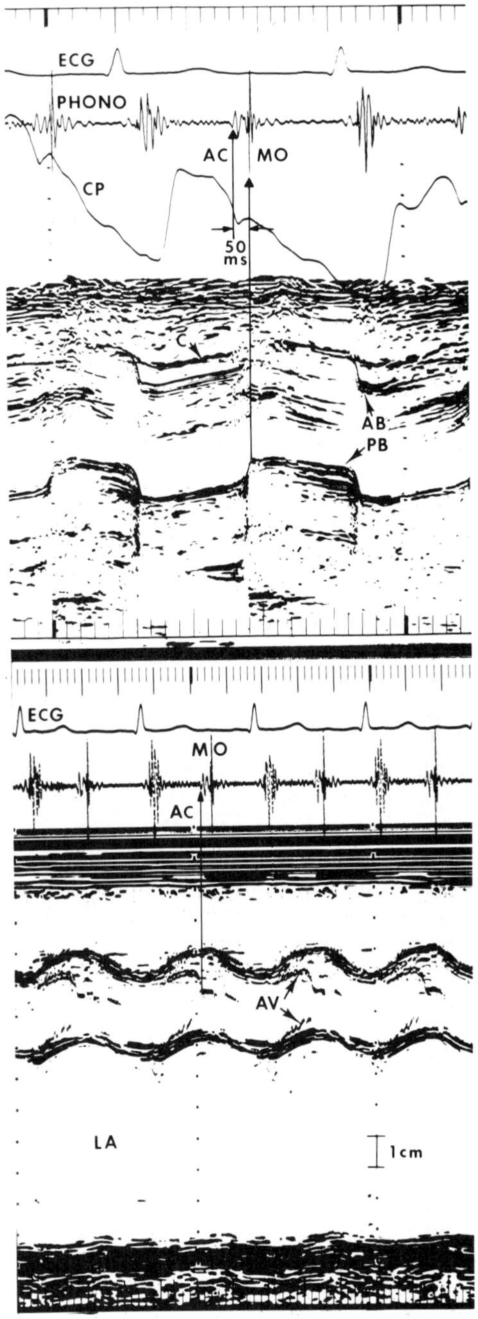

Fig 2-49 Leaking Starr-Edwards mitral ball-cage prosthesis with shortened interval between aortic valve closure and mitral valve opening. **Upper,** mitral valve prosthesis echophonocardiogram showing aortic valve closure-mitral valve opening interval of 50 msec (paper speed, 100 mm/sec). **Lower,** relationship between aortic valve closure on echocardiogram and aortic valve closure sound on phonocardiogram (paper speed, 50 mm/sec). Interval between vertical time lines is 40 msec. *AB,* anterior surface of ball; *AC,* aortic valve closure; *AV,* aortic valve; *C,* cage; *CP,* carotid pulse; *LA,* left atrium; *MO,* mitral valve opening; *PB,* posterior surface of ball. (From Cunha CLP, Giuliani ER, Callahan JA, et al: Echophonocardiographic findings in patients with prosthetic heart valve malfunction. *Mayo Clin Proc* 55:231-242, 1980. By permission, Mayo Foundation.)

with atrial fibrillation this variability should not exceed 30 msec before malfunction is considered.

There should be no mitral pansystolic apical murmur audible in patients with mitral valve ball prostheses. If one becomes audible, then malfunctioning of this prosthesis is the explanation and most often is due to a perivalvular leak. Systolic murmurs, however, often are heard in patients with mitral valve ball prostheses and originate in the left ventricular outflow tract or represent tricuspid valve regurgitation. In patients with mitral ball-cage prostheses, a systolic ejection type of murmur may be audible along the left sternal border and radiating into the neck. The genesis of this murmur is thought to be the cage extending into the left ventricular outflow tract and producing turbulence of blood flow.

The right-sided cardiac murmurs are due to tricuspid valve regurgitation. Many of these patients have far-advanced mitral valve disease when the mitral valve is implanted, and they often will have residual tricuspid valve insufficiency. The increase in intensity of this murmur with inspiration and other associated clinical findings should allow one to identify the source of this murmur. Mitral valve diastolic murmurs are not heard in a normally functioning prosthetic ball-cage mitral valve.

Disk valves. Disk valves placed in a mitral position produce a crisp, distinct closing sound,[131] a high-frequency sound best heard at the apex. Although tilting-disk valves seldom produce an audible opening sound, the central occluded type of disk valve does produce one.[132] Systolic murmurs originating from the mitral valve orifice are not normally heard. Systolic murmurs that are audible in patients with mitral disk prostheses can be best explained on the same basis as for mitral valve ball-cage prostheses. Mitral diastolic murmurs are audible in a normal-functioning disk valve.[133] The cause of this murmur is probably turbulent blood flow across an orifice area that is considerably less than the area of a normal valve orifice.

Absence of a closure sound in a patient with sinus rhythm is distinctly abnormal. An aortic valve closure sound–mitral valve opening sound interval less than 50 or more than 90 msec[133] suggests malfunction of the mitral valve. This interval can be measured by simultaneous phonoechocardiographic studies.

Tissue valves. The closing sound is audible in most patients and is heard best along the left sternal border. This sound is less intense than that from either ball-cage or disk valves. An opening sound of the mitral bioprosthesis is heard in the majority of cases. The interval between aortic valve closure and mitral valve opening normally is between 70 and 110 msec.[134] Midsystolic apical murmurs are present in the majority of these patients.[135] The frequency of heart sounds in patients with degenerated porcine bioprosthetic valves becomes abnormally increased when degeneration is accompanied by fibrosis or calcification.[136] Both musical and nonmusical murmurs are present in patients with porcine valve dysfunction.[137,138] The mechanism responsible for this murmur is unknown. Diastolic flow murmurs similar to those described for the disk valve are present in many patients and do not imply malfunction.[139]

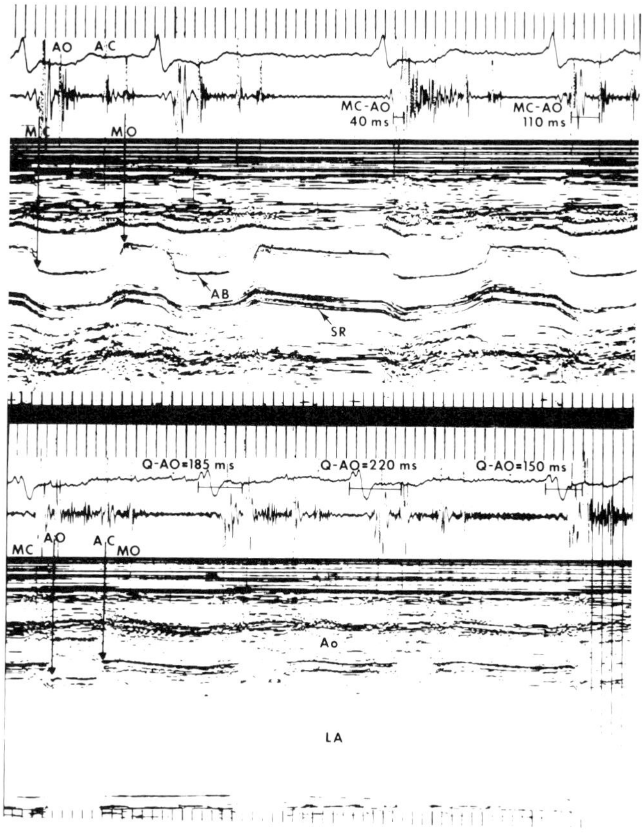

Fig 2-50 Thrombosed Magovern-Cromie aortic valve ball-cage prosthesis and normal Starr-Edwards mitral valve ball-cage prosthesis. Note variability of timing for opening of aortic valve prosthesis. **Upper,** mitral valve echogram with variable interval between mitral valve closing and aortic valve opening *(MC-AO).* **Lower,** aortic valve prosthesis echogram with variable interval between Q wave and aortic opening *(Q-AO).* Time between vertical lines was 40 msec. *AB,* anterior surface of ball; *AC,* aortic valve closing; *AO,* aortic valve opening; *Ao,* aortic root; *LA,* left atrium; *MC,* mitral valve closing; *MO,* mitral valve opening; *SR,* sewing ring. (From Cunha CLP, Giuliani ER, Callahan JA, et al: Echophonocardiographic findings in patients with prosthetic heart valve malfunction. *Mayo Clin Proc* 55:231-242, 1980. By permission, Mayo Foundation.)

Aortic valves

Ball-cage valves. The opening sound of an aortic valve ball prosthesis is crisp, distinct, easily heard, and separated from the first heart sounds by approximately 70 msec. At times, multiple midsystolic sounds are heard and may be explained by the poppet vibrating against the struts during systolic ejection.[140] Variability of timing of the opening sound occurs with malfunction (Fig 2-50). These high-frequency crisp sounds are heard best at the apex but are widely transmitted and are heard over the entire precordium. The closure sound of this prosthesis is of less intensity than the opening sound but is easily heard. A systolic crescendo-decrescendo, harsh, somewhat musical

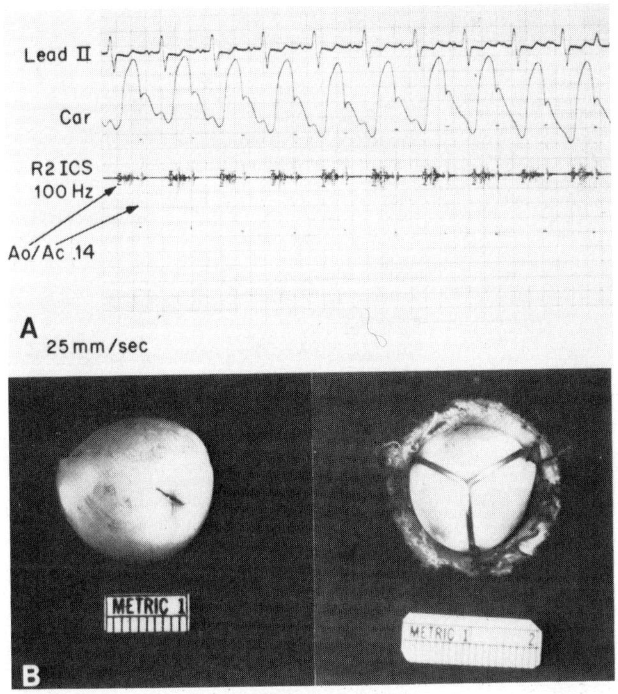

Fig 2-51 **A,** phonocardiograph analysis in patient with Starr-Edwards model 1000 aortic ball-valve prosthesis. Note abnormal Ao/Ac ratio of 0.14. Ao/Ac ratio on tracing obtained 2 years earlier was 0.70. *Car,* carotid; *R2ICS,* right second intercostal space; *Ao,* aortic opening; *Ac,* aortic closure. **B,** valve removed from patient. (From Brandenburg RO, Fuster V, Giuliani ER, et al: Postoperative follow-up of the cardiac surgical patient. *Cardiovasc Clin* 10 No 3:231-240, 1980. By permission of FA Davis Company.)

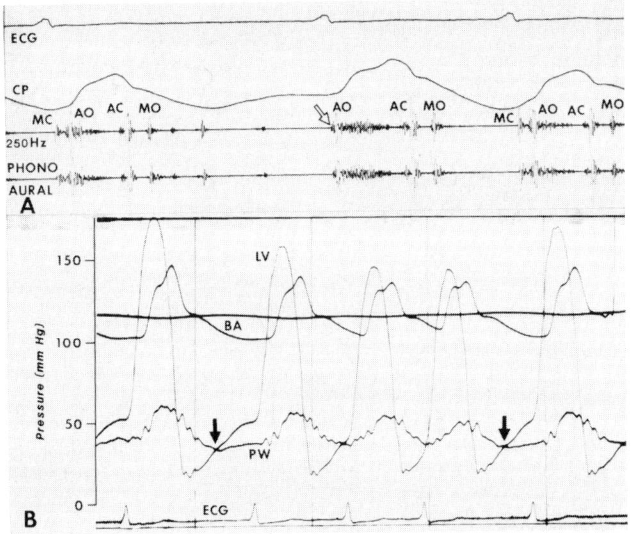

Fig 2-52 Leaking aortic valve ball-cage prosthesis in a 43-year-old man with Braunwald-Cutter prostheses in mitral and aortic positions. **A,** phonocardiogram showing absence of mitral valve closure sound after a long diastolic period *(arrow).* This finding was attributed to premature mitral valve closure secondary to increased left ventricular end-diastolic pressure. Paper speed was 125 mm/sec. **B,** pressure tracings showing that end-diastolic left ventricular pressure was higher than pulmonary wedge pressure during long diastolic periods *(arrow). AC,* aortic valve closing; *AO,* aortic valve opening; *BA,* brachial artery; *CP,* external carotid pulse; *LV,* left ventricle; *MC,* mitral valve closing; *MO,* mitral valve opening; *PW,* pulmonary capillary wedge. (From Cunha CLP, Giuliani ER, Callahan JA, et al: Echophonocardiographic findings in patients with prosthetic heart valve malfunction. *Mayo Clin Proc* 55:231-242, 1980. By permission, Mayo Foundation.)

murmur usually is heard from a ball-cage prosthesis in this position.[141] This is due to turbulence of flow around the ball which produces a persistent transvalvular gradient.

Alteration in the intensity of the opening or closing sound of this prosthesis should suggest malfunction and most often is due to fibrosis or thrombus formation at the apex or the base of the valve. The relative amplitudes of the opening and closing sounds are helpful in identifying the malfunctioning prosthetic valve, particularly in the Starr-Edwards 1000 and 1200 series (Fig 2-51). The ratio of opening sound to closing sound is obtained by phonocardiography and is normally 0.5 or greater.[142] This is particularly helpful if this ratio changes in the same patient.[143] Diastolic murmurs normally are not audible. In patients with aortic and mitral valve prostheses, the development of severe incompetence of the aortic valve prosthesis may alter the intensity of the closing sound of the mitral valve prosthesis (Fig 2-52).

Disk valves. Disk valves produce clear, crisp closing sounds. Opening sounds of the disk valve in the aortic position, however, are often not audible but can be recorded by phonocardiography. Normally this sound follows the first high-frequency component of the first sound by approximately 40 msec. A midsystolic crescendo-decrescendo murmur is frequently heard. Diastolic murmurs, however, should not be present. Malfunction of an aortic disk valve should be considered whenever there is a diminution or absence of the closure sound or a significant change in the quality, character, and length of the systolic murmur or the appearance of an aortic diastolic murmur. When multiple valves are present, correlative phonoechocardiographic studies are useful (Fig 2-53).

Tissue valves. The opening sound of a tissue valve in the aortic position is part of the first heart sound and is not readily appreciated. The closing sound is prominent, distinct, and heard best in the right second parasternal area. Frequently, a brief midsystolic crescendo-decrescendo murmur is audible. Normally, a diastolic murmur should not be heard. Malfunction of this valve is usually indicated by the appearance of a diastolic murmur or loss of a previously audible closure sound.

AUSCULTATION: CARDIAC MURMURS

In considering the patient with a murmur we have arbitrarily divided the evaluation into innocent murmurs

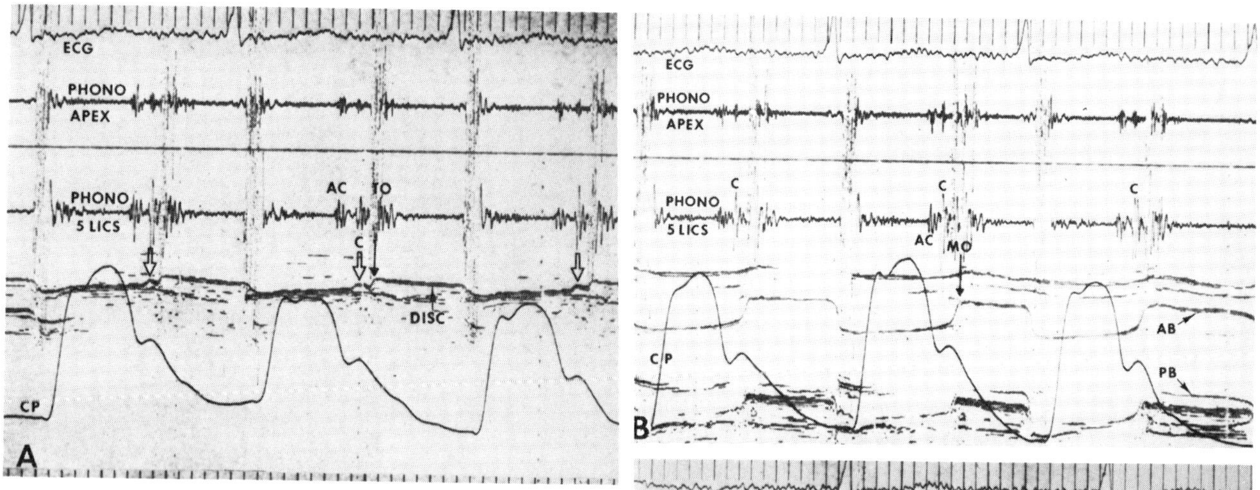

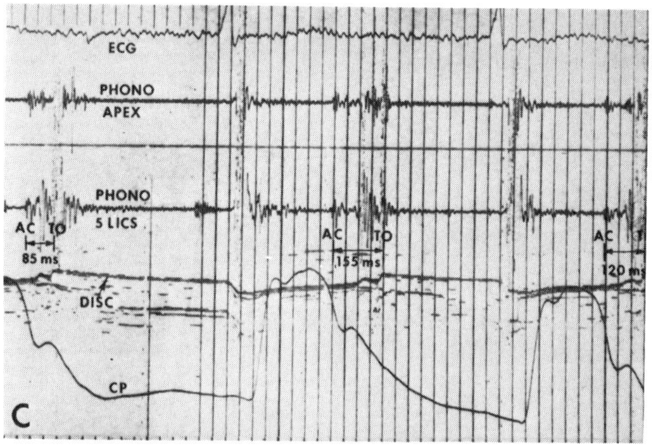

Fig 2-53 Smeloff-Cutter mitral valve ball-cage prosthesis and Beall-Surgitool tricuspid disk valve prosthesis. At operation, tricuspid valve disk was sticking and thrombus involved both disk and stents. **A,** echophonocardiogram shows interrupted opening of tricuspid valve prosthesis. Note extra click coincident with partial opening *(open arrow).* **B,** mitral echophonocardiogram shows that "extra click" was not mitral valve prosthesis opening sound. **C,** variable intervals between aortic valve closure and tricuspid valve sound. *AB,* anterior surface of ball; *AC,* aortic valve closing; *C,* click; *CP,* carotid pulse; MO, mitral valve opening; *PB,* posterior surface of ball; *TO,* tricuspid valve opening; *5 LICS,* fifth left intercostal space. (From Cunha CLP, Giuliani ER, Callahan JA, et al: Echophonocardiographic findings in patients with prosthetic heart valve malfunction. *Mayo Clin Proc* 55:231-242, 1980. By permission, Mayo Foundation.)

and organic murmurs. Because of the value of the Valsalva maneuver in localizing murmurs to the right or left heart, we have further divided organic murmurs into right and left heart murmurs (Table 2-7).

General considerations

Every patient should be examined in the sitting, supine, and left lateral recumbent positions. Additional positions and maneuvers are determined by the findings obtained from these. After the examiner has listened during normal respiration with the patient in the sitting position, the patient should be asked to expel all air and lean forward; the stethoscope diaphragm should be applied firmly at the left sternal border to allow detection of faint murmurs such as aortic diastolic murmurs. The supine semi-upright position is best for evaluation of tricuspid murmurs because the examining table can be readily adjusted to permit viewing of the jugular venous and arterial pulses while one listens to the heart. While the patient is in the left lateral recumbent position one should listen at the point of maximal impulse, with the bell applied lightly to the chest wall. This procedure enhances hearing faint diastolic rumbles of the mitral valve.

Auscultation should begin at the right second parasternal interspace, with the diaphragm. The loudest sound, with rare exceptions, is the second sound. Events following the first sound and preceding the second sound are systolic, and those following the second sound and preceding the first sound are diastolic. From this point, the examiner moves to the left second interspace, where the two components of the second sound are usually heard best. Examination then proceeds along the left sternal border to the apex.

Multiple factors influence murmur intensity, including the quantity and velocity of blood flow, distance from the stethoscope, and ability of the intervening tissue to transmit sound. A murmur will be louder in a young, thin-chested child than in a patient who is obese or an adult with emphysema. Murmurs are louder in hyperdynamic states and softer in hypodynamic states.

In grading cardiac murmur intensity, the system of Levine and Harvey[61] is used. A grade 1 murmur is the faintest murmur that can be heard. Initially, on listening to the chest no murmur is heard; it is only after the examiner concentrates closely that a faint murmur is appreciated. A grade 2 murmur can be detected immediately on placing the stethoscope to the chest. A grade 6 murmur is a murmur that can be heard with the stethoscope removed from the chest wall; indeed, at times

Table 2-7 Classification of cardiovascular murmurs

- Innocent murmurs
  - Systolic
    - In children and young adults
    - In the elderly
  - Diastolic
  - Continuous
    - Venous hum
    - Mammary souffle
- Organic murmurs
  - Right heart
    - Systolic
      - Outflow
        - Left-to-right shunts
        - Right ventricular outflow obstruction
          - Valvular
          - Supravalvular
          - Subvalvular
      - Regurgitant
        - Tricuspid regurgitation
    - Diastolic
      - Pulmonary valve insufficiency
      - Tricuspid valve stenosis
        - Organic
        - Relative (i.e., increased flow)
  - Left heart
    - Systolic
      - Outflow
        - Aortic valve stenosis
        - Localized subaortic stenosis
        - Hypertrophic obstructive cardiomyopathy
        - Supravalvular stenosis
        - Coarctation of aorta
      - Regurgitant
        - Mitral regurgitation
    - Diastolic
      - Aortic insufficiency
      - Mitral valve stenosis
        - Organic
        - Relative (i.e., increased flow)
  - Continuous
    - Patent ductus arteriosus
    - Coronary arteriovenous fistula
    - Ruptured aneurysm of sinus of Valsalva
    - Aortopulmonary window
    - Anomalous left coronary artery
    - Proximal coronary artery stenosis
    - Pulmonary artery branch stenosis
    - Small atrial septal defect
    - Pulmonary arteriovenous fistula
    - Intercostal AV fistula
  - Pericardial friction rubs

the murmur can be heard at the opposite end of a room as in the case of systolic prolapse of the mitral valve. A grade 5 murmur is the loudest murmur that can be heard but requires the aid of a stethoscope. Grade 3 and 4 murmurs are loud murmurs; a grade 4 murmur is distinguished by an associated thrill. Other systems have been proposed.[144]

The murmurs must be timed and their length in the cardiac cycle as well as their configuration and intensity noted. Radiation of a murmur is determined mainly by the direction of blood flow, but intensity and origin also play a role.[145] Murmur quality is described as being musical, high- or low-pitched, blowing, harsh, or rumbling. Murmurs altered in characteristic by valve vibration may be musical or honking.

The examination of the patient should take into account the effect of respiration, postural and position changes, Valsalva maneuver, and vasoactive drugs (Table 2-8). All can be readily performed in the physician's office.

Bedside maneuvers

Changing from the standing to the recumbent position (e.g., with legs elevated) increases venous return which increases first right ventricular volume and then, a few cycles later, left ventricular volume. Initially, the second sound splits due to delay in pulmonary valve closure, right-sided ejection sounds occur earlier, and right-sided third and fourth sounds are louder. A few cycles later, the left-sided filling sounds are augmented. Because the change from recumbent to standing allows more expeditious examination than the reverse, this position change is usually utilized and reverses the above findings.

Respiration. Venous return increases with inspiration because the increase in negative intrathoracic pressure is transmitted in both the right atrium and right ventricle. This augmentation of right heart filling results in a higher right ventricular stroke volume and some prolongation of right ventricular ejection. Goldblatt and associates[146] have shown that transient pulmonary blood pooling during the inspiratory phase of respiration results in a transient decreased return to the left heart, producing a lower left ventricular stroke volume and a slight decrease in left ventricular ejection time. These transitory changes explain in part the narrowed interval between the two components of the second heart sound during expiration and their separation during inspiration (see Fig 2-31). This increase in venous return also increases the intensity of the murmurs and heart sounds generated within the right side of the heart. Thus, the murmurs of pulmonary valve stenosis, tricuspid incompetence, pulmonary valve incompetence, and tricuspid stenosis as well as right ventricular third and fourth heart sounds are usually louder during the inspiratory phase of respiration.[146] An exception to this is the pulmonary ejection sound, which decreases in intensity during inspiration (see Fig 2-40).

In patients with severe heart failure in whom the right atrial and ventricular chambers are already distended, inspiration does not substantially change the filling of the right side of the heart, and therefore changes in intensity of the murmurs and sounds cannot be anticipated.

The murmurs and heart sounds generated in the left side of the heart decrease on inspiration and are best heard during expiration. This is due both to the augmented left ventricular filling during expiration[147] and to decreased lung volume between the heart and the stethoscope.

In mitral valve prolapse, the inspiratory decrease in left ventricular volume may accentuate the prolapse; conse-

Table 2-8 Effects of maneuvers and amyl nitrite on cardiac murmurs in various conditions*

Condition	Inspiration	During Valsalva	After Valsalva†	Amyl nitrite inhalation
Aortic stenosis	↓	↓	Late	
Hypertrophic obstructive cardiomyopathy	↓	↑	Late	↑
Mitral valve insufficiency	↓	↓	Late	↓
Mitral valve prolapse	⇅	⇵	Late	⇅
Ventricular septal defect without pulmonary hypertension	...	↓	Late	↓
Pulmonary valve stenosis	↑	↓	Early	↑
Pulmonary valve insufficiency	↑	↑	Early	...
Tricuspid valve insufficiency	↑	↑	Early	...

* ↑, intensification; ↓, reduction; ..., no significant effect.
†Timing after return to baseline.

quently, the systolic murmur may become accentuated. In this situation, both the murmur and the nonejection click occur earlier in systole.[148]

The intensity of the normal first and second heart sounds also varies with respiration. During normal, quiet respiration, the intensity of both increases during expiration. Auscultatory evaluation of the intensity of heart sounds should be performed carefully, with the respiratory changes kept in mind.[149]

Isometric exercise. These exercises can be done easily and reproducibly by using a calibrated handgrip device. Handgrip should be sustained for 30 to 40 sec, but a Valsalva maneuver during the handgrip must be avoided. The physiologic responses to isometric exercise include increased resistance to left ventricular output due to an increase in systemic arterial pressure and increases in left ventricular filling pressure and left ventricular volume. In patients with compromised left ventricular function, third and fourth heart sounds originating from the left side of the heart appear or, if already present, they become accentuated. The systolic murmur of aortic stenosis is diminished; the diastolic murmur of aortic regurgitation, the systolic murmurs of rheumatic mitral regurgitation and ventricular septal defect, and the diastolic murmur of mitral stenosis become louder.

Valsalva maneuver. The Valsalva maneuver is a routine part of the examination of any patient with a systolic murmur. The response of the murmur is best assessed during the held phase of the maneuver (phase 2). During this time, the intrathoracic pressure exceeds the pressure in the great veins, thus preventing venous return to the heart. This results in decreases in cardiac output and systemic arterial pressure with narrowing of the pulse pressure and reflex increase in heart rate. Attention is then directed to the return of these murmurs after release. Murmurs originating in the right side of the heart will return within one to three beats after release; those originating in the left heart return five to seven beats later.

Vasoactive drugs

Amyl nitrite. Amyl nitrite is inexpensive, safe, and easy to administer. The patient inhales the drug during normal respiration. The onset of tachycardia, identified by the patient's pulse or by ECG monitoring or by facial flush, signals that an adequate dose has been administered, and the drug is discontinued. Although the circulatory effects of the drug are brief (15 to 30 sec), the patients are advised to stay recumbent for several minutes and are allowed to walk only after the examiner has helped the patient to the sitting and then the standing position. The major effect of amyl nitrite is a decrease in peripheral vascular resistance and consequently a decrease in systemic arterial pressure. This is followed by a reflex tachycardia and increases in stroke volume and venous return.[150-153]

The role of amyl nitrite inhalation in identifying the genesis of murmurs is summarized in Table 2-8. Its value in specific clinical situations will be discussed with those situations.

Phenylephrine. Phenylephrine increases systemic pressure and is associated with a reflex bradycardia and a slight decrease in cardiac output. A 0.5-mg dose given intravenously produces a significant increase in systolic pressure within 5 min.[151] The effect on the intensity of the cardiac sounds is variable, but generally the first and second sounds become softer.

Systolic murmurs originating in the left ventricular outflow tract decrease in intensity. In dynamic left ventricular outflow obstruction, this is the consequence of increased left ventricular volume; in fixed obstruction, it is due to a decrease in stroke volume.[154] The regurgitant murmurs of aortic regurgitation and mitral regurgitation are augmented as a result of an increase in systemic pressure. The continuous murmurs of arteriovenous fistula and patent ductus arteriosus become louder.[155,156] This procedure is used infrequently because it requires IV injection. A similar effect can be obtained by having the patient squat.

Innocent murmurs

Most innocent murmurs are systolic. Although occasionally diastolic murmurs and in certain circumstances continuous murmurs may be benign, they generally indicate some cardiovascular abnormality.

Systolic murmurs. Innocent systolic murmurs are frequently heard in the child and adolescent but become less frequent in adulthood.[157-162] The murmurs are usually soft—grade 1 to 2 and only on rare occasions grade 3. They are short, occur early in systole, and occasionally extend into midsystole. The innocent murmur usually is heard best along the mid-left sternal border and in the pulmonic area. The second heart sound is physiologically split, and abnormal sounds are not present (see Fig 2-34).

Although innocent murmurs can originate from the left ventricle,[163,164] if the murmur is right-sided it is more likely to be an innocent murmur. In the patient with an innocent systolic murmur, all other auscultatory events, physical findings, chest radiograph, ECG, and echocardiogram are normal. Innocent murmurs secondary to systemic conditions such as fever, severe anemia, or pregnancy are common and usually readily identified.

If an ejection click is heard in systole, the murmur must be considered to be pathologic. If the second sound is abnormally split, particularly if there is persistent splitting throughout the respiratory cycle in the absence of right bundle-branch block, the murmur is pathologic and likely to be due to an atrial septal defect. Also, if the murmur is pansystolic, one can be certain that an organic lesion such as mitral incompetence, tricuspid incompetence, or a ventricular septal defect is present. Finally, if there is a diastolic component, the murmur is not a benign murmur. Occasionally, a small muscular ventricular septal defect will produce a grade 1 to 3 systolic ejection murmur that may resemble an innocent murmur. This murmur, however, is loudest at the lower left sternal border. It is transmitted well across the sternum to the right sternal border and usually is decrescendo in configuration. The murmur of acute mitral incompetence also is early and mainly decrescendo, ending before the second heart sound because in late systole the pressure produced in the nondistensible left atrium approaches left ventricular pressure.

It is important that the patient or parent or both be advised that a murmur has been detected and that it is likely to be heard on subsequent examinations. It is equally important that the individual be advised of the benign nature of the murmur. Too often, these patients have been classified as having significant heart disease. The patient should be informed that there are no restrictions on physical activity.

Systolic brachiocephalic bruits are also very common in childhood; in one study of more than 1,000 normal subjects, carotid bruits were present in almost 90%.[165] Hyperabduction of the shoulders obliterates most brachiocephalic bruits. This bruit usually disappears in adult life.

In elderly individuals, a grade 1 to 2 short systolic crescendo-decrescendo murmur frequently is audible at the second right interspace. This murmur is due to sclerotic changes in the aortic valve cusps. That the murmur is of no clinical significance is supported by its short duration, normal carotid upstroke, normal apical impulse, normal second sound, and absence of an aortic diastolic murmur. Examination of these patients by two-dimensional sector scan shows each cusp to be thickened but without restriction in aortic valve opening.

Diastolic murmurs. When diastolic murmurs are heard, they must be considered to be pathologic. In certain clinical states, however, misinterpretation of diastolic events may lead to an erroneous diagnosis of organic heart disease. In young patients with hyperkinetic states, often the result of anxiety due to examination by a new physician, a normal third heart sound is followed by a series of low-frequency sounds that at times may be erroneously interpreted as a diastolic rumble. In patients with advanced renal disease, the diastolic component of a venous hum has been heard below the clavicle and has been misinterpreted as a murmur of aortic valve insufficiency. Infrequently, in pregnant patients an apical diastolic murmur has been noted, attributed to increased flow across tricuspid and mitral valves.

Continuous murmurs. A venous hum is frequently heard in young children and adolescents.[61,166] This is heard best with the bell of the stethoscope positioned over the supraclavicular fossa, the patient in a sitting, upright position, and the patient's head turned away from the side of the stethoscope. It usually is heard better on the right side than on the left. The venous hum usually is obliterated by putting the patient in a supine position or by applying pressure over the jugular vein.

In pregnant women, a continuous murmur (mammary souffle) can be heard over the breast. It is most often heard in the latter part of pregnancy and in the postpartum stage in the mother who nurses her child. Simple reexamination of the patient at an appropriate interval will identify this as a benign murmur.

Right heart murmurs

Atrial septal defect. This is the most common congenital defect that causes a right-sided organic outflow murmur in adults. The auscultatory findings will be influenced by the presence of pulmonary hypertension and associated congenital and acquired cardiac defects. In an uncomplicated secundum atrial septal defect, the auscultatory findings include abnormalities in sounds and the presence of murmurs (see Fig 2-37).

SOUNDS. The first heart sound in patients with secundum atrial septal defect is normal.[58] The wide persistent splitting of the second sound in a patient with an atrial septal defect and low pulmonary vascular resistance is due to delay in the pulmonary component secondary to increased capacitance in the pulmonary vascular bed.[167-171] This abnormality of the second sound was first reported by Leatham.[159] The relationship of the two components of the second sound may be normal in neonates, in patients with small shunts, in older patients who develop severe pulmonary hypertension, and in some patients with uncomplicated atrial septal defect.[172]

Castle and associates[171] emphasized the importance of

the patient's position. In the supine position, a normal person may demonstrate wide splitting of the second sound throughout the respiratory cycle but, when examined sitting, the second sound may be entirely normal. Changing from a supine to a sitting or standing position causes a decrease in systemic venous return. This results in decreased right ventricular volume, failure of pulmonary vascular impedance to decrease, and hence an earlier pulmonary closure sound.

The two components of the second heart sound are of normal intensity in the absence of associated anomalies.

A pulmonary ejection sound may be present and is heard best in the second left parasternal interspace. This sound decreases in intensity and moves closer to the first heart sound during inspiration.[75] Rarely, an early diastolic sound is audible. This is heard best along the lower sternal borders and is considered to be an opening snap of the tricuspid valve.[173] Clicks not associated with ejection are heard rarely.[174]

The murmur of atrial septal defect is heard along the left sternal border; it is scratchy in quality and crescendo-decrescendo in configuration (see Fig 2-37). The murmur is seldom louder than grade 3 and usually is best appreciated in the second left interspace.[173] Occasionally, the murmur is transmitted to the apex[57] or, rarely, to the back. The origin of this murmur is the right ventricular outflow tract. It is produced by rapid ejection of a large right ventricular stroke volume into a dilated pulmonary artery.

In uncomplicated atrial septal defect, a tricuspid diastolic flow murmur is present frequently in children and less often in adults. This murmur is heard best along the lower sternal borders or over the xiphoid. It is a soft, short murmur of mixed frequencies and has a noisy or scratchy characteristic. It may have some of the features of a pericardial rub. Rarely, a pericardial rub is present because there is an increased incidence of pericardial disease in patients with atrial septal defect.[175,176] The flow murmur is typically middiastolic and, when present, indicates a large left-to-right shunt.[174,177] The murmur is enhanced or may be heard only during inspiration when venous flow to the right heart is enhanced. Occasionally, murmurs may be presystolic.[177,178]

Rarely, a soft diminuendo diastolic murmur is heard along the left sternal border. In the absence of pulmonary hypertension, the pulmonary diastolic murmur is thought to be secondary to a dilated pulmonary artery causing pulmonary valve incompetence.[179]

Presystolic murmurs may be heard. However, because they can be detected in various clinical situations including normal, their presence does not aid in the diagnosis.[178] When an atrial septal defect is small, the higher left atrial pressure results in blood flow throughout the cardiac cycle, and consequently a continuous murmur may be heard.[180] This is more likely to occur if the patient has some obstruction to flow at the mitral level.[181]

The left-to-right shunt decreases with the development of pulmonary hypertension. As a result, the tricuspid diastolic flow murmur disappears and the right ventricular systolic outflow murmur becomes softer and shorter and, ultimately, also disappears. In their place, the holosystolic murmur of functional tricuspid incompetence will develop. This may be followed by the clinical findings of right ventricular failure.

ASSOCIATED CARDIAC DEFECTS. The frequency with which mitral regurgitation is associated with secundum atrial septal defect is debated. The cause of this most often is mitral valve prolapse.[182-186] Rarely, an opening mitral diastolic sound is heard in patients with severe mitral valve incompetence.

Congenital or acquired mitral stenosis may accompany an atrial septal defect, a complex known as Lutembacher's syndrome. The altered hemodynamics produced by mitral stenosis in patients with uncomplicated atrial septal defect include an increase in the left-to-right shunt, resulting in a decrease in transmitral flow and a decreased gradient between left atrium and left ventricle. These hemodynamic changes account for the masking of the findings of mitral stenosis in many instances.[187] In some patients the findings of atrial septal defect as well as the classic findings of mitral stenosis are present.[170]

ATRIOVENTRICULAR CANAL "PRIMUM" DEFECTS. These defects include a varying combination of abnormalities involving the atrial septum, ventricular septum, and the two AV valves[188-194] (see part VIII).

The auscultatory findings will depend on the structure involved and the magnitude of the defect. In addition, complications such as pulmonary hypertension or associated anomalies will influence the findings. The most frequent combination, particularly in adults, is an atrial ostium primum defect associated with a cleft in a mitral valve leaflet.[195-197] In this clinical state the findings are essentially those described for uncomplicated secundum atrial septal defect plus the murmur of mitral incompetence.[198,199] If the regurgitant jet is directed into the right atrial cavity, the murmur will be transmitted to the right of the sternum where it may be associated with a thrill. Mid-diastolic flow murmurs are common, resulting from an increase in flow across an AV valve because of either a large left-to-right shunt or mitral valve incompetence.

In the complete form of AV canal defects, the auscultatory signs are complex and reflect the underlying pathophysiology.[197]

Right ventricular outflow obstruction. Congenital obstruction of the right ventricular outflow tract may be valvular,[200,201] subvalvular,[200,202,203] supravalvular,[204-206] or a combination of valvular and subvalvular. Acquired causes of right ventricular outflow obstruction are very uncommon and include right-sided infections and tumors.[207]

The response of the murmur of right ventricular outflow obstruction to respiration and to the Valsalva maneuver (see above) will be similar, regardless of the level of obstruction. There are additional auscultatory and clinical findings that allow localization of the obstruction as well as quantitation of the obstruction. Noninvasive techniques including chest radiography, electrocardiography, and Doppler echocardiography are extremely useful; however, cardiac catheterization is often required for preoperative assessment.

Pulmonary valve stenosis

SOUNDS. The first heart sound is usually normal. An ejection sound (see Fig 2-38) is frequently heard in patients with pulmonary valve stenosis.[77] It is rarely present in uncomplicated subvalvular or supravalvular obstruction.[208] The presence of a right-sided ejection sound is important in identifying pulmonary valve stenosis.[77] This sound is related to the abrupt termination of the opening motion of the pulmonary valve and occurs when the valve reaches its limit of motion. The timing of the sound in systole is helpful in estimating the severity of the stenosis. In mild stenosis there is an appreciable interval between the first heart sound and the opening click.[77] As the stenosis becomes more severe, the sound moves closer to the first heart sound; in severe stenosis, it is engulfed by the first sound.[209]

Evaluation of the second heart sound is also helpful in assessing the severity of pulmonary valve stenosis.[77] The greater the stenosis, the greater the gradient and the more prolonged is right ventricular ejection, leading to a delay in pulmonary valve closure. Therefore, the more severe the stenosis, the more widely split the second sound will be (see Fig 2-38). The intensity of the pulmonary valve closure sound varies from normal to inaudible. Generally, the more severe the stenosis, both valvular and subvalvular, the more difficult it is to hear pulmonary valve closure.

MURMURS. The systolic murmur of pulmonary stenosis is crescendo-decrescendo in configuration and is heard best along the left upper sternal border. It radiates to the base of the neck and to the left shoulder. There is no significant relationship between the intensity of the murmur and the severity of the stenosis. However, mild stenoses generally are accompanied by a soft murmur, whereas severe stenoses have louder murmurs and systolic thrills. The duration of the murmur is a better guide to the severity of the stenosis in the presence of an intact ventricular septum (see Fig 2-38). In the presence of normal right ventricular function the severity of obstruction is the major determinant of right ventricular ejection time. This in turn determines the duration of the systolic murmur. In patients with mild pulmonary stenosis, right ventricular ejection is only slightly prolonged. The systolic murmur that is crescendo-decrescendo in configuration is midsystolic in timing and symmetric in shape.[210] As the obstruction increases, the murmur lengthens and peaks later in systole.[210,211]

When the obstruction is below the pulmonary valve, the maximum intensity of the murmur usually is heard lower along the left sternal border.[212] This plus absence of a pulmonic ejection sound is a clue to the correct location of the obstruction.

Rarely, diastolic murmurs are present. A decrescendo diastolic murmur heard best along the left sternal border is considered to be due to pulmonary valve incompetence[77] and is present more often in patients with the more severe forms of obstruction.[213] A presystolic murmur has also been described, low in frequency and best heard at the second left interspace. This murmur is attributed to premature pulmonary valve opening.[210,213] This requires that the right ventricular pressure late in diastole exceeds pulmonary arterial pressure and could occur with a powerful right atrial contraction.

Obstruction distal to the pulmonary valve produces murmurs that usually are systolic and crescendo-decrescendo in configuration;[208] however, continuous murmurs do occur, although less frequently.[214] The location of the murmur on the chest wall is determined by the location of the pulmonary artery stenosis. If the murmur is systolic, then it must be distinguished from systolic murmurs of other origin, particularly pulmonary valve stenosis. In pulmonary artery stenosis, a pulmonary ejection sound is rarely present, the components of the second heart sound are normally related, and the pulmonary component is of normal intensity. If the murmur is continuous, it must be differentiated from other conditions. If anterior in location, it may be confused with patent ductus arteriosus.[215]

Tricuspid insufficiency. Tricuspid valve incompetence rarely is an isolated lesion. The most frequent cause is dilatation of the tricuspid annulus as a result of right ventricular failure. This is usually secondary to left heart disease: mitral valve disease or left ventricular myocardial disease. Less often it is secondary to pulmonary disease. In these clinical situations, the coexistent entities dominate the clinical picture and the findings of tricuspid insufficiency may be overlooked.

Occasionally, tricuspid insufficiency is an isolated lesion. Congenital abnormalities of the tricuspid valve that produce isolated tricuspid insufficiency include prolapse of one or more leaflets and Ebstein's malformation. Acquired lesions include infective endocarditis, right ventricular infarction, right-sided cardiac tumors involving the tricuspid valve or interfering with its function, and traumatic disruption of the valve or supporting structures.

MURMURS. The murmur of tricuspid insufficiency is heard best over the xiphoid or along the fourth and fifth left parasternal areas.[216,217] At times the murmur is heard best over the right subcostal areas, particularly in patients with chronic obstructive pulmonary disease.[218] The murmur is usually pansystolic[219,220] and high-pitched, and it often has a scratchy or superficial quality.[221,222] It is loudest in early and midsystole.[223] When the murmur is due to prolapse of one of the leaflets, it is usually midsystolic or late systolic in timing. Regardless of cause, the murmur increases in intensity with inspiration. This was first recognized and described by Rivero Carvallo[224,225] and is a diagnostic feature of tricuspid insufficiency.[226] This increase in intensity is the result of an increase in systemic venous return during inspiration with increased flow across the tricuspid valve. If right ventricular failure is present, the right ventricle will be functioning at peak capacity and be unable to augment flow across the tricuspid valve during inspiration.[52] The murmur then will not change with inspiration. It is important that the patient avoid a Valsalva maneuver during this evaluation, and therefore this is best evaluated with the patient breathing through the mouth slowly, quietly, and deeply, while sitting or standing. The murmur of tricuspid insufficiency is rarely accompanied by a systolic thrill.

A diastolic murmur occasionally occurs in the presence of severe tricuspid insufficiency and is due to increased diastolic flow across the tricuspid valve—i.e., relative tricuspid stenosis. This murmur is heard best along the left lower sternal border and, although it may be of low frequency,[216] it is most often high-pitched, scratchy, and squeaky in its characteristics.[221] This murmur also increases in intensity during the inspiratory phase of respiration and often is heard only at this time.

At times it is difficult to distinguish between the murmurs of mitral insufficiency and tricuspid insufficiency.[221,227] This is particularly true in patients with marked dilation of the right ventricle and displacement of the cardiac structures within the chest. The murmur of tricuspid insufficiency more frequently varies in intensity in patients with atrial fibrillation and varying cycle lengths, becoming louder after long R-R intervals.[216] The reason for this is the lower systolic pressure of the right ventricle compared with the left so that changes in right ventricular filling cause relatively greater pressure gradients between the right atrium and right ventricle during systole.

Amyl nitrite is helpful in distinguishing between mitral and tricuspid insufficiencies: it increases venous return and thus augments a murmur of tricuspid regurgitation due to increased flow across the tricuspid valve during the few beats before the flow across the mitral valve also increases. Inspiration may have the same effect. On the other hand, by producing an increase in systemic resistance, phenylephrine tends to increase the intensity of the murmur of mitral insufficiency and has no effect on the murmur of tricuspid regurgitation. Acute hypoxemia (breathing a mixture of 10% oxygen and 90% nitrogen) augments the regurgitant cardiac murmurs of right-sided origin. Left-sided murmurs either are unaltered by hypoxemia or change in a direction opposite to that of the equivalent murmur on the right side. Acute hypoxemia also markedly decreases murmurs due to left-to-right shunts and thus permits differentiation between the murmur of ventricular septal defect and the systolic murmur of tricuspid regurgitation.[228]

Pulmonary valve insufficiency. Pulmonary valve insufficiency may be associated with normal pulmonary artery pressure or with pulmonary hypertension.

When the pulmonary artery pressure is normal, congenital defects are usually responsible and include congenital absence or inadequacy of pulmonary valve tissue[229,230] and idiopathic dilatation of the pulmonary artery.[231] Rarely, pulmonary insufficiency accompanies severe pulmonary valve stenosis. Infective endocarditis or trauma[232] may also be responsible.

SOUNDS. Congenital absence of the pulmonary valve is usually associated with other cardiac defects, particularly tetralogy of Fallot.[233] In these patients the auscultatory findings of the associated lesions dominate the clinical picture. When it is an isolated finding,[234] the auscultatory findings are distinctive.[235] The first heart sound is normal. No ejection sound is heard. The relationship of the two components of the second heart sound and the intensity of the pulmonary component are determined by the magnitude of the valve deficiency, the magnitude of the regurgitant fraction, or the presence or absence of delayed activation of the right ventricle (right bundle-branch block). If the pulmonary valve is absent, the pulmonary component of the second sound will be absent and the second sound will be single. If a rudimentary valve is present, the sound will be muffled and may be delayed.[236] A significant regurgitant fraction will prolong right ventricular systole and thereby delay the pulmonary component of the second heart sound.[237] This can occur in the absence of right bundle-branch block.

MURMURS. The murmur that results from inadequacy of pulmonary valve tissue is characteristic. It is diastolic in timing, crescendo-decrescendo in configuration, low in frequency, and relatively short in duration. It is heard best along the left second and third parasternal areas and is accompanied by a diastolic thrill.[213,238] Systolic ejection murmurs, when present, are due to rapid ejection of a large stroke volume and do not imply true pulmonary stenosis.[238]

A diastolic murmur of low to medium frequency occasionally is heard in patients with idiopathic pulmonary artery dilatation.[229] The associated clinical findings, localized systolic pulsation in the second left interspace, ejection sound, and persistent splitting of the second sound allow one to distinguish this abnormality from congenital deficiency of pulmonary valve tissue. Because of the wide splitting of the second sound, this condition must be distinguished from pulmonary stenosis and atrial septal defect.[239]

Pulmonary hypertension of any cause may lead to the development of pulmonary valve incompetence. The clinical findings that dominate will be those secondary to the defects causing pulmonary hypertension, either congenital or acquired. The characteristic auscultatory findings common to all (Fig 2-54) include the presence of a pulmonary ejection sound, a fourth heart sound, accentuation of the pulmonary component of the second sound (which often is palpable), and a decrescendo pulmonic diastolic murmur. In contrast to low-pressure pulmonary valve incompetence, pulmonary arterial hypertension produces a high pulmonary artery-to-right ventricle diastolic gradient. This generates a high-velocity regurgitant flow, often throughout diastole.[240] The resultant murmur, which is best heard along the left sternal border, is of high frequency and may be holodiastolic.[75]

Tricuspid stenosis. Tricuspid stenosis is frequently undetected or misdiagnosed, primarily because this lesion rarely occurs as an isolated defect. For this reason, the examination of the jugular venous pulse and precordial pulsations is important in identifying this lesion. In patients with sinus rhythm there is a large "a" wave or presystolic pulsation that usually is appreciated best at the base of the neck. Accompanying this dominant wave is a slow or gentle x descent. Following the v wave is a slow y descent. In patients with atrial fibrillation or flutter, a systolic wave is prominent and occurs slightly after the arterial pulse. Although difficult to identify in some patients, the slow y descent is a diagnostic feature of tricuspid stenosis.

SOUNDS. The first and second heart sounds are normal in uncomplicated tricuspid valve disease. Rarely, nonejec-

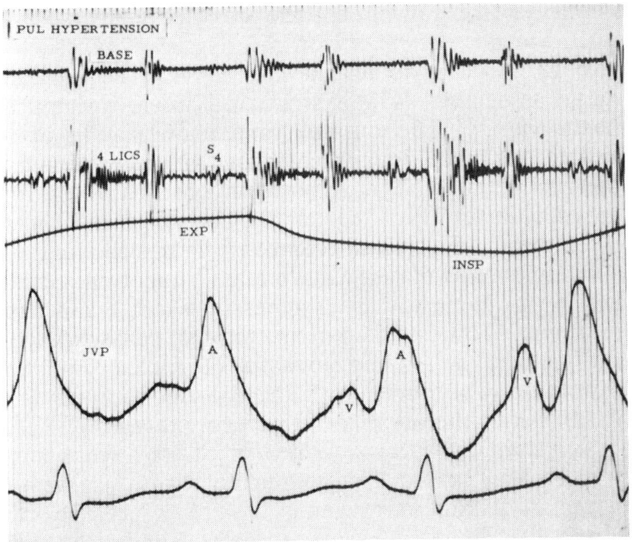

Fig 2-54 Primary pulmonary hypertension in 18-year-old man, showing prominent "a" wave in the neck. With inspiration, there is an increase in the amplitude of the "a" wave and in the right atrial diastolic gallop, as seen at the fourth left intercostal space *(4 LICS). JVP,* jugular venous pressure. (From Shaver JA: Innocent murmurs. *Hosp Med* 14:8-35, April 1978. By permission of Hospital Publications.)

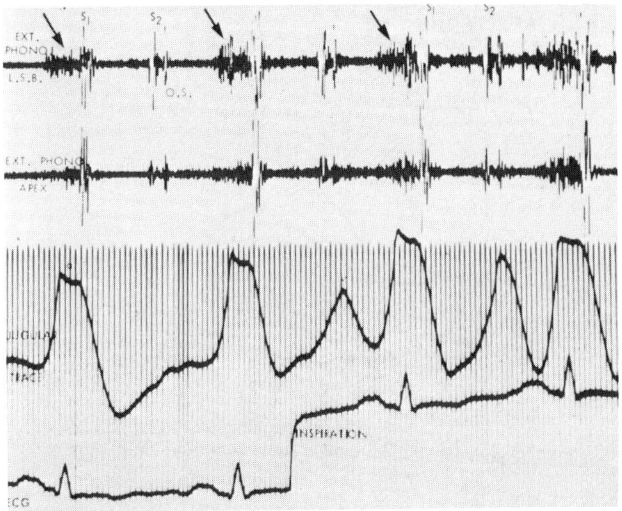

Fig 2-55 Mitral stenosis and severe tricuspid stenosis with normal sinus rhythm. Note the marked "a" wave and the increased intensity of the presystolic rumble at the left sternal border. *O.S.,* opening snap. (From Shaver JA: Current uses of phonocardiography in clinical practice. *Cardiol Update,* 1981, pp 327-378. By permission of Elsevier Science Publishing Company.)

tion sounds are heard in patients with tricuspid valve prolapse. In patients with tricuspid stenosis, the tricuspid opening snap may be recorded but seldom is heard.

MURMURS. The murmur of tricuspid stenosis is diastolic in timing (Fig 2-55), is of high frequency, and is heard best along the left fourth and fifth parasternal edges. Rarely, it can be heard best over the lower sternum and to the right of the sternum. In patients with sinus rhythm, this presystolic murmur begins before the presystolic murmur of mitral stenosis. The murmur contains a higher mixed-frequency component. It is crescendo-decrescendo in its configuration and terminates before the first heart sound. The murmur increases in intensity during inspiration; in fact, it may be heard only during inspiration.

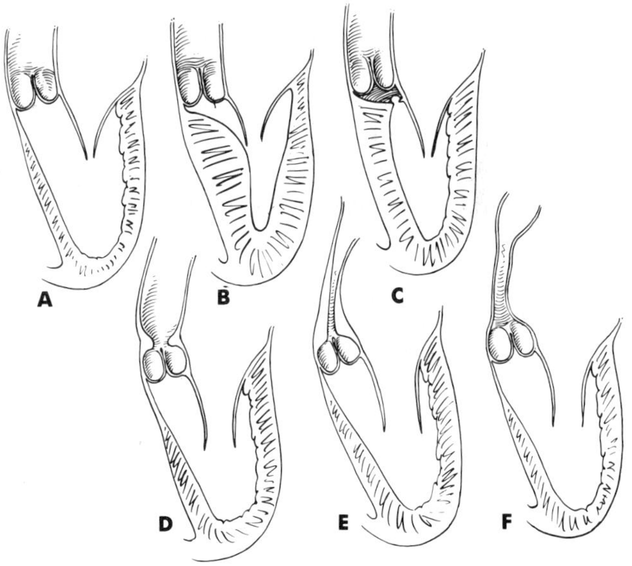

Fig 2-56 Anatomic sites of left ventricular outflow obstruction. **A,** normal. **B,** muscular subvalvular. **C,** localized subvalvular. **D, E,** and **F,** supravalvular.

Left heart systolic murmurs

Left ventricular outflow murmurs. Obstruction to left ventricular outflow occurs at three levels: supravalvular, valvular, and subvalvular (Fig 2-56). Obstruction above the valve level is congenital in origin and is rare. Valvular obstruction is the most common type in adolescents and adults. Subvalvular disease may be a localized fibromuscular membrane or secondary to hypertrophic cardiomyopathy.

Aortic valve disease

SOUNDS. The first heart sound in aortic valve stenosis is usually normal. The aortic component of the second heart sound may be normal in mild aortic stenosis. When the cusps retain their mobility, thus allowing the aortic component to be heard, the relationship of the two components of the second sound varies and is related to the severity of the obstruction. With severe obstruction, left ventricular systole is prolonged, delaying the aortic component of the second heart sound beyond the pulmonic component and producing paradoxic splitting of

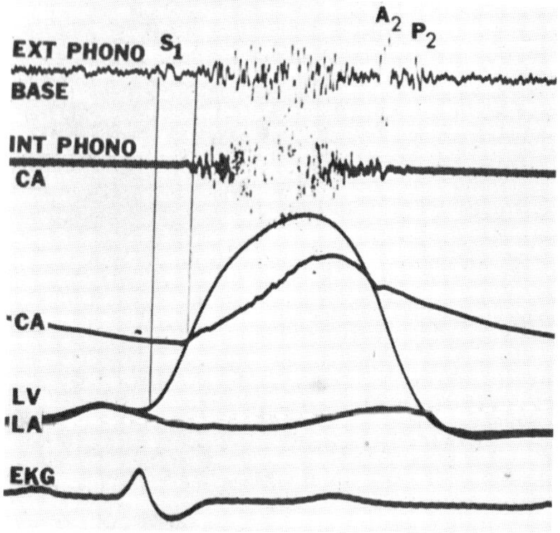

Fig 2-57 Sound pressure correlates of aortic valve stenosis as recorded with a catheter-tip micromanometer in the left atrium *(LA),* left ventricle *(LV),* and central aorta *(CA).* Note that the murmur is crescendo-decrescendo in configuration. Also, the murmur does not begin until after onset of ejection. It is delayed from the first heart sound by the duration of the isometric contraction time. (Courtesy of James A. Shaver, M.D.)

the second heart sound. When this is present in the absence of left bundle-branch block, severe aortic stenosis can be predicted.[241] As the valve thickens and becomes immobile, the aortic component becomes muted and eventually disappears, and only a single pulmonary closure sound is audible. The pulmonary component is normal in intensity. However, phonocardiography reveals that the ratios of intensity of both the pulmonary and the aortic component to that of the first heart sound decrease.[242]

An atrial sound is not a feature of mild obstruction but does indicate significant obstruction when present in the adolescent or young adult. The atrial sound is the result of a forceful atrial contraction in the presence of a left ventricle that is thickened and relatively noncompliant.[109] In adults, an atrial sound is less helpful because of the frequent association of coronary artery disease and myocardial disease.[243] A third heart sound is not a feature of aortic stenosis and, when audible, it implies significant left ventricular dysfunction.

An ejection sound is frequently present in young patients with congenitally bicuspid valves. It may precede the appearance of a murmur and gradient by years. This sound implies mobility of the aortic cusps. As the obstruction progresses, this sound moves closer to the first heart sound.

MURMURS. The murmur of aortic valve stenosis begins after the first sound or after the ejection sound if one is present (Fig 2-57). It is crescendo and decrescendo in its configuration and ends before the second heart sound. The murmur is characteristically harsh in its quality. It is heard best at the base of the heart, with radiation into the carotid arteries and along the left sternal border and to the apex where it may have a more musical quality.[211] The intensity of the murmur and the presence of an associated thrill are not dependent on the degree of obstruction, although generally when the murmur is grade 4 or more and is associated with a systolic thrill, there is significant obstruction.[244] The duration and configuration of the systolic murmur do not correlate with the degree of obstruction as well as they do in obstruction to right ventricular outflow.[245] Generally, the softer and shorter the murmur, the less significant is the obstruction.[246] A soft diminuendo diastolic murmur is frequently associated with aortic stenosis. This is generally a soft, grade 1 to 2 murmur and is best heard in the third left interspace while the patient is leaning forward in forced and held expiration. The duration of the diastolic murmur is an indication of the severity of the regurgitation.

Supravalvular aortic stenosis. Supravalvular aortic stenosis may be localized, segmental, or diffuse with an hourglass-shaped narrowing.

SOUNDS. The first and second heart sounds are usually normal. An ejection sound is rarely audible.

MURMURS. The systolic murmur has the characteristics and distribution described for aortic valve stenosis. An interesting observation is a very marked systolic supramanubrium thrill that is present in the majority of patients. This is in contrast to a basal precordial thrill present in patients with valvular obstruction and the low precordial and apical thrill felt in patients with subvalvular disease. An aortic diastolic murmur is present only occasionally.[247]

Associated clinical findings often are abnormal facial features, abnormalities in dentition, differences in amplitude of right and left radial pulse and blood pressure (more than 20 mm Hg systolic), and continuous murmurs of pulmonary branch stenosis; these readily differentiate this level of obstruction from valvular and subvalvular obstruction.

Subvalvular discrete stenosis

SOUNDS. The first and second heart sounds are usually normal. An ejection click may be present. The appearance of diastolic filling sounds implies impaired ventricular functions.

MURMURS. The systolic murmur of a subvalvular fibromuscular membrane has the same characteristics of timing, quality, and configuration as the murmur of aortic valve stenosis (Fig 2-58). At times, the murmur may be heard best in the first right interspace and may be transmitted selectively to the right carotid.[248] The radiation of this murmur corresponds to the jet of blood that is directed toward the head and right shoulder. A soft, high-frequency, diminuendo murmur of valvular incompetence is frequently an accompaniment of discrete subvalvular stenosis.[249] This insufficiency likely is secondary to fibrosis of the aortic cusp produced by the impact of the high-velocity jet.

Hypertrophic cardiomyopathy. Although investigators agree that a gradient is present in the subvalvular region in some patients with hypertrophic cardiomyopathy, there is considerable disagreement regarding the significance of this gradient.[250,251] For the purposes of this discussion, we will use the terms "subvalvular gradient" and "subvalvular diffuse muscular obstruction" interchangeably.

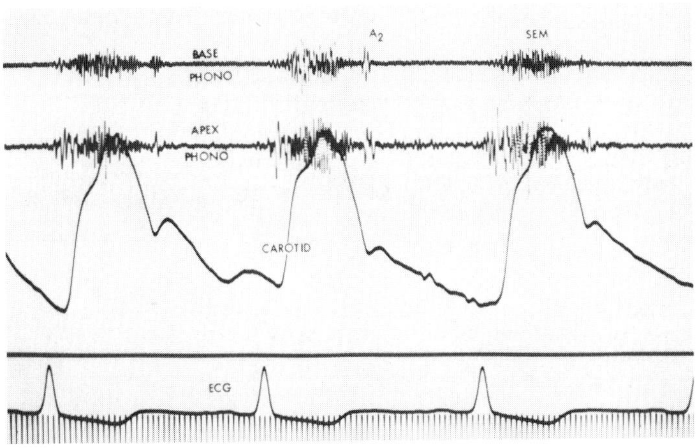

Fig 2-58 Congenital subvalvular aortic stenosis with fixed orifice due to fixed obstruction. Note absence of valvular ejection sound, crescendo-decrescendo nature of murmur, and prolonged ejection time on the indirect carotid pulse. *SEM,* systolic ejection murmur. (From Paley HW: Left ventricular outflow tract obstruction: heart sounds and murmurs. In *Physiologic Principles of Heart Sounds and Murmurs* [American Heart Association Monograph No 46]. Edited by DF Leon, JA Shaver. New York, American Heart Association, 1975, pp 107-117. By permission.)

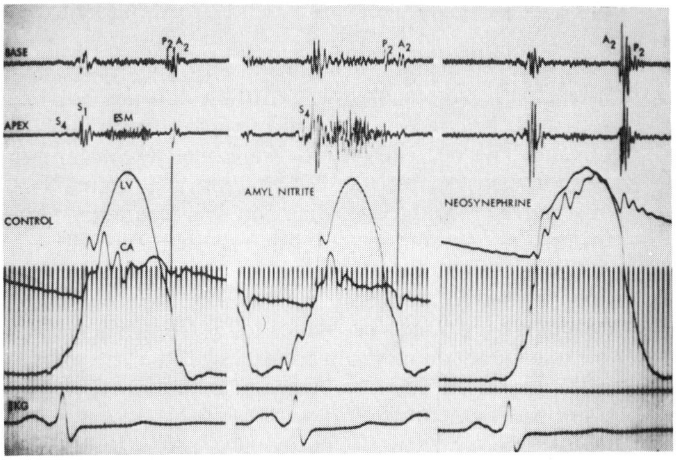

Fig 2-59 Hypertrophic cardiomyopathy with a gradient at rest. *Central panel* shows effect of amyl nitrite on intensity of murmur and on gradient. Paradoxic splitting of the second heart sound is produced. *Right panel* shows murmur and gradient obliterated by infusion of phenylephrine. *ESM,* ejection systolic murmur; *LV,* left ventricle. (From Reddy PS, Shaver JA, Leonard JJ: Cardiac systolic murmurs: pathophysiology and differential diagnosis. *Prog Cardiovasc Dis* 14:1-37, 1971. By permission of Grune & Stratton.)

SOUNDS. The first heart sound is often accent. The relationship of the two components of the second sound is usually normal. However, in approximately 20% of the patients the second sound is paradoxically split because of prolongation of left ventricular mechanical systole. The outflow tract gradient in these patients is consistently greater than in those with normal splitting of the second sound.[252] Both components of the second sound are usually audible, although the splitting may be narrowed.[131] This finding is helpful in distinguishing hypertrophic obstructive cardiomyopathy from severe aortic valve stenosis in which the second heart sound is often single. A third heart sound (see Fig 2-39) is present in approximately 40% of patients[252] but does not have the same ominous significance that it does in aortic stenosis. A fourth heart sound (see Fig 2-39) is heard in 40% to 70% of patients.[154,253] Opening and closing clicks are rare and, when present, suggest associated valvular disease.

MURMURS. The auscultatory hallmark of hypertrophic obstructive cardiomyopathy[252-254] is a high-frequency systolic ejection murmur which is heard best along the left sternal border and at the apex. It begins after the first heart sound, and it does not radiate to the carotid arteries. Characteristically, the murmur varies in intensity during physiologic maneuvers and pharmacologic interventions. In 20% to 30% of the patients[154] it is detected between birth and 5 years of age. This murmur increases in intensity when the left ventricular outflow tract gradient is increased, which occurs when left ventricular chamber size decreases (Fig 2-59). This decrease in left ventricular size occurs during diminished venous return with the Valsalva maneuver[255-257] or vasodilation with nitrates.[255] The murmur increases in intensity also when the force of contraction is increased, as in the beat following a premature ventricular contraction,[258] and by inotropic agents such as digitalis[259] and other similarly acting agents.[260,261] In contrast, the murmur decreases in intensity or disappears with reduction in severity of left ventricular outflow tract gradient when the left ventricular diameter is increased. These changes occur by facilitating venous return during squatting or a Mueller maneuver[262] and when afterload is increased by isometric muscular exertion[263] or drugs such as phenylephrine.[263] An increase in the systolic murmur with carotid sinus pressure is characteristic. The mechanisms involved are multifactorial.[264]

When the patient has primarily right-sided hypertrophic cardiomyopathy, the right ventricular volume increases and the intensity of the systolic murmur decreases.[265] The variability in intensity of the ejection systolic murmur is useful clinically in substantiating the diagnosis in this disease.[256] The latter is especially valuable in children, because in 60% of cases the diagnosis of hypertrophic obstructive cardiomyopathy is confused with congenital cardiac anomalies such as ventricular septal defect and congenital mitral regurgitation, which predominate in the pediatric age group.[254]

Some patients have mitral regurgitation ranging from mild to severe; the mechanism for this is controversial.[266] The regurgitation may be due either to malalignment of the mitral valve apparatus in a disproportionately small outflow tract or to abnormal traction on the free edges of the mitral valve leaflets or to both.[266,267] Whatever the mechanism, the presence of mitral regurgitation is detected by an apical pansystolic murmur extending toward the axilla.

Diastolic murmurs are uncommon in hypertrophic obstructive cardiomyopathy, and their absence has been used as a diagnostic aid. Early decrescendo diastolic murmurs have been described rarely, but these occur more commonly postoperatively, due to operative trauma to the aortic valve.[252] Mid to late diastolic, low-frequency, apical murmurs are present more frequently than early diastolic murmurs, although the genesis of both is unexplained. Such murmurs may result from a decreased rate of left atrial emptying due to resistance to left ventricular filling. This may be secondary to increased wall thickness, which results in decreased left ventricular compliance.[268,269] or to impaired opening of the mitral valve secondary to massive left ventricular hypertrophy.

The classic response to the various maneuvers—e.g., Valsalva, squatting, etc.—is not always present[257] and may be altered by the use of β-blockers or by the appearance of a complication such as a myocardial infarction.[270]

Mitral insufficiency. Mitral insufficiency is the result of a developmental or an acquired abnormality of the mitral leaflets, supporting structures of the mitral valve, mitral valve annulus, or left ventricular myocardium. Normal AV depolarization, with its subsequent synchronous mechanical responses, is also necessary for normal mitral valve function. When one or more of these structures is abnormal, the valve may become incompetent, resulting in a systolic regurgitant murmur. On rare occasions, mitral insufficiency without a systolic regurgitant murmur has been described.[271]

SOUNDS. The first heart sound varies in intensity[16] and is influenced by the underlying defect. The first sound is accentuated when associated with mitral valve stenosis or when there is an increased rate of ventricular contraction. The intensity of the first sound varies inversely with the duration of the preceding diastolic filling period.[272] In uncomplicated mitral insufficiency the first sound is either faint or inaudible. This is considered to be a consequence of partial closure of the mitral valve during ventricular filling because the intensity of the first sound is determined in part by the location of the mitral leaflets at the onset of ventricular systole.

Tei et al.[273] evaluated the amplitude of the first heart sound compared to the aortic second sound in patients with mitral insufficiency. In patients with nonrheumatic mitral regurgitation, the first sound was loud with a holosystolic mitral valve prolapse, normal with middle to late systolic prolapse, and soft or absent with a flail mitral leaflet. This suggests that the intensity of the first sound may be an auscultatory clue to aid in differentiation of patients with flail mitral leaflets with severe mitral regurgitation from those with prolapse.

In uncomplicated mitral insufficiency, the second heart sound is usually normal, although inspiratory splitting may be increased due to early aortic valve closure. Rarely, paradoxic splitting of the second sound will occur in severe mitral insufficiency. With the development of pulmonary vascular obstructive disease and pulmonary hypertension, the pulmonary component of the second sound becomes accentuated. An opening snap occasionally occurs in pure mitral insufficiency. This sound is not as loud as the opening snap of mitral stenosis and occurs in the same time interval in diastole as the opening snap of mitral stenosis.[274]

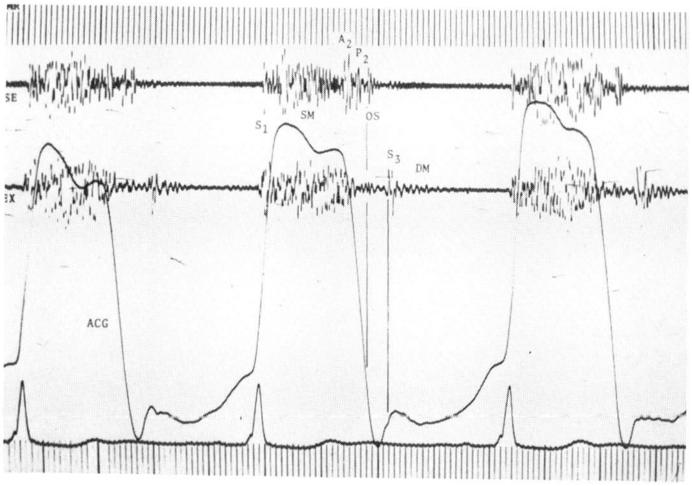

Fig 2-60 Pansystolic murmur of mitral insufficiency. Apexcardiogram *(ACG)* shows loud gallop coincident with rapid filling phase followed by a short diastolic flow rumble. Wide splitting of the second heart sound is seen as well as an early opening snap *(OS)*. This patient had rheumatic heart disease. *DM,* diastolic murmur; *SM,* systolic murmur. (From Shaver JA: Current uses of phonocardiography in clinical practice. *Cardiol Update,* 1981, pp 327-378. By permission of Elsevier Science Publishing Company.)

A fourth heart sound is frequently heard in acute mitral insufficiency.[275] but seldom in patients with chronic mitral insufficiency, particularly those with rheumatic mitral valve disease. The absence of this sound is considered to be due to a dilated noncompliant left atrium that is unable to contract vigorously.[273]

A third heart sound is frequently present in all forms of mitral insufficiency if the regurgitation is significant (Fig 2-60). The sound often is quite prominent in patients with mild to moderate insufficiency but is less intense in patients with severe mitral insufficiency. It usually is secondary to increased rate and volume of ventricular filling rather than to ventricular failure.

Nonejection sounds are heard in patients with mitral valve prolapse. Their intensity and relation to the first heart sound are variable and can be altered by a number of bedside maneuvers and pharmacologic agents.

MURMURS. Both systolic and diastolic murmurs are heard in patients with mitral insufficiency. The presence, quality, duration, and radiation of these murmurs are determined by: (a) severity of the regurgitation, (b) extent of the disease process, (c) duration of the disease process, (d) location of the disease process (Table 2-9), and (e) associated intra- and extracardiac defects.

The typical murmur of mitral insufficiency is a soft, blowing, systolic murmur that starts with the first heart sound and remains at constant intensity throughout

Table 2-9 Integrity of mitral valve function

Valve leaflets
Chordae tendineae
Papillary muscle
Ventricular myocardium
Annulus
Electrical pathways

systole, ending at or after the aortic component of the second heart sound (see Fig 2-60). The murmur is medium to high pitched and is rarely accompanied by a systolic apical thrill. This murmur is usually transmitted to the left and cephalad toward the posterior axillary line.

The systolic murmur in patients with nonrheumatic mitral insufficiency is more musical in quality, holosystolic if the regurgitation is severe, and often accompanied by a systolic thrill. The transmission of the murmur is dependent on the disease process. If the posterior leaflet is incompetent due to ruptured chordae, it may act as a baffle, directing the jet of blood anteriorly and medially, where it strikes the anterior atrial wall adjacent to the aorta and therefore is transmitted well anteriorly to the base and to the aorta[276] (Fig 2-61). If the anterior leaflet is incompetent, it directs the jet posteriorly (Fig 2-62), where it strikes the posterior atrial wall adjacent to the thorax and vertebral column.[20] The murmur is transmitted posteriorly toward the left axilla and also along the thoracic spine, where it may be accompanied by a systolic thrill.[277]

Mitral valve prolapse. Little attention has been given to the first heart sound in mitral valve prolapse, presumably because of the many other auscultatory findings in this condition. Tei et al.[273] reported, on the basis of 52 patients, that the intensity of the first heart sound expressed as a ratio of its amplitude to that of the second sound may provide a clue to the type and timing of mitral valve prolapse. A decreased ratio was found in patients with flail leaflets; in patients who generally have severe regurgitation, the second heart sound usually is normal.

A late systolic murmur, either isolated or accompanied by a nonejection click, is now considered to be the classic finding of mitral valve prolapse (Fig 2-63). A mid-late systolic murmur is present commonly in association with a number of specific cardiac lesions including hypertrophic cardiomyopathy,[278] coarctation of the aorta,[279] pericarditis,[93] and coronary heart disease.[280-282] In the past, isolated late apical systolic murmurs or clicks were considered to be benign and extracardiac in origin. After Barlow and Bosman's[94] description of the prolapsed mitral valve, we now recognize that nonejection clicks and late systolic murmurs are due to mitral valve prolapse. The mitral origin of these auscultatory findings was confirmed by intracardiac phonocardiographic studies.[96,97,283,284] as well as echocardiography and pulsed-wave Doppler echocardiography.[285]

This section deals only with those patients who have

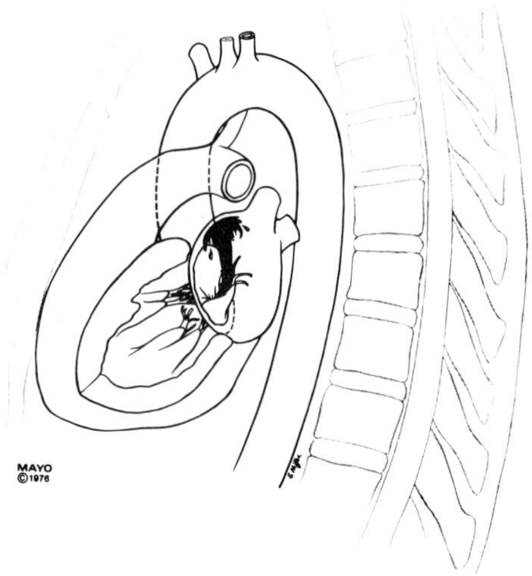

Fig 2-61 Sketch showing flail posterior mitral leaflet acting as baffle and directing jet anteriorly. (From Giuliani ER, Brandenburg RO, Fuster V: Evaluation of cardiac murmurs. *Cardiovasc Clin* 10 No 3:1-18, 1980. By permission, Mayo Foundation.)

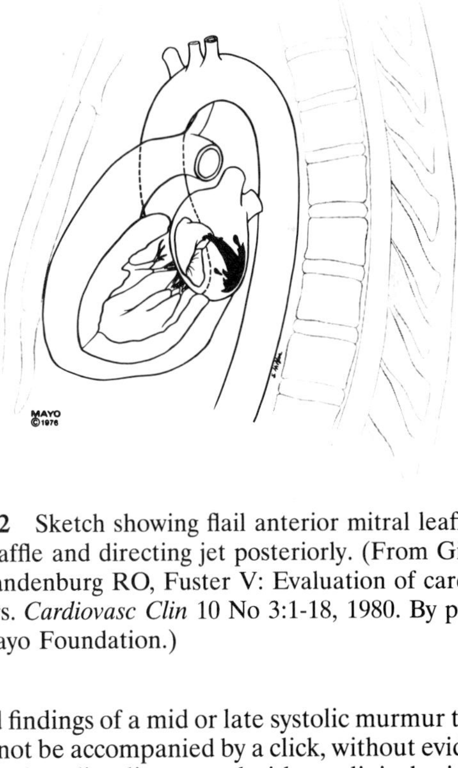

Fig 2-62 Sketch showing flail anterior mitral leaflet acting as baffle and directing jet posteriorly. (From Giuliani ER, Brandenburg RO, Fuster V: Evaluation of cardiac murmurs. *Cardiovasc Clin* 10 No 3:1-18, 1980. By permission, Mayo Foundation.)

isolated findings of a mid or late systolic murmur that may or may not be accompanied by a click, without evidence of associated cardiac disease and without clinical evidence of connective tissue disease. The murmur may be crescendo or decrescendo, with maximum intensity occurring in the middle of the murmur.[286] The murmur is often soft and crescendo but begins in midsystole or late systole and ends with the second sound.[287] It often is initiated by a click or may precede the nonejection sounds.[288] The murmur in each case always extends to the aortic component of the second sound and, in some patients, extends beyond this

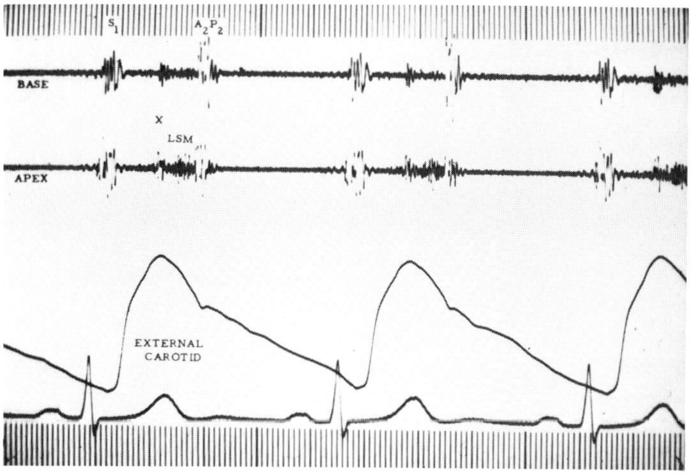

Fig 2-63 Midsystolic click initiating a late systolic murmur *(LSM)*. (Courtesy of James A. Shaver, M.D.)

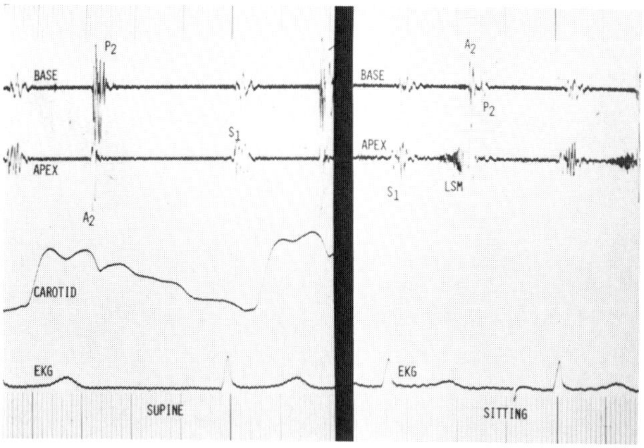

Fig 2-64 **Left,** supine: no evidence of murmur or click. **Right,** when patient is in the sitting position, a late systolic murmur *(LSM)* typical of mitral valve prolapse is demonstrated. (Courtesy of James A. Shaver, M.D.)

sound. In a number of patients, a pansystolic murmur may be heard.[289-291] In general, a late systolic murmur signifies mild mitral regurgitation whereas a pansystolic murmur often is a manifestation of significant mitral insufficiency. The late systolic murmur is usually loudest at the apex and often is well localized to this area; it is usually soft, grade 2 or 3. The transmission of this murmur depends on the leaflet and scallop involved.

An important characteristic of this murmur is its variation in terms of onset and intensity with various body positions (Fig 2-64). In normal subjects, proper spatial relationships are maintained among the papillary muscle, myocardium, chordae tendineae, mitral valve leaflets, and mitral valve annulus. Failure to maintain this proper relationship at varying systolic volumes will result in prolapse of one or both mitral valve leaflets.

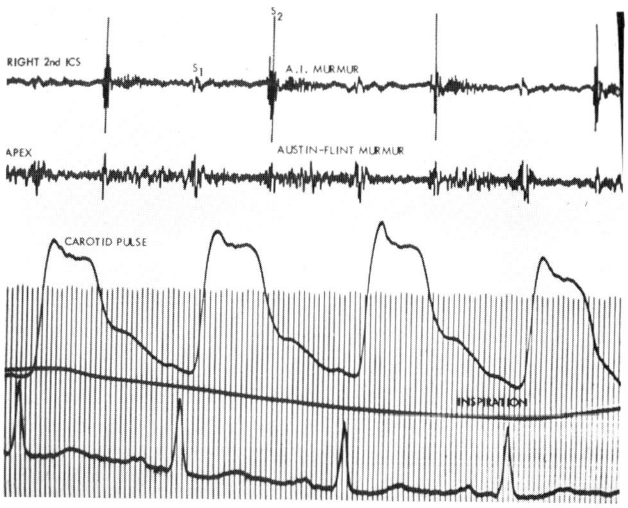

Fig 2-65 Severe acute aortic valve insufficiency. Note soft first heart sound due to preclosure of the mitral valve as well as diastolic aortic insufficiency *(A.I.)* murmur and Austin Flint murmur recorded at the apex. *ICS,* intercostal space. (Courtesy of James A. Shaver, M.D.)

Left heart diastolic murmurs

Aortic valve insufficiency. Aortic valve insufficiency may be congenital or acquired. It may be caused by abnormalities of the aortic cusps, aortic annulus, or aortic root. In this clinical situation, then, there is diastolic communication between the aortic root and left ventricle, with a diastolic pressure gradient causing regurgitation of blood and producing a murmur.

SOUNDS. The first heart sound may be normal or muted (Fig 2-65). If the aortic insufficiency is significant, the first sound is soft to absent due to presystolic partial closure of the mitral valve. In some cases it is due in part to prolongation of the P-R interval. The aortic component of the second sound may be normal, soft, or accentuated. The relationship of the two components of the second sound usually is normal. Rarely, if there is significant regurgitation, the systolic volume can be large enough to prolong systolic emptying and therefore delay the appearance of the aortic component of the second sound. An ejection sound may be present and is thought to be due to a sudden deceleration of the dilated arterial wall. This sound (usually 100 msec after the QRS by phonocardiography) is common in moderate or severe aortic regurgitation.

Rarely, midsystolic nonejection sounds are audible and are related to a bisferiens pulse. This sound is not produced by the mitral valve, and it may imply severe aortic valve insufficiency.[292]

The pulmonic component of the second sound is accentuated when left heart failure and pulmonary hypertension complicate long-standing aortic regurgitation.

A fourth heart sound frequently is associated with aortic valve insufficiency of moderate degree and usually is present when the insufficiency is severe. This sound reflects abnormal left ventricular compliance.

A third heart sound is common in aortic regurgitation and is heard before symptoms from aortic regurgitation appear.[293]

MURMURS. The classic murmur of aortic insufficiency begins with the aortic component of the second heart sound (see Fig 2-65). It is a high-frequency murmur that starts at maximal intensity and gradually decreases in decrescendo fashion, reflecting the decrease in the pressure gradient from aorta to left ventricle during diastole. The intensity of the regurgitant murmur due to rheumatic valvulitis or to bicuspid aortic valve disease is usually maximal in the left second to fourth intercostal spaces.

The high-pitched quality and the softness of the aortic diastolic murmur make it one of the most difficult to identify, particularly in patients with rheumatic valvulitis or a bicuspid aortic valve. The likelihood of missing a soft aortic diastolic murmur is minimized if the patient leans forward during held maximal expiration and the diaphragm of the stethoscope is pressed hard enough to leave a mark on the chest wall[294] or if the patient assumes a knee-elbow position.[295]

In patients with nonrheumatic aortic insufficiency (associated with dilated aorta), the intensity of the murmur along the right sternal border may be equal to or greater than that along the left sternal border.[294] This is best explained by the change in direction of the regurgitant jet. To evaluate this properly, the patient should be sitting or lying supine and the third and fourth parasternal interspaces should be auscultated.

Patients with long-standing hypertension frequently develop mild aortic valve regurgitation. The characteristics of this murmur are as described above. However, except in rare instances,[296] when a patient with known hypertension experiences chest pain and develops a new decrescendo diastolic murmur of aortic insufficiency, best heard along the right sternal border, the most likely diagnosis is dissection of the aorta.

When the murmur is musical, is low in frequency, or has a "seagull sound," then other causes of aortic insufficiency should be considered, including rupture of a valve cusp, eversion of a cusp, or perforation of a cusp by infective endocarditis.[279,297-300]

Thrills rarely accompany aortic diastolic murmurs but may occur in patients with aortic cusp rupture, cusp eversion or perforation, aortic dissection, or aneurysmal dilatation of the ascending aorta. A systolic crescendo-decrescendo murmur heard over the base of the chest and radiating into the neck is almost invariably present. It usually is moderately harsh in quality. In the original description of this murmur, Corrigan considered it characteristic of aortic valve disease.[118] The presence of the murmur and the intensity of the murmur are related to the severity of the regurgitation. The most likely explanation is that this is a flow murmur—i.e., a large stroke volume exiting through a fixed orifice.

When the aortic incompetence is severe and long-standing or is associated with left ventricular enlargement and dysfunction, an apical pansystolic murmur of mitral regurgitation may develop in association with dilatation of the mitral valve annulus.

Occasionally, a low-frequency, mid or late diastolic, apical murmur is present in patients with aortic insufficiency. When present in the absence of mitral stenosis, this murmur is referred to as the Austin Flint murmur[301] (see Fig 2-65). The frequency with which this murmur is present is debatable;[302,303] however, it is present in most patients with moderate to severe aortic regurgitation. The cause of the Austin Flint murmur remains controversial. One theory is that the aortic regurgitant jet restricts the opening of the anterior mitral leaflet, thus producing a functional mitral stenosis.[37,304] A study suggested that the Austin Flint murmur is caused by the turbulence created through mixing of the antegrade mitral flow stream with the retrograde aortic flow.[305] In patients with aortic insufficiency who develop severe left ventricular failure, the diastolic murmur may be markedly attenuated or may even disappear due to the high left ventricular diastolic pressure.

Mitral valve stenosis. This is caused by chronic rheumatic valvulitis, except for the rare instances in which it is congenital in origin. The patient with mitral stenosis presents with clinical and auscultatory findings that allow a precise diagnosis and semiquantitation of the severity of the defect at the bedside. Duroziez[306] is credited with being the first to describe the crescendo presystolic murmur of mitral stenosis.

SOUNDS. The first heart sound characteristically is very loud, often is palpable, and implies mobility of the belly of the mitral valve leaflets, primarily the anterior leaflet. The intensity of the first sound is not influenced significantly by the preceding cycle length,[272,307] in contrast to atrial fibrillation without mitral valve disease. The loud first sound in mitral valve stenosis is the result of two factors: (1) thickened chordae which are less elastic than normal and therefore cause a more abrupt termination of valve motion, and (2) the mitral valve is close to being maximally open at the onset of systole. These two factors produce a sudden deceleration of intracavitary columns of blood and thus the loud first sound. The first sound normally occurs within 50 msec of the onset of the QRS. Because of the delay in mitral valve closure, the mitral component of the first sound is delayed (Fig 2-66). In mitral stenosis, it is usually delayed 70 msec or more.[308] The delay of the first sound depends on the duration of the preceding cycle.[309] Wells[116] devised a formula for estimating the severity of the mitral stenosis based on the delay in the first sound and the interval between the second sound and the opening snap of the mitral valve: the more severe the stenosis, the greater the Q-to-first sound interval and the shorter the second sound-to-opening snap interval. In calcific mitral stenosis, the first sound may be softer than normal, and then the opening snap is usually absent.

The second heart sound usually is normal in patients with mitral stenosis. However, one must identify both components of the second sound and separate them from the opening snap before one can reliably define the qualities of these components. With severe mitral stenosis and the appearance of pulmonary hypertension, the pulmonary component of the second sound will increase in intensity.

Although an opening snap is present in a few patients

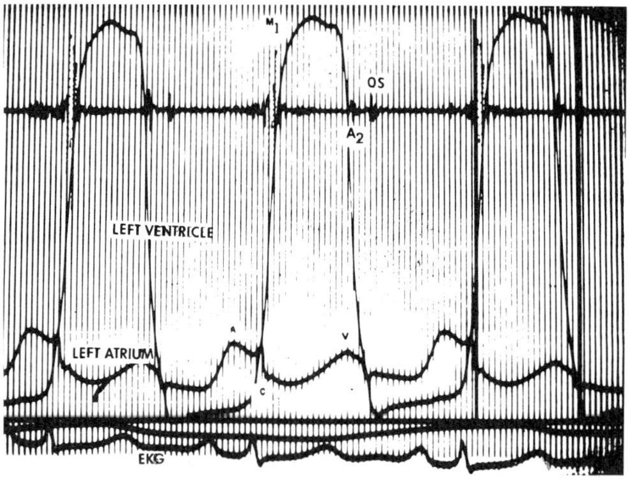

Fig 2-66 Simultaneous external sound and high-fidelity left ventricular and left atrial pressure in a patient with pure mitral stenosis and normal sinus rhythm. The mitral component of the first heart sound is delayed and coincident with the c wave; the opening snap *(OS)* is coincident with a notch on the y descent of the v wave. (Courtesy of James A. Shaver, M.D.)

with pure mitral insufficiency, an opening snap is an important auscultatory sign of mitral stenosis.[310] As with a loud first sound, the opening snap implies mobility of the valve, particularly of the anterior leaflet. This sound is heard between 30 and 120 msec after the aortic component of the second sound and occurs when left ventricular pressure drops below left atrial pressure in early diastole.

The timing of this sound is influenced by both the pressure gradient and the flow from left atrium to left ventricle, permitting a clinical estimation of the severity of the obstruction. In general, the wider the interval between the second sound and the opening snap, the milder the stenosis. In patients with hypertension, severe mitral stenosis can occur with a relatively shorter A_2-to-opening snap interval because of the longer time necessary for left ventricular pressure to fall below left atrial pressure in the presence of systemic hypertension. With some practice, one can estimate the second sound-to-opening snap interval within 20 msec. The patient should be examined both at rest and with exercise in order to estimate the severity of the stenosis properly.[311] The opening snap must be differentiated from the pulmonary component of the second sound, particularly when pulmonary hypertension complicates severe mitral stenosis.

Atrial filling sounds are not common in mitral stenosis. When a presystolic impulse or its counterpart, the fourth heart sound, is present, severe mitral stenosis is excluded unless it can be shown to originate from the right ventricle, as in patients with coexisting pulmonary hypertension. Left ventricular filling sounds also are uncommon in mitral stenosis.[312-314] They may be present in patients with combined mitral stenosis and insufficiency and, when present, indicate that the dominant lesion is insufficiency, not stenosis. They may be due to coexistent significant aortic regurgitation or right ventricular dysfunction.

MURMURS. The characteristic murmur of mitral stenosis is a low-frequency diastolic rumble heard best with the bell applied lightly to the skin over the cardiac apex. The murmur varies in length and may be only presystolic, middiastolic, or holodiastolic with presystolic accentuation. The presystolic accentuation is often, but not always, lost with the appearance of atrial fibrillation. The diastolic murmur results from the rapid turbulent flow through a rigid, narrowed mitral orifice. This rate of flow is accelerated during atrial contraction. When present alone and particularly when associated with a loud first sound, the presystolic murmur is highly suggestive of mitral stenosis but not pathognomonic for it (see Fig 2-45). If limited to presystole, the murmur is heard in the milder form of mitral stenosis. It may be difficult to hear, and often the patient must exercise before it is clearly audible. This component of the murmur then may disappear with the onset of atrial fibrillation. A typical presystolic murmur may be heard in pure aortic valve insufficiency with a normal mitral valve (Austin Flint murmur).[315] The most characteristic murmur of mitral stenosis is one that begins immediately after the opening snap of the mitral valve, extends throughout diastole with presystolic accentuation, and ends with a loud first sound.[316]

Diastolic flow murmurs usually are limited to early to middiastole, occur in the absence of true stenosis, and are caused by an increased flow through a normal mitral valve. They may occur in conditions such as thyrotoxicosis and anemia.[317] Severe mitral insufficiency or left-to-right shunts occurring downstream from the AV valves are also associated with mitral diastolic flow murmurs.

"Silent" mitral stenosis has been reported and is explained on the basis of severe pulmonary hypertension and decreased cardiac output. It has also been related to the presence of associated aortic valve disease or heavy calcification of the mitral valve. With careful auscultation, however, a faint diastolic rumble usually can be heard,[318,319] especially after exercise or administration of amyl nitrite.

A systolic murmur is commonly heard in patients with mitral stenosis. This may be due to associated significant mitral insufficiency, but it may be heard in cases of "pure" mitral stenosis.[320] The murmur also may be due to an associated tricuspid insufficiency. This murmur should be distinguished from that of mitral insufficiency by its inspiratory increase in intensity and the character of the jugular venous pulse form.[321,322]

A murmur that is occasionally heard in association with pure mitral stenosis is a systolic crescendo-decrescendo murmur that originates in the right ventricular outflow tract. The murmur has a scratchy quality, is maximal along the left sternal border, and is frequently associated with an ejection click. In these patients there is some degree of pulmonary hypertension and dilatation of the pulmonary artery. This click and murmur distinguishes these findings from those of an atrial septal defect (patients with mitral stenosis occasionally are misdiagnosed as having an atrial septal defect).

Finally, in the presence of pulmonary hypertension complicating mitral stenosis, pulmonary valve incompetence will develop. This is associated with a high-pitched decrescendo diastolic murmur heard best along the left sternal border (Graham Steele murmur). When this murmur is present, it is associated with a loud pulmonary component of the second sound that usually is palpable and implies severe mitral stenosis. The frequent occurrence of mild aortic insufficiency and mitral stenosis[323] makes the diagnosis of pulmonary valve insufficiency difficult. This diagnosis should not be made without the ancillary evidence of severe mitral stenosis—i.e., a loud palpable pulmonary component of the second heart sound and right ventricular hypertrophy.

Continuous murmurs

Continuous murmurs begin in systole and continue through the second heart sound into diastole. They are produced whenever a high-pressure system is connected to a low-pressure system. They include aortopulmonary fistula, coronary arteriovenous connections, and peripheral arteriovenous contractions. A continuous murmur originating from the accelerated blood flow passing through a small atrial septum in a patient with Lutembacher's syndrome has been reported.[324] These murmurs also may occur with disturbance of flow patterns in arteries or veins. The location of the murmur will be determined by the location of the anomaly.

Patent ductus arteriosus. Of the causes of a continuous murmur (see Table 2-7), patent ductus arteriosus is one of the most frequent and most important defects. The ductus can be long and narrow or relatively short and wide.[325] The auscultatory findings will be influenced in part by the length, width, and tortuosity of the ductus and also by the presence or absence of pulmonary hypertension.

SOUNDS. In uncomplicated patent ductus the first and second heart sounds are usually normal. Occasionally, an ejection sound from either the dilated aorta or the pulmonary trunk is present.[326] Paradoxic splitting of the second sound can be detected occasionally when there is a large left-to-right shunt. This is caused by a combination of prolonged left ventricular ejection and shortened right ventricular ejection.[82,327] The relationship of the two components of the second sound is difficult to appreciate because the sounds are engulfed by the continuous murmur. Occasionally, when there is compromised right ventricular function causing delay in right ventricular emptying, the second sound may be persistently and widely split. With the development of pulmonary hypertension, the pulmonic component increases in intensity. The sounds then become narrowly split.

MURMURS. The classic murmur of patent ductus, first described by Skoda in 1849, is frequently referred to as Gibson's murmur.[328] It is heard best in the left infraclavicular area and second left intercostal space. The important feature of the murmur is that it peaks in late systole, engulfs the second sound, and then gradually decreases in intensity during the remainder of diastole.[329,330] In the neonatal period, the murmur is only systolic in timing because the high pulmonary artery pressure prevents significant diastolic flow across the defect. Occasionally, the murmur will decrease significantly in intensity due to a spontaneous decrease in the size of the lumen of the ductus,[331] or the murmur will disappear with spontaneous closure of the defect.[331,332] In some patients, the murmur may be intermittent. This is believed to be due to interruption of blood flow caused by angulation of the ductus or to the presence of a flutter valve within the duct.[333,334] The timing, length, and configuration of the murmur are influenced by the flow patterns within the ductus. With the onset of systole, the flow through the pulmonary trunk is primarily via the right ventricle. As systole progresses, flow from the aorta through the ductus increases. During diastole, the flow into the pulmonary artery is all from the aorta.

Rarely, a murmur of pulmonary valve incompetence develops in patients with a large uncomplicated ductus. When present, it is due to a dilated pulmonary artery.[335] Apical diastolic murmurs are often heard due to the increased flow across the mitral valve in patients with large left-to-right shunts.[75]

If a patient develops pulmonary vascular obstructive disease with subsequent pulmonary hypertension, the diastolic component of the murmur diminishes and disappears, and the pulmonary component of the second sound becomes loud. Subsequently, these patients develop pulmonary valve incompetence with the associated decrescendo diastolic murmur of high-pressure pulmonary valve incompetence.

Coronary artery anomalies. The murmurs of coronary arteriovenous connections may be systolic or diastolic.[336,337] The murmur of coronary artery fistula is generally heard lower on the chest (mid or lower sternum) than the murmur of patent ductus arteriosus and, as a rule, the murmur does not peak in late systole as does the murmur of patent ductus arteriosus. The systolic component is usually of lesser intensity than the diastolic component, and often only a diastolic murmur is heard. This is probably due to decreased systolic flow related to the increase in intramural pressure in the left ventricular wall during ventricular contraction.[336]

The holosystolic murmur of mitral incompetence, if present, is an important feature in patients with anomalous origin of the left coronary artery from the pulmonary artery and represents dysfunction of one or both of the left ventricular papillary muscles along with the surrounding myocardium. The radiation of this murmur allows one to identify which mitral leaflet is unsupported. If the posterior mitral leaflet is incompetent, the regurgitant jet is directed anteriorly and medially and into the carotids.[337] Thus, although of maximal intensity at the apex, the murmur is well transmitted to the base of the sternum and into the neck. If dysfunction is associated with incompetence of the anterior mitral leaflet, the resultant jet will be directed posteriorly and the murmur can be heard in the axilla and the dorsal spine.[338] This murmur may be associated with a systolic thrill.[277]

Pericardial friction rubs

These are observed in patients with inflammation (irritation) of the serous membranes enveloping the heart. The mechanism of production of a pericardial rub is unclear, but it is believed to be caused by the friction of the roughened pericardial surfaces across each other and is

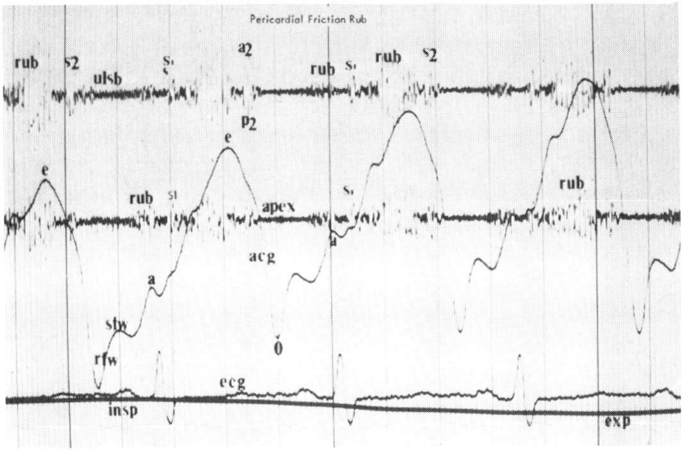

Fig 2-67 Pericardial friction rub and apexcardiogram *(acg)* in patient with renal failure and pericardial effusion. *rfw,* rapid-filling wave; *sfw,* slow-filling wave; *ulsb,* upper left sternal border. (Courtesy of James A. Shaver, M.D.)

heard in the majority of patients with acute pericarditis.[339] A pericardial friction rub is heard in the early phase of myocardial infarction and is related to the presence of regional ventricular dilatation.[340]

Pericardial rubs are heard in patients with small, moderate, or large pericardial effusions.[341] It is well known that pericardial friction rubs are fleeting. The frequency with which a rub is heard depends on the frequency and completeness of the auscultation. Pericardial rubs are related to the cardiac rhythm, and the components of the rub occur during those phases of the cardiac cycle in which there is maximal movement of the heart in the pericardial sac[342,343] (Fig 2-67). The classic rub has three components which occur during atrial systole, ventricular systole, and rapid phase of ventricular filling. The rub may have only two components, and occasionally it occurs with only one component. In this latter instance, it is difficult to be certain of the genesis of this sound.

The rub is best described as a superficial, scratchy, rough sound, occasionally with a coarse, leathery quality, which is heard best when the patient is holding his breath or, occasionally, only during inspiration (diaphragm of the stethoscope held firmly over the left third and fourth interspaces, close to the sternum). If it is not heard in one position and the diagnosis is suspected clinically, then the patient's position should be changed and the examination repeated at intervals.

A rub may be audible for a few hours only, but may at times be present intermittently for days, weeks, or even months. Persistent rubs are usually detected in patients with malignant pericardial disease.

Ischemic heart disease

Myocardial ischemia. The changes in the physical findings that occur as a result of transient cardiac ischemia have received little attention. In part, this is due to the short duration of the ischemic "anginal" attack, so that the physician seldom has the opportunity to examine the patient while the patient is experiencing pain. However, this opportunity presents itself frequently to the hospital residency staff and to the physician who is performing an exercise test. An important initial observation is the response of the patient to the pain. This may allow separation of ischemic distress from symptoms due to anxiety.[344] Pain due to organic disease is usually accompanied by increases in pulse rate and blood pressure and diaphoresis. The degree of change in general is proportional to the severity of pain. The hysteric, on the contrary, often describes excruciating distress with a smile, and there is little or no change in cardiovascular findings.

Pallor and diaphoresis, particularly involving the upper torso, are common findings in patients who are experiencing severe ischemic pain.[345] This probably represents a sympathetic response to the pain. The facial expression often will be one of concern, anxiety, or fear.

Increases in blood pressure preceding the onset of spontaneous angina have been noted for years.[346,347] In patients with coronary artery disease, pain may be precipitated by exercise that produces an increase in blood pressure, and the pain can be prevented by preventing the increase in blood pressure.[348]

More information is available regarding the pulse rate during spontaneous angina.[346,349] Heberden[344] observed that the pulse may not change during pain. However, Parry[350] noted that the pulse invariably increased or changed in quality. In our experience, the pulse rate invariably is altered—either an increase in rate or a change in rhythm. In the majority of the patients, blood pressure and pulse rate increase, and the product of the two values (pulse rate × systolic blood pressure) has been shown to be a reasonably constant guide to the pain threshold for a given individual.[351]

During an anginal attack, an occasional patient will develop a diffuse left precordial pulsation that disappears when ischemia is relieved. The outward impulse is located medial and superior to the apex and is due to dyssynergy of the anterolateral ventricular wall.[61]

Rhythm disorders, both supraventricular and ventricular, frequently complicate acute ischemic events. For clinical recognition, the reader is referred to excellent reviews.[61,352-354]

The first heart sound is often loud. This increase in intensity is attributed to the tachycardia that accompanies the pain. With myocardial infarction and resultant decrease in left ventricular function, the intensity of the first sound may be diminished. The two components of the second sound show no change in intensity, but they may show an abnormal relationship. Occasionally, paradoxic splitting of the second sound is present. The mechanism may be either transient left bundle-branch block[355] or significant transient reduction in left ventricular systolic function[83] prolonging systolic ejection and thereby delaying the aortic component of the second sound. Atrial and ventricular diastolic sounds may occur and reflect altered ventricular compliance. These are significant only when they appear during the episodes of pain. Systolic clicks have not been reported. Transient systolic murmurs are occasionally heard during episodes of angina and are due to transient mitral valve regurgitation associated with left ventricular and papillary muscle dysfunction.[356] When heard, these murmurs are soft, mid to late systolic in timing, and blowing in character. They share some of the features of prolapse of the mitral valve.

Bedside maneuvers are also helpful in the evaluation of chest pain. If the pain is cardiac in origin, relief occurs with slowing of heart rate during carotid sinus pressure.[357,358] In order to evaluate the effects of this maneuver, the patient is told that the pressure on the neck might indeed aggravate the pain, and if it does, the pressure will be terminated. The rapidity with which pain relief is obtained when pain is due to myocardial ischemia is impressive, and, despite the advice of their physician, patients will occasionally use carotid sinus pressure for the relief of recurrent angina. The exact mechanism of this effect is unknown.[358] Many patients are in the older age group with associated carotid artery occlusive disease, and caution should be used in performing this maneuver.

Myocardial infarction. Patients who have clinical evidence of myocardial necrosis (myocardial infarction) demonstrate findings similar to those described above for patients with myocardial ischemia.[359,360] However, an abnormal precordial pulsation may persist after recovery from an acute myocardial infarction, suggesting the presence of significant residual dyskinesis of the anterior ventricular wall.[354,361] The changes in cardiac sounds are similar to those described in transient cardiac ischemic attacks.[362] Systolic murmurs, however, are much more frequent. In patients followed closely in a coronary care unit, more than 50% will develop a soft, blowing, apical systolic murmur of mitral insufficiency. The majority of these murmurs, however, disappear by day 5 to 7. In patients who receive thrombolytic therapy, the incidence of pericardial friction rub is low (about 5%). Rubs occur more frequently in patients with anterior wall infarctions, higher frequency of three-vessel disease, and power failure.[363]

COMPLICATIONS. The most frequent complications of myocardial infarctions are the cardiac arrhythmias. These rhythms can be diagnosed at the bedside by inspection, palpation, and auscultation of the precordium and neck vessels.[61,354] However, because electrocardiography is so readily available and more accurate, time should not be spent in making the diagnosis on the basis of clinical findings.

The mechanical complications that are amenable to surgical intervention include rupture of the interventricular septum, disruption of the supporting structures of the mitral valve to produce mitral valve incompetence, ventricular aneurysms (true and false), and chronic left ventricular failure. Finally, rupture of the free wall into the pericardial sac to produce cardiac tamponade has been identified only rarely and has been approached successfully surgically.

RUPTURE OF INTERVENTRICULAR SEPTUM. This complication of acute myocardial infarction seldom occurs within the first 24 hours; it is seen most commonly between the second and sixth days of infarction. Less frequently, it occurs from day 7 to day 14.[364] Proper management of this complication rests on early recognition and differentiating it from acute mitral regurgitation (Table 2-10).

Table 2-10 Clinical differential diagnosis: ruptured interventricular septum or disruption of mitral apparatus

Ruptured septum	Mitral disruption
Patient recumbent	Patient sitting
Active precordium	Dynamic apical impulse
Venous pressure increased	Venous pressure normal
Systolic murmur: coarse; crescendo-decrescendo in quality; radiates well to right precordium	Systolic murmur: pansystolic; usually radiates to left axilla and back (anterior leaflet) or to base and anterior chest (posterior leaflet) (see text)
Systolic thrill present in 90%; location, low sternum	Systolic thrill present in 25%; location, apical
Diastolic tricuspid flow murmur	Diastolic mitral flow murmur
Systolic murmur of tricuspid insufficiency	. . .
Right-sided third and fourth sounds	Left-sided third and fourth sounds
Lungs clear	Pulmonary rales

Suppose that the patient is doing well clinically but suddenly deteriorates hemodynamically. Simultaneously with this deterioration is the appearance of a loud systolic murmur. This indicates either a perforation of the ventricular septum or disruption of the supporting structures to the mitral valve. With ruptured septum, there are no significant alterations in the heart sounds. Increased jugular venous pressure is common.[365] Right-sided atrial and ventricular gallops do appear. Although a patient with severe hemodynamic impairment without a murmur has been reported, the clue to the correct diagnosis is the appearance, character, and distribution of the systolic murmur. The murmur is very harsh in character, is crescendo and decrescendo in its configuration, is maximal along the left lower sternal border, and radiates well into the right hemithorax. With few exceptions (patients in profound heart failure or shock), there is an associated systolic thrill felt best over the lower sternum.

In the patient with involvement of the mitral valve supporting structures, the outcome will depend entirely on the extent and location of the infarction and of damage to the chordae and papillary muscles. Patients with mitral regurgitation are generally older, female, and nonwhite and have a history of previous infarction.[366] The clinical setting is similar to the one described for rupture of the interventricular septum. However, the clinical findings differ (see Table 2-10). The murmur is midsystolic to late systolic in timing. The transmission of the murmur is dependent on the leaflet that is inadequately supported (discussed earlier under "Mitral valve prolapse"). At times, the murmur may be pansystolic. Usually, the patients are able to tolerate this insult quite well. However, in other patients there may be rupture of the tip or the body of the papillary muscle. In these situations, the extent of the myocardial infarction will determine the clinical course. The auscultatory findings include a harsh, pansystolic, musical murmur that is maximal over the apex and radiates toward the left axilla. In a minority of cases, an apical systolic thrill is present. Left-sided atrial and ventricular gallops are common. No significant alteration in intensity of the second heart sound is present unless pulmonary hypertension develops, in which case the pulmonary component becomes accentuated. Occasionally, a middiastolic low-frequency murmur is audible. This is present only in patients with severe mitral regurgitation and indicates a flow murmur of relative mitral stenosis. In contrast to the patient with ruptured ventricular septum, bibasilar rales are present. Diffuse wheezing may be present and represents peribronchial edema with compromise of the bronchial lumen.

VENTRICULAR ANEURYSMS. The hallmark of a ventricular aneurysm on examination is the paradoxic systolic bulge of the left chest, medial and above the apex. The auscultatory findings of a ventricular aneurysm are usually due to associated mitral regurgitation, related in part to papillary muscle dysfunction.

REFERENCES

1. Conn RD, Cole JS: The cardiac apex impulse: clinical and angiographic correlations. *Ann Intern Med* 75:185-191, 1971

2. Eilen SD, Crawford MH, O'Rourke RA: Accuracy of precordial palpation for detecting increased left ventricular volume. *Ann Intern Med* 99:628-630, 1983

3. Romhilt DW, Bove KE, Norris RJ, et al: A critical appraisal of the electrocardiographic criteria for the diagnosis of left ventricular hypertrophy. *Circulation* 40:185-195, 1969

4. Chikos PM, Figley MM, Fisher L: Correlation between chest film and angiographic assessment of left ventricular size. *AJR* 128:367-373, 1977

5. Kearns TP, Sayre GP: Retinitis pigmentosa, external ophthalmoplegia, and complete heart block. *Arch Ophthalmol* 60:280-289, 1958

6. Braunwald E (ed): *Heart Disease: A Textbook of Cardiovascular Medicine.* Vol. 1. Philadelphia, WB Saunders Company, 1980, pp 13-38

7. Tavel ME: *Clinical Phonocardiography and External Pulse Recording.* Third edition. Chicago, Year Book Medical Publishers, 1978

8. Hurst JW, Schlant RC: Examination of the arteries and their pulsation. In *The Heart, Arteries and Veins.* Fourth edition. Edited by JW Hurst, New York, McGraw-Hill Book Company, 1978, pp 183-192

9. O'Rourke RA: Physical examination of the arteries and veins. In *The Heart, Arteries and Veins.* Fifth edition. Edited by JW Hurst. New York, McGraw-Hill Book Company, 1982, pp 188-198

10. Cintron GB, Hernandez E, Linares E, et al: Bedside recognition, incidence and clinical course of right ventricular infarction. *Am J Cardiol* 47:224-227, 1981

11. Hurst JW, Schlant RC: Examination of the veins and their pulsation. In *The Heart, Arteries and Veins.* Fourth edition. Edited by JW Hurst. New York, McGraw-Hill Book Company, 1978, pp 193-201

12. Ewy GA: The abdominojugular test: technique and hemodynamic correlates. *Ann Intern Med* 109:456-460, 1988

13. Wann LS, Morris SN, Tavel ME: Effects of cardiopulmonary bypass on the jugular venous pulse. *Am Heart J* 94:262-264, 1977

14. Ghiringhelli S, Onofri M, Mortarino G, et al: Echocardiographic findings in patients with a positive jugular venous pulse tracing. *Acta Cardiol (Brux)* 41:215-217, 1986

15. Reddy PS, Curtiss EI: Cardiac tamponade. *Cardiol Clin* 8:627-637, 1990

16. Craige E: Heart sounds: phonocardiography; carotid, apex, and jugular venous pulse tracings; and systolic time intervals. In *Heart Disease: A Textbook of Cardiovascular Medicine.* Vol. 1. Edited by E Braunwald. Philadelphia, WB Saunders Company, 1980, pp 39-69

17. Spodick DH: Kussmaul's sign (letter to the editor). *N Engl J Med* 293:1047-1048, 1975

18. *Dorland's Illustrated Medical Dictionary.* Twenty-sixth edition. Philadelphia, WB Saunders Company, 1981

19. Fairbairn JF II, Bernatz PE: Arteriovenous fistulas. In *Allen-Barker-Hines Peripheral Vascular Diseases.* Fourth edition. Edited by JF Fairbairn II, JL Juergens, JA Spittell Jr. Philadelphia, WB Saunders Company, 1972, pp 303-325

20. Nunn SL: Recognition and treatment of the cardiodynamic effects of atherosclerotic coronary artery disease. *Adv Intern Med* 17:393-408, 1971

21. Eddleman EE Jr: Examination of precordial movements. In *The Heart, Arteries and Veins.* Fourth edition. Edited by JW Hurst. New York, McGraw-Hill Book Company, 1978, pp 201-217

22. Craige E: Inspection and palpation of the precordium. In *The Heart, Arteries and Veins.* Fifth edition. Edited by JW Hurst. New York, McGraw-Hill Book Company, 1982, pp 199-202

23. Craige E, Ozawa Y, Smith D: Origin of the third heart sound. *Acta Cardiol (Brux)* 38:263-265, 1983

24. Reddy PS: The third heart sound. *Int J Cardiol* 7:213-221, 1985

25. Chun PKC, Dunn BE: Clinical clue of severe aortic stenosis: simultaneous palpation of the carotid and apical impulses. *Arch Intern Med* 142:2284-2288, 1982

26. Benchimol A, Harris CL, Desser KB: Midsystolic carotid pulse wave retraction in subjects with prolapsed mitral valve leaflets. *Chest* 62:614-615, 1972

27. Luisada AA, MacCanon DM, Kumar S, et al: Changing views on the mechanism of the first and second heart sounds. *Am Heart J* 88:503-514, 1974

28. Di Bartolo G, Nunez-Dey D, Muiesan G, et al: Hemodynamic correlates of the first heart sound. *Am J Physiol* 201:888-892, 1961

29. Rushmer RF: *Cardiovascular Dynamics.* Second edition. Philadelphia, WB Saunders Company, 1961

30. Renner WF, Renner GW: The quality of resonance of the first heart sound after myocardial infarction: clinical significance. *Circulation* 59:1144-1148, 1979

31. Gupta RC, Bhargava A, Sharma SK: Exercise and the amplitude of first heart sound in ischemic heart disease and normal subjects. *Indian Heart J* 32:349-354, 1980

32. Hearn TC, Mazumdar J, Mahar LJ: First heart sound spectra in relation to anterior mitral-leaflet closing velocity. *Med Biol Eng Comput* 20:466-472, 1982

33. Leatham A, Leech G: Observations on relation between heart sounds and valve movements by simultaneous echo- and phonocardiography (abstract). *Br Heart J* 37:557, 1975

34. Dock W: Mode of production of the first heart sound. *Arch Intern Med* 51:737-746, 1933

35. Waider W, Craige E: First heart sound and ejection sounds: echocardiographic and phonocardiographic correlation with valvular events. *Am J Cardiol* 35:346-356, 1975

36. Brooks N, Leech G, Leatham A: Factors responsible for normal splitting of first heart sound: high-speed echophonocardiographic study of valve movement. *Br Heart J* 42:695-702, 1979

37. Craige E: Echocardiography in studies of the genesis of heart sounds and murmurs. *Prog Cardiol* 4:1-21, 1975

38. Luisada AA: The first heart sound in normal and pathological conditions. *Jpn Heart J* 28:143-156, 1987

39. Hada Y, Takenaka K, Ishimitsu T, et al: Echophonocardiographic study of the initial low frequency component of the first heart sound. *J Am Coll Cardiol* 2:445-451, 1983

40. Leatham A: Splitting of the first and second heart sounds. *Lancet* 2:607-614, 1954

41. Katz LN: The asynchronism of right and left ventricular contractions and the independent variations in their duration. *Am J Physiol* 72:655-681, 1925

42. Potain: Note sur les dédoublements normaux des bruits du coeur. *Bull Soc Med Hop Paris* 3:138-168, 1866

43. Wolferth CC, Margolies A: Asynchronism in contraction of the ventricles in the so-called common type of bundle-branch block: its bearing on the determination of the side of the significant lesion and on

the mechanism of split first and second heart sounds. *Am Heart J* 10:425-452, 1935

44. Dalla-Volta S, Battaglia G, Vincenzi M: Paradoxical splitting of the first heart sound. *Cardiologia (Basel)* 40:33-47, 1962

45. Haber E, Leatham A: Splitting of heart sounds from ventricular asynchrony in bundle-branch block, ventricular ectopic beats, and artificial pacing. *Br Heart J* 27:691-696, 1965

46. Tajik AJ, Gau GT, Giuliani ER, et al: Echocardiogram in Ebstein's anomaly with Wolff-Parkinson-White preexcitation syndrome, type B. *Circulation* 47:813-818, 1973

47. Weiss O, Joachim G: Registrierung von Herztönen und Herzgeräuschen mittels des Phonoskops und ihre Beziehungen zum Elektrokardiogramm. *Z Klin Med* 73:240-256, 1911

48. Hultgren HN, Leo TF: The tricuspid component of the first heart sound in mitral stenosis. *Circulation* 18:1012-1016, 1958

49. Shah PM, Kramer DH, Gramiak R: Influence of the timing of atrial systole on mitral valve closure and on the first heart sound in man. *Am J Cardiol* 26:231-237, 1970

50. Burggraf GW, Craige E: The first heart sound in complete heart block: phono-echocardiographic correlations. *Circulation* 50:17-24, 1974

51. Mann T, McLaurin L, Grossman W, et al: Assessing the hemodynamic severity of acute aortic regurgitation due to infective endocarditis. *N Engl J Med* 293:108-113, 1975

52. McKusick VA: *Cardiovascular Sound in Health and Disease.* Baltimore, Williams & Wilkins Company, 1958, pp 310-321

53. Mills PG, Chamusco RF, Moos S, et al: Echophonocardiographic studies of the contribution of the atrioventricular valves to the first heart sound. *Circulation* 54:944-951, 1976

54. Stept ME, Heid CE, Shaver JA, et al: Effect of altering P-R interval on the amplitude of the first heart sound in the anesthetized dog. *Circ Res* 25:255-263, 1969

55. Renner WF, Renner GW: The quality of S_1 as an indicator of left ventricular performance. *Md State Med J* 28:60-61, July 1979

56. Dashkoff N, Fortuin NJ, Hutchins GM: Clinical features of severe mitral regurgitation due to floppy mitral valve (abstract). *Circulation* 50 Suppl 3:60, 1974

57. Leatham A, Gray I: Auscultatory and phonocardiographic signs of atrial septal defect. *Br Heart J* 18:193-208, 1956

58. Kitapci H, Portaluppi F, Luisada AA: First heart sound in atrial septal defect. *Angiology* 32:846-854, 1981

59. Luisada AA, Portaluppi F: Peculiarities of the first heart sound in bundle branch blocks: a new interpretation based on graphic analysis. *Jpn Heart J* 22:729-738, 1981

60. Burggraf GW: The first heart sound in left bundle branch block: an echophonocardiographic study. *Circulation* 63:429-435, 1981

61. Levine SA, Harvey WP: *Clinical Auscultation of the Heart.* Second edition. Philadelphia, WB Saunders Company, 1959

62. Wolferth CC, Margolies A: Certain effects of auricular systole and prematurity of beat on the intensity of the first heart sound. *Trans Assoc Am Physicians* 45:44-48, 1930

63. Rytand DA: The variable loudness of the first heart sound in auricular fibrillation. *Am Heart J* 37:187-204, 1949

64. Leech G, Brooks N, Green-Wilkinson A, et al: Mechanism of influence of PR interval on loudness of first heart sound. *Br Heart J* 43:138-142, 1980

65. Shaver JA, Nadolny RA, O'Toole JD, et al: Sound pressure correlates of the second heart sound: an intracardiac sound study. *Circulation* 49:316-325, 1974

66. Perloff JK: The physiologic mechanisms of cardiac and vascular physical signs. *J Am Coll Cardiol* 1:184-198, 1983

67. Shaver JA: The second heart sound: hemodynamic determinants. *Acta Cardiol (Brux)* 40:7-18, 1985

68. Harris A, Sutton G: Second heart sound in normal subjects. *Br Heart J* 30:739-742, 1968

69. Boyer SH, Chisholm AW: Physiologic splitting of the second heart sound. *Circulation* 18:1010-1011, 1958

70. Sabbah HN, Stein PD: Investigation of the theory and mechanism of the origin of the second heart sound. *Circ Res* 39:874-882, 1976

71. Hirschfeld S, Liebman J, Borkat G, et al: Intracardiac pressure-sound correlates of echographic aortic valve closure. *Circulation* 55:602-604, 1977

72. Chandraratna PAN, Lopez JM, Cohen LS: Echocardiographic observations on the mechanism of production of the second heart sound. *Circulation* 51:292-296, 1975

73. Anastassiades PC, Quinones MA, Gaasch WH, et al: Aortic valve closure: echocardiographic, phonocardiographic, and hemodynamic assessment. *Am Heart J* 91:228-232, 1976

74. Sutton G, Harris A, Leatham A: Second heart sound in pulmonary hypertension. *Br Heart J* 30:743-756, 1968

75. Perloff JK: Auscultatory and phonocardiographic manifestations of pulmonary hypertension. *Prog Cardiovasc Dis* 9:303-340, 1967

76. Stein PD, Sabbah HN, Anbe DT, et al: The pulmonary component of the second sound in right ventricular failure. *Henry Ford Hosp Med J* 28:79-84, 1980

77. Leatham A, Weitzman D: Auscultatory and phonocardiographic signs of pulmonary stenosis. *Br Heart J* 19:303-317, 1957

78. Vogelpoel L, Schrire V: Pulmonary stenosis with intact ventricular septum and Fallot's tetralogy: assessment of postoperative results by auscultation and phonocardiography. *Am Heart J* 59:645-666, 1960

79. Beck W, Schrire V, Vogelpoel L: Splitting of the second heart sound in constrictive pericarditis, with observations on the mechanism of pulsus paradoxus. *Am Heart J* 64:765-778, 1962

80. Brigden W, Leatham A: Mitral incompetence. *Br Heart J* 15:55-73, 1953

81. Leatham A, Segal B: Auscultatory and phonocardiographic signs of ventricular septal defect with left-to-right shunt. *Circulation* 25:318-327, 1962

82. Gray IR: Paradoxical splitting of the second heart sound. *Br Heart J* 18:21-28, 1956

83. Yurchak PM, Gorlin R: Paradoxical splitting of the second heart sound in coronary heart disease. *N Engl J Med* 269:741-743, 1963

84. Shaver JA, Kroetz FW, Leonard JJ, et al: The effect of steady-state increases in systemic arterial pressure on the duration of left ventricular ejection time. *J Clin Invest* 47:217-230, 1968

85. Strickland NH, Gibson DG: Reversed splitting of the second heart sound due to tricuspid regurgitation. *Int J Cardiol* 20:412-415, 1988

86. Hultgren HN, Reeve R, Cohn K, et al: The ejection click of valvular pulmonic stenosis. *Circulation* 40:631-640, 1969

87. Leatham A, Vogelpoel L: The early systolic sound in dilatation of the pulmonary artery. *Br Heart J* 16:21-33, 1954

88. Mills P, Amara I, Fujii J, et al: Dual echocardiographic right ventricular isovolumic contraction in estimation of pulmonary artery pressure (abstract). *Circulation* 56 Suppl 3:67, 1977

89. Curtiss EI, Reddy PS, O'Toole JD, et al: Alterations of right ventricular systolic time intervals by chronic pressure and volume overloading. *Circulation* 53:997-1003, 1976

90. Whittaker AV, Shaver JA, Gray S III, et al: Sound-pressure correlates of the aortic ejection sound: an intracardiac sound study. *Circulation* 39:475-486, 1969

91. Hancock EW: Origin of the ejection sound in aortic stenosis (abstract). *Clin Res* 13:209, 1965

92. Leatham A: Auscultation of the heart. *Lancet* 2:703-708, 1958

93. Humphries JO'N, McKusick VA: The differentiation of organic and "innocent" systolic murmurs. *Prog Cardiovasc Dis* 5:152-171, 1962

94. Barlow JB, Bosman CK: Aneurysmal protrusion of the posterior leaflet of the mitral valve: an auscultatory-electrocardiographic syndrome. *Am Heart J* 71:166-178, 1966

95. Harvey WP: Some newer or poorly recognized findings on clinical auscultation. *Mod Concepts Cardiovasc Dis* 37:85-88, 1968

96. Luisada AA, Portaluppi F: Considerations on the mechanism of the systolic click of mitral valve prolapse. *Acta Cardiol (Brux)* 40:301-305, 1985

97. Ronan JA, Perloff JK, Harvey WP: Systolic clicks and the late systolic murmur: intracardiac phonocardiographic evidence of their mitral valve origin. *Am Heart J* 70:319-325, 1965

98. Ozawa Y, Smith D, Craige E: Origin of the third heart sound. II. Studies in human subjects. *Circulation* 67:399-404, 1983

99. Vancheri F, Gibson D: Relation of third and fourth heart sounds to blood velocity during left ventricular filling. *Br Heart J* 61:144-148, 1989

100. Van de Werf F, Geboers J, Kesteloot H, et al: The mechanism of disappearance of the physiologic third heart sound with age. *Circulation* 73:877-884, 1986

101. Ishmail AA, Wing S, Ferguson J, et al: Interobserver agreement by auscultation in the presence of a third heart sound in patients with congestive heart failure. *Chest* 91:870-873, 1987

102. Leonard JJ, Weissler AM, Warren JV: Observations on the mechanism of atrial gallop rhythm. *Circulation* 17:1007-1012, 1958

103. Erikssen J, Rasmussen K: Prevalence and significance of the fourth heart sound (S4) in presumably healthy middle-aged men, with particular relation to latent coronary heart disease. *Eur J Cardiol* 9:63-75, 1979

104. Rectra EH, Khan AH, Pigott VM, et al: Audibility of the fourth heart sound: a prospective, "blind" auscultatory and polygraphic investigation. *JAMA* 221:36-41, 1972

105. Benchimol A, Desser KB: The fourth heart sound in patients without demonstrable heart disease. *Am Heart J* 93:298-301, 1977

106. Spodick DH, Quarry VM: Prevalence of the fourth heart sound by phonocardiography in the absence of cardiac disease. *Am Heart J* 87:11-14, 1974

107. Renfro NL, Leonard JJ, deGroot WJ, et el: Auscultatory and phonocardiographic observations in hyperthyroidism (abstract). *Circulation* 22:799, 1960

108. Harvey WP, Stapleton J: Clinical aspects of gallop rhythm with particular reference to diastolic gallops. *Circulation* 18:1017-1024, 1958

109. Goldblatt A, Aygen MM, Braunwald E: Hemodynamic-phonocardiographic correlations of the fourth heart sound in aortic stenosis. *Circulation* 26:92-98, 1962

110. Harvey WP, Segal JP, Gurel T: The clinical spectrum of primary myocardial disease. *Prog Cardiovasc Dis* 7:17-42, 1964

111. Homma S, Bhattacharjee D, Gopal A, et al: Relationship of auscultatory fourth heart sound to the quantitated left atrial filling fraction. *Clin Cardiol* 14:671-674, 1991

112. Perloff JK: Recognition and differential diagnosis of pulmonary stenosis. In *The Theory and Practice of Auscultation* (The 9th Hahnemann Symposium). Edited by BL Segal. Philadelphia, FA Davis Company, 1964, pp 216-229

113. Jordan MD, Taylor CR, Nyhuis AW, et al: Audibility of the fourth heart sound: relationship to presence of disease and examiner experience. *Arch Intern Med* 147:721-726, 1987

114. Mounsey P: The opening snap of mitral stenosis. *Br Heart J* 15:135-142, 1953

115. Barrington WW, Boudoulas H, Bashore T, et al: Mitral stenosis: mitral dome excursion at M_1 and the mitral opening snap—the concept of reciprocal heart sounds. *Am Heart J* 115:1280-1290, 1988

116. Wells B: The assessment of mitral stenosis by phonocardiography. *Br Heart J* 16:261-266, 1954

117. Stefadouros MA, Little RC: The cause and clinical significance of diastolic heart sounds. *Arch Intern Med* 140:537-541, 1980

118. Connolly DC, Mann RJ: Dominic J. Corrigan (1802-1880) and his description of the pericardial knock. *Mayo Clin Proc* 55:771-773, 1980

119. Potain: Adhérence du péricarde; triple bruit du coeur; impulsion diastolique—observation recueillie. *Bull Soc Anat Paris* 31:378-385, 1856

120. Mounsey P: The early diastolic sound of constrictive pericarditis. *Br Heart J* 17:143-152, 1955

121. Ichiyasu H, Nabeyama S, Takasugi M, et al: Pseudo-knock sound in a patient with nephrotic syndrome and massive ascites. *Jpn Heart J* 23:137-145, 1982

122. LaSala AF, Fieldman A: Clicks due to Swan-Ganz catheter. *Chest* 74:92-94, 1978

123. Isner JM, Horton J, Ronan JA Jr: Systolic click from a Swan-Ganz catheter: phonoechocardiographic depiction of the underlying mechanism. *Am J Cardiol* 43:1046-1048, 1979

124. Mintz GS, Carlson EB, Kotler MN: Comparison of noninvasive techniques in evaluation of the nontissue cardiac valve prosthesis. *Am J Cardiol* 49:39-44, 1982

125. Reisner SA, Meltzer RS: Normal values of prosthetic valve Doppler echocardiographic parameters: a review. *J Am Soc Echocardiography* 1:201-210, 1988

126. Cooper DM, Stewart WJ, Schiavone WA, et al: Evaluation of normal prosthetic valve function by Doppler echocardiography. *Am Heart J* 114:576-582, 1987

127. Jacobs LE, Parry WR, Kotler MN: Pulsed, continuous, and color flow Doppler echocardiographic assessment of normal and abnormal Ionescu-Shiley pericardial valves. *J Cardiac Surg* 3 Suppl:429-435, 1988

128. Nellessen U, Masuyama T, Appleton CP, et al: Mitral prosthesis malfunction: comparative Doppler echocardiographic studies of mitral prostheses before and after replacement. *Circulation* 79:330-336, 1989

129. Taams MA, Gussenhoven EJ, Cahalan MK, et al: Transesophageal Doppler color flow imaging in the detection of native and Björk-Shiley mitral valve regurgitation. *J Am Coll Cardiol* 13:95-99, 1989

130. Currie PJ, Calafiore P, Steward WJ, et al: Transesophageal echo in mitral prosthetic dysfunction: echo-surgical correlation (abstract). *J Am Coll Cardiol* 13:69A, 1989

131. Chandraratna PAN, Lopez JM, Hildner FJ, et al: Diagnosis of Björk-Shiley aortic valve dysfunction by echocardiography. *Am Heart J* 91:318-324, 1976

132. Vardan S, Warner R, Mookherjee S, et al: Echo- and phonocardiographic studies in patients with Lillehei-Kaster aortic valve prostheses. *Jpn Heart J* 20:277-288, 1979

133. Kupari M, Harjula A, Mattila S: Auscultatory characteristics of normally functioning Lillehei-Kaster, Björk-Shiley, and St Jude heart valve prostheses. *Br Heart J* 55:364-370, 1986

134. Raizada V, Benchimol A, Desser KB, et al: Echocardiographic features of normally functioning Hancock porcine heterograft in the mitral position (abstract). *Clin Res* 25:144A, 1977

135. Horowitz MS, Goodman DJ, Hancock EW, et al: Noninvasive diagnosis of complications of the mitral bioprosthesis. *J Thorac Cardiovasc Surg* 71:450-475, 1976

136. Stein PD, Sabbah HN, Lakier JB, et al: Frequency spectra of the first heart sound and of the aortic component of the second heart sound in patients with degenerated porcine bioprosthetic valves. *Am J Cardiol* 53:557-561, 1984

137. Stein PD, Sabbah HN, Lakier JB: Origin and clinical relevance of musical murmurs. *Int J Cardiol* 4:103-112, 1983

138. Kinney EL, Machado H, Cortada X: Cooing intracardiac sound in a perforated porcine mitral valve detected by pulsed Doppler echocardiography. *Am Heart J* 112:420-423, 1986

139. Cotter L, Miller HC: Clinical and haemodynamic evaluation of mounted porcine heterograft in mitral position. *Br Heart J* 41:412-417, 1979

140. Kotler MN, Segal BL, Parry WR: Echocardiographic and phonocardiographic evaluation of prosthetic heart valves. *Cardiovasc Clin* 9 No 2:187-207, 1978

141. Hultgren HN, Hubis H: A phonocardiographic study of patients with the Starr-Edwards mitral valve prosthesis. *Am Heart J* 69:306-319, 1965

142. Hylen JC, Kloster FE, Herr RH, et al: Sound spectrographic diagnosis of aortic ball variance. *Circulation* 39:849-858, 1969

143. Brandenburg RO, Fuster V, Giuliani ER, et al: Postoperative follow-up of the cardiac surgical patient. *Cardiovasc Clin* 10 No 3:231-240, 1980

144. Sharma RS: Measurement of intensity of heart sounds and murmurs. *Lancet* 2:612, 1981

145. Boicourt OW, Nagle RE, Mounsey JPD: The clinical significance of systolic retraction of the apical impulse. *Br Heart J* 27:379-391, 1965

146. Goldblatt A, Harrison DC, Glick G, et al: Studies on cardiac dimensions in intact, unanesthetized man. II. Effects of respiration. *Circ Res* 13:448-467, 1963

147. Rios JC, Massumi RA, Breesmen WT, et al: Auscultatory features of acute tricuspid regurgitation. *Am J Cardiol* 23:4-11, 1969

148. Fontana ME, Wooley CF, Leighton RF, et al: Postural changes in left ventricular and mitral valvular dynamics in the systolic click–late systolic murmur syndrome. *Circulation* 51:165-173, 1975

149. Ishikawa K, Tamura T: Study of respiratory influence on the intensity of heart sound in normal subjects. *Angiology* 30:750-755, 1979

150. Barlow J, Shillingford J: The use of amyl nitrite in differentiating mitral and aortic systolic murmurs. *Br Heart J* 20:162-166, 1958

151. Beck W, Schrire V, Vogelpoel L, et al: Hemodynamic effects of amyl nitrite and phenylephrine on the normal human circulation and their relation to changes in cardiac murmurs. *Am J Cardiol* 8:341-349, 1961

152. Schrire V, Vogelpoel L, Beck W, et al: The effects of amyl nitrite and phenylephrine on the intracardiac murmurs of small ventricular septal defects. *Am Heart J* 62:225-236, 1961

153. Vogelpoel L, Schrire V, Nellen M, et al: The use of amyl nitrite in the differentiation of Fallot's tetralogy and pulmonary stenosis with intact ventricular septum. *Am Heart J* 57:803-819, 1959

154. Delman AJ, Stein E: *Dynamic Cardiac Auscultation and Phonocardiography: A Graphic Guide.* Philadelphia, WB Saunders Company, 1979, pp 559-792

155. Criscitiello MG: Physiologic and pharmacologic aids in cardiac auscultation. In *Cardiac Diagnosis and Treatment.* Second edition. Edited by NO Fowler. Hagerstown, Maryland, Harper & Row, Publishers, 1976, pp 173-188

156. Crevasse L: The use of a vasopressor agent as a diagnostic aid in auscultation. *Am Heart J* 58:821-826, 1959
157. Contratto AW: Significance of systolic cardiac murmurs in college students. N Engl J Med 228:499-501, 1943
158. Kram NE: Innocent murmurs of childhood. *J Am Osteopath Assoc* 82:32-37, 1982
159. Leatham A: Systolic murmurs. *Circulation* 17:601-611, 1958
160. Groom D, Chapman W, Francis WW, et al: The normal systolic murmur. *Ann Intern Med* 52:134-144, 1960
161. Cotter L, Logan RL, Poole A: Innnocent systolic murmurs in healthy 40-year-old men. *J R Coll Physicians Lond* 14:128-129, 1980
162. Kulangara RJ, Strong WB, Miller MD: Differential diagnosis of heart murmurs in children. *Postgrad Med* 72:219-228, August 1982
163. Stein PD, Sabbah HN: Aortic origin of innocent murmurs. *Am J Cardiol* 39:665-671, 1977
164. Gardiner HM, Joffe HS: Genesis of Still's murmurs: a controlled Doppler echocardiographic study. *Br Heart J* 66:217-220, 1991
165. Hammond JH, Eisinger RP: Carotid bruits in 1,000 normal subjects. *Arch Intern Med* 109:563-565, 1962
166. Jones FL Jr: Frequency, characteristics and importance of the cervical venous hum in adults. *N Engl J Med* 267:658-660, 1962
167. DuShane JW, Weidman WH, Brandenburg RO, et al: Differentiation of interatrial communications by clinical methods: ostium secundum, ostium primum, common atrium, and total anomalous pulmonary venous connection. *Circulation* 21:363-371, 1960
168. Barber JM, Magidson O, Wood P: Atrial septal defect: with special reference to the electrocardiogram, the pulmonary artery pressure and the second heart sound. *Br Heart J* 12:277-292, 1950
169. Boyer SH, Chisholm AW: Second heart sound in atrial septal defect (abstract). *Circulation* 18:697, 1958
170. Evans JR, Rowe RD, Keith JD: The clinical diagnosis of atrial septal defect in children. *Am J Med* 30:345-356, 1961
171. Castle RF, Hedden CA, Davis NP II: Variables affecting splitting of the second heart sound in normal children. *Pediatrics* 43:183-191, 1969
172. Russo R, Calabrese S, Bortolotti U, et al: Difetto del setto interatriale tipo "ostium secundum": descrizione di un caso con reperto ascoltatorio atipico. *G Ital Cardiol* 11:850-854, 1981
173. Dimond EG, Benchimol A: Phonocardiography in atrial septal defect: correlation between hemodynamics and phonocardiographic findings. *Am Heart J* 58:343-356, 1959
174. Ong LS, Nanda NC, Falkoff MD, et al: Interatrial septal aneurysm, systolic click and atrial tachyarrhythmia—a new syndrome? *Ultrasound Med Biol* 8:691-693, 1982
175. Just H, Mattingly TW: Interatrial septal defect and pericardial disease: a coincidence or causal relationship? *Am Heart J* 76:157-167, 1968
176. Semler HJ, Brandenburg RO, Kirklin JW: Congenital intracardiac defects plus pericardial disease: clinical and surgical findings in six cases. *Dis Chest* 39:293-298, 1961
177. Nadas AS, Ellison RC: Phonocardiographic analysis of diastolic flow murmurs in secundum atrial septal defect and ventricular septal defect. *Br Heart J* 29:684-688, 1967
178. Ishikawa K, Ide Y, Ishikawa M, et al: Critical evaluation of atrial presystolic murmur. *Chest* 77:656-661, 1980
179. Rogers WM, Harrison JS, Malm JR, et al: Phonocardiographic criteria in the diagnosis of atrial and ventricular septal defects: an experimental and clinical study. *J Cardiovasc Surg* 7:29-33, 1966
180. Ross J Jr, Braunwald E, Mason DT, et al: Interatrial communication and left atrial hypertension: a cause of continuous murmur. *Circulation* 28:853-860, 1963
181. Goldfarb B, Wang Y: Mitral stenosis and left to right shunt at the atrial level: a broadened concept of the Lutembacher syndrome. *Am J Cardiol* 17:319-326, 1966
182. Hynes KM, Frye RL, Brandenburg RO, et al: Atrial septal defect (secundum) associated with mitral regurgitation. *Am J Cardiol* 34:333-338, 1974
183. Radtke WE, Tajik AJ, Gau GT, et al: Atrial septal defect: echocardiographic observations; studies in 120 patients. *Ann Intern Med* 84:246-253, 1976
184. Nagata S, Nimura Y, Sakakibara H, et al: Mitral valve lesion associated with secundum atrial septal defect: analysis by real time two dimensional echocardiography. *Br Heart J* 49:51-58, 1983
185. Angel J, Soler-Soler J, Garcia del Castillo H, et al: The role of reduced left ventricular enddiastolic volume in the apparently high prevalence of mitral valve prolapse in atrial septal defect. *Eur J Cardiol* 11:341-355, 1980
186. Pugliese P, Murzi B, Tommasini G, et al: Difetto del setto interatriale tipo ostium secundum associato a cleft della valvola mitrale. *G Ital Cardiol* 12:264-269, 1982
187. Espino-Vela J: Rheumatic heart disease associated with atrial septal defect: clinical and pathologic study of 12 cases of Lutembacher's syndrome. *Am Heart J* 57:185-202, 1959
188. Blount SG Jr, Balchum OJ, Gensini G: The persistent ostium primum atrial septal defect. *Circulation* 13:499-509, 1956
189. Cooley DA, McNamara DG: Ostium primum and atrioventricularis communis defects: clinical manifestations and surgical treatment. *Prog Cardiovasc Dis* 1:89-101, 1958
190. Ellis FH Jr, McGoon DC, Kirklin JW: Surgical management of persistent common atrioventricular canal. *Am J Cardiol* 6:598-604, 1960
191. Kiely B, Adams P Jr, Anderson RC, et al: The ostium primum syndrome. *Am J Dis Child* 96:381-403, 1958
192. Torgersen J: Morphology of the persistent foramen primum. *Acta Chir Scand* 128:565-573, 1964
193. Wakai CS, Edwards JE: Developmental and pathologic considerations in persistent common atrioventricular canal. *Proc Staff Meet Mayo Clin* 31:487-500, 1956
194. Wakai CS, Edwards JE: Pathologic study of persistent common atrioventricular canal. *Am Heart J* 56:779-794, 1958
195. Weyn AS, Bartle SH, Nolan TB, et al: Atrial septal defect—primum type. *Circulation* 32 Suppl 3:13-23, 1965
196. Shumacker HB Jr, King H: Septum primum atrial septal defects. *J Thorac Cardiovasc Surg* 43:366-371, 1962
197. Paul MH: Endocardial cushion defects: persistent common atrioventricular canal and persistent ostium primum. *Pediatr Clin North Am* November 1958, pp 1011-1028
198. Giuliani ER, Brandenburg RO, Fuster V: Evaluation of cardiac murmurs. *Cardiovasc Clin* 10 No 3:1-18, 1980
199. Somerville J: Clinical assessment of the function of the mitral valve in atrioventricular defects related to the anatomy. *Am Heart J* 71:701-711, 1966
200. Edwards JE: Pulmonary stenosis with intact ventricular septum. In *Pathology of the Heart.* Second edition. Edited by SE Gould. Springfield, Illinois, Charles C Thomas, Publisher, 1960, pp 391-397
201. Koretzky ED, Moller JH, Korns ME, et al: Congenital pulmonary stenosis resulting from dysplasia of valve. *Circulation* 40:43-53, 1969
202. Blount SG Jr, Vigoda PS, Swan H: Isolated infundibular stenosis. *Am Heart J* 57:684-700, 1959
203. Perloff JK, Ronan JA Jr, de Leon AC: Ventricular septal defect with the "two-chambered right ventricle." *Am J Cardiol* 16:894-900, 1965
204. Oppenheimer EH: Partial atresia of the main branches of the pulmonary artery occurring in infancy and accompanied by calcification of the pulmonary artery and aorta. *Bull Johns Hopkins Hosp* 63:261-277, 1938
205. Gale GE, Heimann KW, Barlow JB: Double-chambered right ventricle: a report of five cases. *Br Heart J* 31:291-298, 1969
206. Franch RH, Gay BB Jr: Congenital stenosis of the pulmonary artery branches: a classification, with postmortem findings in two cases. *Am J Med* 35:513-529, 1963
207. Giuliani ER, Nasser FN: Two-dimensional echocardiography in acquired heart diseases—Part II. *Curr Probl Cardiol* 5:1-54, March 1981
208. Rios JC, Walsh BJ, Massumi RA, et al: Congenital pulmonary artery branch stenosis. *Am J Cardiol* 24:318-325, 1969
209. Vogelpoel L, Schrire V: Auscultatory and phonocardiographic assessment of pulmonary stenosis with intact ventricular septum. *Circulation* 22:55-72, 1960
210. Vogelpoel L, Schrire V: Auscultatory and phonocardiographic assessment of Fallot's tetralogy. *Circulation* 22:73-89, 1960
211. Gamboa R, Hugenholtz PG, Nadas AS: Accuracy of the phonocardiogram in assessing severity of aortic and pulmonic stenosis. *Circulation* 30:35-46, 1964
212. Abrahams DG, Wood P: Pulmonary stenosis with normal aortic root. *Br Heart J* 13:519-548, 1951
213. Holmes JC, Fowler NO, Kaplan S: Pulmonary valvular insufficiency. *Am J Med* 44:851-862, 1968
214. Luan LL, D'Silva JL, Gasul BM, et al: Stenosis of the right main pulmonary artery: clinical, angiocardiographic, and catheterization findings in ten patients. *Circulation* 21:1116-1125, 1960
215. Gyllenswärd Å, Lodin H, Lundberg A, et al: Congenital, multiple

peripheral stenoses of the pulmonary artery. *Pediatrics* 19:399-410, 1957
216. Lucas D: Auscultatory features of tricuspid stenosis and regurgitation. In *The Theory and Practice of Auscultation* (The 9th Hahnemann Symposium.) Edited by BL Segal. Philadelphia, FA Davis Company, 1964, pp 411-426
217. Salazar E, Levine HD: Rheumatic tricuspid regurgitation: the clinical spectrum. *Am J Med* 33:111-129, 1962
218. Verel D, Sandler G, Mazurkie SJ: Tricuspid incompetence in cor pulmonale. *Br Heart J* 24:441-444, 1962
219. Müller O, Shillingford J: Tricuspid incompetence. *Br Heart J* 16:195-207, 1954
220. Ahn AJ, Segal BL: Isolated tricuspid insufficiency: clinical features, diagnosis and management. *Prog Cardiovasc Dis* 9:166-193, 1966
221. Schilder DP, Harvey WP: Confusion of tricuspid incompetence with mitral insufficiency—a pitfall in the selection of patients for mitral surgery. *Am Heart J* 54:352-367, 1957
222. Segal JP, Harvey WP, Corrado MA: The Austin Flint murmur: its differentiation from the murmur of rheumatic mitral stenosis. *Circulation* 18:1025-1033, 1958
223. Leatham A: Auscultation of the heart. *Lancet* 2:757-766, 1958
224. Rivero Carvallo JM: Signo para el diagnóstico de las insuficiencias tricuspideas. *Arch Inst Cardiol Mex* 16:531-537, 1946
225. Rivero Carvallo JM: El diagnóstico de la estenosis tricuspidea. *Arch Inst Cardiol Mex* 20:1-11, 1950
226. Leon DF, Leonard JJ, Lancaster JF, et al: Effect of respiration on pansystolic regurgitant murmur as studied by biatrial intracardiac phonocardiography. *Am J Med* 39:429-441, 1965
227. Uricchio JF, Bentivoglio L, Gilman R, et al: Tricuspid regurgitation masquerading as mitral regurgitation in patients with pure mitral stenosis. *Am J Med* 25:224-230, 1958
228. Curiel R, Tortoledo F, Rodriguez L, et al: The cardiovascular effects of acute hypoxemia as a diagnostic aid. *Chest* 81:159-165, 1982
229. Cortes FM, Jacoby WJ: Isolated congenital pulmonary valvular insufficiency. *Am J Cardiol* 10:287-290, 1962
230. D'Cruz IA, Lendrum BL, Novak K: Congenital absence of the pulmonary valve. *Am Heart J* 68:728-740, 1964
231. Gold MMA: Congenital dilatation of the pulmonary arterial tree: relation to Ayerza's disease and primary pulmonary arteriosclerosis. *Arch Intern Med* 78:197-209, 1946
232. Lindgren KM, McShane K, Roberts WC: Acute rupture of the pulmonic valve by a balloon-tipped catheter producing a musical diastolic murmur. *Chest* 81:251-253, 1982
233. Miller RA, Lev M, Paul MH: Congenital absence of the pulmonary valve: the clinical syndrome of tetralogy of Fallot with pulmonary regurgitation. *Circulation* 26:266-278, 1962
234. Smith RD, DuShane JW, Edwards JE: Congenital insufficiency of the pulmonary valve: including a case of fetal cardiac failure. *Circulation* 20:554-560, 1959
235. Chandraratna PA, Wilson D, Imaizumi T, et al: Invasive and noninvasive assessment of pulmonic regurgitation: clinical, angiographic, phonocardiographic, echocardiographic, and Doppler ultrasound correlations. *Clin Cardiol* 5:360-365, 1982
236. Jacoby WJ Jr, Tucker DH, Sumner RG: The second heart sound in congenital pulmonary valvular insufficiency. *Am Heart J* 69:603-609, 1965
237. Levin HS, Runco V, Wooley CF, et al: Pulmonic regurgitation following staphylococcal endocarditis: an intracardiac phonocardiographic study. *Circulation* 30:411-416, 1964
238. Criscitiello MG, Harvey WP: Clinical recognition of congenital pulmonary valve insufficiency. *Am J Cardiol* 20:765-772, 1967
239. Ford AB, Hellerstein HK, Wood C, et al: Isolated congenital bicuspid pulmonary valve: clinical and pathologic study. *Am J Med* 20:474-486, 1956
240. Miyatake K, Okamoto M, Kinoshita N, et al: Pulmonary regurgitation studied with the ultrasonic pulsed Doppler technique. *Circulation* 65:969-976, 1982
241. Gorlin R, McMillan IKR, Medd WE, et al: Dynamics of the circulation in aortic valvular disease. *Am J Med* 18:855-870, 1955
242. Portaluppi F, Vadlamudi LS, Atluri VL, et al: The pulmonary component of the second heart sound in acquired aortic stenosis. *Jpn Heart J* 22:527-536, 1981
243. Flohr KH, Weir EK, Chesler E: Diagnosis of aortic stenosis in older age groups using external carotid pulse recording and phonocardiography. *Br Heart J* 45:577-582, 1981
244. Johnson GR, Adolph RJ, Campbell DJ: Estimation of the severity of aortic valve stenosis by frequency analysis of the murmur. *J Am Coll Cardiol* 1:1315-1323, 1983
245. Bentivoglio LG, Sagarminaga J, Uricchio J, et al: Congenital bicuspid aortic valves: a clinical and haemodynamic study. *Br Heart J* 22:321-330, 1960
246. Wooley CF, Hosier DM, Booth RW, et al: Supravalvular aortic stenosis: clinical experiences with four patients including familial occurrence. *Am J Med* 31:717-725, 1961
247. Logan WFWE, Jones EW, Walker E, et al: Familial supravalvular aortic stenosis. *Br Heart J* 27:547-559, 1965
248. Vogel JHK, Blount SG Jr: Clinical evaluation in localizing level of obstruction to outflow from left ventricle: importance of early systolic ejection click. *Am J Cardiol* 15:782-792, 1965
249. Shem-Tov A, Schneeweiss A, Motro M, et al: Clinical presentation and natural history of mild discrete subaortic stenosis: follow-up of 1-17 years. *Circulation* 66:509-512, 1982
250. Pierce GE, Morrow AG, Braunwald E: Idiopathic hypertrophic subaortic stenosis. III. Intraoperative studies of the mechanism of obstruction and its hemodynamic consequences. *Circulation* 30 Suppl 4:152-213, 1964
251. Murgo JP, Alter BR, Dorethy JF, et al: Dynamics of left ventricular ejection in obstructive and nonobstructive hypertrophic cardiomyopathy. *J Clin Invest* 66:1369-1382, 1980
252. Shaver JA, Alvares RF, Reddy PS, et al: Phonoechocardiography and intracardiac phonocardiography in hypertrophic cardiomyopathy. *Postgrad Med J* 62:537-543, 1986
253. Hardarson T, de la Calzada CS, Curiel R, et al: Prognosis and mortality of hypertrophic obstructive cardiomyopathy. *Lancet* 2:1462-1467, 1973
254. Fiddler GI, Tajik AJ, Weidman WH, et al: Idiopathic hypertrophic subaortic stenosis in the young. *Am J Cardiol* 42:793-799, 1978
255. Braunwald E, Oldham HN Jr, Ross J Jr, et al: The circulatory response of patients with idiopathic hypertrophic subaortic stenosis to nitroglycerin and to the Valsalva maneuver. *Circulation* 29:422-431, 1964
256. Rosenblum R, Delman AJ: Valsalva's maneuver and the systolic murmur of hypertrophic subaortic stenosis: a bedside diagnostic test. *Am J Cardiol* 15:868-870, 1965
257. LeJemtel TH, Ribner HS, Strom JA, et al: Lack of accentuation by the Valsalva maneuver of the murmur of idiopathic hypertrophic subaortic stenosis: importance of monitoring the pulse. *Can Med Assoc J* 126:48-50, 1982
258. Kramer DS, French WJ, Criley JM: The postextrasystolic murmur response to gradient in hypertrophic cardiomyopathy. *Ann Intern Med* 104:772-776, 1986
259. Braunwald E, Brockenbrough EC, Frye RL: Studies on digitalis. V. Comparison of the effects of ouabain on left ventricular dynamics in valvular aortic stenosis and hypertrophic subaortic stenosis. *Circulation* 26:166-173, 1962
260. Braunwald E, Ebert PA: Hemodynamic alterations in idiopathic hypertrophic subaortic stenosis induced by sympathomimetic drugs. *Am J Cardiol* 10:489-495, 1962
261. Braunwald E, Brockenbrough EC, Morrow AG: Hypertrophic subaortic stenosis: a broadened concept (editorial). *Circulation* 26:161-165, 1962
262. Buda A, MacKenzie G, Wigle D: The Mueller Maneuver in muscular subaortic stenosis (abstract). *Circulation* 56 Suppl 3:38, 1977
263. Harrison DC, Braunwald E, Glick G, et al: Effects of beta adrenergic blockade on the circulation, with particular reference to observations in patients with hypertrophic subaortic stenosis. *Circulation* 29:84-98, 1964
264. Klein HO, DiSegni E, Dean H, et al: Increased intensity of the murmur of hypertrophic obstructive cardiomyopathy with carotid sinus pressure. *Chest* 93:814-820, 1988
265. Ishikawa K, Hirata F, Hirata S, et al: Reversed Rivero-Carvallo's sign in right-sided hypertrophic obstructive cardiomyopathy. *Chest* 83:694-696, 1983
266. Chandraratna PAN, Aronow WS: Genesis of the systolic murmur of idiopathic hypertrophic subaortic stenosis: phonocardiographic, echocardiographic, and pulsed Doppler ultrasound correlations. *Chest* 83:638-642, 1983
267. Simon AL, Ross J Jr, Gault JH: Angiographic anatomy of the left ventricle and mitral valve in idiopathic hypertrophic subaortic stenosis. *Circulation* 36:852-867, 1967

268. Stewart S, Mason DT, Braunwald E: Impaired rate of left ventricular filling in idiopathic hypertrophic subaortic stenosis and valvular aortic stenosis. *Circulation* 37:8-14, 1968

269. St John Sutton MG, Tajik AJ, Gibson DG, et al: Echocardiographic assessment of left ventricular filling and septal and posterior wall dynamics in idiopathic hypertrophic subaortic stenosis. *Circulation* 57:512-520, 1978

270. Come PC, Riley MF: Hypertrophic cardiomyopathy: disappearance of auscultatory, carotid pulse, and echocardiographic manifestations of obstruction following myocardial infarction. *Chest* 82:451-454, 1982

271. Schrire V, Vogelpoel L, Nellen M, et al: Silent mitral incompetence. *Am Heart J* 61:723-732, 1961

272. Hultgren HN: Intensity of the first heart sound in mitral stenosis with atrial fibrillation (abstract). *Clin Res* 6:84-85, 1958

273. Tei C, Shah PM, Cherian G, et al: The correlates of an abnormal first heart sound in mitral-valve-prolapse syndromes. *N Engl J Med* 307:334-339, 1982

274. Hultgren H, Leo T: Phonocardiographic features of combined mitral stenosis and insufficiency. *Medicine (Baltimore)* 38:103-118, 1959

275. Cohen LS, Mason DT, Braunwald E: Significance of an atrial gallop sound in mitral regurgitation: a clue to the diagnosis of ruptured chordae tendineae. *Circulation* 35:112-118, 1967

276. Osmundson PJ, Callahan JA, Edwards JE: Ruptured mitral chordae tendineae. *Circulation* 23:42-54, 1961

277. Guiliani ER: Mitral valve incompetence due to flail anterior leaflet: a new physical sign. *Am J Cardiol* 20:784-788, 1967

278. Braunwald E, Morrow AG, Cornell WP, et al: Idiopathic hypertrophic subaortic stenosis: clinical, hemodynamic and angiographic manifestations. *Am J Med* 29:924-945, 1960

279. Wells BG, Rappaport MB, Sprague HB: The sounds and murmurs in coarctation of the aorta: a study of auscultation and phonocardiography. *Am Heart J* 38:69-79, 1949

280. Castex MR: Les souffles méso-systoliques. *Arch Mal Coeur* 26:444-457, 1933

281. Jeresaty RM: Mitral valve prolapse-click syndrome. *Prog Cardiovasc Dis* 15:623-652, 1973

282. Jeresaty RM: Etiology of the mitral valve prolapse-click syndrome (editorial). *Am J Cardiol* 36:110-113, 1975

283. Segal BL, Likoff W: Late systolic murmur of mitral regurgitation. *Am Heart J* 67:757-763, 1964

284. Criley JM, Lewis KB, Humphries JO'N, et al: Prolapse of the mitral valve: clinical and cine-angiocardiographic findings. *Br Heart J* 28:488-496, 1966

285. Veyrat C, Kalmanson D, Gourtchiglouian C, et al: Localization of the origin of systolic clicks using echo-pulsed Doppler technique. *Angiology* 32:266-276, 1981

286. Barlow JB, Bosman CK, Pocock WA, et al: Late systolic murmurs and non-ejection ("mid-late") systolic clicks: an analysis of 90 patients. *Br Heart J* 30:203-218, 1968

287. O'Rourke RA, Crawford MH: The systolic click-murmur syndrome: clinical recognition and management. *Curr Probl Cardiol* 1:1-60, April 1976

288. Devereux RB, Perloff JK, Reichek N, et al: Mitral valve prolapse. *Circulation* 54:3-14, 1976

289. Bittar N, Sosa JA: The billowing mitral valve leaflet: report on fourteen patients. *Circulation* 38:763-770, 1968

290. Cooley DA, Frazer OH, Norman JC: Mitral leaflet prolapse: surgical treatment using a posterior annular collar prosthesis. *Cardiovasc Dis Bull Texas Heart Inst* 3:438-443, 1976

291. McKay R, Yacoub MH: Clinical and pathological findings in patients with "floppy" valves treated surgically. *Circulation* 48 Suppl 3:63-73, 1973

292. Robertson WS, Tavel ME: Mid-systolic sound associated with aortic insufficiency and bisferiens pulse. *Chest* 83:141-143, 1983

293. Abdulla AM, Frank MJ, Erdin RA Jr, et al: Clinical significance and hemodynamic correlates of the third heart sound gallop in aortic regurgitation: a guide to optimal timing of cardiac catheterization. *Circulation* 64:464-471, 1981

294. Harvey WP: Personal communication

295. Kohn D, Flatau E, Schiller D, et al: Knee-elbow position to detect the aortic diastolic murmur of regurgitation (letter to the editor). *Am J Cardiol* 51:918, 1983

296. Waller BF, Zoltick JM, Rosen JH, et al: Severe aortic regurgitation from systemic hypertension (without aortic dissection) requiring aortic valve replacement: analysis of four patients. *Am J Cardiol* 49:473-477, 1982

297. Bushong BB: Traumatic rupture of the aortic valve: report of two cases, one a proved and the other a probable example of this condition. *Ann Intern Med* 26:125-129, 1947

298. Gelfand D, Bellet S: The musical murmur of aortic insufficiency: clinical manifestations; based on a study of 18 cases. *Am J Med Sci* 221:644-654, 1951

299. Stembridge VA, Hejtmancik MR, Herrmann GR: Unusual musical murmurs of anterior cusp aortic regurgitation: report of ten cases. *Am Heart J* 48:163-172, 1954

300. Kohno K, Hiroki T, Arakawa K: Aortic regurgitation with dove-coo murmur with special references to the mechanism of its generation using dual echocardiography. *Jpn Heart J* 22:861-869, 1981

301. Flint A: On cardiac murmurs. *Am J Med Sci* 44:29-54, 1862

302. Laubry C, Pezzi C: *Les syndromes cardiaques: les rhythmes de galop.* Paris, G Doin & Cie, 1926

303. Luisada AA: On the apical sounds and murmurs in aortic regurgitation. *Am Heart J* 28:156-166, 1944

304. Gouley BA: The aortic valvular lesion associated with the Austin Flint murmur. *Am Heart J* 22:208-218, 1941

305. Laniado S, Yellin EL, Yoran C, et al: Physiologic mechanisms in aortic insufficiency. I. The effect of changing heart rate on flow dynamics. II. Determinants of Austin Flint murmur. *Circulation* 66:226-235, 1982

306. Duroziez P: Essai sur les maladies du coeur: du rhythme pathognomonique du rétrécissement mitral. *Arch Gen Med* 110:385-401, 1862

307. Longhini C, Baracca E, Aggio S, et al: The first heart sound in mitral stenosis. *Acta Cardiol* 46:73-77, 1991

308. Kelly JJ Jr: Diagnostic value of phonocardiography in mitral stenosis: mode of production of first heart sound. *Am J Med* 19:862-868, 1955

309. Messer AL, Counihan TB, Rappaport MB, et al: The effect of cycle length on the time of occurrence of the first heart sound and the opening snap in mitral stenosis. *Circulation* 4:576-580, 1951

310. Margolies A, Wolferth CC: The opening snap *(claquement d'ouverture de la mitrale)* in mitral stenosis, its characteristics, mechanism of production and diagnostic importance. *Am Heart J* 7:443-470, 1932

311. Schillig S: The significance of the rate and output related variations in the A_2-OS interval. *Am Heart J* 66:644-649, 1963

312. Gamble WH, Reddy PS: Preservation of the third heart sound in mitral stenosis. N Engl J Med 308:498-502, 1983

313. Reddy PS, Meno F, Curtiss EI, et al: The genesis of gallop sounds: investigation by quantitative phono- and apexcardiography. *Circulation* 63:922-933, 1981

314. Boone JA, Levine SA: The prognosis in "potential rheumatic heart disease" and "rheumatic mitral insufficiency." *Am J Med Sci* 195:764-770, 1938

315. Rahko PS: Doppler and echocardiographic characteristics of patients having an Austin Flint murmur. *Circulation* 83:1940-1950, 1991

316. Elkeles A: Disseminated ossified nodules in the lungs associated with mitral stenosis. *Proc R Soc Med* 40:405-408, 1947

317. Davis FW Jr, Scarborough WR, Mason RE, et al: The ballistocardiogram in mitral stenosis. *Circulation* 7:503-510, 1953

318. Decker JP, Hawn CVZ, Robbins SL: Rheumatic "activity" as judged by the presence of Aschoff bodies in auricular appendages of patients with mitral stenosis. I. Anatomic aspects. *Circulation* 8:161-169, 1953

319. Fuchs RM, Fisher J, Schuster EH, et al: The systolic murmur of mitral stenosis. *Johns Hopkins Med J* 151:220-221, 1982

320. Clark RM, Anderson W: Rheumatic activity in auricular appendages removed at mitral valvoplasty. *Am J Pathol* 31:809-819, 1955

321. Clawson BJ, Bell ET, Hartzell TB: Valvular diseases of the heart: with special reference to the pathogenesis of old valvular defects. *Am J Pathol* 2:193-234, 1926

322. Barber H, Osborn GR: A case of mitral stenosis the result of trauma. *Guys Hosp Rep* 87:510-515, 1937

323. Baronofsky ID, Skinner A: Ligation of left auricular appendage for recurrent embolization. *Surgery* 27:848-852, 1950

324. Iga K, Tomonaga G, Hori K: Continuous murmur in Lutembacher syndrome analyzed by Doppler echocardiography. *Chest* 101: 565-566, 1992

325. Edwards JE, Carey LS, Neufeld HN, et al: *Congenital Heart Disease: Correlation of Pathologic Anatomy and Angiocardiography.* Vols. 1 and 2. Philadelphia, WB Saunders Company, 1965

326. Hubbard TF, Neis DD: The sounds at the base of the heart in cases of patent ductus arteriosus. *Am Heart J* 59:807-815, 1960
327. Rudolph AM, Scarpelli EM, Golinko RJ, et al: Hemodynamic basis for clinical manifestations of patent ductus arteriosus. *Am Heart J* 68:447-458, 1964
328. Gibson GA: Clinical lectures on circulatory affections. I. Persistence of the arterial duct and its diagnosis. *Edinburgh Med J* 8:1-10, 1900
329. Haring OM, Luisada AA, Gasul BM: Phonocardiography in patent ductus arteriosus. *Circulation* 10:501-510, 1954
330. Neill C, Mounsey P: Auscultation in patent ductus arteriosus: with a description of two fistulae simulating patent ductus. *Br Heart J* 20:61-75, 1958
331. Campbell M: Natural history of persistent ductus arteriosus. *Br Heart J* 30:4-13, 1968
332. Powell ML: Patent ductus arteriosus in premature infants. *Med J Aust* 2:58-60, 1963
333. Keith TR, Sagarminaga J: Spontaneously disappearing murmur of patent ductus arteriosus: a case report. *Circulation* 24:1235-1238, 1961
334. Kohler CM, McNamara DG: Elongated patent ductus arteriosus with intermittent shunting. *Pediatrics* 39:446-448, 1967
335. Calne DB, Raftery EB: Patent ductus arteriosus in an elderly man. *Br Heart J* 28:716-717, 1966
336. Rudolph AM, Gootman NL, Kaplan N, et al: Anomalous left coronary artery arising from the pulmonary artery with large left-to-right shunt in infancy. *J Pediatr* 63:543-549, 1963
337. Liebman J, Hellerstein HK, Ankeney JL, et al: The problem of the anomalous left coronary artery arising from the pulmonary artery in older children: report of three cases. *N Engl J Med* 269:486-494, 1963
338. Usman A, Fernandez B, Uricchio JF, et al: Aberrant origin of left coronary artery combined with mitral regurgitation in an adult. *Am J Cardiol* 8:130-134, 1961
339. Spodick DH: Acoustic phenomena in pericardial disease. *Am Heart J* 81:114-124, 1971
340. Sugiura T, Iwasaka T, Yuasa F, et al: Clinical significance of pericardial rub with regional ventricular dilatation. *Chest* 100:128-130, 1991
341. Markiewicz W, Brik A, Brook G, et al: Pericardial rub in pericardial effusion: lack of correlation with amount of fluid. *Chest* 77:643-646, 1980
342. Cossio P, Berconsky I, Dambrosi RG: Auricular and ventricular pericardial frictions. *Am Heart J* 24:223-229, 1942
343. Spodick DH: Pericardial rub: prospective, multiple observer investigation of pericardial friction in 100 patients. *Am J Cardiol* 35:357-362, 1975
344. Heberden W: Some account of a disorder of the breast. *Med Trans Coll Physicians Lond* 2:59-67, 1772
345. Lewis T: *Diseases of the Heart: Described for Practitioners and Students.* New York, Macmillan & Company, 1933
346. Roughgarden JW, Newman EV: Circulatory changes during the pain of angina pectoris: 1772-1965 – a critical review. *Am J Med* 41:935-946, 1966
347. Forrester JS, Chatterjee K, Swan JC: Hemodynamic monitoring in patients with acute myocardial infarction. *JAMA* 226:60-61, 1973
348. Georgopoulos AJ, Sones FM Jr, Page IH: Relationship between arterial pressure and exertional angina pectoris in hypertensive patients. *Circulation* 23:892-900, 1961
349. Maseri A, Severi S, De Nes M, et al: "Variant" angina: one aspect of a continuous spectrum of vasospastic myocardial ischemia; pathogenetic mechanisms, estimated incidence and clinical and coronary arteriographic findings in 138 patients. *Am J Cardiol* 42:1019-1035, 1978
350. Parry CH: *An Inquiry Into the Symptoms and Causes of the Syncope Anginosa, Commonly Called Angina Pectoris.* London, Cadell and Davies, 1799
351. Robinson BF: Cited by Epstein SE, Braunwald E: Beta-adrenergic receptor blocking drugs: mechanisms of action and clinical applications. *N Engl J Med* 275:1106-1112, 1966
352. Harvey WP: Tachycardias: diagnosis and treatment. *DM* December 1961, pp 1-45
353. Harvey WP, Corrado MA: Multiple sounds in paroxysmal ventricular tachycardia: an aid in diagnosis by auscultation. *N Engl J Med* 257:325-327, 1957
354. Chizner MA: Bedside diagnosis of the acute myocardial infarction and its complications. *Curr Probl Cardiol* 7:1-86, December 1982
355. Adolph RJ: Second heart sound: the role of altered electromechanical events. In *Physiologic Principles of Heart Sounds and Murmurs* (American Heart Association Monograph No. 46). Edited by DF Leon, JA Shaver. New York, American Heart Association, 1975, pp 45-57
356. Burch GE, De Pasquale NP, Phillips JH: Clinical manifestations of papillary muscle dysfunction. *Arch Intern Med* 112:112-117, 1963
357. Levine SA, Harvey WP: Temporary relief of anginal pain by carotid sinus stimulation. *Trans Assoc Am Physicians* 60:255-258, 1947
358. Levine SA: Carotid sinus massage: a new diagnostic test for angina pectoris. *JAMA* 182:1332-1334, 1962
359. Hurst JW, Blackard E: Inspection and palpation of pulsations on the front of the chest (editorial). *Am Heart J* 56:159-164, 1958
360. Eddleman EE Jr, Langley JO: Paradoxical pulsation of the precordium in myocardial infarction and angina pectoris. *Am Heart J* 63:579-581, 1962
361. Hurst JW, Schlant RC: *Examination of the Heart.* Part 3. New York, American Heart Association, 1972
362. Butterworth JS, Reppert EH Jr: Auscultatory findings in myocardial infarction. *Circulation* 22:448-452, 1960
363. Wall TC, Califf RM, Harrelson-Woodlief L, et al: Usefulness of a pericardial friction rub after thrombolytic therapy during acute myocardial infarction in predicting amount of myocardial damage. *Am J Cardiol* 66:1418-1421, 1990
364. Griffith GC, Hegde B, Oblath RW: Factors in myocardial rupture: an analysis of two hundred and four cases at Los Angeles County Hospital between 1924 and 1959. *Am J Cardiol* 8:792-798, 1961
365. Selzer A, Gerbode F, Kerth WJ: Clinical, hemodynamic, and surgical considerations of rupture of the ventricular septum after myocardial infarction. *Am Heart J* 78:598-607, 1969
366. Barzilai B, Davis VG, Stone PH, et al: Prognostic significance of mitral regurgitation in acute myocardial infarction. *Am J Cardiol* 65:1169-1175, 1990

CHAPTER

3

Electrocardiography

A. Standard electrocardiography and vectorcardiography

Gerald T. Gau, M.D.

ELECTROCARDIOGRAPHY (ECG) is as useful and important a tool in clinical diagnosis now as it was 4 to 6 decades ago. Since the 1930s and the development of Wilson's unipolar leads, the standard 12-lead scalar ECG has been and still is the primary method for graphic display of the heart's electrical activity.[1-4]

It is important to remember that the ECG is only a graphic display of cardiac electrical events and thus requires much careful clinical correlation. All ECGs should be read twice: once for the changes present (descriptive abnormalities) and a second time by the clinician caring for the patient in light of the clinical situation. Similar ECG patterns can be provoked by different clinical problems. The necessary differential diagnoses are reviewed in the clinical discussion of these patterns.

ECG, a relatively new (since the 1900s) and continually evolving method, is not exact or always accurate, and it has many limitations. The heart is not equidistant from all leads of the recording system, and the body is not a homogeneous electrical volume conductor. Standard ECG recordings may have a left arm dominance because the heart is located in the left anterior chest. Precordial lead proximity effects and changes due to variations in torso shape and heart location may introduce variations from individual to individual. All this is complicated by possible inaccurate electrode positioning due to technical placement error, and many graphic artifacts can be produced.

Despite all these limitations, the ECG is remarkably useful and clinically valuable. As with any laboratory test, however, it must be integrated with the clinical picture, and if it does not conform, its interpretation should be carefully reevaluated or the tracing repeated.

Since the 1930s, efforts to overcome some of these discrepancies in ECG recording have led to the development of three-dimensional recording systems, or vectorcardiograms (VCGs). These orthogonal (mutually perpendicular) lead systems (X, Y, and Z leads) have many theoretical advantages. Use of resistor-corrected lead systems reduces distortion from body torso changes and heart location, proximity changes, or left arm dominant effects. The three-dimensional (X,Y,Z) recording systems also give more accurate information in the direction assumed by initial forces and better timing information. X,Y,Z data display the ECG events in the format of either graphic X,Y,Z leads or of planar loops. This format is clearer than the traditional 12-lead scalar presentation, much as a graph is clearer than a table. Because of this, in the discussion that follows, both scalar and VCG presentations of the major diagnostic categories will be discussed.

The author is indebted to the late Dr. Raymond D. Pruitt for his significant input to this chapter.

CARDIAC ELECTROPHYSIOLOGIC EVENTS

The clinical ECG provides a graphic record of potential changes induced at the surface of the body by forces generated by the myocardial fibers as they undergo depolarization and repolarization during the spread of the excitation process.[1,2,4] The P wave, P-R interval, QRS complex, ST segment, T wave, and U wave are identified in Figure 3A-1. Relative dimensions of these deflections can be assessed in this figure. Precise measurements will be given in the discussion of individual components.

Genesis of the QRS complex

In the resting state the potential difference across the myocardial cell membrane is approximately 85 to 90 mV (interior of the cell negative to the outer surface). This potential is maintained by active transport mechanisms that produce different ion concentrations across the cell membrane. The interior of the cell has a higher potassium concentration than the exterior surface of the cell, which is immersed in a medium having a higher sodium concentration than the interior.

In the heart are specialized cells—pacemaker cells—

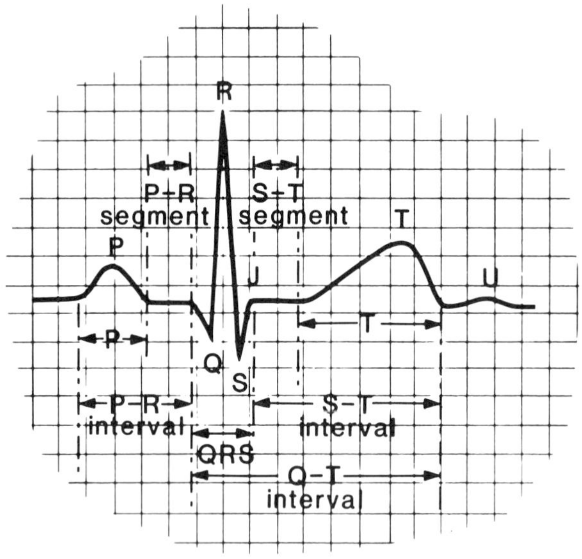

Fig 3A-1 Components of the scalar electrocardiogram with standard wave labeling (P, Q, R, S, T, U) and clinically useful interval and segment measurements.

Table 3A-1 Conduction velocities in human heart

Region	Tissue	Velocity, cm/sec
Atria	Normal	75
	Muscle from patient with mitral stenosis and atrial fibrillation	10-20
Ventricles	Normal muscle:	
	Transmural	30
	Parallel with fibers	50-60
	Acute ischemia	*
Specific conduction system	Normal large branches	250
Subendocardial	Normal	50-75
Purkinje system	Diseased	20-25

*Slow—a few centimeters per second or less.

which are distinguished by their property of slow alteration in the diastolic component of cell membrane potential. In this process there is a progressive decrease in resting transmembrane potential from −85 to −60 mV to achieve a potential that results in spontaneous depolarization of the cell membrane. This electrical event is associated with a cation flux across the cell membrane, first discharging and then restoring the potential difference across the cell membrane. This process moves along the cell membrane as a wavefront, the discharge phase being rapid compared with the restorative phase. The flow of current is from the discharged (negative) to the charged (positive) resting polarized membrane.

The excitation process spreads through the myocardium of the ventricle much more slowly than through the Purkinje system: at 400 mm/sec and up to 4,000 mm/sec, respectively[5,6] (Table 3A-1). This wave of excitation traverses rapidly through specialized conducting pathways of the heart and then spreads more slowly over the contracting myocardial fibers, causing their depolarization. This electrical phenomenon in turn initiates an electrochemical mechanical event—contraction of the myocardial fibers.

The path that the electrical chain of events takes depends on the location of the pacemaker that generates the impulse. The pacemaker tissue in the heart that has the most rapid diastolic membrane depolarization determines the site of origin of the rhythm of the heart. This area is usually the sinoatrial node. When the sinoatrial node initiates electrical events, it suppresses all other pacemaker sites by depolarizing them as the excitation process spreads through the heart. With the sinoatrial node located in the high right atrium and the path of depolarization following special conducting pathways through the heart with each heartbeat, the potential field generated thereby determines the character of the deflection recorded at the body surface in conventional 12-lead ECGs or in VCGs derived from one of the established lead systems.

Electrical axis of the heart

Whether produced by an isolated muscle strip, by an exposed heart, or by a heart maintained in its normal relationship to other body structures, an electromotive force is a vectoral quantity in that it has both direction and magnitude, in contrast to a scalar quantity which has only magnitude. It is apparent that the electromotive force developed during the spread of the excitation over a single cell thus may be represented vectorally (Fig 3A-2). The magnitude of these forces is expressed by the length of the arrow and their orientation, by the direction of the head. The head of the arrow points toward the positive component of the electrical field.

To transpose the concepts of this illustration to a vectoral description of the electromotive forces produced by the heartbeat, it is necessary to consider the course followed by the wave of excitation as it spreads over the ventricle. From a theoretical approach, the potential difference between two extremities may be derived when the instantaneous electrical axis is known. In practice, the known and unknown factors are reversed. The potential difference between any two extremities can be recorded with a galvanometer and, from these data, the mean or the instantaneous electrical axis of the heart can be derived.

It is essential to this calculation to know the potential difference, at any one instant, between one of three extremities (right arm [R], left arm [L], or left leg [F]) and each of the other two. This information can be derived from a record on which two of the standard limb leads are inscribed simultaneously. In Figure 3A-3, complexes from leads I and III are represented. A line perpendicular to the isoelectric line can be drawn through any portion of

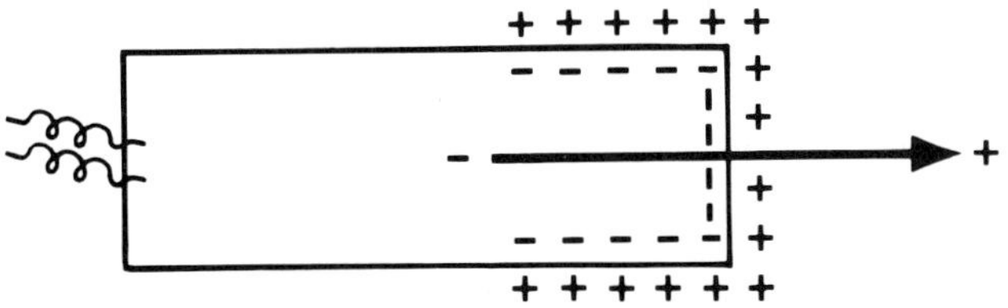

Fig 3A-2 Direction *(arrowhead)* and magnitude (length of arrow) of electromotive force from a single myocardial cell.

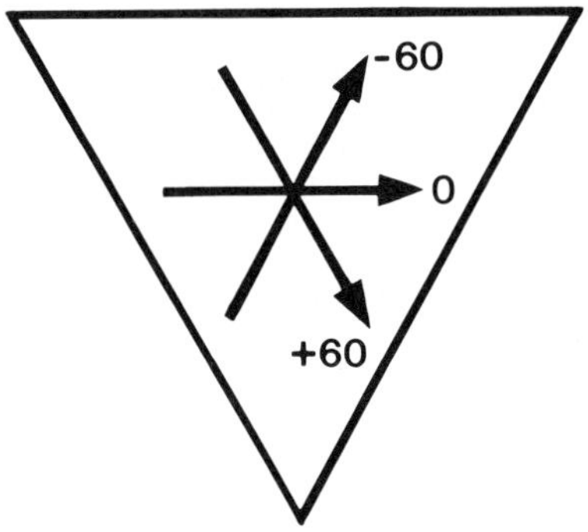

Fig 3A-4 Triaxial reference system. The three sides of Einthoven's triangle are arranged so as to bisect one another, showing axis polarity and direction (see text).

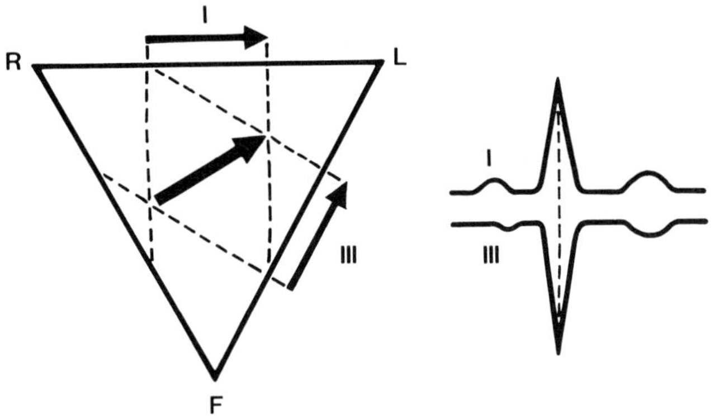

Fig 3A-3 Instantaneous electrical axis derived from potential differences recorded in leads I and III and plotted on the Einthoven equilateral triangle (see text).

the QRS complex. The distance between the isoelectric line and the point at which the perpendicular crosses the QRS deflection can be measured. Lines equivalent to this distance are plotted along the appropriate side of the equilateral triangle (see Fig 3A-3), and perpendiculars are erected from the terminal points of these lines. The intersection of these perpendiculars from the two sides defines the limits of the line representing the instantaneous electrical axis.

An instantaneous electrical axis derived in this manner in an approximation in two respects:

1. Because the electromotive forces produced by the heartbeat create an electrical field in which potential differences decrease as distance from the heart increases, the potential differences between the extremities are only a fraction of those developed in the corresponding plane at the surface of the heart. Hence, the electrical axis derived from potential differences between extremities is an index only of the direction and not of the absolute magnitude of cardiac forces.
2. Because only those components of the electrical forces produced by the heartbeat that are parallel to the frontal plane affect the potential of the extremities, it is only these components of the true electrical axis that are manifest in an electrical axis derived from limb lead ECGs.

For the most accurate computation of the mean electrical axis, precise determination of the areas of the QRS complexes in two of the three standard limb leads would be a preliminary procedure. In practice it is expedient and, in most instances, reasonably accurate to measure the height of the R waves and depth of the S waves in complexes from two limb leads. The algebraic sum of the R and S waves in each of these leads is plotted along the appropriate side of the equilateral triangle, and the mean electrical axis is derived in the same manner as the instantaneous axis. In fact, because of the nature of the complexes and the disposition of the perpendicular line in Fig 3A-3, the mean electrical axis would correspond to the particular instantaneous electrical axis selected for illustrative purposes.

To permit definition of the electrical axis in concise terms, Einthoven proposed the following conventions:

1. When the vectoral representation of the forces produced by the heart is parallel to lead I, the electrical axis is zero (Fig 3A-4).
2. Rotation of the vector in a counterclockwise fashion produces an electrical axis of negative sign.
3. Rotation of the vector in a clockwise fashion produces an electrical axis of positive sign.

For application of these conventions to the description of a clinical state, axis deviations may be defined by these criteria: *(a)* an axis between 0° and +90° lies within the normal range; *(b)* an axis of −1° or less lies in the range of left-axis deviation; and *(c)* an axis of +90° or more lies in the range of right-axis deviation. The same procedures may be applied in computing the axis of P waves and T waves.

The use of the Einthoven triangle to compute a frontal plane mean electrical axis is based on certain assumptions:[7]

1. The heart is a material point in a homogeneous medium.
2. The heart is equidistant from the points to which the electrodes are attached.
3. By virtue of assumptions 1 and 2, the resistances between these points and the heart are equal.

The question of whether or not these assumptions are valid for practical use, if not perfectly so, has generated much controversy.

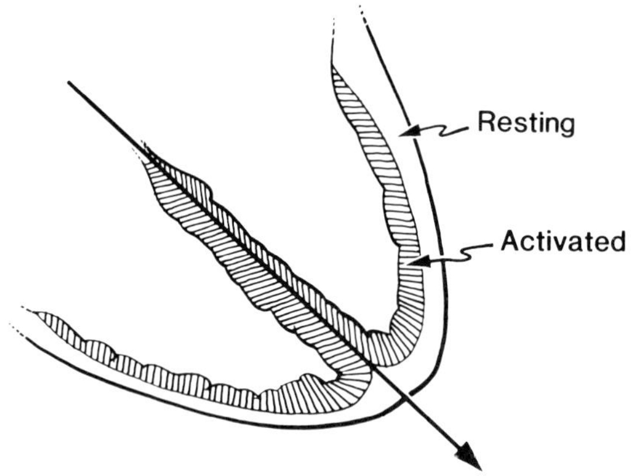

Fig 3A-5 Instantaneous electrical QRS axis. *Arrow* represents summation of component electromotive forces (see text).

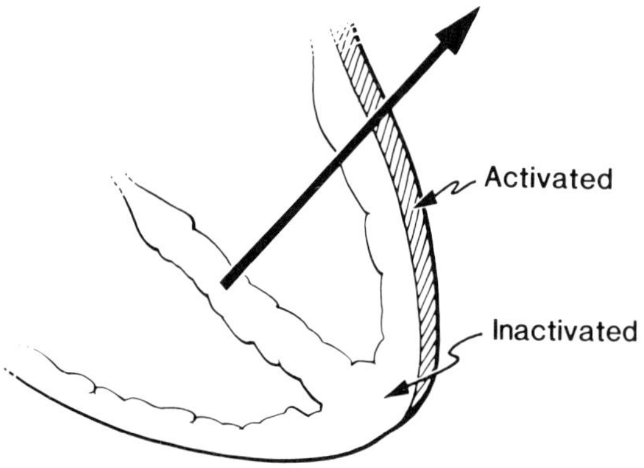

Fig 3A-6 Instantaneous electrical QRS axis in later phase of ventricular myocardial muscle activation. *Arrow* represents summation of component electromotive forces (see text).

The septal forces develop first, and the forces in the base of the free wall of the left ventricle develop last. But, because of the high speed at which endocardial activation occurs compared with myocardial, myocardial excitation in the basal region will have begun before the deeper-lying septal tissues are activated. At this stage in the spread of the wave of excitation, the relationship between activated and resting tissues might have a distribution as is represented in Fig 3A-5. The vectoral summation of all the component electromotive forces existing at this stage would then be represented by an arrow which, in turn, may be held to indicate the electrical axis of the heart at this particular moment. Such a vector is commonly designated "the instantaneous electrical axis." At a later phase in the spread of excitation, the relationship of activated to inactivated tissue might be as represented in Fig 3A-6. The instantaneous electrical axis at this time would have the direction indicated by the arrow.

The mean electrical axis of the heart is derived from the component instantaneous electrical axes. If events transpired as in Figures 3A-5 and 3A-6, the mean electrical axis for this heart would occupy a position represented by the thick arrow in Figure 3A-7. A loop linking the tips of these several instantaneous electrical axes would form a frontal plane ventricular VCG.

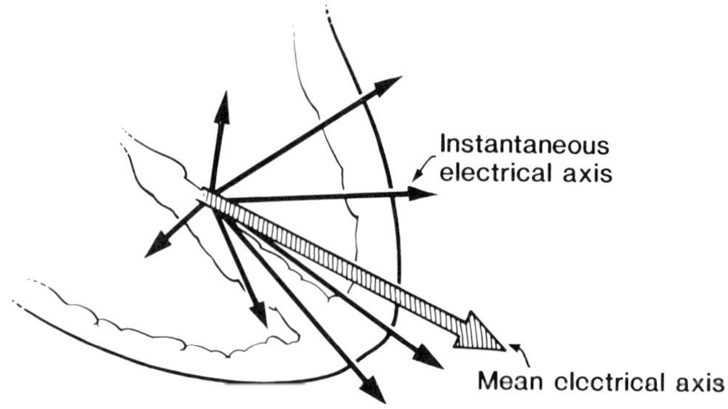

Fig 3A-7 Mean electrical QRS axis *(hatched arrow)* derived from multiple instantaneous electrical axes. Tip of arrow indicates direction; length of arrow indicates voltage or magnitude. Line joining all arrow tips in sequence makes a frontal plane vector loop (VCG).

According to the postulates of the Einthoven triangle hypothesis, the heart may be regarded as a point, and the electrical forces associated with the heartbeat may be represented by a dipole. The direction of the instantaneous electrical axis is determined by the orientation in the conducting medium of this dipole. The potentials of the extremities represent the potentials at sites approximately equidistant from this dipole, and these sites may be disposed relative to the dipole as are the apices of an equilateral triangle with respect to the central point of the triangle. If the postulates of the triangle hypothesis are valid, then the potential differences produced between the extremities by the electromotive force represented vectorally in the instantaneous electrical axis may be derived by projecting onto each side of an equilateral triangle the component of electrical axis that is parallel to that side. This may be achieved by erecting perpendiculars from each side of the triangle to the ends of the centrally disposed vector (Fig 3A-8).

Genesis of the T wave

The electromotive forces that accompany depolarization of the myocardium are represented in the QRS deflections of the ECG; those forces that develop during repolarization are manifested in the T wave. The process of repolarization appears to differ from that of depolarization in at least two respects:

1. The time consumed in restoring the potential difference across the cell membrane is greater than that required for its resolution. This conclusion is based on the fact that the T wave usually is a broader deflection of lower amplitude than is the QRS complex that precedes it. It is supported also by the form of the curves recorded in experiments in which

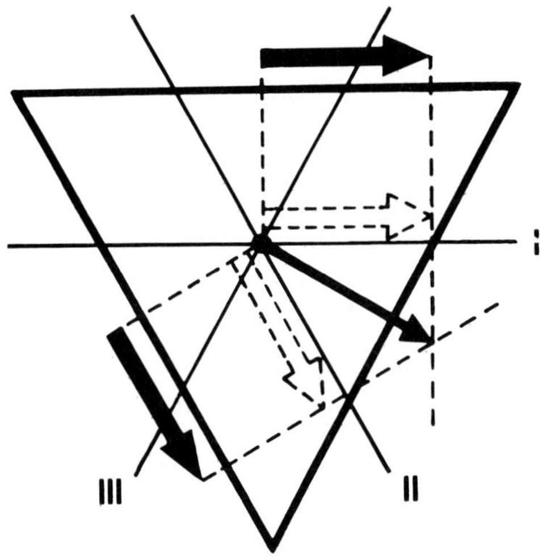

Fig 3A-8 Einthoven triangle and triaxial reference. Method of determining instantaneous electrical axis.

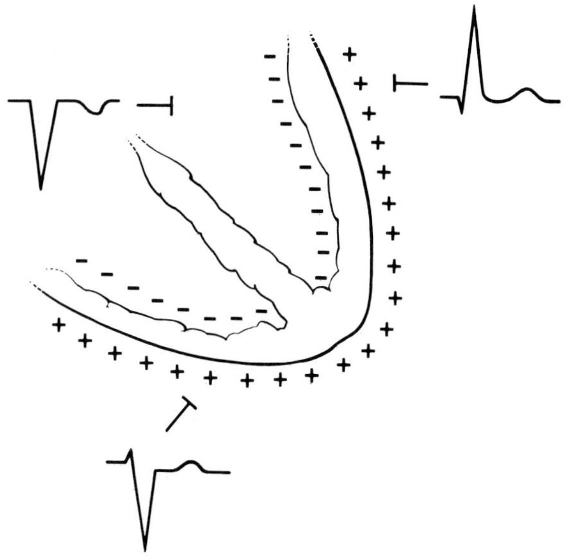

Fig 3A-9 Ventricular repolarization (see text).

changes in the potential difference across a cell membrane are measured directly.

2. Whereas in the normally activated heart the excitatory process consistently moves across any small portion of the ventricular wall from the endocardial to the epicardial surface, the process of repolarization follows no fixed course. This inconstancy is an expression of variations, among fibers in different portions of the heart, in the time interval that separates the onset of depolarization and the completion of repolarization.

"If all the ventricular muscle passed through the period of excitation in the same time and in the same way, the area of QRS and the area of T would be equal in absolute magnitude, but opposite in sign, and the area of QRST would be zero."[8] This precise relationship between QRS and T wave areas does not obtain consistently in ECGs recorded in clinical or experimental studies. In explanation of these deviations, Wilson and associates[8] proposed that among the myocardial fibers a gradient exists in the duration of the excited state: restitution of the potential difference across the cell membrane begins relatively sooner in some fibers and is completed relatively earlier.

Therefore, the direction and form of the T wave will be an expression of two factors: (1) The net area of the QRS complex. All else being equal, an R wave of large area will be followed by an inverted T wave of equal area. (2) Deviations from this relationship are an expression of a gradient among the myocardial fibers in the duration of the excited state. In regard to factor 1, those T wave changes that occur as a consequence of variations from normal in the net area of the QRS complex, as in bundle-branch block, may be regarded as secondary to alterations in another and antecedent process, excitation. T-wave changes that result from alterations in the gradient are an expression of changes in the process of repolarization itself and, therefore, are classed as primary.

In the normal heart, there is a gradient that results in the process of repolarization being at a more advanced stage in the epicardial cells than in the endocardial fibers at the same instant in time. The orientation of the electromotive force across the ventricular walls under these circumstances will be as indicated in Figure 3A-9. The intensity of these forces waxes and wanes, being greatest at the instant when the peak of the T wave is formed. No dipoles have been placed along the line representing the ventricular septum because in repolarization, as in depolarization, the forces developed within one side of the septum cancel a major portion of those produced by the other side.

MODERN LEAD SYSTEMS

The system used at the Mayo Clinic utilizes 14 leads to record both the Frank X,Y,Z and the standard ECG 12-lead system (Fig 3A-10). The limb leads and the standard V_1-V_6 leads are placed as for all ECG recording. The four additional electrodes are E electrode, in the fifth intercostal space, midline anterior over the lower sternum; I electrode, at the level of the fifth intercostal space, in the right midaxillary line; M electrode, at the level of the fifth intercostal space, midline posterior; and H electrode, anterior, on the right or left side of the neck. Precordial electrodes V_4 and V_6 and the left leg electrodes are shared by the X,Y,Z and standard lead systems.

Lead X consists of a right V_6 opposite the standard left V_6, thus providing a left-right reference axis which is positive to the left. X resembles V_6 in configuration but assays the information contained in V_4 and V_6. Thus, increased voltage in X suggests left ventricular hypertrophy, a pathologic Q wave suggests lateral wall infarction, and a deep dominant S wave (rS complex) suggests both right ventricular hypertrophy and probable right-axis deviation. The axis of the X lead, or left-to-right plane, is at the level of V_6, which is considerably lower than the left-to-right planes of leads I and aV_L. These have their respective positive poles at left shoulder level and hence face the high lateral wall of the left ventricle, whereas X

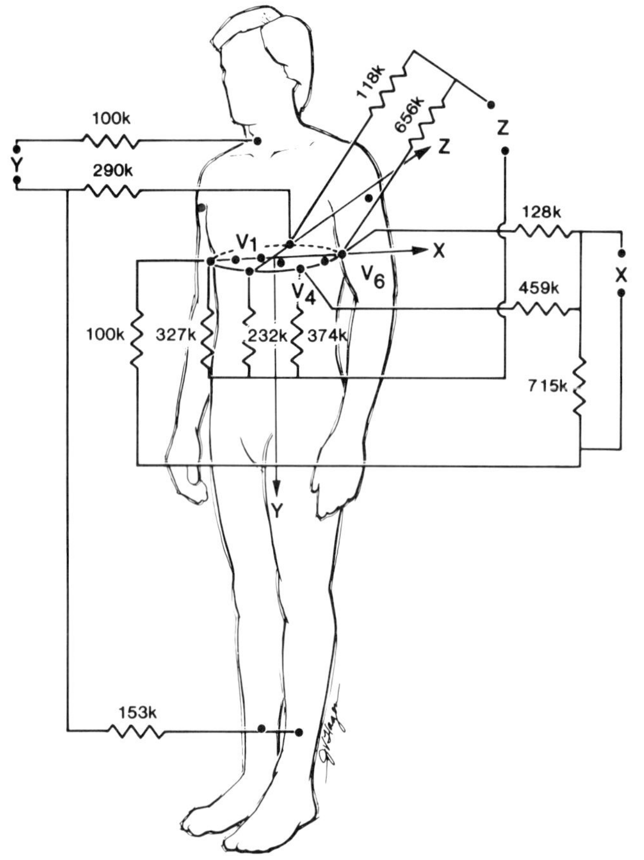

Fig 3A-10 Electrode positions for combined standard ECG and Frank lead VCG.

faces the lateral and apical portions of the left ventricle. Therefore, an infarct involving only the high lateral wall (I and aV_L) would be unseen (electrically silent) in X. This represents an area of poor coverage by the Frank orthogonal lead system, whereas the posterior wall is the problem area in the standard 12-lead ECG.

Lead Y, which represents the inferior-superior axis, consists of a standard left leg lead shared by II, III, and aV_F and the neck electrode and is positive in an inferior direction. Displaying this polarity similar to that of aV_F allows Y to have a configuration similar to that of lead aV_F. Lead Y is critical in the diagnosis of left-axis deviation, inferior wall myocardial infarction, retrograde P waves, and the presence of atrial flutter. It contains the information present in leads II, III, and aV_F on the standard ECG.

Lead Z consists of an electrode placed over the sternum and another placed at the same level posteriorly, over the spine. The positive pole in lead Z is posterior. Z resembles an inverted V_1 or V_2 in the standard ECG. It is a much more sensitive lead for the presence or absence of anterior force than either V_1 or V_2 because both of these are angulated and to the right and left, respectively, of the true anterior-posterior axis and thus suffer from proximity and angulation effects. Therefore, the diagnosis of an anteroseptal myocardial infarction is more reliable from the Z lead than from either the V_1 or V_2, especially in borderline situations such as low anterior force, the presence of left bundle-branch block, and the presence of left ventricular hypertrophy.

Simultaneous plotting of any two orthogonal leads against one another determines a specific plane, and the display then shifts from scalar P, QRS, and T waves to the P, QRS, and T loops.

1. X vs. Z—horizontal plane
2. X vs. Y—frontal plane
3. Y vs. Z—sagittal plane

Vectorcardiography (VCG) is particularly helpful for the following: (1) detection of right ventricular hypertrophy when the ECG is normal or equivocal; (2) differentiation of left bundle-branch block from left ventricular hypertrophy or their coexistence; (3) detection of right ventricular hypertrophy in the presence of right bundle-branch block; (4) diagnosis of true posterior myocardial infarction; (5) diagnosis of an old inferior wall infarction when the ECG is equivocal; (6) detection of anterior or posterior myocardial infarction in the presence of right bundle-branch block; and (7) differentiation of primary from secondary T-wave changes.

The deficiencies of VCG loops include the absence of information regarding rate and rhythm and the difficulty in timing and measuring complexes. These are overcome by using computer technology to analyze X,Y,Z data; the duration and timing information of these data is more precise than it is from standard ECG tracings. With use of the constricted form of the computer-derived 12-lead ECG, X,Y,Z Holter data provide additional information for the more accurate diagnosis of arrhythmias.[9] There is some lack of clarity of P and T loops because of magnification, and of course there is the potential electrical silence of the high lateral wall. Further small but important ECG changes, such as a slight deviation of an ST segment or slight reduction in the height of a T wave, often are impossible to record or are not recognized well on the VCG loop representation. The proximity magnification of standard ECG for these minor changes sometimes is beneficial and calls attention to these events when they are localized. It is thought that use of X,Y,Z data adds about 15% to the diagnostic accuracy of standard 12-lead tracings.

NORMAL ELECTROCARDIOGRAM AND VECTORCARDIOGRAM

The term "a normal ECG" may be somewhat misleading. The identification of a normal ECG tracing is based on a statistical study of apparently normal males and females. It is well recognized that greater than 70% of American men over the age of 22 have gross evidence of coronary artery disease at the time of autopsy. Unrecognized heart disease undoubtedly was present in these men, and the term "normal" therefore is misleading. Recognizing this deficiency, a "characteristic normal pattern" can be recognized, however, and it does give a basis against which the more dramatic abnormalities related to specific organic heart problems can be contrasted.

In the normal ECG, electrical activation begins in the

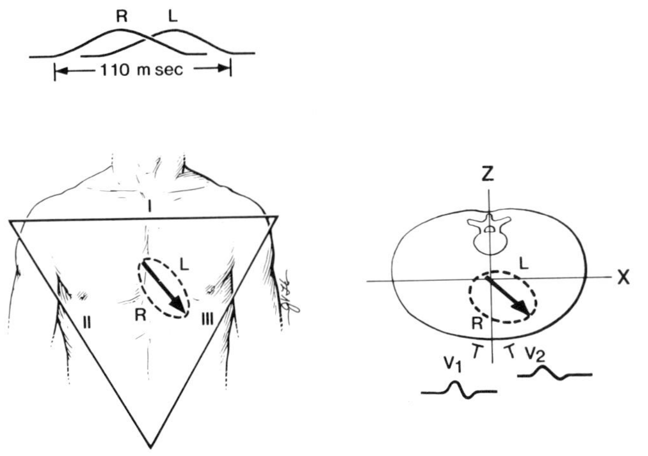

Fig 3A-11 **Upper left,** surface electrical tracing of right and left atrial activities showing time sequence of P wave components and normal activation time. **Lower left,** frontal plane P-wave loop with mean axis paralleling lead II. **Lower right,** horizontal plane P-wave loop and mean axis illustrating surface V_1 and V_2 precordial P wave patterns in normal ECG.

sinoatrial node, traverses special conducting pathways through the atria to the atrioventricular (AV) node, where there is electrical delay, and then enters the bundle of His and the right and left bundle branches to produce depolarization of the lower chambers and the surface ECG. This pathway is similar with each heartbeat, so there is a characteristic surface potential that is generated and this characteristic potential is recognized as the normal ECG. As long as the electrodes are placed in the same position each time the recording is made, there should be a characteristic normal pattern for a specific person.

Atrial activation is initiated by the sinoatrial node in the high right atrial area. The activation begins on the right side and then spreads through the special conducting pathways to the left side; during most of the process, activation occurs simultaneously in the right and left atria (except for initiation and completion being later on the left). This activation generates the P wave (Fig 3A-11). The total duration of the P wave from the beginning of right atrial activation to the end of left atrial activation is less than 110 msec. A slight dip exists between the right and left activations, but the resolution of the present recording system is not adequate to pick up this notch at the top of a normal P wave. The atrial muscle is thin and does not generate a large potential, and therefore the P wave voltage is small – a normal P wave is less than 2.5 mm on the recording paper. The usual P vector is directed in a downward, leftward, and inferior direction, parallel to lead II. Lead II is often selected for rhythm strip analysis because of this parallel relationship to the P frontal axis. Atrial electrical activity is away from lead aV_R and results in an upright P wave in all limb leads except aV_R, in which it is inverted. The P wave is biphasic in leads V_1 and V_2 (see Fig 3A-11). After atrial activity traverses the special conducting pathways through the atria and the atrial muscle, it reaches the area of the AV node where there is a delay. The normal duration from the onset of the P wave to the beginning of the QRS complex is 120 to 200 msec.

After the impulse traverses the AV node and enters the bundle of His, there is rapid activation of the special conducting pathways through the ventricle, down the right and left bundle branches.[10] Activity begins first at the left side of the septum where the early branches from the left conducting system traverse the septum in a left-to-right direction. Because the septum is located at a 45° angle to the anterior chest wall and in a slightly oblique position with the left lower than the right side, the activation going from the left to the right has a slightly superior orientation. This means that the initial depolarizing force of the ventricular muscle is due to electrical activation of the interventricular septum oriented spatially to the right and anteriorly and is slightly superior in direction. The left ventricle, being electrically dominant (10 times the strength of the right), controls the major electrical potential, and the right ventricle is essentially silent in a normal ECG.

As electrical activation spreads over the endocardial surface of the left ventricle and the right ventricle, after septal depolarization the anterior and posterior septa are involved, generating forces moving posteriorly, anteriorly, and down slightly to the left which is the direction of the plane of the left ventricle. This orients the electrical potential in a downward and leftward direction, bringing the main body of the loop activation of the free wall oriented to the left, slightly posterior and inferior to the E point. The terminal portion of the loop in the remaining ventricle to be activated is the base of the wall, which is oriented posteriorly and inferiorly. The inscription of the loop is always counterclockwise in the horizontal plane and clockwise in the sagittal plane; in the frontal plane it is either clockwise or counterclockwise with a narrow configuration (Fig 3A-12,A).

The VCG and ECG representation of septal depolarization is depicted by an initial upward R wave in precordial electrodes V_1 and V_2, while septal activation recorded from the left precordial electrode is depicted as a small Q wave in lead V_6. Because of the orientation of the forces and the location of leads V_1-V_6 over the left ventricle, the voltage increases and the R wave increases from V_1 to V_6 (Fig 3A-12,B). In the normal ECG the septal Q wave is less than 40 msec in duration and less than 25% of the total R wave. Normally there should be Q waves present in left precordial leads and also in leads III and aV_F in recordings from hearts with vertical position orientation. The R wave voltage is 5 to 16 mm in the standard limb leads, 5 to 12 mm in leads aV_L and aV_F, and 15 to 30 mm in leads V_1-V_6. The intrinsicoid deflection (the time from Q wave to the peak of the R wave) is less than 30 msec in leads V_1-V_3 and less than 45 msec in leads V_4-V_6. The normal QRS is less than 120 msec in duration; the average QRS lasts 80 to 90 msec.

Electrical activation of the ventricle begins in the endocardial surface and spreads into the ventricular septum and through the free wall of the ventricle to the epicardial surface, where final activation occurs at the

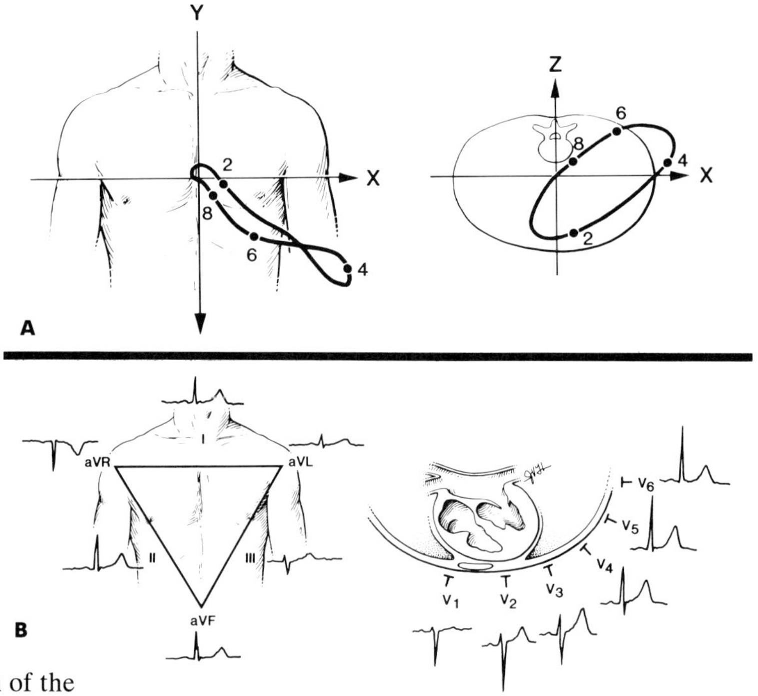

Fig 3A-12 **A,** normal ECG frontal and horizontal plane loops. Sequential numbers indicate speed and direction of loop inscription (see text). **B,** normal ECG showing surface standard 12-lead morphology (see text).

posterobasal portion of the heart. After activation of the left ventricle, repolarization or recovery occurs. Recovery begins in the outer surface of the myocardium and moves inward. The inner depolarized myocardium remains negative compared to the recovering outer myocardium—orientation of repolarization is oriented predominately in an epicardium-to-endocardium direction, from the negative to positive, and so produces upward T waves in leads recorded by precordial electrodes.[11]

A general rule of thumb is that the normal T wave is upright in all leads that have an upright R wave; it is inverted in lead aV_R as are the P wave and QRS complex. The T wave may be inverted in leads V_1 and V_2 with their downward S deflections. The T-wave amplitude is generally about one-fifth that of the R wave, its form is elliptical, and its long axis lies anteriorly, inferiorly, and medially to the long axis of the QRS loop. The spatial angle between the two loops rarely exceeds 45°. The direction of the inscription of the T loop is the same as that of the QRS loop.

If the following lead polarity rules are kept in mind, the recorded waveform information from any unipolar direct or semidirect electrode will indicate the direction and alteration of any electrical events that are under that electrode location.

1. By convention, the exploring δ electrode is attached to the galvanometer so that positivity (i.e., leading aspect of excitation process) produces a positive deflection.
2. In all unipolar leads, relative positivity produces an upward deflection.
3. Limb leads I, II, and III give upright deflections when the direction of the P-QRS-T electrical axis is to the left and inferior.
4. Any potential wavefront moving away from an exploring electrode produces a downward deflection.

The interpretation of an ECG/VCG proceeds in three steps. The first step is determination of rhythm and heart rate and measurements of P wave, P-R interval, QRS duration, Q-T interval, T wave, and frontal plane axis. The second step in ECG analysis involves interpretation of the graphic information on the tracing itself. A diagnosis is deduced from the graphic information, and a preliminary report is generated. The final step in interpretation is made by the clinician who is caring for the patient. The clinical correlation with the preliminary report is the most important and useful step in ECG analysis because it brings into clinical context the graphic information and the diagnoses suggested.

The following section will review, in an orderly fashion, abnormalities of rate and rhythm, P wave, P-R interval, QRS complex, ST-T abnormalities, and U waves. However, even though a tracing may be presented in a discussion of a specific topic, such as myocardial infarction, it may have broader applications of clinical relevance—e.g., an ECG displaying changes that are relics of an old anteroseptal myocardial infarction can also exhibit left ventricular hypertrophy from long-standing hypertension, bifascicular block due to infarction, and left ventricular aneurysm. If the patient is on digitalis therapy, the ST segment will be deformed; if a hypokalemic state has been produced by long-term diuretic therapy, prominent U waves also may be present.

CLINICAL APPLICATIONS OF ELECTROCARDIOGRAPHY AND VECTORCARDIOGRAPHY

Rate and rhythm

A detailed description of cardiac rhythm analysis and physiology is given in chapter 22. The concept of pacing tissue in the heart, the specialized conducting pathways, and the mechanisms of abnormal cardiac rhythms will not be reviewed here.

The sinus node is the dominant cardiac impulse generator and has a normal rate of 60 to 100 beats/min. Heart rates originating from the sinus node in excess of 100 beats/min are called "sinus tachycardia"; when less than 60 beats/min they are called "sinus bradycardia." The extremes of sinus rates, fast or slow, may represent either appropriate or inappropriate (abnormal) cardiac sinus responses, depending on the clinical situation—for example, sinus bradycardia to 30 to 40 beats/min in a trained athlete or in the presence of acute myocardial infarction.

Sinus arrhythmia with variation in the rate of impulses generated by the sinus node, either in phase with respiration or unrelated to respiration, is a normal variant of normal sinus function. This is more commonly seen in younger persons and persons with slower heart rates.

Malfunction of the sinus node with sinoatrial block (failure to form impulse) or exit block (failure of the impulse to get out of the sinus node) producing a dropped P-QRS-T cycle and sinus pauses (failure to produce a sinus impulse for variable periods) represent abnormal sinus rhythm.

Sick sinus syndrome with inappropriate rate responses (bradycardia, tachycardia, sinus pauses, and intermittent atrial tachyarrhythmias, usually atrial fibrillations) represents a disease process that affects all of the heart's conducting tissue. The definition of normal rhythm from infancy to old age remains uncertain. Studies have shown atrial and ventricular premature contractions, supraventricular tachycardia, junctional rhythm, atrial fibrillation, variable heart block, and nonsustained ventricular tachycardia in supposedly healthy subjects.[12-15]

P wave

P-wave electrical potential begins in the high right atrium and spreads in an inferior anterior direction. Its electrical axis is directed in an inferior, slightly anterior, right-to-left direction, producing a P wave that is upright in standard leads I and II, positive or biphasic in lead III, upright in lead aV_F, and inverted in lead aV_R. It tends to be biphasic in lead aV_L. In the frontal plane the P axis lies between +45° and +65°. However, there can be considerable variation in the P axis, −30° to a +80° orientation. It is rare to have a P axis that is +90° or greater; an axis of this orientation suggests the diagnosis of dextrocardia. The normal P-wave duration is less than 110 msec (Fig 3A-13). It begins with right atrial activation, followed by left atrial activation, combined activation through the middle of the P wave, and left atrial activation ending after right atrial activation has been completed.

On the ECG the P wave appears to have a rounded peak without a visible notch. The normal amplitude is less than 2.5 mV.

In analyzing abnormalities of the P wave, one looks first at the electrical axis to determine the origin of activation. Then, one determines the duration of the P wave, assesses the morphology, and notes the voltage.[16]

Left atrial enlargement. This term is preferred to "left atrial hypertrophy" although hypertrophy is usually present when left atrial enlargement is present. Left atrial enlargement occurs when there is disease involving the left heart and there is additional stretch and increased pressure in the left atrium that causes enlargement of that chamber and secondary hypertrophy. In mitral valve disease there are characteristic P-wave abnormalities that can be detected on the ECG. Because the left atrium is located posterior and to the left of the right atrium, with enlargement there is a greater shift of electrical forces in a posterior leftward direction and, because of the enlarged area that needs to be covered by the excitation process, there is a delay in electrical events that occur through the left atrium. The beginning of the P wave is activation of the right atrium, as it is in the normal P wave. The latter portion of the P wave is due to left atrial activity and is prolonged because of the larger area of the dilated chamber. This increases the duration to more than 110 msec, which is the first criterion of left atrial enlargement—atrial conduction delay (see Fig 3A-13).

A second feature of the P wave related to the prolonged activation of the left atrium is the presence of a later voltage peak separate from the right atrial voltage peak. This is manifested by a dip between right atrial and left atrial deflections—i.e., a notch at the top of the P wave called "P mitrale." This is commonly seen in patients with mitral valve disease. The electrical axis of the P wave tends to lie in a more leftward direction, usually between +45° and −30°. We therefore would expect to see a broadly notched P wave, with duration greater than 110 msec, in standard lead I. Because of the posterior leftward orientation of the atrial conduction delay that is present, we would expect to see a more slurred, later component of the P wave registered in leads V_1 and V_2 attended by a sagging terminal segment. Morris and colleagues[17] have

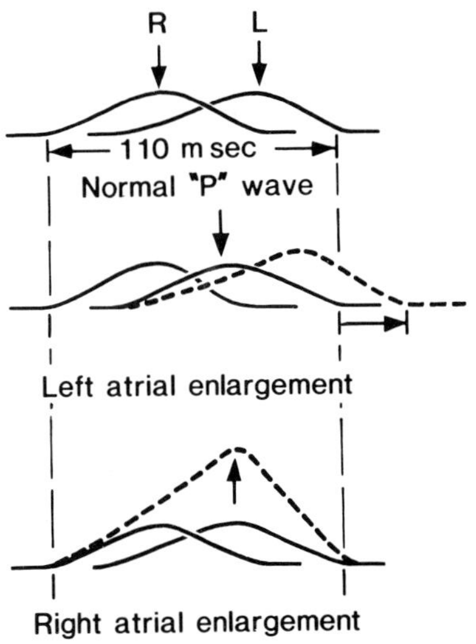

Fig 3A-13 **Top,** normal surface P-wave morphology, illustrating right and left atrial activation sequence and normal duration. **Middle,** left atrial enlargement *(broken line),* illustrating delayed peak and left atrial activation time producing a prolonged P-wave duration and notched P-wave morphology. **Bottom,** right atrial enlargement *(broken line),* illustrating effective combined right and left atrial voltage peaks occurring at the same time with resulting tall peaked P waves.

used the product of the duration of the terminal segment and the depth of the negative terminal portion of the P wave in leads V_1 to identify left atrial enlargement. A product equal to or more negative than -0.04 mm · s has been found to be useful in detecting left atrial enlargement (Morris index). The classic P mitrale configuration is more characteristic of mitral stenosis than of mitral insufficiency, but any condition that is associated with left atrial dilatation results in changes meeting the described criteria:

1. Shift in the electrical axis of the P wave to a more leftward position, between $+45°$ and $-30°$.
2. Increased duration of the P wave, to more than 110 msec, due to prolonged activation of the enlarged left atrial chamber
3. Notched P wave due to separation of right atrial and left atrial peak potentials
4. ECG changes indicative of the posterior leftward shift of atrial activity, producing a downward-sagging terminal P potential in anterior precordial leads

These criteria and their clinical utility have been reviewed by Alpert and Munuswamy[18] and have been found to be both specific and predictive by echocardiographic correlation.[19]

Right atrial hypertrophy (P pulmonale or P congenitale). With congenital or acquired cardiac defects attended by increased pressure on the right side of the heart, dilatation of the atrial chamber and secondary hypertrophy cause characteristic ECG changes. Excitation times are prolonged because of the dilated and hypertrophied chamber wall. Since the initial component of the P wave is produced by right atrial activation and the latter portion by left atrial activation, a delay in right atrial activation generally does not lengthen the P wave. Both right atrial and left atrial excitation are occurring simultaneously, and so their voltages are added, producing a tall, peaked P wave (see Fig 3A-13). A voltage of more than 2.5 mV indicates right atrial hypertrophy. Because the right atrium is located anteriorly and to the right of the left atrium and, when enlarged, has a more prominent influence on the direction of manifest atrial vectors, there tends to be a shift in the P wave frontal axis into a more vertical direction, usually from $+65°$ to $+90°$ but rarely exceeding $+90°$.

Therefore, the criteria for right atrial enlargement would be

1. Axis shift toward the vertical position, of $+65°$ to $+90°$
2. Normal duration of the P wave
3. Tall, peaked P wave with voltage more than 2.5 mV

The presence of the prominent upright P wave in the vertically oriented ECG leads is a common early manifestation in cor pulmonale resulting from emphysema or chronic obstructive lung disease.

Another ECG feature that suggests right atrial enlargement is the pattern of a QR, qR, or Qr deflection over the right precordial leads, suggesting a cavity potential as a result of a prominent dilated underlying right atrial chamber.

Combined atrial enlargement. A high-peaked P wave associated with a longer duration suggests that there is combined atrial enlargement. Another feature that suggests combined atrial enlargement is the presence of tall, peaked P waves in vertically oriented ECG leads II, III, and aV_F associated with a prominent large biphasic P wave in the anterior precordial leads V_1 and V_2.

Atrial infarction. The ECG diagnosis of atrial infarction is difficult to make. The association of sinus node dysfunction and atrial arrhythmias in the presence of an underlying myocardial infarction may suggest atrial infarction. Deviation of the P-R interval with either elevation or depression is compatible with atrial infarction. In cases of ventricular myocardial infarction, one should look for alterations in P-wave morphology, P-R baseline changes, and the presence of associated sinus dysfunction as evidence of possible atrial infarction.[20] However, there is no definite diagnostic ECG manifestation of atrial infarction that can be recognized diagnostically from the ECG.

P-R interval

The normal P-R interval, representing the time from the beginning of the P wave to the beginning of the QRS complex, is 120 to 200 msec. The delay from atrial activation to the beginning of ventricular activation varies from individual to individual and represents different delays through the AV node tissue, until activation spreads rapidly through the specialized conducting tissue in the ventricles. The P-R interval also varies depending on heart rate—persons with slower heart rates have slightly longer P-R intervals. An abnormally short P-R interval suggests rapid atrial to ventricular excitation and little delay in the AV node. It can be a normal finding in some, and it can suggest accessory conduction pathways from atrium to ventricle in others. This will be considered below under normal QRS duration with abnormal AV excitation.

Prolongation of the P-R interval to more than 200 msec can be associated with varying degrees of AV block. This will be discussed under abnormal QRS duration. The mechanism of delay in AV conduction can occur at several levels and can include inherent disease in the conducting tissue itself, secondary ischemia affecting the conducting tissue, or drugs or extraneous vagal influence on the AV node or the lower conducting tissue.

QRS complex

Myocardial infarction. The ECG recognition of myocardial infarction in the past was thought to be related to the extent and location of the myocardial lesion—epicardial, endocardial, or transmural. It was believed that epicardial and endocardial lesions produced alterations in ST-T waves but did not produce the Q waves that were thought to be the hallmark of transmural infarction. It is now recognized that there is no clear relationship between the extent of necrosis into the thickness of the ventricular wall and the presence or absence of a Q wave.[21-24] For this reason, the terms "subendocardial myocardial infarction" and "transmural myocardial infarction" have been replaced with "non-Q-wave myocardial infarction" and "Q-wave myocardial infarction." (See chapter 30.) Freifeld et al.[25] have shown that the extent of

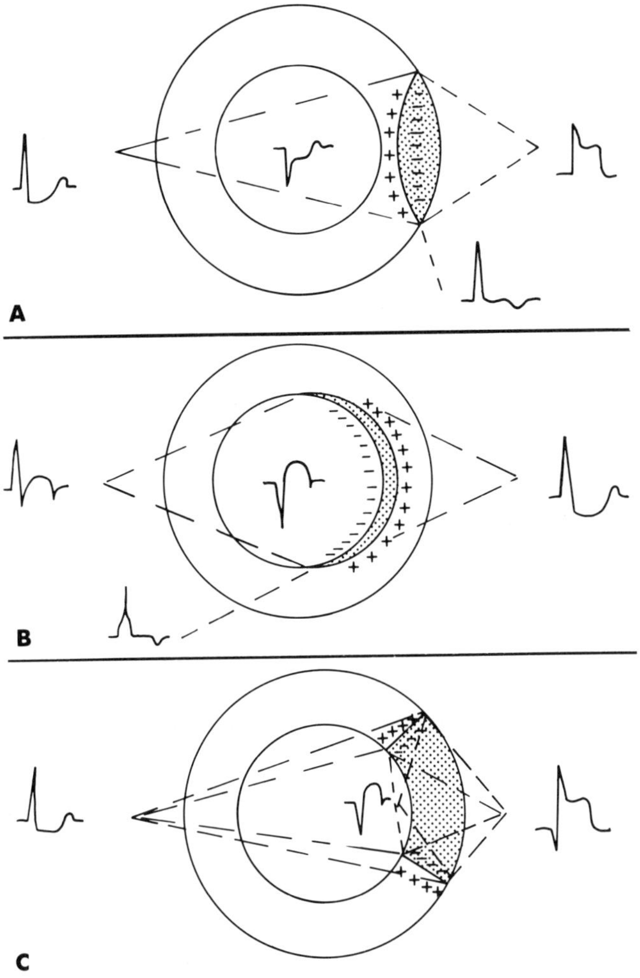

Fig 3A-14 QRS and T wave morphology as seen by exploring electrode placed at different sites with respect to myocardial lesion. Injured area depicted (−) as opposed to (+) normal cell polarity, producing current of injury. **A,** epicardial lesion. **B,** endocardial lesion. **C,** transmural lesion.

the necrosis in relation to the Q wave, although not entirely consistent, holds as a concept, because nontransmural myocardial infarction has a 10% to 20% incidence of Q waves, whereas transmural myocardial infarctions that extend all the way through the myocardium at one point (mixed lesions) or involve large areas of full wall thickness have Q waves in 80% to 87%. To understand the ECG changes, the anatomic concept of nontransmural and transmural is still useful and will be discussed. Since non-Q-wave myocardial infarctions and Q-wave myocardial infarctions are so clinically different,[26] we advise adherence to this new concept.

The ST-T changes produced by cell injury and ischemia are complex.[27,28] Figure 3A-14 illustrates the types of ST-T changes recorded in unipolar leads when the exploring electrode is placed at different sites with respect to the lesions. Electrical current always flows from negative (injured cells) to positive (normal cells) and so produces a "current of injury" that is responsible for the ST injury shift that is noted. This current flow induces a positive electrical field in the direction of the myocardial lesion, with opposing reciprocal changes in areas directly opposite to it.

EPICARDIAL INJURY–PERICARDITIS. The characteristic changes of the ECG in pericarditis depend on the existence of a myocardial injury which, although localized to the epicardium, is widely distributed over the surfaces of the ventricles. Because of this epicardial localization, significant QRS deformities are not present. Because of the diffuse surface involvement, the ST segment shows a similar upward displacement in leads from sites overlying widely separated portions of the epicardium (Fig 3A-15). A vector of injury can be drawn representing the mean effect of those forces developed within the damaged tissues during the period of ST inscription in the ECG. This vector can be projected onto the sides of the Einthoven triangle, and the effect of the injury on the ST segments of the standard leads can be derived in this manner. It is apparent that the vector of injury may rotate in space just as does the mean electrical axis; the direction and degree of the segmental displacement in leads I, II, and III will be influenced by the position of the heart as well as by the distribution of the epicardial lesion.

SUBENDOCARDIAL INJURY. Perhaps the most patent manifestations of subendocardial injury are the ECG alterations that accompany it. Whereas in the presence of pericarditis and myocardial infarction gross morphologic changes are readily identified at certain phases in the

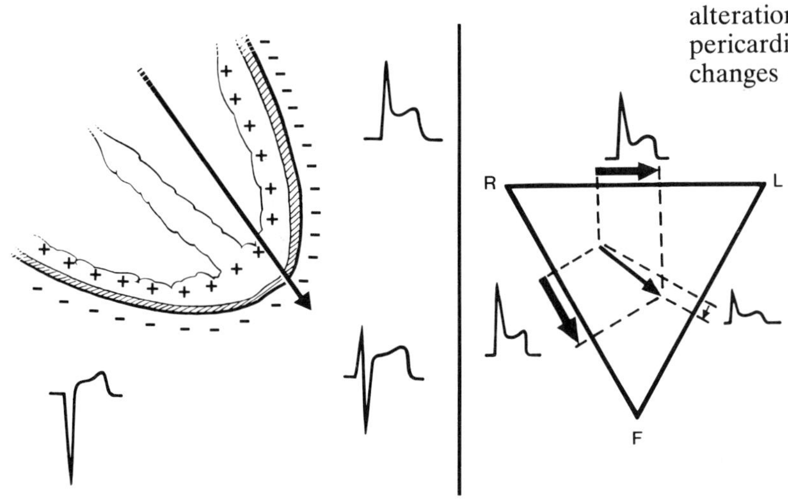

Fig 3A-15 Effect of pericarditis on ECG. *Arrows* illustrate mean vector of injury, but with diffuse pericarditis ST elevation is produced in leads over widely separated areas of the myocardium.

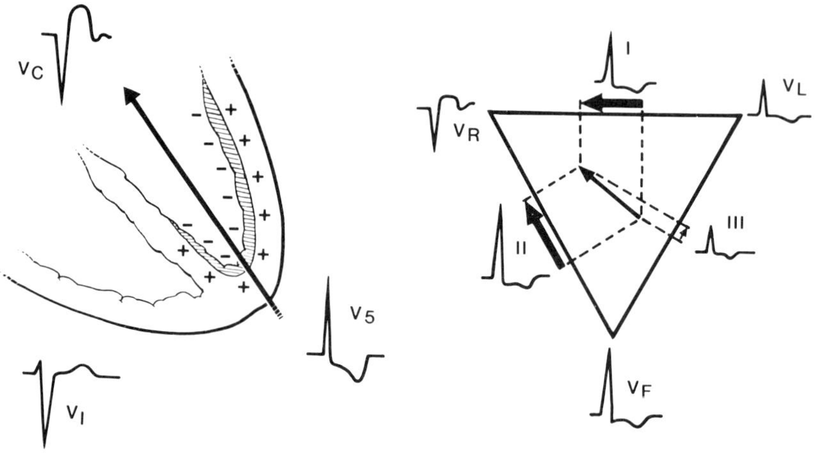

Fig 3A-16 Effect of subendocardial injury on ECG. *Arrows* indicate mean vector of injury (current of injury) induced by subendocardial injury. Diagram illustrates resting polarized state after QRS inscription.

evolution of the lesion, subendocardial injury may be attended by few changes in myocardial structure and may leave no gross scars. This peculiarity of subendocardial injury probably is related to the transient character of the injury state and, in turn, this evanescence is dependent upon the fact that the origin of the trauma lies in a temporary disparity between the metabolic requirements of the subendocardial myocardium and the functional capacity of the coronary circulation to these tissues.

ECG changes are encountered commonly in tracings recorded from patients during an attack of angina pectoris or during oxygen deprivation studies on patients with disease of the coronary arteries.[29-31] In such ECGs, the ST segment is depressed in leads recorded with the exploring electrode over the area most involved. Similar depression is encountered also in the segment of one or more of the standard limb leads. In such records, elevation of the ST segment may occur in the unipolar lead from the right arm (V_R). Some evidence has been presented to indicate a basic similarity in the form of curves recorded in V_R leads and those obtained from an electrode introduced into the right ventricular cavity (Fig 3A-16). The electric field set up by a diffuse subendocardial injury is similar to one that would be produced if, at the end of the QRST interval, the injured muscle were polarized in the sense indicated in the diagram.

TRANSMURAL INJURY. When transmural myocardial infarction is acute, three zones of compromised ventricular myocardium may be distinguished: a central core of necrosis, a surrounding zone of ischemic injury, and a peripheral zone of ischemia. The necrotic core produces the pathologic Q wave in the leads overlying the infarct and identifies a transmural myocardial infarction. The zone of ischemic injury results in ST-segment elevation in the leads overlying the infarct, and the peripheral zone of ischemia produces an inverted T wave.

As a consequence of acute myocardial infarction the QRS complex is altered in four ways: (1) the Q wave becomes abnormal in both amplitude and width (40 msec); (2) the R wave is diminished or entirely obliterated; (3) the ST segment is elevated in those leads overlying the infarct and reciprocally depressed in leads opposite to a transmural infarct; and (4) T-wave inversion over ischemic zones and reciprocal elevation of that deflection may occur in zones remote from the ischemic myocardium. The usual order of appearance of changes is ST-segment elevation, R-wave loss simultaneous with the appearance of pathologic Q waves, and, finally, T-wave changes as ischemic zones evolve, followed by regression of the ST-segment deviations. Although this sequence is the typical one, there are many variations of it that can occur in patients experiencing acute myocardial infarction.

From a VCG approach, myocardial infarction alters the direction of the initial forces such that they point away from the infarct zone (vector direction corresponds to the Q wave), the ST injury vector points toward the infarct, and the altered T-wave vector points away from the infarct and opposite in direction to the QRS changes. Especially when there is scarring of the inferior and posterior ventricular walls, vectorial analysis with orthogonal leads at this late stage is consistently more sensitive in identifying residual changes inasmuch as major ST- and T-wave abnormalities are likely to have been resolved in both scalar and vectoral leads and diagnostic Q waves in scalar leads are either diminished or absent[32] (see below, in discussion of specific healed infarcts).

The diagnosis of a transmural myocardial infarction can be made by ECG in 85% to 90% of cases when both scalar and VCG criteria are applied. In contrast, nontransmural or subendocardial infarction cannot be diagnosed consistently and reliably from the ECG alone and requires other corroborative clinical evidence. But, even in transmural infarction the diagnosis can become difficult or impossible when there are coexisting ECG abnormalities such as those of left bundle-branch block,[33] ventricular preexcitation of the Wolff-Parkinson-White type, cor pulmonale, left ventricular hypertrophy,[34] or previous old infarction or when a transmural infarct is localized to the posterior wall[35] and no pathologic Q wave is present or the infarct is restricted to the high lateral wall and the pathologic Q wave is confined to leads I and aV_L and thus often is overlooked.

In analyzing the ECG of a patient with a transmural myocardial infarction, three clinically important decisions are required: (1) the age of the infarct—acute, recent, or remote; (2) location of the infarct—anterior, inferior, posterior, lateral, or some combination; and (3) identification of associated problems—including rhythm disturbances, bundle-branch block, fascicular blocks, ventricu-

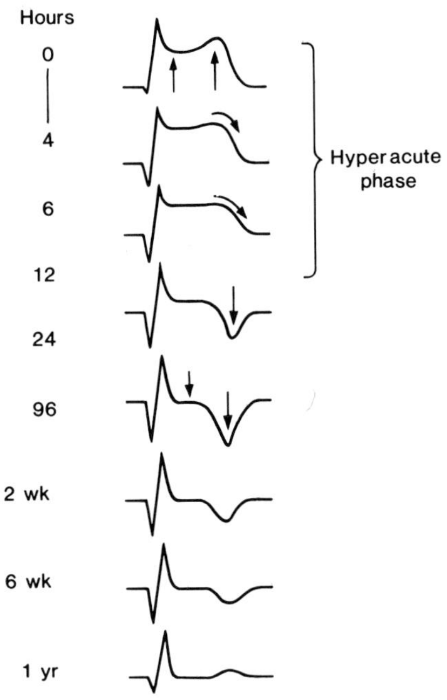

Fig 3A-17 Evolution of ECG changes in myocardial infarction. Serial morphological typical QRST changes with time after transmural myocardial infarction are depicted. See text for details of hyperacute, evolving, and healed phases of the myocardial infarction.

lar conduction delay in the zone of infarction, and, if remote, the possibility of a ventricular aneurysm.

Determining the age of an infarct is related primarily to the serial analysis of the ST-T-segment changes (Fig 3A-17). In the hyperacute stage (first several hours) the characteristic finding is ST-segment elevation (convex upward) with an upright T wave recorded in leads overlying the infarct and corresponding ST-segment depression in leads opposite to the infarct (reciprocal changes) (Fig 3A-18). The degree of ST-segment depression must be equal to or less than the degree of ST-segment elevation to be considered a reciprocal phenomenon. If the ST-segment depression is greater in depth and duration opposite the area of infarction, it indicates primary ischemia in the subendocardial wall of the heart opposite the area of infarction and is related to significant coronary stenosis in the coronary vessels supplying the area of myocardium opposite the area of myocardial infarction.[36] This finding then unmasks more significant coronary artery disease. The T wave, which initially is upright, undergoes gradual inversion during a period ranging from minutes to hours, and deep symmetric T-wave inversion evolves and dominates the infarct pattern over the next 7 to 10 days (Fig 3A-19). By day 4 the ST-segment elevation usually, but not always, returns to baseline. This evolving transition identifies the infarct as being recent (4 to 10 days). From an ECG standpoint, absence of evolving changes in the ST segment or of serial changes in the T wave makes determination of the age of the infarct impossible—it could range from 1 week to several years. If the ST segment remains elevated beyond 6 weeks, an underlying ventricular aneurysm or a large dyskinetic segment is suggested.

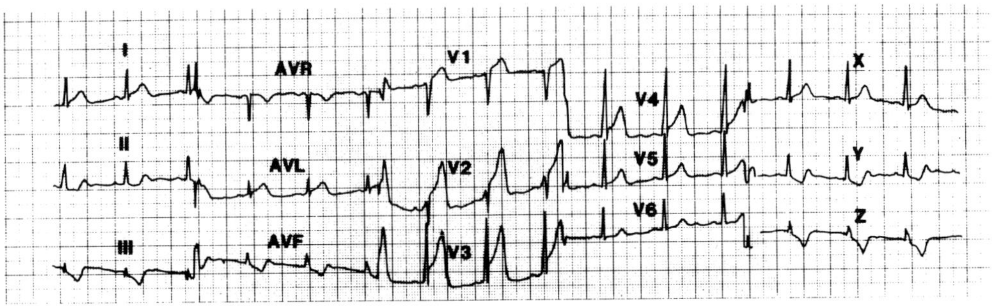

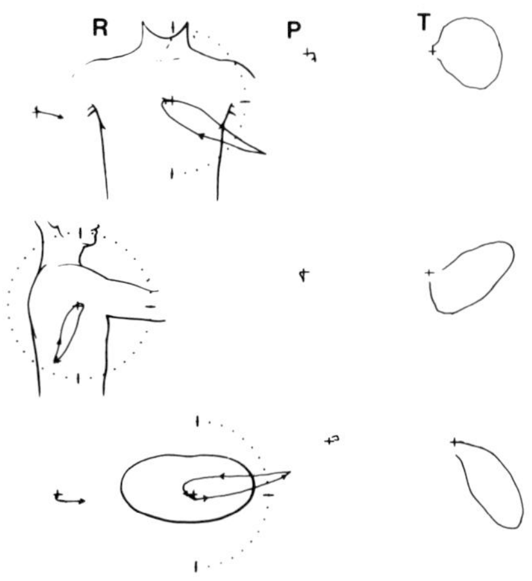

Fig 3A-18 Typical acute changes seen in anteroseptal myocardial infarction. Note the ST-segment elevation in leads V_1, V_2, V_3, and V_4 with reciprocal ST-segment displacement in II, III, and aV_F. The T wave is upright in precordial leads V_1 through V_4, with marked ST elevation and no evidence of Q-wave formation at this stage. This is the hyperacute pattern.

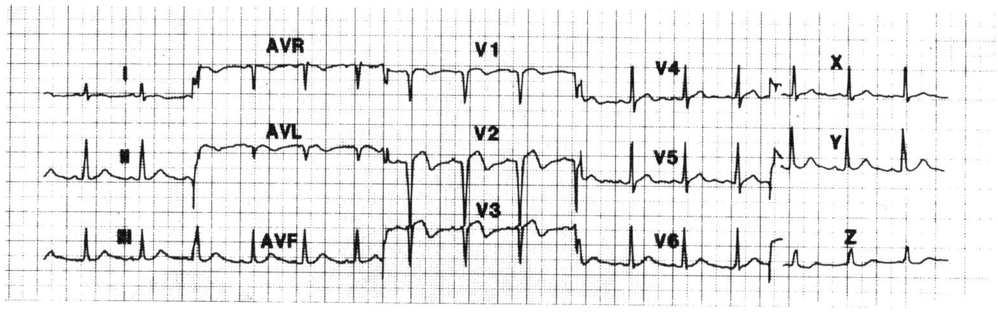

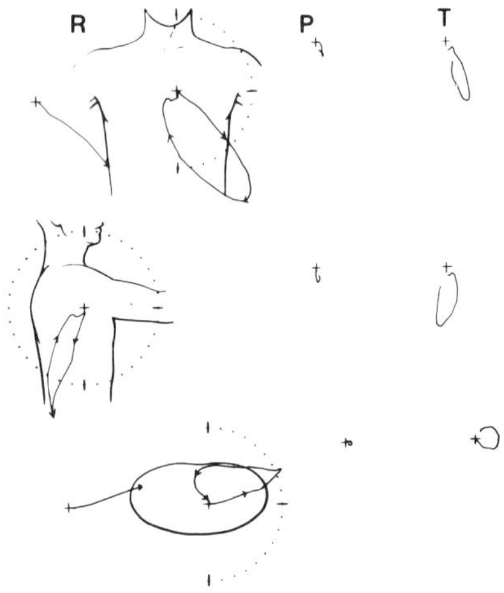

Fig 3A-19 ECG recorded 24 hours after that in Figure 3A-18 demonstrates the expected evolution pattern with an anteroseptal infarction: loss of R wave in V_1, V_2, and V_3 and development of new Q waves in V_1, V_2, and V_3 with persistent ST elevation in these leads. The T wave has rounded down and inverted in the anterior precordial leads. The vector loop representation shows loss of anterior force with a shift of the loop posteriorly in the horizontal plane, consistent with loss of anteroseptal wall as a result of the transmural myocardial necrosis. This correlates with the development of the Q waves in the anterior precordial leads.

The hallmark of the diagnosis of a transmural myocardial infarction in 80% to 87% of cases is the presence of a pathologic Q wave. The Q wave begins to develop over the first few hours of myocardial necrosis and gradually increases in size over several hours (see Fig 3A-17). Because scar tissue has a tendency to shrink, the Q wave on the ECG over the passage of months to years will become smaller (13%) and will show total regression (42%), obscuring the diagnosis of prior myocardial infarction on the ECG.[37]

Until recently, abnormal Q waves were thought to represent the transmission of negative cavity potentials through a "window" of dead myocardium. However, vector analysis suggests that, at least in part, the Q wave is the product of an abnormally directed mean vector evoked by distortion in the activation sequence of the myocardium adjacent to the infarct. This abnormal resultant vector is usually confined to the initial 40 msec of the QRS, but altered forces of excitation can be present in late components of the QRS complex in true posterior and posterobasal infarction. For example, in inferior wall infarction, activation of the inferior wall would be blocked by the infarcted muscle, and thus all early forces, now unopposed, would be directed superiorly away from the inferior wall. In posterior myocardial infarction, there is no scalar lead over the posterior wall, but infarcted muscle in that zone negates initial posterior forces so that septal and right ventricular activation forces anteriorly are now unopposed, producing the abnormal anterior forces (R > S) in the anterior leads held to be typical for the ECG diagnosis of infarction involving the posterior wall and septum.

It is important to realize that a pathologic Q wave may be absent when a transmural infarct is present. "True" posterior infarction affords the classic example of such a circumstance, but infarction of the inferior and lateral walls also may occur without diagnostic Q waves. It is in these atypical presentations that the true VCG has been most helpful.

Criteria for the diagnosis of infarction by location are as follows:

A. Inferior (diaphragmatic) myocardial infarction
   1. Scalar
      a. Q wave ≥40 msec in leads II, III, and aV_F; Q wave amplitude ≥25% of R wave amplitude
      b. QS pattern in leads II, III, and aV_F
   2. Vectorcardiographic (Fig. 3A-20)
      a. Initial superior forces in lead Y ≥40 msec
      b. Frontal plane QRS loop directed superiorly for 25 msec and turning clockwise, extending at least 0.25 mV from the null point, and finally remaining above +15° in the frontal plane in the Frank system
      c. Initial inferior rightward forces, followed by a superiorly directed clockwise loop, as in *b,* seen when lateral wall infarction accompanies inferior wall infarction
      d. "Bites" in the afferent limb of the frontal plane QRS loop
B. Anterior infarction
   1. Scalar
      a. Q wave in leads V_1-V_3 (anteroseptal)
      b. QS pattern in leads V_1-V_3 (anteroseptal)
      c. Q wave in leads V_2-V_4 (anterior)

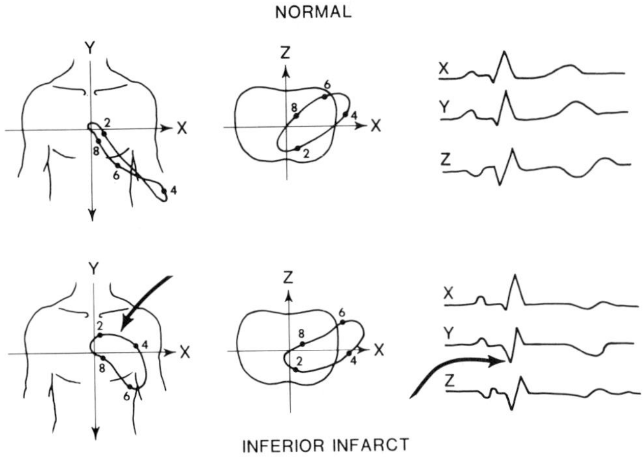

Fig 3A-20 Frontal and horizontal plane vector loop display and X,Y,Z data from which vector loops are generated. **Upper,** normal VCG. **Lower,** pattern of inferior infarction. *Arrows* point to characteristic changes.

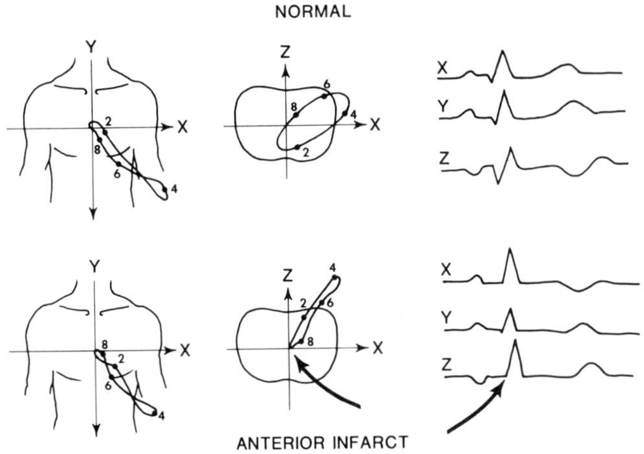

Fig 3A-21 Frontal and horizontal plane vector loop display with X,Y,Z data from which vector loops are generated. **Upper,** normal VCG. **Lower,** VCG pattern in anterior infarction. *Arrows* indicate absence of all anterior force.

d. QS pattern in leads V_2-V_4 (anterior)
e. Loss of r wave from V_1 progressively through V_4 with no Q wave—suggesting anterior infarct

2. Vectorcardiographic (Fig 3A-21)
   a. No anterior force in lead Z and no Q in lead X when definite anteroseptal myocardial infarction exists
   b. Immediate posterior displacement of horizontal plane QRS loop (initial 20 msec) being directed into left posterior quadrant
   c. Notching of initial 40-msec portion of horizontal QRS loop
   d. Inscription of clockwise loop in horizontal plane when anterolateral infarction is present

C. Lateral wall infarction
   1. Scalar
      a. Q wave ≥40 msec in leads V_4-V_6; amplitude ≥25% of R wave amplitude
      b. QS pattern in leads V_4-V_6
      c. Loss of R wave progressively from leads V_4-V_6
   2. Vectorcardiographic
      a. Q wave or QS pattern in lead X
      b. Clockwise rotation of horizontal plane loop
      c. Shift of frontal plane loop to right (pseudo-right-axis deviation)

D. Posterior wall infarction
   1. Scalar
      a. Prominent R wave ≥ S wave in leads V_1 and V_2 together with positive T wave in these leads
      b. Abrupt shift of R wave voltage from leads V_1 and V_2 of more than 7 mV (suggestive)
      c. Normal RS relationship in leads V_1 and V_2 with serial loss of S wave in serial tracings (suggestive)
   2. Vectorcardiographic
      a. R wave ≥ S wave in lead Z or serially observed progressive loss of S wave
      b. Horizontal plane QRS loop (≥75%) displaced anteriorly and usually leftward
      c. Isolated elevation of terminal (afferent limb) of QRS loop in frontal plane, reflecting posterobasal infarct

E. High lateral wall infarction
   1. Scalar
      a. Q wave ≥40 msec in leads I and aV_L; amplitude ≥25% of R wave
      b. QS pattern in leads I and aV_L
   2. Vectorcardiographic
      None—lead X is too low (V_6 level) to record electric activity from high lateral wall of left ventricle, which is then electrically silent in Frank X,Y,Z system leads

Myocardial infarction can involve more than one area simultaneously and, in fact, usually does (Fig 3A-22). Also, two separate infarcts—both old, or one old and one acute—can coexist. Common clinical patterns that are frequently seen include

1. Extension of inferior wall myocardial infarct to lateral wall and also toward base, giving four common clinical presentations for an inferior infarct
   a. Confined to inferior wall
   b. Inferolateral
   c. Inferoposterior
   d. Inferoposterolateral
2. Extension of anterior wall myocardial infarct to lateral wall, high lateral wall, or inferior wall, giving five clinical presentations
   a. Anterior alone
   b. Anterolateral (V_1-V_3 plus V_4-V_6 or Z plus X)
   c. Antero-high lateral (V_1-V_3 plus I and aV_L)
   d. Anterolateral plus high lateral (*b* plus *c*)
   e. Anterior-inferior simultaneously when left anterior descending coronary artery descends over apex onto diaphragmatic surface, producing a pattern of both anterior and inferior infarct (uncommon)

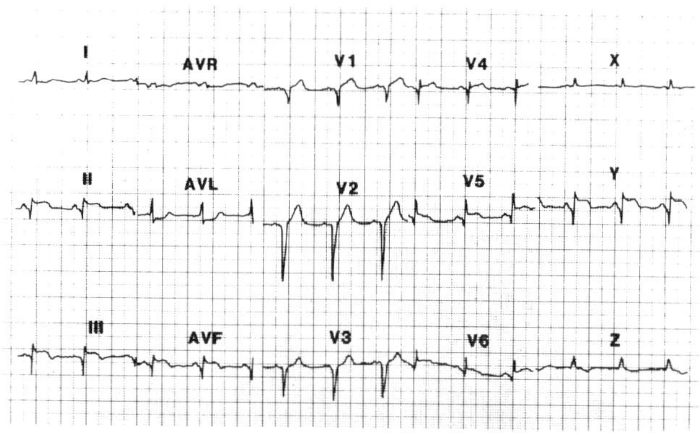

Fig 3A-22 ECG from 52-year-old man with history of anteroseptal myocardial infarction, manifested on this tracing by Q waves in V_1, V_2, and V_3 and extending into V_4 and V_5. The ST segment is flat in these leads with upright T waves, consistent with the presence of an old scar. Also on this tracing is ST elevation in leads II, III, aV_F, V_5, and V_6 with reciprocal ST depression noted in leads I and aV_L. This is consistent with the acute evolving inferior infarction. This tracing was made on day 2 of the infarction. It shows the pattern of the old anteroseptal scar with the new inferior evolving transmural scar. Q waves are present in inferolateral leads, consistent with the transmural nature of this inferolateral myocardial necrosis.

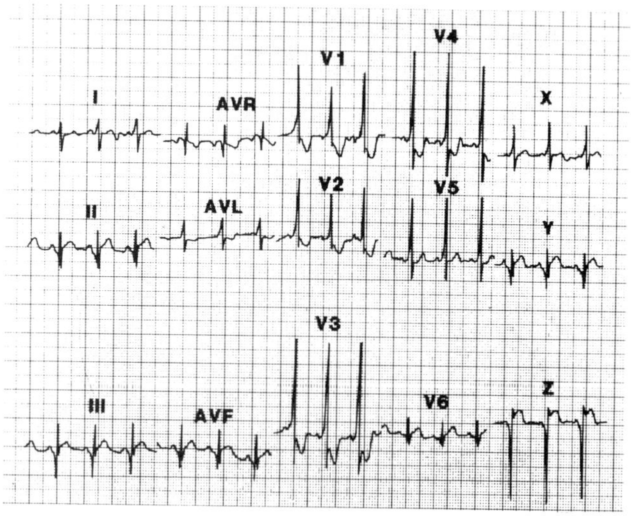

Fig 3A-23 Pattern of Wolff-Parkinson-White syndrome with short P-R interval and δ wave with upright configuration in lead I (so-called type A configuration). This configuration can mimic a true posterior infarction with prominent anterior force and Q waves noted in leads II, III, and aV_F related to the anomalous AV expectation and the δ wave. Careful attention to the short P-R interval, presence of the δ wave, and widened QRS will allow the diagnosis of an accelerated AV excitation and avoid the error of calling this finding an infarction.

3. Posterior wall infarction is usually associated with either inferior or high lateral wall infarct, or both; clinical presentation will consist of
   a. True posterior
   b. Inferoposterior (*a* and *b*, usually right coronary artery lesions)
   c. Postero-high lateral
   d. Postero-high lateral-inferior
   e. Postero-high later-lateral-inferior (*c* through *e*, usually left circumflex lesions)
4. High lateral wall infarct
   a. Exists alone—often missed; leads I and aV_L often overlooked
   b. Can be associated with either posterior or anterior myocardial infarction (see above)

Several excellent studies have demonstrated the comparative values of the ECG and the VCG in the diagnosis of transmural myocardial infarction. Hugenholtz et al.[38] studied 247 patients with conclusive clinical evidence of myocardial infarction and noted VCG confirmation in virtually all of the patients, but by scalar ECG criteria confirmation was not obtained in 30 patients. Gunnar and associates[39] did a similar analysis in an autopsy series of 200 cases. Ninety of the patients had autopsy evidence of myocardial infarction, and 69 (77%) were correctly identified by VCG criteria compared to 66% by scalar criteria. False positives in this series included 31% for the VCG and 35% for the scalar ECG criteria. The findings in these and other similar studies not only emphasize the impressive addition that VCG has made to our diagnostic capability in myocardial infarction but also reconfirm the concept that critical information is provided by both systems and the ability to confirm a difficult diagnosis is lost to the clinician who depends solely on just one of the systems.[40]

Differential diagnosis of myocardial infarction. There are a number of ECG entities that can mimic the patterns of myocardial infarction. Common pseudoinfarct patterns are seen in the following circumstances.

1. Wolff-Parkinson-White syndrome in its type A form can mimic inferior-posterior (Fig 3A-23) and, at times, high lateral infarction; in its type B form, it can mimic anteroseptal infarction (Fig 3A-24).
2. Idiopathic hypertrophic subaortic stenosis can mimic both inferior and posterior myocardial infarctions and, on occasion, also lateral wall infarction.
3. Severe left ventricular hypertrophy can so diminish anterior forces in right precordial leads V_1-V_3 and Z that anteroseptal myocardial infarction may be thought to exist.[34]
4. Left bundle-branch block can diminish anterior forces in leads V_1-V_3 and Z, suggesting anteroseptal myocardial infarction.[33]
5. Right ventricular hypertrophy from any cause can mimic posterior wall myocardial infarction.[35]
6. Left anterior fascicular block, when marked and severe (more than −60°), might suggest inferior infarction or mask high lateral infarction by increasing the voltage of the R wave in lead aV_L.[41]
7. Chronic obstructive pulmonary disease can mimic inferior wall myocardial infarction.[40]

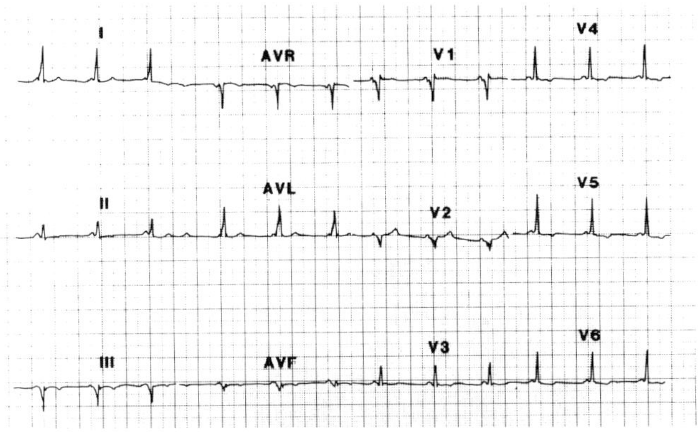

Fig 3A-24 Pattern of anomalous AV excitation, type B, with a downward δ wave noted in anterior precordial lead V_1. With this downward δ wave, frequently the pattern of an anteroseptal infarction can be mimicked, as illustrated here. Again, attention to the short P-R interval, presence of the δ wave, and widened QRS will make the diagnosis clear.

8. Cardiomyopathy can mimic virtually any infarction pattern.[42]
9. Chest deformity, straight back syndrome, or pectus excavatum can produce changes suggestive of anteroseptal myocardial infarction.
10. A normal variant can produce a pattern consistent with either anteroseptal or posterior wall myocardial infarction.
11. Acute pulmonary embolism can mimic acute inferior wall myocardial infarction.
12. Acute pericarditis can produce diffuse ST-segment elevation without reciprocal segmental shifts or pathologic Q waves. ECG changes in pericarditis are produced by epicardial injury.
13. Central nervous system disorders can be associated with marked T-wave changes.
14. Hyperkalemia can produce peaked T waves and bizarre widening of the QRS, suggestive of myocardial damage.
15. Mitral valve prolapse can produce abnormal T waves predominantly in the inferolateral leads, suggesting ischemic injury inferolaterally.

RIGHT VENTRICULAR INFARCTION. Infarction of the right ventricle, sometimes in association with acute inferior or posterior infarction, is characterized by elevated right-sided filling pressures disproportionate to those of the left ventricle, thus mimicking either an acute pulmonary embolism or cardiac tamponade. Unfortunately, the potential changes induced by right ventricular excitation are masked by those induced by the left ventricle to a degree that there are no easily recognizable diagnostic ECG or VCG criteria for infarction of the right ventricular wall. Correct ECG diagnosis of such an infarct may be possible in the presence of right bundle-branch block, in instances in which the late terminal anterior and rightward forces of the classic type I QRS loop (see below, "Right Bundle-Branch Block") are serially and progressively distorted and diminished (see chapter 30).

The findings of ST segment elevation and a QS or QR pattern in right precordial leads (V_3R-V_6R) have been reported to have significant predictive value in the detection of right ventricular infarction in patients with acute inferior infarction. Recording these leads in addition to the standard 12-lead ECG may be helpful.[43]

Bundle-branch block in myocardial infarction.[44,45] The presence of right bundle-branch block does not preclude the diagnosis of myocardial infarction because the initial forces of ventricular excitation critical to the diagnosis of infarction are undisturbed (see below, "Right Bundle-Branch Block"). The only exception is in true posterior wall infarction in which the presence of the right bundle-branch block pattern in leads V_1-V_3 may obscure the diagnosis. But the anterior displacement of the forces in lead Z and an atypical horizontal plane loop characterized by anterior displacement to the left with diminished or absent posterior forces may permit identification of the infarct even in the presence of bundle-branch block.

On the other hand, left bundle-branch block does distort the initial forces and thereby interferes significantly with the diagnosis of myocardial infarction, especially when age of the infarct is indeterminate or the lesion is known to be an ancient one. In acute infarction, when serial records are available, the ST-T changes may permit their identification as primary in character. The following are suggestive, but not diagnostic, of age-indeterminate or old infarcts in the presence of left bundle-branch block.[46]

1. QS pattern in leads II, III, and aV_F in the absence of severe left-axis deviation
2. Q waves, even small, in leads V_4-V_6 and X or a QS pattern in leads V_4-V_6 and X, which would strongly suggest the presence of a lateral wall infarct
3. Asymmetry of ventricular conduction delay associated with a QRS interval of 160 msec or more localized to leads suggestive of anterior, inferior, lateral, or high lateral infarction whereas the QRS duration in other leads is only 110 to 120 msec
4. Progressive loss of R-wave voltage in leads V_1-V_4
5. Loss of R-wave voltage progressively from leads V_4-V_6
6. Atypical left bundle-branch block loops in the horizontal plane suggestive of anteroseptal or anterolateral myocardial infarction (see "Left Bundle-Branch Block," below)
7. QR pattern of ventricular premature contraction in lead V_1

However, left bundle-branch block can either mimic myocardial infarction or mask its presence.

Complications of myocardial infarction. From the ECG standpoint, the important complications of myocardial infarction include (1) rhythm disturbances, (2) appearance of bundle-branch block and fascicular blocks, (3) asymmetric ventricular conduction delay in the zone of infarction, and (4) ventricular aneurysm.

RHYTHM DISTURBANCES. These occur in virtually all patients who sustain a myocardial infarction, and accurate assessment and management of these arrhythmias were powerful motivating elements in the development of the coronary care units in this country and elsewhere.[47-49] Proper and prompt control of potentially lethal rhythm disturbances by pharmacologic and electronic means has resulted in a significant decrease in the in-hospital mortality rate among patients with acute myocardial infarction, from approximately 30% to its current level of 15% or less.

Rhythm disturbances in acute myocardial infarction can be divided along the usual classic lines of tachyarrhythmias and bradyarrhythmias.

Of all the rhythms associated with myocardial infarction, ventricular premature beats are the most common and the most consequential to improved care because ectopic beats usually precede the more malignant sustained ventricular arrhythmias.[50]

Essentially stable ventricular rhythms that also occur in the setting of myocardial infarction include parasystolic ventricular premature beats and accelerated idioventricular rhythm. In the former, an independent ventricular focus with its own inherent rhythmicity, not readily suppressible by antiarrhythmia drugs, appears in either the acute or chronic postinfarction phase and ordinarily is transient and benign. Treatment is usually unnecessary. The same is true of accelerated idioventricular rhythm which is a rhythm virtually confined to the setting of acute myocardial infarction, especially inferior wall infarction.[51] Whenever the sinus rhythm or basic rhythm slows to a critical rate, a wide ventricular QRS appears and occurs repetitively in competition with the normal pacemaker. Numerous fusion beats are seen, and the heart tends to go into and out of the rhythm intermittently. As long as the patient remains hemodynamically stable, the situation can simply be observed because lethal ventricular rhythms are not easily triggered by this specific disturbance. The usual range of this rhythm is 60 to 90 beats/min, but it can reach up to 120 beats/min.

Common supraventricular tachycardias that occur during acute myocardial infarction include paroxysmal supraventricular tachycardia, atrial flutter, and atrial fibrillation.[52-54]

A comment should be made with regard to nonparoxysmal junctional tachycardia.[55] Although this primarily is a rhythm produced by digitalis excess, it can also arise as a result of ischemic insult of the junctional tissues. Thus, a junctional pacemaking site (ectopic focus) is stimulated and driven at a rate faster than 60 beats/min (usual range, 60 to 120 beats/min). This is atypical of a junctional escape rhythm, which is usually in the range of 40 to 55 beats/min, and it may usurp the role of the sinus node intermittently or continuously, producing AV dissociation which mimics complete heart block except for the accelerated rate.

Atrioventricular conduction disturbances produced by myocardial infarction occur primarily at two levels: the AV node, and below the common bundle of His at the bifurcation of the bundle branches.[56] Compromise of AV node conduction is primarily due to inferoposterior myocardial infarction because the right coronary artery supplies the AV node in 90% of humans. Rarely, a dominant left circumflex lesion producing a high lateral wall infarct, together with involvement of the inferior and posterior walls, can also result in compromise of AV node conduction. Distal involvement of the bundle branches at the level of the bifurcation most commonly is the result of anteroseptal myocardial infarction with a very proximal block in the first septal perforator branch which supplies both the ventricular septum and the bundle branches, especially the left anterior fascicle and right bundle branch. A far less common conduction disturbance with inferior wall myocardial infarction due to right coronary artery obstruction involves the appearance of right bundle-branch block (right coronary artery supplies the initial portion of the right bundle) and posterior fascicular block (supplied by the posterior descending coronary artery, a branch of the right coronary artery). However, clinically it is important to recall that infra-His block can occur with an inferior infarct.

Proximal block in the AV node results in (1) first-degree heart block; (2) second-degree heart block, predominantly of Mobitz type I (Wenckebach), although transient periods of high-grade 2:1 and 3:1 second-degree block may be seen; and (3) complete heart block. The vast majority of patients who have second- or third-degree heart block due to AV node compromise have it in the first 72 hours, many in the initial hour or hours of the inferior infarction. Most remain hemodynamically stable or respond to small doses of atropine; few require prophylactic pacing (usually for a very slow rate or increased ventricular ectopy). Even in complete heart block, most patients exhibit a stable escape focus from the junctional area (narrow QRS) with a rate of 40 to 55 beats/min. The block is transient and abates over 3 to 7 days. In hemodynamically stable patients, the presence or absence of block does not appear to affect mortality, but in those patients with significant pump failure or cardiogenic shock the outcome may be influenced favorably by pacing at a more physiologic rate for those in whom a trial evokes a desirable response.

Block at the level of the bundle branches in association with acute myocardial infarction is far less common than AV node block, and it appears later because necrosis of the involved conducting tissue is a prerequisite. The usual presentation involves the appearance of left anterior fascicular block and right bundle-branch block in the course of an acute anteroseptal myocardial infarction which then slowly or suddenly degenerates into trifascicular block manifested by (1) intermittent dropped beats (Mobitz II), (2) high-grade second-degree heart block, (3) complete heart block with a slow distal ventricular escape focus, inherently unstable, at rates of 25 to 35 beats/min, or (4) asystole.

The results of a multicenter study of the significance of bundle-branch block complicating myocardial infarction, involving 432 patients without cardiogenic shock, indicated that these patients could be divided into low-, medium-, and high-risk groups for the development of high-grade block or asystole on the basis of (1) the presence of first-degree AV block (P-R >20 msec), (2) the appearance of new bundle-branch block in the course of the infarction, and (3) the development of bifascicular block or bilateral bundle-branch block in the course of infarction.[57] The risk of high-grade block or asystole was 35% in those who had a bifascicular or bilateral bundle-branch block, 20% in those with uncomplicated block of a single bundle, and 11% in those with first-degree heart block without accompanying fascicular or bundle-branch block. Temporary pacing was recommended for those at great risk, but the hospital mortality was not affected substantially by pacing because of the high association of significant pump failure in these patients as a result of the high incidence among them of proximal obstruction of the left anterior descending coronary artery. Permanent pacemakers were inserted in those who did survive and did have high-grade block, and follow-up at 1 year revealed a significantly decreased incidence of high-grade block and sudden death—10% vs. 65% in the unpaced group. No clear role for permanent pacing has been established for those who did not develop high-grade block or for those with an inferoposterior infarct with high-grade heart block.

Conduction delay below the bifurcation of the bundle branches is manifested in three patterns: (1) widening of the QRS to 120 msec or more in the zone of infarct, mimicking left bundle-branch block but actually representing a ventricular conduction delay due to slowing of conduction in the infarct zone; (2) appearance of fascicular blocks, left anterior or posterior fascicular block, or right bundle-branch block or a combination thereof due to the infarct, sometimes proceeding to high-grade AV block; (3) a combination of *1* and *2*. Thus, conduction delay may result from ventricular conduction delay secondary to infarction or from discrete fascicular, bifascicular, or trifascicular disease, or both. Such a description is more precise and clinically more accurate than the old and somewhat confusing terms "peri-infarction block" and "parietal block."

Persistence of ST-segment elevation in leads overlying the infarct beyond the acute phase of myocardial infarction or for longer than 6 weeks is strongly suggestive of left ventricular aneurysm. This is not an uncommon complication of myocardial infarction, especially in extensive anterior wall infarction. The mechanism responsible for the production of this ECG finding is unknown. It is important to recognize that, when localized, such ST-segment elevation is suggestive of aneurysm but could represent a superimposed reinfarction or Prinzmetal's angina—two other causes of localized ST-segment elevation.

Finally, in the weeks after myocardial infarction, the patient may experience recurrence of chest pain, but more pleuritic in nature than ischemic, associated with diffuse ST-segment elevation without reciprocal changes typical of acute pericarditis. This is the postmyocardial-infarction syndrome (Dressler's syndrome) and is similar to the postcardiotomy syndrome seen after heart surgery, after penetrating trauma to the chest or blunt trauma, or, on occasion, at the time of insertion of an artificial pacemaker.

The use of the ECG to detect myocardial reperfusion in the patient with acute myocardial injury has been evaluated. A 20% or greater decrease in total ST-segment elevation during intravenous thrombolytic therapy has been shown to be both sensitive and specific in determining myocardial reperfusion.[58] Sevilla et al.,[59] in using this criterion, found that sensitivity was 79% and specificity 70% with intravenous therapy and that sensitivity was 90% with intracoronary therapy.

SUMMARY. The ECG and VCG criteria for the diagnosis of myocardial infarction vary, depending on the location and extent of the damaged area. Because myocardial necrosis manifests itself by predominantly distorting the initial depolarizing forces, the "Q wave" or the vector display during the initial 30 to 40 msec of the QRS is utilized in the diagnosis and location of the infarct. The ST-segment and T-wave changes of ischemia and injury permit classifying the infarct as hyperacute (<24 hours), acute (first 4 days), recent (days 4 to 10), or indeterminate (2 weeks to years). Care must be exercised in assessing the ECG and VCG for evidence of problems induced by the infarction, acute or healed—namely, rhythm disturbances, conduction defects (bundle-branch block or fascicular blocks), ventricular conduction delay localized to the infarct zone, and ventricular aneurysm.

Abnormal QRS duration

Recognition of the ECG patterns of ventricular conduction defects requires (1) a clear understanding of the normal activation sequence of both the left and right ventricles via the specialized ventricular conduction system (bundle of His, left and right bundle branches, and the fascicles or radiations); (2) realization that conduction defects in any part of the system may be permanent (anatomic) or intermittent (functional); (3) implicit acceptance of a quadrafascicular ventricular activation apparatus including the right bundle and three left ventricular fascicles (namely, anterior-superior, posterior-inferior, and septal), which is clinically useful, although existence of an anatomically distinct and electrocardiographically unique septal cluster of fascicles is controversial; and (4) recognition of the fact that bundle-branch patterns can result from abnormalities in the common bundle of His, in the bundle branches, in the fascicles, or at the junction of the Purkinje fibers with ventricular muscle.[60,61]

It is important to note that the bundle branches and the radiations are separated, functionally and anatomically, from the myocardium by dense connective tissue. Therefore, endocardial activation does not occur along the course of the bundle branches but occurs at the Purkinje-ventricular myocardial junction. In the right ventricle, initial activation occurs at the apex and spreads rapidly from that site via the moderator band to the lower portion of the ventricular septum and from there over the endocardial surface of the free wall and septum. The earliest site of activation in the left ventricle is in the midseptal area and the anterior and posterior paraseptal areas of the left ventricular free wall. The first ECG representation of this process is septal activation, in an anteriorly oriented left-to-right direction, followed by excitation of the free walls of the left and right ventricles.

Excitation of the endocardial aspect of the left side of the ventricular septum normally precedes excitation of comparable sites on the right by 1.5 msec[62] to produce, as the earliest vector of excitation, one directed from left to right. After the rapid spread of the excitation process over the left and right subendocardia, a slower spread with a predominant endocardial-to-epicardial excitation takes place. Ordinarily, the epicardium at the base of the left ventricle posteriorly is the last region to be reached by excitation. Electrocardiographically, potential generated in the right ventricle is obscured by the predominance of forces generated in the left ventricle.

From this concept of activation of the ventricles and the ECG predominance of left ventricular activation come the predominant features of right and left bundle-branch block. In bundle-branch block, the impulse will be conducted by the intact bundle branch so that the ventricle with the bundle-branch block will be activated later. This asynchronous activation of the ventricles will lengthen total ventricular activation time to more than 120 msec (QRS duration); uncover right ventricular activation, usually electrocardiographically silent, in right bundle-branch block by delaying right ventricular depolarization until after left ventricular activation is completed; and alter the direction and amplitude of septal activation and prolong left ventricular activation in the case of left bundle-branch block.

ECG diagnostic features will be described for each of the following conduction defects: right bundle-branch block, left bundle-branch block, fascicular blocks, bilateral bundle-branch blocks, and nonspecific ventricular conduction delay.

Right bundle-branch block. The right bundle branch is a continuation of the His bundle. It arises distal to the septal leaflet of the tricuspid valve. Its length is 40 to 55 mm, and its diameter averages 1 to 2 mm. It can be divided into three segments: the first segment is subendocardial, begins just proximal to the point of origin of the left bundle fibers, and lies along the membranous portion of the ventricular septum; the second is intramyocardial and courses along the muscular septum; and the third is subendocardial and extends from the septum to the base of the anterior papillary muscle of the right ventricle. From that point the various divisions of the right bundle fan out to the right ventricular free wall and septal musculature. Because of this anatomic arrangement, catheter manipulation along the right side of the septum can result in transient right bundle-branch block, as can an operative procedure that involves the septum or produces a transverse or vertical right ventriculotomy scar that interrupts the radiations of the right bundle.[63]

The blood supply to the right bundle branch is dual. The AV node artery, a branch of the right coronary artery, supplies the first segment of the right bundle branch. The second and third segments are supplied by perforating septal branches of the left anterior descending coronary artery. Knowledge of the vascular supply is critical to understanding right bundle-branch block in the setting of acute or chronic ischemic heart disease.

Diagnostic ECG features of right bundle-branch block include

1. Scalar (Fig 3A-25)
   a. QRS duration ≥120 msec
   b. Terminal QRS delay
      (1) Late r′ or R′ wave in leads aV_R, V_1, and V_2, producing a triphasic RSR′ pattern
      (2) Late broad S wave in leads I, aV_L, V_5, and V_6
   c. Secondary ST-T wave changes in leads V_1-V_3, in which the T-wave direction is opposite that of the QRS (secondary T-wave changes)
   d. Normal mean electrical axis

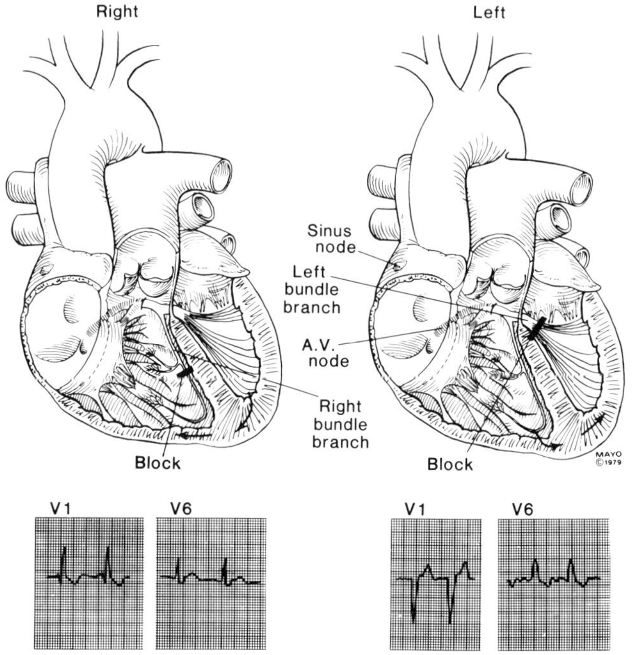

Fig 3A-25 Drawings of heart show location of right bundle-branch block with the characteristic V_1 and V_6, scalar ECG changes RSR′, and terminal sagging of S wave **(left)** and left bundle-branch block with the characteristic scalar ECG changes in V_1 and V_6, deep S waves, and broad notched wide QRS **(right).**

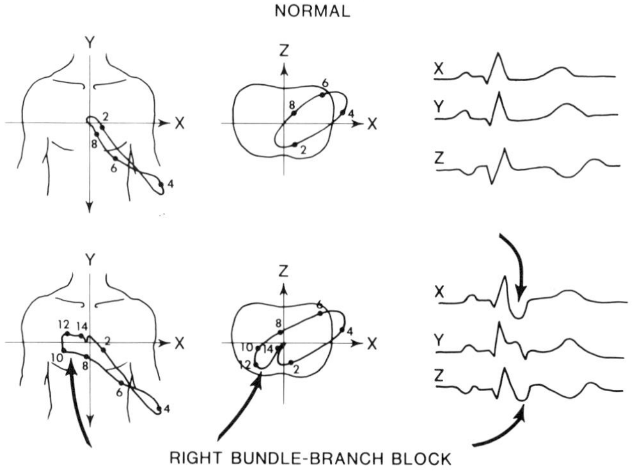

Fig 3A-26 Frontal and horizontal plane vector loop display with X,Y,Z data from normal VCG **(upper)** and from patient with right bundle-branch block **(lower).** *Arrows* show characteristic late terminal QRS delay to the right and anterior.

2. Vectorcardiographic (Fig 3A-26)
   a. r′ or R′ in lead Z; duration ≥120 msec
   b. S wave in lead X
   c. Horizontal plane loop which shows terminal delay with the terminal forces displaced into the right anterior quadrant, demonstrating late activation of the right ventricle (Fig 3A-27)

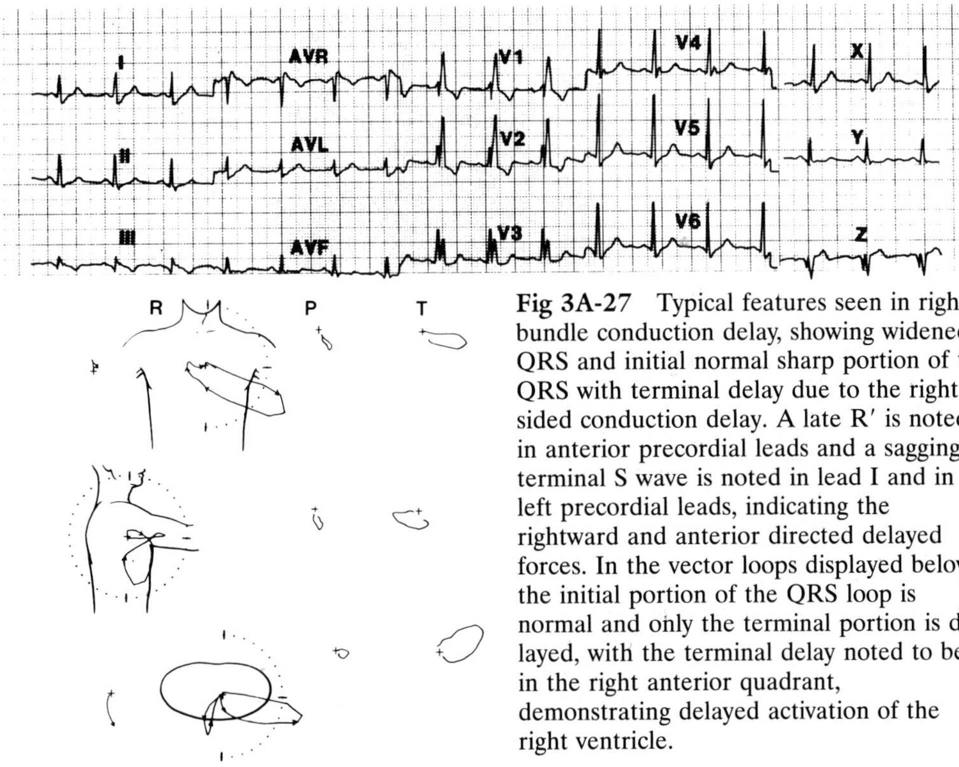

Fig 3A-27 Typical features seen in right bundle conduction delay, showing widened QRS and initial normal sharp portion of the QRS with terminal delay due to the right-sided conduction delay. A late R′ is noted in anterior precordial leads and a sagging terminal S wave is noted in lead I and in left precordial leads, indicating the rightward and anterior directed delayed forces. In the vector loops displayed below, the initial portion of the QRS loop is normal and only the terminal portion is delayed, with the terminal delay noted to be in the right anterior quadrant, demonstrating delayed activation of the right ventricle.

Analysis of these criteria, especially the effect of right bundle-branch block on the ventricular activation sequence, produces several points. First, the ECG hallmark of right bundle-branch block is terminal delay such that the potential changes induced by right ventricular activation that ordinarily are obscured by left ventricular forces become manifest. The terminal R′ wave in the right precordial leads (V_1, V_2, Z), the terminal S wave in the left precordial leads (I, aV_L, V_4-V_6), and the horizontal loop displacement terminally into the right anterior quadrant all identify the delayed activation of the right ventricle. However, this late activation of the right ventricle does not disturb left ventricular activation, which proceeds normally. Note in Figure 3A-26 that, if the terminal R′ wave or S wave is deleted from leads X and Z or the terminal right anterior projection of the horizontal loop is obliterated, the resultant QRS and horizontal loop would then be within normal limits, simulating normal left ventricular excitation.

Because left ventricular excitation proceeds normally in the presence of right bundle-branch block, the initial septal excitation is normal, and hence the right bundle-branch block does not obscure the diagnosis of myocardial infarction that characteristically alters the initial forces. Excitation of the left ventricle proceeds on time so that, again, the ECG finding from any lead is a "normal" QRS until the terminal forces induced by right bundle-branch block appear and define the presence of right bundle-branch block. This pattern of terminal delay can be seen in most leads, and hence the S waves in leads I, aV_L, and V_6 are as characteristic of right bundle-branch block as is the classic RSR′ pattern in lead V_1.

The diagnostic evidence of right bundle-branch block, then, can be recognized in virtually any lead, and the dependence on the RSR′ pattern in V_1 or lead Z is obviated. Finally, with the normal excitation of the left ventricle, in the presence of right bundle-branch block, the QRS axis in the frontal plane remains normal. Aberration is induced, however, by coincident fascicular block, right ventricular hypertrophy, or lateral wall infarction. Thus, the presence of an abnormal mean electrical axis requires consideration of an additional ECG diagnosis.

Right bundle-branch block usually reflects a specific anatomic lesion and therefore is permanent. At times, however, it appears intermittently as rate-dependent or simple intermittent right bundle-branch block. In rate-dependent right bundle-branch block, the supraventricular rate exceeds the capacity of the right bundle to conduct (still refractory), and right bundle-branch block appears and persists until the heart rate again slows to a level below this critical rate.

Rate-dependent right bundle-branch block, the "Ashman phenomenon," and atrial premature beats with right ventricular conduction delay are examples of this situation. Rarely, right bundle-branch block may appear paradoxically in association with a slowing of the ventricular rate, fulfilling the criteria for a bradycardia-dependent right bundle-branch block. Finally, right bundle-branch block may appear intermittently and unrelated to rate change and justifiably be termed "rate-independent right bundle-branch block." From a clinical standpoint, right bundle-branch block may be present in apparently normal persons. In those with cardiac problems, right bundle-branch block can be associated with a wide spectrum of problems.

Left bundle-branch block. The left bundle branch arises perpendicularly from a 10- to 15-mm segment of the terminal portion of the bundle of His. The undivided band then descends from the septal crest to the left side of the ventricular septum. It is a relatively broad structure, compared with the right bundle, which later proceeds as a diminutive counterpart of the common bundle. At its point of origin, the left bundle branch lies adjacent to the membranous septum near the right and noncoronary cusps of the aortic valve, and calcification involving these cusps can readily involve the main left bundle branch and produce left bundle-branch block, a not uncommon clinical situation. At its distal end, before breaking into its fascicular radiations, the main left bundle branch can be injured easily by surgical procedures involving the left side of the septum, especially myotomy or myomectomy in the treatment of hypertrophic cardiomyopathy.[64]

At a level variably located between the upper and middle ventricular septa, and still occupying a subendocardial position, the left bundle branch divides into two discrete fascicles—the anterosuperior and the posteroinferior—and an interlacing midseptal network. The posteroinferior fascicle is broader and shorter than the anterosuperior fascicle. It arises at a right angle to the common bundle and proceeds from its subaortic origin toward the posterior papillary muscle where it branches into a dense Purkinje network. The anterosuperior fascicle, thinner and longer, crosses the left ventricular outflow tract toward the anterior papillary muscle of the left ventricle. The existence of an anatomically and functionally discrete midseptal division of the left branch is disputed, and there are individual variations in the disposition of the septal Purkinje fibers. Functionally, its role for the most part is that of a network. Peripherally, fibers from all three fascicles intertwine. Satisfaction of distinctive ECG criteria for anterior and for posterior fascicular specific lesions, particularly the latter, probably entails not only single or multiple lesions within the given fascicle but also interruption of conduction through fascicles that interlace with the primary fascicle, suggesting conceptually that fascicular block is a manifestation of diffuse disease rather than a single discrete lesion.[65,66]

Blood supply to the common bundle of His is dual and comes from the AV node artery (a branch of the right coronary artery in 90% of patients) and from septal perforators of the left anterior descending coronary artery. The left main bundle and the continuing portion of the posteroinferior fascicle receive blood from septal perforators of the left anterior descending coronary artery and from several branches of the posterior descending coronary artery. In some individuals, supply has been restricted to either the AV node artery or the left anterior descending septal perforators. The anterior fascicle is supplied exclusively by septal perforators of the left anterior descending coronary artery. Vascular supply to the septal network is usually dual: the left anterior descending and posterior descending coronary arteries.

A diagnosis of left bundle-branch block usually should focus attention on the possible presence of some disease that compromises left ventricular conduction within the short, broad, left main bundle, either anatomically or functionally. Evidence on whether lesions within the common bundle of His involving fibers destined to become part of the left main bundle can result in a left bundle-branch block is conflicting.[67] Clearly, block of the left main bundle or a process blocking both the anterior and posterior fascicles can result in a left bundle-branch block pattern. Finally, myocardial infarction, left ventricular hypertrophy, or hyperkalemia can slow conduction at the Purkinje-left ventricular musculature junction, locally (infarct) or diffusely (hyperkalemia), and thereby evoke a pattern of left bundle-branch block. Just as in right bundle-branch block, the appearance of a left bundle-branch block on the ECG can result from interruption of conduction through the main left bundle branch, its principal subdivisions, or the fascicles or at the junction of the Purkinje fibers and ventricular muscle.

Diagnostic criteria of left bundle-branch block are

1. Scalar (see Fig 3A-25)
   a. QRS duration >120 msec
   b. No septal Q waves in leads I, aV_L, and V_4-V_6
   c. Delayed intrinsicoid deflections in leads I, aV_L, and V_4-V_6, with broad R waves or RSR′ patterns in those leads (conduction delay throughout entire QRS)
   d. Broad r-S waves in leads V_1-V_3
   e. Secondary ST-T wave changes in leads I, aV_L, and V_4-V_6, with T-wave orientation opposite to QRS
   f. Normal mean QRS axis
2. Vectorcardiography
   a. Abnormal septal activation, right-to-left and anteriorly
   b. Horizontal QRS loop displaced posteriorly and medially and rotating slowly throughout its midportion (30 to 80 msec) and creating a narrow, tight-turn loop terminally that usually can be covered by an ordinary pen
   c. Normal counterclockwise movement of the loop into the left posterior quadrant after initial abnormal septal activation (Fig 3A-28).

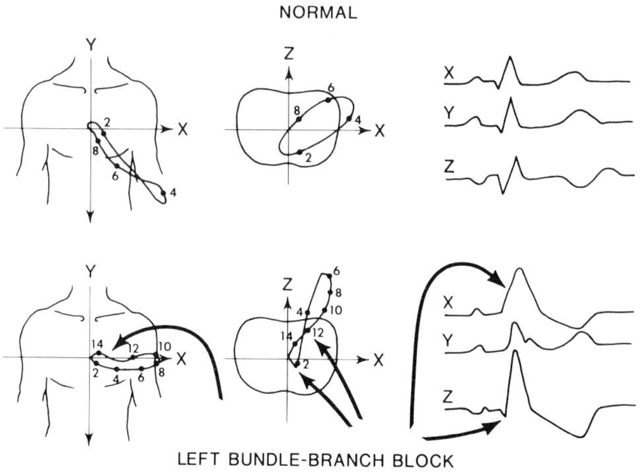

Fig 3A-28 Frontal and horizontal plane vector loop display and X,Y,Z data for normal VCG **(upper)** and from patient with left bundle-branch block **(lower)**. *Arrows* show initial right-to-left anterior force with typical figure-of-8 loop in left posterior quadrant.

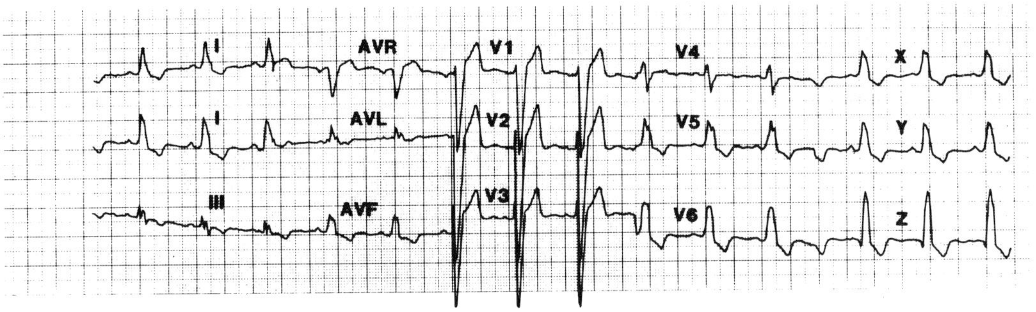

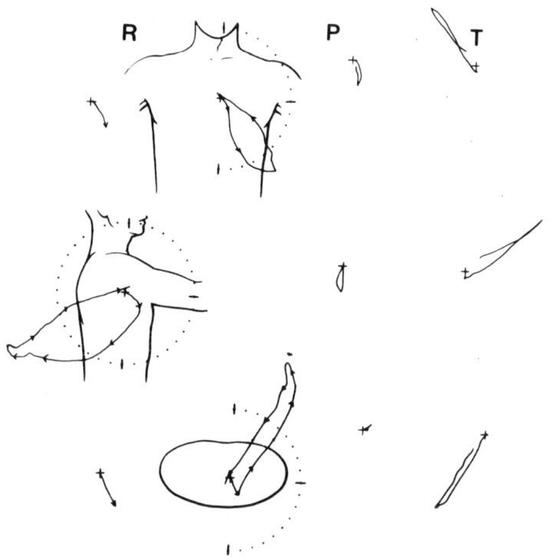

Fig 3A-29 Typical features seen in left bundle conduction delay with widened QRS produced by conduction delay throughout the QRS development. Septal activation is abnormal, now going from right to left, with the loop being narrowed and located in the posterior left quadrant. The delay in the forces is directed toward the left and posterior, producing deep S waves across the anterior precordial leads and a notched, slowly evolving QRS in the left precordial leads. The abnormal depolarization is associated with abnormal repolarization—downward displaced ST segments, and inverted T waves over the left precordial leads.

Left bundle-branch block both distorts and delays left ventricular excitation (Fig 3A-29). Abnormal septal activation from right to left eliminates the septal Q waves normally present in left-sided leads I, aV_L, V_4-V_6, and X and hence alters the initial 20- to 40-msec forces, making the diagnosis of an old myocardial infarct difficult. The left ventricle is activated slowly via ordinary ventricular myocardium rather than via the specialized left bundle-branch system. This accounts for the tightness and slow turning of the counterclockwise horizontal QRS loop in the posterior quadrant. In addition, the greatest mass of activated muscle at any one time will be medial near the septum where first activation took place, and the resultant vector horizontal loop will be pulled posteriorly and medially compared with the normal loop. This distortion of left ventricular excitation often masks the diagnosis of associated left ventricular hypertrophy because the predominance of medial activation over lateral activation enhances S wave depth in leads V_1-V_3 but severely diminishes R wave amplitude in leads V_5 and V_6. Finally, secondary T-wave changes are always present in leads I, aV_L, V_4-V_6, and X and consist of inverted T waves that are 180° discordant to the QRS. The T-wave changes are always difficult to interpret in the left precordial leads, and distinguishing among ischemia, left ventricular hypertrophy, electrolyte problems, and changes due solely to altered excitation produced by left bundle-branch block is not easy. The total distortion of left ventricular depolarization and repolarization produced by complete left bundle-branch block often makes other important diagnoses quite difficult.

The axis in the frontal plane is usually normal in uncomplicated left bundle-branch block. When left-axis deviation does occur, it usually implies more diffuse disease with involvement of both the left main bundle branch and the left anterior-superior fascicle or both the anterior and posterior fascicles, with the greater conduction delay being in the anterior rather than the posterior fascicle. Mortality is higher in patients with left bundle-branch block and left axis deviation than in those with a normal QRS axis.[68] Right-axis deviation is very rare and usually indicates involvement of both of the fascicles, with the conduction delay being greatest in the posterior fascicle. Alternative explanations of right-axis deviation include the presence of right ventricular hypertrophy and a lateral wall infarct.

VCG has been helpful in getting around the masking effects of left bundle-branch block on associated critical diagnoses in three situations: (1) anteroseptal myocardial infarction, (2) lateral wall infarction, and (3) associated left ventricular hypertrophy. When the Z lead is used, in left bundle-branch block a total absence of all anterior force and right-to-left initial QRS activation with marked posterior displacement of the initial 20-msec vector strongly suggests anteroseptal infarction. Abnormal clockwise movement of the horizontal loop in its course toward the posterior quadrant indicates a significant loss of lateral force secondary to a lateral wall infarct. Finally, a three-dimensional maximal spatial R vector > 2.7 mV is reliable evidence of the coexistence of left ventricular hypertrophy and left bundle-branch block.

Just as in right bundle-branch block, functional left bundle-branch block may occur intermittently when the ventricular rates are rapid (rate-dependent left bundle-branch block) or slow (bradycardia-dependent left bundle-branch block) or it can be rate-independent left bundle-branch block.

Differential diagnosis of left bundle-branch block includes

1. Nonspecific ventricular conduction delay in which the QRS is >120 msec but without diagnostic features of either left or right bundle-branch block
2. Wolff-Parkinson-White syndrome type B in which a QS pattern in leads V_1, V_2, and Z mimics left bundle-branch block but the short P-R interval and δ wave permit the correct diagnosis
3. Anteroseptal, lateral, or inferior myocardial infarction producing an asymmetric ventricular conduction delay suggestive of left bundle-branch block except that the asymmetric nature of the conduction delay is inconsistent with typical left bundle-branch block
4. Accelerated idioventricular rhythm and ventricular tachycardia or ventricular escape focus
5. Artificially paced rhythm with an endocardial lead in the right ventricle
6. Left ventricular hypertrophy associated with left anterior fascicular block producing a ventricular conduction delay suggestive of left bundle-branch block

Left bundle-branch block is seen in patients without demonstrable heart disease, but in most instances it indicates a diseased heart, especially one affected by ischemic or hypertensive heart disease or by one of the primary cardiomyopathies.

Left anterior-superior fascicular block. A conduction block involving a left anterior-superior fascicle results, during the early phase, in excitation proceeding inferiorly and posteriorly over the intact posterior fascicle, inducing myocardial excitation with inferior and posterior orientation. The forces generated thereby produce an initial r wave in leads II, III, and aV_F and a q wave in leads I and aV_L; however, the presence of a q wave in these leads is not essential to the diagnosis. Late excitation of the anterior-superior portion of the left ventricular myocardium produces left-axis deviation ($\geq -30°$) reflected in tall R waves in leads I and, especially, aV_L together with deep S waves terminally in leads II, III, and aV_F. The QRS duration is prolonged by only 5 to 17 msec. A wider QRS ($\geq$120 msec) suggests an additional problem, such as left ventricular hypertrophy, associated right bundle-branch block, myocardial disease, or bifascicular (anterior and posterior fascicular) block. From a VCG standpoint, the hallmarks of left anterior-superior fascicular block are a qR pattern in lead Y, which is the inverse of lead aV_F, and a counterclockwise QRS loop in the frontal plane, which moves first inferiorly and then left and superiorly, in sharp contrast to the superior-directed loop produced by an inferior wall myocardial infarction (see section on inferior infarct).

From an ECG standpoint, left anterior-superior fascicular block may generate the following problems: (1) The initial inscription of inferior and posterior forces in the inferior leads may mask an old inferior infarct; (2) the sharply superior sweep of forces resulting in prominent R waves in leads I and aV_L may render unreadable the voltage criteria for left ventricular hypertrophy; however, a new criterion (S-wave III + [R + S]) in the maximal precordial lead ≥ 30 mm has been shown to be very sensitive and specific for left ventricular hypertrophy in the presence of left anterior fascicular block;[69] and (3) the later superiorly directed activation may diminish lateral R-wave voltage in leads X and V_4-V_6, suggesting loss of lateral wall forces.

Left anterior fascicular block is encountered more commonly than posterior fascicular block. The "exposure to risk" of block in the longer anterior fascicle compared with that in the posterior fascicle affords a possible explanation. A further contributing factor may be exposure of the anterior fascicle to the high pressure of the left ventricular outflow tract. There is an increase in prevalence of left anterior-superior fascicular block with advancing age, and in older patients there often is very little evidence of significant organic heart disease, although any one of diverse causes (coronary artery disease, calcific aortic stenosis, Lenegre's disease, and cardiomyopathy) may be present. However, it should be noted that left anterior-superior fascicular block can appear acutely in the course of an anteroseptal myocardial infarction and also can appear functionally as a rate-dependent phenomenon.[70-72] In a retrospective study, left anterior hemiblock in asymptomatic aviators was not associated with syncope or sudden incapacitation and was not the forerunner of left bundle-branch block or complete heart block. Left anterior hemiblock does not modify an aviator's fitness qualification.[73]

Differential diagnosis of left anterior fascicular block includes inferior wall myocardial infarction with entirely superiorly directed forces, suggesting pseudo left-axis deviation, left-axis deviation seen in chronic obstructive pulmonary disease, and malformation or absence of the anterior-superior fascicle as often occurs in an ostium primum atrial septal defect.

Left posterior fascicular block. A conduction block involving a left posterior fascicle would result in (1) initial left ventricular activation occurring leftward anteriorly and superiorly, thus producing an rR wave in leads I and aV_L and a q wave in leads II, III, and aV_F; (2) late activation of the inferior-posterior wall of the left ventricle, resulting in an rS pattern in leads I and aV_L and a qR pattern in leads II, III, and aV_F; and (3) right-axis deviation terminally from the posterior-inferior sweep of the delayed forces. From a VCG standpoint, lead Y would show an rS pattern, and the frontal plane loop would be clockwise, initially superior and then finally inferior and rightward. The initial superior forces recorded in the frontal plane loop and representing the reciprocal of the Q waves inscribed in the inferior leads commonly have a duration and configuration not adequate to suggest inferior wall myocardial infarction.

The key feature suggestive of left posterior fascicular block is right-axis deviation in the frontal plane. However, for this diagnosis to be entertained, more common causes of right-axis deviation must be excluded, such as right ventricular hypertrophy, chronic obstructive pulmonary disease, and lateral wall infarction.

Isolated block of the posterior fascicle is rare, presumably due to its large size, its relationship to the low-pressure inflow tract of the left ventricle, and its dual blood supply. When it does appear clinically, it is associated with right bundle-branch block or posterior wall myocardial infarction. It has also been encountered, again rarely, in association with disease associated with left anterior fascicular block and left bundle-branch block.

Left septal fascicle. The ECG pattern of conduction block in the left septal fascicle is not well defined and, in fact, no such pattern may exist. Absence of the septal r wave, appearance of a q wave in the right precordial leads, and prominent anterior forces unrelated to right ventricular hypertrophy, idiopathic hypertrophic subaortic stenosis, and posterior infarct all have been reported as consistent with the diagnosis of left septal fascicle block but are patently lacking in specificity.

Bifascicular block. The term "bifascicular block" is used when there is ECG evidence of simultaneous block in two fascicles. From a clinical standpoint, bifascicular block may present as left anterior fascicular block plus right bundle-branch block, as left posterior fascicular block plus right bundle-branch block, as left anterior fascicular block plus left posterior fascicular block, and as left bundle-branch block itself, by definition. Marked left-axis deviation would define the first combination, and right-axis deviation would define the second. The terminal delay of right bundle-branch block does not obscure conduction abnormalities (fascicular blocks) and infarct patterns, diagnostic features of which are manifested by distortion of early components of the excitation process (early QRS). The combination of left anterior fascicular block and left posterior fascicular block results in complete left bundle-branch block, and, unless the axis is shifted toward the more involved fascicle, the abnormality of the excitation process will be indistinguishable from that of left main bundle-branch block.

Clinically, bifascicular block most commonly involves the right bundle branch and the anterior-superior fascicle of the left bundle branch. Left posterior fascicular block is very rare as an isolated finding and is also uncommon in combination with right bundle-branch block. Left bundle-branch block is common but can represent a conduction problem at four different levels—the common bundle of His, the left main bundle, the fascicles, and the Purkinje muscle interface—although clinically the left main bundle lesions are the most common.

Trifascicular block (bilateral bundle-branch block). This term is used to delineate a block that simultaneously involves the three major fascicles—the right bundle branch and the anterior and posterior fascicles of the left bundle branch. "Bilateral bundle-branch block" also refers to those instances in which tracings from an individual patient show features diagnostic of right bundle-branch block on one tracing and of left bundle-branch block on another, or the two abnormalities may appear in alternation on the same tracing. If block is complete and involves all three fascicles, a slow escape ventricular rhythm ensues.

Clinically, a trifascicular block usually is identified as such only when the block falls short of complete AV block and is manifested by bifascicular block plus ECG evidence of compromise in the remaining fascicle. Common presentations include (1) alternating left and right bundle-branch block; (2) left or right bundle-branch block with Mobitz II block or marked first-degree heart block (without apparent AV node cause); (3) right bundle-branch block with posterior fascicular block on one occasion and anterior fascicular block on another; (4) Mobitz II block with a normal QRS (intra-His block); and (5) complete heart block with idioventricular escape rhythm or syncope (asystole–Stokes-Adams spells).

Nonspecific ventricular conduction delay. At times, a diffuse conduction delay may produce a QRS of 120 msec or more without characteristic findings of either right or left bundle-branch block. Most often it will resemble left bundle-branch block, but characteristic features of left bundle-branch block, especially those related to abnormal septal activation, may be absent. The term "nonspecific ventricular conduction defect" has been applied to this abnormality in ventricular excitation.

Preexcitation syndrome. Under normal circumstances, the sinus impulse reaches the ventricles via the specialized AV conduction system—the AV node, His bundle, bundle branches, and Purkinje network. Ventricular preexcitation occurs when a supraventricular impulse activates all or a part of the ventricular myocardium earlier than would be expected because of the presence of an accessory conduction pathway.[74-77] This accessory AV pathway may connect the atrium with the distal part of the AV node (James fiber), the atrium with the His bundle (Brechenmacher fiber), the AV node or the His bundle with the ventricular myocardium (Mahaim fiber), or, most commonly, the atrium with the ventricular myocardium (Kent bundle). Currently, the use of proper names for these various fibers and connections is being dropped in favor of characterizing them by their connecting points. By this convention, "Kent bundle" becomes "AV bypass tract."

The ECG manifestation of AV conduction via a James or Brechenmacher fiber is a short P-R interval (≤ 120 msec) and a normal QRS complex without a δ wave.[78] Such patients are prone to paroxysms of supraventricular tachycardia and atrial flutter-fibrillation and are referred to as having the Lown-Ganong-Levine syndrome. However, a short P-R interval with a normal QRS also may be encountered when there is a normal AV node with enhanced conducting ability or a small or immature AV node.

The Wolff-Parkinson-White syndrome is the most common preexcitation syndrome. AV conduction occurs simultaneously by way of an accessory AV pathway (Kent bundle) and a normal AV pathway (AV node-His-Purkinje system). This dual conduction produces a fusion beat characterized by a short P-R interval (≤ 120 msec) and a broad QRS complex with initial slurring (δ wave). Patients so afflicted are also prone to paroxysms of both supraventricular tachycardia and atrial flutter-fibrillation.[79,80] In 85% of the supraventricular tachycardias the QRS is normal because conduction is retrograde over the bypass tract from ventricle to atrium and antegrade over the normal AV node conduction system during the tachycardia, so that recognition of the Wolff-Parkinson-White syndrome is usually confined to the period when the patient exhibits sinus rhythm.

Commonly, the Wolff-Parkinson-White syndrome is divided electrocardiographically into two types: type A (positive δ wave in leads V_1 and V_2 with anteriorly directed precordial QRS forces, often with prominent Q waves in leads II, III, and aV_F or in I and aV_L) (see Fig 3A-23), and type B (negative δ wave in QRS complex in leads V_1 and V_2, often with positive δ waves in the left precordial leads) (see Fig 3A-24). However, this classification of anomalous AV conduction in the Wolff-Parkinson-White syndrome on the basis of the vector of the δ wave as recorded in conventional surface leads does not always correlate with the anticipated anatomic site of preexcitation. It is not possible to discern with the ECG the difference in anterior wall, anteroseptal, and midseptal accessory pathways.[81] General separation into type A and type B helps in understanding whether bypass pathways are anterior or posterior but will not identify those in between. The anatomic site must be determined by intracardiac electrophysiologic studies and by epicardial mapping at the time of surgical treatment, especially when multiple accessory pathways are present.[82] Although lacking in anatomic precision, classification into subgroups A and B has some merit in that type A includes the vast majority of cases with unusual AV conduction, especially in the presence of atrial flutter or fibrillation, in which rates in excess of 250 beats/min are common. Atrial flutter is not common in Wolff-Parkinson-White syndrome, whereas atrial fibrillation is present in 15% to 20% of cases.[79] Depending on the length of the refractory period of the accessory pathway, rates up to 300/min can result, leading to the danger of ventricular fibrillation and sudden death.

The differentiation of ECG abnormalities induced by anomalous ventricular excitation of the Wolff-Parkinson-White type from those resulting from myocardial infarction has been discussed above.

Summary. Ventricular conduction defects include left bundle-branch block, right bundle-branch block, fascicular blocks, nonspecific ventricular conduction delay, and abnormalities induced by preexcitation. An important concept in interpretation of right and left bundle-branch blocks is that this ECG pattern could be produced not only by a conduction delay proximally placed but also by one placed distally in either bundle branch. For example, a typical left bundle-branch block pattern could be produced by a lesion within the common bundle of His, in the proximal left main bundle, in both the left anterior and posterior fascicles of that bundle, or, finally, at the Purkinje-myocardial muscle interface focally or diffusely within the left ventricle. Block at comparable sites can exist in the right bundle. Thus, bundle-branch block is not always the product of a discrete proximal anatomic lesion.

Data derived from various sources may contribute to the determination of the nature and location of the lesion responsible for delay. The fascicular blocks become manifest not in conduction delay per se but primarily in shift of the mean electrical axis. Left anterior fascicular block is the most common and is a common cause of marked left-axis shift. Left posterior fascicular block is not easily diagnosed. It is a far less-common cause of right-axis deviation than right ventricular hypertrophy and lateral wall infarction, both of which must be excluded before considering seriously the possibility of a posterior fascicular block. Finally, combinations of fascicular blocks (bifascicular or trifascicular) may occur and be associated with complete heart block or syncopal spells.

Abnormal QRS voltage

The ECG and VCG diagnosis of left and right ventricular hypertrophy may rest on any one of several different patterns, including

1. Increased amplitude of the R wave or maximal R wave vector in leads overlying the hypertrophied ventricle, as a consequence of the increased thickness of the wall muscle
2. Delayed intrinsicoid deflection of the QRS, probably related to increased muscle mass, and thus increased QRS duration
3. ST-segment depression in leads from points overlying the hypertrophied ventricle, particularly in systolic overload situations
4. Repolarization beginning in the subendocardial area and proceeding toward the epicardium of the hypertrophied chamber in systolic overload situations, producing T-wave inversion in the leads overlying the hypertrophied chamber
5. An inverse relationship of leads opposite or away from the hypertrophied chambers to the leads overlying the hypertrophied ventricle—namely, a small r wave, a deep S wave, and an upright T wave
6. A shift in the mean electrical axis of the heart produced by hypertrophy: (1) with right ventricular hypertrophy, vertical or right axis with transition zone displaced to the left (V_4 or V_5); (2) with left ventricular hypertrophy, horizontal or left-axis deviation with transitional zone displaced to the right (V_2)

With use of standard criteria for ventricular hypertrophy, the ECG has limited ability to detect either left or right ventricular hypertrophy in patients with morbid obesity.[83]

Left ventricular hypertrophy. Clinically apparent left ventricular hypertrophy results in exaggeration of the normal ECG relationship between left and right ventricles. In normal depolarization, the right ventricular activation process is electrically silent, although it does mute somewhat the predominant left-sided activation vectors. With appearance of left ventricular hypertrophy, the S waves in the right precordial leads (V_1, V_2, and Z) become deeper, and the R waves in the left precordial leads (V_5, V_6, and X) become taller. In the VCG the amplitude of the QRS loop is increased and the loop is displaced more leftward and posteriorly.

Scalar ECG criteria for left ventricular hypertrophy include[84-86]

1. Voltage
   a. R wave in lead V_5 or V_6 and S wave in lead V_1 or V_2 ≥ 35 mm
   b. R wave in lead V_5 or V_6 ≥ 26 mm

c. R wave in lead I and S wave in lead III ≥25 mm
d. R wave
(1) ≥15 mm in lead I
(2) ≥13 mm in lead aV_L
(3) ≥20 mm in lead II, III, or aV_F
2. Secondary ST-T changes in leads overlying the left ventricle
3. QRS mean axis shows leftward shift
4. QRS duration >90 msec
5. Intrinsicoid deflection delayed >45 msec

Of these criteria, the most reliable are the voltage wave criterion (S wave V_1 or V_2 + R wave V_5 or V_6 >35 mm) and marked ST-T abnormality in left precordial leads. Application of these criteria permits recognition of approximately 41% of anatomically proven left ventricular hypertrophy with 8% false-positive diagnoses.

The ST-T abnormalities with left ventricular hypertrophy can be mild, moderate, or marked in degree. The term "LV strain" refers to ST-segment depression with T-wave inversion in leads over the left ventricle. Since this finding tends to be labile in the ECG, it is better to refer to ST-T abnormalities as mild, moderate, or marked in degree.

One of the best and most practical ways of determining left ventricular hypertrophy is by use of the Estes Scoring System[86] (Table 3A-2). By scoring points for each criterion for left ventricular hypertrophy, one can realize a more consistent, clinically useful determination of left ventricular hypertrophy.

VCG criteria (Fig 3A-30) for left ventricular hypertrophy include[87,88]

1. Maximal R vector, horizontal plane increased to >1.8 mV with leftward and posterior displacement of QRS loop
2. Delayed time of inscription of maximal QRS vector
3. ST vector and T loop often displaced in an anterior and rightward direction opposite the QRS

These criteria, taken as an aggregate, result in recognition of approximately 50% of anatomically proved left ventricular hypertrophy with a false-positive risk of approximately 11%. Thus, the VCG and the ECG are essentially comparable in their ability to discern clinically verified left ventricular hypertrophy. Continued efforts to improve ECG diagnostic accuracy in left ventricular hypertrophy include the product of QRS voltage and QRS duration as an approximate time voltage integral of the QRS complex. Using a 12-lead product criterion, Molloy et al.[89] accurately diagnosed left ventricular hypertrophy in 45% of patients, whereas success with standard ECG criteria was 31%. Detection of early left ventricular hypertrophy by ECG criteria remains difficult.

Table 3A-2 Estes scoring system for left ventricular hypertrophy

1. Voltage criterion present	3
2. ST-T abnormality	
Without digitalis	3
With digitalis	(1)
3. Left-axis deviation ≥ −15°	2
4. QRS duration ≥0.09 sec	1
5. Intrinsicoid deflection in V_5 or V_6 ≥0.04 sec	1
Total	10

4 points = probable left ventricular hypertrophy.
5 or more points = left ventricular hypertrophy.

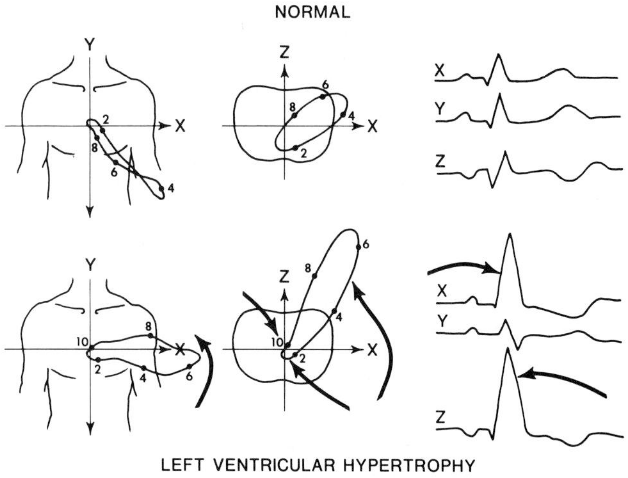

Fig 3A-30 Frontal and horizontal plane vector loop display and X,Y,Z data for normal VCG **(upper)** and characteristic VCG loop changes produced by left ventricular hypertrophy **(lower),** with loop displacement to the posterior left quadrant and delayed activation time, increased voltage, and leftward frontal QRS axis shift. *Arrows* indicate significant changes described.

Two types of left ventricular hypertrophy appear clinically and electrocardiographically: (1) systolic overload type left ventricular hypertrophy, of which systemic hypertension is the most common cause but which also includes aortic stenosis, hypertrophic cardiomyopathy, and coarctation of the aorta; and (2) diastolic overload type left ventricular hypertrophy, which includes aortic insufficiency, mitral incompetence, and high-flow left-to-right shunts. Increased QRS voltage tends to be more prominent in diastolic overload, but the most distinctive feature is the tall, upright T waves in left precordial leads V_4-V_6 and X, in contrast to the strain pattern that is typical of systolic overload (Fig 3A-31).

Right ventricular hypertrophy. Because changes in potential produced by excitation of the left ventricle normally exceed those produced by right ventricular excitation, mild to moderate right ventricular hypertrophy may go undetected by either ECG or VCG. In fact, both are relatively insensitive to this morphological state and, when right ventricular hypertrophy is recognizable, it usually is of severe degree.

Scalar ECG criteria for right ventricular hypertrophy include[90]

1. Voltage
a. R/S ratio >1 in lead V_1
b. R in lead V_1 >7 mm
c. R in lead aV_R >5 mm
d. S in lead V_1 <2 mm
e. R in lead V_1 and S in lead V_5 or V_6 >10.5 mm

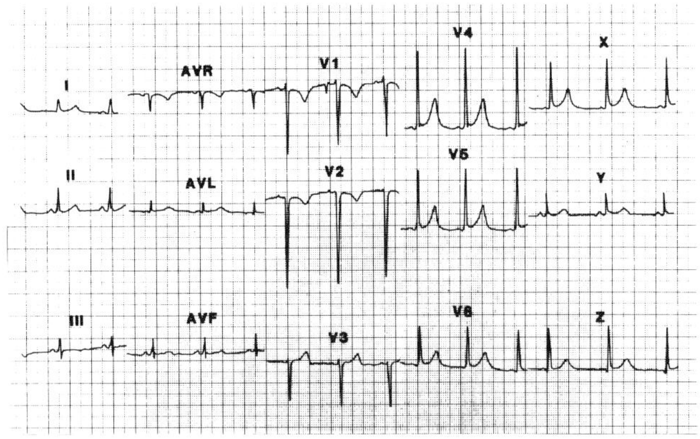

Fig 3A-31 Features of left ventricular hypertrophy with prominent QRS voltages and prominent upright T waves in the left precordial leads, consistent with the diastolic overload pattern seen in left ventricular volume overload. This tracing was taken from a patient with aortic insufficiency.

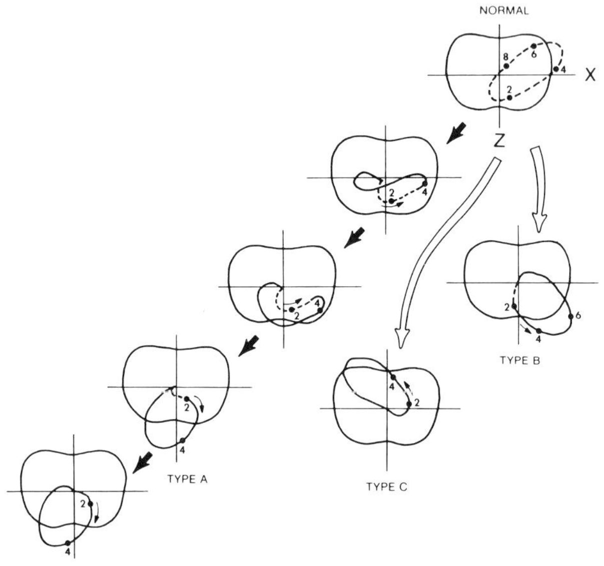

Fig 3A-32 Types of right ventricular hypertrophy. Types B and C are less common. Type C tends to be seen in patients with pulmonary disease with secondary right ventricular hypertrophy. There is evidence that figure-of-8 horizontal loops are less likely to represent right ventricular hypertrophy. These loops start left anterior, rotate counterclockwise, turn posterior, cross their own paths, and end in the right anterior quadrant, rotating clockwise.

2. ST-T abnormalities (over right ventricle) in leads V_1-V_3, II, III, and aV_F
3. QRS mean axis showing right axis deviation
4. QRS duration normal
5. QRS intrinsicoid deflection in lead V_1 delayed >35 msec

A combination of several of these criteria usually is required to establish a diagnosis of right ventricular hypertrophy because a prominent R wave in lead V_1 may be seen in posterior wall myocardial infarction,[91] Wolff-Parkinson-White syndrome type A, posterior septal infarction, septal fascicular block, and idiopathic hypertrophic subaortic stenosis; as a normal variant; and occasionally with muscular dystrophies, particularly Duchenne's muscular dystrophy. Right-axis deviation may be produced by left posterior fascicular block, and it also can be induced by a major lateral wall myocardial infarction.

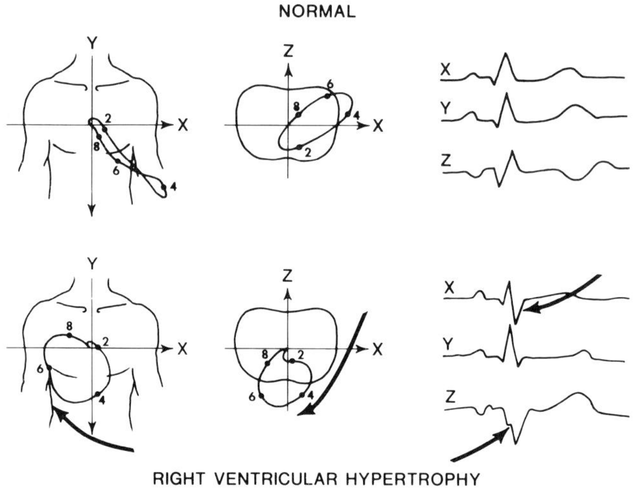

Fig 3A-33 Frontal and horizontal plane vector loop display and X,Y,Z data for normal VCG (**upper**) and characteristic VCG loop changes produced by type A right ventricular hypertrophy (**lower**). The loop includes clockwise horizontal rotation with displacement to the right and anterior with right axis in frontal plane.

In the VCG,[92-94] the increased right ventricular forces displace the horizontal QRS loop anteriorly or posteriorly to the right. Three types of horizontal QRS loops have been described (Fig 3A-32). Type A consists of an anterior rightward-oriented loop inscribed clockwise. This type of loop usually is associated with ventricular hypertrophy (Figs 3A-33 and 3A-34). The type B loop consists of a leftward and anteriorly displaced counterclockwise loop. It is typical of acquired heart disease with severe right ventricular hypertrophy, but it also can be seen with posterior wall myocardial infarction and Wolff-Parkinson-White syndrome type A. The type C loop is a posterior and rightward displacement of the terminal portion of a normally inscribed counterclockwise horizontal plane loop. On occasion, in this type the terminal portion may be displaced anteriorly to the right, at which point it resembles a typical right bundle-branch block loop but without an increase in ventricular excitation time to 120 msec or more. This type C loop usually is seen in patients who have cor pulmonale, but it also has been reported in patients with mitral stenosis or atrial septal defect with significant right ventricular hypertrophy.

To increase the sensitivity of vector analysis of right ventricular hypertrophy, Chou and associates[94] proposed the following criteria:

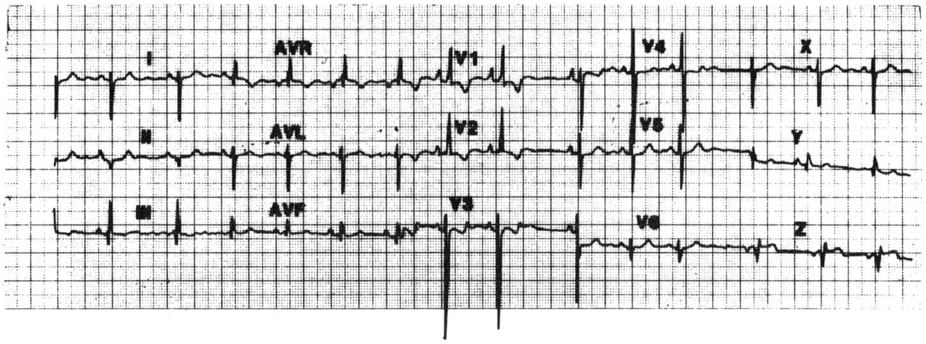

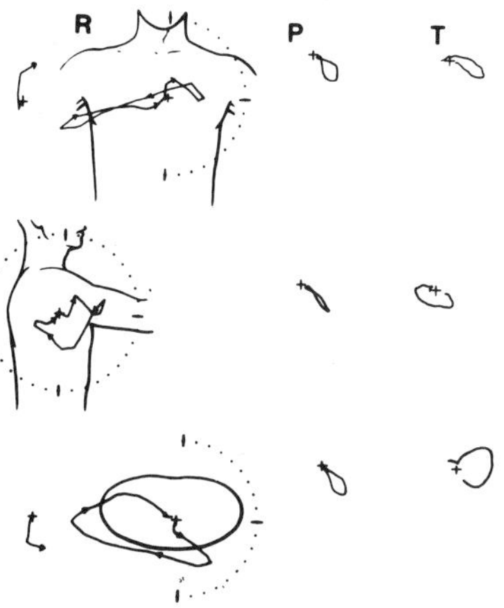

Fig 3A-34 Characteristic features of type A right ventricular hypertrophy. The horizontal plane vector loop courses clockwise, anterior, and to the right. In the standard ECG the presence of right-axis deviation and prominent upright R waves with R/S ratio >1 and R wave in lead V_1 >7 mm, with ST-T changes over the right ventricle, makes the diagnosis of right ventricular hypertrophy.

1. In a horizontal plane, the rightward and anterior QRS loop area occupies >70% of the total area, or the area in the left posterior quadrant is <30% of the total.
2. In a horizontal plane, the QRS loop in the right posterior quadrant is >20% of the total.
3. In a horizontal plane, the area of the QRS loop in the right anterior quadrant of a counterclockwise-turning loop is <20% of the total.

When these criteria were tested in 97 patients with atrial septal defect, mitral stenosis, and chronic obstructive pulmonary disease with pulmonary hypertension, Chou et al.[94] noted that one or more of the criteria were met in 83% of the patients compared with 66% meeting the standard scalar criteria. Cowdery et al.[95] further refined the diagnosis of right ventricular hypertrophy, utilizing the Frank system and a simple linear VCG analysis that is helpful in those patients with a type C loop. This linear analysis suggested that the maximal QRS magnitude had to be <1.8 mV in the horizontal plane and either the amplitude at −45° (horizontal plane) had to be <0.3 mV or at −45° the maximum anterior amplitude plus the maximum rightward amplitude (anterior or posterior) must be ≥0.5 mV. The specificity of these criteria (96%) was significantly better than that of the VCG criteria (83%) found by Chou et al.[94] Despite the improved sensitivity and specificity of these criteria, only 60% of the patients with moderate to severe right ventricular hypertrophy were properly identified. This emphasizes the insensitivity of the ECG and VCG to the presence of acquired right ventricular hypertrophy.

Just as in left ventricular hypertrophy, right ventricular hypertrophy may be displayed as a systolic overload type with an ST-T segment manifesting a strain pattern in leads V_1 and V_2 (this occurs in such conditions as tetralogy of Fallot, pulmonic stenosis, mitral stenosis with pulmonary hypertension, and cor pulmonale) or a diastolic overload pattern (encountered in atrial septal defect and tricuspid insufficiency).

The diagnosis of right ventricular hypertrophy in coexistence with right bundle-branch block is often difficult. The dilemma usually is easily resolved in those cases in which all of the forces are displaced anteriorly in lead Z and in the horizontal plane loop, suggesting an atypical right bundle-branch block loop likely to have been induced by a complicating lesion (see "Right Bundle-Branch Block" above). The situation is more difficult when there is a combination of a typical type I right bundle-branch block loop and right ventricular hypertrophy. Recognition of right ventricular hypertrophy under these circumstances is best accomplished by applying to the right bundle-branch block loop the criteria of Chou et al.[94] and Cowdery et al.[95] (see above). In general, right ventricular hypertrophy should be suspected when the anterior and rightward forces in a right bundle-branch block loop are considerably greater than the posterior and leftward forces induced by left ventricular activation. In most typical right bundle-branch block loops, there is a balance between the anterior and rightward-directed terminal forces and the posterior and leftward left ventricular forces, but when right ventricular hypertrophy coexists, a definite distortion suggestive of right hypertrophy usually is evident.

Biventricular hypertrophy. This is uncommon and usually is found only in congenital heart disease or in a cardiomyopathy. The following suggest such hypertrophy:

1. Pattern of left ventricular hypertrophy in the precordial leads with right-axis deviation (without left posterior fascicular block) and right atrial hypertrophy in the limb leads
2. Pattern of right ventricular hypertrophy in the precordial leads associated with marked left-axis deviation
3. Katz-Wachtle phenomenon (prominent anterior right ventricular and posterior left ventricular forces in the same patient, typical of a ventricular septal defect with pulmonary hypertension)
4. Transverse plane QRS loops indicative of increased anterior forces plus diagnostically significant maximal R vector in the posterior left quadrant
5. R wave plus S wave in mid precordial lead > 45 mm

QRS axis

The electrical depolarization of the atrial and ventricular muscle and the subsequent repolarization take a characteristic pathway with each heartbeat. Because the electrical activity begins in the sinoatrial node of the right atrium and spreads in a right-to-left and superior-to-inferior direction, there is an individual electrical axis of the P wave, the QRS complex, and the T wave. This electrical axis has some diagnostic usefulness, and calculation of this axis should be an integral part of ECG analysis. For diagnostic purposes, the electrical axes of the heart are calculated only in the frontal plane. The horizontal axes are of less diagnostic significance.

By convention, the electrical axis in the frontal plane is plotted within a circle that has been transected into a 180° inferior arc that is designated positive and a superior 180° arc that is negative. For diagnostic purposes, the electrical axis of the QRS complex is the most useful.

The electrical axis can be derived by using the triaxial reference system or the hexaxial reference system.[96] In the triaxial reference system the three limbs of the Einthoven triangle are arranged in such a manner that the lines formed by leads I, II, and III bisect one another in the middle. Addition of the three unipolar limb leads to this system in a similar manner produces the hexaxial reference system. The depolarization of the ventricular muscle can be represented by a mean QRS vector plotted on this reference system. By use of any two limb leads, the magnitude and direction of this mean manifest QRS vector can be determined.

To plot the axis, the net area enclosed under the QRS in each of the limb leads is calculated. For practical purposes, it is not necessary to calculate the area accurately—subtracting the negative QRS deflection from the positive deflection gives a value that can be used in plotting the mean manifest QRS axis. However, the algebraic summation of the negative and positive areas enclosed under the QRS reflects the mean manifest QRS axis with greater accuracy. The deflections in the two

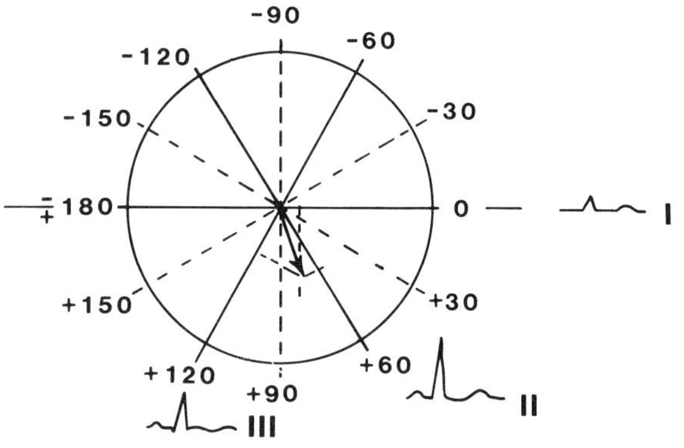

Fig 3A-35 Frontal plane QRS axis according to hexaxial reference system (see text).

standard leads selected then can be plotted on the triaxial or hexaxial reference system (Fig 3A-35). The point of intersection of the perpendiculars drawn from the points representing the algebraic summation of positive and negative QRS areas is connected with the central 0 point of the reference system to identify the mean manifest QRS axis. A normal QRS axis is said to lie in the left lower quadrant when it is between 0° and +90°. It has been found, however, that a normal axis may lie between −30° and +110°, and this broader range should be considered the normal QRS axis range. In older patients, the QRS axis tends to become more horizontal and shifts into the left upper quadrant area.[97] Left-axis deviation is said to exist when the axis lies between −30° and −90°. Right-axis deviation exists when the axis is between +110° and +180°. A mean manifest QRS axis that lies between −90° and ±180° may represent either marked left-axis deviation or marked right-axis deviation.

Calculation of the mean manifest QRS axis has little diagnostic value in itself. The variation in normal individuals is wide (from −30° to +110°), and in most abnormal ECG settings the axis is in the normal range. However, when the QRS axis falls outside of the normal range, it may provide information of considerable value in identifying abnormalities. In right ventricular hypertrophy, the presence of a right mean QRS axis is one of the supportive criteria. Similarly, in left ventricular hypertrophy, a leftward shift in the QRS axis may contribute to accurate assessment of the diagnosis. A shift of the QRS axis in a leftward or a rightward direction may reflect an alteration in the spread of excitation of the ventricles, as discussed above under QRS changes—e.g., left anterior hemiblock produces marked left-axis deviation. In congenital heart disease, calculation of the mean manifest QRS axis has some value in separating certain entities, such as primary from secondary atrial septal defects. Myocardial infarction may induce a shift in the frontal QRS axis consequent to localized loss of muscle mass.

In summary, calculation of the mean manifest QRS axis has some diagnostic usefulness and should be done routinely. The gross determination based on superior deflection minus inferior deflection plotted on the triaxial or hexaxial reference system ordinarily suffices.

ST-T wave

Under usual physiologic conditions, the repolarization process proceeds from epicardium to endocardium, resulting in an upright T wave in the left precordial leads concordant with the QRS. This relationship persists as long as depolarization is normal, but it may be altered in two ways. One way is prolonged depolarization in such situations as ventricular hypertrophy (right or left), bundle-branch block (right or left), or Wolff-Parkinson-White syndrome or in the presence of a ventricular focus (ventricular premature contraction or ventricular escape focus); the course of timing of repolarization is altered, and T-wave polarity commonly is discordant with that of the QRS, producing so-called secondary T-wave changes. In the other way, the depolarization process is normal; a discordant T wave (i.e., opposite to the QRS) is considered primary and reflects changes resulting from an altered myocardial state induced by ischemia, myocarditis, electrolyte disorder, or neurologic disorder.

Ischemia. From a physiologic point of view, in relation to demand the coronary blood flow to the epicardial portion of the left ventricular myocardium is greater than that to the subendocardial portion. This discrepancy is dependent in part on the fact that, within the ventricular wall, the pressure to which the coronary vasculature is subjected is greater in the inner than in the outer layer. This greater pressure in the subendocardial region tends to collapse the vessels and decrease the flow during systole, especially in patients with systemic hypertension or left ventricular outflow obstruction. Thus, in general, subendocardial ischemia is both more common and produced more easily than subepicardial ischemia.

In subendocardial ischemia, slow repolarization in the subendocardial region—which even under physiologic circumstances is the region with the longest refractory period—results in prolongation of the Q-T interval. Ischemia in this region does not alter the epicardium-to-endocardium direction of repolarization, but the slow recovery in the subendocardial region augments the magnitude of the T wave because repolarization persists in this zone as repolarization subsides in the epicardial layer. Thus, the characteristic finding of subendocardial ischemia is tall upright T waves.[98,99] In those leads overlying the ischemic zone, these changes may mimic those produced by hyperkalemia or quinidine.

Ischemia involving the subepicardial region slows the repolarization process so much that its mean direction is from endocardium to epicardium. As a result, discordant or inverted T waves appear in leads overlying the ischemic zone.

When the clinical setting is compatible with the diagnosis, primary T waves suggest myocardial ischemia. The presence or absence of myocardial injury can be proved only with additional evidence provided by enzyme studies because the T waves in themselves reflect only the ischemia, not myocardial injury per se. A special variety of myocardial ischemia is so-called variant angina or Prinzmetal's angina in which there is marked ST elevation suggestive of myocardial injury but no pathologic T waves appear; with resolution of the patient's pain, the ECG returns to normal.

Electrolyte imbalance. Various electrolyte changes have a significant influence on cardiac output and on cardiac impulse formation and conduction. The two electrolytes that produce major ECG changes are potassium and calcium. However, although the ECG provides a rapid means of detecting abnormalities of these two electrolytes, it is important to recognize several modifying factors.

First, the ECG changes reflect alterations of the potassium or calcium concentration within the myocardium, and although this is usually represented in the serum concentration, changes in the serum may occur so rapidly that the myocardial changes may lag behind. Thus, the ECG may be normal with abnormal serum concentrations of the electrolytes or abnormal with a normal serum concentration.[100]

Drugs that the patient is taking may alter the ECG by either masking the electrolyte changes or mimicking them. In this regard, digitalis simulates hypokalemia, and often the two are present together. The effects of tricyclic antidepressants mimic the changes seen with hypercalcemia. Similarly, intrinsic cardiac disease such as coronary artery disease, hypertension, or cardiomyopathy can obscure the presence of electrolyte imbalance.

From a clinical standpoint, combined electrolyte problems are more common than the isolated imbalance of a single electrolyte.[101] In patients with renal insufficiency, the combination of hyperkalemia and hypocalcemia is common. In this instance, the presence of hypocalcemia enhances the AV node and the interventricular conduction disturbances produced by hyperkalemia and also increases the risk of a major ventricular arrhythmia.[102] Another combination occurring in renal insufficiency and secondary hyperparathyroidism is hypercalcemia plus hyperkalemia. In this situation, the two electrolytes block each other so that the AV node and interventricular conduction disturbances are lessened and the risk of ventricular arrhythmia is diminished. Hypernatremia also modifies the manifestations of hyperkalemia, whereas hyponatremia and hypermagnesemia augment them. Also, digitalis-induced toxic rhythm disturbances are enhanced by the presence of hypokalemia, hypercalcemia, and hypomagnesemia.

Potassium is the predominant intercellular cation, and its relative intercellular and extracellular concentrations play a significant role in the repolarization effect induced in the ECG. As the potassium concentration begins to increase above the normal value and approaches the range of 7 mEq/L, the first effect is a peaking of the T waves to produce tall, tented T waves.[103,104] As the serum potassium concentration continues to increase, the peaking of the T waves is associated with development of first-degree AV block, some initial widening of the QRS, and depression of the ST segment. The amplitude of the atrial P wave is decreased, and with increase of the potassium value into the range of 9 to 10 mEq/L, atrial standstill occurs. With these high levels of potassium, ventricular conduction is disturbed, and the QRS becomes widened, with the T wave surpassing the R wave in amplitude. QRS widening is associated with depression of the ST segment, with the QRS and the T-wave unit

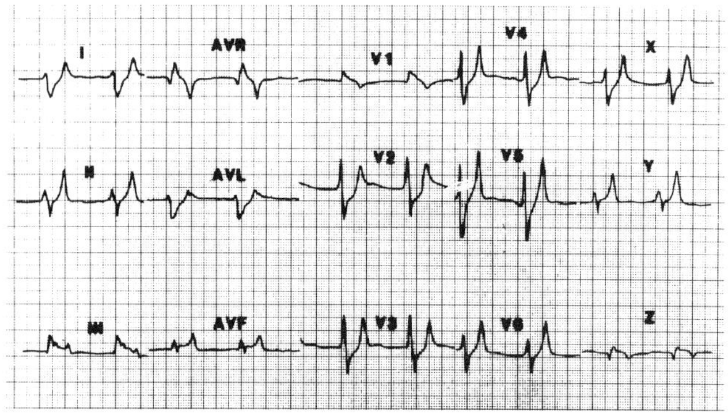

Fig 3A-36 Typical changes in hyperkalemia, with tall, peaked T waves, widening of the QRS, and apparent atrial standstill. As the potassium value increases, the T wave begins to surpass the R wave in amplitude, and with the widening of the QRS and the beginning of the T waves, it develops a sine-wave configuration.

producing a biphasic wave. At this stage, ventricular conduction is depressed and the heart is approaching standstill. Ectopic ventricular rhythms are likely to develop, and ventricular fibrillation may be the terminal event (Fig 3A-36).

The effects of hypokalemia are seen more commonly than hyperkalemia because of the widespread use of diuretics in the management of cardiovascular conditions. As the serum potassium concentration falls below the normal range, the first change usually noted on the ECG is a more prominent U wave following the T wave. The T wave becomes lower in amplitude and more rounded in configuration. As the potassium value falls below 3 mEq/L, the U wave becomes higher than the T wave, and the T wave becomes flat. With continued lowering of the potassium value into the range of 2 mEq/L, the ST segment becomes depressed, the T wave goes flat, and the U wave becomes the prominent signal of repolarization.[105] Unless hypocalcemia coexists with hypokalemia, the Q-T interval remains normal. The Q-U interval is what appears to be prolonged. Less characteristically seen in hypokalemia is a slight prolongation of the P-R interval and more prominent P waves. The ECG effect of change in serum calcium concentration is primarily related to the Q-T interval, which varies inversely with the calcium level in the blood: when the calcium level is high, the Q-T interval is short; when the level is low, the Q-T interval is prolonged.

Endocrine changes. Endocrine abnormalities produce ECG alterations mainly by their effects on the concentration of one or more of the serum electrolytes or on associated abnormal cardiovascular conditions. For example, Cushing's syndrome produces hypokalemia and the associated hypokalemic changes in the ECG. Addison's disease, on the other hand, produces hyperkalemia and its changes in the ECG.

The effects of thyroid hormone on the heart are more complex. Hyperthyroidism tends to make an underlying cardiovascular disease manifest. In the presence of significant coronary disease, hyperthyroidism may foster cardiac arrhythmias, produce myocardial infarction, and result in multiple ECG abnormalities. The more common consequences of hyperthyroidism are atrial arrhythmias (e.g., atrial fibrillation and atrial flutter), sinus tachycardia, and nonspecific ST-T changes. On the other hand, hypothyroidism with myxedema induces bradycardia, a prolonged P-R interval, a decrease in the voltage of the QRS complex, and low-voltage or inverted T waves. With correction of the myxedema, the T waves return to their normal height and the QRS voltage increases. Bradycardia disappears.

All of the ECG findings associated with endocrine disorders are nonspecific, at times supporting the clinical diagnosis but not diagnostic of it per se.

Drug changes. Various commonly used drugs can produce ECG abnormalities. Those associated with a high incidence of ECG abnormalities are discussed here.

QUINIDINE.[106,107] Clinically, the pharmacologic and electrophysiologic problems produced by quinidine can result in prolongation of the Q-T interval, which predisposes the patient to ventricular tachycardia/fibrillation as a consequence of unsuppressed premature ventricular beats extending the vulnerable period. By increasing the concentration of digoxin in the serum, quinidine may induce digitalis toxicity and its attendant rhythm disturbances. Slowing of the flutter rate from 300/min to 220/min or less may permit 1:1 conduction through the AV node, sometimes attended by clinical deterioration. From a purely ECG standpoint, quinidine toxicity is suggested by sinoatrial block or broadening of the P wave (intra-atrial conduction delay), by widening of the QRS to more than 50% of control, and by lengthening of both P-R and Q-T intervals. Similar findings, although usually not as severe, are seen with other type I drugs such as procainamide and isopyramide phosphate.

DIGITALIS.[108,109] The ECG findings of digitalis excess consist primarily of significant rhythm disturbances, including ventricular premature beats, often in bigeminy, or fixed coupling in the presence of atrial fibrillation; nonparoxysmal junctional tachycardia; atrial tachycardia with block; significant compromise of AV node conduction, including complete heart block with a slow junctional escape rhythm; and bidirectional ventricular tachycardia. These rhythm disturbances are to be distinguished from the digitalis effect on the ECG, which consists of lengthening of the P-R interval (first-degree heart block) and a characteristic rounding and sagging of the ST segment.

PHENOTHIAZINES.[110,111] From a cardiovascular standpoint, the phenothiazine group of drugs acts centrally to depress blood pressure and peripherally through α-adrenergic blockade to cause peripheral vasodilation and, at times, symptomatic hypotension. The membrane effects are similar to those of quinidine, and therefore electrocardiographically the toxic effects of these drugs are similar to those produced by quinidine.

TRICYCLIC ANTIDEPRESSANTS. These drugs can block the uptake of norepinephrine by the heart and can induce a negative inotropic effect on the heart. They also have antiarrhythmia properties similar to those of quinidine, but toxicity is usually manifested by sinus or atrial tachycardia with widening of the QRS and decreased T-wave amplitude. The Q-T interval remains normal.

CLOFIBRATE. Although the precise mechanism by which clofibrate produces cardiac arrhythmias is unknown, it is clear that this drug can provoke frequent ectopic beats, both atrial and ventricular. In addition, paroxysmal supraventricular tachycardia has been initiated in association with use of the drug, and, on occasion, so has ventricular tachycardia. Most of the patients who have had arrhythmia with this drug also had known symptomatic coronary artery disease, and it may be that the interplay between the drug and the disease is critical to the presence and frequency of rhythm disturbances.

DOXORUBICIN (ADRIAMYCIN). This anthrocycline antibiotic, used primarily for the treatment of lymphomas and leukemias, has been reported to have significant cardiotoxic effects. It appears to have a direct toxic effect on the functioning myocardium, resulting in a cardiomyopathic picture with cardiac enlargement, mural thrombi, and biventricular failure after 1 to 5 months of therapy. Use of the drug often results in the appearance of supraventricular tachydysrhythmias, ventricular premature contractions, and diffuse ST-T wave changes on the ECG. These clinical and ECG changes eventuate in a cardiomyopathy, emphasizing the poor tolerance of the myocardium for this drug.

Miscellaneous patterns

Long Q-T interval syndrome. This exists as a familial condition in two forms: (1) as the Jervell and Lange-Nielsen syndrome, with deaf mutism, often iron-deficiency anemia, and an autosomal recessive inheritance pattern; and (2) as the Romano-Ward syndrome, with normal hearing and an autosomal dominant inheritance pattern.[112,113] Both forms have a long Q-T interval associated with arrhythmias, syncope, and sudden death. The reason for the Q-T prolongation is unclear at this time, but death usually is related to ventricular fibrillation initiated by an "R on T" phenomenon produced by a ventricular premature beat.

Juvenile T-wave pattern. Inversion of the T waves in leads V_1-V_3 in young healthy individuals, predominantly females, is common and is termed the "juvenile T-wave pattern." The reason for this variation is unknown, but it is important to recognize it in order to avoid erroneously interpreting the ECG as showing anterior wall ischemia.

Early repolarization pattern. In healthy persons, usually those under age 35, it is not uncommon to see ST-segment elevation, predominantly J-point elevation, most often in the inferior (II, III, aV_F) and left precordial (V_4-V_6) leads. This early repolarization pattern is a normal variant and is quite common in black males and Eskimo children. It is important to distinguish these changes from those of acute myocardial injury produced by acute pericarditis or an early stage of myocardial infarction.

U wave

The U wave on the ECG, first mentioned by Einthoven in 1906,[114] is a normal finding on the standard 12-lead tracing. It follows the T wave and is upright in anterior precordial leads. In general, the U-wave vector has the same polarity as the T wave and usually is most prominent in precordial leads V_2 and V_3. The normal U-wave amplitude averages up to 25% of the T-wave amplitude and tends to be larger with slower heart rates.[115] The genesis of the U wave is not clearly known. One hypothesis is that it includes an afterpotential of ventricular repolarization, repolarization of the ventricular Purkinje system. A second hypothesis suggests that the U wave is the product of a family of cells with an unusually long repolarization cycle. Many factors are known to alter the U wave, the most common being hypokalemia, which increases its height.

Abnormally inverted U waves have been recognized since 1939 as being associated with patients who have heart disease.[116] Inverted U waves have been found in patients with left ventricular hypertrophy, significant hypertension, or coronary heart disease.[117,118] The development of U-wave inversion during exercise stress testing has been described as an indicator of coronary artery disease. In 1979, Gerson et al.[119] reported their experience with 36 patients who had exercise-induced U-wave inversion among 248 patients who underwent cineangiographic studies and exercise evaluations. Of these 36, 35 had greater than 75% stenosis of one or more of the major coronary vessels. The proximal left anterior descending or left main coronary artery was involved in 33 of the 36. Exercise-induced U-wave inversion was observed in the absence of an induced abnormal ST-segment response in 8 of 176 patients with coronary artery disease (4.5%) but only in 1 of 82 patients without significant coronary artery disease. They concluded that exercise-induced inversion of the U wave was highly predictive of significant coronary artery disease and, more specifically, of disease in the proximal left anterior descending coronary system.

SPECIAL CLINICAL PROBLEMS

Congenital heart disease

Certain ECG patterns are highly suggestive, but not pathognomonic, of a specific congenital cardiac anomaly. The following are representative.

Right bundle-branch block is uniformly present in atrial septal defect and Ebstein's anomaly, and the association of left-axis deviation with right bundle-branch block in a child is strongly suggestive of an ostium primum type of atrial septal defect.

Left ventricular hypertrophy with a systolic overload pattern is seen in congenital aortic stenosis, coarctation of aorta, and hypertrophic cardiomyopathy, whereas a diastolic overload pattern is common in large left-to-right shunts (ventricular septal defect and patent ductus arteriosus).

Right ventricular hypertrophy with a systolic overload pattern is common in pulmonic stenosis, whereas a diastolic overload pattern is typical of an atrial septal defect.

Supraventricular tachyarrhythmias are most common in mitral valve prolapse, atrial septal defect, and Ebstein's anomaly. The Wolff-Parkinson-White syndrome is asso-

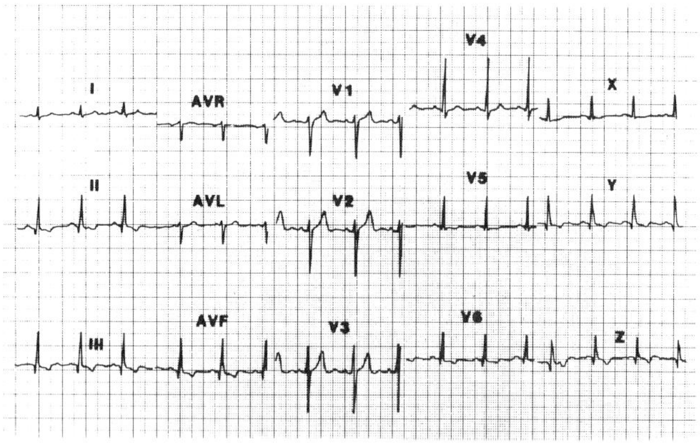

Fig 3A-37 ECG showing nonspecific T-wave abnormalities in leads II, III, and aV_F in a patient with mitral valve prolapse. Typically, as the patient lies down, these T-wave changes become upright. They are quite labile and vary with the position of the patient during recording of the tracing.

ciated with Ebstein's anomaly and hypertrophic cardiomyopathy.

First-degree heart block is common in Ebstein's anomaly, atrial septal defect, ventricular septal defect, and patent ductus arteriosus.

P congenitalis (right atrial hypertrophy) is common in cyanotic congenital heart disease and pulmonic stenosis. Extremely large or tall P waves are seen in Ebstein's anomaly and tricuspid atresia.

A normal ECG does not exclude a congenital heart lesion, and no ECG finding can be termed pathognomonic of a specific anomaly. Distinctive and suggestive patterns in certain common congenital anomalies are as follows:

1. Mitral valve prolapse. In approximately 15% to 20% of patients with mitral valve prolapse, the ECG includes abnormal T-wave inversion in the inferior leads (II, III, aV_F, Y and a lateral precordial lead (V_5, V_6, X)[120] (Fig 3A-37). In addition, ectopic atrial or ventricular premature beats and frequent runs of supraventricular tachycardia are common. Left ventricular hypertrophy is uncommon.
2. Congenital aortic stenosis and coarctation of the aorta. In both of these lesions there is systolic overload of the left ventricle, which results in significant left ventricular hypertrophy and left ventricular conduction delay; when severe, this delay satisfies criteria for left bundle-branch block.
3. Ventricular septal defect. In a small muscular septum with a ventricular septal defect (maladie de Roger type), the ECG is normal despite spectacular auscultatory findings of a harsh pansystolic lower left sternal border murmur. Rarely, left ventricular hypertrophy is present. When the defect is moderate or large, biventricular hypertrophy appears, and the Katz-Wachtle phenomenon—namely, large, equal R-S complexes in leads V_2-V_4—is common.
4. Atrial septal defect.[121] There are four clinically apparent types of atrial septal defect: secundum, primum, sinus venosus, and coronary sinus. In more than 90% the ECG and VCG show right bundle-branch block or right ventricular conduction delay (QRS > 100 msec). The right bundle-branch block reflects hypertrophy of the crista supraventricularis and enlargement of the right ventricle; hence, it is a peripheral conduction defect and not a true proximal right bundle-branch block. The axis in the frontal plane is normal or slightly to the right in all forms of atrial septal defect, except that in the ostium primum variety, congenital left anterior fascicular block produces marked left-axis deviation. If right ventricular hypertrophy supervenes due to pulmonary hypertension, appropriate ECG changes may appear. Atrial fibrillation is common later in the disease process, usually with the appearance of pulmonary hypertension. In ostium primum defects, biventricular hypertrophy is common because of the right ventricular overload and mitral incompetence.
5. Patent ductus arteriosus. When small, this defect can be associated with a normal ECG, but with large shunts, left ventricular hypertrophy with a diastolic overload pattern appears initially. If pulmonary hypertension develops, biventricular hypertrophy supervenes.
6. Pulmonary stenosis. This defect produces outflow obstruction from the right ventricle, and the systolic overload of the right ventricle is manifested electrocardiographically by right ventricular hypertrophy, P congenitale, and vertical or right axis. Leads V_1, V_2, and Z resemble lead V_6 in the setting of significant aortic stenosis—tall R wave with an ST-T "strain" pattern.
7. Tetralogy of Fallot.[122] In a physiologic sense, tetralogy of Fallot consists of a large ventricular septal defect and pulmonic stenosis. The severity of the latter determines the amount of right-to-left shunting across the former; if shunting is greater than a critical level, the patient is cyanotic from birth. The axis is right, and right ventricular hypertrophy is present but is not as severe as in pure pulmonary stenosis with an intact septum, because the septal defect tends to decompress the right ventricle. P congenitale is also less marked. Right bundle-branch block may be induced by therapeutic right ventriculotomy or, less commonly, in the course of repair of the defect.
8. Ebstein's anomaly.[123] This congenital defect consists of the displacement of one or more of the tricuspid leaflets downward into the right ventricle. This displacement induces the development of tricuspid insufficiency, reduces the functional capacity, distorts the anatomy of the right ventricle, and alters the right side of the AV ring in a manner favorable to development of the bypass tract (Kent bundle). The ECG findings in this situation are large, peaked P waves in leads II, III, and aV_F, at times of amplitude virtually equal to that of the QRS; right bundle-branch block with a bizarre configuration and a QRS interval of 160 msec or more; and high incidence of Wolff-Parkinson-White syndrome type B and, consequently, frequent supraventricular tachyarrhythmias.

9. Tricuspid atresia. This rare lesion is distinguished electrocardiographically as the only congenital cardiac lesion in which cyanosis and left ventricular hypertrophy, in association with left-axis deviation, are present from birth. Most other cyanotic congenital lesions have normal or right-axis deviation.
10. Dextrocardia. Two forms are found. One form is mirror-image dextrocardia with situs inversus in which other congenital lesions are not common and in which the ECG shows inversion of the P, QRS, and T waves in lead I; leads II, III, aV_R, and aV_L are reversed, changes similar to those produced by reversal of the right and left leads. The other form is dextrocardia, associated with other complex congenital defects, including D-transposition, tetralogy of Fallot, truncus arteriosus, single ventricle, and ventricular septal defect. The ECG reflects the underlying defect, but the P wave in lead I is inverted.
11. Pulmonary vascular obstructive disease (Eisenmenger's complex). This term describes the situation in which a left-to-right shunt, such as a large ventricular septal defect or patent ductus arteriosus or, less commonly, an atrial septal defect, results in the development of reactive pulmonary hypertension such that the shunting is halted or reversed. When this happens, right ventricular hypertrophy or biventricular hypertrophy will become apparent, the axis will be vertical or right, and right atrial hypertrophy will be present.
12. Congenital complete heart block.[124] This is most commonly associated with a slow, regular heart rate that speeds somewhat with exercise in an essentially asymptomatic patient who has no other evidence of congenital heart defect. The ECG reveals a narrow AV junctional escape focus and a slow sinus rate, indicating that the patient is tolerating the situation reasonably well. Pacing usually is withheld until the patient becomes symptomatic. Sudden death is rare, but the natural history of this defect is not yet well-defined. Block is at the level of the AV junction where the escape focus is located. When congenital complete heart block is associated with another congenital cardiac problem, that problem usually is a common AV canal or a corrected transposition. In the former, failure to unite the atrial and ventricular septa often produces a gap in the conduction system; in the latter, rotation of the interventricular septum compromises the common bundle of His and the bundle branch connections.

Pericarditis

The major ECG finding during the early stage of acute pericarditis is ST-segment elevation in all leads except aV_R and possibly leads I and aV_L, the leads that face the endocardial aspect of the ventricular wall. Characteristically, there are no reciprocal shifts of the ST segment in leads I, II, and III as occur in acute myocardial infarction. Sinus tachycardia usually is present. This typical pattern of acute pericarditis applies not only to idiopathic or viral pericarditis but to all forms, including postpericardiotomy and myocardial infarction (Dressler's) syndromes[125,126] (Fig 3A-38).

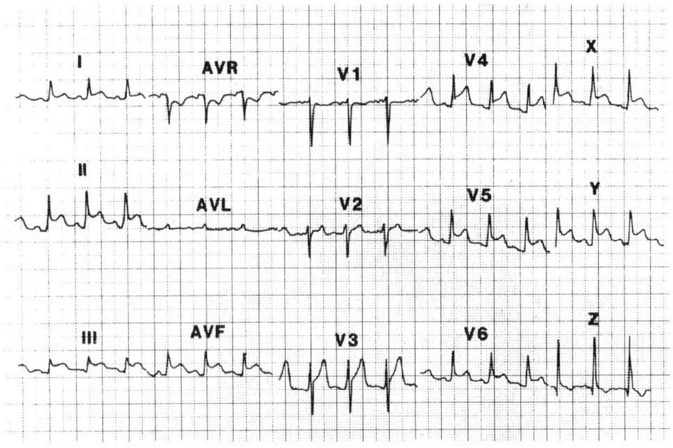

Fig 3A-38 ECG illustrating ST-segment elevation in virtually all leads without localizing pattern. This is the characteristic finding in acute, nonspecific pericarditis.

During recovery or the chronic phase, the ST segment returns to the isoelectric line and the T wave undergoes inversion, usually shallow. The duration of inversion reflects the speed of resolution of the pericarditis, and in smoldering or recurring cases of the disease it may persist for months.

Certain features characterize specific involvement. Low-voltage QRS complexes in the conventional 12-lead ECG occur in chronic constrictive pericarditis, pericardial effusion, and especially myxedematous pericardial effusion; in the last state the QRS may be barely discernible. Electrical alternans involving the QRS only or, at times, the P and T waves as well usually is associated with a rapidly accumulating pericardial effusion produced most commonly by extension of a malignancy (from the breast or lung is most frequent) to the pericardium.[127]

Myocarditis

There are no definite ECG findings associated with myocarditis, but involvement of the epicardium in an acute inflammatory process may induce changes in the ST-T wave that are characteristic of pericarditis. Transient episodes of first- or second-degree heart block may occur as may nonspecific intraventricular conduction delay. Interpretation of these changes depends heavily on the associated clinical signs and symptoms of myocarditis.

Abnormal QRS complexes with pseudoinfarction and left bundle-branch block are markers of poor prognosis independent of initial left and right ventricular function.[128]

Pulmonary embolism[129]

The most common ECG findings reported with pulmonary embolism are (1) sinus tachycardia or atrial fibrillation; (2) shift in mean electrical axis to the right from that of the preembolic status, and at times definite right-axis deviation; (3) inverted T waves in leads V_1-V_3, suggesting

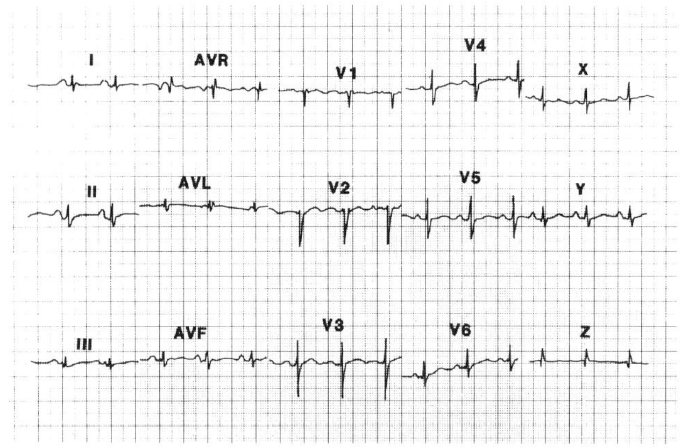

Fig 3A-39 ECG pattern in patient admitted to the hospital with acute thrombophlebitis involving her left leg. The tracing shows low anterior voltage and nonspecific repolarization changes but otherwise is unremarkable.

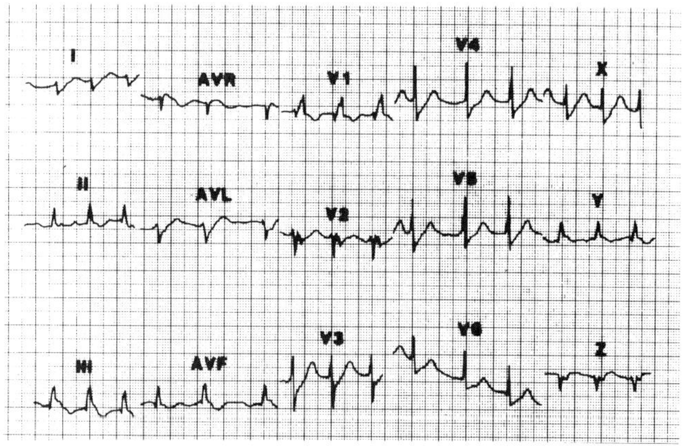

Fig 3A-40 ECG taken 3 days after that in Figure 3A-39, after an acute episode of shortness of breath with associated chest pain. It shows a shift of the axis to the right with an S_1, Q_3 pattern, development of a right bundle conduction delay, and ST changes over the right ventricle. All of these changes are consistent with a diagnosis of acute pulmonary embolism with right heart strain.

right ventricular strain; (4) abrupt onset of right ventricular conduction delay or right bundle-branch block; (5) Q waves in leads III and aV_F suggesting an inferior infarction, but no Q wave in lead II; (6) an S_1, S_2, S_3 pattern or an S_1, Q_3 pattern; and (7) P pulmonale. None of these abnormalities is diagnostic; most are transient (24 to 48 hours) and require correlation with the clinical situation (Figs 3A-39 and 3A-40).

Central nervous system disorders

The association of striking ECG abnormalities with various neurologic diseases has been well-known since the reports by Byer et al.[130] in 1947 and Burch et al.[131] in 1954. The neurologic problems have included cerebrovascular accidents, head injuries, and neoplasms. However, the existing evidence suggests that ECG abnormalities occur more frequently in association with subarachnoid hemorrhage than with any other central nervous system lesion.

Large, broad, inverted T waves, present in most of the conventional leads and associated with Q-T prolongation, are thought to be the typical pattern of subarachnoid hemorrhage. For unexplained reasons, ST-segment elevation may occur before the more typical ECG pattern at the onset of the hemorrhage. In other neurologic disorders, ST-segment elevation, T-wave changes, prolonged Q-T, wide Q waves, and various supraventricular tachycardias all have been reported; all are nonspecific and unexplained. These changes can mimic both acute pericarditis and myocardial infarction.[132]

Hypothermia

In patients with subnormal body temperatures, characteristic ECG changes occur,[133,134] the most striking being an elevation of the proximal portion of the ST segment or J point such that the downstroke of the S wave is notched or slurred similar to a δ wave (Wolff-Parkinson-White syndrome). This distortion of the S wave has been called the "Osborne wave." In addition, these patients often exhibit increased duration of the P-R interval, QRS complex, and Q-T interval. Sinus bradycardia, atrial flutter, or atrial fibrillation may be present.

Cocaine abuse

The intense vessel spasm with thrombosis in cocaine users can be associated with ECG changes typical of Q-wave or non-Q-wave infarction. With chronic abuse of "crack" cocaine, ECG abnormalities were present in 29% of patients: nonspecific ST-T abnormalities in 15%, ST-segment elevation in 10%, old inferior infarction in 2%, old anterior infarction in 2%, and poor R-wave progression in 10%.[135]

Thoracic bony abnormalities

Pectus excavatum and the straight back syndrome both significantly decrease the anterior-posterior diameter of the chest, compress the heart, augment the magnitude of deflections by virtue of proximity effects in the precordial leads, and simulate various ECG abnormalities. These include: anteroseptal infarction, especially with pectus excavatum, because of the angulation of leads V_1 and V_2; and inferior infarction, because of changes suggestive of chronic cor pulmonale evoked by both. When severe, kyphoscoliosis can lead to such significant ventilation-perfusion abnormalities within the lung that hypoxemia, pulmonary hypertension, and ECG evidence of cor pulmonale result.

REFERENCES

1. Marriott HJL: *Practical Electrocardiography.* Seventh edition. Baltimore, Williams & Wilkins, 1983

2. Chou T-C: Clinical aspects of vectorcardiography. In *Cardiac Diagnosis.* Edited by NO Fowler. New York, Harper & Row, Publishers, 1968, pp 75-102

3. Krikler DM, Macfarlane PW: Standards for electrocardiographs (editorial). *Br Heart J* 36:945-947, 1974

4. Lipman BS, Massie E, Kleiger RE: *Clinical Scalar Electrocardiography.* Sixth edition. Chicago, Year Book Medical Publishers, 1972

5. Lewis T: *The Mechanism and Graphic Registration of the Heart Beat.* Third edition. Chicago, Chicago Medical Book Company, 1925, p 96

6. Durrer D, van der Tweel LH: Excitation of the left ventricular wall of the dog and goat. *Ann NY Acad Sci* 65:779-803, 1957

7. Wilson FN, Johnston FD, Rosenbaum FF, et al: On Einthoven's triangle, the theory of unipolar electrocardiographic leads, and the interpretation of the precordial electrocardiogram. *Am Heart J* 32:277-310, 1946

8. Wilson FN, Macleod AG, Barker PS, et al: The determination and the significance of the areas of the ventricular deflections of the electrocardiogram. *Am Heart J* 10:46-61, 1934

9. Denes P: The importance of derived 12-lead electrocardiography in the interpretation of arrhythmias detected by Holter monitor recording. *Am Heart J* 124:905-911, 1992

10. Narula OS (ed): *His Bundle: Electrocardiography and Clinical Electrophysiology.* Philadelphia, FA Davis Company, 1975

11. Massie E, Walsh TJ: *Clinical Vectorcardiography and Electrocardiography.* Chicago, Year Book Medical Publishers, 1960

12. Clarke JM, Hamer J, Shelton JR, et al: The rhythm of the normal human heart. *Lancet* 2:508-512, 1976

13. Southall DP, Richards J, Mitchell P, et al: Study of cardiac rhythm in healthy newborn infants. *Br Heart J* 43:14-20, 1980

14. Talan DA, Bauernfeind RA, Ashley WW, et al: Twenty-four hour continuous ECG recordings in long-distance runners. *Chest* 82:19-24, 1982

15. Fleg JL, Kennedy HL: Cardiac arrhythmias in a healthy elderly population: detection by 24-hour ambulatory electrocardiography. *Chest* 81:302-307, 1982

16. Thomas P, Dejong D: The P wave in the electrocardiogram in the diagnosis of heart disease. *Br Heart J* 16:241-254, 1954

17. Morris JJ Jr, Estes EH Jr, Whalen RE, et al: P-wave analysis in valvular heart disease. *Circulation* 29:242-252, 1964

18. Alpert MA, Munuswamy K: Electrocardiographic diagnosis of left atrial enlargement. *Arch Intern Med* 149:1161-1165, 1989

19. Hazen MS, Marwick TH, Underwood DA: Diagnostic accuracy of resting electrocardiogram in detection and estimation of left atrial enlargement: an electrocardiographic correlation in 551 patients. *Am Heart J* 122:823-828, 1991

20. Liu CK, Greenspan G, Piccirillo RT: Atrial infarction of the heart. *Circulation* 23:331-338, 1961

21. Savage RM, Wagner GS, Ideker RE, et al: Correlation of postmortem anatomic findings with electrocardiographic changes in patients with myocardial infarction: retrospective study of patients with typical anterior and posterior infarcts. *Circulation* 55:279-285, 1977

22. Sullivan W, Vlodaver Z, Tuna N, et al: Correlation of electrocardiographic and pathologic findings in healed myocardial infarction. *Am J Cardiol* 42:724-732, 1978

23. Raunio H, Rissanen V, Romppanen T, et al: Changes in the QRS complex and ST segment in transmural and subendocardial infarctions. A clinicopathologic study. *Am Heart J* 98:176-184, 1979

24. André-Fouet X, Pillot M, Leizorovicz A, et al: "Non-Q wave" alias "nontransmural," myocardial infarction: a specific entity. *Am Heart J* 117:892-902, 1989

25. Freifeld AG, Schuster EH, Bulkley BH: Nontransmural versus transmural myocardial infarction: a morphologic study. *Am J Med* 75:423-432, 1983

26. Kouvaras G, Chronopoulos G, Cokkinos DV: Q and non-Q wave myocardial infarction: current views. *Angiology* 39:333-340, 1988

27. Hecht HH: Concepts of myocardial ischemia. *Arch Intern Med* 84:711-729, 1949

28. Tominaga S, Strasser T, Blackburn H: Serial electrocardiographic changes in myocardial infarction. *Am J Cardiol* 29:767-781, 1972

29. Pruitt RD, Burchell HB, Barnes AR: The anoxia test in the diagnosis of coronary insufficiency: a study of 289 cases. *JAMA* 128:839-845, 1945

30. Pruitt RD, Valencia F: The immediate electrocardiographic effects of circumscribed myocardial injuries: an experimental study. *Am Heart J* 35:161-197, 1948

31. Pruitt RD, Burchell HB, Essex HE: Deviations of the RS-T segment in acute subendocardial injuries. *Circulation* 4:108-110, 1951

32. Young E, Levine HD, Vokonas PS, et al: The frontal plane vectorcardiogram in old inferior myocardial infarction. II. Mid-to-late QRS changes. *Circulation* 42:1143-1162, 1970

33. DePasquale N, Burch GE: The spatial vectorcardiogram in left bundle branch block and myocardial infarction, with autopsy studies. *Am J Med* 29:633-639, 1960

34. Hugenholtz PG, Ryan TJ, Woerner T, et al: Recognition of anterior wall infarction in patients with left ventricular hypertrophy: a study of the Frank vectorcardiogram. *Circulation* 27:386-396, 1963

35. Mathur VS, Levine HD: Vectorcardiographic differentiation between right ventricular hypertrophy and posterobasal myocardial infarction. *Circulation* 42:883-894, 1970

36. Kyriakidis M, Antonopoulos A, Barbetseas J, et al: Correlation of reciprocal ST-segment depression after acute myocardial infarction with coronary angiographic findings. *Int J Cardiol* 36:163-168, 1992

37. Marcus EB, Yano K, MacLean CJ: Regression of Q waves following acute myocardial infarction. *Am J Epidemiol* 129:105-111, 1989

38. Hugenholtz PG, Forkner CE Jr, Levine HD: A clinical appraisal of the vectorcardiogram in myocardial infarction. II. The Frank system. *Circulation* 24:825-850, 1961

39. Gunnar RM, Winslow EBJ, Cabin GI, et al: Autopsy correlation of vectorcardiographic criteria for the diagnosis of myocardial infarction. In *Vectorcardiography 2 (XIth International Symposium).* Edited by I Hoffman, RI Hamby, E Glassman. Amsterdam, North-Holland Publishing Company, 1971, pp 333-342

40. Murata K, Matsushita S, Kurihara H, et al: Some pitfalls of vectorcardiographic diagnosis of myocardial infarction with particular respect to emphysema. *Circulation* 35:172-177, 1967

41. Benchimol A, Desser KB, Massey BJ: Coexisting left anterior hemiblock and inferior wall myocardial infarction: vectorcardiographic features. *Am J Cardiol* 29:7-14, 1972

42. Gau GT, Goodwin JF, Oakley CM, et al: Q waves and coronary arteriography in cardiomyopathy. *Br Heart J* 34:1034-1041, 1972

43. Robalino BD, Whitlow PL, Underwood DA, et al: Electrocardiographic manifestations of right ventricular infarction. *Am Heart J* 118:138-144, 1989

44. Lie KI, Wellens HJ, Schuilenburg RM: Bundle branch block and acute myocardial infarction. In *The Conduction System of the Heart: Structure, Function and Clinical Implications.* Edited by HJJ Wellens, KI Lie, MJ Janse. Philadelphia, Lea & Febiger, 1976, pp 662-672

45. Hindman MC, Wagner GS, JaRo M, et al: The clinical significance of bundle branch block complicating acute myocardial infarction. 2. Indications for temporary and permanent pacemaker insertion. *Circulation* 58:689-699, 1978

46. Hands ME, Cook EF, Stone PH, et al: Electrocardiographic diagnosis of myocardial infarction in the presence of complete left bundle branch block. *Am Heart J* 116:23-31, 1988

47. Pantridge JF, Adgey AAJ, Geddes JS, et al: *The Acute Coronary Attack.* New York, Grune & Stratton, 1975

48. Wit AL, Bigger JT Jr: Possible electrophysiological mechanisms for lethal arrhythmias accompanying myocardial ischemia and infarction. *Circulation* 52 Suppl 3:96-115, 1975

49. Kimball JT, Killip T: Aggressive treatment of arrhythmias in acute myocardial infarction: procedures and results. *Prog Cardiovasc Dis* 10:483-504, 1968

50. Bigger JT Jr, Dresdale RJ, Heissenbuttel RH, et al: Ventricular arrhythmias in ischemic heart disease: mechanisms, prevalence, significance, and management. *Prog Cardiovasc Dis* 19:255-300, 1977

51. Norris RM, Mercer CJ: Significance of idioventricular rhythms in acute myocardial infarction. *Prog Cardiovasc Dis* 16:455-468, 1974

52. James TN: Myocardial infarction and atrial arrhythmias. *Circulation* 24:761-776, 1961

53. DeSanctis RW, Block P, Hutter AM Jr: Tachyarrhythmias in myocardial infarction. *Circulation* 45:681-702, 1972

54. Danzig R, Alpern H, Swan HJC: The significance of atrial rate in patients with atrioventricular conduction abnormalities complicating acute myocardial infarction. *Am J Cardiol* 24:707-712, 1969

55. Rosen KM: Junctional tachycardia: mechanisms, diagnosis, differential diagnosis, and management. *Circulation* 47:654-664, 1973

56. Friedberg CK, Cohen H, Donoso E: Advanced heart block as a complication of acute myocardial infarction: role of pacemaker therapy. *Prog Cardiovasc Dis* 10:466-481, 1968

57. Rotman M, Wagner GS, Waugh RA: Significance of high degree atrioventricular block in acute posterior myocardial infarction: the importance of clinical setting and mechanism of block. *Circulation* 47:257-262, 1973

58. Clemmensen P, Ohman EM, Sevilla DC, et al: Changes in standard electrocardiographic ST-segment elevation predictive of successful reperfusion in acute myocardial infarction. *Am J Cardiol* 66:1407-1411, 1990

59. Sevilla DC, Wagner NB, Pieper KS, et al: Use of the 12-lead ECG to detect myocardial reperfusion and salvage during acute myocardial infarction. *J Electrocardiol* 25:281-286, 1992

60. Massing GK, James TN: Anatomical configuration of the His bundle and proximal bundle branches in the human heart (abstract). *Circulation* 44 Suppl 2:64, 1971

61. Titus JL: Normal anatomy of the human cardiac conduction system. *Mayo Clin Proc* 48:24-30, 1973

62. Scher AM, Young AC: Ventricular depolarization and the genesis of QRS. *Ann NY Acad Sci* 65:768-778, 1957

63. Krongrad E, Hefler SE, Bowman FO Jr, et al: Further observations on the etiology of right bundle branch block pattern following right ventriculotomy. *Circulation* 50:1105-1113, 1974

64. Lev M, Unger PN, Rosen KM, et al: The anatomic substrate of complete left bundle branch block. *Circulation* 50:479-486, 1974

65. Rosenbaum MB, Elizari MV, Lazzari JO: *The Hemiblocks: New Concepts of Intraventricular Conduction Based on Human Anatomical, Physiological and Clinical Studies.* Oldsmar, Florida, Tampa Tracings, 1970

66. Watt TB Jr, Pruitt RD: Electrocardiographic findings associated with experimental arborization block in dogs. *Am Heart J* 69:642-654, 1965

67. Watt TB Jr, Pruitt RD: Focal lesions in the canine bundle of His: their effect on ventricular excitation. *Circ Res* 31:531-545, 1972

68. Flowers NC: Left bundle branch block: a continuously evolving concept. *J Am Coll Cardiol* 9:684-697, 1987

69. Gertsch M, Theler A, Foglia E: Electrocardiographic detection of left ventricular hypertrophy in the presence of left anterior fascicular block. *Am J Cardiol* 61:1098-1101, 1988

70. Watt TB Jr, Murao S, Pruitt RD: Left axis deviation induced experimentally in a primate heart. *Am Heart J* 70:381-389, 1965

71. Watt TB Jr, Pruitt RD: Left posterior fascicular block in canine and p¬imate hearts: an electrocardiographic study. *Circulation* 40:677-685, 1969

72. Watt TB Jr, Freud GE, Durrer D, et al: Left anterior arborization block combined with right bundle branch block in canine and primate hearts: an electrocardiographic study. *Circ Res* 22:57-63, 1968

73. Canaveris G, Halpern S, Elizari MV: Intraventricular conduction disturbances in civilian flying personnel: left anterior hemiblock. *Aviat Space Environ Med* 63:292-298, 1992

74. Wolff L: Syndrome of short P-R interval with abnormal QRS complexes and paroxysmal tachycardia (Wolff-Parkinson-White syndrome). *Circulation* 10:282-291, 1954

75. Wolff L: Wolff-Parkinson-White syndrome: historical and clinical features. *Prog Cardiovasc Dis* 2:677-690, 1960

76. Wolff L, Parkinson J, White PD: Bundle-branch block with short P-R interval in healthy young people prone to paroxysmal tachycardia. *Am Heart J* 5:685-704, 1930

77. Durrer D, Wellens HJ: The Wolff-Parkinson-White syndrome anno 1973. *Eur J Cardiol* 1:347-367, 1974

78. Lown B, Ganong WF, Levine SA: The syndrome of short P-R interval, normal QRS complex and paroxysmal rapid heart action. *Circulation* 5:693-706, 1952

79. Wellens HJJ, Farré J, Bär FWHM: The Wolff-Parkinson-White syndrome. In *Cardiac Arrhythmias: Their Mechanisms, Diagnosis, and Management.* Edited by WJ Mandel. Philadelphia, JB Lippincott Company, 1980, pp 342-365

80. Benditt DG, Pritchett ELC, Gallagher JJ: Spectrum of regular tachycardias with wide QRS complexes in patients with accessory atrioventricular pathways. *Am J Cardiol* 42:828-838, 1978

81. Scheinman MM, Wang Y-S, Van Hare GF, et al: Electrocardiographic and electrophysiologic characteristics of anterior, midseptal and anterior free wall accessory pathways. *J Am Coll Cardiol* 20:1220-1229, 1992

82. Gallagher JJ, Svenson RH, Sealy WC, et al: The Wolff-Parkinson-White syndrome and the preexcitation dysrhythmias: medical and surgical management. *Med Clin North Am* 60:101-123, January 1976

83. Nath A, Alpert MA, Terry BE, et al: Sensitivity and specificity of electrocardiographic criteria for left and right ventricular hypertrophy in morbid obesity. *Am J Cardiol* 62:126-130, 1988

84. Toshima H, Koga Y, Kimura N: Correlations between electrocardiographic, vectorcardiographic, and echocardiographic findings in patients with left ventricular overload. *Am Heart J* 94:547-556, 1977

85. Sokolow M, Lyon TP: The ventricular complex in left ventricular hypertrophy as obtained by unipolar precordial and limb leads. *Am Heart J* 37:161-186, 1949

86. Estes EH Jr: Examinations by means of electrocardiography. A. Electrocardiography and vectorcardiography. In *Heart, Arteries, and Veins.* Edited by JW Hurst, RB Logue, RC Schlant, et al. Third edition. New York, McGraw-Hill Book Company, 1974, pp 297-313

87. Mazzoleni A, Wolff R, Wolff L: The vectorcardiogram in left ventricular hypertrophy. *Am Heart J* 58:648-662, 1959

88. Bristow JD, Porter GA, Griswold HE: Observations with the Frank system of vectorcardiography in left ventricular hypertrophy. *Am Heart J* 62:621-633, 1961

89. Molloy T, Okin PM, Devereux RB, et al: Electrocardiographic detection of left ventricular hypertrophy by simple QRS voltage-duration product. *J Am Coll Cardiol* 20:1180-1186, 1992

90. Sokolow M, Lyon TP: The ventricular complex in right ventricular hypertrophy as obtained by unipolar precordial and limb leads. *Am Heart J* 38:273-294, 1949

91. Mathur VS, Levine HD: Vectorcardiographic differentiation between right ventricular hypertrophy and posterobasal myocardial infarction. *Circulation* 42:883-894, 1970

92. McCaughan D, Koroxenidis GT, Hopff LG, et al: New vectorcardiographic criteria for the diagnosis of acquired right ventricular hypertrophy: comparison with standard electrocardiographic criteria (abstract). *Circulation* 28:766, 1963

93. Lal S, Fletcher E, Binnion P: Frank vectorcardiogram correlated with haemodynamic measurements: quantitative analysis. *Br Heart J* 31:15-20, 1969

94. Chou T-C, Masangkay MP, Young R, et al: Simple quantitative vectorcardiographic criteria for the diagnosis of right ventricular hypertrophy. *Circulation* 48:1262-1267, 1973

95. Cowdery CD, Wagner GS, Starr JW, et al: New vectorcardiographic criteria for diagnosing right ventricular hypertrophy in mitral stenosis: comparison with electrocardiographic criteria. *Circulation* 62:1026-1032, 1980

96. Grant RP: *Clinical Electrocardiography: The Spatial Vector Approach.* New York, Blakiston Division, 1957

97. Bachman S, Sparrow D, Smith LK: Effect of aging on the electrocardiogram. *Am J Cardiol* 48:513-516, 1981

98. Freundlich J: The diagnostic significance of tall upright T waves in the chest leads. *Am Heart J* 52:749-767, 1956

99. Wachtel FW, Teich EM: Tall precordial T waves as the earliest sign of diaphragmatic wall infarction. *Am Heart J* 51:91-97, 1956

100. Surawicz B: Electrolytes and the electrocardiogram. *Mod Concepts Cardiovasc Dis* 33:875-880, 1964

101. Bradlow BA, Levin NW: Combined abnormal serum potassium and calcium levels: effect on the electrocardiogram. *Geriatrics* 24:119-128, January 1969

102. Fisch C: Relation of electrolyte disturbances to cardiac arrhythmias. *Circulation* 47:408-419, 1973

103. Arnsdorf MF: Electrocardiogram in hyperkalemia: electrocardiographic pattern of anteroseptal myocardial infarction mimicked by hyperkalemia-induced disturbance of impulse conduction. *Arch Intern Med* 136:1161-1163, 1976

104. Ettinger PO, Regan TJ, Oldewurtel HA: Hyperkalemia, cardiac conduction, and the electrocardiogram: a review. *Am Heart J* 88:360-371, 1974

105. Surawicz B: The interrelationship of electrolyte abnormalities and arrhythmias. In *Cardiac Arrhythmias: Their Mechanisms, Diagnosis, and Management.* Edited by WJ Mandel. Philadelphia, JB Lippincott Company, 1980, pp 83-106

106. Kaplinsky E, Yahini JH, Barzilai J, et al: Quinidine syncope: report of a case successfully treated with lidocaine. *Chest* 62:764-766, 1972

107. Shub C, Gau GT, Sidell PM, et al: The management of acute quinidine intoxication. *Chest* 73:173-178, 1978

108. Chung EK: Digitalis-induced cardiac arrhythmias: a report of 180 cases. *Jpn Heart J* 10:409-427, 1969

109. Beller GA, Smith TW, Abelmann WH, et al: Digitalis intoxication: a prospective clinical study with serum level correlations. *N Engl J Med* 284:989-997, 1971

110. Alexander CS, Niño A: Cardiovascular complications in young patients taking psychotropic drugs: a preliminary report. *Am Heart J* 78:757-769, 1969

111. Davis JM, Bartlett E, Termini BS: Overdosage of psychotropic drugs: a review. I. Major and minor tranquilizers. II. Antidepressants and other psychotropic agents. *Dis Nerv Syst* 29:157-164; 246-256, 1968

112. Mathews EC Jr, Blount AW Jr, Townsend JI: Q-T prolongation and ventricular arrhythmias, with and without deafness, in the same family. *Am J Cardiol* 29:702-711, 1972

113. Schwartz PJ, Periti M, Malliani A: The long Q-T syndrome. *Am Heart J* 89:378-390, 1975

114. Einthoven W: Le télécardiogramme. *Arch Intern Physiol* 4:132-164, 1906

115. Chou T-C: *Electrocardiography in Clinical Practice.* New York, Grune & Stratton, 1979

116. Nahum LH, Hoff HE: The interpretation of the U wave of the electrocardiogram. *Am Heart J* 17:585-598, 1939

117. Lepeschkin E: The U wave of the electrocardiogram. *Mod Concepts Cardiovasc Dis* 38:39-45, 1969

118. Georgopoulos AJ, Proudfit WL, Page IH: Relationship between arterial pressure and negative U waves in electrocardiograms. *Circulation* 23:675-680, 1961

119. Gerson MC, Phillips JF, Morris SN, et al: Exercise-induced U-wave inversion as a marker of stenosis of the left anterior descending coronary artery. *Circulation* 60:1014-1020, 1979

120. Swartz MH, Teichholz LE, Donoso E: Mitral valve prolapse: a review of associated arrhythmias. *Am J Med* 62:377-389, 1977

121. Forfang K: Electrocardiographic findings before and after surgery for atrial septal defect of the secundum type in middle-aged patients. *Cardiology* 63:94-106, 1978

122. Roberts DL, Wagner HR, Lambert EC: The electrocardiogram in tetralogy of Fallot. *J Electrocardiol* 5:155-161, 1972

123. Lev M, Gibson S, Miller RA: Ebstein's disease with Wolff-Parkinson-White syndrome: report of a case with histopathologic study of possible conduction pathways. *Am Heart J* 49:724-741, 1955

124. Lev M: Pathogenesis of congenital atrioventricular block. *Prog Cardiovasc Dis* 15:145-157, 1972

125. Spodick DH: *Acute Pericarditis.* New York, Grune & Stratton, 1959

126. Engle MA, Zabriskie JB, Senterfit LB, et al: Postpericardiotomy syndrome: a new look at an old condition. *Mod Concepts Cardiovasc Dis* 44:59-64, 1975

127. Spodick DH: Electric alternation of the heart: its relation to the kinetics and physiology of the heart during cardiac tamponade. *Am J Cardiol* 10:155-165, 1962

128. Morgera T, Di Lenarda A, Dreas L, et al: Electrocardiography of myocarditis revisited: clinical and prognostic significance of electrocardiographic changes. *Am Heart J* 124:455-467, 1992

129. McIntyre KM, Sasahara AA, Littmann D: Relation of the electrocardiogram to hemodynamic alterations in pulmonary embolism. *Am J Cardiol* 30:205-210, 1972

130. Byer E, Ashman R, Toth LA: Electrocardiograms with large, upright T waves and long Q-T intervals. *Am Heart J* 33:796-806, 1947

131. Burch GE, Meyers R, Abildskov JA: A new electrocardiographic pattern observed in cerebrovascular accidents. *Circulation* 9:719-723, 1954

132. Nakamura Y, Kaseno K, Kubo T: Transient ST-segment elevation in subarachnoid hemorrhage. *J Electrocardiol* 22:133-137, 1989

133. Clements SD Jr, Hurst JW: Diagnostic value of electrocardiographic abnormalities observed in subjects accidentally exposed to cold. *Am J Cardiol* 29:729-734, 1972

134. Emslie-Smith D, Sladden GE, Stirling GR: The significance of changes in the electrocardiogram in hypothermia. *Br Heart J* 21:343-351, 1959

135. Chakko S, Fernandez A, Mellman TA, et al: Cardiac manifestations of cocaine abuse: a cross-sectional study of asymptomatic men with a history of long-term abuse of "crack" cocaine. *J Am Coll Cardiol* 20:1168-1174, 1992

CHAPTER

3

Electrocardiography

B. Exercise testing

William T. Bardsley, M.D., Harold T. Mankin, M.D., and Todd D. Miller, M.D.

NORMAL PHYSIOLOGIC RESPONSE TO EXERCISE

Hemodynamic and autonomic factors

Cardiac output is the product of heart rate and stroke volume. The normal increase in stroke volume is from 95 ± 22 mL at rest to 144 ± 31 mL at maximal exercise before rigorous training in athletes. After training, stroke volumes show a dramatic increase from 112 ± 26 mL at rest to 176 ± 39 mL at maximal exercise. This training effect, which enhances the very efficient volume work of the heart, has been shown to be directly related to an increase in preload or diastolic volume.[1] Even without the benefit of cardiovascular training, the sedentary heart also increases its diastolic volumes with exercise, and this demonstrates the importance of preload and the Starling mechanism in increasing cardiac output.

The peripheral vascular adaptations to exercise act to increase blood return to the heart[2] and include pronounced vasodilatation in exercising muscles, rhythmic muscular contractions in the limbs, abdomen, and thorax, and splenic contraction to increase red blood cell circulatory mass. Resistance increases in the renal and mesenteric vascular beds and is especially elevated in heart block. A threefold increase in extraction of oxygen from the circulating blood to support aerobic muscle metabolism effectively triples the oxygen utilization at a given cardiac output and is helped by a rightward displacement of the hemoglobin-oxygen dissociation curve.

The heart rate can triple as a result of a decrease in vagal tone and an increase in sympathetic activity, both as an effect of circulatory catecholamines and from direct cardiac sympathetic innervation. Of interest is the observation that in racing greyhounds with denervated hearts or in human cardiac transplant recipients, the heart rate can increase substantially in spite of the absence of neural control.[3] In addition, direct sympathetic stimulation of the heart muscle during exercise increases the contractile state and stroke volume independently of heart rate and preload. The increase of cardiac output usually exceeds the decrease in peripheral resistance, and this results in an increase in systolic pressure of 60 to 80 mm Hg. Diastolic pressure normally decreases by 10 to 20 mm Hg during upright treadmill exercise.

Electrocardiographic (ECG) changes

The ECG changes with exercise in a normal heart include shortening of the P-Q and Q-T intervals as heart rate increases. There is an increase in the magnitude of the P wave without a shift in direction, consistent with an increase in right atrial volume. The septal Q wave in lateral leads increases in magnitude. The magnitude of the maximal depolarization decreases slightly above heart rates of 120 to 130 beats/min and shifts only slightly posteriorly. The magnitude of the J point increases slightly, and the ST segment shifts superiorly and rightward; these changes are reflected in inferior and lateral leads as depression of the J point with rapidly upsloping ST segments[4] (Fig 3B-1). Within 30 seconds of recovery after exercise, the T wave becomes much broader and increases in magnitude. This feature has made computer measurements of the ST segment at J + 60 msec or J + 80 msec unreliable in the immediate postexercise period. These changes have usually returned to baseline by the time of the 3-minute postexercise tracing.

Aerobic capacity

Aerobic capacity is defined as the product of cardiac output and arteriovenous oxygen difference and represents the simultaneous total body aerobic work. This useful parameter can be measured directly by expired gas analysis and by simultaneous measurement of cardiac output and arterial and venous oxygen content or indirectly by the use of its linear relationship to heart rate or workload. Most often, calibrated treadmill exercise protocols, consisting of a series of stages of increasing aerobic work and standardized by direct aerobic measurements in thousands of volunteers, are used to approximate aerobic work of a given patient. Highly useful protocols include those of Bruce et al,[5] Naughton and Haider,[6] Ellestad,[7] and Balke and Ware.[8] Regression equations[5,9] for aero-

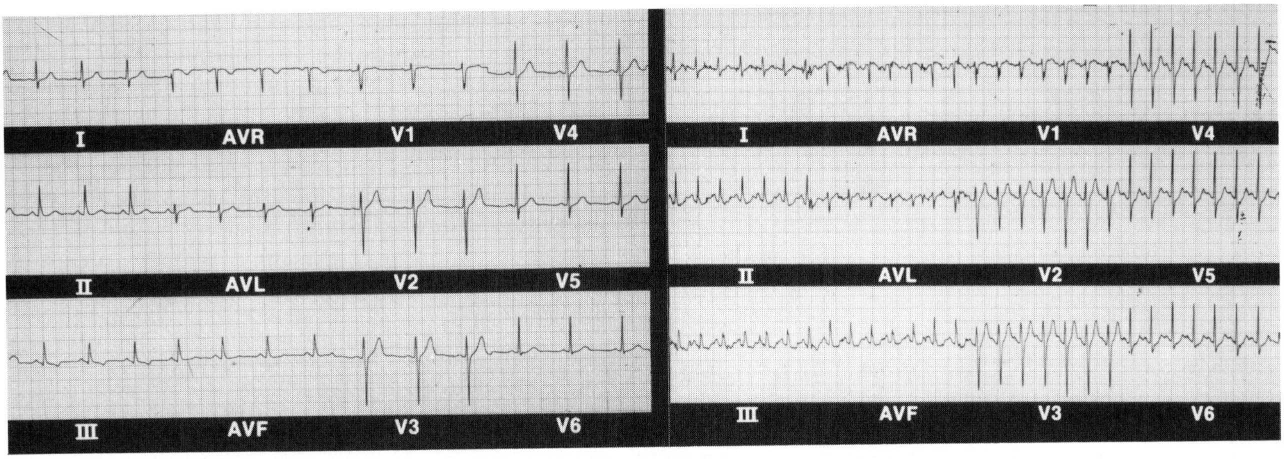

Fig 3B-1 Normal 28-year-old man with no cardiovascular disease. **Left,** at rest. **Right,** during exercise. The left precordial leads demonstrate depression of the J junction with an upsloping ST-segment typical of a normal exercise ECG.

bic capacity are supplied for specific times on the Bruce and Balke protocols. Rigid guidelines must be followed strictly with regard to the patient's posture and in not allowing him or her to hold on to the rails during the exercise. Aerobic capacity calculated from the workload achieved during bicycle ergometry is very accurate; however, fewer muscles are brought into full exertion, which makes the total aerobic capacity measured by this technique less than that with maximal treadmill testing. The relative lack of bicycle exercise in American adults results in early fatigue of the quadriceps muscles as well. Aerobic capacity varies with the sex, age, and training of the individual. Norms have been well established and are useful for assessing a given patient's total performance. It is our practice to relate all symptoms and signs observed to the simultaneous level of aerobic capacity in order to provide a semiquantitative assessment of the level of incapacity.

Using indirect methods of aerobic measurements can be quite misleading in patients with *chronic* congestive heart failure. In these patients, adaptive mechanisms have evolved to enhance anaerobic metabolism and to allow tolerance to high preloads, and this masks the usual *acute* signs and symptoms of left ventricular dysfunction, including dyspnea, fatigue, and low exercise tolerance. This distinction between acute and chronic left ventricular dysfunction is the key to the interpretation of exercise tolerance. In chronic left ventricular dysfunction, such as in the dilated cardiomyopathies, the direct measurement of left ventricular function during exercise by radionuclide angiography is more sensitive in detecting myocardial dysfunction than is the indirect estimation of aerobic capacity by means of exercise protocols, which may be nearly normal.[10] There is no correlation between exercise duration and resting left ventricular ejection fraction in patients with chronic congestive heart failure. Impaired exercise tolerance in these patients has been related to altered skeletal muscle metabolism and also possibly to abnormal myocardial diastolic function rather than systolic dysfunction.[11]

ISCHEMIC RESPONSE TO EXERCISE

Supply and demand

Patients with stable angina can regularly expect to accomplish simple tasks of everyday life without creating a disparity between supply and demand with respect to oxygen needs of the myocardium. If they hurry through the task or there is an added emotional component, their incapacity may be magnified. Exercise tests in patients with stable angina give results that are generally reproducible from day to day, and so the same workload, heart rate, and blood pressure will induce angina and the typical ECG indications of ischemia. This implies fixed coronary artery obstruction that limits exercise capabilities in a predictable fashion.

The New York Heart Association (NYHA) classification of cardiac capacity is simple and useful in the evaluation of such patients (see chapter 29B.) Problems develop in the interpretation of the history, and this weakens the classification. Adaptations of life-style by the patient may cause a class III patient to appear to be in class I. Distinction between classes II and III may be murky, defy resolution, and lack objectivity. Still, the differentiation is of clinical importance, and exercise testing will allow a clearer definition of the various classes. Patients with chronic congestive heart failure may be more accurately classified on the basis of peak oxygen consumption during exercise than on clinical symptoms.[12]

The supply/demand ratio may be markedly altered by the design of the exercise protocol. Multistage continuous exercise protocols such as the Bruce protocol[5] start at 4 METS (1 metabolic equivalent = 1 MET = Vo_2 of 3.5 mL O_2/[kg · min] while patient is sitting) for stage I, and in 3 minutes the workload increases to 6.6 METS. This gives little time for a warm-up to reduce systemic arterial resistance and would be too much work for class III and class IV patients but is ideal for healthy or class I and class II patients. The Naughton protocol[6] begins at slightly more than 1 MET and adds an additional 1 MET every 2 minutes. This provides an opportunity to reduce systemic resistance and thereby to reduce the demand while allowing time to restabilize the supply/demand ratio.

Hemodynamic factors

Two hemodynamic parameters are available in the noninvasive exercise laboratory: heart rate and blood pressure. The product of heart rate times systolic blood pressure, or "double product" (pressure-pulse product), is an index of myocardial oxygen consumption. Factors of physical deconditioning may result in an excessive heart rate response to exercise, which would increase the double product and the myocardial oxygen need disproportionately for the work performed. In other words, work performance is diminished by an excessive chronotropic (heart rate) response. Physical conditioning tends to modulate the heart rate response to the same workload and thus evokes a lower chronotropic response, a lower double product, a lower myocardial oxygen need, and an increased tolerance for activity for any given coronary obstruction. Systemic hypertension also incurs both an increased double product and an increased myocardial oxygen demand, which reduce the tolerance for physical activity.

On the other hand, exercise-induced hypotension has been shown to correlate with both advanced coronary artery disease and poor prognosis.[13,14] Among 2,036 patients who exercised on a treadmill during a 3-year period in one study,[15] 6.4% had a hypotensive blood pressure during exercise. A decrease in systolic blood pressure below the standing preexercise level was associated with an increased risk (3.2-fold) of cardiac events in patients who had had previous myocardial infarction or who had associated signs or symptoms of cardiac ischemia. Exertional hypotension is associated with a 40- to 50-fold risk of complex ventricular dysrhythmias during exercise.[16] However, not all patients with exercise-induced hypotension have coronary artery disease. Hypotension developing early in exercise (within 5 minutes) is usually due to severe coronary artery disease, whereas hypotension occurring later can be due to other causes, including valvular heart disease, cardiomyopathy, and medications.[17] Systolic blood pressure that remains elevated in the early recovery period, resulting in an abnormal ratio of recovery systolic blood pressure to peak exercise systolic blood pressure, has also been shown to be a marker of coronary artery disease.[18] An increase in diastolic pressure after exercise is a potent indicator of coronary artery disease even in the absence of ST-segment changes.[19]

ECG changes

Introduction. The first exercise ECGs were published by Einthoven[20] in 1908 (Fig 3B-2). The ECG responses to exercise have not provided clear-cut "yes or no" answers in all subjects tested as to the presence of ischemic disease. The sensitivity of the test (percentage of tests yielding a positive result in patients with disease) has been 65% to 70% in many laboratories. The specificity (percentage of tests yielding a negative result in subjects without disease) of the exercise ECG ordinarily is about 90% in men and 70% in women. An appreciation of methodologic problems encountered in ECG-monitored exercise testing for coronary artery disease has been provided by Philbrick and associates.[21] In a review of 33 published studies comprising 7,501 patients, they found the range of sensitivity to be 33% to 88% and that of specificity to be 41% to 100%. They expressed the belief that methodologic problems could explain the diversity of results from the various workers in the field.

More recent meta-analyses reached similar conclusions. Again, there was wide variability in test sensitivity and specificity among studies. The reported sensitivities and specificities were found to be related to selected exercise test variables, but the wide variability in reported test accuracy nonetheless could not be explained by the information provided in the medical literature, because

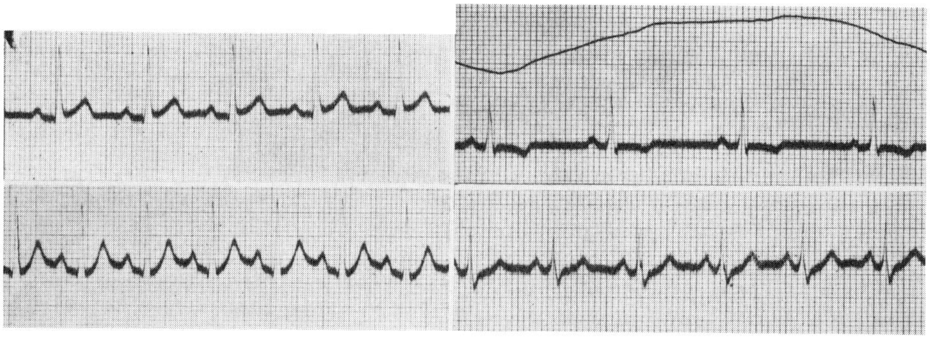

Fig 3B-2 **Left,** Einthoven's ECGs from a normal subject at rest **(upper)** and after exercise **(lower).** The heart rate increased from 91 to 120 beats/min. The lead is II. **Right,** Einthoven's patient. Note pseudonormalization of the inverted T wave at rest **(upper)** to an upright T wave during exercise **(lower),** a finding whose clinical significance is not certain even now. The lead is III; a pneumogram is shown in the rest tracing. (From Einthoven W: Weiteres über das Elektrokardiogramm. *Arch Gesamte Physiol* 122:517-584, 1908.)

patient characteristics and technical factors were underreported.[22,23] Another potential explanation of the limited accuracy of the exercise ECG is the imprecise correlation between anatomic coronary artery disease measured by angiography and coronary flow reserve. Wilson et al.[24] reported that exercise ECG is more accurate at predicting the physiologic than the anatomic significance of a coronary stenosis. Additionally, true myocardial ischemia develops in some patients with normal epicardial coronary arteries and positive exercise ECGs when sophisticated measures are used to detect abnormal coronary flow reserve. This condition is referred to as microvascular angina, or syndrome X.[25] Although patients with normal coronary arteries or "insignificant" coronary artery disease assessed angiographically who have positive exercise ECGs are considered to have false-positive responses, true ischemia does in fact develop in some.

Test results are limited to three categories of interpretation: (1) negative for ischemia, (2) positive for ischemia, and (3) abnormal—not diagnostic of ischemia. A preoccupation with changes in the ST segment detracts from other ECG and exercise parameters,[26] as will be noted below. Criteria for test results are useful but inevitably are arbitrary. The clinicians who will make the ultimate interpretation will use all data at their disposal, from pretest risk of disease[27] to other tests that have diagnostic significance for ischemic disease.[28] Probability calculations by means of the Bayes theorem provide diagnostic accuracy in test interpretations.[29] Application of the multivariate analysis approach is also capable of enhancing the accuracy of treadmill stress testing for myocardial ischemia. For example, Greenberg et al.[30] improved sensitivity from 73% to 88% by using multivariate analysis but did not enhance specificity (from 93% to 87%).

Ischemic waveforms. Depression of the ST segment is associated with subendocardial ischemia (Figs 3B-3 through 3B-7). Elevation of the ST segment suggests more severe—that is, transmural—ischemia (Figs 3B-8 and 3B-9). The lead in which the ST-segment depression occurs maximally is not a reliable detector of the portion of the myocardium that has been rendered ischemic, because subendocardial ischemia is often circumferential and not localized. ST-segment elevation is often localized to a certain set of leads, such as the inferior, anteroseptal, or lateral. It is a good predictor of the area of myocardial ischemia and, by deduction, of the location of the coronary artery lesion.[31] ST-segment elevation may also occur in the setting of exercise-induced coronary artery spasm and in leads over a dyskinetic portion of myocardium, as in ventricular aneurysm.[26] Prolonged ST-segment elevation that develops during exercise and extends into the

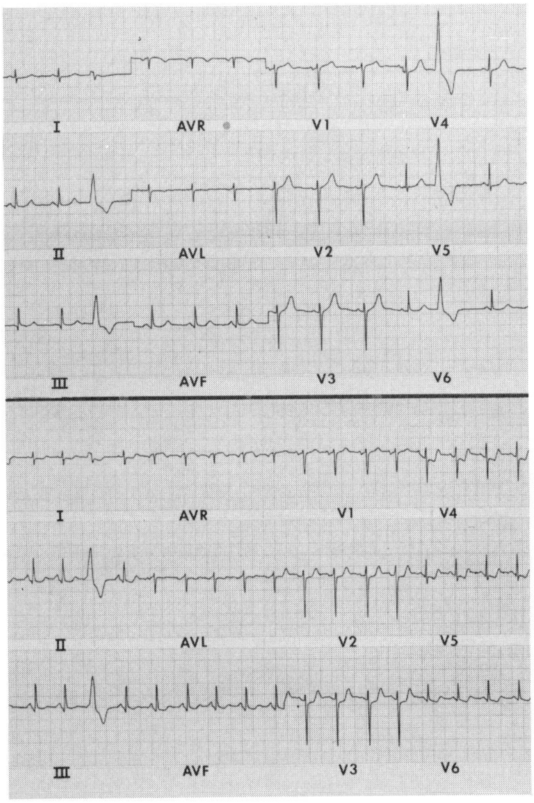

Fig 3B-3 Ischemic response in 62-year-old man with documented coronary artery obstructive disease. Note 1.0-mm sagging ST-segment depression. Random ventricular ectopic activity is present. **Upper,** at rest. **Lower,** immediately after exercise.

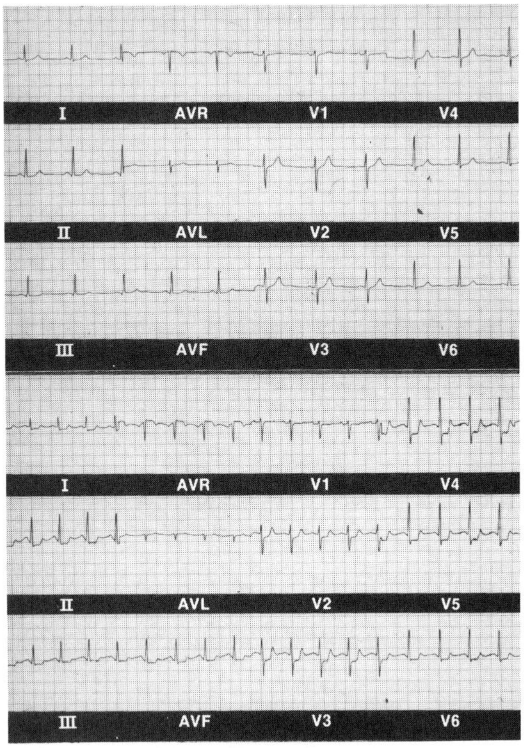

Fig 3B-4 Patient with 100% occlusion of left anterior descending coronary artery. Note 3.0-mm ST-segment depression with a horizontal contour. This readily qualifies as an ischemic response to exercise. **Upper,** at rest. **Lower,** exercise.

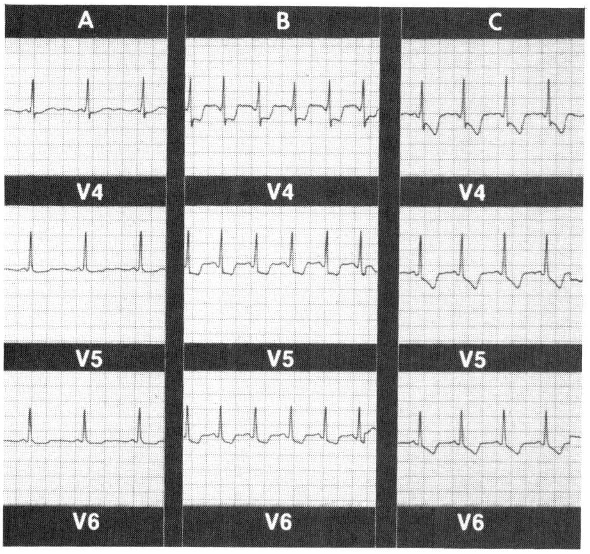

Fig 3B-5 Example of 3.0-mm ST-segment depression with sagging contour in 63-year-old man with prior inferior myocardial infarction, known 100% obstruction in right coronary artery, and 90% obstruction in first diagonal of left anterior descending coronary artery. **A,** control. **B,** during exercise. **C,** recovery period.

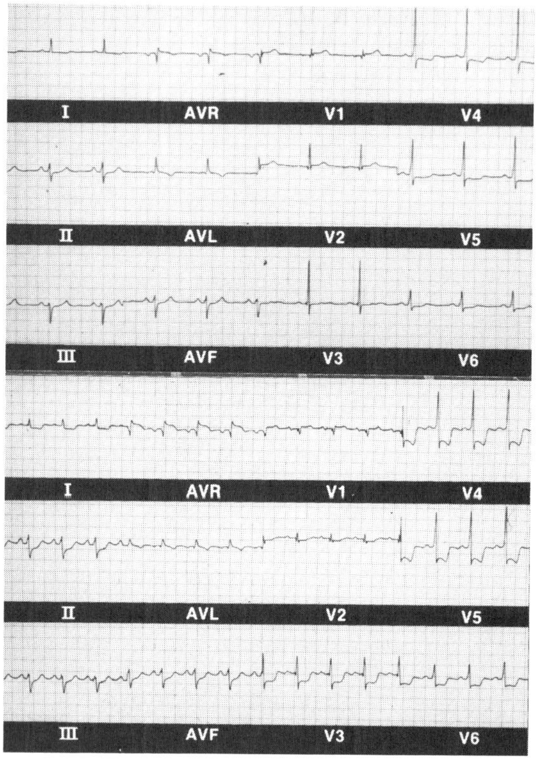

Fig 3B-6 Ischemic response in patient with 100% occlusion of both left anterior descending and left circumflex coronary arteries and 90% occlusion of right coronary artery. **Upper,** resting control, with 1.0-mm ST-segment depression before exercise. **Lower,** additional 4.0-mm ST-segment depression at 1 minute into the recovery period after exercise.

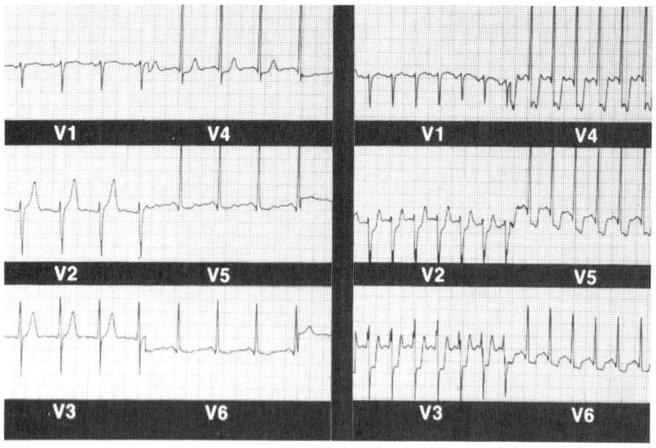

Fig 3B-7 Triple-vessel disease and ruptured chordae to the posterior leaflet of the mitral valve in 61-year-old man. **Left,** at rest. **Right,** exercise evoked a 9.0-mm ST-segment depression in V_4.

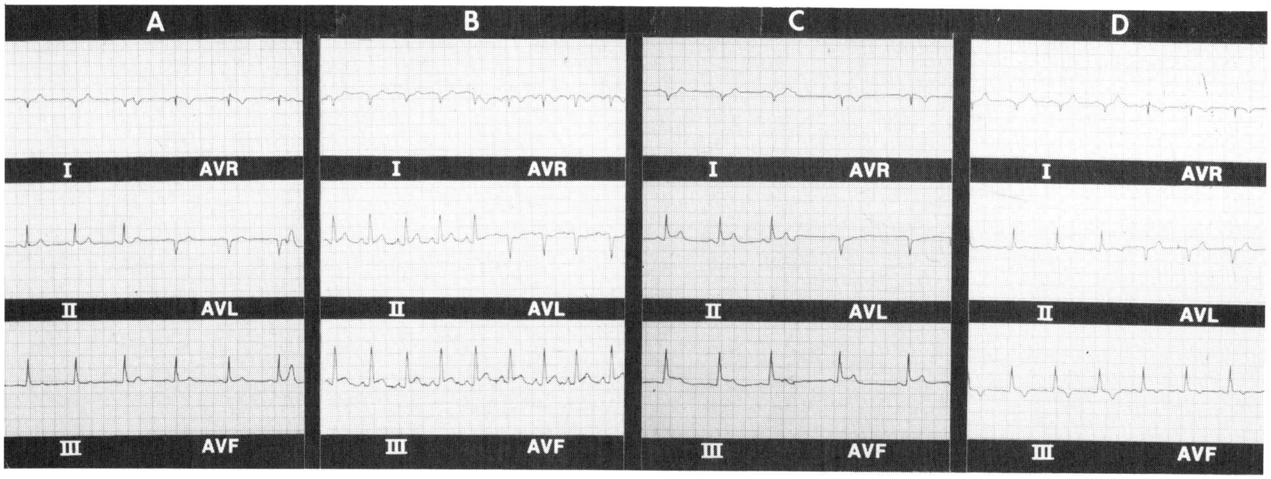

Fig 3B-8 This 46-year-old man with angina at rest and 100% obstruction of the right coronary artery demonstrated inferior ST-segment elevation and T-wave inversion in the inferior leads at 6 minutes of recovery from exercise. **A,** control. **B,** during exercise. **C,** recovery, 1 minute. **D,** recovery, 6 minutes.

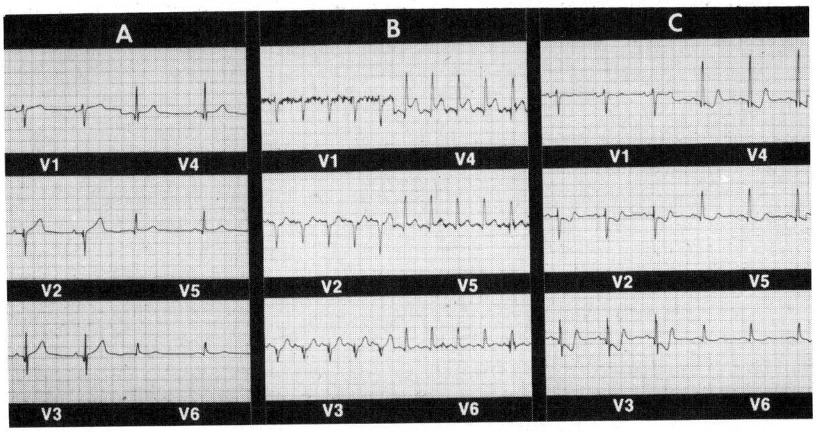

Fig 3B-9 Severe triple-vessel disease in 65-year-old man. **A,** control. **B,** during exercise, demonstrating ST-segment elevation consistent with transmural myocardial ischemia. **C,** early recovery, with sagging ST-segment depression indicative of subendocardial ischemia.

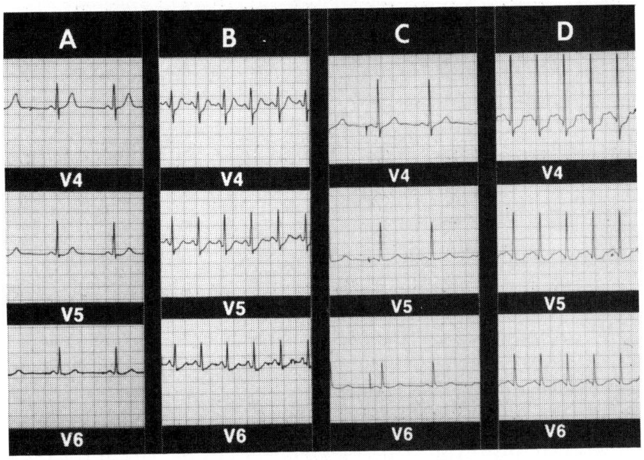

Fig 3B-10 **A** and **B,** normal subject at rest **(A)** and exercising **(B)**, demonstrating J-junctional and ST-segment depression with an upsloping ST-segment. This is not an ischemic response because at 80 msec from the J point the ST segment is not 2.0 mm below the isoelectric line. **C** and **D,** patient with 90% obstruction of the obtuse marginal branch of the left circumflex coronary artery and 80% obstruction of the right posterior descending coronary artery at rest **(C)** and exercising **(D)**, demonstrating ischemic response with exercise. In V_4 there is a positive ST-segment slope with a J-junctional depression of 3.7 mm; at 80 msec from this point, the ST segment is 2.8 mm below the isoelectric line. This fulfills the criteria of the positive slope method of detecting an ischemic response.

recovery period has been shown to correlate with poor prognosis.[32]

Repolarization abnormalities are apt to be displayed more markedly in the lead having the greatest R-wave voltage. This is often found in lead V_5 or a bipolar lead, CM_5 (manubrial, V_5) or CS_5 (right scapular, V_5). The Frank lead system allows computer recognition of an R max waveform.[33]

The classic criterion for an ischemic ST-segment response is a 1-mm (0.1 mV) horizontal or downsloping depression persisting for 80 msec beyond the J junction in any lead during exercise. This is strongly fortified if the abnormal morphology persists for 3 minutes into the recovery period. ST-segment elevation of 1 mm for 80 msec beyond the J point is also a marker for an ischemic response. A positive slope criterion has been receiving some acceptance. This would be described as a J-junctional depression of such magnitude that the ST segment is 2 mm or more below the baseline 80 msec beyond the J junction (Fig 3B-10). Ischemic ECG changes occurring late in exercise or during recovery only were initially thought to represent false-positive tracings. More recent studies have shown that a high percentage of these patients have coronary artery disease.[34,35] Exercise-induced ST-segment depression generally persists much longer after exercise than does mechanical evidence of ischemia measured by radionuclide angiography.[36]

In patients with ST-segment depression on the resting ECG, the specificity of 1 mm of ST depression for identifying patients without previous myocardial infarction who have coronary artery disease or patients with previous myocardial infarction who have severe (left main or three-vessel) coronary artery disease is low. Specificity and overall test accuracy can be improved by defining an ischemic response in these patients as an additional 2 mm of ST depression during exercise.[37] ST-segment analysis is unreliable in patients with left bundle-branch block. In patients with right bundle-branch block, ST-segment analysis should include leads V_4 to V_6 but not leads V_1 to V_3.[38]

Elamin et al.[39] made an innovative contribution to wave-form analysis. Only patients with angina were studied. Analysis of the maximal rate of progression of ST-segment depression relative to increases in heart rate (maximal change in ST/HR slope) is thought to provide accurate assessment of the presence and severity of coronary artery disease. There was no overlap in the data from trivial, single-vessel, double-vessel, or triple-vessel disease, and there were no false-positive, false-negative, or indeterminate results. The importance of using a modified exercise protocol to keep the rate of increase in heart rate to approximately 10 beats/min has been demonstrated[39] with this measurement.

Other investigators, primarily Kligfield et al.[40] and Okin et al.,[41,42] have also reported improved accuracy of the stress ECG for general diagnostic purposes, for identification of extensive coronary artery disease, and for prognostic purposes by using heart rate adjustment of ST-segment depression. Various heart-rate-adjusted ST-segment parameters have been evaluated: the ST/HR index, the simplest parameter, calculated by dividing the magnitude of change in ST-segment depression during exercise by change in heart rate; the ST/HR slope, based on linear regression analysis and requiring precise ST-segment measurements in multiple leads and multiple mathematical calculations as well as a modified exercise protocol with small workload increments between stages; the rate-recovery loop, the pattern of ST depression as a function of heart rate during exercise and recovery; and the ST-HR integral, the time-voltage integral of ST-segment depression divided by exercise-induced change in heart rate. It has not been conclusively shown if one parameter is superior to the others. Importantly, several investigators have been unable to show improved accuracy of heart rate adjustment over that with standard ST-segment measurement.[43] Further validation of heart rate adjustment is necessary before widespread application is advised.

Alterations in T-wave morphology have not been valuable in the diagnosis of ischemic disease. They are often determined by autonomic factors that are altered by body position, respiration, and hyperventilation. This is usually seen in the young and may simulate an ischemic response, but it is likely to be a false-positive result because the clinical model is inappropriate. Pseudonormalization of T waves (inverted at rest and becoming upright with exercise) may be a marker for ischemia[44] (Fig 3B-11). Prolongation of the Q-T interval in ischemic states has been difficult to quantify because of the TUP fusion wave that occurs at high heart rates. U-wave inversion with exercise, even in the absence of ST-segment abnormalities, correlates with left main or left anterior descending coronary artery disease if seen in the anterolateral leads. It is a rather insensitive marker for ischemic disease but quite specific if present.[45] The waveforms are difficult to appreciate at high heart rates (Fig 3B-12).

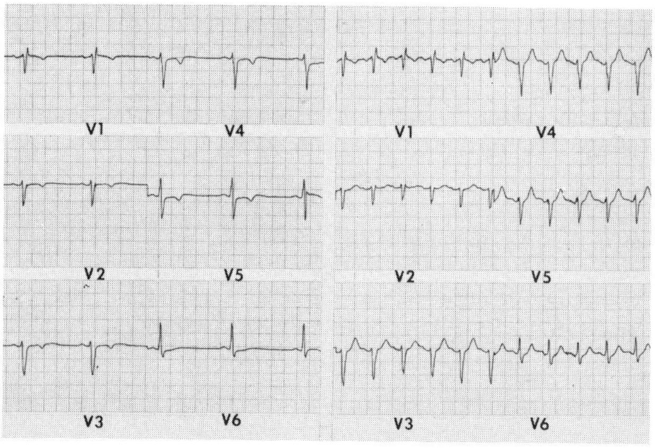

Fig 3B-11 Severe three-vessel coronary obstructive disease in 55-year-old man, displaying pseudonormalization of T waves (inverted at rest **[left]** and normalized with exercise **[right]**). This is a frequent finding and is probably an ischemic response.

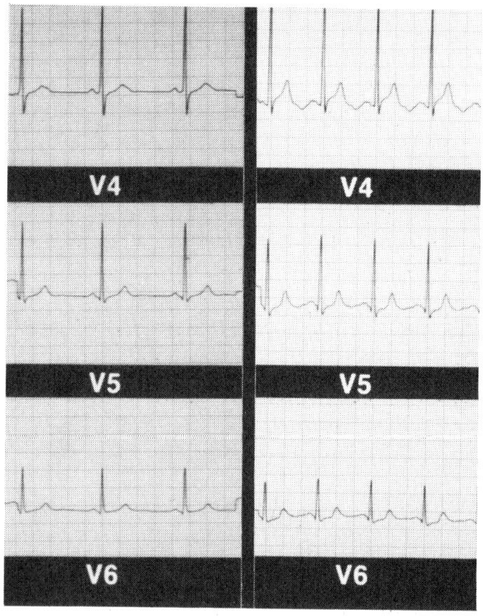

Fig 3B-12 Inversion of the U wave with exercise has been considered a marker of ischemic response. **Left,** control. **Right,** immediately after exercise, showing U-wave inversion (V_4) and a positive test for ischemia in a 51-year-old man.

Observations of septal Q-wave morphology during exercise testing may reduce the number of false-positive tests encountered. Morales-Ballejo et al.[46] noted Q-wave amplitudes in a CM_5 lead in normal subjects and in patients with ischemic heart disease; low Q voltage and its failure to increase after exercise implied abnormal septal activation, as would be present in ischemic disease. An increase in Q-wave amplitude with exercise identified a false-positive ST segment deviation in 75% of the cases. Absence of the Q wave in lead CM_5 with depression of ST segment after exercise identified a true-positive indication of disease in 100% of patients.

R-wave amplitude tends to decrease with high heart rates achieved at maximal exercise. However, there is a large variation in this response, and although initial studies indicated that an increase in R-wave voltage with exercise[47] was associated with high sensitivity and specificity of coronary artery disease, subsequent investigators[48-54] expanded these initial observations, and the current consensus is that R-wave amplitude changes do not have independent predictive value.[55]

Conclusions. All ECG changes that occur with exercise must be interpreted by the clinician in their proper context. No criterion or set of criteria will supplant the responsibility to match the exercise ECG with the clinical model that is in need of categorization.

Aerobic capacity

Determination of a person's functional aerobic capacity is based on the maximal oxygen uptake achieved by normal men and women of varying age groups who submitted to a symptom-limited test. Bruce's group[5] has provided a useful and practical nomogram (see Fig 3B-29) for estimating functional aerobic capacity from data obtained during clinical treadmill exercise testing with the use of a continuous multistage exercise test. Functional aerobic capacity allows anticipation before testing of the time that a trained or untrained subject may exercise. It also provides comparison with the patient's peer group. The ability to objectify the functional aerobic status is of practical value in assessing the value of therapeutic interventions and whether there is a need to embark on new approaches in management.

RESPONSES TO EXERCISE NOT DUE TO CORONARY ARTERY DISEASE

Hypertension

Hypertension is known to evoke false-positive ST-T changes in the exercising subject. The resting ECG may be normal and devoid of any criteria for left ventricular hypertrophy or "strain." Exercise intervention commonly provokes a pronounced hypertensive response, increased left ventricular pressure, and reduced subendocardial perfusion and thereby alters the sequence of repolarization of the ventricle. This results in ST-segment depression mimicking coronary obstruction. Frequent blood pressure recordings should be made during exercise to ensure that a reasonable limit, 250 to 280 mm Hg systolic, is not exceeded.

Cardiomyopathy

Cardiomyopathies may be of the dilated, restrictive, or hypertrophic type. No exercise-induced ECG morphologies can be considered typical of these clinical presentations (Fig 3B-13).

Dilated cardiomyopathies tend to cause rate-dependent left bundle-branch block and ventricular ectopic activity. These disturbances may provide the impetus for the patient to seek medical advice long before symptoms of left ventricular dysfunction occur. The conduction system disease or ventricular ectopy might be evident on a routine physical examination and ECG. Exercise testing is useful for objectively establishing the functional classification of these patients. It can reveal latent conduction system disease, as in rate-dependent left bundle-branch block, or unmask atrioventricular (AV) block, such as second-degree type II or third-degree AV block. Complex ventricular ectopic activity, which is a common terminal event in dilated cardiomyopathy, may become apparent with exercise testing.

Restrictive cardiomyopathies have no special features on the exercise ECG. Limited functional aerobic capacity is present, as is an excessive chronotropic response to exercise because of the limited stroke volume that can be achieved.

Hypertrophic cardiomyopathies may exhibit several exercise-induced responses of interest. Postexercise syncope is a feature of this type of disease. Septal Q waves present in the left precordial leads may undergo considerable enhancement with exercise. A "strain" pattern of ST-T depression may develop with exercise, similar to that observed in patients with systemic hypertension or aortic valve stenosis.

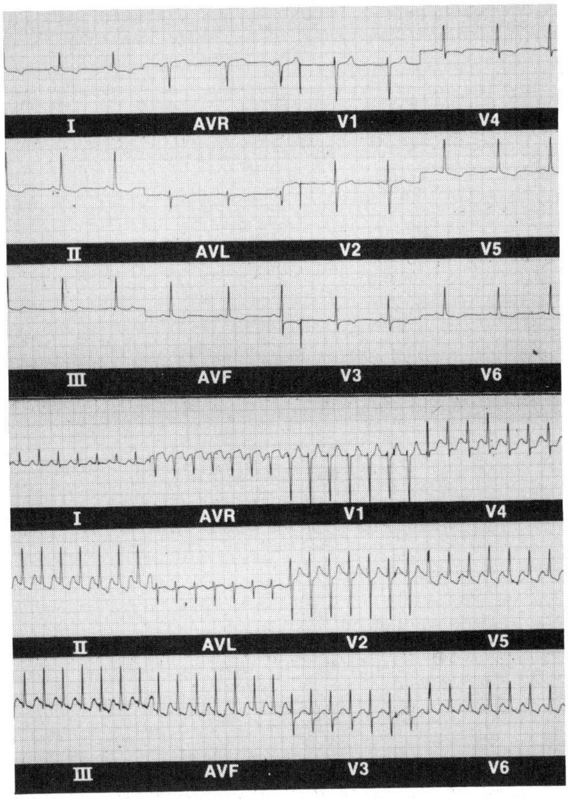

Fig 3B-13 Pattern false-positive for ischemia in 18-year-old man with a dilated cardiomyopathy and normal coronary arteries. **Upper,** resting (64 beats/min) pattern demonstrates widespread repolarization abnormalities. **Lower,** with exercise (165 beats/min) additional ST-T depression is noted. In this example, ischemia and digitalis are not factors.

Neurocirculatory asthenia or hyper-β-adrenergic states

There is a group of young to middle-aged men and women who display an excessive chronotropic response to exercise. They are not physically deconditioned but appear to have an excessive sympathetic discharge, influencing not only heart rate responses to simple interventions such as hyperventilation and changes in body position but also repolarization changes known to be altered by autonomic discharges. These consist of T-wave lability and ST-T changes in the absence of coronary obstructive disease, coronary vasomotion, or symptoms and signs of heart disease (Fig 3B-14).

Valvular heart disease

Many patients with valvular disease have no symptoms at rest but show effort-induced incapacitation. The history

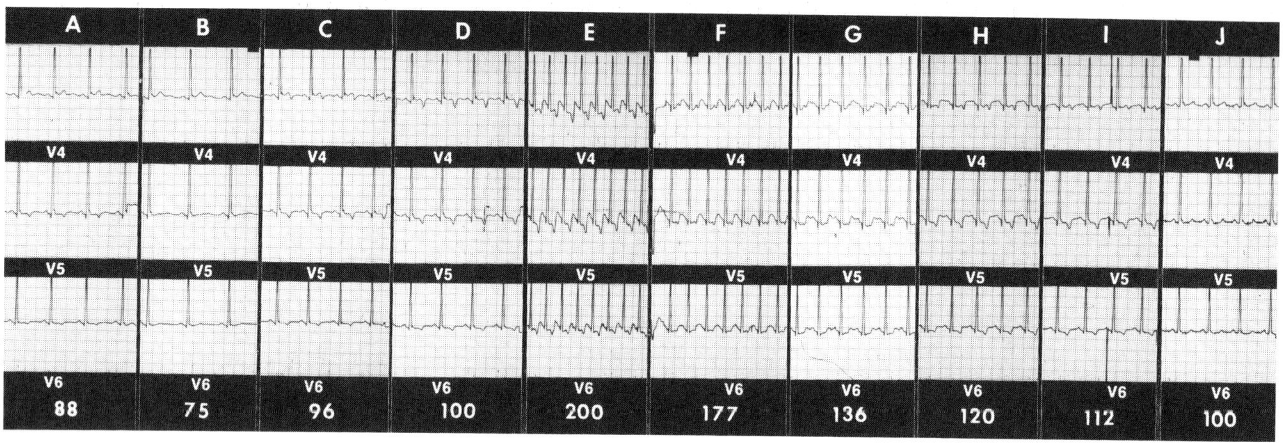

Fig 3B-14 Hyper-β-adrenergic state, or neurocirculatory asthenia, in a normal 32-year-old man. **A,** sitting control. **B,** supine. **C,** abrupt stand; T waves become inverted. **D,** after 45 seconds of hyperventilation, insufficient to induce hypocapnea but evoking a sympathomimetic response inverting the T waves. **E,** exercise, increasing the circulating catecholamines and causing a further displacement of the T wave and ST segment. The heart rate was excessive for the work performed—4.2 mph up a 16% grade. **F,** immediately after exercise. **G,** at 1 minute after exercise. **H,** at 3 minutes after exercise. **I,** at 6 minutes after exercise. (**H** and **I** show morphologies that, in a patient with angina, could be interpreted as ischemic in type.) **J,** after the Valsalva maneuver in the bradycardia phase, which will frequently normalize labile T waves and thereby avoid conveying an inappropriate interpretation of an ischemic response. *Numerals* give heart rate in beats/min.

may be too vague to allow classification of a patient's functional capacity. An alteration in the patient's lifestyle may allow accommodation to the worsening disease process. Using a variety of available exercise testing protocols, the clinician may ascribe an exact level of functional aerobic capacity and properly place the patient in NYHA functional class I, II, III, or IV. This is extremely useful in deciding the optimal time for surgical or catheter-based intervention.

Young patients with aortic valve stenosis can be exercised cautiously to obtain helpful information. Severe gradients across the aortic valve may exist with no evidence of left ventricular hypertrophy or strain in the resting ECG. The exercise ECG is likely to demonstrate a left ventricular strain pattern if the gradient is 50 mm Hg or more. Adult patients with aortic valve stenosis are prone to syncope and complex ventricular ectopic activity with exercise. They are difficult to resuscitate because of the limitations on cardiac output imposed by the stenotic valve. There are documented adverse experiences in this group of patients. Severe aortic stenosis is considered an absolute contraindication to exercise testing. In asymptomatic patients with borderline severe hemodynamics (i.e., mean aortic gradient around 50 mm Hg), low-level exercise testing can cautiously be performed to more accurately determine functional class.[56] In patients who claim to be asymptomatic, angina, severe dyspnea, or presyncope occasionally will develop or an abnormal blood pressure response may become evident, thereby aiding the decision for surgical intervention.

Routine treadmill testing is generally safe in patients with aortic and mitral valve regurgitation. Previously, it was hoped that the radionuclide angiographic response to exercise could be used to determine optimal timing for valve replacement. For aortic insufficiency, it has now been shown that patients with an abnormal angiographic response to exercise (which includes most of these patients) still have a favorable outcome after valve replacement as long as the resting ejection fraction remains in a normal range preoperatively.[57] Exercise duration preoperatively does help predict reversibility of systolic dysfunction and survival postoperatively.[58]

Digitalis

Effort has been directed toward separating resting and exercise-induced changes in repolarization produced by digitalis from those produced by ischemia. These efforts have failed, and not all repolarization abnormalities seen in the presence of digitalis may be construed as ischemia, regardless of the presence of known coronary obstructive disease (Figs 3B-15 and 3B-16). Patients with normal coronary arteries who are taking digitalis usually demonstrate no greater than 2 mm of ST-segment depression during exercise, but occasionally 4 mm or more of ST-segment depression can develop. When exercise testing is being performed for diagnosis in patients receiving digitalis, administration should be discontinued, if possible, 2 weeks before testing.

Arrhythmias

Arrhythmias inducible by exercise include the entire gamut from sinus node dysfunction to ventricular fibril-

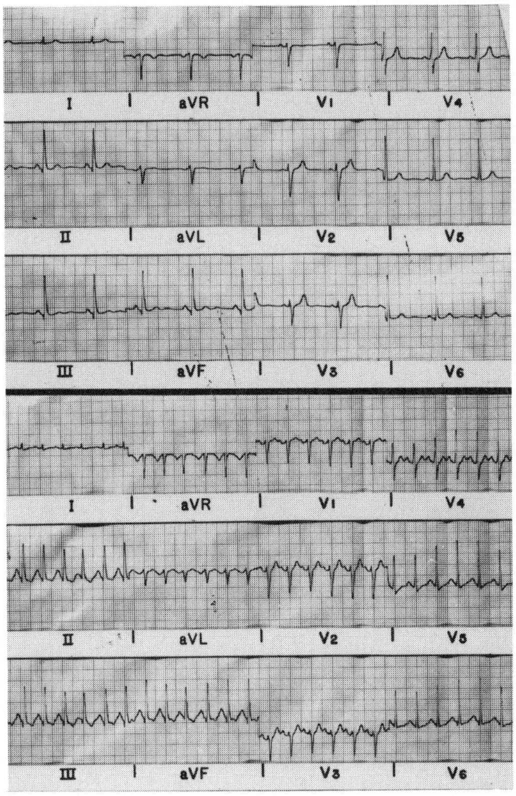

Fig 3B-15 Normal exercise response in 61-year-old man with paroxysmal atrial fibrillation who is not taking digitalis. Coronary angiograms were normal. **Upper,** at rest. **Lower,** exercise. See Figure 3B-16 for response when same patient was digitalized.

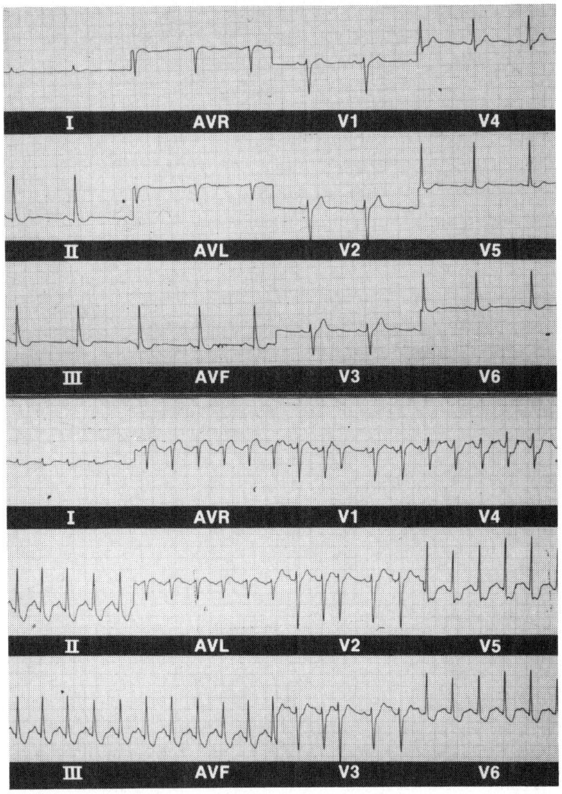

Fig 3B-16 Abnormal exercise response in 61-year-old man with paroxysmal atrial fibrillation who is taking digitalis. **Upper,** at rest. **Lower,** exercise. Compare this ST-T response to that in Figure 3B-15.

lation. Many attempts have been made to correlate their occurrence with specific disease states, such as ischemic heart disease, but with a notable lack of success. Exercise testing may make manifest important arrhythmias such as ventricular ectopic activity or may suppress them as with overdrive atrial pacing. Exercise testing is an important method of gaining an appreciation for the risks that may be encountered in an exercise program for a patient undergoing cardiac rehabilitation. It can test the adequacy of medical or surgical therapy in a given clinical model. It complements, rather than supplants, long-term ECG recording (Holter) in the detection of arrhythmias.

Supraventricular arrhythmias. Chronotropic incompetence is defined by Ellestad[7] as a slow resting pulse that fails to accelerate normally with exercise. In the absence of β-adrenergic blockade, chronotropic incompetence can be an indicator of poor prognosis. Sinus node deceleration, defined as an initial increase followed by subsequent decrease in heart rate during continued exercise, is a marker of right coronary artery disease.[59] The development of a prolonged P-R interval with exercise, with or without bradycardia, suggests conduction system disease, which may occur at any level of the system. Type I (Wenckebach) AV block is rare with exercise and suggests the possibility of digitalis intoxication. Type II AV block in response to an increasing atrial rate is consistent with distal conduction system disease. The occurrence of third-degree AV block with exercise is a dramatic event and is usually associated with incapacitation. In patients with narrow QRS congenital heart block, exercise is very useful for determining whether they are approaching the need for a pacemaker (Fig 3B-17). Rapid junctional rhythms may be induced by exercise and supplant a lower rate of sinus node activity. When bradycardia occurs, a junctional rhythm is seen as an escape mechanism in the postexercise period. Sinus node dysfunction is frequently the cause for a junctional rhythm to emerge (Fig 3B-18).

Atrial ectopic activity is frequent in exercise testing and may take the form of atrial premature beats singly or in runs and as a supraventricular tachycardia (Figs 3B-19 and 3B-20). Bursts of atrial fibrillation or flutter (Fig 3B-21) may result from an exercise-stressed noncompliant ventricle with an increased filling pressure. Exercise-induced junctional ectopic activity has not been related to any specific clinical state.

Ventricular arrhythmias. Ventricular ectopic activity associated with exercise (Figs 3B-22 and 3B-23) has not been helpful in specifically identifying patients with or without ischemic heart disease. Ventricular tachycardia, defined as ≥ 3 premature ventricular beats in a row, is infrequent ($<5\%$ of patients referred for exercise test-

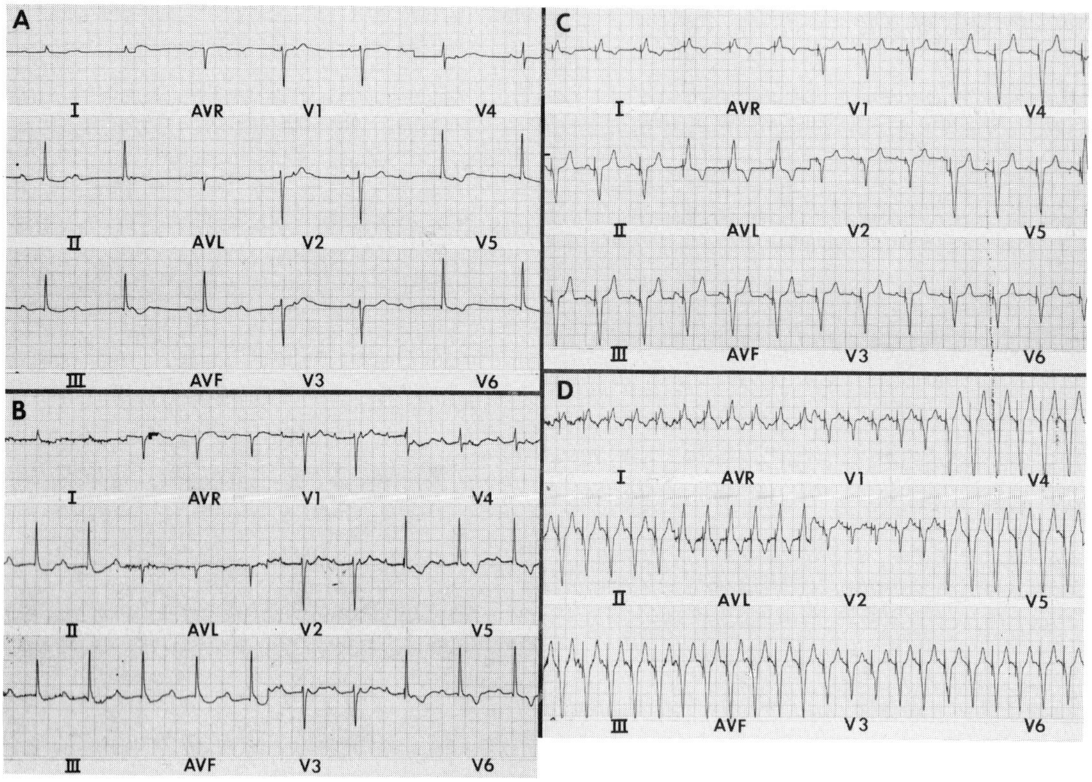

Fig 3B-17 Congenital complete heart block in 54-year-old woman. **A** and **B,** without pacemaker. **A,** at rest: atrial rate, 64 beats/min; ventricular rate, 43 beats/min. **B,** exercise: atrial rate, 136 beats/min; ventricular rate, 67 beats/min. **C** and **D,** with a VDD (P synchronous) permanent pacemaker. (Choice at this time would be a DDD, VVIR, or DDDR pacemaker.) **C,** at rest: paced ventricular rate, 72 beats/min. **D,** immediately after exercise: atrial rate, 134 beats/min; ventricular rate, 134 beats/min.

Fig 3B-18 Tracings from 62-year-old man with prior myocardial infarction who went into an accelerated junctional rhythm with AV dissociation during exercise. **A,** control: atrial rate, 62 beats/min; ventricular rate, 62 beats/min; normal AV conduction. **B,** V_5 rhythm strip. **C,** the 12-lead recovery tracing. **B** and **C** show AV dissociation with an atrial rate slightly greater than the junctional rate. Note exercise-induced hyperacute ischemic pattern in the inferior leads.

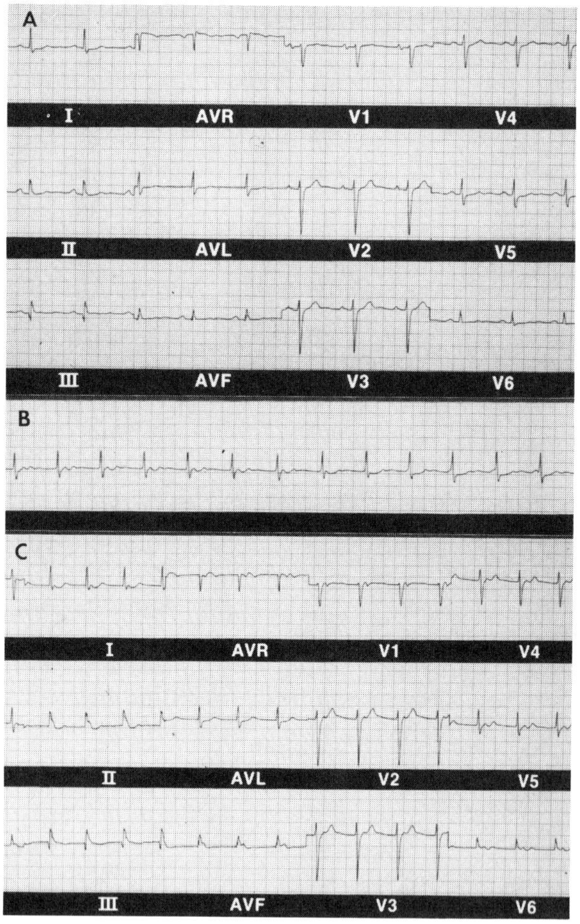

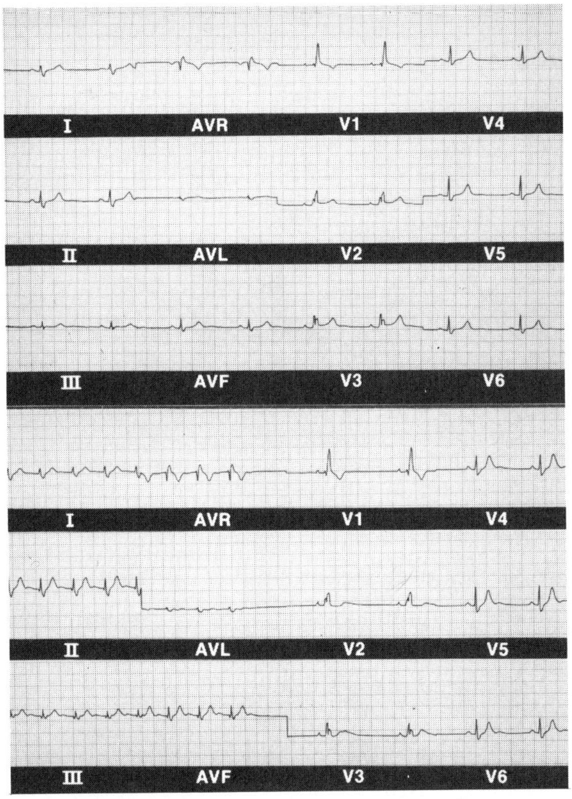

Fig 3B-19 Exercise-induced supraventricular tachycardia. **Upper,** control, sinus rhythm. **Lower,** exercise. Tachycardia apparent in leads I through aV_F. The tachycardia terminated by a pause and emergence of sinus bradycardia that accelerated over several beats in typical fashion.

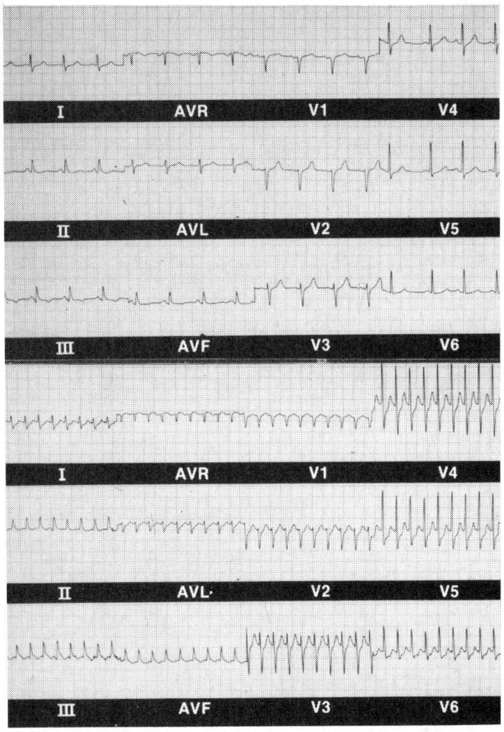

Fig 3B-20 Exercise-induced paroxysmal supraventricular tachycardia in a 56-year-old man with no known heart disease but with tobacco and alcohol abuse. **Upper,** at rest. **Lower,** exercise.

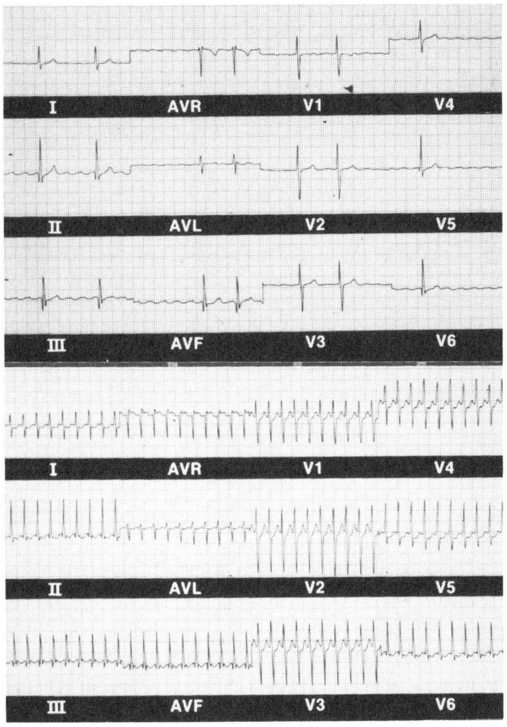

Fig 3B-21 Atrial flutter in 36-year-old man with varying block at rest (digitalized). **Upper,** at rest. **Lower,** exercise-enhanced AV conduction, to achieve a ventricular rate of 240 beats/min.

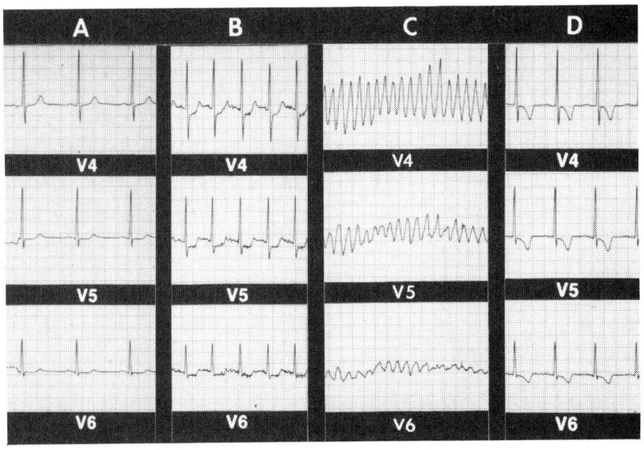

Fig 3B-22 Ventricular tachycardia-flutter-fibrillation with exercise in a 73-year-old man with triple-vessel disease. **A,** control. **B,** during exercise. **C,** exercise-induced arrhythmia. **D,** at 9 minutes of recovery after two electroversion shocks.

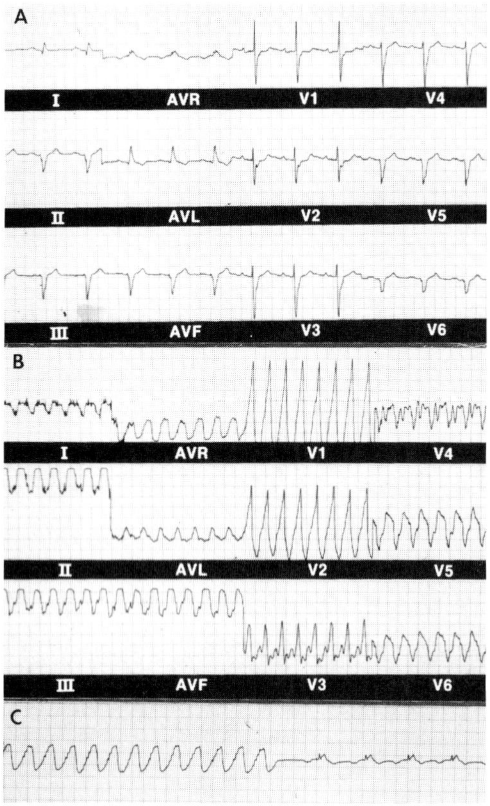

Fig 3B-23 Recurrent exercise-induced ventricular tachycardia in 54-year-old man after ventricular aneurysmectomy. **A,** control tracing shows interoapical infarction relic. **B,** during exercise, ventricular tachycardia occurred. **C,** aV_R tracing at rest, showing spontaneous termination.

ing). Ventricular tachycardia in subjects without evident structural heart disease is of no prognostic significance.[60,61] Exercise-induced ventricular ectopic activity in the ischemic patient may result from a focus in an underperfused portion of the myocardium. However, this explanation fits poorly with a host of observations. Patients who have ischemic heart disease may have ectopy at rest, or ectopy may be suppressed by exercise but become frequent during recovery. The significance of ventricular tachycardia in patients with coronary artery disease is uncertain, with some studies reporting this finding as an adverse prognostic sign and others not. A small subset of patients with coronary artery disease have symptoms suggestive of exercise-induced arrhythmias. It may not be possible to induce these arrhythmias during an electrophysiologic study. Exercise testing is indicated in these patients both for diagnosis and for assessment of the efficacy of antiarrhythmic therapy.[62] Recent documentation of exercise-induced ventricular tachycardia in some patients receiving flecainide has made treadmill testing useful before dismissal in patients requiring flecainide and other class 1C agents. In patients with no evident cardiac disease, effort-induced ventricular tachycardia with or without symptoms may develop.[63]

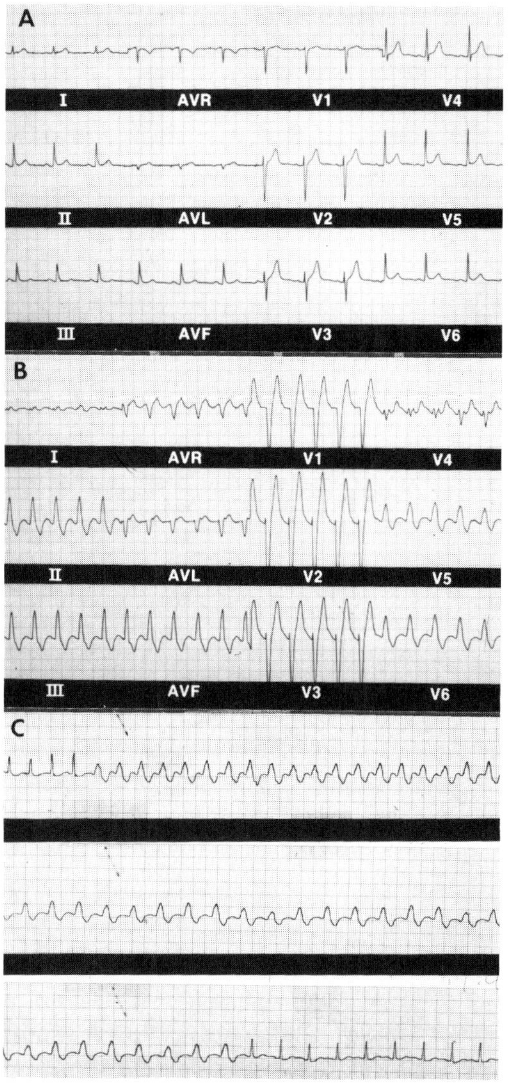

Fig 3B-24 Symptomatic rate-dependent left bundle-branch block in 60-year-old man with normal coronary arteries. **A,** at rest. **B,** exercise. **C,** rhythm strips showing onset (167 beats/min) and ending (124 beats/min) of left bundle-branch block. The cardiac output routinely decreases at the onset of this block but is rarely perceived by patients. An exception is this patient, who would become very lightheaded.

Conduction abnormalities. The most commonly encountered exercise-induced conduction abnormality is rate-dependent left bundle-branch block (Figs 3B-24 and 3B-25). Right bundle-branch block with effort is relatively rare (Fig 3B-26). Prolongation of the P-R interval is common. Exercise-induced Wenckebach phenomenon (type I block) is rare. Type II block is far more common, and third-degree block is encountered with variable frequency, depending on the test population. All such information is of exceptional value when one attempts to document mechanisms of disturbed consciousness, especially if they are related to effort. Such testing may obviate

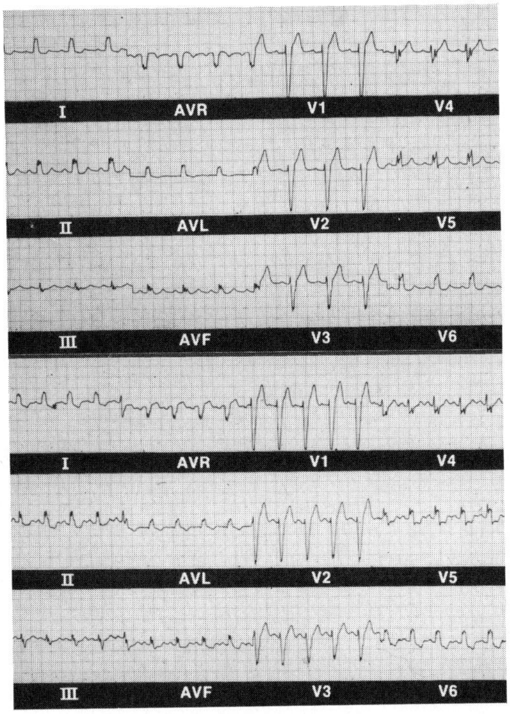

Fig 3B-25 In a 71-year-old man with ischemic heart disease, chronic left bundle-branch block, and concordant repolarization at rest **(upper),** which has been suggested[64] as a marker for ischemia, exercise **(lower)** induced discordant T-wave inversions (V_4, V_5, V_6) and ST-segment depression. This interesting phenomenon may be consistent with an ischemic morphology but lacks adequate documentation. It may be the counterpart of the exercise-induced pseudonormalization of T waves occasionally seen in the left precordial leads in patients with ischemic heart disease.

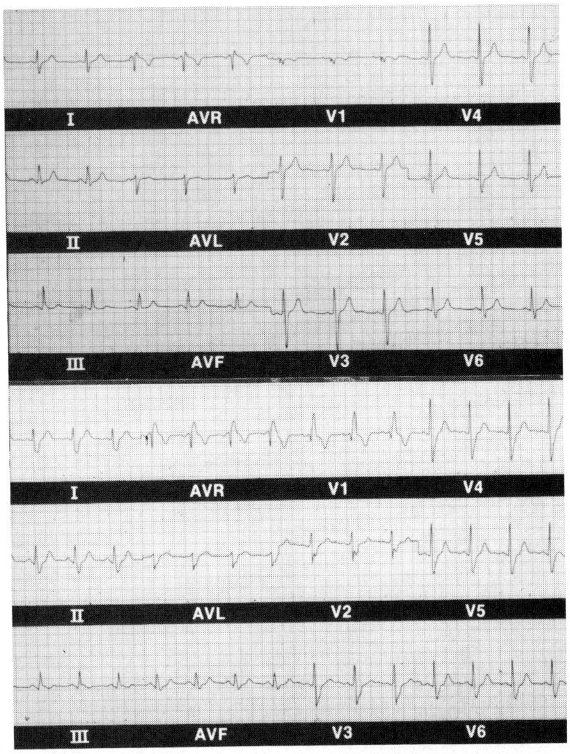

Fig 3B-26 Rate-dependent right bundle-branch block in 55-year-old man who had a right intraventricular conduction defect at rest. This is uncommon compared to the frequency of rate-dependent left bundle-branch block. **Upper,** at rest; rate, 68 beats/min. **Lower,** after exercise; rate, 83 beats/min.

multiple Holter recordings, long periods in a monitored unit, or electrophysiologic study.

Preexcitation states. In patients with Wolff-Parkinson-White syndrome, atrial pacing that increases AV nodal refractoriness will enhance conduction via the bypass tract and increase the delta content of the QRS complex. Exercise causes elaboration of catecholamines which enhance AV nodal conduction and may increase AV conduction to the exclusion of bypass conduction. Therefore, exercise may produce a rate in excess of the bypass tract refractory period and block it to oncoming impulses. This results in a narrow QRS with a normal P-R interval and normal repolarization (Fig 3B-27). Many bypass tracts have such a short refractory period that exercise-induced tachycardias of 180 to 200 beats/min will not render them inoperative. Generally, a patient with the Wolff-Parkinson-White syndrome and no history of tachycardia will have a long bypass refractory period and may with exercise acquire normal AV conduction devoid of a delta wave and with normal repolarization. Patients with Wolff-Parkinson-White syndrome who have a history of tachycardia usually have a short refractory period in the bypass tract, and normal pure AV conduction cannot be induced at heart rates usually attained with exercise testing (Fig 3B-28).

PRINCIPAL TECHNIQUES OF EXERCISE TESTING

Physicians who supervise exercise testing should satisfy minimum training requirements. A task force recommended that physicians participate in at least 50 procedures during training and perform at least 25 procedures a year to maintain competence.[65] Supervising physicians must possess a wide range of cognitive skills to competently perform exercise testing (Table 3B-1).

Treadmill exercise testing requires preparation for both the physician and the patient. The physician should be familiar with the patient's history, physical examination, and resting ECG. This allows the physician to formulate the major purpose for testing the patient, to make a pretest prediction of the limits of heart rate and workload that would be safe and appropriate, and to pay special attention to signs and symptoms relevant to the purpose of testing. An asymptomatic patient whose physical examination and resting ECG are normal may be tested in order to measure the patient's functional aerobic

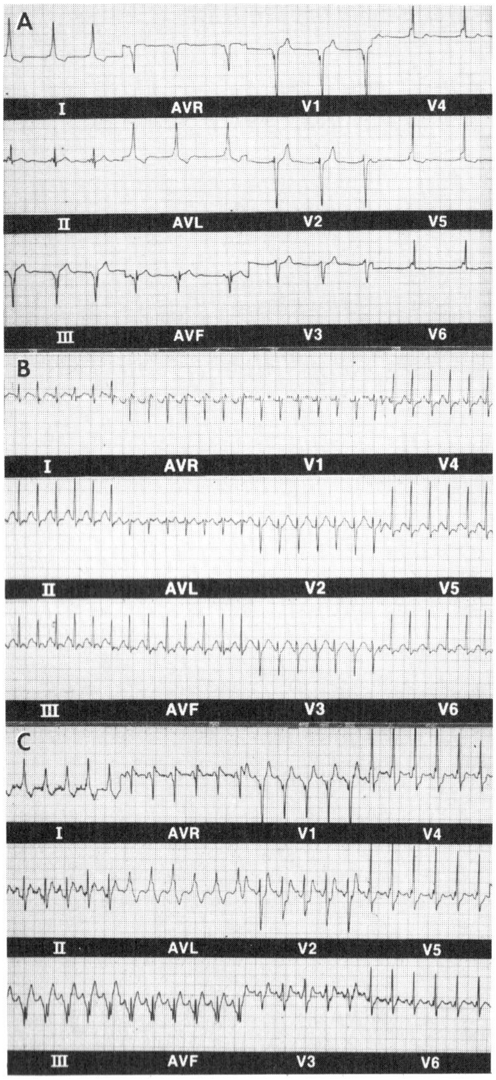

Fig 3B-27 Type B Wolff-Parkinson-White syndrome in patient with left posterior atrial septal bypass tract. During bouts of paroxysmal supraventricular tachycardia, the antegrade pathway was via the AV node and the retrograde pathway was via the bypass tract. **A,** resting control. **B,** immediately after exercise. The R-R interval of 340 msec has exceeded the refractory period of the bypass tract, causing pure conduction via the AV node-His pathway. This normalizes the QRS by eliminating the delta wave. **C,** at 1 minute after exercise, R-R interval is 430 msec, which fails to exceed the refractory period of the bypass tract, and the delta wave reappears.

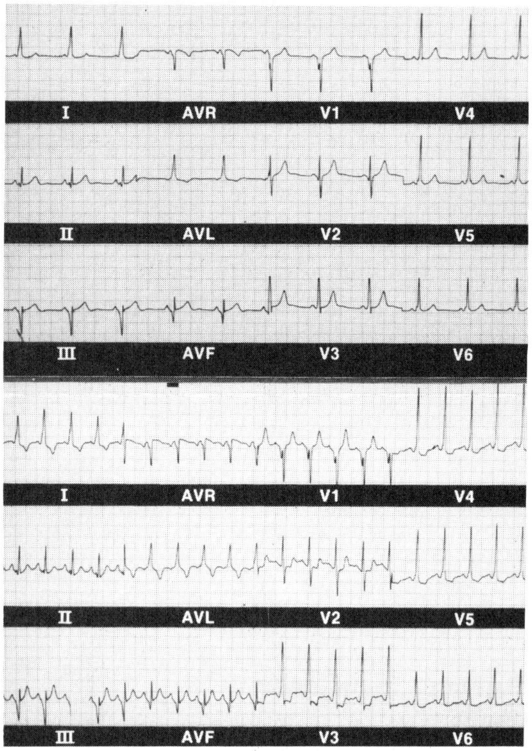

Fig 3B-28 Type B Wolff-Parkinson-White syndrome in 26-year-old man with history of tachycardia. **Upper,** at rest prior to exercise. **Lower,** at 1 minute after exercise (heart rate, 125 beats/min; R-R interval, 440 msec). During an electrophysiologic study it was found that the refractory period of the bypass tract was 300 msec. During exercise the patient was unable to elevate his heart rate to 200 beats/min, which would have been required to achieve an R-R interval of 300 msec and exceed the refractory period of the bypass tract, thereby creating normal AV conduction and normal repolarization. The persistence of the abnormal depolarization creates abnormal repolarization and a false-positive test.

capacity or to develop a prescription for exercise. The predicted limits of heart rate and time of exercise on the Bruce or similar calibrated protocol are determined on the basis of the patient's age, sex, and training before testing. Symptoms of fatigue appearing at the anaerobic threshold—usually at about 75% of the predicted aerobic capacity—are anticipated. The patient is instructed to report the onset of any symptoms to the physician. Frequent communication with the patient is wise to assess any adverse symptoms that might necessitate premature cessation of exercise and also to assess the patient's subjective level of exertion based on the Borg scale of perceived exertion.[66] The test is terminated at the point of fatigue and moderate dyspnea in a healthy patient who exercises beyond the anaerobic threshold.

In contrast, the purpose of testing the patient who has had a recent myocardial infarction is to detect evidence of ischemia and left ventricular dysfunction not present at rest, to ensure electrical stability at low levels of exercise, and to establish a target heart rate for an exercise prescription. A protocol of up to 5 METS, such as with the Naughton protocol, is used. The physician must be aware of any complications that have occurred as a result of the myocardial infarction. Also, if the patient is taking medications that will affect the relative heart rate response, conduction, or depolarization and repolarization (β-blockers, calcium-entry blockers, digitalis), these may affect the physician's interpretation of the patient's

Table 3B-1 Cognitive skills needed to perform exercise tests competently

Knowledge of
- Appropriate indications for exercise testing
- Appropriate contraindications and risks of testing
- How to promptly recognize and treat complications of exercise testing
- Specificity, sensitivity, and diagnostic accuracy of exercise testing in different patient populations
- How to apply Bayes theorem to interpret test results
- Various exercise protocols (Bruce, Naughton, Balke-Ware, USAFSAM, etc.) and indications for each
- Basic cardiovascular and exercise physiology, including blood pressure and heart rate response to exercise
- Electrocardiography and changes in the ECG that may result from exercise, hyperventilation, ischemia, hypertrophy, conduction disorders, electrolyte disturbances, and drugs
- Cardiac arrhythmias and treatment of serious arrhythmias
- Cardiovascular drugs and how they can affect exercise performance, hemodynamics, and the ECG
- Conditions and circumstances that can cause false-positive, indeterminate, or false-negative test results
- The effects of age and disease on hemodynamic and ECG responses to exercise
- Principles and details of exercise testing, including proper lead placement and skin preparation
- Prognostic value of exercise testing
- Alternative diagnostic procedures to exercise testing
- End points of exercise testing and indications to terminate exercise testing
- The concept of metabolic equivalent (MET) and estimation of exercise intensity in different modes of exercise

Competence in cardiopulmonary resuscitation and successful completion of an AHA-sponsored course in advanced cardiac life support.

Ability and commitment to communicate diagnostic accuracy, risks, and results of the test to the patient, the medical record, and other physicians so that appropriately informed patient consent can be obtained.

Modified from Schlant RC, Friesinger GC, Leonard JJ: Clinical competence in exercise testing: a statement for physicians from the ACP/ACC/AHA Task Force on Clinical Privileges in Cardiology. *Circulation* 82:1884-1888, 1990. By permission of American Heart Association.

heart rate, rhythm, or ST changes. Thus, for a postmyocardial infarction patient who is receiving β-blockers, the end point of testing should be 4 to 5 METS of work rather than a heart rate of 120 to 130 beats/min. A patient with atrial fibrillation who is taking digitalis may show a faster heart rate response and nonspecific ST changes. A patient having concomitant valvular disease after myocardial infarction may have to stop sooner at lower workloads so that the left ventricle is not excessively stressed.

Patients who have nonspecific ST-T abnormalities on the resting ECG, who are taking digitalis, or who have left bundle-branch block or pacemakers have less specific ECG changes and might better be tested by radionuclide angiography during bicycle ergometry or by thallium scintigraphy. Patients with severe arteriosclerosis obliterans whose claudication may prevent adequate evaluation by treadmill exercise may tolerate handcrank ergometry that approximates 300 kiloponds. If the resting ECG is normal, exercise electrocardiography alone is almost as accurate as exercise radionuclide angiography for correctly identifying patients with severe (left main or triple-vessel, or both) coronary artery disease,[67] and for predicting outcome.[68]

The key to obtaining a good ECG is optimal skin preparation. The skin electrical resistance should be lowered to less than 5,000 Ω by cleansing and gentle abrasion with emery paper and then by cleansing with an alcohol swab. This resistance can be measured directly with an impedance meter but is often considered acceptable if the signal generated from the electrode has little noise even with tapping of the electrode. Fluid-column silver-silver chloride electrodes with strong adhesive and firm, nonstressed wire connections are essential. Many new disposable electrodes satisfy these requirements and can be applied and removed quickly. The Mason-Likar[69] 12-lead system is recommended because it allows good sensitivity in diagnostic stress testing, although many excellent medical centers have found a bipolar system with a negative electrode at the right scapula (CS_5) or right anterior axillary line at the fifth intercostal space (CS_5) and a positive electrode in the V_5 position to be quite adequate, faster, and more economical. Blackburn and Katigbak[70] demonstrated that 80 of 100 patients with abnormal ST changes during exercise were detected with the V_5 lead. An additional 11% were detected with the inferior leads (II, III, aV_F). The added sensitivity for detecting ST changes provided by the use of more leads is partially offset by a decrease in specificity, especially because of ST depression occurring inferiorly in normal women. One would expect that the other criteria of ischemia, including symptoms, work capacity, and decrease in septal force, would help keep specificity high in multiple lead systems.

The ECG recorder should meet American Heart Association specifications[71] and have an adequate frequency response (usually 0 to 100 Hz) to avoid distortion or loss of information. A three-channel recorder is especially helpful in analyzing disturbances in rhythm and in monitoring ST-segment changes in orthogonal X, Y, and Z leads or V_1, V_5, and aV_F Wilson leads. A video screen with memory capacity and a direct writer recording any single lead help in monitoring rhythm changes from a distance and can be conveniently wired to allow the physician to record an arrhythmia as it appears on the monitor. Averaging programs to remove extraneous muscle artifacts through high-speed microprocessors are now available commercially. The person interpreting the exercise ECG, however, should be aware that commercially available programs that display smoothed, "averaged" beats can occasionally produce tracings that appear to significantly exaggerate abnormalities seen on the real-time tracing, so that the tendency is to produce false-positive tracings.[72] Great care must be taken in selecting the best software to prevent distortion of the ECG signal. We have found a digital template-averaging technique that utilizes three simultaneous leads to be satisfactory.[73] Once the onset of the QRS, R wave, and J point have been defined, measurements of the ST segment 40 to 80 msec beyond the J point can be made in each lead. Because of the immediate postexercise widening of the T wave, measurement of the ST at 60 to 80 msec beyond the J point is often on the ascending limb of the T wave, and this persists for 1 to 2 minutes immediately after exercise. ST-segment slopes can also be calculated during exercise. Printed reports of the stress test, including sequential analog ECG changes, graphic demonstrations of ST changes, and heart rate, are available. We believe that the interpretation of these changes is best done by the primary physician supervising the exercise test.

Total-body oxygen consumption can be measured directly by expiratory gas analysis (mass spectrometer, Haldane method, oxygen electrode). Previously, this measurement was made only for research purposes in specialized exercise laboratories. Refinements in technology have permitted the commercial production of metabolic carts at reasonable cost, so that expiratory gas analysis is now available for clinical use. Measurement of ventilatory status during exercise can be combined with data available from standard exercise testing to provide more physiologic information on cardiovascular and pulmonary function. Mancini et al.[74] reported that directly measured peak exercise oxygen uptake during exercise testing was the best predictor of survival among several variables tested in patients with severely reduced left ventricular function. These authors suggested that cardiac transplantation can be safely deferred in these patients if peak exercise oxygen uptake exceeds 14 mL/kg per minute. Theoretical advantages of obtaining this extra information are more accurate classification of patients with heart failure, more objective determination of disability status, more critical assessment of patient response to interventional therapy, and enhancement of the sensitivity and specificity of standard exercise electrocardiography. Additionally, expiratory gas analysis potentially allows the clinician to determine whether a patient who presents with exertional dyspnea or fatigue is limited predominantly by a cardiovascular or a pulmonary disorder.[12,75,76]

Oxygen consumption can also be calculated indirectly from the percentage grade and speed with the equations in Table 3B-2. Myocardial oxygen consumption is proportional to the product of heart rate and systolic blood pressure. When myocardial oxygen consumption exceeds myocardial oxygen supply, the patient experiences symptoms or signs of myocardial ischemia; this necessitates premature cessation of exercise short of the predicted maximal total body aerobic capacity and indicates functional aerobic impairment.

Table 3B-2 Indirect estimation of aerobic capacity[77]

Condition	Aerobic, $\dot{V}O_2$ = mL O_2/(kg · min)
Walking (1.9 to 3.7 mph*)	
Horizontal	(0.1)(speed)† + 3.5
Incline	[0.1 + (1.8 × % incline)] (speed)† + 3.5
Jogging (>5 mph)	
Horizontal	(0.2)(speed)† + 3.5
Incline (outdoors)	[0.2 + (1.8 × % incline)] (speed)† + 3.5
Incline (treadmill)	[0.2 + (0.9 × % incline)] (speed)† + 3.5
Bicycle ergometry	(2.11 × kg · m/min) + 267

*1 mph = 26.8 m/min = 1.6 km/hr
†Speed is in m/min.

Protocols

Several protocols are currently in use to define the temporal increase in speed and grade of the treadmill. The practicing physician should select a protocol that is consistent with the physical capacity of the patient and the purpose of the test. The Bruce protocol,[5] for example, is a widely accepted format (Table 3B-3). It begins at 1.7 mph and a 10% grade, a level of approximately 4 METS, with increments in speed and grade every 3 minutes that allow total-body aerobic work to increase at approximately 1 MET for every minute of exercise. The 3-minute stages allow approximate equilibration to be attained by the end of the interval in most patients, so that it is convenient to measure blood pressure during the last minute of each stage. Predicted normal exercise time on this protocol is dependent on age, sex, and training and can be determined from a nomogram (Fig 3B-29) prior to testing. The end point that limits the test is usually a symptom or sign. For lower levels of work, the Naughton protocol[6] (Table 3B-4), often used to stress myocardial infarction patients before hospital dismissal, begins at 1 mph and 0% grade, increases to 2 mph and 0% grade, and then increases 3.5% in grade every 2 minutes, or approximately 1 MET every 2 minutes. The end point in myocardial infarction patients is usually 5 METS or a heart rate maximum of 120 to 130 beats/min when tested 8 to 14 days after infarction. Other useful calibrated protocols include those of Balke and Ware[8] and Ellestad.[7] Available studies suggest that peak oxygen uptake, maximal heart rate, and myocardial ischemic threshold are similar between protocols using different work-rate increments.[78,79]

Table 3B-3 Bruce protocol[5]

Time, min	Speed, mph	Grade, %	$\dot{V}O_2$, mL/(kg · min) Normal men	Normal women	Cardiac men	Mean METS*
1	1.7	10	12.4 ± 2.2	9.0 ± 1.7	10.5 ± 2.4	3.0
2			16.7 ± 1.8	15.4 ± 1.5	15.8 ± 3.1	4.6
3			17.4 ± 1.4	16.9 ± 1.5	17.8 ± 2.7	5.0
4	2.5	12	19.6 ± 2.1	19.2 ± 2.0	19.9 ± 3.7	6.0
5			24.1 ± 1.2	21.7 ± 1.7	22.1 ± 2.6	6.5
6			24.8 ± 2.1	23.2 ± 1.8	23.1 ± 2.9	6.8
7	3.4	14	28.6 ± 2.4	25.8 ± 1.8	25.4 ± 2.1	7.6
8			32.6 ± 2.4	29.9 ± 2.8	30.2 ± 3.0	8.8
9			34.3 ± 3.3	32.2 ± 3.2	31.8 ± 2.3	9.4
10	4.2	16	38.3 ± 3.6	39.0 ± 4.2	35.0 ± 3.0	10.7
11			42.3 ± 1.9	46.1 ± 6.2		12.6
12			43.8 ± 4.0	49.1 ± 5.4		13.3
13	5.0	18				
14						
15			56.9†			16.3
16	5.5	20				
17						
18			68.2†			19.5
19	6.0	22				
20						
21			79.6†			22.7

*Metabolic equivalent, defined as multiples of O_2 consumption of 3.5 mL/(kg · min) by patient in sitting position.
†$\dot{V}O_2$ = 0.19 + 3.78 (min); r = 0.906; n = 44.

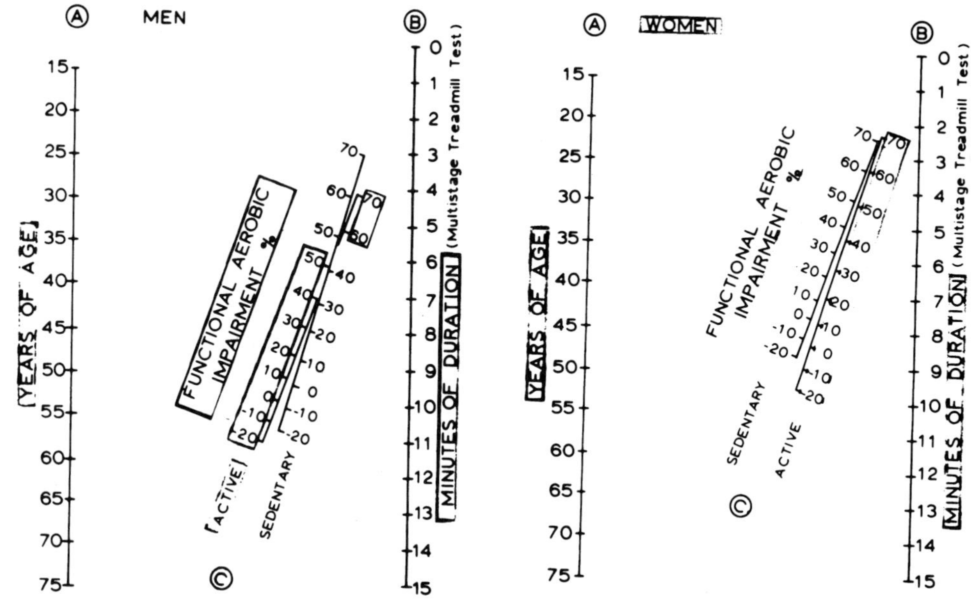

Fig 3B-29 Nomograms for predicting normal exercise time. (From Bruce RA, Kusumi F, Hosmer D: Maximal oxygen intake and nomographic assessment of functional aerobic impairment in cardiovascular disease. *Am Heart J* 85:546-562, 1973. By permission of Mosby–Year Book.)

Table 3B-4 Naughton rehabilitation protocol[6]

Time, min	Speed, mph	Grade, %	METS
1	1	0	
2			1.6
3	2	0	
4			2.0
5	2	3.5	
6			3.0
7	2	7.0	
8			4.0
9	2	10.5	
10			5.0
11	2	14	
12			6.0

Table 3B-5 Equations* for predicting maximal aerobic capacity during treadmill testing[5]

Subject	$\dot{V}O_2$, mL/(kg · min)
Active men†	69.7 − (0.612 × age)
Sedentary men	57.8 − (0.445 × age)
Active women†	44.4 − (0.343 × age)
Sedentary women	41.2 − (0.343 × age)

*Age is in years.
†"Active" means frequent aerobic exercise or sufficient exertion at least once a week to cause perspiring.

Bicycle ergometry is a quantitative tool for accurately increasing workload relatively independent of body weight.[80a] Bicycle ergometers have increased in use in stress testing for nuclear imaging during gated radionuclide angiography because of the relative lack of motion of the chest. Protocols usually increase by 300 kilograms · meters per minute (kg · m/min) every 3 minutes. Maximal predicted aerobic capacity and kg · m/min can be predicted for a patient prior to testing. Studies have shown that upright and supine bicycle aerobic capacities are 94% and 84% of those measured for uphill running.[80b] Maximal predicted aerobic capacities are most accurate when corrected for age, sex, and training (Table 3B-5) and have been well documented for treadmill testing.[5] To calculate predicted maximal bicycle aerobic capacity, use the proper equation from Table 3B-5 and multiply $\dot{V}O_2$ by the patient's weight in kilograms and the correction factor 0.94 for upright or 0.84 for supine bicycle exercise. This will give the corrected ergometric maximal predicted aerobic capacity in mL O_2/min. To convert to kg · m/min, subtract 267 and divide by 2.11 (see Table 3B-2). For example, a healthy 60-year-old, 70-kg, active man has a predicted maximal aerobic capacity of 2,366 mL O_2/min. For supine bicycle exercise, multiplying by 0.84 gives 1,987 mL O_2/min. Subtracting 267 and dividing by 2.11 gives a predicted maximal kg · m/min load of 815. If the patient stops at 600 kg · m/min = 1,533 mL O_2/min (see Table 3B-2), 1,533/1,987 = 77% of maximal predicted capacity.

ECGs are usually taken in four conditions—sitting, supine, abrupt standing, and after hyperventilation—before exercise. This allows pretest assessment of the effect of changes in position and ventilation on ST-T waves and also interpretation of a baseline ECG. Patients are regularly asked whether they are experiencing any symptoms. Signs of fatigue, left ventricular dysfunction, and ischemia and lack of cerebral perfusion are carefully observed and recorded.

Indications for stopping the exercise

The indications for stopping an exercise test depend on the purpose of the test, the discretion of the physician, the maximal predicted heart rate and aerobic capacity, and the patient.

For patients with known ischemic heart disease, the purpose of stress testing is not to rediagnose the disease but to measure its threshold, the degree of impairment, the rapidity of recovery, and the response to treatment. The test provides an objective extension of the resting examination by documenting the threshold heart rate and the product of the heart rate times the systolic blood pressure (double product) at the onset of either angina or ST depression. Signs or symptoms of left ventricular dysfunction, such as excessive dyspnea, decrease in systolic blood pressure, cerebral hypoxia, and vasoconstricted or cool extremities, are important. Extending the test beyond any of these end points in a patient with obvious ischemic heart disease serves no good purpose and, in fact, may cause complications. Patients with myocardial infarction who are exercised within 14 days after the event should not be taken beyond 5 METS. A rapid rate of ST-segment depression with respect to heart rate, $\Delta ST/\Delta HR$, especially at low workloads (fewer than 4 METS; heart rate, <120 beats/min; systolic blood pressure, <130 mm Hg), has been associated with severe three-vessel disease and is a good reason for stopping the test.

For the patient with atypical chest pain syndromes, the goal is to clarify, for both the patient and the physician, the patient's pathophysiologic limitations. To this end, symptoms (angina, excessive fatigue implying that the anaerobic threshold has been exceeded, or excessive dyspnea) or pathologic signs (flat ST depression of 1 mm or more at 80 msec beyond the J point, arrhythmia, or decreasing systolic pressure) are needed for the proper diagnosis of ischemia. As long as signs and symptoms remain stable, the patient is encouraged to continue to exercise until a symptom- or sign-limited end point is achieved or until the normal end point of 100% or more of predicted aerobic capacity is reached. Some protocols use 3 minutes at 85% or more of maximal age-predicted heart rate as a normal end point. However, the heart rate criteria are based on data showing a standard deviation of ±17 beats/min; hence, 95% confidence limits include a wide range—±34 beats/min. In addition, β-blocking drugs, deconditioning, obesity, hypovolemia, temperature, certain calcium-blocking agents, and digitalis all affect heart rate response to exercise directly or indirectly.

For patients with valvular disease, the purpose is to measure safely the aerobic capacity at which signs and symptoms of cardiac dysfunction appear. This allows both a NYHA classification and a quantitative assessment of aerobic impairment, both of which are relevant to understanding the patient's absolute and relative functional impairment. The common fallacy is to determine only the NYHA classification, which is independent of age, sex, and training. For example, a trained 25-year-old man with a bicuspid aortic valve and aortic valve insufficiency who must stop at 6 minutes on the Bruce protocol because of excessive dyspnea and fatigue is class I (more than 6 METS before symptoms) by NYHA criteria. In fact, he has a 50% aerobic impairment in comparison with his normal trained male peer group of the same age. Although this patient may be asymptomatic with normal activity by comparison with standards for older persons (up to 6 METS), he is actually very much impaired by his aortic valve insufficiency.

To determine "level of fitness" for a healthy asymptomatic patient or a marathon runner, a maximal symptom-limited test, preferably with a plateauing of the oxygen consumption as the workload increases, defines the maximal aerobic capacity. Stopping short of this plateau because of fatigue prevents a precise determination of maximal aerobic capacity but is adequate to determine that patient's symptom- or sign-limited end point.

CLINICAL APPLICATIONS

Indications

Persons in NYHA classes I to III are, by definition, asymptomatic at rest. In these patients, use of exercise-intervention provides an opportunity to observe physiologic and ECG parameters that are not apparent in the resting state. The symptom- or sign-limited test is useful in providing clinical data for decision making.

The Subcommittee on Exercise Testing of the American College of Cardiology/American Heart Association Task Force on Assessment of Cardiovascular Procedures published guidelines for exercise testing.[62] These guidelines grade the appropriateness and usefulness of performing exercise testing in a variety of clinical situations. Exercise testing is generally indicated (1) to aid in the diagnosis in patients with suspected coronary artery disease; (2) to help assess disease severity and prognosis in patients with known coronary artery disease, both during stable disease and soon after uncomplicated myocardial infarction; (3) to determine the success of coronary artery revascularization by angioplasty or surgery; and (4) to evaluate patients with symptoms suggestive of exercise-induced arrhythmias. Situations in which exercise testing is commonly performed but in which its usefulness is controversial: (1) to follow serially patients with known coronary artery disease, (2) to evaluate the response to medical therapy in patients with angina or heart failure, (3) to screen selected asymptomatic subjects for coronary artery disease, (4) to determine functional capacity in selected patients with valvular heart disease, (5) to evaluate patients with coronary artery spasm, and (6) to evaluate the blood pressure response during exercise in physically active patients with treated hypertension.

Contraindications

Absolute contraindications. The class IV patient with ischemic heart disease who has angina of effort and angina decubitus is at high risk of incapacitation and of myocardial infarction during exercise testing. Patients with unstable illnesses such as endocarditis, acute infarction, serious ventricular dysrhythmias, pulmonary emboli, pericarditis, and myocarditis should not be exercised.

Relative contraindications. Orthopedic and neurologic limitations may make exercise testing hazardous. The cardiovascular system may not be adequately challenged under these circumstances.

Psychologic unsuitability for testing may exist in patients who have considerable anxiety due to psychosomatic or psychotic disorders.

Symptomatic adults with high-grade aortic valve stenosis are at risk during exercise testing because of the potential for syncope or ventricular ectopic activity. The resuscitation potential for these incapacitated patients is small.

Effort-induced bradycardia or tachycardia does not preclude exercise testing and may be the only means of documenting the arrhythmia. However, such patients require special preparation in the laboratory and the presence of adequate personnel to provide for any resuscitative effort that may be required.

STATISTICAL CONSIDERATIONS IN THE DIAGNOSIS OF ISCHEMIC HEART DISEASE

Sensitivity in relation to the diagnosis of coronary artery disease is defined as the percent of adequately stressed patients with coronary artery disease who have a positive test. Coronary artery disease is usually defined as a lesion obstructing more than 70% of the diameter of at least one major coronary artery. An adequate stress is one that produces an increase in myocardial oxygen demand that results in signs or symptoms of decreased myocardial oxygen supply. This usually implies that the double product (heart rate × systolic blood pressure) be more than 24,000 or that objective signs or symptoms of ischemia require termination of the testing. A positive test has been defined as a flat ST depression of 1 mm or more at 80 msec beyond the J point.

It must be remembered that we are using a functional test to predict anatomic coronary obstruction, with coronary arteriography being used as the standard. The ST segment alone is only one indicator of myocardial ischemia. The presence of a large amount of ischemic muscle due to multivessel disease, a lack of collaterals, a high level of stress, and the use of multiple leads have all

Table 3B-6 Noncoronary causes of ST-segment depression

Ischemic
Increased impedance due to
Aortic stenosis
Muscular obstruction as in hypertrophic cardiomyopathy
Hypertension
Increased wall stress due to left ventricular dilatation, including
Volume overload states of aortic insufficiency
Mitral insufficiency
Left-to-right shunts
Arteriovenous fistulas
Decreased oxygen supply, as in
Anemia
Abnormal oxygen-binding affinity of hemoglobin, e.g., hemoglobin Malmö, left shift of oxygen-hemoglobin dissociation curve
Competitive binding to hemoglobin of nonoxygen compounds such as carbon monoxide
Low-output states, such as mitral stenosis
Desaturation of hemoglobin due to chronic obstructive pulmonary disease, right-to-left shunts
Membrane repolarization abnormalities due to
Digitalis
Glucose-potassium shifts after meals
Hypokalemia and electrolyte disorders
Toxic states and drugs, including diazepam
Hyperadrenergic syndrome
Abnormal depolarization with left bundle-branch block, pacemaker, right bundle-branch block, preexcitation
Cardiomyopathies
Left ventricular hypertrophy
Hyperventilation
Idiopathic mechanisms— mitral prolapse
Miscellaneous—artifact from inadequate recording equipment

been shown to increase sensitivity. But, in any case, experienced physicians do not depend solely on a change in the ST segment to diagnose ischemic heart disease. They use the combination of pretest risk factors (including history of angina, age, and sex), rate of ST change, associated angina during stress, rate of ST-segment normalization, septal Q-wave evolution, R-wave progression, T-wave changes, ventricular ectopy, and aerobic capacity to decide whether the test is positive for ischemia.

From a diagnostic viewpoint, *specificity* in coronary artery disease is defined as the percentage of patients with normal coronary arteries who have a negative test. Normal coronary arteries are usually defined as having stenosis of less than 70% of the diameter. A negative test is defined as ST depression of less than 1 mm at 80 msec beyond the J point with adequate stress. However, multivessel lesions, each lesion involving 50% of the diameter, could cause mild myocardial ischemia at high workloads. The correlation between coronary flow reserve and percentage of diameter stenosis is low, particularly in lesions with a moderate degree (30% to 70% diameter narrowing) of stenosis.[81] Changes in the ST-T wave are not limited to coronary disease but can occur in numerous other situations that must be considered by the physician (Table 3B-6). Normal women are known to have more ST-segment depression in the inferior leads than normal men. Morales-Ballejo and colleagues[46] showed that many of these "false-positive" tests can be properly classified if the normal evolution of the septal force is observed. Absence of the Q wave in lead CM_5 with ST depression after exercise identified a true-positive ST-segment response to stress in 100% of patients in their series; however, an *increase* in Q-wave amplitude with exercise identified a false-positive ST-segment response in 75% of their cases. Right bundle-branch block may cause slightly increased changes in the ST-T wave. Digitalis will certainly cause ST-T changes that mimic those in ischemia (see Figs 3B-15 and 3B-16).

The most useful concept for interpreting the meaning of a "positive" or "negative" test as defined above is the predictive value of the test. The predictive value of a positive test is the percentage of patients with a positive test who *do* have "significant" coronary artery disease. The predictive value of a negative test is the percentage of patients with a negative test who *do not* have "significant" coronary artery disease.

The predictive value of a test depends on the prevalence of the disease in the population studied. Useful prevalence data based on historical symptoms of typical angina, atypical angina, and noncardiac chest pain[82] and asymptomatic patients[4,83] of a given age and sex are available (Tables 3B-7 and 3B-8). Compare a positive test in a population of 30-year-old asymptomatic men with that in a population of 45-year-old men with typical angina by using the same sensitivity of 70% and specificity of 90% (see Table 3B-7). Note that a positive test in an asymptomatic population has a predictive value of only 27%, whereas a positive test in the 45-year-old male population with typical angina has a predictive value of 98%. The post-test probabilities in Tables 3B-7 and 3B-8 are based on the Bayes theorem:

post-test odds of disease with positive ST-segment response =

$$\text{pretest odds} \times \frac{\text{\% of patients with disease with abnormal test}}{\text{\% of patients without disease with abnormal test}}$$

or

$$\text{pretest odds of disease} \times \frac{\text{sensitivity}}{1 - \text{specificity}}$$

A low prevalence of disease increases the proportion of false-positive tests in spite of identical testing procedures, equipment, sensitivity, specificity, and physicians and therefore decreases the predictive value of a positive test.

For a negative ST-segment response:

post-test odds of *no* coronary artery disease = pretest odds of

$$\textit{no}\ \text{disease} \times \frac{\text{\% without disease with normal test}}{\text{\% with disease with normal test}}$$

or

$$\text{pretest odds of } \textit{no} \text{ disease} \times \frac{\text{specificity}}{1 - \text{sensitivity}}$$

Table 3B-7 Coronary artery disease prevalence in men with stable chest pain and no history of myocardial infarction and post-test risk of disease by Bayesian analysis

Age, yr	No.	% With one or more vessels with >70% lesion or left main stenosis ≥50%[82]	Calculated predictive value, %	
			Positive ST change*	Normal ST
Definite angina				
30-39	66	83	97	38
40-49	402	88	98	29
50-59	840	94	99	16
60-69	539	95	99	14
≥70	67	97	99	8
Total	1,914			
Probable angina				
30-39	171	46	86	78
40-49	568	57	90	69
50-59	919	71	94	55
60-69	434	78	96	46
≥70	46	94	99	16
Total	2,138			
Nonspecific chest pain				
<30	51	0	0	100
30-39	249	3.2	19	99
40-49	391	12	49	96
50-59	440	18	60	93
60-69	129	27	72	89
≥70	22	63	92	64
Total	1,282			
Asymptomatic				
≤40		5	27(26)†[4]	98
>40	105[83]	15	55(63)†[83]	94

*Assumes 70% sensitivity, 90% specificity for 1-mm flat ST depression at 80 msec beyond the J point.
†Numbers in parentheses are reported values.

Table 3B-9 shows applications to population subsets. A high prevalence of disease increases the proportion of false-negative results and diminishes the predictive value of a negative test. Thus, a negative test in a 45-year-old man with typical angina by history has a predictive value of only 29%, but a negative test in a 30-year-old asymptomatic man has a predictive value of 98%.

This Bayesian approach to interpretation of the results of stress testing has the advantage of considering pretest odds of disease, including age, sex, symptoms, and risk factors, and combining these with multiple signs and symptoms during the stress test to calculate the post-test odds of disease. Such a program is commercially available[84] and has been used extensively by its originators at Cedars-Sinai Hospital in Los Angeles. The analysis can be applied to serial types of testing but assumes that all variables are mutually independent. This approach can be used in spite of unknown variables. For example, post-treadmill odds of disease can be calculated even if coronary calcification was not examined.

The downside risk of using Bayesian analysis is the assumption of universal values of sensitivity and specificity for a given ST change. ST change depends on voltage, is a continuous variable, and is only one of many exercise risk variables. Rozanski and associates[85] discussed the declining specificity of radionuclide ventriculography in terms of pretest referral bias and post-test referral bias, and these arguments also apply to treadmill testing. Pretest referral bias refers to the trend of exercising patients with a higher pretest risk of coronary artery disease. These patients are more likely to have a positive test result. Since there is a tendency to do coronary angiography because of positive test results (post-test referral bias) and not in patients with normal results, more patients with false-positive tests are identified from the treadmill population than patients with true-negative results. Specificity drops because of the decreasing ratio of true-negatives to false-positives in the population undergoing angiography. Diamond[86] described contributory factors affecting calculated sensitivity and specificity in various studies, and he[87] and others[88] successfully tested a correcting algorithm.

An alternative to the Bayesian analysis is multivariate analysis utilizing logistical regression-derived algorithms, and such a program has been derived by Greenberg and associates[89] at Memorial Hospital Medical Center, Long Beach, Calif. The variables for males and females are listed in Table 3B-10. Data concerning all variables are

Table 3B-8 Coronary artery disease prevalence in women with stable chest pain and no history of myocardial infarction and post-test risk of disease by Bayesian analysis

Age, yr	No.	% With one or more vessels with >70% lesion or left main stenosis ≥50%[82]	Predictive value, %: Positive ST change*	Predictive value, %: Normal ST
Definite angina				
30-39	10	70	85	50
40-49	70	56	75	65
50-59	161	68	83	52
60-69	137	81	91	35
≥70	23	96	99	9
Total	401			
Probable angina				
30-39	39	20	37	90
40-49	257	31	51	84
50-59	414	30	50	84
60-69	264	48	68	72
≥70	34	56	75	65
Total	1,008			
Nonspecific chest pain				
<30	14	0	0	100
30-39	135	4	9	98
40-49	425	4	9	98
50-59	585	6	13	97
60-69	215	10	21	95
≥70	23	0	†	†
Total	1,397			

*Assumes 70% sensitivity, 70% specificity for 1-mm flat ST depression at 80 msec beyond the J point.
†Because of small sample size, we recommend assuming that values for previous decade apply.

Table 3B-9 Bayes' theorem: clinical application to ST changes

Situation*	Pretest odds: CAD† $\frac{\rho}{100-\rho}$	Pretest odds: No CAD $\frac{100-\rho}{\rho}$	×	Odds of CAD based on sensitivity, specificity of ST change: Positive test	Odds of CAD based on sensitivity, specificity of ST change: Negative test	=	Post-test odds $\frac{a}{b}$	Predictive value, % $\frac{a}{a+b} \times 100$
Typical angina pectoris, 45-year-old man	$\frac{88}{12}$		×	$\frac{7}{1}$		=	$\frac{51}{1}$	$\frac{51}{52} = 98$
$\rho = 88\%$		$\frac{12}{88}$	×		$\frac{3}{1}$	=	$\frac{0.41}{1}$	$\frac{0.41}{1.41} = 29$
Atypical angina, 65-year-old woman	$\frac{48}{52}$		×	$\frac{2.33}{1}$		=	$\frac{2.2}{1}$	$\frac{2.2}{3.2} = 68$
$\rho = 48\%$		$\frac{52}{48}$	×		$\frac{2.33}{1}$	=	$\frac{2.5}{1}$	$\frac{2.5}{3.5} = 72$
Noncardiac chest pain, 65-year-old woman	$\frac{1}{9}$		×	$\frac{2.33}{1}$		=	$\frac{.26}{1}$	$\frac{.26}{1.26} = 21$
$\rho = 10\%$		$\frac{9}{1}$	×		$\frac{2.33}{1}$	=	$\frac{21}{1}$	$\frac{21}{22} = 95$
Asymptomatic, 30-year-old man	$\frac{1}{19}$		×	$\frac{7}{1}$		=	$\frac{7}{19}$	$\frac{7}{26} = 27$
$\rho = 5\%$		$\frac{19}{1}$	×		$\frac{3}{1}$	=	$\frac{57}{1}$	$\frac{57}{58} = 98$

*ρ is prevalence of CAD.
†CAD, greater than 70% stenosis in one or more coronary arteries.

Table 3B-10 Multivariate analysis variables

Males	Females
Test duration	ST depression at rest, mm
R-wave change, mm	Presence or absence of downsloping ST segment
Age	R-wave change, mm
% maximal heart rate achieved	Age
Maximal heart rate achieved	Use of estrogen (yes/no)
Presence or absence of abnormal ECG at rest	ST depression with exercise, mm
ST depression with exercise, mm	Test duration
Presence or absence of anginal pain during test	Presence or absence of angina during test

required to calculate a post-test probability of disease, but no assumption is made as to their mutual independence. Arbitrary cut points of post-test probability are selected to best distinguish normal subjects from patients with coronary disease. A comparison of a new multivariate logistical regression approach with the Cadenza analysis[84] has been accomplished, and both methods offer an advantage of quantitating many relevant clinical variables rather than having to rely on the single interpretation of any given parameter. The sensitivity and specificity of these approaches have been found to be comparable to or better than accepted results with the use of ST-segment analysis.[90]

The problems created by analysis of a single sign—the change in the ST segment—are being solved by use of a more holistic statistical perspective of many exercise signs and symptoms along with pretest risk and epidemiologic factors. The value of the test and its importance to the patient depend principally on the physician's interpretation, which should put the variables into a useful perspective for reduction of risk, safe conditioning, and reassurance for patients at low risk for disease. For patients who are at high risk, optimal education and treatment and frequent supportive follow-up can be emphasized. For those with intermediate risk, the variables of left ventricular function are very important in determining prognosis and should be most useful in directing follow-up and therapy.

It bears emphasizing that most patients with an obvious history of angina are not stress-tested for the purpose of a diagnosis of coronary artery disease but rather to determine prognosis and to provide a baseline measurement of functional status and severity of ischemia. The literature tends to confuse these purposes and reports a lack of significant change from pretest to post-test probability of disease. Medical management can be tailored to a given patient's response, and stress testing is often repeated to demonstrate efficacy of the management. If deterioration and left ventricular dysfunction are evident on sequential tests, coronary angiography and surgical consultation are then considered.

Erikssen et al.[83] have drawn attention to subsets of asymptomatic males who have a higher prevalence of coronary artery disease, about 15%, and a predictive value of significant coronary stenosis of 65% based on exercise testing (positive ST-segment change). This observation has been documented epidemiologically in men more than 40 years old, and there seems to be little change in this number as patients age. This finding is relevant when one considers that, of those men who are having their first symptom of coronary heart disease, 55% die suddenly or have myocardial infarction.[91]

PROGNOSIS

The proper interpretation of an exercise test includes an assessment of the prognosis for each patient. The Framingham Study showed that a "positive" stress test is the strongest risk factor in predicting future cardiac events.[92] It has become clear that the prognostic information from a patient's stress test is multivariate and that it should be synthesized from symptoms and signs of ischemia as well as from measurements of ventricular function. Age, sex, previous myocardial infarction, chronotropic response, pretest symptoms, and conventional risk factors are also statistically important clinical variables in the final synthesis.

Asymptomatic men

Bruce and colleagues[93] analyzed 2,365 healthy men (mean age, 45.5 years) in the Seattle Heart Watch for an average follow-up of 5 years. The annual incidence of primary coronary heart disease events (myocardial infarction, cardiac death, angina pectoris, saphenous vein bypass grafting) was 0.36%. Above age 55, the rate was significantly higher ($P < 0.05$). This analysis revealed that if one or more conventional risk factors were present and if any two exercise risk predictors were present, the risk of future primary coronary heart disease events was 33 times greater than in 99% of this population who had no risk factors. The risk factors were positive family history of cardiac death or infarct in a relative less than 70 years of age, blood pressure more than 140/90 mm Hg, cholesterol concentration more than 250 mg/dL, and cigarette smoking. The exercise risk predictors were exercise duration less than 6 minutes on the Bruce protocol, chest pain with maximal exercise, failure to achieve 90% of age-predicted maximal heart rate, and postexertional ST-segment depression of 1 mm or more for at least 1 minute if horizontal or downsloping or at least 3 minutes if upsloping.

This type of evaluation of an *asymptomatic* population clearly demonstrates the importance of a multivariate interpretation and minimizes the problem of interpreting false-positive ST depression in the absence of other risk factors. The average predictive value of a positive ST-segment change in four prospective studies that screened asymptomatic men was only 26%.[4] The exercise risk factors used were of limited predictive value but were powerful when they coexisted with the conventional risk factors.

Asymptomatic women

Asymptomatic women have a two to three times higher incidence of positive ST-segment changes than men do (24% to 35% in women compared with 12% in men).[94] Hence, the specificity of a 1-mm depression of the ST segment is much lower than in men. Careful multivariate analysis is needed for asymptomatic women. Allen and associates[95] showed that exercise for less than 3 minutes on the Ellestad protocol correlated highly with subsequent coronary events in 311 asymptomatic women, although ST-segment depression and R-wave response did not. In 30.8% of these women who exercised less than 3 minutes, a subsequent event occurred in the next 5 years. Exercise duration of less than 3 minutes is an indirect measure of left ventricular dysfunction and in this study had a prognostic sensitivity of only 40% but was highly specific (96.9% of women free of subsequent events exercised for more than 3 minutes). In the same study, in 577 men a positive ST-segment response, an increase or no change in R-wave voltage, and a duration of exercise of 5 minutes or less were highly correlated to subsequent events. In five patients, all three criteria were present and all five experienced subsequent events, for a predictive value of 100%.

Atypical chest pain

In patients with atypical chest pain, the diagnostic predictive value of a positive stress test is much greater than that in the asymptomatic population. In middle-aged men with atypical angina, the probability of coronary artery disease with a normal ST response to symptom-limited exercise is about 25%, but this increases to 88% if the ST-segment change is positive. Long-term follow-up studies specifically limited to atypical angina in men are difficult to find; however, the multivariate approach should be useful in considerations of data already collected for the asymptomatic and known coronary artery disease populations.

Known coronary heart disease

In patients with known coronary heart disease, the risk of secondary coronary events has been well studied. Bruce[96] found that the most frequent secondary event within the first 3 years was death (195 of 1,852 subjects). In the Seattle Heart Watch experience, 59% of these deaths were sudden. Neither age nor conventional risk factors were predictive of secondary events. Left ventricular dysfunction—as measured by cardiomegaly, duration of exercise less than 3 minutes, and peak systolic blood pressure less than 130 mm Hg—was the most important predictor of mortality. In the absence of these three factors of left ventricular dysfunction, the annual coronary heart disease mortality was 20 per 1,000. When one or more criteria were present, the annual rate increased dramatically, to a high of 884 per 1,000 when all three were present. A low annual mortality (21.6 per 1,000) occurred in the largest subgroup (42.5%) of men with coronary heart disease who had no exertional ischemic changes. The mortality was higher (53 per 1,000) in a small subgroup (16.9%) with ST-segment depression. This annual risk gradient, which was obtained noninvasively and at low risk and cost, was equivalent to that of invasive diagnostic (albeit resting) studies in patients followed for 5 years at the Cleveland Clinic.[97]

The presence of angina, lack of decrease of R-wave voltage, absence of increase in septal Q waves, early onset of ST-segment depression, flat ST-segment depression of more than 1 mm, and poor chronotropic response to exercise have all been shown to correlate with higher incidence of subsequent coronary heart disease events.[7] An interesting study on the rate of ST-segment depression with respect to heart rate showed a definite correlation with the number of vessels diseased.[98] Podrid et al.[99] disputed the inference that the magnitude of ST-segment depression alone (more than 2 mm) is a dangerous prognostic sign in a selected population referred with the diagnosis of myocardial ischemia. Certainly both left ventricular function and signs and symptoms of ischemia are needed for accurate prognostic assessment. In a review of the Coronary Artery Surgery Study (CASS) data, survival of 4,083 patients over 5 years was found to depend both on the magnitude of the ST change and on the final exercise stage.[100] Mark et al.[101] used the variables exercise duration and magnitude of ST-segment depression along with a treadmill angina index to calculate a treadmill exercise score. A low score identified patients at low risk of death.

Several studies in postinfarction patients have demonstrated the prognostic value of stress testing in the prediction of secondary events. Of note, patients referred for testing have considerably lower mortality than patients not referred for testing, which is attributable to clinical judgment in excluding high-risk patients from testing.[102] Bruce[103] reported a decreased prevalence of ST-segment changes, especially in anterior infarction. Ellestad[7] showed that a positive ST-segment change alone after an infarction is associated with a 91% likelihood of having progression of angina, infarction, or death over the subsequent 5 years, compared with 34% in those without previous infarction. Even a negative ST-segment result after infarction was associated with an 80% likelihood of subsequent events. Early postinfarct studies[104-108] with ST depression of 1 mm or more gave an average risk of 36% for subsequent events and 16% for cardiac death in patients with 11 to 21 months of follow-up. A negative ST result was associated with a risk of subsequent coronary events of 16% and of death of 4%. Angina, premature ventricular complexes, and ventricular function were not included in this analysis. Although patients with ST depression have traditionally been considered to be at higher risk,[62] a meta-analysis by Klein et al.[109] of 24 studies performed before 1986 determined that ST-segment depression did not predict outcome. Exercise systolic blood pressure and exercise duration were significant predictors.[102] The failure of ST-segment depression to consistently predict increased risk has been attributed to differences in the baseline ECG. ST-segment depression has considerable predictive power in patients with non-Q-wave myocardial infarcts but minimal value in patients with Q-wave myocardial infarction.[109]

The prognostic value of exercise testing in patients who have received thrombolytic therapy remains to be determined. It is likely that the predictive value will be very low, because the prevalence of multivessel disease is low and the prognosis generally favorable in these patients. In the Thrombolysis in Myocardial Infarction II study, only 30% of patients had two- or three-vessel coronary artery disease (compared with 70% to 80% in studies from the prethrombolytic era), and the combined death and nonfatal reinfarction rate after hospital dismissal at 1 year was 7%.[110]

Data from CASS on 4,083 patients who underwent exercise testing and coronary and left ventricular angiography were analyzed. Significant independent predictors of mortality were the clinical congestive heart failure score (treadmill time < 3 minutes on Bruce protocol, S_3 gallop, cardiomegaly) and peak heart rate in single-vessel disease, the congestive heart failure score in patients with two-vessel disease, and the final exercise stage in patients with three-vessel disease.[100] This again emphasized the necessity of considering left ventricular function to provide optimal prognostic conclusions from stress testing.

Exercise testing can be useful in patients with coronary artery disease not only for its ability to help determine prognosis in patients treated medically but also for its ability to identify patients whose survival is improved by revascularization, even among patients with similar coronary anatomy. Weiner and colleagues[111] compared the results of surgical therapy with those of medical therapy in 1,249 nonrandomized patients in the CASS registry who had three-vessel disease and had undergone exercise testing. In patients with preserved left ventricular function, those with ≥1 mm ST-segment depression or exercise capacity ≤ stage II Bruce protocol had improved survival with surgical treatment. Among patients with impaired left ventricular function, surgery was associated with improved survival in most subsets except those with exercise tolerance ≥ stage III Bruce protocol, especially when combined with the absence of ST-segment depression. Exercise testing may play a role in clinical decision-making even when the two most important prognostic indicators, left ventricular function and anatomic extent of disease, are known. In a different randomized CASS subset of patients,[112] most of whom had three-vessel disease and impaired left ventricular function, the presence of exercise-induced angina identified patients who had a survival advantage if assigned to surgery, but ST segment change or exercise stage failed to show any difference in 7-year survival.

EXERCISE TESTING IN THE EVALUATION OF THE APPARENTLY HEALTHY PATIENT

The role of exercise testing in screening healthy populations for the detection of occult coronary artery disease is controversial. It is generally agreed that there is little need for exercise testing for this purpose in patients under the age of 40. There may be a place for screening men over the age of 40 who meet one of these criteria: (1) special occupations, such as airline pilot; (2) two or more risk factors for coronary artery disease; and (3) sedentary lifestyle with plans to enter a vigorous exercise program.[62] Concerning the third indication, a study from the Lipid Research Clinics Coronary Primary Prevention Trial showed that a positive exercise test result was associated with an increased risk of acute cardiac events during physical activity; nonetheless, the usefulness of the test for this purpose was limited because of low test sensitivity (only 37%).[113]

Errors previously have been made in the diagnosis of coronary artery disease on the basis of a positive ST-segment change alone. The prevalence of disease in the asymptomatic population is low, ranging from less than 5% up to 15%, depending on age and presence of other risk factors. A multivariate approach has a higher predictive value than a change in the ST segment alone. Table 3B-7 demonstrates that in the asymptomatic group, a positive change in the ST segment gives a predictive value of coronary artery disease of only 27%. This means that 73% of patients with a positive change in the ST segment (1 mm or more) would have no coronary artery disease. These figures are based on outcome in patients in studies that included the development of angina as an end point. In studies with outcome limited to the "harder" cardiac events of death and myocardial infarction, the positive predictive value of an abnormal test result is only 5%.[102] Most persons with positive test results who have undergone further evaluation, either thallium imaging[114] or coronary angiography,[115] have been shown to have normal studies. The wise physician would consider the low predictive value of the ST change alone and incorporate into the decision-making process conventional risk factors and the other symptoms and signs occurring during the patient's stress test. These should include functional aerobic capacity, chest pain, dyspnea, change in septal force, R wave, blood pressure response, cardiac risk factors, heart rate response, age, sex, and nonischemic causes of ST changes. Attempts to computerize this synthesis of variables may offer a precise predictive value.[90,116]

As mentioned, Bruce et al.[93] have shown that a positive exercise ECG by itself fails to identify subjects who subsequently suffer coronary events but can predict increased risk when associated with clinical risk factors and other abnormalities during exercise testing. Epstein and colleagues[117] pointed out that because of limitations with sensitivity and specificity of exercise testing, there is a "double irony" in screening the asymptomatic population: the large majority (95%) of the population with negative test results still contains the largest number of subjects destined to die suddenly (estimated annual mortality, 0.06%), whereas the mortality is higher but still low (estimated to be 0.72% per year) in the group with positive test results who in fact do have coronary disease (50% of those with positive results). Furthermore, screening large numbers of people can be expensive, and the question of cost-effectiveness has been raised. Sox et al.[118] estimated that screening 60-year-old men at average risk would increase their life expectancy only 12 days, with even less benefit for screening women and younger men.

Routine exercise testing of the general population

cannot be recommended for the purpose of detecting occult coronary artery disease. Nonetheless, exercise testing continues to be commonly performed in the asymptomatic population, probably for a number of reasons. Occasionally, an entirely asymptomatic patient is detected who has severe coronary artery disease. Although this discovery occurs infrequently, the identification of these patients certainly impresses the clinicians involved in their care. Secondly, large companies who require that their employees undergo exercise testing as part of an executive health examination may consider the procedure to be worthwhile in view of their extensive financial investment in these persons. Even though the yield of testing is small, coronary artery disease remains the main cause of mortality in our society, and there clearly are limitations to history-taking and physical examination alone for disease detection. Thirdly, patients occasionally specifically request to undergo treadmill testing, even after a discussion of recommended guidelines and reassurance about the low likelihood of disease based on their clinical profile. A negative treadmill test result provides further reassurance for these individuals.

Previous reports have emphasized the excellent prognosis in patients with good functional aerobic capacity without angina, regardless of ST-segment changes.[119] It seems proper not to alarm an asymptomatic patient about an ST-segment change alone if the test reveals 100% of predicted aerobic capacity without angina. Instead, one repeats the test in 1 year, or sooner if the patient experiences any symptoms of cardiac disease. The patient should be offered a frank discussion of the statistical considerations and of modifiable cardiac risk factors.

COMPLICATIONS RESULTING FROM EXERCISE TESTING

At least three broad surveys have studied complications related to exercise testing and have provided encouraging data showing a halving in mortality rate during the past decade. This decline has occurred in spite of greater utilization of testing by a growing and diverse group of clinicians and physiologists. The good safety record has improved even with the greater use of symptom-limited testing. In a survey of 170,000 exercise tests performed in 73 medical institutions,[120] mortality was 1 per 10,000 and morbidity 3 per 10,000. In another review[121] of 518,448 exercise tests, mortality was 0.5 per 10,000 tests and morbidity 8.35. Despite more symptom-limited and, therefore, more maximal testing, there was no greater mortality but a slight increase in morbidity.[122]

Starling et al.[107] found that early testing of 130 patients with uncomplicated myocardial infarction was safe and without complications in their test group being evaluated a mean of 15 days after their coronary event. Even earlier testing may be safe and useful in carefully selected patients after aggressive treatment. In a small study of 53 patients without complications given reperfusion (thrombolysis or angioplasty) therapy, exercise testing performed 3 days after the onset of myocardial infarction was not associated with any significant complications and, in combination with thallium imaging, identified patients at risk for in-hospital complications.[123] Rod et al.[124] demonstrated that symptom-limited graded exercise testing can be carried out soon after surgical myocardial revascularization without complications. They tested 86 consecutive ambulatory male patients without complications 11.1 ± 2.6 days after operation and found the procedure to be safe.

Complications of exercise testing may be categorized into minor (producing transient or no incapacitation) and major (producing incapacitation or death) (Table 3B-11).

Table 3B-11 Complications of exercise testing

Minor complications
Supraventricular tachycardia
Chronotropic incompetence
Inotropic incompetence
Excessive chronotropic response
Excessive inotropic response
Ventricular ectopic activity
Congestive heart failure
Focal or global cerebrovascular ischemia
Major complications
Supraventricular tachycardia
Ventricular tachycardia-fibrillation
Stroke
Myocardial infarction
Death

Minor complications

Supraventricular tachycardias, such as atrial fibrillation, atrial flutter, and AV nodal reentrant tachycardias, may be transient or persistent, and they produce minor incapacitation. However, electroversion or other interventions, such as intravenous verapamil, may be required. Exercise-induced and catecholamine-dependent tachycardias that utilize an accessory pathway are usually brief, not incapacitating, and self-limiting.

Chronotropic incompetence is indicated by an inadequate or absent heart rate response to an increasing workload during exercise. This failure in heart rate response may be due to sinus node dysfunction or to drug therapy such as β-adrenergic blockade. It could be caused by second-degree AV block. Exercise-induced type I (Wenckebach) second-degree AV block is rare and is usually asymptomatic. Exercise-induced type II second-degree block is more common and may become degraded to third-degree block. These responses are ordinarily symptomatic but transient; they are corrected by rest, which reduces the atrial rate and allows the AV node a longer recovery time and thereby restores normal conduction.

Inotropic incompetence is usually due to left ventricular dysfunction, which has ominous implications. It is suspected during exercise testing by a failure of the systolic blood pressure to increase with increasing workloads. This plateau blood pressure response during graded exercise testing (failure of systolic blood pressure to increase and the diastolic pressure to decrease, or widening of the pulse pressure) may be followed by a decrease in mean blood pressure and syncope. During exercise, as the skeletal muscle imposes increasing demands for cardiac output, the ischemic myocardium is unable to keep pace with these demands, and so a relative decrease in cardiac output results. This leads to hypotension, a further decrease in coronary perfusion, and acidosis, and this vicious circle is conducive to the occurrence of complications. Such a hypotensive response to exercise is aggravated by depletion of intravascular volume.

Exercise-induced hypotension has been shown to correlate with both severe angiographic disease[13] and poor prognosis,[15] especially when defined as a decrease in systolic blood pressure during exercise below the standing preexercise value. Occasionally, normal persons have a decrease in systolic blood pressure at or near peak exercise without any associated adverse consequences. Additionally, 15% to 20% of patients experience a decrease ≥ 10 mm Hg during symptom-limited postinfarction tests. When this finding occurs as an isolated variable without other evidence for exercise-induced ischemia, it resolves in most patients during future testing and is not associated with an adverse prognosis.[62]

Excessive chronotropic responses are usually seen in patients who are severely deconditioned, have a markedly diminished stroke volume as a result of left ventricular dysfunction, or have vasoregulatory asthenia (hyper-β-adrenergic syndrome). These patients suffer premature incapacitation with exercise but experience no permanent disability.

Excessive inotropic responses to exercise are ordinarily seen in patients with systemic hypertension during the resting state. Laboratories have arbitrarily imposed systolic blood pressure limits beyond which they will terminate the test. These limits are prudent but are not based on scientific analysis. If the blood pressure rises above 250 mm Hg, the clinician should consider terminating the test.

Ventricular ectopic activity often complicates exercise testing. When it is present in control tracings and consists of a complex type, such as bigeminy or pairs of ventricular premature beats, one may elect to avoid exercising the patient. If ventricular ectopy of a complex type occurs with exercise, the test should be terminated. The most troublesome reactions may occur in the postexercise period and consist of complex ectopy (bigeminy, ventricular premature complexes in pairs or triplets), frank ventricular tachycardia, or ventricular fibrillation. These complications of exercise testing will occur most often in patients who have ischemic heart disease, but they are not unknown in apparently healthy persons with normal coronary arteriograms. Exercise-induced syncope in otherwise healthy persons should raise the consideration of effort-induced ventricular tachycardia, and the subjects should be studied in a controlled situation.

Congestive heart failure on a small scale is possibly induced in all patients who experience angina during exercise testing. It is known that in patients with ischemic disease, exercise causes an increase in left ventricular end-diastolic pressure, a loss of ventricular compliance, an increase in filling pressure, and an increase in pulmonary wedge pressure; this response may be considered to be a minor degree of left ventricular failure. It is not difficult to conceive that, if this sequence of events were sustained, it would provoke overt left ventricular failure and congestive heart failure. This complication is ordinarily managed by a reduction in the intravascular volume.

Focal or global cerebrovascular ischemia during exercise occurs from failure of the systemic output to increase adequately in a patient with an already compromised cerebral vasculature. It does not occur in patients with normal cerebral circulation.

Major complications

Supraventricular tachycardias produce incapacitation in the patient who has severe left ventricular dysfunction or valvular heart disease that requires an enhanced ventricular filling pressure or a long diastolic filling period, as in mitral valve stenosis. Ventricular tachycardia-flutter-fibrillation that is sustained will occur in approximately 1 in 5,000 exercise tests (0.02%) and is 50 times greater in populations in which the systolic blood pressure fails to increase. The ventricular rate, age of the patient, and degree of cardiac incapacitation determine the outcome of such an event. This complication will ordinarily advance a patient who is in NYHA class I to class II, a class II patient to class III, and a class IV patient to death. Time and intravenous lidocaine or electroversion will resolve the problem. Electromechanical dissociation may occur, and that is the ultimate complication.

Stroke induced by exercise is rare and will remain so if individuals responsible for monitoring patients during testing pay attention to the blood pressure responses and to symptoms of cerebrovascular insufficiency. Patients with known cerebrovascular insufficiency may be exercised only to a level commonly tolerated in their everyday lives. An appreciation of retinal artery pressure or oculoplethysmography studies will help identify persons who might suffer focal or global cerebral ischemia during testing, especially if their systemic blood pressure fails to increase with exercise. Any patient with recent transient cerebral ischemic attacks should not be exercised.

Myocardial infarction occurs randomly in the population being tested, since the patient's presence in the exercise laboratory does not confer any immunity from such a coronary event. Two precautions should reduce the likelihood of an infarction: (1) The patient should be questioned about the anginal history during the interval since the initial history and physical examination were carried out. Does angina occur more readily, and especially has there been any rest angina in the days or hours leading up to the test? Unstable angina has been a marker for impending myocardial infarction, and exercise in such a patient could precipitate the infarction. (2) Careful review of the control tracings may reveal new repolarization abnormalities compared with earlier resting ECGs. This finding could suggest that a subendocardial myocardial infarction had occurred in the recent past, and this would be a setting in which exercise could precipitate a transmural event.

REFERENCES

1. Rerych SK, Scholz PM, Sabiston DC Jr, et al: Effects of exercise training on left ventricular function in normal subjects: a longitudinal study by radionuclide angiography. *Am J Cardiol* 45:244-252, 1980
2. Guyton AC: *Textbook of Medical Physiology.* Sixth edition. Philadelphia, WB Saunders Company, 1981, pp 158-161
3. Donald DE, Milburn SE, Shepherd JT: Effect of cardiac denervation on the maximal capacity for exercise in the racing greyhound. *J Appl Physiol* 19:849-852, 1964
4. Koppes G, McKiernan T, Bassan M, et al: Treadmill exercise testing. Parts I and II. *Curr Probl Cardiol* 2:1-44, November; 1-45, December 1977
5. Bruce RA, Kusumi F, Hosmer D: Maximal oxygen intake and nomographic assessment of functional aerobic impairment in cardiovascular disease. *Am Heart J* 85:546-562, 1973
6. Naughton J, Haider R: Methods of exercise testing. In *Exercise Testing and Exercise Training in Coronary Heart Disease.* Edited by J Naughton, HK Hellerstein. New York, Academic Press, 1973, pp 79-91
7. Ellestad MH: *Stress Testing: Principles and Practice.* Third edition. Philadelphia, FA Davis Company, 1986, pp 107; 316-325
8. Balke B, Ware RW: An experimental study of "physical fitness" of Air Force personnel. *US Armed Forces Med J* 10:675-688, 1959
9. Pollock ML, Bohannon RL, Cooper KH, et al: A comparative analysis of four protocols for maximal treadmill stress testing. *Am Heart J* 92:39-46, 1976
10. Litchfield RL, Kerber RE, Benge JW, et al: Normal exercise capacity in patients with severe left ventricular dysfunction: compensatory mechanisms. *Circulation* 66:129-134, 1982
11. Packer M: Abnormalities of diastolic function as a potential cause of exercise intolerance in chronic heart failure. *Circulation* 81 Suppl 3:78-86, 1990
12. Weber KT, Janicki JS (eds): *CardioPulmonary Exercise Testing: Physiologic Principles and Clinical Applications.* Philadelphia, WB Saunders Company, 1986
13. Gibbons RJ, Hu DC, Clements IP, et al: Anatomic and functional significance of a hypotensive response during supine exercise radionuclide ventriculography. *Am J Cardiol* 60:1-4, 1987
14. Hammermeister KE, DeRouen TA, Dodge HT, et al: Prognostic and predictive value of exertional hypotension in suspected coronary heart disease. *Am J Cardiol* 51:1261-1266, 1983
15. Dubach P, Froelicher VF, Klein J, et al: Exercise-induced hypotension in a male population: criteria, causes, and prognosis. *Circulation* 78:1380-1387, 1988
16. Irving JB, Bruce RA: Exertional hypotension and postexertional ventricular fibrillation in stress testing. *Am J Cardiol* 39:849-851, 1977
17. Watson G, Mechling E, Ewy GA: Clinical significance of early vs late hypotensive blood pressure response to treadmill exercise. *Arch Intern Med* 152:1005-1008, 1992
18. Amon KW, Richards KL, Crawford MH: Usefulness of the postexercise response of systolic blood pressure in the diagnosis of coronary artery disease. *Circulation* 70:951-956, 1984
19. Sheps DS, Ernst JC, Briese FW, et al: Exercise-induced increase in diastolic pressure: indicator of severe coronary artery disease. *Am J Cardiol* 43:708-712, 1979
20. Einthoven W: Weiteres über das Elektrokardiogramm. *Arch Gesamte Physiol* 122:517-584, 1908
21. Philbrick JT, Horwitz RI, Feinstein AR: Methodologic problems of exercise testing for coronary artery disease: groups, analysis and bias. *Am J Cardiol* 46:807-812, 1980
22. Gianrossi R, Detrano R, Mulvihill D, et al: Exercise-induced ST depression in the diagnosis of coronary artery disease: a meta-analysis. *Circulation* 80:87-98, 1989
23. Detrano R, Gianrossi R, Mulvihill D, et al: Exercise-induced ST segment depression in the diagnosis of multivessel coronary disease: a meta analysis. *J Am Coll Cardiol* 14:1501-1508, 1989
24. Wilson RF, Marcus ML, Christensen BV, et al: Accuracy of exercise electrocardiography in detecting physiologically significant coronary arterial lesions. *Circulation* 83:412-421, 1991
25. Epstein SE, Cannon RO III, Bonow RO: Exercise testing in patients with microvascular angina. *Circulation* 83 Suppl 3:73-76, 1991
26. Nosratian FJ, Froelicher VF: ST elevation during exercise testing. *Am J Cardiol* 63:986-988, 1989
27. Rifkin RD, Hood WB Jr: Bayesian analysis of electrocardiographic exercise stress testing. *N Engl J Med* 297:681-686, 1977
28. Diamond GA, Forrester JS: Analysis of probability as an aid in the clinical diagnosis of coronary-artery disease. *N Engl J Med* 300:1350-1358, 1979
29. Hlatky M, Botvinick E, Brundage B: Diagnostic accuracy of cardiologists compared with probability calculations using Bayes' rule. *Am J Cardiol* 49:1927-1931, 1982
30. Greenberg PS, Bible M, Ellestad MH: Prospective application of the multivariate approach to enhance the accuracy of the treadmill stress test. *J Electrocardiol* 15:143-147, 1982
31. Mark DB, Hlatky MA, Lee KL, et al: Localizing coronary artery obstructions with the exercise treadmill test. *Ann Intern Med* 106:53-55, 1987
32. Bruce RA, Fisher LD, Pettinger M, et al: ST segment elevation with exercise: a marker for poor ventricular function and poor prognosis: Coronary Artery Surgery Study (CASS) confirmation of Seattle Heart Watch results. *Circulation* 77:897-905, 1988
33. Bardsley WT, Mankin HT, Zimmerman I: A lead in the right direction – the maximal depolarization vector in stress testing. Presented at the Aerospace Medical Association Scientific Program, Las Vegas, Nevada, May 9-12, 1977. Program preprints, pp 4-5
34. Lachterman B, Lehmann KG, Abrahamson D, et al: "Recovery only" ST-segment depression and the predictive accuracy of the exercise test. *Ann Intern Med* 112:11-16, 1990
35. Ellestad MH, Thomas L, Ong R, et al: The predictive value of the time course of ST segment depression during exercise testing in patients referred for coronary angiograms. *Am Heart J* 123:904-908, 1992
36. Vatterott PJ, Hanley PC, Mankin HT, et al: The divergent recovery of ST-segment depression and radionuclide angiographic indicators of myocardial ischemia. *Am J Cardiol* 66:296-301, 1990
37. Miranda CP, Lehmann KG, Froelicher VF: Correlation between resting ST segment depression, exercise testing, coronary angiography, and long-term prognosis. *Am Heart J* 122:1617-1628, 1991
38. Wangsnes KM, Gibbons RJ: Optimal interpretation of the supine exercise electrocardiogram in patients with right bundle branch block. *Chest* 98:1379-1382, 1990
39. Elamin MS, Boyle R, Kardash MM, et al: Accurate detection of coronary heart disease by new exercise test. *Br Heart J* 48:311-320, 1982
40. Kligfield P, Ameisen O, Okin PM: Heart rate adjustment of ST segment depression for improved detection of coronary artery disease. *Circulation* 79:245-255, 1989
41. Okin PM, Kligfield P, Ameisen O, et al: Identification of anatomically extensive coronary artery disease by the exercise ECG ST segment/heart rate slope. *Am Heart J* 115:1002-1013, 1988
42. Okin PM, Anderson KM, Levy D, et al: Heart rate adjustment of exercise-induced ST segment depression: improved risk stratification in the Framingham offspring study. *Circulation* 83:866-874, 1991
43. Bobbio M, Detrano R: A lesson from the controversy about heart rate adjustment of ST segment depression. *Circulation* 84:1410-1413, 1991
44. Lavie CJ, Oh JK, Mankin HT, et al: Significance of T-wave pseudonormalization during exercise: a radionuclide angiographic study. *Chest* 94:512-516, 1988
45. Gerson MC, Phillips JF, Morris SN, et al: Exercise-induced U-wave inversion as a marker of stenosis of the left anterior descending coronary artery. *Circulation* 60:1014-1020, 1979
46. Morales-Ballejo H, Greenberg PS, Ellestad MH, et al: Septal Q wave in exercise testing: angiographic correlation. *Am J Cardiol* 48:247-251, 1981
47. Bonoris PE, Greenberg PS, Castellanet MJ, et al: Significance of changes in R wave amplitude during treadmill stress testing: angiographic correlation. *Am J Cardiol* 41:846-851, 1978
48. Brody DA: A theoretical analysis of intracavitary blood mass influence on the heart-lead relationship. *Circ Res* 4:731-738, 1956
49. Battler A, Froelicher V, Slutsky R, et al: Relationship of QRS amplitude changes during exercise to left ventricular function and volumes and the diagnosis of coronary artery disease. *Circulation* 60:1004-1013, 1979
50. Wolthuis RA, Froelicher VF, Hopkirk A, et al: Normal electrocardiographic waveform characteristics during treadmill exercise testing. *Circulation* 60:1028-1035, 1979
51. Christison GW, Bonoris PE, Greenberg PS, et al: Predicting coronary artery disease with treadmill stress testing: changes in R-wave amplitude compared with ST segment depression. *J Electrocardiol* 12:179-185, 1979

52. Wagner S, Cohn K, Selzer A: Unreliability of exercise-induced R wave changes as indexes of coronary artery disease. *Am J Cardiol* 44:1241-1246, 1979

53. Yiannikas J, Marcomichelakis J, Taggart P, et al: Analysis of exercise-induced changes in R wave amplitude in asymptomatic men with electrocardiographic ST-T changes at rest. *Am J Cardiol* 47:238-243, 1981

54. Boudoulas H, Dervenagas S, Lewis RP, et al: Adrenergic stimulation and R-wave magnitude. *J Cardiac Rehabil* 1:108-114, 1981

55. Hopkirk JAC, Uhl GS, Hickman JR Jr, et al: Limitation of exercise-induced R wave amplitude changes in detecting coronary artery disease in asymptomatic men. *J Am Coll Cardiol* 3:821-826, 1984

56. Fletcher GF, Froelicher VF, Hartley LH, et al: Exercise standards: a statement for health professionals from the American Heart Association. *Circulation* 82:2286-2322, 1990

57. Bonow RO, Picone AL, McIntosh CL, et al: Survival and functional results after valve replacement for aortic regurgitation from 1976 to 1983: impact of preoperative left ventricular function. *Circulation* 72:1244-1256, 1985

58. Bonow RO, Borer JS, Rosing DR, et al: Preoperative exercise capacity in symptomatic patients with aortic regurgitation as a predictor of postoperative left ventricular function and long-term prognosis. *Circulation* 62:1280-1290, 1980

59. Miller TD, Gibbons RJ, Squires RW, et al: Sinus node deceleration during exercise as a marker of significant narrowing of the right coronary artery. *Am J Cardiol* 71:371-373, 1993

60. Busby MJ, Shefrin EA, Fleg JL: Prevalence and long-term significance of exercise-induced frequent or repetitive ventricular ectopic beats in apparently healthy volunteers. *J Am Coll Cardiol* 14:1659-1665, 1989

61. Mont L, Seixas T, Brugada P, et al: Clinical and electrophysiologic characteristics of exercise-related idiopathic ventricular tachycardia. *Am J Cardiol* 68:897-900, 1991

62. Schlant RC, Froelicher VF Jr, Blomqvist CG, et al: Guidelines for exercise testing: a report of the American College of Cardiology/American Heart Association Task Force on Assessment of Cardiovascular Procedures (Subcommittee on Exercise Testing) *J Am Coll Cardiol* 8:725-738, 1986

63. Podrid PJ, Venditti FJ, Levine PA, et al: The role of exercise testing in evaluation of arrhythmias. *Am J Cardiol* 62:24H-33H, 1988

64. Besoaín-Santander M, Gómez-Ebensperguer G: Electrocardiographic diagnosis of myocardial infarction in cases of complete left bundle branch block. *Am Heart J* 60:886-897, 1960

65. Schlant RC, Friesinger GC II, Leonard JJ: Clinical competence in exercise testing: a statement for physicians from the ACP/ACC/AHA Task Force on Clinical Privileges in Cardiology. *J Am Coll Cardiol* 16:1061-1065, 1990

66. Borg GAV: Perceived exertion: a note on "history" and methods. *Med Sci Sports* 5:90-93, 1973

67. Gibbons RJ, Zinsmeister AR, Miller TD, et al: Comparison of exercise electrocardiography and radionuclide angiography in the identification of severe coronary artery disease. *Ann Intern Med* 112:743-749, 1990

68. Simari RD, Miller TD, Zinsmeister AR, et al: Capabilities of supine exercise electrocardiography versus exercise radionuclide angiography in predicting coronary events. *Am J Cardiol* 67:573-577, 1991

69. Mason RE, Likar I: A new system of multiple-lead exercise electrocardiography. *Am Heart J* 71:196-205, 1966

70. Blackburn H, Katigbak R: What electrocardiographic leads to take after exercise? *Am Heart J* 67:184-185, 1964

71. American Heart Association Committee Report: Recommendations for standardization of leads and of specifications for instruments in electrocardiography and vectorcardiography. *Circulation* 52:11-31, 1975

72. Milliken JA, Abdollah H, Burggraf GW: False-positive treadmill exercise tests due to computer signal averaging. *Am J Cardiol* 65:946-948, 1990

73. Marquette Case Averaging Software, Marquette Electronics, Milwaukee, Wisconsin, 1978

74. Mancini DM, Eisen H, Kussmaul W, et al: Value of peak exercise oxygen consumption for optimal timing of cardiac transplantation in ambulatory patients with heart failure. *Circulation* 83:778-786, 1991

75. Wasserman K, Hansen JE, Sue DY, et al: *Principles of Exercise Testing and Interpretation.* Philadelphia, Lea & Febiger, 1987

76. Neuberg GW, Friedman SH, Weiss MB, et al: Cardiopulmonary exercise testing: the clinical value of gas exchange data. *Arch Intern Med* 148:2221-2226, 1988

77. American College of Sports Medicine: *Guidelines for Graded Exercise Testing and Exercise Prescription.* Second edition. Philadelphia, Lea & Febiger, 1980, pp 137-151

78. Myers J, Buchanan N, Walsh D, et al: Comparison of the ramp versus standard exercise protocols. *J Am Coll Cardiol* 17:1334-1342, 1991

79. McInnis KJ, Balady GJ, Weiner DA, et al: Comparison of ischemic and physiologic responses during exercise tests in men using the standard and modified Bruce protocols. *Am J Cardiol* 69:84-89, 1992

80. Åstrand P-O, Rodahl K: *Textbook of Work Physiology: Physiological Bases of Exercise.* Second edition. New York, McGraw-Hill Book Company, 1977, a, 337; b, 335

81. White CW, Wright CB, Doty DB, et al: Does visual interpretation of the coronary arteriogram predict the physiologic importance of a coronary stenosis? *N Engl J Med* 310:819-824, 1984

82. Chaitman BR, Bourassa MG, Davis K, et al: Angiographic prevalence of high-risk coronary artery disease in patient subsets (CASS). *Circulation* 64:360-367,1981

83. Erikssen J, Enge I, Forfang K, et al: False positive diagnostic tests and coronary angiographic findings in 105 presumably healthy males. *Circulation* 54:371-376, 1976

84. Diamond GA, Forrester JS, Hirsch M, et al: Application of conditional probability analysis to the clinical diagnosis of coronary artery disease. *J Clin Invest* 65:1210-1221, 1980

85. Rozanski A, Diamond GA, Berman D, et al: The declining specificity of exercise radionuclide ventriculography. *N Engl J Med* 309:518-522, 1983

86. Diamond GA: Monkey business (editorial). *Am J Cardiol* 57:471-475, 1986

87. Diamond GA: Off Bayes: effect of verification bias on posterior probabilities calculated using Bayes' theorem. *Med Decis Making* 12:22-31, 1992

88. Begg CB, Greenes RA: Assessment of diagnostic tests when disease verification is subject to selection bias. *Biometrics* 39:207-215, 1983

89. Greenberg PS, Cangiano B, Leamy L, et al: Use of the multivariate approach to enhance the diagnostic accuracy of the treadmill stress test. *J Electrocardiol* 13:227-236, 1980

90. Morise AP, Duval RD, Detrano R, et al: Comparison of logistic regression and Bayesian-based algorithms to estimate posttest probability in patients with suspected coronary artery disease undergoing exercise ECG. *J Electrocardiol* 25:89-99, 1992

91. Gordon T, Kannel WB: Multiple risk functions for predicting coronary heart disease: the concept, accuracy, and application. *Am Heart J* 103:1031-1039, 1982

92. McGee D: The probability of developing certain cardiovascular diseases in eight years at specified values of some characteristics. In The Framingham Study: An Epidemiological Investigation of Cardiovascular Disease (DHEW Publication No [NIH] 74-618), Section 28. Washington DC, Government Printing Office, 1973

93. Bruce RA, DeRouen T, Peterson DR, et al: Noninvasive predictors of sudden cardiac death in men with coronary heart disease: predictive value of maximal stress testing. *Am J Cardiol* 39:833-840, 1977

94. Koppes G, McKiernan T, Bassan M, et al: Treadmill exercise testing. Part II. *Curr Probl Cardiol* 2:32-33, December 1977

95. Allen WH, Aronow WS, Goodman P, et al: Five year follow-up of maximal treadmill stress test in asymptomatic women and men (abstract). *Am J Cardiol* 45:419, 1980

96. Bruce RA: Exercise testing for evaluation of ventricular function. *N Engl J Med* 296:671-675, 1977

97. Bruschke AVG, Proudfit WL, Sones FM Jr: Progress study of 590 consecutive nonsurgical cases of coronary disease followed 5-9 years. II. Ventriculographic and other correlations. *Circulation* 47:1154-1163, 1973

98. Elamin MS, Mary DASG, Smith DR, et al: Prediction of severity of coronary artery disease using slope of submaximal ST segment/heart rate relationship. *Cardiovasc Res* 14:681-691, 1980

99. Podrid PJ, Graboys TB, Lown B: Prognosis of medically treated patients with coronary-artery disease with profound ST-segment depression during exercise testing. *N Engl J Med* 305:1111-1116, 1981

100. Weiner DA, Ryan TJ, McCabe CH, et al: Prognostic importance of a clinical profile and exercise test in medically treated patients with coronary artery disease. *J Am Coll Cardiol* 3:772-779, 1984

101. Mark DB, Shaw L, Harrell FE Jr, et al: Prognostic value of a treadmill exercise score in outpatients with suspected coronary artery disease. *N Engl J Med* 325:849-853, 1991

102. Detrano R, Froelicher VF: Exercise testing: uses and limitations considering recent studies. *Prog Cardiovasc Dis* 31:173-204, 1988

103. Bruce RA: Exercise testing of patients with coronary heart disease: principles and normal standards for evaluation. *Ann Clin Res* 3:323-332, 1971

104. Smith JW, Dennis CA, Gassmann A, et al: Exercise testing three weeks after myocardial infarction. *Chest* 75:12-16, 1979

105. Sami M, Kraemer H, DeBusk RF: The prognostic significance of serial exercise testing after myocardial infarction. *Circulation* 60:1238-1246, 1979

106. Théroux P, Waters DD, Halphen C, et al: Prognostic value of exercise testing soon after myocardial infarction. *N Engl J Med* 301:341-345, 1979

107. Starling MR, Crawford MH, Kennedy GT, et al: Exercise testing early after myocardial infarction: predictive value for subsequent unstable angina and death. *Am J Cardiol* 46:909-914, 1980

108. Weld FM, Chu K-L, Bigger JT Jr, et al: Risk stratification with low-level exercise testing 2 weeks after acute myocardial infarction. *Circulation* 64:306-314, 1981

109. Klein J, Froelicher VF, Detrano R, et al: Does the rest electrocardiogram after myocardial infarction determine the predictive value of exercise-induced ST depression? A 2 year follow-up study in a veteran population. *J Am Coll Cardiol* 14:305-311, 1989

110. Rogers WJ, Babb JD, Baim DS, et al: Selective versus routine predischarge coronary arteriography after therapy with recombinant tissue-type plasminogen activator, heparin and aspirin for acute myocardial infarction. *J Am Coll Cardiol* 17:1007-1016, 1991

111. Weiner DA, Ryan TJ, McCabe CH, et al: Value of exercise testing in determining the risk classification and the response to coronary artery bypass grafting in three-vessel coronary artery disease: a report from the Coronary Artery Surgery Study (CASS) registry. *Am J Cardiol* 60:262-266, 1987

112. Ryan TJ, Weiner DA, McCabe CH, et al: Exercise testing in the Coronary Artery Surgery Study randomized population. *Circulation* 72 Suppl 5:31-38, 1985

113. Siscovick DS, Ekelund LG, Johnson JL, et al: Sensitivity of exercise electrocardiography for acute cardiac events during moderate and strenuous physical activity: The Lipid Research Clinics Coronary Primary Prevention Trial. *Arch Intern Med* 151:325-330, 1991

114. Miller TD, Gibbons RJ, Allison TG, et al: Results of thallium-201 isotope imaging in asymptomatic patients with positive screening treadmill tests (abstract). *J Cardiopulmonary Rehabil* 9:419, October 1989

115. Uhl GS, Troxler RG, Hickman JR Jr, et al: Relation between high density lipoprotein cholesterol and coronary artery disease in asymptomatic men. *Am J Cardiol* 48:903-910, 1981

116. Morise AP, Detrano R, Bobbio M, et al: Development and validation of a logistic regression-derived algorithm for estimating the incremental probability of coronary artery disease before and after exercise testing. *J Am Coll Cardiol* 20:1187-1196, 1992

117. Epstein SE, Quyyumi AA, Bonow RO: Myocardial ischemia—silent or symptomatic. *N Engl J Med* 318:1038-1043, 1988

118. Sox HC Jr, Littenberg B, Garber AM: The role of exercise testing in screening for coronary artery disease. *Ann Intern Med* 110:456-469, 1989

119. Margolis JR: Treadmill stage as a predictor of medical & surgical survival in coronary disease (abstract). *Circulation* 52 Suppl 2:109, 1975

120. Rochmis P, Blackburn H: Exercise tests: a survey of procedures, safety, and litigation experience in approximately 170,000 tests. *JAMA* 217:1061-1066, 1971

121. Stuart RJ Jr, Ellestad MH: National survey of exercise stress testing facilities. *Chest* 77:94-97, 1980

122. Atterhög J-H, Jonsson B, Samuelsson R: Exercise testing: a prospective study of complication rates. *Am Heart J* 98:572-579, 1979

123. Topol EJ, Juni JE, O'Neill WW, et al: Exercise testing three days after onset of acute myocardial infarction. *Am J Cardiol* 60:958-962, 1987

124. Rod JL, Squires RW, Pollock ML, et al: Symptom-limited graded exercise testing soon after myocardial revascularization surgery. *J Cardiac Rehabil* 2:199-205, 1982

CHAPTER

3

Electrocardiography

C. Noninvasive evaluation of patients with arrhythmias: ambulatory and transtelephonic electrocardiographic monitoring and cardiac functional testing

Michael B. Mock, M.D., and David R. Holmes, Jr., M.D.

THIS chapter provides an overview of the use of the 24-hour ambulatory electrocardiographic (ECG) recording, transtelephonic ECG recording, and exercise testing as clinical tools for the documentation of symptomatic and asymptomatic arrhythmias and episodes of ischemia. In the clinical use of these techniques, it is critical to correlate the patient's symptoms with the ECG findings. The physician who evaluates the reports from these tests must remember that although abnormalities are most often found in persons with heart disease, dramatically wide ranges of heart rates and rhythms have been reported in the ambulatory recordings of physically normal persons.[1-4] Ogawa et al.[5] reported that ventricular pauses averaged 2.2 seconds in athletes on 24-hour monitoring and that no symptoms appeared in 3 years of follow-up, even when the pauses measured 3 seconds or more. The true range of normal variation in the ambulatory ECG recording has not yet been determined. Thus, the physician using ambulatory ECG recordings must consider the normal and age-related variations of heart rate and rhythm. But the physician must also be aware of the limitations of our current knowledge, not only concerning the occurrence of arrhythmias in normal persons but also with regard to the varying prognostic implications of ECG changes in different phases of cardiovascular disease.

CLINICAL HISTORY

The variable clinical presentation depends on (1) the hemodynamic consequence of the arrhythmia, (2) associated clinical problems, and (3) the unique awareness that each patient has of himself or herself. The hemodynamic consequences of the arrhythmia are in turn dependent on (1) the heart rate during the arrhythmia, (2) the presence or absence of atrioventricular (AV) synchrony, (3) the effect on coronary blood flow, (4) the effect on cerebral blood flow, (5) the duration of the arrhythmia, (6) the effect of reflex responses to the arrhythmia, and (7) associated cardiac or extracardiac abnormalities.

Perhaps palpitations are the most common symptom in patients who present with arrhythmias. Although physicians define palpitations as a change in heart rate, rhythm, or contractility, patients are not bound by such a definition and more often describe their symptoms as flip-flops, fluttering, or skipping. It is helpful in this regard to have the patient illustrate the cadence of his or her specific complaint by tapping it out. Alternatively, the physician may tap out several cadences and have the patient describe and select the appropriate one. This, with specific questioning concerning the rapidity of onset and offset, duration, and regularity or irregularity, helps the experienced clinician narrow the etiologic possibilities.

In patients who present with episodic complaints other than palpitations, such as chest pain, dyspnea, dizziness, or syncope, a high degree of alertness is required to document the presence of an arrhythmia. In these patients, careful attention must be paid to specific questions as to the presence or absence of associated palpitations.

If a cardiac arrhythmia is present, specific attention must then be directed at the clinical setting in which it occurs, the presence of precipitating factors, and associated clinical problems. The presence of reproducible precipitating factors, such as exercise or caffeine or alcohol, has important implications not only in terms of cause of the rhythm disturbance but also in terms of evaluation and management. It is essential to identify all drugs that the patient is taking, including both prescription and over-the-counter medications. Sympathomimetic drugs, antihistamines, and diuretics, when taken to correct other medical problems, may precipitate arrhythmias. Treatment under these circumstances is obviously best aimed at eliminating the triggering agent if possible.

PHYSICAL EXAMINATION

The physical examination of patients with a history that is consistent with a cardiac arrhythmia should be used to supplement historical information. Attention should be directed to the detection of associated cardiac, central nervous system, and pulmonary conditions that may affect the arrhythmia.

Less commonly, patients may be evaluated during the occurrence of a cardiac rhythm disturbance, at which time valuable information can be obtained concerning the functional consequences of the arrhythmia, the response of the arrhythmia to maneuvers such as carotid sinus massage and the Valsalva maneuver, and clues as to the cause of the arrhythmia and its specific type.

Valuable information can be obtained from observation of the jugular venous pressure because it reflects atrial activity. The presence of cannon "a" waves may be a clue to AV dissociation. In the setting of bradycardia, cannon "a" waves that are constant but unrelated to the carotid or arterial pulse suggest complete AV block. In the setting of tachycardia, the presence of cannon "a" waves is also helpful in that it indicates AV dissociation.

Examination of the arterial pulse during tachycardia is also helpful. Specific attention must be paid to the rate and regularity as well as the relationship to the jugular venous pressure waveforms. Careful observation in these situations can help to narrow the diagnostic possibilities and facilitate the correct diagnosis.

LABORATORY TESTING

Selection of tests for patients with cardiac arrhythmias depends in part on the nature of the presentation. The evaluation of a patient with a life-threatening ventricular arrhythmia must obviously be quite different from that of a young, otherwise healthy patient with palpitations but without sustained tachycardia. Selection of the proper tests must take this into account, along with cost, specificity and sensitivity of the tests, and risks of the tests. The optimal test is one that documents the rhythm disturbance that is associated with the patient's symptoms.

Electrocardiography

Twelve-lead ECG with long rhythm strips has been labeled the Rosetta stone of arrhythmia analysis.[6] The ECG diagnosis of the various arrhythmias is dealt with in chapter 3A. During the initial evaluation, it is important to determine whether the patient has ever had an ECG recorded during a symptomatic arrhythmia. Obtaining ECG documentation in this manner may obviate further testing and facilitate selection of the proper treatment regimen.

Transtelephonic ECG monitoring

Because of the intermittent nature of arrhythmias, there has been considerable interest in the development of event recorders that could be used for long-term monitoring.[7-12] Several commercial systems are available, including the use of transmitters that are provided for patients receiving pacemakers.[11,12] The most important advantage of this system is that the ECG can be recorded during the time the patient has symptoms (Figs 3C-1 to 3C-3). Judson et al.[8] found that this technique provided more information than did conventional Holter monitoring. Of interest in their series, 28% of patients who transmitted during a typical spell had a normal ECG. This finding is of great help in counseling these patients. Transtelephonic monitoring systems have also been useful in identifying postmyocardial infarction patients who have ventricular ectopy.[9]

This technique does have limitations. Some systems are cumbersome and employ either wrist or axillary electrodes, which may be difficult to use. The patient must be able to detect the arrhythmia and then have some time to transmit it. This requires access to a receiving center. For patients who rapidly suffer serious hemodynamic consequences such as syncope soon after the onset of the arrhythmia, the transtelephonic monitoring system is obviously not helpful. Also, in patients with spells of very short duration, the system may not be beneficial.

Reiffel et al.[13] recently reported on the optimal time for a patient to keep the transtelephonic monitoring equipment. In their study of 5,052 patients and 20,590 calls, 95% of the calls documenting arrhythmia were made within 5 weeks.

Transtelephonic ECG monitoring has also been used to monitor exercise rehabilitation performed at a remote site, such as the patient's home or a small community hospital, without an on-site cardiovascular rehabilitation program. In addition to the single-channel ECG, two-way voice communication is possible.[14]

Monitoring systems with a memory loop are now available. These can be activated by the patient, and the data can then be transmitted to a receiving center. These and other advances have increased the role that transtelephonic monitoring plays in the evaluation of arrhythmias.

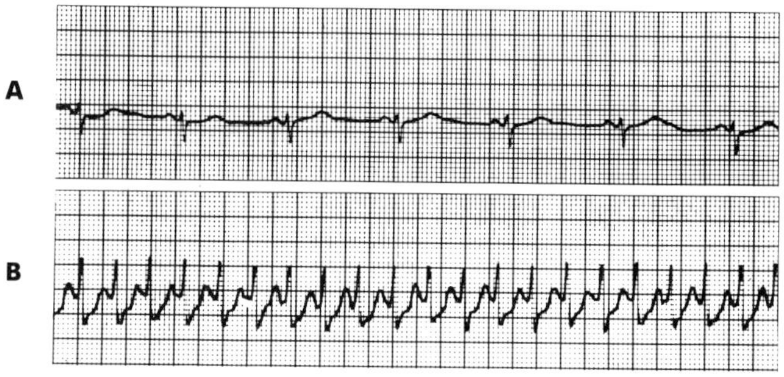

Fig 3C-1 **A,** transtelephonic monitoring system documenting baseline normal sinus rhythm. **B,** transmission at the time of palpitations documents rapid supraventricular tachycardia. (From Hammill SC, Holmes DR Jr, Wood DL: Cardiac arrhythmias. In *Current Diagnosis 7.* Edited by RB Conn. Philadelphia, WB Saunders Company, 1985, pp 405-433. By permission.)

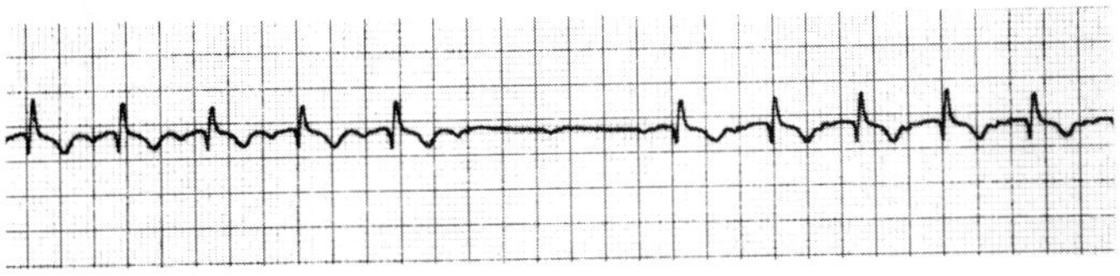

Fig 3C-2 Transtelephonic rhythm strip recorded during an episode of high-grade AV block. (From Hammill SC, Holmes DR Jr, Wood DL: Cardiac arrhythmias. In *Current Diagnosis 7.* Edited by RB Conn. Philadelphia, WB Saunders Company, 1985, pp 405-433. By permission.)

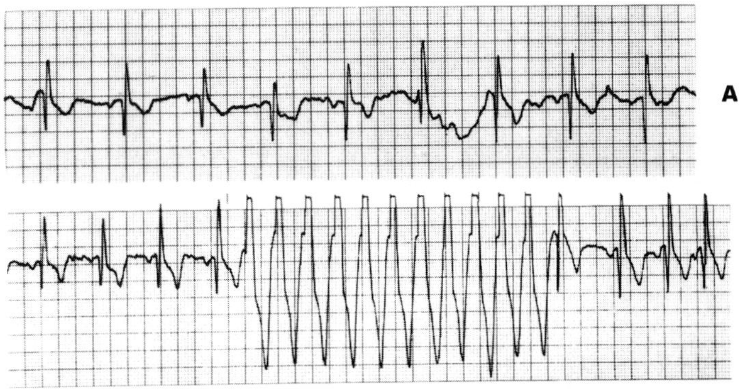

Fig 3C-3 **A,** baseline normal sinus rhythm. **B,** telephone transmission during an episode of palpitations documents nonsustained rapid ventricular tachycardia.

Ambulatory monitoring

At present, major indications for ambulatory monitoring include (1) documentation of symptomatic and asymptomatic rhythm disturbances; (2) documentation of the cardiac rhythm during symptoms that could be related to a cardiac origin, such as fainting spells; (3) documentation of the effect of treatment regimens on rhythm disturbances; (4) evaluation of pacemaker function; and (5) evaluation of the risk of subsequent cardiac events in patient subgroups—for example, post-myocardial infarction patients.[15]

Present systems make use of multiple channels that aid in differentiating artifacts and QRS and P-wave morphology (Fig 3C-4). In addition, combined blood pressure and ambulatory monitoring systems are available that can provide hemodynamic information on the effect of arrhythmias and also may elucidate whether fainting spells are related to arrhythmia or to hypotension alone.[16]

In the application of ambulatory ECG recording in patients with rhythm disturbances, three major factors must be kept in mind: (1) the intermittent nature of symptoms and rhythm disturbances, (2) spontaneous variability in rhythm disturbances, and (3) the wide range of normal findings.

Because of the intermittent nature of patients' symptoms, the standard diagnostic ambulatory monitoring is not practical in all patients.[7,8] This makes estimation of the sensitivity of the technique difficult. Johansson[17] found that 25% of patients with a history consistent with Stokes-Adams attacks have symptoms during the initial 24 hours of monitoring and also that, if recording is extended to 5 to 21 days, 75% will have symptoms. Goldberg et al.[18] found that increasing the duration of monitoring to more than 24 hours results in detection of additional significant arrhythmias in 31% of patients. Other authors have also

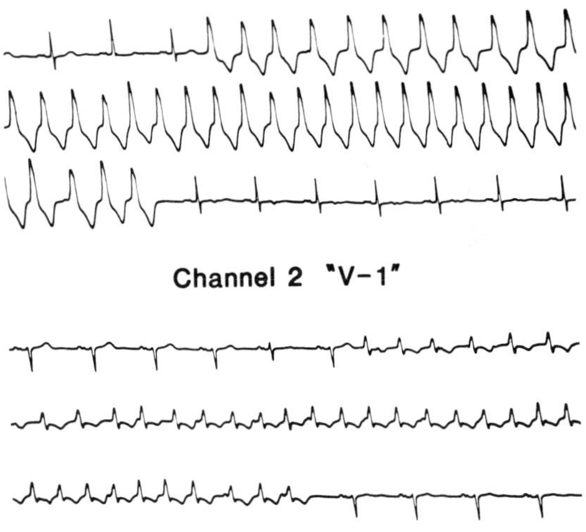

Fig 3C-4 Short run of nonsustained ventricular tachycardia recorded during ambulatory monitoring. Complex ventricular ectopy has been found to be more reproducible with less spontaneous variability than is simple ventricular ectopy.

documented the potential importance of prolonged monitoring.[19]

The reproducibility of the findings of ambulatory monitoring has stimulated considerable interest. This affects the design of clinical trials and also the confidence of documentation of an effective drug in any given patient. Several studies have documented significant variability not only from day to day but also throughout the day and even from hour to hour.[20-24] Although there is variability

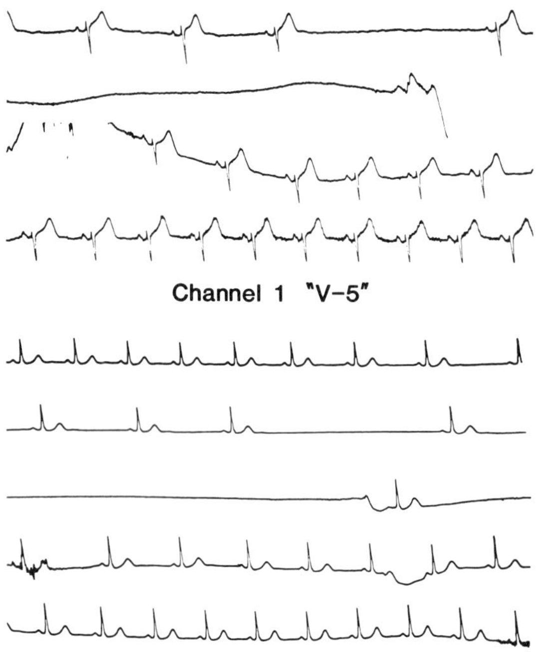

Fig 3C-5 Ambulatory recording during an episode of sinus arrest with failure of adequate subsidiary pacemaker. (From Hammill SC, Holmes DR Jr, Wood DL: Cardiac arrhythmias. In *Current Diagnosis 7.* Edited by RB Conn. Philadelphia, WB Saunders Company, 1985, pp 405-433. By permission.)

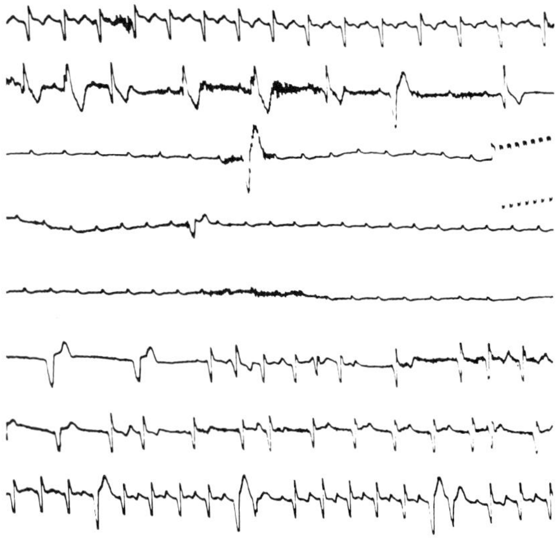

Fig 3C-6 Ambulatory recording during an episode of intermittent complete AV block.

in both simple and complex ventricular ectopy, several authors have found that the latter is more reproducible. The problem of documenting the effect of a drug in the face of the pronounced spontaneous variability is obvious. This problem can be circumvented by increasing the duration of monitoring from 24 to 48 hours or requiring a pronounced decrease in ventricular ectopy before ascribing the change to drug effect. Several studies have estimated that a 75% to 85% decrease in ventricular ectopy is necessary to document a drug effect.[21,23,24] Because there is less spontaneous variability in complex ventricular ectopy, smaller degrees of reduction may be needed to document drug efficacy in comparison with single ventricular ectopy.[23,24] In patients with sustained ventricular tachycardia or ventricular fibrillation, suppression of the sustained disturbance in ventricular rhythm is the important clinical end point, not suppression of isolated ventricular premature contractions. Indeed, in some patients ventricular ectopy may not be suppressed; however, sustained ventricular tachycardia or recurrent cardiac arrest is abolished.[25]

In patients undergoing evaluation of Stokes-Adams attacks, the finding of complete heart block or prolonged sinus arrest at the time of syncope during a 24-hour monitoring period permits an easy clinical decision to be made (Figs 3C-5 and 3C-6). When the same patient has evidence of only simple ventricular ectopy, and syncope does not occur during the study, the decision is considerably more difficult. Ambulatory monitoring in persons without apparent heart disease has documented a relatively wide range of arrhythmias. Brodsky et al.[1] demonstrated a striking variability in the heart rates of healthy male medical students. The range was 37 to 180 beats/min during waking periods and 33 to 115 beats/min during sleep. Twenty-four percent of the subjects had heart rates of 40 beats/min or slower during sleeping periods. Sinus pauses of more than 1.75 seconds were also noted in 28%. Transient second-degree AV block has been documented in 2% to 6% of trained athletes and young, otherwise healthy males and females.[1,26-28] These arrhythmias often occur during sleep and appear to be vagally mediated.[29] Supraventricular and ventricular extrasystoles are also often found in healthy control subjects, although the absolute number in any specific person is low.[1,30] In these studies the frequency of some arrhythmias was found to increase with increasing age.[31,32] Hinkle et al.[33] documented asymptomatic arrhythmias and conduction defects in 93% of patients during ambulatory monitoring—supraventricular arrhythmias in 76% and ventricular arrhythmias in 62%. These findings must be kept in mind during the evaluation of a given patient, and the results of ambulatory monitoring must be placed in the context of the patient's clinical condition.

In addition to relating the findings on ambulatory monitoring to age, it is essential to place them in the context of the patient's cardiovascular disorder. There has been extensive investigation in several patient groups, including patients with arteriosclerotic heart disease, mitral valve prolapse, and hypertrophic obstructive cardiomyopathy.

EQUIPMENT FOR AMBULATORY ECG RECORDINGS

Recording system

The recording system for the ambulatory ECG is a portable, lightweight, battery-operated tape recording unit that is attached to the patient. The recording units have a frequency response comparable to that of a standard 12-lead ECG machine. The tape on which the recording is made is either a small cassette or a reel-to-reel tape. Most units are activated by the technician when the recorder is attached. The unit then continues to operate over a 24-hour period, and this permits the recording to be made both during daily activities and for sleep cycles. Most recorder units have an event marker that can be activated by the patient if any symptoms occur. This feature, along with the symptoms recorded in the patient's diary, enhances the physician's ability to correlate ECG phenomena with clinical symptoms.

A recent modification of the recording format for ambulatory ECGs is the development of a noncontinuous event-recording unit. The event recorder may be activated by the patient in response to the occurrence of symptoms or, in the more sophisticated units, the unit automatically records selected ECG events. These event recorders have their greatest applicability in documenting clinical episodes that occur at infrequent intervals but may require that the patient wear the recorder for long periods. In a comparison study between one "real-time" analysis system and conventional ambulatory recording, Kennedy and co-workers[34] found that sensitivity of the real-time system for some ventricular and supraventricular arrhythmias was lower but overall technical and patient applicability was similar.

Most current ambulatory ECG recorders can record two ECG leads simultaneously throughout the recording period. With two channels of simultaneous ECG recordings from two different leads available for analysis, it is at times easier to identify ectopic ventricular activity and abnormal deviation of the ST segment. Kennedy and co-workers[35] showed that the use of two-channel recording has increased the reliability of the recorded ECG data and has improved the identification and recognition of cardiac arrhythmias and the detection of ST-T wave changes of myocardial ischemia. In some units, the additional channels may also be used to record other data, such as pacemaker spikes in patients wearing implanted pacemaker units or voice recordings describing symptoms.

Electrodes and attachment of electrodes

The most frequently used lead systems for ambulatory ECG recordings are a modified "V_1-like lead system" and "V_5-like lead system." This lead facilitates the identification of ectopic beat patterns, since it has a well-defined P wave, which helps to identify atrial activity. The QRS pattern in this lead also facilitates the differentiation of right and left bundle-branch block. This aids in distinguishing supraventricular ectopic beats with aberrant conduction from ventricular ectopic beats. The "V_5-like lead system" is the lead most often used in identifying ischemia during exercise ECG testing.

Although the proper high-input impedance of modern ambulatory ECG recording equipment has reduced the noise caused by skin impedance in ambulatory ECG recordings, the skin must still be properly prepared before the electrodes are applied. Producing slight skin abrasion before applying the electrode gel helps to maintain the optimal conducting properties of the electrode.

It is vital that the electrodes for 24-hour ambulatory ECG recording remain adequately attached for the entire 24-hour period; therefore, electrode adhesiveness and flexibility are major considerations in the selection of electrodes. It is equally important to use electrodes with adequate polarization and impedance properties in order to avoid distortion or loss of the ECG signal by interference from extraneous electrical noise. Silver-silver chloride electrodes have proved to be the most resistant to polarization, and they also minimize distortion or loss of the ECG signal.

Each laboratory must standardize the maintenance of its equipment, attachment of the electrodes to the patient, attachment of the recorder to the patient, and calibration of the ECG signals and recording of baseline ECG strips in various body positions.

ANALYSIS OF THE AMBULATORY ECG RECORDING

Each 24-hour recorded ambulatory ECG tape contains approximately 100,000 QRS complexes. Thus, the analysis system requires an ability to analyze the tape at a much higher speed than real time. Most ambulatory ECG tapes are still analyzed by trained technicians, who usually identify abnormalities of the ECG and manually prepare printouts in real time by means of a manually operated high-speed scanner. Advances in computer technology have made possible partial automation of the analysis system for ambulatory ECGs. In these systems, computer programs help to distinguish normal from abnormal complexes, and this automated system catalogues the abnormal complexes and creates families of QRS complexes which can then be counted by the system. Most of these systems have a 5% to 10% error rate when compared with records that are scanned by a trained technician on a beat-by-beat basis. The clinician should realize that the most reliable data currently analyzed on ambulatory ECG tapes are based on the ventricular complexes. Most systems do not adequately evaluate P-wave activity or the relationship of the P wave to the QRS complexes.

A number of commercial scanning services have been developed that utilize sophisticated digital computers to process ambulatory ECG recordings that are mailed to the center from physicians, often from great distances. The ordering physician receives a descriptive report and a pulse rate report that characterize the ECG rhythms on the patient's tape. The physician is also provided with ECG rhythm strips taken at various time intervals, in addition to rhythm strips taken at any time that the patient has noted a symptom in the diary he or she is asked to keep or when there is any deviation from the normal rhythm or ECG pattern. The report may also include a comprehensive record of the entire 24-hour ECG. A major disadvantage of using a commercial service is the lack of a frequent interactive relationship between the physician and the technician analyzing the tape. Thus, the physician must rely on the assurance of ongoing quality-control procedures used by the scanning service. The large number of tapes that are analyzed by the commercial systems allows the scanning technician to achieve optimal technical competency, and, of course, the volume permits improved cost economy.

The alternative to the commercial scanning services is an in-house analysis system—hospital based, clinic based, or in the individual physician's office. It is imperative that an in-house system involve a physician with adequate knowledge in electrocardiography, technical expertise with the equipment used, and experience in clinical cardiology to make the necessary clinical correlations. In addition to developing the reports for ambulatory ECG tapes, this physician must take responsibility for training and supervising the technicians who perform the tape scanning. The supervising physician must also provide an ongoing quality-control protocol for the equipment that the scanning technicians use.

The latest generation of analysis systems is increasingly automated through the use of computers. However, these systems still require an expert technician to interact with the equipment for proper labeling of normal and abnormal complexes. In most of these systems, the operator ultimately makes the decision whether a complex is labeled a ventricular premature complex, a supraventricular premature complex, a normal complex, or an artifact. Once the operator labels the complex, the computer can then quickly and often very accurately make a count of all such complexes that are present on the tape, but there is still some question of the ability of the equipment to identify all other similar but not identical complexes. It is unlikely that we will soon have a totally automated analytic system. Rather, an equipment-operator interactive system will permit an integrated approach in which the machine is used to extract and display all the different QRS complexes, ST-T wave changes, rate changes, and P-wave changes and a skilled operator edits these results and determines the precise abnormalities. The equipment should be able to quantitate on an hour-by-hour basis the occurrence of all of the selected ECG events and also any variability in rate that occurs over the course of the recording.[36,37]

The clinician who orders ambulatory ECGs must be aware of the current limitations and problems inherent in all available analysis systems but particularly inadequacies of the analysis system to which the patients' ambulatory ECG tapes are submitted. Each ambulatory ECG laboratory should be able to provide to the clinicians who use its services meaningful data on the performance specifications of their equipment and also data on the reproducibility of readings.

PATIENT DIARY AND CORRELATION OF SYMPTOMS WITH ECG EVENTS

It is important first of all that the patient keep a diary of his or her experience with the rhythm problem and then that the physician who has ordered the test take a particular interest in attempting to correlate the symptoms and events recorded in the patient's diary with the ECG data provided from the analyzed tape. To this end, the ordering physician should review the diary with the patient when the ECG rhythm strips are available.

The ability to make meaningful correlations between symptoms and arrhythmias is enhanced when ambulatory ECG tapes are analyzed as quickly as possible. Expediting turn-around time is usually more likely with in-house scanning systems than with commercial scanning services.

It is not uncommon to find poor correlation between symptoms and ECG disorders. When this occurs, the physician cannot readily tell whether the problem was a timing error on the tape, the patient neglected to make an entry in the diary, or the ECG disorder was indeed asymptomatic. The ordering physician must determine whether any symptoms recorded in the diary can be associated with any recorded ECG abnormalities. That physician must also determine whether the symptoms recorded in the patient's diary are the same as those that prompted the ordering of the ambulatory ECG recording.

THE AMBULATORY ECG AS A CLINICAL TOOL

If we must compare the ambulatory ECG recording with the standard routine multilead ECG, we may say that the standard ECG study is a still portrait of the electrical activity of the heart taken in a very brief time in multiple poses or views. With modern multichannel machines, recording time may be reduced to 15 seconds. The ambulatory ECG can be compared to a moving picture of the electrical activity of the heart, since it records, on one or two leads, the electrical activity of the heart over 6, 12, 24, or more than 24 hours while the subject carries out the daily activities of living. Because of the high cost of the recording and analyzing equipment and the longer time required for interpretation, the cost of the ambulatory ECG is many times greater than that of the standard ECG. Therefore, the physician should have a specific goal in mind when ordering the ambulatory ECG recording. In addition to knowing the clinical indications for ambulatory ECG recording, the physician must be aware of the wide range of normal values for the ambulatory ECG and the variability in ECG abnormalities that can occur in any individual patient. The ambulatory ECG does not take the place of the routine ECG or the exercise ECG. In an occasional patient, the physician may wish to take advantage of the complementary aspects of these various ECG tests in helping to arrive at the correct clinical diagnosis or in formulating the proper therapeutic plan.[38]

In some patients with a history of widely spaced symptoms that may be due to cardiac arrhythmias that are sustained for several minutes or longer, the use of the transtelephonic monitoring unit, often used in the follow-up of implanted pacemakers, may prove more useful in documenting an ECG diagnosis than ambulatory ECG 24-hour recordings. This test may also be more economical.[7]

Event recorders are used when an arrhythmia does not last long enough to be relayed by a telephone transmitter. These recorders are worn 24 hours a day and may be activated retrospectively whenever a symptom or arrhythmia occurs. Current data indicate that a 24-hour duration of ambulatory ECG recording is sufficient for the usual evaluation. Bigger et al.,[39] in comparing ECG recordings of various lengths to identify patients with complex ventricular premature beats, reported that the detection of ventricular premature beats increased nonlinearly with the duration of the recording. The rate of detection for complex multifocal ventricular premature beats, paired ventricular premature beats, and R-on-T phenomena showed a rate of first detection that was much greater in the first 6 to 12 hours than in the additional hours of recording. However, the occurrence of ventricular tachycardia was detected in a more linear relationship during additional time. In investigating patients with sporadic syncopal or near-syncopal episodes, more than 24 hours of ECG recording may be necessary. The Beta-Blocker Heart Attack Trial reported that less than 24 hours of monitoring may be sufficient to help predict subsequent sudden death and total death.[40]

In the usual clinical practice setting, the inconvenience to the patient and the additional costs of repeated 24-hour ambulatory ECG recordings must be considered. In such a setting, if the symptoms persist for an adequate period, the telephone ECG transmitter discussed above can offer a logical alternative diagnostic approach if 24 hours of ambulatory recording does not reveal an ECG abnormality to account for the clinical symptoms. A new recording device, the continuous cardiac loop ambulatory ECG recorder, provides prolonged ambulatory monitoring and can identify the cardiac rhythm at the time of a syncopal spell. Cumbee et al.[41] reported identifying the cause of syncope as cardiac in 36% of 48 patients; median duration was 28 days, and the average charge was $180.

NORMAL VALUES FOR ECG RECORDING

Important cardiac arrhythmias may often be asymptomatic and may occur in persons who have no signs or laboratory evidence of cardiovascular disease. Clarke and co-workers[30] reported on ambulatory ECG recordings in a group of "normal persons" age 16 to 65 years. Twelve percent of the recordings had complex ventricular ectopic beats and significant bradyarrhythmias and tachyarrhythmias, yet no symptoms had been noted by the subjects. Kostis et al.,[42] in a provocative study involving 100 men and women, reported that of 46% of these persons who had premature ventricular beats recorded, 20% had more than 10 ventricular premature beats in 24 hours and a surprising 5% had more than 100 ventricular premature beats on the 24-hour tape. Kennedy et al.[43] described a group of subjects with normal coronary arteries demonstrated by angiography who had frequent multiform ventricular premature beats. These authors emphasized that most ventricular premature beats had a right ventricular focus and were suppressed by increasing pulse rates. As will be developed later, supraventricular arrhythmias occur frequently in apparently healthy persons and appear to increase in frequency with aging.[32] The physical condition of a normal person may be reflected in the range of the heart rate over a 24-hour period. Also, bradyarrhythmias are very common in apparently healthy persons.[1] From a study of cardiac rhythm in 168 healthy men aged 19 to 30, Viitasalo et al.[44] reported that 29 of the sinus pauses and 83% of the second-degree AV blocks were associated with short-term rapid change in heart rate, presumably as a result of an autonomic activator. Cardiologists who interpret clinical ambulatory ECG recordings must remember that the range of normal has not been definitively determined, and they should keep in mind that wide variations in heart rate and significant alterations in the rhythm occur in apparently normal persons without any associated symptoms.

AMBULATORY ECG RECORDINGS FOR EVALUATION OF PALPITATIONS OR SUSPECTED CARDIAC ARRHYTHMIA

When a patient presents with a history of frequent palpitations, episodes of rapid or slow pulse, episodic severe dizziness and lightheadedness, or chest pain associated with a pulse disorder, the differential diagnosis must always include a possible cardiac arrhythmia. In these clinical settings, the ambulatory ECG recording is a most useful tool. Particularly when a physical examination and neurologic examination and the standard 12-lead ECG are normal, the ambulatory ECG recording may be the most useful method of documenting an ECG disorder as the cause of the symptoms reported by the patient. From its earliest clinical use, the ambulatory ECG has been applied to the study of patients with transient symptoms compatible with paroxysmal rhythm disturbance.[45] Today, the predominant use of the ambulatory ECG recording remains the study of such patients; although more complete descriptions and discussions of cardiac arrhythmias are presented in chapters 22B and 22C, we will review here the most common arrhythmias encountered on the ambulatory ECG recording—namely, those seen in relation to palpitations, syncope, and chest pain.

Palpitations

The most frequent presenting complaint that prompts the clinician to order an ambulatory ECG is palpitations. Krasnow and Bloomfield[46] reported that approximately one-third of the patients they studied by ambulatory ECG recording had this complaint. In the patient with symptoms of palpitations, the ambulatory ECG will often demonstrate supraventricular or atrial ectopic beats (Fig 3C-7,A). As discussed in chapter 22B, supraventricular or atrial ectopic beats are thought to arise from an irritable

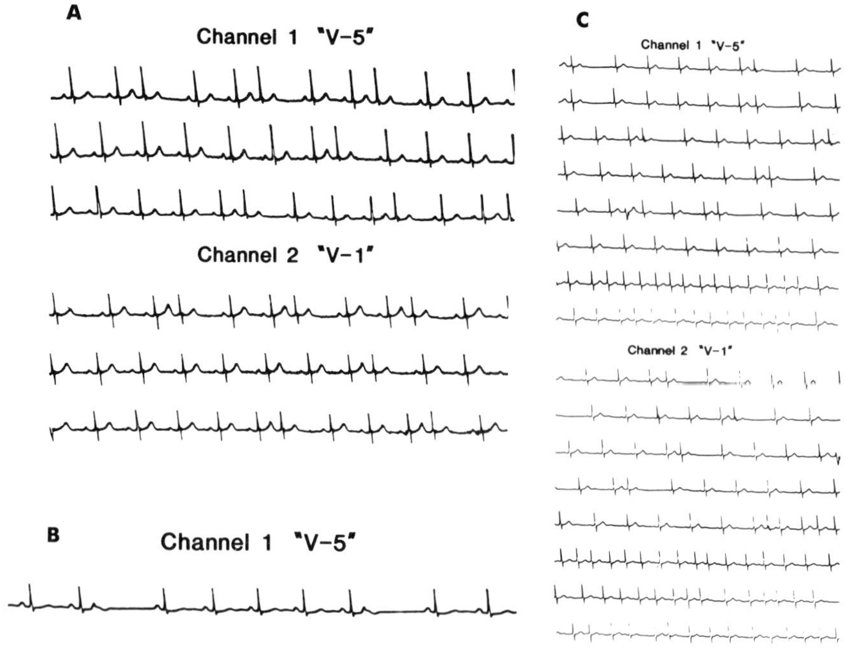

Fig 3C-7 Typical supraventricular arrhythmias commonly encountered on ambulatory ECG recordings. **A,** atrial premature beats. **B,** nonconducted atrial premature beats. These are a common cause of pauses noted on ambulatory ECG recordings. Intermittent supraventricular tachycardias are often encountered on ambulatory ECG recordings and can be correlated with the patient's symptoms. **C,** intermittent atrial fibrillation. Note that multifocal atrial premature beats preceded and followed the brief period of atrial fibrillation.

focus in the atrium or the AV junctional areas and are characterized by a QRS complex that is identical or similar to the normal QRS complex. These ectopic beats may have no preceding P wave or have a normal or abnormal P wave preceding or superimposed on or following the QRS complex. The normal QRS and P-wave pattern may be undisturbed. Occasionally, the atrial extrasystoles will not be conducted because they occur before the electrical recovery of the ventricular myocardium. These ectopic beats will present as nonconducted P waves and manifest themselves as a pause of the normal heartbeat (Fig 3C-7,B). Nonconducted atrial extrasystoles are the most frequent cause of pauses in the regular heart rhythm. Paroxysmal supraventricular tachycardias are characterized by repeated supraventricular ectopic beats usually due to a reentry mechanism. These arrhythmias are manifested on the ECG by the sudden appearance of normal-looking QRS complexes at a rapid rate, preceded by normal or abnormal P waves. The rhythms often have an abrupt onset and cessation. Supraventricular premature complexes may be followed by an abnormal QRS complex, the result of aberrant ventricular conduction. The distinction between aberrantly conducted supraventricular beats and ventricular ectopic beats is often difficult. Paroxysmal atrial fibrillation (Fig 3C-7,C) is another common supraventricular arrhythmia leading to symptoms, particularly palpitations.

As stated earlier, asymptomatic supraventricular arrhythmias have been detected on ambulatory ECG recordings in a high percentage of normal subjects. Clarke and co-workers[47] described asymptomatic supraventricular arrhythmias in almost half of their normal adults studied by 24-hour ambulatory ECG recordings. Asymptomatic supraventricular arrhythmias without clinical evidence of cardiac disease appear to increase with age.[4,31] Almost all normal subjects studied by ambulatory ECG recording showed some degree of sinus arrhythmia.

Ambulatory ECG recording is often used for the diagnosis and management of ventricular arrhythmias, since it provides the clinician with a tool to document and quantify the occurrence of ventricular arrhythmias outside the hospital setting. The impact of the activities of daily living, including occupational tasks, can be related to the occurrence of ventricular arrhythmias. Even when frequent ventricular ectopic beats are detected on the standard 12-lead ECG, the ambulatory ECG recording can be useful in quantitating the occurrence of these arrhythmias throughout the day and during awake and sleep cycles. Bjerregaard et al.[48] reported from a long-term follow-up study of 260 patients that either more than 900 ventricular premature beats or a run of more than three beats of ventricular tachycardia in apparently healthy subjects may predict the subsequent development of ischemic heart disease.

As discussed in more detail in chapter 22C, ventricular premature beats are characterized by a bizarre, widened QRS complex, and the ST segment and T wave also often show deviation from the normal (Fig 3C-8,A). The ventricular premature beat is usually caused by a reentry mechanism. This process can lead to a continuous run of

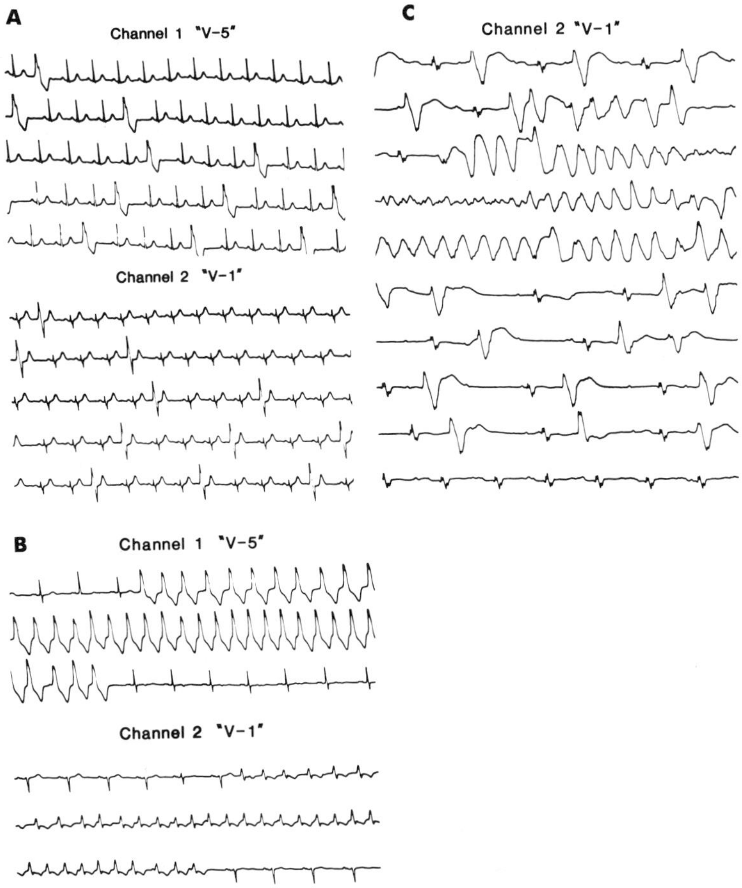

Fig 3C-8 Ventricular arrhythmias recorded on ambulatory ECG recordings. **A,** the most commonly encountered ventricular arrhythmia—isolated uniform ventricular premature beats. The detection of potentially life-threatening ventricular arrhythmias is an important clinical application of ambulatory ECG recordings. **B,** period of ventricular tachycardia with abrupt onset and termination. **C,** the most serious arrhythmia that can be recorded by ambulatory ECG recordings—ventricular fibrillation. This arrhythmia is infrequently recorded and even less often shows spontaneous remission, as in this example.

ventricular ectopic beats, and when three or more ventricular ectopic beats are sustained in a row, this is termed, by definition, ventricular tachycardia. In sustained ventricular tachycardia, the rate is usually 100 to 200 beats/min (Fig 3C-8,B). Ventricular tachycardia can degenerate into ventricular fibrillation. Ventricular fibrillation is a disorganized electrical rhythm that shows a chaotic pattern without any of the characteristics of the normal ECG pattern of P, QRS, and T (Fig 3C-8,C). Ventricular fibrillation is the major mechanism of sudden cardiac death and therefore is infrequently encountered on ambulatory ECG recordings. Savage and co-workers[49] reported 14 episodes of sudden cardiac death in 58,000 patients having an ambulatory ECG recording. They noted increasing isolated premature ventricular complexes and couplets and runs of ventricular tachycardia and return of ST-segment changes toward normal preceding tachyarrhythmic arrest.

Certain complex ventricular premature beats as recorded on ambulatory ECG recordings of patients with chronic ischemic heart disease have been associated with an increased incidence of ventricular fibrillation and sudden death.[50] These patterns include multiform ventricular premature beats, paired ventricular premature beats, and bigeminal patterns of ventricular premature beats[51] (Fig 3C-9). Lown and Wolf[52] developed an early classification for chronic ventricular ectopy. They identified five grades of ventricular ectopic beats, which they considered as having progressive prognostic value for warning of later recurrence of ventricular fibrillation. These grades were as follows: grade 0, absence of ventricular arrhythmias; grade I, fewer than two ectopic beats/min or 30/hour; grade II, two or more ectopic beats/min or more than 30/hour; grade III, multiform ventricular ectopic beats; grade IVA, couplets of ventricular ectopic beats; grade IVB, three or more consecutive ectopic beats (ventricular tachycardia); grade V, early-cycle ventricular ectopic beats with R-on-T phenomena. There have also been reports indicating that a significant number of patients may have ventricular fibrillation

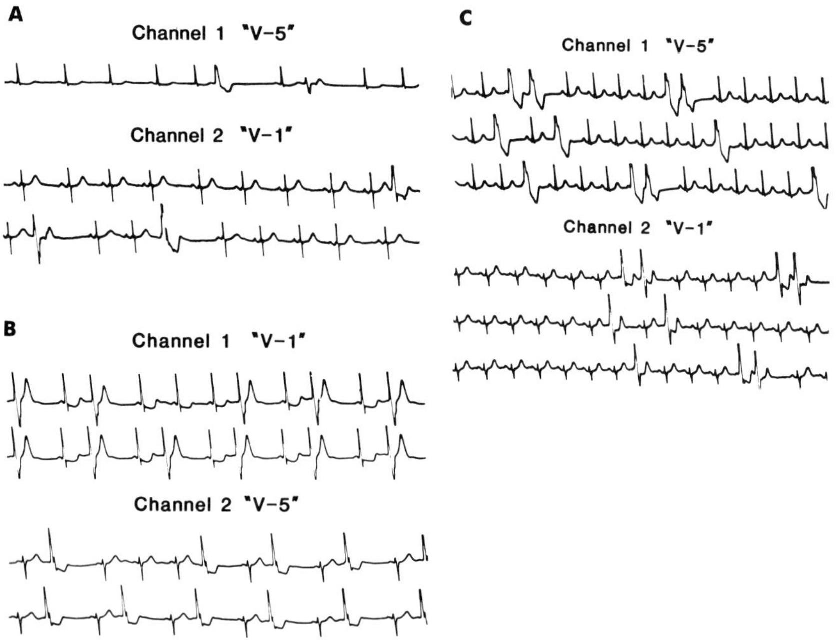

Fig 3C-9 Ventricular premature beat patterns that have been associated with a high frequency of life-threatening arrhythmias. **A,** isolated multiform ventricular premature beats. **B,** bigeminy pattern of ventricular premature beats. **C,** ventricular premature beats occurring in pairs (couplets).

without demonstrating these early warning grades of ventricular ectopic beats.[53,54] McCollam and Parker[55] recently proposed an overall approach for evaluating and treating ventricular arrhythmias based on objective monitoring criteria and emphasizing the potential adverse effects of treatment from the Cardiac Arrhythmia Suppression Trial.

Prolonged ECG monitoring of patients after acute myocardial infarction is often continued in step-down coronary care by means of either a telemetry monitoring unit or ambulatory ECG recording. The latter may be used early after dismissal from the hospital. The prognostic significance of the occurrence of ventricular ectopic beats varies considerably with the time relation of these ectopic beats to the acute myocardial infarction. Ventricular ectopic beats in the initial 48 hours after the onset of acute myocardial infarction do not always predict the occurrence of later ventricular arrhythmias during the hospitalization or after dismissal from the hospital. Moss and co-workers[56] carried out a prospective study of almost 1,000 patients after acute myocardial infarction with the use of ambulatory ECG recording. They subsequently followed these patients for a 2-year period. They reported that the risk of mortality with early-cycle or multiform ventricular premature beats was roughly twice the risk with uniform, late-cycle contractions. They further found that the frequency or the repetitive or bigeminal patterns of ventricular premature beats were not prognostic for death. From their data analysis, they proposed a two-level categorization of the prognostic value of ventricular ectopic beats. They identified a *high-risk group,* composed of patients with either *multiform ventricular premature beats* or *early-cycle ventricular premature beats* (combined presence of these two events is not associated with a significantly higher risk), and a *low-risk group,* comprising patients with *uniform ventricular premature beats* or *late-cycle ventricular premature beats.* In this simplified classification, the frequency of the beats or the occurrence of bigeminal or repetitive patterns was not taken into account, since they were not found to be independent predictors of mortality. The prognostic significance of ventricular premature beats can simply be based on the degree of prematurity and the consistency of the configurational characteristics of the beats. Early-cycle ventricular premature beats appear to be better indicators of electrical instability than late-cycle premature beats. The occurrence of multiform ventricular premature beats probably indicates more extensive areas of electrical instability, providing more locations for the generation of reentry phenomena. The prognostic significance of multiform ventricular premature beats underscores the clinical importance of using two-channel recorders, which increase the probability of accurately identifying such beats. It has not yet been fully documented whether the grading scheme proposed by Moss and colleagues[56] has wider clinical implications beyond the evaluation of patients in the subacute stage of a myocardial infarction.

Before it is appropriate to recommend routine ambulatory ECG recordings shortly after dismissal from the hospital for all patients who have recently had an acute myocardial infarction, we must have more evidence that treating and abolishing asymptomatic high-risk ventricular premature beats prevents or decreases sudden cardiac death or morbidity. Currently, there is no definitive evidence that the suppression of ventricular arrhythmias prevents sudden cardiac death or, on the other hand, that identified high-risk ventricular premature beats can be ignored with impunity.

The most effective treatment for improving survival in patients with recurrent ventricular fibrillation or ventricular tachycardia and cardiac arrest is the implantable cardioverter-defibrillator.[57] The ambulatory ECG has been used to evaluate the clinical performance of this new device. Maloney et al.[58] studied 23 patients with ambulatory ECG monitoring and documented 101 discharges. There were 68 discharges for sustained ventricular tachycardia and 20 for nonsustained ventricular tachycardia. The patients reported that symptoms preceded the firing of the defibrillator in 53% of the sustained episodes and 65% of the nonsustained episodes. All eight discharges for ventricular fibrillation were associated with loss of consciousness. Supraventricular tachycardia and sinus tachycardia triggered five discharges. This ambulatory monitoring of the ECG documented that the implantable device administered clinically appropriate discharges in 75% of the detected arrhythmias.[58]

Syncope

Patients presenting with syncope, near-syncope, or dizziness are often a diagnostic dilemma for the clinician (see chapter 23 for more details). Since these symptoms can often be a manifestation of a disorder of cardiac rhythm, ambulatory ECG recording is a valuable tool in the evaluation of these patients. On occasion, syncope, near-syncope, or dizziness can be due to tachyarrhythmias, and these rhythm disorders have already been described above. When bradyarrhythmia is associated with an alteration in consciousness, the clinical term "Adams-Stokes attack" is used to describe the episode. A great variability in symptoms is reported by patients experiencing Adams-Stokes attacks. The primary feature is the paroxysmal nature of these episodes. Presenting symptoms range from loss of consciousness accompanied by generalized convulsions and incontinence of the bladder and bowel to a brief period of unsteadiness or a feeling of uneasiness. Between these two extremes, patients may present with symptoms of dizziness, confusion, altered vision, or a brief period of weakness. Since transient ischemic attacks due to disorders of the cerebrovascular supply or related to a neurologic disorder may produce identical symptoms, the ambulatory ECG recording has been demonstrated to be an effective method of documenting a cardiac origin of these symptoms.[59,60]

There have been reports of a high incidence of cardiac arrhythmias producing symptoms that suggest transient ischemic attacks and thus masquerade as focal cerebrovascular insufficiency.[61-63] Orthostatic hypotension can produce similar symptoms. Thus, it is important to ask the patient whether the symptoms appear only in the standing or the sitting position and to check the supine and standing blood pressures. In such cases, combining continuous ECG and blood pressure recordings (Avionics) can be most helpful. The physical examination may reveal diminished carotid pulses or carotid bruits, which may indicate underlying obstruction of a carotid artery as the cause of the symptoms. On occasion, the clinical 12-lead ECG may reveal abnormalities, although the symptoms may occur paroxysmally. Clues for a cardiac cause of underlying symptoms may be minor degrees of AV block, evidence of transient periods of asystole, or the presence of alternating bundle-branch block. However, in most cases, the standard ECG does not reveal any clues. The only way to document the cardiac cause of such symptoms is to *record abnormal ECG findings that occur in coincidence with the clinical manifestations.* When this can be shown to occur on several separate occasions, the conclusions can be made with even more conviction. Johansson[63] studied with ambulatory ECG recordings a number of patients presenting with alteration of consciousness, in an attempt to demonstrate any abnormalities in the cardiac rhythm. Johansson reported that 25% of the study group suspected of having Adams-Stokes syncope had experienced their symptoms during the 24 hours of ambulatory ECG recording. In the usual case, he found little additional value of extending the recording for longer periods. In an occasional complicated case, it may be useful to continue the long-term ECG recording until symptoms appear but to analyze only the tape made on the day that symptoms were noted. In some patients it may be impractical or impossible to obtain an ECG recording during the period of alteration of consciousness. In such cases, an alternative diagnostic approach is the use of the telephone transmitter, if the symptoms are of long enough duration and the patient is capable of activating the telephone transmitting equipment. In the occasional patient, if ECG documentation of the cardiac arrhythmia while the patient experiences the symptom is impossible and yet the symptom is a serious one, clinical judgment must be used in deciding whether a pacemaker should be implanted on an empiric basis. However, in these cases, it must be noted that the disappearance of symptoms after implantation of a pacemaker may be coincidental rather than the result of the implanted unit. Johansson[17] reported the spontaneous disappearance of symptoms in 36 patients with syncope or dizziness in which ambulatory ECG could not document an arrhythmia and in whom an artificial pacemaker had not been implanted. Ringqvist and associates[64] reported that ambulatory ECG monitoring was of diagnostic value in 66% of patients with dizziness and 24% of patients presenting with syncope. They stressed that the occurrence of symptoms at least 1 week before the study predicted the occurrence of symptoms during the study.

In many cases of syncope, it is unclear whether the cause is cardiac or neurologic. Beauregard et al.[65] used combined ambulatory ECG and electroencephalographic recording to evaluate 45 patients in whom the cause could be either cardiac or neurologic. Isolated cardiac abnormalities were discovered in 21 patients and isolated electroencephalographic changes in 11; five electroencephalographic abnormalities were consistent with a seizure disorder. Simultaneous ECG and electroencephalographic changes were recorded in four patients, uncovering a seizure disorder as the cause for syncope in a patient with the diagnosis of heart disease and sinus pauses causing syncope in a patient with a previously diagnosed seizure disorder.

One of the most commonly demonstrated disorders is the sinus pause (see chapter 22A). Minor degrees of sinoatrial node abnormalities may be recorded in many otherwise normal persons without their experiencing symptoms (Fig 3C-10,A).

Oddone et al.[66] reported 70 syncopal events during ECG ambulatory monitoring of 10 patients. In four patients, the events were sudden, whereas prodromal symptoms were recorded in four patients. The R-R pause varied from 4.5 to 15 seconds. Results of subsequent electrophysiologic study were normal in seven patients.

In a study of 6,470 consecutive ambulatory monitorings, Hilgard and co-workers[67] found only 52 patients with pauses of three seconds or longer, and only 10% of these patients reported symptoms during the pause. Despite the low incidence of symptoms, 50% of the patients received permanent pacemakers. The subsequent 3-year survival was 78% in the paced group and 85% in the unpaced group. The authors concluded that asymptomatic pauses of 3 seconds or longer do not predict a poor prognosis or require pacing.

In the occasional patient, disorders of sinus node function will alternate with sinus tachycardia. The resulting bradycardia and tachycardia phenomena have been termed the "sick sinus syndrome" or "bradytachy syndrome." The standard 12-lead ECG is usually not of much assistance in diagnosing this not uncommon cardiac disorder, but ambulatory ECG recording has proved most useful in documenting it.[17,68] The sick sinus syndrome has been shown to occur more often in the elderly patient, and the needs for therapy of this arrhythmia have greatly increased the insertion of implanted artificial pacemakers.[69,70]

Disorders of the AV conduction system have often been termed AV block. In the patient presenting with disorders of consciousness or dizziness, the ambulatory ECG has been used to document paroxysmal disturbances of AV conduction as the cause of the symptoms. As discussed in chapter 23, first-degree AV block is characterized by prolonged P-R interval preceding the QRS complex. A prolonged P-R interval can occur on the ambulatory ECG recordings of healthy persons without known cardiac disease during sleep and also when awake if vagal tone is increased, such as with bowel movements or vomiting. This is particularly true in physically conditioned persons. Two types of second-degree AV block have been described – Mobitz type I (Wenckebach) and Mobitz type II. In Mobitz type I block, there is progressive prolongation of the P-R interval until a QRS complex is dropped or blocked (Fig 3C-10,B). In Mobitz type II, the P-R interval remains constant, but not all P waves are followed by a QRS complex. The AV conduction disorder most commonly correlated by the ambulatory ECG recording with symptoms of syncope or dizziness is complete or third-degree AV block (Fig 3C-10,C). Also, as discussed in more detail in chapter 23, in this disorder no P waves are

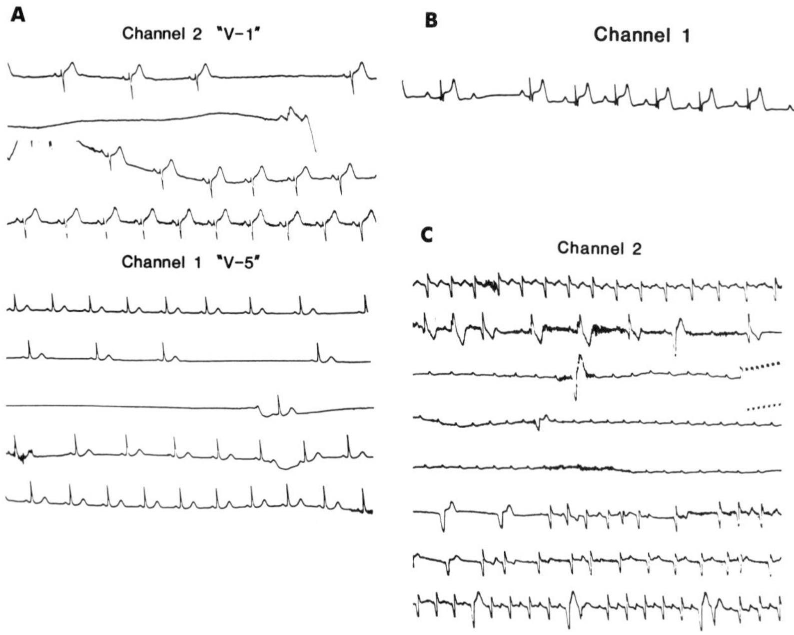

Fig 3C-10 Typical bradyarrhythmias that are recorded on ambulatory ECG recordings and often correlated with symptoms. **A,** sinus arrest. **B,** Mobitz type I AV block. Note that there is progressive prolongation of the P-R interval preceding the blocked QRS complexes. Elevation of the ST segment consistent with ischemia is also demonstrated. **C,** ambulatory ECG finding commonly correlated with syncope. This recording demonstrates intermittent complete (third-degree) heart block. Note in the third line of the recording that the marker was activated before the patient experienced syncope.

conducted from atrium to ventricle, and there is complete independence between the rhythms of atrial depolarizations. On evaluation of the atrial and ventricular ECG complexes, no fixed temporal relationship between the two is found. In a patient with complete AV block, the ventricular pacemaker may arise in the junctional nodal tissue and display a normal-appearing QRS complex. This usually occurs when the site of block is in the AV node. More often, however, the site of the disorder producing the AV block is in the distal bundle of His system, and thus the ventricular pacemaker arises in the distal Purkinje system or cardiac muscle and results in a wide, bizarre QRS complex and a ventricular rate of 25 to 45 beats/min. In many cases of complete third-degree AV block, the standard 12-lead ECG reveals the disorder and is diagnostic. The ambulatory ECG is required when this disorder is intermittent or paroxysmal or when a second-degree AV block intermittently or paroxysmally progresses to a third-degree or complete AV block.

Occasionally, the patient with an implanted artificial pacemaker has a recurrence of syncopal or dizzy spells. In these patients, if the telephonic ECG transmissions fail to reveal an abnormality in pacemaker function, the ambulatory ECG recording may be helpful in attempting to document dysfunction of the pacemaker as a cause of the recurrent symptoms. The most frequent cause of recurrent dizziness or syncope in a patient with an implanted artificial pacemaker is intermittent or paroxysmal failure to pace (Fig 3C-11). These symptoms in the patient with

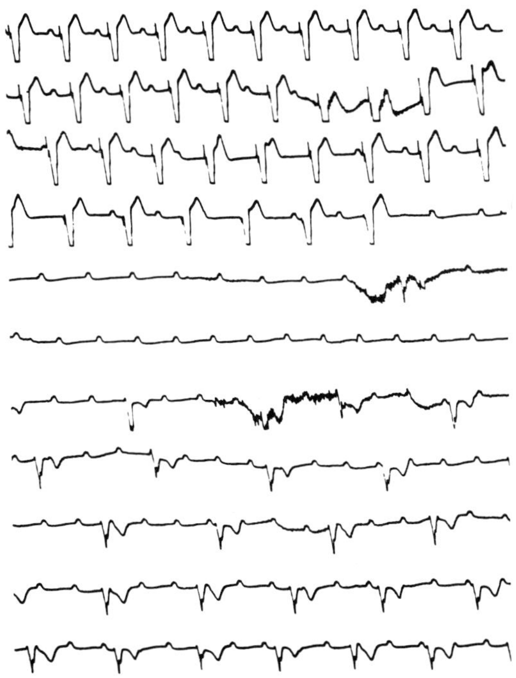

Fig 3C-11 Ambulatory ECG recordings can be useful in evaluating the recurrence of syncopal spells after the insertion of an implantable pacemaker. This recording reveals the intermittent failure of the pacemaker unit in a pacemaker-dependent patient with complete (third-degree) heart block.

an implanted pacemaker, however, may result from intercurrent ventricular tachyarrhythmias occurring in spite of normal function of the pacemaker, and this situation may be revealed by ambulatory ECG monitoring.

When the physician orders an ambulatory ECG recording for a patient with an implanted artificial pacemaker, it is imperative that complete information be provided on the type of implanted pacemaker and model and, if applicable, the mode of programming. In some models of multichannel ambulatory ECG recorders, one channel may be used to record the pacemaker activation spikes. This capability can be useful in evaluating rhythms in patients with an implanted artificial pacemaker.

In a report of 100 consecutive patients with implanted cardiac pacemakers with ambulatory ECG recordings for pacemaker evaluation, Bleifer[71] found that 63 patients noted symptoms of dizziness, lightheadedness, syncope, or palpitations during the recording period. On analysis of the ECG tape, only 17 of these 63 patients with symptoms demonstrated ECG evidence of pacemaker failure, usually failure in sensing. The symptoms that were most likely to be correlated with ECG evidence of pacemaker failure were dizziness and syncope. Janosik and associates[72] reported that in 100 patients on the first day after pacemaker insertion, 42% of the dual-chamber devices and 27% of the single-chamber devices had pacemaker dysfunction on the ambulatory ECG.

Chest pain

The most common presenting complaint of patients who consult a cardiologist is chest pain. In Holter's[73] original report on ambulatory ECG recording, he described the documentation of transient ST-segment changes in patients with chest pain. However, in the early recording instruments, the low-frequency response of the equipment was inadequate, and thus many false-positive ST-T wave deviations occurred; therefore, the usefulness of the ambulatory ECG recording in documenting ischemic ST-T changes was questioned. Current recording units meet the American Heart Association requirements for an adequate low-frequency response (less than 0.05 Hz); thus, they can be used to record ST changes reliably. Silber et al.[74] compared the accuracy of digital ambulatory monitoring with that of analog recording for ischemia and reported that the analog method can overestimate the degree and duration of the ischemic episode. The clinician's first choice of a diagnostic test in a patient with the complaint of chest pain that causes suspicion of ischemic heart disease is often the exercise ECG test. Crawford and colleagues[75] reported on 70 patients evaluated by both treadmill exercise ECG testing and ambulatory ECG recording who subsequently had the extent of their obstructive coronary artery disease documented by coronary angiography. They reported that the exercise ECG was the more sensitive test—67% compared with a sensitivity of 65% for ambulatory ECG recording. The specificity was likewise greater with the exercise ECG—75% compared with 61% for the ambulatory ECG recording. When both tests were utilized,

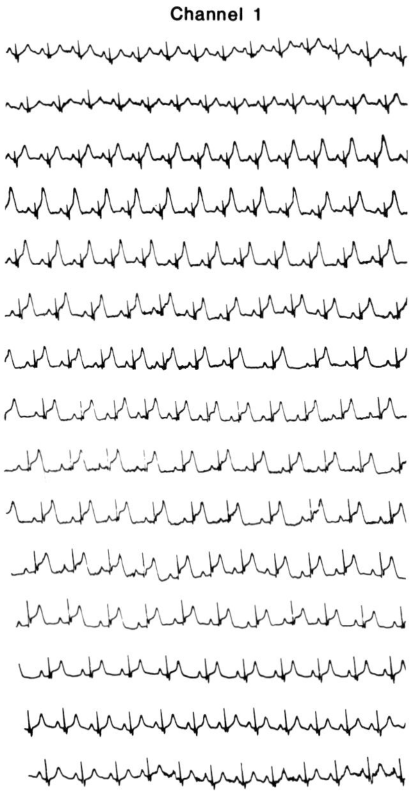

Fig 3C-12 Significant ST elevation that was correlated with chest pain occurring at rest. Note that the normal ST segment before and after persisted for most of the 24-hour period when the patient was free of chest pain.

the sensitivity increased to 85% but specificity decreased to 52%.

The ambulatory ECG recording is likely to be most helpful in evaluating the patient with rest angina or nocturnal angina or episodes of angina precipitated by emotion.[76,77] Araki and colleagues[78] reported that coronary spasms occurring in the early morning are more likely symptomatic. They also reported that complex dysrhythmias can occur during asymptomatic episodes of ischemia and tend to occur when the elevated ST segment is returning toward normal and thus may occur during the "reperfusion period." Angina caused by coronary artery spasm, or "variant angina," is characterized on the ambulatory ECG recording by ST elevation that returns to baseline with the cessation of the pain (Fig 3C-12). It has been estimated that 10% of the angina occurring in patients with coronary artery disease may be due to transient coronary artery spasm. It is important for the cardiologist who is interpreting ambulatory ECG recordings, however, to be aware that transient ST elevations have been described in the ambulatory ECG recordings of normal young persons, and these ECG changes have not been associated with chest pain.[79]

With the current use of calcium blocking agents for the therapy of angina, there has been increasing interest in evaluating the incidence of variant angina that can effectively be treated by these agents. On the other hand, β-blocking agents, which are most often used for the treatment of exertional angina, have also been found to be effective in reducing episodes of ischemia occurring at rest. Thus, ambulatory ECG recording may be of value in evaluating some of these therapeutic interventions.

Ambulatory ECG recordings may also be of use in evaluating the patient with known ischemic heart disease who is having an increase in the frequency or duration of episodes of chest pain during daily activities at home or at work. Schang and Pepine[80] reported the frequent occurrence of ambulatory ECG evidence of episodes of myocardial ischemia which were often asymptomatic and occurred at rest and during physical activities or were precipitated by emotional stress. Ambulatory ECG recordings to detect ischemia may also be valuable for patients in whom the frequency and duration of anginal episodes may contraindicate the performance of an exercise ECG treadmill test or for the physically disabled patient who may be unable to perform an exercise ECG test.

Just as the ambulatory ECG recording has been shown to document the effectiveness of medical or surgical treatment in patients with cardiac arrhythmias, it can also be used to evaluate the effectiveness of treating ischemic heart disease. When the physician uses the ambulatory ECG recording to evaluate ischemic ST-T changes, it is important to determine that the position of the body does not affect the ST segment at the time the equipment is attached to the patient. It must also be realized that just as multiple leads have increased the effectiveness of the exercise ECG test, so also may the availability of multiple ECG leads increase the sensitivity of the ambulatory ECG recording in detecting and localizing the presence of ischemia.

Mitral valve prolapse

Detection of arrhythmias in patients with mitral valve prolapse has received considerable attention because these patients often present with palpitations and also because sudden death, ventricular tachycardia, and ventricular fibrillation have been documented. A wide variety of arrhythmias have been seen, including both supraventricular and ventricular tachycardia and also bradycardia.[81-86] Frequent or complex ventricular arrhythmias have been documented in up to 50% of patients with mitral valve prolapse who have symptomatic palpitations.[81,82] The value of ambulatory monitoring for the purpose of detecting patients without symptoms who are at risk for sudden cardiac death remains uncertain, considering the large number of patients with mitral valve prolapse and the infrequent occurrence of sudden death. In addition, sudden death may occur in patients who have no complex ventricular ectopy. Of course, in patients with palpitations, ambulatory monitoring is very useful for documenting the arrhythmia and directing the treatment.

Hypertrophic cardiomyopathy

The association of sudden death and hypertrophic cardiomyopathy and the lack of specific anatomic or hemodynamic predictors of death has focused attention on arrhythmias in these patients.[87-94] Ambulatory monitoring has documented supraventricular tachycardia or paroxysmal atrial fibrillation in approximately half of these patients.[91] The arrhythmia may be asymptomatic or may be associated with palpitations or cardiac decompensation, particularly if the rate is rapid or the left ventricular outflow obstruction is severe. Ventricular ectopy is also very common, being seen in the majority of patients who undergo ambulatory monitoring. Frequent and complex ventricular arrhythmias are also common, having been identified in 43% to 66% of patients.[90,91,93] In three studies, approximately 20% to 25% of patients had ventricular tachycardia during ambulatory monitoring.[90,91,93] This was often asymptomatic, but its presence did identify a patient population with a significantly increased risk of sudden death.

Patients with symptoms suggestive of arrhythmias

Ambulatory monitoring has been used in patients with episodic dizziness, lightheadedness, syncope, and palpitations in an attempt to correlate symptoms with the ECG.[7,8,38,95,96] The results of ambulatory monitoring in these patients are quite variable, depending in part on the selection of patients for evaluation, the specific complaint, and the frequency of the episodes. Lipski et al.[38] documented significant arrhythmias, particularly bradyarrhythmias, in 55% of patients with syncope, palpitations, or dizziness. In a larger series of 119 patients with presyncope or syncope, Boudoulas et al.[95] documented cardiac arrhythmias considered to be the probable cause of symptoms in 64%. In this regard, it is important to note that symptoms such as dizziness and palpitations may not correlate with arrhythmias and, conversely, that major cardiac arrhythmias may, in fact, be asymptomatic.[96]

EXERCISE TESTING

Exercise testing is often used in the detection of arrhythmias. The major indications include (1) in patients with exercise-induced palpitations or exercise-induced symptoms consistent with a primary rhythm disturbance; (2) for evaluation of the effect of exercise on supraventricular and ventricular ectopy documented during 12-lead electrocardiography or during ambulatory monitoring; and (3) for detection and classification of ventricular ectopy in specific patient subsets, including those with coronary artery disease, hypertrophic obstructive cardiomyopathy, and mitral valve prolapse.

With the use of this technique, several important aspects must be kept in mind: (1) the recording system and exercise protocol used; (2) the type, frequency, and significance of arrhythmias detected during exercise testing in normal and abnormal patients; and (3) spontaneous variability and reproducibility of exercise-induced arrhythmias.

Technical aspects of the recording system play an important role in the detection and evaluation of exercise-induced arrhythmias. The capability of monitoring multiple leads can add information that is of particular importance in distinguishing aberration from ventricular ectopy.[97] In addition, some authors have found that continuous monitoring or real-time playback review of analog tape recordings may increase the yield of arrhythmia detection during exercise testing.[97,98] The amount of exercise performed also affects the yield of arrhythmias. The incidence of arrhythmias has been found to increase during maximal or near-maximal exercise testing.[99,100]

Exercise-induced arrhythmias are common in both normal controls and patients with a variety of cardiovascular diseases. Both supraventricular arrhythmias with atrial ectopy and short paroxysms of atrial tachycardia are seen, as are a wide range of ventricular arrhythmias.[100-106] The prevalence depends on the population studied. In general, the incidence of both supraventricular and ventricular arrhythmias increases with increasing age.[97,105,106] Asymptomatic supraventricular arrhythmias are not associated with increased mortality and morbidity and are seen as often in normal subjects as in patients with cardiovascular disease[106] (Fig 3C-13).

Ventricular arrhythmias have been documented in 20% to 60% of patients undergoing exercise testing.[97,100,102,104,105,107-110] This wide range relates to differences in patient population studied and protocol used. Blackburn et al.[100] documented that the frequency of exercise-induced ventricular premature complexes, the total number detected, and number of patients with ventricular premature complexes increased as the work-

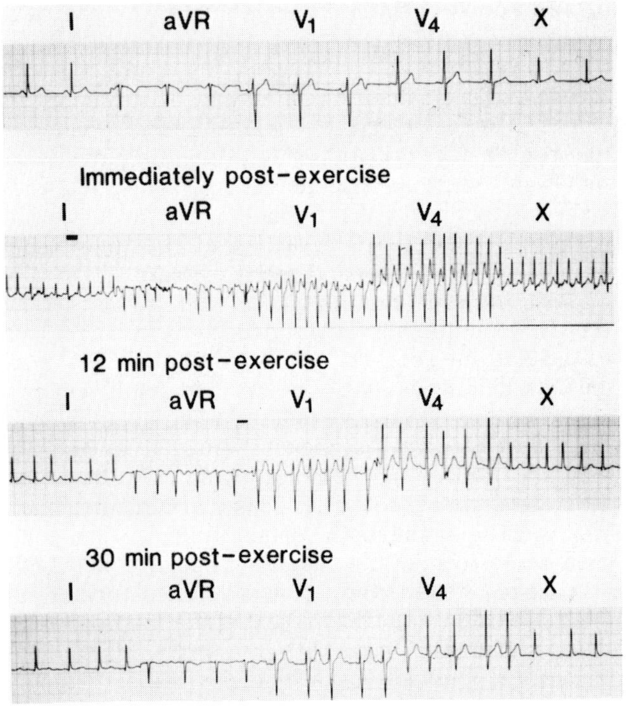

Fig 3C-13 Sinus rhythm documented during exercise test **(top).** As shown in the remaining tracings, immediately after exercise, the patient experienced atrial fibrillation with a rapid ventricular response; the atrial fibrillation persisted at 30 minutes after exercise.

load increased. They found that approximately 50% of symptom-free but high-risk middle-aged men had ventricular premature contractions at a heart rate of more than 173 beats/min. Froelicher et al.[102] and Faris et al.[110] found that 35% and 37% of symptom-free airmen and Indiana state policemen, respectively, had ventricular ectopy with maximal treadmill testing. In patients with normal coronary arteries or in normal young control subjects, the prevalence of exercise-induced ventricular ectopy is lower, ranging from 11% to 16%.[104,107] This contrasts with exercise testing in patients with established coronary artery disease, in whom as many as about 60% have ventricular ectopy.[109] In these patients with coronary artery disease, increased ventricular ectopy is often associated with more extensive coronary artery disease, left ventricular dysfunction, and exercise-induced ischemia with ST depression.[104,107,109]

The frequency of exercise-induced ventricular ectopy in symptom-free patients and normal controls makes the use of this technique suboptimal for identification of patients with occult coronary artery disease. There are some features of ventricular ectopy, however, that can be used to improve its discriminant function. In patients with coronary artery disease, the ventricular ectopy definitely appears at lower rates (< 130 beats/min). In addition, the ventricular ectopy is more frequent and more severe.[97,99,103,107,109]

Ventricular tachycardia or ventricular fibrillation is uncommon during treadmill exercise testing.[108,111] In a study of 7,500 patients undergoing maximal exercise testing, Detry et al.[112] documented ventricular fibrillation or ventricular tachycardia in 46 (0.6%). Ventricular tachycardia may occur either during exercise testing or in the recovery period.[108,113] Usually the ventricular tachycardia is of short duration, but it may be sustained[111,112] (Figs 3C-14 and 3C-15). Irving and Bruce[114] pointed out that ventricular fibrillation may be seen in patients with significant exertional hypotension. Although ventricular tachycardia or ventricular fibrillation may be documented in persons without overt heart disease, it is most usually associated with coronary artery disease.[108,111,112] Of interest, the short-term prognosis with exercise-induced ventricular fibrillation or sustained ventricular tachycardia is relatively poor—a 5-year survival of 43%.[112] Small, uncontrolled series have documented improvement in and abolition of exercise-induced ventricular tachycardia in patients after saphenous vein bypass graft surgery.[108,113,115] A frequent indication for exercise testing is the evaluation of ventricular ectopy documented during 12-lead ECG or ambulatory monitoring. An early goal of exercise testing in this situation was to see whether exercise resulted in suppression of ventricular ectopy and might indicate a more favorable or different prognosis for the patient. This hope has not been substantiated, because suppression of resting ventricular ectopy by exercise does not reliably indicate the absence of significant coronary artery disease.[97,99,104,105,107,109]

Exercise testing has also been used in other patient groups, such as those with hypertrophic obstructive cardiomyopathy and mitral valve prolapse, in an attempt to document arrhythmias and to identify patients who are

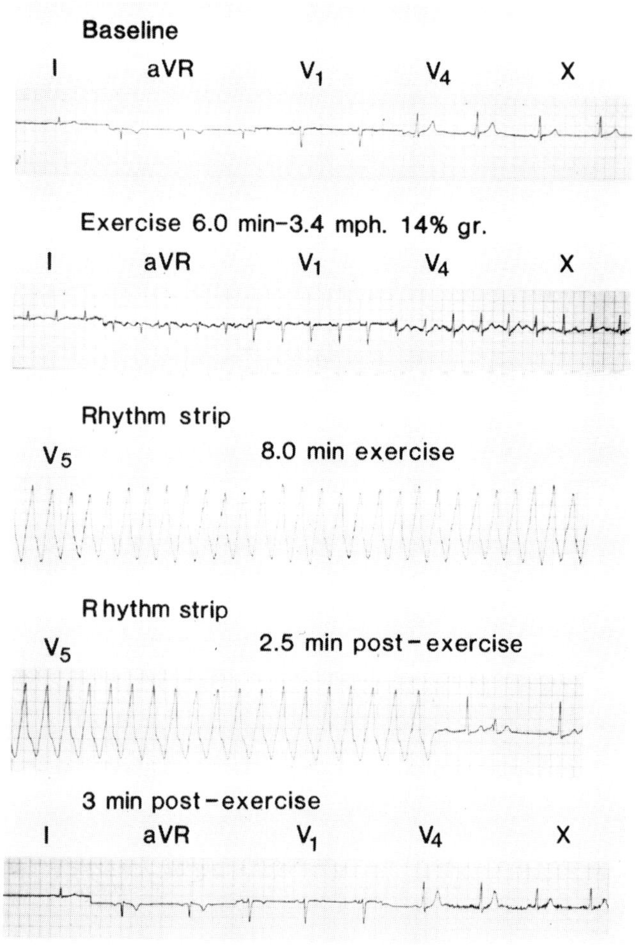

Fig 3C-14 Exercise test with sinus rhythm at baseline. At 8 minutes of exercise the patient experienced hemodynamically stable ventricular tachycardia, which terminated spontaneously 2.5 minutes after exercise.

at risk for sudden death. In patients with hypertrophic obstructive cardiomyopathy, both supraventricular and ventricular arrhythmias are common during exercise. Approximately 50% of selected patients with hypertrophic obstructive cardiomyopathy undergoing exercise testing experience supraventricular arrhythmias; 60% have ventricular arrhythmias, and 28% in this group have complex ventricular ectopy.[90,91] Similarly, in patients with mitral valve prolapse, a wide variety of both symptomatic and asymptomatic ventricular and supraventricular arrhythmias have been documented in up to 75% to 85% of patients.[81,116]

Finally, exercise testing has been used in patients with conduction defects such as sinus node dysfunction and AV block to determine the response to exercise[117-121] (Fig 3C-16). It may be possible to identify the level of AV block. Block occurring at the level of the AV node and related to increased vagal tone improves during exercise, whereas infranodal block usually does not.

Spontaneous variability and the reproducibility of exercise-induced arrhythmias are important factors to be considered in the evaluation of exercise testing. Sheps

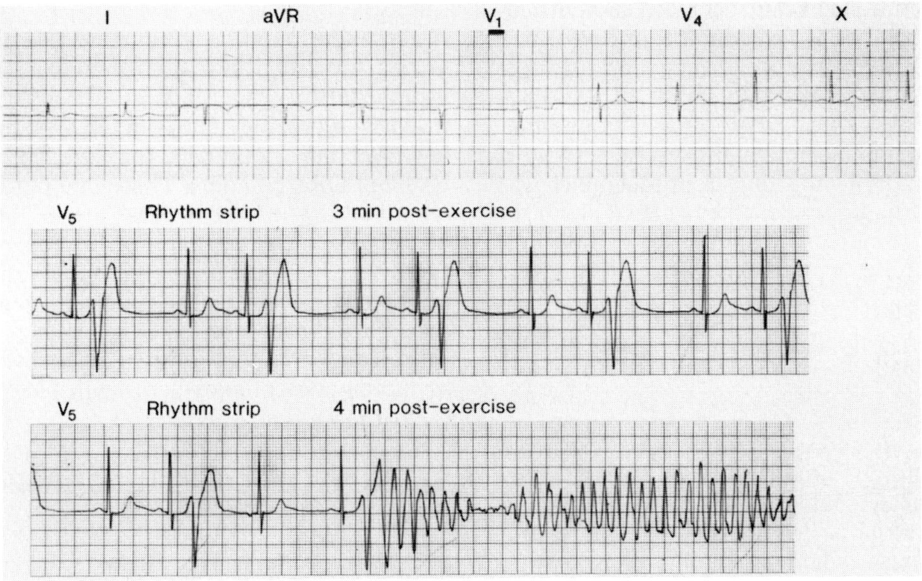

Fig 3C-15 Treadmill exercise test with normal sinus rhythm at baseline. Three minutes after exercise, the patient had ventricular trigeminy and then torsades de pointes. (From Hammill SC, Holmes DR Jr, Wood DL: Cardiac arrhythmias. In *Current Diagnosis 7.* Edited by RB Conn. Philadelphia, WB Saunders Company, 1985, pp 405-433. By permission.)

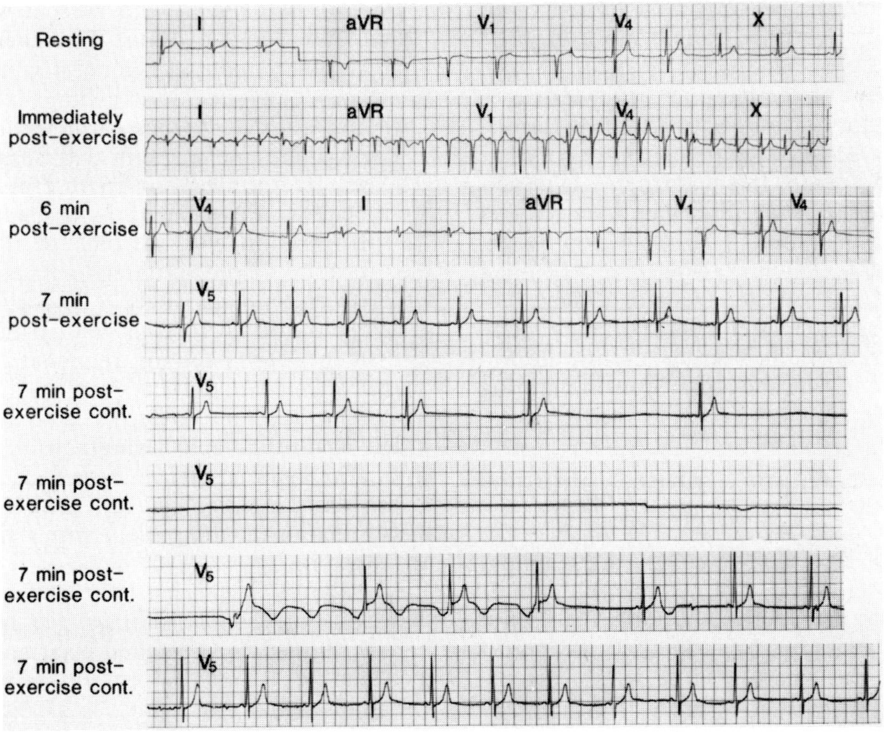

Fig 3C-16 Results of treadmill exercise test in a patient with sinus node dysfunction. Continuous strip starting at 7 minutes after exercise documents sinus arrest and asystole. (From Hammill SC, Holmes DR Jr, Wood DL: Cardiac arrhythmias. In *Current Diagnosis 7.* Edited by RB Conn. Philadelphia, WB Saunders Company, 1985, pp 405-433. By permission.)

et al.[122] documented a significant decrease in ventricular ectopy in the second of two treadmill tests performed 45 minutes apart. This was confirmed in a longer longitudinal study of the reproducibility of exercise-induced ventricular arrhythmias. Faris et al.[110] found that of 543 patients undergoing treadmill exercise tests at a mean of 2.9 years apart, individual reproducibility was only slightly higher than occurrence by chance alone. In patients with symptomatic arrhythmias that can be reliably induced by exercise, reproducibility from test to test may be higher.

Ambulatory monitoring vs. treadmill exercise testing

Ambulatory monitoring and treadmill exercise tests have specific strengths and potential weaknesses. Ambulatory monitoring results in a higher yield of ventricular arrhythmias and also of atrial arrhythmias.[123-130] There are, however, some patients in whom treadmill exercise testing will provoke arrhythmias that are not seen during ambulatory monitoring. In addition, important information on exercise tolerance, blood pressure response to exercise, and ST-segment changes is also available with treadmill exercise tests.[128-130] The pathophysiology of arrhythmias provoked by exercise may, of course, be different from that of arrhythmias seen with ordinary activity. This may affect the natural history of these arrhythmias and mandate different treatment strategies, such as the use of β-blockade in patients with exercise-induced arrhythmias. The two methods may provide different prognostic information. Ivanova et al.[129] found that in patients with arteriosclerotic heart disease, the absence of frequent or complex ventricular extrasystoles during ambulatory monitoring after myocardial infarction identifies a subset of patients with a very low risk of sudden cardiac death. In similar patients undergoing treadmill exercise testing, documentation of frequent ventricular arrhythmias, ST-segment depression, and reduced maximal exercise heart rate identified patients with a high risk of sudden cardiac death. In identifying certain subsets of patients with coronary artery disease who are at risk for future cardiac events, the two techniques of exercise testing and ambulatory monitoring may be complementary.

Ambulatory monitoring vs. transtelephonic event recording

Limited information is available comparing ambulatory monitoring with telephone transmitter event recorders. Judson et al.,[8] in a select group of patients referred for evaluation of palpitations, found that the transtelephonic method was more useful in documenting intermittent symptomatic arrhythmias. Certainly, an event recorder with a memory loop has significant advantages, because it can record the onset of an arrhythmia or a spell. In addition, the cost of an event recorder is significantly lower than that of ambulatory monitoring.

SIGNAL-AVERAGED ECG

A new and expanding noninvasive test to identify patients at risk for ventricular arrhythmias is the use of signal-averaged ECG (see chapter 3D).[131,132] This technique involves averaging multiple QRS complexes to expose low-level late potentials that are contiguous with the terminal QRS complex. These late potentials are usually identified in the border zones around areas of infarction or fibrosis in ventricular myocardium. Identification of these late potentials, therefore, identifies the electrophysiologic substrate for reentrant ventricular arrhythmias. Signal-averaged ECG is now being used in patient subsets at risk for ventricular arrhythmias, including asymptomatic complex ventricular ectopy and postmyocardial infarction.

SELECTION OF THE MEANS OF EVALUATION

Selection of the most effective means of evaluating disturbances in cardiac rhythm involves attention to the nature, severity, and frequency of the complaints and the relative merits, strengths, and weaknesses of each of the options discussed. Very few studies have compared all of the diagnostic options. Some comparative information is available, however (Table 3C-1).

SUMMARY AND CONCLUSIONS

The detection of any arrhythmia is only one step in the evaluation of patients who present with cardiovascular complaints. The arrhythmia must then be placed in the context of the patient's general condition. Often, the prognosis of any specific arrhythmia is related specifically to the patient's underlying cardiovascular disease.

The evaluation of patients with suspected arrhythmias requires careful attention to several specific areas: (1) identification of associated disease states that may affect the presentation and outcome of the arrhythmia, (2) identification of precipitating causes and results of previous treatment regimens, (3) documentation of the arrhythmia and correlation with patient symptoms, (4) assessment of the need for treatment and selection of the proper regimen, and (5) documentation of success of the treatment. Several well-proved diagnostic modalities are widely available, each having advantages and disadvantages. The combination of these tests plus careful use of invasive electrophysiologic testing has done much to aid in the evaluation of the patient with "flip-flops, fluttering, and skipping."

Ambulatory ECG is most likely to be clinically useful in the following clinical settings: (1) for patients whose history suggests the repeated occurrence of disorders in the heartbeat in the form of palpitations or other symptoms, (2) for patients with transient episodes of syncope or near-syncope, and (3) for patients with transient episodes of chest pain that are not related to exertion or that awaken the patient from sleep, suggesting the possibility of coronary artery spasm. Before ordering the ambulatory ECG recording, the physician should

Table 3C-1 Comparison of techniques for noninvasive evaluation of arrhythmias

	Transtelephonic monitoring system	Ambulatory monitoring	Exercise testing	Signal-averaged ECG
Application	Documentation of intermittent palpitations or dizziness Analysis of pacemaker function Detection of asymptomatic ventricular ectopy after myocardial infarction	Documentation of intermittent palpitations or dizziness Detection of ventricular ectopy after myocardial infarction and in specific patient subsets Documentation of symptomatic and asymptomatic rhythm disturbances Assessment of drug efficacy Analysis of pacemaker function	Documentation of exercise or catecholamine-induced spells Detection of arrhythmias during exercise testing for evaluation of chest pain Detection of arrhythmias during recovery from acute myocardial infarction	Identification of patients who will have inducible, sustained monomorphic ventricular tachycardia at the time of electrophysiologic testing Patient subsets: asymptomatic complex ventricular ectopy, history of sustained ventricular tachycardia, syncope, history of wide-complex tachycardia, post-myocardial infarction, follow-up of patients after electrosurgery
Advantages	Correlation of rhythm disturbances at the precise time of patient symptoms Very useful for infrequent spells Inexpensive	Detection of both symptomatic and asymptomatic arrhythmias Correlation of symptoms with heart rhythm (patient diary) Ability to record the onset and termination of spells Multichannel recorder	Documentation of associated physiologic parameters such as heart rate response to exercise, maximum workload achieved, blood pressure response to exercise, and ST-T abnormalities Multichannel to allow for documentation of ventricular ectopy vs. aberration Facilitates assessment of the effect of ischemia on arrhythmias	Identification of substrate for arrhythmias Identification of patients at risk for arrhythmias Inexpensive
Disadvantages	Not useful in patients with syncope or pronounced hemodynamic compromise during their spells No memory loop for the onset of ECG abnormalities and symptoms Symptoms must be of sufficient duration to allow transmission Access to 24-hour monitoring necessary Technique cannot detect asymptomatic rhythm disturbances	Expensive Standard equipment not practical in patients with very intermittent or infrequent spells; these patients require newer and more costly event recorders, which must be worn for prolonged periods Special equipment needed for analysis Prolonged monitoring difficult	Expensive Requires special equipment Not as sensitive for arrhythmias as Holter monitoring Limited window of observation for spell detection	Limited utility in patients with bundle-branch block Low positive predictive accuracy

consider whether there is reasonable likelihood that some ECG clues to the patient's symptoms may be revealed by the procedure.

In utilizing the ambulatory ECG for evaluating ventricular arrhythmias, we must keep in mind that many questions about the prognostic meaning of the occurrence of asymptomatic ventricular premature beats or their suppression with drugs have not been resolved. Still, the ambulatory ECG recording remains a valuable clinical tool for documenting the occurrence and variety of ventricular arrhythmias in patients with cardiovascular disease, in both the home and the workplace.[133] Ambulatory ECG recordings can also be useful in documenting the effect of exercise, sleep-awake cycles, and the efficacy of both medical and surgical therapeutic interventions on the occurrence of ventricular arrhythmias in patients with cardiac disorders.

The uses for ambulatory recording of the ECG will likely expand in the future as continued clinical research defines additional roles for this technique. Developmental work is being carried out on the use of an esophageal lead system during ambulatory ECG recording for better study of supraventricular arrhythmias.

REFERENCES

1. Brodsky M, Wu D, Denes P, et al: Arrhythmias documented by 24 hour continuous electrocardiographic monitoring in 50 male medical students without apparent heart disease. *Am J Cardiol* 39:390-395, 1977
2. Dickinson DF, Scott O: Ambulatory electrocardiographic monitoring in 100 healthy teenage boys. *Br Heart J* 51:179-183, 1984
3. Romhilt DW, Chaffin C, Choi SC, et al: Arrhythmias on ambulatory electrocardiographic monitoring in women without apparent heart disease. *Am J Cardiol* 54:582-586, 1984
4. Kantelip J-P, Sage E, Duchene-Marullaz P: Findings on ambulatory electrocardiographic monitoring in subjects older than 80 years. *Am J Cardiol* 57:398-401, 1986
5. Ogawa S, Tabata H, Ohishi S, et al: Prognostic significance of long ventricular pauses in athletes. *Jpn Circ J* 55:761-766, 1991
6. Shapiro E: The electrocardiogram and the arrhythmias: historical insights. In *Cardiac Arrhythmias: Their Mechanisms, Diagnosis, and Management.* Edited by WJ Mandel. Philadelphia, JB Lippincott Company, 1980, pp 1-11
7. Grodman RS, Capone RJ, Most AS: Arrhythmia surveillance by transtelephonic monitoring: comparison with Holter monitoring in symptomatic ambulatory patients. *Am Heart J* 98:459-464, 1979
8. Judson P, Holmes DR, Baker WP: Evaluation of outpatient arrhythmias utilizing transtelephonic monitoring. *Am Heart J* 97:759-761, 1979
9. Tuttle WB, Lee DW, Schoenfeld CD: Daily transtelephonic electrocardiographic monitoring of convalescent myocardial infarction patients (abstract). *Am J Cardiol* 41:399, 1978
10. Hasin Y, David D, Rogel S: Diagnostic and therapeutic assessment by telephone electrocardiographic monitoring of ambulatory patients. *Br Med J* 2:609-612, 1976
11. Furman S, Escher DJW: Transtelephone pacemaker monitoring: five years later. *Ann Thorac Surg* 20:326-337, 1975
12. Rubin JW, Ellison RG, Moore HV, et al: Influence of telephone surveillance on pacemaker patient care. *J Thorac Cardiovasc Surg* 79:218-226, 1980
13. Reiffel JA, Schulhof E, Joseph B, et al: Optimum duration of transtelephonic ECG monitoring when used for transient symptomatic event detection. *J Electrocardiol* 24:165-168, 1991
14. Squires RW, Miller TD, Harn T, et al: Transtelephonic electrocardiographic monitoring of cardiac rehabilitation exercise sessions in coronary artery disease. *Am J Cardiol* 67:962-964, 1991
15. ACC/AHA Task Force: Guidelines for ambulatory electrocardiography: a report of the American College of Cardiology/American Heart Association Task Force on Assessment of Diagnostic and Therapeutic Cardiovascular Procedures (Subcommittee on Ambulatory Electrocardiography). *Circulation* 79:206-215, 1989
16. Sheps SG, Elveback LR, Close EL, et al: Evaluation of the Del Mar Avionics automatic ambulatory blood pressure-recording device. *Mayo Clin Proc* 56:740-743, 1981
17. Johansson BW: Evaluation of alteration of consciousness and palpitations. In *Ambulatory Electrocardiographic Recording.* Edited by NK Wenger, MB Mock, I Ringqvist. Chicago, Year Book Medical Publishers, 1981, pp 321-330
18. Goldberg AD, Raftery EB, Cashman PMM: Ambulatory electrocardiographic records in patients with transient cerebral attacks or palpitation. *Br Med J* 4:569-571, 1975
19. Kennedy HL, Chandra V, Sayther KL, et al: Effectiveness of increasing hours of continuous ambulatory electrocardiography in detecting maximal ventricular ectopy: continuous 48 hour study of patients with coronary heart disease and normal subjects. *Am J Cardiol* 42:925-930, 1978
20. Harrison DC, Fitzgerald JW, Winkle RA: Contribution of ambulatory electrocardiographic monitoring to antiarrhythmic management. *Am J Cardiol* 41:996-1004, 1978
21. Morganroth J, Michelson EL, Horowitz LN, et al: Limitations of routine long-term electrocardiographic monitoring to assess ventricular ectopic frequency. *Circulation* 58:408-414, 1978
22. Winkle RA: Antiarrhythmic drug effect mimicked by spontaneous variability of ventricular ectopy. *Circulation* 57:1116-1121, 1978
23. Michelson EL, Morganroth J: Spontaneous variability of complex ventricular arrhythmias detected by long-term electrocardiographic recording. *Circulation* 61:690-695, 1980
24. Morganroth J: Evaluation of arrhythmias in clinical trials: relationship to the spontaneous variability of ventricular arrhythmias. In *Ambulatory Electrocardiographic Recording.* Edited by NK Wenger, MB Mock, I Ringqvist. Chicago, Year Book Medical Publishers, 1981, pp 285-298
25. Myerburg RJ, Conde C, Sheps DS, et al: Antiarrhythmic drug therapy in survivors of prehospital cardiac arrest: comparison of effects on chronic ventricular arrhythmias and recurrent cardiac arrest. *Circulation* 59:855-863, 1979
26. Rosen KM, Brodsky M, Mayer J, et al: Arrhythmias in individuals without apparent heart disease. In *Ambulatory Electrocardiographic Recording.* Edited by NK Wenger, MB Mock, I Ringqvist. Chicago, Year Book Medical Publishers, 1981, pp 273-284
27. Meytes I, Kaplinsky E, Yahini JH, et al: Wenckebach A-V block: a frequent feature following heavy physical training. *Am Heart J* 90:426-430, 1975
28. Sobotka PA, Mayer JH, Bauernfeind RA, et al: Arrhythmias documented by 24-hour continuous ambulatory electrocardiographic monitoring in young women without apparent heart disease. *Am Heart J* 101:753-759, 1981
29. Gambetta M, Denes P, Childers RW: Vagally induced second degree A-V block Mobitz type I, and the hyporeactive SA node. *Chest* 62:152-155, 1972
30. Clarke JM, Hamer J, Shelton JR, et al: The rhythm of the normal human heart. *Lancet* 2:508-512, 1976
31. Camm AJ, Evans KE, Ward DE, et al: The rhythm of the heart in active elderly subjects. *Am Heart J* 99:598-603, 1980
32. Glasser SP, Clark PI, Applebaum HJ: Occurrence of frequent complex arrhythmias detected by ambulatory monitoring: findings in an apparently healthy asymptomatic elderly population. *Chest* 75:565-568, 1979
33. Hinkle LE Jr, Carver ST, Stevens M: The frequency of asymptomatic disturbances of cardiac rhythm and conduction in middle-aged men. *Am J Cardiol* 24:629-650, 1969
34. Kennedy HL, Sprague MK, Shriver KK, et al: Real-time analysis ambulatory electrocardiography—clinical evaluation of cardiac arrhythmias by the Aegis system. *J Electrocardiol* 20:247-254, 1987
35. Kennedy HL, Underhill SJ, Warbasse JR: Practical advantages of two-channel electrocardiographic Holter recordings. *Am Heart J* 91:822-823, 1976
36. Campbell RW, Gardiner P, Murray A: Automatic analysis of ambulatory ECG records. *Eur Heart J* 5 Suppl B:31-34, 1984
37. Kennedy HL, Ratcliff JW: Ambulatory electrocardiography and computer technology—practical advantages. *Am Heart J* 113:186-193, 1987
38. Lipski J, Cohen L, Espinoza J, et al: Value of Holter monitoring in assessing cardiac arrhythmias in symptomatic patients. *Am J Cardiol* 37:102-107, 1976
39. Bigger JT Jr, Heller CA, Wenger TL, et al: Risk stratification after acute myocardial infarction. *Am J Cardiol* 42:202-210, 1978

40. Davis BR, Friedman LM, Lichstein E: Are 24 hours of ambulatory ECG monitoring necessary for a patient after infarction? *Am Heart J* 115:83-91, 1988

41. Cumbee SR, Pryor RE, Linzer M: Cardiac loop ECG recording: a new noninvasive diagnostic test in recurrent syncope. *South Med J* 83:39-43, 1990

42. Kostis JB, Moreyra AE, Natarajan N, et al: Ambulatory electrocardiography: what is normal? (abstract.) *Am J Cardiol* 43:420, 1979

43. Kennedy HL, Pescarmona JE, Bouchard RJ, et al: Coronary artery status of apparently healthy subjects with frequent and complex ventricular ectopy. *Ann Intern Med* 92:179-185, 1980

44. Viitasalo M, Halonen L, Partinen M, et al: Sleep and cardiac rhythm in healthy men. *Ann Med* 23:135-139, 1991

45. Corday E, Bazika V, Lang T-W, et al: Detection of phantom arrhythmias and evanescent electrocardiographic abnormalities: use of prolonged direct electrocardiocording. *JAMA* 193:417-421, 1965

46. Krasnow AZ, Bloomfield DK: The relationship between subjective symptomatology and objective findings from ambulatory ECG monitoring studies in a large unselected population. In *Ambulatory ECG Monitoring: A Monograph.* Edited by S Stern. Chicago, Year Book Medical Publishers, 1978, pp 149-169

47. Clarke JM, Hamer J, Shelton JR, et al: The rhythm of the normal human heart. *Lancet* 2:508-512, 1976

48. Bjerregaard P, Sorensen KE, Molgaard H: Predictive value of ventricular premature beats for subsequent ischaemic heart disease in apparently healthy subjects. *Eur Heart J* 12:597-601, 1991

49. Savage HR, Kissane JQ, Becher EL, et al: Analysis of ambulatory electrocardiograms in 14 patients who experienced sudden cardiac death during monitoring. *Clin Cardiol* 10:621-632, 1987

50. Lewis BH, Antman EM, Graboys TB: Detailed analysis of 24 hour ambulatory electrocardiographic recordings during ventricular fibrillation or torsades de pointes. *J Am Coll Cardiol* 2:426-436, 1983

51. Ruberman W, Weinblatt E, Goldberg JD, et al: Ventricular premature beats and mortality after myocardial infarction. *N Engl J Med* 297:750-757, 1977

52. Lown B, Wolf M: Approaches to sudden death from coronary heart disease. *Circulation* 44:130-142, 1971

53. El-Sherif N, Myerburg RJ, Scherlag BJ, et al: Electrocardiographic antecedents of primary ventricular fibrillation: value of R-on-T phenomenon in myocardial infarction. *Br Heart J* 38:415-422, 1976

54. Bigger JT Jr, Wenger TL, Heissenbuttel RH: Limitations of the Lown grading system for the study of human ventricular arrhythmias. *Am Heart J* 93:727-729, 1977

55. McCollam PL, Parker RB: Evaluation and treatment of ventricular arrhythmias: an update. *Clin Pharm* 10:195-205, 1991

56. Moss AJ, Davis HT, DeCamilla J, et al: Ventricular ectopic beats and their relation to sudden and nonsudden cardiac death after myocardial infarction. *Circulation* 60:998-1003, 1979

57. Saksena S: Current application of implantable cardioverter-defibrillators in the management of malignant ventricular tachyarrhythmias. *Cardiology* 77:181-194, 1990

58. Maloney J, Masterson M, Khoury D, et al: Clinical performance of the implantable cardioverter defibrillator: electrocardiographic documentation of 101 spontaneous discharges. *PACE* 14:280-285, 1991

59. Kapoor WN, Karpf M, Wieand S, et al: A prospective evaluation and follow-up of patients with syncope. *N Engl J Med* 309:197-204, 1983

60. Kapoor WN: Diagnostic evaluation of syncope. *Am J Med* 90:91-106, 1991

61. McAllen PM, Marshall J: Cardiac dysrhythmia and transient cerebral ischaemic attacks. *Lancet* 1:1212-1214, 1973

62. Walter PF, Reid SD Jr, Wenger NK: Transient cerebral ischemia due to arrhythmia. *Ann Intern Med* 72:471-474, 1970

63. Johansson BW: Adams-Stokes syndrome: a review and follow-up study of forty-two cases. *Am J Cardiol* 8:76-93, 1961

64. Ringqvist I, Jonason T, Nilsson G, et al: Diagnostic value of longterm ambulatory ECG in patients with syncope, dizziness or palpitations. *Clin Physiol* 9:47-55, 1989

65. Beauregard L-A, Fabiszewski R, Black CH, et al: Combined ambulatory electroencephalographic and electrocardiographic recordings for evaluation of syncope. *Am J Cardiol* 68:1067-1072, 1991

66. Oddone D, Brignole M, Menozzi C, et al: Spontaneous occurrence of the induced cardioinhibitory vasovagal reflex. *PACE* 14:415-419, 1991

67. Hilgard J, Ezri MD, Denes P: Significance of ventricular pauses of three seconds or more detected on twenty-four-hour Holter recordings. *Am J Cardiol* 55:1005-1008, 1985

68. Szatmáry LJ: Autonomic blockade and sick sinus syndrome. New concept in the interpretation of electrophysiological and Holter data. *Eur Heart J* 5:637-648, 1984

69. Ferrer MI: The sick sinus syndrome. *Circulation* 47:635-641, 1973

70. Gann D, Tolentino A, Samet P: Electrophysiologic evaluation of elderly patients with sinus bradycardia: a long-term follow-up study. *Ann Intern Med* 90:24-29, 1979

71. Bleifer SB: Evaluation of implanted pacemaker function. In *Ambulatory Electrocardiographic Recording.* Edited by NK Wenger, MB Mock, I Ringqvist. Chicago, Year Book Medical Publishers, 1981, pp 341-351

72. Janosik DL, Redd RM, Buckingham TA, et al: Utility of ambulatory electrocardiography in detecting pacemaker dysfunction in the early postimplantation period. *Am J Cardiol* 60:1030-1035, 1987

73. Holter NJ: New method for heart studies: continuous electrocardiography of active subjects over long periods is now practical. *Science* 134:1214-1220, 1961

74. Silber S, Bajaj RK, Kirk KA, et al: Accuracy of digital Holter monitoring of extent and duration of ischemic episodes compared to analog recording. *Am J Cardiol* 65:383-388, 1990

75. Crawford MH, Mendoza CA, O'Rourke RA, et al: Limitations of continuous ambulatory electrocardiogram monitoring for detecting coronary artery disease. *Ann Intern Med* 89:1-5, 1978

76. Stern S, Tzivoni D: Dynamic changes in the ST-T segments during sleep in ischemic heart disease. *Am J Cardiol* 32:17-20, 1973

77. Maseri A, L'Abbate A, Pesola A, et al: Coronary vasospasm in angina pectoris. *Lancet* 1:713-717, 1977

78. Araki H, Koiwaya Y, Nakagaki O, et al: Diurnal distribution of ST-segment elevation and related arrhythmias in patients with variant angina: a study by ambulatory ECG monitoring. *Circulation* 67:995-1000, 1983

79. Stern S, Tzivoni D: Evaluation for ischemic ST-T changes. In *Ambulatory Electrocardiographic Recording.* Edited by NK Wenger, MB Mock, I Ringqvist. Chicago, Year Book Medical Publishers, 1981, p 358

80. Schang SJ Jr, Pepine CJ: Transient asymptomatic S-T segment depression during daily activity. *Am J Cardiol* 39:396-402, 1977

81. Winkle RA, Lopes MG, Fitzgerald JW, et al: Arrhythmias in patients with mitral valve prolapse. *Circulation* 52:73-81, 1975

82. DeMaria AN, Amsterdam EA, Vismara LA, et al: Arrhythmias in the mitral valve prolapse syndrome: prevalence, nature, and frequency. *Ann Intern Med* 84:656-660, 1976

83. Winkle RA, Lopes MG, Popp RL, et al: Life-threatening arrhythmias in the mitral valve prolapse syndrome. *Am J Med* 60:961-967, 1976

84. Wei JY, Bulkley BH, Schaeffer AH, et al: Mitral-valve prolapse syndrome and recurrent ventricular tachyarrhythmias: a malignant variant refractory to conventional drug therapy. *Ann Intern Med* 89:6-9, 1978

85. Jeresaty RM: Sudden death in the mitral valve prolapse-click syndrome (editorial). *Am J Cardiol* 37:317-318, 1976

86. Leichtman D, Nelson R, Gobel FL, et al: Bradycardia with mitral valve prolapse: a potential mechanism of sudden death. *Ann Intern Med* 85:453-457, 1976

87. Maron BJ, Roberts WC, Edwards JE, et al: Sudden death in patients with hypertrophic cardiomyopathy: characterization of 26 patients without functional limitation. *Am J Cardiol* 41:803-810, 1978

88. Goodwin JF, Krikler DM: Arrhythmia as a cause of sudden death in hypertrophic cardiomyopathy. *Lancet* 2:937-940, 1976

89. Maron BJ, Lipson LC, Roberts WC, et al: "Malignant" hypertrophic cardiomyopathy: identification of a subgroup of families with unusually frequent premature death. *Am J Cardiol* 41:1133-1140, 1978

90. Savage DD, Seides SF, Maron BJ, et al: Prevalence of arrhythmias during 24-hour electrocardiographic monitoring and exercise testing in patients with obstructive and nonobstructive hypertrophic cardiomyopathy. *Circulation* 59:866-875, 1979

91. McKenna WJ, Chetty S, Oakley CM, et al: Arrhythmia in hypertrophic cardiomyopathy: exercise and 48 hour ambulatory electrocardiographic assessment with and without beta adrenergic blocking therapy. *Am J Cardiol* 45:1-5, 1980

92. Canedo MI, Frank MJ, Abdulla AM: Rhythm disturbances in hypertrophic cardiomyopathy: prevalence, relation to symptoms and management. *Am J Cardiol* 45:848-855, 1980

93. Maron BJ, Savage DD, Wolfson JK, et al: Prognostic significance of 24 hour ambulatory electrocardiographic monitoring in patients with hypertrophic cardiomyopathy: a prospective study. *Am J Cardiol* 48:252-257, 1981
94. Ingham RE, Rossen RM, Goodman DJ, et al: Ambulatory electrocardiographic monitoring in idiopathic hypertrophic subaortic stenosis (abstract). *Circulation* 52 Suppl 2:93, 1975
95. Boudoulas H, Schaal SF, Lewis RP, et al: Superiority of 24 hour output monitoring over multistage exercise testing for the evaluation of syncope. *J Electrocardiol* 12:103-108, 1979
96. Zeldis SM, Levine BJ, Michelson EL, et al: Cardiovascular complaints: correlation with cardiac arrhythmias on 24-hour electrocardiographic monitoring. *Chest* 78:456-462, 1980
97. Faris JV, Morris SN: Detection, prevalence, and significance of arrhythmias during exercise. *Heart Lung* 10:644, 1981
98. Antman E, Graboys TB, Lown B: Continuous monitoring for ventricular arrhythmias during exercise tests. *JAMA* 241:2802-2805, 1979
99. Morris SN, McHenry PL: Cardiac arrhythmias during exercise testing and exercise conditioning. *Cardiovasc Clin* 9 No 3:57-68, 1978
100. Blackburn H, Taylor HL, Hamrell B, et al: Premature ventricular complexes induced by stress testing: their frequency and response to physical conditioning. *Am J Cardiol* 31:441-449, 1973
101. Gooch AS: Exercise testing for detecting changes in cardiac rhythm and conduction. *Am J Cardiol* 30:741-746, 1972
102. Froelicher VF Jr, Thomas MM, Pillow C, et al: Epidemiologic study of asymptomatic men screened by maximal treadmill testing for latent coronary artery disease. *Am J Cardiol* 34:770-776, 1974
103. Goldberg AN: Exercise stress testing in the uncovering of dysrhythmias. *Med Clin North Am* 60:315-324, March 1976
104. Goldschlager N, Cake D, Cohn K: Exercise-induced ventricular arrhythmias in patients with coronary artery disease: their relation to angiographic findings. *Am J Cardiol* 31:434-440, 1973
105. Udall JA, Ellestad MH: Predictive implications of ventricular premature contractions associated with treadmill stress testing. *Circulation* 56:985-989, 1977
106. McHenry PL, Fisch C, Jordan JW, et al: Cardiac arrhythmias observed during maximal treadmill testing in clinically normal men. *Am J Cardiol* 29:331-336, 1972
107. McHenry PL, Morris SN, Kavalier M, et al: Comparative study of exercise-induced ventricular arrhythmias in normal subjects and patients with documented coronary artery disease. *Am J Cardiol* 37:609-616, 1976
108. Talbot S, Kilpatrick D, Krikler D, et al: Ventricular tachycardia due to cardiac ischaemia: assessment by exercise electrocardiography. *Br Med J* 2:733-736, 1978
109. Helfant RH, Pine R, Kabde V, et al: Exercise-related ventricular premature complexes in coronary heart disease: correlations with ischemia and angiographic severity. *Ann Intern Med* 80:589-592, 1974
110. Faris JV, McHenry PL, Jordan JW, et al: Prevalence and reproducibility of exercise-induced ventricular arrhythmias during maximal exercise testing in normal men. *Am J Cardiol* 37:617-622, 1976
111. Codini MA, Sommerfeldt L, Eybel CE, et al: Clinical significance and characteristics of exercise-induced ventricular tachycardia (abstract). *Circulation* 60 Suppl 2:264, 1979
112. Detry JM, Abouantoun S, Wyns W: Incidence and prognostic implications of severe ventricular arrhythmias during maximal exercise testing. *Cardiology* 68 Suppl 2:35-43, 1981
113. Codini MA, Sommerfeldt L, Eybel CE, et al: Efficacy of coronary bypass grafting in exercise-induced ventricular tachycardia. *J Thorac Cardiovasc Surg* 81:502-506, 1981
114. Irving JB, Bruce RA: Exertional hypotension and postexertional ventricular fibrillation in stress testing. *Am J Cardiol* 39:849-851, 1977
115. Bryson AL, Parisi AF, Schechter E, et al: Life-threatening ventricular arrhythmias induced by exercise: cessation after coronary bypass surgery. *Am J Cardiol* 32:995-999, 1973
116. Gooch AS, Vicencio F, Maranhao V, et al: Arrhythmias and left ventricular asynergy in the prolapsing mitral leaflet syndrome. *Am J Cardiol* 29:611-620, 1972
117. Abbott JA, Hirschfeld DS, Kunkel FW, et al: Graded exercise testing in patients with sinus node dysfunction. *Am J Med* 62:330-338, 1977
118. Gooch AS, McConnell D: Analysis of transient arrhythmias and conduction disturbances during submaximal treadmill exercise testing. *Prog Cardiovasc Dis* 13:293-307, 1970
119. Bakst A, Goldberg B, Schamroth L: Significance of exercise-induced second degree atrioventricular block. *Br Heart J* 37:984-986, 1975
120. DeMaria AN, Vera Z, Amsterdam EA, et al: Disturbances of cardiac rhythm and conduction induced by exercise: diagnostic, prognostic and therapeutic implications. *Am J Cardiol* 33:732-736, 1974
121. Rozanski JJ, Castellanos A, Sheps D, et al: Paroxysmal second-degree atrioventricular block induced by exercise. *Heart Lung* 9:887-890, 1980
122. Sheps DS, Ernst JC, Briese FR, et al: Decreased frequency of exercise-induced ventricular ectopic activity in the second of two consecutive treadmill tests. *Circulation* 55:892-895, 1977
123. Ryan M, Lown B, Horn H: Comparison of ventricular ectopic activity during 24-hour monitoring and exercise testing in patients with coronary heart disease. *N Engl J Med* 292:224-229, 1975
124. Crawford M, O'Rourke RA, Ramakrishna N, et al: Comparative effectiveness of exercise testing and continuous monitoring for detecting arrhythmias in patients with previous myocardial infarction. *Circulation* 50:301-305, 1974
125. Kosowsky BD, Lown B, Whiting R, et al: Occurrence of ventricular arrhythmias with exercise as compared to monitoring. *Circulation* 44:826-832, 1971
126. Poblete PF, Kennedy HL, Caralis DG: Detection of ventricular ectopy in patients with coronary heart disease and normal subjects by exercise testing and ambulatory electrocardiography. *Chest* 74:402-407, 1978
127. Møller M, Thayssen P: Ventricular arrhythmias during exercise testing and 24-hour ECG tape recording in patients with ischaemic heart disease and in normal individuals. *Acta Med Scand* 208:65-68, 1980
128. Kennedy HL: Comparison of ambulatory electrocardiography and exercise testing. *Am J Cardiol* 47:1359-1365, 1981
129. Ivanova LA, Mazur NA, Smirnova TM, et al: Electrocardiographic exercise testing and ambulatory monitoring to identify patients with ischemic heart disease at high risk of sudden death. *Am J Cardiol* 45:1132-1138, 1980
130. DeBusk RF, Davidson DM, Houston N, et al: Serial ambulatory electrocardiography and treadmill exercise testing after uncomplicated myocardial infarction. *Am J Cardiol* 45:547-554, 1980
131. Vatterott PJ, Hammill SC, Bailey KR, et al: Signal-averaged electrocardiography: a new noninvasive test to identify patients at risk for ventricular arrhythmias. *Mayo Clin Proc* 63:931-942, 1988
132. Vatterott PJ, Bailey KR, Hammill SC: Improving the prediction ability of the signal-averaged electrocardiogram with a linear logistic model incorporating clinical variables. *Circulation* 81:797-804, 1990
133. Vlay SC, Kallman CH, Reid PR: Prognostic assessment of survivors of ventricular tachycardia and ventricular fibrillation with ambulatory monitoring. *Am J Cardiol* 54:87-90, 1984

CHAPTER

3

Electrocardiography

D. Signal-averaged electrocardiography

Stephen C. Hammill, M.D.

Signal averaging of the surface electrocardiogram (ECG) is a new noninvasive, computerized method of analyzing ECG signals that identifies patients at risk for ventricular tachycardia.[1,2] This technique averages multiple QRS complexes and with filter methods minimizes noise and exposes signals of the microvolt level that are normally hidden in the noise. Late potentials have been recognized as microvolt signals that are fractionated and delayed beyond the QRS duration in border zones surrounding the scar of a previous myocardial infarction. These areas of delayed activation have been shown to act as the substrate for reentry ventricular tachycardia.[3,4] The areas can be measured by direct endocardial catheters (invasive) or by surface signal-averaged microvolt signals (noninvasive).

Signal-averaged ECG recordings can be performed with commercially available equipment consisting of X,Y,Z ECG leads, an amplifier, an analog-to-digital converter, and a personal computer with software to average the ECG waveforms and store the data. Care in lead preparation to obtain a noise-free recording is important. Using the computer technique to average multiple signals of a repetitive QRS waveform (typically, 200 QRS cycles) reduces random noise. The low-frequency ST segment is removed by the use of a high-pass filter to further clarify the signals late or after the QRS. Computer software then computes a vector-magnitude function that helps in identifying the QRS end points. The final function enlarges the complex 200 to 300 times for visual inspection.[2]

For identification of the late potentials, three features are measured by the computer.

1. The QRS duration is measured and is increased by late potentials, since they are contiguous with the end of the QRS.
2. The root-mean-square voltage of the last 40 msec of the QRS complex is computed. Since the late potentials are low-amplitude signals, the root-mean-square voltage is much smaller if late potentials are present.
3. The duration of the low-amplitude signal at the end of the QRS complex that lies below the 40-μV level (low-amplitude signal duration) is determined (Figs 3D-1 through 3D-3).

This technique has been studied in several patient populations. In patients with complex ventricular ectopy, Winters et al.[5] found that signal-averaged ECGs had a sensitivity of 92% and a specificity of 75% for predicting electrophysiologic test results and subsequent prognosis. In the subgroup with coronary artery disease, the sensitivity was 91% and the specificity 56%. Vatterott et al.[2] at the Mayo Clinic found a 95% sensitivity and a 48% specificity for predicting electrophysiologic test results in a similar population of patients.

Probably the greatest application of the signal-averaged ECG will be in the management of patients after myocardial infarction.[6-10] In 1987, Gomes et al.[10] reported that a positive signal-averaged ECG combined with an ejection fraction of less than 40% and Holter evidence of more than 10 ventricular premature contractions per hour was associated with an arrhythmic event rate of 50%. If two of these three factors were present, the arrhythmic event rate was 35% to 37%, and when all three features were normal, the event rate was 0%. Using the signal-averaged ECG as a single test to assess risk for arrhythmic events after acute myocardial infarction gives excellent negative predictive accuracy (95%) but low positive predictive accuracy (15%).[7] In patients with inferior myocardial infarction, late potentials are very sensitive but not as specific for predicting events. In patients with anterior wall myocardial infarction, some sensitivity is lost but specificity is very good. It should be remembered that the signal-averaged ECG can predict arrhythmic events but not ischemic events.

For patients with syncope, the high negative predictive accuracy of 97% should preclude invasive electrophysiologic testing in certain patients.[2] Multivariate analysis in patients with syncope of unknown origin identified late potentials and ejection fraction as risk factors for induction of sustained monomorphic ventricular tachycardia at electrophysiologic study.[11]

The value of signal-averaged ECGs in patients without coronary artery disease remains largely unknown at this time.

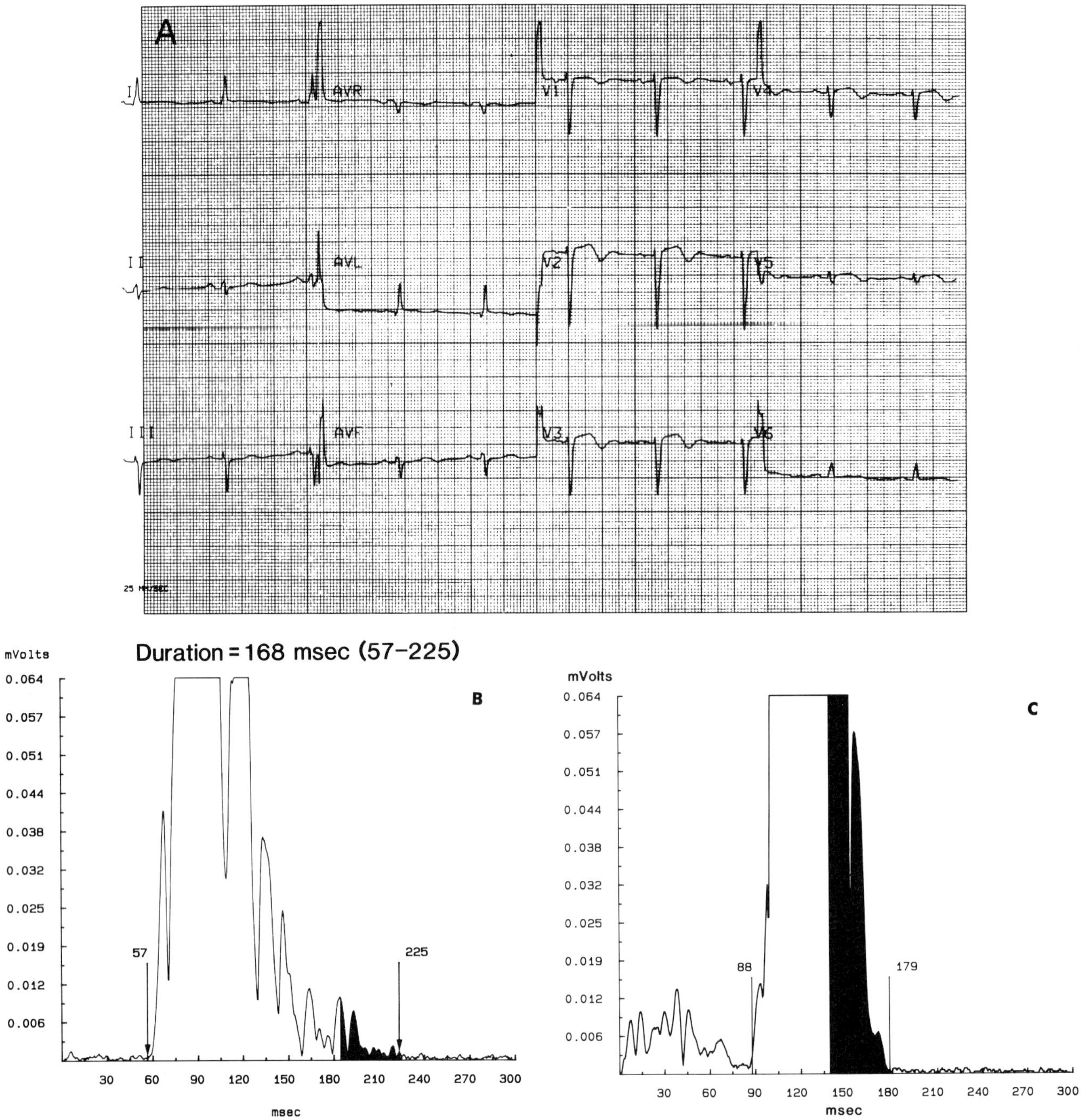

Fig 3D-1 Studies in a 71-year-old woman with a history of anteroseptal myocardial infarction and ventricular tachycardia (**A** and **B**) and in a patient with no cardiac abnormalities (**C**). **A,** standard 12-lead ECG, showing QRS duration of 110 msec. **B,** signal-averaged ECG, demonstrating additional presence of low-level late potentials (vector-magnitude QRS duration of 168 msec). This average was filtered with a 40-Hz bidirectional filter and enlarged 300 times. **C,** for comparison, a normal signal-averaged ECG from a patient with normal results at electrophysiologic testing. This average was filtered with a 40-Hz bidirectional filter and enlarged 300 times. Vector-magnitude QRS duration = 91 msec; root-mean-square voltage of QRS terminal 40 msec = 96 μV; and duration of low-amplitude signal <40 μV = 18 msec. (From Vatterott PJ, Hammill SC, Bailey KR, et al: Signal-averaged electrocardiography: a new noninvasive test to identify patients at risk for ventricular arrhythmias. Mayo Clin Proc 63:931-942, 1988. By permission, Mayo Foundation for Medical Education and Research.)

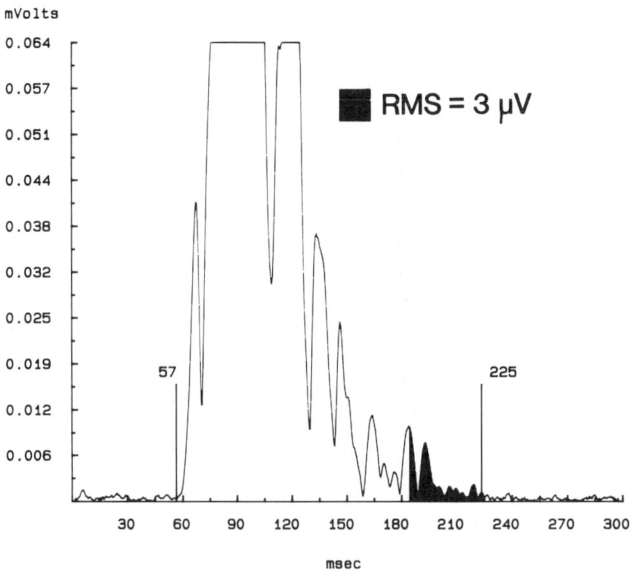

Fig 3D-2 Computer calculates the root-mean-square (RMS) voltage of vector-magnitude QRS terminal 40 msec *(shaded region).* Low levels of RMS voltage measurement are consistent with presence of late potentials, and high RMS values are normal (see Fig 3D-1, **C**). (From Vatterott PJ, Hammill SC, Bailey KR, et al: Signal-averaged electrocardiography: a new noninvasive test to identify patients at risk for ventricular arrhythmias. *Mayo Clin Proc* 63:931-942, 1988. By permission, Mayo Foundation for Medical Education and Research.)

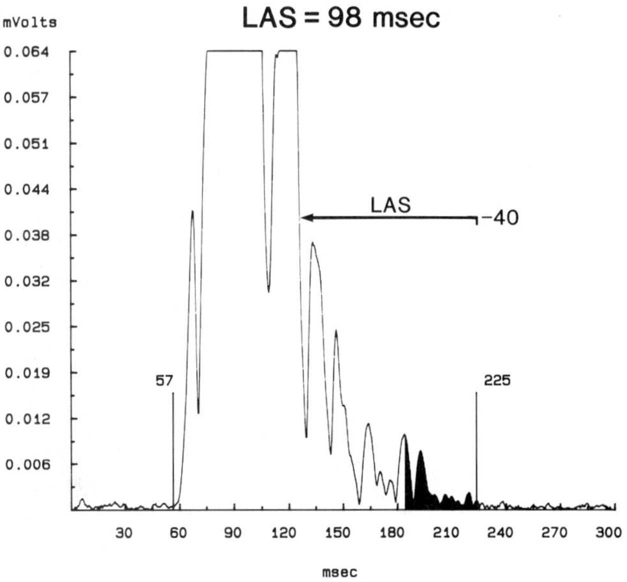

Fig 3D-3 To measure duration of low-amplitude signal (LAS), computer software program determines QRS offset and moves backward in time (to the left) until vector-magnitude QRS complex attains the 40-μV level. This point is then marked, and a determination is made of how much of the terminal vector-magnitude QRS complex (in milliseconds) lies below the 40-μV level. (From Vatterott PJ, Hammill SC, Bailey KR, et al: Signal-averaged electrocardiography: a new noninvasive test to identify patients at risk for ventricular arrhythmias. *Mayo Clin Proc* 63:931-942, 1988. By permission, Mayo Foundation for Medical Education and Research.)

In patients with positive signal-averaged ECG test results, intervention with aneurysmectomy guided by endocardial mapping during ventricular tachycardia can eliminate the late potentials. Antiarrhythmic therapy does not eliminate late potentials,[12] and coronary artery bypass surgery has little effect on late potentials. After an acute myocardial infarction, patients with a patent infarct-related artery have fewer late potentials than those with an occluded artery.[8]

Use of a model incorporating clinical variables, including ejection fraction, with signal-averaged ECG variables improved the predictive accuracy, identifying patients at risk for ventricular tachycardia.[13] Standard time-domain signal-averaged ECG techniques are not helpful in patients with bundle-branch block and nonspecific intraventricular conduction delay. Spectral analysis of the signal-averaged ECG may improve the predictive accuracy in patients with conduction delay.[14]

The criteria for a positive signal-averaged ECG in patients without bundle-branch block on the standard ECG (QRS <118 msec) are two of the following three factors.[15]

1. QRS duration of $\geq$ 120 msec.
2. Root-mean-square voltage of terminal 40 msec of ≤ 20 μV.
3. Low-amplitude signal duration of ≥ 38 msec.

REFERENCES

1. Breithardt G, Cain ME, El-Sherif N, et al: Standards for analysis of ventricular late potentials using high-resolution or signal-averaged electrocardiography: a statement by a task force committee of the European Society of Cardiology, the American Heart Association, and the American College of Cardiology. *Circulation* 83:1481-1488, 1991
2. Vatterott PJ, Hammill SC, Bailey KR, et al: Signal-averaged electrocardiography: a new noninvasive test to identify patients at risk for ventricular arrhythmias. *Mayo Clin Proc* 63:931-942, 1988
3. Kuchar DL, Rosenbaum DS, Ruskin J, et al: Late potentials on the signal-averaged electrocardiogram after canine myocardial infarction: correlation with induced ventricular arrhythmias during the healing phase. *J Am Coll Cardiol* 15:1365-1373, 1990
4. El-Sherif N, Gomes JAC, Restivo M, et al: Late potentials and arrhythmogenesis. *PACE* 8:440-462, 1985
5. Winters SL, Steward D, Targonski A, et al: Role of signal averaging of the surface QRS complex in selecting patients with nonsustained ventricular tachycardia and high grade ventricular arrhythmias for programmed ventricular stimulation. *J Am Coll Cardiol* 12:1481-1487, 1988
6. Farrell TG, Bashir Y, Cripps T, et al: Risk stratification for arrhythmic events in postinfarction patients based on heart rate variability, ambulatory electrocardiographic variables and the signal-averaged electrocardiogram. *J Am Coll Cardiol* 18:687-697, 1991
7. Steinberg JS, Regan A, Sciacca RR, et al: Predicting arrhythmic events after acute myocardial infarction using the signal-averaged electrocardiogram. *Am J Cardiol* 69:13-21, 1992
8. Vatterott PJ, Hammill SC, Bailey KR, et al: Late potentials on

signal-averaged electrocardiograms and patency of the infarct-related artery in survivors of acute myocardial infarction. *J Am Coll Cardiol* 17:330-337, 1991

9. Gomes JA, Winters SL, Ergin A, et al: Clinical and electrophysiologic determinants, treatment and survival of patients with sustained malignant ventricular tachyarrhythmias occurring late after myocardial infarction. *J Am Coll Cardiol* 17:320-326, 1991

10. Gomes JA, Winters SL, Steward D, et al: A new noninvasive index to predict sustained ventricular tachycardia and sudden death in the first year after myocardial infarction: based on signal-averaging electrocardiogram, radionuclide ejection fraction and Holter monitoring. *J Am Coll Cardiol* 10:349-357, 1987

11. Moazez F, Peter T, Simonson J, et al: Syncope of unknown origin: clinical, noninvasive and electrophysiologic determinants of arrhythmia induction and symptom recurrence during long-term follow up. *Am Heart J* 121:81-88, 1991

12. Steinberg JS, Freedman RA, Bigger JT Jr: Antiarrhythmic drug therapy and the signal-averaged electrocardiogram. In *High-Resolution Electrocardiography.* Edited by N El-Sherif, G Turitto. Mount Kisco, New York, Futura Publishing Company, 1992, pp 569-590

13. Vatterott PJ, Bailey KR, Hammill SC: Improving the predictive ability of the signal-averaged electrocardiogram with a linear logistic model incorporating clinical variables. *Circulation* 81:797-804, 1990

14. Kelen GJ, Henkin R, Starr A-M, et al: Spectral turbulence analysis of the signal-averaged electrocardiogram and its predictive accuracy for inducible sustained monomorphic ventricular tachycardia. *Am J Cardiol* 67:965-975, 1991

15. Hammill SC, Tchou PJ, Kienzle MG, et al: Establishment of signal-averaged electrocardiographic criteria with Frank XYZ leads and spectral filter used alone and in combination with ejection fraction to predict inducible ventricular tachycardia in coronary artery disease. *Am J Cardiol* 70:316-320, 1992

CHAPTER

4

The chest roentgenogram

Thomas T. Schattenberg, M.D., Barry L. Karon, M.D., Robert O. Brandenburg, M.D., and Paul R. Julsrud, M.D.

IN the diagnosis and management of heart disease, the standard chest roentgenogram is one of our most useful and important adjuncts. In patients with known or suspected heart disease, careful attention to the cardiac size and shape, configuration of the great vessels, and pulmonary vascular markings often allows a specific categorization of the patient's disease and its severity. The maximum information is obtained by a meticulous examination in three specific areas.

First is the overall size of the heart in comparison with the chest itself and, when possible, a delineation of the sizes of the specific chambers and great vessels, their locations, and their configuration.

The second area of interest is calcific deposits, which may involve valves, intracardiac masses, myocardium, pericardium, and walls of the coronary arteries.

The third major area of interest is the lungs and the thoracic cage, including careful consideration of the pulmonary vascular pattern.

The serial examination of repeated chest roentgenograms forms an important part of the long-term evaluation of the patient. Changes in appearance may suggest the need to initiate medical therapy, change medical therapy, or first consider surgical treatment. Study of serial films also assists in assessing the results of medical and surgical treatment and in estimating prognosis.

A standard chest roentgenogram is considered part of the basic cardiac examination and is universally employed as a baseline for subsequent evaluations of cardiac status. The exposures are made with the patient standing during sustained inspiration, with the anterior chest in immediate proximity to the film. The x-rays emanate from a source 6 ft behind the patient. More parallel rays are obtained if the x-ray tube is positioned 8 or 10 ft away from the film cassette. The more distant tube placement results in less magnification. Caution is therefore necessary in comparing serial films obtained by different methods. Error in comparison of cardiac size can be avoided by observing differences in widths of the entire chest, not just the cardiac silhouette.

Fluoroscopy, utilizing a modern image-intensifier tube, allows continuous viewing of the x-ray image and thus provides real-time observation of thoracic contents during positional and respiratory manipulations. The advent of echocardiography has drastically limited the indications for cardiac fluoroscopy. Fluoroscopy is primarily useful for assessing diaphragmatic excursion and for the functional assessment of a prosthetic cardiac valve.

Chapter 10A discusses the additional information that can be obtained by injection of contrast medium during filmed (cine) fluoroscopy.

PROJECTIONS

Posteroanterior (frontal) view

The posteroanterior view is the most useful view because of its reproducibility and the general familiarity with its virtues and limitations. The distinct lung-to-heart interface created by the different tissue densities of these organs produces an easily visualized cardiac silhouette, which may itself provide diagnostic information.

Every x-ray film should be interpreted in a systematic fashion, beginning with a critical analysis of the techniques of exposure. Proper exposure permits good visualization of the progressively branching pulmonary vessels and bronchi; these blend into a homogeneous haze at the periphery of the lungs, whereas the thoracic spine is barely visible through the cardiac shadow (Fig 4-1). The patient is properly positioned for the exposure if the heads of the clavicles are equidistant from the midpoint of the spine. Because of their greater calcium content, the posterior ribs are better seen than the anterior ribs, whereas the costal cartilages and the sternum are seldom visualized. The scapulae should have been rotated out so that they do not overlie the lung fields, and the hemidiaphragms should be down at least to the level of the 10th rib posteriorly. The right hemidiaphragm is normally 1 or 2 cm higher than the left;[1,2] pronounced elevation of one leaf of the diaphragm indicates possible ipsilateral phrenic nerve paralysis. Both costophrenic angles should be included on the film. The stomach bubble can often be seen; in situs solitus, it lies just beneath the left diaphragm. Free air beneath the diaphragm indicates perforated abdominal viscus, whereas a very hazy, diffuse abdominal opacity may indicate the presence of ascites.

Particular attention is given to the cardiac silhouette (Fig 4-2). The right mediastinal border is primarily formed by the superior vena cava superiorly and the lateral wall of the right atrium inferiorly. At the level of the junction between the superior vena cava and the right atrium, the

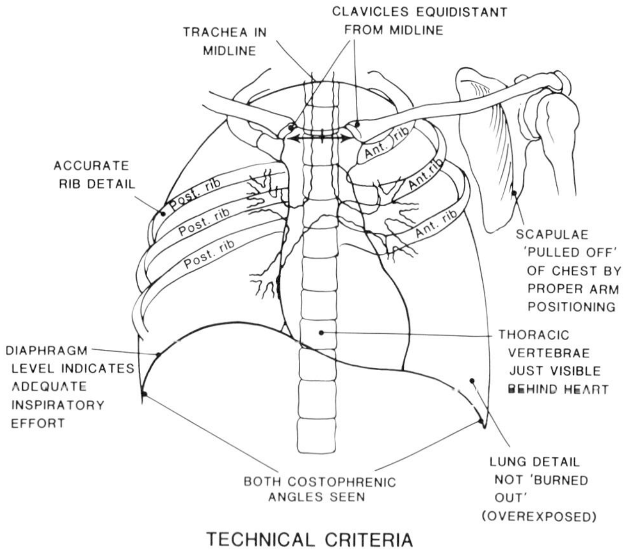

Fig 4-1 Proper technique for exposure of posteroanterior chest x-ray film. (From Schattenberg TT: Chest x-ray films in heart disease. In *Clinical Medicine.* Vol. 6. *Cardiovascular Diseases.* Edited by JA Spittell Jr. Philadelphia, Harper & Row, Publishers, 1982, chap 33, pp 1-13. By permission.)

ascending aorta may protrude enough to the right to form a portion of the border. The contribution to the right cardiac silhouette by the ascending aorta becomes more prominent with advancing age because of the normal increase in length and tortuosity of the aorta which occurs. A bulging ascending aorta may dominate the right upper heart border in the presence of ectasia, aortic dissection, and aortic stenosis with poststenotic aortic dilatation. A small portion of the inferior vena cava may be seen angling from the right diaphragm into the right atrium.

Dilatation of the great veins (superior vena cava and inferior vena cava) results from increased central venous pressure or flow, as in right ventricular failure or in the presence of anomalous pulmonary venous connection to the great veins. Right atrial enlargement results in expansion of the right heart border into the right lung field and is best observed on the posteroanterior view. Right atrial enlargement can result from tricuspid valve disease (Fig 4-3), right ventricular failure, and atrial septal defects. Left atrial enlargement causes a second shadow of density just within and parallel to the right margin in the cardiac silhouette (Fig 4-4).

The left mediastinal border is composed, from superiorly downward, of aortic arch, descending aorta, main and left pulmonary arteries, left atrial appendage, and left ventricle. Since the sternum limits the extent of anterior displacement, progressive right ventricular enlargement can result eventually in the right ventricle's overlapping the left ventricle to form the left heart border, and occasionally the right ventricle represents the entire left heart border. A thin rim of calcium in the aortic arch may be the first manifestation of atherosclerosis. The descend-

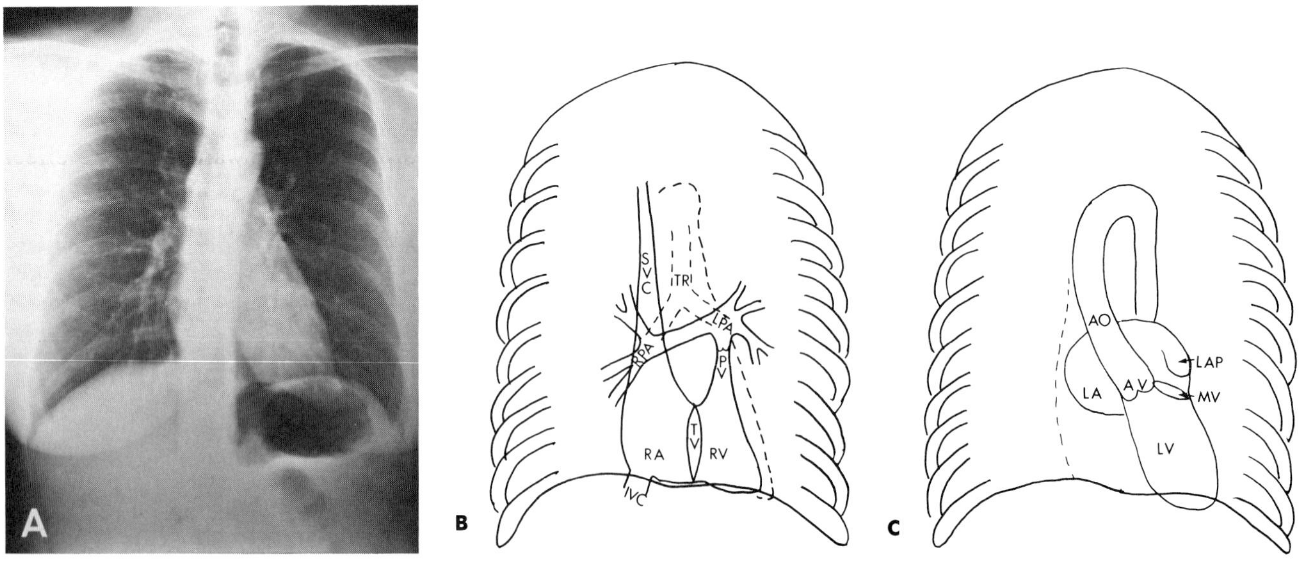

Fig 4-2 **A,** normal posteroanterior chest x-ray film. **B,** outline of right-sided chambers and vessels as they contribute to the cardiac silhouette. RA, right atrium; RV, right ventricle; TV, tricuspid valve; PV, pulmonary valve; LPA, left pulmonary artery; RPA, right pulmonary artery; TR, trachea; IVC, inferior vena cava; SVC, superior vena cava. **C,** outline of left-sided heart chambers and vessels related to the cardiac silhouette. LV, left ventricle; LA, left atrium; AV, aortic valve; MV, mitral valve; LAA, left atrial appendage; AO, aorta.

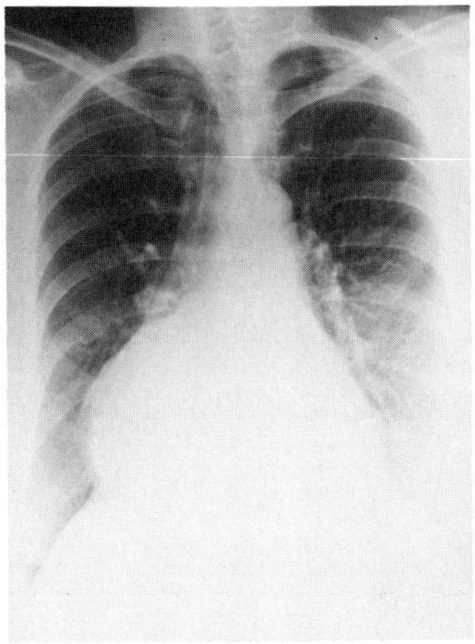

Fig 4-3 Right atrial enlargement. This patient underwent closed mitral commissurotomy several years previously and obtained relief of left-sided symptoms. Organic tricuspid disease persisted, resulting in massive right atrial enlargement.

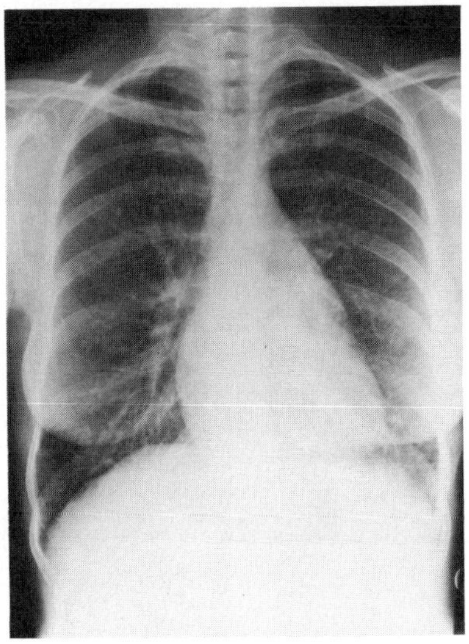

Fig 4-4 Mitral stenosis. The double shadow within the right heart border and the prominent left atrial appendage indicate left atrial enlargement. Cephalization of the pulmonary flow pattern and Kerley B lines are noted on the posteroanterior x-ray film. The left ventricle is not enlarged. (From Schattenberg TT: Chest x-ray films in heart disease. In *Clinical Medicine.* Vol. 6. *Cardiovascular Diseases.* Edited by JA Spittell Jr. Philadelphia, Harper & Row, Publishers, 1982, chap 33, pp 1-13. By permission.)

ing aorta can be identified behind the heart near the midline; it often becomes tortuous in the elderly. The main pulmonary artery courses superiorly and leftward and bifurcates near the left cardiac border; this allows the left pulmonary artery to contribute to the left cardiac silhouette. In contrast, the proximal right pulmonary artery is obscured by the overlying heart and aorta and is not normally visualized on the posteroanterior chest roentgenogram until after it gives off its upper lobe branch and emerges into the right lung. The right pulmonary artery at the hilus lies about 1 cm inferiorly as compared with the left pulmonary artery at the hilus (see Fig 4-2, B).

Lateral view

This view is named according to the side of the chest, commonly the left, that is in contact with the x-ray film. As a result of parallax, the leaf of the diaphragm that is closer to the film is less magnified and in better focus. The right ventricle forms the anterior border of the heart and is usually enlarged if more than half of the anterior cardiac silhouette is in contact with the sternum (Fig 4-5). However, the same appearance may occur in the absence of right ventricular enlargement if left atrial enlargement displaces the entire heart anteriorly. Thus, right ventricular enlargement, whether due to dilatation or hypertrophy or both, causes the heart to bulge anteriorly (Fig 4-6). Overdistention of emphysematous lungs may result in posterior displacement of the heart away from the sternum, whereas a pectus excavatum deformity or a straight back syndrome results in a closer approximation of the heart to the sternum (Figs 4-7 and 4-8). Calcification of the aortic valve may be observed in the center of the cardiac shadow, about one-third of the way posteriorly from the anterior diaphragmatic attachment.

Left atrial enlargement in the lateral projection is evidenced by posterior extension of the upper half of the cardiac silhouette (Fig 4-9). Occasionally, the enlarging left atrium will expand laterally more than posteriorly.

Left ventricular size is determined in the lateral view by noting the relationship of the lower posterior heart border and the inferior vena cava. Normally, the lower cardiac border crosses the posterior margin of the inferior vena cava 2 cm above the diaphragm. When the left ventricle is dilated, its apex is displaced downward, with the effect that the intersection between the ventricular border and the inferior vena cava moves closer to the diaphragm.[3] Aneurysms of the pulmonary artery may present as middle mediastinal masses (Fig 4-10), whereas pericardial cysts may present in either the anterior or the middle mediastinum.

CARDIAC SIZE

Cardiac enlargement detected by x-ray study is often the first evidence of heart disease, but of course heart disease may be present in the absence of enlargement. The heart is considered to be enlarged when its transverse diameter on the posteroanterior view exceeds half the transverse diameter of the bony thoracic cage—that is, the cardiothoracic ratio exceeds 50% (abbreviated as $C/T > 0.5$). The use of the value 0.6 as the upper limit of normal for this ratio has been suggested to reduce false-positive results.[4] Attempts at estimating heart volume by mathematical analysis of cardiac dimensions by roentgenogram are less accurate than those derived by echocardiographic

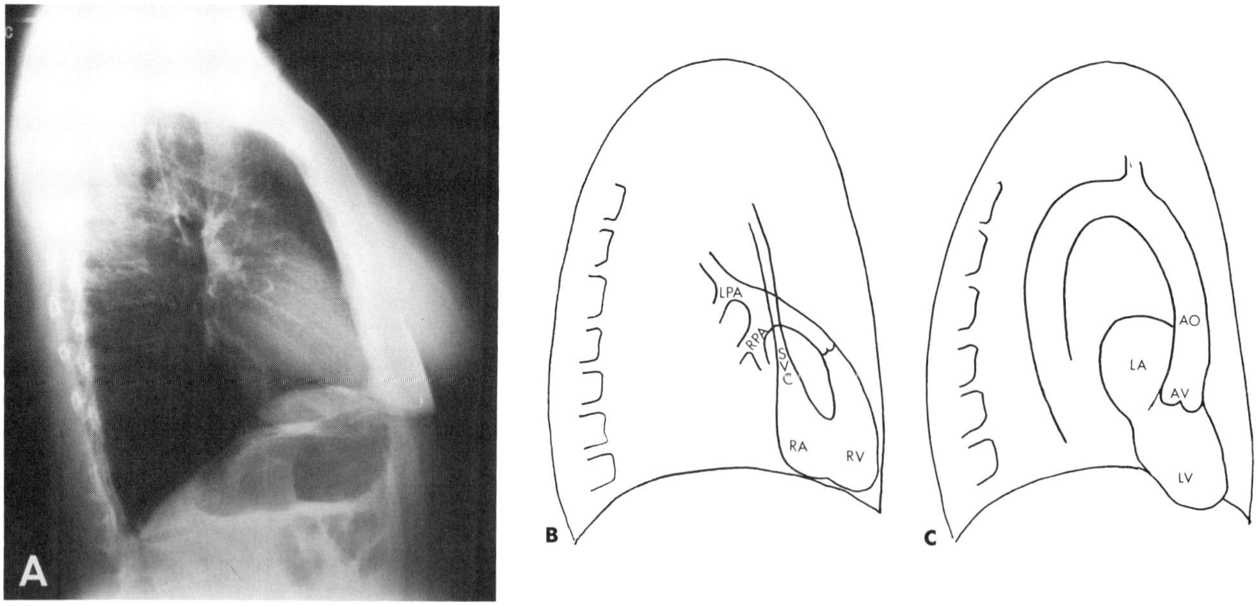

Fig 4-5 **A,** normal lateral x-ray film. **B,** right-sided chambers and vessels as they contribute to the lateral film. **C,** left-sided chambers and vessels related to the lateral film. **B** and **C,** abbreviations are as in Figure 4-2.

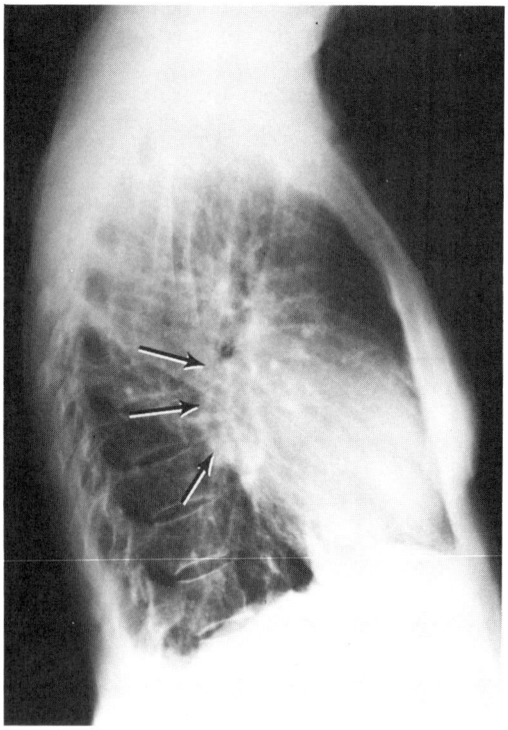

Fig 4-6 Lateral x-ray film of a patient with mitral stenosis (same patient as in Figure 4-4). Right ventricular enlargement with impingement on the sternum and left atrial enlargement posteriorly are noted *(arrows).* (From Schattenberg TT: Chest x-ray films in heart disease. In *Clinical Medicine.* Vol. 6. *Cardiovascular Diseases.* Edited by JA Spittell Jr. Philadelphia, Harper & Row, Publishers, 1982, chap 33, pp 1-13. By permission.

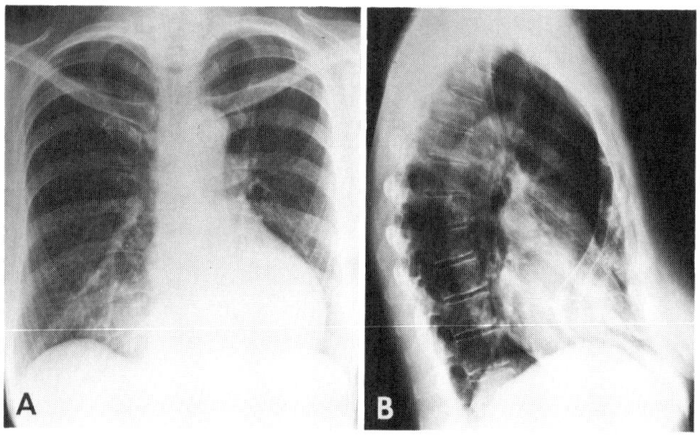

Fig 4-7 Pectus excavatum. Posteroanterior x-ray film **(A)** shows parallel configuration of the ribs, prominent supraclavicular lung fields, and displacement of the cardiac silhouette to the left. The lateral film **(B)** explains the finding of displacement of the silhouette, showing the very small space available between the lower sternum and the thoracic spine. (From Schattenberg TT: Chest x-ray films in heart disease. In *Clinical Medicine.* Vol. 6. *Cardiovascular Diseases.* Edited by JA Spittell Jr. Philadelphia, Harper & Row, Publishers, 1982, chap 33, pp 1-13. By permission.)

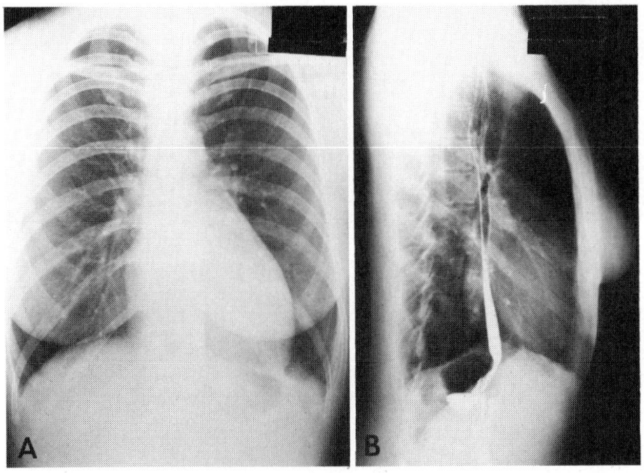

Fig 4-8 **A** and **B,** straight back syndrome. Unusually erect habitus due to loss of thoracic curve is evident on the lateral chest x-ray film **(B).** The cardiac silhouette is normal despite the presence of mitral valve prolapse in this patient.

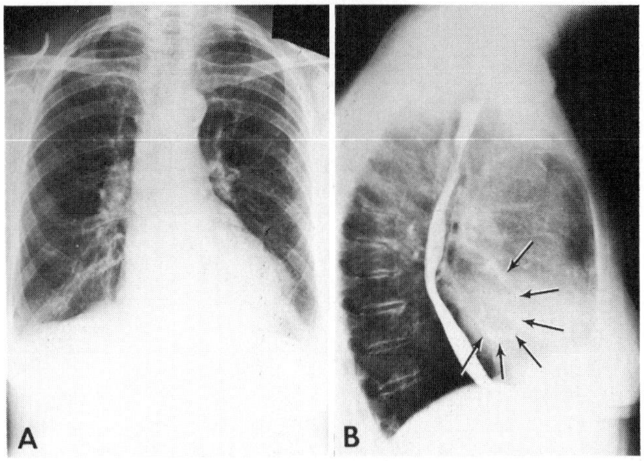

Fig 4-9 Calcified mitral annulus. The finding is barely visible on the posteroanterior x-ray film **(A)** but can be seen on the lateral view **(B)** *(arrows),* which shows posterior displacement of the esophagus by a slightly enlarged left atrium. Note blunted costophrenic angles due to pleural effusions.

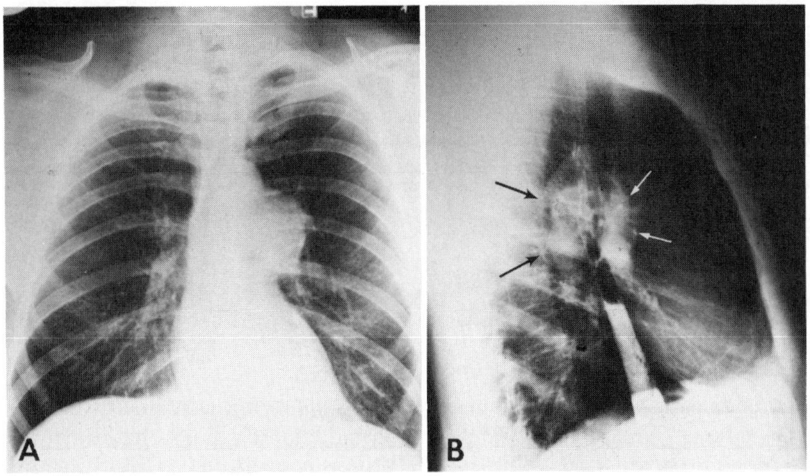

Fig 4-10 **A** and **B,** pulmonary artery aneurysm. A middle mediastinal mass is evident on both views as a rounded density in the region of the left hilus *(arrows).* Catheterization showed a gradient of 35 mm Hg across the pulmonary valve. (From Schattenberg TT: Chest x-ray films in heart disease. In *Clinical Medicine.* Vol. 6. *Cardiovascular Diseases.* Edited by JA Spittell Jr. Philadelphia, Harper & Row, Publishers, 1982, chap 33, pp 1-13. By permission.)

measurements. However, such estimates are helpful in following patients for comparative changes in heart size. It is important to note certain mechanical and anatomic factors that affect apparent heart size.

The degree of inspiration plays a major role in determining the apparent heart size. A maximal inspiratory effort should lower the diaphragm to the 10th rib posteriorly. If it lowers the diaphragm less than this, the transverse diameter of the heart will be increased. Large stroke volumes can also cause problems, as in severe valvular incompetence, in complete heart block, or in a trained athlete, since there may be significant differences in heart size between diastole and systole in these situations. Because x-ray films are exposed in a random fashion with respect to the timing in the cardiac cycle, errors in comparative interpretation may result[5] (Fig 4-11). The heart is magnified on portable bedside films because only 3 ft separate the tube from the film, rather than the usual 6-foot distance on a routine posteroanterior chest film.

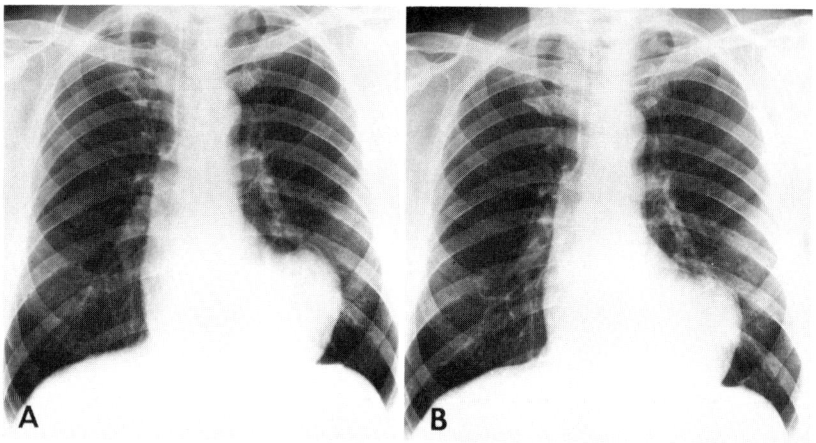

Fig 4-11 Left ventricular aneurysm. Stereoscopic matched x-ray films were obtained at the same sitting but at systole in **A** and at diastole in **B**, emphasizing the difference in cardiac silhouette in relation to temporal events.

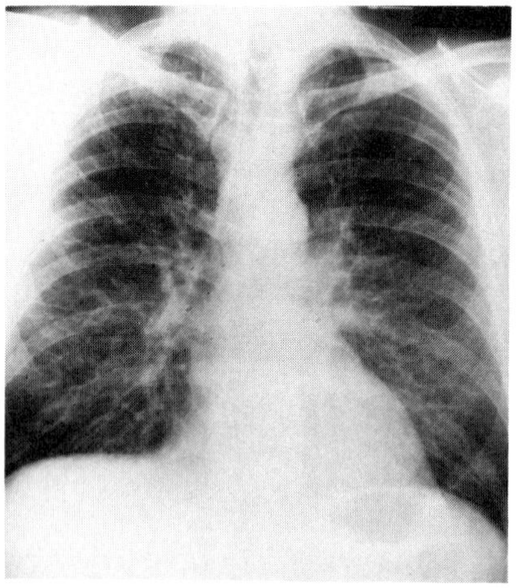

Fig 4-12 Acute pulmonary edema. A butterfly configuration of increased pulmonary markings is seen in a patient with acute myocardial infarction and absence of cardiomegaly.

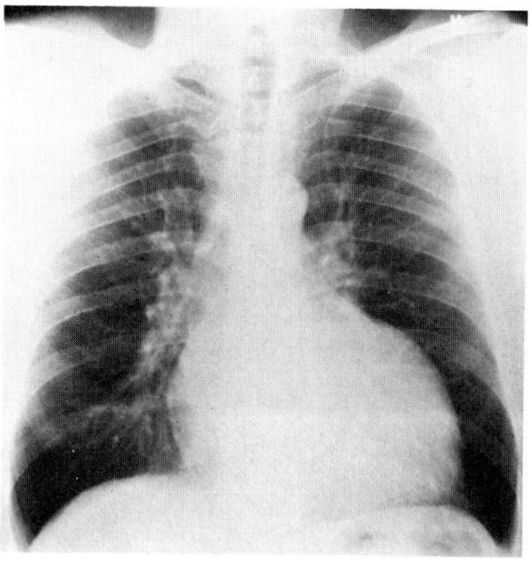

Fig 4-13 Chronic congestive heart failure in a patient with dilated cardiomyopathy, cardiomegaly, and pulmonary venous congestion.

Unusually small hearts may be seen in Addison's disease (adrenal insufficiency), whereas cardiomegaly eventually occurs in many types of cardiac disease. Acute cardiac failure, such as from myocardial infarction, may result in pulmonary edema while the heart size remains normal (Fig 4-12). Ruptured mitral chordae with acute, severe mitral regurgitation and acute aortic valve insufficiency from infective endocarditis may also be present without cardiomegaly. With long-standing congestive cardiac failure the heart usually enlarges, and pulmonary venous congestion may be accompanied by pleural effusion(s). The stepwise sequence of chamber enlargement may give clues to the cause of cardiac failure. As an example, the cardiomyopathic left ventricle will progressively enlarge, followed by left atrial enlargement, pulmonary venous congestion, and, finally, right-sided chamber enlargement (Fig 4-13).

Volume overload is a cause of cardiomegaly. The chamber upstream from a regurgitant valve is typically the first to enlarge. Thus, left atrial enlargement due to mitral regurgitation will precede left ventricular enlargement. Similarly, in left-to-right shunts, the chambers that are moving the additional blood will eventually enlarge; for example, right atrial and right ventricular dimensions are increased in atrial septal defects, and the pulmonary artery may be enlarged in left-to-right shunts at whatever level.

Pericardial effusion increases the cardiac silhouette. Normally, some 20 mL of fluid acts as a lubricant between the pericardial layers. When the effusion increases to 100

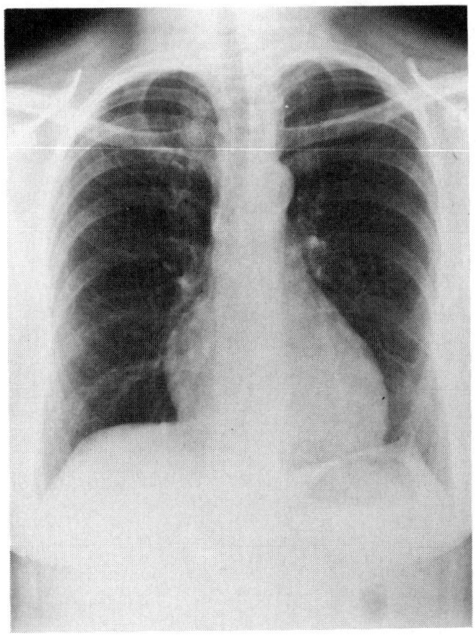

Fig 4-14 Idiopathic pericardial effusion. Mild globular cardiomegaly is present with normal lung fields. (From Schattenberg TT: Chest x-ray films in heart disease. In *Clinical Medicine.* Vol. 6. *Cardiovascular Diseases.* Edited by JA Spittell Jr. Philadelphia, Harper & Row, Publishers, 1982, chap 33, pp 1-13. By permission.)

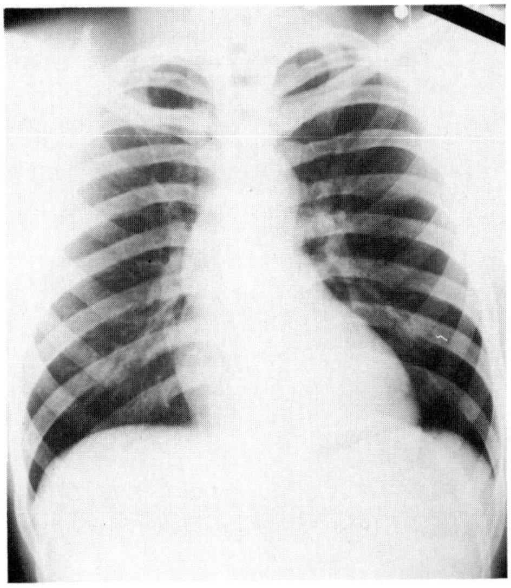

Fig 4-15 Left ventricular hypertrophy. Note the prominent ascending aorta and the left ventricular border extending beneath the left leaf of the diaphragm. The patient had bicuspid aortic stenosis with bacterial endocarditis. (From Schattenberg TT: Chest x-ray films in heart disease. In *Clinical Medicine.* Vol. 6. *Cardiovascular Diseases.* Edited by JA Spittell Jr. Philadelphia, Harper & Row, Publishers, 1982, chap 33, pp 1-13. By permission.)

Table 4-1 Globular cardiomegaly: differential diagnostic features

	Disorder			
Physical feature	**Dilated cardiomyopathy**	**Multivalvular disease**	**Pericardial effusion**	**Ebstein's anomaly**
Cardiophrenic angles	Obtuse – that is, cardiac silhouette slants downward and outward toward lateral diaphragm	More likely acute – that is, cardiac silhouette slants toward medial diaphragm	More likely acute	Acute
Cardiac waist	Normal or increased	Wide	Normal	Narrow
Intracardiac calcium	None	Possible aortic or mitral valve calcium	None	None
Pulmonary vasculature	Normal or venous congestion	Venous congestion	Normal	Normal

or 200 mL of fluid, the cardiac silhouette is expanded and becomes globular, usually unaccompanied by pulmonary congestion (Fig 4-14). Table 4-1 may be helpful in identifying other causes of globular cardiomegaly.

CARDIAC SHAPE

Left ventricular hypertrophy

Increased afterload on the left ventricle, as in isolated aortic stenosis or systemic hypertension, results in concentric hypertrophy of the left ventricle. The apex is pushed downward, and this shift carries the left heart border through the diaphragm and occasionally even into the stomach bubble (Fig 4-15). Initially, the cardiothoracic ratio remains normal.

Left ventricular dilatation

Chronic volume overloading or myocardial disease due to ischemia or other causes may result in left ventricular dilatation, with or without associated hypertrophy. The end stage of volume overloading cannot be distinguished radiographically from other forms of dilated cardiomyopathies. The x-ray findings are similar to those of left

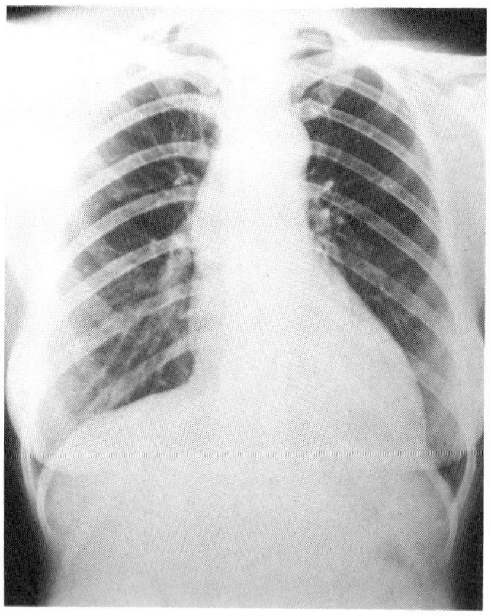

Fig 4-16 Left ventricular enlargement. In this patient with aortic insufficiency, the left ventricular border approaches the left lateral chest wall.

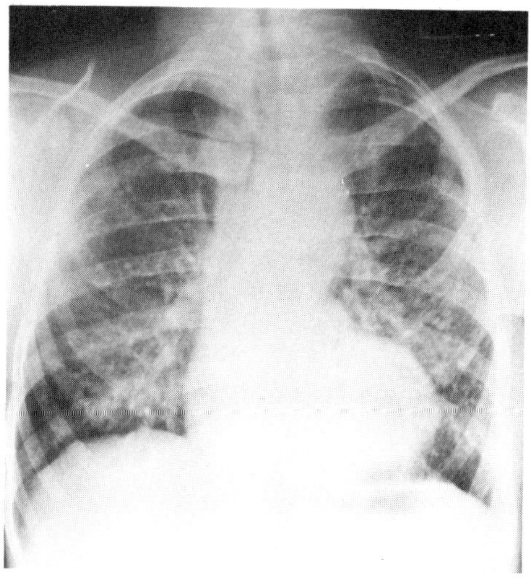

Fig 4-17 Tetralogy of Fallot. Indentation in the region of the left pulmonary artery and elevation of the apex due to right ventricular hypertrophy give rise to a "boot-shaped" contour, typical for this condition. (From Schattenberg TT: Chest x-ray films in heart disease. In *Clinical Medicine.* Vol. 6. *Cardiovascular Diseases.* Edited by JA Spittell Jr. Philadelphia, Harper & Row, Publishers, 1982, chap 33, pp 1-13. By permission.)

ventricular hypertrophy but more exaggerated. In advanced dilatation, the left heart border approaches or even encounters the lateral chest wall (Fig 4-16).

Right ventricular hypertrophy

Since the right ventricle does not form a portion of the silhouette on the posteroanterior chest x-ray film, hypertrophy or dilatation cannot usually be detected in this view. However, right ventricular hypertrophy can elevate the cardiac apex, as seen in the typical "coeur en sabot" of tetralogy of Fallot (Fig 4-17). This "boot-shaped" contour is augmented by the usually associated hypoplastic pulmonary arterial segment.

Right ventricular dilatation

Right ventricular dilatation is usually best appreciated on the lateral and right anterior oblique films by bulging of its outflow tract into the retrosternal space.

Left atrial enlargement

Although the left atrium is predominantly a posteriorly located chamber, its enlargement imparts a characteristic appearance to the posteroanterior film, seen as a prominence of the appendage just below the left pulmonary artery; also, a double shadow extends within the right heart border. An uncommon entity is the giant left atrium, which can extend beyond the right atrium and form part, or all, of the right cardiac border. In these cases, the margin of the right atrium is seen within the cardiac silhouette. The pulmonary venous congestion associated with left atrial enlargement is identified by (1) prominence and thickening, due to edema and dilated lymphatics, of the interlobular pulmonary septa, which become visible in either costophrenic angle (Kerley B lines); and (2) cephalization, or prominence, of the pulmonary vascular markings at the apices ("antler sign"). In view of the posterior location of the left atrium, its enlargement is best seen in the lateral view. Mitral valve disease is the most common cause of these findings. If mitral regurgitation is the dominant lesion, left ventricular enlargement also occurs (Fig 4-18).

Right atrial enlargement

Enlargement of the right atrium is usually due to disease of the tricuspid valve, right ventricular failure, or an atrial septal defect. Right atrial enlargement is more easily noted on the posteroanterior view, since the right atrium protrudes laterally, displacing the right lung. In extreme cases, the right heart border can approach the lateral chest wall in the frontal view and may be seen to overlap the lower esophagus on the right anterior oblique view.

Aortic anomalies

Since the aortic root is well within the cardiac silhouette, its enlargement cannot be perceived radiographically without dye injection. However, dilatation of the ascending aorta, such as occurs with aortic stenosis, may distort the right heart border. Even more pronounced widening of the cephalad portion of the right heart border may occur from aortic dissection. Syphilitic aortitis results in "eggshell" calcification of the ascending aorta, which is virtually pathognomonic. The aorta may descend along the right side of the spine and provide the indication that a right aortic arch is present (Fig 4-19). Although a right

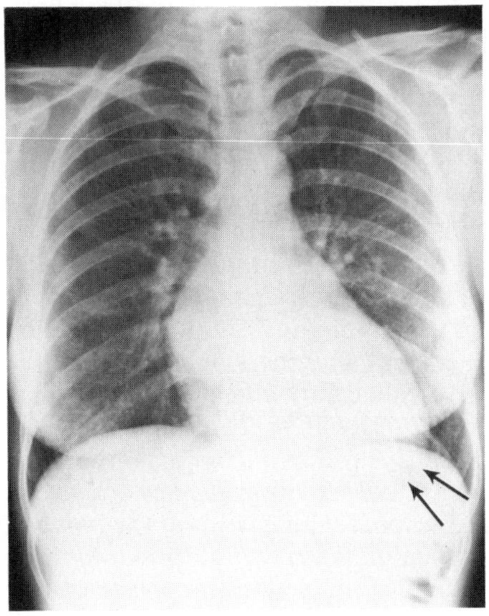

Fig 4-18 Mitral regurgitation. Note the double shadow of the enlarged left atrium and the prominent left ventricular margin extending beneath the left diaphragm *(arrows)*. (From Schattenberg TT: Chest x-ray films in heart disease. In *Clinical Medicine.* Vol. 6. *Cardiovascular Diseases.* Edited by JA Spittell Jr. Philadelphia, Harper & Row, Publishers, 1982, chap 33, pp 1-13. By permission.)

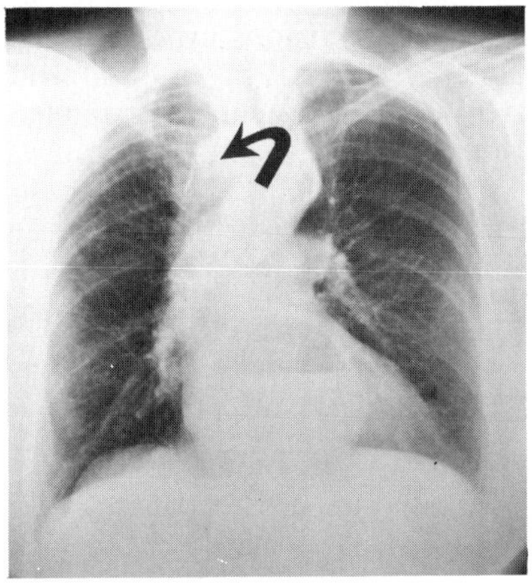

Fig 4-19 Tortuous aorta with right aortic arch *(arrow)*. No other cardiac defects were present in this 78-year-old patient, who has a large diaphragmatic hernia behind the cardiac silhouette.

aortic arch is usually associated with an otherwise normal cardiovascular system, its incidence is highest in the presence of one of the "four *ts*"—tetralogy of Fallot, transposition of the great arteries, truncus arteriosus, or tricuspid atresia.[6] Poststenotic dilatation of the descending aorta beyond a typical coarctation (usually just below the origin of the left subclavian artery) may produce a characteristic "3 sign," as seen in Figure 4-20.[7] This may or may not be associated with notching of the lower edges of the ribs as a result of dilated or tortuous

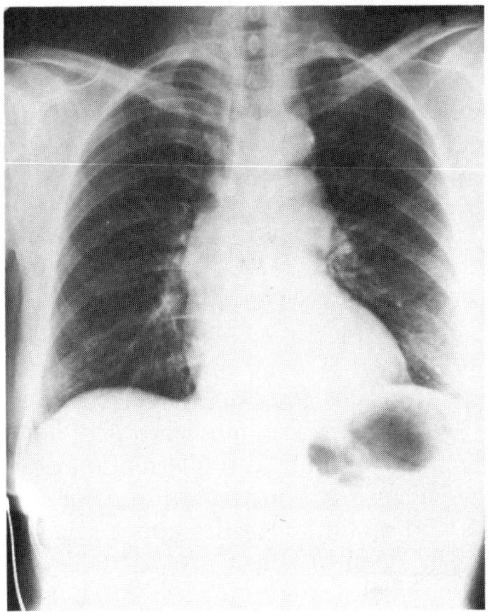

Fig 4-20 Coarctation of the aorta. The "3 sign" is present distal to the aortic arch on the left side, with poststenotic dilatation beyond the point of coarctation. No rib notching is present. (From Schattenberg TT: Chest x-ray films in heart disease. In *Clinical Medicine.* Vol. 6. *Cardiovascular Diseases.* Edited by JA Spittell Jr. Philadelphia, Harper & Row, Publishers, 1982, chap 33, pp 1-13. By permission.)

intercostal arteries carrying collateral flow. A saccular aneurysm just beyond the origin of the left subclavian artery is usually due to prior aortic rupture resulting from a rapid deceleration (closed chest) injury.

Pulmonary arterial anomalies

Even a small gradient across a stenotic pulmonary valve may cause aneurysmal dilatation of the pulmonary trunk.[8] Because of its left hilar location, nearly round contour, and relatively high density, such an aneurysm may be mistaken for bronchogenic carcinoma. Similarly, a pulmonary arteriovenous fistula may resemble a pulmonary neoplasm or metastasis and require angiography for accurate diagnosis.

PULMONARY VASCULATURE

From the cardiovascular standpoint, interest in the lungs is directed primarily to the pulmonary vasculature rather than the parenchyma. The pulmonary vasculature has the unique quality of being visible on a conventional chest x-ray film without the need for invasive procedures or injection of contrast medium. The pulmonary vessels, both arteries and veins, branch in an orderly fashion and progressively decrease in size as they pass from the hilus of the lung to the periphery. The size of the vessels reflects the volume of blood within them, accounting for the larger size of vessels in the lung bases in the erect patient; thus, flow is normally greater in the dependent portion of the lungs. A specific unique pulmonary vascular pattern is present when (1) pulmonary venous pressure is increased, (2) pulmonary arterial pressure is increased, (3) pulmonary blood flow is increased, and (4) pulmonary blood flow is decreased. It should be recognized that variations in the degree and combinations of these changes may make interpretation troublesome.

Pulmonary venous hypertension

The initial change caused by pulmonary venous hypertension is dilatation of venous channels, especially in the dependent portion of each lung, as a result of gravity effect. Later, in the presence of elevated pulmonary venous pressure (for example, mitral stenosis or left ventricular failure), there is redistribution of pulmonary blood flow because of constriction of veins in the lower lung fields and dilatation in the upper regions. Initially, this results in equalization of vascularity between upper and lower lung fields when the elevation in pressure is in the range of 10 to 15 mm Hg. Eventually, at levels of 15 to 20 mm Hg, there is reversal of blood flow, with "cephalization"—that is, larger flow to upper lung fields. Since the veins of the dependent portion of the lung are subject to gravitational effects plus the elevated left atrial pressure, transudation of fluid into the perivascular tissue occurs first in dependent areas. At levels above 25 mm Hg, transudation into the perivascular space results in interstitial edema and formation of Kerley B lines, seen typically in the costophrenic angles. Frank pulmonary edema occurs when pressures exceed 30 mm Hg. In this instance, the differential pressure between the intra-alveolar space and the alveolar capillaries exceeds the oncotic pressure of the blood, resulting in transudation of fluid into the alveolus and the development of edema. Air in the alveoli is replaced by fluid. If the edema develops acutely, it is of the alveolar type and results in the characteristic butterfly distribution of confluent lung density.[10,11] This type of edema usually follows, but may precede, the appearance of interstitial edema.[12] It may be much greater on one side than the other, but is almost always bilateral. The involvement is patchy, involves especially the dependent portion of the lung, and, when acute, tends to spare the periphery. Chest roentgenograms reliably identify pulmonary venous hypertension and congestive failure,[13] although the ability to quantitate hemodynamic parameters is limited.[14,15]

Edema resulting from more chronic elevation of pulmonary venous pressure is usually interstitial and is due to inability of the lymphatic system to clear interstitial fluid. Such edema causes haziness and blurring of the vascular shadows—so-called bronchial cuffing.[16] When fluid collects in the interlobar septa of the lung, the so-called Kerley B lines develop (see Fig 4-4). These lines lie perpendicular to the pleural surface and are usually seen best in the peripheral lung fields at the bases.[17] Occasionally, fluid accumulates in the interlobar fissures and forms a "pseudotumor," as seen in the posteroanterior view; in the lateral view, it can be seen to be simply fluid in a fissure (Fig 4-21).

Pleural effusion will develop in varying amounts in chronic heart failure and is indicative of right heart failure with or without left heart failure.

Pulmonary arterial hypertension

Elevation in pulmonary arterial pressure is often secondary to pulmonary venous hypertension—that is, postcapillary pulmonary hypertension. Thus, pulmonary vascular changes of pulmonary venous hypertension may also be present. Pulmonary arterial hypertension due to pulmonary venous hypertension is characterized by dilatation of the main pulmonary artery and the right and left main branches. In the postcapillary type of pulmonary arterial hypertension, pulmonary systolic pressure is usually less than 60 mm Hg.

Pulmonary hypertension may also occur in the absence

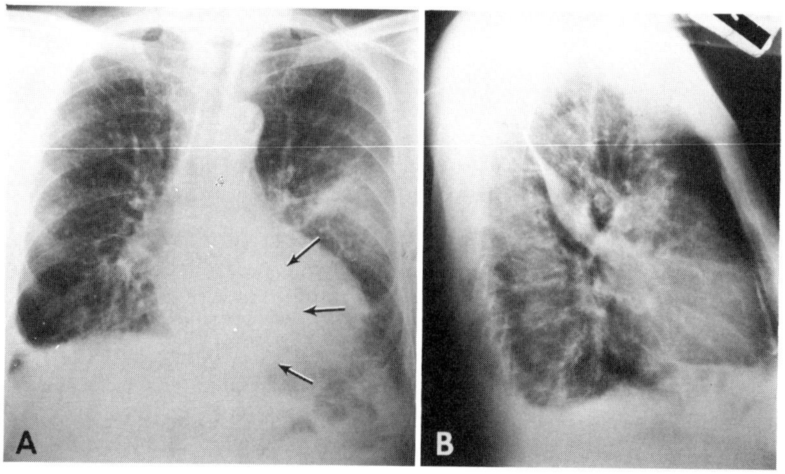

Fig 4-21 **A** and **B**, "vanishing tumor." Cardiomegaly with bilateral interstitial infiltrates and fluid in the left major fissure is confirmed on the lateral view (**B**). Both posterior costophrenic angles are blunted by fluid. Note the tortuous aorta behind cardiac silhouette *(arrows)*.

of postcapillary hypertension and is due to an increase in resistance to blood flow in the pulmonary arterioles—that is, precapillary pulmonary hypertension. This is most commonly associated with left-to-right shunts at whatever level. As the pulmonary artery pressure increases, there is further distention of the main pulmonary artery and its branches, while peripheral pulmonary arteries become attenuated, tortuous, or even indistinguishable, the so-called pruning of pulmonary arteries seen in Eisenmenger's syndrome.

Increased and decreased pulmonary blood flow

Increased pulmonary blood flow (pulmonary flow two times or more than systemic flow) is characterized by a symmetric increase in the size of the proximal and distal pulmonary arteries and veins. The usual disparity in the size of the vessels between upper and lower lung disappears as vessels throughout the lung become dilated. Some centers quantify pulmonary artery–bronchus ratios as an adjunct to discriminating pulmonary vascular plethora from congestive heart failure.[18]

Decreased pulmonary flow, as is present in significant right-to-left intracardiac shunts, is characterized by smaller than usual arterial and venous vascular shadows. Hilar shadows are smaller than usual, and the area along the left cardiac silhouette of the pulmonary artery shadow is often concave.

Acute pulmonary embolism

A well-made chest roentgenogram may appear normal in the presence of significant pulmonary embolism, and in a very ill patient only a portable bedside film of unsatisfactory quality may be available. Despite these problems, the chest x-ray film should show an alteration in over 50% of patients with clinically significant pulmonary embolism.[19]

In the Urokinase Pulmonary Embolism Trial conducted by the National Heart, Lung, and Blood Institute, the two most common alterations on the plain chest x-ray film in patients with pulmonary embolism were elevation of the diaphragm and pulmonary consolidation on the affected side.[20] These were seen in a select group of patients with severe arterial obstruction, however. In the Prospective Investigation of Pulmonary Embolism Diagnosis (PIOPED) trial, the most common findings in patients with pulmonary embolism were atelectasis or parenchymal areas of increased opacity in the lower lung zones and pleural effusions. However, only oligemia occurred significantly more frequently in patients with pulmonary embolism than in those without. The radiologic changes associated with pulmonary embolism are often subtle. They include (1) enlargement of the proximal pulmonary arteries, especially the descending portion of the right pulmonary artery—a comparison with an earlier film would be most helpful for this interpretation; (2) a distal, underperfused segment of lung causing hyperlucency of this lung segment; (3) pleural effusion and splinting of one diaphragm; (4) parenchymal infiltrates (due to infarction), seen most often in the costophrenic sulcus but also evident in the interlobar fissures; and (5) in chronic pulmonary artery pressure elevation, enlargement and dilatation not only of the pulmonary arteries but also of the right ventricle, right atrium, superior vena cava, and azygos vein. Certain radiologic abnormalities in acute pulmonary embolism may be predictive of the severity of pulmonary hypertension.[21] Any roentgenographic changes observed in a case of suspected pulmonary embolism should be correlated with perfusion and ventilation lung scans. Computed tomography and magnetic resonance imaging can be helpful, but pulmonary arteriography may be required for a definitive diagnosis.

CARDIAC CALCIFICATION

Valvular calcification

Valvular calcification involves the mitral and aortic valves and, rarely, the right heart valves. In the posteroanterior view, the aortic valve is slightly more cranial and closer to the spine, and the mitral valve is slightly lower and to the left. The line drawn from the origin of the left main bronchus to the anterior costophrenic sulcus on a lateral film separates the two valves, with the mitral valve below the line and the aortic valve anteriorly and above the line.

Nonvalvular calcification

Left atrial calcification occurs most commonly in association with long-standing mitral valve disease and develops either in an organized thrombus or in the wall of the left atrium. It is usually on the posterolateral aspect of the atrial wall and is linear and curved in shape.

Calcification occasionally occurs in an atrial myxoma. Differentiation from a calcified thrombus is difficult by roentgenography but usually can be made by echocardiography.

Ventricular myocardial calcifications are usually due to previous myocardial infarction, particularly if the myocardial infarction resulted in a left ventricular aneurysm. Such calcium is most commonly seen in the region of the apex of the left ventricle.

Pericardial calcification may be found in patients without symptoms and without evidence of cardiac constriction as well as in the classic patient with constrictive pericarditis. Calcification is most commonly seen along the diaphragmatic aspect of the ventricles, but it may extend from there to the region of the atria (Fig 4-22). It is best seen in the lateral view. Fewer than one-quarter of patients with clinical constrictive pericarditis have associated pericardial calcification, however.[22]

Coronary artery calcification characteristically occurs as two parallel lines or as irregular nodules of calcium arranged in a tubular form. The more dense the calcium and the younger the patient, the more it is likely that significant coronary artery stenosis exists. The left coronary artery is most commonly involved.

CONCLUSION

Roentgenographic examination is one of the most important means of study of the heart. Chest roentgenograms

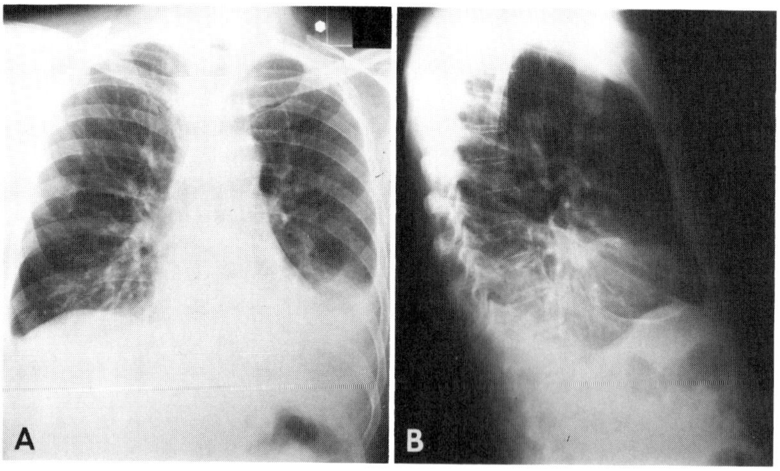

Fig 4-22 Calcified pericardium. Bilateral pleural effusions are present, larger on the left, with a normal heart size on the posteroanterior x-ray film (**A**). Calcification over the diaphragmatic surface of the ventricles, extending over the apex and lower anterior surface, is evident on the lateral film (**B**) but not on the posteroanterior film.

have the important additional attributes of being noninvasive and relatively low in cost. A significant amount of information can be obtained regarding cardiac size and shape; individual chamber enlargement; valvular, pericardial, coronary, and intracavitary calcification; and pulmonary arterial and venous abnormalities associated with the heart disease.

REFERENCES

1. Carlson HC, Kincaid OW, Ongley PA: Some observations on the relative influence of the heart and liver on the position of the diaphragm. *Proc Staff Meet Mayo Clin* 37:25-27, 1962
2. Wittenborg MH, Aviad I: Organ influence on the normal posture of the diaphragm: a radiological study of inversions and heterotaxies. *Br J Radiol* 36:280-288, 1963
3. Hoffman RB, Rigler LG: Evaluation of left ventricular enlargement in the lateral projection of the chest. *Radiology* 85:93-100, 1965
4. Glover L, Baxley WA, Dodge HT: A quantitative evaluation of heart size measurements from chest roentgenograms. *Circulation* 47: 1289-1296, 1973
5. Gammill SL, Krebs C, Meyers P, et al: Cardiac measurements in systole and diastole. *Radiology* 94:115-119, 1970
6. Stewart JR, Kincaid OW, Titus JL: Right aortic arch: plain film diagnosis and significance. *AJR* 97:377-389, 1966
7. Figley MM: Accessory roentgen signs of coarctation of the aorta. *Radiology* 62:671-686, 1954
8. Holman E: On circumscribed dilation of an artery immediately distal to a partially occluding band: poststenotic dilatation. *Surgery* 36:3-24, 1954
9. Simon M: The pulmonary vessels: their hemodynamic evaluation using routine radiographs. *Radiol Clin North Am* 1 No 2:363-376, 1963
10. Fishman AP, Renkin EM: *Pulmonary Edema.* Bethesda, American Physiological Society, 1979
11. Fleischner FG: The butterfly pattern of acute pulmonary edema. *Am J Cardiol* 20:39-46, 1967
12. Chait A: Interstitial pulmonary edema. *Circulation* 45:1323-1330, 1972
13. Spinar J, Vitovec J, Blaha M, et al: Radiologic changes in chronic heart failure. *Cor Vasa* 34:88-99, 1992
14. Herman PG, Khan A, Kallman CE, et al: Limited correlation of left ventricular end-diastolic pressure with radiographic assessment of pulmonary hemodynamics. *Radiology* 174:721-724, 1990
15. Connors AE, Cohen AM, Crass JR, et al: Can the chest radiograph enable prediction of cardiac status in patients with acute diagnosis? (Abstract.) *Radiology* 177 (Scientific Program):230, 1990
16. Don C, Johnson R: The nature and significance of peribronchial cuffing in pulmonary edema. *Radiology* 125:577-582, 1977
17. Rabin CB, Baron MG: *Radiology of the Chest.* Baltimore, Williams & Wilkins Company, 1979
18. Woodring JH: Pulmonary artery–bronchus ratios in patients with normal lungs, pulmonary vascular plethora, and congestive heart failure. *Radiology* 179:115-122, 1991
19. Worsley DF, Alavi A, Aronchick JM, et al: Chest radiographic findings in patients with acute pulmonary embolism: observations from the PIOPED Study. *Radiology* 189:133-136, 1993
20. Sasahara AA [Chairman]: Design of the trial. *Circulation* 47 Suppl II:18-21, 1973
21. Stein PD, Athanasoulis C, Greenspan RH, et al: Relation of plain chest radiographic findings to pulmonary arterial pressure and arterial blood oxygen levels in patients with acute pulmonary embolism. *Am J Cardiol* 69:394-396, 1992
22. Shanks SC, Kerley P (eds): *A Textbook of X-ray Diagnosis.* Vol. 2. Fourth edition. Philadelphia, WB Saunders Company, 1972, p 353

CHAPTER

5

Echocardiography

A. Two-dimensional echocardiography

Sylvia A. Mamby, M.D.

At no time in the history of ultrasound imaging have its applications to cardiovascular medicine been more innovative or intriguing. Since the advent of basic single-dimensional, or M-mode, imaging, echocardiography has evolved into a multifaceted technique with great utility to many aspects of cardiovascular disease and has largely replaced the need for invasive procedures for data acquisition.

The versatility of echocardiography now allows greater quality and diversity of cardiac imaging, with the added feature of functional assessment. Doppler echocardiography supplies a myriad of physiologic data, and transesophageal echocardiography, with its expanded "window," provides tremendous resolution and is often the sole determinant for surgical intervention. Stress echocardiography has become quite successful at accurately assessing myocardial ischemia.

In this and the following chapters, each of these techniques is reviewed. This chapter focuses on the basis of all ultrasonic cardiovascular imaging studies, the standard two-dimensional echocardiogram.

PRINCIPLES OF ULTRASOUND

To aid in the interpretive skills of clinical ultrasound, some basic knowledge of the physical principles of ultrasound is useful. Sound is a waveform, requiring a medium through which to travel, and is transmitted through a series of alternating compressions and rarefactions. Amplitude describes the degree of compressions and rarefactions, and wavelength indicates the distance between two consecutive compressions or rarefactions. A cycle represents a consecutive wave compression and rarefaction.

Sound is characterized by frequency, or the number of cycles per unit of time (hertz), by which 1 Hz equals 1 cycle/sec. Frequencies of sound greater than 20,000 Hz, which are beyond human perception, are referred to as "ultrasound." In general, ultrasound imaging ranges from 1 million to 10 million Hz, that is, up to 10 MHz.

Ultrasonic waves are generated from a source or transducer to a subject. Since sound follows the principles of reflection and refraction, reflected waves return to the source, are processed, and create an image. The velocity at which sound travels through a medium is the product of its frequency and wavelength. Velocity is proportional to the density of the medium through which sound travels. A relationship exists between the density of the medium and its acoustic impedance, so that acoustic impedance is the product of the density of the medium and the velocity of the sound wave. As sound travels through one medium and approaches the interface of another medium of a different acoustic impedance, alterations occur, so that reflected waves, or echoes, travel back to the transducer and transmitted waves are refracted into the medium.

Ultrasound waves are emitted from the transducer at a known rate, or pulse repetition frequency. The transducer not only is the genesis of the sound wave but also behaves as a recipient of the reflected waves. The time interval between emitted and received waves is measured, and knowing the speed of ultrasound transmission through human tissue (approximately 1,540 m/sec) allows calculation of the depth of a given object. The strength of a given object's reflection or signal intensity is also analyzed by the ultrasound source.

Multiple ultrasound images of aligned segments are summated to create a cross-sectional image, or two-dimensional echocardiogram. The requirements to produce an ultrasound image, therefore, are an ultrasound transducer to generate and receive waves, a system to analyze and reconstruct reflected waves, and a monitor to create an image.

EXAMINATION OF THE NORMAL HEART

The standard echocardiographic examination encompasses M-mode, two-dimensional, and conventional and color-flow Doppler imaging. Doppler echocardiography is reviewed in chapter 5B.

A pertinent medical history provides a focus for each echocardiographic study; however, the specific question to be answered by the study must be elicited. Single-dimensional, or M-mode, echocardiography had its greatest use 20 to 30 years ago. Currently, it is largely a supplement that seldom yields information not provided

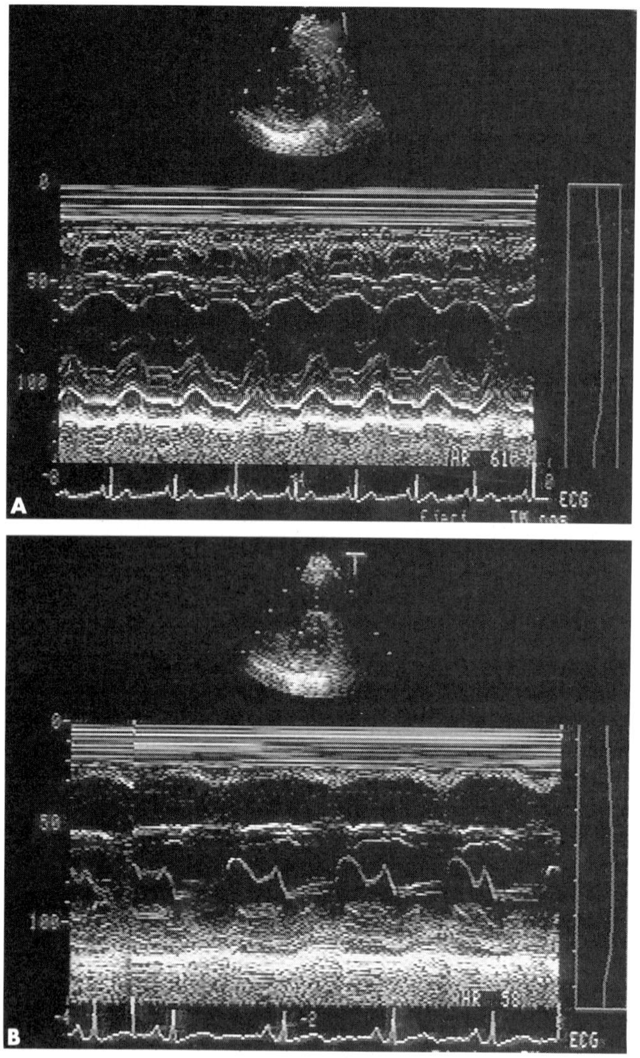

Fig 5A-1 M-mode echocardiograms of the left ventricle in cross section **(A)** and the mitral valve **(B)**.

by two-dimensional imaging. Typically, a two-dimensional transducer is used to obtain M-mode data (Fig 5A-1). Although frequently subject to errors of angulation, M-mode tracings are still occasionally used for determination of chamber dimension and measurement of left ventricular wall thickness. Fine movement definition of valve structure is also well appreciated.

In addition to M-mode imaging, the sonographer obtains multiple two-dimensional images of the heart from a series of standard orthogonal planes or windows. The four basic imaging planes are the parasternal long- and short-axis planes and the apical two- and four-chamber planes. The more comprehensive examination includes suprasternal and subcostal images as well. Two-dimensional imaging typically uses phased-array transducers in which the ultrasonic beam moves in a sector generated by multiple elements.

The patient lies in the left lateral decubitus position. Parasternal long-axis images are obtained with the transducer placed between the second and the fifth intercostal spaces. The imaging plane is parallel to the long axis of the left ventricle (Fig 5A-2). This orientation displays the right and left ventricles, aortic and mitral valves, and left atrium. Gentle counterclockwise rotation of the transducer with angulation toward the right atrium and tricuspid valve creates the right ventricular inflow view (Fig 5A-3). Clockwise rotation of the transducer from the parasternal long-axis view by approximately 90° produces the parasternal short-axis view. This demonstrates the left ventricle in cross section and with gentle angulation allows an inspection of the left ventricular myocardium from basal to apical levels (Fig 5A-4). Short-axis images at the level of the aortic valve allow visualization of the right ventricular outflow tract and pulmonary artery bifurcation.

Apical images are obtained by placing the transducer over the cardiac apex and directing it toward the patient's right shoulder. The apical four-chamber view allows simultaneous visualization of all four cardiac chambers, the atrial and ventricular septa, and the two atrioventricular valves (Fig 5A-5). The junction of the two septa and atrioventricular valves is the crux of the heart. The slightly more apical insertion of the septal tricuspid valve leaflet than of the anterior mitral valve leaflet readily identifies the right ventricle. The apical four-chamber view demonstrates ventricular structure and function, mural thrombi or other cardiac masses, aneurysm formation, and abnormalities of atrioventricular valve structure. In the apical four-chamber view, the septal and lateral walls of the left ventricle are visualized. With clockwise rotation of the transducer, the apical two-chamber view is demonstrated, allowing assessment of the left atrium and anterior and inferior walls of the left ventricle (Fig 5A-6). Slight anterior angulation from this image generates the apical long-axis view. This modification of the two-chamber image allows visualization of the anteroseptal and inferolateral walls of the left ventricle. Subcostal orientation of the transducer can also achieve four-chamber and short-axis images. This window, on occasion, may embody most of the echocardiographic study in patients who have hyperinflated lungs or in whom imaging is otherwise difficult from more standard planes. This view also allows the best demonstration of the atrial septum and lends itself well to caliber determination of the abdominal aorta, inferior vena cava, and hepatic veins (Fig 5A-7).

Placing the transducer in the suprasternal notch creates the suprasternal view, allowing visualization of the aortic arch and, occasionally, the brachiocephalic and left common carotid arteries. With good resolution, the pulmonary artery may also be seen in cross section (Fig 5A-8).

EVALUATION OF CARDIAC PERFORMANCE

Although in every echocardiographic study a specific question is the directive for the evaluation, an assessment of left ventricular structure and function is fundamental to all examinations.

Two-dimensional echocardiography addresses several

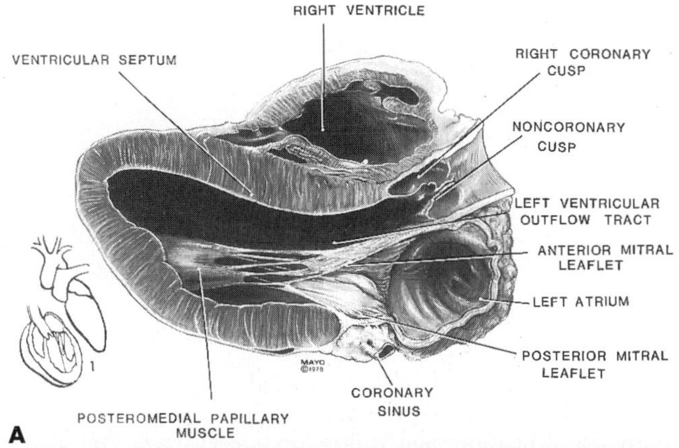

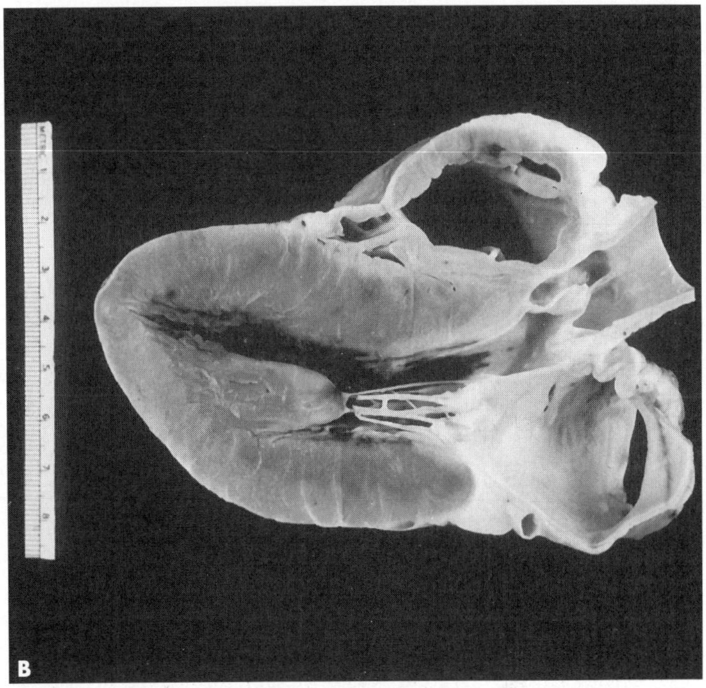

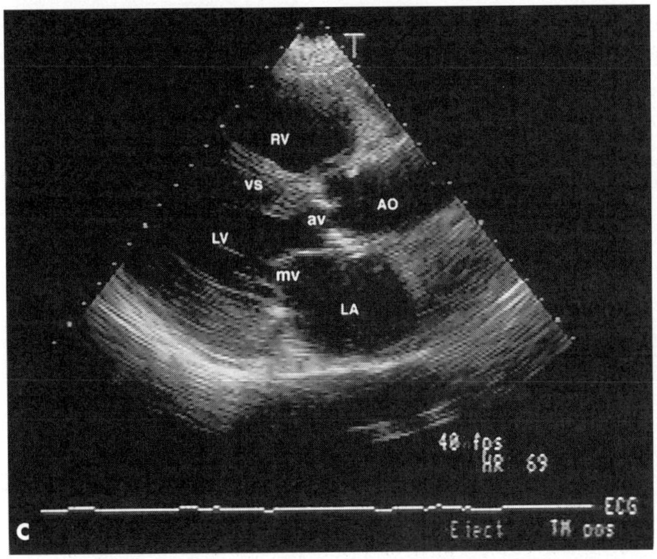

Fig 5A-2 Drawing of the parasternal long-axis view of the heart **(A)** is compared with the corresponding anatomic specimen **(B)** and two-dimensional echocardiographic image **(C)**. This imaging plane is parallel to the long axis of the left ventricle and provides evaluation of the left ventricle *(LV),* right ventricle *(RV),* left atrium *(LA),* and mitral *(mv)* and aortic *(av)* valves. The ventricular septum *(vs)* and descending thoracic aorta *(AO)* are also demonstrated. (**A** and **B** from Tajik AJ, Seward JB, Hagler DJ, et al: Two- dimensional real-time ultrasonic imaging of the heart and great vessels: technique, image orientation, structure identification, and validation. *Mayo Clin Proc* 53:271-303, 1978. By permission, Mayo Foundation.)

features of left ventricular structure, including cavity dimension, wall thickness, and mass determination. Two-dimensional echocardiography provides a more accurate determination of cavity size than does M-mode echocardiography. End-diastolic dimension of the left ventricle can be measured with the onset of the QRS or the peak of the R wave as the reference point.[1]

Echocardiography provides a good quantitative assessment of wall mass. Formerly, left ventricular mass was determined by taking manual M-mode or two-dimensional measurements of septal and posterior wall thicknesses and applying the formula

$$\text{left ventricular mass} = 1.04\,[(\text{LVID} + \text{PWT} + \text{IVST}^3) - \text{LVID}^3] - 13.6\text{ g}$$

in which LVID is left ventricular internal dimension, PWT is posterior wall thickness, and IVST is interventricular septal wall thickness.[2] Currently, however, many echocardiographic computer systems can create similar data from two-dimensional echocardiography by providing a tracing of the epicardial and endocardial surfaces of the left ventricular myocardium. Left ventricular hypertrophy is present when myocardial mass is greater than 125 g/m^2 in men and 110 g/m^2 in women.[3]

Imaging parameters of global left ventricular systolic function are either volume-dependent or volume-independent. Volume-dependent calculations are those for ejection fraction and stroke volume. Ejection fraction traditionally uses the difference between the square of end-diastolic and end-systolic dimensions divided by the

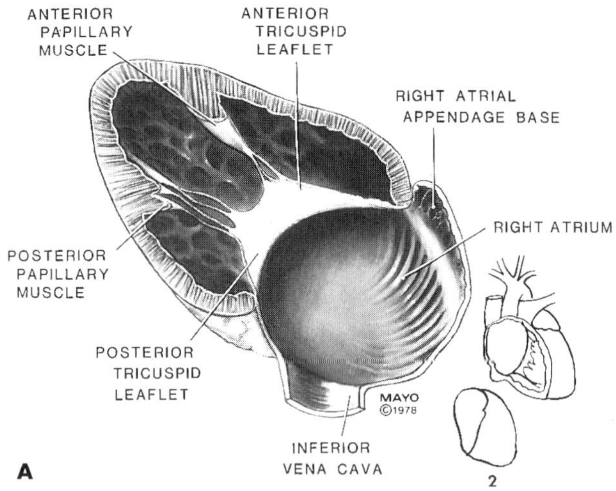

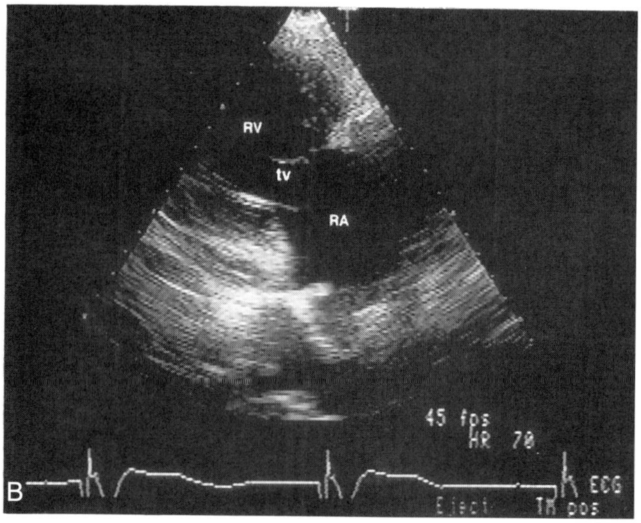

Fig 5A-3 Drawing (**A**) and two-dimensional echocardiographic image (**B**) of the right ventricular inflow view of the heart. This view allows visualization of the right atrium *(RA),* right ventricle *(RV),* and tricuspid valve *(tv).* (**A** from Tajik AJ, Seward JB, Hagler DJ, et al: Two-dimensional real-time ultrasonic imaging of the heart and great vessels: technique, image orientation, structure identification, and validation. *Mayo Clin Proc* 53:271-303, 1978. By permission, Mayo Foundation.)

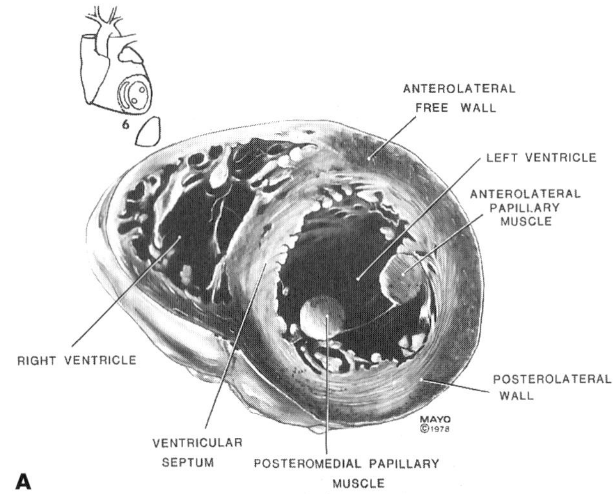

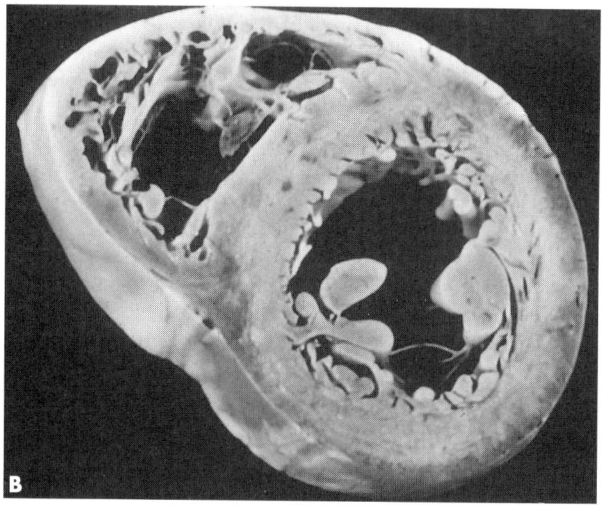

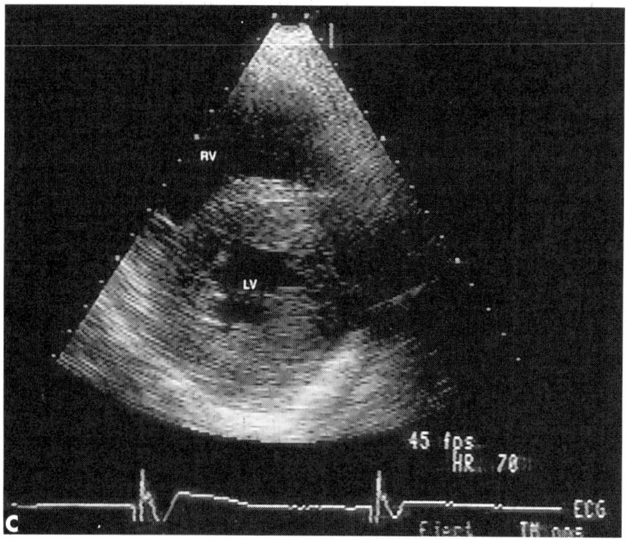

Fig 5A-4 Parasternal short-axis view of the heart by drawing (**A**), anatomic section (**B**), and two-dimensional echocardiographic image (**C**). Clockwise 90° rotation of the transducer from the parasternal long-axis view creates this image. The left *(LV)* and right *(RV)* ventricles can be assessed in cross section. (**A** and **B** from Tajik AJ, Seward JB, Hagler DJ, et al: Two-dimensional real-time ultrasonic imaging of the heart and great vessels: technique, image orientation, structure identification, and validation. *Mayo Clin Proc* 53:271-303, 1978. By permission, Mayo Foundation.)

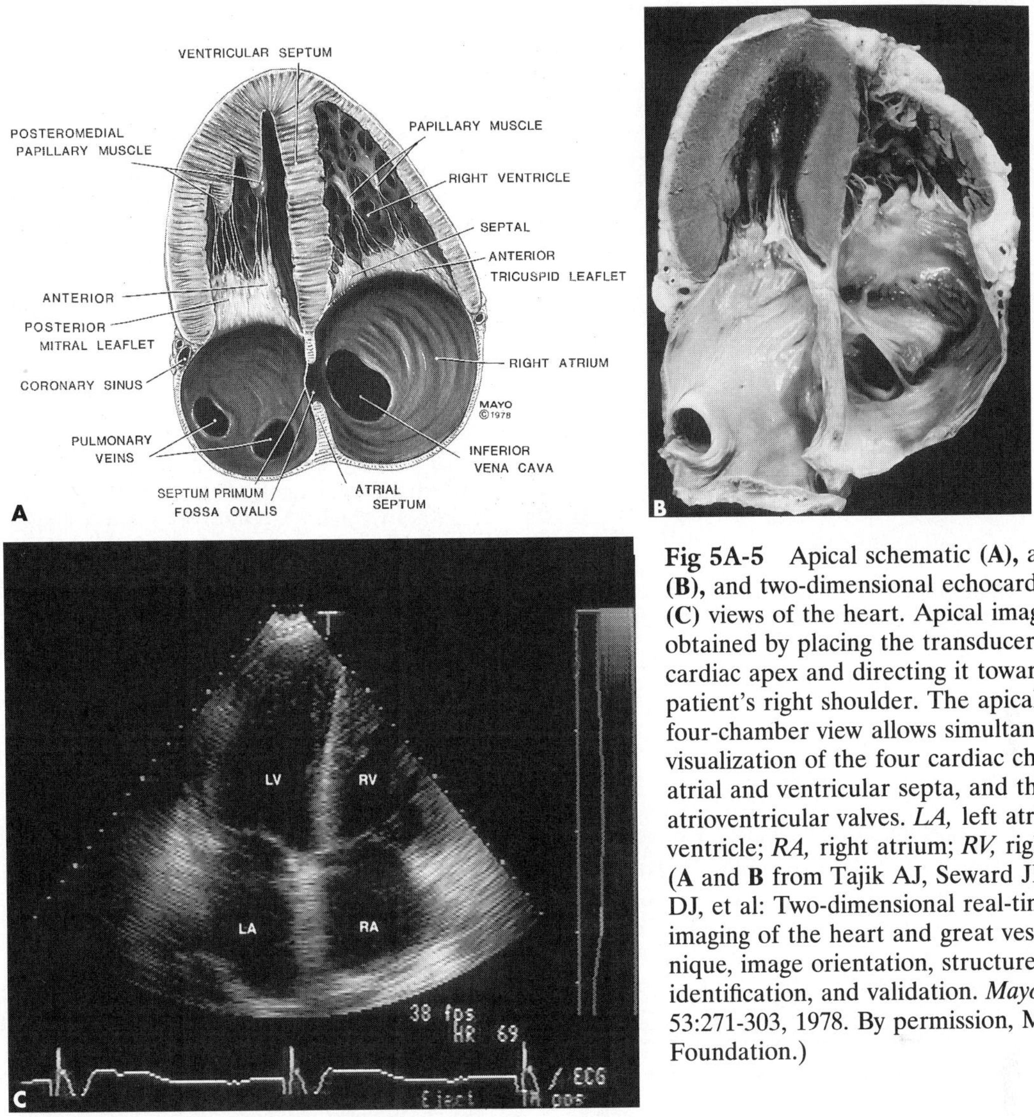

Fig 5A-5 Apical schematic (**A**), anatomic (**B**), and two-dimensional echocardiographic (**C**) views of the heart. Apical images are obtained by placing the transducer over the cardiac apex and directing it toward the patient's right shoulder. The apical four-chamber view allows simultaneous visualization of the four cardiac chambers, the atrial and ventricular septa, and the two atrioventricular valves. *LA,* left atrium; *LV,* left ventricle; *RA,* right atrium; *RV,* right ventricle. (**A** and **B** from Tajik AJ, Seward JB, Hagler DJ, et al: Two-dimensional real-time ultrasonic imaging of the heart and great vessels: technique, image orientation, structure identification, and validation. *Mayo Clin Proc* 53:271-303, 1978. By permission, Mayo Foundation.)

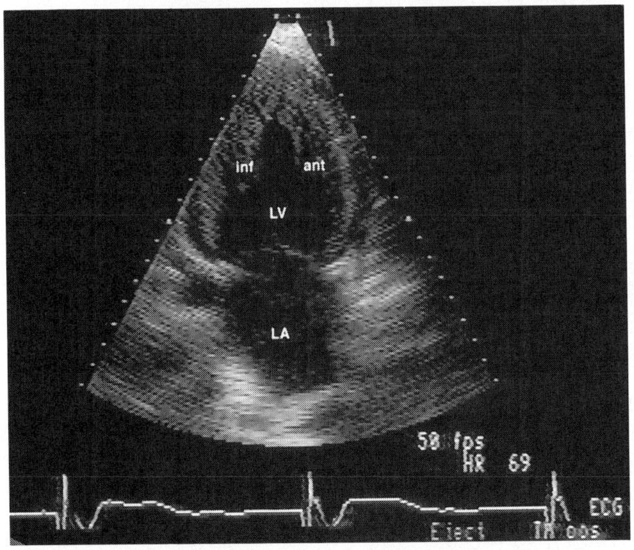

Fig 5A-6 Clockwise rotation of the transducer from the apical four-chamber view produces the apical two-chamber view. This view provides evaluation of the left atrium *(LA)* and the anterior *(ant)* and inferior *(inf)* walls of the left ventricle *(LV).*

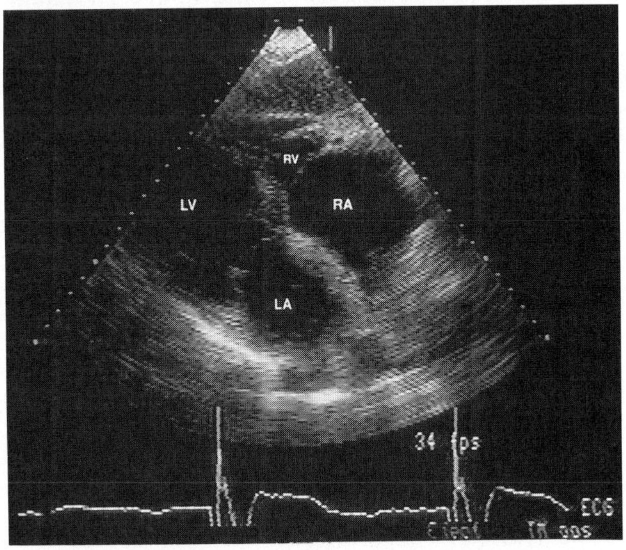

Fig 5A-7 A subcostal two-dimensional echocardiographic image displays the four-chamber view. *LA,* left atrium; *LV,* left ventricle; *RA,* right atrium; *RV,* right ventricle.

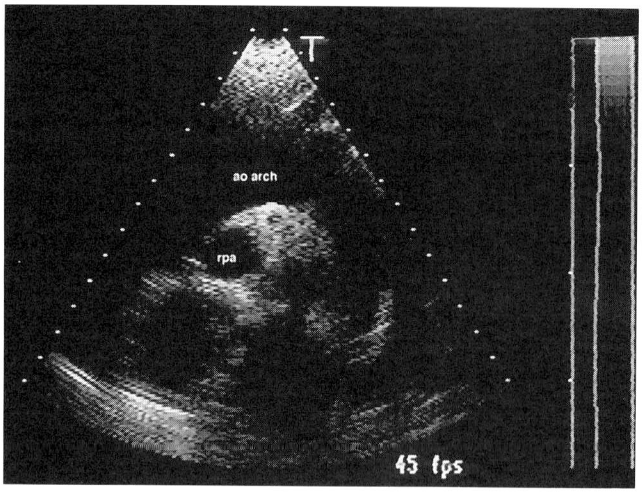

Fig 5A-8 The suprasternal image allows visualization of the aortic arch *(ao arch)* and the proximal portions of its branches. The right pulmonary artery *(rpa)* may also be seen.

square of the end-diastolic dimension. A more accurate assessment can be made with the modified Simpson method (or method of discs).[4] This method, favored by the American Society of Echocardiography, creates a measurement of left ventricular volume by tracing the left ventricular endocardium in the apical two- and four-chamber views. The cavity is divided into multiple slices of equal thickness, and computer summation establishes left ventricular volumes at end-systole and end-diastole. An accurate measurement depends on an apical image of good quality that does not foreshorten the left ventricular cavity.

Volume-independent parameters of left ventricular systolic performance are mean rate of circumferential fiber shortening, separation of E point and septum, and fractional shortening. Mean rate of circumferential fiber shortening (Vcf) is measured in circumferences per second:

$$\text{Vcf} = \frac{\text{EDD} - \text{ESD}}{\text{EDD} \times \text{LVET}}$$

in which EDD is left ventricular end-diastolic dimension, ESD is left ventricular end-systolic dimension, and LVET is left ventricular ejection time.[5] The added effort of left ventricular ejection time can be avoided by calculating percentage of fractional shortening (%FS).[6] The method is quick, reproducible, and comparable with Vcf:

$$\%\text{FS} = \frac{\text{EDD} - \text{ESD}}{\text{EDD}} \times 100\%$$

The margin of error increases with paradoxical septal wall motion. Mitral E point-septal separation has been a useful predictor of an abnormal ejection fraction.[7] This M-mode calculation measures the distance from the mitral E point to the left ventricular border of the septum. A reduced ejection fraction is predicted by a separation of greater than 10 mm. The mitral-septal angle has also been shown to correlate well with ejection fraction.[8] Measured in the apical four-chamber plane, the angle is the narrowest one during early diastole between the anterior mitral valve leaflet and the ventricular septum. An angle of less than 30° suggests a normal ejection fraction. Mitral annular excursion during left ventricular systole has also been used to assess left ventricular function. Reduced annular excursion suggests impaired left ventricular systolic function.

Future assessment of left ventricular volume and ejection fraction calculation may involve the acoustic quantification method developed by Hewlett Packard. Endocardial borders are detected by specific labeling of the blood-myocardium interface, creating a beat-to-beat evaluation of left ventricular volume and ejection. Although early in development at this time, the technique promises to provide a highly accurate assessment of left ventricular function.

REFERENCES

1. Friedman MJ, Roeske WR, Sahn DJ, et al: Accuracy of M mode echocardiographic measurements of the left ventricle. *Am J Cardiol* 49:716-723, 1982
2. Devereux RB, Reichek N: Echocardiographic determination of left ventricular mass in man: anatomic validation of the method. *Circulation* 55:613-618, 1977
3. Devereux RB, Alonso DR, Lutas EM, et al: Echocardiographic assessment of left ventricular hypertrophy: comparison to necropsy findings. *Am J Cardiol* 57:450-458, 1986
4. Schiller NB, Shah PM, Crawford M, et al: Recommendations for quantitation of the left ventricle by two-dimensional echocardiography. *J Am Soc Echocardiogr* 2:358-367, 1989
5. Cooper RH, O'Rourke RA, Karliner JS, et al: Comparison of ultrasound and cineangiographic measurements of the mean rate of circumferential fiber shortening in man. *Circulation* 46:914-923, 1972
6. Rosenblatt A, Clark R, Burgess J, et al: Echocardiographic assessment of the level of cardiac compensation in valvular heart disease. *Circulation* 54:509-518, 1976
7. Massie BM, Schiller NB, Ratshin R, et al: Mitral-septal separation: new echocardiographic index of left ventricular function. *Am J Cardiol* 39:1008-1016, 1977
8. Abinader EG, Kuo LC, Rokey R, et al: Mitral-septal angle: a new two-dimensional echocardiographic index of left ventricular performance. *Am Heart J* 110:381-386, 1985

CHAPTER

5

Echocardiography

B. Doppler echocardiography

Rick A. Nishimura, M.D., and Mark J. Callahan, M.D.

TWO-DIMENSIONAL echocardiography is a noninvasive modality that provides anatomic information by real-time imaging of the heart in multiple tomographic planes.[1] Doppler echocardiography is a valuable adjunct to two-dimensional echocardiography because it provides information about blood flow velocity within the cardiac chambers, across valves, and in the great vessels.[2,3] Application of Doppler principles allows calculation of pressure gradients, intracardiac pressures, and volumetric flow as well as semiquantitative information about regurgitant lesions, intracardiac shunts, and diastolic function. The result is a noninvasive, hemodynamic assessment of the heart by echocardiography. Doppler echocardiography, however, is an operator-dependent technique with its own inherent limitations and pitfalls, which must be understood for proper clinical interpretation.

THE DOPPLER PRINCIPLE

In the 19th century, Christian Doppler offered an explanation for the observation that a star would appear to change colors when viewed from the earth. According to his theory, all stars emitted a pure spectrum white light, but the different colors appeared because movement of the star toward or away from the earth changed the frequency of light being received on earth. This phenomenon, termed the "Doppler effect," refers to the frequency shift that occurs when the source and receiver of a wave are moving with respect to each other. The frequency shift is proportional to the relative movement between the emitter and the receiver (Fig 5B-1).

In Doppler echocardiography, a transducer emits an ultrasound wave of a certain frequency toward the cardiac structures. When this wave reflects off a stationary structure, the backscattered wave is the same frequency as the transmitted one. However, when the beam is reflected off moving red blood cells, there is a change in the frequency of the wave that is proportional to the velocity of the moving red blood cells.

The Doppler shift frequency is the difference between the transmitted frequency and the reflected frequency.

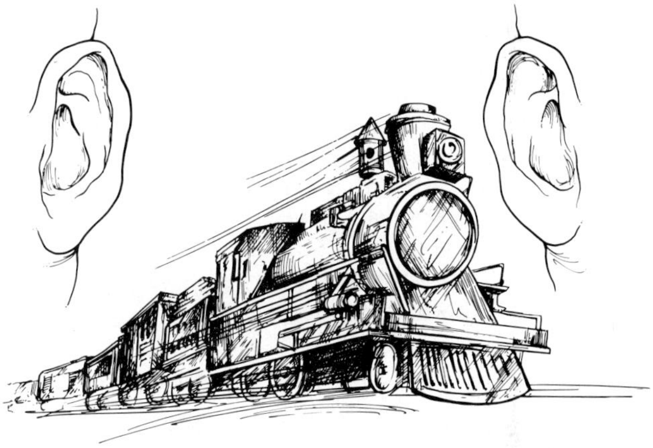

Fig 5B-1 Schematic diagram illustrating the Doppler principle. When a sound beam of a certain frequency is emanating from a moving object (train), the received sound beam has a different frequency. The change in frequency (Doppler shift) is proportional to the velocity of the moving object.

The Doppler equation relates the frequency shift to velocity.

$$\Delta f = \frac{2fo \times v \times \cos\theta}{c} \qquad \textbf{[5B-1]}$$

in which Δf is the Doppler shift, v is the velocity of moving red blood cells, θ is the angle between the Doppler beam and the velocity vector, fo is the frequency of the transmitted sounds, and c is the velocity of sound in tissue (1,560 cm/sec).

From Equation 5B-1, Equation 5B-2 can be derived, which directly calculates the velocity of the moving red blood cells.

$$v = \frac{c}{2fo} \times \frac{f}{\cos\theta} \qquad \textbf{[5B-2]}$$

For an accurate measurement of velocity of blood flow, it is essential that the Doppler beam be placed as parallel as possible to the jet of moving red blood cells ($\cos\theta = 1$). If the angle between the jet and the Doppler beam is large, the velocity will be greatly underestimated (e.g., an angle of greater than 60° causes a greater than 50% underestimation of the velocity). However, if θ is less than 25°, the underestimation will be less than 10%.

PULSED-WAVE, CONTINUOUS-WAVE, AND COLOR-FLOW IMAGING

Currently, three techniques are used in Doppler echocardiography: pulsed-wave, continuous-wave, and color-flow imaging. The velocities obtained by pulsed-wave and continuous-wave Doppler echocardiography are registered on a spectral display in which the velocity is on the y-axis and time is on the x-axis. Shades of gray are used to indicate the intensity of the Doppler signal. By convention, a signal above the baseline indicates a velocity directed toward the transducer, and a signal below the baseline indicates velocity away from the transducer. Color-flow imaging displays the Doppler velocities by superimposing color-encoded blood velocity and direction on a real-time two-dimensional echocardiographic image. Each of these three modalities provides unique information about the intracardiac blood flow velocities. For a complete Doppler evaluation, it is necessary to use information from all three techniques in conjunction with the information provided by M-mode and two-dimensional echocardiography.

Pulsed-wave Doppler echocardiography

In pulsed-wave Doppler echocardiography, a single ultrasound crystal serves as the emitter and the receiver of the reflected ultrasound beams. Bursts of ultrasound are emitted at a frequency called the "pulse-repetition frequency," and the reflected wave is received during the interval between the transmitted pulses. The time delay from the transmission to the reception is proportional to the depth at which the ultrasound beam is being reflected. "Time-gating" the returning signals defines a "sample volume" at a specific depth along the ultrasound beam, allowing interrogation of blood velocity in this region. By using a simultaneous two-dimensional echocardiographic image, one can position the sample volume within various cardiac chambers to determine the location at which blood flow is interrogated (Fig 5B-2).

The principal limitation of pulsed-wave Doppler echocardiography is that there is a limit to the maximal frequency shift that can be measured. This frequency shift, termed the "Nyquist limit," is equal to half the pulse repetition frequency. The farther away the sample volume is placed, the lower is the Nyquist limit. If the velocity of blood flow is greater than the Nyquist limit, "aliasing" occurs: the velocity spectrum folds over on itself. This distortion of the spectral display signal prohibits the determination of the maximal velocity of blood flow. If the blood flow is turbulent, multiple velocity vectors in different directions are present, and the spectral display consists of a broad band of Doppler signals, termed "spectral broadening" (Fig 5B-3).

Pulsed-wave Doppler echocardiography provides two basic types of clinical information. When laminar flow of low velocity is present, pulsed-wave Doppler echocardiography is an ideal modality for determining the instantaneous velocities. This study is used to determine volumetric flow[4,5] and to form the basis for evaluating diastolic filling of the heart.[6,7] When blood flow is turbulent, the pulsed-wave Doppler examination can serve as a "mapping" technique in which placement of the sample volume is used to interrogate the presence and extent of turbulence. This provides the diagnosis and a semiquantitative measurement of the degree of valvular regurgitation and intracardiac shunts.[8,9] The development of color-flow imaging, however, has obviated pulsed-wave mapping in most instances.

Electronic techniques have been developed to increase the usefulness of pulsed-wave mapping. Pulsed-wave Doppler echocardiography with a high frequency of pulse repetition raises the Nyquist limit by increasing the pulse repetition frequency. This reduces the range specificity by adding one, two, or three sample volumes. Although helpful for measurement of slight increases in blood velocities, high pulse repetition frequency significantly underestimates high velocities. The second development that has been built into many Doppler echocardiographic machines is "angle correction." Since the Doppler beam in a pulsed-wave system cannot be directed parallel to a jet in some instances, angle correction allows incorporation of a predetermined angle into the Doppler equation. Angle correction is useful for examination of the peripheral circulation, in which flow is parallel to the long axis of the vascular structure. However, it has not been of clinical utility when applied to intracardiac velocities.

Continuous-wave Doppler echocardiography

In a continuous-wave Doppler system, there are two crystals on the transducer. One of the crystals continuously emits an ultrasound beam, and the second crystal continuously receives the backscattered signal. High velocities are accurately measured, and aliasing does not occur in clinical practice (see Fig 5B-3). The disadvantage of the continuous-wave Doppler system is that the velocities are measured along the entire Doppler beam, so that range ambiguity results.

Continuous-wave Doppler echocardiography is used for quantitation of pressure gradients. In most clinical situations, the origin of the high-velocity jets can be localized to a specific valve or shunt on the basis of the timing and the appearance on the spectral display. By measurement of these high velocities, information about gradients and intracardiac pressures can be accurately and reliably obtained.

Various electronic developments, such as duplex scanning (combination of two-dimensional and continuous-wave Doppler modes), angle correction, and steerable Doppler beams, are available. However, the experienced echocardiographer should perform the continuous-wave Doppler examination with a small, nonimaging transducer

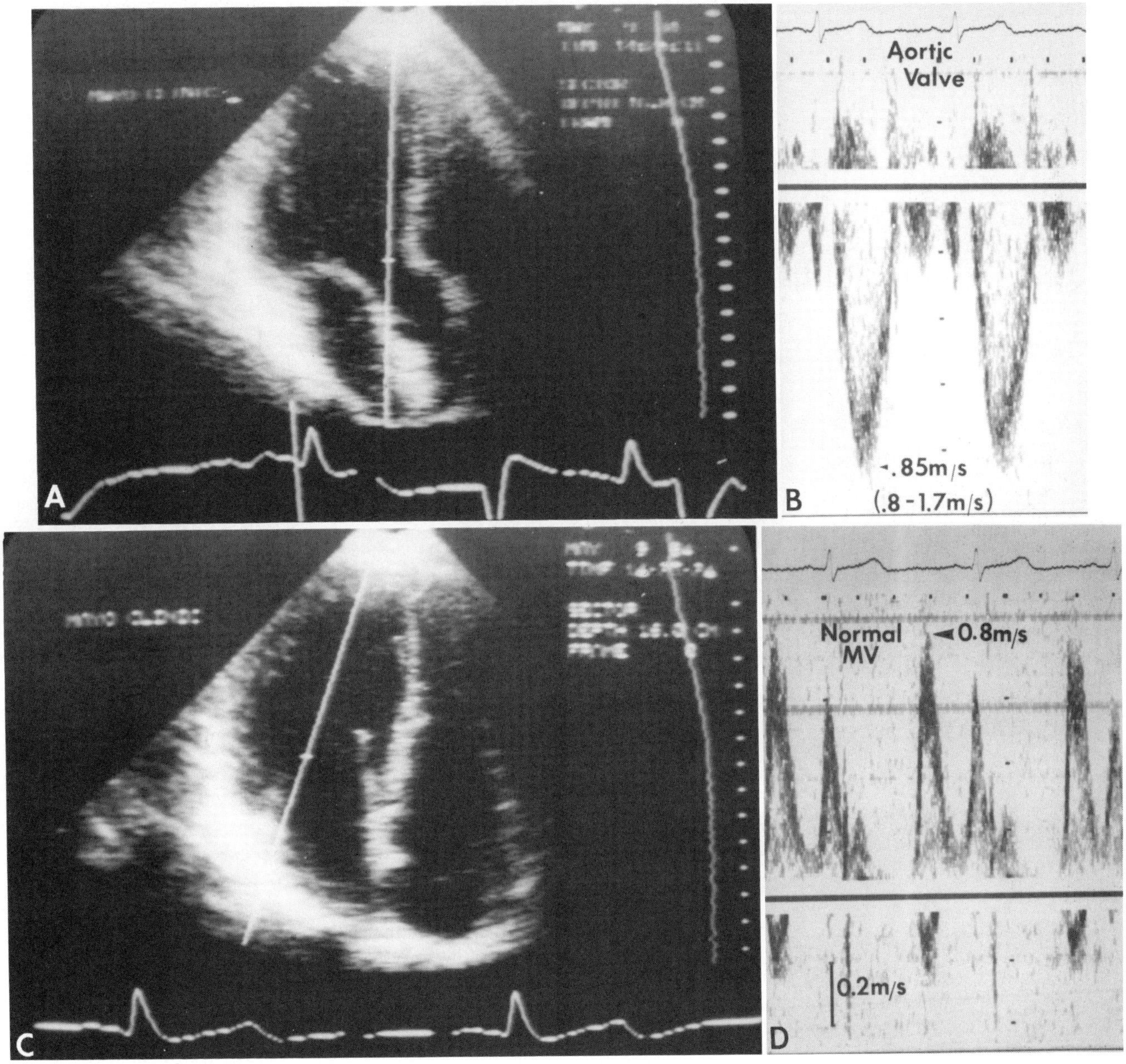

Fig 5B-2 Pulsed-wave Doppler velocity curves across normal valves. **A** and **B,** sample volume placed at the level of the aortic valve from the view demonstrating a systolic velocity below the baseline. **C** and **D,** pulsed-wave sample volume placed at the level of the mitral valve (MV) from the apical view demonstrating an early peak velocity, a rapid deceleration, and a velocity atrial contraction. *Continued.*

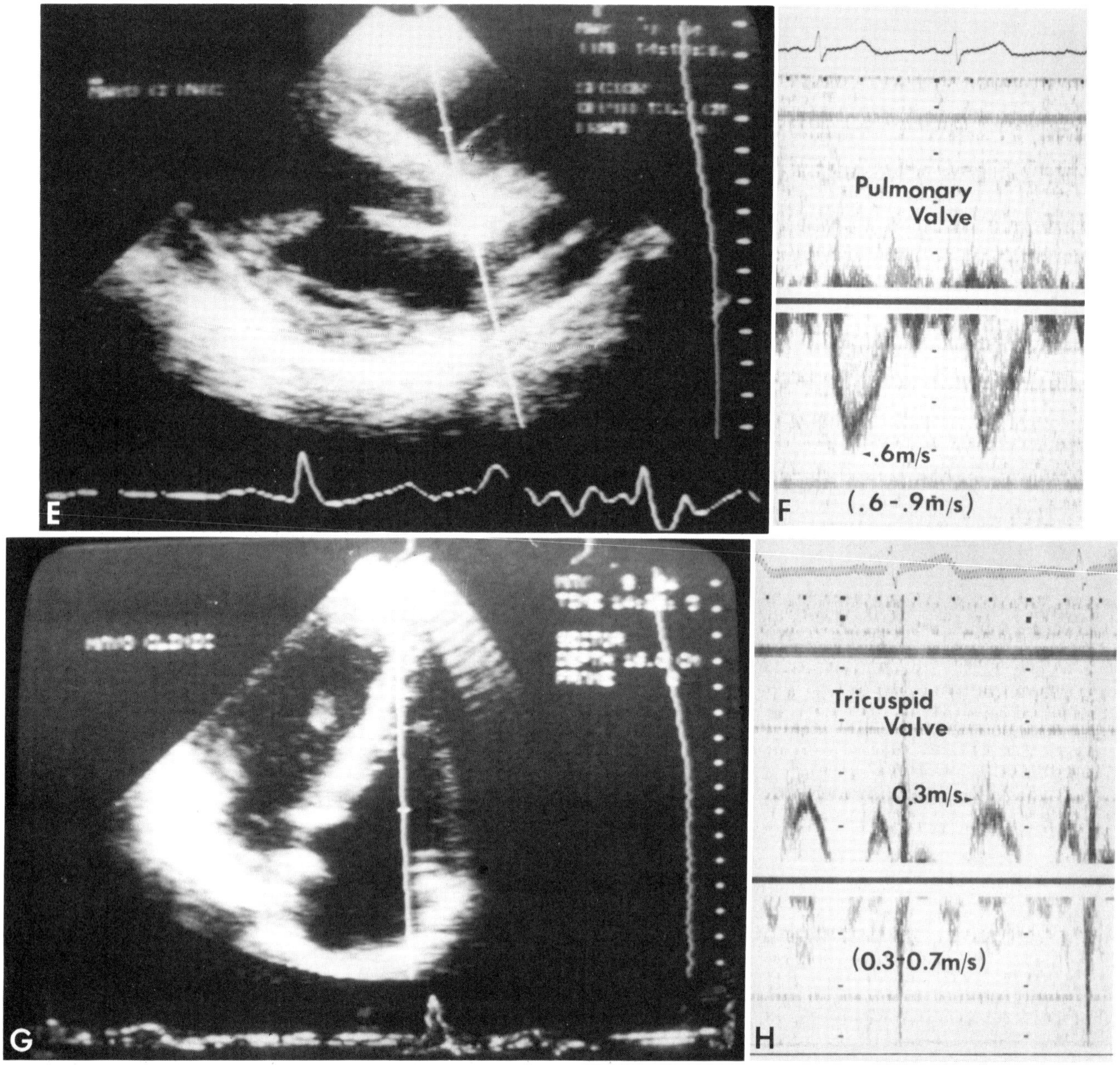

Fig 5B-2, cont'd. **E** and **F**, pulsed-wave sample of volume placed at the level of the pulmonary valve from the parasternal view demonstrating a systolic velocity below the baseline. **G** and **H**, pulsed-wave sample of volume placed at a level of the tricuspid valve from the modified low parasternal view demonstrating the same velocity curve as the mitral valve but with a lower velocity. Normal values (in m/sec) are displayed in parentheses.

(2 to 2.5 MHz, 1- to 1.5-cm diameter). Although a blind approach is necessary, the Doppler beam can usually be aligned nearly parallel to the maximal velocity jet when guided by the audio signal and spectral display alone.[2,3] The small acoustic aperture required allows placement of the transducer in echocardiographic windows not accessible by the larger duplex transducers.

Color-flow imaging

Color-flow imaging allows real-time visualization of intracardiac blood flow superimposed on a two-dimensional echocardiographic image[10,11] (Fig 5B-4). This has been made possible by the development of color-encoded, digital, multigated Doppler flow analysis. By convention, flow toward the transducer is depicted as red and flow

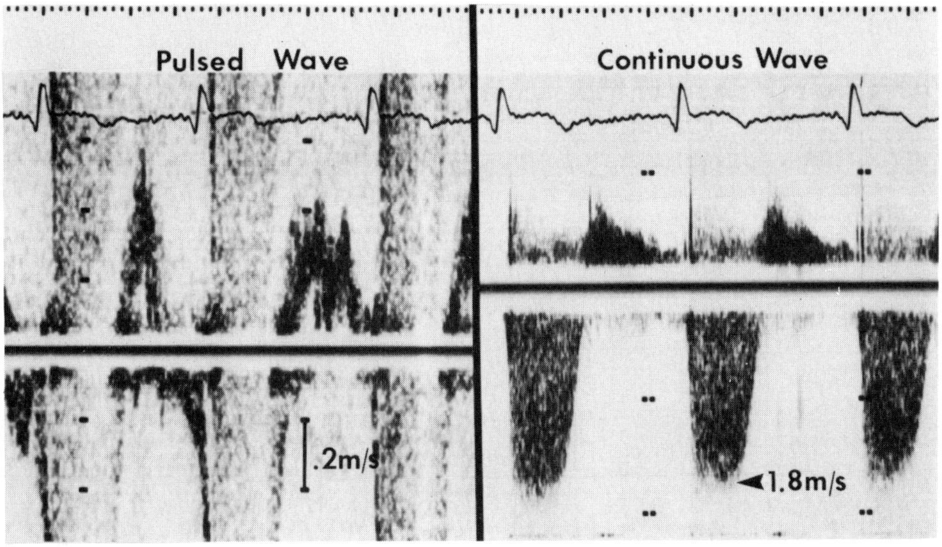

Fig 5B-3 Pulsed-wave and continuous-wave tracings from a patient with tricuspid regurgitation. **Left,** pulsed-wave tracing demonstrating "aliasing" in which the velocity is higher than the Nyquist limit. The velocity "wraps around" the spectral display such that the maximum velocity cannot be determined. **Right,** in continuous-wave Doppler tracing from the same patient, the maximum velocity can be clearly delineated.

away from the transducer as blue. The relative velocities are represented by eight shades of these colors. The lighter the shade, the higher the velocity. In areas of turbulent flow, green may be added, forming a mosaic pattern.

Color-flow imaging can be looked on simply as a method of displaying a multitude of pulsed-wave sample volumes superimposed on a real-time two-dimensional image. This facilitates the ability to detect and "map out" areas of abnormal blood flow. Since this is a pulsed-wave system, a Nyquist limit is present and high velocities cannot be measured. Velocities exceeding the Nyquist limit but remaining less than twice this value are displayed as "reversal" of color flow, such that blue would be substituted for red and vice versa. If velocities are exceedingly high with turbulence, a blue, red, and green mosaic pattern is present. In the normal cardiac chambers and great vessels, the velocities are laminar and do not exceed two times the Nyquist limit of the color-flow imaging modality. Therefore, areas of high velocity and turbulence can be well outlined (Fig 5B-5).

A three-dimensional "reconstruction" of a maximal jet area of high velocity and turbulent flow is possible through the use of two orthogonal planes or multiple cross-sectional tomographic planes through the jet. This method detects valvular regurgitation and intracardiac shunts and provides a semiquantitative estimate of the severity of regurgitation and the size of the shunts.[10,11] The accuracy of color-flow imaging in providing this information depends on image resolution. If the two-dimensional echocardiographic image is poor, the quality of the color-flow imaging will also be suboptimal. Interrogation of chambers in the far field of an echocardiographic image may result in suboptimal color imaging because of poor penetration of the ultrasound beam. A jet of abnormal velocity is a three-dimensional structure, and conventional two-dimensional echocardiographic images may not fully display the maximal jet area. Color-flow imaging depends on gain requiring optimization of instrument settings. Color-flow imaging for semiquantitation has theoretic limitations, as will be discussed later.

Color-flow imaging may be used to direct a pulsed-wave or continuous-wave Doppler interrogation. By visualizing the velocity jet, one can place a pulsed- or continuous-wave Doppler beam in the jet parallel to flow to minimize the angle of θ (Fig 5B-6).

Comprehensive examination

A comprehensive echocardiographic evaluation uses both two-dimensional and Doppler modalities. A complete two-dimensional examination should be performed before the Doppler examination for anatomic information. This provides the basis for a goal-directed Doppler examination, in which an abnormality on two-dimensional echocardiography can be thoroughly investigated by Doppler echocardiography. It is usually necessary to use all three Doppler modalities (pulsed-wave, continuous-wave, and color-flow imaging) during the evaluation.

Doppler echocardiography is an operator-dependent procedure with a steep learning curve. Even when the operator is experienced, in some instances the Doppler examination will not provide adequate information, such

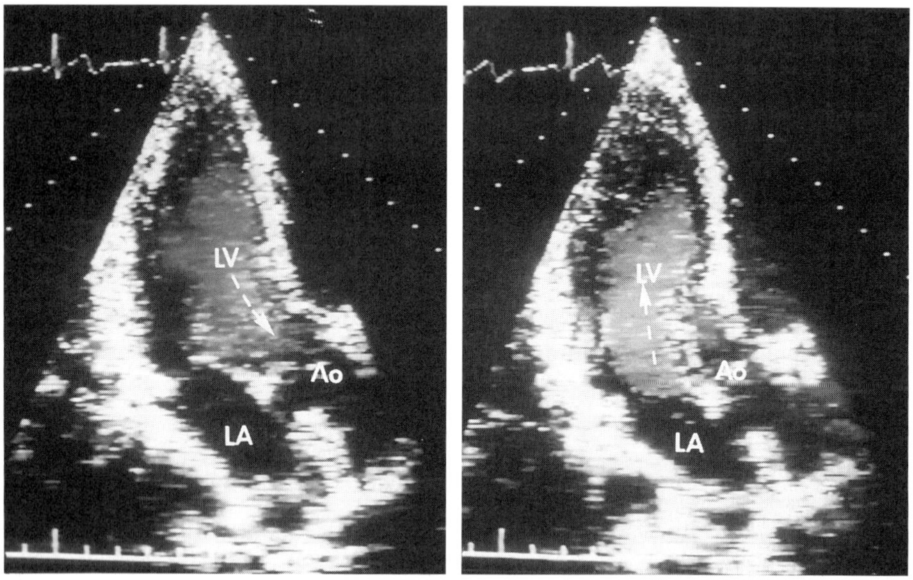

Fig 5B-4 (see color plate after page 200) Color-flow imaging of a normal heart. Two-dimensional apical long-axis views during systole **(left)** and diastole **(right)**. Velocity toward the transducer is depicted as red, and velocity away from the transducer is depicted as blue.

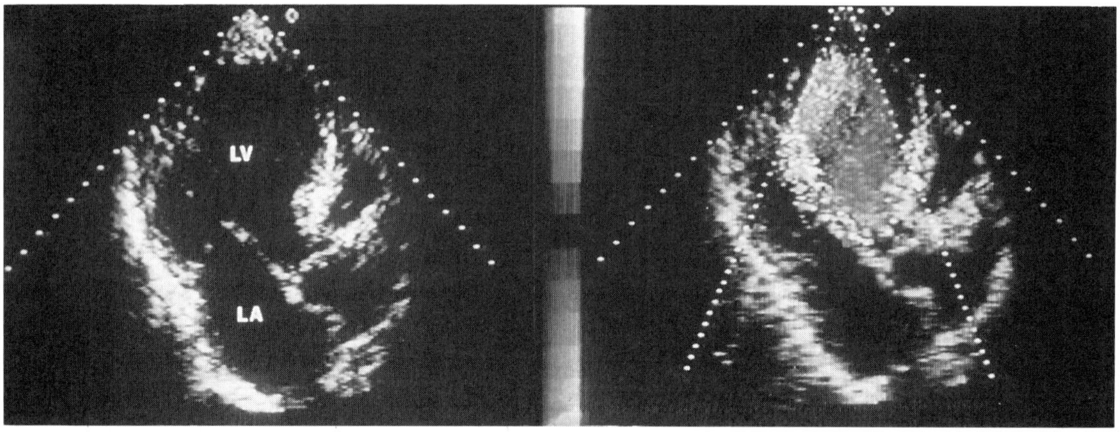

Fig 5B-5 (see color plate after page 200) Color-flow imaging still frame from a patient with aortic regurgitation during diastole. A mosaic pattern jet emanating from the aortic valve into the left ventricular outflow tract indicates aortic regurgitation.

as when the Doppler beam is not directed parallel to the velocity jet (in continuous-wave or pulsed-wave Doppler) or when image resolution is inadequate (as in color-flow imaging). Proper interpretation of a Doppler examination requires that incomplete or unreliable information be reported as such. A distinction must also be made between objective quantitative data (e.g., valve gradients, cardiac pressures) and subjective qualitative data (e.g., regurgitation severity, shunt size).

Despite these limitations, both structural and hemodynamic information about the heart can be obtained from most patients by two-dimensional and Doppler echocardiography. Over the past decade, this information has supplanted the need for cardiac catheterization in many instances of congenital and valvular heart disease.[12] In addition, Doppler echocardiography has the unique ability to measure intracardiac blood flow velocities noninvasively, thus providing the mechanism by which many of the pathophysiologic processes in various disease entities have been elucidated.

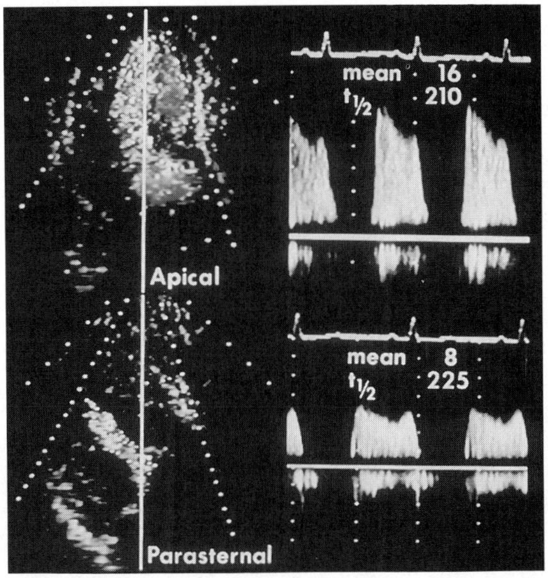

Fig 5B-6 (see color plate after page 200) Utility of color-flow imaging in directing a continuous-wave Doppler beam. **Top,** the continuous-wave Doppler beam is directed along the velocity jet depicted by a mosaic pattern on color-flow imaging (left). The resultant mean gradient and diastolic half-time ($t_{1/2}$) are accurately measured from the spectral display (right). **Bottom,** the continuous-wave Doppler beam is shown to be at a large angle from the velocity jet on color-flow imaging (left), resulting in an underestimation of the mean pressure gradient.

CLINICAL PRINCIPLES (TABLE 5B-1)

Pressure gradients

Continuous-wave Doppler echocardiography has been found to be an accurate and reliable method of measuring pressure gradients noninvasively across stenotic valves.[13-18] When a constant volume of blood is passing through a narrowed site (across the stenotic valve), the blood flow is accelerated in proportion to the degree of the stenosis. On the basis of Bernoulli hydrodynamics, the decrease in pressure across the stenotic valve can be related to the velocity of blood flow.

$$P_1 - P_2 = \frac{1}{2}\rho\left(V_2^2 - V_1^2\right) + R\frac{d\bar{v}}{dt} \times d\bar{s} + R(v) \qquad \textbf{[5B-3]}$$

$$\left(\begin{matrix}\text{Pressure}\\ \text{decrease}\end{matrix} = \begin{matrix}\text{convective}\\ \text{acceleration}\end{matrix} + \begin{matrix}\text{flow}\\ \text{acceleration}\end{matrix} + \begin{matrix}\text{viscous}\\ \text{friction}\end{matrix}\right)$$

in which P_1 is the pressure before stenosis, P_2 is the pressure after stenosis, ρ is the mass density of blood, V_1 is the velocity before stenosis, V_2 is the velocity after stenosis, $d\bar{v}$ is the change in velocity during valve opening, dt is the time for valve opening, $d\bar{s}$ is the pressure drop distance, R is the viscous resistance, and v is the velocity of flow.

This equation can be simplified for the flows encountered in clinical situations. The pressure decrease is related to three factors: (1) convective acceleration, (2) flow acceleration, and (3) viscous friction. In clinical situations, the contributions from the flow acceleration and viscous friction are frequently negligible. In addition,

Table 5B-1 Clinical applications of Doppler echocardiography

Continuous-wave	Pulsed-wave	Color-flow imaging
Pressure gradients	Volumetric flow	Regurgitation lesions
Valve stenoses	Cardiac output	Jet area
Subvalvular obstruction	Regurgitation fractions	Jet width
Prosthetic valves	Qp:Qs	PISA
Large-vessel stenoses	Detection turbulence	Shunts
Conduit stenoses	Regurgitation lesions	Intracardiac velocities
Intracardiac pressures	Shunts	Location
Pulmonary pressure	Diastolic function	Timing
Systolic	Atrioventricular valve	
Diastolic	Pulmonary vein	
LA, LVEDP	Hepatic vein, SVC	
dp/dt	Regurgitation lesions	
Tau	Regurgitation fraction	
Valve area	Indirect clues	
Continuity equation	Pulmonary vein	
Diastolic half-time	Hepatic vein	
Regurgitation lesions	Descending aorta	
Detection		
Signal intensity (semiquantitation)		

LA, left atrium; LVEDP, left ventricular end-diastolic pressure; PISA, proximal isovelocity surface area; SVC, superior vena cava.

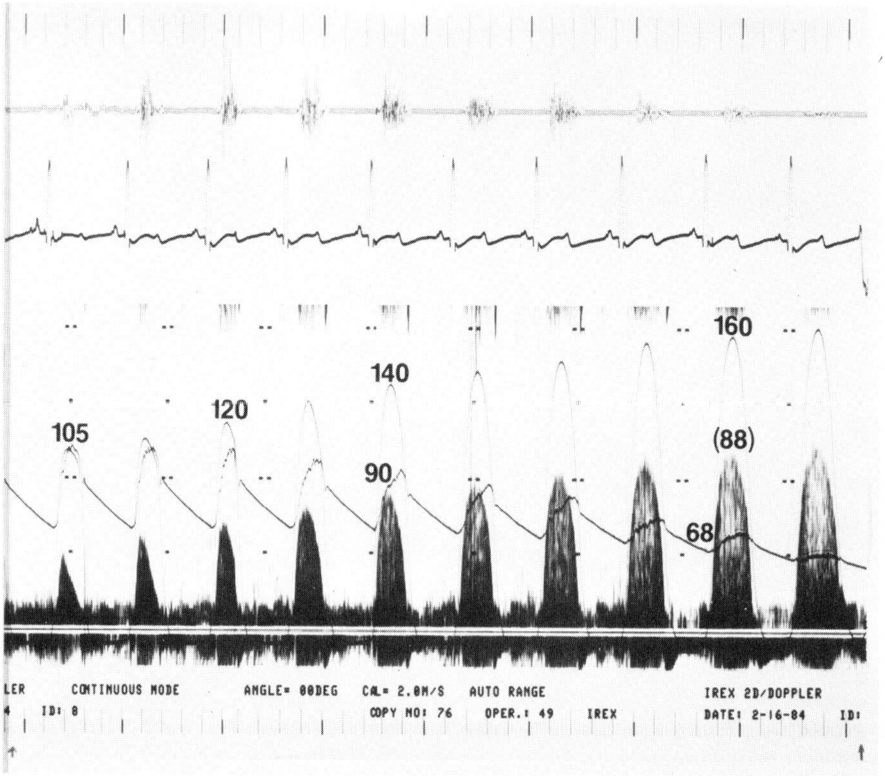

Fig 5B-7 Simultaneous pressure gradients and Doppler velocities in an animal model of aortic stenosis. The relationship is demonstrated over a wide range of pressure gradients. (From Callahan MJ, Tajik AJ, Su-Fan Q, et al: Validation of instantaneous pressure gradients measured by continuous-wave Doppler in experimentally induced aortic stenosis. *Am J Cardiol* 56:989-993, 1985. By permission of Cahners Publishing Company, a Division of Reed Publishing USA.)

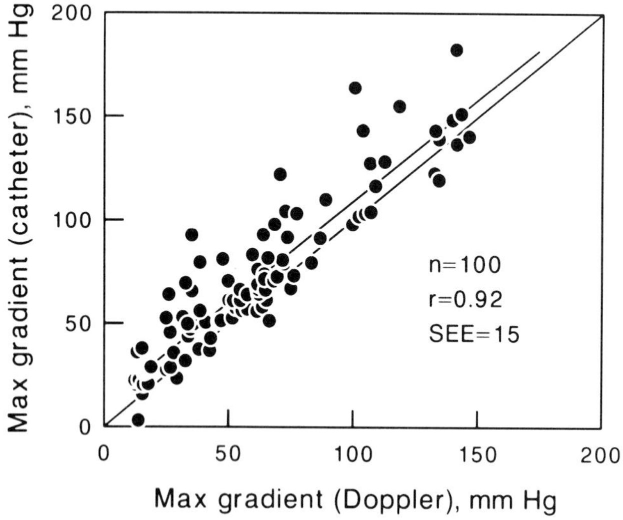

Fig 5B-8 Correlation of the maximum aortic valve gradients between Doppler echocardiography and cardiac catheterization. (From Currie PJ, Seward JB, Reeder GS, et al: Continuous-wave Doppler echocardiographic assessment of severity of calcific aortic stenosis: a simultaneous Doppler-catheter correlative study in 100 adult patients. *Circulation* 71:1162-1169, 1985. By permission of the American Heart Association.)

the square of the proximal velocity is usually negligible in comparison to the square of the distal velocity. Since $\frac{1}{2}\rho$ is approximately 4 for moving red blood cells, the Bernoulli equation can be simplified to Equation 5B-4.

$$P_1 - P_2 = 4V^2 \qquad \textbf{[5B-4]}$$

This simplified Bernoulli equation is the mainstay on which all hemodynamic measurements are made. For a stenotic valve, the simplified Bernoulli equation can be applied to the velocity across the valve to accurately determine the instantaneous pressure gradient (Fig 5B-7). This has been validated for aortic stenosis[13,15,16,18] (Fig 5B-8), mitral stenosis,[14,15] right ventricular outflow obstruction,[17] dynamic left ventricular outflow obstruction,[19,20] prosthetic valves,[21] and conduit obstructions.[22] The clinical utility of Doppler echocardiography for these lesions is discussed in their respective chapters.

There is an important difference between the maximum instantaneous gradient, which is derived from the peak velocity of a Doppler tracing, and gradients derived from cardiac catheterization (Fig. 5B-9). The maximum instantaneous gradient, which is the highest gradient that occurs across the stenotic valve at one point in time, has not been routinely measured at cardiac catheterization. The commonly used gradient by cardiac catheterization has been the peak-to-peak gradient, which is the difference between the proximal pressure and the distal pressure. The peak-to-peak gradient is a nonphysiologic measurement, since these two peak pressures do not occur at the same time and are generally lower than the maximum instantaneous gradient.

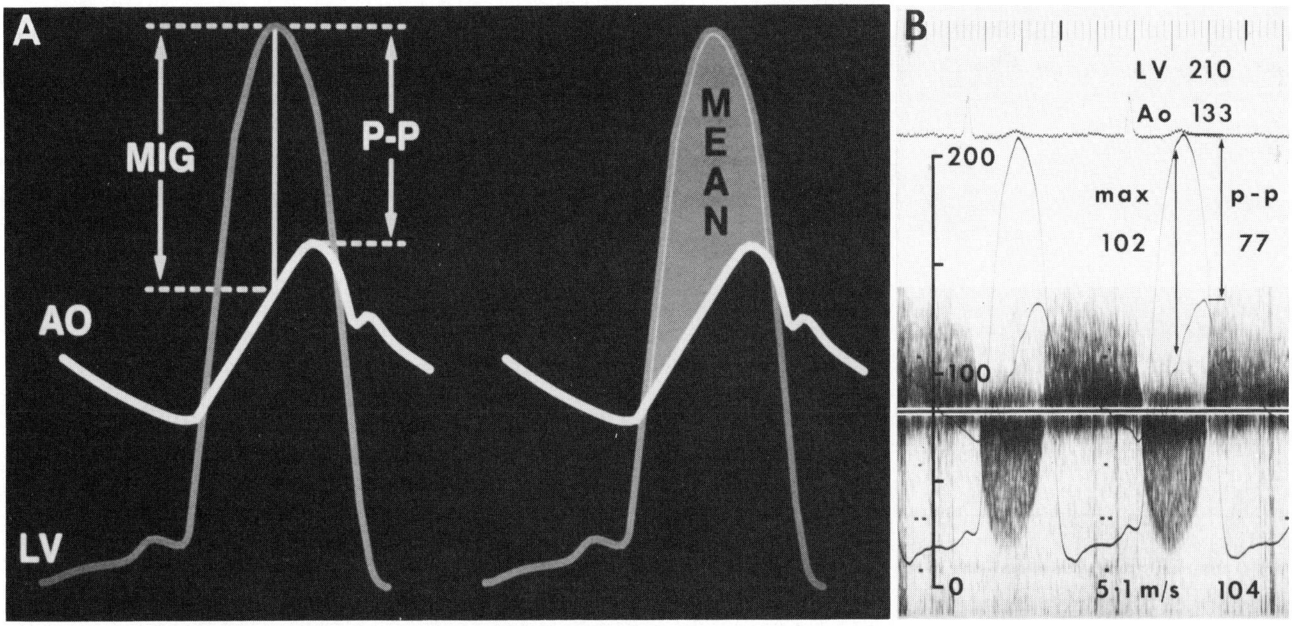

Fig 5B-9 **A,** Schematic ilustration of left ventricular *(LV)* and aortic *(AO)* pressure curves in a patient with aortic stenosis demonstrates the differences among the maximum instantaneous gradient *(MIG),* peak-to-peak gradient *(P-P),* and mean gradient. **B,** simultaneous tracing of the cardiac catheterization pressures and Doppler velocities in a patient with aortic stenosis. The maximum gradient of 104 mm Hg calculated from the Doppler velocity of 5.1 m/sec correlates with the catheter-derived maximum gradient of 102 mm Hg. The peak-to-peak gradient of 77 mm Hg by cardiac catheterization is lower than the maximum instantaneous gradient (**B,** from Currie PJ, Seward JB, Reeder GS, et al: Continuous-wave Doppler echocardiographic assessment of severity of calcific aortic stenosis: a simultaneous Doppler-catheter correlative study in 100 adult patients. *Circulation* 71:1162-1169, 1985. By permission of the American Heart Association.)

The mean gradient is the most representative of the degree of obstruction across a stenotic valve. It is derived by planimetering the area between the proximal pressure curve and the distal pressure curve recorded during cardiac catheterization. With use of continuous-wave Doppler echocardiography, several points in time along the spectral display envelope are converted to a gradient and averaged to obtain the mean gradient. Measurement packages on most Doppler equipment allow calculation of the mean gradient at the time of the study.

There are limitations in applying the simplified Bernoulli equation in clinical practice. Equation 5B-2 shows that the relationship between the recorded Doppler frequency shift and the actual blood flow velocity is dependent on the angle of incidence between the Doppler beam and the velocity jet. If the Doppler beam is parallel to the velocity jet (angle cosine = 0°), the calculated velocity equals the true velocity. If the angle of incidence is larger, the true jet velocity is underestimated. The cosine function allows small variations in the Doppler beam and velocity axis to result in minor changes in the calculated velocity (Fig 5B-10). However, if the angle θ becomes greater than 30°, the resultant calculated velocity is underestimated by more than 15% and may not be acceptable for clinical practice. Thus, a continuous-wave Doppler examination for pressure gradients is a highly operator-dependent technique, and the reliability of a derived pressure gradient depends on the meticulousness and experience of the examiner.

Other problems with the simplified Bernoulli equation may arise in the clinical realm and must be identified for accurate interpretation. The simplified Bernoulli equation makes several assumptions that may not hold up in all clinical circumstances. The velocity proximal to a stenosis is assumed to be negligible in comparison with the distal velocity. However, when there is a high output state (anemia, sepsis, thyrotoxicosis) or significant coexistent regurgitation, the proximal velocity may not be negligible. In addition, when there are stenoses in series, such as those with a coexistent subvalvular and valvular obstruction, the velocity proximal to the second stenosis may be significantly increased, and the modified Bernoulli equation should not be applied in this instance. The contribution from viscous friction may not be negligible in patients with abnormalities of blood viscosity (polycythemia, anemia) or with long, tubular stenoses.

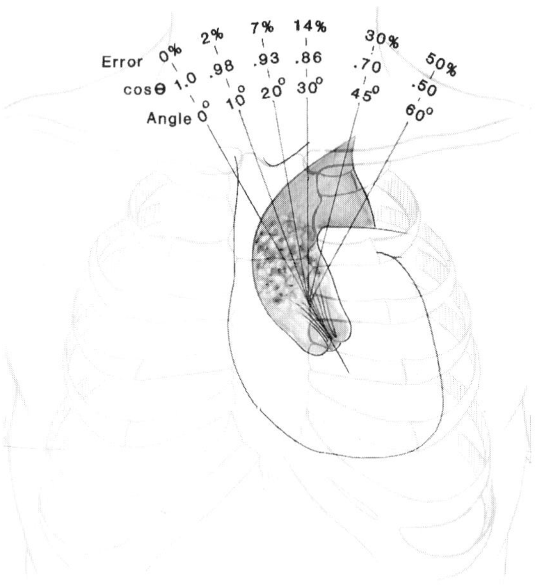

Fig 5B-10 Diagram of the relationship between the Doppler beam and the true velocity jet. CosΘ equals the angle of incidence between the Doppler beam and the true velocity jet. Shown are the percentages of underestimation of the true velocity at these angles of incidence. (From Nishimura RA, Miller FA Jr, Callahan MJ, et al: Doppler echocardiography: theory, instrumentation, technique, and application. *Mayo Clin Proc* 60:321-343, 1985. By permission, Mayo Foundation.)

There may be a discrepancy between Doppler- and catheter-derived gradients in selected circumstances because of a concept called "pressure recovery."[23,24] The pressure in a stenotic lesion is lowest when the velocity is highest (at the vena contracta) and increases again distal to the stenosis. The degree at which the pressure returns depends on the amount of energy lost at the stenosis because of viscous and turbulent energy loss. Doppler echocardiography measures the highest velocity at the site of the stenosis, which may be higher than the catheter gradient when the distal measurement is made downstream from the valve. This effect may apply when there are long, tubular stenoses and has also been shown in vitro to apply to certain types of valve prostheses.[25,26]

Intracardiac pressures

The modified Bernoulli equation can be applied to regurgitant lesions to calculate intracardiac pressures.[27] If a pressure is assumed in one chamber, a pressure can be determined in the unknown chamber. A useful application of this principle in clinical practice has been in the estimation of right ventricular systolic pressure by use of the tricuspid regurgitation peak systolic velocity.[28,29] The peak systolic velocity of a tricuspid regurgitation jet is converted to the pressure gradient between the right ventricle and right atrium by the modified Bernoulli equation. By assuming a right atrial pressure, one estimates a right ventricular systolic pressure from the pressure gradient. In the absence of right ventricular outflow obstruction, this provides a measurement of the pulmonary artery systolic pressure.

$$\begin{aligned} RVSP - RA &= 4 \times (TR_{vel})^2 \\ RVSP &= 4 \times (TR_{vel})^2 + RA \end{aligned} \qquad [5B\text{-}5]$$

in which RVSP is right ventricular systolic pressure, RA is assumed right atrial pressure, and TR_{vel} is peak systolic velocity of the tricuspid regurgitation signal. The assumed right atrial pressure can be derived from examination of the inferior vena cava in conjunction with the tricuspid regurgitation velocity.[30] Sophisticated sonospirometry with measurements of the inferior vena cava diameter is possible.[31] A useful, practical approach is shown in Table 5B-2. When the intensity of the tricuspid regurgitation signal is weak, injection of an agitated saline solution into a brachial vein enhances the signal, so that an accurate peak velocity can be measured[32] (Fig 5B-11).

The pulmonary artery diastolic pressure can be calculated from the pulmonary regurgitation velocity curve.[33] The end-diastolic velocity can be converted to the end-diastolic gradient between the pulmonary artery and the right ventricle. Assuming a right ventricular diastolic pressure (the same as an assumed right atrial pressure if tricuspid stenosis is absent), the pulmonary artery end-diastolic pressure is obtained.

$$\begin{aligned} PADP - RVDP &= 4 \times (PR_{vel})^2 \\ PADP &= 4 \times (PR_{vel})^2 + RVDP \end{aligned} \qquad [5B\text{-}6]$$

in which PADP is pulmonary artery end-diastolic pressure, RVDP is assumed right ventricular diastolic pressure, and PR_{vel} is pulmonary regurgitation end-diastolic velocity. Thus, it is frequently possible to calculate

Table 5B-2 Assumed right atrial pressure (for calculation of pulmonary artery pressures)

Tricuspid regurgitation velocity, m/sec	Inferior vena cava: Diameter (cm)	Inferior vena cava: Change with inspiration (%)	Assumed right atrial pressure, mm Hg
<2.5	<2	>50	5
2.5-4.0	2-3	≤50	10
≥2.5	>3	No collapse	20

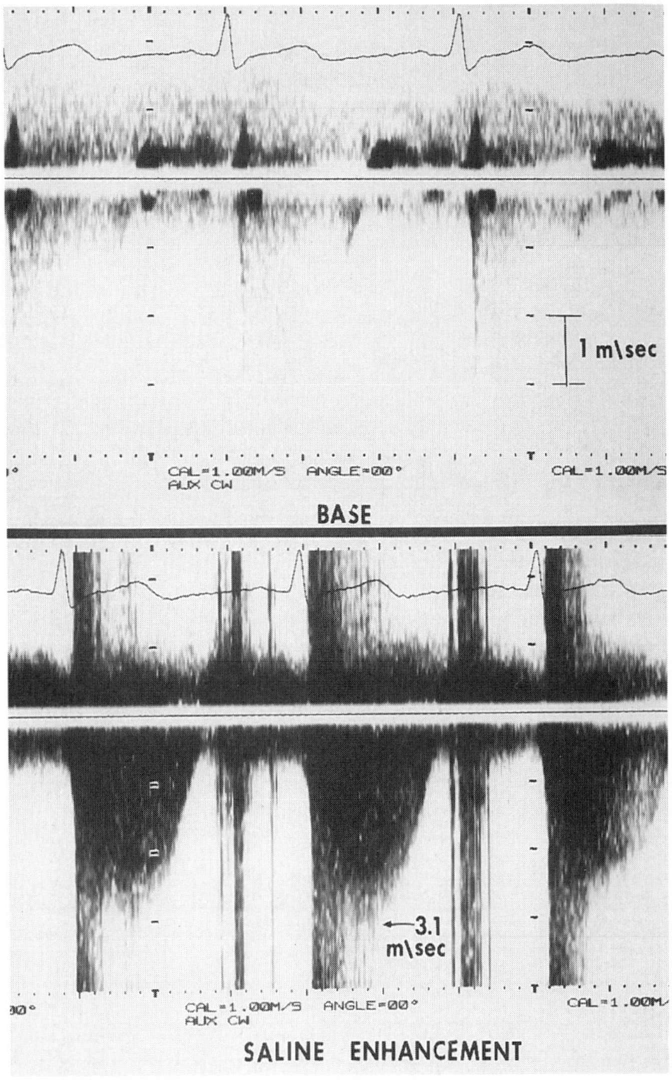

Fig 5B-11 Continuous-wave Doppler recording of a patient with tricuspid regurgitation. In the baseline state, there is a very weak signal, and the peak velocity cannot be assessed. However, during injection of agitated saline solution into a brachial vein, the signal is enhanced, with a peak velocity of 3.7 m/sec.

pulmonary artery systolic and diastolic pressures noninvasively from Doppler echocardiography.

In aortic regurgitation, the instantaneous gradient between the aorta and the left ventricle during diastole can be calculated from the aortic regurgitation jet.[34] A gross estimate of left ventricular end-diastolic pressure can be obtained if the aortic-diastolic pressure is measured. Of greater clinical usefulness is the slope of the aortic regurgitation jet, which reflects the rate of decline of the aortic-left ventricular pressure gradient and can be used as an indirect measurement of hemodynamics. The finding of a very rapid slope indicates a rapidly rising left ventricular end-diastolic pressure and a fast decrease in aortic pressure[35] (Fig 5B-12).

The mitral regurgitation velocity curve reflects the instantaneous gradient between the left atrium and the left ventricle during systole.[34] A gross estimation of left atrial pressure can be obtained if the systolic-aortic pressure is measured in the absence of aortic stenosis (Fig 5B-13). Other valuable information about left ventricular function can be obtained from examining the rate of change of the mitral regurgitation curve. If left atrial pressure is assumed to be constant during isovolumic contraction, the rate of increase of the mitral regurgitation velocity can be used to determine left ventricular dp/dt, an intrinsic measure of systolic contractility[36-38] (Fig 5B-14). A simple measure is the rate of pressure rise (RPR), which divides the pressure change (ΔP) between 1 and 2 m/sec (i.e., 32 mm Hg) into the time interval between 1 and 3 m/sec on the mitral regurgitation Doppler velocity curve (Δt).

$$\text{RPR} = \Delta P/\Delta t \text{ at 1 to 3 m/sec} \qquad \textbf{[5B-7]}$$

$$\text{RPR} = 32/\Delta t$$

Normal RPR is greater than 1,200 mm Hg/sec. An RPR of 800 to 1,200 mm Hg/sec is consistent with a moderate decrease in left ventricular function, and an RPR of less than 800 mm Hg/sec is consistent with severe depression in left ventricular systolic function. The descending limb of the mitral regurgitation curve can similarly be used to calculate the rate of left ventricular pressure decay.[39,40] Therefore, tau, the time constant of relaxation, can be calculated noninvasively from the mitral regurgitation curve by fitting a monoexponential equation to the derived left ventricular pressure decay. Tau provides a direct measurement of left ventricular relaxation in the evaluation of diastolic function (Fig 5B-15).

Volumetric flow

Doppler echocardiography is an accurate modality for measuring volumetric flow through a valve orifice or a great vessel[4,5] (Fig 5B-16). This measurement is based on the hydrodynamic principle of flow through a rigid tube: volumetric flow (Q) can be determined from the time velocity integral (TVI) of flow and cross-sectional area of the tube (A).

$$Q = A \times \text{TVI} \qquad \textbf{[5B-8]}$$

This method incorporates three assumptions: that the cross-sectional area of an orifice is constant throughout the period of measurement, that all the blood flowing through an orifice has a flat velocity profile, and that there will be a small angle of θ in the Doppler measurement.

Despite these assumptions, Doppler echocardiography has been shown to be an accurate measurement of cardiac output when the following sites are used: ascending aorta, pulmonary outflow tract, mitral valve annulus, mitral valve orifice, tricuspid valve orifice, and left ventricular outflow tract.[4,5,41-43] Because of the relatively flat velocity profile and constant annulus area, the left ventricular outflow tract is the most accurate site for measurement of cardiac output[4] (Fig 5B-17). The ascending aorta is a clinically useful measurement site because of its ease of accessibility through a small nonimaging transducer in the suprasternal notch. Although absolute cardiac output is less accurate in this instance, serial changes in cardiac output

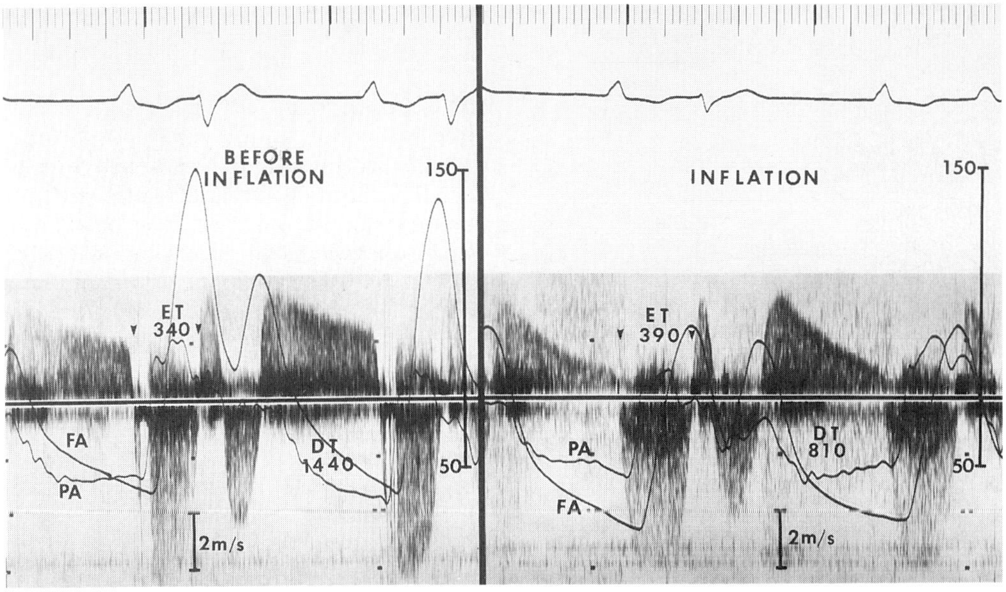

Fig 5B-12 Aortic regurgitation velocity curve before **(left)** and during **(right)** percutaneous aortic balloon valvuloplasty. During the valvuloplasty, there is a significant increase in the rate of decline of the aortic regurgitation velocity slope. This indicates a rapidly increasing left ventricular diastolic pressure and rapidly decreasing aortic pressure, consistent with severe aortic regurgitation. *DT,* deceleration time; *ET,* ejection time; *FA,* femoral artery; *PA,* pulmonary artery. (From Nishimura RA, Holmes DR Jr, Reeder GS, et al: Doppler echocardiographic observations during percutaneous aortic balloon valvuloplasty. *J Am Coll Cardiol* 11:1219-1226, 1988. By permission of American College of Cardiology.)

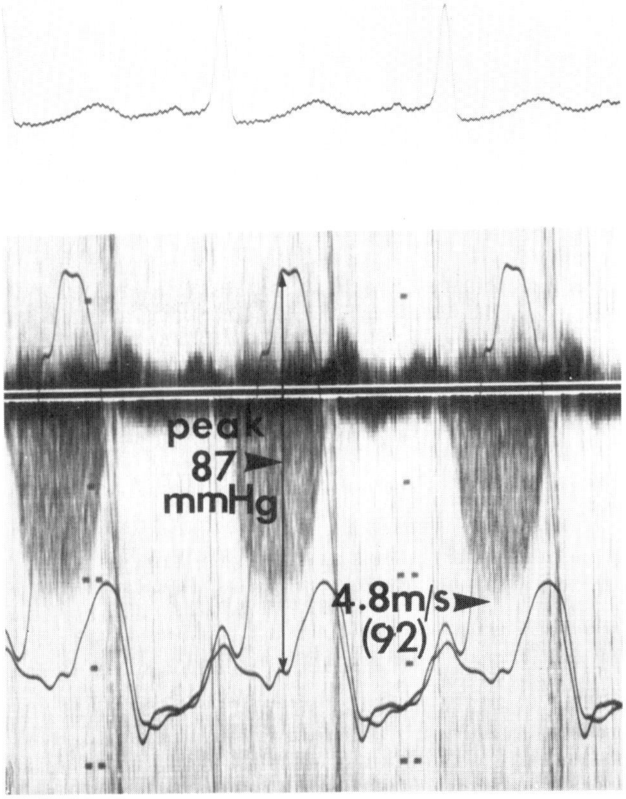

Fig 5B-13 Simultaneous catheter pressures in the left atrium and left ventricle with the mitral regurgitation Doppler velocity curve. The Doppler velocity can be used to determine the instantaneous pressure between the left atrium and the left ventricle. (From Nishimura RA, Tajik AJ: Determination of left-sided pressure gradients by utilizing Doppler aortic and mitral regurgitant signals: validation by simultaneous dual catheter and Doppler studies. *J Am Coll Cardiol* 11:317-321, 1988. By permission of the American College of Cardiology.

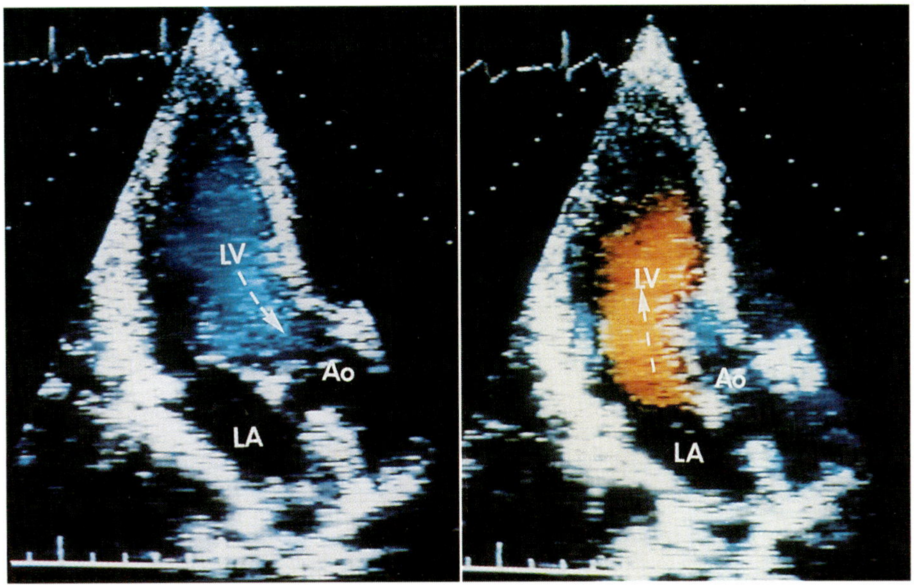

Fig 5B-4 See page 194

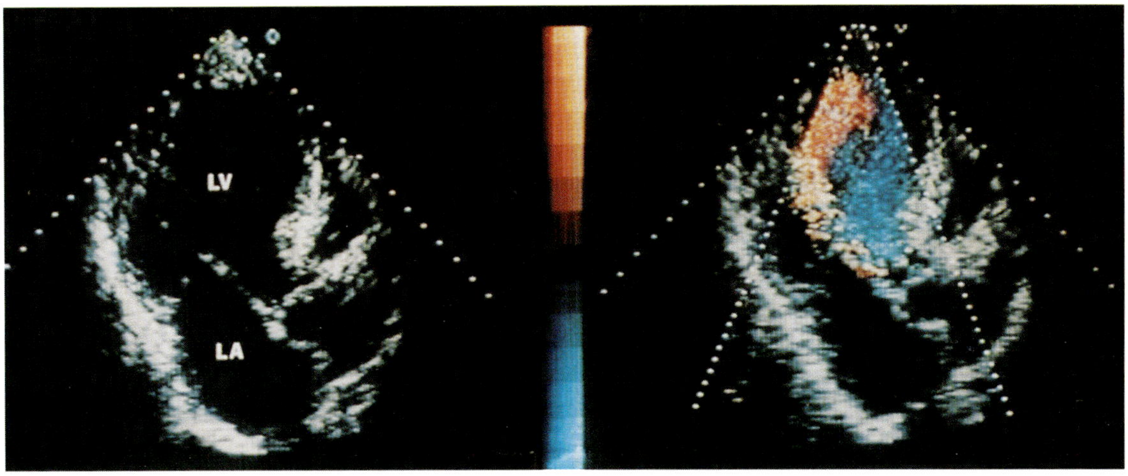

Fig 5B-5 See page 194

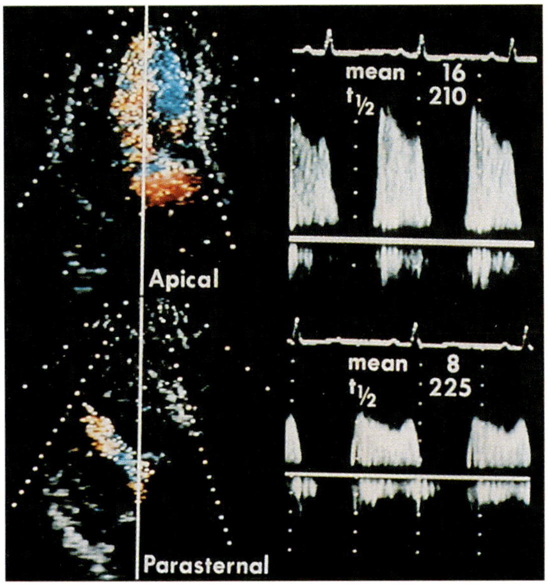

Fig 5B-6 See page 195

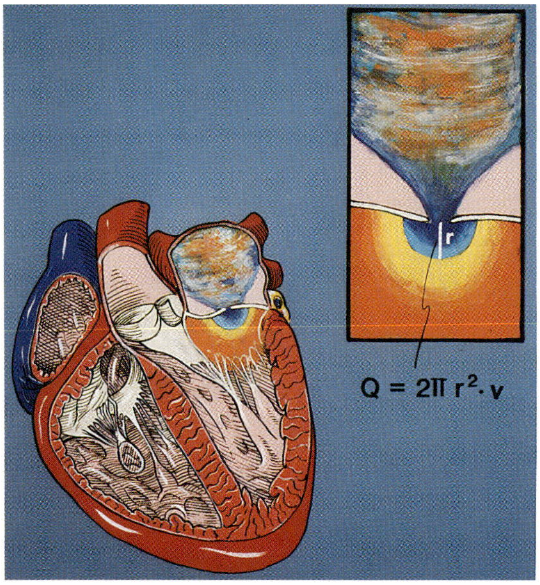

Fig 5B-24 See page 205

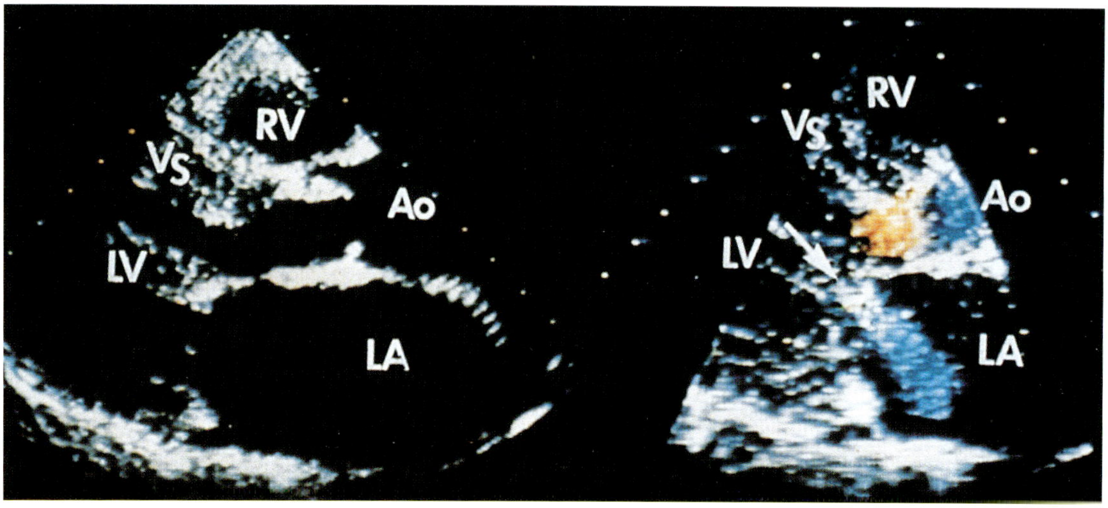

Fig 5B-21 See page 204

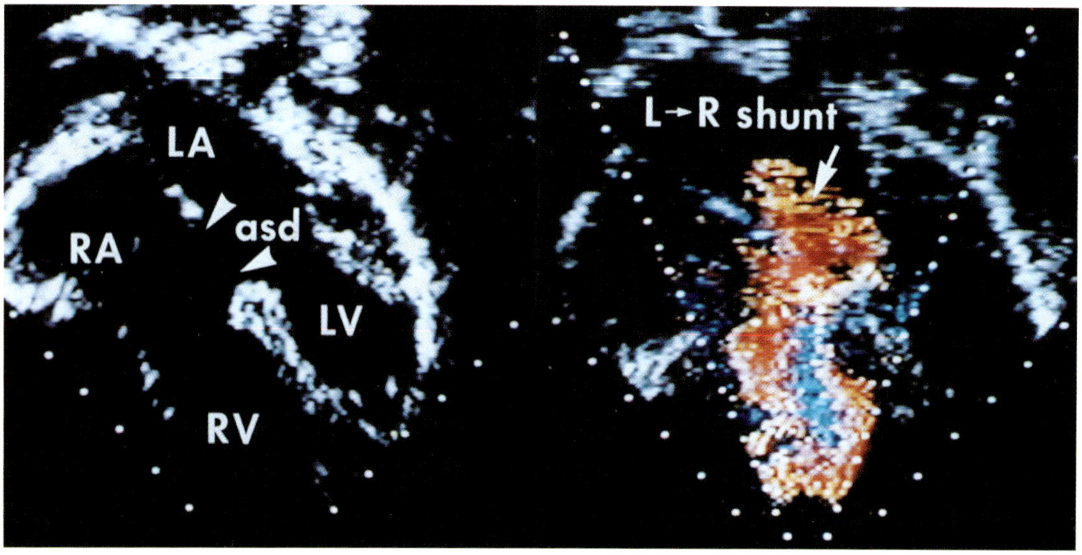

Fig 5B-25 See page 205

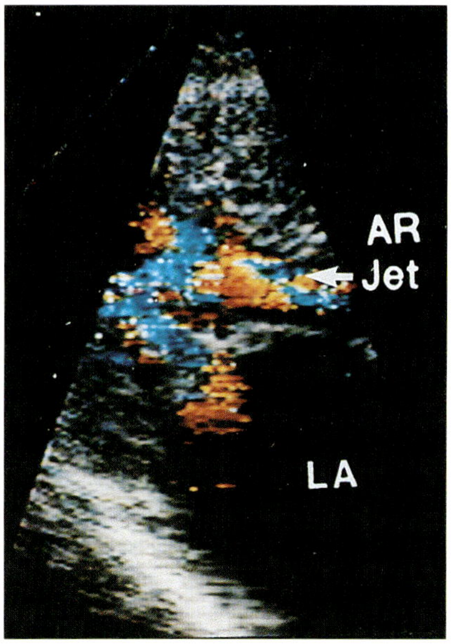

Fig 33-12 See page 1427

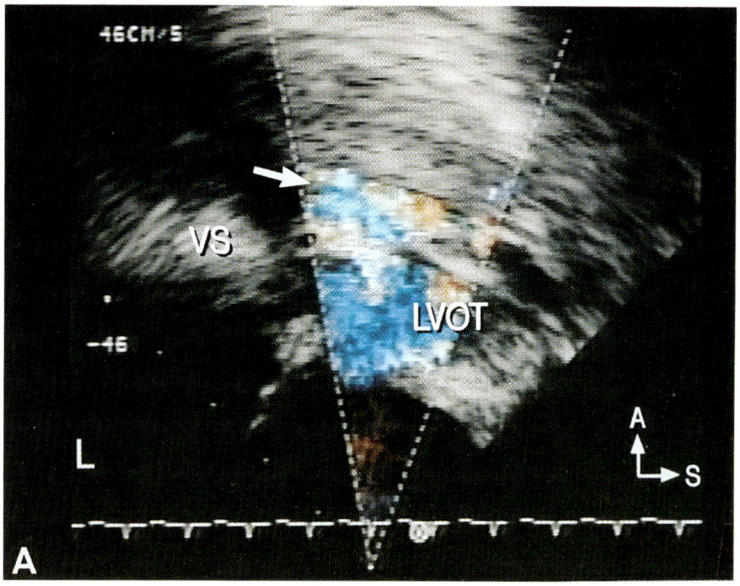

Fig 39-28 See page 1522

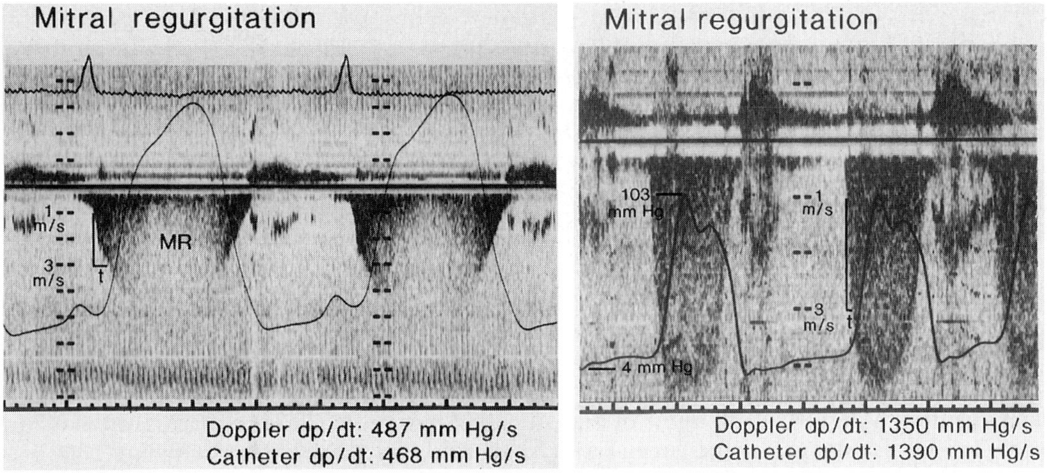

Fig 5B-14 Mitral regurgitation velocity curves with simultaneous high-fidelity left ventricular pressure curves in two patients. The dp/dt between 1 and 3 m/sec is shown for the cardiac catheterization and the Doppler-derived velocity curves. (From Chung N, Nishimura RA, Holmes DR Jr, et al: Measurement of left ventricular dp/dt by simultaneous Doppler echocardiography and cardiac catheterization. *J Am Soc Echocardiogr* 5:147-152, 1992. By permission of the American Society of Echocardiography.)

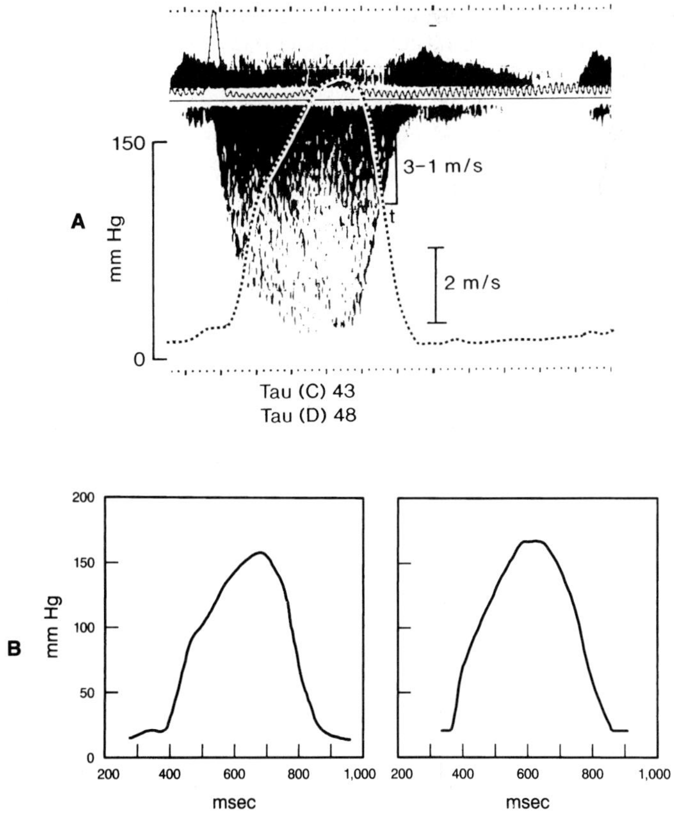

Fig 5B-15 **A,** the Doppler mitral regurgitation velocity curve and high-fidelity manometer-tipped left ventricular pressure curve in a patient with mitral regurgitation. The time constant of relaxation (Tau) is calculated from applying a monoexponential equation to the left ventricular pressure decrease during isovolumic relaxation. **B,** reconstructed digitized left ventricular pressure curves directly from the left ventricular pressure *(left panel)* and from the mitral regurgitation curve *(right panel)* by use of the modified Bernoulli equation. (Modified from Nishimura RA, Schwartz RS, Tajik AJ, et al: Noninvasive measurement of rate of left ventricular relaxation by Doppler echocardiography: validation with simultaneous cardiac catheterization. *Circulation* 88:146-155, 1993)

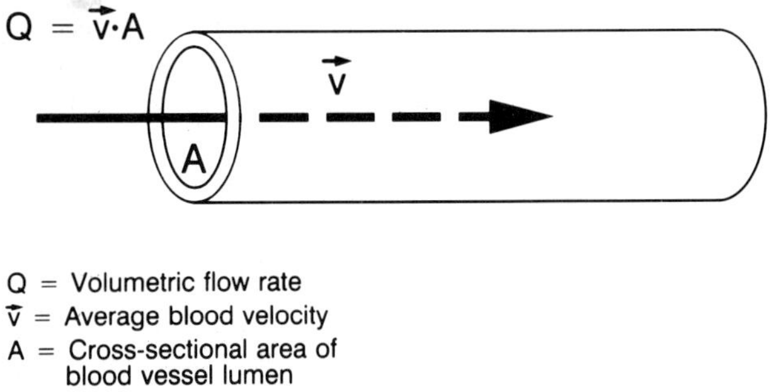

Fig 5B-16 Schematic diagram illustrating the hydrodynamic principle of flow through a rigid tube, which can be applied to the Doppler echocardiogram. The cross-sectional area (A) of an orifice or great vessel multiplied by the time velocity integral (v) obtained by pulsed-wave Doppler echocardiography results in a measurement of volumetric flow (Q).

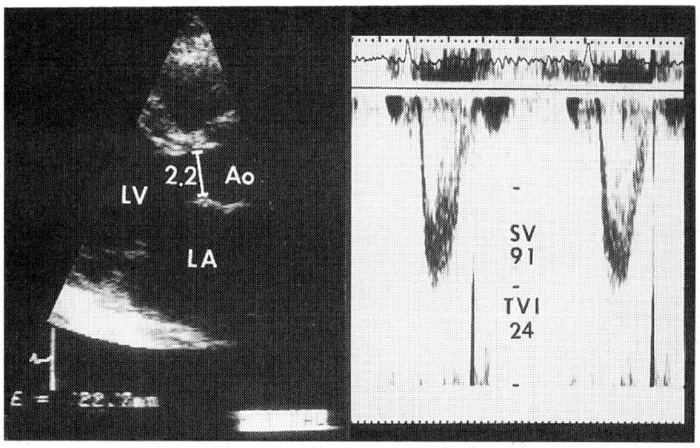

Fig 5B-17 Use of the left ventricular outflow tract for calculating volumetric flow rates. **Left,** a still frame of the left ventricular outflow tract in the parasternal long-axis view. The diameter of the tract is 2.2 cm. **Right,** a pulsed-wave sample volume is placed in the left ventricular outflow tract from the apical long-axis view, and the left ventricular outflow velocity is recorded. The time velocity integral *(TVI)* equals 24 cm, for a calculated stroke volume *(SV)* of 91 mL. *Ao,* aorta; *LA,* left atrium; *LV,* left ventricle. (From Loutfi H, Nishimura RA: Quantitative evaluation of left ventricular systolic function by Doppler echocardiographic techniques. *Echocardiography* 11:305-314, 1994. By permission of Futura Publishing Company.)

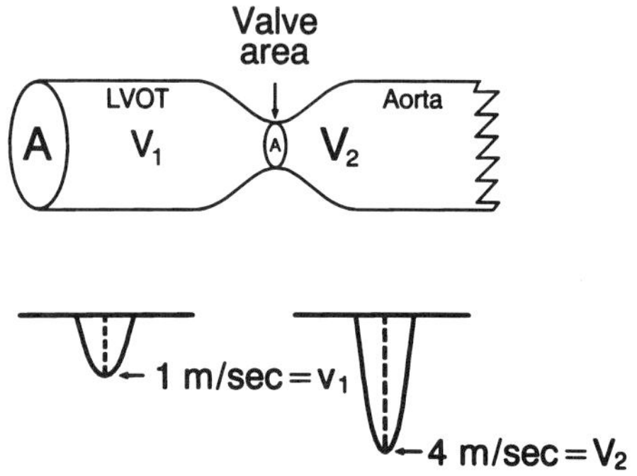

Fig 5B-18 Diagram of the mechanism of calculation of the continuity equation. Large *A,* area of left ventricular outflow tract *(LVOT);* small *A,* area of aortic valve; V_1, time velocity integral of velocity in LVOT; V_2, time velocity integral of velocity across aortic valve.

are rapidly and reliably measured.[41,42] Cardiac output has been measured by transesophageal echocardiography. The most accurate location of cardiac output measurement by this technique is the right ventricular outflow tract from a short-axis monoplane view.[44]

Continuity equation

The gradient across a stenotic valve is determined not only by the degree of stenosis but also by the flow through the valve. Therefore, severe stenosis of a valve may produce a low gradient if cardiac output is low. To circumvent this problem, "valve area" has been applied. The valve area was initially determined from a hydraulic equation by cardiac catheterization.[45] The continuity principle was introduced with the advent of Doppler echocardiography, which is an accurate modality for noninvasively measuring valve area.[46-49]

The continuity equation is based on the calculation of volumetric flow through two orifices (Fig 5B-18). In aortic stenosis, the continuity equation uses flow through (1) the left ventricular outflow tract and (2) the aortic valve. Since volumetric flow through the left ventricular outflow tract equals volumetric flow through the aortic valve, Equation 5B-9 can be derived.

$$A_1 \times V_1 = A_2 \times V_2 \qquad \text{[5B-9]}$$

in which A_1 is the area of left ventricular outflow tract, V_1 is the time velocity integral of the velocity in the left ventricular outflow tract, A_2 is the area of aortic valve, and V_2 is the time velocity integral of the velocity across the aortic valve.

Both V_1 and V_2 are obtained from Doppler echocardiography. V_1 uses the Doppler velocity from a pulsed-wave sample volume placed in the left ventricular outflow tract. V_2 incorporates the continuous-wave Doppler velocity across the aortic valve. The area of the left ventricular outflow tract (A_1) can be obtained from two-dimensional echocardiography by measurement of the diameter in the parasternal long-axis view. The aortic valve area (A_2) can then be calculated.[46-49] In aortic stenosis, V_1 and V_2 have similar velocity envelopes, and a simplified valve area can be measured if peak velocities are used instead of time-velocity integrals.[49] The continuity equation for aortic valve area is more accurate than cardiac catheterization in situations such as coexistent valvular regurgitation, low-output states, and irregular rhythms.

The continuity equation can be used for calculation of valve areas in other sites, such as in mitral stenosis.[50] When the continuity equation is used for these other valves, a site remote from the valve is selected for calculation of the known volumetric flow rate, usually the left ventricular outflow tract. This then requires the assumption that there is no significant regurgitation or shunt present.

Diastolic half-time

Since the velocity curve across a valve represents the instantaneous gradient between two adjacent chambers or a chamber and a great vessel, the rate of fall of the velocity can be used as a measure of the rate of decline of the pressure gradient. This provides another method of determining the severity of mitral stenosis[51] as well as the severity of aortic regurgitation.[52]

In mitral stenosis, the rate of fall of the gradient between the left ventricle and the left atrium is determined by the severity of the stenosis. It has been shown in the cardiac catheterization laboratory that the pressure "half-time," which is the time it takes for the peak pressure gradient to drop by 50%, is an accurate assessment of the severity of mitral stenosis.[53] The Doppler spectral display of a mitral stenotic jet also is a measure of the diastolic half-time. Since there is an exponential relationship between velocity and gradient, the initial peak velocity must first be converted to pressure gradient. The pressure gradient is then divided by half and reconverted to velocity. The time it takes for the velocity to fall to this calculated velocity is the diastolic half-time.

A simplified method of determining the diastolic half-time uses "deceleration time." The deceleration time is measured by extrapolating a line from the fall in velocity to the baseline. The time from the initial peak velocity to the intercept with the baseline is known as the deceleration time (Fig 5b-19). Multiplying the deceleration time by 0.29 equals the half-time.

In mitral stenosis, the diastolic half-time is divided into 220 to obtain a mitral valve area.[51] This is an accurate measurement of mitral valve area, except in instances of abnormal left atrial or left ventricular compliance.[54,55]

The diastolic half-time is also used in assessing severity of aortic regurgitation.[52] Since the rate of decline of pressure between the aorta and the left ventricular diastolic pressure reflects the severity of aortic regurgitation, the diastolic half-time is an indirect measurement of severity. In very severe aortic regurgitation, there is a rapid rate of rise in left ventricular diastolic pressure and a rapid fall in aortic diastolic pressure, culminating in a short diastolic half-time (less than 300 msec) (Fig 5B-20). In patients with very mild aortic regurgitation, there is a slower rate of rise in left ventricular pressure and a slower fall in aortic pressure, resulting in a prolonged diastolic half-time (greater than 800 msec).

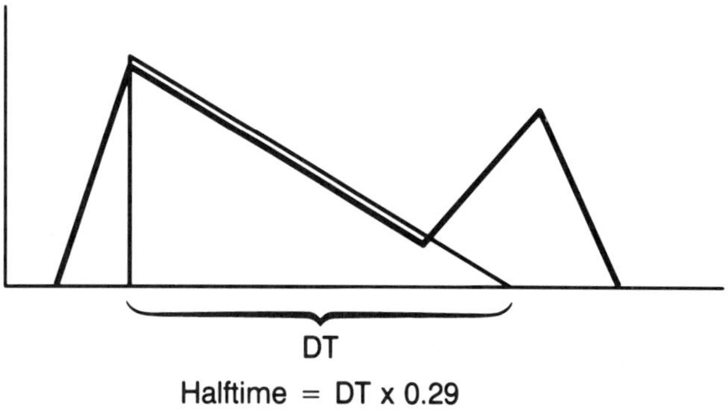

Fig 5B-19 Measurement of deceleration time (DT) from the mitral flow velocity curve in mitral stenosis. A line is drawn from the peak initial E velocity along the deceleration velocity. The line is then extrapolated down to the baseline. The deceleration time is the period fromthe initial E velocity to the point where the extrapolated line reaches the baseline. The diastolic half-time can be calculated by multiplying the deceleration time by 0.29.

Regurgitation lesions

Semiquantitation of the severity of valvular regurgitation is possible by Doppler echocardiography. Initially, pulsed-wave mapping was used to determine the extent of a regurgitation jet into the receiving chamber.[8,9] With the advent of color-flow imaging, a maximal jet area can be obtained from interrogation in multiple tomographic planes (Fig 5B-21). In the middle to late 1980s, several studies demonstrated an excellent correlation between the severity of valvular regurgitation assessed by cardiac catheterization and the maximum jet area divided by the receiving chamber area[11,56,57] (Fig 5B-22). However, subsequent studies have shown that there is a wide scatter for a single jet area measurement in predicting regurgitation severity[58] (Fig 5B-23).

There are several reasons why a single jet area by color-flow imaging does not necessarily correlate with the severity of regurgitation. The Doppler mapping technique examines the velocity, direction, and magnitude of the regurgitation jet rather than the true volume of regurgitation. Thus, many factors other than the regurgitation volume determine the jet area. These include the velocity of a regurgitation jet, compliance of the receiving chambers, size of the receiving chambers, and systolic function.[59-61] In addition, machine factors, such as color gain, frame rate, scanning direction, Doppler angle, color processing, color map, and sector angle, may significantly change a color jet area.[59,60,62,63] Color-flow imaging may not accurately display the extent of regurgitation jet if there is poor image resolution, eccentric jets, or reflectance off structures such as prosthetic valves. Transesoph-

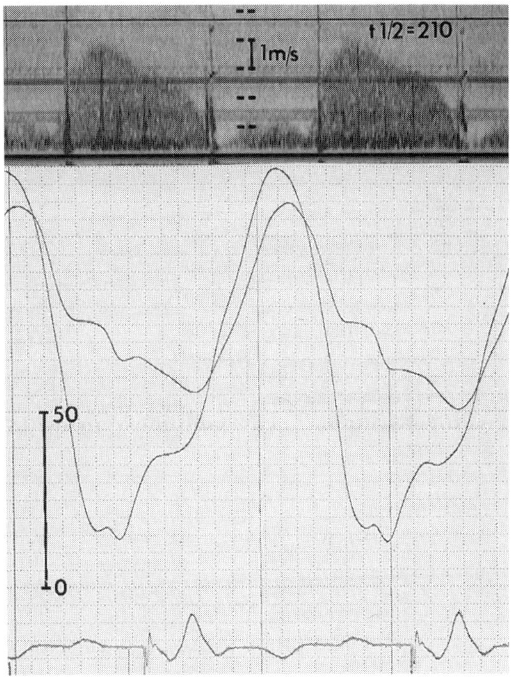

Fig 5B-20 Simultaneous Doppler velocity curve of an aortic regurgitation jet and the left ventricular and femoral artery curve by cardiac catheterization. There is severe aortic regurgitation with a marked increase in left ventricular diastolic pressure, resulting in a significant abbreviation of the diastolic half-time to 210 msec. (From Nishimura RA, Tajik AJ: Quantitative hemodynamics by Doppler echocardiography: a noninvasive alternative to cardiac catheterization. *Prog Cardiovasc Dis* 36:309-342, 1994. By permission of WB Saunders Company.)

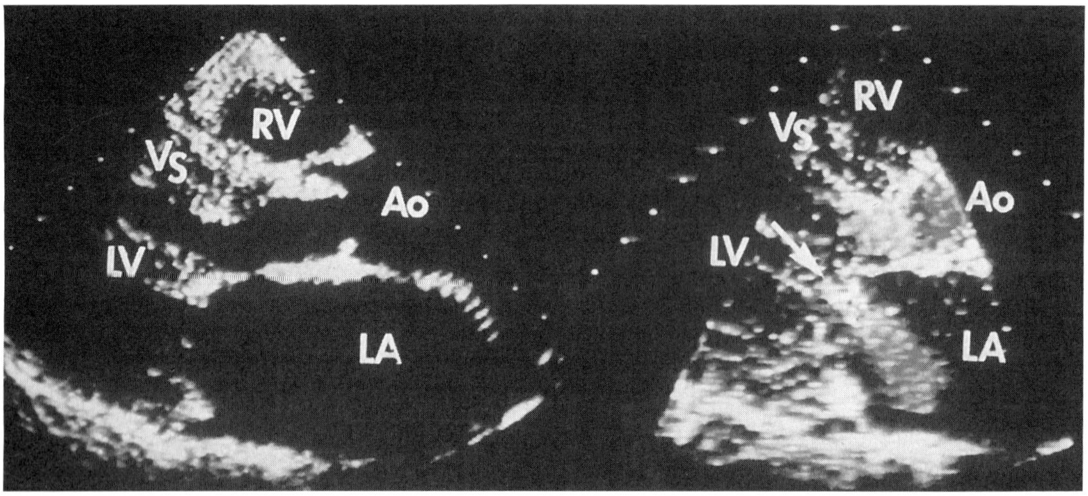

Fig 5B-21 (see color plate after page 200) Color-flow image from a patient with mitral regurgitation. The extent of the blue jet *(arrow)* into the left atrium *(LA)* is used as a semiquantitative estimate of the severity of mitral regurgitation. *Ao,* aorta; *LV,* left ventricle; *RV,* right ventricle; *VS,* ventricular septum. (From Nishimura RA, Miller FA Jr, Callahan MJ, et al: Doppler echocardiography: theory, instrumentation, technique, and application. *Mayo Clin Proc* 60:321-343, 1985. By permission, Mayo Foundation.)

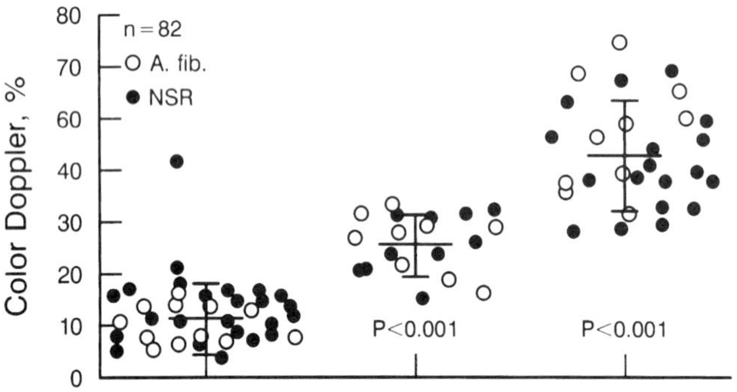

Fig 5B-22 One of the initial studies demonstrating an excellent correlation between the regurgitation jet area and the severity of regurgitation assessed by cardiac catheterization in patients with mitral regurgitation *(MR). A. fib.,* atrial fibrillation; *NSR,* normal sinus rhythm. (From Helmcke F, Nanda NC, Hsiung MC, et al: Color Doppler assessment of mitral regurgitation with orthogonal planes. *Circulation* 75:175-183, 1987. By permission of American Heart Association.)

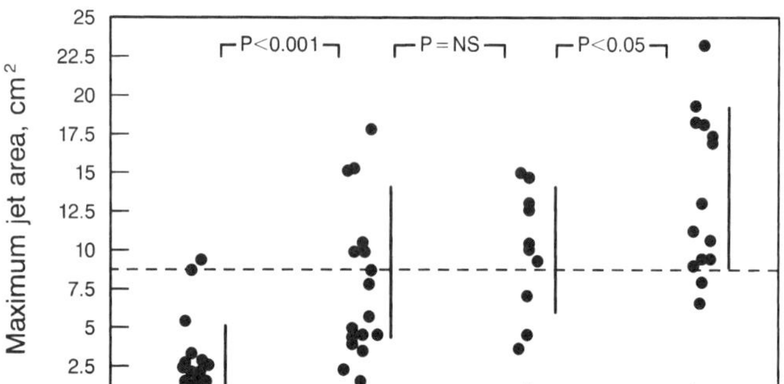

Fig 5B-23 Another study of patients with mitral regurgitation shows the correlation between the jet area and the severity of regurgitation assessed by cardiac catheterization. In this study, there is a wide scatter for a single jet area measurement in predicting the regurgitation severity. (Modified from Spain MG, Smith MD, Grayburn PA, et al: Quantitative assessment of mitral regurgitation by Doppler color flow imaging: angiographic and hemodynamic correlations. *J Am Coll Cardiol* 13:585-590, 1989.)

ageal echocardiography may overcome some of the technical problems, such as image resolution, but even with this high-resolution imaging technique, the jet area alone does not always correlate with the severity of regurgitation.

Other echocardiographic findings need to be analyzed in the color-flow imaging jet area when the severity of regurgitation lesions is assessed. Information provided by color-flow imaging other than jet area can be used, including jet width and the flow convergence region proximal to the orifice[64,65] (Fig 5B-24). Regurgitation volumes can be calculated from volumetric flow through different valve orifices.[66] Indirect clues from two-dimensional echocardiography (e.g., chamber size, chamber function, valve morphology) and Doppler echocardiography (proximal antegrade velocities, diastolic half-times, intensity of continuous-wave signals, velocity curves in the aorta and veins) all provide additional information about the severity of regurgitation and are discussed in detail in their specific chapters.

Intracardiac shunts

Two-dimensional echocardiography is able to identify large intracardiac shunts. In both atrial septal defects and ventricular septal defects, large shunts are visualized by echo dropouts. However, if the shunt is small, the resolution of the two-dimensional image is such that it will not be detected. Most shunts, however, have abnormal blood flow and turbulence at the site of the abnormal connection. Therefore, Doppler echocardiography is an ideal modality in diagnosing these shunts. Pulsed-wave mapping was initially used to detect these shunts. The advent of color-flow imaging greatly facilitates the ability to detect intracardiac shunts.[67] (Fig 5B-25). The high resolution of transesophageal echocardiography with both two-dimensional imaging and color-flow imaging has made echocardiography the procedure of choice in the diagnosis of atrial septal defects.

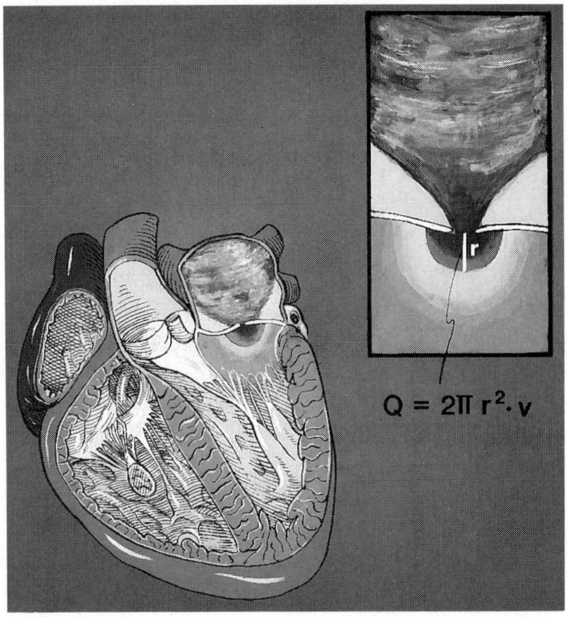

Fig 5B-24 (see color plate after page 200) Diagram of the flow convergence region that occurs proximal to a regurgitation orifice. There is semihemispheric region of solid blue, the boundaries of which equal a known velocity *(v)*. The size of this hemispheric region is proportional to the regurgitation volume *(Q)*.

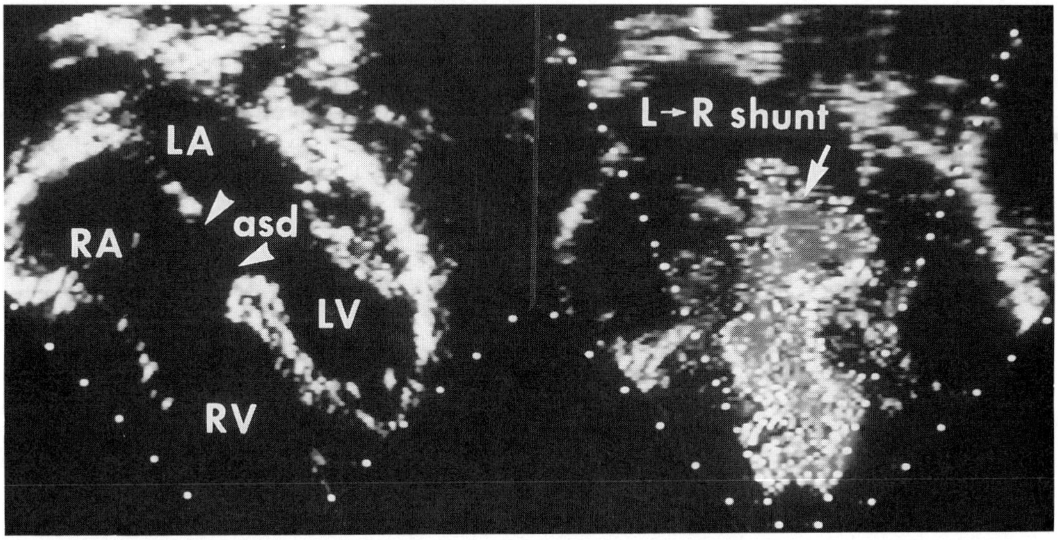

Fig 5B-25 (see color plate after page 200) **Left,** black-and-white still frame from a patient with an atrial septal defect *(asd)*. **Right,** color-flow image demonstrating flow going from the left atrium to the right atrium through the secundum atrial septal defect. *L,* left; *LA,* left atrium; *LV,* left ventricle; *R,* right; *RA,* right atrium; *RV,* right ventricle.

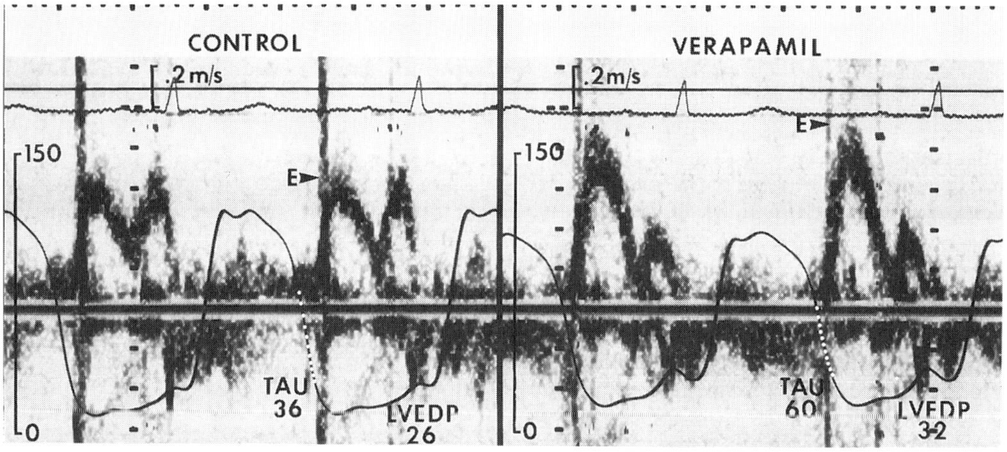

Fig 5B-26 Transmitral Doppler velocity curves and simultaneous high-fidelity left ventricular pressure measurements in a patient with abnormal relaxation. **Left,** the baseline, demonstrating a low E velocity, high A velocity, and elevation of the left ventricular end-diastolic pressure *(LVEDP).* **Right,** after intravenous administration of verapamil, there is "normalization" of the mitral velocity curves. Simultaneously, however, LVEDP is increased and the time constant of relaxation *(TAU),* is prolonged, signs that left ventricular diastolic function has deteriorated. (From Nishimura RA, Schwartz RS, Holmes DR Jr, et al: Failure of calcium channel blockers to improve ventricular relaxation in humans. *J Am Coll Cardiol* 21:182-188, 1993. By permission of the American College of Cardiology.)

Quantitation of shunts is possible. It has been proposed that the width of the color-flow disturbance at the site of the shunt is proportional to the size of the shunt, especially when transesophageal echocardiography is used. In children and young adults, a Qp:Qs ratio can be calculated by use of volumetric flow rates across the right-sided chambers and left-sided chambers.[68,69]

Diastolic function

In recent years, emphasis has been placed on evaluation of diastolic filling of the heart.[70,71] Because of the complexity of the multiple interrelated factors that compose diastole, investigation was limited in the past to the invasive hemodynamic laboratory. The advent of Doppler echocardiography has provided a noninvasive method for assessing diastolic filling of both the left and right ventricles.[6,7,72-75]

Initial studies evaluating diastolic filling of the heart concentrated on the velocity across the mitral valve, using it as a measure of volumetric flow rate.[74,75] A bimodal distribution of peak filling rates was described from these volumetric flow rates. Abnormally low peak filling rates were found in patients with left ventricular hypertrophy due to hypertension, aortic stenosis, coronary artery disease, and hypertrophic cardiomyopathy.[76-80] It was proposed that a low peak filling rate indicated an abnormality of ventricular relaxation. However, peak filling rates are related to multiple factors in addition to the rate of left ventricular relaxation. As shown in Figure 5B-26, there can be "normalization" of abnormally low peak filling rates by certain interventions despite a deterioration in diastolic filling of the heart.[81] For proper interpretation of diastolic filling of the left ventricle, the mitral flow velocity curves should be looked on not as representing volumetric flow rates but rather as indicating the instantaneous changes between the left atrial and the left ventricular pressures.[6,7,82,83]

As the left ventricular pressure falls below the left atrial pressure because of continued myocardial relaxation and diastolic suction, acceleration of flow begins across the mitral valve, culminating in an early peak velocity (E wave). As the viscoelastic forces of the myocardium begin to interact with other factors, such as pericardial restraint and ventricular interaction, a rise in left ventricular pressure causes deceleration of flow. During mid-diastole, forward flow continues in the absence of a pressure gradient because of inertial forces. At end-diastole, atrial contraction causes a rise in the velocity of flow (A wave). The normal values measured are E velocity (0.85 $\pm$ 0.20 msec), A wave (0.65 $\pm$ 0.20 msec), and deceleration time (200 $\pm$ 40 msec).

The mitral flow velocity curves depend on multiple factors, including heart rate, loading conditions of the left ventricle, and even the age of the patient.[6,7,73,84-87] However, mitral flow velocity curves can be placed in several basic categories when they are examined in clinical practice[6,7,88,89] (Fig 5B-27): "Abnormal relaxation" consists of low E velocity, prolonged deceleration time, and low E-to-A ratio. This is present when there is prolongation of the rate of decrease of left ventricular pressure in conjunction with relatively low filling pressures. These are the earlier diastolic abnormalities in various disease states. Frequently, the patient is asymptomatic at rest, but dyspnea may develop because of high left atrial pressures at fast heart rates or with loss of atrial contraction due to onset of atrial fibrillation. In "restriction to filling," high initial E velocity, short deceleration time, and high E-to-A ratio are present. This mitral velocity contour is due to a high initial left atrial pressure at mitral valve opening as well as a rapid, early increase in left ventricular pressure from abnormally low compliance of the left ventricle. When restriction to filling is present, frequently there is end-stage disease with significant heart failure symptoms at rest or with minimal activity.

An important concept in interpreting the mitral flow velocity curves is the "pseudonormalization" pattern that occurs in patients who have a baseline abnormality of relaxation[7] (Fig 5B-28). In this instance, there is deterioration of diastolic filling superimposed on an abnormal relaxation pattern. This causes an increase in the initial driving pressure across the mitral valve due to higher left atrial pressure, so that the E velocity increases. In addition, deceleration time is shortened by decreased effect of left ventricular compliance, so that deceleration time as measured may actually be in the normal range. This pattern of pseudonormalization can be differentiated from the normal mitral flow velocity curve by examination of other variables. In pseudonormalization, the termination of the A velocity is abbreviated as left ventricular pressure rapidly rises and exceeds left atrial pressure during early atrial contraction (Fig 5B-29). Pulmonary

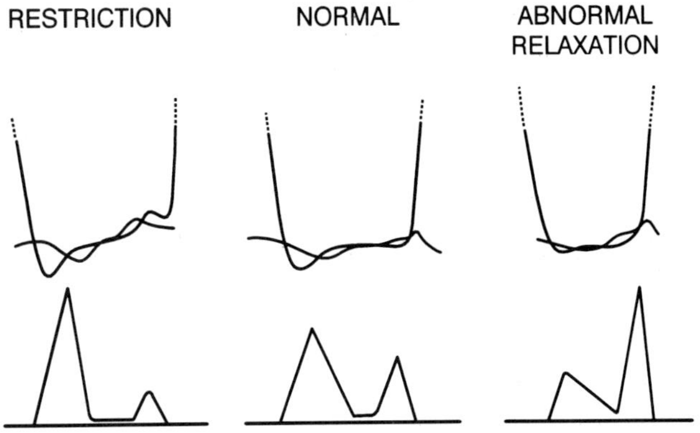

Fig 5B-27 Schematic diagram of the three different types of mitral flow velocity curves with the left atrial and left ventricular pressure shown above. **Left,** restriction to filling in which there is a high initial E velocity, a short deceleration time, and a high E-to-A ratio. **Center,** normal mitral flow velocity curve. **Right,** abnormal relaxation in which there is a low initial E velocity, a prolongation of the deceleration time, and a low E-to-A ratio. (From Nishimura RA, Abel MD, Hatle LK, et al: Assessment of diastolic function of the heart: background and current applications of Doppler echocardiography. Part II. Clinical studies. *Mayo Clin Proc* 64:181-204, 1989. By permission, Mayo Foundation for Medical Education and Research.)

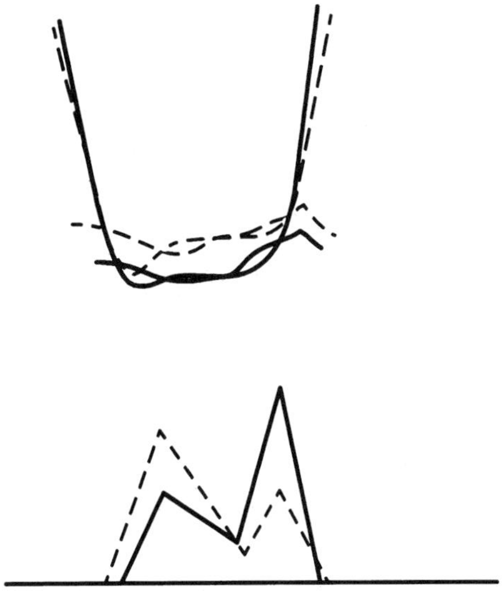

Fig 5B-28 Diagram of the mitral flow velocity curve and simultaneous left atrial and left ventricular pressures. The broken lines equal the baseline state of abnormal relaxation. The solid lines indicate a "pseudonormalization pattern" (see text). (From Nishimura RA, Abel MD, Hatle LK, et al: Assessment of diastolic function of the heart: background and current applications of Doppler echocardiography. Part II. Clinical studies. *Mayo Clin Proc* 64:181-204, 1989. By permission of Mayo Foundation for Medical Education and Research.)

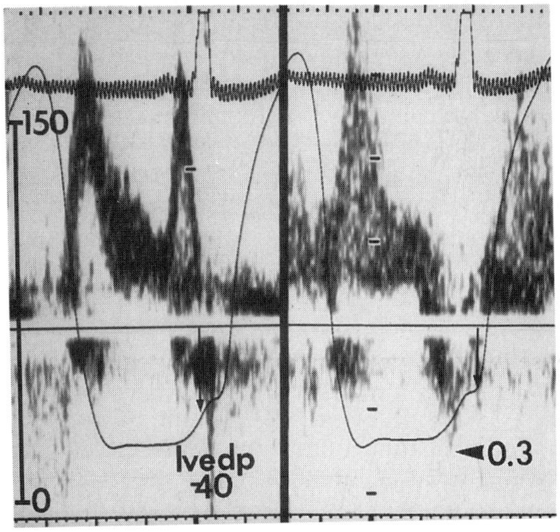

Fig 5B-29 A left ventricular high-fidelity, manometer-tipped pressure tracing demonstrating a high left ventricular end-diastolic pressure of 40 mm Hg. **Left,** the mitral flow velocity curve is shown with a normal E-to-A ratio and normal deceleration time. However, an abbreviation of termination of the A velocity *(long arrow)* occurs before the onset of the QRS pattern. **Right,** the simultaneous pulmonary vein velocity curve demonstrating a high reversal at atrial contraction. The termination of the pulmonary vein velocity *(arrow)* is much later than the mitral A velocity, indicating a high left ventricular end-diastolic pressure.

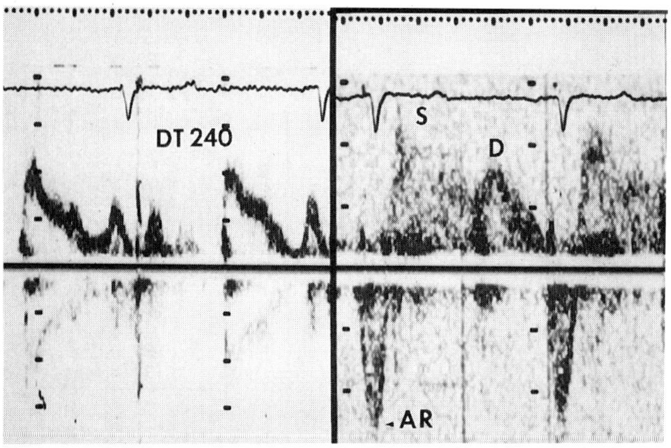

Fig 5B-30 The mitral flow velocity curve **(left)** and pulmonary vein velocity curve **(right)** in a patient with hypertrophic cardiomyopathy. The mitral flow velocity curve appears normal. In the pulmonary vein velocity curve, however, the atrial reversal *(AR)* is significantly elevated to 0.5 m/sec, an indication of pseudonormalization. **D,** diastolic forward flow; *DT,* deceleration time; *S,* systolic forward flow.

vein flow velocities can also be obtained by Doppler echocardiography and contribute further to interpretation of the mitral flow velocity curves.[90-92] If left ventricular end-diastolic pressure is high, an increase in the reversal of velocity at atrial contraction will occur, further aiding in differentiating pseudonormalization from a normal mitral flow velocity curve[91] (Fig 5B-30).

Doppler echocardiography can also be used to measure time intervals, such as the isovolumic relaxation time. In addition, flow on the right side of the heart, such as that in the hepatic vein, superior vena cava, and tricuspid valve, can be interrogated.[7] Disease processes in which ventricular interaction is increased, such as cardiac tamponade[93] and constrictive pericarditis,[94] can be diagnosed by examining the changes in both left- and right-sided velocities during the respiratory cycle.

There is much to be learned about the use of Doppler echocardiography in the evaluation of diastolic filling of the heart. This concept has great potential in providing a method for evaluating a large number of patients noninvasively in a serial manner.

SUMMARY

Doppler echocardiography is a valuable adjunct to two-dimensional echocardiography in the evaluation of the cardiac patient. By noninvasively measuring flow across valves within cardiac chambers and the great vessels, the Doppler examination provides valuable hemodynamic information as an adjunct to the anatomic information of two-dimensional echocardiography. Significant limitations must be understood when Doppler studies are interpreted. However, experienced echocardiographers can obtain a complete hemodynamic assessment in most patients with heart disease.

REFERENCES

1. Tajik AJ, Seward JB, Hagler DJ, et al: Two-dimensional real-time ultrasonic imaging of the heart and great vessels: technique, image orientation, structure identification, and validation. *Mayo Clin Proc* 53:271-303, 1978
2. Hatle L, Angelsen B: *Doppler Ultrasound in Cardiology: Physical Principles and Clinical Applications.* Philadelphia, Lea & Febiger, 1982
3. Nishimura RA, Miller FA Jr, Callahan MJ, et al: Doppler echocardiography: theory, instrumentation, technique, and application. *Mayo Clin Proc* 60:321-343, 1985
4. Zoghbi WA, Quinones MA: Determination of cardiac output by Doppler echocardiography: a critical appraisal. *Herz* 11:258-268, 1986
5. Huntsman LL, Stewart DK, Barnes SR, et al: Noninvasive Doppler determination of cardiac output in man: clinical validation. *Circulation* 67:593-602, 1983
6. Nishimura RA, Housmans PR, Hatle LK, et al: Assessment of diastolic function of the heart: background and current applications of Doppler echocardiography. Part I. Physiologic and pathophysiologic features. *Mayo Clin Proc* 64:71-81, 1989
7. Nishimura RA, Abel MD, Hatle LK, et al: Assessment of diastolic function of the heart: background and current applications of Doppler echocardiography. Part II. Clinical studies. *Mayo Clin Proc* 64:181-204, 1989
8. Miyatake K, Kinoshita N, Nagata S, et al: Intracardiac flow pattern in mitral regurgitation studied with combined use of the ultrasonic pulse Doppler technique and cross-sectional echocardiography. *Am J Cardiol* 45:155-162, 1980
9. Quinones MA, Young JB, Waggoner AD, et al: Assessment of pulsed Doppler echocardiography in detection and quantification of aortic and mitral regurgitation. *Br Heart J* 44:612-620, 1980
10. Omoto R (ed): *Color Atlas of Real-Time Two-Dimensional Doppler Echocardiography.* Tokyo, Shindan-To-Chiryo Company, 1984
11. Miyatake K, Okamoto M, Kinoshita N, et al: Clinical applications of a new type of real-time two-dimensional Doppler flow imaging system. *Am J Cardiol* 54:857-868, 1984
12. Alboliras ET, Seward JB, Hagler DJ, et al: Impact of two-dimensional and Doppler echocardiography on care of children aged two years and younger. *Am J Cardiol* 61:166-169, 1988
13. Hatle L, Angelsen BA, Tromsdal A: Non-invasive assessment of aortic stenosis by Doppler ultrasound. *Br Heart J* 43:284-292, 1980
14. Hatle L, Brubakk A, Tromsdal A, et al: Noninvasive assessment of pressure drop in mitral stenosis by Doppler ultrasound. *Br Heart J* 40:131-140, 1978
15. Stamm RB, Martin RP: Quantification of pressure gradients across stenotic valves by Doppler ultrasound. *J Am Coll Cardiol* 2:707-718, 1983
16. Currie PJ, Seward JB, Reeder GS, et al: Continuous-wave Doppler echocardiographic assessment of severity of calcific aortic stenosis: a simultaneous Doppler-catheter correlative study in 100 adult patients. *Circulation* 71:1162-1169, 1985
17. Currie PJ, Hagler DJ, Seward JB, et al: Instantaneous pressure gradient: a simultaneous Doppler and dual catheter correlative study. *J Am Coll Cardiol* 7:800-806, 1986
18. Callahan MJ, Tajik AJ, Su-Fan Q, et al: Validation of instantaneous pressure gradients measured by continuous-wave Doppler in experimentally induced aortic stenosis. *Am J Cardiol* 56:989-993, 1985
19. Sasson Z, Yock PG, Hatle LK: Doppler echocardiographic determination of the pressure gradient in hypertrophic cardiomyopathy. *J Am Coll Cardiol* 11:752-756, 1988
20. Stewart WJ, Schiavone WA, Salcedo EE, et al: Intraoperative Doppler echocardiography in hypertrophic cardiomyopathy: correlations with the obstructive gradient. *J Am Coll Cardiol* 10:327-335, 1987
21. Burstow DJ, Nishimura RA, Bailey KR, et al: Continuous-wave Doppler echocardiographic measurement of prosthetic valve gradients: a simultaneous dual-catheter correlative study. *Circulation* 80:504-514, 1989
22. Reeder GS, Currie PJ, Hagler DJ, et al: Use of Doppler techniques (continuous-wave, pulsed-wave, and color flow imaging) in the noninvasive hemodynamic assessment of congenital heart disease. *Mayo Clin Proc* 61:725-744, 1986
23. Levine RA: Pressure recovery distal to a stenosis: potential cause of gradient "overestimation" by Doppler echocardiography. *J Am Coll Cardiol* 13:706-715, 1989
24. Yoganathan AP, Valdes-Cruz LM, Schmidt-Dohna J, et al:

Continuous-wave Doppler velocities and gradients across fixed tunnel obstructions: studies in vitro and in vivo. *Circulation* 76:657-666, 1987

25. Baumgartner H, Khan S, DeRobertis M, et al: Discrepancies between Doppler and catheter gradients in aortic prosthetic valves in vitro: a manifestation of localized gradients and pressure recovery. *Circulation* 82:1467-1475, 1990.

26. Yoganathan AP, Corcoran WH: Pressure drops across prosthetic aortic heart valves under steady and pulsatile flow—*in vitro* measurements. *J Biomechanics* 12:153-164, 1979

27. Nishimura RA, Tajik A. Measurement of intracardiac pressures: state of the art—1986. *Herz* 11:283-290, 1986

28. Yock PG, Popp RL: Noninvasive estimation of right ventricular systolic pressure by Doppler ultrasound in patients with tricuspid regurgitation. *Circulation* 70:657-662, 1984

29. Currie PJ, Seward JB, Chan K-L, et al: Continuous wave Doppler determination of right ventricular pressure: a simultaneous Doppler-catheterization study in 127 patients. *J Am Coll Cardiol* 6:750-756, 1985

30. Kircher BJ, Himelman RB, Schiller NB: Noninvasive estimation of right atrial pressure from the inspiratory collapse of the inferior vena cava. *Am J Cardiol* 66:493-496, 1990

31. Simonson JS, Schiller NB: Sonospirometry: a new method for noninvasive estimation of mean right atrial pressure based on two-dimensional echographic measurements of the inferior vena cava during measured inspiration. *J Am Coll Cardiol* 11:557-564, 1988

32. Himelman RB, Stulbarg M, Kircher B, et al: Noninvasive evaluation of pulmonary artery pressure during exercise by saline-enhanced Doppler echocardiography in chronic pulmonary disease. *Circulation* 79:863-871, 1989

33. Masuyama T, Kodama K, Kitabatake A, et al: Continuous-wave Doppler echocardiographic detection of pulmonary regurgitation and its application to noninvasive estimation of pulmonary artery pressure. *Circulation* 74:484-492, 1986

34. Nishimura RA, Tajik AJ: Determination of left-sided pressure gradients by utilizing Doppler aortic and mitral regurgitant signals: validation by simultaneous dual catheter and Doppler studies. *J Am Coll Cardiol* 11:317-321, 1988

35. Nishimura RA, Holmes DR Jr, Reeder GS, et al: Doppler echocardiographic observations during percutaneous aortic balloon valvuloplasty. *J Am Coll Cardiol* 11:1219-1226, 1988

36. Bargiggia GS, Bertucci C, Recusani F, et al: A new method for estimating left ventricular dP/dt by continuous wave Doppler echocardiography: validation studies at cardiac catheterization. *Circulation* 80:1287-1292, 1989

37. Pai RG, Bansal RC, Shah PM: Doppler-derived rate of left ventricular pressure rise: its correlation with the postoperative left ventricular function in mitral regurgitation. *Circulation* 82:514-520, 1990

38. Chung N, Nishimura RA, Holmes DR Jr, et al: Measurement of left ventricular dp/dt by simultaneous Doppler echocardiography and cardiac catheterization. *J Am Soc Echocardiogr* 5:147-152, 1992

39. Chen C, Thomas JD, Anconina J, et al: Impact of impinging wall jet on color Doppler quantification of mitral regurgitation. *Circulation* 84:712-720, 1991

40. Chen C, Rodriguez L, Levine RA, et al: Noninvasive measurement of the time constant of left ventricular relaxation using the continuous-wave Doppler velocity profile of mitral regurgitation. *Circulation* 86:272-278, 1992

41. Nishimura RA, Callahan MJ, Schaff HV, et al: Noninvasive measurement of cardiac output by continuous-wave Doppler echocardiography: initial experience and review of the literature. *Mayo Clin Proc* 59:484-489, 1984

42. Fisher DC, Sahn DJ, Friedman MJ, et al: The mitral valve orifice method for noninvasive two-dimensional echo Doppler determinations of cardiac output. *Circulation* 67:872-877, 1983

43. Chandraratna PA, Nanna M, McKay C, et al: Determination of cardiac output by transcutaneous continuous-wave ultrasonic Doppler computer. *Am J Cardiol* 53:234-237, 1984

44. Muhiudeen IA, Kuecherer HF, Lee E, et al: Intraoperative estimation of cardiac output by transesophageal pulsed Doppler echocardiography. *Anesthesiology* 74:9-14, 1991

45. Gorlin R, Gorlin SG: Hydraulic formula for calculation of the area of the stenotic mitral valve, other cardiac valves, and central circulatory shunts. I. *Am Heart J* 41:1-29, 1951

46. Skjaerpe T, Hegrenaes L, Hatle L: Noninvasive estimation of valve area in patients with aortic stenosis by Doppler ultrasound and two-dimensional echocardiography. *Circulation* 72:810-818, 1985

47. Otto CM, Pearlman AS, Comess KA, et al: Determination of the stenotic aortic valve area in adults using Doppler echocardiography. *J Am Coll Cardiol* 7:509-517, 1986

48. Oh JK, Taliercio CP, Holmes DR Jr, et al: Prediction of the severity of aortic stenosis by Doppler aortic valve area determination: prospective Doppler-catheterization correlation in 100 patients. *J Am Coll Cardiol* 11:1227-1234, 1988

49. Zoghbi WA, Farmer KL, Soto JG, et al: Accurate noninvasive quantification of stenotic aortic valve area by Doppler echocardiography. *Circulation* 73:452-459, 1986

50. Nakatani S, Masuyama T, Kodama K, et al: Value and limitations of Doppler echocardiography in the quantification of stenotic mitral valve area: comparison of the pressure half-time and the continuity equation methods. *Circulation* 77:78-85, 1988

51. Hatle L, Angelsen B, Tromsdal A: Noninvasive assessment of atrioventricular pressure half-time by Doppler ultrasound. *Circulation* 60:1096-1104, 1979

52. Teague SM, Heinsimer JA, Anderson JL, et al: Quantification of aortic regurgitation utilizing continuous wave Doppler ultrasound. *J Am Coll Cardiol* 8:592-599, 1986

53. Libanoff AJ, Rodbard S: Atrioventricular pressure half-time: measure of mitral valve orifice area. *Circulation* 38:144-150, 1968

54. Thomas JD, Wilkins GT, Choong CYP, et al: Inaccuracy of mitral pressure half-time immediately after percutaneous mitral valvotomy: dependence on transmitral gradient and left atrial and ventricular compliance. *Circulation* 78:980-993, 1988

55. Thomas JD, Weyman AE: Doppler mitral pressure half-time: a clinical tool in search of theoretical justification. *J Am Coll Cardiol* 10:923-929, 1987

56. Perry GJ, Helmcke F, Nanda NC, et al: Evaluation of aortic insufficiency by Doppler color flow mapping. *J Am Coll Cardiol* 9:952-959, 1987

57. Helmcke F, Nanda NC, Hsiung MC, et al: Color Doppler assessment of mitral regurgitation with orthogonal planes. *Circulation* 75:175-183, 1987

58. Spain MG, Smith MD, Grayburn PA, et al: Quantitative assessment of mitral regurgitation by Doppler color flow imaging: angiographic and hemodynamic correlations. *J Am Coll Cardiol* 13:585-590, 1989

59. Sahn DJ: Instrumentation and physical factors related to visualization of stenotic and regurgitant jets by Doppler color flow mapping. *J Am Coll Cardiol* 12:1354-1365, 1988

60. Simpson IA, Valdes-Cruz LM, Sahn DJ, et al: Doppler color flow mapping of simulated in vitro regurgitant jets: evaluation of the effects of orifice size and hemodynamic variables. *J Am Coll Cardiol* 13:1195-1207, 1989

61. Bolger AF, Eigler NL, Pfaff JM, et al: Computer analysis of Doppler color flow mapping images for quantitative assessment of in vitro fluid jets. *J Am Coll Cardiol* 12:450-457, 1988

62. Utsunomiya T, Ogawa T, King SW, et al: Pitfalls in the display of color Doppler jet areas: combined variability due to Doppler angle, frame rate, and scanning direction. *Echocardiography* 7:739-745, 1990

63. Rao SR, Richardson SG, Simonetti J, et al: Problems and pitfalls in the performance and interpretation of color Doppler flow imaging: observations based on the influences of technical and physiological factors on the color Doppler examination of mitral regurgitation. *Echocardiography* 7:747-762, 1990

64. Utsunomiya T, Ogawa T, Doshi R, et al: Doppler color flow "proximal isovelocity surface area" method for estimating volume flow rate: effects of orifice shape and machine factors. *J Am Coll Cardiol* 17:1103-1111, 1991

65. Recusani F, Bargiggia GS, Yoganathan AP, et al: A new method for quantification of regurgitant flow rate using color Doppler flow imaging of the flow convergence region proximal to a discrete orifice: an in vitro study. *Circulation* 83:594-604, 1991

66. Rokey R, Sterling LL, Zoghbi WA, et al: Determination of regurgitant fraction in isolated mitral or aortic regurgitation by pulsed Doppler two-dimensional echocardiography. *J Am Coll Cardiol* 7:1273-1278, 1986

67. Khandheria BJ, Shub C, Tajik AJ, et al: Utility of color flow imaging for visualizing shunt flow in atrial septal defect. *Int J Cardiol* 23:91-98, 1989

68. Valdes-Cruz LM, Horowitz S, Mesel E, et al: A pulsed Doppler echocardiographic method for calculating pulmonary and systemic blood flow in atrial level shunts: validation studies in animals and initial human experience. *Circulation* 69:80-86, 1984

69. Dittmann H, Jacksch R, Voelker W, et al: Accuracy of Doppler echocardiography in quantification of left to right shunts in adult patients with atrial septal defect. *J Am Coll Cardiol* 11:338-342, 1988
70. Gaasch WH, Cole JS, Quinones MA, et al: Dynamic determinants of left ventricular diastolic pressure-volume relations in man. *Circulation* 51:317-323, 1975
71. Brutsaert DL, Rademakers FE, Sys SU: Triple control of relaxation: implications in cardiac disease (editorial). *Circulation* 69: 190-196, 1984
72. DeMaria AN, Wisenbaugh T: Identification and treatment of diastolic dysfunction: role of transmitral Doppler recordings. *J Am Coll Cardiol* 9:1106-1107, 1987
73. Labovitz AJ, Pearson AC: Evaluation of left ventricular diastolic function: clinical relevance and recent Doppler echocardiographic insights. *Am Heart J* 114:836-851, 1987
74. Rokey R, Kuo LC, Zoghbi WA, et al: Determination of parameters of left ventricular diastolic filling with pulsed Doppler echocardiography: comparison with cineangiography. *Circulation* 71: 543-550, 1985
75. Kitabatake A, Inoue M, Asao M, et al: Transmitral blood flow reflecting diastolic behavior of the left ventricle in health and disease: a study by pulsed Doppler technique. *Jpn Circ J* 46:92-102, 1982
76. Hanrath P, Mathey DG, Siegert R, et al: Left ventricular relaxation and filling pattern in different forms of left ventricular hypertrophy: an echocardiographic study. *Am J Cardiol* 45:15-23, 1980
77. Bonow RO, Bacharach SL, Green MV, et al: Impaired left ventricular diastolic filling in patients with coronary artery disease: assessment with radionuclide angiography. *Circulation* 64:315-323, 1981
78. Poliner LR, Farber SH, Glaeser DH, et al: Alteration of diastolic filling rate during exercise radionuclide angiography: a highly sensitive technique for detection of coronary artery disease. *Circulation* 70:942-950, 1984
79. Inouye I, Massie B, Loge D, et al: Abnormal left ventricular filling: an early finding in mild to moderate systemic hypertension. *Am J Cardiol* 53:120-126, 1984
80. Fifer MA, Borow KM, Colan SD, et al: Early diastolic left ventricular function in children and adults with aortic stenosis. *J Am Coll Cardiol* 5:1147-1154, 1985
81. Nishimura RA, Schwartz RS, Holmes DR Jr, et al: Failure of calcium channel blockers to improve ventricular relaxation in humans. *J Am Coll Cardiol* 21:182-188, 1993
82. Nishimura RA, Abel MD, Hatle LK, et al: Significance of Doppler indices of diastolic filling of the left ventricle: comparison with invasive hemodynamics in a canine model. *Am Heart J* 118:1248-1258, 1989
83. Nishimura RA, Abel MD, Housmans PR, et al: Mitral flow velocity curves as a function of different loading conditions: evaluation by intraoperative transesophageal Doppler echocardiography. *J Am Soc Echocardiography* 2:79-87, 1989
84. Courtois M, Kovacs SJ Jr, Ludbrook PA: Transmitral pressure-flow velocity relaxation: importance of regional pressure gradients in the left ventricle during diastole. *Circulation* 78:661-671, 1988
85. Ishida Y, Meisner JS, Tsujioka K, et al: Left ventricular filling dynamics: influence of left ventricular relaxation and left atrial pressure. *Circulation* 74:187-196, 1986
86. Choong CY, Abascal VM, Thomas JD, et al: Combined influence of ventricular loading and relaxation on the transmitral flow velocity profile in dogs measured by Doppler echocardiography. *Circulation* 78:672-683, 1988
87. Choong CY, Herrmann HC, Weyman AE, et al: Preload dependence of Doppler-derived indexes of left ventricular diastolic function in humans. *J Am Coll Cardiol* 10:800-808, 1987
88. Appleton CP, Hatle LK, Popp RL: Relation of transmitral flow velocity patterns to left ventricular diastolic function: new insights from a combined hemodynamic and Doppler echocardiographic study. *J Am Coll Cardiol* 12:426-440, 1988
89. Appleton CP, Hatle LK, Popp RL: Demonstration of restrictive ventricular physiology by Doppler echocardiography. *J Am Coll Cardiol* 11:757-768, 1988
90. Nishimura RA, Abel MD, Hatle LK, et al: Relation of pulmonary vein to mitral flow velocities by transesophageal Doppler echocardiography: effect of different loading conditions. *Circulation* 81:1488-1497, 1990
91. Kuecherer HF, Muhiudeen IA, Kusumoto FM, et al: Estimation of left atrial pressure from transesophageal pulsed Doppler echocardiography of pulmonary venous flow. *Circulation* 82:1127-1139, 1990
92. Keren G, Meisner JS, Sherez J, et al: Interrelationship of mid-diastolic mitral valve motion, pulmonary venous flow, and transmitral flow. *Circulation* 74:36-44, 1986
93. Appleton CP, Hatle LK, Popp RL: Cardiac tamponade and pericardial effusion: respiratory variation in transvalvular flow velocities studied by Doppler echocardiography. *J Am Coll Cardiol* 11:1020-1030, 1988
94. Hatle LK, Appleton CP, Popp RL: Differentiation of constrictive pericarditis and restrictive cardiomyopathy by Doppler echocardiography. *Circulation* 79:357-370, 1989

CHAPTER

5

Echocardiography

C. Stress echocardiography

Patricia A. Pellikka, M.D., Barbara A. Nichols, R.N., R.D.C.S., and Jae K. Oh, M.D.

In 1990, the American College of Cardiology endorsed stress echocardiography as "a valid, clinically useful and accepted procedure in the diagnosis of ischemic heart disease."[1]

Echocardiography, because of its relatively low cost, availability, and noninvasiveness, has been recognized since 1979 as a useful imaging modality to combine with the stress test.[2,3] However, the technique was not widely utilized until more recently because of technical limitations, which have generally been resolved.

Stress-induced myocardial ischemia results in abnormalities in regional wall motion and thickening, and ejection fraction may decrease or fail to increase. Mechanical evidence of ischemic dysfunction has been shown to develop before angina pectoris and electrocardiographic evidence of ischemia.[4] These abnormalities are readily detected by two-dimensional echocardiography.[2,5]

Stress echocardiography has been performed with a variety of methods of stress, including treadmill or bicycle exercise, isometric exercise, cold pressor stress, atrial pacing,[6-8] and pharmacologic stress. For the patient able to perform isometric exercise, information on workload, functional aerobic capacity, and double product is valuable to the clinician, so that treadmill or bicycle is the preferred modality for stress echocardiography. In patients unable to perform an adequate exercise test, echocardiography combined with atrial pacing or with pharmacologic stress produced by dobutamine, dipyridamole, or adenosine has been shown to be useful in evaluating coronary artery disease. Because respiratory artifacts are avoided, the likelihood of obtaining high-quality images is slightly better than with exercise echocardiography. Because imaging is continuous during nonexercise stress echocardiography, these techniques are not subject to the limitation of rapid recovery of regional wall motion abnormalities that may reduce sensitivity of postexercise imaging with treadmill exercise echocardiography.

METHODS

Treadmill exercise echocardiography

Treadmill exercise echocardiography is the most widely used form of exercise echocardiography. In contrast to bicycle exercise, with treadmill exercise more muscle groups are recruited, more adults are familiar with the type of exercise, and maintaining a constant work rate in following a specific protocol is less dependent on subject cooperation. Therefore, a higher workload and greater maximal heart rate are typically achieved with treadmill exercise and, in turn, ischemia is more apt to be induced in a patient with coronary artery disease.

Images are obtained before and immediately after treadmill exercise. The performance of exercise echocardiography typically adds 10 minutes to the duration of the treadmill test (Table 5C-1). Attention is directed toward assessment of regional wall motion and determination of ejection fraction. With the use of digital image acquisition, four views—parasternal long-axis and short-axis and apical four-chamber and two-chamber—are acquired. Alternatively, subcostal views may be acquired if this window provides better visualization of endocardium. Digital acquisition systems trigger automatically off the R wave of the electrocardiogram. Eight successive images at 50-msec intervals are captured during systole, beginning at the R wave and including the next 350 msec of the cardiac cycle. In this way, the entire systole and a portion of early diastole of a single cardiac cycle are stored and may be reviewed in a cine-loop format.

After treadmill exercise, the patient is promptly returned to the left lateral decubitus position for acquisition of postexercise images. Continuous videotape recording of the postexercise study is valuable for analysis. In addition, the images are acquired and stored by a digital acquisition system. All postexercise views should be captured as quickly as possible within 1½ minutes of cessation of exercise, because exercise-induced regional wall motion abnormalities may normalize rapidly. If exercise-induced abnormalities are detected, imaging may

Table 5C-1 Exercise echocardiography protocol

1. A resting electrocardiogram is obtained and blood pressure is measured. Resting two-dimensional echocardiographic images are obtained, with four standard views digitized by use of cine-loop technology.
2. A symptom-limited treadmill exercise test is performed during usual blood pressure and electrocardiographic monitoring.
3. The patient is promptly returned to the examining table after exercise, and standard echocardiographic views (parasternal long-axis and short-axis and apical four-chamber and two-chamber) are obtained within the first 1½ minutes of recovery. These views are digitized.
4. Images before and after exercise are displayed on a four-part screen in cine-loop fashion for comparison.
5. A videotape of the entire postexercise study is available for comparison.

be continued during recovery to observe their resolution. After completion of imaging, the best in quality and most representative image for each of the four views is selected, and preexercise and postexercise views are displayed side by side with use of a quad-screen format (Fig 5C-1). Left ventricular volumes and ejection fractions may be determined by previously described techniques.[9,10]

Feasibility studies have shown that with stress echocardiography performed in conjunction with treadmill exercise, interpretable images can be obtained in more than 90% of patients.[9,11,12] Feasibility of stress echocardiography is enhanced by the application of digital technology. In our initial experience of 2,000 consecutive exercise echocardiographic studies, images of diagnostic quality were obtained in 95% of cases.[13]

Bicycle exercise echocardiography

An alternative method of performing exercise echocardiography uses supine or upright bicycle exercise. Bicycle exercise offers the advantage that echocardiographic imaging can be performed through the apical window during exercise. Imaging in the four standard views is also performed before and after exercise with the patient in the left lateral decubitus position. Imaging during peak exercise may improve the sensitivity of the test in detecting coronary artery disease.[14] Bicycle exercise testing with peak exercise imaging may be particularly useful when both two-dimensional echocardiography and Doppler measurements are desired at or near peak exercise, such as in the evaluation of the patient with

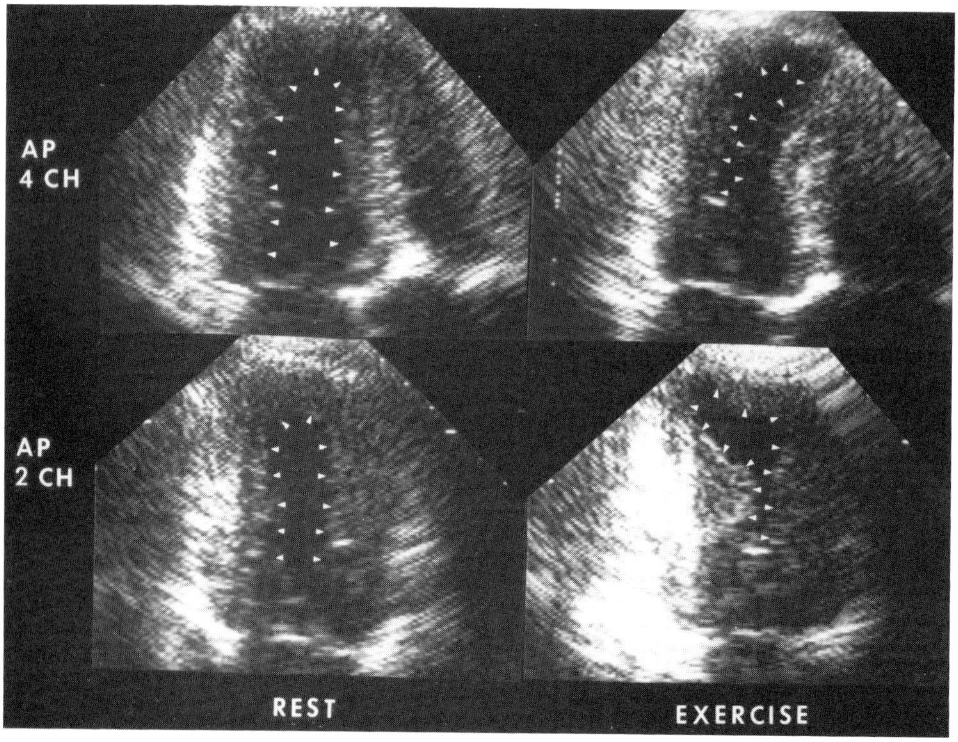

Fig 5C-1 Quad screen display of apical four-chamber *(top)* and two-chamber *(bottom)* images of the left ventricle in systole. Preexercise images are shown on the left and postexercise images on the right. Although basal left ventricular function became hyperdynamic after exercise, the apex became dyskinetic. The patient had high-grade stenoses of the mid-left anterior descending coronary artery and mid-right coronary artery at angiography. *Arrowheads* outline endocardial borders. *AP,* apical; *CH,* chamber.

Table 5C-2 Protocol for dobutamine stress echocardiography

Steps
1. The patient is allowed nothing by mouth except medications for 3 hours before the test.
2. An intravenous line is placed.
3. A premixture of 250 mg of dobutamine in 250 mL of isotonic saline or D5W is infused at a beginning rate of 5 μg/kg per minute.
4. At 3-minute intervals, the infusion rate is increased to 10, 20, 30, and 40 μg/kg per minute. If another end point is reached, the test may be terminated before the maximum dose is accomplished.
5. If no end point is reached, atropine, 0.5 mg, may be administered intravenously at the peak infusion rate to increase heart rate. Additional doses of 0.25 to 0.5 mg may be repeated at 1-minute intervals to a maximum dose of 2 mg or until an end point is reached. Alternatively, the infusion rate may be increased to 50 μg/kg per minute.
6. Heart rate and electrocardiogram are recorded each minute, and blood pressure at each stage of infusion.
7. Images are digitized at baseline, low dose (usually 10 μg/kg per minute), prepeak dose, and peak dose. A quad-screen format is used for each of the four standard views.
8. Esmolol at a dose of 0.5 mg/kg may be administered intravenously should it be necessary to reverse the β-adrenergic effects of dobutamine.

End points
1. New or worsening wall motion abnormalities
2. Target heart rate (85% of age-predicted maximum or 70% after recent myocardial infarction)
3. Peak infusion rate
4. Significant arrhythmia
5. Unacceptable side effects
6. Horizontal or downsloping ST-segment depression ≥2 mm

both valvular disease and suspected coronary artery disease.

Dobutamine echocardiography

Dobutamine is predominantly a β_1-adrenergic stimulating agent with lesser effects on β_2 and α_1 receptors. In experimental studies in open-chest dogs with a critical coronary stenosis, dobutamine was more effective than dipyridamole[15] or dopamine[16] in inducing echocardiographically detectable myocardial ischemia. Dobutamine increases cardiac output by an inotropic effect and by an increase in heart rate, especially at doses above 20 μg/kg per minute.[17,18] Dobutamine is not effective orally, and since its half-life in plasma is approximately 2 minutes, it must be administered by continuous intravenous infusion. A typical protocol for dobutamine stress echocardiography is provided in Table 5C-2.

The normal response to dobutamine infusion is a marked decrease in end-systolic volume and increase in ejection fraction with development of hyperdynamic function of all walls. In regions supplied by a stenosed coronary artery, myocardial oxygen demand exceeds supply and wall motion abnormalities occur. Although dobutamine stress echocardiography is generally well tolerated, side effects include arrhythmia, nausea, tremulousness, dyspnea, headache, hypertension and hypotension. Angina pectoris is occasionally produced. A decrease in blood pressure during dobutamine stress echocardiography may occur without regional wall motion abnormalities and in this situation does not indicate significant coronary artery disease or portend a poor prognosis.[19] Dynamic intracavitary obstruction as a result of hyperdynamic left ventricular function may be detected with Doppler echocardiography in approximately 20% of patients during dobutamine stress echocardiography and may account for a decrease in blood pressure during the test without evidence of ischemia.[20]

Side effects can be rapidly reversed by termination of dobutamine infusion or by administration of a short-acting β-blocker, such as esmolol. Contraindications to the test include uncontrolled hypertension, hypotension, and uncontrolled arrhythmia. The experience with dobutamine stress echocardiography in large numbers of patients has been described,[21,22] and the procedure appears feasible, safe, and accurate in the evaluation of patients with coronary artery disease.[23-25]

Dipyridamole echocardiography

Dipyridamole is a coronary vasodilator, the effects of which are mediated by increased interstitial levels of endogenous adenosine. Dipyridamole decreases coronary vascular resistance and increases coronary blood flow but appears to have little effect on vascular resistance in ischemic areas where small vessels are already maximally dilated.[26] Wall motion abnormalities may develop in regions subtended by a stenosed coronary artery. Dipyridamole infusion typically produces a 20% to 40% increase in heart rate and a mild decrease in blood pressure.[27]

Dipyridamole echocardiography, with an intravenous infusion of dipyridamole at doses of 0.56 mg/kg over 4 minutes, followed by 0.28 mg/kg over 2 minutes, has been demonstrated to be useful in evaluating the presence and extent of coronary artery disease.[28,29] Side effects include lightheadedness, headache, nausea, hypotension, chest pain, and heart block; they can be reversed by termination of the infusion and administration of aminophylline. Contraindications include severe obstructive lung disease, significant bronchospastic airways disease, severe carotid artery disease, aminophylline use, and allergy to dipyridamole.

Adenosine echocardiography

Like dipyridamole, adenosine is a vasodilator that offers the advantages of greater coronary vasodilation and a shorter half-life (< 10 seconds). Although side effects are frequently more frequent and intense, they resolve quickly.[30,31] Adenosine is infused at a rate of 50 μg/kg per minute, which is increased every minute to 75, 100, and 140 or 180 μg/kg per minute. The highest dose is maintained for 4 minutes. All myocardial segments are imaged throughout the infusion. Indications for discontinuing the adenosine infusion include third-degree atrioventricular block, ST-segment depression greater than 2 mm from baseline, severe symptoms, and hypotension unresponsive to dose reduction.

INTERPRETATION OF THE STRESS ECHOCARDIOGRAM

The normal response to stress is the development of hyperdynamic wall motion, decreased end-systolic volume, and increased ejection fraction, which can be appreciated echocardiographically.[2,32] Wall motion is assessed in each of 16 segments in accordance with the model recommended by the American Society of Echocardiography.[33] Failure of a wall to become hyperdynamic and development of new hypokinesis, akinesis, or dyskinesis are markers of various degrees of coronary insufficiency.[9,11] Regional wall motion abnormalities correlate well with coronary artery anatomy,[9] and anatomic distribution of coronary artery stenosis can be determined. An increase in left ventricular volume and decrease in ejection fraction with exercise echocardiography are other markers of significant coronary artery disease.[12]

Decrease in global left ventricular function during dobutamine stress appears to be a less sensitive marker of ischemia than development of regional wall motion abnormalities.[34] This finding may reflect exaggerated hyperkinesis of normal segments in these patients as well as the effects of dobutamine on the peripheral vasculature.

CLINICAL APPLICATIONS

Stress echocardiography is valuable in the diagnosis of ischemic heart disease in patients in whom the electrocardiographic diagnosis of ischemia may be difficult, such as patients receiving digoxin and patients with left ventricular hypertrophy or resting ST-T wave abnormalities. Exercise echocardiography is useful in those who have an increased incidence of false-positive electrocardiographic changes with exercise, such as women[35] and patients with mitral valve prolapse.

Stress echocardiography may be used to determine the extent and location of coronary artery disease.[23,36] Exercise echocardiography has been demonstrated to add independent and incremental information to clinical and exercise test variables for identifying multivessel coronary artery disease.[37] Coronary stenosis severity measured by quantitative angiography is closely related to wall motion abnormalities detected by exercise echocardiography, and exercise echocardiography may be used to assess the physiologic significance of coronary artery lesions.[38] The heart rate at which a regional wall motion abnormality occurs with dobutamine stress echocardiography has been correlated with the severity of coronary artery disease.[39] A positive test result at a heart rate less than or equal to 125 beats/min indicates a high probability of multivessel coronary artery disease.

Prognostic applications of stress echocardiography have been demonstrated. A normal exercise echocardiogram in a patient with good exercise capacity was predictive of an excellent prognosis during a mean follow-up of 28 months.[40] Among survivors of acute myocardial infarction who underwent submaximal treadmill exercise testing within 3 weeks, exercise echocardiography was more accurate in predicting subsequent cardiac events than were clinical characteristics and treadmill electrocardiographic findings. Exercise-induced development of new wall motion abnormalities, marked worsening of wall motion in an area remote from the infarcted area, or decrease in ejection fraction identified patients prone to early new ischemic events.[41-43] In 539 consecutive patients undergoing dipyridamole echocardiography, transient wall motion abnormality was found to be a valuable predictor of subsequent events.[44] Dobutamine stress echocardiography appears to be useful in preoperative cardiac risk assessment before noncardiac surgery; stress-induced wall motion abnormalities during dobutamine infusion identify patients with increased risk of experiencing perioperative cardiac events.[45-48] Furthermore, the test was noted to be superior to clinical assessment in identifying patients at increased risk.[45]

The efficacy of interventional therapy may be assessed with stress echocardiography. Stress echocardiography is useful in demonstrating the functional impact of coronary angioplasty on rest and exercise left ventricular regional wall motion and can be used to identify coronary restenosis.[49-51] Exercise echocardiography after coronary artery bypass surgery permits detection of graft stenosis.[52,53]

Dobutamine stress echocardiography has been used to identify viable myocardium in patients with ventricular dysfunction. Regions of severely hypokinetic or akinetic myocardium that improve in contractility with low-dose dobutamine infusion (5 to 10 μg/kg per minute) correlate with areas of viability identified by positron emission tomography[54] or thallium perfusion imaging.[55] Furthermore, improvement in function with a low dose of dobutamine appears to predict recovery of function after revascularization.[55-57]

Stress color-flow and Doppler echocardiography may have roles in evaluation of the extent and functional significance of valvular heart disease.[58,59] Stress-induced changes in the severity of mitral regurgitation and in the pressure gradient across a stenotic valve may be measured. The role of such techniques merits further investigation.

VALIDATION AND COMPARISON WITH OTHER TECHNIQUES

The reproducibility of exercise echocardiography, including interobserver, intraobserver, and temporal variability, has been evaluated. Oberman et al.[60] examined the reproducibility of two-dimensional exercise echocardiography, performing duplicate studies in the same patients a median of 14 days apart. A high degree of interobserver agreement was found in evaluation of both ejection fraction measurements, as determined by the biplane Simpson method, and preexercise and postexercise wall motion score index. Ejection fractions and wall motion scores were highly correlated between the two tests ($r = 0.92$ and 0.98, respectively). Readings for ejection fraction immediately after exercise on different days could be estimated within 4% of the values measured in the first test; wall motion score index was within 6% of that in the first test. Determinations of both ejection fraction and regional wall motion were reproducible and suitable for serial evaluation of patients.

Exercise echocardiography substantially improves the sensitivity and specificity of exercise electrocardiography in detecting coronary artery disease.[11,12,61,62] In studies involving a general referral population of patients, exercise echocardiography had a sensitivity of from 71% to 97% and a specificity of from 64% to 96% in identifying significant coronary artery stenosis, defined as 50% or greater stenosis of the diameter by angiography (Table 5C-3). False-positive results occurred in patients with non-ischemic cardiomyopathy and in those in whom coronary artery disease was misdiagnosed on the basis of wall motion abnormalities at rest. False-negative findings were associated with failure to achieve maximal exercise, single-vessel coronary artery disease, and moderate (50% to 70% of diameter) coronary stenosis. If patients with evidence of previous myocardial infarction were excluded, the sensitivity for detection of coronary artery disease was 80%.[3] In patients with normal wall motion at rest, the development of regional wall motion abnormalities after exercise was highly specific (100%) for the detection of coronary artery disease. In these patients, exercise echocardiography was significantly more sensitive than exercise electrocardiography in detecting single-vessel disease.[11]

The sensitivity and specificity of nonexercise stress echocardiography have also been reported. Among 85 patients who underwent dobutamine stress echocardiography and quantitative coronary angiography, the sensitivity of the technique for the detection of significant coronary artery disease ($\geq 50\%$ diameter stenosis) was 95%; specificity was 82%. In 55 patients with normal wall motion at baseline, dobutamine echocardiography had an 89% sensitivity and an 85% specificity.[23] The sensitivity was 81% in those with single-vessel disease and 100% in those with multivessel or left main coronary artery disease. Similarly, a favorable clinical experience was reported for vasodilator stress echocardiography.[28-30] However, in comparative studies, a higher sensitivity was obtained with dobutamine than with adenosine and dipyridamole.[31,66]

Exercise echocardiography compares favorably with exercise radionuclide angiography in the diagnosis and evaluation of coronary artery disease.[9,67] Exercise echocardiography allows visualization of all cardiac walls; with exercise radionuclide angiography, a left anterior oblique projection is usually the only view obtained during exercise.

Stress-induced asynergy detected by echocardiography has been demonstrated to correlate well with stress-induced perfusion defects.[31,68-71] In an analysis of 292 patients, exercise echocardiography and thallium single-photon-emission computed tomography (SPECT) had 82% concordance in detecting the same finding (ischemia, infarction, or normal) within the regions analyzed.[69] In a study of 217 patients without previous myocardial infarction examined by simultaneous dobutamine stress echocardiography and technetium-99m methoxyisobutyl isonitrile (MIBI) SPECT, the sensitivities of dobutamine echocardiography and MIBI SPECT were 72% and 76%, respectively (not significant).[71] In the 75 patients without angiographically significant disease, specificity was 83% for dobutamine echocardiography and 67% for scintigraphy ($P = 0.05$). The better specificity of dobutamine echocardiography was most marked in the patients with left ventricular hypertrophy.

ADVANTAGES

Stress echocardiography holds several advantages over currently available noninvasive techniques for assessment of coronary artery disease (Table 5C-4). Many similarities to radionuclide techniques are obvious, and its accuracy appears comparable.[31, 69-71] Stress echocardiography provides information about regional function of all segments of myocardium. In addition, global left ventricular function and its response to stress may be assessed. Stress echocardiography is relatively inexpensive. Echocardiography is convenient for the patient, who does not need to return for delayed images, and with exercise echocardiography no intravenous catheter is required. Radiation hazard is avoided. No time-consuming processing of data is required; results are available immediately. The equipment is portable and compact and can be used with any treadmill. Digital technology permits ready side-by-side comparison of serial studies. Furthermore, stress echocardiography is extremely versatile. In addition to providing information about left ventricular function and wall motion and the response to exercise, it permits determination of chamber size and wall thickness and serves as a screening tool for other abnormalities, such as mitral valve prolapse, other valvular disease, pericardial effusion, left ventricular hypertrophy, and intracardiac masses and thrombi.

LIMITATIONS

Although the ability to obtain diagnostic information has been greatly enhanced by the use of computer-based analysis systems, in a small percentage of patients

Table 5C-3 Accuracy of exercise echocardiography for detection of stenosis of 50% or more of the diameter of an artery or major branch

Year	Study	No. of patients	Exercise modality	Sensitivity, %	Specificity, %
1993	Ryan et al.[63]	309	Bicycle	91	78
1993	Pellikka[64]	114	Treadmill	86	80
1992	Marwick et al.[61]	179	Treadmill	84	86
1991	Crouse et al.[62]	228	Treadmill	97	64
1991	Pozzoli et al.[65]	75	Bicycle	71	96
1987	Armstrong et al.[36]	123	Treadmill	86	86

Table 5C-4 Advantages and disadvantages of stress echocardiography

Advantages	Disadvantages
Similar sensitivity and specificity to nuclear studies	Failure rate in 3% to 8%
Cost-effective	Skilled sonographers and physicians
Global and regional function	Imaging generally postexercise rather than at peak
Patient convenience	Requires end effect of ischemia
No radiation	Requires digital equipment
Versatile	
Portable	
Immediate results	
Comparison of serial studies practical	

satisfactory images cannot be obtained. In addition, because postexercise rather than peak-exercise imaging is usually performed, exercise echocardiography may fail to detect some abnormalities that normalize rapidly. Data suggest that lack of detection occurs in only a small number of patients, who have predominantly milder coronary lesions.[14] In contrast to perfusion imaging, stress echocardiography requires the end effect of ischemia, that is, the wall motion abnormality. Because wall motion abnormalities may be present in cardiomyopathy as well as in coronary artery disease, the specificity of stress echocardiography will be lower in patients with resting abnormalities of wall motion. Importantly, a high degree of physician and sonographer expertise in the performance and interpretation of two-dimensional echocardiography is required. Whether this expertise will be widely obtainable is unknown.

CONCLUSION

Advances in echocardiographic instrumentation and computer technology have made stress echocardiography practical and effective. It has been validated in representative patient populations and has an accuracy comparable to that of radionuclide techniques. Stress echocardiography is a relatively inexpensive, efficient, and highly versatile noninvasive technique. It will continue to evolve into a widely applicable tool for the evaluation of ischemic heart disease.

REFERENCES

1. American College of Cardiology. Policy statement: stress echocardiography, Oct. 14, 1990
2. Mason SJ, Weiss JL, Weisfeldt ML, et al: Exercise echocardiography: detection of wall motion abnormalities during ischemia. *Circulation* 59:50-59, 1979
3. Armstrong WF, O'Donnell J, Dillon JC, et al: Complementary value of two-dimensional exercise echocardiography to routine treadmill exercise testing. *Ann Intern Med* 105:829-835, 1986
4. Upton MT, Rerych SK, Newman GE, et al: Detecting abnormalities in left ventricular function during exercise before angina and ST-segment depression. *Circulation* 62:341-349, 1980
5. Ginzton LE, Laks MM, Brizendine M, et al: Noninvasive measurement of the rest and exercise peak systolic pressure/end-systolic volume ratio: a sensitive two-dimensional echocardiographic indicator of left ventricular function. *J Am Coll Cardiol* 4:509-516, 1984
6. Chapman PD, Doyle TP, Troup PJ, et al: Stress echocardiography with transesophageal atrial pacing: preliminary report of a new method for detection of ischemic wall motion abnormalities. *Circulation* 70:445-450, 1984
7. Lambertz H, Kreis A, Trümper H, et al: Simultaneous transesophageal atrial pacing and transesophageal two-dimensional echocardiography: a new method of stress echocardiography. *J Am Coll Cardiol* 16:1143-1153, 1990
8. Iliceto S, Sorino M, D'Ambrosio G, et al: Detection of coronary artery disease by two-dimensional echocardiography and transesophageal atrial pacing. *J Am Coll Cardiol* 5:1188-1197, 1985
9. Limacher MC, Quinones MA, Poliner LR, et al: Detection of coronary artery disease with exercise two-dimensional echocardiography: description of a clinically applicable method and comparison with radionuclide ventriculography. *Circulation* 67:1211-1218, 1983
10. Gordon EP, Schnittger I, Fitzgerald PJ, et al: Reproducibility of left ventricular volumes by two-dimensional echocardiography. *J Am Coll Cardiol* 2:506-513, 1983
11. Ryan T, Vasey CG, Presti CF, et al: Exercise echocardiography: detection of coronary artery disease in patients with normal left ventricular wall motion at rest. *J Am Coll Cardiol* 11:993-999, 1988
12. Berberich SN, Zager JRS, Plotnick GD, et al: A practical approach to exercise echocardiography: immediate postexercise echocardiography. *J Am Coll Cardiol* 3:284-290, 1984
13. Roger VL, Pellikka PA, Oh JK, et al: Stress echocardiography. Part I. Exercise echocardiography: techniques, implementation, clinical applications, and correlations. *Mayo Clin Proc* 70:5-15, 1995
14. Presti CF, Armstrong WF, Feigenbaum H: Comparison of echocardiography at peak exercise and after bicycle exercise in the evaluation of patients with known or suspected coronary artery disease. *J Am Soc Echocardiography* 1:119-126, 1988

15. Fung AY, Gallagher KP, Buda AJ: The physiologic basis of dobutamine as compared with dipyridamole stress interventions in the assessment of critical coronary stenosis. *Circulation* 76:943-951, 1987

16. McGillem MJ, DeBoe SF, Friedman HZ, et al: The effects of dopamine and dobutamine on regional function in the presence of rigid coronary stenoses and subcritical impairments of reactive hyperemia. *Am Heart J* 115:970-977, 1988

17. Tuttle RR, Mills J: Dobutamine: development of a new catecholamine to selectively increase cardiac contractility. *Circ Res* 36:185-196, 1975

18. Weiner N: Norepinephrine, epinephrine, and the sympathomimetic amines. In *The Pharmacological Basis of Therapeutics.* Edited by AG Gilman, LS Goodman, TW Rall, et al. New York, Macmillan Publishing Company, 1985, pp 145-180

19. Rosamond TL, Vacek JL, Hurwitz A, et al: Hypotension during dobutamine stress echocardiography: initial description and clinical relevance. *Am Heart J* 123:403-407, 1992

20. Pellikka PA, Oh JK, Bailey KR, et al: Dynamic intraventricular obstruction during dobutamine stress echocardiography: a new observation. *Circulation* 86:1429-1432, 1992

21. Mertes H, Sawada SG, Ryan T, et al: Symptoms, adverse effects, and complications and associated with dobutamine stress echocardiography. Experience in 1118 patients. *Circulation* 88:15-19, 1993

22. Pellikka PA, Roger VL, Oh JK, et al: Stress echocardiography. Part II. Dobutamine stress echocardiography: techniques, implementation, clinical applications, and correlations. *Mayo Clin Proc* 70:16-27, 1995

23. Sawada SG, Segar DS, Ryan T, et al: Echocardiographic detection of coronary artery disease during dobutamine infusion. *Circulation* 83:1605-1614, 1991

24. Berthe C, Pierard LA, Hiernaux M, et al: Predicting the extent and location of coronary artery disease in acute myocardial infarction by echocardiography during dobutamine infusion. *Am J Cardiol* 58:1167-1172, 1986

25. Mazeika PK, Nadazdin A, Oakley CM: Dobutamine stress echocardiography for detection and assessment of coronary artery disease. *J Am Coll Cardiol* 19:1203-1211, 1992

26. Needleman P, Carr PB, Johnson EM Jr: Drugs used for the treatment of angina: organic nitrates, calcium channel blockers, and β-adrenergic antagonists. In *The Pharmacological Basis of Therapeutics.* Edited by AG Gilman, LS Goodman, TW Rall, et al. New York, Macmillan Publishing Company, 1985, pp 806-826

27. Albro PC, Gould KL, Westcott RJ, et al: Noninvasive assessment of coronary stenoses by myocardial imaging during pharmacologic coronary vasodilatation. III. Clinical trial. *Am J Cardiol* 42:751-760, 1978

28. Picano E, Lattanzi F, Masini M, et al: Comparison of the high-dose dipyridamole-echocardiography test and exercise two-dimensional echocardiography for diagnosis of coronary artery disease. *Am J Cardiol* 59:539-542, 1987

29. Bolognese L, Sarasso G, Aralda D, et al: High dose dipyridamole echocardiography early after uncomplicated acute myocardial infarction: correlation with exercise testing and coronary angiography. *J Am Coll Cardiol* 14:357-363, 1989

30. Zoghbi WA, Cheirif J, Kleiman NS, et al: Diagnosis of ischemic heart disease with adenosine echocardiography. *J Am Coll Cardiol* 18:1271-1279, 1991

31. Marwick T, Willemart B, D'Hondt A-M, et al: Selection of the optimal nonexercise stress for the evaluation of ischemic regional myocardial dysfunction and malperfusion: comparison of dobutamine and adenosine using echocardiography and ^{99m}Tc-MIBI single photon emission computed tomography. *Circulation* 87:345-354, 1993

32. Zwehl W, Gueret P, Meerbaum S, et al: Quantitative two dimensional echocardiography during bicycle exercise in normal subjects. *Am J Cardiol* 47:866-873, 1981

33. American Society of Echocardiography Committee on Standards, Subcommittee on Quantitation of Two-Dimensional Echocardiograms: Recommendations for quantitation of the left ventricle by two-dimensional echocardiography. *J Am Soc Echocardiogr* 2:358-367, 1989

34. Attenhofer CH, Pellikka PA, Sohn DW, et al: Left ventricular cavity dilatation: the unreliable sign for severe ischemic heart disease in dobutamine stress echocardiography (abstract). *Circulation* 90 Suppl 1:660, 1994

35. Sawada SG, Ryan T, Fineberg NS, et al: Exercise echocardiographic detection of coronary artery disease in women. *J Am Coll Cardiol* 14:1440-1447, 1989

36. Armstrong WF, O'Donnell J, Ryan T, et al: Effect of prior myocardial infarction and extent and location of coronary disease on accuracy of exercise echocardiography. *J Am Coll Cardiol* 10:531-538, 1987

37. Roger VL, Pellikka PA, Oh JK, et al: Identification of multivessel coronary artery disease by exercise echocardiography. *J Am Coll Cardiol* 24:109-114, 1994

38. Sheikh KH, Bengston JR, Helmy S, et al: Relation of quantitative coronary lesion measurements to the development of exercise-induced ischemia assessed by exercise echocardiography. *J Am Coll Cardiol* 15:1043-1051, 1990

39. Segard D, Brown SE, Sawada SG, et al: Dobutamine stress echocardiography: correlation with coronary lesion severity as determined by quantitative angiography. *J Am Coll Cardiol* 19:1197-1202, 1992

40. Sawada SG, Ryan T, Conley MJ, et al: Prognostic value of a normal exercise echocardiogram. *Am Heart J* 120:49-55, 1990

41. Ryan T, Armstrong WF, O'Donnell JA, et al: Risk stratification after acute myocardial infarction by means of exercise two-dimensional echocardiography. *Am Heart J* 114:1305-1316, 1987

42. Jaarsma W, Visser CA, Funke Kupper AJ, et al: Usefulness of two-dimensional exercise echocardiography shortly after myocardial infarction. *Am J Cardiol* 57:86-90, 1986

43. Applegate RJ, Dell'italia LJ, Crawford MH: Usefulness of two-dimensional echocardiography during low-level exercise testing early after uncomplicated acute myocardial infarction. *Am J Cardiol* 60:10-14, 1987

44. Picano E, Severi S, Michellassi C, et al: Prognostic importance of dipyridamole-echocardiography test in coronary artery disease. *Circulation* 80:450-457, 1989

45. Pellikka PA, Oh JK, Bailey KR, et al: Prognostic role of dobutamine stress echocardiography before noncardiac surgery (abstract). *J Am Coll Cardiol* 19 Suppl A:100, 1992

46. Lane RT, Sawada SG, Segar DS, et al: Dobutamine stress echocardiography for assessment of cardiac risk before noncardiac surgery. *Am J Cardiol* 68:976-977, 1991

47. Dávila-Román VG, Waggoner AD, Sicard GA, et al: Dobutamine stress echocardiography predicts surgical outcome in patients with an aortic aneurysm and peripheral vascular disease. *J Am Coll Cardiol* 21:957-963, 1993

48. Poldermans D, Fioretti PM, Forster T, et al: Dobutamine stress echocardiography for assessment of perioperative cardiac risk in patients undergoing major vascular surgery. *Circulation* 87:1506-1512, 1993

49. Broderick T, Sawada S, Armstrong WF, et al: Improvement in rest and exercise-induced wall motion abnormalities after coronary angioplasty: an exercise echocardiographic study. *J Am Coll Cardiol* 15:591-599, 1990

50. Picano E, Pirelli S, Marzilli M, et al: Usefulness of high-dose dipyridamole echocardiography test in coronary angioplasty. *Circulation* 80:807-815, 1989

51. Mertes H, Erbel R, Nixdorff U, et al: Exercise echocardiography for the evaluation of patients after nonsurgical coronary artery revascularization. *J Am Coll Cardiol* 21:1087-1093, 1993

52. Sawada SG, Judson WE, Ryan T, et al: Upright bicycle exercise echocardiography after coronary artery bypass grafting. *Am J Cardiol* 64:1123-1129, 1989

53. Crouse LJ, Vacek JL, Beauchamp GD, et al: Exercise echocardiography after coronary artery bypass grafting. *Am J Cardiol* 70:572-576, 1992

54. Piérard LA, DeLandsheere CM, Berthe C, et al: Identification of viable myocardium by echocardiography during dobutamine infusion in patients with myocardial infarction after thrombolytic therapy: comparison with positron emission tomography. *J Am Coll Cardiol* 15:1021-1031, 1990

55. Marzullo P, Parodi O, Reisenhofer B, et al: Value of rest thallium-201/technetium-99m sestamibi scans and dobutamine echocardiography for detecting myocardial viability. *Am J Cardiol* 71:166-172, 1993

56. Barilla F, Gheorghiade M, Alam M, et al: Low-dose dobutamine in patients with acute myocardial infarction identifies viable but not contractile myocardium and predicts the magnitude of improvement in wall motion abnormalities in response to coronary revascularization. *Am Heart J* 122:1522-1531, 1991

57. Cigarroa CG, deFilippi CR, Brickner ME, et al: Dobutamine stress echocardiography identifies hibernating myocardium and predicts recovery of left ventricular function after coronary revascularization. *Circulation* 88:430-436, 1993

58. Fehrenbacher G, Paumer L, Bommer W: Exercise induced mitral regurgitation in patients with coronary artery disease. *Circulation* 78 Suppl 2:273, 1988

59. Sagar KB, Wann LS, Paulson WJH, et al: Role of exercise Doppler echocardiography in isolated mitral stenosis. *Chest* 92:27-30, 1987

60. Oberman A, Fan P-H, Nanda NC, et al: Reproducibility of two-dimensional exercise echocardiography. *J Am Coll Cardiol* 14:923-928, 1989

61. Marwick TH, Nemec JJ, Pashkow FJ, et al: Accuracy and limitation of exercise echocardiography in a routine clinical setting. *J Am Coll Cardiol* 19:74-81, 1992

62. Crouse LJ, Harbrecht JJ, Vacek JL, et al: Exercise echocardiography as a screening test for coronary artery disease and correlation with coronary arteriography. *Am J Cardiol* 67:1213-1218, 1991

63. Ryan T, Segar DS, Sawada SG, et al: Detection of coronary artery disease with upright bicycle exercise echocardiography. *J Am Soc Echocardiogr* 6:186-197, 1993

64. Pellikka PA: Stress echocardiography: is there an optimal type of stress? *J Am Soc Echocardiogr* 6:198-199, 1993

65. Pozzoli MMA, Fioretti PM, Salustri A, et al: Exercise echocardiography and technetium-99m MIBI single-photon emission computed tomography in the detection of coronary artery disease. *Am J Cardiol* 67:350-355, 1991

66. Martin TW, Seaworth JF, Johns JP, et al: Comparison of adenosine, dipyridamole, and dobutamine in stress echocardiography. *Ann Intern Med* 116:190-196, 1992

67. Crawford MH, Petru MA, Amon KW, et al: Comparative value of 2-dimensional echocardiography and radionuclide angiography for quantitating changes in left ventricular performance during exercise limited by angina pectoris. *Am J Cardiol* 53:42-46, 1984

68. Maurer G, Nanda NC: Two dimensional echocardiographic evaluation of exercise-induced left and right ventricular asynergy: correlation with thallium scanning. *Am J Cardiol* 48:720-727, 1981

69. Quiñones MA, Verani MS, Haichin RM, et al: Exercise echocardiography versus ^{201}Tl single-photon emission computed tomography in evaluation of coronary artery disease: analysis of 292 patients. *Circulation* 85:1026-1031, 1992

70. Forster T, McNeill AJ, Salustri A, et al: Simultaneous dobutamine stress echocardiography and technetium-99m isonitrile single-photon emission computed tomography in patients with suspected coronary artery disease. *J Am Coll Cardiol* 21:1591-1596, 1993

71. Marwick T, D'Hondt A-M, Baudhuin T, et al: Optimal use of dobutamine stress for the detection and evaluation of coronary artery disease: combination with echocardiography or scintigraphy, or both? *J Am Coll Cardiol* 22:159-167, 1993

CHAPTER

5

Echocardiography

D. Invasive echocardiography: transesophageal, intravascular, and other innovative echocardiographic technologies

James B. Seward, M.D.

THE echocardiographic laboratory no longer merely obtains images.[1] A comprehensive cardiovascular ultrasound imaging and hemodynamic laboratory is capable of performing many functions heretofore equated with an invasive catheterization laboratory. These include (1) anatomic assessment; (2) cardiac function, such as ejection fraction, ventricular volumes, and muscle mass; (3) hemodynamics, including gradient, pressure, flow, and valve area; and (4) an angiographic substitute in the form of Doppler color-flow imaging. Additionally, special echocardiographic applications and technologies have evolved. These procedures include (1) contrast echocardiography,[2-4] (2) echocardiographically directed pericardiocentesis,[5] (3) exercise and pharmacologic stress echocardiography[6,7] (see chapter 5C), (4) transesophageal echocardiography,[8-10] (5) vascular[11] and intravascular[12] (see chapter 27B) echocardiography, and (6) echocardiography with implantable and catheter-tipped devices.[13,14] The wide application of echocardiographic technology also includes (1) fetal[15] (see chapter 57), (2) congenital[16] (see chapter 39), and (3) intraoperative[17] echocardiography. Innovations expected to come into clinical application in the future include (1) three- and four-dimensional echocardiography,[18] (2) tissue characterization,[19] (3) ultrasonic tomography,[20] and (4) intracardiac echocardiography.[21,22] Many of these techniques, applications, and technologies are described or alluded to elsewhere in this textbook. This chapter is intended to describe some of the newer invasive clinical echocardiographic techniques, particularly transesophageal echocardiography and intravascular echocardiography.

TRANSESOPHAGEAL ECHOCARDIOGRAPHY

Transesophageal echocardiography (TEE) was initially introduced in the late 1970s but did not mature or receive wide clinical use until the introduction of high-frequency transducers (5 MHz) incorporating pulsed-wave Doppler and color-flow imaging.[8] Since approximately 1988, TEE has made an increasing impact and is now considered a routine extension of a comprehensive precordial surface echocardiographic examination. Clinical indications for TEE are evolving; however, superior information is obtained in patients with (1) prosthetic valves, particularly mitral prostheses; (2) native mitral valve regurgitation; (3) critical illness thought to be caused by cardiac complications (e.g., after infarction or trauma); (4) endocarditis; (5) cardiac tumors, thrombus, and masses, all potential sources for embolism; (6) congenital heart disease; and (7) thoracic aortic diseases, including dissection, aneurysm, and atherosclerosis. Also, TEE can complement precordial echocardiographic examinations that are technically difficult or yield results of poor quality.

Equipment

A conventional endoscope without optics or suction is fitted with a phased-array or mechanical ultrasound transducer at its tip. A 90° tomographic plane of section was initially available. Transducers now have two orthogonally related arrays (i.e., biplane) or a rotatable plane capable of obtaining a continuum of plane in an 80° arc (i.e., multiplane). The tip has 90° or more of operator-controlled forward and reverse flexibility and approximately 70° of lateral manipulatability. A wide selection of adult- and pediatric-sized transducers is available, ranging from approximately 5 to 13 mm in diameter. A thermocouple within the transducer is incorporated into most instruments to monitor temperature and potential electrical hazards.

Physician training

Physicians are trained to master esophageal intubation and learn tomographic esophageal anatomy. Esophageal intubation is best accomplished under the tutelage of an

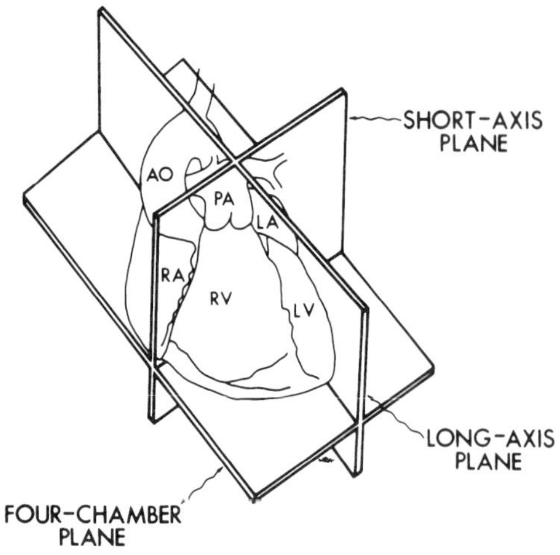

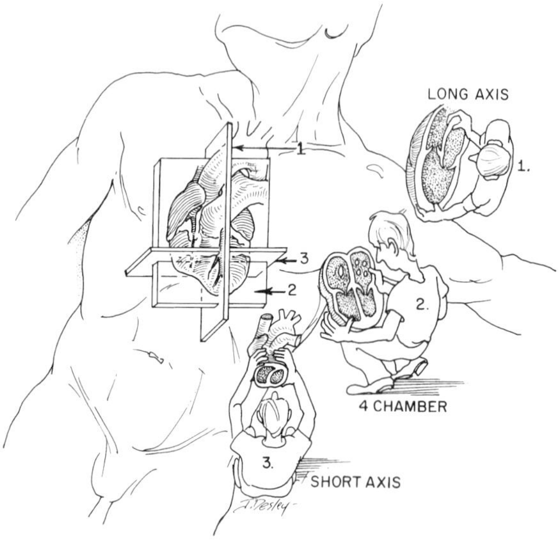

Fig 5D-1 Two-dimensional echocardiographic imaging planes. **Top,** diagram of the three orthogonal imaging planes of the heart used to visualize the heart with two-dimensional echocardiography. Note: In the original American Society of Echocardiography document on standards (1980), designation of transducer position is not specified. The document only recommends tomographic presentation of cardiac structures, as follows: (1) the short axis is to be viewed from apex toward base, (2) the long axis is to be viewed from the left side toward the right, and (3) the four chambers can be viewed in two formats—option 1, apex down, viewing from the anterior surface toward the posterior surface; and option 2, apex up, viewing from the heart's posterior surface toward the anterior surface. *AO,* aorta; *LA,* left atrium; *LV,* left ventricle; *PA,* pulmonary artery; *RA,* right atrium; *RV,* right ventricle. **Bottom,** characterization of the recommended orientation for tomographic planes of the heart. The heart can be cut in three primary planes: long-axis, four-chamber, and short-axis. Note that there is no designation of transducer position. Also note that the patient is depicted recumbent, as though lying on an examination table (for catheterization, physical examination, operation, etc.). *1.* In the *long-axis* anatomy and accompanying tomographic image, the heart is viewed from left to right. *2.* The *four-chamber* plane is easiest to appreciate with the apex down (i.e., American Society of Echocardiography option 1). In option 2, apex up, the heart is viewed from the posterior surface of the patient's chest looking anteriorly. *3. Short-axis* views are presented as though one were looking from the cardiac apex toward the base. (**Top** from Henry WL, DeMaria A, Gramiak R, et al: Report of the American Society of Echocardiography Committee on Nomenclature and Standards in Two-dimensional Echocardiography. *Circulation* 62:212-217, 1980. By permission of American Heart Association. **Bottom** from Seward JB: Transesophageal echocardiographic anatomy. In *Transesophageal Echocardiography.* Edited by WK Freeman, JB Seward, BK Khandheria, et al. Boston, Little, Brown and Company, 1994, pp 55-128. By permission, Mayo Foundation.)

experienced gastroenterologist. We believe that from 25 to 30 esophageal intubations are a necessary prerequisite. With this experience, it usually takes an additional 30 to 50 esophageal examinations to become familiar with transesophageal tomographic anatomy. It is imperative that the echocardiographer or physician be familiar with potential pitfalls, limitations, and complications associated with TEE.[23]

Patient preparation

The patient should abstain from oral intake for approximately 4 hours before the procedure. A brief drug and allergy history as well as a history of any dysphagia or esophageal disease should be elicited. Dentures or other oral prostheses are removed. The echocardiographic physician performs the imaging examination, and a trained nurse assistant monitors and cares for the patient's comfort, airway, and the like.

Medications commonly used are (1) topical anesthetic to the oral pharynx (lidocaine), (2) anticholinergic (glycopyrrolate) to reduce salivation, and (3) an anxiolytic (benzodiazepine) to decrease anxiety and provide transient amnesia for the procedure. Endocarditis prophylaxis is recommended only for patients at high risk of endocarditis:[24] those with prosthetic valves, conduits, or previous endocarditis.

Within the procedure room, other recommended equipment includes (1) oral suction capability, (2) personnel and equipment for cardiac resuscitation, (3) pulsed oximeter to monitor changing oxygen saturation, and (4) echocardiographic instrumentation that accommodates electrocardiographic monitoring and a transesophageal transducer.

The complication rate of TEE is very low. However, transient arrhythmias, hypoxia, worsening congestive heart failure, cardiac arrest, esophageal perforation, and death have been reported with esophageal examination.[23] An appropriate environment and patient selection with adequate support of personnel and equipment are abso-

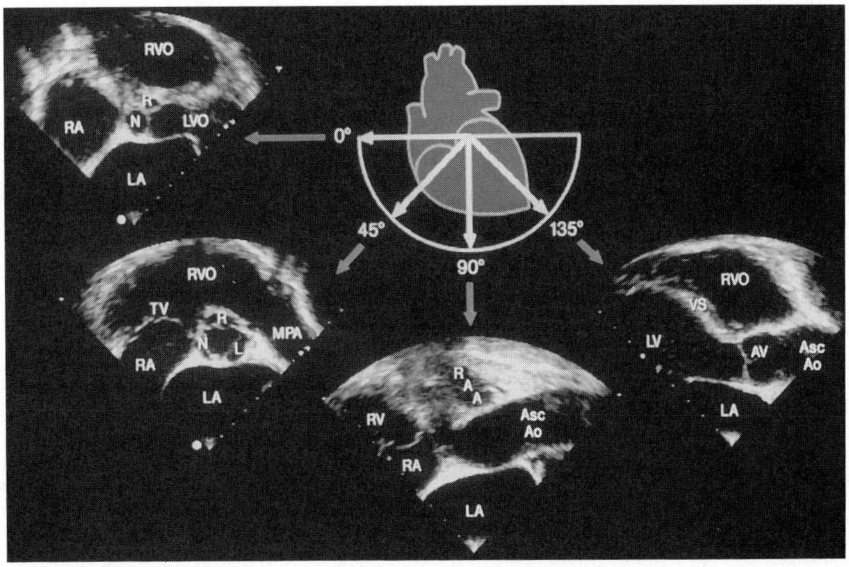

Fig 5D-2 With the transducer tip in midesophagus and posterior to the left atrium, a sequence of short- and long-axis views can be obtained (the ultrasound images are described from left to right). 0°: The array is in a transverse (short-axis) orientation to the body (i.e., *biplane,* transverse plane without tip manipulation; *multiplane* array set at 0°). The heart (aortic valve) is cut obliquely. Only the right coronary *(R)* and noncoronary *(N)* cusps of the aortic valve are appreciated. 45°: The array has been manipulated to lie in the basal short axis of the heart (i.e., *biplane,* medial flexion of the longitudinal plane or lateral flexion of the transverse plane; *multiplane,* rotation of the array to 45°). The three cusps of the aortic valve are optimally visualized in short axis. 90°: The array is in the longitudinal (long-axis) orientation to the body (i.e., *biplane,* longitudinal plane without tip flexion; *multiplane,* array rotated to 90°). The array is parallel to the long axis of the endoscope shaft. Note that the image is oblique to the long axis of the left ventricle but is in the long axis of the ascending aorta *(AscAo)* and other basal and upper mediastinal structures. 135°: The array is in the long axis of the heart (i.e., *biplane,* lateral flexion of the longitudinal plane or, rarely, far medial flexion [and left-to-right image reversal] of the transverse plane; *multiplane,* array rotated to 135°). The left ventricular outflow and mitral inflow are simultaneously imaged. This view is identical to a parasternal long-axis view of the left ventricle. *AV,* aortic valve; *L,* left coronary cusp; *LA,* left atrium; *LV,* left ventricle; *LVO,* left ventricular outflow; *MPA,* main pulmonary artery; *RA,* right atrium; *RAA,* right atrial appendage; *RV,* right ventricle; *RVO,* right ventricular outflow; *TV,* tricuspid valve; *VS,* ventricular septum. (From Seward JB: Transesophageal echocardiographic anatomy. In *Transesophageal Echocardiography.* Edited by WK Freeman, JB Seward, BK Khandheria, et al. Boston, Little, Brown and Company, 1994, pp 55-128. By permission, Mayo Foundation.)

lutely necessary for the safe performance of this newest echocardiographic examination.

Anatomic correlations

A comprehensive transesophageal examination entails a sequence of transducer positions and tomographic planes of section.[25] A step-by-step approach is suggested that can be altered on the basis of clinical situations.[9] During the TEE examination, two distinct tomographic examinations are performed—namely, of the *heart* and of the *thoracic aorta*. Transverse (short-axis), longitudinal (long-axis), frontal (four-chamber), and off-axis images of the heart and associated thoracic structures can be obtained.[9,25] A standardized anatomic orientation of the resultant images is preferred—an orientation identical to the accepted surface echocardiographic standard[26] (Fig 5D-1).

Midesophagus short (horizontal) and long (longitudinal) views

After the ultrasound endoscope is advanced into the midesophagus (25 to 30 cm from the incisors), short-axis and long-axis scans of the heart can be uniformly obtained (Fig 5D-2). The transducer is intimately adjacent and posterior to the left atrial cavity. The image orientation corresponds to a familiar echocardiographic presentation of the heart.[9,25] However, because the transducer is posterior to the heart within the esophagus, the electronic display places the transducer artifact ("bang") at the

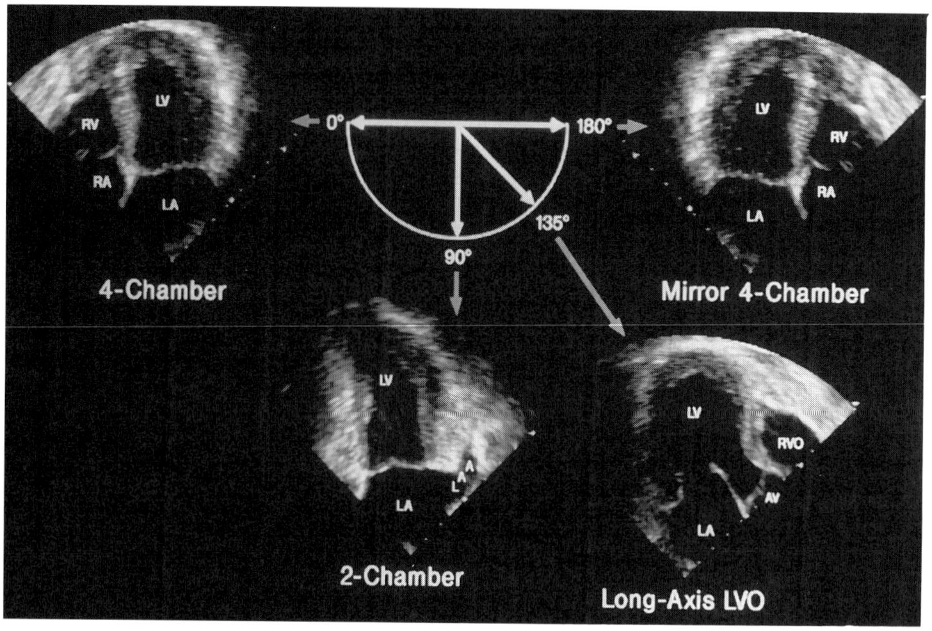

Fig 5D-3 Midesophageal four-chamber views. Apex-up long-axis views of the heart. From the viewer's left to right in this collage, a series of images can be obtained with either biplane or multiplane transesophageal echocardiography. *Four-chamber:* With the transverse plane of a biplane endoscope or a multiplane array at 0°, the endoscope tip is retroflexed and usually slightly withdrawn. A conventional apex-up four-chamber view of the heart is obtained. *Two-chamber:* With the endoscope tip continuously retroflexed, the multiplane array is rotated to 90°, or with a biplane endoscope, a switch is made to the longitudinal plane. When the biplane instrument is used, sometimes medial tip flexion is also required. *Long-axis left ventricular outflow:* With the endoscope tip continuously retroflexed, the multiplane array is rotated to 135° to obtain a long-axis view of the left ventricular outflow *(LVO).* If the biplane endoscope is used, retroflexion of the longitudinal plane is maintained during lateral flexion of the endoscope tip. *Mirror image four-chamber:* With overrotation of the transducer array (180°), a mirror image orientation of the four-chamber view is obtained. The same effect can be obtained from the precordial examination by manually overrotating the transducer. *Apex-down* four-chamber views are obtained by electronic inversion of the image (i.e., the same maneuver required when doing a surface echocardiogram when apex-down orientation is preferred). *AV,* aortic valve; *LA,* left atrium; *LAA,* left atrial appendage; *LV,* left ventricle; *RA,* right atrium; *RV,* right ventricle; *RVO,* right ventricular outflow. (From Seward JB, Khandheria BK, Freeman WK, et al: Multiplane transesophageal echocardiography: image orientation, examination technique, anatomic correlations, and clinical applications. *Mayo Clin Proc* 68:523-551, 1993. By permission, Mayo Foundation for Medical Education and Research.)

bottom of the image throughout the examination.[9] The only exception is the four-chamber plane, which may preferably be displayed with the apex downward. With this display convention, anterior structures are to the top of the image, posterior structures to the bottom, and left-sided structures to the viewer's right. Important anatomic landmarks are the aortic root and aortic valve cusps, proximal coronary arteries, atrial appendages, superior vena cava, atrial septum, pulmonary veins, pulmonary valve, and proximal pulmonary arteries.

Four-chamber (frontal) views

With the endoscope in the midesophagus (approximately 30 cm from the incisors), retroflexion of the endoscope tip images the four-chamber frontal planes of the heart (Fig 5D-3). An electronic inversion of the image, similar to a surface examination, is required to display these views with the cardiac apex oriented downward. These views image the atrioventricular valves and support apparatus, ventricles, left ventricular outflow tract, and coronary sinus. With the apex down, the left ventricle is to the right on the video screen.

Transgastric short-axis scans

With advancement of the endoscope tip into the fundus of the stomach (approximately 35 or 40 cm from the incisors), anteflexion of the transducer tip images the heart from the stomach and through the left lobe of the

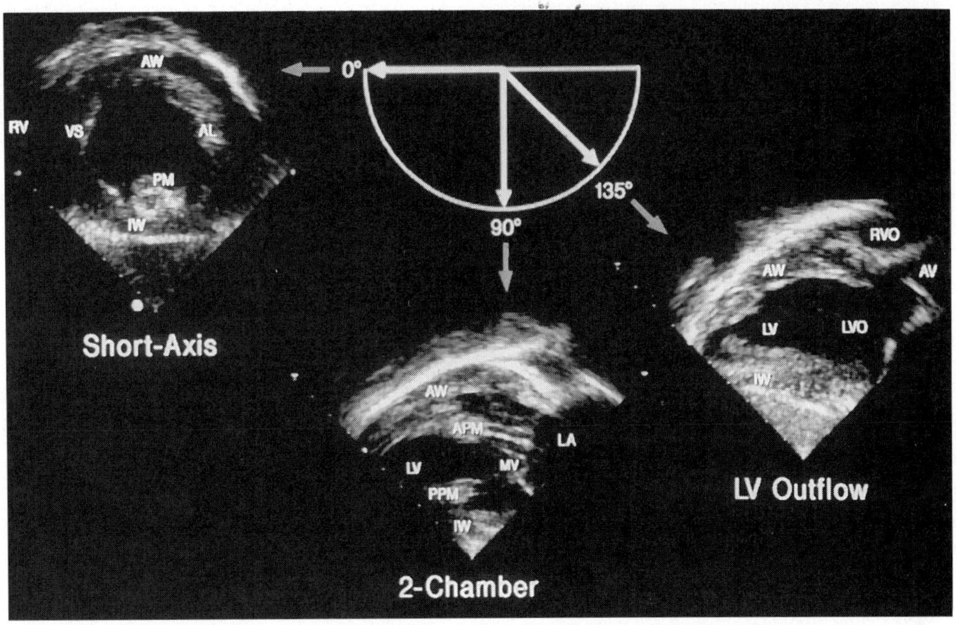

Fig 5D-4 Transgastric short- and long-axis views. *Short-axis:* The transducer tip is in the fundus of the stomach. The transverse plane of the biplane endoscope or 0° rotation of the multiplane array is used to obtain this view. The transducer is posterior to the heart and adjacent to the left ventricular inferior wall *(IW)*. The anterior wall *(AW)* is at the top of the image. The posteromedial *(PM)* and anterolateral *(AL)* papillary muscles are visualized. The right ventricle *(RV)* is to the viewer's left. The heart is being viewed from apex toward base. *Two-chamber:* The longitudinal plane of the biplane endoscope or the multiplane array at 90° rotation obtains this view. The left ventricle *(LV)* and left atrium *(LA)* are simultaneously viewed. This is an excellent view for assessing the mitral support apparatus. *Left ventricular outflow:* This view is obtained by lateral flexion of the biplane endoscope tip during imaging in the longitudinal plane. Alternatively, the multiplane array is rotated to approximately 135° without endoscope tip manipulation. The aortic valve *(AV)* and left ventricular outflow *(LVO)* are imaged from the left ventricle. The transducer is posterior to the inferior wall of the left ventricle. *APM,* anterior papillary muscle; *MV,* mitral valve; *PPM,* posterior papillary muscle; *RVO,* right ventricular outflow; *VS,* ventricular septum. (From Seward JB: Transesophageal echocardiographic anatomy. In *Transesophageal Echocardiography.* Edited by WK Freeman, JB Seward, BK Khandheria, et al. Boston, Little, Brown and Company, 1994, pp 55-128. By permission, Mayo Foundation.)

liver (i.e., transgastric view of the heart) (Fig 5D-4). This view is best used to assess ventricular function and morphology. Short- and long-axis scans and, occasionally, four-chamber views can be obtained from this transducer position.

Examination of the thoracic aorta

Throughout the vertical extent of the thorax, the esophagus and thoracic aorta are intimately related, so that imaging of the entire thoracic aorta from the esophagus is possible in nearly every patient (Fig 5D-5). The aortic root, ascending aorta, transverse aortic arch, left carotid and left subclavian arteries, entire descending thoracic aorta, and upper abdominal aorta can be consistently imaged. With multiplanar TEE, there is no longer a significant difficulty in imaging the upper ascending aorta.

Multiplanar and biplanar transesophageal imaging

Endoscopic transducers now allow biplanar[10] or multiplanar[9] imaging. These devices have markedly improved the ability to obtain not only the standard short, long, and four-chamber views but also the off-axis intermediate views (see Figs 5D-2 through 5D-4). All transesophageal views are best oriented in accordance with the established recommendations of the American Society of Echocardiography tomographic display of ultrasound images.[26]

Clinical applications of TEE

TEE has made an increasing impact in clinical cardiology and now should be considered a logical extension of the transthoracic surface echocardiographic examination. Most laboratories report that approximately 7% to 10% of

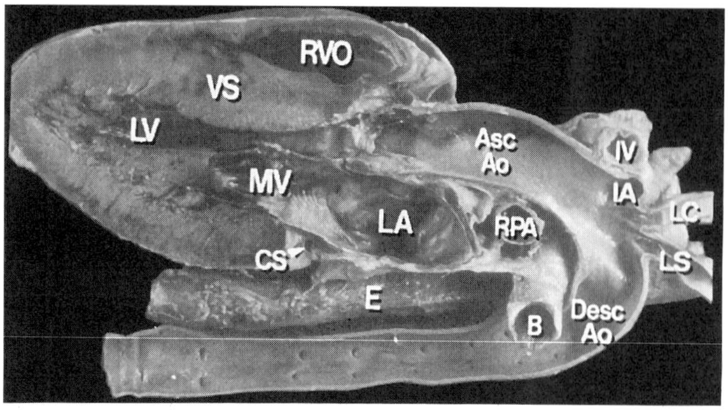

Fig 5D-5 Thoracic aorta. The entire thoracic aorta has been cut in a tomographic manner. The relationship of the esophagus *(E)* and aorta is appreciated. (The esophagus is anterior to the aorta in the low thorax, medial in the middle thorax, and posterior in the upper thorax). The aorta at the level of the right pulmonary artery *(RPA)* is consistently visualized from a high esophageal transducer position. Thus, potentially only a very small segment of the upper ascending aortic or proximal aortic arch may be obscured by the air-filled bronchial tree. *AscAo,* ascending aorta; *B,* left bronchus; *CS,* coronary sinus; *DescAo,* descending aorta; *IA,* innominate artery; *IV,* innominate vein; *LA,* left atrium; *LC,* left common carotid artery; *LS,* left subclavian artery; *LV,* left ventricle; *MV,* mitral valve; *RVO,* right ventricular outflow; *VS,* ventricular septum. (From Seward JB: Transesophageal echocardiographic anatomy. In *Transesophageal Echocardiography.* Edited by WK Freeman, JB Seward, BK Khandheria, et al. Boston, Little, Brown and Company, 1994, pp 55-128. By permission, Mayo Foundation.)

all transthoracic studies also have a transesophageal examination. Although the clinical indications for TEE are still expanding and evolving, there now are well-accepted indications for both outpatient and operating room examinations.[25]

Outpatient TEE

MITRAL VALVE AND PROSTHESIS. The transesophageal approach allows an unimpeded view of the left atrium. When it is combined with color-flow imaging, further semiquantitation of the degree of mitral regurgitation is obtainable.[27,28] The underlying pathologic condition causing the mitral regurgitation, such as ruptured chordae, mitral valve prolapse, rheumatic mitral valve disease, papillary muscle rupture, or leaflet tears, can also be assessed.[29] Because of the high echo reflectance of prostheses, precordial echocardiography has been inadequate in evaluating a patient with a suspected dysfunctional mitral prosthesis.[30] Although mitral valve stenosis is best diagnosed by precordial continuous-wave Doppler echocardiography, the severity of prosthetic mitral valve regurgitation has been difficult to diagnose and predict. By imaging the heart posteriorly, TEE best visualizes the left atrium without interference and the posterior surface of the prosthetic valve. Transesophageal two-dimensional echocardiography and color-flow imaging provide superior assessment of prosthetic and periprosthetic mitral regurgitation.[31-33]

AORTA AND AORTIC DISEASE. The entire thoracic aorta is adjacent to the esophagus, and high-resolution images of this structure can be predictably obtained. Aortic dissection appears as an intimal flap in the thoracic aorta. Color-flow imaging helps in determining the point of entry and differentiating the true lumen from the false lumen. In a multicenter study, TEE was more sensitive (99% compared with 88%) and more specific (98% compared with 94%) in the diagnosis of aortic dissection than conventional aortography.[34,35] Biplane and multiplane TEE have increased the sensitivity and specificity of this cost-effective bedside examination.

INFECTIVE ENDOCARDITIS.[36-38] High-resolution TEE images can detect vegetations not seen by transthoracic echocardiography. One study showed that TEE had a 90% detection rate, compared with a 58% detection rate by transthoracic echocardiography. The procedure is especially of value in patients with small vegetations, in patients who have poor-quality images by the transthoracic approach, and in patients with prosthetic valves. TEE is also useful in detecting complications of infective endocarditis, such as abscess formation, fistula formation, and valve dehiscence.

SOURCE OF SYSTEMIC EMBOLISM.[39-42] Visualization of the left atrium allows detection of left atrial thrombi and tumors (Fig 5D-6) not routinely seen by transthoracic echocardiography.[43,44] This is especially true in the area of the left atrial appendage, which can be predictably imaged by TEE. Other abnormalities, such as small vegetations, tumors, and right-to-left shunts, can be detected by TEE. With the high-resolution transducers, "swirling" blood is seen in the left atrium (i.e., spontaneous echo contrast). This has been shown to be associated with low-output states and an increased risk of systemic embolic events.[41]

LEFT ATRIUM. Atrial septal defects of all types are better assessed with TEE.[25,45] Other atrial abnormalities, such as tumors (e.g., myxoma),[44] cor triatriatum,[46] and vegetations or thrombi on indwelling catheters, can be diagnosed by this approach.

OTHER. TEE provides high-resolution images in nearly all patients. It obtains information about cardiac structures in patients in whom the transthoracic examination is suboptimal. This is especially relevant in the critical care unit, where the transthoracic approach is frequently inadequate.[47] The cause of hemodynamic deterioration can be safely determined by the transesophageal approach in the critically ill patient. Pathophysiologic processes that can be elucidated include hypovolemia, severe left ventricular dysfunction, mechanical complications of myocardial infarction,[47,48] and acute valvular regurgitation. TEE can be safely used in the critical care setting, even in patients who are on mechanical ventilation.

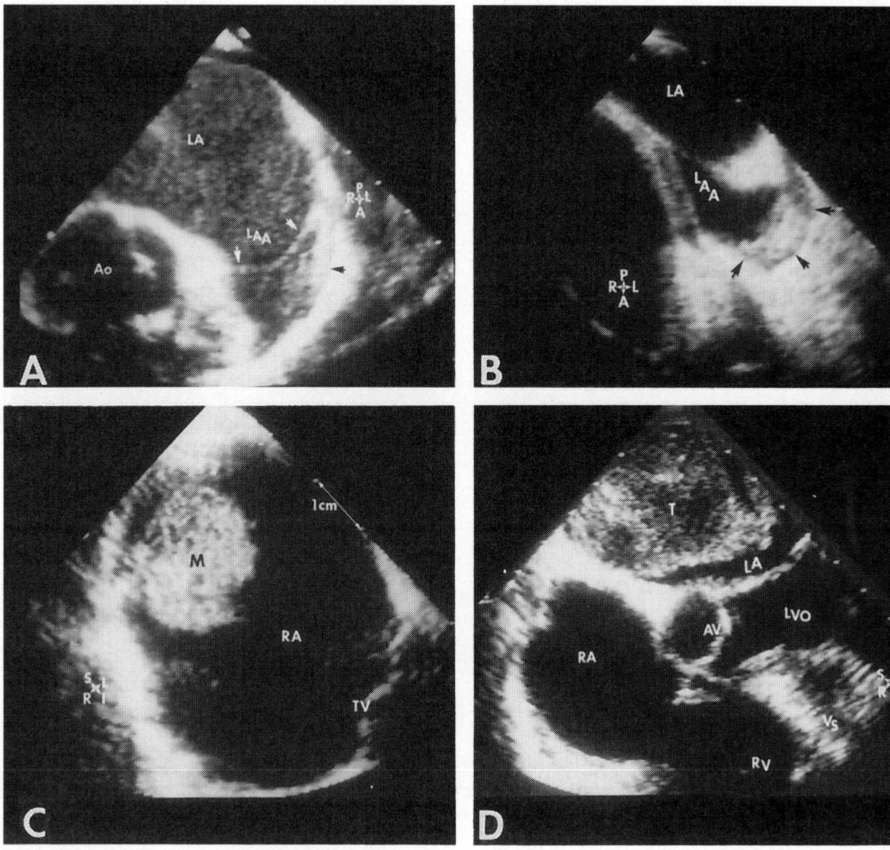

Fig 5D-6 Examples of the clinical utility of transesophageal echocardiography in patients with cardiac masses. **A,** magnified view of the left atrium *(LA)* in a patient with severe mitral valve dysfunction. Spontaneous contrast effect (i.e., visualization of blood without contrast medium) seen throughout the left atrium is indicative of low flow. In the left atrial appendage *(LAA),* the blood is particularly stagnant *(arrows)* and appears as slow-moving currents. This phenomenon has a high association with embolic embolism. **B,** low output state and thrombus *(arrows)* in the left atrial appendage. Thrombus in the left atrial appendage is rarely diagnosed by precordial echocardiography. **C,** multiple recurrent atrial myxoma. On precordial echocardiography, there was a suggestion of a small ovoid mass on the free wall of the right atrium. Transesophageal echocardiography was performed to better elucidate the possible mass. A distinct pedunculated tumor *(M)* (myxoma), 2.5 by 2.0 cm, was visualized on the free wall of the right atrium *(RA).* **D,** metastatic melanoma in a patient with breathlessness. On precordial echocardiography, there was a slight suggestion of a filling defect in the left atrium. On transesophageal echocardiography, a large tumor *(T)* nearly filled the left atrium and was observed to be emanating from the right upper pulmonary vein. This picture was compatible with metastatic melanoma to the heart. *Ao,* aortic root; *AV,* aortic valve; *LVO,* left ventricular outflow; *RV,* right ventricle; *TV,* tricuspid valve; *VS,* ventricular septum. Directional axis: *A,* anterior; *I,* inferior; *L,* left; *P,* posterior; *R,* right; *S,* superior. (**B** and **C** from Seward JB: Cardiac tumors and thrombus: transesophageal echocardiographic experience. In *Transesophageal Echocardiography: a New Window to the Heart,* Edited by R Erbel, BK Khandheria, R Brennecke, et al. Berlin, Springer-Verlag Berlin Heidelberg, 1989, pp 120-128. By permission.)

Intraoperative TEE. Today intraoperative TEE is most frequently used for mitral valve repair for significant mitral valve regurgitation. TEE provides excellent assessment of the adequacy of the mitral valve repair before the patient leaves the operating room.[49,50] Intraoperative TEE has also been shown to be useful in assessing the results of other cardiac procedures, such as myectomy for hypertrophic cardiomyopathy,[51] repair of intracardiac shunts,[52] and diagnosis of intracardiac masses.[25,44]

TEE has also been used during both cardiac and noncardiac surgery to evaluate the function of the left ventricle.[53-57] A transgastric short-axis approach allows continuous imaging of the left ventricle at its midcavitary level throughout the operative procedure. Relative changes in left ventricular volume and contractility can be assessed. Demonstration of new regional wall motion abnormalities has been found to be an early and sensitive indicator of cardiac ischemia. Wall motion changes occur before the onset of electrocardiographic changes or pulmonary capillary wedge changes and may aid in alerting the anesthesiologist and surgeon to myocardial ischemia, which may be correctable.

TEE has also been used by neurosurgical anesthesiologists to detect air embolism.[58-60] In upright neurosurgical procedures, air embolus frequently occurs from decompression of the cervical veins during the operation. Occasionally, the air embolism shunts right to left through a patent foramen ovale, and this movement can cause a devastating neurologic outcome. TEE is the only available means to detect both the entry of air embolus into the right side of the heart and passage of the air embolus from the right-sided chambers into the left-sided chambers.[58-60] During orthopedic surgery, fat embolism may occur, producing severe hemodynamic deterioration. It is thought that TEE can aid in detecting the occurrence of this event.[61]

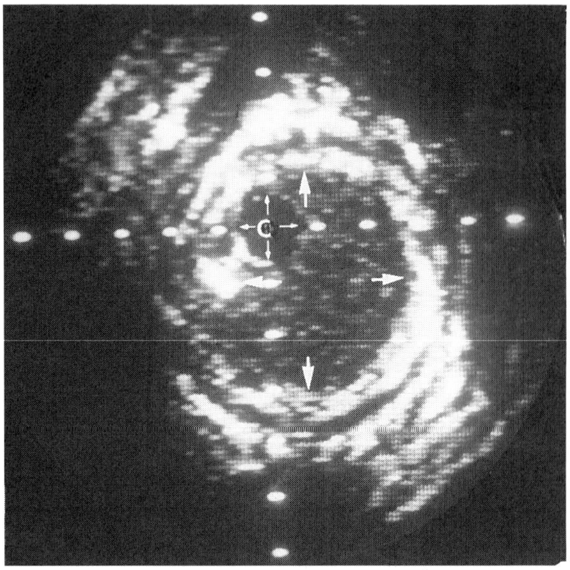

Fig 5D-7 Intravascular echocardiography: A 2.5-mm catheter *(C)* with a 20-MHz transducer at its tip permits imaging of the vessel lumen and wall *(arrows).* Vascular dimension and pathophysiology can be elucidated by this ultrasound innovation. (Courtesy of Rick A. Nishimura, M.D.)

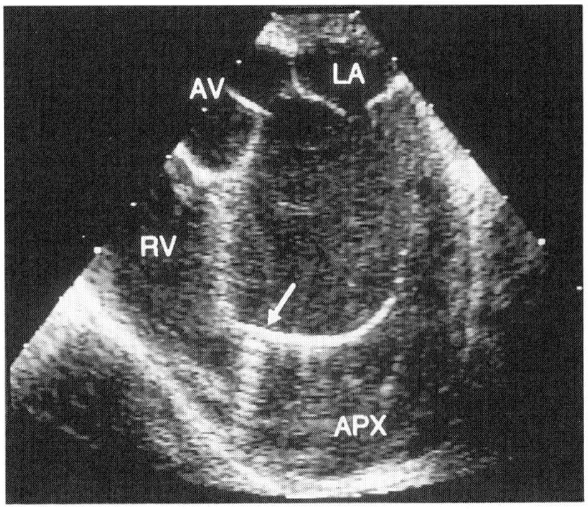

Fig 5D-8 Intracardiac echocardiographic monitoring of an experimental left ventricular ablation *(arrow)* procedure. An intracardiac ultrasound imaging catheter is placed in the right atrium. A resultant frontal image of the heart displays the aortic valve *(AV),* left atrium *(LA),* left ventricular apex *(APX),* and a portion of the right ventricle *(RV).* An ablation catheter, introduced across the aortic valve, is moved under ultrasound guidance in such a way that the tip of the catheter lies at the apical ventricular septum. Exact placement of the ablation catheter is possible by this invasive use of echocardiography.

OTHER INVASIVE ECHOCARDIOGRAPHIC APPLICATIONS

Intravascular imaging (see chapter 27B)

Transducer-tipped catheters have been investigated ever since the M-mode era. More recently, miniaturization of two-dimensional transducer catheters has generated enthusiasm for imaging from within a blood vessel.[12,62] A rotating 360° scanning intravascular transducer can be used to characterize luminal dimensions and vessel wall characteristics (Fig 5D-7). Intracoronary scanning appears promising as a means of characterizing luminal disease, such as plaque morphology, and the pathophysiology of interventional therapeutics, such as balloon angioplasty. A Doppler transducer mounted on a guide wire also appears to be a useful device for the assessment of coronary flow and velocity.[63]

Intracardiac echocardiography

With the emergence of transesophageal and intravascular echocardiography, a third application of echocardiography will surely develop in the near future. Transducer-tipped catheters that have the capability of imaging beyond the vessel wall show great clinical promise. Blood vessels are a unique ultrasonic conduit to many areas within the body. For the cardiologist, transvascular echocardiography (imaging the heart or contiguous structures from blood vessels)[22] and intracardiac echocardiography (imaging the heart from within the cardiac chambers)[21] are natural extensions of evolving technology (Fig 5D-8). Because blood is echogenic and a potential conduit, such imaging applications appear most promising. The invasive investigation of intracardiac pathophysiology, such as valvular disease or myocardial disease, may be better elucidated with high-frequency, high-resolution transducer-tipped catheters.

COMMENT

The advent of the unique ultrasound imaging transducers has greatly enhanced the capability of the cardiologist to investigate innovative applications of cardiovascular imaging. With these new ultrasound devices, the heart and related anatomy can be imaged with predictable clarity. Transesophageal, intravascular, transvascular, and intracardiac echocardiography all hold tremendous potential. The horizons of diagnostic ultrasonography continue to expand, and the modality shows great promise not only for noninvasive but also for invasive imaging.

REFERENCES

1. Seward JB: Cardiovascular ultrasound imaging and hemodynamic laboratory (echocardiography). *Curr Opin Cardiol* 3:912-921, 1988
2. Seward JB, Tajik AJ, Spangler JG, et al: Echocardiographic contrast studies: initial experience. *Mayo Clin Proc* 50:163-192, 1975
3. Vandenberg BF: Myocardial perfusion and contrast echocardiography: review and new perspectives. *Echocardiography* 8:65-75, 1991
4. Quiñones MA, Cheirif J: New perspectives for perfusion imaging in echocardiography. *Circulation* 83 Suppl 3:104-110, 1991
5. Callahan JA, Seward JB, Nishimura RA, et al: Two-dimensional echocardiographically guided pericardiocentesis: experience in 117 consecutive patients. *Am J Cardiol* 55:476-479, 1985
6. Ryan T, Vasey CG, Presti CF, et al: Exercise echocardiography: detection of coronary artery disease in patients with normal left ventricular wall motion at rest. *J Am Coll Cardiol* 11:993-999, 1988
7. Bach DS, Armstrong WF: Dobutamine stress echocardiography. *Am J Cardiol* 69:90H-96H, 1992
8. Seward JB, Khandheria BK, Oh JK, et al: Transesophageal echocardiography: technique, anatomic correlations, implementation, and clinical applications. *Mayo Clin Proc* 63:649-680, 1988
9. Seward JB, Khandheria BK, Freeman WK, et al: Multiplane transesophageal echocardiography: image orientation, examination technique, anatomic correlations, and clinical applications. *Mayo Clin Proc* 68:523-551, 1993
10. Seward JB, Khandheria BK, Edwards WD, et al: Biplanar transesophageal echocardiography: anatomic correlations, image orientation, and clinical applications. *Mayo Clin Proc* 65:1193-1213, 1990
11. Jacobs NM, Grant EG, Schellinger D, et al: The role of duplex carotid sonography, digital subtraction angiography, and arteriography in the evaluation of transient ischemic attack and the asymptomatic carotid bruit. *Med Clin North Am* 68:1423-1450, November 1984
12. Pandian NG, Kreis A, Brockway B, et al: Ultrasound angioscopy: real-time, two-dimensional, intraluminal ultrasound imaging of blood vessels. *Am J Cardiol* 62:493-494, 1988
13. Matre K, Segadal L, Engedal H: Continuous measurement of aortic blood velocity, after cardiac surgery, by means of an extractable Doppler ultrasound probe. *J Biomed Eng* 7:84-88, 1985
14. Sibley DH, Millar HD, Hartley CJ, et al: Subselective measurement of coronary blood flow velocity using a steerable Doppler catheter. *J Am Coll Cardiol* 8:1332-1340, 1986
15. Copel JA, Pilu G, Green J, et al: Fetal echocardiographic screening for congenital heart disease: the importance of the four-chamber view. *Am J Obstet Gynecol* 157:648-655, 1987
16. Seward JB, Tajik AJ, Edwards WD, et al (eds): *Two-Dimensional Echocardiographic Atlas. Vol 1. Congenital Heart Disease.* New York, Springer-Verlag, 1987
17. Drexler M, Erbel R, Dahm M, et al: Assessment of successful valve reconstruction by intraoperative transesophageal echocardiography (TEE). *Int J Card Imaging* 2:21-30, 1986
18. Belohlavek M, Foley DA, Gerber TC, et al: Three- and four-dimensional cardiovascular ultrasound imaging: a new era for echocardiography. *Mayo Clin Proc* 68:221-240, 1993
19. Vered Z, Barzilai B, Mohr GA, et al: Quantitative ultrasonic tissue characterization with real-time integrated backscatter imaging in normal human subjects and in patients with dilated cardiomyopathy. *Circulation* 76:1067-1073, 1987
20. Seward JB, Khandheria BK, Tajik AJ: Wide-field transesophageal echocardiographic tomography: feasibility study. *Mayo Clin Proc* 65:31-37, 1990
21. Pandian NG, Kumar R, Katz SE, et al: Real-time, intracardiac, two-dimensional echocardiography. *Echocardiography* 8:407-422, 1991
22. Seward JB, Khandheria BK, McGregor CGA, et al: Transvascular and intracardiac two-dimensional echocardiography. *Echocardiography* 7:457-464, 1990
23. Seward JB, Khandheria BK, Oh JK, et al: Critical appraisal of transesophageal echocardiography: limitations, pitfalls, and complications. *J Am Soc Echocardiogr* 5:288-305, 1992
24. Steckelberg JM, Khandheria BK, Anhalt JP, et al: Prospective evaluation of the risk of bacteremia associated with transesophageal echocardiography. *Circulation* 84:177-180, 1991
25. Freeman WK, Seward JB, Khandheria BK, et al (eds): *Transesophageal Echocardiography*. Boston, Little, Brown and Company, 1994
26. Henry WL, DeMaria A, Gramiak R, et al: Report of the American Society of Echocardiography Committee on Nomenclature and Standards in Two-dimensional Echocardiography. *Circulation* 62:212-217, 1980
27. Castello R, Fagan L Jr, Lenzen P, et al: Comparison of transthoracic and transesophageal echocardiography for assessment of left-sided valvular regurgitation. *Am J Cardiol* 68:1677-1680, 1991
28. Kamp O, Dijkstra J-W, Huitink H, et al: Transesophageal color flow Doppler mapping in the assessment of native mitral valvular regurgitation: comparison with left ventricular angiography. *J Am Soc Echocardiogr* 4:598-606, 1991
29. Sochowski RA, Chan K-L, Ascah KJ, et al: Comparison of accuracy of transesophageal versus transthoracic echocardiography for the detection of mitral valve prolapse with ruptured chordae tendineae (flail mitral leaflet). *Am J Cardiol* 67:1251-1255, 1991
30. Daniel WG, Mügge A, Grote J, et al: Comparison of transthoracic and transesophageal echocardiography for detection of abnormalities of prosthetic and bioprosthetic valves in the mitral and aortic positions. *Am J Cardiol* 71:210-215, 1993
31. Khandheria BK, Seward JB, Oh JK, et al: Value and limitations of transesophageal echocardiography in assessment of mitral valve prostheses. *Circulation* 83:1956-1968, 1991
32. Nellessen U, Schnittger I, Appleton CP, et al: Transesophageal two-dimensional echocardiography and color Doppler flow velocity mapping in the evaluation of cardiac valve prostheses. *Circulation* 78:848-855, 1988
33. Mohr-Kahaly S, Kupferwasser I, Erbel R, et al: Value and limitations of transesophageal echocardiography in the evaluation of aortic prostheses. *J Am Soc Echocardiogr* 6:12-20, 1993
34. Mohr-Kahaly S, Erbel R, Rennollet H, et al: Ambulatory follow-up of aortic dissection by transesophageal two-dimensional and color-coded Doppler echocardiography. *Circulation* 80:24-33, 1989
35. Erbel R, Engberding R, Daniel W, et al: Echocardiography in diagnosis of aortic dissection. *Lancet* 1:457-461, 1989
36. Daniel WG, Schröder E, Mügge A, et al: Transesophageal echocardiography in infective endocarditis. *Am J Card Imaging* 2:78-85, 1988
37. Erbel R, Rohmann S, Drexler M, et al: Improved diagnostic value of echocardiography in patients with infective endocarditis by transesophageal approach. A prospective study. *Eur Heart J* 9:43-53, 1988
38. Mügge A, Daniel WG, Frank G, et al: Echocardiography in infective endocarditis: reassessment of prognostic implications of vegetation size determined by the transthoracic and the transesophageal approach. *J Am Coll Cardiol* 14:631-638, 1989
39. Daniel WG, Schröder E, Nellessen U, et al: Diagnosis of intra- and extracardiac masses by echocardiography: comparison between the transthoracic and transesophageal approach (abstract). *Circulation* 76 Suppl 4:38, 1987
40. Aschenberg W, Schlüter M, Kremer P, et al: Transesophageal

two-dimensional echocardiography for the detection of left atrial appendage thrombus. *J Am Coll Cardiol* 7:163-166, 1986

41. Daniel WG, Nellessen U, Schröder E, et al: Left atrial spontaneous echo contrast in mitral valve disease: an indicator for an increased thromboembolic risk. *J Am Coll Cardiol* 11:1204-1211, 1988

42. Nellessen U, Daniel WG, Matheis G, et al: Impending paradoxical embolism from atrial thrombus: correct diagnosis by transesophageal echocardiography and prevention by surgery. *J Am Coll Cardiol* 5:1002-1004, 1985

43. Seward JB: Cardiac tumors and thrombus: transesophageal echocardiographic experience. In *Transesophageal Echocardiography: a New Window to the Heart*. Edited by R Erbel, BK Khandheria, R Brennecke, et al. Berlin, Springer-Verlag Berlin Heidelberg, 1989, pp 120-128

44. Reeder GS, Khandheria BK, Seward JB, et al: Transesophageal echocardiography and cardiac masses. *Mayo Clin Proc* 66:1101-1109, 1991

45. Hanrath P, Schlüter M, Langenstein BA, et al: Detection of ostium secundum atrial septal defects by transoesophageal cross-sectional echocardiography. *Br Heart J* 49:350-358, 1983

46. Schlüter M, Langenstein BA, Thier W, et al: Transesophageal two-dimensional echocardiography in the diagnosis of cor triatriatum in the adult. *J Am Coll Cardiol* 2:1011-1015, 1983

47. Oh JK, Seward JB, Khandheria BK, et al: Transesophageal echocardiography in critically ill patients. *Am J Cardiol* 66:1492-1495, 1990

48. Koenig K, Kasper W, Hofmann T, et al: Transesophageal echocardiography for diagnosis of rupture of the ventricular septum or left ventricular papillary muscle during acute myocardial infarction. *Am J Cardiol* 59:362, 1987

49. Sheikh KH, de Bruijn NP, Rankin JS, et al: The utility of transesophageal echocardiography and Doppler color flow imaging in patients undergoing cardiac valve surgery. *J Am Coll Cardiol* 15:363-372, 1990

50. Reichert SLA, Visser CA, Moulijn AC, et al: Intraoperative transesophageal color-coded Doppler echocardiography for evaluation of residual regurgitation after mitral valve repair. *J Thorac Cardiovasc Surg* 100:756-761, 1990

51. Stanley TE III, Rankin JS: Idiopathic hypertrophic subaortic stenosis and ischemic mitral regurgitation: the value of intraoperative transesophageal echocardiography and Doppler color flow imaging in guiding operative therapy. *Anesthesiology* 72:1083-1085, 1990

52. Stümper O, Kaulitz R, Sreeram N, et al: Intraoperative transesophageal versus epicardial ultrasound in surgery for congenital heart disease. *J Am Soc Echocardiogr* 3:392-401, 1990

53. Smith JS, Cahalan MK, Benefiel DJ, et al: Intraoperative detection of myocardial ischemia in high-risk patients: electrocardiography versus two-dimensional transesophageal echocardiography. *Circulation* 72:1015-1021, 1985

54. Abel MD, Nishimura RA, Callahan MJ, et al: Evaluation of intraoperative transesophageal two-dimensional echocardiography. *Anesthesiology* 66:64-68, 1987

55. Gewertz BL, Kremser PC, Zarins CK, et al: Transesophageal echocardiographic monitoring of myocardial ischemia during vascular surgery. *J Vasc Surg* 5:607-613, 1987

56. Clements FM, de Bruijn NP: Perioperative evaluation of regional wall motion by transesophageal two-dimensional echocardiography. *Anesth Analg* 66:249-261, 1987

57. Beaupre PN, Kremer PF, Cahalan MK, et al: Intraoperative detection of changes in left ventricular segmental wall motion by transesophageal two-dimensional echocardiography. *Am Heart J* 107: 1021-1023, 1984

58. Cucchiara RF, Nugent M, Seward JB, et al: Air embolism in upright neurosurgical patients: detection and localization by two-dimensional transesophageal echocardiography. *Anesthesiology* 60:353-355, 1984

59. Cucchiara RF, Seward JB, Nishimura RA, et al: Identification of patent foramen ovale during sitting position craniotomy by transesophageal echocardiography with positive airway pressure. *Anesthesiology* 63:107-109, 1985

60. Glenski JA, Cucchiara RF, Michenfelder JD: Transesophageal echocardiography and transcutaneous O_2 and CO_2 monitoring for detection of venous air embolism. *Anesthesiology* 64:541-545, 1986

61. Ereth MH, Weber JG, Abel MD, et al: Cemented versus noncemented total hip arthroplasty—embolism, hemodynamics, and intrapulmonary shunting. *Mayo Clin Proc* 67:1066-1074, 1992

62. Liebson PR, Klein LW: Intravascular ultrasound in coronary atherosclerosis: a new approach to clinical assessment. *Am Heart J* 123:1643-1660, 1992

63. Doucette JW, Corl D, Payne HM, et al: Validation of a Doppler guide wire for intravascular measurement of coronary artery flow velocity. *Circulation* 85:1899-1911, 1992

CHAPTER

6

Nuclear cardiology

Raymond J. Gibbons, M.D.

PRINCIPLES OF NUCLEAR CARDIOLOGY

Photons and gamma rays

A complete understanding of the entire course of events between the injection of an isotope, or radionuclide, into a patient and the display of a nuclear cardiology study for interpretation involves a considerable knowledge of nuclear physics, radiation principles, and instrumentation. Although a complete description is beyond the scope of this chapter, some appreciation of the principles of physics and instrumentation involved in this complex series of events is vital for a proper understanding of the potential and limitations of the use of radionuclides in cardiology and will be offered here. More detailed reviews of this subject are available for the interested reader.[1-3]

All nuclear cardiology studies depend on the injection into the patient of an isotope that will emit photons that can be detected outside the patient. Photons can best be described as "units" or "packets" of energy in the form of electromagnetic radiation. Photons come in many forms, including visible light, x-rays, and gamma rays. Gamma rays are the particular photons that are most often employed in nuclear cardiology studies. Gamma rays originate during radioactive decay when the nucleus of an isotope changes from one energy level to a lower one. Different gamma rays are generally distinguished from one another by their particular energy content. The energy content of gamma rays and other photons is generally described in units of electron volts. An electron volt is equivalent to the amount of energy acquired by an electron when it is acted on by an electric field with a potential difference of 1 V. It is a tiny quantity of energy; an ordinary 60-W light bulb consumes 3.8×10^{20} electron volts of energy in 1 second. The gamma rays emitted by the commonly used radionuclides have energies of between 50,000 and 200,000 electron volts—usually abbreviated as 50 keV and 200 keV.

Fate of the photon

All nuclear medicine procedures must deal with an important basic limitation: namely, not all photons emitted by an injected radionuclide are detected outside the patient. This is true because a substantial portion of the photons emitted by the radionuclide do not leave the patient's body. In addition, a portion of the photons that do leave the patient's body are not detected by the imaging device. Photons emitted by an injected radiopharmaceutical have three different fates in passing through the patient's chest wall: (1) they may pass through uneventfully to the outside of the patient's body; (2) they may be absorbed by the soft tissue or bone of the chest wall; and (3) they may be scattered by the same soft tissue or bone of the chest wall.

The energy levels of the photons emitted by thallium-201 (^{201}Tl) and technetium-99m (^{99m}Tc), the two isotopes commonly used in nuclear cardiology, are such that scattering is considerably more important than absorption. Scattering, more properly known as "Compton scattering," involves the deflection of a photon from its original path by an electron of an atom within the patient. The angle of deflection is related to the wavelength, or energy, of the original photon and the wavelength, or energy, of the photon after it undergoes interaction with the electron of the atom. The angle of deflection, θ, can be determined from the formula

$$\text{cosine } \theta = (1 - \lambda' + \lambda)$$

in which λ' is the wavelength of the photon after interaction and λ is the wavelength of the photon before interaction (Fig 6-1). A fairly small change in energy involves a rather large angle of deflection. For example, a 10% loss of energy from the 140-keV photon of ^{99m}Tc involves a 54° scattering angle.

A large proportion of the photons emitted from ^{201}Tl or ^{99m}Tc undergo Compton scattering before they leave the patient. A relatively small number of the original photons leave the patient in a straight line. It is therefore vitally important that the detection system have some means of distinguishing photons that have been scattered from those that have traveled through the patient in a straight line. As we shall see below in the discussion of detecting systems, the various angles at which scattered photons travel and the various energies that they have are both used to help distinguish unscattered (and therefore "good") photons from those that have been scattered (and are therefore "bad").

A certain proportion of photons emitted from the radionuclide undergo a different process, known as "photoelectric absorption." This absorption involves the

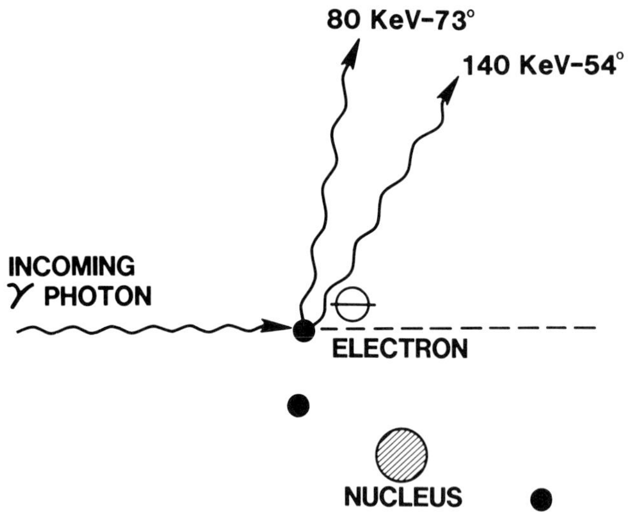

Fig 6-1 Compton scattering deflects a photon by an angle, theta (θ), that depends on the energy of the incoming photon and the energy of the outgoing photon. The outgoing photons shown have undergone a 10% energy loss.

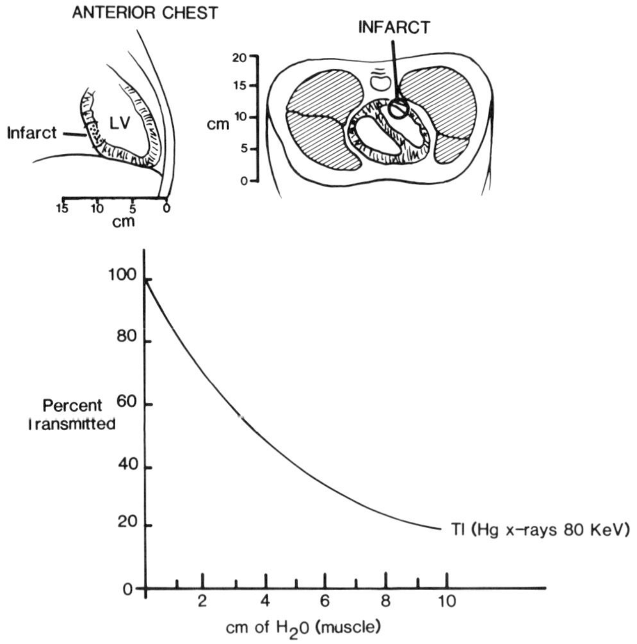

Fig 6-2 Attenuation of photons depends on the thickness of tissue between the source of the photons and the body surface. It obeys the equation $N(x) = N_o e^{-\mu x}$, in which x is tissue thickness. See text also. *LV,* left ventricle.

total annihilation of the photon, with a transfer of its energy to an atom within the patient. This transfer of energy leads to the release of an electron from the atom. Whether a photon will undergo photoelectric absorption depends on both its energy and the atomic number of the material through which it is passing. Higher-energy photons are less likely to undergo photoelectric absorption. Materials with higher atomic numbers, such as calcium in bone, completely absorb more photons than materials with lower atomic numbers, such as water and soft tissue. The photons of ^{201}Tl and ^{99m}Tc have sufficient energy and, in general, body tissues have sufficiently low atomic numbers that the photoelectric interaction is relatively unimportant for the photons used in nuclear cardiology.

The overall effect of both Compton scattering and the photoelectric interaction is that only a fraction of the photons emitted from a radionuclide ever leave the body. The amount of absorption of these photons within the body is dependent upon the photon energy. The number of photons leaving any material of thickness *x* is dependent upon the number of photons entering that material *(N_o)* in an exponential fashion:

$$N(x) = N_o e^{-\mu x}$$

in which μ is a property of the material called the "attenuation coefficient." The magnitude of the attenuation coefficient decreases with increasing energy of the photons. For example, the attenuation coefficient of tissue for the 80-keV photons emitted by ^{201}Tl is 0.18 cm^{-1}, so that after 5.6 cm the number of photons is reduced to 1/e, or approximately 37%, of the original number of photons. Thus, photons that have their origin closer to the detector—for example, the anterior surface of the heart—will be quantitatively considerably more important than photons that have their origin farther away from the detector—for example, the posterior surface of the heart (Fig 6-2).

Detection of photons

Nuclear cardiology procedures generally employ one of two commonly available devices to detect photons that are emitted from radionuclides and eventually leave the patient. These two devices are the conventional gamma camera and the so-called multicrystal camera. The gamma camera consists of a series of components that convert the energy present in the incoming photon into an electrical current. A complete description of the process by which this occurs is beyond the scope of this text, but some understanding of the process is important. The incoming photon strikes a sodium iodide crystal, where it undergoes a photoelectric interaction that gives off visible light energy (Fig 6-3). These visible light photons then strike the photocathode of a photomultiplier tube. The photocathode consists of a phosphor that releases an electron when it is struck by the incoming photon. This electron is then accelerated by a series of dynodes to a measurable electrical pulse.

A gamma camera consists of a single large sodium iodide crystal with a sizable number of connected photomultiplier tubes (usually 37). The sodium iodide crystal is covered by a lead shield known as a collimator. This shield is used basically to prevent photons from outside the organ of interest from reaching the crystal of the camera (Fig 6-4). The collimator consists of a solid piece of lead with a series of holes through it to permit photons that

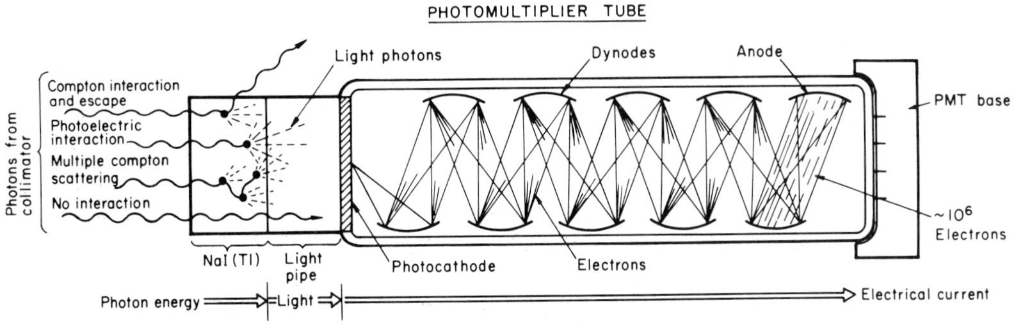

Fig 6-3 Basic system for detecting a photon. A sodium iodide crystal is coupled to a photomultiplier tube *(PMT).* (From Budinger TF, Rollo FD: Physics and instrumentation. *Prog Cardiovasc Dis* 20:19-53, 1977. By permission of WB Saunders Company.)

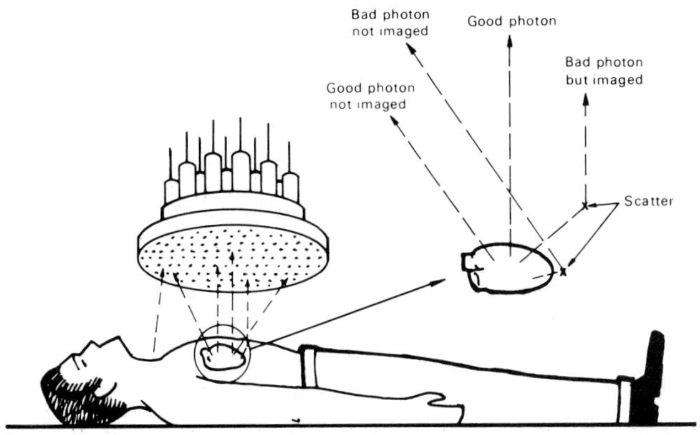

Fig 6-4 A collimator is a lead shield that prevents photons from outside the organ of interest from reaching the crystal of the camera. (From Budinger TF, Rollo FD: Physics and instrumentation. *Prog Cardiovasc Dis* 20:19-53, 1977. By permission of WB Saunders Company.)

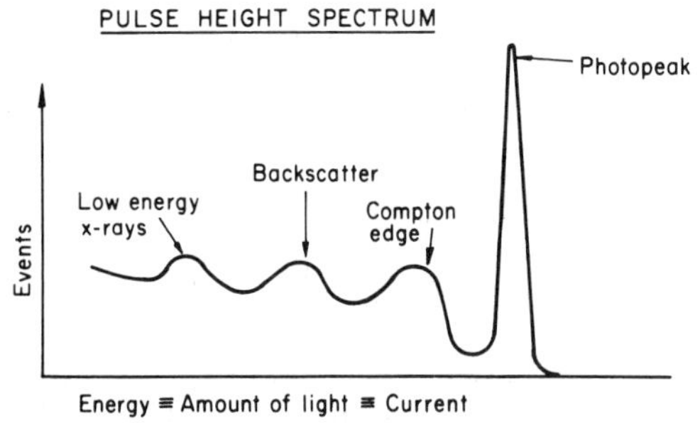

Fig 6-5 Output from the photomultiplier tube is dependent upon the energy of the incoming photon. Photons that are not scattered produce the strongest signals (the photopeak). Weaker signals from scattered photons can be excluded from consideration. (From Budinger TF, Rollo FD: Physics and instrumentation. *Prog Cardiovasc Dis* 20:19-53, 1977. By permission of WB Saunders Company.)

strike the collimator at a 90° angle to pass through but to prevent those that strike the camera at a different angle from reaching the crystal. The thickness of the collimator, the energy of the photons being imaged, and the size of the septa between the collimator holes all influence how well the collimator admits "good" photons and how well it excludes "bad" photons. The generally poor transmission of a lead collimator is one of the major limitations of all nuclear medicine studies. It is not uncommon for only 1 in 1,000 or 1 in 10,000 of the photons emitted by ^{99m}Tc or ^{201}Tl to pass successfully through the collimator. However, collimation is vitally important to obtain reasonable resolution in an image of any organ when a radionuclide is used.

Since some scattered photons may accidentally strike the collimator at the correct angle to pass through to the crystal itself, further efforts must be made to obtain an accurate image. These efforts involve the use of an "energy window." Since the output of the photomultiplier tubes is dependent upon the energy of the incoming photon, and since scattered photons lose a percentage of their original energy, scattered photons will produce generally lower energy pulses from the photomultiplier tube (Fig 6-5). These lower-energy pulses can be excluded from consideration by the use of a device known as a pulse-height analyzer. In practice, this device is set to consider only those electrical impulses from the photomultiplier tube which fall within a set percentage of the pulses expected from a given radionuclide (the "photopeak"). The electrical pulses that are accepted by this pulse-height analyzer can be stored by a computer for further analysis or displayed on either photographic film or a cathode-ray tube.

The overall efficiency of a gamma camera is basically the product of the efficiencies of its various components, including the collimator, the crystal, the photomultiplier tubes, and the electronics. Although a complete discussion of the technical aspects of this process is not possible here, it should be apparent from the above discussion that the overall efficiency of such a system is low.

The other detector system often used in nuclear cardiology studies is the multicrystal camera. Instead of a single large sodium crystal, this camera consists of 200 small sodium iodide crystals, each 1 by 2 cm in area. Each crystal is scored in the middle to essentially create 400 crystals arranged in a square array 20 by 20 cm. In contrast to a conventional gamma camera, which has a single large crystal connected to 30 to 60 photomultiplier tubes, the multicrystal camera has approximately one photomultiplier tube for every four crystals. A decoding scheme using groups of four photomultiplier tubes allows the system to localize a light pulse to a given crystal. Hence, this multicrystal camera has an intrinsic resolution of 1 cm.

The collimators for this camera consist of 1,600 holes, 4 for each crystal. The poor intrinsic resolution and coarse collimation used with this type of gamma camera result in poor overall resolution. However, the electronic arrangement of one photomultiplier tube for every four crystals results in very rapid determination of event location, so that much higher count rates are possible on this camera than with most conventional gamma cameras. The high temporal and poor spatial resolution limit the applications of this type of gamma camera to first-pass techniques outlined below. The modern multicrystal camera is a small mobile unit costing approximately half as much as a conventional gamma camera. Its small size and portability make it ideal for exercise and rest first-pass studies.

Some of the modern single-crystal gamma cameras can perform high-resolution tomographic studies and also perform first-pass studies at count rates approaching those achievable with the multicrystal camera.

Radioisotopes

As mentioned, the two most important radioisotopes in nuclear cardiology currently are ^{99m}Tc and ^{201}Tl.

^{99m}Tc is formed from molybdenum-99 (^{99}Mo). ^{99}Mo can be easily transported because of its relatively long half-life (66 hours), and ^{99}Mo-to-^{99m}Tc generators are commercially available. The generator system basically consists of a column of ^{99}Mo that is adsorbed to aluminum oxide. A sodium chloride solution is passed through the column in order to elute the ^{99m}Tc that is constantly being formed from the ^{99}Mo. The amount of ^{99}Mo contained in the eluate must be carefully controlled. These generators may typically cost several hundred dollars but will produce several curies of ^{99m}Tc, so that the basic cost of a typical 30-mCi dose of ^{99m}Tc is about $5.00. To this cost must be added, of course, the cost of maintaining a qualified radiopharmacy for handling the isotope in the appropriate fashion.

^{99m}Tc is given the designation "m" because it is metastable. (A metastable state is an unstable nuclear state that has a half-life sufficiently long to be observed.) It decays by a change in the energy level of its nucleus to ^{99}Tc with a half-life of 6 hours and releases a 140-keV photon. Its short half-life helps keep the radiation dose to the patient low. Its 140-keV photons are less likely to be absorbed or scattered than are photons of lower energy.

The other isotope commonly used in nuclear cardiology studies is ^{201}Tl. ^{201}Tl is cyclotron-produced and is available from several commercial suppliers in this country. It has a half-life of 73 hours and can thus be transported by air with relatively little decay. A 2-mCi to 4-mCi dose of ^{201}Tl required for a nuclear cardiology study costs approximately $50 to $125. Thus, in contrast to ^{99m}Tc, the cost of the isotope is a major portion of the cost of a ^{201}Tl study.

The decay scheme of ^{201}Tl is relatively complex. Ninety-three percent of the photons emitted are at the range of 69 to 83 keV and for convenience are thought of as 80-keV photons; there are additional 135-keV and 167-keV emissions with lower intensity. The relatively low-energy 80-keV photons emitted by ^{201}Tl are less desirable for imaging than the 140-keV photons of ^{99m}Tc, for they are more subject to scattering and absorption. Because of the long half-life of ^{201}Tl, the total body radiation dose to the patient from 2 mCi of ^{201}Tl approximates that from 30 mCi of ^{99m}Tc.

IMPORTANT TECHNIQUES

Knowledge of the principles of radiation physics and instrumentation outlined in the previous section is necessary for a better understanding of the testing techniques currently utilized in nuclear cardiology. This section describes the techniques most commonly utilized in nuclear cardiology. Each of these techniques is described along with its technical advantages and disadvantages, the important underlying physiologic principles, and the basic data acquired from each. Additional imaging techniques, such as tomographic equilibrium radionuclide angiography, are currently under study but are not yet widely utilized in clinical cardiology practice and therefore are not discussed here.

Equilibrium radionuclide angiography

Equilibrium radionuclide angiography, also known as multiple-gated blood pool imaging, is useful for the noninvasive assessment of ventricular function. It involves the imaging of ^{99m}Tc-labeled albumin or red blood cells, which are uniformly distributed throughout the blood volume. Early studies that made use of this technique generally relied on human serum albumin that was labeled with ^{99m}Tc and was then injected intravenously. More than 95% of the ^{99m}Tc was bound to albumin; it was therefore not filtered by the kidneys and remained in the circulating blood volume. More recently, alternative methods employing ^{99m}Tc-labeled red blood cells have been used because these have been shown to maintain the radionuclide in the blood pool for a longer period.[4] Blood cells may be labeled with ^{99m}Tc by one of three methods – in vitro,[5,6] in vivo,[7,8] or modified in vivo.[9]

The in vitro[5,6] method of labeling requires the withdrawal of a small quantity of blood from the patient. This blood is gently agitated with stannous citrate for 5 minutes. The red blood cells are then centrifuged, mixed with ^{99m}Tc, and incubated for an additional 5 minutes. The red blood cells become labeled with ^{99m}Tc during this time; they are then injected into the patient and allowed to distribute throughout the blood volume. This method is time-consuming and technically demanding. In contrast, the in vivo method is rapid and technically simple. Several milligrams of stannous pyrophosphate is injected intravenously and allowed to circulate for approximately 30 minutes. During this time, the stannous ion binds to red blood cells. The patient then receives an injection of 20 to 30 mCi of [^{99m}Tc]pertechnetate, which labels the red blood cells in the next 5 minutes. A major disadvantage of this method is that a significant portion of the injected radionuclide dose is distributed to the thyroid gland, stomach, and kidneys before binding to the red blood cells. This method has reduced labeling efficiency in some patients, presumably because ^{99m}Tc has not remained within the blood pool long enough to permit satisfactory labeling.

The third method used to label red blood cells is the modified in vivo method first described by Callahan et al.[9] This method combines the speed of the in vivo method with the labeling efficiency of the in vitro method. The initial step is an intravenous injection of stannous pyrophosphate, as in the in vivo method. Approximately 30 minutes later, 30 to 50 mL of the patient's blood is withdrawn through a three-way stopcock into a heparinized syringe. [^{99m}Tc]pertechnetate, which is attached to the other port of the stopcock, is then injected into the syringe containing the patient's blood. After gentle agitation for 5 minutes, the mixture is injected into the patient. Although time-consuming and technically demanding, this method results in uniformly high labeling efficiency and virtually eliminates background activity in the stomach.

Once the red blood cells have been labeled by any of these methods, they have a biologic half-life of approximately 20 hours;[10] the major determinant of blood pool activity is therefore the 6-hour half-life of ^{99m}Tc. Depending on the patient's body habitus, high-quality images are generally feasible for at least 3 to 5 hours.

The basic equipment required to perform an equilibrium radionuclide angiogram includes a standard gamma camera, an electrocardiographic (ECG) monitoring device capable of transmitting a signal triggered by the ECG R wave, and a computer to acquire, organize, analyze, and display the study data. An equilibrium radionuclide angiographic study basically creates an image of the cardiac chambers and great vessels by adding together counts acquired over many cardiac cycles. The R-wave trigger mentioned above performs the vital function of indicating the timing of each cardiac cycle. The computer then divides each cardiac cycle into a designated number of "frames," usually between 16 and 32. Data collected during the same frame of successive cardiac cycles are added together, usually over several hundred cardiac cycles (Fig 6-6). The result is a series of images of the cardiac chambers and great vessels, each taken at a particular point in the cardiac cycle. These images can then be displayed individually or in a motion picture format for analysis and review. Multiple views of the left ventricle, including an anterior, a 45° left anterior oblique, and a steeper left anterior oblique or left lateral view,[11] can be performed at rest and examined for an assessment of wall motion. However, quantitative measurements can be made only on a left anterior oblique view, which avoids overlap of the right and left ventricles.

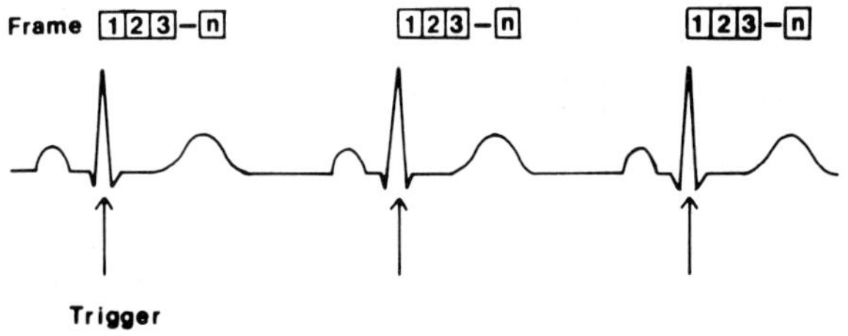

Fig 6-6 Data acquisition is gated to the patient's ECG. Each R-R interval is divided into a designated number of frames. Data collected during the same frame of successive cycles are added together. (From Burow RD, Strauss HW, Singleton R, et al: Analysis of left ventricular function from multiple gated acquisition cardiac blood pool imaging: comparison to contrast angiography. *Circulation* 56:1024-1028, 1977. By permission of American Heart Association.)

Equilibrium radionuclide angiography can also be performed during bicycle ergometer exercise. The subject must be maintained in a reasonably steady state of exercise for approximately 2 minutes to permit acquisition of a satisfactory number of counts for statistical validity. In practice, this generally requires that the patient exercise in 3-minute stages with an acquisition during the last 2 minutes of each stage. As a means of minimizing patient movement during the 2-minute acquisition, supine bicycle exercise has most often been employed. A few institutions have designed exercise systems that restrict patient movement and permit upright exercise testing, and exercise equipment designed for this purpose is now commercially available. Cold pressor testing may be used as an alternative to stress exercise testing, but it is less sensitive.[12]

A single left anterior oblique view is generally obtained with exercise. Visualization of the anterior wall of the left ventricle during exercise will usually require a second acquisition, although the use of a bifocal collimator has been reported.[13] In addition, the relatively long times required for acquisition will sometimes prevent data acquisition at absolutely peak exercise. Premature ventricular contractions and other arrhythmias should ideally be absent for the complete acquisition period to permit the addition of similar cardiac cycles.

Information that may be obtained from equilibrium radionuclide angiography is listed in Table 6-1. One of the first measurements made from these studies was that of left ventricular ejection fraction. This is usually obtained by means of a semiautomated, operator-assisted method that finds the border of the left ventricle throughout the cardiac cycle and computes the left ventricular ejection fraction from the formula

$$(\text{end-diastolic counts} - \text{end-systolic counts}) \div \text{end-diastolic counts}$$

Table 6-1 Information obtained by equilibrium radionuclide angiography

- Left ventricle
  - Ejection fraction
  - Regional wall motion (subjective and quantitative)
  - Volume
  - Diastolic filling
  - Output (cardiac output in the absence of regurgitation)
- Right ventricle
  - Ejection fraction
  - Regional wall motion (subjective)
  - Volume
- Other
  - Regurgitant fraction
  - Pulmonary blood volume changes

Table 6-2 Left ventricular ejection fraction: correlation between contrast ventriculography and equilibrium radionuclide angiography

Investigators	No. of patients	Correlation coefficient
Green et al.[17]	39	0.92
Pfisterer et al.[19]	24	0.92
Folland et al.[16]	30	0.84
Secker-Walker et al.[14]	16	0.87
Burow et al.[15]	17	0.93
Berman et al.[18]	27	0.93
Wackers et al.[20]	26	0.84

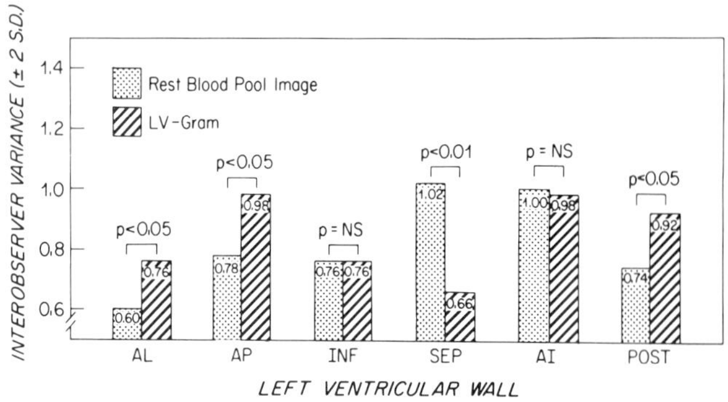

Fig 6-7 Left ventricular regional wall motion was assessed on a five-point scoring system with the use of contrast left ventriculography *(LV-Gram)* and equilibrium radionuclide angiography (Rest Blood Pool Image). The walls are anterolateral *(AL)*, apical *(AP)*, inferior *(INF)*, septal *(SEP)*, apical-inferior *(AI)*, and posterior *(POST)*. The interobserver variance of the two techniques is comparable. *NS* = not significant. (From Okada RD, Kirshenbaum HD, Kushner FG, et al: Observer variance in the qualitative evaluation of left ventricular wall motion and the quantitation of left ventricular ejection fraction using rest and exercise multigated blood pool imaging. *Circulation* 61:128-136, 1980. By permission of American Heart Association.)

Both end-diastolic and end-systolic counts are corrected for background. It should be noted that this calculation does not rely on any assumption concerning the geometry of the left ventricle. Although some investigators have employed a fixed-region-of-interest method, in which the left ventricular border is defined only in the initial frame, the most common technique makes use of a variable region of interest in which the left ventricular borders are defined in each frame through the cardiac cycle. Numerous investigators have found that left ventricular ejection fractions obtained in this fashion correlate well with those obtained with contrast ventriculography over a wide range of left ventricular function[14-20] (Table 6-2) and have an acceptable interobserver variability.[20-23]

Equilibrium radionuclide angiography also yields valuable information concerning regional wall motion. Regional wall motion is usually evaluated visually from a video display of images throughout the cardiac cycle in an endless-loop motion picture format. Multiple views of the ventricle may be examined at rest, but usually only a left anterior oblique view is examined at exercise. The assessment of regional wall motion in this fashion has been shown to correlate quite well with the subjective assessment of regional wall motion by contrast ventriculography.[23,24] The interobserver variance of this method is comparable to that of contrast ventriculography in the assessment of right anterior oblique and left anterior oblique images[23] (Fig 6-7). Assessment at rest of inferior wall motion has been shown to be slightly less reliable by this technique, probably because of right ventricular overlap. The interobserver variance of this method at exercise is somewhat worse than that at rest. In particular, whether there is a change in regional wall motion with exercise is more difficult to judge in the septum than in the lateral wall.

Several different methods have been devised for the quantitation of regional wall motion at rest.[25-27] These methods have divided the left ventricular diastolic frame in the left anterior oblique view into several regions. The change in counts in each region during the cardiac cycle can be used to determine a regional "ejection fraction." These measurements have correlated well with quantitative measurements on contrast ventriculograms. One study has suggested that these methods can be applied to exercise studies as well.[28]

Left ventricular volume can also be assessed by equilibrium radionuclide angiography. The simplest technique is a count-based method with no geometric assumptions.[29,30] The formula employed in this method is shown in Table 6-3. The counts recorded from the ventricular region of interest are corrected for the time of acquisition and the activity of a blood sample of known volume. A regression equation has been developed by comparing the

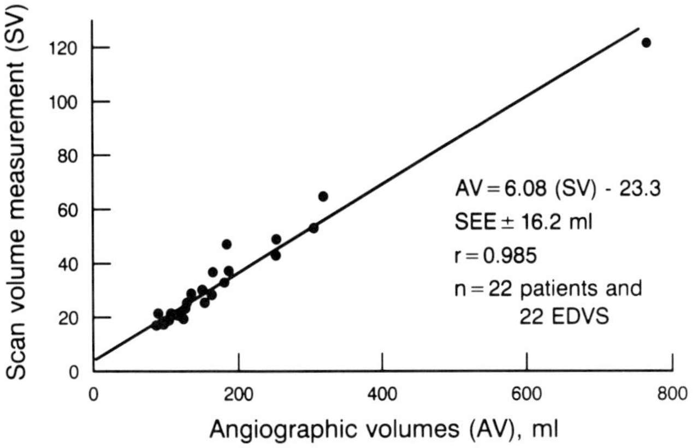

Fig 6-8 Left ventricular end-diastolic volumes *(EDVS)* measured by equilibrium radionuclide angiography *(SV)* and contrast ventriculography *(AV)*. Comparable results were obtained for end-systolic volume. *SEE,* standard error of estimate. (From Dehmer GJ, Lewis SE, Hillis LD, et al: Non-geometric determination of left ventricular volumes from equilibrium blood pool scans. *Am J Cardiol* 45:293-300, 1980. By permission of Cahners Publishing Company, a Division of Reed Publishing USA.)

Table 6-3 Formula for measuring left ventricular volumes by means of equilibrium radionuclide angiography

$$\text{Volume} = k \frac{\text{left ventricular counts}}{\text{number of cycles} \times \frac{\text{time}}{\text{frame}} \times \text{blood activity}}$$

k, regression coefficient relating radionuclide angiographic volume units to contrast ventriculographic volumes

volume "units" determined in this fashion with volumes determined by contrast ventriculography. It is generally advised that each nuclear cardiology facility develop its own regression equation to account for slight differences in equipment and technique. Ventricular volume measurements obtained in this fashion have correlated very well with those obtained from contrast ventriculography. The correlation coefficient reported originally by Dehmer et al.[29] was 0.98, with an average error of the estimate of 16 mL for end-diastolic volume and 15 mL for end-systolic volume (Fig 6-8).

These results have since been duplicated by other investigators.[30] However, since the regression equation developed to relate volumes obtained by this method to volumes obtained by contrast ventriculography attempts to account for chest wall attenuation, and since chest wall attenuation will obviously vary according to body geometry, more substantial errors can be expected from this method in very thin and very obese patients. Alternative methods for measuring volumes have been proposed. The simplest is a count-proportional reference volume method that does not require blood sampling or attenuation correction.[31] Other investigators have developed methods that calculate attenuation in individual patients by measuring the actual distance from the detector to the center of the left ventricle.[32-34] The most careful analysis of the contribution of Compton-scattered photons to volume measurements found that attenuation correction, interpolative background subtraction, and a 50% count threshold region of interest were required for accurate volume determination without correction for Compton scatter.[35] The incremental clinical value of this more tedious approach has not been clearly demonstrated.

Despite the limitations of count-based ventricular volume measurements, they remain very useful for making repeat measurements over time in the same person, because attenuation remains relatively constant in the absence of significant changes in body weight. Changes in resting left ventricular volume over time in the same patient can, therefore, be estimated using this method, as can changes in volume between rest and different levels of exercise.[36-38] However, blood activity will change during exercise if labeling is done by the in vivo method.[39] Although the modified in vivo method has produced contradictory findings,[40,41] blood activity probably increases to a modest degree with this method as well. Multiple blood samples are therefore required for accurate volume determinations during exercise.

Two studies have applied similar techniques to the measurement of right ventricular volume.[42,43] The absence of an accepted ventriculographic "standard" for right ventricular volume has presented an obstacle to the validation of these measurements. However, the right ventricular stroke volume measured by this approach does agree closely with that derived from thermodilution cardiac output measurements.[42]

Other measurements that can be made from equilibrium radionuclide angiography are of interest in specific clinical situations. The severity of mitral or aortic regurgitation can be assessed by the noninvasive determination of a regurgitant fraction. This determination depends on the calculation of the stroke counts from the right ventricle and the left ventricle.[44,45] The ratio of left to right ventricular stroke counts has been shown to be near unity in control patients without evidence of left-sided regurgitation. In patients with mitral or aortic regurgitation (or both), this ratio will exceed unity and may be as high as 5.[44] There is generally good agreement between the stroke count ratio obtained in this fashion and the qualitative angiographic assessment of regurgitation. The regurgitant fraction calculated from this stroke count ratio has been demonstrated to correlate well with the regurgitant fraction obtained from the difference of angiographic and Fick cardiac output determinations.[45]

Right ventricular ejection fraction can also be determined from equilibrium radionuclide angiography by the use of techniques similar to those applied for the left ventricle. The major technical difficulties are related to the determination of the tricuspid and pulmonic valve planes and to the presence of right atrial overlap. Regions of interest can be drawn manually around the right ventricular region of interest in end-systole and end-diastole. The right ventricular ejection fraction determined in this fashion agrees reasonably well with other methods and has acceptable interobserver and intraobserver reproducibility.[46-48] However, a more accurate determination of right ventricular ejection fraction can be obtained by gating the first-pass transit of ^{99m}Tc through the heart.[49] Although such studies can be performed with standard gamma cameras, they require in vivo labeling and significant incremental technologist and camera time. We therefore perform such studies only on selected patients.

Left ventricular output can also be estimated by the use of equilibrium radionuclide angiography. This output is derived from the product of ejection fraction, end-diastolic volume, and heart rate. The first two quantities can be determined from the procedures already outlined. Ventricular outputs determined in this fashion have correlated well ($r = 0.97$) with thermodilution cardiac outputs in patients without aortic or mitral regurgitation.[50,51] On the other hand, left ventricular outputs determined in this fashion in patients with aortic and mitral regurgitation consistently exceed the Fick cardiac output, as expected. These same outputs can be used to calculate a regurgitant fraction, which has been shown to correlate with the severity of regurgitation assessed angiographically.[52]

The measurement of changes in pulmonary blood volume during exercise by means of equilibrium radionuclide angiography has also been described.[53] This measurement has been validated as a noninvasive indicator of the changes that occur in pulmonary capillary wedge pressure with exercise.[54]

Diastolic changes in ventricular volume have also been examined with the use of equilibrium radionuclide angiography.[55-57] The peak rate of diastolic filling and the time at which this occurs have been utilized as indices of diastolic function. The diastolic portion of the radionuclide left ventricular volume curve may be combined with simultaneous intracardiac micromanometer pressure recordings to assess diastolic pressure-volume relationships.[58]

First-pass radionuclide angiography

First-pass radionuclide angiography is an alternative method for the noninvasive assessment of ventricular function. Although this technique yields information that is very similar to that provided by equilibrium radionuclide angiography, there are a number of technical differences between the two techniques.

As implied in its name, first-pass radionuclide angiography involves the recording of the movement of a bolus of radionuclide during its "first pass" through the central circulation. Unlike equilibrium radionuclide angiography, no labeling of red blood cells is required. Almost any radionuclide could therefore be used for imaging purposes, although [^{99m}Tc]pertechnetate is currently utilized because of its ready availability, low cost, and relatively short half-life. The saline eluate from a ^{99}Mo generator is generally used directly to permit maximum concentration of the isotope. Ten to 15 mCi of [^{99m}Tc]pertechnetate is injected into a short length of intravenous (IV) tubing and delivered into the circulation as a discrete bolus by forceful injection of 15 to 20 mL of isotonic saline. Although some laboratories have administered the isotope through an antecubital vein, more consistent delivery of the radionuclide into the central circulation as a discrete bolus is achieved through an external jugular vein. Gold-195m (^{195m}Au) is an acceptable alternative to ^{99m}Tc when multiple studies are required in a short time. Its very short half-life (30.5 seconds) permits rapid sequential imaging with less radiation exposure and residual background.[59-61]

The passage of the radioisotope through the right atrium, right ventricle, pulmonary circulation, left atrium, left ventricle, and ascending aorta is recorded with a multicrystal camera as described above. (A gamma camera may be employed, but the count rates achieved are less satisfactory.) The high count rates achieved by this camera permit accurate temporal definition of the passage of the bolus. This temporal resolution is utilized to identify the various cardiac chambers, including the left ventricle. It is therefore vitally important that the radionuclide arrive at the right atrium in fairly concentrated form—that is, as a "tight" bolus. Commercially available software can be utilized for accurate definition of the left ventricular border. The change in counts within this border during the passage of the bolus through the left ventricle reflects the effect of individual heartbeats (Fig 6-9). Several such beats can be added together to provide high count-rate images reflecting left ventricular wall motion during a typical cardiac cycle.[62-64] This wall motion can be visualized in a dynamic cine format or in a static two-image (end-systole and end-diastole) format.

The principal advantage of the first-pass technique is the short acquisition time required for performance of this study. The injected bolus of ^{99m}Tc will generally complete its passage through the left ventricle within 30 seconds. This shorter acquisition time permits the performance of upright bicycle exercise, in contrast to the supine bicycle exercise that is most often utilized for equilibrium studies. The second advantage of this technique is that it can provide an anterior or right anterior oblique view[65] of the ventricle at exercise, for it does not rely on spatial resolution for the separation of the right and left ventricles. As a result, a more direct assessment of anterior wall motion with exercise should certainly be possible. This advantage, however, is somewhat offset by the major disadvantage of this technique, which is the decreased resolution of the multicrystal camera. As a result, the assessment of ventricular wall motion by this technique is probably not as sensitive as that achieved by equilibrium radionuclide angiography, although there are no definitive studies to compare the two techniques in this respect. In addition, the first-pass technique is not applicable in situations in which the injected bolus becomes "strung out"—that is, diluted—before reaching the left heart phase. The most common clinical situations in which this occurs are tricuspid regurgitation and severe pulmonary hypertension.

As mentioned above, the basic data acquired from

first-pass radionuclide angiography are quite similar to those obtained from equilibrium radionuclide angiography. Left ventricular ejection fraction is calculated from the end-diastolic and end-systolic counts from several cardiac cycles during the passage of the bolus through the left ventricle.[62-64] This involves determination of the left ventricular border by means of a computer algorithm and a determination of background. The most commonly used technique of background subtraction relies on a determination of the spatial distribution of counts during the appearance of the radionuclide in the left atrium and before its entry into the left ventricle. A computer algorithm determines this point in the bolus passage, and it is confirmed by the operator by examination of a visual display. Left ventricular ejection fractions determined in this fashion have correlated well with those obtained by contrast ventriculography.[62,63,66] The interobserver variability in the determination of ejection fraction has been reported to be 2.0% ± 1.5% at rest and 2.1% ± 1.0% during exercise[67]—which compares very favorably with similar values determined from contrast ventriculography.[68]

Left ventricular volumes are determined by utilization of the left ventricular border defined at end-diastole. The aortic valve plane is identified both from dynamic images and from the zone in which counts do not change between end-systole and end-diastole. The end-diastolic image determined in this fashion is used to calculate an end-diastolic volume by the area-length method of Sandler and Dodge.[69] The radionuclide end-diastolic volume correlates well with the end-diastolic volume obtained by contrast ventriculography,[66] although the radionuclide volume does tend to underestimate the contrast ventriculographic volume systematically. This systematic underestimation can be corrected by means of a regression equation. The stroke volume can be determined by multiplying the end-diastolic volume by the ejection fraction, and when multiplied by the heart rate, the stroke volume can be utilized to obtain a cardiac output. The cardiac output so obtained correlates well with that obtained from simultaneous dye-dilution curves.[66] The interobserver variability in end-diastolic volumes and the variability of end-diastolic volume between studies on different days have both been carefully studied;[67] they are generally less than the comparable variabilities obtained with the use of contrast ventriculography.[68,70]

Left ventricular wall motion may be assessed on the display of static end-diastolic and end-systolic images or from a real-time, continuous-loop cine display, which is similar to a left ventriculogram with contrast. Most laboratories utilize a subjective assessment of wall motion from these images. This assessment has been found to correlate reasonably well with findings at left ventriculography,[62,63] but its reproducibility has not been well established. Others have utilized quantitative methods for the examination of regional function,[71] but these methods have not been well validated.

Right ventricular ejection fractions have been determined from first-pass radionuclide angiograms with techniques analogous to those employed for determination of left ventricular ejection fraction.[72,73] These determinations are reportedly reproducible,[72] and one laboratory has confirmed that they agree favorably with ejection fractions obtained by contrast ventriculograms with an approach involving Simpson's rule.[73]

The initial passage of the radionuclide through the pulmonary circulation can be used to construct tracer dilution curves that are analogous to the dye-dilution curves obtained with the injection of indocyanine green. Curves constructed in this fashion can be employed to quantitate left-to-right shunting in patients with congenital heart disease. Their use in this regard is long-standing and well validated.[74-76] The determination of similar curves from the region of the carotid arteries has permitted quantification of right-to-left shunts noninvasively.[77]

Other measurements that can be made with first-pass radionuclide angiography include regurgitant fractions[78] and diastolic filling.[79]

Thallium-201 myocardial scintigraphy

Another important nuclear cardiology technique is that of ^{201}Tl myocardial scintigraphy, which has been widely used in the clinical evaluation of ischemic heart disease. ^{201}Tl is a metal in group III-A of the periodic table, and it has properties similar to, but not identical with, those of potassium. Although the energies of the photons that it emits are somewhat lower than ideal for gamma camera imaging, this energy range does permit imaging with greater resolution than is possible with potassium, rubidium, or cesium. In addition, ^{201}Tl is very highly extracted by the myocardium, and this feature permits a better target-to-noise ratio.

The principal role of ^{201}Tl has been in conjunction with exercise testing. The use of ^{201}Tl in this setting is highly dependent upon its kinetics. This complex topic has been well reviewed elsewhere.[80] The initial regional distribution of ^{201}Tl in the myocardium after IV administration depends both on delivery of the pharmaceutical to the myocardium—that is, on regional blood flow—and on the extraction of the isotope by the myocardium. The fraction of the tracer extracted by the myocardium is quite high and is relatively constant under various physiologic and metabolic conditions. Hypoxia and acidosis have been shown to reduce the extraction fraction slightly.[81] Insulin, propranolol, and acetylstrophanthidin do not appear to alter the myocardial extraction of ^{201}Tl.

The regional distribution of ^{201}Tl has been shown to be generally linearly related to regional blood flow.[82] Experimental preparations using acute coronary occlusion have consistently demonstrated a close relationship between distribution of ^{201}Tl and regional myocardial blood flow for flow magnitudes at control levels or lower. Although some studies have suggested that the distribution of ^{201}Tl may not be linearly related to regional blood flow at flows above normal values,[82,83] experiments employing radioisotope-labeled microspheres in an exercising dog model have clearly demonstrated a very high correlation between ^{201}Tl activity and myocardial blood flow over a wide range of blood flow (up to seven times the control value)[84] (Fig 6-10). Thus, when ^{201}Tl is injected during

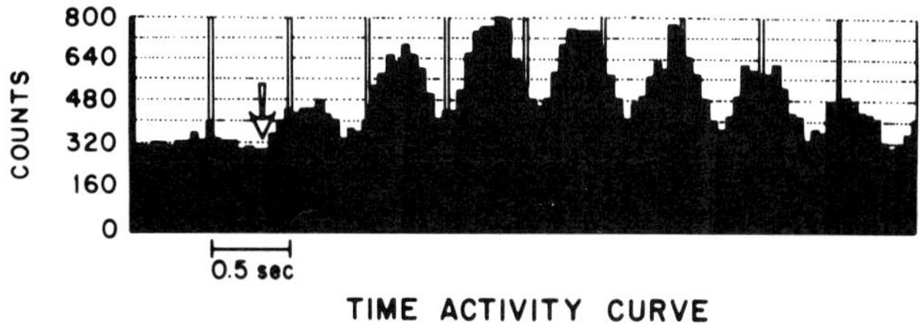

Fig 6-9 Time-activity curve obtained over the left ventricle from a first-pass radionuclide angiogram in a normal patient. The *arrow* indicates the selection of the background frame. The peaks occur during diastole, and the troughs occur during systole. (From Marshall RC, Berger HJ, Costin JC, et al: Assessment of cardiac performance with quantitative radionuclide angiocardiography: sequential left ventricular ejection fraction, normalized left ventricular ejection rate, and regional wall motion. *Circulation* 56:820-829, 1977. By permission of American Heart Association.)

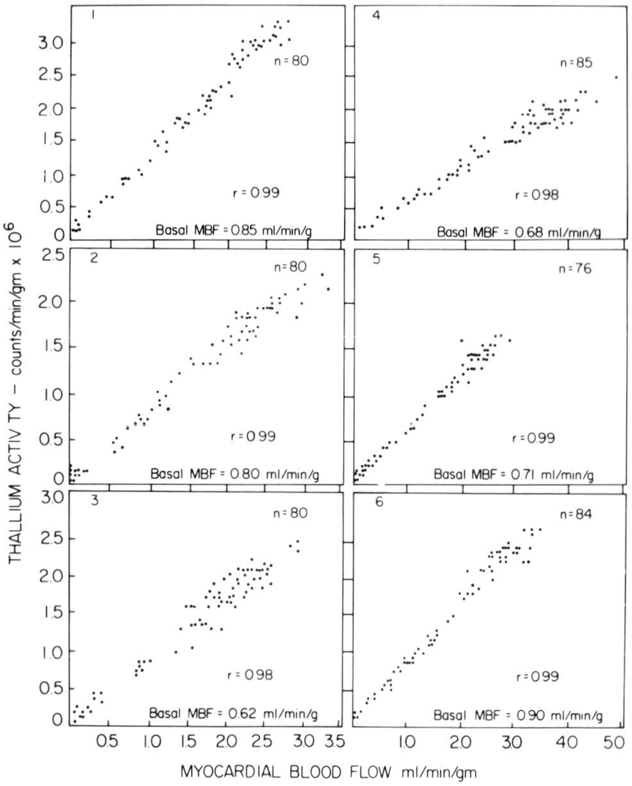

Fig 6-10 Relationship between ^{201}Tl activity and myocardial blood flow *(MBF)* measured by microspheres in six dogs with circumflex coronary artery occlusion during exercise. n = number of myocardial samples from each dog. (From Nielson AP, Morris KG, Murdock R, et al: Linear relationship between the distribution of thallium-201 and blood flow in ischemic and nonischemic myocardium during exercise. *Circulation* 61:797-801, 1980. By permission of American Heart Association.)

exercise, the initial myocardial distribution parallels regional myocardial blood flow. Regions of the myocardium that are supplied by significantly stenosed coronary arteries will not increase their blood flow appropriately with exercise. They will therefore have less ^{201}Tl distributed to them and will appear as defects on the initial ^{201}Tl scan. Animal experiments suggest that hypoperfused zones as small as 5 g may be detected.[85]

After the initial uptake of ^{201}Tl by the myocardium, its distribution changes continuously as a function of time. This process is generally referred to as "redistribution." It involves the continuous exchange of ^{201}Tl among the blood pool, myocardium, and other organs. The other body organs generally serve as a large reservoir of ^{201}Tl, which can be exchanged with the myocardium via the blood pool.[80]

The process of redistribution generally reflects the balance between two competing processes. The first of these is the input of ^{201}Tl into the myocardium on a continuing basis from the blood pool. Although the concentration of ^{201}Tl in the blood falls abruptly after IV administration, a low concentration of ^{201}Tl persists in the blood for many hours. It is therefore continuously delivered to the myocardium and distributed according to the prevailing pattern of regional blood flow. At the same time, ^{201}Tl continuously washes out of the myocardium. The myocardial washout rate depends directly on myocardial perfusion. The intrinsic ^{201}Tl washout has a half-life of approximately 1 hour in normally perfused areas, but this half-life is dramatically increased in areas that are poorly perfused.[86] The local concentration of ^{201}Tl continues to change over time until there is an equilibrium condition in which input from the blood pool and output from the intrinsic myocardial washout rate are approximately constant. The net difference between these two processes can be termed the "net myocardial washout rate." It is much longer than the intrinsic washout rate because of the continuous replacement of ^{201}Tl from the blood pool and is about 7 hours.[87-90]

Repeat assessment of the myocardial distribution of ^{201}Tl after its initial distribution will reflect the effects of the redistribution process. In the presence of viable myocardium, ^{201}Tl will tend to accumulate in the previously underperfused areas and will tend to wash out from the previously normally perfused area. As a result, the concentration of ^{201}Tl will tend to equalize in all areas containing viable myocardium (Fig 6-11). In contrast, areas of myocardial scar will have no further uptake of ^{201}Tl from the blood pool over time; therefore, these areas will persist as defects on ^{201}Tl images made hours after the initial injections.[80] The reversibility of ^{201}Tl defects seen on the initial distribution can therefore be used as an indicator of myocardial viability[91-93] (Table 6-4).

Exercise ^{201}Tl myocardial imaging is generally performed simultaneously with exercise electrocardiography. Routine resting ECGs are obtained both supine and upright before the test is begun. The patient is then exercised on either a bicycle ergometer or a treadmill to maximum capacity. Continuous monitoring of the ECG is necessary to ensure the patient's safety. At peak exercise, 2.0 to 4.0 mCi of ^{201}Tl is injected intravenously, and the

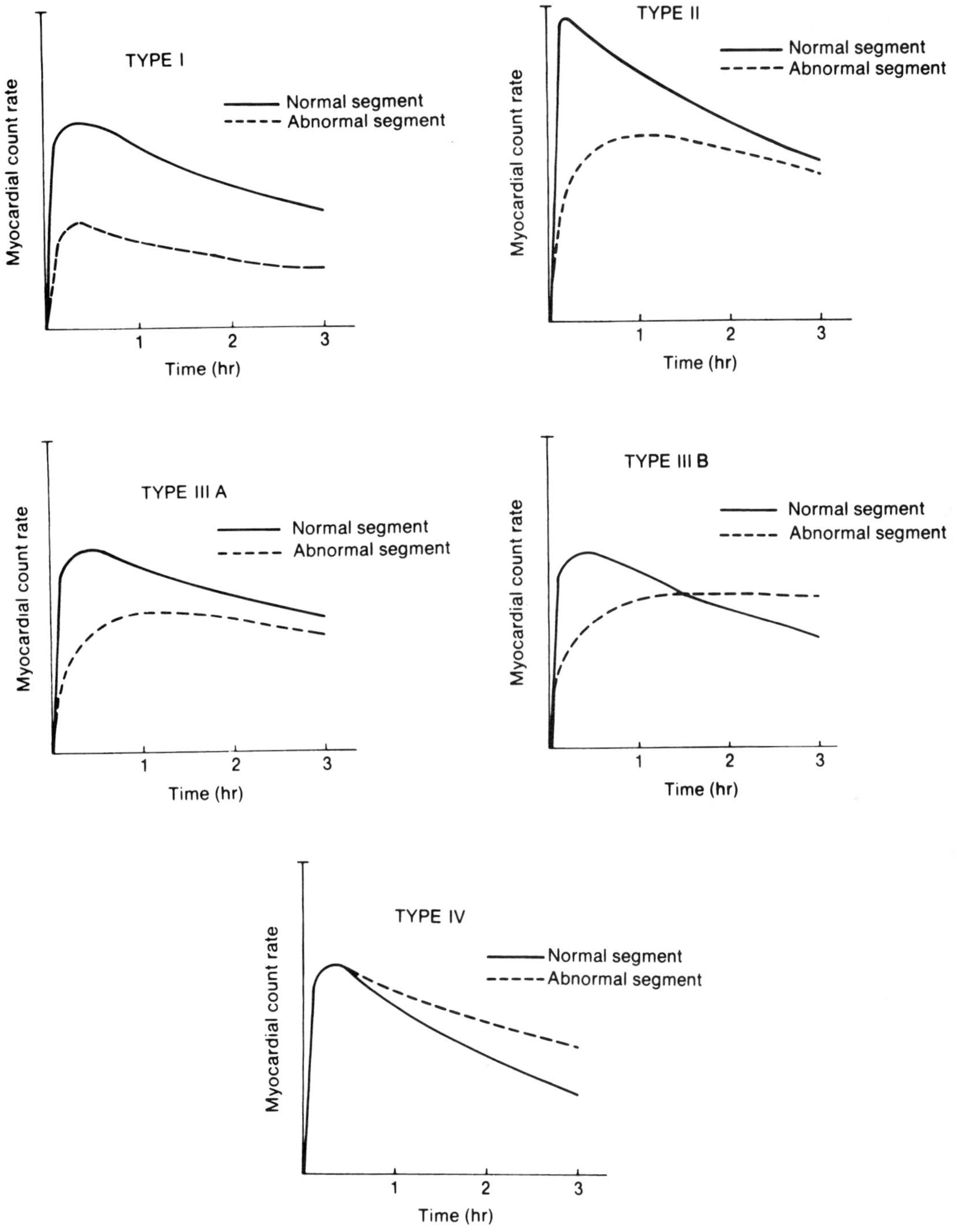

Fig 6-11 Patterns of $^{201}Tl^{+}$ uptake in patients with coronary artery disease. Idealized time-activity curves are shown for normal and ischemic segments. (From Beller GA, Watson DD, Pohost GM: Kinetics of thallium distribution and redistribution: clinical applications in sequential myocardial imaging. In *Cardiovascular Nuclear Medicine.* Second edition. Edited by HW Strauss, B Pitt. St Louis, CV Mosby Company, 1979, pp 225-242. By permission.)

Table 6-4 Comparison of ^{201}Tl redistribution pattern with postoperative wall motion response in 72 asynergic segments*

Postoperative wall motion	Preoperative ^{201}Tl redistribution	
	Normal	Abnormal
Improved	35	4
Not improved	8	25

*From Rozanski A, Berman DS, Gray R, et al: Use of thallium-201 redistribution scintigraphy in the preoperative differentation of reversible and nonreversible myocardial asynergy. *Circulation* 64:936-944, 1981. By permission of American Heart Association.

patient is exercised for an additional minute. This additional exercise minute ensures that the ^{201}Tl will be distributed according to the regional blood flow pattern at peak exercise. Ideally, the patient should not have taken propranolol within 48 hours of testing, for this has been shown to reduce the sensitivity.[94] In addition, adequate exercise is definitely necessary, because intermediate levels of exercise reveal less abnormality.[95]

Pharmacologic stress may be used as an alternative to exercise stress in association with ^{201}Tl imaging.[96-98] The first pharmacologic stress agent used in nuclear cardiology studies was intravenously delivered dipyridamole. Dipyridamole is usually administered rapidly over 4 minutes at a total dose of 0.56 mg/kg of body weight. At the blood levels achieved with this rapid infusion, dipyridamole usually promotes a near-maximum coronary vasodilatation and an increase in coronary blood flow of 300% to 400%. The mechanism of the vasodilatation is thought to rely primarily on the inhibition of reuptake of adenosine by the myocardial cell.[99] The increase in coronary blood flow is less than normal in areas of the myocardium supplied by hemodynamically significant coronary arterial stenoses, because these stenoses create a fixed resistance that does not change in response to dipyridamole.[100] In such areas of the myocardium, the administration of dipyridamole tends to redistribute coronary blood flow away from the endocardium toward the epicardium, because the epicardial arterioles have a greater capacity for vasodilatation.[101] As a result, if significant coronary artery disease is present, inhomogeneities will occur in myocardial perfusion and ^{201}Tl uptake. These inhomogeneities generally do not require a true "coronary steal," although this occasionally occurs in response to dipyridamole.

Although clearly useful as an alternative to exercise, pharmacologic stress with IV dipyridamole should be used only with an adequate understanding of the differences between dipyridamole and exercise and appropriate attention to issues of safety. Continuous monitoring of the ECG throughout the pharmacologic infusion and for at least 6 minutes thereafter is necessary to ensure the patient's safety. In contrast to exercise, IV dipyridamole usually provokes a mild decrease in systemic blood pressure and a mild reflex increase in heart rate. Many side effects have been reported;[102] the most common are light-headedness, headache, and nausea. More severe side effects can occur, including profound hypotension, chest pain, and ECG changes. Prolonged ischemia,[103] cardiac arrest,[104] and respiratory arrest[105] have been reported after IV administration of dipyridamole. IV aminophylline directly reverses the effects of IV dipyridamole and should be immediately available. Absolute contraindications to IV dipyridamole are allergy to dipyridamole, allergy to aminophylline or current aminophylline use, unstable angina, and severe asthma. Relative contraindications are resting hypotension, aortic stenosis, mitral stenosis, and mild bronchospasm.

In recent years, intravenously administered adenosine has also been used for pharmacologic stress testing.[106-108] The mechanism of action of adenosine is very similar to that described previously for dipyridamole. Exogenous adenosine has an extremely short half-life (less than 10 seconds). A continuous infusion at a dose of 140 μg/kg per minute provokes maximal or near-maximal coronary vasodilatation in most patients. The short half-life of adenosine permits rapid control of the infusion and its effects. Although side effects, including headache, flushing, dyspnea, and chest pain, are common, they are generally well tolerated and disappear quickly after the infusion is discontinued. High-degree atrioventricular block occurs rarely but also is usually fleeting. The potential advantages of adenosine over dipyridamole are its more easily controlled infusion and side effects and a more uniform maximal vasodilatation at the standard dose. In a small series of patients studied with coronary Doppler flow catheters, adenosine provoked a greater coronary vasodilatation than dipyridamole, but the ratio of flow in the normal to abnormal areas was not significantly different for the two agents.[109] The contraindications to IV administration of adenosine are similar to those for dipyridamole and include chronic obstructive pulmonary disease, current aminophylline use, unstable angina, asthma, second- or third-degree atrioventricular block, and current dipyridamole use. Relative contraindications are resting hypotension, aortic stenosis, and mitral stenosis.

Dobutamine given intravenously has also been used as a pharmacologic stress agent in association with perfusion imaging.[110,111] This agent was used initially for stress radionuclide angiography and subsequently for echocardiography. It provokes a 1.5- to 2.5-fold increase in coronary blood flow by increasing heart rate, systolic blood pressure, and contractility. Preliminary studies suggest that dobutamine perfusion scintigraphy has reasonable sensitivity and specificity for the detection of coronary artery disease.[110] It is a promising alternative to dipyridamole or adenosine for patients in whom dipyridamole and adenosine are contraindicated by, for example, asthma or aminophylline therapy.

Pharmacologic stress should be considered in patients who are unable to exercise adequately because of orthopedic limitations, peripheral vascular disease, or general physical condition. Pharmacologic stress with dipyridamole[112,113] or adenosine[114] is also preferable for patients with fixed or exercise-induced left bundle-branch block (or ventricular pacing), in whom exercise may provoke perfusion abnormalities without coronary artery disease.[115-118] Patients receiving β-adrenergic receptor blockers frequently have a limited exercise heart rate (and therefore myocardial oxygen demand). In such patients, dipyridamole or adenosine stress may be preferable. Dobutamine infusion at the usual dosage may not be able to overcome the effects of β-adrenergic receptor blockade.

After exercise or pharmacologic stress, ^{201}Tl imaging may be performed by either standard planar methods or the more recently developed approach of single-photon-emission computed tomography. Planar imaging techniques have been in widespread use for more than a decade. With these techniques, ^{201}Tl imaging should begin quickly, since redistribution of the ^{201}Tl begins almost immediately. Images should be acquired for a constant period (generally 6 to 10 minutes) in several different projections. Those most commonly used are the anterior, a 45° left anterior oblique, and either a 70° left anterior oblique or a left lateral. After the initial series of images has been completed, the patient is instructed to return to the laboratory for repeat images in approximately 4 hours. During this period, it is advisable that the patient not eat heavily or exercise substantially to avoid disturbing the continuous ^{201}Tl exchange throughout the body. Repeat images are then obtained 4 hours after exercise in the same set of projections for the same period of time.

In some patients, ^{201}Tl redistribution may not be present on the 4-hour images despite viable myocardium. In such instances, absent or incomplete redistribution at 4 hours may incorrectly imply myocardial infarction.[119,120] Redistribution of ^{201}Tl may depend on both the severity of the stress-induced perfusion abnormality and the subsequent levels of thallium in the blood. The reinjection of an additional dose of thallium several hours after stress may result in enhanced thallium uptake in apparently irreversible defects.[121,122] Enhanced thallium uptake after reinjection has been associated with preserved metabolic activity on positron-emission computed tomography[123] and with improved regional wall motion after revascularization.[121] Repeat imaging after additional time, usually 24 hours, also facilitates the detection of thallium redistribution and the identification of viable myocardium.[119,120] The reinjection of thallium may be performed in several different ways: (1) on a selective basis after 4-hour imaging if redistribution is not present, (2) on a selective basis after 24-hour imaging if redistribution is not evident, and (3) on a routine basis 15 to 20 minutes before 4-hour imaging. Each of these approaches has potential advantages and disadvantages. We prefer the third approach, because it enhances the detection of redistribution on the 4-hour images and often obviates a third set of images (Fig 6-12). The disadvantage of this approach is the potential problem of differential uptake of the reinjected thallium if regional perfusion is reduced because of critically stenosed or occluded coronary arteries.[124] Such differential uptake may conceivably mask redistribution and change the interpretation of the defect from reversible to fixed. This problem occurs very infrequently because an almost exact balance is required

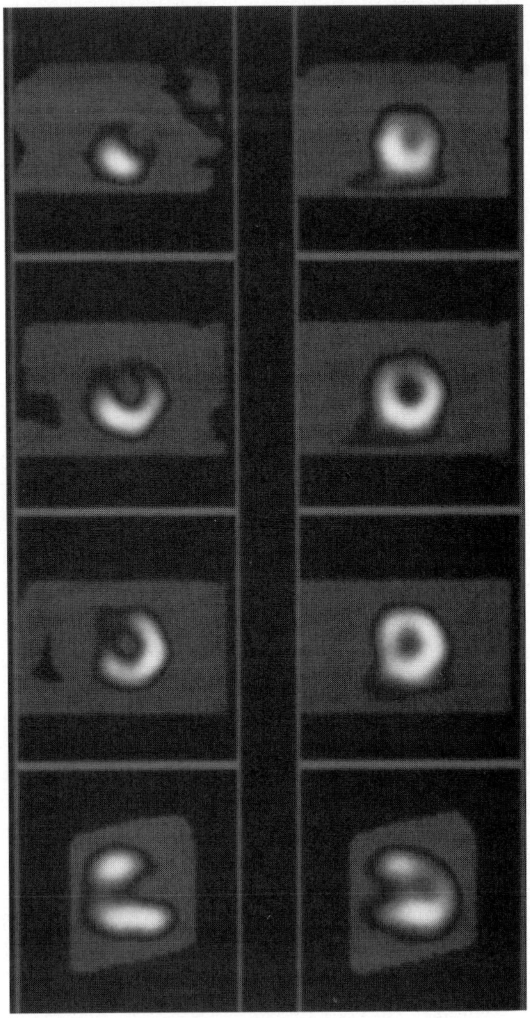

Fig 6-12 Tomographic thallium images obtained after exercise (**left column**) and 4 hours later after thallium reinjection (**right column**) in a 62-year-old woman with typical angina. Three pairs of short-axis tomographic slices were obtained at different levels—apex *(first row),* midventricle *(second row),* and base *(third row).* A single pair of vertical long-axis images was obtained at the midventricle *(fourth row).* The images obtained immediately after exercise show a large perfusion defect in the anterior wall, anterior septum, and apex. The images obtained after reinjection show nearly complete resolution of this defect.

between the magnitude of thallium redistribution after the stress study and the regional differences in perfusion at rest. We have used 24-hour imaging to detect such regions. Our experience has been that this phenomenon does not occur when redistribution is entirely absent on the reinjection images but that it may occur when insignificant redistribution appears to be present on the reinjection images.[125]

Imaging with ^{201}Tl may also be performed at rest. This technique was once used to detect myocardial ischemia.[91,126] Resting ^{201}Tl imaging with subsequent redistribution imaging may be used to detect hibernating myocardium.[127-130] In occasional patients, the major goal of imaging is to detect hibernating myocardium rather than coronary lesions that are flow-limiting during stress. In such patients, rest redistribution thallium imaging is the preferred technique, because it avoids the potential compounding effects of exercise or pharmacologic stress on ^{201}Tl kinetics.

Planar ^{201}Tl images may be displayed in several different ways and interpreted subjectively or quantitatively. Although computer processing using background subtraction and quantification is common, the images may be interpreted subjectively on either Polaroid or transparent film. Areas of reduced ^{201}Tl uptake are identified visually in each view. The possible effects of soft tissue attenuation from the diaphragm and breast tissue must be taken into account, as must the smaller amount of myocardium present at the apex. Defects should generally be investigated in more than one view if they reflect a true decrease in ^{201}Tl uptake.[131] The images obtained 4 hours (or 24 hours) after exercise, generally referred to as "redistribution images," should be compared with the initial image to determine whether a defect initially seen is still present ("fixed") or has disappeared ("reversible").

Computer background subtraction is often used to improve image quality and therefore the detection of defects. The two most commonly employed methods involve either a simple threshold or a bilinear interpolative background subtraction. Caution must be exercised with either method because oversubtraction of background may create spurious defects.

Observer agreement in the subjective assessment of planar ^{201}Tl images has been studied. The same observer will identify a study as normal or as abnormal on two different occasions approximately 90% of the time.[132] Interobserver agreement is not as good. Three of four observers will identify the same study as normal or as abnormal approximately 70% of the time.[132] Interobserver agreement on the location of defects is poorer, particularly in the posterior and lateral walls.[132]

A number of methods have been developed for the quantitation of ^{201}Tl images.[133-136] Background subtraction is usually required in these methods. These methods have generally employed both spatial quantitation of the uptake of ^{201}Tl in specific myocardial regions and temporal quantitation of the changes in ^{201}Tl distribution in the same region over time. Some investigators have found that quantification of ^{201}Tl images improves the detection of abnormal images.[137] Others have found that the overall classification of images as normal or abnormal is not definitely improved but that the ability to identify individual myocardial segments as abnormal is enhanced.[138] It is likely, but unproven, that the degree of improvement in interpretation provided by quantification of ^{201}Tl images is inversely related to the experience of the observer. Quantification clearly improves interobserver agreement and increases confidence in image interpretation. Quantitative methods developed at one institution can be applied in other laboratories with similar accuracy.[139]

Tomographic imaging with ^{201}Tl has become increasingly popular. Tomographic reconstruction has a theoretical advantage, because it can limit the superimposition of adjacent myocardial layers and background activity. Early efforts in this regard used a seven-pinhole collimator.[140,141] Later studies of this technique did not demonstrate any significant advantage over planar imaging.[142-145] Subsequent efforts focused on the use of single-photon-emission computed tomography (SPECT).[146] This technique is theoretically similar to x-ray computed tomography. A gamma camera rotates 180° or 360° around the patient, taking a series of images; these images are then reconstructed with use of standard back-projection algorithms. This approach is clearly superior to seven-pinhole collimation.[147] SPECT imaging requires greater attention to quality control, as there are many more potential sources of false-positive studies. Collimator integrity, detector uniformity, and a correct center of rotation are all very important for SPECT imaging.[148] SPECT acquisitions are also subject to false-positive results from patient motion[149] and upward movement of the heart during acquisition due to a decrease in depth of respiration.[150] None of these problems is insurmountable, but they do require greater attention to detail than is the case for planar imaging.

When SPECT imaging is performed properly, the results appear to be superior to those of planar imaging. Prior myocardial infarction can be more easily detected[151,152] and its size more accurately estimated.[153] SPECT provides improved identification of normal and abnormal vascular regions, with improved detection of multivessel coronary artery disease.[154-157] It appears to offer a relatively greater advantage in male patients and in patients with milder forms of coronary artery disease.[157] Although some authorities continue to favor planar imaging with quantification, others have argued strongly that SPECT imaging is the technique of choice.[148]

Interpretation of planar or tomographic ^{201}Tl images should also include assessment of both lung and right ventricular uptake. An increase in ^{201}Tl uptake during its first transit through the lung has been shown to develop in patients with left heart failure, possibly on the basis of an increase in left atrial pressure and a prolonged transit time.[158] Increased lung uptake of ^{201}Tl during exercise correlates with the development of exercise-induced left ventricular dysfunction.[159] The evaluation of lung activity during exercise may be performed on an anterior planar image either subjectively[160] or quantitatively.[161] Many laboratories that perform SPECT imaging do a separate anterior planar view for this purpose, although a quantitative method to assess pulmonary uptake during SPECT imaging has been reported.[162]

With planar imaging, right ventricular uptake is often visualized on the left anterior oblique view during exercise but is usually not well defined on the redistribution image. Right ventricular uptake on the redistribution image implies right ventricular hypertrophy.[163] Right ventricular uptake is often seen on SPECT imaging on both the exercise and the redistribution images. Standards for its interpretation are less well defined.

Technetium-99m myocardial scintigraphy

The low energy and long half-life of ^{201}Tl make it less than ideal from an imaging standpoint despite the excellent

correlation between its uptake and myocardial blood flow. Over the past decade, extensive efforts have been made to develop radiopharmaceuticals that use ^{99m}Tc for the assessment of myocardial perfusion. The higher energy and more favorable radiation dosimetry of ^{99m}Tc should provide higher count rates with a higher resolution per count, permitting improved image quality.

Two such agents have already been approved for general clinical use: ^{99m}Tc teboroxime[164,165] and ^{99m}Tc sestamibi (^{99m}Tc hexakis-2-methoxy-2-methylpropyl-isonitrile).[166,167] The latter radiopharmaceutical has been more extensively evaluated and used clinically. Like ^{201}Tl, ^{99m}Tc sestamibi is taken up in the myocardium in proportion to myocardial blood flow.[166] Unlike ^{201}Tl, this agent is bound within the mitochondria and demonstrates little myocardial washout or redistribution. Separate stress and rest injections are therefore necessary to distinguish areas of infarction and ischemia. This agent provides higher count rates, which permit first-pass radionuclide angiography and gated tomographic imaging as part of a single myocardial perfusion study. This agent also facilitates the use of high-resolution collimation in association with tomographic imaging. This feature further enhances image quality, which is clearly superior to that achieved with ^{201}Tl, particularly in obese patients (Fig 6-13). Somewhat surprisingly, the published studies of use of this radiopharmaceutical have generally not demonstrated superior diagnostic results to thallium perfusion imaging despite improved image quality.[168-171] One study in which this radiopharmaceutical and SPECT imaging were used reported that it was superior in the detection of disease in individual coronary arteries.[169] The published comparisons are generally based on small numbers of patients and qualitative analysis.

Because of the minimal redistribution of ^{99m}Tc sestamibi, it can be administered in the emergency room during acute myocardial infarction, with delayed imaging hours later to determine the distribution of myocardial perfusion at the time of administration. The amount of myocardium "at risk" in acute infarction can be assessed without any delay in reperfusion therapy. The change in myocardial perfusion determined by ^{99m}Tc sestamibi before and after acute reperfusion therapy may be a superior measurement for the assessment of the efficacy of acute intervention.[172-174] This radiopharmaceutical can also be administered to patients with unstable angina during episodes of spontaneous chest pain.[175,176]

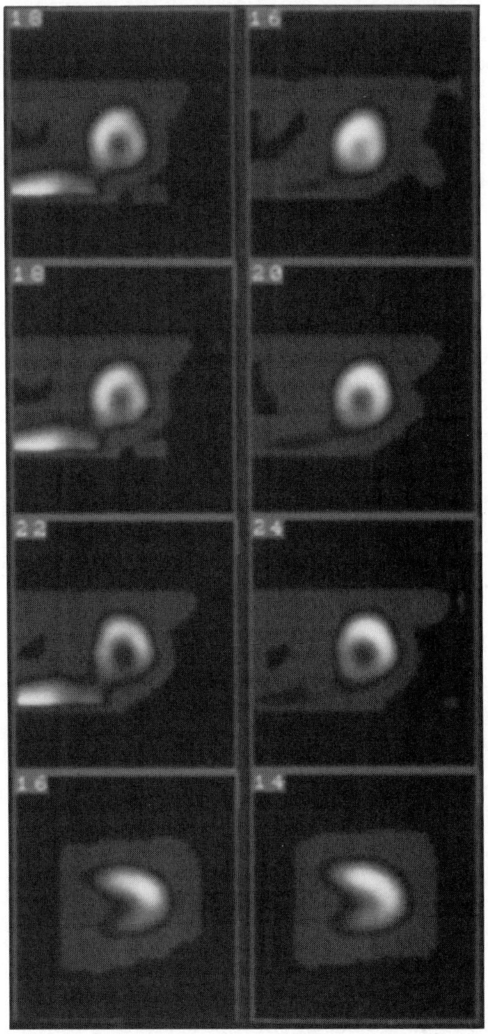

Fig 6-13 Technetium-99m sestamibi tomographic images obtained after adenosine infusion **(left column)** and 4 hours later after thallium reinjection **(right column)** in a 65-year-old woman. Three pairs of short-axis images and a single pair of vertical long-axis images are displayed in the same format as that in Figure 6-12. The patient was 162 cm tall and weighed 106 kg. The quality of the images is good despite her obesity. A moderate perfusion defect in the inferior wall and a mild perfusion defect in the lateral wall on the earlier images redistribute nearly completely after thallium reinjection.

Infarct-avid imaging

Another technique utilized in nuclear cardiology is infarct-avid imaging with ^{99m}Tc pyrophosphate (^{99m}Tc PP). Extensive reviews of this procedure are available.[177,178] ^{99m}Tc PP was first proposed as a potential agent for the imaging of acute myocardial infarcts because of the observation that calcium accumulates in irreversibly damaged muscle cells. The exact mechanism by which the isotope accumulates in necrotic myocardial cells has not been entirely established. The uptake of the ^{99m}Tc PP is dependent upon both myocardial necrosis and residual myocardial blood flow.[179,180] The isotope seems to accumulate in areas with elevated calcium levels, but a consistent correlation between calcium levels and concentration of the isotope has not been demonstrated. It was initially thought that the isotope concentrated in mitochondria, but cell fractionation studies subsequently demonstrated concentration of the isotope and calcium in the soluble supernate and membrane-debris fraction of infarcted myocardium.[180] The concentration of ^{99m}Tc PP in necrotic myocardial tissue is thought to be a result of elective adsorption of the isotope on various forms of tissue calcium stores and of complexing with denatured protein and other organic macromolecules. The isotope uptake does appear to be limited to necrotic myocardial cells.[180]

The imaging procedure involves the IV injection of 10 to 15 mCi of ^{99m}Tc PP into the patient. Imaging is then carried out at least 3 hours later in the anterior, left anterior oblique, and left lateral views. Each view is generally timed to collect a set number of counts, perhaps 400,000 to 600,000.[177,178] Multiple views are performed to permit accurate infarct localization and to help differentiate isotope uptake in the myocardium from uptake in bone.

^{99m}Tc PP uptake is demonstrable within 4 hours after acute myocardial infarction, but in some patients uptake will not be evident until 12 to 24 hours after infarction.[181] Peak uptake of ^{99m}Tc PP is present 48 to 72 hours after myocardial infarction. The concentration of the isotope in infarcted myocardium will generally decline after that time. Imaging is generally not feasible beyond 1 week after acute infarction, although some patients will have increased myocardial uptake of the isotope for an indefinite period.[177]

There are several different schemes for the interpretation of ^{99m}Tc PP scans.[182,183] Quality control in the interpretation of these images would appear to be vitally important.

CLINICAL APPLICATIONS

Chronic ischemic heart disease

The techniques described in the previous section may be employed in a wide variety of clinical settings. This section outlines a number of different clinical settings and describes the potential utility of nuclear cardiology procedures in each (Table 6-5).

Diagnosis. One of the major applications of nuclear cardiology testing has been in the noninvasive diagnosis of the presence or absence of coronary artery disease. The differential diagnosis of chest pain is a frequent and often difficult clinical problem. The patient's age, sex, description of the pain, and resting ECG all provide important clinical clues as to whether coronary artery disease is responsible for the patient's chest pain. However, even after these factors have been considered, there will be considerable uncertainty in a reasonable number of patients, leading to the need for further testing to help establish the diagnosis.

The key question when such a noninvasive diagnostic test has been performed is, What is the probability that significant coronary artery disease is present in this *individual* patient? In statistical terms, this is what is known as the "post-test probability."[184-186] It is a function of the prevalence of the disease in the population being tested, the sensitivity of the test, and the specificity of the test. The importance of the prevalence of the disease in the population will be discussed later in this section. The sensitivity of the test is defined as the percentage of patients with the disease who have a positive test result. The specificity of the test is defined as the percentage of patients without disease who have a negative test result. These test characteristics, sensitivity and specificity, are employed to evaluate and compare different noninvasive procedures.

Many different studies have compared gated equilibrium angiography, first-pass radionuclide angiography,

Table 6-5 Clinical applications of nuclear cardiology procedures

Chronic ischemic heart disease
Diagnosis
Screening for severe disease
Prognosis
Functional assessment
Complications–aneurysm, right ventricular infarction, reversible asynergy, and myocardial viability
Therapeutic interventions
Acute ischemic heart disease
Diagnosis
Response to therapy
Prognosis
Valvular heart disease
Left ventricular size and function
Timing of valve replacement
Assessment of effects of valve replacement
Cardiomyopathy
Left ventricular function
Potential clues to etiology
Follow-up
Congenital heart disease
Detection and quantification of shunts
Ventricular function
Other
Preoperative screening
Chronic obstructive pulmonary disease
Differential diagnosis of dyspnea
Cardiotoxic drugs
Clinical investigation

and ^{201}Tl exercise testing for the diagnosis of coronary artery disease. A summary of these studies is shown in Tables 6-6 and 6-7.[187-208] Radionuclide angiography has generally been found to have a much higher sensitivity and a slightly lower specificity than exercise ECG testing; ^{201}Tl exercise testing has had a higher sensitivity and specificity than exercise ECG studies. It is important to note that these comparisons have often omitted patients with "inadequate" or "uninterpretable" results of treadmill tests. If such treadmill results were counted as negative, the difference in sensitivity between nuclear cardiology studies and treadmill tests would widen considerably.

Relatively few studies have directly compared the various nuclear cardiology procedures with respect to their diagnostic accuracy. The few studies that are available are summarized in Table 6-8.[205-208] The pooled data suggest that radionuclide angiography is more sensitive but less specific than ^{201}Tl exercise testing. However, these previously published results may no longer be applicable to current clinical practice. The interpretation of the radionuclide angiograms was generally based on the change in ejection fraction, which is not optimal (see below). The interpretation of the thallium studies was performed subjectively without either quantification or tomography, which are now commonly used. There is no published comparison between radionuclide

Table 6-6 Comparison of planar ^{201}Tl exercise imaging and ECG exercise testing in the diagnosis of coronary artery disease*

		^{201}Tl		ECG	
Investigators	No.	Sensitivity	Specificity	Sensitivity	Specificity
Ritchie et al.[187]	101	58/76	23/25	50/76	21/25
Rosenblatt et al.[188]	18	14/15	3/3	6/15	3/3
Carrillo et al.[189]	55	34/39	16/16	21/39	12/16
Turner et al.[190]	64	23/34	29/30	25/34	23/30
Ritchie et al.[191]	190	115/148	37/42	62/148	37/42
Dash et al.[192]	96	66/81	15/15	30/81	12/15
Okada et al.[193]	49	27/38	10/11	23/38	10/11
Bodenheimer et al.[194]	95	55/73	20/22	41/73	19/22
Botvinick et al.[195]	46	23/27	17/19	18/27	12/19
McCarthy et al.[196]	128	81/95	26/33	61/95	30/33
Bailey et al.[197]	83	46/63	20/20	26/63	20/20
Verani et al.[198]	82	38/48	33/34	31/48	26/34
Blood et al.[199]	87	55/62	20/25	40/62	22/25
Boucher et al.[159]	210	141/162	36/48	81/162	37/48
Iskandrian et al.[200]	121	75/91	28/30	39/91	25/30
Overall	1,425	851/1,052 (81%)	333/373 (89%)	554/1,052 (53%)	309/373 (83%)

*Earliest reported series to avoid subsequent referral bias.

Table 6-7 Comparison of radionuclide angiography and ECG exercise testing in the diagnosis of coronary artery disease*

		Radionuclide angiography		ECG	
Investigators	No.	Sensitivity	Specificity	Sensitivity	Specificity
Borer et al.[201]	84	60/63	21/21	43/63	20/21
Berger et al.[202]	73	52/60	13/13	33/60	13/13
Jengo et al.[203]	19	11/11	8/8	4/11	8/8
Jones et al.†[204]	248	151/183	43/65	103/183	56/65
Overall		274/317 (86%)	85/107 (79%)	183/317 (58%)	97/107 (91%)

*Modified from Okada RD, Boucher CA, Strauss HW, et al: Exercise radionuclide imaging approaches to coronary artery disease. *Am J Cardiol* 46:1188-1204, 1980.
†Inadequate tests counted as negative.

Table 6-8 Comparison of ^{201}Tl exercise tests and radionuclide angiography in the diagnosis of coronary artery disease

		^{201}Tl		Radionuclide angiography	
Investigators	No.	Sensitivity	Specificity	Sensitivity	Specificity
Johnstone et al.[205]	48	30/39	9/9	35/39	9/9
Jengo et al.[206]	58	39/42	15/16	41/42	16/16
Bodenheimer et al.[207]	75	46/56	17/19	46/56	15/19
Caldwell et al.[208]	52	35/41	11/11	38/41	6/11
Overall	233	150/178 (84%)	52/55 (95%)	160/178 (90%)	46/55 (84%)

angiography and ^{201}Tl scintigraphy as currently practiced.

Some studies have cast doubt on earlier estimates of specificity for both radionuclide angiography and ^{201}Tl testing.[94,209] The largest reported series of patients with chest pain and normal coronary arteriograms who underwent first-pass radionuclide angiography found that many such patients had abnormal first-pass radionuclide angiograms without any evidence of cardiovascular abnormality.[209] This suggested that the earlier estimates of specificity for this test may have been erroneously high. Similarly, in the largest single series of patients with chest pain and normal coronary arteriograms who underwent ^{201}Tl exercise testing, the specificity was only 75%.[94] This was again considerably lower than the previously reported figures. Both of these studies suggest that the previously reported high specificities may have been clinically unrealistic because they were generally based on normal volunteers rather than on patients with chest pain. These normal volunteers were generally not representative of a patient population in terms of age, sex, and exercise capacity, and therefore they may have performed better on these tests. However, the estimates of specificity made in the two series mentioned above were probably falsely low, for the decision to have these patients undergo cardiac catheterization was influenced by the abnormal results on their nuclear cardiology studies. There were probably many additional patients with normal nuclear cardiology studies who did not undergo cardiac catheterization in these institutions and were, therefore, not included in the estimates of specificity. The use of the results of nuclear cardiology studies to select patients for cardiac catheterization has become more frequent in recent years.[210] This "post-test referral bias" has resulted in declining estimates of specificity that are spuriously low. One reasonably simple approach to the estimation of specificity in the face of such referral bias is the use of patients who have a low likelihood of coronary artery disease on clinical grounds.[211] More complex analytic techniques are available.[212,213] In a series of 120 patients with a low likelihood of coronary artery disease, the specificity (or "normalcy rate") of radionuclide angiography was 82%.[214] Thus, the true specificity of nuclear cardiology studies is probably between the earlier optimistic estimates and the later pessimistic ones.

The proper clinical application of these tests requires a basic knowledge of Bayes' theorem and its importance in clinical decision-making. As mentioned above, the issue of paramount importance to the clinician is the probability that an individual patient will have coronary artery disease after a particular test result. This post-test probability is a function of both the characteristics of the test and the prevalence of the disease in the population being tested.[184-186] In other words, it is a combination of the probability that a given patient had disease before a test and the results of that test. Figure 6-14 displays the effect of nuclear cardiology testing on the chances that a patient has coronary artery disease. A test with 80% sensitivity and 90% specificity is presumed. The lower curve represents the post-test probability after a negative test, and the upper curve represents the probability after a positive test. The dotted line represents the line of identity when no test

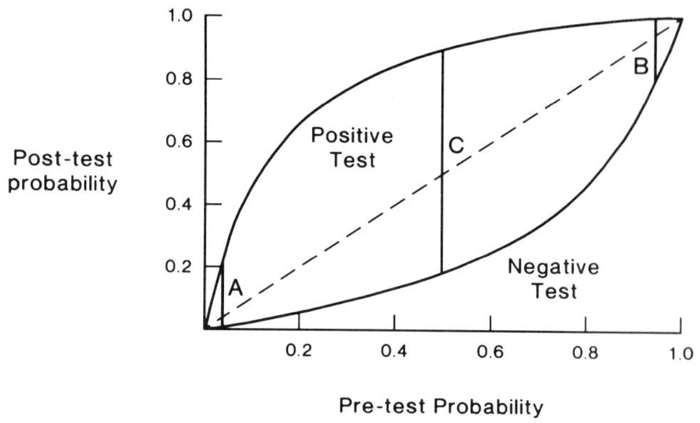

Fig 6-14 Relationship between pretest probability and post-test probability for a test with an 80% sensitivity and a 90% specificity. The *lower curve* indicates the effect of a negative test. The *upper curve* indicates the effect of a positive test. Vertical lines *A, B,* and *C* are discussed in the text.

has been performed. The vertical lines display the effects of nuclear cardiology testing in three typical clinical situations.

The first example (line A) is that of a 45-year-old woman with chest pain that was thought to be nonanginal. Population studies estimated that her pretest probability of disease was approximately 3%. A negative nuclear cardiology study would decrease the likelihood of her having disease to approximately 0.7%, as shown on the lower curve. A positive test in this patient would raise the likelihood of her having disease to only 20%. A positive test in such a patient would therefore most likely represent a "false-positive" and therefore should not affect patient management.

The second case (line B) represents a problem at the other end of the spectrum of coronary artery disease. A 65-year-old white male patient with chest pain that was thought to be typical angina would have a 95% chance of having coronary artery disease. A positive nuclear cardiology study in this patient would increase the likelihood of disease to 99%; however, a negative test would decrease the likelihood to only 81%. A negative test would, therefore, most likely represent a "false-negative" and should therefore have little impact on patient management.

The proper role for diagnostic nuclear cardiology testing is exemplified by the third example (line C). A 50-year-old man with pain that was thought to be atypical angina would have a 50% chance of having coronary artery disease. A positive nuclear cardiology test in this patient would increase the likelihood of his having significant coronary artery disease to 89%, and a negative test would reduce the probability of coronary artery disease to 18%. Thus, the difference in post-test likelihood between a positive and a negative test would be considerable, and very different approaches to the subsequent management of this patient would be justified. The major diagnostic benefit of nuclear cardiology testing is, therefore, in patients whose age, sex, and type of pain suggest an intermediate pretest likelihood of coronary artery disease. Nuclear cardiology testing in these patients will have a meaningful effect on clinical management.

For the purpose of diagnosis, nuclear cardiology studies should ideally move a significant number of patients from an "uncertain" pretest probability to an "acceptably certain" post-test probability. The definition of "acceptable certainty" is a matter of individual clinical judgment. Several studies have used criteria of post-test probabilities of less than 10% and greater than 90% for definitive diagnosis. With such criteria, both radionuclide angiography and ^{201}Tl exercise testing have been shown to move a significant number of patients to an "acceptably certain" post-test probability.[215-217] However, significant numbers of patients, particularly those with a low or intermediate pretest probability, will remain in an uncertain category in which further testing is necessary.

The criteria used to label a radionuclide angiogram "abnormal" have been a matter of some controversy. Many studies have required an increase in ejection fraction of 0.05 from rest to exercise to label a result "normal."[202,203,205,208] Subsequent studies showed that the change in ejection fraction from rest to exercise is a complex response that is influenced by many physiologic and pathologic variables.[209,218,219] The influences of rest ejection fraction[209] and patient gender[209,220,221] are particularly important. A detailed analysis of 736 patients, the largest series reported in the literature, found that the peak exercise ejection fraction was a better indicator for the detection of coronary artery disease.[216] Other series have confirmed the superiority of this factor, not only for a diagnosis[214,222] but also for the identification of severe disease[223-225] and for prognosis.[226-228]

The proper interpretation of the results of both radionuclide angiography and ^{201}Tl exercise testing requires careful consideration of all the information from the exercise portion of the test, including hemodynamics,[223-225,229,230] symptoms,[216] and ECG changes during exercise.[215,216,225] The level of myocardial oxygen demand achieved during exercise, as reflected in the heart rate and blood pressure, and the presence of symptomatic or ECG evidence of ischemia during exercise are complementary to radionuclide findings.

Screening for severe disease. The functional assessment of coronary artery disease during exercise by radionuclide methods may also provide noninvasive assessment of the extent of coronary artery disease. In particular, these techniques may be used to screen patients for left main or three-vessel coronary artery disease.

A number of studies have examined the ability of ^{201}Tl exercise imaging to noninvasively identify patients with left main or three-vessel coronary artery disease.[192,231,232] The initial results with subjective interpretation of planar imaging were somewhat disappointing, because less than half of the patients with severe coronary artery disease were identified by ^{201}Tl imaging. This result was not surprising, since the subjective interpretation of ^{201}Tl images relies on the detection of inhomogeneities of perfusion. In the absence of any normal vessels, it is difficult to identify vessels with less severe stenoses as being abnormal. Much better results were demonstrated with the quantitative analysis of planar images[138,233] and tomographic methods.[154,155] The largest study using tomographic methods found that the magnitude of ST depression, diabetes mellitus, number of abnormal thallium segments, and product of peak exercise heart rate and blood pressure were independently predictive of severe coronary artery disease.[234] Clinically useful estimates of the likelihood of left main and three-vessel coronary artery disease could be easily obtained (Fig 6-15).

Radionuclide angiography has also been proven to be useful in noninvasive screening for left main and three-vessel coronary artery disease.[224,225,229] The largest study,[225] of 681 patients, found that magnitude of ST-segment depression, peak exercise ejection fraction, peak exercise heart rate and blood pressure product, and patient gender were all independently predictive of severe coronary artery disease (Fig. 6-16). Previous studies have demonstrated the ability of exercise ECG testing to screen for severe coronary artery disease.[235,236] In patients with a normal resting ECG, exercise ECG testing is nearly as effective as radionuclide angiography or thallium scintigraphy in the identification of severe coronary artery disease.[237]

Prognosis. Resting left ventricular function is recognized as a major determinant of prognosis in coronary artery disease. The prognostic value of the resting ejection fraction measured by contrast ventriculography has been well demonstrated.[238,239] Given the close correlation between ejection fraction measurements by contrast ventriculography and radionuclide angiography, it is not surprising that the resting ejection fraction measured by radionuclide angiography is also a major predictor of patient outcome, both after acute myocardial infarction[240-242] and in patients with chronic ischemic heart disease.[227]

Exercise radionuclide angiography and exercise ^{201}Tl scintigraphy are both important noninvasive tools that provide prognostic information that is complementary to resting function. In patients undergoing exercise radionuclide angiography, the exercise ejection fraction is the single most important predictor of subsequent nonfatal myocardial infarction or cardiovascular death. An exercise ejection fraction above 0.50 is associated with a favorable short-term prognosis; as the exercise ejection fraction falls below 0.50, the percentage of patients who die or have a nonfatal infarction during the next 8 years increases greatly[243] (Fig 6-17). These results, obtained by first-pass radionuclide angiography, have also been confirmed by equilibrium techniques.[227] Exercise ^{201}Tl scintigraphy has also been shown to be highly effective for noninvasive prognosis (Table 6-9). Gill et al.[160] found that increased lung uptake on an exercise ^{201}Tl study was more important than any clinical, ECG, or other scintigraphic measurement for the prediction of subsequent cardiac events. However, their analysis did not include the resting ejection fraction. Kaul et al.[251] found that the number of segments demonstrating redistribution on delayed ^{201}Tl images was the single most important noninvasive predictor of future cardiac events, even when the resting ejection fraction was taken into account (Fig 6-18).

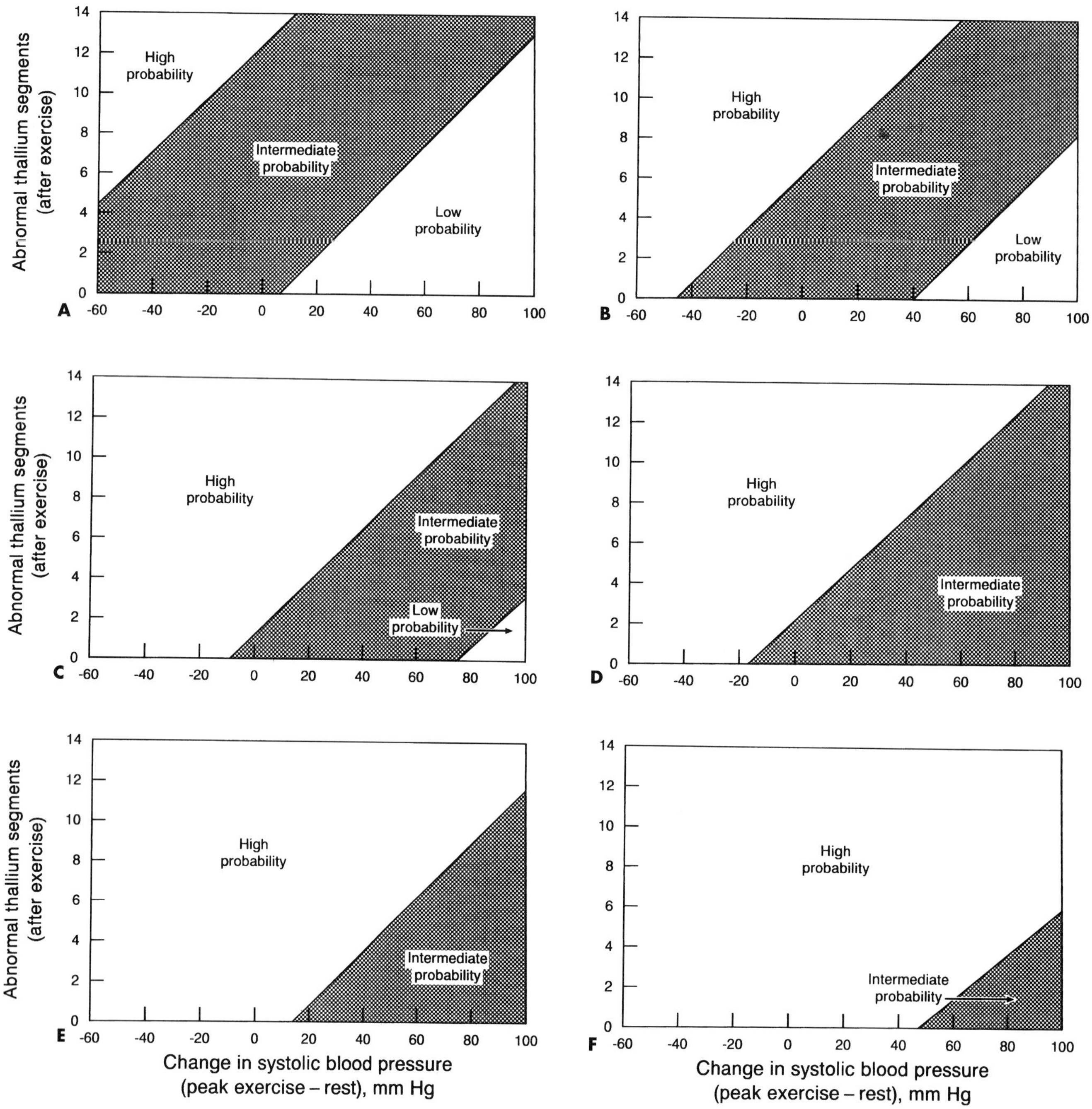

Fig 6-15 Estimated probability of left main or three-vessel coronary artery disease for nondiabetic patients with ST-segment depression of **(A)** < 1, **(B)** 1 to 1.9, and **(C)** ≥ 2 mm and for diabetic patients with ST-segment depression of **(D)** < 1, **(E)** 1 to 1.9, and **(F)** ≥ 2 mm. Zones of different probabilities are shown. (From Christian TF, Miller TD, Bailey KR, et al: Noninvasive identification of severe coronary artery disease using exercise tomographic thallium-201 imaging. *Am J Cardiol* 70:14-20, 1992. By permission of Cahners Publishing Company, a Division of Reed Publishing USA.)

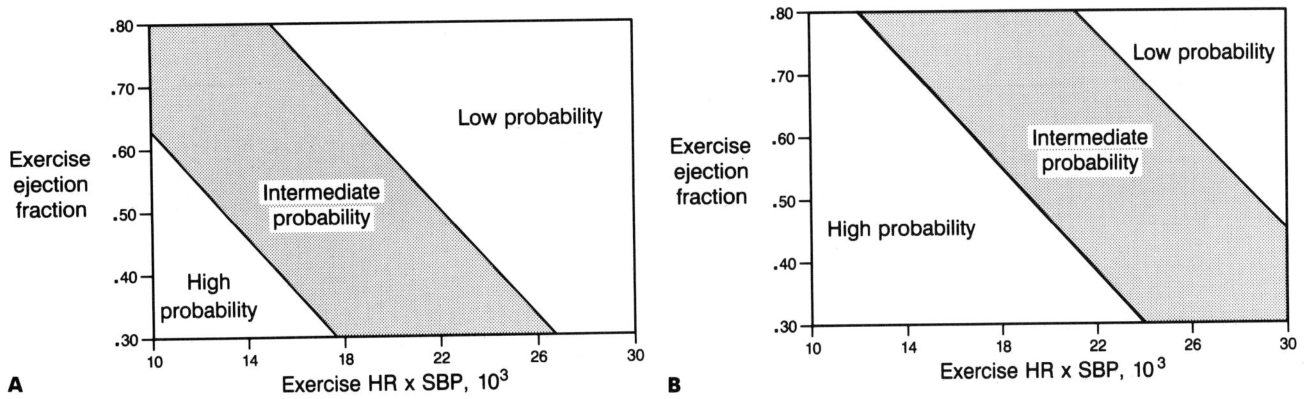

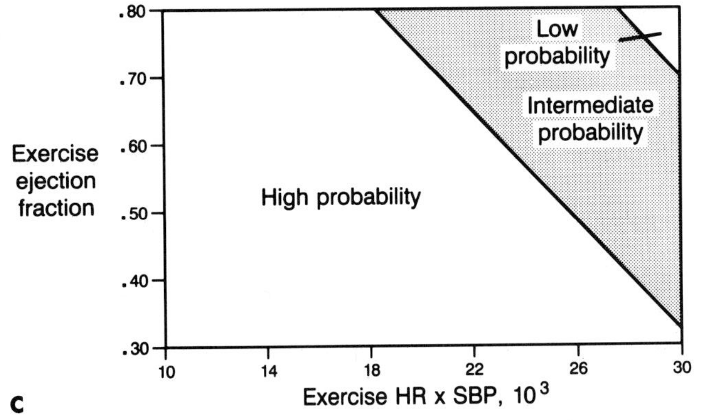

Fig 6-16 Estimated probability of left main or three-vessel coronary artery disease for men with **(A)** less than 1 mm, **(B)** 1.0 mm, and **(C)** 2.0 mm of ST-segment depression. Zones of different probability are shown. Exercise heart rate (HR) × systolic blood pressure (SBP) = exercise heart rate and systolic blood pressure product. (From Gibbons RJ, Fyke FE III, Clements IP, et al: Noninvasive identification of severe coronary artery disease using exercise radionuclide angiography. *J Am Coll Cardiol* 11:28-34, 1988. By permission of the American College of Cardiology.)

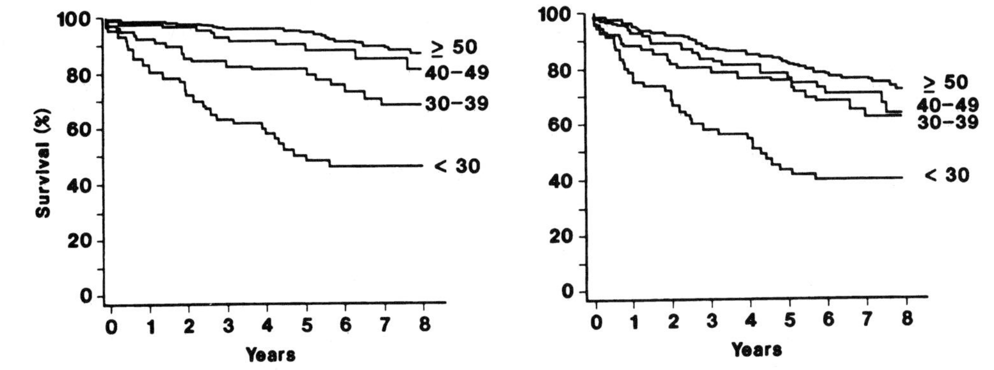

≥ 50	318	262	213	148	85
40–49	107	83	69	41	19
30–39	83	65	55	38	21
< 30	63	45	33	21	8

≥ 50	318	250	199	133	75
40–49	107	80	64	36	18
30–39	83	62	53	36	20
< 30	63	42	31	20	8

Fig 6-17 Kaplan-Meier curves for cardiovascular survival **(left panel)** and infarction-free survival **(right panel)** for groups of patients stratified by exercise ejection fraction. For each exercise ejection fraction subgroup (i.e., <30, 30-39, 40-49, and ≥50), the number of patients free of events and followed at least k years (for k = 0, 2, 4, 6, and 8) is displayed below abscissa. (From Lee KL, Pryor DB, Pieper KS, et al: Prognostic value of radionuclide angiography in medically treated patients with coronary artery disease: a comparison with clinical and catheterization variables. *Circulation* 82:1705-1717, 1990. By permission of American Heart Association.)

Table 6-9 Prognostic value of ^{201}Tl imaging in patients with known or suspected coronary artery disease

Study	Type of stress	No. of patients	Mean follow-up (mo)	Catheterization data	Cardiac events	Multivariate predictors of cardiac events: ^{201}Tl	Multivariate predictors of cardiac events: Other
Brown et al.[244]	Ex	100	46	+	Death, MI	Number of RD	None
Ladenheim et al.[245]	Ex	1,689	12	0	Death, MI, CABG	Number of RD, severity of SD	%MPHR
Staniloff et al.[246]	Ex	819	12	0	Death, MI, CABG	Severity of SD, presence of RD, number of SD, number of RD	ST $\downarrow$, Ex duration
Iskandrian et al.[247]	Ex	743	13	0	Death, MI	Number of SD	None
Iskandrian et al.[248]	Ex	196	15	0	Death, MI	Number of SD	None
Felsher et al.[249]	Ex	123	21	0	Death, MI	Abnormal scan	None
Iskandrian et al.[250]	Ex	449	25	0	Death, MI	SD, MRD	None
Gill et al.[160]	Ex	467	91	0	Death, MI, CABG	$\uparrow$ Lung uptake	Typical AP Prior MI ST $\downarrow$
Kaul et al.[161]	Ex	293	64	+	Death, MI, CABG	Lung:heart ratio	Diseased vessels Gender Δ Hr
Kaul et al.[251]	Ex	383	55	+	Death, MI, CABG	Number of RD	Diseased vessels Δ Hr VEA w/Ex β-blocker use
Younis et al.[252]	DP	107	14	+	Death, MI Death, MI, UA, CABG	Combined RD & FD RD	None None
Hendel et al.[253]	DP	516	21	0	Death, MI	SD, RD, >1 segment with RD, combined RD & FD	CHF, DM
Shaw et al.[254]	DP	348	23	0	Death, MI	RD, FD	CHF, prior MI

AP, angina pectoris; CABG, coronary artery bypass graft surgery; CHF, congestive heart failure; DM, diabetes mellitus; DP, dipyridamole-induced coronary vasodilation; Ex, exercise; FD, fixed defect; Δ Hr, change in heart rate during exercise; MI, myocardial infarction; MPHR, maximal predicted heart rate; MRD, multiple reversible defects; RD, reversible defects; SD, stress defect; ST $\downarrow$, ST segment depression; UA, unstable angina; VEA, ventricular ectopic activity.

Modified from Brown KA: Prognostic value of thallium-201 myocardial perfusion imaging: a diagnostic tool comes of age. Circulation 83:363-381, 1991.

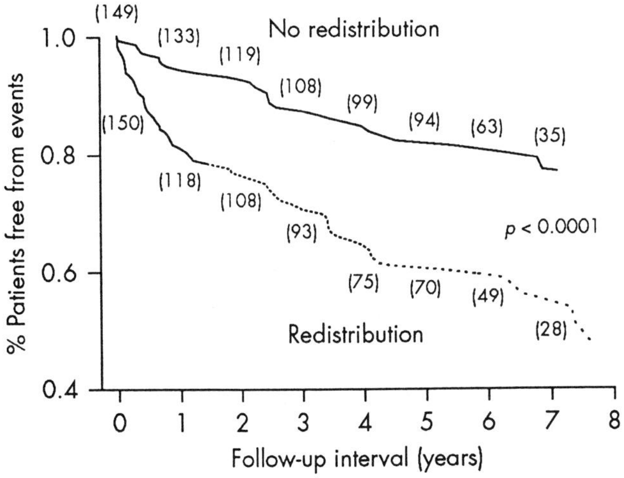

Fig 6-18 Event-free survival according to the presence or absence of redistribution on planar thallium 201 exercise scintigraphy. The numbers in parentheses indicate the number of patients in each subgroup available for analysis at each time point. (From Kaul S, Lilly DR, Gascho JA, et al: Prognostic utility of the exercise thallium-201 test in ambulatory patients with chest pain: comparison with cardiac catheterization. *Circulation* 77:745-758, 1988. By permission of American Heart Association.)

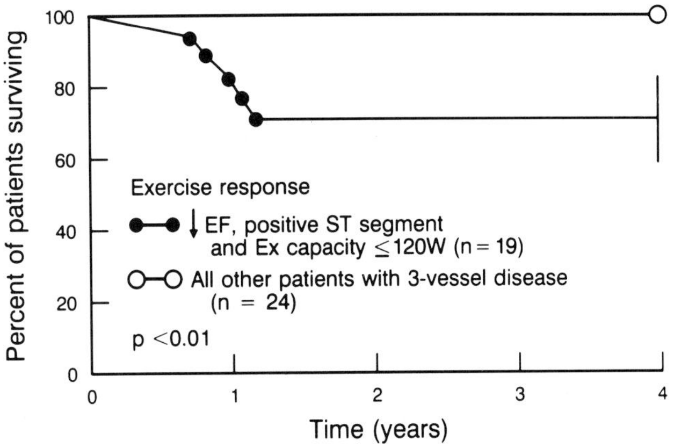

Fig 6-19 Survival as a function of a markedly abnormal exercise response in 43 patients from the National Institutes of Health with three-vessel disease and resting ejection fraction *(EF)* greater than 0.40. Patients with marked ischemia had a poor prognosis. (From Bonow RO, Kent KM, Rosing DR, et al: Exercise-induced ischemia in mildly symptomatic patients with coronary-artery disease and preserved left ventricular function: identification of subgroups at risk of death during medical therapy. *N Engl J Med* 311:1339-1345, 1984. By permission of the Journal.)

A more important issue is whether nuclear cardiology studies provide prognostic information that adds to our ability to predict subsequent outcome in an individual patient once the coronary anatomy and resting ejection fraction are known. Bonow et al.[255] reported the first data addressing this issue (Fig 6-19). In patients with three-vessel disease and normal or near-normal resting left ventricular ejection fraction, exercise-induced ischemia on exercise equilibrium radionuclide angiography was highly predictive of subsequent cardiac death. These results, obtained in patients who were all asymptomatic or mildly symptomatic, were not reproduced in a subsequent study of more symptomatic patients with three-vessel disease.[227] However, in the largest study reported to date, first-pass radionuclide angiography clearly provided incremental prognostic information to both clinical and catheterization variables[243] (Table 6-10). The exercise ejection fraction further stratified prognosis in patients with three-vessel disease and in patients with three-vessel disease and abnormal resting ventricular function (Fig 6-20). Two additional studies in patients with one-vessel or two-vessel disease[256,257] and abnormal resting ventricular function (Fig 6-21) confirmed the finding that exercise radionuclide angiography provides important prognostic information that is complementary to that provided by cardiac catheterization.

Several studies have demonstrated that exercise ^{201}Tl scintigraphy also provides prognostic information that is complementary to clinical and cardiac catheterization variables.[161,251,258] Kaul et al.[251] found that the combina-

Table 6-10 Relative prognostic importance of radionuclide angiography, clinical, and catheterization variables

Variable	Number of variables* (df)	Total model χ^2: CV death	Total model χ^2: Total CV events
Clinical	6	71	48
Catheterization	6	102	64
RNA	3	104	66
Clinical plus RNA	9	120	78
Clinical plus catheterization	12	124	82
Clinical plus catheterization plus RNA	15	138	93

CV, cardiovascular; df, degrees of freedom; RNA, radionuclide angiography.
From Lee KL, Pryor DB, Pieper KS, et al: Prognostic value of radionuclide angiography in medically treated patients with coronary artery disease: a comparison with clinical and catheterization variables. *Circulation* 82:1705-1717, 1990. By permission of the American Heart Association.

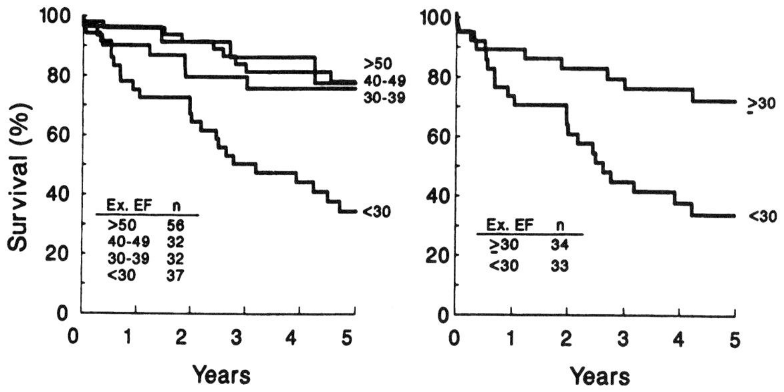

Fig 6-20 Kaplan-Meier survival curves for patients with three-vessel coronary disease stratified into four subgroups according to exercise ejection fraction (Ex. EF) **(left panel)** and patients with three-vessel disease and angiographic ejection fraction equal to or less than 45 stratified into two Ex. EF subgroups **(right panel).** (From Lee KL, Pryor DB, Pieper KS, et al: Prognostic value of radionuclide angiography in medically treated patients with coronary artery disease: a comparison with clinical and catheterization variables. *Circulation* 82:1705-1717, 1990. By permission of American Heart Association.)

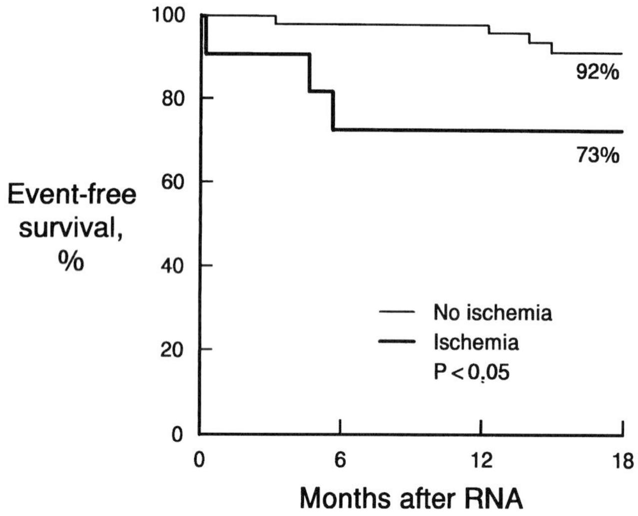

Fig 6-21 Event-free survival curves for patients with and without severe ischemia on exercise radionuclide angiograms *(RNA)*. (From Miller TD, Taliercio CP, Zinsmeister AR, et al: Risk stratification of single or double vessel coronary artery disease and impaired left ventricular function using exercise radionuclide angiography. *Am J Cardiol* 65:1317-1321, 1990. By permission of Excerpta Medica.)

tion of both catheterization and exercise ^{201}Tl data was clearly superior to the data from either alone in the prediction of future cardiac events. Exercise ^{201}Tl data appeared to be superior for predicting subsequent nonfatal myocardial infarction. In a separate study from a different institution, Kaul et al.[161] found that exercise ^{201}Tl data were slightly superior to cardiac catheterization data for the prediction of subsequent patient outcome. In the most rigorous published study, Pollock et al.[258] found that redistribution on thallium imaging added independent prognostic information to clinical and stress test information. However, the lung-heart ratio provided even greater incremental prognostic information (Fig 6-22). When the clinical, stress test, and lung-heart ratio values were known, coronary angiography did not provide any additional prognostic information. Pollock et al. also demonstrated that models developed at one institution could predict survival in unrelated but similar patients at another institution.

These studies also help predict the symptomatic response of patients to coronary revascularization. Patients with anatomic coronary disease and exercise-induced ischemia experience a much greater symptomatic improvement with surgical therapy than with medical therapy. In the absence of exercise-induced ischemia, patients with anatomic coronary disease do not benefit symptomatically from surgical revascularization compared with medical therapy.[259] As a result, third-party payers have increasingly required demonstration of exercise-induced ischemia before authorizing payment for elective coronary artery bypass grafting.

Functional assessment. Both radionuclide angiography and ^{201}Tl exercise testing may be utilized to assess the physiologic importance of anatomic coronary artery disease. The limitations of coronary arteriography in predicting physiologic status are well established;[260] functional assessment and coronary arteriography are therefore complementary. For example, radionuclide angiography or ^{201}Tl exercise testing may provide valuable information for clinical patient management when coronary arteriography demonstrates atherosclerotic lesions that appear to be of borderline hemodynamic

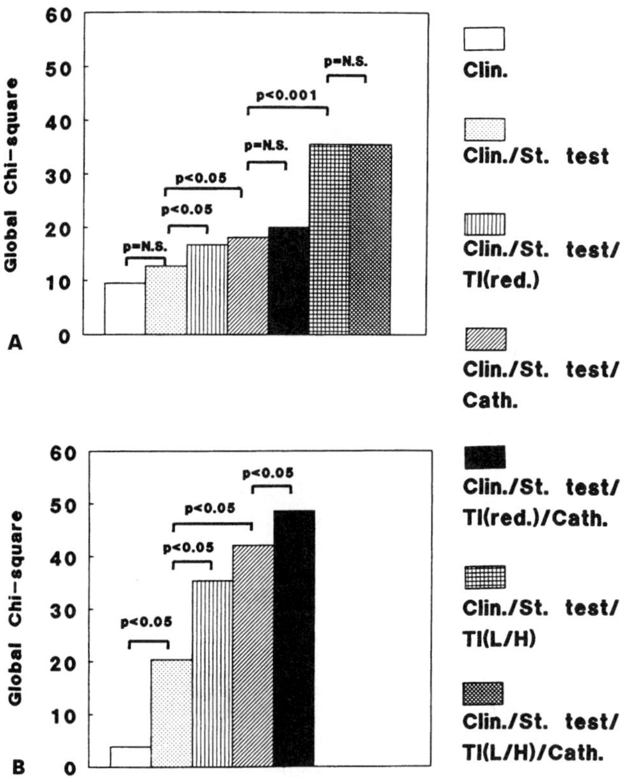

Fig 6-22 Incremental prognostic value (depicted by χ^2 value on y axis) of tests performed in a hierarchical order at Massachusetts General Hospital (**A**) and the University of Virginia (**B**). Clin., clinical; St., stress; Tl (red.), redistribution on ^{201}Tl imaging; T1 (L/H), lung/heart ^{201}Tl ratio; Cath., coronary angiography at cardiac catheterization. (From Pollock SG, Abbott RD, Boucher CA, et al: Independent and incremental prognostic value of tests performed in hierarchical order to evaluate patients with suspected coronary artery disease: validation of models based on these tests. *Circulation* 85:237-248, 1992. By permission of American Heart Association.)

significance—for example, a 50% narrowing in diameter in one of the major coronary arteries. Unequivocal evidence of exercise-induced ischemia in such a patient would confirm the hemodynamic significance of the lesion and prompt a more aggressive therapeutic approach. On the other hand, an entirely negative radionuclide angiogram or ^{201}Tl exercise study at a good level of exercise would indicate that the lesion was not of hemodynamic significance and probably would lead to more conservative clinical management. In addition, there are often clinical situations in which a patient's symptoms of chest pain seem to be out of proportion to the atherosclerotic lesion seen on coronary arteriography. In such a situation, radionuclide angiography or ^{201}Tl exercise testing would help to provide objective evidence that the patient's symptoms were due to myocardial ischemia.

^{201}Tl exercise testing is particularly useful in the evaluation of single-vessel disease. Multiple planar views or tomographic slides provide an opportunity to assess nearly all regions of the myocardium. Early studies using the subjective interpretation of planar ^{201}Tl images found that sensitivity was relatively poor for the detection of left circumflex coronary artery disease.[261] Subsequent reports using the quantification of planar ^{201}Tl images[138] and tomographic imaging[262] showed improvement in the detection of left circumflex disease, although left circumflex disease may still not be optimally detected. Although no formal studies have been published, ^{201}Tl scintigraphy is probably superior to radionuclide angiography for the detection of left anterior descending or right coronary artery disease. However, exercise equilibrium radionuclide angiography appears to be more sensitive than ^{201}Tl exercise testing for the detection of left circumflex disease,[263] presumably because it uses a left anterior oblique view that directly visualizes the lateral wall. In contrast to ^{201}Tl exercise testing, radionuclide angiography has the ability to assess ventricular performance at intermediate levels of exercise and thereby to determine whether functional evidence of ischemia is present at low levels of exercise (and, presumably, low levels of myocardial oxygen consumption).

Complications and therapy. Radionuclide angiography may be utilized to define further the extent and nature of the anatomic effects of coronary artery disease. It can specifically confirm the presence or absence of left ventricular aneurysm,[264,265] false left ventricular aneurysm,[266-268] and right ventricular infarction.[269-273] One of the earlier studies employing radionuclide angiography demonstrated its value as a noninvasive means of diagnosing the presence of left ventricular aneurysm. Although radionuclide angiography appears promising for this indication,[265] neither its sensitivity for the detection of left ventricular aneurysm nor its capabilities in relation to other modalities, such as two-dimensional echocardiography, are well documented. We have found the following three criteria to be most useful in the diagnosis of left ventricular aneurysm by radionuclide angiography: (1) distortion of the end-diastolic silhouette, (2) presence of a dyskinetic (or less often akinetic) segment, and (3) well-maintained residual motion in other segments, suggesting a "neck." When these criteria are used, a sizable majority of left ventricular aneurysms can be identified noninvasively by radionuclide angiography. In addition, the ejection fraction calculated from radionuclide angiography in such patients is often more reliable than that calculated from contrast ventriculography, because of the pronounced distortion of the cardiac silhouette in these cases and its effects on the geometric assumptions inherent in area-length methods.

Radionuclide angiography may also be employed to identify and quantitate right ventricular involvement in myocardial infarction, in both the acute and the chronic settings.[269-271] Both first-pass and equilibrium techniques have been successfully employed for the measurement of right ventricular ejection fraction in the setting of acute myocardial infarction. Several studies have demonstrated that the right ventricle is often involved in inferior myocardial infarction and that it is uncommonly involved in anterior myocardial infarction.[269,270] The presence of a right ventricular ejection fraction below normal limits in a patient with coronary artery disease, particularly in the presence of regional wall motion abnormalities of the left ventricle which suggest inferior myocardial infarction, is perhaps the best method available for the diagnosis of prior right ventricular infarction in patients with chronic ischemic heart disease. In extreme cases in which the myocardial infarction affects predominantly the right ventricle, this finding may have important therapeutic implications.

Myocardial viability. The differentiation of ischemic but viable myocardium from irreversible myocardial fibrosis in patients with abnormal global or regional ventricular function is an important issue in patients with chronic ischemic heart disease. The identification of such viable myocardium may influence the decision to proceed with coronary revascularization with either percutaneous transluminal coronary angioplasty or coronary artery bypass surgery. Although clinicians often assume that the degree of wall motion abnormality predicts the degree of myocardial fibrosis, autopsy studies have clearly demonstrated that there is often considerable discordance between the amount of fibrosis and the degree of regional wall motion revealed by contrast ventriculography,[274] radionuclide angiography,[275] or echocardiography.[276] Although radionuclide angiography with nitroglycerin[272,273] and with post-exercise imaging[277] has been used for this purpose, ^{201}Tl imaging generally provides better information about myocardial viability. Regions that demonstrate abnormal ^{201}Tl uptake immediately after exercise and complete or nearly complete redistribution by 4 hours are primarily composed of viable myocardium. If there is abnormal regional wall motion in these regions, it is very likely to improve after coronary artery bypass grafting.[93,278] Regions of initially abnormal ^{201}Tl uptake that did not demonstrate redistribution on 4-hour images were initially thought to represent myocardial fibrosis. However, many of these defects were demonstrated to have improved regional wall motion and ^{201}Tl uptake after coronary artery bypass grafting.[93,278] (Fig 6-23). Twenty-four-hour delayed imaging,[104,105] repeat imaging after thallium reinjection,[121,122] and rest thallium studies[127,128] help better differentiate areas of fibrosis from areas of viable myocardium. Even if a defect appears fixed, only mild or moderate reduction in thallium uptake indicates viable myocardium. If the area of viable myocardium is large enough and revascularization of this area is feasible, significant improvement in ventricular function can be expected after revascularization[128] (Fig 6-24).

Positron-emission tomography seems to be the best technique available for the determination of myocardial viability. Preserved myocardial uptake of fluorine-18-deoxyglucose, a tracer of exogenous glucose uptake, has been shown to be a reliable indicator of myocardial viability. Abnormal regional wall motion in regions in which glucose uptake is preserved will usually improve after coronary artery bypass grafting.[279] Several studies have demonstrated that positron-emission tomography is clearly superior to both planar and tomographic ^{201}Tl images that are obtained 4 hours after exercise stress.[280-282] When such 4-hour images are followed by reinjection of thallium and reimaging, the advantage of positron-emission tomography is considerably smaller. Thallium defects that are still fixed after reinjection usually contain viable myocardium if they are only mild or moderate in severity and generally do not contain viable myocardium if they are severe. When the severity of the fixed defect after reinjection is taken into account, the advantage of positron-emission tomography over thallium imaging is quite modest.

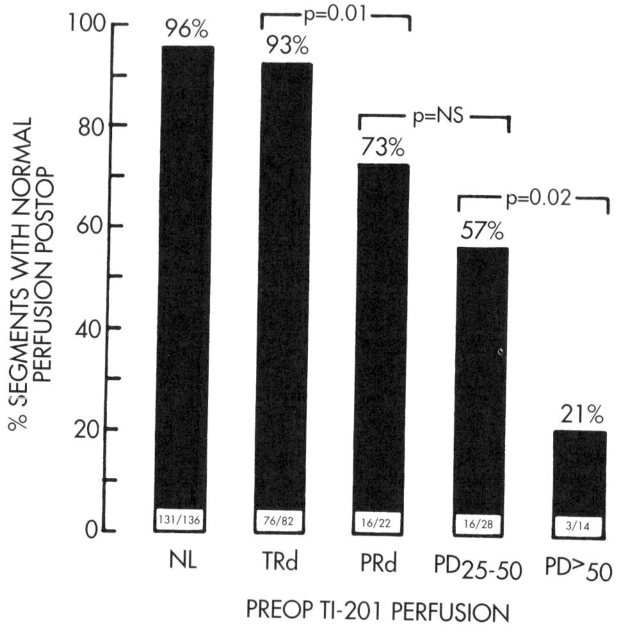

Fig 6-23 As preoperative perfusion abnormalities become progressively more severe (abscissa), the probability of restoring thallium uptake and washout to normal postoperatively (ordinate) becomes progressively less likely. NL, normal; NS, not significant; P, probability; PD, persistent defect; PRd, partial redistribution; TRd, total redistribution. (From Gibson RS, Watson DD, Taylor GJ, et al: Prospective assessment of regional myocardial perfusion before and after coronary revascularization surgery by quantitative thallium-201 scintigraphy. *J Am Coll Cardiol* 1:804-815, 1983. By permission of American College of Cardiology.)

Assessment of therapy. The final general area in which nuclear cardiology studies are potentially useful in the management of patients with chronic ischemic heart disease is in the assessment of therapeutic interventions. The most common intervention in such cases is the use of medical therapy, including long-acting nitrates and β-blocking agents. Radionuclide angiography may be employed with exercise before and after such therapy to assess its impact. Nitroglycerin reduces exercise-induced regional wall abnormalities and increases the ejection fraction achieved during exercise in patients with coronary artery disease.[273] Oral propranolol has also been shown to improve peak exercise left ventricular ejection fraction in patients with coronary artery disease.[283,284] Aortocoronary bypass grafting is obviously also commonly used in patients with chronic ischemic heart disease.

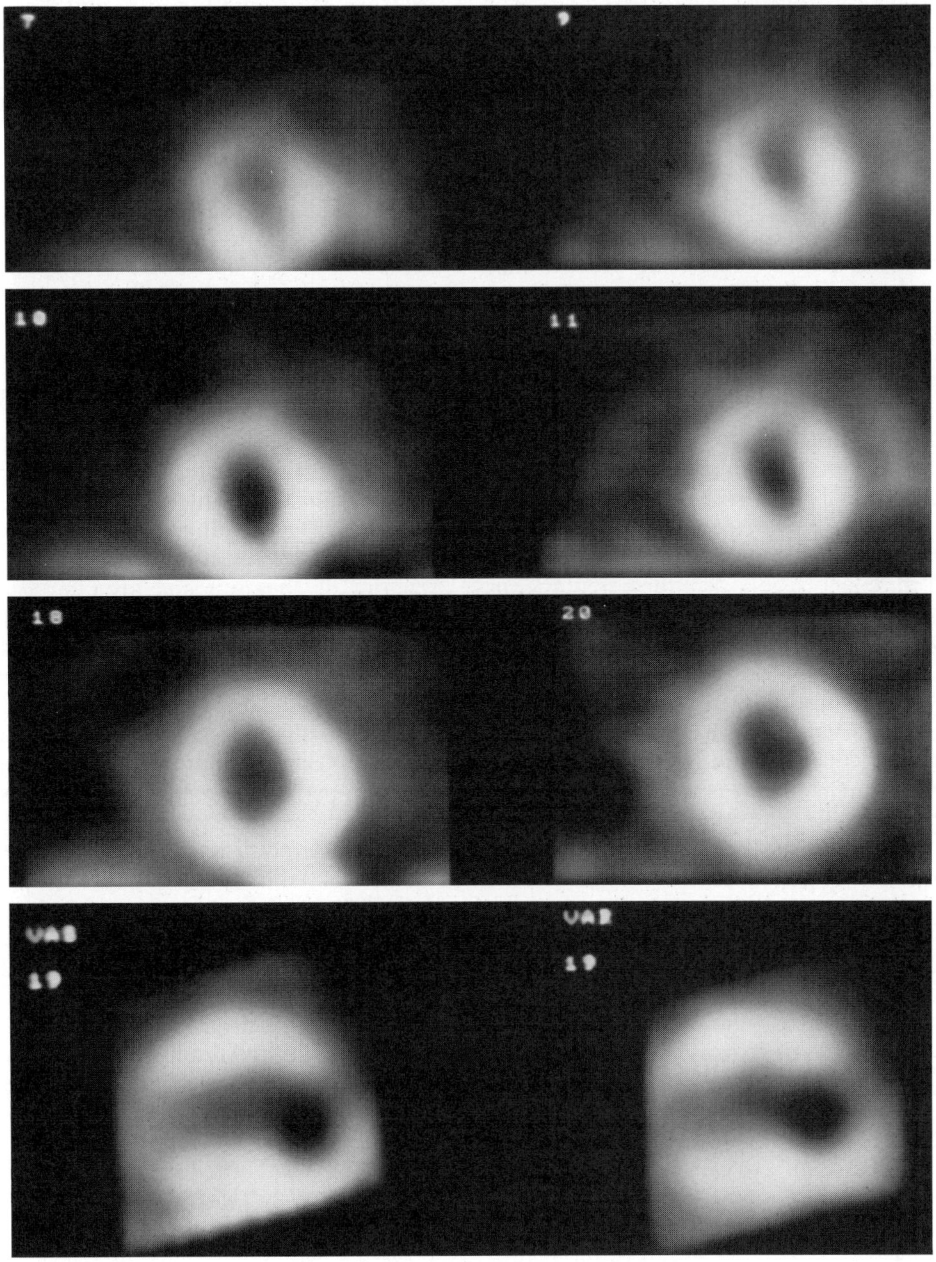

Fig 6-24 Tomographic thallium images obtained 30 minutes after resting injection **(left column)** and 7 hours later **(right column)** in a 66-year-old man with fatigue and severe left ventricular dysfunction. Three pairs of short-axis slices and a single pair of vertical long-axis slices are displayed in the same format as that in Figure 6-12. Uptake in the apex and in the anterior wall toward the apex is moderately decreased on both sets of images. After coronary artery bypass grafting, the patient's fatigue resolved and his resting ejection fraction improved from 23% to 33%. (From Patel TC, Gibbons RJ, Mullany CJ: Resting thallium-201 scintigraphy for identifying viable myocardium in a patient with severe left ventricular dysfunction. *Mayo Clin Proc* 68:63-67, 1993. By permission, Mayo Foundation.)

Radionuclide angiography has been employed before and after surgery to assess the effects of surgery on exercise ventricular function.[285-287] Patients who improve symptomatically after bypass grafting have generally been found to have pronounced improvement in their exercise ventricular function in comparison with their preoperative performance. On the other hand, in patients who continue to have symptoms despite coronary artery bypass grafting, the exercise left ventricular performance is virtually unchanged from that found preoperatively. Thus, radionuclide angiography may be employed to document the effects of coronary artery bypass grafting on exercise left ventricular function and to assess objectively the presence or absence of ischemia in patients whose symptoms continue after such surgery. ^{201}Tl may be used in the same setting to assess the patency of bypass grafts.[288,289] Finally, percutaneous transluminal coronary angioplasty is used as frequently as surgery in patients with chronic ischemic heart disease. Radionuclide angiography and ^{201}Tl exercise testing have been utilized to assess the effect of percutaneous transluminal coronary angioplasty on exercise ventricular function and exercise coronary blood flow, respectively.[290-292] Thallium exercise testing has been increasingly used to detect restenosis after percutaneous transluminal coronary angioplasty. In the first few weeks after angioplasty, an abnormal thallium exercise test result does not necessarily indicate restenosis, because many patients continue to have abnormal flow reserve early after angioplasty,[293,294] although there is some controversy about this point.[295] For this reason, it is generally best to defer the use of thallium exercise testing for at least 3 or 4 weeks after angioplasty.

Acute ischemic heart disease

Diagnosis. Although it has long been recognized that resting ^{201}Tl studies may demonstrate defects in the first 6 hours after an acute ischemic event,[296-299] they have not been widely employed in the diagnosis of acute myocardial infarction because of their expense and the absence of any clear advantage over more conventional methods (clinical history, ECG, and cardiac enzyme determinations). More recent studies of myocardial perfusion imaging using ^{99m}Tc sestamibi have demonstrated the ability of this technique to identify patients without ECG ST elevation who have severe perfusion defects consistent with coronary occlusion.[300] Such occlusions often involve a left circumflex coronary artery territory, which is relatively silent on ECG examination. Although this approach is promising because patients may benefit from thrombolytic therapy, its clinical value has yet to be demonstrated. ^{99m}Tc PP scanning, on the other hand, does have a definite, though limited, role in the diagnosis of acute myocardial infarction. It is most often employed in patients in whom a definitive diagnosis cannot be made by more conventional means.[301,302] This may occur in the following settings: (1) the presence of otherwise equivocal data; (2) the presence of ECG abnormalities, such as permanent pacing or left bundle-branch block, which prevents useful ECG analysis; (3) the evaluation of a patient 3 to 7 days after an acute myocardial event, when cardiac enzymes are unlikely to provide a definitive diagnosis but when ^{99m}Tc PP scanning may still be positive; and (4) immediately after coronary artery bypass grafting, when both the ECG and the cardiac enzymes are likely to demonstrate relatively nonspecific abnormalities.

The sensitivity of the technique in series of consecutive patients approaches 90%,[178] but its sensitivity for the detection of nontransmural infarction is considerably lower.[182,303] Increased uptake may be seen in a wide variety of other conditions, including unstable angina, valvular calcification, cardioversion, and myocardial contusion.[178]

As mentioned above, radionuclide angiography may be used in the setting of acute myocardial infarction for the purpose of the noninvasive identification of right ventricular infarction. The diagnosis of right ventricular infarction in the acute setting, however, will often be made from invasive hemodynamic measurements.[304,305]

Although patients with rest angina often have diagnostic ECG changes during chest pain, many do not. There is early evidence that myocardial perfusion imaging may be of value in such patients for the diagnosis of ischemic heart disease and the delineation of the extent and severity of the ischemic area.[175,176] Grégoire et al.[175] injected ^{99m}Tc sestamibi during episodes of spontaneous chest pain in a series of 45 patients. The ability of perfusion defects on subsequent tomographic imaging to identify significant coronary artery disease was clearly superior to that of the resting ECG obtained during pain. Follow-up images after a repeat injection when the patient was no longer having pain usually showed improvement, although some patients still had a residual perfusion defect. This approach has been used clinically at Mayo in patients with uninterpretable ECGs and to better define the "culprit" angiographic lesion for revascularization.

Response to therapy. As discussed elsewhere, multiple randomized trials have now demonstrated that acute thrombolytic therapy reduces mortality in myocardial infarction.[306-308] Attempts to demonstrate that thrombolytic therapy reduces infarct size have produced less consistent results.[308-317] Infarct size has been assessed by the resting ejection fraction measured after infarction,[308-315] the size of the ^{201}Tl defect after infarction,[315-317] and the change in resting ejection fraction measured during and after infarction.[309,314] These measurements have obviously frequently involved nuclear cardiology studies. However, these end points do not easily permit an assessment of treatment benefit in an individual patient, as they do not accurately measure the amount of myocardium that is at risk.

^{99m}Tc sestamibi has properties well suited to the measurement of myocardium at risk.[166,167] Although its initial uptake by normal myocardium is directly proportional to myocardial blood flow, it has a very slow washout independent of blood flow and, therefore, demonstrates minimal redistribution over time. Patients with acute infarction can, therefore, receive an injection of ^{99m}Tc sestamibi at the time of initial presentation, be subsequently treated with thrombolytic agents or percutaneous transluminal coronary angioplasty (or both), and then undergo imaging hours later to provide an accurate assessment of myocardial blood flow at the time of presentation.[172-174] The 140-keV emission and the 30-mCi administered dose of this agent provide high-count density images that can be readily quantitated. Phantom studies using tomographic imaging with this radiopharmaceutical have demonstrated that it is highly accurate for the measurement of perfusion defects.[318] In animal models of coronary occlusion, there is a close agreement between the perfusion defect measured by tomographic ^{99m}Tc sestamibi imaging and the subsequent quantitation of histologic infarction.[319] In animal models of coronary reperfusion, a perfusion defect measured by ^{99m}Tc sestamibi imaging correlates closely with the angiographic area at risk when sestamibi is injected during coronary occlusion, and the perfusion defect measured by sestamibi imaging correlates closely with histologic infarct size when the agent is injected after reperfusion.[320] Thus, these studies suggest that the isotope may be injected during occlusion to measure area at risk and after reperfusion to measure final infarct size. The difference between these two measurements is presumably a measure of myocardial salvage, or treatment efficacy.

The initial case report of the use of ^{99m}Tc sestamibi in acute infarction suggested that this technique offered great promise.[172] Subsequent series using both planar[173]

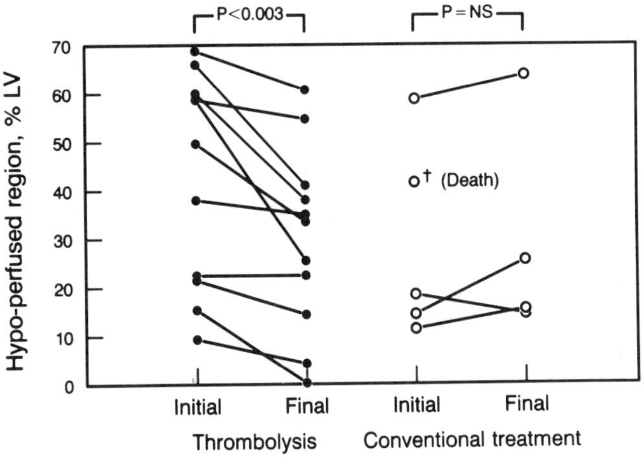

Fig 6-25 The change in hypoperfused myocardium as a percentage of the left ventricle *(% LV)* in patients with acute myocardial infarction, as measured by ^{99m}Tc sestamibi. Injections for the initial study were performed before acute therapy. The final study was performed 6 to 14 days later. Patients treated with IV thrombolysis had a significant improvement in hypoperfused myocardium between the initial and final images. Patients treated with conventional treatment did not. *NS,* not significant. (From Gibbons RJ, Verani MS, Behrenbeck T, et al: Feasibility of tomographic technetium-99m-hexakis-2-methoxy-2-methylpropyl-isonitrile imaging for the assessment of myocardial area at risk and efficacy of thrombolytic therapy in acute myocardial infarction. *Circulation* 80:1277-1286, 1989. By permission of American Heart Association.)

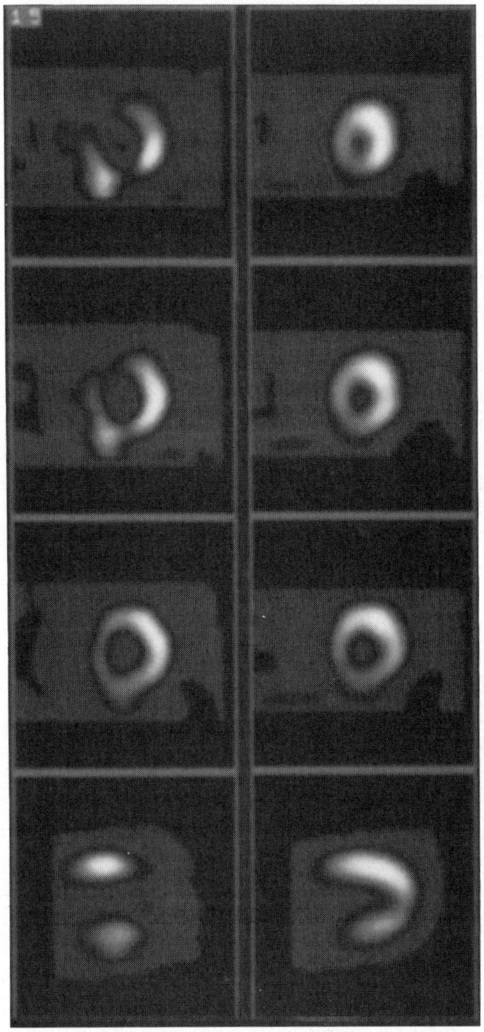

Fig 6-26 Tomographic technetium-99m sestamibi images obtained after injection in the emergency room **(left column)** and 1 week later **(right column)** in a 76-year-old man with acute anterior myocardial infarction. Three sets of short-axis images and one set of vertical long-axis images are displayed in the same format at that in Figure 6-12. The images obtained after injection in the emergency room showed a large perfusion defect, measuring 47% of the left ventricle, involving the anterior wall, anterior septum, and apex. The patient was treated successfully with direct coronary angioplasty after severe chest pain lasting 4 hours. The images obtained 1 week later are within normal limits. Final infarct size measured from these images was 0% of the left ventricle.

and tomographic[174] imaging have demonstrated that the change in perfusion defect between the initial images and follow-up images (typically obtained before dismissal) is a sensitive measurement tool for the assessment of the efficacy of acute therapy (Figs 6-25 and 6-26). This tool has provided a number of important insights:

1. Myocardium at risk varies widely, even for patients with a similar coronary occlusion.[321] This ob-

servation parallels previous observations in animal models.

2. The extent of the late perfusion defect 6 to 10 days after infarction appears to reflect the extent of infarction, because it correlates with ejection fraction at dismissal,[174] 6 weeks,[322] and 1 year,[323] with regional wall motion at dismissal[174] and 6 weeks,[322] and with end-systolic volume index at 1 year.[323]
3. The effectiveness of acute therapy can be assessed in individual patients as well as in groups of patients. Most of the variability in final infarct size can be explained by myocardium at risk, collateral flow, and time to reperfusion.[324]
4. Discrepancies between perfusion and mechanical function at dismissal may be related to both stunning and hyperkinesia.[322] The assessment of mechanical function at dismissal may therefore provide misleading information about infarct size in many patients.
5. Myocardium at risk and final infarct size are much greater for anterior infarction than for inferior infarction.[325] The absolute benefit of treating inferior infarction is therefore greater, although there is no intrinsic difference in the response to therapy in anterior and inferior infarctions.

Prognosis. Nuclear cardiology techniques have been used widely for the assessment of patient prognosis after acute myocardial infarction. There are several consistent themes in the voluminous literature from the prethrombolytic era. The first is that the extent of myocardial infarction is a major determinant of subsequent patient outcome.[242,326] Infarct size may be assessed by either radionuclide angiography[242] or myocardial perfusion imaging.[326] Resting ejection fraction measured by radionuclide angiography at dismissal is a powerful predictor of mortality[242] (Fig 6-27). It provides information that is complementary to clinical data and predictive of both short-term and long-term outcome. Patients with an ejection fraction of less than 20% have a 1-year cardiac mortality that approaches 50%. The extent of the ^{201}Tl perfusion defect on a resting planar ^{201}Tl scan within 15 hours of admission for an acute ischemic event is also a powerful predictor of subsequent patient mortality.[326] The 1-year survival exceeds 90% in patients with a low-risk scan. The 1-year survival is less than 20% in patients with a high-risk scan. A comparison of the prognostic value of the dismissal resting ejection fraction and resting planar ^{201}Tl perfusion defect size found that perfusion defect size was almost twice as powerful as the left ventricular ejection fraction for the prediction of subsequent mortality.[327] The ability of tomographic ^{201}Tl perfusion defect size to accurately quantitate infarct size has been demonstrated in several animal studies.[328,329] This technique has been used as an end point in several trials of thrombolytic therapy.[315-317]

The second consistent theme on patient outcome after acute myocardial infarction is the importance of the presence and extent of exercise-induced ischemia. The prognostic value of exercise radionuclide angiography performed in the first few weeks after acute myocardial infarction was demonstrated by Corbett et al.[330] They found that 95% of patients whose ejection fraction did not increase with exercise had cardiac events within 6 months, compared with 9% of patients whose ejection fraction increased with exercise. These results were subsequently confirmed by other investigators.[241,331] The value of planar exercise ^{201}Tl testing has also been clearly demonstrated (Table 6-11). Gibson et al.[332] found that ^{201}Tl was significantly more effective than the exercise ECG or the coronary angiogram in the identification of patients at low risk for subsequent cardiac events (Fig 6-28). All three modalities were similar in their ability to identify high-risk patients. Several other studies have confirmed these findings. In patients who are unable to exercise, dipyridamole ^{201}Tl scintigraphy is a useful alternative.[335] Multiple studies have demonstrated that reversible ^{201}Tl defects after administration of dipyridamole are associated with an increased risk of subsequent cardiac events. Two studies[339,340] suggested that dipyridamole may be used for risk stratification as early as 3 days after the acute event. Adenosine ^{201}Tl scintigraphy performed 5 days after acute infarction predicts cardiac events during the initial hospitalization.[343] Exercise ^{201}Tl scintigraphy and exercise radionuclide angiography have been directly compared in very few studies. In a study of 117 patients, Hung et al.[331] found that the single best predictor of subsequent cardiac events was the exercise-induced change in ejection fraction at a limited bicycle workload. The only other variable that added independent prognostic information was peak treadmill workload. ^{201}Tl findings were important on a univariate basis but did

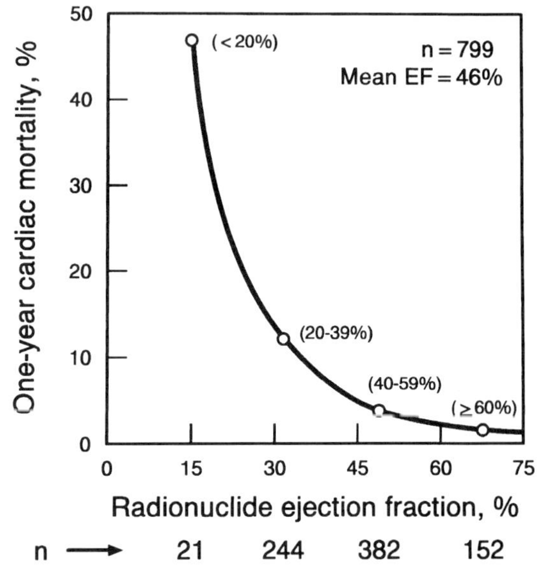

Fig 6-27 One-year cardiac mortality after dismissal following acute myocardial infarction as a function of the resting ejection fraction *(EF)* determined by equilibrium radionuclide angiography before dismissal. *n,* number of patients in each category and the total population. (From The Multicenter Postinfarction Research Group: Risk stratification and survival after myocardial infarction. *N Engl J Med* 309:331-336, 1983. By permission of the Journal.)

Table 6-11 Prognostic value of ^{201}Tl imaging after myocardial infarction

Study	Types of stress	No. of patients	Mean time after MI (days)	Mean follow-up (mo)	Catheterization data	RNA	Cardiac events	Significant multivariate predictors of cardiac events: ^{201}Tl	Other
Gibson et al.[332]	Submax ex	140	11	15	+	0	Death, MI, UA	RD, MSD, ↑ lung uptake	2 or 3 DV, ST ↓, AP
Hung et al.[331]	Max ex	117	21	12	0	+	Death, MI, VF	Extent of RD,* extent of SD*	Δ LVEF, peak workload
Abraham et al.[333]	Max ex	103	24	12	+	0	Death, MI, VF, UA	NIZ SD*	ST ↓ *
Wilson et al.[334]	Submax ex	97	11	39	+	0	Death, MI, UA	Number of RD*	None
Leppo et al.[335]	DP	51	10-16	19	0	+	Death, MI	RD*	None
Pirelli et al.[336]	DP	35	9	11	0	0	Death, MI, new AP	RD	None
Younis et al.[337]	DP	77	9	12	+	0	Death, MI, UA, CABG	RD	Number of DV
							Death, MI	RD	Number of DV, LVEF
Gimple et al.[338]	DP, submax ex, max ex	40	NA	6	0	+	Death, MI, VF, UA	NIZ RD*	None
Brown et al.[339]	DP	50	2.6	12	+	0	Death, MI, UA	IZ RD	None
Bosch et al.[340]	DP	76	3	NA	0	0	Death, MI, CABG	RD*	None
Gibson et al.[341]	Submax ex	241	10	30	+	+	Death, MI, CABG	IZ RD*	NA
Brown et al.[342]	Max ex	61	10 mo	37	+	0	Death, MI	IZ RD	None
							Death, MI, UA	IZ RD	None
							Death, MI, UA, CABG	Any RD	2 or 3 DV

AP, angina pectoris; CABG, coronary artery bypass graft surgery; DP, dipyridamole; DV, diseased vessels; ex, exercise; IZ, infarct zone; LVEF, left ventricular ejection fraction; max, maximal; MI, myocardial infarction; MSD, multiple stress defects; NA, not available; NIZ, noninfarct zone; RD, reversible defects; RNA, radionuclide angiogram; SD, stress defect; ST ↓, ST segment depression; submax, submaximal; UA, unstable angina; VF, ventricular fibrillation.

*In some studies, multivariate analysis was not performed; variables listed are significant univariate predictors. In one study, univariate ^{201}Tl predictors are included, although they were not multivariate predictors when other data were available.

Modified from Brown KA: Prognostic value of thallium-201 myocardial perfusion imaging; a diagnostic tool comes of age. *Circulation* 83:363-381, 1991.

not add any information once the change in ejection fraction was known.

It has been increasingly recognized that application of these data from the prethrombolytic era to current patients who have been treated with thrombolysis is problematic. The current patient population is clearly changing. One study from our laboratory[344] found that there were highly significant trends over time in multiple clinical variables in patients at predismissal exercise testing, suggesting that previously published results may no longer apply to current patient populations. Patients in whom predismissal testing is performed after thrombolysis are certainly different. There is increasing use of early β-blockade, intravenous thrombolysis, and early coronary angiography. As a result, patients in the current era who receive predismissal testing are a low-risk group with a much lower long-term event rate. Early studies suggest that our ability to predict subsequent cardiac events in such patients with a low likelihood of subsequent events is quite limited.[345,346]

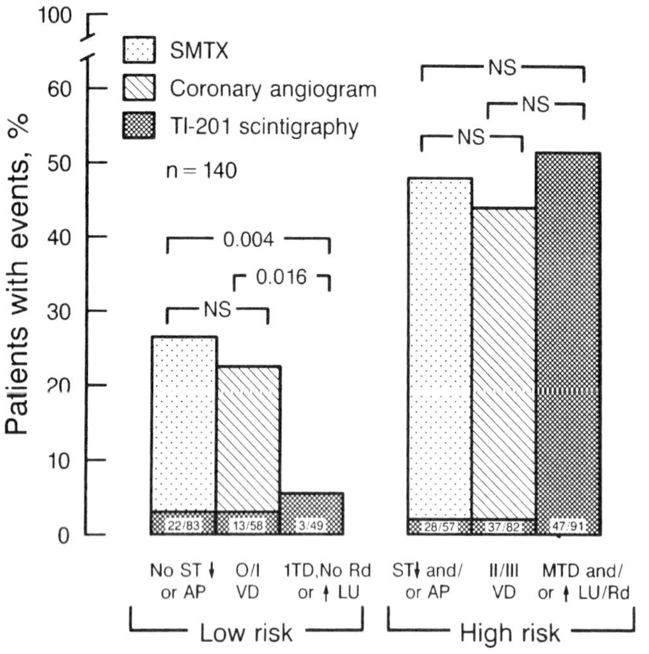

Fig 6-28 Cardiac event rate after myocardial infarction in high-risk and low-risk subgroups of patients defined by the results of submaximal treadmill exercise testing *(SMTX),* coronary angiography, and planar thallium 201 *(Tl-201)* exercise scintigraphy. The high-risk subgroups identified by each test had a similar incidence of subsequent events. The low-risk subgroup identified by thallium 201 scintigraphy had a significantly lower incidence of subsequent events. *AP,* angina pectoris; *↑ LU,* increased lung uptake; *MTD,* multiple thallium defects; *NS,* not significant; *Rd,* redistribution; *ST ↓*, ST segment depression; *TD,* thallium defect; *VD,* diseased vessels. (From Gibson RS, Watson DD, Craddock GB, et al: Prediction of cardiac events after uncomplicated myocardial infarction: a prospective study comparing predischarge exercise thallium-201 scintigraphy and coronary angiography. *Circulation* 68:321-336, 1983. By permission of American Heart Association.)

Valvular heart disease

Nuclear cardiology procedures have little place at this time in the assessment of stenotic valvular lesions other than the noninvasive assessment of coexistent coronary artery disease. The principal role of nuclear cardiology procedures in valvular heart disease is the use of equilibrium radionuclide angiography to assess left-sided regurgitant lesions, that is, mitral and aortic insufficiency, although the use of radionuclide angiography to assess tricuspid insufficiency has also been reported.[347]

In patients with mitral or aortic insufficiency (or both), radionuclide angiography can be used to measure resting left ventricular size and resting left ventricular ejection fraction. Left ventricular volume estimates obtained by radionuclide angiography in such patients with large left ventricles are subject to greater than usual error because of the increased attenuation of counts from the distant portions of the left ventricle. In addition, previously published studies validating volume measurements have included relatively few patients with very large hearts. Despite these potential limitations in the measurement of absolute volumes, measurements of changes in volume in the same patient remain highly accurate; these changes in volume have been used to assess the response to exercise[348-355] and the long-term response to medical therapy.[37]

Measurements of resting ejection fraction in patients with aortic insufficiency are highly accurate by equilibrium radionuclide angiography. Although the measurement of ejection fraction by contrast ventriculography may be somewhat inaccurate in patients with severe left ventricular dilatation, such dilatation increases the counts within the left ventricle, thereby improving the accuracy of equilibrium radionuclide angiography. Unfortunately, this increase in accuracy due to reduced statistical fluctuation may be offset by an increased degree of left atrial and left ventricular overlap in patients with mitral insufficiency. Although this overlap can be reduced somewhat by increased caudal-cranial angulation of the gamma camera, it can usually not be eliminated when there is severe left atrial enlargement.

As described above, left-sided regurgitation can be quantitated by measurement of the regurgitant fraction and left ventricular output. Such measurements are primarily useful when the magnitude of regurgitation is not readily evident on clinical assessment. This is particularly true when mitral regurgitation is associated with severe left ventricular enlargement and the magnitude of mitral regurgitation is not readily apparent.

Radionuclide angiography can contribute important information to the timing of valve replacement in patients with severe left-sided regurgitation. Patients with aortic regurgitation remain asymptomatic for many years despite substantial volume overload of the left ventricle. After symptoms appear, patients treated medically often decline rapidly. For that reason, there is general agreement that symptomatic patients with aortic insufficiency should undergo aortic valve replacement.[356] The timing of aortic valve replacement in asymptomatic or minimally symptomatic patients is much more controversial. The long-term results of aortic valve replacement in patients with chronic insufficiency are somewhat disappointing, with many late postoperative deaths related to chronic congestive heart failure.[357] These late deaths presumably reflect the development of irreversible left ventricular dysfunction from long-standing volume overload. There has been great interest, therefore, in the identification of such patients earlier in the natural history of their disorder, when aortic valve replacement may prevent development of irreversible left ventricular dysfunction. The benefit of earlier aortic valve replacement must, however, outweigh the risks of surgery as well as the subsequent risk of a prosthetic heart valve.

The timing of aortic valve replacement in aortic insufficiency has been the subject of a series of studies from the National Institutes of Health.[356-361] Preoperative ventricular function, as determined by the measurement

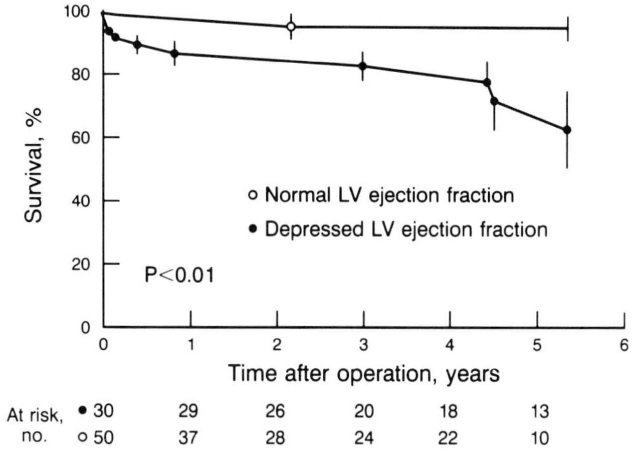

Fig 6-29 Survival of patients with aortic insufficiency following aortic valve replacement. Preoperative resting left ventricular *(LV)* ejection fraction is a major determinant of postoperative survival. (From Bonow RO, Picone AL, McIntosh CL, et al: Survival and functional results after valve replacement for aortic regurgitation from 1976 to 1983: impact of preoperative left ventricular function. *Circulation* 72:1244-1256, 1985. By permission of American Heart Association.)

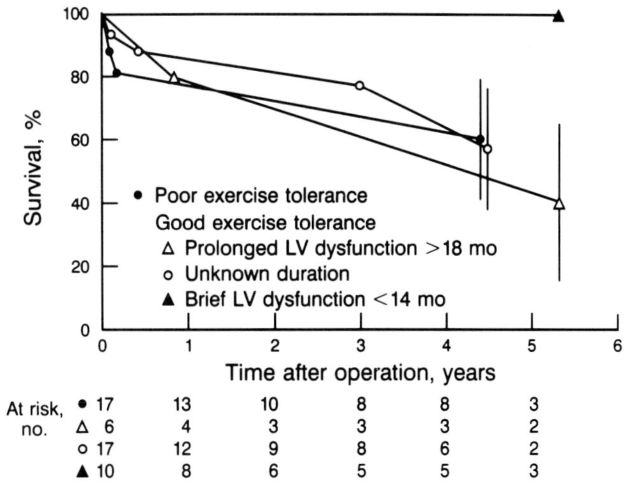

Fig 6-30 Survival of patients with aortic insufficiency and abnormal preoperative resting left ventricular *(LV)* ejection fraction following aortic valve replacement. Preoperative exercise tolerance and the duration of preoperative left ventricular dysfunction are determinants of survival. (From Bonow RO, Picone AL, McIntosh CL, et al: Survival and functional results after valve replacement for aortic regurgitation from 1976 to 1983: impact of preoperative left ventricular function. *Circulation* 72:1244-1256, 1985. By permission of American Heart Association.)

of resting ejection fraction by equilibrium radionuclide angiography, is clearly associated with postoperative survival (Fig 6-29). Patients with a normal preoperative ejection fraction had a far better long-term survival rate than patients with an abnormal preoperative ejection fraction. In patients with an abnormal preoperative ejection fraction, two other factors are associated with postoperative death—the duration of abnormal left ventricular function and exercise tolerance (Fig 6-30). Poor exercise tolerance and abnormal resting function that had been present for at least 18 months are both associated with poor postoperative survival (see Fig 6-30). On the basis of these findings, the periodic measurement of resting ejection fraction in patients with asymptomatic or minimally symptomatic aortic insufficiency appears reasonable. Patients with a progressive decline in systolic function are more likely to require operative intervention.[361] In most cases, aortic valve replacement can be safely postponed until the resting ejection fraction becomes abnormal or until symptoms develop. With this strategy, relatively few patients require aortic valve replacement each year, and preoperative death is rare.[359] More importantly, postoperative resting function returns to normal and postoperative survival is excellent.[360]

Earlier studies[349] had suggested that an abnormal ejection fraction response to exercise might be an early sign of impending irreversible left ventricular dysfunction. The ejection fraction response to exercise is clearly influenced by the marked changes in ventricular loading that occur in patients with aortic insufficiency. The change in ejection fraction with exercise correlates with end-systolic pressure volume ratio[362] and with resting systolic wall stress[363,364] but not with left ventricular filling pressure.[365] Changes in ventricular volumes and ejection fraction during exercise are highly variable and depend on when patients are studied in the natural history of their disease.[350,355,362] In patients with an increase in ejection fraction during exercise, left ventricular dysfunction or symptoms are unlikely to develop during the next few years. However, the magnitude of decrease in ejection fraction with exercise does not appear to predict the subsequent course. Thus, although exercise radionuclide angiography can identify a subgroup of patients who are unlikely to warrant aortic valve replacement in the next few years, its routine use for follow-up cannot be justified.

Radionuclide angiography may also be used to assess the effects of aortic valve replacement on left ventricular function at rest and during exercise.[366,367] It must be recognized that altered loading conditions in the early postoperative period may cause a decrease in resting ejection fraction, but this does not necessarily reflect a decline in contractility.

The use of radionuclide angiography in patients with severe mitral regurgitation has received far less attention.[368-370] Resting right ventricular ejection fraction has been clearly associated with exercise tolerance.[368] Both resting right ventricular ejection fraction and resting left ventricular ejection fraction have been shown to predict survival in patients treated medically. Further studies are clearly warranted.

Cardiomyopathy

Nuclear cardiology studies are useful in the evaluation of patients with suspected congestive cardiomyopathy. Resting radionuclide angiography alone can provide objective documentation of left ventricular size and ejection fraction. In patients with severe left ventricular dysfunction, a nongeometric measurement of ejection fraction by this technique has clear advantages over contrast ventriculography or echocardiography, both of which rely on geometric assumptions. The radionuclide angiographic measurements of ejection fraction in a low ejection fraction range are highly reproducible because the increased counts within the left ventricle minimize statistical fluctuation in the measurement. Accurate measurements of left ventricular ejection fraction below 0.25 have great prognostic significance.[371,372] The common belief that there is little prognostic difference between an ejection fraction of 0.15 and one of 0.20 is clearly erroneous. The curve relating patient survival to ejection fraction in this range is quite steep, so that a difference in ejection fraction between 0.15 and 0.20 is much more prognostically important than a difference between 0.45 and 0.50. The prognostic importance of ejection fraction measurements in the low ejection fraction range has been clearly demonstrated in several studies[371,372] (Fig 6-31).

Both resting radionuclide angiography and ^{201}Tl perfusion scans can provide clues about the cause of the cardiomyopathy. Regional wall motion abnormalities that are substantially greater in one segment than in another are more likely in patients with ischemic cardiomyopathy, although they may occur in congestive cardiomyopathy as well.[373] Right ventricular dilatation is more common in patients with congestive cardiomyopathy. These clues on cause from radionuclide angiography usually do not

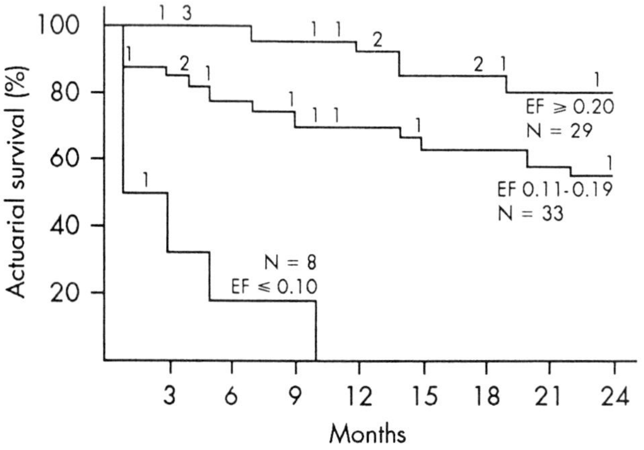

Fig 6-31 Actuarial survival in idiopathic cardiomyopathy according to ejection fraction (EF) on radionuclide scan. Group 1, left ventricular EF ≤ 0.10 (n = 8); group 2, left ventricular EF 0.11 to 0.19 (n = 33); group 3, left ventricular EF ≥ 0.20 (n = 29). (From Keogh AM, Freund J, Baron DW, et al: Timing of cardiac transplantation in idiopathic dilated cardiomyopathy. *Am J Cardiol* 61:418-422, 1988. By permission of Cahners Publishing Company, a Division of Reed Publishing USA.)

permit a definite diagnosis. However, ^{201}Tl perfusion scans, performed either at rest or as part of a stress study after thallium reinjection, may permit better differentiation of ischemic cardiomyopathy from congestive cardiomyopathy.[374] Large, severe perfusion defects are present in most patients with ischemic cardiomyopathies and are rare in congestive cardiomyopathies.[375,376] Patients with ejection fractions below 0.20 on an ischemic basis usually have severe perfusion defects that involve more than one-half of the left ventricle. When the perfusion defects are less severe and less extensive despite other evidence supporting an ischemic cause (known myocardial infarction, occluded coronary arteries, definite redistribution on stress or rest perfusion imaging), the possibility of hibernating myocardium should be entertained. Even when both radionuclide angiography and ^{201}Tl perfusion scintigraphy are performed, a definite cause cannot be established noninvasively in some patients. Coronary angiography frequently provides a definitive diagnosis in such patients. However, a subset of patients remains with significant coronary artery disease in whom left ventricular dysfunction appears to be out of proportion to the severity of the coronary artery disease. It is often difficult to establish whether such patients have had previous myocardial infarction due to plaque rupture at the site of mild coronary stenoses that later recanalized or have a second contributing condition, such as alcohol abuse.

Radionuclide angiography may obviously give assistance in the medical management and follow-up of patients with congestive cardiomyopathy. Since the clinical course of these patients is quite variable, radionuclide angiography may be used as an objective means of assessing any temporal change in left ventricular size or function. The response to therapeutic interventions, such as vasodilator therapy, abstention from alcohol, and corticosteroids in selected cases, may also be objectively assessed in this fashion.[377,378] Such information may be of great benefit in the clinical management of these patients.

Congenital heart disease

Nuclear cardiology studies have a limited role in patients with congenital heart disease.

The most common indication for radionuclide angiography in a patient with congenital heart disease is the detection and quantification of a left-to-right shunt. This is done by employing a first-pass study. As mentioned earlier, such studies are optimally performed with multicrystal cameras that provide very high count rates. In the absence of such cameras, however, studies for this purpose may be generally performed satisfactorily with a standard gamma camera. The technique employed was first described by Maltz and Treves[379] in 1973. The basic requirement is the development of a time-activity histogram from the passage of the radioactive bolus through the pulmonary circulation. This pulmonic flow curve is then fitted with a gamma variate function, for which a least-squares method is used.[74-76,380] The main difficulty in this approach is the determination of whether the gamma variate function fitted to the original raw data is satisfactory. It is important that the bolus entering the heart be "tight," and so injection in an external jugular vein or a central vein through a long indwelling catheter is preferred. Experience is required to obtain accurate and reproducible results with this method. The reported correlation between the $\dot{Q}p:\dot{Q}s$ ratio obtained by this technique and that obtained at cardiac catheterization is excellent; Askenazi et al.[76] reported a correlation coefficient of 0.94 in 105 patients.

The assessment of left and right ventricular function is also often useful in patients with congenital heart disease. The validity of measurements of right and left ventricular ejection fractions in a pediatric population has been demonstrated.[381] Patients with congenital mitral or aortic insufficiency may be evaluated at rest and with exercise as described previously. Radionuclide angiography has also been employed in the assessment of right heart function in patients with complex congenital heart disease, and it offers a technique by which right heart function can be serially measured noninvasively after operative repair of complex congenital lesions.[382,383] Both exercise radionuclide angiography and stress thallium perfusion imaging may be used in patients with suspected or proven congenital anomalies of a coronary artery. Such testing often establishes that perfusion or function is inadequate in response to exercise and thereby influences patient management.

Preoperative assessment for noncardiac surgery

Nuclear cardiology techniques have been widely studied for the preoperative assessment of patients undergoing noncardiac surgery, particularly major vascular surgical procedures.[384-388] Such patients are at increased risk for general anesthesia for several reasons. First, peripheral vascular disease is a well-recognized marker for coronary artery disease. Second, the cardiac stress associated with peripheral vascular procedures is greater, particularly because of aortic cross-clamping. Third, patients with peripheral vascular disease are often unable to exercise. As a result, they may have few, if any, symptoms of angina despite having very severe underlying coronary artery disease. In patients who can still exercise, exercise radionuclide angiography may be of value. Limited exercise capacity on such a study indicates that the patient is at increased cardiac risk, although the ejection fraction and regional wall motion measurements performed on such studies have not been shown to add any significant additional information.[384] Because many patients scheduled to undergo vascular surgery cannot exercise, myocardial perfusion imaging with pharmacologic stress has become the preferred modality for preoperative assessment. Most of the published data are based on IV administration of dipyridamole in association with thallium perfusion scintigraphy, although more recent studies have used adenosine and sestamibi scintigraphy, with apparently similar results.[389,390] The published studies of dipyridamole ^{201}Tl scintigraphy for preoperative assessment have generally shown that redistribution on dipyridamole imaging is associated with a high risk of perioperative cardiac events (Table 6-12). Patients with normal dipyridamole images or fixed perfusion defects have a very low risk (less than 5%) of perioperative cardiac events. One published study was unable to confirm these findings;[394] however, the cardiac event rate in this study was unusually low, suggesting that patient selection may have contributed to this discrepancy.

Dipyridamole ^{201}Tl imaging appears to be complementary to clinical assessment for preoperative risk stratification. Eagle et al.[387,388] have published several studies demonstrating the importance of an integrated approach that incorporates both clinical assessment and ^{201}Tl imaging. They have advocated an approach that uses clinical assessment as the first level of screening. If clinical variables that predict an increased level of cardiac risk (history of angina, ventricular ectopy requiring treatment, Q waves, diabetes, and age greater than 70) are absent, the risk of perioperative cardiac events is low and ^{201}Tl imaging does not appear to be cost-effective. With three or more such clinical risk factors, the perioperative risk is high regardless of the ^{201}Tl results, although patients with such high risk are uncommon. ^{201}Tl imaging appears to be most appropriate in patients with one or two clinical risk factors (Fig 6-32). Redistribution on ^{201}Tl imaging in such patients is associated with a risk of perioperative cardiac events that is nine times greater than that in patients without redistribution.

Several studies have suggested that the extent and severity of reversible defects should also be incorporated into clinical decision-making. Lane et al.[393] found that the perioperative risk of cardiac events in diabetic patients undergoing vascular surgery was directly related to the number of reversible ^{201}Tl defects. Patients with a large number of reversible defects had a threefold greater increase in the rate of perioperative cardiac events than patients with a small number of reversible defects. Lette et al.[391] found that the extent and severity of reversible ^{201}Tl defects could identify a significant subgroup of patients with a very high rate of perioperative death and myocardial infarction. At the Mayo Clinic, we have found that the rate of perioperative cardiac events is still low for a single small, reversible perfusion defect. Such a defect is generally not a cause for great concern and is not sufficient to warrant further evaluation with coronary angiography. During the past decade, we have followed a strategy of clinical assessment with very selective use of nuclear cardiology studies, coronary angiography, and coronary revascularization before vascular surgery. This strategy has been highly successful. The perioperative mortality in 2,452 patients was only 2.9%.[395]

Other indications

Radionuclide angiography may be employed in a variety of other clinical situations, which will be briefly outlined in this section.

Patients with severe chronic obstructive pulmonary disease may ultimately experience cor pulmonale. The early diagnosis of this condition is difficult by any means. The measurement of right ventricular ejection fraction by radionuclide angiography, both at rest and with exercise, may provide evidence of early cor pulmonale. Berger and

Table 6-12 Value of dipyridamole and ^{201}Tl imaging for perioperative risk stratification

Study	No. of patients	Types of surgery	Cardiac events	Significant multivariate predictors of cardiac events: ^{201}Tl	Significant multivariate predictors of cardiac events: Other	Frequency of perioperative cardiac events: RD No.	RD %	No RD No.	No RD %
Boucher et al.[385]	48	AA, LEV	Death, MI, UA	RD*		8/16	50	0/32	0
Leppo et al.[386]	89	AA, LEV	Death, MI	RD		14/42	33	1/47	2
Eagle et al.[387]	111	AA	Death, MI, UA, IPE	RD	Q waves	16/48	33	2/69	3
Eagle et al.[388]	200	AA, LEV, CE	Death, MI, UA, IPE	RD, DP-ST ↓	Q waves, age, Hx AP, DM, VEA	25/82	30	5/118	4
			Death, MI	RD*, DP-ST ↓ *	Hx AP,* CHF, DM,* S_3G*	13/82	16	2/118	2
Lette et al.[391,392]	66	AA, LEV, major general surgery	Death, MI	RD,* number of RD*	None	9/21	43	0/39	0
Lane et al.[393]	101	AA, LEV, CE	Death, MI, UA, CHF	Number of RD*	Hx AP,* Goldman score*	10/71	14	1/30	3
Total						82/280	29	9/335	3

AA, abdominal aortic surgery; CE, carotid endarterectomy; CHF, congestive heart failure; DM, diabetes mellitus; DP-ST ↓, dipyridamole-induced ST segment depression; Hx AP, history of angina pectoris; IPE, ischemic pulmonary edema; LEV, lower extremity vascular surgery; MI, myocardial infarction; RD, transient defects; S_3G, S_3 gallop; UA, unstable angina; VEA, ventricular ectopic activity.
*Univariate analysis only.

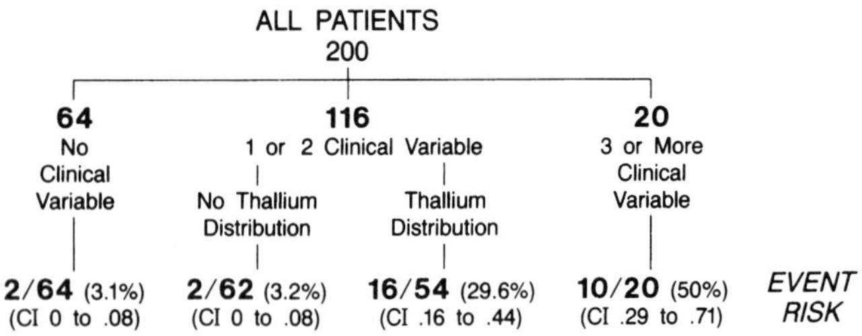

Fig 6-32 Relation of risk of perioperative cardiac event to presence and number of clinical risk factors and presence or absence of ^{201}Tl redistribution. CI, confidence interval. (From Eagle KA, Coley CM, Newell JB, et al: Combining clinical and thallium data optimizes preoperative assessment of cardiac risk before major vascular surgery. *Ann Intern Med* 110:859-866, 1989. By permission of American College of Physicians.)

Matthay and their associates[72,396] have demonstrated that patients with known chronic obstructive pulmonary disease may have depressed right ventricular function in the absence of clinical cor pulmonale. The identification of this dysfunction in earlier stages may lead to more intensive therapy at a time when there is at least some reversible component.

The differential diagnosis of dyspnea on exertion includes both cardiac and pulmonary causes. Although this differentiation can usually be made on clinical grounds alone, there are often circumstances in which the coexistence of possible cardiac and pulmonary problems in a patient presents considerable difficulty to the clinician. The chest x-ray film and the ECG are less useful indicators of cardiac problems in the setting of severe chronic obstructive pulmonary disease. Radionuclide angiography at exercise offers an objective assessment of cardiac function that may uncover clinically occult dysfunction in some patients and focus attention more appropriately on the pulmonary component of disease in other situations. We at the Mayo Clinic have found this to be a very useful application of the test, one that has received little attention in the literature.

Radionuclide angiography has been employed to monitor for cardiotoxic effects of antitumor agents such as doxorubicin. Measurements of ejection fraction in these patients correlate with clinical manifestations of cardiotoxicity. The adjustment of drug dosage on the basis of ejection fraction measurements may make it possible to prevent congestive heart failure in these patients.[397,398]

Finally, rest and exercise radionuclide angiography is a very valuable tool for the clinical investigation of a wide variety of pathophysiologic mechanisms and pharmacologic interventions. It has been employed widely in the study of drug interventions in coronary artery disease, for which it provides useful objective data regarding the effects of the intervention on exercise left ventricular function.[277,283,284,399] It has been used to study aspects of the aging process[400] and the effects of physical training.[401,402]

CONCLUSION

The past 2 decades have witnessed tremendous growth in the field of nuclear cardiology. Radionuclide procedures are now available for the noninvasive assessment of many aspects of the cardiovascular system that were previously approachable only by invasive means, if at all. These techniques are now available to the clinical cardiologist for routine use. It should be evident from this chapter that radionuclide techniques offer great promise in many different areas, but their exact clinical role is still under refinement. The proper utilization of these tests by the practicing clinician demands an effort by him or her to keep abreast of the many new developments in this burgeoning field.

REFERENCES

1. Budinger TF, Rollo FD: Physics and instrumentation. *Prog Cardiovasc Dis* 20:19-53, 1977
2. Budinger TF: Physiology and physics of nuclear cardiology. *Cardiovasc Clin* 10:9-78, 1979
3. Wagner HN Jr: Basic principles: instrumentation, radiopharmaceuticals, and dosimetry. In *Nuclear Cardiology.* Edited by DS Berman, DT Mason. New York, Grune & Stratton, 1981, pp 28-45
4. Thrall JH, Freitas JE, Swanson D, et al: Clinical comparison of cardiac blood pool visualization with technetium-99m red blood cells labeled in vivo and with technetium-99m human serum albumin. *J Nucl Med* 19:796-803, 1978
5. Eckelman W, Richards P, Hauser W, et al: Technetium-labeled red blood cells. *J Nucl Med* 12:22-24, 1971
6. Smith TD, Richards P: A simple kit for the preparation of ^{99m}Tc-labeled red blood cells. *J Nucl Med* 17:126-132, 1976
7. Pavel DG, Zimmer AM, Patterson VN: In vivo labeling of red blood cells with ^{99m}Tc: a new approach to blood pool visualization. *J Nucl Med* 18:305-308, 1977
8. Stokely EM, Parkey RW, Bonte FJ, et al: Gated blood pool imaging following ^{99m}Tc stannous pyrophosphate imaging. *Radiology* 120:433-434, 1976
9. Callahan RJ, Froelich JW, McKusick KA, et al: A modified method for the in vivo labeling of red blood cells with Tc-99m: concise communication. *J Nucl Med* 23:315-318, 1982
10. Berger HJ, Zaret BL: Nuclear cardiology. *N Engl J Med* 305:855-864, 1981
11. Kelly MJ, Giles RW, Simon TR, et al: Multigated equilibrium radionuclide angiocardiography: improved detection of left ventricular wall motion abnormalities and aneurysms by the addition of the left lateral view. *Radiology* 139:167-173, 1981
12. Manyari DE, Nolewajka AJ, Purves P, et al: Comparative value of the cold-pressor test and supine bicycle exercise to detect subjects with coronary artery disease using radionuclide ventriculography. *Circulation* 65:571-579, 1982
13. Boucher CA, Strauss HW, Okada RD, et al: The bifocal diverging collimator: a means of simultaneous biplane imaging of the heart during equilibrium radionuclide ventriculography. *J Nucl Med* 21:71-76, 1980
14. Secker-Walker RH, Resnick L, Kunz H, et al: Measurement of left ventricular ejection fraction. *J Nucl Med* 14:798-802, 1973
15. Burow RD, Strauss HW, Singleton R, et al: Analysis of left ventricular function from multiple gated acquisition cardiac blood pool imaging: comparison to contrast angiography. *Circulation* 56:1024-1028, 1977
16. Folland ED, Hamilton GW, Larson SM, et al: The radionuclide ejection fraction: a comparison of three radionuclide techniques with contrast angiography. *J Nucl Med* 18:1159-1166, 1977
17. Green MV, Brody WR, Douglas MA, et al: Ejection fraction by count rate from gated images. *J Nucl Med* 19:880-883, 1978
18. Berman DS, Salel AF, DeNardo GL, et al: Clinical assessment of left ventricular regional contraction patterns and ejection fraction by high-resolution gated scintigraphy. *J Nucl Med* 16:865-874, 1975
19. Pfisterer ME, Ricci DR, Schuler G, et al: Validity of left-ventricular ejection fractions measured at rest and peak exercise by equilibrium radionuclide angiography using short acquisition times. *J Nucl Med* 20:484-490, 1979
20. Wackers FJT, Berger HJ, Johnstone DE, et al: Multiple gated cardiac blood pool imaging for left ventricular ejection fraction: validation of the technique and assessment of variability. *Am J Cardiol* 43:1159-1166, 1979
21. Pfisterer ME, Battler A, Swanson SM, et al: Reproducibility of ejection-fraction determinations by equilibrium radionuclide angiography in response to supine bicycle exercise: concise communication. *J Nucl Med* 20:491-495, 1979
22. Slutsky R, Karliner J, Battler A, et al: Reproducibility of ejection fraction and ventricular volume by gated radionuclide angiography after myocardial infarction. *Radiology* 132:155-159, 1979
23. Okada RD, Kirshenbaum HD, Kushner FG, et al: Observer variance in the qualitative evaluation of left ventricular wall motion and the quantitation of left ventricular ejection fraction using rest and exercise multigated blood pool imaging. *Circulation* 61:128-136, 1980
24. Okada RD, Pohost GM, Nichols AB, et al: Left ventricular regional wall motion assessment by multigated and end-diastolic, end-systolic gated radionuclide left ventriculography. *Am J Cardiol* 45:1211-1218, 1980
25. Maddox DE, Wynne J, Uren R, et al: Regional ejection fraction: a quantitative radionuclide index of regional left ventricular performance. *Circulation* 59:1001-1009, 1979
26. Papapietro SE, Yester MV, Logic JR, et al: Method for quantitative analysis of regional left ventricular function with first pass and gated blood pool scintigraphy. *Am J Cardiol* 47:618-625, 1981
27. Steckley RA, Kronenberg MW, Born ML, et al: Radionuclide ventriculography: evaluation of automated and visual methods for regional wall motion analysis. *Radiology* 142:179-185, 1982
28. Gibbons RJ, Morris KG, Lee K, et al: Assessment of regional left ventricular function using gated radionuclide angiography. *Am J Cardiol* 54:294-300, 1984
29. Dehmer GJ, Lewis SE, Hillis LD, et al: Nongeometric determination of left ventricular volumes from equilibrium blood pool scans. *Am J Cardiol* 45:293-300, 1980
30. Clements IP, Brown ML, Smith HC: Radionuclide measurement of left ventricular volume. *Mayo Clin Proc* 56:733-739, 1981
31. Massardo T, Gal RA, Grenier RP, et al: Left ventricular volume calculation using a count-based ratio method applied to multigated radionuclide angiography. *J Nucl Med* 31:450-456, 1990
32. Links JM, Becker LC, Shindledecker JG, et al: Measurement of absolute left ventricular volume from gated blood pool studies. *Circulation* 65:82-90, 1982
33. Starling MR, Dell'Italia LJ, Walsh RA, et al: Accurate estimates of absolute left ventricular volumes from equilibrium radionuclide angiographic count data using a simple geometric attenuation correction. *J Am Coll Cardiol* 3:789-798, 1984
34. Petru MA, Sorensen SG, Chaudhuri TK, et al: Attenuation correction of equilibrium radionuclide angiography for noninvasive quantitation of cardiac output and ventricular volumes. *Am Heart J* 107:1221-1228, 1984
35. Levy WC, Cerqueira MD, Matsuoka DT, et al: Four radionuclide methods for left ventricular volume determination: comparison of a manual and an automated technique. *J Nucl Med* 33:763-770, 1992
36. Brown ML, Vaqueiro M, Clements IP, et al: Stability of radionuclide left ventricular volume measurements. *Nucl Med Commun* 9:117-122, 1988
37. Greenberg B, Massie B, Bristow JD, et al: Long-term vasodilator therapy of chronic aortic insufficiency: a randomized double-blinded, placebo-controlled clinical trial. *Circulation* 78:92-103, 1988

38. Warren SE, Royal HD, Markis JE, et al: Time course of left ventricular dilation after myocardial infarction: influence of infarct-related artery and success of coronary thrombolysis. *J Am Coll Cardiol* 11:12-19, 1988.
39. Konstam MA, Tu'meh S, Wynne J, et al: Effect of exercise on erythrocyte count and blood activity concentration after technetium-99m in vivo red blood cell labeling. *Circulation* 66:638-642, 1982
40. Vatterott PJ, Gibbons RJ, Hu DCK, et al: Assessment of left ventricular volume changes during exercise radionuclide angiography in coronary artery disease. *Am J Cardiol* 61:912-914, 1988
41. Levy WC, Cerqueira MD, Veith R, et al: Factors influencing serial measurements of cardiac volumes by count-based methods: effects of elevated catecholamines, position, and exercise on technetium-99m-blood radioactivity concentration. *J Nucl Med* 33:1324-1329, 1992
42. Dehmer GJ, Firth BG, Hillis LD, et al: Nongeometric determination of right ventricular volumes from equilibrium blood pool scans. *Am J Cardiol* 49:78-84, 1982
43. Slutsky R, Ashburn W, Karliner J: A method for the estimation of right ventricular volume by equilibrium radionuclide angiography. *Chest* 80:471-477, 1981
44. Rigo P, Alderson PO, Robertson RM, et al: Measurement of aortic and mitral regurgitation by gated cardiac blood pool scans. *Circulation* 60:306-311, 1979
45. Sorensen SG, O'Rourke RA, Chaudhuri TK: Noninvasive quantitation of valvular regurgitation by gated equilibrium radionuclide angiography. *Circulation* 62:1089-1098, 1980
46. Maddahi J, Berman DS, Matsuoka DT, et al: A new technique for assessing right ventricular ejection fraction using rapid multiple-gated equilibrium cardiac blood pool scintigraphy. *Circulation* 60:581-589, 1979
47. Korr KS, Gandsman EJ, Winkler ML, et al: Hemodynamic correlates of right ventricular ejection fraction measured with gated radionuclide angiography. *Am J Cardiol* 49:71-77, 1982
48. Holman BL, Wynne J, Zielonka JS, et al: A simplified technique for measuring right ventricular ejection fraction using the equilibrium radionuclide angiocardiogram and the slant-hole collimator. *Radiology* 138:429-435, 1981
49. Rezai K, Weiss R, Stanford W, et al: Relative accuracy of three scintigraphic methods for determination of right ventricular ejection fraction: a correlative study with ultrafast computed tomography. *J Nucl Med* 32:429-435, 1991
50. Dehmer GJ, Firth BG, Lewis SE, et al: Direct measurement of cardiac output by gated equilibrium blood pool scintigraphy: validation of scintigraphic volume measurements by a nongeometric technique. *Am J Cardiol* 47:1061-1067, 1981
51. Sorensen SG, Ritchie JL, Caldwell JH, et al: Serial exercise radionuclide angiography: validation of count-derived changes in cardiac output and quantitation of maximal exercise ventricular volume change after nitroglycerin and propranolol in normal men. *Circulation* 61:600-609, 1980
52. Konstam MA, Wynne J, Holman BL, et al: Use of equilibrium (gated) radionuclide ventriculography to quantitate left ventricular output in patients with and without left-sided valvular regurgitation. *Circulation* 64:578-585, 1981
53. Okada RD, Pohost GM, Kirshenbaum HD, et al: Radionuclide-determined change in pulmonary blood volume with exercise: improved sensitivity of multigated blood-pool scanning in detecting coronary-artery disease. *N Engl J Med* 301:569-576, 1979
54. Okada RD, Osbakken MD, Boucher CA, et al: Pulmonary blood volume ratio response to exercise: a noninvasive determination of exercise-induced changes in pulmonary capillary wedge pressure. *Circulation* 65:126-133, 1982
55. Bacharach SL, Green MV, Borer JS, et al: Left-ventricular peak ejection rate, filling rate, and ejection fraction-frame rate requirements at rest and exercise: concise communication. *J Nucl Med* 20:189-193, 1979
56. Bonow RO, Bacharach SL, Green MV, et al: Impaired left ventricular diastolic filling in patients with coronary artery disease: assessment with radionuclide angiography. *Circulation* 64:315-323, 1981
57. Clements IP, Nelson MA, O'Connor MK, et al: Diastolic measurements from alternate R-wave gating of radionuclide angiograms. *Am Heart J* 116:113-117, 1988
58. Magorien DJ, Shaffer P, Bush CA, et al: Assessment of left ventricular pressure-volume relations using gated radionuclide angiography, echocardiography, and micromanometer pressure recordings: a new method for serial measurements of systolic and diastolic function in man. *Circulation* 67:844-853, 1983
59. Wackers FJ, Giles RW, Hoffer PB, et al: Gold-195m, a new generator-produced short-lived radionuclide for sequential assessment of ventricular performance by first pass radionuclide angiocardiography. *Am J Cardiol* 50:89-94, 1982
60. Dymond DS, Elliott AT, Flatman W, et al: The clinical validation of gold-195m: a new short half-life radiopharmaceutical for rapid, sequential, first pass angiocardiography in patients. *J Am Coll Cardiol* 2:85-92, 1983
61. Fazio F, Gerundini P, Margonato A, et al: Quantitative radionuclide angiocardiography using gold-195m. *Am J Cardiol* 53:1442-1446, 1984
62. Marshall RC, Berger HJ, Costin JC, et al: Assessment of cardiac performance with quantitative radionuclide angiocardiography: sequential left ventricular ejection fraction, normalized left ventricular ejection rate, and regional wall motion. *Circulation* 56:820-829, 1977
63. Jengo JA, Mena I, Blaufuss A, et al: Evaluation of left ventricular function (ejection fraction and segmental wall motion) by single pass radioisotope angiography. *Circulation* 57:326-332, 1978
64. Rerych SK, Scholz PM, Newman GE, et al: Cardiac function at rest and during exercise in normals and in patients with coronary heart disease: evaluation by radionuclide angiocardiography. *Ann Surg* 187: 449-463, 1978
65. Bodenheimer MM, Banka VS, Fooshee CM, et al: Quantitative radionuclide angiography in the right anterior oblique view: comparison with contrast ventriculography. *Am J Cardiol* 41:718-725, 1978
66. Scholz PM, Rerych SK, Moran JF, et al: Quantitative radionuclide angiocardiography. *Cathet Cardiovasc Diagn* 6:265-283, 1980
67. Upton MT, Rerych SK, Newman GE, et al: The reproducibility of radionuclide angiographic measurements of left ventricular function in normal subjects at rest and during exercise. *Circulation* 62:126-132, 1980
68. Cohn PF, Levine JA, Bergeron GA, et al: Reproducibility of the angiographic left ventricular ejection fraction in patients with coronary artery disease. *Am Heart J* 88:713-720, 1974
69. Sandler H, Dodge HT: The use of single plane angiocardiograms for the calculation of left ventricular volume in man. *Am Heart J* 75:325-334, 1968
70. Chaitman BR, DeMots H, Bristow JD, et al: Objective and subjective analysis of left ventricular angiograms. *Circulation* 52:420-425, 1975
71. Bodenheimer MM, Banka VS, Fooshee CM, et al: Detection of coronary heart disease using radionuclide determined regional ejection fraction at rest and during handgrip exercise: correlation with coronary arteriography. *Circulation* 58:640-648, 1978
72. Berger HJ, Matthay RA, Loke J, et al: Assessment of cardiac performance with quantitative radionuclide angiocardiography: right ventricular ejection fraction with reference to findings in chronic obstructive pulmonary disease. *Am J Cardiol* 41:897-905, 1978
73. Steele P, Kirch D, LeFree M, et al: Measurement of right and left ventricular ejection fractions by radionuclide angiocardiography in coronary artery disease. *Chest* 70:51-56, 1976
74. Anderson PAW, Jones RH, Sabiston DC Jr: Quantitation of left-to-right cardiac shunts with radionuclide angiography. *Circulation* 49:512-516, 1974
75. Alderson PO, Jost RG, Strauss AW, et al: Radionuclide angiocardiography: improved diagnosis and quantitation of left-to-right shunts using area ratio techniques in children. *Circulation* 51:1136-1143, 1975
76. Askenazi J, Ahnberg DS, Korngold E, et al: Quantitative radionuclide angiocardiography: detection and quantitation of left-to-right shunts. *Am J Cardiol* 37:382-387, 1976
77. Peter CA, Armstrong BE, Jones RH: Radionuclide quantitation of right-to-left intracardiac shunts in children. *Circulation* 64:572-577, 1981
78. Janowitz WR, Fester A: Quantitation of left ventricular regurgitant fraction by first pass radionuclide angiocardiography. *Am J Cardiol* 49:85-92, 1982
79. Reduto LA, Wickemeyer WJ, Young JB, et al: Left ventricular diastolic performance at rest and during exercise in patients with coronary artery disease: assessment with first-pass radionuclide angiography. *Circulation* 63:1228-1237, 1981
80. Pohost GM, Alpert NM, Ingwall JS, et al: Thallium redistribution: mechanisms and clinical utility. *Semin Nucl Med* 10:70-93, 1980
81. Weich HF, Strauss HW, Pitt B: The extraction of thallium-201 by the myocardium. *Circulation* 56:188-191, 1977
82. Strauss HW, Harrison K, Langan JK, et al: Thallium-201 for

myocardial imaging: relation of thallium-201 to regional myocardial perfusion. *Circulation* 51:641-645, 1975.

83. Hamilton GW, Narahara KA, Yee H, et al: Myocardial imaging with thallium-201: effect of cardiac drugs on myocardial images and absolute tissue distribution. *J Nucl Med* 19:10-16, 1978

84. Nielsen AP, Morris KG, Murdock R, et al: Linear relationship between the distribution of thallium-201 and blood flow in ischemic and nonischemic myocardium during exercise. *Circulation* 61:797-801, 1980

85. Mueller TM, Marcus ML, Ehrhardt JC, et al: Limitations of thallium-201 myocardial perfusion scintigrams. *Circulation* 54:640-646, 1976

86. Grunwald AM, Watson DD, Holzgrefe HH Jr, et al: Myocardial thallium-201 kinetics in normal and ischemic myocardium. *Circulation* 64:610-618, 1981

87. Beller GA, Watson DD, Ackell P, et al: Time course of thallium-201 redistribution after transient myocardial ischemia. *Circulation* 61:791-797, 1980

88. Gewirtz H, O'Keefe DD, Pohost GM, et al: The effect of ischemia on thallium-201 clearance from the myocardium. *Circulation* 58:215-219, 1978

89. Pohost GM, Zir LM, Moore RH, et al: Differentiation of transiently ischemic from infarcted myocardium by serial imaging after a single dose of thallium-201. *Circulation* 55:294-302, 1977

90. Bradley-Moore PR, Lebowitz E, Greene MW, et al: Thallium-201 for medical use. II. Biologic behavior. *J Nucl Med* 16:156-160, 1975

91. Berger BC, Watson DD, Burwell LR, et al: Redistribution of thallium at rest in patients with stable and unstable angina and the effect of coronary artery bypass surgery. *Circulation* 60:1114-1125, 1979

92. Bodenheimer MM, Banka VS, Fooshee C, et al: Relationship between regional myocardial perfusion and the presence, severity and reversibility of asynergy in patients with coronary heart disease. *Circulation* 58:789-795, 1978

93. Rozanski A, Berman DS, Gray R, et al: Use of thallium-201 redistribution scintigraphy in the preoperative differentiation of reversible and nonreversible myocardial asynergy. *Circulation* 64:936-944, 1981

94. Pohost GM, Boucher CA, Zir LM, et al: The thallium stress test: the qualitative approach revisited (abstract). *Circulation* 60 Suppl 2:149, 1979

95. McLaughlin PR, Martin RP, Doherty P, et al: Reproducibility of thallium-201 myocardial imaging. *Circulation* 55:497-503, 1977

96. Gould KL: Noninvasive assessment of coronary stenoses by myocardial perfusion imaging during pharmacologic coronary vasodilatation. I. Physiologic basis and experimental validation. *Am J Cardiol* 41:267-278, 1978

97. Gould KL, Westcott RJ, Albro PC, et al: Noninvasive assessment of coronary stenoses by myocardial imaging during pharmacologic coronary vasodilatation. II. Clinical methodology and feasibility. *Am J Cardiol* 41:279-287, 1978

98. Albro PC, Gould KL, Westcott RJ, et al: Noninvasive assessment of coronary stenoses by myocardial imaging during pharmacologic coronary vasodilatation. III. Clinical trial. *Am J Cardiol* 42:751-760, 1978

99. Kalsner S: Adenosine and dipyridamole actions and interactions on isolated coronary artery strips of cattle. *Br J Pharmacol* 55:439-445, 1975

100. Feldman RL, Nichols WW, Pepine CJ, et al: Acute effect of intravenous dipyridamole on regional coronary hemodynamics and metabolism. *Circulation* 64:333-344, 1981

101. Meerdink DJ, Okada RD, Leppo JA: The effect of dipyridamole on transmural blood flow gradients. *Chest* 96:400-405, 1989

102. Homma S, Gilliland Y, Guiney TE, et al: Safety of intravenous dipyridamole for stress testing with thallium imaging. *Am J Cardiol* 59:152-154, 1987

103. Lewen MK, Labovitz AJ, Kern MJ, et al: Prolonged myocardial ischemia after intravenous dipyridamole thallium imaging. *Chest* 92: 1102-1104, 1987

104. Blumenthal MS, McCauley CS: Cardiac arrest during dipyridamole imaging. *Chest* 93:1103-1104, 1988

105. Lette J, Cerino M, Laverdiere M, et al: Severe bronchospasm followed by respiratory arrest during thallium-dipyridamole imaging. *Chest* 95:1345-1347, 1989

106. Verani MS, Mahmarian JJ, Hixson JB, et al: Diagnosis of coronary artery disease by controlled coronary vasodilation with adenosine and thallium-201 scintigraphy in patients unable to exercise. *Circulation* 82:80-87, 1990

107. Nishimura S, Mahmarian JJ, Boyce TM, et al: Quantitative thallium-201 single-photon emission computed tomography during maximal pharmacologic coronary vasodilation with adenosine for assessing coronary artery disease. *J Am Coll Cardiol* 18:736-745, 1991

108. Iskandrian AS, Heo J, Nguyen T, et al: Left ventricular dilatation and pulmonary thallium uptake after single-photon emission computed tomography using thallium-201 during adenosine-induced coronary hyperemia. *Am J Cardiol* 66:807-811, 1990

109. Rossen JD, Quillen JE, Lopez JAG, et al: Comparison of coronary vasodilation with intravenous dipyridamole and adenosine. *J Am Coll Cardiol* 18:485-491, 1991

110. Pennell DJ, Underwood SR, Swanton RH, et al: Dobutamine thallium myocardial perfusion tomography. *J Am Coll Cardiol* 18:1471-1479, 1991

111. Zellner JL, Elliott BM, Robison JG, et al: Preoperative evaluation of cardiac risk using dobutamine-thallium imaging in vascular surgery. *Ann Vasc Surg* 4:238-243, 1990

112. Burns RJ, Galligan L, Wright LM, et al: Improved specificity of myocardial thallium-201 single-photon emission computed tomography in patients with left bundle branch block by dipyridamole. *Am J Cardiol* 68:504-508, 1991

113. Larcos G, Brown ML, Gibbons RJ: Role of dipyridamole thallium-201 imaging in left bundle branch block. *Am J Cardiol* 68:1097-1098, 1991

114. O'Keefe JH Jr, Bateman TM, Silvestri R, et al: Safety and diagnostic accuracy of adenosine thallium-201 scintigraphy in patients unable to exercise and those with left bundle branch block. *Am Heart J* 124:614-621, 1992

115. Hirzel HO, Senn M, Nuesch K, et al: Thallium-201 scintigraphy in complete left bundle branch block. *Am J Cardiol* 53:764-769, 1984

116. DePuey EG, Guertler-Krawczynska E, Robbins WL: Thallium-201 SPECT in coronary artery disease patients with left bundle branch block. *J Nucl Med* 29:1479-1485, 1988

117. Braat SH, Brugada P, Bär FW, et al: Thallium-201 exercise scintigraphy and left bundle branch block. *Am J Cardiol* 55:224-226, 1985

118. Larcos G, Gibbons RJ, Brown ML: Diagnostic accuracy of exercise thallium-201 single-photon emission computed tomography in patients with left bundle branch block. *Am J Cardiol* 68:756-760, 1991

119. Kiat H, Berman DS, Maddahi J, et al: Late reversibility of tomographic myocardial thallium-201 defects: an accurate marker of myocardial viability. *J Am Coll Cardiol* 12:1456-1463, 1988

120. Cloninger KG, DePuey EG, Garcia EV, et al: Incomplete redistribution in delayed thallium-201 single photon emission computed tomographic (SPECT) images: an overestimation of myocardial scarring. *J Am Coll Cardiol* 12:955-963, 1988

121. Dilsizian V, Rocco TP, Freedman NMT, et al: Enhanced detection of ischemic but viable myocardium by the reinjection of thallium after stress-redistribution imaging. *N Engl J Med* 323:141-146, 1990

122. Rocco TP, Dilsizian V, McKusick KA, et al: Comparison of thallium redistribution with rest "reinjection" imaging for the detection of viable myocardium. *Am J Cardiol* 66:158-163, 1990

123. Bonow RO, Dilsizian V, Cuocolo A, et al: Identification of viable myocardium in patients with chronic coronary artery disease and left ventricular dysfunction: comparison of thallium scintigraphy with reinjection and PET imaging with ^{18}F-fluorodeoxyglucose. *Circulation* 83:26-37, 1991

124. Dilsizian V, Bonow RO: Differential uptake and apparent ^{201}Tl washout after thallium reinjection: options regarding early redistribution imaging before reinjection or late redistribution imaging after reinjection. *Circulation* 85:1032-1038, 1992

125. McCallister BD Jr, Clemments IP, Hauser MF, et al: The limited value of 24-hour images following 4-hour reinjection thallium imaging (abstract). *Circulation* 84 Suppl 2:533, 1991

126. Gewirtz H, Beller GA, Strauss HW, et al: Transient defects of resting thallium scans in patients with coronary artery disease. *Circulation* 59:707-713, 1979

127. Mori T, Minamiji K, Kurogane H, et al: Rest-injected thallium-201 imaging for assessing viability of severe asynergic regions. *J Nucl Med* 32:1718-1724, 1991

128. Ragosta M, Beller GA, Watson DD, et al: Quantitative planar rest-redistribution ^{201}Tl imaging in detection of myocardial viability and prediction of improvement in left ventricular function after coronary bypass surgery in patients with severely depressed left ventricular function. *Circulation* 87:1630-1641, 1993

129. Iskandrian AS, Hakki A-H, Kane SA, et al: Rest and redistribution thallium-201 myocardial scintigraphy to predict improvement in

left ventricular function after coronary artery bypass grafting. *Am J Cardiol* 51:1312-1316, 1983

130. Patel TC, Gibbons RJ, Mullany CJ: Resting thallium-201 scintigraphy for identifying viable myocardium in a patient with severe left ventricular dysfunction. *Mayo Clin Proc* 68:63-67, 1993

131. Dunn RF, Wolff L, Wagner S, et al: The inconsistent pattern of thallium defects: a clue to the false positive perfusion scintigram. *Am J Cardiol* 48:224-232, 1981

132. Atwood JE, Jensen D, Froelicher V, et al: Agreement in human interpretation of analog thallium myocardial perfusion images. *Circulation* 64:601-609, 1981

133. Burow RD, Pond M, Schafer AW, et al: "Circumferential profiles": a new method for computer analysis of thallium-201 myocardial perfusion images. *J Nucl Med* 20:771-777, 1979

134. Garcia E, Maddahi J, Berman D, et al: Space/time quantitation of thallium-201 myocardial scintigraphy. *J Nucl Med* 22:309-317, 1981

135. Watson DD, Campbell NP, Read EK, et al: Spatial and temporal quantitation of plane thallium myocardial images. *J Nucl Med* 22:577-584, 1981

136. Wackers FJT, Fetterman RC, Mattera JA, et al: Quantitative planar thallium-201 stress scintigraphy: a critical evaluation of the method. *Semin Nucl Med* 15:46-66, 1985

137. Berger BC, Watson DD, Taylor GJ, et al: Quantitative thallium-201 exercise scintigraphy for detection of coronary artery disease. *J Nucl Med* 22:585-593, 1981

138. Maddahi J, Garcia EV, Berman DS, et al: Improved noninvasive assessment of coronary artery disease by quantitative analysis of regional stress myocardial distribution and washout of thallium-201. *Circulation* 64:924-935, 1981

139. Van Train KF, Berman DS, Garcia EV, et al: Quantitative analysis of stress thallium-201 myocardial scintigrams: a multicenter trial. *J Nucl Med* 27:17-25, 1986

140. Vogel RA, Kirch DL, LeFree MT, et al: Thallium-201 myocardial perfusion scintigraphy: results of standard and multi-pinhole tomographic techniques. *Am J Cardiol* 43:787-793, 1979

141. Rizi HR, Kline RC, Thrall JH, et al: Thallium-201 myocardial scintigraphy: a critical comparison of seven-pinhole tomography and conventional planar imaging. *J Nucl Med* 22:493-499, 1981

142. Ritchie JL, Williams DL, Caldwell JH, et al: Seven-pinhole emission tomography with thallium-201 in patients with prior myocardial infarction. *J Nucl Med* 22:107-112, 1981

143. Bateman T, Garcia E, Maddahi J, et al: Clinical evaluation of seven-pinhole tomography for the detection and localization of coronary artery disease: comparison with planar imaging using quantitative analysis of myocardial thallium-201 distribution and washout after exercise. *Am Heart J* 106:263-271, 1983

144. Massie BM, Wisneski JA, Hollenberg M, et al: Quantitative analysis of seven-pinhole tomographic thallium-201 scintigrams: improved sensitivity and estimation of the extent of coronary involvement by evaluation of radiotracer uptake and clearance. *J Am Coll Cardiol* 3:1178-1186, 1984

145. Massie BM, Wisneski JA, Inouye IK, et al: Detection and quantification of previous myocardial infarction by exercise-redistribution tomographic thallium-201 scintigraphy. *Am J Cardiol* 53:1244-1249, 1984

146. Holman BL, Hill TC, Wynne J, et al: Single-photon transaxial emission computed tomography of the heart in normal subjects and in patients with infarction. *J Nucl Med* 20:736-740, 1979

147. Tamaki N, Mukai T, Ishii Y, et al: Clinical evaluation of thallium-201 emission myocardial tomography using a rotating gamma camera: comparison with seven-pinhole tomography. *J Nucl Med* 22:849-855, 1981

148. Kiat H, Berman DS, Maddahi J: Comparison of planar and tomographic exercise thallium-201 imaging methods for the evaluation of coronary artery disease. *J Am Coll Cardiol* 13:613-616, 1989

149. Friedman J, Berman DS, Van Train K, et al: Patient motion in thallium-201 myocardial SPECT imaging: an easily identified frequent source of artifactual defect. *Clin Nucl Med* 13:321-324, May 1988

150. Friedman J, Van Train K, Maddahi J, et al: "Upward creep" of the heart: a frequent source of false-positive reversible defects on Tl-201 stress-redistribution SPECT (abstract). *J Nucl Med* 27:899-900, 1986

151. Ritchie JL, Williams DL, Harp G, et al: Transaxial tomography with thallium-201 for detecting remote myocardial infarction: comparison with planar imaging. *Am J Cardiol* 50:1236-1241, 1982

152. Maublant J, Cassagnes J, Le Jeune JJ, et al: A comparison between conventional scintigraphy and emission tomography with thallium-201 in the detection of myocardial infarction: concise communication. *J Nucl Med* 23:204-208, 1982

153. Tamaki S, Nakajima H, Murakami T, et al: Estimation of infarct size by myocardial emission computed tomography with thallium-201 and its relation to creatine kinase-MB release after myocardial infarction in man. *Circulation* 66:994-1001, 1982

154. Nohara R, Kambara H, Suzuki Y, et al: Stress scintigraphy using single-photon emission computed tomography in the evaluation of coronary artery disease. *Am J Cardiol* 53:1250-1254, 1984

155. Tamaki N, Yonekura Y, Mukai T, et al: Segmental analysis of stress thallium myocardial emission tomography for localization of coronary artery disease. *Eur J Nucl Med* 9:99-105, 1984

156. DePasquale EE, Nody AC, DePuey EG, et al: Quantitative rotational thallium-201 tomography for identifying and localizing coronary artery disease. *Circulation* 77:316-327, 1988

157. Fintel DJ, Links JM, Brinker JA, et al: Improved diagnostic performance of exercise thallium-201 single photon emission computed tomography over planar imaging in the diagnosis of coronary artery disease: a receiver operating characteristic analysis. *J Am Coll Cardiol* 13:600-612, 1989

158. Bingham JB, Strauss HW, Pohost GM, et al: Mechanisms of lung uptake of Tl-201 (abstract). *Circulation* 58 Suppl 2:62, 1978

159. Boucher CA, Zir LM, Beller GA, et al: Increased lung uptake of thallium-201 during exercise myocardial imaging: clinical, hemodynamic and angiographic implications in patients with coronary artery disease. *Am J Cardiol* 46:189-196, 1980

160. Gill JB, Ruddy TD, Newell JB, et al: Prognostic importance of thallium uptake by the lungs during exercise in coronary artery disease. *N Engl J Med* 317:1485-1489, 1987

161. Kaul S, Finkelstein DM, Homma S, et al: Superiority of quantitative exercise thallium-201 variables in determining long-term prognosis in ambulatory patients with chest pain: a comparison with cardiac catheterization. *J Am Coll Cardiol* 12:25-34, 1988

162. Kahn JK, Carry MM, McGhie I, et al: Quantitation of postexercise lung thallium-201 uptake during single photon emission computed tomography. *J Nucl Med* 30:288-294, 1989

163. Khaja F, Alam M, Goldstein S, et al: Diagnostic value of visualization of the right ventricle using thallium-201 myocardial imaging. *Circulation* 59:182-188, 1979

164. Seldin DW, Johnson LL, Blood DK, et al: Myocardial perfusion imaging with technetium-99m SQ30217: comparison with thallium-201 and coronary anatomy. *J Nucl Med* 30:312-319, 1989

165. Meerdink D, Moring A, Leppo J: Comparative myocardial transport of technetium labeled SQ 30,217 (Cardiotec) and thallium-201 (abstract). *J Am Coll Cardiol* 9 Suppl A:137, 1987

166. Okada RD, Glover D, Gaffney T, et al: Myocardial kinetics of technetium-99m-hexakis-2-methoxy-2-methylpropyl-isonitrile. *Circulation* 77:491-498, 1988

167. Li Q-S, Frank TL, Franceschi D, et al: Technetium-99m methoxyisobutyl isonitrile (RP30) for quantification of myocardial ischemia and reperfusion in dogs. *J Nucl Med* 29:1539-1548, 1988

168. Kiat H, Maddahi J, Roy LT, et al: Comparison of technetium 99m methoxy isobutyl isonitrile and thallium 201 for evaluation of coronary artery disease by planar and tomographic methods. *Am Heart J* 117:1-11, 1989

169. Kahn JK, McGhie I, Akers MS, et al: Quantitative rotational tomography with 201Tl and 99mTc 2-methoxy-isobutyl-isonitrile. A direct comparison in normal individuals and patients with coronary artery disease. *Circulation* 79:1282-1293, 1989

170. Hassan IM, Mohammed MMJ, Constantinides C, et al: Segmental analysis of SPECT ^{99m}Tc-methoxy isobutyl isonitrile and ^{201}Tl myocardial imaging in ischaemic heart disease. *Eur J Nucl Med* 16:705-711, 1990

171. Iskandrian AS, Heo J, Kong B, et al: Use of technetium-99m isonitrile (RP-30A) in assessing left ventricular perfusion and function at rest and during exercise in coronary artery disease, and comparison with coronary arteriography and exercise thallium-201 SPECT imaging. *Am J Cardiol* 64:270-275, 1989

172. Kayden DS, Mattera JA, Zaret BL, et al: Demonstration of reperfusion after thrombolysis with technetium-99m isonitrile myocardial imaging. *J Nucl Med* 29:1865-1867, 1988

173. Wackers FJ, Gibbons RJ, Verani MS, et al: Serial quantitative planar technetium-99m isonitrile imaging in acute myocardial infarction:

efficacy for noninvasive assessment of thrombolytic therapy. *J Am Coll Cardiol* 14:861-873, 1989

174. Gibbons RJ, Verani MS, Behrenbeck T, et al: Feasibility of tomographic ^{99m}Tc-hexakis-2-methoxy-2-methylpropyl-isonitrile imaging for the assessment of myocardial area at risk and the effect of treatment in acute myocardial infarction. *Circulation* 80:1277-1286, 1989

175. Grégoire J, Théroux P: Detection and assessment of unstable angina using myocardial perfusion imaging: comparison between technetium-99m sestamibi SPECT and 12-lead electrocardiogram. *Am J Cardiol* 66:42E-46E, 1990

176. Bilodeau L, Théroux P, Grégoire J, et al: Technetium-99m sestamibi tomography in patients with spontaneous chest pain: correlations with clinical, electrocardiographic and angiographic findings. *J Am Coll Cardiol* 18:1684-1691, 1991

177. Wynne J, Holman BL, Lesch M: Myocardial scintigraphy by infarct-avid radiotracers. *Prog Cardiovasc Dis* 20:243-266, 1978

178. Holman BL, Wynne J: Infarct avid (hot spot) myocardial scintigraphy. *Radiol Clin North Am* 18:487-499, Dec. 1980

179. Buja LM, Parkey RW, Stokely EM, et al: Pathophysiology of technetium-99m stannous pyrophosphate and thallium-201 scintigraphy of acute anterior myocardial infarcts in dogs. *J Clin Invest* 57:1508-1522, 1976

180. Buja LM, Tofe AJ, Kulkarni PV, et al: Sites and mechanisms of localization of technetium-99m phosphorus radiopharmaceuticals in acute myocardial infarcts and other tissues. *J Clin Invest* 60:724-740, 1977

181. Holman BL, Lesch M, Alpert JS: Myocardial scintigraphy with technetium-99m pyrophosphate during the early phase of acute infarction. *Am J Cardiol* 41:39-42, 1978

182. Berman DS, Amsterdam EA, Hines HH, et al: New approach to interpretation of technetium-99m pyrophosphate scintigraphy in detection of acute myocardial infarction: clinical assessment of diagnostic accuracy. *Am J Cardiol* 39:341-346, 1977

183. Cuarón A, Acero AP, Cárdenas M, et al: Interobserver variability in the interpretation of myocardial images with Tc-99m-labeled diphosphonate and pyrophosphate. *J Nucl Med* 21:1-9, 1980

184. Diamond GA, Forrester JS: Analysis of probability as an aid in the clinical diagnosis of coronary-artery disease. *N Engl J Med* 300:1350-1358, 1979

185. Diamond GA, Forrester JS, Hirsch M, et al: Application of conditional probability analysis to the clinical diagnosis of coronary artery disease. *J Clin Invest* 65:1210-1221, 1980

186. Rifkin RD, Hood WB Jr: Bayesian analysis of electrocardiographic exercise stress testing. *N Engl J Med* 297:681-686, 1977

187. Ritchie JL, Trobaugh GB, Hamilton GW, et al: Myocardial imaging with thallium-201 at rest and during exercise: comparison with coronary arteriography and resting and stress electrocardiography. *Circulation* 56:66-71, 1977

188. Rosenblatt A, Lowenstein JM, Kerth W, et al: Post-exercise thallium-201 myocardial scanning: a clinical appraisal. *Am Heart J* 94:463-470, 1977

189. Carrillo AP, Marks DS, Pickard SD, et al: Correlation of exercise ^{201}thallium myocardial scan with coronary arteriograms and the maximal exercise test. *Chest* 73:321-326, 1978

190. Turner DA, Battle WE, Deshmukh H, et al: The predictive value of myocardial perfusion scintigraphy after stress in patients without previous myocardial infarction. *J Nucl Med* 19:249-255, 1978

191. Ritchie JL, Zaret BL, Strauss HW, et al: Myocardial imaging with thallium-201: a multicenter study in patients with angina pectoris or acute myocardial infarction. *Am J Cardiol* 42:345-350, 1978

192. Dash H, Massie BM, Botvinick EH, et al: The noninvasive identification of left main and three-vessel coronary artery disease by myocardial stress perfusion scintigraphy and treadmill exercise electrocardiography. *Circulation* 60:276-284, 1979

193. Okada RD, Raessler KL, Woolfenden JM, et al: Clinical value of the thallium-201 stress test: sensitivity and specificity in the detection of coronary artery disease. *Int J Nucl Med Biol* 5:211-221, 1978

194. Bodenheimer MB, Banka VS, Fooshee CM, et al: Extent and severity of coronary heart disease: determinations by thallous chloride Tl 201 myocardial perfusion scanning and comparison with stress electrocardiography. *Arch Intern Med* 139:630-634, 1979

195. Botvinick EH, Taradash MR, Shames DM, et al: Thallium-201 myocardial perfusion scintigraphy for the clinical clarification of normal, abnormal and equivocal electrocardiographic stress tests. *Am J Cardiol* 41:43-51, 1978

196. McCarthy DM, Blood DK, Sciacca RR, et al: Single dose myocardial perfusion imaging with thallium-201: application in patients with nondiagnostic electrocardiographic stress tests. *Am J Cardiol* 43:899-906, 1979

197. Bailey IK, Griffith LSC, Rouleau J, et al: Thallium-201 myocardial perfusion imaging at rest and during exercise: comparative sensitivity to electrocardiography in coronary artery disease. *Circulation* 55:79-87, 1977

198. Verani MS, Marcus ML, Razzak MA, et al: Sensitivity and specificity of thallium-201 perfusion scintigrams under exercise in the diagnosis of coronary artery disease. *J Nucl Med* 19:773-782, 1978

199. Blood DK, McCarthy DM, Sciacca RR, et al: Comparison of single-dose and double-dose thallium-201 myocardial perfusion scintigraphy for the detection of coronary artery disease and prior myocardial infarction. *Circulation* 58:777-788, 1978

200. Iskandrian AS, Segal BL, Haaz W, et al: Effects of coronary artery narrowing, collaterals, and left ventricular function on the pattern of myocardial perfusion. *Cathet Cardiovasc Diagn* 6:159-172, 1980

201. Borer JS, Kent KM, Bacharach SL, et al: Sensitivity, specificity and predictive accuracy of radionuclide cineangiography during exercise in patients with coronary artery disease: comparison with exercise electrocardiography. *Circulation* 60:572-580, 1979

202. Berger HJ, Reduto LA, Johnstone DE, et al: Global and regional left ventricular response to bicycle exercise in coronary artery disease: assessment by quantitative radionuclide angiocardiography. *Am J Med* 66:13-21, 1979

203. Jengo JA, Oren V, Conant R, et al: Effects of maximal exercise stress on left ventricular function in patients with coronary artery disease using first pass radionuclide angiocardiography: a rapid, noninvasive technique for determining ejection fraction and segmental wall motion. *Circulation* 59:60-65, 1979

204. Jones RH, McEwan P, Newman GE, et al: Accuracy of diagnosis of coronary artery disease by radionuclide measurement of left ventricular function during rest and exercise. *Circulation* 64:586-601, 1981

205. Johnstone DE, Sands MJ, Berger HJ, et al: Comparison of exercise radionuclide angiocardiography and thallium-201 myocardial perfusion imaging in coronary artery disease. *Am J Cardiol* 45:1113-1119, 1980

206. Jengo JA, Freeman R, Brizendine M, et al: Detection of coronary artery disease: comparison of exercise stress radionuclide angiocardiography and thallium stress perfusion scanning. *Am J Cardiol* 45:535-541, 1980

207. Bodenheimer MM, Banka VS, Fooshee CM, et al: Comparative sensitivity of the exercise electrocardiogram, thallium imaging and stress radionuclide angiography to detect the presence and severity of coronary heart disease. *Circulation* 60:1270-1278, 1979

208. Caldwell JH, Hamilton GW, Sorensen SG, et al: The detection of coronary artery disease with radionuclide techniques: a comparison of rest-exercise thallium imaging and ejection fraction response. *Circulation* 61:610-619, 1980

209. Gibbons RJ, Lee KL, Cobb F, et al: Ejection fraction response to exercise in patients with chest pain and normal coronary arteriograms. *Circulation* 64:952-957, 1981

210. Rozanski A, Diamond GA, Berman D, et al: The declining specificity of exercise radionuclide ventriculography. *N Engl J Med* 309:518-522, 1983

211. Rozanski A, Diamond GA, Forrester JS, et al: Alternative referent standards for cardiac normality: implications for diagnostic testing. *Ann Intern Med* 101:164-171, 1984

212. Diamond GA, Rozanski A, Forrester JS, et al: A model for assessing the sensitivity and specificity of tests subject to selection bias: application to exercise radionuclide ventriculography for diagnosis of coronary artery disease. *J Chronic Dis* 39:343-355, 1986

213. Goris ML, Bretille J, Askienazy S, et al: Validation of diagnostic procedures on stratified populations: application on the quantification of thallium myocardial perfusion scintigraphy. *Am J Physiol Imaging* 4:11-15, 1989

214. Gibbons RJ, Clements IP, Zinsmeister AR, et al: Exercise response of the systolic pressure to end-systolic volume ratio in patients with coronary artery disease. *J Am Coll Cardiol* 10:33-39, 1987

215. Currie PJ, Kelly MJ, Harper RW, et al: Incremental value of clinical assessment, supine exercise electrocardiography, and biplane exercise radionuclide ventriculography in the prediction of coronary artery disease in men with chest pain. *Am J Cardiol* 52:927-935, 1983

216. Gibbons RJ, Lee KL, Pryor D, et al: The use of radionuclide angiography in the diagnosis of coronary artery disease—a logistic regression analysis. *Circulation* 68:740-746, 1983

217. Detrano R, Yiannikas J, Salcedo EE, et al: Bayesian probability analysis: a prospective demonstration of its clinical utility in diagnosing coronary disease. *Circulation* 69:541-547, 1984

218. Dehmer GJ, Lewis SE, Hillis LD, et al: Exercise-induced alterations in left ventricular volumes and the pressure-volume relationship: a sensitive indicator of left ventricular dysfunction in patients with coronary artery disease. *Circulation* 63:1008-1018, 1981

219. Gibbons RJ, Lee KL, Cobb FR, et al: Ejection fraction response to exercise in patients with chest pain, coronary artery disease, and normal resting ventricular function. *Circulation* 66:643-648, 1982

220. Higginbotham MB, Morris KG, Coleman RE, et al: Sex-related differences in the normal cardiac response to upright exercise. *Circulation* 70:357-366, 1984

221. Hanley PC, Zinsmeister AR, Clements IP, et al: Gender-related differences in cardiac response to supine exercise assessed by radionuclide angiography. *J Am Coll Cardiol* 13:624-629, 1989

222. Clements IP, Gibbons RJ, Mankin HT, et al: Guidelines for the interpretation of the exercise radionuclide ventriculogram for diagnosing coronary artery disease. *Am J Cardiol* 60:1265-1268, 1987

223. DePace NL, Iskandrian AS, Hakki A-H, et al: Value of left ventricular ejection fraction during exercise in predicting the extent of coronary artery disease. *J Am Coll Cardiol* 1:1002-1010, 1983

224. DePace NL, Hakki A-H, Weinreich DJ, et al: Noninvasive assessment of coronary artery disease. *Am J Cardiol* 52:714-720, 1983

225. Gibbons RJ, Fyke FE III, Clements IP, et al: Noninvasive identification of severe coronary artery disease using exercise radionuclide angiography. *J Am Coll Cardiol* 11:28-34, 1988

226. Pryor DB, Harrell FE Jr, Lee KL, et al: Prognostic indicators from radionuclide angiography in medically treated patients with coronary artery disease. *Am J Cardiol* 53:18-22, 1984

227. Taliercio CP, Clements IP, Zinsmeister AR, et al: Prognostic value and limitations of exercise radionuclide angiography in medically treated coronary artery disease. *Mayo Clin Proc* 63:573-582, 1988

228. Lee KL, Pryor DB, Pieper KS, et al: Exercise radionuclide angiography yields prognostic information equivalent to cardiac catheterization (abstract). *J Am Coll Cardiol* 13 Suppl A:126, 1989

229. Weintraub WS, Schneider RM, Seelaus PA, et al: Prospective evaluation of the severity of coronary artery disease with exercise radionuclide angiography and electrocardiography. *Am Heart J* 111:537-542, 1986

230. Gibbons RJ, Hu DC, Clements IP, et al: Anatomic and functional significance of a hypotensive response during supine exercise radionuclide ventriculography. *Am J Cardiol* 60:1-4, 1987

231. Massie BM, Botvinick EH, Brundage BH: Correlation of thallium-201 scintigrams with coronary anatomy: factors affecting region by region sensitivity. *Am J Cardiol* 44:616-622, 1979

232. Rigo P, Bailey IK, Griffith LSC, et al: Value and limitations of segmental analysis of stress thallium myocardial imaging for localization of coronary artery disease. *Circulation* 61:973-981, 1980

233. Maddahi J, Abdulla A, Garcia EV, et al: Noninvasive identification of left main and triple vessel coronary artery disease: improved accuracy using quantitative analysis of regional myocardial stress distribution and washout of thallium-201. *J Am Coll Cardiol* 7:53-60, 1986

234. Christian TF, Miller TD, Bailey KR, et al: Noninvasive identification of severe coronary artery disease using exercise tomographic thallium-201 imaging. *Am J Cardiol* 70:14-20, 1992

235. McNeer JF, Margolis JR, Lee KL, et al: The role of the exercise test in the evaluation of patients for ischemic heart disease. *Circulation* 57:64-70, 1978

236. Weiner DA, McCabe CH, Ryan TJ: Identification of patients with left main and three vessel coronary disease with clinical and exercise test variables. *Am J Cardiol* 46:21-27, 1980

237. Gibbons RJ, Zinsmeister AR, Miller TD, et al: Supine exercise electrocardiography compared with exercise radionuclide angiography in noninvasive identification of severe coronary artery disease. *Ann Intern Med* 112:743-749, 1990

238. Rigo P, Murray M, Strauss HW, et al: Left ventricular function in acute myocardial infarction evaluated by gated scintiphotography. *Circulation* 50:678-684, 1974

239. Hammermeister KE, DeRouen TA, Dodge HT: Variables predictive of survival in patients with coronary disease: selection by univariate and multivariate analyses from the clinical, electrocardiographic, exercise, arteriographic, and quantitative angiographic evaluations. *Circulation* 59:421-430, 1979

240. Corbett JR, Dehmer GJ, Lewis SE, et al: The prognostic value of submaximal exercise testing with radionuclide ventriculography before hospital discharge in patients with recent myocardial infarction. *Circulation* 64:535-544, 1981

241. Dewhurst NG, Muir AL: Comparative prognostic value of radionuclide ventriculography at rest and during exercise in 100 patients after first myocardial infarction. *Br Heart J* 49:111-121, 1983

242. Multicenter Postinfarction Research Group: Risk stratification and survival after myocardial infarction. *N Engl J Med* 309:331-336, 1983

243. Lee KL, Pryor DB, Pieper KS, et al: Prognostic value of radionuclide angiography in medically treated patients with coronary artery disease: a comparison with clinical and catheterization variables. *Circulation* 82:1705-1717, 1990

244. Brown KA, Boucher CA, Okada RD, et al: Prognostic value of exercise thallium-201 imaging in patients presenting for evaluation of chest pain. *J Am Coll Cardiol* 1:994-1001, 1983

245. Ladenheim ML, Pollock BH, Rozanski A, et al: Extent and severity of myocardial hypoperfusion as predictors of prognosis in patients with suspected coronary artery disease. *J Am Coll Cardiol* 7:464-471, 1986

246. Staniloff HM, Forrester JS, Berman DS, et al: Prediction of death, myocardial infarction, and worsening chest pain using thallium scintigraphy and exercise electrocardiography. *J Nucl Med* 27:1842-1848, 1986

247. Iskandrian AS, Hakki A-H, Kane-Marsch S: Prognostic implications of exercise thallium-201 scintigraphy in patients with suspected or known coronary artery disease. *Am Heart J* 110:135-143, 1985

248. Iskandrian AS, Hakki A-H, Kane-Marsch S: Exercise thallium-201 scintigraphy in men with nondiagnostic exercise electrocardiograms: prognostic implications. *Arch Intern Med* 146:2189-2193, 1986

249. Felsher J, Meissner MD, Hakki A-H, et al: Exercise thallium imaging in patients with diabetes mellitus: prognostic implications. *Arch Intern Med* 147:313-317, 1987

250. Iskandrian AS, Heo J, Decoskey D, et al: Use of exercise thallium-201 imaging for risk stratification of elderly patients with coronary artery disease. *Am J Cardiol* 61:269-272, 1988

251. Kaul S, Lilly DR, Gascho JA, et al: Prognostic utility of the exercise thallium-201 test in ambulatory patients with chest pain: comparison with cardiac catheterization. *Circulation* 77:745-758, 1988

252. Younis LT, Byers S, Shaw L, et al: Prognostic importance of silent myocardial ischemia detected by intravenous dipyridamole thallium myocardial imaging in asymptomatic patients with coronary artery disease. *J Am Coll Cardiol* 14:1635-1641, 1989

253. Hendel RC, Layden JJ, Leppo JA: Prognostic value of dipyridamole thallium scintigraphy for evaluation of ischemic heart disease. *J Am Coll Cardiol* 15:109-116, 1990

254. Shaw L, Chaitman BR, Hilton TC, et al: Prognostic value of dipyridamole thallium-201 imaging in elderly patients. *J Am Coll Cardiol* 19:1390-1398, 1992

255. Bonow RO, Kent KM, Rosing DR, et al: Exercise-induced ischemia in mildly symptomatic patients with coronary-artery disease and preserved left ventricular function: identification of subgroups at risk of death during medical therapy. *N Engl J Med* 311:1339-1345, 1984

256. Mazzotta G, Bonow RO, Pace L, et al: Relation between exertional ischemia and prognosis in mildly symptomatic patients with single or double vessel coronary artery disease and left ventricular dysfunction at rest. *J Am Coll Cardiol* 13:567-573, 1989

257. Miller TD, Taliercio CP, Zinsmeister AR, et al: Prognostic value of exercise-induced ischemia in patients with single or double vessel disease and left ventricular dysfunction (abstract). *Circulation* 78 Suppl 2:110, 1988

258. Pollock SG, Abbott RD, Boucher CA, et al: Independent and incremental prognostic value of tests performed in hierarchical order to evaluate patients with suspected coronary artery disease: validation of models based on these tests. *Circulation* 85:237-248, 1992

259. Jones RH, Floyd RD, Austin EH, et al: The role of radionuclide angiocardiography in the preoperative prediction of pain relief and prolonged survival following coronary artery bypass grafting. *Ann Surg* 197:743-753, 1983

260. White CW, Wright CB, Doty DB, et al: Does visual interpretation of the coronary arteriogram predict the physiologic importance of a coronary stenosis? *N Engl J Med* 310:819-824, 1984

261. Rigo P, Bailey IK, Griffith LSC, et al: Stress thallium-201 myocardial scintigraphy for the detection of individual coronary arterial lesions in patients with and without previous myocardial infarction. *Am J Cardiol* 48:209-216, 1981

262. Maddahi J, Van Train KF, Wong C, et al: Comparison of Tl-201 single photon emission computerized tomography (SPECT) and planar imaging for evaluation of coronary artery disease (abstract). *J Nucl Med* 27:999, 1986

263. Dilsizian V, Perrone-Filardi P, Cannon RO III, et al: Comparison of exercise radionuclide angiography with thallium SPECT imaging for detection of significant narrowing of the left circumflex coronary artery. *Am J Cardiol* 68:320-328, 1991

264. Rigo P, Murray M, Strauss HW, et al: Scintiphotographic evaluation of patients with suspected left ventricular aneurysm. *Circulation* 50:985-991, 1974

265. Dymond DS, Jarritt PH, Britton KE, et al: Detection of post-infarction left ventricular aneurysms by first pass radionuclide ventriculography using a multicrystal gamma camera. *Br Heart J* 41:68-78, 1979

266. Perkins PJ: Radioisotopic diagnosis of false left ventricular aneurysm. *AJR* 132:117-119, 1979

267. Botvinick EH, Shames D, Hutchinson JC, et al: Noninvasive diagnosis of a false left ventricular aneurysm with radioisotope gated cardiac blood pool imaging: differentiation from true aneurysm. *Am J Cardiol* 37:1089-1093, 1976

268. Sweet SE, Sterling R, McCormick JR, et al: Left ventricular false aneurysm after coronary bypass surgery: radionuclide diagnosis and surgical resection. *Am J Cardiol* 43:154-157, 1979

269. Rigo P, Murray M, Taylor DR, et al: Right ventricular dysfunction detected by gated scintiphotography in patients with acute inferior myocardial infarction. *Circulation* 52:268-274, 1975

270. Reduto LA, Berger HJ, Cohen LS, et al: Sequential radionuclide assessment of left and right ventricular performance after acute transmural myocardial infarction. *Ann Intern Med* 89:441-447, 1978

271. Tobinick E, Schelbert HR, Henning H, et al: Right ventricular ejection fraction in patients with acute anterior and inferior myocardial infarction assessed by radionuclide angiography. *Circulation* 57:1078-1084, 1978

272. Salel AF, Berman DS, DeNardo GL, et al: Radionuclide assessment of nitroglycerin influence on abnormal left ventricular segmental contraction in patients with coronary heart disease. *Circulation* 53:975-982, 1976

273. Borer JS, Bacharach SL, Green MV, et al: Effect of nitroglycerin on exercise-induced abnormalities of left ventricular regional function and ejection fraction in coronary artery disease: assessment by radionuclide cineangiography in symptomatic and asymptomatic patients. *Circulation* 57:314-320, 1978

274. Ideker RE, Behar VS, Wagner GS, et al: Evaluation of asynergy as an indicator of myocardial fibrosis. *Circulation* 57:715-725, 1978

275. Cabin HS, Clubb KS, Vita N, et al: Regional dysfunction by equilibrium radionuclide angiocardiography: a clinicopathologic study evaluating the relation of degree of dysfunction to the presence and extent of myocardial infarction. *J Am Coll Cardiol* 10:743-747, 1987

276. Shen W-K, Khandheria BK, Edwards WD, et al: Value and limitations of two-dimensional echocardiography in predicting myocardial infarct size. *Am J Cardiol* 68:1143-1149, 1991

277. Rozanski A, Berman D, Gray R, et al: Preoperative prediction of reversible myocardial asynergy by postexercise radionuclide ventriculography. *N Engl J Med* 307:212-216, 1982

278. Gibson RS, Watson DD, Taylor GJ, et al: Prospective assessment of regional myocardial perfusion before and after coronary revascularization surgery by quantitative thallium-201 scintigraphy. *J Am Coll Cardiol* 1:804-815, 1983

279. Tillisch J, Brunken R, Marshall R, et al: Reversibility of cardiac wall-motion abnormalities predicted by positron tomography. *N Engl J Med* 314:884-888, 1986

280. Brunken R, Schwaiger M, Grover-McKay M, et al: Positron emission tomography detects tissue metabolic activity in myocardial segments with persistent thallium perfusion defects. *J Am Coll Cardiol* 10:557-567, 1987

281. Tamaki N, Yonekura Y, Senda M, et al: Value and limitation of stress thallium-201 single photon emission computed tomography: comparison with nitrogen-13 ammonia positron tomography. *J Nucl Med* 29:1181-1188, 1988

282. Brunken RC, Kottou S, Nienaber CA, et al: PET detection of viable tissue in myocardial segments with persistent defects at Tl-201 SPECT. *Radiology* 172:65-73, 1989

283. Marshall RC, Berger HJ, Reduto LA, et al: Assessment of cardiac performance with quantitative radionuclide angiocardiography: effects of oral propranolol on global and regional left ventricular function in coronary artery disease. *Circulation* 58:808-814, 1978

284. Battler A, Ross J Jr, Slutsky R, et al: Improvement of exercise-induced left ventricular dysfunction with oral propranolol in patients with coronary heart disease. *Am J Cardiol* 44:318-324, 1979

285. Newman GE, Rerych SK, Jones RH, et al: Noninvasive assessment of the effects of aorta-coronary bypass grafting on ventricular function during rest and exercise. *J Thorac Cardiovasc Surg* 79:617-624, 1980

286. Freeman MR, Gray RJ, Berman DS, et al: Improvement in global and segmental left ventricular function after coronary bypass surgery. *Circulation* 64 Suppl 2:34-39, 1981

287. Kent KM, Borer JS, Green MV, et al: Effects of coronary-artery bypass on global and regional left ventricular function during exercise. *N Engl J Med* 298:1434-1439, 1978

288. Ritchie JL, Narahara KA, Trobaugh GB, et al: Thallium-201 myocardial imaging before and after coronary revascularization: assessment of regional myocardial blood flow and graft patency. *Circulation* 56:830-836, 1977

289. Greenberg BH, Hart R, Botvinick EH, et al: Thallium-201 myocardial perfusion scintigraphy to evaluate patients after coronary bypass surgery. *Am J Cardiol* 42:167-176, 1978

290. Sigwart U, Grbic M, Essinger A, et al: Improvement of left ventricular function after percutaneous transluminal coronary angioplasty. *Am J Cardiol* 49:651-657, 1982

291. Kent KM, Bonow RO, Rosing DR, et al: Improved myocardial function during exercise after successful percutaneous transluminal coronary angioplasty. *N Engl J Med* 306:441-446, 1982

292. Ganz W, Buchbinder N, Marcus H, et al: Intracoronary thrombolysis in evolving myocardial infarction. *Am Heart J* 101:4-13, 1981

293. Wilson RF, Johnson MR, Marcus ML, et al: The effect of coronary angioplasty on coronary flow reserve. *Circulation* 77:873-885, 1988

294. Manyari DE, Knudtson M, Kloiber R, et al: Sequential thallium-201 myocardial perfusion studies after successful percutaneous transluminal coronary artery angioplasty: delayed resolution of exercise-induced scintigraphic abnormalities. *Circulation* 77:86-95, 1988

295. Iskandrian AS, Lemlek J, Ogilby JD, et al: Early thallium imaging after percutaneous transluminal coronary angioplasty: tomographic evaluation during adenosine-induced coronary hyperemia. *J Nucl Med* 33:2086-2089, 1992

296. DiCola VC, Downing SE, Donabedian RK, et al: Pathophysiological correlates of thallium-201 myocardial uptake in experimental infarction. *Cardiovasc Res* 11:141-146, 1977

297. Wackers FJT, Sokole EB, Samson G, et al: Value and limitations of thallium-201 scintigraphy in the acute phase of myocardial infarction. *N Engl J Med* 295:1-5, 1976

298. Wackers FJT, Lie KI, Liem KL, et al: Potential value of thallium-201 scintigraphy as a means of selecting patients for the coronary care unit. *Br Heart J* 41:111-117, 1979

299. Berger HJ, Gottschalk A, Zaret BL: Dual radionuclide study of acute myocardial infarction: comparison of thallium-201 and technetium-99m stannous pyrophosphate imaging in man. *Ann Intern Med* 88:145-154, 1978

300. Christian TF, Clements IP, Gibbons RJ: Noninvasive identification of myocardium at risk in patients with acute myocardial infarction and nondiagnostic electrocardiograms with technetium-99m-sestamibi. *Circulation* 83:1615-1620, 1991

301. Lyons KP, Olson HG, Aronow WS: Sensitivity and specificity of Tc-99m-pyrophosphate myocardial scintigraphy for the detection of acute myocardial infarction. *Clin Nucl Med* 5:8-12, 1980

302. Hung J, Kelly DT, McLaughlin AF, et al: Preoperative and postoperative technetium-99m pyrophosphate myocardial scintigraphy in the assessment of operative infarction in coronary artery surgery. *J Thorac Cardiovasc Surg* 78:68-73, 1979

303. Massie BM, Botvinick EH, Werner JA, et al: Myocardial scintigraphy with technetium-99m stannous pyrophosphate: an insensitive test for nontransmural myocardial infarction. *Am J Cardiol* 43:186-192, 1979

304. Cohn JN, Guiha NH, Broder MI, et al: Right ventricular infarction: clinical and hemodynamic features. *Am J Cardiol* 33:209-214, 1974

305. Rackley CE, Russell RO Jr: Right ventricular function in acute myocardial infarction (editorial). *Am J Cardiol* 33:927-929, 1974

306. Gruppo Italiano per lo Studio della Streptochi-nasi nell'Infarto Miocardico (GISSI): Long-term effects of intravenous thrombolysis in acute myocardial infarction: final report of the GISSI study. *Lancet* 2:871-874, 1987

307. ISIS Steering Committee: Intravenous streptokinase given within 0-4 hours of onset of myocardial infarction reduced mortality in ISIS-2. *Lancet* 1:502, 1987

308. Kennedy JW, Martin GV, Davis KB, et al: The Western Washington Intravenous Streptokinase in Acute Myocardial Infarction Randomized Trial. *Circulation* 77:345-352, 1988

309. O'Rourke M, Baron D, Keogh A, et al: Limitation of myocardial infarction by early infusion of recombinant tissue-type plasminogen activator. *Circulation* 77:1311-1315, 1988

310. Rentrop KP, Feit F, Blanke H, et al: Effects of intracoronary streptokinase and intracoronary nitroglycerin infusion on coronary angiographic patterns and mortality in patients with acute myocardial infarction. *N Engl J Med* 311:1457-1463, 1984

311. Khaja F, Walton JA Jr, Brymer JF, et al: Intracoronary fibrinolytic therapy in acute myocardial infarction: report of a prospective randomized trial. *N Engl J Med* 308:1305-1311, 1983

312. Leiboff RH, Katz RJ, Wasserman AG, et al: A randomized, angiographically controlled trial of intracoronary streptokinase in acute myocardial infarction. *Am J Cardiol* 53:404-407, 1984

313. Simoons ML, Serruys PW, van den Brand M, et al: Early thrombolysis in acute myocardial infarction: limitation of infarct size and improved survival. *J Am Coll Cardiol* 7:717-728, 1986

314. Guerci AD, Gerstenblith G, Brinker JA, et al: A randomized trial of intravenous tissue plasminogen activator for acute myocardial infarction with subsequent randomization to elective coronary angioplasty. *N Engl J Med* 317:1613-1618, 1987

315. Ritchie JL, Davis KB, Williams DL, et al: Global and regional left ventricular function and tomographic radionuclide perfusion: the Western Washington Intracoronary Streptokinase in Myocardial Infarction Trial. *Circulation* 70:867-875, 1984

316. Ritchie JL, Cerqueira M, Maynard C, et al: Ventricular function and infarct size: the Western Washington Intravenous Streptokinase in Myocardial Infarction Trial. *J Am Coll Cardiol* 11:689-697, 1988

317. De Coster PM, Melin JA, Detry J-MR, et al: Coronary artery reperfusion in acute myocardial infarction: assessment by pre- and post-intervention thallium-201 myocardial perfusion imaging. *Am J Cardiol* 55:889-895, 1985

318. O'Connor MK, Hammell T, Gibbons RJ: In vitro validation of a simple tomographic technique for estimation of % myocardium "at risk" using technetium-99m methoxyisobutyl isonitrile (sestamibi). *Eur J Nucl Med* 17:69-76, 1990

319. Verani MS, Jeroudi MO, Mahmarian JJ, et al: Quantification of myocardial infarction during coronary occlusion and myocardial salvage after reperfusion using cardiac imaging with technetium-99m hexakis 2-methoxyisobutyl isonitrile. *J Am Coll Cardiol* 12:1573-1581, 1988

320. Sinusas AJ, Trautman KA, Bergin JD, et al: Quantification of area at risk during coronary occlusion and degree of myocardial salvage after reperfusion with technetium-99m methoxyisobutyl isonitrile. *Circulation* 82:1424-1437, 1990

321. Gibbons RJ: Technetium 99m sestamibi in the assessment of acute myocardial infarction. *Semin Nucl Med* 21:213-222, 1991

322. Christian TF, Behrenbeck T, Pellikka PA, et al: Mismatch of left ventricular function and infarct size demonstrated by technetium-99m isonitrile imaging after reperfusion therapy for acute myocardial infarction: identification of myocardial stunning and hyperkinesia. *J Am Coll Cardiol* 16:1632-1638, 1990

323. Christian TF, Behrenbeck T, Gersh BJ, et al: Relation of left ventricular volume and function over one year after acute myocardial infarction to infarct size determined by technetium-99m sestamibi. *Am J Cardiol* 68:21-26, 1991

324. Christian TF, Schwartz RS, Gibbons RJ: Determinants of infarct size in reperfusion therapy for acute myocardial infarction. *Circulation* 86:81-90, 1992

325. Christian TF, Gibbons RJ, Gersh BJ: The effect of infarct location on myocardial salvage assessed by technetium-99m isonitrile. *J Am Coll Cardiol* 17:1303-1308, 1991

326. Silverman KJ, Becker LC, Bulkley BH, et al: Value of early thallium-201 scintigraphy for predicting mortality in patients with acute myocardial infarction. *Circulation* 61:996-1003, 1980

327. Hakki A-H, Nestico PF, Heo J, et al: Relative prognostic value of rest thallium-201 imaging, radionuclide ventriculography and 24 hour ambulatory electrocardiographic monitoring after acute myocardial infarction. *J Am Coll Cardiol* 10:25-32, 1987

328. Caldwell JH, Williams DL, Harp GD, et al: Quantitation of size of relative myocardial perfusion defect by single-photon emission computed tomography. *Circulation* 70:1048-1056, 1984

329. Prigent F, Maddahi J, Garcia EV, et al: Quantification of myocardial infarct size by thallium-201 single-photon emission computed tomography: experimental validation in the dog. *Circulation* 74:852-861, 1986

330. Corbett JR, Nicod P, Lewis SE, et al: Prognostic value of submaximal exercise radionuclide ventriculography after myocardial infarction. *Am J Cardiol* 52:82A-91A, 1983

331. Hung J, Goris ML, Nash E, et al: Comparative value of maximal treadmill testing, exercise thallium myocardial perfusion scintigraphy and exercise radionuclide ventriculography for distinguishing high- and low-risk patients soon after acute myocardial infarction. *Am J Cardiol* 53:1221-1227, 1984

332. Gibson RS, Watson DD, Craddock GB, et al: Prediction of cardiac events after uncomplicated myocardial infarction: a prospective study comparing predischarge exercise thallium-201 scintigraphy and coronary angiography. *Circulation* 68:321-336, 1983

333. Abraham RD, Freedman SB, Dunn RF, et al: Prediction of multivessel coronary artery disease and prognosis early after acute myocardial infarction by exercise electrocardiography and thallium-201 myocardial perfusion scanning. *Am J Cardiol* 58:423-427, 1986

334. Wilson WW, Gibson RS, Nygaard TW, et al: Acute myocardial infarction associated with single vessel coronary artery disease: an analysis of clinical outcome and the prognostic importance of vessel patency and residual ischemic myocardium. *J Am Coll Cardiol* 11:223-234, 1988

335. Leppo JA, O'Brien J, Rothendler JA, et al: Dipyridamole-thallium-201 scintigraphy in the prediction of future cardiac events after acute myocardial infarction. *N Engl J Med* 310:1014-1018, 1984

336. Pirelli S, Inglese E, Suppa M, et al: Dipyridamole-thallium 201 scintigraphy in the early post-infarction period. (Safety and accuracy in predicting the extent of coronary disease and future recurrence of angina in patients suffering from their first myocardial infarction.) *Eur Heart J* 9:1324-1331, 1988

337. Younis LT, Byers S, Shaw L, et al: Prognostic value of intravenous dipyridamole thallium scintigraphy after an acute myocardial ischemic event. *Am J Cardiol* 64:161-166, 1989

338. Gimple LW, Hutter AM Jr, Guiney TE, et al: Prognostic utility of predischarge dipyridamole-thallium imaging compared to predischarge submaximal exercise electrocardiography and maximal exercise thallium imaging after uncomplicated acute myocardial infarction. *Am J Cardiol* 64:1243-1248, 1989

339. Brown KA, O'Meara J, Chambers CE, et al: Ability of dipyridamole-thallium-201 imaging one to four days after acute myocardial infarction to predict in-hospital and late recurrent myocardial ischemic events. *Am J Cardiol* 65:160-167, 1990

340. Bosch X, March R, Magriña J, et al: Prediction of in-hospital cardiac events using dipyridamole perfusion scintigraphy early after myocardial infarction (abstract). *Circulation* 80 Suppl 2:307, 1989

341. Gibson RS, Beller GA, Gheorghiade M, et al: The prevalence and clinical significance of residual myocardial ischemia 2 weeks after uncomplicated non-Q wave myocardial infarction: a prospective natural history study. *Circulation* 73:1186-1198, 1986

342. Brown KA, Weiss RM, Clements JP, et al: Usefulness of residual ischemic myocardium within prior infarct zone for identifying patients at high risk late after acute myocardial infarction. *Am J Cardiol* 60:15-19, 1987

343. Mahmarian JJ, Pratt CM, Nishimura S, et al: Quantitative adenosine ^{201}Tl single-photon emission computed tomography for the early assessment of patients surviving acute myocardial infarction. *Circulation* 87:1197-1210, 1993

344. Lavie CJ, Gibbons RJ, Zinsmeister AR, et al: Interpreting results of exercise studies after acute myocardial infarction altered by thrombolytic therapy, coronary angioplasty or bypass. *Am J Cardiol* 67:116-120, 1991

345. Tilkemeier PL, Guiney TE, LaRaia PJ, et al: Prognostic value of predischarge low-level exercise thallium testing after thrombolytic treatment of acute myocardial infarction. *Am J Cardiol* 66:1203-1207, 1990

346. Sutton JM, Topol EJ: Significance of a negative exercise thallium test in the presence of a critical residual stenosis after thrombolysis for

acute myocardial infarction. *Circulation* 83:1278-1286, 1991

347. Handler B, Pavel DG, Pietras R, et al: Equilibrium radionuclide gated angiography in patients with tricuspid regurgitation. *Am J Cardiol* 51:305-310, 1983

348. Boucher CA, Kanarek DJ, Okada RD, et al: Exercise testing in aortic regurgitation: comparison of radionuclide left ventricular ejection fraction with exercise performance at the anaerobic threshold and peak exercise. *Am J Cardiol* 52:801-808, 1983

349. Borer JS, Bacharach SL, Green MV, et al: Exercise-induced left ventricular dysfunction in symptomatic and asymptomatic patients with aortic regurgitation: assessment with radionuclide cineangiography. *Am J Cardiol* 42:351-357, 1978

350. Huxley RL, Gaffney FA, Corbett JR, et al: Early detection of left ventricular dysfunction in chronic aortic regurgitation as assessed by contrast angiography, echocardiography, and rest and exercise scintigraphy. *Am J Cardiol* 51:1542-1550, 1983

351. Iskandrian AS, Hakki A-H, Kane SA, et al: Quantitative radionuclide angiography in assessment of hemodynamic changes during upright exercise: observations in normal subjects, patients with coronary artery disease and patients with aortic regurgitation. *Am J Cardiol* 48:239-246, 1981

352. Dehmer GJ, Firth BG, Hillis LD, et al: Alterations in left ventricular volumes and ejection fraction at rest and during exercise in patients with aortic regurgitation. *Am J Cardiol* 48:17-27, 1981

353. Steingart RM, Yee C, Weinstein L, et al: Radionuclide ventriculographic study of adaptations to exercise in aortic regurgitation. *Am J Cardiol* 51:483-488, 1983

354. Iskandrian AS, Hakki A-H, Manno B, et al: Left ventricular function in chronic aortic regurgitation. *J Am Coll Cardiol* 1:1374-1380, 1983

355. Johnson LL, Powers ER, Tzall WR, et al: Left ventricular volume and ejection fraction response to exercise in aortic regurgitation. *Am J Cardiol* 51:1379-1385, 1983

356. Bonow RO, Rosing DR, Kent KM, et al: Timing of operation for chronic aortic regurgitation. *Am J Cardiol* 50:325-336, 1982

357. Bonow RO, Picone AL, McIntosh CL, et al: Survival and functional results after valve replacement for aortic regurgitation from 1976 to 1983: impact of preoperative left ventricular function. *Circulation* 72:1244-1256, 1985

358. Bonow RO, Borer JS, Rosing DR, et al: Preoperative exercise capacity in symptomatic patients with aortic regurgitation as a predictor of postoperative left ventricular function and long-term prognosis. *Circulation* 62:1280-1290, 1980

359. Bonow RO, Rosing DR, McIntosh CL, et al: The natural history of asymptomatic patients with aortic regurgitation and normal left ventricular function. *Circulation* 68:509-517, 1983

360. Bonow RO, Rosing DR, Maron BJ, et al: Reversal of left ventricular dysfunction after aortic valve replacement for chronic aortic regurgitation: influence of duration of preoperative left ventricular dysfunction. *Circulation* 70:570-579, 1984

361. Bonow RO, Lakatos E, Maron BJ, et al: Serial long-term assessment of the natural history of asymptomatic patients with chronic aortic regurgitation and normal left ventricular systolic function. *Circulation* 84:1625-1635, 1991

362. Schuler G, von Olshausen K, Schwarz F, et al: Noninvasive assessment of myocardial contractility in asymptomatic patients with severe aortic regurgitation and normal left ventricular ejection fraction at rest. *Am J Cardiol* 50:45-52, 1982

363. Lewis SM, Riba AL, Berger HJ, et al: Radionuclide angiographic exercise left ventricular performance in chronic aortic regurgitation: relationship to resting echographic ventricular dimensions and systolic wall stress index. *Am Heart J* 103:498-504, 1982

364. Goldman ME, Packer M, Horowitz SF, et al: Relation between exercise-induced changes in ejection fraction and systolic loading conditions at rest in aortic regurgitation. *J Am Coll Cardiol* 3:924-929, 1984

365. Boucher CA, Wilson RA, Kanarek DJ, et al: Exercise testing in asymptomatic or minimally symptomatic aortic regurgitation: relationship of left ventricular ejection fraction to left ventricular filling pressure during exercise. *Circulation* 67:1091-1100, 1983

366. Borer JS, Rosing DR, Kent KM, et al: Left ventricular function at rest and during exercise after aortic valve replacement in patients with aortic regurgitation. *Am J Cardiol* 44:1297-1305, 1979

367. Boucher CA, Bingham JB, Osbakken MD, et al: Early changes in left ventricular size and function after correction of left ventricular volume overload. *Am J Cardiol* 47:991-1004, 1981

368. Hochreiter C, Niles N, Devereux RB, et al: Mitral regurgitation: relationship of noninvasive descriptors of right and left ventricular performance to clinical and hemodynamic findings and to prognosis in medically and surgically treated patients. *Circulation* 73:900-912, 1986

369. Schuler G, Peterson KL, Johnson A, et al: Temporal response of left ventricular performance to mitral valve surgery. *Circulation* 59:1218-1231, 1979

370. Lavie CJ, Lam JB, Gibbons RJ: Effects of exercise on left ventricular volume and output changes in severe mitral regurgitation: a radionuclide angiographic study. *Chest* 96:1086-1091, 1989

371. Keogh AM, Freund J, Baron DW, et al: Timing of cardiac transplantation in idiopathic dilated cardiomyopathy. *Am J Cardiol* 61:418-422, 1988

372. Keogh AM, Baron DW, Hickie JB: Prognostic guides in patients with idiopathic or ischemic dilated cardiomyopathy assessed for cardiac transplantation. *Am J Cardiol* 65:903-908, 1990

373. Bulkley BH, Hutchins GM, Bailey I, et al: Thallium 201 imaging and gated cardiac blood pool scans in patients with ischemic and idiopathic congestive cardiomyopathy: a clinical and pathologic study. *Circulation* 55:753-760, 1977

374. Dunn RF, Uren RF, Sadick N, et al: Comparison of thallium-201 scanning in idiopathic dilated cardiomyopathy and severe coronary artery disease. *Circulation* 66:804-810, 1982

375. Chikamori T, Doi YL, Yonezawa Y, et al: Value of dipyridamole thallium-201 imaging in noninvasive differentiation of idiopathic dilated cardiomyopathy from coronary artery disease with left ventricular dysfunction. *Am J Cardiol* 69:650-653, 1992

376. Tauberg SG, Orie JE, Bartlett BE, et al: Usefulness of thallium-201 for distinction of ischemic from idiopathic dilated cardiomyopathy. *Am J Cardiol* 71:674-680, 1993

377. Hindman MC, Slosky DA, Peter RH, et al: Rest and exercise hemodynamic effects of oral hydralazine in patients with coronary artery disease and left ventricular dysfunction. *Circulation* 61:751-758, 1980

378. O'Connell JB, Robinson JA, Henkin RE, et al: Immunosuppressive therapy in patients with congestive cardiomyopathy and myocardial uptake of gallium-67. *Circulation* 64:780-786, 1981

379. Maltz DL, Treves S: Quantitative radionuclide angiocardiography: determination of Qp:Qs in children. *Circulation* 47:1049-1056, 1973

380. Hurwitz RA, Treves S, Keane JF, et al: Current value of radionuclide angiocardiography for shunt quantification and management in patients with secundum atrial septal defect. *Am Heart J* 103:421-425, 1982

381. Parrish MD, Graham TP Jr, Born ML, et al: Radionuclide evaluation of right and left ventricular function in children: validation of methodology. *Am J Cardiol* 49:1241-1247, 1982

382. Rosing DR, Borer JS, Kent KM, et al: Long-term hemodynamic and electrocardiographic assessment following operative repair of tetralogy of Fallot. *Circulation* 58 Suppl 1:209-217, 1978

383. Reduto LA, Berger HJ, Johnstone DE, et al: Radionuclide assessment of right and left ventricular exercise reserve after total correction of tetralogy of Fallot. *Am J Cardiol* 45:1013-1018, 1980

384. Gerson MC, Hurst JM, Hertzberg VS, et al: Cardiac prognosis in noncardiac geriatric surgery. *Ann Intern Med* 103:832-837, 1985

385. Boucher CA, Brewster DC, Darling RC, et al: Determination of cardiac risk by dipyridamole-thallium imaging before peripheral vascular surgery. *N Engl J Med* 312:389-394, 1985

386. Leppo J, Plaja J, Gionet M, et al: Noninvasive evaluation of cardiac risk before elective vascular surgery. *J Am Coll Cardiol* 9:269-276, 1987

387. Eagle KA, Singer DE, Brewster DC, et al: Dipyridamole-thallium scanning in patients undergoing vascular surgery: optimizing preoperative evaluation of cardiac risk. *JAMA* 257:2185-2189, 1987

388. Eagle KA, Coley CM, Newell JB, et al: Combining clinical and thallium data optimizes preoperative assessment of cardiac risk before major vascular surgery. *Ann Intern Med* 110:859-866, 1989

389. Shaw L, Miller DD, Kong BA, et al: Determination of perioperative cardiac risk by adenosine thallium-201 myocardial imaging. *Am Heart J* 124:861-869, 1992

390. Stratmann HG, Tamesis BR, Wittry MD, et al: Dipyridamole stress technetium-99m sestamibi myocardial tomography: an independent predictor of adverse outcome in patients following acute ischemic events. *J Nucl Med* 34 Suppl:85P, 1993

391. Lette J, Waters D, Lapointe J, et al: Usefulness of the severity and extent of reversible perfusion defects during thallium-dipyridamole imaging for cardiac risk assessment before noncardiac surgery. *Am J Cardiol* 64:276-281, 1989

392. Lette J, Waters D, Lassonde J, et al: Postoperative myocardial infarction and cardiac death: predictive value of dipyridamole-thallium imaging and five clinical scoring systems based on multifactorial analysis. *Ann Surg* 211:84-90, 1990

393. Lane SE, Lewis SM, Pippin JJ, et al: Predictive value of quantitative dipyridamole-thallium scintigraphy in assessing cardiovascular risk after vascular surgery in diabetes mellitus. *Am J Cardiol* 64:1275-1279, 1989

394. Mangano DT, London MJ, Tubau JF, et al: Dipyridamole thallium-201 scintigraphy as a preoperative screening test: a reexamination of its predictive potential. *Circulation* 84:493-502, 1991

395. Elmore JR, Hallett JE Jr, Gibbons RJ, et al: Myocardial revascularization before abdominal aortic aneurysmorrhaphy: effect of coronary angioplasty. *Mayo Clin Proc* 68:637-641, 1993

396. Matthay RA, Berger HJ, Loke J, et al: Effects of aminophylline upon right and left ventricular performance in chronic obstructive pulmonary disease: noninvasive assessment by radionuclide angiocardiography. *Am J Med* 65:903-910, 1978

397. Alexander J, Dainiak N, Berger HJ, et al: Serial assessment of doxorubicin cardiotoxicity with quantitative radionuclide angiocardiography. *N Engl J Med* 300:278-283, 1979

398. Gottdiener JS, Mathisen DJ, Borer JS, et al: Doxorubicin cardiotoxicity: assessment of late left ventricular dysfunction by radionuclide cineangiography. *Ann Intern Med* 94:430-435, 1981

399. Okada RD, Boucher CA, Strauss HW, et al: Exercise radionuclide imaging approaches to coronary artery disease. *Am J Cardiol* 46:1188-1204, 1980

400. Port S, Cobb FR, Coleman RE, et al: The effects of age on the response to the left ventricular ejection fraction to exercise. *N Engl J Med* 303:1133-1137, 1980

401. Jensen D, Atwood JE, Froelicher V, et al: Improvement in ventricular function during exercise studied with radionuclide ventriculography after cardiac rehabilitation. *Am J Cardiol* 46:770-777, 1980

402. Cobb FR, Williams RS, McEwan P, et al: Effects of exercise training on ventricular function in patients with recent myocardial infarction. *Circulation* 66:100-108, 1982

CHAPTER

7

Cardiac magnetic resonance imaging

Jerome F. Breen, M.D., and Paul R. Julsrud, M.D.

In the first edition of this textbook, the topic of cardiac magnetic resonance imaging (MRI) was discussed in a few paragraphs, and it was stated that "the dimensions of its capability as a diagnostic tool have not yet been defined." MRI of the heart and great vessels has since evolved into a modality of proven clinical utility, yet as this third edition goes to press, the statement remains accurate and appropriate. Because of continuing technologic advances, the potential capability of MRI in the routine evaluation of cardiovascular diseases is likely to continue to expand. This chapter outlines areas in which MRI has acquired a role for clinical imaging and examines some of the potential future applications. Excellent reviews of the principles of MRI can be found in the literature.[1-4]

CARDIAC IMAGING

Technical considerations

A standard spin-echo MR image results from many repetitions of the nuclear magnetic resonance phenomenon and is not simply a "snapshot." Acquisition of the signal data must therefore be gated to the electrocardiogram.[5-7] An irregular rhythm can seriously degrade image quality in standard MRI techniques. Even with regular rhythms, a recognizable QRS complex may be difficult to obtain because of induced electrical potentials in the leads produced by the changing magnetic gradients, the radio frequency pulses, and the beating heart in the strong external magnetic field.[8] Thus, some experimentation of lead placement may be necessary to obtain a satisfactory signal tracing.[9] Similarly, because of induced voltages, pacemaker function can be affected by the MR environment, so that pacemaker presence is a contraindication to imaging by this method.[10,11]

Imaging time with standard spin-echo techniques is relatively long. Although multiple levels spanning the entire heart can be obtained simultaneously, the need for many separate signal acquisitions for adequate spatial resolution (typically 128 to 192 steps, or views) and adequate signal-to-noise ratio (usually two excitations per view) results in a scan time of 4 or 5 minutes for someone with an average heart rate. Several acquisitions are performed in most studies, depending on the need for multiple imaging planes, the spatial resolution required, and the signal-to-noise ratio necessary for diagnostic information.[12-15]

Although spin-echo technique is the mainstay of morphologic cardiac imaging because it provides high spatial resolution, functional information imaging is provided by "fast" MR techniques. One of these techniques, known as "cine MRI," uses very rapid excitations and signal measurement sequences (gradient-recalled echo techniques) that markedly increase the number of images that can be obtained at a given anatomic location during a single acquisition.[16-18] Standard spin-echo imaging results in only one cardiac phase per tomographic level, with each level being at a different phase in the cardiac cycle. Cine MRI can yield up to 64 images per level, which are reviewed in a real-time-like loop fashion. Standard cine MRI uses retrospective gating with acquisition times in the range of 3 to 5 minutes for a typical two-level study. The time to image the entire heart with this method depends on the spatial and temporal resolution desired.

Recent development of "ultrafast" cine and spin-echo sequences permits images to be obtained in one held breath on standard MRI imaging equipment.[19-21] These techniques provide high-resolution images, reduce acquisition times, and eliminate respiratory motion artifacts.

An MRI method known as "echo planar technique" uses rapidly changing gradients after the initial radio frequency pulse and can acquire complete "snapshot" cardiac images in as little as 30 msec.[22,23] Cardiac gating is not required, and image quality is not degraded by arrhythmias or respiratory motion. Currently, echo planar imaging is not in routine use, as it requires expensive equipment modification to standard MR imagers.

Contraindications and safety

No known biologic ill effects have been shown to occur with current MR techniques.[24] Although there are no demonstrable effects, imaging of pregnant patients should be done only after judicious consideration of the options.

MRI is contraindicated in patients with pacemakers, internal cardiac defibrillators, or ferromagnetic cerebral aneurysm clips.[10,11,25] The presence of surgical clips, vascular coils, sternotomy wires, and metallic orthopedic implants is not a contraindication; however, all may produce some or many artifacts on the images. Several prosthetic heart valves have been shown to experience some attractive force when placed in the bore of an MR imager, but the force generated is small compared with that experienced by valves during normal cardiac contraction. With the exception of patients with an older Starr-Edwards (pre-6000) valve and suspected dehiscence of that valve, we use MRI in all patients with prosthetic valves.[26,27]

CARDIAC ANATOMY

Spin-echo MRI techniques produce high-quality, detailed static images of the heart and great vessels. The inherent contrast is provided by the high-intensity signal from fat, the low-intensity signal from fibrous tissues, and the intermediate-intensity signal from myocardium. Rapidly flowing blood yields a low signal, therefore providing natural contrast between the blood pool and cardiovascular structures. The cardiac cavities, great vessels, and pericardium are well demarcated and can be imaged in any chosen plane. Spatial relationships are easily recognized because of the all-encompassing large field of view available (Fig 7-1).

Cine MRI produces images in which the blood pool appears as a bright signal. Continuous reexcitement of the same slice by rapid radio frequency pulses results in partial saturation of relatively stationary tissue and enhancement of the signal of blood flowing into the imaging slice. Turbulent blood flow returns no signal with cine techniques, allowing visualization of flow disturbance secondary to shunts, stenoses, and regurgitant jets as areas of signal void (Fig 7-2).

Additional anatomic and functional information can be obtained by displaying cine MRI information in a manner that maps the velocities of structures moving in and through the imaging plane.[28-30] MR signals have both magnitude and phase information, and the conventional image is a display of the magnitude of signal returned from each point. The phase of an emitted signal depends on the velocity of the nuclei at that point, with stationary tissue having zero phase. Flowing blood has a phase shift that can be displayed to depict the velocity and direction of flow. Mapping velocities in a region of interest in a manner analogous to placement of a Doppler probe allows for similar quantitative information to be obtained. Pressure gradients, shunt calculations, regurgitant volumes, and cardiac output measurements are all possible by this technique.[31-34] An advantage of this gray-scale equivalent of color-flow Doppler imaging is the ability to place an "MR electronic electromagnetic flowmeter" anywhere in the body without the need for an adequate acoustic window to the site of interest (Fig 7-3).

CURRENT CLINICAL CARDIAC MAGNETIC RESONANCE IMAGING

Congenital heart disease

Since cardiovascular anatomy is clearly demonstrated by MRI, it is very helpful in diagnosing congenital heart diseases. Fortunately, because patients with these diseases often are seen at a young age and are relatively small, MRI can be done with smaller fields of view, which result in increased spatial resolution. Patients younger than 6 years routinely are given chloral hydrate to minimize motion during the examination, which usually requires 45 to 60 minutes.

Most physicians involved in diagnosing congenital heart diseases currently consider echocardiography to be the primary imaging modality. Therefore, it seems prudent to discuss MRI's diagnostic abilities as they compare with those of echocardiography, highlighting those instances in which MRI proves advantageous. Consequently, in the following discussion, an attempt is made to indicate not only MRI's capability to demonstrate a certain anomaly but also its clinical usefulness vis-à-vis echocardiography.

Septal defects. Intracardiac lesions involving defects of the atrial or ventricular septum can be demonstrated by MRI.[35-38] Figure 7-4,A illustrates the MRI findings in a secundum atrial septal defect. The dropout of MRI signal due to absence of the septum is analogous to the signal dropout used by an echocardiographer to diagnose an atrial septal defect (Fig 7-4,B). However, Doppler interrogation and color-flow imaging can also be used by the echocardiographer to assess the hemodynamic consequences of an interatrial septal defect (see Fig 7-4,B). Although cine MRI techniques can also depict blood flow, MRI does not appear to offer any major advantage over echocardiography in diagnosing secundum or primum atrial septal defects. However, there is more difficulty recognizing sinus venosus atrial septal defects with conventional precordial echocardiography.[39] MRI, on the other hand, has been extremely reliable in demonstrating this defect, which is located in the superior aspect of the interatrial septum (Fig 7-5).

As mentioned above, MRI can also demonstrate ventricular septal defects. However, current echocardiographic techniques are quite accurate in identifying these defects.[40,41] Consequently, MRI's use in ventricular septal defect has been primarily confirmatory. Figure 7-6 illustrates a large malalignment ventricular septal defect in a patient with tetralogy of Fallot. Figure 7-7 shows the findings on cine MRI of a restrictive ventricular septal defect in a patient with univentricular heart who is a candidate for the Fontan procedure. The lack of signal due to turbulent flow just beyond the ventricular septal defect during systole on the cine MRI examination indicates the obstructive nature of this defect (see Fig 7-7,B).

Conotruncal abnormalities. In addition to demonstrating the ventricular septal defect in patients with tetralogy of Fallot, MRI can elucidate some of the clinically relevant malformations of the great arteries and pulmonary outflow tract that are due to the conotruncal

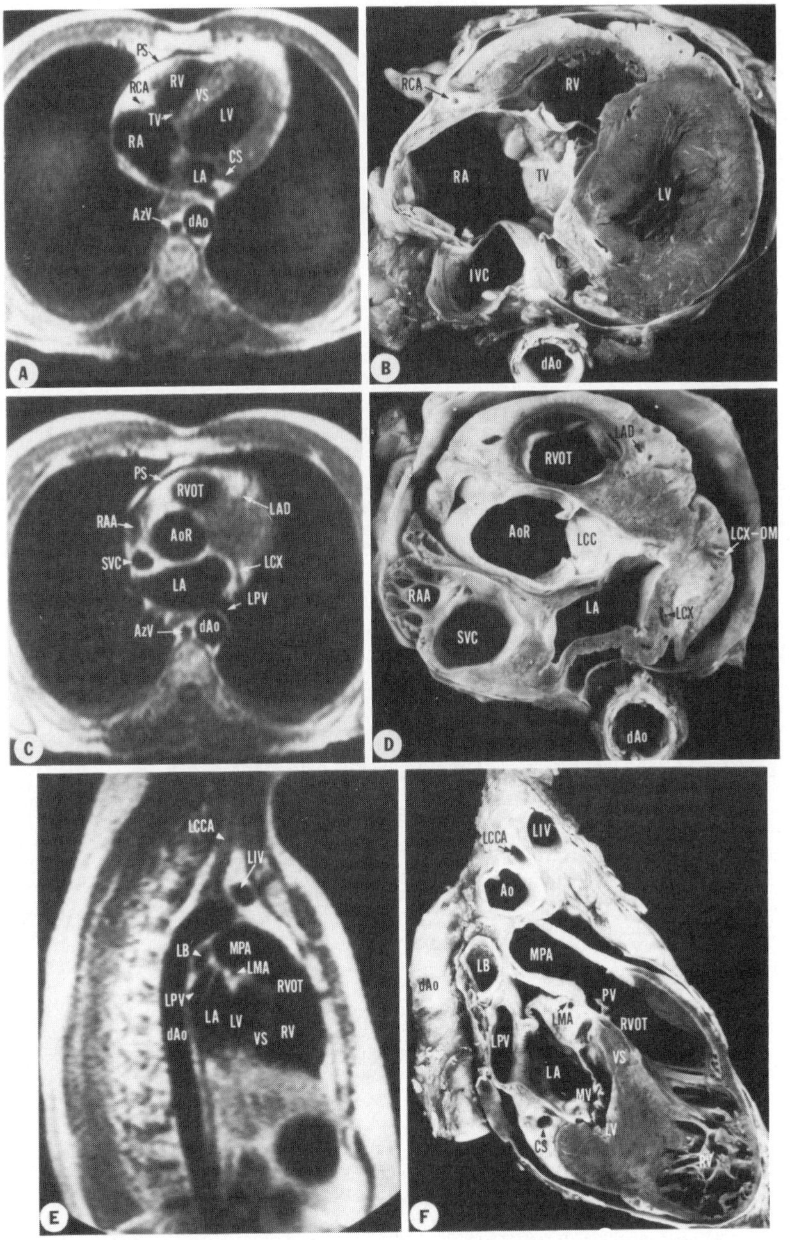

Fig 7-1 Transverse (**A** through **D**), sagittal (**E** through **H**), and coronal (**I** through **L**) planes of the heart shown in analogous magnetic resonance images (at left) and anatomic sections (at right). *aAo,* ascending aorta; *Ao,* aortic arch; *AoR,* aortic root; *AV,* aortic valve; *AzV,* azygos vein; *CS,* coronary sinus; *dAo,* descending thoracic aorta; *IA,* innominate artery; *LA,* left atrium; *LAA,* left atrial appendage; *LAD,* left anterior descending coronary artery; *LB,* left bronchus; *LCC,* left coronary cusp; *LCCA,* left common carotid artery; *LCX,* left circumflex coronary artery; *LCX-OM,* left circumflex coronary artery, obtuse marginal branch; *LIV,* left innominate vein; *LLPV,* left lower pulmonary vein; *LMA,* left main coronary artery; *LPA,* left pulmonary artery; *LPV,* left pulmonary vein; *LSA,* left subclavian artery; *LSV,* left subclavian vein; *LUPV,* left upper pulmonary vein; *LV,* left ventricle; *MPA,* main pulmonary artery; *MV,* mitral valve; *PS,* pericardial sac; *PV,* pulmonary valve; *RA,* right atrium; *RAA,* right atrial appendage; *RCA,* right coronary artery; *RCCA,* right common carotid artery; *RIV,* right innominate vein; *RJV,* right internal jugular vein; *RPA,* right pulmonary artery; *RSV,* right subclavian vein; *RV,* right ventricle; *RVOT,* right ventricular outflow tract; *SVC,* superior vena cava; *T,* trachea; *TV,* tricuspid valve; *VS,* ventricular septum. (From Nazarian GK, Julsrud PR, Ehman RL, et al: Correlation between magnetic resonance imaging of the heart and cardiac anatomy. *Mayo Clin Proc* 62:573-583, 1987. By permission, Mayo Foundation.) (Continued on next page.)

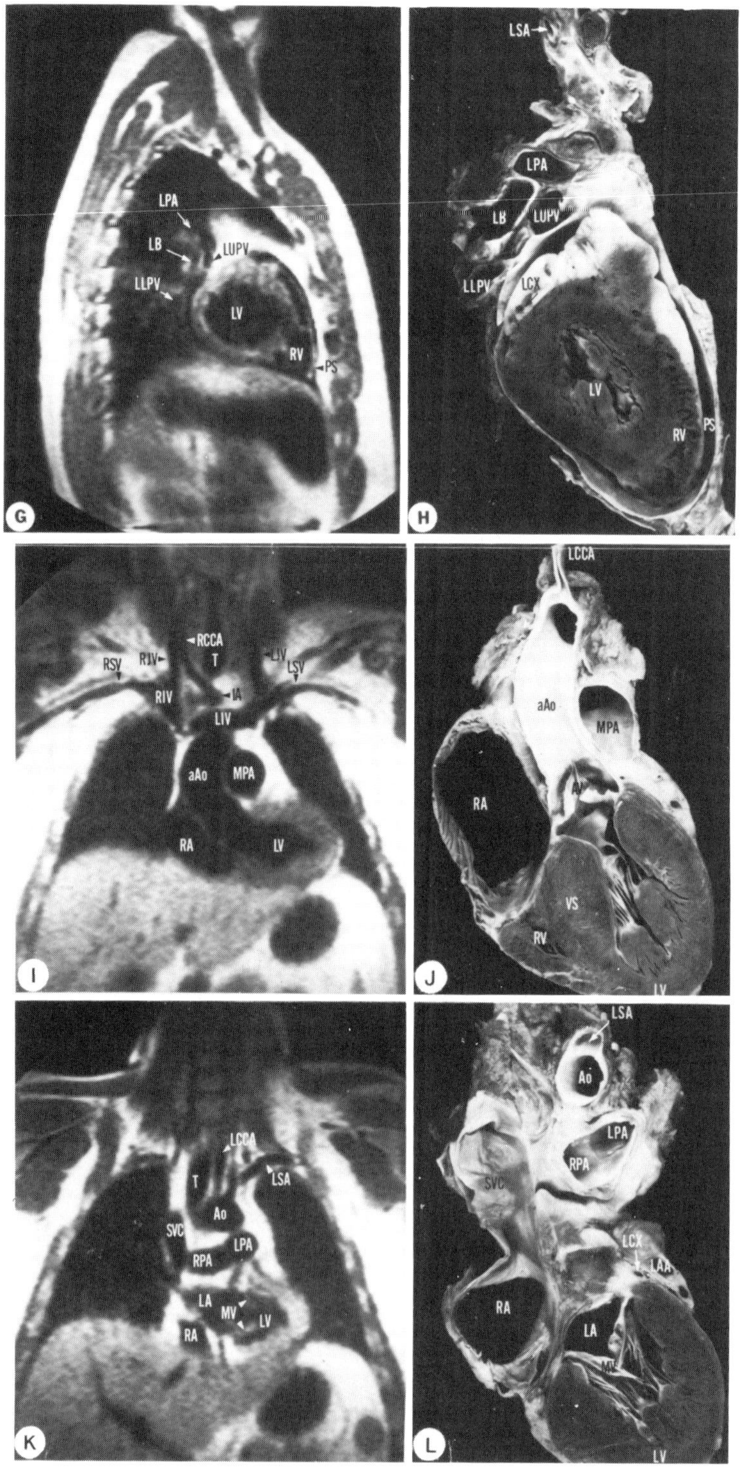

Fig 7-1, cont'd. For legend see p. 277.

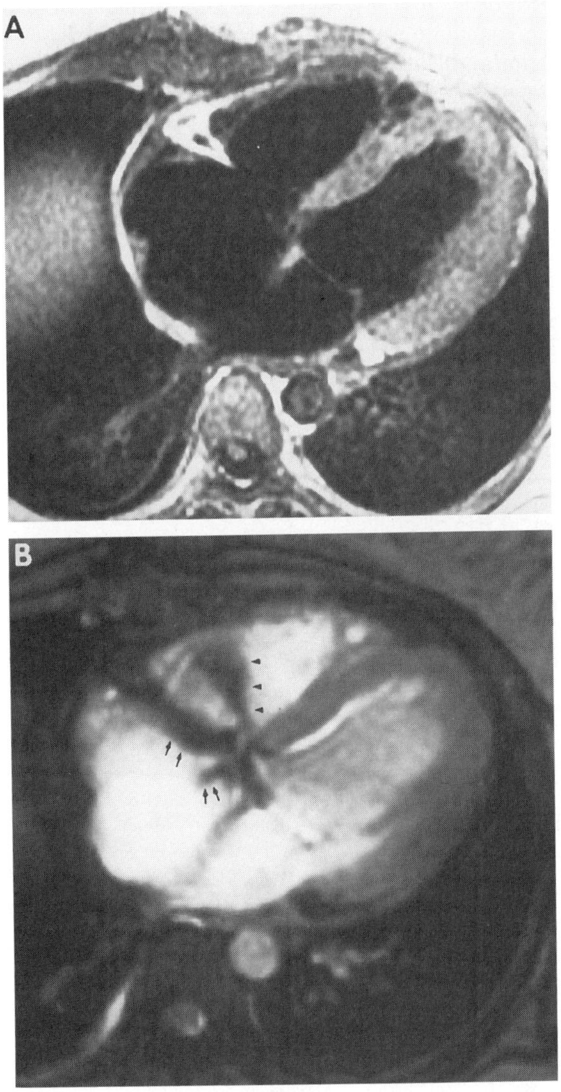

Fig 7-2 After insertion of an aortic valve prosthesis and repair of a ventricular septal defect secondary to subacute bacterial endocarditis with perivalvular abscess in a 28-year-old woman, echocardiography demonstrated a fistula from the left ventricle to the right atrium through the ventricular septal defect patch. **A,** spin-echo image appears normal. **B,** gradient-echo image demonstrates two turbulent jets *(arrows)* from the left ventricle to the right atrium and a larger shunt *(arrowheads)* from the left ventricle to the right ventricle.

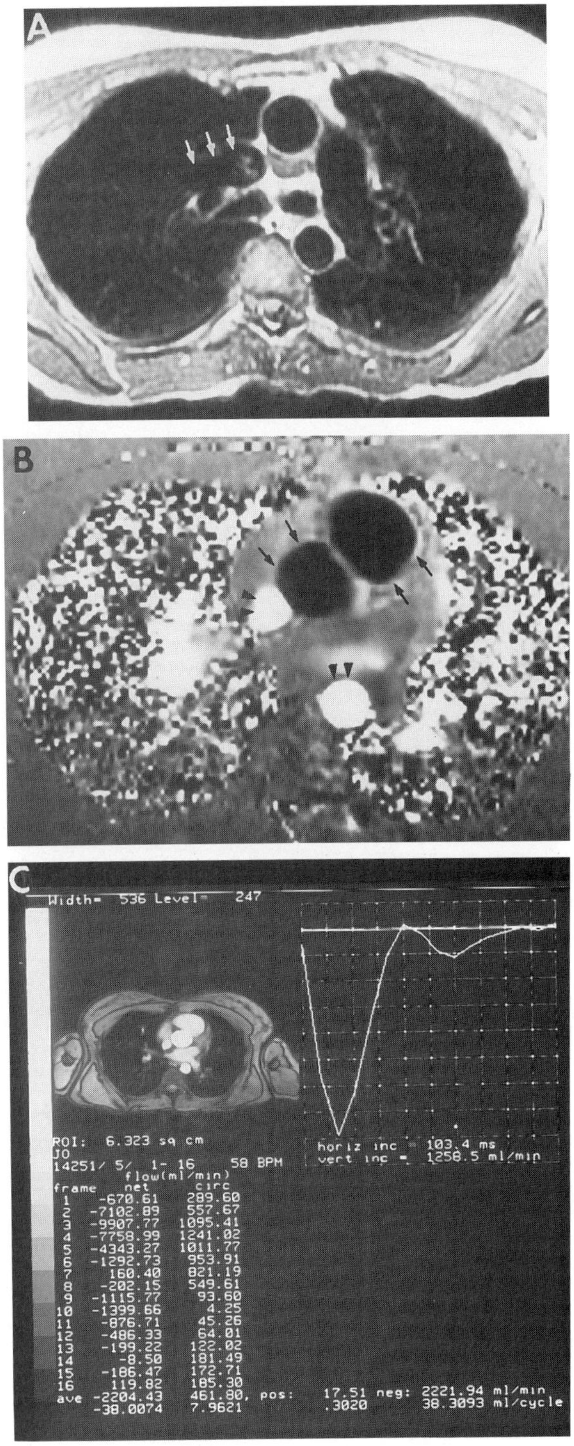

Fig 7-3 Partial anomalous pulmonary venous return in a 42-year-old woman. **A,** the right upper pulmonary vein enters the superior vena cava *(arrows)*. **B,** phase image at the level of the proximal ascending aorta and pulmonary artery with flow toward the head is displayed as black *(arrows)*. Caudal flow in the descending aorta and superior vena cava is white *(arrowheads)*. **C,** region of interest measurement of flow through the aorta during systole and diastole. Similar measurement of pulmonary flow gave a Qp:Qs ratio of 1.5.

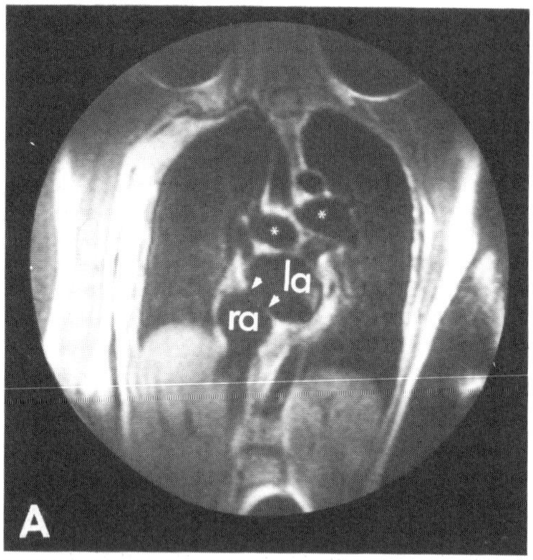

Fig 7-4 Secundum atrial septal defect. **A,** MR image in coronal plane demonstrates secundum atrial septal defect (*small arrowheads* identify edges of defect). Note enlargement of pulmonary arteries *(asterisks)* due to the left-to-right shunt. **B,** echocardiogram in same patient demonstrates atrial septal defect in coronal plane (*larger arrowheads* identify edges of defect). Color-flow Doppler examination in right panel shows left-to-right shunting through the atrial septal defect. *la* and *LA,* left atrium; *ra* and *RA,* right atrium.

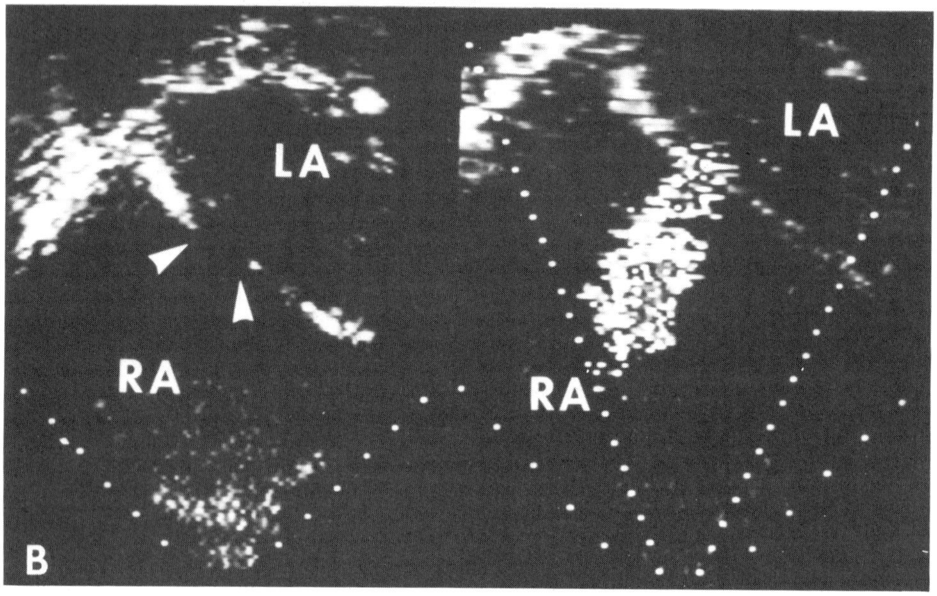

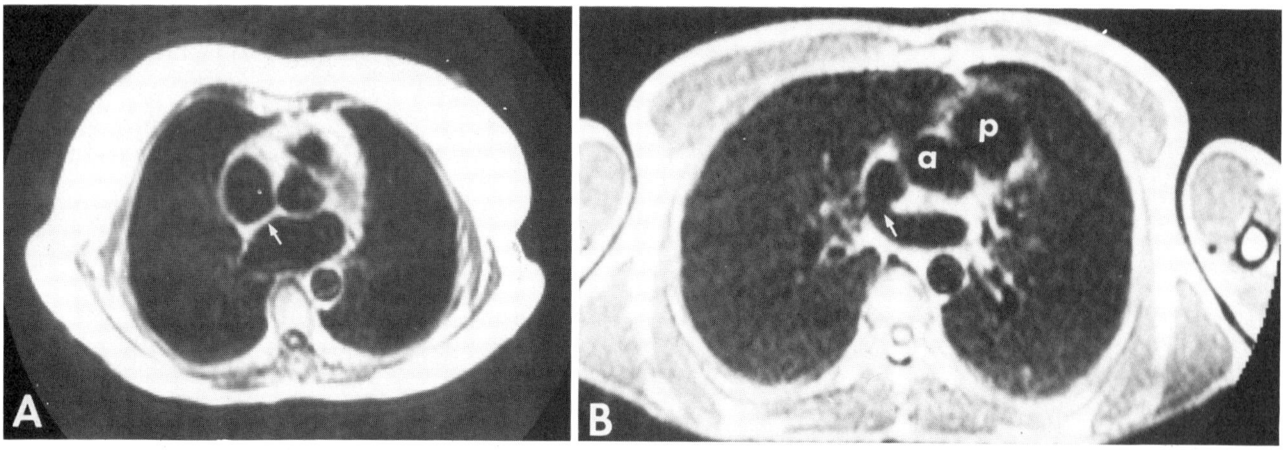

Fig 7-5 Sinus venosus atrial septal defect. **A,** MR image appearance of superior aspect of intact interatrial septum *(arrow)* in transverse plane. Image is viewed from below, so that arrow is located in left atrium and points anteriorly and to the patient's right.
B, transverse MR image of sinus venosus atrial septal defect *(arrow).* Note the dilated pulmonary outflow tract of the right ventricle, located anteriorly. *a,* aorta; *p,* pulmonary outflow tract of right ventricle.

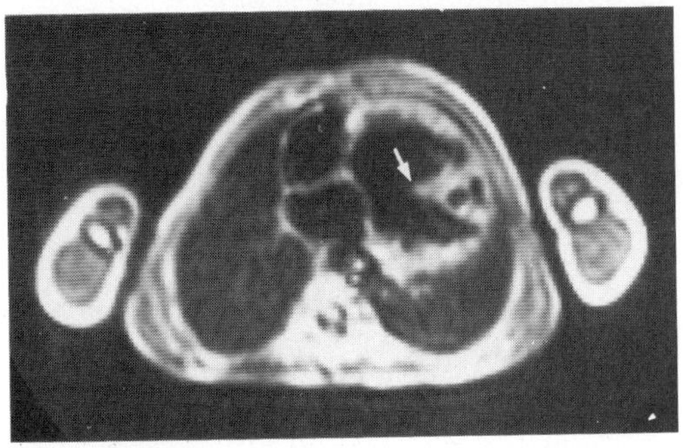

Fig 7-6 Ventricular septal defect. Transverse MR image at level of both atria and ventricles. Note the large defect in the interventricular septum in a patient with tetralogy of Fallot. (*Arrow* identifies the edge of the interventricular septum.) (From Ehman RL, Julsrud PR: Magnetic resonance imaging of the heart: current status. *Mayo Clin Proc* 64:1134-1146, 1989. By permission, Mayo Foundation for Medical Education and Research.)

developmental abnormalities of this anomaly[42] (Fig 7-8). MRI can also depict the ventricle and great vessel relationships that characterize other congenital heart abnormalities due to conotruncal maldevelopment, such as truncus arteriosus communis, double-outlet right ventricle, and the transposition complexes[42,43] (Fig 7-9). In addition to revealing the spatial locations and connections of the aorta and main pulmonary artery in transposition of the great vessels, MRI has been useful in evaluating the adequacy of the surgically created systemic and pulmonary intracardiac venous pathways in patients who have had interatrial baffle procedures (see Fig 7-9). Although echocardiography with Doppler augmentation has also been helpful in demonstrating these pathways, MRI provides an additional means of acquiring a noninvasive evaluation of this difficult clinical situation.[44]

Pulmonary arteries. The proximal right and left pulmonary arteries and their branches, at least to slightly beyond the hilar level, are well demonstrated by MRI. On the other hand, echocardiography frequently has difficulty visualizing pulmonary artery anatomy because of the air-filled lungs, which limit the acoustical window. The echocardiographic examination of the pulmonary arteries is usually even more difficult postoperatively. Unfortunately, this is precisely the situation in which one may be especially interested in excluding iatrogenic distortion or narrowing of the pulmonary arteries. Therefore, it is particularly fortunate that even in the patient who has been operated on, MRI is extremely good at demonstrating this anatomy. Figure 7-10 illustrates the hypoplastic (7 mm) proximal right and left pulmonary arteries in a patient who had had previous banding of the main pulmonary artery. MRI reveals the additional discrete stenosis at the origin of the right pulmonary artery and a ductal diverticulum protruding from the proximal left pulmonary artery. Figure 7-11 documents MRI's ability to detect distortion and narrowing of pulmonary arteries secondary to previously placed shunts between systemic and pulmonary arteries. Cephalad "tenting" of the proximal right pulmonary artery with associated narrowing is due to placement of a right Blalock-Taussig shunt. In Figure 7-11,C, a patent left Blalock-Taussig shunt to a left pulmonary artery does not deform the artery.

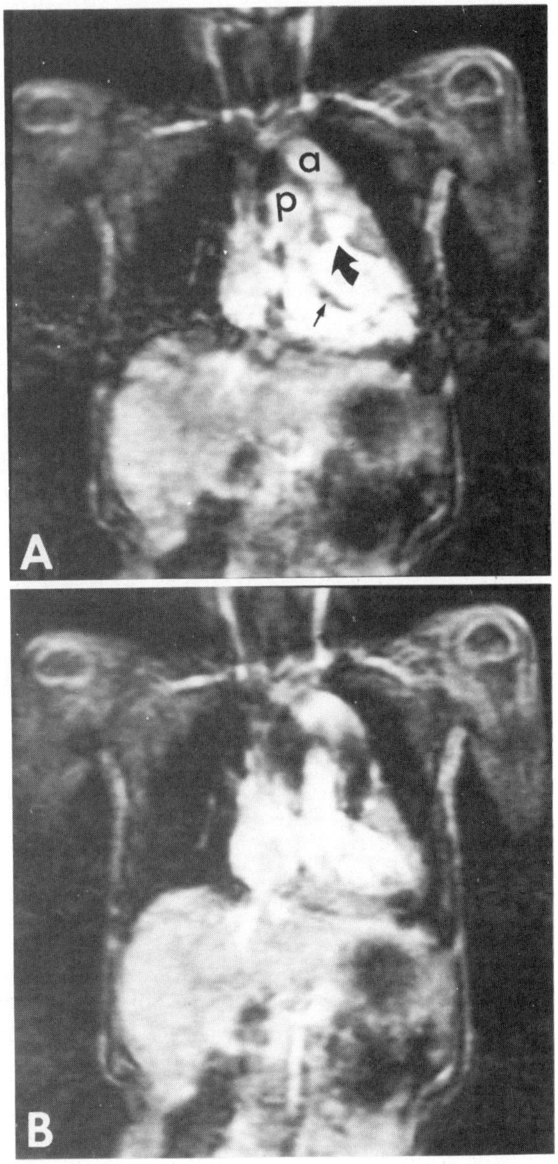

Fig 7-7 Cine MR images in coronal plane demonstrating restrictive ventricular septal defect in a patient with univentricular heart and transposition of the great vessels. **A,** diastolic phase of cardiac cycle. Note small size of ventricular septal defect *(curved arrow)* and regurgitant "jet" due to insufficiency of the pulmonary valve *(smaller straight arrow).* **B,** systolic phase of cardiac cycle. Note lack of MRI signal from blood flowing through ventricular septal defect and immediately "downstream" in the aortic root due to turbulent flow secondary to the stenosis. The systolic gradient across the ventricular septal defect was 20 mm Hg at surgery. *a,* aorta; *p,* pulmonary artery.

Gradient-refocused echo techniques have expanded MRI's ability to decipher difficult situations involving pulmonary artery anatomy. When blood flow is too slow to create a good signal void with routine spin-echo image

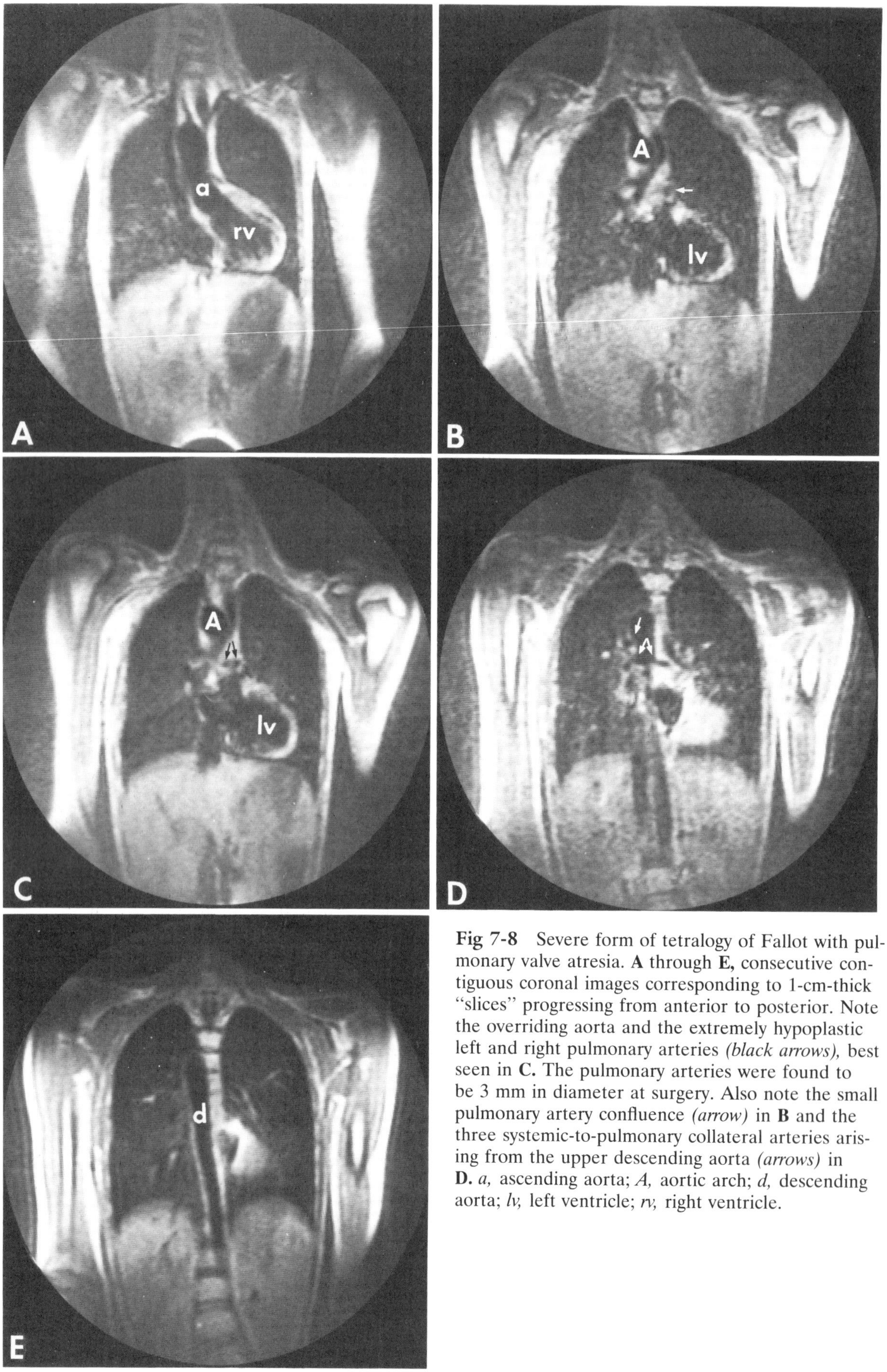

Fig 7-8 Severe form of tetralogy of Fallot with pulmonary valve atresia. **A** through **E,** consecutive contiguous coronal images corresponding to 1-cm-thick "slices" progressing from anterior to posterior. Note the overriding aorta and the extremely hypoplastic left and right pulmonary arteries *(black arrows),* best seen in **C.** The pulmonary arteries were found to be 3 mm in diameter at surgery. Also note the small pulmonary artery confluence *(arrow)* in **B** and the three systemic-to-pulmonary collateral arteries arising from the upper descending aorta *(arrows)* in **D.** *a,* ascending aorta; *A,* aortic arch; *d,* descending aorta; *lv,* left ventricle; *rv,* right ventricle.

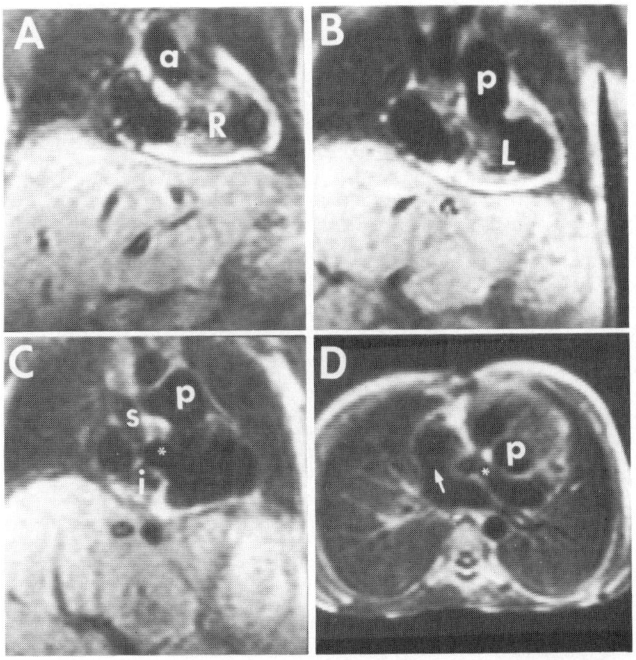

Fig 7-9 MR images of D-transposition of the great arteries after the Mustard procedure. **A** through **C,** coronal images progressing from anterior to posterior. **D,** transverse image at level of interatrial baffle. Note narrowing at the junction between both the superior and the inferior venae cavae and the surgically created systemic venous atrium in **C.** The anatomy of the interatrial baffle is best displayed on the transverse image of **D.** *a,* aorta; *i,* inferior vena cava; *L,* left ventricle; *p,* pulmonary artery; *R,* right ventricle; *s,* superior vena cava; *arrow,* pulmonary venous atrium; *asterisk,* systemic venous atrium.

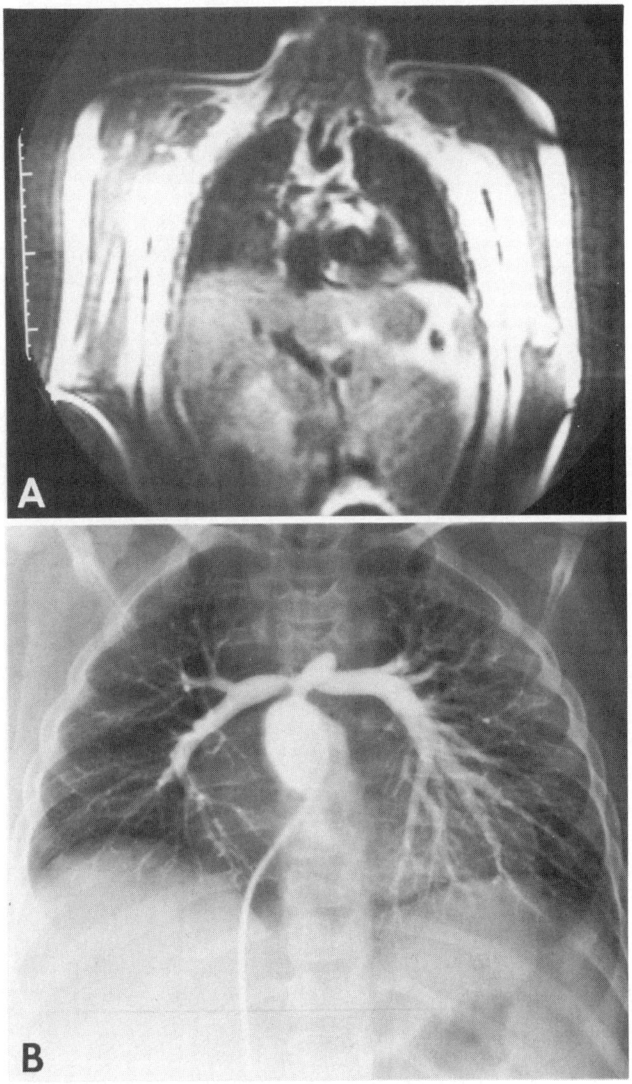

Fig 7-10 Hypoplastic pulmonary arteries with stenosis at the origin of the right pulmonary artery and a ductal diverticulum arising from the proximal left pulmonary artery. **A,** coronal MR image. **B,** pulmonary angiogram for correlation. (See text.)

sequences, these "faster" sequences, which are more motion sensitive, can be used to elicit information about blood flow. Figure 7-12 illustrates a case in which this MRI technique proved advantageous in demonstrating a small central left pulmonary artery; it was confirmed at surgery and measured 4 mm in diameter.

Pulmonary veins. The importance of accurately assessing the pulmonary venous system is perhaps best exemplified in patients with anomalous pulmonary venous connections. Physiologically, these patients have left-to-right atrial-level shunts as a result of a variety of anomalies of pulmonary venous anatomy. The anomalous venous pathways can be difficult to demonstrate echocardiographically. For this reason, cardiac catheterization, with a detailed angiographic assessment, has often been necessary to definitely establish the nature of anomalous pulmonary venous connection. However, MRI has been shown to be an ideal noninvasive method to assess anomalies of pulmonary venous connection.[45] Furthermore, experience in patients considered to be candidates for the Fontan procedure has confirmed the initial impression that MRI was extremely good at visualizing abnormalities of pulmonary venous return. One article reported a sensitivity of 91% and a specificity of 100% for the MRI diagnosis of anomalous pulmonary venous connections in Fontan candidates.[46] The importance of preoperatively detecting anomalies of pulmonary venous connection in Fontan candidates becomes obvious when one considers that postoperatively such an anomalous connection would result in equalization of pulmonary arterial and venous pressures. This unfortunate outcome has been reported, and it led to stasis of pulmonary blood flow and pulmonary infarction.[47] Figures 7-13 and 7-14 illustrate MRI's ability to visualize pulmonary venous connections. The transverse and coronal imaging planes are complementary, because the normal lower pulmonary veins are best demonstrated in the transverse plane and the upper pulmonary veins are usually visualized in the coronal plane.

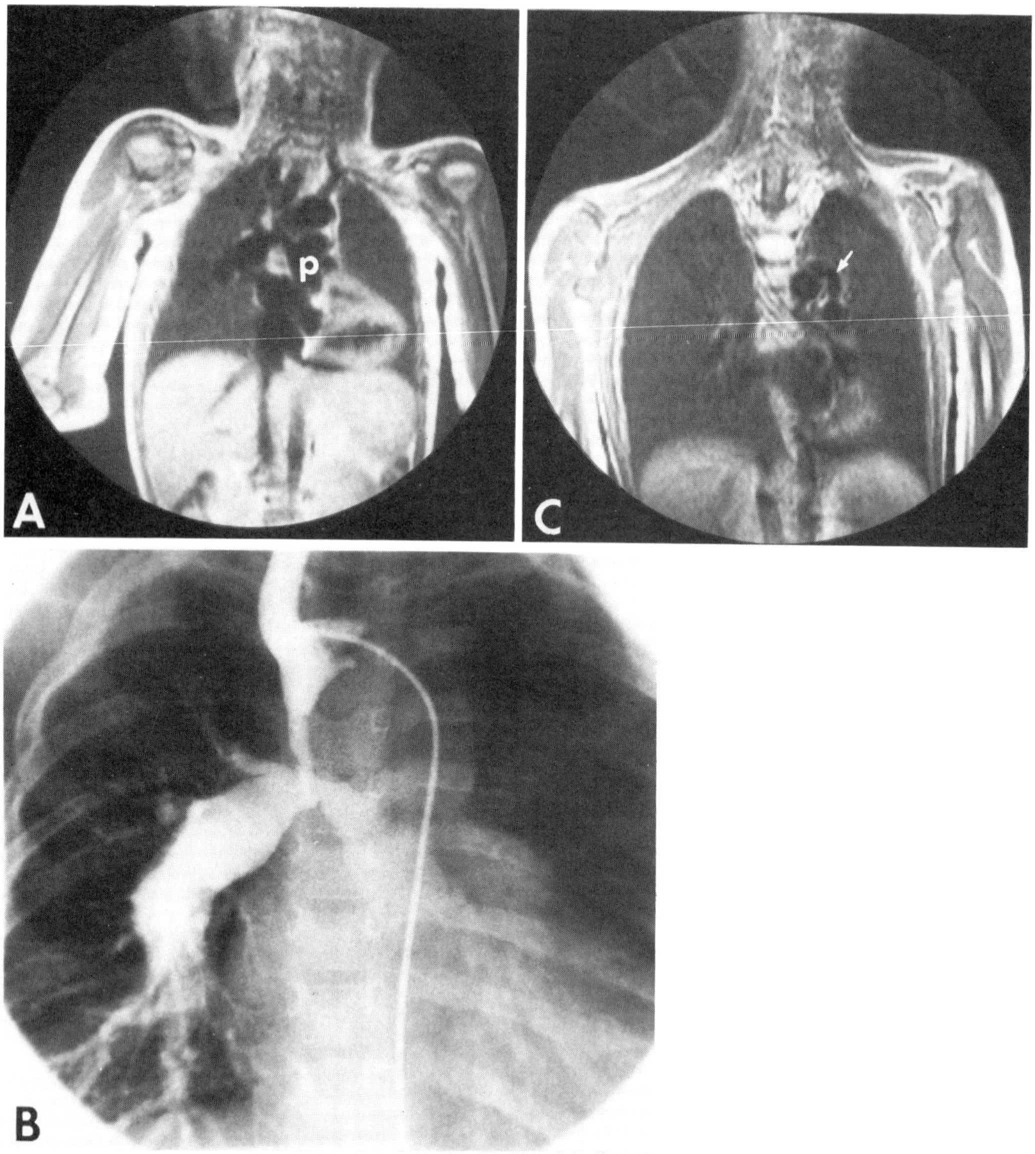

Fig 7-11 Shunts from systemic to pulmonary arteries. **A,** coronal MR image demonstrates narrowing and distortion of the proximal right pulmonary artery due to a right Blalock-Taussig shunt. **B,** angiogram of the right Blalock-Taussig shunt for correlation. **C,** coronal MR image in patient with a left Blalock-Taussig shunt to good-sized, nondistorted left pulmonary artery. *Arrow* points to left subclavian artery, which connects inferiorly to the left pulmonary artery. *p,* main pulmonary artery.

Systemic veins. Although most congenital abnormalities of the systemic venous system are clinically silent, certain circumstances change this situation dramatically. One such situation is illustrated in patients who undergo a modification of the Fontan procedure in which the coronary sinus drains to the systemic side of the circulation after the operation. If a left superior vena cava is present and it connects to the coronary sinus, as it usually does, an obligatory right-to-left shunt will be present postoperatively. Since there is a potential for such a right-to-left shunt to increase in size over time, it is particularly important to exclude even a small left superior vena cava in these patients. MRI has been found extremely effective in evaluating whether a left superior vena cava is present, with one study citing 100% specificity and sensitivity.[46] Echocardiography, on the other hand, is reported to miss about one-third of the left superior vena cava.[48] In this series of 73 patients with proven left superior vena cava, the addition of color-flow Doppler imaging did not improve accuracy. Figure 7-15 documents MRI's ability to demonstrate a small left superior vena cava; it was confirmed at surgery and measured 3 mm in diameter.

Aortic arch anomalies. Perhaps the clearest example

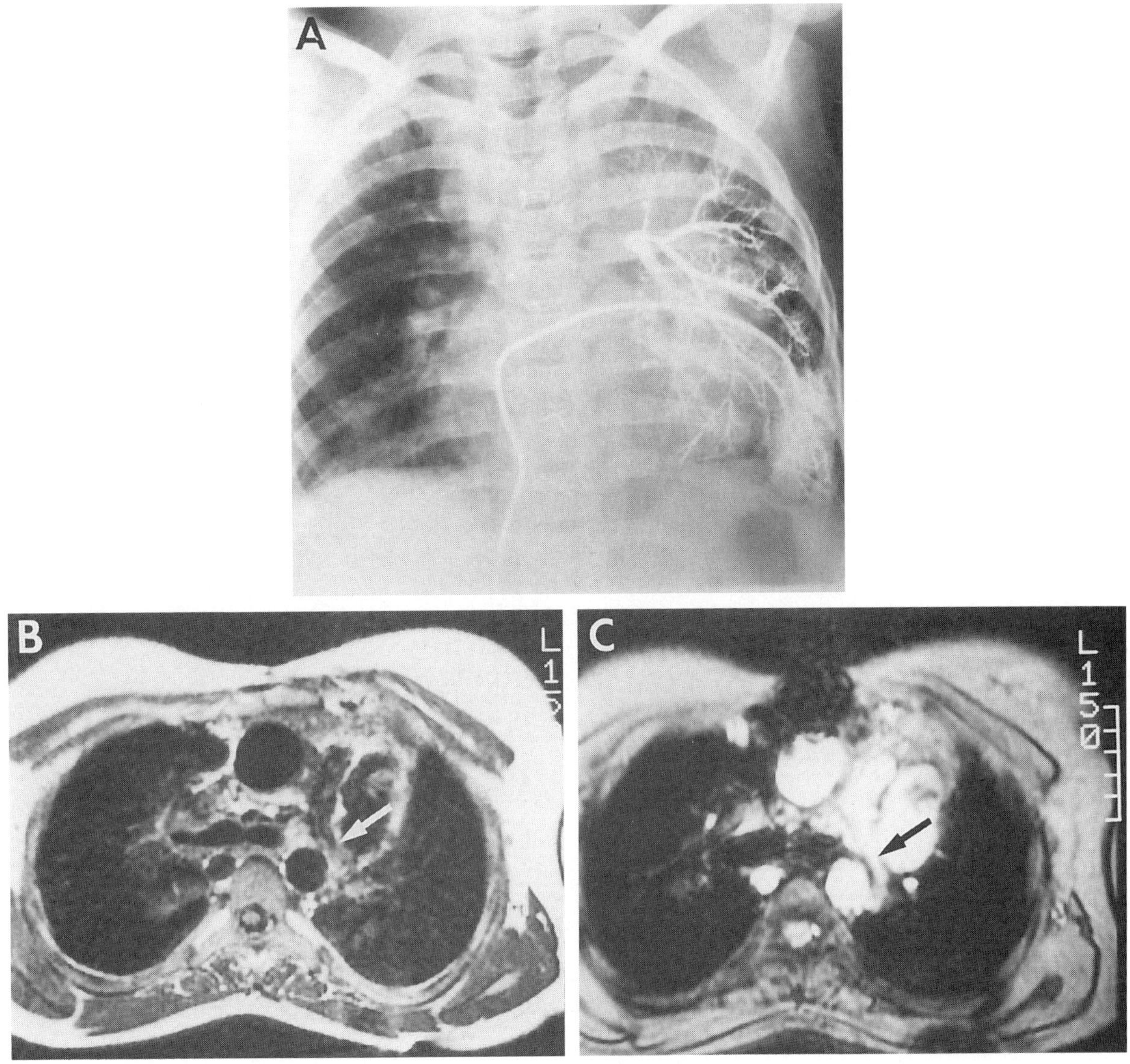

Fig 7-12 **A,** pulmonary vein wedge angiogram with failure to identify the central portion of the left pulmonary artery. **B,** transverse MR image using spin-echo technique fails to demonstrate convincingly a central left pulmonary artery *(white arrow)*. **C,** transverse MR image using gradient-refocused echo technique at the same level as **B** demonstrates a patent central left pulmonary artery *(black arrow)*.

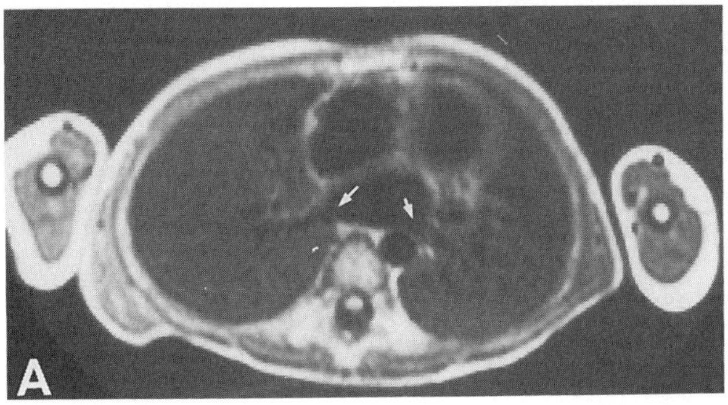

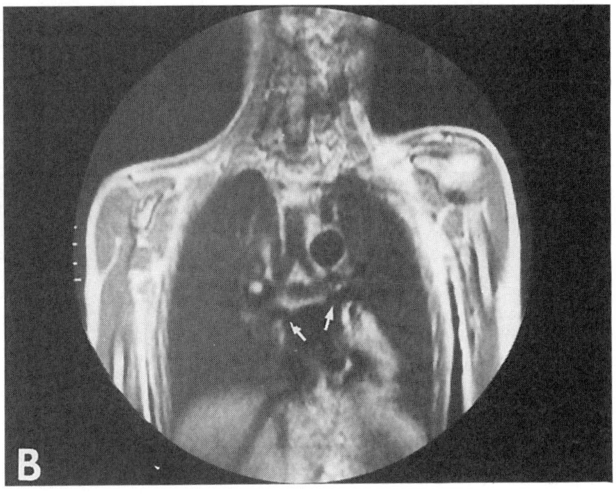

Fig 7-13 MR images of normally connecting pulmonary veins. **A,** transverse image demonstrates right and left lower pulmonary veins entering the posterior aspect of the left atrium. **B,** coronal image shows right and left upper pulmonary veins entering the superior aspect of the left atrium. *Arrows* indicate points of entrance of pulmonary veins.

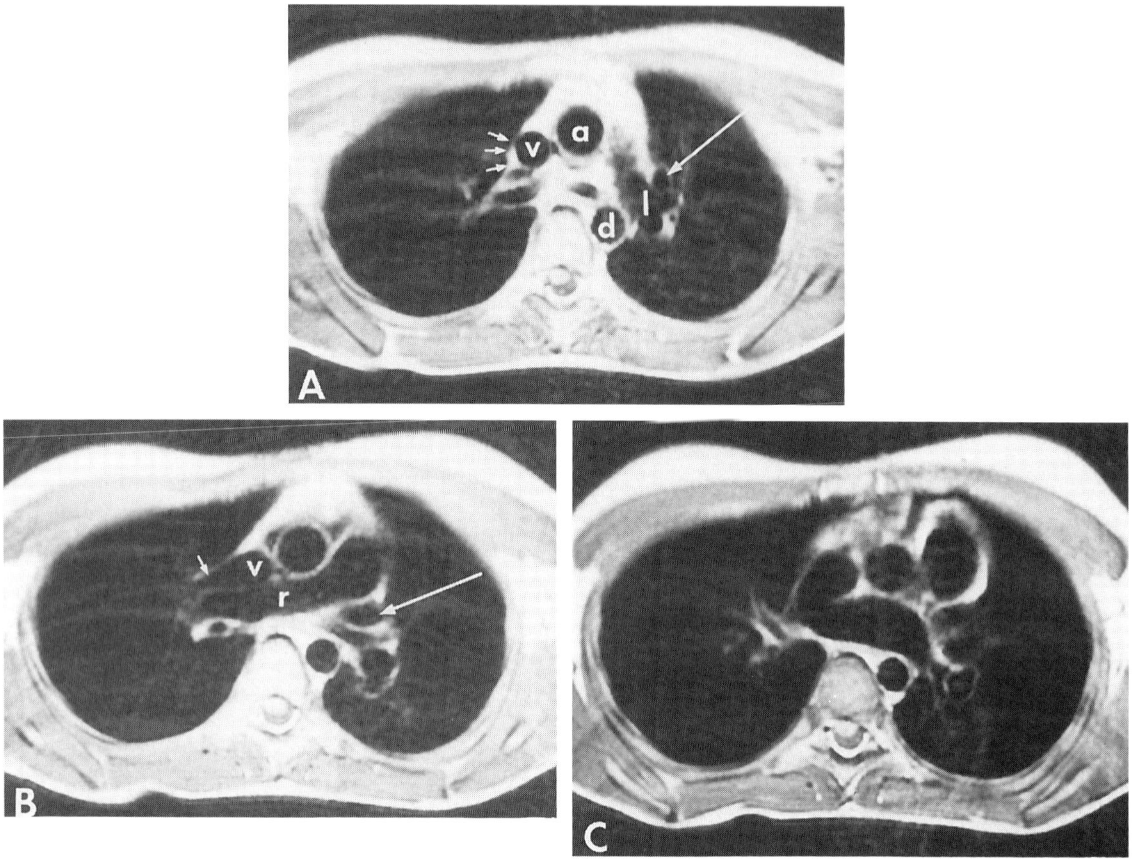

Fig 7-14 MR images of anomalously connecting pulmonary veins. **A,** transverse image at level at which left pulmonary artery crosses over left main-stem bronchus. Multiple *small arrows* indicate normal "complete ring," appearance of superior vena cava above entrance of anomalously connecting pulmonary veins. *Long arrow* points to left upper pulmonary vein. **B,** transverse image 1 cm below level depicted in **A.** Note "broken ring" appearance of superior vena cava due to entrance of anomalously connecting right upper pulmonary vein *(short arrow). Long arrow* points to left upper pulmonary vein as it courses anterior to the left main-stem bronchus. **C,** transverse image from same patient is located 1 cm below level depicted in **B.** Note the sinus venosus atrial septal defect, which is frequently associated with partial anomalous pulmonary venous connections to the superior vena cava (see Fig 7-5 for comparison). *a,* ascending aorta; *d,* descending aorta; *l,* left pulmonary artery; *r,* right pulmonary artery; *v,* superior vena cava.

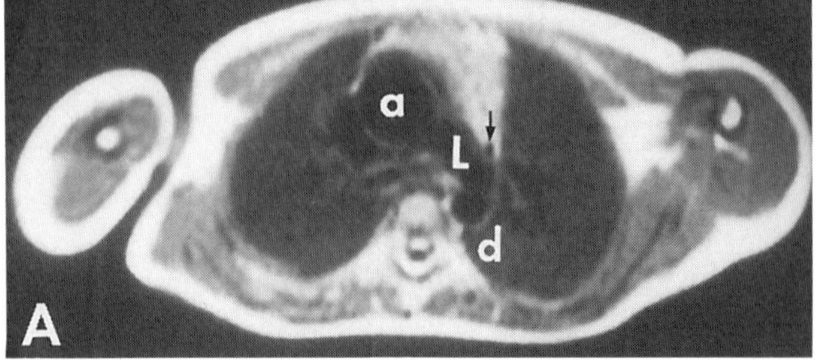

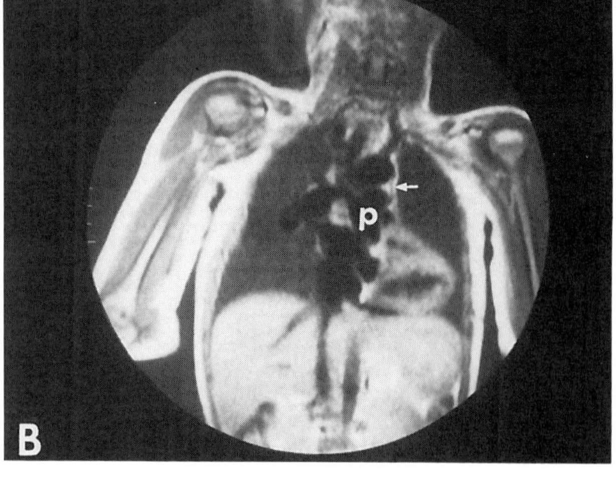

Fig 7-15 Small left superior vena cava demonstrated by MRI in same patient as that in Fig 7-11, A and B. **A,** transverse image at level of pulmonary artery; *black arrow* indicates the left superior vena cava. **B,** coronal image; *white arrow* indicates left superior vena cava. *a,* ascending aorta; *d,* descending aorta; *L,* left pulmonary artery; *p,* main pulmonary artery.

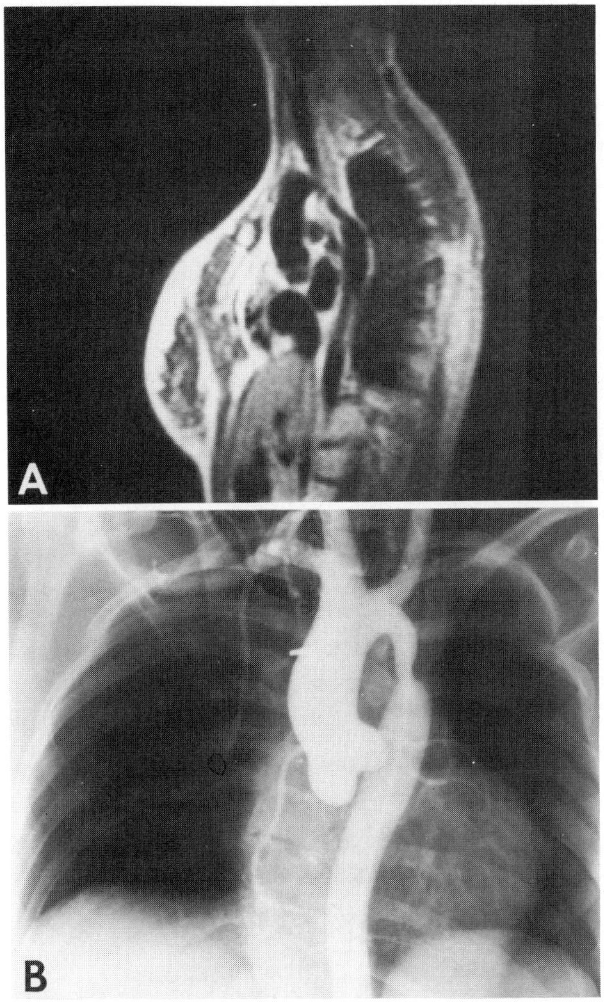

Fig 7-16 Recoarctation of the aorta after a coarctation repair with a subclavian flap angioplasty in infancy. **A,** oblique longitudinal MR image demonstrates the entire sweep of the thoracic aorta. Note narrowed periductal segment at aortic isthmus, revealng recoarctation site. **B,** aortic angiogram in same patient for correlation.

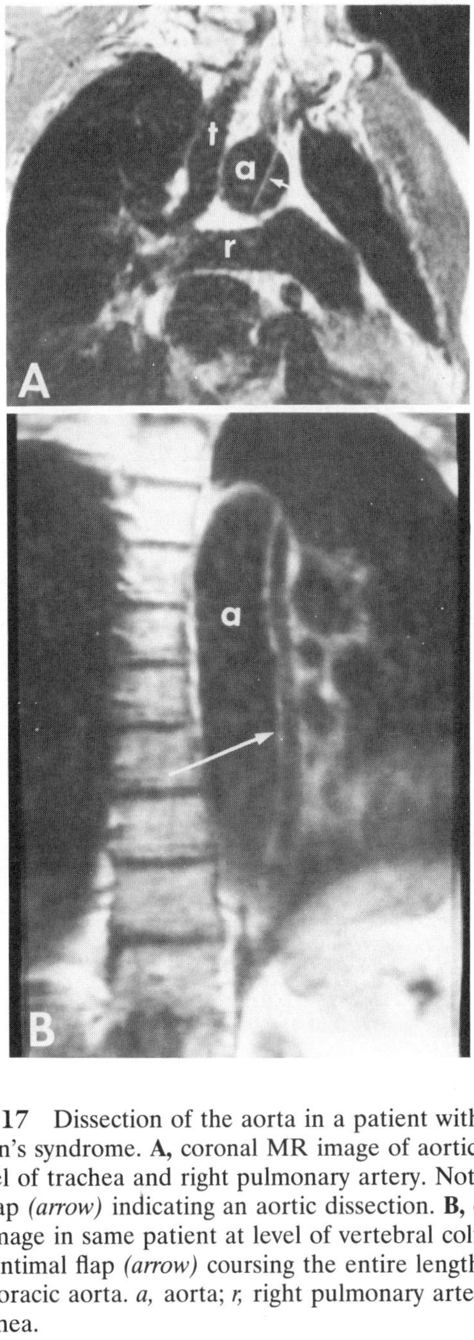

Fig 7-17 Dissection of the aorta in a patient with Marfan's syndrome. **A,** coronal MR image of aortic arch at level of trachea and right pulmonary artery. Note intimal flap *(arrow)* indicating an aortic dissection. **B,** coronal MR image in same patient at level of vertebral column. Note intimal flap *(arrow)* coursing the entire length of the thoracic aorta. *a,* aorta; *r,* right pulmonary artery; *t,* trachea.

of the advantage gained by use of MRI to elucidate cardiovascular abnormalities is its ability to delineate aortic arch anomalies. Most would agree that MRI is currently the noninvasive technique of choice to image the aortic arch and the proximal portions of its branches. MRI has been particularly useful in demonstrating the pertinent structural abnormalities associated with coarctation of the aorta (Fig 7-16), aortic dissections (Fig 7-17), and vascular rings (Fig 7-18).[49,50]

Postoperative evaluations. Although the use of MRI to evaluate patients postoperatively has been briefly alluded to for assessment of intra-atrial baffling of venous pathways and iatrogenic distortion of pulmonary arteries secondary to shunt procedures, we would be remiss if we did not more fully discuss this use of MRI in congenital heart disease. As mentioned above, it is frequently more difficult in this situation for an echocardiographer to accomplish an adequate examination. Figure 7-18 shows MR images of a 15-year-old patient who 5 years previously had had a Rastelli repair for double-outlet right ventricle. At that time, a 25-mm valved conduit was placed from the right ventricle to the main pulmonary artery. His postoperative course was complicated by an infected substernal sinus tract, which required debridement of the anterior mediastinum 3½ months after the Rastelli procedure. At the time of his 4-year routine postoperative evaluation, an echocardiographic study identified tricuspid valve insufficiency and elevation of the right ventricular pressure.

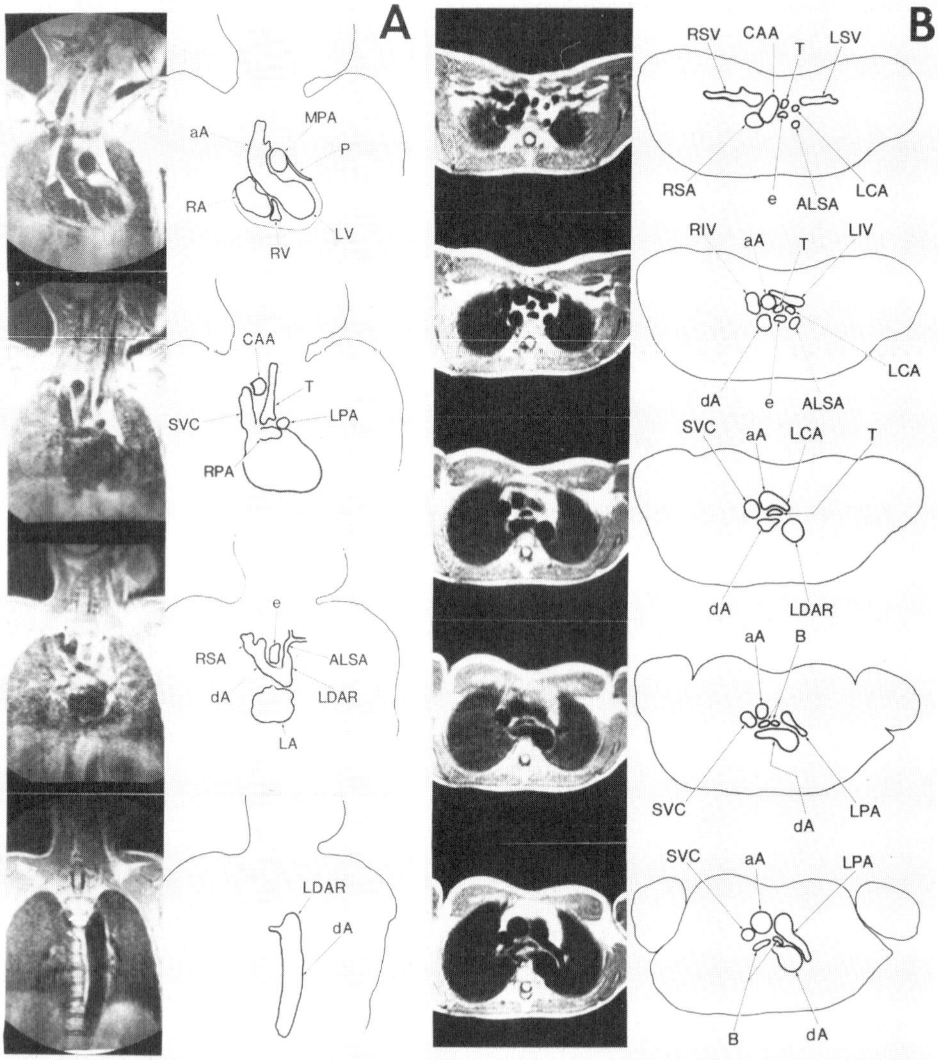

Fig 7-18 MR images demonstrating vascular ring. **A,** coronal plane images viewed from front illustrate sequentially more posterior sections, beginning with top image. In third panel, note upper descending aorta *(dA)* as it courses obliquely posterior to the esophagus to continue as left-sided descending aorta. **B,** transverse plane images viewed from below illustrate sequentially more inferior sections, beginning with top image. In last image, note close approximation of left pulmonary artery *(LPA)* to descending aorta at level of left ligamentum arteriosum, which completes vascular ring. *aA,* ascending aorta; *ALSA,* aberrant left subclavian artery; *B,* bronchi; *CAA,* cervical aortic arch; *e,* esophagus; *LA,* left atrium; *LCA,* left common carotid artery; *LDAR,* left dorsal aortic root; *LIV,* left innominate vein; *LSV,* left subclavian vein; *LV,* left ventricle; *MPA,* main pulmonary artery; *P,* pericardium; *RA,* right atrium; *RIV,* right innominate vein; *RPA,* right pulmonary vein; *RSA,* right subclavian artery; *RSV,* right subclavian vein; *RV,* right ventricle; *SVC,* superior vena cava; *T,* trachea. (From Julsrud PR, Ehman RL: Magnetic resonance imaging of vascular rings. *Mayo Clin Proc* 61:181-185, 1986. By permission, Mayo Foundation.)

However, adequate visualization by echocardiography of the conduit from the right ventricle to the pulmonary artery was not possible. Therefore, at the examination a year later, MRI was done in an attempt to clarify the status of the extracardiac conduit. Figure 7-19 illustrates the MRI findings in this patient, including a narrowed extracardiac conduit. This conduit narrowing was confirmed by subsequent cardiac catheterization. At catheterization, the right ventricular pressure was also found to be at systemic levels, an indication that reoperation was needed to replace the stenotic conduit.

Summary. Diagnostic capabilities in patients with

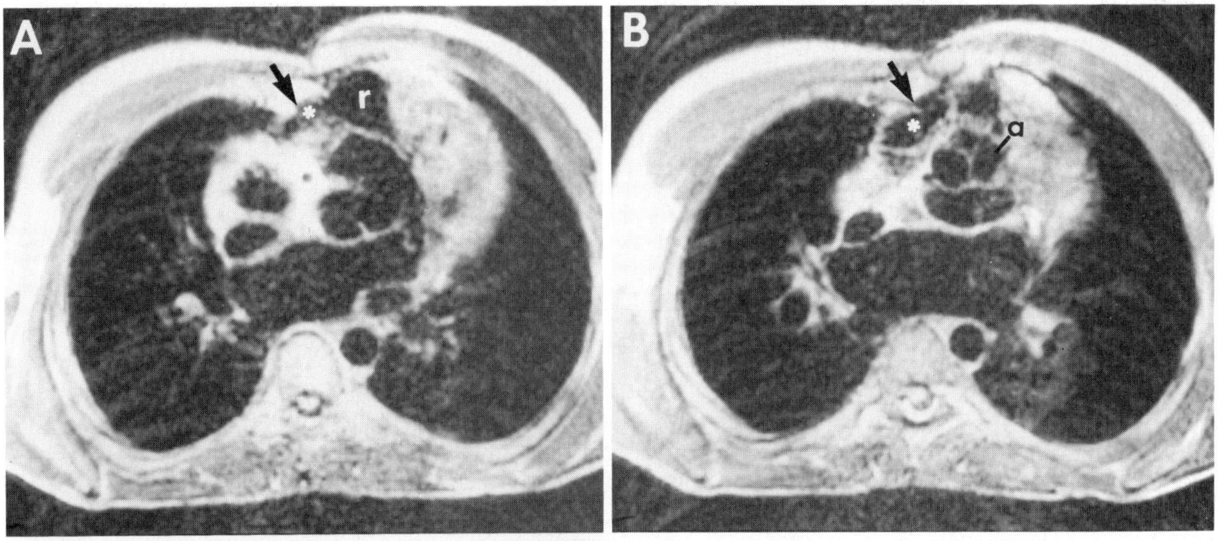

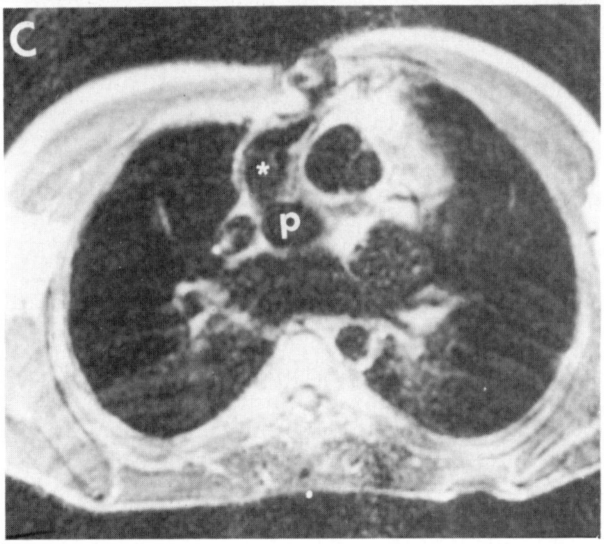

Fig 7-19 Narrowing of extracardiac conduit demonstrated by MRI. **A,** transverse image at level of proximal conduit anastomosis to right ventricle. Note narrowed segment of conduit *(arrow).* **B,** transverse image located immediately above that depicted in **A** at level of aortic valve. Note that conduit narrowing is also present at this level *(arrow).* **C,** transverse image located immediately above that depicted in **B** at level of distal conduit anastomosis to main pulmonary artery. Note that conduit is not narrowed at this level. *a,* aortic root at level of sinuses of Valsalva; *p,* main pulmonary artery; *r,* right ventricle; *asterisk,* conduit.

congenital heart disease have been expanded by the introduction of MRI into our imaging armamentarium. Since echocardiography is usually the initial imaging examination, MRI may be thought of as an extension of the noninvasive assessment of these patients. In some instances, such as defining pulmonary artery anatomy, aortic arch anomalies, systemic and pulmonary venous return, and cardiac tumors, the MRI examination will complement echocardiography by supplying additional information. In other situations, MRI will be confirmatory, reevaluating an abnormality detected by an echocardiographer. The importance of the latter role should not be underestimated, as we all know of situations when we would like another noninvasive "look" at a questionable lesion. Finally, since technological advances in MRI are continuing at a rapid pace, its usefulness for diagnosing congenital anomalies of the cardiovascular system may increase. Therefore, physicians responsible for the evaluation of these patients should stay abreast of the progress in all potentially useful imaging modalities. In this way, they will be in a position to use them appropriately and determine their clinical efficacy.

Cardiac masses

A proven use of MRI is in the morphologic evaluation of primary myocardial, intracardiac, and pericardial masses.[51-53] Indeed, if on a radiograph of the chest a primary cardiac or pericardial mass is suspected, MRI, if available, should be the first imaging choice and may be the only modality required. In this situation, the distinct advantage of MRI over echocardiography is its ability to image a wide field of view and provide definition of tumor extent (Figs 7-20 through 7-22). MRI is superior to computed tomography in demonstrating soft tissue contrast, typically without the need for intravenous administration of contrast medium. Occasionally, the use of intravenous contrast increases the conspicuity of a mass (Fig 7-23) and, when combined with rapid imaging and bolus administration, helps differentiate intracardiac and pericardial tumors, thrombus, and perfused myocardium by their perfusion patterns.[54] The capability to image in any plane provides useful anatomic information for surgical planning. Although catheterization may still occasionally be required to define the coronary anatomy before any resection, no other imaging technique can provide such a comprehensive picture to determine possible surgical options for primary and pericardial masses.

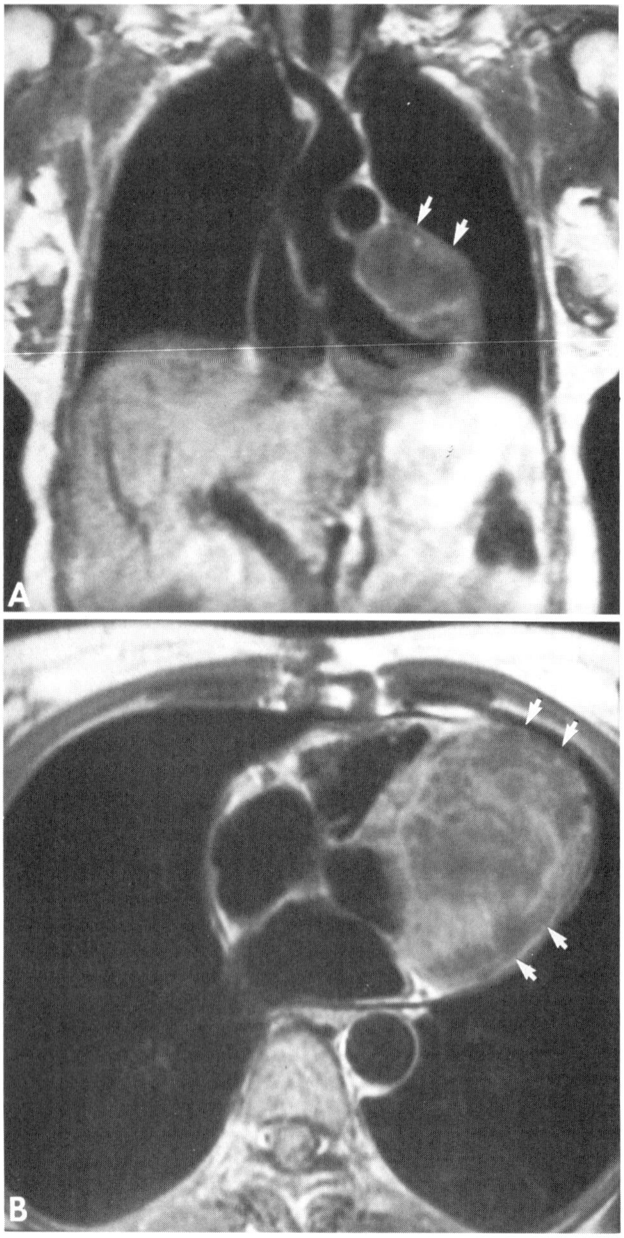

Fig 7-20 Coronal (**A**) and transverse (**B**) images clearly demonstrate extent of residual tumor *(arrows)* in left ventricular wall of a 46-year-old man who had undergone partial resection of a cardiac fibroma.

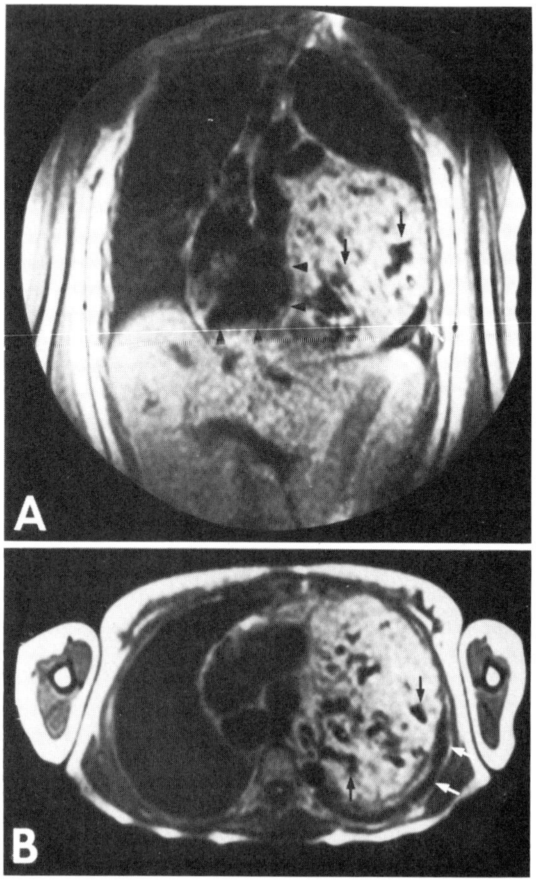

Fig 7-21 In a 41-year-old woman with chest pain and enlarged cardiac silhouette on chest radiograph, coronal (**A**) and transverse (**B**) images reveal an extremely vascular, unresectable tumor distorting and displacing the left ventricle *(arrowheads)*. Numerous vessels are evident because of the flow-void phenomenon *(black arrows)*. A small pericardial effusion is present *(white arrows)*.

Intracavitary masses are often detected by echocardiography, which remains the technique of choice in their initial evaluation. MRI has been shown to have a beneficial complementary role in the evaluation of detected or suspected intracavitary lesions[55,56] (Figs 7-24 and 7-25). In the case of surgical lesions that have not been clearly shown to represent classic myxomas or thrombi, MRI should strongly be considered to ensure that there is no extension outside the cavity of interest.[57,58]

In addition to its morphologic role, the natural contrast provided by MRI yields opportunities for qualitative tissue characterization (Figs 7-26 and 7-27). Relative tissue intensity characteristics of fat, fibrous tissue, hemorrhage, and cyst fluid have been shown to allow a degree of specificity in the MRI diagnosis of some cardiac lesions, such as lipomatous hypertrophy of the atrial septum, fibroma, thrombus, pericardial cyst, and pericardial fat pad.[51-54,56-63]

Cine MRI acquisitions can demonstrate the functional significance of a cardiac mass, including valvular outflow tract obstructions and ventricular dysfunction, in a manner similar to that of echocardiography.[64,65] MRI is operator-independent and therefore allows excellent reproducibility for serial examinations evaluating the efficacy of treatment of masses or for simple clinical observation.

Ischemic heart disease

Initial experience in the evaluation of ischemic heart disease with MRI has demonstrated excellent sensitivity in the detection of morphologic abnormalities due to

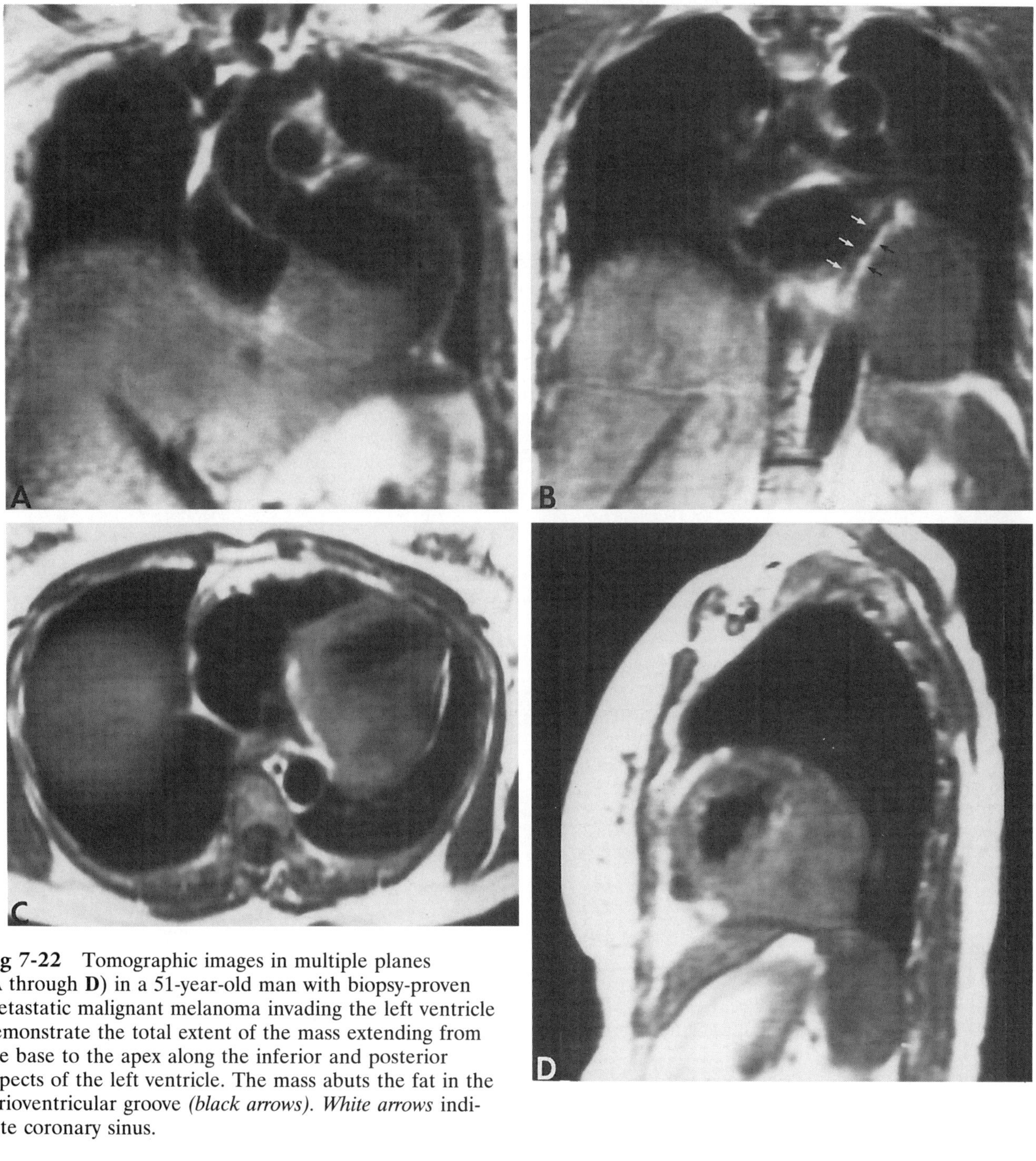

Fig 7-22 Tomographic images in multiple planes (**A** through **D**) in a 51-year-old man with biopsy-proven metastatic malignant melanoma invading the left ventricle demonstrate the total extent of the mass extending from the base to the apex along the inferior and posterior aspects of the left ventricle. The mass abuts the fat in the atrioventricular groove *(black arrows)*. *White arrows* indicate coronary sinus.

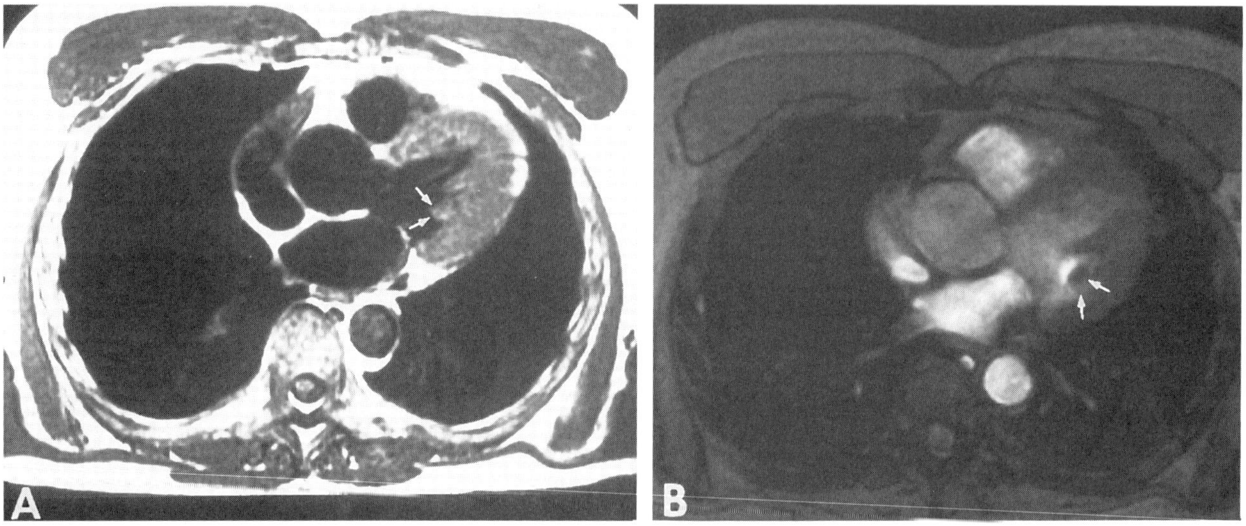

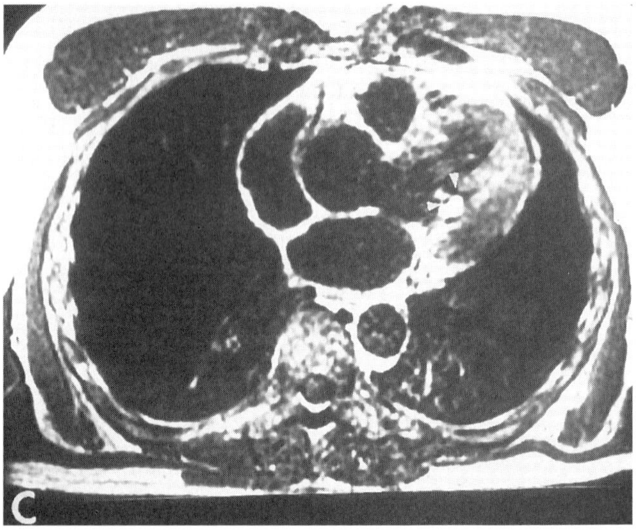

Fig 7-23 Small mass adjacent to the anterolateral papillary muscle in a 38-year-old man. Spin-echo (**A**) and gradient-echo (**B**) images demonstrate the mass *(arrows),* but it is isointense with the myocardium on these sequences and could be confused with a bifid papillary muscle. After intravenous administration of gadolinium contrast agent, spin-echo image (**C**) shows marked enhancement of the small mass *(arrowheads),* which was a myxoma.

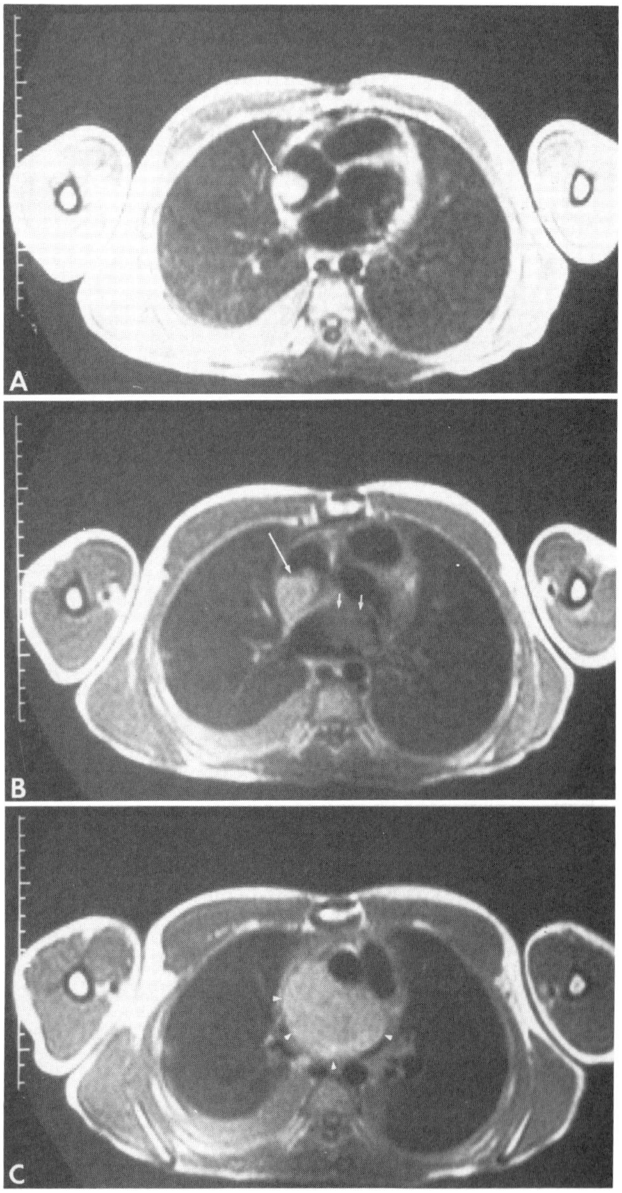

Fig 7-24 Transverse images in a 17-year-old boy with recurrence of a pericardial malignant mesothelioma show total extent of the tumor. Progressing cephalad, **A** through **C** show tumor within the right atrium *(long arrows)* and extending into the roof of the left atrium *(short arrows),* with the bulk of the mass in the transverse sinus of the pericardium *(arrowheads).*

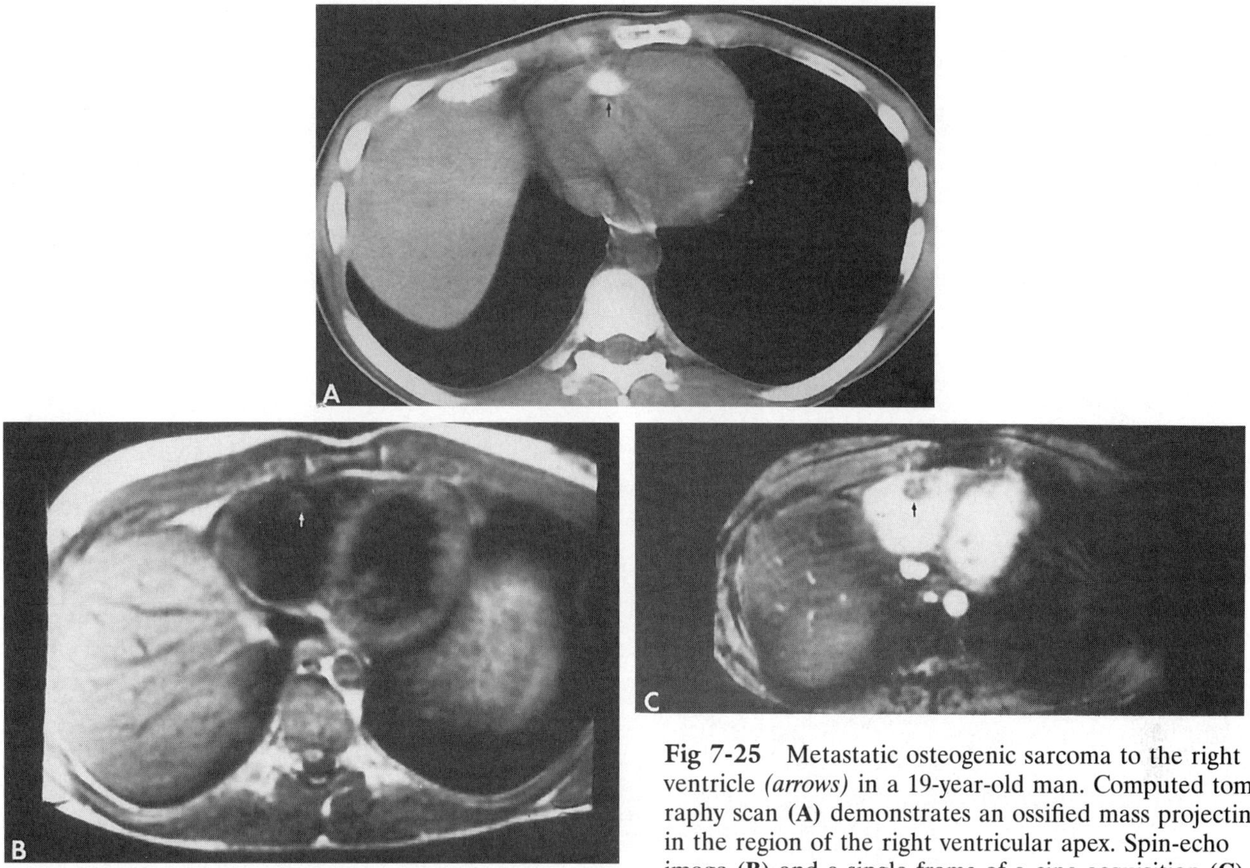

Fig 7-25 Metastatic osteogenic sarcoma to the right ventricle *(arrows)* in a 19-year-old man. Computed tomography scan (**A**) demonstrates an ossified mass projecting in the region of the right ventricular apex. Spin-echo image (**B**) and a single frame of a cine acquisition (**C**) show the mass to be intracavitary.

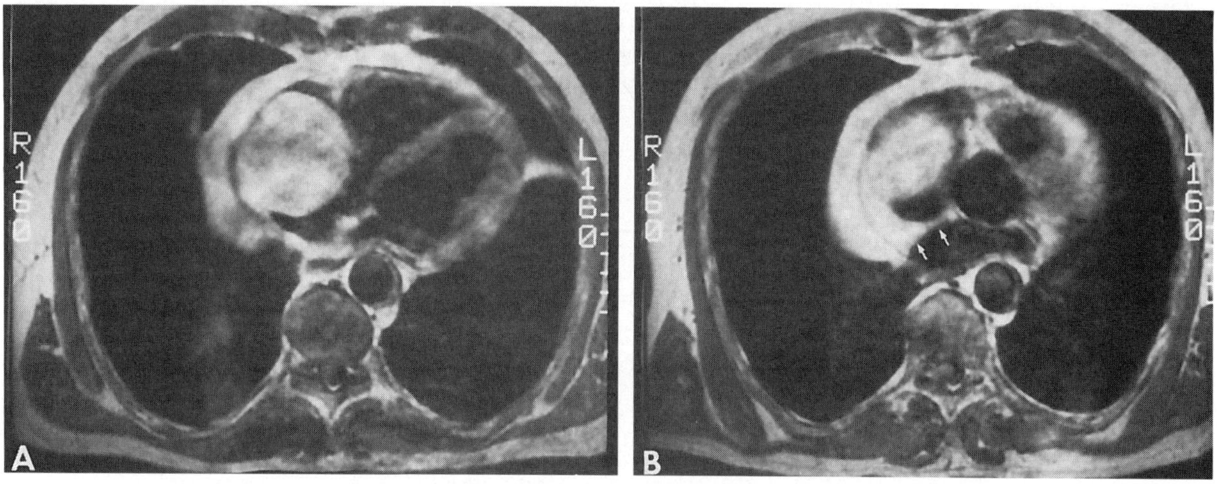

Fig 7-26 Right atrial mass on echocardiogram obtained during workup for angina in a 70-year-old man. The high signal intensity on these gated, partial-saturation, spin-echo images of the mass exactly matching that of the epicardial fat leads to the diagnosis of lipoma (confirmed at surgery). A generous amount of fat extends into the atrial septum *(arrows)*.

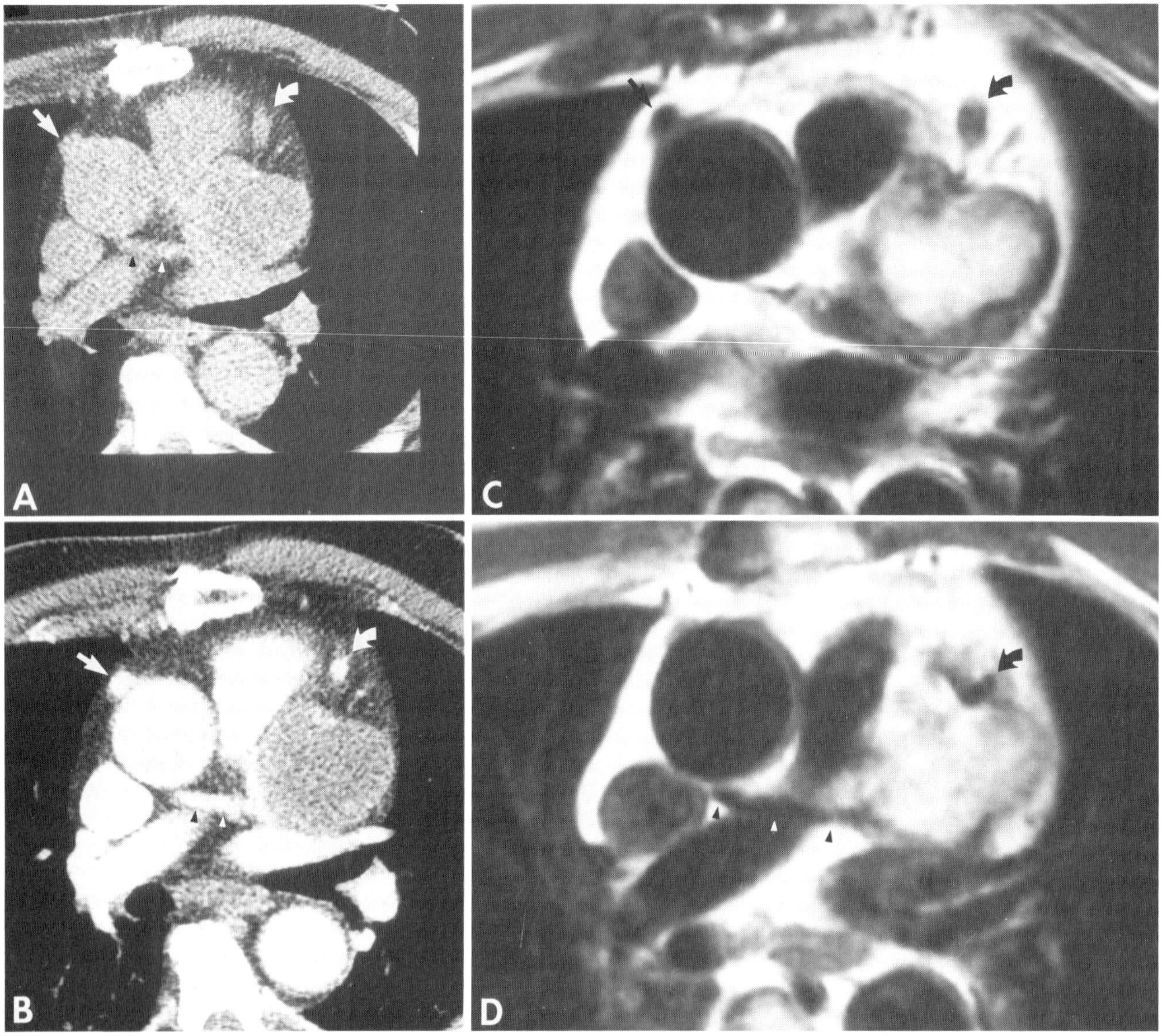

Fig 7-27 Imaging studies in a 60-year-old man with recurrent angina after three-vessel coronary artery bypass grafting. The left anterior descending coronary artery *(curved arrows)* and right coronary grafts *(straight arrows)* are patent, as shown by contrast enhancement on computed tomography images (**A** and **B**) and flow void on spin-echo images (**C** and **D**). The graft to an obtuse marginal vessel *(arrowheads)* is patent proximally but leads to a mass. The high signal centrally in the mass establishes the diagnosis of thrombus, likely in a pseudoaneurysm.

previous myocardial infarction, such as ventricular aneurysms and segmental wall thinning.[66-69] Animal and human studies have demonstrated signal changes within acutely infarcted myocardium, allowing quantification of infarction size relative to noninfarcted myocardium.[70-72] Acutely infarcted myocardium has an increased signal intensity on T2-weighted spin-echo images. Such changes have been reported within hours to days of coronary occlusion and most likely reflect regional edema. Chronic infarcts have a decreased signal intensity, which is attributed to fibrotic tissue, on spin-echo images. Increased signal intensity of T2-weighted images is not, however, specific for acute infarction. Ischemic, clinically noninfarcted myocardium in patients with unstable angina has been shown to give increased signal on T2-weighted images. Motion artifacts can also decrease the specificity of increased signal.

Despite the somewhat limited specificity, MRI has shown the potential for characterizing severely ischemic tissue, and this may have prognostic importance and therapeutic implications. The use of intravascular paramagnetic contrast agents can improve MR visualization

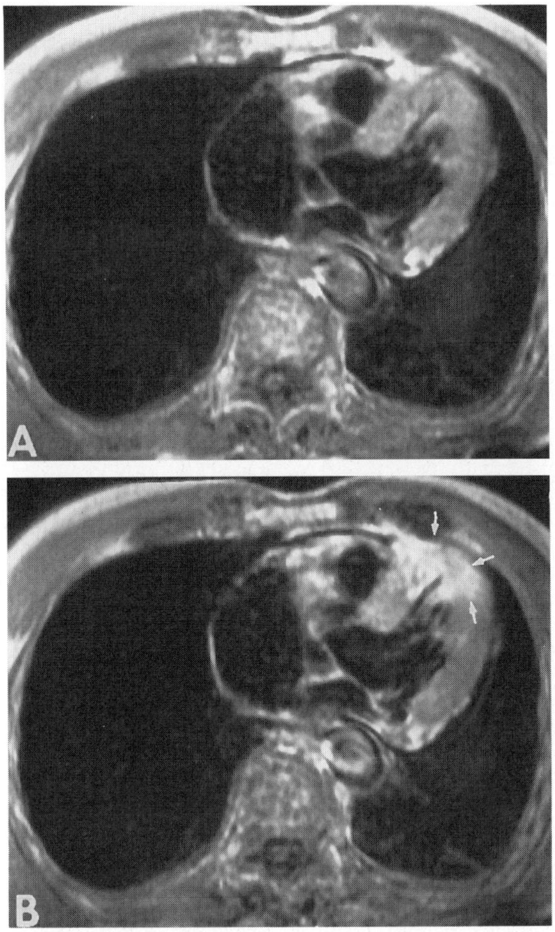

Fig 7-28 MRI examination in a 58-year-old man 7 days after anterior infarction. **A,** spin-echo image without contrast enhancement is unremarkable. **B,** after gadolinium administration, image shows marked enhancement *(arrows)* in the anterior wall and anterior septum.

and detection of acute infarction in humans and has shown potential in discrimination between reperfused and occlusive infarcts[73-81] (Fig 7-28). Resting and pharmacologically stressed perfusion abnormalities seen on contrast-enhanced rapid MR imaging have shown excellent correlation with two-dimensional echocardiographic wall motion and nuclear perfusion studies with single photon emission computed tomography.

Accurate estimation of functional extent of acute and remote infarction by MRI has been greatly aided by the development of fast imaging techniques.[82-84] Although echocardiography and radionuclide angiography remain the noninvasive techniques most commonly used to follow segmental ventricular wall motion and overall contractile dysfunction, the reproducibility on serial examinations, relative operative independence, and more accurate quantitative measurements afforded by MRI's independence of geometric assumptions make its use in risk stratification and monitoring of therapies potentially a powerful tool in patients with the diagnosis of coronary artery disease.

The natural contrast of flowing blood in MRI provides a noninvasive means of establishing coronary artery bypass graft patency[85,86] (see Fig 7-27). Cine MRI has demonstrated a sensitivity of greater than 90% in determining bypass graft patency, and although current spatial resolution cannot exclude significant stenoses in a graft, an accurate noninvasive means of demonstrating patency in the early postoperative period often provides valuable clinical information.[87,88]

Valvular disease

Echocardiography with Doppler techniques is currently the modality of choice in evaluation of valvular disease; however, many aspects of valvular disease are well demonstrated by MRI.[89-95] Chamber volumes, especially those of right-sided chambers, are more completely and more reproducibly visualized by MRI.[96,97] Cine MRI techniques demonstrate regurgitant (Fig 7-29) and stenotic jets as discrete areas of low signal intensity extending from the involved valve into the respective chamber or the ascending aorta with an accuracy comparable to that of color-flow imaging.[98-100] The spatial resolution of valve leaflets is not yet equal to that of transesophageal echocardiography, but moderately thickened mitral and bicuspid valves are readily identified by cine techniques.

Pericardial disease

MRI depicts the pericardial anatomy clearly.[101,102] The normal pericardium is seen as a low-intensity curvilinear line between the high-intensity epicardial fat and medium-intensity myocardium (Fig 7-30). Although echocardiography is the method of choice for the diagnosis of pericardial effusion, MRI clearly demonstrates effusions (Figs 7-31 and 7-32) and can often distinguish organizing and hemorrhagic effusions from the adjacent pericardium. MRI is superior in detecting pericardial thickening and transpericardial invasion by tumor. The lack of interference from overlying bone and lung can enable a more complete assessment of epicardial borders, especially anteriorly and about the apex.[101,103-105]

FUTURE APPLICATIONS OF MAGNETIC RESONANCE IMAGING

Magnetic resonance spectroscopy

In vivo MR spectroscopy of the myocardium holds great potential for investigative noninvasive interrogation of cardiac metabolism. Phosphorus-31 MR spectroscopy has been used to study high-energy phosphate metabolism in normal, ischemic, and infarcted hearts.[106-110] Potential differentiation of reperfused but viable myocardium from reperfused but infarcted muscle has been shown. The ratio of phosphocreatine to adenosine triphosphate may be a sensitive measure of depressed left ventricular function due to underperfusion. Unfortunately, formidable technical problems associated with these techniques must be overcome before MR spectroscopy can be established as a clinically relevant tool.[111,112] Efficient and

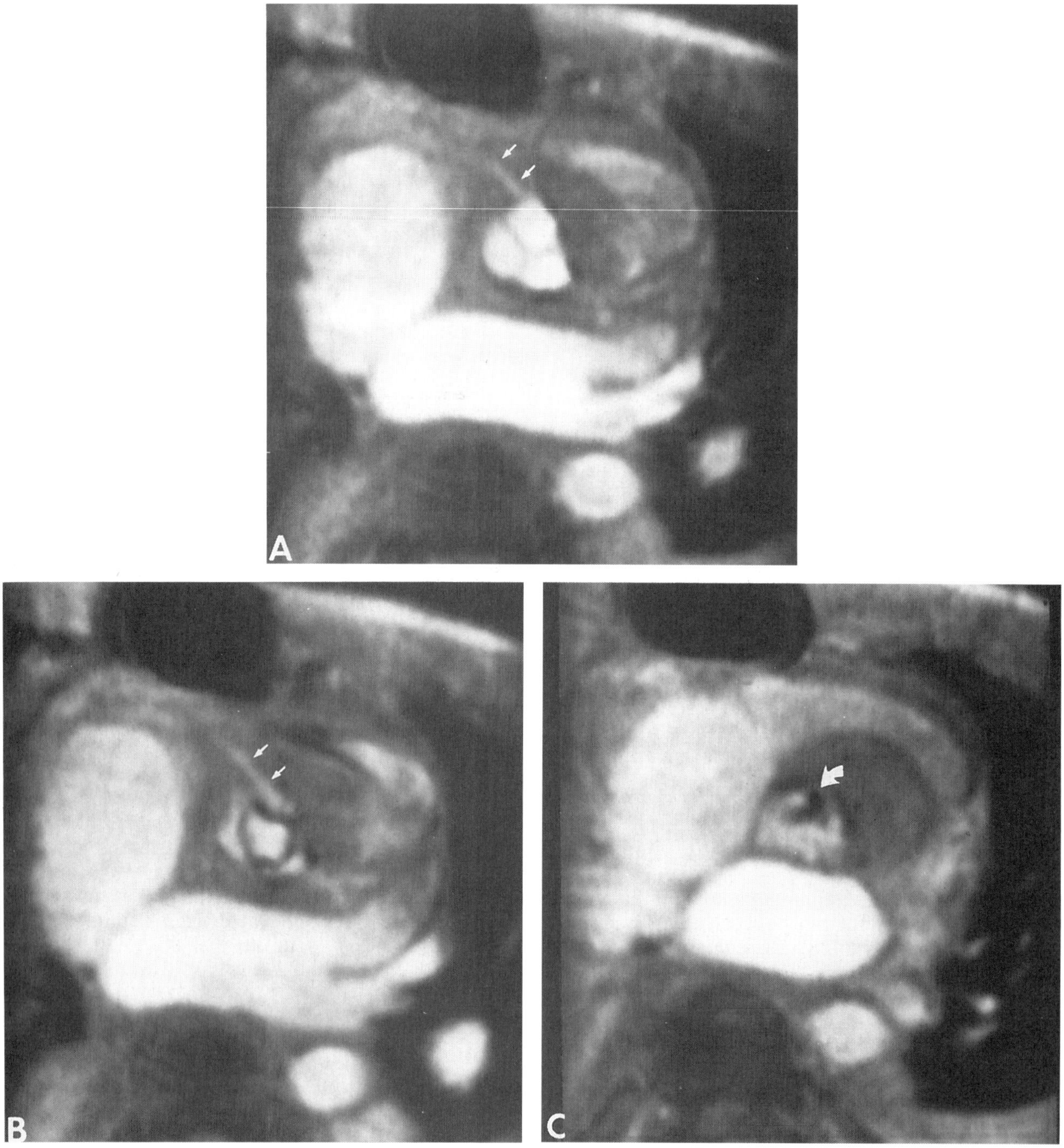

Fig 7-29 Short-axis cine MR images at (**A** and **B**) and just caudal to (**C**) the aortic valve level in a patient with recent aortic valve homograft placement for subacute bacterial endocarditis. The opening of the valve is clearly demonstrated. A regurgitant jet extending down from the right coronary artery is evident by the flow void *(curved arrow)*. This was secondary to *Candida* endocarditis, which rapidly progressed, necessitating repeat valve replacement. *Short arrows* point to right coronary artery.

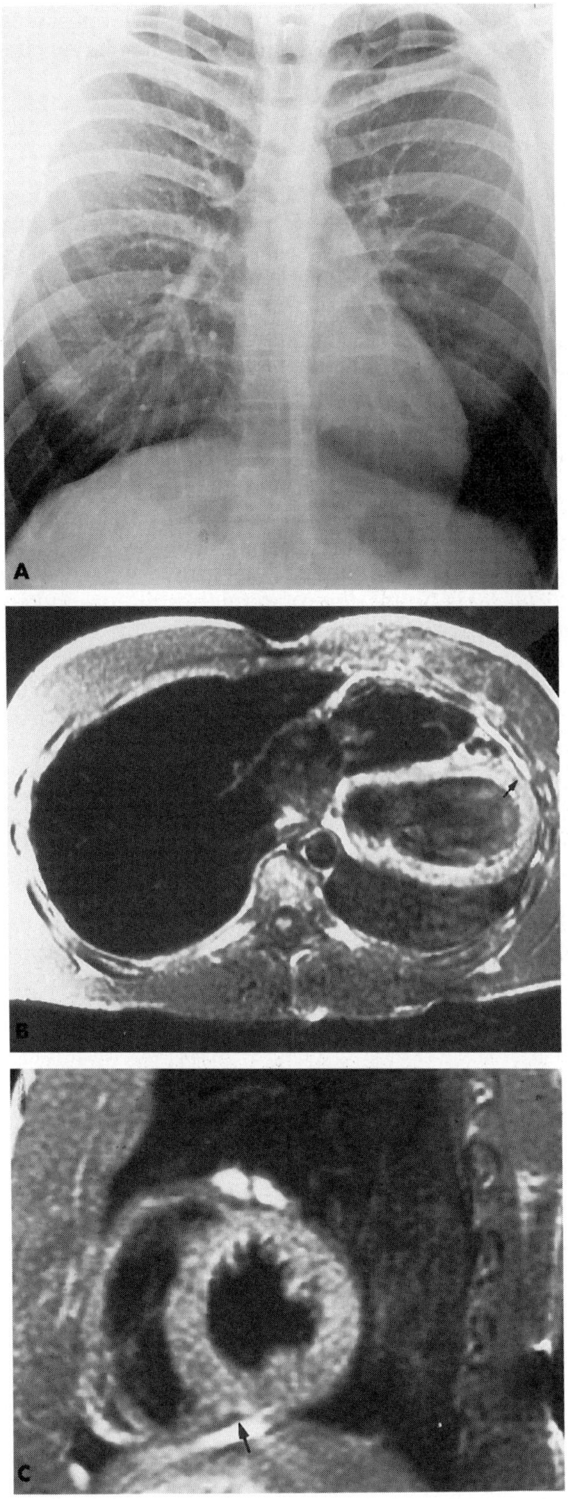

Fig 7-30 Abnormally positioned heart on chest radiograph (**A**) in a 25-year-old asymptomatic man. Axial (**B**) and sagittal (**C**) images demonstrate abrupt end to the pericardium over the left side of the heart *(arrows).*

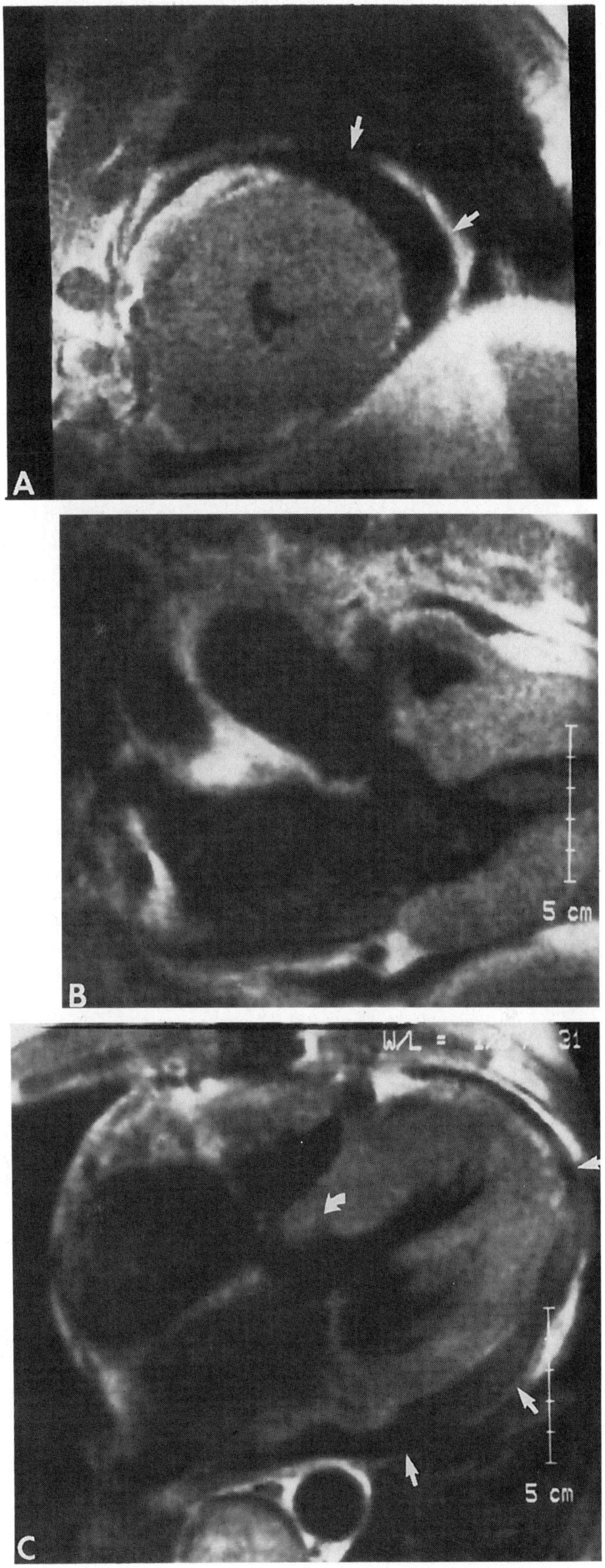

Fig 7-31 Postoperative pericardial effusion *(straight arrows)* in a 32-year-old patient who had recent myotomy and myectomy for hypertrophic obstructive cardiomyopathy. **A,** short-axis view demonstrates marked left ventricular hypertrophy. **B,** long-axis view nicely demonstrates the left ventricular outflow tract. **C,** the surgical defect in the interventricular septum *(curved arrow)* is best seen on transverse images.

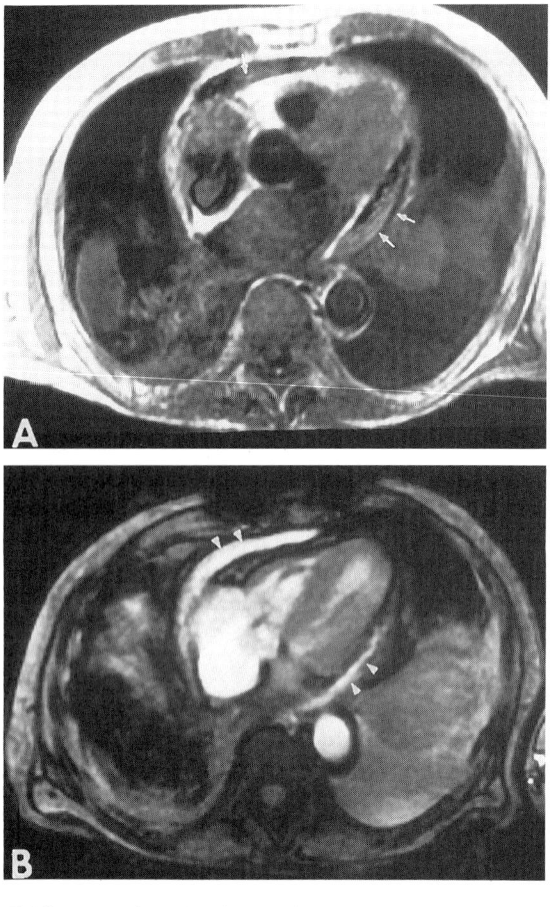

Fig 7-32 **A,** spin-echo image in a 45-year-old man with symptoms of constrictive pericarditis demonstrates areas of low and medium signal intensity within the pericardial space, possibly because of organizing effusion *(arrows).* **B,** a single frame from the gradient-echo cine acquisition scan shows that most of the pericardial space is free fluid, indicated by the high signal of moving fluid. There is moderate thickening of the pericardium *(arrowheads).*

reliable localization of the spectral acquisition both temporally and spatially to ensure accuracy of the spectra is a major technical limitation currently.

Cardiac transplantation

Endomyocardial biopsy is the standard technique for the diagnosis of transplant rejection.[113] MRI has demonstrated a potential role as a noninvasive method in the detection and monitoring of acute rejection. Excellent morphologic detail provided by MRI allows accurate and reproducible measurements of the increased myocardial wall thickness associated with acute rejection.[114] Preliminary studies have indicated that rejection is accompanied by changes in relaxation times.[115,116] Although accurate measurements of relaxation times in the beating heart have important limitations, serial measurements of T2 relaxation times to identify patients with acute rejection and myocardial edema have obvious potential.[117-119]

The use of paramagnetic contrast agents such as gadolinium-DTPA has demonstrated intense T1-weighted image enhancement associated with biopsy-proven rejection in animals.[120,121] Promising preliminary animal work has also been performed in the use of phosphorus MR spectroscopy in the assessment of rejection.[122-124] The practical routine use of both imaging and spectroscopic MR techniques awaits large clinical trials.

Magnetic resonance coronary angiography

Clinical applications of MR angiography are well established. The procedure is most commonly used during neurologic imaging of the head and neck but has many body and peripheral vascular applications as well. The relatively small size and nearly constant motion of coronary arteries make coronary MR angiography a more formidable task. Current techniques can identify the proximal coronary arteries; with existing technology, however, it may be impossible to visualize distal branches and collateral vessels with detail approaching that of conventional contrast angiography.[125] Quantification of flow in bypass grafts and native coronary segments has been accomplished, and recent imaging developments on current imagers have displayed impressive coronary detail.[126,127] Combining the anatomic resolution and functional information currently available with further advancements in perfusion and coronary imaging, MRI may soon have a major role in evaluation of ischemic heart disease, providing the "one-stop" comprehensive examination.

REFERENCES

1. Pykett IL, Newhouse JH, Buonanno FS, et al: Principles of nuclear magnetic resonance imaging. *Radiology* 143:157-168, 1982
2. Mansfield P, Morris PG: *NMR Imaging in Biomedicine.* Suppl 2: *Advances in Magnetic Resonance.* Edited by JS Waugh. New York, Academic Press, 1982
3. Mills CM, Brant-Zawadzke M, Crooks LE, et al: Nuclear magnetic resonance: principles of blood flow imaging. *AJR* 142:165-170, 1984
4. Fullerton GD: Magnetic resonance imaging signal concepts. *Radiographics* 7:579-596, 1987
5. Lanzer P, Botvinick EH, Schiller NB, et al: Cardiac imaging using gated magnetic resonance. *Radiology* 150:121-127, 1984
6. Crooks LE, Barker B, Chang H, et al: Magnetic resonance imaging strategies for heart studies. *Radiology* 153:459-465, 1984
7. Lanzer P, Barta C, Botvinick EH, et al: ECG-synchronized cardiac MR imaging: method and evaluation. *Radiology* 155:681-686, 1985
8. van Genderingen HR, Sprenger M, De Ridder JW, et al: Carbon-fiber electrodes and leads for electrocardiography during MR imaging. *Radiology* 171:872, 1989
9. Dimick RN, Hedlund LW, Herfkens RJ, et al: Optimizing electrocardiograph electrode placement for cardiac-gated magnetic resonance imaging. *Invest Radiol* 22:17-22, 1987
10. Pavlicek W, Geisinger M, Castle L, et al: The effects of nuclear magnetic resonance on patients with cardiac pacemakers. *Radiology* 147:149-153, 1983
11. Holmes DR Jr, Hayes DL, Gray JE, et al: The effects of magnetic resonance imaging on implantable pulse generators. *PACE* 9:360-370, 1986
12. Feiglin DH, George CR, MacIntyre WJ, et al: Gated cardiac magnetic resonance structural imaging: optimization by electronic axial rotation. *Radiology* 154:129-132, 1985
13. Higgins CB: MR of the heart: anatomy, physiology, and metabolism. *AJR* 151:239-248, 1988

14. Dinsmore RE, Wismer GL, Levine RA, et al: Magnetic resonance imaging of the heart: positioning and gradient angle selection for optimal imaging planes. *AJR* 143:1135-1142, 1984

15. Dinsmore RE, Wismer GL, Miller SW, et al: Magnetic resonance imaging of the heart using image planes oriented to cardiac axes: experience with 100 cases. *AJR* 145:1177-1183, 1985

16. Haase A, Frahm J, Matthaei D, et al: FLASH imaging. Rapid NMR imaging using low flip-angle pulses. *J Magn Reson* 67:258-266, 1986

17. Sechtum U, Pflugfelder PW, White RD, et al: Cine MR imaging: potential for the evaluation of cardiovascular function. *AJR* 148:239-246, 1987

18. Pflugfelder PW, Sechtem UP, White RD, et al: Noninvasive evaluation of mitral regurgitation by analysis of left atrial signal loss in cine magnetic resonance. *Am Heart J* 117:1113-1119, 1989

19. Matthaei D, Haase A, Henrich D, et al: Cardiac and vascular imaging with an MR snapshot technique. *Radiology* 177:527-532, 1990

20. Atkinson DJ, Edelman RR: Cineangiography of the heart in a single breath hold with a segmented turboFLASH sequence. *Radiology* 178:357-360, 1991

21. Henrich D, Haase A, Matthaei D: 3D-snapshot flash NMR imaging of the human heart. *Magn Reson Imaging* 8:377-379, 1990

22. Rzedzian RR, Pykett IL: Instant images of the human heart using a new, whole-body MR imaging system. *AJR* 149:245-250, 1987

23. Chapman B, Turner R, Ordidge RJ, et al: Real-time movie imaging from a single cardiac cycle by NMR. *Magn Reson Med* 5:246-254, 1987

24. Budinger T: Nuclear magnetic resonance (NMR) *in vivo* studies: known thresholds for health effects. *J Comput Assist Tomogr* 5:800-811, 1981

25. New PF, Rosen BR, Brady TJ, et al: Potential hazards and artifacts of ferromagnetic and nonferromagnetic surgical and dental materials and devices in nuclear magnetic resonance imaging. *Radiology* 147:139-148, 1983

26. Soulen RL, Budinger TF, Higgins CB: Magnetic resonance imaging of prosthetic heart valves. *Radiology* 154:705-707, 1985

27. Randall PA, Kohman LJ, Scalzetti EM, et al: Magnetic resonance imaging of prosthetic cardiac valves in vitro and in vivo. *Am J Cardiol* 62:973-976, 1988

28. Moran PR: A flow velocity zeugmatographic interlace for NMR imaging in humans. *Magn Reson Imaging* 1:197-203, 1982

29. von Schulthess GK, Higgins CB: Blood flow imaging with MR: spin-phase phenomena. *Radiology* 157:687-695, 1985

30. Firmin DN, Nayler GL, Klipstein RH, et al: In vivo validation of MR velocity imaging. *J Comput Assist Tomogr* 11:751-756, 1987

31. Mohiaddin RH, Amanuma M, Kilner PJ, et al: MR phase-shift velocity mapping of mitral and pulmonary venous flow. *J Comput Assist Tomogr* 15:237-243, 1991

32. Kondo C, Caputo GR, Semelka R, et al: Right and left ventricular stroke volume measurements with velocity-encoded cine MR imaging: in vitro and in vivo validation. *AJR* 157:9-16, 1991

33. Søndergaard L, Thomsen C, Ståhlberg F, et al: Mitral and aortic valvular flow: quantification with MR phase mapping. *J Magn Reson Imaging* 2:295-302, 1992

34. Dulce MC, Mostbeck GH, O'Sullivan M, et al: Severity of aortic regurgitation: interstudy reproducibility of measurements with velocity-encoded cine MR imaging. *Radiology* 185:235-240, 1992

35. Jacobstein MD, Fletcher BD, Goldstein S, et al: Evaluation of atrioventricular septal defect by magnetic resonance imaging. *Am J Cardiol* 55:1158-1161, 1985

36. Diethelm L, Déry R, Lipton MJ, et al: Atrial-level shunts: sensitivity and specificity of MR in diagnosis. *Radiology* 162:181-186, 1987

37. Fletcher BD, Jacobstein MD, Nelson AD, et al: Gated magnetic resonance imaging of congenital cardiac malformations. *Radiology* 150:137-140, 1984

38. Didier D, Higgins CB, Fisher MR, et al: Congenital heart disease: gated MR imaging in 72 patients. *Radiology* 158:227-235, 1986

39. Shub C, Dimopoulos IN, Seward JB, et al: Sensitivity of two-dimensional echocardiography in the direct visualization of atrial septal defect utilizing the subcostal approach: experience with 154 patients. *J Am Coll Cardiol* 2:127-135, 1983

40. Sutherland GR, Smyllie JH, Ogilvie BC, et al: Colour flow imaging in the diagnosis of multiple ventricular septal defects. *Br Heart J* 62:43-49, 1989

41. Helmcke F, De Souza A, Nanda NC, et al: Two-dimensional and color Doppler assessment of ventricular septal defect of congenital origin. *Am J Cardiol* 63:1112-1116, 1989

42. Mirowitz SA, Gutierrez FR, Canter CE, et al: Tetralogy of Fallot: MR findings. *Radiology* 171:207-212, 1989

43. Guit GL, Bluemm R, Rohmer J, et al: Levotransposition of the aorta: identification of segmental cardiac anatomy using MR imaging. *Radiology* 161:673-679, 1986

44. Rees S, Somerville J, Warnes C, et al: Comparison of magnetic resonance imaging with echocardiography and radionuclide angiography in assessing cardiac function and anatomy following Mustard's operation for transposition of the great arteries. *Am J Cardiol* 61:1316-1322, 1988

45. Julsrud PR, Ehman RL: The "broken ring" sign in magnetic resonance imaging of partial anomalous pulmonary venous connection to the superior vena cava. *Mayo Clin Proc* 60:874-879, 1985

46. Julsrud PR, Ehman RL, Hagler DJ, et al: Extracardiac vasculature in candidates for Fontan surgery: MR imaging. *Radiology* 173:503-506, 1989

47. Downing TP, Danielson GK, Ritter DG, et al: Pulmonary artery thrombosis associated with anomalous pulmonary venous connection: an unusual complication following the modified Fontan procedure. *J Thorac Cardiovasc Surg* 90:441-447, 1985

48. Zellers TM, Hagler DJ, Julsrud PR: Accuracy of two-dimensional echocardiography in diagnosing left superior vena cava. *J Am Soc Echocardiography* 2:132-138, 1989

49. Julsrud PR, Ehman RL: Magnetic resonance imaging of vascular rings. *Mayo Clin Proc* 61:181-185, 1986

50. Gomes AS, Lois JF, George B, et al: Congenital abnormalities of the aortic arch: MR imaging. *Radiology* 165:691-695, 1987

51. Winkler M, Higgins CB: Suspected intracardiac masses: evaluation with MR imaging. *Radiology* 165:117-122, 1987

52. Lund JT, Ehman RL, Julsrud PR, et al: Cardiac masses: assessment by MR imaging. *AJR* 152:469-473, 1989

53. Brown JJ, Barakos JA, Higgins CB: Magnetic resonance imaging of cardiac and paracardiac masses. *J Thorac Imaging* 4 No. 2:58-64, 1989

54. Semelka RC, Shoenut JP, Wilson ME, et al: Cardiac masses: signal intensity features on spin-echo, gradient-echo, gadolinium-enhanced spin-echo, and TurboFLASH images. *J Magn Reson Imaging* 2:415-420, 1992

55. Conces DJ Jr, Vix VA, Klatte EC: Gated MR imaging of left atrial myxomas. *Radiology* 156:445-447, 1985

56. Go RT, O'Donnell JK, Underwood DA, et al: Comparison of gated cardiac MRI and 2D echocardiography of intracardiac neoplasms. *AJR* 145:21-25, 1985

57. Barakos JA, Brown JJ, Higgins CB: MR imaging of secondary cardiac and paracardiac lesions. *AJR* 153:47-50, 1989

58. Freedberg RS, Kronzon I, Rumancik WM, et al: The contribution of magnetic resonance imaging to the evaluation of intracardiac tumors diagnosed by echocardiography. *Circulation* 77:96-103, 1988

59. Applegate PM, Tajik AJ, Ehman RL, et al: Two-dimensional echocardiographic and magnetic resonance imaging observations in massive lipomatous hypertrophy of the atrial septum. *Am J Cardiol* 59:489-491, 1987

60. Gomes AS, Lois JF, Child JS, et al: Cardiac tumors and thrombus: evaluation with MR imaging. *AJR* 149:895-899, 1987

61. Menegus MA, Greenberg MA, Spindola-Franco H, et al: Magnetic resonance imaging of suspected atrial tumors. *Am Heart J* 123:1260-1268, 1992

62. Jungehülsing M, Sechtem U, Theissen P, et al: Left ventricular thrombi: evaluation with spin-echo and gradient-echo MR imaging. *Radiology* 182:225-229, 1992

63. Tuna IC, Julsrud PR, Click RL, et al: Tissue characterization of an unusual right atrial mass by magnetic resonance imaging. *Mayo Clin Proc* 66:498-501, 1991

64. Higgins CB, Holt W, Pflugfelder P, et al: Functional evaluation of the heart with magnetic resonance imaging. *Magn Reson Med* 6:121-139, 1988

65. Deutsch H-J, Smolorz J, Sechtem U, et al: Cardiac function by magnetic resonance imaging. *Int J Card Imaging* 3:3-11, 1988

66. Akins EW, Hill JA, Sievers KW, et al: Assessment of left ventricular wall thickness in healed myocardial infarction by magnetic resonance imaging. *Am J Cardiol* 59:24-28, 1987

67. Johnston DL, Liu P: Evaluation of myocardial ischemia and infarction by nuclear magnetic resonance techniques. *Can J Cardiol* 4:116-129, 1988

68. McNamara MT, Higgins CB: Magnetic resonance imaging of chronic myocardial infarcts in man. *AJR* 146:315-320, 1986
69. Baer FM, Smolarz K, Jungehülsing M, et al: Chronic myocardial infarction: assessment of morphology, function, and perfusion by gradient echo magnetic resonance imaging and ^{99m}Tc-methoxyisobutyl-isonitrile SPECT. *Am Heart J* 123:636-645, 1992
70. Caputo GR, Sechtem U, Tscholakoff D, et al: Measurement of myocardial infarct size at early and late time intervals using MR imaging: an experimental study in dogs. *AJR* 149:237-243, 1987
71. Matheijssen NAA, de Roos A, van der Wall EE, et al: Acute myocardial infarction: comparison of T2-weighted and T1-weighted gadolinium-DTPA enhanced MR imaging. *Magn Reson Med* 17:460-469, 1991
72. Thompson RC, Liu P, Brady TJ, et al: Serial magnetic resonance imaging in patients following acute myocardial infarction. *Magn Reson Imaging* 9:155-158, 1991
73. De Roos A, Doornbos J, van der Wall EE, et al: MR imaging of acute myocardial infarction: value of Gd-DTPA. *AJR* 150:531-534, 1988
74. McNamara MT, Tscholakoff D, Revel D, et al: Differentiation of reversible and irreversible myocardial injury by MR imaging with and without gadolinium-DTPA. *Radiology* 158:765-769, 1986
75. van Dijkman PRM, van der Wall EE, de Roos A, et al: Gadolinium-enhanced magnetic resonance imaging in acute myocardial infarction. *Eur J Radiol* 11:1-9, 1990
76. de Roos A, Matheijssen NAA, Doornbos J, et al: Myocardial infarct size after reperfusion therapy: assessment with Gd-DTPA-enhanced MR imaging. *Radiology* 176:517-521, 1990
77. Van Rossum AC, Visser FC, Van Eenige MJ, et al: Value of gadolinium-diethylene-triamine pentaacetic acid dynamics in magnetic resonance imaging of acute myocardial infarction with occluded and reperfused coronary arteries after thrombolysis. *Am J Cardiol* 65:845-851, 1990
78. Manning WJ, Atkinson DJ, Grossman W, et al: First-pass nuclear magnetic resonance imaging studies using gadolinium-DTPA in patients with coronary artery disease. *J Am Coll Cardiol* 18:959-965, 1991
79. Pennell DJ, Underwood SR, Ell PJ, et al: Dipyridamole magnetic resonance imaging: a comparison with thallium-201 emission tomography. *Br Heart J* 64:362-369, 1990
80. Baer FM, Smolarz K, Jungehülsing M, et al: Feasibility of high-dose dipyridamole-magnetic resonance imaging for detection of coronary artery disease and comparison with coronary angiography. *Am J Cardiol* 69:51-56, 1992
81. Pennell DJ, Underwood SR, Manzara CC, et al: Magnetic resonance imaging during dobutamine stress in coronary artery disease. *Am J Cardiol* 70:34-40, 1992
82. Gaudio C, Tanzilli G, Mazzarotto P, et al: Comparison of left ventricular ejection fraction by magnetic resonance imaging and radionuclide ventriculography in idiopathic dilated cardiomyopathy. *Am J Cardiol* 67:411-415, 1991
83. van der Wall EE, de Roos A, van Voorthuisen AE, et al: Magnetic resonance imaging: a new approach for evaluating coronary artery disease? *Am Heart J* 121:1203-1220, 1991
84. Meese RB, Spritzer CE, Negro-Vilar R, et al: Detection, characterization and functional assessment of reperfused Q-wave acute myocardial infarction by cine magnetic resonance imaging. *Am J Cardiol* 66:1-9, 1990
85. Gomes AS, Lois JF, Drinkwater DC Jr, et al: Coronary artery bypass grafts: visualization with MR imaging. *Radiology* 162:175-179, 1987
86. White RD, Caputo GR, Mark AS, et al: Coronary artery bypass graft patency: noninvasive evaluation with MR imaging. *Radiology* 164:681-686, 1987
87. White RD, Pflugfelder PW, Lipton MJ, et al: Coronary artery bypass grafts: evaluation of patency with cine MR imaging. *AJR* 150:1271-1274, 1988
88. Aurigemma GP, Reichek N, Axel L, et al: Noninvasive determination of coronary artery bypass graft patency by cine magnetic resonance imaging. *Circulation* 80:1595-1602, 1989
89. Schiebler M, Axel L, Reichek N, et al: Correlation of cine MR imaging with two-dimensional pulsed Doppler echocardiography in valvular insufficiency. *J Comput Assist Tomogr* 11:627-632, 1987
90. Utz JA, Herfkens RJ, Heinsimer JA, et al: Valvular regurgitation: dynamic MR imaging. *Radiology* 168:91-94, 1988
91. Sechtem U, Pflugfelder PW, Cassidy MM, et al: Mitral or aortic regurgitation: quantification of regurgitant volumes with cine MR imaging. *Radiology* 167:425-430, 1988
92. Aurigemma G, Reichek N, Schiebler M, et al: Evaluation of mitral regurgitation by cine magnetic resonance imaging. *Am J Cardiol* 66:621-625, 1990
93. Higgins CB, Wagner S, Kondo C, et al: Evaluation of valvular heart disease with cine gradient echo magnetic resonance imaging. *Circulation* 84 Suppl 1:198-207, 1991
94. Cranney GB, Lotan CS, Pohost GM: Nuclear magnetic resonance imaging for assessment and follow-up of patients with valve disease. *Circulation* 84 Suppl 1:216-227, 1991
95. Akins EW, Slone RM, Wiechmann BN, et al: Perivalvular pseudoaneurysm complicating bacterial endocarditis: MR detection in five cases. *AJR* 156:1155-1158, 1991
96. Turnbull LW, Ridgway JP, Biernacki W, et al: Assessment of the right ventricle by magnetic resonance imaging in chronic obstructive lung disease. *Thorax* 45:597-601, 1990
97. Boxt LM, Katz J, Kolb T, et al: Direct quantitation of right and left ventricular volumes with nuclear magnetic resonance imaging in patients with primary pulmonary hypertension. *J Am Coll Cardiol* 19:1508-1515, 1992
98. Deutsch HJ, Bachmann R, Sechtem U, et al: Regurgitant flow in cardiac valve prostheses: diagnostic value of gradient echo nuclear magnetic resonance imaging in reference to transesophageal two-dimensional color Doppler echocardiography. *J Am Coll Cardiol* 19:1500-1507, 1992
99. Aurigemma G, Reichek N, Schiebler M, et al: Evaluation of aortic regurgitation by cardiac cine magnetic resonance imaging: planar analysis and comparison to Doppler echocardiography. *Cardiology* 78:340-347, 1991
100. Casolo GC, Zampa V, Rega L, et al: Evaluation of mitral stenosis by cine magnetic resonance imaging. *Am Heart J* 123:1252-1260, 1992
101. Sechtem U, Tscholakoff D, Higgins CB: MRI of the abnormal pericardium. *AJR* 147:245-252, 1986
102. Hoit BD: Imaging the pericardium. *Cardiol Clin* 8:587-600, 1990
103. Soulen RL, Stark DD, Higgins CB: Magnetic resonance imaging of constrictive pericardial disease. *Am J Cardiol* 55:480-484, 1985
104. Mulvagh SL, Rokey R, Vick GW III, et al: Usefulness of nuclear magnetic resonance imaging for evaluation of pericardial effusions, and comparison with two-dimensional echocardiography. *Am J Cardiol* 64:1002-1009, 1989
105. Masui T, Finck S, Higgins CB: Constrictive pericarditis and restrictive cardiomyopathy: evaluation with MR imaging. *Radiology* 182:369-373, 1992
106. Bottomley PA, Herfkens RJ, Smith LS, et al: Altered phosphate metabolism in myocardial infarction: P-31 MR spectroscopy. *Radiology* 165:703-707, 1987
107. Grist TM, Kneeland JB, Rilling WR, et al: Gated cardiac MR imaging and P-31 MR spectroscopy in humans at 1.5 T: work in progress. *Radiology* 170:357-361, 1989
108. Rehr RB, Tatum JL, Hirsch JI, et al: Effective separation of normal, acutely ischemic, and reperfused myocardium with P-31 MR spectroscopy. *Radiology* 168:81-89, 1988
109. Auffermann W, Chew WM, Wolfe CL, et al: Normal and diffusely abnormal myocardium in humans: functional and metabolic characterization with P-31 MR spectroscopy and cine MR imaging. *Radiology* 179:253-259, 1991
110. Hardy CJ, Weiss RG, Bottomley PA, et al: Altered myocardial high-energy phosphate metabolites in patients with dilated cardiomyopathy. *Am Heart J* 122:795-801, 1991
111. Willis RJ, Clarke K: The ^{31}P-nuclear magnetic resonance spectrum of heart: will it be of diagnostic use in clinical cardiology? *Cardiology* 74:182-195, 1987
112. Schaefer S: Clinical nuclear magnetic resonance spectroscopy: insight into metabolism. *Am J Cardiol* 66:45F-50F, 1990
113. Billingham ME: Diagnosis of cardiac rejection by endomyocardial biopsy. *Heart Transplant* 1:25-30, 1981
114. Revel D, Chapelon C, Mathieu D, et al: Magnetic resonance imaging of human orthotopic heart transplantation: correlation with endomyocardial biopsy. *J Heart Transplant* 8:139-146, 1989
115. Tscholakoff D, Aherne T, Yee ES, et al: Cardiac transplantations in dogs: evaluation with MR. *Radiology* 157:697-702, 1985
116. Eugene M, Lechat P, Hadjiisky P, et al: Nuclear magnetic

resonance and proton relaxation times in experimental heterotopic heart transplantation. *J Heart Transplant* 5:39-45, 1986

117. Wisenberg G, Pflugfelder PW, Kostuk WJ, et al: Diagnostic applicability of magnetic resonance imaging in assessing human cardiac allograft rejection. *Am J Cardiol* 60:130-136, 1987

118. Lund G, Morin RL, Olivari MT, et al: Serial myocardial T2 relaxation time measurements in normal subjects and heart transplant recipients. *J Heart Transplant* 7:274-279, 1988

119. Doornbos J, Verwey H, Essed CE, et al: MR imaging in assessment of cardiac transplant rejection in humans. *J Comput Assist Tomogr* 14:77-81, 1990

120. Konstam MA, Aronovitz MJ, Runge VM, et al: Magnetic resonance imaging with gadolinium-DTPA for detecting cardiac transplant rejection in rats. *Circulation* 78 Suppl 3:87-94, 1988

121. Nishimura T, Sada M, Sasaki H, et al: Cardiac transplantation in dogs: evaluation with gated MRI and Gd-DTPA contrast enhancement. *Heart Vessels* 3:141-145, 1987

122. Fraser CD Jr, Chacko VP, Jacobus WE, et al: Metabolic changes preceding functional and morphologic indices of rejection in heterotopic cardiac allografts. A 31P nuclear magnetic resonance study. *Transplantation* 46:346-351, 1988

123. Haug CE, Shapiro JI, Chan L, et al: P-31 nuclear magnetic resonance spectroscopic evaluation of heterotopic cardiac allograft rejection in the rat. *Transplantation* 44:175-178, 1987

124. Bottomley PA, Weiss RG, Hardy CJ, et al: Myocardial high-energy phosphate metabolism and allograft rejection in patients with heart transplants. *Radiology* 181:67-75, 1991

125. Paulin S, von Schulthess GK, Fossel E, et al: MR imaging of the aortic root and proximal coronary arteries. *AJR* 148:665-670, 1987

126. Manning WJ, Li W, Boyle N, et al: Magnetic resonance coronary angiography (abstract). *Circulation* 86 Suppl 1:476, 1992

127. Poncelet BP, Wedeen VJ, Weisskoff RM, et al: Quantification of the LAD coronary flow with magnetic resonance echo-planar imaging (abstract). *Circulation* 86 Suppl 4:476, 1992

CHAPTER

8

Use of ultrafast (cine) x-ray computed tomography in cardiac and cardiovascular imaging

John A. Rumberger, Ph.D., M.D., Patrick F. Sheedy, M.D., and Jerome F. Breen, M.D.

EVALUATIONS by radionuclide angiography, cardiac perfusion field imaging, transthoracic and transesophageal echocardiography, magnetic resonance imaging (MRI), and conventional x-ray computed tomography (CT) are now routine in clinical practice. Ultrafast x-ray computed tomography (UFCT) (also termed "cine-CT"), facilitated by three-dimensional image registration, has emerged as yet another means to examine and define cardiovascular anatomy, function, and flow in patients with a variety of diseases of the heart, pericardium, and great vessels. Ultrasound and nuclear medicine methods are described in chapters 5 and 6 and MRI of the heart in chapter 7. The purposes of this chapter are to examine the applications of UFCT to the practice of cardiovascular medicine and to discuss clinically appropriate uses of this advanced cardiac imaging modality.

ULTRAFAST CT SCANNER DESIGN AND OPERATION

Clinical application of UFCT to define cardiovascular anatomy, function, and flow requires comprehension of the inherent versatility of the instrument. Additionally, it involves knowledge of proper methods for administration of iodinated contrast medium.

Scanner design

Conventional CT scanners are of several designs but basically involve mechanical rotation of a single x-ray source about the patient in concert with a stationary or rotating collimator-detector combination.

In 1979 Boyd and colleagues,[1] working at the University of California, San Francisco, and Robb et al.,[2] working at the Mayo Clinic, nearly simultaneously introduced x-ray scanners designed specifically to image the beating heart. The Boyd scanner, first introduced commercially in 1983 and now called "ultrafast CT" (Imatron C-100, South San Francisco, CA), uses a stationary x-ray source-detector pair coupled to a unique electron beam scanning technology. X-rays are produced as the rotating electron beam is swept across a series of one to four semicircular (210°) tungsten targets situated beneath the subject (Fig 8-1). Thus, the system has no moving parts, and imaging through the cardiac cycle or from adjacent cardiac sites is possible in rapid succession. This technology acquires images from an electrocardiographic (ECG) "trigger"; scans are acquired prospectively at multiple times during the cardiac cycle or, alternatively, from one tomographic plane to the other. As originally designed, up to 8 cm of the myocardium could be scanned nearly simultaneously. In 1986, a "high-resolution" scanning procedure was introduced, and all scanners were retrofitted with a circular collimator to allow for traditional body CT examinations of the thorax and abdomen.

In contrast, the Mayo Clinic's unique Dynamic Spatial Reconstructor used conventional transmission x-ray and fluoroscopic technology but in such a way that true thoracic volume images were acquired repeatedly at a rate of up to 60 frames/sec. An excellent review of the imaging physics of both of these instruments was recently given by Robb and Morin.[3]

Ultrafast CT scanner operation

Current UFCT scanning options include an ECG-triggered, rapid-sequence, multislice (2 to 12 levels), 50-msec scan acquisition for studies requiring information from temporal sequences (e.g., cardiac function and flow) and a single-slice, 100- to 1,400-msec acquisition (in steps of 100 msec) for studies requiring improved density and spatial resolution from static images (e.g., pericardial detail, aortic dissection, coronary artery calcification). The tomographic slice thickness is nominally 0.8 cm for the 50-msec images but can be 0.15, 0.3, 0.6, or 1.0 cm for the 100-msec images. The sequential scan repetition rate is 17 frames/sec for the multislice mode and 8 frames/sec for the single-slice mode. The specifications of the scanner

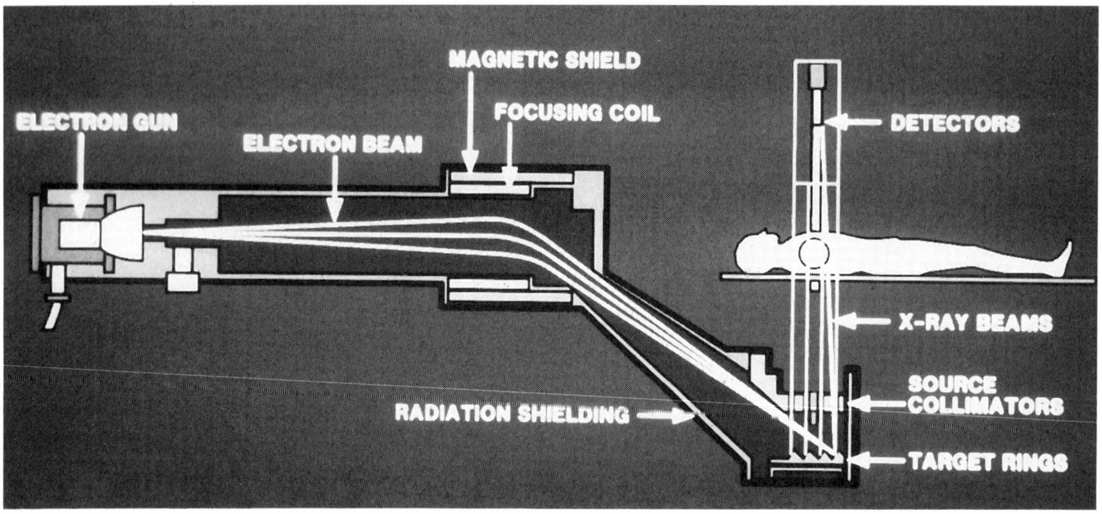

Fig 8-1 Schematic illustration of ultrafast computed tomographic scanner (see text for details of operation).

Table 8-1 Specifications for ultrafast computed tomography

	Multilevel mode	Single-slice mode
Number of detectors per tomographic level	432	864
Number of levels per scan	2	1
Number of levels per study	2-12	1-40
Scan time (seconds)	0.05	0.1-1.4
Slice thickness (mm)	8.0	3.0, 6.0, 10.0
Matrix size (number of pixels)	256^2, 360^2	512^2
Nominal pixel dimension (mm) (for 35-cm reconstruction size)	1.4, 0.97	0.68
Maximum number of images per study	80	40

and the scanning options are given in Table 8-1. Pixel (short for "picture element") size is the smallest single display element for the image. Pixel dimensions are fundamental to the spatial resolution of the image and depend on the dimensions of the reconstructed image field. Matrix size defines how many pixels are used to describe the field of the image. For reconstruction of an image encompassing 35 cm of the thorax (the "field-of-view" size used for most adult cardiac studies), the pixel dimensions vary from 1.4 mm by 1.4 mm for a matrix of 256 by 256 pixels to 0.68 mm by 0.68 mm for a matrix of 512 by 512 pixels. Routine matrix size in our laboratory is 360 by 360 for multilevel (i.e., cardiac) studies and 512 by 512 for single-slice (high-resolution) studies.

Prospective ECG triggering (as opposed to manual triggering) is preferred for cardiac imaging and commences at 0%, 40%, or 80% of the measured ECG R-R interval. An analog ECG signal and the timing of each scan are recorded with the scan file header during each acquisition and can be viewed and analyzed independently of the tomographic image data. Scanning is performed in one of three modes: cine, flow, and volume. An example of ECG triggering on the R wave (i.e., 0% of the R-R interval) for each of the three scanning modes is shown in Figure 8-2. An outline of these modes and the scanning variables that govern the use of each mode is given in Table 8-2. Basically, the cine mode is used to define time-dependent cardiac cavity and muscle motion (i.e., endocardial motion and wall thickening), the flow mode to follow time-dependent changes in regional vascular opacification that correspond to measurements of local blood flow, and the volume mode to define static anatomic information, with or without the use of iodinated contrast medium.

Scanning planes for cardiovascular images

Standard CT images of the aorta and other great vessels are generally obtained from a standard transaxial plane by acquiring images perpendicular to the long axis of the body. Since the position of the heart within the thorax is not parallel to the transaxial plane, an alteration from the standard thorax-body imaging plane is usually advantageous for most cardiac studies. In two-dimensional echocardiography, the apical four-chamber (apical long-axis) and parasternal short-axis views generally allow for identification of all surfaces of the left ventricle and are

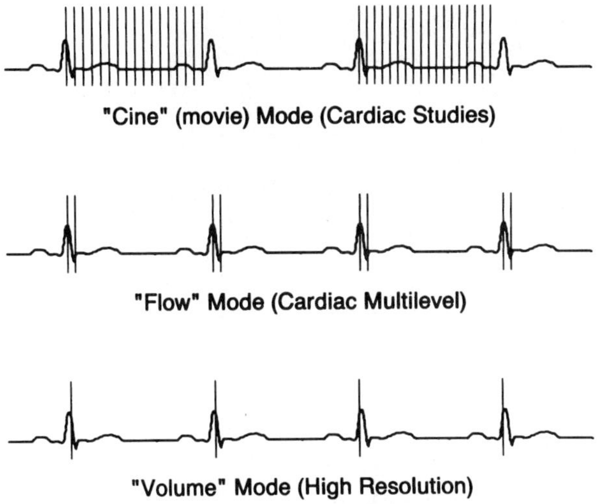

Fig 8-2 ECG-triggered scanning modes used by UFCT for cardiac studies. "Cine" images are acquired rapidly and in succession after the trigger signal from the patient's ECG. After imaging from one target ring, the electron beam moves quickly to imaging in the cine mode from an adjacent target ring. "Flow" images are acquired at a predesignated time during the cardiac cycle, and imaging at multiple target rings occurs nearly simultaneously. For both cine and flow mode acquisitions, the scanning table remains fixed. "Volume" mode scans are also acquired at a preset time during the cardiac cycle, but images are taken from only one target ring. After acquisition of an image, the scanning table is moved a preset distance and imaging repeated. (From Rumberger JA: Ultrafast computed tomography scanning modes, scanning planes and practical aspects of contrast administration. In *Ultrafast Computed Tomography in Cardiac Imaging: Principles and Practice.* Edited by W Stanford, JA Rumberger. Mount Kisco, New York, Futura Publishing Company, 1992, pp 17-24. By permission.)

complementary in the evaluation of cardiac structure and function.[4] Nearly identical orthogonal views of the left ventricle are routinely obtained by UFCT and are properly termed "horizontal long axis" and "short axis," respectively. This nomenclature is in accord with criteria put forward by both the American Heart Association and the American College of Cardiology for displays from advanced cardiac imaging devices.[5] An example of a midventricular short- and long-axis image pair in a normal person is shown in Figure 8-3.

The scanning platform (table) can be slewed to the patient's left or right for up to 25°, and the body can be tilted directly up to 17° from the horizontal. The method to facilitate short-axis images was adapted from animal studies[6,7] and later modified to provide long-axis images in patients.[8] Examples of some indications for scanning in the short and long axes are given in Table 8-3. Indications for use of UFCT in the high-resolution mode are listed in Table 8-4.

Aspects of scanning and contrast administration

The basic scanning protocol for cardiovascular studies is usually tailored to the clinical question or specific problem to be addressed. In most patients, however, the following procedures are used.

No premedications are given before scanning under usual circumstances. For all cardiac studies and most examinations of the great vessels, standard ECG electrodes are placed on the patient's chest for continuous monitoring and for triggering the CT exposures. An intravenous catheter is placed in either an antecubital vein or, when this is not possible, a hand vein. Rarely is it necessary to insert a "central" venous catheter for a

Table 8-2 Scanning modes in ultrafast computed tomography

	Mode		
	Cine	Flow	Volume
Contrast medium injection	Infusion (1-3 mL/sec)	Bolus (5-15 mL/sec)	Infusion (0.5-3 mL/sec)
ECG triggering (% of R-R interval)	0, 40, 80, *or* manual	0, 40, 80, *or* manual	Move table after each scan
Levels scanned	2, 4, 6, 8, or 12	2, 4, 6, or 8	Up to 40
Clinical use	Cardiac anatomy or function	Cardiac flow	Cardiac or vascular anatomy
Reconstruction time per image (seconds)	5	5	10
Time required to complete a single study	8-level scan completed in 7 cardiac cycles	8-level scan at every other cardiac cycle for 10 images per level; completed in 19 cardiac cycles	40-level scan completed in approximately 80 cardiac cycles (two separate held breaths)
Images per tomographic level in a single scan	10 for 8-level 13 for 6-level 20 for 4-level 40 for 2-level	Same as cine-mode scanning	1

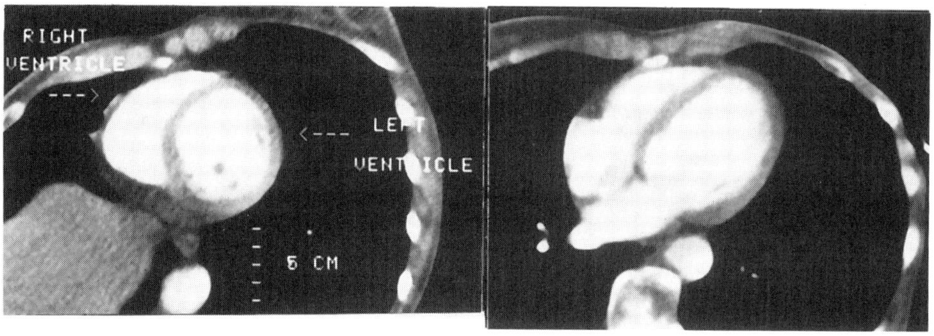

Fig 8-3 Representative short- and long-axis images at the midventricular position in a patient without known cardiac disease. Note the details of both the right and the left ventricular cavities as well as of other cardiac chambers. (All CT studies are presented in the standard format, with the left ventricle on the right side of the image, viewed as if one were looking up from the patient's feet.)

Table 8-3 Indications for ultrafast computed tomography scanning in the long and short cardiac axes

Long axis
Simultaneous imaging of all four cardiac chambers
Visualization of atrioventricular valve motion
Evaluation of left ventricular apex for thrombi or tumor
Evaluation of pericardial disease (thickening, effusion)
Quantitation of the extent of left ventricular and apical aneurysm
Evaluation of global left ventricular function
Evaluation of interatrial septum
Examination of left and right atria
Evaluation for pericardial disease
Short axis
Simultaneous evaluation of anterior, lateral, posterior, and ventricular septal walls of the left ventricle
Quantitation of left ventricular mass and chamber volumes
Evaluation of the proximal aorta and aortic valve
Quantitation of segmental left ventricular function
Quantitation of right ventricular chamber volumes and function
Evaluation of the extent of left ventricular posterior aneurysm

Table 8-4 Indications for high-resolution, single-slice scanning

Detailed right ventricular muscle mass
Right ventricular anatomy
Evaluation of the aorta
Evaluation of the pulmonary artery

routine examination. Initial multilevel, end-diastolic localization scans are taken without the use of contrast medium to determine the anatomic position of the cardiac apex. An assessment of the "circulation time" (i.e., the time for contrast material to travel from the injection site to the systemic circulation) is made by injection of 0.2 mg of indocyanine dye and detection of the time between injection and appearance of the dye in the systemic circulation as shown by the deflection from baseline of a tracing from an earlobe oximeter (Waters Instruments, Rochester, MN). Alternatively, circulation time can be assessed by injecting a bolus of 0.1 mg of magnesium sulfate intravenously and asking the patient to note when a warm flush sensation appears over the face and body.

Quantitative cardiac imaging of the cardiac chambers and vasculature with UFCT requires intravascular administration of iodinated contrast medium, and definition of the circulation time allows precise timing between the administration of medium and the commencement of image acquisition. For assessment of the great vessels, an estimation of circulation time is often not mandatory, except for studies of pulmonary embolism (see later).

After quantitation of circulation time, the patient is requested to suspend respiration at a comfortable mid-inspiratory level for a few seconds before and during scanning. For both flow and cine studies, the scanning sequence usually encompasses images at all ventricular levels. Scan acquisition in the volume mode is usually easily accomplished with the patient in the standard transaxial position, since serial movements of the scanning table are required during acquisition. For routine studies of the great vessels within the thorax, images are obtained from the top of the aortic arch through the first portion of the abdominal aorta.

Usually, routine complete apex-to-base short- and long-axis images of the heart can be obtained with less than 1.5 mL/kg of contrast medium administered intravenously by a powered injector. For studies of cardiac function, we use only nonionic contrast material because, given intravenously, it has little effect on baseline cardiac dynamics.[7,9]

In our laboratory, a 20-second infusion of contrast medium with scanning commencing at or 1 to 3 seconds after the predefined circulation time provides excellent multilevel cine images for definition of right and left ventricular function during the cardiac cycle. The injection of contrast medium may have to be prolonged if the circulation time is much beyond 25 seconds (approximate range of normal is 8 to 15 seconds). Such instances frequently arise in patients with congestive heart failure.

A bolus injection of contrast material (nominally, 10 mL/sec) is best for flow studies. Scanning is triggered at a predesignated phase of the ECG R-R interval for each of the multiple tomographic levels. To capture vascular opacifications on the left side of the circulation (e.g., for bypass graft patency or myocardial perfusion), scanning should commence at a time approximately one-half the time for maximum opacification on the left side (i.e., at one-half the "circulation time"). For preferential definition of flow on the right side of the circulation (e.g., definition of left-to-right shunt), scanning should commence just preceding or simultaneous with the injection of the contrast medium.

Prolonged infusions—lasting from 20 to 40 seconds (at rates of approximately 1.5 mL/sec)—are appropriate for volume mode scans (e.g., for aortic dissection), with scanning commencing at or about the time of circulation.

SCANNING PROCEDURES

Cardiac images

A complete cardiac examination should include both short- and long-axis multilevel images from the left ventricular apex and caudad through the base of the left ventricle and the right ventricular outflow tract. After placement of the intravenous catheter, the subject is positioned in the scanner to facilitate acquisition of short-axis (transverse cardiac) images from apex to base.[8,10] A noncontrast localization scan is performed to determine the level of the left ventricular apex. The subject is then mechanically moved into the scanner to assure that the most caudad tomographic image is obtained at the level of the cardiac apex.

Commencing image acquisition at the "circulation time" for studies of cardiac dynamics guarantees excellent opacification of both the left and the right ventricular cavities at all levels scanned. Imaging, initiated at the ECG R wave, consists of 13 consecutive frames through the cardiac cycle at six tomographic levels. Studies of cardiac output or myocardial perfusion require commencing the serial imaging at about one-half the circulation time. After 2 to 5 minutes, the scanning table is moved (with the patient lying still) 6.0 cm and the scanning sequence repeated. The normal human left ventricle is roughly 10 to 12 cm from the tip of the epicardial apex, through the origin of the aortic root, just cephalad to the aortic valve. Thus, for most patients, two scan series (encompassing 12 cm of the heart) are sufficient to image the entire heart; however, for many patients with isolated aortic valvular insufficiency or ventricular dilatation (cardiomyopathy), three consecutive and contiguous scan series (now spanning 18 cm from apex to base) may be necessary to examine the entire heart (i.e., all left *and* right ventricular surfaces).

Imaging of the great vessels

Because UFCT does not rely on mechanical motion of the x-ray tube, it does not encounter problems of heat loading, and, therefore, multilevel images can be acquired over a short period, usually during a single held breath. For imaging of the great vessels, the scanner is used in the single-slice, high-resolution mode. The ability to obtain a single scan in a short time (100 msec) has provided excellent image quality by decreasing motion blurring of any object that might move during scan acquisition. This is of particular importance in the thorax, since most structures move coincident with the cardiac cycle.

Currently, up to 40 tomographic images can be obtained continuously during an acquisition in the single-slice (high resolution, 100 msec) mode. Acquisition can usually be accomplished during two separate held breaths of approximately 35 seconds. Most studies of the thoracic great vessels are done with 6-mm tomograms spaced roughly 6 mm to 1.0 cm apart. Studies of coronary artery calcification acquire 3-mm contiguous tomograms.

Although UFCT can be used for evaluation of abdominal disease, the scan times are increased to four to six consecutive 100-msec images (without ECG triggering), thus confounding the temporal resolution advantage of the system. The exception is studies of renal parenchymal volume or mass and renal perfusion (see later).

CLINICAL USE OF ULTRAFAST CT FOR IMAGING OF THE CARDIOVASCULAR SYSTEM

In selected patients, UFCT offers the potential to assess such anatomic and functional information during a single session. Relative, but not absolute, contraindications are allergy to contrast media (with premedication essential) and renal insufficiency (usually a serum creatinine value of > 2.0 mg/dL). As stated previously, the methods of data acquisition, the orientation of the imaging planes, and the analysis of the images are designed specifically to answer the clinical questions posed for each subject.

Anatomy

Right and left ventricular muscle mass. Quantitation of global left ventricular muscle mass (and, simultaneously, of left ventricular volumes) involves definition of the cardiac borders at each tomographic imaging plane and summation across all ventricular levels, from apex to base. A schema of the analysis is shown in Figure 8-4 (modified Simpson's rule).

Comparison between left ventricular mass ex vivo and that calculated from UFCT in vivo is shown in Figure 8-5.[6] Correlations are excellent ($r = 0.99$), and the standard error of the mean is 4.1 g (about 5% of the mean). Additionally, interobserver and intraobserver variability were assessed and the data found to be highly reproducible. Feiring et al.[10] also extended these observations to

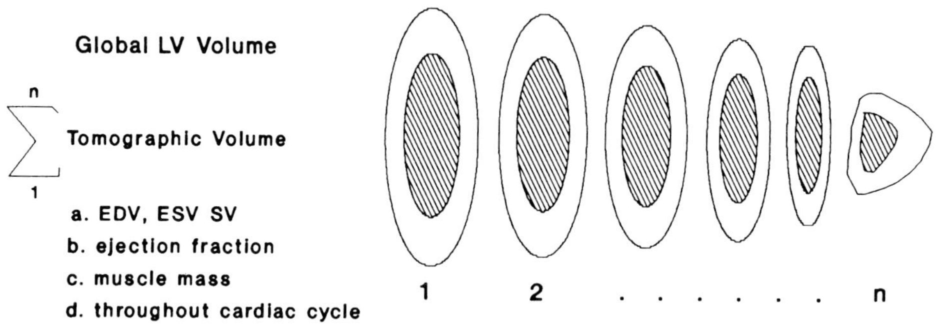

Fig 8-4 Schematic illustration of determination of global left ventricular (LV) volumes, ejection fraction, and muscle mass by UFCT. The total value for global volumes is defined by the sum of the individual tomographic volumes at each level of the heart (modified Simpson's rule). *EDV,* end-diastolic volume; *ESV,* end-systolic volume; *SV,* stroke volume. (From Rumberger JA: Ultrafast computed tomographic assessment of left ventricular function at rest: applications in myocardial infarction, cardiomyopathy and aneurysm. In *Ultrafast Computed Tomography in Cardiac Imaging: Principles and Practice.* Edited by W Stanford, JA Rumberger. Mount Kisco, New York, Futura Publishing Company, 1992, pp 117-137. By permission.)

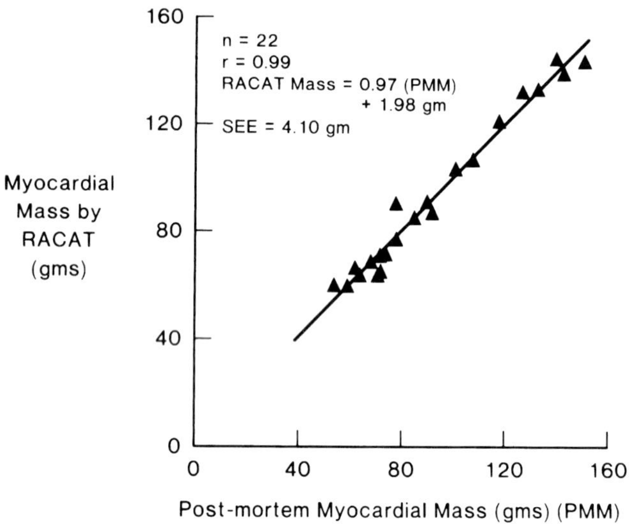

Fig 8-5 Comparison of postmortem myocardial mass with calculations made by UFCT *(RACAT)* in 22 animals. Note the precision with which the measurements are determined and the very small standard error of the estimate *(SEE).* (From Feiring AJ, Rumberger JA, Reiter SJ, et al: Determination of left ventricular mass in dogs with rapid-acquisition cardiac computed tomographic scanning. *Circulation* 72:1355-1364, 1985. By permission of American Heart Association.)

determination of left ventricular mass in a group of normal individuals and found that the clinical application of these methods also provided an excellent correlation with normal values determined by other methods, including autopsy. The reproducibility of such means for determination of left ventricular mass in man was shown by Roig et al.,[11] who found a less than 1% to 2% difference in calculations of left ventricular muscle mass in a group of patients who had three separate UFCT scans within a 24-hour period.

UFCT remains the imaging modality of choice to provide definition of right ventricular size and function (see later section), but Hajduczok et al.[12] recently extended this application to quantitation of right ventricular muscle mass. For quantitation of left ventricular muscle mass or volume by UFCT, tomograms 8 mm in thickness are acquired from multiple tomographic planes and the total cardiac volume is calculated by a modified Simpson ("stack of coins") rule. The nominal spatial resolution of 1.0 to 1.4 mm/pixel is sufficient to define left ventricular wall thickness. However, to define right ventricular muscle mass, UFCT imaging must be done with contiguous 3-mm, high-spatial-resolution tomograms (nominal resolution of 0.7 mm/pixel) because of the need to resolve the thickness of the normally very thin right ventricular wall. Using this approach, Hajduczok et al. found an excellent correlation between ECG-triggered UFCT scanning and autopsy definitions of right ventricular muscle mass.

Congenital heart disease. The high-resolution imaging mode (single slice) along with the multislice cine mode for UFCT provides exquisite anatomic and functional details of the heart, surrounding great vessels, and extracardiac conduits in patients with existing or surgically corrected congenital heart disease. High-resolution (anatomic) imaging is appropriate even in infants and, because overall image registration is rapid, can be done with little or no sedation, which is necessary in many of the conventional CT examinations and virtually all the MRI examinations. Husayni[13] recently reported on the use of UFCT in series of patients with a variety of congenital heart diseases and several hundred examinations over a 3-year period. The general imaging procedures are similar to those mentioned previously in the evaluation of cardiac anatomy by UFCT. However, in patients weighing less

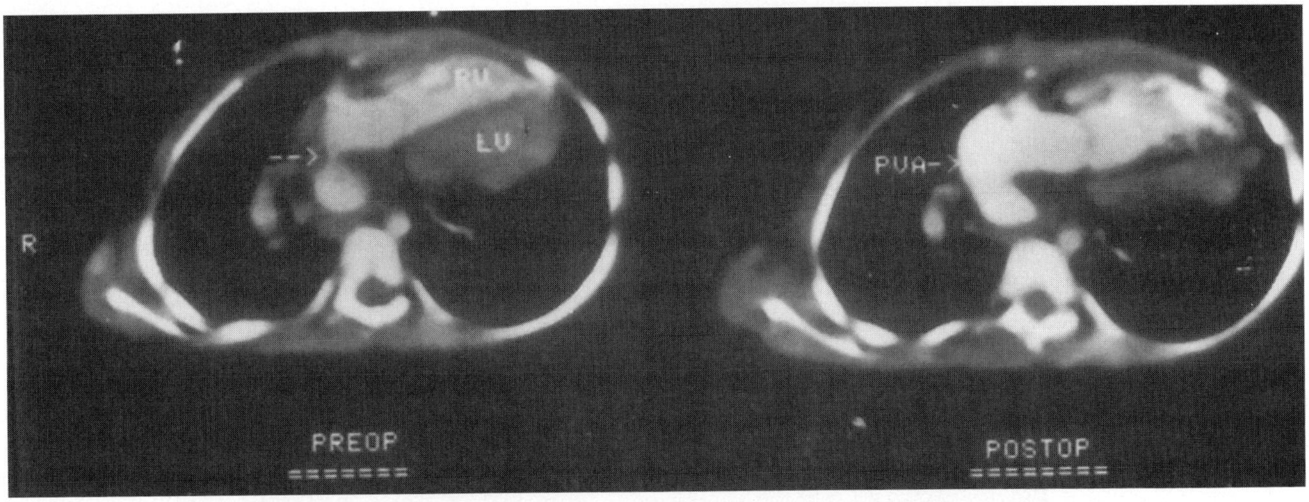

Fig 8-6 UFCT long-axis images from a 5-year-old child with severe obstruction of the pulmonary venous atrium *(PVA)* (*arrow,* left image) 4 years after Mustard repair of transposition of the great vessels. The images were obtained before **(left)** and after **(right)** a second operation to relieve the obstruction. *LV,* left ventricle; *RV,* right ventricle. (From Husayni TS: Ultrafast computed tomographic imaging in congenital heart disease. In *Ultrafast Computed Tomography in Cardiac Imaging: Principles and Practice.* Edited by W Stanford, JA Rumberger. Mount Kisco, New York, Futura Publishing Company, 1992, pp 311-336. By permission.)

than 40 kg, the infusion rates and total amount of contrast medium are modified to account for a smaller distribution of the intravascular agents.

Three-dimensional displays of congenital defects with use of off-line commercially available software afford an additional means to provide anatomic diagnoses or follow serial progression after palliative or corrective surgery. An example of UFCT imaging is shown in Figure 8-6: in a 5-year-old who had obstruction of the pulmonary venous atrium 4 years after Mustard repair, UFCT images were obtained before and after surgical correction of the obstruction.

Diseases of the great vessels. Specific CT examinations of the aorta are usually performed because of suspicion of disease such as atherosclerotic aneurysm, aortic dissection, postoperative problems associated with a peripheral bypass graft, post-trauma problems, or symptoms that suggest a rupture or atheromatous ulcer with hematoma. Additionally, examinations are performed as a convenient means of following progression of known disease. Although most of these examinations are accomplished with conventional CT, UFCT allows quick evaluation of multiple tomographic sections during peak contrast enhancement. Reduction of examination time is particularly important in the ill, uncomfortable, or uncooperative patient. The availability of programmable, high-volume, low-flow-rate automatic powered injections for contrast media administration has led to the development of many different protocols, which can be tailored to the individual patient.

Although conventional CT produces excellent diagnostic images of the thoracic great vessels, scan times of 1 to 2 seconds mean that fine details can often be missed or are blurred because of significant motion of the great vessels during the cardiac cycle. Various "streak artifacts" can be appreciated in such images. Acquiring adjacent anatomic images of the great vessels at the same time during the cardiac cycle by ECG-triggered scanning reduces errors due to variable volume averaging of structures reconstructed in a tomographic format. The UFCT examination also has the advantage of using variable slice thicknesses.

At present, the UFCT scanner allows for 40 consecutive slices during peak opacification of the aorta. This ability, coupled with the significant limitation of motion artifacts, greatly facilitates the diagnosis or exclusion of significant aortic disease. Although the high-resolution mode of scanning is most frequently used for assessment of great vessel disease, imaging in the cardiac "flow" mode can allow for rapid separation of true lumen from false lumen in patients with aortic dissection (Fig 8-7).

Aneurysms can be clearly differentiated from other vascular structures, such as abundant mediastinal fat, large lymph nodes, and a variety of discrete "masses" that might contain fat, fluid, or necrotic debris. With selective opacification of the vasculature, separation of vascular and avascular structures is relatively straightforward.

Specific applications include detection and extent of atherosclerotic aneurysm or dissecting aneurysm as well as specific clinical questions associated with postoperative status of peripheral bypass grafts, aortic deceleration injuries (i.e., post-trauma), or symptoms that suggest rupture or atheromatous ulcer with hematoma formation. In these situations, both noncontrast and contrast studies must be done; the noncontrast scans can show existence of hemorrhage or hematoma that might not be as obvious on scans done with contrast only. Differentiation of

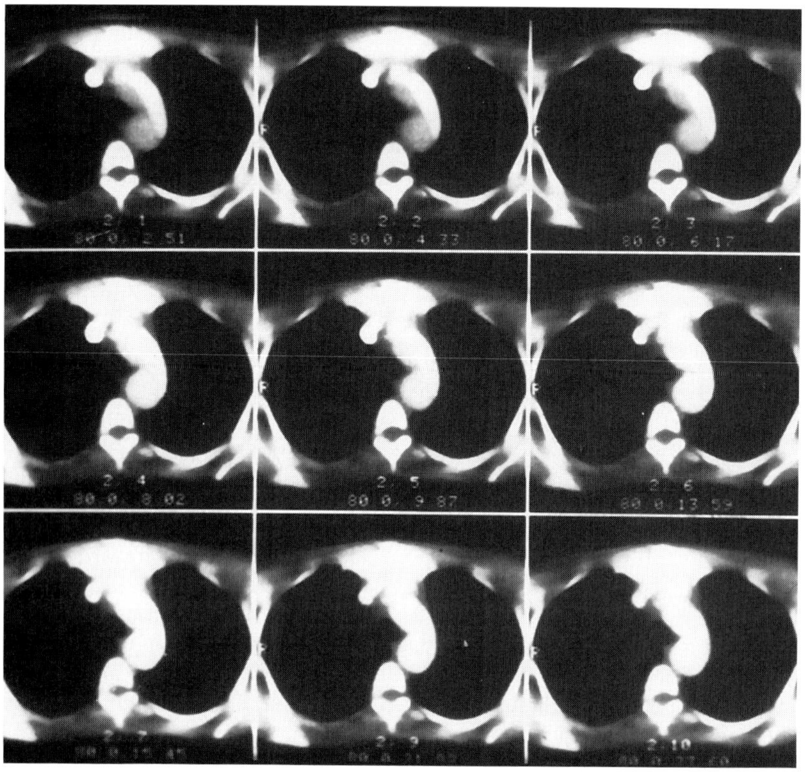

Fig 8-7 UFCT images from the aortic arch in a patient with proximal dissection of the aorta. Shown are a series of time sequence "flow" studies (left to right, top to bottom) demonstrating initial contrast opacification of the true aortic lumen and then, later, opacification of the false aortic (dissection) channel.

penetrating ulcer from dissection is important, because treatment for patients with dissection of the descending thoracic aorta alone is often medical, whereas penetrating ulcer with or without hematoma formation may be best treated surgically.

Although conventional CT provides some anatomic details of the pulmonary arteries, whether intraluminal filling defects are absent or present is rarely determined by this method. However, UFCT may be of considerable benefit here because overall image quality in the proximal pulmonary vasculature is improved over that with conventional devices.

A pilot investigation in 50 patients at the Mayo Clinic compared high-resolution UFCT imaging of the pulmonary arteries for pulmonary thromboembolism with direct pulmonary angiography. The comparison was encouraging for use of UFCT to screen rapidly, safely, and conveniently for thromboembolism of the pulmonary artery trunk, right and left main pulmonary arteries, and secondary branches. A prospective trial in 100 patients is under way. Recent studies by Geraghty et al.[14] suggest that UFCT can potentially detect thrombi in the second through fourth branches of the pulmonary division. A high-resolution UFCT image from a patient with pulmonary embolism documented by direct angiography is shown in Figure 8-8.

Three-dimensional anatomy. Several modes for three-dimensional displays can facilitate recognition of cardiac surfaces (Fig 8-9) or define details of a particular region of the heart. As an example of the latter, Figure 8-10 shows a volume-rendered image set from UFCT images (3-mm, 100-msec, high-resolution scans) of a cadaver heart whose coronary arteries had been filled with barium. By selective reconstruction of the cardiac volume for densities in the barium-filled heart, a reasonable three-dimensional display of the complete coronary artery tree can be made by use of a variety of commercially available software packages.

Although three-dimensional surface and cavity displays are often dramatic, they frequently are not of the image quality of the original tomographic scans and must be used with caution or interpreted in conjunction with the original tomographic images.

Diseases of the pericardium. UFCT can be used to define the entire anatomy of the pericardium and may be of particular value in localization of effusions in the posterior portions of the heart and, in particular, on the right side of the cardiac circulation (Fig 8-11).

High-resolution UFCT images can define the anatomic localization and extent of pericardial thickening (Fig 8-12). Scans before and immediately after administration of contrast material are particularly helpful here. Because of similarities in baseline CT density (i.e., x-ray attenuation), noncontrast CT examination of the pericardium frequently cannot separate thickening of the pericardium from effusions. Since the pericardium has its own vascular

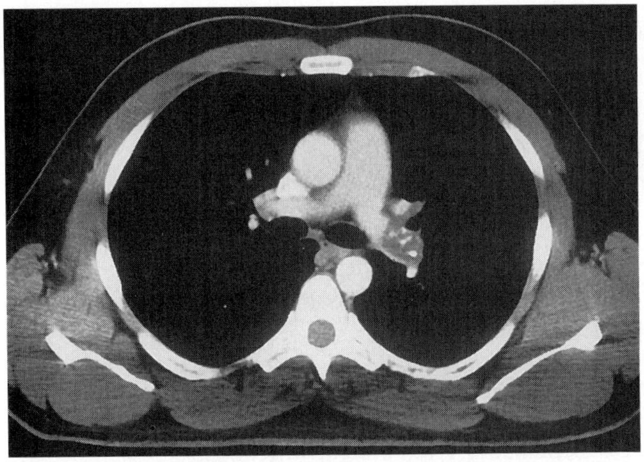

Fig 8-8 High-resolution UFCT scan, enhanced by iodinated contrast medium, at the base of the pulmonary artery bifurcation. Note the absence of contrast opacification in the left main pulmonary artery (right lower portion of the image), identifying a pulmonary thrombosis. Scattered calcification within the thrombus suggests a chronic situation.

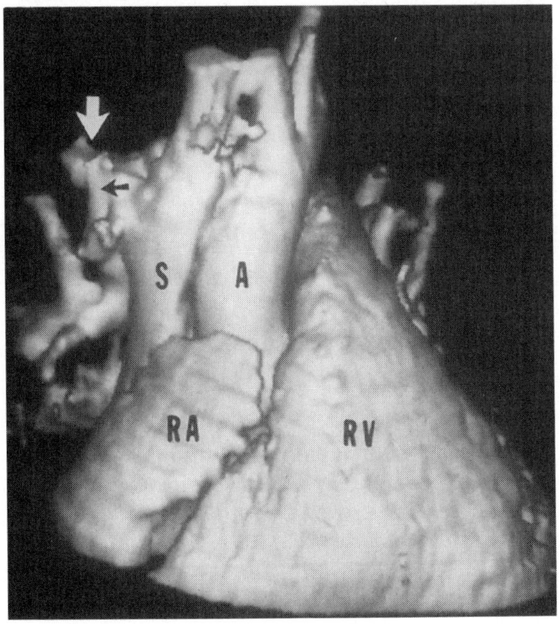

Fig 8-9 Three-dimensional reconstruction from a multilevel, high-resolution study with UFCT of the heart in a 12-year-old patient. The *white arrow* identifies a right upper pulmonary vein draining to the superior vena cava *(S)*. A pulmonary artery branch crosses in front of the anomalous pulmonary vein *(black arrow)*. *A,* aorta; *RA,* right atrium; *RV,* right ventricle. (From Husayni TS: Ultrafast computed tomographic imaging in congenital heart disease. In *Ultrafast Computed Tomography in Cardiac Imaging: Principles and Practice.* Edited by W Stanford, JA Rumberger. Mount Kisco, New York, Futura Publishing Company, 1992, pp 311-336. By permission.)

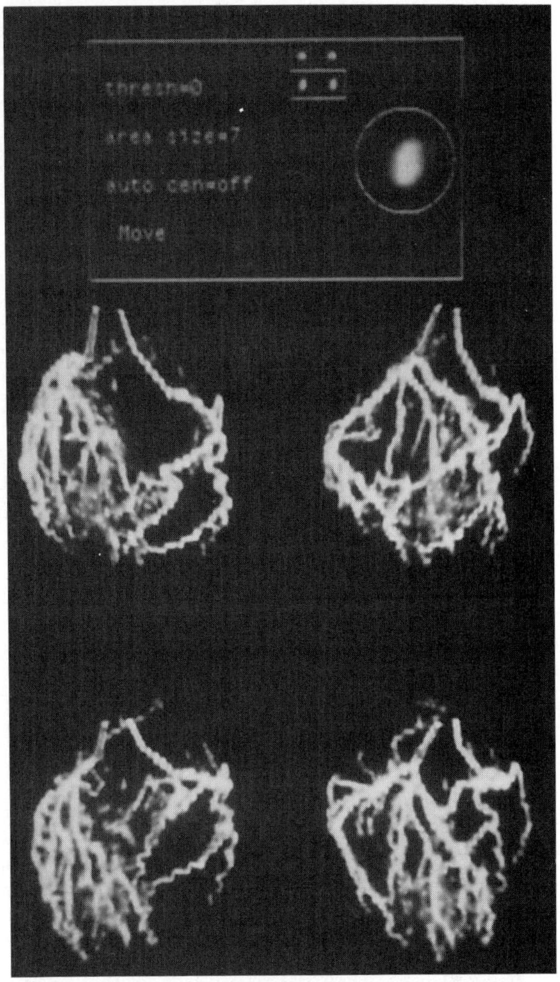

Fig 8-10 Three-dimensional reconstructions from various angles of the epicardial coronary arteries from a multilevel, high-resolution UFCT scan. The study is from an autopsy specimen of a human heart prefilled with barium to simulate the opacification possible with injection of iodinated contrast medium. The image within the box is a further reconstruction of a single 3-mm section of a coronary artery derived from reformatting the three-dimensional imaging parallel to the vessel lumen.

supply, however, it can be selectively opacified and then conveniently separated in the image from an adjacent pericardial effusion.

Additional information on the physiologic consequences of pericardial constriction may be provided from analysis of the character of the right or left ventricular time-dependent volume data when the conventional high-resolution examination is coupled with a cine study of left and right ventricular function and motion. Figure 8-13 shows a global left ventricular volume curve defined by UFCT in a patient with a thickened pericardium and diastolic equilibration of right and left ventricular pressures during cardiac catheterization (see later discussion on studies of diastolic function). Note that the pattern of early diastolic filling is distinctly different from that in a normal person, who has a "square root" pattern.

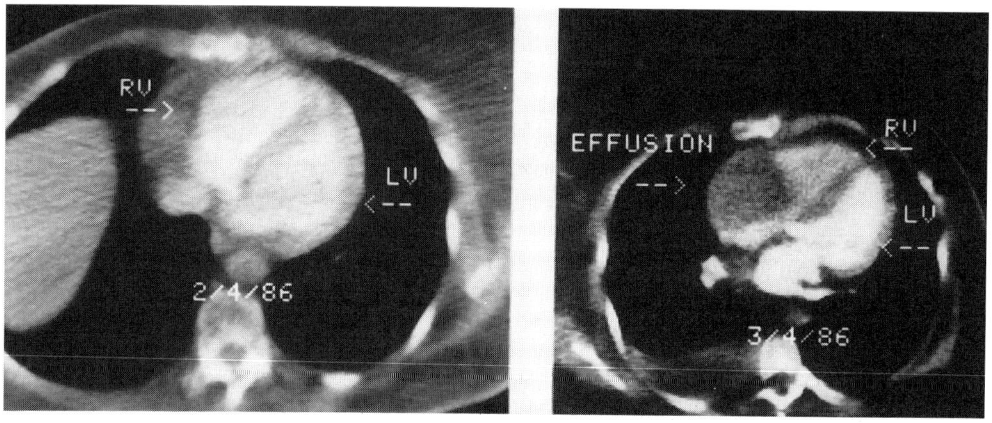

Fig 8-11 Serial midventricular long-axis UFCT examinations in a patient with an isolated right-sided pericardial effusion. The patient was stable at the time of the study shown on the **left;** within 1 month **(right image),** however, the patient presented with clinical signs and symptoms of right-sided cardiac tamponade. After the UFCT study, drainage of the pericardium at surgical intervention completely relieved the hemodynamic compromise. *LV,* left ventricle; *RV,* right ventricle.

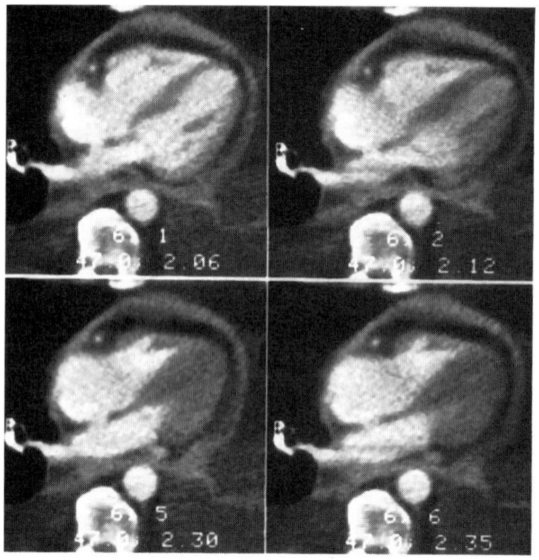

Fig 8-12 Multilevel studies at end-diastole from UFCT examination in a patient with thickened pericardium. Despite the thickened pericardium, the patient did not have other UFCT criteria consistent with the diagnosis of constrictive pericarditis. See text for details.

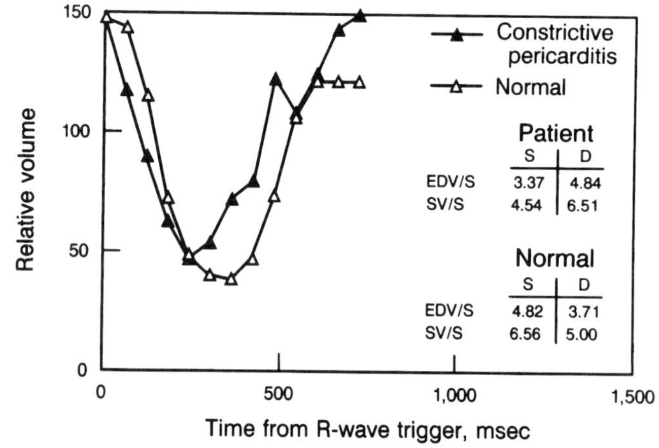

Fig 8-13 Time-dependent left ventricular volume in a normal person compared with that in a patient with constrictive pericarditis proved by catheterization. Note that in the patient with pericardial disease, there is a distinct abnormality in the early left ventricular filling. See text for details. *D,* peak filling rate during diastole; *EDV,* end-diastolic volume; *S,* peak emptying rate during systole; *SV,* stroke volume.

Bypass graft patency. Bolus intravenous injections of iodinated contrast medium and serial ECG-triggered UFCT scanning of the proximal aorta in the "flow" mode of image acquisition allow for temporal resolution of vascular opacifications, thus providing an expeditious means to determine coronary artery bypass graft patency (Fig 8-14). Nominally, scanning is done on every or every other cardiac cycle at the ECG R-wave trigger. Results of a multicenter trial comparing UFCT with angiographic assessment of bypass graft patency have been reported. A total of 127 separate grafts (saphenous and internal mammary) were evaluated; the sensitivity, specificity, and accuracy of the determination of bypass graft patency by CT compared with invasive selective graft angiography were 93.4%, 88.9%, and 92.1%, respectively.[15] Subsequent improvements in methodology and scanning techniques have shown that the overall sensitivity to detect a patent graft is from 94% to 96%.

Flow information on the bypass graft may be evaluated by graphic displays of time-density data (i.e., clearance of contrast material) from each graft. Comparisons of the

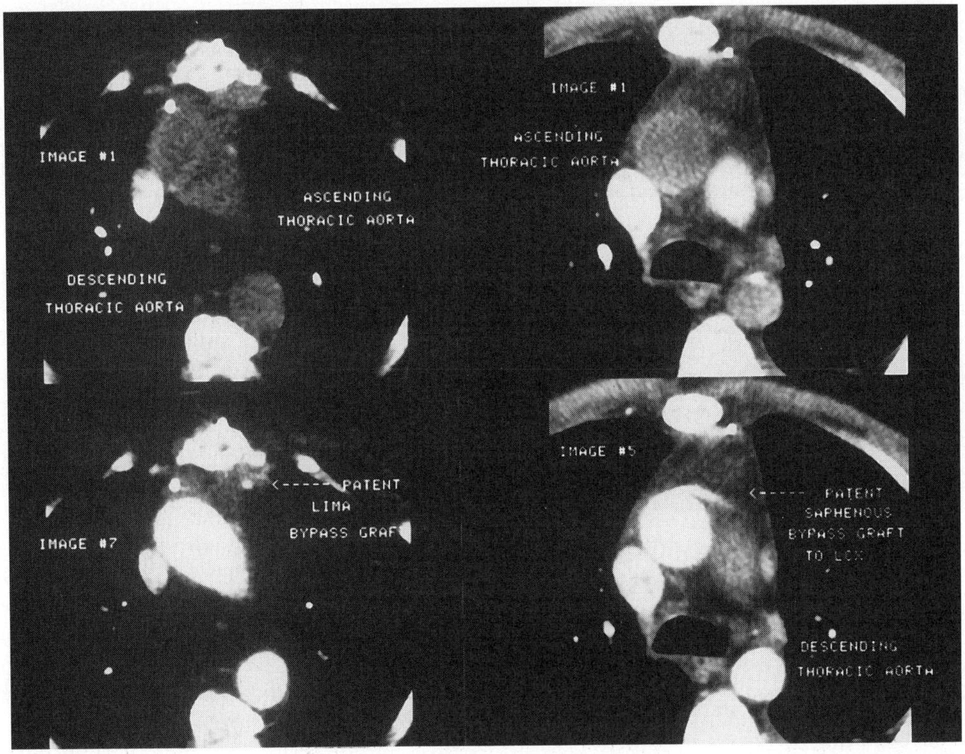

Fig 8-14 UFCT images from two patients with patent bypass grafts to the coronary arteries. **Top left,** imaging at the root of the aorta before arrival of contrast medium to the systemic circulation. **Bottom left,** image obtained approximately 10 seconds later at the same anatomic level shows simultaneous opacification of a left internal mammary graft *(LIMA)* and the ascending thoracic aorta. **Right,** similar sequencing in a patient with a patent saphenous bypass graft to the left circumflex coronary artery *(LCX).* These studies were obtained with a 40-mL injection of contrast medium into a brachiocephalic vein and serial imaging in the "flow" mode.

time for peak opacification in the graft with that in the aorta allow for qualitative statements on individual graft flow rates at rest. Studies on quantitation of bypass graft flow rates or flow reserve in animals[16] and in selected patients[17] before and after intravenous injection of dipyridamole have been encouraging, but additional studies are indicated before this aspect of graft patency studies can be considered a clinical tool.

Coronary artery calcification. One of the newest and most interesting applications for UFCT adopts concepts that have been used clinically for decades, that is, the diagnosis of focal coronary artery disease by the detection of discrete calcification of the involved coronary arteries. Detection of coronary artery calcium by fluoroscopy has been shown to have prognostic value for future coronary syndromes;[18] however, conventional CT has a greater sensitivity for detecting discrete coronary artery calcification.[19]

Three aspects of UFCT technology make it ideal for detecting coronary arterial calcification in patients. First, because of rapid acquisition time and ECG triggering (1/100 sec), motion of the epicardial coronary arteries is "frozen" at end-diastole (triggering on R wave of ECG), so that blurring of the vessel borders due to motion artifact is minimal. Second, the x-ray tomographic imaging process is particularly germane because imaged opacities (densities) are accurately localized in three-dimensional space. Calcific deposits in arterial walls demonstrate relatively high CT densities (measured on the relative Hounsfield scale), from 2 to 10 times higher than surrounding tissue, depending on the tomographic "volume" (or thickness) of the calcification. The sensitivity for identifying areas of high CT density in and around the proximal epicardial coronary arteries with use of UFCT is further aided by the low CT density of fat normally found in the surrounding atrioventricular and interventricular grooves. The appearance of intramural coronary calcium deposits of relatively high CT density adjacent to lower density soft tissue and surrounding fat makes visual identification of these abnormalities in the coronary arteries quite apparent, even to untrained observers (Fig 8-15). Finally, imaging can be accomplished in as little as 40 seconds with three-dimensionally registered images, without gaps, from the base of the aorta to the level of the posterior descending coronary artery.

Simons et al[20] performed UFCT scanning on dissected coronary vessels from autopsy hearts and compared the extent of coronary artery calcification on a segment-by-

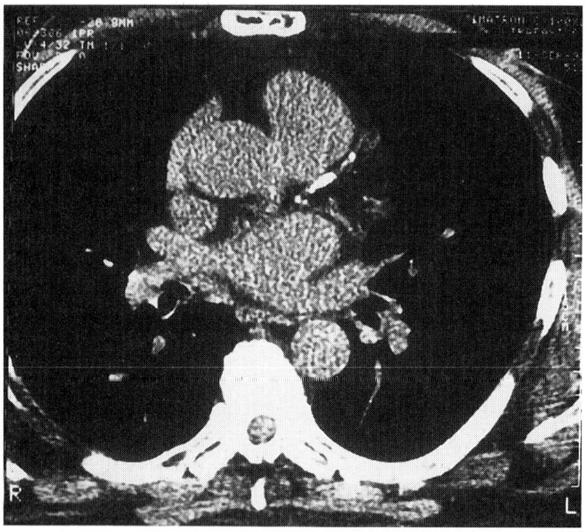

Fig 8-15 High-resolution, noncontrast UFCT examination at the origin of the left coronary artery system. Note that distinct areas of calcification (high-density material [white], right of center) along the distal portion of the left main and proximal portion of the left anterior descending coronary arteries.

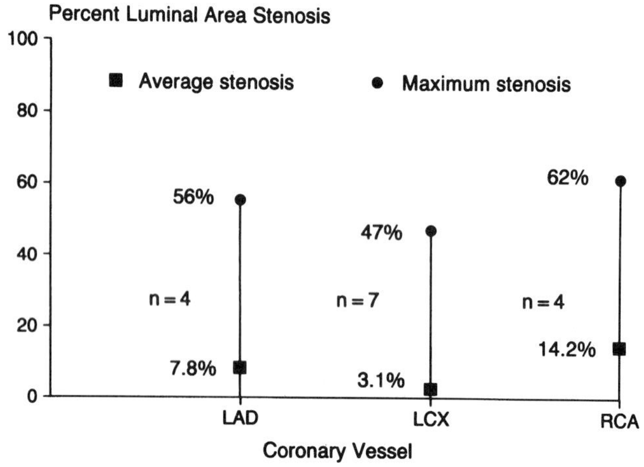

Fig 8-16 Results from subanalysis of UFCT studies of coronary artery calcification in pathologic hearts. Analysis of coronary artery narrowing in whole arterial segments failed to show any evidence of epicardial coronary artery calcification by UFCT along the entire vessel. For each major vessel is shown the maximum luminal area stenosis at any point and the average luminal stenosis along the vessel. Note that when no coronary artery calcification is positively identified by UFCT along an entire epicardial vessel, no stenoses are identified that would be classified as obstructive (i.e., >75% area stenosis). *LAD,* left anterior descending artery; *LCX,* left circumflex artery; *RCA,* right coronary artery. (From Simons DB, Schwartz RS, Edwards WD, et al: Noninvasive definition of anatomic coronary artery disease by ultrafast computed tomographic scanning: a quantitative pathologic comparison study. *J Am Coll Cardiol* 20:1118-1126, 1992. By permission of American College of Cardiology.)

segment basis with histologic sectioning. From this study, when UFCT detection of *any* coronary artery calcification was applied to defining the presence (positive) or absence (negative) of *any* discrete atheromatous disease in the same coronary segment, the positive and negative predictive values were 87% and 68%, respectively, for 525 separate coronary sections examined.

Despite the potential for use of UFCT to define coronary artery calcification, it may actually be too sensitive to facilitate definition of the extent of coronary disease between or among calcified coronary segments. However, a totally negative study may have important clinical implications. Preliminary data from the Mayo Clinic, in a group of patients in whom the coronary anatomy was known, suggest that the absence of identifiable coronary calcification by UFCT may be virtually diagnostic of the absence of hemodynamically significant coronary artery disease (i.e., no lesions >50% diameter stenosis;[21] negative predictive value of 100%). This observation has also been confirmed in studies of noncalcified coronary segments in the aforementioned study in autopsy hearts.[22] Here, "significant" coronary disease was found in only 2% of the coronary segments without detectable calcification by UFCT scanning. When the entire coronary artery distribution (i.e., the left anterior descending, left circumflex, or right coronary artery) had no calcification by UFCT scanning, *no* significant coronary artery disease was to be found in any segment within that artery (negative predictive value of 100%) (Fig 8-16).

However, despite the encouraging results of these early studies, more definitive studies are necessary to define the long-term consequences of a totally negative scan or the clinical implications of a positive scan for coronary calcification before this method can be advocated as a general screening tool for coronary artery disease.

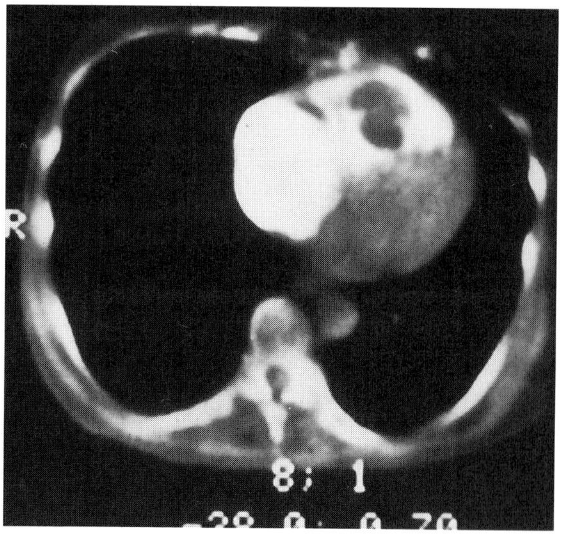

Fig 8-17 End-diastolic UFCT scan in the long axis demonstrating a mass in the right ventricle in a patient who presented with pulmonary embolism.

Tumors and thrombi. Orthogonal (short- and long-axis) UFCT contrast images allow for identification of nonopacified intracardiac thrombi and tumors with, in particular, excellent resolution of the left atrial appendage. UFCT provides spatially excellent images of all cardiac chambers and can identify structures as small as 1 to 2 mm. Figure 8-17 shows a long-axis UFCT scan in a patient who presented with multiple pulmonary emboli. A right ventricular myxoma was found at the time of surgery.

UFCT can additionally be of assistance in defining thrombi or occult occlusion of the venae cavae and other right-sided structures. Minor et al.[23] recently reported a case study of UFCT used to define biventricular apical thrombi in a patient with idiopathic dilated cardiomyopathy. The thrombi were well appreciated in the left ventricular apex by transthoracic echocardiography, but incomplete interrogation of the right ventricle led to the diagnostic UFCT examination.

Renal parenchymal volume. Assessment of the volume (or mass) of one or both kidneys may be useful in the evaluation of patients with hypertension with or without cardiac disease. Commonly, changes in the renal parenchyma occur with renal artery stenosis, hydronephrosis, and nephrosclerosis secondary to diabetes. Lerman et al.[24] recently evaluated the use of UFCT to quantitate total as well as medullary and cortical volumes of the kidney.

Estimation of in vivo renal volumes in the high-resolution imaging mode before and after intravenous administration of contrast medium in the canine showed excellent agreement with actual postmortem renal volumes (r = 0.86; SEE, 4.7 mL). Estimates of cortical and medullary volumes, however, showed a definite but less favorable correlation.

Function

Right and left ventricular stroke volumes and ejection fraction. UFCT can be used to quantitate left ventricular systolic function and muscle mass in patients with no contraindication to the use of iodinated contrast medium. A disadvantage of the UFCT approach to calculations of ventricular volumes and global function is that a "quasi-steady" assumption must be used. This requires that the individual multilevel tomographic information, which is acquired not simultaneously but from consecutive cardiac cycles, be an accurate representation so that the sum across all tomograms is appropriate for the ventricle as a whole. Thus, quantitative information about systolic function must be limited to patients in normal sinus rhythm with fairly constant ECG R-R intervals during the study. Scanning during premature atrial or ventricular depolarizations significantly limits the quantitative data. UFCT performed in patients with various atrial dysrhythmias during the examination is quantitative for cardiac anatomy, but calculations of cardiac volumes must be viewed only as qualitative under these circumstances.

Figure 8-3 shows end-diastolic mid-left ventricular short- and long-axis images in a patient with normal right and left ventricular function. For comparison, Figure 8-18 shows mid-left ventricular short- and long-axis images from a patient with functional class IV congestive heart failure. Note the dilatation of the left and right ventricles in the latter patient.

Normal values by UFCT have been established for left ventricular mass (98 ± 18 g/m^2), end-diastolic volume (73 ± 19 mL/m^2), end-systolic volume (24 ± 8 mL/m^2), and stroke volume (48 ± 11 mL/m^2).[10] Comparison of quantitation of left ventricular ejection fraction by UFCT with that obtained in the same patients by radionuclide angiography is shown in Figure 8-19 for patients with a variety of cardiac abnormalities. UFCT, like radionuclide angiography, makes no assumptions regarding left ventricular shape for calculation of ejection fractions or volumes (as is necessary with two-dimensional echocardiography).

Left ventricular aneurysm. Preliminary studies allowing for preoperative "digital resection" of a left ventricular aneurysm have been encouraging for estimation of postoperative residual left ventricular function. Such studies may define patients at high or low risk for

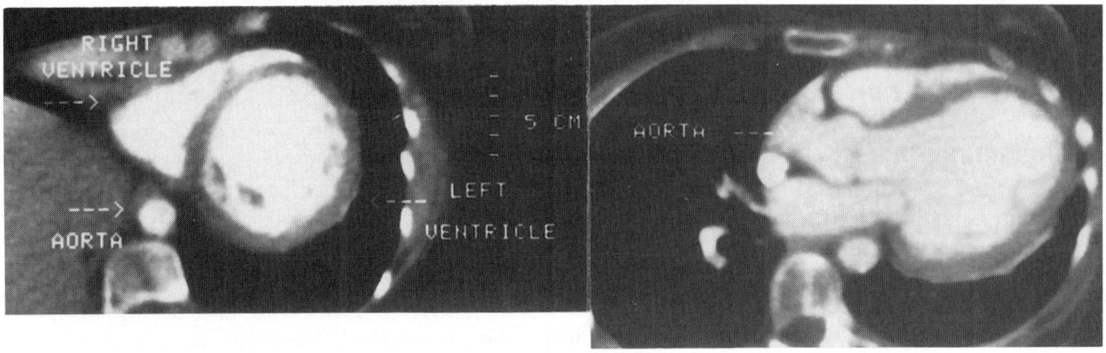

Fig 8-18 Representative short- and long-axis UFCT images at the midventricular position in a patient with functional class IV congestive heart failure. Note that the left ventricle is significantly dilated.

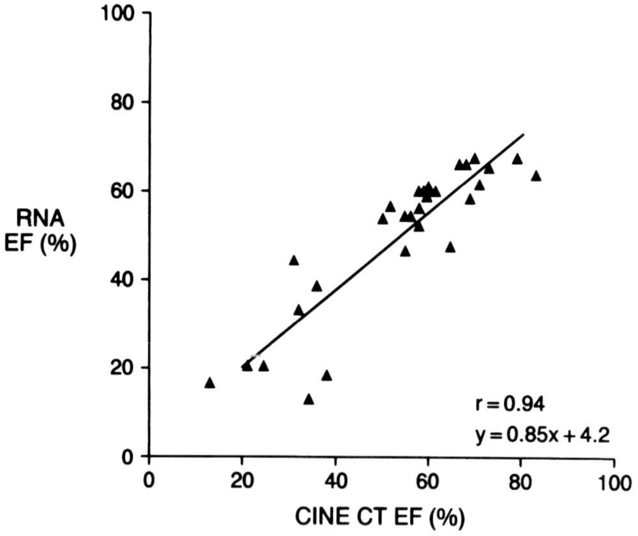

Fig 8-19 Comparison between determinations of ejection fraction *(EF)* by radionuclide angiography *(RNA)* and UFCT (cine CT). Note that there is an excellent correlation across a very broad range of values for left ventricular function.

postaneurysmectomy congestive heart failure. Figure 8-20 shows a multilevel UFCT examination in a patient before (left) and after (right) aneurysmectomy for refractory congestive heart failure. Figure 8-21 shows the quantitation of the left ventricular volumes and ejection fraction before surgery, after preoperative "digital resection" and estimation of residual postsurgical myocardium (by defining the three-dimensional anatomic extent between the aneurysm hinge points and functional myocardium in the preoperative images), and after the operation. UFCT and three-dimensional cardiac imaging have recently been used to define the details of regional systolic function in patients with fibrous left ventricular aneurysms.[25]

Regional left ventricular function. Because of the multitomographic approach offered by UFCT, regional left ventricular function can be defined both qualitatively and quantitatively. This approach is facilitated by definition of both chamber and myocardium on the same image.

Quantification of regional left ventricular systolic function by UFCT requires use of a coordinate system from which one region can be compared with another or, most importantly, compared with "normal" regional function defined by the same coordinate system. Setup of this coordinate system is facilitated by the previously defined border recognition algorithms first described by Feiring et al.[6] However, definition of cardiac contraction within a given tomographic plane must account for translation and rotation of the left ventricle across and parallel to that plane. The most commonly applied method is to define a "centroid," or center of gravity, within the tomogram from either the epicardial or the endocardial surfaces and to fix a fiducial reference point on a boundary that moves with the heart during contraction.

In 11 normal patients, Feiring et al.[10] defined systolic function at multiple short-axis imaging planes with both endocardial and epicardial centroids and a fiducial reference point at the anterior junction of the left and right ventricular surfaces. An example of such a reference system using an epicardially defined centroid is shown in Figure 8-22. Here, the left ventricular cavity and myocardium can be divided into 12 or more regions from which can be derived estimates of regional ejection fraction or regional wall thickening. From these methods, Feiring et al. defined the normal ranges of tomographic endocardial (cavity) motion at multiple left ventricular short-axis levels. However, certain differences in regional ejection fraction can be calculated, depending on the reference coordinate system chosen and the location of the centroid (i.e., epicardial center or endocardial center). Although the debate about the appropriate method to quantitate regional wall motion continues, the most important point to keep in mind is that the *same* reference coordinate system should be used in differentiating abnormal from normal left ventricular regional systolic function, regardless of the choice of imaging modality.

Figure 8-23 shows end-diastolic (peak of R wave, 0% R-R interval) and end-systolic (smallest cavity volume during the cardiac cycle) mid-left ventricular short-axis scans in a patient after anterior wall myocardial infarction. The images are divided into 12 30° pie-wedged segments to allow for assessment of regional endocardial motion and wall thickening. A graphic display of regional contraction demonstrates akinesis and hypokinesis (reduced regional endocardial contraction and systolic wall thickening) from 0° to about 180° (corresponding to the anterior and inferior septum and part of the posterior wall).

Definition of regional left ventricular systolic wall thickening by UFCT has been examined by Lanzer et al.[26] and Farmer et al.[27] during administration of various adrenergic drugs and during ischemia, respectively. These data provide insight into details of mechanics of regional ventricular function and the applicability of CT for these evaluations. Psomas et al.[28] defined regional wall thickening and thicknesses in normals by use of an epicardial floating point reference method in six contiguous left ventricular short-axis slices and found a surprising degree of homogeneity in function from apex to base. These data facilitate investigations into the details of serial changes in regional function and muscle mass during early and late changes in ventricular size, shape, and mass after transmural left ventricular infarction[29,30] and may be useful in conjunction with provocative exercise testing (see later section).

As with echocardiography, visual scoring of the UFCT multilevel images to analyze systolic function can be performed in a straightforward fashion (see chapter 5A). The advantage of UFCT here is that multiple, parallel imaging planes can be evaluated rather than the limited two or three levels used in routine two-dimensional echocardiography.

Dynamics of ventricular emptying and early diastolic filling. Most clinical information defining ventricular function by UFCT or other imaging modalities has been derived from images acquired at end-diastole

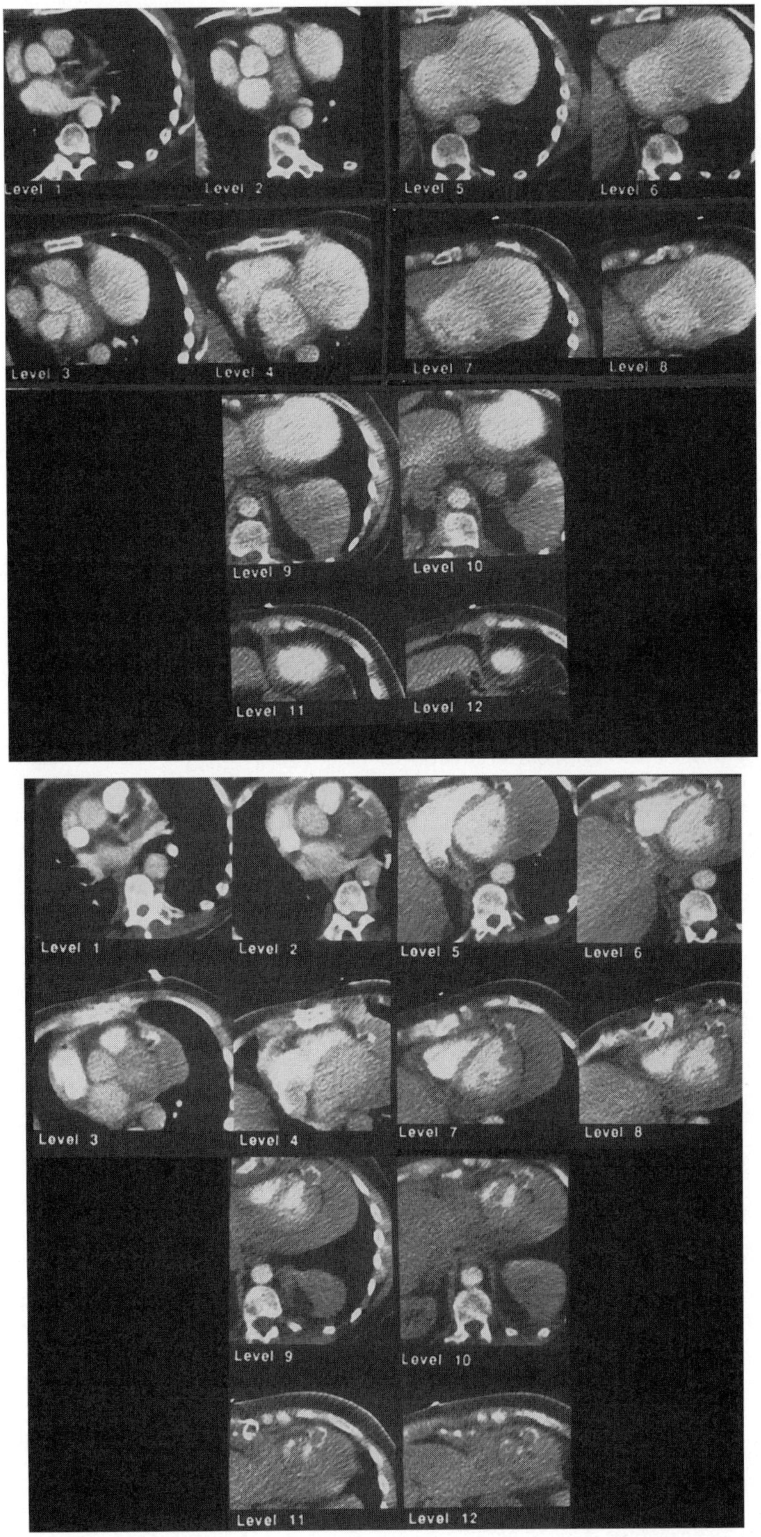

Fig 8-20 Representative multi-level end-diastolic, short-axis UFCT study in a patient with a large left ventricular aneurysm. **Top,** preoperative images. Note the details of the size and position of the aneurysm in relation to other structures within the cardiac silhouettes (level 1, aortic root; level 12, ventricular apex). **Bottom,** postoperative images. The images are at roughly the same ventricular levels as those in the preoperative study. Note the position from base to apex of the pledget used by the surgeon to join the viable myocardial surfaces after aneurysmectomy.

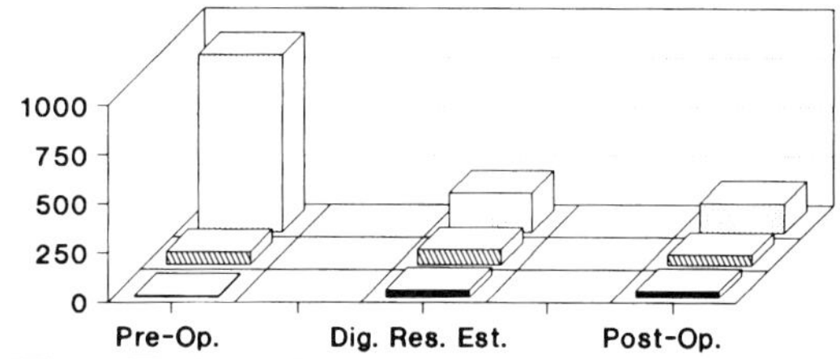

	Pre-Op.	Dig. Res. Est.	Post-Op.
EDV (cc)	904	200	150
Stroke Volume (cc)	65	78	52
EF (%)	7	39	35

Fig 8-21 Analysis of left ventricular volumes *(EDV)*, stroke volume, and ejection fraction *(EF)* from UFCT study shown in Figure 8-20. The preoperative CT study was analyzed by excluding those portions of the left ventricular cavity that included the aneurysm and including only cavity confined to areas within functioning myocardium (digital resection method). The digital resection estimations *(Dig. Res. Est.)* of the postoperative volumes and ejection fraction were similar to the actual volumes and ejection fraction found after analysis of the postoperative scans. (From Rumberger JA: Ultrafast computed tomographic assessment of left ventricular function at rest: applications in myocardial infarction, cardiomyopathy and aneurysm. In *Ultrafast Computed Tomography in Cardiac Imaging: Principles and Practice.* Edited by W Stanford, JA Rumberger. Mount Kisco, New York, Futura Publishing Company, 1992, pp 117-137. By permission.)

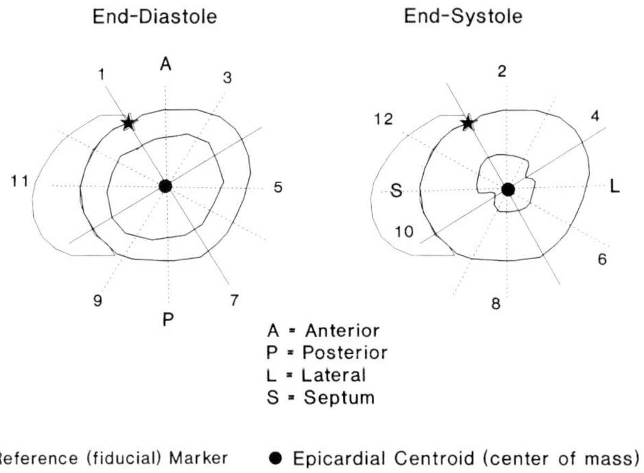

Fig 8-22 Schema of division of left ventricular surfaces at end-diastole and end-systole into regions for regional analysis of systolic function. An epicardial centroid was chosen as the reference coordinate system. Selection of a predefined fiducial point on both the end-diastolic and the end-systolic images (usually at the anatomic junction of the left and right ventricular surfaces) facilitates identification of the same anatomic regions on both images by accounting for any rotation or translation of the heart during contraction. (From Rumberger JA: Ultrafast computed tomographic assessment of left ventricular function at rest: applications in myocardial infarction, cardiomyopathy and aneurysm. In *Ultrafast Computed Tomography in Cardiac Imaging: Principles and Practice.* Edited by W Stanford, JA Rumberger. Mount Kisco, New York, Futura Publishing Company, 1992, pp 117-137. By permission.)

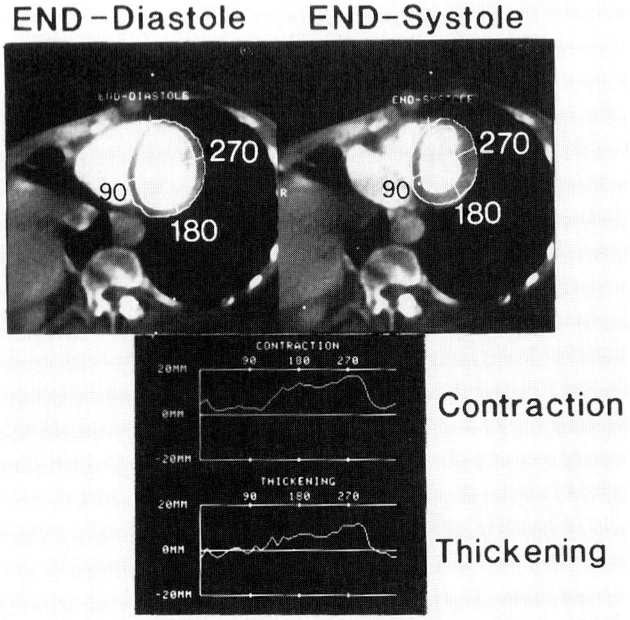

Fig 8-23 Example of quantitative analysis of regional systolic function at the mid-left ventricle in a patient with a prior anteroseptal myocardial infarction. Note the absence of wall thickening and contraction in an area defined by the left ventricular septum (0° through 180°).

and end-systole only; however, characterization of the "path" from end-diastole to end-systole (ventricular emptying) and from end-systole through the rapid-filling phase of the cardiac cycle (early diastolic filling) can also provide additional insight into cardiac function. Quantitation of ventricular peak emptying rate or peak early diastolic filling rate has been shown by radionuclide angiography,[31,32] contrast angiography,[33] Doppler echocardiography,[34,35] and UFCT.[36-38]

For definition of left ventricular time-dependent emptying or early diastolic filling, UFCT images are acquired in the traditional short-axis (transverse cardiac) plane. Scanning sequences are designed to allow for acquisition of images through the cardiac cycle, as previously described, to facilitate analysis of both systolic and diastolic images from the same data set. Practical experience has shown that 13 scans over six cardiac levels yield data from end-diastole through end-systole and up to at least diastasis in most patients. For patients with lower heart rates, it may be necessary to use four-level scans at 20 images per level. Generally, to define a global assessment of the rates of ventricular emptying and early diastolic filling, it is necessary to acquire two separate six-level scans so that a complete set of images is available from the left ventricular apex through the aortic outflow tract.

Tomographic volumes can be determined by defining

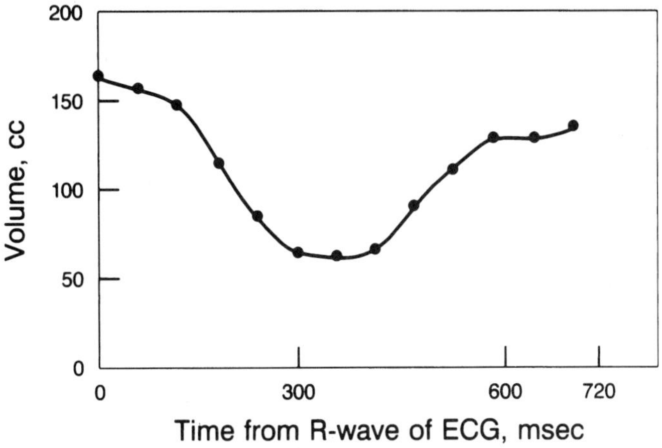

Fig 8-24 Time-dependent curve of global left ventricular volume during the cardiac cycle as determined by UFCT in a normal patient. See text for details. *ECG,* electrocardiogram.

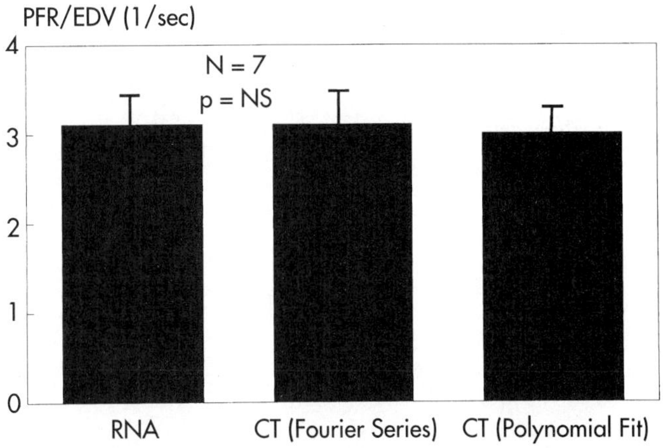

Fig 8-25 Comparison of use of conventional radionuclide angiographic *(RNA)* techniques and UFCT (polynomial curve-fitting method[35] and Fourier harmonic analysis[39]) to measure left ventricular peak early diastolic filling rate *(PFR)* (normalized to end-diastolic volume, *EDV*) in a group of normal persons. Note that at normal resting heart rates, there is no statistical difference between radionuclide and UFCT measurements. (From Rumberger JA: Use of ultrafast computed tomography to assess early diastolic filling in man. In *Ultrafast Computed Tomography in Cardiac Imaging: Principles and Practice.* Edited by W Stanford, JA Rumberger. Mount Kisco, New York, Futura Publishing Company, 1992, pp 161-175. By permission.)

the borders of the endocardial surfaces from each level according to standardized methods, as previously discussed; afterward, the volumes are inscribed and recorded (tomographic area multiplied by slice thickness) through each image obtained during the cardiac cycle. This process is repeated at all left or right ventricular levels. In our laboratory, these data are automatically entered into a database, but they can conveniently be recorded onto a common spreadsheet program with time from end-diastole (R wave trigger) as column 1 and the time-dependent tomographic volumes per level recorded in parallel as the adjacent columns. These data can then be reviewed in graphic form from any particular tomographic level for regional analysis or summed across rows (modified Simpson's rule) to define global time-dependent changes in cavity volume during the cardiac cycle. The construction of such a table facilitates analyses of both systolic and diastolic function.

An example of a ventricular volume curve obtained by UFCT from a normal subject is shown in Figure 8-24. Note that this resembles a left ventricular volume curve as described either during direct left ventricular angiography or, indirectly, by radionuclide angiography. Generally, imaging by UFCT using the protocols described does not include diastasis unless the heart rate is greater than 75 to 80 beats/min; however, the imaging sequence is adequate to quantitate the peak rates of emptying and filling unless the heart rate is less than 52 beats/min.

The rates of ventricular emptying and filling can be defined by two basic methods. Both methods are direct extensions of methods previously established for analysis of the dynamics of left ventricular function by radionuclide angiography. The initial method used by our laboratory involved a third-order polynomial curve fit to the data from end-systole through the rapid filling phase and, if necessary, up to the initial portion of diastasis.[36,37] The other method, now preferred in our laboratory, involves the direct application of a Fourier interpolator to the entire data set.[39,40] To satisfy the Nyquist limit, an 8-harmonic Fourier series is used to sample the CT data acquired at the predefined rate of 17 frames/sec. The advantages of this approach are that data on rates of systolic emptying are also available and that, since all time-dependent data during the cardiac cycle are used, the results are reproducible and not as dependent on minor errors in individual volume calculations in the image analysis set as in the polynomial methods. However, careful application of either method yields essentially the same results. Figure 8-25 shows comparisons for left ventricular peak filling rate (normalized to left ventricular end-diastolic volume) in a group of normal patients as determined by standardized radionuclide angiography and UFCT using the polynomial method and the Fourier interpolator method. Note that each is equivalent to the other.

From analyses of the time-dependent volume data, one can derive the time to peak emptying from end-diastole or time to peak filling rate from end-systole, peak emptying or filling rate (the maximum rate of dynamics volume change occurring during this phase of the cardiac cycle), and filling fraction (that portion of total diastolic filling—i.e., the stroke volume—that has occurred by the time of peak filling). Additional measurements needed to define dynamic function are normalization of peak emptying rate or peak filling rate for absolute end-diastolic volume and stroke volume (tomographic or global).

Valvular disease. Reiter et al.[41] demonstrated that UFCT can be used to quantitate regurgitant fractions and

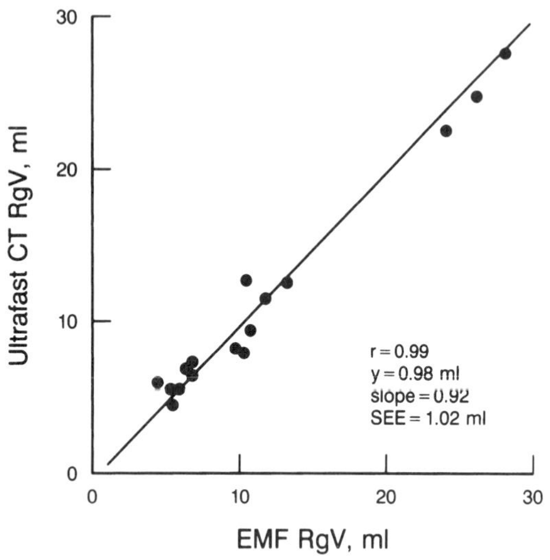

Fig 8-26 Comparison of absolute aortic regurgitant volumes *(RgV)* quantitated by an electromagnetic flowmeter *(EMF)* with simultaneous measurements made by UFCT in animals. Determination of regurgitant volume by CT was defined as the difference between forward left ventricular and right ventricular stroke volumes. (From Reiter SJ, Rumberger JA, Stanford W, et al: Quantitative determination of aortic regurgitant volume in dogs by ultrafast computed tomography. *Circulation* 76:728-735, 1987. By permission of American Heart Association.)

regurgitant volumes in animals with acute aortic regurgitation. Perhaps one of the more attractive uses of UFCT for evaluation of aortic regurgitation is the potential for serial assessment of patients for quantitation of the amount of regurgitation and changes in left ventricular size and in systolic and diastolic function. In clinical practice, the actual calculation of univalvular regurgitation is assessed by determination of absolute right and left ventricular stroke volumes.[7,40,42] The differences between right and left ventricular stroke volumes represent the regurgitant volume (Fig 8-26).

Dynamic and pharmacologic stress testing. Normal left ventricular regional systolic function before and after infusion of dobutamine, a potent β-agonist, has been demonstrated in normal volunteers.[43] Characterization of normal response demonstrated not only an increase in global ejection fraction but also an increase in regional ejection fraction at multiple ventricular levels (Fig 8-27). The normal response to provocation by catecholamine congeners is characterized not only by a significant increase in global left ventricular ejection fraction but also by a more uniform regional pattern of contraction at all ventricular levels.

Roig et al.[44] reported the first use of UFCT technology for exercise testing during supine bicycle ergometry. In that study, 27 patients undergoing cardiac catheterization for diagnosis of coronary artery disease had UFCT examinations at rest followed immediately by repeat scanning during symptom-limited bicycle ergometry. Fourteen (93%) of the 15 patients with significant coronary disease in any vessel had a reduction in the global left ventricular ejection fraction during exercise, whereas, in comparison, global ejection fraction increased more than 5% in 10 (83%) of the 12 patients with normal coronary arteries. Analysis of regional ventricular function used the method of Feiring et al.[10] to examine cardiac motion in 12 pie-wedged sectors of each tomographic left ventricular section. From this analysis, 11 of the 12 patients (92%) with normal coronary arteries had normal wall motion during exercise. Of particular importance was the finding that no patient with ischemic heart disease in whom both analyses (i.e., global ejection fraction *and* quantitation of regional ejection fraction) were done had normal ejection fractions either at rest or during exercise. By combining *quantitation* of both global and regional function, the UFCT method may provide for a more specific and sensitive test than conventional exercise imaging, during which, although quantitation of global function is done, only qualitative assessments of regional function are usually examined.

Flow

For studies to assess flow phenomena, scanning is done by acquisition of a single image (or images from multiple adjacent tomograms) on consecutive cardiac cycles at the same phase of the cardiac cycle. Contrast medium now is given as a rapidly injected bolus, either intravenously or intra-arterially, rather than as a slow infusion. When these images are viewed as a closed-loop motion picture, there is no cardiac motion (since all images were acquired at the same phase of successive cardiac cycles) but the contrast opacification of the cardiac chambers, great vessels, and myocardium increases and then decreases as the contrast bolus travels with the blood flow. Subsequent analysis of contrast density at any operator-defined region of interest within the tomogram allows for registration of a contrast clearance (or "indicator dilution") curve from that region.

Cardiac output. Although one can conveniently define left ventricular cardiac output from the product of stroke volume and heart rate, certain clinical and UFCT scanning conditions may limit this application. For instance, it is inconvenient to evaluate regional myocardial perfusion (discussion to follow) with a bolus injection of contrast medium and imaging in the "flow" mode and then to evaluate cardiac output with additional contrast medium and scanning in the "movie" mode (in perhaps a totally different imaging plane). Additionally, ventricular stroke volume information must be viewed in the context of competency of the aortic and mitral valves. Although definition of right ventricular stroke volume in isolated aortic insufficiency can be used to determine total forward cardiac output with UFCT,[45] the question of concomitant tricuspid regurgitation must be entertained.

In situations such as those discussed above, cardiac output can be defined by UFCT with use of classic indicator dilution theory.[46] With these principles, cardiac output (CO, in liters per minute) is defined as

$$CO = k \times (Q/A) \times 60/1{,}000$$

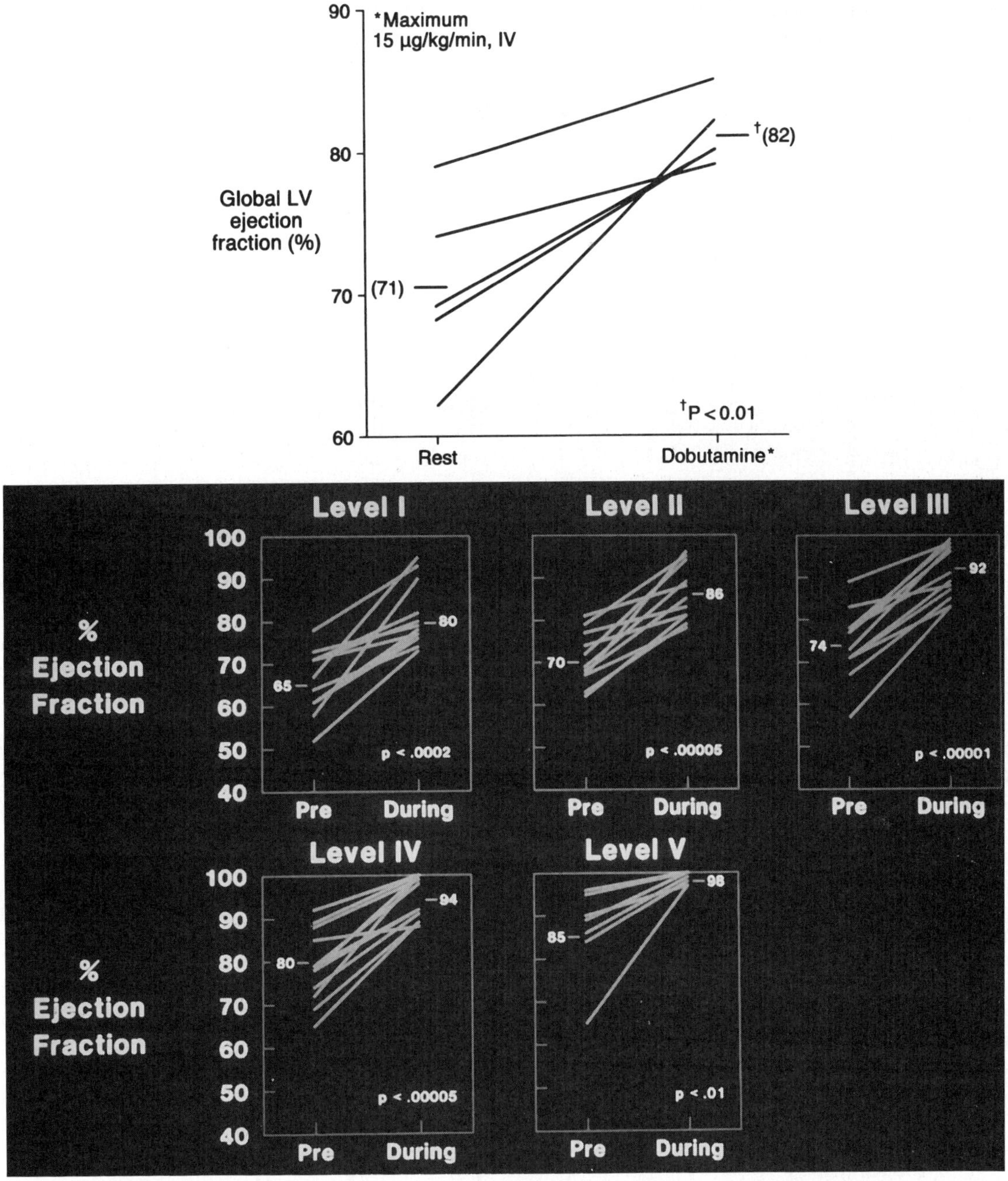

Fig 8-27 Results from analysis of UFCT studies in a group of normal subjects before and during intravenous administration of dobutamine. Shown are the values at rest and with dobutamine infusion for global left ventricular *(LV)* ejection fraction **(top)** and regional ejection fraction **(bottom)** at six adjacent left ventricular levels. Note that the normal response is for global and regional ejection fractions to increase during pharmacologic stress testing.

in which Q is the amount of indicator (i.e., contrast medium) injected (in milligrams of iodine), k is a "calibration" factor relating iodine concentration to CT density (in Hounsfield units per milligram of iodine), A is the area under the contrast clearance curve in the aorta or pulmonary artery (in Hounsfield units-seconds), and 60/1,000 is a conversion factor.

Using these concepts and contrast clearance kinetics, Garrett et al.[47] defined cardiac output in animals and compared the results with standard thermodilution measurements for the reference standard. Results from this study showed excellent correlations ($r = 0.92$). Thus, cardiac output can be defined by UFCT to a high degree of accuracy by two different methods: definition of stroke volume in the "movie" mode and definition of cardiac output with indicator dilution methods. The choice of the method depends on the scanning conditions and the protocols defined by the operator.

Myocardial perfusion. Wang et al.,[48] using the Dynamic Spatial Reconstructor, validated the application of UFCT to quantitation of regional myocardial perfusion in the dog. Aortic root injections of nonionic contrast material and application of classic indicator dilution kinetics showed that this approach can define regional flow rates across the entire physiologic range. Rumberger et al.[9] and later Wolfkiel et al.[49] used intravenous injection methods to apply UFCT to quantitation of regional myocardial perfusion. A preliminary application of this method to evaluation of regional myocardial flow reserve in man has also been presented.[50] An extensive review of the theory, application, and limitations to assessing regional myocardial perfusion by UFCT has recently been published.[51]

Efforts to modify methods originally designed in the animal laboratory so that they can be applied to man are currently under way at several medical centers. Preliminary studies at the Mayo Clinic, however, suggest that clinically useful data on regional myocardial perfusion can be obtained by use of a central venous injection of contrast medium and careful accounting for dynamic changes in regional myocardial vascular volumes. Bell et al.[52] extended the measurement method to evaluation of regional myocardial perfusion at rest and during intravenous infusion of adenosine (to produce maximum coronary vasodilation) in 10 normal volunteers. By limiting the amount of contrast material injected intravenously, modifying patient orientation within the scanner to significantly reduce imaging artifacts, and properly accounting for dynamic changes in intramyocardial vascular volume, these investigators showed that maximal regional flow rates up to 450 mL/100 g per minute can be determined (resting myocardial flow is about 100 mL/100 g per minute).[53] However, the ultimate clinical use of UFCT for the assessment of regional myocardial perfusion in patients with known coronary artery disease remains to be defined.

Renal perfusion. Using methods derived from the studies of regional myocardial perfusion, Lerman et al.[54] demonstrated the feasibility of quantifying perfusion to both the medullary and the cortical regions of the kidney with UFCT. Central venous injection of a bolus of nonionic contrast material is followed by sequential multilevel "flow" imaging over the abdominal aorta and kidneys timed to record the entrance and exit of contrast medium through the renal circulation. Differences between renal perfusion to both kidneys can be compared by direct off-line analysis of the image sequences with use of classic indicator dilution principles. Values of renal parenchymal flow have been shown by Taler et al.[55] to correlate very well with values of renal vein renin, reflecting increases in renin when renal hypoperfusion is present in patients with renovascular hypertension. This approach, coupled with studies of renal parenchymal volumes (i.e., mass), offers an excellent means to define the nature and extent of renal diseases in patients undergoing evaluations for cardiac disease.

Intracardiac shunts. Individual cardiac chamber size, location, volume, and function can be assessed by UFCT and previously mentioned methods in patients with congenital heart disease. In addition, with proper injection of contrast medium, right-to-left and left-to-right intracardiac shunting can be localized.

ISSUES AND CONSIDERATIONS IN THE USE OF ULTRAFAST CT

UFCT offers a quantitative means to define global and regional cardiac anatomy, ventricular function, and myocardial and renal perfusion noninvasively. Additionally, in the high-resolution mode it can be used to define great vessel anatomy, identify discrete calcification of the coronary arteries, and define renal parenchymal volume. However, the attributes must be weighed against some of the drawbacks. Subjects are exposed to radiation, and most imaging requires the intravenous administration of iodinated contrast medium.

The radiation exposure profile for UFCT is in Figure 8-28. Since the radiation source enters from the patient's back through an angle of only 210° and is not circumferential, as is required with conventional CT, the exposure is greatest to the skin near the spine and least to the anterior thorax and sternal bone marrow. The average integrated body dose of radiation for a complete cardiac study is similar to that received from a standard abdominal CT. A study for coronary calcification involves a single 100-msec image at contiguous levels of the heart; thus, the skin entry dose is about 1.0 rad total, about twice that of a standard posteroanterior chest x-ray examination.

The issue of the use of intravenous contrast medium is often discussed, but the risk to the patient is small if consideration is given to screening patients with diabetes and increased creatinine concentration or patients with a

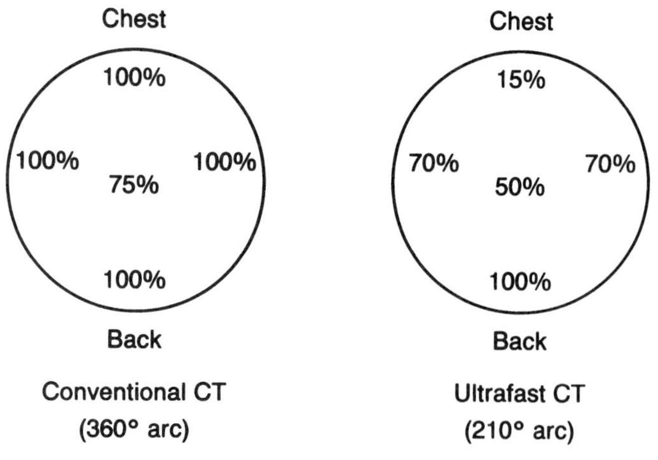

Fig 8-28 Profile of radiation dosing from UFCT compared with that from conventional CT. Note that because UFCT images across an arc of 210° rather than the 360° arc of conventional CT, radiation dosing is spatially heterogeneous. The total integrated dose from UFCT is slightly less than that from conventional scanners.

history of contrast allergy. The limitations to UFCT, however, must be weighed against the high likelihood of completion of a satisfactory examination (>90% in our laboratory) and the convenience to the patient (most examinations can be completed in 10 to 30 minutes with only moderate cooperation and minor discomfort).

CONCLUSIONS

UFCT offers a noninvasive means to provide quantitative information on cardiac and extracardiac anatomy, function, and flow. Additionally, it offers some advantages over conventional CT for studies of the great vessels. This chapter has outlined the current clinical uses of the device.

Diagnostic UFCT in cardiovascular medicine is complementary to conventional methods and offers versatility in unique applications for imaging of the heart and great vessels. These positive attributes must be weighed against the use of radiation and the need for intravenous administration of contrast medium.

Given these considerations, it is proper to use UFCT, not in the unnecessary duplication of examinations by two-dimensional echocardiography, radionuclide angiography, perfusion imaging, or conventional CT, but as a complementary examination in selected patients to determine left ventricular anatomy or function, as a primary noninvasive imaging tool in circumstances that involve unique applications (right ventricular size and function, bypass graft patency and flow), and as a means to obviate multiple cardiac imaging methods (such as evaluation of thoracic disease and cardiac size and function).

REFERENCES

1. Boyd DP, Gould RG, Quinn JR, et al: A proposed dynamic cardiac 3-D densitometer for early detection and evaluation of heart disease. *IEEE Trans Nucl Sci* 26:2724-2739, 1979
2. Robb RA, Ritman EL, Gilbert BK, et al: The DSR: a high-speed three-dimensional x-ray computed tomography system for dynamic spatial reconstruction of the heart and circulation. *IEEE Trans Nucl Sci* 26:2713-2717, 1979
3. Robb RA, Morin RL: Principles and instrumentation for dynamic x-ray computed tomography. In *Cardiac Imaging: a Companion to Braunwald's Heart Disease*. Edited by ML Marcus, HR Schelbert, DJ Skorton, et al. Philadelphia, WB Saunders Company, 1991, pp 634-668
4. Feigenbaum H: *Echocardiography*. Philadelphia, Lea & Febiger, 1986, pp 127-187
5. ACC/AHA/SNM Policy Statement: Standardization of cardiac tomographic imaging. *J Am Coll Cardiol* 20:255-256, 1992
6. Feiring AJ, Rumberger JA, Reiter SJ, et al: Determination of left ventricular mass in dogs with rapid-acquisition cardiac computed tomographic scanning. *Circulation* 72:1355-1364, 1985
7. Reiter SJ, Rumberger JA, Feiring AJ, et al: Precision of measurements of right and left ventricular volume by cine computed tomography. *Circulation* 74:890-900, 1986
8. Rees MR, Feiring AJ, Rumberger JA, et al: Heart evaluation by cine CT: use of two new oblique views. *Radiology* 159:804-806, 1986
9. Rumberger JA, Feiring AJ, Lipton MJ, et al: Use of ultrafast computed tomography to quantitate regional myocardial perfusion: a preliminary report. *J Am Coll Cardiol* 9:59-69, 1987
10. Feiring AJ, Rumberger JA, Reiter SJ, et al: Sectional and segmental variability of left ventricular function: experimental and clinical studies using ultrafast computed tomography. *J Am Coll Cardiol* 12:415-425, 1988
11. Roig E, Georgiou D, Chomka EV, et al: Reproducibility of left ventricular myocardial volume and mass measurements by ultrafast computed tomography. *J Am Coll Cardiol* 18:990-996, 1991
12. Hajduczok ZD, Weiss RM, Stanford W, et al: Determination of right ventricular mass in humans and dogs with ultrafast cardiac computed tomography. *Circulation* 82:202-212, 1990
13. Husayni TS: Ultrafast computed tomographic imaging in congenital heart disease. In *Ultrafast Computed Tomography in Cardiac Imaging: Principles and Practice*. Edited by W Stanford, JA Rumberger. Mount Kisco, New York, Futura Publishing Company, 1992, pp 311-336
14. Geraghty JJ, Stanford W, Galvin JR, et al: Ultrafast CT in the diagnosis of pulmonary embolism (abstract). *Radiology* 177 Suppl:163, 1990
15. Stanford W, Brundage BH, MacMillan R, et al: Sensitivity and specificity of assessing coronary bypass graft patency with ultrafast computed tomography: results of a multicenter study. *J Am Coll Cardiol* 12:1-7, 1988
16. Rumberger JA, Feiring AJ, Hiratzka LF, et al: Quantification of coronary artery bypass flow reserve in dogs using cine-computed tomography. *Circ Res* 61 Suppl 2:117-123, 1987
17. Rumberger JA, Rossen JD, Simonetti I, et al: Determination of bypass graft flow reserve by ultrafast-CT (abstract). *Circulation* 76 Suppl 4:5, 1987
18. Margolis JR, Chen JTT, Kong Y, et al: The diagnostic and prognostic significance of coronary artery calcification: a report of 800 cases. *Radiology* 137:609-616, 1980
19. Reinmuller R, Lipton MJ: Detection of coronary artery calcification by computed tomography. *Dynamic Cardiovasc Imaging* 1:139-145, 1987
20. Simons DB, Schwartz RS, Edwards WD, et al: Noninvasive definition of anatomic coronary artery disease by ultrafast computed tomographic scanning: a quantitative pathologic comparison study. *J Am Coll Cardiol* 20:1118-1126, 1992
21. Breen JF, Sheedy PF II, Schwartz RS, et al: Coronary artery calcification detected with ultrafast CT as an indication of coronary artery disease: works in progress. *Radiology* 185:435-439, 1992
22. Agatston AS, Janowitz WR, Hildner FJ, et al: Quantification of coronary artery calcium using ultrafast computed tomography. *J Am Coll Cardiol* 15:827-832, 1990
23. Minor RL Jr, Oren RM, Stanford W, et al: Biventricular thrombi and pulmonary emboli complicating idiopathic dilated cardiomyopathy: diagnosis with cardiac ultrafast CT. *Am Heart J* 122:1477-1481, 1991
24. Lerman LO, Bentley MD, Bell MR, et al: Quantitation of the in vivo kidney volume with cine computed tomography. *Invest Radiol* 25:1206-1211, 1990
25. Lessick J, Sideman S, Azhari H, et al: Regional three-dimensional geometry and function of left ventricles with fibrous aneurysms: a cine-computed tomography study. *Circulation* 84:1072-1086, 1991
26. Lanzer P, Garrett J, Lipton MJ, et al: Quantitation of regional myocardial function by cine computed tomography: pharmacologic changes in wall thickness. *J Am Coll Cardiol* 8:682-692, 1986
27. Farmer D, Lipton MJ, Higgins CB, et al: In vivo assessment of left ventricular wall and chamber dynamics during transient myocardial ischemia using cine computed tomography. *Am J Cardiol* 55:560-565, 1985
28. Psomas MP, Rumberger JA, Reed JE, et al: Global and segmental ventricular wall thickening in normal subjects with ultrafast computed tomography (abstract). *Circulation* 80 Suppl 2:109, 1989
29. Rumberger JA, Reed JE, Behrenbeck T: Serial changes in regional infarct and non-infarct wall thickness after anterior wall myocardial infarction (abstract). *Circulation* 84 Suppl 2:475, 1991
30. Rumberger JA, Behrenbeck T, Breen JR, et al: Nonparallel changes in global left ventricular chamber volume and muscle mass during the first year after transmural myocardial infarction in humans. *J Am Coll Cardiol* 21:673-682, 1993
31. Bonow RO, Bacharach SL, Green MV, et al: Impaired left ventricular diastolic filling in patients with coronary artery disease: assessment with radionuclide angiography. *Circulation* 64:315-323, 1981
32. Miller TR, Goldman KJ, Sampathkumaran KS, et al: Analysis of cardiac diastolic function: application to coronary artery disease. *J Nucl Med* 24:2-7, 1983
33. Hammermeister KE, Warbasse JR: The rate of change of left ventricular volume in man. II. Diastolic events in health and disease. *Circulation* 49:739-741, 1974

34. Upton MT, Gibson DG, Brown DJ: Echocardiographic assessment of abnormal left ventricular relaxation in man. *Br Heart J* 38:1001-1009, 1976

35. Rokey R, Kuo LC, Zoghbi WA, et al: Determination of parameters of left ventricular diastolic filling with pulsed-Doppler echocardiography: comparison with cine angiography. *Circulation* 71: 543-555, 1985

36. Rumberger JA, Weiss RM, Feiring AJ, et al: Patterns of regional diastolic function in the normal human left ventricle: an ultrafast computed tomographic study. *J Am Coll Cardiol* 14:119-126, 1989

37. Rumberger JA, Bell MR, Sheedy PF, et al: Use of ultrafast computed tomography to assess early diastolic filling of the left ventricle in humans. *Am J Card Imaging* 4:130-137, 1990

38. Marzullo P, L'Abbate A, Marcus ML: Patterns of global and regional systolic and diastolic function in the normal right ventricle assessed by ultrafast computed tomography. *J Am Coll Cardiol* 17:1318 1325, 1991

39. Lipton MJ, Rumberger JA: The assessment of left ventricular systolic and diastolic function by ultrafast computed tomography. *Am J Card Imaging* 5:318-327, 1991

40. Rumberger JA, Reed JE: Quantitative dynamics of left ventricular emptying and filling as a function of heart size and stroke volume in pure aortic regurgitation and in normal subjects. *Am J Cardiol* 70:1045-1050, 1992

41. Reiter SJ, Rumberger JA, Stanford W, et al: Quantitative determination of aortic regurgitant volume in dogs by ultrafast computed tomography. *Circulation* 76:728-735, 1987

42. Nishimura RA, Vonk GD, Rumberger JA, et al: Semiquantitation of aortic regurgitation by different Doppler echocardiographic techniques and comparison with ultrafast computed tomography. *Am Heart J* 124:995-1001, 1992

43. Rumberger JA: Quantifying left ventricular regional and global systolic function using ultrafast computed tomography. *Am J Cardiol* 5:29-37, 1991

44. Roig E, Chomka EV, Castaner A, et al: Exercise ultrafast computed tomography for the detection of coronary artery disease. *J Am Coll Cardiol* 13:1073-1081, 1989

45. MacMillan RM, Rees MR, Lumia FJ, et al: Preliminary experience in the use of ultrafast computed tomography to diagnose aortic valve stenosis. *Am Heart J* 115:665-671, 1988

46. Zierler KL: A simplified explanation of the theory of indicator-dilution for measurement of fluid flow and volume and other distributive phenomena. *Bull Johns Hopkins Hosp* 103:199, 1958

47. Garrett JS, Lanzer P, Jaschke W, et al: Measurement of cardiac output by cine computed tomography. *Am J Cardiol* 56:657-661, 1985

48. Wang T, Wu X, Chung N, et al: Myocardial blood flow estimated by synchronous, multislice, high-speed computed tomography. *IEEE Trans Med Imaging* 8:70-77, 1989

49. Wolfkiel CJ, Ferguson JL, Chomka EV, et al: Measurement of myocardial blood flow by ultrafast computed tomography. *Circulation* 76:1262-1273, 1987

50. Rumberger JA, Stanford W, Marcus ML: Quantitation of regional myocardial perfusion by ultrafast CT: promises and pitfalls. *Am J Card Imaging* 4:336-343, 1987

51. Rumberger JA, Bell ML, Feiring AJ, et al: Measurement of myocardial perfusion using fast computed tomography. In *Cardiac Imaging: a Companion to Braunwald's Heart Disease*. Edited by ML Marcus, HR Shelbert, DJ Skorton, et al. Philadelphia, WB Saunders Company, 1991, pp 688-702

52. Bell MR, Rumberger JA, Lerman LO, et al: Influence of intramyocardial blood volume in the quantitation of myocardial perfusion using external densitometric measurements (abstract). *J Am Coll Cardiol* 15 Suppl A:161, 1990

53. Bell MR, Rumberger JA, Stanson AW, et al: Rapid and minimally invasive measurement of myocardial flow reserve in man with ultrafast CT (abstract). *Circulation* 84 Suppl 2:678, 1991

54. Lerman LO, Taler SJ, Textor SC, et al: Ultrafast CT determination of global and intrarenal blood flow in renovascular and essential hypertensive patients. *J Am Soc Nephrol* 2:508, 1991

55. Taler SJ, Lerman LO, Textor SC, et al: Ultrafast CT derived global and intrarenal blood flow correlate with renal vein renin ratio in patients with renovascular and essential hypertension (abstract). *Am J Hypertens* 5 Suppl A:132, 1992

CHAPTER

9

Positron-emission tomography

Donald L. Johnston, M.D., Michael K. O'Connor, Ph.D., and Lee A. Forstrom, M.D.

TECHNICAL CONSIDERATIONS

Positrons

Radioactive decay by an unstable nucleus can occur in a variety of ways. Elements with an excess number of protons may undergo either electron capture or positron decay (β^+). In the latter process, a proton in the atomic nucleus is transformed into a neutron and a positively charged electron (positron). Some of the excess energy from the decay process is transferred to the positron as kinetic energy, and the positron is ejected from the nucleus. In soft tissue, the positron rapidly ($<10^{-9}$ sec) loses its kinetic energy over a range of a few millimeters and combines with an electron in an annihilation event in which the masses of the two particles are converted into energy. This energy is released in the form of two 511-keV gamma rays that are emitted in opposite directions (180° apart). Since it is impossible to detect the positrons themselves in vivo, their locations are determined by detecting the two 511-keV gamma rays emitted after their annihilation. This unique feature of positron decay permits detection by coincidence counting (Fig 9-1) and, as discussed later in this chapter, is the basis for all commercially available positron-emission tomography (PET) scanners. Table 9-1 lists the physical properties of the most commonly used positron-emitting radionuclides

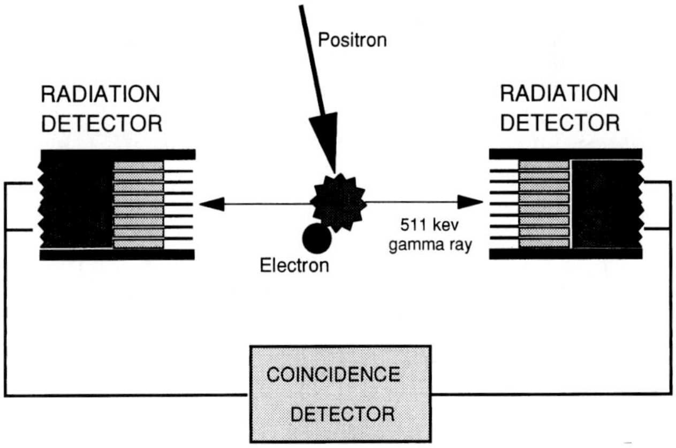

Fig 9-1 Principle of coincidence counting. The positron and electron combine in an annihilation event, which results in the emission of two 511-keV gamma rays. The coincidence detector records this event only when two 511-keV gamma rays are simultaneously recorded by opposing detectors.

Table 9-1 Physical properties of some positron-emitting radionuclides used in the study of the heart

Nuclide	Produced by	Half-life (min)	Maximum $\beta+$ energy (MeV)	Range* in water (mm)
Carbon ^{11}C	Cyclotron	20.0	0.96	4.1
Oxygen ^{15}O	Cyclotron	2.1	1.72	8.2
Nitrogen ^{13}N	Cyclotron	10.0	1.19	5.4
Fluorine ^{18}F	Cyclotron	110.0	0.64	2.4
Rubidium ^{82}Rb	Generator	1.3	3.15	16.5
Potassium ^{38}K	Cyclotron	7.7	2.68	13.3
Gallium ^{68}Ga	Generator	68.1	1.90	9.0
Copper ^{62}Cu	Generator	9.7	2.91	14.5

*Maximum $\beta+$ range in water.
Data from *Radiological Health Handbook.* Rockville, Maryland, Bureau of Radiological Health, United States Department of Health, Education, and Welfare, 1970.

as well as the range of positrons in soft tissue. Positron range refers to the distance the positrons travel in soft tissue before they come to rest and undergo annihilation. This is an important factor from an imaging perspective, as it places a limit on the resolution with which a given radionuclide can be localized in soft tissue.[1]

Production of positron-emitting radionuclides

Accelerator-produced radionuclides. From Table 9-1, it can be seen that most of the medically useful radionuclides have half-lives of minutes or less and, therefore, with the possible exception of fluorine-18 (^{18}F), must be produced on-site. The on-site production of radionuclides is achieved by bombarding the appropriate target materials with high-energy particles (usually protons or deuterons) to change the elemental composition of the target material into that of the appropriate radionuclide. This process is performed in a small-particle accelerator, either a cyclotron or a linear accelerator. Until recently, most accelerators were designed and built for research in physics and nuclear chemistry, with the production of medical radionuclides as a sideline. Over the past 5 years, significant advances in the design of accelerators have resulted in the availability today of small, easy-to-use, compact cyclotrons and linear accelerators suitable for use in a hospital.[2]

Figure 9-2 shows a cross-sectional view through the central chamber of a modern cyclotron. The entire chamber is placed under a high vacuum, and charged particles (hydrogen ions) are introduced into the center of the chamber. A high-frequency, alternating-current voltage is applied to the two hollow electrodes (called "dees" because of their letter "D" shape) that accelerate the hydrogen ions back and forth between each other. The entire chamber is positioned between the poles of a large electromagnet, which forces the hydrogen ions to follow a circular path as they are accelerated from dee to dee. With each acceleration between the dees, the ions gain energy and the radius of their orbit increases. The ions follow an outwardly spiral path until they strike the beam extractor and are swung out of the chamber to hit a small target containing the material to be bombarded.[2] In modern compact linear accelerators, the hydrogen ions are accelerated in a straight line from one end of the machine to the other, where they hit the target. Hence, on shutoff, radioactivity is present only in the target. This feature permits the construction of self-shielded accelerators that can easily be located in the hospital without the need for a concrete vault, as was required with the older cyclotrons and linear accelerators.

A variety of nuclear reactions can be used for the production of carbon-11 (^{11}C), nitrogen-13 (^{13}N), oxygen-15 (^{15}O), and ^{18}F. The most appropriate target material and production reaction depend on the desired radiochemical to be produced. Currently, a number of automated "black box" devices are available to produce the most commonly used radiochemicals, such as [^{18}F]2-fluoro-2-deoxyglucose (FDG). Many different types of amino acids, amines, amides, carboxylic acids, alcohols, sugars, nitrites, and steroids have been successfully labeled with ^{11}C or ^{18}F.[3] Table 9-2 lists the most commonly used positron-emitter-labeled compounds for clinical use in PET studies.

Currently, most medical cyclotrons and linear accelerators are capable of accelerating protons up to energies of 4 to 17 megaelectron volts (MeV). This permits the production of adequate quantities of ^{11}C, ^{13}N, ^{15}O, and ^{18}F for clinical studies. Although higher energy cyclotrons (30 to 40 MeV) can produce additional positron-emitting radionuclides, such as beryllium-68 (^{68}Be), together with

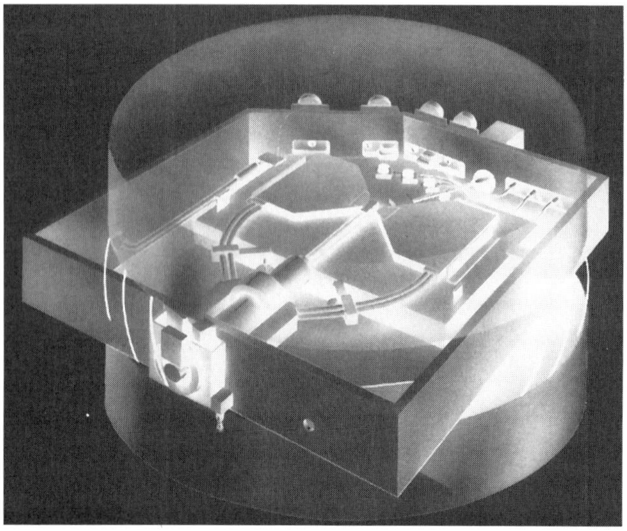

Fig 9-2 Cross-sectional view through the central chamber of a modern negative-ion cyclotron. (Courtesy of Siemens Medical Systems.)

Table 9-2 Some commonly used positron-emitting radiochemicals in studies of the heart*

Purpose	Labeled compounds
Myocardial metabolic tracers	[^{11}C]palmitate
	[^{11}C]acetate
	[^{18}F]fluorodeoxyglucose
	[^{11}C]lactic acid
	[^{13}N]glutamate
	[^{11}C]pyruvic acid
Myocardial blood flow	[^{13}N]ammonia
	[^{15}O]water
	^{82}Rb (rubidium)
Blood pool imaging agents	^{11}CO
	$C^{15}O$ (bound to red blood cells)

*See reference 3 for an exhaustive review of positron-emitter-labeled compounds

radionuclides such as thallium-201 (^{201}Tl), the size and complexity of these machines prohibit their use in the usual clinical environment.

Non-accelerator-produced radionuclides. Certain positron-emitting radionuclides can be produced in a generator. A generator is essentially a radionuclide with a long half-life, typically days or weeks, that decays to produce the required radionuclide. This is an attractive alternative to an accelerator because of its lower cost and ease of use. Although it is not possible to produce radionuclides of carbon, oxygen, nitrogen, or fluorine, a number of important radionuclides can be obtained in this manner. The most useful of these is rubidium-82 (^{82}Rb), with a half-life of 1.25 minutes. Rubidium is an alkali metal analogue of potassium and has similar chemical and biologic properties.[4] It is obtained from the decay of its parent radionuclide, strontium-82 (^{82}Sr), which has a half-life of 25 days. Hence, a generator of ^{82}Sr can produce useful quantities of ^{82}Rb for 1 to 2 months.

An $^{82}Sr/^{82}Rb$ generator consists of an elution column containing ^{82}Sr absorbed onto hydrous SnO_2. The ^{82}Rb produced from the decay on the ^{82}Sr can be extracted by passing isotonic saline through the column. This process can be repeated after approximately four half-lives of ^{82}Rb, allowing repeat elutions of ^{82}Rb from the generator every 5 minutes. Because of the short half-life of ^{82}Rb, current $^{82}Sr/^{82}Rb$ generators are designed to be installed in a special cart that controls the activity to be eluted from the generator, the injected volume, the dose, and the flow rate to the patient.[4,5]

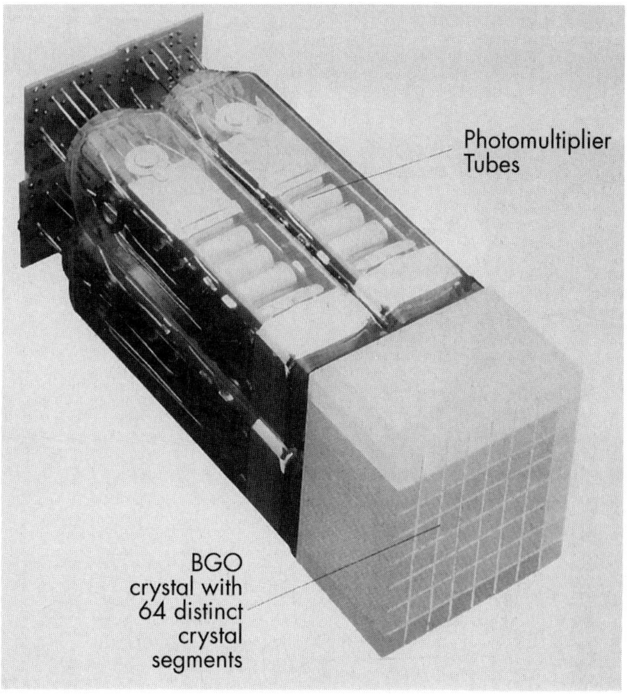

Fig 9-3 Detector block unit consisting of four photomultiplier tubes connected to 64 bismuth germinate (BGO) crystals. (Courtesy of Siemens Medical Systems.)

PET instrumentation

The modern PET scanner operates on the principle of coincidence detection. If two radiation detectors are placed on opposite sides of a positron-emitting radionuclide, a coincidence circuit can be established that records an event only when both detectors simultaneously record annihilation photons. When an event is recorded, it is assumed to have occurred somewhere along the line of sight (coincidence line) between the two detectors. This type of electronic collimation gives a PET scanner two major advantages over a conventional gamma camera. First, since no physical collimation is required, sensitivity is typically about 10^4 times greater. Second, the sensitivity with which an annihilation event is detected is a constant along the coincidence line, and this has important consequences for quantitative analysis of radionuclide distribution in the body.

In all commercial PET scanners, the radiation detector is similar to that used in gamma cameras, consisting of a scintillating crystal and a photomultiplier tube. Unlike the gamma camera, which consists of 30 to 90 photomultiplier tubes coupled to a single large crystal, the PET scanner may contain thousands of small crystals, with two to eight crystals coupled to a single photomultiplier tube (Fig 9-3). These small detectors are arranged in a ring geometry around the object to be imaged, with each detector linked by a coincidence circuit to a number of detectors on the other side of the ring. Since a single crystal is typically 4 to 6 mm square, a single ring of such crystals can image only a 4- to 6-mm longitudinal segment of the body. Hence, modern PET scanners may have more than 20 detector rings, giving them a longitudinal or axial field of view of between 10 and 15 cm (Fig 9-4). The total number of detectors, the number of detector rings, their configuration, and the type of crystal used in the detectors vary according to the design of the PET scanner. All these factors affect the resolution, sensitivity, and count-rate capability of a PET scanner, which in turn determine the types of clinical studies that can be performed on such machines. The advantages and disadvantages of the current commercial PET scanners have been the subject of several studies.[6-10]

Spatial resolution is determined by the range of positrons in tissue (short range gives higher resolution) (see Table 9-1) and by the size of the crystal detectors. High spatial resolution can be achieved through the use of small rectangular or square crystals packed in ring arrays.[11] Crystals of high density and high atomic number are needed to ensure that the 511-keV photons can be absorbed within the crystal. For this reason, most commercial PET scanners use bismuth germanate.[12] Currently, the best commercial scanners can achieve an in-plane resolution of 5 to 7 mm in clinical cardiac studies.

Count-rate capability refers to the speed at which a PET scanner can collect data without saturation of the system. This capability is determined by the number of crystals per photomultiplier tube and by the electronics and becomes important for dynamic studies involving the very high count rates that can be achieved with ^{15}O and ^{82}Rb.[13,14]

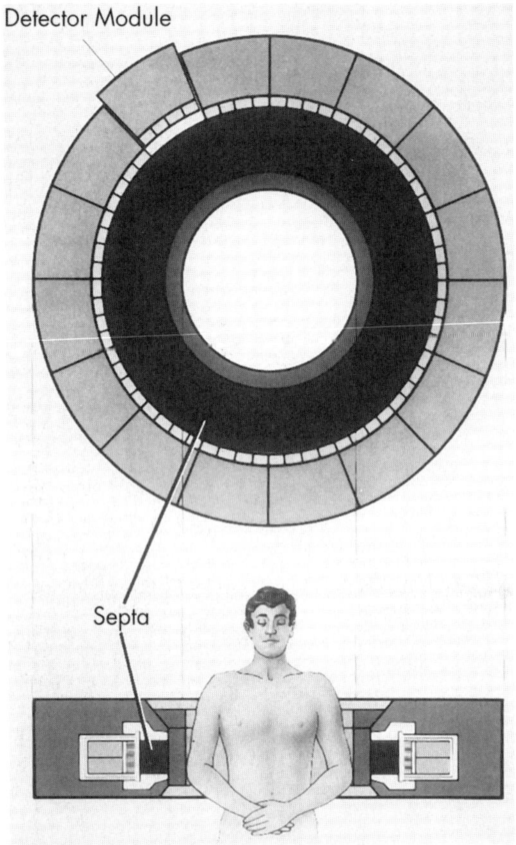

Fig 9-4 Diagram of PET scanner. Each detector module contains four block units, shown in Figure 9-3. Septa placed between the rings of crystals limit detection to gamma rays emitted in the transaxial plane. (Courtesy of Siemens Medical Systems.)

Sensitivity refers to the ability of a system to detect as many true events as possible for a given amount of radioactivity in the field of view. Sensitivity is inversely proportional to the size of the crystal, so that a larger crystal has high sensitivity but poorer spatial resolution.[14] Hence, for all PET scanners, instrument design is a trade-off among these three variables. If the primary application is imaging ^{18}F- or ^{11}C-labeled compounds, spatial resolution is of paramount importance. At the other end of the spectrum, dynamic studies with ^{15}O or ^{82}Rb require good temporal resolution (high count-rate capability), with spatial resolution being of secondary importance.

Quantitative PET

PET offers the capability of performing quantitative measurements of myocardial blood flow that cannot be achieved with existing single-photon-emission computed tomography (SPECT) techniques. The primary reasons for this are, first, the ability to perform accurate attenuation correction and, second, the small contribution of scattered radiation to PET images (10% to 15%) compared with SPECT (30% to 40%).[15] An inherent characteristic of a PET scanner is that for a given line of coincidence between two opposing detectors, the recorded counts are independent of the depth of a source in tissue.[1] This permits the correction of the measured counts for the effects of tissue attenuation. This attenuation correction map is obtained in a manner analogous to a CT scan, by performing a transmission scan with a rotating source of gallium-68 (^{68}Ga) fitted to the inside of the gantry.[16] Until recently, it was necessary to perform the transmission scan before injection of the PET radiopharmaceutical. This increased procedure time and could lead to misregistration errors between transmission and emission data because of patient motion. Recent advances in hardware and software now permit the simultaneous acquisition of emission and transmission data.[17,18]

Once the data have been corrected for attenuation, the next step in the quantitation of activity is the calibration of the detector efficiency. A PET scanner detects only a fraction of the radiation emitted by a radionuclide. The detection efficiency of a given scanner can be determined by scanning a large, uniform cylindrical source. Counts from a given image volume on the PET images can be compared with a known aliquot of activity taken from the phantom and counted in a well counter. This calculation yields a conversion factor to convert image counts to microcuries per milliliter.[19] The ability to convert counts to microcuries per milliliter or microcuries per gram of tissue may be of little practical use in itself; however, such a calibrated system can now be used to measure myocardial blood flow.

A number of techniques are available with PET for the measurement of regional myocardial blood flow. These techniques are based either on the use of labeled particles, such as ^{11}C-labeled microspheres, or on the use of extractable tracers that diffuse into the myocyte, such as ^{82}Rb.

Non-diffusible tracers. An ideal PET tracer for the quantitative measurement of myocardial perfusion should be entirely dependent on coronary flow, with a constant extraction fraction independent of flow rate, and have an extraction fraction of 100% on a single pass through the coronary circulation. Radiolabeled microspheres exhibit such characteristics, and animal studies with ^{68}Ga or ^{11}C microspheres have demonstrated the feasibility of quantitatively analyzing regional myocardial blood flow with PET.[20,21]

Microspheres labeled with either ^{68}Ga or ^{11}C are injected directly into the left atrium or coronary arteries. With a calibrated scanner, the absolute number of microspheres in the heart can be obtained from the image data and converted to blood flow by comparison with arterial blood samples. Regional myocardial blood flow (RMBF) is given by the equation

$$RMBF = BF_A \cdot A_H / A_A$$

in which BF_A is the rate in milliliters per minute at which arterial blood is sampled, A_H is activity in the heart, expressed in microcuries per gram of tissue, and A_A is total activity in the arterial blood sample, stated in microcuries. Although the microsphere method is considered the reference standard with which all other techniques are compared, its main disadvantage is the need to catheterize the left heart for the injection of the microspheres and the need for arterial blood samples.[22]

Diffusible tracers. Another method of measuring myocardial blood flow is to use extractable tracers that diffuse into the myocyte and can be injected into a peripheral vein. Nitrogen-13-ammonia, ^{15}O-labeled water ($H_2{}^{15}O$), and ^{82}Rb are currently used diffusible tracers. Two of these tracers, [^{13}N]ammonia and ^{82}Rb, are influenced by the metabolic status of the myocardium, which can alter tracer retention and activity.[23,24] Additionally, both tracers show a nonlinear relationship between tracer-derived flow and microspheres because of decreasing extraction-retention at high flow rates.[25-28] Although [^{13}N]ammonia can still be used to quantify regional myocardial blood flow if minor modifications are made to the equation shown above,[29] its suitability for this purpose remains the subject of much discussion.[23,30-32] More recently, studies have focused on initial uptake of [^{13}N]ammonia in the heart, rather than retention, as a way of measuring blood flow.[33] These methods have used a slow bolus injection with dynamic acquisition of [^{13}N]ammonia uptake in the heart. No arterial blood samples are required, because the arterial input function can be obtained from a region of interest placed in the left ventricular chamber.[34,35] Time activity curves generated from this arterial region, together with those from regions placed over various parts of the myocardium, are analyzed by a three-compartment model, with correction for the nonlinear nature of the extraction fraction, to yield the ammonia uptake rate constant (K value). From this constant, the myocardial blood flow in milliliters per minute per gram can be obtained.[33]

Although ^{82}Rb has been used extensively for qualitative assessment of myocardial blood flow,[4] absolute quantitation with this radiotracer raises some serious technical limitations. The tracers described above all have extraction fractions of greater than 90%. The extraction fraction for ^{82}Rb is approximately 50% and decreases with increasing blood flow.[36] Hence, ^{82}Rb is far from the ideal blood flow tracer. Nevertheless, because it is generator-produced and therefore more widely available than cyclotron-produced agents, there have been renewed efforts at developing more accurate mathematical models to permit this tracer to be used for quantitative measurement of myocardial blood flow.[37,38] Further work is needed to determine if these models will be applicable in the clinical setting.

Oxygen-15-labeled water has been used extensively in animal research for many years and more recently has been successfully used in clinical studies to estimate regional myocardial blood flow.[39,40] From a theoretical point of view, $H_2{}^{15}O$ appears to be the ideal blood flow agent. It is metabolically inactive and freely diffusible, with an extraction factor approaching unity. Furthermore, this extraction factor does not vary with either flow rate or the metabolic state of the myocardium.[41] It has a short half-life (2.1 minutes), which makes it possible to obtain repeated blood flow measurements, and a rest-stress (dipyridamole) study can be performed in approximately 1 hour. A bolus injection of $H_2{}^{15}O$ is administered intravenously, and image data are acquired dynamically. The arterial input function to the heart can be obtained from arterial samples, or, more recently, from a region of interest placed over the left atrium.[34,35] Time activity curves are obtained from regions over the myocardium, and the uptake rate constant for the myocardial regions is obtained by fitting the curves to a single-compartment tracer kinetic model.[42] A number of technical problems are associated with the use of this radiotracer. Inhalation of 40 to 50 mCi of ^{15}O-labeled carbon monoxide ($C^{15}O$) is required to allow subtraction of the ^{15}O-labeled blood pool. This is necessary because of the rapid clearance of $H_2{}^{15}O$ from the myocardium with little difference between the ventricular blood pool and the myocardium. Subtraction of the $C^{15}O$ data from the $H_2{}^{15}O$ data increases the statistical noise and leads to errors in the estimation of blood flow.[41]

Although $H_2{}^{15}O$ and [^{13}N]ammonia have technical and physiologic limitations as blood flow tracers for quantitative measurements, both have been used for quantitative purposes with considerable success in the research environment. In bringing these techniques into the clinical environment, the choice of a tracer may depend on the expertise within a given laboratory, together with the count-rate and spatial resolution characteristics of the PET scanner.[43-45]

CLINICAL APPLICATIONS

Myocardial blood flow

Background. The favorable imaging characteristics of PET allow quantification of regional myocardial blood flow, a measurement that cannot be obtained with SPECT imaging because of variable photon attenuation, depth-dependent resolution, effect of scatter radiation, and superimposition of radioactivity from overlying myocardium and noncardiac structures. Exercise PET is difficult to perform because of the transient nature of positron-emitting perfusion agents. By the time the patient is properly positioned in the imaging system, the radionuclide previously injected at peak exercise has largely decayed. Consequently, pharmacologic stress PET imaging is generally performed, most frequently with dipyridamole. Adenosine may become more widely used because of the convenience of its extremely short half-life.

Rubidium was the first positron-labeled agent to be used for the measurement of myocardial flow in man.[46] Because of the convenient production characteristics and short half-life of the positron isotope ^{82}Rb, this radionuclide became the focus of subsequent studies designed to measure myocardial perfusion.[5,26] Rubidium-82 does not require a cyclotron for production and is readily obtained from a commercially available, on-site $^{82}Sr/^{82}Rb$ generator. It substitutes for potassium at the cellular level and is actively transported across the sarcolemmal membrane. Its use was reported in man in 1982 to detect significant coronary artery stenosis during exercise.[26] A decrease in tracer activity in the area supplied by the stenotic coronary artery contrasted with homogeneous regional myocardial uptake in the normal subjects.

The remaining positron-labeled myocardial flow tracers in clinical use require a cyclotron for production.

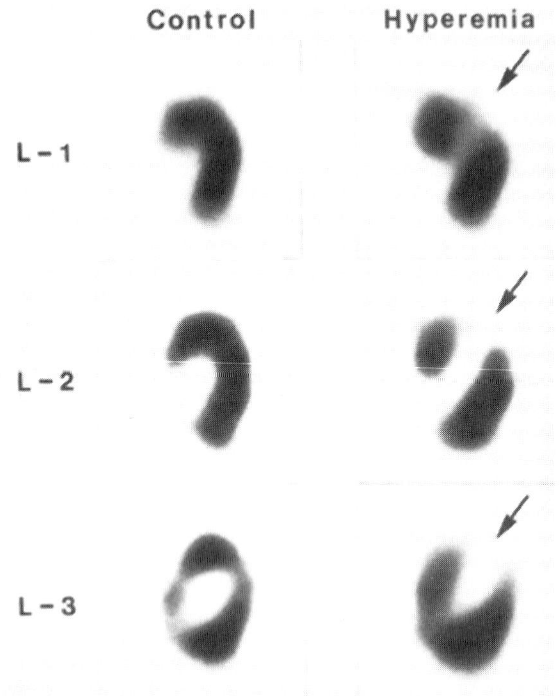

Fig 9-5 Control and hyperemic (dipyridamole) PET images of the heart demonstrating ^{13}N-ammonia distribution in a patient with 100% stenosis of the proximal left anterior descending coronary artery. Beginning superiorly and progressing inferiorly, three tomographic levels (L-1, 2, 3) are shown. The control images reveal uniform ^{13}N activity throughout the left ventricle, suggesting adequate collateral blood flow to the anterior wall at rest. During hyperemia, ^{13}N activity in the anterior wall is greatly reduced *(arrow)*. Image orientation: *top,* anterior; *bottom,* posterior; *right,* lateral; *left,* septum. (From Schelbert HR, Wisenberg G, Phelps ME, et al: Noninvasive assessment of coronary stenoses by myocardial imaging during pharmacologic coronary vasodilation. VI. Detection of coronary artery disease in human beings with intravenous N-13 ammonia and positron computed tomography. *Am J Cardiol* 49:1197-1207, 1982. By permission of Excerpta Medica.)

Nitrogen-13-labeled ammonia has been shown to be a reliable indicator of myocardial perfusion,[28] but extraction and retention within the myocardium are not exclusively dependent on flow, and quantitation may not be reliable.[23,30,31] Transport across the cellular membrane is by passive diffusion. It was first administered, in 1982, to normal subjects and patients during dipyridamole stress[47] (Fig 9-5). Sensitivity and specificity for detecting coronary disease were 97% and 100%, respectively. Although technically more challenging, administration of [^{13}N]ammonia during exercise may also be done.[48] More recently, in a study of 193 patients, variation in regional PET tracer activity (^{82}Rb or [^{13}N]ammonia) during pharmacologic stress with dipyridamole was shown to correlate with the severity of coronary stenosis as defined by the reduction in coronary flow reserve on quantitative coronary angiography.[49] Spatial resolution of images obtained with ^{82}Rb is less than that with [^{13}N]ammonia, but the shorter imaging time with ^{82}Rb and its availability from an on-site generator make its use attractive. Whether a reduction in image detail is significant compared with the effect of cardiac motion on image quality remains to be determined.

Oxygen-15-labeled water possesses characteristics that permit accurate quantification of flow and effectively measures regional myocardial blood flow.[40,41,50] A lipophilic copper (II) complex of derivatives of pyruvaldehyde bis (thiosemicarbazone) called "^{62}Cu-PTSM" labeled with a positron-emitting isotope of copper has also been shown in animal models to be a reliable measure of myocardial flow.[51] It diffuses passively into the cell and has a long clearance half-time while clearing from the blood quickly. Distinct myocardial retention indicates that high-quality images can be obtained several hours after injection. This would allow exercise studies to be performed without the need for immediate imaging as currently required with PET imaging. The tracer is conveniently available from a generator but is unlikely to be suitable for quantitative flow measurements.

Comparison of PET with ^{201}Tl. An ideal study comparing PET imaging with stress scintigraphy has not been conducted. However, at least four studies have been performed in which the two tests have been compared in some fashion.[52-55] A study involving 51 patients with known coronary artery disease compared exercise [^{13}N]ammonia PET with exercise ^{201}Tl SPECT.[52] Sensitivities for the detection of significant coronary stenosis with ^{201}Tl and PET imaging were 81% and 88%, respectively. Classification of myocardial segments into normal, transient defects, and fixed defects showed concordance of 79% for the two methods. PET detected transient defects in 9% of segments reported to have fixed defects on ^{201}Tl imaging. Neither reinjection of ^{201}Tl nor 24-hour imaging was performed to enhance detection of ^{201}Tl redistribution. Another study (202 patients) included patients with normal coronary arteries and permitted calculation of specificity.[53] Both ^{201}Tl and ^{82}Rb were injected during a single dipyridamole infusion (Figs 9-6 and 9-7). Sensitivity and specificity of ^{201}Tl SPECT for the diagnosis of coronary disease were 76% and 80%, respectively, and for ^{82}Rb, 93% and 78%, respectively. A significant improvement in sensitivity was found with PET over that with ^{201}Tl. In 21 of the 27 patients with significant coronary artery stenosis by coronary angiography and negative ^{201}Tl results, PET detected the disease, with most defects involving the inferior and posterior walls. Improved image quality due to less scatter fraction with 511-keV annihilation photons than with the 60- to 80-keV photons of ^{201}Tl may have contributed to the enhanced sensitivity. This factor may also have contributed to a greater detection of mild to moderate coronary artery disease and greater specificity with PET imaging.[49] Attenuation correction with PET may also have contributed to the improved specificity. A study of 81 patients examined because of chest pain showed a sensitivity and specificity of 84% and 53%, respectively, for ^{201}Tl and 84%

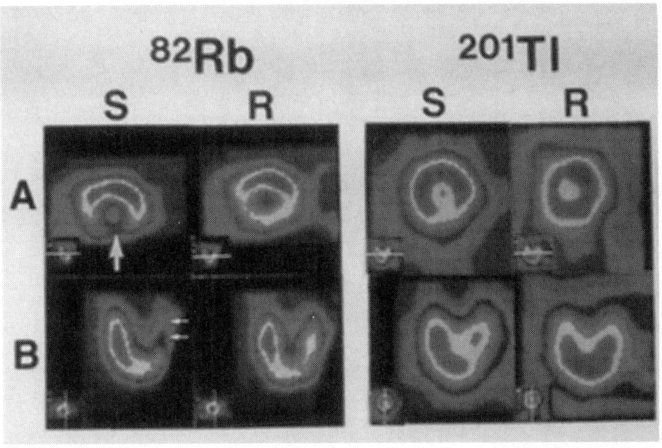

Fig 9-6 Comparison of dipyridamole rubidium-82 (^{82}Rb) and thallium-201 (^{201}Tl) imaging in a patient with inferior wall hypoperfusion *(arrows)* during stress *(S)*. Short-axis images are shown in the *top row (A),* and vertical long-axis images are in the *bottom row (B).* Rubidium-82 images show a reversible decrease in activity in the inferior wall. The amount of reduction in ^{201}Tl activity is less pronounced. *R,* rest. (From Go RT, Marwick TH, MacIntyre WJ, et al: A prospective comparison of rubidium-82 PET and thallium-201 SPECT myocardial perfusion imaging utilizing a single dipyridamole stress in the diagnosis of coronary artery disease. *J Nucl Med* 31:1899-1905, 1990. By permission of the Society of Nuclear Medicine.)

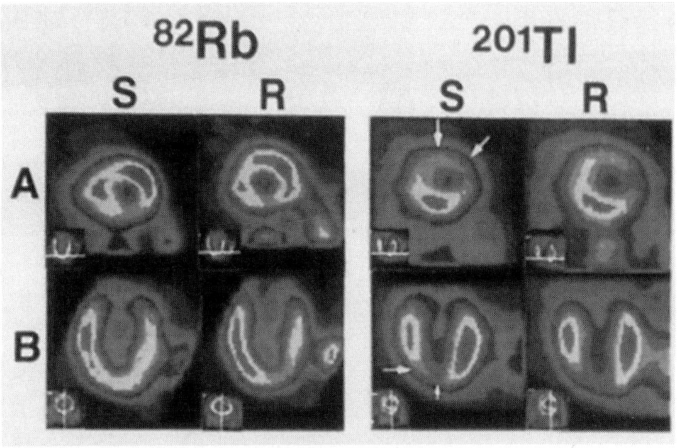

Fig 9-7 Comparison of dipyridamole rubidium-82 (^{82}Rb) and thallium-201 (^{201}Tl) imaging in a patient with a fixed anterior wall defect *(arrows)* that appears only in the ^{201}Tl images. The ^{82}Rb images show normal anterior wall radionuclide uptake and diaphragmatic attenuation. The ^{201}Tl defect is most likely due to breast attenuation. The coronary angiogram was normal. *Top row (A),* short-axis images; *bottom row (B),* vertical long-axis images. *S,* stress; *R,* rest. (From Go RT, Marwick TH, MacIntyre WJ, et al: A prospective comparison of rubidium-82 PET and thallium-201 SPECT myocardial perfusion imaging utilizing a single dipyridamole stress in the diagnosis of coronary artery disease. *J Nucl Med* 31:1899-1905, 1990. By permission of the Society of Nuclear Medicine.)

and 88%, respectively, for PET.[55] An American Heart Association special report on PET concluded that PET imaging data do not yet demonstrate a clear superiority of PET over other currently accepted, more readily available, and less expensive techniques for the routine diagnosis of coronary artery disease or for determining the functional significance of coronary stenosis in patients with established coronary artery disease.[56]

Quantitative myocardial perfusion. Quantitative assessment of regional myocardial flow with $H_2{}^{15}O$ PET provides information not available with SPECT imaging, which cannot provide quantitative data (Figs 9-8 and 9-9). Measurement of flow can be helpful in myocardial diseases in which global flow may be altered.[57,58] Also, by quantifying regional flow, therapeutic interventions aimed at improving myocardial perfusion can be directly compared among patients.[39,59] When PET was used to calculate global myocardial flow, normal subjects had a mean blood flow of 0.9 ± 0.22 mL/g per minute at rest, which increased to 3.55 ± 1.15 mL/g per minute with dipyridamole.[42] In 17 patients presenting with ischemic-like chest pain and angiographically normal coronary arteries, nearly half had diminished myocardial perfusion in a homogeneous manner without regional disparity during dipyridamole stress.[58] Flow was 2.26 mL/g per minute in the group with chest pain, compared with 4.62 mL/g per minute in normal subjects. A two-compartment kinetic model of [^{13}N]ammonia described by Krivokapich et al.[57] was used to quantitatively estimate myocardial perfusion in recipients of cardiac transplants without transplant-related coronary arteriopathy. Blood flow measured during exercise in the transplant recipients doubled to 1.7 ± 0.6 mL/g per minute; this result was similar to that in normal subjects, whose flow increased to 1.56 ± 0.71 mL/g per minute.

Use of $H_2{}^{15}O$ may provide a better understanding of regional coronary flow response after percutaneous transluminal coronary angioplasty.[39] Five days after the procedure, dipyridamole stress PET imaging demonstrated hyperemic myocardial perfusion similar to perfusion of remote normal segments. Flow increased from 1.5 mL/g per minute at rest to 4.36 mL/g per minute with stress. Approximately 7 months after angioplasty in patients with no clinical evidence of restenosis, dipyridamole-induced hyperemia was only slightly less (3.23 mL/g per minute).

Regional myocardial blood flow can also be quantitatively measured with $C^{15}O$ inhalation in humans.[43] The advantages of this tracer include complete extraction from the blood over a wide range of flows during its first pass through the heart, lack of metabolic activity, and a very short half-life. Potential advantages of this agent over $H_2{}^{15}O$ include its ease of production and handling and the relatively long period of inhalation (3.5 minutes) that provides a slow input function and reduces artifacts from scanner dead time that occur with bolus injections of $H_2{}^{15}O$. An obvious disadvantage of both $C^{15}O$ and $H_2{}^{15}O$ is the high level of activity in the cardiac chambers, which interferes with tracer detection in the myocardium.

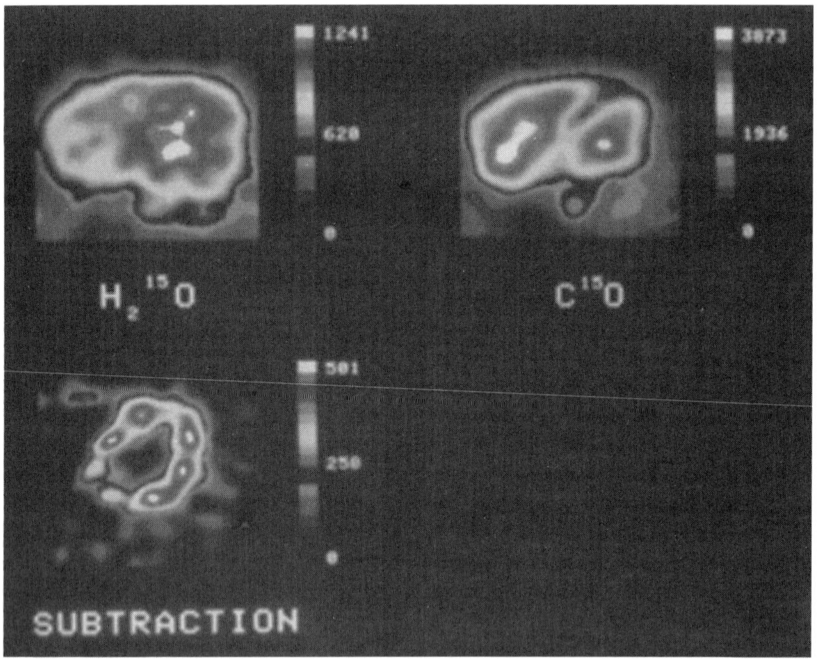

Fig 9-8 Normal myocardial $H_2{}^{15}O$ content during dipyridamole hyperemia. *Upper left,* midventricular image after infusion of $H_2{}^{15}O$. Increase in counts in the center of the image is attributable to blood pool activity. *Upper right,* blood pool image at the same anatomic level after inhalation of $C^{15}O$. *Lower left,* myocardial $H_2{}^{15}O$ content after blood pool subtraction. (From Walsh MN, Bergmann SR, Steele RL, et al: Delineation of impaired regional myocardial perfusion by positron emission tomography with $H_2{}^{15}O$. *Circulation* 78:612-620, 1988. By permission of American Heart Association.)

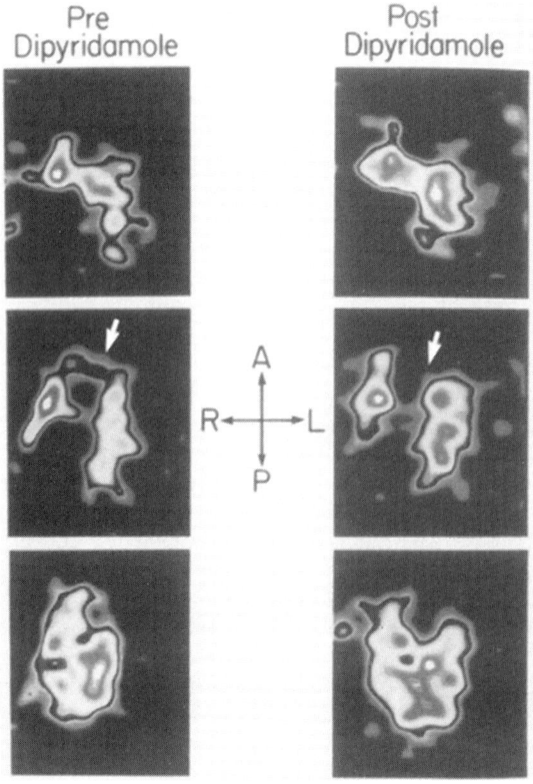

Fig 9-9 Images of an $H_2{}^{15}O$ perfusion study in a patient with a high-grade stenosis of the left anterior descending coronary artery. The pre-dipyridamole (rest), midventricular tomogram *(middle left image)* demonstrates a decrease in activity in the anterior wall *(arrow)* consistent with resting hypoperfusion. This defect worsens with dipyridamole stress *(middle right image).* The *top* and *bottom images* show different levels of the left ventricle. *A,* anterior; *L,* left; *P,* posterior; *R,* right. (From Walsh MN, Bergmann SR, Steele RL, et al: Delineation of impaired regional myocardial perfusion by positron emission tomography with $H_2{}^{15}O$. *Circulation* 78:612-620, 1988. By permission of American Heart Association.)

Myocardial viability

Background. The heart preferentially uses free fatty acids in the fasting, postabsorptive state.[60] Fatty acid uptake is governed largely by circulating nonesterified fatty acid levels and the rate of cellular utilization. Diffusion has long been thought to account for fatty acid transport across the myocyte sarcolemma, although a carrier protein has been identified.[61] On entering the cell, fatty acids are bound to a fatty-acid-binding protein. The acyl-CoA-carnitine transferase system then transports the fatty acid into the mitochondria for β-oxidation and subsequent entry into the energy-producing tricarboxylic acid (TCA) cycle. As an alternative means of metabolism, fatty acids may be converted to triglycerides for substrate storage. The largest determinant of free fatty acid uptake is the plasma insulin concentration. With an increase in insulin production, tissue lipolysis is inhibited and free fatty acid utilization is greatly diminished.

Glucose is freely transported into the cell according to a concentration gradient and is regulated by a stereospecific-dependent glucose carrier system. Once in the cell, it is phosphorylated to glucose-6-phosphate under the control of the enzyme hexokinase. During glycolysis, glucose-6-phosphate produces two molecules of pyruvate and adenosine triphosphate molecules. Lactate is produced under anaerobic conditions (anaerobic glycolysis), whereas entry of pyruvate into the TCA cycle through acetyl-CoA proceeds under aerobic conditions (aerobic glycolysis). Free fatty acids and metabolic products of fat metabolism inhibit glycolysis and decrease TCA cycle utilization of pyruvate from glucose.

Glycolysis accelerates when myocardial perfusion is mildly reduced. Phosphofructokinase enzyme activity is stimulated by low cellular content of adenosine triphosphate and citrate and high inorganic phosphate. As ischemia worsens, products of anaerobic glycolysis, including protons, lactate, and $NADH_2$, inhibit glycolysis. If coronary flow is maintained but hypoxia is present, the inhibitors wash out and anaerobic glycolysis is maintained. Mild resting ischemia is associated with hypocontractility (hibernating myocardium) and increased glucose uptake relative to blood flow. When myocardial perfusion is restored to normal after ischemia (stunned myocardium), fatty acid is the preferred substrate,[62] whereas the role of glycolysis has not been clearly defined.[63]

Fatty acid imaging. Carbon-11-palmitate is a positron-labeled substrate suitable for PET imaging.[64,65] Studies performed in animal models have demonstrated the value of positron-labeled fatty acids, primarily [^{11}C]palmitate, for assessing myocardial metabolism.[66-70] The lack of fatty acid uptake indicates scar, whereas uptake and slow clearance occur in the ischemic myocardium. Slow clearance presumably represents diminished β-oxidation of the fatty acid within the ischemic or postischemic myocardium. After a 20-minute coronary artery occlusion and reperfusion in the dog, [^{11}C]palmitate clearance remained slow for at least 3 hours, paralleling the recovery of wall motion.[71,72] Slowed palmitate clearance is associated with an increase in the appearance of lipid droplets in hypoperfused zones surrounding the central necrotic myocardium.[73]

Only a few studies with positron-induced fatty acid have been performed in human subjects. Patients with ischemic cardiomyopathy and multiple infarctions have a severe, homogeneous reduction in tracer activity distributed in multiple regions[74,75] (Fig 9-10). Those with nonischemic (dilated) cardiomyopathy display marked spatial heterogeneity (variation in tracer activity within a region) in palmitate accumulation throughout the entire left ventricle. Early after acute myocardial infarction, palmitate accumulation has been shown to increase in the infarcted area when patients are given nifedipine orally.[76] These patients have a high incidence of postinfarction chest pain, suggesting that palmitate serves as a marker of jeopardized myocardium. Carbon-11-labeled palmitate is identical to physiologically available palmitate and is dispersed throughout multiple metabolic pathways. Also, a considerable portion of labeled fatty acid diffuses back into the blood without being metabolized.[77] Diffusion of free fatty acid and the amount of fatty acid incorporated into lipid storage increase during ischemia, although neither can be separately identified by PET imaging. Unfortunately, these factors greatly complicate assessment of intracellular fatty acid function and have resulted in diminished enthusiasm for [^{11}C]palmitate PET imaging. Currently, positron-emission imaging with FDG is widely preferred for the assessment of tissue viability.

Glucose imaging. Radiolabeled 2-deoxyglucose was initially used to measure regional glucose utilization in the brain.[78] Subsequently, FDG was produced for PET imaging. FDG is transported into the cell like glucose and is phosphorylated by hexakinase to FDG-6-phosphate. This compound is metabolically trapped and does not proceed through glycolysis and is not converted to glycogen. Although [^{11}C]glucose is metabolically indistinguishable from glucose, its rapid utilization and appearance in multiple metabolic substances would not only require rapid imaging techniques but also make it difficult to determine which labeled substrate was being imaged.

Early PET studies measured rates of glucose metabolism in myocardium in animal models.[79-81] More recently, measurement of myocardial FDG uptake has been used to assess tissue viability in hypokinetic myocardial segments with the patient at rest (Fig 9-11). An increase in glucose uptake in mildly to moderately ischemic myocardium implies the occurrence of anaerobic glucose metabolism in living myocytes, whereas the loss of metabolic activity indicates infarction. As a means of enhancing image quality by increasing tracer activity in the myocardium, patients are usually given a glucose meal before FDG injection. This increases glucose uptake in normal myocardium but somewhat reduces the difference in radioactivity between normal and ischemic myocardium.

To establish standards for tissue viability, FDG activity and [^{13}N]ammonia activity are normalized relative to the highest [^{13}N]ammonia uptake; normal mean values and standard deviations are established for multiple sectors of short-axis tomographic images. Similar values are established for the difference between flow and uptake of FDG. Myocardium is identified as infarcted if both flow and uptake of FDG are more than two standard deviations below the normal mean values for that sector. Myocardium is identified as ischemic if the difference between FDG uptake and flow exceeds normal by two standard deviations. Although FDG uptake may be decreased relative to normal myocardium, the segment is regarded as ischemic if flow is significantly lower than FDG activity. Using these methods, Marshall et al.[82] identified five of nine patients with Q-wave infarction who

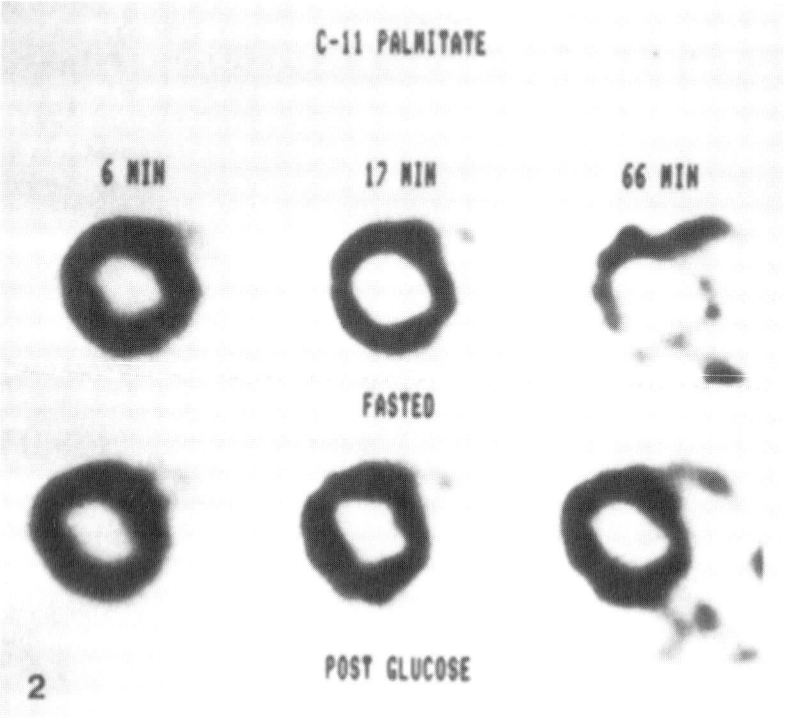

Fig 9-10 Serial [^{11}C]palmitate images at one level of the heart in a patient with dilated cardiomyopathy and moderate depression of left ventricular function. *Top row,* fasting; *bottom row,* glucose loading. Utilization of [^{11}C]palmitate is heterogeneous in the fasting state and is best demonstrated in the image obtained at 66 minutes after [^{11}C]palmitate injection. After glucose loading *(bottom row),* [^{11}C]palmitate is retained and not metabolized, because of a shift to glucose utilization. (From Sochor H, Schelbert HR, Schwaiger M, et al: Studies of fatty acid metabolism with positron emission tomography in patients with cardiomyopathy. *Eur J Nucl Med* 12 Suppl:S66-S69, 1986. By permission of Springer-Verlag GmbH & Company).

had glucose utilization consistent with ischemic but viable myocardium in the region of the infarction. Metabolism and perfusion mismatches were also found in zones remote from the infarction. Similarly, Brunken et al.[83] studied 20 patients with previous Q-wave infarction and found that only 10 of 31 infarcted segments had concordant reduction in perfusion and FDG uptake. The remaining 21 segments showed metabolic activity consistent with viable myocardium. Since the patients were studied before the widespread use of thrombolytic therapy, salvage was most likely due to the early development of coronary collaterals or spontaneous reperfusion. Fudo et al.[84] examined the relationship between resting regional wall motion abnormalities and glucose uptake. Mildly hypokinetic segments in the region of a previous anterior wall myocardial infarction had increased FDG uptake. Eight of the 15 patients with dyskinetic or akinetic segments had concordant decreases in perfusion and FDG uptake in the central infarction zone, whereas the remaining 7 patients had metabolism-perfusion mismatch consistent with viability.

PET provides a method of predicting left ventricular contractile recovery after coronary revascularization. Akinetic segments with metabolism-perfusion mismatches indicating viable or hibernating myocardium should respond to an increase in perfusion. Tillisch et al.[85] studied 17 patients with preoperative wall motion abnormalities after FDG infusion who subsequently underwent coronary bypass surgery. Eighty-five percent of hypokinetic segments with preserved FDG uptake or a metabolism-perfusion mismatch more than two standard deviations above normal had improved regional function after successful coronary artery bypass surgery. Twenty-seven regions were predicted to be scar tissue preoperatively, and only two improved postoperatively. Others have reported similar results.[86] After myocardial infarction in humans, FDG uptake has been shown to be associated with an open coronary artery.[87] Despite the impressive preliminary data, a cautionary note on the interpretation of FDG PET images is required.[88] Uptake of FDG is significantly affected by physiologic factors that alter glucose metabolism. Variations in glucose utilization incurred with insulin in dogs have been shown to significantly alter myocardial FDG uptake, and adrenergic stimulation with dopamine decreases FDG uptake despite normal myocardial perfusion.

A depressed metabolic effect has been described in patients immediately after exertional angina in whom FDG uptake is increased in postischemic segments despite normal regional myocardial blood flow.[89] FDG

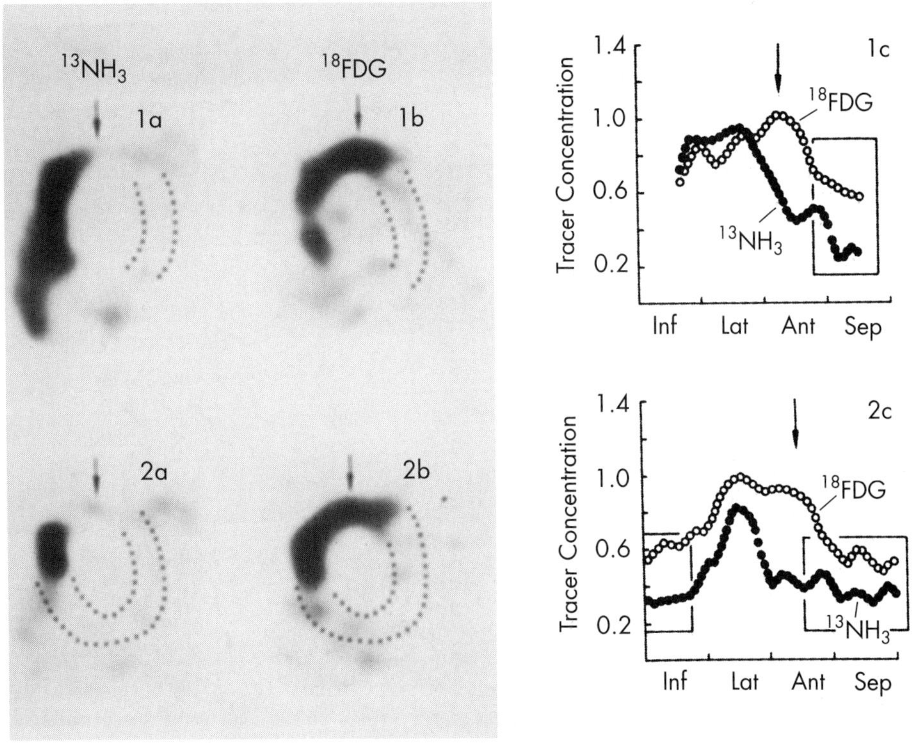

Fig 9-11 Resting regional myocardial perfusion evaluated with [^{13}N]ammonia ($^{13}NH_3$) *(1a, 2a)* and [^{18}F]fluorodeoxyglucose (^{18}FDG) *(1b, 2b)* at two levels of the heart (*top images,* superior; *bottom images,* inferior) in a patient with a recent anterior and remote inferior infarction, postinfarction angina, and known proximal three-vessel coronary artery disease. Uptake of $^{13}NH_3$ is decreased in the anterior and inferior segments and septum. Uptake of ^{18}FDG in the anterior segment *(1b, 2b, arrows)* indicates that the myocardium is viable. Absence of ^{18}FDG and $^{13}NH_3$ in the inferior wall is consistent with infarction. Count profile curves *(1c, 2c)* are shown to the right of the images. The *arrows* indicate the anterior wall. Image orientation: *top,* anterior *(Ant)*; *bottom,* inferior *(Inf)*; *left,* lateral *(Lat)*; *right,* septum *(Sep)*. (From Marshall RC, Tillisch JH, Phelps ME, et al: Identification and differentiation of resting myocardial ischemia and infarction in man with positron computed tomography, ^{18}F-labeled fluorodeoxyglucose and N-13 ammonia. *Circulation* 67:766-778, 1983. By permission of American Heart Association.)

uptake is also increased at rest after percutaneous transluminal coronary angioplasty in patients with unstable or stable angina before the revascularization procedure.[90] The number of patients in these studies is small, and additional studies will be required to confirm the findings.

Comparison of PET with other imaging modalities for the detection of viability. Fixed ^{201}Tl defects have typically been associated with myocardial scar. In contrast, redistribution after stress has been attributed to ischemia and viable tissue.[91] After revascularization, however, function of segments with fixed perfusion defects has frequently improved, a suggestion that viable myocardium may be present in regions without ^{201}Tl redistribution.[92] In a comparison with PET imaging, 58% of fixed defects had FDG uptake and 64% with partial redistribution had uptake.[93] In another study, 73% of fixed ^{201}Tl defects at 4 hours had FDG uptake.[94] To unmask viable myocardium in fixed ^{201}Tl defects, 1 mCi of ^{201}Tl was injected immediately after redistribution imaging.[95] With reinjection imaging, 49% of fixed ^{201}Tl defects display redistribution. The severity of exercise ^{201}Tl hypoperfusion correlates with the degree of FDG uptake. Nearly all fixed defects with mild-to-moderate reduction in ^{201}Tl activity at the time of redistribution imaging have FDG uptake, and most of these segments have redistribution after reinjection of 1 mCi of ^{201}Tl.[94] However, fewer (51%) fixed ^{201}Tl defects with severely reduced ^{201}Tl activity have glucose uptake, and 51% have redistribution with reinjection.[94] Detection of scar and viable myocardium is concordant in 88% of segments. The greater the change in ^{201}Tl activity after reinjection (relative to the 4-hour redistribution study), the more likely that FDG uptake will be found.[96] Finally, it has been shown that with 24-hour redistribution imaging after stress-reinjection imaging, the likelihood of detecting viable myocardium is similar to that of stress-redistribution-reinjection imaging at 4 hours.[97] Although these reports require confirmation in larger numbers of patients, they suggest the possibility that ^{201}Tl imaging

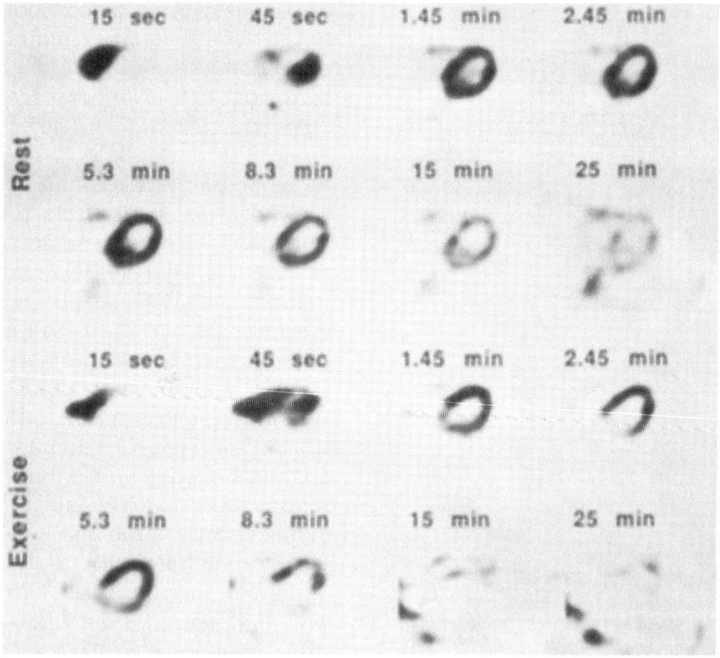

Fig 9-12 Sequential midventricular images of myocardial ^{11}C activity obtained after bolus intravenous administration of [^{11}C]acetate. Times above the images are midacquisition times. Images one and two in the first and third rows depict tracer accumulation in the right and left ventricular chambers. The remaining images show ^{11}C uptake by the left ventricular myocardium. Acetate washout from the myocardium takes place much faster with exercise than with rest. Image orientation: *left,* septum; *right,* lateral; *top,* anterior; *bottom,* inferior. (From Armbrecht JJ, Buxton DB, Brunken RC, et al; Regional myocardial oxygen consumption determined noninvasively in humans with (1-^{11}C)acetate and dynamic positron tomography. *Circulation* 80:863-872, 1989. By permission of American Heart Association.)

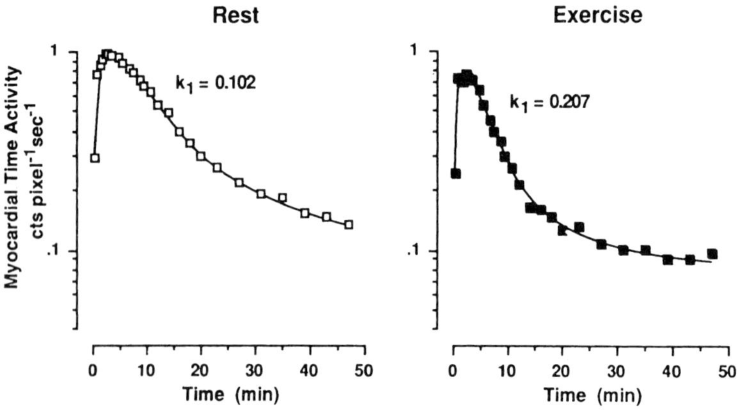

Fig 9-13 Myocardial time-activity curves derived from the serial images in Figure 9-12. Note that the [^{11}C]acetate clearance curve is steeper with exercise than at rest, as indicated by a higher k_1 value. (From Armbrecht JJ, Buxton DB, Brunken RC, et al: Regional myocardial oxygen consumption determined noninvasively in humans with (1-^{11}C)acetate and dynamic positron tomography. *Circulation* 80:863-872, 1989. By permission of American Heart Association.)

provides the same information about tissue viability as PET imaging, a more cumbersome and expensive imaging technology.

Useful indicators of transmural myocardial infarction on echocardiography include regional wall thinning and increased ultrasound density. Another recently described echocardiographic indicator of tissue viability is wall thickening during low-dose dobutamine infusion (5 to 10 μg/kg per minute).[98] The results assessing viability with low-dose dobutamine infusion and FDG uptake on PET imaging were concordant in patients immediately after acute myocardial infarction and at delayed imaging a mean of 9 months after infarction. When segmental perfusion was normal early after infarction, evidence of viability by both methods persisted at 9 months. When perfusion was decreased and glucose uptake was high initially, delayed imaging at 9 months revealed loss of wall thickening with dobutamine stimulation and reduced glucose uptake. Infusion of a higher dose of dobutamine in patients with a high-grade coronary stenosis may result in loss of wall thickening.

Myocardial oxygen consumption

For a positron-labeled tracer to serve as a marker of myocardial oxygen consumption, it must be the preferred substrate under a variety of physiologic and pathophysiologic conditions. Acetate is one such substrate. It is readily oxidized to carbon dioxide upon entry into the TCA cycle, exhibiting single-pathway metabolism in the myocardium. Carbon-14-acetate is extracted under a variety of metabolic conditions and coronary flows in the isolated rabbit heart.[99] When detected externally, positron-labeled [^{11}C]acetate activity correlates closely with myocardial oxygen consumption under the same conditions. Data derived from in vivo-acquired PET images in the dog demonstrate that [^{11}C]acetate clearance correlates with myocardial oxygen consumption under different work conditions.[100] Norepinephrine increases systolic blood pressure and accelerates acetate utilization, whereas pharmacologically induced hypotension decreases acetate utilization. The rate constant for the initial phase of $^{14}CO_2$ clearance correlates well with myocardial oxygen consumption in the isolated rat heart.[101] The rate constant also correlates with normoxic regional myocardial oxygen consumption, although slight changes occur depending on the substrate utilized. The rate constant for [^{11}C]acetate clearance derived from monoexponential curve fitting shows a close correlation with rate-pressure product in normal human subjects.[102] To demonstrate the feasibility of calculating TCA cycle flux from [^{11}C]acetate clearance measurements in ischemic heart disease, Armbrecht et al.[103] subjected dogs to coronary occlusion and reperfusion and intracoronary injection of [^{11}C]acetate (Figs 9-12 and 9-13). Externally measured carbon-11 clearance was linearly related to myocardial oxygen consumption in ischemic and reperfused tissue. Acetate clearance was not affected by a fourfold change in blood flow induced by dipyridamole but was altered slightly by substrate (lactate and free fatty acid) availability. Refinements in tracer kinetic modeling enhance calculation of TCA flux over that with conventional monoexponential fitting of [^{11}C]acetate myocardial kinetics.[104] Noninvasive measurement of oxidative metabolism and estimation of TCA cycle flux with PET may provide useful information about myocardial viability. However, the benefits of this type of evaluation over FDG PET imaging remain to be determined.

REFERENCES

1. Hoffman EJ, Phelps ME: Positron emission tomography: principles and quantitation. In *Positron Emission Tomography and Autoradiography: Principles and Applications for the Brain and Heart.* Edited by ME Phelps, JC Mazziotta, HR Schelbert. New York, Raven Press, 1986, pp 237-286
2. Tilyou S: The evolution of positron emission tomography. *J Nucl Med* 32 (4):15N-26N, 1991
3. Fowler JS, Wolf AP: Positron emitter-labeled compounds: priorities and problems. In *Positron Emission Tomography and Autoradiography: Principles and Applications for the Brain and Heart.* Edited by ME Phelps, JC Mazziotta, HH Schelbert. New York, Raven Press, 1986, pp 391-450
4. Gould KL: PET perfusion imaging and nuclear cardiology. *J Nucl Med* 32:579-606, 1991
5. Yano Y, Cahoon JL, Budinger TF: A precision flow-controlled Rb-82 generator for bolus or constant-infusion studies of the heart and brain. *J Nucl Med* 22:1006-1010, 1981
6. Batchelor S, Blake GM, Saunders JE: A comparison of three commercially available PET imaging systems. *Nucl Med Commun* 13:20-27, 1992
7. Spinks TJ, Jones T, Gilardi MC, et al: Physical performance of the latest generation of commercial positron scanner. *IEEE Trans Nucl Sci* 35:721-725, 1989
8. Evans AC, Thompson CJ, Marrett S, et al: Performance evaluation of the PC-2048: a new 15-slice encoded-crystal PET scanner for neurological studies. *IEEE Trans Med Imaging* 10:90-98, 1991
9. Spinks TJ, Guzzardi R, Bellina CR: Performance characteristics of a whole-body positron tomograph. *J Nucl Med* 29:1833-1841, 1988
10. Trebossen R, Mazoyer B: Count rate performances of TTV03: the CEA-LETI time-of-flight positron emission tomograph. *IEEE Trans Med Imaging* 10:261-266, 1991
11. Muehllehner G, Karp JS: Positron emission tomography imaging—technical considerations. *Semin Nucl Med* 16:35-50, 1986
12. Wong W-H: PET camera performance design evaluation for BGO and BAF_2 scintillators (non-time-of-flight). *J Nucl Med* 29:338-347, 1988
13. Hoffman EJ, Phelps ME, Huang S-C: Performance characteristics of a positron tomograph designed for brain imaging. *J Nucl Med* 24:245-257, 1983
14. Volkow ND, Mullani NA, Bendriem B: Positron emission tomography instrumentation: an overview. *Am J Phys Imaging* 3:142-153, 1988
15. Jordan K, Knoop BO: Cardiac nuclear medicine tomographic systems. *Eur J Nucl Med* 13:612-618, 1988
16. Carroll LR, Kretz P, Orcutt G: The orbiting rod source: improving performance in PET transmission correction scans. In *Emission Computed Tomography: Current Trends.* Edited by PD Esser. New York, Society of Nuclear Medicine, 1983, pp 235-247
17. Carson RE, Daube-Witherspoon ME, Green MV: A method for postinjection PET transmission measurements with a rotating source. *J Nucl Med* 29:1558-1567, 1988
18. Thompson CJ, Ranger NT, Evans AC: Simultaneous transmission and emission scans in positron emission tomography. *IEEE Trans Nucl Sci* 36:1011-1016, 1989
19. Schelbert HR, Schwaiger M: PET studies of the heart. In *Positron Emission Tomography and Autoradiography: Principles and Applications for the Brain and Heart.* Edited by ME Phelps, JC Mazziotta, HR Schelbert. New York, Raven Press, 1986, pp 581-661
20. Wilson RA, Shea MJ, De Landsheere CM, et al: Validation of quantitation of regional myocardial blood flow in vivo with ^{11}C-labeled human albumin microspheres and positron emission tomography. *Circulation* 70:717-723, 1984

21. Wisenberg G, Schelbert HR, Hoffman EJ, et al: In vivo quantitation of regional myocardial blood flow by positron-emission computed tomography. *Circulation* 63:1248-1258, 1981

22. Geltman EM, Bergmann SR, Sobel BE: Cardiac positron emission tomography. In *Positron Emission Tomography*. Edited by M Rievich, A Alavi. New York, Alan R Liss, 1985, pp 345-385

23. Bergmann SR, Hack S, Tewson T, et al: The dependence of accumulation of $^{13}NH_3$ by myocardium on metabolic factors and its implications for quantitative assessment of perfusion. *Circulation* 61:34-43, 1980

24. Goldstein RA, Mullani NA, Marani SK, et al: Myocardial perfusion with rubidium-82. II. Effects of metabolic and pharmacologic interventions. *J Nucl Med* 24:907-915, 1983

25. Fukuyama T, Nakamura M, Nakagaki O, et al: Reduced reflow and diminished uptake of ^{82}Rb after temporary coronary occlusion. *Am J Physiol* 234:H724-H729, 1978

26. Selwyn AP, Allan RM, L'Abbate A, et al: Relation between regional myocardial uptake of rubidium-82 and perfusion: absolute reduction of cation uptake in ischemia. *Am J Cardiol* 50:112-121, 1982

27. Rauch B, Helus F, Grunze M, et al: Kinetics of ^{13}N-ammonia uptake in myocardial single cells indicating potential limitations in its applicability as a marker of myocardial blood flow. *Circulation* 71:387-393, 1985

28. Schelbert HR, Phelps ME, Huang S-C, et al: N-13 ammonia as an indicator of myocardial blood flow. *Circulation* 63:1259-1272, 1981

29. Shah A, Schelbert HR, Schwaiger M, et al: Measurement of regional myocardial blood flow with N-13 ammonia and positron-emission tomography in intact dogs. *J Am Coll Cardiol* 5:92-100, 1985

30. Krivokapich J, Huang S-C, Phelps ME, et al: Dependence of $^{13}NH_3$ myocardial extraction and clearance on flow and metabolism. *Am J Physiol* 242:H536-H542, 1982

31. Bianco JA: Quantitation of regional myocardial blood flow: oxygen-15-water versus nitrogen-13-ammonia (letter to the editor). *J Nucl Med* 31:1431, 1990

32. Schelbert HR, Czernin J, Huang S-C: Quantitation of regional myocardial blood flow: oxygen-15-water versus nitrogen-13-ammonia (reply). *J Nucl Med* 31:1431-1433, 1990

33. Hutchins GD, Schwaiger M, Rosenspire KC, et al: Noninvasive quantification of regional myocardial blood flow in the human heart using N-13 ammonia and dynamic positron emission tomographic imaging. *J Am Coll Cardiol* 15:1032-1042, 1990

34. Gambhir SS, Schwaiger M, Huang S-C, et al: Simple noninvasive quantification method for measuring myocardial glucose utilization in humans employing positron emission tomography and fluorine-18-deoxyglucose. *J Nucl Med* 30:359-366, 1989

35. Weinberg IN, Huang SC, Hoffman EJ, et al: Validation of PET-acquired input functions for cardiac studies. *J Nucl Med* 29: 241-247, 1988

36. Wilson RA, Shea M, De Landsheere C, et al: Rubidium-82 myocardial uptake and extraction after transient ischemia: PET characteristics. *J Comput Assist Tomogr* 11:60-66, 1987

37. Herrero P, Markham J, Shelton ME, et al: Noninvasive quantification of regional myocardial perfusion with rubidium-82 and positron emission tomography: exploration of a mathematical model. *Circulation* 82:1377-1386, 1990

38. Herrero P, Markham J, Shelton ME, et al: Implementation and evaluation of a two-compartment model for quantification of myocardial perfusion with rubidium-82 and positron emission tomography. *Circ Res* 70:496-507, 1992

39. Walsh MN, Geltman EM, Steele RL, et al: Augmented myocardial perfusion reserve after coronary angioplasty quantified by positron emission tomography with $H_2{}^{15}O$. *J Am Coll Cardiol* 15:119-127, 1990

40. Iida H, Kanno I, Takahashi A, et al: Measurement of absolute myocardial blood flow with $H_2{}^{15}O$ and dynamic positron-emission tomography: strategy for quantification in relation to the partial-volume effect. *Circulation* 78:104-115, 1988

41. Bergmann SR, Fox KAA, Rand AL, et al: Quantification of regional myocardial blood flow in vivo with $H_2{}^{15}O$. *Circulation* 70:724-733, 1984

42. Bergmann SR, Herrero P, Markham J, et al: Noninvasive quantitation of myocardial blood flow in human subjects with oxygen-15-labeled water and positron emission tomography. *J Am Coll Cardiol* 14:639-652, 1989

43. Araujo LI, Lammertsma AA, Rhodes CG, et al: Noninvasive quantification of regional myocardial blood flow in coronary artery disease with oxygen-15-labeled carbon dioxide inhalation and positron emission tomography. *Circulation* 83:875-885, 1991

44. Soufer R, Zaret BL: Positron emission tomography and the quantitative assessment of regional myocardial blood flow. *J Am Coll Cardiol* 15:128-130, 1990

45. Schelbert HR, Czernin J: Noninvasive quantification of regional myocardial blood flow: assessment of myocardial perfusion reserve and collateral circulation (editorial). *J Nucl Med* 31:271-273, 1990

46. Bing RJ, Bennish A, Bluemchen G, et al: The determination of coronary flow equivalent with coincidence counting technic. *Circulation* 29:833-846, 1964

47. Schelbert HR, Wisenberg G, Phelps ME, et al: Noninvasive assessment of coronary stenoses by myocardial imaging during pharmacologic coronary vasodilation. VI. Detection of coronary artery disease in human beings with intravenous N-13 ammonia and positron computed tomography. *Am J Cardiol* 49:1197-1207, 1982

48. Tamaki N, Yonekura Y, Senda M, et al: Myocardial positron computed tomography with ^{13}N-ammonia at rest and during exercise. *Eur J Nucl Med* 11:246-251, 1985

49. Demer LL, Gould KL, Goldstein RA, et al: Assessment of coronary artery disease severity by positron emission tomography: comparison with quantitative arteriography in 193 patients. *Circulation* 79:825-835, 1989

50. Knabb RM, Fox KAA, Sobel BE, et al: Characterization of the functional significance of subcritical coronary stenoses with $H_2{}^{15}O$ and positron-emission tomography. *Circulation* 71:1271-1278, 1985

51. Shelton ME, Green MA, Mathias CJ, et al: Kinetics of copper-PTSM in isolated hearts: a novel tracer for measuring blood flow with positron emission tomography. *J Nucl Med* 30:1843-1847, 1989

52. Tamaki N, Yonekura Y, Senda M, et al: Value and limitation of stress thallium-201 single photon emission computed tomography: comparison with nitrogen-13 ammonia positron tomography. *J Nucl Med* 29:1181-1188, 1988

53. Go RT, Marwick TH, MacIntyre WJ, et al: A prospective comparison of rubidium-82 PET and thallium-201 SPECT myocardial perfusion imaging utilizing a single dipyridamole stress in the diagnosis of coronary artery disease. *J Nucl Med* 31:1899-1905, 1990

54. Marwick TH, Go RT, MacIntyre WJ, et al: Myocardial perfusion imaging with positron emission tomography and single photon emission computed tomography: frequency and causes of disparate results. *Eur Heart J* 12:1064-1069, 1991

55. Stewart RE, Schwaiger M, Molina E, et al: Comparison of rubidium-82 positron emission tomography and thallium-201 SPECT imaging for detection of coronary artery disease. *Am J Cardiol* 67:1303-1310, 1991

56. Bonow RO, Berman DS, Gibbons RJ, et al: Cardiac positron emission tomography: a report for health professionals from the Committee on Advanced Cardiac Imaging and Technology of the Council on Clinical Cardiology, American Heart Association. *Circulation* 84:447-454, 1991

57. Krivokapich J, Stevenson LW, Kobashigawa J, et al: Quantification of absolute myocardial perfusion at rest and during exercise with positron emission tomography after human cardiac transplantation. *J Am Coll Cardiol* 18:512-517, 1991

58. Geltman EM, Henes G, Senneff MJ, et al: Increased myocardial perfusion at rest and diminished perfusion reserve in patients with angina and angiographically normal coronary arteries. *J Am Coll Cardiol* 16:586-595, 1991

59. Walsh MN, Bergmann SR, Steele RL, et al: Delineation of impaired regional myocardial perfusion by positron emission tomography with $H_2{}^{15}O$. *Circulation* 78:612-620, 1988

60. Camici P, Ferrannini E, Opie LH: Myocardial metabolism in ischemic heart disease: basic principles and application to imaging by positron emission tomography. *Prog Cardiovasc Dis* 32:217-238, 1989

61. Stremmel W: Fatty acid uptake by isolated rat heart myocytes represents a carrier-mediated transport process. *J Clin Invest* 81:844-852, 1988

62. Lopaschuk GD, Spafford MA, Davies NJ, et al: Glucose and palmitate oxidation in isolated working rat hearts reperfused following a period of transient global ischemia. *Circ Res* 66:546-553, 1990

63. Schelbert HR, Buxton D: Insights into coronary artery disease gained from metabolic imaging. *Circulation* 78:496-505, 1988

64. Hoffman EJ, Phelps ME, Weiss ES, et al: Transaxial tomographic

imaging of canine myocardium with ^{11}C-palmitate acid. *J Nucl Med* 18:57-61, 1977

65. Weiss ES, Hoffman EJ, Phelps ME, et al: External detection and visualization of myocardial ischemia with ^{11}C-substrates in vitro and in vivo. *Circ Res* 39:24-32, 1976

66. Schön HR, Schelbert HR, Robinson G, et al: C-11 labeled palmitic acid for the noninvasive evaluation of regional myocardial fatty acid metabolism with positron-computed tomography. I. Kinetics of C-11 palmitic acid in normal myocardium. *Am Heart J* 103:532-547, 1982

67. Schön HR, Schelbert HR, Najafi A, et al: C-11 labeled palmitic acid for the noninvasive evaluation of regional myocardial fatty acid metabolism with positron-computed tomography. II. Kinetics of C-11 palmitic acid in acutely ischemic myocardium. *Am Heart J* 103:548-561, 1982

68. Schelbert HR, Henze E, Schön HR, et al: C-11 palmitate for the noninvasive evaluation of regional myocardial fatty acid metabolism with positron computed tomography. III. In vivo demonstration of the effects of substrate availability on myocardial metabolism. *Am Heart J* 105:492-504, 1983

69. Schelbert HR, Henze E, Keen R, et al: C-11 palmitate for the noninvasive evaluation of regional myocardial fatty acid metabolism with positron-computed tomography. IV. In vivo evaluation of acute demand-induced ischemia in dogs. *Am Heart J* 106:736-750, 1983

70. Lerch RA, Ambos HD, Bergmann SR, et al: Localization of viable, ischemic myocardium by positron-emission tomography with ^{11}C-palmitate. *Circulation* 64:689-699, 1981

71. Schwaiger M, Schelbert HR, Keen R, et al: Retention and clearance of C-11 palmitic acid in ischemic and reperfused canine myocardium. *J Am Coll Cardiol* 6:311-320, 1985

72. Schwaiger M, Schelbert HR, Ellison D, et al: Sustained regional abnormalities in cardiac metabolism after transient ischemia in the chronic dog model. *J Am Coll Cardiol* 6:336-347, 1985

73. Schwaiger M, Fishbein MC, Block M, et al: Metabolic and ultrastructural abnormalities during ischemia in canine myocardium: noninvasive assessment by positron emission tomography. *J Mol Cell Cardiol* 19:259-269, 1987

74. Sochor H, Schelbert HR, Schwaiger M, et al: Studies of fatty acid metabolism with positron emission tomography in patients with cardiomyopathy. *Eur J Nucl Med* 12 Suppl: S66-S69, 1986

75. Eisenberg JD, Sobel BE, Geltman EM: Differentiation of ischemic from nonischemic cardiomyopathy with positron emission tomography. *Am J Cardiol* 59:1410-1414, 1987

76. Jaffe AS, Biello DR, Sobel BE, et al: Enhancement of metabolism of jeopardized myocardium by nifedipine. *Int J Cardiol* 15:77-89, 1987

77. Rosamond TL, Abendschein DR, Sobel BE, et al: Metabolic fate of radiolabeled palmitate in ischemic canine myocardium: implications for positron emission tomography. *J Nucl Med* 28:1322-1329, 1987

78. Sokoloff L, Reivich M, Kennedy C, et al: The [^{14}C] deoxyglucose method for the measurement of local cerebral glucose utilization: theory, procedure, and normal values in the conscious and anesthetized albino rat. *J Neurochem* 28:897-916, 1977

79. Phelps ME, Hoffman EJ, Selin C, et al: Investigation of [^{18}F]2-fluoro-2-deoxyglucose for the measure of myocardial glucose metabolism. *J Nucl Med* 19:1311-1319, 1978

80. Krivokapich J, Huang S-C, Phelps ME, et al: Estimation of rabbit myocardial metabolic rate for glucose using fluorodeoxyglucose. *Am J Physiol* 243:H884-H895, 1982

81. Ratib O, Phelps ME, Huang S-C, et al: Positron tomography with deoxyglucose for estimating local myocardial glucose metabolism. *J Nucl Med* 23:577-586, 1982

82. Marshall RC, Tillisch JH, Phelps ME, et al: Identification and differentiation of resting myocardial ischemia and infarction in man with positron computed tomography, ^{18}F-labeled fluorodeoxyglucose and N-13 ammonia. *Circulation* 67:766-778, 1983

83. Brunken R, Tillisch J, Schwaiger M, et al: Regional perfusion, glucose metabolism, and wall motion in patients with chronic electrocardiographic Q wave infarctions: evidence for persistence of viable tissue in some infarct regions by positron emission tomography. *Circulation* 73:951-963, 1986

84. Fudo T, Kambara H, Hashimoto T, et al: F-18 deoxyglucose and stress N-13 ammonia positron emission tomography in anterior wall healed myocardial infarction. *Am J Cardiol* 61:1191-1197, 1988

85. Tillisch J, Brunken R, Marshall R, et al: Reversibility of cardiac wall-motion abnormalities predicted by positron tomography. *N Engl J Med* 314:884-888, 1986

86. Tamaki N, Yonekura Y, Yamashita K, et al: Positron emission tomography using fluorine-18 deoxyglucose in evaluation of coronary artery bypass grafting. *Am J Cardiol* 64:860-865, 1989

87. Schwaiger M, Brunken RC, Krivokapich J, et al: Beneficial effect of residual anterograde flow on tissue viability as assessed by positron emission tomography in patients with myocardial infarction. *Eur Heart J* 8:981-988, 1987

88. Merhige ME, Ekas R, Mossberg K, et al: Catecholamine stimulation, substrate competition, and myocardial glucose uptake in conscious dogs assessed with positron emission tomography. *Circ Res* 61 Suppl 2:124-129, 1987

89. Camici P, Araujo LI, Spinks T, et al: Increased uptake of ^{18}F-fluorodeoxyglucose in postischemic myocardium of patients with exercise-induced angina. *Circulation* 74:81-88, 1986

90. Nienaber CA, Brunken RC, Sherman CT, et al: Metabolic and functional recovery of ischemic human myocardium after coronary angioplasty. *J Am Coll Cardiol* 18:966-978, 1991

91. Rozanski A, Berman DS, Gray R, et al: Use of thallium-201 redistribution scintigraphy in the preoperative differentiation of reversible and nonreversible myocardial asynergy. *Circulation* 64:936-944, 1981

92. Liu P, Kiess MC, Okada RD, et al: The persistent defect on exercise thallium imaging and its fate after myocardial revascularization: Does it represent scar or ischemia? *Am Heart J* 110:996-1001, 1985

93. Brunken R, Schwaiger M, Grover-McKay M, et al: Positron emission tomography detects tissue metabolic activity in myocardial segments with persistent thallium perfusion defects. *J Am Coll Cardiol* 10:557-567, 1987

94. Bonow RO, Dilsizian V, Cuocolo A, et al: Identification of viable myocardium in patients with chronic coronary artery disease and left ventricular dysfunction: comparison of thallium scintigraphy with reinjection and PET imaging with ^{18}F-fluorodeoxyglucose. *Circulation* 83:26-37, 1991

95. Dilsizian V, Rocco TP, Freedman NMT, et al: Enhanced detection of ischemic but viable myocardium by the reinjection of thallium after stress-redistribution imaging. *N Engl J Med* 323:141-146, 1990

96. Dilsizian V, Freedman NMT, Bacharach SL, et al: Regional thallium uptake in irreversible defects: magnitude of change in thallium activity after reinjection distinguishes viable from nonviable myocardium. *Circulation* 85:627-634, 1992

97. Dilsizian V, Bonow RO: Differential uptake and apparent ^{201}Tl washout after thallium reinjection: options regarding early redistribution imaging before reinjection or late redistribution imaging after reinjection. *Circulation* 85:1032-1038, 1992

98. Piérard LA, De Landsheere CM, Berthe C, et al: Identification of viable myocardium by echocardiography during dobutamine infusion in patients with myocardial infarction after thrombolytic therapy: comparison with positron emission tomography. *J Am Coll Cardiol* 15:1021-1031, 1990

99. Brown M, Marshall DR, Sobel BE, et al: Delineation of myocardial oxygen utilization with carbon-11-labeled acetate. *Circulation* 76:687-696, 1987

100. Brown MA, Myears DW, Bergmann SR: Noninvasive assessment of canine myocardial oxidative metabolism with carbon-11 acetate and positron emission tomography. *J Am Coll Cardiol* 12:1054-1063, 1988

101. Buxton DB, Schwaiger M, Nguyen A, et al: Radiolabeled acetate as a tracer of myocardial tricarboxylic acid cycle flux. *Circ Res* 63:628-634, 1988

102. Armbrecht JJ, Buxton DB, Brunken RC, et al: Regional myocardial oxygen consumption determined noninvasively in humans with (1-^{11}C)acetate and dynamic positron tomography. *Circulation* 80:863-872, 1989

103. Armbrecht JJ, Buxton DB, Schelbert HR: Validation of (1-^{11}C)acetate as a tracer for noninvasive assessment of oxidative metabolism with positron emission tomography in normal, ischemic, postischemic, and hyperemic canine myocardium. *Circulation* 81:1594-1605, 1990

104. Buck A, Wolpers HG, Hutchins GD, et al: Effect of carbon-11-acetate recirculation on estimates of myocardial oxygen consumption by PET. *J Nucl Med* 32:1950-1957, 1991

CHAPTER

10

Cardiac catheterization and angiography

A. Coronary arteriography

Malcolm R. Bell, M.B., B.S., Hugh C. Smith, M.D., and Guy S. Reeder, M.D.

HISTORICAL PERSPECTIVE

The first selective coronary arteriogram in a human was performed in 1959 by F. Mason Sones.[1] In the prior 15 years, nonselective coronary visualization during retrograde aortography had been attempted with use of pharmacologic and mechanical interventions designed to provide a satisfactory concentration of dye entering the coronary ostia, but the images of the coronary circulation lacked sufficient detail and resolution to be reliable. Utilizing a brachial arteriotomy and a catheter designed to engage the coronary ostia, Sones and Shirey[2] had performed and reported on 1,000 cases by 1962. From 1962 to 1969, Ricketts and Abrams,[3] Judkins,[4] Amplatz et al.,[5] and Bourassa et al.[6] developed, refined, and reported femoral percutaneous methods of coronary arteriography, the most commonly utilized approach today.

Along with accurate delineation of coronary anatomy came the evolution of coronary artery bypass surgery. In 1962, Vineberg[7] reported internal mammary artery myocardial implants and demonstrated collateral filling to diseased vessels. Favaloro[8] is generally credited with performing the first large series of saphenous vein bypass graft operations five years later, in 1967. (The first saphenous vein bypass graft was performed in 1964 by Dr. Edward Garrett.) Over the ensuing years, rapid advances in scientific and clinical knowledge about coronary artery disease—its pathogenesis, detection, and therapy—have occurred. Thus, a thorough understanding of coronary arteriography is essential in today's practice of cardiology.

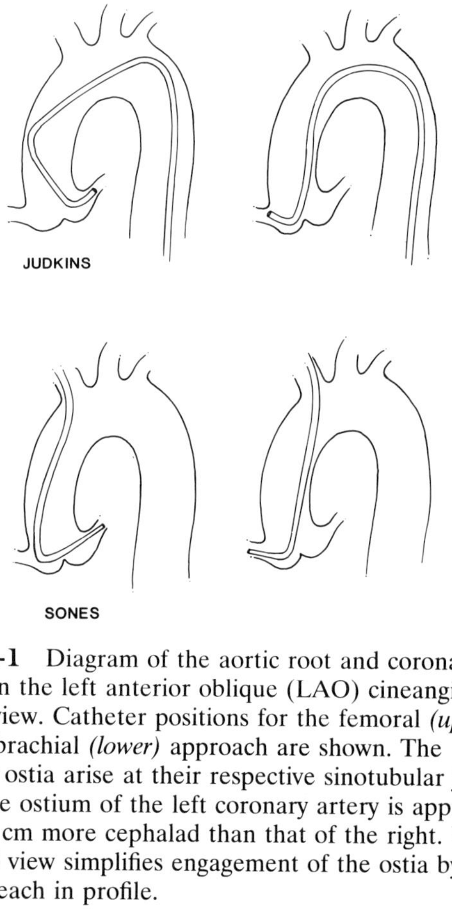

Fig 10A-1 Diagram of the aortic root and coronary ostia as seen in the left anterior oblique (LAO) cineangiographic view. Catheter positions for the femoral *(upper)* and the brachial *(lower)* approach are shown. The coronary ostia arise at their respective sinotubular junctions. The ostium of the left coronary artery is approximately 1 cm more cephalad than that of the right. Use of the LAO view simplifies engagement of the ostia by showing each in profile.

CORONARY ARTERY ANATOMY

The following is a description of coronary artery anatomy as it pertains to angiography. For a more detailed anatomic description, the reader is referred to several excellent sources.[9-11]

The coronary ostia are usually located at the junction of the sinus of Valsalva with the ascending aorta (sinotubular junction). Because of the oblique orientation of the ascending aorta in the chest, the right sinotubular junction lies about 1 cm more caudal than the left (Fig 10A-1). In the left anterior oblique (LAO) view, the left coronary ostium is rightward and slightly superior, and the right coronary ostium is leftward and inferior. Use of this radiographic position simplifies selective engagement of the ostia by presenting them in full profile from the aorta.

The left coronary artery originates as the left main segment. The left main vessel is usually large (5 to 10 mm in diameter), is of variable length (up to 4 cm long), and is buried in epicardial fat as it passes behind the pulmonary trunk and under the left atrial appendage. Before reaching the anterior interventricular groove, the left main segment gives rise to the left anterior descending (LAD) and circumflex arteries. Although often termed a "bifurcation," the termination of the left main artery is sometimes seen as a trifurcation; the third vessel is an intermediate one with the course of an obtuse marginal artery.

The LAD follows the anterior interventricular sulcus, passes around the cardiac apex, and ascends along the posterior interventricular sulcus a variable distance; its terminal branches anastomose with those of the posterior descending branch of the right coronary artery. Septal perforating branches serve the anterior two-thirds and the apical inferior portions of the ventricular septum. These features usually make angiographic identification of the LAD straightforward. Occasionally, identification may be more difficult if the LAD terminates before reaching the apex (usually associated with a large diagonal vessel or unusually large posterior descending branch) or major septal perforators arise from a diagonal branch (uncommon). Besides perforating branches, the LAD supplies vessels to the free surfaces of both ventricles. The right ventricular branches are small and form an anastomotic network with similar branches from the proximal right coronary artery. The left ventricular branches of the LAD course along the anterolateral free wall of the left ventricle in a diagonal fashion—hence, their name, diagonals. Usually, two major diagonals are present, although occasionally a number of smaller vessels may be seen.

The circumflex coronary artery arises from the left main artery at an acute angle, traveling in the epicardial fat beneath the left atrial appendage to its location in the left atrioventricular (AV) sulcus. Important branches include one to three obtuse marginals that supply the posterolateral left ventricular wall and the AV groove artery, which is the distal continuation of the circumflex. This artery is of variable length; in 90% of hearts, it reaches but does not pass the crux cordis. In 10% of hearts—those with so-called left dominant distribution—the AV groove branch is large and gives rise to posterolaterals and a left posterior descending branch. Coronary dominance is defined by the artery from which the posterior descending branch originates. Ninety percent of the time this is the right coronary artery.

The right coronary artery originates in the right sinus of Valsalva and follows the right AV sulcus around the acute margin of the heart, after which it bifurcates into its two distal branches, the posterior descending artery and the right posterolateral artery. The first branch of the right coronary artery is the conus artery; about 50% of the time this small vessel arises from a separate ostium rather than as a branch of the right coronary artery. This vessel is angiographically important for two reasons: first, in engaging the right coronary, the catheter may inadvertently enter the ostium of the conus artery; second, the conus artery may serve as an important collateral vessel to the LAD when the latter is occluded proximally. The second branch of the right coronary artery is often the artery to the sinoatrial node. This artery arises from the proximal right coronary artery 55% of the time and from the proximal circumflex artery 45% of the time. The acute marginal branches of the right coronary artery supply the right ventricular free wall and anastomose with similar small branches of the LAD. The posterior descending artery arises at an acute angle from the distal right coronary artery and follows the posterior interventricular sulcus toward the apex, where it anastomoses with the distal branches of the LAD. The posterolateral branch continues in the AV sulcus to the crux of the heart, where it has a characteristic inverted "U" shape seen in the LAO projection. At this point, the AV nodal artery may be seen as a small twig heading cephalad. The posterolateral artery usually terminates in two or three posterolateral branches, which course toward the cardiac apex. In a left-dominant circulation, the posterior descending and posterolateral vessels arise from the AV groove branch of the circumflex; the right coronary artery is then a small vessel that terminates at the acute margin of the heart (Fig 10A-2).

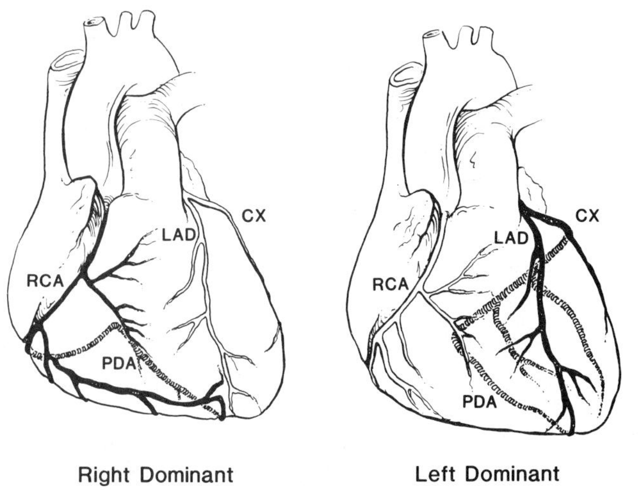

Fig 10A-2 Coronary artery dominance. Coronary dominance is defined by the coronary artery from which the posterior descending branch *(PDA)* arises. In right coronary dominance, the posterior descending branch arises from the right coronary artery *(RCA)*. In left dominance, the right coronary artery is a diminutive vessel, and the posterior descending artery arises as a continuation of the left atrioventricular groove artery, a branch of the circumflex *(CX)* system. *LAD,* left anterior descending artery.

The venous drainage of the heart is provided by three systems: (1) tiny thebesian veins, which empty directly into the underlying cardiac chamber (the total flow is minimal); (2) anterior cardiac veins, which drain the right ventricle (these originate on the anterior surface of the heart and drain into the right atrium); and (3) the coronary sinus and its tributaries, which arise on the surface of the left ventricle, generally in parallel to the coronary arterial branches. The anterior intraventricular branch parallels the LAD, becoming the great cardiac vein as it turns to enter the AV groove. It courses posteriorly to become the coronary sinus, which enters the right atrium adjacent to the tricuspid valve. Other branches include those from the lateral and anterior walls and the posterior interventricular branch, which runs parallel to the posterior descending artery.

Coronary artery anomalies

Coronary artery anomalies represent significant variations of normal coronary anatomy in terms of origin, distribution, and number of coronary arteries as well as coronary artery fistulae. The incidence of coronary artery anomalies from angiographic series ranges from 0.6% to 1.6%.[12] Most anomalies are noted as incidental findings during coronary angiography, and if they are not recognized, erroneous diagnoses of occluded vessels may be made. Less frequently, anomalies are associated with symptoms of angina, congestive heart failure, arrhythmias, myocardial infarction, syncope, or cardiac arrest.

The largest and one of the most complete series of coronary artery anomalies was reported by Yamanaka and Hobbs[12] from a total of 126,595 patients undergoing coronary angiography (Table 10A-1). The incidence of coronary artery anomalies in their series was 1.3%. Eighty-seven percent of the anomalies were associated with an abnormal origin and distribution of a coronary artery, and the remainder were associated with coronary artery fistulae.

Coronary anomalies are most usefully divided into those considered to be benign and those considered to be potentially serious or associated with symptoms. The vast majority of anomalies are considered to be benign. Separate "side-by-side" origins of the LAD and circumflex arteries occur in approximately 0.4% to 1.0% of hearts and may be associated with a bicuspid aortic valve. The ostia are usually adjacent to each other, and selective catheter engagement of one vessel generally fails to opacify the other. The distributions of the LAD and circumflex are otherwise normal. The next most frequent anomaly is the origin of the circumflex system from the right coronary sinus or proximal right coronary artery (Fig 10A-3). Although not a rare anomaly, it can be missed during routine angiography and result in nonvisualization of the circumflex system. The retroaortic course of the anomalous vessel may place it at risk for damage during aortic and mitral valve replacement if the surgeon is unaware of its presence.[13] Occasionally, the angiographer cannot engage either the left main coronary artery or the right coronary artery in the sinuses of Valsalva. When faced with this difficulty, one should immediately withdraw the catheter above the sinotubular junction to search for an aortic origin of these vessels. A far rarer form of

Table 10A-1 Coronary artery anomalies among 126,595 angiograms

Type of anomaly	Incidence (%)	Anomalies (%)
Benign (80%)		
Separate, adjacent LAD and LCx ostia	0.41	30.4
LCx origin from RSV or RCA	0.37	27.7
Anomalous origin from PSV	0.004	0.3
Anomalous origin from aorta		
LMCA	0.01	1.0
RCA	0.15	11.2
Absent LCx	0.003	0.2
Small fistulae	0.12	9.7
Potentially serious (20%)		
Origin of coronary artery from opposite aortic sinus		
LMCA from RSV	0.02	1.3
LAD from RSV	0.03	2.3
RCA from LSV	0.11	8.1
Anomalous origin from pulmonary artery		
LMCA	0.008	0.6
LAD or RCA	0.003	0.2
Single coronary artery	0.05	3.3
Multiple or large coronary fistulae	0.05	3.7

LAD, left anterior descending; LCx, left circumflex; LMCA, left main coronary artery; LSV, left sinus of Valsalva; PSV, posterior sinus of Valsalva; RCA, right coronary artery; RSV, right sinus of Valsalva.
Modified from Yamanaka O, Hobbs RE: Coronary artery anomalies in 126,595 patients undergoing coronary arteriography. *Cathet Cardiovasc Diagn* 21:28-40, 1990.

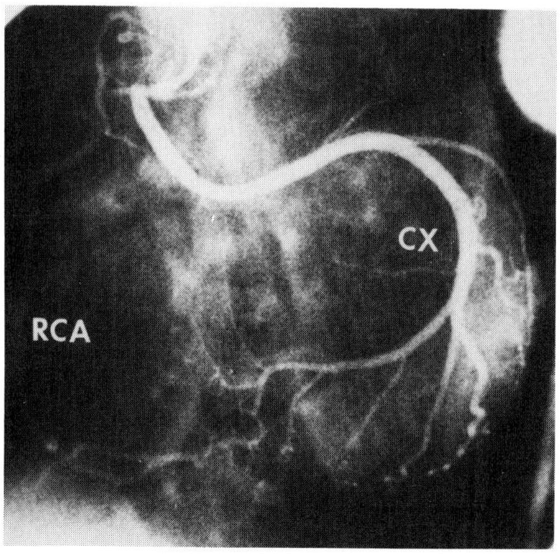

Fig 10A-3 Anomalous origin of the circumflex coronary artery *(CX)* from the right coronary artery *(RCA)*. This anomaly occurs in 0.5% of cases. The circumflex branch arises from or near the ostium of the right coronary artery and courses posteriorly to supply the obtuse margin of the heart.

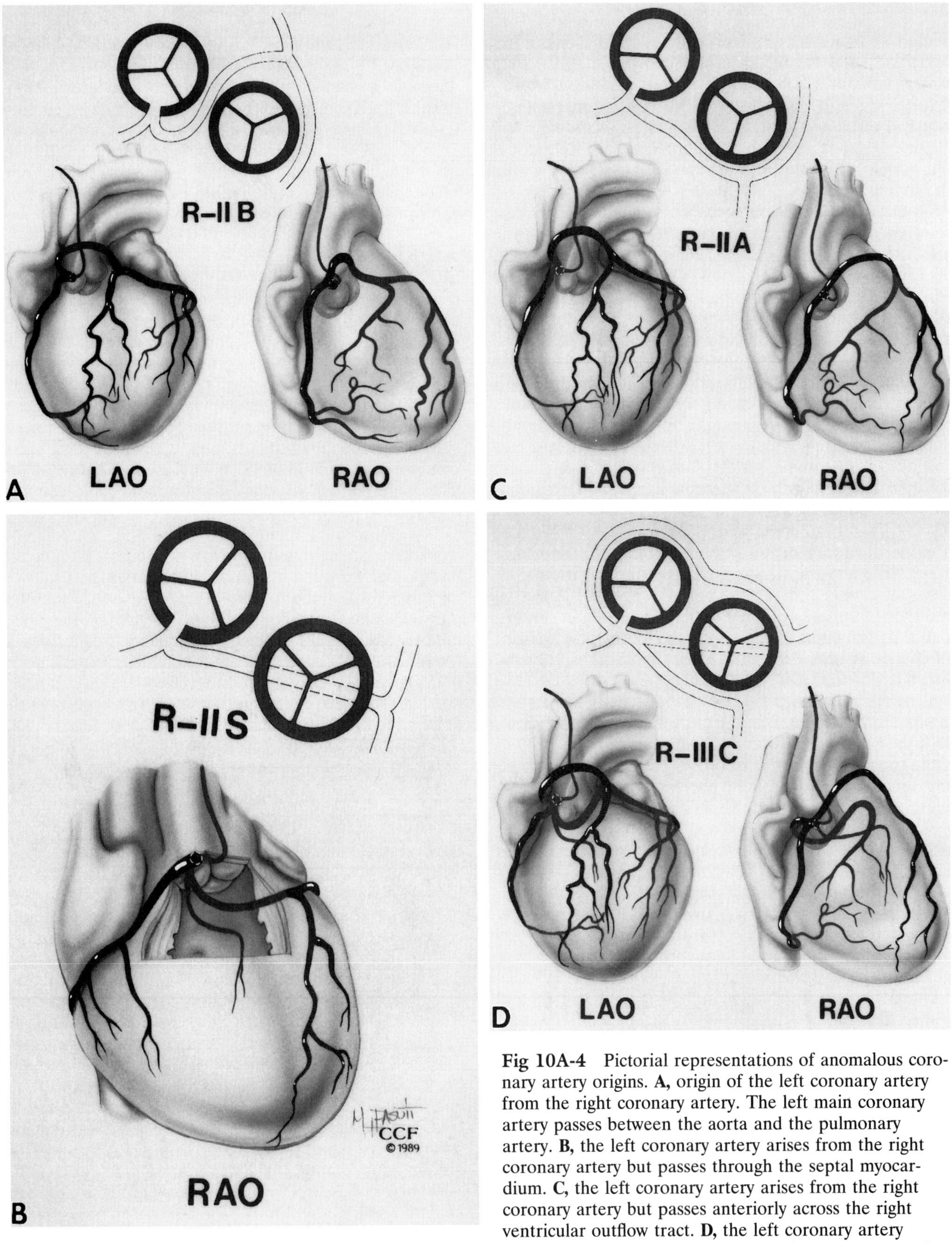

Fig 10A-4 Pictorial representations of anomalous coronary artery origins. **A,** origin of the left coronary artery from the right coronary artery. The left main coronary artery passes between the aorta and the pulmonary artery. **B,** the left coronary artery arises from the right coronary artery but passes through the septal myocardium. **C,** the left coronary artery arises from the right coronary artery but passes anteriorly across the right ventricular outflow tract. **D,** the left coronary artery arises from the right coronary artery but passes posteriorly behind the aorta. (From Yamanaka O, Hobbs RE: Coronary artery anomalies in 126,595 patients undergoing coronary arteriography. *Cathet Cardiovasc Diagn* 21:28-40, 1990. By permission of Cleveland Clinic Foundation.)

benign anomaly is complete absence of the circumflex vessel with the entire posterolateral wall supplied by a superdominant right coronary artery. Small coronary fistulae are also considered to be benign anomalies.[12] None of the above-described anomalies, including small fistulae, requires any specific therapy unless it is clear that the patient has symptoms attributable to disease within the vessels.

Of the more significant coronary anomalies,[12] the most common are related to coronary artery origins from the opposite aortic sinus, such as the left main coronary artery or LAD from the right sinus of Valsalva or the right coronary artery from the left sinus of Valsalva (Fig 10A-4). For these anomalies, it is important to be able to define how the course of the anomalous vessel is related to the aorta and pulmonary artery and whether the course is "septal" (intramyocardial). A "septal" course of the left main coronary artery after its origin from the right sinus of Valsalva is the most common variation but generally does not cause any symptoms if atherosclerotic disease is absent. In the more serious variation, the left main coronary artery passes between the aorta and the pulmonary artery, and the result may be symptoms of angina or myocardial infarction as well as ventricular arrhythmias, syncope, or sudden death. If the left main coronary artery passes anterior or posterior to the great vessels, symptoms generally do not occur.

Origin of the right coronary artery from the left sinus of Valsalva, the most common of the potentially serious anomalies involving origin of a coronary artery from the opposite aortic sinus, is potentially very serious because the artery almost invariably passes between the aorta and the pulmonary artery, and symptoms similar to those described above can occur. If symptoms are associated with the more serious forms or if perfusion abnormalities are detected on subsequent nuclear scintigraphic stress tests, surgical correction is indicated. In tetralogy of Fallot, the LAD originates from the right coronary sinus in 4% of cases.[14] Preoperative knowledge of this condition is important to prevent inadvertent transection of this vessel at the time of surgical repair.

Origin of a coronary artery from the pulmonary artery is a very serious problem but is only rarely seen. In this situation, flow is antegrade in the normal coronary vessel, and after the vessel communicates by way of collaterals, flow appears to be retrograde in the anomalous vessel and is seen to drain into the pulmonary artery. Consequently, left-to-right shunting is present. The anomalous vessel is usually the left main coronary artery, but in rare cases, it can be the LAD alone or the right coronary artery. Symptoms of angina, heart failure, or acute myocardial infarction are usually associated with this condition.[15] Ninety percent of patients with this condition die during infancy, so that this finding is very rare during adult coronary angiography. Multiple surgical approaches to treat this condition have been tried; most involve either ligation and bypass grafting of this vessel or reanastomosis of the anomalous vessel to the aorta or subclavian artery.

Identification of the course of anomalous coronary arteries during angiography is often very difficult. However, with careful examination in the right anterior oblique (RAO) and LAO views, often combined with ventriculography in the RAO projection, the course of most anomalous vessels can be determined accurately. Angiographic and pictorial representations of the most common anomalies have been well illustrated by Yamanaka and Hobbs.[12] When angiographic interpretation is problematic, alternative imaging techniques, such as magnetic resonance imaging and electron beam computed tomography, have been helpful.

Coronary artery bridging

The major coronary arteries and their branches are epicardial in location, usually buried in the epicardial fat. Occasionally, a coronary segment will take an intramyocardial course for several centimeters. Less commonly, aberrant epicardial muscle fibers may "bridge" over the vessel and tether it to the cardiac surface. In either case, contraction of the myocardium produces a transient systolic narrowing of the bridged segment. It occurs most commonly in the middle portion of the LAD (Fig 10A-5). The angiographic incidence of bridging has been estimated at 0.5% to 0.9%.[16,17]

The significance of myocardial bridging remains controversial. Some investigators have found evidence of myocardial ischemia in symptomatic patients with bridging but no associated coronary artery disease[16,18] who had improvement after surgical correction. Others have been unable to document evidence of ischemia.[17] Since flow in the left coronary artery is a predominantly diastolic event, one logically might expect little effect from a transient systolic reduction in lumen diameter, and, clinically, this appears to be the usual case. However, with long bridged segments and severe systolic compromise (>75%), the possibility of ischemia should be considered.

Coronary artery collaterals

Intercoronary arterial anastomoses exist in normal hearts from birth and commonly reach sizes of 200 to 300 μm in luminal diameter,[19] which is within the range of resolution of coronary arteriography. However, these collateral vessels are virtually never seen angiographically unless high-grade arterial obstructions are present. Collaterals may enlarge greatly after occlusion or high-grade stenosis of a coronary artery, often reaching 1 to 2 mm in diameter. Epicardial, intramyocardial, and subendocardial anastomotic networks occur. Clinically important and commonly observed collaterals occur between the distal LAD and distal posterior descending arteries, right posterolateral and distal left circumflex arteries, septal perforators of the LAD and posterior descending arteries, conus branch of the right coronary artery and proximal LAD, and communications among diagonals, marginals, and LAD. Although all hearts possess a collateral anastomotic network, the degree to which the coronary collateral circulation develops and its physiologic protective role may vary from one heart to another, even though similar degrees of coronary atherosclerosis are present. Clinical studies[20-24] have provided evidence that, at least in some patients, angiographically definable collaterals are asso-

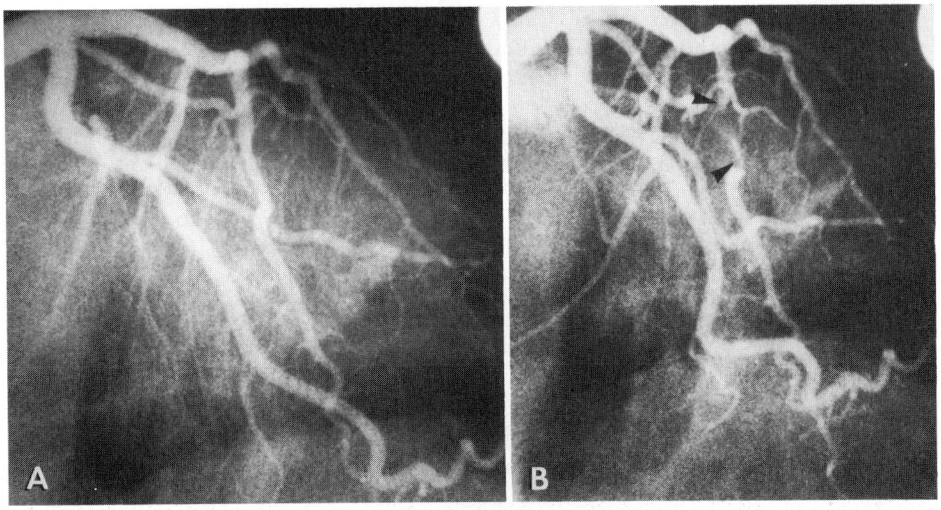

Fig 10A-5 Coronary artery bridging. **A,** RAO view of the left coronary artery in diastole. The LAD is only minimally narrowed. **B,** systolic frame showing obliteration of the middle LAD *(arrows)* due to muscular bridging.

ciated with preservation of regional wall motion, less histologic fibrosis, a lower incidence of transmural infarction, and less evidence of exercise-induced ischemia. Other patients have extensive myocardial damage despite angiographically demonstrable collateral vessels.

Unfortunately, studies of the clinical importance of collaterals have been hampered by the fact that the vast majority of human collaterals are subendocardial and are beyond the resolution of modern angiographic imaging (<100 μm). For this reason, the true importance of coronary collaterals remains speculative in many instances. Recently, myocardial contrast echocardiography has been advocated as a useful technique to measure and assess the functional significance of collaterals. This technique involves intracoronary injections of sonicated contrast material and mapping of the area of perfusion with two-dimensional echocardiography. Its applicability to assessing the functional significance of collaterals in patients with myocardial infarction appears promising.[25,26]

Coronary nomenclature

Several systems of coronary artery nomenclature exist; our system (virtually identical to that used by the multicenter Coronary Artery Surgery Study—CASS[27]) is demonstrated in Figure 10A-6. The left coronary artery segments consist of the left main, proximal LAD (up to the first septal perforator), middle LAD (first septal to second diagonal), distal LAD, first and second diagonals, proximal circumflex (to the first marginal vessel), distal circumflex, AV groove branch, and one to three marginal vessels. The right coronary segments include proximal (to the first acute marginal branch), middle (to the acute margin), and distal (to the bifurcation of the posterior descending and posterolateral arteries). The use of this type of standardized nomenclature facilitates film interpretation, computer coding, and data storage.

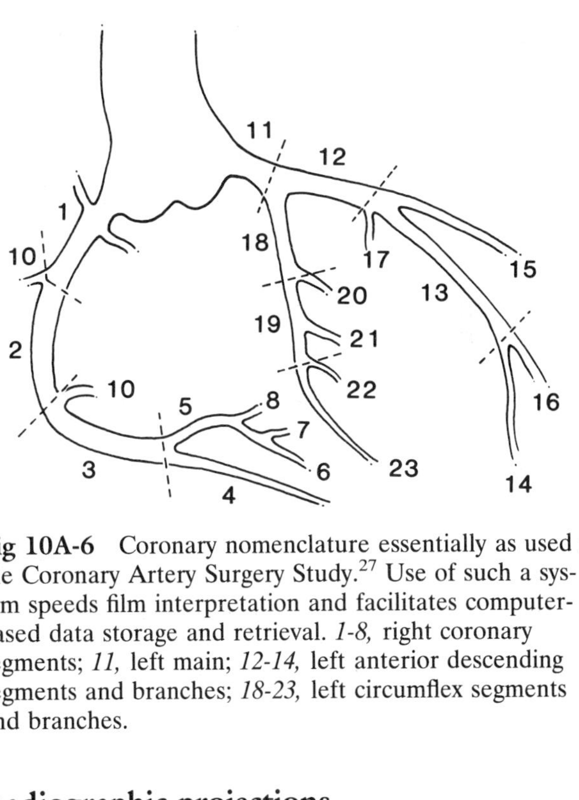

Fig 10A-6 Coronary nomenclature essentially as used in the Coronary Artery Surgery Study.[27] Use of such a system speeds film interpretation and facilitates computer-based data storage and retrieval. *1-8,* right coronary segments; *11,* left main; *12-14,* left anterior descending segments and branches; *18-23,* left circumflex segments and branches.

Radiographic projections

Current cineangiographic techniques use two-dimensional images to display the three-dimensional anatomy of the coronary arteries. As a result, serious limitations may occur because of vessel superimposition, angular foreshortening, and misrepresentation of true luminal size due to eccentric lesions. To minimize these limitations, multiple views from a variety of angles are obtained to image each vessel as completely as possible. This requires not only RAO and LAO rotations but also hemiaxial cranial and caudal angulation of the x-ray beam to separate overlapping vessels and reduce errors due to foreshortening.[28-30] Each patient's anatomy is unique and requires individual attention to selection of optimal views (Fig 10A-7).

Left coronary artery. The LAO projection (see Fig 10A-7,A) allows interpretation of coronary dominance and offers good views of the middle and distal segments of the LAD and circumflex arteries. The proximal portions of these vessels lie obliquely in relation to the x-ray beam and are severely foreshortened in this view; with 25° to 30° of cranial angulation (see Fig 10A-7,B, cranial LAO), this problem is reduced and the proximal portions of these vessels and also the origin of the diagonals are well imaged. A steep (50° to 60°) LAO projection with

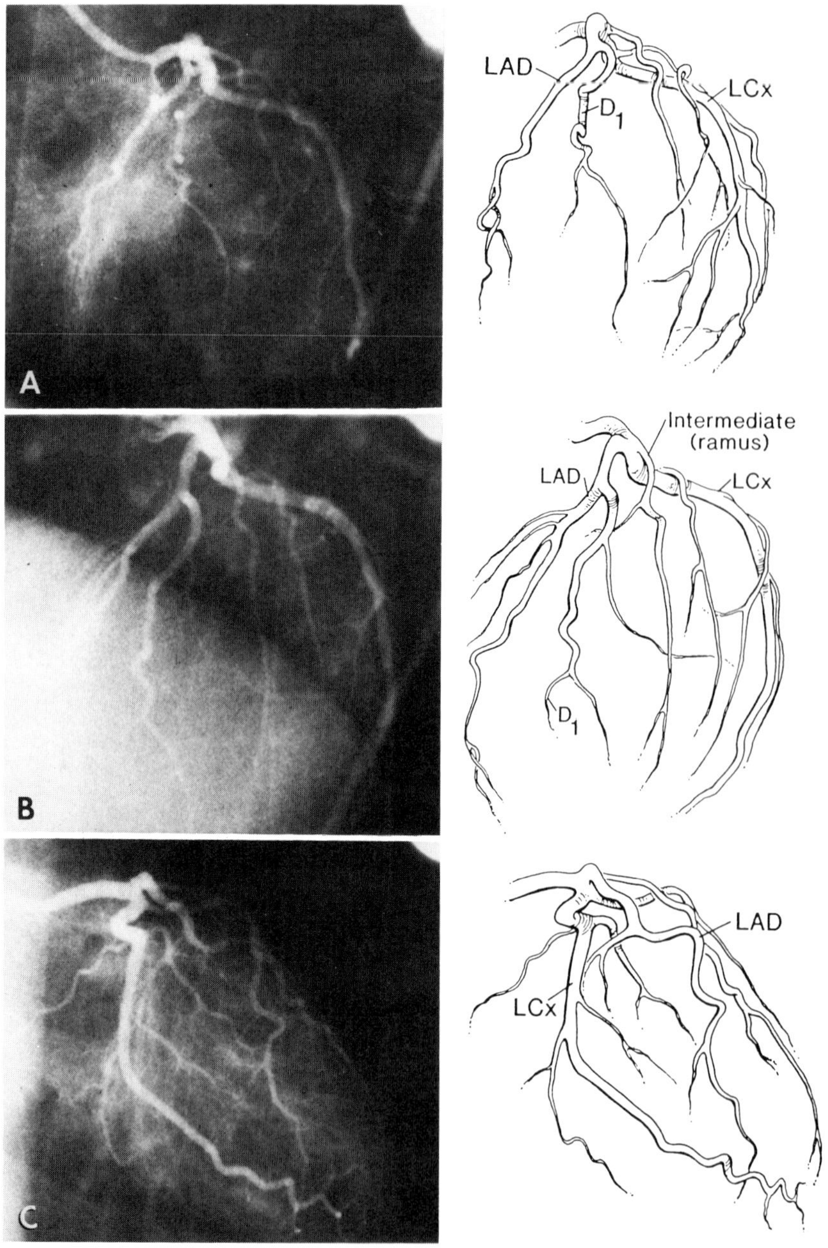

Fig 10A-7 Coronary projections. **A,** left coronary artery, LAO view. Coronary dominance is easily appreciated in this view. Proximal portions of the left coronary artery, including the origin of the diagonal vessels, are severely foreshortened, so lesions in this region may be missed. **B,** left coronary LAO view with cranial angulation. Addition of cranial angulation reduces foreshortening and allows excellent visualization of the proximal left anterior descending and diagonal vessels. **C,** left coronary artery, RAO projection. Portions of the left coronary artery and its branches are displayed in this view. Overlap among left anterior descending artery, diagonal branches, and obtuse marginal branches may cause masking of lesions in these vessels.

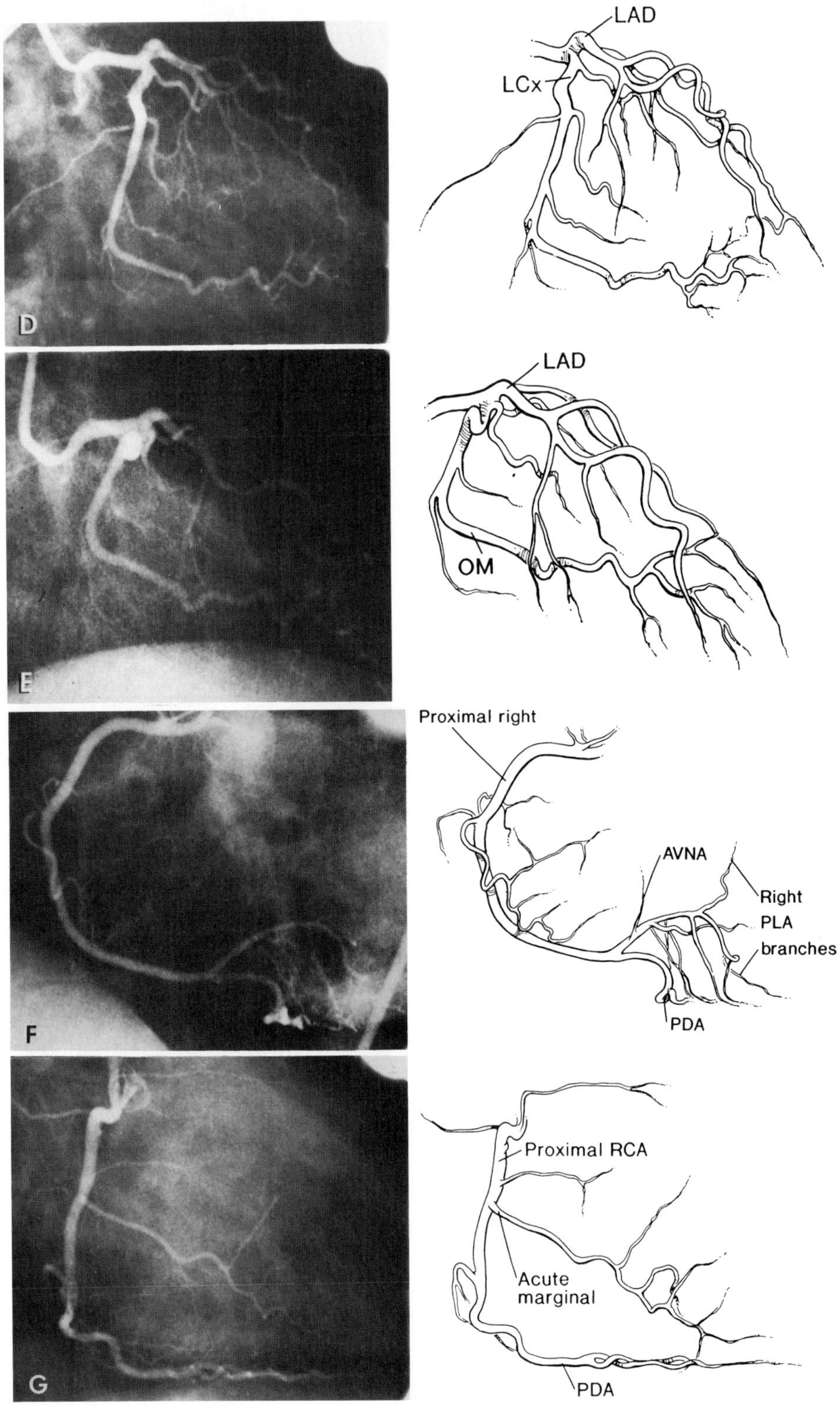

Fig 10A-7, cont'd **D,** left coronary artery on RAO view with caudal angulation. The proximal portion of the circumflex artery is less foreshortened in this view than in **C.** Superimposition of vessels may be reduced. **E,** left coronary artery, RAO view with cranial angulation. This view often shows the proximal and middle left anterior descending segments free of superimposition of diagonal and obtuse marginal branches. (With views **A-D** above, the left coronary system is usually optimally imaged.) **F,** right coronary artery, LAO projection. The course of the right coronary artery, including its termination in posterior descending and posterolateral branches, is easily seen in this view. **G,** right coronary artery, RAO projection. The proximal middle and distal portions of the right coronary artery are well seen, but the posterolateral and posterior descending branches show considerable overlap. Caudal or cranial angulation may be added to this view to separate branches further if there is a question of masking of lesions. *AVNA,* atrioventricular nodal artery; D_1, first diagonal; *LAD,* left anterior descending; *LCx,* left circumflex; *OM,* obtuse marginal; *PDA,* posterior descending artery; *PLA,* posterolateral artery; *RCA,* right coronary artery.

approximately 20° of caudal angulation often provides an excellent view of the left main coronary artery and its relation to the proximal segments of the LAD, circumflex, and intermediate vessels ("spider" view). The RAO projection (see Fig 10A-7,C) with 20° to 30° of caudal angulation (see Fig 10A-7,D) and approximately 25° of cranial angulation (see Fig 10A-7,E) usually affords complete visualization of the left coronary system and reduces problems of vessel overlap. In addition, the RAO caudal view is excellent for lesions involving the proximal circumflex artery. The RAO cranial view provides optimal visualization of the proximal LAD and diagonal vessels.

Right coronary artery. The right coronary artery and its branches are usually well visualized with LAO and RAO views (see Fig 10A-7,F and G). Again, individual differences in anatomy may require steeper or shallower rotation to ensure that the artery is not superimposed over the spine. Occasionally, caudally or cranially angled projections may be required for the best display of a lesion in the posterior descending and posterolateral arteries.

TECHNIQUES OF CORONARY ARTERIOGRAPHY

General requirements of the coronary arteriography laboratory

Specific standards of performance for laboratories performing coronary angiography have been recommended by the American College of Cardiology/American Heart Association task force on cardiac catheterization.[31] Reiteration of these recommendations is beyond the scope of this chapter; however, certain points deserve comment. Ideally, the laboratory should be specifically designed for performance of coronary arteriography. Ancillary support facilities such as a coronary care unit and the availability of cardiac surgery are highly desirable for greatest patient safety and urgent treatment of potential complications.

Recently, freestanding or mobile catheterization laboratories have rapidly proliferated. Although these are designed specifically for ambulatory care patients, good data on their overall performance and safety are not available. The American College of Cardiology/American Heart Association joint task force has declined to endorse such facilities until patient need and overall safety performance are demonstrated.[32]

X-ray equipment, probably the most expensive single component of the laboratory, should be designed specifically for high-quality coronary imaging and should have capabilities for angulated projections, simultaneous biplane angiography, and in-room television fluoroscopy replay (videotape or digital). To maintain standards of quality, daily testing of the x-ray generator, cine camera, and optical chain should be performed by photographing a calibrated test grid or phantom. Regular preventive maintenance to ensure quality images[33] and to minimize equipment downtime is important. Periodic inspection of the equipment by a radiation physicist for radiation leaks and daily wearing of radiation badges by physicians and staff are important to keep exposure below currently acceptable limits, 5 rem/year. Specific performance criteria should be optimized; they include input radiation dose

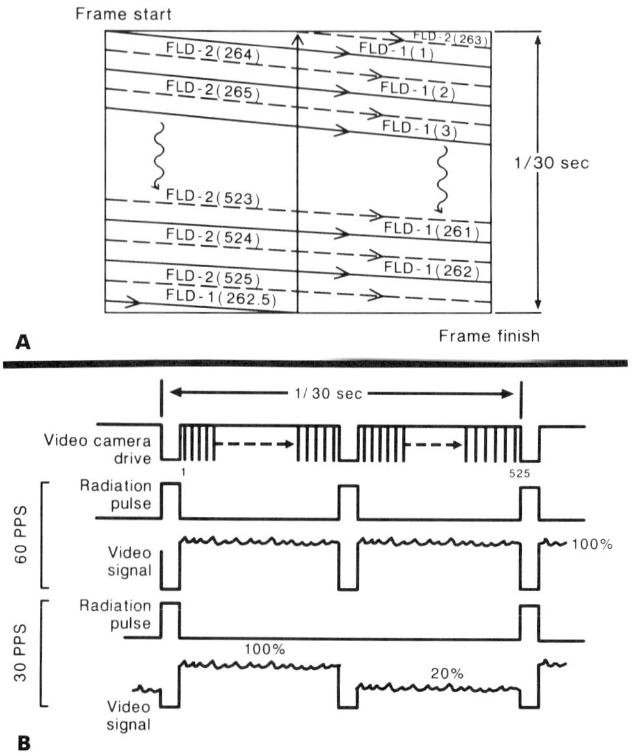

Fig 10A-8 Conventional interlaced scanning. **A,** a 525-line video frame is scanned from top to bottom in 1/30 sec. Each frame is composed of two fields, each containing 262.5 horizontal lines. The starting point for scanning is line 1 of field 1 (FLD-1[1]). The line scans from left to right on alternate lines until it reaches the middle of the image at the bottom (FLD-1[262.5]). The scan then shifts back to the middle of the image at the top (FLD-2[263]). For field 2, the remaining lines are scanned *(dashed lines)* to complete the frame. **B,** the radiation and video timing for interlaced scanning at 60 pps are shown in the second and third waveforms. If the radiation is pulsed at 30 pps (fourth waveform), image brightness is decreased. (From Holmes DR Jr, Bove AA, Wondrow MA, et al: Video x-ray progressive scanning: new technique for decreasing x-ray exposure without decreasing image quality during cardiac catheterization. *Mayo Clin Proc* 61:321-326, 1986. By permission, Mayo Foundation.)

to the input phosphor, cine and video spatial resolution, focal spot size, and automatic brightness control. Manually operated collimators should always be available.

High-quality fluoroscopic video images have assumed increasing importance in diagnostic and therapeutic catheterization. Along with the need for increased spatial and temporal resolution, limitation of radiation to the patient and laboratory staff is desirable. These somewhat disparate goals are achievable with pulsed-progressive scanning[34] (Fig 10A-8 and 10A-9). There are several advantages to this system. First, the high-definition images are flicker-free on replay, even though recorded at 30 frames per second. Second, because each image is progressively scanned rather than interlaced, no blurring of rapidly moving objects is seen on freeze-frame stop action. Third, because the x-ray pulses only once instead of twice each 1/30 of a second, radiation doses and exposure are cut by 50%. Image clarity is enhanced, and signal-to-noise ratio is improved over conventional video. Figure 10A-10 shows a schematic drawing of the progressive biplane video imaging system currently in use in our catheterization laboratory. Figure 10A-11 shows the improvement in stop-frame images obtained with progressive scanning compared with conventional interlaced scanning.

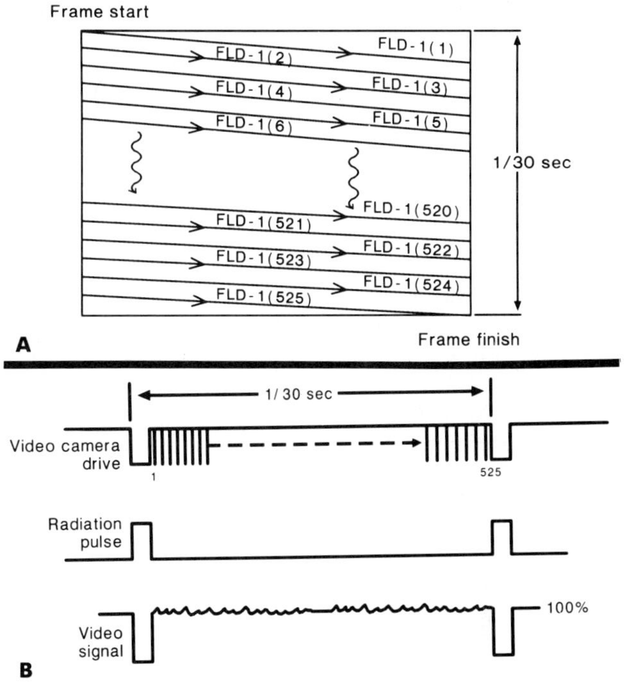

Fig 10A-9 Progressive video scanning. The entire field is scanned in 1/30 sec. **A,** each frame is composed of a single scan (field). **B,** radiation can be pulsed at 30 pps with no degradation in image quality. (From Holmes DR Jr, Bove AA, Wondrow MA, et al: Video x-ray progressive scanning: new technique for decreasing x-ray exposure without decreasing image quality during cardiac catheterization. *Mayo Clin Proc* 61:321-326, 1986. By permission, Mayo Foundation.)

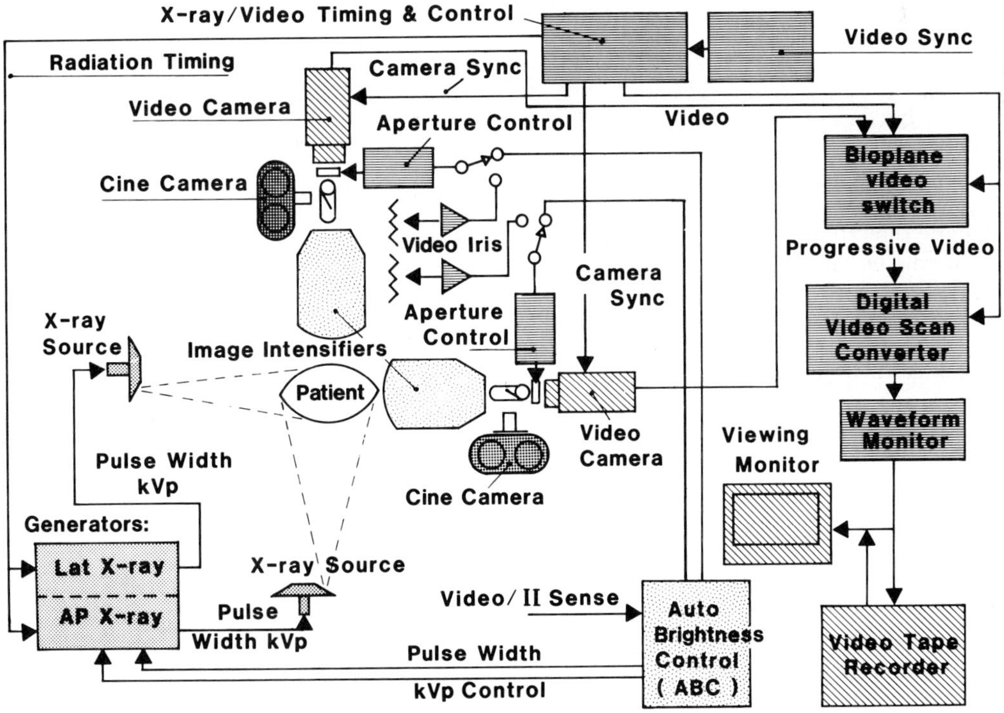

Fig 10A-10 Block diagram of a cardiac-biplane video/cine imaging system. A common video-synchronizing generator drives a timing-and-control device. This is necessary to achieve synchronization and also is essential for progressive scanning. (From Julsrud PR, Wondrow MA, Stears JG, et al: X-ray equipment. In *Interventional Cardiology.* Edited by DR Holmes JR, RE Vlietstra. Philadelphia, FA Davis Company, 1989, pp 30-41. By permission, Mayo Foundation.)

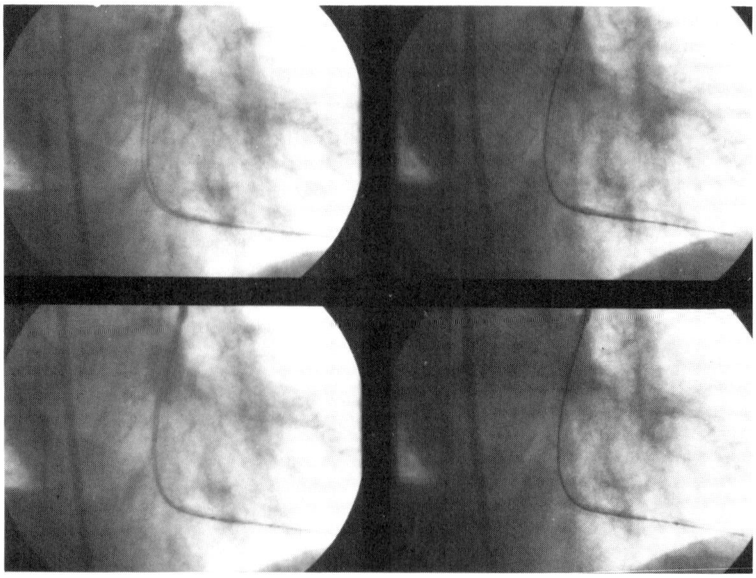

Fig 10A-11 Right anterior oblique images from a 74-kg patient undergoing dilation of the right coronary artery. The images were recorded at identical angles with interlaced scanning (**left**) and progressive scanning (**right**). Two distinct guide wires are seen with conventional recording. Because of the snapshot effect in progressive scanning, only a single wire is seen, and image quality is improved. (From Holmes DR Jr, Bove AA, Wondrow MA, et al: Video x-ray progressive scanning: new technique for decreasing x-ray exposure without decreasing image quality during cardiac catheterization. *Mayo Clin Proc* 61:321-326, 1986. By permission, Mayo Foundation.)

Further improvements in stop-frame and real-time video images have been achieved by a 1,023-line display system. Image acquisition with a 1,023-line system is no better and perhaps subjectively less satisfactory than the standard 525-line video acquisition, primarily because of a degrading of signal-to-noise ratio related to the low-intensity video signal.[35,36] However, when images are recorded in the standard 525-line format and then reprocessed ("upscanned") in a 1,023-line display, both stop-frame and real-time images are smoother and subjectively more pleasing and interference from superimposed raster-lines is eliminated.[37] Enhancement of displayed television images can also be achieved with various digital filters; digital subtraction may also occasionally be useful.

Cineangiography continues to be the standard method for coronary imaging (cine film). Many commercial x-ray systems now feature digital imaging capabilities, and there are growing indications that this technology will replace cineangiography as a standard for recording coronary angiographic images. A complete description of digital imaging technology is beyond the scope of this chapter, but a brief summary should provide a satisfactory introduction to the concept, features, and potential advantages of digital imaging.

The analog signal obtained with the television camera is converted into a digital matrix by an analog-to-digital converter. Most digital matrices consist of 512 by 512 picture elements (pixels). Each pixel is quantified into a gray scale based on 256 levels (8-bit resolution) or 1,024 levels (10-bit resolution). This information is stored and processed in a computer; the image can then be redisplayed on a television monitor by a digital-to-analog converter, undergo image enhancement, be available for quantitative analysis, or be transmitted to a digital (or analog) archiving system.

The major advantages of digital coronary angiography are (1) instantaneous image review capability with slow motion, forward and backward review, and "cine loop" display; (2) image enhancement with digital filtering, zoom, and rove functions; (3) computer-assisted quantification of coronary stenoses in addition to the potential to measure myocardial perfusion; and (4) potential for mass storage on computer disks, optical laser disks, or digital tapes. The major impediment to the widespread utilization and acceptance of digital imaging over conventional cineangiography lies in the unresolved issue of selecting a standardized archival system. A standardized archival system, particularly for each patient's diagnostic record, will be essential to facilitate the transfer and review of angiographic images from one laboratory to another.

Patient preparation

Before proceeding with diagnostic coronary angiography, the cardiologist should review the patient's pertinent cardiac history, especially information on previous catheterization procedures, contrast-medium allergy, medication, and previous vascular surgical procedures (including coronary revascularization). Pertinent physical findings, including the state of the peripheral pulses, and auscultatory findings should be noted. Finally, the important laboratory results to note include the electrocardiogram, serum creatinine and potassium concentrations, and prothrombin time (or international normalized ratio) if anticoagulants have been used.

Particular note of the patient's renal function is essential because of the possibility of contrast medium-induced acute renal failure, which has been estimated to occur in 0.15% of procedures.[38] The pathogenesis is uncertain and probably multifactorial but likely relates to the hyperosmolality of contrast agents. Risk factors for the development of renal failure include age over 60 years, preexisting renal insufficiency, diabetes mellitus with nephropathy, and dehydration.[39] When angiography is essential in such patients, adequate hydration should be ensured by intravenous administration of fluid, and the

Table 10A-2 Clinical characteristics of patients considered unsuitable for ambulatory catheterization

General agreement

Geographic remoteness from laboratory, with inadequate or unreliable follow-up available in next 24 hours
Percutaneous transluminal coronary angioplasty or valvuloplasty
Transient cerebral ischemic episodes or recent stroke (< 1 month before)
Suspected severe pulmonary hypertension
Severe peripheral vascular disease
Severe insulin-dependent diabetes
Noninvasive testing with results suggestive of severe coronary artery disease (e.g., left main stenosis, three-vessel disease, or severely depressed left ventricular function)

Relative contraindication

History of contrast allergy
Age > 75 years
Severe obesity
Generalized debility or dementia
Frequent ventricular arrhythmias
Renal insufficiency (serum creatinine value > 2 mg/dL)

Data from Pepine CJ, Allen HD, Bashore TM, et al: ACC/AHA guidelines for cardiac catheterization and cardiac catheterization laboratories: American College of Cardiology/American Heart Association Ad Hoc Task Force on Cardiac Catheterization. *J Am Coll Cardiol* 18:1149-1182, 1991.

dosage of contrast agent should be limited. This can also be achieved by performing biplane angiography.

If provocative pharmacologic testing for coronary spasm is contemplated, nitrates and other vasoactive therapy should be withheld for 24 hours preceding the test; this is inadvisable, however, in a patient who has frequent or uncontrolled rest angina. The patient should be in a fasting state with some preprocedure sedation (such as diazepam). Intramuscular injections should be avoided because they cause discomfort and might cause an increase of serum creatine kinase values.

Cardiac catheterization and coronary arteriography can be safely performed on an outpatient basis.[40-44] In general, results and complications do not differ significantly from those reported for inpatient studies. Because one of the major causes of catheterization-related mortality is the presence of significant left main stenosis, patients with suspected left main lesions or profound exercise-induced ischemia (or both) are best served by hospitalization and stabilization, before the catheterization procedure. The American College of Cardiology/American Heart Association joint task force has provided general criteria for exclusion from ambulatory catheterization (Table 10A-2).[31] According to the 1990 report of the Registry of the Society for Cardiac Angiography and Interventions, 19% of 59,792 diagnostic cardiac catheterizations from 63 laboratories were performed on an outpatient basis.[32]

Access to the arterial circulation

The percutaneous femoral approach with use of a modified Seldinger technique[45] is performed as follows. The right (or left) groin is shaved, painted with povidone-iodine solution, and draped. The inguinal ligament is located and the femoral pulse palpated. Approximately 2 cm below the ligament, a transverse skin crease marks the ideal location for arterial puncture. Alternatively, the skin incision site can be located by use of fluoroscopy to identify the inferior border of the femoral head; both approaches generally ensure that the common femoral artery is punctured below the inguinal ligament. The area is infiltrated with 1% lidocaine, and an 18-gauge, thin-walled needle is advanced into the femoral artery. A soft-tipped guide wire is advanced through the needle into the femoral artery and beyond the iliac bifurcation to the aorta. The needle is removed; a dilator (and sheath if necessary) is advanced over the wire to enlarge the puncture hole. Angiographic catheters may then be advanced over the wire into the arterial circulation and the wire may be withdrawn. The catheter must be cleared of air bubbles or possible platelet-fibrin thrombi by aspiration before any injections.

In many laboratories, heparin (2,500 to 5,000 units) is administered intravenously once the catheter is in place. Changes in catheters require reintroduction of the guide wire. Although Teflon coating and heparinization make the occurrence of thromboembolism rare, it is prudent to minimize the time that the exposed guide wire lies in the ascending aorta. Usually, Judkins catheters are used with the femoral approach; occasionally, various preformed catheters, such as the Schoonmaker (multipurpose) or Amplatz catheters, are required. At the end of the procedure, the catheters are removed, protamine (25 mg) is administered if heparin was used, and firm pressure is applied for 15 to 30 minutes over the puncture site. When bleeding has stopped, the distal pulses are checked, and the patient is returned to his or her room.

With use of smaller (5F or 6F) catheters, ambulation earlier than the traditional 6 to 8 hours is possible and permits early dismissal of ambulatory patients undergoing outpatient catheterization. Results of a prospective multicenter trial demonstrated that, among 260 patients undergoing attempted diagnostic angiography with 5F catheters who were ambulated in less than 3 hours, small hematomas developed in 20 (3 of whom had 6F sheaths placed), although none required surgical therapy.[46] The femoral approach should not be utilized when very severe atherosclerotic disease of lower limb peripheral arteries, of distal aorta, or of iliac arteries is present. Presence of aortoiliac grafts or abdominal aortic aneurysms may also be a reason to avoid a femoral artery approach.

The brachial cutdown approach (Sones technique) is performed as follows. The right arm is painted with povidone-iodine and draped. After infiltration with 1% lidocaine, an incision is made transversely over the brachial pulse in the antecubital fossa. The artery lies in a vascular sheath beneath the insertion of the bicipital aponeurosis; localization and isolation of the vessel are achieved with blunt dissection. Rubber ligatures are passed around the artery above and below the site of arteriotomy, which is made transversely with a scalpel blade. Heparin, 1,000 units, is infused into the distal vessel, and the catheter (usually NIH, Sones, or brachial preformed type) is introduced. When the procedure is finished, the catheter is withdrawn, and the artery is allowed to bleed freely for one or two seconds, heparin is again injected distally, and the arteriotomy is closed. If a good radial pulse is present, the skin is closed; if the pulse is more than slightly diminished, Fogarty embolectomy may be required.

Coronary angiography by the brachial cutdown approach is usually a more lengthy procedure and requires somewhat more skill and experience than the femoral percutaneous technique. In experienced hands, both techniques are equally safe. We usually reserve the brachial cutdown for patients who have lower extremity atherosclerosis, particularly if coronary angioplasty is likely to be performed at the same time, or for whom exercise (supine bicycle) is planned. The well-trained angiographer is thoroughly versed in both techniques.

Percutaneous puncture of the brachial artery appears to be an acceptable alternative to a cutdown procedure.[47,48] Although it can be performed with 7F catheters, we prefer to use 5F or 6F catheters in this situation and find that multipurpose brachial preformed catheters provide satisfactory coronary engagement and visualization in most cases. When necessary, the left brachial artery approach can also be used with Judkins catheters;[48] this approach is particularly useful when a left internal mammary artery needs to be visualized. In the aforementioned 1990 registry report, 83% of diagnostic angiographic procedures were performed via the femoral route.[32]

Left ventriculography

The assessment of left ventricular myocardial abnormalities by left ventriculography should be part of the evaluation of the patient who is undergoing coronary arteriography. A catheter is advanced to the aortic root and the pressure recorded. The aortic valve is then crossed in a 30° RAO projection and the catheter placed in a stable position in the body of the left ventricle, care being taken that it lies free.

Conventionally, 7F or 8F catheters have been used to minimize catheter recoil during contrast ventriculography, but with more patients undergoing outpatient catheterizations, 5F or 6F catheters are now more commonly used. Unfortunately, these smaller catheters suffer from two problems. First, they are often difficult to advance across the aortic valve and often require a guide wire to facilitate passage into the left ventricle,[49] increasing procedure time and potentially exposing the patient to an increased risk of thromboembolism. Second, high injection rates (above 14 mL/sec) may result in catheter recoil and ventricular ectopy.

Catheters should always be of the type with multiple side holes; this feature reduces catheter recoil during injection and minimizes extrasystoles and myocardial staining. We usually use a pigtail catheter from the leg and an NIH (Rodriguez) or pigtail catheter from the arm. A test injection of 5 to 10 mL allows adjustment of the catheter position.

Usual injection volumes are 40 to 50 mL of contrast medium injected at a rate of 10 to 15 mL/sec. The contrast agent is delivered into the catheter by a power injector with a pressure-sensitive shutoff circuit for safety. Biplane (30° RAO, 60° LAO) cineangiographic images are then recorded (Fig 10A-12).

Contrast material for left ventriculography is hypertonic and has calcium-chelating properties, features that are responsible for various hemodynamic changes after injection. The calcium-chelating properties cause peripheral vasodilation with resultant transient hypotension, reflex tachycardia, and increased cardiac output. The hypertonicity of the medium causes transient hypervolemia which, along with a direct myocardial depressant effect, produces elevation of left ventricular end-diastolic pressure.

Standard contrast material for left ventriculography and coronary angiography has been aqueous *N*-methylglucamine diatrizoate (Renografin, Angiovist). The osmolality of 1,560 is approximately five times that of normal plasma. Several agents with markedly lower osmolality have been developed in an attempt to avoid these hemodynamic perturbations (Table 10A-3). Although they are called "low-osmolality" contrast agents, it is important to realize that the osmolality of these newer agents is still over twice that of normal plasma, whereas their iodine content is very close to that of diatrizoate. Numerous studies have documented less alteration of myocardial contractility, cardiac output, and left ventricular pressures; fewer ventricular arrhythmias; and better patient acceptance of these low-osmolality agents.[50-59]

The only major drawback to the use of lower osmolality agents is their extraordinary cost compared with that of the diatrizoate-based compounds. The choice of a contrast agent must be made with the patient's safety

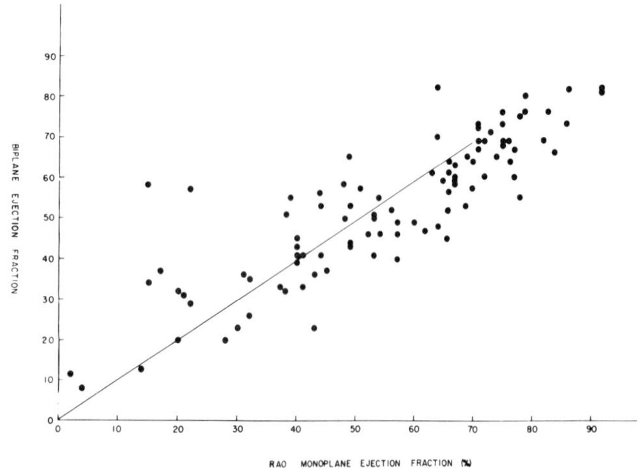

Fig 10A-12 In general, there is a fairly good correlation between monoplane and biplane ejection fractions, especially at the higher end of this spectrum. The monoplane technique may underestimate left ventricular function at lower ejection fractions.

Table 10A-3 Comparative osmolality of contrast media

	mOsm/kg of water	Iodine content (mg/mL)
Diatrizoate	1,560	320
Ioxaglate	600	320
Iohexol	672	300
Iopamidol	616	300

From Higgins CB: Coronary angiography: a decade of advances. *Am J Cardiol* 62:7K-10K, 1988. By permission of Cahners Publishing Company, a Division of Reed Publishing USA.

foremost in mind and be based on knowledge of data on the use of such agents.[60,61] However, these criteria do not imply that low-osmolality agents be used for all patients; rather, these agents should be used for patients at higher risk. In general, low-osmolality contrast agents should be considered for patients with moderate or severe left ventricular dysfunction whether or not symptoms are present, with severe aortic stenosis, with unstable angina or suspected severe left main coronary artery stenosis, with significant renal impairment, or with a history of anaphylaxis to contrast agents. Most other patients are considered to be at low risk and can safely undergo coronary angiography with conventional agents.

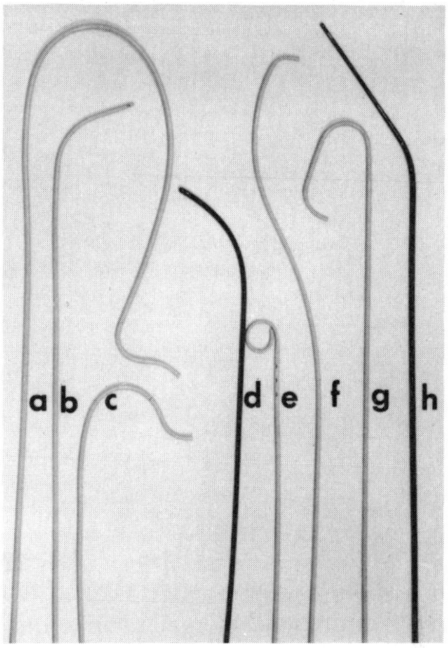

Fig 10A-13 Coronary and left ventriculographic catheters. This is a selection of commonly used catheters: *a,* Amplatz right coronary catheter; *b,* Schoonmaker multipurpose catheter; *c,* brachial preformed left coronary catheter; *d,* NIH left ventriculography catheter; *e,* Judkins pigtail left ventriculography catheter; *f,* Judkins right coronary catheter; *g,* Judkins left coronary catheter; *h,* Sones catheter.

Coronary arteriography

In selected patients, diagnostic catheterization can be satisfactorily completed with 5F or 6F catheters. However, technical problems with torquability and problems with image quality do occur in some patients.[62-64] Situations in which diagnostic accuracy may be potentially compromised or the procedure unnecessarily prolonged should prompt the operator to immediately change to a larger size catheter.

The LAO projection places the right coronary ostium on the left of the monitoring screen and the left coronary ostium on the right. The left Judkins coronary catheter (Fig 10A-13) has a double bend which causes the tip to be directed along the minor curve of the aorta. Various-sized curves are available to "fit" small or dilated aortic roots. With continuous pressure monitoring, the left coronary catheter is gently advanced until it engages the left ostium. A test injection of 1 to 2 mL of dye helps to ensure that the ostium is engaged and allows positioning of the patient for optimal coronary imaging.

After multiple views of the left coronary artery have been taken and reviewed by video or digital replay, the catheter is withdrawn and exchanged for a right Judkins catheter. The right coronary ostium is engaged by placing the tip of the catheter medially in the right sinus of Valsalva and then pulling back while turning clockwise on the catheter to rotate the tip laterally up to the orifice. The catheter springs into the right coronary artery as it engages the vessel. When two or three views of the right coronary artery have been obtained and judged adequate, the catheter is withdrawn. Because 5F catheters are often more difficult to torque into the right coronary ostium and can also dive deeply into the proximal segment, some operators prefer to use a modified right Amplatz catheter or a Williams (no-torque) catheter.

The Sones catheter is often utilized with the brachial artery approach. For engagement of the left coronary ostium, the tip of the catheter is placed in the left coronary cusp and slowly advanced until the tip is in the region of the ostium. The catheter may have to be rotated until the tip lies in or close to the ostium. A sudden, smooth withdrawal on the catheter or a series of back-and-forth movements to expand the loop usually seats the tip in the ostium and allows a stable position for injection. When adequate examination of the left coronary artery has been completed, the catheter can be withdrawn into the left coronary cusp of the aorta, with the tip above the level of the commissures. Clockwise torque allows the tip to rotate medially across the cusp margin into the right sinus of Valsalva. Gentle withdrawal may be needed to drop the tip to the level of the right coronary artery orifice.

Occasionally, it is necessary to utilize other catheters because of anatomic variations, catheter damping, or the presence of anomalous vessels. Useful catheters are the Amplatz femoral, Schoonmaker multipurpose femoral, and brachial preformed catheters. Coronary artery bypass grafts are most easily engaged with a special graft catheter

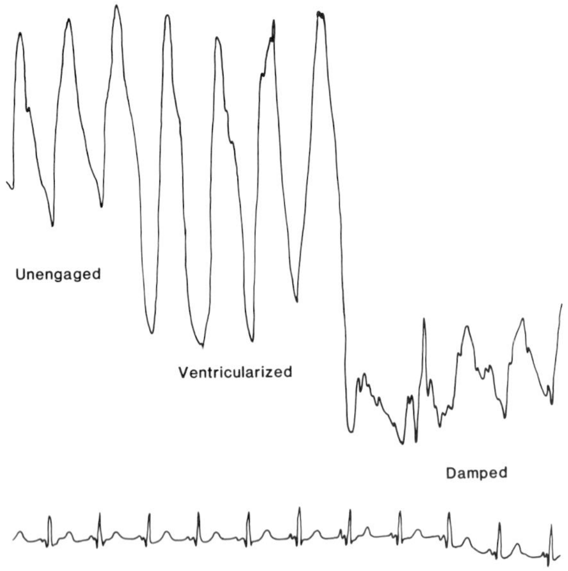

Fig 10A-14 Pressure monitoring. During coronary catheter manipulation, continuous monitoring of the catheter tip should be performed. Pressure damping occurs when the catheter tip is partially obstructed by the arterial wall, a coronary lesion, or intraluminal thrombotic material. Ventricularization of pressure occurs when the catheter tip is wedged into the coronary artery without obstructing the catheter lumen.

from the leg. It may also be necessary to image the internal mammary arteries, for which a special mammary graft catheter (or "headhunter" visceral angiography catheter) is most useful.

Problems encountered with coronary arteriography

Catheter damping. Catheter damping (Fig 10A-14) occurs when there is obstruction to the transmission of arterial pressure through the catheter. This may result from thrombus formation in the catheter or, more commonly, from impaction of the tip against the vessel wall or a lesion. A damped catheter should immediately be withdrawn from the coronary ostium so that it lies free in the aorta. If damping persists, the catheter should be drawn back to the descending aorta before aspiration, flushing, or catheter exchange occurs. Injecting through a damped catheter may cause embolization or coronary dissection by directing a jet of contrast material subintimally.

Pressure ventricularization. Ventricularization of pressure occurs when the catheter is wedged into a coronary ostium but not damped. The tip of the catheter measures, in essence, left ventricular intracavitary pressure transmitted through the coronary bed to the catheter. Thus, the systolic pressure is not diminished, but the diastolic pressure falls below aortic diastolic pressure, since no blood flow enters the artery in diastole. A ventricularized catheter results in lack of blood flow, myocardial ischemia, and increased risk of serious arrhythmias.

Subselective injections. Injections are subselective when the catheter tip is advanced beyond the origin of a branch vessel. The operator must exclude this entity before deciding that the circumflex or LAD artery is totally occluded at its origin. Withdrawal of the catheter and slight rotation may allow visualization of the other vessel. This is most common in cases in which the left main coronary artery is very short or absent.

Inappropriate rates of coronary injections. Six to eight milliliters of contrast material is injected by hand into the coronary artery for each angiographic projection; less may be used in smaller vessels, such as a nondominant right coronary artery. For maximal opacification of the vessel, the injection should be rapid enough to eliminate phasic washout of contrast medium by blood during diastole. Because of laminar blood flow in the vessel, slower rates of injection may allow the contrast medium to layer along one side of the artery; this produces a false appearance of luminal narrowing or failure to visualize vessel branches. On the other hand, too vigorous an injection usually causes contrast material to spill retrogradely into the aortic sinuses of Valsalva and may obscure the proximal coronary vessels. The risks of coronary artery dissection, myocardial staining, and bradycardia are also increased when injection is too vigorous, particularly if the catheter is partially wedged in the coronary artery.

Catheter-induced spasm. Catheter-induced spasm (Fig 10A-15) should be suspected when a smooth narrowing of the proximal artery begins near the tip of the catheter in the vessel. This most commonly occurs at the ostium of the right coronary artery. Less commonly, catheter-induced spasm may involve the LAD, circumflex, or middle right coronary artery without spasm more proximally. Use of sublingual nitroglycerin will usually relieve the spasm; if not, withdrawing the catheter, administering additional nitrates, and waiting several minutes before performing flush injections near the ostium of the artery may be required to discriminate between catheter-induced spasm and a proximal fixed lesion.

Dilated aortic root. Moderate degrees of aortic dilatation pose little problem for engagement of the coronary arteries. When the transverse aortic diameter exceeds 6 cm, standard preformed catheters are usually inadequate, and Sones catheters may be difficult to control. In these circumstances, larger (6- to 9-cm curve) left Judkins catheters may be necessary to engage the left coronary artery; larger right Judkins catheters are also available. Multipurpose or Amplatz II or III catheters are also useful in this situation.

Aortic dissection. In dissection of the ascending aorta, the intimal flap may interfere with engagement of the coronary ostia. Occasionally, the coronary ostia may arise from the false lumen, or the catheter be passed retrogradely into the false lumen. Hand injection in the region of the ostia may partially visualize the vessels; sometimes the coronary arteries cannot be imaged except by aortic root injection.

Orifice lesions. Occasionally, discrete, very proximal lesions of the left main or right coronary artery may go unrecognized because the catheter tip slides past the lesion into a normal-caliber distal vessel. Catheter damp-

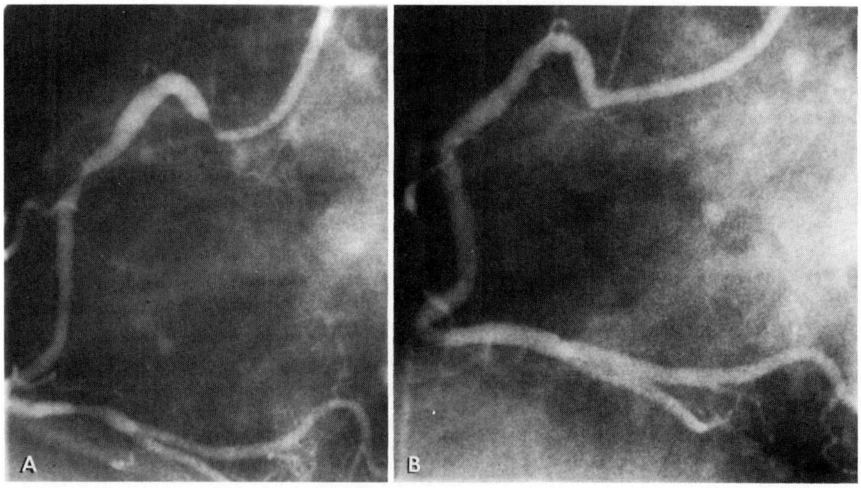

Fig 10A-15 Catheter-induced spasm. **A,** spasm of the proximal coronary artery of severe degree. Additional areas of narrowing are visible in the middle and distal segments. The patient did not experience chest pain. **B,** after the catheter was withdrawn and nitroglycerin was administered, the spasm subsided.

ing or ventricularization may be a clue to this problem. Observing the pattern of contrast medium as it retrogradely opacifies the proximal vessel and ostia will usually show the lesion. Then aortic cusp flushes can be used to document its presence further with views perpendicular to the coronary artery origin from the aorta.

Risks and complications

Death, myocardial infarction, and stroke are the most important of the major complications associated with coronary arteriography. The incidence of these complications appears to be inversely related to the experience of the arteriographer and the number of cases performed yearly and directly proportional to the number of patients with severe coronary heart disease studied. Major complications reported in the 1990 Registry of the Society for Cardiac Angiography and Interventions occurred in 1.7% of patients and included death in 0.11%, acute myocardial infarction in 0.05%, and neurologic events in 0.07%.[32] Complication rates are known to be significantly higher in the presence of left main coronary artery or three-vessel disease and with reduction of the ejection fraction below 30%.

Minor complications, such as local vascular damage, hematoma, ventricular fibrillation, and severe bradycardia, occur in about 1% of procedures and can be corrected promptly.

Ventricular fibrillation. Ventricular arrhythmias may also occur during cardiac angiography and appear to be related to the sodium and calcium content of the radiocontrast material. The incidence of ventricular fibrillation is very low for both high-osmolar ionic contrast agents and nonionic agents. In a series of 4,630 patients who underwent cardiac angiography with high-osmolar ionic contrast agents, the incidence of ventricular fibrillation was 0.2%.[65] In a series of almost twice as many patients who received nonionic contrast material, the incidence of ventricular fibrillation or tachycardia was 0.1%.[66] Ventricular fibrillation appears to occur slightly more commonly after injection in the right coronary artery than in the left, particularly if the conus branch is inadvertently selectively engaged. A forceful cough from the patient can occasionally revert the fibrillation to sinus rhythm, but generally, direct current defibrillation is required. Should ventricular fibrillation occur, the catheter must be immediately withdrawn from the ostium of the coronary artery to ensure that adequate antegrade flow is restored.

Bradycardia. Mild bradycardia commonly occurs during coronary artery injection both as a result of the Bezold-Jarisch reflex and because of direct depression of sinoatrial nodal automaticity due to the calcium-chelating properties of contrast material.[67-70] Chemoreceptors in the left ventricular inferior wall are stimulated by contrast medium, activating a cholinergic reflex arc that results in bradycardia and peripheral vasodilation. The reflex can be partially blocked by administering atropine. Occasionally, transient severe bradycardia or asystole occurs, more commonly with right coronary artery injections, which may result in syncope. Instructing the patient to cough forcefully several times at the onset of bradycardia is sufficient in almost all instances to break this slowing and to restore normal rhythm. Seldom is intravenously administered atropine needed. Significant bradycardias are only rarely seen today in laboratories exclusively using nonionic contrast agents for angiography.

Allergic reaction. Allergy to contrast medium occurs in about 5% of procedures, usually manifesting itself as hives and occasionally as mild angioedema. Severe anaphylactic reactions are fortunately rare but when they occur may require aggressive treatment for shock and laryngeal obstruction. For patients suspected of having contrast allergy, premedication with corticosteroids and antihistamine prior to the procedure lessens the risk of a serious problem.[71,72]

Nephropathy. Contrast agent-induced renal failure accounts for approximately 10% of all patients with hospital-acquired acute renal failure. In one study,[39] it occurred in 23% of patients undergoing left ventriculography and coronary arteriography with baseline creatinine levels of 2 mg/dL or greater. Independent predictors of contrast media nephropathy included class IV heart failure, more than one radiocontrast study within a 72-hour period, and insulin-dependent diabetes mellitus. The dose of radiocontrast material used was also important. A 2% incidence of nephropathy occurred in patients who received less than 125 mL of contrast agent and a 19% incidence in those given 125 mL or more.

A recent randomized study from our institution of high-risk patients (serum creatinine concentration ≥1.5 mg/dL) undergoing cardiac angiography found that iopamidol was significantly less nephrotoxic than diatrizoate. However, this difference did not appear to be of any major clinical significance in most of these patients and, interestingly, could not be documented in patients with insulin-dependent diabetes.[73] Whether low-osmolality contrast agents are safer in patients with very advanced renal impairment is not known; however, we generally avoid the use of high-osmolality contrast agents in such patients.

In high-risk patients, avoidance of dehydration and reduction of contrast agent load are suggested. In such cases, we often do not perform ventriculography but rely instead on two-dimensional echocardiography or radioisotope analysis of left ventricular function; total contrast load can also be reduced by performing coronary arteriography with biplane imaging.

Radiation protection. The major goal for cardiac angiographers should be to obtain images of the highest quality while ensuring patient safety. Unfortunately, this is achieved only with the use of ionizing radiation, of which no level, either to the operating personnel or to the patient, can be considered safe. Several important publications pertaining to the use of x-ray equipment and radiation exposure are available from the National Council on Radiation Protection. Well-maintained x-ray imaging equipment along with optimization of all paths of the imaging chain, from the x-ray pulse generator to the television display of images, helps reduce the amount of radiation exposure. Diagnostic x-ray equipment is expected to conform to federal performance standards, which are to be regulated even more strictly in the near future. Whereas patients are exposed to the primary beam of radiation, operating personnel are exposed mostly to scattered radiation.

Angiographers should be cognizant of the basic principles of radiation physics and the optimal use of angiography equipment, and they should conscientiously promote the observance of radiation safety in the laboratory. Every laboratory should have a radiation safety program that includes the monitoring of exposure to all laboratory personnel. Approaches to decreasing the amount of radiation exposure are summarized in Table 10A-4.

Table 10A-4 Approaches to decreasing the amount of radiation exposure to operating personnel in the cardiac catheterization laboratory

- Increase distance from x-ray source
- Avoid unnecessary fluoroscopy ("light foot")
- Use shielding devices, lead aprons
- Collimate the field
- Avoid unnecessary magnification
- Reduce frame rate if practical
- Improve procedural efficiency
- Increase x-ray tube filtration
- Remove antiscatter grid (not recommended for cineangiography)
- Inspect and maintain x-ray equipment regularly
- Display and record cumulative fluoroscopic time
- Educate physician and other personnel

Special interventions

In patients with variant angina[74,75] or with exertional angina[76,77] and minimal coronary artery lesions, it may be useful to attempt provocation of coronary artery spasm. This has been accomplished in the past by the intravenous injection of ergonovine maleate[78] (Fig 10A-16), which has recently been withdrawn from the United States market. Methylergonovine maleate (Methergine) has proven to be a suitable substitute for ergonovine maleate, and administration of a weight-adjusted dose has been well described and appears to be safe.[79] This test should be avoided in patients with uncontrolled hypertension, severe peripheral vascular disease, cerebrovascular disease, or severe fixed coronary obstructions. After review of the coronary arteriogram to exclude any severe fixed lesions, a record of the blood pressure, heart rate, and electrocardiogram is made. With continuous electrocardiographic monitoring, methylergonovine maleate is administered in sequential doses until symptoms occur or until the maximum dose has been given. Usually, the systolic blood pressure will increase 20 to 30 mm Hg, and the heart rate will slow reflexly. Repeat coronary injections are made, note being taken of any severe or focal spasm; then one or two sublingual nitroglycerin tablets are given to reverse the effects of the drug. In rare instances, it may be necessary to administer intracoronary nitroglycerin to reverse severe spasm, and the test should not be performed without the immediate availability of this drug and calcium-entry blocking agents.

The exact mechanism(s) of provoked or spontaneous coronary spasm remains unclear. Whatever the cause, a localized hypersensitivity of coronary smooth muscle allows abnormal tonic contraction in response to various stimuli. Methylergonovine maleate is thought to act by stimulating 5-hydroxytryptamine receptors,[80] but methacholine,[81] hyperventilation and tromethamine buffer,[82] hand immersion in ice water,[83] and exercise[76,77] all have been shown to precipitate spasm in susceptible subjects.

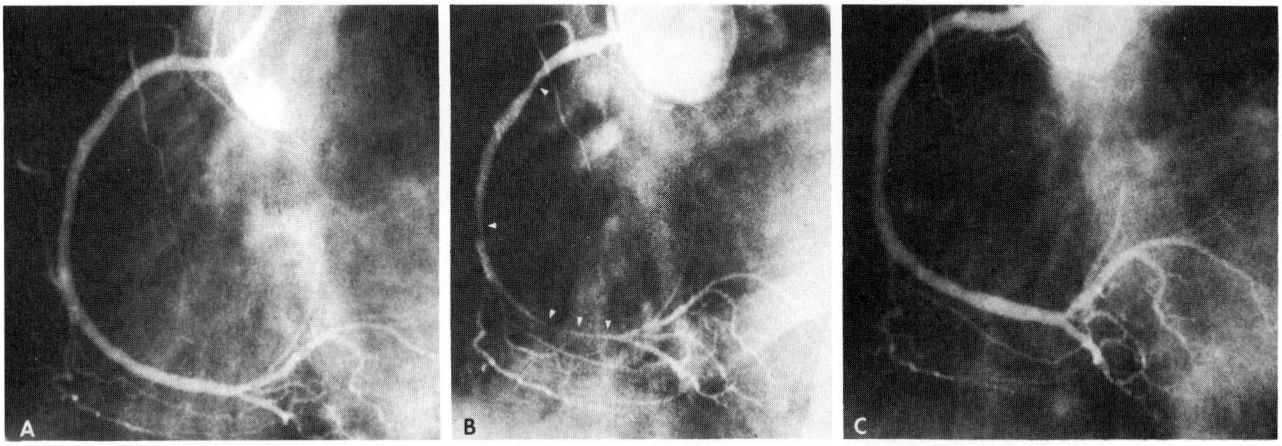

Fig 10A-16 Ergonovine-induced coronary artery spasm. **A,** right coronary artery injection demonstrating mild luminal irregularities but no severe stenosing disease. **B,** after intravenous administration of ergonovine maleate, multiple areas of narrowing were noted, most severe in the distal portion of the right coronary artery, where the luminal diameter is approximately 95% reduced. At that time the patient experienced chest pain, and inferior ST-segment elevation occurred. **C,** after the administration of nitroglycerin, the spasm subsided, and the artery again appeared only mildly abnormal.

Unlike normal subjects, who show mild reduction of vessel caliber, positive responders usually have luminal diameter narrowing greater than 75%, often localized to a vessel segment involved by modest atherosclerotic disease. Ischemic pain and ST-segment shift usually accompany provoked spasm. In a series of 862 patients,[84] there were 110 positive responders (13%), all of whom had variant angina pectoris. In another group of 429 patients, spasm was provoked in 16%; almost all with clinical variant angina responded.

More recently, the direct intracoronary infusion of acetylcholine to provoke coronary arterial spasm in patients with variant angina has been advocated as a more sensitive and safer technique than intravenous administration of ergonovine.[85] Since the technique involves direct intracoronary injection of acetylcholine, the induction of spasm can be studied separately in the left and right coronary arteries and may be safer for the investigation of patients with multivessel spasm.[86] Although intracoronary infusion of acetylcholine appears to be highly sensitive and specific for the detection of coronary artery spasm, research continues into whether it is specific for patients with variant angina or whether induced spasm is simply a nonspecific consequence of atherosclerotic endothelium.

In recent years, we have witnessed the emergence of intracoronary imaging with intravascular ultrasound catheters and fiber-optic angioscopic catheters. Intravascular ultrasonography allows a detailed cross-sectional examination of the arterial vessel wall, whereas angioscopy provides excellent visualization of the lumen and the luminal surface of the vascular wall. Imaging with both techniques is possible throughout almost the entire epicardial coronary tree. These two techniques are discussed in chapter 27B.

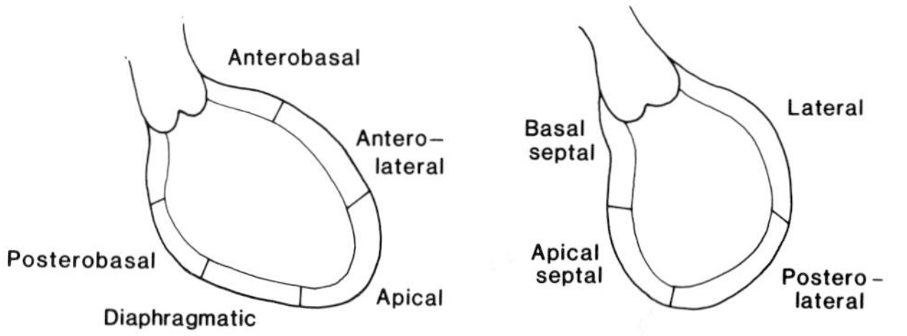

Fig 10A-17 Analysis of left ventricular wall motion. The outline of the left ventricular cavity in the RAO *(left)* and LAO *(right)* views is demonstrated. The RAO view shows anterobasal, anterolateral, apical, diaphragmatic, and posterobasal segments. The LAO view shows lateral, posterolateral, apical septal, and basal septal segments.

INTERPRETATION OF RESULTS
Assessment of left ventricular function

Assessment of left ventricular function includes a visual analysis of regional endocardial wall motion and systolic thickening and objective measures of global left ventricular function. Wall motion analysis involves dividing the outline of the left ventricular cavity into segments, usually five in the RAO view and three or four in the LAO view (Fig 10A-17). Inward systolic endocardial motion of each segment toward the center of the ventriculographic image should occur in a smooth, concentric fashion (Fig 10A-18). Regional wall motion abnormalities are present when a reduction in systolic wall thickening is noted along with various degrees of hypokinesis, akinesis, or dyskinesis (Fig 10A-19). When several contiguous dyskinetic segments

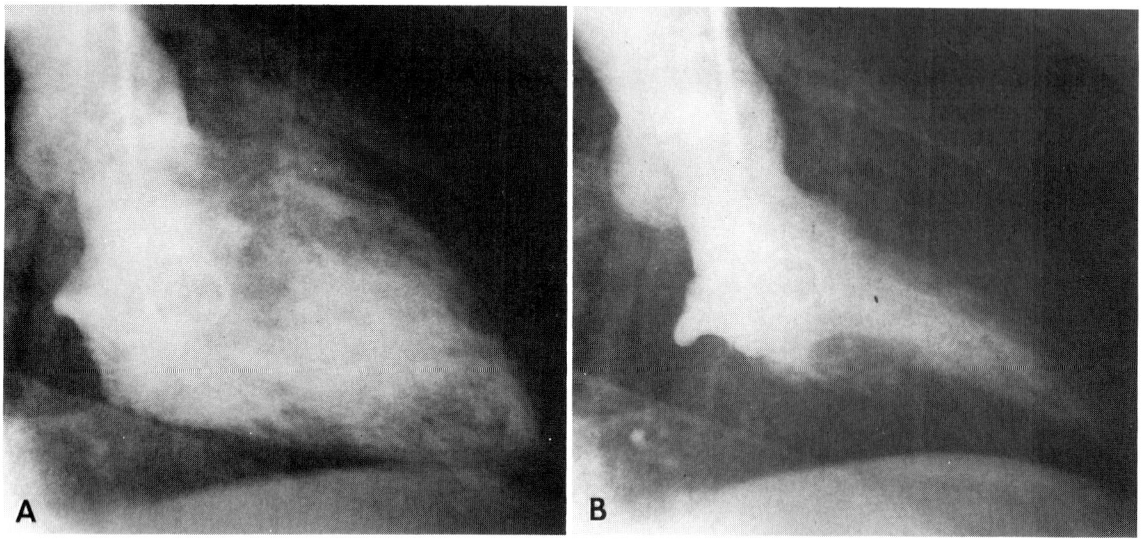

Fig 10A-18 Normal left ventriculogram in RAO projection. **A,** diastolic frame. **B,** systolic frame. Concentric inward motion of wall segments occurs. Compare with Figure 10A-20.

Fig 10A-19 Wall motion analysis. Various degrees of anteroapical wall motion abnormalities are demonstrated. The *solid line* illustrates the ventriculographic border in diastole, and the *dotted line* depicts systole.

are seen, an aneurysm is often present (Fig 10A-20). Regional analysis of left ventricular function allows correlation of prior ischemic myocardial damage with the angiographic anatomy of the vessels supplying these segments. An appraisal of the myocardium at risk can also be made. For example, a 90% LAD lesion associated with anteroapical dyskinesis implies prior infarction and probably a small amount of residual ischemic myocardium at risk; the same lesion supplying a mildly hypokinetic anteroapical area implies more myocardium at risk. Such observations, along with results of exercise testing, may help in the decision among clinical management options.

Global left ventricular function may be similarly assessed. The angiographer can obtain a subjective impression of left ventricular performance by visually integrating the function of all left ventricular segments. Alternatively, a scoring system (LV score)[27] has been developed to summate degrees of segmental dysfunction. The lower the overall number, the better is the left ventricular function. This score has shown high correlation with long-term survival.

The left ventricular ejection fraction is the most commonly used objective measure of left ventricular function. Ejection fraction is defined as stroke volume divided by end-diastolic volume. A number of mathematical formulae exist for converting the measurements of systolic and diastolic angiographic dimensions into approximations of systolic and diastolic volumes. All rely on the assumption that the shape of the ventricular cavity approximates that of a geometric figure, usually an ellipsoid in revolution. The area-length method of Dodge is probably the most widely used.[87] Outlines of the left ventricular cavity are traced in systole and diastole, in both RAO and LAO views. The left ventricular long axis is measured directly as the longest apex-to-base distance. With the use of a hand (or computer-assisted) planimeter, the area of each "ellipse" (left ventricular outline) is determined in each view. The minor axes can then be calculated by substitution of area *(A)* and major axis length *(L)* into the formula for an ellipse, $A = \pi DL/4$, and solving for the minor axis *(D)*. When the minor axes in both RAO $(D)_1$ and LAO (D_2) views are determined, the ventricular volume is calculated by substitution of these data into the formula for the volume of an ellipsoid

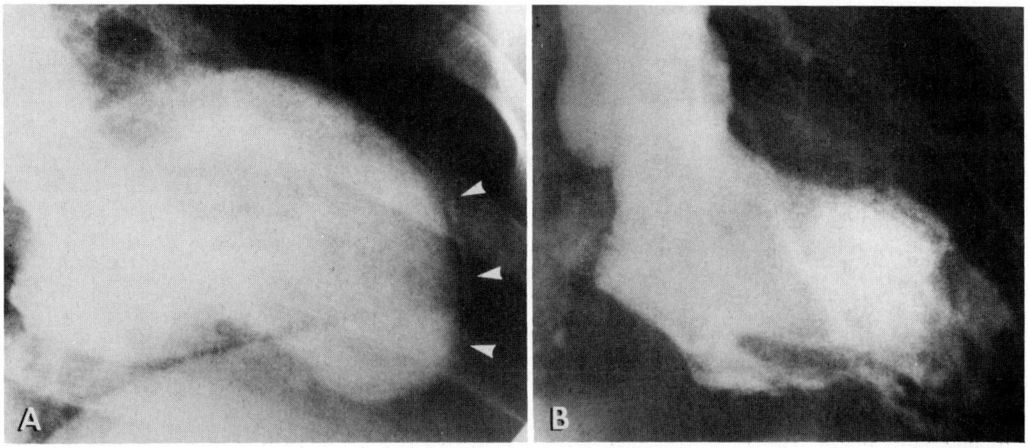

Fig 10A-20 **A,** left ventriculogram in the RAO projection. A large anteroapical left ventricular aneurysm is present. A thin rim of calcification *(arrows)* is present along the anterolateral wall. The posterobasal and anterobasal segments showed systolic inward motion, but the remaining segments were dyskinetic. **B,** anteroapical aneurysm with extensive apical mural thrombus.

$$V = \frac{4\pi}{3}\frac{(L)}{(2)}\frac{(D_1)}{(2)}\frac{(D_2)}{(2)},$$

and, from the systolic and diastolic volumes, the ejection fraction can be obtained. If absolute volumes are needed, correction for image magnification must be performed, usually by the use of a calibrated grid or nomogram. If ejection fraction is all that is wanted, the systematic error of magnification cancels out in the equation. Similar formulae are available for single-plane angiography;[88] in most circumstances, the ejection fraction values obtained with single-plane (RAO) ventriculography correlate well with those obtained by biplane imaging.

At our institution, we also use a method[89] based on a modification of Simpson's rule. Biplane (30° RAO and 60° LAO) orthogonal angiograms are recorded on high-quality videotape, and stop-action images in systole and diastole are oriented so that their long axes are parallel. An operator-interactive computer contouring system identifies the endocardial border of the ventricular cavity, and the dimensions of each video scan line in RAO are computed. These dimensions represent major and minor axes of an ellipse with the depth equal to one video scan line. The computer summates the total number of lines contributing to the ventricular image, adding the volumes of all the ellipses to calculate a total ventricular volume and, from this, an ejection fraction. Volumes determined in this manner correlate well with left ventricular casts of known volume and also with other validated methods of ejection fraction determination.

Despite the common use and proved accuracy of ejection fraction determinations, problems may occur in the calculation or interpretation of ejection fraction results. Errors in measurements may produce values that do not match subjective impressions of left ventricular function. Selection of ectopic or postectopic beats will spuriously reduce or increase measured ejection fractions, respectively. Acute increases or decreases in afterload will reduce or increase measured ejection fractions, respectively.[90] The ventricle with reduced afterload (such as occurs with chronic severe mitral regurgitation) may have an ejection fraction that overestimates left ventricular function. Finally, pathologic states that distort the normal left ventricular geometry, such as left ventricular aneurysm or even severe left ventricular dilatation, cause disparity between the true left ventricular shape and the ellipsoid assumption and thus increase the inaccuracy of ejection fraction measurements when the elliptic formula is employed.

In addition to derangements in regional and global left ventricular function, the left ventriculogram may reveal other abnormalities. Coronary artery, pericardial, valvular, and myocardial calcification are important. A well-demarcated, large dyskinetic area of myocardial thinning denotes the presence of a left ventricular aneurysm. True aneurysms are usually anteroapical in location, and their walls are composed of thinned, scarred myocardium. False aneurysms, or pseudoaneurysms, occur with left ventricular free-wall perforation and formation of a localized hemopericardium; they may be located anterolaterally or posterolaterally, and they tend to have a narrower "neck" than true aneurysms. Pathologically, their walls are composed of fibrous tissue, pericardium, and thrombus. The distinction between these is important because false aneurysms, unlike true aneurysms, have a propensity to rupture, with resultant cardiac tamponade and death.[91] Left ventricular mural thrombus is often seen as a filling defect within aneurysms or filling the apex of poorly contracting ventricles. Old laminated thrombi may calcify and form an apical crescentic density (see Fig 10A-20).

Mitral regurgitation (and aortic regurgitation with aortic root angiography) is subjectively measured by a four-grade system (Table 10A-5). Contrast load, ventricular function, heart rate, and rate of dye injection all may

Table 10A-5 Severity of valvular regurgitation from contrast angiography

Grade	Mitral regurgitation	Aortic regurgitation
+	"Whiff"; mild LA opacification; rapidly cleared	Incomplete LV opacification; cleared each beat
+ +	Moderate LA opacification; LA < LV density	Faint but complete LV opacification; LV < aortic density; incomplete clearance
+ + +	Moderate and complete LA opacification; LA = LV density	Rapid LV opacification; LV = aortic density; slow clearance
+ + + +	Rapid (1 beat) LA opacification; LA > LV density; opacification of pulmonary veins	Rapid (1 beat) LV opacification, persistent; LV > aortic density; slow clearance

LA, left atrium; LV, left ventricle.
Regurgitant grade + + + or + + + + may be accompanied by enlargement of the chamber receiving the regurgitant volume in patients with chronic regurgitation.

affect the apparent severity of regurgitation. Premature ventricular contractions during angiography can produce mitral regurgitation through a competent mitral valve and can cause erroneous appraisals of mitral valve incompetence.

Grading of coronary lesions

Grading of obstructive lesions is a subjective process in which an experienced angiographer usually compares the diameter of the narrowed segment with the diameter of the nearest "normal" segment of the same vessel, the difference being expressed as a percentage of normal. Thus, a segment reduced to 20% of normal diameter represents an 80% stenosis (Fig 10A-21). In addition, it is useful to note whether the obstruction is localized and discrete or longer and tubular or diffuse; the longer stenosis has more profound implications with respect to reduction of coronary flow. The characteristics of the vessel distal to the obstruction are important. Is the vessel diseased and small or of sufficient size to allow reasonable assurance that a bypass graft will remain patent? In general, a vessel 2 mm or larger in diameter is desirable. By comparing the vessel diameter with the known diameter of the catheter, one can assess the size of the distal vessel. For each arterial segment, we routinely note these features: percentage of obstruction, type of lesion (discrete, tubular, diffuse), size and extent of disease of the distal vessel, and collateralization when present. In evaluating stenoses for possible intracoronary therapeutic procedures, such as coronary angioplasty, we also take note of the degree of eccentricity, presence or absence of thrombus, and calcification. Attempts to "quantify" degrees of stenoses more accurately by direct measurement or by computer-assisted methods have been advocated. Although these objective measurements provide greater accuracy, at present they are expensive and time-consuming and are not generally employed for routine angiographic interpretation (see below).

Several inherent limitations of coronary arteriography exist. One major problem occurs in relating stenoses to the size of adjacent uninvolved vessels. Often these "uninvolved" segments are found at autopsy to be diffusely narrowed by atherosclerotic disease, so that the stenotic areas actually were more severe than they appeared angiographically (Fig 10A-22). This primarily accounts for the finding that, in general, coronary arteriography underestimates the degree of narrowing when compared with postmortem examination.[92,93] This is a common problem in assessing the severity of narrowing in cardiac transplant recipients, in whom diffuse narrowing of the entire coronary tree can occur.

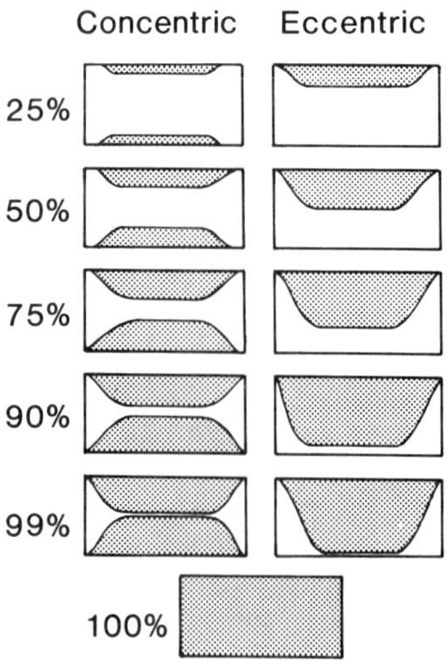

Fig 10A-21 Coronary artery lesions. Various degrees of coronary arterial narrowing are depicted. A 25% lesion obstructs the vessel by 25% in comparison with the adjacent normal vessel diameter, and so on. Because visual estimates are made and the adjacent "normal" vessel may actually be diseased, significant interobserver and anatomic-pathologic variability with respect to the true severity of the lesion can occur.

A second major problem is related to eccentric lesions, which account for approximately 70% of apparent stenoses. Depending on the angle of projection, the lesion may appear severe, mild, or even normal. Multiple

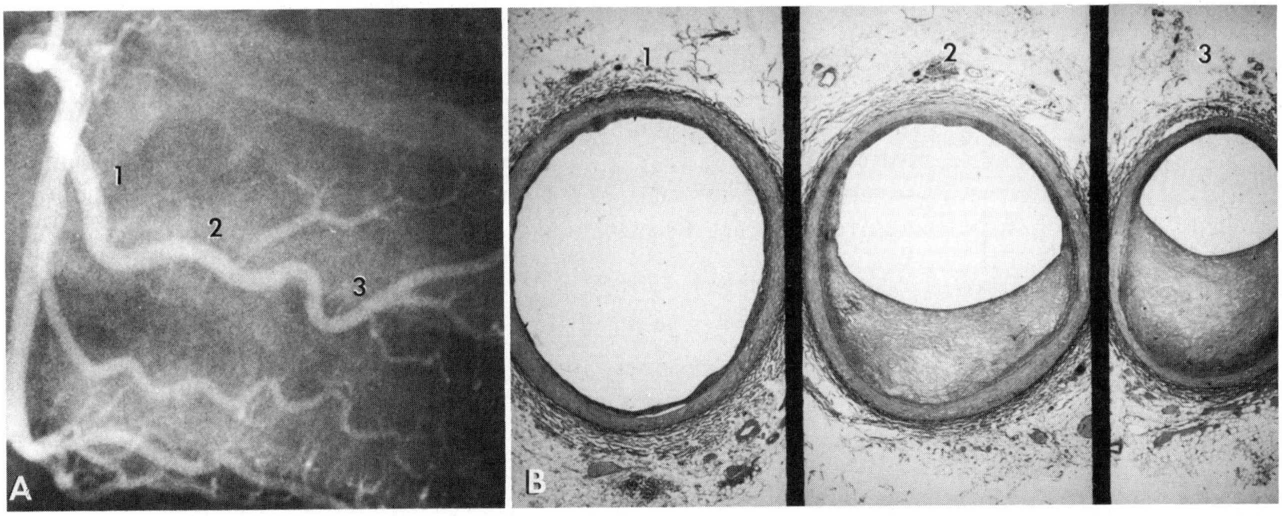

Fig 10A-22 Angiographic-anatomic correlation. **A,** the first obtuse marginal branch of this circumflex coronary artery was interpreted as being essentially normal. However, the patient subsequently died. **B,** at autopsy, artery cross sections corresponding to numbered positions **(A)** showed an eccentric narrowing of the lumen of more than 60%. Because of the lesion's eccentricity and the fact that it involved the artery in a gradually increasing fashion, it was not detected by angiography. Angiography generally underestimates the degree of luminal narrowing as seen on pathologic examination.

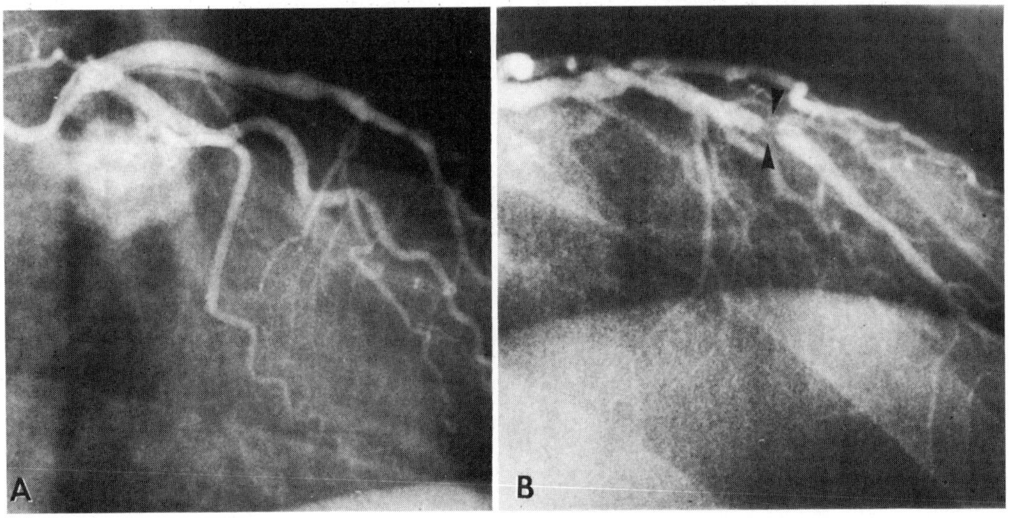

Fig 10A-23 **A,** RAO view of left coronary artery. There are multiple luminal irregularities involving the proximal and middle LAD arteries, but no critical lesion is visible. A diagonal vessel overlaps the middle LAD. **B,** addition of cranial angulation. The diagonal vessel is shown superiorly. A subtotal middle LAD lesion (with luminal thrombus) can now be visualized *(arrows)*. Use of cranial and caudal angulation is of utmost importance in reducing vessel overlap and demonstrating "hidden" lesions.

projections of each coronary segment minimize errors due to eccentric lesions. When one is faced with a markedly different appearance of a stenosis in different views, it is best to rely on the most severe appearance and to assume that an eccentric lesion is present.

A third problem occurs when stenoses are missed because of superimposition of other vessels (Fig 10A-23). The proximal LAD, diagonals, and first obtuse marginal arteries often overlap in RAO views. Routine use of hemiaxial views reduces this problem, and it also reduces the masking of lesions that is a result of foreshortening.

In addition to technical limitations of angiography, there are significant interobserver variations in interpretation of the severity of lesions.[94] Lesions at either end of

Table 10A-6 Guidelines for coronary angiography from the American College of Cardiology/American Heart Association Task Force:[97] summary of conditions for which there is general agreement that coronary angiography is justified in patients with known or suspected coronary heart disease

A. Asymptomatic patients
   1. Evidence of high risk, such as left main or multivessel coronary artery disease or impaired left ventricular function, on noninvasive testing
   2. Individuals with occupations involving the safety of others (e.g., airline pilots, bus drivers); persons such as firefighters, police officers, and athletes
   3. After successful resuscitation from cardiac arrest in patients with a reasonable possibility of coronary artery disease
B. Symptomatic patients
   1. Angina pectoris unresponsive to medical treatment, percutaneous transluminal angioplasty, thrombolytic therapy, or coronary bypass surgery
   2. Unstable angina pectoris
   3. Variant angina pectoris
   4. Angina pectoris in association with any of the following:
      a. Evidence of high risk indicated by noninvasive testing
      b. Coexistence of history of myocardial infarction, hypertension, and ST-segment depression on electrocardiogram
      c. Intolerance of medical therapy
      d. Occupational or lifestyle considerations
      e. Episodic pulmonary edema without obvious cause
   5. Preceding major vascular surgery in patients with angina pectoris or objective evidence of myocardial ischemia on noninvasive testing
   6. After resuscitation from cardiac arrest if acute myocardial infarction is absent
C. Atypical chest pain of uncertain origin
   1. Atypical chest pain when electrocardiographic or radionuclide stress tests indicate the possibility of high-risk coronary artery disease
   2. Atypical chest pain suggestive of coronary artery spasm
   3. Pain accompanied by symptoms or signs of left ventricular dysfunction
D. Convalescent myocardial infarction
   1. Angina pectoris occurring at rest or with minimal activity
   2. Development of left ventricular dysfunction, particularly when associated with recurrent myocardial ischemia or with significant ventricular arrhythmias
   3. Objective evidence of myocardial ischemia on noninvasive testing
   4. Non-Q-wave myocardial infarction
E. Valvular heart disease
   1. Contemplated valve surgery in adult with chest discomfort or electrocardiographic changes suggestive of coronary artery disease
   2. Contemplated valve surgery in male patients 35 years old or older or in postmenopausal patients
F. Known or suspected congenital heart disease
   1. Evaluation of patients with congenital heart disease who have signs or symptoms suggestive of coronary artery disease
   2. Suspected congenital coronary anomalies if aortography is not diagnostic
   3. Contemplated corrective open heart surgery for male patients older than 40 or for postmenopausal patients
G. Other conditions
   1. Diseases affecting the aorta (e.g., ascending aortic aneurysm, aortic dissection, arteritis)
   2. Left ventricular failure without obvious cause and with adequate left ventricular systolic function
   3. Male patients older than 35 or postmenopausal patients who have hypertrophic cardiomyopathy with angina pectoris in whom medical therapy has failed or outflow tract obstruction surgery is planned

Data from Ross J Jr, Fisch C (Chairmen): Guidelines for coronary angiography: a report of the American College of Cardiology/American Heart Association Task Force on Assessment of Diagnostic and Therapeutic Cardiovascular Procedures (Subcommittee on Coronary Angiography). *J Am Coll Cardiol* 10:935-950, 1987.

the spectrum (that is, 0% to 10% or 90% to 100% stenosed) are interpreted similarly by separate observers; most discrepancies occur in the range of 40% to 70% stenosis.

Given that the angiographic interpretation is accurate, what constitutes a significant lesion? In general, lesions 50% or more in diameter (approximately 75% cross-sectional narrowing) are considered capable of producing reduction in flow with exercise; lesions more than 85% in diameter may cause reduced blood flow at rest. These values are derived from animal models in which resting and hyperemia-enhanced coronary flow are measured after various degrees of coronary constriction.[95] In the presence of a series of stenoses of fairly similar degree, the effects on blood flow are additive. In a series of lesions of greatly differing degree, the more severe lesion predominates. Finally, tubular lesions produce a greater decrease in flow than do discrete lesions of identical percentage narrowing.[96] Thus, it is likely that a long tubular 50% lesion or two discrete 50% lesions in series may reduce blood flow to the same extent or more than a single 70% discrete lesion does. The presence of distal collateral vessels implies a hemodynamically significant proximal stenosis. This finding may help decide whether a borderline lesion is significant; however, the lack of apparent collateralization does not exclude a significant stenosis.

Quantitative coronary angiography

With the increase in interventional procedures over the past decade, including intracoronary thrombolysis, percutaneous transluminal coronary angioplasty, coronary atherectomy, laser angioplasty, and intracoronary stent placement, a more accurate, rigorous, and quantitative analysis of coronary artery narrowings is required. Visual estimation of coronary artery narrowings is no longer acceptable for the reporting of scientific studies in which these data are reported. With computer-assisted techniques, a number of approaches for quantitative analysis of coronary angiograms have been developed. These include both off-line (from videotape or cineangiographic recording) and on-line capabilities when digital imaging systems are being used. Although many computer software packages are available for quantitative coronary angiography with various automated edge-detection techniques, two general approaches are used. Geometric sizing requires edge detection, and sizing of a stenosis is determined by reference to the adjacent normal vessel. Densitometric approaches, on the other hand, measure the change in contrast density along a vessel segment and are of use when the edges of the lumen are indistinct. Although not currently performed routinely in most laboratories, quantitative coronary angiography is expected to be used more widely with the growth of digital imaging systems.

INDICATIONS FOR CORONARY ARTERIOGRAPHY

In general, coronary arteriography is indicated to establish the presence of coronary artery disease, its distribution, and its severity. These data then can be used for prognostication of risk and selection of management strategies. Published specific indications for coronary arteriography vary, depending on the author. Ultimately, each physician must develop his or her own philosophy of practice. Guidelines to indications for arteriography recommended by the joint task force of the American College of Cardiology and the American Heart Association should be reviewed by all who practice coronary arteriography[97] (Table 10A-6).

REFERENCES

1. Sones FM Jr: Acquired heart disease. Presented at the Eighth Scientific Session of the Symposium on Present and Future of Cineangiocardiography, Philadelphia, May 29, 1959
2. Sones FM Jr, Shirey EK: Cine coronary arteriography. *Mod Concepts Cardiovasc Dis* 31:735-738, 1962
3. Ricketts HJ, Abrams HL: Percutaneous selective coronary cine arteriography. *JAMA* 181:620-624, 1962
4. Judkins MP: Selective coronary arteriography. I. A percutaneous transfemoral technic. *Radiology* 89:815-824, 1967
5. Amplatz K, Formanek G, Stanger P, et al: Mechanics of selective coronary artery catheterization via femoral approach. *Radiology* 89:1040-1047, 1967
6. Bourassa MG, Lespérance J, Campeau L: Selective coronary arteriography by the percutaneous femoral artery approach. *AJR* 107:377-388, 1969
7. Vineberg A: Surgery of coronary artery disease. *Prog Cardiovasc Dis* 4:391-418, 1962
8. Favaloro R: Cited by Sones FM Jr: Indications and value of coronary arteriography. *Adv Cardiol* 8:67-75, 1973
9. James TN: *Anatomy of the Coronary Arteries.* New York, Paul B Hoeber, 1961
10. Vlodaver Z, Neufeld HN, Edwards JE: *Coronary Arterial Variations in the Normal Heart and in Congenital Heart Disease.* New York, Academic Press, 1975
11. McAlpine WA: *Heart and Coronary Arteries: An Anatomical Atlas for Clinical Diagnosis, Radiological Investigation, and Surgical Treatment.* Berlin, Springer-Verlag, 1975
12. Yamanaka O, Hobbs RE: Coronary artery anomalies in 126,595 patients undergoing coronary arteriography. *Cathet Cardiovasc Diagn* 21:28-40, 1990
13. Roberts WC, Morrow AG: Compression of anomalous left circumflex coronary arteries by prosthetic valve fixation rings. *J Thorac Cardiovasc Surg* 57:834-838, 1969
14. Fellows KE, Freed MD, Keane JF, et al: Results of routine preoperative coronary angiography in tetralogy of Fallot. *Circulation* 51:561-566, 1975
15. Wesselhoeft H, Fawcett JS, Johnson AL: Anomalous origin of the left coronary artery from the pulmonary trunk: its clinical spectrum, pathology, and pathophysiology, based on a review of 140 cases with seven further cases. *Circulation* 38:403-425, 1968
16. Noble J, Bourassa MG, Petitclerc R, et al: Myocardial bridging and milking effect of the left anterior descending coronary artery: normal variant or obstruction? *Am J Cardiol* 37:993-999, 1976
17. Greenspan M, Iskandrian AS, Catherwood E, et al: Myocardial bridging of the left anterior descending artery: evaluation using exercise thallium-201 myocardial scintigraphy. *Cathet Cardiovasc Diagn* 6:173-180, 1980
18. Faruqui AMA, Maloy WC, Felner JM, et al: Symptomatic myocardial bridging of coronary artery. *Am J Cardiol* 41:1305-1310, 1978
19. Gensini GG, da Costa BCB: The coronary collateral circulation in man. *Am J Cardiol* 24:393-400, 1969
20. Schwarz F, Schaper J, Becker V, et al: Coronary collateral vessels: their significance for left ventricular histologic structure. *Am J Cardiol* 49:291-295, 1982
21. Fuster V, Frye RL, Kennedy MA, et al: The role of collateral circulation in the various coronary syndromes. *Circulation* 59:1137-1144, 1979

22. Newman PE: The coronary collateral circulation: determinants and functional significance in ischemic heart disease. *Am Heart J* 102:431-445, 1981

23. Gregg DE, Patterson RE: Functional importance of the coronary collaterals. *N Engl J Med* 303:1404-1406, 1980

24. Kolibash AJ, Bush CA, Wepsic RA, et al: Coronary collateral vessels: spectrum of physiologic capabilities with respect to providing rest and stress myocardial perfusion, maintenance of left ventricular function and protection against infarction. *Am J Cardiol* 50:230-238, 1982

25. Sabia PJ, Powers ER, Ragosta M, et al: An association between collateral blood flow and myocardial viability in patients with recent myocardial infarction. *N Engl J Med* 327:1825-1831, 1992

26. Sabia PJ, Powers ER, Jayaweera AR, et al: Functional significance of collateral blood flow in patients with recent acute myocardial infarction: a study using myocardial contrast echocardiography. *Circulation* 85:2080-2089, 1992

27. Mock MB, Ringqvist I, Fisher LD, et al: Survival of medically treated patients in the Coronary Artery Surgery Study (CASS) registry. *Circulation* 66:562-568, 1982

28. Bunnell IL, Greene DG, Tandon RN, et al: The half-axial projection: a new look at the proximal left coronary artery. *Circulation* 48:1151-1156, 1973

29. Aldridge HE, McLoughlin MJ, Taylor KW: Improved diagnosis in coronary cinearteriography with routine use of 110° oblique views and cranial and caudal angulations: comparison with standard transverse oblique views in 100 patients. *Am J Cardiol* 36:468-473, 1975

30. Frederick PR, Fry WH, Russell JG, et al: Longitudinal angulation in coronary arteriography: apparatus and evaluation. *Cathet Cardiovasc Diagn* 3:305-311, 1977

31. Pepine CJ, Allen HD, Bashore TM, et al: ACC/AHA guidelines for cardiac catheterization and cardiac catheterization laboratories: American College of Cardiology/American Heart Association Ad Hoc Task Force on Cardiac Catheterization. *J Am Coll Cardiol* 18:1149-1182, 1991

32. Noto TJ Jr, Johnson LW, Krone R, et al: Cardiac catheterization 1990: a report of the Registry of the Society for Cardiac Angiography and Interventions (SCA&I). *Cathet Cardiovasc Diagn* 24:75-83, 1991

33. Levin DC, Dunham LR, Stueve R: Causes of cine image quality deterioration in cardiac catheterization laboratories. *Am J Cardiol* 52:881-886, 1983

34. Wondrow MA, Bove AA, Holmes DR Jr, et al: Technical consideration for a new x-ray video progressive scanning system for cardiac catheterization. *Cathet Cardiovasc Diagn* 14:126-134, 1988

35. Holmes DR Jr, Smith HC, Gray JE, et al: Clinical evaluation and application of cardiac laboratory high-definition video systems. *Cathet Cardiovasc Diagn* 10:63-71, 1984

36. Gray JE, Wondrow MA, Smith HC, et al: Technical considerations for cardiac laboratory high-definition video systems. *Cathet Cardiovasc Diagn* 10:73-86, 1984

37. Holmes DR Jr, Wondrow MA, Reeder GS, et al: Optimal display of the coronary arterial tree with an upscan 1,023-line video display system. *Cathet Cardiovasc Diagn* 18:175-180, 1989

38. Byrd L, Sherman RL: Radiocontrast-induced acute renal failure: a clinical and pathophysiologic review. *Medicine (Baltimore)* 58:270-279, 1979

39. Taliercio CP, Vlietstra RE, Fisher LD, et al: Risks for renal dysfunction with cardiac angiography. *Ann Intern Med* 104:501-504, 1986

40. Klinke WP, Kubac G, Talibi T, et al: Safety of outpatient cardiac catheterizations. *Am J Cardiol* 56:639-641, 1985

41. Mahrer PR, Young C, Magnusson PT: Efficacy and safety of outpatient cardiac catheterization. *Cathet Cardiovasc Diagn* 13:304-308, 1987

42. Fighali S, Krajcer Z, Gonzales-Camid F, et al: Safety of outpatient cardiac catheterization. *Chest* 88:349-351, 1985

43. Rogers WF, Moothart RW: Outpatient arteriography and cardiac catheterization: effective alternatives to inpatient procedures. *AJR* 144:233-234, 1985

44. Clements SD Jr, Gatlin S: Outpatient cardiac catheterization: a report of 3,000 cases. *Clin Cardiol* 14:477-480, 1991

45. Seldinger SI: Catheter replacement of the needle in percutaneous arteriography: a new technique. *Acta Radiol (Stockh)* 39:368-376, 1953

46. Kern MJ, Cohen M, Talley JD, et al: Early ambulation after 5 French diagnostic cardiac catheterization: results of a multicenter trial. *J Am Coll Cardiol* 15:1475-1483, 1990

47. Lupon-Rosés J, Domingo E, Angel J, et al: Percutaneous right brachial artery approach with 5F catheters for studying coronary artery disease. *Cathet Cardiovasc Diagn* 22:47-51, 1991

48. Eugster GS, Reisig AH, Ugaldea CT: Percutaneous left brachial catheterization using 5-French preformed (Judkins) catheters. *Cathet Cardiovasc Diagn* 12:274-276, 1986

49. Brown RIG, MacDonald AC: Use of 5 French catheters for cardiac catheterization and coronary angiography: a critical review. *Cathet Cardiovasc Diagn* 13:214-217, 1987

50. Dawson P, Grainger RG, Pitfield J: The new low-osmolar contrast media: a simple guide. *Clin Radiol* 34:221-226, 1983

51. Morris TW, Fischer HW: The pharmacology of intravascular radiocontrast media. *Annu Rev Pharmacol Toxicol* 26:143-160, 1986

52. Sacks BA, Ellison HP, Bartek S, et al: A comparison of Hexabrix and Renografin 60 in peripheral arteriography. *Invest Radiol* 19 Suppl:S320-S322, 1984

53. Wolf GL: A double-blind clinical comparison of the electrophysiologic adverse effects of Hexabrix and Renografin-76. *Invest Radiol* 19: Suppl:S328-S332, 1984

54. Svenson RH: Comparison of the hemodynamic effects of Hexabrix and Renografin-76 following left ventriculography and coronary arteriography. *Invest Radiol* 19 Suppl:S333-S334, 1984

55. Dawson P: Chemotoxicity of contrast media and clinical adverse effects: a review. *Invest Radiol* 20 Suppl:S84-S91, 1985

56. Hirshfeld JW Jr, Laskey W, Martin JL, et al: Hemodynamic changes induced by cardiac angiography with ioxaglate: comparison with diatrizoate. *J Am Coll Cardiol* 2:954-957, 1983

57. Cooper MW, Reed PJ: Comparison of ionic and non-ionic contrast agents in cardiac catheterization: the effects of ventriculography and coronary arteriography on hemodynamics, electrocardiography, and serum creatinine. *Cathet Cardiovasc Diagn* 22:267-277, 1991

58. Soiva M, Hekali P, Keto P, et al: Iohexol, ioxaglate and iopamidol in coronary angiography: a double-blind comparative study of 300 patients. *Australas Radiol* 35:109-111, 1991

59. Matthai WH Jr, Hirshfeld JW Jr: Choice of contrast agents for cardiac angiography: review and recommendations based on clinically important distinctions. *Cathet Cardiovasc Diagn* 22:278-289, 1991

60. Steinberg EP, Moore RD, Powe NR, et al: Safety and cost effectiveness of high-osmolality as compared with low-osmolality contrast material in patients undergoing cardiac angiography. *N Engl J Med* 326:425-430, 1992

61. Barrett BJ, Parfrey PS, Vavasour HM, et al: A comparison of nonionic, low-osmolality radiocontrast agents with ionic, high-osmolality agents during cardiac catheterization. *N Engl J Med* 326:431-436, 1992

62. Kohli RS, Vetrovec GW, Lewis SA, et al: Study of the performance of 5 French and 7 French catheters in coronary angiography: a functional comparison. *Cathet Cardiovasc Diagn* 18:131-135, 1989

63. Hui WKK, Klinke WP, Kubac G, et al: Comparison of 5F and 7/8F catheters for left ventricular and coronary angiography. *Cathet Cardiovasc Diagn* 19:84-86, 1990

64. Hirshfeld JW Jr: Low-osmolality contrast agents—who needs them? *N Engl J Med* 326:482-484, 1992

65. Hirshfeld JW Jr, Kussmaul WG, Di Battiste PM, et al: Safety of cardiac angiography with conventional ionic contrast agents. *Am J Cardiol* 66:355-361, 1990

66. Davidson CJ, Mark DB, Pieper KS, et al: Thrombotic and cardiovascular complications related to nonionic contrast media during cardiac catheterization: analysis of 8,517 patients. *Am J Cardiol* 65:1481-1484, 1990

67. Eckberg DL, White CW, Kioschos JM, et al: Mechanisms mediating bradycardia during coronary arteriography. *J Clin Invest* 54:1455-1461, 1974

68. Zelis R, Caudill CC, Baggette K, et al: Reflex vasodilation induced by coronary angiography in human subjects. *Circulation* 53:490-493, 1976

69. Perez-Gomez F, Garcia-Aguado A: Origin of ventricular reflexes caused by coronary arteriography. *Br Heart J* 39:967-973, 1977

70. Zucker IH, Cornish KG: The Bezold-Jarisch reflex in the conscious dog. *Circ Res* 49:940-948, 1981

71. Greenberger PA, Patterson R, Tapio CM: Prophylaxis against repeated radiocontrast media reactions in 857 cases: adverse experience with cimetidine and safety of β-adrenergic antagonists. *Arch Intern Med* 145:2197-2200, 1985

72. Greenberger PA, Patterson R: Adverse reactions to radiocontrast media. *Prog Cardiovasc Dis* 31:239-248, 1988

73. Taliercio CP, Vlietstra RE, Ilstrup DM, et al: A randomized comparison of the nephrotoxicity of iopamidol and diatrizoate in high risk patients undergoing cardiac angiography. *J Am Coll Cardiol* 17:384-390, 1991

74. Prinzmetal M, Kennamer R, Merliss R, et al: Angina pectoris. I. A variant form of angina pectoris: preliminary report. *Am J Med* 27:375-388, 1959

75. Luchi RJ, Chahine RA, Raizner AE: Coronary artery spasm. *Ann Intern Med* 91:441-449, 1979

76. Waters DD, Chaitman BR, Dupras G, et al: Coronary artery spasm during exercise in patients with variant angina. *Circulation* 59:580-585, 1979

77. Yasue H, Omote S, Takizawa A, et al: Circadian variation of exercise capacity in patients with Prinzmetal's variant angina: role of exercise-induced coronary arterial spasm. *Circulation* 59:938-948, 1979

78. Heupler FA Jr, Proudfit WL, Razavi M, et al: Ergonovine maleate provocative test for coronary arterial spasm. *Am J Cardiol* 41:631-640, 1978

79. Bory M, Joly P, Bonnet J-L, et al: Methergin® testing with angiographically normal coronary arteries. *Am J Cardiol* 61:298-302, 1988

80. Müller-Schweinitzer E: The mechanism of ergometrine-induced coronary arterial spasm: *in vitro* studies on canine arteries. *J Cardiovasc Pharmacol* 2:645-655, 1980

81. Endo M, Hirosawa K, Kaneko N, et al: Prinzmetal's variant angina: coronary arteriogram and left ventriculogram during angina attack induced by methacholine. *N Engl J Med* 294:252-255, 1976

82. Yasue H, Nagao M, Omote S, et al: Coronary arterial spasm and Prinzmetal's variant form of angina induced by hyperventilation and Tris-buffer infusion. *Circulation* 58:56-62, 1978

83. Raizner AE, Chahine RA, Ishimori T, et al: Provocation of coronary artery spasm by the cold pressor test: hemodynamic, arteriographic and quantitative angiographic observations. *Circulation* 62:925-932, 1980

84. Heupler FA Jr: Provocative testing for coronary arterial spasm: risk, method and rationale (editorial). *Am J Cardiol* 46:335-337, 1980

85. Okumura K, Yasue H, Matsuyama K, et al: Sensitivity and specificity of intracoronary injection of acetylcholine for the induction of coronary artery spasm. *J Am Coll Cardiol* 12:883-888, 1988

86. Okumura K, Yasue H, Horio Y, et al: Multivessel coronary spasm in patients with variant angina: a study with intracoronary injection of acetylcholine. *Circulation* 77:535-542, 1988

87. Dodge HT, Sandler H, Ballew DW, et al: The use of biplane angiocardiography for the measurement of left ventricular volume in man. *Am Heart J* 60:762-776, 1960

88. Sandler H, Dodge HT: The use of single plane angiocardiograms for the calculation of left ventricular volume in man. *Am Heart J* 75:325-334, 1968

89. Ritman EL, Sturm RE, Wood EH: Biplane roentgen videometric system for dynamic (60/sec) studies of the shape and size of circulatory structures, particularly the left ventricle. *Am J Cardiol* 32:180-187, 1973

90. Tsakiris AG, Vandenberg RA, Banchero N, et al: Variations of left ventricular end-diastolic pressure, volume, and ejection fraction with changes in outflow resistance in anesthetized intact dogs. *Circ Res* 23:213-222, 1968

91. Martin RH, Almond CH, Saab S, et al: True and false aneurysms of the left ventricle following myocardial infarction. *Am J Med* 62:418-424, 1977

92. Grondin CM, Dyrda I, Pasternac A, et al: Discrepancies between cineangiographic and postmortem findings in patients with coronary artery disease and recent myocardial revascularization. *Circulation* 49:703-708, 1974

93. Schwartz JN, Kong Y, Hackel DB, et al: Comparison of angiographic and postmortem findings in patients with coronary artery disease. *Am J Cardiol* 36:174-178, 1975

94. Zir LM, Miller SW, Dinsmore RE, et al: Interobserver variability in coronary angiography. *Circulation* 53:627-632, 1976

95. Gould KL, Lipscomb K, Hamilton GW: Physiologic basis for assessing critical coronary stenosis: instantaneous flow response and regional distribution during coronary hyperemia as measures of coronary flow reserve. *Am J Cardiol* 33:87-94, 1974

96. Gould KL, Lipscomb K: Effects of coronary stenoses on coronary flow reserve and resistance. *Am J Cardiol* 34:48-55, 1974

97. Ross J Jr, Fisch C (Chairmen): Guidelines for coronary angiography: a report of the American College of Cardiology/American Heart Association Task Force on Assessment of Diagnostic and Therapeutic Cardiovascular Procedures (Subcommittee on Coronary Angiography). *J Am Coll Cardiol* 10:935-950, 1987

CHAPTER

10

Cardiac catheterization and angiography

B. Interventional cardiac therapy

Kirk N. Garratt, M.D., Guy S. Reeder, M.D., and David R. Holmes, Jr., M.D.

SINCE Forssmann[1] performed the first human cardiac catheterization on himself in 1929, the role of cardiac catheterization has been primarily a diagnostic one. Therapeutic use of intravascular catheters began in 1965, when Rashkind and Miller[2] performed the first atrial septostomy using a handmade balloon catheter. Today, catheter therapy is routinely used in four general cardiovascular areas: vascular occlusion, selective delivery of drugs, electrical stimulation, and stenosis enlargement.

Vascular occlusion is of great interest to pediatric cardiologists. The Rashkind ductal occluder, for instance, has been used to percutaneously close patent ductus arterioses with low morbidity and essentially no mortality.[3] In both children and adults, clamshell occluders may be used to close atrial and ventricular septal defects, and they also appear promising for closure of perivalvular leaks.[4,5] Umbrella or bird's nest filters can partially occlude the inferior vena cava to prevent recurrent pulmonary emboli in patients with deep venous thrombi.[6] Selective occlusion of some vessels, such as arterioles supplying vascular tumors or arteriovenous malformations, can be accomplished with copper coils, autologous blood, collagen, or silicone balloons.

Infusion of most cardioactive drugs is accomplished through the relatively unselective venous route. However, selective infusion of thrombolytic drugs into peripheral or coronary arteries has been used extensively. In the past, intracoronary thrombolysis was a first line of therapy for acute myocardial infarction; this has been supplanted by the success of intravenous thrombolysis. Prolonged infusion of thrombolytic drugs before intervention appears to have reduced the frequency of abrupt closures with dilatations.[7]

Electrical stimulation of the heart from catheter tip electrodes forms the basis of cardiac pacing. This important subject is discussed in chapter 25. Application of sufficient energy to cause injury permits electrophysiologists to ablate atrioventricular bypass tracts in patients with Wolff-Parkinson-White syndrome and atrioventricular nodes in patients with intractable atrioventricular nodal reentrant arrhythmias and to create focal areas of injury to disrupt reentrant pathways in patients with ventricular tachycardia.

The chief utility of catheter therapy to adult cardiologists is in enlarging stenotic lesions in coronary and peripheral arteries. Balloon catheters have also been used for enlarging stenotic valves – balloon valvuloplasty – with variable success. This chapter focuses on techniques currently used for the treatment of occlusive arterial and valvular disease.

PERCUTANEOUS TRANSLUMINAL CORONARY ANGIOPLASTY

Historical perspective

On Sept. 16, 1977, the first percutaneous transluminal coronary angioplasty (PTCA) procedure was performed by Andreas Grüntzig in Zurich. In 15 years, PTCA became the most common catheter therapy applied to adult patients with cardiac disease. More than 350,000 PTCA procedures are estimated to have been performed in the United States in 1992, and some analysts predict that more than 600,000 PTCAs will be done annually by the end of the decade. Figure 10B-1 compares the use of balloon angioplasty and isolated coronary artery bypass surgery since the inception of the interventional program at the Mayo Clinic in 1979; it is apparent that more PTCA procedures are now done than coronary artery bypass operations.

This remarkable technique was built on concepts more than 150 years old: the first balloon dilatation of a urethra was performed in 1819,[8] and noninflatable dilators for the urologic and gastrointestinal tracts preceded this by centuries.[9] Charles Dotter[10] was the first to apply the concept of dilatation to vascular stenoses, although his first dilatation was, by his own account, an accident: an

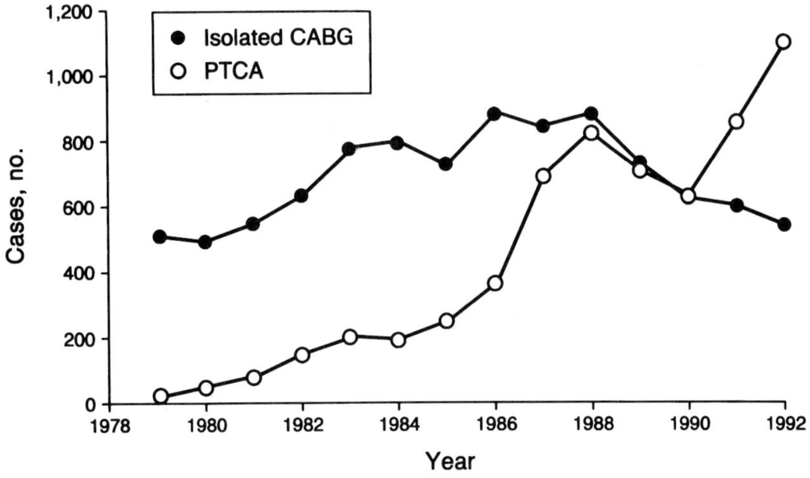

Fig 10B-1 Increasing use of percutaneous transluminal coronary angioplasty (PTCA) at the Mayo Clinic. Although the frequency of isolated coronary artery bypass surgery (CABG) increased in tandem with PTCA during the early 1980s, CABG has recently been performed less often and PTCA use continues to rise (1992 CABG figures are estimates).

angiographic catheter was inadvertently passed through an occluded iliac artery into the abdominal aorta. This stimulated the idea of purposefully enlarging stenotic arterial segments with catheters. A year later, in 1964, Dotter and Judkins[11] reported the first successful transluminal dilatation of a popliteal artery stenosis. A coaxial catheter system was used in which a small guiding catheter was positioned across the stenosis, and dilating catheters of various sizes could then be introduced over the guide to enlarge the stenotic area. The "Dotter technique" never achieved wide application in this country but was used and refined in Europe.

Early attempts to design a balloon catheter were unsuccessful, in part because of a lack of appropriate materials for the balloon. However, in 1974, Grüntzig successfully developed a polyvinyl chloride balloon catheter and applied it to peripheral arterial stenoses, with good results. Encouraged by this success, he modified the system for use in the coronary arteries and tested it in canine coronary arteries and in the autopsy room. He and Richard Myler then tried this small balloon catheter intraoperatively in patients undergoing saphenous vein bypass graft surgery; they demonstrated that human coronary narrowings could be enlarged in this manner. By 1977, the catheter system had undergone sufficient refinement to allow percutaneous use for dilation of human coronary arteries, and in 1978, Grüntzig[12] published the results in the first five patients. Since then, many investigators have further refined the technique of PTCA. Improvements in catheter design and materials are now allowing high success rates and the applicability of the technique to a wide spectrum of coronary disease.

Technical considerations

For the performance of PTCA, the American College of Cardiology, the American Heart Association, the American College of Physicians, and the Society for Cardiac Angiography and Intervention agree that additional, dedicated training and a reasonable continuing case load are necessary to achieve and maintain competency (Table 10B-1). Their recommendations have been published.[11,12]

Table 10B-1 Catheterization and angioplasty training guidelines

Level one:	Clinical cardiologist 4 to 6 months, catheterization of ≥ 100 patients
Level two:	Diagnostic angiographer 12 months, catheterization of ≥ 300 patients, 200 as primary operator
Level three:	Interventionalist Additional 12 months, angioplasty of ≥ 125 patients, 75 as primary operator; specialized training in use of newer interventional devices

Catheter systems used for PTCA consist of three major elements: guiding equipment, the balloon-tipped dilating catheter, and an inflation device. A large variety of guide catheters are available. For PTCA, 8F (2.6 mm) diameter guides are generally used, although 7F (2.3 mm) and smaller guides are used with increasing frequency. A wide variety of guide catheter shapes, most of which are patterned after successful diagnostic catheter shapes, are available. The internal dimensions of guide catheters have steadily improved with advances in guide catheter design and material developments. Guide wires are used to direct dilating catheters into the coronary arterial tree. They are available in sizes ranging from 0.009 to 0.021 inch in diameter. All guide wires possess a forming ribbon at the distal tip that allows the wire to be shaped; the shaping of a guide wire greatly enhances the operator's ability to steer the wire into place across a coronary stenosis. An important consideration in the selection of a guide wire is its axial rigidity, or stiffness. Very stiff wires have greater ability to cross high-grade lesions or total occlusions but may pose greater risk of intimal dissection or coronary perforation.

Many dilating balloon catheters are now available. Important characteristics of balloon catheters are a low deflated profile, known balloon compliance response to various inflation pressures, minimal friction for passage of tight stenoses, "pushability" (sufficient longitudinal rigidity so that movement of the shaft produces a proportional movement of the distal catheter tip), "trackability" (the ability of the balloon catheter to slide along the guide wire to the stenosis), and steering. Many balloons are made of polyethylene terephthalate, a plastic that can achieve a very low balloon profile and that is minimally compliant even at high inflation pressures. Other polymers, such as polyethylene and polyolefin copolymer, have a compliant response to varying inflation pressures. Various coatings are used to improve lubriciousness. Most catheters require use of a separate guide wire ("over-the-wire" systems), although a few catheters have integral, nonremovable wires ("fixed-wire" systems). Over-the-wire catheters are slightly larger in profile but benefit from the enhanced steering that results from use of an independent guide wire. Since exchange wires and devices are available for nearly all over-the-wire systems, these catheters can be removed and exchanged without surrendering the guide wire position. Fixed-wire systems have an extremely low profile and are slightly longer than over-the-wire catheters, but steering requires movement of the entire catheter rather than just a guide wire; hence, torque tends to be somewhat less efficiently transmitted to the catheter tip. Also, these catheters do not currently have a reliable, convenient mechanism for making catheter exchanges.

Balloon inflation is carried out with a handheld pressure manometer that displays the inflation pressure in both atmospheres (bars) and pounds of pressure per square inch. Because some fibrocalcific stenoses may require very high pressure for full dilatation, some inflation devices are capable of providing pressures of 20 atmospheres or more. Automated inflation devices have been used, but they offer little benefit.

High-quality video and x-ray systems are also essential during PTCA. These permit the detailed assessment of coronary anatomy necessary for appropriate patient selection and for safely navigating the coronary vessels during the procedure. Characteristics of the imaging systems used for angioplasty at the Mayo Clinic are described in chapter 10A.

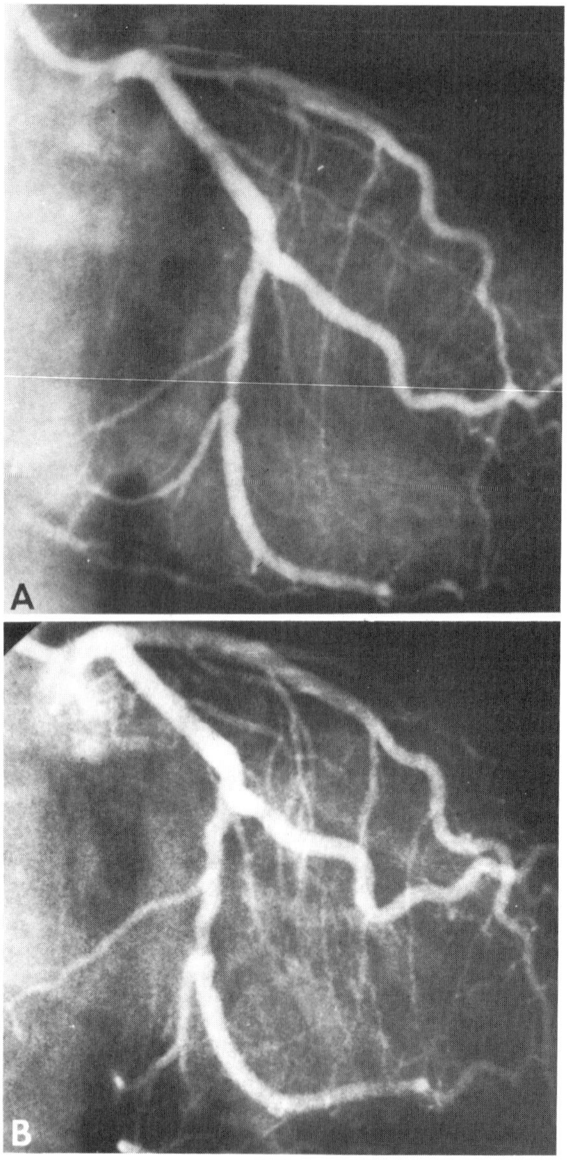

Fig 10B-2 **A,** after angioplasty, large dissection in proximal left anterior descending artery. **B,** 6 months later; no residual dissection is apparent. (From Vlietstra RE, Bresnahan JF, Holmes DR Jr: Coronary balloon angioplasty. In *Interventional Cardiology.* Edited by DR Holmes Jr, RE Vlietstra. Philadelphia, F. A. Davis Company, 1989, pp 55-72. By permission, Mayo Foundation.)

Mechanism of dilation

The mechanism of balloon dilation was established in the animal laboratory[13-16] and in postmortem human studies.[17-20] In normal vessels, balloon inflation produces endothelial cell denudation; this exposes the collagen-rich subendothelial matrix, which is rapidly covered by a platelet-fibrin meshwork.[14] As inflation continues, there is stretching of the intima, media, and adventitia without disruption of these layers. However, if gross overdilation occurs, arterial rupture may result.

Atherosclerotic plaques are intimal accumulations of smooth muscle cells, lipids, and fibrous tissue, and they are often eccentrically located in the artery wall. The mechanisms of dilation of these lesions include plaque element shearing and splitting, with formation of one or more intimal clefts. If the lesion is noncircumferential, the adjacent normal vessel wall may also be stretched to enhance the result further. Localized intimal or medial dissection can occur; occasionally, this is of sufficient degree to cause partial or total occlusion of the vessel lumen. Over time, remodeling of successfully dilated lesions occurs (Fig 10B-2), with retraction of the separated plaque elements and reendothelialization.[16] Figure 10B-3 shows pathologic findings after angioplasty.

Patient selection

Initially, PTCA was limited to patients with recent onset of disabling angina who had proximal noncalcified sin-

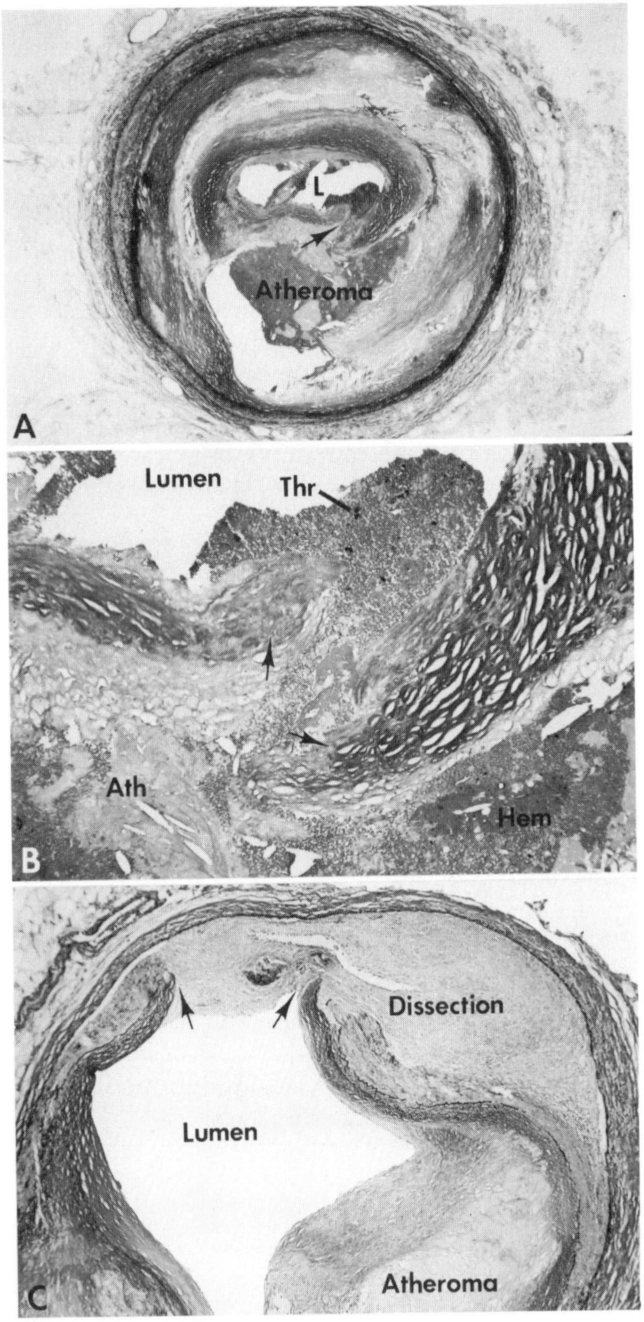

Fig 10B-3 Coronary arterial lesion after angioplasty. **A,** disruption of intima *(arrow)* allows communication between lumen *(L)* and atheroma. **B,** close-up view of **A** shows site of intimal tear *(arrows),* hemorrhage *(Hem)* into atheroma *(Ath),* and fresh thrombus *(Thr)* along rupture tract 1 day after procedure. **C,** intimal tear *(arrows)* along wall opposite atheroma is associated with intramedial dissection and plugging of false channel by granulation tissue 3 weeks after procedure. (From Bresnahan DR: Mechanism of action. In *PTCA, Percutaneous Transluminal Coronary Angioplasty.* Edited by RE Vlietstra, DR Holmes Jr. Philadelphia, F. A. Davis Company, 1987, pp 19-33. By permission, Mayo Foundation.)

Table 10B-2 Selection criteria for PTCA

Myocardial ischemia (symptoms or demonstrated on functional testing)
Revascularization necessary (or preferable to medical treatment)
Lesions approachable with PTCA
High likelihood of success
Absence of factors in favor of surgery: left main artery disease, older bypass, diffuse disease, chronic total occlusion, high-risk anatomy, etc.

Additional indications

Cardiogenic shock
Salvage of failed thrombolysis
Primary therapy in acute myocardial infarction

gle coronary stenoses and were considered candidates for surgical revascularization. By these criteria, from 1% to 15% of patients undergoing bypass appeared to be candidates for PTCA.[21-24] However, with increasing physician experience and improvements in catheter design, the criteria for angioplasty have broadened. Although the original criteria still identify the "ideal" patient, successful angioplasty of multiple lesions in multiple vessels,[25] calcified lesions,[26] and saphenous vein graft stenoses[27] has been reported. Angioplasty has been used in patients with unstable angina,[28] for management of total coronary occlusions,[29] and intraoperatively to improve distal runoff in patients undergoing saphenous vein bypass surgery.[30]

Selection criteria for angioplasty are shown in Table 10B-2. Myocardial ischemia must be present, either demonstrated by functional testing or manifested by symptoms. Second, revascularization should be judged either necessary or strongly preferable to medical therapy. Third, all significant lesions should be approachable with angioplasty techniques. Fourth, the likelihood of successful dilatation should be high. Fifth, there should be absence of factors directly favoring surgery, such as unprotected left main coronary artery disease, severe diffuse multivessel disease, chronic total occlusion subtending a viable area of myocardium, or anatomic features that would allow inadvertent occlusion of the dilated vessel to jeopardize an unduly large area of myocardium. Additional indications include acute myocardial infarction, especially in patients who are in cardiogenic shock or in whom intravenous thrombolytic therapy has failed to open an occluded artery.

PTCA is contraindicated in certain situations (Table 10B-3). Patients with such little disease that PTCA is unlikely to improve blood flow and patients with such severe disease that bypass surgery would provide superior benefit or safety should not undergo PTCA.

To assist in determining the risk of PTCA, the American College of Cardiology and the American Heart Association have jointly published estimates of success and complications of PTCA based on lesion morphol-

Table 10B-3 Contraindications to PTCA

Unprotected left main stenosis
Nondilatable lesion with large area of ischemia
Revascularization unnecessary
Many lesions (surgery preferable)
Low anticipated success rate
Borderline stenosis (<60%)
Variant angina with mild fixed stenoses
Other surgical cardiac disease

ogy.[31] According to these guidelines, lesions can be classified as type A, B, or C on the basis of the angiographic appearance and a few essential historical facts (such as the age of a saphenous vein graft or approximate duration of a total occlusion). These estimates are intended to facilitate a risk:benefit analysis for each patient referred for PTCA (Table 10B-4). An early test of the validity of these guidelines indicated that they were reasonable approximations of risk and success,[32] but recent studies have called into question the accuracy of the figures with current technology.[33,34] In addition, even if abrupt closure (the most serious complicating event during angioplasty) occurs, it can usually be managed with further balloon inflations or use of bailout devices such as intracoronary stents.

PTCA in patients with poor left ventricular function remains controversial. Most published reports indicate a higher rate of acute and long-term complications if the left ventricular ejection fraction is 35% or less,[35,36] and a matched case-control study performed at the Mayo Clinic suggests that surgery may offer a superior outcome for these patients, probably as a result of more complete revascularization.[37] Several large randomized trials comparing PTCA with coronary bypass surgery for multivessel coronary disease are under way; these are likely to clarify the relative benefit of each strategy for many patient subsets.

Patient preparation

Patients are evaluated in an outpatient setting before elective PTCA, at which time routine laboratory studies are done. Patients in otherwise good health are admitted on the morning of the procedure, whereas those with significant concomitant illness (such as poorly controlled hypertension or diabetes mellitus, significant electrolyte disturbance, or coagulation abnormality) are admitted on the evening before PTCA.

Before the procedure, the angioplasty operator reviews the goals and risks with the patient and family, including the likelihood of procedural success and the risks involved, namely, acute occlusion, myocardial infarction, emergency operation, and death. Review of the case with a cardiovascular surgeon is done at our institution if there is an increased likelihood of complications or uncertainty in selecting between angioplasty and surgery. Administration of aspirin, 325 mg daily, is begun, preferably 1 to 2 days before angioplasty. Antiplatelet therapy has been shown to reduce the occurrence of acute closure at the time of angioplasty.[38,39]

Technique

Fasting patients are taken to the catheterization suite, and arterial access is obtained either by the femoral percuta-

Table 10B-4 American College of Cardiology and American Heart Association angioplasty guidelines: lesion-specific characteristics of type A, B, and C lesions

Type A lesions (high success, >85%; low risk)	
• Discrete (<10 mm long)	• Little or no calcification
• Concentric	• Less than totally occlusive
• Readily accessible	• Nonostial in location
• Nonangulated segment, <45°	• No major branch involvement
• Smooth contour	• Absence of thrombus
Type B lesions (moderate success, 60% to 85%; moderate risk)	
• Tubular (10 to 20 mm long)	• Moderate to heavy calcification
• Eccentric	• Total occlusions <3 months old
• Moderate tortuosity of proximal segment	• Ostial in location
• Moderately angulated segment, >45°, <90°	• Bifurcation lesions requiring double guide wires
• Irregular contour	• Some thrombus present
Type C lesions (low success, <60%; high risk)	
• Diffuse (>2 cm long)	• Total occlusions >3 months old
• Excessive tortuosity of proximal segment	• Inability to protect major side branches
• Extremely angulated segments, >90°	• Degenerated vein grafts with friable lesions

From Ryan TJ (Chairman): Guidelines for percutaneous transluminal coronary angioplasty. *J Am Coll Cardiol* 12:529-545, 1988. By permission of American College of Cardiology.

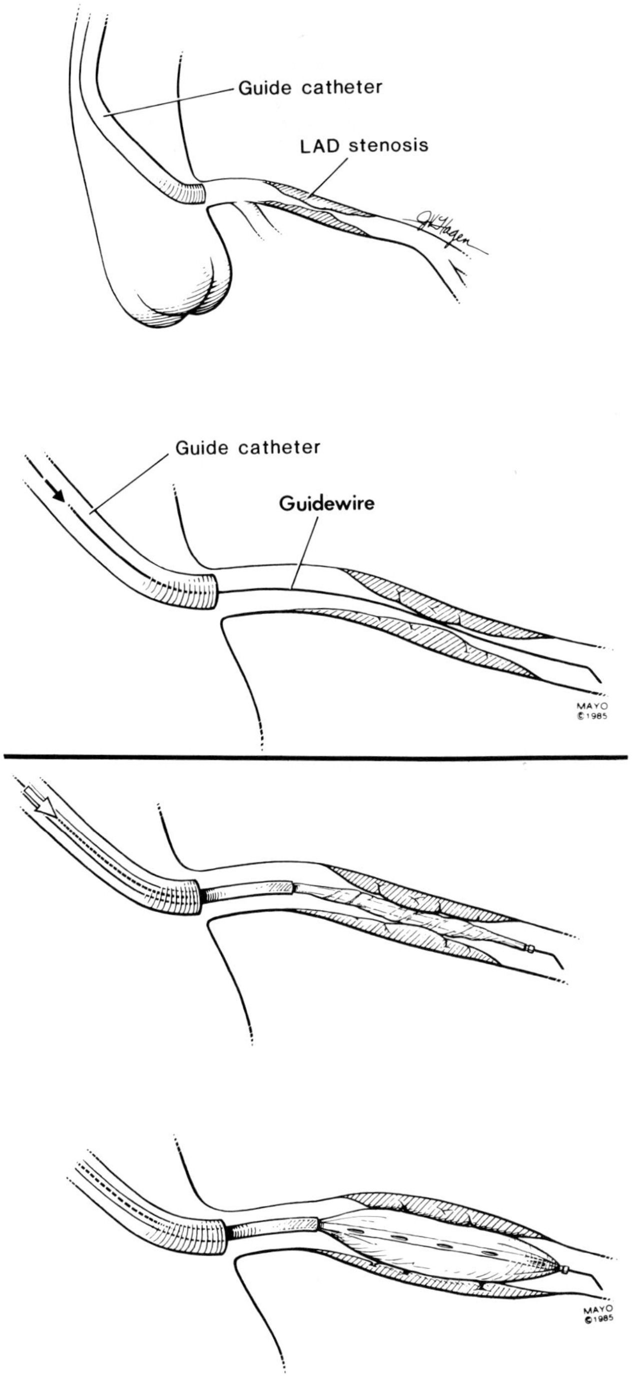

Fig 10B-4 Technique of PTCA. See text for details of the procedure. *LAD,* left anterior descending coronary artery. (From Shepherd RFJ, Vlietstra RE: The history of balloon angioplasty. In *PTCA, Percutaneous Transluminal Coronary Angioplasty.* Edited by RE Vlietstra, DR Holmes Jr. Philadelphia, F. A. Davis Company, 1987, pp 1-17. By permission, Mayo Foundation.)

neous (modified Seldinger) technique or by a brachial artery cutdown approach (Sones technique). If a prolonged procedure is anticipated or if intraluminal thrombus is evident before PTCA, a continuous infusion of heparin is begun. Anticoagulation is guided by monitoring the activated clotting time.[40] A calcium blocker, such as nifedipine, 10 mg sublingually, and nitrates are administered. A guiding catheter is selected on the basis of the anatomy of the aortic root and coronary ostium (Fig 10B-4). A dilating catheter system is selected on the basis of size and location of the stenosis, lesion severity, presence of tortuosity, or branching proximal to or involving the lesion itself. Balloon size is selected according to the estimated or measured diameter of the nearest normal vessel segment. Undersizing the balloon is likely to leave an inadequate dilatation, with a higher risk of restenosis, whereas oversizing the balloon carries a higher risk of acute complications and does not reduce the restenosis risk.[41] Low-profile catheters are selected in very tight lesions, and over-the-wire systems are preferred when the need for catheter exchanges is envisioned. Usually, a guide wire with a very flexible tip is selected to reduce the possibility of distal arterial trauma or inadvertent guide-wire dissection. For total occlusions, a large-diameter wire with increased stiffness may be necessary to cross the occluded segment.

In general, the guide wire is placed across the lesion first and test injections are made in multiple views to ensure the intraluminal passage of the wire. The dilating catheter is advanced across the stenosis. In the past, a transstenotic pressure gradient was measured routinely. However, the physiologic significance of the lesion is usually apparent from its angiographic appearance, and many of the commonly used low-profile balloon catheters are unable to accurately measure distal pressures. A new guide wire incorporating a Doppler ultrasound transducer is available[42] that permits measurement of distal blood velocities and flow profiles before and after PTCA and may also be of use in assessing coronary blood flow reserve.

After the catheter is positioned across the target lesion, balloon inflations are performed until an adequate result is obtained, which generally means a residual stenosis of 30% or less (Fig 10B-5). Sometimes selection of larger balloon sizes, a balloon of higher pressure, or multiple balloons and wires may be necessary, for example, in the case of a bifurcation stenosis. When an adequate result has been obtained, catheters are removed and the arterial sheath is sewn in place. If a small residual stenosis with a smooth angiographic appearance is obtained, no additional heparin is given and the vascular sheath is removed at the earliest time possible. However, if the residual stenosis is substantial, if the lesion has a shaggy or hazy angiographic appearance, or if frank intraluminal thrombus is evident, a continuous infusion of heparin is maintained overnight. Repeat limited angiography may be performed the following day to assure that the lesion is stable before removal of the vascular sheath.

Initial results

Successful PTCA reduces the stenosis, abolishes or lessens demonstrable myocardial ischemia, and is not associated with major complications, such as myocardial infarction, emergency bypass surgery, and death. At least

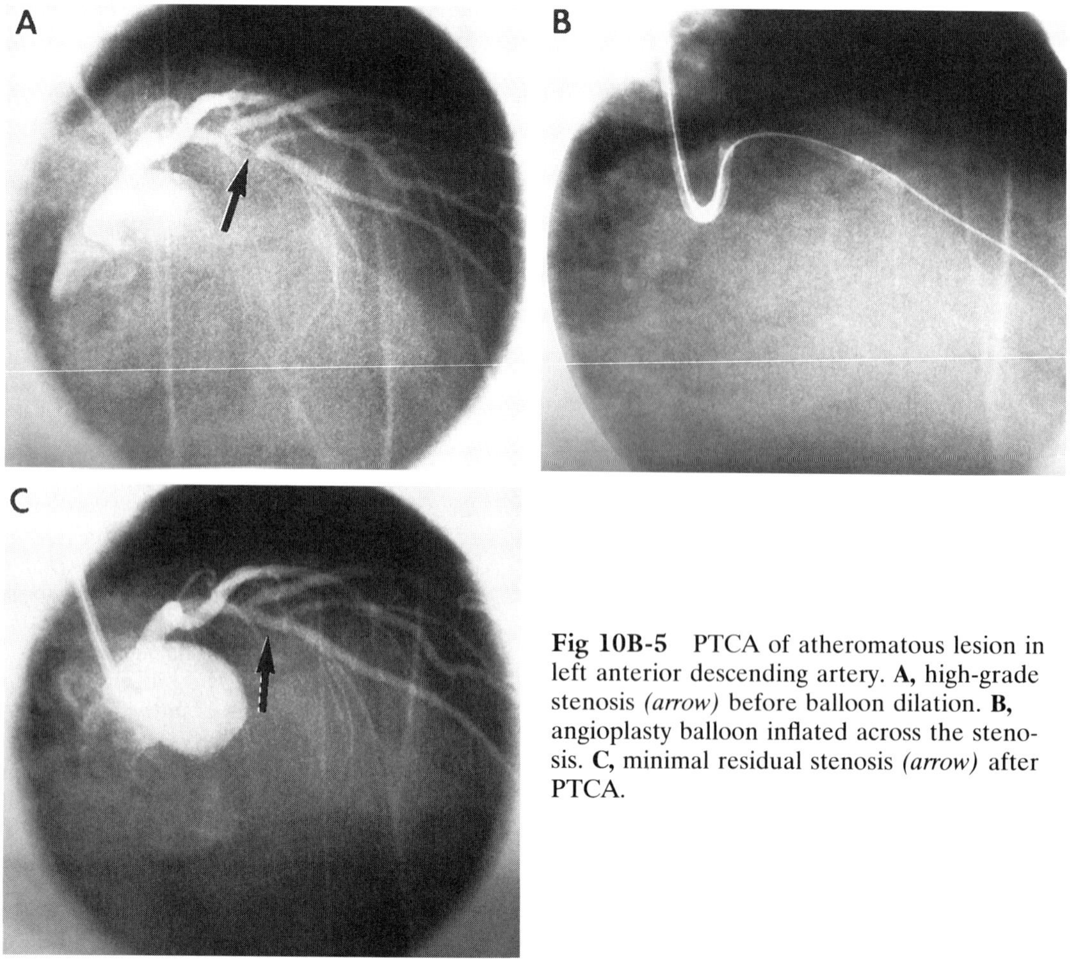

Fig 10B-5 PTCA of atheromatous lesion in left anterior descending artery. **A,** high-grade stenosis *(arrow)* before balloon dilation. **B,** angioplasty balloon inflated across the stenosis. **C,** minimal residual stenosis *(arrow)* after PTCA.

20% improvement in stenosis diameter must occur for a procedure to be judged successful.

The National Heart, Lung, and Blood Institute (NHLBI) PTCA Registry reported outcome data on angioplasty between 1977 and 1981 and for 1985 and 1986.[43,44] These results are shown in Table 10B-5. Most centers currently performing angioplasty should be able to conform to the results shown for 1985 and 1986—namely, a success rate of approximately 90%, mortality of 1% or less, nonfatal infarction of 5% or less, and need for urgent coronary bypass operation of 5% to 6.1%.

A variety of angiographic patterns are seen after successful angioplasty. A hazy "ground glass" appearance of the dilated segment is frequent and probably represents contrast medium filling small intimal fissures and slits. Intimal flaps are also seen, which vary from thin linear densities to spiral dissections with persistent staining of contrast medium within the wall. The spiral dissections may result in significant luminal compromise. The significance of angiographic patterns in relation to long-term results remains unclear. Interestingly, on follow-up angiography, large intimal slits or flaps have often totally resolved.

In addition to clinical improvement with reduced angina and improved exercise performance and angiographic findings demonstrating increased vessel lumen and reduced transstenotic gradient, other evidence of physiologic benefit has been documented in patients with successful dilation. Increases in coronary sinus blood flow and myocardial lactate extraction occur. Also, exercise-induced thallium-201 (^{201}Tl) perfusion defects improve or

Table 10B-5 Results of PTCA according to NHLBI PTCA registry

	1977-1981, %	1985-1986, %
One or more lesions reduced ≥20%	67.5	90.7
All lesions attempted reduced >20%; no death, infarction, or bypass	61.0	78.3
Death	1.2	1.0
Nonfatal infarction	4.9	4.3
Coronary bypass	26.5	5.6

Data from Detre K, Holubkov R, Kelsey S, et al: Percutaneous transluminal coronary angioplasty in 1985-1986 and 1977-1981: the National Heart, Lung, and Blood Institute Registry. *N Engl J Med* 318:265-270, 1988.

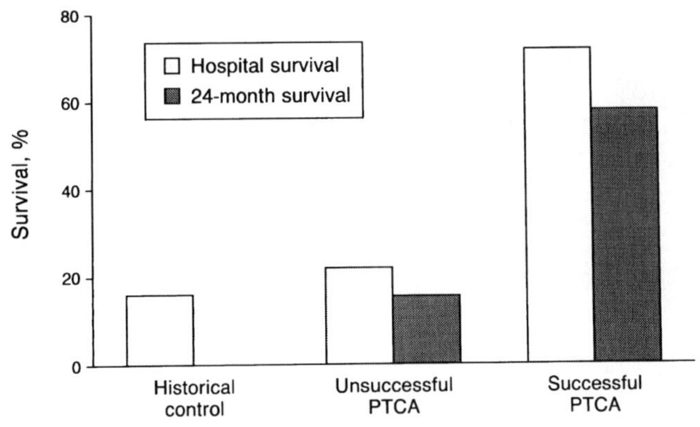

Fig 10B-6 Effect of PTCA on survival of patients with cardiogenic shock. Patients have an expected 15% survival with conventional care, whereas successful PTCA results in about 70% survival. Unsuccessful angioplasty is still associated with a poor outcome. Long-term survival is also improved. (Data from Lee L, Erbel R, Brown TM, et al: Multicenter registry of angioplasty therapy of cardiogenic shock: initial and long-term survival. *J Am Coll Cardiol* 17:599-603, 1991.)

disappear, and improvement in exercise-induced regional wall motion abnormalities after successful dilation has been noted.

Patients in cardiogenic shock are the only subset known to have better survival with PTCA than with standard therapy.[45-48] Patients with acute myocardial infarction and Killip class 4 shock are expected to have a hospital mortality of about 85%, but such patients successfully treated with a strategy of direct PTCA have a much lower hospital mortality (Fig 10B-6). PTCA has been reported to be successful in only two-thirds of patients, however, and mortality remains high when PTCA fails.

The first randomized trial to show a clinical benefit for patients treated with PTCA was the Angioplasty Compared to Medicine (ACME) trial.[49] In this study, patients at Veterans Administration hospitals who had single-vessel coronary artery disease and good left ventricular function were randomized to receive medical therapy alone or in combination with PTCA. The end point of the trial was performance during exercise treadmill testing 6 months after entry into the trial. Although patients treated with PTCA had administration of cardiac drugs held before the follow-up treadmill test, they still performed significantly better than those randomized to medical therapy.

Long-term results

From the initial Zurich experience, 133 patients with successful angioplasty were followed up for a mean of 72 months. Survival was 96% at 7 years, and 79% were free from death, myocardial infarction, and subsequent bypass surgery. Twenty-seven patients underwent repeat angioplasty, and 19 had bypass surgery. At follow-up, approximately three-fourths were in functional class I.[50]

These results, as well as those from other centers, demonstrate the excellent outcome from angioplasty in patients with predominantly single-vessel disease. Although the results are gratifying, critics are quick to point out that the prognosis in most patients with single-vessel disease is excellent with medical therapy alone.

Multivessel disease

Angioplasty has been applied increasingly in patients with multivessel disease[51-64] (Fig 10B-7). Although initial success rates of 80% to 90% have been demonstrated, comparison of results from different centers is open to question because of differences in classification of lesions; differentiation among single-lesion, multilesion, and multivessel dilation; and differences in selection criteria for angioplasty and even for single-vessel and multivessel disease. It seems clear, however, that the results of angioplasty are less favorable as coronary disease becomes more advanced. Table 10B-6 shows the complications of angioplasty related to the severity of disease in 1,802 patients forming the 1985-1986 NHLBI PTCA Registry cohort. Although the incidence of procedural death was only 0.2% in single-vessel disease, it rose to 2.8% in triple-vessel disease. Likewise, the incidences of myocardial infarction of 5.2%, emergency coronary bypass of 4.4%, and acute occlusion of 7.9% found with triple-vessel disease are all substantially higher than figures reported for double- or single-vessel disease. The incidence of restenosis on a per-patient basis is also higher for patients with multivessel angioplasty, although the true incidence remains unknown because of incomplete angiographic follow-up in these studies.

Completeness of revascularization has been shown to be important in patients with multivessel disease undergoing bypass surgery.[65,66] Most patients with multivessel disease have at least one vessel that does not readily lend itself to angioplasty. This has led to the concept of selective, or "culprit"-vessel, angioplasty, in which an attempt is made to identify and dilate the principal lesion thought responsible for the patient's symptoms.[67,68] Although complete revascularization seems intuitively desirable, many factors besides completeness of revascularization probably affect outcome in patients with multivessel disease.[69]

Because the long-term results of multivessel angioplasty are not established, substantial controversy remains about selection of PTCA over elective coronary bypass surgery for multivessel disease. To address this issue, several multicenter investigations are under way that aim to compare PTCA with coronary artery bypass graft surgery (Table 10B-7). Although entry criteria differ for each study, each randomly assigned patients with single-vessel or multivessel disease to undergo PTCA or coronary artery bypass graft surgery. In some, patients who refused randomization were followed in a registry. The Bypass Angioplasty Revascularization Investigation (BARI) is the largest trial.[70,71] This trial, sponsored by the NHLBI, randomized over 1,800 patients at medical centers in the United States, Canada, and Europe. Clinical outcome will be measured at 5 years after randomization; recruitment into the study was completed in June 1992. Other trials are

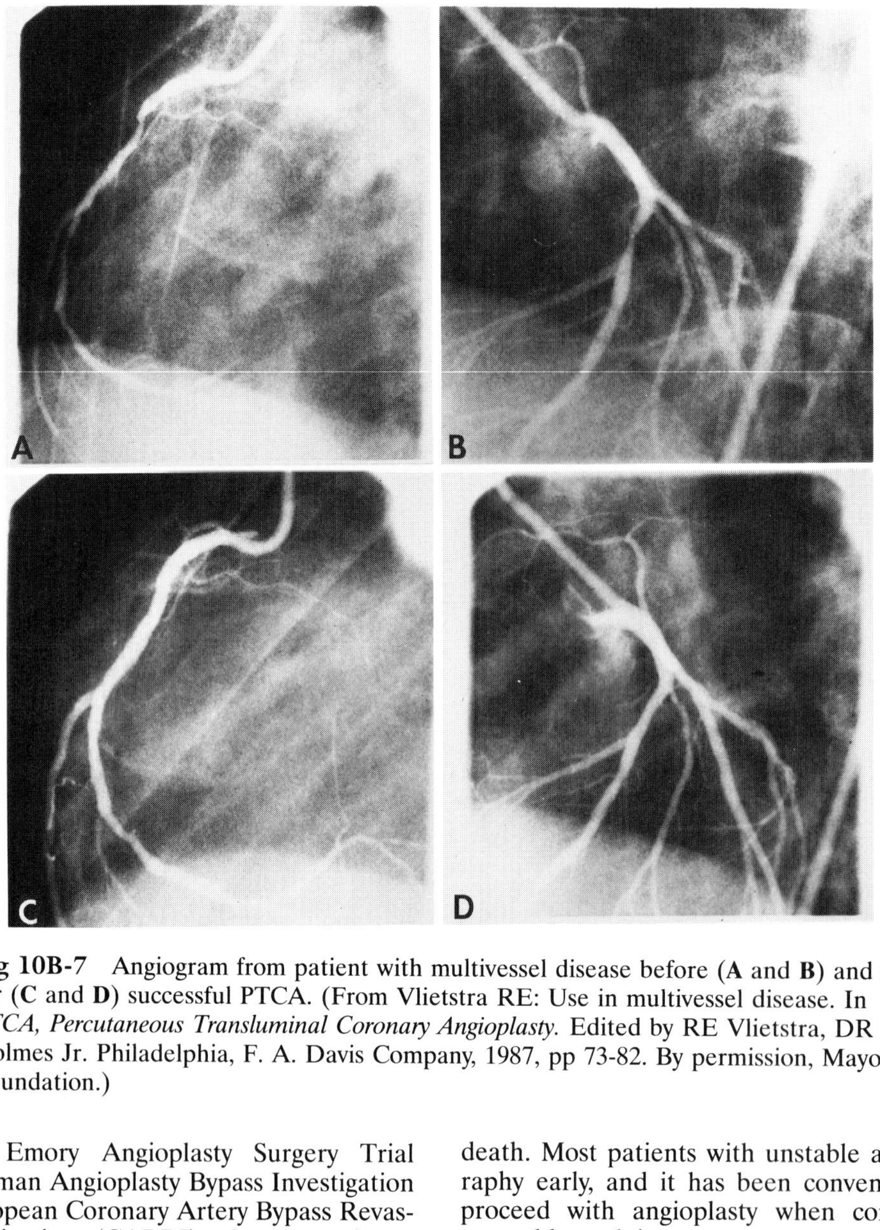

Fig 10B-7 Angiogram from patient with multivessel disease before (**A** and **B**) and after (**C** and **D**) successful PTCA. (From Vlietstra RE: Use in multivessel disease. In *PTCA, Percutaneous Transluminal Coronary Angioplasty.* Edited by RE Vlietstra, DR Holmes Jr. Philadelphia, F. A. Davis Company, 1987, pp 73-82. By permission, Mayo Foundation.)

the single-center Emory Angioplasty Surgery Trial (EAST),[72] the German Angioplasty Bypass Investigation (GABI),[73] the European Coronary Artery Bypass Revascularization Investigation (CABRI), the Argentinean ERACI trial,[74] and the English Randomised Interventional Treatment of Angina (RITA). These trials demonstrate that as initial treatment strategies, both PTCA and coronary artery bypass grafting yield similar clinical benefits. Hospital stays and initial morbidity are greater after coronary artery bypass grafting, but because of higher rates of incomplete revascularization and restenosis, recurrent angina and the need for additional revascularization procedures are greater after PTCA.

Unstable angina

Unstable angina is associated with an increased risk of continuing angina, myocardial infarction, and death. Observational studies have described the use of angioplasty for patients with unstable angina.[75-77] The objectives in such patients are twofold: the relief of ischemic episodes and the prevention of infarction or cardiac death. Most patients with unstable angina have angiography early, and it has been convenient and logical to proceed with angioplasty when coronary anatomy is amenable to doing so.

Table 10B-8 shows the success and complication rates in angioplasty performed in patients with unstable angina. In general, success rates are slightly lower than in elective procedures, and complication rates are slightly higher. Comparison of these results with those for coronary artery bypass surgery in patients with unstable angina is not possible because of substantial differences in patient selection. Most unstable patients undergoing angioplasty have single- or double-vessel disease with relatively preserved left ventricular function, whereas patients in most surgical series have a higher prevalence of three-vessel disease and impaired ventricular function.

Patients undergoing PTCA for unstable angina are likely to have irregular, high-grade, complex stenoses (Fig 10B-8) with associated intraluminal thrombus and secondary coronary spasm—all features that decrease the changes of success and increase complications with

Table 10B-6 Complications of PTCA according to Second (1985-1986) NHLBI PTCA Registry (n = 1,802)

	Complications, %				
Vessels diseased	Death	Myocardial infarction	Emergency coronary bypass	Acute occlusion
Single	0.2	3.5	2.9	3.9
Double	0.9	5.2	3.9	4.5
Triple	2.2	5.2	4.4	7.9
Left main	8.1	2.7	2.7	2.7
Total	0.9	4.3	3.5	4.9
P	<0.001	NS	NS	<0.01

From Holmes DR Jr, Holubkov R, Vlietstra RE, et al: Comparison of complications during percutaneous transluminal coronary angioplasty from 1977 to 1981 and from 1985 to 1986: the National Heart, Lung, and Blood Institute Percutaneous Transluminal Coronary Angioplasty Registry. *J Am Coll Cardiol* 12:1149-1155, 1988. By permission of the American College of Cardiology.

PTCA. At the Mayo Clinic, an attempt is made to stabilize the patient medically before angiography. If angiography demonstrates left main disease or extensive three-vessel disease, patients are referred for surgical treatment, particularly if left ventricular function is impaired. If an obvious "culprit" lesion is apparent, PTCA of just that lesion may be undertaken, with treatment of other lesions (if necessary) deferred to a later time.

Acute myocardial infarction

For patients with acute myocardial infarction, PTCA can be used as primary therapy to restore vessel patency, as an adjunct to intravenous thrombolysis, or as secondary therapy for spontaneous or exercise-induced myocardial ischemia after the acute phase of myocardial infarction.

Observational studies have shown that PTCA for acute myocardial infarction achieves vessel patency in more patients than would be expected with thrombolytic therapy[90-99] (Table 10B-9). Only recently have randomized studies compared direct PTCA and thrombolytic therapy with subsequent conservative management. A small study in 1989 indicated that PTCA compared favorably with streptokinase therapy.[92] The results of three important randomized trials were published in 1993[101-103] (Table 10B-10). All showed high rates of PTCA success (93%-98%). One study, conducted at the Mayo Clinic,[101] found that both therapies were effective in salvaging myocardium at jeopardy of infarction (Fig 10B-9). Infarct-related artery patency was greater with PTCA than with streptokinase treatment, and recurrent ischemic events were less frequent in patients with PTCA than in those with streptokinase or tissue plasminogen activator therapy. Recurrent ischemia, myocardial infarction, death, hospital readmissions, need for repeat catheter procedures and angioplasty, and follow-up costs were all lower for patients treated with PTCA. High-risk patients appeared to receive the greatest benefit from an invasive treatment strategy. One study[103] showed superior resting and exercise left ventricular performance in patients receiving PTCA therapy. Although direct PTCA may be the treatment of choice for some patient subsets,[104] the limitation of catheterization facilities to fewer than one-fifth of hospitals in the United States[105] and the logistics of having the necessary catheterization and surgical resources available around the clock preclude this therapy from becoming a practical reality for most patients.

Angioplasty as an adjunct to thrombolytic therapy has been well studied in three large-scale randomized trials.[106-108] All showed conclusively that after successful intravenous thrombolytic therapy with tissue plasminogen activator, angioplasty produced no measurable benefits of survival, left ventricular function, or reduction of postinfarct complications and, in fact, increased the risk of bleeding and emergency surgery (Table 10B-11). The current consensus is that angioplasty is not indicated routinely in patients who have successful reperfusion after thrombolytic therapy. In these patients, it now seems most appropriate to consider delayed angioplasty (or bypass surgery), depending on the results of functional testing and coronary angiographic morphology determined in the late postinfarction hospitalization phase.

For patients in whom thrombolysis has failed, however, salvage PTCA has merit.[100,109-114] Salvage PTCA has been shown to be effective (Table 10B-12), although success rates may be lower than those reported for primary PTCA. Reocclusion has been a problem for these patients, probably because of the volume of intraluminal thrombus present at the time of PTCA. This assumption is supported by the Thrombolysis and Angioplasty in Myocardial Infarction (TAMI) I and II data, since salvage PTCA was more effective in patients treated with tissue plasminogen activator and urokinase than in those treated with tissue plasminogen activator alone; the addition of the non-fibrin-specific urokinase was associated with much greater levels of fibrinogen degradation products, which have known thrombus and platelet inhibitory effects.[120,121]

Ventricular myocardium may be salvaged after relatively long periods of vessel occlusion; in such cases, the myocytes are thought to be "stunned" or "hibernating" rather than infarcted[122-125] (see chapter 27A). A recent report indicated that restoring patency several weeks after an infarct can result in substantial improvement in the performance of the infarcted zone.[126] Data from animal models of chronic coronary occlusion support the concept that a patent infarct-related artery is superior to a closed one, independent of myocardial cell survival.[127] This "open artery hypothesis" argues that late reperfusion may be of benefit by enhancing late healing characteristics, thereby reducing the likelihood of sequelae to myocardial infarction, such as ventricular arrhythmias, cardiac rupture, thromboembolic events, and left ventricular dilatation.[128,129]

Table 10B-7 Multicenter trials comparing outcome of PTCA with that of coronary artery bypass grafting

	Clinical eligibility criteria				
	Severe angina	Unstable angina	Myocardial infarction	Mild angina	Silent ischemia
RITA	Revascularization judged necessary				
GABI	Class III	No	>4 wk	No	No
EAST	>5 days Revascularization judged necessary and positive exercise stress test				
CABRI	>1 mo Revascularization judged necessary and objective evidence of ischemia				
BARI	Yes	Yes	Yes	If EF <50%, severe ischemia, or prior MI	If prior MI or angina

BARI, Bypass Angioplasty Revascularization Investigation; CABRI, Coronary Artery Bypass Revascularization Investigation; EAST, Emory Angioplasty Surgery Trial; EF, ejection fraction; GABI, German Angioplasty Bypass Investigation; LV, left ventricular; MI, myocardial infarction; RITA, Randomised Interventional Treatment of Angina.

Table 10B-8 Percutaneous transluminal coronary angioplasty in unstable angina

Study	Year	Comment	Pt, no.	Success, %
Meyer et al.[78]	1983	a	50	74
de Feyter et al.*[79]	1985	a,c	88	92
Plokker et al.[80]	1988	a	469	88
Haraphongse et al.[81]	1988	a	29	85
de Feyter et al.*[82]	1988	a	114	90
		b	86	88
Szatmáry et al.[83]	1988	a	236	87
Perry et al.[84]	1988		105	87
Holt et al.[77]	1988	d	69	80
Kamp et al. *[85]	1989		334	87
Morrison[86]	1990	a,d	66	88
Morrison[87]	1990	a,e	34	94
Ilia et al.[88]	1992		149	95
Bauters et al.[89]	1993	f	50	90

CABG, coronary artery bypass grafting surgery; FU, follow-up; MI, myocardial infarction.
Comments:
a. Unstable angina pectoris refractory to medical therapy.
b. Unstable angina pectoris stabilized with medical therapy.
c. Emergency coronary angioplasty.
d. Post-myocardial infarction angina.
e. Post-coronary artery bypass surgery patients only.
f. Post-angioplasty restenosis patients only.

*May include some of the same patients.
†5-year actuarial death rate.

Age, yr	Angiographic criteria	Follow-up registry for all eligible patients	Clinic follow-up schedule	Major end points
...	1, 2, or 3 vessels >50% stenotic; equivalent revascularization feasible	Yes	1 and 6 mo; 1, 2, 3, 4, and 5 yr	Death, MI, severity of angina, exercise test performance, subsequent employment, LV function, and additional revascularization procedures
≤75	2 or 3 vessels ≥70% stenotic	...	3, 6, and 12 mo	Severity of angina and dyspnea, exercise test performance, MI, and death
...	2 or 3 vessels ≥50% stenotic	Yes	1 and 3 yr	Angiographically defined revascularization status and thallium-201 perfusion, death, cardiovascular events, additional revascularization procedures, and quality of life
...	2 or 3 vessels ≥50% stenotic	Yes	6 mo and 2 yr	Relief of angina, treadmill exercise and thallium perfusion, death, MI, recurrent angina, heart failure, and angiographic assessment
17-79	2 or 3 vessels ≥50% stenotic (by electronic calipers) supplying 2 or 3 of the major myocardial territories	Yes	6 wk; 1, 3, and 5 yr	Mortality and MI at 5 yr, severity of angina, treadmill exercise performance and ischemia, heart failure, coronary angiographic assessment, LV function, subsequent revascularization procedures, resource utilization, and quality of life

Initial complications, %				Late complications, %		
Death	MI	CABG	Mean FU, mo	Death	MI	Angina
0	4	2	6	0	0	36
0	6	8	12	2	2	15
1	2	3	19	6†	...	...
0	0	3	...	...	...	...
1	4	5	12	1	2	12
0	4	5	12	1	1	12
3	3	2	14	4	3	6
2	9	4	...	...	...	...
2	...	12	21	0	4	24
0	9	10	25	5	14	...
3	3	3	14	7	...	14
0	0	3	6 to 36	6	6	...
0	2	2	...	...	...	...
0	4	2	6	2	...	16

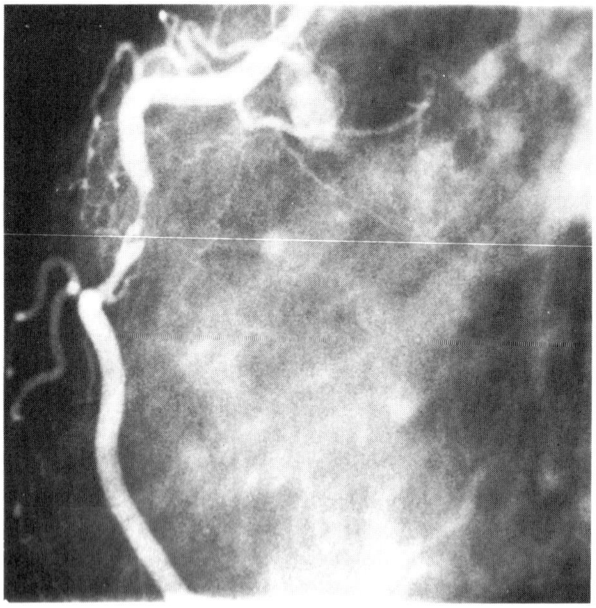

Fig 10B-8 Left anterior oblique view of right coronary artery. Immediately distal to severe proximal stenosis is an intraluminal filling defect consistent with coronary arterial thrombus. This finding identifies patients at increased risk of occlusion during attempted dilation. (From Mabin TA, Holmes DR Jr, Smith HC, et al: Intracoronary thrombus: role in coronary occlusion complicating percutaneous transluminal coronary angioplasty. *J Am Coll Cardiol* 5:198-202, 1985. By permission of the American College of Cardiology.)

Table 10B-9 Success of primary PTCA for acute myocardial infarction

Study	Year	Patients, no.	Success, % of pt
Kimura et al.[90]	1986	58	88
O'Neill et al.[92]	1986	29	83
Rothbaum et al.[93]	1987	151	87
Miller et al.[94]	1987	81	92
Marco et al.[95]	1987	43	95
Zolnick et al.[96]	1988	61	85
O'Keefe et al.[97]	1989	500	94
Kahn et al.[99]	1990	250	96
Juliard et al.[98]	1992	40	90
Ellis et al.[100]	1994	78	92

From Holmes DR Jr, Gersh BJ: The role of percutaneous transluminal coronary angioplasty in acute myocardial infarction. In *Acute Myocardial Infarction.* Edited by BJ Gersh, SH Rahimtoola. New York, Elsevier, 1991, pp 371-385. By permission of Chapman & Hall.

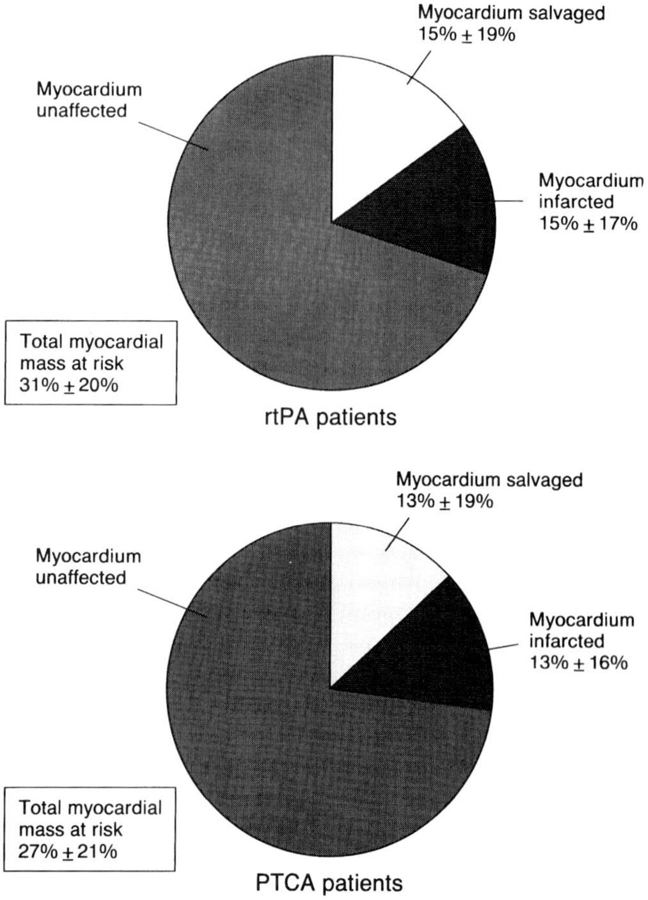

Fig 10B-9 Myocardial salvage with recombinant tissue-type plasminogen activator *(rtPA)* or PTCA. Total ventricular myocardial mass at risk, salvaged, and infarcted (determined using serial technetium-99 sestamibi scans) was not significantly different between patients treated with intravenous thrombolysis and those receiving direct angioplasty. (Data from Gibbons RJ, Holmes DR, Reeder GS, et al: Immediate angioplasty compared with the administration of a thrombolytic agent followed by conservative treatment for myocardial infarction. *N Engl J Med* 328:685-691, 1993.)

Table 10B-10 Summary of results of three randomized trials comparing direct angioplasty with intravenous thrombolysis for acute myocardial infarction

Characteristic	Thrombolysis	PTCA	*P*
	Gibbons et al.[101]*		
No. of patients	56	47	...
Recurrent ischemia, %	36	15	0.017
Death, %	3.6	4.3	NS
Additional PTCA, %	31	2.4	<0.001
CABG surgery, %	14	14	NS
LVEF at rest, %	50 ± 11	53 ± 12	NS
Hospital days, no.	10.6 ± 8.1	7.7 ± 2.9	0.01
Death or MI within 6 mo, %	3.7	2.2	NS
CABG surgery or PTCA within 6 mo, %	22.2	8.9	0.07
Hospital costs, × $1,000	21.4 ± 14.8	16.8 ± 8.8	0.09
Follow-up costs, × $1,000	2.7 ± 7.7	0.5 ± 3.1	0.03
Hospital readmissions, %	18	4	0.04
	Grines et al.[102]†		
No. of patients	200	195	...
Recurrent ischemia, %	28	10	<0.001
Reinfarction, %	6.5	2.6	0.06
Death, %	6.5	2.6	0.06
Death or nonfatal MI, %	12	5.1	0.02
Hospital days, no.	8.4 ± 4.6	7.5 ± 3.3	0.03
Additional PTCA, %	36	6.2	<0.001
Abnormal exercise ECG, %	8.6	2.9	0.04
Abnormal exercise thallium, %	38	27	0.06
LVEF at rest, %	53 ± 13	53 ± 13	NS
LVEF with exercise, %	56 ± 13	56 ± 14	NS
Death within 6 mo, %	7.9	3.7	0.08
Death or nonfatal MI within 6 mo, %	16.8	8.5	0.02
	Zijlstra et al.[103]‡		
No. of patients	70	72	...
Any complication, %	26	14	0.07
Recurrent ischemia, %	38	9	<0.001
Death, heart failure, or reocclusion, %	17	19	0.001
Additional PTCA, %	31	4	<0.001
Infarct artery patency after therapy, %	68	91	0.001
LVEF at rest, %	45 ± 12	51 ± 11	0.004
LVEF with exercise, %	46 ± 15	52 ± 14	0.02

CABG, coronary artery bypass graft; ECG, electrocardiogram; LVEF, left ventricular ejection fraction by radionuclide angiography; MI, myocardial infarction; PTCA, percutaneous transluminal coronary angioplasty.
*Thrombolytic agent was double-chain tissue plasminogen activator. Patients < 80 years, chest pain for < 12 hours, shock excluded, β-blockers routine, calcium antagonists avoided.
†Thrombolytic agent was tissue plasminogen activator. Patients any age, chest pain < 12 hours, shock excluded, left bundle-branch block excluded, diltiazem used uniformly, β-blocker use variable.
‡Thrombolytic agent was streptokinase. Patients < 76 years, chest pain < 6 hours (up to 24 hours if evidence of continued ischemia), shock included, β-blocker and calcium antagonist use variable.

Complications

Abrupt total occlusion is the most common serious complication of PTCA. The usual cause is an occlusive intracoronary thrombus with or without underlying arterial dissection. This complication tends to occur within the first 6 hours after PTCA, and the presentation is usually that of acute myocardial infarction. Use of a continuous heparin infusion for 24 hours after PTCA may reduce the frequency of thrombotic occlusion, but the benefit must be balanced against the risk of bleeding and the prolonged hospital stay that this approach entails. Aspirin before and after PTCA is critical to limit platelet aggregation,[130] and inhibition of the platelet glycoprotein complex IIb-IIIa with a chimeric antibody appears to improve the safety of complex angioplasty procedures.[39] When occlusion occurs, an attempt is made to recross the lesion and redilate. If extensive thrombus is evident, adjunctive intravenous or intracoronary thrombolysis is frequently useful.[131] Use of an autoperfusion catheter that can maintain some distal blood flow during balloon inflations has been very

Table 10B-11 Results from three randomized trials comparing emergency and delayed or no coronary angioplasty for acute myocardial infarction

	No. of patients	Hospital mortality, %	Reinfarction, %	Reocclusion rate, %	Dismissal LVEF
Thrombolysis and Angioplasty in Myocardial Infarction trial[108]					
Emergency	99	4	NR	11	53.2
Delayed	98	1	NR	13	56.4
European Cooperative Study Group for TPA[107]					
Emergency	183	7	4	14	51.0
Medical management	184	3	7	12	51.0
Thrombolysis in Myocardial Infarction trial, IIA[106]					
Emergency	195	7.2	6.7	17	50.3
Delayed	194	5.7	4.1	15	49.0

LVEF, left ventricular ejection fraction; *NR,* not reported; *TPA,* tissue plasminogen activator.
From Chaitman BR: More on the saga of routine emergency coronary angioplasty for acute myocardial infarction. *J Am Coll Cardiol* 13:1260-1261, 1989. By permission of the American College of Cardiology.

Table 10B-12 Results of rescue PTCA after failed thrombolysis

Study	Agents	Patients, no.	Success, %	Reocclusion, %	Mortality, %
Califf et al.[112]	tPA	96(86)*	73	29	10.4
Topol et al.[115]	tPA + UK	27(22)*	86	4	0
Baim et al.[116]	tPA	37	...	26	5.4
Fung et al.[117]	SK	13	92	16	7.6
O'Connor et al.[111]	SK	90	89	14	17.0
Grines et al.[118]	tPA + SK	10	90	...	...
Holmes et al.[119]	SK	34	71	...	3.0
Abbottsmith et al.[109]	tPA, UK, tPA + UK, or tPA + Ilo	192	88	29	5.9
Juliard et al.[98]	Alt, SK, Ani, or Alt + UK	19	95	12.5	5.0

Ani, anistreplase; Alt, alteplase; Ilo, iloprost (nonthrombolytic prostaglandin analogue); SK, streptokinase; tPA, tissue-type plasminogen activator (including recombinant forms); UK, urokinase.
*Analysis of intention to treat; number of patients actually receiving rescue angioplasty in parentheses.
Modified from Topol EJ: Mechanical interventions for acute myocardial infarction. In *Textbook of Interventional Cardiology.* Edited by EJ Topol. Philadelphia, WB Saunders Company, 1990, pp 269-299. By permission.

Table 10B-13 Probability of successful resolution of abrupt closure when the mechanism of closure is dissection, thrombus, or indeterminate

	Indeterminate		Dissection		Thrombus		
Treatment	*n*	Success rate, %	*n*	Success rate, %	*n*	Success rate, %	Overall success rate, %
Thrombolytic agents only	4	0	1	0	2	0	0
Other Rx with thrombolytic agents	19	58	5	40	12	50	53
Other Rx without thrombolytic agents	28	46	24	38	3	67	44
Inflations of standard duration	30	3	17	6	10	10	5
Prolonged inflations	37	54	22	41	14	43	48
Intracoronary stent	4	75	3	100	2	50	78
Directional atherectomy	1	100	1	100			100

Rx, treatment.
From Lincoff AM, Popma JJ, Ellis SG, et al: Abrupt vessel closure complicating coronary angioplasty: clinical, angiographic and therapeutic profile. *J Am Coll Cardiol* 19:926-935, 1992. By permission of American College of Cardiology.

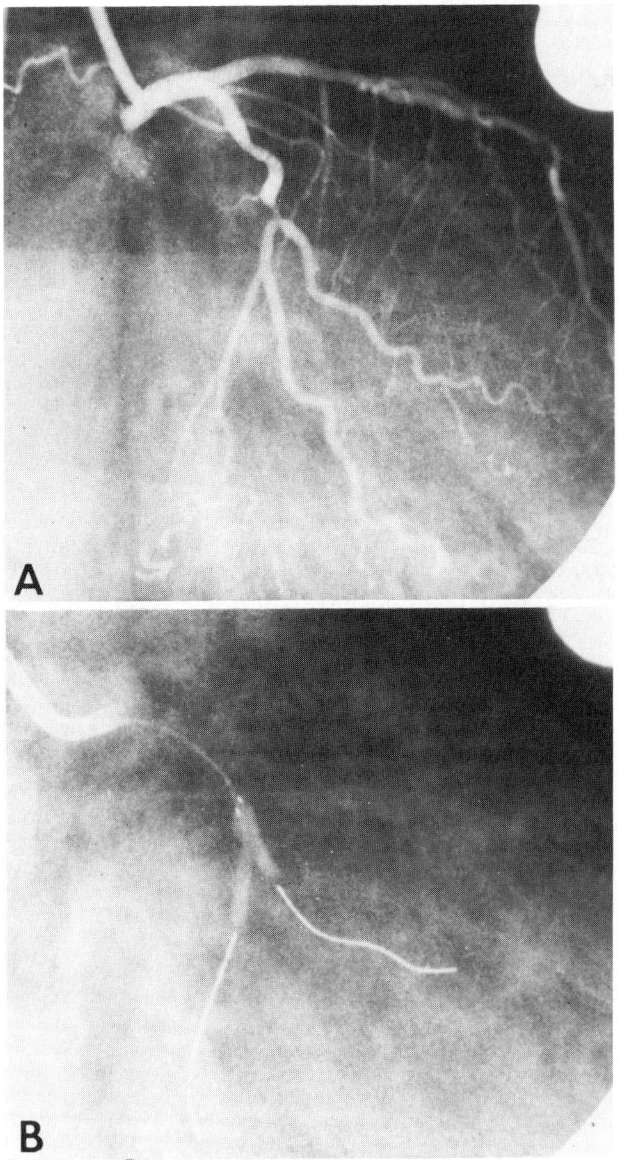

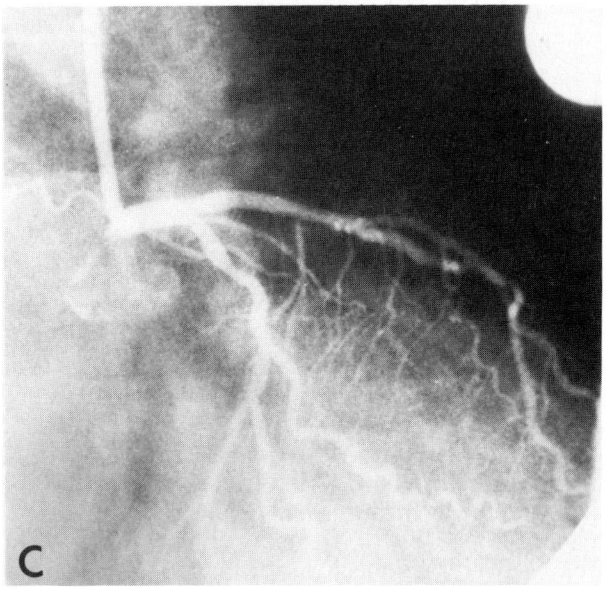

Fig 10B-10 Dual-probe technique for dilation of bifurcation stenosis. **A,** bifurcation lesion of circumflex is visualized. **B,** low-profile dilation catheters lie across stenosis with tips in respective branches, and simultaneous inflation is performed. **C,** angiographic result obtained with this technique is shown. (From O'Keefe JH Jr, Holmes DR Jr, Reeder GS, et al: A new approach for dilation of bifurcation stenoses: the dual probe technique. *Mayo Clin Proc* 64:277-281, 1989. By permission, Mayo Foundation.)

satisfying, because prolonged balloon inflations can sometimes "tack up" obstructive intimal tears.[132] These catheters can also be used as bailout devices that can preserve some anterograde coronary flow while arrangements are made for emergency surgery in patients with refractory coronary occlusion.[133] Other new technologies have had an effect on the frequency and consequences of abrupt closure, as discussed below, and a combined approach that integrates old and new technologies offers the best outcome (Table 10B-13).

Branch vessel occlusion is a problem better prevented than treated. Complex angioplasty often involves dilating lesions at branch points. If the branching vessel is itself involved at its origin by the stenosis, the risk of occluding that vessel is increased after angioplasty. The operator may wish to place guide wires down both branches and perform sequential inflations in each branch. With the use of lower profile balloon catheters, it is possible also to simultaneously inflate balloons in both branches, thus avoiding inadvertent compromise[134] (Fig 10B-10). If unexpected branch vessel occlusion occurs in the absence of a preplaced guide wire, it is sometimes possible to cross the occlusion to restore patency.

Coronary spasm is frequently seen in the dilated vessel, often distal to the area of dilatation. Pretreatment with calcium-entry blockers, nitrates, and aspirin usually prevents significant spasm from causing vascular occlusion. Intracoronary nitroglycerin is occasionally necessary to reverse significant spasm that limits blood flow.

Distal embolization of thrombus is occasionally seen during dilation in patients with acute myocardial infarction or by diagnostic angiography in patients with unstable angina. When distal embolization occurs, passing a guide wire or balloon catheter into the embolus may serve to disrupt and disperse the thrombus and improve blood flow. Adjunctive intracoronary thrombolysis is also of benefit.

Restenosis

The problem of restenosis continues to elude a definitive cure. Restenosis is a response to arterial injury occurring at the time of PTCA. It almost always occurs within 3 to 6 months, although rare late restenosis has been observed; 13 years after the procedure, we found recurrent stenosis within the treated arterial segment in the first patient to undergo PTCA at the Mayo Clinic (Fig 10B-11). Clinical restenosis occurs in 25% to 30% of patients, although angiographic renarrowing may be found in a substantially higher proportion of treated patients.[135-138] A study from Japan[139] in which more than 200 patients with mixed clinical syndromes underwent serial angiography suggests that angiographic restenosis may occur in about 45% of patients at 6 months (Fig 10B-12). Increasingly greater emphasis is being given to clinical rather than angiographic restenosis, in recognition of the fact that the ultimate aim is to improve patient well-being, not achieve an arbitrary angiographic goal.

Recent work has helped define some of the mechanisms involved in restenosis. The final expression of restenosis is a fibrocellular mass,[140] but as demonstrated by Chesebro et al.[141,142] and Harker,[143] early thrombus deposition appears pivotal in the process (Fig 10B-13). Rheologic factors,[141] coronary artery spasm,[144] and local characteristics of the arterial segment[32] contribute, probably through their influence on the deposition and incorporation of thrombus. The original thrombus is believed to mediate the release of platelet- and macrophage-derived mitogens and growth factors that result in the migration and proliferation of smooth muscle cells.[145] Barotrauma to the underlying media may stimulate medial smooth muscle cells, enhancing their sensitivity to growth factors. However, recent data from

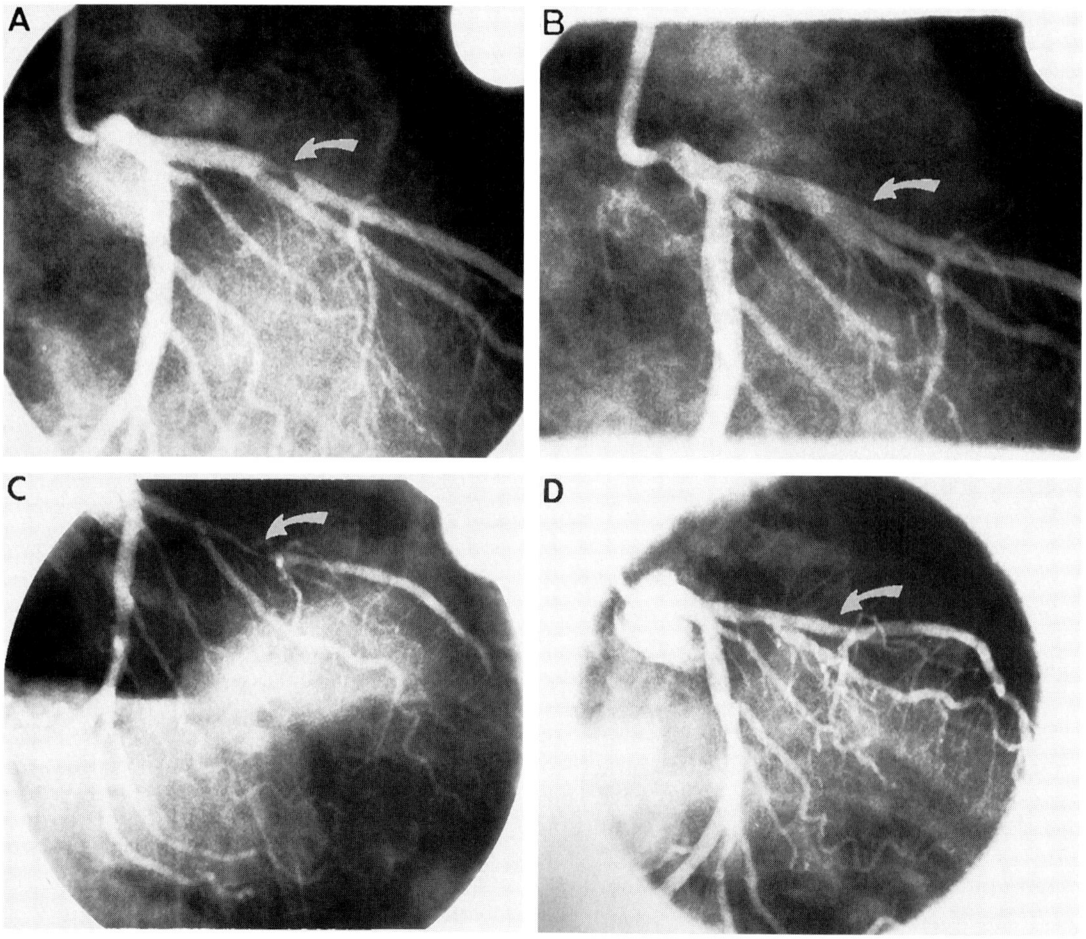

Fig 10B-11 Late restenosis in the first patient to undergo PTCA at the Mayo Clinic. **A,** severe stenosis *(arrow)* in proximal left anterior descending artery. **B,** excellent result *(arrow)* from PTCA. **C,** recurrent severe stenosis *(arrow)* in coronary segment treated with PTCA after 13 symptom-free years. **D,** excellent result *(arrow)* from repeat PTCA.

Schwartz et al.[146] and Schwartz and Edwards[147] suggest that smooth muscle cells appearing in the fibrotic restenosis lesion may originate from distant sites. Adverse vascular remodeling appears to play an important role in development of restenosis.[148]

Certain clinical features have been identified that seem to carry an increased risk of restenosis (Table 10B-14), but it has not been possible in a given patient to predict whether restenosis will occur. Although use of fish oils[149] and sharp reductions in serum cholesterol[150] seemed promising, no drug or combination of drugs has been shown to consistently alter the rates of restenosis in humans.

Restenosis is generally signaled by recurrent exertional angina rather than myocardial infarction or sudden death. Usually, it is best managed with repeat balloon dilation. This strategy has found favor because of the high success rate and low complication rate associated with dilation of restenosis lesions and the observation that repeat PTCA results in a lasting favorable result in many patients.[151] Patients requiring several PTCA procedures are referred for coronary bypass surgery, although newer technologies hold some promise for "repeat restenosers."

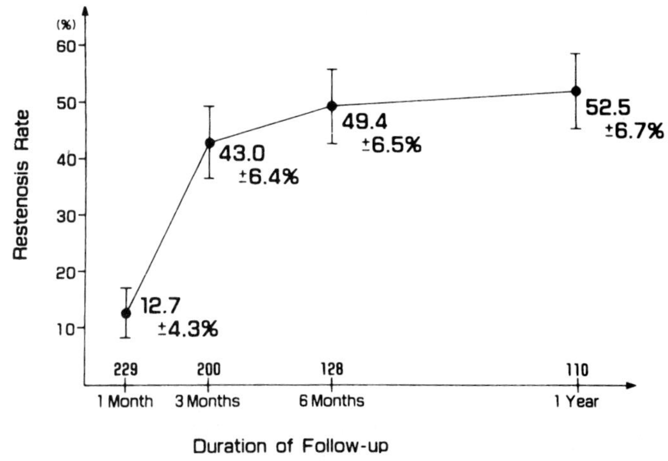

Fig 10B-12 Angiographic restenosis among 229 patients undergoing PTCA and serial angiography. (From Nobuyoshi M, Kimura T, Nosaka H, et al: Restenosis after successful percutaneous transluminal coronary angioplasty: serial angiographic follow-up of 229 patients. *J Am Coll Cardiol* 12:616-623, 1988. By permission of American College of Cardiology.)

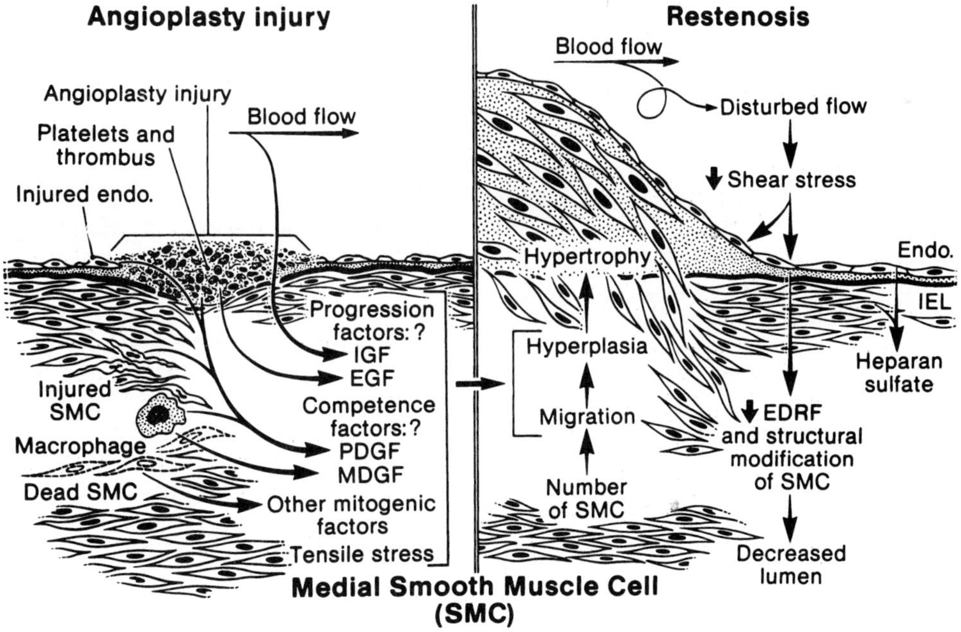

Fig 10B-13 A model of restenosis. Angioplasty injury promotes platelet and thrombus deposition with release of growth factors (progression, competence, and mitogenic factors). Injured smooth muscle cells and macrophages also contribute. These factors, combined with altered blood flow dynamics, promote cellular migration and replication, which narrow the vascular lumen. The process is regulated by endothelial cell-derived heparan sulfate and other homeostatic factors. EDRF, endothelium-derived relaxation factor; EGF, endothelial growth factor; Endo., endothelium; IEL, internal elastic lamina; IGF, insulin-like growth factor; MDGF, macrophage-derived growth factor; PDGF, platelet-derived growth factor. (From Liu MW, Roubin GS, King SB III: Restenosis after coronary angioplasty: potential biologic determinants and role of intimal hyperplasia. *Circulation* 79:1374-1387, 1989. By permission of American Heart Association.)

Table 10B-14 Factors having consistent, occasional, or no relationship to restenosis after PTCA

	Association with restenosis		
Characteristics	**Often**	**Occasionally**	**None**
Patient	Male sex Diabetes Variant angina New onset angina	Unstable angina Anginal class No previous MI Cholesterol	Age Hypertension
Angiographic	Severe stenoses Prox. LAD stenoses Spasm Chronic occlusions Branch point stenoses SVG ostial or graft body lesions	Eccentric stenoses	Stenosis length Dist. anastomosis Multivessel disease LV function
Procedural	High residual stenosis High initial gradient High final gradient Absence of int. tear	Low balloon-artery ratio Inflation duration	Number of balloon inflations Inflation pressure
Post-PTCA		Smoking	Calcium antagonists Warfarin Heparin Aspirin

Dist., distal; int., intimal; LAD, left anterior descending artery; LV, left ventricular; MI, myocardial infarction; Prox., proximal; SVG, saphenous vein bypass graft.
Modified from Rose B, Pepine CJ: Restenosis following coronary artery angioplasty: patterns, recognition, and results of repeat angioplasty. *Cardiovasc Clin* 19 No. 2:233-251, 1988.

CORONARY ATHERECTOMY

Atherectomy refers to the actual removal of atheromatous material from the diseased vessel; this technique is accomplished percutaneously with catheter-based systems (Fig 10B-14). Unlike angioplasty, which stretches the vessel and fissures plaque material, atherectomy has the potential to "resect" the atheromatous lesion. This is appealing from several theoretical perspectives. First, the removal of atheromatous material might reduce the thrombogenesis that can occur with plaque disruption after angioplasty, and this reduction, in turn, may conceivably reduce the incidence of acute vessel closure. Second, the incidence of dissection appears to be lower, and this reduction also may translate clinically to a lower rate of acute closure. Third, even with excellent angioplasty results, a residual stenosis nearly always remains, and this may exert adverse rheologic effects leading to platelet activation and release of growth factor substances in regions of lower shear stress. The larger lumen that can be achieved with atherectomy may reduce these undesirable factors and might help to reduce restenosis. Finally, analysis of material removed at atherectomy may allow morphologic and metabolic studies to further elucidate cellular events in the restenosis process.

Most experience has been gathered with the directional atherectomy catheter (Fig 10B-15). This device consists of a hollow metal cylinder with a window cut into one side. Within the cylinder, a cup-shaped cutter is attached to a torque cable, which is connected to a hand-held motor. When activated, the motor spins the cutter at about 2,000 rpm. The cylinder is advanced into the coronary artery or vein graft and positioned such that the window faces the atheroma to be resected. A low-pressure balloon on the side of the cylinder opposite the window is inflated to ensure firm engagement of the atheroma. As the cutter is activated and advanced across the lesion, the resected tissue is collected into the distal nose cone. The directional atherectomy device uses standard angioplasty guide wires, but because of the larger dimensions of the device (5F, 6F, and 7F), special 10F and 11F guide catheters are necessary.

The short-term results with directional atherectomy have been favorable.[152-155] At the Mayo Clinic, the device was used successfully in about 90% of the first 200 patients treated, with complication rates similar to those associated with PTCA. These results are similar to those reported by other large-volume centers. Directional atherectomy appears effective in treating many lesions with morphologic characteristics unfavorable for PTCA, including highly eccentric lesions,[156] saphenous vein graft lesions,[157] and thrombotic lesions.[158]

The Coronary Angioplasty Versus Excisional Atherectomy Trial (CAVEAT) compared long-term outcomes in 1,000 patients with primary atheromatous lesions in native coronary arteries who were randomly assigned to receive PTCA or directional atherectomy. As such, it was the first trial to randomize patients between two methods of percutaneous revascularization. The primary end point

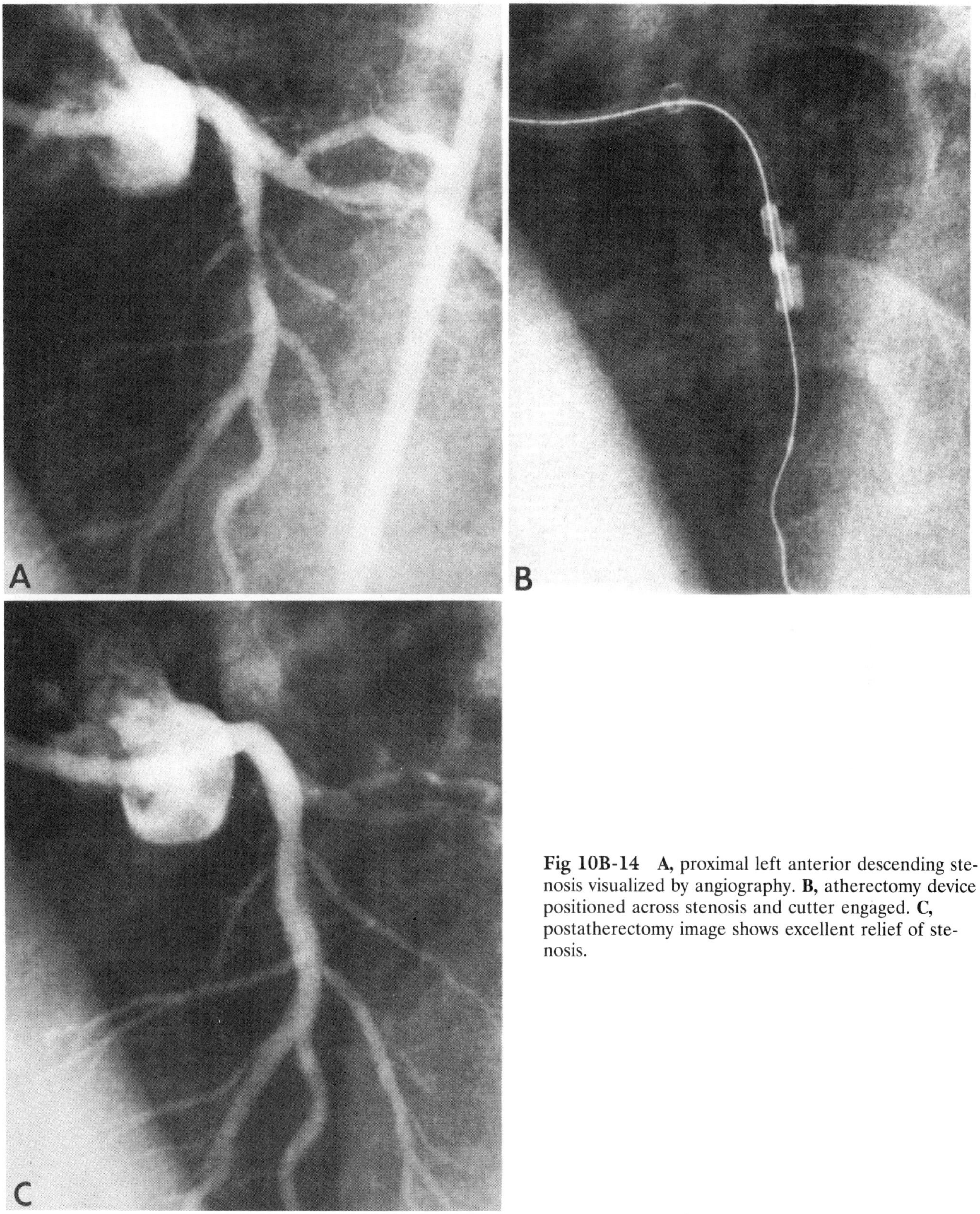

Fig 10B-14 **A,** proximal left anterior descending stenosis visualized by angiography. **B,** atherectomy device positioned across stenosis and cutter engaged. **C,** postatherectomy image shows excellent relief of stenosis.

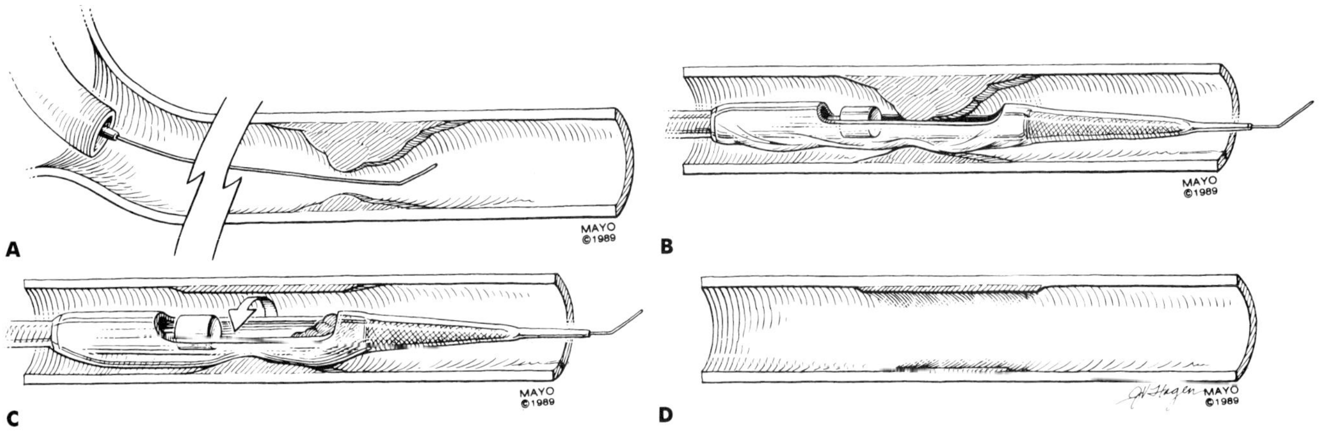

Fig 10B-15 Directional coronary atherectomy device (AtheroCath). **A,** guide wire is placed across the coronary lesion. **B,** atherectomy catheter is positioned at the atheroma to be treated. A low-pressure balloon holds the cutter housing against the lesion while the cutter resects tissue, which is pushed into a distal collecting nose cone. **C,** the catheter can be rotated to direct the housing window toward other aspects of the artery (hence, a directional device). **D,** a smooth luminal surface is the expected result. (By permission, Mayo Foundation.)

was angiographic restenosis at 6 months after the procedure. The trial found that restenosis tended to be lower with directional atherectomy than with PTCA, although the rate of angiographic restenosis was surprisingly high for both groups (50% and 57%; $P = 0.055$).[159] The greatest restenosis benefit was seen among proximal left anterior descending artery lesions (51% and 63%; $P = 0.04$). The difference in angiographic restenosis did not equate to a clinical benefit; in fact, more adverse clinical events were observed among patients treated with atherectomy, with significantly greater frequencies of abrupt closure and myocardial infarction (Table 10B-15). The vessels treated tended to be smaller than ideal (<3.0 mm), and about two-thirds of the patients had unstable angina; these factors are believed to increase restenosis and clinical complications.

The Canadian Coronary Atherectomy Trial (CCAT) also compared atherectomy and balloon angioplasty, but only lesions within the proximal two-thirds of the left anterior descending artery were randomized.[160] This study found that despite significantly larger vessel dimensions after atherectomy, restenosis (stenosis ≥50% within 6 months of treatment) occurred in equal proportions of patients treated by balloon angioplasty and atherectomy. Clinical results within 6 months of treatment were similar in the two patient groups.

Does directional atherectomy offer any substantial benefit over balloon angioplasty? Or if restenosis rates are similar and complication rates may be lower with balloon angioplasty, should directional atherectomy be abandoned? Although the data from these randomized trials may be interpreted several ways, it is reasonable to conclude that if a lesion is suitable for either directional atherectomy or balloon angioplasty, angioplasty is preferable. However, lesions that are at high risk for complications or failure with balloon angioplasty, such as very eccentric, thrombus-laden, or ostial lesions, may be better treated with atherectomy.[161,162] Also, the immediate postprocedure minimal lumen diameter is inversely related to restenosis rates, regardless of the technique used to achieve luminal enlargement.[163,164] However, significant residual stenoses (20% to 30%) remained after atherectomy in these randomized studies. Some investigators believe that similarities in restenosis rates between angioplasty and atherectomy in these trials can be explained by the "large" residual stenoses left after atherectomy.[165,166] "Near zero" residual stenoses may be necessary to significantly reduce restenosis. Since directional atherectomy can achieve larger lumens than can usually be attained with balloon angioplasty, atherectomy should be associated with less restenosis when it is used to achieve an optimal procedural result. This theory is being tested currently in a small pilot trial, the Optimal Atherectomy Restenosis Study (OARS), and a larger study, the Balloon Angioplasty Versus Optimal Atherectomy Trial (BOAT).

CAVEAT, CCAT, OARS, and BOAT were designed to compare treatment of lesions within native coronary arteries. In the Second Coronary Angioplasty Versus Excisional Atherectomy Trial (CAVEAT II), lesions within saphenous vein grafts were randomized to therapy with angioplasty or atherectomy.[167] Restenosis rates were slightly lower with atherectomy (45.5% versus 50%), and there was no difference in rates of Q-wave myocardial infarction, repeat coronary bypass surgery, and death between the two treatment groups. Interestingly, the need for repeat target vessel revascularization (bypass surgery or catheter intervention) within 6 months of treatment was lower for the atherectomy-treated patients (13% versus 24%).

There is some debate about the importance of deep arterial resection with directional atherectomy. In our early experience, recovery of media or adventitia with atherectomy was not associated with an increase in acute

Table 10B-15 Clinical and angiographic characteristics in the Coronary Angioplasty Versus Excisional Atherectomy Trial (CAVEAT)

Characteristic	DCA	PTCA
Patients, no.	512	500
Median age, yr	59	59
Males, %	75	70
Presenting symptom, %		
Unstable angina	65	70
Myocardial infarction	11	9
Success (≤50% stenosis), %	89	80
Restenosis at 6 months,* %	48.6	57.3
In-hospital complications, %		
Death	0	0.4
Myocardial infarction	6	3
CABG	3	2
Cardiac arrest	1	1
Stroke	0.4	0.2
Abrupt closure	6	3
Clinical events within 6 months,† %		
Death	1.6	0.6
Myocardial infarction	7.6	4.4
CABG	8.2	6.8
Percutaneous intervention	21	24
Event-free	63	66

CABG, coronary artery bypass grafting; DCA, directional coronary atherectomy; PTCA, percutaneous transluminal coronary angioplasty.
*Primary study end point.
†Each patient appears only once in the worst category, in the order that the end points appear in the table.
Compiled from data read at the meeting of the CAVEAT Investigators, November 1992, New Orleans, Louisiana, and Topol EJ, Leya F, Pinkerton CA, et al: A comparison of directional atherectomy with coronary angioplasty in patients with coronary artery disease. *N Engl J Med* 329:221-227, 1993.

adverse events[168] but did seem to be related to a tendency for greater restenosis, particularly in vein grafts and in restenosis lesions after balloon angioplasty.[169] Others have not observed this trend,[154] and a systematic evaluation of tissue specimens submitted in the CAVEAT study to a core laboratory group revealed no apparent relationship between resection of medial or adventitial tissue and restenosis.[170] Variability in the amount of adventitia removed and the character of the injury done during atherectomy may explain these disparate observations. There does appear to be a tendency toward late development of coronary aneurysms when adventitia is removed;[171] the long-term outcome of such aneurysms is unknown.

Several other atherectomy devices have recently been approved for general use.[172,173] The rotational atherectomy device (Fig 10B-16) consists of a diamond-coated burr that spins at about 200,000 rpm. This high-speed atherectomy tool can micropulverize noncompliant materials that come into contact with the burr.[174-176] In the coronary circulation, the debris that is formed is sufficiently small (80% less than 10 μm) that it

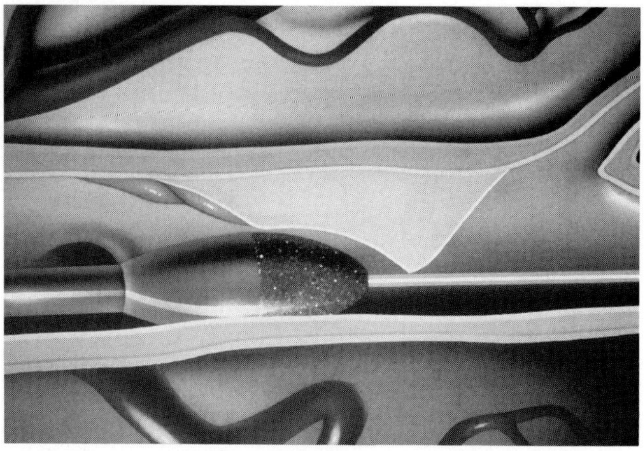

Fig 10B-16 High-speed rotational atherectomy device (Rotablator). The olive-shaped tip, which is coated with industrial diamond chips, rotates at high speed. Relatively rigid coronary atheroma is micropulverized, but the compliant normal vessel wall is not injured. Microscopic debris can pass through distal capillary beds. (Courtesy of Heart Technologies.)

can pass through capillaries. Poor distal flow observed with this device may be related to accumulation of particulate debris or microcavitations formed by the spinning burr.[177,178] Initial success rates are high, although adjunctive balloon angioplasty is often required and restenosis rates have not been reduced with use of this technique.[175,176] Randomized trials (STRATAS and DART studies) are under way to determine if this device can be used to improve patient outcomes or reduce restenosis.

The transluminal extraction-endarterectomy catheter (Fig 10B-17) is also a rotational atherectomy catheter, but it rotates at a slower speed. The distal blades pulverize atheromatous material into macroscopic fragments that are aspirated through a vacuum port. Success rates are generally good, although complication and restenosis rates are reported to be high with this device[179-181] and may reflect its frequent use in the treatment of friable vein grafts with extensive disease.[179,182] Several other atherectomy catheter designs are currently under study.

INTRAVASCULAR STENTS

Stents are intraluminal devices placed to maintain patency of a biologic tube. Stents have been used extensively to treat biliary and ureteral stenoses and are under investigation in urethral obstruction due to prostatic hypertrophy. Recently, stents have been placed into vascular conduits (Table 10B-16).

Stents may find their greatest application in the treatment of abrupt closure after PTCA (Fig 10B-18). Myocardial infarction may occur in 26% to 66% of patients treated with emergency bypass surgery for abrupt closure, and mortality for these patients is about 6%.[183,184] These events are probably related to the time required to restore coronary flow, which may be in excess of an hour, even in large medical centers with

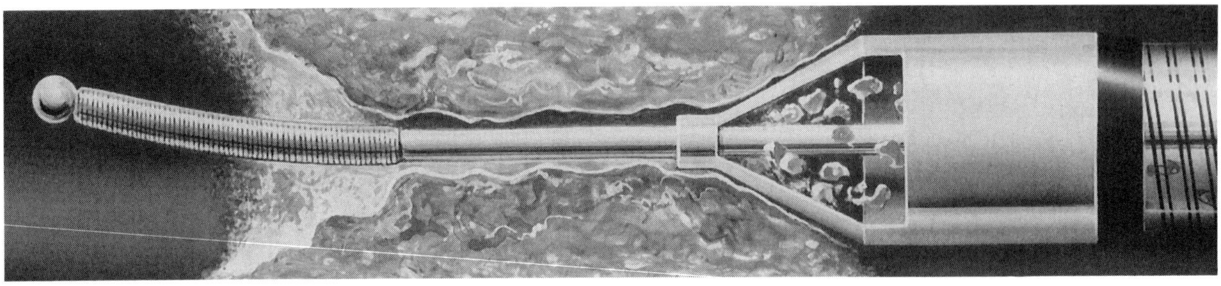

Fig 10B-17 Transluminal extraction-endarterectomy (TEC) atherectomy device. The rotating tip pulverizes atheroma but creates fragments too large to pass through distal capillary beds. The treated area is flushed with saline, and the saline and debris are aspirated through a vacuum port at the catheter tip. (Courtesy of Interventional Technology.)

Table 10B-16 Stent designs under clinical investigation in North America

Stent	Design	Material	Length, mm	Flexible?
Gianturco-Roubin	Reflecting coil	SSS	12 & 20	Yes
Wiktor	Interlocking coil	Tantalum	15	Yes
Schatz-Palmaz	Slotted tube	SSS	15	No*
Microstent	Zigzag hoop	SSS	4.2-7.2	Yes
Wallstent	Wire mesh	SSS	8-29	Yes
Cordis	Interlocking coil	Tantalum	18	Yes
Act-One	Slotted tube	Nitinol	15	No

SSS, surgical stainless steel.
*Flexibility enhanced by use of articulation design.

surgical backup. Stents offer the opportunity to restore coronary flow within a few minutes of the occlusion. Stents may also be of benefit in the treatment of restenosis; at least one stent is currently involved in a randomized trial to assess this potential.

The first coronary stent placed into humans was the Wallstent (Schneider, Minneapolis, MN),[185] a catheter-deployed, self-expanding stainless steel stent (Fig 10B-19). Because this stent continues to exert an outward expanding force after placement, the vessel lumen may actually enlarge over time.[186] Initial results with this stent were mixed, with subacute thrombosis posing the greatest risk.[187] More recent experience with this stent has been excellent, with very low restenosis rates reported.[188] Used in England and Europe, the Wallstent is entering clinical trials in America.

The Schatz-Palmaz stent (Johnson & Johnson, Warren, NJ)[189] is a rigid, slotted steel tube that is placed by expanding the stent with a balloon catheter (Fig 10B-20). Results with this stent have been excellent,[190] although it has primarily been placed under elective circumstances in large coronary arteries—conditions that probably favor a good outcome. Two large international, randomized studies, the Stent Restenosis Study (STRESS)[191] and the Belgium-Netherlands Stent Study (BENESTENT),[192] have been conducted to compare 6-month restenosis rates after implantation of this stent with rates after conventional balloon angioplasty.[193] Both studies showed a significant reduction in restenosis with stent implantation at 6 months, although stent recipients had longer hospital stays and more bleeding complications.

The Gianturco-Roubin stent (Cook, Bloomington, IN)[194] is a balloon-expandable stainless steel stent (Fig 10B-21). Because it is more flexible than the Schatz-Palmaz stent, the Gianturco-Roubin stent may be more easily placed through tortuous vascular segments. Most of these stents have been placed for treatment of intimal tears after PTCA that caused, or threatened to cause, vessel occlusion. Immediate efficacy has been excellent.[195,197] Bleeding and stent thrombosis are problems,[198] but both are declining with greater experience.

Other metallic stents are in the early stages of investigation. The Wiktor stent (Medtronic, Minneapolis, MN)[199] and the Cordis stent (Cordis, Miami, FL)[200] are made of tantalum, an alloy with physical properties similar to steel but with greater radiodensity, which enhances fluoroscopic visualization. Most stents are between 12 and 20 mm in length, and placement of one or two is intended to provide full support. The Microstent (Applied Vascular Engineering, Santa Rosa, CA) is another steel stent undergoing clinical study in the U.S.

Several synthetic and biologic polymers may be suitable alternatives to metal. Polymeric stents may have the ability to autolyse and absorb over a predetermined period and thus obviate concerns about the long-term effects of an indwelling coronary prosthesis. They may also be saturated with drugs and act to deliver anticoagulants or cell growth modifiers. Impregnating polymeric

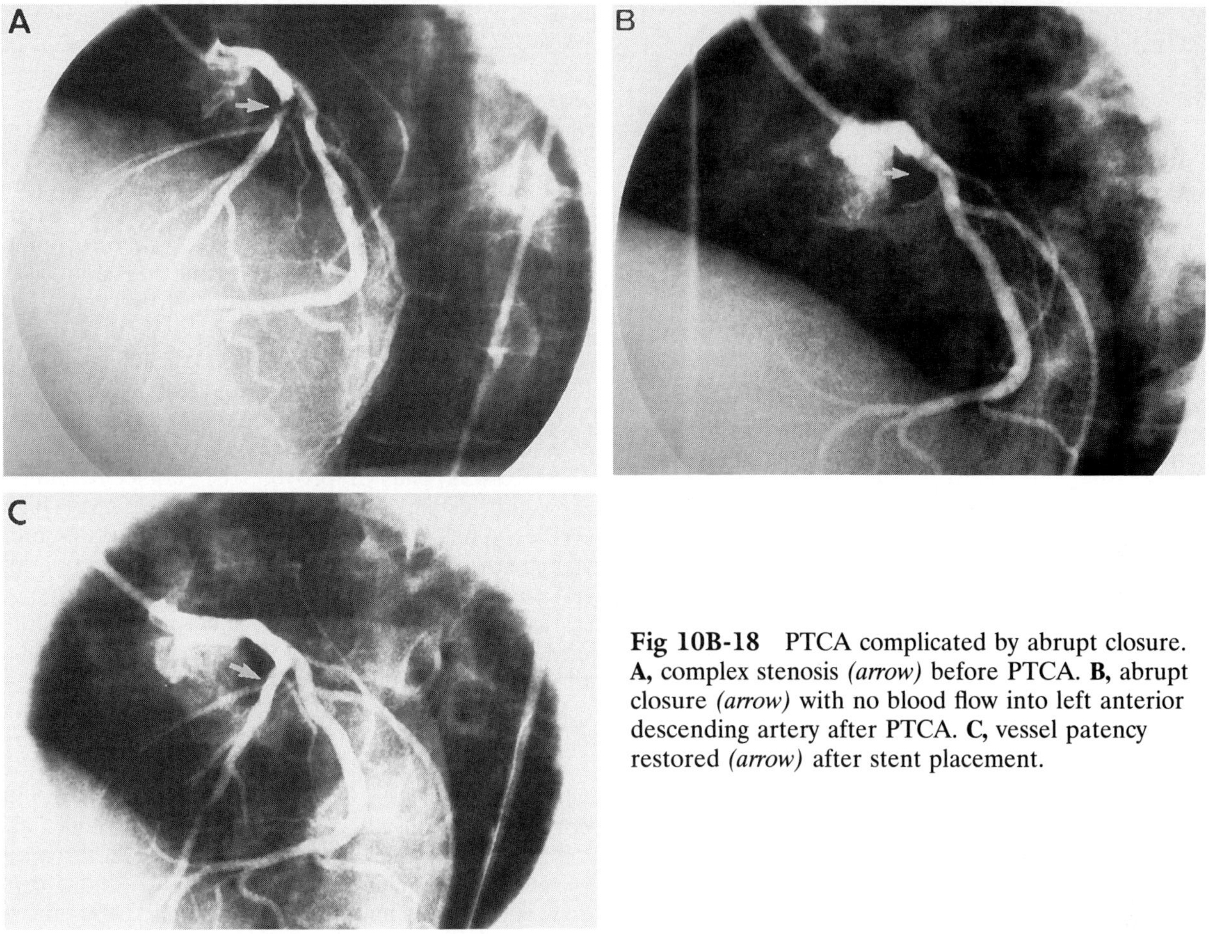

Fig 10B-18 PTCA complicated by abrupt closure. **A,** complex stenosis *(arrow)* before PTCA. **B,** abrupt closure *(arrow)* with no blood flow into left anterior descending artery after PTCA. **C,** vessel patency restored *(arrow)* after stent placement.

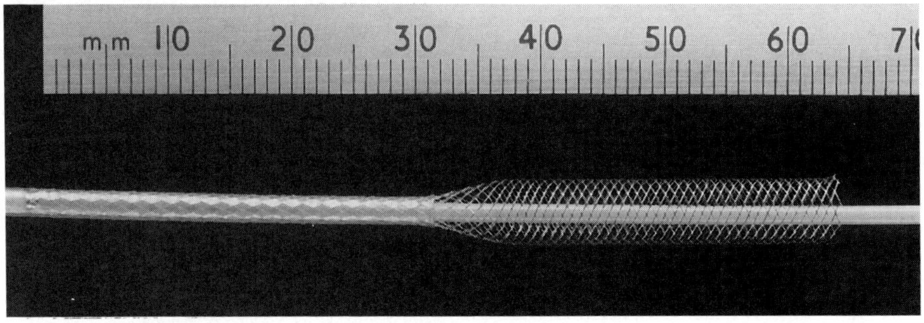

Fig 10B-19 The Wallstent. The first stent placed in humans, this self-expanding wire mesh is placed by retracting a protective sleeve. (Courtesy of Schneider-Shiley, U.S.A.)

stents with microspheres having known decay properties could help control drug delivery. Finally, coating of stents with endothelial cells[201] or even autologous venous segments[202] may promote the benign incorporation of stents into the vessel wall.

Vascular stents are used with excellent results in peripheral arteries. A variation of the stent theme is endoluminal paving, in which a tube of synthetic material is laid down onto the arterial surface.[203] Although this has found limited success in coronary arteries, a percutaneously placed aortic tube has been successfully used to treat abdominal aortic aneurysms[204] and dissections.[205]

Temporary stents that may be retrieved after some period have been constructed of steel and tantalum; these must remain attached to a retrieval wire or catheter while in place.[206,207] A stent made of nitinol can be expanded with a balloon and then made to resume its original collapsed shape by brief exposure to fluid at 50° to 60°C.

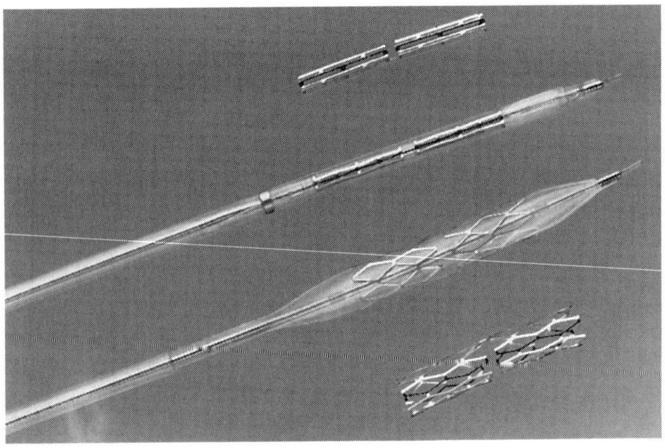

Fig 10B-20 The Schatz-Palmaz stent. The stent consists of slotted stainless steel tubing that is manually placed onto a delivery balloon catheter. The rectangular slots assume a diamond latticework configuration when the stent is expanded. Flexibility has been improved by creating interruptions in the tubing, with segments connected by short articulations. (Courtesy of Johnson and Johnson Interventional Systems Company.)

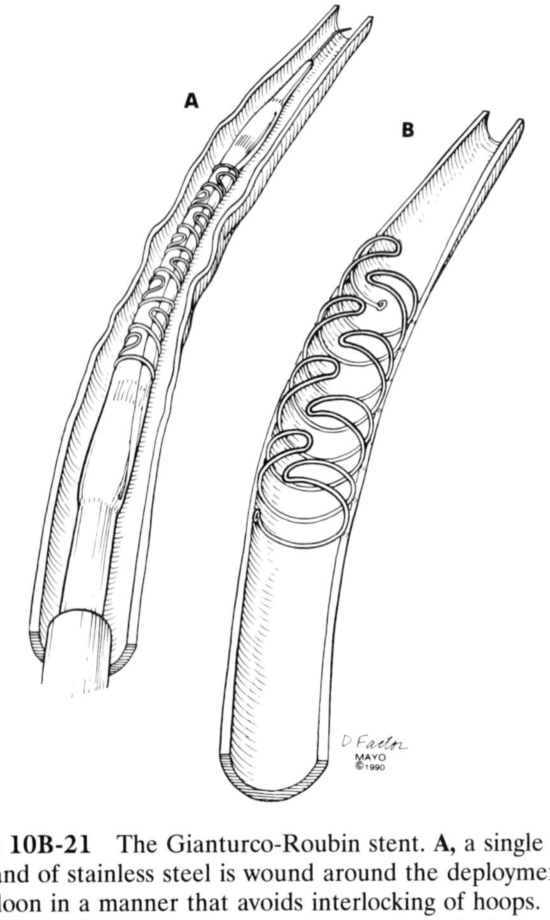

Fig 10B-21 The Gianturco-Roubin stent. **A,** a single strand of stainless steel is wound around the deployment balloon in a manner that avoids interlocking of hoops. **B,** this flexible design does not shorten along the long axis during balloon expansion. (By permission, Mayo Foundation.)

When made to collapse over a retrieval catheter, this heat-activated, recoverable temporary stent can be removed.[208]

CORONARY LASERS

Laser energy can be used to burn tissue (hot lasers) or to ablate it (cold lasers); in the latter instance, laser energy is thought to excite electrons sufficiently to break covalent bonds and literally "atomize" tissue. The ultraviolet (308 nm wavelength) excimer xenon-chloride cold laser has received restricted FDA approval for use in long or diffuse coronary lesions, where it is thought to offer most benefit. Procedural success has been achieved in about 90% of cases,[209,210] despite limited operator experience and treatment of complex coronary disease, but adjunctive PTCA is frequently necessary. A directional laser fiber (Fig 10B-22) has improved the ability to approach eccentric lesions. Laser use has allowed more high-risk lesions to be treated safely. Restenosis rates do not seem to be improved by use of the laser, but this observation has not yet been tested in a randomized fashion.

Hot lasers may be useful as probes in total or near-total occlusions. Transparent contact probes connected to neodymium:yttrium-aluminum-garnet (Nd:YAG) lasers (about 1,060 nm wavelength) attain temperatures of up to 1,000°C;[211] such probes cause thermal remodeling rather than plaque ablation.[212] A laser-assisted PTCA device, which applied Nd:YAG laser energy through an inflated coronary balloon, was effective in sealing intimal tears and desiccating thrombus,[213] but its use was discontinued because of a high rate of restenosis. A more compact solid-state holmium hot laser (about 2,100 nm wavelength) is associated with somewhat less thermal injury.[214,215] A truly novel use of laser was reported by Japanese investigators, who used lasers to cut holes into the endocardial surface of ischemic regions of the left ventricle; the percolation of blood into the tissue appeared to relieve ischemia.[216]

Complications with laser use have generally been similar in type and frequency to those reported for PTCA,[210,213,217] except for a higher rate of perforations.[218] There is also concern that laser-generated debris may cause platelet activation distal to the lesion.[219]

OTHER ADJUNCTS TO CORONARY INTERVENTION

Percutaneous intra-aortic balloon pump

Counterpulsation with a percutaneous intra-aortic balloon pump (IABP) provides temporary mechanical circulatory support for patients with potentially reversible severe cardiac dysfunction. By means of a percutaneous technique, a balloon catheter system is positioned in the upper part of the descending thoracic aorta. The balloon is phasically inflated and deflated in time with the cardiac cycle to augment diastolic perfusion and reduce systolic impedance. A reduction in myocardial oxygen demand and an increase in blood pressure and cardiac output

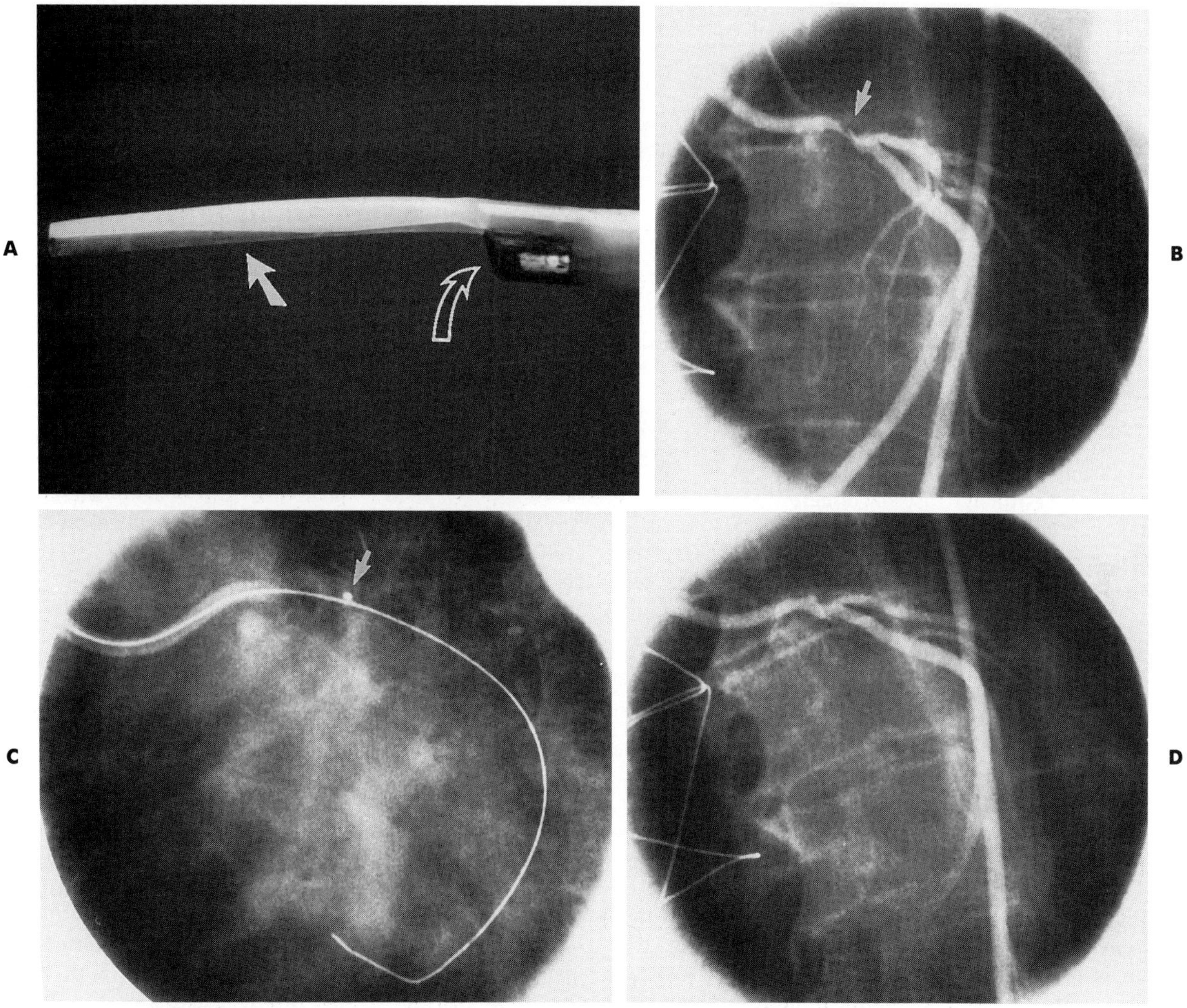

Fig 10B-22 The directional excimer laser fiber. **A,** a guiding protrusion *(solid arrow)* tends to orient the laser tip *(hollow arrow)* toward the lesion, away from the less diseased vascular wall, in eccentric lesions. **B,** an eccentric lesion *(arrow)* in the left main artery before treatment. **C,** application of laser energy by the directional excimer fiber. Note that the laser tip *(arrow)* is directed toward the lesion. **D,** lesion substantially improved after laser therapy.

usually result (Table 10B-17). IABP may be utilized for days or for a week or more while improvement in cardiac function is awaited.

The catheter is prepared by evacuating all air from the balloon to minimize its profile. A large arterial sheath (9.5F to 12F) is inserted into a femoral artery; some IABP catheters can be inserted without a sheath. A guide wire is inserted through a central lumen and used to direct the insertion of the IABP catheter under fluoroscopy. The IABP catheter is positioned in such a way that the distal catheter tip lies just distal to the origin of the left subclavian artery. The inflation port of the IABP catheter is connected to a pumping unit, and counterpulsation is commenced. Helium gas is used to inflate the balloon. The

Table 10B-17 Determinants of myocardial oxygen supply and demand

Supply	Demand
Severity of coronary obstruction	Heart rate
Length of diastole (heart rate)	Inotropic state
Diastolic perfusion pressure*	Wall tension (left ventricular volume,* afterload*)

*Factors improved by balloon counterpulsation.

Table 10B-18 Indications for use of balloon counterpulsation

Cardiogenic shock due to myocardial infarction
Shock due to acute, severe mitral regurgitation
Medically uncontrollable unstable angina
Inability to wean from cardiopulmonary bypass postoperatively

Table 10B-19 Contraindications to use of balloon counterpulsation

Significant valvular aortic insufficiency
Severe aortoiliac obstructive vascular disease
Abdominal or thoracic aortic aneurysm
Severe nonremediable left ventricular dysfunction

supported pressure waveform can be analyzed to ensure that the timing of inflation and deflation provides optimal hemodynamic benefits.

IABP counterpulsation has been used most to support patients with cardiogenic shock due to myocardial infarction (Table 10B-18). Untreated, this hemodynamic state is nearly always fatal. In a review of 251 patients treated with IABP, 70 (28%) survived to hospital dismissal.[220] It is important to emphasize that IABP placement is a temporizing maneuver; with medical therapy alone, a few patients may recover enough myocardial function to survive, but in most patients the IABP is used to provide support until other catheter techniques or surgery can be used to restore independent hemodynamic stability.

The IABP catheter is also used to treat refractory angina pectoris and acute severe mitral regurgitation with pulmonary edema and to support hemodynamically tenuous patients after cardiac surgery. Some surgeons and anesthesiologists prefer placement of an IABP before cardiac surgery in unstable patients to prevent hemodynamic collapse during induction of anesthesia. As an adjunct to PTCA, IABP catheters have been demonstrated to prevent reocclusion and to enhance recovery of left ventricular performance in patients undergoing direct PTCA for acute myocardial infarction,[221] and some investigators advise prophylactic placement before high-risk PTCA procedures.[222]

Aortoiliac disease that may make catheter insertion or counterpulsation hazardous and aortic valve insufficiency that may be worsened by augmented diastolic aortic pressures preclude use of an IABP (Table 10B-19).

Coronary sinus retroperfusion

It is possible to perfuse coronary capillary beds retrogradely through the cardiac venous system. Synchronized coronary sinus retroperfusion requires placement into the coronary sinus of a balloon catheter that is similar in concept to the IABP, except that with each balloon inflation, autologous blood (or a substitute oxygen carrier) is perfused into the cardiac veins. Although this system limits myocardial dysfunction and chest pain,[223,224] it has found only limited practical use outside the operating room.

Extracorporeal cardiopulmonary bypass and support devices

Percutaneous extracorporeal cardiopulmonary bypass systems that can provide total hemodynamic support for patients with little or no forward cardiac output have been used to support patients with cardiovascular collapse in (or near) the catheterization laboratory and have been used electively to support patients undergoing high-risk PTCA. Morbidity with these devices has been high, in part related to the large arterial and venous cannulae used; in a registry of 14 American centers using one system, some serious vascular complications developed in 39% of 363 patients, and 43% required blood transfusion.[225]

Other support devices (Table 10B-20) include a catheter-based left ventricular assist device that propels blood out of the left ventricle[226] and a percutaneous partial left heart bypass system that draws blood from the left atrium (accessed transseptally) and returns it into a femoral artery.[227]

Special medical adjuncts

Heparin and aspirin are the mainstays of antithrombin and antiplatelet therapy. However, abrupt closure, which essentially always involves some degree of thrombosis, still occurs in about 5% of PTCA cases, an indication of the insufficiencies of these drugs. Hirudin, a specific antithrombin protein found in the saliva of the European leech, is now manufactured through recombinant technology. Extensive laboratory studies[228-230] have shown its superiority to heparin, and clinical trials with hirudin have begun. Other thrombin inhibitors, both natural and synthetic, are also under study.

Platelet adhesion to an area of endothelial injury involves the participation of three platelet receptors: glycoprotein Ia, which binds to subendothelial collagen; glycoprotein Ib, which binds von Willebrand's factor; and glycoprotein IIb-IIIa, which binds von Willebrand's factor, fibrinogen, and fibronectin;[231] this last receptor is also key in platelet aggregation. Monoclonal antibodies against these receptors and their related adhesive macromolecules have shown some promise in reducing thrombosis after arterial injury.[39] Other platelet inhibitors, such as ticlopidine and the prostaglandin analogue iloprost, also show early promise.

There is interest in synthetic oxygen vehicles, such as perfluorochemical emulsions, which may provide better support than whole blood for distal myocardium during coronary intervention, but studies have not been entirely in agreement on the efficacy of these drugs.[232-234]

Reperfusion injury is defined as paradoxical deterioration in myocardial metabolism, architecture, or performance on restoration of blood flow after a period of severe

Table 10B-20 Percutaneous support devices

Device	Size, F	Advantages	Disadvantages	Applications
Intraaortic balloon counterpulsation	10.5	↓ Myocardial oxygen demand Ease of placement in 90% of patients Prolonged treatment duration possible	Requires a stable cardiac rhythm and output 9% to 43% incidence of vascular complications	Prophylactic placement in selected high-risk patients Support before CABG with complicated PTCA
Anterograde coronary perfusion (autoperfusion) catheter	4.5	Improved myocardial oxygen supply Hemoperfusion or fluosol perfusion possible	Large-profile catheter Ischemia of side branches involving the stenosis Removal of guide wire needed Thrombosis risk	Prolonged balloon inflations expected Placement before bypass surgery with abrupt closure
Coronary sinus retroperfusion	8.5	Maintains perfusion to branches compromised by PTCA No specialized PTCA catheter	Perfusion improvement documented only in LAD distribution Incomplete protection from ischemia Complex apparatus and additional arterial and venous access	Prolonged balloon inflations in high-risk patients; investigational
Cardiopulmonary support	18-20	Independent of LV function or rhythm ↓ Myocardial oxygen demand	No improvement in coronary perfusion 40% vascular complications	Prophylactic placement in very high risk patients Severe hemodynamic compromise after complicated PTCA
Other devices				
Hemopump	21	Direct LV decompression Use up to 14 days possible Independent of LV function or rhythm	Requires arteriotomy and adequate femoral artery size for placement Arrhythmogenic LV cannula Potential for dislodgment from LV	Investigational
Partial left heart bypass	14-20	No oxygenator required May decompress LV	Requires large bore transseptal cannulation	Investigational

CABG, coronary artery bypass surgery; LAD, left anterior descending artery; LV, left ventricle, left ventricular; PTCA, percutaneous transluminal coronary angioplasty; ↓, decreased.
From Lincoff AM, Popma JJ, Ellis SG, et al: Percutaneous support devices for high risk or complicated coronary angioplasty. *J Am Coll Cardiol* 17:770-780, 1991. By permission of American College of Cardiology.

ischemia (see chapter 27A). Several potential mechanisms have been offered to explain this phenomenon, and it may be possible to limit the deleterious consequences of reperfusion injury through use of drugs that interfere with these mechanisms of injury. There is great interest in adenosine, an endogenous purine nucleotide that may limit reperfusion injury through multiple mechanisms.[235-238] The beneficial effects of some drugs that limit reperfusion injury may, in part, be mediated by endogenous adenosine release.[239] Despite a large volume of encouraging animal work, few data on limitation of reperfusion injury in humans yet exist.

BALLOON VALVULOPLASTY

Given the increased use of balloon dilatation in coronary and other vascular disease, it is not surprising that balloons have been used to dilate stenotic valvular lesions.

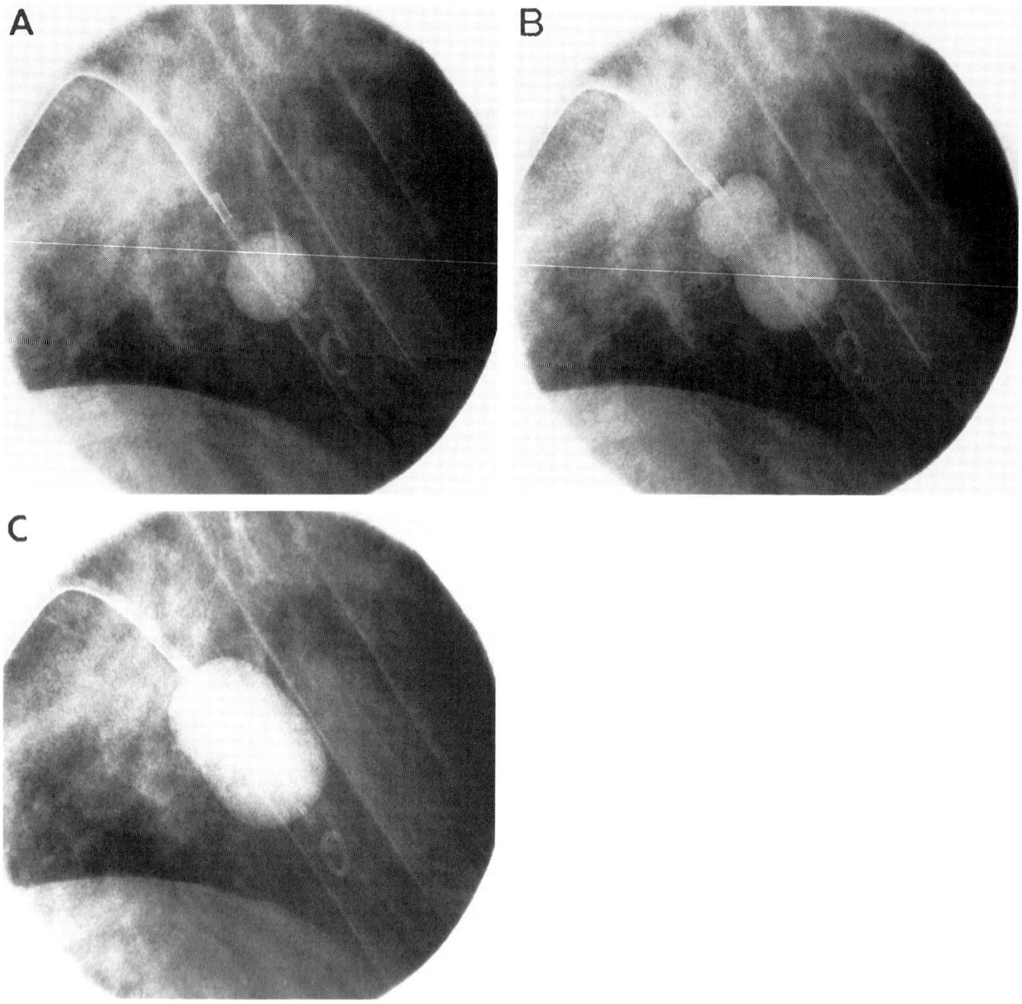

Fig 10B-23 The Inoue mitral valvuloplasty balloon catheter. **A,** the catheter is passed transseptally from the left atrium to the left ventricle. The distal (ventricular) portion of the balloon inflates first. **B,** further inflation causes the proximal (atrial) portion to expand, so that the catheter is positioned across the mitral valve. **C,** further pressure effects dilation of the mitral valve.

Although the approach varies according to the valve to be treated, the basic technique is similar for all balloon valvuloplasty. The valve and its annulus are first assessed with echocardiography and catheter techniques. Access to the valve is achieved transluminally; an anterograde venous approach is used for pulmonic and tricuspid valves, and an anterograde transseptal approach can be used for mitral and aortic valves, although the retrograde arterial approach is preferred for aortic valvuloplasty. A guide wire is passed across the stenotic valve, and the valvuloplasty balloon is advanced into position. The balloon is rapidly inflated and deflated; because valvuloplasty interrupts forward cardiac blood flow, inflations of more than 10 to 15 seconds are poorly tolerated. To reduce vascular injury caused by withdrawal of single large balloons, multiple smaller balloons can be used to achieve large final valve dimensions.[240]

Most valvuloplasty balloons are made of relatively noncompliant materials. An interesting exception to this is the mitral valvuloplasty balloon designed by Inoue.[241] This balloon consists of a double-layered rubber tube with a synthetic mesh inserted between the layers that results in variable compliance along the length of the balloon: roughly, the distal one-third is the most compliant, the proximal one-third the next most compliant, and the middle one-third the least compliant. When this balloon is passed transseptally across the mitral valve and inflated, the distal portion of the balloon inflates first; the balloon can then be pulled back to ensure firm engagement of the mitral valve. Further pressure causes the proximal portion to inflate, so that the balloon stabilizes itself on the atrial and ventricular sides of the valve. Finally, the middle portion inflates and dilates the valve (Fig 10B-23).

For discussion of tricuspid balloon valvuloplasty, see chapter 36; pulmonary balloon valvuloplasty, chapter 47; mitral balloon valvuloplasty, chapter 34; and aortic balloon valvuloplasty, chapter 32.

REFERENCES

1. Forssmann W: Die Sondierung des rechten Herzens. *Klin Wochenschr* 8:2085–2087, 1929
2. Rashkind WJ, Miller WW: Creation of an atrial septal defect without thoracotomy: a palliative approach to complete transposition of the great arteries. *JAMA* 196:991–992, 1966
3. Hosking MCK, Benson LN, Musewe N, et al: Transcatheter occlusion of the persistently patent ductus arteriosus: forty-month follow-up and prevalence of residual shunting. *Circulation* 84:2313-2317, 1991
4. Lock JE, Cockerham JT, Keene JF, et al: Transcatheter umbrella closure of congenital heart defects. *Circulation* 75:593-599, 1987
5. Benton JP, Barker KS: Transcatheter closure of ventricular septal defect: a nonsurgical approach to the care of the patient with acute ventricular septal rupture. *Heart Lung* 21:356-364, 1992
6. Mobin-Uddin K, Callard GM, Bolooki H, et al: Transvenous caval interruption with umbrella filter. *N Engl J Med* 286:55-58, 1972
7. Laskey MA, Deutsch E, Hirshfeld JW Jr, et al: Influence of heparin therapy on percutaneous transluminal coronary angioplasty outcome in patients with coronary arterial thrombus. *Am J Cardiol* 65:179-182, 1990
8. Arnott J: *A Treatise on Stricture of the Urethra, Containing an Account of Improved Methods of Treatment, With an Appendix Noticing the Application of a New Instrument to the Treatment of Enlarged Prostate Gland, Gleet, Fistula, and Other Diseases of the Urethra, Oesophagus, and Rectum.* London, Burgess & Hill, 1819
9. Abele JE: Balloon catheters and transluminal dilatation: technical considerations. *AJR* 135:901-906, 1980
10. Dotter CT: Transluminal angioplasty: a long view. *Radiology* 135:561-564, 1980
11. Dotter CT, Judkins MP: Transluminal treatment of arteriosclerotic obstruction: description of a new technic and a preliminary report of its application. *Circulation* 30:654-670, 1964
12. Grüntzig A: Transluminal dilatation of coronary-artery stenosis (letter to the editor). *Lancet* 1:263, 1978
13. Jensen R, Olin T: Complications at balloon catheter angiography: experiments in rabbits and dogs. *Acta Radiol [Diagn] (Stockh)* 20:593-605, 1979
14. Pasternak RC, Baughman KL, Fallon JT, et al: Scanning electron microscopy after coronary transluminal angioplasty of normal canine coronary arteries. *Am J Cardiol* 45:591-598, 1980
15. Block PC, Baughman KL, Pasternak RC, et al: Transluminal angioplasty: correlation of morphologic and angiographic findings in an experimental model. *Circulation* 61:778-785, 1980
16. Block PC, Fallon JT, Elmer D: Experimental angioplasty: lessons from the laboratory. *AJR* 135:907-912, 1980
17. Lee G, Ikeda RM, Joye JA, et al: Evaluation of transluminal angioplasty of chronic coronary artery stenosis: value and limitations assessed in fresh human cadaver hearts. *Circulation* 61:77-83, 1980
18. Castaneda-Zuniga WR, Formanek A, Tadavarthy M, et al: The mechanism of balloon angioplasty. *Radiology* 135:565-571, 1980
19. Block PC, Myler RK, Stertzer S, et al: Morphology after transluminal angioplasty in human beings. *N Engl J Med* 305:382-385, 1981
20. Baughman KL, Pasternak RC, Fallon JT, et al: Transluminal coronary angioplasty of postmortem human hearts. *Am J Cardiol* 48:1044-1047, 1981
21. Grüntzig AR, Senning Å, Siegenthaler WE: Nonoperative dilatation of coronary-artery stenosis: percutaneous transluminal coronary angioplasty. *N Engl J Med* 301:61-68, 1979
22. Vlietstra RE, Holmes DR Jr: Coronary balloon angioplasty: has its importance been over-inflated? *Cardiovasc Rev Rep* 4:245-252, 1983
23. Berger SM, Gorfinkel HJ: Candidates for transluminal coronary angioplasty (letter to the editor). *Am J Cardiol* 48:810, 1981
24. Hamby RI: Candidates for transluminal coronary angioplasty (reply to letter to the editor). *Am J Cardiol* 48:810, 1981
25. Hartzler GO, Rutherford BD, McConahay DR: "Non-investigational" experience with percutaneous transluminal coronary angioplasty in a clinical center (abstract). *Am J Cardiol* 49:916, 1982
26. Roubin GS, Gruentzig AR: Percutaneous transluminal coronary angioplasty: state of the art and future directions. *Int J Card Imaging* 1:143-154, 1985
27. Ford WB, Wholey MH, Zikria EA, et al: Percutaneous transluminal dilation of aortocoronary saphenous vein bypass grafts. *Chest* 79:529-535, 1981
28. Williams DO, Riley RS, Singh AK, et al: Evaluation of the role of coronary angioplasty in patients with unstable angina pectoris. *Am Heart J* 102:1-9, 1981
29. LeVeau PJ, Remetz MS, Cabin HS, et al: Predictors of success in percutaneous transluminal coronary angioplasty of chronic total occlusions. *Am J Cardiol* 64:1264-1269, 1989
30. Wallsh E, Franzone AJ, Clauss RH, et al: Transluminal coronary angioplasty: use during saphenous coronary bypass surgery. *NY State J Med* 80:630-631, 1980
31. American College of Cardiology/American Heart Association Task Force on Assessment of Diagnostic and Therapeutic Cardiovascular Procedures (Subcommittee on Percutaneous Transluminal Coronary Angioplasty): Guidelines for percutaneous transluminal coronary angioplasty. *J Am Coll Cardiol* 12:529-545, 1988
32. Ellis SG, Vandormael MG, Cowley MJ, et al: Coronary morphologic and clinical determinants of procedural outcome with angioplasty for multivessel coronary disease: implications for patient selection. *Circulation* 82:1193-1202, 1990
33. Myler RK, Shaw RE, Stertzer SH, et al: Lesion morphology and coronary angioplasty: current (1990-91) experience (abstract). *J Am Coll Cardiol* 19 Suppl A:23, 1992
34. Ellis SG, Cowley MJ, Vandormael M, et al: Coronary revascularization in 1986-87 and 1991 – dramatically improved acute phase results using percutaneous technologies (abstract). *Circulation* 86 Suppl 1:373, 1992
35. Kohli RS, DiSciascio G, Cowley MJ, et al: Coronary angioplasty in patients with severe left ventricular dysfunction. *J Am Coll Cardiol* 16:807-811, 1990
36. Taylor GJ, Rabinovich E, Mikell FL, et al: Percutaneous transluminal coronary angioplasty as palliation for patients considered poor surgical candidates. *Am Heart J* 111:840-844, 1986
37. Munger TM, Garratt KN, Gersh BJ, et al: Percutaneous transluminal coronary angioplasty compared with coronary artery bypass surgery in patients with severely depressed left ventricular function. *Mayo Clin Proc* (submitted for publication)
38. Schwartz L, Bourassa MG, Lespérance J, et al: Aspirin and dipyridamole in the prevention of restenosis after percutaneous transluminal coronary angioplasty. *N Engl J Med* 318:1714-1719, 1988
39. The EPIC Investigators: Use of a monoclonal antibody directed against the platelet glycoprotein IIb/IIIa receptor in high-risk coronary angioplasty. *N Engl J Med* 330:956-961, 1994
40. Hattersley PG: Activated coagulation time of whole blood. *JAMA* 196:436-440, 1966
41. Roubin GS, Hutchison N, Douglas JS Jr, et al: Influence of balloon size on complications and late restenosis after coronary angioplasty: a prospective randomized trial (abstract). *Circulation* 76 Suppl 4:215, 1987
42. Segal J, Kern MJ, Scott NA, et al: Alterations of phasic coronary artery flow velocity in humans during percutaneous coronary angioplasty. *J Am Coll Cardiol* 20:276-286, 1992
43. Kent KM, Bentivoglio LG, Block PC, et al: Percutaneous transluminal coronary angioplasty: report from the registry of the National Heart, Lung, and Blood Institute. *Am J Cardiol* 49:2011-2018, 1982
44. Detre K, Holubkov R, Kelsey S: Percutaneous transluminal coronary angioplasty in 1985-1986 and 1977-1981: the National Heart, Lung, and Blood Institute Registry. *N Engl J Med* 318:265-270, 1988
45. Meyer J, Merx W, Dörr R, et al: Successful treatment of acute myocardial infarction shock by combined percutaneous transluminal coronary recanalization (PTCR) and percutaneous transluminal coronary angioplasty (PTCA). *Am Heart J* 103:132-134, 1982
46. Lee L, Erbel R, Brown TM, et al: Multicenter registry of angioplasty therapy of cardiogenic shock: initial and long-term survival. *J Am Coll Cardiol* 17:599-603, 1991
47. Lee L, Walton JA, Bates E, et al: Cardiogenic shock complicating acute myocardial infarction: changing therapies and prognosis. *Circulation* 74 Suppl 2:276, 1986
48. Moosvi AR, Khaja F, Villanueva L, et al: Early revascularization improves survival in cardiogenic shock complicating acute myocardial infarction. *J Am Coll Cardiol* 19:907-914, 1992
49. Parisi AF, Folland ED, Hartigan P, et al: A comparison of angioplasty with medical therapy in the treatment of single-vessel coronary artery disease. *N Engl J Med* 326:10-16, 1992
50. Gruentzig AR, King SB III, Schlumpf M, et al: Long-term follow-up after percutaneous transluminal coronary angioplasty: the early Zurich experience. *N Engl J Med* 316:1127-1132, 1987
51. Vlietstra RE, Holmes DR Jr, Reeder GS, et al: Balloon angioplasty in multivessel coronary artery disease. *Mayo Clin Proc* 58:463-467, 1983

52. Dorros G, Stertzer SH, Cowley MJ, et al: Complex coronary angioplasty: multiple coronary dilatations. *Am J Cardiol* 53 Suppl:126C-130C, 1984

53. Cowley MJ, Vetrovec GW, DiSciascio G, et al: Coronary angioplasty of multiple vessels: short-term outcome and long-term results. *Circulation* 72:1314-1320, 1985

54. Mata LA, Bosch X, David PR, et al: Clinical and angiographic assessment 6 months after double vessel percutaneous coronary angioplasty. *J Am Coll Cardiol* 6:1239-1244, 1985

55. Vandormael MG, Chaitman BR, Ischinger T, et al: Immediate and short-term benefit of multilesion coronary angioplasty: influence of degree of revascularization. *J Am Coll Cardiol* 6:983-991, 1985

56. Hartzler GO: Percutaneous coronary angioplasty in patients with multivessel disease. In *Angioplasty*. Edited by GD Jang. New York, McGraw-Hill Book Company, 1986, pp 321-336

57. Dorros G, Lewin RF, Janke L: Multiple lesion transluminal coronary angioplasty in single and multivessel coronary artery disease: acute outcome and long-term effect. *J Am Coll Cardiol* 10:1007-1013, 1987

58. Finci L, Meier B, De Bruyne B, et al: Angiographic follow-up after multivessel percutaneous transluminal coronary angioplasty. *Am J Cardiol* 60:467-470, 1987

59. Myler RK, Topol EJ, Shaw RE, et al: Multiple vessel coronary angioplasty: classification, results, and patterns of restenosis in 494 consecutive patients. *Cathet Cardiovasc Diagn* 13:1-15, 1987

60. Vandormael MG, Deligonul U, Kern MJ, et al: Multilesion coronary angioplasty: clinical and angiographic follow-up. *J Am Coll Cardiol* 10:246-252, 1987

61. Deligonul U, Vandormael MG, Kern MJ, et al: Coronary angioplasty: a therapeutic option for symptomatic patients with two and three vessel coronary disease. *J Am Coll Cardiol* 11:1173-1179, 1988

62. DiSciascio G, Cowley MJ, Vetrovec GW, et al: Triple vessel coronary angioplasty: acute outcome and long-term results. *J Am Coll Cardiol* 12:42-48, 1988

63. Holmes DR Jr, Reeder GS, Vlietstra RE: Role of percutaneous transluminal coronary angioplasty in multivessel disease. *Am J Cardiol* 61:9G-14G, 1988

64. Reeder GS, Vlietstra RE, Mock MB, et al: Comparison of angioplasty and bypass surgery in multivessel coronary artery disease. *Int J Cardiol* 10:213-221, 1986

65. Jones EL, Craver JM, Guyton RA, et al: Importance of complete revascularization in performance of the coronary bypass operation. *Am J Cardiol* 51:7-12, 1983

66. Bell MR, Gersh BJ, Schaff HV, et al: Effect of completeness of revascularization on long-term outcome of patients with three-vessel disease undergoing coronary artery bypass surgery: a report from the Coronary Artery Surgery Study (CASS) Registry. *Circulation* 86:446-457, 1992

67. Wohlgelernter D, Cleman M, Highman HA, et al: Percutaneous transluminal coronary angioplasty of the "culprit lesion" for management of unstable angina pectoris in patients with multivessel coronary artery disease. *Am J Cardiol* 58:460-464, 1986

68. de Feyter PJ, Serruys PW, Arnold A, et al: Coronary angioplasty of the unstable angina related vessel in patients with multivessel disease. *Eur Heart J* 7:460-467, 1986

69. Reeder GS, Holmes DR Jr, Detre K, et al: Degree of revascularization in patients with multivessel coronary disease: a report from the National Heart, Lung, and Blood Institute Percutaneous Transluminal Coronary Angioplasty Registry. *Circulation* 77:638-644, 1988

70. American Heart Association: Protocol for the Bypass Angioplasty Revascularization Investigation. *Circulation* 84 Suppl 5:1-27, 1991

71. Dimas AP, Healy B: Coronary artery bypass surgery vs coronary angioplasty: from antithesis to synthesis. *Eur Heart J* 10 Suppl H:85-91, 1989

72. King SB III, Lembo NJ, Weintraub WS, et al: A randomized trial comparing coronary angioplasty with coronary bypass surgery. Emory Angioplasty versus Surgery Trial (EAST). *N Engl J Med* 331:1044-1050, 1994

73. Hamm CW, Reimers J, Ischinger T, et al: A randomized study of coronary angioplasty compared with bypass surgery in patients with symptomatic multivessel coronary disease. German Angioplasty Bypass Surgery Investigation (GABI). *N Engl J Med* 331:1037-1043, 1994

74. Rodriguez A, Boullon F, Perez-Balino N, et al: Argentine randomized trial of percutaneous transluminal coronary angioplasty versus coronary artery bypass surgery in multivessel disease (ERACI): in-hospital results and 1-year follow-up. *J Am Coll Cardiol* 22:1060-1067, 1993

75. Faxon DP, Detre KM, McCabe CH, et al: Role of percutaneous transluminal coronary angioplasty in the treatment of unstable angina: report from the National Heart, Lung, and Blood Institute Percutaneous Transluminal Coronary Angioplasty and Coronary Artery Surgery Study Registries. *Am J Cardiol* 53:131C-135C, 1984

76. de Feyter PJ, Serruys PW, van den Brand M, et al: Percutaneous transluminal coronary angioplasty for unstable angina. *Am J Cardiol* 68:125B-135B, 1991

77. Holt GW, Gersh BJ, Holmes DR Jr, et al: Results of percutaneous transluminal coronary angioplasty for angina pectoris early after acute myocardial infarction. *Am J Cardiol* 61:1238-1242, 1988

78. Meyer J, Schmitz HJ, Kiesslich T, et al: Percutaneous transluminal coronary angioplasty in patients with stable and unstable angina pectoris: analysis of early and late results. *Am Heart J* 106:973-980, 1983

79. de Feyter PJ, Serruys PW, van den Brand M, et al: Emergency coronary angioplasty in refractory unstable angina. *N Engl J Med* 313:342-346, 1985

80. Plokker HWT, Ernst SMPG, Bal ET, et al: Percutaneous transluminal coronary angioplasty in patients with unstable angina pectoris refractory to medical therapy: long-term clinical and angiographic results. *Cathet Cardiovasc Diagn* 14:15-18, 1988

81. Haraphongse M, Tymchak W, Rossall RE: Coronary angioplasty at the time of initial diagnostic coronary angiography in patients with unstable angina. *Cathet Cardiovasc Diagn* 14:73-75, 1988

82. de Feyter PJ, Suryapranata H, Serruys PW, et al: Coronary angioplasty for unstable angina: immediate and late results in 200 consecutive patients with identification of risk factors for unfavorable early and late outcome. *J Am Coll Cardiol* 12:324-333, 1988

83. Szatmáry LJ, Marco J, Fajadet J, et al: Actuality in the treatment of unstable angina pectoris. *Acta Med Hung* 45:23-34, 1988

84. Perry RA, Seth A, Hunt A, et al: Coronary angioplasty in unstable angina and stable angina: a comparison of success and complications. *Br Heart J* 60:367-372, 1988

85. Kamp O, Beatt KJ, De Feyter PJ, et al: Short-, medium-, and long-term follow-up after percutaneous transluminal coronary angioplasty for stable and unstable angina pectoris. *Am Heart J* 117:991-996, 1989

86. Morrison DA: Coronary angioplasty for medically refractory unstable angina within 30 days of acute myocardial infarction. *Am Heart J* 120:256-261, 1990

87. Morrison DA: Coronary angioplasty for medically refractory unstable angina in patients with prior coronary bypass surgery. *Cathet Cardiovasc Diagn* 20:174-181, 1990

88. Ilia R, Kolansky D, Setaro J, et al: Percutaneous transluminal coronary angioplasty in unstable and stable angina pectoris: a comparison of immediate success and complications. *Cardiology* 81:245-250, 1992

89. Bauters C, Lablanche J-M, McFadden EP, et al: Repeat percutaneous coronary angioplasty; clinical and angiographic follow-up in patients with stable or unstable angina pectoris. *Eur Heart J* 14:235-239, 1993

90. Kimura T, Nosaka H, Ueno K, et al: Role of coronary angioplasty in acute myocardial infarction (abstract). *Circulation* 74 Suppl 2:22, 1986

91. Pepine CJ, Prida X, Hill JA, et al: Percutaneous transluminal coronary angioplasty in acute myocardial infarction. *Am Heart J* 107:820-822, 1984

92. O'Neill W, Timmis GC, Bourdillon PD, et al: A prospective randomized clinical trial of intracoronary streptokinase versus coronary angioplasty for acute myocardial infarction. *N Engl J Med* 314:812-818, 1986

93. Rothbaum DA, Linnemeier TJ, Landin RJ, et al: Emergency percutaneous transluminal coronary angioplasty in acute myocardial infarction: a 3 year experience. *J Am Coll Cardiol* 10:264-272, 1987

94. Miller PF, Brodie BR, Weintraub RA, et al: Emergency coronary angioplasty for acute myocardial infarction: results from a community hospital. *Arch Intern Med* 147:1565-1570, 1987

95. Marco J, Caster L, Szatmary LJ, et al: Emergency percutaneous transluminal coronary angioplasty without thrombolysis as initial therapy in acute myocardial infarction. *Int J Cardiol* 15:55-63, 1987

96. Zolnick MR, Gersh BJ, Holmes DR Jr: Long term follow-up after percutaneous transluminal coronary angioplasty during acute myocardial infarction (abstract). *Circulation* 78 Suppl 2:634, 1988

97. O'Keefe JH Jr, Rutherford BD, McConahay DR, et al: Early and late results of coronary angioplasty without antecedent thrombolytic therapy for acute myocardial infarction. *Am J Cardiol* 64:1221-1230, 1989

98. Juliard J-M, Steg PG, Himbert D, et al: A patency-oriented strategy for early management of acute myocardial infarction using emergency coronary angiography and selective coronary angioplasty. *Am J Cardiol* 69:1383-1388, 1992
99. Kahn JK, Rutherford BD, McConahay DR, et al: Catheterization laboratory events and hospital outcome with direct angioplasty for acute myocardial infarction. *Circulation* 82:1910-1915, 1990
100. Ellis SG, da Silva ER, Heyndrickx G, et al: Randomized comparison of rescue angioplasty with conservative management of patients with early failure of thrombolysis for acute anterior myocardial infarction. *Circulation* 90:2280-2284, 1994
101. Gibbons RJ, Holmes DR, Reeder GS, et al: Immediate angioplasty compared with the administration of a thrombolytic agent followed by conservative treatment for myocardial infarction. *N Engl J Med* 328:685-691, 1993
102. Grines CL, Browne KF, Marco J, et al: A comparison of immediate angioplasty with thrombolytic therapy for acute myocardial infarction. *N Engl J Med* 328:673-679, 1993
103. Zijlstra F, de Boer MJ, Hoorntje JCA, et al: A comparison of immediate coronary angioplasty with intravenous streptokinase in acute myocardial infarction. *N Engl J Med* 328:680-684, 1993
104. Stone GW, Grines CL, Vlietstra RE, et al: Primary angioplasty is the preferred therapy for women and the elderly with acute myocardial infarction: results of the Primary Angioplasty in Myocardial Infarction (PAMI) Trial (abstract). *J Am Coll Cardiol* 21 Suppl A:330, 1993
105. Facilities and services in the United States. In *Hospital Statistics*. 1992-93 edition. Chicago, American Hospital Association, 1992, pp 208-209
106. The TIMI Research Group: Immediate vs delayed catheterization and angioplasty following thrombolytic therapy for acute myocardial infarction: TIMI II A results. *JAMA* 260:2849-2858, 1988
107. Simoons ML, Arnold AE, Betriu A, et al: Thrombolysis with tissue plasminogen activator in acute myocardial infarction: no additional benefit from immediate percutaneous coronary angioplasty. *Lancet* 1:197-203, 1988
108. Topol EJ, Califf RM, George BS, et al: A randomized trial of immediate versus delayed elective angioplasty after intravenous tissue plasminogen activator in acute myocardial infarction. *N Engl J Med* 317:581-588, 1987
109. Abbottsmith CW, Topol EJ, George BS, et al: Fate of patients with acute myocardial infarction with patency of the infarct-related vessel achieved with successful thrombolysis versus rescue angioplasty. *J Am Coll Cardiol* 16:770-778, 1990
110. Belenkie I, Traboulsi M, Hall CA, et al: Rescue angioplasty during myocardial infarction has a beneficial effect on mortality: a tenable hypothesis. *Can J Cardiol* 8:357-362, 1992
111. O'Connor CM, Mark DB, Hinohara T, et al: Rescue coronary angioplasty after failure of intravenous streptokinase in acute myocardial infarction: in-hospital and long-term outcomes. *J Intervent Cardiol* 1:85-95, 1989
112. Califf RM, Topol EJ, George BS, et al: Characteristics and outcome of patients in whom reperfusion with intravenous tissue-type plasminogen activator fails: results of the Thrombolysis and Angioplasty in Myocardial Infarction (TAMI) I trial. *Circulation* 77:1090-1099, 1988
113. The CORAMI Study Group: Outcome of attempted rescue coronary angioplasty after failed trhombolysis for acute myocardial infarction. *Am J Cardiol* 74:172-174, 1994
114. Ellis SG, Lincoff AM, George BS, et al: Randomized evaluation of coronary angioplasty for early TIMI 2 flow after thrombolytic therapy for the treatment of acute myocardial infarction: a new look at an old study. The Thrombolysis and Angioplasty in Myocardial Infarction (TAMI) Study Group. *Coron Artery Dis* 5:611-615, 1994
115. Topol EJ, Califf RM, George BS, et al: Coronary artery thrombolysis with combined intravenous recombinant tissue-type plasminogen activator and urokinase in patients with acute myocardial infarction. *Circulation* 77:1100-1107, 1988
116. Baim DS, Diver DJ, Knatterud GL, et al: PTCA "salvage" for thrombolytic failures—implications from TIMI II-A (abstract). *Circulation* 78 Suppl 2:112, 1988
117. Fung AY, Lai P, Topol EJ, et al: Value of percutaneous transluminal coronary angioplasty after unsuccessful intravenous streptokinase therapy in acute myocardial infarction. *Am J Cardiol* 58:686-691, 1986
118. Grines CL, Nissen SE, Booth DC, et al: Efficacy, safety and cost effectiveness of a new thrombolytic regimen for acute myocardial infarction using half-dose tPA with full dose streptokinase (abstract). *Circulation* 78 Suppl 2:304, 1988
119. Holmes DR Jr, Gersh BJ, Bailey KR, et al: Emergency "rescue" percutaneous transluminal coronary angioplasty after failed thrombolysis with streptokinase: early and late results. *Circulation* 81 Suppl 4:51-56, 1990
120. Thorsen LI, Brosstad F, Gogstad G, et al: Competitions between fibrinogen with its degradation products for interactions with the platelet-fibrinogen receptor. *Thromb Res* 44:611-623, 1986
121. Wilson PA, McNicol GP, Douglas AS: Effect of fibrinogen degradation products on platelet aggregation. *J Clin Pathol* 21:147-153, 1968
122. Rahimtoola SH: The hibernating myocardium. *Am Heart J* 117:211-221, 1989
123. Kloner RA, Przyklenk K: Stunned and hibernating myocardium. *Annu Rev Med* 42:1-8, 1991
124. Trevi GP, Sheiban I: Chronic ischaemic ('hibernating') and postischaemic ('stunned') dysfunctional but viable myocardium. *Eur Heart J* 12 Suppl G:20-26, 1991
125. Braunwald E, Rutherford JD: Reversible ischemic left ventricular dysfunction: evidence for the "hibernating myocardium." *J Am Coll Cardiol* 8:1467-1470, 1986
126. Montalescot G, Faraggi M, Drobinski G, et al: Myocardial viability in patients with Q wave myocardial infarction and no residual ischemia. *Circulation* 86:47-55, 1992
127. Hochman JS, Choo H: Limitation of myocardial infarct expansion by reperfusion independent of myocardial salvage. *Circulation* 75:299-306, 1987
128. Hale SL, Kloner RA: Left ventricular topographic alterations in the completely healed rat infarct caused by early and late coronary artery reperfusion. *Am Heart J* 116:1508-1513, 1988
129. Warren SE, Royal HD, Markis JE, et al: Time course of left ventricular dilation after myocardial infarction: influence of infarct-related artery and success of coronary thrombolysis. *J Am Coll Cardiol* 11:12-19, 1988
130. Barnathan ES, Schwartz JS, Taylor L, et al: Aspirin and dipyridamole in the prevention of acute coronary thrombosis complicating coronary angioplasty. *Circulation* 76:125-134, 1987
131. Lincoff AM, Popma JJ, Ellis SG, et al: Abrupt vessel closure complicating coronary angioplasty: clinical, angiographic and therapeutic profile. *J Am Coll Cardiol* 19:926-935, 1992
132. Stack RS, Quigley PJ, Collins G, et al: Perfusion balloon catheter. *Am J Cardiol* 61:77G-80G, 1988
133. Hinohara T, Simpson JB, Phillips HR, et al: Transluminal intracoronary reperfusion catheter: a device to maintain coronary perfusion between failed coronary angioplasty and emergency coronary bypass surgery. *J Am Coll Cardiol* 11:977-982, 1988
134. O'Keefe JH Jr, Holmes DR Jr, Reeder GS, et al: A new approach for dilation of bifurcation stenoses: the dual probe technique. Mayo Clin Proc 64:277-281, 1989
135. Holmes DR Jr, Vlietstra RE, Smith HC, et al: Restenosis after percutaneous transluminal coronary angioplasty (PTCA): a report from the PTCA Registry of the National Heart, Lung, and Blood Institute. *Am J Cardiol* 53:77C-81C, 1984
136. Leimgruber PP, Roubin GS, Hollman J, et al: Restenosis after successful coronary angioplasty in patients with single-vessel disease. *Circulation* 73:710-717, 1986
137. McBride W, Lange RA, Hillis LD: Restenosis after successful coronary angioplasty: pathophysiology and prevention. *N Engl J Med* 318:1734-1737, 1988
138. Serruys PW, Luijten HE, Beatt KJ, et al: Incidence of restenosis after successful coronary angioplasty: a time-related phenomenon. A quantitative angiographic study in 342 consecutive patients at 1, 2, 3, and 4 months. *Circulation* 77:361-371, 1988
139. Nobuyoshi M, Kimura T, Nosaka H, et al: Restenosis after successful percutaneous transluminal coronary angioplasty: serial angiographic follow-up of 229 patients. *J Am Coll Cardiol* 12:616-623, 1988
140. Wolinsky H: Insights into coronary angioplasty-induced restenosis from examination of atherogenesis. *Am J Cardiol* 60:65B-67B, 1987
141. Chesebro JH, Lam JYT, Badimon L, et al: Restenosis after arterial angioplasty: a hemorrheologic response to injury. *Am J Cardiol* 60:10B-16B, 1987
142. Chesebro JH, Webster MWI, Zoldhelyi P, et al: Thrombosis and restenosis after angioplasty. In *Coronary Restenosis*. Edited by RS Schwartz. Boston, Blackwell Scientific Publications, 1992, pp 219-237

143. Harker LA: Role of platelets and thrombosis in mechanisms of acute occlusion and restenosis after angioplasty. *Am J Cardiol* 60:20B-28B, 1987

144. Rensing BJ, Hermans WRM, Beatt KJ, et al: Quantitative angiographic assessment of elastic recoil after percutaneous transluminal coronary angioplasty. *Am J Cardiol* 66:1039-1044, 1990

145. Forrester JS, Fishbein M, Helfant R, et al: A paradigm for restenosis based on cell biology: clues for the development of new prevention therapies. *J Am Coll Cardiol* 17:758-769, 1991

146. Schwartz RS, Holmes DR Jr, Topol EJ: The restenosis paradigm revisited: an alternative proposal for cellular mechanisms. *J Am Coll Cardiol* 20:1284-1293, 1992

147. Schwartz RS, Edwards WD: Cellular mechanisms of restenotic neointima in a porcine coronary model. In *Coronary Restenosis*. Edited by RS Schwartz. Boston, Blackwell Scientific Publications, 1992, pp 205-218

148. Currier JW, Faxon DP: Restenosis after percutaneous transluminal coronary angioplasty: have we been aiming at the wrong target? (Editorial.) *J Am Coll Cardiol* 25:516-520, 1995

149. Dehmer GJ, Popma JJ, van den Berg EK, et al: Reduction in the rate of early restenosis after coronary angioplasty by a diet supplemented with n-3 fatty acids. *N Engl J Med* 319:733-740, 1988

150. Sahni R, Maniet AR, Voci G, et al: Prevention of restenosis by lovastatin (abstract). *Circulation* 80 Suppl 2:65, 1989

151. Deligonul U, Vandormael M, Kern MJ, et al: Repeat coronary angioplasty for restenosis: results and predictors of follow-up clinical events. *Am Heart J* 117:997-1002, 1989

152. Garratt KN, Holmes DR Jr, Bell MR, et al: Results of directional atherectomy of primary atheromatous and restenosis lesions in coronary arteries and saphenous vein grafts. *Am J Cardiol* 70:449-454, 1992

153. Safian RD, Gelbfish JS, Erny RE, et al: Coronary atherectomy: clinical, angiographic, and histological findings and observations regarding potential mechanisms. *Circulation* 82:69-79, 1990

154. Fishman RF, Kuntz RE, Carrozza JP Jr, et al: Long-term results of directional atherectomy: predictors of restenosis. *J Am Coll Cardiol* 20:1101-1110, 1992

155. Umans V, Haine E, Renkin J, et al: One hundred and thirteen attempts at directional coronary atherectomy: the early and combined experience of two European centres using quantitative angiography to assess their results. *Eur Heart J* 13:918-924, 1992

156. Hinohara T, Rowe MH, Robertson GC, et al: Effect of lesion characteristics on outcome of directional coronary atherectomy. *J Am Coll Cardiol* 17:1112-1120, 1991

157. Kaufmann UP, Garratt KN, Vlietstra RE, et al: Transluminal atherectomy of saphenous vein aortocoronary bypass grafts. *Am J Cardiol* 65:1430-1433, 1990

158. Holmes DR Jr, Ellis SG, Garratt KN: Directional coronary atherectomy for thrombus containing lesions: improved outcome (abstract). *Circulation* 84 Suppl 2:26, 1991

159. Topol EJ, Leya F, Pinkerton CA, et al: A comparison of directional atherectomy with coronary angioplasty in patients with coronary artery disease. *N Engl J Med* 329:221-227, 1993

160. Adelman AG, Cohen EA, Kimball BP, et al: A comparison of directional atherectomy with balloon angioplasty for lesions of the left anterior descending coronary artery. *N Engl J Med* 329:228-233, 1993

161. Simonton CA: Lesion-specific technique considerations in directional coronary atherectomy. *Cathet Cardiovasc Diagn* 1 Suppl:3-9, 1993

162. Whitlow PL, Franco I: Indications for directional coronary atherectomy: 1993. *Am J Cardiol* 72:21E-29E, 1993

163. Kuntz RE, Safian RD, Carrozza JP, et al: The importance of acute luminal diameter in determining restenosis after coronary atherectomy or stenting. *Circulation* 86:1827-1835, 1992

164. Baim DS, Kuntz RE: Directional coronary atherectomy: How much lumen enlargement is optimal? *Am J Cardiol* 72:65E-70E, 1993

165. Safian RD: Coronary atherectomy versus angioplasty (letter to the editor). *N Engl J Med* 329:1891, 1993

166. Safian RD, Freed M, Lichtenberg A, et al: Are residual stenoses after excimer laser angioplasty and coronary atherectomy due to inefficient or small devices? Comparison with balloon angioplasty. *J Am Coll Cardiol* 22:1628-1634, 1993

167. Holmes DR, Topol EJ, Califf RM, et al: A multicenter, randomized trial of coronary angioplasty versus directional atherectomy for patients with saphenous vein bypass graft lesions. *Circulation* 91:1966-1974, 1995

168. Garratt KN, Kaufmann UP, Edwards WD, et al: Safety of percutaneous coronary atherectomy with deep arterial resection. *Am J Cardiol* 64:538-540, 1989

169. Garratt KN, Holmes DR Jr, Bell MR, et al: Restenosis after directional coronary atherectomy: differences between primary atheromatous and restenosis lesions and influence of subintimal tissue resection. *J Am Coll Cardiol* 16:1665-1671, 1990

170. Isner J: Read at the meeting of the CAVEAT Investigators, New Orleans, Louisiana, November, 1992

171. Bell MR, Garratt KN, Bresnahan JF, et al: Relation of deep arterial resection and coronary artery aneurysm after directional coronary atherectomy. *J Am Coll Cardiol* 20:1474-1481, 1992

172. Bertrand ME, LaBlanche JM, Fourrier JL, et al: Percutaneous coronary rotary ablation. *Herz* 15:285-291, 1990

173. Pavlides GS, Hauser AM, Grines CL, et al: Clinical, hemodynamic, electrocardiographic and mechanical events during nonocclusive, coronary atherectomy and comparison with balloon angioplasty. *Am J Cardiol* 70:841-845, 1992

174. Dietz U, Erbel R, Rupprecht H-J, et al: High frequency rotational ablation: an alternative in treating coronary artery stenoses and occlusions. *Br Heart J* 70:327-336, 1993

175. Safian RD, Niazi KA, Strzelecki M, et al: Detailed angiographic analysis of high-speed mechanical rotational atherectomy in human coronary arteries. *Circulation* 88:961-968, 1993

176. Stertzer SH, Rosenblum J, Shaw RE, et al: Coronary rotational ablation: initial experience in 302 procedures. *J Am Coll Cardiol* 21:287-295, 1993

177. Zotz RJ, Erbel R, Philipp A, et al: High-speed rotational angioplasty-induced echo contrast in vivo and in vitro optical analysis. *Cathet Cardiovasc Diagn* 26:98-109, 1992

178. Zotz R, Stähr P, Erbel R, et al: Analysis of high-frequency rotational angioplasty-induced echo contrast. *Cathet Cardiovasc Diagn* 22:137-144, 1991

179. Safian RD, Grines CL, May MA, et al: Clinical and angiographic results of transluminal extraction coronary atherectomy in saphenous vein bypass grafts. *Circulation* 89:302-312, 1994

180. Popma JJ, Satler LF, Pichard AD, et al: Vascular complications after balloon and new device angioplasty. *Circulation* 88:1569-1578, 1993

181. Safian RD, May MA, Lichtenberg A, et al: Detailed clinical and angiographic analysis of transluminal extraction coronary atherectomy for complex lesions in native coronary arteries. *J Am Coll Cardiol* 25:848-854, 1995

182. Popma JJ, Leon MB, Mintz GS, et al: Results of coronary angioplasty using the transluminal extraction catheter. *Am J Cardiol* 70:1526-1532, 1992

183. Schaff HV: Role of the surgeon in interventional cardiology. In *Interventional Cardiology*. Edited by DR Holmes Jr, RE Vlietstra. Philadelphia, F. A. Davis Company, 1989, pp 42-52

184. Connor AR, Vlietstra RE, Schaff HV, et al: Early and late results of coronary artery bypass after failed angioplasty. Actuarial analysis of late cardiac events and comparison with initially successful angioplasty. *J Thorac Cardiovasc Surg* 96:191-197, 1988

185. Sigwart U, Puel J, Mirkovitch V, et al: Intravascular stents to prevent occlusion and restenosis after transluminal angioplasty. *N Engl J Med* 316:701-706, 1987

186. Puel J, Juilliere Y, Bertrand ME, et al: Early and late assessment of stenosis geometry after coronary arterial stenting. *Am J Cardiol* 61:546-553, 1988

187. Serruys PW, Strauss BH, Beatt KJ, et al: Angiographic follow-up after placement of a self-expanding coronary-artery stent. *N Engl J Med* 324:13-17, 1991

188. Strauss BH, Serruys PW, Bertrand ME, et al: Quantitative angiographic follow-up of the coronary Wallstent in native vessels and bypass grafts (European experience – March 1986 to March 1990). *Am J Cardiol* 69:475-481, 1992

189. Schatz RA: Introduction to intravascular stents. *Cardiol Clin* 6:357-372, 1988

190. Schatz RA, Goldberg S, Leon M, et al: Clinical experience with the Palmaz-Schatz coronary stent. *J Am Coll Cardiol* 17 Suppl B:155-159, 1991

191. Fischman DL, Leon MB, Baim DS, et al: A randomized comparison of coronary-stent placement and balloon angioplasty in the treatment of coronary artery disease. Stent Restenosis Study Investigators. *N Eng J Med* 331:496-501, 1994

192. Serruys PW, de Jaegere P, Kiemeneij F, et al: A comparison of balloon-expandable-stent implantation with balloon angioplasty in

patients with coronary artery disease. Benestent Study Group. *N Engl J Med* 331:489-495, 1994

193. Yellayi SS, Schatz RA: Indications and use of the Palmaz-Schatz coronary stent. *Cardiol Clin* 12:651-663, 1994

194. Roubin GS, King SB III, Douglas JS Jr, et al: Intracoronary stenting during percutaneous transluminal coronary angioplasty. *Circulation* 81 Suppl 4:92-100, 1990

195. Garratt KN, Holmes DR Jr, Roubin GS: Early outcome after placement of a metallic intracoronary stent: initial Mayo Clinic experience. *Mayo Clin Proc* 66:268-275, 1991

196. Roubin GS, Cannon AD, Agrawal SK, et al: Intracoronary stenting for acute and threatened closure complicating percutaneous transluminal coronary angioplasty. *Circulation* 85:916-927, 1992

197. George BS, Voorhees WE III, Roubin GS, et al: Multicenter investigation of coronary stenting to treat acute or threatened closure after percutaneous transluminal coronary angioplasty: clinical and angiographic outcomes. *J Am Coll Cardiol* 22:135-143, 1993

198. Sutton JM, Ellis SG, Roubin GS, et al: Major clinical events after coronary stenting. The multicenter registry of acute and elective Gianturco-Roubin stent placement. The Gianturco-Roubin Intracoronary Stent Investigator Group. *Circulation* 89:1126-1137, 1994

199. Buchwald A, Unterberg C, Werner G, et al: Initial clinical results with the Wiktor stent: a new balloon-expandable coronary stent. *Clin Cardiol* 14:374-379, 1991

200. Zidar JP, Jackman JD Jr, Virmani R, et al: Long term angiographic and histopathologic results of a new tantalum stent (abstract). *Circulation* 86 Suppl 1:732, 1992

201. Dichek DA, Neville RF, Zwiebel JA, et al: Seeding of intravascular stents with genetically engineered endothelial cells. *Circulation* 80:1347-1353, 1989

202. Stefanadis C, Karayannako SP, Kallikazaros I, et al: Transluminal vascular stenting using autologous vein grafts: an experimental study (abstract). *Circulation* 86 Suppl 1:732, 1992

203. Slepian MJ: Polymeric endoluminal paving and sealing: therapeutics at the crossroad of biomechanics and pharmacology. In *Textbook of Interventional Cardiology*. Edited by EJ Topol. Philadelphia, WB Saunders Company, 1990, pp 647-670

204. Parodi JC, Palmaz JC, Barone HD: Transfemoral intraluminal graft implantation for abdominal aortic aneurysms. *Ann Vasc Surg* 5:491-499, 1991

205. Yoshida H, Kakino T, Kajitani M, et al: Transcatheter placement of an intraluminal prosthesis for the thoracic aorta: a new approach to aortic dissections. *ASAIO Trans* 37:M272-M273, 1991

206. Cannon AD, Chou CY, Bilodeau L, et al: Initial experience with a removable tantalum coil stent in dog coronary arteries (abstract). *Circulation* 86 Suppl 1:731, 1992

207. Muller DWM, White CJ, Friedman HZ, et al: Temporary coronary "splinting" for abrupt closure post-PTCA: initial in vivo studies (abstract). *J Am Coll Cardiol* 17 Suppl A:235, 1991

208. Khorsandi MJ, Eigler NL, Lambert T, et al: Temporary stenting with the heat activated recoverable temporary stent: implantations up to six weeks (abstract). *Circulation* 86 Suppl 1:800, 1992

209. Cook SL, Eigler NL, Shefer A, et al: Percutaneous excimer laser coronary angioplasty of lesions not ideal for balloon angioplasty. *Circulation* 84:632-643, 1991

210. Sanborn TA, Bittl JA, Hershman RA, et al: Percutaneous coronary excimer laser-assisted angioplasty: initial multicenter experience in 141 patients. *J Am Coll Cardiol* 17 Suppl B:169-173, 1991

211. Verdaasdonk RM, Holstege FC, Jansen ED, et al: Temperature along the surface of modified fiber tips for Nd:YAG laser angioplasty. *Lasers Surg Med* 11:213-222, 1991

212. Vincent GM, Fox J, Johnson MD, et al: Thermal laser probe angioplasty: influence of constant tip temperature, plaque composition, and probe/vessel diameter ratio. *Lasers Surg Med* 10:420-426, 1990

213. Spears JR, Reyes VP, Wynne J, et al: Percutaneous coronary laser balloon angioplasty: initial results of a multicenter experience. *J Am Coll Cardiol* 16:293-303, 1990

214. Haase KK, Baumbach A, Wehrmann M, et al: Potential use of Holmium lasers for angioplasty: evaluation of a new solid-state laser for ablation of atherosclerotic plaque. *Lasers Surg Med* 11:232-237, 1991

215. Heuser RR, Mehta SS: Holmium laser angioplasty after failed coronary balloon dilation: use of a new solid-state, infrared laser system. *Cathet Cardiovasc Diagn* 23:187-189, 1991

216. Okada M, Shimizu K, Ikuta H, et al: A new method of myocardial revascularization by laser. *Thorac Cardiovasc Surg* 39:1-4, 1991

217. Baumbach A, Bittl JA, Fleck E, et al: Acute complications of coronary excimer laser angioplasty: analysis of two multicenter registries (abstract). *Circulation* 86 Suppl 1:510, 1992

218. Ellis SG, Arnold AZ, Raymond RE, et al: Increased coronary perforation in the new device era: incidence, classification, management and outcome (abstract). *Circulation* 86 Suppl 1:787, 1992

219. Scriven AJI, Lidbury PS, Nathan AW: Effects of laser-generated tissue debris on aggregation of human platelets. *Am Heart J* 122:802-808, 1991

220. Amsterdam EZ, Awan NA, Lee G, et al: Intra-aortic balloon counterpulsation: rationale, application and results. *Cardiovasc Clin* 11 No. 3:79-96, 1981

221. Ishihara M, Sato H, Tateishi H, et al: Intraaortic balloon pumping as the postangioplasty strategy in acute myocardial infarction. *Am Heart J* 122:385-389, 1991

222. Lincoff AM, Popma JJ, Ellis SG, et al: Percutaneous support devices for high risk or complicated coronary angioplasty. *J Am Coll Cardiol* 17:770-780, 1991

223. Kar S, Drury JK, Hajduczki I, et al: Synchronized coronary venous retroperfusion for support and salvage of ischemic myocardium during elective and failed angioplasty. *J Am Coll Cardiol* 18:271-282, 1991

224. Constantino C, Sampaolesi A, Serra CM, et al: Coronary venous retroperfusion support during high risk angioplasty in patients with unstable angina: preliminary experience. *J Am Coll Cardiol* 18:283-292, 1991

225. Vogel RA, Shawl FA: Report of the National Registry of Elective Supported Angioplasty: comparison of the 1988 and 1989 results (abstract). *Circulation* 82 Suppl 3:653, 1990

226. Frazier OH, Nakatani T, Duncan JM, et al: Clinical experience with the Hemopump. ASAIO Trans 35:604-606, 1989

227. Babic UU, Grujicic S, Djurisic Z, et al: Percutaneous left atrial-aortic bypass with a roller pump (abstract). *Circulation* 80 Suppl 2:272, 1989

228. Heras M, Chesebro JH, Penny WJ, et al: Effects of thrombin inhibition on the development of acute platelet-thrombus deposition during angioplasty in pigs: heparin versus recombinant hirudin, a specific thrombin inhibitor. *Circulation* 79:657-665, 1989

229. Kaiser B, Simon A, Markwardt F: Antithrombotic effects of recombinant hirudin in experimental angioplasty and intravascular thrombolysis. *Thromb Haemost* 63:44-47, 1990

230. Ip JH, Fuster V, Israel D, et al: The role of platelets, thrombin and hyperplasia in restenosis after coronary angioplasty. *J Am Coll Cardiol* 17 Suppl B:77-88, 1991

231. Hawiger J: Formation and regulation of platelet and fibrin hemostatic plug. *Hum Pathol* 18:111-122, 1987

232. Forman MB, Perry JM, Wilson BH, et al: Demonstration of myocardial reperfusion injury in humans: results of a pilot study utilizing acute coronary angioplasty with perfluorochemical in anterior myocardial infarction. *J Am Coll Cardiol* 18:911-918, 1991

233. Cleman M, Jaffee CC, Wohlgelerntner D: Prevention of ischemia during percutaneous transluminal coronary angioplasty by transcatheter infusion of oxygenated Fluosol DA 20%. *Circulation* 74:555-562, 1986

234. Bell MR, Nishimura RA, Holmes DR Jr, et al: Does intracoronary infusion of fluosol-DA 20% prevent left ventricular diastolic dysfunction during coronary balloon angioplasty? *J Am Coll Cardiol* 16:959-966, 1990

235. Sollevi A: Cardiovascular effects of adenosine in man: possible clinical implications. *Prog Neurobiol* 27:319-349, 1986

236. Hori M, Kitakaze M: Adenosine, the heart, and coronary circulation. *Hypertension* 18:565-574, 1991

237. Olafsson B, Forman MB, Puett DW, et al: Reduction of reperfusion injury in the canine preparation by intracoronary adenosine: importance of the endothelium and no-reflow phenomenon. *Circulation* 76:1137-1145, 1987

238. Pitarys CJ II, Virmani R, Vildibill HD Jr, et al: Reduction of myocardial reperfusion injury by intravenous adenosine administered during the early reperfusion period. *Circulation* 83:237-247, 1991

239. Ely SW, Berne RM: Protective effects of adenosine in myocardial ischemia. *Circulation* 85:893-904, 1992

240. Mullins CE, Nihill MR, Vick GW III, et al: Double balloon technique for dilation of valvular or vessel stenosis in congenital and acquired heart disease. *J Am Coll Cardiol* 10:107-114, 1987

241. Inoue K, Hung J-S: Percutaneous transvenous mitral commissurotomy (PTMC): the Far East experience. In *Textbook of Interventional Cardiology*. Edited by EJ Topol. Philadelphia, WB Saunders Company, 1990, pp 887-899

CHAPTER

11

Assessment and use of cardiovascular tests in clinical prediction

Arnold M. Weissler, M.D.

"The theory of probability is at bottom nothing but common sense reduced to calculation."

Pierre Simon de LaPlace (1749-1829)[1]

THE cardiologist must commonly venture clinical predictions on the basis of a probabilistic interpretation of cardiovascular test data. In seeking a better understanding of probability analysis in the literature, this physician encounters unfamiliar terms and symbols that convey an incomplete perception of their clinical application. As a consequence, the cardiologist often forsakes the probabilistic jargon for an intuitive interpretation of test results. As implied above in the incisive quotation of the French mathematician LaPlace,[1] medical probability theory is nothing more than an adaptation of basic mathematics to clinical prediction. When detailed in clinical terms, probability estimates can be eminently understood and of practical value in clinical decision-making.

The purpose of this chapter is to present a basic rationale for assessing the quality of cardiovascular tests and their use in clinical prediction and to do so in a perspective and language familiar to the clinician.

HISTORIC REVIEW

The rationale for the contemporary application of probability theory to the prediction of cardiac disease and clinical outcome is rooted in the historic dissertations of the 18th century mathematicians Jakob Bernoulli, Abraham DeMoivre, and Reverend Thomas Bayes.[2] The ideas of these early contributors were elaborated and popularized during the 19th century by LaPlace in his renowned thesis *Théorie Analytique des Probabilités.*[3] It is to Reverend Thomas Bayes that modern authors give credit for conceiving the equations adapted to the calculation of the probability of disease after a given test result. Bayes' dissertation entitled "An Essay Towards Solving a Problem in the Doctrine of Chances" was presented posthumously by his esteemed colleague Richard Price in 1763.[2] Bayes' basic design, as quoted by Price, was "to find out a method by which we might judge concerning the probability that an event has to happen, in given circumstances, upon supposition that we know nothing concerning it, but that, under the same circumstances, it has happened a certain number of times, and failed a certain number of times." A unique and less often emphasized contribution of the Bayes essay is his solution to the following problem. "Given the number of times in which an unknown event has happened and failed: Required the chance that the probability of its happening in a single trial lies somewhere between any two degrees of probability that can be named." In devising equations for the solution of these problems, Bayes elucidated two of the most commonly applied probabilistic formulations of modern medicine, that of predicting the probability of a disease or disorder from specific experiential data (the principle of conditional probability) and that of designating specific limits for such predictions (the principle of confidence limits).

EVALUATING TEST PERFORMANCE IN AN INDEX POPULATION

Test performance indices

Cardiovascular tests are designed with two primary purposes in mind: (1) to judge the presence or absence of cardiovascular disease and (2) to predict the occurrence or absence of future events (clinical outcome). In subsequent discussions in this chapter, the term "disease" refers generically to any cardiovascular disease, disorder, or dysfunction; the term "no disease" refers to the status of normal, no disease, without disease, or disease absence. The potential quality or accuracy of a cardiovascular test in providing predictive information in a clinically representative patient group termed the *index population* is generally evaluated in four performance indices of the test, namely, sensitivity, specificity, positive predictive accuracy, and negative predictive accuracy. The *sensitivity (Se)** is the proportion of the subpopulation with disease that has a positive test result, and the *specificity (Sp)* is the proportion of the subpopulation with no disease that has a negative test result. The *positive predictive accuracy* [$(+)PA_c$] is the proportion of the subpopulation with a positive test result that has disease, and the *negative predictive accuracy* [$(-)PA_c$] is the proportion of the subpopulation with a negative test result that has no disease. Alternative terms for predictive accuracy are *positive predictive value* and *negative predictive value*. The test performed on an index population is referred to as an *index test*. The Se and Sp are hence estimates of the quality or accuracy of an index test in classifying individuals as having (positive) and not having (negative) disease. The $(+)PA_c$ and $(-)PA_c$ are estimates of the quality or accuracy of an index test in predicting the presence or absence of disease.

The unit complements of Se and Sp are often used in estimating test error. Thus, *insensitivity (1 − Se)* refers to the proportion of the subpopulation with disease that has a negative test result, and *nonspecificity (1 − Sp)* refers to the proportion of the subpopulation with no disease that has a positive test result. Some authors refer to Se as the *true-positive rate* and Sp as the *true-negative rate* of a test. By this definition, the insensitivity is the *false-negative rate* and the nonspecificity the *false-positive rate*.

Population characteristics

Of critical significance to the evaluation of an index test is knowledge of the prevalence of disease and of the frequency or fraction of the index population with positive and negative test results. The *prevalence of disease (PD)* is the proportion of the total index population with disease determined by an accepted standard (commonly referred to as the "gold standard" for the disease). The *prevalence of normality (PN)*, which is the complement of PD, is the proportion of the total index population without disease. The *positive fraction* [$(+)F$] is the proportion of the total index population with positive test results. The *negative fraction* [$(-)F$], which is the complement of $(+)F$, is the proportion of the total index population with negative test results.

In subsequent discussions of test performance indices and population characteristics, we adopt the convention that measures of prevalence, predictive accuracy, and probability are expressed in percentage and that those of sensitivity, specificity, and population fraction are expressed in decimals.

Test characteristics and the probability spectrum

As a primary step preparatory to the determination of test performance indices, it is practical to subdivide the index population into four subsets, or *test characteristics*, expressed in percentage. These test characteristics are determined by the association of two sets of variables: (1) the presence of a positive (abnormal) or negative (normal) test result with respect to the test threshold and (2) the presence or absence of disease as determined by the "gold standard." An alternative term for the test threshold is "cutoff point." A true test result is an appropriately matched test; a false test result is an inappropriately matched test.

	Disease present		Disease absent	
Test result	+	−	−	+
Characteristics	TP	FN	TN	FP
Patients, no.	390	210	332	68
Total population, %	39	21	33	7

Fig 11-1 Probability spectrum format for presentation of test results in an index population of 1,000 patients. The test characteristics reported in numbers of patients or percentage of total population facilitate calculation of population characteristics and test performance indices. *FN*, false negative; *FP*, false positive; *TN*, true negative; *TP*, true positive.

The four index test characteristics are as follows: (1) *true positives* (TP), individuals with disease who test positively; (2) *true negatives* (TN), individuals with no disease who test negatively; (3) *false positives* (FP), individuals with no disease who test positively; and (4) *false negatives* (FN), individuals with disease who test negatively.

A convenient tabular format for display of the primary data from an index population, which the author refers to as the *probability spectrum*, is displayed in Figure 11-1. All test and population characteristics and test performance indices can be calculated from this spectrum. The data from a model study are illustrated. In the figure, the index population of 1,000 patients is divided into four subgroups according to the test characteristics. The data are presented in numbers of individuals and in percentage of total index population.

The presentation of the test characteristics in percentage of total index population facilitates the calculation of the population characteristics. The prevalence of disease in the index population is calculated, in percent, as the sum of the true positives and false negatives ($PD\% = TP\% + FN\% = 60\%$). The prevalence of normality is calculated in percent as the sum of the true negatives and the false positives ($PN\% = TN\% + FP\% = 40\%$). The PD and PN are 100% complements. The positive fraction for the index population is calculated in decimals as the sum of the true-positive and false-positive subgroups divided by 100, [$(+)F = (TP\% + FP\%)/100 = 0.46$]. The negative fraction for the index population is calculated in decimals as the sum of the true-negative and false-negative subgroups divided by 100, [$(-)F = (TN\% + FN\%)/100 = 0.54$]. The $(+)F$ and $(-)F$ are unit complements.

With use of the four test characteristics, the calculations

*A glossary of abbreviations appears at the end of the chapter.

of Se and Sp for an index test, expressed in decimals, are as follows:

$$Se = \frac{TP\%}{TP\% + FN\%} = \frac{39}{39 + 21} = 0.65 \quad [11\text{-}1]$$

$$Sp = \frac{TN\%}{TN\% + FP\%} = \frac{33}{33 + 7} = 0.83 \quad [11\text{-}2]$$

With use of the four test characteristics, the calculations for $(+)PA_c$ and $(-)PA_c$ for an index test, expressed in percent, are as follows:

$$(+)PA_c = \frac{TP\%}{TP\% + FP\%} \times 100 = \frac{39}{39 + 7} \times 100 = 85\% \quad [11\text{-}3]$$

$$(-)PA_c = \frac{TN\%}{TN\% + FN\%} \times 100 = \frac{33}{33 + 21} \times 100 = 61\% \quad [11\text{-}4]$$

A useful calculation in presenting probability data clinically is the *predictive accuracy of disease for patients with a negative test result,* that is, the proportion of the subpopulation with a negative test result that has disease, expressed in percent. This is calculated as the 100% complement of the $(-)PA_c$ as follows:

$$100 - (-)PA_c = 100 - \left[\frac{TN\%}{TN\% + FN\%} \times 100\right] \quad [11\text{-}5]$$

$$100 - \left[\frac{TN\%}{TN\% + FN\%} \times 100\right] =$$

$$100 - \left[\frac{33}{33 + 21} \times 100\right] = 39\%$$

An alternative calculation for the 100% complement of $(-)PA_c$ is

$$100 - (-)PA_c = \frac{FN\%}{TN\% + FN\%} \times 100 \quad [11\text{-}6]$$

$$\frac{FN\%}{TN\% + FN\%} \times 100 = \frac{21}{33 + 21} \times 100 = 39\%$$

Another approach to the calculation of the test performance indices for an index test is to apply the absolute numbers of individuals in each test characteristic to Equations 11-1 through 11-6, retaining the appropriate expression in percent or decimals for the test performance indices.

Although the format of the probability spectrum offers a convenient means for displaying the test characteristics preparatory to the calculation of test performance indices, it does not afford a graphic or visual picture of the distribution of the test scores for the index population. Such a graphic plot of the distribution of test scores for groups of individuals with disease and without disease is illustrated in Figure 11-2. In this illustration, the test

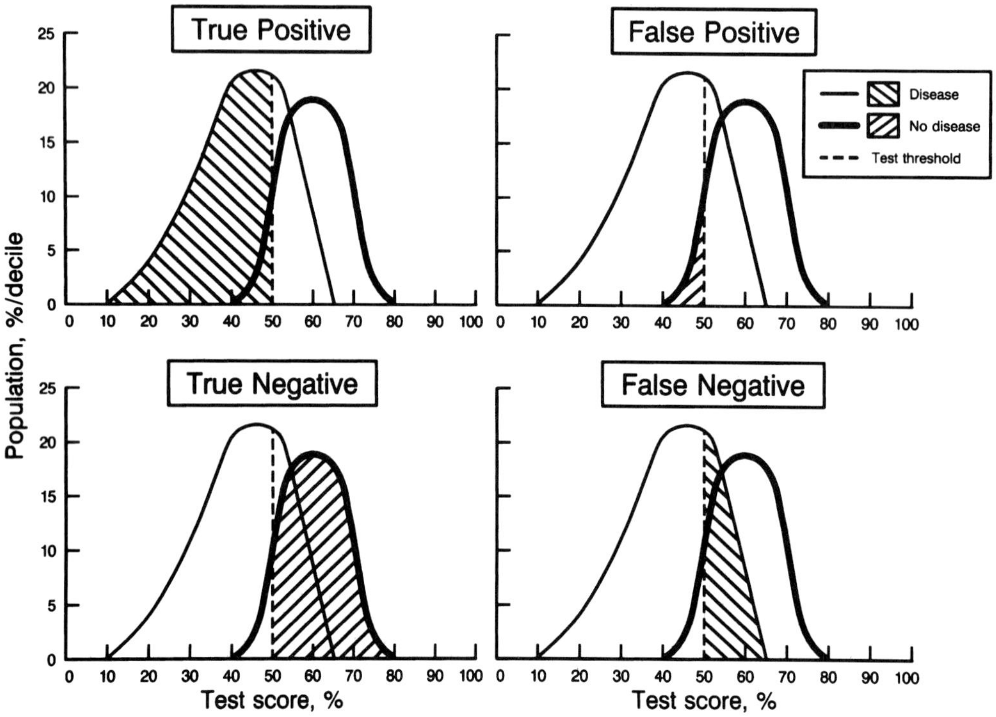

Fig 11-2 Distribution of test scores relative to test threshold among patient subgroups with and without disease. The data in each subgroup are plotted as percentage of total population for each decile of test scores. The dashed vertical line at test score 50% is the normal threshold; scores at levels below 50% are designated abnormal.

scores are distributed in a theoretic range from 0% to 100%. The test threshold for normality is set at 50%, and abnormal test scores are those below 50%. The distribution of the subpopulations with and without disease is plotted as percent of the total index population per decile of test score. The sum of the areas under the curves of distribution of test scores for the subpopulations with and without disease is equivalent to 100%. The illustration is divided into four panels to highlight (shaded areas) the subpopulations encompassed by each of the test characteristics. It is apparent that the overlapping of populations with and without disease relative to the test threshold determines the four test characteristics. *True positive* defines the subpopulation with disease and test scores in the abnormal range. *True negative* defines the subpopulation without disease and test scores in the normal range. *False positive* defines the subpopulation without disease and test scores in the abnormal range. *False negative* defines the subpopulation with disease and test scores in the normal range. The subareas, in percent of total index population for each test characteristic, correspond to the percent distribution of the test characteristics in the probability spectrum displayed in Figure 11-1.

USE OF TESTS IN CLINICAL PREDICTION

The mathematical basis for the use of test performance indices in predicting the presence or absence of disease in individuals is founded on a basic tenet of probability, enunciated by Richard Price in his introductory comments to the essay by Thomas Bayes:[2] "Common sense is indeed sufficient to show us that from the observation of what has in former instances been the consequence of a certain cause or action, one may make a judgement what is likely to be the consequence of it another time, and that the larger the number of experiments we have to support a conclusion, so much the more reason we have to take it for granted." Thus, having validated test performance indices on an index population, it is simple logic that the same test performance should be repeatable in future studies on populations of the same composition.

In contemporary clinical practice, this probability principle has been extended to the proposition that once the Se and Sp of a test have been established for one or more index populations of known disease prevalence, the Se and Sp may be extended to the estimation of the post-test probability of that disease for a population of any pretest prevalence. In a further extension of the probability theory in current practice, the Se and Sp derived from an index study are used in predicting the post-test probability of disease for an individual in whom the pretest probability is derived on the basis of the disease prevalence in populations with clinical characteristics similar to those of that individual. When such an assumed pretest prevalence is interpreted as the probability of disease for an individual, it is termed the *pretest probability of disease (PPD)* for that individual. The 100% complement of the assumed PPD is the *pretest probability of normality or no disease (PPN)* for that individual.

The overall principle on which the post-test prediction for the presence or absence of disease in an individual is made on the basis of a preestablished Se and Sp and an assumed PPD is referred to as *conditional probability*. The post-test predictions are formulated on two commonly calculated post-test predictive indices, the *post-test probability of disease for a positive test result [(+)PTPD]*, defined as the probability of disease in an individual with a positive test result based on conditional probability estimation, and the *post-test probability of disease for a negative test result [(−)PTPD]*, defined as the probability of disease in an individual with a negative test result based on conditional probability estimation. (The terms *pretest likelihood* and *post-test likelihood* are often used interchangeably with pretest and post-test probability.) In the following paragraphs, the rationale and method for the calculation of (+)PTPD and (−)PTPD are outlined, and a discussion of the value and limitations of such predictive determinations follows.

Calculation of post-test probability of disease: the Bayesian equations

Equations 11-7, 11-8, and 11-9 in Figure 11-3, which are used in calculating (+)PTPD and (−)PTPD for an individual, are referred to as the Bayesian equations for conditional probability testing. The Bayesian equations are based on the same principles underlying the equations cited previously for the calculation of the $(+)PA_c$ (see Equation 11-3) and the 100% complement of the $(-)PA_c$ (see Equations 11-5 and 11-6). The Bayesian equations provide a mathematical model for calculating the (+)PTPD and (−)PTPD, in which the predicted post-test characteristics (*TP, FN, TN, FP*)*are expressed in terms of (1) the Se and Sp for an index test and (2) the level of PPD and PPN assumed from clinical evaluation as follows:

$$TP = \text{Se} \times \text{PPD} \quad \textbf{[11-10]}$$

$$FN = (1 - \text{Se}) \times \text{PPD} \quad \textbf{[11-11]}$$

$$TN = \text{Sp} \times \text{PPN} \quad \textbf{[11-12]}$$

$$FP = (1 - \text{Sp}) \times \text{PPN} \quad \textbf{[11-13]}$$

The relationships of the Bayesian equations expressed in terms of Se, Sp, PPD, and PPN to the same equations expressed in terms of the predicted post-test characteristics are illustrated in Figure 11-4. The (+)PTPD and (−)PTPD in these equations are expressed in percent.

A key factor in the calculation of Bayesian post-test estimates of disease probability is the determination of the PPD and its 100% complement, the PPN. In clinical practice, the pretest probability estimate is derived from prevalence studies on large populations of patients classified according to clinical characteristics wherein disease is documented by established standards. Figure 11-5 is a useful graphic representation of the probability of coronary artery disease relative to risk factors, age, sex, and the clinical character of chest discomfort that is applicable to individual prediction. It is modified slightly from the original illustration by Patterson and Horowitz[4]

*Italicized to emphasize predicted post-test characteristics.

THE BAYESIAN EQUATIONS

$$(+)\,PTPD = \frac{Se \times PPD}{Se \times PPD + (1\text{-}Sp) \times PPN} \times 100 \quad [11\text{-}7]$$

$$(-)\,PTPD = 100 - \left[\frac{Sp \times PPN}{Sp \times PPN + (1\text{-}Se) \times PPD} \times 100\right] \quad [11\text{-}8]$$

$$(-)\,PTPD = \frac{(1\text{-}Se) \times PPD}{Sp \times PPN + (1\text{-}Se) \times PPD} \times 100 \quad [11\text{-}9]$$

Fig 11-3 The Bayesian equations for calculation of post-test probability of disease for a positive test result [(+)PTPD] and for a negative test result [(−)PTPD]. The bracketed section of 11-8 is the equation for the post-test probability of no disease for a negative test, (−)PTPN. The (−)PTPD is hence the 100% complement of the (−)PTPN. Equation 11-9 is a simplification of 11-8. *PPD,* pretest probability of disease; *PPN,* pretest probability of normality (no disease); *Se,* sensitivity; *Sp,* specificity.

Post-test probability	Bayesian equation	Post-test characteristics
(+) PTPD	$\frac{Se \times PPD}{Se \times PPD + (1\text{-}Sp) \times PPN} \times 100$	$\frac{TP}{TP + FP} \times 100$
(−) PTPD	$100 - \left[\frac{Sp \times PPN}{Sp \times PPN + (1\text{-}Se) \times PPD} \times 100\right]$	$100 - \left[\frac{TN}{TN + FN} \times 100\right]$
(−) PTPD	$\frac{(1\text{-}Se) \times PPD}{Sp \times PPN + (1\text{-}Se) \times PPD} \times 100$	$\frac{FN}{TN + FN} \times 100$

Fig 11-4 Relationship of Bayesian equations to predicted post-test characteristics. *FN,* false negative; *FP,* false positive; *TN,* true negative; *TP,* true positive. Other abbreviations are explained in Figure 11-3 legend.

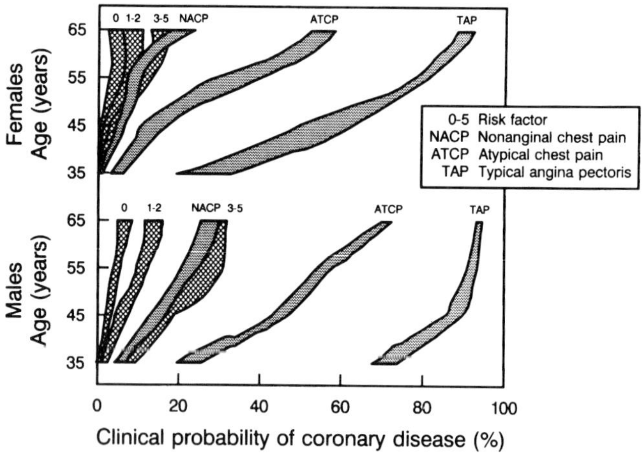

Fig 11-5 Use of clinical data to estimate the probability of coronary artery disease. Clinical data include sex (women, *upper panel,* men, *lower panel*), age (vertical axis), number of risk factors for persons without symptoms (none to five [0, 1-2, 3-5] of the following: diabetes, hyperlipidemia, hypertension, smoking, and at rest electrocardiographic abnormality of ST-T waves). Symptoms are defined as nonanginal chest pain, atypical chest pain, and typical angina pectoris. The probability of coronary artery disease increases from left to right, and the 95% confidence intervals are shown as the widths of the bars. (From Patterson RE, Horowitz SF. Importance of epidemiology and biostatistics in deciding clinical strategies for using diagnostic tests: a simplified approach using examples from coronary artery disease. *J Am Coll Cardiol* 13:1653-1665, 1989. By permission of the American College of Cardiology.)

and is based on data from the landmark Framingham study of 1968[5] and the extensive prevalence base compiled by Diamond and Forrester[6] and Diamond et al.[7]

Value of post-test probability calculations

A common format for illustrating the application of the principle of conditional probability is that shown in Figure 11-6,A, in which the calculated (+)PTPD and (−)PTPD for levels of assumed PPD from 0% to 100% are plotted for three tests: (1) a test of relatively high Se and Sp (0.90), (2) a test of relatively low Se and Sp (0.70), and (3) a test of Se 0.50 and Sp 0.50. For the third test, the post-test probability of disease equals the pretest probability.

Figure 11-6,B is an alternative plot of the absolute increment and decrement in post-test probability of disease relative to the assumed PPD after a positive result and a negative result. In this format, the influence of the level of Se and Sp on post-test probability throughout the range of PPD is more readily apparent. This illustration highlights several important probabilistic implications when conditional probability testing is applied.

1. Relative to the PPD, the increment in the (+)PTPD and the decrement in the (−)PTPD depends on the level of PPD and follows a curvilinear pattern. For tests of Se and Sp greater than 0.50, the maximal increment in (+)PTPD occurs in the estimated PPD range of 10% to 50%, whereas the maximal decrement in (−)PTPD occurs in the estimated PPD range of 50% to 90%.
2. The magnitude of the increment in (+)PTPD and the decrement in (−)PTPD increases directly with Se and Sp.
3. In the highest range of PPD (≥90%), a positive test result provides little increment in (+)PTPD and a negative test result yields a modest decrement in (−)PTPD. In the lowest range of PPD (≤10%), a negative test result provides little decrement in (−)PTPD and a positive test result yields a modest increment in (+)PTPD.

These relationships among (+)PTPD, (−)PTPD, and PPD have several important clinical implications when the Bayesian equations are used in calculating post-test probability on the basis of individualized estimates of pretest probability.

1. Clinical tests of high sensitivity and specificity (≥0.90) offer the most significant augmentation of

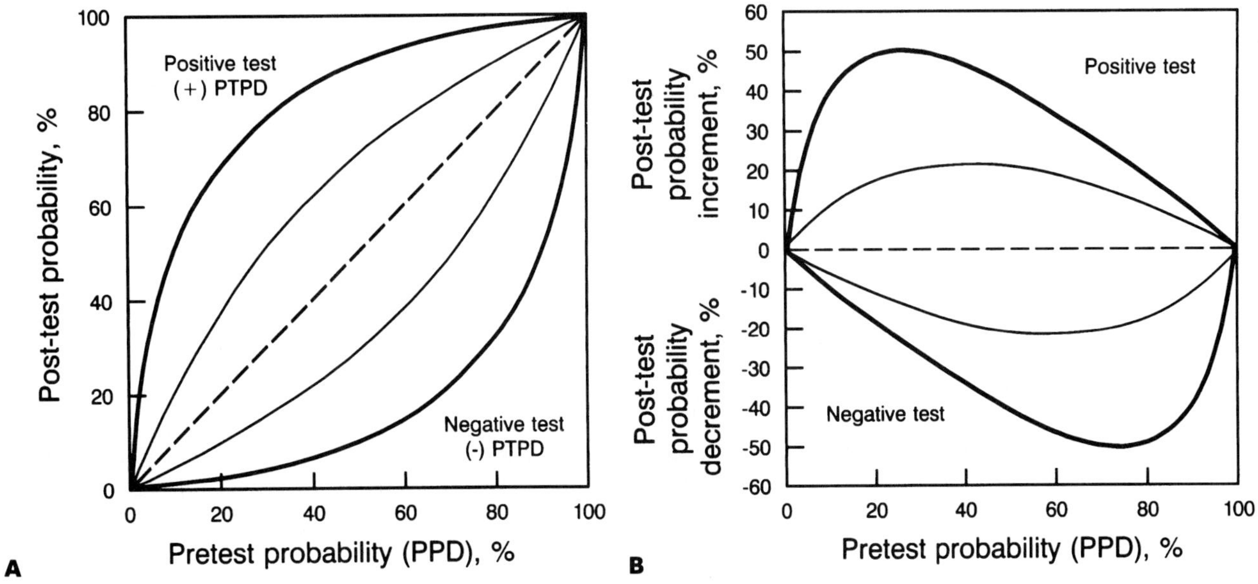

Fig 11-6 **A,** relationship of post-test probability of disease for a positive test result [(+)PTPD] and for a negative test result [(−)(PTPD] to pretest probability of disease (PPD) for tests of sensitivity and specificity of 0.50 (dashed line), 0.70 (thin solid line), and 0.90 (thick solid line). **B,** relationship of the increment in post-test probability of disease for a positive result and the decrement in post-test probability of disease for a negative result to the pretest probability of disease (PPD) for tests of sensitivity and specificity of 0.50 (dashed line), 0.70 (thin solid line), and 0.90 (thick solid line).

the pretest estimates of disease probability when the PPD is in the uncertain range, that is, PPD >10% to <90%.

In a 65-year-old man with nonanginal chest discomfort and an estimated PPD for coronary disease of 27% (see Fig 11-5), a positive test of Se and Sp 0.90 revises the estimated probability of coronary disease significantly upward to a (+)PTPD of 77%. A negative test revises the estimated probability of coronary disease significantly downward to a (−)PTPD of 4%.

In a 60-year-old woman with atypical chest discomfort and an estimated PPD for coronary disease of 48% (see Fig 11-5), a positive test of Se and Sp 0.90 revises the estimate of coronary disease significantly upward to a (+)PTPD of 89%; a negative test of the same Se and Sp revises the estimate of probability of disease significantly downward to a (−)PTPD of 9%.

2. In patients with very high or very low PPD (≥90% and ≤10%), even tests of high Se and Sp are of little value in augmenting the clinical estimate.

In a 55-year-old man with typical angina pectoris and an estimated PPD of 94%, the upward revision in prediction of coronary disease by a positive test of Se 0.81 and Sp 0.89 (e.g., thallium scintigraphy) is to a (+)PTPD of 99%, a relatively minor increment from the high pretest probability of disease. For an unexpected negative test, the downward revision in probability of coronary disease is a modest decrement, from 94% to 77%.

In a 45-year-old woman with nonanginal chest discomfort and an estimated probability of coronary disease of 6%, the downward revision in probability of coronary disease after a negative test of Se 0.81 and Sp 0.89 is to a (−)PTPD of 1.3%, a clinically minor change from the very low pretest estimate. For an unexpected positive test, the upward revision in probability of coronary artery disease is a modest increment in the pretest estimate, from 6% to 32%.

3. Single tests of a relatively low order of sensitivity and specificity (i.e, Se and Sp ≤ 0.75) have little value in augmenting probability estimates of disease and may obfuscate clinical decision-making.

In a 40-year-old man with nonanginal chest pain and an estimated PPD for coronary disease of 12%, a positive test of Se and Sp 0.70 yields a (+)PTPD of 24%. The probability that the positive test result is a false positive is 76% [100% complement of (+)PTPD].

In a 45-year-old woman with nonanginal chest pain and an estimated PPD for coronary disease of 4%, a positive test of Se and Sp 0.70 yields a (+)PTPD of 9%. The probability that the positive test is a false positive is 91% [100% complement of (+)PTPD].

4. In populations of patients with extremely low disease prevalence (≤5%), even the most powerful cardiovascular tests (Se and Sp ≥ 0.95) have little power in detecting disease. Results of screening tests among individuals in these low prevalence ranges are commonly misleading.

In a 40-year-old man without symptoms who had an estimated pretest probability of coronary disease of 5% on the basis of risk factors, a positive cardiac screening test of highest putative potency (Se 0.95 and Sp 0.95) yields a (+)PTPD of 50%. The probability that a positive test is a false positive is 50% [100% complement of (+)PTPD].

In a 50-year-old woman with an estimated pretest coronary disease probability of 4%, the same test has a (+)PTPD of

44%. The probability that the positive test is a false positive is 56% [100% complement of (+)PTPD].

The value of multiple tests

Among the most clinically opportune applications of conditional probability is its use in predicting the post-test results for sequential or combined determinations. This approach is of special advantage when the estimated pretest probability of disease leaves considerable uncertainty about the presence of disease. In light of the graphic illustration of the relationship of pretest probability to post-test probability of disease presented in Figure 11-6,A, one can estimate the sequential changes in post-test probability of disease by entering the calculated post-test probability estimate from the first test as the pretest probability for a sequential test. With concordant sequential positive or negative test results (+ + or − −), there is augmentation of the probability estimate for the presence or absence of disease. With mixed sequential test results (+ − or − +), augmentation is minimized or indeterminate, and the probability estimate of disease commonly remains indecisive.

The calculated sequential estimates in post-test probability of coronary artery disease after two tests for a patient with a PPD of 30% are illustrated in Figure 11-7. The final PTPD estimates that follow test 1 (exercise electrocardiography [ECG], Se 0.53, Sp 0.83) and test 2 (thallium scintigraphy, Se 0.81, Sp 0.89) are derived by entering as pretest probability (1) the assumed PPD before test 1 and (2) the calculated (+)PTPD and (−)PTPD after test 1 (labeled PTPD-1) as the assumed PPD for test 2. The calculated estimates of probability of disease for the four possible test combinations following the sequential tests (labeled PTPD-2) are illustrated. The calculated predicted fraction of the population responding positively and negatively in each of the tests is shown in the parentheses. (The method for calculation of the population subfractions is described in Appendix 1.) The fraction of the whole population for each test combination after the sequential tests is calculated as the product of the population subfractions in the sequential positive and negative test arms of the test protocol.

As shown in the illustration, the post-test probability of disease for sequential positive tests (+ +) is 91% and for sequential negative tests (− −) 5%. In this illustration, the sequentially concordant tests yield significant revision in the initial PPD for 68% of all individuals tested (sum of subfractions of 0.14 and 0.54 for concordant tests, expressed in percent of total population). The sequentially discordant tests yield a modest revision in estimated probability of disease from the initial PPD to 22% for (+ −) and 65% for (− +). Thus, for discordant tests, a limited and indecisive revision in estimated probability occurs in 32% of the population (sum of discordant subfractions of 0.14 and 0.18, expressed in percent of total population).

In applying conditional probability to multiple tests, it is necessary to adhere to the principle of functional independence of sequential tests. Thus, the consecutive tests must be based on independent predictive functions. If one were to apply the same test repeatedly in calculating conditional probability sequences, an obviously erroneous multiplying effect on the determination of (+)PTPD and (−)PTPD would result. In a similar manner, the application of sequential tests that measure the same or overlapping disease characteristics, for example, cardiac contractile function, would produce a cascading error in the estimate of (+)PTPD or (−)PTPD.

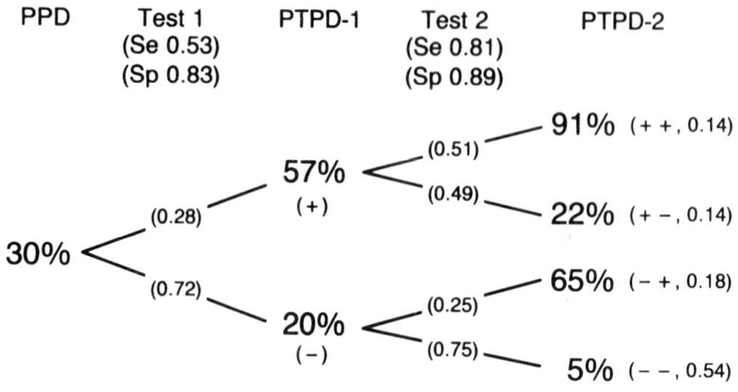

Fig 11-7 Conditional probability testing with a sequential two-test protocol in a population of patients with 30% pretest probability of disease (PPD). The sequential tests have sensitivity (Se) and specificity (Sp) as shown. PTPD-1 is the post-test probability for positive (+) and negative (−) test results after test 1; PTPD-2 is the post-test probability for (+ +), (+ −), (− +), and (− −) test results after sequential testing. Parenthetical numbers interrupting lines are subpopulation fractions for positive or negative results; numbers in parentheses under PTPD-2 represent the respective fraction of the total population for each combined result. See text for additional details.

Odds ratio form of the Bayesian equations

The probability of disease is often expressed in the familiar terminology of the odds ratio, which is conveniently calculated as the quotient of probability divided by its complement as follows:

$$\text{Odds} = \frac{\text{Probability}}{100 - \text{Probability}} \qquad \textbf{[11-14]}$$

in which probability is in percent (in the range 0 to 100) and odds may be expressed as a fraction or relative to unity.

Thus, in a population of disease prevalence of 60%, the pretest odds ratio of disease (POD) is 60:40. The pretest odds ratio for disease expressed relative to unity in this population is 1.5:1. In this same population, the prevalence of normality (no disease) is 40%. The pretest odds ratio for no disease (PON) in this population is 40:60. The pretest odds ratio for no disease expressed relative to unity is 0.67:1. As is evident, the odds ratio for disease is the inverse of the odds ratio for no disease and vice versa.

The same principle for odds calculation from probability data is applicable to converting post-test probability data to post-test odds. When (+)PTPD is 75%, the post-test odds ratio for disease after a positive test result [(+)PTOD] is 75:25, or 3:1; when the (−)PTPD is 5%, the post-test odds ratio for disease after a negative test result [(−)PTOD] is 5:95, or 0.053:1.

The odds ratio form of the Bayesian equations allows calculation of the post-test odds of disease for positive and negative test results from the estimated pretest odds of disease and the Se and Sp of a test. For positive and negative test results of established Se and Sp and an estimated POD, the equations are as follows:

$$(+)\text{PTOD} = \frac{\text{Se}}{1 - \text{Sp}} \times \text{POD} \qquad [11\text{-}15]$$

$$(-)\text{PTOD} = \frac{1 - \text{Se}}{\text{Sp}} \times \text{POD} \qquad [11\text{-}16]$$

in which (+)PTOD is the post-test odds of disease for a positive test result and (−)PTOD is the post-test odds of disease for a negative test result. As will be discussed in the section on test comparison, the quotient Se/1 − Sp is the likelihood ratio for a positive test result, and 1 − Se/Sp is the inverse of the likelihood ratio for a negative result. In this context, Equations 11-15 and 11-16 may be referred to as the odds-likelihood form of the Bayesian equations.

It is often desirable to convert expressions of odds to probability. This can be readily accomplished through use of the following general equation:

$$\frac{\text{Odds}}{1 + \text{Odds}} \times 100 = \text{Probability (\%)} \qquad [11\text{-}17]$$

Conversion of odds to probability by Equation 11-17 is most directly accomplished by expressing the odds relative to unity. Thus, when (+)PTOD is 3:1, the (+)PTPD is 75%; when (−)PTOD is 0.05:1, the (−)PTPD is 4.8%.

The application of these concepts in deriving post-test probability of coronary disease after exercise stress testing is discussed in chapter 3B.

Limitations in conditional probability assumptions

Clinical application of conditional probability estimates depends on the validity of four assumptions: (1) that test performance standards can be reproduced equivalently in all laboratories, (2) that the Se and Sp of a test remain constant through all ranges of PPD, (3) that PPD can be accurately estimated from clinical characteristics, and (4) that the prediction of (+)PTPD and (−)PTPD derived from representative populations is applicable to an individual. Let us examine these assumptions on the basis of the formulations relevant to the prediction of post-test probability of disease discussed previously.

The *assumption of equivalence in test performance standards* implies that all tests meet the same standards for quality of instrumentation, procedural technique, test threshold, and subjective interpretation of test results. To date, such standardization of test performance among cardiovascular laboratories has not been achieved for any of the cardiovascular diagnostic tests currently in vogue.

The theoretical variation in Se and Sp that may result from variation in one standard of test performance, the

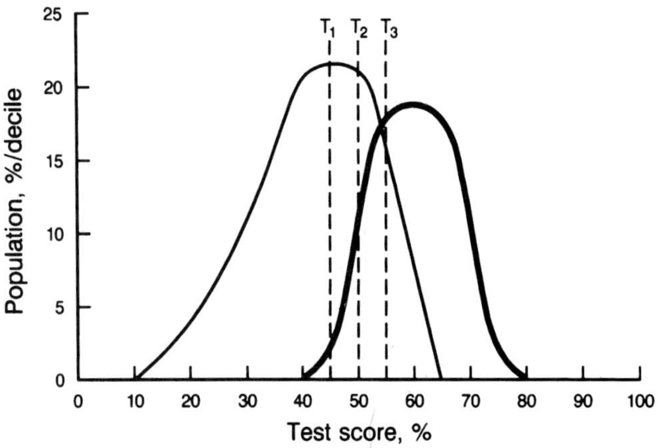

	PD, %	Se	Sp
T_1	60	0.48	0.97
T_2	60	0.65	0.83
T_3	60	0.81	0.60

Fig 11-8 Effect of variation in test threshold on the distribution of test scores and on the sensitivity (Se) and specificity (Sp) of an index test in a population of constant prevalence. The calculated Se and Sp for each test threshold is shown. Solid lines represent patients with disease (thin lines) and patients without disease (thick lines). PD, prevalence of disease; T_1, T_2, T_3, test thresholds. See text for additional details.

test threshold, is illustrated graphically in Figure 11-8. The area under the thin line is the PD for the index population; the area under the thick line is the PN. The calculated variation in Se and Sp induced by changes in test threshold is illustrated. As is evident, variations in test threshold (from T_1 to T_3) at constant disease prevalence and test score distribution can result in a major difference in the apportionment of test characteristics and hence in the estimated Se and Sp for the test.

Similar variation in test Se and Sp is to be expected for variation in other test standards. Most cogent in this regard are variations in the standard definition for the extent of coronary artery occlusive disease.[8-11] An emerging factor that will have a key influence in the future evaluation of test Se and Sp in coronary disease is the variation in the definition of myocardial ischemia that occurs when a physiologic rather than an anatomic end point is selected.[12,13] Such variation in test standards can account for significant differences in Se and Sp between laboratories and between what is reported in the literature and what is applied in clinical practice.

The *assumption that the Se and Sp for a given test remain constant* for all ranges of disease prevalence is the most challengeable of the assumptions in applying conditional probability among patients with cardiovascular disease. It implies that the Se and Sp estimate has been previously established from a complete and unbiased selection of patients with the disease in question. On theoretical grounds, one could establish such an unbiased estimate of Se and Sp, provided that the index population were large, randomly selected, and representative of the breadth of variation that exists among all individuals who have the disease. In practice, however, index cardiovascular tests from which the Se and Sp are derived are not performed on large populations selected in a random fashion. The tests are in fact biased by preselection of populations of patients who are referred to a cardiovascular center. Such populations do not encompass the full range of disease encountered in clinical practice. Under such circumstances, the postulate that an Se and Sp determined in a population of referred patients can provide an unbiased estimate applicable to all populations is difficult, if not impossible, to accept. On this basis alone, the assumption that the Se and Sp determined on a sample of patients referred to any one laboratory can be applied to all tested populations must remain tenuous.

The assumption of constancy in test Se and Sp can be challenged in a practical sense by the marked variation evident in the reported Se and Sp for such widely used cardiovascular tests as exercise ECG, radionuclide angiography, and thallium perfusion scintigraphy[14-17] (see chapter 6). Several studies have documented that differences in clinical characteristics are a major source for such reported variation in Se and Sp.[15,18,19] Reduction in the Sp of radionuclide ventriculography over time has been documented when patients with increasing severity of disease or increasing frequency of prereferral positivity are referred to the same center during a period when test performance standards have remained constant.[20] Variation in selection of normal referent populations has been shown to be a potentially major determinant of variation in the Sp of the radionuclide ventriculogram.[21] Such variation in Se and Sp determined by the characteristics of the population referred for testing has been termed *referral bias*.

Among the assumptions related to clinical use of Bayesian conditional probability strategy, the *assumption of pretest probability of disease* on the basis of clinical indicators appears to have the greatest validity, particularly for the diagnosis of coronary artery disease. Diamond and Forrester[6] and Diamond et al.[7] published tables of pretest prevalence of coronary artery disease in men and women with symptoms (typical angina, atypical angina, nonanginal chest pain) and without symptoms for age deciles from 30 to 69 years. These data were established on the basis of a literature review of studies of 4,952 patients with symptoms in whom coronary arterial disease was verified by coronary arteriography and of studies reporting autopsy verification of atherosclerotic coronary disease among 23,996 persons who did not have symptoms of cardiac disease. A graphic representation of the prevalence of coronary artery disease by age, sex, clinical presentation, and risk factors compiled by Patterson and Horowitz[4] (see Fig 11-5) is applicable to pretest probability estimates of coronary disease. Tables of coronary artery disease prevalence by age and sex in patients without symptoms and among those with stable chest pain syndromes without a history of myocardial infarction are presented in chapter 3B.

The *assumption that estimates of (+)PTPD and (−)PTPD can be applied to individuals* is open to reservations similar to those expressed above for the assumption of constancy in Se and Sp for all prevalence groups. When one considers the compounded variance for estimates of the multiple variables entered into the predictive equation, including the pretest prevalence and the Se and Sp of the predictive test, the potential range of variation for individualized post-test probability can be exceedingly wide (see section on confidence limits and Appendix 3).

Additional limitations in conditional probability prediction

Additional factors responsible for variability in Se and Sp among laboratories include any study design variations or workup biases that preclude independence between the determination of test results and the definition of disease. The role of such factors has been discussed critically by Detrano et al.[15] and Ransohoff and Feinstein.[22] Another significant factor that influences the Se and Sp of an index test is the sample size. Because of the potential variation in clinical expression, severity, and test performance among individuals with disease and the variations that occur in nondiseased populations, only studies encompassing numbers large enough to represent the entire spectrum of disease and normality should be accepted in formulating estimates of test Se and Sp. Most studies purporting to evaluate the Se and Sp of current cardiovascular tests have in fact compiled data on groups of fewer than 100 patients with or without disease.[15-17] On this basis alone, our current estimates of Se and Sp for common cardiovascular tests must be applied conservatively and with due caution for their potential error.

Current status of clinical prediction in cardiovascular disease

The use of quantitative prediction in clinical practice must take into account the major limitations posed by the assumptions underlying conditional probability estimates. Although the use of sequential testing generally enhances the accuracy of prediction, the breadth of the confidence range for such compounded predictive estimates remains wide. As our tests are perfected and our estimates of Se and Sp advance to consistently high levels for all prevalence groups, ideally approaching a level of 0.95, post-test prediction in cardiology will gain enormous value. For the present, predictions of diagnosis and outcome based on interpretation of cardiovascular tests must remain an artful exercise and must be insinuated wisely into the panorama of clinical observations that lead to clinical decisions.

COMPARING TESTS

The single-threshold test

It is common practice in cardiovascular medicine to express test results as positive or negative relative to a single test threshold. Comparisons of Se and Sp for tests applied to such dichotomous distributions provide a basis for comparison of their relative accuracy in discriminating the presence or absence of disease. In attempting such comparisons of single-threshold tests, one must recognize that the Se and Sp are both test- and population-dependent. For valid comparison of two single-threshold tests performed on different populations, the studied populations must be virtually identical in distribution of severity of disease and in the characteristics of the population without disease. The "gold standard" for judging disease must of course be the same for the two tests. On theoretical grounds, comparisons of Se and Sp for single-threshold tests can be made if these variables are strictly controlled. In practice, such population control is rarely attainable. On this basis, the most accurate approach to comparing the quality of contrasting single-threshold tests is to submit them in parallel to all subjects of a single population. For such comparisons, when one test yields significantly higher levels of Se or Sp in the same population, the observed differences can be accepted as valid for that population. Comparisons of such single-threshold stress tests as the exercise ECG, radionuclide angiography, and thallium-201 myocardial perfusion scan are well illustrated in the section of this chapter on the likelihood ratio and in chapter 6.

Multiple-threshold tests: the receiver operating characteristic curve

An alternative practice for comparing tests is made available when test results are expressed in a continuous range of values. Such continuous data form the basis for a unique analytic method referred to as the receiver operating characteristic (ROC) curve. Given a series of continuous test results, one can plot the covariance in Se and Sp for test thresholds ranging from highest to lowest. The ROC curve so derived provides two useful measures of test performance for that population: (1) an estimate of the intrinsic quality of the test throughout its range of thresholds, expressed in the shape of the ROC curve, and (2) an estimate of the optimal test threshold. Further, the ROC curve provides a powerful tool for comparing continuous test results for two or more tests performed on the same population.

To understand the use of the ROC curve as a basis for evaluating test quality, one should consider the distribution of test scores for populations of individuals with and without disease for a perfect test, an indiscriminate test, and an imperfect test (Fig 11-9). The *perfect test* is one in which at least one test threshold completely separates the continuous range of scores without overlap between individuals with disease and those without disease, as illustrated in the lower left panel of Figure 11-9. For such a threshold, there are no false-negative or false-positive results. The distribution of test scores in the subpopulations may be symmetrical (as shown) or asymmetrical. A graphic plot of Se versus Sp for a full range of potential test thresholds for a perfect test is shown in the upper left panel of Figure 11-9. In this illustration, a threshold of 50% yields complete separation of the subpopulation with disease (below threshold 50%) from that with no disease (above threshold 50%). The graphic plot of Se versus Sp for increasing thresholds in the range of test scores from

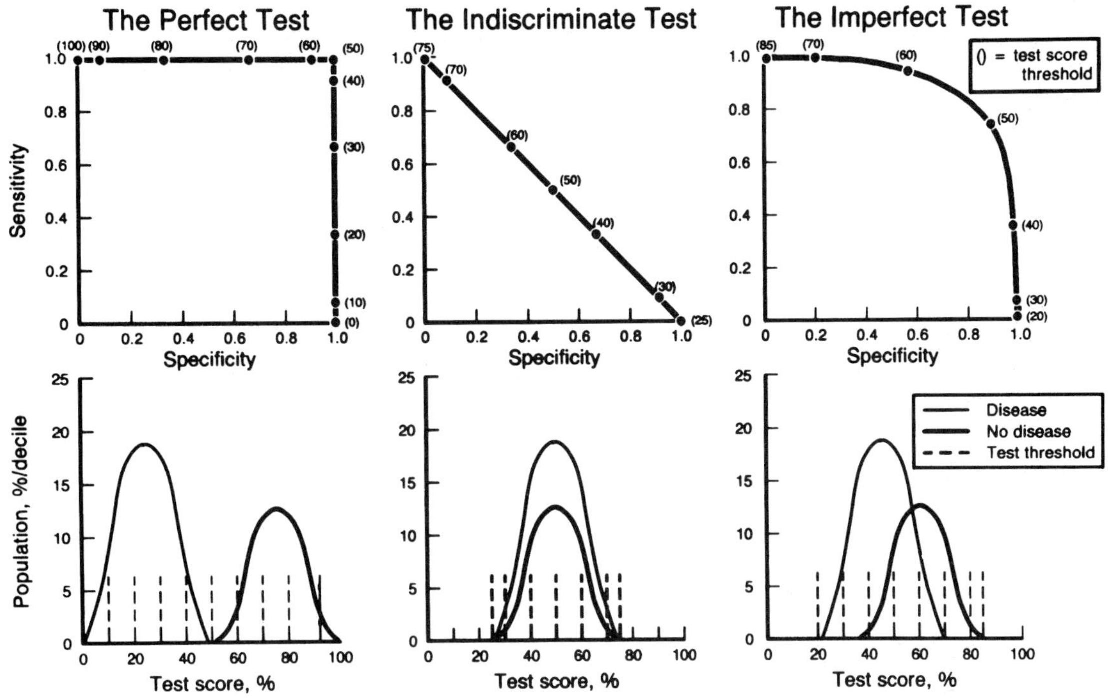

Fig 11-9 The derivation of receiver operating characteristic curves for a perfect test *(left panels),* an indiscriminate test *(middle panels),* and an imperfect test *(right panels).* The sensitivity levels are plotted against the specificity levels at various test thresholds (in parentheses) for a theoretical range of test scores from 0% to 100%. See text for additional details.

0% to 50% is a vertical line at Sp 1.0. The plot of Se versus Sp for increasing thresholds in the range of test scores from 50% to 100% is a horizontal line at Se 1.0. The two lines intersect at Se 1.0, Sp 1.0. Thus, the ROC curve of Se versus Sp for a perfect test is a square wave plot with the apex at the point Se 1.0, Sp 1.0. The more closely an ROC curve derived from any series of continuous data thresholds approximates this square wave relationship, the more closely the test approaches perfection.

The *indiscriminate test* is one in which there is perfect symmetry of overlap in test results, as illustrated in the lower middle panel of Figure 11-9. As test thresholds increase from test scores of 0% to 100%, the Se and Sp remain in a complementary relationship for all thresholds. The curve of Se versus Sp follows a straight line plot connecting coordinates Se 1.0, Sp 0.0 with Se 0.0, Sp 1.0. The more closely an ROC curve approximates this straight line diagonal plot, the closer the test approaches nondiscrimination.

The *imperfect test*, illustrated in the lower right panel, is one with partially overlapping distributions. The subpopulations with and without disease may be symmetrically or asymmetrically distributed with respect to the test scores. The ROC curve lies below the square wave plot of the perfect test. It may lie above or below the diagonal plot of the indiscriminate test. For thresholds in which the ROC curve is above the diagonal line, the test yields incremental post-test probability relative to the pretest probability. For thresholds that are below the diagonal line, the test yields decremental post-test probability relative to the pretest probability. Clinical cardiologic tests in contemporary practice are universally of the imperfect classification.

Figure 11-10 illustrates ROC curves constructed for two tests performed on the same population. These ROC curves depict the shapes of two imperfect tests in which the graphic plot lies between curves of the perfect test and the indiscriminate test. The numbers in parentheses are the various thresholds selected for calculation of Se and Sp. The ROC curve for test 1 bows toward the right; the maximal combined Se and Sp is in the range of test threshold of 50% to 55%. The curve for test 2 bows only gently and approximates the diagonal line of the indiscriminate test. There is no distinct optimal Se and Sp. The ROC curve for test 1 is shifted rightward with respect to the curve for test 2. On the basis of the ROC curves, test 1 has more discriminating quality than test 2.

The shape of the ROC curve hence serves as an independent expression of the quality of a test throughout the continuous range of test results. In depicting levels of Se and Sp throughout the threshold range, the ROC curve allows identification of test thresholds yielding maximal combined Se and Sp, that is, the point or area on the curve that most closely approximates Se 1.0, Sp 1.0. A comparison of the curves for two or more tests allows selection of the test with higher discriminating quality.

The principles underlying test analysis by the ROC curve can be applied to a variety of additional graphic plots, including Se versus (1 − Sp), Sp versus (1 − Se), and (1 − Se) versus (1 − Sp).

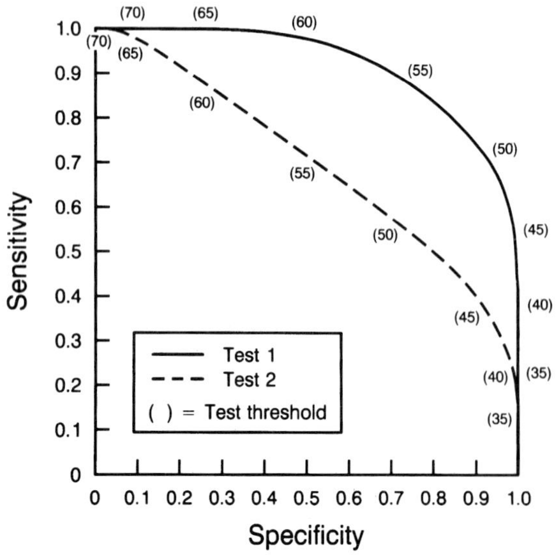

Fig 11-10 Receiver operating characteristic curves for two imperfect tests in the same population. The test of higher discriminating power (Test 1) approaches the configuration of a perfect test; the test of low discriminating power (Test 2) approaches the configuration of an indiscriminate test.

The likelihood ratio

Among the mathematical instruments for comparison of the quality of cardiovascular tests, the likelihood ratio determination is among the most easily derived and useful expressions. Like the ROC curve, the likelihood ratios encompass the Se and Sp measures and can be applied in test comparisons for single- or multiple-threshold tests.

In clinical applications, it is convenient to differentiate the likelihood ratios for positive and negative test results, known as the *positive likelihood ratio* [(+)LR] and the *negative likelihood ratio* [(−)LR]. The positive and negative likelihood ratios are calculated from the Se and Sp of a test as follows:

$$(+)\text{LR} = \frac{\text{Se}}{1 - \text{Sp}} \qquad \textbf{[11-18]}$$

$$(-)\text{LR} = \frac{\text{Sp}}{1 - \text{Se}} \qquad \textbf{[11-19]}$$

The value of the (+)LR and (−)LR as measures of relative test quality becomes evident in a consideration of the odds ratio form of the Bayesian equations (Equations 11-15 and 11-16). If Equation 11-16 is transformed into its inverse form, that is, solving for (−)PTON in terms of (−)LR and PON, these equations can be written as follows:

$$(+)\text{PTOD} = (+)\text{LR} \times \text{POD} \qquad \textbf{[11-15A]}$$

and

$$(-)\text{PTON} = (-)\text{LR} \times \text{PON} \qquad \textbf{[11-16A]}$$

in which (+)PTOD is post-test odds of disease for a positive test result, POD is pretest odds of disease,

(−)PTON is post-test odds of no disease for a negative test result, and PON is pretest odds of no disease. Solving for (+)LR and (−)LR, Equations 11-15A and 11-16A take the following form:

$$(+)\text{LR} = \frac{(+)\text{PTOD}}{\text{POD}} \quad \textbf{[11-15B]}$$

and

$$(-)\text{LR} = \frac{(-)\text{PTON}}{\text{PON}} \quad \textbf{[11-16B]}$$

In this form, it is evident that (+)LR is the ratio of post-test odds of disease for a positive test result to the pretest odds of disease and that (−)LR is the ratio of post-test odds of no disease for a negative test result to the pretest odds of no disease. The likelihood ratios are hence direct measures of the potential predictive power of positive and negative tests expressed as odds ratios.

In a clinical idiom, the likelihood ratio can be considered a measure of the rule-in or rule-out power of a test result. The higher the (+)LR of a test, the greater the post-test odds of disease relative to the pretest estimate of disease and, hence, the higher the rule-in power of a positive test result. The higher the (−)LR of a test, the greater the post-test odds of no disease relative to the pretest estimate of no disease and, hence, the higher the rule-out power for a negative test result.

Figure 11-11,A depicts the influence of the (+)LR on the relationship of post-test probability of disease to the pretest probability of disease for a positive test result. Figure 11-11,B depicts the influence of the (−)LR on the relationship of post-test probability of no disease to the pretest probability of no disease for a negative test result. These relationships assume constancy of the (+)LR and (−)LR throughout the range of pretest probability. For levels of (+)LR or (−)LR greater than 1.0, the post-test probability of disease for a positive test result and the post-test probability of no disease for a negative test result exceed the respective pretest probability estimates. For levels of (+)LR or (−)LR less than 1.0, the post-test probability of disease and post-test probability of no disease for positive and negative test results are less than the respective pretest probability estimates. For tests in which the (+)LR and (−)LR equal 1.0, a positive or negative test result has no predictive power. The display of the likelihood ratio curves in this manner permits comparison of the relative predictive power of tests with different (+)LR and (−)LR.

Figure 11-11 illustrates a potential application of the (+)LR and (−)LR in estimating the range of pretest probability in which a test acquires 90% post-test predictive probability, as depicted in the shaded areas. Thus, at (+)LR 20, post-test probability of disease is 90% or greater for a positive test result at all levels of pretest probability of disease equal to or above 31%. For (−)LR 20, the post-test probability of no disease is 90% or greater for a negative test result at all levels of pretest probability of no disease equal to or above 31%. The range of pretest probability in which a 90% post-test predictive probability can be achieved narrows as levels of (+)LR and (−)LR decrease. This format can be applied to any other desired level of post-test probability, for example, 95% or 99%.

The computations of the post-test probability of disease after a positive test result [(+)PTPD] or the post-test

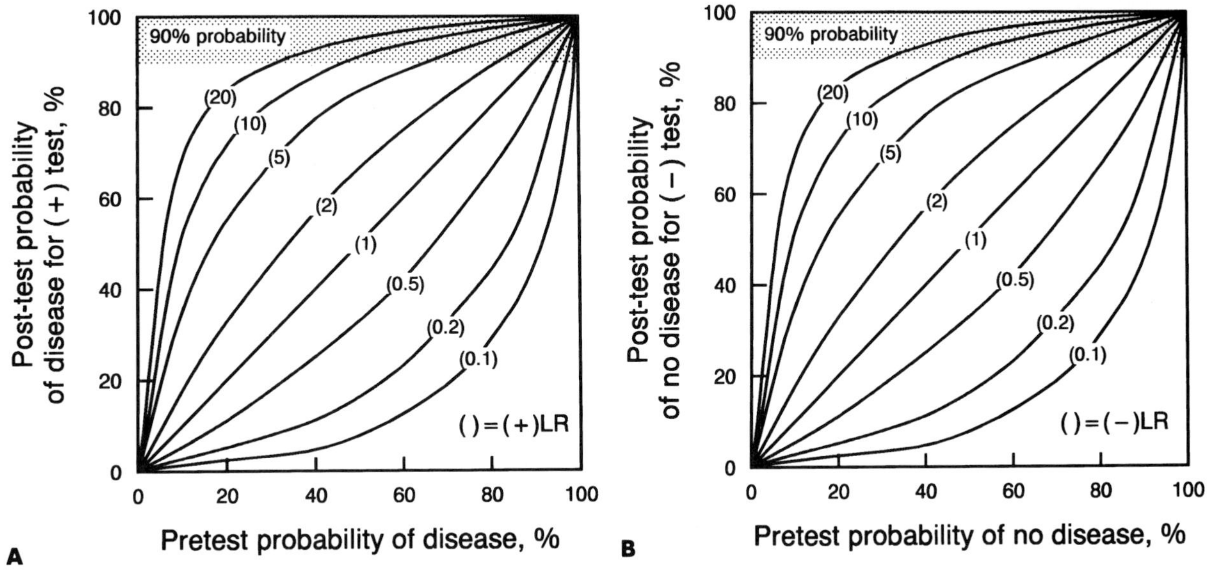

Fig 11-11 **A,** influence of the positive likelihood ratio [(+)LR] in the range 0.1 to 20 on the relationship of post-test probability of disease after a positive test result to the pretest probability of disease. The band of 90% probability of disease for a positive test is shown. **B,** influence of the negative likelihood ratio [(−)LR] in the range 0.1 to 20 on the relationship of post-test probability of no disease after a negative test result to the pretest probability of no disease. The band of 90% probability of no disease for a negative test is shown.

probability of no disease after a negative test result [(−)PTPN] are facilitated by use of the following likelihood ratio transformations of the Bayesian equations:

$$(+)\text{PTPD}(\%) = \frac{\text{PPD}}{\text{PPD} + \text{PPN}/(+)\text{LR}} \times 100 \quad [11\text{-}20]$$

and

$$(-)\text{PTPN}(\%) = \frac{\text{PPN}}{\text{PPN} + \text{PPD}/(-)\text{LR}} \times 100 \quad [11\text{-}21]$$

in which PPD is pretest probability of disease and PPN is pretest probability of no disease (calculated as 100 − PPD).

The (+)LR and (−)LR have their most useful application in the comparison of the relative potency of two or more tests performed on the same population. In chapter 6, there is a summary of data from studies in which the three most commonly applied laboratory tests for the detection of coronary artery disease—exercise ECG, thallium-201 scintigraphy (^{201}Tl), and radionuclide angiography (RNA)—are contrasted by paired observation on the same population. A meta-analysis of the data designed to illustrate the value of (+)LR and (−)LR in comparing tests derived from the same population is summarized in Table 11-1. The reported average Se and Sp are weighted for numbers of patients in each study. The (+)LR and (−)LR are calculated from the average Se and Sp. The standard deviations and confidence limits for the averaged data are calculated according to the principles outlined in the section on confidence limits at the end of this chapter.

On the basis of the likelihood data and the overlap in their 95% confidence limits, the following conclusions can be drawn for this series of studies: (1) the (+)LR and (−)LR are significantly greater for ^{201}Tl than for exercise ECG; (2) the (−)LR is significantly greater for RNA than for exercise ECG; there is no significant difference in (+)LR between RNA and exercise ECG; (3) neither (+)LR nor (−)LR is significantly different for the ^{201}Tl and RNA tests; and (4) the (+)LR is significantly greater than the (−)LR for the exercise ECG test. There is a trend for higher (+)LR than (−)LR for the ^{201}Tl test.

On the basis of this meta-analysis of paired tests for the prediction of coronary artery disease, the following clinical inferences can be drawn: (1) the ^{201}Tl test is significantly superior to the ECG stress test in ruling in and ruling out coronary artery disease; (2) the RNA test is significantly superior to the ECG stress test in ruling out but not in ruling in coronary artery disease; (3) there is no significant difference in the predictive capacity of the ^{201}Tl and RNA stress tests; and (4) the ECG stress test has significantly higher rule-in than rule-out diagnostic power; the ^{201}Tl test tends to have higher rule-in than rule-out diagnostic power.

Table 11-1 Comparison of exercise stress tests for the diagnosis of coronary artery disease by meta-analysis of paired tests on the same population*

Test	Studies (no.)	Patients (no.)	PD (%) Mean	PD (%) Range	Se†	Sp†	(+)LR‡	(-)LR‡
ECG					0.53 (.015)	0.83 (.019)	3.1 (2.4-4.2)	1.8 (1.6-2.0)
vs.	15	1,425	74	53-84				
^{201}Tl					0.81 (.012)	0.89 (.016)	7.4§ (5.5-10.7)	4.7§ (4.1-5.4)
ECG					0.58 (.028)	0.91) (.028)	6.4 (3.5-18.7)	2.2 (1.8-2.7)
vs.	4	424	75	58-82				
RNA					0.86 (.019)	0.79 (.040)	4.1 (2.8-6.9)	5.6§ (4.0-8.5)
^{201}Tl					0.84 (.027)	0.95 (.029)	16.8 (7.3-∞)	5.9 (4.2-9.4)
vs.	4	233	76	52-75				
RNA					0.90 (.022)	0.84 (.049)	5.6 (3.3-15.2)	8.4 (5.2-16.8)

PD, prevalence of disease; Se, sensitivity; Sp, specificity; (+)LR, positive likelihood ratio; (-)LR, negative likelihood ratio; ECG, exercise electrocardiography; ^{201}Tl, exercise thallium perfusion scintigraphy; RNA, exercise radionuclide angiography.

*Data from Gibbons RJ: Rest and exercise radionuclide angiography for diagnosis in chronic ischemic heart disease. *Circulation* 84 Suppl 1:93-99, 1991, and chapter 6.

†Se and Sp averages are weighted for number of patients. Standard deviation levels (in parentheses) are derived by the method of Galen and Gambino.[23]

‡(+)LR and (-)LR are calculated by Equations 11-18 and 11-19. Parenthetical values are 95% confidence limits.

§No overlap in 95% confidence limits with paired test.

The inferences above are based on studies in a limited range of coronary artery disease prevalence and on a limited number of studies comparing RNA with exercise ECG and ^{201}Tl tests. Additional studies in a wider prevalence range are necessary for a more definitive positioning of the relative predictive power of these diagnostic tests.

Comparing risk factors

The principles related to the derivation of test Se and Sp from index test results in a given population are readily transferable to the evaluation of cardiovascular risk factors. Expressed in terms of mortality and survival, the *risk sensitivity (RSe)* is the estimated proportion of individuals who succumb during a given follow-up time who were preclassified as high risk. The *risk specificity (RSp)* is the estimated proportion of survivors during a given follow-up time who were preclassified as low risk. The RSe and RSp can be calculated similarly for nonfatal morbid events. The RSe and RSp are expressed in decimals.

To compute the RSe for any follow-up time from reported data, one must acquire three basic mortality measures: (1) the cumulative or standard mortality (in percent) for the high-risk subgroup (CM_h), (2) the high-risk fraction (HRF) of the population (in decimals) at the inception of the follow-up, and (3) the cumulative mortality (in percent) for the whole population (CM_p).

The RSe at any follow-up time in terms of these three variables is calculated as

$$RSe = \frac{CM_h \times HRF}{CM_p} \qquad [11\text{-}22]$$

To compute the RSp for any follow-up time, one must acquire three basic survival measures: (1) the cumulative or standard survival (in percent) for the low-risk subgroup (CS_l), (2) the low-risk fraction (LRF) of the population (in decimals) at the inception of follow-up, and (3) the cumulative survival (in percent) for the whole population (CS_p). The RSp in terms of these three variables is as follows:

$$RS_p = \frac{CS_l \times LRF}{CS_p} \qquad [11\text{-}23]$$

The CM_h and CS_l in Equations 11-22 and 11-23 are derived from the reported survival or mortality data for the designated high- and low-risk subgroups. The following complementary relationships permit ready conversion of the mortality and survival data within each risk subgroup:

$$CS_h = 100 - CM_h \qquad [11\text{-}24]$$

and

$$CS_l = 100 - CM_l \qquad [11\text{-}25]$$

in which CS_h is cumulative survival for the high-risk subgroup and CM_l is cumulative mortality for the low-risk subgroup. The cumulative mortality and survival data for the total population are similarly complementary as follows:

$$CM_p = 100 - CS_p \qquad [11\text{-}26]$$

The high- and low-risk fractions are unit complements and hence are readily interconvertible as follows:

$$HRF = 1.0 - LRF \qquad [11\text{-}27]$$

The derivation of Equations 11-22 and 11-23 in terms of the principles applied to diagnostic test performance indices is detailed in Appendix 2.

Among the most useful applications of the determination of RSe and RSp, yet one infrequently used, is the comparison of risk factors as predictors of clinical events. Application of this approach is illustrated in an analysis of the relative potency of three mortality risk factors studied in the screening cohort of the Multiple Risk Factor Intervention Trial (MRFIT).[24,25] This study encompassed a 6-year follow-up of 356,222 men, aged 35 to 57 years, who were free of myocardial infarction at baseline. Table 11-2 summarizes the reported data pertinent to the computation of the RSe, RSp, high-risk likelihood ratio [(+)LR], and low-risk likelihood ratio [(−)LR] for three risk factors: (1) serum cholesterol concentration (abnormal threshold, 203 mg/dL), (2) smoking (abnormal threshold, one cigarette or more per day), and (3) diastolic blood pressure (abnormal threshold, 90 mm Hg). The 6-year coronary heart disease mortality rate for the entire cohort was 0.634%. The risk indicators are listed in column 1. The number of individuals reported in each risk subgroup is indicated in column 2.

The risk fractions indicated in column 3 are calculated from the numbers in column 2. The 6-year mortality rate, calculated in percent, for each risk group is shown in column 4. The survival rate for each risk group, calculated as the 100% complement of the mortality rate, is shown in column 5. The RSe and RSp in columns 6 and 7 are calculated by Equations 11-22 and 11-23. The calculated (+)LR in column 8 is the high-risk likelihood ratio [(+)LR = RSe/1 − RSp]. The calculated (−)LR in column 9 is the low-risk likelihood ratio [(−)LR = RSp/1 − RSe]. The (+)LR applied to mortality risk for coronary heart disease is a measure of the relative power of the presence of a risk factor in predicting mortality during a given follow-up time; the (−)LR is a measure of the relative power of the absence of the risk factor in predicting survival during the same follow-up time.

The RSe, RSp, and risk likelihood data for the 6-year follow-up period in Table 11-2 conform with reported epidemiologic trends for serum cholesterol, smoking, and diastolic arterial pressure. The average likelihood ratios cluster in a restricted low range (1.22 to 1.65), reflecting the relatively low predictive power of each of the risk factors. The large number of subjects in the study yields narrow confidence limits for the (+)LR and (−)LR levels. Of the three risk factors, the serum cholesterol at a threshold of 203 mg/dL and smoking exhibit significantly higher (−)LR than diastolic pressure, evidencing their slightly greater potency as indicators of low mortality risk in this male population. The presence of smoking exhibits a significantly higher (+)LR than cholesterol or diastolic

Table 11-2 Risk sensitivity, risk specificity, and likelihood ratios for cardiac mortality risk*

1 Risk factor	2 Enrollees† (no.)	3 HRF LRF	4 MR‡ (%)	5 SR§ (%)	6 RSe‖	7 RSp‖	8 (+)LR¶	9 (−)LR¶
Cholesterol ≥203 mg/dL	214,046	0.601	0.80	99.20	0.758 (0.001)	0.400 (0.0008)	1.26 (1.23-1.30)	1.65 (1.53-1.79)
Cholesterol <203 mg/dL	142,176	0.399	0.37	99.63				
Smokers	131,082	0.368	1.03	98.97	0.598 (0.010)	0.633 (0.0008)	1.63 (1.57-1.69)	1.57 (1.50-1.56)
Nonsmokers	225,140	0.632	0.43	99.57				
DBP ≥90 mm Hg	100,032	0.281	0.93	99.07	0.412 (0.010)	0.720 (0.0008)	1.47 (1.39-1.53)	1.22 (1.18-1.27)
DBP <90 mm Hg	256,190	0.719	0.52	99.48				

HRF, high-risk fraction; LRF, low-risk fraction; MR, mortality rate; SR, survival rate; RSe, risk sensitivity; RSp, risk specificity; (+)LR, high-risk likelihood ratio; (−)LR, low-risk likelihood ratio; DBP, diastolic blood pressure.

*Data from Stamler J, Wentworth D, Neaton JD: Is relationship between serum cholesterol and risk of premature death from coronary artery disease continuous and graded? Findings in 356 222 primary screenees of the Multiple Risk Factor Intervention Trial (MRFIT). *JAMA* 256:2823-2828, 1986, and Stamler J: Epidemiology, established major risk factors, and the primary prevention of coronary heart disease. In *Cardiology*. Vol. 2: *Cardiovascular Disease*. Chap 1. Edited by WW Parmley, K Chatterjee. Philadelphia, JB Lippincott Company, 1988, pp 1-41. Six-year follow-up for enrollees in Multiple Risk Factor Intervention Trial. RSe, RSp, HRF, and LRF are carried to three decimals because of sample size.

†Men screened in study.

‡Six-year age-standardized coronary heart disease death rates derived by weighted averaging of reported subgroup mortality rates. Six-year population mortality rate is 0.634%.

§Derived from calculated mortality rates for the respective subgroups.

‖RSe and RSp are calculated by Equations 11-22 and 11-23. Parenthetical values are standard deviations.

¶(+)LR and (−)LR are calculated by Equations 11-18 and 11-19 from RSe and RSp. Parenthetical values are 95% confidence limits.

pressure, evidencing its slightly greater relative potency among the three factors as an indicator of high mortality risk in this male population.

Of pertinence to the cardiologist in this analysis is the potential clinical value of these risk factors in predicting mortality in individuals. Notable is the observation in Table 11-2 that the maximal (+)LR for any single risk factor is 1.63 and the maximal (−)LR for any single risk factor is 1.65. Rearranging the terms of Equations 11-20 and 11-21, one can calculate, for any risk factor of known (+)LR or (−)LR, the minimum pretest probability (based on independent information) required to predict 90% post-test mortality or survival. The closer this calculated pretest probability is to the post-test estimate of 90%, the weaker is the predictive power of the risk factor. At the above (+)LR, a probability of 90% 6-year mortality for a positive test result could be estimated only for individuals with a minimum pretest probability of mortality based on independent risk factors (such as age, sex, and clinical characteristics) of 85% or greater. At the above (−)LR for a negative test result, a post-test probability for survival of 90% in 6 years could be estimated only for individuals with a pretest survival probability on the basis of independent risk factors of 85% or greater (i.e., pretest mortality probability of 15% or less). Assuming independence of each factor, the cumulative (+)LR for the presence of three risk factors could be calculated as the product of their respective (+)LR levels. For the three risk factors above, the cumulative (+)LR level derived from the data in Table 11-2 is 3.02. At that level of (+)LR, an estimate of 90% post-test probability of coronary disease mortality in 6 years would require a minimum pretest probability of mortality based on other factors of 75%.

On the basis of the computed levels of RSe and RSp and the likelihood ratio data in Table 11-2, one can conclude that the epidemiologic associations of cholesterol, smoking, and diastolic hypertension with coronary artery disease mortality at the thresholds tested are not sufficiently powerful to permit individualized prediction of 6-year outcome among men in the age range of 35 to 57 years.

Confidence limits for probability estimates

Probabilistic relationships are expressed in proportions that are in fact estimates of the predicted association between a test result and the presence or absence of disease. Such proportions have a statistical range of reproducibility, knowledge of which provides valuable information relevant to their precision as predictive indices. By convention, such estimates of error for a single proportion are expressed in terms of its confidence limits, the calculation of which is based on the determination of the standard error of a proportion.[23] The *standard error of a proportion (SE_p)* is calculated from the relationship

$$SE_p = \sqrt{\frac{p \times (1 - p)}{n}} \quad \textbf{[11-28]}$$

in which p is the proportion (in decimals), (1 − p) is the complement of p, and n is the number of subjects from which the proportion was determined. For data reported in percent, p and (100 − p) are entered in percent. The SE_p so calculated is equivalent statistically to a standard deviation measure.

A practical estimate of the limits of certainty for a proportion is provided in the determination of p ± (1.96 × SE_p) as the upper and lower bounds of 95% confidence for repeated estimates for that proportion, that is, 95% of repeated measures on the same population are expected to lie within this range. The upper and lower bounds are commonly termed the *95% confidence limits*. The *95% confidence range* is the range of proportions between the lower and the upper confidence limits. When the 95% confidence limits for proportions derived for different tests on the same population do not overlap, it may be concluded that the differences are significant at a 95% level of probability.

Because the 95% confidence limits are an approximation of the clustering to the mean of repeated measures, the confidence limits provide an estimate of the reproducibility or precision of the proportion. The wider the confidence interval, the less precise the proportion; the more narrow the confidence interval, the more precise the proportion.

Confidence limits may be calculated for any desired range of probability depending on the level of certainty one wants to achieve in estimating a difference between proportions. The coefficients 1.65, 1.96, and 2.58 are the multiples of the SE_p that encompass the 90%, 95%, and 99% range of repeated estimates of a proportion, respectively, when such repeated estimates are derived from a normal distribution.

For convenience, the 95% limits of confidence are usually calculated as ±2 × SE_p. Appendix 3 details the calculation of 95% confidence limits for tests with simple proportions, such as the Se and Sp, and with complex proportions, such as (+)PTPD and (−)PTPD.

Alternative sources for determining the 95% confidence limits for a proportion are published reference tables[26] derived by more exact formulations than the SEp method outlined herein. For the range of proportions from 0.20 to 0.99 (20% to 99%) and sample size of 100 or greater, the upper and lower bounds of confidence calculated by the SEp method described above are within 5.0% of those in the reference tables. For proportions less than 0.20 or greater than 0.99 and for sample sizes less than 100, the reference tables should be consulted.

Appendix 1

DERIVATION OF POSITIVE AND NEGATIVE POST-TEST FRACTION FROM PRETEST AND POST-TEST PROBABILITY DATA AND THE Se AND Sp OF A TEST*

The fraction of a post-test population with a positive test result [(+)F] can be calculated from a transformation of the Bayesian equation for (+)PTPD:

$$(+)\text{PTPD} = \frac{\text{Se} \times \text{PPD}}{\text{Se} \times \text{PPD} + (1 - \text{Sp}) \times \text{PPN}} \times 100 \qquad \textbf{[11-7]}$$

The terms of the denominator of Equation 11-7 can be converted to the post-test TP and FP as follows:

$$\text{Se} \times \text{PPD} = \text{TP}$$

$$(1 - \text{Sp}) \times \text{PPN} = \text{FP}$$

Substituting post-test TP and FP for the terms in the denominator, Equation 11-7 can be expressed as

$$(+)\text{PTPD}\% = \frac{\text{Se} \times \text{PPD}}{\text{TP} + \text{FP}} \times 100$$

By definition, the post-test TP + FP = (+)F × 100, in which (+)F is the post-test positive fraction (see section on test characteristics). Equation 11-7 can thus be expressed as

$$(+)\text{PTPD} = \frac{\text{Se} \times \text{PPD}}{(+)\text{F} \times 100} \times 100$$

Transposing terms, canceling 100, and solving for post-test (+)F:

$$(+)\text{F} = \frac{\text{Se} \times \text{PPD}}{(+)\text{PTPD}}$$

in which Se is the test sensitivity, PPD the pretest probability of disease, and (+)PTPD the calculated post-test probability for a positive test result. Since (+)F and (−)F are unit complements, (−)F for the post-test population is calculated from (+)F as

$$(-)\text{F} = 1 - (+)\text{F}$$

*Author's derivation.

Appendix 2

DERIVATION OF THE EQUATION FOR RISK SENSITIVITY (RSe) IN AN INDEX POPULATION*

The diagnostic sensitivity of a test in an index population is defined as

$$Se = \frac{TP}{TP + FN} \quad [11\text{-}1]$$

in which Se is expressed in decimals and TP and FN are expressed either in percent or in number of subjects in the total population.

Expressing TP and TP + FN in terms of test performance indices and population characteristics for an index population:

$$TP = (+)PA_c \times (+)F$$

$$TP + FN = PD$$

in which $(+)PA_c$ and PD are expressed in percent and (+)F in decimals.

Thus, Equation 11-1 expressed in terms of $(+)PA_c$, (+)F, and PD for an index population becomes

$$Se = \frac{(+)PA_c \times (+)F}{PD} \quad [11\text{-}1A]$$

The $(+)PA_c$, (+)F, and PD for an index population have the following equivalent expressions in mortality data:

1. $(+)PA_c$ expressed in mortality terminology is equivalent to the cumulative (or standard) mortality for high-risk patients (CM_h) at a specific follow-up time.
2. (+)F expressed in mortality terminology is equivalent to the high-risk fraction (HRF) of the whole population at time of entry.
3. PD in mortality terminology is equivalent to the cumulative (or standard) mortality for the total population (CM_p) at a specific follow-up time.

Transforming Equation 11-1A to risk mortality terms, the risk sensitivity (RSe) at a given follow-up time becomes

$$RSe = \frac{CM_h \times HRF}{CM_p} \quad [11\text{-}22]$$

The RSe, so calculated, is the estimated proportion of all deaths during a given follow-up time that were preclassified as high risk at the inception of follow-up.

*Author's derivation.

DERIVATION OF THE EQUATION FOR RISK SPECIFICITY (RSp) FOR AN INDEX POPULATION*

The diagnostic specificity for a test in an index population is defined as

$$Sp = \frac{TN}{TN + FP} \quad [11\text{-}2]$$

in which Sp is expressed in decimals and TN and FP are expressed either in percent or in number of subjects in the total population.

Expressing TN and TN + FP in terms of test performance indices and population characteristics for an index population:

$$TN = (-)PA_c \times (-)F$$

and

$$TN + FP = PN$$

Thus, Equation 11-2 expressed in terms of $(-)PA_c$, (−)F, and PN for an index population is:

$$Sp = \frac{(-)PA_c \times (-)F}{PN} \quad [11\text{-}2A]$$

The $(-)PA_c$, (−)F, and PN for an index population have the following equivalent expressions in survival data:

1. $(-)PA_c$ expressed in survival terminology is equivalent to cumulative (or standard) survival in the low-risk population (CS_l) at a specific follow-up time.
2. (−)F expressed in survival terminology is equivalent to the low-risk fraction (LRF) of the whole population at time of entry.
3. PN in survival terminology is equivalent to cumulative (or standard) survival for the total population (CS_p) at a specific follow-up time.

Transforming Equation 11-2A to survival terms, risk specificity (RSp) at a given follow-up time becomes

$$RSp = \frac{CS_l \times LRF}{CSp} \quad [11\text{-}23]$$

The RSp, so calculated, is the estimated proportion of all survivors during a given follow-up time who were preclassified as low risk at the inception of follow-up.

Appendix 3

CALCULATION OF 95% UPPER AND LOWER LIMITS FOR POST-TEST PROBABILITY

Let us assume that among 100 unselected patients with symptoms in whom coronary artery disease has been independently diagnosed, a given noninvasive test yields a positive result in 80. The Se of the test is 0.80. The standard error (SE_p) of the Se is determined from Equation 11-28 as

$$SE_p = \sqrt{\frac{0.80 \times 0.20}{100}} = 0.04$$

The 95% confidence limits for the Se are calculated as

$$0.80 \pm (2 \times 0.04) = 0.72 \text{ to } 0.88$$

Let us assume that among 100 additional unselected patients with symptoms in whom coronary artery disease has been independently ruled out, the result of the same test is negative in 90. The Sp of the test is 0.90. The standard error of the Sp is determined as

$$SE_p = \sqrt{\frac{0.90 \times 0.10}{100}} = 0.03$$

The 95% confidence limits for Sp are calculated as

$$0.90 \pm (2 \times 0.03) = 0.84 \text{ to } 0.96$$

For individualized probability estimates expressed in compounded proportions, the determination of confidence limits must encompass the SE_p range for each of the components. Let us assume that we want to determine the (+)PTPD and confidence limits for an individual whose estimated PPD is 32% with an SE_p of 3.0%. When the Se and Sp determinations derived from the index population are used, the (+)PTPD calculated by the Bayesian equation is

$$(+)\text{PTPD} = \frac{\text{Se} \times \text{PPD}}{\text{Se} \times \text{PPD} + (1 - \text{Sp}) \times \text{PPN}} \times 100 \qquad [11\text{-}7]$$

$$(+)\text{PTPD} = \frac{(0.8 \times 32)}{(0.8 \times 32) + (0.1 \times 68)} \times 100 = 79\%$$

To calculate the 95% confidence limits for the (+)PTPD estimate, one must determine the 95% upper and lower confidence limits for each term of the (+)PTPD equation as follows:

For Se 0.80 ± 0.04, upper limit 0.88, lower limit 0.72

For Sp 0.90 ± 0.03, upper limit 0.96, lower limit 0.84

For PPD 32% ± 3.0%, upper limit 38, lower limit 26

When the 95% upper limit estimates for Se, Sp, and PPD are used, the calculation of the upper limit for (+)PTPD from Equation 11-7 is

$$(+)\text{PTPD} = \frac{(0.88 \times 38)}{(0.88 \times 38) + [(1 - 0.96) \times 62]} \times 100 = 93\%$$

in which 0.88 is the upper limit for Se, 0.96 is the upper limit for Sp, 38% is the upper limit for PPD, and 62% is the lower limit of PPN. The lower limit of PPN is derived as the 100% complement of the upper limit for PPD.

When the 95% lower limit estimates for Se, Sp, and PPD are used, the calculation of the lower 95% limit of (+)PTPD is

$$(+)\text{PTPD} = \frac{(0.72 \times 26)}{(0.72 \times 26) + [(1 - 0.84) \times 74]} \times 100 = 61\%$$

in which 0.72 is the lower limit for Se, 0.84 is the lower limit for Sp, and 26 is the lower limit for PPD. The upper limit of PPN of 74 is derived as the 100% complement of the lower limit for PPD.

Thus, the estimate for a (+)PTPD of 79% is made with a 95% confidence interval of 93% to 61%.

Similar calculations provide 95% upper and lower limits for (−)PTPD from the same data base.

*Author's derivation.

Glossary of abbreviations

Abbreviation	Term	Definition	Unit*
Evaluating test performance in an index population			
(+)	Positive	A test result within the abnormal range of test scores.	. . .
(−)	Negative	A test result within the normal range of test scores.	. . .
Se	Sensitivity	Proportion of the subpopulation with disease that has a (+) test result. True-positive rate.	D
Sp	Specificity	Proportion of the subpopulation with no disease that has a (−) test result. True-negative rate.	D
1 − Se	Insensitivity	Proportion of the subpopulation with disease that has a (−) test result. False-negative rate.	D
1 − Sp	Nonspecificity	Proportion of subpopulation with no disease that has a (+) test result. False-positive rate.	D
$(+)PA_c$	Positive predictive accuracy	Proportion of the subpopulation with a (+) test result that has disease.	P
$(-)PA_c$	Negative predictive accuracy	Proportion of the subpopulation with a (−) test result that has no disease.	P
PD	Prevalence of disease	Proportion of total index population with disease.	P
PN	Prevalence of normality (no disease)	Proportion of total index population with no disease. The 100% complement of PD.	P
(+)F	Positive fraction	Proportion of total index population with (+) test result.	D
(−)F	Negative fraction	Proportion of total index population with (−) test result. The unit complement of (+)F.	D
TP	True positive	Proportion of total index population with disease that tests (+).	P
TN	True negative	Proportion of total index population with no disease that tests (−).	P
FP	False positive	Proportion of total index population with no disease that tests (+).	P
FN	False negative	Proportion of total index population with disease that tests (−).	P
Use of tests in clinical prediction			
PPD	Pretest probability of disease for an individual	Assumed pretest probability of disease based on prevalence of disease in a population with clinical characteristics identical to those of the individual.	P
PPN	Pretest probability of normality (no disease) for an individual	The 100% complement of PPD.	P
(+)PTPD	Post-test probability of disease for a (+) test	Probability of disease in an individual with a (+) test result based on conditional probability estimation.	P
(−)PTPN	Post-test probability of no disease for a (-) test	Probability of no disease in an individual with a (−) test result based on conditional probability estimation.	P
(−)PTPD	Post-test probability of disease for a (-) test	Probability of disease in an individual with a (−) test result based on conditional probability estimation. The 100% complement of (−)PTPN.	P
OD	Odds of disease	Quotient of probability of disease divided by its 100% complement.	R
ON	Odds of no disease	Quotient of probability of no disease divided by its 100% complement. The inverse of the odds of disease.	R
POD	Pretest odds of disease	Pretest odds of disease calculated on the basis of prevalence estimates in an index population.	R

Continued.

Glossary of abbreviations—cont'd

Abbreviation	Term	Definition	Unit*
PON	Pretest odds of no disease	Pretest odds of no disease calculated on the basis of prevalence estimates in an index population.	R
(+)PTOD	Post-test odds of disease for a (+) test	Post-test odds of disease in an individual with a (+) test result based on conditional probability estimation.	R
(−)PTON	Post-test odds of no disease for a (−) test	Post-test odds of no disease in an individual with a (−) test result based on conditional probability estimation.	R
(−)PTOD	Post-test odds of disease for a (−) test	Post-test odds of disease in an individual with a (−) test result based on conditional probability estimation. The inverse of (−)PTON.	R
Comparing tests			
ROC curve	Receiver operating characteristic curve	A graphic plot of Se vs. Sp of a test for a continuous range of thresholds. (Alternative plots: Se vs. 1 − Sp, 1 − Se vs. Sp, and 1 − Se vs. 1 − Sp.)	. . .
(+)LR	Likelihood ratio for a (+) test	The ratio of an index test Se to (1 − Sp).	R
(−)LR	Likelihood ratio for a (−) test	The ratio of an index test Sp to (1 − Se).	R
Comparing risk factors			
CM_p	Cumulative mortality for a total population	Cumulative proportion of a total index population that succumbs during a given follow-up time.	P
CS_p	Cumulative survival for a total population	Cumulative proportion of a total index population that survives during a given follow-up time.	P
HRF	High-risk fraction of total population	Proportion of the total index population that was preclassified as high risk at inception of follow-up.	D
LRF	Low-risk fraction of total population	Proportion of the total index population that was preclassified as low risk at inception of follow-up.	D
RSe	Risk sensitivity	Proportion of the subpopulation succumbing during a given follow-up time that was preclassified as high risk at inception of follow-up.	D
RSp	Risk specificity	Proportion of the subpopulation surviving during a given follow-up time that was preclassified as low risk at inception of follow-up.	D
CM_h	Cumulative mortality for high risk	Proportion of the high-risk subpopulation that succumbs during a given follow-up time.	P
CM_l	Cumulative mortality for low risk	Proportion of the low-risk subpopulation that succumbs during a given follow-up time.	P
CS_h	Cumulative survival for high risk	Proportion of the high-risk subpopulation that survives during a given follow-up time.	P
CS_l	Cumulative survival for low risk	Proportion of the low-risk subpopulation that survives during a given follow-up time.	P
SE_p	Standard error of a proportion	Square root of the quotient derived from the product of a proportion and its complement divided by the number of subjects from which the proportion was derived.	P, D

*D, decimals; P, percentage; R, ratio (preferred odds reduction is n : 1).

REFERENCES

1. LaPlace PS: *Essai philosophique sur les probabilités.* Paris, Courcier. Sixth edition, 1840. (English translation in 1902 as *A Philosophical Essay on Probabilities* and edited by FW Trunott, FL Emory.) New York, Dover. Reprinted 1951

2. Bayes T: An essay towards solving a problem in the doctrine of chances. *Philos Trans R Soc Lond* 53:370-418, 1763

3. LaPlace PS: *Théorie Analytique des Probabilités*, 1812. Paris, Courcier. (Third edition, 1820.) Reprinted in *Oeuvres Complètes de LaPlace*, 14 volumes. Paris, Gauthier-Villars, Vol. 7, 1878-1912

4. Patterson RE, Horowitz SF: Importance of epidemiology and biostatistics in deciding clinical strategies for using diagnostic tests: a simplified approach using examples from coronary artery disease. *J Am Coll Cardiol* 13:1653-1665, 1989

5. Kannel WB, Gordon T: *The Framingham Study: an Epidemiological Investigation of Cardiovascular Disease.* Vol. 12. Bethesda, National Heart, Lung and Blood Institute, National Institutes of Health, 1968

6. Diamond GA, Forrester JS: Analysis of probability as an aid in the clinical diagnosis of coronary-artery disease. *N Engl J Med* 300:1350-1358, 1979

7. Diamond GA, Forrester JS, Hirsch M, et al: Application of conditional probability analysis to the clinical diagnosis of coronary artery disease. *J Clin Invest* 65:1210-1221, 1980

8. Burggraf GW, Parker JO: Progress in coronary artery disease: angiographic, hemodynamic, and clinical factors. *Circulation* 51:146-156, 1975

9. Califf RM, Phillips HR III, Hindman MC, et al: Prognostic value of a coronary artery jeopardy score. *J Am Coll Cardiol* 5:1055-1063, 1985

10. Gensini GG: *Coronary Arteriography.* Mount Kisco, New York, Futura Publishing Company, 1975, pp 271-274

11. Friesinger GC, Humphries JO, Ross RS: Prognostic significance of coronary arteriography. In *Coronary Heart Disease.* Edited by M Kaltenbach, P Lichtlen, GC Friesinger. Stuttgart, Georg Thieme Verlag, 1973, pp 132-138

12. White CW, Wright CB, Doty DB, et al: Does visual interpretation of the coronary arteriogram predict the physiologic importance of a coronary stenosis? *N Engl J Med* 310:819-824, 1984

13. Harrison DG, White CW, Hiratzka LF, et al: The value of lesion cross-sectional area determined by quantitative coronary angiography in assessing the physiologic significance of proximal left anterior descending coronary arterial stenoses. *Circulation* 6:1111-1119, 1984

14. Gianrossi R, Detrano R, Mulvihill D, et al: Exercise-induced ST depression in the diagnosis of coronary artery disease: a meta-analysis. *Circulation* 80:87-98, 1989

15. Detrano R, Janosi A, Lyons KP, et al: Factors affecting sensitivity and specificity of a diagnostic test: the exercise thallium scintigram. *Am J Med* 84:699-710, 1988

16. Gibbons RJ: Rest and exercise radionuclide angiography for diagnosis in chronic ischemic heart disease. *Circulation* 84 Suppl 1:93-99, 1991

17. Kotler TS, Diamond GA: Exercise thallium-201 scintigraphy in the diagnosis and prognosis of coronary artery disease. *Ann Intern Med* 113:684-702, 1990

18. Hlatky MA, Pryor DB, Harrell FE Jr, et al: Factors affecting sensitivity and specificity of exercise electrocardiography: multivariable analysis. *Am J Med* 77:64-71, 1984

19. Hlatky MA, Mark DB, Harrell FE Jr, et al: Rethinking sensitivity and specificity. *Am J Cardiol* 59:1195-1198, 1987

20. Rozanski A, Diamond GA, Berman D, et al: The declining specificity of exercise radionuclide ventriculography. *N Engl J Med* 309:518-522, 1983

21. Rozanski A, Diamond GA, Forrester JS, et al: Alternative referent standards for cardiac normality: implications for diagnostic testing. *Ann Intern Med* 101:164-171, 1984

22. Ransohoff DF, Feinstein AR: Problems of spectrum and bias in evaluating the efficacy of diagnostic tests. *N Engl J Med* 299:926-930, 1978

23. Galen RS, Gambino SR: *Beyond Normality: the Predictive Value and Efficiency of Medical Diagnoses.* New York, John Wiley & Sons, 1975, p 129

24. Stamler J, Wentworth D, Neaton JD: Is relationship between serum cholesterol and risk of premature death from coronary artery disease continuous and graded? Findings in 356 222 primary screenees of the Multiple Risk Factor Intervention Trial (MRFIT). *JAMA* 256:2823-2828, 1986

25. Stamler J: Epidemiology, established major risk factors, and the primary prevention of coronary heart disease. In *Cardiology. Vol. 2: Cardiovascular Disease.* Chap 1. Edited by WW Parmley, K Chatterjee. Philadelphia, JB Lippincott Company, 1988, pp 1-41

26. Diem K, Lentner C (eds): *Scientific Tables.* Seventh edition. Basle, Ciba-Geigy, 1970, pp 85-106

CHAPTER

12

Applied anatomy of the heart

William D. Edwards, M.D.

A fundamental knowledge of cardiac anatomy forms the cornerstone of clinical cardiology. Auscultation and percussion of the heart would be meaningless without an appreciation of normal chamber and valvular positions within the thorax. Similarly, an understanding of cardiac anatomy is prerequisite for the proper interpretation of chest roentgenograms, electrocardiograms, and the angiograms obtained at cardiac catheterization. Furthermore, as noninvasive two-dimensional imaging techniques (such as echocardiography and radiographic computed tomography) allow viewing of the heart by many rather unconventional planes, an understanding of detailed three-dimensional cardiac anatomy becomes essential.[1]

The cardiac surgeon, whose operative view of intracardiac structures is often both limited and from unusual angles, has a keen appreciation of the importance of understanding the anatomy of the heart. Several outstanding atlases of cardiac anatomy are available,[2-5] and their popularity underscores the importance of this topic. Techniques for specimen fixation, dissection, and photography have been described in detail.[3,6]

In this chapter, the segmental approach to cardiac anatomy and embryology is employed, since it best facilitates the comparison of analogous right- and left-sided structures, as visualized both morphologically and by clinical imaging techniques. Paragraphs printed in smaller type either emphasize clinical applications of the aforementioned anatomy and embryology or describe how specific disease processes affect certain anatomic sites and thereby alter normal structure and function.

MEDIASTINUM

The mediastinum is bounded anteriorly by the sternum and adjacent ribs, posteriorly by the vertebral column and adjacent ribs, laterally by the medial parietal pleural surfaces of each hemithorax, superiorly by the plane of the first pair of ribs, and inferiorly by the diaphragm (Fig 12-1).

In addition to the heart and great vessels the mediastinum also contains the distal portion of the trachea, right and left bronchi, esophagus, thymus, autonomic nerves (cardiac and splanchnic, left recurrent laryngeal, and bilateral vagal and phrenic), various small arteries (such as bronchial and esophageal) and veins (such as bronchial, azygos, and hemiazygos), lymph nodes, cardiopulmonary lymphatics, and thoracic duct.

Enlargement of a cardiac chamber or great vessel may displace or compress an adjacent noncardiac structure. For example, the enlarged left atrium associated with chronic rheumatic mitral disease may displace the left bronchus superiorly and the esophagus rightward; both structural shifts might be observed by chest roentgenography with barium swallow. Similarly, an aberrant retroesophageal right subclavian artery may indent the esophagus posteriorly and may, in some subjects, cause dysphagia. A markedly dilated heart may compress even the lungs and result in partial atelectasis, particularly of the lingula and left lower lobe; coexistent pleural and pericardial effusions may further compress the lungs.

Conversely, perturbations of noncardiac thoracic structures may affect the configuration or position of adjacent cardiac chambers or the entire heart. For example, mediastinal neoplasms may indent the low-pressure atria or may compress the superior vena cava or pulmonary veins; and after pneumonectomy, all mediastinal structures tend to shift toward the side of resection. Even expansile processes of the abdomen may elevate the diaphragm significantly and thereby alter the position of the heart.

PERICARDIUM

Anatomy

The pericardium surrounds the heart and consists of fibrous and serous portions.[7] The fibrous pericardium forms a flask-shaped, tough outer sac, which envelops the heart and attaches to the great vessels. As a result, the ascending aorta, pulmonary trunk, and terminal 2 to 4 cm of superior vena cava lie within the pericardial cavity; shorter lengths of pulmonary veins and inferior vena cava also are intrapericardial (Fig 12-2). The outer surface of the fibrous pericardium is firmly adherent to the central tendinous portion of the diaphragm and is loosely adherent to the sternum, parietal pleurae, esophagus, and descending thoracic aorta. This layer contains variable amounts of adipose tissue, particularly near the diaphragm, which may contribute to the cardiac silhouette roentgenographically (see Fig 12-1).

The fibrous pericardium is quite inelastic and may effectively limit the diastolic dimensions of the heart. However, with normal cardiac growth or abnormal cardiac enlargement, which develops slowly, the fibrous pericardium grows or stretches to

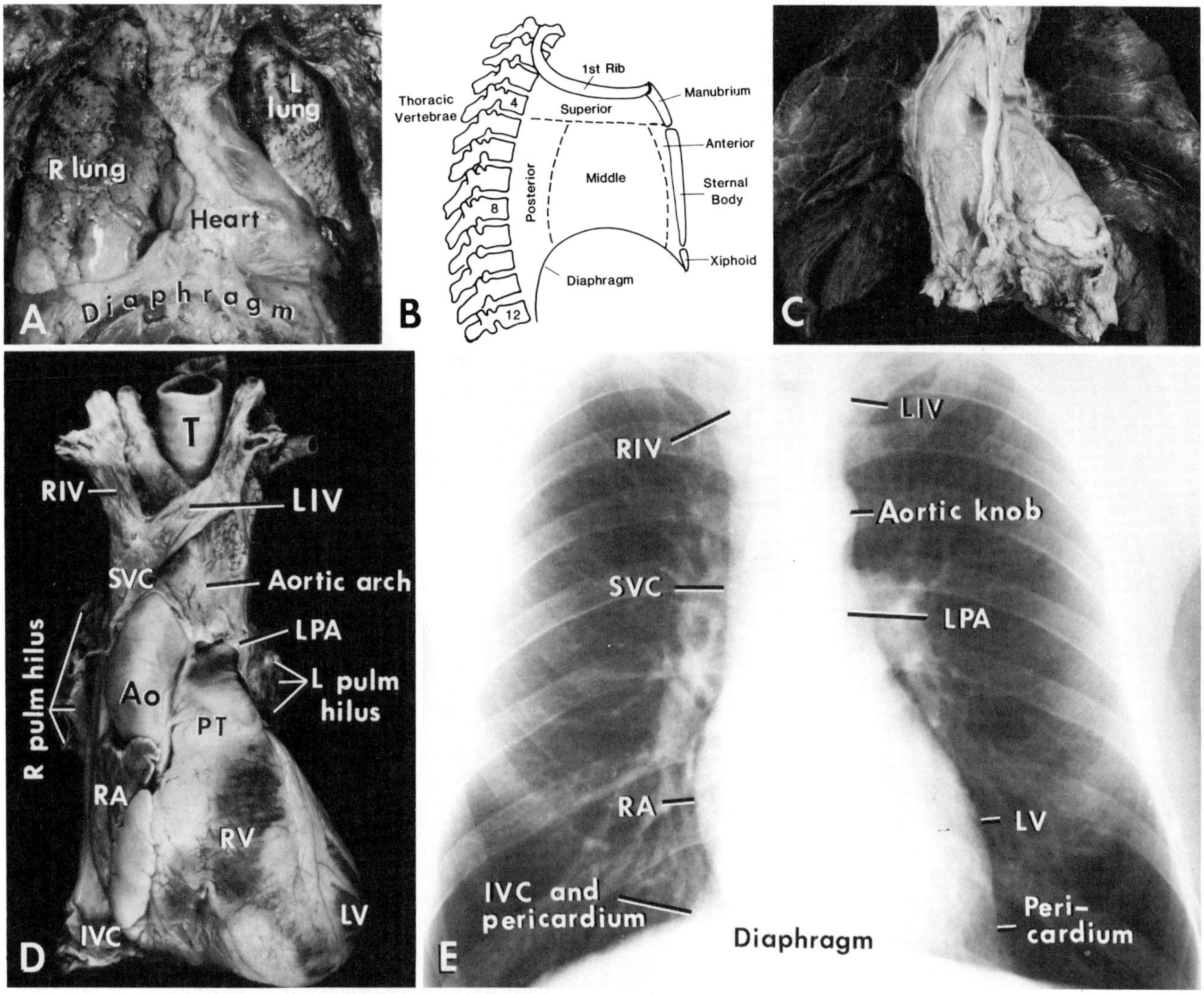

Fig 12-1 **A,** the heart occupies the middle mediastinum (in situ view of the thoracic organs in a 24-year-old man at autopsy). **B,** diagram of the mediastinal components (right lateral view). (Modified from Pansky B, House EL: Review of Gross Anatomy. Second edition. New York, Macmillan Company, 1969, p 285.) **C,** fat along the external surface of the parietal pericardium may contribute to the cardiac silhouette roentgenographically (anterior view, with lungs retracted, from a 27-year-old man). **D,** middle and superior mediastinal structures. (Anterior view, from a 27-year-old man.) **E,** frontal chest roentgenogram, for comparison with anatomic specimens (from a 33-year-old man). (See Appendix, this chapter, for abbreviations.)

accommodate the enlarging heart. A similar expansion may occur with chronic pericardial effusions, which may exceed 1 L (Fig 12-3). However, the fibrous pericardium cannot adequately stretch acutely, and the rapid accumulation of as little as 200 mL of fluid may produce fatal cardiac tamponade. Hemopericardium may result from perforation or rupture of either the heart or the intrapericardial great vessels (see Fig 12-3).

The serous pericardium is a thin and delicate mesothelial layer that lines not only the inner aspect of the fibrous pericardium (parietal pericardium) but also the outer surface of the heart and the intrapericardial great vessels (visceral pericardium). The visceral serous pericardium covering the heart, the epicardium, contains the coronary arteries and veins, autonomic nerves, lymphatic channels, and variable amounts of adipose tissue; the adipose tissue tends to occupy the atrioventricular (AV), interventricular, and interatrial sulci and the acute margin. The fold of Rindfleisch constitutes a prominent fat tag that covers the right aortic sinus and proximal right coronary artery.[2]

In cachectic states, epicardial depot fat may undergo serous atrophy into small gelatinous tissue tags (Fig 12-4). In obese subjects, excessive epicardial depot fat may encase the heart and

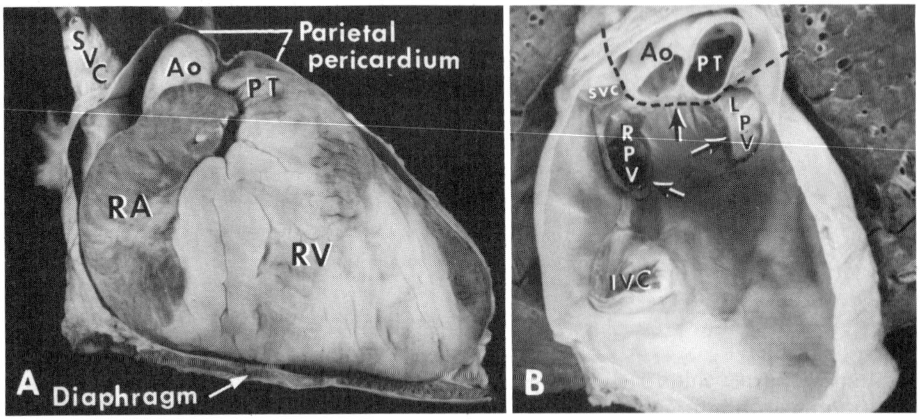

Fig 12-2 Parietal pericardium. **A,** the anterior portion of the parietal pericardium has been removed to show the intrapericardial segments of the great arteries and superior vena cava. (Anterior view from 16-year-old boy.) **B,** the heart has been removed from the posterior portion of the parietal pericardium to show the great vessels, the transverse sinus *(dashed line),* and the oblique sinus *(arrows).* (Anterior view from 13-year-old boy.) (See Appendix for abbreviations.) (**A,** from Edwards WD, Tajik AJ, Seward JB: Standardized nomenclature and anatomic basis for regional tomographic analysis of the heart. *Mayo Clin Proc* 56:479-497, 1981. By permission, Mayo Foundation.)

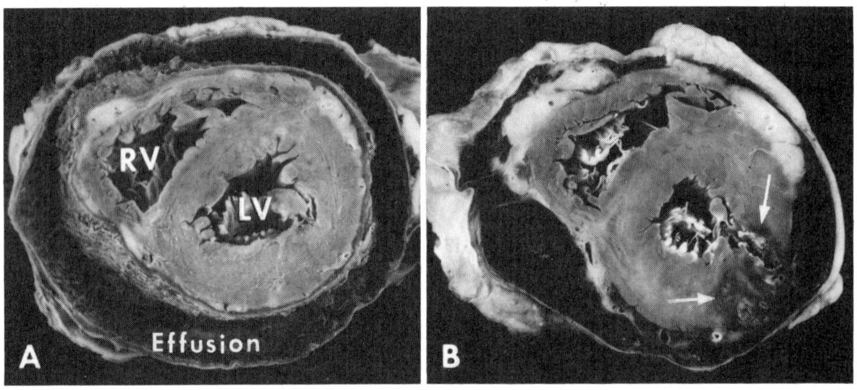

Fig 12-3 Pericardial expansion. **A,** the parietal pericardium has stretched and dilated appreciably with time in this case of chronic pericarditis with a chronic effusion. (Ventricular short-axis view from 61-year-old man.) **B,** in contrast, in this case of acute transmural lateral myocardial infarction (between *arrows*), rupture has produced not only a hemopericardium but also fatal cardiac tamponade because the pericardium could not stretch acutely. (Ventricular short-axis view from 85-year-old man.) (See Appendix for abbreviations.)

may even match the weight of the myocardium (see Fig 12-4); however, since pericardial fat is liquid and easily moldable at body temperature, cardiac motion is generally unhindered. Occasionally, epicardial fat may be misinterpreted tomographically as metastases or ventricular hypertrophy.

Focal epicardial fibrosis along the anterior right ventricle or posterobasal left ventricle (so-called soldiers' patches) may result from old pericarditis or perhaps from the trauma of an enlarged heart's impact against the sternum or calcified descending thoracic aorta.

Along the great vessels, the junction of the visceral and parietal layers forms the pericardial reflection. The reflections along the great veins (venae cavae and pulmonary) are continuous and form an inverted U-shaped posterior cul-de-sac known as the oblique sinus

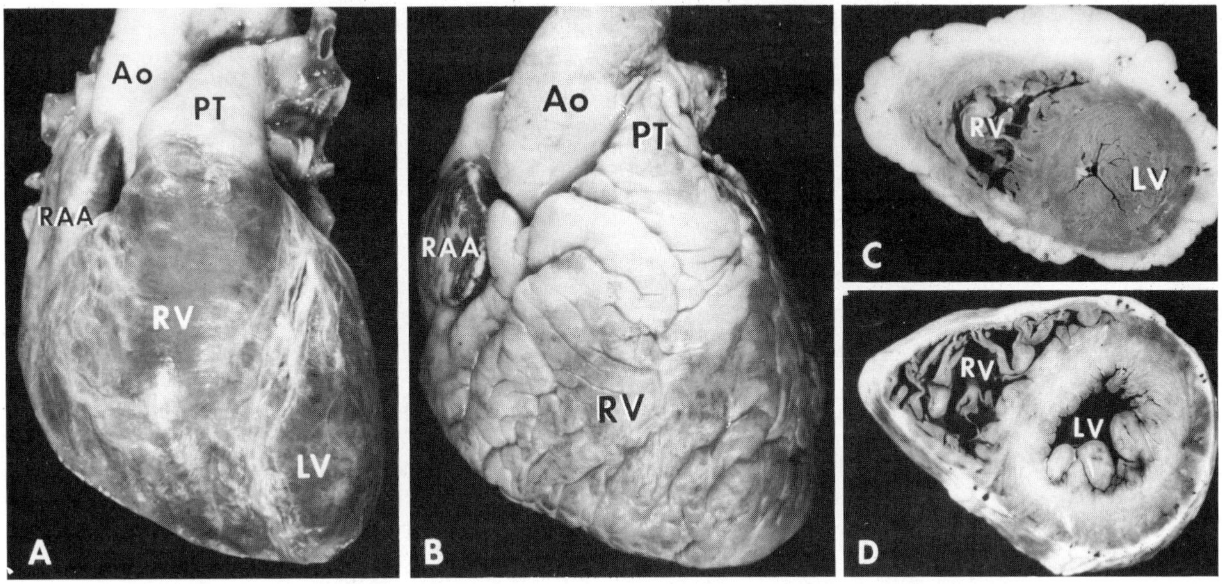

Fig 12-4 Epicardial fat. **A,** marked serous atrophy of epicardial fat, in a case of gastric adenocarcinoma with severe cachexia. (Anterior view from 37-year-old man.) **B,** excessive epicardial fat. (Anterior view from obese 75-year-old woman.) **C,** excessive epicardial fat, approximately 100 g. (Ventricular short-axis view from obese 69-year-old woman.) **D,** normal distribution of epicardial fat, for comparison with **C.** (Ventricular short-axis view from 18-year-old man.) (See Appendix for abbreviations.)

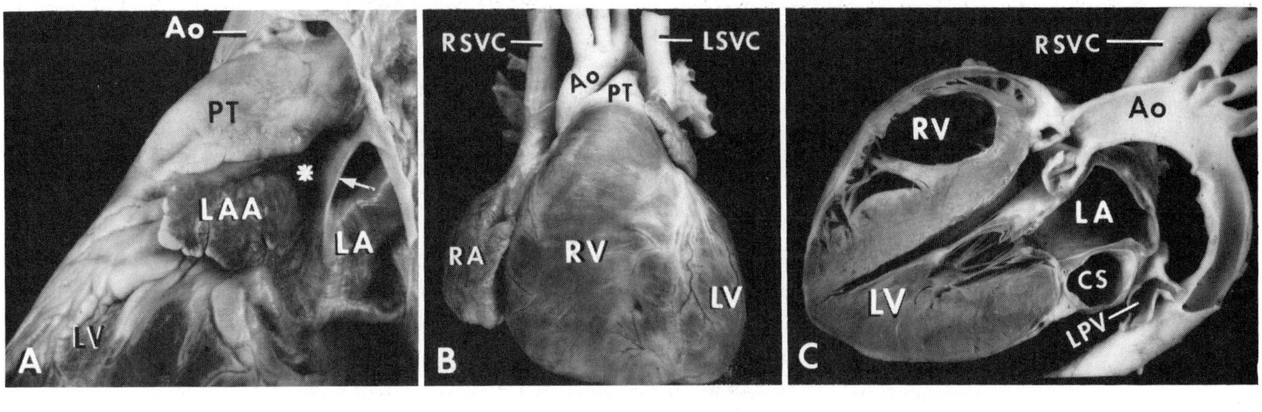

Fig 12-5 Ligament of Marshall. **A,** the ligament of Marshall *(arrow)* lies just posterior to the left border of the transverse sinus (*), and it externally demarcates the level of the orifice of the left atrial appendage. (Left lateral view of the heart and lungs from 27-year-old man.) **B** and **C,** persistent left superior vena cava **(B)** drains into a dilated coronary sinus **(C),** in a case of congenital supravalvular aortic and pulmonary stenoses. By clinical tomography, the dilated coronary sinus may be misinterpreted as the descending thoracic aorta. (Anterior **[B]** and left ventricular-long axis **[C]** views from 5-year-old boy.) (See Appendix for abbreviations.)

(see Fig 12-2). Between the great arteries (aorta and pulmonary trunk) and the atria is a tunnel-like transverse sinus (Figs 12-2 and 12-5). The ligament of Marshall is a pericardial fold that contains the embryonic remnants of the left superior vena cava (see Fig 12-5).

A sequential saphenous vein bypass graft to the left coronary system may be positioned posteriorly through the transverse sinus. In cases of pulmonary atresia, the pulmonary trunk may be hypoplastic, atretic, or absent; at operation, the intrapericardial pulmonary trunk (if present) must lie anterior to a finger or

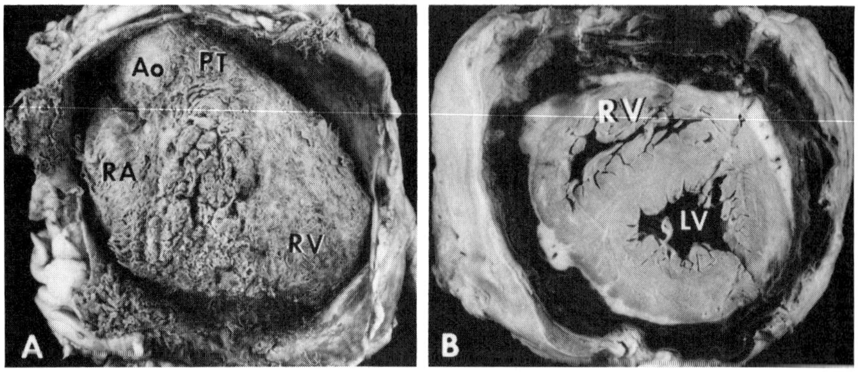

Fig 12-6 Pericarditis. **A,** diffuse fibrinous pericarditis has produced roughened surfaces along the epicardium and parietal pericardium. (Anterior view from 61-year-old man; same patient as in Figure 12-3,A.) **B,** noncalcific constrictive pericarditis due to organization and progressive fibrosis of a chronic fibrinohemorrhagic pericarditis. (Ventricular short-axis view from 36-year-old woman.) (See Appendix for abbreviations.)

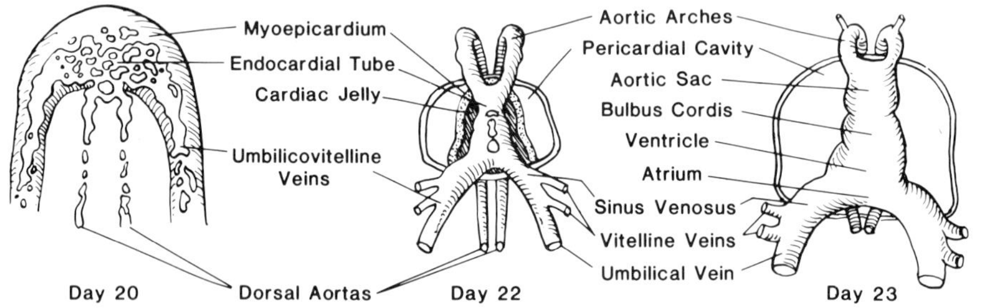

Fig 12-7 Embryology of the heart tube. Fusion of the endocardial tubes forms a midline heart tube, which is surrounded by cardiac jelly and myoepicardium. Dates are approximate. (Modified from Netter FH: Embryology. In *The Ciba Collection of Medical Illustrations. Vol 5, Heart.* Edited by FF Yonkman. Summit, New Jersey, Ciba Pharmaceutical Company, 1969, pp 112-130.)

probe passed through the transverse sinus. When atrial appendages are juxtaposed, the anomalous appendage passes through the transverse sinus. In total anomalous pulmonary venous connection, the oblique and transverse sinuses merge. A persistent left superior vena cava will occupy the expected site of the ligament of Marshall, and conversely, if the ligament of Marshall is identified, a left superior vena cava will not be present.

Between the parietal and visceral layers of the serous pericardium is a potential space, the pericardial cavity, which normally contains 10 to 20 mL of serous fluid. This fluid allows the two tissue surfaces to glide over each other with minimal friction.

The thick and roughened surfaces associated with fibrinous pericarditis (Figs 12-3,A, and 12-6) form the anatomic substrate for the classic auscultatory friction rub, and organization of such an exudate may result in fibrous adhesions between the epicardium and the parietal pericardium. Although focal adhesions are usually unimportant functionally, occasionally they may allow the accumulation of loculated fluid or, rarely, tamponade of an isolated cardiac chamber. After cardiac operation and pericardiotomy, the opened and draining pericardial cavity may become sealed as the parietal pericardium adheres to the sternum; in this setting, the raw pericardial surfaces, which are lined by fibrovascular granulation tissue, may ooze enough blood to produce cardiac tamponade.

Densely fibrotic adhesions, with or without calcification, may hinder cardiac motion and may become progressively restrictive (see Fig 12-6); the pericardium is classically quite thickened in subjects with chronic constriction but not necessarily so in persons with constriction that develops rapidly. In the setting of constrictive pericarditis, surgical excision of only the anterior pericardium (between the phrenic nerves) is often inadequate, since the remaining pericardium surrounds enough of the heart to maintain constriction.

Diffuse postoperative pericardial adhesions are usually functionally unimportant, but they may obscure the location of the coronary arteries at subsequent cardiac operation.

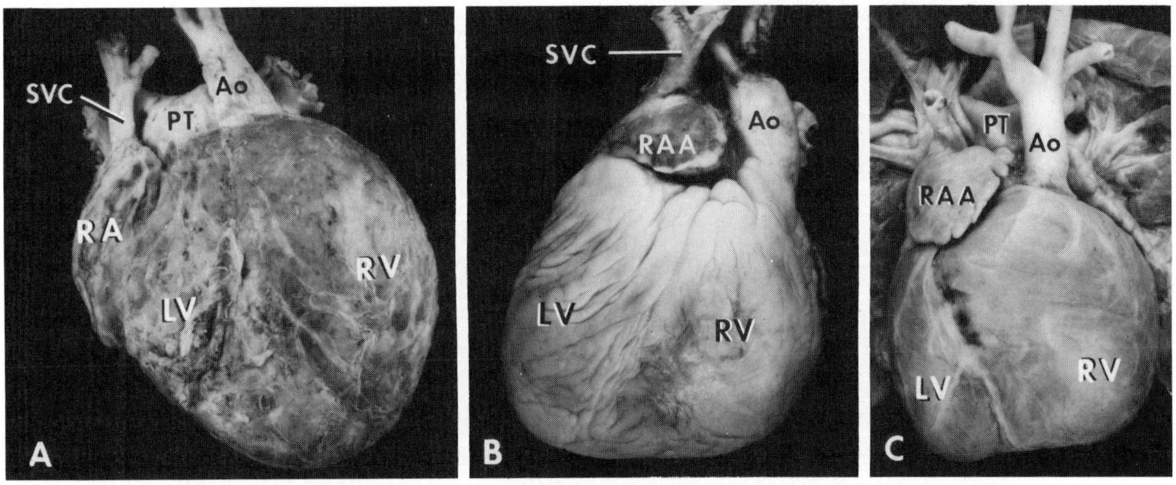

Fig 12-8 Cardiac base-apex axis in three cases of corrected transposition of the great arteries, with AV discordance and left anterior aorta. Anterior view in all. **A,** levocardia (from 19-year-old man). **B,** dextrocardia (from 45-year-old woman). **C,** mesocardia (from 3-month-old girl). (See Appendix for abbreviations.)

Embryology

By the end of the third week (approximately day 20), angiogenic cells from the splanchnopleuric mesoderm form bilateral anterior and posterior clusters of blood islands, which coalesce into a plexus of patent channels containing luminal primitive blood cells.[2] From such channels, bilateral anterior and posterior endothelial tubes develop. These four tubes merge, anterosuperior to the foregut and forebrain, and form the primitive heart tube (Fig 12-7).

The paired anterior endothelial tubes will form the umbilicovitelline veins (umbilicoportal system); the cardinal veins (nonportal systemic veins) will develop later. The paired posterior endothelial tubes will form the aortic arches, paired dorsal aortas, and systemic arteries. The paired endocardial tubes, which are fusing from arterial pole toward venous pole, will form the four-chambered heart.

Posterior to the developing heart tube is a saclike structure, the intraembryonic coelom, which will form the pericardial cavity. As the forebrain expands rapidly, the heart tube and pericardial cavity undergo a 180° flip, which places the heart tube retropericardially. Although the bulboventricular portion soon invaginates and becomes intrapericardial, only later do the atria and sinus venosus attain an intrapericardial position.

The intrapericardial bulboventricular portion of the heart tube contains three layers—namely, a thin luminal endocardium, a thin outer myoepicardial mantle, and an interposed thick layer of amorphous cardiac jelly. The mantle will form not only the epicardium but also the myocardium as cardiac muscle cells infiltrate the cardiac jelly.

The bilateral posterior expansions of the pericardial cavity eventually fuse in the midline to form the dorsal mesocardium. Fenestrations of this tissue result in a tunnel, the transverse sinus, between the future great arteries superiorly and the future atria and great veins inferiorly. The oblique sinus forms as the atria become intrapericardial and as the four pulmonary veins develop.

Congenital cysts or diverticula of the pericardium may form, or the parietal pericardium may be focally deficient or absent. An internally ectopic heart may result from central deficiency of the diaphragm, whereas an externally ectopic heart may result from absence of fusion of the anterior thoracic midline (skin, sternum, and pericardium).

EXTERNAL TOPOGRAPHY

Anatomy

The base of the heart consists of the plane defined by the right and left AV sulci and thereby contains the mitral and tricuspid annuli. The aortic and pulmonary valves are generally depicted in this plane. However, as will be discussed later, the four cardiac valves do not actually lie in the same plane but are somewhat tilted and rotated relative to one another.

The ventricles, being somewhat conical, have a base (at the base of the heart) and an apex. A line drawn from the medial aspect of the AV valve to the ventricular apex defines the base-apex axis of each ventricle. The right and left base-apex axes are normally roughly parallel and are directed leftward, anteriorly, and somewhat inferiorly; this constitutes levocardia (Fig 12-8).

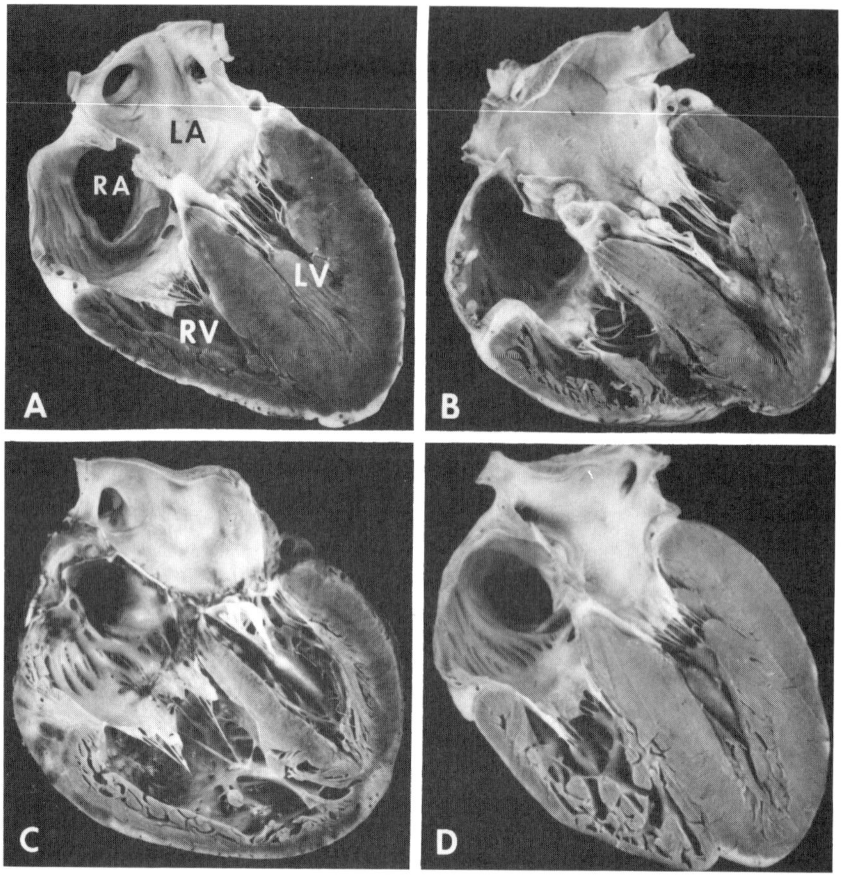

Fig 12-9 Cardiac base-apex length. (Four-chamber view in all.) **A,** equal ventricular lengths (from 21-year-old man). **B,** left ventricular predominance (from 23-year-old man). **C,** right ventricular predominance (from 57-year-old man with a secundum atrial septal defect and right ventricular volume hypertrophy). **D,** biapical heart (from 15-year-old boy). (See Appendix for abbreviations.)

In conditions characterized by an elevated diaphragm (for example, in obesity or the supine position or during infancy), the base-apex axis may be directed more laterally than normal. Similarly, when the diaphragm is lowered (for example, in chronic obstructive pulmonary disease or in a tall, thin subject), the base-apex axis may be directed more inferiorly than normal.

In dextrocardia, the base-apex axis is directed to the right of the midline. In mesocardia, the ventricular mass is often box-shaped, and the base-apex axes are each directed inferiorly and diverge somewhat laterally. Both dextrocardia and mesocardia are usually accompanied by complex congenital heart disease (see Fig 12-8). In some malformed hearts, the right and left base-apex axes are no longer parallel but cross each other and thereby constitute so-called criss-cross hearts.

The left base-apex length is normally greater than the right, such that the left ventricular apex tends to form the major apex of the heart (Fig 12-9). In some normal hearts, but particularly in hearts with prominent right ventricular hypertrophy and dilatation, the right ventricle may form the major cardiac apex. In rare instances, two distinct ventricular apices are present and form a bifid apex. In levocardia, the cardiac apex occupies the midclavicular line at the fourth or fifth intercostal space. However, the clinical point of maximal impulse usually corresponds to the anteroseptal region of the left ventricle rather than to the true cardiac apex.

Between the cardiac chambers are three prominent grooves, or sulci, which are usually filled with epicardial fat (Fig 12-10). The right and left AV sulci delineate atria from ventricles and thereby indicate the levels of the mitral and tricuspid annuli and the course of the right and circumflex coronary arteries. The anterior and inferior interventricular sulci delineate the junction of right and left ventricular free walls, the plane of the ventricular septum, and the course of the anterior descending and posterior (inferior) descending coronary arteries. The interatrial sulcus defines the plane of the atrial septum and the junction of right and left atrial free walls. The crux

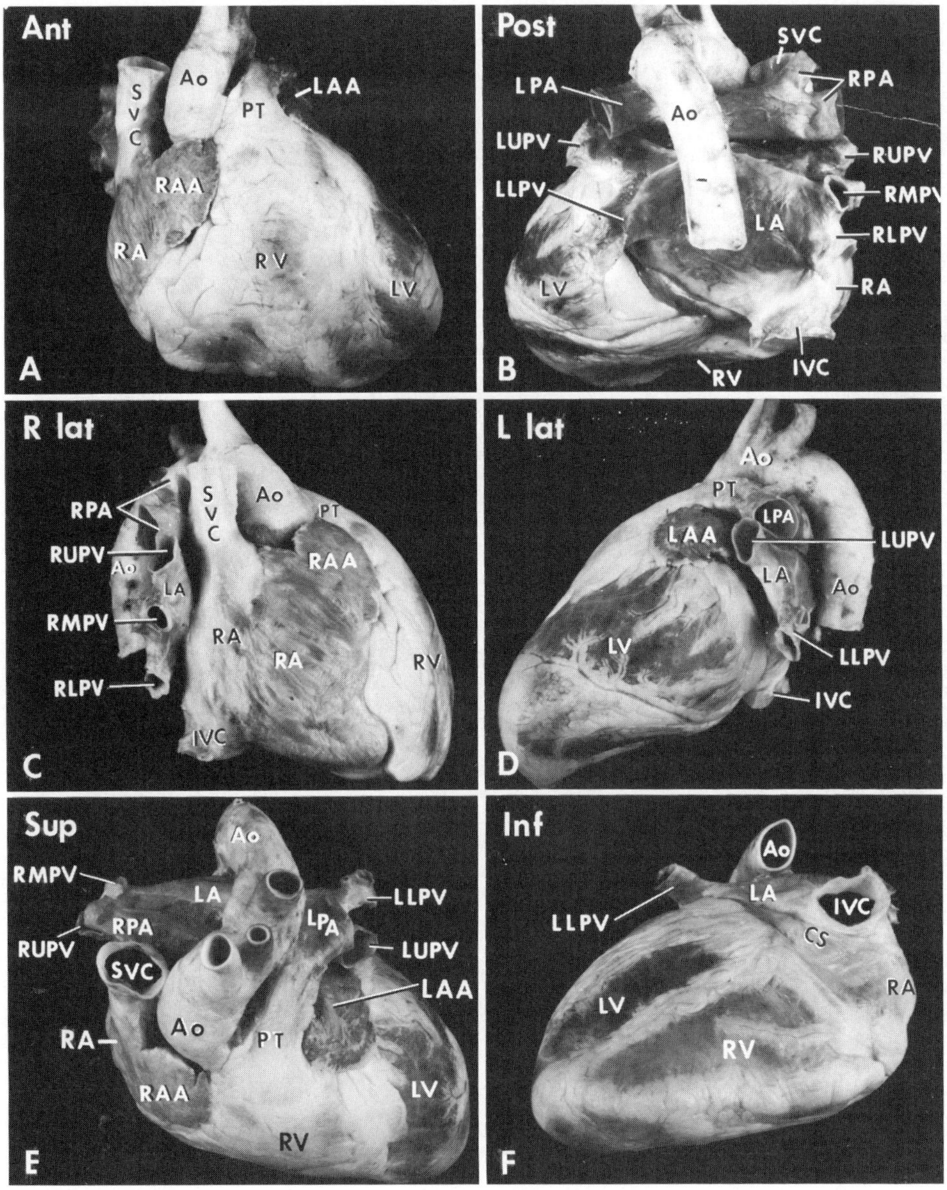

Fig 12-10 External views of the heart and great vessels (from 32-year-old man). **A,** anterior. **B,** posterior. **C,** right lateral. **D,** left lateral. **E,** superior. **F,** inferior.

Continued.

cordis (cross of the heart) is an external landmark along the inferior cardiac surface, which is formed by the intersection of the AV, interatrial, and interventricular sulci (see Fig 12-10); this landmark is used in the definition of coronary artery dominance.

The junction between the anterosuperior and inferior surfaces of the right ventricle forms a rather sharp angle, the acute margin of the heart, which is heavily invested with epicardial fat and contains a prominent marginal branch of the right coronary artery. The rounded lateral wall of the left ventricle forms an ill-defined obtuse margin, which normally contains the obtuse marginal branch of the circumflex coronary artery. The superiorly oriented anterobasal surface of the left ventricle is commonly referred to as the left shoulder of the heart, whereas the junctional angle between the acute margin and the right AV sulcus forms the right shoulder of the heart. The anteriorly bulging right ventricular outflow tract constitutes the conus, or infundibulum, of the heart.

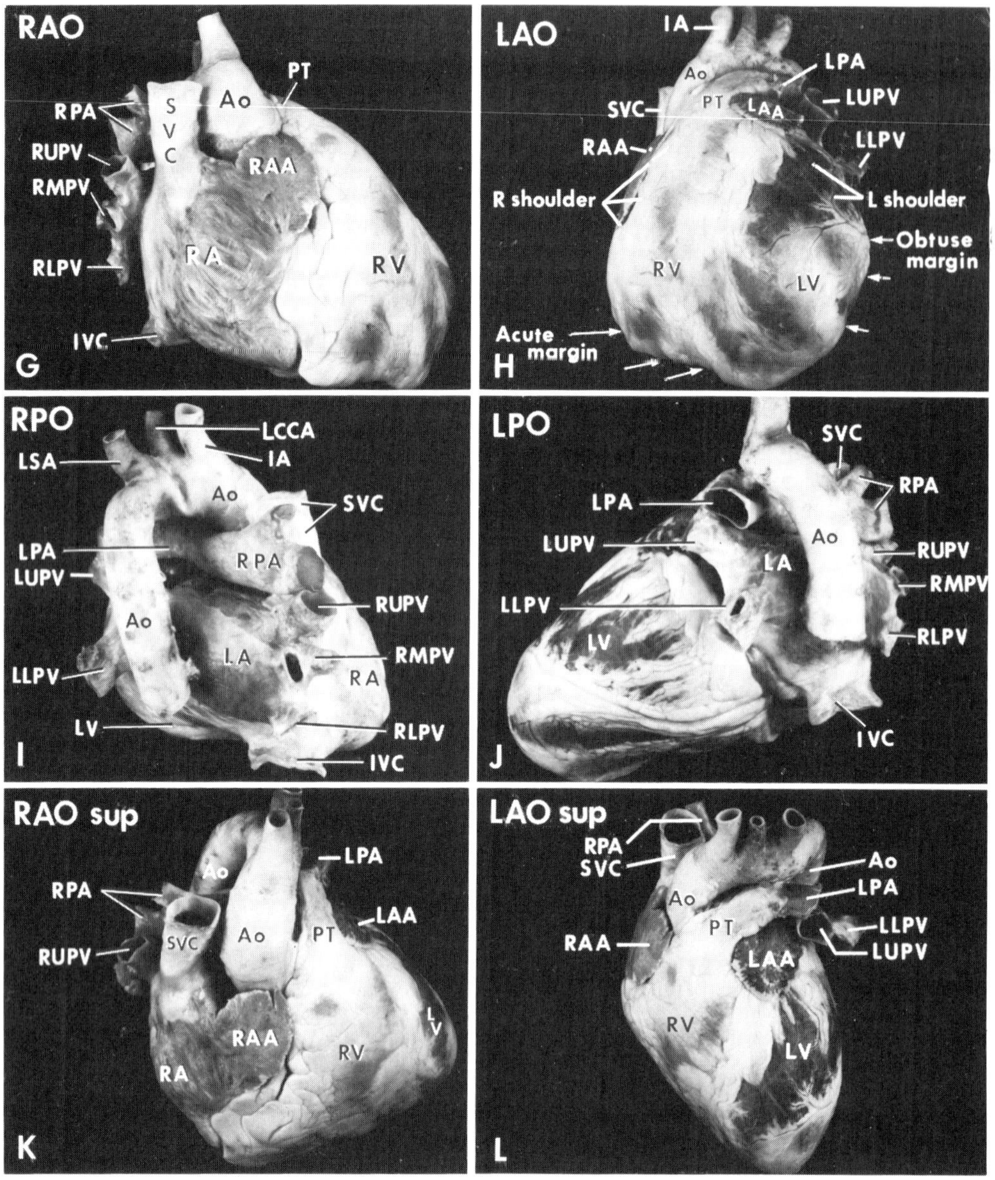

Fig 12-10, cont'd **G,** right anterior oblique. **H,** left anterior oblique. **I,** right posterior oblique. **J,** left posterior oblique. **K,** right anterior oblique with superior (cranial) angulation. **L,** left anterior oblique with superior (cranial) angulation. (See Appendix for abbreviations.)

As the external cardiac surface is examined by a surgeon or pathologist, identification of the cardiac sulci and margins is useful not only for determining the position of the epicardial coronary arteries but also for determining relative chamber size and the expected position of internal cardiac structures.

To understand and properly interpret the various cardiac imaging modalities, one must appreciate not only the normal size and shape of the cardiac chambers and great vessels but also their relative positions in three-dimensional space (see Fig 12-10). The superior and inferior venae cavae lie to the right of the midline, and the right atrium is therefore a right lateral chamber. In contrast, the left atrium is a midline posterior chamber, and the right and left pairs of pulmonary veins are similar in length. The atria are located slightly superiorly relative to the ventricles. The right ventricle is a right anterior chamber, whereas the left ventricle is a left posterior chamber. The aorta arises posteriorly, inferiorly, and to the right of the pulmonary trunk. The cardiac apex is directed leftward, anteriorly, and somewhat inferiorly, and the planes of the ventricular and atrial septa are likewise directed leftward and anteriorly. The plane of the cardiac base is roughly perpendicular to the base-apex axis.

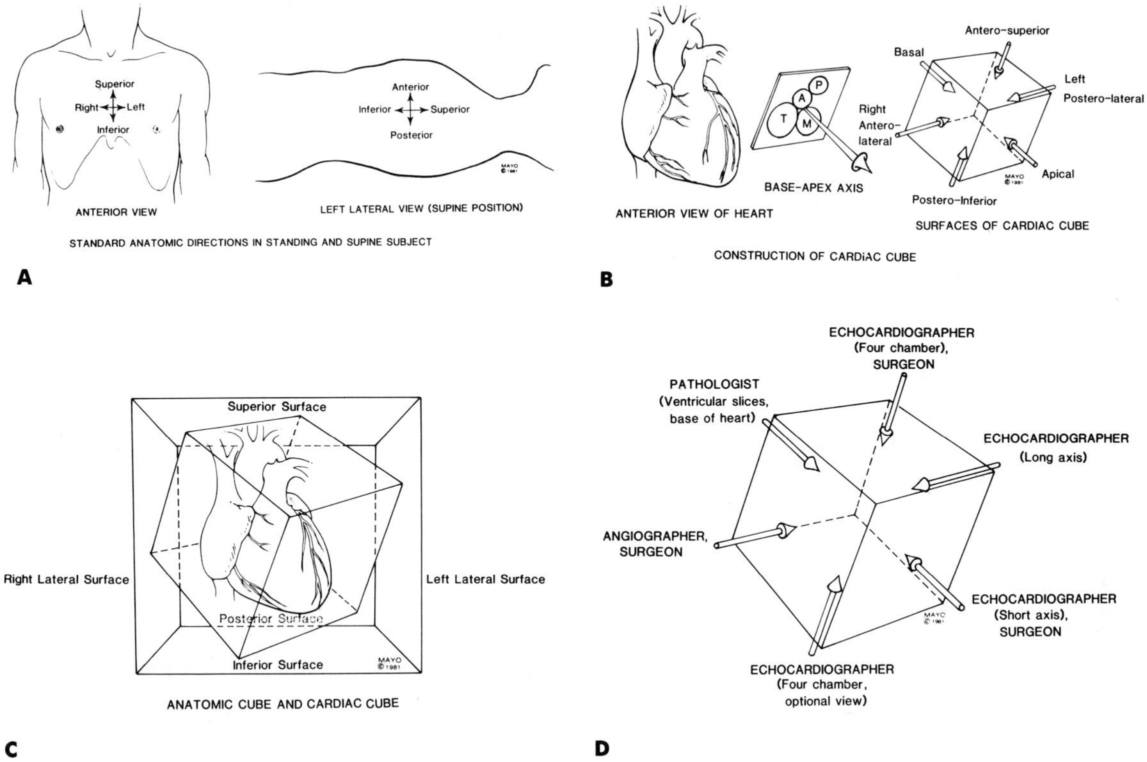

Fig 12-11 Three-dimensional orientation of the heart in the chest. **A,** anatomic directions are always assigned relative to the patient and not relative to the observer. **B,** the cardiac base contains the four cardiac valves (*A,* aortic; *M,* mitral; *P,* pulmonary; *T,* tricuspid). From this plane, one may construct not only the base-apex axis but also the cardiac cube. **C,** the six surfaces of the cardiac cube do not conform to any of the standard anatomic planes. **D,** however, various subspecialists commonly view the heart from the perspective of the cardiac cube rather than the anatomic cube. Any accurate system of cardiac nomenclature must recognize the incongruity of the anatomic and cardiac cubes. (From Edwards WD, Tajik AJ, Seward JB: Standardized nomenclature and anatomic basis for regional tomographic analysis of the heart. *Mayo Clin Proc* 56:479-497, 1981. By permission, Mayo Foundation.)

In the past, cardiac anatomic nomenclature was established by viewing hearts that had been removed from the chest and oriented like a valentine—that is, placed on apex with atria atop and rotated such that the ventricular septum assumed a mid-sagittal plane. This has led to much confusion concerning the orientation and proper terminology of cardiac structures in the living patient.[1] Contributing to this confusion is the fact that the surfaces of the heart fail to conform to any of the standard anatomic planes (Fig 12-11).

Since the ventricular mass is roughly conical and its apex is skewed, and since the ventricular surfaces do not conform well to the standard anatomic planes, the surfaces of the ventricular free walls are difficult and cumbersome to label with accurate anatomic terms. The diaphragmatic ventricular surface is directed primarily inferiorly and is best considered the inferior wall. However, the portion at the cardiac base which is directed more posteriorly could accurately be considered the posterobasal or posterior surface. Although the lateral ventricular walls are actually right anterolateral and left posterolateral surfaces, these are commonly referred to simply as right and left lateral walls. The remaining ventricular surface, the anterosuperior wall (directed anteriorly near the apex and superiorly at the base), is commonly called the anterior wall. It is hoped that the use of this somewhat simplified anatomic terminology to describe complex cardiac surfaces will not lead to confusion concerning the actual position of the heart or individual cardiac chambers within the living patient.

The weight of the adult human heart averages 325 ± 100 g in men and 275 ± 100 g in women. In the adult, heart weight varies with age, gender, and body size (Fig A12-1).[8] In athletic young adults, the heart weight may approach or exceed slightly the upper limit of normal, whereas in the elderly it may approach or fall slightly below the lower limit of normal. Age-related changes in the cardiac weight and other cardiac measurements have been recorded for fetuses, infants, children, and adolescents.[9]

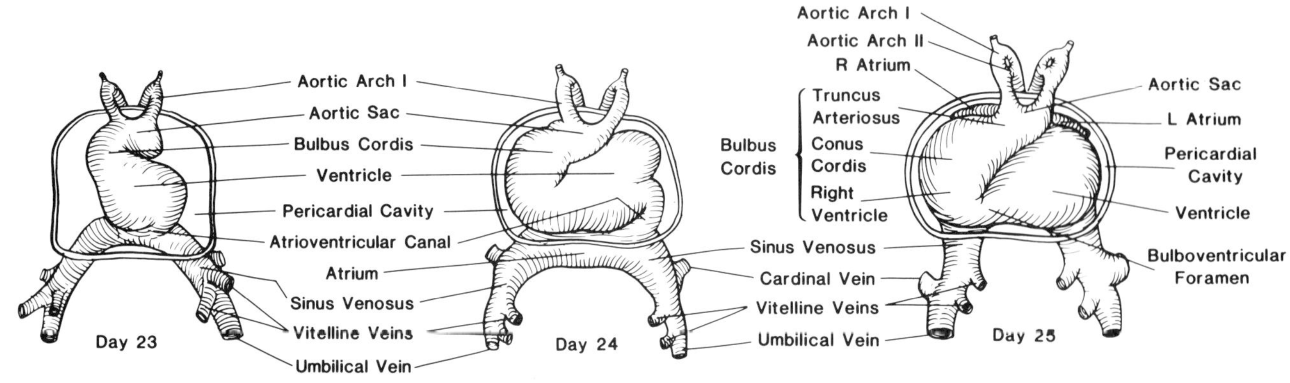

Fig 12-12 Embryology of the heart loop. Rightward looping of the heart tube results in an asymmetric heart in which the ventricles occupy a position similar to that in the adult. Dates are approximate. (Modified from Netter FH: Embryology. In *The Ciba Collection of Medical Illustrations, Vol. 5, Heart.* Edited by FF Yonkman. Summit, New Jersey, Ciba Pharmaceutical Company, 1969, pp 112-130.)

Embryology

By approximately day 23, the heart tube begins to beat, and during the next 2 days the intrapericardial bulboventricular portion, which is anchored at its atrial pole proximally and its aortic pole distally, bends rightward and twists anteriorly (dextro-looping, or D-looping); this complex and incompletely understood process is critically important for the proper positioning of the future ventricles (Fig 12-12). Accordingly, within the bulboventricular loop, the ventricle, which will form the left ventricle, lies posterior and leftward, as in the adult heart. Similarly, the bulbus cordis, which will develop into the right ventricle and infundibulum (conotruncus), is a right anterior structure, analogous to the adult heart. When the atria later become intrapericardial, they will migrate and expand posterosuperiorly and thereby also occupy a position similar to that in the adult heart.

Following the direction of blood flow, the heart loop comprises bilateral sinus venosi and atria, AV canal, ventricle, bulboventricular foramen, bulbus cordis (primitive right ventricle and conus cordis), truncus arteriosus, aortic sac, and bilateral aortic arches and dorsal aortas. The once symmetric heart tube has now become an asymmetric heart loop (see Figs 12-7 and 12-12). As the AV canal, bulboventricular foramen, and conotruncal region shift medially and align with one another, subsequent septation of the atria, ventricles, and conotruncus will produce a four-chambered heart.

The organs that occupy the thoracoabdominal body cavities begin embryologic development as symmetric midline structures but later become asymmetric. As asymmetry is achieved, these organs acquire handedness, or chirality, which may be expressed in terms of situs.[10] Situs solitus implies normal asymmetry, whereas situs inversus designates mirror-image asymmetry. Situs ambiguus describes either indeterminate situs or symmetric situs (for example, bilateral right-sidedness [right isomerism] or bilateral left-sidedness [left isomerism]; these are commonly associated with asplenia and polysplenia syndromes, respectively).

Situs appears to be genetically determined, and abnormalities thereof may affect the entire body (situs inversus totalis) or individual organ systems; accordingly, the situs of the cardiovascular, respiratory, and digestive systems should be stated separately. For example, a person with polysplenia may have indeterminate cardiac situs ambiguus, left pulmonary isomerism, and abdominal situs inversus.

Cardiac situs is based on atrial situs. Thus, the ventricular base-apex axis does not determine cardiac situs. For example, dextrocardia does not imply situs inversus, and levocardia does not necessarily imply situs solitus. However, nonatrial cardiac segments may have abnormal situs (they just are not used in determining the general *cardiac* situs).[10] For example, leftward looping of the heart tube (levo- or L-loop) results in ventricular situs inversus (ventricular inversion) and is most commonly associated with corrected transposition of the great arteries (see Fig 12-8).

GREAT VEINS

Superior vena cava

The bilateral internal jugular veins, which lie anterolateral to the common carotid arteries, and the bilateral subclavian veins, which travel anteroinferiorly to their respective arteries (separated by the anterior scalene muscles), merge to form bilateral innominate (brachiocephalic) veins. Their junction is usually guarded by venous valves.[11] The innominate veins then enter the thoracic cage at the level of the first rib, posterior to the sternoclavicular joint. The left innominate vein is twice to thrice the length of the right innominate vein and lies along the anterosuperior aspect of the aortic arch and its brachiocephalic branches (Figs 12-13 and 12-14). Each of the innominate veins receives a pericardiophrenic and a mammary (internal thoracic) vein, and the left also receives the inferior thyroid vein.

The innominate veins merge to form the superior vena cava, which lies adjacent to the right posterolateral aspect of the proximal ascending aorta and the anterior surface of the right pulmonary artery. The azygos vein arches over the right bronchus and joins the superior vena cava posteriorly. The superior vena cava drains into the superior aspect of the right atrium, and approximately one-third to one-half of its length is intrapericardial (see

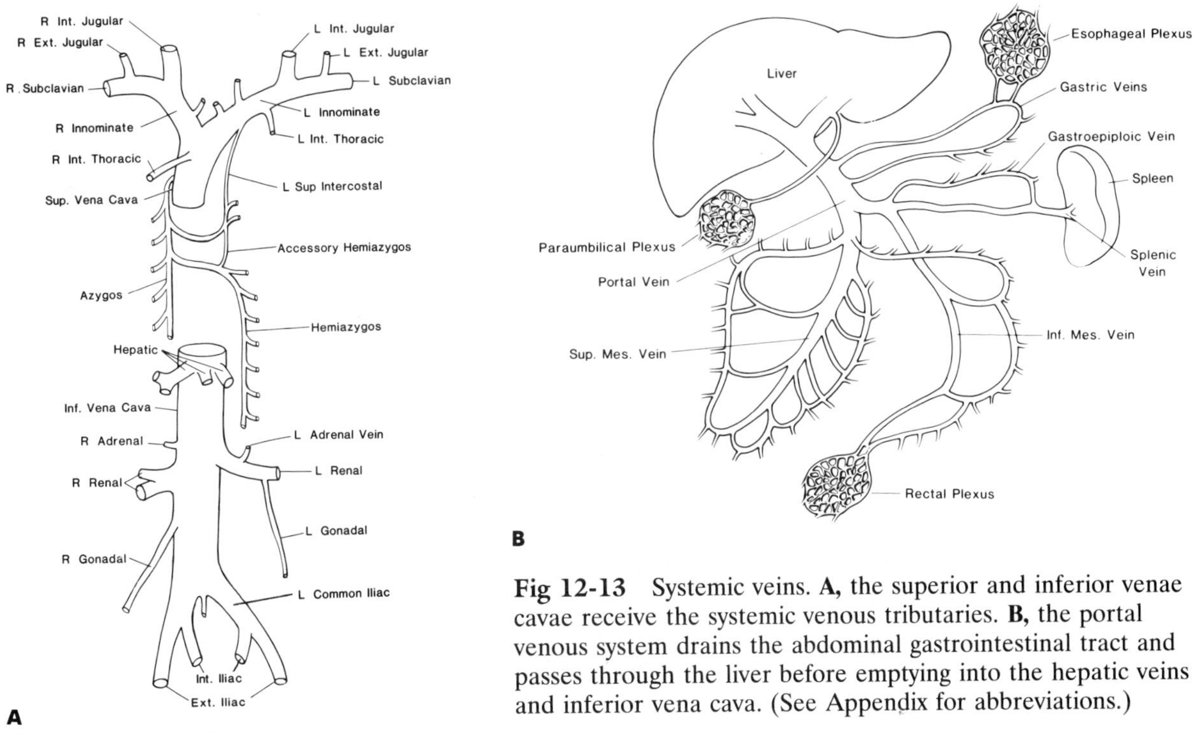

Fig 12-13 Systemic veins. **A,** the superior and inferior venae cavae receive the systemic venous tributaries. **B,** the portal venous system drains the abdominal gastrointestinal tract and passes through the liver before emptying into the hepatic veins and inferior vena cava. (See Appendix for abbreviations.)

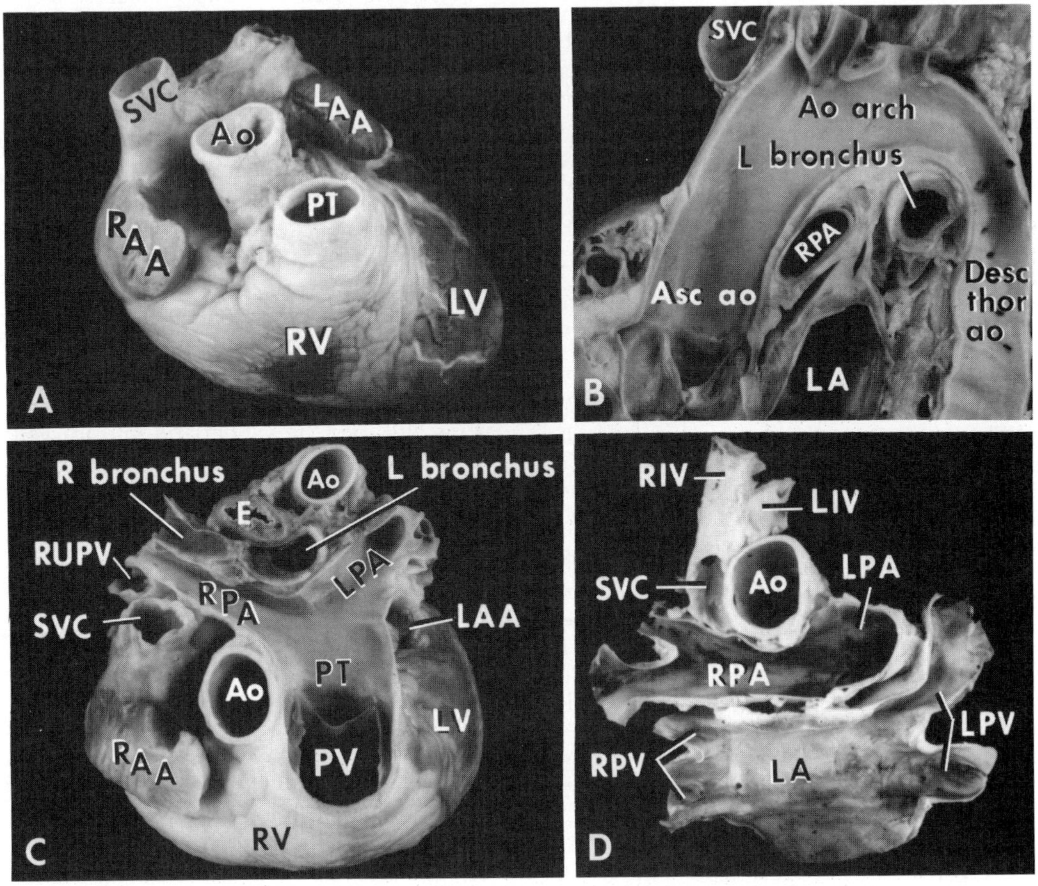

Fig 12-14 Interrelationships of the great vessels. **A,** the superior vena cava, ascending aorta, and pulmonary trunk align in the direction of the base-apex axis, and the right and left atrial appendages embrace the great arteries. (Anterosuperior view from 75-year-old woman.) **B,** the aortic arch travels over the right pulmonary artery, left bronchus, and left atrium. (Left ventricular long-axis view from 15-year-old boy.) **C,** the right pulmonary artery travels under the aortic arch, posterior to the superior vena cava and anterior to the right bronchus. (Superior view of transverse section from 24-year-old woman.) **D,** the right pulmonary artery travels between the aortic arch and the left atrium. (Frontal section from 23-year-old man.) (See Appendix for abbreviations.)

Fig 12-2). As a right lateral structure, it contributes to the right superior border of the frontal cardiac silhouette roentgenographically.

The right internal jugular vein, right innominate vein, and superior vena cava afford a short and relatively straight intravascular route to the right atrium and tricuspid orifice; accordingly, this route may be used for passage of the rather stiff endomyocardial bioptome across the tricuspid valve and into the right ventricular apex. Both temporary and permanent transvenous pacemaker leads are generally inserted into the subclavian veins and are threaded into the right ventricular apex. Right-sided pressure-monitoring catheters may be inserted via either the subclavian or the internal jugular vein.

Catheters and pacemakers within the innominate veins and superior vena cava rather quickly become partially coated with thrombus and may be associated with thrombotic venous obstruction, pulmonary thromboembolism, or secondary infection. Mediastinal neoplasms, fibrosis, and aortic aneurysms may compress the thin-walled veins and result in the superior vena caval syndrome.

Inferior vena cava

The inferior vena cava receives systemic venous drainage from the legs and retroperitoneal viscera and, at the level of the liver, from the intra-abdominal systemic venous drainage (portal circulation) via the hepatic veins (see Fig 12-13). The portal circulation ensures that most ingested substances will be metabolized by the liver before gaining access to the remainder of the body. The suprahepatic inferior vena cava is only 1 to 3 cm long and, after traversing the diaphragm, joins the inferior surface of the right atrium. The vertebral venous plexus drains into the intracranial veins, portal system, and intercostal, lumbar, and lateral sacral veins, rather than directly into the inferior vena cava. Accordingly, metastases or infections may spread to the vertebral bodies or central nervous system via this venous plexus.

The inferior vena cava, which is retroperitoneal, may become trapped and compressed between the vertebral column posteriorly and either an adjacent retroperitoneal structure (for example, an abdominal aortic aneurysm) or an intraperitoneal structure (for example, a neoplasm) and thereby produce the inferior vena caval syndrome.

Venous thrombi in the lower extremities may extend into the inferior vena cava or may become dislodged and embolize to the right heart and pulmonary circulation. Renal cell carcinomas may extend intravascularly within the renal veins and inferior vena cava and may even form tethered intracavitary right-sided cardiac masses. Hepatocellular carcinomas often involve the hepatic veins and occasionally may enter the suprahepatic inferior vena cava or right atrium. Nonobstructive carcinoid plaques may also involve the hepatic veins and suprahepatic inferior vena cava.

Pulmonary veins

The superior and inferior pulmonary veins from each lung join the posterolateral aspects of the midline left atrium (see Fig 12-14). Occasionally, a middle lobe pulmonary vein from the right lung may enter the left atrium separately, whereas in other subjects the superior and inferior pulmonary veins, particularly on the left, may merge and join the left atrium as a single vein. The right and left inferior pulmonary veins are similar in length and travel along the inferior border of the right and left bronchi, respectively. The right and left superior pulmonary veins are likewise similar in length but travel anteriorly to their respective bronchi and, at the pulmonary hilus, are anterior to the right intermediate pulmonary artery and left main pulmonary artery, respectively. Owing to the anterior course of the superior pulmonary veins and the posterior course of the pulmonary arteries (moving from heart to hilus), the veins are posterior to the arteries at the level of the left atrium and anterior to the arteries at the level of the pulmonary hilus.

The proximal 1 to 3 cm of the pulmonary veins contain cardiac muscle within the media and may thereby function somewhat like sphincters during atrial systole as well as when significant mitral valve disease exists.

The rather thin-walled and low-pressure pulmonary veins may be compressed extrinsically by mediastinal neoplasms or fibrosis. Rarely, a primary neoplasm may cause luminal obstruction in the major pulmonary veins.

Embryology

Systemic veins. By approximately day 25, the paired sinus venosus segments have fused and they then comprise a transverse midportion and lateral extensions (right and left sinus horns). The lateral extensions receive drainage from three bilateral venous systems: (1) the vitelline (omphalomesenteric) veins, (2) the umbilical (allantoic) veins, and (3) the cardinal veins.

The umbilicovitelline systems will form the umbilical vein, ductus venosus, entire portal venous system, hepatic veins, and suprahepatic inferior vena cava, and the cardinal system will form the remainder of the systemic veins. The anterior cardinal veins will give rise to the superior vena cava and its tributaries, and the extensions of the posterior cardinal veins (supra-, sub-, and sacrocardinal) will develop into the azygos and hemiazygos veins and into the subhepatic inferior vena cava and its tributaries (Fig 12-15).

The right sinus horn, a vertical structure, will form the smooth-walled intercaval posterior wall of the right atrium. The transverse midportion and the proximal left sinus horn will develop into the coronary sinus, whereas the distal left sinus horn (left superior vena cava) will be represented only by the ligament of Marshall and the left atrial coronary vein.

At the sinoatrial junction, the right and left venous valves develop and merge superiorly to form the septum spurium. Inferiorly, the left venous valve fuses to the atrial septum, but the right venous valve forms the valves of the inferior vena cava and the coronary sinus.

Congenital anomalies of the systemic veins include a persistent left superior vena cava (with or without a left innominate vein) joining the coronary sinus (see Fig 12-5) or, rarely, the left atrium; an unroofed or absent coronary sinus; a large right sinus venosus valve (so-called cor triatriatum dexter); azygos continuity of the inferior vena cava; and bilateral subrenal inferior venae cavae.

In the setting of advanced cirrhosis, dilated paraumbilical venous channels may allow the egress of portal blood into the

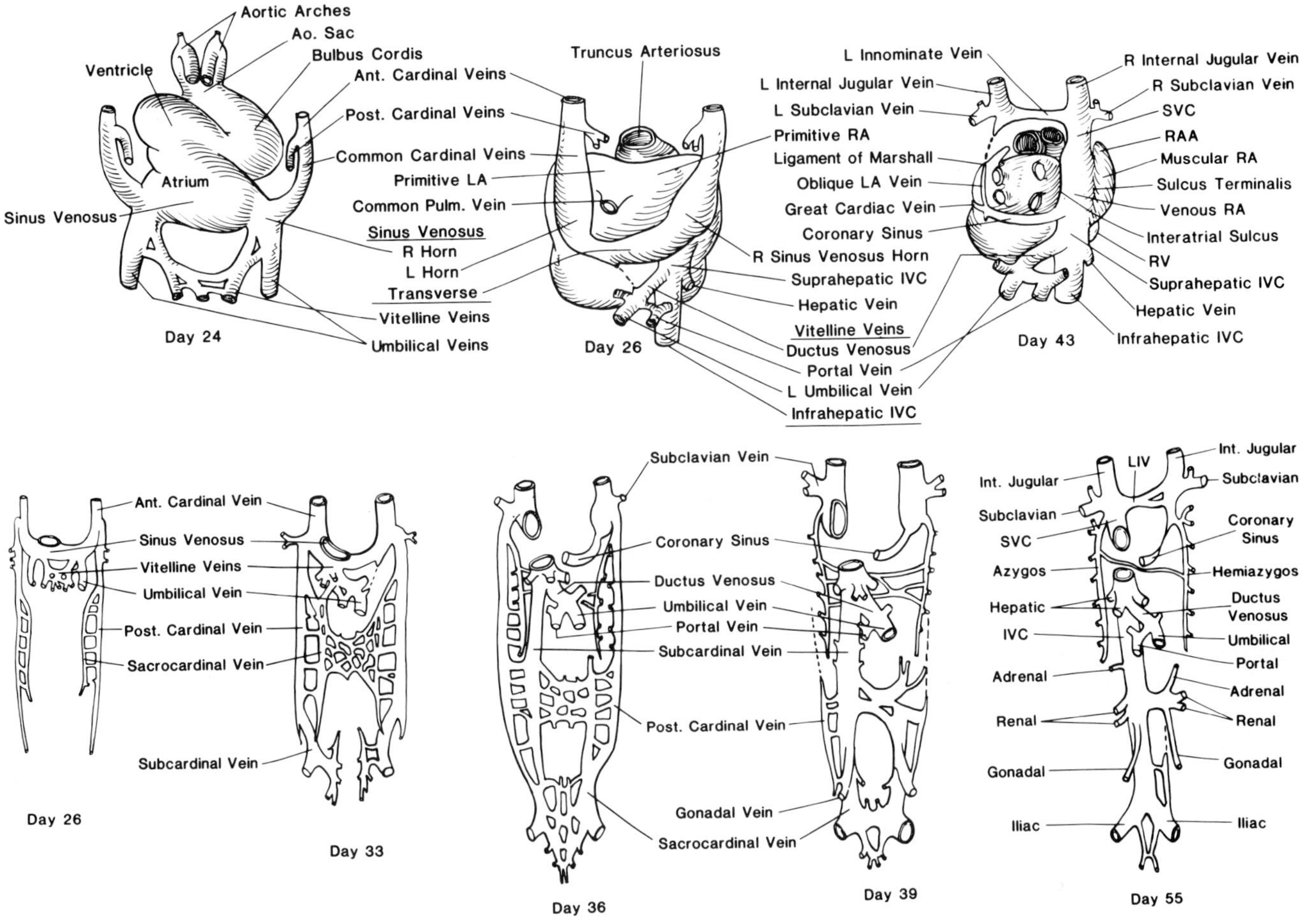

Fig 12-15 Embryology of the systemic veins. **Upper,** posterior view. The sinus venosus forms the posterior right atrial free wall, the coronary sinus, and the ligament of Marshall. **Lower,** anterior view. The umbilicovitelline system forms the umbilical vein, ductus venosus, and hepatoportal venous system, and the cardinal system forms the remainder of the systemic veins. Dates are approximate. (See Appendix for abbreviations.) (Modified from Netter FH: Embryology. In *The Ciba Collection of Medical Illustrations, Vol. 5, Heart.* Edited by FF Yonkman. Summit, New Jersey, Ciba Pharmaceutical Company, 1969, pp 112-130.)

systemic venous system. The resulting tortuous and dilated subcutaneous paraumbilical veins may form the classic caput medusae.

Pulmonary veins. The lung buds, like the remainder of the foregut, initially receive systemic arterial blood and have systemic venous drainage (into the cardinal and umbilicovitelline venous systems). By day 26, the common pulmonary vein develops as an evagination of the posterior left atrial wall and, by day 29, anastomoses with the systemic (splanchnic) plexus of pulmonary veins. At this time, venous drainage from the developing lungs may be via the systemic veins or the common pulmonary vein (Fig 12-16). However, during the next 4 days, the systemic venous channels from the lungs tend to disappear, and by day 33, pulmonary venous drainage is almost exclusively to the left atrium. As the common pulmonary vein dilates and becomes incorporated into the body of the left atrium, it forms the large, smooth-walled portion of this chamber.

In total anomalous pulmonary venous connection, the confluence of pulmonary veins does not join the left atrium but rather maintains connection to derivatives of the cardinal or umbilicovitelline veins, such as the left innominate vein, coronary sinus, or ductus venosus. An interatrial communication must also be present.

In partial anomalous pulmonary venous connection, only some veins (usually from the right lung) lack left atrial connections. Connection of the right pulmonary veins to the right atrium commonly accompanies sinus venosus atrial septal defects, whereas connection of these veins to the suprahepatic inferior vena cava is usually part of the scimitar syndrome.

Cor triatriatum (sinistrum) results when the junction between common pulmonary vein and left atrium is stenotic. A fenestrated membranous or muscular shelf subdivides the left atrium into a posterosuperior chamber, which receives the pulmonary veins, and an anteroinferior chamber, which contains the atrial appendage and mitral orifice.

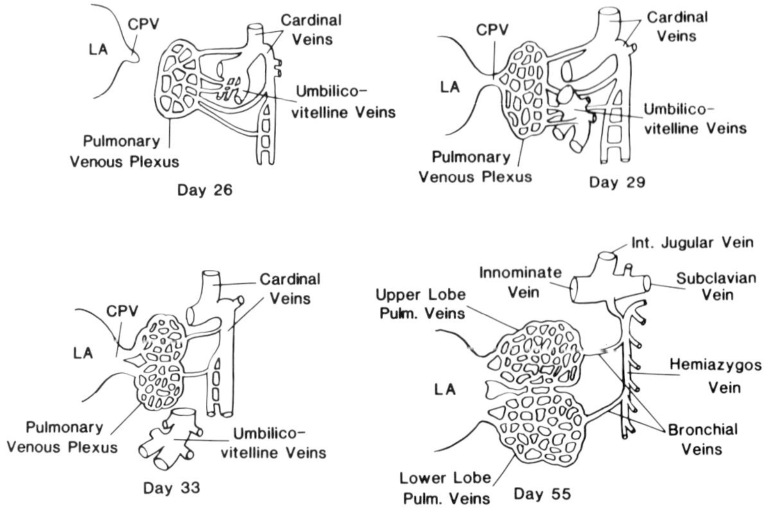

Fig 12-16 Embryology of the pulmonary veins (schematic, left lateral view). Although the pulmonary venous plexus initially drains into the systemic (cardinal and umbilicovitelline) veins, it soon attains left atrial drainage as the common pulmonary vein *(CPV)* anastomoses with this plexus. Later, the systemic venous connections wither and either disappear or persist as bronchial veins, and the common pulmonary vein expands greatly to form most of the left atrial free wall. Dates are approximate.

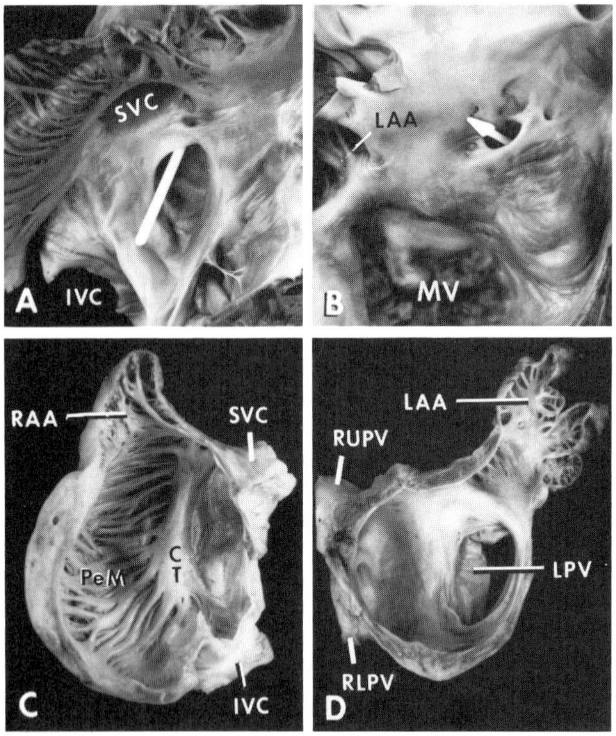

Fig 12-17 Comparison of atria. **A** and **B,** a probe in the patent foramen ovale passes from the right atrium **(A)** to the left atrium **(B).** (Opened atria from 85-year-old man.) The right atrial free wall **(C)** is muscular and contains the crista terminalis and pectinate muscles, whereas the left atrial free wall **(D)** is smooth like a vein. (Excised atrial free walls from 26-year-old woman.) (See Appendix for abbreviations.) (**A** and **B,** from Hagen PT, Scholz DG, Edwards WD: Incidence and size of patent foramen ovale during the first 10 decades of life: an autopsy study of 965 normal hearts. *Mayo Clin Proc* 59:17-20, 1984. By permission, Mayo Foundation.)

ATRIA

Right atrium

The right atrium is a right posterolateral chamber (see Fig 12-10) that, along with the superior vena cava, forms the right lateral border of the frontal cardiac silhouette roentgenographically. It receives the systemic venous return from the superior and inferior venae cavae and receives most of the coronary venous return via the coronary sinus and numerous small thebesian veins. No valvular tissue guards the orifice of the superior vena cava. However, the ostium of the inferior vena cava is bordered anteriorly by a crescentic eustachian valve, which may be large and fenestrated and form a so-called Chiari net. The coronary sinus ostium is partly shielded by a fenestrated thebesian valve. These two valves share a common commissure. From the right atrium, systemic venous blood is expelled across the tricuspid orifice and into the right ventricle. The right atrium consists of free wall and septum.

The right atrial free wall has a smooth-walled (sinus venarum) posterior portion, which receives the venae cavae and coronary sinus, and a muscular lateral portion, which contains a large pyramidal atrial appendage (auricle). These two regions are separated externally by the sulcus terminalis (sulcus intercavarum) and internally by a prominent C-shaped ridge of muscle, the crista terminalis (Fig 12-17). Numerous parallel pectinate muscles arise from this muscle ridge and course anteriorly ("pectinatus" is Latin for comb; the crista terminalis and pectinate muscles may be considered the backbone and teeth of the comb, respectively). The right atrial appendage is large and contains irregular pectinate muscles (the largest of which is the taenia sagittalis); the appendage abuts the right aortic sinus and overlies the proximal right coronary artery. The posterior aortic sinus produces a bulge, the torus aorticus, along the superomedial aspect of the right atrial free wall. Myocytes, particularly those in the right atrium, not only conduct impulses and contract but also serve an endocrine role, with the production and

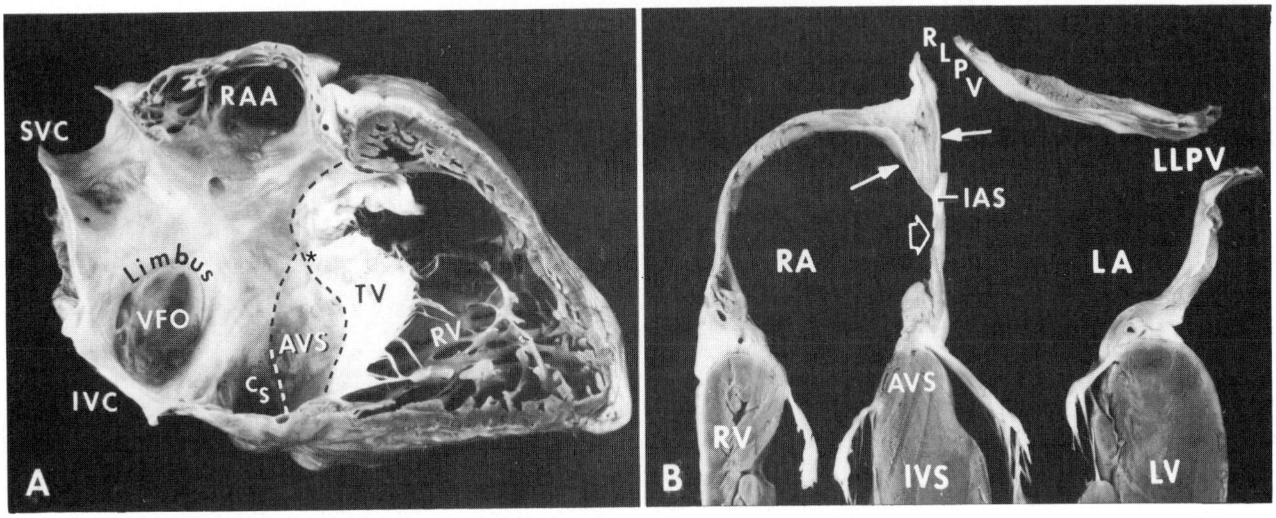

Fig 12-18 Atrioventricular septum. **A,** the AV septum lies between the tricuspid and mitral annuli *(dashed lines),* from the level of the membranous septum (°) to the coronary sinus ostium, and thereby separates the right atrium from the left ventricle. (Right two-chamber view from 56-year-old man.) **B,** the AV septum lies anterior to the interatrial septum and posterior to the interventricular septum; note also the infolded nature of the limbus *(arrow)* and the relative thinness of the valve of the fossa ovalis *(open arrow).* (Four-chamber view from 15-year-old boy.) (See Appendix for abbreviations.)

release of atrial natriuretic factor, which affects total blood volume.[12]

The thickness of the right atrial free wall varies considerably. Although the sinus venarum is rarely thicker than 1 mm, the crista terminalis may be 3 to 6 mm thick, and the pectinate muscles may be 2 to 3 mm thick. However, the atrial wall between the pectinate muscles is paper-thin and could be perforated by a stiff catheter.

When atrial enlargement and stasis to blood flow occur, mural thrombi may form within the recesses between the pectinate muscles, particularly in the atrial appendage. Intracardiac catheters or pacemaker wires tend to injure the endocardium at the cavoatrial junction and are often associated with shallow linear mural thrombi.

The atrial septum has interatrial and AV components (Fig 12-18). The interatrial portion contains the fossa ovalis, which includes an arch-shaped outer muscular rim (the limbus) and a central fibrous membrane (the valve).[13] In contrast to the fossa ovalis, the foramen ovale (which is patent throughout fetal life) represents a potential interatrial passageway, which courses between the anterosuperior limbic rim and the valve of the fossa ovalis and then through the natural valvular perforation (ostium secundum) into the left atrium. In approximately two-thirds of subjects, the foramen ovale closes anatomically during the first year of life as the valve of the fossa ovalis becomes permanently sealed to the limbus. In the remaining third, this flap-valve closes functionally only when left atrial pressure exceeds right atrial pressure; this constitutes the so-called valvular-competent patent foramen ovale (see Fig 12-17). The foramen ovale remains potentially patent in about one-third of persons 1 to 29 years old, about one-fourth of those 30 to 79 years old, and about one-fifth of those older than 80 years.[14] When patent, the foramen ovale averages 5 to 6 mm in maximal potential diameter.

Through a patent foramen ovale, systemic venous emboli may enter the systemic arterial circulation; such paradoxic emboli may be thrombotic (for example, from the legs) or nonthrombotic (for example, air emboli during neurosurgery).

Pronounced atrial dilatation may so stretch the atrial septum that the limbus no longer covers ostium secundum in the valve of the fossa ovalis; as a result, interatrial shunting may occur across the valvular-incompetent patent foramen ovale (acquired atrial septal defect). In some subjects, aneurysms of the valve of the fossa ovalis may develop and may undulate during the cardiac cycle. Atrial dilatation also stimulates the release of natriuretic factor.

The AV component of the atrial septum, which lies anterior to the interatrial component and separates the right atrium from the left ventricle, is primarily muscular but has an anterosuperior membranous region (the AV portion of the membranous septum). The AV septum corresponds to the triangle of Koch, an important anatomic landmark that contains the AV node and bundle; it is bound by the septal tricuspid annulus, the coronary sinus ostium, and the tendon of Todaro. The tendon of Todaro is a subendocardial fibrous cord that extends from the eustachian-thebesian valvular commissure to the anteroseptal tricuspid commissure (at the membranous septum); it very roughly corresponds to the level of the mitral annulus.

The thickness of the atrial septum varies considerably. The valve of the fossa ovalis is a paper-thin translucent membrane at birth but becomes more fibrotic with time and may achieve a thickness of 1 to 2 mm.[15-17] The limbus of the fossa ovalis ranges from 4 to 8 mm in thickness; however, lipomatous hypertrophy may produce bulging masses more than thrice this thickness. The muscular AV septum forms the summit of the ventricular septum and may range from 5 to 10 mm in thickness; this may be greatly increased in the setting of hypertrophic cardiomyopathy or concentric left ventricular hypertrophy. The membranous AV septum generally is less than 1 mm thick.

Left atrium

The left atrium is a posterosuperior midline chamber (see Fig 12-10) that receives pulmonary venous blood and expels it across the mitral orifice and into the left ventricle. The body of the left atrium, by virtue of its posterior position, does not contribute to the frontal cardiac silhouette roentgenographically; however, the lateral left atrial appendage, when enlarged, may form the portion of the left cardiac border between the left ventricle and the pulmonary trunk.

Interposed between the midline left atrium and the vertebral bodies are the esophagus, rightward, and the descending thoracic aorta, leftward. The left pulmonary artery and left bronchus contact the superior surface of the left atrium, and the left and posterior aortic sinuses may slightly indent the atrial wall, as the torus aorticus, just superior to the area of fibrous continuity between mitral and aortic valves. The left atrium consists of free wall and septum.

The left atrial free wall has a posterosuperior dome-shaped body, which receives the pulmonary veins (see Fig 12-14), and a lateral windsock-like appendage (auricle). These two regions are separated externally by the left atrial coronary vein and the ligament of Marshall (see Fig 12-5,A) and internally by the ostium of the appendage. The left atrial body, although infiltrated by cardiac muscle cells, is derived from the embryonic common pulmonary vein and maintains a smooth, veinlike endocardial surface (see Fig 12-17). The endocardium is opaque gray-white and is thicker and less compliant than that in the three other cardiac chambers. The atrial appendage lies in the AV sulcus atop the proximal circumflex coronary artery. Its tortuous lumen contains numerous small pectinate muscles and several blind-ended channels. In the left atrium, there is no crista terminalis, and pectinate muscles are not present outside the appendage. The free wall is 1 to 3 mm thick.

From the left atrial aspect, the atrial septum is entirely interatrial; the AV septum is not observed from this view, since it lies between the left ventricle and the right atrium. The valve of the fossa ovalis, which becomes opaque during the first year, contains one or more anterosuperior fenestrations, representing the embryonic ostium secundum (see Fig 12-17). The limbus of the fossa ovalis is not directly visible from the left atrium.

With chronic obstruction to left atrial emptying (for example, rheumatic mitral stenosis), the dilated left atrium may shift the atrial septum rightward and in severe cases may actually form the right cardiac border roentgenographically (Fig 12-19). Moreover, the esophagus may be shifted rightward, as demonstrated by barium swallow, and the left bronchus may be elevated appreciably. Mural thrombi may develop within the atrial appendage or, less commonly, the atrial body, and in severe cases may virtually fill the chamber except for small channels leading from the pulmonary veins to the mitral orifice (see Fig 12-19). In contrast to left atrial mural thrombi, which tend to involve the free wall, most myxomas arise from the left side of the atrial septum (see Fig 12-19).

Comparison of atria

The volume of the right atrium is 75 to 80 mL, and that of the left atrium is 55 to 65 mL;[18,19] left atrial stroke volume is 20 to 30 mL, and its passive conduit volume is 30 to 50 mL.[20] The limbus of the fossa ovalis forms the anatomic hallmark of the morphological right atrium, and the ostium secundum forms the anatomic landmark of the morphological left atrium (see Fig 12-17). The right atrial free wall contains the crista terminalis and pectinate muscles, whereas the left atrial free wall has no crista terminalis and contains pectinate muscles only within the atrial appendage (see Fig 12-17). The right atrial appendage is large and pyramidal, whereas the left atrial appendage is a small, tortuous, windsock-like projection (see Fig 12-10).

By two-dimensional echocardiography, the limbus and valve of the fossa ovalis may be identified, and the anatomy of the atrial septum may be used to determine atrial morphology. However, since the fossa ovalis cannot readily be identified by angiography, the relative size and shape of the atrial appendages are used to distinguish atrial morphology by this imaging technique. Atrial morphology is important, since it determines both atrial and cardiac situs (that is, solitus, inversus, or ambiguus).

Embryology

Approximately between days 25 and 40, the atrial, ventricular, conotruncal, and aortopulmonary septa develop. A septum may form by several mechanisms, the most common of which involves the proliferation and eventual fusion of two opposing tissue ridges (Fig 12-20). Similarly, a septum may develop by proliferation of a single ridge that eventually fuses with the opposite wall. In contrast to active (proliferative) septal formation, a partition may develop passively, without cell proliferation. For example, a portion of wall may cease growing, while that on either side expands; this will thereby form a relative constriction between the two growing regions. As the two expanding walls fuse to each other behind this constriction, a passive septum develops. The stenotic site, although unchanged in absolute size, will appear to become progressively smaller relative to adjacent structures that are growing. However, cell proliferation is still necessary to close this narrow opening (foramen or ostium) completely. Atrial septation requires both active and passive processes.

By approximately day 25, the atria begin to expand and

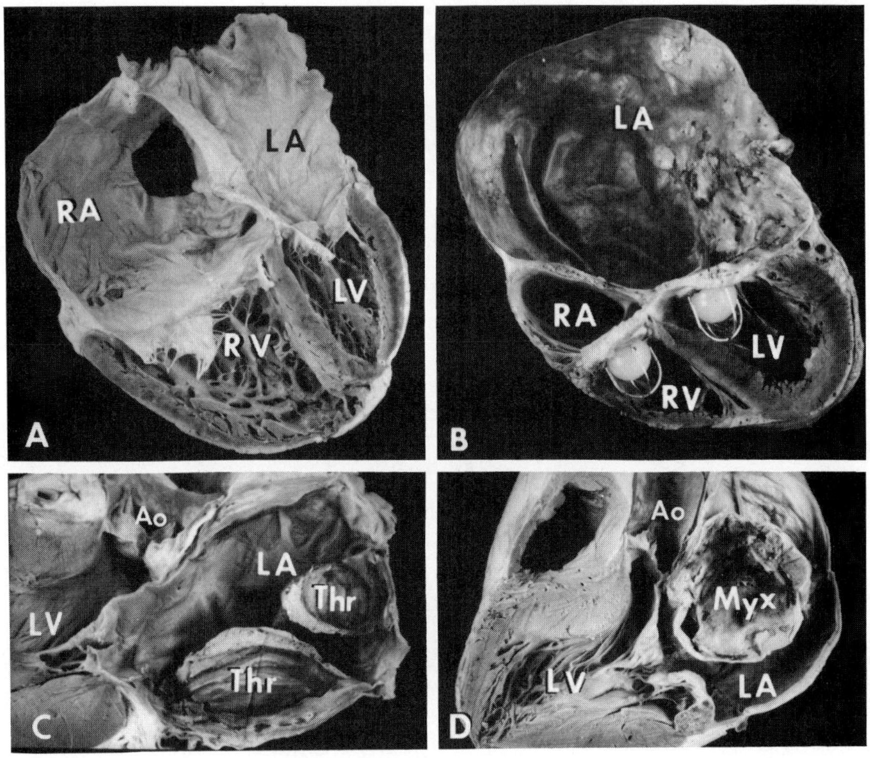

Fig 12-19 Atrial abnormalities. **A,** right, atrial dilatation, tricuspid regurgitation, and right ventricular volume hypertrophy resulting from a secundum atrial septal defect. (Four-chamber view from 76-year-old man.) **B,** giant left atrium resulting from rheumatic mitral insufficiency after recent mitral and tricuspid valve replacements. (Four-chamber view from 57-year-old woman.) **C,** large left atrial mural thrombi *(Thr)* are associated with rheumatic mitral stenosis and permitted only small channels of blood flow from the pulmonary veins to the mitral valve. (Left ventricular long-axis view from 44-year-old woman.) **D,** obstructive left atrial myxoma *(Myx)* mimics mitral stenosis. (Left ventricular long-axis view from 78-year-old woman.) (See Appendix for other abbreviations.)

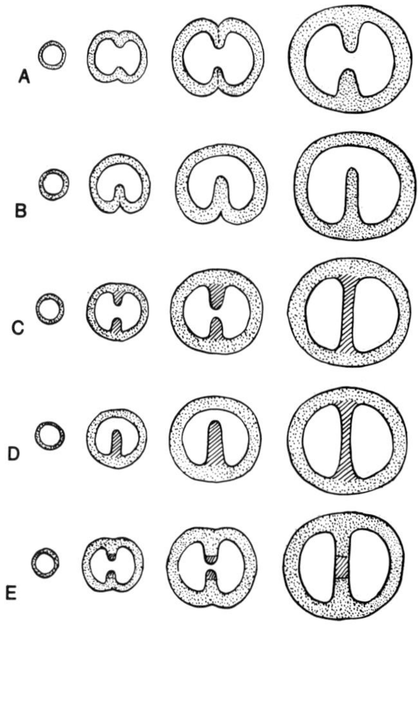

Fig 12-20 Embryology of septum formation. **A** and **B,** with passive septum formation, a communication remains between two regions. **C** and **D,** with active septum formation, two regions may be completely separated from each other. **E,** septation may occur by a combination of passive and active processes.

to ascend into the pericardial cavity. As they become positioned posterior to the heart loop, the overlying truncus arteriosus indents the superior atrial surface and thereby first demarcates the interatrial sulcus and initiates the passive formation of the septum primum (Fig 12-21). The crescentic free edge of this septum overlies the AV canal; the interatrial communication between these two structures is known as the ostium primum. The free edge of the septum primum soon becomes lined by tissue derived from the superior and inferior endocardial

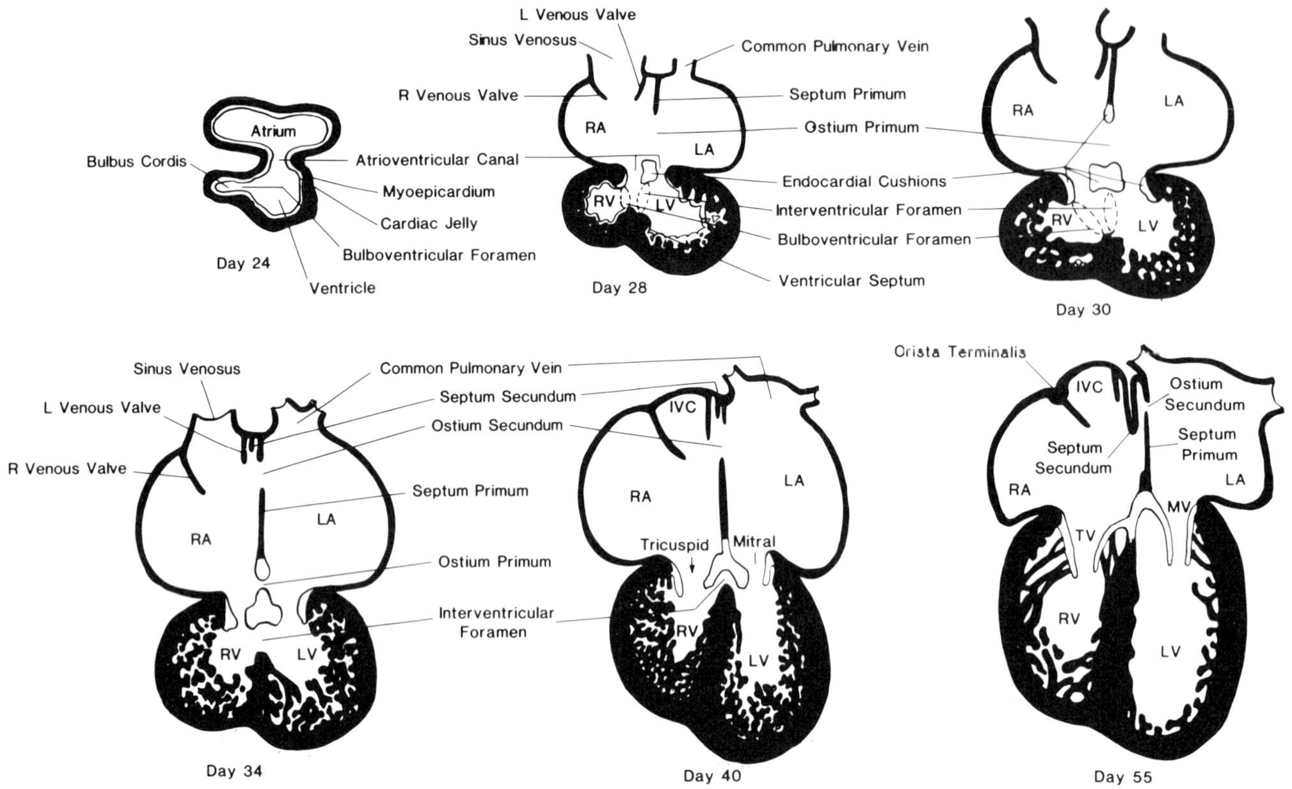

Fig 12-21 Embryology of the atrial septum, AV canal, and muscular interventricular septum. The septum primum forms the valve of the fossa ovalis, and the septum secundum forms the limbus. The endocardial cushions contribute not only to the formation of the AV valves but also to the closure of the ostium primum and the secondary interventricular foramen. Right ventricular trabeculations are more prominent than left ventricular. Dates are approximate. (See Appendix for abbreviations.) (Modified from Netter FH: Embryology. In *The Ciba Collection of Medical Illustrations, Vol. 5, Heart.* Edited by FF Yonkman. Summit, New Jersey, Ciba Pharmaceutical Company, 1969, pp 112-130.)

cushions, and proliferation of this ring of cushion tissue tends to close the ostium primum by day 34. However, by day 32, a second opening has developed in the posterosuperior aspect of the septum primum, as multiple fenestrations coalesce to form the ostium secundum. Later, as the right sinus venosus horn becomes incorporated into the posterior right atrial wall, the ostium secundum will be shifted anterosuperiorly.

At this time, infolding of the atrial wall between the left venous valve and the septum primum initiates the passive formation of the septum secundum (see Fig 12-21). As the right sinus venosus horn becomes incorporated into the right atrium, and as the common pulmonary vein dilates and becomes incorporated into the left atrium, the two atria rapidly expand and contribute significantly to the infolding process that forms the septum secundum (see Fig 12-17,D). This septum is thicker than the septum primum and forms as a tissue arch with its concavity directed toward the orifice of the inferior vena cava. Although the septum secundum soon overlies the ostium secundum in septum primum, the two septa do not fuse, and the passageway between the two (the foramen ovale) will remain patent throughout fetal life. The septum secundum forms the muscular limbus of the fossa ovalis, and the septum primum forms the membranous valve of the fossa ovalis.

As the right horn of the sinus venosus becomes incorporated into the right atrium, two prominent tissue folds (the right and left venous valves) guard the sinoatrial junction (see Fig 12-21). These valves fuse posterosuperiorly and form the septum spurium. Eventually, the left venous valve fuses to the septum secundum, the septum spurium forms the crista terminalis, and the right venous valve forms the eustachian valve of the inferior vena cava and the thebesian valve of the coronary sinus. The right sinus venosus horn forms the smooth-walled veinlike sinus venarum region of the right atrium.

Owing to hemodynamic streaming within the right atrium during intrauterine life, superior vena caval blood is directed toward the tricuspid orifice, and inferior vena caval blood, carrying well-oxygenated placental blood, is directed by the eustachian valve toward the foramen ovale. As a result, the most-well-oxygenated

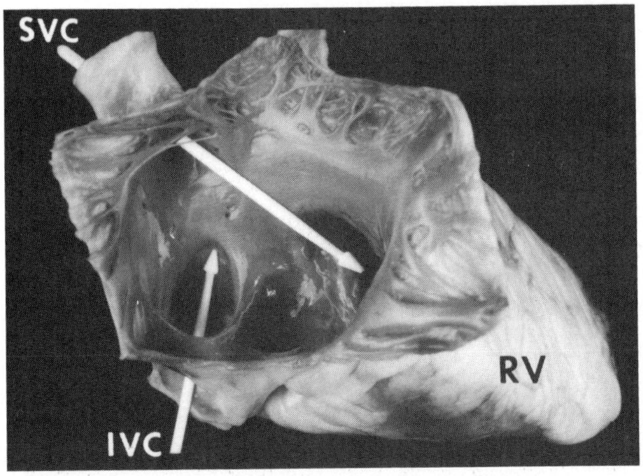

Fig 12-22 Right atrial hemodynamic streaming. Superior vena caval blood is directed toward the tricuspid orifice, and inferior vena caval blood is directed toward the fossa ovalis. (Opened right atrium from 31-year-old man.) (See Appendix for abbreviations.) (From Edwards WD: Anatomy of the cardiovascular system. In *Clinical Medicine.* Vol. 6, Chap. 1. Edited by JA Spittell Jr. Philadelphia, Harper & Row, Publishers, 1984, pp 1-24. By permission.)

blood in the fetal circulation is directed, via the left heart, to the coronary arteries, the upper extremities, and the rapidly developing central nervous system. Even postnatally, the superior vena cava maintains its orientation toward the tricuspid annulus, and the inferior vena cava maintains its orientation toward the atrial septum (Fig 12-22). Accordingly, an endomyocardial biopsy specimen of the right ventricular apex is much more easily obtained via the superior vena caval approach than the inferior vena caval approach. In contrast, the passage of a catheter from the right atrium into the left heart is much more easily performed via an inferior vena caval approach. In subjects in whom the foramen ovale is anatomically sealed, the valve of the fossa ovalis may be perforated (transseptal approach); however, this membrane becomes thicker and more fibrotic with age.[16]

A secundum atrial septal defect involves the fossa ovalis region of the interatrial septum and results from deficiency of the septum primum or the septum secundum or both; it is the most common form of atrial septal defect and often is an isolated anomaly (Fig 12-23). A primum atrial septal defect involves the AV septum and represents a malformation of the endocardial cushions (see Fig 12-23); it is almost invariably associated with mitral and tricuspid abnormalities. A sinus venosus atrial septal defect involves the posterior aspect of the atrial septum and is usually associated with anomalous right atrial connection of the right pulmonary veins (see Fig 12-23). A coronary sinus atrial septal defect is usually associated with an absent coronary sinus and connection of a left superior vena cava to the left atrium (see

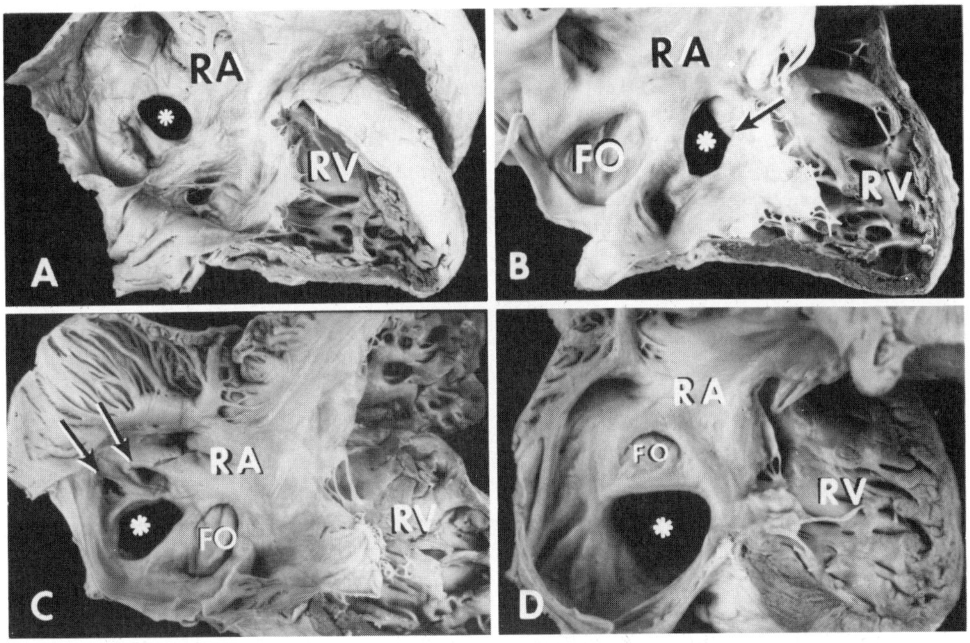

Fig 12-23 Atrial septal defect (ASD). Right atrial view in all. **A,** secundum ASD (*) in 67-year-old man. **B,** primum ASD (*) associated with a cleft anterior mitral leaflet *(arrow)* and mitral regurgitation in 72-year-old man. **C,** sinus venosus ASD (*) accompanied by anomalous connection of the right pulmonary veins *(arrows)* to the right atrium in 41-year-old man. **D,** coronary sinus ASD (*) associated with left atrial connection of a persistent left superior vena cava in 2-year-old girl. (See Appendix for abbreviations.) (**A** and **B,** from Feldt RH, Porter CJ, Edwards WD, et al: Defects of the atrial septum and the atrioventricular canal. In *Moss' Heart Disease in Infants, Children, and Adolescents.* Fourth edition. Edited by FH Adams, GC Emmanouilides, TA Riemenschneider. Baltimore, Williams & Wilkins, 1989, pp 170-189. By permission.)

Fig 12-23). A common atrium results when a primum defect and a huge secundum defect coexist; the only atrial septal remnants are a posterosuperior ridge and a small muscular cord between the two defects.

ATRIOVENTRICULAR VALVES
General features

The right (tricuspid) and left (mitral) AV valves maintain unidirectional blood flow and separate the atria from the ventricles. Each valve has five components, three of which form the valvular apparatus (annulus, leaflets, commissures) and two of which form the tensor apparatus (chordae tendineae and papillary muscles).

The annulus of each AV valve is somewhat saddle-shaped and represents an ill-defined ring of fibrous tissue from which the leaflets arise. As part of the fibrous cardiac skeleton at the base of the heart, each annulus electrically insulates atrium from ventricle. Since the tricuspid annulus is an incomplete fibrous ring, loose connective tissue maintains insulation at the points of annular discontinuity. The mitral annulus, in contrast, constitutes a relatively continuous ring of fibrous tissue. The opening at the annular level constitutes the anatomic valvular orifice.

The leaflets are delicate fibrous tissue flaps that close the anatomic valvular orifice during ventricular systole (Fig 12-24). The leading edge of each leaflet is its free edge, and its serrated appearance results from direct chordal insertions into this border. The closing edge, in contrast, represents a slightly thickened nodular ridge several millimeters above the free edge. When the valve closes, apposing leaflets contact one another along their closing edges, and interdigitation of these nodular ridges ensures a competent seal. The ventricular undersurface of each leaflet constitutes the so-called valve pocket.

Between the free edge and the closing edge, a leaflet is somewhat thick and opaque; this constitutes the rough zone. In contrast, the large expanse of tissue between the rough zone and the annulus forms the thin clear zone of a leaflet.

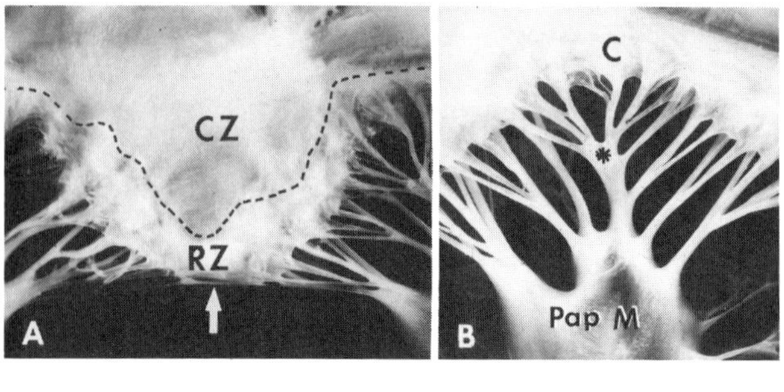

Fig 12-24 Components of an AV valve (from the mitral valve of an 8-year-old girl). **A,** each leaflet has a large clear zone *(CZ)* and a smaller rough zone *(RZ)* between its free edge *(arrow)* and closing edge *(dotted line).* **B,** each commissure (C) separates two leaflets and overlies a papillary muscle *(Pap M);* a fan-like commissural chorda tendinea (*) connects the tip of the papillary muscle to the commissure.

Each leaflet comprises two major layers—namely, the fibrosa, which forms the strong structural backbone of the valve, and the spongiosa, which acts as a shock absorber along the atrial surface, particularly at the closing edge (rough zone), where one leaflet coapts with an adjacent leaflet.[21] Additionally, the atrialis and ventricularis are thin linings along the atrial and ventricular surfaces, respectively. The fibrosa is continuous with the annulus proximally and with the chordae tendineae distally; thereby, structural strength and integrity are maintained between the various valvular components. Since the delicate and compliant valves are attached only at the annulus and papillary muscles, wide and sudden excursion of the leaflets and chordae tendineae is possible and allows rapid opening and closing of the AV valves.

Commissures represent cleftlike splits in the leaflet tissue which represent the sites of separation of one leaflet from its neighboring leaflets (see Fig 12-24). However, in contrast to congenital clefts, a true commissure is always associated with an underlying papillary muscle and an intervening fanlike array of chordae tendineae. Since the commissures generally do not attain the level of the annulus, and since the leaflets form a somewhat funnel-shaped curtain, the cross-sectional area at the annulus may be slightly greater than that along the leaflets distally.

The chordae tendineae are strong, fibrous tendinous cords that act as guide wires to anchor and support the leaflets (see Fig 12-24). They restrict excessive valvular excursion during ventricular systole and thereby prevent valvular prolapse into the atria. Most chordae tendineae branch one or more times, so that generally more than 100 chordae insert into the free edge or ventricular surface of each AV valve.[22,23] By virtue of these numerous chordal insertions, both radially and circumferentially, the force of systolic ventricular blood tends to be evenly distributed throughout the valvular undersurface.

A commissural chorda tendinea has fanlike branching, with insertions into two adjacent leaflets (major commissure) or into two scallops of one leaflet (minor commissure).[24,25] Chordal insertions into the leading edge impart a serrated appearance to the free edge of a leaflet. One thick strut chorda may be found on each side of a semicircular leaflet, particularly the anterior mitral leaflet, and may represent an unusually thick column that contains cardiac muscle and tends to calcify with age.

The papillary muscles, which may have multiple heads, are conical mounds of ventricular muscle that receive the majority of the chordae tendineae. Because of their position directly beneath a commissure, each papillary muscle receives chordae from two adjacent leaflets. As a result, papillary muscle contraction tends to pull the two leaflets toward each other and thereby facilitates valve closure. Ventricular function also affects papillary muscle function.

In the elderly, the AV valves, particularly the mitral, may become altered anatomically by various aging changes (Fig A12-2), which are not to be confused with disease states.[26] Mild annular dilatation may occur, with or without age-related atrial dilatation.[8,27] Leaflets become thicker, with increasing nodularity of the rough zone and with mild hooding deformity of the entire leaflet.[28] Contributing to the latter is a decrease in ventricular base-apex length which makes the thickened chordae appear relatively longer than necessary. Degeneration of collagen in the annulus and fibrosa may be accompanied by lipid accumulation and focal calcification.[27,29-31]

Although the annular plane defines the anatomic valvular orifice, the functional orifice represents the cross-sectional area of the smallest passageway through a maximally opened valve and may exist at the annulus or at some level along the leaflets distally. The principal valvular orifice is nonplanar and is bounded by the free edges of the leaflets, whereas the secondary orifices make up the interchordal spaces. Valvular disorders may affect the principal or secondary orifices and thereby alter the size, shape, and position of the functional valvular orifice. For example, rheumatic mitral disease that is characterized by chordal and commissural fusion results in mitral stenosis, as a result of narrowing of the principal orifice and obliteration of the secondary orifices. In contrast, rheumatic mitral valve disease that is characterized by fibrosis and scar retraction of leaflets and chordae tendineae results in mitral regurgitation, because of insufficient leaflet tissue for complete closure of the functional orifice.

Abnormalities of the AV valves may involve any of the five major components or combinations thereof. The pattern of involvement determines whether valve function is altered and whether the valve becomes stenotic or incompetent, or both.

Tricuspid valve

The plane of the tricuspid annulus faces anteriorly, leftward, and somewhat inferiorly, toward the right ventricular apex. Because of the normal rightward bowing of the ventricular septum, the annulus is shaped somewhat like an inverted D when viewed from the ventricular aspect. Along the free wall, the annulus inserts into the atrioventricular junction, whereas along the septum, it forms the junction between atrioventricular and interventricular portions of the muscular and membranous ventricular septum.

The annular circumference in fixed postmortem specimens averages 11.0 ± 1.5 cm; it is approximately 0.5 cm greater in men than in women and is about 1.0 cm greater in fresh than in fixed specimens[8,32-34] (see Fig A12-2). In the living subject, the annular circumference varies with the cardiac cycle: it is maximum during ventricular diastole and decreases 15% to 23% during ventricular systole; the postmortem values in fixed hearts correspond to the maximum (diastolic) values recorded by two-dimensional echocardiography.[32] Annular area in the living individual ranges from a maximum of 11.3 ± 1.8 cm^2 during ventricular diastole to a minimum of 7.6 ± 1.4 cm^2 during systole;[32] the 29% to 37% reduction in area is presumably due to contraction of the underlying basal right ventricular myocardium, since the incomplete tricuspid annulus cannot adequately constrict by itself.

The three tricuspid leaflets are not always particularly well separated from one another and may have poorly formed major commissures or accessory minor commissures.[35] The septal (medial) leaflet lies parallel to the ventricular septum, and the posterior (inferior) leaflet lies parallel to the inferior, or diaphragmatic, aspect of the right ventricular free wall. In contrast, the anterior (anterosuperior) tricuspid leaflet is not parallel to the ventricular wall but, rather, forms a large sail-like intracavitary curtain that partially separates the inflow tract from the outflow tract (Fig 12-25). At the midleaflet level, the valvular orifice is shaped somewhat like a right triangle, with the right angle between the septal and posterior leaflets (see Fig 12-25).

The anterior leaflet, the most mobile of the three, is semicircular and may have not only a serrated free edge but also small notches or, rarely, an accessory minor commissure. The posterior leaflet is rectangular and may consist of several scallops with interposed minor commissures. The septal leaflet is semicircular and, in part, has an annular attachment to the inferior free wall; as a result, at the angle of junction between septum and free wall this leaflet has a prominent crease or fold. By virtue of its short chordae tendineae and oblique position, the septal leaflet is the least mobile of the three. Chordal length averages 0.7 to 1.7 cm.[24]

The anterior tricuspid papillary muscle is the largest and best formed of the three; it may be single or bifid, and it originates from the acute margin of the right ventricular free wall (see Fig 12-25). From this muscle arise several chordae tendineae, which branch and insert into the anterior and posterior leaflets. The anteroposterior commissure may be shallow or deep, and it receives a fanlike chordal array.

The posterior papillary muscle, which is usually rather small, arises from the inferior right ventricular free wall near its junction with the ventricular septum. The posterior and septal leaflets receive chordae tendineae not only from this muscle but also from numerous trabeculae carneae and small accessory papillary muscles. The posteroseptal commissure is generally quite deep and receives a typical commissural chorda from the major papillary muscle.

The medial (conal) papillary muscle, which is also called the papillary muscle of the conus or the muscle of Lancisi, emanates from the superior aspect of the septal band at the level of the membranous septum[36,37] (see Fig 12-25). It tends to be quite prominent in infants and children, but it often later fuses to the septal band and appears small or absent in adults. The anteroseptal commissure is a deep indentation, and its chorda tendinea has short, broad branches, which may arise from a distinct papillary muscle or directly from the septum.[24] A small triangular veil of valvular tissue often joins this commissure to the underlying membranous septum. In 6% to 15% of hearts, leaflet tissue is deficient at this commissure, and the membranous septum fills the gap of 1 to 7 mm between anterior and septal leaflets.[24,38,39]

Because of differences in leaflet size and chordal length, the excursion of the posterior and septal leaflets is less than that of the anterior leaflet. In the setting of annular dilatation, leaflet excursion may be inadequate to effect central coaptation, and valvular incompetence results. Since the tricuspid annulus is incomplete, and since the basal right ventricular myocardium forms a subjacent muscular ring, dilatation of the right ventricle commonly produces annular dilatation and tricuspid regurgitation (Figs 12-19,A and 12-26). Right atrial dilatation alone, as in constrictive pericarditis, usually does not cause significant tricuspid insufficiency.

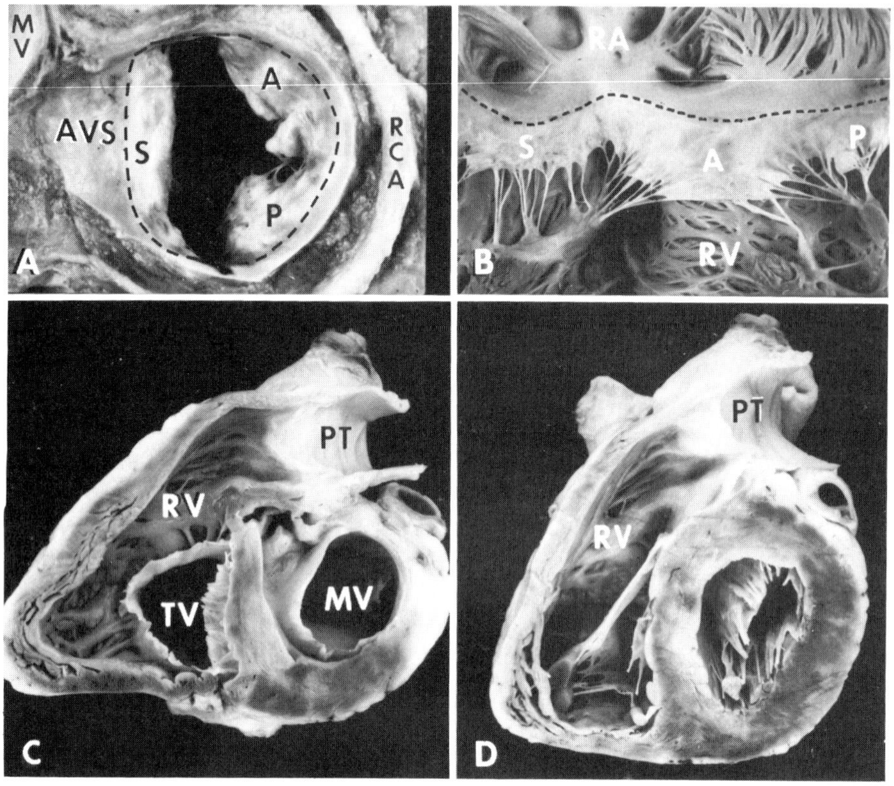

Fig 12-25 Tricuspid valve. **A,** the tricuspid annulus *(dashed line)* is somewhat D-shaped; the septal leaflet attaches to the ventricular septum, whereas the anterior and posterior leaflets attach to the right ventricular free wall. The AV septum lies between the tricuspid and mitral valves. The right coronary artery travels near the lateral tricuspid leaflet. (Atrial view from 62-year-old woman.) **B,** the tricuspid annulus *(dashed line)* is generally planar but dips apically along the septal leaflet. (Opened valve from 22-year-old man; also see Fig 12-18,A.) **C** and **D,** just below the annulus **(C),** the orifice is shaped like a reversed "D," but at the midleaflet level **(D),** the tricuspid orifice becomes more triangular. The inflow and infundibular septa form a right angle **(C),** and the mitral orifice is elliptic **(D).** (Ventricular short-axis views from 15-year-old boy.) (See Appendix for abbreviations.) (**D,** from Edwards WD: Anatomy of the cardiovascular system. In *Clinical Medicine.* Vol. 6, Chap. 1. Edited by JA Spittell Jr. Philadelphia, Harper & Row, Publishers, 1984, pp. 1-24. By permission.)

Valvular incompetence also may be observed in conditions that limit leaflet and chordal excursion (see Fig 12-26), such as rheumatic disease (fibrosis and scar retraction), carcinoid endocardial plaques (thickening and retraction), and eosinophilic endomyocardial diseases (thrombotic adherence to myocardium). Even in normal hearts, trivial degrees of tricuspid regurgitation commonly exist.

In contrast, tricuspid stenosis involves commissural and chordal fusion and may occur in rheumatic or carcinoid heart disease. Combined tricuspid stenosis and incompetence also may develop in these two conditions. Since the tricuspid valve and right atrium lie beneath the right sternal border, and since the right ventricular apex lies beneath the left sternal border, tricuspid murmurs are best heard between these two regions of the anterior chest wall.

Mitral valve

The plane of the mitral annulus faces anteriorly, leftward, and somewhat inferiorly, toward the ventricular apex. The orifice changes shape during the cardiac cycle; it is elliptic during ventricular systole but becomes more circular during diastole.[40] Although the entire annular circumference contacts the overlying left atrium, only a C-shaped portion contacts the underlying left ventricular wall; the remaining 25% to 30% of the annulus is intracavitary and continuous with the aortic valve and the right and left fibrous trigones. Although the mitral annulus per se has limited contractility, contraction of the basal left ventricle may contribute appreciably to cyclic changes in the area of the annular orifice.[41]

In the living subject, the normal mitral annular circumference is maximum during ventricular diastole and decreases 10% to 16% during systole; accordingly, the annular area decreases 23% to 31%, from a maximum ventricular diastolic value of 7.1 ± 1.8 cm^2 to a systolic minimum of 5.2 ± 1.6 cm^2.[40,42] In fixed postmortem specimens, the normal mitral annular circumference averages 9.5 ± 2.0 cm and is about 1.0 to 1.5 cm greater in men than

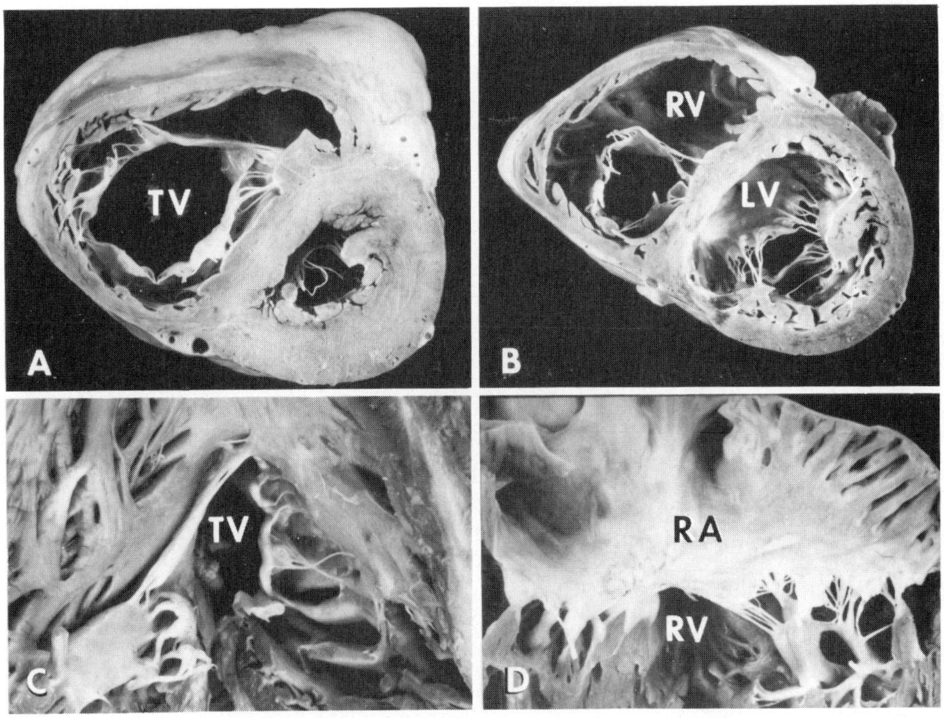

Fig 12-26 Tricuspid valve disease. **A,** right ventricular hypertrophy and dilatation, associated with thromboembolic pulmonary hypertension, has caused tricuspid annular dilatation and valvular incompetence. (Ventricular short-axis view from 58-year-old man.) **B,** idiopathic dilated cardiomyopathy with biventricular dilatation has resulted in tricuspid and mitral regurgitation. (Short-axis view from 50-year-old man.) **C,** rheumatic retraction of leaflets has produced tricuspid insufficiency. (Right ventricular view from 54-year-old woman.) **D,** carcinoid plaques have caused leaflet retraction and fused chordae tendineae, resulting in tricuspid stenosis and insufficiency. (Opened valve from 55-year-old woman.) (See Appendix for abbreviations.) (**D,** from Callahan JA, Wroblewski EM, Reeder GS: Echocardiographic features of carcinoid heart disease. *Am J Cardiol* 50:762-768, 1982. By permission of Technical Publishing Company.)

in women, in fresh than in fixed specimens, and in perfusion-fixed than in routinely fixed specimens.[8,33,34,41] (see Fig A12-2). The annular circumferences in postmortem fixed specimens are similar to the maximum (diastolic) values determined by two-dimensional echocardiography.[40]

Mitral annular calcification almost invariably involves only the posterior leaflet and forms a C-shaped ring of annular and subannular calcium which may impede basal ventricular contraction and thereby produce mitral regurgitation. Similarly, inadequate basal ventricular contraction may contribute to valvular incompetence in the setting of pronounced left ventricular dilatation; however, since only part of the mitral annulus is in direct contact with the basal ventricular myocardium, dilatation of the ventricle rarely increases annular circumference more than 25%.[43,44]

Secondary left atrial dilatation may contribute to the progression of preexisting mitral incompetence by displacing the posterior leaflet and its annulus and thereby hindering the excursion of this taut leaflet.

The mitral leaflets form a continuous funnel-shaped veil with two prominent indentations, the anterolateral and posteromedial commissures. Although the two commissures do not extend entirely to the annulus, they effectively separate the anterior and posterior leaflets. In contrast to the three other cardiac valves, which each comprise three leaflets or cusps, the mitral valve has only two leaflets (Fig 12-27). At midleaflet level, the mitral orifice is elliptic or football-shaped, and its long axis aligns with the two commissures and their papillary muscles (Figs 12-25 and 12-28). Mitral leaflets thicken with age.[28]

The anterior leaflet is semicircular and, by virtue of its intracavitary position, subdivides the left ventricle into inflow and outflow tracts (see Fig 12-28). The posterior leaflet is somewhat rectangular and, in more than 90% of hearts, is subdivided by minor commissures into three semicircular scallops, the largest of which is the middle scallop.[45] The basal portion of the anterior leaflet contains atrial myocardial cells, and their contraction may facilitate valve closure, not only by arching this leaflet atrially but also by shortening the adjacent annulus.[46]

Although the anterior leaflet occupies only 35% to 40% of the annular circumference, its leaflet area, 4.0 to 5.9 cm^2 (mean, 4.9), is almost identical to the area of the posterior leaflet, 4.2 to 6.2 cm^2 (mean, 5.0).[45] The total available leaflet surface area, 9.9 cm^2, therefore, is nearly

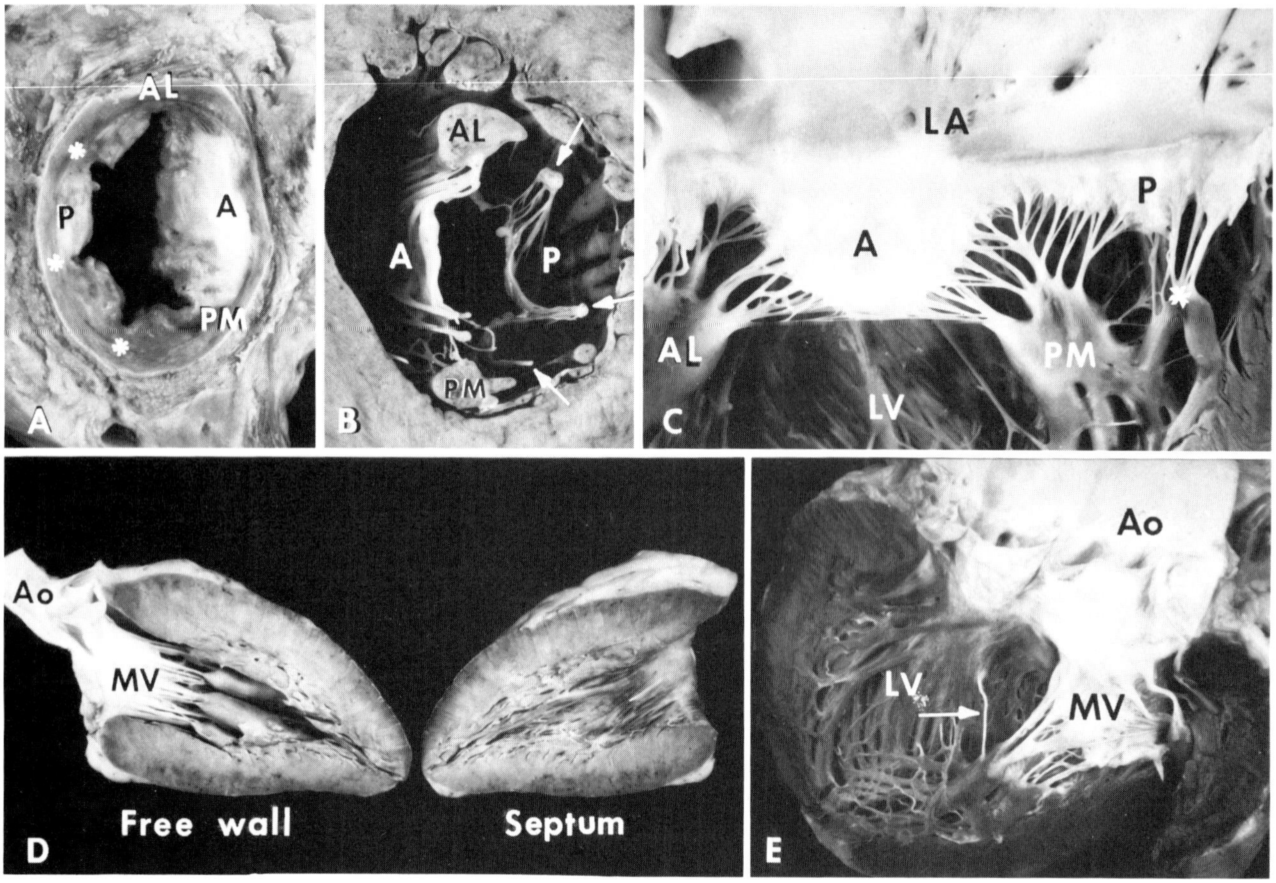

Fig 12-27 Mitral valve. **A** and **B,** unopened mitral valve, viewed from the left atrium **(A)** and left ventricle **(B),** shows the anterior and posterior leaflets and their anterolateral and posteromedial commissures and papillary muscles; furthermore, several minor commissures (*) and their accessory papillary muscles *(arrows)* divide the posterior leaflet into four scallops. (From 67-year-old man.) **C,** opened mitral valve has a large, semicircular anterior leaflet and a shallow, rectangular posterior leaflet; an arch-like accessory papillary muscle (*) is interposed between the two major papillary muscles (From 8-year-old girl.) **D,** because the mitral leaflets normally have no chordal attachments to the septum, the mitral valve and left ventricular free wall (left) may be separated from the ventricular septum (right). (From 16-year-old boy.) **E,** an accessory chorda tendinea (so-called false tendon) *(arrow)* connects the posteromedial mitral papillary muscle to the ventricular septum. (Opened left ventricle from 78-year-old woman.) (See Appendix for abbreviations.)

twice that necessary to close the systolic annular orifice, 5.2 cm^2; however, since some folding and puckering of leaflet tissue is needed to ensure a competent seal, the normal leaflets are not as redundant as might appear.

The floppy mitral valve is characterized by annular dilatation, stretched chordae tendineae, and redundant hooded folds of leaflet tissue, which are prone to prolapse, incomplete coaptation, chordal rupture, and mitral insufficiency (Fig 12-29). In contrast, rheumatic mitral insufficiency results from scar retraction of leaflets and chordae tendineae (see Fig 12-29).

In the setting of infective endocarditis, virulent organisms may perforate the leaflet tissue and produce acute mitral regurgitation (see Fig 12-29). In hypertrophic cardiomyopathy, the anterior leaflet may contact the ventricular septum during systole and contribute both to left ventricular outflow tract obstruction and to mitral incompetence.

In the setting of chronic aortic insufficiency, the regurgitant stream may impact on the anterior mitral leaflet and produce not only a fibrotic jet lesion but also the leaflet flutter and premature valve closure that are so characteristic echocardiographically.

A classic fan-shaped chorda tendinea emanates from the tip of each of the two papillary muscles and inserts into its overlying commissure and into both adjacent leaflets (see Fig 12-24,B). Similarly, a smaller commissural chorda inserts into each minor commissure between posterior scallops. Two particularly prominent chordae insert along each half of the ventricular surface of the anterior mitral leaflet, and these so-called strut chordae may offer

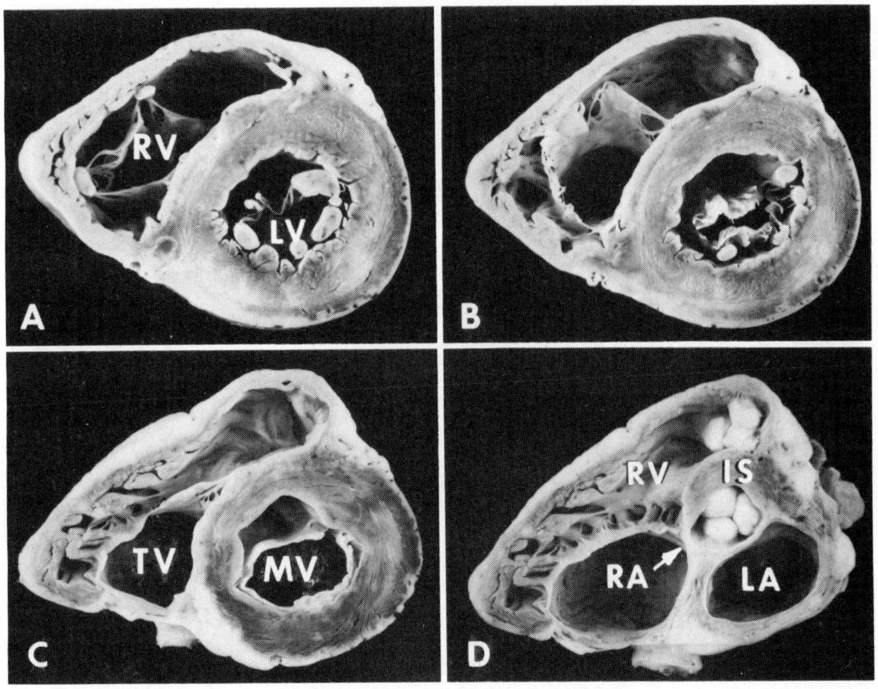

Fig 12-28 Mitral valve. (Ventricular short-axis views from 19-year-old man.) **A,** the mitral papillary muscles arise from the left ventricular free wall. **B** and **C,** the mitral orifice is elliptic at the free edge (**B**) and midportion (**C**) of its leaflets; the anterior mitral leaflet forms an intracavitary curtain that separates the left ventricular inflow and outflow tracts. **D,** at the mitral annulus, the anterior leaflet contacts the left and posterior aortic cusps; in contrast, the tricuspid valve is separated from the pulmonary valve. The aortic valve is tangential to the three other cardiac valves. The infundibular septum separates the aortic and pulmonary valves, and the membranous septum *(arrow)* lies between the aortic and tricuspid valves. (See Appendix for abbreviations.) (From Edwards WD: Anatomy of the cardiovascular system. In *Clinical Medicine.* Vol. 6, Chap. 1. Edited by JA Spittell Jr. Philadelphia, Harper & Row, Publishers, 1984, pp 1-24. By permission.)

additional support for this mid-cavitary leaflet that also forms part of the wall of the left ventricular outflow tract. Chordal length is generally 1.0 to 2.2 cm.[25]

Rheumatic mitral stenosis is characterized by chordal and commissural fusion, which obliterate the secondary interchordal orifices and narrow the primary orifice (Fig 12-30).

Chordal rupture may occur in the floppy valve, the infected valve, or, rarely, the apparently normal valve and lead to acute mitral insufficiency. Minor congenital malformations or focal absence of chordae may contribute to the development of a floppy valve and may impose inordinate chordal stresses, which favor eventual rupture.[47]

Chordae tendineae, particularly basal chordae, may contact the underlying endocardium and adhere to it (for example, rheumatic disease or eosinophilic endomyocardial disease) or may produce linear friction lesions (for example, floppy mitral valve).

The mitral papillary muscles occupy the middle third of the left ventricular base-apex length, not only in the normal heart but also in hypertrophied and dilated hearts.[1] Two prominent muscles (or fused clusters of muscles) originate from the trabeculae carneae of the anterolateral and posteromedial (inferomedial) free wall, beneath their respective mitral commissures, and may have diameters similar to those of the free wall.[23,41,48] The trabeculae carneae not only anchor the papillary muscles but also may form a muscle bridge between the two papillary groups and thereby contribute to valve closure.[49]

Although the papillary muscles may be multiple or single with multiple heads, the anterolateral muscle is a single structure with a midline groove in 70% to 85% of cases, whereas the posteromedial muscle, in contrast, is multiple or is bifid or trifid in 60% to 70%.[23] The anterolateral muscle is generally larger and extends closer to the annulus than the posteromedial muscle. Occasionally, an accessory papillary muscle is interposed between the two major muscles along the free wall (see Fig 12-27,B). No papillary muscles or chordae tendineae originate from the septum and terminate on the mitral leaflets. However, in about 50% of subjects, one or more chordal structures, known as left ventricular false tendons, or pseudotendons, arise from a papillary muscle and insert either onto the septal surface or onto the opposite

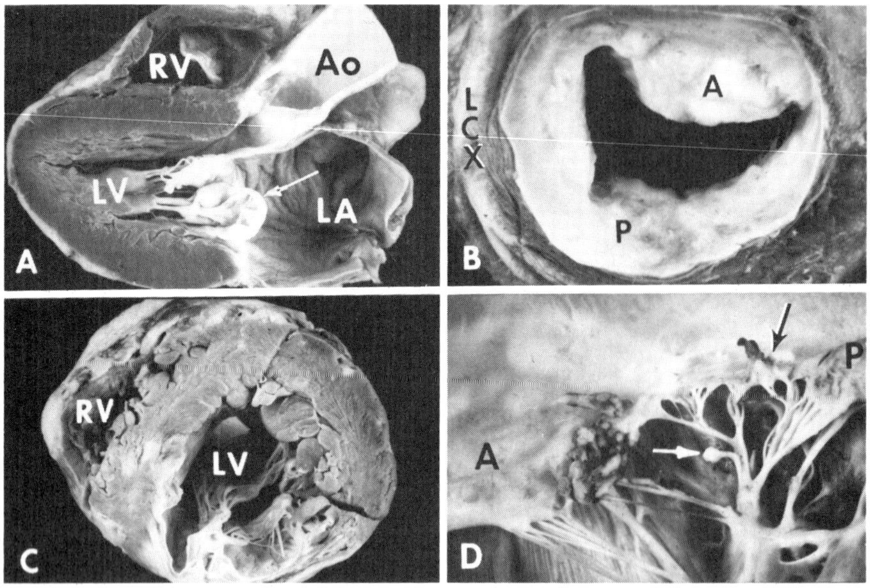

Fig 12-29 Mitral regurgitation. **A,** rupture of a chorda tendinea has caused marked prolapse of the posterior leaflet *(arrow)* of this floppy mitral valve. (Left ventricular long-axis view from 75-year-old man.) **B,** rheumatic fibrosis and scar retraction has prevented the central coaptation of leaflets; calcification and commissural fusion are absent. Note proximity of circumflex coronary artery. (Left atrial view from 62-year-old woman.) **C,** healed transmural myocardial infarction of the inferior left ventricular free wall and the posteromedial mitral papillary muscle has interfered with valve closure. (Ventricular short-axis view from 75-year-old man.) **D,** destruction and rupture of chordae tendineae by bacterial endocarditis *(arrows)* has resulted in unsupported and flail leaflet segments. (Opened valve from 67-year-old man.) (See Appendix for abbreviations.) (**A** and **C,** from Edwards WD, Tajik AJ, Seward JB: Standardized nomenclature and anatomic basis for regional tomographic analysis of the heart. *Mayo Clin Proc* 56:479-497, 1981. By permission, Mayo Foundation.)

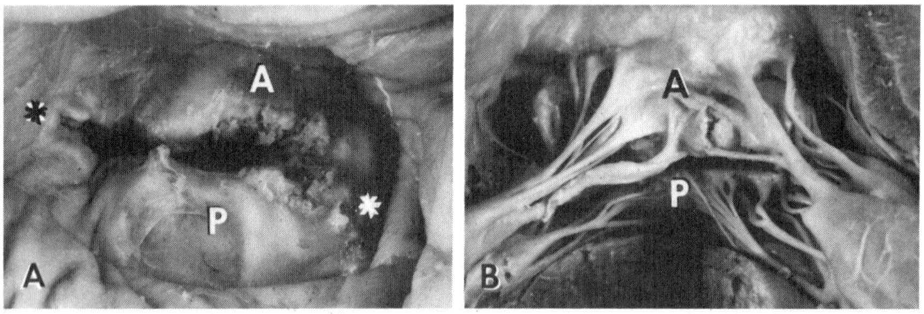

Fig 12-30 Mitral stenosis. Rheumatic fibrocalcific fusion of commissures (*) and chordae tendineae has prevented the valve from opening. (Left atrial **[A]** and left ventricular **[B]** views from 73-year-old woman.) (See Appendix for abbreviations.)

papillary muscle or its chordae tendineae (see Fig 12-27,D).[50]

Chronic postinfarction mitral incompetence is associated with papillary muscle atrophy and scarring, thinning and scarring of the subjacent left ventricular free wall, and left ventricular dilatation (see Fig 12-29). Moreover, infarcted or chronically ischemic papillary muscles may become focally calcified. Acute postinfarction mitral regurgitation may be associated with rupture of a papillary muscle (almost invariably posteromedial) and may involve the entire muscle or only one of its multiple heads.

After operative mitral valve replacement, the papillary muscles atrophy and lose their once parallel arrangement of myocardial cells.

Since the mitral valve annulus lies anterior to the left lateral border of the vertebral column, and since the left ventricular apex occupies the midclavicular line, mitral murmurs are generally detected between the left sternal border and the left anterolateral chest wall. Murmurs of mitral stenosis are usually best heard anteriorly, whereas those of mitral regurgitation may be heard anteriorly or posteriorly. When the regurgitant stream contacts the portion of left atrial wall adjacent to the aortic sinuses, the murmur may be transmitted to the aorta and carotid arteries and may thereby simulate the murmur of aortic stenosis.

Competent function of the mitral valve requires the harmonious interaction of all valvular components, including the left atrium and left ventricle, and is a complex cyclic process that still remains incompletely understood. Valvular lesions may involve individual components or various combinations thereof and may be functionally unimportant or may produce stenosis or insufficiency or both.

Comparison of atrioventricular valves

In contrast to the elliptic mitral annulus, the tricuspid annulus is shaped like an inverted "D" and is larger (7.6 vs. 5.2 cm^2, systolic). Moreover, dilatation of the right ventricle leads to tricuspid annular dilatation, whereas that of the left ventricle generally does not lead to significant mitral annular dilatation. A large right ventricular muscle bundle, the parietal band, separates the tricuspid and pulmonary annuli, whereas the mitral and aortic annuli, in contrast, share direct fibrous continuity (Fig 12-31). Between the membranous septum and the cardiac crux, the mitral annulus becomes increasingly more posterior than the tricuspid annulus as the coronary sinus ostium and AV septum intervene between the two valves (see Fig 12-18).

Although classically the tricuspid valve consists of three leaflets and the mitral valve of two, the anterior and posterior tricuspid leaflets may have poorly developed commissural separation, and the posterior mitral leaflet is usually subdivided by two minor commissures into three scallops. Two features shared by both anterior leaflets are their semicircular shape and their intracavitary position as curtainlike flaps that partially separate the ventricular inflow and outflow tracts (see Figs 12-28 and 12-31). However, the shape of the orifice at midleaflet level differs between the two valves: that of the tricuspid is like a right triangle and that of the mitral is elliptic or football-shaped (see Fig 12-25). The tricuspid leaflets and chordae tend to be thinner and more translucent than the mitral leaflets.

The tricuspid papillary muscles are variable in size and number, and the septal leaflet has numerous insertions directly into the ventricular septum, the most prominent of which is the medial papillary muscle. In contrast, the mitral valve has two large and distinct papillary muscle groups, both of which arise from the left ventricular free wall. The mitral leaflets normally have no septal insertions (see Figs 12-27 and 12-31).

The morphological features that allow distinction, by two-dimensional echocardiography, between tricuspid and mitral

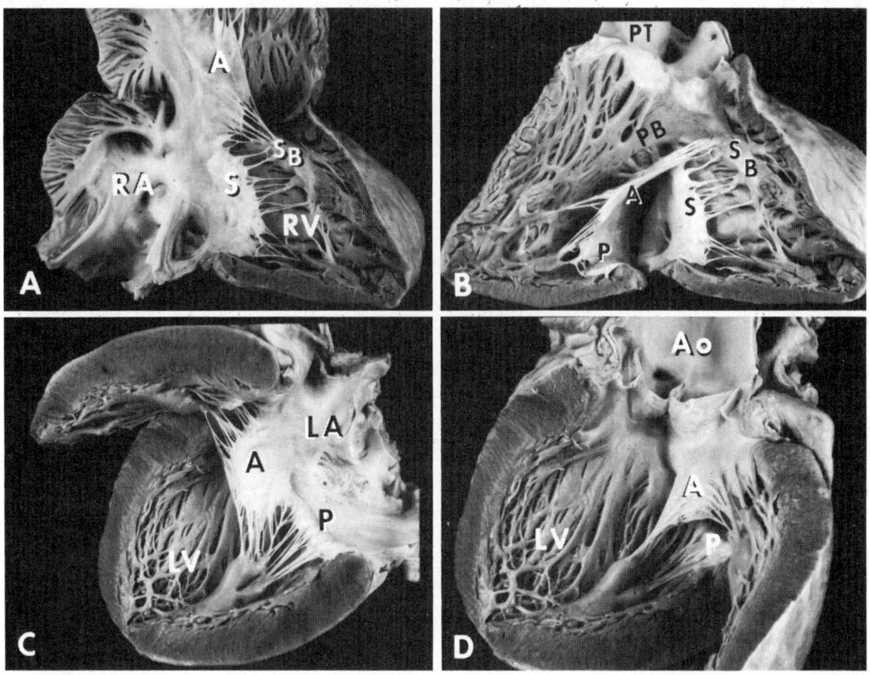

Fig 12-31 Comparison of AV valves and ventricles. The tricuspid valve has septal attachments, but the mitral valve does not. The tricuspid and pulmonary valves are separated by the parietal band, whereas there is fibrous continuity between the mitral and aortic valves. Apical trabeculations are prominent in the crescentic right ventricle and are shallow in the conical left ventricle. (Right ventricular inflow **[A]** and outflow **[B]** views and left ventricular inflow **[C]** and outflow **[D]** views from 22-year-old man.) (See Appendix for abbreviations.)

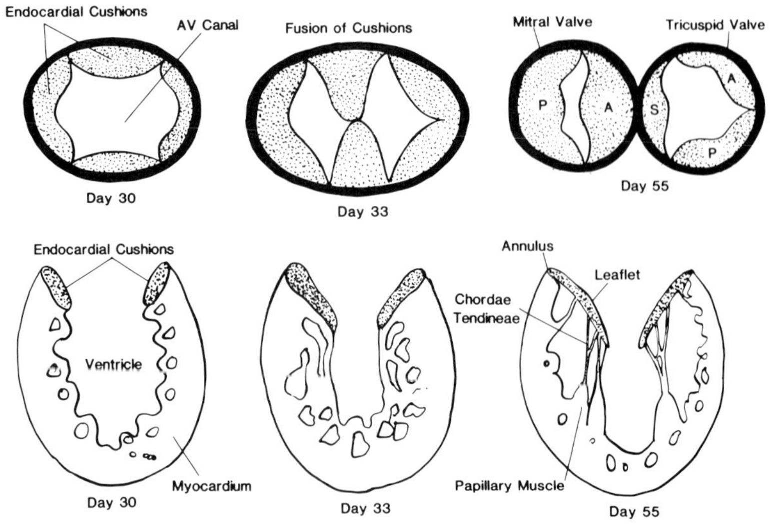

Fig 12-32 Embryology of the AV valves. **Upper,** the mitral and tricuspid valves form as fusion of the superior and inferior endocardial cushions divides the AV canal into two orifices. **Lower,** the leaflets, chordae tendineae, and papillary muscles develop by undermining and diverticulation of the ventricular myocardium. Dates are approximate. (See Appendix for abbreviations.)

valves include differences in the annular level at the cardiac crux, in the shape of the orifice at midleaflet level, and in the size and location of papillary muscles. Angiographically, the tricuspid and mitral valves cannot be differentiated and, therefore, are designated according to the morphology of the ventricle into which they empty.

Embryology

As the junction between the left atrium proximally and the primitive ventricle distally is forming a relatively narrow AV canal, the endocardial cushions proliferate and not only form the tricuspid and mitral valves but also close the ostium primum and the secondary interventricular foramen, between days 29 and 55. These AV endocardial cushions represent bulky mounds of mesenchyme, which function either as a tissue adhesive to seal apposing masses during septal formation or as primitive valves.

By approximately day 29, the bulky superior and inferior endocardial cushions and smaller right and left lateral cushions begin to proliferate and produce an H-shaped AV orifice (Fig 12-32). The apposing superior and inferior cushions grow toward each other and fuse by day 35, and they thereby form two orifices (tricuspid and mitral). Furthermore, tissue from these two cushions extends onto the septum primum along the rim of the ostium primum and actively closes this orifice by day 35 (see Fig 12-21). Along with the conus septum and muscular ventricular septum, ventricular extensions of the superior and inferior endocardial cushions contribute to closure of the secondary interventricular foramen by day 40.

Attenuation and relative absorption of the bulboventricular flange not only effects leftward shifting of the aorta toward the primitive (left) ventricle but also allows rightward shifting of the AV canal with alignment between the tricuspid orifice and the proximal bulbus cordis (right ventricle). Accordingly, the mitral orifice maintains its left ventricular connection, and the tricuspid orifice gains right ventricular connection by day 31 (see Fig 12-21).

As the developing septal tricuspid leaflet shifts rightward and anteriorly, and as the developing anterior mitral leaflet shifts leftward and posteriorly, the intervening cushion tissue arches obliquely and draws posteriorly with it the ventricular septal summit. In this manner, the superior and inferior endocardial cushions contribute much more to the formation of the AV septum than of the interatrial septum.

Only the free-floating anterior leaflets of the tricuspid and mitral valves are derived primarily from the mesenchymal cells of the endocardial cushions, and they develop earlier than the remaining leaflets. The septal tricuspid leaflet and both posterior leaflets form by an undermining and excavating of the ventricular wall; this produces fenestrated muscular flaps, from which the leaflets, chordae tendineae, and papillary muscles will develop between days 35 and 55 (see Fig 12-21). Myocardial cells are subsequently lost from the leaflets and chordae tendineae and are replaced by dense connective tissue.

The superior and inferior endocardial cushions contribute to the formation of the septal tricuspid and anterior mitral leaflets. The right lateral endocardial cushion forms the framework for the anterior and posterior tricuspid leaflets, and the left lateral cushion contributes to the posterior mitral leaflet (see Fig 12-32). The dextrodorsal conus swelling forms the medial portion of the anterior tricuspid leaflet, and the sinistroventral conus swelling forms the medial tricuspid papillary muscle. Since this portion of the tricuspid valve forms early, whereas the adjacent septal leaflet forms quite late, a small gap in the tricuspid annulus may occur at the anteroseptal commissure, adjacent to the membranous septum.

The morphogenesis of an AV valve is greatly influenced by the morphology of the ventricle into which it empties. Accordingly, the valve that joins the morphological right ventricle is almost invariably tricuspid, and that emptying into the morphological left ventricle is almost always mitral.

The complete form of AV canal comprises a common AV valve and a large AV septal defect, which literally represents a

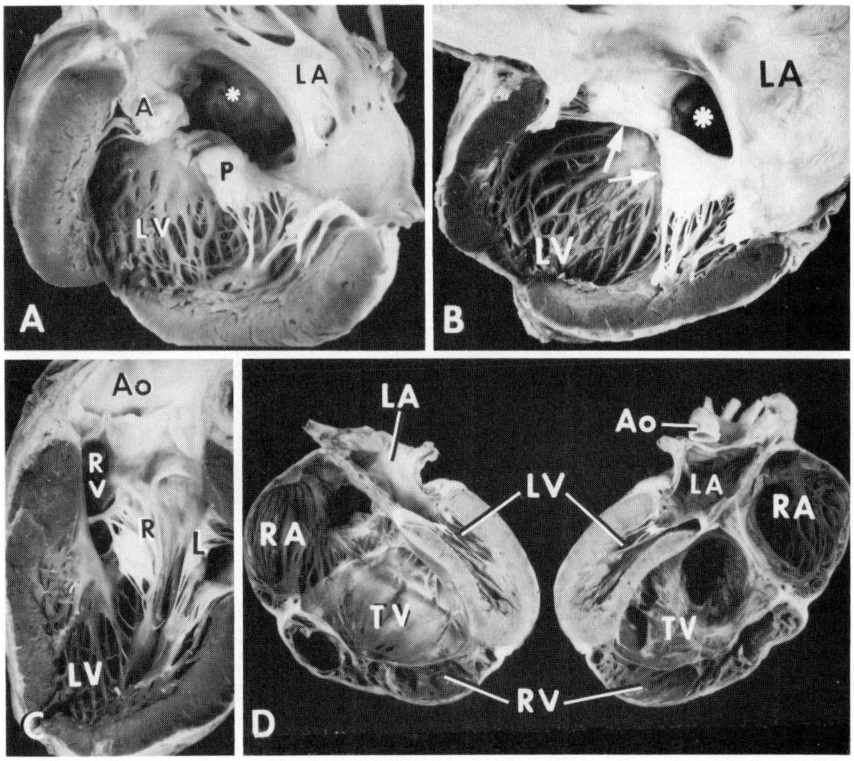

Fig 12-33 Congenital malformations of the AV valves. **A,** complete AV canal is characterized by a common AV valve and a large AV septal defect (*); the anterior and posterior bridging leaflets correspond to the embryonic superior and inferior endocardial cushions. (Left ventricular inflow view from 5-year-old girl.) **B,** this partial AV canal is characterized by a regurgitant cleft in the anterior mitral leaflet *(arrows)* and by a primum atrial septal defect (*). (Left ventricular inflow view from 72-year-old man; same case as in Figure 12-23,B.) **C,** in a double-inlet left ventricle, the right and left AV valves join the left ventricle; the right ventricle is hypoplastic. (Opened left ventricle from 20-year-old woman.) **D,** Ebstein's anomaly is associated with a severely malformed valve *(TV)* and tricuspid regurgitation. (Four-chamber views from 13-year-old boy.) (See Appendix for abbreviations.) (**B,** from Feldt RH, Porter CJ, Edwards WD, et al: Defects of the atrial septum and the atrioventricular canal. In *Moss' Heart Disease in Infants, Children, and Adolescents.* Fourth edition. Edited by FH Adams, GC Emmanouilides, TA Riemenschneider. Baltimore, Williams & Wilkins, 1989, pp 170-189. By permission.)

hole in the center of the heart through which all four cardiac chambers may communicate (Fig 12-33). Associated findings may include a secundum atrial septal defect, a persistent left superior vena cava, and Down's syndrome.

The partial form of AV canal classically comprises a primum atrial septal defect and a cleft anterior mitral leaflet, with mitral incompetence and apical (downward) displacement of the mitral annulus at the cleft (see Fig 12-33). A prominent gap exists at the anteroseptal tricuspid commissure, but this is not a true cleft.

When the AV canal fails to shift rightward, a double-inlet left ventricle (single left ventricle) may result (see Fig 12-33). Similarly, although rarely, the rightward shift is too great, and a double-inlet right ventricle (single right ventricle) develops. Between these two extremes are cases in which the tricuspid or mitral valve may straddle a ventricular septal defect and form papillary muscle attachments within both ventricles. Since the morphology of the valve generally corresponds to the ventricle into which it connects, the double-inlet left ventricle may have two mitral-like valves; the rarer single right ventricle usually receives a common AV valve.

Ebstein's anomaly of the tricuspid valve results from incomplete diverticulation and undermining of the developing valve, so that the septal and posterior leaflets appear partially adherent to the myocardium, and the anterior leaflet is redundant and often fenestrated (see Fig 12-33). The apical (downward) displacement of the functional annulus results in atrialization of a portion of the right ventricular inflow tract and is often associated with severe tricuspid regurgitation and with such conduction disorders as the ventricular preexcitation (Wolff-Parkinson-White) syndrome. In corrected transposition of the great arteries (with inverted ventricles and AV valves), the left-sided tricuspid valve may also exhibit Ebstein's malformation.

Fusion of both groups of mitral papillary muscles or severe hypoplasia of one group may form the so-called parachute mitral valve, in which all mitral chordae insert into a single papillary

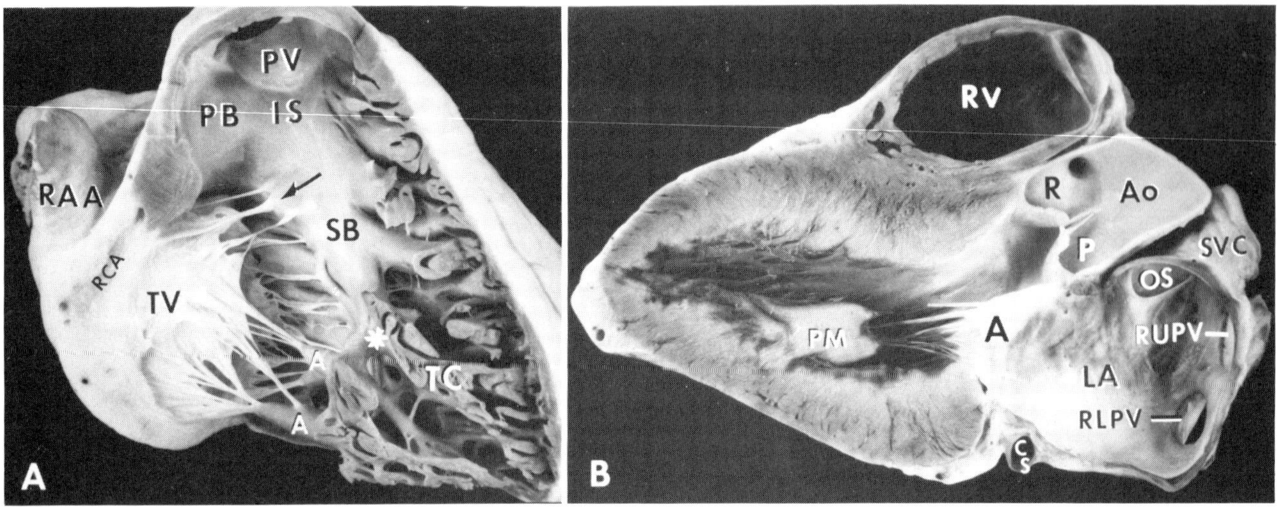

Fig 12-34 Ventricles. **A,** in the right ventricle, the trabeculae carneae are prominent, and the inflow and outflow tracts are separated by the crista supraventricularis (parietal band, infundibular septum, septal band); also note the moderator band (*), the papillary muscle of the conus *(arrow),* and the bifid anterior papillary muscle. (Anterior view of heart with excised right ventricular free wall from 21-year-old man.) **B,** in the left ventricle, the apical trabeculae carneae are shallow, and the anterior mitral leaflet forms part of the wall of the left ventricular outflow tract; also note the ostium secundum, the posteromedial papillary muscle and the right and posterior aortic cusps. (Left ventricular long-axis view from 18-year-old man.) (See Appendix for abbreviations.) (**A,** from Seward JB, Tajik AJ, Hagler DJ, et al: Update on nomenclature, image orientation and anatomic-echocardiographic correlations, with new tomographic views. In *Two-Dimensional Echocardiography.* Edited by JN Schapira, Y Charuzi, RM Davidson. Baltimore, Williams & Wilkins Company, 1982, pp 11-142. By permission.)

muscle. Such valves are almost always stenotic and may form part of a spectrum of congenital left-sided obstructive lesions.

Rarely, the tricuspid or mitral valve may be atretic. The result is a heart with a univentricular AV connection.

VENTRICLES

Right ventricle

The right ventricle is a right anterior chamber (see Fig 12-10), which, by virtue of its position, does not contribute to the borders of the frontal cardiac silhouette roentgenographically. It is bounded by a free wall, a septum, and the tricuspid and pulmonary orifices. The inferior and anterosuperior surfaces of the free wall merge along the acute margin and form an angle of 60° to 90° (see Fig 12-10). The ventricular septum bulges rightward, as if conforming to the surface of an ellipsoid (see Fig 12-28) and thereby produces a crescent-shaped right ventricular chamber when it is viewed from the left anterior oblique perspective. However, from the right anterior oblique view, this chamber appears triangular (Fig 12-34).

The inflow length (from tricuspid annulus to apex) is 6.5 ± 1.0 cm, and the outflow length (from apex to pulmonary annulus) is 8.0 ± 1.0 cm.[33,34] The distance from the cardiac crux to the membranous septum is similar to that from the membranous septum to the pulmonary annulus. The right ventricular chamber has a diastolic volume of 120 ± 20 mL and a systolic volume of 40 ± 10 mL, with a calculated stroke volume of 80 ± 15 mL and an ejection fraction of 65% ± 5%.[51,52] The free wall averages 4 to 6 mm in thickness inferiorly and 2 to 4 mm anterosuperiorly[19,33,34,53,54] (Fig A12-3); the apical thickness, between trabeculae carneae, is only 1 to 2 mm.

Because of the position of both the inflow (tricuspid) valve and the outflow (pulmonary) valve at the base of the heart, blood flow through the right ventricle must follow a V-shaped course. The inflow (base-apex) axis is directed anteriorly, leftward, and somewhat inferiorly; the outflow axis, in contrast, is directed superiorly, leftward, and posteriorly. As a result, the angle between inflow and outflow axes is approximately 45° to 60° and thereby represents a 120° to 135° redirection of blood flow within the right ventricular chamber.

Conditions, such as pulmonary hypertension, that impose a pressure or volume overload on the right ventricle and cause its hypertrophy and dilatation may be attended by straightening of the ventricular septum such that both ventricles attain a D shape on cross section (Fig 12-35). In extreme cases, such as Ebstein's anomaly or total anomalous pulmonary venous connection, leftward bowing of the ventricular septum may result not only in a circular right ventricle and crescentic left ventricle but also in possible obstruction of the left ventricular outflow tract (see Fig

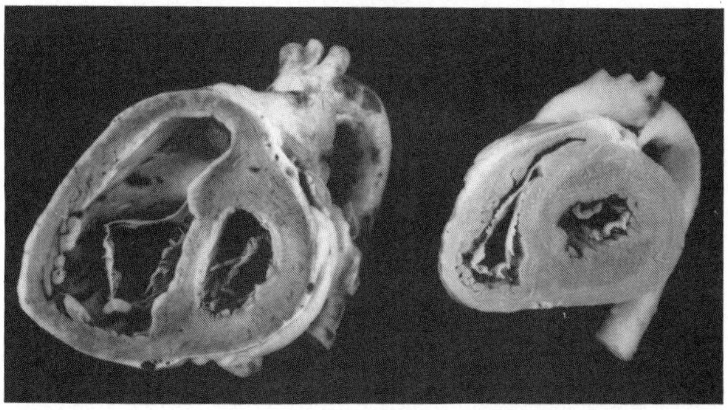

Fig 12-35 Alterations of ventricular shape. Right ventricular hypertrophy and dilatation have produced straightening of the ventricular septum and D-shaped ventricles in a case of chronic thromboembolic pulmonary hypertension. (Ventricular short-axis view from 35-year-old woman.) Normal heart (**right**) is shown for comparison.

12-33,D). This reversal in ventricular shapes is not to be confused with that observed in ventricular situs inversus, which occurs, for example, in corrected transposition of the great arteries.

The right ventricle is divided into an inflow (sinus) portion and an outflow (infundibulum or conus) portion by a nearly circular but nonobstructive ring of prominent muscle bundles, comprising the parietal band, infundibular septum, septal band, and moderator band (see Figs 12-31 and 12-34). The first three form a muscular arch known as the crista supraventricularis.[55] The parietal band, also called the ventriculoinfundibular fold, forms the right posterolateral free wall of the right ventricular outflow tract and is interposed between the tricuspid and pulmonary annuli. The infundibular septum separates the two ventricular outflow tracts beneath the right and left cusps of each semilunar valve and tilts approximately 45° relative to the remainder of the ventricular septum[56] (see Figs 12-25 and 12-34). The parietal band and infundibular septum form a continuous muscle bundle, which is partly free wall and partly septum. The septal band, also called the septomarginal trabecula, is a Y-shaped muscle bundle with a long, broad stem and smaller inferior and anterosuperior limbs; the two limbs cradle the infundibular septum.

The moderator band forms an intracavitary muscular bridge between the septal band and the acute margin of the free wall; accordingly, it originally was called the trabecula septomarginalis (a term that has more recently been applied to the septal band). The moderator band is somewhat variable in size and position but generally inserts into the anterior tricuspid papillary muscle at its free-wall junction (see Fig 12-34). The medial tricuspid papillary muscle emanates from the branching point of the septal band. Furthermore, since the anterior and medial papillary muscles both arise from the ventriculoinfundibular junction, the anterior tricuspid leaflet, which is interposed between these two muscles, forms an intracavitary curtain that partially separates the inflow and outflow tracts during ventricular diastole.

The right ventricular inflow tract extends from the tricuspid annulus to the apex and is separated from the infundibulum by the crista supraventricularis and moderator band. Fleshy columns of muscle, the trabeculae carneae, are present along the septum and free wall. The inflow septum is entirely interventricular and is predominantly muscular, except for a small interventricular portion of the membranous septum near the anteroseptal tricuspid commissure. Along the basal and middle thirds of the septal surface, the trabeculae carneae tend to form muscle bundles parallel to the inferior free wall. In contrast, the apical third of the inflow tract is quite heavily trabeculated by thick muscle bundles which intermesh and form numerous septoparietal bridges; the most prominent of these is the moderator band (see Fig 12-34).

The right ventricular outflow tract extends from the inferior border of the crista supraventricularis to the pulmonary annulus and forms a muscular tube, shaped like an inverted and truncated cone ("conus" and "infundibulum" are Latin for "cone" and "funnel," respectively). The proximal anteroapical portion is heavily trabeculated, whereas the distal anterosuperior portion is relatively smooth-walled along its septal surface and contains shallow, broad-based trabeculae carneae along its free wall. The broad anterosuperior limb of the septal band inserts beneath the left pulmonary cusp, whereas a prominent conical trabecula, arising from the free wall parallel to the parietal band, inserts beneath the right pulmonary cusp; diminutive trabeculae carneae abut the anterior pulmonary cusp. The inflow and outflow tracts of the right ventricle each have distinct and heavily trabeculated apices, which are separated from each other by the septal band. Some authors have conceptualized the tripartite right ventricle, with inlet, trabecular, and outlet components;[55] this approach correlates well with the embryological development of the right ventricle.

During right ventricular endomyocardial biopsy, the bioptome is positioned within the apical half and is directed septally, not only to avoid injury to the cardiac conduction system and tricuspid apparatus but also to prevent possible perforation of the relatively thin free wall; tissue is more often procured from the meshwork of trabeculae carneae than from the septal surface per se.

When permanent transvenous pacemaker electrodes are inserted into the right ventricle, the apical trabeculae tend to entrap the tined tip and thereby prevent its subsequent dislodgment; however, right ventricular perforation may occur.

During vigorous cardiopulmonary resuscitation in which ribs are fractured, the jagged-edged bones may inadvertently be forced through the parietal pericardium, anteriorly, and may lacerate an epicardial coronary artery or may perforate the right atrial or ventricular free wall. Furthermore, if pumping pressure is exerted along the midsternum rather than the xiphoid area, the right ventricular outflow tract may be compressed and this may result in the generation of inordinately high right ventricular pressure, which may produce apical rupture.

Left ventricle

The left ventricle is a left posterior chamber (see Fig 12-10) that forms the left border of the frontal cardiac silhouette roentgenographically. It is bounded by a free wall, a septum, and the mitral and aortic orifices. The lateral free wall forms an ill-defined border known as the oblique margin, and the anterobasal region, subjacent to the left atrial appendage, forms the left shoulder of the heart (see Fig 12-10). The ventricular septum bulges rightward and, from the left anterior oblique view (short-axis cross section), produces a circular left ventricular chamber (see Fig 12-28). However, when viewed from the right anterior oblique (long-axis) perspective, this chamber is bullet shaped, and its three-dimensional shape is best approximated by a truncated ellipsoid (see Fig 12-34). It is of interest that, whereas the spherical chamber (for example, dilated cardiomyopathy) has the least energy expenditure for diastolic filling, and the conical chamber (for example, aortic stenosis) utilizes the least energy for systolic pumping, the normal elliptical left ventricular chamber expends the least sum total of systolic and diastolic energy.[53]

The inflow length (from mitral annulus to apex) and the outflow length (from apex to aortic annulus) each average 7.5 ± 1.0 cm.[33,34] In the living adult patient, the maximum cross-sectional chamber diameter averages 4.5 ± 0.5 cm in diastole and 3.0 ± 0.5 cm in systole.[57] The left ventricular chamber has a diastolic volume of 125 ± 15 mL and a systolic volume of 40 ± 15 mL, with a calculated stroke volume of 80 ± 15 mL and an ejection fraction of 70% ± 10%.[58,59] The diastolic free-wall thickness averages 8 ± 1 mm, and the systolic thickness averages 14 ± 2 mm.[57,60] Moreover, the free wall is thickest basally and tapers toward the apex, the tip of which averages only 1 to 2 mm in thickness, even in hypertrophied hearts.[61] The muscular ventricular septum, which averages 8 ± 2 mm in diastole and 12 ± 2 mm in systole,[57] is thinnest at its basal summit and thickest at its midportion, as a result of the contribution of the right-sided septal band. The membranous septum rarely achieves a thickness of more than 1 mm. Left ventricular septal and free-wall thickness in autopsy specimens, which average 13 ± 2 mm[8,33,34,53] (see Fig A12-3), correlate with antemortem systolic measurements[62] and probably represent the effects of cardiac rigor mortis.[19]

Since both the inflow (mitral) valve and the outflow (aortic) valve occupy the base of the heart, blood flow through the left ventricle must follow a V-shaped course. The inflow (base-apex) axis is directed anteriorly, leftward, and inferiorly; the outflow axis, in contrast, is directed posteriorly, rightward, and superiorly. Although the angle between inflow and outflow axes ranges from 30° to 45°, the outflow axis bends an additional 30° to 45° at the level at which the infundibular septum sharply angles rightward, relative to the remainder of the muscular septum (see Figs 12-25 and 12-34). Accordingly, the inflow and outflow axes diverge by 60° to 90° and thereby represent a 90° to 120° net redirection of blood flow within the left ventricular chamber.

Conditions such as aortic stenosis and chronic hypertension, which impose a pressure overload on the left ventricle, induce concentric left ventricular hypertrophy without appreciable dilatation, and they thereby produce an elongated heart with an increased base-apex length (Fig 12-36). Although the short-axis chamber diameter does not increase significantly, the wall thickness generally increases 25% to 75%, and the heart weight may double or triple (see Fig 12-36).

In contrast, disorders that impose a volume overload on the left ventricle, such as chronic aortic or mitral regurgitation or dilated cardiomyopathy, are attended not only by concentric hypertrophy but also by chamber dilatation, and they thereby produce a globoid heart with increased base-apex and short-axis dimensions (see Fig 12-36). Although the heart weight may double or triple, the left ventricular wall thickness generally remains within the normal range because of the geometry of dilatation.

Accordingly, when the left ventricle is dilated, wall thickness cannot be used as a reliable indicator of hypertrophy (Fig 12-37). Furthermore, since ventricular hypertrophy may occur as rapidly as cardiac dilatation, rarely is a heart dilated but not hypertrophied. Hypertrophy, with or without chamber dilatation, decreases myocardial compliance and may thereby hinder diastolic filling. Recently, the term "eccentric hypertrophy" was recommended for the designation of chambers involved by hypertrophy with dilatation.[63] However, because this term may be misunderstood to imply asymmetric hypertrophy (as in hypertrophic cardiomyopathy or old transmural myocardial infarctions), the term "volume hypertrophy" is favored.

Hypertrophic cardiomyopathy is characterized, in part, by asymmetric (nonconcentric) left ventricular hypertrophy. This disproportionate hypertrophy usually involves the septum (Fig 12-38), although it may involve only part of the septum or may extend onto the free wall, and it results in a ratio of septal to free-wall thickness of more than 1.3. Cardiac amyloid may mimic hypertrophic cardiomyopathy (see Fig 12-36).

Direct fibrous continuity exists between the anterior mitral leaflet and the left and posterior aortic cusps (see Figs 12-31 and 12-34) and is reinforced bilaterally by the left and right fibrous trigones, the latter of which is continuous with the membranous septum.[64] In some individuals, small bundles of myocardial cells may be embedded within this fibrous tissue and afford a minor degree of muscular separation between the two valves;[65] very rarely, a prominent muscle bundle persists between the mitral and aortic valves.

The left ventricle comprises an inflow tract and an outflow tract. The cone-shaped inflow portion extends from the mitral annulus to the apex and is bounded by the anterolateral and inferior portions of the free wall, the inferior (inflow) ventricular septum, and the anterior mitral leaflet. The outflow tract constitutes the remainder of the left ventricular chamber, from apex to aortic annulus, and is bounded by the anterior free wall, the anterior (outflow) ventricular septum, and the anterior mitral leaflet.[66] Owing to rightward septal bowing and infundibular septal angulation, which have collectively been described as the sigmoid or angled septum, the course of the outflow tract is shaped like an inverted S[56] (see Figs 12-25 and 12-34). The basal one-third to one-half of the septal surface is smooth-walled, whereas the remainder is characterized by small, shallow, and irregularly arranged trabeculae carneae; the free wall trabeculae are similar but may become more prominent at the bases of the papillary muscles.

Depending on one's perspective, the ventricular septum may be divided into muscular and membranous components, AV and interventricular components, or inflow and outflow components; the last-named components are in accordance with the position of the right ventricular septal

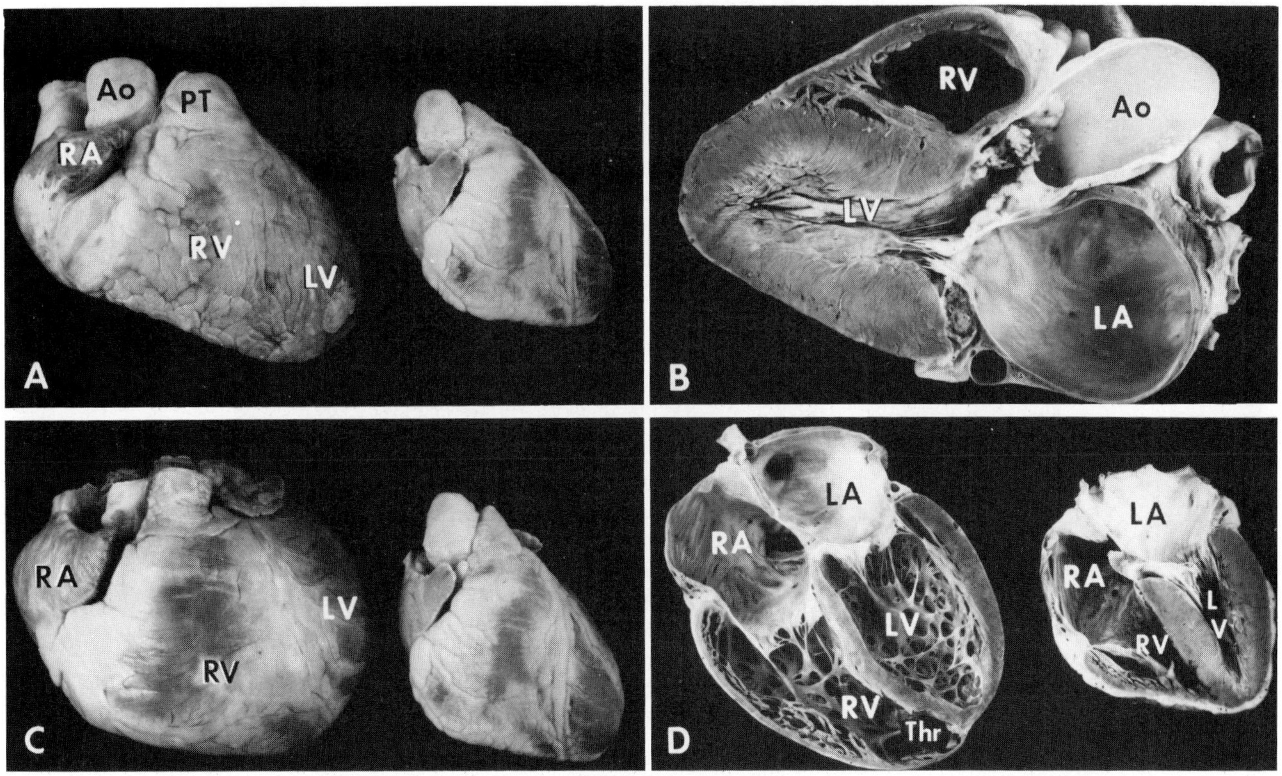

Fig 12-36 Ventricular hypertrophy and dilatation, with normal hearts for comparison. **A** and **B,** aortic stenosis has produced concentric left ventricular hypertrophy and an elongated nondilated heart. (Anterior view **[A]** and left ventricular long-axis view **[B]** from 79-year-old man.) **C** and **D,** idiopathic dilated cardiomyopathy has resulted in biventricular hypertrophy, four-chamber dilatation, and a globoid heart. (**C,** anterior view from 50-year-old man [same case as Figure 12-26,B]; **D,** four-chamber view from 23-year-old man.) (*Thr,* thrombus; see Appendix for other abbreviations.) (**B,** from Edwards WD, Tajik AJ, Seward JB: Standardized nomenclature and anatomic basis for regional tomographic analysis of the heart. *Mayo Clin Proc* 56:479-497, 1981. By permission, Mayo Foundation.)

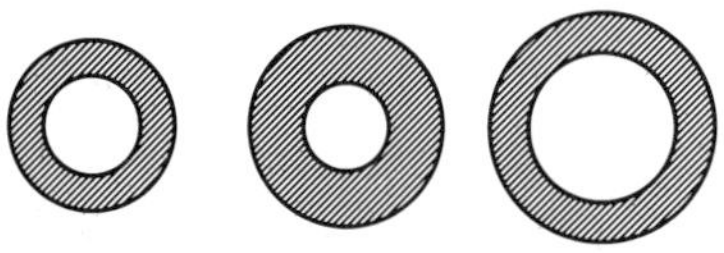

	Normal	Hypertrophy	Hypertrophy and Dilatation
Outer Radius = R_1	3.0 cm	3.2 cm	3.9 cm
Inner Radius = R_2	1.7 cm	1.4 cm	2.6 cm
LV Wall Thickness	1.3 cm	1.8 cm	1.3 cm
Area = $\pi(R_1^2 - R_2^2)$	19.2 cm^2	26.0 cm^2	26.5 cm^2

A

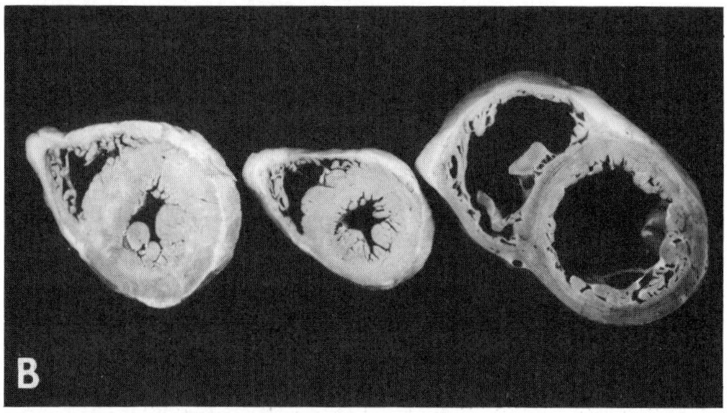

Fig 12-37 Geometry of left ventricular hypertrophy and dilatation (short-axis views). **A,** hypertrophy produces an increase in both wall thickness and surface area. However, when dilatation accompanies hypertrophy, the surface area of the myocardium increases but the wall thickness generally remains normal. Accordingly, when the ventricle is dilated, wall thickness is no longer a reliable indicator of hypertrophy. **B,** compared to the normal heart **(center),** the hypertrophied heart **(left)** has a thick left ventricular wall, but the hypertrophied and dilated heart **(right)** has a normal wall thickness; both hypertrophied hearts weighed more than twice normal. (**Left** from 64-year-old man with aortic stenosis; **right** from 50-year-old man with idiopathic dilated cardiomyopathy; same case as Figure 12-26,B and 12-36,C.)

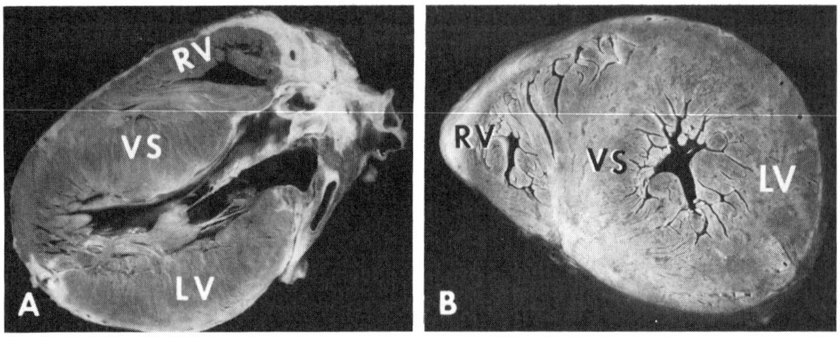

Fig 12-38 Increased ventricular wall thickness. **A,** in hypertrophic cardiomyopathy, both ventricular free walls are thickened, and the ventricular septum is disproportionately hypertrophied. (Left ventricular long-axis view from 13-year-old boy.) **B,** amyloid characteristically produces an increase in ventricular wall thickness and clinically may mimic hypertrophic cardiomyopathy. (Ventricular short-axis view from 72-year-old man.) An increase in wall thickness is not always due to hypertrophy of myocardial cells. (See Appendix for abbreviations.) (**A,** from Edwards WD, Zakheim R, Mattioli L: Asymmetric septal hypertrophy in childhood: unreliability of histologic criteria for differentiation of obstructive and nonobstructive forms. *Hum Pathol* 8:277-284, 1977. By permission of WB Saunders Company.)

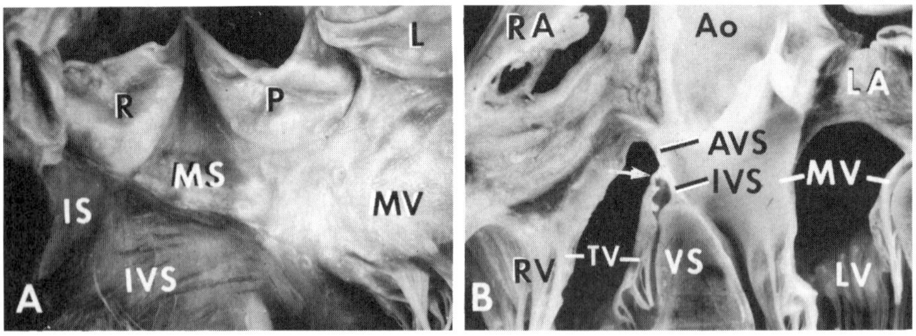

Fig 12-39 Membranous septum. **A,** the membranous septum is bordered by the right and posterior aortic cusps, the anterior mitral leaflet, the muscular interventricular septum, and the infundibular septum. (Opened left ventricular outflow tract from 65-year-old man.) **B,** the septal tricuspid leaflet *(arrow)* inserts along the midportion of the membranous septum and divides it into AV and interventricular components. (Ventricular long-axis view from 30-year-old man.) (See Appendix for abbreviations.)

band. The membranous septum is bordered by the muscular septum, the right and posterior aortic cusps, and the right fibrous trigone[64,67] (Figs 12-28,D and 12-39). It varies considerably in size and tends to be largest in Down's syndrome; the relative contributions by the AV and interventricular components vary inversely and depend on the insertion level of the tricuspid annulus. Between the membranous septum and the cardiac crux, the basal muscular septum is interposed between the left ventricle and the right atrium and thereby constitutes the muscular AV septum (see Fig 12-18). Thus, reference to the entire ventricular septum as the "interventricular septum," which commonly occurs in the medical literature, is anatomically inaccurate.

In the normal geriatric heart, left ventricular geometry becomes altered by various aging changes, which may simulate certain disease states. By virtue of shortening of the base-apex length, the mitral chordae tendineae may appear relatively longer than necessary and may allow mild interchordal hooding, particularly of the posterior leaflet, and thereby simulate a floppy mitral valve. Although the mitral annulus dilates only mildly with advancing age, the aortic annulus tends to dilate appreciably and to increase the maximum distance spanned by the two valves. Moreover, as the infundibular septum shifts rightward and more inferiorly, the dilated aortic orifice tends to tilt more rightward and less posteriorly; this thereby alters the shape and direction of the left ventricular outflow tract. Furthermore, this shift in the infundibular septum not only bulges the subjacent muscular septum into the outflow tract but also, by virtue of its tilting effect

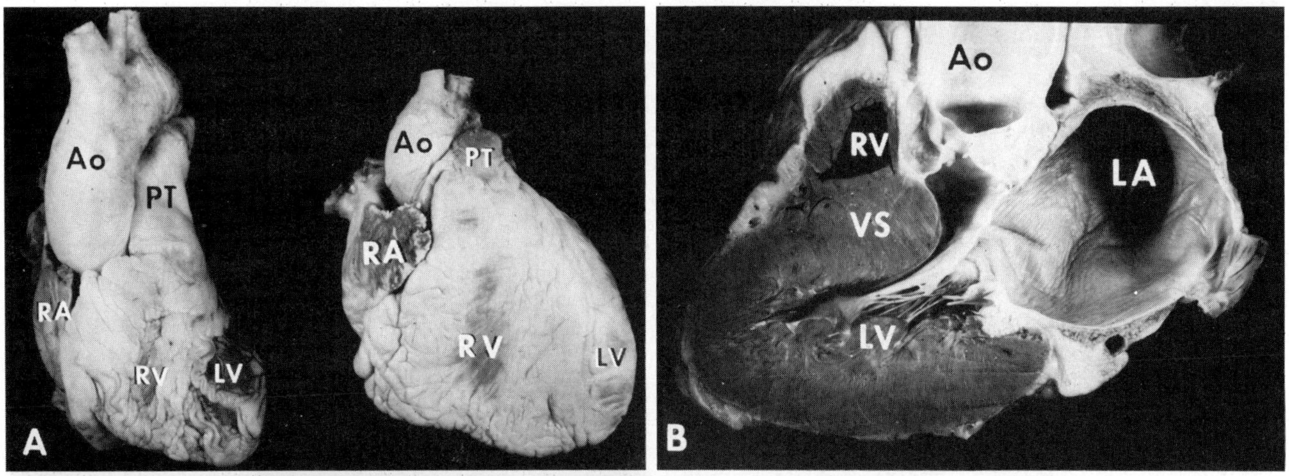

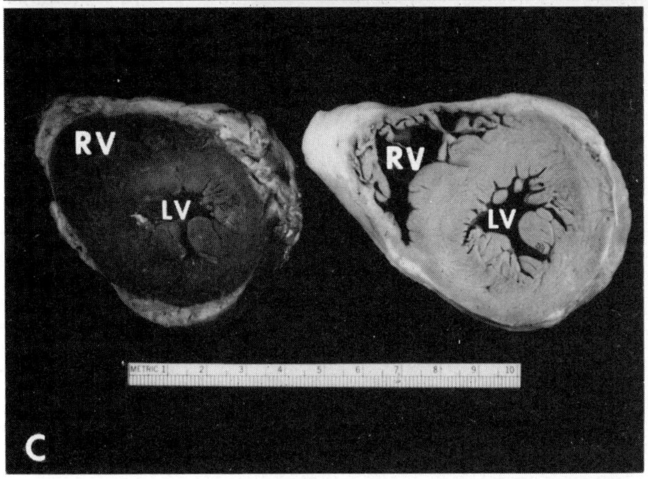

Fig 12-40 Geriatric heart. **A,** normal heart from a 62-year-old woman **(left)** has undergone atrophy of the ventricular myocardium and dilatation of the ascending aorta, compared to the normal heart from a 19-year-old man **(right).** (Anterior views.) **B,** the aortic annulus has dilated and is now similar in size to the mitral annulus, and the ventricular septum protrudes into the left ventricular outflow tract. (Left ventricular long-axis view from 84-year-old man.) Compare with Figure 12-34,B. **C,** the darkened myocardium (so-called brown atrophy) in the normal heart from a 90-year-old woman **(left)** is due to the time-related accumulation of lipofucsin "wear-and-tear" pigment; compare with the normal heart from a 20-year-old man **(right).** (Ventricular short-axis views.) (See Appendix for abbreviations.)

on the aortic valve, tends to draw the mitral annulus medially and bring its anterior leaflet nearer the septum and thereby simulate hypertrophic cardiomyopathy (Fig 12-40). These age-related alterations, acting in concert with mild fibrosis and calcification of the aortic and mitral valves, may contribute to the low-grade systolic ejection murmurs that are so common in the elderly.

Since the trabeculae carneae are small and do not usually form significant septoparietal bridges, permanent apical entrapment of a tined transvenous pacemaker electrode is difficult to achieve and may necessitate the placement of epicardial electrodes (for example, in patients with corrected transposition of the great arteries or with complete transposition of the great arteries and a previous Mustard or Senning operation).

When left ventricular endomyocardial biopsy is performed, care must be taken not to injure the mitral apparatus or left bundle branch and not to perforate the apical thin point; since the trabeculae carneae are small, actual subtrabecular septal tissue is usually procured.

In some persons, apical trabeculae carneae may form a prominent spongy meshwork that may be misinterpreted as apical mural thrombus at angiography or echocardiography. Similarly, prominent ridge-like anteroseptal trabeculae carneae may occasionally occur and may be misinterpreted by these imaging modalities as mural thrombus.[68,69]

Comparison of ventricles

The right ventricle wraps around the left ventricle in such a way that their outflow tracts are nearly perpendicular (see Figs 12-25 and 12-28), and this results in a crescentic right ventricular chamber and a bullet-shaped left ventricular chamber. However, the expected chamber shapes may be altered significantly by disorders associated with straightening or leftward bowing of the ventricular septum. In the normal heart, only the base-apex axis of the left ventricular inflow tract is straight; that of the left ventricular outflow tract is sigmoidal, and both right ventricular axes curve along the septum. Regardless of differences in shape, both ventricles have similar volumes and ejection fractions.[70]

The apical trabeculations of the right ventricle are coarse and form numerous interlacing septoparietal bridges; in contrast, those of the left ventricle are small and shallow (see Figs 12-31 and 12-34). These features of the trabeculae remain distinct, even in markedly hypertrophied or dilated hearts.

The ventricular septum and left ventricular free wall have similar thicknesses and are three to four times as thick as the right ventricular free wall. However, since the

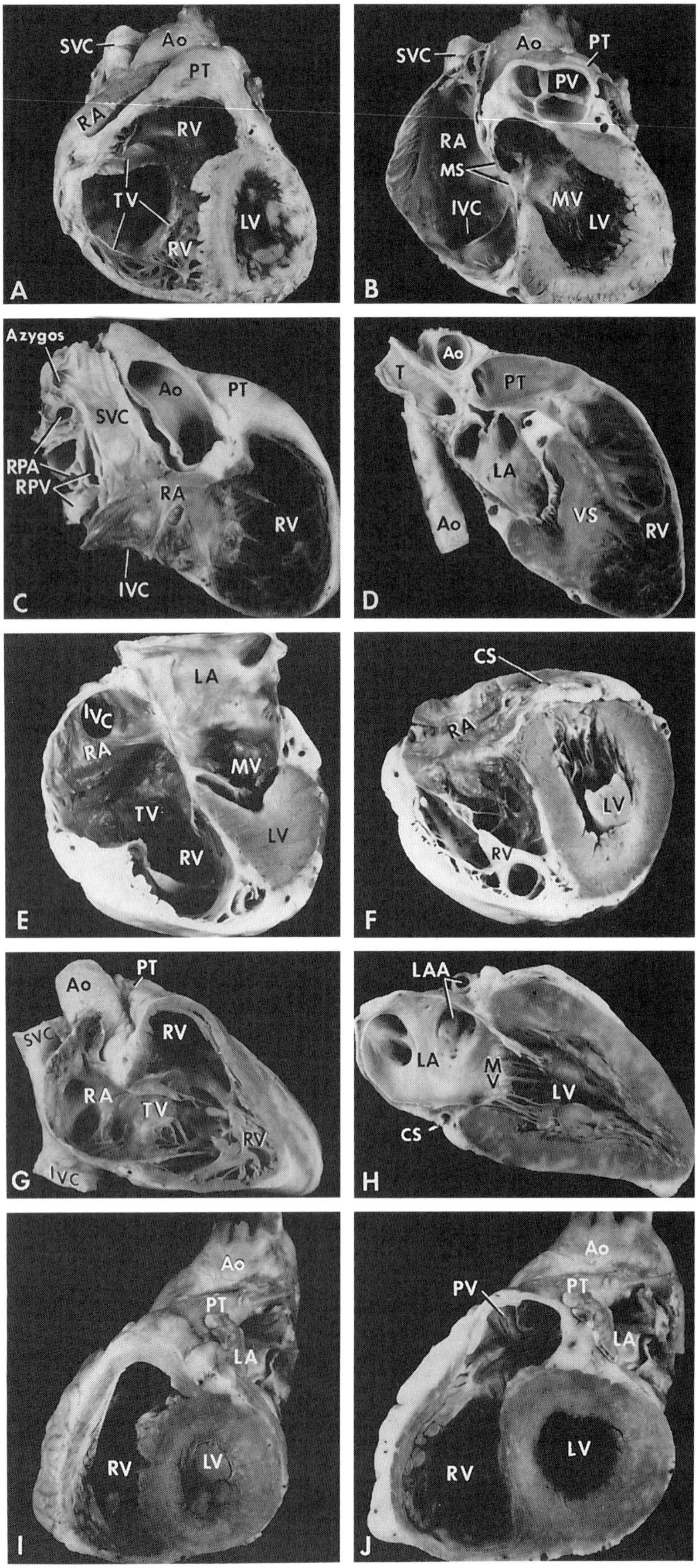
SVC
Ao
PT
RA
RV
TV
RV
LV
A
SVC
Ao
PT
PV
RA
MS
IVC
MV
LV
B
Azygos
Ao
PT
SVC
RPA
RPV
RA
RV
IVC
C
Ao
T
PT
LA
Ao
VS
RV
D
LA
IVC
RA
MV
TV
RV
LV
E
CS
RA
LV
RV
F
Ao
PT
SVC
RV
RA
TV
RV
IVC
G
LAA
LA
M
V
LV
CS
H
Ao
PT
LA
RV
LV
I
Ao
PV
PT
LA
LV
RV
J

Fig 12-41 Tomographic sections. **A** and **B**, frontal views (from 24-year-old man). **C** and **D**, right lateral views (from 20-year-old woman). **E** and **F**, horizontal views (from 24-year-old woman). **G** and **H**, right anterior oblique views (from 20-year-old man). **I** and **J**, left anterior oblique views (from 38-year-old man). (See Appendix for abbreviations.)

hypertrophied right ventricle may attain a wall thickness approaching that of the normal left ventricle, a comparison of wall thicknesses is not always a reliable means of clinically distinguishing ventricular morphology.

The tricuspid and pulmonary valves are separated by the parietal band of the crista supraventricularis, whereas the mitral and aortic valves share fibrous continuity (see Figs 12-31 and 12-34). Since the AV valves almost invariably travel with their respective morphological ventricles, the distinguishing features of these valves may prove helpful in the proper evaluation of ventricular morphology. The tricuspid valve has a triangular orifice and numerous septal insertions, whereas the mitral valve has a football-shaped orifice and has no septal attachments.

By two-dimensional echocardiography, ventricular morphology is best inferred by the morphology of the AV valves, particularly by differences in their annular levels at the cardiac crux (see Fig 12-18); additionally, continuity or discontinuity between AV and semilunar valves may be evaluated, but apical trabeculae are not easily distinguished. Angiographically, the most reliable feature of a morphological right ventricle is the coarse pattern of apical trabeculations. Differences in chamber shapes may be useful criteria for both diagnostic methods.

Tomographic analysis

The noninvasive evaluation of cardiac diseases by two-dimensional imaging techniques is commonplace. Such tools include echocardiography, roentgenographic computed tomography, magnetic resonance imaging, and isotope positron reconstructions of the heart. To understand the pathologic alterations demonstrated by such imaging modalities, one must first understand the tomographic anatomy of the normal heart.

For two-dimensional echocardiography, the five most commonly used views are short-axis, left ventricular long-axis, left ventricular two-chamber, four-chamber, and right ventricular long-axis[1,71,72] (see Figs 12-9, 12-25, 12-28, and 12-34). For other tomographic imaging modalities, cardiac anatomy and pathology may best be displayed by the standard anatomic planes (frontal or coronal, median or sagittal, and horizontal or transverse), by special cardiac views (right anterior oblique or left anterior oblique), or by planes not yet in standard use (Fig 12-41).

Several common cardiac disorders, most notably ischemic heart disease, are characterized by regional, rather than global, disturbances in ventricular structure and function (Fig 12-42), which may be assessed by electrocardiography, angiocardiography, echocardiography, and radionuclide studies. For physicians working in these and other disciplines to be able to evaluate properly and treat patients with such regional myocardial abnormalities and to communicate this information accurately and unambiguously to their colleagues, a standardized and anatomically correct system of regional cardiac nomenclature is necessary.[1]

Accordingly, a system has been recommended that divides the left ventricular base-apex length into thirds and thereby produces basal, midventricular, and apical levels.[73] Each level is then divided into six anatomic segments (Fig 12-43). Since the percentage of total left ventricular mass accounted for by each region has been determined (Table 12-1), the percentage of left ventricular mass that is abnormal may be estimated.

In the clinical setting of acute myocardial infarction, the observation of wall motion abnormalities does not imply either that the process is acute or that the entire wall thickness is involved. Accordingly, when infarct size is estimated tomographically, allowances must be made for areas of old infarction and for viable subepicardial myocardium in the region of acute infarction. Moreover, the nonhomogeneous nature of normal regional contraction and relaxation must be taken into account when wall motion abnormalities are evaluated.[74]

Response to injury

Myocardial cells are highly structured and highly specialized cells whose volume is nearly one-half contractile elements and one-third mitochondria. As a result of this specialization and reliance on oxidative phosphorylation, myocardial cells are exquisitely sensitive to oxygen deprivation, and therefore ischemia represents the most common form of myocardial injury. However, many injurious agents, such as viruses, chemicals, and excessive cardiac workload, also may induce adaptive responses or cause sublethal or lethal cellular injury.

The heart has only a limited response to stress or injury. Adaptive responses include hypertrophy and dilatation, whereas sublethal cellular injury is characterized by various degenerative changes. Necrosis is the histologic hallmark of lethal cellular injury and elicits an inflammatory response and subsequent healing by scar formation.

By light microscopy, the normal myocardial cell is cylindric, often Y-shaped, and has an elongated central nucleus. Its diameter is 12 ± 2 μm in the right ventricle and 14 ± 2 μm in the left ventricle. With advanced age,

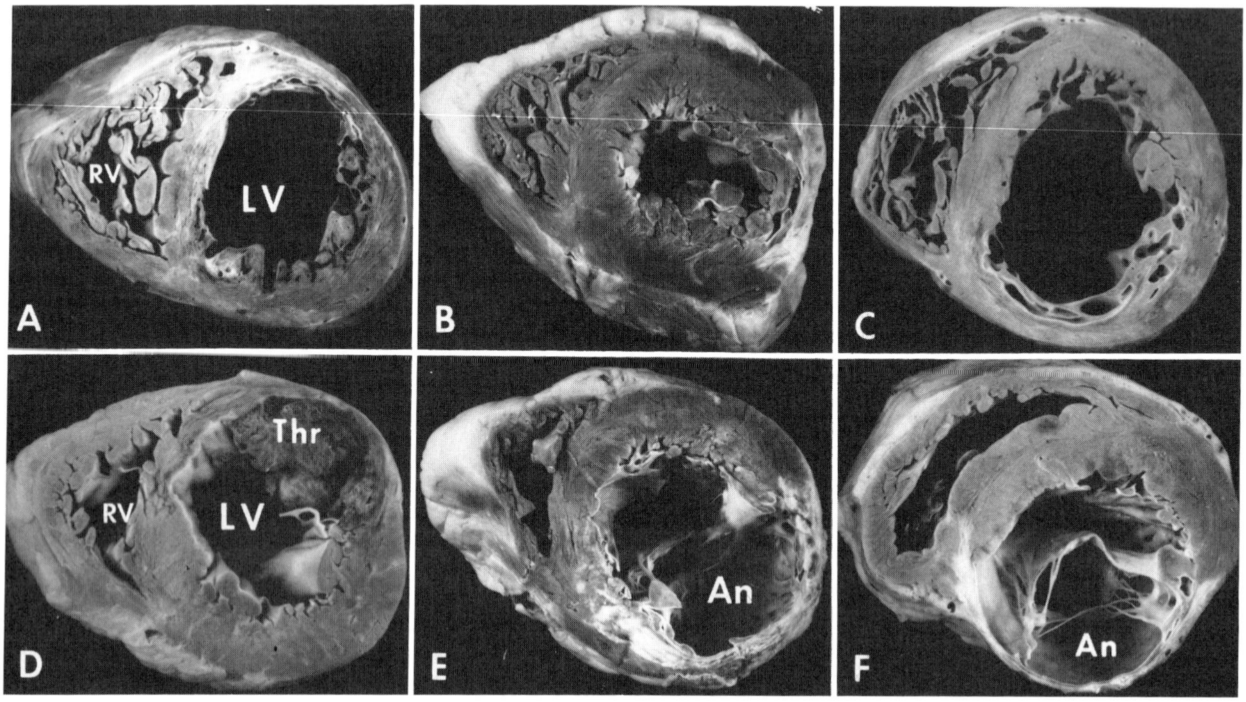

Fig 12-42 Regional left ventricular disorders. (Short-axis views of healed transmural myocardial infarctions.) **A,** anteroseptal (from 62-year-old man). **B,** lateral (from 93-year-old man). **C,** inferior (from 49-year-old man). **D,** anteroseptal aneurysm with mural thrombus *(Thr)* (from 84-year-old woman). **E,** lateral aneurysm *(An)* (from 74-year-old man). **F,** inferior aneurysm *(An)* (from 73-year-old man). (See Appendix for other abbreviations.) (**A,** from Edwards WD, Tajik AJ, Seward JB: Standardized nomenclature and anatomic basis for regional tomographic analysis of the heart. *Mayo Clin Proc* 56:479-497, 1981. By permission, Mayo Foundation.)

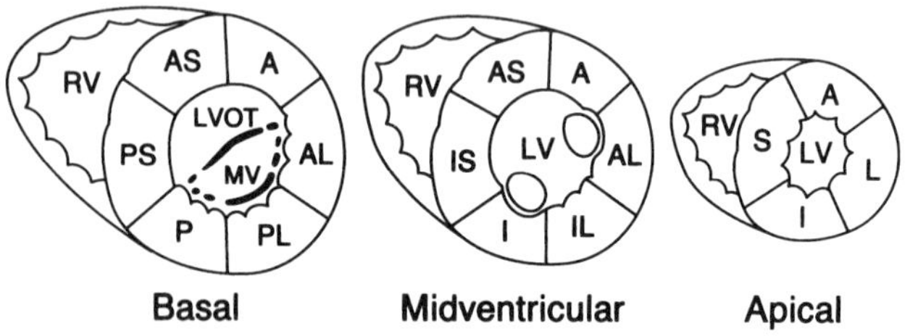

Fig 12-43 Regional analysis of the left ventricle. Short-axis views show 16-segment system. (See Appendix for abbreviations.) (Modified from Schiller NB, Shah PM, Crawford M, et al: Recommendations for quantitation of the left ventricle by two-dimensional echocardiography. *J Am Soc Echocardiogr* 2:358-367, 1989.)

Table 12-1 Percentage of regional left ventricular mass

Level	% LV volume per segment	No. of segments	Total, %
Basal	7.2	6	43
Middle	6.0	6	36
Apical	5.3	4	21

progressive accumulation of perinuclear lipofuscin pigment occurs and may impart a brown discoloration to the heart grossly (so-called brown atrophy) (see Fig 12-40). A discussion of the ultrastructural features of normal myocardial cells is beyond the scope of this chapter, but excellent reviews are available.[75]

In nondilated hearts, hypertrophied myocardial cells are characterized by an increase in length, diameter, and volume, as all sarcoplasmic elements increase in number.[76] On the basis of average cellular diameter, hypertrophy may be graded as mild (16 to 20 μm), moderate (21 to 25 μm), or marked (more than 25 μm). Although nuclei maintain their central position, they become enlarged and hyperchromatic (Fig 12-44) as a result of nuclear polyploidy, and they may assume irregular shapes or even undergo nuclear division (replication). Although most investigators consider myocardial cells incapable of actual cell division (hyperplasia),[77] others are of the opinion that, beyond a heart weight of about 500 g, hyperplasia does occur by longitudinal splitting of cardiac muscle cells.[78]

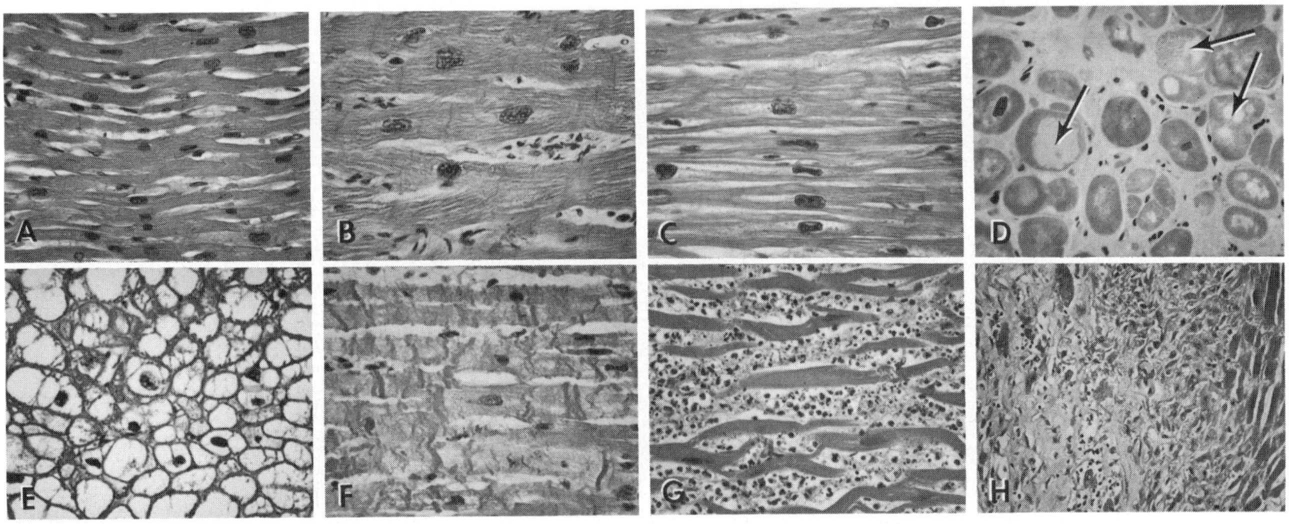

Fig 12-44 Myocardial response to injury (hematoxylin-eosin; ×200). **A,** longitudinal section of normal myocardial cells, for comparison (from 40-year-old woman). **B,** longitudinal section of hypertrophied myocardial cells, showing increased cell diameters and enlarged nuclei (from 16-year-old girl). **C,** longitudinal section of hypertrophied and attenuated myocardial cells, showing nuclear enlargement but normal cell diameters (from 19-year-old man with dilated cardiomyopathy). **D,** cross section of hypertrophied myocardial cells, showing degeneration *(arrows)* and interstitial fibrosis (from 35-year-old man). **E,** cross section of chronic subendocardial myocardial ischemia (from 64-year-old woman). **F,** longitudinal section of acute myocardial ischemia (from 30-year-old man). **G,** longitudinal section of the inflammatory response 5 days after an acute myocardial infarction (from 59-year-old man). **H,** longitudinal section of the reparative response (fibrovascular granulation tissue) several weeks after infarction.

Hypertrophy of cardiac muscle cells, in dilated or nondilated hearts, is accompanied by degenerative changes (see Fig 12-44),[79] by an increase in interstitial collagen,[80] and by a decrease in ventricular compliance.[77]

In dilated hearts, hypertrophied myocardial cells are stretched or attenuated, with increased lengths and volumes but normal or only mildly increased diameters; therefore, neither wall thickness grossly nor cellular diameter microscopically correlates well with hypertrophy (see Figs 12-37 and 12-44). In dilated hearts, the best histologic indicators of hypertrophy are the nuclear alterations, and the best overall hallmark of hypertrophy is a gross increase in heart weight or in ventricular muscle mass. On the basis of the percent increase in weight beyond the expected normal mean, hypertrophy may be graded as mild (up to 50%), moderate (51% to 100%), or marked (more than 100%).

Histologic evidence of chronic sublethal ischemia includes not only sarcoplasmic edema and fat accumulation, which impart a foamy or "chicken-wire" appearance to myocardial cells[81] (see Fig 12-44), but also the earlier typical mitochondrial alterations which may be observed ultrastructurally.[75] The histopathology of nonischemic sublethal injury differs somewhat from ischemic injury and is characterized by sarcoplasmic vacuolization and pale granularity, which correspond ultrastructurally to sarcotubular dilatation and to either myofibrillar loss or mitochondriosis, respectively.[82] Basophilic myocardial degeneration is characterized by sarcoplasmic accumulations of insoluble glycoproteins[83,84] and represents either a nonspecific response to nonischemic injury or an aging change. Whereas chronic ischemia tends to involve patchy areas of subendocardial myocardium, nonischemic injury is more microfocal and is not necessarily restricted to the subendocardium.

Acute myocardial ischemia, either sublethal or lethal, is characterized by intense sarcoplasmic staining with eosin dyes, prominent sarcoplasmic contraction bands, and, occasionally, stretched and wavy myocardial cells[85] (see Fig 12-44). When these ischemic cells are irreversibly injured (by infarction), the changes of coagulative necrosis appear; nuclei may fade away (karyolysis) or fragment (karyorrhexis), and the sarcoplasm may develop a glassy homogeneous appearance, although in many cases the cross striations remain intact for several days. Necrotic myocardium elicits an inflammatory infiltrate of neutrophils and macrophages, which serves histologically to differentiate acute infarction from acute ischemia (see Fig 12-44). Since, in contrast to infarction, the nonischemic forms of lethal injury generally involve individual cells or small clusters of cells rather than large patchy areas of myocardium, the necrotic cells often seem just to fade away and show little, if any, inflammatory cellular infiltrate.

Since myocardial cells cannot replicate, healing is by organization with scar formation rather than by regener-

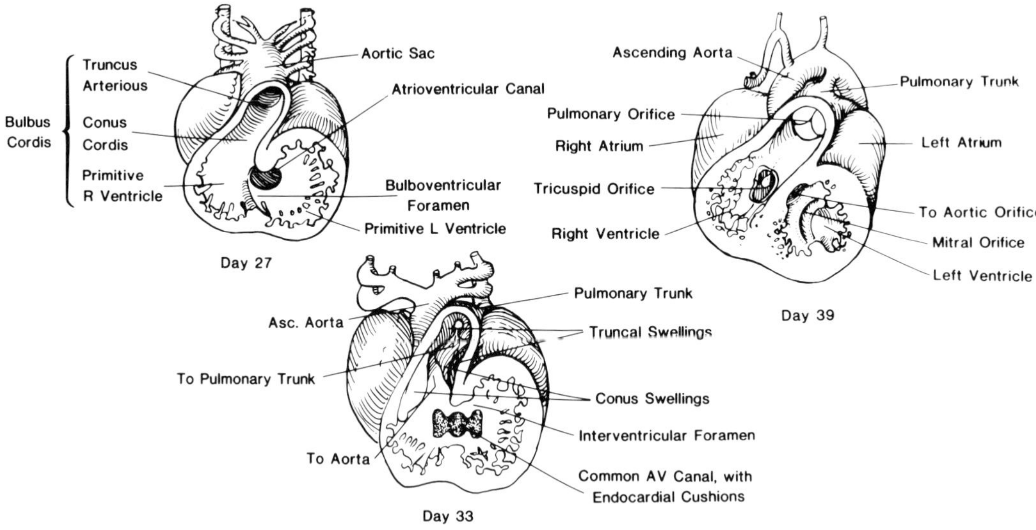

Fig 12-45 Embryology of the ventricular septum. Rightward shift of the AV canal aligns each AV valve with its proper ventricle, and leftward shift of the conotruncus aligns each ventricle with its appropriate great artery. Although the muscular interventricular septum and the conoventricular septum develop passively, conotruncal septation is an active process. Dates are approximate. (See Appendix for abbreviations.) (Modified from Netter FH: Embryology. In *The Ciba Collection of Medical Illustrations, Vol. 5, Heart.* Edited by FF Yonkman. Summit, New Jersey, Ciba Pharmaceutical Company, 1969, pp 112-130.)

ation. Although scars, with time, may retract and diminish wall thickness, they cannot, of course, rhythmically contract and, accordingly, represent not only structural but also functional loss of myocardium (see Fig 12-42). Furthermore, scarring may impart rigidity to the ventricle and thereby hinder diastolic filling; coexistent hypertrophy would further lessen the ventricular compliance.

The greater the loss of myocardial cells, the larger the scar will be. Both chronic ischemia and microfocal nonischemic necrosis may produce delicate interstitial or perivascular fibrosis and small (less than 1 cm) fibrotic patches. Healed myocardial infarctions, in contrast, are associated with large (greater than 1 cm) scars, which may involve less than half the wall thickness (subendocardial or nontransmural) or more than half (transmural). Although dystrophic calcification commonly complicates fibrotic processes in the coronary arteries and cardiac valves, it uncommonly involves fibrotic myocardium, except perhaps in ventricular aneurysms.

Embryology

Although dextro-looping produces an external configuration that resembles an adult heart, the internal luminal pathway is still a single, although tortuous, tube. Along the anterosuperior lesser curvature of the heart loop, a prominent infolded ridge, the bulboventricular fold, develops and forms the superior border of the bulboventricular foramen. As ventricular septation begins, resorption (effacement or growth retardation) of the distal, or posterior, bulboventricular fold allows a rightward shift of the AV canal to bring each AV valve into proper alignment with its respective ventricle, and it allows a leftward shift of the conotruncus to accomplish similar alignment between each ventricle and its appropriate great artery (Figs 12-21 and 12-45). Ventricular septation occurs between days 25 and 40.

The ventricle and proximal bulbus cordis expand and form two outpouchings, the primitive left and right ventricles, respectively. Anteroinferiorly, their two medial walls fuse and passively form the muscular interventricular septum (see Fig 12-21). Anterosuperiorly, the conoventricular septum also develops passively but will become much more heavily trabeculated than the interventricular septum, whose right surface it eclipses and fuses to anteroapically.[86,87] The leading edge of the conoventricular septum is the anterior aspect of the bulboventricular fold and is destined to form the septal and moderator bands at the future ventriculoinfundibular junction (see Fig 12-45).

Diverticulation, undermining, and fenestration of the subendocardial myocardium produce a complex network of intracavitary trabeculations (stratum spongiosum), most of which are eventually resorbed (see Fig 12-21). In this manner, the ventricular outpouchings may expand centrifugally yet maintain a relatively thin solid layer of subepicardial myocardium (stratum compactum). Persistent trabeculations form the trabeculae carneae and tensor apparatus of the AV valves. In the adult heart, the free-wall thickness of the left ventricle is about three-fourths compact myocardium and one-fourth trabeculae, whereas that of the right ventricle often consists of the opposite fractions.

In contrast to the passive formation of inflow and

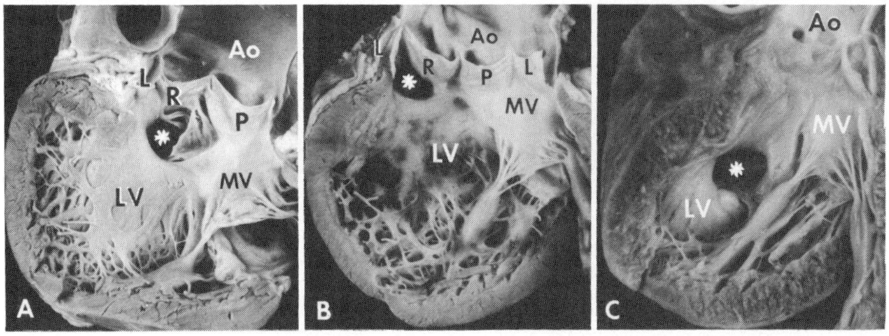

Fig 12-46 Ventricular septal defect (VSD) (left ventricular view in all). **A,** the membranous VSD (*) lies beneath the right and posterior aortic cusps (from 2-year-old girl). **B,** an infundibular VSD (*) lies beneath the left and right aortic cusps (from 18-month-old girl). **C,** a muscular VSD (*) is rimmed entirely by muscle and does not abut against a cardiac valve (from 4-day-old girl). (See Appendix for abbreviations.)

proximal conoventricular septa, the septation of the conotruncus distally is an active process, which is effected by apposing pairs of conal cushions (dextrodorsal and sinistroventral) and truncal cushions (dextrosuperior and sinistroinferior). The growth and fusion of the truncal cushions precede those of the conal cushions and divide the truncus arteriosus into pulmonary and aortic channels (see Fig 12-45). Resorption (effacement or growth retardation) of the distal bulboventricular fold allows the tricuspid orifice to shift rightward; it also allows the aorta to shift leftward and posteroinferiorly, to nestle between the two AV valves and contact the developing anterior mitral leaflet, and thereby to attain left ventricular origin. Fusion of the apposing conal cushions with themselves and their respective truncal cushions produces a gently spiraling partition that separates the two ventricular outflow tracts.[88]

However, at the expected site of the membranous septum, there still remains a small interventricular communication, which has received three distinct names—bulboventricular, primary interventricular, and secondary interventricular foramen—representing the various stages of bulboventricular development (see Fig 12-21). In the nonseptated heart loop, the ventricle and bulbus cordis are separated by a short constricted channel, the bulboventricular foramen. As the right AV valve aligns with the primitive right ventricle, the enlarging bulboventricular foramen tilts rightward and faces the tricuspid orifice more than the primitive left ventricle. Accordingly, the passage between both ventricles is now defined by another aspect of this opening, called the primary interventricular foramen. Then as the endocardial cushions arch atrially and shift leftward to form the anterior mitral leaflet, the primary interventricular foramen likewise enlarges and tilts leftward and now defines the orifice of the distal left ventricular outflow tract, or aortic vestibule. The adjacent remaining interventricular passage—the secondary interventricular foramen—is bordered by the muscular ventricular septum, the conus septum, and the right tubercles of the fused endocardial cushions. Although the bulboventricular and primary interventricular foramina expand and remain widely patent, the secondary interventricular foramen eventually closes, primarily by active extension of the inferior endocardial cushion; only later, as the septal tricuspid leaflet forms, does it attenuate and form the thin membranous septum.[89]

The most common ventricular septal defect, either isolated or associated with other cardiac anomalies, is the membranous (perimembranous) type, which involves the membranous septum and adjacent musculature beneath the right-posterior aortic commissure (Fig 12-46). The infundibular (supracristal; subarterial) ventricular septal defect is commonly encountered in tetralogy of Fallot and truncus arteriosus and involves the infundibular septum beneath the right-left aortic and pulmonary commissures (see Fig 12-46). A malalignment ventricular septal defect of either the membranous or the infundibular type is a result of malalignment between the infundibular septum and the remaining ventricular septum, such that one of the great arteries overrides the septum and attains biventricular origin, or both great arteries arise from one ventricle. Muscular defects (see Fig 12-46) may involve the remainder of the septum and may be solitary or multiple (so-called Swiss cheese septum). A defect of the AV septum is generally considered to be of the AV canal type, and straddling of an AV valve most commonly occurs across a defect of either this type or membranous type.

For an understanding of the pathologic anatomy of certain complex cardiac anomalies, it has been useful to conceptualize the heart as a five-chambered organ with two atria, two ventricles, and an infundibulum.[10] For example, in double-inlet left ventricle, the outlet chamber represents infundibulum, and the right ventricular expansion of the bulbus cordis appears to be very diminutive or absent. Since the infundibulum (outflow tract) lies distal and anterosuperior to the right ventricular inflow tract, the crista supraventricularis in normal hearts has been aptly named, for it does form a crest (crista) just above the right ventricle (supraventricularis) at the ventriculoinfundibular junction. In Ebstein's anomaly (see Fig 12-33,D), the tricuspid and right ventricular abnormalities involve only the inflow tract and do not extend beyond the ventriculoinfundibular junction. The so-called double-chamber right ventricle may result from separation of inflow and outflow tracts by a prominent moderator band or other anomalous muscle bundles.

Within the spectrum of cyanotic congenital heart disease is a group of anomalies that share in common a maldevelopment of the conotruncal septum. Tetralogy of Fallot, the most common

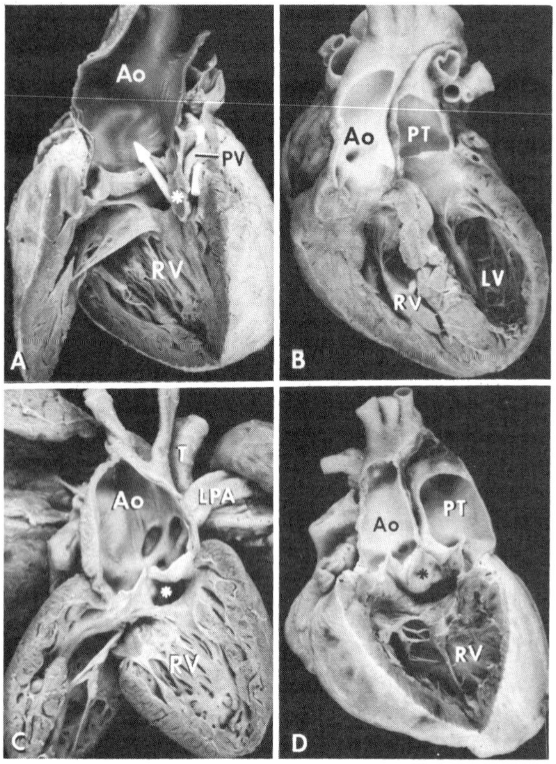

Fig 12-47 Congenital conotruncal anomalies. **A,** tetralogy of Fallot. Displacement of the infundibular septum (*) has produced subpulmonary stenosis (probe), a membranous ventricular septal defect (VSD) *(arrow),* and an overriding aorta with biventricular origin. (Opened right ventricle from 6-year-old boy). **B,** complete transposition of the great arteries. (Biventricular outflow view from 10-month-old boy.) **C,** truncus arteriosus with an infundibular VSD (*). (Opened right ventricle from 2-month-old girl.) **D,** double-outlet right ventricle with malalignment of the infundibular septum (*) and origin of both great arteries from the right ventricle, above the U-shaped VSD. (Right ventricular view from 2-year-old boy.) (See Appendix for abbreviations.) (**B,** from Daskalopoulos DA, Edwards WD, Driscoll DJ, et al: Correlation of two-dimensional echocardiographic and autopsy findings in complete transposition of the great arteries. *J Am Coll Cardiol* 2:1151-1157, 1983. By permission of the American College of Cardiology.) (**C,** from Mair DD, Edwards WD, Julsrud PR, et al: Truncus arteriosus. In *Moss' Heart Disease in Infants, Children, and Adolescents.* Fourth edition. Edited by FH Adams, GC Emmanouilides, TA Riemenschneider. Baltimore, Williams & Wilkins Company, 1989, pp 504-515. By permission.) (**D,** from Hagler DJ, Ritter DG, Puga FJ: Double-outlet right ventricle. In *Moss' Heart Disease in Infants, Children, and Adolescents.* Fourth edition. Edited by FH Adams, GC Emmanouilides. Baltimore, Williams & Wilkins, 1989, pp 442-460. By permission.)

anomaly in this group, results from anterosuperior displacement of the infundibular septum and is characterized by a large malalignment ventricular septal defect, an overriding aorta, and variable degrees of infundibular and valvular pulmonary stenosis (Fig 12-47); when the pulmonary valve is atretic, pulmonary blood flow may be derived from the ductus arteriosus or systemic collateral arteries (analogous to total anomalous pulmonary venous connection).

Complete transposition of the great arteries is associated with abnormal conotruncal septation and parallel rather than intertwined great arteries, such that the aorta arises from the right ventricle and the pulmonary artery emanates from the left ventricle (see Fig 12-47); a ventricular septal defect is present in about one-third of cases. Truncus arteriosus implies absent conotruncal septation and is characterized by a single arterial trunk from which the aorta, pulmonary arteries, and coronary arteries arise (see Fig 12-47); the ventricular septal defect is of membranous or infundibular type. Double-outlet right ventricle is characterized by the origin of both great arteries from the right ventricle, a malalignment ventricular septal defect, and infundibular septal displacement that differs from the type observed in tetralogy (see Fig 12-47); presumably, the distal embryonic bulboventricular fold did not resorb and the aorta could not attain left ventricular origin.

Some investigators have explained cardiac embryogenesis in terms of the concept that ontogeny recapitulates phylogeny. However, it is recognized that congenital cardiac malformations do not represent a state of arrested development and do not resemble the normal cardiac anatomy of lower animals. For example, neither truncus arteriosus nor double-inlet left ventricle (or their combination) resembles the three-chambered heart of an amphibian or lower reptile.

SEMILUNAR VALVES

General features

The right (pulmonary) and left (aortic) semilunar valves maintain unidirectional blood flow and separate the ventricles from the great arteries. In contrast to the AV valves, the arterial valves have no tensor apparatus (see Fig 12-31) and, therefore, are structurally simpler valves, which comprise annulus, cusps, and commissures. Behind each cusp is an outpouching of the arterial root, known as a sinus (of Valsalva); accordingly, there are three aortic sinuses and three pulmonary sinuses, which impart a tribulbous, or cloverleaf, shape to the arterial roots. The junction between the sinus portion of a great artery and its distal tubular portion forms a prominent ridge, the sinotubular junction (Fig 12-48). From the right and left aortic sinuses, proximal to this junction, arise the right and left coronary arteries, respectively.

The annuli of the semilunar valves contribute to the fibrous cardiac skeleton, but unlike the AV valves, they are intact, nonplanar rings of dense collagen. The annulus of each semilunar valve assumes the shape of a triradiate crown, the three points of which attain the level of the sinotubular junction and demarcate the commissures; the commissures represent the sites of lateral separation of one cusp from its adjacent cusps. The opening at the level of the sinotubular junction constitutes the anatomic valvular orifice, and the circumference of a semilunar valve at autopsy is measured at this level rather than along the nonplanar annulus.

The cusps are half-moon-shaped (semilunar), pocket-like flaps of delicate fibrous tissue which close the valvular orifice during ventricular diastole (see Fig 12-48). The leading edge of each cusp is its free edge. The closing edge, in contrast, represents a slightly thickened bi-scalloped ridge that lies a few millimeters below the free

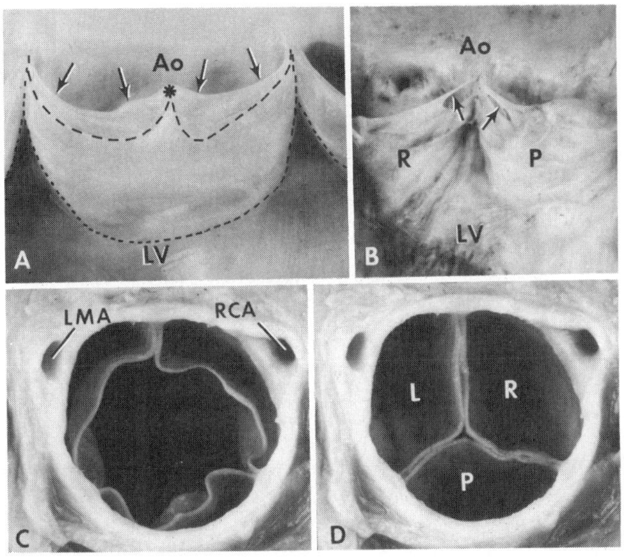

Fig 12-48 Aortic valve. **A,** the closing edge *(long-dashed line)* of a semilunar cusp lies below the free edge *(arrows);* however, at the center of each cusp, the closing and free edges meet at the nodule of Arantius (*); the annulus *(short-dashed line)* is nonplanar. (Opened aortic valve from 18-year-old woman.) **B,** the lunulae lie between the closing and free edges and, with age, may become fenestrated *(arrows)* near the commissures. (Opened aortic valve from 67-year-old man.) **C** and **D,** the free edge length of each cusp is greater than its straight-line intercommissural distance, so that the valve may open during ventricular systole **(C)** and close during diastole **(D);** the cusps do not cover the coronary ostia *(RCA, LMA)* during ventricular systole. (Aortic valve viewed from above from 37-year-old woman.) (See Appendix for abbreviations.)

edge, along the ventricular surface of the cusp. At the center of each cusp, the closing edge meets the free edge and forms a small fibrous mound, the nodule of Arantius. On either side of this nodule, between the free and closing edges of each cusp, are crescentic areas, or lunulae, which are commonly fenestrated, particularly in the aortic valve (see Fig 12-48). When the valve closes, apposing cusps contact one another along their closing edges and lunular surfaces and thereby form a competent seal; the center of the orifice is closed by the interdigitation of the three nodules of Arantius. Since lunular fenestrations lie distal to the closing edge, rarely do they produce valvular incompetence. The arterial surface of each cusp, in conjunction with its arterial sinus, forms the so-called valve pocket.

Like the AV valves, the semilunar valves comprise two major layers histologically.[21] The fibrosa forms the structural backbone of the valve and is continuous with the annulus, whereas the spongiosa acts more as a shock absorber along the ventricular surface, especially at the closing edge. Additionally, the ventricularis and arterialis are thin linings along the ventricular and arterial surfaces, respectively. The cusp contains little elastic tissue and, accordingly, has no appreciable elastic recoil; as a passively mobile structure, it apparently has no memory of shape and, therefore, has no tendency to assume either an open or a closed position.

Since the annulus cannot contract, the opening and closing of the semilunar valves is a passive process, which entails cuspid excursion and annulocuspid hinge-like motion. However, during isovolumetric ventricular contraction, expansion of the arterial root may produce commissural separation and thereby initiate valvular opening.[90] Each cusp, which hangs like a pocket from its U-shaped (parabolic) annular segment,[90] is freely mobile and moves in undulating fashion toward its arterial sinus during ventricular systole and then back toward the center of the arterial lumen during ventricular diastole, as retrograde blood flow fills the valve pocket. When the valve is viewed from above, the linear distance along the closing edge appears much greater than the straight-line distance between commissures (see Fig 12-48), and this extra length of cuspid tissue is necessary for nonstenotic opening and nonregurgitant closure of the valve. Accordingly, the nodules of Arantius traverse a greater distance during the cardiac cycle than any other cuspid region. The orifice of a fully opened semilunar valve assumes a circular or bowed triangular shape (see Fig 12-48).

In the elderly, various aging changes may alter the semilunar valves, particularly the aortic,[27,30] and may result in low-grade systolic ejection murmurs. Beyond the age of 20 years, the annular circumference of the aortic valve (that is, the perimeter of the aortic sinotubular junction) increases linearly[8,91,92] (see Fig A12-2) and is attended by mild cuspid thickening and redundancy (see Fig 12-40).[28] The closing edges become thickened and, along the nodules of Arantius, may form whisker-like projections called Lambl's excrescences. Lunular fenestrations also tend to develop with increasing age. Degeneration of valvular collagen is often accompanied by lipidosis and focal calcification, even in the absence of significant aortic atherosclerosis, and most commonly involves the annulus (annulocuspid hinge), the nodules of Arantius and adjacent closing edges, and the basal portions of the valve pockets.[27,30,93]

Although the sinotubular junction defines the anatomic valvular orifice, the functional orifice represents the cross-sectional area of the smallest passageway through a maximally opened valve and, therefore, may lie in a plane other than this junction. Disease processes that tend to increase cuspid rigidity, such as fibrosis or calcification, or that lead to commissural fusion, such as rheumatic valvulitis, tend to narrow the effective valvular orifice and, as a consequence, produce stenosis. In contrast, processes that straighten the cuspid line between commissures and thereby hold the commissures open, such as arterial root dilatation or rheumatic cuspid scar retraction, tend to produce a regurgitant valvular orifice. The pattern of valvular involvement by a disease process determines whether valvular function will be significantly altered and, if so, whether the valve will be stenotic or insufficient or both.

Pulmonary valve

The plane of the pulmonary annulus faces posteriorly, leftward, and superiorly, toward the left midscapula. In fixed postmortem specimens, the pulmonary annular circumference measures 7.0 ± 1.0 cm and is approximately 0.5 cm greater in men than in women and in fresh than in fixed specimens[19,33,34] (see Fig A12-2). The cusps are usually similar in size (Fig. 12-49), although minor variations are commonly observed. The annular dimen-

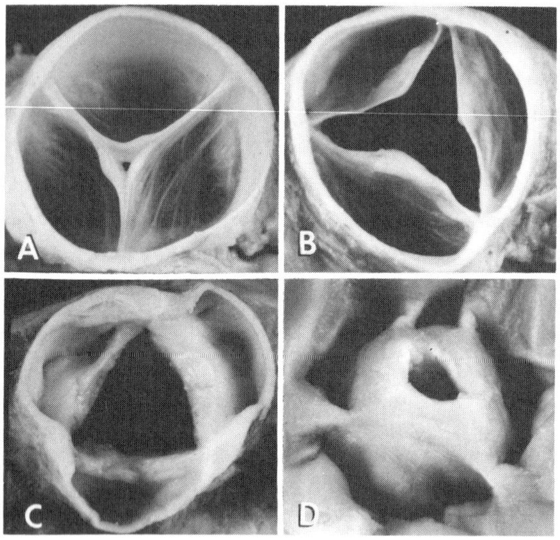

Fig 12-49 Pulmonary valve. (All viewed from above.) **A,** the normal pulmonary cusps are delicate and similar in size (from 68-year-old woman). **B,** in thromboembolic pulmonary hypertension, dilatation has resulted in pulmonary insufficiency (from 20-year-old man). **C,** in carcinoid heart disease, annular constriction and cuspid retraction have produced pulmonary stenosis and incompetence (from 36-year-old man). **D,** a congenitally acommissural dome-shaped pulmonary valve has caused severe pulmonary stenosis (from 4-year-old girl).

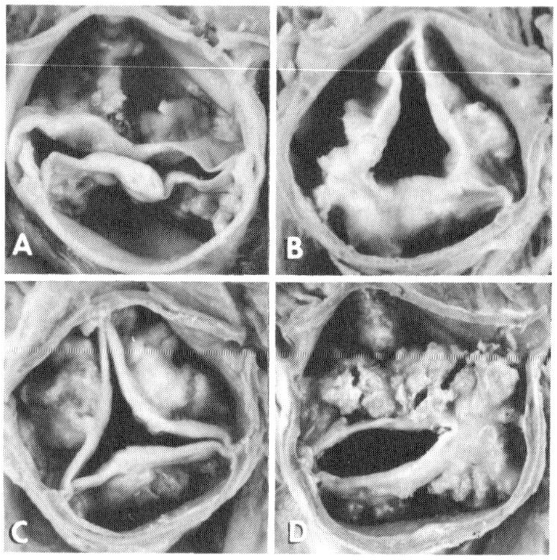

Fig 12-50 Aortic stenosis. (All viewed from above.) **A,** calcification of a congenitally bicuspid aortic valve (63-year-old man). **B,** fibrocalcific rheumatic disease (68-year-old man). **C,** degenerative (senile) calcification (80-year-old woman). **D,** calcification of a congenitally unicommissural aortic valve (from 75-year-old man).

sions of the pulmonary valve also have been measured in children.[8,94]

The infundibular septum lies subjacent to the right-left pulmonary commissure, whereas infundibular free wall subtends the remainder of the valve. A lip of right ventricular myocardium extends onto the pulmonary sinuses, such that the pulmonary valve appears in part buried within the crater of the right ventricular infundibulum. The anterosuperior limb of the septal band extends onto the left pulmonary sinus, and prominent trabeculae parallel to the parietal band insert onto the right pulmonary sinus; trabecular extensions onto the anterior sinus are less prominent.

Pulmonary incompetence may be observed in conditions that produce dilatation of the pulmonary trunk and annulus, such as pulmonary hypertension or heart failure (see Fig 12-49). Combined pulmonary stenosis and incompetence are features of carcinoid heart disease (see Fig 12-49), in which the annulus becomes constricted and stenotic and in which the cusps are also retracted and insufficient. Pure pulmonary stenosis is almost always congenital in origin (see Fig 12-49). Since the pulmonary valve lies anteriorly, near the upper left sternal border, pulmonary murmurs are generally heard best in this area.

Aortic valve

The plane of the aortic valve faces posteriorly, rightward, and superiorly, toward the right shoulder. In the living subject, the normal aortic annular area averages 3.1 ± 0.6 cm^2.[95] In fixed postmortem specimens, the normal aortic annular circumference measures 6.5 ± 1.0 cm and is approximately 0.5 cm greater in men than in women and in fresh than in fixed specimens.[19,33,34] However, annular area and circumference also vary considerably with age and body size[8,91,92] (see Fig A12-3); by the ninth decade, aortic and mitral annular dimensions are similar. Minor degrees of cuspid inequality are the rule.[3] In two-thirds of hearts, either the right or the posterior cusp is larger than the two others; in only 3% to 15% are the cusps truly of equal size.[92,96]

Variations in cuspid size may promote degenerative calcification, not only in native valves but also in porcine bioprostheses. Calcific spurs may extend from the aortic valve onto the anterior mitral leaflet or onto the left bundle branch at the ventricular septal summit.

Unoperated symptomatic aortic stenosis has a worse prognosis than many malignancies. Although it may be produced by a purely fibrotic process, either with or without commissural fusion, the vast majority of stenotic aortic valves are calcified, and many may be recognized roentgenographically. Most commonly, the valve is either congenitally bicuspid or involved by rheumatic disease; less commonly, it may represent degenerative (senile) calcification or a congenitally unicommissural valve (Fig 12-50). Only rarely are heavily calcified valves the site of active infective endocarditis. Subvalvular aortic stenosis may be congenital (discrete or tunnel types) or may be associated with hypertrophic cardiomyopathy. Supravalvular aortic stenosis represents a spectrum of arterial dysplasia that may constrict only the sinotubular junction or may involve most of the aorta; the pulmonary arteries also may be involved.

Chronic aortic incompetence, either with or without coexistent aortic stenosis, is most commonly associated with postrheumatic cuspid retraction, which yields a fixed triangular orifice (Fig 12-51). Similarly, aortic root dilatation may stretch open the commissures (see Fig 12-51) and thereby produce aortic insufficiency in either a tricuspid or a bicuspid valve. Acute

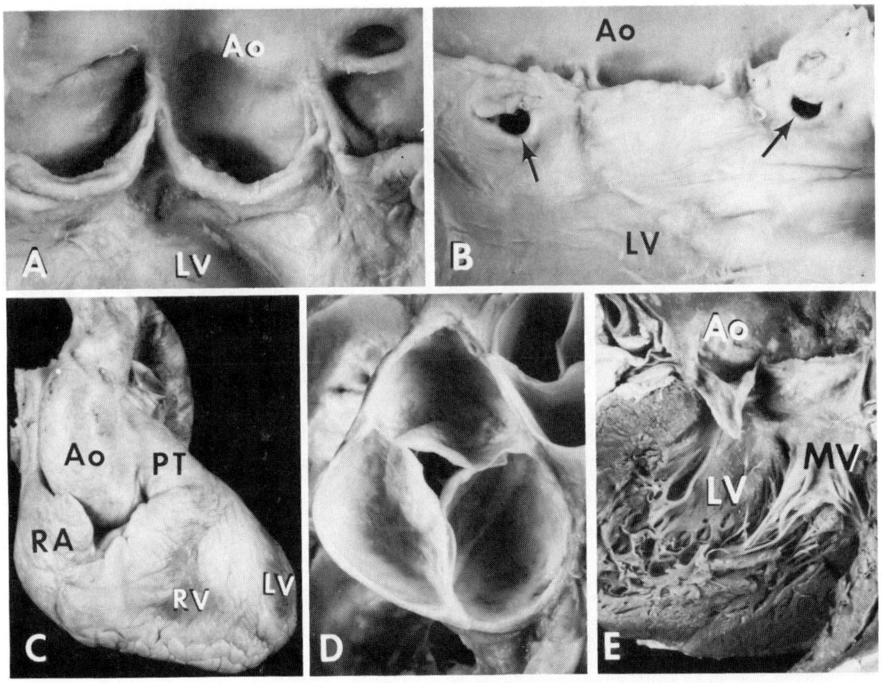

Fig 12-51 Aortic insufficiency. **A,** rheumatic fibrosis and retraction of cusps. (Opened aortic valve from 24-year-old man.) **B,** cuspid perforations *(arrows)* in healed endocarditis. (Opened aortic valve from 33-year-old man.) **C** and **D,** dilatation of the ascending aorta (**C,** anterior view) precludes complete closure of the aortic valve and results in a central triangular regurgitant orifice (**D,** from above). (From 79-year-old man.) **E,** incompetence of a noninfected bicuspid aortic valve is usually associated with annular dilatation or prolapse of the conjoined cusp. (Opened left ventricle from 69-year-old woman.) (See Appendix for abbreviations.)

aortic regurgitation may be produced by infective aortic endocarditis with cuspid perforation (see Fig 12-51) or by acute aortic dissection with commissural prolapse. Since the aortic valve is retrosternal, the murmurs of aortic stenosis and insufficiency are best heard along both upper sternal borders and may radiate toward the neck.

By virtue of its central position within the heart, the aortic valve and its sinuses contact all four cardiac chambers[97] (Fig 12-52). The right aortic cusp and its sinus overlie the anterosuperior ventricular septal summit and the parietal band of the right ventricular outflow tract. The right sinus is shielded by a prominent epicardial fat tag, the fold of Rindfleisch,[2] and may be covered in part by the right atrial appendage. The left aortic cusp and its sinus overlie the anterior left ventricular free wall and part of the anterior mitral leaflet; they abut the epicardium and atrial free wall and are covered in part by the pulmonary trunk. The posterior (noncoronary) aortic cusp and its aortic sinus overlie the posteroinferior ventricular septal summit and a portion of the anterior mitral leaflet; they abut the atrial septum, indent both atrial free walls—as the torus aorticus—and line a portion of the transverse sinus.

Each of the three aortic valve commissures is tangential to one of the three other cardiac valves (see Fig 12-52). The right-left commissure, between right and left aortic cusps, overlies the infundibular septum and is tangential to the right-left commissure of the pulmonary valve. The left-posterior commissure overlies the left ventricular chamber and, via the intervalvular fibrosa, is continuous with the anterior mitral leaflet. The right-posterior commissure overlies the membranous septum and is tangential to the anteroseptal commissure of the tricuspid valve.

Among cases of infective endocarditis, perhaps none presents so varied a clinical spectrum as those associated with aortic annular abscesses. The possible clinical presentations depend to a great extent on the particular cusp(s) involved. Subvalvular extension may involve the anterior mitral leaflet, left bundle branch, or ventricular septal myocardium; involvement of the ventricular septal myocardium may produce a large abscess cavity or result in rupture into a ventricular chamber with the formation of either an aorto-right ventricular or aorto-left ventricular fistula. An annular abscess may expand laterally and enter the pericardial cavity and thereby produce purulent pericarditis or fatal hemopericardium, or it may burrow into adjacent cardiac chambers or vessels and produce various fistulas (aorto-right atrial, aorto-left atrial, or aortopulmonary).

The posterior aortic cusp may be called the "noncoronary aortic cusp," and its sinus may be termed the "noncoronary aortic sinus." However, the term "noncoronary sinus" should not be used, and the expressions "right coronary sinus" and "left coronary sinus" are gross misnomers, since the coronary sinus, of course, is a specific venous structure that drains into the right atrium.

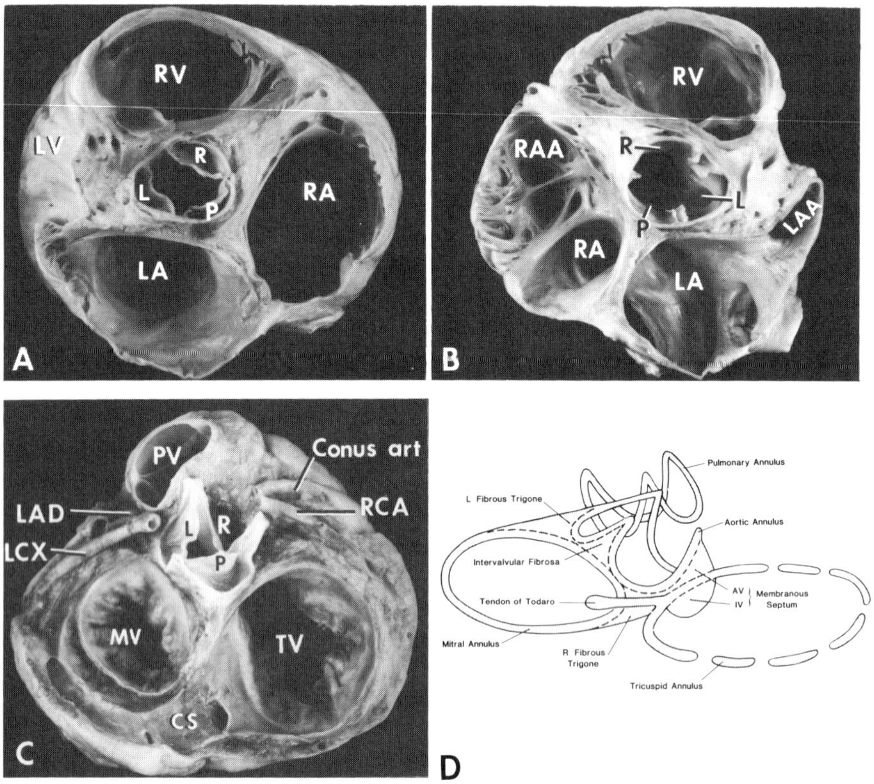

Fig 12-52 Aortic valve and base of heart. **A** and **B,** tomographic sections through the plane of the aortic valve show the adjacent cardiac structures, as viewed from above (**A**) and below (**B**). (From 27-year-old man.) **C,** the atria and great arteries have been removed to expose the four cardiac valves at the base of the heart. (From 26-year-old woman.) **D,** diagram of the fibrous cardiac skeleton. (See Appendix for abbreviations.) (**C,** from Edwards WD, Tajik AJ, Seward JB: Standardized nomenclature and anatomic basis for regional tomographic analysis of the heart. *Mayo Clin Proc* 56:479-497, 1981. By permission, Mayo Foundation.) (**D,** modified from Du Plessis LA, Marchand P: The anatomy of the mitral valve and its associated structures. *Thorax* 19:221-227, 1964.)

Comparison of semilunar valves

Since the ventricular outflow tracts and great arteries are intertwined, the two semilunar valves are likewise not parallel and subtend an angle of 60° to 90° (see Figs 12-28,D, and 12-52,C). The aortic cusps are thicker and more opaque than the pulmonary cusps, and in persons older than 40 years the circumference of the aortic valve is greater than that of the pulmonary valve[8] (see Fig A12-3). Lunular fenestrations are more common in aortic than in pulmonary valves.

With advanced age or aortic root dilatation, the aortic cusps may stretch and begin to prolapse slightly. Accordingly, the functional closing edge may shift toward the free edge; under these specific conditions, lunular fenestrations may produce aortic incompetence.

Unlike the AV valves, which tend to travel with their respective ventricles, the semilunar valves are named according to the great artery into which they empty. For example, in complete transposition of the great arteries, the aortic valve is interposed between the right ventricle and the aorta. By echocardiography and angiography, the proper identification of semilunar valves depends on the correct identification of the great arteries.

Fibrous cardiac skeleton

At the base of the heart (see Fig 12-52), the fibrous cardiac skeleton encircles the four cardiac valves and thereby uniquely guards the only sites of ventricular entry or exit. Furthermore, it comprises not only the four valvular annuli but also their intervalvular collagenous attachments (the right and left fibrous trigones, the intervalvular fibrosa, and the conus ligament) and the membranous septum and tendon of Todaro[98,99] (see Fig 12-52). This fibrous scaffold is firmly anchored to the ventricles but is rather loosely attached to the atria. Accordingly, the cardiac skeleton not only electrically insulates the atria from the ventricles but also supports the cardiac valves and provides a firm foundation against which the ventricles may contract.

The aortic valve forms the cornerstone of the cardiac skeleton, and its fibrous extensions anchor and support the three other valves. The intervalvular fibrosa, or trigone, is interposed between the left-posterior aortic commissure and the anterior mitral leaflet, and its epicardial surface is fused to the left atrial free wall. From the left and posterior aortic annular segments, the left and right fibrous trigones, respectively, project like outstretched arms and embrace the mitral annulus along its anterior leaflet. Accordingly, the left fibrous trigone, intervalvular fibrosa, and right fibrous trigone, in that order, provide direct mitral-aortic continuity between the anterolateral and posteromedial mitral commissures.

Furthermore, the right fibrous trigone, in conjunction with the membranous septum, also joins the right-posterior aortic commissure to the anteroseptal tricuspid commissure and maintains fibrous continuity between the anterior mitral and septal tricuspid leaflets. Therefore, the right fibrous trigone (central fibrous body) welds together the aortic, mitral, and tricuspid valves and forms the largest and strongest component of the cardiac skeleton (see Fig 12-52). The conus ligament, or tendon of Krehl, forms a diminutive connection between the aortic and pulmonary valves, just to the right of their right-left commissures.

Although in schematic drawings the four cardiac valves are generally pictured within a single plane at the cardiac base, they actually do not lie in the same plane or even in parallel planes. The tricuspid and mitral valves are skewed 10° to 15° such that they approach each other at the membranous septum and diverge at the cardiac crux, as the ostium of the coronary sinus interposes. Similarly, a tilt of 60° to 90° is observed between the mitral and aortic valves and between the pulmonary and aortic valves. These angles may vary somewhat during the cardiac cycle and may be altered by advanced age, particularly as the ventricular septum becomes more angulated.

Because of the intervalvular attachments of the fibrous cardiac skeleton, perturbations of one valve may affect the size, shape, position, or relative angulation of its neighboring valves and may affect the adjacent coronary arteries or cardiac conduction system. Such perturbations may be caused by various disease states or by surgical interventions for those valvular disorders. Tricuspid annuloplasty or replacement may be complicated by injury to the right coronary artery or AV conduction tissues, whereas mitral valve replacement may be attended by trauma to the circumflex coronary artery, coronary sinus, or aortic valve. At aortic valve replacement, the anterior mitral leaflet, left bundle branch, or coronary ostia may be injured inadvertently.

Embryology

By approximately day 32, the dextrosuperior and sinistroinferior truncal swellings have fused and have partitioned the truncus arteriosus. Distally, along both sides of the truncal septum, tubercles form from each swelling and are destined to become the right and left cusps and sinuses of the pulmonary and aortic valves. Opposite the septum, between these two pairs of tubercles, arise a pair of intercalated valve swellings, which will form the anterior pulmonary and posterior aortic cusps and sinuses. By a process of excavating and hollowing in a proximal direction, the semilunar cusps and their arterial sinuses are molded, between days 35 and 55 (Fig 12-53).

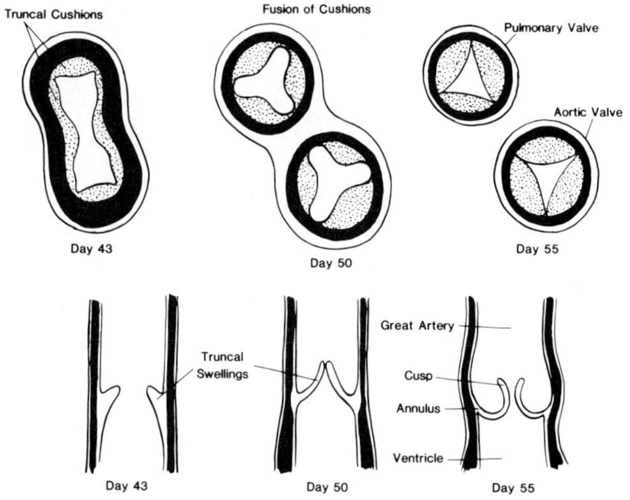

Fig 12-53 Embryology of the semilunar valves. **Upper,** the aortic and pulmonary valves form as fusion of the right superior and left inferior truncal swellings divides the truncus arteriosus into two orifices. **Lower,** the cusps are produced by excavation and hollowing of the valve swellings. Dates are approximate.

The fibrous cardiac skeleton is derived, for the most part, from epicardial connective tissue.[99] Invagination of the AV sulcus contributes to the formation of the tricuspid and mitral annuli, whereas truncal swellings form the pulmonary and aortic annuli. The central fibrous body (right fibrous trigone) is derived from ingrowth of the dorsal mesocardium and the AV sulcus, and the membranous septum develops primarily by attenuation of endocardial cushion tissue that has effected closure of the secondary interventricular foramen.[89] As the distal bulboventricular fold resorbs, the developing aortic and mitral valves make contact, and the intervening AV sulcus tissue, in conjunction with endocardial and truncal cushion tissue, forms the left fibrous trigone and intervalvular fibrosa. Development of the tendon of Todaro is associated with infolding of the sinoatrial junction and subsequent formation of the eustachian and thebesian valves from the right venous valve. The development of the fibrous cardiac skeleton is intimately associated with the formation of the AV conduction system.

Most congenital anomalies of the pulmonary valve are associated with stenosis (see Fig 12-49,D). Isolated pulmonary stenosis is almost always due to a dome-shaped acommissural valve, with congenital fusion of all three commissures. However, forms of pulmonary stenosis which are associated with other cardiac malformations, such as tetralogy of Fallot, usually result from a bicuspid or unicommissural valve (often with a hypoplastic annulus) or from a dysplastic valve with three thickened cusps. Quadricuspid pulmonary valves are more common than quadricuspid aortic valves, but both are usually incidental findings.

Congenitally bicuspid aortic valves affect 1% to 2% of the general population and constitute the most common form of congenital heart disease. Although they usually are neither stenotic nor insufficient at birth (Fig 12-54), most bicuspid valves will become stenotic during adulthood as the cusps calcify (see Fig 12-50,A), and some will become insufficient as a result of

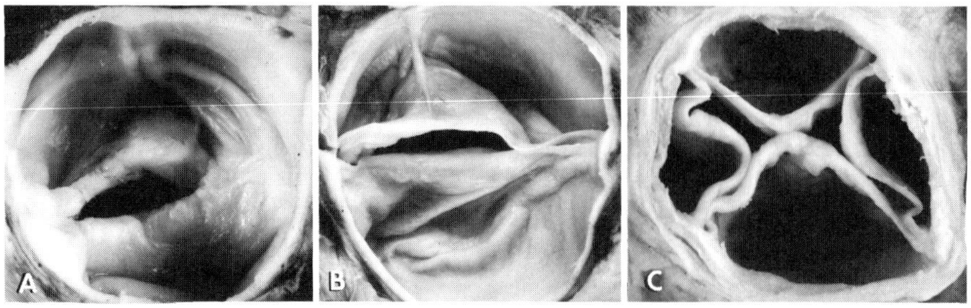

Fig 12-54 Congenital aortic valve anomalies. (All viewed from above.) **A,** this noncalcified unicommissural valve was inherently moderately stenotic. (From 18-year-old woman; compare with Figure 12-50,D.) **B,** this noncalcified and nondilated bicuspid valve was neither stenotic nor incompetent. (From 45-year-old man; compare with Figs 12-50,A, and 12-51,E.) **C,** this noncalcified quadricuspid valve apparently functioned normally and was an incidental finding at autopsy. (From 68-year-old man.)

infective endocarditis or aortic root dilatation (see Fig 12-51,E). In contrast, the congenitally unicommissural aortic valve is usually stenotic at birth (see Fig 12-54) and becomes progressively more obstructive as calcification develops in adulthood (see Fig 12-50,D). Acommissural and dysplastic aortic valves are rare and are usually severely stenotic at birth. Aortic atresia is associated with the hypoplastic left heart syndrome and is usually fatal during the first week of life. All congenital anomalies of the aortic valve are much more common in males than in females.

In truncus arteriosus, the truncal valve most commonly comprises three cusps and resembles a normal aortic valve. However, it may be quadricuspid, bicuspid, or, rarely, pentacuspid and may contain one or more raphes; such nontricuspid valves are often incompetent, particularly if the truncal root is dilated.

GREAT ARTERIES
Pulmonary arteries

The pulmonary trunk emanates from the right ventricle and travels to the left of the ascending aorta. At the bifurcation, the left pulmonary artery and the pulmonary trunk form a smooth arch, whereas the right pulmonary artery, in contrast, arises from the pulmonary trunk at a right angle and then travels beneath the aortic arch and behind the superior vena cava (see Figs 12-10 and 12-14). The pulmonary trunk and left pulmonary artery contribute to the left border of the frontal cardiac silhouette roentgenographically, between the aortic arch and the left atrial appendage (or left shoulder of the heart).

Within the lungs, the pulmonary arteries accompany their respective bronchi, but the pulmonary veins are found in the interlobular septa. In general, pulmonary arteries with a diameter greater than 1 mm are elastic arteries, whereas those that are smaller are muscular arteries. The latter are the true resistance vessels in normal lungs. Since pulmonary arterioles do not normally contain medial smooth muscle,[100] the popular term "arteriolar resistance" is a misnomer. Although the lungs receive 100% of the right cardiac output, the pulmonary circulation is commonly referred to as the "lesser" circulation.

In the adult, the pulmonary trunk is slightly greater in diameter than the ascending aorta, and its wall thickness is roughly half that of the aorta.[101] At birth, however, the wall thicknesses are equal, and the elastic media of the pulmonary trunk attenuates only as pulmonary pressure and resistance diminish during the first few months of life. In the elderly, as both great arteries become ectatic, the pulmonary trunk dilates to a lesser extent than the ascending aorta[8] (see Fig A12-3).

Since neither the tracheobronchial tree nor the pulmonary arterial tree exhibits bilateral mirror-image symmetry, the spatial relationships between the bronchi and the arteries provide the anatomic hallmark for distinguishing a morphological right lung from a morphological left lung. The right pulmonary artery and right upper lobar artery travel anteriorly to their respective bronchi, but the right intermediate pulmonary artery travels superiorly to the bronchus intermedius and posteriorly to the right middle lobar bronchus (Fig 12-55). In contradistinction, the left pulmonary artery arches over the left main bronchus and posteriorly to the left upper lobar bronchus (see Fig 12-55). External patterns of pulmonary lobation are unreliable indicators of pulmonary situs.

Roentgenographically, in pulmonary situs solitus, the distance from the carina to the left upper lobar bronchus is 1.5 to 2.0 times that from the carina to the right upper lobar bronchus. In situs inversus, the opposite pertains. In right or left pulmonary isomerism, the ratio approaches unity, but the absolute length from the carina to the upper lobar bronchi is greater with bilateral morphological left lungs than with right lungs. Pulmonary situs cannot be determined by echocardiography alone.

In the setting of pulmonary hypertension, especially in children with pliable tracheobronchial cartilage, the tense and dilated pulmonary arteries may compress the left bronchus and the left upper and right middle lobar bronchi and thereby contribute to recurrent bronchopneumonia in those lobes. Furthermore, the dilated pulmonary trunk may displace the aortic arch rightward and secondarily produce tracheal indentation and, occasionally, hoarseness as a result of compression of the left recurrent laryngeal nerve. Pulmonary arterial atheromas, in contrast to their counterpart in the aorta, are shallow, nonulcerated, noncalcified, and nonobstructive.

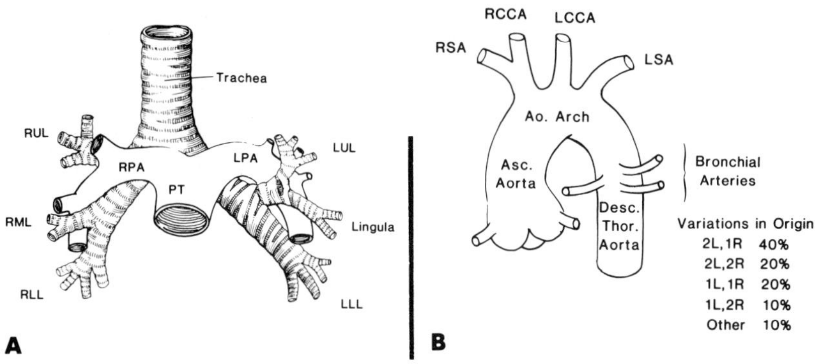

Fig 12-55 Pulmonary and bronchial arteries. **A,** the right and left pulmonary arteries do not exhibit mirror-image symmetry. **B,** the bronchial arteries usually arise from the descending thoracic aorta at the level of the carina. (See Appendix for abbreviations.)

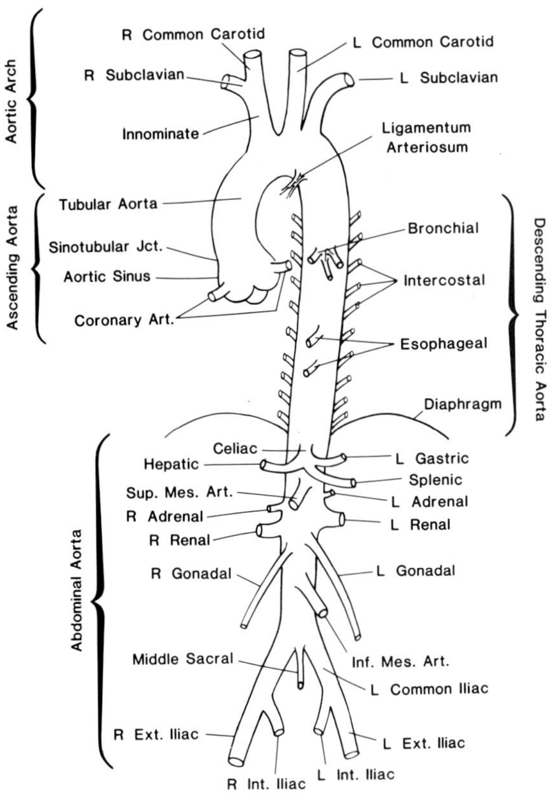

Fig 12-56 Systemic arteries. The aorta may be divided into ascending arch, descending thoracic, and abdominal regions. (See Appendix for abbreviations.)

Aorta

The aorta is the major systemic elastic artery of the body. It arises at the level of the aortic valve annulus and terminates at the aortic bifurcation, approximately at the level of the umbilicus and the fourth lumbar vertebra. The aorta has four major divisions: ascending aorta, aortic arch, descending thoracic aorta, and abdominal aorta (Fig 12-56).

The ascending aorta lies almost entirely within the pericardial sac (see Fig 12-2) and comprises sinus and tubular portions, which are demarcated by the aortic sinotubular junction. The aortic valve is related to the three sinuses, and the right and left coronary arteries arise from the right and left aortic sinuses, respectively. The ascending aorta lies to the right of the pulmonary trunk (see Fig 12-10).

With age or with the development of atherosclerosis, the aortic sinotubular junction may become heavily calcified, particularly above the right cusp, and may produce coronary ostial stenosis. Aortic annular abscesses and congenital aortic sinus aneurysms may perforate into neighboring structures and produce a variety of clinical manifestations. Among the causes of annuloaortic ectasia, perhaps aging, medial degeneration (so-called cystic medial necrosis), and chronic hypertension are the most common and may produce an ascending aortic aneurysm, aortic valvular incompetence, or acute aortic dissection. Acute aortic dissection is commonly associated with an intimal tear above the right aortic cusp (Fig 12-57) and with eventual rupture into the pericardial sac.

The aortic arch travels over the right pulmonary artery and the left bronchus (see Fig 12-14). From its superior aspect emanate the innominate, left common carotid, and left subclavian arteries, in that order (see Fig 12-56). In 11% of subjects, the innominate and left common carotid arteries form a common ostium, and in 5%, the left vertebral artery arises from the aortic arch, between the left common carotid and left subclavian arteries. The ligamentum arteriosum represents the obstructed fibrotic or fibrocalcific remnant of the fetal ductus arteriosus, which joined the proximal left pulmonary artery to the undersurface of the aortic arch. The aortic arch contributes to the left superior border of the frontal cardiac silhouette and thereby forms the roentgenographic aortic knob.

When aortic dissections do not involve the ascending aorta (type III or type B), the intimal tear is commonly near the ligamentum arteriosum or the ostium of the left subclavian artery. By virtue of severe torsional and shear stresses placed on the heart and great vessels during nonpenetrating decelerative chest trauma,

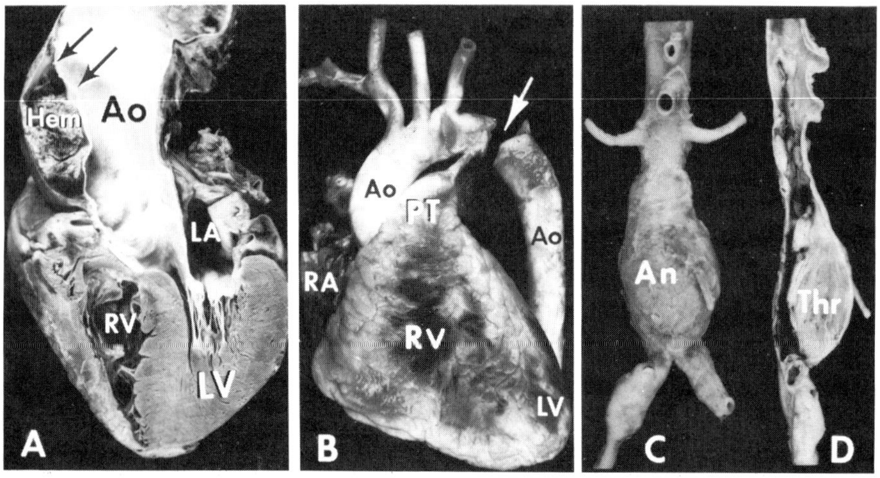

Fig 12-57 Acquired diseases of the aorta. **A,** this acute aortic dissection, with intimal flap *(arrows)* and intramedial hematoma *(Hem),* involved only the ascending aorta; its rupture produced a fatal hemopericardium. (Long-axis view in 78-year-old woman.) **B,** nonpenetrating decelerative blunt chest trauma during an automobile accident resulted in complete transection of the aorta *(arrow)* just distal to the left subclavian artery. (Anterior view in 22-year-old man.) **C** and **D,** an atherosclerotic aneurysm *(An)* of the infrarenal abdominal aorta bulges anteriorly (**C**) and is filled with mural thrombus *(Thr)* (**D**). (Anterior view [**C**] and right lateral view [**D**] of longitudinal section from 64-year-old man.) (See Appendix for other abbreviations.)

as may occur in motor vehicle accidents, the aorta may be transected at the junction between the aortic arch and the descending thoracic aorta (see Fig 12-57). When the tear is incomplete, a posttraumatic pseudoaneurysm may develop with time. Aneurysms of the aortic arch may be associated with hypertension, atherosclerosis, or aortitis or may be idiopathic.

The descending thoracic aorta abuts the left anterior surface of the vertebral column and lies adjacent to the esophagus and the left atrium. Its posterolateral branches are the bilateral intercostal arteries, and its anterior branches include the bronchial, esophageal, mediastinal, pericardial, and superior phrenic arteries (see Fig 12-56). The bronchial arteries, most commonly two left and one right, nourish the bronchial walls and the pulmonary arterial and venous walls[102] (see Fig 12-55). Uncommonly, bronchial arteries may arise from intercostal or subclavian arteries or, rarely, from a coronary artery. The bronchial veins drain not only into the azygos and hemiazygos veins but also into the pulmonary veins.

Pulmonary emboli may cause pulmonary infarction, particularly when shock or heart failure supervenes; adequate bronchial collateral arteries may minimize the extent of infarction. In several forms of pulmonary hypertension, the bronchial arteries may become quite enlarged and tortuous.

Aneurysms of the descending thoracic aorta may be associated with aortic dissection, aortitis, atherosclerosis, hypertension, or trauma. They may or may not extend below the diaphragm.

The abdominal aorta travels along the left anterior surface of the vertebral column and lies adjacent to the inferior vena cava. The major lateral (retroperitoneal) branches include the renal, adrenal, right and left lumbar, and inferior phrenic arteries (see Fig 12-56). The gonadal arteries arise somewhat more anteriorly but remain retroperitoneal. The intraperitoneal branches arise anteriorly and include the celiac artery (with its left gastric, splenic, and hepatic branches) and the superior and inferior mesenteric arteries. The distal aortic branches include the right and left common iliac arteries and the small middle sacral artery.

Atherosclerotic abdominal aortic aneurysms are most commonly infrarenal; they tend to bulge anteriorly and they thereby stretch and compress the gonadal and inferior mesenteric arteries (see Fig 12-57). Such aneurysms are generally filled with laminated thrombus and so their residual lumens may appear normal or even narrowed rather than dilated. Rupture of an atherosclerotic abdominal aortic aneurysm may be associated with extensive retroperitoneal hemorrhage, with or without intraperitoneal hemorrhage.

Embryology

As the forebrain and foregut expand cranially and the primitive heart tube folds down into the developing thorax, between days 20 and 21, the bilateral arterial connections between the heart and the dorsal aortas likewise fold and form the first aortic arches (see Fig 12-7); at this time, dilatation of the truncoaortic junction produces a prominent aortic sac. As paired pharyngeal pouches subsequently develop, five additional pairs of aortic arches will form, as bilateral vascular sprouts from the aortic sac merge with similar vessels arising from the paired dorsal aortas (Fig 12-58). The eventual fate of each

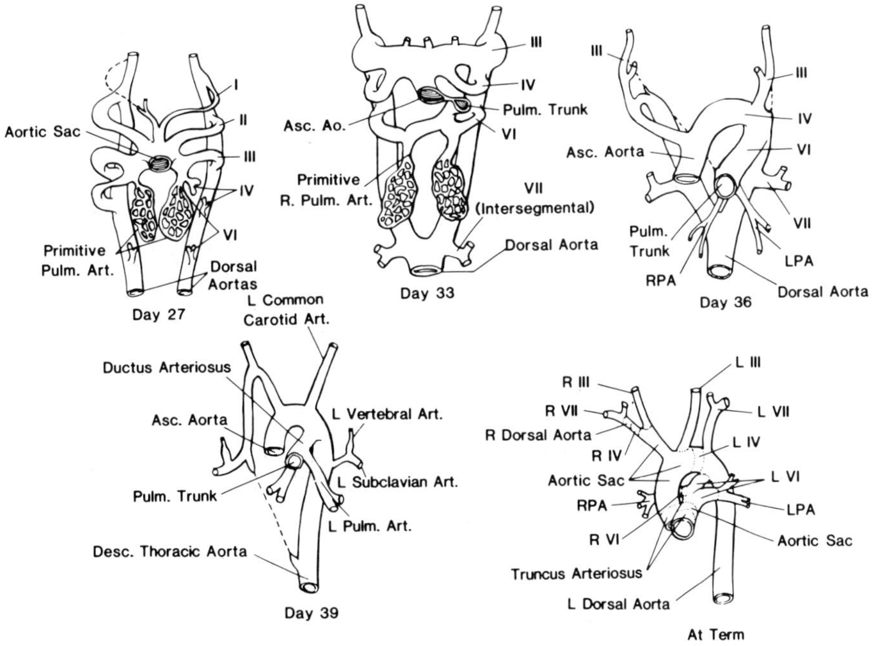

Fig 12-58 Embryology of the aortic arches. The left fourth arch forms the isthmus of the definitive left aortic arch, and the distal left sixth arch forms the (left) ductus arteriosus. Dates are approximate. (See Appendix for abbreviations.) (Modified from Netter FH: Embryology. In *The Ciba Collection of Medical Illustrations, Vol. 5, Heart.* Edited by FF Yonkman. Summit, New Jersey, Ciba Pharmaceutical Company, 1969, pp 112-130.)

pair of arches is different, but generally the distal portion of each arch will wither and disappear; only the left fourth arch will remain intact and form the isthmus of the definitive left aortic arch.

By day 27, the first and second pairs of aortic arches have largely disappeared, and they will persist only as the maxillary and stapedial arteries, respectively. The third pair of aortic arches is prominent and will eventually form the common carotid arteries and proximal portions of the internal carotid arteries. At this time, the fourth and sixth pairs of aortic arches are beginning to form, and already the primitive pulmonary arteries are developing from the proximal (aortic sac) sprouts of the sixth aortic arches. In humans, the fifth aortic arches never develop completely and rapidly disappear.

By day 30, the fourth and sixth pairs of aortic arches have become prominent structures (see Fig 12-58). Proximally, along the aortic sac, the fourth arches shift rightward, and the sixth arches migrate leftward. Accordingly, by the time the truncal septum has formed, on day 32, the sixth aortic arches are aligned with the developing right ventricular outflow tract and the fourth aortic arches are aligned with the left ventricle. The aortopulmonary septum, which forms by invagination of the posterior wall of the aortic sac, bulges anteriorly and fuses with the truncal septum on day 33; it thus separates the ascending aorta from the pulmonary trunk and contributes to the spiral septum that intertwines the great arteries.

By day 35, the portion of the aortic sac which forms the ascending aorta becomes Y-shaped and thereby also forms the innominate artery, on the right, and the aortic arch to the level of the left common carotid artery (left third arch), on the left (see Fig 12-58). The distal third arches and the dorsal aortas between the third and fourth arches have by this time disappeared. Furthermore, the right fourth aortic arch is becoming narrowed, and the distal right sixth aortic arch has withered and disappeared. The distal left sixth arch remains prominent and forms the (left) ductus arteriosus, which normally closes only after birth. In addition, the seventh intersegmental arteries, destined to become the subclavian arteries, migrate up the dorsal aortas toward the fourth aortic arches.

By day 40, the portion of the right dorsal aorta which lies distal to the right seventh intersegmental artery has withered and disappeared. The right fourth aortic arch and the remainder of the right dorsal aorta form the proximal segment of the right subclavian artery, and the right seventh intersegmental artery forms its distal segment and also gives rise to the right vertebral artery. The left intersegmental artery, which forms the left subclavian artery and gives rise to the left vertebral artery, continues migrating superiorly and will eventually achieve the level of the left fourth aortic arch. At this time, the aorta is asymmetric and closely resembles its appearance in the adult (see Fig 12-58).

Since the lungs are foregut derivatives, their blood supply, like that of the esophagus, arises initially from the dorsal aortas. However, by day 27, the arterial branches of

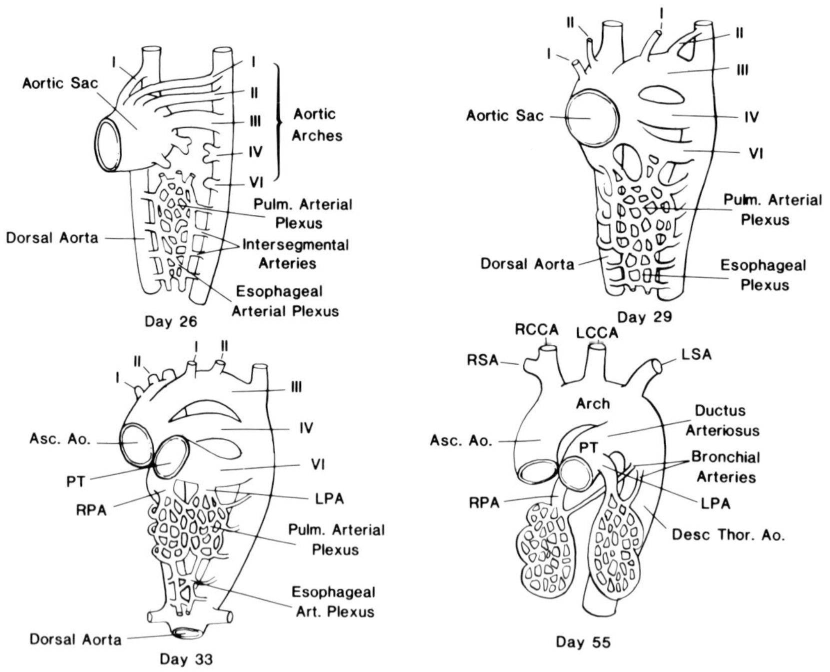

Fig 12-59 Embryology of the pulmonary arteries (schematic left lateral view). Although the pulmonary arterial plexus initially is supplied by intersegmental branches of the paired dorsal (descending thoracic) aortas, this plexus soon develops anastomoses with the right and left pulmonary arteries (proximal sixth aortic arches). Later, the systemic arterial connections wither and either disappear or persist as bronchial arteries. Dates are approximate. (See Appendix for abbreviations.)

the sixth aortic arches anastomose with this pulmonary vascular plexus, and the initial systemic arterial supply to the lungs soon regresses (Fig 12-59). These smaller branches of the descending thoracic aorta will form the bronchial arteries as the lungs develop.

An aortopulmonary septal defect represents a large opening between the ascending aorta and the pulmonary trunk and hemodynamically resembles a patent ductus arteriosus. Rarely, one pulmonary artery may originate from the ascending aorta or ductus arteriosus while the other arises normally from the pulmonary trunk. Congenital stenosis of the pulmonary arteries is usually associated with maternal rubella during the first trimester. In pulmonary atresia with ventricular septal defect, the pulmonary arteries may be derived from the right or left ductus arteriosus and from bronchial or other systemic collateral arteries (analogous to total anomalous pulmonary venous connection).

A variety of anomalies result from faulty development of the aortic arches. A right aortic arch with mirror-image brachiocephalic branching presumably results from persistence of the right fourth aortic arch and disappearance of its left counterpart; although this may be an isolated anomaly, it most commonly accompanies tetralogy of Fallot (Fig 12-60), pulmonary atresia with ventricular septal defect, and truncus arteriosus. A double aortic arch presumably results from persistence of both fourth aortic arches, and an interrupted aortic arch may represent the resorption of both fourth aortic arches. An aberrant retroesophageal right subclavian artery is a relatively common anomaly, which may cause dysphagia (see Fig 12-60); it probably results from persistence of the right dorsal aorta and resorption of the right fourth aortic arch.

The patent ductus arteriosus may be isolated or may accompany other cardiac malformations. A left ductus arteriosus joins the proximal left pulmonary artery to the aortic arch (see Fig 12-60), whereas a right ductus arteriosus joins the proximal right pulmonary artery to the right subclavian artery; in cases of right aortic arch with mirror-image brachiocephalic branching, the opposite pertains. Coarctation of the aorta represents an obstructive infolded ridge just distal to the left subclavian artery and opposite the ductus arteriosus (see Fig 12-60); it is associated with a congenitally bicuspid aortic valve in at least half of the cases.

CORONARY CIRCULATION

Coronary arteries

Coronary atherosclerosis is the major cause of death in industrialized nations today, and its diagnosis and clinical management require a thorough understanding of the common variants of coronary anatomy. To this end, several excellent texts are available.[2,3,103,104]

The coronary ostia arise from the aortic sinuses, midway between the aortic valve commissures and roughly two-thirds of the distance between the aortic annulus and the sinotubular junction (Fig. 12-61). The expanse of the aortic valvular cusps is insufficient to shield the coronary ostia during ventricular systole.

From the right aortic sinus, the right coronary artery arises nearly perpendicularly (see Fig 12-61); its elliptic ostium is 2.4 $\pm$ 0.9 mm high and 3.7 $\pm$ 1.1 mm wide.[3] In 40% to 50% of subjects, one or more conus arteries of

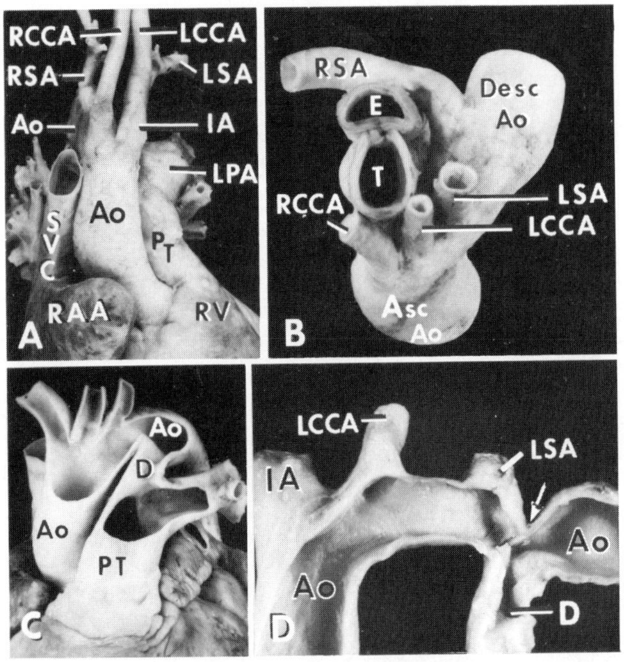

Fig 12-60 Congenital aortic anomalies. **A,** right aortic arch with mirror-image brachiocephalic branching, in atypical tetralogy of Fallot. (Anterior view from 37-year-old woman.) **B,** an anomalous right subclavian artery arises from the lateral surface of the aortic arch, distal to the left subclavian artery, and travels posterior to the trachea and esophagus. (Superior view from elderly man.) **C,** patent ductus arteriosus. (Anterior view from 33-year-old woman.) **D,** coarctation of the aorta *(arrow)*. (Left lateral view from 1-month-old boy.) (See Appendix for abbreviations.)

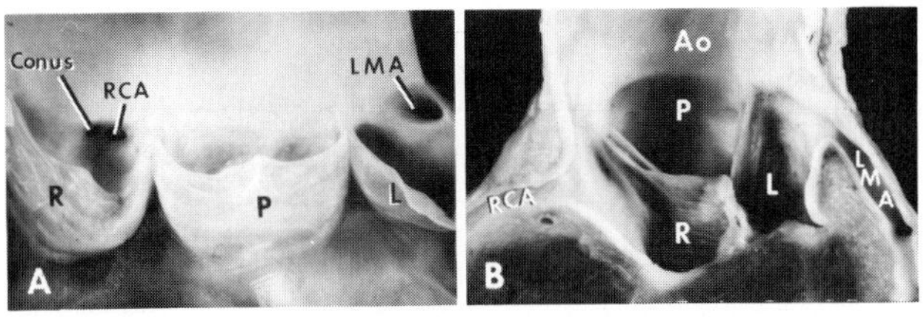

Fig 12-61 Origins of coronary arteries. **A,** the right and left coronary arteries arise from their respective aortic sinuses. When the conus coronary artery arises from the aorta, its ostium is anterior to the right coronary artery. (Opened aortic valve from 18-year-old woman.) **B,** the right coronary artery arises perpendicularly from the aorta, whereas the left main coronary artery arises at an acute angle. (Anterior view from 16-year-old boy.) (See Appendix for abbreviations.)

variable size arise from the right aortic sinus, anterior to the right coronary ostium (see Fig 12-61).[3,104,105] Rarely, the descending septal artery or the sinus nodal artery may originate directly from the aorta, anterior or posterior to the right coronary ostium, respectively.[3,106]

The left coronary artery arises from the left aortic sinus and, in contrast to the right coronary artery, tends to emanate at an acute angle and to travel parallel to the aortic sinus wall (see Fig 12-61); its elliptic ostium measures 3.2 ± 1.1 mm high and 4.7 ± 1.2 mm wide.[4] When the left main artery is exceptionally short, its ostium may assume a double-barrel appearance.

Among the various causes of coronary ostial stenosis, perhaps aortic atherosclerosis is the most common. However, degenerative calcification of the aortic sinotubular junction, which often overlies the right aortic sinus, may also produce ostial obstruction, particularly if an ostium arises near or along this junction. Stenosis of the right coronary ostium occurs six to eight times more often than that of the left. Aortitis associated with syphilis or ankylosing spondylitis also may be complicated by coronary ostial obstruction. Iatrogenic ostial injury may complicate coronary arteriography, intraoperative coronary perfusion, or aortic valve replacement.

The right coronary artery (Fig 12-62), at its origin as it lies between the pulmonary trunk and right atrial appendage, is embedded in the fatty epicardial fold of Rindfleisch, and it remains surrounded by abundant adipose tissue throughout its course within the right AV sulcus.[2] In 50% to 60% of subjects, the first anterior branch is the conus artery, which nourishes the right superolateral aspect of the right ventricular outflow tract; in the remainder, this artery arises independently from the right aortic sinus. An aortic or very proximal right coronary arterial origin of the conus artery may result in its inadequate visualization at coronary arteriography.[107] The descending septal artery, which arises from the proximal right coronary artery or, rarely, from the conus artery or right aortic sinus, supplies the infundibular septum and, in some individuals, the distal AV (His) bundle.[106] Along the acute cardiac margin, from base to apex, courses a prominent acute marginal branch, and between this vessel and the conus artery, several smaller marginal branches arise and travel parallel to the acute margin; these vessels nourish the lateral two-thirds of the anterior right ventricular free wall.

Beyond the acute margin, along the inferior surface of the heart, the length of the right coronary artery varies inversely with that of the circumflex coronary artery. However, in 90% of human hearts, the right coronary artery gives rise not only to the posterior (inferior) descending artery, which travels in the inferior interventricular sulcus, but also to branches that supply the inferior left ventricular free wall[103,104] (see Fig 12-62). Accordingly, these arteries nourish the inferior third of the ventricular septum (the inlet septum), including the right bundle branch and the posterior portion of the left bundle branch, and the inferior left ventricular free wall, including the posteromedial mitral papillary muscle.[48]

In 55% to 65% of individuals, a single main atrial branch arises proximally from the right coronary artery and terminates as the sinus nodal artery (Fig 12-63); the sinus nodal artery in the remainder originates from the circumflex coronary artery.[3,103,104,108] Furthermore, in 90% of human hearts, the distal right coronary artery forms a U-shaped invagination at the cardiac crux which gives rise to the AV nodal artery (see Fig 12-63). Small right atrial branches also supply the most basal aspects of

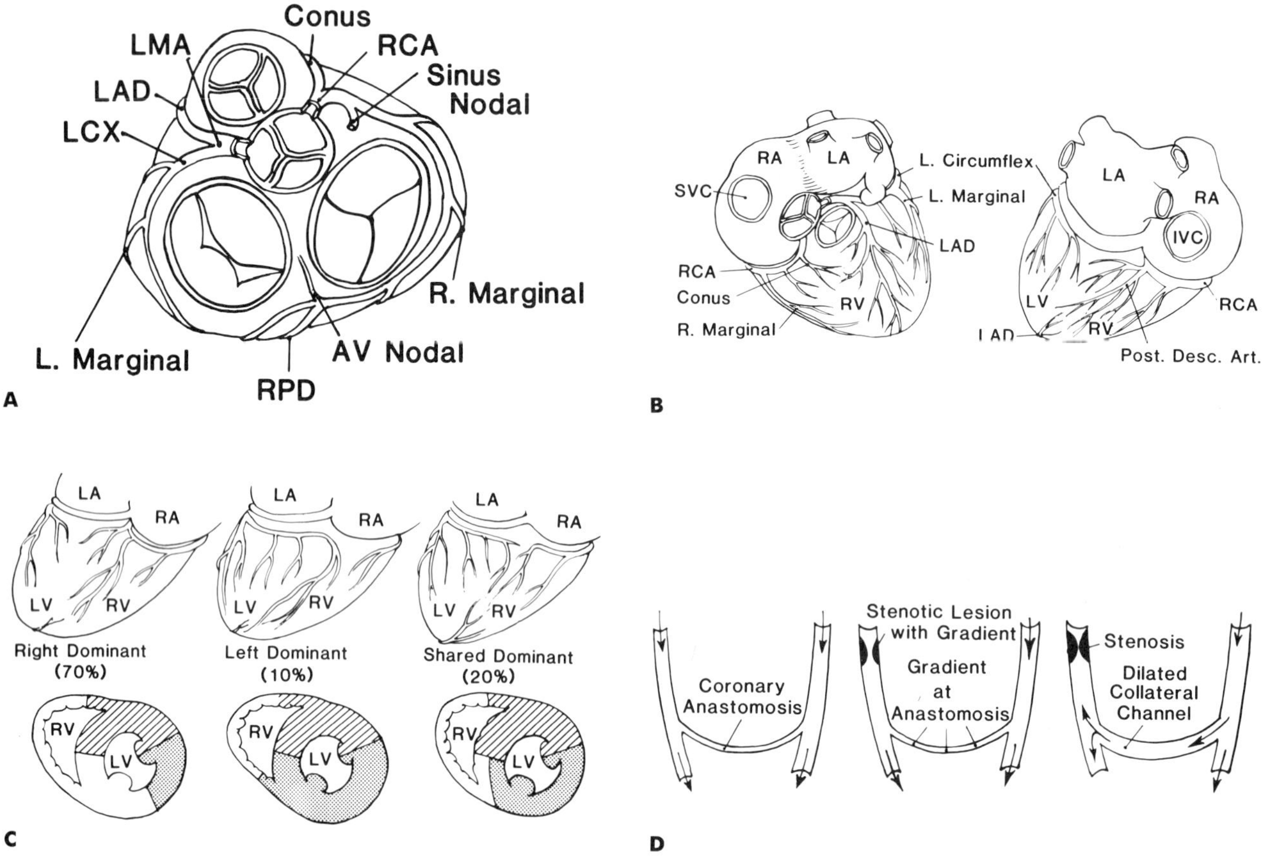

Fig 12-62 Coronary arterial distribution. **A,** the right and circumflex coronary arteries travel in the AV sulcus, adjacent to the tricuspid and mitral valves, respectively (view of base of heart). **B,** the left anterior descending and posterior descending coronary arteries travel in the interventricular sulcus and demarcate the plane of the ventricular septum (superior [left] and inferior [right] views). **C,** coronary dominance is determined by the origin of the posterior descending branch (*white* = LAD distribution; *dotted* = LCX; *striped* = RCA). **D,** stenotic lesions may result in dilatation of coronary collateral channels. (See Appendix for abbreviations.)

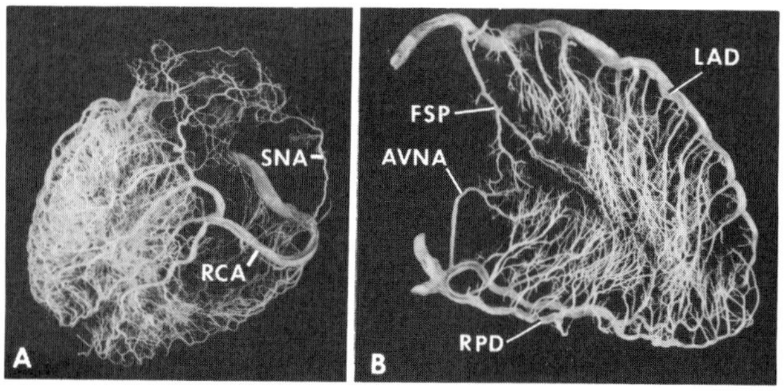

Fig 12-63 Vinyl corrosion cast of normal coronary arteries (from 24-year-old man). **A,** right coronary dominance pertains (inferior view). The sinus nodal artery arises from the right coronary artery and forms small, delicate anastomoses with other atrial branches. **B,** septal perforating branches from the left anterior descending and right posterior descending coronary arteries nourish the ventricular septum. The AV nodal artery supplies the AV node and bundle, and the first septal perforating branch of the left anterior descending artery supplies the AV bundle and proximal left bundle branch. Other septal perforating branches nourish the remainder of the bundle branches (right anterior oblique view). (See Appendix for abbreviations.)

the tricuspid leaflets;[41] the pulmonary cusps contain no blood vessels.

The left main coronary artery ranges in length from 0 to 25 mm, but 75% measure 6 to 15 mm; its diameter averages 3 to 6 mm.[3,103,104] This artery, which is surrounded by epicardial fat, travels between the pulmonary artery and the left atrium and is covered in part by the left atrial appendage. In two-thirds of subjects, it bifurcates into left anterior descending and circumflex branches, and in the remaining one-third, it trifurcates into the aforementioned branches and an intermediate artery, which follows a course similar to that of either the first diagonal or first marginal branch.

The left anterior descending coronary artery travels within the epicardial fat of the anterior interventricular sulcus and, after wrapping around the apex, may ascend a variable distance along the inferior interventricular sulcus (see Fig 12-62). Septal perforating branches nourish not only the anterosuperior two-thirds and entire apical one-third of the ventricular septum (anteroapical trabecular septum) but also the AV (His) bundle and the right and anterior left bundle branches[104,109] (see Fig 12-63). The proximal septal perforators anastomose with the descending septal artery.[106] Epicardial branches, called diagonals, nourish the anterior left ventricular free wall and the medial third of the anterior right ventricular free wall. The first right diagonal branch is analogous to the conus artery and anastomoses with it to form the circle of Vieussens, just below the pulmonary valve.[103] Myocardial bridges may be demonstrated angiographically in 12% of subjects and almost invariably involve the anterior descending artery; they produce critical systolic luminal narrowing in only 1% to 2% of hearts and probably have a benign prognosis in most cases.[110]

The (left) circumflex coronary artery travels within the adipose tissue of the left atrioventricular sulcus and often terminates just beyond the obtuse marginal branch. The intermediate artery, when present, may follow the course of a large marginal branch. The circumflex artery nourishes the lateral left ventricular free wall; however, in the 10% of subjects in whom the circumflex artery gives rise to the posterior descending branch, it also supplies the inferior left ventricular free wall and the inferior third of the ventricular septum. The circumflex and anterior descending arteries nourish the anterolateral mitral papillary muscles, and the circumflex and right coronary arteries supply the posteromedial mitral papillary muscles. In 35% to 45% of subjects, the sinus nodal artery arises from the circumflex coronary artery, either proximally or distally. In 10%, the AV nodal artery has a circumflex origin. Additionally, small left atrial branches supply the most basal aspects of the mitral leaflets;[41] the aortic cusps contain no blood vessels.

The four major epicardial coronary arteries tend to occupy only two planes of the heart. The right and circumflex arteries delineate the plane of the AV sulcus (cardiac base), and the left main artery and anterior and posterior descending arteries delineate the plane of the ventricular septum (see Fig 12-62).

The course of the coronary arteries changes somewhat with variations in heart size. They straighten out in ventricular diastole when the heart is maximally distended, and they tend to pleat loosely, like an accordion, during ventricular systole when the chamber size is much smaller. Similarly, a chronically dilated heart, as in dilated cardiomyopathy, may exhibit stretched coronaries, whereas a small heart, such as a normal heart in an elderly individual, may have very tortuous arteries.

The origin of the posterior descending artery determines the blood supply to the inferior portion of the left ventricle and thereby defines coronary dominance. In 70% of hearts, the right coronary artery crosses the crux and gives rise to this branch, and right coronary dominance pertains. In 10%, the circumflex coronary artery terminates as the posterior descending branch and thereby establishes left coronary dominance. Both the right and circumflex arteries supply the cardiac crux in the remaining 20% and constitute so-called shared coronary dominance. The dominant coronary artery, however, does *not* supply most of the left ventricular myocardium (see Fig 12-62). In subjects with right coronary dominance, for example, the anterior descending artery supplies about 45% of the left ventricle and the circumflex and right coronary arteries nourish about 20% and 35%, respectively.

The blood supply to the cardiac conduction system depends, in part, on coronary dominance. The sinus nodal artery arises from the right coronary artery in 55% to 65% of subjects and from the circumflex artery in 35% to 45%, but its artery of origin does not depend on patterns of coronary arterial dominance. However, the AV nodal artery originates from the dominant artery and, accordingly, arises from the right coronary in 90% and the circumflex in 10%. The AV nodal artery and the first septal perforator of the anterior descending artery offer dual blood supply to the AV (His) bundle (see Fig 12-63). Other septal perforating branches of the anterior descending artery supply the anterior aspect of the left bundle branch, and septal perforators of the posterior descending branch, an extension of the dominant artery, supply the posteroinferior portion of the left bundle branch. The right bundle branch receives a dual blood supply from the septal perforators of the anterior and posterior descending arteries.

The length of the left main coronary artery is influenced by coronary dominance.[111,112] Among subjects with a short left artery (that is, less than 8 mm), the incidence of left coronary dominance is thrice that in the general population. Similarly, the mean length of the left main artery is substantially less in patients with left coronary dominance (7 mm) than in those with right or shared dominance (11 mm). Among subjects with a congenitally bicuspid aortic valve, the incidence of left coronary dominance is 25% to 30%, or nearly thrice that expected, but the length of the left main coronary artery is not significantly shorter than normal.

In the human heart, the major epicardial coronary arteries communicate with one another by means of anastomotic channels 50 to 200 μm in diameter.[103,104] Normally, these small collateral arteries probably afford very little blood flow. However, if arterial obstruction induces a pressure gradient across such a channel, then with time the collateral vessel may dilate and provide an avenue for significant blood flow beyond the stenotic lesion (see Fig 12-62). Such functional collaterals may develop between the terminal extensions of two coronary arteries, between the side branches of two arteries, between branches of the same artery, or within the same branch (via the vasa vasorum). They are most numerous in the ventricular septum (between septal perforators of anterior and posterior descending arteries), in the ventricular apex (between anterior descending septal perforators), in the anterior right ventricular free wall (between anterior descending and right or conus arteries), in the anterolateral left ventricular free wall (between anterior descending diagonals and circumflex marginals), at the cardiac crux (between the right and circumflex arteries), and along the atria (Kugel's artery between right and circumflex arteries).[103,104] Smaller subendocardial anastomoses also exist. Moreover, extracardiac mediastinal arteries may anastomose with the coronary arteries.

Coronary atherosclerosis is a chronic, progressive, multifocal intimal disease that involves only the epicardial arteries. Its basic lesion, the atheroma, may be soft or fibrous and may be complicated by calcification, rupture, hemorrhage, or thrombosis. The relative composition of an atheromatous plaque may determine, in part, whether its dilation by balloon in percutaneous transluminal coronary angioplasty will be successful.

Regardless of the type of plaque or its complications, the major effect is luminal narrowing with decreased coronary blood flow. The residual lumen is often eccentric and either elliptic or crescentic.[113] Several investigators have shown that, before narrowing of an epicardial artery causes more resistance to blood flow than the intramural arteriolar resistance, the luminal cross-sectional area must be reduced by 75%. Obstructions of this magnitude or greater are termed critical stenoses (Fig 12-64). The pathologist evaluates the reduction in cross-sectional area, whereas the angiographer determines the reduction in luminal diameter; the two methods correlate as follows:

↓ Luminal diameter (%)	10	20	30	40	50	60	70	80	90
↓ Cross-sectional area (%)	19	36	51	64	75	84	91	96	99
Grade of stenosis	1	2	3	3	4	4	4	4	4
Noncritical vs. critical	←Noncritical→				←Critical→				

In fatal ischemic heart disease, critical (grade 4) obstruction involves one or, more commonly, two or three of the major epicardial arteries. When critical stenosis of the left main coronary artery is observed, the three other arteries are almost always severely involved also; only rarely is critical left main coronary artery disease an isolated lesion. The most common sites for grade 4 lesions are the proximal one-half of the anterior descending and circumflex arteries and the origin and entire length of the right coronary artery. The distribution and severity of atherosclerotic plaques do not differ significantly among patients with angina pectoris, acute myocardial infarction, end-stage ischemic heart disease, or sudden death. Coronary angiography during the acute phase of evolving myocardial infarctions indicates that acute coronary thrombosis is the precipitating event in most instances, although the underlying plaque is noncritical in about half the cases.

Coronary veins

The venous circulation of the heart comprises a coronary sinus system, an anterior cardiac venous system, and the thebesian venous system[103,104] (Fig 12-65). The great cardiac vein travels in the anterior interventricular sulcus and left AV sulcus, and it receives the left marginal vein and several smaller tributaries before merging with the coronary sinus. Between the great cardiac vein and the coronary sinus (see Figs 12-18 and 12-52), near the junction of the oblique left atrial vein of Marshall, is the characteristic valve of Vieussens. The coronary sinus receives the left posterior and middle cardiac veins and several smaller tributaries, including the small cardiac vein, before it joins the right atrium. It measures 35 ± 20 mm in length and 9 ± 4 mm in diameter.[104]

Along the anterior right ventricular free wall, three or four anterior cardiac veins either drain directly into the right atrium or first join a common collecting vein. Anastomoses occur freely between all coronary venous channels. Finally, many small thebesian veins drain directly into a cardiac chamber, particularly the right atrium or right ventricle; the ostia of these veins are easily recognized along the relatively smooth atrial walls but are difficult to identify in the trabeculated ventricles.

During cardiac electrophysiologic studies among patients with Wolff-Parkinson-White syndrome and left-sided bypass tracts, a catheter electrode may be positioned within the coronary sinus and great cardiac vein, adjacent to the mitral annulus, to localize the aberrant conduction pathways. In the setting of tricuspid insufficiency, blood may regurgitate into the coronary sinus; accordingly, carcinoid plaques have been reported within the

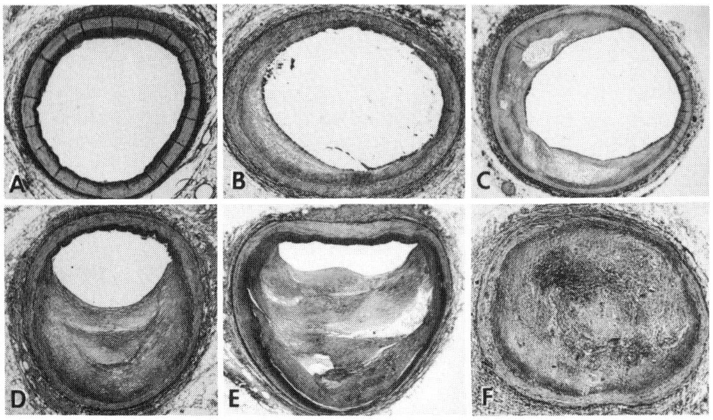

Fig 12-64 Coronary atherosclerosis (cross sections stained with elastic-van Gieson in each case). **A,** grade 0; normal vessel for comparison (from 33-year-old woman). **B,** grade 1 (from 54-year-old woman). **C,** grade 2 (from 54-year-old woman). **D,** grade 3 (from 74-year-old woman). **E,** grade 4; greater than 75% obstruction in cross-sectional area (from 69-year-old man). **F,** grade 5; 100% occlusion (from 62-year-old man).

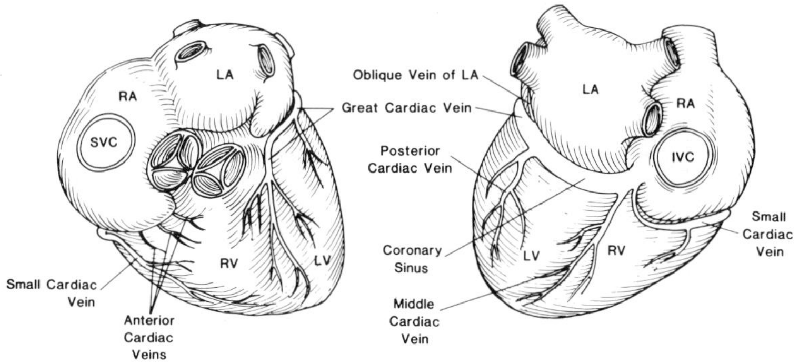

Fig 12-65 Coronary veins. The anterior cardiac veins empty directly into the right atrium, whereas the other major epicardial coronary veins drain into the coronary sinus. (See Appendix for abbreviations.)

coronary sinus and its tributaries in cases of carcinoid heart disease with tricuspid incompetence.

Cardiac lymphatics

The subendocardial, myocardial, and subepicardial lymphatics form an interconnecting network of fine channels within the ventricular myocardium which drain toward the epicardial surface. Here they are joined by lymphatic channels from the sinus node and AV conduction system and also by a few sparse lymphatic vessels from the atria and the valves.[114,115] Along the epicardial surface, the right and left lymphatic channels form and accompany their respective coronary arteries, in retrograde fashion, back to the aortic root. Then, traveling along the ascending aorta beneath the pulmonary trunk, the confluence of right and left lymphatic vessels first reaches the undersurface of the aortic arch and drains into a pretracheal lymph node; continuing superiorly, it next drains into a cardiac lymph node between the superior vena cava and the innominate artery; finally, it empties into the right lymphatic duct. The lymphatics of the parietal pericardium may join either the thoracic duct or the right lymphatic duct.

The coronary veins and cardiac lymphatics work in concert to remove excess fluid from the myocardial interstitium and pericardial sac. Accordingly, obstruction of either system or of both systems may result in myocardial edema and pericardial effusion. For example, chronic heart failure is attended by elevated central venous (and coronary sinus) pressure, which may produce a chronic pericardial effusion. Moreover, metastatic involvement of epicardial lymphatics, as commonly occurs with breast or lung cancer, often produces a malignant pericardial effusion.

Embryology

During the initial stages of cardiac embryogenesis, the heart tube and heart loop are nourished by luminal blood. As ventricular trabeculations produce a somewhat spongy myocardium, luminal blood reaches the subepicardial zones via the intertrabecular sinusoids. These sinusoids produce a rich myocardial plexus of vascular channels, which will later form the intramural coronary circulation. Evaginations from the sinus venosus form numerous venous channels along the ventricular epicardium which will anastomose with the underlying myocardial vascular plexus. As a result, the intramural coronary veins may drain epicardially into the coronary sinus system and anterior cardiac veins or intracamerally via the smaller thebesian channels (myocardial sinusoids).

By day 28, before truncal septation has occurred, two vascular buds evaginate from the truncal root, and their ramifications will eventually form the epicardial coronary arteries[116] (Fig 12-66). The left coronary artery extends along the bulboventricular fold and soon bifurcates; one branch travels along the interventricular sulcus as the anterior descending artery, and the other travels in the left AV sulcus as the circumflex artery. Similarly, the right coronary artery remains in the right AV sulcus. From these arterial stems, an epicardial arterial plexus soon develops that will form the diagonal and marginal branches and their various interconnections. Furthermore, the arterial segments that become trapped in the passively developing ventricular septa will form the septal perforating branches. Consequently, the perforating branches of the anterior descending artery will nourish the trabeculated anteroapical (conoventricular) septum, including the septal and moderator bands and the anterior and medial tricuspid papillary muscles, and those of the posterior descending artery will nourish the inflow (interventricular) septum.

According to an alternative explanation, an epicardial collection of arterial islands forms along the atrioventricular and interventricular sulci and merges to form an epicardial arterial plexus by day 33.[117] These vessels form additional branches along the cardiac surface and within the myocardium; the latter anastomose with the intramural sinusoids. Two buds from the root of the truncus arteriosus evaginate and anastomose with the epicardial arterial plexus by day 42 and thereby establish aortic origin of the coronary arteries.

Congenital malformations of the coronary arteries include anomalous ostial origin, anomalous arterial branching patterns, and anomalous arterial anastomoses. Such anomalies may be isolated or they may be associated with other cardiac malfor-

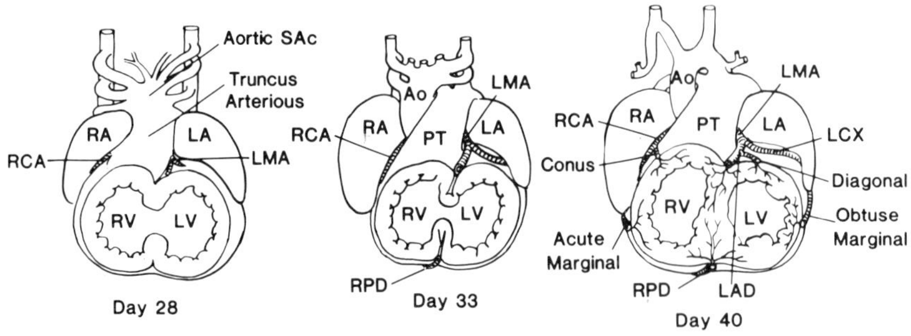

Fig 12-66 Embryology of the coronary arteries. Two vascular buds from the truncal root form the right and left coronary arteries. Septal perforating branches develop during passive ventricular septation. Dates are approximate. (See Appendix for abbreviations.)

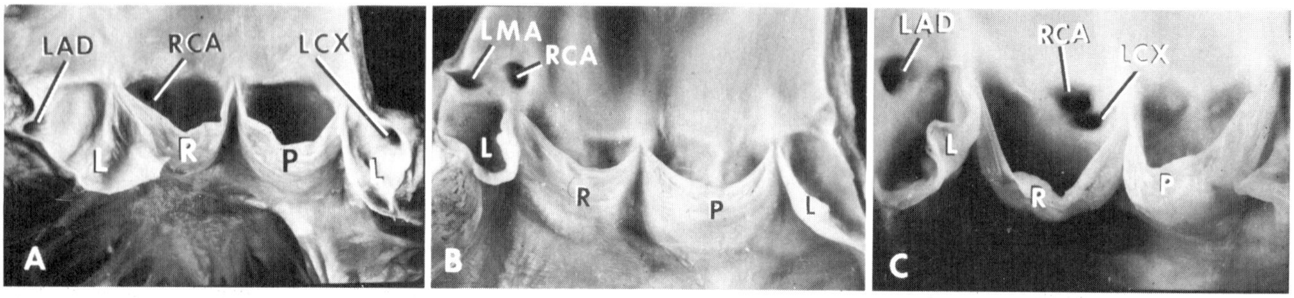

Fig 12-67 Coronary artery anomalies (opened aortic valve in each case). **A,** separate origins of the left anterior descending and circumflex coronary arteries from the left aortic sinus (from 69-year-old woman). **B,** high origins of the right and left coronary arteries, with ectopic origin of the right above the commissure between the right and left aortic cusps (from 10-month-old girl). **C,** ectopic origin of the circumflex coronary artery from the right aortic sinus (from 17-year-old boy). (See Appendix for abbreviations.)

mations, and their importance ranges from trivial to life-threatening. In some forms of congenital heart disease, certain coronary anomalies may limit the surgical options.

A coronary artery may arise close to an aortic commissure or it may arise at or distal to the sinotubular junction (so-called high origin) (Fig 12-67); in the latter condition, calcification of the aortic sinotubular junction is likely to produce ostial stenosis. Rarely, an aortic cusp may be congenitally adherent to the aortic wall and thereby isolate a coronary ostium. A coronary artery may arise from an inappropriate aortic sinus, and origin of the circumflex artery from the right aortic sinus (or proximal right coronary artery) is a relatively frequent anomaly (see Fig 12-67). When an anomalous coronary artery passes between the two great arteries, it may become compressed between their sinuses. Anomalous origin of a coronary artery from the pulmonary trunk results in regional left ventricular ischemia and fibrosis; with the development of functional intercoronary collaterals, the direction of blood flow may change in the anomalous vessel and thereby produce an aortopulmonary fistula. Rarely, a coronary artery may originate from an extracardiac artery such as the subclavian.

Anomalous origin of the anterior descending artery from the proximal right coronary artery, or vice versa, is particularly common in tetralogy of Fallot and alters the surgical approach to right ventricular outflow tract reconstruction. When the entire coronary arterial circulation arises from only one ostium, a single coronary artery exists, and ostial or proximal stenoses may be associated with an especially poor prognosis. Similarly, when either the anterior descending artery or the circumflex artery arises from the right coronary artery, subsequent stenosis of the proximal right artery or its ostium carries the same risk as stenosis of the left main coronary artery in the normal population. Congenital atresia of a proximal coronary arterial segment is associated with retrograde flow of blood into the distal artery via intercoronary anastomoses. Although anomalous coronary branching patterns are relatively common in congenital conotruncal malformations, truncus arteriosus behaves differently and is more often characterized by anomalous ostial origin than by abnormal peripheral coronary distribution.

A coronary artery may form fistulous connections with one of the four cardiac chambers, the coronary sinus, the superior vena cava, or the pulmonary trunk. The right coronary artery is involved in about 60% of cases, and the fistula joins the right atrium or right ventricle in about 70%; along the fistulous coronary artery, saccular aneurysms are common. Isolated congenital aneurysms of the coronary arteries are very rare and should not be confused with acquired aneurysms caused by atherosclerosis, inflammation, or dissection.

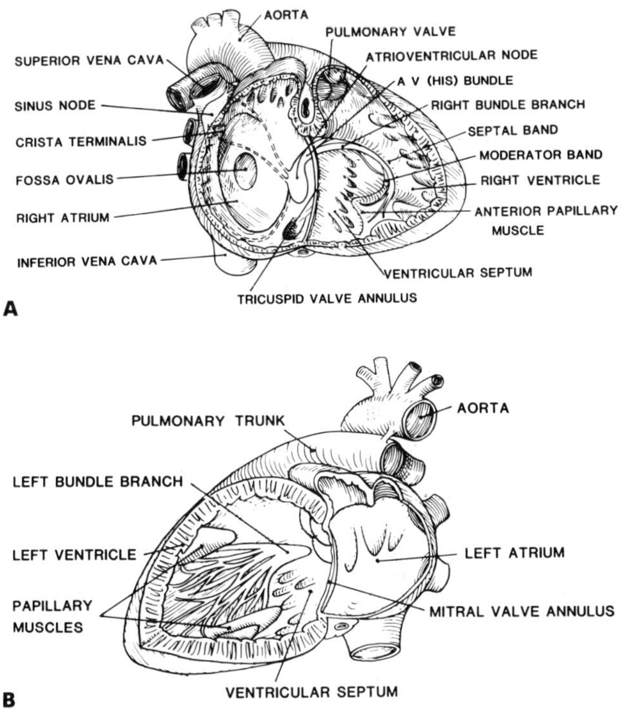

Fig 12-68 Cardiac conduction system. **A,** right heart. The sinus and AV nodes are both right atrial structures. **B,** left heart. The left bundle branch forms a broad sheet that does not divide into distinct anterior and posterior fascicles. (From Edwards WD: Anatomy of the cardiovascular system. In *Clinical Medicine.* Vol. 6, Chap. 1. Edited by JA Spittell Jr., Philadelphia, Harper & Row, Publishers, 1984, pp 1-24. By permission.)

CARDIAC CONDUCTION SYSTEM
Sinus node

The sinus node is the primary pacemaker of the heart. It is an epicardial structure that measures approximately 15 by 5 by 2 mm and is located in the sulcus terminalis (intercavarum) near the superior cavoatrial junction[2,118](Figs 12-68 and 12-69). Through its center passes a relatively large sinus nodal artery;[108] as a result, arterial pulsation and sinus nodal impulse formation may be intimately related. Moreover, sinus nodal function is greatly influenced by humoral substances and by numerous sympathetic and parasympathetic nerves that terminate within its boundaries; paranodal parasympathetic ganglia are also plentiful.

Histologically, the sinus node consists of specialized cardiac muscle cells embedded within a prominent collagenous stroma.[118] Since the collagen increases progressively with age, one must take care not to overdiagnose sinus nodal fibrosis in hearts from the elderly. In accordance with the specialized function of the sinus node, its myocardial cells are smaller than ventricular muscle cells and contain only scant contractile elements. Unlike the parallel arrangement of ventricular muscle cells, nodal cells form a complex interwoven pattern (see Fig 12-69). Ultrastructurally, the sinus node comprises transitional cells and variable numbers of P cells centrally and atrial myocardial cells peripherally.[75,119] Although P cells are thought to be the source of impulse formation, changes in autonomic input may alter the actual pacing site within the node.

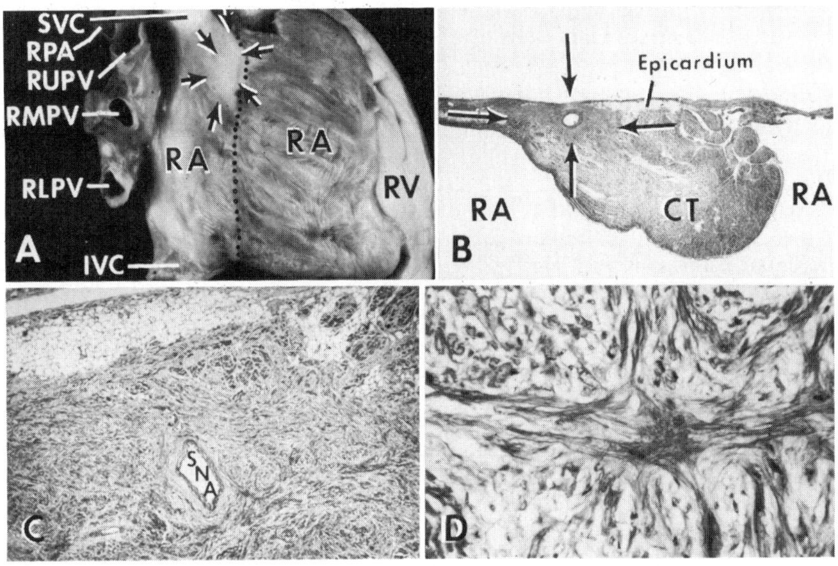

Fig 12-69 Sinus node. **A,** the sinus node *(arrows)* lies in the sulcus terminalis *(dotted line)* near the cavoatrial junction. (Right lateral view from 32-year-old man.) **B,** the sinus node *(arrows)* is a subepicardial structure that overlies the superolateral portion of the crista terminalis. (Trichrome ×5; from 61-year-old man.) **C,** the sinus nodal artery courses through the center of the sinus node. (Trichrome ×20; from 20-year-old man.) **D,** the specialized myocardial cells of the sinus node form an interlacing pattern. (Trichrome ×100; from 20-year-old man.) (See Appendix for abbreviations.)

Because the sinus node occupies an epicardial position, its function may be affected by pericarditis, particularly in the presence of preexisting heart disease. Metastatic neoplasms may infiltrate or obliterate the sinus node but do not necessarily alter nodal function. In the setting of cardiac amyloidosis, the sinus node may be involved by extensive fibrosis or amyloid deposition. Although the sinus node is rarely infarcted, its function may be altered by adjacent atrial infarction, with or without nearby right atrial mural thrombus. Excessive nodal fibrosis with atrial myocardial fibrosis, either idiopathic or associated with chronic ischemia, may underlie the tachybradycardias that characterize the so-called sick sinus syndrome. Similar findings have been reported with other atrial arrhythmias. During open heart surgery, the sinus node may be injured; this most commonly occurs during the Mustard operation for complete transposition of the great arteries.

Internodal tracts

Although most investigators have concluded that, by light microscopy, there are no morphologically distinct conduction pathways between the sinus and the AV nodes, electrophysiologic studies support the concept of functional preferential pathways. These pathways may be related to the geometry of the atrial septum and right atrial free wall and represent three potential internodal tracts[118] (see Fig 12-68). The anterior pathway (of Bachmann) arches leftward along the superior aspect of the crista terminalis and then anteroinferiorly along the atrial septum, in the anterior limb of the fossa ovalis; superiorly, numerous muscle bundles also branch onto the left atrial free wall. The middle pathway (of Wenckebach) arches rightward along the superior aspect of the crista terminalis and then anteroinferiorly along the atrial septum, just posteroinferior to the anterior tract. The posterior internodal pathway (of Thorel) courses rightward and inferiorly along the entire crista terminalis and then follows the tendon of Todaro toward the AV node. By ultrastructural studies, some investigators have observed specialized cardiac muscle cells in these internodal tracts.[120]

Lipomatous hypertrophy of the atrial septum may interfere with internodal conduction and induce a variety of atrial arrhythmias. Since the functional preferential pathways travel only in the limbus and not in the valve of the fossa ovalis, internodal conduction disturbances would not be expected with septal perforation at cardiac catheterization (transseptal approach), with the Rashkind balloon atrial septostomy, or with the Blalock-Hanlon partial (posterior) atrial septectomy. However, with the Mustard operation for complete transposition of the great arteries, in which the entire atrial septum is resected and in which the surgical atriotomy may disrupt the crista terminalis, severe disturbances of internodal conduction may result.

Atrioventricular node

The AV node is a subendocardial right atrial structure that measures approximately 6 by 4 by 1.5 mm.[118] It is located within the triangle of Koch (bordered by the tendon of Todaro, septal tricuspid annulus, and coronary sinus ostium) and abuts the right fibrous trigone (central fibrous body) (Figs 12-68 and 12-70). The AV nodal artery (or several of its branches) courses near the node but not necessarily through it, and venous and lymphatic channels are plentiful.[121] Sympathetic and parasympathetic nerves enter the AV node and may greatly affect its function, and numerous parasympathetic ganglia lie adjacent to the node. Humoral substances also influence AV nodal function.

Like the sinus node, the AV node histologically consists of a complex interwoven pattern of small specialized cardiac muscle cells within a fibrous stroma[118] (see Fig 12-70). With advanced age, the AV node acquires progressively more fibrous tissue, although not as extensively as the sinus node, and may also acquire interstitial adipose tissue. Proximally, at the AV junctional region, the functional myocardial elements are loosely arranged as they receive connections from the atrial myocardium. Centrally, the AV node is quite compact and exhibits a complex interlacing of specialized myocardial cells, whereas distally, bundles of cells begin to align in parallel fashion as the AV (His) bundle is formed. Ultrastructurally, the AV node comprises transitional cells and fewer numbers of atrial myocardial cells proximally and peripherally, P cells centrally, and Purkinje's cells distally.[75]

The so-called mesothelioma of the AV node represents a small and rare primary neoplasm which, by virtue of its position, may produce various arrhythmias and may cause sudden death. Metastatic neoplasms may rarely infiltrate the AV node but do not necessarily alter its function. Likewise, sarcoid granulomas tend to involve the basal ventricular myocardium and may impinge on the AV conduction system. Among persons with potentially life-threatening arrhythmias is a group who would benefit from interruption of the AV conduction pathways; because of its subendocardial position, the AV node may be ablated in such cases by freezing or by electrocoagulation or by laser.

Atrioventricular bundle

The AV (His) bundle arises from the distal portion of the AV node and courses through the central fibrous body to attain the summit of the muscular ventricular septum, adjacent to the membranous septum[118] (see Figs 12-68 and 12-70). As such, it affords the only normal avenue for electrical continuity between the atria and the ventricles. The AV bundle measures 7 to 20 mm in length and 1 to 2 mm in diameter and forms a triangular cord, the apex of which conforms to the septal summit and the two opposite corners of which give rise to the right and left bundle branches. By virtue of its position within the central fibrous body (right fibrous trigone), the AV bundle is closely related to the annuli of the aortic, mitral, and tricuspid valves. It has a dual blood supply—from the AV nodal artery and the first septal perforating branch of the anterior descending artery. In some subjects, the descending septal branch of the proximal right coronary artery also nourishes the AV bundle.[106]

The AV bundle is made up of numerous parallel bundles of specialized cardiac muscle cells, which are separated by delicate fibrous septa. Moreover, for each of these bundles, their final destination in the right or left bundle branches is probably determined proximally by their positions within the main His bundle.[118] The entire AV bundle is insulated by a collagenous sheath. With

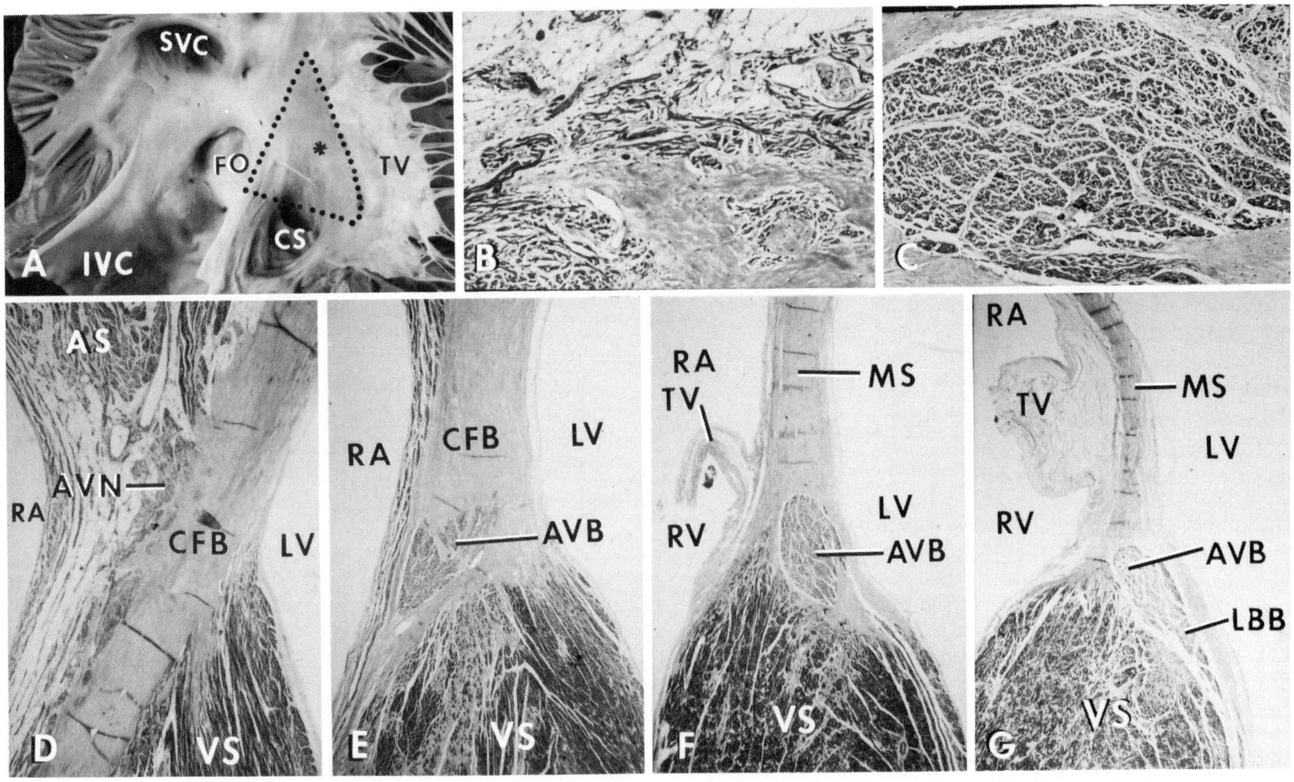

Fig 12-70 Atrioventricular conduction system. **A,** the AV node (*) lies within the triangle of Koch *(dotted lines),* along the right atrial aspect of the AV septum. (Opened right atrium from 32-year-old man.) **B,** the node is characterized by an interlacing pattern of specialized myocardial cells. (Trichrome ×50; from 20-year-old man.) **C,** the AV bundle consists of parallel bundles of specialized myocardial cells (Trichrome ×50; from 20-year-old man.) **D-G,** as the right atrial AV node **(D)** begins to penetrate the central fibrous body, it forms the AV bundle **(E)**. The bundle attains the level of the ventricular septal summit **(F)** and gives rise to the left bundle branch **(G)**. The right bundle branch is not included in these planes of section. **(D-G,** Trichrome ×5 in each; from 20-year-old man.) (See Appendix for abbreviations.)

increasing age, the fibrous septa become thicker, and the functional elements may be partially replaced by adipose tissue. Ultrastructurally, the AV bundle comprises Purkinje's cells and ventricular myocardial cells in parallel arrangement.[75]

In some subjects, alternate conduction pathways exist between the atria and the ventricles, either within the existing AV conduction system or elsewhere along the fibrous cardiac skeleton, and may produce various arrhythmias. Atrionodal bypass tracts (of James) connect the atria to the distal AV node, and atriofascicular tracts (of Breckenmacher) connect the atria to the AV bundle; nodoventricular and fasciculoventricular bypass fibers (of Mahaim) connect the AV node and AV bundle, respectively, to the underlying ventricular septal summit. These bypass fibers are quite commonly observed histologically and are apparently nonfunctional in most persons, although they may produce ventricular preexcitation in some instances.

Ventricular preexcitation is usually associated with aberrant AV bypass tracts that bridge the tricuspid or mitral annuli. These tracts often travel within the adipose tissue of the AV sulcus rather than through a defect in the valvular annuli. Such bypass tracts may be single or multiple and may be identified by electrophysiologic mapping. In contrast, nodules of specialized conduction tissue, representing the bundles of Kent, may be observed in the right lateral AV sulcus, but these usually do not afford a connection between atria and ventricles.[118]

Acquired complete heart block may involve the AV node, AV bundle, or both bundle branches. That occurring with acute myocardial infarction is usually transient and more commonly complicates inferoseptal than anteroseptal infarction; usually the AV node and AV bundle are edematous, and the bundle branches are focally infarcted. Acute heart block may also complicate aortic infective endocarditis. Chronic heart block may be associated with ischemic heart disease or with fibrocalcific disorders of the aortic or mitral valves, but it is most commonly due to idiopathic fibrosis of the AV bundle and bilateral bundle branches. Heart block may also complicate aortic or mitral valve replacement.

Bundle branches

As an extension of the AV bundle, the right bundle branch forms a cordlike structure, approximately 50 mm in length and 1 mm in diameter, which courses along the septal and moderator bands to achieve the level of the anterior tricuspid papillary muscle[118] (see Fig 12-68). The left bundle branch, in contrast, forms a broad fenestrated sheet of conduction fibers which spreads along the septal subendocardium of the left ventricle and separates incompletely and variably into two or three indistinct fascicles (see Fig 12-68). The fascicles travel toward the left ventricular apex and both mitral papillary muscle groups. The bundle branches are nourished by septal perforators arising from the anterior and posterior descending coronary arteries. Histologically, the bundle branches consist of parallel tracts of specialized cardiac muscle cells which are insulated by a delicate fibrous sheath that becomes thicker with increasing age. Ultrastructurally, Purkinje's cells and ventricular myocardial cells form the bundle branches.[75,118]

Right bundle-branch block may be idiopathic or be associated with ischemic heart disease, chronic systemic hypertension, or pulmonary hypertension. Right ventriculotomy usually produces the electrocardiographic features of right bundle-branch block, even though the bundle may not have been transected.

Left bundle-branch block may complicate acute myocardial infarction, particularly of the anteroseptal wall, and is often transient. Chronic left bundle-branch block may be associated with fibrocalcific degeneration of the ventricular septal summit as a result of chronic ischemia, left ventricular hypertension, calcification of the aortic or mitral valves, any form of cardiomyopathy, or aging changes.

Cardiac innervation

Since the embryonic heart tube first forms in the future neck region, its autonomic innervation also arises from this level.[2] From the cervical ganglia originate three pairs of cervical sympathetic cardiac nerves, which intermingle as they join the cardiac plexus, between the great arteries (aortic arch and pulmonary trunk) and the tracheal bifurcation. Several thoracic sympathetic cardiac nerves arise from the upper thoracic ganglia and also join the cardiac plexus. From the parasympathetic vagus nerves emanate the superior and inferior cervical vagal cardiac nerves and the thoracic vagal cardiac nerves, which likewise interweave within the cardiac plexus. The various sympathetic and parasympathetic nerves then descend from this plexus onto the heart and thereby innervate the coronary arteries, cardiac conduction system, and myocardium. Furthermore, afferent nerves concerned with pain and various reflexes ascend from the heart toward the cardiac plexus.

The transplanted human heart represents a completely denervated cardiac preparation that responds only to circulating (humoral) substances and not to autonomic impulses. Similarly, afferent pathways are also lost, including pain tracts and various reflexes. Accordingly, when chronic cardiac transplant rejection produces diffuse coronary arterial obstruction, subsequent myocardial ischemia and infarction may remain undetected, since the telltale symptom, angina pectoris, cannot develop.

Embryology

The embryologic development of the human cardiac conduction system has been reviewed by numerous investigators,[118] but it still remains controversial and incompletely understood. However, all agree that it develops from specialized myocardial cells that originate along the epicardial surface. The final internal disposition of the AV conduction system and its nutrient arteries is explained by tissue invagination that accompanies passive atrial and ventricular septation.

By the time cardiac looping occurs, between days 23 and 25, the sinus node already consists of a discrete elongated structure, which occupies its definitive position at the sinoatrial junction (sulcus terminalis) near the entrance of the right common cardinal vein (future superior vena cava). Between days 35 and 40, the sinus nodal artery develops and becomes surrounded by expanding sinus nodal tissue.

The asplenia syndrome is characterized by bilateral right-sided symmetry and is generally associated with right atrial isomerism, right pulmonary isomerism, abdominal situs ambiguus, and, in some instances, bilateral sinus nodes. In contrast, the sinus node may be congenitally absent or malpositioned in cases of polysplenia with left atrial isomerism.

The AV junction of the developing heart tube becomes encircled by specialized myocardial cells by approximately day 23. At the cardiac crux, proliferation of this tissue forms the compact AV node, and an anterior extension from it produces the AV (His) bundle. Atrial septation and development of the crista terminalis form the anatomic substrates for functional internodal conduction. Concurrently, specialized myocardial cells encircle the bulboventricular junction and proliferate to form the right and left bundle branches as ventricular septation occurs. Cardiac looping and chamber expansion bring the developing AV bundle and bundle branches closer together and thereby facilitate fusion of the two.

Congenital complete heart block may present as persistent bradycardia in utero and may represent an isolated anomaly or may accompany other cardiac malformations. It results from interruption of AV conduction pathways, either at the junction between atrial muscle and the AV node or at the junction between the AV node and the AV bundle. The different embryologic origins of these three regions account for the specific atrionodal and nodofascicular sites of tissue discontinuity.

As AV sulcus tissue participates in the formation of the tricuspid and mitral annuli, all sites of AV muscular continuity normally are disrupted and lost, except for the AV conduction system. Persistence of such connections forms the anatomic substrate for ventricular preexcitation (Wolff-Parkinson-White syndrome). The right anterolateral bundle of Kent may persist as a nodelike structure but usually does not link the right atrium to the right ventricle. However, when the ventricles are inverted, as in corrected transposition of the great arteries and most cases of single (double inlet) left ventricle, an anterior AV node usually joins the bundle branches and may be linked to the posterior (normal) AV node via a sling of AV bundle tissue.

REFERENCES

1. Edwards WD, Tajik AJ, Seward JB: Standardized nomenclature and anatomic basis for regional tomographic analysis of the heart. *Mayo Clin Proc* 56:479-497, 1981

2. Netter FH: Anatomy; Embryology. In *The Ciba Collection of Medical Illustrations,* Vol. 5, *Heart.* Edited by FF Yonkman. Summit, New Jersey, Ciba Pharmaceutical Company, 1969, pp 1-33; 112-4130

3. McAlpine WA: *Heart and Coronary Arteries: An Anatomical Atlas for Clinical Diagnosis, Radiological Investigation, and Surgical Treatment.* Berlin, Springer-Verlag, 1975

4. Walmsley R, Watson H: *Clinical Anatomy of the Heart.* Edinburgh, Churchill Livingstone, 1978

5. Anderson RH, Becker AE: *The Heart: Structure in Health and Disease.* London, Gower Medical Publishing, 1992

6. Edwards WD: Photography of medical specimens: experiences from teaching cardiovascular pathology. *Mayo Clin Proc* 63:42-57, 1988

7. Ishihara T, Ferrans VJ, Jones M, et al: Histologic and ultrastructural features of normal human parietal pericardium. *Am J Cardiol* 46:744-753, 1980

8. Kitzman DW, Scholz DG, Hagen PT, et al: Age-related changes in normal human hearts during the first 10 decades of life. Part II (Maturity): A quantitative anatomic study of 765 specimens from subjects 20 to 99 years old. *Mayo Clin Proc* 63:137-146, 1988

9. Scholz DG, Kitzman DW, Hagen PT, et al: Age-related changes in normal human hearts during the first 10 decades of life. Part I (Growth): A quantitative anatomic study of 200 specimens from subjects from birth to 19 years old. *Mayo Clin Proc* 63:126-136, 1988

10. Van Praagh R, Van Praagh S: Embryology and anatomy: keys to the understanding of complex congenital heart disease. *Coeur* 13:313-337, 1981

11. Harmon JV Jr, Edwards WD: Venous valves in subclavian and internal jugular veins: frequency, position, and structure in 100 autopsy cases. *Am J Cardiovasc Pathol* 1:51-54, 1987

12. Forssman W-G: The endocrine heart. *Prog Clin Biol Res* 295:401-417, 1989

13. Sweeney LJ, Rosenquist GC: The normal anatomy of the atrial septum in the human heart. *Am Heart J* 98:194-199, 1979

14. Hagen PT, Scholz DG, Edwards WD: Incidence and size of patent foramen ovale during the first 10 decades of life: an autopsy study of 965 normal hearts. *Mayo Clin Proc* 59:17-20, 1984

15. Rosenquist GC, Sweeney LJ, Ruckman RN, et al: Atrial septal thickness and area in normal heart specimens and in those with ostium secundum atrial septal defects. *J Clin Ultrasound* 7:345-348, 1979

16. Hutchins GM, Moore GW, Jones JF, et al: Postnatal endocardial fibroelastosis of the valve of the foramen ovale. *Am J Cardiol* 47:90-94, 1981

17. Schwinger ME, Gindea AJ, Freedberg RS, et al: The anatomy of the interatrial septum: a transesophageal echocardiographic study. *Am Heart J* 119:1401-1405, 1990

18. Murray JA, Kennedy JW, Figley MM: Quantitative angiocardiography: II. The normal left atrial volume in man. *Circulation* 37:800-804, 1968

19. Hutchins GM, Anaya OA: Measurements of cardiac size, chamber volumes and valve orifices at autopsy. *Johns Hopkins Med J* 133:96-106, 1973

20. Gutman J, Wang YS, Wahr D, et al: Normal left atrial function determined by 2-dimensional echocardiography. *Am J Cardiol* 51:336-340, 1983

21. Gross L, Kugel MA: Topographic anatomy and histology of the valves in the human heart. *Am J Pathol* 7:445-474, 1931

22. Seccombe JF, Cahill DR, Edwards WD: Quantitative morphology of normal human tricuspid valve: autopsy study of 24 cases. *Clin Anat* 6:203-212, 1993

23. Roberts WC, Cohen LS: Left ventricular papillary muscles: description of the normal and a survey of conditions causing them to be abnormal. *Circulation* 46:138-154, 1972

24. Silver MD, Lam JHC, Ranganathan N, et al: Morphology of the human tricuspid valve. *Circulation* 43:333-348, 1971

25. Lam JHC, Ranganathan N, Wigle ED, et al: Morphology of the human mitral valve. I. Chordae tendineae: a new classification. *Circulation* 41:449-458, 1970

26. Kitzman DW, Edwards WD: Age-related changes in the anatomy of the normal human heart. *J Gerontol* 45:M33-M39, 1990

27. Schenk KE, Heinze G: Age-dependent changes of heart valves and heart size. *Recent Adv Stud Cardiac Struct Metab* 10:617-624, 1975

28. Sahasakul Y, Edwards WD, Naessens JM, et al: Age-related changes in aortic and mitral valve thickness: implications for two-dimensional echocardiography based on an autopsy study of 200 normal human hearts. *Am J Cardiol* 62:424-430, 1988

29. Roberts WC: Ninety-three hearts ≥ 90 years of age. *Am J Cardiol* 71:599-602, 1993

30. Sell S, Scully RE: Aging changes in the aortic and mitral valves: histologic and histochemical studies, with observations on the pathogenesis of calcific aortic stenosis and calcification of the mitral annulus. *Am J Pathol* 46:345-365, 1965

31. Lie JT, Hammond PI: Pathology of the senescent heart: anatomic observations on 237 autopsy studies of patients 90 to 105 years old. *Mayo Clin Proc* 63:552-564, 1988

32. Tei C, Pilgrim JP, Shah PM, et al: The tricuspid valve annulus: study of size and motion in normal subjects and in patients with tricuspid regurgitation. *Circulation* 66:665-671, 1982

33. Eckner FAO, Brown BW, Overll E, et al: Alteration of the gross dimensions of the heart and its structures by formalin fixation: a quantitative study. *Virchows Arch [Pathol Anat]* 346:318-329, 1969

34. Eckner FAO, Brown BW, Davidson DL, et al: Dimensions of normal human hearts: after standard fixation by controlled pressure coronary perfusion. *Arch Pathol* 88:497-507, 1969

35. Wafae N, Hayashi H, Gerola LR, et al: Anatomical study of the human tricuspid valve. *Surg Radiol Anat* 12:37-41, 1990

36. Restivo A, Smith A, Wilkinson JL, et al: The medial papillary muscle complex and its related septomarginal trabeculation: a normal anatomic study on human hearts. *J Anat* 163:231-242, 1989

37. Wenink ACG: The medial papillary complex. *Br Heart J* 39:1012-1018, 1977

38. Restivo A, Smith A, Wilkinson JL, et al: Normal variations in the relationship of the tricuspid valve to the membranous septum in the human heart. *Anat Rec* 226:258-263, 1990

39. Rosenquist GC, Sweeney LJ: Normal variations in tricuspid valve attachments to the membranous ventricular septum: a clue to the etiology of left ventricle-to-right atrial communication. *Am Heart J* 89:186-188, 1975

40. Ormiston JA, Shah PM, Tei C, et al: Size and motion of the mitral valve annulus in man. I. A two-dimensional echocardiographic method and findings in normal subjects. *Circulation* 64:113-120, 1981

41. Silverman ME, Hurst JW: The mitral complex: interaction of the anatomy, physiology, and pathology of the mitral annulus, mitral valve leaflets, chordae tendineae, and papillary muscles. *Am Heart J* 76:399-418, 1968

42. Davis PKB, Kinmonth JB: The movements of the annulus of the mitral valve. *J Cardiovasc Surg* 4:427-431, 1963

43. Bulkley BH, Roberts WC: Dilatation of the mitral anulus: a rare cause of mitral regurgitation. *Am J Med* 59:457-463, 1975

44. Chandraratna PAN, Aronow WS: Mitral valve ring in normal vs dilated left ventricle: cross-sectional echocardiographic study. *Chest* 79:151-154, 1981

45. Ranganathan N, Lam JHC, Wigle ED, et al: Morphology of the human mitral valve. II. The valve leaflets. *Circulation* 41:459-467, 1970

46. Boucek RJ, Boučková B, Levy S: Anatomical arrangement of muscle tissue in the anterior mitral leaflet in man. *Cardiovasc Res* 12:675-680, 1978

47. Becker AE, de Wit APM: Mitral valve apparatus: a spectrum of normality relevant to mitral valve prolapse. *Br Heart J* 42:680-689, 1979

48. Estes EH Jr, Dalton FM, Entman ML, et al: The anatomy and blood supply of the papillary muscles of the left ventricle. *Am Heart J* 71:356-362, 1966

49. Chiechi MA, Lees WM, Thompson R: Functional anatomy of the normal mitral valve. *J Thorac Surg* 32:378-398, 1956

50. Luetmer PH, Edwards WD, Seward JB, et al: Incidence and distribution of left ventricular false tendons: an autopsy study of 483 normal human hearts. *J Am Coll Cardiol* 8:179-183, 1986

51. Lange PE, Onnasch DG, Schaupp GH, et al: Size and function of the human left and right ventricles during growth: normative angiographic data. *Pediatr Cardiol* 3:205-211, 1982

52. Ferlinz J: Right ventricular function in adult cardiovascular disease. *Prog Cardiovasc Dis* 25:225-267, 1982
53. Hutchins GM, Bulkley BH, Moore GW, et al: Shape of the human cardiac ventricles. *Am J Cardiol* 41:646-654, 1978
54. Prakash R, Lindsay P: Determination of right ventricular wall thickness by echocardiogram. *JAMA* 239:638-640, 1978
55. Anderson RH, Becker AE, Van Mierop LHS: What should we call the "crista"? *Br Heart J* 39:856-859, 1977
56. Goor D, Lillehei CW, Edwards JE: The "sigmoid septum": variation in the contour of the left ventricular outlet. *AJR* 107:366-376, 1969
57. Henry WL, Ware J, Gardin JM, et al: Echocardiographic measurements in normal subjects: growth-related changes that occur between infancy and early adulthood. *Circulation* 57:278-285, 1978
58. Kennedy JW, Baxley WA, Figley MM, et al: Quantitative angiocardiography. I. The normal left ventricle in man. *Circulation* 34:272-278, 1966
59. Wynne J, Green LH, Mann T, et al: Estimation of left ventricular volumes in man from biplane cineangiograms filmed in oblique projections. *Am J Cardiol* 41:726-732, 1978
60. Feigenbaum H, Popp RL, Chip JN, et al: Left ventricular wall thickness measured by ultrasound. *Arch Intern Med* 121:391-395, 1968
61. Bradfield JWB, Beck G, Vecht RJ: Left ventricular apical thin point. *Br Heart J* 39:806-809, 1977
62. Maron BJ, Henry WL, Roberts WC, et al: Comparison of echocardiographic and necropsy measurements of ventricular wall thicknesses in patients with and without disproportionate septal thickening. *Circulation* 55:341-346, 1977
63. Frohlich ED, Apstein C, Chobanian AV, et al: The heart in hypertension. *N Engl J Med* 327:998-1008, 1992
64. Rosenquist GC, Sweeney LJ: The membranous ventricular septum in the normal heart. *Johns Hopkins Med J* 135:9-16, 1974
65. Rosenquist GC, Clark EB, Sweeney LJ, et al: The normal spectrum of mitral and aortic valve discontinuity. *Circulation* 54:298-301, 1976
66. Walmsley R: Anatomy of left ventricular outflow tract. *Br Heart J* 41:263-267, 1979
67. Teofilovski PG, Baptista CAC, DiDio LJA, et al: The membranous portion of the interventricular septum and its relationship with the aortic valve in humans. *Surg Radiol Anat* 13:23-28, 1991
68. Wafae N, Wafae M, Vieira MC: Morphological study of one septal trabecula carnea of the left ventricle. *Bull Assoc Anat* 74:33-36, 1990
69. Boyd MT, Seward JB, Tajik AJ, et al: Frequency and location of prominent left ventricular trabeculations at autopsy in 474 normal human hearts: implications for evaluation of mural thrombi by two-dimensional echocardiography. *J Am Coll Cardiol* 9:323-326, 1987
70. Pietras RJ, Kondos GT, Kaplan D, et al: Comparative angiographic right and left ventricular volumes. *Am Heart J* 109:321-326, 1985
71. Tajik AJ, Seward JB, Hagler DJ, et al: Two-dimensional realtime ultrasonic imaging of the heart and great vessels: technique, image orientation, structure identification, and validation. *Mayo Clin Proc* 53:271-303, 1978
72. Henry WL, DeMaria A, Gramiak R, et al: Report of the American Society of Echocardiography Committee on Nomenclature and Standards in Two-Dimensional Echocardiography. *Circulation* 62:212-217, 1980
73. Schiller NB, Shah PM, Crawford M, et al: Recommendations for quantitation of the left ventricle by two-dimensional echocardiography. *J Am Soc Echocardiogr* 2:358-367, 1989
74. Klausner SC, Blair TJ, Bulawa WF, et al: Quantitative analysis of segmental wall motion throughout systole and diastole in the normal human left ventricle. *Circulation* 65:580-590, 1982
75. Ferrans VJ, Rodríguez ER: Ultrastructure of the normal heart. In *Cardiovascular Pathology.* Edited by MD Silver. Vol. 1. Second edition. New York, Churchill Livingstone, 1991, pp 43-101
76. Zak R: Cardiac hypertrophy: biochemical and cellular relationships. *Hosp Pract* 18:85-97, March 1983
77. Moore GW, Hutchins GM, Bulkley BH, et al: Constituents of the human ventricular myocardium: connective tissue hyperplasia accompanying muscular hypertrophy. *Am Heart J* 100:610-616, 1980
78. Hort W: Quantitative morphology and structural dynamics of the myocardium. *Methods Achiev Exp Pathol* 5:3-21, 1971
79. Maron BJ, Ferrans VJ, Roberts WC: Ultrastructural features of degenerated cardiac muscle cells in patients with cardiac hypertrophy. *Am J Pathol* 79:387-430, 1975
80. Fuster V, Danielson MA, Robb RA, et al: Quantitation of left ventricular myocardial fiber hypertrophy and interstitial tissue in human hearts with chronically increased volume and pressure overload. *Circulation* 55:504-508, 1977
81. Geer JC, Crago CA, Little WC, et al: Subendocardial ischemic myocardial lesions associated with severe coronary atherosclerosis. *Am J Pathol* 98:663-679, 1980
82. Dick MR, Unverferth DV, Baba N: The pattern of myocardial degeneration in nonischemic congestive cardiomyopathy. *Hum Pathol* 13:740-744, 1982
83. Roy P-E: Basophilic degeneration of the myocardium: an ultrastructural study. *Lab Invest* 32:729-735, 1975
84. Kosek JC, Angell W: Fine structure of basophilic myocardial degeneration. *Arch Pathol* 89:491-499, 1970
85. Report of a WHO Scientific Group: The pathological diagnosis of acute ischaemic heart disease. *WHO Tech Rep Ser* 441:1-27, 1970
86. Wenink ACG: Embryology of the ventricular septum: separate origin of its components. *Virchows Arch [Pathol Anat]* 390:71-79, 1981
87. Wenink ACG, Gittenberger-de Groot AC: Left and right ventricular trabecular patterns: consequence of ventricular septation and valve development. *Br Heart J* 48:462-468, 1982
88. Bartelings MM, Gittenberger-de Groot AC: The outflow tract of the heart: embryologic and morphologic correlations. *Int J Cardiol* 22:289-300, 1989
89. Allwork SP, Anderson RH: Developmental anatomy of the membranous part of the ventricular septum in the human heart. *Br Heart J* 41:275-280, 1979
90. Thubrikar M, Bosher LP, Nolan SP: The mechanism of opening of the aortic valve. *J Thorac Cardiovasc Surg* 77:863-870, 1979
91. Krovetz LJ: Age-related changes in size of the aortic valve annulus in man. *Am Heart J* 90:569-574, 1975
92. Silver MA, Roberts WC: Detailed anatomy of the normally functioning aortic valve in hearts of normal and increased weight. *Am J Cardiol* 55:454-461, 1985
93. Kim KM, Valigorsky JM, Mergner WJ, et al: Aging changes in the human aortic valve in relation to dystrophic calcification. *Hum Pathol* 7:47-60, 1976
94. Mercer JL: Acceptable size of the pulmonary valve ring in congenital cardiac defects. *Ann Thorac Surg* 20:567-570, 1975
95. Pollick C, Pittman M, Filly K, et al: Mitral and aortic valve orifice area in normal subjects and in patients with congestive cardiomyopathy: determination by two dimensional echocardiography. *Am J Cardiol* 49:1191-1196, 1982
96. Vollebergh FEMG, Becker AE: Minor congenital variations of cusp size in tricuspid aortic valves: possible link with isolated aortic stenosis. *Br Heart J* 39:1006-1011, 1977
97. Sud A, Parker F, Magilligan DJ Jr: Anatomy of the aortic root. *Ann Thorac Surg* 38:76-79, 1984
98. Anderson RH, Devine WA, Ho SY, et al: The myth of the aortic annulus: the anatomy of the subaortic outflow tract. *Ann Thorac Surg* 52:640-646, 1991
99. Van Gils FAW: The fibrous skeleton in the human heart: embryological and pathogenetic considerations. *Virchows Arch [Pathol]* 393:61-73, 1981
100. Takahashi T, Wagenvoort N, Wagenvoort CA: The density of muscularized pulmonary arteries in normal lungs: a morphometric study. *Arch Pathol Lab Med* 107:19-22, 1983
101. Plank L, James J, Wagenvoort CA: Caliber and elastin content of the pulmonary trunk. *Arch Pathol Lab Med* 104:238-241, 1980
102. Cudkowicz L: Bronchial arterial circulation in man: normal anatomy and responses to disease. *Lung Biol Health Dis* 14:111-232, 1979
103. James TN: *Anatomy of the Coronary Arteries.* New York, Paul B Hoeber, 1961
104. Baroldi G, Scomazzoni G: *Coronary Circulation in the Normal Heart and the Pathologic Heart.* Washington DC, Government Printing Office, 1967
105. Edwards BS, Edwards WD, Edwards JE: Aortic origin of conus coronary artery: evidence of postnatal coronary development. *Br Heart J* 45:555-558, 1981

106. Taylor JR: The descending septal artery: its relation to the conduction system of the heart. *Arch Pathol Lab Med* 104:599-602, 1980

107. Levin DC, Beckmann CF, Garnic JD, et al: Frequency and clinical significance of failure to visualize the conus artery during coronary arteriography. *Circulation* 63:833-837, 1981

108. Anderson KR, Ho SY, Anderson RH: Location and vascular supply of sinus node in human heart. *Br Heart J* 41:28-32, 1979

109. James TN: Anatomy of the coronary arteries in health and disease. *Circulation* 32:1020-1033, 1965

110. Kramer JR, Kitazume H, Proudfit WL, et al: Clinical significance of isolated coronary bridges: benign and frequent condition involving the left anterior descending artery. *Am Heart J* 103:283-288, 1982

111. Kronzon I, Deutsch P, Glassman E: Length of the left main coronary artery: its relation to the pattern of coronary arterial distribution. *Am J Cardiol* 34:787-789, 1974

112. Lerer PK, Edwards WD: Coronary arterial anatomy in bicuspid aortic valve: necropsy study of 100 hearts. *Br Heart J* 45:142-147, 1981

113. Brown BG, Bolson EL, Dodge HT: Dynamic mechanisms in human coronary stenosis. *Circulation* 70:917-922, 1984

114. Miller AJ: *Lymphatics of the Heart.* New York, Raven Press, 1982, pp 107-180; 318-325

115. Eliška O, Elišaková M: Lymphatic drainage of the ventricular conduction system in man and in the dog. *Acta Anat* 107:205-213, 1980

116. Vlodaver Z, Neufeld HN, Edwards JE: *Coronary Arterial Variations in the Normal Heart and in Congenital Heart Disease.* New York, Academic Press, 1975, pp 1-134

117. Boucek RJ, Morales AR, Romanelli R, et al: *Coronary Artery Disease: Pathologic and Clinical Assessment.* Baltimore, Williams & Wilkins, 1984, pp 38-46

118. Davies MJ, Anderson RH, Becker AE: *The Conduction System of the Heart.* London, Butterworths, 1983, pp 9-94

119. James TN: The sinus node. *Am J Cardiol* 40:965-986, 1977

120. Sherf L, James TN: Fine structure of cells and their histologic organization within internodal pathways of the heart: clinical and electrocardiographic implications. *Am J Cardiol* 44:345-369, 1979

121. Eliška O, Elišaková M: Venous circulation of the human cardiac conduction system. *Br Heart J* 42:508-513, 1979

Appendix

Abbreviations used in figures

A	Anterior	L	Left
AL	Anterolateral	LA	Left atrium
Ant	Anterior	LAA	Left atrial appendage
Ao	Aorta	LAD	Left anterior descending coronary artery
Art	Artery	LAO	Left anterior oblique
AS	Anteroseptal (Fig 12-43 only)	Lat	Lateral
AS	Atrial septum	LBB	Left bundle branch
Asc	Ascending	LCCA	Left common carotid artery
AV	Atrioventricular	LCX	Left circumflex coronary artery
AVB	AV bundle	LIV	Left innominate vein
AVN	AV node	LLL	Left lower lobe
AVNA	AV nodal artery	LLPV	Left lower pulmonary vein
AVS	AV septum	LMA	Left main coronary artery
CFB	Central fibrous body	LPA	Left pulmonary artery
CS	Coronary sinus	LPO	Left posterior oblique
CT	Crista terminalis	LPV	Left pulmonary veins
D	Ductus arteriosus	LSA	Left subclavian artery
Desc	Descending	LSVC	Left superior vena cava
E	Esophagus	LUL	Left upper lobe
Ext	External	LUPV	Left upper pulmonary vein
FO	Fossa ovalis	LV	Left ventricle
FSP	First septal perforating coronary artery	LVOT	Left ventricular outflow tract
I	Inferior	Mes	Mesenteric
IA	Innominate artery	MS	Membranous septum
IAS	Interatrial septum	MV	Mitral valve
IL	Inferolateral	OS	Ostium secundum
Inf	Inferior	P	Posterior
Int	Internal	PB	Parietal band
IS	Inferoseptal (Fig 12-43 only)	PeM	Pectinate muscles
IS	Infundibular septum	PL	Posterolateral
IVC	Inferior vena cava	PM	Posteromedial
IVS	Interventricular septum	Post	Posterior

Continued.

Appendix – cont'd

Abbreviations used in figures

PS	Posteroseptal	RPV	Right pulmonary veins
PT	Pulmonary trunk	RSA	Right subclavian artery
Pulm	Pulmonary	RSVC	Right superior vena cava
PV	Pulmonary valve	RUL	Right upper lobe
R	Right	RUPV	Right upper pulmonary vein
RA	Right atrium	RV	Right ventricle
RAA	Right atrial appendage	S	Septal
RAO	Right anterior oblique	SB	Septal band
RCA	Right coronary artery	SNA	Sinus nodal artery
RCCA	Right common carotid artery	Sup	Superior
RIV	Right innominate vein	SVC	Superior vena cava
RLL	Right lower lobe	T	Trachea
RLPV	Right lower pulmonary vein	TC	Trabeculae carneae
RML	Right middle lobe	Thor	Thoracic
RMPV	Right middle pulmonary vein	TV	Tricuspid valve
RPA	Right pulmonary artery	VFO	Valve of fossa ovalis
RPD	Right posterior descending coronary artery	VS	Ventricular septum
RPO	Right posterior oblique		

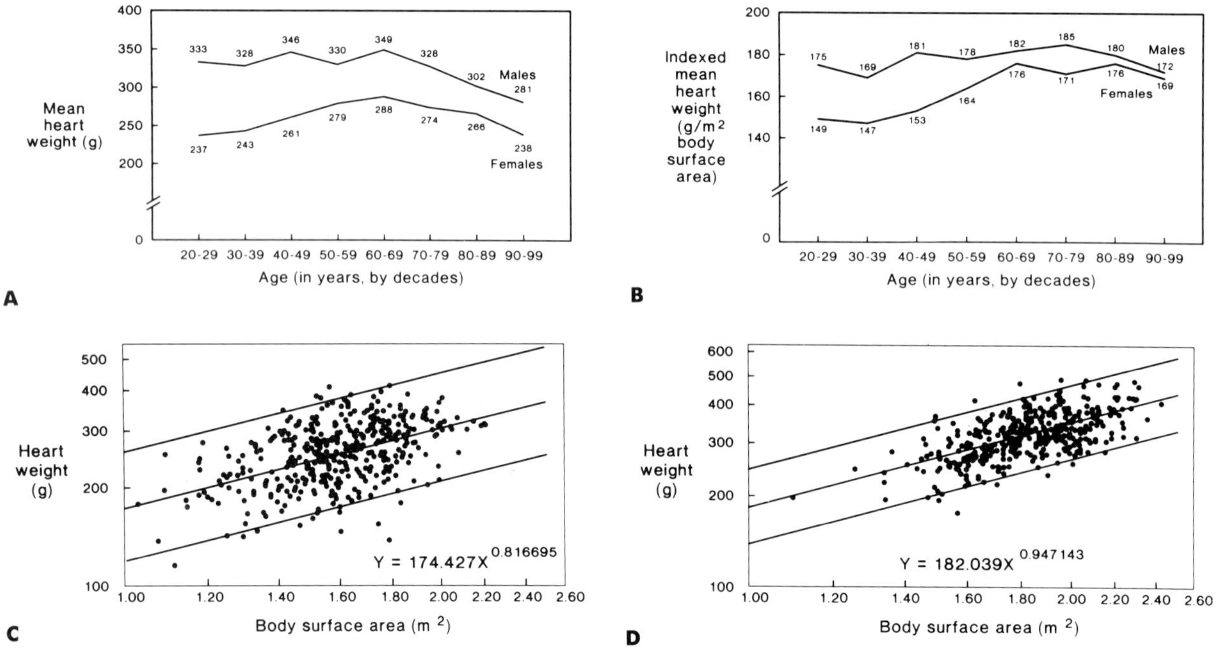

Fig A12-1 Normal heart weights, from 392 females and 373 males. **A** and **B,** mean **(A)** and indexed **(B)** heart weights vs. age. **C** and **D,** heart weight vs. body surface area in women **(C)** and men **(D)**. (See references 8 and 9.)

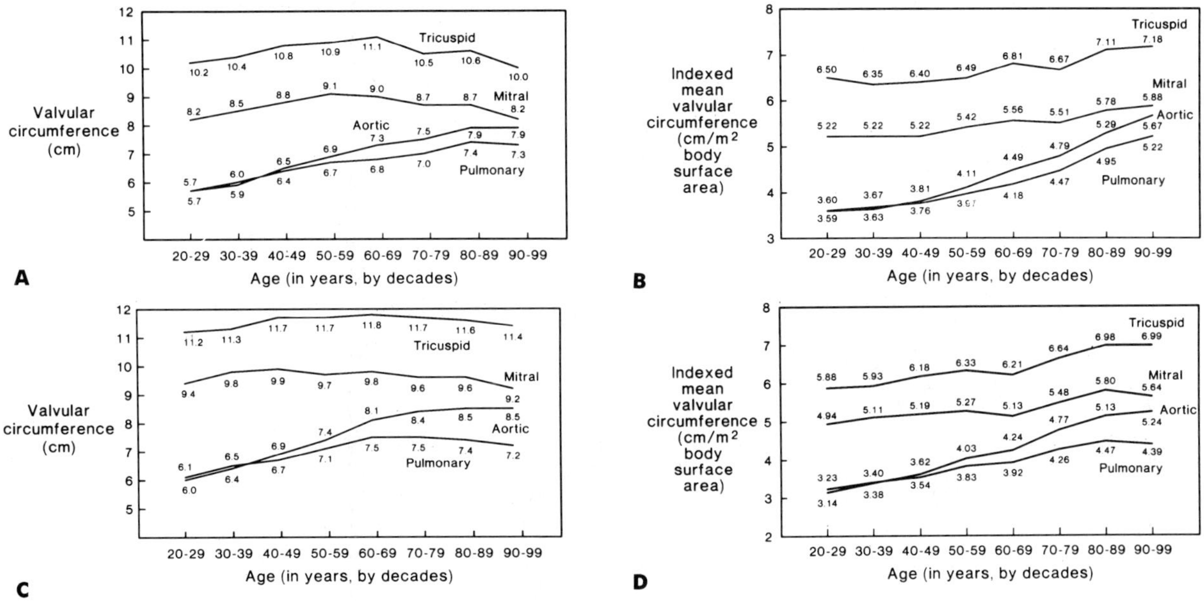

Fig A12-2 Normal valve circumferences. **A** and **B,** mean **(A)** and indexed **(B)** circumferences vs. age in 392 females. **C** and **D,** mean **(C)** and indexed **(D)** circumferences vs. age in 373 males. (See references 8 and 9.)

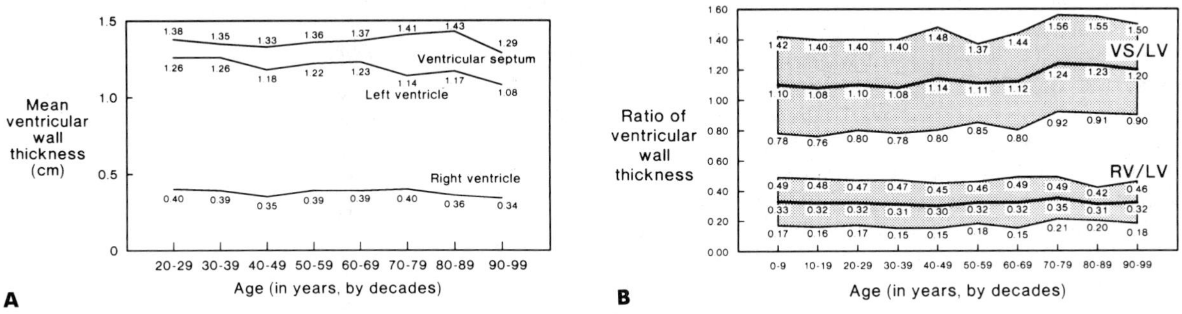

Fig A12-3 Normal ventricular wall thicknesses from 765 cases. **A,** mean ventricular thickness vs. age. **B,** ratios of ventricular thicknesses (mean ± 2 SD) vs. age. (See references 8 and 9.)

CHAPTER

13

Prevention of coronary heart disease

Thomas E. Kottke, M.D., William H. Weidman, M.D., and Tu T. Nguyen, M.D.

When Rudolph Virchow first observed the pathologic changes in the arterial wall that he called "atherosclerosis," he attributed them to substances imbibed from the blood.[1,2] Although others attributed atherosclerosis to degenerative changes of aging, he postulated that these abnormalities were potentially preventable. Aschoff's observation[3] that deaths from coronary heart disease declined during World War I lent credence to the diet-heart disease hypothesis. Studies conducted between the two world wars demonstrated that atherosclerosis also could be induced in animal models,[2] and observations in Scandinavia during World War II corroborated those of Aschoff.[4]

After World War II, Paul Dudley White, Ancel Keys, and Martti Karvonen were among the first to observe that rates of death from coronary heart disease differed tenfold around the world and even within Europe.[5] Keys began his studies of risk factors for atherosclerosis just after World War II,[6] his international studies in Italy and Spain in 1952,[7] and the Seven Countries Study in 1958. About the same time, the first examinations of the Framingham population were initiated.[1] With few exceptions the studies of these and other investigators consistently pointed toward three major risk factors for coronary heart disease: a diet high in saturated fat causing increased serum cholesterol concentration, high blood pressure, and smoking.[8-18] More recently, the risk associated with physical inactivity was identified.[19,20]

Because the association of two factors does not necessarily mean that one factor is the cause of the other and trial data may not be available, Hill[21] developed quality-of-evidence criteria with which to judge the probability that a risk factor associated with a disease actually causes the disease (Table 13-1). When applying these guidelines, it is important not to use these criteria too strictly, since coronary heart disease is known to be a disease of multiple causes with incomplete expression in populations exposed to the risk factors. For further discussion, the reader is encouraged to read Hill's original text and a textbook of epidemiologic methods.[22]

This chapter first describes the observational evidence that diet, smoking, obesity, diabetes, psychosocial conditions, and physical inactivity are causative risk factors for coronary heart disease.* It then reviews the results of the intervention trials and describes clinical approaches to the modification of coronary heart disease risk factors. Finally, the chapter discusses the strategies that the physician must consider when implementing risk factor interventions. The evidence that risk factor modification can cause the regression of coronary heart disease is presented in chapter 14.

DIET

Carefully controlled metabolic studies have demonstrated the influence of dietary cholesterol on total plasma cholesterol concentrations.[23-26] Population studies have reinforced these conclusions.[27] Four studies, in particular, reinforce the intimate relationship of lipids to coronary heart disease. The Seven Countries Study[17] showed a high correlation between the percentage of calories consumed as saturated fat and deaths due to coronary heart disease (Fig 13-1). Unfortunately, intake of dietary cholesterol was not measured directly in this study.

In the Ni Hon San Study,[28,29] intakes of saturated fat calories of Japanese men living in Japan, Hawaii, and San Francisco were estimated to be about 7%, 12%, and 14%, respectively; greater intakes of saturated fats and cholesterol correlated with higher levels of serum cholesterol in these populations. In comparison with Japan, death rates

*The evidence that hypertension is a risk factor for the development of coronary heart disease is discussed in chapter 60.

Table 13-1 Factors to consider when trying to determine whether a risk factor is a cause of a disease

Strength	Is there a large difference in rates between individuals exposed and not exposed to the risk factor?
Consistency	Has the association been observed by different persons, in different places, in different circumstances and times?
Specificity	Are cases limited to individuals exposed to the risk factor?
Relationship in time	Does the disease occur after the exposure to the risk factor?
Biologic gradient	Is a dose-response curve present?
Biologic plausibility effect relationship	Is there a biologic mechanism that can explain a cause-and-effect relationship?
Coherence of the evidence	Is a cause-and-effect interpretation consistent with other knowledge?
Experimental evidence	Can the relationship be produced experimentally?
Reasoning by analogy	Does an association exist between two similar factors?

Data from Hill AB: *Principles of Medical Statistics.* Ninth edition. New York, Oxford University Press, 1971, pp 309-323

from coronary heart disease were 1.7 times higher in Hawaii and 2.8 times higher in San Francisco.

In the Seventh-Day Adventist study,[30] mortality rates among predominantly lacto-ovo-vegetarians were lower in comparison with an age-matched California population; Seventh-Day Adventists had lower serum cholesterol values and smoked less often.

In the Western Electric Study,[31] a positive association between the diet scores of Hegsted et al.[26] and Keys and Parlin[32] and serum cholesterol concentration at the initial examination was positively and prospectively associated with the 19-year risk of death from coronary heart disease. In this study, the relationship among dietary scores, serum cholesterol, and coronary heart disease incidence was maintained after adjustment for confounding factors.

It was once thought that serum lipid levels were irrelevant as predictors of risk in the population over 65. However, data have shown that for both men and women over age 65, serum cholesterol concentration remains a risk factor for coronary heart disease.[33,34]

The evidence in humans that diet is a causal risk factor for coronary heart disease is strong, consistent, coherent, and plausible.[35] It is therefore more reasonable to conclude that a diet high in saturated fat is a cause of coronary heart disease than it is to conclude that there is no relationship between diet and coronary heart disease.

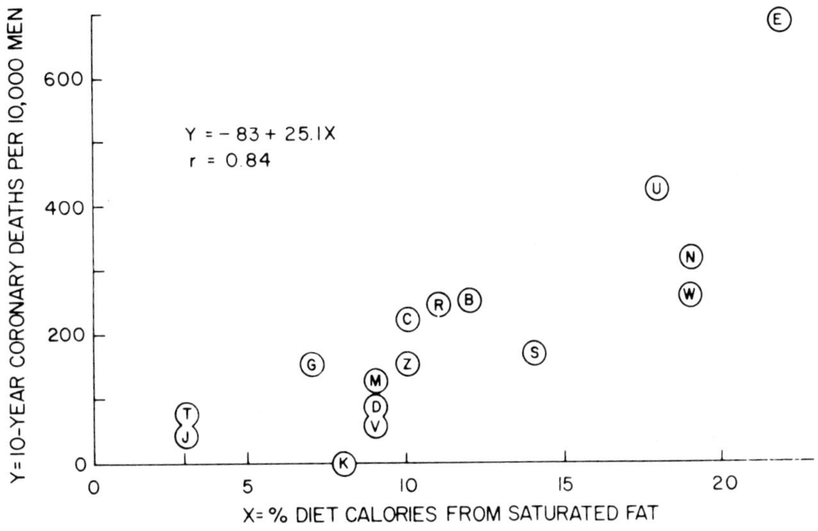

Fig 13-1 Coronary heart disease age-standardized 10-year death rates of the cohorts versus the percentage of calories from saturated fat consumed by the cohorts. All men were judged free of coronary heart disease at entry. The coefficient of correlation is $r = 0.84$. *B,* Belgrade; *C,* Crevalcore; *D,* Dalmatia; *E,* east Finland; *G,* Corfu; *K,* Crete; *M,* Montegiorgio; *N,* Zutphen; *R,* American railroad; *S,* Slavonia; *T,* Tanushimaru; *U,* Ushibuka; *V,* Velika Krsna; *W,* west Finland; *Z,* Zrenjanin. (From Keys A: *Seven Countries: A Multivariate Analysis of Death and Coronary Heart Disease.* Cambridge, Massachusetts, Harvard University Press, 1980. By permission of the President and Fellows of Harvard College.)

LIPIDS, LIPOPROTEINS, AND APOPROTEINS

In this section, we review the current understanding of the biochemistry and cell biology of lipid metabolism and, with the help of diagrams, attempt to offer a rational basis for an understanding of the mechanisms involved in the regulation of lipid metabolism.

Classes of plasma lipids

The major lipids of the plasma include the sterol cholesterol; the esters of cholesterol, formed by the equimolar reaction of cholesterol with various fatty acids; triglycerides, formed by the interaction of three molecules of fatty acids with one molecule of glycerol; and phospholipids, formed by the interaction of phosphatidic acid with two molecules of fatty acids. In the plasma, the specific fatty acids of the triglycerides and phospholipids tend to reflect those present in the diet. Cholesterol is esterified primarily with linoleic acid, and the major phospholipid class is the lecithins. In atherosclerotic lesions, the major cholesterol ester is cholesterol oleate.

Plasma lipoproteins

Since most lipids are insoluble in the aqueous environment of plasma, they occur in the plasma as complex particles called lipoproteins. The major classes of these particles (based on electrophoretic mobility and density) include fatty acid-albumin complexes, the simplest particles formed by the binding of free fatty acids to the hydrophobic sites of this major plasma protein; chylomicrons, the particles formed in the intestinal lymph during the ingestion of dietary fat: very-low-density lipoprotein (VLDL), triglyceride-rich endogenous particles secreted primarily by the liver; low-density lipoprotein (LDL), secreted by the liver and the intestine in part as a product of VLDL catabolism; and high-density lipoprotein (HDL), the smallest of the lipoprotein particles, which are secreted by the liver and intestines and play a critical role in the reverse transport of cholesterol from peripheral cells to the liver.

The association between elevated serum total cholesterol and an increased risk of coronary heart disease is related to elevations of cholesterol in the LDL fraction (LDL cholesterol), a major carrier of serum cholesterol.[36,37] An inverse correlation between the incidence of coronary heart disease and levels of HDL cholesterol has also been noted[38-42] (Fig 13-2). (Factors influencing levels of HDL are listed in Table 13-2.) Inverse relationships between the incidence of coronary heart disease and HDL cholesterol levels are seen when total plasma cholesterol levels are relatively high, but low levels of HDL cholesterol may not increase the risk for coronary heart disease in populations in which concentrations of LDL cholesterol are low[41,43] (Table 13-3). Low levels of both cholesterol-containing particles (LDL and HDL) would not be expected to result in an increase in cellular cholesterol content (that is, cellular cholesterol balance would be normal, with a low input and a low output).

An independent association between triglycerides and the incidence of coronary heart disease has been reported in several studies.[12,44] Although multivariate adjustments for major risk variables have not shown that triglyceride is an independent risk factor in many studies,[11,45-47] other studies have shown that triglyceride levels predict the development of coronary heart disease.[48] The association

Table 13-2 Factors influencing levels of high-density lipoprotein

Relatively high levels	Relatively low levels
Females	Males
Blacks in United States	Whites in United States
Exercise	Diabetes
Estrogen	Hypertriglyceridemia
Alcohol	High-carbohydrate diet
Weight reduction	Obesity
Nicotinic acid	Smoking
Fibric acid derivatives	Progesterone
Chlorinated hydrocarbons	Antihypertensive drugs
Familial hyperalphalipoproteinemia	Polyunsaturated fats
Insulin	Sedentary lifestyle

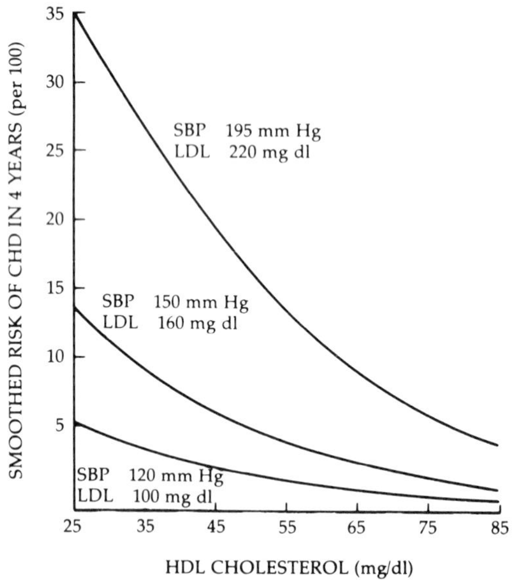

Fig 13-2 Risk of coronary heart disease *(CHD)* according to levels of HDL cholesterol in the Framingham Study. *SBP,* systolic blood pressure. (From Kannel WB, Castelli WP: Prognostic implications of blood lipid measurements. In *Prognosis: Contemporary Outcomes of Disease.* Edited by JF Fries, GE Ehrlich. Bowie, Maryland, The Charles Press Publishers, Division of Robert J. Brady Company, A Prentice-Hall Publishing and Communications Company, 1981, pp 263-267. By permission.)

between increased triglyceride levels and risk of coronary heart disease may have been underestimated in the studies using multivariate analyses because of the wide intraindividual variation in the triglyceride levels. The presence of abnormal lipoprotein particles, which are often associated with hypertriglyceridemia, may also predict risk. Such abnormalities include low levels of HDL cholesterol, increased levels of VLDL cholesterol, dysbetalipoproteinemia (with β-VLDL), and abnormal isoforms of apolipoprotein E.

The particle size, lipid composition, and cellular interaction of these classes of particles depend primarily on the lipid-binding characteristics, the affinity for enzymes, and the cellular receptor-binding affinities of the specific proteins of each class of lipoprotein particles. A lipoprotein in its delipidated state is termed "apolipoprotein." The characteristics of each of the known apolipoproteins of plasma are summarized in Table 13-4. Any specific function in addition to their role as lipid carriers is also listed. Figure 13-3 illustrates the usual composition of the major classes of apolipoproteins.

Lp(a) is an LDL-like lipoprotein that has a large glycoprotein apo(a) bound to apo B by disulfide bonds. Lp(a) is a genetic risk factor for coronary heart disease[49] and seems to exert its pathogenic effect at about 20 to 30 mg/dL. Increased plasma levels of Lp(a) are found in 10% to 15% of the white population. Modified Lp(a) can be taken up by macrophages like modified LDL, leading to foam cell formation. Lp(a) may, in addition, interfere with clot lysis by inhibiting conversion of plasminogen to plasmin.[50]

Table 13-3 Prevalence of coronary heart disease (CHD) by high-density lipoprotein (HDL) level in men*

HDL cholesterol, mg/dL	CHD rate per 1,000
25	180
25-34	124
35-44	95
45-54	78
55-64	78
65-74	79
75	86

*The Cooperative Lipoprotein Phenotyping Study showed a twofold increase in the incidence of coronary heart disease at HDL levels below 45 mg/dL in men ages 50 to 69 years.
Modified from Castelli WP, Doyle JT, Gordon T, et al: HDL cholesterol and other lipids in coronary heart disease: the Cooperative Lipoprotein Phenotyping Study. *Circulation* 55:767-772, 1977.

SMOKING

Converging lines of investigation have identified the adverse consequences of cigarette smoking to health. The relationship between cigarette smoking and excess deaths, predominantly due to coronary heart disease, was initially demonstrated in large prospective studies of white American men.[51,52] Support for these initial observations has been garnered in subsequent studies in Framingham.[53,54] In a large study of United States veterans, middle-aged heavy smokers had a fivefold to tenfold increased risk of death compared with nonsmokers.[55] The risk from cigarette smoking persists at least until the age of 74.[56]

Cigarette smoking is a powerful contributor to coronary heart disease, morbidity, and mortality in men and women. The risk of vascular disease is magnified in young females taking oral contraceptives who also smoke cigarettes.[57,58] The male and female gradients of risk are seen at all levels of cigarette smoking and increase sharply in heavy smokers. The addition of cigarette smoking to elevated cholesterol levels and blood pressure increases the risk of coronary heart disease in excess of the sum of the contributions by the individual risk factors.[59,60]

Smoking predicts the appearance of congestive cardio-

Table 13-4 Major classes of plasma lipoproteins in order of decreasing size

Apolipoproteins	Site of synthesis	Specialized function
A-I	Intestine and liver	Cofactor for lecithin-cholesterol acyltransferase (L-CAT)
A-II	Intestine and liver	Activates hepatic triglyceride lipase
B (two forms: B_{100} and B_{48})	Liver for B_{100} Intestine for B_{48}	B_{100} recognized by LDL (B-E) receptors
C-I	Liver	Activates L-CAT
C-II	Liver	Cofactor for lipoprotein lipase (in vitro and in vivo)
C-III	Liver	Inhibitor of lipoprotein lipase (in vitro)
D	?Liver	Transfer of cholesterol esters between HDL and other lipoproteins
E (three isoforms: E_2, E_3, and E_4)	Liver	Recognized by LDL (B-E) receptors and by remnant (E) receptors
Apo(a)	Liver	May inhibit formation of plasmin and fibrinolysis
CETP	Liver, adipose tissue	Transfers cholesterol esters and triglycerides between lipoproteins and cholesterol esters between lipoprotein and peripheral cells

CETP, cholesterol ester transfer protein.

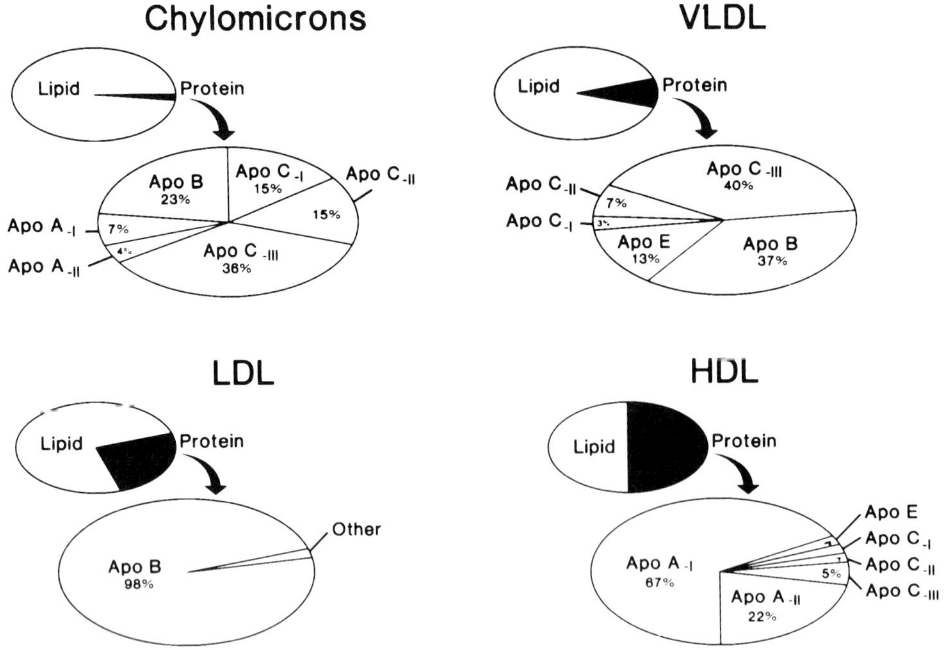

Fig 13-3 Apo composition of lipoprotein particles. The lipid composition of chylomicrons is 90% (expressed as percent of total particle mass) triglycerides, 1% free cholesterol, 4% cholesterol esters, and 4% phospholipids; *VLDL* is 60% triglycerides, 5% free cholesterol, 10% cholesterol esters, and 15% phospholipids; *LDL* is 30% cholesterol esters, 15% free cholesterol, 10% triglycerides, and 20% phospholipids; *HDL* is 15% cholesterol esters, 5% free cholesterol, 27% phospholipids, and 3% triglycerides.

myopathy independent of coronary artery disease.[61] Young women with myocardial infarction are six times as likely to be smokers as are control women.[57] Continued smoking after myocardial infarction is associated with a doubling of death rates,[62-64] and continued smoking predicts recurrence of sudden cardiac arrest.[65] Smoking causes silent ischemia[66] and reduces the antianginal effects of propranolol, atenolol, and nifedepine.[67] Continued smoking results in higher failure rates for femoral-popliteal artery grafts[68] and coronary artery bypass grafts.[69]

The impact of stopping smoking is large relative to other interventions. For example, Gillum et al.[70] demonstrated an improvement in survival between 1970 and 1980 for patients hospitalized with acute myocardial infarction. Further analysis suggests that this improvement is indeed because of medical care.[71] However, on the basis of risk coefficients of the United States railroad cohort of the Seven Countries Study,[7] the estimated effects of a 15% smoking cessation rate among a cohort of middle-aged men in which 30% are smokers are twice as great as the effects observed by Gillum et al.[70] that are attributable to an improvement in medical care.

The association of cigarette smoking with the risk of myocardial infarction or sudden death is independent of other risk factors,[53,72] although the presence of other risk factors greatly amplifies the risk. There are large differences in risk between smokers and nonsmokers. The gradient of risk among cigarette smokers is small; even low levels of cigarette smoking enhance risk. Reports[73] describing heightened risk of nonfatal myocardial infarction with angiographically demonstrated mild, moderate, or severe occlusions suggest that smoking with any grade of atherosclerosis increases risk of coronary occlusion or sudden death.

In the two-factor randomized Oslo trial,[74] a multivariate statistical model was used to separate the effects of cholesterol lowering and cigarette cessation. In this study, changes in serum cholesterol accounted for 60% of the reduction in coronary heart disease mortality, whereas the smoking-cessation factor accounted for 25%. In the Kaiser-Permanente Study,[75] after adjustment for major baseline differences in risk characteristics, the relative risk of dying from coronary heart disease among persistent smokers was 2.2 times that of those who quit smoking. In the Multiple Risk Factor Intervention Trial, those who quit smoking had a significantly lower probability of developing coronary heart disease.[76] Persons who discontinue smoking are at a substantially lower risk of coronary heart disease than those who continue to smoke.[52,63,77-79]

The mechanisms by which cigarette smoking provokes coronary attacks may be related to carbon monoxide or other compounds in cigarette smoke. These chemicals damage arterial endothelium, increase platelet adhesion, release platelet-derived growth factor, and possibly increase the permeability of the endothelium for lipids.[80,81] Carbon monoxide, furthermore, may exert its adverse

Table 13-5 Five-year incidence of death or definite infarction from coronary heart disease estimated from the multiple logistic equation: influence of body mass index (BMI)*

Probability decile	BMI ignored		BMI included	
	Cases	Expected	Cases	Expected
1	0	1.32	0	1.32
2	1	2.20	2	2.19
3	3	2.94	2	2.92
4	5	3.74	4	3.71
5	3	4.70	5	4.66
6	9	5.81	8	5.78
7	9	7.49	8	7.49
8	11	9.80	11	9.86
9	13	13.74	15	13.70
10	24	27.67	23	27.48

*Data are for United States-raised men classified into deciles of probability of risk, on the basis of entry data on age, systolic blood pressure, serum cholesterol, and smoking habit alone and on these data plus BMI.
From Keys A, Aravanis C, Blackburn H, et al: Coronary heart disease: overweight and obesity as risk factors. *Ann Intern Med* 77:15-27, 1972. By permission of the American College of Physicians.

influence through vascular toxic and inflammatory effects, hemostatic changes, and accelerated atherogenesis. The acute effect of cigarette smoking on platelet function, resulting in enhanced platelet adhesiveness with the subsequent release of platelet-derived growth factor, is a major contributing effect.[82] Cigarette smoking mobilizes catecholamines in adrenergic axon terminals within the tissues.[83] A smoking-initiated sympathetic discharge could conceivably lower the ventricular-fibrillation threshold and thus trigger sudden death in an ischemic myocardium.[84]

OVERWEIGHT AND OBESITY

Obesity may not be an independent risk factor for coronary heart disease. In one of the better studies exploring the relationship between relative weight and coronary heart disease (Table 13-5), multivariate analysis, which accounted for age, blood pressure, cholesterol, and smoking, showed that no index of relative weight or fatness made a significant contribution to future coronary heart disease.[85] Multivariate analysis of the Framingham data suggests that relative weight is a risk factor only between ages 40 and 49.[86] No relationship between reciprocal ponderal index and coronary heart disease was found in the Western Collaborative Group Study.[87] Studies of Chicago men[88,89] in whom coronary heart disease developed showed significantly greater skinfold thickness in the diseased cohorts in a univariate analysis. However, the risk disappears when other factors are taken into consideration.

Even so, excess weight is related to hypertension, diabetes, emotional problems, and unintentional trauma. Obesity is also associated with an increased incidence of hypertriglyceridemia with a concomitant increase in levels of VLDL cholesterol and decreased levels of HDL cholesterol. Furthermore, declines in levels of LDL and VLDL and increases in HDL are facilitated by weight reduction.

CARBOHYDRATE INTOLERANCE AND DIABETES MELLITUS

Persons with diabetes mellitus have a mortality three times that of those without diabetes.[90,91] In a 5-year prospective study of 18,000 men, the reported coronary heart disease mortality rate doubled for persons in the highest 2% of the group (2-hour postprandial glucose, 106 to 504 mg/dL) even after exclusion of clinically labeled diabetic patients.[92] Data from coronary angiographic studies also support the observations of epidemiologic data pointing to a greater involvement of vessels with atherosclerotic disease.[93,94] Autopsy studies have shown that the prevalence of coronary heart disease ranges from 18% to 75% among diabetic persons.[95-97] The mechanisms that increase the risk of coronary heart disease in patients with diabetes mellitus are not known[90] but may include increased adhesiveness of platelets, higher prevalence of hyperlipidemias, abnormalities in coagulation, and higher insulin levels. In spite of the controversies surrounding the University Group Diabetes Program,[98] most experts at present believe that close control of hyperglycemia, as is currently advocated, may prove beneficial.

PSYCHOSOCIAL RISK FACTORS

Coronary heart disease has now been linked to indices of social mobility, disrupted social networks, and life stress.[99-103] For example, pioneering studies of acculturation among men of Japanese ancestry in California have suggested that the stable, close-knit Japanese culture may protect against coronary heart disease.[104] These cross-sectional linkages fail to hold up when the incidence of disease is measured in cohorts.[105] Multivariate analysis of incidence rates suggests that measures of acculturation are also significantly associated with many other coronary heart disease risk factors, and this may explain, at least in part, the observed East-to-West gradients of disease. However, there is a cogent and growing body of evidence suggesting that social networks militate against the pathologic effects of stress, including psychiatric and physical morbidity.[106-109]

Contrary to popular opinion, coronary heart disease now appears to be more prominent among working classes. The Whitehall Study[110] confirmed a large preponderance of coronary heart disease among men in the lower employment grades. In England and Wales, increases in mortality from coronary heart disease have been noted among working-class men, whereas mortality rates for professional men have been stable for the past 20 years. Studies in the United States have also shown a greater prevalence of coronary heart disease in the lower social economic strata.[111] It is very probable that these differences are related to differences particularly in smoking behavior but also in lipid levels and hypertension.

Psychologic precursors of coronary heart disease have been reported in numerous studies.[101,102] Prospective studies[112] have shown a relationship between indices of dissatisfaction with life and manifestations of coronary heart disease. Such indices include family problems, dissatisfaction with work, conflicts in finance and family, and interpersonal difficulties with co-workers. Positive associations have also been noted between sleep disturbances and coronary heart disease, implying some involvement of the central nervous system in the causation of this disorder.[102]

The question of life stress has also attracted attention among workers in this field. A prospective study of middle-aged Swedish construction workers with use of standardized measures of life stress[113] found no association between elevated life stress scores and the incidence of myocardial infarction over a short period of observation.[114] Comparisons of life stress scores of men in East Finland, where excess coronary heart disease has been observed, with those of men in West Finland suggest higher life-change scores among the eastern group.[115]

In recent years, patterns of coronary disease-prone behavior have been described by Friedman and Rosenman, whose pioneering studies related behavioral characteristics to the development of coronary heart disease. Subsequently, Jenkins[101,102] provided support for the Friedman-Rosenman hypotheses.[103] He suggested that persons who are more prone to the development of coronary artery disease have a characteristic action-emotion complex exemplified by excessive aggression, hurry, and competitiveness. Friedman[103] defined this behavior pattern as a characteristic action-emotion complex that is exhibited by persons who are engaged in a relatively *long-term struggle* to obtain an *unlimited* number of *poorly defined* things from their environment in the *shortest time* and, if necessary, against the opposing efforts of other persons in the same environment. Such an individual is classified as type A (in contrast to type B persons, who, although interested in achievement, in most instances are relaxed, unhurried, and more easily satisfied with their pace). A review[102] of 24 studies dealing with type A behavior listed 22 of these studies showing positive associations with coronary heart disease. In the Western Collaborative Group Study,[116] the relative risk for men 50 to 59 years old was twofold compared with men classified as type B. The contribution of type A personality is independent of other risk factors.[117] The strength of association approaches that of other standard risk factors. The type A factor is specific and is unrelated to other medical problems, and in at least two studies a continuous positive gradient between the strength of type A personality and the probability of coronary heart disease has been reported.[118,119]

Behavioral characteristics and other psychosocial states may have biologic plausibility in the genesis of coronary heart disease. Acute and chronic arousal may influence blood pressure, serum free fatty acids, lipids, platelet aggregation, clotting mechanisms, and the sympathetic nervous system, although these changes are transient and the relationship to atherogenesis remains unproved. Type A individuals display larger episodic increases in systolic pressure when confronted with stress and greater increases in heart rate.[120] Studies suggest that distinct neuroendocrine responses to cognitive tasks occur among type A individuals.[121] These include hyperresponsivity to norepinephrine and epinephrine and a greater excretion of cortisol (for those with a family history of hypertension) and testosterone. Animal studies suggest that enhanced neuroendocrine and adrenocortical arousal presumably influences accelerated atherogenesis.[122,123]

The relationship of coronary disease-prone behavior to heart disease has been reviewed by expert panels.[124,125] Evidence suggesting that type A personalities may be measured by a structured-interview technique,[126] the Jenkins activity survey,[127] and the Framingham type A behavior scale[128] is generally accepted. It also appears that adverse behavioral characteristics are associated with increased risk of coronary heart disease in middle-aged Americans. This risk is independent of age, elevated values of systolic blood pressure, serum cholesterol levels, and smoking, and it appears to be of the same order of magnitude as the relative risk and comparison with the three other factors.[11,117,129] Data from the Framingham Study show that the associations of type A behavior with angina and coronary heart disease as seen in men are also evident in women.[129] Newer evidence suggests that it is anger and hostility that are the causes of the increased risk of coronary heart disease associated with type A behavior.[130] The structured-interview technique and the Jenkins activity survey employed in other countries have been found to be predictive of coronary heart disease.[131,132]

PHYSICAL INACTIVITY

When Powell et al.[19] reviewed all the articles in the English language that provided sufficient data to calculate a relative risk or odds ratio for coronary heart disease at different levels of physical activity, they observed a consistent inverse association between physical activity and incidence of coronary heart disease. This association was found to be appropriately sequenced, biologically graded, plausible, and coherent with existing knowledge. The reviewers found that it was the better studies that showed the stronger associations, and the relative risk of inactivity appeared to be similar in magnitude to that of hypertension, hypercholesterolemia, and smoking.

In a 22-year follow-up of 3,686 San Francisco longshoremen,[133] high-energy outputs on the job were associated with a diminished risk of fatal heart attacks and sudden death (the risk of sudden death was three times greater in less active longshoremen). In a study of 17,000 Harvard University male alumni,[134] the levels of energy expenditure predicted risk of heart attacks. On the basis of the Harvard data, the authors postulated a reduction of coronary heart disease rates by 26% among sedentary alumni exposed to high levels of habitual physical activity. In the Harvard cohort, beginning moderately vigorous sports activity, quitting cigarette smoking, maintaining normal blood pressure, and avoiding obesity were sepa-

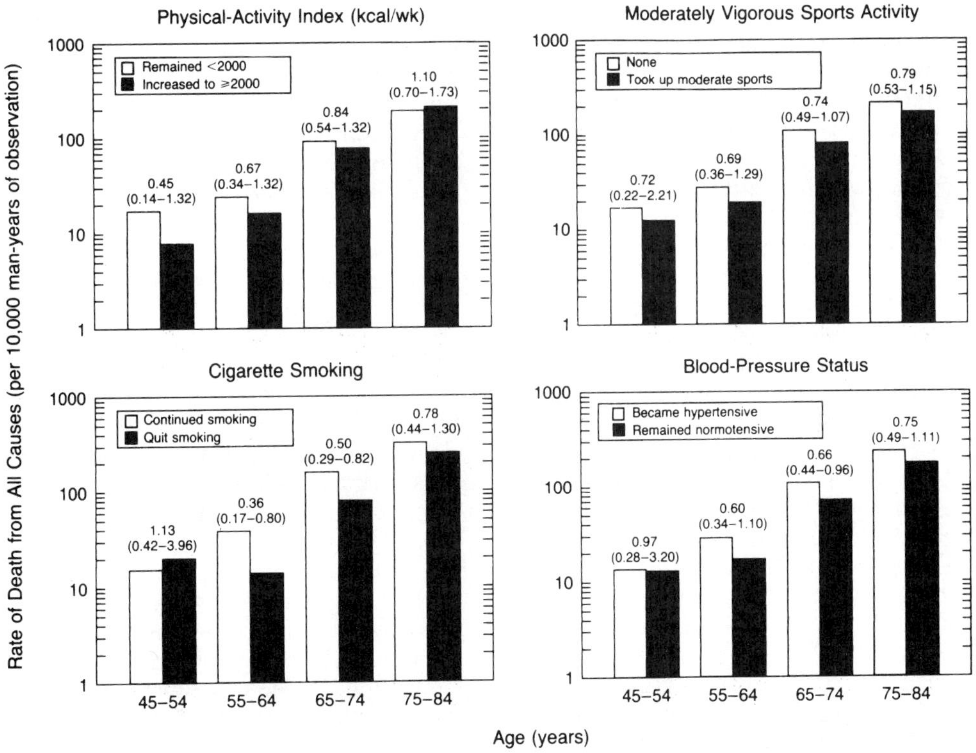

Fig 13-4 Rates and relative risks of death from all causes among 10,269 Harvard alumni, according to age in 1977 and changes in patterns of physical activity and other characteristics between 1962 or 1966 and 1977. Relative risks are expressed in relation to men who did not make the change, as indicated in each panel. The men ranged in age from 45 to 84 years in 1977. The follow-up period, from 1977 through 1985, totaled 90,650 man-years of observation. Relative risks and 95% confidence intervals are shown above the bars. (From Paffenbarger RS Jr, Hyde RT, Wing AL, et al: The association of changes in physical-activity level and other lifestyle characteristics with mortality among men. *N Engl J Med* 328:538-545, 1993. By permission of the journal.)

rately associated with lower rates of death from all causes and from coronary heart disease in middle-aged and older men[135] (Fig 13-4). Sixteen-year follow-up of 1,960 healthy Norwegian men 40 to 59 years of age demonstrated that after adjustment for age, smoking status, serum lipids, blood pressure, resting heart rate, vital capacity, body mass index, level of physical activity, and glucose tolerance, physical fitness was a graded independent predictor of mortality from cardiovascular causes.[136] In addition, the men in the highest fitness quartile experienced lower mortality from any cause. In contrast to these observations, long-term prospective studies in Finland have failed to reveal differences in coronary heart disease mortality or sudden death between men performing work of low or moderate levels of energy output and lumberjacks whose calorie expenditures were much greater.[137] In the Seven Countries Study, Finnish populations showed high rates of coronary heart disease despite high levels of physical activity. However, the high cholesterol content of the Finnish diet needs to be carefully considered in evaluating these findings.

The Harvard alumni data[134] suggest that cardiovascular fitness is increased by expending up to 2,000 kcal per week in vigorous exercise (which would involve running or walking 20 miles per week). If these assumptions of strenuous physical activity were to be tested prospectively, a valid study would require 10,000 marathoners followed for 10 years (with an equal number of controls) to test cardioprotection at a 90% probability level of observing a relative risk different from unity.[138] Reports of coronary heart disease immunity in small groups of marathon runners are therefore premature.[139] Indeed, progressive coronary heart disease has been reported in highly trained marathon runners.[140-144] One interesting insight concerning the risks of jogging comes from calculations of mortality rates among joggers in Rhode Island. In this study, the adjusted death rate among joggers was 1/7,622 joggers per year; even though the risk appears to be small, the mortality among Rhode Island joggers during jogging is seven times the estimated death rate for the more sedentary populations of the state.[145]

Cardiovascular adaptation to exercise may have beneficial effects on health. Several studies report exercise-induced increases in maximal rate of oxygen uptake per minute (Vo_2 max), maximal cardiac output, systemic arterial-venous oxygen differences, increased oxygen extraction by working muscles, lower heart rates during rest, submaximal exercise, and increases in the diastolic phase of coronary flow. Numerous reports suggest that active athletes at all ages have higher stroke volumes, maximum cardiac outputs, and heart volumes than sedentary persons.[146] Exercise-induced increases in cardiac output are primarily a result of increased left ventricular volume.[147]

Augmentation of coronary flow after exercise has not yet been demonstrated in man, although decreases in myocardial infarction seem to occur during training.[148] Exercise results in a negative chronotropism at rest or with submaximal workload in trained persons;[149,150] an increased parasympathetic activity has been implicated in the causation of resting bradycardia.[151]

Exercise also reduces the levels of other risk factors.[20,152-155] Initial studies suggested that pre-β VLDL are most affected by exercise; temporary reductions of triglyceride concentrations return to preexercise levels within a few days. In contrast, total serum cholesterol levels may not be substantially altered in physically conditioned persons.[152,156] Studies suggest that changes in total cholesterol, LDL cholesterol, or triglycerides are not demonstrable with habitual physical activity, but significant increases in HDL cholesterol may occur more consistently.[157-162]

Improved myocardial perfusion over prolonged periods of cardiac activity (with or without increased collateral coronary blood flow) has been demonstrated both in man and in animals.[150,163,164] These relationships in man may not be causal, for it is quite possible that persons with larger coronary arteries tend to become athletes. Recent studies of the effects of exercise in monkeys have shown a general increase in luminal diameter in the coronary arteries of the exercising group. The effects of habitual training on the intrinsic caliber of coronary vessels and on coronary collateralization have more recently been studied in patients with coronary heart disease.[165-168] Serial arteriography in patients with angina pectoris or myocardial infarction who undergo supervised exercise programs has not shown consistent improvement of collaterals.[166-168]

An epidemiologic study of the benefits and risks of running concluded that more than one-third of the respondents who were engaged in regular aerobic exercise suffered musculoskeletal injuries during that span.[20] These injuries were more likely in those who ran longer distances and were severe enough to curtail activity; they were not associated with age, speed, or years of running. Serious hazards of running include dog bites, collisions with vehicles, and injuries from lethal objects thrown at unsuspecting runners. Although sudden death can occur even in the presence of widely patent coronary arteries,[169] pathologic evidence of the cause of sudden death in a number of conditioned joggers has been reported to indicate severe occlusion of the coronary vasculature.[170] Other authors have argued that an enhanced risk of sudden death during or immediately after physical activity, although biologically plausible, is more likely in those with underlying coronary vessel disease, whereas those with no disease of this kind are protected against the risks of sudden death.[171]

About 40% of the United States population is estimated to be predominantly sedentary.[172,173] Therefore, a major change in the epidemiology of coronary heart disease might accrue if this portion of the population could be convinced to walk for 30 minutes three to five times per week.

Without randomized trials, the causal risk of physical inactivity for the subsequent development of coronary heart disease must remain in doubt. However, there are other clear benefits to physical activity, and physical activity programs are integral to the management of obesity, hypertension secondary to obesity, dietary change, and smoking cessation.

OTHER RISK FACTORS

In addition to age and sex, hyperlipidemia, hypertension, cigarette smoking, and psychosocial risks, a number of other risk factors have been implicated in the causation of coronary heart disease. Arcus cornea,[174] diagonal earlobe creases,[175] water softness,[176] mesomorphy,[177] and baldness and early graying[178] have not been confirmed in careful long-term follow-up of large populations. Excessive coffee consumption was not found to be a risk factor for atherosclerotic cardiovascular disease in the Framingham study.[179] The relationship of soft water to mortality from cardiovascular disease[180] requires confirmation.

Low dehydroepiandrosterone (DHEA) levels were found to predict the development of coronary heart disease in a population of men,[181] and DHEA levels were inversely correlated with atherosclerosis and its extent in men in a coronary angiography study.[182] Studies suggest that a low-calorie diet and exercise raise DHEA levels,[183,184] and DHEA has been given to humans.[185] However, efficacy and safety data are not yet available.

Hyperhomocystinuria has been reported to be a risk factor for both coronary artery disease and cerebrovascular disease.[186-188] Because the studies are case-control analyses of individuals with and without disease, however, it is impossible to determine whether the condition is a cause or a consequence of disease. More work will have to be done to define the clinical importance of hyperhomocystinuria.

In case-control studies, deletion polymorphism in the gene for the angiotensin-converting enzyme has been found to be a risk factor for myocardial infarction.[189] Individuals with low body mass index or low apo B who had suffered from myocardial infarction were particularly likely to have the abnormal genotype.

FIRST-GENERATION INTERVENTION TRIALS

Evidence of an etiologic role of risk factors in coronary heart disease is provided by intervention trials. A brief description of the first-generation intervention trials is of historical importance because the results are often cited in support of arguments in favor of dietary modification. Cornfield and Mitchell[190] have summarized the statistical inadequacies of earlier dietary intervention trials.

First-generation dietary intervention trials have focused on attempts to modify the natural history of coronary heart disease by dietary intervention. The New

York Anti-Coronary Club Study[191] and the National Diet-Heart Study[192] suggested that a prudent low-cholesterol and low-fat diet (a ratio of polyunsaturated to saturated fats of 1.25) was acceptable to free-living volunteer populations and effectively lowered total serum cholesterol. The Finnish Mental Hospital Study,[193] employing a crossover design with two periods of 6 years each, reported that a diet low in saturated fats and high in polyunsaturated fats reduced total serum cholesterol levels and caused a decline in coronary heart disease mortality in institutionalized men and women in two mental hospitals in Helsinki, Finland. However, the design of this study and the analysis of its results have been criticized.[194] A similar trial carried out in a Minnesota mental hospital suggested that with a diet low in saturated fats and cholesterol and high in polyunsaturated fats, rates of coronary events were lower in men under 40 years of age, but differences were not seen in groups for older men and women.[195]

Dietary trials at the Veterans Administration domiciliary facility in Los Angeles[196] used double blinding with randomized control groups. An experimental diet low in saturated fats and cholesterol and high in polyunsaturated fats reduced coronary events, although the total death rates in the two experimental groups were the same. This trial has been criticized because of an excessive age at entry (average age, 65.6 years) and mixed intervention among subjects with and without coronary artery disease. Two secondary intervention trials from Oslo have demonstrated reduction in coronary heart disease incidence by means of a diet low in cholesterol and high in polyunsaturated fats.[197]

An adequate trial of the effect of diet on the heart would require at least 60,000 participants followed over a decade of closely standardized study in a controlled population.[192] The costs of such an undertaking make such a trial unlikely in the foreseeable future. The Lipid Research Clinic Study has provided important insights into the magnitude of these problems, which have not been generally appreciated in the planning of such large intervention trials. Protagonists of dietary intervention[198] point to the widespread changes in lifestyle since 1970, which may have led to decreasing mortality from cardiovascular diseases in the United States. Although most observers agree that no single risk factor is the sole cause of coronary heart disease and that multiple causal factors play interrelated roles in the incidence of this disorder, the rationale of dietary recommendations for prevention of coronary heart disease continues to be supported by groups such as the American Heart Association.

The American Heart Association's diet-heart statement is supported by several lines of argument.[199] Vegetarians in a Boston commune whose diet is principally whole grains, beans, and fresh vegetables[200]—a diet totally devoid of cholesterol and animal fat—have total cholesterol and LDL cholesterol values 31% and 38%, respectively, lower than those of age-matched Framingham controls. These findings support the contention that serum lipid levels are influenced by dietary factors.

SECOND-GENERATION INTERVENTION TRIALS

In the 1970s, several major intervention trials explored the health benefits of risk reduction in various populations. Because of differences in entry criteria (age, sex, comorbidity, risk stratification), methodologic rigor, approaches to randomization, and extent of intervention (single or multiple risk-factor intervention), the mortality outcomes described in this chapter are not comparable. Thus, higher mortality rates for trials such as the Multiple Risk Factor Intervention Trial[75] are related to inclusion of high-risk individuals.

Multiple risk-factor intervention trials

Two multiple risk-factor intervention trials can be cited to support the hypothesis that risk reduction in patients with high risk of coronary heart disease is beneficial. The Oslo Study Group[73] randomized 1,232 healthy normotensive men at high risk of coronary heart disease into an intervention group and a control group. (This trial should not be confused with the Oslo Study[201] of mild hypertension.) Men were admitted to the trial if their serum cholesterol level was 290 to 380 mg/dL, coronary risk score (based on cholesterol levels, smoking habits, and blood pressure) was in the upper quartile of the distribution, and systolic blood pressure was less than 150 mm Hg (mean of two measurements). The mean serum cholesterol concentrations were 13% lower and the mean tobacco consumption per man decreased by 45% more in the intervention group. At the end of the observation period, the incidence of myocardial infarction (fatal or nonfatal) and sudden death was 47% lower in the intervention group than in controls. Statistical analysis suggested that reduction of the incidence in the intervention group correlated with the reduction of total cholesterol maximally and to a lesser extent with smoking reduction.

The results of the Multiple Risk Factor Intervention Trial[75] (MRFIT) also support the conclusions of the Oslo Study Group. This trial randomly assigned men to either a special intervention program or the usual sources of health care in the community. In 12,866 high-risk men ages 35 to 57 years (who were followed for 7 years), risk factor levels declined in both groups but to a greater extent for the men in the special intervention group. Although no significant differences in coronary heart disease mortality were initially noted in the two study groups, subgroup data for men who were free of hypertension at baseline suggested that systematic management of hyperlipidemia with diet and reduction of smoking resulted in favorable reduction of coronary heart disease mortality. In this trial, a subset of hypertensive persons with ECG abnormalities had higher mortality rates. However, after medication in the participants was changed from hydrochlorothiazide to chlorthalidone at a daily maximum dose of 50 mg, the death rates for hypertensive men in the special intervention group were significantly lower than the death rates for hypertensive men in the usual care group.[202]

Lipid intervention trials

The Lipid Research Clinics Coronary Primary Prevention Trial (LRC-CPPT)[203] has far-reaching therapeutic implications. In this double-blind, randomized study,[203] 3,806 middle-aged males with type II hypercholesterolemia (plasma cholesterol >265 mg/dL, LDL cholesterol >175 mg/dL, triglycerides <300 mg/dL) were selectively screened from 480,000 age-eligible men and randomized to treatment with cholestyramine plus diet or with diet alone for a mean duration of 7.4 years. At 7 years the life table cumulative incidence of definite coronary heart disease death or definite nonfatal myocardial infarction, or both, was 8.6% in the diet group and 7.0% in the cholestyramine plus diet group. Thus, a 19% reduction in the occurrence of the primary end point ($P < 0.05$) was achieved with cholestyramine treatment. The all-cause mortality was reduced only 7%. The "beneficial" result of cholestyramine treatment correlated best with a differential 9.6% LDL cholesterol reduction and was not significantly correlated with the 3% differential increase in HDL cholesterol. In the actively treated group, decreases of total serum cholesterol (8%) and LDL cholesterol (12%) were accompanied by a 19% decrease in coronary heart disease death or nonfatal myocardial infarction. Thus, the death rates for coronary heart disease decreased from 2% to 1.6%, and rates of nonfatal myocardial infarction decreased from 8.3% to 6.8% during the brief period of observation.

The findings are in contrast to those of the National Heart, Lung, and Blood Institute (NHLBI) type II coronary intervention study,[204] in which the beneficial effect (a reduction of angiographically assessed disease progression) with cholestyramine treatment was correlated to a greater degree with increases of HDL cholesterol than with decreases of LDL cholesterol. Whether the differences were due to differences in the susceptibility of the two groups to cholestyramine or to differences in treatment compliance remains to be determined.

In the Helsinki Heart Study, 4,081 asymptomatic men with primary dyslipidemia were randomized to receive 600 mg of gemfibrozil or a placebo two times a day for 5 years.[205] In the treatment group, mean total serum cholesterol declined from 269.9 to 246.9 mg/dL, mean LDL declined from 189.2 to 173.5 mg/dL, and mean HDL increased from 47.1 to 51.2 mg/dL. There were few changes in serum lipid values among the men in the control group. Over the 5 years of observation, the cumulative rate of cardiac events was 27.3 per 1,000 in the treatment group and 41.4 per 1,000 in the placebo group ($P < 0.02$). The decline in incidence became evident in the second year of the study and persisted throughout the study. Neither the total number of deaths, 45 (21.9/1,000) in the treatment group and 42 (20.7/1,000) in the control group, nor cancer incidence rates were significantly different between the two groups.

A recent secondary prevention trial with simvastatin demonstrated, over the 5.4-year median follow-up period, a relative risk of death of 0.70 (95% confidence interval, 0.58 to 0.85; $P = 0.0003$) in the simvastatin group.[206] Relative risk of a coronary death was 0.58 (95% confidence interval, 0.46 to 0.73) in the simvastatin group. Women and patients of both sexes aged 60 years or older experienced a similar benefit from treatment. There was a 37% reduction ($P < 0.00001$) in the risk of undergoing myocardial revascularization procedures. In a primary prevention trial that enrolled subjects with asymptomatic intimal-medial thickening of the carotid arteries, subjects receiving lovastatin had a significantly lower risk of a major cardiovascular event ($P = 0.04$) or death ($P = 0.02$).[207]

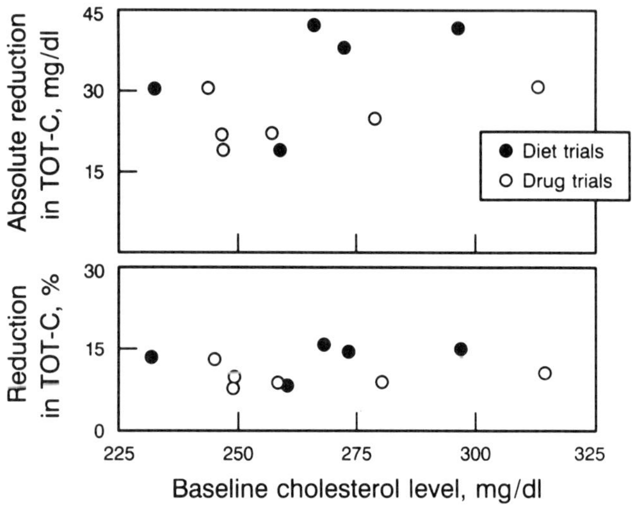

Fig 13-5 In six drug trials and five diet trials, four of the five diet trials had greater lowering of serum cholesterol levels than all of the drug trials. *TOT-C,* total serum cholesterol. (From Tyroler HA: Review of lipid-lowering clinical trials in relation to observational epidemiologic studies. *Circulation* 76:515-522, 1987. By permission of American Heart Association.)

Tyroler[208] reviewed the lipid-lowering clinical trials in relation to observational epidemiologic studies. In comparing the findings of five diet trials and six drug trials, he found that four of the five diet trials resulted in a greater absolute reduction and percentage reduction in total serum cholesterol concentration than all six drug trials (Fig 13-5). He also found that the risk functions were similar for the intervention trials and epidemiologic studies and that the percentage reduction observed with the trials was the same as that predicted from the population experience. These observations imply that when patients lower their lipid profiles to a new level, they acquire the risk characteristics of the new level. The experience from the Scandinavian Simvastatin Survival Study[206] and the Asymptomatic Carotid Artery Progression Study [207] suggests that the lowering takes from 1 to 2 years to become effective.

Antithrombosis trials

Dalen[209] reported that the first clinical trial to prevent coronary heart disease was begun in 1948 by a Glendale, Calif., general practitioner. Since that time, multiple randomized trials have demonstrated the efficacy of

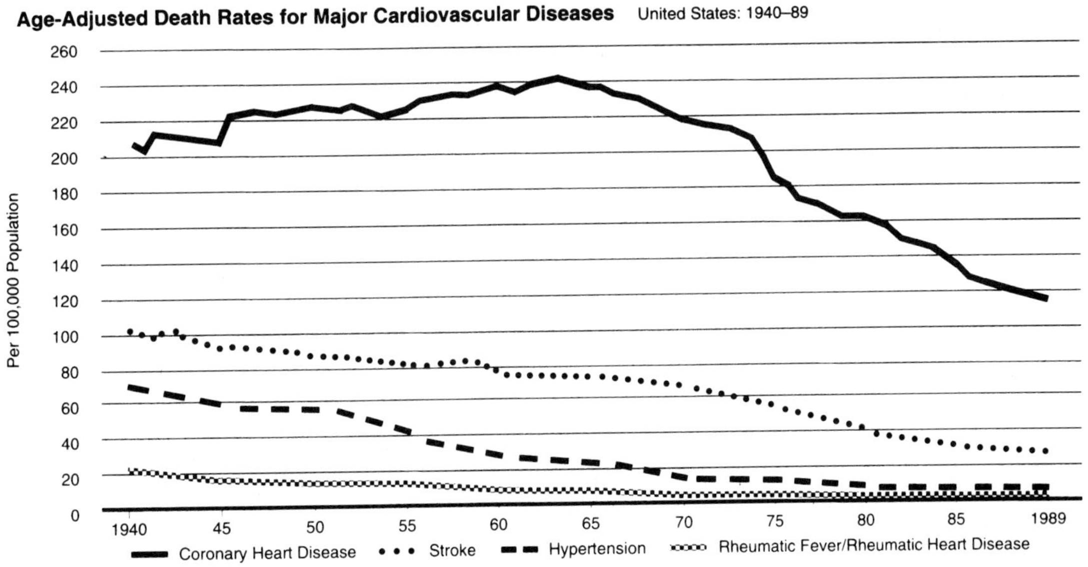

Fig 13-6 Age-adjusted death rates for coronary heart disease, stroke, hypertension, and rheumatic fever/rheumatic heart disease from 1940 to 1989 in the United States. Between 1963 and 1989, age-adjusted death rates from coronary heart disease declined by more than 50%. (From 1993 Heart and Stroke Facts Statistics, American Heart Association. By permission.)

aspirin in preventing complications after acute myocardial infarction,[210] unstable angina,[211] coronary artery bypass grafting,[212] and percutaneous coronary angioplasty.[213] Although aspirin reduced first myocardial infarction in a randomized trial,[214] the hemorrhagic complications offset the benefit of the reduced myocardial infarction rate. Because of the observed hemorrhagic complications, the British Medical Research Council is conducting a study of a low dose of aspirin (75 mg/day) or a low dose of warfarin (titrated to produce an international normalized ratio of 1.5), or both, in men in the top 20% of the risk distribution.[215] For the time being and if there are no contraindications, it is recommended that aspirin be given at a dose of 325 mg/day to all persons with coronary artery disease[216] and at a dose of 1 g/day to all persons with a history of transient ischemic attacks or stroke.[217]

CHANGE IN RISK FACTORS AND DECLINING CORONARY HEART DISEASE RATES

Dramatic declines in cardiovascular mortality have occurred in the United States and elsewhere[218-221] (Fig 13-6). Since 1978, the mortality from coronary heart disease has decreased by more than 40% (in contrast to the trends of earlier years when mortality from this major chronic disease was steadily increasing). Age-adjusted death rates for atherosclerotic heart disease (including coronary heart disease) increased from 185.2 per 100,000 in 1950 to 220.3 per 100,000 in 1963. Between 1950 and 1957, age-adjusted deaths from atherosclerotic heart disease increased by 14%; during 1968 to 1976, a dramatic decline of 27% was recorded. These changes were noted for all sex and race categories. In the 1970s and 1980s, further declines in all major causes of cardiovascular death, including coronary heart disease, were noted.

Although the precise causes underlying the decline in coronary heart disease are uncertain, some conjectures are reasonable. Improved control of hypertension, reduction of cigarette smoking in adult males, increased physical activity, and changes in lipid consumption may underlie these salutary trends.[219,222-224] There is evidence that medical therapeutic regimens may also have altered the course of coronary heart disease.[225-227]

It is also possible that the numerous innovations in the care of patients with acute coronary heart disease after 1973 may be reflected in these vital statistics.[70] The influence of such innovations on coronary heart disease mortality may have played a major role between 1969 and 1973, when new modalities for the prevention and treatment of ventricular fibrillation and other fatal cardiac arrhythmias became available. Evidence from studies in the Boston area suggests that improvement in in-hospital care of patients with acute myocardial infarction is not a major explanation for the nationwide mortality trends between 1973 and 1978.[228] Declines in coronary heart disease mortality experienced in the United States have also been seen in other countries.[229]

CLINICAL APPROACHES TO RISK REDUCTION

Physicians and others in the health care professions frequently assume that patient behavior is primarily motivated by attempts to avoid disease.[230-232] They try to induce behavior change by stressing the risk of disease and the hazards of the patient's behavior. Because strong negative messages can generate hostility and denial and

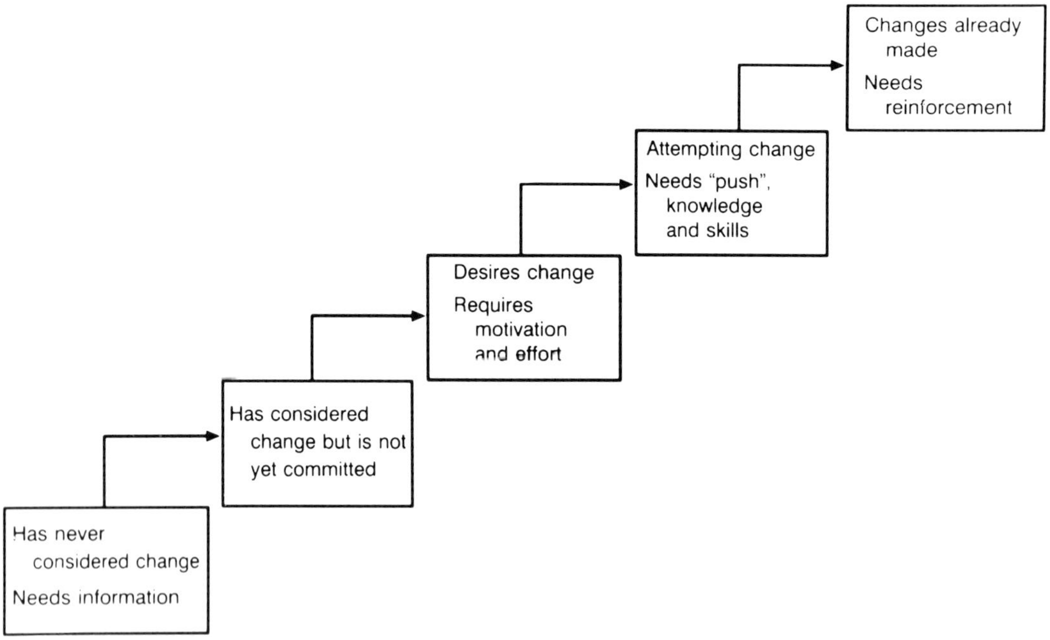

Fig 13-7 Continuum of readiness to change risk factor behaviors. Rather than trying to move patients from one end of the scale to the other in a single session, the physician should set a goal of moving each patient one step closer to ideal risk factor behaviors. This is more feasible than making large changes in behaviors and will be less frustrating to both the physician and the patient. Small changes among all patients will prevent more heart disease than large changes among a small group of patients. (From Kottke TE: Risk factor control in coronary heart disease: Who needs it? *Postgrad Med* 78:233-245, 1985. By permission of McGraw-Hill.)

rarely lead to long-term behavior change, physicians using these techniques find that counseling to change behavior is frustrating and unrewarding.

Research in behavioral medicine has provided a better explanation of patient behavior and suggests a model for patient-physician interaction: all individuals have conflicting needs, and current needs for food, shelter, or social integration can take precedence over considerations of future health.[233] Therefore, patient behavior can appear irrational from the point of maximizing health but explainable from the perspective that the patient is trying to satisfy current needs,[234,235] frequently those defined by the patient's peer group.[236] Rather than emphasize the *health risks of the old behavior,* the physician should emphasize the *social benefits of the new behavior.* The most effective behavior change interventions exhibit consonance and relevance with the patient's goals, are individualized to the patient's needs, provide feedback and reinforcement for the patient, facilitate the patient's behavior change, and use multiple methods of intervention.[237]

As an example, most adult smokers acknowledge that smoking is a health hazard, although they continue to smoke. They learned to smoke from their friends as teenagers and now feel unable to quit smoking. They may use smoking to cope with daily stressors but also find that smoking is triggered by situations that are not perceived as stressful. Most patients will freely acknowledge that their behavior is irrational. Most have also tried to quit many times, but because each relapse has made them feel inadequate, they are not happy about the prospects of trying once again to quit and may be unwilling to try.

Rather than try to induce immediate cessation by a patient who is not yet ready to quit, the physician should set a goal of convincing the patient to consider making a change[238] (Fig 13-7). Likewise, patients at other stages of change can be "nudged" along the continuum one step at a time. Three of the most important skills that a clinician can possess are knowing how to determine where the patient is on the continuum of change, how far the patient is willing to change at present, and how to take "No!" for an answer. Even if the patient is unwilling to make any changes at a given visit, it is important for the physician to give the patient positive reinforcement for any changes made in the past. Without this reinforcement, the patient cannot be expected to maintain newly adopted healthful behaviors.[239] In addition to increasing the patient's resolve to maintain the healthful behaviors, positive reinforcement makes counseling a positive event for both the patient and the physician and increases the likelihood of future change on the part of the patient.

The origins of behavior modification lie in the experimental work of Skinner[239] and are based on social learning theories.[240] The clinical application of this science as a management tool implies a contractual

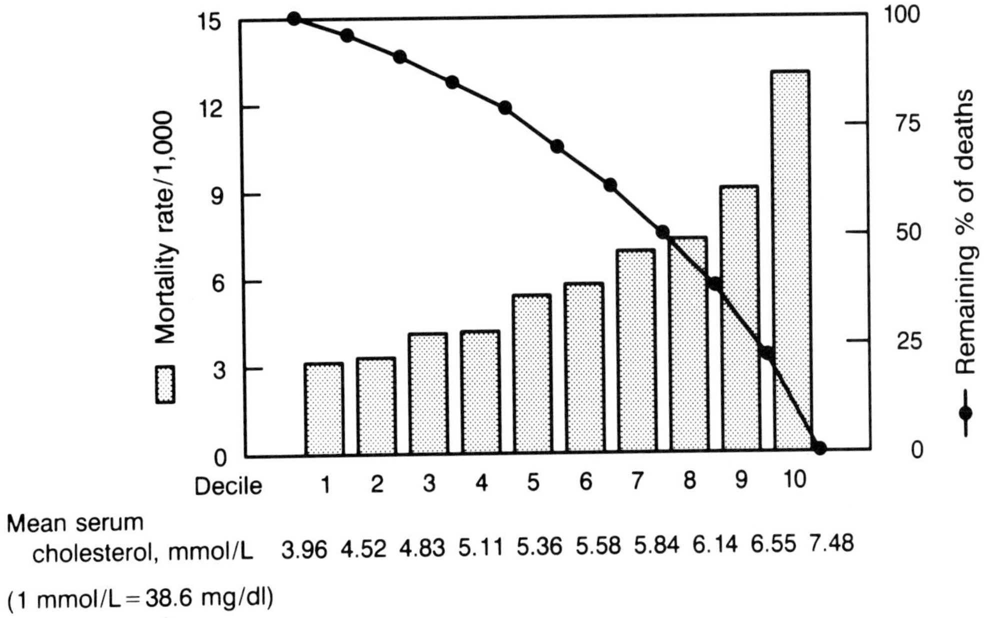

Fig 13-8 Deciles of serum cholesterol values and 6-year coronary heart disease mortality for 356,222 men screened for the Multiple Risk Factor Intervention Trial. The men in deciles 2 through 10 are at above basal risk for death from coronary heart disease. More than 25% of deaths occurred in the lower five deciles of the population, and approximately 50% of the deaths occurred among the men in the lower seven deciles. (Data from Stamler J, Wentworth D, Neaton JD: Is relationship between serum cholesterol and risk of premature death from coronary heart disease continuous and graded? Findings in 356,222 primary screenees of the Multiple Risk Factor Intervention Trial (MRFIT). *JAMA* 256:2823-2828, 1986.)

relationship between the patient and the physician that is the starting point of behavior modification. The essential approaches involve a number of steps:

1. Goal setting. A clear, well-defined goal needs to be developed as a measurable end point for assessing any change in behavior. Often failure occurs because goals are excessively high.
2. Self-monitoring. This requires that the individual maintain a record of his or her behaviors, particularly those that either facilitate or negate successful implementation of goal-seeking strategies.
3. Surveillance. This implies frequent and structured physician supervision for appropriate reinforcement, modification of therapy, tailoring of therapies, and continued support. Such consultations are often problem centered; they are focused more on the individual's needs than on the physician's perceptions of therapy and are modified according to individual perceptions of progress or side effects.
4. Social support and positive reinforcement. These are invariably very important ingredients for the achievement of success. Such reinforcement can often be arranged to involve peer group appreciation, spouse support, and, most important of all, physician reinforcement of positive outcomes. Many intelligent and educated patients will develop token reward systems that serve to reinforce positive behavior.

MANAGEMENT OF RISK FACTORS*

Diet and hyperlipidemia

The National Cholesterol Education Program (NCEP) has outlined the rationale for combining the population and high-risk approaches to the management of elevated blood cholesterol levels.[240] The rationale is based on observations like those from the MRFIT. A 6-year follow-up of more than 350,000 men screened for the MRFIT trial demonstrates that risk of death from coronary heart disease rises progressively from the first to the tenth deciles of total serum cholesterol[241] (Fig 13-8). This means that at least 90% of the population have serum cholesterol levels that place them above basal risk. The data also show that deaths from coronary heart disease are spread widely across the risk gradient. For example, the half of the population at lowest risk of death from coronary heart disease still contributes more than a quarter of all deaths, and only half of the deaths arise from the top 30% of the population. These data are interpreted to mean that all patients should be given advice to consume a low-fat diet unless there is a good reason to believe that the patient would suffer.

Most patients now have a high level of awareness about the implications of serum cholesterol and a diet high in

*Please see chapter 60B for a discussion of the management of hypertension.

Table 13-6 Dietary guidelines for achieving optimal lipid levels*

Emphasize	Rationale
Appropriately combined foods of plant origin: beans, cereal grains, vegetables (cooked and raw), fruits	Good-quality protein; low in fat, saturated fat, and cholesterol; low in sodium; low in refined sugar; complex carbohydrates; high in minerals, vitamins, and fiber; lower calorie intake
Fish, poultry, and lean meats used in small portions and eaten less often as main dish	Good-quality protein; low in fat, saturated fat, and cholesterol; lower calorie intake
Low-fat dairy products for adults	Good-quality protein; high in minerals; low in fat, saturated fat, and cholesterol; lower calorie intake
Fewer oils and fats used in food preparation and as spreads, with preference for liquid vegetable oils	
Deemphasize	**Rationale**
High-fat meats from domestic breeds as principal protein source	High in saturated fat and cholesterol; high calorie intake
High-fat dairy products (whole milk, cream, cheese)	High in saturated fat and cholesterol; high calorie intake
Whole eggs, unless used as a major source of protein	Egg yolks high in cholesterol
Commercially baked products	High in saturated fat; high calorie intake
Alcoholic beverages	High calorie intake; low in nutrients

*Established by the World Health Organization.
From Kottke TE: Risk factor control in coronary heart disease: who needs it? *Postgrad Med* 78:233-245, 1985. By permission of McGraw-Hill.

Table 13-7 Cholesterol and fat content of animal products in three-ounce portions (cooked)

Source	Cholesterol content, mg/3 oz	Total fat content, g/3 oz
Red meats (lean)		
Beef	77	8.7
Lamb	78	8.8
Pork	79	11.1
Veal	128	4.7
Organ meats		
Liver	270	4.0
Pancreas (sweetbreads)	400	2.8
Kidney	329	2.9
Brains	1,746	10.7
Heart	164	4.8
Poultry		
Chicken (without skin)		
Light	72	3.8
Dark	79	8.2
Turkey (without skin)		
Light	59	1.3
Dark	72	6.1
Fish		
Salmon	74	9.3
Tuna, light, canned in water	55	0.7
Shellfish		
Abalone	90	0.8
Clams	57	1.7
Crab meat		
Alaskan king	45	1.3
Blue crab	85	1.5
Lobster	61	0.5
Oysters	93	4.2
Scallops	35	0.8
Shrimp	166	0.9

From The Expert Panel: Report of the National Cholesterol Education Program Expert Panel on Detection, Evaluation, and Treatment of High Blood Cholesterol in Adults. *Arch Intern Med* 148:36-69, 1988.

fat;[242] what they lack is a sense of personal salience. Identification of high-fat items in the diet can be accomplished quite easily by asking the patient to recall the foods that he or she usually consumes throughout the day, starting with breakfast. In addition to the traditional three meals, the physician must ask about midmorning, midafternoon, and evening snacks. One must be alert for ambiguous terms like "a good meal," "a light meal," or "an average diet." When these are encountered, they should be further explored for more concrete meaning. Obtaining this brief history increases the sense of salience for the patient, and it is probably not terribly important in the clinical setting to verify eating patterns unless the patient is genuinely concerned that he or she may unknowingly be eating some high-fat foods. If the patient habitually consumes a diet either high in fat or low in fat and accurately reports consumption, the physician will be able to suggest changes in the high-fat foods and indicate approval of the low-fat foods. Even if the patient lies, the fact that the physician shows interest in the patient's diet will tend to reinforce the importance of dietary habits for the patient.

The authors favor the strategy of encouraging one eating style over another rather than the strategy of carefully trying to estimate the fat in the diet. The physician should encourage the patient to emphasize fruits, vegetables, whole grains, skim milk dairy products, and lean meats and to avoid sausages, lunch meats, bacon, eggs, cheese, breaded foods that are fried, bakery prod-

Table 13-8 Recommended diet modifications to lower blood cholesterol

	The step-one diet	
	Choose	**Decrease**
Fish, chicken, turkey and lean meats	Fish, poultry without skin, lean cuts of beef, lamb, pork, or veal, shellfish	Fatty cuts of beef, lamb, pork; spare ribs, organ meats, regular cold cuts, sausage, hot dogs, bacon, sardines, roe
Skim and low-fat milk, cheese, yogurt and dairy substitutes	Skim or 1% fat milk (liquid, powdered, evaporated), buttermilk	Whole milk (4% fat): regular, evaporated, condensed; cream, half and half, 2% milk, imitation milk products, most non-dairy creamers, whipped toppings
	Nonfat (0% fat) or low-fat yogurt	Whole-milk yogurt
	Low-fat cottage cheese (1% or 2% fat)	Whole-milk cottage cheese (4% fat)
	Low-fat cheeses, farmer or pot cheeses (all of these should be labeled no more than 2 to 6 g of fat per ounce)	All natural cheeses (e.g., blue, Roquefort, Camembert, cheddar, Swiss), low-fat or "light" cream cheese, low-fat or "light" sour cream, cream cheeses, sour cream
	Sherbet, sorbet	Ice cream
Eggs	Egg whites (2 whites equal 1 whole egg in recipes), cholesterol-free egg substitutes	Egg yolks
Fruits and vegetables	Fresh, frozen, canned, or dried fruits and vegetables	Vegetables prepared in butter, cream, or other sauces
Breads and cereals	Homemade baked goods using unsaturated oils sparingly, angel food cake, low-fat crackers, low-fat cookies	Commercial baked goods: pies, cakes, doughnuts, croissants, pastries, muffins, biscuits, high-fat crackers, high-fat cookies
	Rice, pasta	Egg noodles
	Whole-grain breads and cereals (oatmeal, whole wheat, rye, bran, multigrain, etc.)	Breads in which eggs are a major ingredient
Fats and oils	Baking cocoa	Chocolate
	Unsaturated vegetable oils: corn, olive, rapeseed (canola oil), safflower, sesame, soybean, sunflower	Butter, coconut oil, palm oil, palm kernel oil, lard, bacon fat
	Margarine or shortenings made from one of the unsaturated oils listed above, diet margarine	...
	Mayonnaise, salad dressings made with unsaturated oils listed above, low-fat dressings	Dressings made with egg yolk
	Seeds and nuts	Coconut

From The Expert Panel: Report of the National Cholesterol Education Program Expert Panel on Detection, Evaluation, and Treatment of High Blood Cholesterol in Adults. *Arch Intern Med* 148:36-69, 1988.

ucts other than bread, ice cream, and snacks that are high in fat (Table 13-6). The leanness of the particular cut of meat and whether fat is used in the preparation of the meat can be more important than whether the source of the meat is poultry, fish, beef, pork, or lamb (Table 13-7). As is true with meats, the fats used in preparation and presentation are an important determinant of the fat content of nonmeat foods (Table 13-8). The NCEP flow chart for initial assessment is pictured in Figure 13-9.

Almost all patients have made at least some changes in their diets; mean serum cholesterol levels have declined significantly in the United States.[243] The physician should be sure to congratulate the patient for any positive dietary changes. This not only reinforces the behavior of the patient but also reinforces the physician's impression that patients actually do change their eating habits. All patients who are hospitalized for known or suspected coronary heart disease should be seen by a dietitian for an initial prescription or a "booster" session, whichever is appropriate. All patients being seen for initial evaluation of diet or hyperlipidemia as outpatients should also be seen in consultation by a dietitian.

The NCEP has outlined an approach to the management of hyperlipidemia in clinical practice.[244] If the patient's blood cholesterol level is in the "desirable" range (<200 mg/dL) and the HDL value is ≥35 mg/dL, the patient should be instructed in diet (Fig 13-10). The patient who has a "borderline-high" blood cholesterol value (200 to 239 mg/dL), no history of coronary heart disease, and no other risk factors (Table 13-9) should be provided with the dietary intervention described above and be seen in 1 year for a remeasurement of serum cholesterol and reinforcement of a low-fat diet. The patient who has a borderline-high blood cholesterol level,

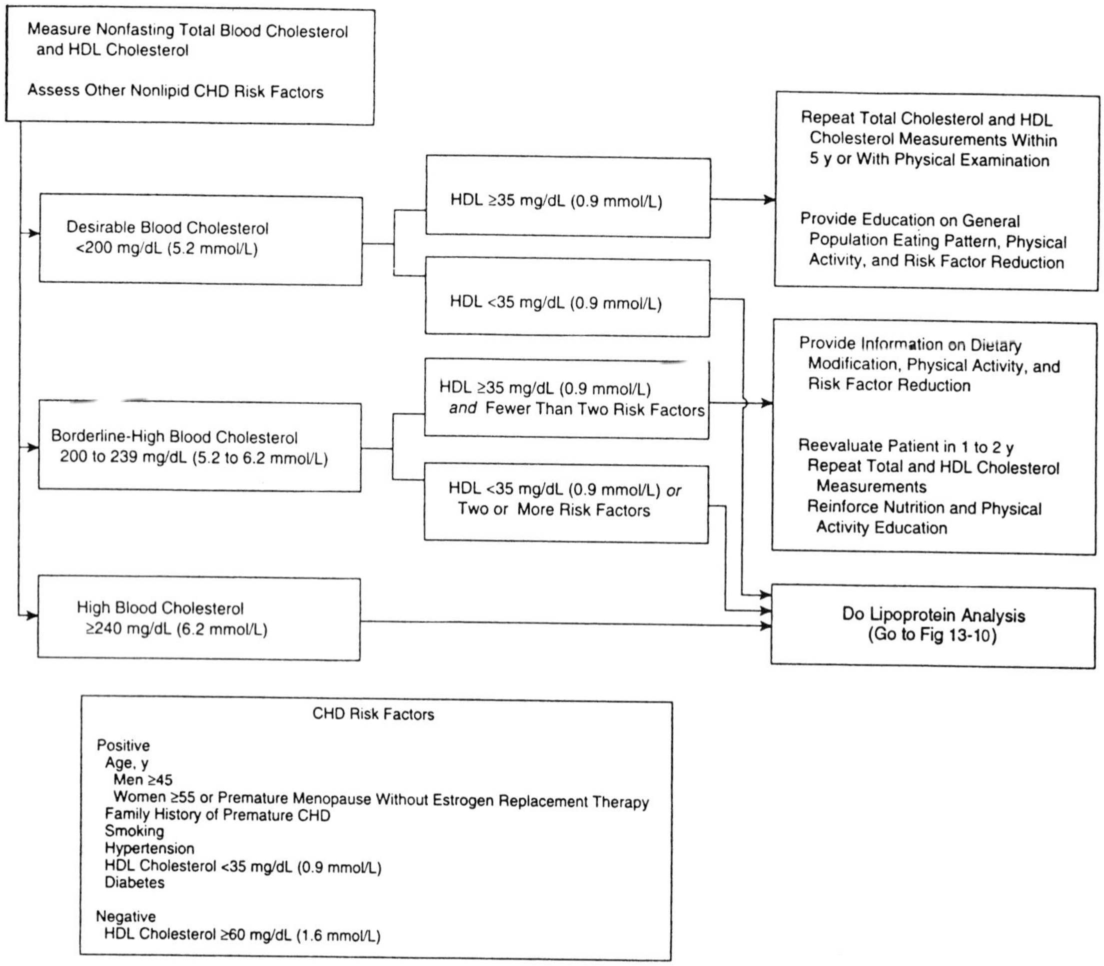

Fig 13-9 Primary prevention in adults without evidence of coronary heart disease *(CHD)*. Initial classification is based on total cholesterol and high-density lipoprotein *(HDL)* cholesterol levels. (From Expert Panel on Detection, Evaluation, and Treatment of High Blood Cholesterol in Adults: Summary of the Second Report of the National Cholesterol Education Program [NCEP] Expert Panel on Detection, Evaluation, and Treatment of High Blood Cholesterol in Adults [Adult Treatment Panel II]. *JAMA* 269:3015-3023, 1993.)

a low HDL (< 35 mg/dL), or two other risk factors and the patient who has a "high" (≥ 240 mg/dL) blood cholesterol value should have a lipoprotein analysis.

The patient without coronary disease who has a serum LDL cholesterol level of < 130 mg/dL should be provided with the dietary intervention described above and should have a measurement of total serum cholesterol repeated within 5 years (see Fig 13-9). The patient who has an LDL cholesterol level between 130 and 159 mg/dL and fewer than two other risk factors should be advised about the intervention described above and have annual reevaluation of diet and lipids. Both the patient with an LDL cholesterol level between 130 and 159 mg/dL who has two other risk factors and the patient with an LDL ≥ 160 mg/dL should be evaluated for secondary causes, familial disorders, and other coronary heart disease risk factors. The goal LDL cholesterol level suggested by the NCEP is < 160 mg/dL if the patient has no history of coronary heart disease and fewer than two risk factors; otherwise, the suggested goal is < 130 mg/dL for the patient without coronary heart disease. The LDL goal for the patient with coronary heart disease is ≤ 100 mg/dL (Table 13-10).

If the goal LDL cholesterol level is achieved at the end of 6 months, long-term monitoring is indicated. If the goal LDL cholesterol level is not achieved, the physician should consider secondary causes of hyperlipidemia (Table 13-11). If there are no secondary causes, the LDL cholesterol level is < 190 mg/dL, and the patient has no history of coronary heart disease and does not have two other risk factors, the NCEP suggests nonpharmacologic approaches, perhaps also with low doses of bile acid sequestrants. It is the authors' preference to add psyllium, oat bran, or long-acting niacin instead of bile acid sequestrants at this point.

Drug therapy for hyperlipidemia

If the patient without coronary heart disease has an LDL cholesterol level ≥ 190 mg/dL or two risk factors and an

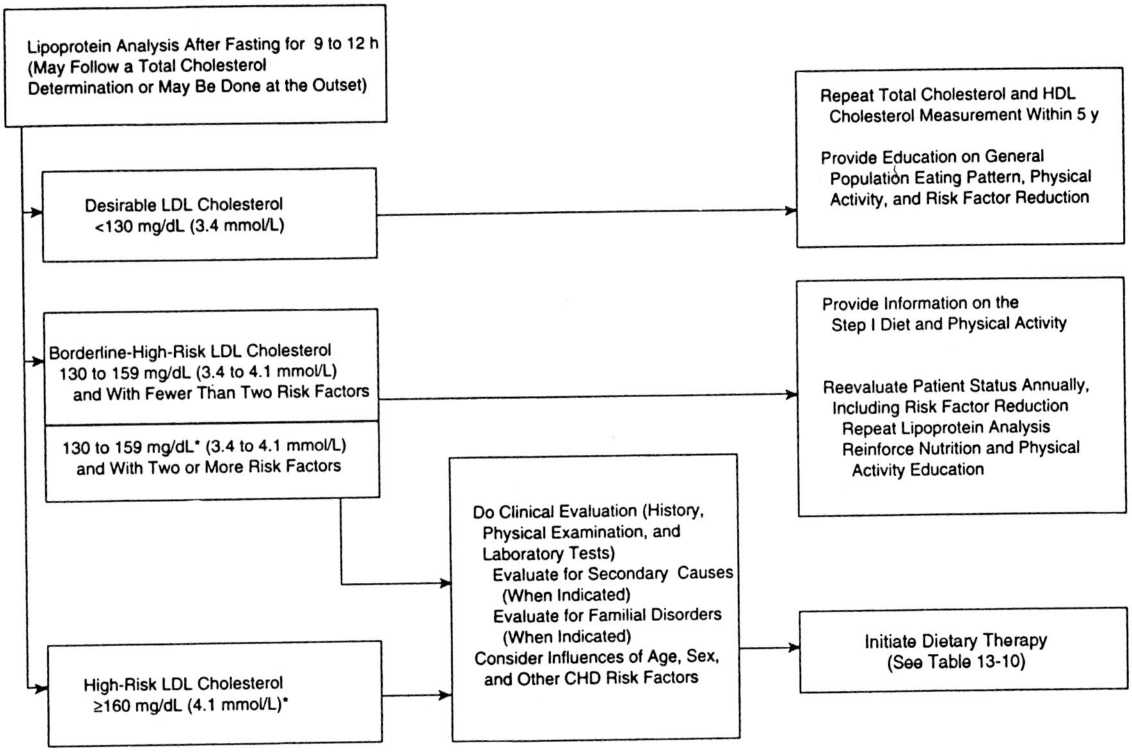

Fig 13-10 Primary prevention in adults without evidence of coronary heart disease *(CHD)*. Subsequent classification is based on low-density lipoprotein *(LDL)* cholesterol level. (From Expert Panel on Detection, Evaluation, and Treatment of High Blood Cholesterol in Adults: Summary of the Second Report of the National Cholesterol Education Program [NCEP] Expert Panel on Detection, Evaluation, and Treatment of High Blood Cholesterol in Adults [Adult Treatment Panel II]. *JAMA* 269:3015-3023, 1993.)

LDL cholesterol level ≥160 mg/dL, drug therapy is suggested. If the patient has coronary heart disease, drug treatment is indicated for an LDL level of > 100 mg/dL or an HDL level of < 35 mg/dL, or both (Fig 13-11). The lipid panel should be measured every 6 weeks for the first 6 months or until the patient's lipid profile is under control. The drugs currently available for the treatment of hyperlipidemia and their dosages, therapeutic effects, costs, and side-effects are listed in Table 13-12.

The bile acid sequestrants currently available include cholestyramine and cholestipol. *Cholestyramine* is dispensed in packets or scoops containing 4 g of an active drug. The usual dosage ranges from 16 to 32 g daily taken with fluids in divided doses. *Cholestipol* is dispensed in 5-g packets. The usual dosage ranges from 15 to 30 g daily in divided doses. These agents are not absorbed. The major side effects are constipation and difficulty in ingesting the agents because of their bulk. Usually, constipation is a problem at the lower dosages and decreases as the dosage is increased. It can be controlled with psyllium. Occasionally, cholestyramine can increase plasma triglyceride levels. This can be controlled with the addition of small doses of triglyceride-lowering agents, e.g., nicotinic acid or gemfibrozil.

The use of nicotinic acid as a cholesterol-lowering agent was first reported by Parsons et al.[245] in 1956. Its mechanism of action is not known. It does not alter bile acid or neutral sterol excretion in patients. The usual dosage for the treatment of hypercholesterolemia ranges from 1.5 to 4 g/day in divided doses. Side effects include cutaneous flushing (which occurs in nearly all patients), gastric irritation, hepatic toxicity (rarely leading to the development of jaundice), and alteration of glucose tolerance. Most patients develop tolerance to the cutaneous flushing up to 1 to 2 weeks after the initiation of therapy or an increase in the therapeutic dose. In addition, the flushing can be greatly reduced by using time-release preparations or the concurrent administration of small doses of aspirin.[246] The starting dose should be 500 mg three times a day or less with meals. Gastric irritation is usually not a major problem and can almost always be avoided by having susceptible patients take their medications with antacids. All patients who are using this agent should have measurements of aspartate aminotransferase (AST) at regular intervals. If the levels of these enzymes become elevated, the dosage should be reduced; often, after a period of reduced dosage, the dosage can be slowly increased to levels below those resulting in hepatic toxicity. With careful attention to detail, the occurrence of jaundice as a complication of this agent is extremely rare. Although glucose intolerance occurs, it rarely leads to hyperglycemia that requires the use of insulin or hypoglycemic agents.

An important benefit of nicotinic acid is its effect in

Table 13-9 Risk status based on presence of coronary heart disease (CHD) risk factors other than low-density lipoprotein cholesterol*

Positive risk factors

Age, years
- Male ≥45
- Female ≥55 or premature menopause without estrogen replacement therapy

Family history of premature CHD (definite myocardial infarction or sudden death before 55 years of age in father or other male first-degree relative or before 65 years of age in mother or other female first-degree relative)

Current cigarette smoking

Hypertension (blood pressure ≥140/90 mm Hg† or taking antihypertensive medication)

Low HDL cholesterol (<35 mg/dL† [0.9 mmol/L])

Diabetes mellitus

Negative risk factor‡

High HDL cholesterol (≥60 mg/dL [1.6 mmol/L])

*High risk, defined as a net of two or more CHD risk factors, leads to more vigorous intervention, shown in Figures 13-9 and 13-10. Age (defined differently for men and women) is treated as a risk factor because rates of CHD are higher in the elderly than in the young and in men than in women of the same age. Obesity is not listed as a risk factor because it operates through other risk factors that are included (hypertension, hyperlipidemia, decreased high-density lipoprotein [HDL] cholesterol, and diabetes mellitus), but it should be considered a target for intervention. Physical inactivity is similarly not listed as a risk factor, but it too should be considered a target for intervention, and physical activity is recommended as desirable for everyone. High risk due to coronary or peripheral atherosclerosis is addressed directly in Figure 13-11.
†Confirmed by measurements on several occasions.
‡If the HDL cholesterol level is ≥60 mg/dL (1.6 mmol/L), subtract one risk factor (because high HDL cholesterol levels decrease CHD risk).
From Expert Panel on Detection, Evaluation, and Treatment of High Blood Cholesterol in Adults: Summary of the Second Report of the National Cholesterol Education Program (NCEP) Expert Panel on Detection, Evaluation, and Treatment of High Blood Cholesterol in Adults (Adult Treatment Panel II). *JAMA* 269:3015-3023, 1993.

raising the levels of HDL cholesterol.[245] It is also relatively inexpensive.

Gemfibrozil has been shown to decrease coronary mortality.[205] Gemfibrozil can be used as first-line therapy in patients with diabetes and concomitant high triglyceride and low HDL levels. Dosage is 600 mg twice a day. It is useful with niacin or resins but should be used with 3-hydroxy-3-methylglutaryl coenzyme A (HMG CoA) reductase inhibitors only with caution. The most common side effect is gastrointestinal intolerance, and myalgia is a rare effect. Gemfibrozil has also been associated with increased lithogenicity.

The mechanism of action of *probucol*[247] has not been established. It has been suggested that it may act by preventing oxidation of LDL particles and by changing the kinetics of the HDL transport system.[248] Trials in which the outcome is survival in humans are now under way. These trials have the potential of greatly increasing our understanding of lipid metabolism and the prevention of atherosclerosis.

The most common side effect is gastrointestinal irritation, especially diarrhea. In monkeys and dogs, serious arrhythmias developed when the drug was used under certain experimental conditions. However, no arrhythmias

Table 13-10 Treatment decisions based on low-density lipoprotein (LDL) cholesterol level

	Initiation level		LDL goal	
Patient category	**mg/dL**	**mmol/L**	**mg/dL**	**mmol/L**
Dietary therapy				
Without CHD and with fewer than two risk factors	≥160	4.1	<160	4.1
Without CHD and with two or more risk factors	≥130	3.4	<130	3.4
With CHD	>100	2.6	≤100	2.6
Drug treatment				
Without CHD and with fewer than two risk factors	≥190	4.9	<160	4.1
Without CHD and with two or more risk factors	≥160	4.1	<130	3.4
With CHD	≥130	3.4	≤100	2.6

CHD, coronary heart disease.
From Expert Panel on Detection, Evaluation, and Treatment of High Blood Cholesterol in Adults: Summary of the Second Report of the National Cholesterol Education Program (NCEP) Expert Panel on Detection, Evaluation, and Treatment of High Blood Cholesterol in Adults (Adult Treatment Panel II). *JAMA* 269:3015-3023, 1993.

Table 13-11 Causes of secondary hyperlipidemia

Hypertriglyceridemia	Hypercholesterolemia
Excessive alcohol or simple sugars	Excessive dietary cholesterol or saturated fats (or both)
Contraceptives, estrogen, pregnancy	Hypothyroidism
Obesity	Obstructive liver disease
Diabetes mellitus	Nephrotic syndrome
Chronic renal failure	Multiple myeloma or dysglobulinemia
Cushing's disease, corticosteroid therapy	Progestational agents and anabolic steroids

From Lavie CJ, Gau GT, Squires RW, et al: Management of lipids in primary and secondary prevention of cardiovascular diseases. *Mayo Clin Proc* 63:605-621, 1988. By permission, Mayo Foundation for Medical Education and Research.

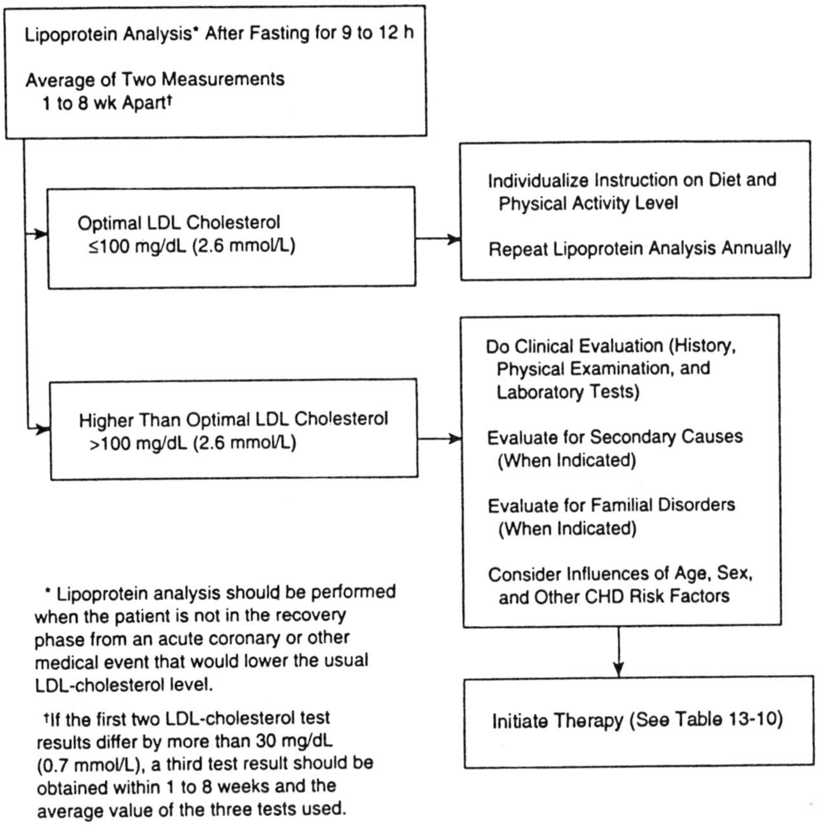

Fig 13-11 Secondary prevention in adults with evidence of coronary heart disease *(CHD).* Classification is based on low-density lipoprotein *(LDL)* cholesterol level. (From Expert Panel on Detection, Evaluation, and Treatment of High Blood Cholesterol in Adults: Summary of the Second Report of the National Cholesterol Education Program [NCEP] Expert Panel on Detection, Evaluation, and Treatment of High Blood Cholesterol in Adults [Adult Treatment Panel II]. *JAMA* 269:3015-3023, 1993.)

in humans have ever been related to the use of this drug.[249] Because of results of the animal studies, use of the drug should be discontinued if prolongation of the Q-T interval develops, and the agent probably should not be used in patients with multifocal or paired extrasystoles.

HMG CoA reductase inhibitors (lovastatin, simvastatin, pravastatin, fluvastatin), alone or in combination with nicotinic acid or bile acid sequestrants, can markedly reduce serum cholesterol levels.[250-252] These agents inhibit the rate-determining step in synthesis of cholesterol and increase LDL receptors. They are well-tolerated, and efficacy in reducing mortality has been demonstrated.[206,207] The drugs are not recommended for women of childbearing age and, because of the risk of myositis and rhabdomyolysis, should be used carefully in patients receiving cyclosporine.[253] They should be used only with care in patients who are receiving gemfibrozil. It is unclear whether differences in hydrophobicity and bioavailability among these agents are clinically important.

Recently, a meta-analysis was performed of all randomized trials of more than 2 years' duration (35 trials) to describe how coronary heart disease, non-coronary-heart-disease, and total mortality are related to cholesterol lowering and to type of intervention.[254] The authors concluded that for every 10 percentage points of cholesterol lowering, coronary heart disease mortality was reduced by 13% ($P < 0.002$) and total mortality by 10% ($P < 0.03$). Fibrates increased non-coronary-heart-disease mortality by about 30% ($P < 0.01$) and total mortality by about 17% ($P < 0.02$). No specific effects due to diet, resins, niacin, statins, or partial ileal bypass independent of cholesterol lowering were found.

Other treatments of hyperlipidemia

In surgical therapy, ileal bypass was first proposed for the treatment of hypercholesterolemia in 1964.[255] After 5 years, overall mortality and mortality due to coronary heart disease were reduced by 20% and 30%, respectively, in the Program on the Surgical Control of the Hyperlipidemias (POSCH).[256] Although these two differences are not significant, the 36% lower overall mortality in the surgery subgroup with an ejection fraction ≥50% is significant ($P = 0.021$). Two patients died of complications of the surgery, and in 5 years of follow-up, 13.5% of surgery-group patients had symptoms of bowel obstruction, and 3.6% required surgery for this problem. Surgical patients averaged more than three bowel movements a day (compared with an average of fewer than 1.5 per day in the control group). The incidence rate of kidney stones in the surgery group was 4% per year (compared with 0.7% in the control group), and 4 control-group and 14

Table 13-12 Drug therapy for lipid disorders*

Drug	Daily dose, g	Cholesterol	Effect on triglycerides	HDL-C	Approximate cost/yr†	Adverse effect
Cholestyramine	12-24	Decrease	No change or increase	No change or increase	$625-1,250	Taste, bloating, nausea, gout, constipation, diarrhea
Colestipol	15-30	Decrease	No change or increase	No change or increase	630-1,260	Same as above
Nicotinic acid (niacin)	1.5-6	Decrease	Decrease	Increase	50-200	Pruritus, flushing, GI distress, glucose intolerance, gout, skin rash, dizziness, liver dysfunction, atrial arrhythmias
Gemfibrozil	600-1,200 mg	Decrease	Decrease	Increase	285-570	Myositis, possibly cholelithiasis, GI distress
Clofibrate	1-2	Decrease	Decrease	No change or increase	258-516	Cholelithiasis, myositis, possible increase in GI malignant lesions
Probucol	500-1,000 mg	Decrease	No change	Decrease	308-616	Diarrhea, prolonged Q-T interval, GI distress
Eicosapentaenoic acid (fish oils)	1-8	Increase, no change, or decrease	Decrease	No change or increase	308-2,460	Weight gain, immune dysfunction
HMG CoA enzyme inhibitors	5-80 mg	Decrease	No change or decrease	No change or increase	520-2,080	Liver function abnormalities, myositis

*GI, gastrointestinal; HDL-C, high-density lipoprotein cholesterol.
†Based on the mean cost from five local pharmacies.
From Lavie CJ, Gau GT, Squires RW, et al: Management of lipids in primary and secondary prevention of cardiovascular diseases. *Mayo Clin Proc* 63:605-621, 1988. By permission, Mayo Foundation for Medical Education and Research.

surgery-group patients underwent cholecystectomy during the first 5 years of follow-up. Although the changes in lipid values are similar to those seen with cholestyramine,[257] compliance after surgery is not a problem. Even so, the clinical role of this procedure has yet to be defined.

Currently, plasmapheresis (3,500 to 4,000 mL) every 2 weeks is the treatment of choice for homozygous familial hypercholesterolemia.[258] Plasma cholesterol levels can be lowered to near normal by this procedure, although they increase significantly during the 2 weeks between procedures. The removed plasma is replaced with human serum albumin or some other plasma protein preparation. This is an extremely expensive form of therapy because of the cost of the replacement protein. To try to lower the cost substantially, we and others have attempted to remove LDL from the patient's plasma by affinity chromatography and thus permit replacement of the patient's own plasma minus the LDL. Such an approach could have the added benefit of maintaining the patient's HDL levels. To date, however, no satisfactory system has been established, although there is a theoretic basis for this approach and with future studies it should become feasible.[259]

Omega-3 fatty acids are polyunsaturated fats that can lower serum triglyceride levels. Their effect on LDL cholesterol and HDL cholesterol is quite variable. In some persons, omega-3 fatty acids may cause increased bleeding time and thrombocytopenia. They may worsen glycemic control in diabetic patients.

Postmenopausal estrogen replacement has been shown to reduce the risk of coronary artery disease for women.[260] Most of this reduction can be attributed to lipoprotein changes, particularly an increase of 10% to 15% in HDL levels.[261] Although estrogen therapy has been shown to increase deaths from coronary heart disease in men,[262] estrogen has been used in the treatment of primary hypercholesterolemia, with a 22% reduction in LDL cholesterol.[263] In postmenopausal women, estrogen replacement, even in combination with medroxyprogesterone, should be considered in the treatment of hypercholesterolemia if there is no contraindication for estrogen use. A potential adverse lipoprotein effect of estrogen is an increase in triglycerides. This adverse effect does not seem to occur with the use of transdermal estrogen.

Modification of type A behavior

The possibility of modifying behavior characteristics associated with coronary heart disease has attracted attention. It is not known whether the results of such efforts reduce the risk of coronary heart disease. Most physicians tend to assume that reduction of stressful environments or improvement of coping responses to inevitable stress may be beneficial for their patients. Evidence to support these contentions is not yet available, and they require much further study.

Changing behavior is in itself a difficult mission and is often poorly understood by physicians. The research techniques that have been employed in small studies have included training in the management of anxiety and visual-motor rehearsal[264] and comprehensive treatment programs such as group psychotherapy, relaxation training, and environmental management.[265] One randomized trial of intervention on type A behavior after myocardial infarction has been successful.[266]

It is important to emphasize that the goal of therapy is to reduce the intensity of an adverse behavioral pattern without compromising the efficiency and productivity of an individual. One starting point is to assess the environmental stressors in a patient's schedule and to recommend possible modifications in stressful environments. Failing such modifications—these circumstances are often not amenable to change—altering an individual's perceptions of the environmental stresses so as to reduce arousal may be useful. Embarking on behavioral change also implies self-observation by type A individuals who are often unaware of their behavior. Such observation might involve the use of a log of incidences that arouse anger, anxiety, frustration, and a sense of time urgency. Effective new habits can often be established, as is true of other behavior modification techniques, by self-contracting strategies that are conducive to a more relaxed lifestyle. Simple changes in lifestyle, including walking at a more relaxed pace, slower driving, providing ample time for completion of work, and using relaxing practices such as muscle relaxation exercises, brisk walking, or programs of regular physical activity, may be useful adjuncts in a continuing commitment to changing adverse daily behavior patterns. Muscular relaxation in particular can be helpful. In certain instances, progressive relaxation can be facilitated by biofeedback.

Association of low blood cholesterol with mortality

A 1990 National Institutes of Health conference explored the association between very low serum cholesterol values and mortality in 19 cohort studies from the United States, Europe, Japan, and Israel.[267] For men, the relation between total serum cholesterol concentration and total mortality was U-shaped. For women, the relation was flat. For both men and women, there was a positive association between death from coronary heart disease and levels of serum cholesterol and an inverse correlation between serum cholesterol values and some cancers. Risk for combined noncardiovascular, noncancer deaths decreased steadily with increasing serum cholesterol values. These associations persisted after exclusion of deaths occurring in the first 5 years of follow-up. Although some have suggested that these findings require the entire rethinking of diet and cholesterol policy,[268] it must be kept in mind that total mortality was increased only for the group with serum cholesterol levels of less than 160 mg/dL. Less than 10% of the United States population has levels this low, and it is expected that very few of the remaining individuals could lower their serum cholesterol levels to this extent with diet alone. More research needs to be directed toward understanding these very interesting associations.

Clinical methods in smoking cessation

Smoking is typical of a lifestyle that a patient must change if physical health is to be optimized.

- Most smokers continue to smoke even while acknowledging that smoking threatens their health.
- Smoking is learned as a social behavior; the addictive effects of nicotine that later become a problem for the veteran smoker who wishes to quit do not affect the novice taking up the habit.
- Eighty-five percent of current smokers have tried to quit or would like to quit smoking, yet 90% will fail on any single cessation attempt.
- Many of the smokers who report that they would like to quit also report that they are afraid of even trying.

Analysis of 39 controlled trials of smoking interventions revealed that successful interventions are based on four properties: multiple intervention modalities, both physicians and nonphysicians working with the patient, multiple contacts with the patient, and contact with the patient over the longest possible period to avoid relapse.[269] Therefore, no single intervention is clearly better for all patients than all others. The task of sorting patient complaints of high acuity into those that represent problems of high severity or low severity tends to distract the physician from attending to the treatment of conditions like smoking that represent future but not acute risk of severe disease. Therefore, an office-based smoking intervention program within a supporting framework allows the physician to maintain appropriate attention to the important task of offering smoking cessation advice and assistance to the patient.[270]

The office-based smoking intervention program. The effective office-based smoking intervention program has five basic elements (Table 13-13). Just as it is irrelevant to ask "Which is most important, muscles, valves, coronary circulation, or conduction system?" it is irrelevant to ask which component of the system is most important.[271] Rather, the question that must be asked is "What is the

Table 13-13 The basic elements of an effective office smoking cessation intervention

1. Screening and labeling
   Routinely identifies at least all adult patients as to use or nonuse of tobacco
   Labels charts for user or nonuser status
   Rescreens users at each office visit for current usage
2. Physician reminders
   Reminds physicians at each visit of user status and current usage
   Reminds physicians of previous tobacco-related encounter attitudes and plans
3. Physician message
   Physician gives message during each visit that is brief, clear, supportive, and specific (negotiates specific plans, assistance, and follow-up)
4. Assistance
   Makes available self-help guides, education, and counseling to those who want or need them
5. Follow-up
   Gives supportive communication (revisit, telephone call, or mail) near a promised quitting date and after quitting
   Reviews previous plans at all visits

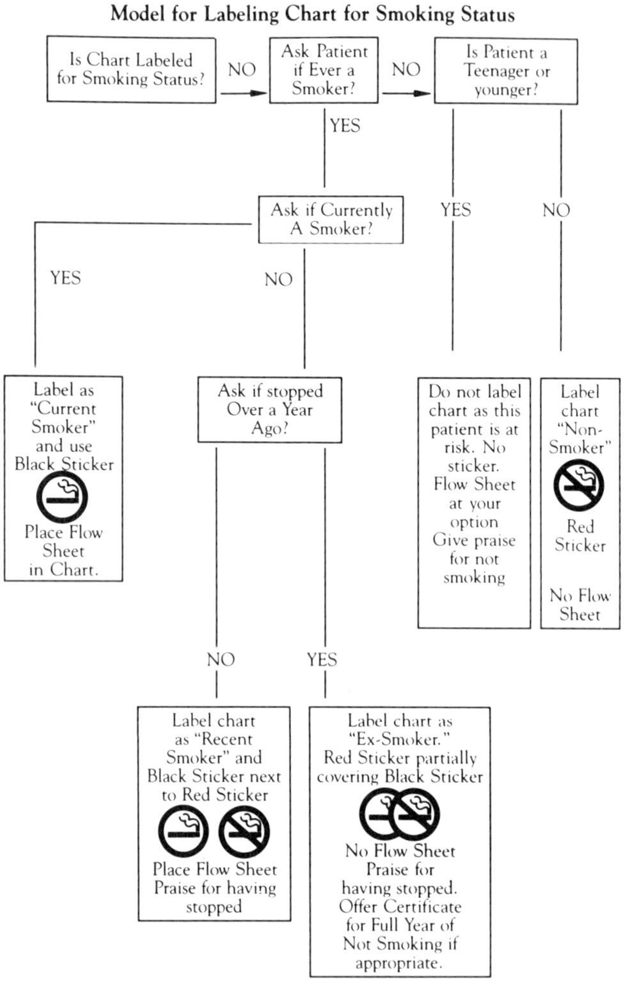

Fig 13-12 Labeling the chart at the time the blood pressure is measured allows the physician to rapidly determine whether the patient has ever been a smoker. If the patient is a current smoker, the physician asks what he or she would like to do about smoking. If the patient is an exsmoker, the physician gives positive verbal reinforcement. (From *AAFP Stop Smoking Program. Physician and Office Staff Manual.* Kansas City, Missouri, American Academy of Family Physicians, 1987. By permission.)

best way to implement each of the components to create a system?" The program can be implemented after 1 to 2 months of planning and a month of pretesting on a limited scale by a team consisting of a physician, an office nurse, and an administrator. The components of the program are described in the following paragraphs.

SCREENING AND LABELING. The successful office-based smoking intervention program identifies all smokers for the purpose of giving the smokers who want to quit the skills to quit and the support they need while they are trying to quit. Figure 13-12, taken from the *Physician and Office Staff Manual* of the American Academy of Family Physicians,[272] gives one example of how the identification of smokers might take place.

PHYSICIAN REMINDERS. The smoke card (Fig 13-13) is placed on the front of the chart of each smoker at the time of registration. It reminds the physician that the patient smokes and that smoking cessation must be discussed. The smoke card also advises the physician of the patient's user status and current usage. Finally, the smoke card enables the physician to recall previous tobacco-related encounter attitudes and plans and build on these past discussions.

PHYSICIAN MESSAGE. The physician's time commitment to the program can be as little as 10 seconds to a maximum of 3 minutes per smoker: "I see that you're smoking, and I would like you to stop. What would you like to do about it?" The physician does not try to convince the patient to stop smoking. Rather, the physician asks the patient to select the category that most closely fits his or her current attitude about smoking cessation (Table 13-14). If the patient wants extensive help, the physician can ask the nurse to spend a few minutes with the patient to describe the intervention options. The physician who wants to spend more time has the option of spending it with the patient to offer reassurance about the problems associated with quitting. The physician then negotiates specific plans, assistance, and follow-up with the patient (Fig 13-14).

ASSISTANCE. The cessation education plan is a joint contract with the patient, the physician, and the cessation educator. The contents of the plan depend on the patient's interest in quitting smoking and the patient's willingness to pay for the intervention. The physician provides the cue to action, the encouragement to try quitting, and reinforcement for not smoking after the

W	S	H	L	↓	?	N	O
Winner	Stop on own	Stop with help	Later	Decrease	Uncertain	No	Omitted

NAME: ________ (last) ________ (first) ________ (chart #) **PHONE: (H)** ________ **(W)** ________

ADDRESS: ________ **BIRTH YEAR:** ________ **SEX:** ________

SMOKE HISTORY: TYPE: ______; **YRS:** ______; **# QUITS:** ______; **LONGEST:** ______; **LATEST:** ______

#'s OF SMOKERS AT HOME ______ **HEALTH PROBLEMS** ________

DATE	AMT.	WHO	HISTORY	CAT.	PLANS	FOLLOW-UP

Fig 13-13 The smoking record is the pivot point of the clinic-based smoking intervention program. At the first visit, a member of the office staff fills out the demographic information, the date of the visit, the amount smoked at that time, and whom the patient visited. The physician writes a brief history, has the patient categorize himself or herself, and records a brief treatment and follow-up plan. The use of the smoking record decreases the time required for intervention while increasing the effectiveness. (From *AAFP Stop Smoking Program. Physician and Office Staff Manual.* Kansas City, Missouri, American Academy of Family Physicians, 1987. By permission.)

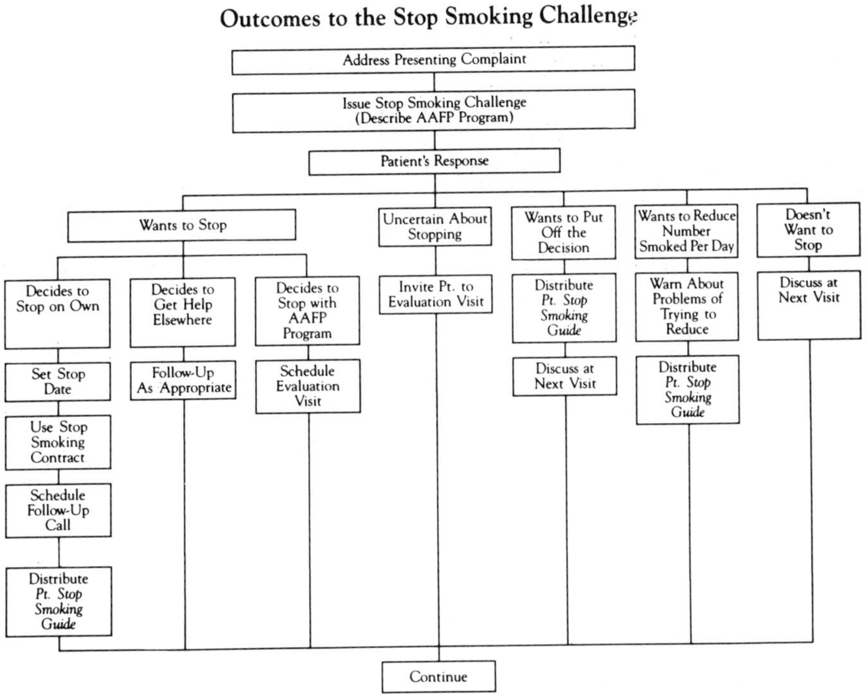

Fig 13-14 After addressing the patient's presenting complaint, the physician asks the patient if he or she is willing to stop smoking. The patient chooses one of the categories, and the physician responds as suggested by the flow chart. The interchange takes less than 3 minutes. (From *AAFP Stop Smoking Program. Physician and Office Staff Manual.* Kansas City, Missouri, American Academy of Family Physicians, 1987. By permission.)

Table 13-14 Self-classification categories for the smoker

Category	Description
W = Winner	A former smoker who is not smoking now
Stop = Stop on own	Agrees to quit but doesn't want help beyond receiving some take-home materials
H = Help with stopping	Agrees to quit and would like some help such as counseling, nicotine gum, a group program
L = Later	Agrees with the need to quit but believes this isn't a good time because of problems like the desire to lose weight first, an acutely stressful situation, or an important event in the near future
T = Taper	Not ready to quit but will try to reduce the amount smoked
? = Uncertain	Either isn't sure it's necessary to quit or isn't sure of sufficient desire to quit
N = No	Patient doesn't want to talk about quitting smoking
O = Omitted	The physician didn't take the opportunity to ask the patient about his or her smoking

Table 13-15 Basic responses to a smoker's fears about smoking

Fear	Response
I've failed before, so I'll probably fail again.	Fewer than 25% of smokers are able to quit on the first try. Most take three or four tries. Stopping smoking is like learning anything new: it takes several tries. Did you learn to ride a bicycle on the first try?
I'll have unbearable cravings.	Most urges last less than 20 minutes. Let's plan what you can do until the urge goes away.
I'll get irritable and frustrated.	Transiently decrease demands on yourself.
I'll have difficulty concentrating.	Quit smoking during your vacation.
I'll get restless.	Take walks or other "time out" periods. Handle objects.
I need the stimulant effect.	Increase activity and begin exercising. Work on getting better sleep (see below).
I'll gain weight.	One-third of exsmokers gain weight, ⅓ lose weight, ⅓ remain at the same weight. Only 10% of those who gain weight keep the increased weight. Let's keep a diet diary while you're quitting. Let's start an exercise program while you're quitting.
I can't sleep.	Use bed only for sleep. Go to bed only when tired. No sleeping during the day. Avoid caffeine at night. If not asleep in 30 minutes, get up. Exercise during the day.

Modified from Hughes JR, Kottke T: Doctors helping smokers: real world tactics. *Minn Med* 69:293-295, 1986.

patient has quit. The trained educator focuses on skills building and reinforcement of smoking cessation attempts.

Self-help guides, education, and counseling are made available to those who want or need them. The physician also offers supportive advice to counter the fears expressed by the patient (Table 13-15). Face-to-face assistance programs are billed to the patient at a rate that reimburses the clinic for its costs. Patients are asked to pay for the service beforehand so that misunderstandings about service fees are eliminated and uncollected fees are kept from becoming a problem.

FOLLOW-UP. Most patients who try to quit smoking will relapse.[273] Therefore, the patient is given supportive telephone calls, visits, or mailings near a promised quitting date and after quitting. Follow-up also includes review of previous cessation plans at all subsequent visits.

The supporting framework for smoking intervention. All successful medical therapy programs exist within a supportive framework. The successful smoking intervention program is no exception. Eight elements are required to support the basic smoking intervention program.

POLICY ESTABLISHMENT. Clinic management clearly and specifically states the goal and time frame of action. It names the individuals with authority to carry out the plan. Because smoking interventions must be systematized like hypertension treatment, endorsement of a smoking intervention program must take place after discussion among the entire medical staff. Staff endorsement can frequently be acquired in a stepwise manner: "We agree that program development should be explored," "We agree that the proposed program should undergo a trial," "We agree that the tested program should be implemented," and so forth. Endorsement clears the way for involvement by administration and the support staff.

The smoking intervention program should include a smoke-free clinic. A smoke-free clinic and hospital are recommended because allowing patients to smoke in health-care facilities reduces their perception of smoking as a threat to their health.[274] Smoking in health-care facilities decreases the effectiveness of interventions and increases practitioner frustration. Smoke-free health-care facilities are feasible. Prestigious institutions like the Mayo Clinic[275] and the Johns Hopkins Medical Center[276] were among the first to become totally smoke-free, and step-by-step instructions have been prepared.[277] A smoke-free plan has become a criterion for certification by the Joint Commission on Accreditation of Health Care Organizations.

STAFF ENDORSEMENT. Although the support staff theoretically takes direction from the clinic physicians, few programs can be successful without the endorsement of the support staff. Because of its responsibility for the day-to-day operation of the program, the support staff usually understands the details of clinic operation more fully than does the physician. Enlisting its advice and help at the time of program development increases the likelihood that the program will both be accepted and fit into clinic routines.

COORDINATION. Both a physician coordinator and a staff coordinator must be identified to implement the policy. Just as each hospital has a physician who coordinates the catheterization laboratory and a physician who coordinates the coronary care unit, the clinic-based smoking intervention program needs a physician who can transmit information back and forth between the staff and other physicians and assure that physicians and staff are oriented and provided with feedback. The physician in charge is also responsible for updating protocols when necessary. Just as each coronary care unit and each catheterization laboratory also has a nurse in charge, the smoking intervention program needs a staff member in charge. The role of this individual is to work closely with the physician in charge and with the administration to see that problems are addressed and that protocols are updated as necessary. In large clinics, a committee or task force is desirable to support the coordinators.

IMPLEMENTATION PLAN. A written plan is devised that identifies how each intervention element is to be performed. This plan includes role definitions, job descriptions, financial impact analyses, scheduling plans, and a timetable for start-up.

ORIENTATION AND TRAINING. All physicians and staff persons affected by the plan are informed of it, given an opportunity to feel involved, and trained in the tasks that will be required of them. A 1-hour orientation program is recommended for the physicians who will be in contact with patients and the program. This allows them to understand and support the goals of the program. It also helps them understand their own roles and tasks. Personnel whose job descriptions include working with the program may benefit from up to 8 hours of orientation. The staff is trained to identify the smoking status of the patient. The staff also is trained to explain the intervention options to the patient after the physician's visit and to provide agreed-on follow-up. The primary requirements for an effective smoking intervention counselor are the willingness to learn from experience and the willingness to work with patients. Many interested nurses find that working with patients to help them stop smoking increases the emotional reward that they receive from their work. They also like the systematized program that clearly defines their role and increases the efficacy of treatment.

RESOURCES. All the materials needed are developed by the clinic or obtained from outside sources and distributed. At a minimum, the program must have self-help materials available. These provide tangible evidence of the physician's commitment to smoking cessation, and they increase the confidence of the physician and staff.[278] *Clearing the Air*[279] is available free of charge from the National Cancer Institute and is an effective intervention tool. Other materials are available from the American Academy of Family Physicians,[280] the American Heart Association, the American Lung Association, and the American Cancer Society. The National Cancer Institute has published an excellent smoking intervention manual for physicians.[281] Referral arrangements for patients requesting group or other special interventions are identified as needed.

AUDIT. Periodic audit assesses the end results and the process for both the overall clinic and the individual physicians and staff members. If the smoke cards are stored in their own box apart from the patients' charts, the success of the program can be evaluated easily and rapidly with movable tabs along the tops of the smoke cards (see Fig 13-13). For example, the results in Figure 13-15 were obtained in about 30 minutes by the nurse coordinator at one clinic. She was able to compare the current status with previous data and found an increase in the proportion of "winners" and a decrease in the proportion of patients who said that they would quit "later." She was also able to document that more than 90% of smokers were asked about their smoking at their last visit.

MAINTENANCE PROGRAM. Without maintenance activities, physicians and staff will lose interest in helping patients stop smoking. Because physicians tend to recall their failures in preventive medicine more strongly than their successes, formal evaluation and feedback are necessary to document program success. The maintenance program features feedback and spirit-building information and events. Feedback may include a poster with the names of the patients who have quit smoking with the program. It can also include periodic posting of audit information in a graph like that in Figure 13-15 to let the staff know how the program is progressing. Repeat orientations and training are needed for both old and new clinic members. The efficacy of this approach for increasing advice to smokers has been documented in a controlled trial.[270]

Prescription of physical activity

Physicians are in a unique position to maximize patient compliance by influencing many of the important determinants of adopting and adhering to an exercise program. Brisk walking should be emphasized for currently inactive patients, because even small differences in physical activity among such persons are associated with a large reduction in risk, and the prescription of brisk walking is more likely to be adhered to than programs requiring more strenuous and intrusive adaptations.[282] An activity like walking still has the characteristics associated with efficacy in disease prevention (weight-bearing, energy expenditure, and contribution to cardiorespiratory fitness) as well as those associated with maximal adoption and adherence (moderate intensity, low perceived exertion, simplicity, convenience, low cost, sociability, etc.) and has minimal risk of adverse effects.[282]

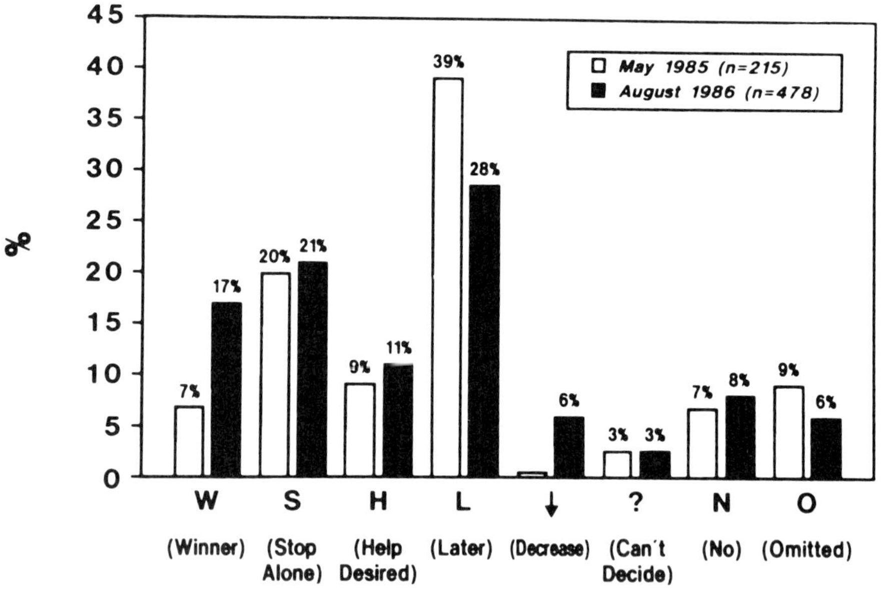

Fig 13-15 Using the smoke charts, the nurse coordinator at the Nokomis Clinic in Minneapolis was able to produce this figure in less than 20 minutes. It summarizes the clinic's experience and tells the staff that 17% of their patients have stopped smoking. It also documents that more than 90% of patients are asked about their smoking at each visit. Periodic posting of updated results gives reinforcement and feedback to the clinic staff. (From Kottke TE, Solberg LI, Brekke ML, et al: Smoking cessation strategies and evaluation. *J Am Coll Cardiol* 12:1105-1110, 1988. By permission of American College of Cardiology.)

Motivation to begin an exercise program depends on knowledge of and belief in the health benefits of exercise, individual risk for conditions associated with inactivity, and good perceived health. However, the reasons for continuing an exercise program primarily concern the enjoyment, convenience, and social support for the activity itself. The key counseling points are related to the regular pattern of exercise activity that can be maintained with minimal disruption of other aspects of life but that will yield the desired benefits, including an increased sense of enjoyment and fulfillment.

Exercise prescription guidelines for patients known to have heart disease are described in chapter 14.

Risk factor intervention in childhood

Attributes present in adults in countries that have a high prevalence of coronary artery disease are present in the children of those countries,[283,284] and the levels of plasma total cholesterol, LDL cholesterol, and HDL cholesterol in children are predictive of the incidence of coronary artery disease in their grandfathers.[285] There is also a positive correlation between parental blood pressure and the blood pressure of these parents' offspring.[286,287]

Although no information is available at present to prove that intervention in childhood will decrease or prevent coronary artery disease in adult years, a strategy to prevent the appearance of risk factors is attractive. Present information strongly suggests that such intervention would be of benefit.[288-291]

The risks that are potentially modifiable in childhood include cigarette smoking, systemic hypertension, diabetes mellitus, sedentary lifestyle, obesity, use of oral contraceptives, and increased plasma LDL.

Smoking. Children begin smoking as a result of peer pressure, and the most successful preventive programs include educational efforts early in school[292] that provide techniques to allow children to resist peer pressure. In addition, the physician who cares for children should set an example by not smoking and by prominently displaying "no smoking" signs in the office. He should realize that failure to discuss the avoidance of smoking may be interpreted by the adolescent as meaning that antismoking campaigns are unimportant. Finally, short-term effects of smoking should be emphasized, because the long-term effects seem less meaningful to the adolescent.

Hypertension. Blood pressure levels "track" in some individuals from childhood to adolescence,[293] and blood pressure levels attained in late adolescence are significantly correlated with subsequent hypertension in adult life.[291] Although more knowledge is continuously being accumulated, for now it is sensible to measure children's blood pressures at least once yearly and to identify possible treatable causes in those who have significant elevations. Also, greater emphasis should be given to the development of healthful lifestyles early in childhood to influence the incidence of significant hypertension in the adolescent and adult. The measures would include a decrease in the currently high level of dietary sodium, prevention and treatment of obesity, and development of a habit of repetitive physical exercise. These recommendations are particularly important in children whose blood pressure is in the upper part of the distributions for age and sex and in those from families in which one or more adults have primary hypertension.

Diabetes mellitus. Diabetic adults appear to be at increased risk for the development of coronary artery disease.[91] This relationship has not been demonstrated as yet in children and adolescents with early-onset diabetes. In the adult, physical activity, body weight, blood lipid levels, and dietary composition appear to affect the coronary artery disease risk of diabetics and this provides a sound rationale for a treatment program of juvenile diabetic patients which includes maintenance of normal weight, increased physical exercise, and a diet restricted in saturated fat, cholesterol, and sodium.

Sedentary lifestyle. The benefits associated with a repetitive physical activity program have been demonstrated in adults. Repetitive exercise is associated with a decrease in plasma total triglycerides, cholesterol, and LDL and an increase in HDL.[294,295] A lowering of blood pressure and an improvement in the maintenance of normal body weight have also been demonstrated. The development of the habit of repetitive physical activity in childhood may be associated with the same benefits and, in addition, result in improved physical fitness, appearance, and mental well-being.

Obesity. The association of obesity with higher blood pressures has been demonstrated in children,[288] and body size has been found to correlate more strongly with systolic pressure in children than does age.[293]

Obesity is a significant medical problem in American children and adolescents in that it is estimated that between 6% and 13% of American children are obese. The obese adolescent stands a far greater chance of becoming an obese adult than does an adolescent of normal weight. In addition, prevention of obesity affords the benefits of improved physical fitness, appearance, and mental well-being. Treatment of obesity in the child and adolescent is an extremely difficult medical problem; however, it is possible that early development of a lifestyle that includes increased physical activity and a healthful diet might help prevent obesity and the associated treatment problems.

Oral contraceptives. Oral contraception is a risk factor for hypertension in some women. Women who use oral contraception have a small but significant increase in blood pressure, and hypertension develops in some.[296] Adolescent girls with blood pressure elevation or a family history of hypertension probably should not use oral contraceptives.

Plasma lipids. Children in countries with a high prevalence of coronary artery disease in the adult population have higher plasma total cholesterol levels than do children from countries in which there is a low risk of coronary artery disease.[283] The mean level of plasma total cholesterol in North American children varies with age, but at 5 to 18 years of age it is 160 ± 24 mg/dL; about 5% of North American children 5 to 18 years old have plasma total cholesterol concentrations exceeding 200 to 220 mg/dL. Epidemiologists in the United States have set the goal of achieving an average plasma total cholesterol level of 160 mg/dL among adults. This is ideal; however, realistically it is thought that 190 mg/dL is achievable. In children, the goal has been set at an average plasma total cholesterol level of < 170 mg/dL and an LDL cholesterol level of < 110 mg/dL.[283]

Although genetic and possibly unknown environmental factors influence the level of plasma cholesterol, what an individual eats is known to affect the level.[297,298] The response of the plasma cholesterol level to dietary nutrients varies from person to person, but a decrease in excess dietary cholesterol and saturated fat will result in a decrease in plasma cholesterol level, more in some than in others.[298] It has not been proved, and cannot be proved in the foreseeable future, that lowering the plasma cholesterol level in children will affect the incidence of coronary artery disease in adulthood; however, there is strong evidence to support the benefit of lower plasma cholesterol levels,[299] and dietary intervention is the first step.

The following are four potential intervention strategies:

1. Plasma lipid levels could be measured in all American children and dietary intervention could be prescribed only in those with high levels.
2. Plasma lipid levels could be measured in all American children, and dietary intervention could be prescribed for all children.
3. Plasma lipid levels could be measured only in children from families in which there were adult members with elevated lipid levels or in which there was a history of premature vascular disease. Dietary intervention could then be prescribed for those with high levels.
4. Finally, plasma lipid levels would not be measured in any children and a recommendation would be made that all American children eat diets that are low in cholesterol and saturated fat.

Most cholesterol is carried on LDL, and it has been shown that the risk of atherosclerosis and coronary artery disease is more strongly associated with the level of LDL cholesterol than with the level of total cholesterol; increased HDL is inversely correlated with coronary artery disease.[283,300]

Since an increased plasma level of LDL cholesterol appears to be the chief atherogenic factor and an increased level of HDL seems to be protective, it is important to know how efficient a screening program that measures plasma total cholesterol would be in identifying children with increased LDL cholesterol. In a study in Rochester, Minn., plasma total cholesterol, total triglyceride, and lipoprotein fractions were measured in 2,421 children. Of these, 94 had plasma total cholesterol levels above the 95th percentile distribution for age and sex and normal triglyceride levels. In 61 of the 94 (65%), the elevations in total plasma cholesterol were due to high levels of LDL, whereas in 33 (35%) the high total levels were a result of high levels of HDL with an associated normal level of LDL.[301] Kwiterovich et al.[302] assessed the measurement of total plasma cholesterol as a screening test for identifying an increased plasma level of LDL cholesterol in 1,325 children and adolescents. Almost one-third of young subjects with elevated plasma levels of LDL were undetected, and 40% of the test results were falsely positive.

It can be concluded from these two studies that the use of plasma total cholesterol levels as a screening test for an increase in LDL in a general population of children results in a relatively large number of false-positive and false-negative tests. Thus, universal screening of all American children is not advisable until an effective, low-cost test is developed.

The second strategy has been advocated by a group of leading physicians in the field of preventive cardiology.[303] Their recommendations are that

a. Universal screening for total cholesterol levels in the blood of all children should be conducted between the ages of 2 and 5 outside school or between 6 and 10 in school as part of a general cardiovascular risk profiling.
b. Healthy children over 2 years of age should adopt the recommended diet.
c. The development of support mechanisms to enhance the adoption of a healthful lifestyle should be encouraged in medical and school systems, by industry, and by the community.
d. Commercial food preparation should be improved in line with the recommended diet.

The major disadvantage of the second strategy is its cost. Resources that could go directly to the education of children and their parents[304,305] would be diverted by the lipid screening program.

The third strategy involves the measurement of plasma lipid levels only in children who are from high-risk families—members with hyperlipidemia or a family history of premature vascular disease. Coronary artery disease clusters in families, and children from families with premature vascular disease tend to have higher levels of plasma total cholesterol.[306] The Rochester study[301] showed that children with elevated plasma levels of LDL came from families with a higher incidence of coronary artery disease. Conversely, children with elevated levels of HDL came from families with a low incidence of coronary artery disease. The correlation of plasma LDL with coronary artery disease in the family was stronger than that of plasma total cholesterol, and the ratio of HDL to total cholesterol in the index children was the strongest correlate (Fig 13-16).[285]

Genetic factors influence cholesterol metabolic pathways; these factors are stronger in some children than in others, and the strongest expression is in the children with familial hypercholesterolemia. In addition, there is evidence to suggest that genetic factors influence the response of plasma lipid levels to environmental influences.[297,298]

A number of genetically transmitted lipid abnormalities have been identified, as has a clustering of specific hyperlipoproteinemias in families.[307,308] Familial hypercholesterolemia (type IIa hyperlipoproteinemia) is the most common and is manifested by an increase in LDL cholesterol. These children are at greater risk of premature vascular disease than is the general population.

Genetically transmitted abnormalities in the lipoprotein metabolic pathway are probably more common in children than was previously believed. Since these abnormalities affect the individual response to environment (diet), it is important that information on lipoprotein levels be obtained in all children who are found to have elevated plasma total cholesterol or triglyceride levels. A complete quantitation of lipoprotein fractions is not usually available, and, in children with hypercholesterolemia, measurements of HDL cholesterol and plasma total triglycerides are indicated. This would allow one to estimate the LDL cholesterol by means of the following formula: LDL cholesterol = total cholesterol − (HDL cholesterol + total triglyceride/5).

There are two disadvantages to measuring lipid levels only in children from high-risk families. Only children in whom an accurate family history is obtainable would be identified, and children who do not have familial hyperlipoproteinemia but have elevated plasma levels of lipids which are largely environmentally induced would be missed.

The fourth strategy would be not to measure plasma lipid levels in any children but to gradually change the diet of all healthy American children more than 2 years old to one recommended by the American Heart Association (Table 13-16). The advantage of this strategy is that such a diet is safe, if the children are healthy and not nutritionally deprived. It is also the least expensive of the four strategies. Although the response of plasma total cholesterol and LDL would be variable, an average

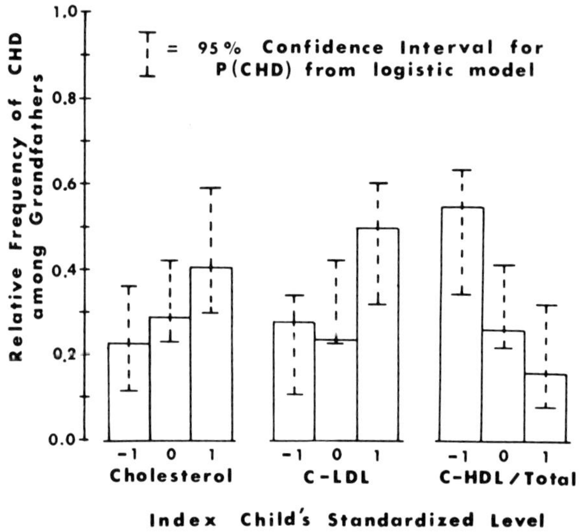

Fig 13-16 The observed frequency of coronary heart disease (CHD) in grandfathers plotted against an index child's standardized cholesterol value. *C-LDL,* low-density lipoprotein cholesterol; *C-HDL/Total,* high-density lipoprotein cholesterol as a fraction of total cholesterol. (From Moll PP, Sing CF, Weidman WH, et al: Total cholesterol and lipoproteins in schoolchildren; prediction of coronary heart disease in adult relatives. *Circulation* 67:127-134, 1983. By permission of American Heart Association.)

Table 13-16 Recommended diet for healthy children

1. Nutritionally adequate diet consisting of a variety of foods
2. Caloric intake based on growth rate, activity level, and content of deposits of subcutaneous fat so as to maintain ideal body weight
3. Total fat intake no more than 30% of calories, with less than 10% from saturated fat, less than 10% from polyunsaturated fat, and the remainder from monounsaturated fat
4. Daily cholesterol intake not to exceed 300 mg. This allows for differences in caloric intake in various age groups
5. Protein intake of about 15% to 20% of calories, derived from varied sources
6. Carbohydrate calories derived primarily from complex carbohydrate sources to provide necessary vitamins and minerals. Thus, the total percentage of calories from carbohydrate would be about 55%.
7. Limitation of most highly salted processed foods and sodium-containing condiments and the elimination of added salt at the table

From Weidman W, Kwiterovich P Jr, Jesse MJ, et al: Diet in the healthy child: Task Force Committee of the Nutrition Committee and the Cardiovascular Disease in the Young Council of the American Heart Association. *Circulation* 67:1411A-1414A, 1983. Reproduced with permission. ©"Diet in the Healthy Child." Copyright American Heart Association.

decrease of about 10% could be expected. On the basis of population studies, such as the Framingham Study, even a 10% overall decrease in plasma total lipids in children would likely be beneficial. The disadvantage of this strategy, of course, is that children with familial hyperlipoproteinemia would not be identified. So it is important to add to the first goal – lowering the average plasma cholesterol level in all children – the goal of identifying children with familial hyperlipoproteinemia, because dietary management is likely to be less successful in those children, and more intensive treatment will usually be necessary.

The authors agree with the American Heart Association[309,310] and the NCEP Expert Panel[283] that the most effective strategy at present is to recommend dietary modification for all healthy children more than 2 years old and to measure plasma lipids only in children from high-risk families.

An important question is whether abnormal levels of plasma cholesterol, triglycerides, and lipoprotein fractions identified in childhood will persist through childhood, adolescence, and adulthood. This question has not been answered. However, in two studies of children, the correlation coefficient of plasma cholesterol level 4 years after an initial survey was 0.61 to 0.68, and the majority of the children in the top deciles of distribution remained in the top deciles over the 4-year period. LDL cholesterol and HDL cholesterol also "tracked" during this period.[311,312]

Table 13-17 Cutpoints for 75th and 90th percentiles of serum cholesterol and diastolic blood pressure (BP) for the U.S. railroad cohort of the Seven Countries Study (n = 2,571) and 40- to 59-year-old men in the baseline cohort of the North Karelia Project (*n* = 3,022)

	U.S. railroad percentile		North Karelia percentile	
Risk factor	**75th**	**90th**	**75th**	**90th**
Cholesterol, mg/dL	268	295	303	337
Diastolic BP, mm Hg	92	101	100	110
Cigarette smoking, no./day	20	30	20	25
Number in cohort with three risk factors above the cutpoint	49	7	79	8

From Kottke TE, Gatewood LC, Wu S-C et al: Preventing heart disease: Is treating the high risk sufficient? *J Clin Epidemiol* 41:1083-1093, 1988. By permission of Pergamon Press.

Intervention strategies

Because only one-quarter of the United States population is defined as hypertensive[313] and a quarter have a serum cholesterol value that places them at high risk for heart disease,[314] the implication seems to be that focusing on this high-risk population to control coronary heart disease may be the most efficient intervention strategy for clinicians. However, this is not necessarily the case. The best intervention strategy depends, in part, on the extent that the disease is limited to an identifiable high-risk subpopulation or is widely dispersed throughout the population as a whole. If the risk factors are tightly clustered in a limited portion of the population, focusing on this population might reduce costs and limit the potential for harmful side effects of intervention. On the other hand, if heart disease risk is widely dispersed throughout the population, creating a social consensus about desired behaviors for the whole population might be the most appropriate strategy. These questions have been addressed in several studies.[315,316] In one study, the data from the United States Railroad cohort of the Seven Countries Study[7] and the North Karelia Project[317] were applied to a Monte Carlo simulation process to evaluate the impact of various interventions.[316]

The potential impact of limiting an intervention to male smokers with serum cholesterol levels and blood pressure readings in the top quarter of the risk distribution was small. Of the 2,571 men in the United States cohort, only 49 had three risk factors at or above the 75th percentile (Table 13-17). Only 79 of the 3,022 men in the baseline cohort of the North Karelia Project had all three risk factors at or above the 75th percentile. Focusing on men

Table 13-18 Distribution of the cohort nonfatal myocardial infarction (MI) rates and coronary heart disease (CHD) death rates and distribution of nonfatal MIs and CHD deaths by number of risk factors in the United States railroad cohort of the Seven Countries Study and 40- to 59-year-old men in the baseline cohort of the North Karelia Project

	Number of risk factors in the highest quartile			
	0	1	2	3
Proportion of population				
U.S. railroad	0.438	0.400	0.143	0.019
North Karelia	0.408	0.403	0.162	0.026
Five-year nonfatal MI rate				
U.S. railroad	0.016	0.033	0.065	0.122
North Karelia	0.021	0.045	0.055	0.101
Five-year CHD death rate				
U.S. railroad	0.010	0.024	0.054	0.143
North Karelia	0.014	0.018	0.041	0.051
Proportion of nonfatal MI attributable to the group				
U.S. railroad	0.220	0.415	0.293	0.073
North Karelia	0.224	0.474	0.233	0.069
Proportion of CHD death rate attributable to the group				
U.S. railroad	0.175	0.397	0.317	0.111
North Karelia	0.270	0.349	0.317	0.063

From Kottke TE, Gatewood LC, Wu S-C, et al: Preventing heart disease: Is treating the high risk sufficient? *J Clin Epidemiol* 41:1083-1093, 1988. By permission of Pergamon Press.

with all three risk factors above the 90th percentile would have an even more limited impact: only seven of the United States men and eight of the Finnish men had all three risk factors at or above the 90th percentile.

The nonfatal myocardial infarction rates for the United States men with all three risk factors in the upper quartile were three times as high as those for men with no risk factors in the upper quartile and twice as high as those for men with two risk factors in the upper quartile (Table 13-18). The nonfatal myocardial infarction rates for high-risk North Karelian men were five times as high as those for men with no risk factors in the upper quartile and twice as high as those for men with two risk factors in the highest quartile.

The rates for death from coronary heart disease for United States railroad men with three risk factors in the upper quartile were 14 times as great as those for men with no risk factors in the highest quartile and 2.6 times as great as those for men with two risk factors in the highest quartile. The rates for death from coronary heart disease for North Karelian men with three risk factors in the upper quartile were 3.6 times as great as the death rates for those with no risk factors in the upper quartile and 25% greater than those for men with two risk factors in the upper quartile.

Only about 7% of nonfatal myocardial infarctions in both cohorts occurred among men with three risk factors in the highest quartile. More than 60% of nonfatal myocardial infarctions occurred among men with no more than one risk factor in the highest quartile.

An intervention that reduced total serum cholesterol by 10%, reduced diastolic blood pressure by 5%, and induced 20% of the smokers to stop smoking (the "high effectiveness" population intervention) would be expected to lower rates of nonfatal myocardial infarction by slightly over 20%. Rates of death from coronary heart disease would be reduced by about one-third. If serum cholesterol were reduced by only 4%, diastolic blood pressure were reduced by 3%, and 15% of the smokers were to quit smoking (the "low effectiveness" intervention), rates of nonfatal myocardial infarction would decrease by about 12% and deaths from coronary heart disease would decrease by about one-fifth.

Single interventions (reducing serum cholesterol concentration to 180 mg/dL, reducing diastolic blood pressure to 80 mm Hg, or eliminating smoking) among the group of men with all three risk factors in the highest quartile would have small effects. The maximum effect would be an 8% decline in deaths from coronary heart disease among the Finnish men. Combining the three interventions would approximately double the effect of any single intervention.

Intervening in the same fashion among men with at least two risk factors in the top quartile would have an effect equal to that of the "low effectiveness" intervention in the whole United States population. Treating all three risk factors for any man with two risk factors in the upper quartile would have approximately the same effect as the "high effectiveness" population-based intervention.

The implications of these and corroborating data[318-321] are that most preventable myocardial infarctions and deaths from cardiovascular disease will occur not among the patients at highest risk but rather among the patients in the middle of the risk distribution. This fact may itself be the reason why clinicians were relatively resistant to accept the concept that cholesterol is a risk factor for coronary heart disease: most events that they see are among patients who are not markedly different from the average "well" patient seen in the office.

There are other reasons for not limiting risk factor interventions to the "high-risk" population. First, targeting this population requires that it be identified. Identification requires screening the entire population. The costs of screening do not accrue just from the testing of cholesterol. If the entire population is to be truly screened, a census must be performed, and a tally of the population screened and not screened must be main-

Table 13-19 Grades of quality of evidence and classification of recommendations of the United States Preventive Services Task Force

Grades of quality of evidence	
I	Evidence obtained from at least one properly randomized, controlled trial
II-1	Evidence obtained from well-designed controlled trials without randomization
II-2	Evidence obtained from well-designed cohort or case-control analytic studies, preferably from more than one center or research group
II-3	Evidence obtained from multiple time series studies with or without the intervention. Dramatic results in uncontrolled experiments (such as the results of the introduction of penicillin in the 1940s) could also be regarded as this type of evidence
III	Opinions of respected authorities based on clinical experience, descriptive studies, or reports of expert committees
Classification of recommendations	
A	There is good evidence to support the recommendation that the condition be specifically considered in a periodic health examination
B	There is fair evidence to support the recommendation that the condition be specifically considered in a periodic health examination
C	There is poor evidence regarding the inclusion of the condition in a periodic health examination, but recommendations may be made on other grounds
D	There is fair evidence to support the recommendation that the condition be excluded from consideration in a periodic health examination
E	There is good evidence to support the recommendation that the condition be excluded from consideration in a periodic health examination

tained. Thus, the cost of screening may be 8 to 10 times the cost of simply implementing a population-wide intervention,[322,323] and screening is less cost-effective than strategies designed to change diet among the members of the community.[316]

Second, targeting an intervention at a subpopulation requires that this group accept behavior that differs from that of the population at large. Although this labeling is necessary for identification, it is not always sufficient to cause behavior change[324] and may stigmatize the target subpopulation.[325,326] There is also evidence that the high-risk subpopulation is no more likely to change than the population as a whole.[327]

Third, the unlabeled portion of the population may incorrectly conclude that because they are unlabeled, they are not at risk of having disease develop. As demonstrated by the data presented above, this conclusion is definitely erroneous.

The high-risk and population interventions complement each other. The behavioral risk factors for coronary heart disease—smoking, eating, and exercise habits—are social behaviors whose appropriateness is defined by the patient's peer group. Community interventions can thus augment the effectiveness of clinical interventions.[328] Community interventions provide priming before the patient receives the heart disease prevention message in the physician's office and reinforce the patient's intentions to change after the physician has given the message. This not only increases the probability that the patient will be able to maintain change but also increases the physician's sense of satisfaction when the patient does change. The physician has many potential sources of support from community agencies, and, in turn, the physician should support the efforts of agencies like the American Heart Association to reduce the burden of cardiovascular disease in the community.

Is it the physician's responsibility to prevent heart disease?

The responsibility of the physician to provide heart disease prevention services is ambiguous on two domains. There is ambiguity about which interventions should be advocated to which patients, and there is ambiguity about the physician's responsibility to the patient. This lack of definition causes misunderstanding and frustration among physicians, their patients, and the public.

The Canadian Task Force on the Periodic Health Examination[329] considerably clarified the first problem when they developed explicit definitions for quality of evidence and the strength of their recommendations. These criteria were adopted by the United States Preventive Services Task Force with slight modifications[330] (Table 13-19). Although the rules have shortcomings, they serve to transmit information about recommendations just as the methods section in a scientific paper transmits information about an experiment or observation. This information helps the physician understand whether a recommendation is firmly based on trial evidence or is based only on speculation.

In the second instance of ambiguity, the physician's claimed responsibility to the patient ranges from the duty to convince the patient to change behavior[331] to no responsibility to even advise the patient about risk factors.[332] An examination of the physician's more general role in society can help reduce the ambiguity and define a preventive cardiology role for the physician that has the potential of being accepted by all parties.[333]

Patient-physician interaction almost exclusively takes the form of a patient (or the patient's guardian) seeking out a physician and asking for help by making a "chief complaint." The physician responds by telling the patient if and how he or she is willing to provide help. Depending on the context, the same action can be desired by the patient but refused by the physician, desired by the physician but refused by the patient, or desired by both the patient and the physician. For example, in one case, a patient may come to a physician seeking a tranquilizer for recreational purposes; it is likely that the physician will refuse to prescribe the drug. In a second case, the physician may wish to prescribe the same tranquilizer for a patient who shows signs of distress but denies feeling unwell; it is not unlikely in this case that the patient will refuse the drug. In a third case, a patient who has experienced a recent death in the family may seek a tranquilizer for treatment of short-term situational distress; in this case, the physician can be expected to prescribe the tranquilizer.

Although society recognizes that physicians can help patients, it also recognizes that physicians can abuse patients with their power. Society therefore attempts to protect patients from unwanted therapy with devices like informed consent. Forced intervention is accepted as justified only when the individual has harmed or will harm others.[334] In only three cases is the physician permitted or obligated to carry out action against the will of the patient: incarceration when the patient is mentally incompetent, quarantine when the patient poses an infective threat to the community, and pediatric immunization. It is thus not without grounds that physicians are uncomfortable when it is suggested that they must convince patients to change their behaviors.

Although the physician should not be expected to coerce or convince a patient to adopt preventive behaviors, patients look to their physicians for advice about health behavior and are disappointed when advice is not forthcoming. It therefore behooves the physician to take responsibility for six tasks related to preventive cardiology: (1) remain knowledgeable about preventive cardiology services, (2) identify the heart disease prevention services needed by each patient, (3) advise each patient of the types of actions that are needed, (4) enable and assist the patient to take action to the extent that the patient expresses interest, (5) reinforce the patient in his or her preventive activities, and (6) establish, support, and maintain a system to facilitate tasks (2) through (5).

Because the physician is subject to the same environmental and personal forces that influence patient behavior, society must financially and psychologically support the physician who fulfills the obligations defined above. If physicians and lay society can face the task of heart disease prevention as a team, it appears that Paul Dudley White's credo of the last generation can become a reality in the next generation: "Heart disease before 80 is our fault, not God's or nature's will."[335]

REFERENCES

1. Dawber TR: *The Framingham Study: the Epidemiology of Atherosclerotic Disease.* Cambridge, Massachusetts, Harvard University Press, 1980
2. Paul O: Background of the prevention of cardiovascular disease. II. Arteriosclerosis, hypertension, and selected risk factors. *Circulation* 80:206-214, 1989
3. Aschoff L: *Lectures on Pathology.* New York, Paul B. Hoeber, 1924
4. Malmros H: The relation of nutrition to health: a statistical study of the effect of the war-time on atherosclerosis, cardiosclerosis, tuberculosis and diabetes. *Acta Med Scand* [*Suppl*] 246:137-153, 1950
5. Blackburn H: The epidemiology and prevention of coronary heart disease. *Excerpta Medica International Congress* Series No 470, 1979, pp 23-32
6. Keys A: Nutrition in relation to the etiology and the course of degenerative diseases. *J Am Diet Assoc* 24:281-285, 1948
7. Keys A: *Seven Countries: A Multivariate Analysis of Death in Coronary Heart Disease.* Cambridge, Massachusetts, Harvard University Press, 1980
8. Goldbourt U, Medalie JH, Neufeld HN: Clinical myocardial infarction over a five-year period. III. A multivariate analysis of incidence, the Israel Ischemic Heart Disease Study. *J Chronic Dis* 28:217-237, 1975
9. Kleinbaum DG, Kupper LL, Cassel JC, et al: Multivariate analysis of risk of coronary heart disease in Evans County, Georgia. *Arch Intern Med* 128:943-948, 1971
10. Kozarević D, Pirc B, Račić Z, et al: The Yugoslavia Cardiovascular Disease Study. II. Factors in the incidence of coronary heart disease. *Am J Epidemiol* 104:133-140, 1976
11. Rosenman RH, Brand RJ, Sholtz RI, et al: Multivariate prediction of coronary heart disease during 8.5 year follow-up in the Western Collaborative Group Study. *Am J Cardiol* 37:903-910, 1976
12. Pelkonen R, Nikkilä EA, Koskinen S, et al: Association of serum lipids and obesity with cardiovascular mortality. *Br Med J* 2:1185-1187, 1977
13. Miller NE, Førde OH, Thelle DS, et al: The Tromsø Heart-Study: high-density lipoprotein and coronary heart disease; a prospective case control study. *Lancet* 1:965-968, 1977
14. Friedman GD, Klatsky AL, Siegelaub AB, et al: Kaiser-Permanente epidemiologic study of myocardial infarction: study design and results for standard risk factors. *Am J Epidemiol* 99:101-116, 1974
15. McGee D, Gordon T: The results of the Framingham Study applied to four other U.S.-based epidemiologic studies of cardiovascular disease. In *The Framingham Study: An Epidemiological Investigation of Cardiovascular Disease* (DHEW Publication No [NIH] 76-1083). Section 31. Edited by WB Kannel, T Gordon. Washington DC, US Department of Health, Education, and Welfare, 1976
16. Pooling Project Research Group: Relationship of blood pressure, serum cholesterol, smoking habit, relative weight and ECG abnormalities to incidence of major coronary events: final report of the Pooling Project. *J Chronic Dis* 31:201-306, 1978
17. Keys A (ed): Coronary heart disease in seven countries. *Circulation* 41 Suppl 1:1-211, 1970
18. Bronte-Stewart B, Keys A, Brock JF: Serum-cholesterol, diet, and coronary heart-disease: an inter-racial survey in the Cape Peninsula. *Lancet* 2:1103-1108, 1955
19. Powell KE, Thompson PD, Caspersen CJ, et al: Physical activity and the incidence of coronary heart disease. *Annu Rev Public Health* 8:253-287, 1987
20. Koplan JP, Powell KE, Sikes RK, et al: An epidemiologic study of the benefits and risks of running. *JAMA* 248:3118-3121, 1982
21. Hill AB; *Principles of Medical Statistics.* Ninth edition. New York, Oxford University Press, 1971, pp 309-323
22. Fletcher RH, Fletcher SW, Wagner EH: *Clinical Epiedemiology: the Essentials.* Second edition. Baltimore, Williams & Wilkins, 1988
23. Keys A, Mickelsen O, Miller EvO, et al: The relation in man between cholesterol levels in the diet and in the blood. *Science* 112:79-81, 1950
24. Mattson FH, Erickson BA, Kligman AM: Effect of dietary cholesterol on serum cholesterol in man. *Am J Clin Nutr* 25:589-594, 1972
25. Keys A, Anderson JT, Grande F: Serum cholesterol response to changes in the diet. II. The effect of cholesterol in the diet. IV. Particular saturated fatty acids in the diet. *Metabolism* 14:759-765; 776-787, 1965

26. Hegsted DM, McGandy RB, Myers ML, et al: Quantitative effects of dietary fat on serum cholesterol in man. *Am J Clin Nutr* 17:281-295, 1965
27. Keys A, Kimura N, Kusukawa A, et al: Lessons from serum cholesterol studies in Japan, Hawaii, and Los Angeles. *Ann Intern Med* 48:83-94, 1958
28. Tillotson JL, Kato H, Nichaman MZ, et al: Epidemiology of coronary heart disease and stroke in Japanese men living in Japan, Hawaii, and California: methodology for comparison of diet. *Am J Clin Nutr* 26:177-184, 1973
29. Kagan A, Harris BR, Winkelstein W Jr, et al: Epidemiologic studies of coronary heart disease and stroke in Japanese men living in Japan, Hawaii, and California: demographic, physical, dietary and biochemical characteristics. *J Chronic Dis* 27:345-364, 1974
30. Wynder EL, Lemon FR, Bross IJ: Cancer and coronary artery disease among Seventh-Day Adventists. *Cancer* 12:1016-1028, 1959
31. Shekelle RB, Shryock AM, Paul O, et al: Diet, serum cholesterol, and death from coronary heart disease: the Western Electric Study. *N Engl J Med* 304:65-70, 1981
32. Keys A, Parlin RW: Serum cholesterol response to changes in dietary lipids. *Am J Clin Nutr* 19:175-181, 1966
33. Harris T, Cook EF, Kannel WB, et al: Proportional hazards analysis of risk factors for coronary heart disease in individuals aged 65 or older: the Framingham Heart Study. *J Am Geriatr Soc* 36:1023-1028, 1988
34. Benfante R, Reed D: Is elevated serum cholesterol level a risk factor for coronary heart disease in the elderly? *JAMA* 263:393-396, 1990
35. Kushi LH, Kottke TE: Dietary fat and coronary heart disease; evidence of a causal relation. In *Preventing Disease: Beyond the Rhetoric.* Edited by RB Goldbloom, RS Lawrence. New York, Springer-Verlag, 1990, pp 385-400
36. Gordon T, Castelli WP, Hjortland MC, et al: Predicting coronary heart disease in middle-aged and older persons: the Framingham Study. *JAMA* 238:497-499, 1977
37. Wilson PW, Garrison RJ, Castelli WP, et al: Prevalence of coronary heart disease in the Framingham Offspring Study: role of lipoprotein cholesterols. *Am J Cardiol* 46:649-654, 1980
38. Barr DP, Russ EM, Eder HA: Protein-lipid relationships in human plasma. II. In atherosclerosis and related conditions. *Am J Med* 11:480-493, 1951
39. Rhoads GG, Gulbrandsen CL, Kagan A: Serum lipoproteins and coronary heart disease in a population study of Hawaii Japanese men. *N Engl J Med* 294:293-298, 1976
40. Castelli WP, Doyle JT, Gordon T, et al: HDL cholesterol and other lipids in coronary heart disease: the Cooperative Lipoprotein Phenotyping Study. *Circulation* 55:767-772, 1977
41. Gwynne JT: HDL and atherosclerosis: an update. *Clin Cardiol* 14 Suppl I:17-24, 1991
42. Mänttäri M, Huttunen JK, Koskinen P, et al: Lipoproteins and coronary heart disease in the Helsinki Heart Study. *Eur Heart J* 11 Suppl H:26-31, 1990
43. Knuiman JT, Hermus RJJ, Hautvast JGAJ: Serum total and high density lipoprotein (HDL) cholesterol concentrations in rural and urban boys from 16 countries. *Atherosclerosis* 36:529-537, 1980
44. Carlson LA, Böttiger LE, Åhfeldt P-E: Risk factors for myocardial infarction in the Stockholm prospective study: a 14-year follow-up focusing on the role of plasma triglycerides and cholesterol. *Acta Med Scand* 206:351-360, 1979
45. Hulley SB, Rosenman RH, Bawol RD, et al: Epidemiology as a guide to clinical decisions: the association between triglyceride and coronary heart disease. *N Engl J Med* 302:1383-1389, 1980
46. Wilhelmsen L, Wedel H, Tibblin G: Multivariate analysis of risk factors for coronary heart disease. *Circulation* 48:950-958, 1973
47. Robertson TL, Kato H, Gordon T, et al: Epidemiologic study of coronary heart disease and stroke in Japanese men living in Japan, Hawaii and California: coronary heart disease risk factors in Japan and Hawaii. *Am J Cardiol* 39:244-249, 1977
48. Welin L, Eriksson H, Larsson B, et al: Triglycerides, a major coronary risk factor in elderly men. A study of men born in 1913. *Eur Heart J* 12:700-704, 1991
49. Brown MS, Goldstein JL: Teaching old dogmas new tricks. *Nature* 330:113-114, 1987
50. Lawn RM: The structure and evolution of apolipoprotein(a), pp 209-211. In Lipoprotein(a) and Atherosclerosis. Moderated by AM Scanu. *Ann Intern Med* 115:209-218, 1991
51. Hammond EC, Horn D: The relationship between human smoking habits and death rates: a follow-up study of 187,766 men. *JAMA* 155:1316-1328, 1954
52. Hammond EC, Horn D: Smoking and death rates: report on forty-four months of follow-up of 187,783 men. I. Total mortality. II. Death rates by cause. *JAMA* 166:1159-1172; 1294-1308, 1958
53. Kannel WB, Castelli WP, McNamara PM: Cigarette smoking and risk of coronary heart disease: epidemiologic clues to pathogenesis; the Framingham Study. *Natl Cancer Inst Monogr* 28:9-20, 1968
54. Doyle JT, Dawber TR, Kannel WB, et al: Cigarette smoking and coronary heart disease: combined experience of the Albany and Framingham studies. *N Engl J Med* 266:796-801, 1962
55. Kahn HA: The Dorn Study of smoking and mortality among U.S. veterans: report on eight and one-half years of observation. *Natl Cancer Inst Monogr* 19:1-27, 1966
56. Benfante R, Reed D, Frank J: Does cigarette smoking have an independent effect on coronary heart disease incidence in the elderly? *Am J Public Health* 81:897-899, 1991
57. Slone D, Shapiro S, Rosenberg L, et al: Relation of cigarette smoking to myocardial infarction in young women. *N Engl J Med* 298:1273-1276, 1978
58. Inman WHW, Vessey MP: Investigation of deaths from pulmonary, coronary, and cerebral thrombosis and embolism in women of child-bearing age. *Br Med J* 2:193-199, 1968
59. Auerbach O, Hammond EC, Garfinkel L: Smoking in relation to atherosclerosis of the coronary arteries. *N Engl J Med* 273:775-779, 1965
60. Report of Inter-Society Commission for Heart Disease Resources: Primary prevention of the atherosclerotic diseases. *Circulation* 42:A-55-A-95, 1970
61. Hartz AJ, Anderson AJ, Brooks HL, et al: The association of smoking with cardiomyopathy. *N Engl J Med* 311:1201-1206, 1984
62. Wilhelmsson C, Vedin JA, Elmfeldt D, et al: Smoking and myocardial infarction. *Lancet* 1:415-420, 1975
63. Salonen JT: Stopping smoking and long-term mortality after acute myocardial infarction. *Br Heart J* 43:463-469, 1980
64. Mulcahy R: Influence of cigarette smoking on morbidity and mortality after myocardial infarction. *Br Heart J* 49:410-415, 1983
65. Hallstrom AP, Cobb LA, Ray R: Smoking as a risk factor for recurrence of sudden cardiac arrest. *N Engl J Med* 314:271-275, 1986
66. Deanfield JE, Shea MJ, Wilson RA, et al: Direct effects of smoking on the heart: silent ischemic disturbances of coronary flow. *Am J Cardiol* 57:1005-1009, 1986
67. Deanfield J, Wright C, Krikler S, et al: Cigarette smoking and the treatment of angina with propranolol, atenolol, and nifedepine. *N Engl J Med* 310:951-954, 1984
68. Myers KA: Relationship of smoking to peripheral arterial disease. *Aust Fam Physician* 8:765-768, 1979
69. Hermanson B, Omenn GS, Kronmal RA, et al: Beneficial six-year outcome of smoking cessation in older men and women with coronary artery disease: results from the CASS registry. *N Engl J Med* 319:1365-1369, 1988
70. Gillum RF, Folsom A, Luepker RV, et al: Sudden death and acute myocardial infarction in a metropolitan area, 1970-1980: the Minnesota Heart Survey. *N Engl J Med* 309:1353-1358, 1983
71. Gomez-Marin O, Folsom AR, Kottke TE, et al: Improvement in long-term survival among patients hospitalized with acute myocardial infarction, 1970 to 1980: the Minnesota Heart Survey. *N Engl J Med* 316:1353-1359, 1987
72. The Health Consequences of Smoking. Cardiovascular Disease: A Report of the Surgeon General. (DHHS Publication No [PHS] 84-50204). Washington, DC, US Department of Health and Human Services, 1984
73. Hartz AJ, Barboriak PN, Anderson AJ, et al: Smoking, coronary artery occlusion, and nonfatal myocardial infarction. *JAMA* 246:851-853, 1981
74. Hjermann I, Velve Byre K, Holme I, et al: Effect of diet and smoking intervention on the incidence of coronary heart disease: report from the Oslo Study Group of a randomised trial in healthy men. *Lancet* 2:1303-1310, 1981
75. Friedman GD, Petitti DB, Bawol RD, et al: Mortality in cigarette smokers and quitters: effect of base-line differences. *N Engl J Med* 304:1407-1410, 1981

76. Multiple Risk Factor Intervention Trial Research Group: Multiple risk factor intervention trial: risk factor changes and mortality results. *JAMA* 248:1465-1477, 1982

77. Gordon T, Kannel WB, McGee D: Death and coronary attacks in men after giving up cigarette smoking: a report from the Framingham Study. *Lancet* 2:1345-1348, 1974

78. Somer AR (ed): *The Kaiser-Permanente Medical Care Program: A Symposium.* New York, The Commonwealth Fund, 1971

79. Ball K, Turner R: Smoking and the heart: the basis for action. *Lancet* 2:822-826, 1974

80. Astrup P, Kjeldsen K, Wanstrup J: Enhancing influence of carbon monoxide on the development of atheromatosis in cholesterol-fed rabbits. *J Atheroscler Res* 7:343-354, 1967

81. Davies RF, Topping DL, Turner DM: The effect of intermittent carbon monoxide exposure on experimental atherosclerosis in the rabbit. *Atherosclerosis* 24:527-536, 1976

82. Levine PH: An acute effect of cigarette smoking on platelet function: a possible link between smoking and arterial thrombosis. *Circulation* 48:619-623, 1973

83. Cryer PE, Haymond MW, Santiago JV, et al: Norepinephrine and epinephrine release and adrenergic mediation of smoking-associated hemodynamic and metabolic events. *N Engl J Med* 295:573-577, 1976

84. Lefkowitz RJ: Smoking, catecholamines, and the heart (editorial). *N Engl J Med* 295:615-616, 1976

85. Keys A, Aravanis C, Blackburn H, et al: Coronary heart disease: overweight and obesity as risk factors. *Ann Intern Med* 77:15-27, 1972

86. Truett J, Cornfield J, Kannel W: A multivariate analysis of the risk of coronary heart disease in Framingham. *J Chronic Dis* 20:511-524, 1967

87. Rosenman RH, Friedman M, Straus R, et al: Coronary heart disease in the Western Collaborative Group Study: a follow-up experience of 4½ years. *J Chronic Dis* 23:173-190, 1970

88. Stamler J, Lindberg HA, Berkson DM, et al: Prevalence and incidence of coronary heart disease in strata of the labor force of a Chicago industrial corporation. *J Chronic Dis* 11:405-420, 1960

89. Paul O, Lepper MH, Phelan WH, et al: A longitudinal study of coronary heart disease. *Circulation* 28:20-31, 1963

90. Ostrander LD Jr, Epstein FH: Diabetes, hyperglycemia and atherosclerosis: new research directions. In *Diabetes Mellitus* (DHEW Publication No [NIH] 76-854). Edited by SS Fajans. Washington DC, Department of Health, Education, and Welfare, 1976

91. Garcia MJ, McNamara PM, Gordon T, et al: Morbidity and mortality of diabetics in the Framingham population: sixteen year follow-up study. *Diabetes* 23:105-111, 1974

92. Fuller JH, McCartney P, Jarrett RJ, et al: Hyperglycaemia and coronary heart disease: the Whitehall Study. *J Chronic Dis* 32:721-728, 1979

93. Hamby RI, Sherman L, Mehta J, et al: Reappraisal of the role of the diabetic state in coronary artery disease. *Chest* 70:251-257, 1976

94. Dortimer AC, Shenoy PN, Shiroff RA, et al: Diffuse coronary artery disease in diabetic patients: fact or fiction? *Circulation* 57:133-136, 1978

95. Goodale F, Daoud AS, Florentin R, et al: Chemico-anatomic studies of arteriosclerosis and thrombosis in diabetics. I. Coronary arterial wall thickness, thrombosis, and myocardial infarcts in autopsied North Americans. *Exp Mol Pathol* 1:353-363, 1962

96. Feldman M, Feldman M Jr: The association of coronary occlusion and infarction with diabetes mellitus: a necropsy study. *Am J Med Sci* 228:53-56, 1954

97. Goldenberg S, Alex M, Blumenthal HT: Sequelae of arteriosclerosis of the aorta and coronary arteries: a statistical study in diabetes mellitus. *Diabetes* 7:98-108, 1958

98. University Group Diabetes Program: A study of the effects of hypoglycemic agents on vascular complications in patients with adult-onset diabetes. II. Mortality results. *Diabetes* 19:785-830, 1970

99. Lehman EW: Social class and coronary heart disease: a sociological assessment of the medical literature. *J Chronic Dis* 20:381-391, 1967

100. Syme SL: Social and psychological risk factors in coronary heart disease. *Mod Concepts Cardiovasc Dis* 44:17-21, 1975

101. Jenkins CD: Psychologic and social precursors of coronary disease. *N Engl J Med* 284:244-255; 307-317, 1971

102. Jenkins CD: Recent evidence supporting psychologic and social risk factors for coronary disease. *N Engl J Med* 294:987-994; 1033-1038, 1976

103. Friedman M: *Pathogenesis of Coronary Artery Disease.* New York, McGraw-Hill Book Company, 1969

104. Marmot MG, Syme SL: Acculturation and coronary heart disease in Japanese-Americans. *Am J Epidemiol* 104:225-247, 1976

105. Reed D, McGee D, Cohen J, et al: Acculturation and coronary heart disease among Japanese men in Hawaii. *Am J Epidemiol* 115:894-905, 1982

106. Brown GW, Harris T: *Social Origins of Depression: A Study of Psychiatric Disorder in Women.* New York, Macmillan, 1978

107. Henderson S, Byrne DG, Duncan-Jones P, et al: Social bonds in the epidemiology of neurosis: a preliminary communication. *Br J Psychiatry* 132:463-466, 1978

108. Klerman GL, Izen JE: The effects of bereavement and grief on physical health and general well-being. *Adv Psychosom Med* 9:63-104, 1977

109. Berkman LF, Syme SL: Social networks, host resistance, and mortality: a nine-year follow-up study of Alameda County residents. *Am J Epidemiol* 109:186-204, 1979

110. Rose G, Marmot MG: Social class and coronary heart disease. *Br Heart J* 45:13-19, 1981

111. Antonovsky A: Social class and the major cardiovascular diseases. *J Chronic Dis* 21:65-106, 1968

112. Medalie JH, Snyder M, Groen JJ, et al: Angina pectoris among 10,000 men: 5 year incidence and univariate analysis. *Am J Med* 55:583-594, 1973

113. Holmes TH, Rahe RH: The social readjustment rating scale. *J Psychosom Res* 11:213-218, 1967

114. Theorell T, Lind E, Flodérus P: The relationship of disturbing life-changes and emotions to the early development of myocardial infarction and other serious illnesses. *Int J Epidemiol* 4:281-293, 1975

115. Rahe RH, Arajärvi H, Arajärvi S, et al: Recent life changes and coronary heart disease in East versus West Finland. *J Psychosom Res* 20:431-437, 1976

116. Rosenman RH, Friedman M, Straus R, et al: A predictive study of coronary heart disease: the Western Collaborative Group Study. *JAMA* 189:15-22, 1964

117. Brand RJ, Rosenman RH, Sholtz RI, et al: Multivariate prediction of coronary heart disease in the Western Collaborative Group Study compared to the findings of the Framingham Study. *Circulation* 53:348-355, 1976

118. Jenkins CD, Rosenman RH, Zyzanski SJ: Prediction of clinical coronary heart disease by a test for the coronary-prone behavior pattern. *N Engl J Med* 290:1271-1275, 1974

119. Jenkins CD, Zyzanski SJ, Rosenman RH: Risk of new myocardial infarction in middle-aged men with manifest coronary heart disease. *Circulation* 53:342-347, 1976

120. Dembroski TM, MacDougall JM, Shields JL: Physiologic reactions to social challenge in persons evidencing the type A coronary-prone behavior pattern. *J Human Stress* 3:2-9, 1977

121. Williams RB Jr, Lane JD, Kuhn C, et al: Type A behavior and elevated physiological and neuroendocrine responses to cognitive tasks. *Science* 218:483-485, 1982

122. Williams JK, Vita JA, Manuck SB, et al: Psychosocial factors impair vascular responses of coronary arteries. *Circulation* 84:2146-2153, 1991

123. Strawn WB, Bondjers G, Kaplan JR, et al: Endothelial dysfunction in response to psychosocial stress in monkeys. *Circ Res* 68:1270-1279, 1991

124. Review Panel on Coronary-Prone Behavior and Coronary Heart Disease: Coronary-prone behavior and coronary heart disease: a critical review. *Circulation* 63:1199-1215, 1981

125. Shepherd JT, Weiss SM (eds): *Conference on Behavioral Medicine and Cardiovascular Disease.* Dallas, American Heart Association, Circulation Monograph Number 6, 1987

126. Brand RJ: Coronary-prone behavior as an independent risk factor for coronary heart disease. In *Coronary-Prone Behavior.* Edited by TM Dembroski, SM Weiss, JL Shields, et al. New York, Springer-Verlag, 1978, pp 11-24

127. Zyzanski SJ: Coronary-prone behavior pattern and coronary heart disease: epidemiological evidence. In *Coronary-Prone Behavior.* Edited by TM Dembroski, SM Weiss, JL Shields, et al. New York, Springer-Verlag, 1978, pp 25-40

128. Haynes SG, Feinleib M, Kannel WB: The relationship of psychosocial factors to coronary heart disease in the Framingham Study.

III. Eight-year incidence of coronary heart disease. *Am J Epidemiol* 111:37-58, 1980

129. Haynes SG, Feinleib M, Levine S, et al: The relationship of psychosocial factors to coronary heart disease in the Framingham Study. II. Prevalence of coronary heart disease. *Am J Epidemiol* 107:384-402, 1978

130. Williams RB: Psychological factors in coronary artery disease: epidemiologic evidence. In *Conference on Behavioral Medicine and Cardiovascular Disease.* Edited by JT Shepherd, SM Weiss. Dallas, American Heart Association, Circulation Monograph Number 6, 1987

131. Jenkins CD: Behavioral risk factors in coronary artery disease. *Annu Rev Med* 29:543-562, 1978

132. Kittel F, Kornitzer M, Zyzanski SJ, et al: Two methods of assessing the type A coronary-prone behavior pattern in Belgium. *J Chronic Dis* 31:147-155, 1978

133. Paffenbarger RS Jr, Hale WE, Brand RJ, et al: Work-energy level, personal characteristics, and fatal heart attack: a birth-cohort effect. *Am J Epidemiol* 105:200-213, 1977

134. Paffenbarger RS Jr, Wing AL, Hyde RT: Physical activity as an index of heart attack risk in college alumni. *Am J Epidemiol* 108:161-175, 1978

135. Paffenbarger RS Jr, Hyde RT, Wing AL, et al: The association of changes in physical-activity level and other lifestyle characteristics with mortality among men. *N Engl J Med* 328:538-545, 1993

136. Sandvik L, Erikssen J, Thaulow E, et al: Physical fitness as a predictor of mortality among healthy, middle-aged Norwegian men. *N Engl J Med* 328:533-537, 1993

137. Punsar S, Karvonen MJ: Physical activity and coronary heart disease in populations from East and West Finland. *Adv Cardiol* 18:196-207, 1976

138. Walter SD: Determination of significant relative risks and optimal sampling procedures in prospective and retrospective comparative studies of various sizes. *Am J Epidemiol* 105:387-397, 1977

139. Bassler TJ: Marathon running and immunity to atherosclerosis. *Ann NY Acad Sci* 301:579-592, 1977

140. Handler JB, Asay RW, Warren SE, et al: Symptomatic coronary artery disease in a marathon runner. *JAMA* 248:717-719, 1982

141. Opie LH: Long-distance running and sudden death (letter to the editor). *N Engl J Med* 293:941-942, 1975

142. Colt E: Coronary-artery disease in marathon runners (letter to the editor). *N Engl J Med* 302:57, 1980

143. Maron BJ, Roberts WC, McAllister HA, et al: Sudden death in young athletes. *Circulation* 62:218-229, 1980

144. Noakes TD, Opie LH, Rose AG, et al: Autopsy-proved coronary atherosclerosis in marathon runners. *N Engl J Med* 301:86-89, 1979

145. Thompson PD, Funk EJ, Carleton RA, et al: Incidence of death during jogging in Rhode Island from 1975 through 1980. *JAMA* 247:2535-2538, 1982

146. Leon AS: Comparative cardiovascular adaptation to exercise in animals and man and its relevance to coronary heart disease. In *Comparative Pathophysiology of Circulatory Disturbances.* Edited by CM Bloor. New York, Plenum Publishing Corporation, 1972, pp 143-174

147. Rerych SK, Scholz PM, Sabiston DC Jr, et al: Effects of exercise training on left ventricular function in normal subjects: a longitudinal study by radionuclide angiography. *Am J Cardiol* 45:244-252, 1980

148. Tomoike H, Franklin D, Ross J Jr: Detection of myocardial ischemia by regional dysfunction during and after rapid pacing in conscious dogs. *Circulation* 58:48-56, 1978

149. Badeer HS: Resting bradycardia of exercise training: a concept based on currently available data. *Recent Adv Stud Cardiac Struct Metab* 10:553-560, 1975

150. Aravanis C: Exercise and the heart. *Cardiovasc Clin* 2 No 3:181-195, 1971

151. Lin Y-C, Horvath SM: Autonomic nervous control of cardiac frequency in the exercise-trained rat. *J Appl Physiol* 33:796-799, 1972

152. Bonanno JA, Lies JE: Effects of physical training on coronary risk factors. *Am J Cardiol* 33:760-764, 1974

153. Lopez-S A, René A, Bell L, et al: Metabolic effects of exercise. I. Effect of exercise on serum lipids and lipogenesis in rats. *Proc Soc Exp Biol Med* 148:640-645, 1975

154. Balart L, Moore MC, Gremillion L, et al: Serum lipids, dietary intakes, and physical exercise in medical students. *J Am Diet Assoc* 64:42-46, 1974

155. Hoffman AA, Nelson WR, Goss FA: Effects of an exercise program on plasma lipids of senior Air Force officers. *Am J Cardiol* 20:516-524, 1967

156. Holloszy JO, Skinner JS, Toro G, et al: Effects of a six month program of endurance exercise on the serum lipids of middle-aged men. *Am J Cardiol* 14:753-760, 1964

157. Erkelens DW, Albers JJ, Hazzard WR, et al: High-density lipoprotein-cholesterol in survivors of myocardial infarction. *JAMA* 242:2185-2189, 1979

158. Streja D, Mymin D: Moderate exercise and high-density lipoprotein-cholesterol: observations during a cardiac rehabilitation program. *JAMA* 242:2190-2192, 1979

159. Havel RJ: High-density lipoproteins, cholesterol transport and coronary heart disease (editorial). *Circulation* 60:1-3, 1979

160. Adner MM, Castelli WP: Elevated high-density lipoprotein levels in marathon runners. *JAMA* 243:534-536, 1980

161. Wood PD, Haskell W, Klein H, et al: The distribution of plasma lipoproteins in middle-aged male runners. *Metabolism* 25:1249-1257, 1976

162. Lopez-S A, Vial R, Balart L, et al: Effect of exercise and physical fitness on serum lipids and lipoproteins. *Atherosclerosis* 20:1-9, 1974

163. Tomanek RJ: Effects of age and exercise on the extent of the myocardial capillary bed. *Anat Rec* 167:55-62, 1970

164. Barnard RJ: Long-term effects of exercise on cardiac function. *Exerc Sport Sci Rev* 3:113-133, 1975

165. Hellerstein HK: A misguided goal or unrealized objective? Introduction. *Bibl Cardiol* No 36:125-135, 1977

166. Bemis CE, Gorlin R, Kemp HG, et al: Progression of coronary artery disease: a clinical arteriographic study. *Circulation* 47:455-464, 1973

167. Kennedy CC, Speikerman RE, Lindsay MI Jr, et al: One-year graduated exercise program for men with angina pectoris: evaluation of physiologic studies and coronary arteriography. *Mayo Clin Proc* 51:231-236, 1976

168. Conner JF, LaCamera F Jr, Swanick EJ, et al: Effects of exercise on coronary collateralization: angiographic studies of six patients in a supervised exercise program. *Med Sci Sports* 8:145-151, Fall 1976

169. Hayashi KD, Lewis ER: Sudden death in a marathon runner with widely patent coronary arteries. *Clin Cardiol* 3:288-291, Aug 1980

170. Thompson PD, Stern MP, Williams P, et al: Death during jogging or running: a study of 18 cases. *JAMA* 242:1265-1267, 1979

171. Siscovick DS, Weiss NS, Hallstrom AP, et al: Physical activity and primary cardiac arrest. *JAMA* 248:3113-3117, 1982

172. Stephens T, Jacobs DR Jr, White CC: A descriptive epidemiology of leisure-time physical activity. *Public Health Rep* 100:147-158, 1985

173. Caspersen CJ, Christenson GM, Pollard RA: Status of the 1990 physical fitness and exercise objectives—evidence from NHIS 1985. *Public Health Rep* 101:587-592, 1986

174. Rosenman RH, Brand RJ, Sholtz RI, et al: Relation of corneal arcus to cardiovascular risk factors and the incidence of coronary disease. *N Engl J Med* 291:1322-1324, 1974

175. Lichstein E, Chadda KD, Naik D, et al: Diagonal ear-lobe crease: prevalence and implications as a coronary risk factor. *N Engl J Med* 290:615-616, 1974

176. Strong JP, Correa P, Solberg LA: Water hardness in atherosclerosis. *Lab Invest* 18:620-622, 1968

177. Paffenbarger RS Jr, Wolf PA, Notkin J, et al: Chronic disease in former college students. I. Early precursors of fatal coronary heart disease. *Am J Epidemiol* 83:314-328, 1966

178. Gertler MM, White PD: *Coronary Heart Disease in Young Adults: a Multidisciplinary Study.* Cambridge, Massachusetts, Harvard University Press, 1954

179. Dawber TR, Kannel WB, Gordon T: Coffee and cardiovascular disease: observations from the Framingham Study. *N Engl J Med* 291:871-874, 1974

180. Crawford MD, Gardner MJ, Morris JN: Changes in water hardness and local death-rates. *Lancet* 2:327-329, 1971

181. Barrett-Connor E, Khaw K-T, Yen SSC: A prospective study of dehydroepiandrosterone sulfate, mortality, and cardiovascular disease. *N Engl J Med* 315:1519-1524, 1986

182. Herrington DM, Gordon GB, Achuff SC, et al: Plasma dehydroepiandrosterone and dehydroepiandrosterone sulfate in patients undergoing diagnostic coronary angiography. *J Am Coll Cardiol* 16:862-870, 1990

183. Hendrikx A, Heyns W, De Moor P: Influence of low-calorie diet and fasting on the metabolism of dehydroepiandrosterone sulfate in adult obese subjects. *J Clin Endocrinol* 28:1525-1533, 1968

184. Šonka J, Gregorová I, Tomsová Z, et al: Plasma androsterone, dehydroepiandrosterone and 11-hydroxycorticoids in obesity: effects of diet and physical activity. *Steroids Lipids Res* 3:65-74, 1972
185. Adlercreutz H, Kerstell J, Schaumann K-O, et al: Plasma lipids and steroid hormones in patients with hypercholesterolaemia or hyperlipaemia during dehydroepiandrosterone sulphate administration. *Eur J Clin Invest* 2:91-95, 1972
186. Boers GHJ, Smals AGH, Trijbels FJM, et al: Heterozygosity for homocystinuria in premature peripheral and cerebral occlusive arterial disease. *N Engl J Med* 313:709-715, 1985
187. Malinow MR: Hyperhomocyst(e)inemia: a common and easily reversible risk factor for occlusive atherosclerosis (editorial). *Circulation* 81:2004-2006, 1990
188. Clarke R, Daly L, Robinson K, et al: Hyperhomocysteinemia: an independent risk factor for vascular disease. *N Engl J Med* 324:1149-1155, 1991
189. Cambien F, Poirier O, Lecerf L, et al: Deletion polymorphism in the gene for angiotensin-converting enzyme is a potent risk factor for myocardial infarction. *Nature* 359:641-644, 1992
190. Cornfield J, Mitchell S: Selected risk factors in coronary disease: possible intervention effects. *Arch Environ Health* 19:382-391, 1969
191. Rinzler SH: Primary prevention of coronary heart disease by diet. *Bull NY Acad Med* 44:936-949, 1968
192. National Diet-Heart Study Research Group: The National Diet-Heart Final Report. *Circulation* 37 Suppl 1:1-421, 1968
193. Miettinen M, Turpeinen O, Karvonen MJ, et al: Effect of cholesterol-lowering diet on mortality from coronary heart-disease and other causes: a twelve-year clinical trial in men and women. *Lancet* 2:835-838, 1972
194. Halperin M, Cornfield J, Mitchell SC: Effects of diet on coronary-heart-disease mortality (letter to the editor). *Lancet* 2:438-439, 1973
195. Frantz ID Jr, Dawson EA, Kuba K, et al: The Minnesota coronary survey: effect of diet on cardiovascular events and deaths (abstract). *Circulation* 52 Suppl 2:4, 1975
196. Dayton S, Pearce ML, Hashimoto S, et al: A controlled clinical trial of a diet high in unsaturated fat in preventing complications of atherosclerosis. *Circulation* 40 Suppl 2:1-63, 1969
197. Leren P: The effect of plasma cholesterol lowering diet in male survivors of myocardial infarction: a controlled clinical trial. *Acta Med Scand [Suppl]* 466:5-92, 1966
198. AHA Committee Report: Risk factors in coronary disease: a statement for physicians. *Circulation* 62:449A-455A, 1980
199. Grundy SM, Bilheimer D, Blackburn H, et al: Rationale of the diet-heart statement of the American Heart Association: Report of Nutrition Committee. *Circulation* 65:839A-854A, 1982
200. Sacks FM, Castelli WP, Donner A, et al: Plasma lipids and lipoproteins in vegetarians and controls. *N Engl J Med* 292:1148-1151, 1975
201. Helgeland A: Treatment of mild hypertension: a five year controlled drug trial. The Oslo Study. *Am J Med* 69:725-732, 1980
202. Multiple Risk Factor Intervention Trial Research Group: Mortality after 10½ years for hypertensive participants in the Multiple Risk Factor Intervention Trial. *Circulation* 82:1616-1628, 1990
203. Lipid Research Clinics Program: The Lipid Research Clinics Coronary Primary Prevention Trial results. I. Reduction in incidence of coronary heart disease. II. The relationship of reduction in incidence of coronary heart disease to cholesterol lowering. *JAMA* 251:351-364; 365-374, 1984
204. Levy RI: The influence of cholestyramine-induced lipid changes on coronary artery disease progression: the NHLBI type II coronary intervention study (abstract). *Circulation* 68 Suppl 3:188, 1983
205. Frick MH, Elo O, Haapa K, et al: Helsinki Heart Study: primary-prevention trial with gemfibrozil in middle-aged men with dyslipidemia; safety of treatment, changes in risk factors, and incidence of coronary heart disease. *N Engl J Med* 317:1237-1245, 1987
206. Scandinavian Simvastatin Study Group: Randomised trial of cholesterol lowering in 4444 patients with coronary heart disease: the Scandinavian Simvastatin Survival Study (4S). *Lancet* 344:1383-1389, 1994
207. Furberg CD, Adams HP Jr, Applegate WB, et al: Effect of lovastatin on early carotid atherosclerosis and cardiovascular events. *Circulation* 90:1679-1687, 1994
208. Tyroler HA: Review of lipid-lowering clinical trials in relation to observational epidemiologic studies. *Circulation* 76:515-522, 1987
209. Dalen JE: An apple a day or an aspirin a day? *Arch Intern Med* 151:1066-1069, 1991
210. Elwood PC, Cochrane AL, Burr ML, et al: A randomized controlled trial of acetyl salicylic acid in the secondary prevention of mortality from myocardial infarction. *Br Med J* 1:436-440, 1974
211. The RISC Group: Risk of myocardial infarction and death during treatment with low dose aspirin and intravenous heparin in men with unstable coronary artery disease. *Lancet* 336:827-830, 1990
212. Goldman S, Copeland J, Moritz T, et al: Improvement in early saphenous vein graft patency after coronary artery bypass surgery with antiplatelet therapy: results of a Veterans Administration Cooperative Study. *Circulation* 77:1324-1332, 1988
213. Barnathan ES, Schwartz JS, Taylor L, et al: Aspirin and dipyridamole in the prevention of acute coronary thrombosis complicating coronary angioplasty. *Circulation* 76:125-134, 1987
214. Steering Committee of the Physicians' Health Study Research Group: Final report on the aspirin component of the ongoing Physicians' Health Study. *N Engl J Med* 321:129-135, 1989
215. Meade TW, Wilkes HC, Stirling Y, et al: Randomized controlled trial of low dose warfarin in the primary prevention of ischaemic heart disease in men at high risk: design and pilot study. *Eur Heart J* 9:836-843, 1988
216. Resnekov L, Chediak J, Hirsh J, et al: Antithrombotic agents in coronary artery disease. *Chest* 95 Suppl:52S-72S, 1989
217. Sherman DG, Dyken ML, Fisher M, et al: Antithrombotic therapy for cerebrovascular disorders. *Chest* 95 Suppl:140S-155S, 1989
218. Cooper R, Stamler J, Dyer A, et al: The decline in mortality from coronary heart disease, U.S.A., 1968-1975. *J Chronic Dis* 31:709-720, 1978
219. Kannel WB, Thom TJ: Implications of the recent decline in cardiovascular mortality. *Cardiovasc Med* 4:983-997, 1979
220. United States Department of Health, Education and Welfare: Vital Statistics of the United States, 1968 to 1975. Vol. 2, Part A, Mortality. Washington DC, Government Printing Office, 1972, 1974, 1974, 1975, 1975, 1976, 1977
221. National Center for Health Statistics: Vital Statistics of the United States, 1978. Vol. 2, Part A, DHHS Publication No (PHS) 83-1101. Public Health Service, Washington DC, US Government Printing Office, 1982
222. Stamler J: George Lyman Duff Memorial Lecture: Lifestyles, major risk factors, proof and public policy. *Circulation* 58:3-19, 1978
223. Stern MP: The recent decline in ischemic heart disease mortality. *Ann Intern Med* 91:630-640, 1979
224. Krishan I: Public health education and the control of hypertension in the United States. *Mayo Clin Proc* 54:794-801, 1979
225. European Coronary Surgery Study Group: Coronary-artery bypass surgery in stable angina pectoris: survival at two years. *Lancet* 1:889-893, 1979
226. Webster JS, Moberg C, Rincon G: Natural history of severe proximal coronary artery disease as documented by coronary cineangiography. *Am J Cardiol* 33:195-200, 1974
227. Reeves TJ, Oberman A, Jones WB, et al: Natural history of angina pectoris. *Am J Cardiol* 33:423-430, 1974
228. Goldman L, Cook F, Hashimoto B, et al: Evidence that hospital care for acute myocardial infarction has not contributed to the decline in coronary mortality between 1973-1974 and 1978-1979. *Circulation* 65:936-942, 1982
229. Beaglehole R: International trends in coronary heart disease: mortality, morbidity, and risk factors. *Epidemiol Rev* 12:1-15, 1990
230. Rosenstock IM: Historical origins of the health belief model. *Health Educ Monogr* 2:328-335, 1974
231. Becker MH, Maiman LA: Sociobehavioral determinants of compliance with health and medical care recommendations. *Med Care* 13:10-24, 1975
232. Janz NK, Becker MH: The health belief model: a decade later. *Health Educ Q* 11:1-47, 1984
233. Mechanic D, Cleary PD: Factors associated with the maintenance of positive health behavior. *Prev Med* 9:805-814, 1980
234. Johnson AW: *Quantification in Cultural Anthropology; An Introduction to Research Design.* Stanford, California, Stanford University Press, 1978, pp 141-157
235. Marlatt GA, Gordon JR: Determinants of relapse: implications for the maintenance of behavior change. In *Behavioral Medicine: Changing Health Lifestyles.* (Banff International Conference on Behavior Modification, 10th, 1978.) Edited by P Davidson, SM Davidson. New York, Brunner/Mazel, 1980, pp 410-452
236. Bandura A: *Social Learning Theory.* Englewood Cliffs, New Jersey, Prentice-Hall, 1977, p 5

237. Mullen PD, Green LW, Persinger GS: Clinical trials of patient education for chronic conditions: a comparative meta-analysis of intervention types. *Prev Med* 14:753-781, 1985

238. Kottke TE: Risk factor control in coronary heart disease: Who needs it? *Postgrad Med* 78:233-245, 1985

239. Skinner BF: *Science and Human Behavior.* New York, Macmillan, 1953

240. National Cholesterol Education Program: Report of the Expert Panel on Population Strategies for Blood Cholesterol Reduction: executive summary. *Arch Intern Med* 151:1071-1084, 1991

241. Stamler J, Wentworth D, Neaton JD: Is relationship between serum cholesterol and risk of premature death from coronary heart disease continuous and graded? Findings in 356, 222 primary screenees of the Multiple Risk Factor Intervention Trial (MRFIT). *JAMA* 256:2823-2828, 1986

242. Whiteside C, Robbins JA: Cholesterol knowledge and practices among patients compared with physician management in a university primary care setting. *Prev Med* 18:526-531, 1989

243. Johnson CL, Rifkind BM, Sempos CT, et al: Declining serum total cholesterol levels among US adults: the National Health and Nutrition Examination Surveys. *JAMA* 269:3002-3008, 1993

244. Expert Panel on Detection, Evaluation, and Treatment of High Blood Cholesterol in Adults: Summary of the Second Report of the National Cholesterol Education Program (NCEP) Expert Panel on Detection, Evaluation, and Treatment of High Blood Cholesterol in Adults (Adult Treatment Panel II). *JAMA* 269:3015-3023, 1993

245. Parsons WB Jr, Achor RWP, Berge KG, et al: Changes in concentration of blood lipids following prolonged administration of large doses of nicotinic acid to persons with hypercholesterolemia: preliminary observations. *Proc Staff Meet Mayo Clin* 31:377-390, 1956

246. Andersson RGG, Åberg G, Brattsand R, et al: Studies on the mechanism of flush induced by nicotinic acid. *Acta Pharmacol Toxicol* 41:1-10, 1977

247. LeLorier J, DuBreuil-Quidoz S, Lussier-Cacan S, et al: Diet and probucol in lowering cholesterol concentrations: additive effects on plasma cholesterol concentrations in patients with familial type II hyperlipoproteinemia. *Arch Intern Med* 137:1429-1434, 1977

248. Steinberg D, Parthasarathy S, Carew TE, et al: Beyond cholesterol: modifications of low-density lipoprotein that increase its atherogenicity. *N Engl J Med* 320:915-924, 1989

249. *Physicians' Desk Reference.* Thirty-fifth edition. Oradell, New Jersey, Medical Economics Company, 1981, pp 858-859

250. Tikkanen MJ, Nikkilä EA: Current pharmacologic treatment of elevated serum cholesterol. *Circulation* 76:529-533, 1987

251. The Lovastatin Study Group II: Therapeutic response to lovastatin (Mevinolin) in nonfamilial hypercholesterolemia: a multicenter study. *JAMA* 256:2829-2834, 1986

252. Malloy MJ, Kane JP, Kunitake ST, et al: Complementarity of colestipol, niacin, and lovastatin in treatment of severe familial hypercholesterolemia. *Ann Intern Med* 107:616-623, 1987

253. Tobert JA: Reply to letters to the editor. *N Engl J Med* 318:48, 1988

254. Gould AL, Rossouw JE, Santanello NC, et al: Cholesterol reduction yields clinical benefit: a new look at old data. *Circulation* 91:2274-2282, 1995

255. Buchwald H: Lowering of cholesterol absorption and blood levels by ileal exclusion: experimental basis and preliminary clinical report. *Circulation* 29:713-720, 1964

256. Buchwald H, Varco RL, Matts JP, et al: Effect of partial ileal bypass surgery on mortality and morbidity from coronary heart disease in patients with hypercholesterolemia: report of the Program on the Surgical Control of the Hyperlipidemias (POSCH). *N Engl J Med* 323:946-955, 1990

257. Grundy SM, Ahrens EH Jr, Salen G: Interruption of the enterohepatic circulation of bile acids in man: comparative effects of cholestyramine and ileal exclusion on cholesterol metabolism. *J Lab Clin Med* 78:94-121, 1971

258. Thompson GR, Lowenthal R, Myant NB: Plasma exchange in the management of homozygous familial hypercholesterolaemia. *Lancet* 1:1208-1211, 1975

259. Barr SI, Kottke BA, Pineda AA, et al: Plasma lipid and apoprotein levels following plasmapheresis in a subject homozygous for familial hypercholesterolemia. *Experientia* 37:114-115, 1981

260. Stampfer MJ, Willett WC, Colditz GA, et al: A prospective study of past use of oral contraceptive agents and risk of cardiovascular diseases. *N Engl J Med* 319:1313-1317, 1988

261. Tikkanen MJ, Kuusi T, Vartianen E, et al: Treatment of post-menopausal hypercholesterolaemia with estradiol. *Acta Obstet Gynecol Scand Suppl* 88:83-88, 1979

262. The Coronary Drug Project Research Group: The Coronary Drug Project: initial findings leading to modifications of its research protocol. *JAMA* 214:1303-1313, 1970

263. Miller VT, Meusing RA, LaRosa JC, et al: Effects of conjugated equine estrogen with and without three different progestogens on lipoproteins, high-density lipoprotein subfractions, and apolipoprotein A-I. *Obstet Gynecol* 77:235-240, 1991

264. Suinn RM, Bloom LJ: Anxiety management training for pattern A behavior. *J Behav Med* 1:25-35, 1978

265. Rosenman RH, Friedman M: Modifying Type A behaviour pattern. *J Psychosom Res* 21:323-331, 1977

266. Friedman M, Thoresen CE, Gill JJ, et al: Alteration of type A behavior and its effect on cardiac recurrences in post myocardial infarction patients: summary results of the Recurrent Coronary Prevention Project. *Am Heart J* 112:653-665, 1986

267. Jacobs D, Blackburn H, Higgins M, et al: Report of the Conference on Low Blood Cholesterol: Mortality Associations. *Circulation* 86:1046-1060, 1992

268. Hulley SB, Walsh JMB, Newman TB: Health policy and blood cholesterol: time to change directions. *Circulation* 86:1026-1029, 1992

269. Kottke TE, Battista RN, DeFriese GH, et al: Attributes of successful smoking cessation interventions in medical practice. A meta-analysis of 39 controlled trials. *JAMA* 259:2883-2889, 1988

270. Kottke TE, Solberg LI, Brekke ML, et al: A controlled trial to integrate smoking cessation advice into primary care practice: doctors helping smokers, Round III. *J Fam Pract* 34:701-708, 1992

271. Kottke TE, Solberg LI, Brekke ML: Beyond efficacy testing: introducing preventive cardiology into primary care. *Am J Prev Med* 6 (suppl 1):77-83, 1990

272. *AAFP Stop Smoking Program. Physician and Office Staff Manual.* Kansas City, Missouri, American Academy of Family Physicians, 1987

273. Kottke TE, Brekke ML, Solberg LI, et al: A randomized trial to increase smoking intervention by physicians: doctors helping smokers, round 1. *JAMA* 261:2101-2106, 1989

274. Kottke TE, Hill C, Heitzig C, et al: Smoke-free hospitals: attitudes of patients, employees, and faculty. *Minn Med* 68:53-55, 1985

275. Hurt RD, Berge KG, Offord KP, et al: The making of a smoke-free medical center. *JAMA* 261:95-97, 1989

276. Becker DM, Connor HF, Waranch HR, et al: Banning smoking in a children's hospital: Are employees supportive? *Prev Med* 18:72-78, 1989

277. Knapp J, Silvis G, Sorensen G, et al: *Clean Air Health Care. A Guide to Establish Smoke-Free Health Care Facilities.* Minneapolis, Minnesota Coalition for a Smoke-Free Society 2000, 1986

278. The impact of providing physicians with quit-smoking materials for smoking patients. *CA* 31:75-78, 1981

279. *Clearing the Air.* (DHHS National Institutes of Health Publication No [PHS] 89-1647.) Bethesda, Maryland, National Cancer Institute, February 1989

280. *AAFP Stop Smoking Program. Patient Stop Smoking Guide.* Kansas City, Missouri, American Academy of Family Physicians, 1987

281. Glynn TJ, Manley MW: *How to Help Your Patients Stop Smoking. A National Cancer Institute Manual for Physicians.* (NIH Publication No 89-3064). Bethesda, Maryland, Smoking, Tobacco, and Cancer Program, Division of Cancer Prevention and Control, National Cancer Institute, 1989

282. Harris SS, Caspersen CJ, DeFriese GH, et al: Physical activity counseling for healthy adults as a primary preventive intervention in the clinical setting: report for the US Preventive Services Task Force. *JAMA* 261:3590-3598, 1989

283. National Cholesterol Education Program: Report of the Expert Panel on Blood Cholesterol Levels in Children and Adolescents. (NIH Publication No 91-2732). Washington DC, US Department of Health and Human Services, 1991

284. Golubjatnikov R, Paskey T, Inhorn SL: Serum cholesterol levels of Mexican and Wisconsin school children. *Am J Epidemiol* 96:36-39, 1972

285. Moll PP, Sing CF, Weidman WH, et al: Total cholesterol and lipoproteins in school children: prediction of coronary heart disease in adult relatives. *Circulation* 67:127-134, 1983

286. Havlik RJ, Garrison RJ, Feinleib M, et al: Blood pressure aggregation in families. *Am J Epidemiol* 110:304-312, 1979

287. Bringgold B, Labarthe DR, Weidman WH: A re-examination of the "tracking" hypothesis in a familial study of blood pressure (abstract). *Circulation* 54 Suppl 2:24, 1976

288. Rames LK, Clarke WR, Connor WE, et al: Normal blood pressures and the evaluation of sustained blood pressure elevation in children: the Muscatine Study. *Pediatrics* 61:245-251, 1978

289. Epstein FH, Lloyd J: Study of atherosclerosis precursors in children. Report of WHO CVD-74.4, Geneva, 1974

290. Heyden S, Bartel AG, Hames CG, et al: Elevated blood pressure levels in adolescents, Evans County, Georgia: seven-year follow-up of 30 patients and 30 controls. *JAMA* 209:1683-1689, 1969

291. Paffenbarger RS, Thorne MC, Wing AL: Chronic disease in former college students. VIII. Characteristics in youth predisposing to hypertension in later years. *Am J Epidemiol* 88:25-32, 1968

292. Arkin RM, Roemhild HF, Johnson CA, et al: The Minnesota Smoking Prevention Program: a seventh-grade health curriculum supplement. *J Sch Health* 51:611-616, 1981

293. Katz SH, Hediger ML, Schall JI, et al: Blood pressure, growth and maturation from childhood through adolescence: mixed longitudinal analyses of the Philadelphia Blood Pressure Project. *Hypertension* 2 Suppl 1:55-69, 1980

294. Wood PD, Klein H, Lewis S, et al: Plasma lipoprotein concentrations in middle-aged runners (abstract). *Circulation* 50 Suppl 3:115, 1974

295. Brownell KD, Bachorik PS, Ayerle RS: Changes in plasma lipid and lipoprotein levels in men and women after a program of moderate exercise. *Circulation* 65:477-484, 1982

296. Fisch IR, Frank J: Oral contraceptives and blood pressure. *JAMA* 237:2499-2503, 1977

297. Tsang RC, Fallat RW, Glueck CJ: Cholesterol at birth and age 1: comparison of normal and hypercholesterolemic neonates. *Pediatrics* 53:458-470, 1974

298. Quivers ES, Driscoll DJ, Garvey CD, et al: Variability in response to a low-fat, low-cholesterol diet in children with elevated low-density lipoprotein cholesterol levels. *Pediatrics* 89:925-929, 1992

299. Nichols AB, Ravenscroft C, Lamphiear DE, et al: Daily nutritional intake and serum lipid levels: the Tecumseh study. *Am J Clin Nutr* 29:1384-1392, 1976

300. Goldstein JL, Brown MS: The low-density lipoprotein pathway and its relation to atherosclerosis. *Annu Rev Biochem* 46:897-930, 1977

301. Ellefson RD, Elveback LR, Hodgson PA, et al: Cholesterol and triglycerides in serum lipoproteins of young persons in Rochester, Minnesota. *Mayo Clin Proc* 53:307-320, 1978

302. Kwiterovich PO Jr, Heiss G, Johnson N, et al: Assessment of plasma total cholesterol as a test to detect elevated low density (beta) lipoprotein cholesterol levels (type IIa hyperlipoproteinemia) in young subjects from a population-based sample. *Am J Epidemiol* 115:192-204, 1982

303. Wynder EL, Berenson GS, Strong WB, et al: Coronary artery disease prevention: cholesterol, a pediatric perspective. *Prev Med* 18:323-409, 1989

304. Perry CL, Luepker RV, Murray DM, et al: Parent involvement with children's health promotion: the Minnesota Home Team. *Am J Public Health* 78:1156-1160, 1988

305. Crockett SJ, Mullis R, Perry CL, et al: Parent education in youth-directed nutrition interventions. *Prev Med* 18:475-491, 1989

306. Schrott HG, Clarke WR, Wiebe DA, et al: Increased coronary mortality in relatives of hypercholesterolemic school children: the Muscatine Study. *Circulation* 59:320-326, 1979

307. Morrison JA, Khoury P, Mellies MJ, et al: Identifying CHD risk factors in children: intrafamilial lipoprotein correlations. *Prev Med* 9:484-495, 1980

308. Morrison JA, Kelly K, Horvitz R, et al: Parent-offspring and sibling lipid and lipoprotein associations during and after sharing of household environments: the Princeton School District Family Study. *Metabolism* 31:158-166, 1982

309. Task Force Committee of the Nutrition Committee and the Cardiovascular Disease in the Young Council of the American Heart Association: Diet in the healthy child. *Circulation* 67 No 6:A-1411-A-1414, 1983

310. Diagnosis and treatment of primary hyperlipidemia in childhood. (A Joint Statement for Physicians by the Committee on Atherosclerosis and Hypertension in Childhood of the Council of Cardiovascular Disease in the Young and the Nutrition Committee, American Heart Association.) *Circulation* 74 No 5:A-1181-A-1188, 1986

311. Clarke WR, Schrott HG, Leaverton PE, et al: Tracking of blood lipids and blood pressures in school age children: the Muscatine Study. *Circulation* 58:626-634, 1978

312. Laskarzewski P, Morrison JA, deGroot I, et al: Lipid and lipoprotein tracking in 108 children over a four-year period. *Pediatrics* 64:584-591, 1979

313. Folsom AR, Luepker RV, Gillum RF, et al: Improvement in hypertension detection and control from 1973-1974 to 1980-1981: the Minnesota Heart Survey experience. *JAMA* 250:916-921, 1983

314. Lipid Metabolism Branch, Division of Heart and Vascular Diseases, National Heart, Lung, and Blood Institute. *The Lipid Research Clinics Population Studies Data Book.* Vol 1. *The Prevalence Study.* (NIH Publication No 80-1527). Washington DC, US Department of Health and Human Services, Public Health Service, National Institutes of Health, 1980

315. Kottke TE, Gatewood LC, Wu S-C, et al: Preventing heart disease: Is treating the high risk sufficient? *J Clin Epidemiol* 41:1083-1093, 1988

316. Kottke TE, Gatewood LC, Park HA: Using serum cholesterol to identify high risk and stimulate behavior change: Will it work? *Ann Med* 21:181-187, 1989

317. Puska P, Nissinen A, Tuomilehto J, et al: The community-based strategy to prevent coronary heart disease: conclusions from the ten years of the North Karelia project. *Annu Rev Public Health* 6:147-193, 1985

318. Rose G: Strategy of prevention: lessons from cardiovascular disease. *Br Med J* 282:1847-1851, 1981

319. Epstein FH, Holland WW: Prevention of chronic diseases in the community – one-disease versus multiple-disease strategies. *Int J Epidemiol* 12:135-137, 1983

320. Martin MJ, Hulley SB, Browner WS, et al: Serum cholesterol, blood pressure, and mortality: implications from a cohort of 361,662 men. *Lancet* 2:933-936, 1986

321. Rose G, Shipley M: Plasma cholesterol concentration and death from coronary heart disease: 10 year results of the Whitehall study. *Br Med J* 293:306-307, 1986

322. Kottke TE, Nissinen A, Puska P, et al: Message dissemination for a community-based cardiovascular disease prevention programme (the North Karelia project). *Scand J Prim Health Care* 2:99-104, 1984

323. Office of Disease Prevention and Health Promotion. Integration of Risk Factor Interventions. Two reports to the Office of Disease Prevention and Health Promotion. Washington, DC, US Department of Health and Human Services (PHS), November 1986

324. Sackett DL, Haynes RB, Gibson ES, et al: Randomised clinical trial of strategies for improving medication compliance in primary hypertension. *Lancet* 1:1205-1207, 1975

325. Haynes RB, Sackett DL, Taylor DW, et al: Increased absenteeism from work after detection and labeling of hypertensive patients. *N Engl J Med* 299:741-744, 1978

326. Polk BF, Harlan LC, Cooper SP, et al: Disability days associated with detection and treatment in a hypertension control program. *Am J Epidemiol* 119:44-53, 1984

327. Salonen JT, Heinonen OP, Kottke TE, et al: Change in health behaviour in relation to estimated coronary heart disease risk during a community-based cardiovascular disease prevention programme. *Int J Epidemiol* 10:343-354, 1981

328. Kottke TE: Reducing community risk of heart disease. *J Am Coll Cardiol* 12:1113-1116, 1988

329. Report of a Task Force to the Conference of Deputy Ministers of Health. *Periodic Health Examination Monograph.* Hull, Quebec, Canadian Publishing Center, 1980

330. Report of the US Preventive Services Task Force. *Guide to Clinical Preventive Services: An Assessment of the Effectiveness of 169 Interventions.* Baltimore, Maryland, Williams & Wilkins, 1989

331. Eraker SA, Becker MH, Strecher VJ, et al: Smoking behavior, cessation techniques, and the health decision model. *Am J Med* 78:817-825, 1985

332. Oppenheim M: Healers. *N Engl J Med* 303:1117-1120, 1980

333. Kottke TE, Solberg LI, Brekke ML: Initiation and maintenance of behavioral change: What is the role of the physician? *J Gen Intern Med* 5 (Suppl 5S):62-67, 1990

334. Freidson E: *Profession of Medicine: a Study of the Sociology of Applied Knowledge.* New York, Dodd, Mead & Company, 1970, p 355

335. White PD: The evolution of our knowledge of the heart and its diseases. In *The Heart, Arteries, and Veins.* Second edition. Edited by JW Hurst, RB Logue. New York, McGraw-Hill Book Company, 1970, pp 3-4

CHAPTER

14

Cardiac rehabilitation and cardiovascular health enhancement

Ray W. Squires, Ph.D., Gerald T. Gau, M.D., Todd D. Miller, M.D., Thomas G. Allison, Ph.D., and Pamela B. Morris, M.D.

Cardiac rehabilitation is a longitudinal form of care designed to develop and maintain a desirable level of physical, social, and psychologic ability in patients with cardiovascular disease.[1] Education, counseling, and exercise are combined to assist patients in returning to a near-normal lifestyle as soon as possible after recognition of the disease or in adapting to the limitations imposed by the disease. Identification of risk factors and their modification form a central theme designed to retard progression of[2,3] or potentially to reverse[4-6] the disease process to reduce the probability of future clinical manifestations.

Because coronary artery disease is a chronic condition, usually requiring decades to reach clinical importance,[7] and because in 30% to 40% of cases sudden cardiac collapse is the first manifestation of the disease,[8] emphasis has been placed on primary prevention by efforts to ameliorate selected risk factors.[9] The welcome decline in coronary mortality in the United States during the past 3 decades corresponds to a time when a sizable segment of the population has adopted a "more healthful" lifestyle, as indicated by a reduction in certain risk factors: cigarette smoking, high-fat diet, elevated serum cholesterol, hypertension, and physical inactivity.[10] Although the positive change in some risk factors has not been established as being responsible for the decline in cardiovascular mortality, the pattern suggests that risk-factor alteration has had an impact.[11]

ADMINISTRATION

The American Association of Cardiovascular and Pulmonary Rehabilitation[12] and the American College of Sports Medicine[13] have published state-of-the-art guidelines for cardiac rehabilitation programs. Certification by the American College of Sports Medicine of the personnel involved with the exercise portion of rehabilitation has become generally accepted.

The primary patient population that may benefit from cardiac rehabilitation consists of selected patients with cardiovascular disease, that is, acute myocardial infarction, angina pectoris, cardiac surgery (bypass grafting, percutaneous coronary angioplasty, laser angioplasty, coronary atherectomy, valve repair or replacement, valvuloplasty, congenital abnormalities, and cardiac or cardiopulmonary transplantation), cardiomyopathy, peripheral vascular disease, hypertension, and angiographically demonstrated but silent disease. Additional patient subgroups may benefit from exercise training and other rehabilitation efforts, such as pacemaker, cardioverter-defibrillator, renal dialysis, renal or renal-pancreatic transplantation, liver transplantation, pulmonary disease, obesity, diabetes mellitus, anxiety and depression, neurologic problems (stroke, spinal cord injury), cancer, and drug dependency.

The current practice in cardiac rehabilitation deals with multiple aspects of a patient's life: risk-factor modification, nutrition, exercise, psychosocial status, family relationships, stress management, vocational adjustment, and understanding of the acute event. The components of the rehabilitation program require individualization, and the primary physician usually cannot allocate sufficient time to supervise each aspect personally. The team approach, utilizing the collective skills and experience of many health professions, has been successful in overcoming the limitations of physician time and attaining the stated rehabilitation goals.[14-17] The interdisciplinary approach allows patient management problems to be addressed in a comprehensive manner (Table 14-1).

Most patients have the potential to benefit from the instructional aspects of the program, such as information regarding the acute event, medications, diet, smoking cessation, stress management, psychosocial adjustment, and group discussion. The exercise portion of the program should be restricted to patients who do not exhibit any absolute contraindication to exercise training (Table 14-2). These conditions, if unresolved, exclude patients from the exercise program.

The primary physician retains the responsibility for the rehabilitation of his or her patients. He or she may elect to utilize the experience of the rehabilitation specialists by referring patients to the program. The patient referral process does not mean that the referring physician is relinquishing control or responsibility. The cardiac reha-

Table 14-1 Cardiac rehabilitation team members

Primary physician	Nurse coordinator
Cardiologist	Physical therapist
Surgeon	Occupational therapist
Psychiatrist	Dietitian
Physiatrist	Cardiac rehabilitation nurse
Exercise physiologist	Primary nurse
Psychologist	Physician extender
Pharmacist	Exercise specialist
Social worker	Nicotine-dependence counselor
Vocational rehabilitation counselor	

Table 14-2 Absolute contraindications to exercise training

Unstable angina pectoris	Thrombophlebitis
Dangerous arrhythmias	Recent systemic or pulmonary embolus
Overt cardiac failure	Severe hypertension
Severe left ventricular outflow tract obstruction	Overt psychoneurotic disturbances
Dissecting aneurysm	Uncontrolled diabetes mellitus
Serious systemic disease	Severe orthopedic limitation
Myocarditis (acute)	

bilitation program is designed to improve patient care and to assist the physician in patient management. The program provides patient surveillance to assist the primary physician in determining the effectiveness of the specific treatment modalities employed. Problems that occur are communicated to the referring physician, and treatment questions are his or her responsibility. An essential component of a well-functioning program is a flow of information to the primary physician regarding the patient's progress.

PROGRAM OVERVIEW (Table 14-3)

Inpatient rehabilitation – phase I

The phase I program begins with admission, is medically supervised, and continues until hospital dismissal. This initial rehabilitation effort includes, but is not limited to, patients with acute myocardial infarction or angina pectoris, those who have undergone revascularization, and cardiac transplant recipients.

Individual patient needs must be addressed, with inclusion of family members and significant others in the rehabilitation process. Program components include patient and family education, group and individual counseling, group discussion sessions, and controlled low-level exercise. The objectives are diverse:

1. To hasten adjustment to the hospital environment and the acute event by providing information regarding cardiac rehabilitation procedures and the recovery process
2. To begin risk-factor assessment, grading, and modification for secondary prevention
3. To prevent potential deleterious effects of prolonged bed rest
4. To facilitate return to physical activity and thereby reduce the feelings of invalidism
5. To provide medical surveillance – that is, to determine the appropriateness of psychologic adaptation and the hemodynamic and ECG responses to exercise
6. To maintain neuromuscular relaxation

Table 14-3 Phases of cardiac rehabilitation

Phase	Type of program	Duration
I	Inpatient	Days
II	Outpatient, immediate post-hospitalization	2-12 wk
III	Late recovery period	Minimum of 6 mo beyond phase II
IV	Maintenance program	Indefinite

The common psychologic responses of a patient to an acute cardiac event have been described.[18,19] Panic and anxiety surface during the first hours after myocardial infarction. Precipitating factors include the stress of illness, unfamiliar surroundings, the threat of death, and discomfort. Depression, probably related to a feeling of loss of physical ability or potential as an individual, may occur as early as 3 days after the event or during the early outpatient phase of recovery. The depression is usually transient and may be characterized by typical somatization complaints of fatigue or nonspecific discomfort. Denial is common and may constitute a beneficial response (that is, complete acceptance of the illness but denial of its seriousness) or may be manifested by complete rejection of the reality of the illness. Beneficial denial is associated with a high potential for rehabilitation and a favorable outcome.[20] Careful education and encouragement are generally all that is necessary, with particular emphasis on the normal psychologic reaction to a cardiac event as well as stress education.

Education is provided by the nursing staff and other health professionals such as physical and occupational therapists, dietitians, and pharmacists. Patient teaching is coordinated by the cardiac rehabilitation nurse.

The topics of medication, proper diet, and cessation of smoking are particularly emphasized. Cardiovascular anatomy and disease along with dismissal plans are discussed. Information regarding community resources for financial assistance and job retraining and placement is included, as needed. A multimedia presentation of information (oral, written, audiovisual) is utilized. Individual and group approaches are used. Education and discussion groups appear to help reduce patient and family anxiety and serve as an outlet for expression of

Table 14-4 Mayo Clinic inpatient cardiac rehabilitation physical activity protocol

Stage	Days of program: 6-day plan	9-day plan	12-day plan	Activity schedule
I	1	1	1	Use bedside commode. Begin physical therapy range-of-motion exercises to each extremity. Sit at side of bed 5-10 min.
		2	2	Sit in chair 5-15 min twice daily. Begin education program at bedside. Continue physical therapy as above.
	2	3	3	Sit in chair up to 30 min twice daily. Continue physical therapy as above.
II	3	4	5	Move to step-down area. Bathe above waist, shave, and comb hair. Begin self-exercise program with physical therapy supervision. Sit in chair 60-120 min twice daily.
		5	7	Continue self-exercise program with physical therapy supervision. Begin ambulation with physical therapist. Sit in chair 90-150 min twice daily. Begin attending education classes and discussion groups.
		6	8	Take wheelchair shower and use bathroom ad lib. Continue physical activity as above.I
III	4	7	9	Move to general cardiovascular ward. Dress in street clothes if desired. Be up and around room as tolerated. Begin climbing stairs with physical therapist.
	5	8	11	Take predismissal graded-exercise test. Continue physical activity as above. Take standing shower.
	6	9	12	Receive final going-home instructions.

Note: A 4-day accelerated plan for selected low-risk patients is also available.

fears and concerns. The peer-group atmosphere reinforces and enhances the learning process. Group discussions provide psychologic support for the patient and family and allow review of material covered in the education program. The goal of patient education is to have the information understood on a level that will result in a change in behavior which will enable the patient to assume some of the responsibility for his or her care.[21] Education has been shown to have a favorable influence on patient adherence to a medical regimen.[22]

The physical activity program follows a step-by-step written protocol (Table 14-4). A step is defined as a specified activity level, and patients typically advance one step each day. Exercise guidelines are similar for all patients and are conservative in intensity and duration. At our institution, three stages of activity are identified. Stage I begins when the patient is hemodynamically and electrically stable in the intensive care unit. This stage commences with passive range-of-motion exercises and sitting at the bedside and in an armchair to maintain vasomotor reflexes that prevent orthostatic hypotension. For some patients after myocardial infarction, the recent severe chest pain and the associated anxiety tend to produce subconscious contraction of the shoulder girdle musculature, and this may result in chest wall myalgia and periarthritis of the shoulder.[23] Range-of-motion exercises are initiated, with emphasis on voluntary relaxation of the shoulder and pelvic girdle musculature.

During stage II, the patient gradually assumes self-care activities, supervised walking, and active motion exercises. An upper-limit heart rate of 20 beats/min above the rate for standing at rest is used. If necessary, the occupational therapist discusses specific techniques of energy conservation with the patient and spouse which will allow greater independence and freedom in the home during recovery.

The safety of low-level inpatient physical activity for both acute myocardial infarction patients[24,25] and coronary bypass surgery patients[26] has been established. Early ambulation does not result in an increase of hospital or follow-up complications such as angina pectoris, recurrent myocardial infarction, sudden cardiac death, ventricular aneurysm, or congestive heart failure.[27] The hemodynamic responses to early exercise are moderate and acceptable. Heart rate responses for active range of motion and ambulation are between 5 and 15 beats/min above resting levels. The systolic blood pressure response is 4 to 14 mm Hg above rest.[28]

Progressive ambulation at 1 to 2 mph for up to 10 minutes three times daily is supervised by the physical therapist during stage III. Stair climbing at a conservative pace is also performed. Throughout stage III, the patient dresses in street clothes. Dismissal plans with respect to medications and diet are discussed. A predismissal or early postdismissal submaximal graded-exercise test using either a rehabilitation treadmill protocol (Naughton) or a nuclear cardiology procedure (radionuclide angiogram or thallium perfusion scan) is usually performed. The purposes of this test include the assessment of multiple factors (ECG or nuclear medicine evidence of ischemia, blood pressure, symptoms, exercise capacity) that may be prognostic of the future clinical course and of the ability of the patient to meet the challenges of daily tasks, determination of a safe level for the home exercise prescription, and instillation of confidence in the patient and family.[29,30] The feasibility and safety of predismissal graded-exercise testing of both myocardial infarction patients[31,32] and coronary bypass surgery patients[30] have been established. Exercise test end points include fatigue or dyspnea, attainment of an exercise intensity of 5 to 6 METs (1 MET = resting energy expenditure equivalent to 3.5 mL $O_2 \cdot kg^{-1} \cdot min^{-1}$), severe angina pectoris, exertional hypotension, and the development of ECG abnormalities (serious arrhythmias, heart block, significant ST-segment displacement).

Théroux et al.[32] pointed out the prognostic value of early post-myocardial-infarction exercise testing in predicting mortality (17 of 64 patients, or 27%, with ST-segment depression vs. 3 of 146 patients, or 2.1%, with no ST-segment abnormality on submaximal exercise testing). Reinfarction or death has been reported to be six times greater in patients with ST-segment depression on predismissal submaximal exercise testing.[33] Patients with exercise-induced ST-segment depression, angina pectoris, or inadequate blood pressure response to exercise have a significantly greater incidence of all cardiac events during follow-up.[34] It is possible that gated cardiac pool scanning with exercise early after a myocardial infarction may add more specific predictive information.[35] Schulze et al.[36] found that all sudden cardiac deaths during a mean of 7 months after myocardial infarction occurred in the group with low ejection fraction (less than 40%) as determined by gated cardiac pool scanning. They also noted that complex ventricular arrhythmias (Lown class III to V) identified those patients who died during the follow-up period. However, the cost-effectiveness of imaging techniques in addition to the standard treadmill exercise test is under evaluation.

A detailed home exercise program is prepared and discussed with the patient and spouse before hospital dismissal. Table 14-5 gives a graduated activity guideline

Table 14-5 Guidelines for graduated activity after dismissal from the hospital following myocardial infarction*

Week 1

METs	mL $O_2 \cdot kg^{-1} \cdot min^{-1}$	kcal/min (70-kg person)
1½-3	5-11	2-4

1. Any light activity that can be done while sitting
2. Walking, 1-2 mph, on level
3. Stationary cycling, minimal resistance
4. Light household work
   - Dishes or meal preparation (alternate with rest periods)
   - Dusting
   - Sweeping
5. Personal hygiene
   - Shaving
   - Showering
   - Dressing

Week 2

METs	mL $O_2 \cdot kg^{-1} \cdot min^{-1}$	kcal/min (70-kg person)
≤4	11-14	4-5

1. More social activity
   - Playing cards at home
   - Visiting neighbors
   - Car riding
2. Walking, 2-3 mph, on level
3. Stationary cycling, slight resistance
4. Increased household work
   - Bedmaking
   - Ironing
   - Minor appliance repair
   - Bench work
   - Supervising farm work
5. Potential return to part-time work

Week 3

METs	mL $O_2 \cdot kg^{-1} \cdot min^{-1}$	kcal/min (70-kg person)
≤5	14-18	5-6

1. Driving with another driver present
2. Household work, vacuuming
3. Resumption of sexual intercourse
4. Social activity
   - Movies
   - Church
   - Concerts
5. Walking, 3.5 mph
6. Stationary cycling, slight resistance
7. Lifting, 10-15 lb

Week 4

METs	mL $O_2 \cdot kg^{-1} \cdot min^{-1}$	kcal/min (70-kg person)
<6	18-21	6-7

1. Driving alone
2. Light gardening
3. Pitch and putt golfing
4. Social group activities
   - Club meetings
   - Parties
   - Dancing
5. Grocery shopping (no heavy lifting)
6. Walking, stationary cycling

*These guidelines should be altered according to the patient's clinical status. Beyond week 4, heavier activity may be added gradually on an individual basis. Return to work may be as soon as week 2, depending on the nature of the work responsibilities and the patient's condition.

for the initial 4 weeks after dismissal from the hospital. Low-level calisthenics and either walking or stationary cycling are prescribed in a graded format; the heart rate measurement is used as an indicator for a desirable level of energy expenditure.

With respect to results of phase I, evaluation of the impact of patient education and exercise for hospitalized cardiac patients includes two levels. First, the short-term information gain may be evaluated by a pretest and a post-test. Second, the more important long-term changes in behavior may be determined. The result of an in-hospital-only rehabilitation program on long-term change in behavior is not clear. As a result of a phase I program, Johnston et al.[16] found favorable behavior changes and outcomes such as adherence to a low-fat diet, exercise program, weight loss, blood pressure control, and cessation of smoking in a majority of patients after approximately 1 year. In contrast, Hayes et al.[37] followed, for up to 3.5 years, patients with myocardial infarction who either did or did not participate in a 2-week multidisciplinary inpatient cardiac rehabilitation program. Mortality was similar in both groups, and no significant differences were found with respect to nonfatal recurrent myocardial infarction, recurrence of angina pectoris, subsequent coronary surgery, return to work, or selected risk factors (diet, smoking, blood pressure). In evaluating follow-up physical activity levels only after coronary bypass surgery, Knapp et al.[38] found that patients who participated in a phase I program reported significantly more habitual exercise at 1 year than did patients from a hospital with no formal inpatient program.

Although the long-term outcomes of phase I participation are questionable, the short-term benefits are well accepted. Potential benefits documented as a result of early rehabilitation efforts include

1. Prevention of the deleterious effects of prolonged bed rest such as orthostatic hypotension, reduced physical work capacity, thromboembolism, reduced joint range of motion, and hypoventilation[39-41]
2. Improved psychologic status during convalescence[18,42]
3. Reduction in disability and an earlier return to work[43]
4. Potential reduction in hospital stay
5. Earlier resumption of previous activities[15]
6. Fewer office visits to the physician[15]
7. Increased sense of well-being[23]

The reduction in physical work capacity observed after 1 to 2 weeks of bed rest is primarily a result of impaired vasomotor reflexes. Convertino et al.[40] demonstrated that, in middle-aged men experiencing 10 days of bed rest, the most important factor limiting exercise ability is orthostatic stress. They recommended intermittent exposure to gravitational stress during the bed rest portion of hospitalization to help eliminate the potential reduction in physical work capacity that follows myocardial infarction.

The recent trend toward shorter periods of hospitalization and more invasive procedures during the hospital stay for cardiac patients has resulted in less time for phase I activities. For patients without complications, hospital dismissal as early as 3 days after myocardial infarction has been advocated.[44] Shortening the inpatient cardiac rehabilitation program is not in the best interests of patient care, but the financial benefits leave no alternative. The importance of a continuation of rehabilitation services during the immediate posthospitalization period emphasizing the critical role of risk-factor modification has resulted from these changes and represents one of the strongest challenges of the next decade. Patients must not assume that because their hospitalization and rehabilitation progress rapidly, their disease is not serious.

Immediate posthospitalization – phase II

Phase II of rehabilitation begins with hospital dismissal and usually continues for 2 weeks to 3 months (Table 14-6). Program length is determined by the need of the patient for both supervised exercise and counseling and education. In many respects, this is the most critical stage of rehabilitation in that patients are most receptive to changes in lifestyle and are motivated by their clear recollections of the acute event. The phase II program, which is directed by a cardiologist and closely supervised by paramedical personnel, consists of carefully prescribed exercise, education, counseling, and risk-factor modification. Referral channels to specialists are established for assistance in dealing with additional patient problems, such as smoking cessation, depression, psychosocial stress, musculoskeletal disease or injury, massive obesity, hypercholesterolemia, hypertension, and diabetes. The objectives of phase II are as follows:

1. To instruct patients in proper exercise procedures and to restore their exercise capacity to a state appropriate to their occupation and lifestyle
2. To provide understanding for both patient and family regarding cardiovascular disease and to continue appropriate risk-factor modification steps
3. To meet the psychosocial needs of patients and families, restore confidence, and reduce anxiety and depression
4. To assist the referring physician in identifying medical problems and to provide surveillance concerning the effectiveness of the therapeutic regimen
5. To assist in the gradual return to occupational and avocational activities

Table 14-6 Phase II (immediate outpatient) cardiac rehabilitation

Duration	2-12 wk, beginning at hospital dismissal
Components	Aerobic and muscle-conditioning exercise, limited game activities, education, risk-factor modification, and counseling
Program locations	Hospital, clinic, community exercise facility, and home
Characteristics	Interdisciplinary approach, close medical supervision, and availability of continuous ECG monitoring

Table 14-7 Phase II routine testing procedures

Procedure	When performed
Graded-exercise test*	At program entry and at 6-8 wk into the program
Body composition (% body fat)	At program entry and exit
Pulmonary function (in smokers and patients with history of pulmonary disease)	At program entry
Knowledge assessment	At program entry
Psychometric tests	At program entry
Occupational readiness assessment	Before return to work

*At entry into the program, most patients who have experienced a recent cardiac event perform a submaximal exercise test. This may be performed either before hospital dismissal or just before they begin phase II. Other patients perform a symptom-limited test at entry. A symptom-limited graded-exercise test is performed at 6-8 weeks into phase II to ascertain the functional capacity and to refine the exercise prescription.

The need for continuing supervision of the rehabilitation program after hospital dismissal is illustrated by the report of Silvidi et al.[45] They surveyed patients 6 weeks after hospitalization, which included a multidimensional rehabilitation program with specific guidelines for home exercise. None of the patients was involved in an outpatient rehabilitation program. It was found that the average patient walked for a shorter time and at a lower heart rate than prescribed. This suggests that patients may not follow directions explicitly and may require additional supervision during rehabilitation.

Cardiac rehabilitation programs are an excellent means of assessing patient tolerance to medication regimens that were started during hospitalization. Orthostatic hypotension, bradycardia, or other signs of medication intolerance are often discovered during cardiac rehabilitation sessions.

In addition to patients who have recently been hospitalized with cardiovascular problems, patients with either severe risk factors or symptoms of cardiovascular disease or patients who require considerable supervision in an exercise and risk-factor-modification program may be considered candidates for the phase II program. Patients who require continuous supervision in exercise and those who would benefit from patient education may be referred.

Entrance to the program is initiated with a review of the patient's medical history. Routine phase II testing procedures are listed in Table 14-7. Graded-exercise testing is helpful to determine patient suitability and for preparation of an exercise prescription. A submaximal predismissal or early outpatient exercise test is appropriate for patients with acute myocardial infarction or cardiac surgery. A symptom-limited graded-exercise test is desirable for most other patient categories. For all patients, a second exercise test (symptom-limited) is performed during the sixth to the eighth week to determine the magnitude of the training effect and for refinement of the exercise prescription. Absolute contraindications for exercise training as given in Table 14-2, if unresolved, eliminate a patient from acceptance into the exercise program. Direct measurement of oxygen uptake is very helpful in the precise determination of aerobic exercise capacity in cardiac patients.[46] Furthermore, measured peak oxygen uptakes of greater than 4 METs in patients with chronic heart failure are indicative of a much better 2-year survival rate (84%) than that in patients with lower peak oxygen uptakes (32%).[47] Persons with extremely limited functional capacities (less than 3 METs) and orthopedic limitations may be admitted if specific care plans have been designed and target outcomes have been stipulated. Nonambulatory patients may benefit from upper-extremity aerobic exercise. For patients with exercise capacities of less than 5 METs, two or three exercise sessions each day may result in improvement in exercise tolerance.[13,48]

Educational needs are assessed by interview with a physician and the paramedical staff. In addition, knowledge assessment via a pencil-and-paper test is carried out at the beginning of phase II. Because of the many disconcerting aspects of hospitalization involving an acute cardiac event, the number of new concepts that are thrust upon patients, and the trend toward shorter hospital stays, the amount of learning that occurs during phase I is not adequate for most patients.[49] Phase II serves to reinforce and amplify the teaching that took place in the hospital. Individual and group session discussions and lectures are used. Every effort is made to ensure consistency with phase I information. Inclusion of the spouse and other family members is desirable in most situations. The normal psychologic responses to an acute cardiac event are discussed. Return to previous activities such as sex, hobbies, and vocation is planned. General information concerning cardiovascular disease, risk-factor modification, and medications is provided. Strategies for making changes in behavior are discussed. Efforts at risk-factor modification are directed toward cessation of smoking, optimization of the blood lipid profile, control of blood pressure and body weight, diet (sodium, total fat, saturated fat, cholesterol, total calories), exercise, and stress management. The dietitian plays the key role in assisting patients in making changes in eating habits to facilitate a lowering of serum cholesterol and triglycerides and in reducing excess body fat. Body composition is assessed with skinfold calipers[50] at entry and exit from phase II. A desirable target weight may then be individualized much more accurately than by the use of a height-weight chart.[50] A review of patient medications by the cardiac rehabilitation nurse helps ensure patient compliance with prescribed therapeutic measures. Stress management through relaxation training is incorporated into the supervised exercise sessions. Patients who require more intense assistance in stress management may be referred for additional treatment such as biofeedback training.

Additional education is provided and emotional issues

in heart disease are addressed in an outpatient and spouse support group. The group is conducted by an exercise physiologist with assistance from cardiac rehabilitation nurses. The format combines presentation of information by group leaders with both directed and open discussion among group participants. Much of the information is presented through the story of a composite fictional patient—a narrative describing the heart attack, subsequent coronary bypass operation, and recovery of the patient and the concurrent reactions of his or her spouse. Through this narrative, common psychologic and emotional concerns, such as denial, anger, depression, and resumption of sexual relationships, are addressed without the need for a didactic presentation or extensive discussion of the cases of individual group participants.

The phase II program is individualized as much as possible to meet specific patient needs. A standard program consists of frequent visits (three per week) for supervised exercise and education and regular home exercise sessions. Patients who live some distance from the medical center may benefit from home exercise sessions with recommended reading supervised by mail or telephone. Transtelephonic transmission of the ECG with voice communication between the patient at home (or at a remote hospital) and cardiac rehabilitation personnel at a regional center is an alternative form of program for selected patients.[51] Occasional clinic visits with home exercise sessions may be an alternative for patients with transportation or financial difficulties. As the program progresses, gradually less frequent supervised sessions may be considered. Favorable patient compliance in programs with infrequent supervision has been reported.[52]

Psychosocial adjustment after an acute cardiac event may be improved by counseling in the rehabilitation program.[53] Return to work after myocardial infarction is also associated with a decline in emotional distress, even when employees return to dissatisfying jobs.[54] The common depression on homecoming, as described by Hackett and Cassem,[55] which is characterized by a generalized feeling of weakness, can be discussed with the patient. Patients should be made aware that this phenomenon is not unexpected and that it usually dissipates within 3 months. The presence of chronic depression is correlated with both the severity of the disease and the complications resulting from the disease.[55] Controversy between the patient and the family regarding the specific meaning of dismissal instructions can be disruptive to patient compliance and a source of contention and anxiety. Clear and precise guidelines for posthospital activities and procedures and the support and repetition provided by team members help to minimize misinterpretation.[53] Return to sexual activity should be discussed early in the program, because a reduction in sexual activity as a result of fear and anxiety is common. Male impotence is common after myocardial infarction and may require counseling or further evaluation.[56] Resumption of physical activity may favorably influence return to sexual activity.[57]

We screen each patient at entry into phase II of rehabilitation with a brief psychometric instrument (Symptom Check List 90-R).[58] The SCL 90-R is a 90-item, self-administered questionnaire that addresses 13 categories of emotional and psychologic function. Depression and somatic anxiety are the principal abnormal findings. Psychologic consultation is arranged for individual patients when needed. Group education sessions provide important psychologic support and education about the normal emotional reactions of patient and spouse to a cardiac event.

Psychosocial factors have recently been identified as important prognostic indicators after the appearance of clinical coronary artery disease. In a study by Case et al.[59] of 1,234 patients between the ages of 25 and 75 years who had no other serious disease, average follow-up was 2.1 years after myocardial infarction. Living alone was an independent factor for recurrent myocardial infarction or cardiac death, with a relative risk of 1.54. Williams et al.[60] studied the relationship of patient economic resources and social support to survival time until cardiovascular death in 1,368 patients with angiographically documented coronary artery disease. Patients with annual incomes of $40,000 or more had an unadjusted 5-year survival rate of 0.91, compared with 0.76 for patients with incomes of $10,000 or less ($P < 0.02$). Patients with social support (spouse or confidant) experienced a 5-year survival rate of 0.82, whereas those without social support had a rate of 0.50. Depression after myocardial infarction is associated independently with a threefold higher mortality over 1.5 years.[61] Whether an intervention such as an extended cardiac rehabilitation program or a support group to provide social support would improve survival in socially isolated patients is not known. Cardiac rehabilitation activities (exercise training and behavioral counseling) have been shown to accelerate recovery by lessening anxiety and depression.[62]

The phase II exercise program is designed to improve cardiovascular fitness (maximum oxygen uptake) to levels that allow resumption of usual activities. Aerobic (endurance) exercise forms the core of the physical activity program, but flexibility, muscle strengthening, and relaxation exercises are included. The prescription of aerobic exercise includes four factors: intensity, duration, frequency, and mode of activity. Initially, exercise is prescribed conservatively—that is, 10 to 15 minutes per session at an energy cost of 1.5 to 2.5 METs. A safe upper limit heart rate is derived from the predismissal graded-exercise test. The perceived exertion scale developed by Borg[63] is used to adjust exercise intensity to a comfortable level for the patient (Table 14-8). Gutmann et al.[64] demonstrated the efficacy of the Borg scale for use by cardiac patients. The perceptions of the patient regarding the relative severity of the exercise is critical in designing a program for optimal patient compliance. The scale is a 15-grade instrument ranging from 6 to 20 with descriptive verbal anchors at each odd number; 6 corresponds to resting conditions and 20, to maximal aerobic exercise. Most patients, once instructed in the proper use of the scale, can use it in an appropriate, meaningful fashion. Ratings of 11 to 14 are appropriate for patients during phase II. Exercise intensity is thus prescribed by means of a combination of factors: heart rate, patient signs and symptoms, estimated energy cost, and perceived exertion.

Table 14-8 Borg rating of perceived exertion scale

Grade	Description
6	
7	Very, very light
8	
9	Very light
10	
11	Fairly light
12	
13	Somewhat hard
14	
15	Hard
16	
17	Very hard
18	
19	Very, very hard
20	

Over the first 3 weeks, the duration of aerobic exercise is gradually increased to approximately 40 continuous minutes during the supervised sessions. Walking and cycle ergometry—forms of exercise that are easily quantifiable and reproducible in terms of energy expenditure—are used as the major modes of aerobic exercise. Other forms of aerobic exercise are available: rowing, arm ergometry, combination arm and leg ergometry, stair-stepping, and cross-country skiing simulator. Exercise frequency is five to six sessions per week for the typical patient who can perform at at least 5 METs on the entry graded-exercise test. For patients with extremely poor functional capacities, multiple daily sessions are recommended.[48] For these patients, exercise duration is kept at 5 to 15 minutes per session. Patients may use an interval approach to exercise, interspersing periods of rest and exercise during the exercise session.[65]

β-Adrenergic-receptor blocking agents lower the heart rate response to a given exercise intensity and have been shown to reduce carbon dioxide production, minute ventilation, and respiratory exchange ratio during exercise.[66] Because of these alterations in the metabolic response to exercise, doubts have been expressed concerning whether cardiac patients who take β-blocking drugs would benefit from exercise training.[66,67] Pratt et al.,[68] however, demonstrated substantial training effects in patients taking these drugs. β-Blocking drugs do not affect perceived exertion ratings in patients, and the use of this feature as a tool with these patients is appropriate.[69]

Patients with left ventricular dysfunction are at higher risk of sudden cardiac death than patients with normal ventricular function,[70,71] and there may be reluctance to include these patients in the exercise portion of the program. However, Lee et al.[72] reported favorable results after several months of exercise training and an increase in physical work capacity in patients with resting ejection fractions below 40%. In these patients, the improvement in fitness was not associated with an improvement in ventricular function. On the other hand, the exercise program did not result in deterioration of ventricular function. Several other investigators have established the safety and efficacy of exercise training for patients with resting left ventricular ejection fractions of less than 25%.[73-75]

A report by Jugdutt et al.[76] urged caution in recommending exercise training for patients with anterior wall myocardial infarctions who exhibit significant akinesia or dyskinesia. They found evidence for increased cardiac shape distortion, wall thinning, infarct expansion, and reduced left ventricular ejection fraction in patients who exercised moderately but not in controls. However, a recent report by Giannuzzi et al.[77] demonstrated that ventricular remodeling occurred over time in patients with anterior wall myocardial infarctions and ejection fractions of less than 40% but that exercise training did not influence the process. Aerobic capacity was improved by exercise training in their patients. Additional studies have demonstrated the safety of exercise training in patients with large myocardial infarctions.[78,79]

Upper extremity exercise is an important consideration, because much of the improvement in exercise tolerance is specific to the muscle groups undergoing exercise training; that is, there is little carryover in adaptive training responses from one muscle group to another.[80] Such exercise allows daily activities requiring arm work to be performed with a lower myocardial oxygen requirement—that is, with a lower elevation of heart rate and systolic blood pressure. Aerobic upper extremity exercise may be accomplished with a standard arm ergometer, a combination arm and leg ergometer, or a rowing machine. Isotonic strengthening exercises that make use of wrist weights and small dumbbells are started at the outset of phase II. A graded program ranging from 1 to approximately 15 lb of resistance with each arm is accomplished over an 8-week period. Specific occupational and recreational goals are addressed, and the strengthening exercise program is adjusted accordingly. Selected patients participate in resistance strength training using standard circuit-weight-training machines. We have demonstrated the safety of weight training with standard machines during phase II rehabilitation.[81] In 13 selected patients, weight training (chest press, shoulder press, two-leg press) began an average of 50 days after the cardiac event. Patients progressed in a few weeks to lifting approximately 40 lb with the arms and 130 lb with the legs. Average heart rate and systolic blood pressure increased a modest 20 beats/min and 21 mm Hg, respectively. No clinical problems occurred. Weight training exercise results in improved strength and augments aerobic training, especially in patients with weak skeletal musculature.[82]

Complex ventricular arrhythmias in patients with coronary artery disease are indicative of an increased risk of sudden cardiac death.[83] In addition, exercise may induce arrhythmias in these patients.[84] Therefore, all coronary artery disease patients receive continuous ECG monitoring during some of their supervised exercise sessions to reduce the probability of untoward events. It is apparent that significant arrhythmias may occur during exercise sessions and may not be detected by either Holter monitoring or graded-exercise testing.[85] Monitoring may provide useful information regarding the effectiveness of antiarrhythmia agents. The optimal length of time for monitoring in the phase II setting is not known.

For most cardiac patients, ECG monitoring during some exercise sessions is appropriate. Prolonged use of ECG monitoring (greater than 4 weeks) should be restricted to patients who are considered high risk for an exercise-related complication. The American College of Cardiology and the American College of Physicians have recommended guidelines for the use of ECG monitoring during cardiac exercise programs.[86,87] The criteria for continuous ECG monitoring include severely depressed left ventricular or congestive heart failure ejection fraction ($\leq 30\%$), complex ventricular arrhythmia, signs of marked exercise-induced ischemia, decrease in systolic blood pressure during exercise testing, survival after sudden cardiac arrest, and the inability to self-monitor heart rate. In addition, the American Association of Cardiovascular and Pulmonary Rehabilitation identifies as high risk patients with exercise capacities of less than 5 METs who have evidence of ischemia during exercise.[12] Ideally, high-risk patients should remain in an ECG-monitored exercise program indefinitely, although this is not standard practice at present because insurance reimbursement is limited. The product of heart rate and systolic blood pressure at which myocardial ischemia first appears (ischemic threshold) is not necessarily constant, presumably because of changes in coronary tone.[88] Therefore, careful monitoring of the ST segments during the initiation of exercise programs for patients with ischemia documented by exercise testing should be performed to reduce the likelihood of exceeding the ischemic threshold during exercise training. Upper extremity exercise results in no more arrhythmias than does lower extremity exercise at matched heart rates.[89]

Exercise training sessions are individualized to prepare patients for the type and amount of physical activity required by their occupations. Before a patient's return to employment, it may be advisable to perform an occupational task physiologic assessment. The hemodynamic and ECG responses to isometric or dynamic arm exercise or specific job tasks may be evaluated and recommendations given. Also important in determining readiness for resumption of occupational tasks are the results of the symptom-limited graded-exercise test. The estimated safe functional capacity in METs may be compared with the estimated energy expenditure requirement of the job. The 8-hour average energy cost of the job should not exceed 30% to 40% of the maximal oxygen uptake for apparently healthy persons.[90] Thus, a cardiac patient with a functional capacity of 7 METs would probably be incapable of performing a job requiring an average energy cost of more than 3 METs for an 8-hour shift. Environmental and mental stress factors must also be evaluated. Occupational rehabilitation or adjustment in work schedule may be necessary for patients in this category.

It is important to identify goals to be met before completion of the program. Individual patient objectives should be discussed. However, certain basic exit criteria should be met before graduation from phase II.[48] Examples of such criteria include

1. Completion of the exercise program with acceptable attendance
2. Completion of the education program with a demonstrated understanding of personal risk factors and medications
3. An estimated functional capacity of at least 5 METs
4. A resting blood pressure of less than 170/100 mm Hg
5. Control of serious arrhythmias
6. Control of angina pectoris—stable and absent at a desirable level of activity for the patient's lifestyle
7. Demonstrated ability to understand and perform proper exercise procedures
8. Satisfactory understanding and performance of dietary and exercise recommendations for control of body weight, blood lipids, and hypertension
9. Satisfactory psychosocial adjustment to the presence of cardiac disease

After completion of the symptom-limited graded-exercise test, usually during the sixth to eighth week of phase II, the exercise prescription for intensity is adjusted and a new upper limit heart rate is calculated. It has been shown that an exercise intensity of 50% to 70% of the functional capacity will result in gains in cardiorespiratory fitness in cardiac patients.[91] In patients who have no symptoms with a normal heart rate, blood pressure, and ECG response to graded exercise, the new heart rate prescription is calculated by the technique described by Karvonen et al.[92] The resting heart rate is subtracted from the peak exercise heart rate, and the difference is referred to as the maximum heart rate reserve or range. Sixty to seventy percent of the heart rate reserve is added to the resting heart rate to yield a heart rate corresponding to 60% to 70% of the functional capacity. This method has the advantage that the percentage of the maximal heart rate reserve correlates closely with the percentage of the maximal METs performed during the graded-exercise test.[91] This is not the case when a given percentage of the maximal heart rate is calculated. Exercise training of low to moderate intensity results in improvement in aerobic capacity for most patients.[93,94] Higher intensity exercise is not necessary for the rehabilitation of most coronary patients.[95]

Because of the unsolved problem of early repeat occlusion, post-myocardial-infarction patients who have undergone percutaneous transluminal coronary angioplasty are best served by a medically supervised exercise program for 2 to 8 weeks after hospital dismissal. Patients at low risk may safely participate in home exercise training exclusively if a medically supervised program is not available or is not a practical alternative, in our opinion Patients at higher risk who cannot be revascularized or whose risk status cannot be otherwise improved are best served by a medically supervised exercise program and close surveillance. For all cardiac patients, participation in at least a brief supervised outpatient exercise program is indicated before participation in an exclusively home activity regimen.

Outpatient late recovery—phase III

Phase III of rehabilitation begins at the completion of phase II and continues for 6 months or more (Table

Table 14-9 Phase III (late recovery) cardiac rehabilitation

Duration	Begins at end of phase II and continues for a minimum of 6 mo
Components	Aerobic and muscle-conditioning exercise, game activities, and education
Program locations	Community exercise facility, hospital, or clinic and home
Characteristics	Medical supervision (less than phase II) and availability of periodic ECG monitoring

Table 14-10 Phase IV (maintenance program) cardiac rehabilitation

Duration	Begins no earlier than 8-10 mo after hospital dismissal and continues indefinitely
Components	Aerobic and muscle-conditioning exercise and selected games; reinforcement of education and concepts of risk-factor modification through community coronary club
Program locations	Community exercise facility and home
Characteristics	No direct medical supervision; not all patients will progress to phase IV

14-9). The program is medically directed but has less direct supervision than phase II. The program consists of either group exercise and education sessions at a community exercise facility, hospital, or clinic with some individual exercise sessions or a purely home exercise program. Patients who are following a purely home exercise program document the specifics of the exercise session and communicate regularly with the rehabilitation staff.

Supervised group exercise sessions may include periodic blood pressure measurement but only intermittent or infrequent ECG monitoring. Education consists of the reinforcement of risk-factor modification and a review of other pertinent topics. Group lectures and individual counseling sessions may be included.

The objectives of phase III are to increase the exercise capacity further, to reinforce steps for risk-factor modification, to provide fun and recreation through game activities, and to provide social interaction and support. The exercise program includes aerobic activities and also flexibility and strengthening exercises. Noncompetitive games are used to improve compliance and to maintain interest.

A formal evaluation of the patient's program occurs at 3, 6, and 9 months. The evaluation includes a review of the progress in exercise, diet, blood lipids, body weight, other risk factors, medications, and previously unsolved problems. At 6 months, a symptom-limited graded-exercise test is performed to ascertain changes in the functional capacity and prognosis.[6] After a period of diet, exercise, and weight loss, patients with an adverse blood lipid profile begin a regimen of lipid-improving medication.[96,97] The cardiac rehabilitation program, with its multidisciplinary team and patient follow-up schedule, is an ideal model for blood lipid management. Long-term (indefinite) follow-up of blood lipids, diet, exercise, and other risk factors occurs for many patients through the rehabilitation program.[98] Blood lipid goals for patients with coronary atherosclerosis recommended by the National Cholesterol Education Program Adult Treatment Panel II include a low-density lipoprotein cholesterol level of 100 mg/dL or less.[99]

Patient exit from phase III is based on the following criteria.[48]

1. The functional capacity should be at least 8 METs.
2. The ECG at rest and during exercise should be stable or improved as compared with entry
3. Angina or dyspnea should be stable and absent at exercise levels adequate for the patient's lifestyle
4. Resting blood pressure and heart rate should not exceed 160/96 mm Hg and 90 beats/min, respectively
5. Patients should understand the basic pathophysiology of their disease, their medications, and the need for continuance of the recommended changes in lifestyle

Maintenance program – phase IV

Phase IV is a nonmedically supervised exercise program designed to maintain the exercise capacity that was developed during phases II and III (Table 14-10). Some patients may continue to improve in cardiorespiratory fitness for more than 1 year after the acute event, however. Generally, phase IV does not begin until after at least 6 months of participation in phase III. Phase IV may be considered as a state-of-the-art adult fitness program. It may be inappropriate for some cardiac patients – that is, those with poor functional capacities, severe hypertension, a history of refractory arrhythmia, chronotropic or inotropic incompetence, or extremely poor left ventricular function – to leave phase III and enter phase IV. These patients may remain in the supervised phase III program on a long-term basis. Patients who are qualified to enter phase IV should have an exercise capacity of at least 8 METs; an understanding of environmental factors such as heat, cold, humidity, wind, altitude, and air quality, which may affect exercise performance; and a firm understanding of their personal exercise prescription.

The program may include an individual exercise program to be carried out at home or at an exercise facility or a supervised adult fitness program at a community complex. The exercise program includes aerobic activities, flexibility and strengthening exercises, and games. Reinforcement of steps toward risk-factor modification and

Table 14-11 Aerobic exercise prescription for cardiac rehabilitation

Phase	Intensity*	Duration	Frequency	Mode
I	RHR + 20; perceived exertion 11 to 13	5-20 min	2-3 times/day	Slow walk or cycle or arm ergometry†
II	RHR + 20 40%-70% of functional capacity;‡ perceived exertion 11 to 14	10-45 min	5-6 times/wk	Walk, cycle or arm ergometry, rowing, stair climbing, cross-country skiing simulator, walk-jog, low-level games
III	50%-75% of functional capacity; perceived exertion 12 to 14	20-45 min	3-6 times/wk	Walk, walk-jog, jog, cycle or arm ergometry or other aerobic equipment, outdoor cycle, games, swimming
IV	50%-80% of functional capacity; perceived exertion 12 to 15	20-45 min	3-6 times/wk	Same as above (III)

*RHR = resting heart rate.
† Arm ergometry during phase I is limited to nonambulatory patients.
‡ Heart rate correlates of percentage of functional capacity are calculated by the heart rate range method of Karvonen et al.[92]

other patient education is accomplished through the community coronary club, which meets monthly.

Aerobic exercise, a component common to all phases of cardiac rehabilitation, is prescribed with increasing intensity and duration as the program continues. The basic components of the aerobic exercise prescription for phases I to IV are presented in Table 14-11. The goal is for patients to expend at least 1,000 kcal/week with exercise by phase IV. This level of energy expenditure has been shown to be an effective stimulus for the development and maintenance of a desirable functional capacity.[100] Yearly medical evaluations, including graded exercise testing, are recommended.

EXPECTATIONS AND LIMITATIONS OF CARDIAC REHABILITATION

An important aspect in the evaluation of the efficacy of outpatient cardiac rehabilitation is the safety of the supervised exercise sessions. Since cardiac patients may have a limited coronary reserve, the increase in myocardial oxygen demand during exercise may result in myocardial ischemia and potentially precipitate cardiac arrest or myocardial infarction. Haskell[101] surveyed 30 North American cardiac rehabilitation programs and found that cardiovascular complications are, fortunately, infrequent. The most frequent complication was cardiac arrest, and nonfatal and fatal rates of occurrence were 1/38,801 and 1/203,704 patient-hours of participation, respectively. Nonfatal and fatal complication rates for myocardial infarction were 1/325,927 and 1/814,816 patient-hours, respectively. Total nonfatal and fatal complication rates for all causes were 1/34,673 and 1/116,402 patient-hours, respectively. Complication rates were lower in programs using continuous ECG monitoring. Supervised exercise for properly selected cardiac patients appears to be reasonably safe. More recently, Van Camp and Peterson[102] reported a rate for cardiac arrest of 1/111,996 hours of patient exercise and rates for myocardial infarction and sudden cardiac death of 1/293,990 and 1/783,972 hours of patient exercise, respectively.

Table 14-12 lists benefits that may result from long-term outpatient cardiac rehabilitation. Therapy prescribed for patients with chronic disease is designed to decrease symptoms and to improve function. For many cardiac patients, rehabilitation achieves these expectations.

Exercise training has been shown to increase physical work capacity and to allow the cardiac patient to exercise to a higher workload before ischemic ECG changes or symptoms such as angina pectoris, dyspnea, and fatigue occur.[67] The maximal oxygen uptake ($\dot{V}O_2max$) may increase 10% to 30% or more in patients.[103,104] Patients with exercise-induced ischemia during graded exercise testing often have a smaller increase in $\dot{V}O_2max$ as a result of training than do other patients.[105,106] In general, for cardiac patients, the magnitude of the improvement in $\dot{V}O_2max$ is inversely proportional to the exercise capacity before training.[107] The rate of improvement is greatest during the first 3 months of exercise training, but the increase in fitness continues for 6 months or more.[108] Elderly patients have relative increases in $\dot{V}O_2max$ similar to those in younger patients.[109] The increased physical work capacity results in utilization of a smaller percentage of the $\dot{V}O_2max$ during routine activities (Fig 14-1). As a result, tasks are performed with less fatigue and dyspnea, and the productivity of the patient may be enhanced. The product of heart rate and systolic blood pressure (double-product) is lowered for a given dynamic workload, and this leads to a reduced myocardial oxygen demand.[103,104,107,108] Increas-

Table 14-12 Benefits resulting from long-term outpatient cardiac rehabilitation

Physiologic*

↑ $\dot{V}O_2$max
↓ $M\dot{V}O_2$ for given workload
↑ Muscle strength and endurance
↑ Blood fibrinolytic activity
↓ Platelet aggregation
↓ Catecholamines
Improved left ventricular function†
Increased resistance to ventricular fibrillation†

Symptomatic

↓ Angina pectoris
↓ Dyspnea
↓ Claudication
↓ Fatigue

Anatomic

↓ Progression of disease†
Regression of disease†
Improved myocardial perfusion†

Psychologic

↓ Anxiety and depression
↑ Confidence and self-esteem
↑ Knowledge

Epidemiologic

↓ Morbidity†
↓ Mortality†

Risk factors

↓ Smoking
↓ Total cholesterol and triglycerides
↑ High-density lipoprotein cholesterol
↓ Obesity
↓ Hypertension
↑ Carbohydrate metabolism

Economic

↑ Patient productivity†
↓ Disability cases†
↓ Physician office visits†
↓ Medications

*$\dot{V}O_2$ max, maximal oxygen uptake; $M\dot{V}O_2$, myocardial oxygen demand.
†Potential benefits.

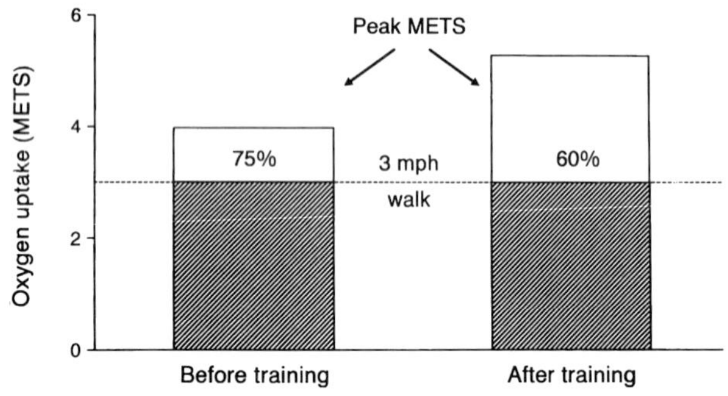

Fig 14-1 Effects of exercise training on peak oxygen uptake in metabolic energy equivalents *(METS)* and relative oxygen uptake for walking 3 mph on a level surface. After exercise training, peak oxygen uptake increased; thus, the relative oxygen cost for the activity decreased. (From Franklin BA, Rubenfire M: Exercise training in coronary heart disease: mechanisms of improvement. *Pract Cardiol* 6:84-99, 1980. By permission of the author.)

ing the muscular strength of the upper extremities results in utilization of a lower percentage of the maximal contractile force during routine tasks and permits activities that require muscular strength to be accomplished at a lower heart rate and blood pressure and thus at a lower myocardial oxygen demand.[110]

Table 14-13 Adaptations to exercise training in cardiac patients*

1. ↑ $\dot{V}O_2$max resulting from:
   a. Skeletal muscle adaptation (↑ $c(a - \bar{v})O_2$)
   b. Improvement in left ventricular function in selected patients (↑ maximal cardiac output)
2. ↓ HR and SBP for a given submaximal exercise intensity resulting from:
   a. ↑ $c(a - \bar{v})O_2$
   b. ↓ Submaximal cardiac output
3. As a result, symptoms of angina pectoris, fatigue, and dyspnea improve

*$\dot{V}O_2$max, maximal oxygen uptake; $c(a - \bar{v})O_2$, difference in oxygen content between the arterial and mixed venous blood; HR, heart rate; SBP, systolic blood pressure.

The observed increases in $\dot{V}O_2$max in cardiac patients after a period of exercise training are a result of adaptations in the skeletal muscle and possibly changes in left ventricular function (Table 14-13). An increase in the oxidative enzyme activity and myoglobin concentration in addition to adjustments in the peripheral circulation allow more oxygen to be extracted from the arterial blood; this results in an increase in arterial-mixed venous oxygen difference.[107] After training, the systemic $\dot{V}O_2$ is higher

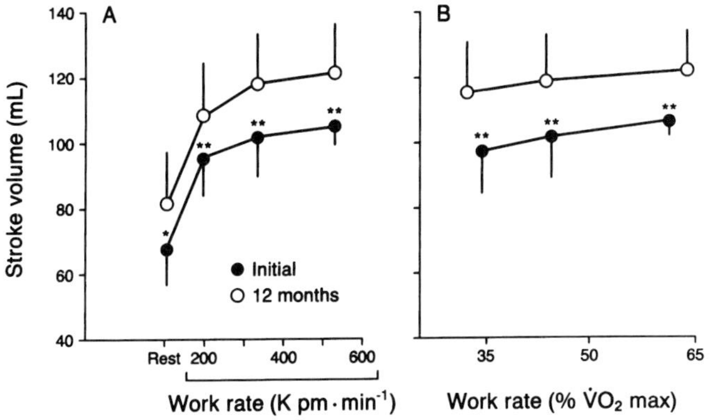

Fig 14-2 Stroke volume at the same absolute work rate (**A**) and the same relative work rate (**B**) before (●—●) and after (○—○) 12 months of exercise training. One asterisk, $P < 0.05$; two asterisks, $P < 0.01$. (From Hagberg JM, Ehsani AA, Holloszy JO: Effect of 12 months of intense exercise training on stroke volume in patients with coronary artery disease. *Circulation* 67:1194-1199, 1983. By permission of American Heart Association.)

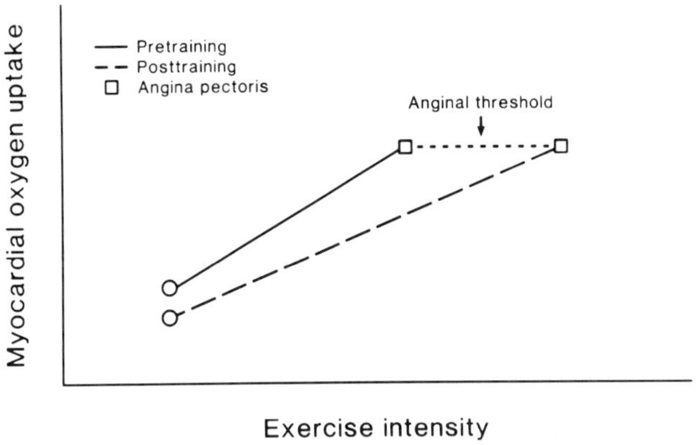

Fig 14-3 Effect of exercise training on exertional angina pectoris. (Modified from Dressendorfer RH, Amsterdam EA, Mason DT: Therapeutic effects of exercise training in angina patients. In *Physical Conditioning and Cardiovascular Rehabilitation.* Edited by LS Cohen, MB Mock, I Ringqvist. New York, John Wiley & Sons, 1981, p 123.)

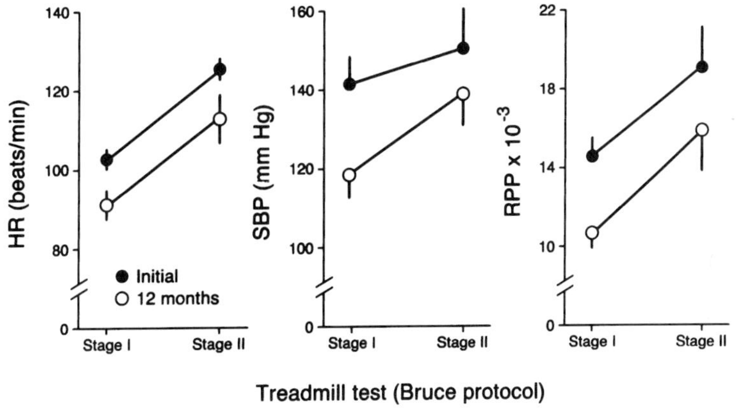

Fig 14-4 Effects of exercise training on heart rate *(HR),* systolic blood pressure *(SBP),* and rate-pressure product *(RPP)* at stages I and II of the Bruce treadmill protocol. All variables after 12 months of exercise training (○—○) were significantly ($P < 0.01$) lower than before training (●—●). (From Ehsani AA, Martin WH III, Heath GW, et al: Cardiac effects of prolonged and intense exercise training in patients with coronary artery disease. *Am J Cardiol* 50:246-254, 1982. By permission of Excerpta Medica.)

for a given cardiac output than before training. Studies evaluating the effects of exercise training on left ventricular function have yielded conflicting results. Some studies have reported improvement in both myocardial perfusion[111,112] and maximal cardiac output,[113] whereas others have reported no such improvement.[114,115] An increase in stroke volume in cardiac patients during submaximal exercise after one year of exercise training has been reported, indicating that myocardial contractility may be improved.[116] The heterogeneity of cardiac patients in rehabilitation programs may obscure cardiac changes that may occur in selected patients.[117] Hagberg et al.[118] demonstrated an increased stroke volume of 18% after 1 year of intense exercise in selected cardiac patients (Fig 14-2).

Figure 14-3 illustrates the effect of exercise training on stable exertional angina pectoris. After a period of exercise training, the myocardial oxygen demand (estimated from the double-product—heart rate times systolic blood pressure) is lower for a given exercise intensity (Fig 14-4). A higher exercise intensity is required to exceed the anginal threshold than before training. In some patients, angina may disappear entirely[104] or appear only at a higher double-product; this finding may indicate that an increase in myocardial perfusion has occurred[119] or that the sensitivity to anginal pain has diminished.[120] Some studies have shown an improvement in ST-segment displacement after exercise training at a fixed double-product; this is consistent with an improvement in myocardial perfusion (Fig 14-5).[121,122] The combination of a low-fat diet and aerobic exercise training resulted in an improvement in thallium perfusion in a report by Schuler et al.[123] However, there is no evidence that exercise training alone improves the coronary collateral circulation.

Exercise training, in sufficient amounts, may retard or reverse coronary atherosclerosis.[124] Serial coronary angiograms separated by year demonstrated minimal progression of disease in patients who expended an average of 1,500 kcal per week in exercise. For patients with a mean weekly energy expenditure of 2,200 kcal, angiographic regression occurred in 28% of subjects.

Patients with peripheral vascular disease and intermittent claudication may improve their ambulatory capacity greatly with an exercise program.[125] Walking to the point of moderate discomfort and continuing for at least 20 minutes has been recommended.[48]

As with all longitudinal forms of treatment, compliance with rehabilitation recommendations is of concern. Lifestyle changes are not easily accomplished by most patients. Although dropouts cannot be accurately predicted, certain factors do increase the chance of noncompliance:[126,127] continued cigarette smoking, depressed mood, blue-collar occupation, poor left ventricular function, and obesity.

Making lasting lifestyle changes is difficult for most patients, even after they have received comprehensive health education and understand the health benefits that will result from a change in habits. A widely accepted model of health behavior change and maintenance is social learning theory.[128] Patient confidence and the ability to make lasting lifestyle changes are enhanced by the following factors:

1. Advice from a health care professional
2. Observation of others performing the behavior (modeling)
3. Practice of the behavior
4. Feedback of the results

Social support and positive reinforcement also appear to be critical elements in a behavioral approach to compliance enhancement.

The efficacy of risk-factor modification in reducing coronary artery disease progression and future morbidity and mortality (secondary prevention) has been established. Progression of disease in the native coronary arteries and in saphenous bypass grafts has been linked to continued cigarette smoking, increased concentration of total serum cholesterol and low levels of high-density lipoprotein cholesterol, hypertension, sedentary lifestyle, and increased fasting blood glucose concentration.[129-132] Low concentrations of high-density lipoprotein cholesterol are strongly predictive of subsequent cardiovascular events in cardiac patients despite normal levels of total cholesterol.[133] Patients with low levels of high-density lipoprotein cholesterol often possess a clustering of other risk factors: insulin resistance, increased triglycerides, increased fibrinogen and hemoglobin, and a history of smoking.[134,135] Drug therapy designed to improve arrhythmia, ischemia, left ventricular function, symptoms, and platelet function provides important secondary prevention benefits. Such benefits have been reviewed elsewhere.[136]

Prospective trials have conclusively demonstrated the importance of control of serum cholesterol concentration in coronary patients. The Scandinavian Simvastatin Survival Study randomized 4,444 patients with coronary artery disease to treatment with a hydroxymethylglutary Co A reductase inhibitor or placebo.[137] After approximately 5 years of follow-up, total mortality was 44% lower in the treatment group. The National Heart, Lung, and Blood Institute Type II Coronary Intervention Study included serial angiography in 116 patients who received either a low-fat and low-cholesterol diet plus placebo or diet plus cholestyramine.[138] Follow-up at 5 years demonstrated progression of coronary disease in 49% of placebo patients compared with 32% of drug-treated patients ($P < 0.05$). Progression of disease was inversely associated with an increase in high-density lipoprotein cholesterol and a decrease in low-density lipoprotein cholesterol concentrations.[139]

The Cholesterol-Lowering Atherosclerosis Study involved 162 nonsmoking men who received diet and drug therapy (colestipol and nicotinic acid) and underwent serial coronary angiographic examinations 2 years apart.[4] Marked improvement in the treatment group's blood lipid profile was achieved (decrease in low-density lipoprotein cholesterol of 43%, increase in high-density lipoprotein cholesterol of 37%) and was associated with less disease progression and more disease regression (16% of treatment patients) than in the control subjects.

Brown et al.[5] in the Familial Atherosclerosis Treatment Study treated men with documented coronary artery disease and increased levels of apolipoprotein B with diet and either lovastatin and colestipol or niacin and colestipol. Blood lipids were markedly improved with treatment. Compared with patients treated conventionally, the patients in the trial had less coronary atherosclerosis progression, increased frequency of regression on serial coronary angiograms 2.5 years apart, and a reduced incidence of cardiovascular events. Cholesterol lowering, in addition to improving the angiographic natural history of coronary atherosclerosis, improves endothelium-dependent coronary vasodilation.[140]

Continued cigarette smoking has a negative effect on the results of surgical or medical therapy.[141] Cigarette smoking continues to predict cardiac-related death after myocardial infarction, and the risk decreases rapidly upon cessation of the habit.[142,143] Cigarette smoking results in many undesirable consequences: increased incidence of thromboembolic events, vasoconstriction, and reduced threshold for ventricular fibrillation.[144-146] Continued cigarette smoking after myocardial infarction is associated with progression of coronary artery disease.[131] Cessation of smoking after myocardial infarction may reduce total mortality by 20% to 50%.[147,148]

No prospective controlled trial has demonstrated that

treatment of hypertension reduces rates of reinfarction or sudden cardiac death. However, Connolly et al.[149] reported epidemiologic data demonstrating better survival in patients with angina pectoris or with myocardial infarction and adequately controlled hypertension than in patients who had uncontrolled or inadequately controlled arterial pressure.

Control of hypertension may improve anginal symptoms and congestive heart failure. The lack of association between blood pressure after infarction and survival may be a result of a reduction in blood pressure due to left ventricular dysfunction or medications such as β-blockers.

Correction of obesity has not been shown to independently lower morbidity and mortality in cardiac patients. However, reduction of excess body fat does reduce anginal and fatigue symptoms and improves established risk factors, such as blood lipid concentrations, hypertension, increased blood glucose values, platelet abnormalities, left ventricular hypertrophy, and a sedentary existence.[150] Apparently, abdominal (or central) obesity, defined as a waist-to-hip ratio of more than 1.0 in men and 0.85 in women, is associated with greater cardiovascular risk than hip and leg obesity.[151,152]

The coronary-prone behavior pattern (type A: high level of ambition, aggressiveness, hostility, competitiveness, and time urgency) was originally identified as an independent risk factor for first myocardial infarction in the Western Collaborative Study.[153] The role of type A characteristics for secondary prevention is controversial. Data from the Recurrent Coronary Prevention Project indicate that intensive counseling can alter type A behavior and result in an improvement in the rates of recurrent myocardial infarction and cardiac death.[154] However, data from the Western Collaborative Study[155] demonstrated that type A behavior is associated with a lower mortality than type B behavior after myocardial infarction. Psychosocial improvement as a result of cardiac rehabilitation has been demonstrated by several investigators.[156-160]

Epidemiologic studies have demonstrated a strong relationship between habitual physical activity and primary coronary artery disease morbidity and mortality.[161,162] Powell et al.[163] examined 47 epidemiologic studies of physical activity and coronary disease published in English and reported a strong (relative risk, 1.9), consistent inverse relationship between habitual physical activity and the incidence of coronary artery disease.

The evidence on the role of habitual physical activity for second or subsequent coronary events is less impressive. Paffenbarger and Hyde,[161] in an elegant epidemiologic study of Harvard alumni, indexed habitual physical activity in 782 alumni with known coronary disease. Over an approximately 12-year study period, more active subjects had a coronary event rate 30% lower than that of the less active alumni. The beneficial effect persisted after adjustment for smoking, blood pressure, body weight, family history of coronary artery disease, and age.

The question of protection versus selection in evaluation of the benefit of exercise in epidemiologic studies is open. Unfortunately, randomized trials have not conclu-

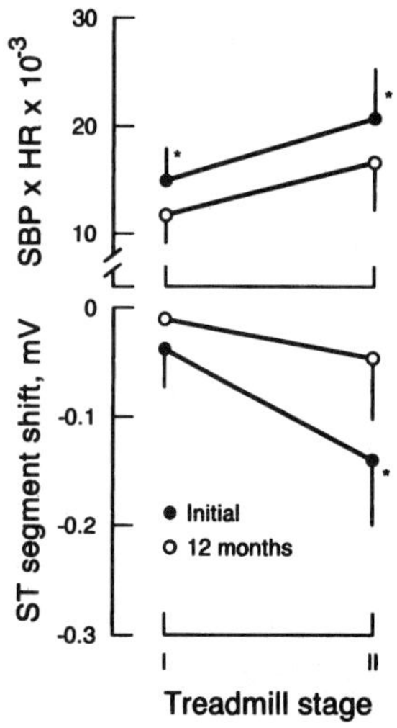

Fig 14-5 Rate-pressure product and extent of ischemic ST-segment depression at two submaximal levels of the Bruce treadmill protocol before (●—●) and after (○—○) 12 months of exercise training. *Asterisk* indicates $P < 0.01$ for difference from before to after training. *HR,* heart rate; *SBP,* systolic blood pressure. (From Ehsani AA, Heath GW, Hagberg JM, et al: Effects of 12 months of intense exercise training on ischemic ST-segment depression in patients with coronary artery disease. *Circulation* 64:1116-1124, 1981. By permission of American Heart Association.)

sively demonstrated a protective effect of exercise training on second coronary events. The most recent meta-analysis by O'Connor et al.[164] pooled data from 22 randomized trials involving 4,554 patients who underwent follow-up for 3 years. Compared with control subjects, these patients experienced total mortality, cardiovascular mortality, and fatal reinfarction rates that were significantly reduced by 20%, 22%, and 25%, respectively. Thus, exercise training may improve survival after myocardial infarction.

Economic evaluations of cardiac rehabilitation have been performed by Levin et al.[165] and Oldridge et al.[166] These analyses have established the cost-effectiveness of rehabilitation services.

CARDIOVASCULAR HEALTH ENHANCEMENT

The Cardiovascular Health Clinic at the Mayo Clinic has been designed to identify persons who are at high risk of developing cardiovascular disease and to make specific recommendations for risk reduction (primary prevention). Potentially, persons at risk of accelerated atherosclerosis may be detected long before the appearance of symptoms such as angina pectoris, sudden cardiac collapse, myocardial infarction, and stroke. Although a general population approach emphasizing public education through the media and schools is desirable and is needed, a personalized risk-factor evaluation with individualized recommendations is an important consideration in preventive medicine. This procedure appears worthwhile when one considers the general lack of preventive measures in standard medical practice and the potential for misinterpretation of information presented through the media.

The program is based on the premise that modification of risk factors will reduce atherosclerosis and its sequelae. This effect has not been demonstrated for all the major risk factors but has been reported for hypertension, cigarette smoking, serum cholesterol, and physical inactivity. The Veterans Administration Study on Antihypertensive Agents demonstrated that treatment for hypertension prolonged life and reduced cardiovascular morbidity compared with untreated hypertensive patients.[167] Cigarette smokers, both men and women, who stop the habit experience a rapid decline in coronary risk (to a relative risk approaching 1.0) over the first 1 to 3 years of abstinence.[168,169] The Oslo Study Group[170] reported results of a 5-year randomized trial in middle-aged healthy normotensive men with elevated serum cholesterol who smoked cigarettes. Compared with the controls, the intervention group, who received instructions on change in diet and cessation of smoking, experienced a 47% lower combined fatal and nonfatal incidence of myocardial infarction over the 5-year period. The intervention group reduced cholesterol by 13%, triglycerides by 20%, and smoking by 45%. The reduction in morbidity and mortality correlated with the decrease in cholesterol and smoking. The Helsinki Heart Study was a 5-year randomized, double-blind primary prevention trial in 4,000 subjects with non-high-density lipoprotein cholesterol levels of 200 mg/dL or greater.[171] The intervention subjects, who were treated with gemfibrozil, had a 34% lower coronary artery disease event incidence than controls. The reduction in risk resulted from both a decrease in low-density lipoprotein cholesterol and an increase in high-density lipoprotein cholesterol. The Multiple Risk Factor Intervention Trial was a primary prevention trial to assess the effect of smoking cessation, dietary treatment of hypercholesterolemia and obesity, and drug treatment of hypertension in high-risk men randomly assigned to the intervention (n = 6,428) or the usual care (n = 6,438) group.[172] At 10.5 years of follow-up (3.8 years after the end of intervention), coronary mortality, all-causes mortality, and death rate from acute myocardial infarction were significantly reduced in the intervention group by 10.6%, 7.7%, and 24%, respectively.

Habitual physical activity has been demonstrated to result in a lower risk of myocardial infarction and cardiac death than sedentary living.[163,173] In nonhuman primates, exercise training retards the development of coronary atherosclerosis in the setting of an atherogenic diet.[2]

The incidence of coronary artery disease increases in women after the age of menopause. Estrogen replacement therapy raises high-density lipoprotein cholesterol levels and potentially may reduce coronary risk in postmenopausal women.[174] Smoking with concurrent use of oral contraceptives is a powerful risk factor for thrombotic complications in premenopausal women.[175]

Although only 2% to 6% of families in the general population have very strong family histories of early coronary artery disease, they account for nearly 50% of all early coronary deaths in the population.[176] High-risk families share genetic (familial hypercholesterolemia, hypertension) and environmental factors. Risk factors such as smoking, depressed levels of high-density lipoprotein cholesterol, and increased triglyceride concentrations cluster in high-risk families. Risk-factor intervention in high-risk families is likely to result in a substantial reduction in coronary mortality. In particular, children from families in which one parent or grandparent has clinically important coronary artery disease before the age of 55 should be screened for hyperlipidemia and hypertension. Dietary change has been shown to improve the blood lipid profile in children from high-risk families.[177]

Table 14-14 Evaluation procedures for cardiovascular health enhancement

Physical examination
Medical history and questionnaire
Chest radiograph
Resting 12-lead ECG
Blood analyses: total cholesterol, high-density lipoprotein cholesterol, low-density lipoprotein cholesterol, triglycerides, glucose
Body composition (% body fat, waist-to-hip ratio)
Graded-exercise test

The procedures included in the cardiovascular health enhancement program evaluation are listed in Table 14-14. A physical examination within the previous year is required. Body composition (percent body fat) is determined with skinfold calipers and standard equations.[50] A waist-to-hip ratio is obtained as a measure of central obesity, which is an independent coronary risk factor for both men and women.[151,178] Cardiorespiratory fitness is assessed by means of a continuous multistage exercise test performed on either a motor-driven treadmill or a cycle ergometer. The test is supervised by a registered nurse or exercise physiologist. Test end points include volitional fatigue and the standard contraindications to continuance of exercise.[58] At least one ECG lead is continuously monitored throughout the test, and the ECG is recorded each minute. Blood pressure and perceived exertion are recorded during the final 30 seconds of each stage. Exercise ECGs with the hallmarks of myocardial ischemia are shown to the cardiologist. The purpose of the test is to evaluate the functional capacity and not to diagnose occult coronary disease. The diagnostic yield of positive tests with this procedure in this population is very low. In our experience, only 2% of subjects have an abnormal exercise ECG when the standard of 1 mm of ST depression is used with the usual criteria.[179] The functional capacity in METs is estimated by means of standard tables.[50] A self-report questionnaire is used to obtain the family history of cardiovascular disease and diabetes mellitus and the personal history of smoking, blood pressure evaluation, and psychosocial stress.

During the counseling session, an exercise physiologist or physician reviews the risk-factor profile (Fig 14-6). The common risk factors are presented as being either modifiable or nonmodifiable. The modifiable risk factors

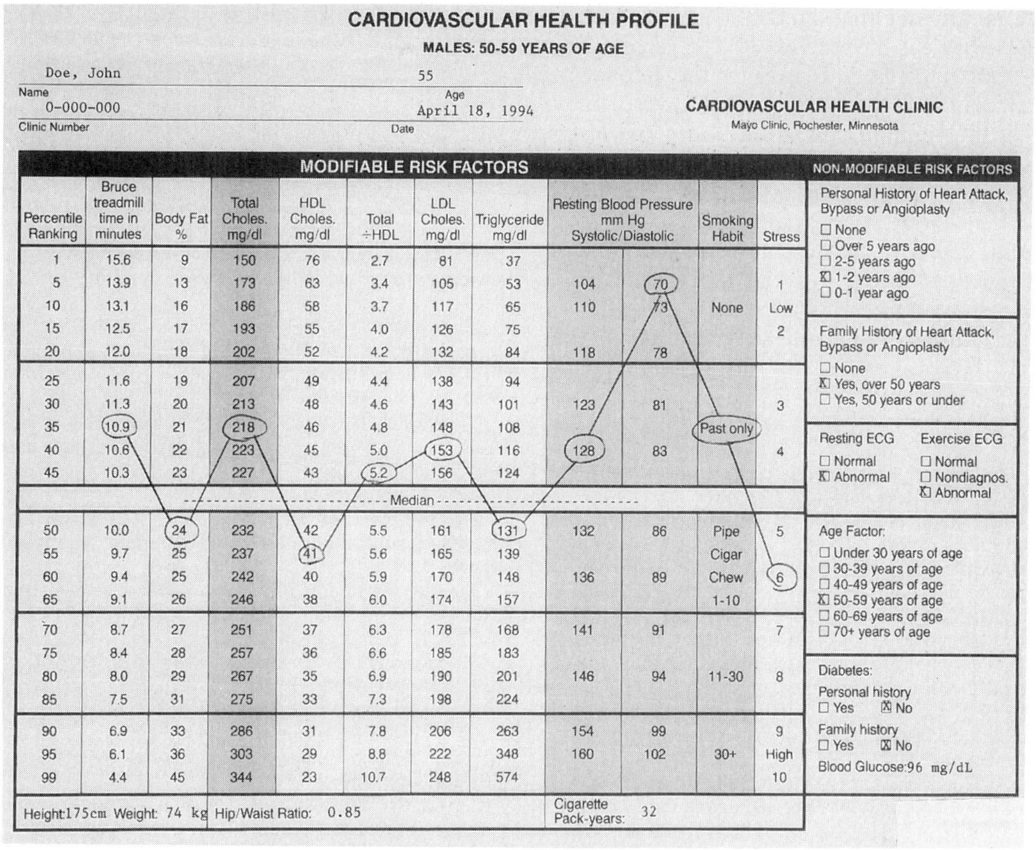

CARDIOVASCULAR HEALTH PROFILE

MALES: 50-59 YEARS OF AGE

Name: Doe, John   Age: 55

Clinic Number: 0-000-000   Date: April 18, 1994

CARDIOVASCULAR HEALTH CLINIC
Mayo Clinic, Rochester, Minnesota

MODIFIABLE RISK FACTORS

Percentile Ranking	Bruce treadmill time in minutes	Body Fat %	Total Choles. mg/dl	HDL Choles. mg/dl	Total ÷HDL	LDL Choles. mg/dl	Triglyceride mg/dl	Resting Blood Pressure mm Hg Systolic/Diastolic		Smoking Habit	Stress
1	15.6	9	150	76	2.7	81	37				
5	13.9	13	173	63	3.4	105	53	104	70		1
10	13.1	16	186	58	3.7	117	65	110	73	None	Low
15	12.5	17	193	55	4.0	126	75				2
20	12.0	18	202	52	4.2	132	84	118	78		
25	11.6	19	207	49	4.4	138	94				
30	11.3	20	213	48	4.6	143	101	123	81		3
35	10.9	21	218	46	4.8	148	108			Past only	
40	10.6	22	223	45	5.0	153	116	128	83		4
45	10.3	23	227	43	5.2	156	124				
Median											
50	10.0	24	232	42	5.5	161	131	132	86	Pipe	5
55	9.7	25	237	41	5.6	165	139			Cigar	
60	9.4	25	242	40	5.9	170	148	136	89	Chew	6
65	9.1	26	246	38	6.0	174	157			1-10	
70	8.7	27	251	37	6.3	178	168	141	91		7
75	8.4	28	257	36	6.6	185	183				
80	8.0	29	267	35	6.9	190	201	146	94	11-30	8
85	7.5	31	275	33	7.3	198	224				
90	6.9	33	286	31	7.8	206	263	154	99		9
95	6.1	36	303	29	8.8	222	348	160	102	30+	High
99	4.4	45	344	23	10.7	248	574				10

Height: 175 cm Weight: 74 kg Hip/Waist Ratio: 0.85 Cigarette Pack-years: 32

NON-MODIFIABLE RISK FACTORS

Personal History of Heart Attack, Bypass or Angioplasty
- ☐ None
- ☐ Over 5 years ago
- ☐ 2-5 years ago
- ☒ 1-2 years ago
- ☐ 0-1 year ago

Family History of Heart Attack, Bypass or Angioplasty
- ☐ None
- ☒ Yes, over 50 years
- ☐ Yes, 50 years or under

Resting ECG
- ☐ Normal
- ☒ Abnormal

Exercise ECG
- ☐ Normal
- ☐ Nondiagnos.
- ☒ Abnormal

Age Factor:
- ☐ Under 30 years of age
- ☐ 30-39 years of age
- ☐ 40-49 years of age
- ☒ 50-59 years of age
- ☐ 60-69 years of age
- ☐ 70+ years of age

Diabetes:

Personal history ☐ Yes ☒ No

Family history ☐ Yes ☒ No

Blood Glucose: 96 mg/dL

Fig 14-6 Cardiovascular health profile for a 55-year-old man. The profile is used to enhance patient education and serves to motivate patients in their efforts to modify risk factors. ECG, electrocardiogram; HDL, high-density lipoprotein; LDL, low-density lipoprotein.

are compared with norms based on age and sex, for which Mayo Clinic data are used. The total relative risk is then discussed. The results of the graded-exercise test are presented and discussed.

Specific recommendations are made for modification of existing risk factors. A dietitian recommends dietary changes to modify obesity, hyperlipidemia, elevated blood glucose, and hypertension.[180] Nutritional guidelines are provided as advised by the American Heart Association two-phase diet plan, with fat intake below 30% of total calories.[181] These recommendations include a reduction in the total amount of calories from fat, particularly saturated fat, an increase in complex carbohydrates, a decrease in sugar, and a reduction in sodium and cholesterol.

Referral to programs for smoking cessation and stress management and classes for risk-factor modification may be appropriate for selected patients. For patients at high risk, a supervised exercise and education program (phase III) may be beneficial.

An aerobic exercise program is designed, and the patient receives instructions in proper exercise principles from exercise specialists and cardiac rehabilitation nurses. The exercise prescription is prepared on the basis of the guidelines suggested for phase IV cardiac rehabilitation/adult fitness programs (see Table 14-11). The patient may participate in one or more staff-supervised exercise sessions to facilitate understanding. The concepts of warm-up and cool-down, pulse taking, and perceived exertion for proper exercise intensity and the advised gradual progression of the exercise program are stressed. An activity log to document progress in the exercise program is presented to the patient. The completed log is returned through the mail and evaluated by the staff. The results of the evaluation are communicated to the patient.

For patients with serious modifiable risk factors, a follow-up appointment is advised. At an interval of 3 to 6 months, the entire risk-factor profile may be repeated or, more simply, the risk factors in question may be reevaluated.

In the future, additional coronary risk factors, such as hyperinsulinemia, Lp(a) excess, increased iron storage, and postprandial lipemia, may be used as part of the coronary risk assessment.[135,182-184] New techniques, such as the detection of coronary artery calcification by electron-beam computed tomography as a marker for early atherosclerosis, may assist greatly in identifying patients who merit aggressive steps in risk-factor modification.[185]

Efforts in primary prevention of cardiovascular disease are of great concern, given the magnitude of the premature mortality and economic loss resulting from the disease. It is encouraging that epidemiologic evidence strongly suggests that cardiovascular disease is preventable. However, our knowledge regarding the impact of risk-factor modification on future morbidity and mortality is not complete. Information concerning both the long-term results with risk-factor intervention and the most beneficial approaches for changing potentially dangerous habits is needed. It is our belief that efforts to improve lifestyle to help control the major risk factors are justifiable and that they warrant more widespread application. We hope that the recent decline in cardiovascular mortality in the United States will be amplified in the coming years.

REFERENCES

1. Report of the Task Force on Cardiovascular Rehabilitation: Needs and Opportunities for Rehabilitating the Coronary Heart Disease Patient (DHEW Publication No. [NIH] 75-750). Washington, DC, National Heart and Lung Institute, 1974, p 3

2. Kramsch DM, Aspen AJ, Abramowitz BM, et al: Reduction of coronary atherosclerosis by moderate conditioning exercise in monkeys on an atherogenic diet. *N Engl J Med* 305:1483-1489, 1981

3. Arntzenius AC, Kromhout D, Barth JD, et al: Diet, lipoproteins, and the progression of coronary atherosclerosis: the Leiden Intervention Trial. *N Engl J Med* 312:805-811, 1985

4. Blankenhorn DH, Nessim SA, Johnson RL, et al: Beneficial effects of combined colestipol-niacin therapy on coronary atherosclerosis and coronary venous bypass grafts. *JAMA* 257:3233-3240, 1987

5. Brown G, Albers JJ, Fisher LD, et al: Regression of coronary artery disease as a result of intensive lipid-lowering therapy in men with high levels of apolipoprotein B. *N Engl J Med* 323:1289-1298, 1990

6. Ornish D, Brown SE, Scherwitz LW, et al: Can lifestyle changes reverse coronary heart disease? The Lifestyle Heart Trial. *Lancet* 336:129-133, 1990

7. Voller RD Jr, Strong WB: Pediatric aspects of atherosclerosis. *Am Heart J* 101:815-836, 1981

8. Wolf FG, Akhtar M: Sudden cardiac death. In *Heart Disease and Rehabilitation.* Edited by ML Pollock, DH Schmidt. Boston, Houghton Mifflin Professional Publishers, 1979, pp 120-139

9. Stamler J: Primary prevention of coronary heart disease: the last 20 years. *Am J Cardiol* 47:722-735, 1981

10. Thom TJ, Kannel WB: Downward trend in cardiovascular mortality. *Annu Rev Med* 32:427-434, 1981

11. Stern MP: The recent decline in ischemic heart disease mortality. *Ann Intern Med* 91:630-640, 1979

12. American Association of Cardiovascular and Pulmonary Rehabilitation: *Guidelines for Cardiac Rehabilitation Programs.* Second Edition. Champaign, Illinois, Human Kinetics Books, 1995

13. American College of Sports Medicine: *Guidelines for Exercise Testing and Prescription.* Fourth edition. Philadelphia, Lea & Febiger, 1991

14. Foxworth GD: Rehabilitation for hospitalized adults after open-heart procedures: the team approach. *Heart Lung* 7:834-839, 1978

15. Gau GT: Cardiac rehabilitation. I. A cardiologist's view. *Psychiatr Ann* 8:31-43, October 1978

16. Johnston BL, Cantwell JD, Fletcher GF: Eight steps to inpatient cardiac rehabilitation: the team effort—methodology and preliminary results. *Heart Lung* 5:97-111, 1976

17. Squires RW, Gau GT, Miller TD, et al: Cardiovascular rehabilitation: status, 1990. *Mayo Clin Proc* 65:731-755, 1990

18. Cassem NH, Hackett TP: Psychological rehabilitation of myocardial infarction patients in the acute phase. *Heart Lung* 2:382-388, 1973

19. Eliot RS, Long DR, Boone JL: Rehabilitation. In *Stress and the Heart: Mechanisms, Measurements, and Management.* Edited by RS Eliot. Mount Kisco, New York, Futura Publishing Company, 1988, pp 185-200

20. Denolin H (ed): Psychological problems before and after myocardial infarction. *Adv Cardiol* 29:1-155, 1982

21. Wenger NK: Patient and family education and counseling: a requisite component of cardiac rehabilitation. In *Controversies in Cardiac Rehabilitation.* Edited by P Mathes, ML Halhuber. New York, Springer-Verlag, 1982, pp 108-114

22. Dunbar JM: Adherence to medication: an intervention study with poor adherers (abstract). *Circulation* 56 Suppl 3:169, 1977

23. Opitz JL: Physical activity following myocardial infarction. *Psychiatr Ann* 8:80-91, October 1978

24. Harpur JE, Kellett RJ, Conner WT, et al: Controlled trial of early mobilisation and discharge from hospital in uncomplicated myocardial infarction. *Lancet* 2:1331-1334, 1971

25. Hutter AM Jr, Sidel VW, Shine KI, et al: Early hospital discharge after myocardial infarction. *N Engl J Med* 288:1141-1144, 1973

26. Dion WF, Grevenow P, Pollock ML, et al: Medical problems and physiologic responses during supervised inpatient cardiac rehabilitation: the patient after coronary artery bypass grafting. *Heart Lung* 11:248-255, 1982

27. Wenger NK: In-hospital rehabilitation after myocardial infarction. In *Physical Conditioning and Cardiovascular Rehabilitation.* Edited by LS Cohen, MB Mock, I Ringqvist. New York, John Wiley & Sons, 1981, pp 139-144

28. Silvidi GE, Squires RW, Pollock ML, et al: Hemodynamic responses and medical problems associated with early exercise and ambulation in coronary artery bypass graft surgery patients. *J Cardiac Rehabil* 2:355-362, 1982

29. Hartman CW, Bartel AG, Call TD, et al: The safety and value of exercise testing soon after coronary artery bypass surgery. *J Cardiac Rehabil* 1:142-145, 1981

30. Rod JL, Squires RW, Pollock ML, et al: Symptom-limited graded exercise testing soon after myocardial revascularization surgery. *J Cardiac Rehabil* 2:199-205, 1982

31. Sivarajan ES, Snydsman A, Smith B, et al: Low-level treadmill testing of 41 patients with acute myocardial infarction prior to discharge from the hospital. *Heart Lung* 6:975-980, 1977

32. Théroux P, Waters DD, Halphen C, et al: Prognostic value of exercise testing soon after myocardial infarction. *N Engl J Med* 301:341-345, 1979

33. Smith JW, Dennis CA, Gassmann A, et al: Exercise testing three weeks after myocardial infarction. *Chest* 75:12-16, 1979

34. Starling MR, Crawford MH, Kennedy GT, et al: Exercise testing early after myocardial infarction: predictive value for subsequent unstable angina and death. *Am J Cardiol* 46:909-914, 1980

35. Sami M, Kraemer H, DeBusk RF: The prognostic significance of serial exercise testing after myocardial infarction. *Circulation* 60:1238-1246, 1979

36. Schulze RA Jr, Strauss HW, Pitt B: Sudden death in the year following myocardial infarction: relation to ventricular premature contractions in the late hospital phase and left ventricular ejection fraction. *Am J Med* 62:192-199, 1977

37. Hayes JR, Gau GT, O'Brien PC: The effect of intensive cardiac rehabilitation on long-term morbidity and mortality after myocardial infarction (abstract). Presented at the II World Congress on Cardiac Rehabilitation, Jerusalem, Israel, November 30-December 3, 1981

38. Knapp D, Gutmann M, Regis S, et al: Follow-up activity level among coronary artery bypass surgery (CABS) patients (abstract). *Med Sci Sports Exerc* 14:178, 1982

39. Broustet JP, Dubecq M, Bouloumie J, et al: Réhabilitation des coronariens: programme de mobilisation à la phase aiguë. *Schweiz Med Wochenschr* 103:57-63, 1973

40. Convertino V, Hung J, Goldwater D, et al: Cardiovascular responses to exercise in middle-aged men after 10 days of bedrest. *Circulation* 65:134-140, 1982

41. Saltin B, Blomqvist G, Mitchell JH, et al: Response to exercise after bed rest and after training: a longitudinal study of adaptive changes in oxygen transport and body composition. *Circulation* 38 Suppl 7:1-78, 1968

42. Naughton J, Bruhn J, Lategola MT, et al: Rehabilitation following myocardial infarction. *Am J Med* 46:725-734, 1969

43. Bloch A, Maeder J-P, Haissly J-C, et al: Early mobilization after myocardial infarction: a controlled study. *Am J Cardiol* 34:152-157, 1974

44. Topol EJ, Burek K, O'Neill WW, et al: A randomized controlled trial of hospital discharge three days after myocardial infarction in the era of reperfusion. *N Engl J Med* 318:1083-1088, 1988

45. Silvidi GE, Squires RW, Pollock ML, et al: Early cardiac rehabilitation: perceptions and compliance (abstract). *Phys Ther* 62:646-648, 1982

46. Neuberg GW, Friedman SH, Weiss MB, et al: Cardiopulmonary exercise testing: the clinical value of gas exchange data. *Arch Intern Med* 148:2221-2226, 1988

47. Mancini DM, Eisen H, Kussmaul W, et al: Value of peak oxygen consumption for optimal timing of cardiac transplantation in ambulatory patients with heart failure. *Circulation* 83:778-786, 1991

48. American College of Sports Medicine: *Guidelines for Graded Exercise Testing and Exercise Prescription.* Second edition. Philadelphia, Lea & Febiger, 1980, pp 1-81

49. Bader CA: Teaching the coronary patient and his family. *Nurs Clin North Am* 7:563-571, 1972

50. Pollock ML, Schmidt DH, Jackson AS: Measurement of cardiorespiratory fitness and body composition in the clinical setting. *Compr Ther* 6:12-27, September 1980

51. Squires RW, Miller TD, Harn T, et al: Transtelephonic electrocardiographic monitoring of cardiac rehabilitation exercise sessions in coronary artery disease. *Am J Cardiol* 67:962-964, 1991

52. Kavanagh T, Shephard RJ: Exercise for postcoronary patients: an assessment of infrequent supervision. *Arch Phys Med Rehabil* 61:114-118, 1980

53. Thoreson RW, Ackerman M: Cardiac rehabilitation: basic principles and psychosocial factors. *Rehabil Counseling Bull* 24:223-257, 1981

54. Rost K, Smith GR: Return to work after an initial myocardial infarction and subsequent emotional distress. *Arch Intern Med* 152:381-385, 1992

55. Hackett TP, Cassem NH: The psychologic reactions of patients in the pre- and post-hospital phases of myocardial infarction. *Postgrad Med* 57:43-46, April 1975

56. Cooper AJ: Myocardial infarction and advice on sexual activity. *Practitioner* 229:575-579, 1985

57. Hellerstein HK, Friedman EH: Sexual activity and the postcoronary patient. *Arch Intern Med* 125:987-999, 1970

58. De Rogatis LR: *The SCL 90R.* Baltimore, Clinical Psychometric Research, 1975

59. Case RB, Moss AJ, Case N, et al: Living alone after myocardial infarction: impact on prognosis. *JAMA* 267:515-519, 1992

60. Williams RB, Barefoot JC, Califf RM, et al: Prognostic importance of social and economic resources among medically treated patients with angiographically documented coronary artery disease. *JAMA* 267:520-524, 1992

61. Frasure-Smith N, Lesperance F, Talajic M: Depression and 18-month prognosis after myocardial infarction. *Circulation* 91:999-1005, 1995

62. Oldridge N, Guyatt G, Jones N, et al: Effects on quality of life with comprehensive rehabilitation after acute myocardial infarction. *Am J Cardiol* 67:1084-1089, 1991

63. Borg GAV: Perceived exertion: a note on "history" and methods. *Med Sci Sports* 5:90-93, 1973

64. Gutmann MC, Squires RW, Pollock ML, et al: Perceived exertion – heart rate relationship during exercise testing and training in cardiac patients. *J Cardiac Rehabil* 1:52-59, 1981

65. Meyer K, Lehmann M, Sünder G, et al: Interval versus continuous exercise training after coronary bypass surgery: a comparison of training-induced acute reactions with respect to the effectiveness of the exercise methods. *Clin Cardiol* 13:851-861, 1990

66. Hossack KF, Bruce RA, Kusumi F: Altered exercise ventilatory responses by apparent propranolol-diminished glucose metabolism: implications concerning impaired physical training benefit in coronary patients. *Am Heart J* 102:378-382, 1981

67. Scheuer J, Greenberg MA, Zohman LR: Exercise training in patients with coronary artery disease. *Mod Concepts Cardiovasc Dis* 47:85-90, 1978

68. Pratt CM, Welton DE, Squires WG Jr, et al: Demonstration of training effect during chronic β-adrenergic blockade in patients with coronary artery disease. *Circulation* 64:1125-1129, 1981

69. Squires RW, Rod JL, Pollock ML, et al: Effect of propranolol on perceived exertion soon after myocardial revascularization surgery. *Med Sci Sports Exerc* 14:276-280, 1982

70. Cobb LA, Baum RS, Alvarez H, et al: Resuscitation from out-of-hospital ventricular fibrillation: 4 years follow-up. *Circulation* 52: Suppl 3:223-228, 1975

71. Oberman A, Ray M, Turner ME, et al: Sudden death in patients evaluated for ischemic heart disease. *Circulation* 52 Suppl 3:170-172, 1975

72. Lee AP, Ice R, Blessey R, et al: Long-term effects of physical training on coronary patients with impaired ventricular function. *Circulation* 60:1519-1526, 1979

73. Squires RW, Lavie CJ, Brandt TR, et al: Cardiac rehabilitation in patients with severe ischemic left ventricular dysfunction. *Mayo Clin Proc* 62:997-1002, 1987

74. Sullivan MJ, Higginbotham MB, Cobb FR: Exercise training in patients with severe left ventricular dysfunction: hemodynamic and metabolic effects. *Circulation* 78:506-515, 1988

75. Coats AJS, Adamopoulos S, Meyer TE, et al: Effects of physical training in chronic heart failure. *Lancet* 335:63-66, 1990

76. Jugdutt BI, Michorowski BL, Kappagoda CT: Exercise training after anterior Q wave myocardial infarction: importance of regional left ventricular function and topography. *J Am Coll Cardiol* 12:362-372, 1988

77. Giannuzzi P, Temporelli PL, Tavassi L, et al: EAMI – exercise training in anterior myocardial infarction: an ongoing multicenter randomized study: preliminary results on left ventricular function and remodeling. *Chest* 101 Suppl:315S-321S, 1992

78. Jetté M, Heller R, Landry F, et al: Randomized 4-week exercise program in patients with impaired left ventricular function. *Circulation* 84:1561-1567, 1991

79. Hedback B, Perk J: Can high-risk patients after myocardial infarction participate in comprehensive cardiac rehabilitation? *Scand J Rehabil Med* 22:15-20, 1990

80. Clausen JP, Trap-Jensen J, Lassen NA: The effects of training on the heart rate during arm and leg exercise. *Scand J Clin Lab Invest* 26:295-301, 1970

81. Squires RW, Muri AJ, Anderson LJ, et al: Weight training during phase II (early outpatient) cardiac rehabilitation: heart rate and blood pressure responses. *J Cardiopulmonary Rehabil* 11:360-364, 1991

82. McCartney N, McKelvie RS, Haslam DRS, et al: Usefulness of weightlifting training in improving strength and maximal power output in coronary artery disease. *Am J Cardiol* 67:939-945, 1991

83. The Coronary Drug Project Research Group: Prognostic importance of premature beats following myocardial infarction: experience in the Coronary Drug Project. *JAMA* 223:1116-1124, 1973

84. Halpern SW, Mandel WJ: The significance of exercise-induced ventricular arrhythmias (editoral). *Chest* 77:1-2, 1980

85. Puntillo R, Pollock ML, Squires R, et al: Comparison of graded exercise testing, Holter monitoring and monitored exercise training in detecting serious dysrhythmias in myocardial revascularization surgery patients (abstract). *Med Sci Sports Exerc* 13:137, 1981

86. American College of Cardiology: Recommendations of the American College of Cardiology on cardiovascular rehabilitation. *J Am Coll Cardiol* 7:451-453, 1986

87. Health and Public Policy Committee, American College of Physicians: Cardiac rehabilitation services. *Ann Intern Med* 109:671-673, 1988

88. Garber CE, Carleton RA, Camaione DN, et al: The threshold for myocardial ischemia varies in patients with coronary artery disease depending on the exercise protocol. *J Am Coll Cardiol* 17:1256-1262, 1991

89. Fardy PS, Doll N, Taylor J, et al: Monitoring cardiac patients: how much is enough? *Physician Sportsmed* 10:146-152, June 1982

90. Åstrand P-O, Rodahl K: *Textbook of Work Physiology: Physiological Bases of Exercise.* Second edition. New York, McGraw-Hill Book Company, 1977, p 460

91. Pollock ML, Ward A, Foster C: Exercise prescription for rehabilitation of the cardiac patient. In *Heart Disease and Rehabilitation.* Edited by ML Pollock, DH Schmidt. Boston, Houghton Mifflin Professional Publishers, 1979, pp 413-445

92. Karvonen MJ, Kentala E, Mustala O: The effects of training on heart rate: a "longitudinal" study. *Ann Med Exp Biol Fenn* 35:307-315, 1957

93. Franklin BA, Gordon S, Timmis GC: Amount of exercise necessary for the patient with coronary artery disease. *Am J Cardiol* 69:1426-1432, 1992

94. Blumenthal JA, Rejeski WJ, Walsh-Riddle M, et al: Comparison of high- and low-intensity exercise training early after acute myocardial infarction. *Am J Cardiol* 61:26-30, 1988

95. Goble AJ, Hare DL, Macdonald PS, et al: Effect of early programmes of high and low intensity exercise on physical performance after transmural acute myocardial infarction. *Br Heart J* 65:126-131, 1991

96. Gotto AM Jr: Therapeutic intervention for hypercholesterolemia. *Clin Cardiol* 15 Suppl III:III-18-III-21, 1992

97. Lavie CJ, Gau GT, Squires RW, et al: Management of lipids in primary and secondary prevention of cardiovascular diseases. *Mayo Clin Proc* 63:605-621, 1988

98. Squires RW, Allison TG, Gau GT, et al: Low-dose, time-release nicotinic acid: effects in selected patients with low concentrations of high-density lipoprotein cholesterol. *Mayo Clin Proc* 67:855-860, 1992

99. Expert Panel on Detection, Evaluation, and Treatment of High Blood Cholesterol in Adults: Summary of the Second Report of the National Cholesterol Education Program (NCEP) Expert Panel on Detection, Evaluation, and Treatment of High Blood Cholesterol in Adults (Adult Treatment Panel II). *JAMA* 269:3015-3023, 1993

100. American College of Sports Medicine: Position statement on the recommended quantity and quality of exercise for developing and maintaining fitness in healthy adults. *Med Sci Sports* 10:vii-xi, 1978

101. Haskell WL: Cardiovascular complications during exercise training of cardiac patients. *Circulation* 57:920-924, 1978

102. Van Camp SP, Peterson RA: Cardiovascular complications of outpatient cardiac rehabilitation programs. *JAMA* 256:1160-1163, 1986

103. Clausen JP, Trap-Jensen J: Effects of training on the distribution of cardiac output in patients with coronary artery disease. *Circulation* 42:611-624, 1970

104. Redwood DR, Rosing DR, Epstein SE: Circulatory and symptomatic effects of physical training in patients with coronary-artery disease and angina pectoris. *N Engl J Med* 286:959-965, 1972

105. Arvan S: Exercise performance of the high risk acute myocardial infarction patient after cardiac rehabilitation. *Am J Cardiol* 62:197-201, 1988

106. Ades PA, Grunvald MH, Weiss RM, et al: Usefulness of myocardial ischemia as predictor of training effect in cardiac rehabilitation after acute myocardial infarction or coronary artery bypass grafting. *Am J Cardiol* 63:1032-1036, 1989

107. Detry J-MR, Rousseau M, Vandenbroucke G, et al: Increased arteriovenous oxygen difference after physical training in coronary heart disease. *Circulation* 44:109-118, 1971

108. Pollock ML, Foster C, Anholm J, et al: Randomized exercise and relaxation trials with myocardial revascularization surgery patients: cardiorespiratory and hemodynamic effects (abstract). *Med Sci Sports Exerc* 13:133, 1981

109. Ades PA, Grunvald MH: Cardiopulmonary exercise testing before and after conditioning in older coronary patients. *Am Heart J* 120:585-589, 1990

110. Fardy PS: Isometric exercise and the cardiovascular system. *Physician Sportsmed* 9:43-56, September 1981

111. Atwood E, Jensen D, Froelicher V, et al: Radionuclide perfusion images before and after cardiac rehabilitation. *Aviat Space Environ Med* 51:892-898, 1980

112. Todd IC, Bradnam MS, Cooke MBD, et al: Effects of daily high-intensity exercise on myocardial perfusion in angina pectoris. *Am J Cardiol* 68:1593-1599, 1991

113. Hindman MC, Wallace AG: Radionuclide exercise studies. In *Physical Conditioning and Cardiovascular Rehabilitation.* Edited by LS Cohen, MB Mock, I Ringqvist. New York, John Wiley & Sons, 1981, pp 33-46

114. Charuzi Y, Vyden J, Berman D, et al: Myocardial perfusion by thallium-201 scintigraphy before and after cardiac rehabilitation (abstract). *Clin Res* 27:158A, 1979

115. Beller GA, Murray GC, ErkenBrack SK: Influence of exercise training soon after myocardial infarction on regional myocardial perfusion and resting left ventricular function. *Clin Cardiol* 15:17-23, 1992

116. Paterson DH, Shephard RJ, Cunningham D, et al: Effects of physical training on cardiovascular function following myocardial infarction. *J Appl Physiol* 47:482-489, 1979

117. Froelicher VF, Brown P: Exercise and coronary heart disease. *J Cardiac Rehabil* 1:277-288, 1981

118. Hagberg JM, Ehsani AA, Holloszy JO: Effect of 12 months of intense exercise training on stroke volume in patients with coronary artery disease. *Circulation* 67:1194-1199, 1983

119. Detry J-M, Bruce RA: Effects of physical training on exertional ST-segment depression in coronary heart disease. *Circulation* 44:390-396, 1971

120. Haskell WL: Mechanisms by which physical activity may enhance the clinical status of cardiac patients. In *Heart Disease and Rehabilitation.* Edited by ML Pollock, DH Schmidt. Boston, Houghton Mifflin Professional Publishers, 1979, pp 276-296

121. Ehsani AA, Heath GW, Hagberg JM, et al: Effects of 12 months of intense exercise training on ischemic ST-segment depression in patients with coronary artery disease. *Circulation* 64:1116-1124, 1981

122. Kattus AA, Jorgensen CR, Worden RE, et al: ST segment depression with near-maximal exercise: its modification by physical conditioning. *Chest* 62:678-683, 1972

123. Schuler G, Schlierf G, Wirth A, et al: Low-fat diet and regular, supervised physical exercise in patients with symptomatic coronary artery disease: reduction of stress-induced myocardial ischemia. *Circulation* 77:172-181, 1988

124. Hambrecht R, Niebauer J, Marburger C, et al: Various intensities of leisure time physical activity in patients with coronary artery disease: effects on cardiorespiratory fitness and progression of coronary atherosclerotic lesions. *J Am Coll Cardiol* 22:468-477, 1995

125. Jonason T, Jonzon B, Ringqvist I, et al: Effect of physical training on different categories of patients with intermittent claudication. *Acta Med Scand* 206:253-258, 1979

126. Blumenthal JA, Williams RS, Wallace AG, et al: Physiological and psychological variables predict compliance to prescribed exercise therapy in patients recovering from myocardial infarction. *Psychosom Med* 44:519-527, 1982

127. Oldridge NB, Spencer J: Exercise habits and perceptions before and after graduation or dropout from supervised cardiac exercise rehabilitation. *J Cardiopulmonary Rehabil* 5:313-319, 1985

128. Taylor CB, Houston-Miller N: The behavioral approach. In *Rehabilitation of the Coronary Patient.* Third edition. Edited by NK Wenger, HK Hellerstein. New York, Churchill Livingstone, 1991, pp 461-477

129. Raichlen JS, Healy B, Achuff SC, et al: Importance of risk factors in the angiographic progression of coronary artery disease. *Am J Cardiol* 57:66-70, 1986

130. Campeau L, Enjalbert M, Lespérance J, et al: The relation of risk factors to the development of atherosclerosis in saphenous-vein bypass grafts and the progression of disease in the native circulation. A study 10 years after aortocoronary bypass surgery. *N Engl J Med* 311:1329-1332, 1984

131. Moise A, Théroux P, Taeymans Y, et al: Factors associated with progression of coronary artery disease in patients with normal or minimally narrowed coronary arteries. *Am J Cardiol* 56:30-34, 1985

132. Selvester R, Camp J, Sanmarco M: Effects of exercise training on progression of documented coronary arteriosclerosis in men. *Ann NY Acad Sci* 301:495-508, 1977

133. Miller M, Seidler A, Kwiterovich PO, et al: Long-term predictors of subsequent cardiovascular events with coronary artery disease and 'desirable' levels of plasma total cholesterol. *Circulation* 86:1165-1170, 1992

134. Luria MH, Erel J, Sapoznikov D, et al: Cardiovascular risk factor clustering and ratio of total cholesterol to high-density lipoprotein cholesterol in angiographically documented coronary artery disease. *Am J Cardiol* 67:31-36, 1991

135. Reaven GM: Role of insulin resistance in human disease. *Diabetes* 37:1595-1607, 1988

136. May GS, Eberlein KA, Furberg CD: Secondary prevention after myocardial infarction: a review of long-term trials. *Prog Cardiovasc Dis* 24:331-352, 1982

137. Scandinavian Simvastatin Survival Study Group: Randomised trial of cholesterol lowering in 4444 patients with coronary heart disease: the Scandinavian Simvastatin Survival Study (4S). *Lancet* 344:1383-1389, 1994

138. Brensike JF, Levy RI, Kelsey SF, et al: Effects of therapy with cholestyramine on progression of coronary arteriosclerosis: results of the NHLBI Type II Coronary Intervention Study. *Circulation* 69:313-324, 1984

139. Levy RI, Brensike FJ, Epstein SE, et al: The influence of changes in lipid values induced by cholestyramine and diet on progression of coronary artery disease: results of the NHLBI Type II Coronary Intervention Study. *Circulation* 69:325-337, 1984

140. Egashira K, Hirooka Y, Kai H, et al: Reduction in serum cholesterol with pravastatin improves endothelium-dependent coronary vasomotion in patients with hypercholesterolemia. *Circulation* 89:2519-2524, 1994

141. Cavender JB, Rogers WJ, Fisher LD, et al: Effects of smoking on survival and morbidity in patients randomized to medical or surgical therapy in the Coronary Artery Surgery Study (CASS): 10-year follow-up. *J Am Coll Cardiol* 20:287-294, 1992

142. Åberg A, Bergstrand R, Johansson S, et al: Cessation of smoking after myocardial infarction: effects on mortality after 10 years. *Br Heart J* 49:416-422, 1983

143. Rosenberg L, Kaufman DW, Helmrich SP, et al: The risk of myocardial infarction after quitting smoking in men under 55 years of age. *N Engl J Med* 313:1511-1514, 1985
144. Vlietsra RE, Frye RL, Kronmal RA, et al: Risk factors and angiographic coronary artery disease: a report from the Coronary Artery Surgery Study (CASS). *Circulation* 62:254-261, 1980
145. Vlietsra RE, Kronmal RA, Frye RL, et al: Factors affecting the extent and severity of coronary artery disease in patients enrolled in the Coronary Artery Surgery Study. *Arteriosclerosis* 2:208-215, 1982
146. Hopkins PN, Williams RR: Identification and relative weight of cardiovascular risk factors. *Cardiol Clin* 4:3-31, Feb 1986
147. Mulcahy R: Influence of cigarette smoking on morbidity and mortality after myocardial infarction. *Br Heart J* 49:410-415, 1983
148. Daly LE, Mulcahy R, Graham I, et al: Long term effect on mortality of stopping smoking after unstable angina and myocardial infarction. *Br Med J [Clin Res]* 287:324-326, 1983
149. Connolly DC, Elveback LR, Oxman HA: Coronary heart disease in residents of Rochester, Minnesota, 1950-1975. III. Effect of hypertension and its treatment on survival of patients with coronary artery disease. *Mayo Clin Proc* 58:249-254, 1983
150. Bray GA: Obesity and the heart. *Mod Concepts Cardiovasc Dis* 56:67-71, 1987
151. Larsson B, Svärdsudd K, Welin L, et al: Abdominal adipose tissue distribution, obesity, and risk of cardiovascular disease and death: 13 year follow up of participants in the study of men born in 1913. *Br Med J [Clin Res]* 288:1401-1404, 1984
152. Vague J: The degree of masculine differentiation of obesities: a factor determining predisposition to diabetes, atherosclerosis, gout, and uric calculous disease. *Am J Clin Nutr* 4:20-34, 1956
153. Rosenman RH, Brand RJ, Sholtz RI, et al: Multivariate prediction of coronary heart disease during 8.5 year follow-up in the Western Collaborative Group Study. *Am J Cardiol* 37:903-910, 1976
154. Friedman M, Thoresen CE, Gill JJ, et al: Alteration of type A behavior and its effect on cardiac recurrences in post myocardial infarction patients: summary results of the Recurrent Coronary Prevention Project. *Am Heart J* 112:653-665, 1986
155. Ragland DR, Brand RJ: Type A behavior and mortality from coronary heart disease. *N Engl J Med* 318:65-69, 1988
156. Sanne H: Rehabilitation after a myocardial infarction. *Acta Med Scand* 712 Suppl:72-78, 1986
157. Roviaro S, Holmes DS, Holmsten RD: Influence of a cardiac rehabilitation program on the cardiovascular, psychological, and social functioning of cardiac patients. *J Behav Med* 7:61-81, 1984
158. Taylor CB, Houston-Miller N, Ahn DK, et al: The effects of exercise training programs on psychosocial improvement in uncomplicated postmyocardial infarction patients. *J Psychosom Res* 30:581-587, 1986
159. Burgess AW, Lerner DJ, D'Agostino RB, et al: A randomized control trial of cardiac rehabilitation. *Soc Sci Med* 24:359-370, 1987
160. van Dixhoorn J, Duivenvoorden HJ, Staal JA, et al: Cardiac events after myocardial infarction: possible effect of relaxation therapy. *Eur Heart J* 8:1210-1214, 1987
161. Paffenbarger RS Jr, Hyde RT: Exercise in the prevention of coronary heart disease. *Prev Med* 13:3-22, 1984
162. Leon AS, Connett J, Jacobs DR Jr, et al: Leisure-time physical activity levels and risk of coronary heart disease and death: the Multiple Risk Factor Intervention Trial. *JAMA* 258:2388-2395, 1987
163. Powell KE, Thompson PD, Caspersen CJ, et al: Physical activity and the incidence of coronary heart disease. *Annu Rev Public Health* 8:253-287, 1987
164. O'Connor GT, Buring JE, Yusuf S, et al: An overview of randomized trials of rehabilitation with exercise after myocardial infarction. *Circulation* 80:234-244, 1989
165. Levin L-Å, Perk J, Hedbäck B: Cardiac rehabilitation—a cost analysis. *J Intern Med* 230:427-434, 1991
166. Oldridge N, Furlong W, Feeny D, et al: Economic evaluation of cardiac rehabilitation soon after acute myocardial infarction. *Am J Cardiol* 72:154-161, 1993
167. Veterans Administration Cooperative Study Group on Antihypertensive Agents: Effects of treatment on morbidity in hypertension: results in patients with diastolic blood pressures averaging 115 through 129 mm Hg. *JAMA* 202:1028-1034, 1967
168. Ockene JK, Kuller LH, Svendsen KH, et al: The relationship of smoking cessation to coronary heart disease and lung cancer in the Multiple Risk Factor Intervention Trial (MRFIT). *J Public Health* 80:954-958, 1990
169. Rosenberg L, Palmer JR, Shapiro S: Decline in the risk of myocardial infarction among women who stop smoking. *N Engl J Med* 322:213-217, 1990
170. Hjermann I, Byre KV, Holme I, et al: Effect of diet and smoking intervention on the incidence of coronary heart disease: report of the Oslo Study Group of a randomised trial in healthy men. *Lancet* 2:1303-1310, 1981
171. Frick MH, Elo O, Haapa K, et al: Helsinki Heart Study: primary-prevention trial with gemfibrozil in middle-aged men with dyslipidemia: safety of treatment, changes in risk factors, and incidence of coronary heart disease. *N Engl J Med* 317:1237-1245, 1987
172. The Multiple Risk Factor Intervention Trial Research Group: Mortality rates after 10.5 years for participants in the Multiple Risk Factor Intervention Trial: findings related to a priori hypotheses of the trial. *JAMA* 263:1795-1801, 1990
173. Paffenbarger RS Jr, Hyde RT, Wing AL, et al: Physical activity, all-cause mortality, and longevity of college alumni. *N Engl J Med* 314:605-613, 1986
174. Corrao JM, Becker RC, Ockene IS, et al: Coronary heart disease risk factors in women. *Cardiology* 77 Suppl 2:8-24, 1990
175. Russell-Briefel R, Ezzati TM, Fulwood R, et al: Cardiovascular risk status and oral contraceptive use: United States, 1976-1980. *Prev Med* 15:352-362, 1986
176. Williams RR, Hopkins PN, Hunt SC, et al: Population-based frequency of dyslipidemia syndromes in coronary-prone families in Utah. *Arch Intern Med* 150:582-588, 1990
177. Quivers ES, Driscoll DJ, Garvey CD, et al: Variability in response to a low-fat, low-cholesterol diet in children with elevated low-density lipoprotein cholesterol levels. *Pediatrics* 89:925-929, 1992
178. Wing RR, Mathews KA, Kuller LH, et al: Waist to hip ratio in middle-aged women: associations with behavioral and psychosocial factors and with changes in cardiovascular risk factors. *Arterioscler Thromb* 11:1250-1257, 1991
179. Gau GT, Lynch JJ, Herrick JM: Assessment of cardiovascular fitness: the value of risk-factor profile and treadmill exercise testing (abstract). Presented at the II World Congress on Cardiac Rehabilitation, Jerusalem, Israel, November 30-December 3, 1981
180. Hartmann G: The role of diet. In *Controversies in Cardiac Rehabilitation.* Edited by P Mathes, MJ Halhuber. New York, Springer-Verlag, 1982, pp 1-5
181. The Expert Panel: Report of the National Cholesterol Education Program Expert Panel on detection, evaluation, and treatment of high blood cholesterol in adults. *Arch Intern Med* 148:36-69, 1988
182. Modan M, Or J, Karasik A, et al: Hyperinsulinemia, sex, and risk of atherosclerotic cardiovascular disease. *Circulation* 84:1165-1175, 1991
183. Genest J Jr, McNamara JR, Ordovas JM, et al: Lipoprotein cholesterol, apolipoprotein A-I and B and lipoprotein (a) abnormalities in men with premature coronary artery disease. *J Am Coll Cardiol* 19:792-802, 1992
184. Salonen JT, Nyyssönen K, Korpela H, et al: High stored iron levels are associated with excess risk of myocardial infarction in eastern Finnish men. *Circulation* 86:803-811, 1992
185. Simons DB, Schwartz RS, Edwards WD, et al: Noninvasive definition of anatomic coronary artery disease by ultrafast computed tomographic scanning: a quantitative pathologic comparison study. *J Am Coll Cardiol* 20:1118-1126, 1992

CHAPTER

15

Pathophysiology of circulatory failure

Richard J. Rodeheffer, M.D., Wayne L. Miller, M.D., and John C. Burnett, Jr., M.D.

TERMINOLOGY

Congestive heart failure refers to a clinical syndrome characterized by symptoms of dyspnea, reduced exercise tolerance, orthopnea, and signs such as tachycardia, rales, gallop rhythm, and edema. The syndrome is a multisystem response to an initial reduction in ventricular function. Although useful in a general descriptive sense, the term "congestive heart failure" lacks pathophysiologic specificity.

The clinical congestive heart failure syndrome may be thought of within a larger anatomic framework (Table 15-1). *Circulatory failure,* a widely encompassing term, refers to the inability of the cardiovascular system to meet the metabolic demands of the body. This term emphasizes the integrated and dynamic coupling between the heart and the peripheral circulation. Circulatory failure may be caused by a central disorder of cardiac pump function that reduces cardiac output; or it may be caused by a disorder of peripheral circulation, such as systemic or pulmonary hypertension, increased vascular capacity (e.g., vasodilatation), or vascular shunts; or it may be the result of reduced oxyhemoglobin (e.g., anemia) or reduced blood volume (e.g., hemorrhage or excessive diuresis).

Cardiac, or heart, failure, a more specific term than "circulatory failure," directs attention to disorders of cardiac pump performance. Cardiac failure may result from abnormal muscle function during systole or diastole, disturbed cardiac rhythm or conduction, valvular disease, pericardial disease, congenital disease, or cardiac tumors. Disordered systolic or diastolic pump function may result from a specific myocardial injury or from a myocardial response to peripheral vascular dysfunction, such as systemic or pulmonary hypertension.

Myocardial failure, a still more narrowly circumscribed term, refers to circulatory failure caused by primary systolic or diastolic dysfunction of cardiac muscle per se. Myocardial failure results from ischemic injury, cardiomyopathy, toxic or metabolic myocyte dysfunction, or inflammatory or infiltrative myocardial disorders.

Therefore, the terms "circulatory failure," "cardiac failure," and "myocardial failure" denote progressively more specific ranges of circulatory dysfunction. Nevertheless, because of the integrated character of the cardiovascular system, even the most focal central or peripheral disorder (e.g., myocardial infarction or arteriovenous shunt) can result in the more general condition of circulatory failure and in the clinical syndrome of congestive heart failure.

Table 15-1 Causes of circulatory failure

Circulatory failure

- I. Vascular regulation disorders
  - A. Systemic hypertension
  - B. Pulmonary hypertension
- II. Volume regulation disorders
  - A. Excessive blood volume
  - B. Reduced blood volume
- III. Inadequate or abnormal oxyhemoglobin
- IV. High-output conditions
- V. **Cardiac failure**
  - A. Pericardial disease
  - B. Valvular disease
  - C. Congenital disease
  - D. Cardiac tumors or trauma
  - E. Cardiac rhythm or conduction disorders
  - F. **Myocardial failure**
    1. Cardiomyopathy: dilated, hypertrophic, restrictive
    2. Ischemia and infarction
    3. Myocardial infiltrative conditions
    4. Myocardial inflammation

Left- and right-sided circulatory failure

Patients are often described as having signs and symptoms of either left or right ventricular dysfunction. Cardiac disorders that predominantly affect left ventricular function are manifest first by symptoms and signs of increased left atrial pressure (dyspnea, rales) and reduced cardiac output (fatigue). In contrast, some patients have predominant evidence of increased right atrial pressure (edema, ascites, hepatic congestion). Although the most common cause of right ventricular failure is left ventricular failure, manifestations of "pure" right-sided dysfunction may occur with pulmonary hypertension, pericardial disease, right-sided valve disease, and restrictive cardiomyopathy.

Systolic and diastolic failure

Depressed systolic ejection has long been recognized as a cause of circulatory failure. Since the 1970s, there has been increasing interest in the complex and dynamic process of diastole. Abnormal diastolic function has now emerged as a distinctly important contributor to the syndrome of congestive heart failure and may be observed in association with pericardial constriction or in myocardial restrictive processes. Abnormal diastolic function is a common concomitant of systolic dysfunction and a pathophysiologic phenomenon in its own right. It is further discussed below.

Compensatory adaptation

The cardiovascular system under stress has a remarkable capacity for compensatory adaptation. In clinical situations, this is apparent when severely depressed systolic function is found incidentally in a patient without symptoms. As depicted in Figure 15-1, compensatory changes involve myocyte structure and function, ventricular geometry, vascular tone, and volume regulation. These mechanisms are considered in greater detail below.

It is important to appreciate the *time course* of these compensatory physiologic alterations. Many are beneficial in acute circulatory failure (hours to days), but in chronic heart failure (months to years), they may contribute to the progressive ventricular and vascular dysfunction typical of the natural history of the congestive heart failure syndrome. Tachycardia and peripheral vasoconstriction are critical immediate responses that maintain blood flow and mean arterial pressure when a decrease in cardiac output is perceived. As sustained responses, however, they result in myocyte dysfunction and increased vascular afterload on an already failing ventricle. Acute dilatation of the left ventricle may augment the stroke volume of an injured ventricle, but long-term dilatation increases ventricular wall stress and may cause further deterioration in pump efficiency. Salt and water retention serve to maintain cardiac preload and are appropriate short-term responses to reduced renal perfusion; over the long term, however,

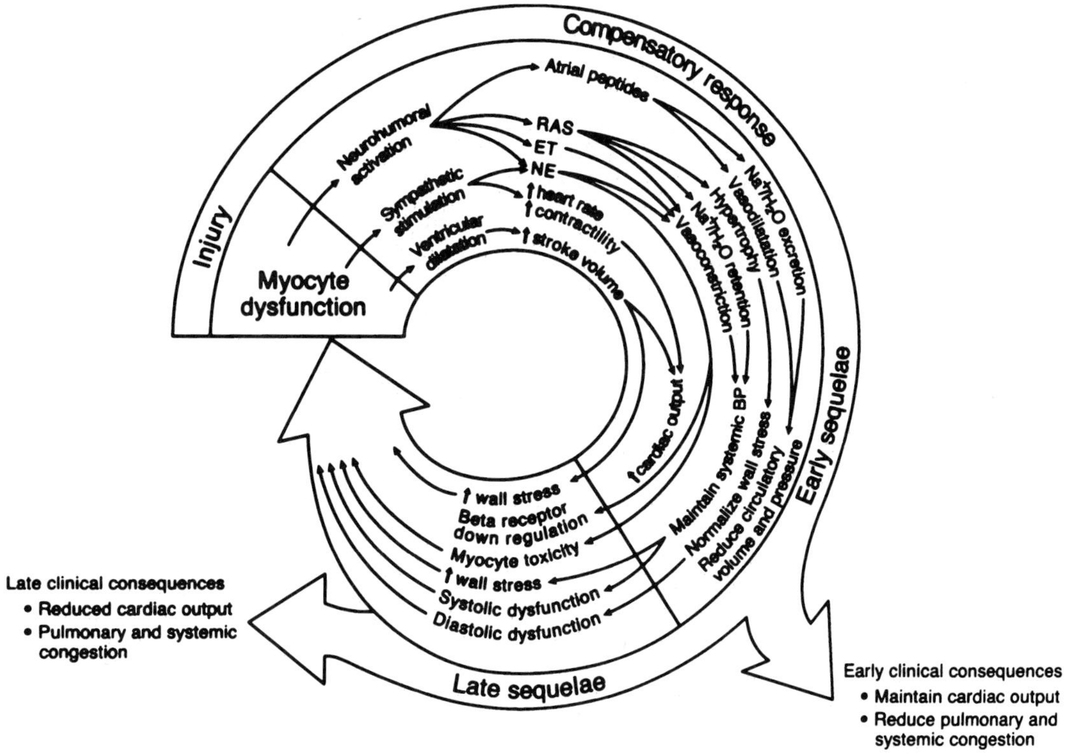

Fig 15-1 The pathophysiology of circulatory failure depicted as a cycle starting with myocyte injury and progressing through early compensatory responses and their long-term unfavorable consequences. *BP,* blood pressure; *ET,* endothelin; *NE,* norepinephrine; *RAS,* renin-angiotensin system.

volume expansion contributes to circulatory volume overload. Activation of neurohormonal systems that acutely increase contractility, circulatory volume, and arterial pressure may chronically promote disadvantageous remodeling of left ventricular architecture. To fully appreciate their significance, therefore, one must view compensatory events in the proper temporal context.

In the following discussion, we consider systolic ventricular performance, diastolic performance, and the systemic and vascular pathophysiology of circulatory failure.

SYSTOLIC FUNCTION AND DYSFUNCTION

Cellular adaptations

Myocardial nutritive supply. Although acute myocardial failure may be precipitated by abrupt reduction in myocardial blood flow (e.g., an acute ischemic insult), chronic myocardial failure does not appear to be primarily a consequence of reduced tissue blood flow and inadequate cellular nutritive support. Although both canine and human studies show that blood flow to failing myocardium is reduced, there is evidence that myocardial oxygen consumption is commensurately diminished.[1-3] Thus, chronic myocardial failure is characterized by reduced energy consumption with reduced blood flow. Such diminished energy requirements could be interpreted as compensatory; that is, they may contribute to a lower rate of metabolic activity and myocyte preservation.[4]

However, in contrast to these metabolic findings is the histologic observation that hypertrophied failing myocardium is characterized by increased intercapillary distance and potential reduction in oxygen diffusion, particularly in the subendocardium.[4] These data suggest an alternative interpretation, that is, that heart failure is characterized in some clinical situations by regional myocardial ischemia. This explanation would be particularly likely in heart failure due to coronary artery disease.[3] Further evidence for chronic ischemia comes from patients with coronary disease but without extensive myocardial infarction who have ventricular dysfunction that is reversible after coronary revascularization, a phenomenon known as "hibernating myocardium."

Mitochondrial function. The role of mitochondrial function in myocardial failure remains uncertain (Fig 15-2). Information on mitochondrial respiratory activity depends on the heart failure model being used (pressure overload models with myocyte hypertrophy have increased mitochondrial mass) and the temporal stage at which heart failure is being studied. Hence, hypertrophied myocardium studied before the onset of heart failure may show increased mitochondrial oxygen consumption, whereas after muscle failure ensues, the external efficiency of this augmented respiration may be diminished.[5,6] Mitochondria from chronic failing human hearts show reduced or normal oxygen uptake.[7,8] Of relevant interest are recent data on murine myocarditis and human dilated cardiomyopathy indicating that the adenosine diphosphate (ADP) and adenosine triphosphate (ATP) carrier, an important mitochondrial transport protein,

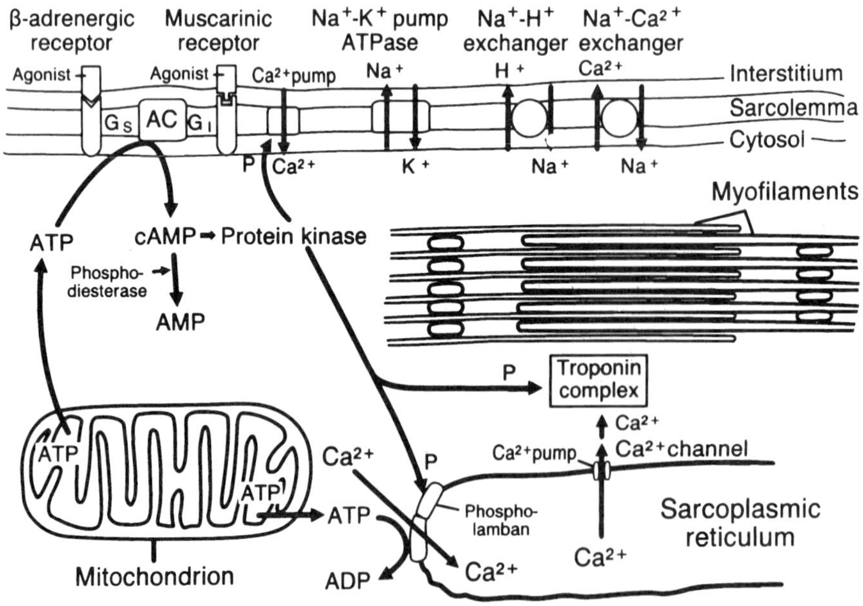

Fig 15-2 The regulation of excitation-contraction coupling. The sarcolemma and sarcoplasmic reticulum modulate cytoplasmic calcium availability, and the troponin-tropomyosin complex regulates responsiveness to cytoplasmic calcium. *AC,* adenylate cyclase; *ADP,* adenosine phosphate; *AMP,* adenosine monophosphate; *ATP,* adenosine triphosphate; *ATPase,* adenosinetriphosphatase; *cAMP,* cyclic adenosine monophosphate; *Gi,* guanine nucleotide-binding regulatory protein that inhibits adenylate cyclase; *Gs,* guanine nucleotide-binding regulatory protein that stimulates adenylate cyclase.

may be the target of antibody-mediated cell injury; impaired function of such a transport protein could be an important mechanism linking myocardial inflammation and impaired contractility.[9,10]

Energy reserve. The importance of myocardial energy reserves in myocardial failure is uncertain. Although there are multiple paths for ATP production in the myocyte, phosphoryl transfer from phosphocreatine, catalyzed by creatine kinase, is thought to be the predominant mechanism.[11,12] To maintain a steady cellular concentration of ATP, the high-energy phosphate turnover must be dynamic, that is, able to respond to changes in demand. Recent data suggest that the cytosolic ratio of phosphocreatine to ATP, normally about 2, is decreased in patients with dilated cardiomyopathy.[13,14] There is also evidence for a decrease in total creatine kinase content and activity, an indicator of in vivo high-energy phosphate turnover, in failing human myocardium.[15] The possibility remains, therefore, that depletion of phosphocreatine content and reduced creatine kinase activity play a role in the contractile abnormalities of chronic myocardial failure by contributing to depression of cellular energy reserves, particularly in circumstances of increased demand.[11] Further substantiation of this hypothesis requires demonstration that absolute reductions of phosphocreatine content and creatine kinase activity result in depression of ATP availability of a magnitude that could explain reduced myocardial performance.

Myofibrils. Myocellular adaptation in heart failure includes changes in contractile proteins. Although cardiac hypertrophy without ventricular failure is characterized by normal or increased myofibrillar elements, myofibril density and adenosinetriphosphatase (ATPase) activity decrease in severe ventricular failure.[16,17] The reason for decreased myofibrillar ATPase activity is unclear, but it could be related to a shift in myosin isoforms in myocardial failure. In the rat model, heart failure induces a switch from the fast adult type a-myosin isoform to a slow fetal type b-myosin isoform with decreased ATPase activity.[18] Such a change would lead to greater contractile efficiency and a reduction in energy demands on mitochondria. There is evidence that such a myosin isoform shift may take place in the failing human heart as well; however, its effects would be more prominent in the human atrium than ventricle (where the principal myosin isoform is already slow b-myosin), and its relevance to human myocardial failure is therefore uncertain.[4,19-24] In addition to changes in the myosin heavy chain, there could be alterations in myosin light chain structure and function or in other proteins, such as actin, troponin, and tropomyosin.[12,25] Studies of changes in contractile proteins in hypertrophy and heart failure have underscored the importance of the genetic modulation of the contractile apparatus and the fundamental significance of gene regulation in adaptive responses.[26]

Myocardial adrenergic receptors. As circulatory failure progresses, there are major changes in the neuroregulation of cardiac and vascular function. These systemic changes, which include increased sympathetic nervous system activity and elevation of plasma catecholamines, are closely associated with altered adrenergic modulation of myocardial function.

Plasma catecholamines, particularly norepinephrine, are increased in circulatory failure, and the degree of elevation is inversely related to the ejection fraction. In contrast, myocardial norepinephrine content is directly related to ejection fraction.[27-30] The cause of this depletion of myocardial norepinephrine content is unclear. Its overall significance is also uncertain; since myocardial norepinephrine content does not appear to correlate with contractile function in vitro, the reduction in cardiac norepinephrine may be an epiphenomenon, rather than a key mechanism, of myocardial failure.[31]

The most striking aspect of relationship between the heart and the increased adrenergic stimulation of circulatory failure appears to be that of myocardial desensitization to adrenergic drive. Down-regulation of myocardial β_1-receptors has been demonstrated in human heart failure in vitro and in vivo and may help protect the heart from excessive adrenergic stimulation.[32-39] The temporal dimension, again, may be important in this compensatory response to circulatory failure.[40] Increased adrenergic stimulation may be of central importance in acute heart failure, supporting cardiac output by increased heart rate and contractility. However, intense adrenergic stimulation may result in myocyte injury and death.[41-46] Hence, down-regulation of myocardial β_1-receptors may protect the heart from catecholamine "toxicity" while concomitantly decreasing the extent to which adrenergic stimulation can support the failing heart.

In addition to alterations in myocardial adrenergic receptor function, there are changes in the reflex-mediated control of the circulation. These changes are discussed below.

The G protein system. Another link in the chain of sympathetic stimulation of the heart is that of the guanine nucleotide-binding protein (G protein) system (see Fig 15-2). These proteins signaling cell membrane association mediate the myocardial response to β-adrenergic stimulation by coupling the beta receptor to the intracellular formation of cyclic adenosine monophosphate (AMP). The G protein complex contains a stimulatory G protein that increases cyclic AMP generation and an inhibitory G protein that reduces cyclic AMP production. Recent data indicate that inhibitory G proteins are increased and stimulatory G proteins are reduced in the failing human heart.[47-50] This change in ratio of stimulatory to inhibitory G proteins may result in a blunted increase in intracellular cyclic AMP as a result of adrenergic stimulation and, therefore, reduced myocyte Ca^{2+} influx or delayed uptake of cytosolic Ca^{2+} by the sarcoplasmic reticulum. This altered G protein function appears to uncouple adrenergic stimulation and cyclic AMP formation in failing myocardium. It is not known whether changes in the G protein complex are a primary defect in heart failure or are a part of the process of compensatory adaptation to sustained increases in adrenergic stimulation.

Cellular calcium dynamics. Control of intracellular calcium concentration is central to excitation-contraction coupling in the myocyte, and considerable effort has been directed toward characterizing cytosolic calcium dynamics in the failing heart. In the normal heart, excitation and depolarization of the cell membrane in the region of the

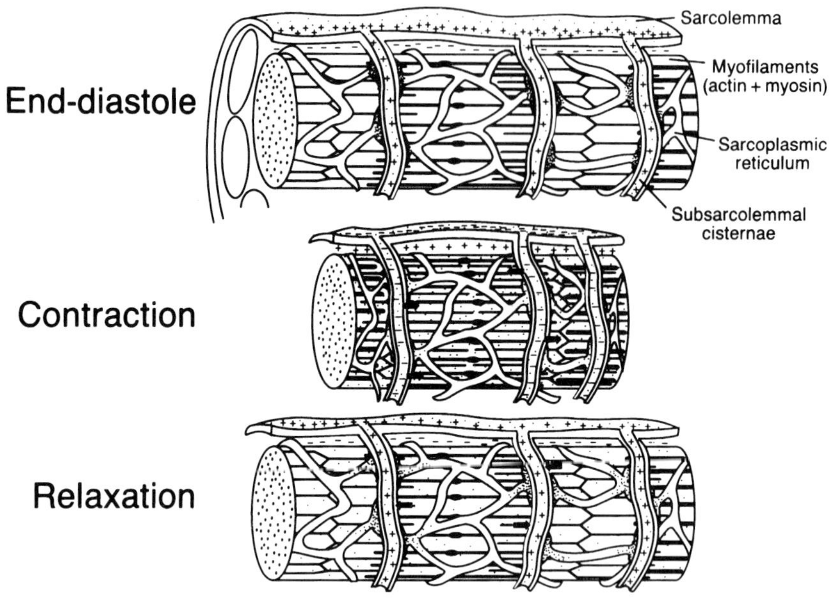

Fig 15-3 The major shifts of calcium ions during myocyte excitation-contraction coupling and relaxation. The dots represent calcium ions, and the positive and negative signs indicate electrical charge across membrane partitions.

sarcotubular system result in rapid influx of extracellular Ca^{2+} into the myocyte and release of intracellular Ca^{2+} stores from the sarcoplasmic reticulum into the cytosol (Figs 15-2 and 15-3). This permits activation of the actin-myosin interaction and mechanical contraction. Disengagement of actin and myosin, and consequent relaxation, can occur only when cytosolic calcium is again taken up by the sarcoplasmic reticulum and pumped back across the cell membrane to the extracellular space. Data from human myocardium indicate that intracellular calcium concentrations are maintained in failing myocardium, and this suggests that altered contractile function is not due to reduced intracellular calcium availability but may be due to altered myofibrillar calcium responsiveness.[51] In addition, inadequate removal of Ca^{2+} from the cytosol might be expected to prolong contraction, impair relaxation, and perhaps contribute to cell injury.[46] Such changes have been observed in human heart failure as well as in animal models of pressure overload.[52-56] Reduced Ca^{2+} uptake by the sarcoplasmic reticulum may also result in a subsequent diminution of Ca^{2+} release during depolarization and, hence, reduced systolic excitation-contraction coupling. The extent to which these changes in cytosolic Ca^{2+} modulation reflect myocardial failure rather than myocyte hypertrophy is unclear.[57]

Taken together, these biochemical and cellular changes produce a two-edged sword. As a form of short-term adaptation, myocardial desensitization to adrenergic stimulation may protect the heart from catecholamine-induced myocellular injury and rhythm disturbance. But over the long term, such adaptation may deprive the heart of the hemodynamic support provided by adrenergic drive.

Alterations in myocardial function

In addition to studies of myocyte biochemistry, there is a large body of information on the performance of normal and failing myocardium derived from in vitro experiments utilizing isolated muscle or isolated whole heart preparations.

Classic experiments in small mammals have focused on the effects of pressure overload on papillary muscle function. Studies of isolated papillary muscle from hearts subjected to chronic pressure overload show that further abrupt increases in pressure load result in depression of the maximum velocity of unloaded muscle contraction (Vmax); the extent of this contractility depression is moderate if hypertrophy has been allowed to develop without gross heart failure but severe if overt heart failure has supervened.[58-60] Similar findings have been made in muscle from the failing human heart studied in vitro[61] and in vivo.[62] When the pressure load is maintained for an extended period, there is evidence indicating that some hearts regain normal contractile function but that further extension of the duration of the pressure load again results in eventual deterioration of force development.[59,63,64] Such observations underscore the time-dependent nature of the relationship between load stress and muscle function, suggesting that an initial compensatory phase stabilizes contractile performance but that sustained stress ultimately overcomes the compensatory mechanisms provided by the induction of cell and muscle hypertrophy.

Volume loading has been assessed in isolated beating heart preparations, and the results are consistent with studies of pressure loading on isolated papillary muscles. The initial responses to volume loading are increases in

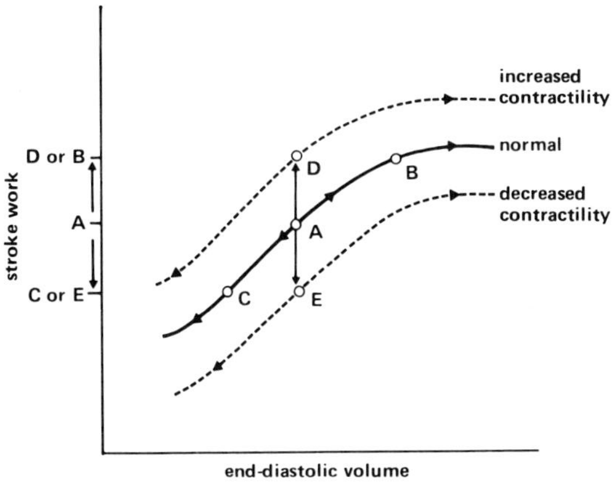

Fig 15-4 Family of ventricular function curves relating output (work) to end-diastolic volume. Output can be varied by changes along a single curve *(A* to *B, A* to *C)* or by shifting to a curve of different contractility. The decreased contractility curve represents a disease state; increased contractility is induced by inotropic agents. (From Katz AM: *Physiology of the Heart.* New York, Raven Press, 1977, p 225. By permission.)

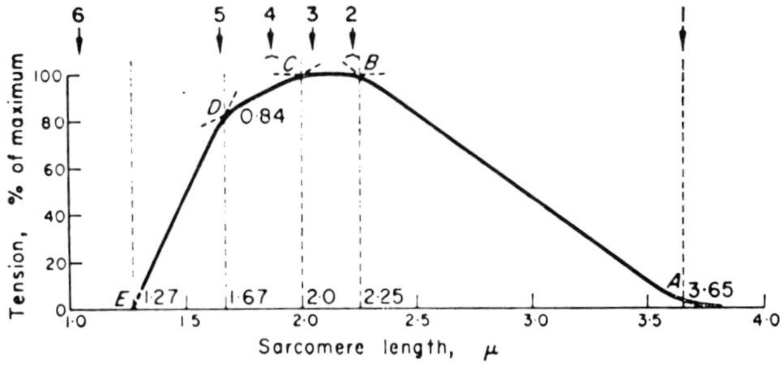

Fig 15-5 Sarcomere length-tension relationship in skeletal muscle fiber. Peak tension is produced at a length of about 2.2 μm. Similar curves have been found for cat papillary muscle and for dog left ventricle. (From Gordon AM, Huxley AF, Julian FJ: The variation in isometric tension with sarcomere length in vertebrate muscle fibres. *J Physiol (Lond)* 184:170-192, 1966. By permission of Physiological Society.)

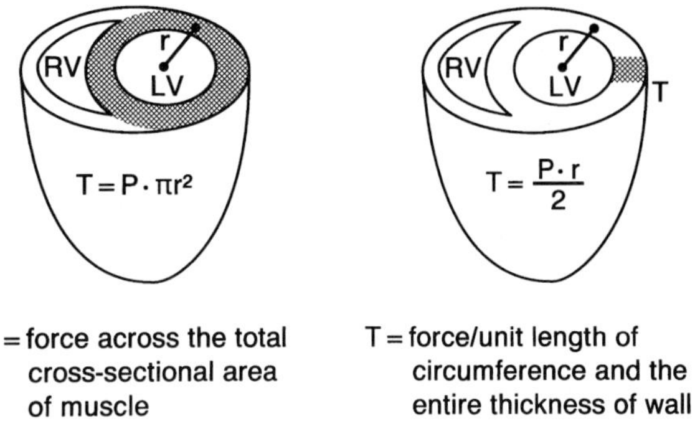

Fig 15-6 Two depictions of the law of Laplace, which describes the relationships among wall tension *(T),* intraventricular pressure *(P),* and left ventricular *(LV)* cavity radius *(r). RV,* right ventricle.

stroke volume, ventricular contractility, and cardiac output (i.e., the Frank-Starling mechanism). Chronic volume stress, however, results in a decline in contractility accompanied by further increases in end-diastolic ventricular volume.[65-67] As depicted in Figure 15-4, the dilated ventricle under chronic volume stress functions on a depressed ventricular function curve. To maintain the same stroke work at a lower state of contractility, the ventricle must operate at a larger end-diastolic volume. This larger ventricular volume results in a further increment in ventricular wall stress (see below), which in turn may contribute to progressive deterioration in contractility. A positive feedback loop, therefore, is established, which characterizes the progressive decline in ventricular performance seen in the chronic phase of circulatory failure.

Alterations in ventricular geometry

As noted above, one initial response to increased load is ventricular dilatation. This phenomenon, known since the classic observations of Starling, is the gross anatomic manifestation of increasing sarcomere length to its optimal range of 2.2 μm[68,69] (Fig 15-5). This augmentation of end-diastolic volume and contractility increases stroke volume. The advantage gained by this mechanism, however, is won at the price of increased ventricular wall tension.[70] By application of the law of Laplace (Fig 15-6), it can be appreciated that increasing ventricular radius necessitates a concomitant increase in wall tension to maintain a constant intraventricular pressure. This increase in wall tension is present not only at the onset of systole but also throughout the ejection period; thus, instantaneous wall stress does not decrease during systole to the extent that it would if contraction commenced at a smaller end-diastolic ventricular radius. Although the Starling mechanism is of great utility in maintaining stroke volume during brief perturbations of cardiac pump function, the untoward consequence of its sustained application—increased wall stress—has significant further implications for ventricular geometry and performance, that is, the development of hypertrophy.

Changes in ventricular geometry and contractile state have classically been expressed by Starling curves (see Fig 15-4). The more recent appreciation of the information contained in left ventricular pressure-volume loops has provided a valuable technique for assessing the relationships between pressure and volume and the performance of muscle during systole and diastole[71-73] (Fig 15-7). As depicted in Figure 15-7,A, pressure-volume loops acquired during a graduated change of loading conditions produce a measurement of end-systolic elastance that is a relatively load-insensitive assessment of ventricular contractility. As in the example in Figure 15-7,B, the slope of this end-systolic pressure-volume relationship is depressed by β-blockade, reflecting the change in contractile state of the myocardium. In addition to providing information about systolic function, pressure-volume loops offer a technique for measuring diastolic compliance of the ventricle[74] (see Fig 15-7,A).

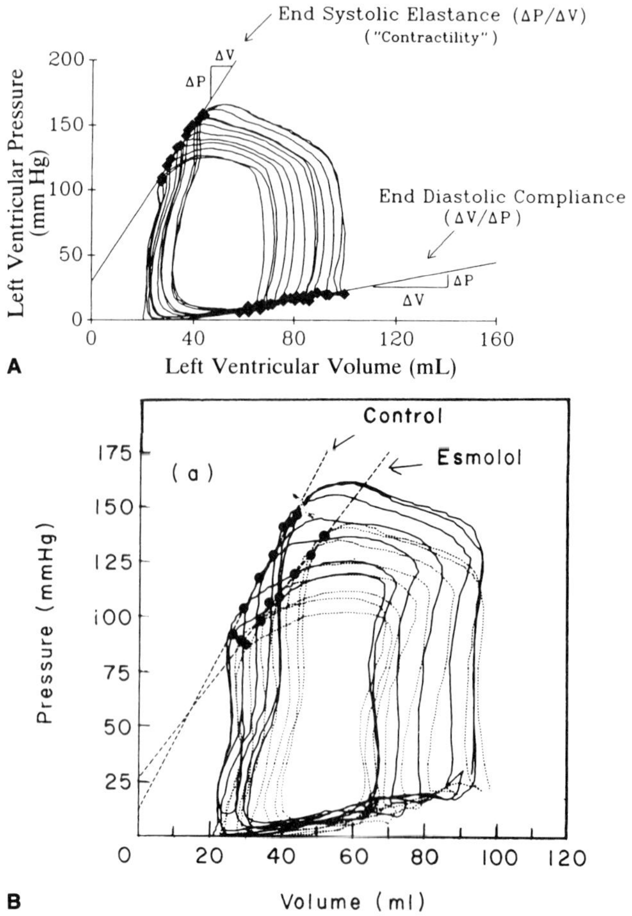

Fig 15-7 **A,** measurement of systolic and diastolic chamber properties from pressure-volume relations loops and relations in humans. Left ventricular pressure-volume data are recorded continuously by conductance catheter during gradual mechanical reduction of inferior vena cava inflow. Several cycles are combined to generate systolic *(upper left corners)* and diastolic *(lower left corners)* pressure-volume boundaries. The systolic boundary is fit by linear regression, and its slope (end-systolic elastance) provides a relatively load-insensitive measure of chamber contractility. This slope has units of millimeters of mercury per milliliter and was 3.02 mm Hg/mL in this patient. The lower boundary, defined by points taken from late diastole, is also fit by linear regression. The slope of the diastolic boundary is also elastance; however, more commonly the inverse slope (compliance) is reported (ΔV/ΔP). This slope was 2.29 mL/mm Hg for this patient. **B,** assessment of systolic function by pressure-volume relations. Pressure-volume loops are obtained during inferior vena cava occlusion by conductance catheter technique both before and after administration of an intravenous β-blocker (esmolol). The end-systolic pressure-volume relation is clearly reduced. (**A,** from Kass DA, Wolff MR, Ting C-T, et al: Diastolic compliance of hypertrophied ventricle is not acutely altered by pharmacologic agents influencing active processes. *Ann Intern Med* 119:466-473, 1993. By permission of American College of Physicians; **B,** from Kass DA: Clinical evaluation of left heart function by conductance catheter technique. *Eur Heart J* 13 Suppl E:57-64, 1992. By permission of The European Society of Cardiology.)

Hypertrophy

Although hypertrophy occurs in response to stress, the molecular mechanisms that result in DNA replication, messenger RNA transcription, and protein synthesis are not fully understood. These molecular responses to stress appear to be requisite for the increases in mitochondria, myofibrils, and interstitial collagen that are characteristic of myocardial hypertrophy.

Hypertrophy of the adult human heart is a direct reflection of an increase in the number of sarcomeres in each cell. The development of hypertrophy serves to normalize the ratio of ventricular wall thickness to chamber radius in the dilated heart, that is, to minimize increases in wall stress[62,70,75] (Fig 15-8). During chronic pressure overload (for example, aortic stenosis or hypertension), marked concentric left ventricular hypertrophy develops without ventricular dilatation; that is, the ratio of wall thickness to chamber radius is increased. In patients with clinically compensated systolic cardiac failure, the combination of ventricular hypertrophy and dilatation results in maintenance of stroke volume with relatively small increases in wall tension. Indeed, the development of an appropriate degree of hypertrophy appears to be important for maintaining pump performance, reducing symptoms of ventricular dysfunction, and possibly improving short- and medium-term survival.[76,77]

In summary, these in vitro findings are consistent with a model in which the initial acute response to increased load is increased contractility generated by augmented adrenergic drive and chamber dilatation (to achieve optimal sarcomere length). This is followed by hypertrophy, which increases the total myocardial mass. These adaptations permit maintenance of overall cardiac pump performance, at least temporarily. If excessive loading conditions become chronic, however, a phase of diminishing myocardial contractility ensues and with it a downward spiral of circulatory function and the clinical syndrome of chronic congestive heart failure.[78]

DIASTOLIC FUNCTION AND DYSFUNCTION

As already noted, the compensatory adaptive response of left ventricular dilatation may have potentially deleterious long-term effects. The same may be said of hypertrophy.

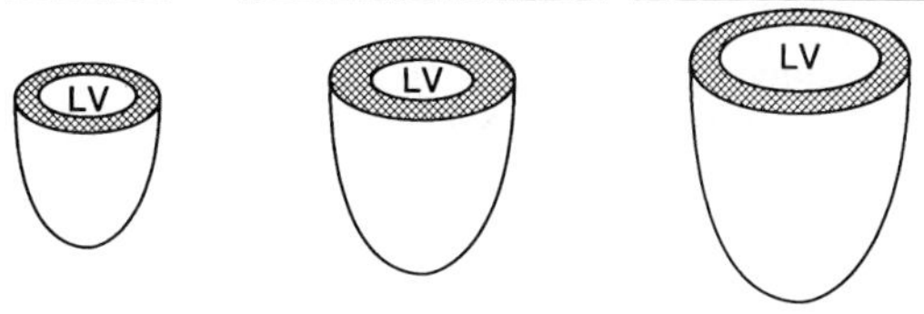

	Normal	Pressure overload	Volume overload
LV pressure (mm Hg)	117 ± 7/10 ± 1	226 ± 6/23 ± 3*	138 ± 7/23 ± 2*
LVMI (gm/m^2)	71 ± 8	206 ± 17*	196 ± 17*
LV wall thickness (mm)	8.2 ± 0.6	15.2 ± 0.9*	10.6 ± 5*
Wall thickness/radius (h/R)	0.34 ± 0.03	0.56 ± 0.05*	0.33 ± 0.02
σ_m (10^3 dynes/cm^2)			
Peak systolic	151 ± 4	161 ± 24	175 ± 7
End diastolic	17 ± 2	23 ± 3	41 ± 3*

*P < 0.01

Fig 15-8 Left ventricular *(LV)* pressure, mass index *(LVMI),* wall thickness to radius ratio *(h/R),* and peak systolic wall tension (σ_m) in 6 normal subjects, 6 patients with pressure overload, and 18 patients with volume overload. Mass increases in both groups but is associated with more marked wall thickening in the pressure overload group. (Data from Grossman W, Jones D, McLaurin LP: Wall stress and patterns of hypertrophy in the human left ventricle. *J Clin Invest* 56:56-64, 1975.)

Although the development of ventricular hypertrophy seems to be beneficial in maintaining stroke volume and normalizing wall stress, it also results in impaired diastolic filling of the ventricle. Thus, diastolic dysfunction may contribute to heart failure alone or, more commonly, in combination with systolic dysfunction.

Broadly considered, diastole may be divided into two components[79,80] (Fig 15-9). The first, *relaxation*, takes place during early diastole and is a dynamic energy-dependent process; it encompasses the phases of isometric relaxation and rapid filling. The second, *diastasis*, occurs later in diastole and reflects the passive properties of ventricular stiffness; it is assessed by examining the pressure-volume relationship of the ventricle after filling has been completed (see Fig 15-7,A).

A number of factors may contribute to disordered *relaxation* and, hence, to diastolic failure.[81] For example, among the earliest effects of ischemia is a prolongation of the energy-dependent aspects of relaxation; diastolic dysfunction is characteristic of ischemic myocardium.[82-84] Also, ventricular hypertrophy such as that seen under the chronic pressure load of aortic stenosis or hypertension results in slowing of early ventricular relaxation.[85-88] This may be related in part to subendocardial ischemia in these conditions. An abrupt increase in ventricular afterload may also produce attenuated relaxation.[89,90] Early diastolic filling may be abnormal in conditions with regional asynchrony of relaxation, such as that observed with ischemic heart disease or altered cardiac conduction.[89,91,92] Finally, disordered control of intracellular Ca^{2+} compartmentalization, as postulated to take place in some hypertrophic cardiomyopathies, may result in delayed relaxation.[93-95]

In addition to these factors contributing to abnormal early relaxation, disorders characterized by increased passive *chamber stiffness* may manifest diastolic dysfunction. Diastolic stiffness, measured at the end of the ventricular filling phase, is the relationship between the change in pressure and the change in volume (see Fig 15-7,A). Chamber stiffness may rise because of an increase in the stiffness of the myocardial tissue (e.g., fibrosis, hypertrophy, amyloid deposition), which effectively means moving to a new and steeper pressure-volume curve, one with a greater pressure for any given volume. The development of ventricular scarring after myocardial infarction is the most clinically common cause of a regional increase in passive chamber stiffness that produces such a shift in the ventricular pressure-volume curve.[96] In sustained pressure overload conditions, such as hypertension or aortic stenosis, hypertrophy results in increased myocardial stiffness.[80,85,87,97,98] Increased myocardial stiffness in chronic pressure overload may be related to increased myocardial mass and to increased deposition of interstitial collagen matrix.[99-102] Myocardial stiffness may also be augmented by chronic volume overload (e.g., left-sided valve regurgitation).[103] Finally, augmented stiffness may be related to extrinsic cardiac factors, such as constrictive or effusive pericardial disease, that result in pericardial restraint and reduced chamber distensibility.

Diastolic dysfunction is now known to have a significant role in the clinical manifestation of circulatory failure. Indeed, among patients referred to tertiary centers with the syndrome of congestive heart failure, 20% to 40% are found to have evidence of diastolic dysfunction with relatively preserved systolic performance.[104-109] A sub-

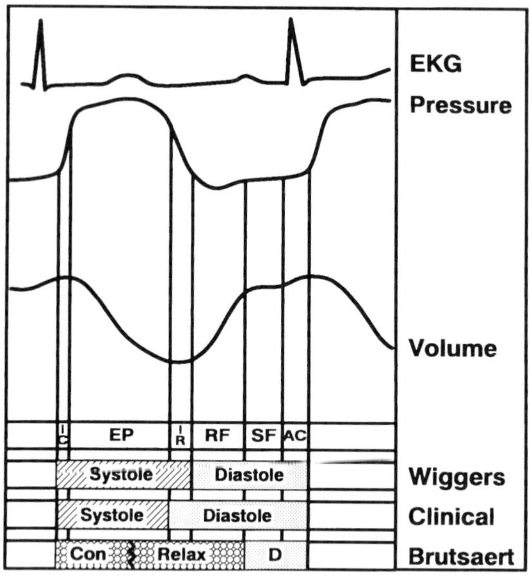

Fig 15-9 Diagram depicting various definitions of diastole that have been proposed, based on left ventricular pressure and volume curves throughout the cardiac cycle. Original definition by Wiggers consisted of time period from mitral valve opening to mitral valve closure. Clinical definition of diastole encompasses a period beginning at aortic valve closure and extending to mitral valve closure. A new physiologic definition of diastole reported by Brutsaert et al.[89] proposes two phases for the cardiac cycle. In the systolic phase, both active contraction *(Con)* and relaxation *(Relax)* occur. Diastasis *(D)* is a passive phase dependent on filling properties of the heart. *EKG,* electrocardiogram; *IC,* isovolumic contraction (mitral closure to aortic valve opening); *EP,* ejection period (aortic valve opening to aortic valve closure); *IR,* isovolumic relaxation (aortic valve closure to mitral valve opening); *RF,* rapid filling; *SF,* slow filling; *AC,* atrial contraction. (From Nishimura RA, Housmans PR, Hatle LK, et al: Assessment of diastolic function of the heart: background and current applications of Doppler echocardiography. Part I. Physiologic and pathophysiologic features. *Mayo Clin Proc* 64:71-81, 1989. By permission, Mayo Foundation for Medical Education and Research.)

stantial number of such patients have hypertension as a risk factor for ventricular dysfunction. Diastolic dysfunction may be severe and, if not diagnosed, can lead to therapeutic maneuvers of preload or afterload reduction that, although appropriate for systolic dysfunction, may be deleterious in advanced diastolic failure.[110] If significant diastolic dysfunction is taken into account, the clinician may direct attention to maintaining adequate ventricular filling pressures, to optimizing the diastolic filling interval by slowing the heart rate, and, when applicable, to restoring normal atrial contraction in patients in whom atrial arrhythmias have developed.

NEUROVASCULAR ADAPTATION AND DYSFUNCTION

Autonomic nervous system

The autonomic nervous system responds to acute reductions in pump function by modulating circulatory function to augment cardiac output and maintain perfusion to vital organs. Increased adrenergic output serves to increase heart rate, increase contractility, and, by selective adjustment of vascular tone, preferentially shunt flow to the most critical circulations.[111-114] With the development of circulatory failure, there are changes in both sympathetic-adrenergic and parasympathetic systems.

Alterations in regional blood flow

In addition to the changes in the distribution of cardiac output occasioned by acute circulatory failure, there are sustained alterations in regional blood flow in chronic circulatory failure.[111] In general, chronic circulatory failure is characterized by preservation of blood flow to the brain and heart at the expense of supply to the renal splanchnic, skeletal muscle, and cutaneous beds[112-117] (Fig 15-10). In mild cases, these regional changes may be evident only when the circulatory system is stressed by exercise. In advanced failure, they are evident at rest, as reflected by oliguria and cool extremities. The reduction in skeletal muscle flow and the intrinsic changes in skeletal muscle structure are important factors in the declining exercise tolerance of circulatory failure.[116,118-123]

Autonomic nervous system activity

Altered distribution of blood flow may result from changes in regional vascular tone mediated by sympathetic nerve activity to afferent arterioles in specific vascular beds.[111] It may also be under the endocrine influence of circulating humoral substances, such as catecholamines, members of the family of atrial peptides, arginine vasopressin, and components of the renin-angiotensin system. Finally, the vascular endothelium produces and releases vasoactive factors that act in a paracrine or autocrine fashion to modulate local vascular tone.

As described above, circulatory failure is marked by increased plasma catecholamines at rest and during exercise.[124,125] Higher plasma concentrations of norepinephrine are a reflection of increased adrenergic nerve activity and norepinephrine release combined with reduced norepinephrine uptake at the neuromuscular junction and reduced norepinephrine clearance.[113,126-128] In general, the degree of plasma norepinephrine elevation correlates with the severity of circulatory failure.[125] Direct measurement of peripheral nerve activity in patients with heart failure demonstrates increased central adrenergic drive, which correlates with plasma norepinephrine, cardiac filling pressures, and stroke volume.[129,130] Such increased sympathetic tone is an important factor producing vasoconstriction in skeletal muscle beds in chronic heart failure.

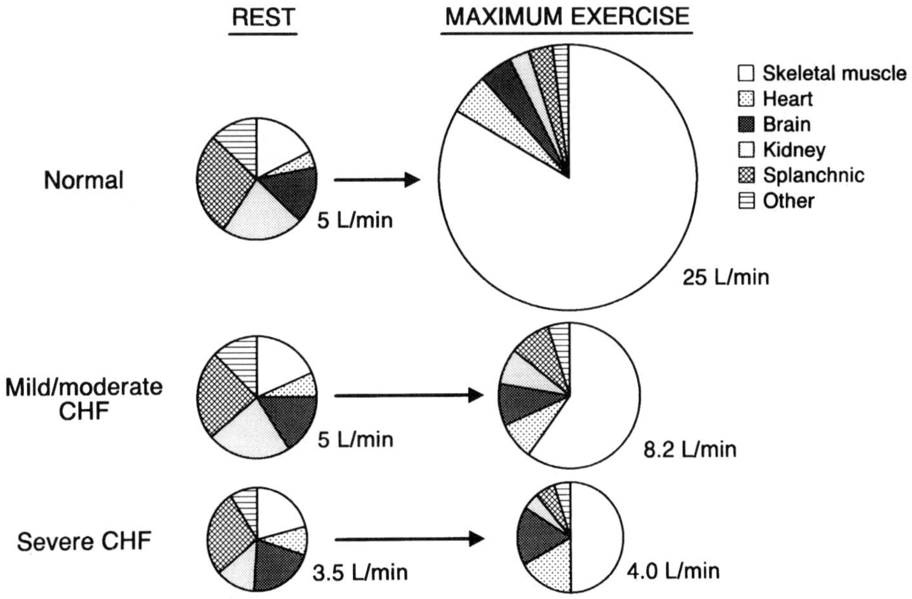

Fig 15-10 Organ distribution of blood flow at rest and during maximum exercise in normal subjects and patients with heart failure *(CHF)*. The total cardiac output declines during heart failure, and the distribution of blood flow to the brain, heart, and kidney is preserved at the expense of flow to skeletal muscle. (Modified from Zelis R, Flaim SF: Alterations in vasomotor tone in congestive heart failure. *Prog Cardiovasc Dis* 24:437-459, 1982.)

Alterations in cardiovascular reflexes are also known to occur in circulatory failure. Studies using pharmacologic hypotension, upright-tilt, or lower body negative pressure have been devised to assess the adequacy of baroreflex-induced tachycardia and peripheral vasoconstriction. These forms of barostress have been shown to result in subnormal tachycardia and peripheral vasoconstriction responses in both patients with heart failure and canine models of congestive heart failure.[131-138] These reflex abnormalities may come into play during upright activity and contribute to orthostatic hypotension and exercise intolerance.[33,131,139] There is uncertainty about the reversibility of these abnormalities of reflex function with improvement in circulatory failure.[140] These derangements in reflex control of cardiac output and arterial pressure may be underlying factors contributing to heightened sympathetic nervous system activity and its associated changes in adrenergic receptor function.[141]

Adrenergic receptors

In addition to abnormalities in the autonomic reflexes that modulate the circulation, heart failure is associated with abnormalities in adrenergic receptor function. There is down-regulation of myocardial β-adrenoreceptors.[35-38] This down-regulation is characterized by a decrease in β-receptor density and in isoproterenol-induced adenylate cyclase and contractile responses. It is believed to be related to sustained exposure to high levels of catecholamines. The impact on the β_2-receptor is primarily a reduction in receptor number, whereas that on the β_1-receptor is one of disrupted coupling of the β_1-receptor and the adenylate cyclase system.[39] Although this down-regulation may be an appropriate response that protects the myocardium from the long-term toxicity of high concentrations of catecholamines, it reduces the effectiveness with which the adrenergic nervous system can acutely or chronically stimulate the circulation in chronic heart failure.

Parasympathetic nervous system

In addition to the alterations in the sympathetic nervous system response to hypotensive barostress described above, circulatory failure is characterized by impaired parasympathetic response to hypertensive barostress.[136,139-143] Canine studies suggest that altered bradycardiac response may be related to a decrease in high-affinity muscarinic receptors in the failing heart.[144] These disturbances in the normal modulation of heart rate contribute to the impaired regulation of cardiac output in circulatory failure.

Atrial volume sensing reflexes

Increased left atrial pressure classically results in an increase in afferent sympathetic impulses leading to inhibition of antidiuretic hormone release, diuresis, reduction of plasma volume, and a reduction in atrial filling pressure.[145,146] In chronic heart failure, there is desensitization of these atrial baroreceptors, with a consequent reduction in this reflex-mediated diuresis, thus contributing to the fluid retention of the syndrome of chronic circulatory failure.[147,148]

NEUROHUMORAL MECHANISMS IN HEART FAILURE

In the syndrome of congestive heart failure, vasoconstrictor-antinatriuretic-mitogenic factors (Table 15-2) may alter peripheral hemodynamic function to increase cardiac afterload and preload and, thus, through hemodynamic mechanisms contribute to progressive ventricular failure. These circulating and local humoral factors may also contribute to coronary endothelial dysfunction and vasoconstriction leading to ischemia. They may have direct toxic actions on the myocyte, which may result in disorders of contraction and lead to myocyte death. Recent studies of the time course of the evolution of circulatory failure have revealed an initial (often chronic) stage in which the patient, despite ventricular dysfunction, is asymptomatic, does not have vasoconstriction, and is not retaining sodium. Evidence indicates that this initial stage of "asymptomatic left ventricular dysfunction" may remain asymptomatic as a consequence of activation of circulating and local vasodilatory-natriuretic-antimitogenic substances (see Table 15-2). On the basis of our understanding of these counterregulatory endocrine systems, therapeutic strategies have evolved that are designed to inhibit or antagonize the factors that mediate vasoconstriction, sodium retention, and remodeling of the heart. These approaches could potentiate vasodilatory and natriuretic systems to delay the progression of asymptomatic left ventricular dysfunction to overt circulatory failure or to reverse established circulatory failure.

Vasodilatory-natriuretic-antimitogenic systems

Natriuretic peptides. In addition to its role as a pump, the heart is an endocrine organ that synthesizes and releases the peptide hormone atrial natriuretic peptide (ANP), which mediates diverse biologic actions. These actions include natriuresis, inhibition of the renin-angiotensin-aldosterone system, modulation of the sympathetic nervous system, increases in capillary permeability, arterial vasodilatation, and inhibition of vascular smooth muscle proliferation.[149] ANP is increased into the circulation within minutes of the onset of ventricular dysfunction by rapid release from myocytes and is maintained at increased concentrations with chronic circulatory failure by enhanced cardiac synthesis and secretion.[150,151]

A dual natriuretic peptide system of cardiac origin may complement ANP. Brain natriuretic peptide (BNP), a second structurally related peptide stored in atrial cells, is a distinct gene product from ANP. BNP circulates at lower concentrations than ANP but may circulate at levels that exceed ANP in advanced circulatory failure. As with ANP, the increase of circulating BNP in heart failure is due to recruitment of the ventricle to synthesize the peptide; thus, the importance of the ventricular myocardium as an endocrine organ in heart failure is underscored.[152]

A third structurally related peptide, C-type natriuretic peptide (CNP), has also been described. In contrast to ANP and BNP, CNP is of endothelial cell origin rather than cardiac origin.[153] CNP is a potent vasoactive peptide that decreases arterial blood pressure, most likely through peripheral vasodilatation.[154] Unlike ANP or BNP, CNP is not natriuretic and does not appear to inhibit the renin-angiotensin-aldosterone system. CNP does inhibit endothelin, an endothelium-derived vasoconstrictor peptide (see below).[155] This action on endothelin release may be linked to the activation of cyclic guanosine monophosphate (GMP), an action shared by ANP and BNP.

The concept of a family of natriuretic and vasoactive peptides is underscored by investigations demonstrating the existence of a family of three natriuretic peptide receptors (NPRs) that interact with these three peptides.[156] Two of these, NPR-A and NPR-B, are members of a newly described family of receptor guanylyl cyclases that are single transmembrane proteins with identical extracellular domains. Both ANP and BNP bind to the A-receptor, whereas CNP binds exclusively to the B-receptor. Binding to these receptors results in activation of cyclic GMP. The NPR-A receptor is highly expressed in endothelial cells and in the kidney, and the NPR-B receptor appears to be highly expressed in vascular smooth muscle. The third member of the natriuretic peptide receptor family, the NPR-C receptor, functions as a clearance receptor that removes the natriuretic peptides from the circulation.

As noted above, ANP, BNP, and CNP (in myocardial tissue) are increased in congestive heart failure.[157] The elevation of these natriuretic peptides may have diagnostic relevance. Recent human studies used increased circulating levels of ANP as a noninvasive clinical predictor for acute congestive heart failure in elderly patients.[158] The risk for development of congestive heart failure increased progressively with increasing ANP levels.

The N-terminus of the ANP molecule (N-ANP) is not biologically active and is cleared more slowly than ANP

Table 15-2 Neurohumoral mechanisms in congestive heart failure

Vasodilatory, natriuretic, and antimitogenic factors	Vasoconstrictive, antinatriuretic, and mitogenic factors
Natriuretic peptides	Renin-angiotensin-aldosterone system
Kallikrein, kinins	Sympathetic nervous system
Prostaglandin	Vasopressin
Dopamine	Thromboxane
Endothelium-derived relaxing factor–nitric oxide	Endothelin
	Cytokines

from the circulation. The potential utility of N-ANP as a sensitive and specific marker for asymptomatic ventricular dysfunction has recently been explored. N-ANP was measured in a population of patients undergoing rest and exercise radionuclide angiography to detect coronary artery disease.[159] In patients with ventricular dysfunction but without symptoms of heart failure, a plasma N-ANP concentration above 54 pmol/L had a sensitivity of 90% and a specificity of 92% for detection of patients with ventricular dysfunction. Thus, N-ANP emerges as a novel and sensitive noninvasive serum marker for diagnosing asymptomatic left ventricular dysfunction.

Two therapeutic strategies are emerging to potentiate the biologic activity of these hormones on the basis of knowledge of their clearance and metabolism. As discussed above, the natriuretic peptides are cleared by a clearance receptor localized to endothelial cells, vascular smooth muscle cells, and the kidney. This receptor-mediated clearance is complemented by an enzymatic clearance pathway for natriuretic peptide metabolism, that is, degradation by the enzyme neutral endopeptidase 24.11 (NEP).[160] NEP is also localized to endothelial cells and vascular smooth muscle cells and is present in highest concentration in the kidney. The concept that inhibition of the clearance receptor may promote increased concentrations of ANP has been demonstrated in studies in experimental canine heart failure.[161] This ANP potentiation was further augmented by inhibition of NEP.[162] Therefore, clearance receptor blockade with or without NEP inhibitors is potentially useful in the treatment of circulatory failure.

Investigations in human heart failure have recently established NEP inhibition as a new approach in the treatment of heart failure. NEP inhibitor therapy in patients with moderately severe congestive heart failure acutely increased plasma ANP levels, suppressed aldosterone, and decreased right atrial and pulmonary capillary wedge pressures.[163] Body weight was reduced, a reflection of chronic natriuretic and diuretic effects, and there was a trend toward increased cardiac index and reduced preload. In a separate investigation, inhibition of ANP degradation was investigated in patients with severe chronic heart failure.[164] This study also demonstrated elevation of ANP with inhibition of NEP; cardiac index increased only transiently, but sodium excretion increased sixfold. Plasma norepinephrine decreased significantly in association with a transient reduction in vasopressin, aldosterone, and plasma renin activity.

The natriuretic peptide system emerges as an important functional vasodilatory, natriuretic, and antimitogenic system that is activated in both early and chronic circulatory failure. The elevations of ANP, BNP, and, perhaps, CNP, when defined, have diagnostic and prognostic significance. On the basis of the knowledge of their clearance and degradation, unique therapeutic strategies have evolved that may be important in potentiating the biologic activity of these peptides in early heart failure to delay the progression of asymptomatic left ventricular dysfunction to overt and irreversible ventricular dysfunction.

Endothelium-derived relaxing factor – nitric oxide. An endothelium-derived relaxing factor (EDRF), which may be nitric oxide (NO), is also capable of stimulating cyclic GMP through activation of soluble guanylate cyclase and is a modulator of vascular tone. The functional significance of EDRF/NO in the regulation of vascular tone and how it is related to heart failure have been advanced by the ability of *N*-monomethyl-L-arginine to inhibit its production. Inhibition of EDRF/NO production by exogenous administration of *N*-monomethyl-L-arginine results in significant increases in systemic, renal, and pulmonary vascular resistances. This finding supports the concept that this endogenous vasodilator has functional importance in the regulation of basal hemodynamic function.[165] Because overt circulatory failure is characterized by peripheral vasoconstriction, abnormalities in the control of vascular tone by the endothelium may contribute to the increased vasomotor tone.[166] Recent investigations have attempted to define whether endothelium-dependent vasodilatation is impaired in the peripheral vasculature of patients with chronic congestive heart failure by examining the local vascular response to intra-arterial infusions of graded concentrations of acetylcholine, an endothelium-dependent vasodilator, and nitroglycerin, a direct-acting vasodilator.[167] Acetylcholine resulted in vasodilatation in normal subjects but was markedly impaired in patients with circulatory failure. The endothelium-independent vasodilator nitroglycerin, which mediated vasodilatation in normal subjects, also resulted in impaired vasodilatation in heart failure. Thus, these studies demonstrated an impairment not only in endothelial function but also in vascular smooth muscle responsiveness in patients with circulatory failure. The impaired response to acetylcholine may be mediated by alterations in the muscarinic receptor or by abnormal synthesis or release of EDRF, or by both. The impaired nitroglycerin response implies that a possible abnormal cyclic GMP mechanism may also be involved in altering vascular tone in circulatory failure.

Recent studies in a canine heart failure model determined that EDRF/NO may be enhanced in selective vascular beds in heart failure.[168] In these experiments, a heterogeneous alteration in endothelial function was observed: α_2-adrenergic pathways of endothelium-dependent relaxation were enhanced in the coronary circulation and to a lesser degree in the renal circulation, whereas a tendency for reduced vascular responsiveness to NO was recorded in the femoral artery. This enhancement in coronary and renal arterial endothelium-dependent vasorelaxation in experimental congestive heart failure was mediated by increased production of EDRF/NO through a G-protein pathway. Thus, congestive heart failure may be characterized by enhanced EDRF/NO production to oppose the actions of endogenous vasoconstrictors activated in heart failure.

Evidence exists that the endothelium of the endocardium also is capable of releasing EDRF/NO.[169] Bioassay experiments suggest that an EDRF/NO-like agent is released that may shorten the duration of contraction. EDRF/NO may also increase myocardial cyclic GMP, which may lead to alterations in myocardial contractility and could also influence myocyte growth. Relevant to the natriuretic peptides, as discussed in the preceding section, is the realization that myocardial cyclic GMP may also increase secondary to these vasodilatory substances; indeed, receptors for the natriuretic peptides exist in both rat and human myocardium.[170] Thus, a paracrine role emerges for local cardiac humoral systems such as EDRF/NO and the natriuretic peptides in the control of cardiac function. A full understanding of their role in heart failure will require further investigation.

Vasoconstrictor-antinatriuretic-mitogenic systems

Evidence of the activation of sympathetic and renin-angiotensin-aldosterone systems in circulatory failure supports the hypothesis that short-term compensatory responses contribute to long-term progression of disease.[171] These vasoconstrictor-antinatriuretic-mitogenic autocrine and paracrine mechanisms, in addition to circulating or systemic mechanisms, mediate the progression of circulatory failure.

These hormonal, autocrine, and paracrine mediators include angiotensin, endothelin, serotonin, thromboxane, cytokines, and peptide growth factors. Sympathetic nervous system activation also promotes vasoconstriction and increases circulating catecholamines, which with chronic stimulation contribute to a "toxic" environment for the myocardium and peripheral vasculature. Collectively, these factors may overwhelm any counterbalancing forces (e.g., ANP, BNP, CNP, and EDRF/NO) and promote cardiac or vascular remodeling, which occurs with chronic circulatory failure. There is now evidence that local mechanisms rather than systemic diffuse mechanisms have a more profound role in the adrenergic abnormalities of failing human heart muscle.[172] Isolated right ventricular failure secondary to primary pulmonary hypertension has been compared with biventricular failure of idiopathic dilated cardiomyopathy and nonfailure in normal organ donor hearts. Despite systemic hormonal activation that occurs with circulatory failure, β-adrenergic neuroeffector abnormalities were present only in the failing right ventricle of hearts from patients with primary pulmonary hypertension and not in the accompanying left ventricle. This finding suggests that the regulatory processes in the failing human heart are predominantly under local rather than systemic control.

Angiotensin II. Angiotensin II, a potent vasoconstrictor peptide, is produced systemically and locally in the heart, kidney, and vascular endothelium because of the abundant production of angiotensin-converting enzyme (ACE). Specifically, angiotensin II is formed in two steps by the action of renin and converting enzyme. Recent studies have documented that angiotensin II binds to three classes of receptors, designated AT1, AT2, and AT3, in which almost all the biologic actions are mediated via the AT1 receptor.[173] This receptor, like other peptide hormone receptors, is linked to G proteins. After binding, angiotensin II activates phospholipase C, and this results in formation of inositol triphosphate and diacylglycerol. These second messengers increase intracellular calcium and mediate the actions of angiotensin II.

Table 15-3 Angiotensin II: sites and actions

Targets	Actions
Heart	Positive inotropism, hypertrophy
Kidney	Renin release, mesangial contraction, sodium reabsorption
Adrenal body	Aldosterone release
Brain	Vasopressin release, thirst, increased sympathetic outflow
Sympathetic nervous system	Norepinephrine release
Vascular smooth muscle	Vasoconstriction, hypertrophy

The biologic actions of angiotensin II are widespread and should be viewed as acute and chronic (Table 15-3). Acute compensatory actions support the circulation and are activated in states of acute hypotension, such as those with hemorrhage or severe volume depletion. Angiotensin II thus serves to maintain blood pressure by vasoconstriction and sodium retention as well as by augmenting myocardial contractility. Chronic elevation of angiotensin II may have trophic actions by mediating the development of myocardial and vascular hypertrophy. Current understanding of the renin-angiotensin system (RAS) recognizes its existence as a circulating humoral system in which renin is released from the kidney and contributes to the increased generation of circulating (i.e., endocrine) angiotensin II. Additionally, because all components of the RAS have been identified in specific tissues, a role is supported for local (i.e., paracrine) RAS activation independent of the circulating RAS.[174] Three specific local renin-angiotensin systems are discussed below.

The kidney is one of the first organs in which a tissue-specific RAS was described. Renin, angiotensinogen, and converting enzyme in the kidney support a local system. Despite lack of activation of circulating angiotensin II in experimental congestive heart failure, increased renal angiotensinogen messenger RNA has been observed in association with improvements in renal hemodynamics reported in response to ACE inhibition.[175] As in the kidney, similar components of the RAS have been identified in the heart, which is one of the most sensitive target organs to angiotensin II. Specifically, angiotensin II exerts potent direct inotropic actions through modulation of intracellular calcium.[176] Angiotensin II generation locally in the heart could also activate myocardial proto-oncogenes to stimulate myocyte hypertrophy. Indeed, ACE inhibition without hypotensive actions reduces myocardial hypertrophy in experimental cardiac remodeling. Lastly, a local RAS may also exist in vasculature.[177] All components of the RAS have been localized to the vessel wall, with reports of local activation in genetic hypertension independent of increases in systemic angiotensin II or renin. Thus, a local vascular RAS activation may contribute to increases in arterial tone as well as to anatomic vascular remodeling. Such locally activated RAS, independent of increases in the circulating RAS, may explain beneficial actions of ACE inhibition in states in which plasma angiotensin II concentrations are normal.

A pathophysiologic role for angiotensin II in circulatory failure is now well established. Although the actions of angiotensin II in part mimic the hallmarks of advanced circulatory failure, that is, vasoconstriction, sodium retention, and hyperaldosteronism, studies have documented the reversibility of these effects.[178] It has been demonstrated in an animal model of circulatory failure that chronic ACE inhibition during the development of circulatory failure leads to a delay in the progression of ventricular dysfunction by preventing an increase in peripheral vascular resistance and by blunting neurohumoral activation.[178] Other studies with chronic ACE inhibition in the canine myocardial infarction model have also demonstrated improvement in left ventricular function with a decrease in ventricular dilatation in association with improved survival.[179]

These studies in experimental circulatory failure have been extended to humans with symptomatic and asymptomatic left ventricular dysfunction in SOLVD (Studies of Left Ventricular Dysfunction). This important human clinical trial was designed to determine whether ACE inhibitor treatment with enalapril reduces mortality in patients with low ejection fractions ($<35\%$)[180,181] These investigations demonstrated that enalapril reduced mortality and morbidity related to worsening circulatory failure. The mechanisms of these beneficial effects of ACE inhibition remain unclear, but they may be due to limitation of the cellular actions of long-term angiotensin II on the heart, vasculature, and kidneys. These important actions in circulatory failure may include decreases in preload and afterload, coronary vasodilatation, direct antiatherogenic and antihypertrophic actions, and opposition to the sodium-retaining actions of angiotensin II within the kidney.

Endothelin. Endothelin, a 21-amino acid peptide, is also a component of the local tissue compensatory mechanisms activated in heart failure.[182] Endothelin is a potent vasoconstrictor of endothelial cell origin with positive inotropic properties. Endothelin, which is released in response to both mechanical and humoral stimulation, functions via at least two receptor subtypes. The endothelin-A receptor, which is highly expressed on vascular smooth muscle and myocardium, mediates the vasoconstrictor and inotropic actions of endothelin. In contrast, the endothelin-B receptor, which is highly expressed in endothelial cells, results in release of EDRF/NO. Endothelin-1 is the mature product of a precursor molecule, big-endothelin, which is cleaved by a converting enzyme. Like angiotensin II, endothelin has growth-promoting and mitogenic potential and, therefore, contributes to cardiac and vascular remodeling. Endothelin also may stimulate renin and aldosterone release and thus function to potentiate angiotensin-like effects in heart failure.

The potential for a positive feedback loop is also evidenced by the demonstration of endothelin gene induction by angiotensin and vasopressin in bovine vascular endothelial cells.[183] This would further contribute to the imbalance in regulatory and counterregulatory mechanisms and favor vasoconstriction and cell proliferation in circulatory failure. Impaired endothelial cell release of EDRF/NO would also contribute to the imbalance in regulatory mechanism. The infusion of *N*-monomethyl-L-arginine, a competitive inhibitor of EDRF/NO generation, increased baseline systemic vascular resistance and decreased cardiac output in a canine circulatory failure model.[184] Also, the inhibition of EDRF/NO significantly enhanced the vasoconstrictor response to endothelin infusion. These findings further support the concept of a dynamic balance between endothelium-derived vasodilating and vasoconstricting factors in the modulation of vascular tone. Furthermore, plasma concentration of endothelin in humans with circulatory failure is increased.[185,186] A correlation of plasma endothelin concentration and severity of circulatory failure has also been demonstrated.

Mechanisms for increased plasma endothelin in circulatory failure include increased production stimulated by either hemodynamic or neurohumoral factors and decreased clearance or metabolism of the peptide. With respect to hemodynamic factors, right and left atrial pressures were independently and significantly correlated with plasma endothelin in experimental circulatory failure.[187] Because recent observations suggest that cardiac and pulmonary production of endothelin occurs, it is tempting to speculate that increased cardiac filling pressures and perhaps chronic cardiac or pulmonary vascular distention are stimuli for endothelin production or secretion, as has been demonstrated for ANP. Recently, angiotensin II was shown to stimulate endothelin production in vitro,[155] and the known elevation of angiotensin II in circulatory failure may contribute to the increase of circulating endothelin in circulatory failure.

It is unlikely that endothelin evolved as a regulator specifically in response to circulatory failure. More likely, this peptide system participates in the regulation of vascular tone, perhaps in response to decreases in cardiac output, as may occur with hemorrhage. A reasonable conclusion from the currently available data is that endothelin has functionally important local and systemic effects that might be activated at either level. At the local level, thrombin, an important mediator released during hemorrhage, is known to stimulate endothelin secretion, raising the possibility that endothelin has the function of maintaining vascular constriction and thus preventing further hemorrhage while local repair and clotting mechanisms attempt to repair damaged tissue. At the systemic level, in association with significant decreases in effective arterial volume, there is marked activation of the RAS. Angiotensin II thus could serve as an obvious and potent stimulus to endothelin secretion.[155] Therefore, endothelin might function systemically during hemorrhage to enhance fluid retention through renal vasoconstriction and activation of the RAS to preserve perfusion pressure. Additionally, the potent effects of venoconstriction would attempt to increase preload, possibly further augmenting cardiac output in this situation.

Because circulatory failure is a low cardiac output state similar to that in significant hemorrhage, it seems likely that endothelin may be increased because of the decrease in effective arterial volume. As in the RAS, the vasoconstricting effects of endothelin may be beneficial early in circulatory failure, augmenting preload by venoconstriction and increasing systemic vascular resistance to maintain perfusion pressure despite offsetting actions of such modulators as EDRF and ANP. With time, however, the chronic effects of endothelin activation most likely become excessive and contribute to a continuing deterioration of circulatory function. This deterioration of circulatory efficiency may also be linked to the remodeling of the heart, with associated ventricular hypertrophy and myocyte loss. Studies in vitro have documented an important action of endothelin on cardiac myocytes, which appear to be mediated by highly expressed and widely distributed cardiac endothelin receptors.[188]

Cytokines. Cytokines, products of immune cells, have recently been implicated in the progression of circulatory failure. Cytokines such as interleukin-1, tissue necrosis factor, and interferon-γ may influence myocardial function directly through negative inotropic effects and indirectly through effects on endothelial cell function.[189] Cytokines may also influence local mechanisms in the development of atherosclerotic lesions, particularly in transplantation-associated atherosclerosis.

Neurohumoral mechanisms to prevent the progression of heart failure: therapeutic strategies (Table 15-4)

Evidence to date supports a role for endogenous circulating and paracrine systems such as the natriuretic peptides and EDRF/NO in maintaining circulatory compensation and delaying the onset of overt circulatory failure. In our attempt to delay the progression of asymptomatic left ventricular dysfunction to overt circulatory failure, we will see the further development of sensitive and specific diagnostic tests, such as N-ANP, to screen for asymptomatic left ventricular dysfunction in addition to strategies to control the risk factors that favor ventricular dysfunction, such as coronary atherosclerosis and hypertension. Early detection would permit administration of pharmacologic agents to delay or prevent the progression to overt circulatory failure.

Once diagnosis of early heart failure is made, agents that potentiate the endogenous vasodilatory-natriuretic-antimitogenic factors, such as neutral endopeptidase inhibitors for ANP or L-arginine to augment synthesis of EDRF/NO, may delay progression. Such agents could complement the ACE inhibition currently known to delay the onset of symptoms and retard cardiac dilatation. Indeed, such a strategy could contribute to a delay in the ventricular remodeling and myocyte death that characterize progressive circulatory failure or could mediate beneficial actions via modulation of peripheral vascular or renal function. Once overt circulatory failure is established, efforts should continue to focus on antagonism or suppression of vasoconstrictor, antinatriuretic, and mitogenic systems. Specifically, the development of inhibitors and antagonists of the RAS as well as those to endothelin may be of value.

Table 15-4 Neurohumoral strategies for the future: therapeutic considerations

Step one:

Aggressive diagnosis and treatment of risk factors, i.e., atherosclerosis, hypertension, and diabetes

Step two:

Early diagnosis of asymptomatic left ventricular dysfunction, i.e., use of the N-terminus of the atrial natriuretic peptide molecule for screening and confirmation of reduced ventricular function by noninvasive imaging

Step three:

Treatment of asymptomatic left ventricular dysfunction by potentiation of endogenous vasodilator, natriuretic, and antimitogenic factors, i.e., enhancement of natriuretic peptides with neutral endopeptidase inhibitors and augmentation of endothelium-derived relaxing factor–nitric oxide with nitric oxide analogues or L-arginine, such agents alone or with antagonists of the renin-angiotensin system

Step four:

Treatment of symptomatic overt congestive heart failure by antagonism of endogenous vasoconstrictor, antinatriuretic, and mitogenic factors, i.e., angiotensin-converting enzyme inhibitors, angiotensin II receptor antagonists or renin inhibitors to oppose the renin-angiotensin system, and endothelin receptor antagonists or endothelin-converting enzyme inhibitors to counteract the endothelin system

REFERENCES

1. Henry PD, Eckberg D, Gault JH, et al: Depressed inotropic state and reduced myocardial oxygen consumption in the human heart. *Am J Cardiol* 31:300-306, 1973
2. Graham TP Jr, Ross J Jr, Covell JW, et al: Myocardial oxygen consumption in acute experimental cardiac depression. *Circ Res* 21:123-138, 1967
3. Parodi O, De Maria R, Oltrona L, et al: Myocardial blood flow distribution in patients with ischemic heart disease or dilated cardiomyopathy undergoing heart transplantation. *Circulation* 88:509-522, 1993
4. Katz AM: Cardiomyopathy of overload. A major determinant of prognosis in congestive heart failure. *N Engl J Med* 322:100-110, 1990
5. Sievers R, Parmley WW, James T, et al: Energy levels at systole vs. diastole in normal hamster hearts vs. myopathic hamster hearts. *Circ Res* 53:759-766, 1983
6. Cooper G IV, Satava RM Jr, Harrison CE, et al: Mechanisms for the abnormal energetics of pressure-induced hypertrophy of cat myocardium. *Circ Res* 33:213-223, 1973
7. Chidsey CA, Weinbach EC, Pool PE, et al: Biochemical studies of energy production in the failing human heart. *J Clin Invest* 45:40-50, 1966
8. Buchwald A, Till H, Unterberg C, et al: Alterations of the mitochondrial respiratory chain in human dilated cardiomyopathy. *Eur Heart J* 11:509-516, 1990
9. Ansari AA, Wang YC, Danner DJ, et al: Abnormal expression of histocompatibility and mitochondrial antigens by cardiac tissue from patients with myocarditis and dilated cardiomyopathy. *Am J Pathol* 139:337-354, 1991

10. Neumann DA, Rose NR, Ansari AA, et al: Induction of multiple heart autoantibodies in mice with coxsackievirus B3- and cardiac myosin-induced autoimmune myocarditis. *J Immunol* 152:343-350, 1994

11. Ingwall JS: Is cardiac failure a consequence of decreased energy reserve? *Circulation* 87 Suppl 7:58-62, 1993

12. Scheuer J: Metabolic factors in myocardial failure. *Circulation* 87 Suppl 7:54-57, 1993

13. Weiss RG, Bottomley PA, Hardy CJ, et al: Regional myocardial metabolism of high-energy phosphates during isometric exercise in patients with coronary artery disease. *N Engl J Med* 323:1593-1600, 1990

14. Hardy CJ, Weiss RG, Bottomley PA, et al: Altered myocardial high-energy phosphate metabolites in patients with dilated cardiomyopathy. *Am Heart J* 122:795-801, 1991

15. Nascimben L, Pauletto P, Pessina AC, et al: Decreased energy reserve may cause pump failure in human dilated cardiomyopathy (abstract). *Circulation* 84 Suppl 2:563, 1991

16. Schwarz F, Schaper J, Kittstein D, et al: Reduced volume fraction of myofibrils in myocardium of patients with decompensated pressure overload. *Circulation* 63:1299-1304, 1981

17. Pagani ED, Alousi AA, Grant AM, et al: Changes in myofibrillar content and Mg-ATPase activity in ventricular tissues from patients with heart failure caused by coronary artery disease, cardiomyopathy, or mitral valve insufficiency. *Circ Res* 63:380-385, 1988

18. Geenen DL, Malhotra A, Scheuer J: Regional variation in rat cardiac myosin isoenzymes and ATPase activity after infarction. *Am J Physiol* 256:H745-750, 1989

19. Gorza L, Mercadier JJ, Schwartz K, et al: Myosin types in the human heart. An immunofluorescence study of normal and hypertrophied atrial and ventricular myocardium. *Circ Res* 54:694-702, 1984

20. Bouvagnet P, Leger J, Dechesne CA, et al: Local changes in myosin types in diseased human atrial myocardium: a quantitative immunofluorescence study. *Circulation* 72:272-279, 1985

21. Bouvagnet P, Mairhofer H, Leger JO, et al: Distribution pattern of alpha and beta myosin in normal and diseased human ventricular myocardium. *Basic Res Cardiol* 84:91-102, 1989

22. Katz AM: Biochemical "defect" in the hypertrophied and failing heart: deleterious or compensatory? *Circulation* 47:1076-1079, 1973

23. Tsuchimochi H, Sugi M, Kuro-o M, et al: Isozymic changes in myosin of human atrial myocardium induced by overload. Immunohistochemical study using monoclonal antibodies. *J Clin Invest* 74:662-665, 1984

24. Kurabayashi M, Komuro I, Tsuchimochi H, et al: Molecular cloning and characterization of human atrial and ventricular myosin alkali light chain cDNA clones. *J Biol Chem* 263:13930-13936, 1988

25. Solaro RJ, Powers FM, Gao L, et al: Control of myofilament activation in heart failure. *Circulation* 87 Suppl 7:38-43, 1993

26. Schwartz K, Carrier L, Mercadier J-J, et al: Molecular phenotype of the hypertrophied and failing myocardium. *Circulation* 87 Suppl 7:5-10, 1993

27. Chidsey CA, Sonnenblick EH, Morrow AG, et al: Norepinephrine stores and contractile force of papillary muscle from the failing human heart. *Circulation* 33:43-51, 1966

28. Chidsey CA, Braunwald E, Morrow AG: Catecholamine excretion and cardiac stores of norepinephrine in congestive heart failure. *Am J Med* 39:442-451, 1965

29. Schofer J, Tews A, Langes K, et al: Relationship between myocardial norepinephrine content and left ventricular function—an endomyocardial biopsy study. *Eur Heart J* 8:748-753, 1987

30. Thomas JA, Marks BH: Plasma norepinephrine in congestive heart failure. *Am J Cardiol* 41:233-243, 1978

31. Spann JF Jr, Sonnenblick EH, Cooper T, et al: Cardiac norepinephrine stores and the contractile state of heart muscle. *Circ Res* 19:317-325, 1966

32. Colucci WS, Ribeiro JP, Rocco MB, et al: Impaired chronotropic response to exercise in patients with congestive heart failure. Role of postsynaptic beta-adrenergic desensitization. *Circulation* 80:314-323, 1989

33. Colucci WS: In situ assessment of α- and β-adrenergic responses in failing human myocardium. *Circulation* 87 Suppl 7:63-67, 1993

34. Bristow MR, Ginsburg R, Minobe W, et al: Decreased catecholamine sensitivity and beta-adrenergic-receptor density in failing human hearts. *N Engl J Med* 307:205-211, 1982

35. Bristow MR: The adrenergic nervous system in heart failure (editorial). *N Engl J Med* 311:850-851, 1984

36. Fowler MB, Laser JA, Hopkins GL, et al: Assessment of the beta-adrenergic receptor pathway in the intact failing human heart: progressive receptor down-regulation and subsensitivity to agonist response. *Circulation* 74:1290-1302, 1986

37. Bristow MR, Anderson FL, Port JD, et al: Differences in beta-adrenergic neuroeffector mechanisms in ischemic versus idiopathic dilated cardiomyopathy. *Circulation* 84:1024-1039, 1991

38. Bristow MR, Hershberger RE, Port JD, et al: Beta 1- and beta 2-adrenergic receptor-mediated adenylate cyclase stimulation in nonfailing and failing human ventricular myocardium. *Mol Pharmacol* 35:295-303, 1989

39. Bristow MR, Kantrowitz NE, Ginsburg R, et al: Beta-adrenergic function in heart muscle disease and heart failure. *J Mol Cell Cardiol* 17 Suppl 2:41-52, 1985

40. Meerson FZ: On the mechanism of compensatory hyperfunction and insufficiency of the heart. Cor Vasa 3:161-177, 1961

41. Lee JC, Downing SE: Ventricular function in norepinephrine-induced cardiomyopathic rabbits. *Am J Physiol* 242:H191-H196, 1982

42. Chen V, Downing SE: Preservation of cardiac metabolic capacity after acute catecholamine injury. *Am J Physiol* 258:H101-H106, 1990

43. Downing SE, Chen V: Myocardial injury following endogenous catecholamine release in rabbits. *J Mol Cell Cardiol* 17:377-387, 1985

44. Reichenbach DD, Benditt EP: Catecholamines and cardiomyopathy: the pathogenesis and potential importance of myofibrillar degeneration. *Hum Pathol* 1:125-150, 1970

45. Haft JI: Cardiovascular injury induced by sympathetic catecholamines. *Prog Cardiovasc Dis* 17:73-86, 1974

46. Fleckenstein A, Janke J, Doring HJ, et al: Ca overload as the determinant factor in the production of catecholamine-induced myocardial lesions. *Recent Adv Stud Cardiac Struct Metab* 2:455-466, 1973

47. Feldman AM, Cates AE, Veazey WB, et al: Increase of the 40,000-mol wt pertussis toxin substrate (G protein) in the failing human heart. *J Clin Invest* 82:189-197, 1988

48. Neumann J, Schmitz W, Scholz H, et al: Increase in myocardial Gi-proteins in heart failure. *Lancet* 2:936-937, 1988

49. Horn EM, Corwin SJ, Steinberg SF, et al: Reduced lymphocyte stimulatory guanine nucleotide regulatory protein and beta-adrenergic receptors in congestive heart failure and reversal with angiotensin converting enzyme inhibitor therapy. *Circulation* 78:1373-1379, 1988

50. Denniss AR, Marsh JD, Quigg RJ, et al: Beta-adrenergic receptor number and adenylate cyclase function in denervated transplanted and cardiomyopathic human hearts. *Circulation* 79:1028-1034, 1989

51. Gwathmey JK, Slawsky MT, Hajjar RJ, et al: Role of intracellular calcium handling in force-interval relationships of human ventricular myocardium. *J Clin Invest* 85:1599-1613, 1990

52. Edes I, Talosi L, Kranias EG: Sarcoplasmic reticulum function in normal heart and in cardiac disease. *Heart Failure* December 1990/January 1991, pp 221-237

53. Mercadier JJ, Lompre AM, Duc P, et al: Altered sarcoplasmic reticulum Ca2(+)-ATPase gene expression in the human ventricle during end-stage heart failure. *J Clin Invest* 85:305-309, 1990

54. de la Bastie D, Levitsky D, Rappaport L, et al: Function of the sarcoplasmic reticulum and expression of its Ca2(+)-ATPase gene in pressure overload-induced cardiac hypertrophy in the rat. *Circ Res* 66:554-564, 1990

55. Gwathmey JK, Copelas L, MacKinnon R, et al: Abnormal intracellular calcium handling in myocardium from patients with end-stage heart failure. *Circ Res* 61:70-76, 1987

56. Harigaya S, Schwartz A: Rate of calcium binding and uptake in normal animal and failing human cardiac muscle. Membrane vesicles (relaxing system) and mitochondria. *Circ Res* 25:781-794, 1969

57. Perreault CL, Williams CP, Morgan JP: Cytoplasmic calcium modulation and systolic versus diastolic dysfunction in myocardial hypertrophy and failure. *Circulation* 87 Suppl 7:31-37, 1993

58. Spann JF Jr, Buccino RA, Sonnenblick EH, et al: Contractile state of cardiac muscle obtained from cats with experimentally produced ventricular hypertrophy and heart failure. *Circ Res* 21:341-354, 1967

59. Cooper G IV, Tomanek RJ, Ehrhardt JC, et al: Chronic progressive pressure overload of the cat right ventricle. *Circ Res* 48:488-497, 1981

60. Spann JF Jr, Covell JW, Eckberg DL, et al: Contractile performance of the hypertrophied and chronically failing cat ventricle. *Am J Physiol* 223:1150-1157, 1972

61. Crozatier B, Hittinger L: Mechanical adaptation to chronic pressure overload. *Eur Heart J* 9 Suppl E:7-11, 1988
62. Spann JF, Bove AA, Natarajan G, et al: Ventricular performance, pump function and compensatory mechanisms in patients with aortic stenosis. *Circulation* 62:576-582, 1980
63. Williams JF Jr, Potter RD: Normal contractile state of hypertrophied myocardium after pulmonary artery constriction in the cat. *J Clin Invest* 54:1266-1272, 1974
64. Williams JF Jr, Mathew B, Hern DL, et al: Myocardial hydroxyproline and mechanical response to prolonged pressure loading followed by unloading in the cat. *J Clin Invest* 72:1910-1917, 1983
65. Legault F, Rouleau JL, Juneau C, et al: Functional and morphological characteristics of compensated and decompensated cardiac hypertrophy in dogs with chronic infrarenal aorto-caval fistulas. *Circ Res* 66:846-859, 1990
66. Carabello BA, Nakano K, Corin W, et al: Left ventricular function in experimental volume overload hypertrophy. *Am J Physiol* 256:H974-H981, 1989
67. Pinsky WW, Lewis RM, Hartley CJ, et al: Permanent changes of ventricular contractility and compliance in chronic volume overload. *Am J Physiol* 237:H575-H583, 1979
68. Patterson SW, Starling EH: On the mechanical factors which determine the output of the ventricles. *J Physiol (Lond)* 48:357-379, 1914
69. Ross J Jr, Sonnenblick EH, Taylor RR, et al: Diastolic geometry and sarcomere lengths in the chronically dilated canine left ventricle. *Circ Res* 28:49-61, 1971
70. Badeer HS: Contractile tension in the myocardium. *Am Heart J* 66:432-434, 1963
71. Sagawa K, Suga H, Shoukas AA, et al: End-systolic pressure/volume ratio: a new index of ventricular contractility. *Am J Cardiol* 40:748-753, 1977
72. Suga H, Kitabatake A, Sagawa K: End-systolic pressure determines stroke volume from fixed end-diastolic volume in the isolated canine left ventricle under a constant contractile state. *Circ Res* 44:238-249, 1979
73. Kass DA: Clinical evaluation of left heart function by conductance catheter technique. *Eur Heart J* 13 Suppl E:57-64, 1992
74. Kass DA, Wolff MR, Ting CT, et al: Diastolic compliance of hypertrophied ventricle is not acutely altered by pharmacologic agents influencing active processes. *Ann Intern Med* 119:466-473, 1993
75. Grossman W, Jones D, McLaurin LP: Wall stress and patterns of hypertrophy in the human left ventricle. *J Clin Invest* 56:56-64, 1975
76. Feild BJ, Baxley WA, Russell RO Jr, et al: Left ventricular function and hypertrophy in cardiomyopathy with depressed ejection fraction. *Circulation* 47:1022-1031, 1973
77. Benjamin IJ, Schuster EH, Bulkley BH: Cardiac hypertrophy in idiopathic dilated congestive cardiomyopathy: a clinicopathologic study. *Circulation* 64:442-447, 1981
78. Meerson FZ: Introduction. *Circ Res* 24 Suppl 2:1-8, 1969
79. Nishimura RA, Housmans PR, Hatle LK, et al: Assessment of diastolic function of the heart: background and current applications of Doppler echocardiography. Part I. Physiologic and pathophysiologic features. *Mayo Clin Proc* 64:71-81, 1989
80. Shepherd RF, Zachariah PK, Shub C: Hypertension and left ventricular diastolic function. *Mayo Clin Proc* 64:1521-1532, 1989
81. Grossman W: Diastolic dysfunction in congestive heart failure. *N Engl J Med* 325:1557-1564, 1991
82. Serizawa T, Carabello BA, Grossman W: Effect of pacing-induced ischemia on left ventricular diastolic pressure-volume relations in dogs with coronary stenoses. *Circ Res* 46:430-439, 1980
83. Hess OM, Osakada G, Lavelle JF, et al: Diastolic myocardial wall stiffness and ventricular relaxation during partial and complete coronary occlusions in the conscious dog. *Circ Res* 52:387-400, 1983
84. Farhi ER, Canty JM Jr, Klocke FJ: Effects of graded reductions in coronary perfusion pressure on the diastolic pressure-segment length relation and the rate of isovolumic relaxation in the resting conscious dog. *Circulation* 80:1458-1468, 1989
85. Fifer MA, Borow KM, Colan SD, et al: Early diastolic left ventricular function in children and adults with aortic stenosis. *J Am Coll Cardiol* 5:1147-1154, 1985
86. Smith VE, Schulman P, Karimeddini MK, et al: Rapid ventricular filling in left ventricular hypertrophy: II. Pathologic hypertrophy. *J Am Coll Cardiol* 5:869-874, 1985
87. Douglas PS, Berko B, Lesh M, et al: Alterations in diastolic function in response to progressive left ventricular hypertrophy. *J Am Coll Cardiol* 13:461-467, 1989
88. Papademetriou V, Gottdiener JS, Fletcher RD, et al: Echocardiographic assessment by computer-assisted analysis of diastolic left ventricular function and hypertrophy in borderline or mild systemic hypertension. *Am J Cardiol* 56:546-550, 1985
89. Brutsaert DL, Rademakers FE, Sys SU: Triple control of relaxation: implications in cardiac disease. *Circulation* 69:190-196, 1984
90. Gillebert TC, Sys SU, Brutsaert DL: Influence of loading patterns on peak length-tension relation and on relaxation in cardiac muscle. *J Am Coll Cardiol* 13:483-490, 1989
91. Heyndrickx GR, Paulus WJ: Effect of asynchrony on left ventricular relaxation. *Circulation* 81 Suppl 3:41-47, 1990
92. Bonow RO: Regional left ventricular nonuniformity: effects on left ventricular diastolic function in ischemic heart disease, hypertrophic cardiomyopathy, and the normal heart. *Circulation* 81 Suppl 3:54-65, 1990
93. Morgan JP, Morgan KG: Calcium and cardiovascular function. Intracellular calcium levels during contraction and relaxation of mammalian cardiac and vascular smooth muscle as detected with aequorin. *Am J Med* 77:33-46, 1984
94. Morgan JP: Abnormal intracellular modulation of calcium as a major cause of cardiac contractile dysfunction. *N Engl J Med* 325:625-632, 1991
95. Wagner JA, Sax FL, Weisman HF, et al: Calcium-antagonist receptors in the atrial tissue of patients with hypertrophic cardiomyopathy. *N Engl J Med* 320:755-761, 1989
96. Diamond G, Forrester JS: Effect of coronary artery disease and acute myocardial infarction on left ventricular compliance in man. *Circulation* 45:11-19, 1972
97. Cuocolo A, Sax FL, Brush JE, et al: Left ventricular hypertrophy and impaired diastolic filling in essential hypertension. Diastolic mechanisms for systolic dysfunction during exercise. *Circulation* 81:978-986, 1990
98. Diver DJ, Royal HD, Aroesty JM, et al: Diastolic function in patients with aortic stenosis: influence of left ventricular load reduction. *J Am Coll Cardiol* 12:642-648, 1988
99. Weber KT, Pick R, Silver MA, et al: Fibrillar collagen and remodeling of dilated canine left ventricle. *Circulation* 82:1387-1401, 1990
100. Weber KT, Jalil JE, Janicki JS, et al: Myocardial collagen remodeling in pressure overload hypertrophy. A case for interstitial heart disease. *Am J Hypertens* 2:931-940, 1989
101. Weber KT, Janicki JS, Shroff SG, et al: Collagen remodeling of the pressure-overloaded, hypertrophied nonhuman primate myocardium. *Circ Res* 62:757-765, 1988
102. Chapman D, Weber KT, Eghbali M: Regulation of fibrillar collagen types I and III and basement membrane type IV collagen gene expression in pressure overloaded rat myocardium. *Circ Res* 67:787-794, 1990
103. Corin WJ, Murakami T, Monrad ES, et al: Left ventricular passive diastolic properties in chronic mitral regurgitation. *Circulation* 83:797-807, 1991
104. Aguirre FV, Pearson AC, Lewen MK, et al: Usefulness of Doppler echocardiography in the diagnosis of congestive heart failure. *Am J Cardiol* 63:1098-1102, 1989
105. Dougherty AH, Naccarelli GV, Gray EL, et al: Congestive heart failure with normal systolic function. *Am J Cardiol* 54:778-782, 1984
106. Echeverria HH, Bilsker MS, Myerburg RJ, et al: Congestive heart failure: echocardiographic insights. *Am J Med* 75:750-755, 1983
107. Soufer R, Wohlgelernter D, Vita NA, et al: Intact systolic left ventricular function in clinical congestive heart failure. *Am J Cardiol* 55:1032-1036, 1985
108. Ghali JK, Kadakia S, Cooper RS, et al: Bedside diagnosis of preserved versus impaired left ventricular systolic function in heart failure. *Am J Cardiol* 67:1002-1006, 1991
109. Marantz PR, Tobin JN, Wassertheil-Smoller S, et al: The relationship between left ventricular systolic function and congestive heart failure diagnosed by clinical criteria. *Circulation* 77:607-612, 1988
110. Topol EJ, Traill TA, Fortuin NJ: Hypertensive hypertrophic cardiomyopathy of the elderly. *N Engl J Med* 312:277-283, 1985
111. Vanhoutte PM: Adjustments in the peripheral circulation in chronic heart failure. *Eur Heart J* 4 Suppl A:67-83, 1983
112. Zelis R, Mason DT, Braunwald E: A comparison of the effects

of vasodilator stimuli on peripheral resistance vessels in normal subjects and in patients with congestive heart failure. *J Clin Invest* 47:960-970, 1968

113. Zelis R, Sinoway LI, Musch TI, et al: Regional blood flow in congestive heart failure: concept of compensatory mechanisms with short and long time constants. *Am J Cardiol* 62:2E-8E, 1988

114. Creager MA, Hirsch AT, Dzau VJ, et al: Baroreflex regulation of regional blood flow in congestive heart failure. *Am J Physiol* 258:H1409-H1414, 1990

115. Zelis R, Mason DT, Braunwald E: Partition of blood flow to the cutaneous and muscular beds of the forearm at rest and during leg exercise in normal subjects and in patients with heart failure. *Circ Res* 24:799-806, 1969

116. Wilson JR, Mancini DM, McCully K, et al: Noninvasive detection of skeletal muscle underperfusion with near-infrared spectroscopy in patients with heart failure. *Circulation* 80:1668-1674, 1989

117. Mancini DM, Coyle E, Coggan A, et al: Contribution of intrinsic skeletal muscle changes to ^{31}P NMR skeletal muscle metabolic abnormalities in patients with chronic heart failure. *Circulation* 80:1338-1346, 1989

118. Wilson JR, Mancini DM: Skeletal muscle metabolic dysfunction: implications for exercise intolerance in heart failure. *Circulation* 87 Suppl 7:104-109, 1993

119. Sullivan MJ, Knight JD, Higginbotham MB, et al: Relation between central and peripheral hemodynamics during exercise in patients with chronic heart failure. Muscle blood flow is reduced with maintenance of arterial perfusion pressure. *Circulation* 80:769-781, 1989

120. Sullivan MJ, Green HJ, Cobb FR: Altered skeletal muscle metabolic response to exercise in chronic heart failure. Relation to skeletal muscle aerobic enzyme activity. *Circulation* 84:1597-1607, 1991

121. Sullivan MJ, Green HJ, Cobb FR: Skeletal muscle biochemistry and histology in ambulatory patients with long-term heart failure. *Circulation* 81:518-527, 1990

122. Kraemer MD, Kubo SH, Rector TS, et al: Pulmonary and peripheral vascular factors are important determinants of peak exercise oxygen uptake in patients with heart failure. *J Am Coll Cardiol* 21:641-648, 1993

123. Wilson JR, Mancini DM, Dunkman WB: Exertional fatigue due to skeletal muscle dysfunction in patients with heart failure. *Circulation* 87:470-475, 1993

124. Chidsey CA, Harrison DC, Braunwald E: Augmentation of the plasma nor-epinephrine response to exercise in patients with congestive heart failure. *N Engl J Med* 267:650-654, 1962

125. Cohn JN, Levine TB, Olivari MT, et al: Plasma norepinephrine as a guide to prognosis in patients with chronic congestive heart failure. *N Engl J Med* 311:819-823, 1984

126. Hasking GJ, Esler MD, Jennings GL, et al: Norepinephrine spillover to plasma in patients with congestive heart failure: evidence of increased overall and cardiorenal sympathetic nervous activity. *Circulation* 73:615-621, 1986

127. Hasking GJ, Esler MD, Jennings GL, et al: Norepinephrine spillover to plasma during steady-stage supine bicycle exercise. Comparison of patients with congestive heart failure and normal subjects. *Circulation* 78:516-521, 1988

128. Davis D, Baily R, Zelis R: Abnormalities in systemic norepinephrine kinetics in human congestive heart failure. *Am J Physiol* 254:E760-E766, 1988

129. Leimbach WN Jr, Wallin BG, Victor RG, et al: Direct evidence from intraneural recordings for increased central sympathetic outflow in patients with heart failure. *Circulation* 73:913-919, 1986

130. Ferguson DW, Berg WJ, Sanders JS: Clinical and hemodynamic correlates of sympathetic nerve activity in normal humans and patients with heart failure: evidence from direct microneurographic recordings. *J Am Coll Cardiol* 16:1125-1134, 1990

131. Kassis E: Cardiovascular response to orthostatic tilt in patients with severe congestive heart failure. *Cardiovasc Res* 21:362-368, 1987

132. Goldstein RE, Beiser GD, Stampfer M, et al: Impairment of autonomically mediated heart rate control in patients with cardiac dysfunction. *Circ Res* 36:571-578, 1975

133. Marin-Neto JA, Pintya AO, Gallo L Jr, et al: Abnormal baroreflex control of heart rate in decompensated congestive heart failure and reversal after compensation. *Am J Cardiol* 67:604-610, 1991

134. Levine TB, Francis GS, Goldsmith SR, et al: The neurohumoral and hemodynamic response to orthostatic tilt in patients with congestive heart failure. *Circulation* 67:1070-1075, 1983

135. Ferguson DW, Abboud FM, Mark AL: Selective impairment of baroreflex-mediated vasoconstrictor responses in patients with ventricular dysfunction. *Circulation* 69:451-460, 1984

136. Higgins CB, Vatner SF, Eckberg DL, et al: Alterations in the baroreceptor reflex in conscious dogs with heart failure. *J Clin Invest* 51:715-724, 1972

137. Creager MA, Creager SJ: Arterial baroreflex regulation of blood pressure in patients with congestive heart failure. *J Am Coll Cardiol* 23:401-405, 1994

138. Wang W, Chen JS, Zucker IH: Carotid sinus baroreceptor sensitivity in experimental heart failure. *Circulation* 81:1959-1966, 1990

139. Stone GW, Kubo SH, Cody RJ: Adverse influence of baroreceptor dysfunction on upright exercise in congestive heart failure. *Am J Med* 80:799-802, 1986

140. White CW: Reversibility of abnormal arterial baroreflex control of heart rate in heart failure. *Am J Physiol* 241:H778-H782, 1981

141. Ferguson DW: Sympathetic mechanisms in heart failure: pathophysiological and pharmacological implications. *Circulation* 87 Suppl 7:68-75, 1993

142. Eckberg DL, Drabinsky M, Braunwald E: Defective cardiac parasympathetic control in patients with heart disease. *N Engl J Med* 285:877-883, 1971

143. Dibner-Dunlap ME, Thames MD: Baroreflex control of renal sympathetic nerve activity is preserved in heart failure despite reduced arterial baroreceptor sensitivity. *Circ Res* 65:1526-1535, 1989

144. Vatner DE, Lee DL, Schwarz KR, et al: Impaired cardiac muscarinic receptor function in dogs with heart failure. *J Clin Invest* 81:1836-1842, 1988

145. Gauer OH, Henry JP: Neurohormonal control of plasma volume. *Int Rev Physiol II* 9:145-190, 1976

146. Henry JP, Gauer OH, Reeves JL: Evidence of the atrial location of receptors influencing urine flow. *Circ Res* 4:85-90, 1956

147. Zucker IH, Earle AM, Gilmore JP: The mechanism of adaptation of left atrial stretch receptors in dogs with chronic congestive heart failure. *J Clin Invest* 60:323-331, 1977

148. Zucker IH, Earle AM, Gilmore JP: Changes in the sensitivity of left atrial receptors following reversal of heart failure. *Am J Physiol* 237:H555-H559, 1979

149. Brandt RR, Wright RS, Redfield MM, et al: Atrial natriuretic peptide in heart failure. *J Am Coll Cardiol* 22 Suppl A:86-92, 1993

150. Perrella MA, Schwab TR, O'Murchu B, et al: Cardiac atrial natriuretic factor during evolution of congestive heart failure. *Am J Physiol* 262:H1248-H1255, 1992

151. Rodeheffer RJ, Naruse M, Atkinson JB, et al: Molecular forms of atrial natriuretic factor in normal and failing human myocardium. *Circulation* 88:364-371, 1993

152. Mukoyama M, Nakao K, Hosoda K, et al: Brain natriuretic peptide as a novel cardiac hormone in humans. Evidence for an exquisite dual natriuretic peptide system, atrial natriuretic peptide and brain natriuretic peptide. *J Clin Invest* 87:1402-1412, 1991

153. Stingo AJ, Clavell AL, Heublein DM, et al: Presence of C-type natriuretic peptide in cultured human endothelial cells and plasma. *Am J Physiol* 263:H1318-H1321, 1992

154. Stingo AJ, Clavell AL, Aarhus LL, et al: Cardiovascular and renal actions of C-type natriuretic peptide. *Am J Physiol* 262:H308-H312, 1992

155. Kohno M, Horio T, Yokokawa K, et al: C-type natriuretic peptide inhibits thrombin- and angiotensin II-stimulated endothelin release via cyclic guanosine 3′, 5′-monophosphate. *Hypertension* 19:320-325, 1992

156. Koller KJ, Goeddel DV: Molecular biology of the natriuretic peptides and their receptors. *Circulation* 86:1081-1088, 1992

157. Wei CM, Heublein DM, Perrella MA, et al: Natriuretic peptide system in human heart failure. *Circulation* 88:1004-1009, 1993

158. Davis KM, Fish LC, Elahi D, et al: Atrial natriuretic peptide levels in the prediction of congestive heart failure risk in frail elderly. *JAMA* 267:2625-2629, 1992

159. Lerman A, Gibbons RJ, Rodeheffer RJ, et al: Circulating N-terminal atrial natriuretic peptide as a marker for symptomless left-ventricular dysfunction. *Lancet* 341:1105-1109, 1993

160. Margulies KB, Burnett JC Jr: Neutral endopeptidase 24.11: a modulator of natriuretic peptides. *Semin Nephrol* 13:71-77, 1993

161. Perrella MA, Aarhus LL, Heublein DM, et al: Biologic role of atrial natriuretic factor clearance receptor in congestive heart failure. *Am J Physiol* 265:H401-H408, 1993

162. Okolicany J, McEnroe GA, Koh GY, et al: Clearance receptor and neutral endopeptidase-mediated metabolism of atrial natriuretic factor. *Am J Physiol* 263:F546-F553, 1992

163. Elsner D, Muntze A, Kromer EP, et al: Effectiveness of endopeptidase inhibition (candoxatril) in congestive heart failure. *Am J Cardiol* 70:494-498, 1992

164. Munzel T, Kurz S, Holtz J, et al: Neurohormonal inhibition and hemodynamic unloading during prolonged inhibition of ANF degradation in patients with severe chronic heart failure. *Circulation* 86:1089-1098, 1992

165. Perrella MA, Edell ES, Krowka MJ, et al: Endothelium-derived relaxing factor in pulmonary and renal circulations during hypoxia. *Am J Physiol* 263:R45-R50, 1992

166. Lerman A, Burnett JC Jr: Intact and altered endothelium in regulation of vasomotion. *Circulation* 86 Suppl 3:12-19, 1992

167. Katz SD, Biasucci L, Sabba C, et al: Impaired endothelium-mediated vasodilation in the peripheral vasculature of patients with congestive heart failure. *J Am Coll Cardiol* 19:918-925, 1992

168. O'Murchu B, Miller VM, Perrella MA, et al: Increased production of nitric oxide in coronary arteries during congestive heart failure. *J Clin Invest* 93:165-171, 1994

169. Henderson AH, Lewis MJ, Shah AM, et al: Endothelium, endocardium, and cardiac contraction. *Cardiovasc Res* 26:305-308, 1992

170. Nunez DJ, Dickson MC, Brown MJ: Natriuretic peptide receptor mRNAs in the rat and human heart. *J Clin Invest* 90:1966-1971, 1992

171. Packer M: The neurohormonal hypothesis: a theory to explain the mechanism of disease progression in heart failure. *J Am Coll Cardiol* 20:248-254, 1992

172. Bristow MR, Minobe W, Rasmussen R, et al: Beta-adrenergic neuroeffector abnormalities in the failing human heart are produced by local rather than systemic mechanisms. *J Clin Invest* 89:803-815, 1992

173. Catt K: Angiotensin II receptors. In *The Renin-Angiotensin System*. Edited by JIS Robertson, M Nicholls. London, Gower Medical Publishing, 1993, pp 12.1-12.14

174. Lee MA, Böhm M, Paul M, et al: Tissue renin-angiotensin systems: their role in cardiovascular disease. *Circulation* 87 Suppl 4:7-13, 1993

175. Schunkert H, Hirsch AT, Mankodi S, et al: Renal angiotensinogen gene expression in experimental heart failure: effect of angiotensin converting enzyme inhibition (abstract). *Clin Res* 37 Suppl A:584, 1989

176. Campbell DJ, Habener JF: Angiotensinogen gene is expressed and differentially regulated in multiple tissues of the rat. *J Clin Invest* 78:31-39, 1986

177. Dzau VJ: Vascular wall renin-angiotensin pathway in control of the circulation. A hypothesis. *Am J Med* 77:31-36, 1984

178. Riegger GA, Liebau G, Holzschuh M, et al: Role of the renin-angiotensin system in the development of congestive heart failure in the dog as assessed by chronic converting-enzyme blockade. *Am J Cardiol* 53:614-618, 1984

179. Pfeffer MA, Pfeffer JM, Steinberg C, et al: Survival after an experimental myocardial infarction: beneficial effects of long-term therapy with captopril. *Circulation* 72:406-412, 1985

180. Yusuf S: Overview of the design and key results of the studies of left ventricular dysfunction. *Heart Failure* 9:28-35, 1993

181. Konstam MA, Kronenberg MW, Rousseau MF, et al: Effects of the angiotensin converting enzyme inhibitor enalapril on the long-term progression of left ventricular dilatation in patients with asymptomatic systolic dysfunction. *Circulation* 88:2277-2283, 1993

182. Yanagisawa M, Kurihara H, Kimura S, et al: A novel potent vasoconstrictor peptide produced by vascular endothelial cells. *Nature* 332:411-415, 1988

183. Imai T, Hirata Y, Emori T, et al: Induction of endothelin-1 gene by angiotensin and vasopressin in endothelial cells. *Hypertension* 19:753-757, 1992

184. Lerman A, Sandok EK, Hildebrand FL Jr, et al: Inhibition of endothelium-derived relaxing factor enhances endothelin-mediated vasoconstriction. *Circulation* 85:1894-1898, 1992

185. Rodeheffer RJ, Lerman A, Heublein DM, et al: Increased plasma concentrations of endothelin in congestive heart failure in humans. *Mayo Clin Proc* 67:719-724, 1992

186. Lerman A, Kubo SH, Tschumperlin LK, et al: Plasma endothelin concentrations in humans with end-stage heart failure and after heart transplantation. *J Am Coll Cardiol* 20:849-853, 1992

187. Margulies KB, Hildebrand FL Jr, Lerman A, et al: Increased endothelin in experimental heart failure. *Circulation* 82:2226-2230, 1990

188. Power RF, Wharton J, Zhao Y, et al: Autoradiographic localization of endothelin-1 binding sites in the cardiovascular and respiratory systems. *J Cardiovasc Pharmacol* 13 Suppl 5:50-56, 1989

189. Libby P: Do vascular wall cytokines promote atherogenesis? *Hosp Pract (Off Ed)* 27:51-58, October 15, 1992

CHAPTER

16

Evaluation of congestive heart failure

Margaret M. Redfield, M.D.

THE National Heart, Lung, and Blood Institute estimates that 2 to 3 million Americans have overt heart failure.[1] This estimate is supported by recent data from the National Health and Nutrition Examination Survey.[2] Worldwide it is estimated that over 15 million people have heart failure.[3] The prevalence and incidence of asymptomatic ventricular dysfunction or unrecognized cardiac dysfunction causing only mild symptoms are unknown but probably are significant,[4,5] and epidemiologic data from Sweden suggest that the prevalence of "latent heart failure," or asymptomatic ventricular dysfunction, approaches that of overt heart failure.[6] The prevalence and incidence of heart failure increase progressively with age, as demonstrated in Figures 16-1 and 16-2 from the Framingham study.[1] The marked increase in the prevalence of heart failure in the elderly is especially important because 13% of the population are currently 65 years old or older, and this figure will increase to 21% by the year 2030. Three percent of the population are currently 80 years old or older, and this will increase to 4.3% of the population (12 million people) by the year 2010.[7] On the basis of the Framingham data, the prevalence of heart failure in this rapidly growing population segment approaches 10%, and thus one can expect an increasing prevalence of heart failure as our population ages.

Heart failure is responsible for more than 900,000 hospitalizations per year.[1] Even in patients with heart failure treated aggressively with angiotensin-converting enzyme (ACE) inhibitors and followed closely as part of the Studies of Left Ventricular Dysfunction (SOLVD) trial, 26% were hospitalized for heart failure at least once and 12% were hospitalized two or more times over a 4-year follow-up period.[8] The rates of hospitalization for heart failure in patients with asymptomatic ventricular dysfunction treated with ACE inhibitors and followed closely as part of the SOLVD prevention trial or Survival and Ventricular Enlargement (SAVE) trial were 9% to 14% over a 3- to 4-year follow-up period.[4,5] In all these trials, the rates of hospitalization for heart failure were much higher in patients not treated with ACE inhibitors and might be as high as 35% of patients per year for patients with symptomatic heart failure.[8] Even patients managed as outpatients require frequent follow-up and monitoring, and standard therapy for heart failure often includes at least five drugs. Thus, the morbidity and costs related to heart failure consume a significant portion of our current health care resources. Indeed, heart failure was recently the most frequent DRG (diagnosis-related group) diagnosis for hospitalized patients older than 65.[7]

Estimates of mortality in patients with heart failure vary widely, depending on the population studied. Although early studies estimated a 2-year mortality rate as high as 70%,[9-12] recent data suggest a much improved prognosis for patients with heart failure. The observed mortality rates in recent multicenter trials of vasodilators in heart failure are shown in Table 16-1. The 2-year mortality rate remains 10% to 15% in patients with asymptomatic ventricular dysfunction treated aggressively and followed closely and still approaches 50% in class IV patients. Recent studies of patients with idiopathic dilated cardiomyopathy suggest that data derived from multicenter drug trials may not be applicable to all populations, because the data are largely from patients treated at referral centers, which are subject to potent referral bias.[17,18] Although recent data from the Framingham study indicate that little progress has been made in reducing the mortality from congestive heart failure (CHF), this study was completed before the widespread use of ACE inhibitors.[19] Other studies of patients with idiopathic dilated cardiomyopathy treated at a tertiary referral center indicate improved survival for patients in whom the diagnosis was made in the 1980s.[18] Nonetheless, mortality remains high despite improvements in diagnosis and treatment, and heart failure continues to be an important and growing health-care problem.

DEFINITION AND CLASSIFICATION OF HEART FAILURE

Mechanistic classification

Systolic and diastolic cardiac dysfunction. Heart failure has classically been defined as the pathophysiologic state in which an abnormality of cardiac function is responsible for failure of the heart to pump blood at a rate commensurate with the requirements of the metabolizing

Age:	50-59	60-69	70-79	80-89
Person-bienniums	20520	19298	8994	2084
Person-bienniums with CHF	166	451	438	190
Percent prevalence	0.8	2.3	4.9	9.1

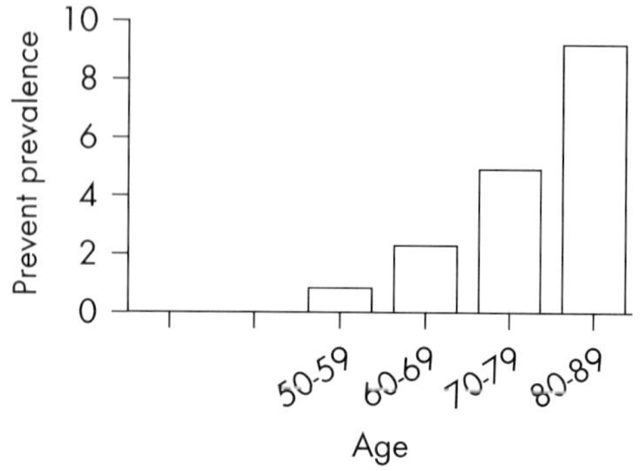

Fig 16-1 Framingham data showing the prevalence of heart failure by age in both men and women. The prevalence increases to approximately 9% in persons older than 80. (From Kannel WB, Belanger AJ: Epidemiology of heart failure. *Am Heart J* 121:951-957, 1991. By permission of Mosby-Year Book.)

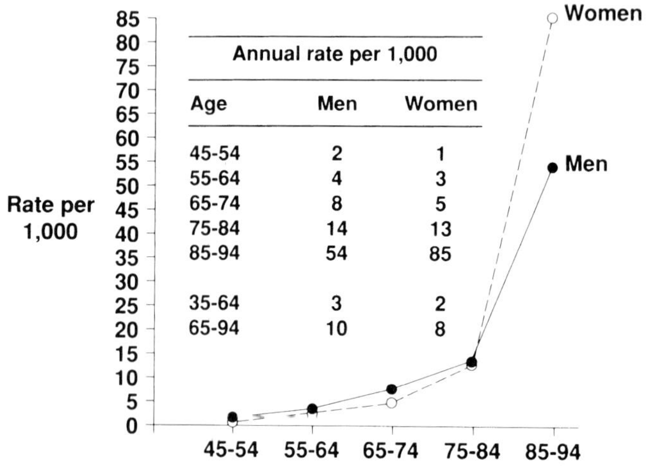

Fig 16-2 Incidence of heart failure by age and sex from the Framingham study. As with the prevalence of heart failure, the incidence increases greatly with age. (From Kannel WB, Belanger AJ: Epidemiology of heart failure. *Am Heart J* 121:951-957, 1991. By permission of Mosby-Year Book.)

Table 16-1 Studies related to prognosis in heart failure and asymptomatic left ventricular dysfunction

Study	Years of study	NYHA functional class	No. of patients	Cause	2 year mortality, %	
V-HeFTI[13]	1980-1985	I-IV	642	All	P	34
					H-I	26
SOLVD prevention[5]	1986-91	I-II	4,200	All	P & E	10
SAVE[4]	1987-90	I	2,200	Post-MI	P	18
					C	15
SOLVD, treatment[8]	1986-89	II-III	2,400	All	P	27
					E	21
V-HeFTII[14]	1986-90	II-III	804	All	H-I	25
					E	18
PROMISE[15]	1989-1990	III-IV	1,008	All	P & M	30*
CONSENSUS[16]	1980s	IV	127	All	P	75
					E	47

C, captopril; CONSENSUS, Cooperative North Scandinavian Enalapril Survival Study; E, enalapril; H-I, hydralazine-isosorbide dinitrate; M, milrinone; MI. myocardial infarction; NYHA, New York Heart Association; P, placebo; PROMISE, Prospective Randomized Milrinone Survival Evaluation; SAVE, Survival and Ventricular Enlargement; SOLVD, Studies of Left Ventricular Dysfunction; V-HeFT, Veterans Administration Cooperative Vasodilator-Heart Failure Trial.
*One-year mortality.

tissues or for pumping that is adequate only from an increased filling pressure.[20] Although valid, these definitions are not as useful in identifying patients clinically, because metabolic requirements and cardiac output are not routinely measured and the depressed cardiac output or increase in filling pressures may be due to greatly different types of cardiac dysfunction with unique pathophysiologic features, natural history, and therapeutic requirements. The recognition that diastolic dysfunction in association with systolic dysfunction or in isolation may produce signs and symptoms of CHF[21-23] has altered the approach to the evaluation of the patient with suspected heart failure and placed the emphasis on symptoms of increased filling pressures as the most consistent feature of symptomatic cardiac dysfunction. Several studies indicate that a significant proportion of patients with signs and symptoms of CHF have preserved systolic function.[24-28] Studies indicate that 30% to 40% of patients with a clinical diagnosis of heart failure have normal systolic function[21-23] and that most patients have symptoms related to increased intracardiac filling pressure due to diastolic dysfunction. Many of the same disease processes that produce systolic dysfunction also produce isolated diastolic dysfunction[22,29] and thus may produce either or both at different stages of the disease process.

High-output and low-output heart failure. Because some patients with significant symptomatic heart failure due to systolic or diastolic dysfunction may have preservation of cardiac output,[30] this classic subclassification is less applicable today and serves primarily to highlight cardiac disorders in which a high-output state is the initial derangement. These disorders are rare and produce a highly variable degree of cardiac dysfunction, in part determined by whether other cardiac disease is present.

High-output heart failure due to arteriovenous fistula has been used to produce experimental heart failure in the dog and the rat. This well-described and fairly reproducible form of experimental heart failure is characterized by increased cardiac output, hypotension, decreased systemic vascular resistance, sodium retention, and neurohumoral activation.[31] In humans, hyperthyroidism, beriberi, Paget's disease, anemia, pregnancy, and arteriovenous fistulas or shunts have been reported to produce high-output heart failure.

Temporal classification of heart failure

Asymptomatic ventricular dysfunction and symptomatic heart failure. An equally important development in the evaluation of patients with "heart failure" is the realization that asymptomatic ventricular dysfunction precedes symptomatic heart failure for a variable but significant period.[4,5] Although they are without symptoms of heart failure, these patients have significant systolic or diastolic dysfunction, activation of compensatory neurohumoral systems, and a tendency for progression to symptomatic "heart failure."[4,5,32-36] The true prevalence of asymptomatic systolic and diastolic dysfunction is unknown, but recent studies have suggested that this condition is not uncommon[6] and that treatment during the asymptomatic phase of systolic dysfunction favorably alters the natural history of the process, delaying the onset of symptomatic heart failure[4,5] and decreasing mortality.[4]

Acute and chronic heart failure. The causes of acute heart failure are relatively few and include ischemia or infarction with acute systolic or diastolic dysfunction or mechanical complications, such as acute mitral regurgitation and ventricular septal defect. Acute mitral regurgitation may also be due to mitral chordal rupture, which sometimes occurs with mitral valve prolapse, endocarditis, or hypertrophic cardiomyopathy, and may produce acute heart failure. Acute aortic valvular regurgitation due to endocarditis or aortic dissection may also be manifested by acute heart failure. Acute myocarditis may progress quickly enough to produce the sudden onset of heart failure. Sepsis has been reported to produce cardiac dilatation or systolic dysfunction,[37] which is often reversible. Acute cardiac tamponade, acute pulmonary emboli, and acute cardiac arrhythmias are other potential causes of sudden heart failure. A much more common manifestation is acute or subacute decompensation in a patient with known cardiac dysfunction. Table 16-2 lists potential precipitating causes of acute decompensation in the patient with ventricular dysfunction. One must consider these possibilities in the patient with an episode of decompensation before attributing the episode to progression of the primary process responsible for the patient's heart failure. Increasingly, nonsteroidal anti-inflammatory agents are being prescribed or obtained over-the-counter for a wide variety of indications. These medications not only promote sodium retention through inhibition of intrarenal prostaglandins but also may have potent deleterious systemic hemodynamic effects and blunt the action of ACE inhibitors.[38,39]

Table 16-2 Causes of acute decompensation in the patient with heart failure

- Patient noncompliance
  - Medications
  - Sodium and fluid restriction
  - Alcohol or cocaine use
- Hemodynamic factors
  - Tachycardia
  - Bradycardia
  - Loss of atrial contribution to filling
  - Hypertension
- Inappropriate medication
  - Agents with negative inotropic properties
    - β-blockers
    - Calcium channel blockers
    - Disopyramide
    - Propafenone
  - Agents that promote sodium retention
    - Nonsteroidal anti-inflammatory agents
    - Hormonal agents
- Ischemia or infarction
- Systemic diseases
  - Anemia
  - Thyroid disease
  - Infection
- Pulmonary embolism

Symptom-focused classification of heart failure

Backward and forward heart failure. Classification of heart failure into "backward" and "forward" heart failure in the past has been useful in focusing attention on manifestations of heart failure due to low cardiac output and those due to pulmonary or systemic venous congestion caused by increases in ventricular diastolic pressures. This classification is still useful in the evaluation of patients with systolic and diastolic dysfunction, because both types of cardiac dysfunction can produce congestive symptoms without decreased cardiac output (backward failure) as well as symptoms due to low cardiac output (forward failure). Even isolated diastolic dysfunction in patients with hypertension and left ventricular hypertrophy can produce unfavorable loading conditions with exercise, so that ejection fraction decreases in response to exercise and the expected increase in cardiac output is blunted in the absence of a primary decrease in contractility.[40] Patients with hypertrophic cardiomyopathy in whom systolic function is preserved can have reductions in resting cardiac output due to marked diastolic dysfunction.[29] Backward and forward heart failure can be manifested in patients with significant mitral regurgitation who have normal systolic function. Profound systolic dysfunction can be associated with normal filling pressures at the expense of cardiac output or with maintenance of cardiac output, with compensation due to tachycardia, dilatation, and increased filling pressures.

Right-sided and left-sided heart failure. This classification scheme was primarily used to emphasize the fact that because the specific cardiac process may not affect both ventricles to the same extent, the manifestations of heart failure may vary to some degree, depending on which ventricle is affected more. Although systolic function may be different in the right and left ventricles, cardiac output is the same, because small differences lead to fluid accumulation behind the low-output side.[41] Right ventricular systolic and diastolic function can be preserved for a significant time in patients who have ischemic left ventricular dysfunction, idiopathic dilated cardiomyopathy, or other disorders, and right-sided filling pressures may remain normal for a time. With progressive left ventricular failure and chronic elevation of left atrial pressures, pulmonary artery hypertension and, eventually, right ventricular dysfunction ensue. Patients with preserved right ventricular systolic function usually have less severe symptoms.[42,43]

Etiologic classification of ventricular dysfunction and heart failure

Systolic dysfunction. In the Framingham heart study, hypertension was the most common precursor for the development of CHF. These studies defined the incidence and outcome of CHF in a population over a period from the late 1940s to the mid 1980s. Seventy-five percent of patients with a clinical diagnosis of CHF had hypertension, and hypertension was the sole cause of heart failure in 24% of patients. Fifty-four percent of patients had coronary artery disease, and 16% of patients had valvular disease without coronary artery disease as the cause of heart failure. Only 7% of patients had "other or unknown" cause, and this category presumably included patients with primary cardiomyopathy.[19] On the basis of the Framingham data, it was concluded that hypertension with or without coronary artery disease was a major precursor of heart failure. More recent large drug trials in patients with heart failure diagnosed by criteria that generally include objective demonstration of reduced ejection fraction reflect a much lower prevalence of hypertension and a higher incidence of coronary artery disease as the presumed cause of ventricular dysfunction (Table 16-3). Indeed, all recent drug trials exclude patients with recent myocardial infarction or unstable or exercise-limiting angina and therefore probably underestimate the importance of coronary artery disease as the cause of systolic dysfunction.

An extensive review of heart failure trials from July 1989 to June 1990 generated a more contemporary list of the causes of heart failure and their relative prevalence (Fig 16-3).[49] On the basis of these more recent studies, approximately 50% to 70% of patients with systolic dysfunction have significant coronary artery disease as the presumed cause of heart failure. "Idiopathic" dilated cardiomyopathy accounts for roughly 10% to 20% of patients, and the remaining patients have valvular disease,

Table 16-3 Etiology of ventricular dysfunction in recent studies of patients with congestive heart failure

Study	History of hypertension, %	Dysfunction, % Ischemic	Dysfunction, % Nonischemic	Idiopathic dilated cardiomyopathy, %
CONSENSUS[44]	19	74	26	16
V-HeFT I[13]	40	44	56	
V-HeFT II[14]	50	54	46	
SOLVD, treatment[8]	42	72	28	18
SOLVD, prevention[5]	37	83	17	10
Quinapril[45]		63	37	
Vesnarinone[46]		51	43	
Hy-C[47]		68	32	25
RADIANCE[48]		52	48	39

CONSENSUS, Cooperative North Scandinavian Enalapril Survival Study; Hy-C, hydralazine-captopril; RADIANCE, Randomized Assesment of (the effect of) Digoxin on Inhibitors of the Angiotensin-Converting Enzyme; SOLVD, Studies of Left Ventricular Dysfunction; V-HeFT, Veterans Administration Cooperative Vasodilator-Heart Failure Trial.

hypertensive heart disease, and a variety of more uncommon cardiomyopathies. The category of dilated cardiomyopathy is broad; the potential causes of dilated cardiomyopathy are reviewed in chapter 19.

Diastolic dysfunction. When a patient presents with signs and symptoms of CHF but noninvasive testing indicates normal or near-normal systolic function, one must consider a number of diagnostic possibilities, as outlined in Table 16-4. Some patients have a condition that impairs diastolic function through either an effect on ventricular relaxation or changes in chamber or myocardial compliance.[22,23] Others have conditions that result in increases in filling pressure without primary alteration of myocardial diastolic function. As with systolic dysfunction, coronary artery disease and arterial hypertension, usually with left ventricular hypertrophy, are the most common underlying causes of diastolic dysfunction. Increased intravascular volume due to renal failure is a very common precipitant of symptoms. In patients with long-standing hypertension or vascular disease who have left ventricular hypertrophy and normal systolic function, symptoms of heart failure frequently develop as renal function deteriorates and volume status is harder to control.

CLINICAL EVALUATION

The goals of evaluation of the patient with ventricular dysfunction are given in Table 16-5. Clinical assessment of the patient should be conducted in a manner that addresses these goals, usually in the order listed.

Make the diagnosis of heart failure or asymptomatic ventricular dysfunction

Clinical assessment of the patient, including history, physical examination, chest radiograph, and electrocardiogram, establishes the diagnosis or suspicion of congestive heart failure or the need to screen for asymptomatic ventricular dysfunction.

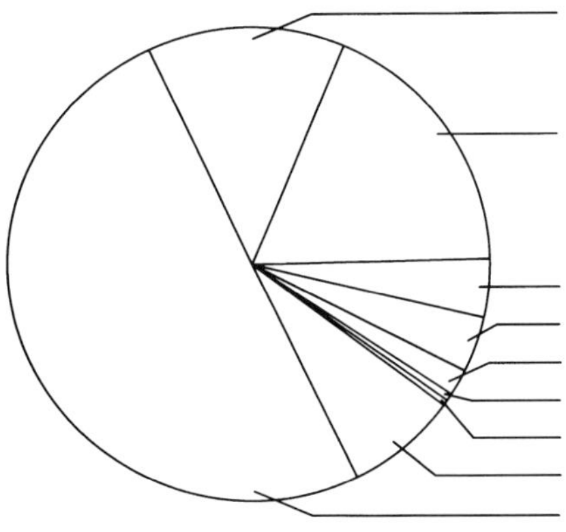

Fig 16-3 Causes of congestive heart failure in 1,861 patients. (Data from Teerlink JR, Goldhaber SZ, Pfeffer MA: An overview of contemporary etiologies of congestive heart failure. *Am Heart J* 121:1852-1853, 1991.)

The history. Although the diagnosis of florid heart failure in a patient without other medical conditions is fairly straightforward, the diagnosis of mild-to-moderate heart failure in patients with other chronic illnesses that may produce similar symptoms is often difficult. Various clinical scoring systems for the diagnosis of heart failure have been developed[25,50] (Table 16-6). However, these criteria are not used in a formal manner by most clinicians and do not assure the accurate diagnosis of systolic dysfunction. The symptoms of heart failure are fatigue, dyspnea on exertion, orthopnea, paroxysmal nocturnal dyspnea, edema, arrhythmias, and cerebral or peripheral emboli. Although not specific for heart failure, these symptoms are suggestive and should prompt formal evaluation of cardiac function.

Fatigue and weakness are prominent but often under-appreciated symptoms of heart failure. Indeed, many patients perceive exertional dyspnea as fatigue.[51] Unfor-

Table 16-4 Underlying processes in patients with heart failure and preserved systolic function

Disease states associated with abnormal diastolic function
Coronary artery disease
Hypertension
Aortic stenosis
Hypertrophic cardiomyopathy
Infiltrative cardiomyopathies
Primary restrictive cardiomyopathies
Exacerbating conditions
Tachycardia
Volume overload
Increased afterload
Mitral regurgitation
Disease states not primarily associated with abnormal diastolic function
Mitral valve disease (stenosis or regurgitation)
Atrial myxoma
Pericardial disease
Pulmonary veno-occlusive disease

Table 16-5 Steps in the evaluation of ventricular dysfunction

Make the diagnosis of heart failure or asymptomatic ventricular dysfunction
Determine the type and severity of the cardiac dysfunction
Determine the cause of the cardiac dysfunction
Determine the patient's prognosis
Provide treatment and follow-up recommendations

Table 16-6 Clinical criteria for the diagnosis of congestive heart failure (CHF)

Framingham criteria[25]

Major criteria
- Paroxysmal nocturnal dyspnea or orthopnea
- Neck vein distention
- Rales
- Cardiomegaly
- Acute pulmonary edema
- S_3 gallop
- Increased venous pressure >16 cm H_2O
- Circulation time >25 sec
- Hepatojugular reflux

Minor criteria
- Ankle edema
- Night cough
- Dyspnea on exertion
- Hepatomegaly
- Pleural effusion
- Vital capacity decreased 1/3 from maximum
- Tachycardia (rate of >120/bpm)

Major or minor criterion
- Weight loss >4.5 kg in 5 days in response to treatment

Definite CHF = 2 major or 1 major and 2 minor criteria

Boston criteria[25]

Criterion	Point value
Category I: history	
Rest dyspnea	4
Orthopnea	4
Paroxysmal nocturnal dyspnea	3
Dyspnea on walking on level	2
Dyspnea on climbing	1
Category II: physical examination	
Heart rate abnormality	1-2
91-110 bpm, 1 point	
>110 bpm, 2 points	
Jugular venous pressure elevation	2-3
>6 cm H_2O, 2 points	
>6 cm H_2O + hepatomegaly or edema, 3 points	
Lung crackles	1-2
Basilar, 1 point	
>Basilar, 2 points	
Wheezing	3
Third heart sound	3
Category III: chest radiography	
Alveolar pulmonary edema	4
Interstitial pulmonary edema	3
Bilateral pleural effusions	3
Cardiothoracic ratio >0.50	3
Upper zone flow redistribution	2

No more than 4 points from each category
Definite CHF: 8-12 points
Possible CHF: 5-7 points
Unlikely CHF: ≤4 points

Duke criteria[50]

I. Cardiomegaly on chest radiograph
II. Third heart sound

The presence of one or both of these criteria identified approximately 50% of patients with coronary artery disease and a left ventricular end-diastolic filling pressure of >15 mm Hg. Adding other clinical findings of CHF identified only 1% more and decreased specificity significantly.

tunately, this complaint is also among the least specific for heart failure. Symptoms of fatigue were traditionally attributed to reduction of cardiac output. However, exercise tolerance correlates poorly with resting ejection fraction, cardiac output, and filling pressures.[51-56] In the treated patient with heart failure, fatigue and muscle weakness can be aggravated by overdiuresis and hypokalemia. Patients whose sleep is disturbed because of orthopnea, paroxysmal nocturnal dyspnea, or frequent urination due to diuretic agents are especially prone to complain of prominent fatigue. Patients with severe heart failure may also have cool extremities due to peripheral vasoconstriction. If right-sided heart failure becomes predominant, the patient may complain more of fatigue and less of dyspnea, as do patients with end-stage mitral valve disease.

Dyspnea on exertion in patients without orthopnea, paroxysmal nocturnal dyspnea, or other symptoms of heart failure is also an extremely nonspecific symptom of heart failure. However, it is often the only complaint of patients with heart failure, so that other symptoms or signs supportive of the diagnosis must be sought. Often the patient with progressive systolic dysfunction gradually and unconsciously decreases his or her level of activity and denies symptoms of exertional dyspnea in activities of daily living. Asking the patient to compare the level of activity routinely engaged in 6 to 24 months earlier often unmasks a significant reduction in functional level. The amount of physical activity performed in daily activities varies widely among patients, and those who are sedentary may report no symptoms with daily activities. The active patient may report severe symptoms despite a functional status greatly exceeding that of sedentary patients; thus, specific tasks performed in daily activities must be specifically questioned.

Classifying the severity of dyspnea and functional limitation in the individual patient in an objective manner to allow serial assessment and comparison with the functional level of other patients with heart failure is difficult. The severity of dyspnea is commonly graded by the New York Heart Association (NYHA) functional class[57] (Table 16-7). Although useful in classification of patients, the NYHA functional class designation is subjective and susceptible to bias from both the patient and the clinician making the assessment. Quality-of-life questionnaires and exercise testing with measurement of gas exchange, increasingly used to stratify patients, provide more objective and reproducible quantification of functional status.[58-61] An alternative to the NYHA functional classification uses impairment in maximal oxygen uptake with exercise ($\dot{V}O_2max$) to grade the limitation of activity[61] (Table 16-8). The level of $\dot{V}O_2max$ also provides further useful prognostic information for patients with severe symptoms.[62-64] Others have suggested that submaximal exercise tolerance correlates better with daily functional status and that functional tests used to determine response to therapy in heart failure should assess submaximal exercise tolerance.[65]

The mechanisms responsible for dyspnea and exercise intolerance are complex. The traditional belief is that increased pulmonary venous pressures result in variable increases in interstitial lung water. The resultant reduction in lung compliance and diffusing capacity as well as ventilation and perfusion mismatch contribute to dyspnea.[51] However, exercise tolerance is not consistently related to pulmonary venous pressures.[66-68] Furthermore, desaturation during exercise is uncommon in heart failure. It is increasingly recognized that abnormalities in pulmonary function and in respiratory and peripheral muscle blood flow and metabolism also contribute importantly to exercise intolerance in heart failure.[51,60,61,69] The interaction of pulmonary, cardiac, and peripheral systems in oxygen delivery and utilization is depicted in Figure 16-4. The role of these interrelated systems in determining functional status and prognosis in heart failure, especially in the interesting subgroup of patients with asymptomatic left ventricular dysfunction, continues to evolve. The reader is referred to chapter 3B for a more detailed discussion of the assessment of cardiopulmonary function by measurement of gas exchange.

Table 16-7 New York Heart Association functional classification[57]

Class I	Patients with cardiac disease but without resulting limitations of physical activity. Ordinary physical activity does not cause undue fatigue, palpitation, dyspnea, or anginal pain.
Class II	Patients with cardiac disease resulting in slight limitation of physical activity. They are comfortable at rest. Ordinary physical activity results in fatigue, palpitation, dyspnea, or anginal pain.
Class III	Patients with cardiac disease resulting in marked limitation of physical activity. They are comfortable at rest. Less than ordinary physical activity causes fatigue, palpitation, dyspnea or anginal pain.
Class IV	Patients with cardiac disease resulting in inability to carry on any physical activity without discomfort. Symptoms of cardiac insufficiency or of the anginal syndrome may be present even at rest. If any physical activity is undertaken, discomfort is increased.

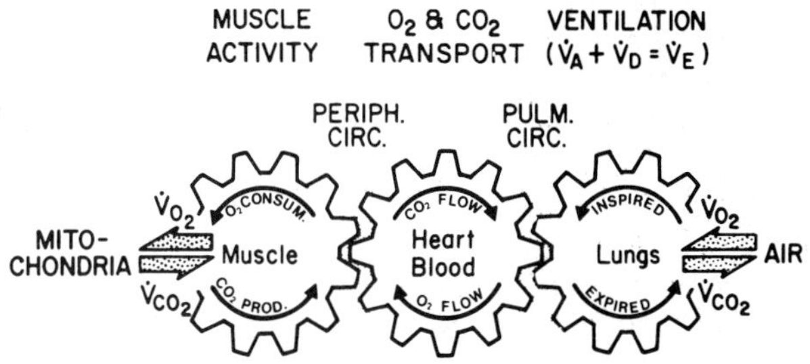

Fig 16-4 Interaction of physiologic mechanisms coupling respiration to cellular metabolic activity. Advanced heart failure is characterized by abnormalities of pulmonary function and muscle metabolic activity in addition to the primary cardiac abnormality. *CIRC,* circulation; *CONSUM.,* consumption; *PERIPH.,* peripheral; *PROD.,* production; *PULM.,* pulmonary; $\dot{V}_A$, alveolar ventilation; $\dot{V}_D$, physiologic dead space ventilation; $\dot{V}_E$, expired ventilation; $\dot{V}O_2$, oxygen uptake; $\dot{V}CO_2$, carbon dioxide output. (From Wasserman K: Measures of functional capacity in patients with heart failure. *Circulation* 81 Suppl 2:1-4, 1990. By permission of American Heart Association.)

Table 16-8 Functional classification for congestive heart failure based on maximal oxygen consumption ($\dot{V}O_2max$)[61]

Class	Severity	$\dot{V}O_2max$, mL/kg/min	Anaerobic threshold, mL/kg/min	Maximal cardiac index, L/min/m^2
A	None to mild	>20	>14	>8
B	Mild to moderate	16-20	11-14	6-8
C	Moderate to severe	10-15	8-11	4-6
D	Severe	6-9	5-8	2-4
E	Very severe	<6	3-4	<2

"Orthopnea" refers to the sensation of dyspnea that worsens with recumbency and is relieved by sitting or standing. Although somewhat more specific than exertional dyspnea as a diagnostic criterion for symptomatic heart failure, orthopnea can also occur in some patients with obstructive lung disease, diaphragmatic dysfunction, ascites, or coronary artery disease without resting systolic dysfunction (angina decubitus). Some patients have recumbency-related cough as an "orthopnea equivalent." Asking the patient the number of pillows used is a poor measure of the extent of orthopnea. A specific change in the posture of sleep in response to recumbency-related dyspnea is required to establish the diagnosis of orthopnea. Patients who have the most severe form state that they need to sleep in a chair or recliner.

Paroxysmal nocturnal dyspnea occurs after the patient has been asleep and recumbent for some time. It is described as a suffocating sensation with or without wheezing that is relieved by sitting or standing, sometimes in front of an open window or fan. Some patients use nitrates or bronchodilators with episodes. This type of dyspnea is usually a late symptom of heart failure and is usually though not always associated with orthopnea.

Edema, a common but inconsistent manifestation of cardiac failure, has the same lack of specificity as other symptoms of CHF. The mechanisms that prevent edema formation or sodium retention in general in some patients with ventricular dysfunction are incompletely understood. The degree of resting left ventricular dysfunction alone is insufficient to account for the disparity in sodium balance and edema formation. Neurohumoral activation, renal function, and peripheral venous, lymphatic, and interstitial factors all affect the propensity to edema formation and sodium retention in general. Edema in the gut wall, ascites, and congestion of the liver contribute to abdominal pain and distention, nausea, and early satiety reported by patients with advanced symptoms and may contribute to cardiac cachexia by limiting caloric intake.

Nocturia is a classic symptom of heart failure, thought to be due to enhanced renal perfusion and central blood volume produced by recumbency. Diuretic doses taken late in the day also contribute to nocturia.

Patients with heart failure frequently complain of symptoms potentially attributable to arrhythmias. Palpitations consistent with frequent premature beats, short runs of supraventricular or ventricular tachycardia, exertional tachycardia, atrial fibrillation, or sustained tachycardia are reported. Sudden episodic worsening of dyspnea, fatigue, or lightheadedness or a more gradual decompensation may be due to increases in ectopy or the onset of atrial fibrillation. Syncope and presyncope may be due to a variety of dysrhythmias but also may be caused primarily by hypotension, vasovagal spells, or neurologic disorders. Sudden death is common in patients with heart failure: 50% die suddenly. Although extremely common, ventricular arrhythmias are not the only cause of sudden death, and some of these episodes are bradycardiac.[70] Other patients may have chronic resting sinus tachycardia, poorly controlled atrial fibrillation, or high-grade ventricular ectopy and be completely unaware of it. Indeed, chronic tachycardia due to a variety of persistent tachycardias, including rapid atrial fibrillation (Grogan's syndrome), is now a well-documented cause of reversible left ventricular dysfunction.[71-74] The frequency of this entity is probably significantly underappreciated. Assessment of the adequacy of rate control in the patient with ventricular dysfunction and atrial fibrillation is imperative and should include a Holter monitor or exercise test. If the heart rate exceeds 110 to 140 bpm for much of the day or if it increases to 120 to 140 bpm in the first 2 minutes of exercise, tachycardia-related cardiomyopathy should be considered. The patient with extremely frequent premature ventricular contractions may not be aware of the ectopy but may still have "symptomatic" ventricular ectopy due to reduction in cardiac output produced by the frequent ectopy. A patient may have a resting heart rate of 80 bpm in bigeminy with little or no stroke volume associated with the premature ventricular beat, so that the effective heart rate is 40 bpm and cardiac output is markedly compromised.

Central and peripheral embolic phenomena are a well-recognized complication of heart failure, though the frequency of such episodes in patients with heart failure and sinus rhythm is somewhat controversial.[75-77] Embolic phenomena include stroke and coronary or peripheral arterial occlusion as well as pulmonary embolism, which is a common and often lethal complication of CHF.[78] The Stroke Prevention in Atrial Fibrillation (SPAF) study demonstrated that a clinical diagnosis of congestive heart failure or echocardiographic evidence of ventricular dysfunction is independently associated with an increased risk of stroke in patients with atrial fibrillation.[79,80] A left ventricular thrombus in dilated cardiomyopathy is not always associated with a greater risk of emboli than that in patients with dilated cardiomyopathy without a thrombus.[81-83] This finding probably reflects the importance of a dilated ventricle and thrombogenic milieu rather than the presence of thrombus at any one time. Several small trials or retrospective reviews have demonstrated that the frequency of emboli is reduced by anticoagulation therapy.[76,77] There are few data on the level of ventricular size or systolic dysfunction at which the incidence of embolic phenomena significantly increases and at what point the risk-benefit ratio of chronic anticoagulation is favorable.[84]

Patients with heart failure often complain of anginal or atypical chest pain, even when the coronary arteries are normal. The cause of chest pain in patients without coronary artery disease is unclear but may be related to subendocardial ischemia due to high left ventricular diastolic pressures that compromise subendocardial perfusion. Since approximately 70% of cases of left ventricular dysfunction are due to coronary artery disease, many patients with heart failure may also have angina.

Whereas patients with symptomatic dysfunction are identified when they are seen for evaluation of symptoms, patients with asymptomatic ventricular dysfunction are identified by screening patients at risk for cardiac dysfunction. Because 50% of patients with asymptomatic left ventricular dysfunction in the SOLVD prevention trial and SAVE trials who later died and 75% of those who had myocardial infarction did not have symptoms before their events, a need clearly exists to identify patients before the onset of symptoms. Therapy with ACE inhibitors before symptoms reduces mortality and the incidence of myocardial infarction.[4,5] As in symptomatic ventricular dysfunction, most patients with asymptomatic ventricular dysfunction have coronary artery disease.[4,5] Other patients at risk are those with inadequately controlled hypertension, valvular disease, excessive alcohol intake, family history of dilated cardiomyopathy, exposure to cardiotoxic drugs, abnormal electrocardiogram or chest radiograph, or symptoms of palpitations or peripheral emboli. Since the true prevalence and incidence of asymptomatic ventricular dysfunction are unknown, the cost-effectiveness of screening is unknown. Clearly, patients with coronary artery disease and hypertension are at risk and should have assessment of systolic function if they have a history consistent with myocardial infarction or abnormalities detected in the clinical examination, electrocardiogram, or chest radiograph.

Because two well-controlled studies have now demonstrated that idiopathic dilated cardiomyopathy is familial in up to 25% of cases, screening of family members of patients with idiopathic dilated cardiomyopathy is warranted.[85,86] In a study by Michels et al.,[85] cardiac disease was not suspected in 44% of relatives found to have idiopathic dilated cardiomyopathy, and asymptomatic ventricular dysfunction was incidentally discovered in 20% of patients with idiopathic dilated cardiomyopathy examined at a referral center.[87] Thus, although most patients with asymptomatic left ventricular dysfunction probably have coronary artery disease, a significant minority have idiopathic or familial dilated cardiomyopathy. Ventricular dilatation may precede ventricular systolic dysfunction, because a significant number of relatives of patients with idiopathic dilated cardiomyopathy have ventricular dilatation,[85,86] and a preliminary study from Hungary demonstrated that radiographic evidence of cardiomegaly preceded the onset of symptoms by 8 to 10 years in patients with familial and idiopathic dilated cardiomyopathy.[88] Thus, once cardiac enlargement is demonstrated, the patient should be reassessed, since ventricular enlargement may predict future systolic dysfunction.

The physical examination. Cardiac cachexia, ascites, marked edema, and tachypnea all may be apparent on general inspection of the patient. The patient with severe heart failure may appear comfortable at rest but may become dyspneic with dressing or even talking. Blood pressure may be increased or extremely low with or without marked orthostatic changes. Assessment of orthostatic changes in blood pressure is extremely important in the patient being treated with diuretics and vasodilators. Equally important is the documentation of whether the patient does or does not have symptoms associated with hypotension, because many patients receiving vasodilators may tolerate low systolic pressures without symptoms, and such asymptomatic hypotension is not an indication for withdrawal of vasodilators. Pulse pressure in advanced heart failure is classically of low volume and correlates with low cardiac output. A proportional pulse pressure [(systolic pressure − diastolic pressure)/systolic pressure] of less than 25% correlates well with a cardiac index of less than 2.2 l/min/m^2.[89] Pulsus alternans may be present in decompensated patients. Heart rate and the frequency of ectopy must be assessed. Observation of the pattern of respiration may reveal tachypnea with minimal exertion, typically in the patient with severe symptoms, and is helpful in assessing functional status. Cheyne-Stokes respiratory pattern is sometimes seen in patients with severe CHF and may contribute to disordered sleep patterns, daytime somnolence, and fatigue.

The specific cardiopulmonary examination should include assessment of carotid pulse volume and contour, as outlined above. Internal jugular venous pressure, waveforms, and respiratory response are carefully assessed. If the internal jugular venous pressure is not increased, the hepatojugular reflux should be assessed. The patient must be cautioned not to change respiratory pattern during abdominal compression, because held respiration and an involuntary Valsalva maneuver will produce a "false-positive" hepatojugular maneuver.[90]

Palpation of the right parasternal area for evidence of right ventricular enlargement and the left upper parasternal area for a palpable pulmonic closure sound indicative of pulmonary hypertension should be performed. The size, location, and quality of the apex are usually abnormal in patients with significant ventricular dilatation and systolic dysfunction. A large inferiorly and laterally displaced apex with a feeble quality is classic for patients with dilated cardiomyopathy and systolic dysfunction. There may be a palpable third or fourth heart sound. Patients with primarily diastolic dysfunction due to hypertrophy may have a smaller, less displaced apex with a forceful, sustained quality and a palpable fourth heart sound. Heart sounds are variable in patients with CHF and are influenced by the rhythm, rate, type, and cause of cardiac dysfunction; associated valvular diseases; and pericardial effusion. Classically, the findings associated with a dilated heart with poor systolic function include a soft first heart sound, a third or fourth heart sound, and a holosystolic murmur of tricuspid or mitral regurgitation. The reader is referred to chapter 2 for further discussion of the physical findings in other specific conditions that may be associated with CHF.

Auscultation of the lung fields may reveal decreased breath sounds and dullness at the bases due to pleural effusion. Rales may be fine and limited to the bases or the dependent side in the recumbent patient and may extend further up the lung fields and become louder with worsening CHF. With acutely decompensated failure and frank pulmonary edema, rales are coarse and bubbling, with wheezing, rhonchi, and production of frothy sputum.

Examination of the abdomen in patients with heart failure should include inspection and palpation for ascites and percussion and palpation for liver size and pulsatility. The liver is enlarged in patients with long-standing elevation of right-sided pressures and may be tender with acute further increases in right-sided pressures in decompensated patients. Severe tricuspid regurgitation may produce a pulsatile liver.

The sacrum and extremities should both be examined for pitting edema. There may be asymmetrical edema due

Table 16-9 Relation of chest radiographic findings to left atrial pressure[91,92]

Increase in pressure		
Degree	**mm Hg**	**Radiographic description**
Mild	13-17	Equalization of apical and basal vessel size
Moderate	18-23	Cephalization with apical > basal vessel size
Moderately severe	20-25	Interstitial edema with Kerley's B lines
Markedly severe	>25	Alveolar edema with perihilar or "butterfly" distribution

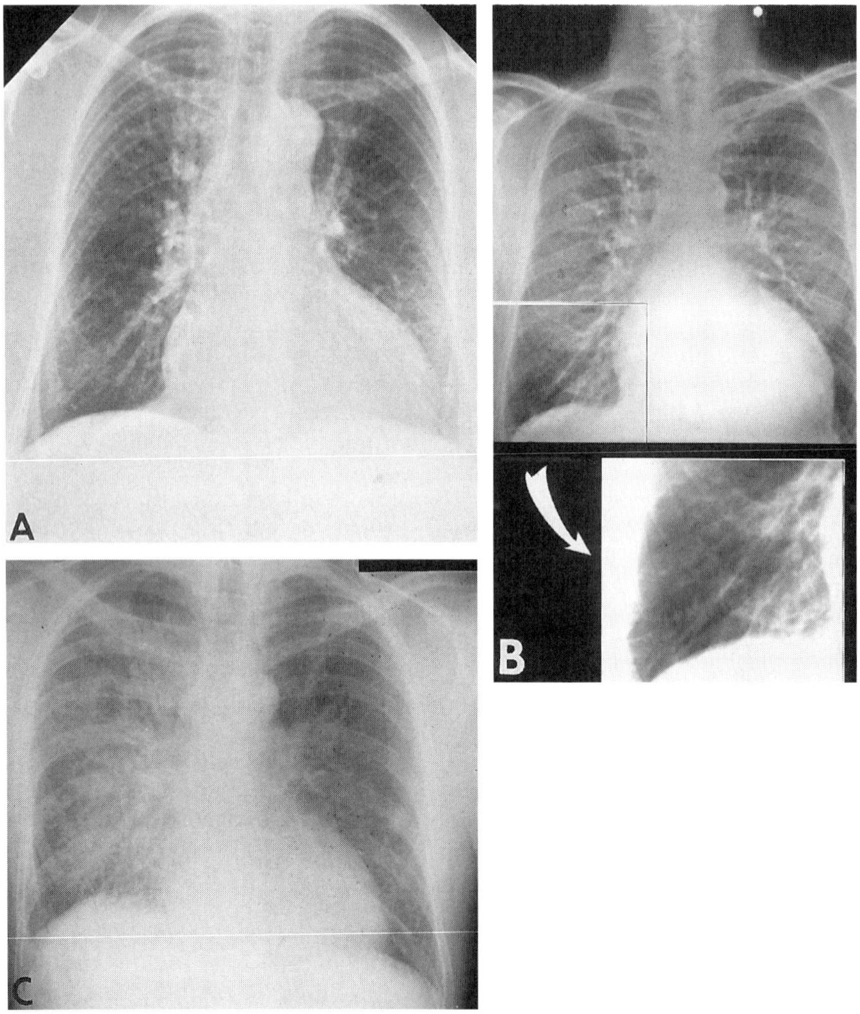

Fig 16-5 **A,** cardiomegaly and significant redistribution or cephalization of the pulmonary venous pattern without any significant interstitial or alveolar edema. The caliber of the upper pulmonary venous vessels is significantly greater than the caliber of those in the lower lung fields. **B,** cardiomegaly and pulmonary venous hypertension as well as interstitial edema shown by Kerley's B lines (see insert) in both bases. **C,** cardiomegaly and diffuse fluffy alveolar pattern consistent with marked pulmonary edema.

to previous venous or musculoskeletal diseases. Edema is an insensitive and nonspecific finding, and if other physical findings or a history of cardiac disease is lacking, it should not be considered highly suggestive of CHF.

Chest radiograph. Cardiomegaly is the most frequent abnormality on chest radiographs in patients with dilated cardiomyopathy and systolic dysfunction but can also be seen frequently in patients with normal systolic function and CHF symptoms due to ventricular hypertrophy and abnormal diastolic function.[28] A thoracic ratio of greater than 0.5 on the chest radiograph is a relatively insensitive measure of ventricular enlargement. The shape of the cardiac silhouette can sometimes indicate specific chamber enlargement, and the reader is referred to chapter 4 for a discussion of the chest radiographic findings in specific chamber enlargement. Pericardial disease should be considered in the patient with CHF symptoms and globular cardiomegaly (pericardial effusion) or a small heart (constrictive pericarditis).

Examination of the pulmonary arterial vasculature may reveal signs of pulmonary hypertension with enlargement of the central pulmonary arteries. Examination of the pulmonary venous pattern and lung fields is helpful in assessing left-sided filling pressures.[91,92] The patterns classically associated with mild to severe increases in left atrial pressures are listed in Table 16-9 and examples of these findings are shown in Figure 16-5. Pleural effusions can be present at any stage and may persist for some time after therapy has lowered filling pressures. As outlined below, these findings are not consistently present in patients with increases in left-sided filling pressures, especially in those with significant obstructive lung disease.

Electrocardiogram. No electrocardiographic findings are specific for CHF, but the electrocardiogram is usually abnormal in patients with significant cardiac disease. Although the abnormalities may suggest a cause for CHF, they are extremely nonspecific (Table 16-10). Importantly, the electrocardiogram may assist in the exclusion of asymptomatic systolic dysfunction; in one study, 95% of patients with chest pain and suspected coronary artery disease who had normal electrocardiographic results had a normal ejection fraction.[93]

Laboratory examination. The standard laboratory examination in a patient with suspected CHF should include a hematology group to exclude anemia as a factor precipitating decompensation. Serum electrolytes should be assessed to exclude hyponatremia. Hyponatremia is induced by diuretics and consumption of excess free water. Activation of the renin-angiotensin-aldosterone system and arginine vasopressin both contribute to the hyponatremia by stimulating thirst centers and altering free water clearance. Hyponatremia is a poor prognostic factor, and although it usually is relieved by ACE inhibitor therapy, hyponatremic patients often have an excessive hypotensive response to the initiation of ACE inhibitor therapy. Serum potassium concentration may be decreased because of potassium-wasting diuretics or increased because of renal dysfunction, which may be exacerbated by ACE inhibitors.

Assessment of renal function with serum creatinine findings must be interpreted cautiously; one should remember that mild renal dysfunction may be greatly worsened by ACE inhibitors and that a significant increase in serum creatinine concentration may be reversible with withdrawal of ACE inhibitors or improvement in renal perfusion because of improvement in cardiac output. Short-term inotropic therapy with intravenously administered dobutamine can sometimes be used to assess the reversibility of renal dysfunction in patients with severe CHF in whom cardiac transplantation is being considered.

Liver function test results are often abnormal in patients with increased right-sided pressures and chronic hepatic congestion. Increases in hepatic enzymes, hepatobiliary enzymes, and prothrombin time due to compromise of hepatic synthetic function are common. Serum aspartate aminotransferase or alanine aminotransferase values may increase to 5 to 10 times normal with a severe episode of decompensation and will return to normal with successful treatment. Mild hyperbilirubinemia and increased alkaline phosphatase concentration are common. In rare instances, chronic hepatic congestion can lead to cardiac cirrhosis and impaired synthetic function with hypoalbuminemia and greatly increased prothrombin time. Close attention to hepatic and renal function is important during selection and follow-up of drug therapy in patients with CHF, because many agents affect renal and hepatic function or are predominantly cleared

Table 16-10 Electrocardiographic findings in specific cardiac diseases associated with heart failure

Idiopathic dilated cardiomyopathy	Atrial fibrillation Intraventricular conduction defect (especially LBBB) in 60% Left ventricular hypertrophy
Coronary artery disease	Q waves ST- and T-wave abnormalities Intraventricular conduction defect
Hypertension	Left ventricular hypertrophy
Hypertrophic cardiomyopathy	Intraventricular conduction delay Q waves (pseudoinfarct) ST- and T-wave abnormalities
Tachycardia-related cardiomyopathy	Atrial fibrillation with poorly controlled ventricular response Other incessant tachycardias
Amyloidosis	Low voltage, Q waves (pseudo infarct)
Hypothyroidism	Low voltage
Pericardial disease	Low voltage ST- and T-wave abnormalities

LBBB, left bundle-branch block.

through these mechanisms, and significant impairment of hepatic or renal function can potentiate drug actions and side effects.

Limitations of the clinical assessment of heart failure. The symptoms of CHF are straightforward but to some extent nonspecific. Dyspnea and fatigue are extremely common complaints, and determining the relative role of ventricular dysfunction in conjunction with obesity, deconditioning, pulmonary disease, and other systemic illnesses in producing these symptoms is sometimes difficult. The difficulty of selecting clinical criteria considered diagnostic of heart failure is underscored by the diagnostic heterogeneity in clinical trials of heart failure.[94] Studies may rely on symptoms, physical findings, chest x-ray findings, or various levels of ejection fraction, and there is no consensus on the best set of clinical criteria for the diagnosis of heart failure.

Recent studies have focused on systolic dysfunction assessed by echocardiography or radionuclide or contrast angiography with or without symptoms of heart failure as the basis for inclusion in studies of heart failure. This trend appropriately reflects the importance of asymptomatic ventricular dysfunction as a precursor of overt heart failure and recognizes the frequency of symptomatic heart failure due to diastolic dysfunction in patients with normal systolic function. The inconsistent correlation between systolic function and symptomatic status has long been recognized, as discussed above. This factor and others are reflected in a study that examined the poor correlation between the clinical diagnosis of heart failure assessed by various heart failure diagnostic criteria and the presence or absence of systolic dysfunction defined as an ejection fraction of less than 40% as determined by radionuclide angiography. Of 153 patients with an ejection fraction of less than 40%, 20% met none of the criteria for CHF, and of 204 patients with an ejection fraction over 50%, 51% met at least one of the criteria.[25] In separate studies, Stevenson and Perloff[89] and Chakko et al.[95] demonstrated that clinical and radiographic signs of heart failure were often absent in patients with increased left ventricular end-diastolic pressure (LVEDP) and depressed systolic function. Other studies documented significant interobserver variability among clinicians in the detection of the clinical signs of heart failure and demonstrated a poor correlation between the clinical signs of heart failure and measures of ventricular volume and systolic performance.[96]

Intraobserver and interobserver variability are also common in the assessment of signs of CHF on the chest radiograph,[97] and the ability of the chest radiograph to predict LVEDP is limited. Herman et al.[98] demonstrated that 38% of patients with an LVEDP over 20 mm Hg had no signs of heart failure on the chest radiograph. Mahdyoon et al.[99] reported similar findings in 68% of patients with end-stage heart failure, severe systolic dysfunction, and significant increase in LVEDP who had minimal or no evidence of pulmonary congestion on the chest radiograph.

Thus, although a careful history, physical examination, and chest radiograph allow the diagnosis of heart failure and its severity in many patients, the symptoms are nonspecific and the physical examination and chest x-ray findings are not completely reliable indicators of hemodynamics or systolic performance. In the near future, one may be able to screen for cardiac dysfunction with serum markers that indicate increased filling pressures or cardiac hypertrophy.[100,101]

Determine the nature and severity of the cardiac dysfunction

Once a clinical suspicion of the syndrome of CHF or of a significant risk of asymptomatic ventricular dysfunction exists, the nature and severity of the cardiac dysfunction must be established. As discussed above, the limitations of the clinical evaluation alone in correctly establishing the diagnosis of systolic or diastolic dysfunction and the realization that as many as 40% of patients with a firm clinical diagnosis of CHF have diastolic dysfunction with preserved systolic function make objective assessment of cardiac function essential. The optimal method of quantifying cardiac function varies with the resources available to the clinician, the clinician's familiarity with different technologies, and the clinical situation. Cost-containment issues increasingly influence the selection of studies to quantify cardiac function, and studies that give information about cause or concomitant conditions may be preferred. Table 16-11 characterizes the data *potentially* available with each method. The availability and quality of some of the data potentially available with these tests vary considerably among laboratories, and it is essential that the clinician be aware of the strengths and weaknesses of the laboratories utilized.

Two-dimensional Doppler echocardiography allows quantification of global and regional left and right ventricular systolic function through a variety of quantitative and semiquantitative techniques. It provides a detailed assessment of chamber dimensions and allows the detection of valvular disease, which may be the cause or the result of ventricular dilatation and systolic dysfunction, and assessment of its severity. Ventricular wall thickness can be determined and ventricular mass calculated to assess the existence and severity of ventricular hypertrophy or infiltration that may produce systolic or diastolic dysfunction. One can identify patients with thrombus formation, which may indicate an increased risk of peripheral embolization. In many echocardiographic laboratories, Doppler technology can provide an increasingly comprehensive hemodynamic evaluation, which routinely includes cardiac output, pulmonary artery systolic and diastolic pressure, and valvular gradients.

The analysis of diastolic function is increasingly sophisticated, and abnormal Doppler patterns correlated with abnormalities in ventricular relaxation and compliance have been characterized[36] (Fig 16-6). Diastolic function may be abnormal without evidence of systolic dysfunction (diastolic heart failure) and is usually abnormal in patients with systolic dysfunction. Patients with well-compensated systolic dysfunction or with abnormalities of ventricular relaxation without systolic dysfunction usually have an "abnormal relaxation" pattern on Doppler evaluation of left ventricular diastolic filling. As atrial

Table 16-11 Techniques to detect systolic and diastolic ventricular dysfunction

	Systolic function	Diastolic function	Ventricular wall morphology	Valve disease	Coronary artery disease	Strengths & weaknesses	
						Cost	Other
Echocardiography	E	E	E	E	S*	Moderate	Noninvasive, dependent on laboratory & patient
Radionuclide ventriculography	E	S	L	L	S*	Moderate	Noninvasive, dependent on laboratory & patient
Sestamibi first-pass imaging	L	N	L	N	S*	Moderate-high	Noninvasive, limited availability
Contrast ventriculography, LVEDP, and coronary angiography	E	E	L	E	E	High	Invasive, radiation, limited availability
Ultrafast CT	E	S	E	S	S	Moderate	Limited availability, radiation
Cardiac MRI	S	S	E	S	S	Moderate-high	Limited availability

E, extensive information; S, some information; L, limited information; N, no information.
CT, computed tomography; LVEDP, left ventricular end-diastolic pressure; MRI, magnetic resonance imaging.
*With exercise.

pressures become increasingly high from fluid retention or alterations in ventricular compliance, the mitral inflow pattern progresses through a "pseudonormal" phase and finally a "restrictive" phase. Assessment of the pattern of pulmonary venous filling can augment the information obtained from the mitral inflow pattern and allow one to separate out a normal pattern of ventricular filling from a "pseudonormal" one. Many investigators now believe that analysis of the mitral inflow and pulmonary venous signal can provide a valid estimate of LVEDP in many patients.[102,103] Alteration of atrial pressures with diuretics and vasodilators results in marked variability in these patterns, and in an acutely decompensated patient, it is not unusual for a restrictive pattern to revert to abnormal relaxation or normal pattern as filling pressures are reversed with therapy. It is especially important that the patient with suspected CHF due to diastolic dysfunction be examined during acute decompensation, as filling patterns may normalize after aggressive diuresis and it may not be possible to firmly establish that diastolic function is abnormal and to attribute the patient's dyspnea to the abnormality.

Echocardiography can also exclude other causes of heart failure with normal systolic function, such as "silent" mitral stenosis, mitral regurgitation, aortic valve disease, pericardial disease, restrictive cardiomyopathy (in some cases), and hypertrophic cardiomyopathy. Stress echocardiography with exercise or pharmacologic agents can provide noninvasive assessment of coronary artery disease. The reader is referred to chapters 5B, 5C, and 5D for a more complete discussion of the use of echocardiographic Doppler techniques to evaluate systolic function, diastolic function, hemodynamics, and valvular disease, to detect coronary artery disease, and to assess myocardial viability.

Radionuclide angiography routinely provides information on ventricular volumes and global and regional left ventricular function. Some laboratories can also analyze diastolic filling and right ventricular function. Combined with exercise, radionuclide angiography is a well-established adjuvant to the diagnosis of significant coronary artery disease. Although regurgitant fractions can be calculated to quantify mitral regurgitation, this capability is not routinely available in all laboratories. Some laboratories can assess ejection fraction by first-pass analysis of sestamibi perfusion imaging. This combination is especially useful in the patient with suspected ischemic systolic or diastolic dysfunction and may also provide information on viability. The reader is referred to chapter 6 for a more complete discussion of the use of radionuclide angiography and sestamibi perfusion imaging to assess systolic and diastolic function and coronary artery disease.

Cardiac catheterization with contrast ventriculography and measurement of left ventricular diastolic pressures provides assessment of global and regional systolic function, mitral regurgitation, and extent of coronary artery disease. Increased filling pressures without systolic dysfunction is the standard definition of diastolic dysfunction, although as with echocardiography, normalization of filling pressures after extensive diuresis can produce false-negative results. In patients considered for cardiac transplantation, cardiac hemodynamics are routinely assessed during pharmacologic intervention to exclude

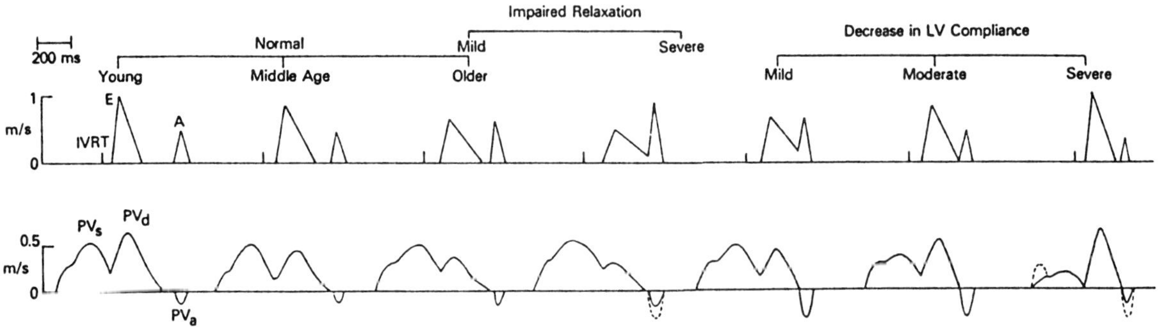

Fig 16-6 Natural history of left ventricular filling assessed by Doppler echocardiography. The diagram shows the hypothetical progression of changes in mitral and pulmonary inflow velocities. These progressive changes are believed to occur with aging and in many cardiac disease states. Labeled variables include the aortic valve closure click *(Ac),* the time interval from Ac to the start of mitral flow (left ventricular [*LV*] isovolumic relaxation time, *IVRT*), mitral deceleration time *(Mdt),* peak mitral flow velocity in early diastole (*E*), peak mitral flow velocity at atrial contraction (*A*) and peak pulmonary flow velocity during ventricular systole *(PV_s),* during ventricular diastole *(PV_d),* and at atrial contraction *(PV_a).* The mitral and pulmonary flow velocities are staggered, so that early diastolic flow of both is approximately aligned. Width and spacing of mitral and pulmonary vein flow velocity components vary because of changes in LV IVRT interval and Mdt. In young adults, most LV filling takes place in early diastole and the LV IVRT and Mdt are relatively short. PV_s and PV_d are approximately equal, or sometimes PV_d predominates. With aging, LV relaxation slows and E-wave velocity and PV_d progressively decrease, while LV IVRT, Mdt, and PV_s all increase. The result is that the proportion of LV filling that occurs with atrial contraction increases. Similar changes are seen at an earlier age than normal in patients with many types of cardiac disease that cause a slowing (impairment) of LV relaxation. Reverse flow in the pulmonary veins may be normal (*solid line*) or increased (*dashed line*) at this stage, depending on whether left atrial and LV compliance is normal and how much atrial pressure increases with atrial contraction. With abnormally slow LV relaxation and a mild decrease in LV compliance, left atrial volume and pressure begin to increase. The higher left atrial pressure at mitral valve opening results in a shortening of the IVRT and an increase in E and PV_d velocities back toward normal. As the LV compliance decreases further, left atrial volume and pressure continue to increase, and the changes in the variables described above become more pronounced. Pulmonary venous flow in systole decreases as atrial compliance decreases and is usually less than diastolic flow velocity. At this stage, the LV filling pattern may appear normal. However, the increase in atrial size, decrease in atrial compliance, and increased flow reversal in the pulmonary veins with atrial contraction all indicate that abnormalities in diastolic function are present. With a severe decrease in LV compliance, the left atrium dilates and fails and filling pressures are markedly elevated. The early diastolic mitral flow velocity is much larger than velocity at atrial contraction, the IVRT is very short, and the mitral deceleration time is less than 160 msec—features that are characteristic of "restrictive" ventricular physiology and its abrupt, premature cessation of filling. Pulmonary venous flow velocity in diastole is also increased and demonstrates an abrupt deceleration of flow. Pulmonary venous flow in systole is markedly reduced because of marked decrease in atrial compliance and, in some cases, because of depressed atrial systolic function. (From Appleton CP, Hatle LK: The natural history of left ventricular filling abnormalities: assessment by two-dimensional and Doppler echocardiography. *Echocardiography* 9:437-457, 1992. By permission of Futura Publishing Company.)

"fixed" pulmonary hypertension (see chapter 18). The usefulness of endomyocardial biopsy is controversial (see chapter 19B). If a patient with obvious CHF and angina or multiple risk factors for coronary artery disease is a potential candidate for revascularization, valve surgery, or transplantation, cardiac catheterization with ventriculography and limited hemodynamics may be the most cost-effective procedure of first choice. Patients in whom the diagnosis and suspected cause are less clear are often best served by echocardiography or other noninvasive assessment of systolic and diastolic function to establish presence, type, and severity of cardiac dysfunction. If coronary artery disease is later thought to be a strong possibility, limited coronary angiography can be performed. The cost of these combined procedures is not greatly increased over that of ventriculography and hemodynamic assessment combined with coronary angiography.

Ultrafast computed tomography and magnetic resonance imaging gated to the cardiac cycle are now available at many institutions and can provide information on systolic and diastolic function in patients undergoing these studies for other indications (pericardial disease, cardiac tumors, aortic disease, or pulmonary vascular disease). The information obtainable with these modalities is discussed in detail in their respective chapters.

Determine the cause of the cardiac dysfunction

A decision on the probable cause of the cardiac dysfunction (systolic or diastolic) is usually possible after the initial clinical evaluation. Because coronary artery disease is the most common cause of both systolic and diastolic dysfunction, a careful estimate of the probability of this disease is a major goal of the initial evaluation, and coronary artery disease must always be excluded in the patient older than 40 years. A history of risk factors for coronary artery disease, possible or proven myocardial infarction, and angina should be carefully reviewed and the electrocardiogram and chest radiograph reviewed for supporting evidence.

Because revascularization can preserve and restore systolic function in patients with systolic dysfunction and "hibernating," or "stunned," myocardium even if anginal symptoms are absent[104] and since patients with three-vessel disease and ventricular dysfunction obtain the greatest mortality benefit with revascularization, an aggressive approach to angiography and revascularization is warranted in patients who are otherwise surgical candidates. Angiography is usually required to establish the diagnosis of coronary artery disease, since noninvasive assessment of coronary artery disease is sometimes difficult in the patient with heart failure. An intraventricular conduction delay, frequently present, can affect both perfusion studies and imaging techniques. Nonischemic cardiomyopathies can often demonstrate patchy defects on perfusion studies and regional wall motion abnormalities on imaging studies. Patients with heart failure often are unable to exercise to a level considered adequate to exclude ischemia. Multivessel percutaneous transluminal coronary angioplasty may expand the patient population that can benefit from angiography and revascularization. Even in patients not considered candidates for revascularization, it is essential to establish the extent of coronary disease, because medical therapy for the patient with heart failure worsened by ischemic episodes may benefit from β-blocking agents or calcium channel antagonists, agents not traditionally thought to be of benefit in CHF.

Often, patients have mild-to-moderate coronary artery disease that seems insufficient to explain ventricular dysfunction. In general, if one or more major epicardial arteries have a fixed stenosis of 50% or greater, a diagnosis of nonischemic cardiomyopathy is not made, although with single-vessel disease it is difficult to attribute significant global systolic dysfunction to coronary artery disease. When significant coronary artery disease is present and appears appropriate for bypass surgery, one needs to attempt to assess the viability of the myocardium and the potential for improvement in symptoms and systolic function with revascularization. If the patient has a clear history of massive or multiple myocardial infarctions and clear-cut scar or aneurysm on noninvasive imaging in most of the left ventricle, significant areas of viability are unlikely. However, studies have demonstrated marked improvement in functional class and systolic function with revascularization, even in patients with large areas of akinesis, and there is active investigation into noninvasive techniques to assess myocardial viability.[105,107] This subject is reviewed in chapter 6.

Determine prognosis

Because CHF is a highly lethal condition, an assessment of each patient's prognosis is important for decisions on referral for cardiac transplantation, for other standard and investigational surgical and medical treatments, and for patient counseling. Although multiple clinical and laboratory indicators provide excellent prognostic information when applied to large numbers of patients with a broad spectrum of disease severity, determining prognosis in individuals with the most severe disease is considerably more difficult. Those variables demonstrated to have prognostic value are listed in Table 16-12. Functional class provides a quick and universally available estimate of risk; prognosis associated with each functional class in large populations of patients enrolled in multicenter drug trials is noted in Table 16-1. Patients with coronary artery disease as the cause of CHF are generally[11,109] but not universally[9,121] thought to have a poorer prognosis than patients with nonischemic cardiomyopathies. Ejection fraction is another widely available and important prognostic indicator;[113] however, since the average ejection fraction in patients with heart failure of all functional classes is 25% or less, its value in many patients is limited. Enlarged cardiac size, regardless of how measured, consistently indicates increased mortality.[112]

If a patient is considered at high risk, that is, class III or IV, on the basis of this initial basic clinical assessment, has a dilated ventricle with an ejection fraction of less than 25%, or has a history of symptomatic arrhythmias, more

Table 16-12 Prognostic indicators in congestive heart failure

Clinical	
NYHA functional class[108]	
Ischemic cause[11,109]	
Syncope or symptomatic ventricular arrhythmias[108,110]	
Third heart sound[108]	
Atrial fibrillation[111]	
Laboratory	
Hemodynamic	
Degree of cardiomegaly (by multiple techniques)[108,112]	
Ejection fraction[113]	
Filling pressures[108,111,114]	
Right ventricular dilatation and dysfunction[42]	
Diastolic function ("restrictive pattern")[115]	
Biochemical	
Hyponatremia[116]	
Neurohumoral activation	
Norepinephrine[113]	
Atrial natriuretic peptide[117]	
N-terminal atrial natriuretic peptide[118]	
Renin-angiotensin-aldosterone system[108]	
Peak oxygen consumption[62-64]	
Electrical	
Ventricular tachycardia on Holter monitoring[108]	
Signal-averaged electrocardiogram[119]	
Anatomic	
Extent of myocardial fibrosis[120]	

specific prognostic information may be of value. Many tests demonstrated to generate data with prognostic value can be ordered, but one of the most useful is the measurement of peak oxygen uptake. Peak oxygen uptake predicts short-term survival in patients with low ejection fractions and severe symptoms who are being considered for cardiac transplantation and is increasingly used to assign priority for transplantation.[62-64] Although indicating increased risk for sudden death,[110] asymptomatic complex arrhythmias have been of limited prognostic value in the nontransplant population because the ability to reduce mortality with drug therapy is controversial. Newer therapies with transvenous defibrillators may increase the importance of arrhythmias as a marker of potentially preventable future events. Reduction in serum sodium concentration is a poor prognostic marker in the patient with severe symptoms and is associated with extremely poor short-term survival.[116] The clinical value of neurohumoral assessment for determining prognosis is controversial, although its use as a diagnostic tool may be expanding. In general, a thorough clinical assessment supplemented by measurement of systolic and diastolic function, cardiac size, and oxygen uptake can provide most of the prognostic information that is clinically useful. Specialized, more specific assessments may be warranted in some patients who are potential candidates for transplantation.

Provide follow-up for the patient with heart failure or asymptomatic ventricular dysfunction

The optimal frequency of follow-up for a patient with heart failure varies widely, depending on the severity of heart failure and ability of the patient to follow a medical regimen. Few studies address the optimal timing of follow-up. Patients with asymptomatic left ventricular dysfunction should be seen once or twice a year to ensure compliance with medication, as most authorities support the use of ACE inhibition in these patients, some of whom may need anticoagulation. Other measures are careful assessment for the development of subtle symptoms (especially embolic symptoms, which may require specific therapy), review of risk factor modification if coronary artery disease is present, assessment of possible deleterious conditions, such as tachycardia and hypertension, and review of the principles of exercise and dietary therapy. Because 10% to 25% of patients with nonischemic cardiomyopathy may experience marked improvement in systolic function, intermittent assessment of cardiac size and function is reasonable.[122] Patients with symptoms need closer follow-up, depending on the stability of their symptoms, the complexity of their medical regimen, and the extent of their coexisting medical conditions. Close monitoring of renal function and electrolytes is especially important in older patients with vascular disease who are treated with ACE inhibitors, digoxin, and diuretics. One must always reassess previous decisions about revascularization, antiarrhythmic therapy, anticoagulation, and referral for transplantation during long-term follow-up, because the patient's disease progresses and treatment options improve.

REFERENCES

1. Kannel WB, Belanger AJ: Epidemiology of heart failure. *Am Heart J* 121:951-957, 1991
2. Schocken DD, Arrieta MI, Leaverton PE, et al: Prevalence and mortality rate of congestive heart failure in the United States. *J Am Coll Cardiol* 20:301-306, 1992
3. Geltman EM: Mild heart failure: diagnosis and treatment. *Am Heart J* 118:1277-1291, 1989
4. Pfeffer MA, Braunwald E, Moyé LA, et al: Effect of captopril on mortality and morbidity in patients with left ventricular dysfunction after myocardial infarction: results of the Survival and Ventricular Enlargement trial. *N Engl J Med* 327:669-677, 1992
5. The SOLVD Investigators: Effect of enalapril on mortality and the development of heart failure in asymptomatic patients with reduced left ventricular ejection fractions. *N Engl J Med* 327:685-691, 1992
6. Eriksson H, Svärdsudd K, Larsson B, et al: Risk factors for heart failure in the general population: the study of men born in 1913. *Eur Heart J* 10:647-656, 1989
7. Wenger NK: Cardiovascular disease in the elderly. *Curr Probl Cardiol* 17:615-690, 1992
8. The SOLVD Investigators: Effect of enalapril on survival in patients with reduced left ventricular ejection fractions and congestive heart failure. *N Engl J Med* 325:293-302, 1991
9. Wilson JR, Schwartz JS, Sutton MSJ, et al: Prognosis in severe heart failure: relation to hemodynamic measurements and ventricular ectopic activity. *J Am Coll Cardiol* 2:403-410, 1983

10. Massie B, Ports T, Chatterjee K, et al: Long-term vasodilator therapy for heart failure: clinical response and its relationship to hemodynamic measurements. *Circulation* 63:269-278, 1981

11. Franciosa JA, Wilen M, Ziesche S, et al: Survival in men with severe chronic left ventricular failure due to either coronary heart disease or idiopathic dilated cardiomyopathy. *Am J Cardiol* 51:831-836, 1983

12. McKee PA, Castelli WP, McNamara PM, et al: The natural history of congestive heart failure: the Framingham Study. *N Engl J Med* 285:1441-1446, 1971

13. Cohn JN, Archibald DG, Ziesche S, et al: Effect of vasodilator therapy on mortality in chronic congestive heart failure: results of a Veterans Administration Cooperative Study. *N Engl J Med* 314:1547-1552, 1986

14. Cohn JN, Johnson G, Ziesche S, et al: A comparison of enalapril with hydralazine-isosorbide dinitrate in the treatment of chronic congestive heart failure. *N Engl J Med* 325:303-310, 1991

15. Packer M, Carver JR, Rodeheffer RJ, et al: Effect of oral milrinone on mortality in severe chronic heart failure. *N Engl J Med* 325:1468-1475, 1991

16. Kjekshus J, Swedberg K, Snapinn S, et al: Effects of enalapril on long-term mortality in severe congestive heart failure. *Am J Cardiol* 69:103-107, 1992

17. Sugrue DD, Rodeheffer RJ, Codd MB, et al: The clinical course of idiopathic dilated cardiomyopathy: a population-based study. *Ann Intern Med* 117:117-123, 1992

18. Redfield MM, Gersh BJ, Bailey KR, et al: Natural history of idiopathic dilated cardiomyopathy: effect of referral bias and secular trend. *J Am Coll Cardiol* 22:1921-1926, 1993

19. Ho KKL, Anderson KM, Kannel WB, et al: Survival after the onset of congestive heart failure in Framingham Heart Study subjects. *Circulation* 88:107-115, 1993

20. Braunwald E: Pathophysiology of heart failure. In *Heart Disease: a Textbook of Cardiovascular Medicine.* Edited by E Braunwald. Third edition. Philadelphia, WB Saunders Company, 1988, pp 426-448

21. Grossman W: Diastolic dysfunction and congestive heart failure. *Circulation* 81 Suppl 3:1-7, 1990

22. Shah PM, Pai RG: Diastolic heart failure. *Curr Probl Cardiol* 17:787-845, 1992

23. Brutsaert DL, Sys SU, Gillebert TC: Diastolic failure: pathophysiology and therapeutic implications. *J Am Coll Cardiol* 22:318-325, 1993

24. Ghali JK, Kadakia S, Cooper RS, et al: Bedside diagnosis of preserved versus impaired left ventricular systolic function in heart failure. *Am J Cardiol* 67:1002-1006, 1991

25. Marantz PR, Tobin JN, Wassertheil-Smoller S, et al: The relationship between left ventricular systolic function and congestive heart failure diagnosed by clinical criteria. *Circulation* 77:607-612, 1988

26. Aguirre FV, Pearson AC, Lewen MK, et al: Usefulness of Doppler echocardiography in the diagnosis of congestive heart failure. *Am J Cardiol* 63:1098-1102, 1989

27. Dougherty AH, Naccarelli GV, Gray EL, et al: Congestive heart failure with normal systolic function. *Am J Cardiol* 54:778-782, 1984

28. Echeverria HH, Bilsker MS, Myerburg RJ, et al: Congestive heart failure: echocardiographic insights. *Am J Med* 75:750-755, 1983

29. Bonow RO, Udelson JE: Left ventricular diastolic dysfunction as a cause of congestive heart failure. *Ann Intern Med* 117:502-510, 1992

30. Starling EH: *The Linacre Lecture on the Law of the Heart: Given at Cambridge, 1915.* London, Longmans, 1918

31. Villarreal D, Freeman RH, Davis JO, et al: Atrial natriuretic factor secretion in dogs with experimental high-output heart failure. *Am J Physiol* 252:H692-H696, 1987

32. Francis GS, Benedict C, Johnstone DE, et al: Comparison of neuroendocrine activation in patients with left ventricular dysfunction with and without congestive heart failure: a substudy of the studies of left ventricular dysfunction (SOLVD). *Circulation* 82:1724-1729, 1990

33. Cohn JN: The prevention of heart failure—a new agenda (editorial). *N Engl J Med* 327:725-727, 1992

34. Klein AL, Hatle LK, Taliercio CP, et al: Serial Doppler echocardiographic follow-up of left ventricular diastolic function in cardiac amyloidosis. *J Am Coll Cardiol* 16:1135-1141, 1990

35. Klein AL, Hatle LK, Taliercio CP, et al: Prognostic significance of Doppler measures of diastolic function in cardiac amyloidosis: a Doppler echocardiography study. *Circulation* 83:808-816, 1991

36. Appleton CP, Hatle LK: The natural history of left ventricular filling abnormalities: assessment by two-dimensional and Doppler echocardiography. *Echocardiography* 9:437-457, 1992

37. Parrillo JE, Parker MM, Natanson C, et al: Septic shock in humans: advances in the understanding of pathogenesis, cardiovascular dysfunction, and therapy. *Ann Intern Med* 113:227-242, 1990

38. Dzau VJ, Packer M, Lilly LS, et al: Prostaglandins in severe congestive heart failure: relation to activation of the renin-angiotensin system and hyponatremia. *N Engl J Med* 310:347-352, 1984

39. Dzau VJ, Swartz SL, Creager MA: The role of prostaglandins in the pathophysiology of and therapy for congestive heart failure. *Heart Failure* February/March 1986, pp 6-13

40. Cuocolo A, Sax FL, Brush JE, et al: Left ventricular hypertrophy and impaired diastolic filling in essential hypertension: diastolic mechanisms for systolic dysfunction during exercise. *Circulation* 81:978-986, 1990

41. Rushmer RF: *Cardiovascular Dynamics.* Fourth edition. Philadelphia, WB Saunders Company, 1976, pp 532-567

42. Lewis JF, Webber JD, Sutton LL, et al: Discordance in degree of right and left ventricular dilation in patients with dilated cardiomyopathy: recognition and clinical implications. *J Am Coll Cardiol* 21:649-654, 1993

43. Baker BJ, Wilen MM, Boyd CM, et al: Relation of right ventricular ejection fraction to exercise capacity in chronic left ventricular failure. *Am J Cardiol* 54:596-599, 1984

44. The CONSENSUS Trial Study Group: Effects of enalapril on mortality in severe congestive heart failure: results of the Cooperative North Scandinavian Enalapril Survival Study (CONSENSUS). *N Engl J Med* 316:1429-1435, 1987

45. Pflugfelder PW, Baird MG, Tonkon MJ, et al: Clinical consequences of angiotensin-converting enzyme inhibitor withdrawal in chronic heart failure: a double-blind, placebo-controlled study of quinapril. *J Am Coll Cardiol* 22:1557-1563, 1993

46. Feldman AM, Bristow MR, Parmley WW, et al: Effects of vesnarinone on morbidity and mortality in patients with heart failure. *N Engl J Med* 329:149-155, 1993

47. Fonarow GC, Chelimsky-Fallick C, Stevenson LW, et al: Effect of direct vasodilation with hydralazine versus angiotensin-converting enzyme inhibition with captopril on mortality in advanced heart failure: the Hy-C Trial. *J Am Coll Cardiol* 19:842-850, 1992

48. Packer M, Gheorghiade M, Young JB, et al: Withdrawal of digoxin from patients with chronic heart failure treated with angiotensin-converting-enzyme inhibitors. *N Engl J Med* 329:1-7, 1993

49. Teerlink JR, Goldhaber SZ, Pfeffer MA: An overview of contemporary etiologies of congestive heart failure. *Am Heart J* 121:1852-1853, 1991

50. Harlan WR, Oberman A, Grimm R, et al: Chronic congestive heart failure in coronary artery disease: clinical criteria. *Ann Intern Med* 86:133-138, 1977

51. Kraemer MD, Kubo SH, Rector TS, et al: Pulmonary and peripheral vascular factors are important determinants of peak exercise oxygen uptake in patients with heart failure. *J Am Coll Cardiol* 21:641-648, 1993

52. Franciosa JA, Park M, Levine TB: Lack of correlation between exercise capacity and indexes of resting left ventricular performance in heart failure. *Am J Cardiol* 47:33-39, 1981

53. Tischler MD, Niggel J, Borowski DT, et al: Relation between left ventricular shape and exercise capacity in patients with left ventricular dysfunction. *J Am Coll Cardiol* 22:751-757, 1993

54. Meiler SEL, Ashton JJ, Moeschberger ML, et al: An analysis of the determinants of exercise performance in congestive heart failure. *Am Heart J* 113:1207-1217, 1987

55. Benge W, Litchfield RL, Marcus ML: Exercise capacity in patients with severe left ventricular dysfunction. *Circulation* 61:955-959, 1980

56. Myers J, Froelicher VF: Hemodynamic determinants of exercise capacity in chronic heart failure. *Ann Intern Med* 115:377-386, 1991

57. Goldman L, Hashimoto B, Cook EF, et al: Comparative reproducibility and validity of systems for assessing cardiovascular functional class: advantages of a new specific activity scale. *Circulation* 64:1227-1234, 1981

58. Rector TS, Cohn JN, with the Pimobendan Multicenter Research Group: Assessment of patient outcome with the Minnesota Living with Heart Failure questionnaire: reliability and validity during a randomized, double-blind, placebo-controlled trial of pimobendan. *Am Heart J* 124:1017-1025, 1992

59. Rector TS, Kubo SH, Cohn JN: Validity of the Minnesota Living with Heart Failure questionnaire as a measure of therapeutic response to enalapril or placebo. *Am J Cardiol* 71:1106-1107, 1993

60. Wasserman K: Measures of functional capacity in patients with heart failure. *Circulation* 81 Suppl 2:1-4, 1990

61. Weber KT, Janicki JS (eds): *CardioPulmonary Exercise Testing: Physiologic Principles and Clinical Applications.* Philadelphia, WB Saunders Company, 1986

62. Mancini DM, Eisen H, Kussmaul W, et al: Value of peak exercise oxygen consumption for optimal timing of cardiac transplantation in ambulatory patients with heart failure. *Circulation* 83:778-786, 1991

63. Cohn JN, Ziesche S, Archibald DG, et al: Quantitative exercise tolerance as a predictor of mortality in congestive heart failure: the V-HeFT Study (abstract). *Circulation* 74 Suppl 2:447, 1986

64. Sevenson LW, Steimle AE, Chelimsky-Fallick C, et al: Outcomes predicted by peak oxygen consumption during evaluation of 333 patients with advanced heart failure (abstract). *Circulation* 88 Suppl 1:94, 1993

65. Zelis R, Musch TI, Sinoway LI: The maximal stress test: Does it have any value in heart failure? *J Am Coll Cardiol* 15:62-63, 1990

66. Gibbs JSR, Keegan J, Wright C, et al: Pulmonary artery pressure changes during exercise and daily activities in chronic heart failure. *J Am Coll Cardiol* 15:52-61, 1990

67. Szlachcic J, Massie BM, Kramer BL, et al: Correlates and prognostic implication of exercise capacity in chronic congestive heart failure. *Am J Cardiol* 55:1037-1042, 1985

68. Fink LI, Wilson JR, Ferraro N: Exercise ventilation and pulmonary artery wedge pressure in chronic stable congestive heart failure. *Am J Cardiol* 57:249-253, 1986

69. Wilson JR, Mancini DM, Dunkman WB: Exertional fatigue due to skeletal muscle dysfunction in patients with heart failure. *Circulation* 87:470-475, 1993

70. Middlekauff HR, Stevenson WG, Stevenson LW, et al: Syncope in advanced heart failure: high risk of sudden death regardless of origin of syncope. *J Am Coll Cardiol* 21:110-116, 1993

71. Grogan M, Smith HC, Gersh BJ, et al: Left ventricular dysfunction due to atrial fibrillation in patients initially believed to have idiopathic dilated cardiomyopathy. *Am J Cardiol* 69:1570-1573, 1992

72. Packer DL, Bardy GH, Worley SJ, et al: Tachycardia-induced cardiomyopathy: a reversible form of left ventricular dysfunction. *Am J Cardiol* 57:563-570, 1986

73. Giorgi LV, Hartzler GO, Hamaker WR: Incessant focal atrial tachycardia: a surgically remediable cause of cardiomyopathy. *J Thorac Cardiovasc Surg* 87:466-469, 1984

74. McLaran CJ, Gersh BJ, Sugrue DD, et al: Tachycardia induced myocardial dysfunction: a reversible phenomenon? *Br Heart J* 53:323-327, 1985

75. Fuster V, Halperin JL: Left ventricular thrombi and cerebral embolism (editorial). *N Engl J Med* 320:392-394, 1989

76. Dunkman WB, Johnson GR, Cohn JN, et al: Incidence of thromboembolic events in congestive heart failure: the V-HeFT Study (abstract). *Circulation* 78 Suppl 2:617, 1988

77. Kyrle PA, Korninger C, Gössinger H, et al: Prevention of arterial and pulmonary embolism by oral anticoagulants in patients with dilated cardiomyopathy. *Thromb Haemost* 54:521-523, 1985

78. Roberts WC, Siegel RJ, McManus BM: Idiopathic dilated cardiomyopathy: analysis of 152 necropsy patients. *Am J Cardiol* 60:1340-1355, 1987

79. The Stroke Prevention in Atrial Fibrillation Investigators: Predictors of thromboembolism in atrial fibrillation: I. Clinical features of patients at risk. *Ann Intern Med* 116:1-5, 1992

80. The Stroke Prevention in Atrial Fibrillation Investigators: Predictors of thromboembolism in atrial fibrillation: II. Echocardiographic features of patients at risk. *Ann Intern Med* 116:6-12, 1992

81. Gottdiener JS, Gay JA, VanVoorhees L, et al: Frequency and embolic potential of left ventricular thrombus in dilated cardiomyopathy: assessment by 2-dimensional echocardiography. *Am J Cardiol* 52:1281-1285, 1983

82. Ciaccheri M, Castelli G, Cecchi F, et al: Lack of correlation between intracavitary thrombosis detected by cross sectional echocardiography and systemic emboli in patients with dilated cardiomyopathy. *Br Heart J* 62:26-29, 1989

83. Falk RH, Foster E, Coats MH: Ventricular thrombi and thromboembolism in dilated cardiomyopathy: a prospective follow-up study. *Am Heart J* 123:136-142, 1992

84. Falk RH: A plea for a clinical trial of anticoagulation in dilated cardiomyopathy. *Am J Cardiol* 65:914-915, 1990

85. Michels VV, Moll PP, Miller FA, et al: The frequency of familial dilated cardiomyopathy in a series of patients with idiopathic dilated cardiomyopathy. *N Engl J Med* 326:77-82, 1992

86. Keeling PJ, Gang Y, Seo H, et al: Familial dilated cardiomyopathy in the UK (abstract). *Circulation* 88 Suppl 1:212, 1993

87. Redfield MM, Gersh BJ, Bailey KR, et al: The natural history of incidentally discovered, asymptomatic idiopathic dilated cardiomyopathy (abstract). *J Am Coll Cardiol* 21 Suppl A:20, 1993

88. Hógye M, Bali I, Forster T, et al: Natural course of biopsy-confirmed dilated cardiomyopathies with particular respect to the onset of cardiomegaly (abstract). *J Heart Failure* Vol 1, May 1993

89. Stevenson LW, Perloff JK: The limited reliability of physical signs for estimating hemodynamics in chronic heart failure. *JAMA* 261:884-888, 1989

90. Butman SM, Ewy GA, Standen JR, et al: Bedside cardiovascular examination in patients with severe chronic heart failure: importance of rest or inducible jugular venous distension. *J Am Coll Cardiol* 22:968-974, 1993

91. Baumstark A, Swensson RG, Hessel SJ, et al: Evaluating the radiographic assessment of pulmonary venous hypertension in chronic heart disease. *AJR* 142:877-884, 1984

92. Spindola-Franco H: Plain film diagnosis of congestive heart failure. *J Med Soc NJ* 75:783-784, 1978

93. O'Keefe JH Jr, Zinsmeister AR, Gibbons RJ: Value of normal electrocardiographic findings in predicting resting left ventricular function in patients with chest pain and suspected coronary artery disease. *Am J Med* 86:658-662, 1989

94. Marantz PR, Alderman MH, Tobin JN: Diagnostic heterogeneity in clinical trials for congestive heart failure. *Ann Intern Med* 109:55-61, 1988

95. Chakko S, Woska D, Martinez H, et al: Clinical, radiographic, and hemodynamic correlations in chronic congestive heart failure: conflicting results may lead to inappropriate care. *Am J Med* 90:353-359, 1991

96. Gadsbøll N, Høilund-Carlsen PF, Nielsen GG, et al: Symptoms and signs of heart failure in patients with myocardial infarction: reproducibility and relationship to chest x-ray, radionuclide ventriculography and right heart catheterization. *Eur Heart J* 10:1017-1028, 1989

97. Henriksson L, Sundin A, Smedby Ö, et al: Assessment of congestive heart failure in chest radiographs: observer performance with two common film-screen systems. *Acta Radiol* 31:469-471, 1990

98. Herman PG, Khan A, Kallman CE, et al: Limited correlation of left ventricular end-diastolic pressure with radiographic assessment of pulmonary hemodynamics. *Radiology* 174:721-724, 1990

99. Mahdyoon H, Klein R, Eyler W, et al: Radiographic pulmonary congestion in end-stage congestive heart failure. *Am J Cardiol* 63:625-627, 1989

100. Lerman A, Gibbons RJ, Rodeheffer RJ, et al: Circulating N-terminal atrial natriuretic peptide as a marker for symptomless left-ventricular dysfunction. *Lancet* 341:1105-1109, 1993

101. Haug C, Metzele A, Kochs M, et al: Plasma brain natriuretic peptide and atrial natriuretic peptide concentrations correlate with left ventricular end-diastolic pressure. *Clin Cardiol* 16:553-557, 1993

102. Kuecherer HF, Muhiudeen IA, Kusumoto FM, et al: Estimation of mean left atrial pressure from transesophageal pulsed Doppler echocardiography of pulmonary venous flow. *Circulation* 82:1127-1139, 1990

103. Rossvoll O, Hatle LK: Pulmonary venous flow velocities recorded by transthoracic Doppler ultrasound: relation to left ventricular diastolic pressures. *J Am Coll Cardiol* 21:1687-1696, 1993

104. Elefteriades JA, Tolis G Jr, Levi E, et al: Coronary artery bypass grafting in severe left ventricular dysfunction: excellent survival with improved ejection fraction and functional state. *J Am Coll Cardiol* 22:1411-1417, 1993

105. Ragosta M, Beller GA, Watson DD, et al: Quantitative planar rest-redistribution ^{201}Tl imaging in detection of myocardial viability and prediction of improvement in left ventricular function after coronary bypass surgery in patients with severely depressed left ventricular function. *Circulation* 87:1630-1641, 1993

106. Dilsizian V, Bonow RO: Current diagnostic techniques of assessing myocardial viability in patients with hibernating and stunned myocardium. *Circulation* 87:1-20, 1993

107. Ragosta M, Beller GA: The noninvasive assessment of myocardial viability. *Clin Cardiol* 16:531-538, 1993

108. Francis GS, Kubo SH: Prognostic factors affecting diagnosis and treatment of congestive heart failure. *Curr Probl Cardiol* 14:631-671, 1989

109. Likoff MJ, Chandler SL, Kay HR: Clinical determinants of mortality in chronic congestive heart failure secondary to idiopathic dilated or to ischemic cardiomyopathy. *Am J Cardiol* 59:634-638, 1987

110. De Maria R, Gavazzi A, Caroli A, et al: Ventricular arrhythmias in dilated cardiomyopathy as an independent prognostic hallmark. *Am J Cardiol* 69:1451-1457, 1992

111. Middlekauff HR, Stevenson WG, Stevenson LW: Prognostic significance of atrial fibrillation in advanced heart failure: a study of 390 patients. *Circulation* 84:40-48, 1991

112. Lee TH, Hamilton MA, Stevenson LW, et al: Impact of left ventricular cavity size on survival in advanced heart failure. *Am J Cardiol* 72:672-676, 1993

113. Cohn JN, Rector TS: Prognosis of congestive heart failure and predictors of mortality. *Am J Cardiol* 62:25A-30A, 1988

114. Griffin BP, Shah PK, Ferguson J, et al: Incremental prognostic value of exercise hemodynamic variables in chronic congestive heart failure secondary to coronary artery disease or to dilated cardiomyopathy. *Am J Cardiol* 67:848-853, 1991

115. Pinamonti B, DiLenarda A, Sinagra G, et al: Restrictive left ventricular filling pattern in dilated cardiomyopathy assessed by Doppler echocardiography: clinical, echocardiographic and hemodynamic correlations and prognostic implications. *J Am Coll Cardiol* 22:808-815, 1993

116. Lee WH, Packer M: Prognostic importance of serum sodium concentration and its modification by converting-enzyme inhibition in patients with severe chronic heart failure. *Circulation* 73:257-267, 1986

117. Gottlieb SS, Kukin ML, Ahern D, et al: Prognostic importance of atrial natriuretic peptide in patients with chronic heart failure. *J Am Coll Cardiol* 13:1534-1539, 1989

118. Hall C, Rouleau JL, Klein M, et al: N-terminal proatrial natriuretic factor (PRO-ANF)—a uniquely powerful predictor of long term outcome after myocardial infarction (abstract). *J Am Coll Cardiol* 21 Suppl A:270, 1993

119. Mancini DM, Wong KL, Simson MB: Prognostic value of an abnormal signal-averaged electrocardiogram in patients with nonischemic congestive cardiomyopathy. *Circulation* 87:1083-1092, 1993

120. Figulla HR, Rahlf G, Nieger M, et al: Spontaneous hemodynamic improvement or stabilization and associated biopsy findings in patients with congestive cardiomyopathy. *Circulation* 71:1095-1104, 1985

121. Gradman A, Deedwania P, Cody R, et al: Predictors of total mortality and sudden death in mild to moderate heart failure. *J Am Coll Cardiol* 14:564-570, 1989

122. Grogan M, McGoon MD, Smith HC, et al: Reversible cardiomyopathy: marked improvement in left ventricular function in patients with idiopathic dilated cardiomyopathy (abstract). *Circulation* 88 Suppl 1:212, 1993

CHAPTER

17

Pharmacotherapy of congestive heart failure

Lyle J. Olson, M.D., and Wayne L. Miller, M.D., Ph.D.

Congestive heart failure has become the most important cardiovascular public health problem in the United States. It affects 4 million Americans, and 400,000 new diagnoses are made annually.[1] In patients over age 65 it is the most frequent hospital dismissal diagnosis, and 10% of the population over age 75 are affected.[2,3] It is the only major cardiovascular disorder of increasing incidence and prevalence.

The treatment of congestive heart failure that has no underlying remediable cause may be by either pharmacotherapy or replacement of the heart. However, heart transplantation is severely limited for lack of donors, and major advances in immunology are required before xenografting will be feasible.[4,5] Similarly, a practical mechanical replacement seems unlikely in the near future. Hence, pharmacotherapy remains the mainstay of therapy.

Previously, the aim of pharmacotherapy for the patient with congestive heart failure was limited to palliation of symptoms by a diuretic and digitalis. In the past decade, strategies for pharmacotherapy were dramatically altered commensurate with completion of large, multicenter, prospective, controlled trials demonstrating improved survival for patients with heart failure treated with vasodilators. Accordingly, though symptom relief remains a primary goal, improved survival and alteration of the natural history of the disorder have become equally important.

Although symptom palliation and prognosis have been improved in the past decade for the patient with heart failure, mortality remains unacceptably high (Table 17-1). Hence, the search for new agents and new applications of existing drugs in the treatment of chronic congestive heart failure continues. This chapter reviews current treatment of congestive heart failure due to predominant systolic dysfunction.

GENERAL PRINCIPLES OF THERAPY

Spectrum of disease

Rational selection of drugs for the treatment of the patient with chronic congestive heart failure requires recognition that the syndrome has a wide spectrum of severity and many underlying causes of different natural history and that the natural history may vary greatly among individual patients. It is customary to categorize patients with chronic congestive heart failure on the bases of cause and functional class, as this aids the clinician in prognostication and therapeutic strategies (see chapter 16). The physician managing the patient with heart failure must appreciate that the state is dynamic and that no simple algorithm exists for its management. Basic principles for the medical management of congestive heart failure include establishment of the primary cause, correction of the cause if feasible, and elimination and prevention of precipitating factors (see chapter 16).

Pathophysiology

An appreciation of the pathophysiology of heart failure is necessary to understand the rationale for pharmacotherapeutic intervention (see chapter 15). The pathophysiologic hallmark of heart failure is edema as a consequence of decreased cardiac output and reduced renal excretion of sodium and water. Associated aberrant neurohumoral responses and altered function of the autonomic nervous system yield increased circulating catecholamines, activation of the renin-angiotensin-aldosterone system, and blunted reflex–baroreceptor function, which promote sodium and water retention.[6-14] Although these alterations of neurohormonal and nervous system function are appropriate short-term adaptations to preserve perfusion of vital organs, in the long term these responses may be maladaptive, because they exacerbate sodium and water retention and promote tachycardia, vasoconstriction, increased myocardial contractility, and adverse ventricular remodeling.

Neurohormonal antagonism

Pharmacotherapy directed at characteristic pathophysiologic aberrations has been demonstrated to favorably modify the heart failure state and its natural history.[15-17] Moreover, neurohormonal antagonism with angiotensin-converting enzyme (ACE) inhibitor therapy has been demonstrated to prevent the progression of subclinical left ventricular dysfunction to overt heart

Table 17-1 Survival in congestive heart failure mortality trials

Trial	Follow-up, mo	Mortality, % Placebo	Mortality, % Drug	Difference, %
V-HeFT I	36	47	36	36
CONSENSUS	6	44	26	40
	12	52	36	31
*V-HeFT II	24	25	18	28
SOLVD	41	40	35	16

*No placebo arm.

failure and to prevent adverse ventricular remodeling in established heart failure.[18] Hence, the former limited strategy of intervention for palliation of symptoms has been replaced by a proactive approach of neurohormonal antagonism to prevent the development or progression of heart failure.

Efficacy and therapeutic end points

The clinical assessment of drug efficacy requires identification of therapeutic end points. Routinely monitored end points are symptom relief, physical signs of congestion, measurement of resting or exercise cardiac function, specific drug and drug-dose requirements to achieve therapeutic end points, and survival. Drug therapy is adjusted for each individual to obtain an optimal clinical response.

Adjunctive therapy

Nonpharmacologic measures are an important facet of therapy to be applied concurrently with drug intervention. For the patient with decompensated heart failure, the work of the heart must be reduced. This requires decreased physical activity and for patients with advanced heart failure often requires hospitalization with bed rest, which enhances diuresis. Coexistent medical problems that increase the work of the heart may include obesity and hypertension and require appropriate management. Isometric work increases systemic blood pressure, and this increase tends to decrease cardiac output and should generally be avoided. For this reason, activity should be restricted until the patient is optimally treated. Activity may then be gradually increased as tolerated and the patient encouraged to be active within the limits of dyspnea and fatigue.

Patients with heart failure should be instructed to reduce dietary salt intake to 2 to 3 g/day. This goal is achieved in most by eliminating table salt and foods that contain excessive amounts of sodium. More severe sodium restriction is generally not necessary, because sodium and water retention may be effectively treated by a diuretic. In patients with dilutional hyponatremia, restriction of water may be necessary. In patients with refractory heart failure, mechanical removal of fluid by thoracentesis or paracentesis may be helpful, as may ultrafiltration, especially if coexisting renal dysfunction impairs the ability to excrete a sodium and water load.

Improvement in cardiac hemodynamic function may be achieved in some patients by nonpharmacologic means. Therapy that may improve cardiac performance includes supplemental oxygen in the hypoxic patient and pacemaker implantation to treat bradycardia, restore atrioventricular (AV) synchrony, or optimize cardiac hemodynamics (see chapter 25A).

Pharmacotherapy

In most patients, first-line drug therapy comprises widely varying doses of specific pharmacotherapeutic agents from each of four classes: (1) diuretics, (2) ACE inhibitors or other vasodilators, (3) digitalis glycosides, and (4) antithrombotic drugs.

DIURETICS

Diuretics are ion-transport inhibitors that act on the renal tubules to enhance sodium and water excretion. The role of diuretics in the management of heart failure is related to the importance of the kidney as a target organ for many of the neurohumoral adaptations to heart failure that promote sodium and water retention (see chapter 15). Despite widespread use, no diuretic agent has been primarily evaluated for the treatment of heart failure. This class of drugs has been approved for the treatment of edema but not specifically evaluated for safety and efficacy in the treatment of heart failure. However, all major trials evaluating the treatment of established heart failure have used diuretics as standard therapy. Although diuretic therapy is necessary and remains a mainstay in the treatment of the patient with chronic congestive heart failure, the effect of diuretics on long-term mortality is unknown.

Classification

Diuretics are classified according to mechanism and site of action within the nephron (Fig 17-1). The proximal tubule consists of a convoluted tubule and a straight portion. Most sodium and water reabsorption occurs in the proximal tubule. The loop of Henle is formed by a descending limb and a thin and thick ascending limb; these segments also have a substantial capacity for reabsorption of sodium. The distal tubules coalesce to form the collecting system within the cortex; only a small fraction of filtered sodium is reabsorbed within the cortex. The cortical collecting ducts descend into the medulla to form the medullary and papillary collecting ducts, which open on the surface of the papilla. This segment is important in determination of the final concentration of urine under the influence of antidiuretic hormone.

Loop agents

The prototype loop diuretic is furosemide, which inhibits active chloride reabsorption in the ascending limb of the

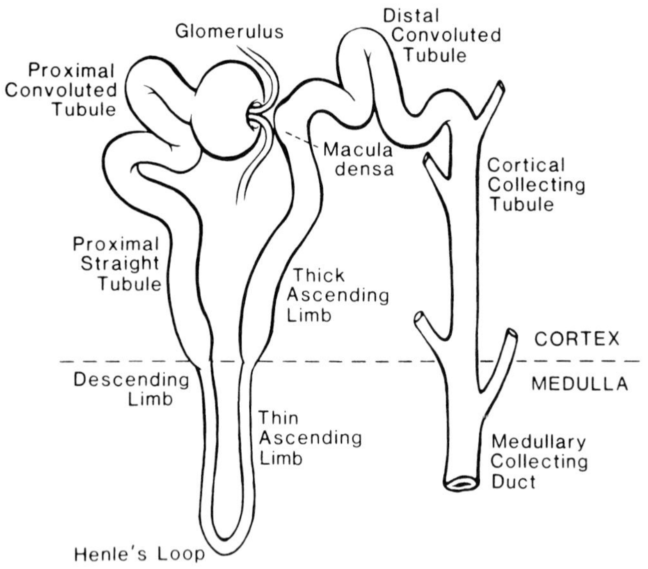

Fig 17-1 Functional anatomy of nephron.

Table 17-2 Thiazide diuretics

Drug	Trade name	Dose, mg	Duration of action, hours
Hydrochlorothiazide	HydroDIURIL Esidrix Thiuretic	25-100	6-12
Chlorthalidone	Hygroton Thalitone	12.5-50	48-72
Chlorothiazide	Diuril	250-1,000	6-12
Indapamide	Lozol	2.5	12-36
Metolazone	Zaroxolyn Diulo	5-20	18-24

loop of Henle.[19] Furosemide is a sulfonamide and is structurally similar to the thiazides. Ethacrinic acid has a similar mechanism, duration of action, and side effects but is less widely used because of greater ototoxicity.[20] Bumetanide is similar to furosemide in structure, mechanism, and duration of action. Approximately 1 mg of bumetanide is equivalent to 40 mg of furosemide.[21] Furosemide and bumetanide may be given either intravenously or orally.

The loop diuretics are extracted and concentrated by the renal tubule, which accounts for potency as well as utility in patients with decreased glomerular filtration rate, offering a distinct advantage over the thiazides. The loop agents decrease renal vascular resistance and promote increased renal blood flow; these hemodynamic changes may be mediated by prostaglandins, because the renal excretion of prostaglandin E is increased by furosemide, whereas inhibitors of prostaglandin synthetase attenuate furosemide-induced renal vasodilatation and may exacerbate heart failure.[22,23]

The loop agents also have systemic hemodynamic effects that promote an acute increase in venous capacitance that promptly relieves pulmonary edema by reduction in preload and decreased blood flow to the left side of the heart.[24] This action is independent of the kidney and may occur before or without diuresis. Symptomatic improvement is also due to improved pulmonary function. Through the actions of diuresis and reduction of preload with concomitant decrease of pulmonary artery wedge pressure, pulmonary water is reduced, pulmonary compliance is improved, and resistance to airflow and respiratory work is decreased.[25]

Diuretics have also been demonstrated to have vasodilatory properties, an action that has been attributed to reduction of arterial and interstitial sodium content, with improved vascular compliance.[26-28] However, studies of short-term therapy with diuretics have also described an apparent vasoconstrictor action.[29] This action has been ascribed to activation of neurohormonal pathways, particularly the renin-angiotensin-aldosterone pathway.[30-33] Over a period of days, the initially favorable hemodynamic and renal response is diminished.

The dose range for furosemide is wide (40 to 1,000 mg per day). Given orally, the drug has an onset of action within 30 to 60 minutes and a duration of action of approximately 6 to 8 hours (4 to 6 hours for bumetanide). The onset of action is rapid with intravenous administration, and the duration of action is 2 to 3 hours for furosemide.[34] Because of the potency and effectiveness of loop diuretics administered orally, as well as a steep dose-response curve, rapid onset, and relatively short duration of action, these agents are widely used in the treatment of congestive heart failure.[35]

Thiazides

The thiazides are less potent than the loop diuretics. Like the loop agents, these drugs are also sulfonamide derivatives; there are several structural variants, including chlorthalidone and metolazone (Table 17-2). All thiazides inhibit sodium chloride reabsorption in the distal tubule and thereby prevent dilution of the tubular fluid. Hence, these agents result in concentration but not dilution of urine. Thiazides inhibit reabsorption of sodium chloride by acting on the distal convoluted tubule to decrease membrane permeability to sodium and chloride.[36,37] Kaliuresis also occurs from a direct effect on potassium secretion as well as increased delivery of sodium to the distal nephron. There is also decreased proximal reabsorption, most likely due to carbonic anhydrase inhibition.

Thiazides are administered orally and have an onset of action of 1 to 2 hours and a duration of action of 6 to 24 hours. The longer duration of action of some of these agents (chlorthalidone, quinethazone, and metolazone) does not allow the kidney to recover and reclaim potassium or excrete retained urate; hence, they are more frequently associated with hypokalemia and hyperuricemia.

Metolazone has characteristics of both loop and thiazide diuretics. The onset of action of metolazone occurs in approximately 1 hour, with a peak action at 2 to 4 hours that persists for 24 to 48 hours.[38] Like the loop agents, it is effective in patients with low glomerular filtration rate.[39] Long-term daily use is not advised because of associated electrolyte disturbances, including hyponatremia, hypokalemia, hypochloremia, alkalosis, and dehydration.

Potassium-sparing agents

The potassium-sparing diuretics include spironolactone, amiloride, and triamterene. Spironolactone is a synthetic steroid and competitive antagonist of aldosterone.[40] Accordingly, the site of action is the distal tubule and cortical collecting duct, and action depends on aldosterone being present.[41]

Triamterene and amiloride directly block the secretion of potassium and reabsorption of sodium in the distal convoluted tubule and in the cortical collecting duct.[42,43] In contrast to spironolactone, both triamterene and amiloride are effective in the absence of aldosterone. Triamterene and amiloride action is observed within 2 hours and absent within 12 to 24 hours. The onset of action of spironolactone is typically several days, and its effects persist for 2 to 3 days.

This diuretic class is considered weak in comparison with the loop and thiazide diuretics. The major application of these agents is in the treatment of hypertension. They are seldom indicated in patients with congestive heart failure who are on concomitant therapy with ACE inhibitors, because ACE inhibition blocks release of aldosterone by inhibition of the renin-angiotensin-aldosterone system. Furthermore, the use of these drugs in combination with an ACE inhibitor may cause life-threatening hyperkalemia.

Carbonic anhydrous inhibitors

The carbonic anhydrous inhibitors block reabsorption of sodium bicarbonate in the proximal tubule.[44] They also decrease the proximal reabsorption of sodium and chloride. Acetazolamide is the only drug of this class in routine clinical use. Like the potassium-sparing agents, it has limited usefulness in patients with heart failure because of low potency. However, the bicarbonaturia induced by acetazolamide can be helpful in management of metabolic alkalosis in patients with chronic congestive heart failure.[45]

Complications of diuretic therapy

Hypokalemia. The rate of potassium secretion by the renal tubules increases as sodium delivery and urine flow rate increase. Diuretic therapy also promotes a state of hyperaldosteronism as a result of volume depletion, and the excess mineralocorticoid further enhances distal tubular secretion of potassium.[46] Diuretic-induced metabolic alkalosis additionally stimulates distal secretion of potassium.[47]

In patients with heart failure, potassium depletion may promote cardiac arrhythmia, especially in those receiving concurrent digitalis therapy. Other consequences of potassium depletion are carbohydrate intolerance, myalgias, and generalized malaise. Potassium depletion may be avoided in some patients by simultaneous use of ACE inhibitors, which are potassium-sparing. However, in patients who require high doses of loop diuretics, oral potassium supplementation is generally required if renal dysfunction is absent.

Hyperkalemia. Patients with heart failure and decreased renal function are at risk for hyperkalemia, especially if they are receiving an ACE inhibitor. Other agents predisposing to hyperkalemia are β-blockers and prostaglandin synthetase inhibitors. Diuretic-induced hyperkalemia is confined to the potassium-sparing agents. For this reason, the combination of these agents and ACE inhibitors should generally be avoided.

Hyponatremia. Sodium depletion with associated volume depletion is a common complication of diuretic use; the more potent loop diuretics are the usual cause. Diuretic-induced hyponatremia is caused by inability to adequately dilute the urine and by concurrent increased serum vasopressin and angiotensin II, which in turn stimulate excessive thirst. Volume depletion may cause azotemia, orthostatic hypotension, syncope, metabolic alkalosis, and exacerbation of heart failure by excessive reduction of preload and hence cardiac output.

Loop and thiazide diuretics decrease the formation of free water by the kidney. Furthermore, antidiuretic hormone release induced by volume depletion causes increased reabsorption of water in the collecting duct. Hyponatremia occurs if ingestion of water exceeds the ability of the kidneys to dilute the urine. Coexistent hypokalemia may promote diuretic-induced hyponatremia.[48] Management of diuretic-induced hyponatremia begins with fluid restriction (typically <1.5 L/day). In patients with severe (<120 mEq/L) hyponatremia, restoration of serum sodium levels toward normal may require intravenous administration of normal saline in combination with a loop diuretic.

Hypomagnesemia. The urinary excretion of magnesium is increased by loop diuretics and thiazides.[49] Hypomagnesemia, because it can be associated with hypocalcemia and may promote cardiac arrhythmias and exacerbation of heart failure, should be routinely monitored.[50] Concurrent therapy with ACE inhibitors tends to prevent hypomagnesemia; some patients require oral magnesium supplementation.

Acid-base abnormalities. Metabolic alkalosis is commonly observed with diuretic therapy in chronic congestive heart failure. The coexistence of volume depletion, excess mineralocorticoid effect, and depletion of potassium contributes to the cause of metabolic alkalosis.[51] The alkalosis is maintained by increased renal tubular reabsorption of sodium bicarbonate in association with volume depletion. The alkalosis can be corrected by reduction of diuretic dose and restoration of extracellular fluid volume with sodium chloride. Potassium supplementation may also expedite restoration of normal acid-base balance. Metabolic acidosis may occur when acetazolamide or spironolactone is used as monotherapy.

Miscellaneous. Other side effects of diuretic therapy are hyperuricemia, disordered serum calcium regulation, hyperglycemia, hyperlipidemia, gynecomastia, renal calculi, and ototoxicity. Thiazides, furosemide, and ethacrynic acid have been associated with hyperuricemia because of increased reabsorption of urate by the proximal tubule.[52] Urate levels to 10 mg/dL probably have no deleterious effects on renal function.[53] Dosage reduction of diuretic often corrects hyperuricemia. In patients with gouty arthritis or nephropathy, allopurinol is indicated to decrease production of uric acid by inhibition of xanthine oxidase. Thiazides decrease the renal excretion of calcium and thereby promote hypercalcemia. Hypocalcemia may also be seen with diuretic therapy, especially with the loop diuretics.[54,55]

Thiazides,[56] furosemide,[57] and ethacrynic acid[58] have also been associated with carbohydrate intolerance. The mechanism for hyperglycemia is not well understood, although it may be related to diuretic-induced potassium depletion, thereby inhibiting release of insulin. Thiazide diuretics have also been observed to have an unfavorable effect on the lipid profile, producing hypercholesterolemia and hypertriglyceridemia.[59-61] The magnitude of lipid increment is generally low (a 5% increase in total cholesterol), and the potential effect on cardiovascular morbidity is unknown. Since most patients with heart failure have ischemic heart disease, it is prudent to carefully monitor the lipid profile in this group and manage it accordingly.

Spironolactone and furosemide have been associated with gynecomastia. Decreased libido and irregular menses have also been reported with the use of spironolactone, which has a steroid structure that may inhibit or antagonize androgen production and action.[62]

Nephrolithiasis can be precipitated or exacerbated by diuretic use through volume depletion, hyperuricemia, hypercalcemia, and renal tubular acidosis. Triamterene may precipitate as stones within the urinary tract.[63,64]

Ototoxicity with hearing loss has been observed with administration of furosemide and ethacrynic acid. It is typically observed in patients with coexistent renal dysfunction receiving high doses of diuretic and is exacerbated by coadministration of aminoglycoside antibiotics.[65] Ototoxicity is usually reversible, although irreversible hearing loss has been described.[66]

Application of diuretics for heart failure

Diuretics are extremely effective in reversing sodium and water retention and relieve symptoms of pulmonary and systemic congestion rapidly within hours to days. Intravenous diuretic therapy is used to treat pulmonary edema and patients with symptomatic congestive heart failure in whom the response to oral therapy is suboptimal.[67] In this situation, furosemide is generally the drug of choice because of its prompt hemodynamic, natriuretic, and diuretic actions.

For long-term maintenance therapy, a thiazide or low-dose loop diuretic may be used in the patient with mild sodium retention and normal renal function. In patients with more advanced heart failure or coexistent renal dysfunction, a loop diuretic is indicated. Patients in more advanced stages of heart failure may initially require large doses of diuretic to promote diuresis and then smaller doses for long-term maintenance therapy. Diuretic requirements may also be altered when the patient becomes upright (because there is more sodium retention in the upright posture), especially if the patient becomes active as an outpatient. Concurrent therapy with an ACE inhibitor is advanced incrementally to a target or maximum tolerated dose over a period of several weeks. During this time, the requirements for diuretic may decrease, because ACE inhibitors are diuretic-sparing.[68,69]

Although diuretics reduce edema and intravascular pressure, they may exacerbate the pathophysiology of heart failure, because cardiac output may decline and the renin-angiotensin-aldosterone system and sympathetic nervous system may be activated. These alterations of neurohormonal function may contribute to the progression of disease as well as cause or exacerbate azotemia. When a strategy for treatment is developed, diuretics generally must be used as the initial intervention, because most patients present with signs and symptoms of congestion. For long-term therapy, however, they should be used in combination with other agents and in minimum dose.

Some patients with left ventricular dysfunction without clinical signs of salt and water overload can be managed without diuretic therapy, and, when feasible, diuretic therapy should be omitted. When combined with the ACE inhibitors, diuretics are associated with fewer adverse neurohormonal and metabolic abnormalities. The risk of progression of symptoms is reduced when diuretics are combined with digitalis or ACE inhibitor.[70]

Diuretic resistance

The patient with heart failure is considered resistant to diuretic when moderate doses of a loop agent do not decrease edema. There are many potential causes of diuretic resistance[71] (Table 17-3). Resistance to diuretic may be due to ingestion of excess sodium chloride in the diet. In this case, restriction of dietary salt intake is indicated. When diuretic resistance persists or continues despite adequate sodium restriction, other causes of diuretic resistance should be sought. Regular diuretic administration may lead to decreased urine volume due to decreased intravascular volume, which promotes enhanced renal tubular sodium and water reabsorption. Other mechanisms for diuretic resistance are low cardiac output with decreased renal blood flow, diuretic-induced activation of the renin-angiotensin-aldosterone system, and electrolyte disturbances, including hyponatremia, hypokalemia, and hypomagnesemia. In patients using thiazide diuretics, a more potent loop agent may be indicated; in patients with intrinsic renal disease, the thiazide diuretics generally are not effective if the glomerular infiltration rate is less than 20 mL/min. An important drug interaction that antagonizes diuretics is the effect of the nonsteroidal anti-inflammatory agents, including aspirin.[72,73]

Excessive hypotension associated with use of vasodila-

Table 17-3 Diuretic resistance

Causes	
Noncompliance	
	Not taking drug
	Excessive dietary salt
Impaired bioavailability	
Drug-drug interaction	
	NSAID
	Vasodilators
Renal disease	
Management strategies	
Assess compliance	
	Diet
	Medications
Consider drug-drug interactions	
	NSAID
	Vasodilators
Alter diuretic program	
Change to loop agent	
	Intravenous therapy
	Diuretic combinations
Give renal dose of dopamine	

tors or overdiuresis may decrease renal blood flow, thereby reducing urine formation. In diuretic therapy, reduced renal blood flow is also associated with decreased delivery of the drug to the tubular lumen. The absorption of oral furosemide may be delayed in heart failure[74] and the action of a given concentration of furosemide within the renal tubule attenuated.[67] Clinically, these problems may be overcome in the short term with intermittent intravenous therapy.

Combination therapy using agents with different mechanisms of action to enhance diuresis can be helpful in patients with refractory edema. Combination therapy with metolazone and a loop diuretic can be especially useful in patients with refractory edema when either a loop or a thiazide diuretic alone does not promote diuresis.[39,75] However, such therapy is potentially hazardous, because marked diuresis with electrolyte losses may ensue. For this reason, in the patient with refractory edema due to heart failure, it is generally advisable that therapy be started in the hospital under close observation. Dopaminergic doses of dopamine given intravenously are also effective in promoting diuresis (see "Dopamine," below).

INOTROPIC AGENTS

Inotropic drugs improve left ventricular function by augmenting myocardial contractility and thus increasing cardiac output and reducing left ventricular end-diastolic pressure and volume. Increased cardiac output increases renal blood flow and reduces intracardiac filling pressures, and these effects yield reduced systemic and pulmonary venous congestion.

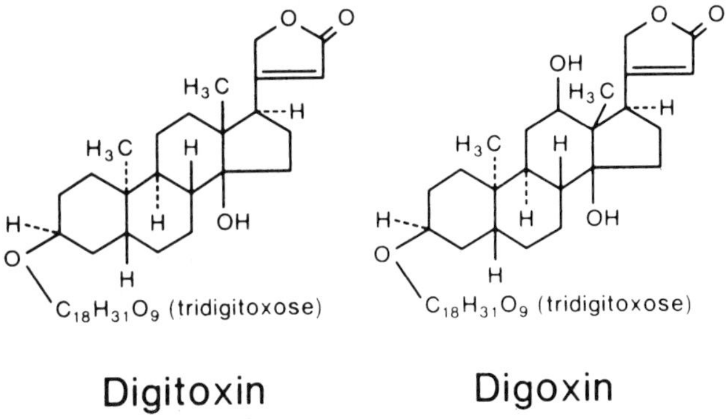

Fig 17-2 Chemical structures of digitoxin and digoxin.

Digitalis glycosides

The digitalis glycosides have been in clinical use for over 200 years.[76] Digoxin remains the only orally administered inotrope approved for the treatment of heart failure. Moreover, despite many years of investigation and numerous trials of investigational agents, the digitalis glycosides have not been displaced as the oral inotropic agents of choice for the treatment of chronic congestive heart failure. The digitalis glycosides have properties other than promotion of increased myocardial contractility that contribute to therapeutic benefit for patients with heart failure.

Physiologic actions

INOTROPY. The digitalis glycosides have a steroid structure with an unsaturated lactone ring at C-17 and a carbohydrate moiety at C-3 (Fig 17-2). The steroid and unsaturated lactone portion of the molecule is referred to as "genin" or "aglycone." This structure is essential for the pharmacologic activity of the digitalis glycosides.[77-79]

The sarcolemmal-bound Na^+, K^+-ATPase pump is the pharmacologic receptor for the digitalis glycosides that specifically inhibit pump activity[80,81] (Fig 17-3). The transmembrane Na^+ influx that occurs during phase 0 of the action potential, associated with diminished outward Na^+ pumping due to inhibition of the Na^+, K^+-ATPase pump, yields increased intracellular Na^+ available for transmembrane ion exchange. The primary consequence of the rise in intracellular Na^+ is a secondary rise in intracellular Ca^{2+} available for binding to the contractile elements mediated through enhanced exchange of intracellular Na^+ for extracellular Ca^{2+}. Microelectrode studies have demonstrated increased intracellular Na^+ associated with the use of digitalis, a direct confirmation that Na^+, K^+-ATPase pump inhibition yields increased intracellular Na^+.[82,83] Experiments utilizing the Ca^{2+}-dependent, bioluminescent photoprotein aequorin demonstrate a rapid initial rise in light intensity due to a calcium-transient associated with increased tension consistent with rapid mobilization of Ca^{2+} and subsequent binding to the contractile elements[84] (Fig 17-4).

ELECTROPHYSIOLOGY. The 90-mV transmembrane resting action potential of cardiac cells is maintained by Na^+ and K^+ transmembrane ionic gradients. Intracellular concentration of Na^+ increases and that of K^+

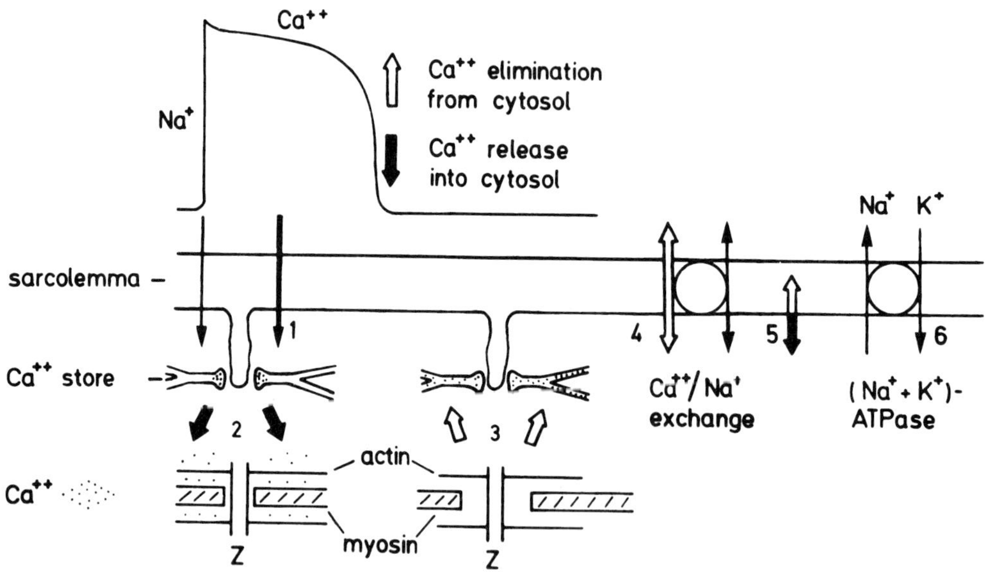

Fig 17-3 Slow Ca^{++} inward current via the sarcolemma *(1)* augments intracellular Ca^{++} stores for subsequent release *(2)*, with increased Ca^{++} concentration at the contractile proteins. Ca^{++} reuptake in the sarcoplasmic reticulum *(3)* replenishes Ca^{++} stores for next cardiac cycle. The sarcolemma *(5)* also serves as a site for release and uptake of Ca^{++}. Digoxin binds to Na^{+}, K^{+}-ATPase receptors *(6)*, which results in increased Na^{+} available for Ca^{++}/Na^{+} exchange *(4)*, yielding increased cytosolic Ca^{++} for augmentation of myocardial contractility. (From Scholz H: Inotropic drugs and their mechanisms of action. *J Am Coll Cardiol* 4:389-397, 1984. By permission of American College of Cardiology.)

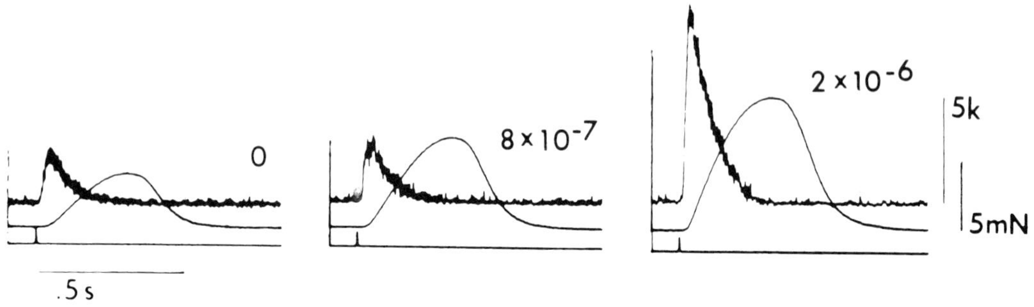

Fig 17-4 Influence of acetylstrophanthidin on tension development and aequorin luminescence.

decreases because of Na^{+}, K^{+}-ATPase pump inhibition by digitalis. Pump inhibition is dose-dependent, and a progressive decrease in transmembrane potential is observed because of decreased intracellular K^{+}. The changes in ionic gradients yield predictable effects on the transmembrane electrical potential[85] (Fig 17-5).

Excitability of the cardiac cell is increased by digitalis because the transmembrane resting potential is reduced to a point nearer to threshold potential. However, marked reduction in membrane potential causes diminished excitability as a result of inactivation of the rapid inward Na^{+} current by the increased intracellular Na^{+} concentration and reduced gradient for ion flow.[86] Refractoriness and automaticity are also altered by digitalis because of changes in K^{+} conductance.[87,88] Transmembrane permeability to K^{+} is increased during phase 2 and phase 3 of the cardiac action potential. These effects of digitalis shorten the duration of action potential, and as a consequence, refractoriness is decreased. The decline in K^{+} conductance characteristic of pacemaker cells is augmented and yields an increased slope of phase 4, which in association with reduced transmembrane potential promotes increased automaticity. These alterations of refractoriness and automaticity are a substrate for digitalis-induced toxic rhythm disturbances. Digitalis also shortens the refractory period of the cardiac cell, which

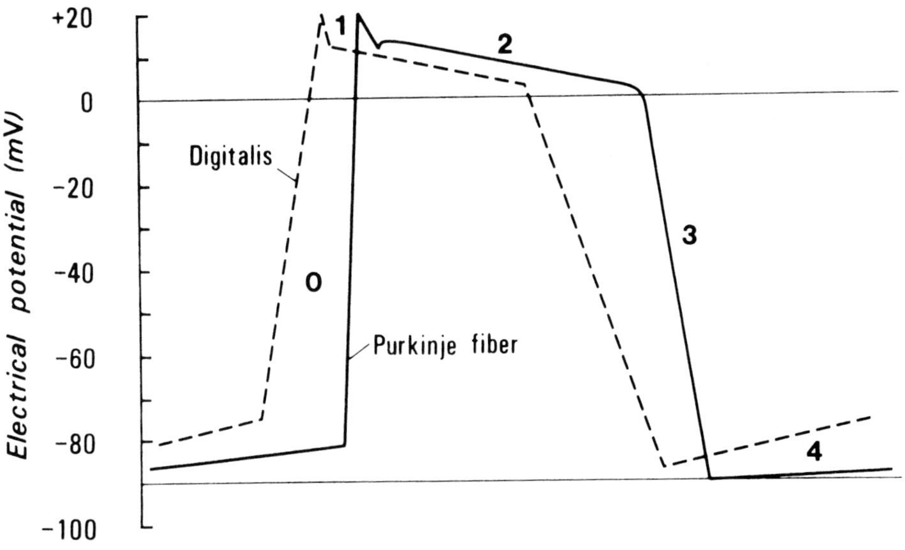

Fig 17-5 Four phases of cardiac action potential and modification by digitalis. An initial rapid influx of Na^+ (phase *0*) yields a rapid decrease in transmembrane potential and is followed by an early rapid repolarization (phase *1*) due to an inward C1- flux and then by a period of relative isoelectricity (phase *2*) with an associated slow inward Ca^{++} movement. Final repolarization (phase *3*) is associated with an efflux of K^+. In myocardial cells with pacemaker activity, a decline in K^+ efflux occurs in diastole with a decrease in membrane potential (phase *4*) until threshold is reached, initiating another action potential. Digitalis affects the action potential of a Purkinje fiber by increasing intracellular Na^+ concentration and decreasing K^+ concentration by Na^+, K^+-ATPase inhibition. As a consequence, resting membrane potential is reduced, the duration of the action potential is shortened, and the slope of phase 4 is increased. The changes in ion currents underlying the action potential account for enhanced membrane excitability, decreased refractoriness, and increased automaticity.

may be clinically manifested by increased atrial flutter rate or conversion of atrial flutter to atrial fibrillation.[89,90]

Clinically, the most important electrophysiologic actions of the cardiac glycosides are slowed conduction velocity and prolonged refractoriness of the AV node mediated via enhanced parasympathetic tone. Slowing of the ventricular rate in atrial fibrillation and atrial flutter and termination and prevention of AV node reentrant tachycardia are results of these actions.

AUTONOMIC NERVOUS SYSTEM. The clinically relevant actions of digitalis are not limited to the heart. Digitalis affects noncardiac excitable tissue, including the autonomic nervous system, which modulates both therapeutic and toxic manifestations.[91]

The heart failure state is characterized by altered autonomic tone. Stimulation of aortic and carotid baroreceptors inhibits sympathetic outflow as well as renin and vasopressin release and increases parasympathetic activity. Desensitization of baroreflex activity is characteristic of heart failure and is associated with increased sympathetic neural outflow as well as vasopressin release and renin secretion[92,93] (Fig 17-6). The short-term effect of increased sympathetic outflow leads to the adaptive responses of increased stroke volume and cardiac output in the failing heart; however, the long-term consequences are tachycardia, vasoconstriction, and salt and water retention.[94,95]

Sympathetic neural recordings obtained in patients with heart failure have demonstrated that digitalis produces sympathoinhibitory actions.[96] It has been suggested that this action may result from afferent activation of baroreceptors by digitalis. There is evidence from animal investigation that attenuation of baroreceptor discharge sensitivity from the carotid sinus is related to augmented Na^+, K^+-ATPase activity and that cardiac glycosides may resensitize this mechanism, resulting in restoration of normal autonomic tone.[97]

The effects of digitalis glycosides on the sympathetic nervous system are dose-dependent. With therapeutic doses, sympathetic tone is decreased, primarily as a result of baroreceptor activation. At large doses, however, sympathetic tone is increased as a result of stimulation of central and possibly peripheral sympathetic centers, which may promote tachyarrhythmia.[98]

HEMODYNAMICS. Cardiac output and other hemodynamic measurements of ventricular performance are determined by preload and afterload as well as by myocardial contractility. Alteration of autonomic tone has important modulating effects on cardiac output in both normal and failing hearts. The hemodynamic actions of

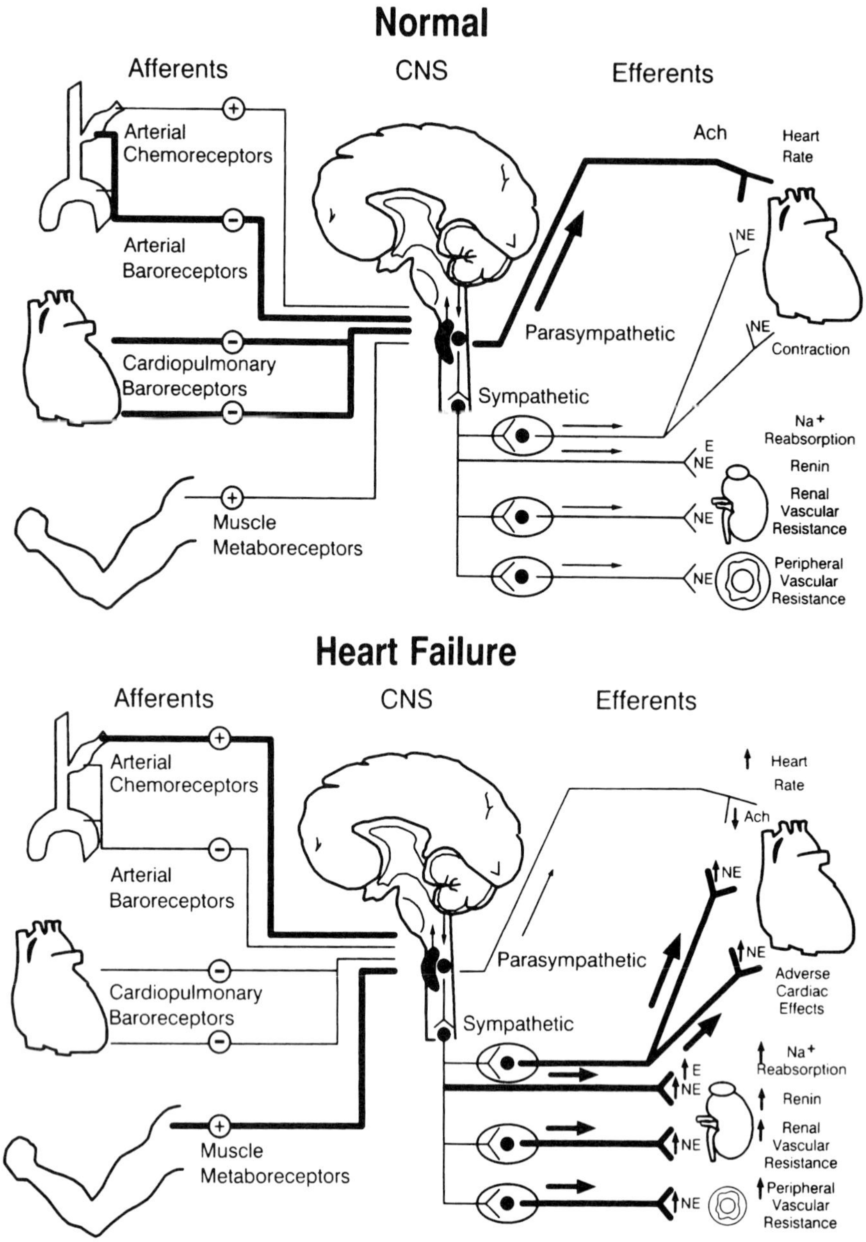

Fig 17-6 Sympathetic activation and parasympathetic withdrawal characteristic of heart failure promote increased sodium retention and increased peripheral vascular resistance. *Ach,* acetylcholine; *CNS,* central nervous system; *E,* epinephrine; *NE,* norepinephrine. (From Floras JS: Clinical aspects of sympathetic activation and parasympathetic withdrawal in heart failure. *J Am Coll Cardiol* 22 Suppl A:72-84, 1993. By permission of American College of Cardiology.)

digitalis are due to direct myocardial effects as well as to actions on the peripheral vasculature and autonomic nervous system. The net hemodynamic effect of digitalis on the nonfailing heart is different from that on the failing heart because of differences in digitalis action on the peripheral vessels and nervous system.

In the nonfailing heart, digitalis decreases venous return and increases peripheral vascular resistance, and these effects tend to negate inotropic effects, so that cardiac output is not increased and may actually decrease.[99-101] In contrast, in patients with heart failure, there is a net reduction in peripheral resistance because of reduced sympathetic tone.[102] Hence, when digitalis is given to patients with heart failure, it produces vasodilatation instead of vasoconstriction. This action has been presumed to be related to increased cardiac output attributed to the inotropic action of digitalis as well as direct baroreflex-mediated withdrawal of sympathetic vasoconstriction due to resensitization of baroreflexes.[93-98] Accordingly, the ventricular function curve is shifted, so that for a given ventricular end-diastolic pressure, cardiac output is increased. Hemodynamically, this is manifested as a reduction in end-diastolic volume and pressure and an increase in cardiac output. Clinically, this is associated with decreased pulmonary and systemic venous pressure.

MYOCARDIAL OXYGEN CONSUMPTION. Myocardial oxygen consumption is determined by heart rate, contractility, and myocardial wall tension.[103] The net effect of the administration of digoxin on myocardial oxygen consumption depends on the effect of digoxin on each of these determinants. In the normal or nonfailing heart, digitalis has little effect on heart rate but increases contractility and systemic vascular resistance, producing a proportional net increase in myocardial oxygen consumption.[104] In contrast, in the failing heart, left ventricular dilatation is associated with markedly increased myocardial wall tension, and sympathetic stimulation increases heart rate and peripheral vascular resistance. Through its action to decrease ventricular volume and pressure, digitalis reduces wall tension, and by effecting withdrawal of sympathetic tone, it also decreases heart rate and peripheral resistance. The favorable effects on these factors more than offset augmented contractility associated with digitalis, with a resulting net decrease in myocardial oxygen consumption.[105]

Bioavailability and pharmacokinetics. Digoxin is the predominant glycoside preparation used in clinical practice, primarily because of flexibility in route of administration and duration of action. The major factor determining digoxin bioavailability is absorption from the gut. Absorption occurs primarily in the upper small intestine and occurs rapidly, with peak levels achieved approximately 30 to 60 minutes after ingestion.[107] Absorption is incomplete, and there is considerable individual variation. Administration with meals delays the rate but not the extent of absorption. Bioavailability of digoxin tablets ranges from 50% to 78% of that of an intravenous dose, with aqueous solutions providing higher bioavailability.[108,109] The soft gelatin capsules of digoxin in solution in polyethylene glycol (Lanoxicaps) provide bioavailability approaching 100%.[110,111] Bioavailability of orally administered digitoxin also approaches 100%.[112,113] Similar to digoxin, digitoxin is rapidly absorbed in the proximal gut, with peak levels achieved in approximately 1 hour.[114]

Digoxin undergoes hepatic metabolism to active and inactive metabolites, with the major route of excretion via the kidneys.[108,115] The half-life is approximately 36 to 48 hours in individuals with normal renal function. Renal excretion is directly proportional to glomerular filtration rate. Most of the drug is excreted as digoxin in the urine, and the remainder is excreted as dihydrodigoxin, which arises via biotransformation in the gut. Biliary excretion of digoxin also occurs, although the total amount excreted in the stool is negligible because of enterohepatic recycling.

Tissue-binding affinity for digitoxin is high, and large amounts are concentrated in the liver, where the drug is metabolized and excreted. Another major difference between digoxin and digitoxin is the extent of protein binding; more than 90% of digitoxin is bound to albumin, and higher serum levels result.[116] The principal pathway for elimination of digitoxin is metabolism, and relatively small amounts of the drug are excreted unchanged in the urine and feces. There is significant individual variation in the rate of hepatic metabolism, and hence the plasma half-life of digitoxin is also variable; half-life typically averages 4 to 7 days.[117] Renal excretion is the second major route of elimination.

Conditions altering the pharmacokinetics of digitalis glycosides. A great variety of conditions may alter the bioavailability and pharmacokinetics of digitalis glycosides and thereby affect clinical management.[118] A few of the more important conditions are summarized.

RENAL INSUFFICIENCY. The most frequent disorder affecting digoxin pharmacokinetics is renal dysfunction. Decreased renal function results in prolongation of digoxin elimination and half-life, which increases the digoxin level. In patients with renal dysfunction, the plasma digoxin level for a given dose of drug is higher, and hence both loading dose and maintenance dose need to be adjusted downward. Dialysis is generally ineffective in removing significant amounts of digoxin from the body because of tissue binding.[119] Urinary excretion of digitoxin decreases in patients with renal dysfunction, but total clearance is maintained, consistent with an increase in hepatic metabolism.[120,121]

HEPATIC INSUFFICIENCY. Moderate or even severe liver dysfunction generally has little effect on digoxin elimination.[122] Similarly, significant liver dysfunction either has no effect or decreases digitoxin plasma half-life; this suggests altered protein binding or enhanced renal excretion.[121]

THYROID DISEASE. Digitalis pharmacokinetics are altered in both hyperthyroidism and hypothyroidism. Serum levels of the cardiac glycosides are decreased in hyperthyroidism and increased in hypothyroidism.[123] The volume of distribution for digoxin is increased in hyperthyroidism and decreased in hypothyroidism.[123,124]

AGING. The major tissue-binding site for cardiac glycosides is skeletal muscle, which decreases with age.[125,126] Glomerular filtration rate also decreases steadily with age, and as a consequence, digoxin excretion declines.[127] Together these factors prolong plasma half-life and increase plasma level for a given dose, and they probably underlie the observed greater prevalence of digitalis toxicity in the elderly. Limited data suggest that digitoxin excretion is not significantly altered by age.[128]

Drug interactions. Administration of digitalis with other classes of drugs may cause clinically significant alterations of glycoside pharmacokinetics and pharmacologic action. Examples of various drug interactions are summarized in Table 17-4. Known drug interactions with digoxin are too numerous to cover comprehensively within the scope of this chapter, and the reader is referred elsewhere.[128]

Table 17-4 Drug interactions that alter digoxin and digitoxin pharmacokinetics

	Effect on plasma level		
Drug	**Digoxin**	**Digitoxin**	**Mechanism**
Drugs that alter absorption			
Antacids			
Magnesium trisilicate	↓	?	
Magnesium carbonate	↓	?	
Aluminum hydroxide	↓	?	
Antibiotics			
Neomycin	↓	?	
p-Aminosalicylic acid	↓	?	
Sulfasalazine	↓	?	
Tetracycline	↑ *	?	
Erythromycin	↑ *	?	
Binding agents			
Cholestyramine	↓	↓	
Colestipol	↓	↓	
Activated charcoal	↓	↓	
Drugs affecting GI motility			
Metoclopramide	↓	?	
Propantheline	↑	?	
Kaolin-pectin	↓	?	
Paregoric	↑	?	
Diphenoxylate with atropine	↑	?	
Cytotoxic agents	↓	? ↓	
Drugs that alter distribution, metabolism, or excretion			
Antiarrhythmia agents			
Quinidine	↑	↑	↓ V_d and renal excretion of digoxin
Verapamil	↑	?	↓ renal and nonrenal clearance of digoxin
Amiodarone	↑	?	↓ total body clearance ? ↑ bioavailability
Diuretics			
Spironolactone	↑	?	↓ renal tubular secretion, assay interference
Triamterene	↑	?	?
Miscellaneous			
Barbiturates	→	↓	↑ hepatic clearance by microsomal enzyme induction
Phenytoin	→	↓	↑ hepatic clearance by microsomal enzyme induction
Phenylbutazone	→	↓	↑ hepatic clearance by microsomal enzyme induction
Quinine	↑	?	↓ nonrenal excretion

Symbols: ↑ increase; ↓ decrease; → no significant change; ?, unknown.
*In patients with significant digoxin metabolism by gut flora.

PHARMACOLOGIC DRUG INTERACTION. Pharmacologic drug interactions result from alterations of myocardial sensitivity to digitalis or from synergistic drug actions. An example of the former is the enhancement of glycoside effects by hypokalemia associated with the use of diuretics. An example of the latter is the potentiation of glycoside action on sinoatrial and AV nodes by β-adrenergic blockers or calcium blockers. Many classes of drugs, including sympathomimetic agents, succinylcholine, and parenteral calcium, have been implicated in decreasing the threshold for digitalis toxicity.[129]

ALTERED BIOAVAILABILITY. Several classes of drugs decrease digitalis bioavailability by impairing absorption of the drug. Liquid antacids, especially those containing magnesium trisilicate, may adsorb digoxin and digitoxin and cause reduced bioavailability. Other drugs that bind digitalis glycosides in the gut are the antidiarrheal agent kaolin-pectin, activated charcoal, and the cholesterol-lowering agents cholestyramine and colestipol, all of which absorb the drug and thereby reduce the amount available for absorption.[130]

Numerous antibiotics, including neomycin and sulfasalazine, have been demonstrated to inhibit digoxin absorption through an unknown mechanism.[131,132] In a small subset of patients receiving digoxin who are concomitantly treated with broad-spectrum antibiotics, an increase in serum digoxin level has been attributed to suppression of gut flora important in the metabolism of digoxin.[133] Cytotoxic drugs have been demonstrated to interfere transiently with absorption of digoxin, presumably by damaging the intestinal mucosa.[134] Drugs that alter gastrointestinal motility may also influence absorption of digoxin; agents that reduce motility, including propantheline and paregoric, tend to increase absorption,[135,136] whereas agents that increase motility, such as metoclopramide, tend to decrease absorption.[135]

ALTERED DISTRIBUTION, METABOLISM, OR EXCRETION. The most important and most frequently encountered clinical drug interaction occurs with quinidine. Quinidine causes significant increases in serum digoxin level by reduction in both renal and nonrenal elimination of digoxin and also appears to decrease the volume of distribution.[137,138]

The observed frequency of the quinidine-digoxin interaction is approximately 90%.[137,139,140] Interaction occurs rapidly, because increased serum digoxin concentrations are detected within 6 hours of quinidine administration. With maintenance doses of quinidine, the serum digoxin level increases gradually and plateaus in 4 to 7 days.[140-142] In general, standard doses of quinidine double the steady-state serum digoxin level. However, marked individual variation is observed.[143]

The mechanism of the interaction appears to be a change in the tissue binding of digoxin that produces a decrease in the volume of distribution and a decrease in total body clearance.[142,144] Renal excretion appears to be impaired primarily by inhibition of tubular secretion, because no decrement in glomerular filtration has been demonstrated.[145] Whether the increase in serum digoxin level correlates with an increased digitalis effect at the Na^+, K^+-ATPase receptor or myocardium is unclear. In general, the maintenance dose of digoxin should be decreased by half when quinidine therapy is commenced and the patient closely monitored for digitalis toxicity.

A second important antiarrhythmic agent that alters digoxin metabolism is amiodarone. Like quinidine, amiodarone approximately doubles the serum digitalis concentration and thereby promotes bradyarrhythmia.[146,147] The mechanism appears to be reduction in total body clearance of digoxin. Hence, as with quinidine, digoxin doses should be decreased by half when given concurrently with amiodarone.

The calcium blocker verapamil has also been shown to increase digoxin levels through a nonrenal effect on the clearance of digoxin.[148] The dose of verapamil should be decreased when administered with digoxin. Studies of other calcium blockers, including diltiazem, nifedipine, and nicardipine, have not demonstrated increased risk of digitalis toxicity.[149]

A pharmacokinetic interaction in which serum digoxin concentration is increased occurs when spironolactone and digoxin are used concurrently. The mechanism of the increased serum digoxin concentration is related to two separate actions; spironolactone and its metabolites interfere with radioimmunoassays for digoxin, yielding a falsely increased level and reducing renal tubular secretion and the volume of distribution of digoxin.[150,151]

Altered cardiac sensitivity to digitalis. A number of conditions have been associated with altered sensitivity to digitalis. Altered sensitivity may be manifested as either an increased or a decreased threshold to digitalis toxicity (Table 17-5).

ELECTROLYTE DISTURBANCES. The most clinically important electrolyte abnormalities altering sensitivity to digitalis are hypokalemia and hyperkalemia. In experimentally induced hypokalemia, the amount of digitalis required to produce toxic arrhythmias is decreased.[152,153] These observations have been corroborated by general clinical experience.[154] Hypokalemia produces ectopy and conduction disturbances similar to those observed for digitalis toxicity and is associated with inhibition of the activity of the Na^+, K^+-ATPase pump.[155] These observations indicate that the electrophysiologic disturbances

Table 17-5 Factors affecting myocardial sensitivity to digitalis

Electrolyte disturbances
Hypokalemia
Hyperkalemia
Hypercalcemia
Hypomagnesemia
Organic heart disease
Pulmonary disease
Hyperthyroidism
Hypothyroidism
Autonomic nervous system status

From Bresnahan JF, Vlietstra RE: Series on pharmacology in practice. 3. Digitalis glycosides. *Mayo Clin Proc* 54:675-684, 1979. By permission, Mayo Foundation.

of hypokalemia and digitalis toxicity are similar and may be synergistic. In contrast, hyperkalemia antagonizes the effect of digitalis on the heart, and larger doses of digitalis are required to produce toxicity.[156]

Hypomagnesemia also predisposes to development of digitalis toxicity.[157-159] The mechanism by which this occurs is uncertain, although it has been reported that hypomagnesemia enhances myocardial uptake of the cardiac glycosides.[160] As with hypokalemia, hypomagnesemia is most likely to be encountered in the patient receiving diuretic therapy.

Experimental hypercalcemia induces digitalis toxicity, but calcium levels commonly encountered in clinical practice probably seldom promote toxicity.[161] However, calcium therapy with a parenteral bolus should probably be avoided in patients receiving digitalis.

PULMONARY DISEASE. Patients with chronic obstructive pulmonary disease appear to be at increased risk for digitalis toxicity. The reasons for the increased sensitivity have not been identified. Assessment of the cause of apparent increased sensitivity is confounded by comorbid conditions that predispose to the development of rhythm abnormalities characteristic of digitalis intoxication; hypoxia may be a contributing factor.[162,163]

UNDERLYING HEART DISEASE. The type and severity of underlying heart disease affect the manifestations of digitalis toxicity and lower the threshold for toxicity.[164] In normal subjects who ingest toxic quantities of digitalis, the predominant rhythm disturbances consist of increased degrees of sinoatrial and AV nodal block; ventricular ectopy is generally a late phenomenon.[165] However, in patients with organic heart disease, ventricular ectopy is frequently the primary manifestation of toxicity. The differences observed in sensitivity to digitalis toxicity are presumably related to disease-induced alteration of the electrophysiologic substrate for arrhythmia.

THYROID DISEASE. Hyperthyroidism appears to confer resistance to digitalis toxicity, whereas hypothyroidism is associated with increased sensitivity, which may be mediated by receptor density.[166,167]

Clinical utility of serum digitalis level. Because the diagnosis of digitalis toxicity is clinical, no specific serum value clearly separates toxic from nontoxic levels; levels are supporting data rather than definitive diagnostic tests. Although the usefulness of the serum digitalis level is limited in the diagnosis of drug toxicity, levels are important in the prevention of toxicity and are also beneficial in the general use of digitalis glycosides.

The ratio of toxic to therapeutic levels for cardiac glycosides is small. Generally, serum levels between 0.8 and 2 ng/mL for digoxin are regarded as therapeutic and of low risk for toxicity; the risk of toxicity progressively increases with levels greater than 2 ng/mL. Mean serum digoxin concentrations are generally threefold higher in patients with toxicity, although considerable overlap exists in digitalis levels between toxic and nontoxic states.[168-173] In a large prospective investigation, 29% of patients with digitalis toxicity had levels considered therapeutic and 15% of patients without toxicity had levels beyond this range.[169] The risk of toxicity for digitoxin increases progressively with levels greater than 25 ng/mL.[174]

The clinical interpretation of serum digitalis levels requires consideration of the timing of dose, assay method, protein-binding, therapeutic response, and coexistent factors that may alter sensitivity to digitalis toxicity. Venipuncture to assess digitalis levels should not be performed within 8 to 12 hours of digoxin dosing or 12 hours for digitoxin. Spironolactone or other steroid compounds may interfere with the radioimmunoassay and decrease the accuracy of determination.[151,175] For assessment of serum digitoxin levels, it is necessary to know the serum albumin concentration. To further complicate the issue, digitalis-like immunoreactive substances have been identified in patients with renal and hepatic dysfunction as well as in neonates and pregnant women.[176] Levels as high as 4 ng/mL have been reported in patients not receiving digoxin.

Digitalis toxicity. Digitalis toxicity has been reported in up to 29% of patients hospitalized for the treatment of heart failure.[169] Despite long clinical experience and the availability of a reliable serum assay, digitalis intoxication remains a pervasive clinical problem; therefore, the clinician must remain vigilant to establish the diagnosis. Symptoms are both cardiac and noncardiac; gastrointestinal and neurologic symptoms predominate and include nausea, vomiting, anorexia, malaise, headache, insomnia, altered color perception, photophobia, visual scotoma, and drowsiness. In 80% of patients, anorexia and nausea are the earliest symptoms of toxicity.[174] The gastrointestinal symptoms of digitalis toxicity are mediated via chemoreceptors located in the area postrema of the medulla.[177] Toxic doses of digitalis glycosides have been associated with increased central and peripheral sympathetic nerve activity, and a close temporal relationship has been demonstrated between onset of ventricular arrhythmias and increase in sympathetic neural traffic.[178-181] Drugs that interfere with formation of sympathetic impulses both centrally and peripherally (for example, propranolol and phenytoin) increase the threshold for toxicity.[178,181]

Disorders of cardiac rhythm are the most important manifestations of digitalis toxicity. The most commonly observed rhythm disturbances are those attributable to increased automaticity of the atrial, junctional, and ventricular pacemakers and decreased conduction of the sinoatrial and AV nodes. Table 17-6 is a compilation of rhythm disturbances in 769 patients with digitalis intoxication.[182]

There are no specific electrocardiographic features that identify digitalis toxic rhythms from arrhythmias due to intrinsic cardiac disease. However, rhythms that demonstrate both increased automaticity of ectopic pacemakers and impaired conduction, including paroxysmal atrial tachycardia with AV block, are highly suggestive of digitalis toxicity. Other characteristic rhythm abnormalities are ventricular tachycardia, nonparoxysmal junctional tachycardia, and regularization of ventricular response in patients with atrial fibrillation or group beating.

Many patients with digitalis intoxication have normal or only modestly increased serum digitalis levels. Less commonly, digitalis toxicity is a manifestation of massive overdose. The approach to the patient with massive

Table 17-6 Most frequent arrhythmias in 769 patients with digitalis intoxication

Arrhythmia type*	No.
Premature ventricular beats (608 patients)	349
Second- and third-degree heart block	176
Atrioventricular junctional tachycardia	172
Atrioventricular junctional escape beats	122
Atrial tachycardia with block	98
Ventricular tachycardia	77
Sinoatrial block, sinus arrest	22

*Other arrhythmias occurred but were less frequent.
From Ewy GA, Marcus FI, Fillmore SJ, et al: Digitalis intoxication: diagnosis, management and prevention. *Cardiovasc Clin* 6 No. 2:153-174, 1974. By permission of FA Davis Company.

overdose has been greatly altered in recent years because of the availability of digoxin-specific Fab fragments, which can be administered intravenously and rapidly reverse the manifestations of toxicity.[183-185] Generally, this management is reserved for patients with life-threatening disease. A wide experience with the use of digoxin-specific Fab fragments has demonstrated that this therapy is highly efficacious in digoxin or digitoxin toxicity.

In the patient with suspected nonmassive digitalis intoxication, initial therapy requires discontinuation of the drug and rhythm monitoring. Predisposing conditions, including electrolyte disturbances, pulmonary dysfunction, drug interactions, and altered renal function, should be aggressively sought and managed. In many cases, sinoatrial or AV node depression without hemodynamic compromise can be observed. In more advanced degrees of sinus node dysfunction or heart block, atropine is useful for short-term intervention. High-grade AV block and ventricular arrhythmias should be treated with digoxin-specific antibody fragments. Supportive measures that may be useful until digoxin-specific antibody fragments are given include administration of potassium and magnesium. Potassium is useful in the suppression of ventricular ectopy, especially when there is coexistent hypokalemia. However, it should be used cautiously in patients with AV block, as it may further decrease AV conduction, and should not be administered if levels are increased or if heart block is prominent.[186,187] Magnesium sulfate should be administered when hypomagnesemia is documented, as it appears to have antiarrhythmic properties in digitalis intoxication.[188]

Other possible pharmacologic antiarrhythmic interventions include administration of lidocaine, phenytoin, and β-blockers. Lidocaine is particularly efficacious in the treatment of ventricular arrhythmias; its utility is related to a lack of deleterious effect on hemodynamics, sinus node automaticity, AV conduction, and the autonomic nervous system.[189] Phenytoin is comparable to lidocaine in therapeutic efficacy for control of digitalis-induced ventricular ectopy, probably because of an action on the central nervous system to reduce sympathetic neural activity.[190]

The β-blockers decrease automaticity, shorten the refractory period of atrial and ventricular muscle and Purkinje fibers, and slow conduction velocity. If this therapeutic intervention is implemented, a short-acting drug, such as esmolol, is preferred. Generally, β-blockers should be avoided in patients with AV block.[191]

Utility of digitalis for heart failure. The use of the digitalis glycosides for the treatment of patients with chronic congestive heart failure became controversial in the decade of the 1980s because of several uncontrolled trials that reported an apparent lack of efficacy.[192-194] However, more recent prospective randomized trials support the use of digoxin for the treatment of class II-IV symptoms of heart failure when use is combined with either diuretic or vasodilator therapy.

Digoxin has been demonstrated to improve functional capacity and quality of life,[195,196] hemodynamics,[197] and left ventricular ejection fraction[198] and to delay progression of symptoms, as assessed by diuretic requirements, hospitalizations, and emergency room visits.[70] Prospective, controlled studies have demonstrated improved exercise performance and quality of life when digoxin is used with either diuretic[194,199] or ACE inhibitor.[200] When added to a regimen including a diuretic and the ACE inhibitor captopril, digoxin is associated with improved functional capacity, hemodynamic parameters, and exercise performance as well as decreased plasma norepinephrine and aldosterone.[200-204]

Prospective, placebo-controlled trials have also used randomized drug withdrawal to demonstrate the efficacy of digoxin in patients with heart failure. In the PROVED (Prospective Randomized Study of Ventricular Failure and Efficacy of Digoxin)[205] and RADIANCE (Randomized Assessment of Digoxin on Inhibitors of Angiotensin-Converting Enzyme)[206] trials, patients with stable class II or III congestive heart failure were evaluated for the effects of digoxin withdrawal. No patient in the PROVED trial was receiving an ACE inhibitor, whereas all patients in the RADIANCE trial were treated concurrently with diuretic and ACE inhibitor in stable doses. In each trial, patients withdrawn to placebo had a significantly higher rate of clinical deterioration, manifested as decreased exercise capacity, increased need for diuretic or vasodilator therapy, death, or hospital admission.

Digoxin has also been shown to be efficacious in patients with more advanced (class III or IV) heart failure. In the milrinone-digoxin trial,[207] patients were randomized to receive placebo, digoxin, milrinone, or a combination of both drugs in addition to diuretic therapy. Patients who received digoxin had increased ejection fraction and improved exercise tolerance as well as less frequent clinical decompensation compared with patients who received placebo or milrinone.

The efficacy of digoxin is less clear in mild (class I or II) heart failure than in more advanced heart failure. In the digoxin-xamoterol trial, 87% of patients had mild symptoms of heart failure. The partial β-agonist xamoterol was compared with placebo or digoxin for efficacy; patients treated with digoxin and xamoterol had less severe symptoms than patients receiving placebo.[208] In the captopril-digoxin trial, 300 patients receiving diuretic were randomized to placebo, captopril, or digoxin; 85% of patients had mild congestive heart failure. Although only captopril significantly increased exercise duration, digoxin increased left ventricular ejection fraction and was as effective as captopril in the reduction of diuretic requirements, hospitalization, and emergency room visits.[70] Cardiac glycosides have not yet been demonstrated to improve survival in patients with congestive heart failure. A prospective, randomized, and placebo-controlled Digitalis Investigators Group (DIG) trial will assess the effect of digoxin on survival in patients with chronic congestive heart failure.

The optimal dose of digitalis in heart failure depends on the clinical response of the patient. When the clinical response is suboptimal or suggests toxicity, serum digoxin levels may assist in the clinical assessment of problems related to compliance, bioavailability, and altered metabolism. Serum levels are particularly useful in guiding the clinician in regulating dosage in patients who have disorders of renal function or who use medications that alter digitalis pharmacokinetics. A good correlation between serum digoxin level and hemodynamic benefit has been demonstrated;[200] hence, incremental hemodynamic benefit may be obtained by titrating digoxin dose, using levels to guide therapy.

Many formulas and nomograms have been described to aid the clinician in selection of the optimal dose of digitalis glycoside.[209-211] Although in principle these methods may be helpful, they are infrequently used in clinical practice. Moreover, clinical judgment with or without the assistance of a computer program has been shown to be similarly effective in prediction of digoxin levels.[212]

In previously undigitalized patients, a single dose of 0.5 to 0.75 mg of digoxin may be given for a discernible effect in approximately 2 hours and maximal effect in 2 to 6 hours. Additional doses of 0.125 mg may be given at 6- to 8-hour intervals to a total dose of 1.0 to 1.25 mg for a 70-kg patient.

In principle, the maintenance dose is based on the proportion of body stores lost each day, primarily through renal excretion. Renal dysfunction slows elimination and therefore necessitates a decreased maintenance dose. The maintenance dose may be estimated by the following formula:

$$\text{maintenance dose} = \text{loading dose} \times \frac{\%\ \text{daily loss}}{100}$$

$$(\%\ \text{daily loss} = 14 + \text{Ccr}/5)$$

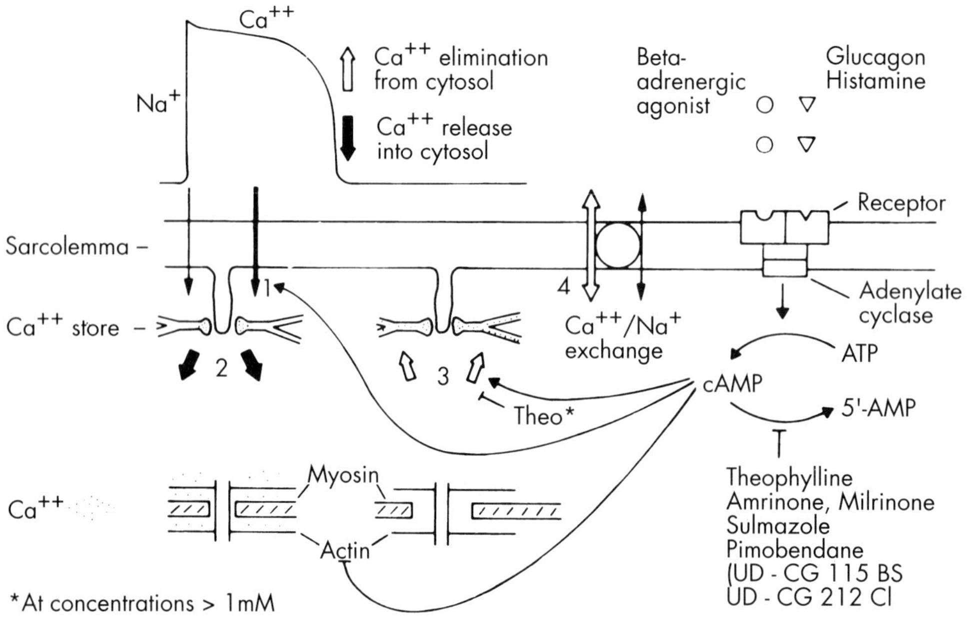

Fig 17-7 Second messenger system for β-adrenoreceptor agonists. The levels of cyclic adenosine monophosphate (cAMP) are increased either through increased cAMP formation or decreased cAMP degradation. Increased cAMP levels promote increased slow Ca^{++} inward current *(1)* and increased filling of intracellular Ca^{++} stores for subsequent release. Increased Ca^{++} release *(2)* increases Ca^{++} concentration at the contractile proteins, augmenting the force of contraction. cAMP also promotes uptake of Ca^{++} into the sarcoplasmic reticulum *(3)* and decreases the sensitivity of the contractile proteins to Ca^{++}, producing a decrease in the duration of contraction. Increased cAMP levels do not act directly on Ca^{++}/Na^{+} exchange *(4)*. *ATP,* adenosine triphosphate. (From Scholz H, Meyer W: Phosphodiesterase-inhibiting properties of newer inotropic agents. *Circulation* 73 Suppl 3:99-106, 1986. By permission of American Heart Association.)

in which Ccr is creatinine clearance corrected to 70 kg of body weight. In adult men, creatinine clearance may be estimated on the basis of serum creatinine (Scr) as (140 − age)/Scr. For women, the preceding formula is multiplied by a factor of 0.85 to arrive at the approximate maintenance dose.

Nonglycoside inotropes

The utility of nonglycoside inotropes is primarily for the short-term hemodynamic support of patients with refractory congestive heart failure. Long-term use of these agents has generally been limited by side effects, hemodynamic tolerance, or excess mortality.

Sympathomimetic amines. Catecholamines and sympathomimetic amines stimulate myocardial β-receptors to increase inotropy as well as chronotropy (Fig 17-7). The main use of these agents has been for the short-term management of hospitalized patients with cardiogenic shock after recent cardiac surgery or myocardial infarction. For chronic congestive heart failure, the clinical use of β-adrenergic agonists has been limited by tachycardia, proarrhythmia, and rapid tachyphylaxis with hemodynamic tolerance.

DOPAMINE. Dopamine is a neurotransmitter and the immediate precursor of norepinephrine in catecholamine synthesis. Its actions include direct β_1-adrenoreceptor agonist activity as well as stimulation of norepinephrine release from sympathetic neurons, which then activates β_1, β_2, and α receptors. Direct dopaminergic receptor activation promotes vasodilatation of the coronary, renal, mesenteric, and cerebrovascular beds.[213,214]

Activation of the various adrenoreceptor subtypes by dopamine is dose dependent; observed hemodynamic actions are related to the infusion rate of the drug.[214,215] At low rates of infusion (1 to 5 μg/kg per minute), dopaminergic and β_1-receptor stimulation predominate, yielding decreased peripheral vascular resistance and increased cardiac output. There is also preferential dilatation of renal cortical vessels, which promotes diuresis. In patients with heart failure, low doses of dopamine increase sodium excretion.[216] Dopamine-induced diuresis, a prominent and clinically important action in patients with heart failure, is due to a combination of inotropic and selective renal vasodilator effects. At low rates of infusion, there is typically little or no change in left ventricular filling pressures or heart rate. At higher rates of infusion, α-adrenergic receptor stimulation becomes more prominent. Cardiac output is increased, but there is concurrent increased afterload promoted by α-receptor-mediated arteriolar vasoconstriction, which may be associated with decreased renal blood flow.[217]

Dopamine administration is associated with increased coronary blood flow to meet increased myocardial oxygen consumption related to increased cardiac work. Direct vasodilatation mediated through dopaminergic receptors is an additional mechanism of augmented coronary flow. At high doses, dopamine causes myocardial ischemia due to imbalance between myocardial oxygen utilization and coronary flow. Increases in heart rate, contractility, and arterial pressure increase myocardial oxygen requirements.[218] However, reduced peripheral resistance and reduction in cardiac size at low doses may reduce myocardial oxygen utilization.[219] Hence, in patients with congestive heart failure, dopamine may exert favorable hemodynamic and renal actions with careful dose titration.

DOBUTAMINE. Dobutamine is a synthetic sympathomimetic amine that directly stimulates β_1, β_2, and α adrenoreceptors.[220] Dobutamine does not act on dopaminergic receptors and does not release norepinephrine from adrenergic neurons. Dobutamine augments myocardial contractility through stimulation of β and α receptors, and its peripheral action yields minimal change in vascular resistance or arterial pressure. At higher doses, however, left ventricular filling pressures and peripheral vascular resistance tend to decrease, perhaps because of β_2-receptor stimulation. In the usual therapeutic range of 2.5 to 15 mg/kg per minute, increases in heart rate are generally not significant. The usefulness of dobutamine for short-term inotropic support of the failing left ventricle has been well demonstrated.[221-223]

Sinus tachycardia and other cardiac arrhythmias are limiting adverse effects associated with the use of dopamine and dobutamine. The electrophysiologic properties of these agents include acceleration of spontaneous depolarization of sinoatrial cells, promoting increased heart rate; enhanced diastolic depolarization and automaticity; shortening of the refractory period of atrial and ventricular muscle; and speeding of AV conduction. These actions tend to promote ventricular arrhythmia and to precipitate myocardial ischemia.

Neither dopamine nor dobutamine is active orally. Either agent may be used for short-term administration to ameliorate refractory symptoms in patients with chronic congestive heart failure. Dobutamine administered by continuous infusion for 48 to 72 hours has been shown to improve exercise performance and clinical status.[224-228] However, although dobutamine infusion may significantly increase treadmill exercise time and decrease symptoms, it may also promote lethal arrhythmia.[229] Establishment of the utility and duration of this type of therapy for long-term management requires further investigation.

Orally active sympathomimetic amines generally appear to have side effects similar to those of catecholamines, and long-term use has been associated with rapid development of hemodynamic tolerance.[230-232]

Phosphodiesterase inhibitors. This class of agents exerts positive inotropic and vasodilator actions by the inhibition of phosphodiesterase III (PDE III). The membrane-bound enzyme system PDE III is responsible for the metabolism of the intracellular second messenger cyclic adenosine monophosphate (AMP). Inhibition of PDE III raises intracellular concentration of cyclic AMP, which promotes increased myocardial contractility. Inhibitors of adenylate cyclase interfere with the positive inotropic action of these agents, supporting the hypothesized mechanism of action. A great many agents from this class have been tested clinically. However, long-term, large-scale controlled studies have been reported for relatively few agents, including amrinone, milrinone, and enoximone.

AMRINONE. Amrinone is a bipyridine derivative approved for intravenous therapy in patients with refractory heart failure. Amrinone yields dose-dependent increases in cardiac output and reduces right- and left-sided filling pressures and systemic vascular resistance. At a low dose, the positive inotropic action is predominant, whereas at higher doses, a direct vasodilatory action is observed.[233-235]

The peak effect of a single intravenous dose occurs within 5 to 10 minutes of administration, and duration of action is 30 minutes to 2 hours. The drug is metabolized in the liver and excreted in the urine. In contrast to the sympathomimetic amines, amrinone is not associated with tolerance.[236] Amrinone therapy has been shown to increase ejection fraction, effective renal plasma flow, and glomerular filtration rate without significantly changing heart rate and mean arterial pressure.[234-238] In patients with atrial fibrillation, amrinone may accelerate AV conduction and increase the ventricular response rate.

Amrinone produces hemodynamic benefits comparable to those of dobutamine in patients with severe heart failure. At comparable levels of hemodynamic effect, sympathomimetic amines may not be as well tolerated because of nausea and tachycardia. The hemodynamic actions of the drug are synergistic with both sympathomimetics and digitalis glycosides. For myocardial oxygen demand, the vasodilating action tends to offset the effects of the positive inotropic action; hence, amrinone generally does not intensify ischemia in patients with coronary artery disease.[239,240]

Administered intravenously as an initial bolus of 0.75 mg/kg, the drug is infused at a rate of 5 to 10 μg/kg per minute. To avoid an excessive decrease in left ventricular filling pressure during infusion, diuretic and vasodilator therapy are generally reduced or stopped before administration of the drug. Invasive hemodynamic monitoring assists in optimal dose titration and in deciding whether to use diuretic therapy and other vasodilators.

Reported side effects include gastrointestinal upset with nausea, vomiting, cramps, diarrhea, and anorexia with prolonged use; thrombocytopenia, which is dose-related and reversible, can be managed by reducing the dose.[237,238,241,242]

Orally administered amrinone is well absorbed from the gastrointestinal tract, and its hemodynamic actions are similar to those with intravenous infusion. However, the agent has not proved suitable for long-term use because of the high incidence of adverse side effects and lack of efficacy when compared with a placebo in multicenter, randomized, double-blind, controlled studies. End points of the studies included control of heart failure, symptoms, treadmill exercise capacity, and noninvasive measurements of left ventricular function.[239,240]

MILRINONE. Milrinone, structurally related to amrinone, is approximately 20 times more potent and has similar pharmacologic and hemodynamic actions, including vasodilator and positive inotropic effects.[243,244] Consistent with these actions, it improves exercise capacity, maximum oxygen consumption, and anaerobic threshold; improved exercise performance is maintained during long-term oral therapy.[245] Like amrinone, however, it is approved only for intravenous therapy of refractory heart failure.

In a prospective, double-blind, randomized trial of 230 patients in sinus rhythm who had moderately severe heart failure, the subjects were assigned to treatment with continuation of digoxin, substitution of milrinone for digoxin, addition of milrinone to digoxin, or double placebo; exercise tolerance and symptoms were evaluated for 12 weeks. Milrinone significantly increased exercise tolerance and reduced the frequency of worsened heart failure in comparison with placebo. However, milrinone or the combination of milrinone and digoxin offered no advantage over digoxin alone.[207]

The Prospective Randomized Milrinone Survival Evaluation (PROMISE) trial evaluated the effect of milrinone on survival in 1,088 patients with chronic class III-IV heart failure despite therapy with digoxin, diuretics, and converting enzyme inhibitor.[246] The study was terminated because overall mortality was increased 28% over that with placebo (with a 58% increased mortality in class IV patients).[246] Because of the demonstrated detrimental effect on patient survival, use of the drug as a long-term oral agent has been abandoned.

ENOXIMONE. An imadazol compound, enoximone is dissimilar in structure from the bipyridines amrinone and milrinone but has similar biochemical and pharmacologic actions owing to its inhibition of PDE III. The drug has been tested in clinical trials by both oral and intravenous administration. Long-term oral administration of enoximone improves hemodynamics in patients with heart failure.[247,248] However, at high doses (3 to 6 μg/kg per dose, administered three times a day) serious side effects may occur, including nausea, diarrhea, headache, thrombocytopenia, and liver function test abnormalities.

Similar to the trial with milrinone, a large multicenter, prospective, placebo-controlled trial of orally administered enoximone demonstrated increased mortality in patients randomized to enoximone.[249]

Calcium-sensitizing positive inotropic agents. Inotropes of this class are investigational; they exert a positive inotropic action primarily by increasing the sensitivity of the myocardial contractile elements to the calcium ion. Pimobendan (a benzimidazole derivative) and vesnarinone (a quinolone derivative) have been shown to increase calcium sensitivity in isolated myocardial tissue from normal and failing hearts.[250,251] They also tend to produce minor phosphodiesterase inhibition. In principle, these agents may be superior to sympathomimetics and phosphodiesterase inhibitors for the treatment of heart failure, because increased calcium sensitivity may increase contractility without the toxic effects that otherwise accompany increased intracellular cyclic AMP or calcium ion.

VESNARINONE. Vesnarinone, orally or intravenously administered, improves hemodynamic variables and exercise capacity and has class III antiarrhythmic properties.[252-255] Three randomized, placebo-controlled trials have demonstrated improved quality of life and reduced cardiovascular morbidity or mortality at a dose of 60 mg per day.[256-258] Notably, a dose of 120 mg per day has been associated with a markedly increased risk of death, suggesting a very narrow therapeutic window.[258] This agent remains investigational pending results of a placebo-controlled survival study.

PIMOBENDAN. Similar to vesnarinone, pimobendan exerts relatively little phosphodiesterase inhibition. Pimobendan increases the affinity of troponin C of the cardiac myofilaments for calcium ion, thereby increasing contractility; it is also a peripheral vasodilator.[250,251,259] Experience in clinical trials has generally been favorable because of sustained symptomatic and hemodynamic benefits.[260] However, no controlled survival trials have been performed, and this agent has not recently been available for clinical investigation in the United States.

VASODILATOR THERAPY

The concept that cardiac performance may be improved by alteration of the resistance and capacitance of the peripheral circulation originated from hemodynamic investigations of vasodilator agents. Infusion of nitroprusside in patients with left ventricular dysfunction decreased elevated left ventricular filling pressures and increased cardiac output with minimal change in mean arterial pressure or heart rate. Similar responses were observed with other vasodilator drugs, and the specific hemodynamic action was related to the relative action of drug on venous or arterial vascular smooth muscle. In acute hemodynamic studies, vasodilators produce beneficial hemodynamic effects through either increased venous capacitance, yielding reduced preload, or reduced impedance (afterload) to left ventricular ejection (Fig 17-8).

Classification

Vasodilator drugs are classified according to mechanism and site of action. Direct-acting drugs exert dose-dependent vasodilatory effects on peripheral vessels, producing favorable hemodynamic changes in nearly all patients.[261] Neurohormonal antagonist drugs inhibit the action of endogenous vasoconstrictor hormones.

Drug efficacy

Hemodynamic values do not differentiate abnormalities of myocardial dysfunction from excessive peripheral vasoconstriction. Moreover, favorable short-term hemodynamic response does not reliably predict long-term patient benefit.[262-264] These observations indicate that improvement in hemodynamic abnormalities characteristic of left ventricular dysfunction should not be considered the standard by which long-term drug efficacy is judged.[265]

The degree of neurohormonal activation has been considered a possible guide to the selection of efficacious therapy for heart failure. Increased plasma catecholamine

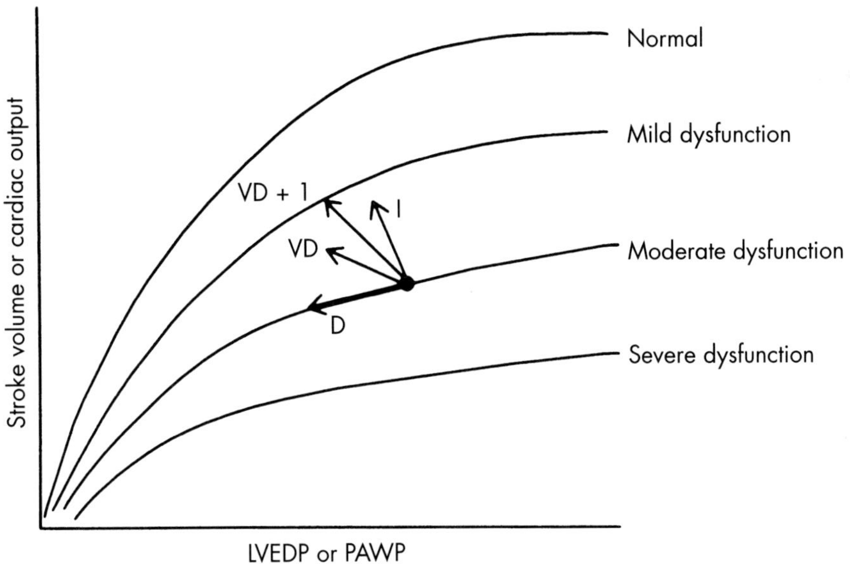

Fig 17-8 Hemodynamic benefit of vasodilator therapy with shift to a more favorable pressure-volume relationship (Frank-Starling curves). Diuretic *(D)* alone lowers left ventricular end-diastolic pressure *(LVEDP)*, yielding less pulmonary congestion but also lowering cardiac output. Inotropes *(I)* augment myocardial contractility, raising the ventricular function curve and yielding increased cardiac output. Vasodilators *(VD)* lower LVEDP and promote increased cardiac output through lowered impedance to ejection. The actions of VD and I are synergistic. *dysf.*, dysfunction; *PAWP*, pulmonary artery wedge pressure.

levels have been associated with a poor prognosis and may serve as an indicator of favorable response to vasodilator therapy.[8,9,17,266,267] Increased plasma renin activity has also been evaluated as a predictor of drug efficacy. However, long-term clinical hemodynamic responses have not been consistently predicted by pretreatment plasma renin activity.[268-273] The suboptimal correlation between plasma levels of neurohormones and the clinical and hemodynamic responses to antagonists of neurohormonal activity is not unexpected, since plasma levels of neurohormonal substances do not directly correspond to tissue receptor activity.[268,274]

The most useful approach to the selection of vasodilator drug therapy for patients with heart failure is based on results of clinical trials. In addition to digoxin and a diuretic, converting enzyme inhibition and the combination of hydralazine and isosorbide dinitrate are of demonstrated benefit. Although other agents result in hemodynamic changes that closely resemble those with digoxin, converting enzyme inhibitors, or the combination of hydralazine and nitrates, no other agents have proven superior to placebo in randomized, controlled trials. Successful therapies incorporate strategies for modulation of neurohormonal activity as well as hemodynamic variables in patients with heart failure. In the discussion that follows, vasodilator drug therapies are presented in two basic categories, direct-acting vasodilators and neurohormonal antagonists.

Direct-acting venous vasodilators

Nitrates were among the first vasodilators used for oral treatment in patients with severe heart failure. These agents primarily affect venous smooth muscle tone by activation of guanylate cyclase, which increases cyclic guanosine monophosphate and promotes vasorelaxation.

Systemic and right atrial pressures are acutely decreased with nitrate administration. The first dose of isosorbide dinitrate has also been shown to decrease resting and exercise systemic and pulmonary arterial pressures and pulmonary capillary wedge pressures but has not been shown to improve maximum exercise hemodynamics or exercise capacity.[275-278] Isosorbide dinitrate is the only direct-acting venodilator that produces a sustained decrease in left ventricular filling pressure and is the direct-acting agent least likely to be associated with activation of endogenous neurohormonal systems.[279] Long-term administration of isosorbide dinitrate, unlike that of placebo, has been demonstrated to improve long-term hemodynamics and exercise capacity and relieve symptoms in patients with moderate to severe heart failure.[276] Similar observations have been reported for patients with severe heart failure.[279]

Rest and exercise systemic blood pressures and vascular resistance return to pretreatment values during long-term administration of isosorbide dinitrate. However, pulmonary blood pressures, vascular resistance, and capillary wedge pressure remain improved. Hence, nitrate tolerance develops to the arterial but not to the systemic or pulmonary venous action. Because of the lack of chronic systemic arterial effects and the lack of direct myocardial or neurohumoral activating effects, nitrates may benefit patients with pulmonary hypertension.

Nitrates should be considered adjunctive therapy; converting enzyme inhibitors are the drugs of choice given the survival benefit demonstrated in clinical trials such as the second Veterans Administration Cooperative Vasodilator-Heart Failure Trial (V-HeFT II) (see below).[16] In patients for whom converting enzyme inhibitors are contraindicated, the combination of isosorbide dinitrate and hydralazine is indicated.[280]

Direct-acting arterial vasodilators

In general, clinically relevant decreases in left ventricular filling pressure or volumes are not sustained by arterial vasodilators. The loss of vasodilator action is due to tolerance or activation of endogenous neurohormonal vasoconstrictor mechanisms that counter hemodynamic improvement by promotion of peripheral vasoconstriction. Intracardiac filling pressures may actually increase because of sodium retention induced by arterial vasodilators. Utility is limited by the relatively high incidence of side effects, including headache, gastrointestinal upset, tachycardia, and edema.

Hydralazine. Hydralazine is an orally active, direct-acting agent that produces primarily arteriolar dilatation. The afterload-reducing effect yields an increase in cardiac output, with minor reduction of ventricular filling and arterial pressure and a small increase in heart rate in patients with heart failure. The usual dosage range is 25 to 100 mg three or four times per day, with onset within 30 minutes and duration of approximately 6 hours. There is significant first-pass hepatic metabolism via acetylation, which affects the bioavailability of the drug. Bioavailability is approximately 30% in patients with rapid acetylation and 50% in those with slow acetylation. The absorption of hydralazine taken with food is increased.

Drug-specific tolerance to hydralazine occurs in approximately 30% of patients in whom the hemodynamic response is initially favorable. There is no observed benefit to increased doses in this situation. Sustained hemodynamic effect generally is indicative of long-term clinical benefit.[281] At high doses, hydralazine may exert an inotropic action.

Four general types of adverse reactions have been described with hydralazine. The first is headache, flushing, and palpitations, occurring in approximately one-third of patients, which may be severe but typically are of short duration and seldom require withdrawal of medication. A second type is nausea and vomiting, which are the most common indications to discontinue therapy. The third is provocation of myocardial ischemia, which may occur in 25% of patients with ischemic left ventricular dysfunction.[282] The fourth category of adverse reaction is systemic lupus erythematosus or lupus-like syndrome, generally not observed in patients receiving less than 200 mg per day. Both the lupus-like syndrome and a peripheral neuropathy secondary to pyridoxine deficiency are more likely to develop in patients who have slow acetylation.[282] Drug-induced lupus subsides when medication is discontinued.

Hydralazine used in combination with nitrates has been

shown to improve exercise tolerance and ejection fraction and improve survival in patients with mild to moderate heart failure.[16,280,283] In the first Veterans Administration Cooperative Vasodilator-Heart Failure Trial (V-HeFT I) study, male patients with impaired cardiac function and reduced exercise capacity were assigned to treatment with placebo, hydralazine (300 mg per day) and isosorbide dinitrate (160 mg per day), or prazosin (20 mg per day). Mortality at 3 years of follow-up was reduced from approximately 47% in the placebo group to 36% in the group treated with hydralazine and isosorbide dinitrate; no benefit was observed for the placebo or prazosin groups. Other studies have not clearly demonstrated a difference between hydralazine and placebo in the long-term treatment of heart failure.

Minoxidil. Minoxidil is an orally administered, direct-acting arterial vasodilator with actions on arterial smooth muscle comparable to those of hydralazine. Its duration of action is relatively long, with hemodynamic effects after a single dose persisting up to 8 hours.[284,285] Virtually all orally administered minoxidil is recovered in the urine. Dosage adjustment is not necessary for patients with renal failure. Short- and long-term hemodynamic responses are similar to those in patients treated with hydralazine.[284,286-288] Symptomatic improvement appears to correlate with hemodynamic improvement.[287,288] Most patients have a response to a dose of 20 mg twice a day.[284]

Minoxidil has not been widely used in therapy for patients with heart failure. The greater frequency of adverse effects with minoxidil than with other direct-acting vasodilators limits its usefulness.[281,286-289] Like hydralazine, minoxidil yields increased catecholamines and plasma renin activity.[286] Fluid retention, pericardial effusion with or without tamponade, and pericarditis have been reported in hypertensive patients;[290] angina or hypotension may also occur with minoxidil.[286,290] Hypertrichosis is often observed and may be particularly prominent around the face, arms, and back. This drug should be considered a third-line agent to be used only if patients are unable to tolerate converting enzyme inhibitors or the combination of hydralazine and isosorbide dinitrate.

Calcium channel antagonists

The extent of calcium channel blocker use in the treatment of patients with chronic congestive heart failure is not known. Recent published trials suggest that more than 30% of patients enrolled in the Studies of Left Ventricular Dysfunction (SOLVD) were treated with calcium blockers at enrollment.[15,17] However, available data demonstrate no survival or symptom benefit and increased morbidity associated with first-generation calcium antagonists for patients with left ventricular dysfunction. Hemodynamic and clinical deterioration have been demonstrated, and there has been an increase in the incidence of cardiovascular morbidity and mortality after myocardial infarction in patients with heart failure. Despite the anti-ischemic effects of calcium channel antagonists, unfavorable effects of these drugs in patients with chronic heart failure after myocardial infarction and in patients with heart failure due to chronic coronary artery disease suggest that first-generation calcium channel antagonists are detrimental for patients with chronic heart failure, including those with ischemic heart disease.[291-293]

Two randomized trials of the long-term effects of nifedipine in patients with heart failure have been reported. In one study, the effects of captopril and nifedipine given for 8 weeks were compared in a double-blind crossover design in patients with dilated cardiomyopathy who were treated with digoxin and diuretics.[294] Functional and symptomatic improvement and enhancement of exercise tolerance occurred with captopril but not with nifedipine. Another study compared the long-term administration of isosorbide dinitrate, nifedipine, and a combination of the two agents in patients with mild to moderate heart failure.[295] Results were unfavorable for nifedipine therapy, because a significantly higher incidence of deterioration requiring increased diuretic therapy or hospitalization was associated with nifedipine alone or in combination with isosorbide dinitrate.

The Multicenter Diltiazem Postinfarction Trial[296] provided information on long-term use of diltiazem in patients with heart failure (Fig 17-9). This study compared the efficacy of diltiazem at 240 mg per day with that of placebo on mortality and reinfarction in approximately 1,200 patients 3 to 15 days after myocardial infarction. The results showed that chronic heart failure was more likely to develop during follow-up in patients with pulmonary congestion, anterolateral Q-wave myocardial infarction, or ejection fraction of less than 40% than in comparably treated patients without these clinical characteristics. Additionally, an inverse relationship was demonstrated between diltiazem-associated development of chronic heart failure and severity of left ventricular dysfunction. Experience with verapamil has been similar to that reported for nifedipine and diltiazem.

The cause of clinical deterioration associated with calcium channel antagonists in patients with heart failure is unclear. Acute hemodynamic deterioration most likely is related to negative inotropic effects.[295,297-302] Clinical deterioration despite hemodynamic improvement has also been observed and suggests detrimental neurohormonal activation. Activation of the sympathetic nervous system, renin-angiotensin-aldosterone system, and vasopressin systems has been demonstrated with calcium channel blockers.[301,303,304] Another potential adverse action of calcium channel antagonists may be increased blood volume associated with congestion.

Felodipine, a calcium channel antagonist of the dihydropyridine group, has negligible negative inotropic effects and a relatively high selectivity for vascular smooth muscle.[305] The third Veterans Administration Cooperative Vasodilator-Heart Failure Trial (V-HeFT III) will compare the efficacy of felodipine and placebo on morbidity and mortality in patients with mild to moderate heart failure. Background therapy will include diuretics, ACE inhibitors, and digoxin. The Prospective Randomized Amlodipine Survival Evaluation (PRASE) trial is comparing amlodipine, a vasoselective calcium channel antagonist, with placebo for the effect on survival in

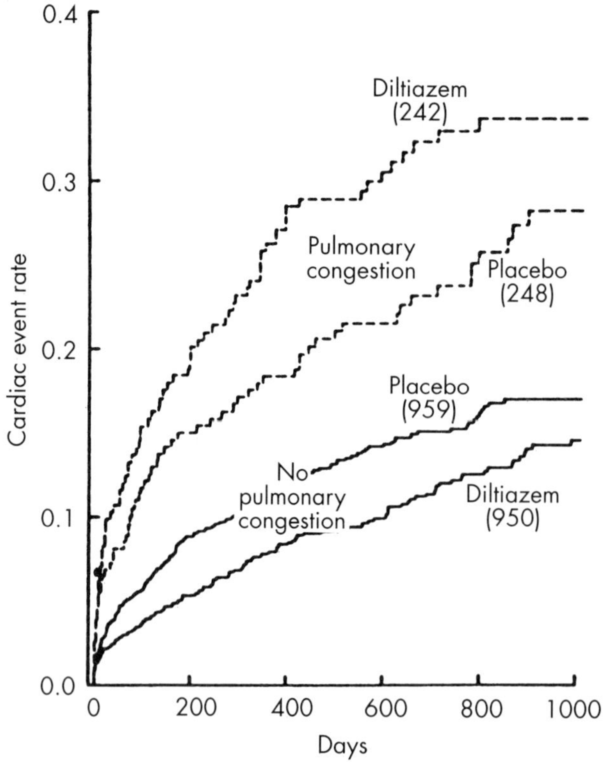

Fig 17-9 Cumulative rate of recurrent cardiac events in patients with and without pulmonary congestion (chest radiograph) after blind randomization to diltiazem or placebo therapy. (From The Multicenter Diltiazem Postinfarction Trial Research Group: The effect of diltiazem on mortality and reinfarction after myocardial infarction. *N Engl J Med* 319:385-392, 1988. By permission of the journal.)

patients with classes III and IV heart failure. These studies will provide information necessary to determine whether calcium channel antagonists have a place in the treatment of chronic heart failure secondary to left ventricular systolic dysfunction when used in combination with neurohormonal antagonists.

NEUROHORMONAL ANTAGONIST THERAPY

Converting enzyme inhibitors

The greatest success in the treatment of heart failure has been with the converting enzyme inhibitors. ACE inhibitors approved for the treatment of heart failure include captopril, enalapril, and lisinopril. Only captopril and enalapril have demonstrated survival benefit. Evidence to support the efficacy of converting enzyme inhibition in patients with heart failure has been demonstrated for all functional classes, including asymptomatic left ventricular dysfunction.[15,16,18,70,306-319] Converting enzyme inhibitors have been shown to improve symptoms, increase exercise tolerance, prolong life, attenuate progressive left ventricular enlargement after myocardial infarction, and delay onset of symptoms and frequency of hospitalizations in patients with asymptomatic left ventricular dysfunction (Fig 17-10).

Although converting enzyme inhibitors differ in structure and pharmacokinetics, efficacy and general mechanisms of action are comparable. The major mechanism of action of the orally active agents captopril, enalapril, and lisinopril is the inhibition of ACE, which converts inactive angiotensin I to angiotensin II. The ACE is also responsible for inactivating bradykinin and other kinins that exert direct vasodilator effects and stimulate endogenous synthesis and release of vasoactive prostaglandins, particularly in the kidney. Potentiation of bradykinin may be responsible for several actions of the converting enzyme inhibitors. Converting enzyme inhibitors also decrease plasma aldosterone and plasma catecholamine levels with long-term therapy.[308] Long-term benefits of reducing increased catecholamine levels may contribute to the improved prognosis in patients with heart failure.[320]

In patients with severe heart failure and hyponatremia, the hyponatremia can often be corrected without fluid restriction by initiation of converting enzyme inhibition therapy and by continued therapy with a diuretic such as furosemide.[69,321,322] The correction of hyponatremia with converting enzyme inhibition is consistent with suppression of angiotensin production, since angiotensin impairs renal free water clearance by stimulating release of antidiuretic hormone[323] and decreasing renal blood flow and glomerular filtration rate.[324] Angiotensin also

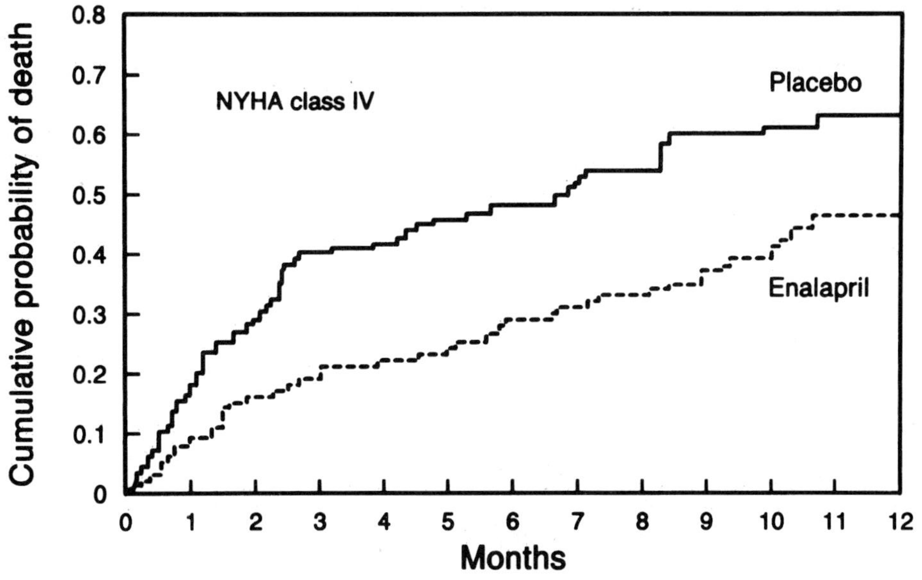

Fig 17-10 Benefit of converting enzyme inhibition therapy on cumulative probability of death in patients with heart failure randomized to placebo or enalapril therapy in the Cooperative North Scandinavian Enalapril Survival Study (CONSENSUS I). *NYHA,* New York Heart Association. (From The CONSENSUS Trial Study Group: Effects of enalapril on mortality in severe congestive heart failure. Results of the Cooperative North Scandinavian Enalapril Survival Study (CONSENSUS). *N Engl J Med* 316:1429-1435, 1987. By permission of the journal.)

increases free water accumulation by stimulating the hypothalamic thirst center.[325] Hence, converting enzyme inhibitors facilitate correction of hyponatremia by decreasing thirst and water intake, improving renal function, and decreasing the release of antidiuretic hormone.

Captopril. The absorption of captopril is rapid, with peak blood levels observed in 30 to 90 minutes. In the fasting state, absorption is improved to 75% of the administered dose. Food in the gastrointestinal tract decreases absorption by 40%. Captopril is rapidly metabolized; the half-life of unchanged drug in normal subjects is less than 2 hours.[326] Higher peak plasma concentrations of captopril occur in patients with renal insufficiency, and dose reduction is necessary.

The hemodynamic effects of converting enzyme inhibitors are related to inhibition of angiotensin II.[327] In patients with heart failure, the decrease in mean arterial pressure is greater than that with direct vasodilator agents.[328] Captopril has also been reported to produce a greater decrease in pulmonary capillary wedge pressure than nitroprusside, perhaps because of increased ventricular compliance by inhibition of angiotensin II.[328] Hemodynamic tolerance is not observed, because reduced left ventricular filling pressure at rest and during exercise and decreased systemic vascular resistance are sustained.[262,329]

Symptomatic hypotension after the first dose of converting enzyme inhibitor is more likely to develop in patients with heart failure complicated by severe hyponatremia than in patients with normal serum sodium levels.[330] Acute hypotension appears to be due to decreased arterial vasoconstriction by angiotensin and may be potentiated by the withdrawal of the positive inotropic effect of angiotensin.[331] An acute hypotensive response to administration of converting enzyme inhibitor can be eliminated or substantially attenuated by withholding diuretic therapy for 12 hours before beginning converting enzyme inhibitor therapy. Symptomatic hypotension occurring more than 1 week after initiation of therapy most likely is due to excessive reduction in left ventricular filling pressure.[330] Other adverse effects of converting enzyme inhibitors are azotemia and hyperkalemia, which can be avoided or minimized by reductions of diuretic dose, often without the need to reduce the dose of converting enzyme inhibitor.

The captopril dose in most randomized, controlled trials associated with improved exercise tolerance and survival has ranged from 150 to 300 mg per day in three divided doses.[307,310,314] It cannot be assumed that low doses produce optimal improvement in exercise tolerance and survival. On the basis of results of large clinical trials (described below), the choice favors captopril at 150 mg per day in three divided doses. Additionally, observations from clinical trials support the necessity of suppressing neurohormonal overactivation with higher doses ($>$75 mg per day) of captopril, as reflected by sequential neurohormonal plasma measurements.[332]

The action of captopril is attenuated by indomethacin and other cyclooxygenase inhibitors.[333] In patients with heart failure, prostaglandin synthetase inhibition by aspirin has been reported to counteract the vasodilator action of captopril.[334] This action of aspirin may limit the benefit of converting enzyme inhibitor therapy for patients with heart failure or patients who have reduced left ventricular function after myocardial infarction.

Other ACE inhibitors. The dose of enalapril used in large randomized clinical trials has ranged from 20 to 40 mg per day in two divided doses. Once-a-day dose preparations of lisinopril and ramipril are also being evaluated for clinical efficacy in large trials. Acute once-a-day oral administration of ACE inhibitor has not demonstrated an increased incidence of hypotension over that with multidose preparations. Three to 6 months of treatment are required before the full therapeutic effect of converting enzyme inhibition is apparent.[314,335]

Side effects with converting enzyme inhibitor therapy include maculopapular rash, which may be accompanied by pruritus, fever, and eosinophilia; it is usually transient, occurring during the first several weeks of therapy or when the dose is advanced. Symptoms and findings often resolve within 7 to 10 days after dose reduction. Rash and dysgeusia are observed with all converting enzyme inhibitors, most frequently with captopril. Cough and angioneurotic edema occur with a similar frequency for all converting enzyme inhibitors and may be related to the accumulation of tissue kinins. Cough may be especially prominent in patients with advanced heart failure and be difficult to discriminate from pulmonary congestion due to heart failure. Agranulocytosis has been reported, most often in severely ill patients receiving multiple drug regimens, and is reversible with discontinuation of the medication.[336] Ageusia is drug-related and usually transient with continued administration but has been reported to occur in approximately 6% of patients.[337]

β-Adrenergic receptor blockers

β-Adrenergic blockade is an investigational therapy for heart failure and is not appropriate for acute or decompensated heart failure. Clinical and hemodynamic deterioration can occur abruptly, with dire consequences. In investigational trials of heart failure, 10% to 20% of patients have not tolerated β-blocker therapy.[338] However, increasing evidence indicates that β-blocker therapy will eventually play a role in the management of patients with heart failure. The benefits of β-blocker therapy require a minimum of 3 to 6 months to be realized and may be preceded by transient deterioration in the early phase of therapy. Fatigue and shortness of breath with exertion are common complaints.

β-Blockers are of demonstrated usefulness in the reduction of mortality and sudden death in patients with congestive heart failure after myocardial infarction.[339-343] β-Blockers may also reduce mortality in patients with chronic heart failure of nonischemic cause.[344,345] Evidence from several studies, including V-HeFT I, suggests that prognosis is significantly worse with ischemia than with a nonischemic cause of impaired left ventricular function.[280,346] Lichstein[340] examined the relationship among correlates of left ventricular function (ejection fraction, rales, S_3 gallop, pulmonary congestion), probability of congestive heart failure developing, and β-blocker use in patients with ischemic left ventricular dysfunction. The results of this study of approximately 1,000 patients indicated that the risk of congestive heart failure and death was less for patients receiving β-blocker therapy. The benefit of β-blocker therapy was greatest among the patients with the most severely impaired left ventricular function. Data from the Metoprolol in Acute Myocardial Infarction (MIAMI) trial[342] and the Beta-Blocker Heart Attack Trial (BHAT) (propranolol)[339] also supported significant benefit in high-risk patients with congestive heart failure after infarction. A benefit of β-blockers in decreasing ventricular ectopy and sudden death has also been shown in patients with impaired left ventricular function.[339,347,348]

β-Blocker therapy has also been associated with functional and hemodynamic improvement, particularly in nonischemic heart disease.[344,349-354] Engelmeier et al.[355] used a double-blind, randomized, placebo-controlled design to demonstrate improvement in exercise capacity, functional class, and left ventricular ejection fraction in patients with idiopathic dilated cardiomyopathy treated with metoprolol. Subsequent studies confirmed hemodynamic improvement, including increased ejection fraction and stroke work in association with reduced filling pressures, after long-term treatment with metoprolol in patients with idiopathic dilated cardiomyopathy.[344,356] Heilbrunn et al.[356] demonstrated that graded doses of the β-agonist dobutamine (2 to 8 μg/kg per minute) during β-blocker treatment produced increased responsiveness and that metoprolol withdrawal resulted in clinical deterioration.

Woodley et al.[357] conducted a double-blind, randomized, placebo-controlled trial of bucindolol in patients with both ischemic and nonischemic heart failure. Patients were assessed by right heart catheterization, echocardiography, exercise testing, and plasma catecholamine levels. Compared with baseline values obtained before randomization, left ventricular dimension, ejection fraction, stroke work, and filling pressures improved. However, the observed benefits occurred primarily in the subgroup of patients without coronary artery disease.

Cause-specific response to β-blockade in heart failure was also observed in the study of Anderson et al.,[358] in which hemodynamic and myocardial metabolism at rest and during exercise were studied in 21 patients with either ischemic or nonischemic left ventricular dysfunction. Patients received long-term therapy with metoprolol (mean, 14 months). Those with nonischemic cardiomyopathy had significant clinical improvement, whereas the group with ischemia-related ventricular dysfunction did not have improvement. Although hemodynamic and clinical improvement with long-term β-adrenergic blockade have been demonstrated, the mechanism of these favorable actions is not understood. Neurohormonal antagonism with β-blocker therapy tends to reduce myocardial oxygen consumption through decreased heart rate and blood pressure and to directly antagonize the actions of catecholamines at the myocardium and peripheral vasculature.

Down-regulation of β_1-receptor density occurs with heart failure and generally is in proportion to severity.[359] Up-regulation (restoration of receptor density) occurs with β-blocker therapy and has been associated with restoration of the contractile response to catecholamines.[344,356,360] However, no conclusive cause-and-effect relationship exists between up-regulation of β-receptor density and clinical response to β-blockade.[356,361] β-Receptor up-regulation occurs within hours to days, but the clinical and hemodynamic benefits of β-blocker therapy are delayed. Additional mechanisms must be considered to explain the clinical benefit of β-blocker therapy.[362]

The type of β-blocking agent is also an issue in a large number of reported studies using the B_1-selective agent metoprolol. Nonselective β-blockers antagonize all β-receptors and have the potential of permitting unopposed vasoconstriction modulated by α-receptors.

Bucindolol and carvedilol are investigational nonselective β-blockers that possess peripheral vasodilating properties. Bucindolol improved ejection fraction and functional class and stabilized exercise performance in double-blind, placebo-controlled short-term (3 months)[363] and long-term (2 years)[358] studies. Evidence of improved myocardial contractility and diastolic relaxation has also been reported for bucindolol.[364] After 3 months of therapy (100 mg b.i.d. titrated from 12.5 mg b.i.d. over 5 weeks), two load-independent indices of contractility, end-systolic elastance and positive dp/dt, increased. Bucindolol also reduced pulmonary artery pressure and pulmonary artery resistance.

α-Adrenergic blockers

α-Adrenergic receptor blockade for treatment of heart failure has been attempted to antagonize catecholamine-mediated peripheral vasoconstriction. Acute hemodynamic benefit has been observed with the nonselective α-blockers phentolamine and phenoxybenzamine; prazosin, a selective postsynaptic α_1-adrenergic antagonist, also produces short-term hemodynamic benefit in patients with heart failure.[365-367] However, the development of tolerance has limited the long-term benefit of α-adrenergic antagonists in patients with heart failure. Hemodynamic tolerance may occur as early as 24 to 48 hours after initiation of therapy.[367-374] Double-blind, placebo-controlled trials evaluating prazosin and other α-adrenergic blocking agents have not demonstrated sustained therapeutic benefit despite lower mean arterial pressure.[280,368-373,375] Moreover, the randomized, placebo-controlled V-HeFT I trial demonstrated no survival benefit or improvement in left ventricular function.[280]

Central adrenergic inhibitors

Clonidine, methyldopa, and guanabenz are adrenergic inhibitors that act within the central nervous system by stimulating α_2-adrenergic receptors. These agents decrease plasma catecholamine levels; however, the favorable neurohormonal action does not result in significant hemodynamic effects. In patients with heart failure, these agents generally reduce mean arterial pressure and heart rate rather than increase cardiac output.[376,377] The reduction in blood pressure and heart rate probably results from a decrease in positive inotropic and chronotropic actions mediated by the sympathetic nervous system. Because of the frequent disabling sedation and unfavorable hemodynamic side effects, there has been little enthusiasm for long-term trials with centrally acting adrenergic inhibitors in patients with left ventricular dysfunction.

CLINICAL TRIALS OF VASODILATOR THERAPY

Symptomatic left ventricular dysfunction

The first large, randomized, double-blind trial of vasodilator therapy to assess mortality from symptomatic congestive heart failure was the Veterans Administration heart failure trial (V-HeFT I). The results of this trial demonstrated that the combination of hydralazine and isosorbide dinitrate added to baseline therapy consisting of digitalis and diuretics improved survival of patients with classes II and III heart failure.[280] The results of the Cooperative North Scandinavian Enalapril Survival Study (CONSENSUS) trial were reported 1 year later[309] (see Fig 17-10) and demonstrated that the addition of enalapril to conventional therapy in patients with class IV congestive heart failure also relieved symptoms and reduced mortality; after 6 months of therapy with converting enzyme inhibitor, the difference in mortality between the placebo group (conventional therapy; mortality rate, 44%) and the enalapril-treated group (6-month mortality rate, 26%) was highly significant. The beneficial effect on mortality was shown to be due to a reduction in death from progression of heart failure.

The SOLVD studies were undertaken to determine whether mortality could be reduced by the ACE inhibitor enalapril in patients with symptomatic (treatment trial) and asymptomatic (prevention trial) left ventricular dysfunction (Fig 17-11). The primary end point was all-cause mortality, and the secondary end points were cardiovascular mortality, sudden death, myocardial infarction, and cerebrovascular accident. Hospital admissions for congestive heart failure and quality of life were also assessed. For the patients in the prevention arm, the onset of symptomatic congestive heart failure was determined. The results of the treatment arm[15] indicated that enalapril in a dose of 10 mg twice a day compared with placebo had a survival benefit in patients with New York Heart Association classes II and III heart failure. The incidence of recurrent myocardial infarction was also reduced, and virtually all survival benefit was due to reduction of progressive heart failure.

The second Veterans Administration heart failure trial (V-HeFT II) (Fig 17-12) was designed to provide a direct comparison of enalapril and the combination of hydralazine and isosorbide dinitrate in patients with classes II and III heart failure.[16] Patients were randomly assigned to either enalapril (10 mg b.i.d.) or hydralazine (75 mg q.i.d.) and isosorbide dinitrate (40 mg t.i.d.). A significant survival benefit of enalapril over the combination of hydralazine and isosorbide dinitrate was observed at 2-year follow-up. In long-term follow-up, the hydralazine-isosorbide dinitrate combination produced a more signif-

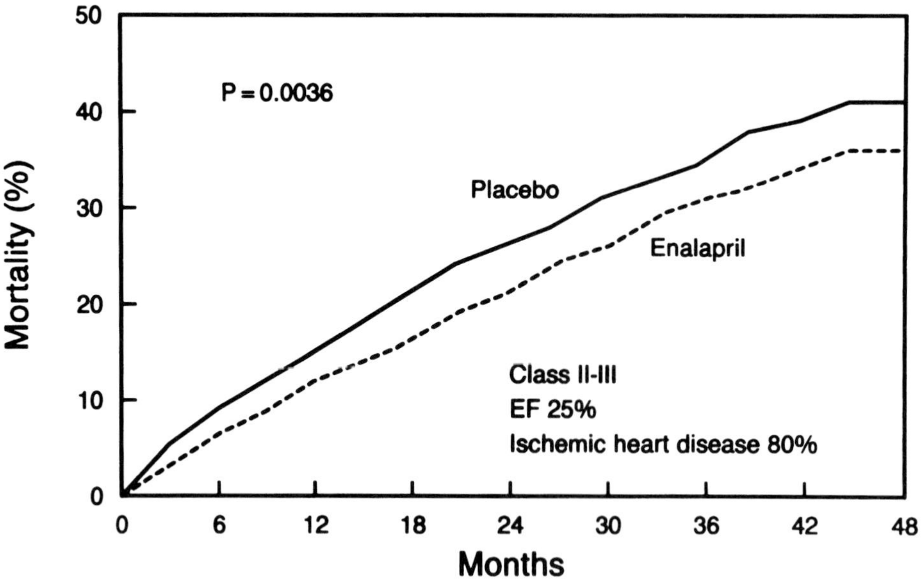

Fig 17-11 Benefit of enalapril therapy on cumulative mortality in patients with heart failure in the Studies of Left Ventricular Dysfunction (SOLVD). *EF,* ejection fraction. (From The SOLVD Investigators: Effect of enalapril on survival in patients with reduced left ventricular ejection fractions and congestive heart failure. *N Engl J Med* 325:293-302, 1991. By permission of the journal.)

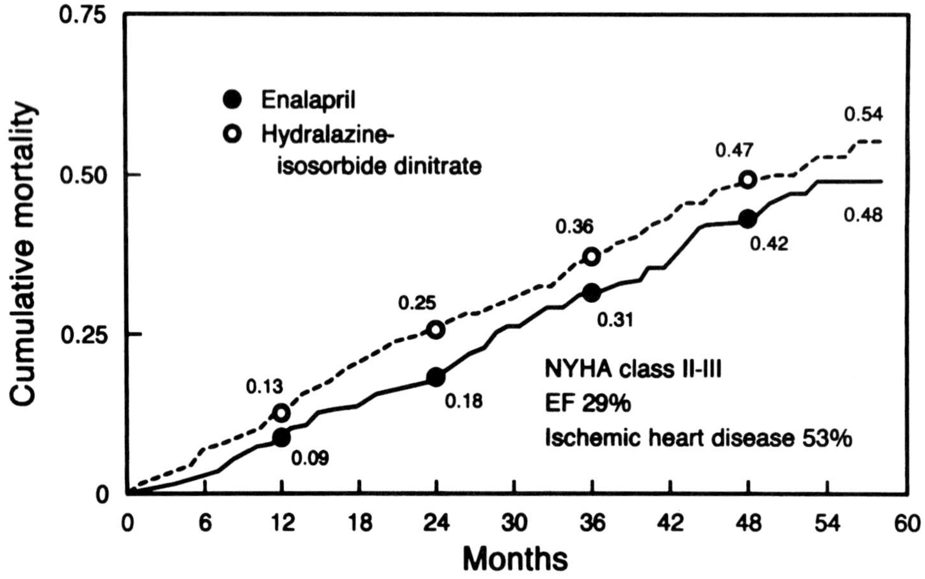

Fig 17-12 Comparative benefit of converting enzyme inhibition treatment and hydralazine-isosorbide dinitrate therapy on cumulative mortality in patients with heart failure in the Second Veterans Administration Cooperative Vasodilator-Heart Failure Trial (V-HeFT II). *EF,* ejection fraction; *NYHA,* New York Heart Association. (From Cohn JN, Johnson G, Ziesche S, et al: A comparison of enalapril with hydralazine-isosorbide dinitrate in the treatment of chronic congestive heart failure. *N Engl J Med* 325:303-310, 1991. By permission of the journal.)

icant improvement in peak exercise oxygen consumption and left ventricular ejection fraction than did enalapril. However, the 2-year mortality rate was significantly lower in the enalapril-treated patients. In contrast to the finding of the SOLVD trial, nearly all survival benefit for patients in V-HeFT II was due to a reduction in sudden death. These observations suggest that vasodilator drugs and ACE inhibitors may act through a different mechanism to improve prognosis in heart failure.

V-HeFT II demonstrated that enalapril therapy was associated with significantly lower plasma and norepinephrine concentration than that associated with the combination of hydralazine and isosorbide dinitrate and with less frequent emergence of ventricular tachycardia on serial Holter monitoring.[268] These observations suggest that direct-acting vasodilators and converting enzyme inhibitors used in combination may be more efficacious than either agent alone. V-HeFT III will test this hypothesis by use of the vasoselective calcium antagonist felodipine in combination with enalapril.

The Hy-C Trial[315] compared captopril with hydralazine, with both groups receiving isosorbide dinitrate (88% of the hydralazine-treated patients and 84% of the captopril-treated patients). The hemodynamic improvements were comparable for each treatment regimen. However, actuarial survival at 1 year was 81% for the captopril-treated patients and 51% for the hydralazine-treated patients. As in the V-HeFT II study, the improved survival with captopril resulted from a decrease in sudden death.[315]

Asymptomatic left ventricular dysfunction and progression of left ventricular dysfunction

The SAVE (Survival and Ventricular Enlargement) trial assessed the efficacy of captopril and placebo for the prevention of heart failure in asymptomatic patients with myocardial infarction and an ejection fraction of less than 40%. Administration of captopril began 3 to 16 days after myocardial infarction, with titration as tolerated to 50 mg twice a day. Patients assigned to captopril had a 19% reduction in death. The survival benefits were evident in patients who received thrombolytic therapy, aspirin, and β-blockers and in those who did not receive such therapy.[316]

A second study assessing the efficacy of converting enzyme inhibitor therapy for the prevention of heart failure in patients with asymptomatic left ventricular dysfunction was in the prevention arm of the SOLVD.[18] In this trial, enalapril significantly reduced the incidence of heart failure and hospitalizations over that with placebo. However, for a relatively short duration of follow-up, enalapril did not benefit survival. The SAVE trial and prevention arm of the SOLVD indicate a role for the use of converting enzyme inhibitors in the prevention of congestive heart failure.

The CONSENSUS II trial demonstrated no clear survival benefit when intravenous administration of enalaprilat was followed by oral administration of enalapril during the acute (<24 hours) phase of myocardial infarction.[317] Because the initial follow-up in the trial was 6 months, a longer period may be necessary to demonstrate that converting enzyme inhibition benefits patients who have had acute myocardial infarction.

The impact of converting enzyme inhibition on the progression of chronic heart failure was studied in the Munich Mild Heart Failure Trial,[378] in which 170 patients with New York Heart Association functional class II status and a mean ejection fraction of 35% were randomized to double-blind treatment with captopril (25 mg twice a day) or placebo in addition to baseline therapy with digoxin, diuretic, and vasodilator. Progression of heart failure to class IV status occurred in 10.8% of patients treated with captopril and 26.4% receiving placebo. Fewer deaths caused by progressive heart failure were noted in the captopril group than in the placebo group, but similar numbers of sudden deaths occurred in each group. Progressive heart failure was the cause of death in 18.2% of all patients in the captopril group and 50% in the placebo group at the end of a median observation period of 2.7 years. In long-term follow-up, the captopril group had a significant reduction in death due to progressive heart failure; the incidence of death due to pump failure was 7% in this group and 28% in the placebo group at 5 years.[378] The results of this study suggest that the benefit of converting enzyme inhibition is mediated primarily through prevention of progression of heart failure. As in CONSENSUS I and the SOLVD trials, there was no treatment benefit on sudden death in the Munich Mild Heart Failure Trial.

The CONSENSUS I study, in which the 1-year mortality in patients with severe (class IV) heart failure was 47% despite converting enzyme inhibition therapy, demonstrates that mortality remains high when therapy is administered at a late stage of disease. Results of more recent trials suggest that converting enzyme inhibition therapy and perhaps additional vasodilator therapy have a favorable influence in patients with progressive heart failure. Hence, an emphasis on identification of patients with asymptomatic left ventricular dysfunction is critical to maximize the benefit of pharmacotherapy on improving survival and quality of life in this patient population.

ANTITHROMBOTIC THERAPY

Chronic congestive heart failure is associated with an increased risk for venous and arterial thromboembolism. Hence, patients with chronic congestive heart failure should have prophylactic anticoagulation with either intravenous heparin or warfarin. Long-term follow-up of patients with idiopathic dilated cardiomyopathy demonstrated that systemic thromboemboli were confined to patients not receiving an oral anticoagulant regimen.[379] Systemic thromboembolism occurred in 18% of patients (3.5 events per 100 patient-years) not receiving anticoagulant therapy and in no patient receiving anticoagulant orally; the risk of systemic thromboembolism was increased with coexistent atrial fibrillation. Deep venous thromboembolism of the lower extremities and pulmonary embolism are also common in patients with chronic congestive heart failure and can be prevented.

Hence, long-term oral anticoagulation therapy should

be administered to patients with heart failure associated with a dilated left ventricle and an ejection fraction of less than 35% unless such therapy is contraindicated. All patients with heart failure and atrial fibrillation should have anticoagulation regardless of the ejection fraction.[380] The therapeutic range of anticoagulation should be 1.3 to 1.8 times control (international normalized ratio, 2.0 to 4.0). The prothrombin time should be monitored approximately monthly for as long as the patient is receiving therapy.

PHARMACOTHERAPY OF VENTRICULAR ARRHYTHMIA

Sudden death remains a major cause of mortality in patients with chronic congestive heart failure; it is estimated that 40% to 50% of patients with chronic heart failure die suddenly, presumably because of ventricular arrhythmia.[381,382] Ambulatory electrocardiographic monitoring identifies patients at increased risk through the detection of complex ventricular ectopy.[383] Although patients at increased risk may be identified, no satisfactory management approach has yet been described for those with asymptomatic ventricular ectopy and left ventricular dysfunction (see chapters 22C and 24A). Prophylactic empiric antiarrhythmic therapy in this group has been associated with an unacceptably high incidence of proarrhythmia.[382] Furthermore, antiarrhythmic drugs have negative inotropic actions, which tend to exacerbate heart failure.[384] Sustained symptomatic ventricular tachycardia in this patient group can be managed successfully when aided by invasive electrophysiologic testing; therapy may be by drugs, cardioverter-defibrillator, or surgery (see chapters 22C and 22D).

PHARMACOTHERAPY OF DIASTOLIC VENTRICULAR DYSFUNCTION

Therapeutic strategies for patients with chronic congestive heart failure due to primary diastolic dysfunction differ considerably from those used in the management of systolic dysfunction.[385] If there is no underlying remediable cause (see chapter 16), pharmacotherapy is directed at relief of pulmonary and systemic venous congestion. This is generally achieved through the judicious use of diuretics. Diuretic therapy should be commenced in a low dose in the outpatient setting to avoid hypotension, because these patients typically require increased intracardiac filling pressures to sustain adequate cardiac output. Nitrates are also useful in the reduction of preload and thereby relieve symptoms of pulmonary venous congestion.

Digoxin and arterial vasodilators should generally be avoided. In principle, digoxin therapy may increase diastolic ventricular wall stiffness by increasing cytosolic calcium, and increased myocardial contractility may predispose to dynamic left ventricular outflow obstruction in patients with hypertensive heart disease. Arterial vasodilators (e.g., hydralazine) may also produce dynamic left ventricular outflow obstruction in patients by excessively reducing left ventricular impedance.

Calcium antagonists may be of some use in these patients, because positive lusitropic actions of the calcium blockers may enhance ventricular filling and thereby relieve pulmonary congestion. Maintenance of sinus rhythm is particularly important in this subgroup of patients, as loss of atrial ventricular synchrony is often associated with a significant reduction of cardiac output and symptoms of pulmonary congestion. Similarly, if sinus tachycardia is present, slowing the sinus rate with either β-blockers or calcium blockers may ameliorate symptoms by increasing diastolic filling time. ACE inhibitor therapy has an uncertain role, but it may be beneficial in the hypertensive patient because it may facilitate regression of left ventricular hypertrophy and improve ventricular compliance.

REFERENCES

1. Massie BM, Packer M: Congestive heart failure: current controversies and future prospects. *Am J Cardiol* 66:429-430, 1990
2. National Center for Health Statistics: Inpatient utilization of short-stay hospitals by diagnosis: United States, 1968-1980. Rockville and Hyattville, Maryland: National Center for Health Statistics, 1974-1984; DHEW and DHHS publications. *Vital Health Stat [13]*
3. Graves EJ: Detailed diagnoses and procedures, National Hospital Discharge Survey, 1989. Hyattsville, Maryland: National Center for Health Statistics 1991; DHHS Publication no. (PHS) 91-1769. *Vital Health Stat [13]* no. 108
4. Benenson E (ed): *United Network of Organ Sharing Bulletin.* Vol. 8. Richmond, Virginia, 1993
5. Hastillo A, Hess ML: Heart xenografting: a route not yet to trod (editorial). *J Heart Lung Transplant* 12:3-4, 1993
6. Francis GS, Goldsmith SR, Levine TB, et al: The neurohumoral axis in congestive heart failure. *Ann Intern Med* 101:370-377, 1984
7. Hirsch AT, Dzau VJ, Creager MA: Baroreceptor function in congestive heart failure: effect on neurohumoral activation and regional vascular resistance. *Circulation* 75 Suppl 4:36-48, 1987
8. Swedberg K, Eneroth P, Kjekshus J, et al: Hormones regulating cardiovascular function in patients with severe congestive heart failure and their relation to mortality. CONSENSUS Trial Study Group. *Circulation* 82:1730-1736, 1990
9. Cohn JN, Levine TB, Olivari MT, et al: Plasma norepinephrine as a guide to prognosis in patients with chronic congestive heart failure. *N Engl J Med* 311:819-823, 1984
10. Cohn JN, Simon A, Johnson G for the V-HeFT Study Group: Relationship of plasma norepinephrine and plasma renin activity to mortality in heart failure (abstract). *Circulation* 84 Suppl 2:310, 1991
11. Massie BM: Is neurohormonal activation deleterious to the long-term outcome of patients with congestive heart failure? I. Introduction. *J Am Coll Cardiol* 12:547-550, 1988
12. Daly PA, Sole MJ: Myocardial catecholamines and the pathophysiology of heart failure. *Circulation* 82 Suppl 2:35-43, 1990
13. Viquerat CE, Daly P, Swedberg K, et al: Endogenous catecholamine levels in chronic heart failure. Relation to the severity of hemodynamic abnormalities. *Am J Med* 78:455-460, 1985
14. Ferguson DW, Berg WJ, Roach PJ, et al: Effects of heart failure on baroreflex control of sympathetic neural activity. *Am J Cardiol* 69:523-531, 1992
15. The SOLVD Investigators: Effect of enalapril on survival in patients with reduced left ventricular ejection fractions and congestive heart failure. *N Engl J Med* 325:293-302, 1991
16. Cohn JN, Johnson G, Ziesche S, et al: A comparison of enalapril with hydralazine-isosorbide dinitrate in the treatment of chronic congestive heart failure. *N Engl J Med* 325:303-310, 1991
17. Francis GS, Benedict C, Johnstone DE, et al: Comparison of neuroendocrine activation in patients with left ventricular dysfunction with and without congestive heart failure. A substudy of the Studies of Left Ventricular Dysfunction (SOLVD). *Circulation* 82:1724-1729, 1990
18. The SOLVD Investigators: Effect of enalapril on mortality and

the development of heart failure in asymptomatic patients with reduced left ventricular ejection fractions. *N Engl J Med* 327:685-691, 1992

19. Burg M, Stoner L, Cardinal J, et al: Furosemide effect on isolated perfused tubules. *Am J Physiol* 225:119-124, 1973

20. Burg M, Green N: Effect of ethacrynic acid on the thick ascending limb of Henle's loop. *Kidney Int* 4:301-308, 1973

21. Carriere S, Dandavino R: Bumetanide, a new loop diuretic. *Clin Pharmacol Ther* 20:424-438, 1976

22. Stein JH, Lameire NH, Earley LE: Renal hemodynamic factors in the regulation of sodium excretion. In *Physiology of Membrane Disorders.* Edited by TE Andreoli, JR Hoffman, DD Fanestil. New York, Plenum Press, 1978, pp 739-772

23. Abe K, Yasujima M, Chiba S, et al: Effect of furosemide on urinary excretion of prostaglandin E in normal volunteers and patients with essential hypertension. *Prostaglandins* 14:513-521, 1977

24. Larsen FF: Haemodynamic effects of high or low doses of furosemide in acute myocardial infarction. *Eur Heart J* 9:125-131, 1988

25. Biddle TL, Yu PN: Effect of furosemide on hemodynamics and lung water in acute pulmonary edema secondary to myocardial infarction. *Am J Cardiol* 43:86-90, 1979

26. Dikshit K, Vyden JK, Forrester JS, et al: Renal and extrarenal hemodynamic effects of furosemide in congestive heart failure after acute myocardial infarction. *N Engl J Med* 288:1087-1090, 1973

27. Ikram H, Chan W, Espiner EA, et al: Haemodynamic and hormone responses to acute and chronic frusemide therapy in congestive heart failure. *Clin Sci (Colch)* 59:443-449, 1980

28. Zelis R, Delea CS, Coleman HN, et al: Arterial sodium content in experimental congestive heart failure. *Circulation* 41:213-216, 1970

29. Francis GS, Siegel RM, Goldsmith SR, et al: Acute vasoconstrictor response to intravenous furosemide in patients with chronic congestive heart failure. Activation of the neurohumoral axis. *Ann Intern Med* 103:1-6, 1985

30. Knight RK, Miall PA, Hawkins LA, et al: Relation of plasma aldosterone concentration to diuretic treatment in patients with severe heart disease. *Br Heart J* 42:316-325, 1979

31. Nicholls MG, Espiner EA, Donald RA, et al: Aldosterone and its regulation during diuresis in patients with gross congestive heart failure. *Clin Sci Mol Med* 47:301-315, 1974

32. Kubo SH, Clark M, Laragh JH, et al: Identification of normal neurohormonal activity in mild congestive heart failure and stimulating effect of upright posture and diuretics. *Am J Cardiol* 60:1322-1328, 1987

33. Bayliss J, Norell M, Canepa-Anson R, et al: Untreated heart failure: clinical and neuroendocrine effects of introducing diuretics. *Br Heart J* 57:17-22, 1987

34. Brater DC, Chennavasin P, Day B, et al: Bumetanide and furosemide. *Clin Pharmacol Ther* 34:207-213, 1983

35. Brater DC, Day B, Burdette A, et al: Bumetanide and furosemide in heart failure. *Kidney Int* 26:183-189, 1984

36. Kunau RT Jr, Weller DR, Webb HL: Clarification of the site of action of chlorothiazide in the rat nephron. *J Clin Invest* 56:401-407, 1975

37. Costanzo LS, Windhager EE: Calcium and sodium transport by the distal convoluted tubule of the rat. *Am J Physiol* 235:F492-F506, 1978

38. Sheth UK, Mehta JM, Paul T, et al: Clinical experience with metolazone--a new diuretic--in cases of edema and ascites due to hepatic cirrhosis, C.C.F., and malnutrition. *J Postgrad Med* 23:147-155, 1977

39. Kiyingi A, Field MJ, Pawsey CC, et al: Metolazone in treatment of severe refractory congestive cardiac failure. *Lancet* 335:29-31, 1990

40. Edelman IS, Fimognari GM: On the biochemical mechanism of action of aldosterone. *Recent Prog Horm Res* 24:1-44, 1968

41. O'Neil RG, Helman SI: Transport characteristics of renal collecting tubules: influences of DOCA and diet. *Am J Physiol* 233:F544-F558, 1977

42. Gross JB, Kokko JP: Effects of aldosterone and potassium-sparing diuretics on electrical potential differences across the distal nephron. *J Clin Invest* 59:82-89, 1977

43. Stoner LC, Burg MB, Orloff J: Ion transport in cortical collecting tubule; effect of amiloride. *Am J Physiol* 227:453-459, 1974

44. Malnic G, Giebisch G: Mechanism of renal hydrogen ion secretion. *Kidney Int* 1:280-296, 1972

45. Hanly PJ, Millar TW, Steljes DG, et al: The effect of oxygen on respiration and sleep in patients with congestive heart failure. *Ann Intern Med* 111:777-782, 1989

46. Chonko AM, Bay WH, Stein JH, et al: The role of renin and aldosterone in the salt retention of edema. *Am J Med* 63:881-889, 1977

47. Seldin DW, Rector FC Jr: The generation and maintenance of metabolic alkalosis. *Kidney Int* 1:306-321, 1972

48. Fichman MP, Vorherr H, Kleeman CR, et al: Diuretic-induced hyponatremia. *Ann Intern Med* 75:853-863, 1971

49. Agus ZS, Wasserstein A, Goldfarb S: Disorders of calcium and magnesium homeostasis. *Am J Med* 72:473-488, 1982

50. Iseri LT, Freed J, Bures AR: Magnesium deficiency and cardiac disorders. *Am J Med* 58:837-846, 1975

51. Cogan MG, Rector FC Jr, Seldin DW: Acid-base disorders. In *The Kidney.* Vol. 1. Second edition. Edited by BM Brenner, FC Rector Jr. Philadelphia, WB Saunders Company, 1981, p 888

52. Steele TH, Oppenheimer S: Factors affecting urate excretion following diuretic administration in man. *Am J Med* 47:564-574, 1969

53. Berger L, Yu TF: Renal function in gout. IV. An analysis of 524 gouty subjects including long-term follow-up studies. *Am J Med* 59:605-613, 1975

54. Koppel MH, Massry SG, Shinaberger JH, et al: Thiazide-induced rise in serum calcium and magnesium in patients on maintenance hemodialysis. *Ann Intern Med* 72:895-901, 1970

55. Stote RM, Smith LH, Wilson DM, et al: Hydrochlorothiazide effects on serum calcium and immunoreactive parathyroid hormone concentrations. Studies in normal subjects. *Ann Intern Med* 77:587-591, 1972

56. Goldner MG, Zarowitz H, Akgun S: Hyperglycemia and glycosuria due to thiazide derivatives administered in diabetes mellitus. *N Engl J Med* 262:403-405, 1960

57. Weller JM, Borondy M: Effect of furosemide on glucose metabolism. *Metabolism* 16:532-536, 1967

58. Andersen OO, Persson I: Carbohydrate metabolism during treatment with chlorthalidone and ethacrynic acid. *Br Med J* 2:798-801, 1968

59. Raftery EB: The metabolic effects of diuretics and other antihypertensive drugs: a perspective as of 1989. *Int J Cardiol* 28:143-150, 1990

60. Thompson WG: An assault on old friends: thiazide diuretics under siege. *Am J Med Sci* 300:152-158, 1990

61. Goldman AI, Steele BW, Schnaper HW, et al: Serum lipoprotein levels during chlorthalidone therapy. A Veterans Administration-National Heart, Lung, and Blood Institute cooperative study on antihypertensive therapy: mild hypertension. *JAMA* 244:1691-1695, 1980

62. Loriaux DL, Menard R, Taylor A, et al: Spironolactone and endocrine dysfunction. *Ann Intern Med* 85:630-636, 1976

63. Werness PG, Bergert JH, Smith LH: Triamterene urolithiasis: solubility, pK, effect on crystal formation, and matrix binding of triamterene and its metabolites. *J Lab Clin Med* 99:254-262, 1982

64. White DJ, Nancollas GH: Triamterene and renal stone formation. *J Urol* 127:593-597, 1982

65. Mathog RH, Klein WJ Jr: Ototoxicity of ethacrynic acid and aminoglycoside antibiotics in uremia. *N Engl J Med* 280:1223-1224, 1969

66. Davies DL, Wilson GM: Diuretics: mechanism of action and clinical application. *Drugs* 9:178-226, 1975

67. Brater DC, Chennavasin P, Seiwell R: Furosemide in patients with heart failure: shift in dose-response curves. *Clin Pharmacol Ther* 28:182-186, 1980

68. Kelly RA, Wilcox CS, Mitch WE, et al: Response of the kidney to furosemide. II. Effect of captopril on sodium balance. *Kidney Int* 24:233-239, 1983

69. Dzau VJ, Hollenberg NK: Renal response to captopril in severe heart failure: role of furosemide in natriuresis and reversal of hyponatremia. *Ann Intern Med* 100:777-782, 1984

70. The Captopril-Digoxin Multicenter Research Group: Comparative effects of therapy with captopril and digoxin in patients with mild to moderate heart failure. *JAMA* 259:539-544, 1988

71. Brater DC: Resistance to loop diuretics. Why it happens and what to do about it. *Drugs* 30:427-443, 1985

72. Webster J: Interactions of NSAIDs with diuretics and beta-blockers. Mechanisms and clinical implications. *Drugs* 30:32-41, 1985

73. Wilson TW, McCauley FA, Wells HD: Effects of low-dose aspirin on responses to furosemide. *J Clin Pharmacol* 26:100-105, 1986

74. Brater DC, Seiwell R, Anderson S, et al: Absorption and disposition of furosemide in congestive heart failure. *Kidney Int* 22:171-176, 1982

75. Oster JR, Epstein M, Smoller S: Combined therapy with

thiazide-type and loop diuretic agents for resistant sodium retention. *Ann Intern Med* 99:405-406, 1983

76. Withering W: *An Account of the Foxglove, and Some of Its Medical Uses: With Practical Remarks on Dropsy and Other Diseases.* London, GGJ and J Robinson, 1785
77. Tamm C: The stereochemistry of the glycosides in relation to biological activity. In *Proceedings of the First International Pharmacological Meeting.* Vol. 3. Edited by B Uvnäs. Oxford, Pergamon Press, 1963, pp 11-26
78. Thomas R, Brown L, Boutagy J, et al: The digitalis receptor. Inferences from structure-activity relationship studies. *Circ Res* 46 Suppl 1:167-172, 1980
79. Yoda A, Yoda S: Structure-activity relationships of cardiotonic steroids for the inhibition of sodium- and potassium-dependent adenosine triphosphatase. V. Dissociation rate constants of digitoxin acetates. *Mol Pharmacol* 11:653-662, 1975
80. Okita GT: Dissociation of Na^+, K^+-ATPase inhibition from digitalis inotropy. *Fed Proc* 36:2225-2230, 1977
81. Peters T, Raben RH, Wassermann O: Evidence for a dissociation between positive inotropic effect and inhibition of the Na^+-K^+-ATPase by ouabain, cassaine and their alkylating derivatives. *Eur J Pharmacol* 26:166-174, 1974
82. Eisner DA, Lederer WJ, Vaughan-Jones RD: The quantitative relationship between twitch tension and intracellular sodium activity in sheep cardiac Purkinje fibres. *J Physiol (Lond)* 355:251-266, 1984
83. Lee CO: 200 years of digitalis: the emerging central role of the sodium ion in the control of cardiac force. *Am J Physiol* 249:C367-C378, 1985
84. Allen DG, Blinks JR: Calcium transients in aequorin-injected frog cardiac muscle. *Nature* 273:509-513, 1978
85. Hoffman BF, Singer DH: Effects of digitalis on electrical activity of cardiac fibers. *Prog Cardiovasc Dis* 7:226-260, 1964
86. Moe GK, Méndez R: The action of several cardiac glycosides on conduction velocity and ventricular excitability in the dog heart. *Circulation* 4:729-734, 1951
87. Bissett JK, de Soyza ND, Kane JJ, et al: Effect of digitalis on human ventricular refractoriness. *Cardiovasc Res* 12:288-293, 1978
88. Méndez R, Méndez C: The action of cardiac glycosides on the refractory period of heart tissues. *J Pharmacol Exp Ther* 107:24-36, 1953
89. Gillis RA: Digitalis: a neuroexcitatory drug. *Circulation* 52:739-742, 1975
90. Gillis RA: Cardiac sympathetic nerve activity: changes induced by ouabain and propranolol. *Science* 166:508-510, 1969
91. Gillis RA, Quest JA: The role of the nervous system in the cardiovascular effects of digitalis. *Pharmacol Rev* 31:19-97, 1979
92. Porter TR, Eckberg DL, Fritsch JM, et al: Autonomic pathophysiology in heart failure patients. Sympathetic-cholinergic interrelations. *J Clin Invest* 85:1362-1371, 1990
93. Creager MA, Hirsch AT, Dzau VJ, et al: Baroreflex regulation of regional blood flow in congestive heart failure. *Am J Physiol* 258:H1409-1414, 1990
94. Osterziel KJ, Dietz R, Manthey J, et al: Haemodynamic changes caused by alteration of autonomic activity in patients with heart failure. *Br Heart J* 63:221-224, 1990
95. Rea RF, Berg WJ: Abnormal baroreflex mechanisms in congestive heart failure. Recent insights. *Circulation* 81:2026-2027, 1990
96. Ferguson DW, Berg WJ, Sanders JS, et al: Sympathoinhibitory responses to digitalis glycosides in heart failure patients. Direct evidence from sympathetic neural recordings. *Circulation* 80:65-77, 1989
97. Wang W, Chen J-S, Zucker IH: Carotid sinus baroreceptor sensitivity in experimental heart failure. *Circulation* 81:1959-1966, 1990
98. McLain PL: Effects of cardiac glycosides on spontaneous efferent activity in vagus and sympathetic nerves of cats. *Int J Neuropharmacol* 8:379-387, 1969
99. Braunwald E, Bloodwell RD, Goldberg LI, et al: Studies on digitalis. IV. Observations in man on the effects of digitalis preparations on the contractility of the non-failing heart and on total vascular resistance. *J Clin Invest* 40:52-59, 1961
100. Sonnenblick EH, Williams JF Jr, Glick G, et al: Studies on digitalis. XV. Effects of cardiac glycosides on myocardial force-velocity relations in the nonfailing human heart. *Circulation* 34:532-539, 1966
101. Daggett WM, Weisfeldt ML: Influence of the sympathetic nervous system on the response of the normal heart to digitalis. *Am J Cardiol* 16:394-405, 1965
102. Mason DT, Braunwald E: Studies on digitalis. X. Effects of ouabain on forearm vascular resistance and venous tone in normal subjects and in patients with heart failure. *J Clin Invest* 43:532-543, 1964
103. Braunwald E: Control of myocardial oxygen consumption: physiologic and clinical considerations. *Am J Cardiol* 27:416-432, 1971
104. Sonnenblick EH, Ross J Jr, Braunwald E: Oxygen consumption of the heart. Newer concepts of its multifactorial determination. *Am J Cardiol* 22:328-336, 1968
105. Covell JW, Braunwald E, Ross J Jr, et al: Studies on digitalis. XVI. Effects on myocardial oxygen consumption. *J Clin Invest* 45:1535-1542, 1966
106. Doherty JE, de Soyza N, Kane JJ, et al: Clinical pharmacokinetics of digitalis glycosides. *Prog Cardiovasc Dis* 21:141-158, 1978
107. Beermann B, Hellström K, Rosén A: The absorption of orally administered [12α-^{3}H]digoxin in man. *Clin Sci* 43:507-518, 1972
108. Greenblatt DJ, Duhme DW, Koch-Weser J, et al: Evaluation of digoxin bioavailability in single-dose studies. *N Engl J Med* 289:651-654, 1973
109. Huffman DH, Manion CV, Azarnoff DL: Intersubject variation in absorption of digoxin in normal volunteers. *J Pharm Sci* 64:433-437, 1975
110. Johnson BF, Bye C, Jones G, et al: A completely absorbed oral preparation of digoxin. *Clin Pharmacol Ther* 19:746-751, 1976
111. Mallis GI, Schmidt DH, Lindenbaum J: Superior bioavailability of digoxin solution in capsules. *Clin Pharmacol Ther* 18:761-768, 1975
112. Weissler AM, Snyder JR, Schoenfeld CD, et al: Assay of digitalis glycosides in man. *Am J Cardiol* 17:768-780, 1966
113. Storstein L, Johnsgard M: Studies on digitalis. 15. Bioavailability of digitoxin. *Acta Med Scand Suppl* 645:91-95, 1981
114. Beermann B, Hellstrom K, Rosen A: Fate of orally administered ^{3}H-digitoxin in man with special reference to the absorption. *Circulation* 43:852-861, 1971
115. Doherty JE, Perkins WH: Studies with tritiated digoxin in human subjects after intravenous administration. *Am Heart J* 63:528-536, 1962
116. Lukas DS, De Martino AG: Binding of digitoxin and some related cardenolides to human plasma proteins. *J Clin Invest* 48:1041-1053, 1969
117. Lukas DS: Some aspects of the distribution and disposition of digitoxin in man. *Ann N Y Acad Sci* 179:338-361, 1971
118. Reuning RH, Sams RA, Notari RE: Role of pharmacokinetics in drug dosage adjustment. I. Pharmacologic effect kinetics and apparent volume of distribution of digoxin. *J Clin Pharmacol New Drugs* 13:127-141, 1973
119. Ackerman GL, Doherty JE, Flanigan WJ: Peritoneal dialysis and hemodialysis of tritiated digoxin. *Ann Intern Med* 67:718-723, 1967
120. Storstein L: Studies on digitalis. II. The influence of impaired renal function on the renal excretion of digitoxin and its cardioactive metabolites. *Clin Pharmacol Ther* 16:25-34, 1974
121. Ochs HR, Greenblatt DJ, Bodem G, et al: Disease-related alterations in cardiac glycoside disposition. *Clin Pharmacokinet* 7:434-451, 1982
122. Marcus FI, Kapadia GG: The metabolism of tritiated digoxin in cirrhotic patients. *Gastroenterology* 47:517-524, 1964
123. Doherty JE, Perkins WH: Digoxin metabolism in hypo- and hyperthyroidism. Studies with tritiated digoxin in thyroid disease. *Ann Intern Med* 64:489-507, 1966
124. Shenfield GM, Thompson J, Horn DB: Plasma and urinary digoxin in thyroid dysfunction. *Eur J Clin Pharmacol* 12:437-443, 1977
125. Forbes GB, Reina JC: Adult lean body mass declines with age: some longitudinal observations. *Metabolism* 19:653-663, 1970
126. Cusack B, Kelly J, O'Malley K, et al: Digoxin in the elderly: pharmacokinetic consequences of old age. *Clin Pharmacol Ther* 25:772-776, 1979
127. Ewy GA, Kapadia GG, Yao L, et al: Digoxin metabolism in the elderly. *Circulation* 39:449-453, 1969
128. Donovan MA, Castleden CM, Pohl JE, et al: The effect of age on digitoxin pharmacokinetics. *Br J Clin Pharmacol* 11:401-402, 1981
129. Brown DD, Spector R, Juhl RP: Drug interactions with digoxin. *Drugs* 20:198-206, 1980
130. Binnion PF: Absorption of different commercial preparations of digoxin in the normal human subject and the influence of antacid, anti-diarrheal, and ion-exchange agents. In *Symposium on Digitalis.* Edited by O Storstein. Oslo, Norway, Gyldendal Norsk Forlag, 1973, pp 216-224

131. Lindenbaum J, Maulitz RM, Butler VP Jr: Inhibition of digoxin absorption by neomycin. *Gastroenterology* 71:399-404, 1976

132. Juhl RP, Summers RW, Guillory JK, et al: Effect of sulfasalazine on digoxin bioavailability. *Clin Pharmacol Ther* 20:387-394, 1976

133. Lindenbaum J, Rund DG, Butler VP Jr, et al: Inactivation of digoxin by the gut flora: reversal by antibiotic therapy. *N Engl J Med* 305:789-794, 1981

134. Kuhlmann J, Zilly W, Wilke J: Effects of cytostatic drugs on plasma level and renal excretion of β-acetyldigoxin. *Clin Pharmacol Ther* 30:518-527, 1981

135. Manninen V, Apajalahti A, Melin J, et al: Altered absorption of digoxin in patients given propantheline and metoclopramide. *Lancet* 1:398-400, 1973

136. Brown DD, Juhl RP: Altered bioavailability of digoxin produced by gastrointestinal medications (abstract). *Clin Res* 27:610, 1979

137. Leahey EB Jr, Reiffel JA, Drusin RE, et al: Interaction between quinidine and digoxin. *JAMA* 240:533-534, 1978

138. Ejvinsson G: Effect of quinidine on plasma concentrations of digoxin. *Br Med J* 1:279-280, 1978

139. Leahey EB Jr, Reiffel JA, Giardina EG, et al: The effect of quinidine and other oral antiarrhythmic drugs on serum digoxin. A prospective study. *Ann Intern Med* 92:605-608, 1980

140. Doering W: Quinidine-digoxin interaction: pharmacokinetics, underlying mechanism and clinical implications. *N Engl J Med* 301:400-404, 1979

141. Mungall DR, Robichaux RP, Perry W, et al: Effects of quinidine on serum digoxin concentration: a prospective study. *Ann Intern Med* 93:689-693, 1980

142. Leahey EB Jr, Bigger JT Jr, Butler VP Jr, et al: Quinidine-digoxin interaction: time course and pharmacokinetics. *Am J Cardiol* 48:1141-1146, 1981

143. Bigger JT Jr, Leahey EB Jr: Quinidine and digoxin. An important interaction. *Drugs* 24:229-239, 1982

144. Hager WD, Fenster P, Mayersohn M, et al: Digoxin-quinidine interaction: pharmacokinetic evaluation. *N Engl J Med* 300:1238-1241, 1979

145. Ochs HR, Bodem G, Greenblatt DJ: Impairment of digoxin clearance by coadministration of quinidine. *J Clin Pharmacol* 21:396-400, 1981

146. Oetgen WJ, Sobol SM, Tri TB, et al: Amiodarone-digoxin interaction. Clinical and experimental observations. *Chest* 86:75-79, 1984

147. Nademanee K, Kannan R, Hendrickson J, et al: Amiodarone-digoxin interaction: clinical significance, time course of development, potential pharmacokinetic mechanisms and therapeutic implications. *J Am Coll Cardiol* 4:111-116, 1984

148. Johnson BF, Wilson J, Marwaha R, et al: The comparative effects of verapamil and a new dihydropyridine calcium channel blocker on digoxin pharmacokinetics. *Clin Pharmacol Ther* 42:66-71, 1987

149. Rodin SM, Johnson BF: Pharmacokinetic interactions with digoxin. *Clin Pharmacokinet* 15:227-244, 1988

150. Steiness E: Renal tubular secretion of digoxin. *Circulation* 50:103-107, 1974

151. Waldorff S, Andersen JD, Heeboll-Nielsen N, et al: Spironolactone-induced changes in digoxin kinetics. *Clin Pharmacol Ther* 24:162-167, 1978

152. Kunin AS, Surawicz B, Sims EAH: Decrease in serum potassium concentrations and appearance of cardiac arrhythmias during infusion of potassium with glucose in potassium-depleted patients. *N Engl J Med* 266:228-233, 1962

153. Kleiger RE, Vitale J, Lown B: Clinical and experimental relationships between digitalis and potassium. *Proc N Engl Cardiovasc Soc* 23:19-21, 1965

154. Steiness E, Olesen KH: Cardiac arrhythmias induced by hypokalaemia and potassium loss during maintenance digoxin therapy. *Br Heart J* 38:167-172, 1976

155. Fisch C: Relation of electrolyte disturbances to cardiac arrhythmias. *Circulation* 47:408-419, 1973

156. Allen JC, Schwartz A: Effects of potassium, temperature and time on ouabain interaction with the cardiac Na^+, K^+-ATPase: further evidence supporting an allosteric site. *J Mol Cell Cardiol* 1:39-45, 1970

157. Seller RH, Cangiano J, Kim KE, et al: Digitalis toxicity and hypomagnesemia. *Am Heart J* 79:57-68, 1970

158. Kleiger RE, Seta K, Vitale JJ, et al: Effects of chronic depletion of potassium and magnesium upon the action of acetylstrophanthidin on the heart. *Am J Cardiol* 17:520-527, 1966

159. Beller GA, Hood WB Jr, Smith TW, et al: Correlation of serum magnesium levels and cardiac digitalis intoxication. *Am J Cardiol* 33:225-229, 1974

160. Goldman RH, Kleiger RE, Schweizer E, et al: The effect on myocardial ^{3}H-digoxin of magnesium deficiency. *Proc Soc Exp Biol Med* 136:747-749, 1971

161. Nola GT, Pope S, Harrison DC: Assessment of the synergistic relationship between serum calcium and digitalis. *Am Heart J* 79:499-507, 1970

162. Doherty JE, Kane JJ, Phillips JR, et al: Digitalis in pulmonary heart disease (cor pulmonale). *Drugs* 13:142-151, 1977

163. Harrison DC, Robinson MD, Kleiger RE: Role of hypoxia in digitalis toxicity. *Am J Med Sci* 256:352-359, 1968

164. Green LH, Smith TW: Factors influencing individual sensitivity to cardiac glycosides. *Adv Manage Clin Heart Dis* 3:161-187, 1978

165. Smith TW, Willerson JT: Suicidal and accidental digoxin ingestion. Report of five cases with serum digoxin level correlations. *Circulation* 44:29-36, 1971

166. Lawrence JR, Sumner DJ, Kalk WJ, et al: Digoxin kinetics in patients with thyroid dysfunction. *Clin Pharmacol Ther* 22:7-13, 1977

167. Kim D, Smith TW: Effects of thyroid hormone on sodium pump sites, sodium content, and contractile responses to cardiac glycosides in cultured chick ventricular cells. *J Clin Invest* 74:1481-1488, 1984

168. Smith TW: Digitalis toxicity: epidemiology and clinical use of serum concentration measurements. *Am J Med* 58:470-476, 1975

169. Beller GA, Smith TW, Abelmann WH, et al: Digitalis intoxication. A prospective clinical study with serum level correlations. *N Engl J Med* 284:989-997, 1971

170. Carruthers SG, Kelly JG, McDevitt DG: Plasma digoxin concentrations in patients on admission to hospital. *Br Heart J* 36:707-712, 1974

171. Evered DC, Chapman C: Plasma digoxin concentrations and digoxin toxicity in hospital patients. *Br Heart J* 33:540-545, 1971

172. Fogelman AM, La Mont JT, Finkelstein S, et al: Fallibility of plasma-digoxin in differentiating toxic from non-toxic patients. *Lancet* 2:727-729, 1971

173. Smith TW, Haber E: Digoxin intoxication: the relationship of clinical presentation to serum digoxin concentration. *J Clin Invest* 49:2377-2386, 1970

174. Lely AH, van Enter CH: Large-scale digitoxin intoxication. *Br Med J* 3:737-740, 1970

175. Kramer WG, Kinnear NL, Morgan HK: Variability among commercially available digoxin radioimmunoassay kits in cross reactivity to dihydrodigoxin. *Clin Chem* 24:155-157, 1978

176. Hastreiter AR, John EG, van der Horst RL: Digitalis, digitalis antibodies, digitalis-like immunoreactive substances, and sodium homeostasis: a review. *Clin Perinatol* 15:491-522, 1988

177. Borison HL, Wang SC: Physiology and pharmacology of vomiting. *Pharmacol Rev* 5:193-230, 1953

178. Gillis RA, Raines A, Sohn YJ, et al: Neuroexcitatory effects of digitalis and their role in the development of cardiac arrhythmias. *J Pharmacol Exp Ther* 183:154-168, 1972

179. McLain PL: Effects of ouabain on spontaneous afferent activity in the aortic and carotid sinus nerves of cats. *Neuropharmacology* 9:399-402, 1970

180. Lathers CM, Kelliher GJ, Roberts J, et al: Nonuniform cardiac sympathetic nerve discharge: mechanism for coronary occlusion and digitalis-induced arrhythmia. *Circulation* 57:1058-1065, 1978

181. Helke CJ, Gillis RA: Centrally mediated protective effects of dopamine agonists on digitalis-induced ventricular arrhythmias. *J Pharmacol Exp Ther* 207:263-270, 1978

182. Ewy GA, Marcus FI, Fillmore SJ, et al: Digitalis intoxication—diagnosis, management and prevention. *Cardiovasc Clin* 6:153-174, 1974

183. Wenger TL, Butler VP Jr, Haber E, et al: Treatment of 63 severely digitalis-toxic patients with digoxin-specific antibody fragments. *J Am Coll Cardiol* 5 Suppl A:118-123, 1985

184. Smith TW, Butler VP Jr, Haber E, et al: Treatment of life-threatening digitalis intoxication with digoxin-specific Fab antibody fragments: experience in 26 cases. *N Engl J Med* 307:1357-1362, 1982

185. Smith TW: Digitalis. Mechanisms of action and clinical use. *N Engl J Med* 318:358-365, 1988

186. Fisch C, Martz BL, Priebe FH: Enhancement of potassium-

induced atrioventricular block by toxic doses of digitalis drugs. *J Clin Invest* 39:1885-1893, 1960

187. Citrin D, Stevenson IH, O'Malley K: Massive digoxin overdose: observations on hyperkalaemia and plasma digoxin levels. *Scott Med J* 17:275-277, 1972

188. Szekely P, Wynne NA: The effects of magnesium on cardiac arrhythmias caused by digitalis. *Clin Sci* 10:241-253, 1951

189. Hilmi KI, Regan TJ: Relative effectiveness of antiarrhythmic drugs in treatment of digitalis-induced ventricular tachycardia. *Am Heart J* 76:365-369, 1968

190. Garan H, Ruskin JN, Powell WJ Jr: Centrally mediated effect of phenytoin on digoxin-induced ventricular arrhythmias. *Am J Physiol* 241:H67-H72, 1981

191. Gibson D, Sowton E: The use of beta-adrenergic receptor blocking drugs in dysrhythmias. *Prog Cardiovasc Dis* 12:16-39, 1969

192. Boman K, Allgulander S, Skoglund M: Is maintenance digoxin necessary in geriatric patients? *Acta Med Scand* 210:493-495, 1981

193. Fonrose HA, Ahlbaum N, Bugatch E, et al: The efficacy of digitalis withdrawal in an institutional aged population. *J Am Geriatr Soc* 22:208-211, 1974

194. Johnston GD, McDevitt DG: Is maintenance digoxin necessary in patients with sinus rhythm? *Lancet* 1:567-570, 1979

195. Lee DC, Johnson RA, Bingham JB, et al: Heart failure in outpatients: a randomized trial of digoxin versus placebo. *N Engl J Med* 306:699-705, 1982

196. Guyatt GH, Sullivan MJ, Fallen EL, et al: A controlled trial of digoxin in congestive heart failure. *Am J Cardiol* 61:371-375, 1988

197. Gheorghiade M, St Clair J, St Clair C, et al: Hemodynamic effects of intravenous digoxin in patients with severe heart failure initially treated with diuretics and vasodilators. *J Am Coll Cardiol* 9:849-857, 1987

198. Arnold SB, Byrd RC, Meister W, et al: Long-term digitalis therapy improves left ventricular function in heart failure. *N Engl J Med* 303:1443-1448, 1980

199. Davies RF, Beanlands DS, Nadeau C, et al: Enalapril versus digoxin in patients with congestive heart failure: a multicenter study. Canadian Enalapril Versus Digoxin Study Group. *J Am Coll Cardiol* 18:1602-1609, 1991

200. Gheorghiade M, Hall V, Lakier JB, et al: Comparative hemodynamic and neurohormonal effects of intravenous captopril and digoxin and their combination in patients with severe heart failure. *J Am Coll Cardiol* 13:134-142, 1989

201. Ribner HS, Zucker MJ, Stasior C, et al: Vasodilators as first-line therapy for congestive heart failure: a comparative hemodynamic study of hydralazine, digoxin, and their combination. *Am Heart J* 114:91-96, 1987

202. Cantelli I, Vitolo A, Lombardi G, et al: Combined haemodynamic effects of digoxin and captopril in patients with congestive heart failure. *Curr Ther Res* 36:323-331, 1984

203. Sullivan M, Atwood JE, Myers J, et al: Increased exercise capacity after digoxin administration in patients with heart failure. *J Am Coll Cardiol* 13:1138-1143, 1989

204. Pugh SE, White NJ, Aronson JK, et al: Clinical, haemodynamic, and pharmacological effects of withdrawal and reintroduction of digoxin in patients with heart failure in sinus rhythm after long term treatment. *Br Heart J* 61:529-539, 1989

205. Young JB, Uretsky BF, Shahidi E, et al: Multicenter, double-blind, placebo-controlled randomized withdrawal trial of the efficacy and safety of digoxin in patients with mild to moderate chronic heart failure not treated with converting enzyme inhibitors (abstract). *J Am Coll Cardiol* 19 Suppl A:259, 1992

206. Packer M, Gheorghiade M, Young JB, et al: Withdrawal of digoxin from patients with chronic heart failure treated with angiotensin-converting-enzyme inhibitors. RADIANCE Study. *N Engl J Med* 329:1-7, 1993

207. DiBianco R, Shabetai R, Kostuk W, et al: A comparison of oral milrinone, digoxin, and their combination in the treatment of patients with chronic heart failure. *N Engl J Med* 320:677-683, 1989

208. The German and Austrian Xamoterol Study Group: Double-blind placebo-controlled comparison of digoxin and xamoterol in chronic heart failure. *Lancet* 1:489-493, 1988

209. Sheiner LB, Rosenberg B, Melmon KL: Modeling of individual pharmacokinetics for computer-aided drug dosage. *Comput Biomed Res* 5:441-459, 1972

210. Jelliffe RW, Brooker G: A nomogram for digoxin therapy. *Am J Med* 57:63-68, 1974

211. Jusko WJ: Clinical pharmacokinetics of digoxin. In *Symposium on Clinical Pharmacokinetics.* Edited by G Levy. Washington DC, Academy of Pharmaceutical Sciences, 1974, pp 31-43

212. Peck CC, Sheiner LB, Martin CM, et al: Computer-assisted digoxin therapy. *N Engl J Med* 289:441-446, 1973

213. Goldberg LI: Cardiovascular and renal actions of dopamine: potential clinical applications. *Pharmacol Rev* 24:1-29, 1972

214. Goldberg LI, Hsieh YY, Resnekov L: Newer catecholamines for treatment of heart failure and shock: an update on dopamine and a first look at dobutamine. *Prog Cardiovasc Dis* 19:327-340, 1977

215. Beregovich J, Bianchi C, Rubler S, et al: Dose-related hemodynamic and renal effects of dopamine in congestive heart failure. *Am Heart J* 87:550-557, 1974

216. McDonald RH Jr, Goldberg LI, McNay JL, et al: Effects of dopamine in man: augmentation of sodium excretion, glomerular filtration rate, and renal plasma flow. *J Clin Invest* 43:1116-1124, 1964

217. Allwood MJ, Ginsburg J: Peripheral vascular and other effects of dopamine infusions in man. *Clin Sci* 27:271-281, 1964

218. Brooks HL, Stein PD, Matson JL, et al: Dopamine-induced alterations in coronary hemodynamics in dogs. *Circ Res* 24:699-704, 1969

219. Crexells C, Bourassa MG, Biron P: Effects of dopamine on myocardial metabolism in patients with ischaemic heart disease. *Cardiovasc Res* 7:438-445, 1973

220. Ruffolo RR Jr, Spradlin TA, Pollock GD, et al: Alpha and beta adrenergic effects of the stereoisomers of dobutamine. *J Pharmacol Exp Ther* 219:447-452, 1981

221. Akhtar N, Mikulic E, Cohn JN, et al: Hemodynamic effect of dobutamine in patients with severe heart failure. *Am J Cardiol* 36:202-205, 1975

222. Loeb HS, Khan M, Klodnycky ML, et al: Hemodynamic effects of dobutamine in man. *Circ Shock* 2:29-35, 1975

223. Gillespie TA, Ambos HD, Sobel BE, et al: Effects of dobutamine in patients with acute myocardial infarction. *Am J Cardiol* 39:588-594, 1977

224. Leier CV, Webel J, Bush CA: The cardiovascular effects of the continuous infusion of dobutamine in patients with severe cardiac failure. *Circulation* 56:468-472, 1977

225. Unverferth DV, Magorien RD, Lewis RP, et al: Long-term benefit of dobutamine in patients with congestive cardiomyopathy. *Am Heart J* 100:622-630, 1980

226. Applefeld MM, Newman KA, Sutton FJ, et al: Outpatient dobutamine and dopamine infusions in the management of chronic heart failure: clinical experience in 21 patients. *Am Heart J* 114:589-595, 1987

227. Liang CS, Sherman LG, Doherty JU, et al: Sustained improvement of cardiac function in patients with congestive heart failure after short-term infusion of dobutamine. *Circulation* 69:113-119, 1984

228. Leier CV, Huss P, Lewis RP, et al: Drug-induced conditioning in congestive heart failure. *Circulation* 65:1382-1387, 1982

229. Dies F, Krell MJ, Whitlow P, et al: Intermittent dobutamine in ambulatory outpatients with chronic cardiac failure (abstract). *Circulation* 74 Suppl 2:38, 1986

230. Weber KT, Andrews V, Janicki JS, et al: Pirbuterol, an oral beta-adrenergic receptor agonist, in the treatment of chronic cardiac failure. *Circulation* 66:1262-1267, 1982

231. Roubin GS, Choong CY, Devenish-Meares S, et al: Beta-adrenergic stimulation of the failing ventricle: a double-blind, randomized trial of sustained oral therapy with prenalterol. *Circulation* 69:955-962, 1984

232. Lambertz H, Meyer J, Erbel R: Long-term hemodynamic effects of prenalterol in patients with severe congestive heart failure. *Circulation* 69:298-305, 1984

233. Farah AE, Alousi AA: New cardiotonic agents: a search for digitalis substitute. *Life Sci* 22:1139-1147, 1978

234. Benotti JR, Grossman W, Braunwald E, et al: Hemodynamic assessment of amrinone. A new inotropic agent. *N Engl J Med* 299:1373-1377, 1978

235. LeJemtel TH, Keung E, Sonnenblick EH, et al: Amrinone: a new non-glycosidic, non-adrenergic cardiotonic agent effective in the treatment of intractable myocardial failure in man. *Circulation* 59:1098-1104, 1979

236. Malacoff RF, Curfman GD, Wynne J, et al: Inotropic effect of

amrinone in severe congestive heart failure: lack of attenuation with sequential doses (abstract). *Am J Cardiol* 45:433, 1980

237. LeJemtel TH, Keung E, Ribner HS, et al: Sustained beneficial effects of oral amrinone on cardiac and renal function in patients with severe congestive heart failure. *Am J Cardiol* 45:123-129, 1980

238. Wynne J, Malacoff RF, Benotti JR, et al: Oral amrinone in refractory congestive heart failure. *Am J Cardiol* 45:1245-1249, 1980

239. DiBianco R, Shabetai R, Silverman BD, et al: Oral amrinone for the treatment of chronic congestive heart failure: results of a multicenter randomized double-blind and placebo-controlled withdrawal study. *J Am Coll Cardiol* 4:855-866, 1984

240. Massie B, Bourassa M, DiBianco R, et al: Long-term oral administration of amrinone for congestive heart failure: lack of efficacy in a multicenter controlled trial. *Circulation* 71:963-971, 1985

241. Kinney EL, Carlin B, Ballard JO, et al: Clinical experience with amrinone in patients with advanced congestive heart failure. *J Clin Pharmacol* 22:433-440, 1982

242. Leier CV, Dalpiaz K, Huss P, et al: Amrinone therapy for congestive heart failure in outpatients with idiopathic dilated cardiomyopathy. *Am J Cardiol* 52:304-308, 1983

243. Alousi AA, Stankus GP, Stuart JC, et al: Characterization of the cardiotonic effects of milrinone, a new and potent cardiac bipyridine, on isolated tissues from several animal species. *J Cardiovasc Pharmacol* 5:804-811, 1983

244. Maskin CS, Sinoway L, Chadwick B, et al: Sustained hemodynamic and clinical effects of a new cardiotonic agent, WIN 47203, in patients with severe congestive heart failure. *Circulation* 67:1065-1070, 1983

245. Baim DS, McDowell AV, Cherniles J, et al: Evaluation of a new bipyridine inotropic agent—milrinone—in patients with severe congestive heart failure. *N Engl J Med* 309:748-756, 1983

246. Packer M, Carver JR, Rodeheffer RJ, et al: Effect of oral milrinone on mortality in severe chronic heart failure. The PROMISE Study Research Group. *N Engl J Med* 325:1468-1475, 1991

247. Uretsky BF, Generalovich T, Verbalis JG, et al: MDL 17,043 therapy in severe congestive heart failure: characterization of the early and late hemodynamic, pharmacokinetic, hormonal and clinical response. *J Am Coll Cardiol* 5:1414-1421, 1985

248. Shah PK, Amin DK, Hulse S, et al: Inotropic therapy for refractory congestive heart failure with oral fenoximone (MDL-17,043): poor long-term results despite early hemodynamic and clinical improvement. *Circulation* 71:326-331, 1985

249. Uretsky BF, Jessup M, Konstam MA, et al: Multicenter trial of oral enoximone in patients with moderate to moderately severe congestive heart failure. Lack of benefit compared with placebo. Enoximone Multicenter Trial Group. *Circulation* 82:774-780, 1990

250. Rüegg JC: Effects of new inotropic agents on Ca^{++} sensitivity of contractile proteins. *Circulation* 73 Suppl 3:78-84, 1986

251. Solaro RJ, Fujino K, Sperelakis N: The positive inotropic effect of pimobendan involves stereospecific increases in the calcium sensitivity of cardiac myofilaments. *J Cardiovasc Pharmacol* 14 Suppl 2:7-12, 1989

252. Rapundalo ST, Lathrop DA, Harrison SA, et al: Cyclic AMP-dependent and cyclic AMP-independent actions of a novel cardiotonic agent, OPC-8212. *Naunyn Schmiedebergs Arch Pharmacol* 338:692-698, 1988

253. Inoue M, Kim BH, Hori M, et al: Oral OPC-8212 for the treatment of congestive heart failure: hemodynamic improvement and increased exercise capacity. *Heart Vessels* 2:166-171, 1986

254. Sasayama S, Inoue M, Asanoi H, et al: Acute hemodynamic effects of a new inotropic agent, OPC-8212, on severe congestive heart failure. *Heart Vessels* 2:23-28, 1986

255. Feldman AM, Becker LC, Llewellyn MP, et al: Evaluation of a new inotropic agent, OPC-8212, in patients with dilated cardiomyopathy and heart failure. *Am Heart J* 116:771-777, 1988

256. OPC-8212 Multicenter Research Group: A placebo-controlled, randomized, double-blind study of OPC-8212 in patients with mild chronic heart failure. *Cardiovasc Drugs Ther* 4:419-425, 1990

257. Feldman AM, Baughman KL, Lee WK, et al: Usefulness of OPC-8212, a quinolinone derivative, for chronic congestive heart failure in patients with ischemic heart disease or idiopathic dilated cardiomyopathy. *Am J Cardiol* 68:1203-1210, 1991

258. Feldman AM, Bristow MR, Parmley WW, et al: Effects of vesnarinone on morbidity and mortality in patients with heart failure. Vesnarinone Study Group. *N Engl J Med* 329:149-155, 1993

259. Verdouw PD, Hartog JM, Duncker DJ, et al: Cardiovascular profile of pimobendan, a benzimidazole-pyridazinone derivative with vasodilating and inotropic properties. *Eur J Pharmacol* 126:21-30, 1986

260. Kubo SH, Gollub S, Bourge R, et al: Beneficial effects of pimobendan on exercise tolerance and quality of life in patients with heart failure. Results of a multicenter trial. The Pimobendan Multicenter Research Group. *Circulation* 85:942-949, 1992

261. Francis GS, Cohn JN: Heart failure: mechanisms of cardiac and vascular dysfunction and the rationale for pharmacologic intervention. *FASEB J* 4:3068-3075, 1990

262. Packer M, Medina N, Yushak M, et al: Hemodynamic patterns of response during long-term captopril therapy for severe chronic heart failure. *Circulation* 68:803-812, 1983

263. Massie B, Ports T, Chatterjee K, et al: Long-term vasodilator therapy for heart failure: clinical response and its relationship to hemodynamic measurements. *Circulation* 63:269-278, 1981

264. Franciosa JA, Wilen M: Relationship between acute hemodynamic responses to vasodilators and long-term efficacy in heart failure (abstract). *J Am Coll Cardiol* 1:712, 1983

265. Packer M: Vasodilator and inotropic drugs for the treatment of chronic heart failure: distinguishing hype from hope. *J Am Coll Cardiol* 12:1299-1317, 1988

266. Chidsey CA, Harrison DC, Braunwald E: Augmentation of the plasma nor-epinephrine response to exercise in patients with congestive heart failure. *N Engl J Med* 267:650-654, 1962

267. Francis GS, Rector TS, Cohn JN: Sequential neurohumoral measurements in patients with congestive heart failure. *Am Heart J* 116:1464-1468, 1988

268. Fletcher RD, Cintron GB, Johnson G, et al: Enalapril decreases prevalence of ventricular tachycardia in patients with chronic congestive heart failure. The V-HeFT II VA Cooperative Studies Group. *Circulation* 87 Suppl 6:49-55, 1993

269. Levine TB, Franciosa JA, Cohn JN: Acute and long-term response to an oral converting-enzyme inhibitor, captopril, in congestive heart failure. *Circulation* 62:35-41, 1980

270. Faxon DP, Halperin JL, Creager MA, et al: Angiotensin inhibition in severe heart failure: acute central and limb hemodynamic effects of captopril with observations on sustained oral therapy. *Am Heart J* 101:548-556, 1981

271. Davis R, Ribner HS, Keung E, et al: Treatment of chronic congestive heart failure with captopril, an oral inhibitor of angiotensin-converting enzyme. *N Engl J Med* 301:117-121, 1979

272. Ader R, Chatterjee K, Ports T, et al: Immediate and sustained hemodynamic and clinical improvement in chronic heart failure by an oral angiotensin-converting enzyme inhibitor. *Circulation* 61:931-937, 1980

273. Awan NA, Evenson MK, Needham KE, et al: Efficacy of oral angiotensin-converting enzyme inhibition with captopril therapy in severe chronic normotensive congestive heart failure. *Am Heart J* 101:22-31, 1981

274. Packer M, Meller J, Medina N, et al: The first dose response to captopril is superior to the pretreatment plasma renin activity in predicting its long-term hemodynamic effects in severe heart failure (abstract). *Am J Cardiol* 49:989, 1982

275. Franciosa JA, Goldsmith SR, Cohn JN: Contrasting immediate and long-term effects of isosorbide dinitrate on exercise capacity in congestive heart failure. *Am J Med* 69:559-566, 1980

276. Leier CV, Huss P, Magorien RD, et al: Improved exercise capacity and differing arterial and venous tolerance during chronic isosorbide dinitrate therapy for congestive heart failure. *Circulation* 67:817-822, 1983

277. Stephens J, Camm J, Spurrell R: Improvement in exercise haemodynamics by isosorbide dinitrate in patients with severe congestive cardiac failure secondary to ischaemic heart disease. *Br Heart J* 40:832-837, 1978

278. Franciosa JA, Cohn JN: Effect of isosorbide dinitrate on response to submaximal and maximal exercise in patients with congestive heart failure. *Am J Cardiol* 43:1009-1014, 1979

279. Franciosa JA, Nordstrom LA, Cohn JN: Nitrate therapy for congestive heart failure. *JAMA* 240:443-446, 1978

280. Cohn JN, Archibald DG, Ziesche S, et al: Effect of vasodilator

therapy on mortality in chronic congestive heart failure. Results of a Veterans Administration Cooperative Study. *N Engl J Med* 314:1547-1552, 1986

281. Stein L: Randomized comparison of minoxidil and hydralazine in severe chronic congestive heart failure (abstract). *J Am Coll Cardiol* 1:713, 1983

282. Reece PA, Zacest R: Hydralazine. In *Cardiovascular Drug Therapy.* Edited by FH Messerli. Philadelphia, WB Saunders Company, 1990, pp 834-848

283. Packer M: Effect of vasodilator and inotropic drugs on clinical symptoms and long-term survival in chronic congestive heart failure. *Eur Heart J* 9 Suppl H:105-108, 1988

284. Franciosa JA, Cohn JN: Effects of minoxidil on hemodynamics in patients with congestive heart failure. *Circulation* 63:652-657, 1981

285. Pluss RG, Orcutt J, Chidsey CA: Tissue distribution and hypotensive effects of minoxidil in normotensive rats. *J Lab Clin Med* 79:639-647, 1972

286. Markham RV Jr, Gilmore A, Pettinger WA, et al: Central and regional hemodynamic effects and neurohumoral consequences of minoxidil in severe congestive heart failure and comparison to hydralazine and nitroprusside. *Am J Cardiol* 52:774-781, 1983

287. Nathan M, Rubin SA, Siemienczuk D, et al: Effects of acute and chronic minoxidil administration on rest and exercise hemodynamics and clinical status in patients with severe, chronic heart failure. *Am J Cardiol* 50:960-966, 1982

288. McKay CR, Chatterjee K, Ports TA, et al: Minoxidil therapy in chronic congestive heart failure: acute plus long-term hemodynamic and clinical study. *Am Heart J* 104:575-580, 1982

289. Packer M, Meller J, Medina N, et al: Sustained effectiveness of minoxidil in heart failure after development of tolerance to other vasodilator drugs. *Am J Cardiol* 48:375-379, 1981

290. Martin WB, Spodick DH, Zins GR: Pericardial disorders occurring during open-label study of 1,869 severely hypertensive patients treated with minoxidil. *J Cardiovasc Pharmacol* 2 Suppl 2:217-227, 1980

291. Dawson JR, Whitaker NH, Sutton GC: Calcium antagonist drugs in chronic stable angina. Comparison of verapamil and nifedipine. *Br Heart J* 46:508-512, 1981

292. Mueller HS, Chahine RA: Interim report of multicenter double-blind, placebo-controlled studies of nifedipine in chronic stable angina. *Am J Med* 71:645-657, 1981

293. Gerstenblith G, Ouyang P, Achuff SC, et al: Nifedipine in unstable angina: a double-blind, randomized trial. *N Engl J Med* 306:885-889, 1982

294. Agostoni PG, De Cesare N, Doria E, et al: Afterload reduction: a comparison of captopril and nifedipine in dilated cardiomyopathy. *Br Heart J* 55:391-399, 1986

295. Elkayam U, Amin J, Mehra A, et al: A prospective, randomized, double-blind, crossover study to compare the efficacy and safety of chronic nifedipine therapy with that of isosorbide dinitrate and their combination in the treatment of chronic congestive heart failure. *Circulation* 82:1954-1961, 1990

296. The Multicenter Diltiazem Postinfarction Trial Research Group: The effect of diltiazem on mortality and reinfarction after myocardial infarction. *N Engl J Med* 319:385-392, 1988

297. Kulick DL, McIntosh N, Campese VM, et al: Central and renal hemodynamic effects and hormonal response to diltiazem in severe congestive heart failure. *Am J Cardiol* 59:1138-1143, 1987

298. Packer M, Lee WH, Medina N, et al: Comparative negative inotropic effects of nifedipine and diltiazem in patients with severe left ventricular dysfunction (abstract). *Circulation* 72 Suppl 3:275, 1985

299. Elkayam U, Weber L, McKay C, et al: Spectrum of acute hemodynamic effects of nifedipine in severe congestive heart failure. *Am J Cardiol* 56:560-566, 1985

300. Elkayam U, Weber L, Torkan B, et al: Comparison of hemodynamic responses to nifedipine and nitroprusside in severe chronic congestive heart failure. *Am J Cardiol* 53:1321-1325, 1984

301. Fifer MA, Colucci WS, Lorell BH, et al: Inotropic, vascular and neuroendocrine effects of nifedipine in heart failure: comparison with nitroprusside. *J Am Coll Cardiol* 5:731-737, 1985

302. Packer M, Lee WH, Medina N, et al: Prognostic importance of the immediate hemodynamic response to nifedipine in patients with severe left ventricular dysfunction. *J Am Coll Cardiol* 10:1303-1311, 1987

303. Barjon JN, Rouleau JL, Bichet D, et al: Chronic renal and neurohumoral effects of the calcium entry blocker nisoldipine in patients with congestive heart failure. *J Am Coll Cardiol* 9:622-630, 1987

304. Elkayam U, Roth A, Hsueh W, et al: Neurohumoral consequences of vasodilator therapy with hydralazine and nifedipine in severe congestive heart failure. *Am Heart J* 111:1130-1138, 1986

305. Ljung B: Vascular selectivity of felodipine. *Drugs* 29 Suppl 2:46-58, 1985

306. Packer M: Therapeutic options in the management of chronic heart failure. Is there a drug of first choice? *Circulation* 79:198-204, 1989

307. Cleland JG, Dargie HJ, Hodsman GP, et al: Captopril in heart failure. A double blind controlled trial. *Br Heart J* 52:530-535, 1984

308. Cleland JG, Dargie HJ, Ball SG, et al: Effects of enalapril in heart failure: a double blind study of effects on exercise performance, renal function, hormones, and metabolic state. *Br Heart J* 54:305-312, 1985

309. The CONSENSUS Trial Study Group: Effects of enalapril on mortality in severe congestive heart failure. Results of the Cooperative North Scandinavian Enalapril Survival Study (CONSENSUS). *N Engl J Med* 316:1429-1435, 1987

310. Newman TJ, Maskin CS, Dennick LG, et al: Effects of captopril on survival in patients with heart failure. *Am J Med* 84:140-144, 1988

311. Kleber FX, Laube A, Osterkorn K, et al: Captopril in mild to moderate heart failure over 18 months. Effects on morbidity and mortality (abstract). *J Am Coll Cardiol* 9 Suppl A:42, 1987

312. Sharpe N, Murphy J, Smith H, et al: Treatment of patients with symptomless left ventricular dysfunction after myocardial infarction. *Lancet* 1:255-259, 1988

313. Pfeffer MA, Lamas GA, Vaughan DE, et al: Effect of captopril on progressive ventricular dilatation after anterior myocardial infarction. *N Engl J Med* 319:80-86, 1988

314. Captopril Multicenter Research Group: A placebo-controlled trial of captopril in refractory chronic congestive heart failure. *J Am Coll Cardiol* 2:755-763, 1983

315. Fonarow GC, Chelimsky-Fallick C, Stevenson LW, et al: Effect of direct vasodilation with hydralazine versus angiotensin-converting enzyme inhibition with captopril on mortality in advanced heart failure: the Hy-C trial. *J Am Coll Cardiol* 19:842-850, 1992

316. Pfeffer MA, Braunwald E, Moye LA, et al: Effect of captopril on mortality and morbidity in patients with left ventricular dysfunction after myocardial infarction. Results of the Survival and Ventricular Enlargement trial. The SAVE Investigators. *N Engl J Med* 327:669-677, 1992

317. Swedberg K, Held P, Kjekshus J, et al: Effects of the early administration of enalapril on mortality in patients with acute myocardial infarction. Results of the Cooperative New Scandinavian Enalapril Survival Study II (CONSENSUS II). *N Engl J Med* 327:678-684, 1992

318. The Acute Infarction Ramipril Efficacy (AIRE) Study Investigators: Effect of ramipril on mortality and morbidity of survivors of acute myocardial infarction with clinical evidence of heart failure. *Lancet* 342:821-828, 1993

319. Kleber FX, Niemoller L, Doering W: Impact of converting enzyme inhibition on progression of chronic heart failure: results of the Munich Mild Heart Failure Trial. *Br Heart J* 67:289-296, 1992

320. Clough DP, Collis MG, Conway J, et al: Interaction of angiotensin-converting enzyme inhibitors with the function of the sympathetic nervous system. *Am J Cardiol* 49:1410-1414, 1982

321. Packer M, Medina N, Yushak M: Correction of dilutional hyponatremia in severe chronic heart failure by converting-enzyme inhibition. *Ann Intern Med* 100:782-789, 1984

322. Hamilton RW, Buckalew VM Jr: Sodium, water, and congestive heart failure. *Ann Intern Med* 100:902-904, 1984

323. Bonjour JP, Malvin RL: Stimulation of ADH release by the renin-angiotensin system. *Am J Physiol* 218:1555-1559, 1970

324. Hollenberg NK, Williams GH, Burger B, et al: Blockade and stimulation of renal, adrenal, and vascular angiotensin II receptors with 1-Sar, 8-Ala angiotensin II in normal man. *J Clin Invest* 57:39-46, 1976

325. Johnson AK, Mann JF, Rascher W, et al: Plasma angiotensin II concentrations and experimentally induced thirst. *Am J Physiol* 240: R229-R234, 1981

326. Kripalani KJ, McKinstry DN, Singhvi SM, et al: Disposition of captopril in normal subjects. *Clin Pharmacol Ther* 27:636-641, 1980

327. Alderman EL, Glantz SA: Acute hemodynamic interventions shift the diastolic pressure-volume curve in man. *Circulation* 54:662-671, 1976

328. Packer M, Meller J, Medina N, et al: Quantitative differences in the hemodynamic effects of captopril and nitroprusside in severe chronic heart failure. *Am J Cardiol* 51:183-188, 1983

329. Kramer B, Topic N, Massie B: Acute and long-term effects of captopril on exercise cardiac performance and exercise capacity in congestive heart failure. *Br J Clin Pharmacol* 14 Suppl 2:143-151, 1982

330. Packer M, Medina N, Yushak M: Relation between serum sodium concentration and the hemodynamic and clinical responses to converting enzyme inhibition with captopril in severe heart failure. *J Am Coll Cardiol* 3:1035-1043, 1984

331. Foult J-M, Tavolaro O, Antony I, et al: Direct myocardial and coronary effects of enalaprilat in patients with dilated cardiomyopathy: assessment by a bilateral intracoronary infusion technique. *Circulation* 77:337-344, 1988

332. Pacher R, Globits S, Bergler-Klein J, et al: Clinical and neurohumoral response of patients with severe congestive heart failure treated with two different captopril dosages. *Eur Heart J* 14:273-278, 1993

333. Swartz SL, Williams GH: Angiotensin-converting enzyme inhibition and prostaglandins. *Am J Cardiol* 49:1405-1409, 1982

334. Hall D, Zeitler H, Rudolph W: Counteraction of the vasodilator effects of enalapril by aspirin in severe heart failure. *J Am Coll Cardiol* 20:1549-1555, 1992

335. Massie BM, Kramer BL, Topic N: Long-term captopril therapy for chronic congestive heart failure. *Am J Cardiol* 53:1316-1320, 1984

336. Staessen J, Fagard R, Lijnen P, et al: Captopril and agranulocytosis (letter to the editor). *Lancet* 1:926-927, 1980

337. Richardson A, Bayliss J, Scriven AJ, et al: Double-blind comparison of captopril alone against frusemide plus amiloride in mild heart failure. *Lancet* 2:709-711, 1987

338. Eichhorn EJ: The paradox of beta-adrenergic blockade for the management of congestive heart failure. *Am J Med* 92:527-538, 1992

339. Chadda K, Goldstein S, Byington R, et al: Effect of propranolol after acute myocardial infarction in patients with congestive heart failure. *Circulation* 73:503-510, 1986

340. Lichstein E: Why do beta-receptor blockers decrease mortality after myocardial infarction? *J Am Coll Cardiol* 6:973-975, 1985

341. Lichstein E, Hager WD, Gregory JJ, et al: Relation between beta-adrenergic blocker use, various correlates of left ventricular function and the chance of developing congestive heart failure. The Multicenter Diltiazem Post-Infarction Research Group. *J Am Coll Cardiol* 16:1327-1332, 1990

342. The MIAMI Trial Research Group: Metoprolol in acute myocardial infarction. Mortality. *Am J Cardiol* 56:15G-22G, 1985

343. Yusuf S, Peto R, Lewis J, et al: Beta blockade during and after myocardial infarction: an overview of the randomized trials. *Prog Cardiovasc Dis* 27:335-371, 1985

344. Waagstein F, Caidahl K, Wallentin I, et al: Long-term beta-blockade in dilated cardiomyopathy. Effects of short- and long-term metoprolol treatment followed by withdrawal and readministration of metoprolol. *Circulation* 80:551-563, 1989

345. Swedberg K, Hjalmarson A, Waagstein F, et al: Adverse effects of beta-blockade withdrawal in patients with congestive cardiomyopathy. *Br Heart J* 44:134-142, 1980

346. Warner-Stevenson L, Tillisch JH, Hamilton M, et al: Importance of hemodynamic response to therapy in predicting survival with ejection fraction less than or equal to 20% secondary to ischemic or nonischemic dilated cardiomyopathy. *Am J Cardiol* 66:1348-1354, 1990

347. Lichstein E, Morganroth J, Harrist R, et al: Effect of propranolol on ventricular arrhythmia. The beta-blocker heart attack trial experience. *Circulation* 67 Suppl 1:5-10, 1983

348. Brodsky MA, Allen BJ, Bessen M, et al: Beta-blocker therapy in patients with ventricular tachyarrhythmias in the setting of left ventricular dysfunction. *Am Heart J* 115:799-808, 1988

349. Waagstein F, Hjalmarson A, Varnauskas E, et al: Effect of chronic beta-adrenergic receptor blockade in congestive cardiomyopathy. *Br Heart J* 37:1022-1036, 1975

350. Swedberg K, Hjalmarson A, Waagstein F, et al: Prolongation of survival in congestive cardiomyopathy by beta-receptor blockade. *Lancet* 1:1374-1376, 1979

351. Swedberg K, Hjalmarson A, Waagstein F, et al: Beneficial effects of long-term beta-blockade in congestive cardiomyopathy. *Br Heart J* 44:117-133, 1980

352. Anderson JL, Lutz JR, Gilbert EM, et al: A randomized trial of low-dose beta-blockade therapy for idiopathic dilated cardiomyopathy. *Am J Cardiol* 55:471-475, 1985

353. Andersson B, Blomstrom-Lundqvist C, Hedner T, et al: Exercise hemodynamics and myocardial metabolism during long-term beta-adrenergic blockade in severe heart failure. *J Am Coll Cardiol* 18:1059-1066, 1991

354. Alderman J, Grossman W: Are beta-adrenergic-blocking drugs useful in the treatment of dilated cardiomyopathy? *Circulation* 71:854-857, 1985

355. Engelmeier RS, O'Connell JB, Walsh R, et al: Improvement in symptoms and exercise tolerance by metoprolol in patients with dilated cardiomyopathy: a double-blind, randomized, placebo-controlled trial. *Circulation* 72:536-546, 1985

356. Heilbrunn SM, Shah P, Bristow MR, et al: Increased beta-receptor density and improved hemodynamic response to catecholamine stimulation during long-term metoprolol therapy in heart failure from dilated cardiomyopathy. *Circulation* 79:483-490, 1989

357. Woodley SL, Gilbert EM, Anderson JL, et al: Beta-blockade with bucindolol in heart failure caused by ischemic versus idiopathic dilated cardiomyopathy. *Circulation* 84:2426-2441, 1991

358. Anderson JL, Gilbert EM, O'Connell JB, et al: Long-term (2 year) beneficial effects of beta-adrenergic blockade with bucindolol in patients with idiopathic dilated cardiomyopathy. *J Am Coll Cardiol* 17:1373-1381, 1991

359. Bristow MR, Ginsburg R, Umans V, et al: Beta 1- and beta 2-adrenergic-receptor subpopulations in nonfailing and failing human ventricular myocardium: coupling of both receptor subtypes to muscle contraction and selective beta 1-receptor down-regulation in heart failure. *Circ Res* 59:297-309, 1986

360. Bristow MR, Port JD, Sandoval AB, et al: Beta-adrenergic receptor pathways in the failing human heart. *Heart Failure* 5:77-90, 1989

361. Gilbert EM, Olsen SL, Mealey P, et al: Is β-receptor up-regulation necessary for improved LV function in dilated cardiomyopathy? (Abstract.) *Circulation* 84 Suppl 2:469, 1991

362. Bohm M, Gierschik P, Jakobs KH, et al: Increase of $G_{i\alpha}$ in human hearts with dilated but not ischemic cardiomyopathy. *Circulation* 82:1249-1265, 1990

363. Gilbert EM, Anderson JL, Deitchman D, et al: Long-term beta-blocker vasodilator therapy improves cardiac function in idiopathic dilated cardiomyopathy: a double-blind, randomized study of bucindolol versus placebo. *Am J Med* 88:223-229, 1990

364. Eichhorn EJ, Bedotto JB, Malloy CR, et al: Effect of beta-adrenergic blockade on myocardial function and energetics in congestive heart failure. Improvements in hemodynamic, contractile, and diastolic performance with bucindolol. *Circulation* 82:473-483, 1990

365. Weber KT, Kinasewitz GT, West JS, et al: Long-term vasodilator therapy with trimazosin in chronic cardiac failure. *N Engl J Med* 303:242-250, 1980

366. Packer M, Meller J, Gorlin R, et al: Hemodynamic and clinical tachyphylaxis to prazosin-mediated afterload reduction in severe chronic congestive heart failure. *Circulation* 59:531-539, 1979

367. Leier CV, Patterson SE, Huss P, et al: The hemodynamic and clinical responses to terazosin, a new alpha blocking agent, in congestive heart failure. *Am J Med Sci* 292:128-135, 1986

368. Harper RW, Claxton H, Middlebrook K, et al: The acute and chronic haemodynamic effects of prazosin in severe congestive cardiac failure. *Med J Aust* 2 Suppl: 36-38, 1980

369. Higginbotham MB, Morris KG, Bramlet DA, et al: Long-term ambulatory therapy with prazosin versus placebo for chronic heart failure: relation between clinical response and left ventricular function at rest and during exercise. *Am J Cardiol* 52:782-788, 1983

370. Markham RV Jr, Corbett JR, Gilmore A, et al: Efficacy of prazosin in the management of chronic congestive heart failure: a 6-month randomized, double-blind, placebo-controlled study. *Am J Cardiol* 51:1346-1352, 1983

371. Kirlin PC, Das S, Pitt B: Chronic alpha-adrenoceptor blockade with trimazosin in congestive heart failure. *Int J Cardiol* 8:89-92, 1985

372. Reifart N, Schmidt-Moritz AD, Nadj M, et al: Lack of symptomatic and long-term hemodynamic effects of prazosin in chronic heart failure. Double-blind, randomized study over one year. *Z Kardiol* 74:205-212, 1985

373. Leier CV, Binkley PF, Randolph PH, et al: Long-term indoramin therapy in congestive heart failure: a double-blind, randomized, parallel placebo-controlled trial. *J Am Coll Cardiol* 9:426-432, 1987

374. Packer M, Medina N, Yushak M: Role of the renin-angiotensin system in the development of hemodynamic and clinical tolerance to long-term prazosin therapy in patients with severe chronic heart failure. *J Am Coll Cardiol* 7:671-680, 1986

375. Colucci WS, Williams GH, Braunwald E: Clinical, hemodynamic, and neuroendocrine effects of chronic prazosin therapy for congestive heart failure. *Am Heart J* 102:615-621, 1981

376. Kirlin PC, Das S, Grekin R, et al: Sympathetic inhibition with methyldopa in heart failure. *J Cardiovasc Pharmacol* 8:1092-1100, 1986

377. Hermiller JB, Magorien RD, Leithe ME, et al: Clonidine in congestive heart failure: a vasodilator with negative inotropic effects. *Am J Cardiol* 51:791-795, 1983

378. Kleber FX, Niemoller L: Long-term survival in the Munich Mild Heart Failure Trial (MHFT). *Am J Cardiol* 71:1237-1239, 1993

379. Fuster V, Gersh BJ, Giuliani ER, et al: The natural history of idiopathic dilated cardiomyopathy. *Am J Cardiol* 47:525-531, 1981

380. Stroke Prevention in Atrial Fibrillation Study Group Investigators: Preliminary report of the Stroke Prevention in Atrial Fibrillation Study. *N Engl J Med* 322:863-868, 1990

381. Packer M: Sudden unexpected death in patients with congestive heart failure: a second frontier. *Circulation* 72:681-685, 1985

382. Parmley WW, Chatterjee K: Congestive heart failure and arrhythmias: an overview. *Am J Cardiol* 57:34B-37B, 1986

383. Holmes J, Kubo SH, Cody RJ, et al: Arrhythmias in ischemic and nonischemic dilated cardiomyopathy: prediction of mortality by ambulatory electrocardiography. *Am J Cardiol* 55:146-151, 1985

384. Wilson JR: Use of antiarrhythmic drugs in patients with heart failure: clinical efficacy, hemodynamic results, and relation to survival. *Circulation* 75 Suppl 4:64-73, 1987

385. Litwin SE, Grossman W: Diastolic dysfunction as a cause of heart failure. *J Am Coll Cardiol* 22 Suppl A:49-55, 1993

CHAPTER

18

Cardiac transplantation

Brooks S. Edwards, M.D., Richard J. Rodeheffer, M.D., and Christopher G. A. McGregor, M.D.

End-stage congestive heart failure carries with it the grim prognosis of both an impaired lifestyle and a limited life expectancy.[1] Despite recent advances in the medical treatment of severe congestive heart failure,[2] cardiac transplantation offers the greatest potential for both alleviating symptoms and markedly prolonging survival.[3] Cardiac replacement has been a goal since early in this century and has now been clinically applied for over 25 years.[4] As early as 1933, Frank D. Mann of the Mayo Foundation reported on the behavior of the transplanted dog heart and described the physiologic and morphologic alterations that occur with allograft rejection.[5]

The modern era of cardiac transplantation began in 1960 with the description by Lower and Shumway[6] of the techniques and short-term success with orthotopic cardiac transplantation in the dog. Over several years, these workers refined the surgical techniques and immunosuppressive protocols required to allow the clinical application of cardiac transplantation. On the basis of the extensive laboratory work of Shumway and co-workers, Barnard[4] performed the first human cardiac transplantation in December 1967. One month later, Shumway and associates performed their first cardiac transplantation. Early successes and the straightforward surgical techniques encouraged a number of centers to perform cardiac transplantation. In 1968, a total of 101 cardiac transplantations were performed worldwide. Unfortunately, the short-term success initially enjoyed in most centers was replaced with long-term complications, including infection and rejection. Only in centers where a dedicated team paid exquisite attention to detail was cardiac transplantation initially successful.

In the 1970s, cyclosporine, a novel immunosuppressive compound, was isolated from a soil fungus. This agent exhibits a selective and sensitive inhibition of T-cell-mediated activation. Since its clinical introduction in 1980, there has been a dramatic improvement in both graft and patient survival and a reduction in infectious complications.[7] Cyclosporine therapy has revolutionized solid organ transplantation, and in combination with other immunosuppressive agents, cyclosporine has become the standard agent for the prevention of rejection. The availability of cyclosporine has allowed cardiac transplant programs to achieve 1-year survival rates in excess of 80% and 5-year survival rates in excess of 60%[8] (Fig 18-1).

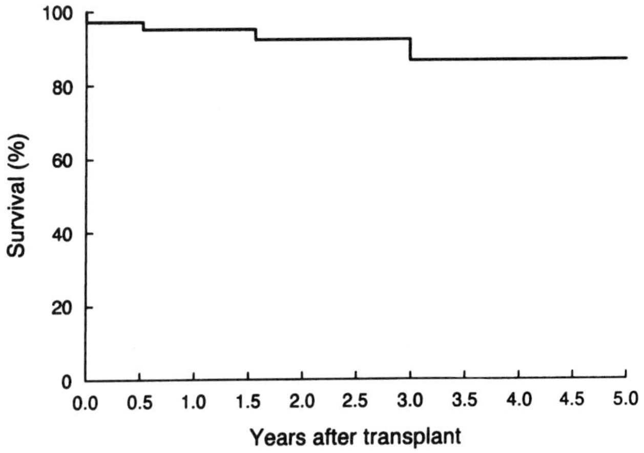

Fig 18-1 Actuarial Kaplan-Meier survival curve for 71 consecutive cardiac transplantations at the Mayo Clinic. The 1-year survival is 95.1% ± 2.8%, and the 5-year survival is 87.2% ± 6.3%.

SELECTION OF RECIPIENTS

Because of the extreme shortage of donor organs in the United States and abroad, recipients must be carefully selected to ensure the best utilization of this limited resource. The ideal candidate for cardiac transplantation is a young person with severe and irreversible cardiac dysfunction[9,10] (Table 18-1). Prognostic factors suggesting a poor short-term outcome without cardiac transplantation include an ejection fraction of less than 15%, complex ventricular ectopy, activation of the sympathetic nervous system, and impairment in exercise capacity with a reduction in maximum oxygen consumption below 14 mL/kg per minute.[10]

Most cardiac transplantations are performed for treatment of either ischemic heart disease or idiopathic dilated cardiomyopathy. Fewer transplantations have been done for persons with severe hypertrophic or restrictive cardiomyopathy, valvular disease, or congenital heart disease.[8]

Initially, transplantation was restricted to persons younger than 50 years. However, it now appears that transplantation may be successful even in patients in their middle 60s.[11] Coexistent systemic disease that limits the

Table 18-1 Selection criteria for cardiac transplantation

Irreversible cardiac disease
Life expectancy of less than 2 years
Medically compliant
Motivated for transplantation
Absence of contraindications

Table 18-2 Contraindications to cardiac transplantation

Fixed pulmonary hypertension >6 Wood units
Recent pulmonary infarction
Active infection
Noncardiac disease significantly limiting life expectancy
Unresolved drug or alcohol abuse
Extreme obesity
Inability to adhere to a regimented lifestyle

life expectancy of the candidate should be considered a contraindication to transplantation (Table 18-2). A generally favorable outcome has been achieved, however, in selected patients with cardiac disease who underwent transplantation after curative therapy for neoplastic disease. A history of neoplastic disease in a patient with severe cardiac failure should not be considered an absolute contraindication to transplantation.[12]

Diabetes mellitus may be aggravated by steroid therapy after transplantation.[13] In persons with juvenile-onset (type I) diabetes mellitus, transplantation is relatively contraindicated because of the systemic nature of this disease and the likelihood that coexistent organ systems (notably the kidney) will be diseased and ultimately will limit the patient's survival. In young diabetic patients with severe cardiac disease, consideration may be given to multiorgan transplantation (i.e., heart and pancreas or heart, kidney, and pancreas) if the remainder of their vasculature is not highly diseased. In individuals with adult-onset diabetes, even those using insulin, successful cardiac transplantation can be accomplished, but additional attention must be paid to the maintenance of a euglycemic state.[14]

Cardiac transplantation in patients with fixed pulmonary hypertension is contraindicated, since the donor heart may be unable to immediately generate the right ventricular systolic pressure needed to maintain adequate cardiac output. Persons with pulmonary hypertension should receive nitroprusside, prostacyclin, or PGE_1 during right heart catheterization to assess the reversibility of the pulmonary vascular disease.[15,16] The risk of transplantation in patients with pulmonary hypertension is a continuum: even in those with mild pulmonary hypertension, the risk increases with increasing pulmonary vascular resistance.[17] In patients with fixed and severe pulmonary hypertension (pulmonary vascular resistance >8 Wood units), orthotopic cardiac transplantation carries a significantly increased risk. They may, however, be candidates for heterotopic transplantation ("piggyback heart") or combined heart-lung transplantation,[18] although the expected results after these operations are lower than those of simple orthotopic transplantation.[8]

Recent and unresolved pulmonary infarction should be considered a contraindication to transplantation because of the substantial risk of an abscess developing in the necrotic pulmonary tissue. Once the pulmonary infarction has resolved, transplantation can be successfully accomplished.

Active infection in the patient awaiting transplantation should be treated, and the infectious process should have resolved before cardiac transplantation. In patients with unresolved infection, the risk of systemic sepsis after immunosuppressive therapy begins is high.

Among patients with idiopathic dilated cardiomyopathy is a group with severely impaired ventricular function (stroke volume <40 mL/beat) and minimal symptoms (the patient is "too well" for transplantation). In a retrospective analysis it appears that despite the lack of symptoms survival is markedly reduced, and these patients may benefit from transplantation[19] or more aggressive conventional medical therapy. On the other end of the spectrum are patients in whom functional impairment is so severe that they require inotropic support or a mechanical assist device. These patients were once regarded as "too sick" for transplantation; however, results in a carefully selected group of patients demonstrate acceptable postoperative survival for these critically ill patients, similar to that in ambulatory patients undergoing transplantation.[20-23]

In addition to the tangible selection criteria, patient motivation for cardiac transplantation is paramount. The potential recipient must be willing to follow a regimented lifestyle that includes daily medications with frequent and lifelong medical follow-up, including rejection surveillance with regular endomyocardial biopsies. A supportive and stable home life assists in the successful rehabilitation of patients after cardiac transplantation. The potential recipient should be educated in depth to develop realistic expectations for the results and limitations of cardiac transplantation.

SELECTION OF DONORS

Proper selection of potential cardiac donors is vital to successful cardiac transplantation. Donors may be procured locally or regionally.[24,25] Current techniques of cardioplegia allow for a maximum of 4 to 6 hours of cold ischemia. Variations in techniques of cardioplegia may eventually allow for prolongation of acceptable ischemic time.

Before organ donation is considered, the potential donor should be declared legally dead by two physicians not affiliated with the transplantation team. The legal requirements for brain death vary from state to state. The potential donor's closest relatives should be consulted and informed consent obtained for organ donation. Donors should undergo a general physical examination, and any history of cardiac or noncardiac disorders should be elicited from family members. The donors should be young persons with no history of cardiovascular disorders. Because of the prevalence of coronary artery disease in the Western Hemisphere, we prefer women donors under age 45 and men donors under 35 years of age. Persons beyond these ages may be acceptable donors, but coronary angiography should be considered before acceptance. An electrocardiogram should be free of pathologic Q waves. Isolated T-wave abnormalities may be related to central nervous disorders and are not in isolation a contraindication to organ donation. If the electrocardiogram is abnormal or cardiac contusion may have occurred, transthoracic or transesophageal echocardiography should be performed. The potential donor may require intravenous inotropic support, but high doses required over a prolonged period should alert the physician to the possibility of intrinsic cardiac dysfunction as well as to the risk of catecholamine-induced myocardial necrosis.

Before acceptance, the donor should have ABO blood typing performed along with determination of human immunodeficiency virus and hepatitis serology. For future use, toxoplasma and cytomegalovirus immune status should be determined.

The donor heart should be matched with a recipient who is ABO compatible and of similar body size. In general, the donor may be 20% smaller or 50% larger than the recipient. If the recipient has preexisting pulmonary hypertension, a larger donor heart may be beneficial.

SURGICAL TECHNIQUES

Donor procedure

Distant organ procurement of the heart was introduced in 1977 at Stanford, and the vast majority of donor hearts are now harvested at a site distant from the recipient. The maximum acceptable ischemic time of a donor heart remains 4 to 6 hours, although shorter preservation times result in better early hemodynamic performance and a significantly lower 30-day mortality.[8] The surgical techniques are straightforward, do not require cardiopulmonary bypass, and therefore may be performed in any standard hospital operating room. Donors are placed on a heating blanket to avoid systemic hypothermia that can occur after dissection of the liver, pancreas, and kidneys with the chest and abdomen open. Measurement of central venous pressure and arterial blood pressure is important to optimize hemodynamics during the donor procedure. The cardiac excision takes approximately 20 minutes, but with the simultaneous retrieval of liver, kidney, and pancreas, a donor operation can take 4 to 6 hours. Crossmatch of 3 units of blood is advisable to replace potential blood loss in the abdomen.

A median sternotomy incision is made, and the heart and great vessels are carefully inspected and palpated. The cavae and ascending aorta are dissected and encircled with tapes. The cardiac team then waits until the abdominal surgeons have completed their dissection and placed their cannulae. Systemic heparinization is carried out. Both cavae are clamped or tied, and after the heart is allowed to empty for a few beats, the ascending aorta is cross-clamped and cold (4°C) crystalloid cardioplegic solution infused into the aortic root. The heart is then decompressed by division of the inferior pulmonary veins and inferior vena cava. Simultaneous supplemental topical cooling with cold (4°C) saline is performed. At the end of the cardioplegic infusion, the heart is excised by division of the superior vena cava, the remaining pulmonary veins, the right and left pulmonary arteries, and the aorta. The heart is then placed in a solution of cold (4°C) saline or cardioplegic solution within two sealed containers surrounded by ice in a standard cooler. In heart transplantation for congenital heart disease, a more generous excision is carried out in the donor to include the innominate vein and the arch of the aorta so that extra tissue is provided for insertion into the recipient.

Recipient procedure

Orthotopic heart transplantation is the procedure of choice in the vast majority of cases and has changed little since the original description by Lower and Shumway[6] (Fig 18-2). The only significant deviation from this description, introduced by Barnard,[26] is the more curvilinear right atrial incision away from the region of the sinoatrial node to avoid donor sinus node dysfunction. A median sternotomy incision is used, and cardiopulmonary bypass is instituted. The recipient heart is excised by dividing the aorta and pulmonary artery 1 cm distal to the valves to allow their use for allograft valve replacement after cryopreservation. The right and left atria are then excised close to the atrioventricular ring, so that most of the interatrial septum is left in place. Thus, a generous cuff of both right and left atrium (including the pulmonary veins) is available for suturing.

The donor heart is brought onto the operating table, and the left atrium is opened between the pulmonary veins. The left atrial anastomosis is performed first with a single continuous 54-in. 3-0 polypropylene (Prolene) suture, beginning in the region of the left superior pulmonary vein in the recipient and the base of the left atrial appendage in the donor (Fig 18-2,A). External pericardial cold irrigation is begun during this anastomosis, and when it is complete, a bubble-free cold line is inserted through the left atrial appendage. Cold saline is allowed to perfuse the interior of the left ventricle, both to cool it and to expel any air contained therein. A curvilinear incision is then made in the right atrium from the inferior vena cava to the base of the right atrial appendage (Fig 18-2,B). The right atrial anastomosis is accomplished with a suture similar to that used for the left atrium. Rewarming of the patient is begun. The aortic anastomosis is created with a single continuous 4-0 polypropylene suture (Fig 18-2,C).

When the anastomosis is complete, external pericardial irrigation is stopped and de-airing of the heart is done before the aortic cross-clamp is removed. The left atrial cold line is removed. After removal of the aortic clamp, the pulmonary arterial anastomosis is completed (Fig 18-2,D). If necessary, the heart is defibrillated. Pacing wires are inserted. Cardiopulmonary bypass is discontinued while the patient receives a continuous infusion of isoproterenol, used both for its chronotropic and for its inotropic effects. In uncompli-

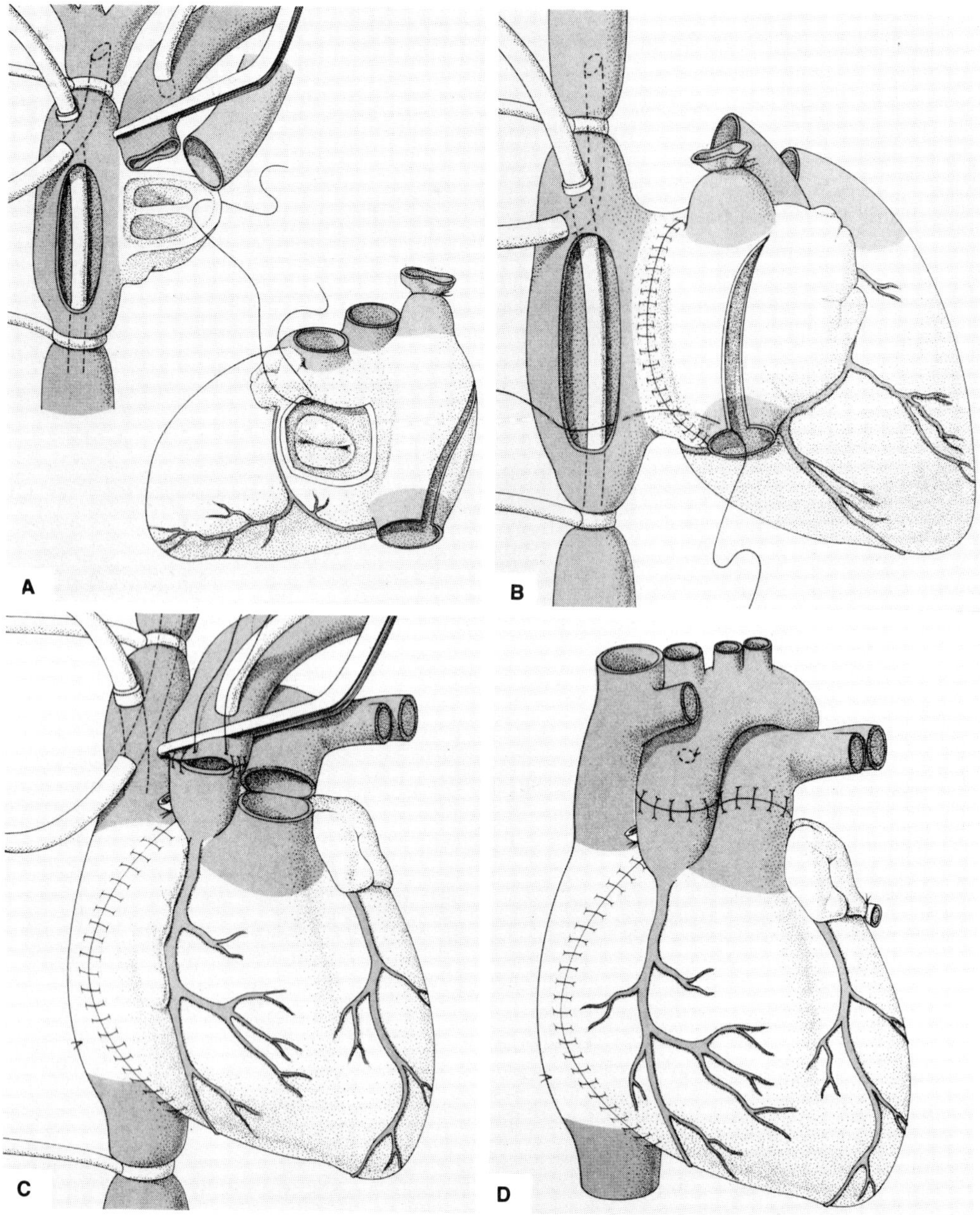

Fig 18-2 **A** to **D**, surgical techniques of orthotopic cardiac transplantation (see text for details). (From McGregor CGA: Current state of heart transplantation. *Br J Hosp Med* 37:310-318, 1987. By permission of Mark Allen Publishing.)

cated cases, the entire procedure is complete in approximately 3 hours, and the patient can usually be extubated within 12 hours.

CARE AND REHABILITATION AFTER TRANSPLANTATION

In the week after transplantation, patients should be monitored closely. The heart rate of the allograft initially requires support by isoproterenol infusion or cardiac pacing. We prefer isoproterenol because of the concomitant beneficial hemodynamic and inotropic effects of β-receptor stimulation. Isoproterenol may be withdrawn gradually as a sinus node recovers and heart rates approach 90 beats/min.[27] Some patients may experience a long delay in sinus node recovery, requiring prolonged isoproterenol stimulation. In unusual circumstances, permanent cardiac pacing may be required, but in most cases administration of isoproterenol with gradual tapering obviates permanent pacing.[28]

The patient should be extubated as soon as possible and mobilized early. Physical therapy, consisting at first of passive range of motion and stretching exercises, should begin early. Monitored use of a stationary bicycle is frequently beneficial, and this can be accomplished in the patient's room to minimize the exposure to nosocomial infections during the period of maximal immunosuppression.

Education of the patient and family, which began in the pretransplantation period, should be continued and intensified during the postoperative period. The patient should be instructed in the use of a sphygmomanometer and gradually, while in the hospital, self-administration of oral medications should begin.

Long-term successful exercise training can be accomplished in most transplant recipients. Since the transplanted heart lacks vagal innervation, the resting heart rate is increased. Elegant studies by Wilson et al.[29] have documented gradual sympathetic reinnervation in many patients 1 year or more after transplantation. After surgical recovery, patients typically have a resting sinus tachycardia of 90 to 110 beats/min. Exercise results in a delayed increase in heart rate, since the sinus node depends on circulating catecholamines for stimulation. The maximum heart rate obtained at peak exercise ranges from 140 to 150 beats/min, or approximately 20% less than that in age-matched control patients.[30-32] Despite the impaired heart rate response, it has been demonstrated that arterial baroreceptor sensitivity, which is attenuated in heart failure, normalizes rapidly after transplantation.[33] The effect of the reset baroreceptors may affect vascular tone, but it does not modify the rate of the denervated heart. During dynamic exercise, cardiac output increases initially because of increasing stroke volume, but as exercise progresses, with circulating catecholamine stimulation, an increase in heart rate also contributes to the increase in cardiac output. At rest, intracardiac pressures are usually normal, but with exercise, they tend to increase to a greater degree than that observed in normal patients.[34] This suggests that the transplanted heart may exhibit some element of diastolic dysfunction.[35] Whether this dysfunction is related to cyclosporine-induced interstitial fibrosis, the effect of transplant-related ischemia, or other factors is unknown. Despite these abnormalities, the motivated transplant recipient may participate in, and be successful at, even the highest level of competitive athletics.

Recent studies have demonstrated progressive left ventricular remodeling after transplantation, with an increase in left ventricular cavity size and a reduction in mass. This process maintains a normal ejection fraction and increases wall stress from an initially low level to the normal range.[36]

IMMUNOSUPPRESSION AND REJECTION SURVEILLANCE

Mechanisms of rejection

Rejection of the allograft may occur at any time after coronary perfusion is established. The highest risk for allograft rejection occurs during the first 6 months after transplantation.

Hyperacute rejection may occur in the operating room or within the first postoperative hours. This rare form of rejection may result in immediate loss of the grafted organ. Hyperacute rejection occurs when the recipient has preformed antibodies against donor tissue. This may occur in an ABO-incompatible match or in a recipient who has received multiple previous transfusions or prior transplantation. To screen for and prevent this catastrophic reaction, serum from all potential recipients is tested against a panel of 50 to 100 random lymphocyte samples to detect preformed antibodies. Should the recipient serum react to a significant number of these random lymphocyte samples, a direct lymphocytotoxic cross matching between recipient serum and donor cells should be performed before accepting the donor heart. Avoidance of ABO-incompatible matches requires strict attention to the donor and recipient blood groups.

Table 18-3 Mayo Clinic surveillance biopsy schedule

Time after transplantation	Biopsy frequency
0 to 6 weeks	Weekly
6 to 12 weeks	Biweekly
3 to 9 months	Monthly
9 months and later	Quarterly

The classic form of cardiac rejection results from T-cell activation with a cellular myocardial infiltrate and activation of lymphokines. Before the widespread availability and use of cyclosporine, cell-mediated rejection occurred precipitously and was associated with distinct clinical signs, including fever, rales, a third heart sound, and elevation of jugular venous pressure. Coincident with the development of myocardial edema, the electrocardiogram showed a loss of voltage, and cardiomegaly was observed on a chest radiograph. Cyclosporine has modified the cellular response so that a more indolent form of rejection occurs. The recipient receiving cyclosporine therapy may have a low-grade fever or complain of general malaise; clinical signs of rejection are often subtle or absent until overwhelming rejection is present. Therefore, right ventricular endomyocardial biopsy continues to be used to assess the presence and severity of rejection in otherwise asymptomatic patients.

Rejection surveillance and pathology

Transvenous endomyocardial biopsy is routinely performed as an outpatient procedure[37] (see chapter 19B). In most laboratories, right ventricular endomyocardial biopsy is performed from a right internal jugular approach; however, adequate biopsy samples can be obtained by a subclavian or femoral venous approach. At least five biopsy specimens should be obtained from each patient to minimize the possibility of sampling error. Since rejection is a diffuse process, in most cases left ventricular biopsy adds little additional useful information. In unusual circumstances, however, in which isolated left ventricular dysfunction is a predominant problem, a left ventricular biopsy should be obtained.

Because the risk of allograft rejection is greatest during the first 6 months after transplantation, the frequency of obtaining surveillance biopsies is highest during this period (Table 18-3). Evidence of rejection requires repeat biopsy in 7 to 14 days. Myocardial biopsy specimens should be obtained at times other than those prescheduled if there is clinical suspicion of allograft rejection or

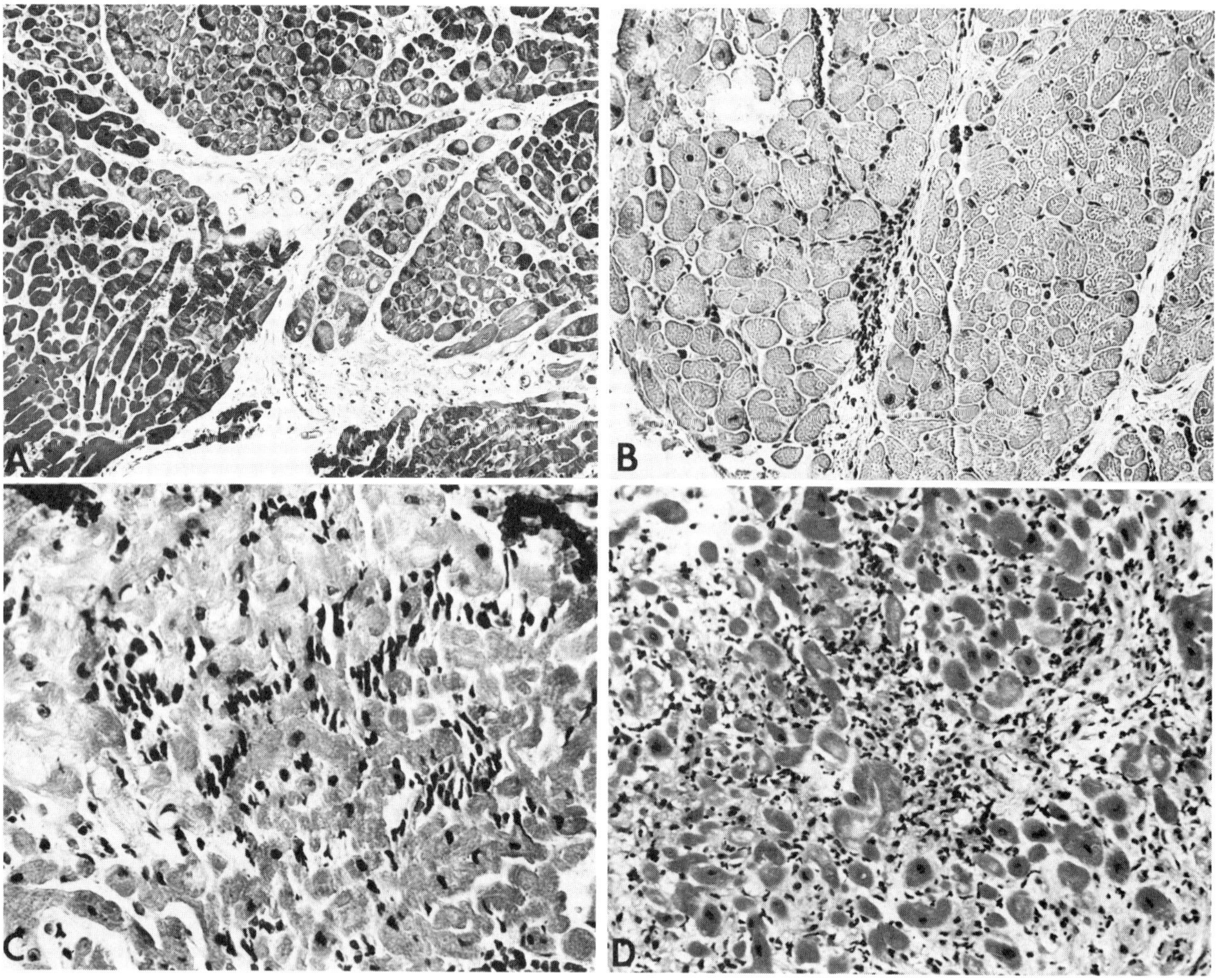

Fig 18-3 Right ventricular endomyocardial biopsy. **A,** no evidence of rejection. (×25.) **B,** mild cellular rejection characterized by a perivascular lymphocytic infiltrate (grade 1A). (×40.) **C,** moderate cellular rejection with lymphocytic infiltration and cellular necrosis (grade 3B). (×40.) **D,** severe rejection with a dense lymphocytic infiltrate, extensive myocyte necrosis, and edema (grade 4). (**D,** courtesy of M. Billingham, M.D., Stanford, CA.)

concern that the allograft is involved by an infectious process. Risk factors for more aggressive rejection include multiparous female recipients, female donors (even into female recipients), and HLA mismatches.[38]

Interpretation of the cardiac biopsy specimen must be made by a pathologist thoroughly familiar with cardiac transplantation (Fig 18-3). Many classifications of rejection have been proposed, including the Billingham criteria,[39] the Texas Heart Institute classification,[40] and the Hanover classification.[41] Under the leadership of the International Society for Heart and Lung Transplantation, a study group recently proposed a working formulation for the standardization of nomenclature in the classification of cardiac allograft rejection[42] (Table 18-4). This standardized formulation has been widely accepted by most transplantation centers and has enhanced the ability for intergroup comparison and outcome analysis.

The current biopsy specimen should be compared with previous specimens. By comparison, a rejection episode may be classified as *ongoing* if it shows no evidence of resolution from the last biopsy, *resolving* if the rejection is still present but improved, and *resolved* if cellular infiltration is absent or confined to areas of fibrous tissue.

The pathologist and clinician must be aware of the so-called rejection look-alikes that may be seen on biopsy. Infectious infiltrates such as those occurring with cytomegalovirus or toxoplasmosis may be confused with cellular rejection. The *Quilty phenomenon* is an endocardial collection of lymphocytes with extensive vascular spaces.[43] These lymphocytes may extend into the subjacent myocardium, and there may even be evidence of myocyte damage in the vicinity of the Quilty infiltrate. Cutting the biopsy sample tangentially may give the false appearance of an intramyocardial collection of activated lymphocytes consistent with mild or moderate rejection. Utilizing the polymerase chain reaction, we identified

Table 18-4 Standardized cardiac biopsy grading scheme*

Grade	Nomenclature: "New" (ISHLT)	Nomenclature: "Old"
0	No rejection	No rejection
1A	Focal (perivascular or interstitial) infiltrate without necrosis	Mild rejection
1B	Diffuse but sparse infiltrate without necrosis	
2	One focus only with aggressive infiltration or focal myocyte damage, or both	"Focal" moderate rejection
3A	Multifocal aggressive infiltrates or myocyte damage, or both	"Low" moderate rejection
3B	Diffuse inflammatory process with necrosis	"Borderline severe" rejection
4	Diffuse aggressive polymorphous infiltrate with or without edema, hemorrhage, and vasculitis and with necrosis	"Severe acute" rejection

ISHLT, International Society for Heart and Lung Transplantation.
*"Resolving" rejection is denoted by a lesser grade. "Resolved" rejection is denoted by grade 0.
From Billingham ME, Cary NRB, Hammond ME, et al: A working formulation for the standardization of nomenclature in the diagnosis of heart and lung rejection: Heart Rejection Study Group. *J Heart Transplant* 9:587-593, 1990. By permission of International Society for Heart and Lung Transplantation.

sequences of the Ebstein-Barr virus genome in biopsy specimens demonstrating the Quilty phenomenon.[44] The classic Quilty phenomenon has not been treated as rejection and typically follows a benign course.

Because rejection may take 7 to 14 days to resolve after treatment, tissue obtained too early may be classified as showing ongoing rejection when in fact the process is resolving. Complications of biopsy are unusual but include damage to vascular structures, cardiac arrhythmias, cardiac perforation, right ventricular-coronary artery fistulae, and infection.[45-47]

Attempts have been made to devise noninvasive markers for acute rejection.[48-50] Two-dimensional echocardiography has proved too insensitive for mild or moderate degrees of rejection. Doppler evaluation of diastolic function has been reported to correlate well with rejection in the early post-transplantation period;[51] however, the ultimate usefulness of Doppler ultrasound in detecting rejection will require further validation.[52,53]

Prevention and treatment of rejection

Currently available immunosuppressive therapy is considered antigen-nonspecific immunosuppression. In the future, there may be an opportunity to inhibit the immune response to a specific antigen or group of antigens.

Cyclosporine. Cyclosporine is a peptide derivative of the fungus *Trichoderma polysporum.* Cyclosporine acts to inhibit the production of the lymphokine interleukin-2 (IL-2).[7] IL-2 is produced by helper T cells when the T-cell receptor is bound to a foreign antigen. IL-2 is essential in promoting T-cell division and allowing for amplification of the immune response. In addition, IL-2 stimulates B-cell growth and activates monocytes and natural killer cells.

Cyclosporine is orally active and has a narrow toxic to therapeutic range. To ensure appropriate dosing of the agent, circulating levels of cyclosporine must be monitored.[54] Currently available techniques to monitor cyclosporine include both radioimmunoassay techniques and high-performance liquid chromatography. The most common radioimmunoassay currently available uses a polyclonal antibody to cyclosporine and measures both metabolites and active cyclosporine. Monoclonal antibodies for cyclosporine may be used to assay cyclosporine. The liquid chromatography technique measures only cyclosporine. Cyclosporine is highly lipophilic and readily diffuses into erythrocytes, so that concentrations of cyclosporine within circulating red blood cells are high. The cyclosporine in erythrocytes is not in equilibrium with plasma cyclosporine and is therefore not available for immunosuppression. Because of this, results of measurement of cyclosporine in whole blood may vary with changes in the hematocrit.

In the early period after transplantation, trough plasma cyclosporine, as determined by radioimmunoassay, should be kept in the range of 150 to 300 ng/mL. Because the risk of rejection declines with time, cyclosporine levels may be safely reduced. By 60 days after transplantation, most patients can be maintained with trough serum levels of 75 to 150 ng/mL. The precise level needs to be individualized for each patient on the basis of rejection history and renal function. Cyclosporine is hepatically metabolized and is excreted both by the gastrointestinal tract and by the kidney. Dose adjustments are required for both hepatic and renal insufficiency. Important drug-drug interactions may occur and result in clinically important changes in circulating cyclosporine. Drugs that compete for cytochrome P-450 activity, including erythromycin, ketoconazole, and calcium channel blockers, all increase circulating levels of cyclosporine. Drugs that induce cytochrome P-450 result in enhanced metabolism and reduced circulating concentration of cyclosporine. Administration of isoniazid, rifampin, phenytoin, and phenobarbital requires an increase in the dose of cyclosporine to maintain adequate circulating levels. In addition, bile acid binding resins may impair cyclosporine absorption.

The syndrome of post-transplantation lymphoproliferative disorders is characterized by the occurrence of a malignant B-cell lymphoma serologically associated with Epstein-Barr virus infection.[55] This syndrome occurred with considerable frequency when high doses of cyclosporine were initially used as monotherapy. With current combined immunosuppressive protocols, fewer cases of post-transplantation lymphoproliferative disorder are encountered. Often, post-transplantation lymphoma responds dramatically to a reduction in immunosuppression.

Cyclosporine acts by binding to a specific cytosolic binding protein, cyclophilin. Recent studies have identified a new immunosuppressive agent, FK 506. This agent acts by binding to a specific cytosolic binding protein known as "FK 506 binding protein." Studies are under way comparing cyclosporine with FK 506. Although it was initially hoped that patients treated with FK 506 would have less nephrotoxicity and hypertension than those receiving cyclosporine, these problems persist. The ultimate usefulness and indication for the agent will be resolved by further investigation.

Corticosteroids. Corticosteroids have been the mainstay of immunosuppressive therapy since the first clinical cardiac transplantations. Although steroids appear to inhibit the cell-mediated limb of the immune system more than the humoral limb, the mechanisms of action responsible for immunosuppressive effects of corticosteroids are incompletely understood. Steroids are known to impair the production of interferon-γ and block the effects of the lymphokine migration inhibitory factor, thereby preventing the accumulation of macrophages at the site of an immune response. In addition, glucocorticoids inhibit phospholipase A and thereby decrease the formation of prostaglandin and derivatives of arachidonic acid.[56]

Traditionally, glucocorticoids have been used intraoperatively and in high doses during the first 6 weeks after cardiac transplantation. For most patients, long-term maintenance dosage is 0.1 to 0.2 mg of prednisone per kilogram of body weight per day. Episodes of moderate or severe rejection are treated with either intravenously administered methylprednisolone (1 g daily for 3 days) or an increase in the oral dose of prednisone (50 mg twice daily) followed by tapering over approximately 2 weeks. New protocols using cyclosporine and azathioprine alone or in combination with a third agent, such as vincristine, have demonstrated that 40% to 80% of patients may tolerate complete withdrawal of steroids.[57-59] Because of the many steroid-induced side effects, it has been considered desirable to markedly reduce or totally eliminate the long-term use of corticosteroids after cardiac transplantation. It is currently unknown, however, whether the long-term benefits of avoiding corticosteroids will exceed the potential risks of chronic rejection and the possible toxicity from increased immunosuppression with other agents.

Steroid-induced side effects are not unique in the transplantation population. They include glucose intolerance, hypercholesterolemia, weight gain, osteoporosis, avascular necrosis, cushingoid facies, and impaired immunity.

Azathioprine. Azathioprine is a purine analogue of 6-mercaptopurine. The drug was originally synthesized with the hope that it would be an effective antineoplastic agent. Although this has not been the case, azathioprine is recognized as an immunosuppressive agent.[60] As a purine analogue, azathioprine is incorporated into intracellular DNA and interferes with cell replication and proliferation. Although azathioprine inhibits proliferation of T and B lymphocytes, it also acts nonspecifically to suppress all bone marrow elements. The dose of azathioprine needs to be titrated according to the patient's leukocyte count, with a goal of suppressing the total count to approximately 4,000 cells/mL^3. The dose can gradually be increased to 1.5 to 2.5 mg/kg per day, depending on the bone marrow response. Great care should be exercised to avoid the concomitant administration of allopurinol with azathioprine. Azathioprine is metabolized by xanthine oxidase, and if the enzyme is inhibited by allopurinol, dangerous and potentially lethal bone marrow suppression may occur.

Methotrexate. Methotrexate is a folic acid analogue initially used in systemic chemotherapy for neoplastic disease. Recent clinical studies have demonstrated its potency as an immunosuppressive agent[61-63] for treatment of both recalcitrant rejection[61] and persistent mild rejection.[62] Toxicity is often related to leukopenia and requires careful monitoring. Long-term exposure may lead to hepatic fibrosis and liver failure. Short-term (2 to 10 weeks) use of the drug has been associated with sustained immunosuppression and an improved rejection profile.

Antilymphocytic antibody therapy. Antilymphocytic antibodies raised in xenotypic animals have been used to destroy or disable lymphocytes and thereby prevent or treat allograft rejection. Early preparations were polyclonal antibodies directed against many leukocytic antigens. These polyclonal antibody preparations include antilymphocyte globulin and antithymocyte globulin. More recently, cell hybridization techniques have been used to raise monoclonal antibodies against specific T-cell membrane antigens. OKT3 is a murine monoclonal preparation raised against the pan T-cell antigen CD3. The cell surface protein CD3 is linked to the T-cell antigen receptor, and binding of CD3 with OKT3 antibody renders the T cell nonfunctional.[64] Monoclonal antibodies raised against other pan T-cell antigens structurally remote from the T-cell receptor may not result in modulation of the immune response. Additional classes of monoclonal antibodies raised against other specific surface markers may increase the specificity and efficacy of monoclonal antibody therapy. One such antibody raised against IL-2 receptor shows great promise as an effective modulator of cell-mediated immunity.[65-67] Additionally, an antibody directed against the CD4 cell (helper T cell) has been shown in the rat to induce specific immune tolerance.[68]

A 10- to 14-day course of antilymphocytic antibody therapy has been successfully used both as rejection prophylaxis in the early transplantation period and as

Table 18-5 Mayo Clinic approach for calculating the daily dose of OKT3 (milligrams) after heart or lung transplantation

Absolute CD3 cell count	CD3 receptors/cell <5	6-10	>10
≤50	0	0	0
51-100	0	2.5	2.5
101-200	2.5	2.5	5
>200	2.5	2.5	5

treatment for steroid-resistant (refractory) rejection.[69-72] Initial dosing may be associated with the release of lymphokines and result in fever, chills, bronchospasm, diarrhea, pulmonary capillary leak syndrome, and hypotension. Pretreatment of the patient with administration of antihistamines and steroids may attenuate this reaction, and after the first or second dose, the agents are usually well tolerated. Interestingly, the anti-IL-2 antibody does not produce this anaphylactoid reaction.

Although the standard dose of OKT3 for induction therapy has been 5 mg/day for 10 to 14 days, we have attempted to modify the dose according to the CD3 cell count and receptor density (Table 18-5). This approach has allowed us to achieve adequate immunosuppression while minimizing the total dose of OKT3, often to less than 25 mg for the entire induction period. We believe that this modification has helped limit overimmunosuppression and reduce the total cost of OKT3 therapy.

In approximately 10% of treated patients, antibodies to the antilymphocytic antibody preparation develop and thereby limit the utility of these agents for subsequent use. Patients treated with OKT3 should have antibody titers to the OKT3 determined after each course of therapy. Before a course of polyclonal therapy is repeated, skin testing should be done.

Total lymphoid irradiation. It has been recognized that after radiation therapy for neoplastic disease, the absolute lymphocyte count may be suppressed. Long-term suppression occurs primarily in the T-cell line, with a secondary and compensatory increase in circulating B cells. Remaining T cells demonstrate an impairment in function, with reduced proliferation in response to a mitogenic stimulation.[73] These alterations in cell-mediated function have been used as immunosuppressive therapy in transplantation. Low levels of total lymphoid irradiation (2 to 8 Gy) may alter T-cell number and function with little or no radiation toxicity.[74] Studies have demonstrated that total lymphoid irradiation may be successfully used to treat recurrent and resistant cardiac rejection and in some cases may avoid the necessity of retransplantation.[75-77] In a limited series of renal transplant recipients, total lymphoid irradiation was used as induction or prophylactic therapy to avoid early rejection and allow for the potential development of immune tolerance.[78] In several cardiac transplant recipients undergoing total lymphoid irradiation, we observed cytomegalovirus activation coincident with the initiation of total lymphoid irradiation therapy. The clinical experience with total lymphoid irradiation in cardiac transplantation is currently limited, and subsequent investigations will be required to fully understand its uses and limitations.

COMPLICATIONS OF CARDIAC TRANSPLANTATION

Infectious complications

Since the addition of cyclosporine to the routine immunosuppressive protocol, the frequency and nature of both rejection and infection have changed. Infection is still the leading cause of post-transplantation morbidity and mortality. Virtually any microorganism may be responsible for disease in these immunosuppressed patients; however, in the post-transplantation state, certain pathogens are distinctly more common.[79]

Viral infections may occur early or late after transplantation. Cytomegalovirus (CMV) may result from transplantation of a CMV-seropositive donor heart into a CMV-seronegative recipient or from reactivation of a recipient's latent CMV infection. Manifestations of CMV infections may range from a self-limited nonspecific febrile illness to an overwhelming CMV pneumonia, myocarditis, enteritis, or hepatitis. Typical intranuclear inclusions can be seen on biopsy of the affected organ. Commonly, the patient in the post-transplantation period may shed CMV in urine and saliva without evidence of invasive CMV infection. Studies have suggested a link between CMV infections and development of coronary artery disease in the graft.[80] It is hoped that antiviral agents, including hyperimmune globulin and ganciclovir, may lessen the severity and frequency of CMV illnesses.[81,82]

Cyclosporine-mediated inhibition of helper T-cell function has resulted in an increased incidence of *Pneumocystis* pneumonia. This may be manifested by fever, pulmonary infiltrates, and hypoxemia. The risk of *Pneumocystis* infections correlates closely with the degree of immunosuppression. Diagnosis is often made by bronchoalveolar lavage; rarely, open lung biopsy is necessary. Fortunately, prophylactic treatment with daily oral trimethoprim-sulfamethoxazole or monthly inhaled pentamidine appears to markedly reduce the frequency of *Pneumocystis* infections.[83-85]

Systemic fungal infections, including *Candida* septicemia (often related to an indwelling catheter) and aspergillosis, may occur in the immunocompromised patient. Therapy has generally been disappointing, but if success is to be obtained, early and aggressive antifungal treatment is necessary.[86] Oral candidiasis occurs frequently and may be successfully treated or altogether avoided with a regular topical antifungal regimen that includes nystatin. For resistant cases, fluconazole may be effective.

Legionella pneumonia is now recognized with increased frequency in heart transplant recipients. Diagnosis depends on positive staining of sputum or bronchoalveolar lavage fluid with the direct fluorescent antibody technique. Empiric therapy with erythromycin may be required before a positive diagnosis can be made. If erythromycin is given, care should be taken to reduce the cyclosporine dose, since erythromycin increases cyclosporine levels.

Although a controlled study has never been performed, most transplantation centers have recommended that patients follow American Heart Association recommendations for prophylaxis of subacute bacterial endocarditis.

Nephrotoxicity

Cyclosporine therapy may adversely affect both short-term and long-term renal function after transplantation.[87,88] Immediately after cardiac transplantation, renal function may be impaired by multiple insults, including preexisting heart failure, a prolonged period of cardiopulmonary bypass, and cyclosporine therapy. Usually, this early renal insufficiency is reversible but requires careful attention to the administration of cyclosporine and other nephrotoxic agents. Early use of OKT3 has allowed for a delay in the introduction of cyclosporine. Hence, renal function may have time to recover after cardiopulmonary bypass before additional nephrotoxic insults occur. In the long-term follow-up of heart transplant recipients, serum creatinine concentration tends to gradually increase coincident with a decrease in glomerular filtration rate and renal blood flow.[89-91] The degree of renal impairment is usually mild or moderate, but renal function must be followed closely and use of nephrotoxic agents should be minimized. The mechanism of cyclosporine-induced nephrotoxicity is incompletely understood, but increases in renal vascular resistance with secondary renal interstitial fibrosis appear to be involved in the pathogenesis of this syndrome.[92] In the early post-transplantation period, the potent peptide vasoconstrictor endothelin may be activated and result in renal vasoconstriction and impaired excretory function.[93,94] Recent studies have demonstrated a synergistic interaction between endothelin and cyclosporine that may further impair renal function.[95] Although long-term administration of cyclosporine may have variable effects on plasma endothelin, it is likely that local or regional levels are more important.[96,97]

Post-transplantation systemic hypertension

Post-transplantation systemic arterial hypertension, a relatively uncommon occurrence before the introduction of cyclosporine, has now become a ubiquitous problem. In as many as 92% of patients, hypertension develops within 6 months of transplantation.[98] The presence of hypertension does not correlate with cyclosporine levels, circulating norepinephrine, or serum creatinine. Systemic vascular resistance is increased, whereas resting cardiac output is normal.[99] The mechanism of systemic vasoconstriction is incompletely understood but may be related to activation or enhanced sensitivity of the vasculature to systemic vasoconstrictors such as angiotensin II[100] and endothelin.[93,94] The systemic and renal vasodilator atrial natriuretic factor is increased after transplantation.[101] Although the mechanism for this increase is incompletely understood, atrial natriuretic factor may be activated as a compensatory response to systemic vasoconstriction.

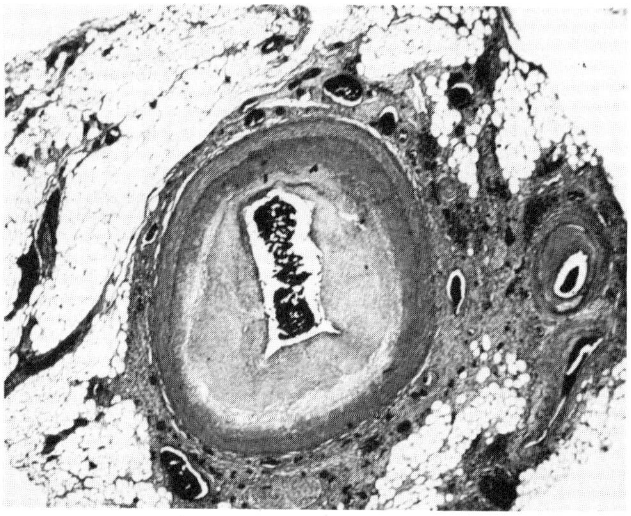

Fig 18-4 Graft-related coronary artery disease. Extensive fibrous intimal proliferation in the left anterior descending coronary artery and in a diagonal artery years after transplantation. (×5.)

Graft-related coronary artery disease

Development of diffuse, severe, and progressive coronary artery disease is a recognized long-term complication of cardiac transplantation. It is estimated that as many as 44% of transplant recipients may have angiographic evidence of coronary artery disease 3 years after transplantation.[102] Utilization of intracoronary ultrasonography greatly increases the ability to diagnose the disorder and hence increases the prevalence of the disorder. Graft-related coronary artery disease is now the leading indication for retransplantation.[103,104]

Pathologically, the coronary arteries may display diffuse or focal intimal proliferation with or without atheromas[105-107] (Fig 18-4). Because of the unique pathologic and angiographic appearance, the disease should not be considered classic atherosclerosis. Some have observed subintimal inflammatory cells and have correlated rejection episodes with the development of graft-related coronary artery disease, suggesting that an immune mechanism may be responsible for this entity.[102] However, Gao et al.[106] found no correlation between development of coronary artery disease and rejection episodes during the first year after transplantation, nor was there a correlation between coronary disease and HLA mismatches, steroid doses, fasting blood sugar level, or serum cholesterol value. There was only a weak correlation favoring the development of coronary artery disease in patients with increased plasma triglycerides and increasing age of the donor heart. A strong correlation was observed between cytomegalovirus infection and subsequent development of coronary artery disease.[80,108]

Since all coronary arteries may be symmetrically involved, with little development of collateral flow, clinical techniques that evaluate relative myocardial perfusion, such as thallium perfusion scanning, may be insensitive in identifying severe graft-related coronary artery disease.[109]

SPECIAL CONSIDERATIONS

Transplantation in infants and children

Cardiac transplantation has been successfully performed in children from the neonatal period to the teenage years. Indications for heart transplantation include inoperable congenital heart disease; dilated, restrictive, or hypertrophic cardiomyopathy; and various forms of specific heart muscle diseases, including daunorubicin-induced cardiomyopathy.[12,110-112] In addition to the technical limitations associated with transplantation in small children, special preoperative attention needs to be given to the status of the pulmonary vasculature. Pulmonary arteriolar resistance should be measured preoperatively and should be indexed to body surface area. Congenital lesions associated with left-to-right shunts may eventually lead to irreversible pulmonary hypertension, necessitating combined heart-lung transplantation. In children with congenital heart disease, previous palliative shunting procedures may distort the intrathoracic anatomy and increase the complications associated with transplantation. Immunosuppressive regimens that do not include corticosteroids have been demonstrated to decrease or eliminate long-term complications of growth retardation and glucose intolerance.

Successful transplantation is possible in newborns with the hypoplastic left heart syndrome.[110] In these infants, noninvasive assessments of allograft function have been used to monitor for rejection, thereby eliminating or markedly reducing the necessity for endomyocardial biopsies. Because of the immature status of the immune system in the newborn, some degree of immune tolerance to the graft may occur and allow prolonged survival with less immunosuppression or eventually allow for successful xenotransplantation.[113] Transplantation in older children with various forms of cardiomyopathy is highly successful, and the overall prognosis is similar to that observed in adults undergoing transplantation.

Xenografts

In parallel with the development of the permanent artificial heart, progress is being made in transplantation across species lines (xenotransplantation).[114-116] Survival of 20 days has been reported in a human infant with a transplanted baboon heart used as a bridge to transplantation.[113] Long-term survival in that situation was limited by humoral rejection, but cell-mediated rejection was controlled. Although genetic similarities might favor use of primates as donors for xenotransplantation, this course has resulted in considerable societal controversy. Nonprimate donors (porcine or bovine) have elicited less public concern. The development of potent and targeted immunosuppression will be necessary for this line of therapy to become successful. Work is continuing on the development of genetically modified xenotypic donors that could perhaps elicit a less intense immune response. In the future, new tools of immunobiology may allow the induction of immune tolerance for xenotransplantation, so that cross-species grafts can become a realistic and exciting alternative.

REFERENCES

1. Schroeder JS, Hunt S: Cardiac transplantation: update 1987. *JAMA* 258:3142-3145, 1987
2. The CONSENSUS Trial Study Group: Effects of enalapril on mortality in severe congestive heart failure: results of the Cooperative North Scandinavian Enalapril Survival Study (CONSENSUS). *N Engl J Med* 316:1429-1435, 1987
3. Edwards BS: Recent advances in cardiac transplantation. *Curr Opin Cardiol* 5:295-299, 1990
4. Barnard CN: A human cardiac transplant: an interim report of a successful operation performed at Groote Schuur Hospital, Cape Town. *South Afr Med J* 41:1271-1274, 1967
5. Mann FC, Priestley JT, Markowitz J, et al: Transplantation of the intact mammalian heart. *Arch Surg* 26:219-224, 1933
6. Lower RR, Shumway NE: Studies on orthotopic homotransplantation of the canine heart. *Surg Forum* 11:18-19, 1960
7. Kahan BD: Immunosuppressive therapy with cyclosporine for cardiac transplantation. *Circulation* 75:40-56, 1987
8. Kaye MP: The Registry of the International Society for Heart and Lung Transplantation: Tenth Official Report—1993. *J Heart Lung Transplant* 12:541-548, 1993
9. Copeland JG, Emery RW, Levinson MM, et al: Selection of patients for cardiac transplantation. *Circulation* 75:2-9, 1987
10. Mudge GH, Goldstein S, Addonizio LJ, et al: 24th Bethesda Conference: Cardiac Transplantation. Task Force 3: Recipient guidelines/prioritization. *J Am Coll Cardiol* 22:21-31, 1993
11. Aravot DJ, Banner NR, Khaghani A, et al: Cardiac transplantation in the seventh decade of life. *Am J Cardiol* 63:90-93, 1989
12. Edwards BS, Hunt SA, Fowler MB, et al: Cardiac transplantation in patients with preexisting neoplastic diseases. *Am J Cardiol* 65:501-504, 1990
13. Ladowski JS, Kormos RL, Uretsky BF, et al: Posttransplantation diabetes mellitus in heart transplant recipients. *J Heart Transplant* 8:181-183, 1989
14. Rhenman MJ, Rhenman B, Icenogle T, et al: Diabetes and heart transplantation. *J Heart Transplant* 7:356-358, 1988
15. Costard A, Hill IR, Schroeder JS, et al: Nitroprusside effect on pulmonary vascular resistance and systolic blood pressure predicts early transplant patient survival (abstract). *J Heart Transplant* 8:108, 1989
16. Addonizio LJ, Gersony WM, Robbins RC, et al: Elevated pulmonary vascular resistance and cardiac transplantation. *Circulation* 76 Suppl 5:52-55, 1987
17. Kirklin JK, Naftel DC, Kirklin JW, et al: Pulmonary vascular resistance and the risk of heart transplantation. *J Heart Transplant* 7:331-335, 1988
18. Nakatani T, Frazier OH, Lammermeier DE, et al: Heterotopic heart transplantation: a reliable option for a select group of high-risk patients. *J Heart Transplant* 8:40-46, 1989
19. Stevenson LW, Fowler MB, Schroeder JS, et al: Poor survival of patients with idiopathic cardiomyopathy considered too well for transplantation. *Am J Med* 83:871-876, 1987
20. O'Connell JB, Renlund DG, Robinson JA, et al: Effect of preoperative hemodynamic support on survival after cardiac transplantation. *Circulation* 78 Suppl 3:78-82, 1988
21. Hardesty RL, Griffith BP, Trento A, et al: Mortally ill patients and excellent survival following cardiac transplantation. *Ann Thorac Surg* 41:126-129, 1986.
22. Copeland JG, Smith R, Icenogle T, et al: Orthotopic total artificial heart bridge to transplantation: preliminary results. *J Heart Transplant* 8:124-137, 1989
23. Pae WE Jr, Pierce WS: Combined registry for the clinical use of mechanical ventricular assist pumps and the total artificial heart: second official report—1987. *J Heart Transplant* 8:1-4, 1989
24. Emery RW, Cork RC, Levinson MM, et al: The cardiac donor: a six-year experience. *Ann Thorac Surg* 41:356-361, 1986
25. Hetzer R, Warnecke H, Schüler S: The donor heart: procurement, selection, and preservation. *Transplant Proc* 18 Suppl 3:27-30, 1986

26. Barnard CN: What we have learned about heart transplants, *J Thorac Cardiovasc Surg* 56:457-468, 1968
27. Stinson EB, Caves PK, Griepp RB, et al: Hemodynamic observations in the early period after human heart transplantation. *J Thorac Cardiovasc Surg* 69:264-270, 1975
28. Scott CD, Omar I, McComb JM, et al: Long-term pacing in heart transplant recipients is usually unnecessary. *PACE* 14:1792-1796, 1991
29. Wilson RF, Christensen BV, Olivari MT, et al: Evidence for structural sympathetic reinnervation after orthotopic cardiac transplantation in humans. *Circulation* 83:1210-1220, 1991
30. Kavanagh T, Yacoub MH, Mertens DJ, et al: Cardiorespiratory responses to exercise training after orthotopic cardiac transplantation. *Circulation* 77:162-171, 1988
31. Quigg RJ, Rocco MB, Gauthier DF, et al: Mechanism of the attenuated peak heart rate response to exercise after orthotopic cardiac transplantation. *J Am Coll Cardiol* 14:338-344, 1989
32. Hidalgo R, Alegriá E, Castelló R, et al: Stress testing in patients one year after orthotopic cardiac transplantation. *Angiology* 40:650-655, 1989
33. Ellenbogen KA, Mohanty PK, Szentpetery S, et al: Arterial baroreflex abnormalities in heart failure: reversal after orthotopic cardiac transplantation. *Circulation* 79:51-58, 1989
34. Stinson EB, Griepp RB, Schroeder JS, et al: Hemodynamic observations one and two years after cardiac transplantation in man. *Circulation* 45:1183-1194, 1972
35. Hausdorf G, Banner NR, Mitchell A, et al: Diastolic function after cardiac and heart-lung transplantation. *Br Heart J* 62:123-132, 1989
36. Vigneswaran WT, Rodeheffer RJ, Breen JF, et al: Left ventricular remodeling after orthotopic cardiac transplantation (abstract). *J Am Coll Cardiol* 21:142A, 1993
37. Caves PK, Stinson EB, Billingham ME, et al: Diagnosis of human cardiac allograft rejection by serial cardiac biopsy. *J Thorac Cardiovasc Surg* 66:461-466, 1973
38. Miller LW, Schlant RC, Kobashigawa J, et al: 24th Bethesda Conference: Cardiac Transplantation. Task Force 5: Complications. *J Am Coll Cardiol* 22:41-54, 1993
39. Billingham ME: Diagnosis of cardiac rejection by endomyocardial biopsy. *Heart Transplant* 1:25-30, 1981
40. McAllister HA Jr, Schnee MJM, Radovančevič B, et al: A system for grading cardiac allograft rejection. *Texas Heart Inst J* 13:1-3, 1986
41. Kemnitz J, Cohnert T, Schäfers H-J, et al: A classification of cardiac allograft rejection: a modification of the classification of Billingham. *Am J Surg Pathol* 11:503-515, 1987
42. Billingham ME, Cary NRB, Hammond ME, et al: A working formulation for the standardization of nomenclature in the diagnosis of heart and lung rejection: Heart Rejection Study Group. *J Heart Transplant* 9:587-593, 1990
43. Billingham ME: Endomyocardial biopsy detection of acute rejection in cardiac allograft recipients. *Heart Vessels Suppl* 1:86-90, 1985
44. Telenti A, Tazelaar HD, Smith TF, et al: Detection of Epstein-Barr virus in endomyocardial biopsies of heart transplant recipients (abstract). *J Heart Lung Transplant* 10:191, 1991
45. Sandhu JS, Uretsky BF, Zerbe TR, et al: Coronary artery fistula in the heart transplant patient: a potential complication of endomyocardial biopsy. *Circulation* 79:350-356, 1989
46. Henzlova MJ, Nath H, Bucy RP, et al: Coronary artery to right ventricle fistula in heart transplant recipients: a complication of endomyocardial biopsy. *J Am Coll Cardiol* 14:258-261, 1989.
47. Nippoldt TB, Edwards WD, Holmes DR Jr, et al: Right ventricular endomyocardial biopsy: clinicopathologic correlates in 100 consecutive patients. *Mayo Clin Proc* 57:407-418, 1982
48. Carlquist JF, Hammond EH, Anderson JL: Propagation and characterization of lymphocytes from rejecting human cardiac allografts. *J Heart Transplant* 7:397-406, 1988
49. Revel D, Chapelon C, Mathieu D, et al: Magnetic resonance imaging of human orthotopic heart transplantation: correlation with endomyocardial biopsy. *J Heart Transplant* 8:139-146, 1989
50. Cosson C, Myara I, Guillemain R, et al: Serum prolactin as a rejection marker in heart transplantation. *Clin Chem* 35:492-493, 1989
51. Valantine HA, Fowler MB, Hunt SA, et al: Changes in Doppler echocardiographic indexes of left ventricular function as potential markers of acute cardiac rejection. *Circulation* 76 Suppl 5:86-92, 1987
52. Forster T, McGhie J, Rijsterborgh H, et al: Can we assess the changes of ventricular filling resulting from acute allograft rejection with Doppler echocardiography? *J Heart Transplant* 7:430-434, 1988
53. Valantine HA: Rejection surveillance by Doppler echocardiography (editorial). *J Heart Lung Transplant* 12:422-426, 1993
54. Kahan BD: Pharmacokinetics and pharmacodynamics of cyclosporine. *Transplant Proc* 21 Suppl 1:9-15, 1989
55. Nalesnik MA, Jaffe R, Starzl TE, et al: The pathology of post-transplant lymphoproliferative disorders occurring in the setting of cyclosporine A-prednisone immunosuppression. *Am J Pathol* 133:173-192, 1988
56. Haynes RC Jr, Murad F: Adrenocorticotropic hormone; adrenocortical steroids and their synthetic analogs; inhibitors of adrenocortical steroid biosynthesis. In *Goodman and Gilman's The Pharmacological Basis of Therapeutics.* Edited by AG Gilman, LS Goodman, TW Rall, et al. Seventh edition. New York, Macmillan Publishing Company, 1985, pp 1459-1489
57. Esmore DS, Spratt PM, Keogh AM, et al: Cyclosporine and azathioprine immunosuppression without maintenance steroids: a prospective randomized trial. *J Heart Transplant* 8:194-199, 1989
58. Renlund DG, Bristow MR, Crandall BG, et al: Hypercholesterolemia after heart transplantation: amelioration by corticosteroid-free maintenance immunosuppression. *J Heart Transplant* 8:214-219, 1989
59. Crandall BG, Gilbert EM, Menlove RL, et al: Immunosuppressive efficacy of vincristine in cardiac transplantation: decreased rejection frequency and increased removal from steroids (abstract). *J Heart Transplant* 8:95, 1989
60. Calabresi P, Parks RE Jr: Antiproliferative agents and drugs used for immunosuppression. In *Goodman and Gilman's The Pharmacological Basis of Therapeutics.* Edited by AG Gilman, LS Goodman, TW Rall, et al. Seventh edition. New York, Macmillan Publishing Company, 1985, pp 1276-1277
61. Costanzo-Nordin MR, Grusk BB, Silver MA, et al: Reversal of recalcitrant cardiac allograft rejection with methotrexate. *Circulation* 78 Suppl 3:47-57, 1988
62. Olsen SL, O'Connell JB, Bristow MR, et al: Methotrexate as an adjunct in the treatment of persistent mild cardiac allograft rejection. *Transplantation* 50:773-775, 1990
63. Bouchart F, Gundry SR, Van Schaack-Gonzales J, et al: Methotrexate as rescue/adjunctive immunotherapy in infant and adult heart transplantation. *J Heart Lung Transplant* 12:427-433, 1993
64. O'Connell JB, Renlund DG, Lee HR, et al: Newer techniques of immunosuppression in cardiac transplantation. *Cardiac Surg* 2:607-615, 1988
65. Sakagami K, Ohsaki T, Ohnishi T, et al: The effect of antiinterleukin 2 monoclonal antibody treatment on the survival of rat cardiac allograft. *J Surg Res* 46:262-266, 1989
66. Kupiec-Weglinski JW, Tilney NL, Stunkel KG, et al: Agonistic and antagonistic interactions of anti-interleukin 2 receptor monoclonal antibodies in rat recipients of cardiac allografts. *Transplantation* 47:11-16, 1989
67. Lorberboum-Galski H, Barrett LV, Kirkman RL, et al: Cardiac allograft survival in mice treated with IL-2-PE40. *Proc Natl Acad Sci U S A* 86:1008-1012, 1989
68. Flavin TF III, Seydel C, Shizuru J, et al: Selective T-cell depletion with Ox-38 anti-CD4 monoclonal antibody prevents cardiac allograft rejection in rats (abstract). *J Heart Transplant* 8:97, 1989
69. O'Connell JB, Renlund DG, Gay WA Jr, et al: Efficacy of OKT3 retreatment for refractory cardiac allograft rejection. *Transplantation* 47:788-792, 1989
70. Starnes VA, Oyer PE, Stinson EB, et al: Prophylactic OKT3 used as induction therapy for heart transplantation. *Circulation* 80 Suppl 3:79-83, 1989
71. Macris MP, Frazier OH, Lammermeier D, et al: Clinical experience with muromonab-CD3 monoclonal antibody (OKT3) in heart transplantation. *J Heart Transplant* 8:281-287, 1989
72. Hosenpud JD, Norman DJ, Pantely GA, et al: OKT3-induced hypotension in heart allograft recipients treated for steroid-resistant rejection. *J Heart Transplant* 8:159-165, 1989
73. Fuks Z, Strober S, Bobrove AM, et al: Long term effects of radiation on T and B lymphocytes in peripheral blood of patients with Hodgkin's disease. *J Clin Invest* 58:803-814, 1976
74. Strober S, Modry DL, Hoppe RT, et al: Induction of specific unresponsiveness to heart allografts in mongrel dogs treated with total lymphoid irradiation and anti-thymocyte globulin. *J Immunol* 132:1013-1018, 1984

75. Levin B, Bohannon L, Warvariv V, et al: Total lymphoid irradiation (TLI) in the cyclosporine era – use of TLI in resistant cardiac allograft rejection. *Transplant Proc* 21:1793-1795, 1989

76. Hunt S, Strober S, Hoppe R, et al: Use of total lymphoid irradiation for therapy of intractable cardiac allograft rejection (abstract). *J Heart Transplant* 8:104, 1989

77. Evans MA, Schomberg PJ, Rodeheffer RJ, et al: Total lymphoid irradiation: a novel and successful therapy for resistant cardiac allograft rejection. *Mayo Clin Proc* 67:785-790, 1992

78. Strober S, Dhillon M, Schubert M, et al: Acquired immune tolerance to cadaveric renal allografts. A study of three patients treated with total lymphoid irradiation. *N Engl J Med* 321:28-33, 1989

79. Gentry LO, Zeluff BJ: Diagnosis and treatment of infection in cardiac transplant patients. *Surg Clin North Am* 66:459-465, 1986

80. Grattan MT, Moreno-Cabral CE, Starnes VA, et al: Cytomegalovirus infection is associated with cardiac allograft rejection and atherosclerosis. *JAMA* 261:3561-3566, 1989

81. Erice A, Jordan MC, Chace BA, et al: Ganciclovir treatment of cytomegalovirus disease in transplant recipients and other immunocompromised hosts. *JAMA* 257:3082-3087, 1987

82. Freeman R, Gould FK, McMaster A: Management of cytomegalovirus antibody negative patients undergoing heart transplantation. *J Clin Pathol* 43:373-376, 1990

83. Hughes WT, Kuhn S, Chaudhary S, et al: Successful chemoprophylaxis for *Pneumocystis carinii* pneumonitis. *N Engl J Med* 297:1419-1426, 1977

84. Hughes WT, Rivera GK, Schell MJ, et al: Successful intermittent chemoprophylaxis for *Pneumocystis carinii* pneumonitis. *N Engl J Med* 316:1627-1632, 1987

85. Conte JE Jr, Hollander H, Golden JA: Inhaled or reduced-dose intravenous pentamidine for *Pneumocystis carinii* pneumonia: a pilot study. *Ann Intern Med* 107:495-498, 1987

86. McHenry MC, Duchesneau PM, Keys TF, et al: Vertebral osteomyelitis presenting as spinal compression fracture: six patients with underlying osteoporosis. *Arch Intern Med* 148:417-423, 1988

87. Greenberg A, Egel JW, Thompson ME, et al: Early and late forms of cyclosporine nephrotoxicity: studies in cardiac transplant recipients. *Am J Kidney Dis* 9:12-22, 1987

88. Myers BD: What is cyclosporine nephrotoxicity? *Transplant Proc* 21:1430-1432, 1989

89. Moran M, Tomlanovich S, Myers BD: Cyclosporine-induced chronic nephropathy in human recipients of cardiac allografts. *Transplant Proc* 17 Suppl 1:185-190, 1985

90. Myers BD, Sibley R, Newton L, et al: The long-term course of cyclosporine-associated chronic nephropathy. *Kidney Int* 33:590-600, 1988

91. Nizze H, Mihatsch MJ, Zollinger HU, et al: Cyclosporine-associated nephropathy in patients with heart and bone marrow transplants. *Clin Nephrol* 30:248-260, 1988

92. Kopp JB, Klofman PE: Cellular and molecular mechanisms of cyclosporin nephrotoxicity. *J Am Soc Nephrol* 1:162-179, 1990

93. Edwards BS, Anderson LM: Endothelin may mediate the acute hemodynamic effects of cyclosporine. *Circulation* 82 Suppl III: 630, 1990

94. Lerman A, Click RL, Narr BJ, et al: Elevation of plasma endothelin associated with systemic hypertension in humans following orthotopic liver transplantation. *Transplantation* 51:646-650, 1991

95. Edwards BS, Lloyd MA, Anderson LM: The synergistic effects of cyclosporine and endothelin: demonstration of an important cardiopressor action. *Transplantation* 55:8-11, 1993

96. Edwards BS, Hunt SA, Fowler MB, et al: Circulating endothelin is independent of cyclosporine therapy following cardiac transplantation (abstract). *Am J Hypertens* 3:82A, 1990

97. Haas GJ, Wooding-Scott M, Binkley PF, et al: Effects of successful cardiac transplantation on plasma endothelin. *Am J Cardiol* 71:237-240, 1993

98. Olivari M-T, Antolick A, Ring WS: Arterial hypertension in heart transplant recipients treated with triple-drug immunosuppressive therapy. *J Heart Transplant* 8:34-39, 1989

99. Greenberg ML, Uretsky BF, Reddy PS, et al: Long-term hemodynamic follow-up of cardiac transplant patients treated with cyclosporine and prednisone. *Circulation* 71:487-494, 1985

100. Bellet M, Cabrol C, Sassano P, et al: Systemic hypertension after cardiac transplantation: effect of cyclosporine on the renin-angiotensin-aldosterone system. *Am J Cardiol* 56:927-931, 1985

101. Edwards BS, Goldenberg IF, Pritzker MR, et al: Persistent elevation of atrial natriuretic factor following cardiac transplantation (abstract). *Circulation* 76 Suppl 4:136, 1987

102. Uretsky BF, Murali S, Reddy PS, et al: Development of coronary artery disease in cardiac transplant patients receiving immunosuppressive therapy with cyclosporine and prednisone. *Circulation* 76:827-834, 1987

103. Gao SZ, Schroeder JS, Hunt S, et al: Retransplantation for severe accelerated coronary disease in heart transplant recipients. *Am J Cardiol* 62:876-881, 1988.

104. Dein JR, Oyer PE, Stinson EB, et al: Cardiac retransplantation in the cyclosporine era. *Ann Thorac Surg* 48:350-355, 1989

105. Griepp RB, Stinson EB, Bieber CP, et al: Control of graft atherosclerosis in human heart transplant recipients. *Surgery* 81:262-269, 1977

106. Gao SZ, Schroeder JS, Alderman EL, et al: Clinical and laboratory correlates of accelerated coronary artery disease in the cardiac transplant patient. *Circulation* 76 Suppl 5:56-61, 1987

107. Gao S-Z, Alderman EL, Schroeder JS, et al: Accelerated coronary vascular disease in the heart transplant patient: coronary arteriographic findings. *J Am Coll Cardiol* 12:334-340, 1988

108. McDonald K, Rector T, Braunlin E, et al: Allograft atherosclerosis in cardiac transplant recipients is associated with cytomegalovirus infection (abstract). *J Heart Transplant* 8:105, 1989

109. Nitkin RS, Hunt SA, Schroeder JS: Accelerated atherosclerosis in a cardiac transplant patient. *J Am Coll Cardiol* 6:243-245, 1985

110. Bailey LL, Nehlsen-Cannarella SL, Doroshow RW, et al: Cardiac allotransplantation in newborns as therapy for hypoplastic left heart syndrome. *N Engl J Med* 315:949-951, 1986

111. Chartrand C, Dumont L, Stanley P: Pediatric cardiac transplantation. *Transplant Proc* 21:3349-3350, 1989

112. Starnes VA, Bernstein D, Oyer PE, et al: Heart transplantation in children. *J Heart Transplant* 8:20-26, 1989

113. Bailey LL, Nehlsen-Cannarella SL, Concepcion W, et al: Baboon-to-human cardiac xenotransplantation in a neonate. *JAMA* 254:3321-3329, 1985

114. Reichenspurner H, Human PA, Boehm DH, et al: Optimalization of immunosuppression after xenogeneic heart transplantation in primates. *J Heart Transplant* 8:200-207, 1989

115. Sadeghi A, Drinkwater D, Laks H, et al: Heart-lung xenotransplantation in primates (abstract). *J Heart Transplant* 8:91, 1989

116. Costanzo-Nordin MR, Cooper DKC, Jessup M, et al: 24th Bethesda Conference: Cardiac Transplantation. Task Force 6: Future developments. *J Am Coll Cardiol* 22:54-64, 1993

PART IV *Myocardial Disease*

CHAPTER

19

Cardiomyopathy and biopsy

A. Dilated cardiomyopathy and the myocarditides

Richard J. Rodeheffer, M.D., and Bernard J. Gersh, M.B.,Ch.B., D.Phil.

DILATED CARDIOMYOPATHY

Cardiomyopathies are defined as "heart muscle diseases of unknown cause."[1] They are subdivided into three types (Fig 19A-1): dilated cardiomyopathy, hypertrophic cardiomyopathy (see chapter 20), and restrictive cardiomyopathy (see chapter 21).

In dilated cardiomyopathy there is dilatation of the right ventricle or left ventricle or both, with a variable degree of hypertrophy. Systolic and diastolic contractile function are impaired, and congestive failure is a frequent complication. Atrial or ventricular arrhythmias are frequent, and death may occur at any stage. In most cases, no clear cause can be determined and the classification "idiopathic dilated cardiomyopathy" is applied. Other terms previously applied to dilated cardiomyopathy are "congestive cardiomyopathy" and "primary cardiomyopathy."

Despite large gaps in our knowledge of etiology and pathogenesis, certain pathogenetic concepts are relevant to understanding dilated cardiomyopathy. One of these is the concept of variation of individual susceptibility to heart muscle disease. A second concept is that there may be multiple etiologic factors, such as genetic, environmental, and immunologic factors, converging to produce disease. A third concept is that of an initial insult producing an illness of wide-ranging severity that is followed by apparent partial or complete recovery, which in turn is followed by a short or long latent period, after which heart muscle disease may again be manifest but need not be similar to the initial event.

Idiopathic dilated cardiomyopathy

Incidence. Epidemiologic studies by Torp[2,3] in a defined population in Sweden revealed, by clinical criteria, 5.3 cases per 100,000 population per year, whereas postmortem study detected 7.5 cases per 100,000 population per year. Population-based studies in Olmsted County, Minn., confirmed these data, with an incidence of 6 per 100,000.[4] The disease was three times as common in men as in women, and there was a steady increase over a period of at least 10 years. In New York City[5] idiopathic dilated cardiomyopathy was found in 0.34% of admissions to municipal hospitals and in 0.12% of admissions to voluntary hospitals; even after exclusion of alcoholics, the incidence was still twice as great in an indigent population. Recent studies in an urban biracial community showed independent associations between idiopathic dilated cardiomyopathy and black race, low annual income, and a history of asthma.[6] It is estimated that idiopathic dilated cardiomyopathy is one-tenth to one-fourth as common as ischemic left ventricular dysfunction.[7] The clinical incidence of idiopathic dilated cardiomyopathy may be significantly underestimated.

Pathology. Hearts of patients dying with idiopathic dilated cardiomyopathy are usually heavy, weighing from 400 to more than 1,000 g.[8] All cardiac chambers are dilated and the myocardium is pale and flabby[9] (Fig 19A-2). The atrial and ventricular wall dimensions are often normal in spite of hypertrophy, because the dilatation masks the hypertrophy. The degree of hypertrophy appears to be related to the length of survival.[10] There is nonspecific thickening of the endocardium of the atria and ventricles, and the atrioventricular (AV) valves may be white and thickened when there is valvular insufficiency. Approximately 60% of autopsy cases have superimposed mural thrombi, most frequently in the apex.[2] On transverse section of the ventricles, areas of fibrous replacement may be seen, predominantly in the inner third of the myocardial wall. The extent of fibrosis appears to be

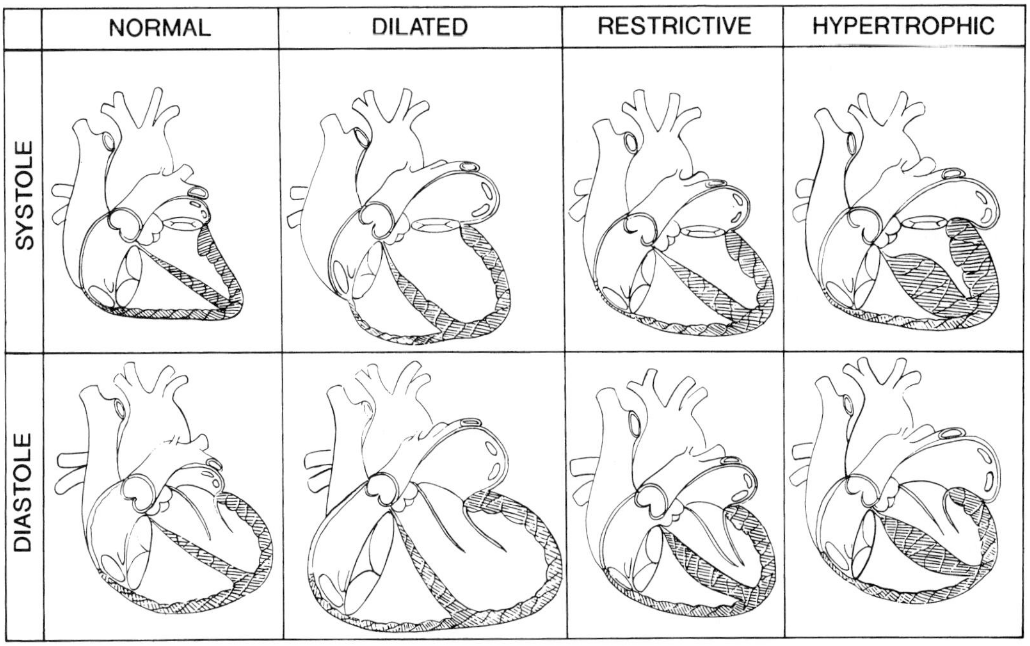

Fig 19A-1 Diagrams of 50° left anterior oblique view of heart in different types of cardiomyopathy at end-systole and end-diastole.

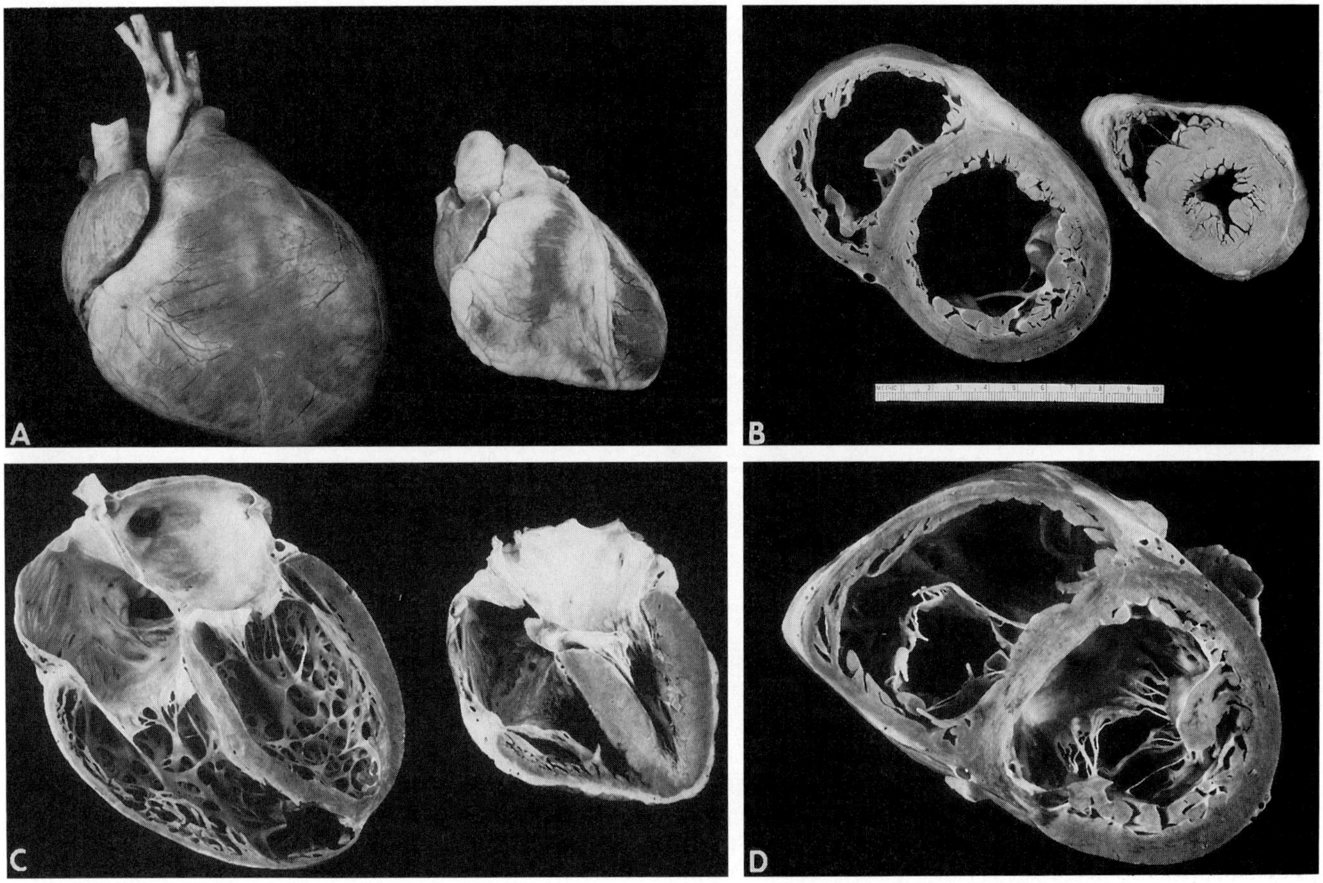

Fig 19A-2 Gross appearance of heart with dilated cardiomyopathy (left on **A, B,** and **C**) compared with normal heart (right on **A, B,** and **C**). **A,** anterior view. **B,** short-axis view. **C,** four-chamber view. **D,** short-axis view of cardiac base. (From Edwards WD: Cardiomyopathies. *Hum Pathol* 18:625-635, 1987. By permission of WB Saunders Company.)

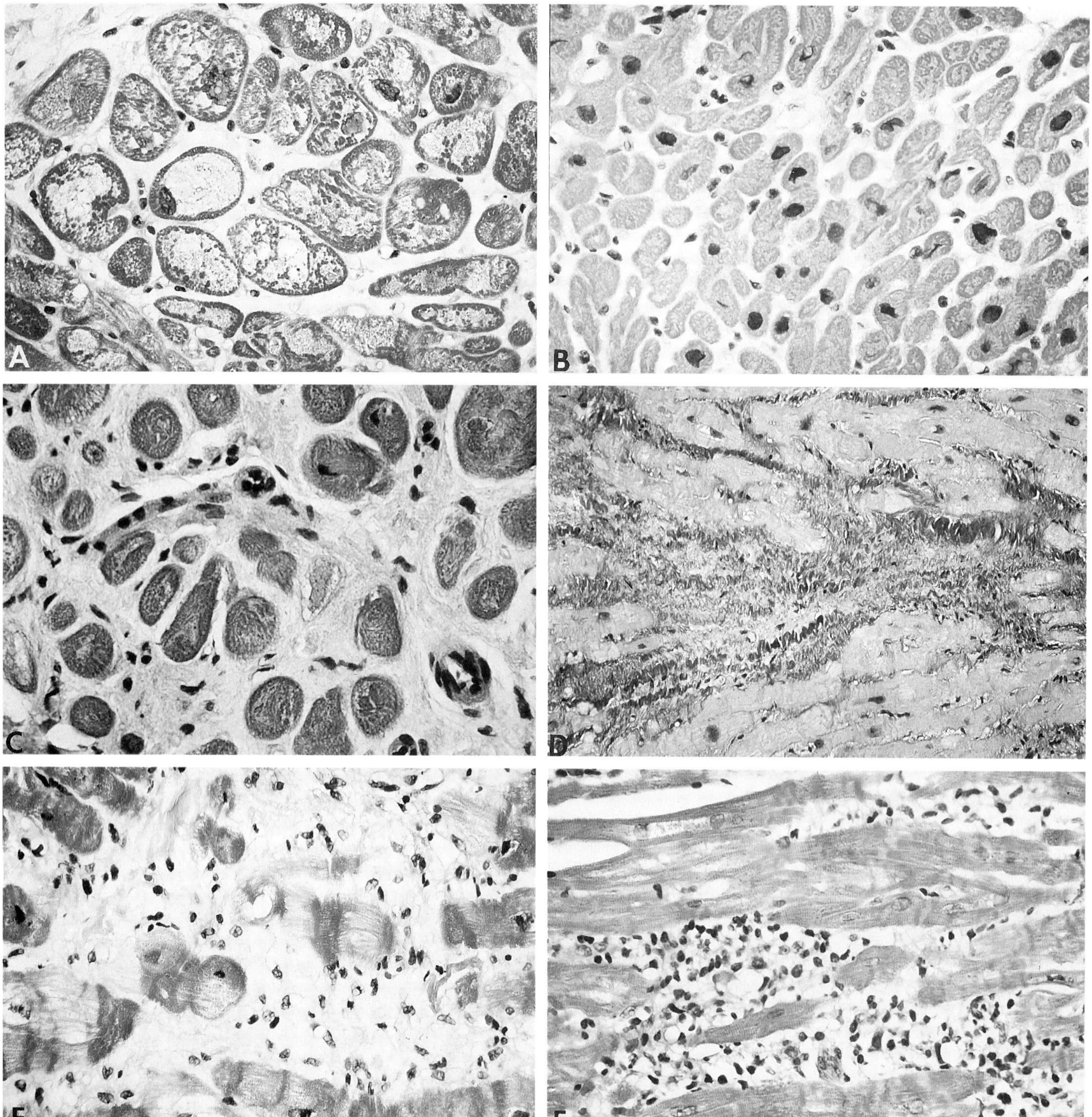

Fig 19A-3 Microscopic features of idiopathic dilated cardiomyopathy. **A,** myocytes are hypertrophied and show focal sarcoplasmic degeneration, with loss of contractile elements. **B,** myocytes are both hypertrophied and attenuated (compare with cell diameters in **A** and **C**). **C,** interstitial fibrosis is pericellular in distribution. **D,** interstitium is involved by patchy replacement fibrosis. **E,** early fibrosis, with noninflammatory interstitial hypercellularity, should not be misinterpreted as myocarditis. **F,** focal myocarditis is characterized by lymphocytic infiltrate and adjacent myocyte injury (compare with **E**). (**A** through **C,** hematoxylin and eosin; original magnification, ×360. **D,** sulfated alcian blue; original magnification, ×180.) (From Edwards WD: Cardiomyopathies. *Hum Pathol* 18:625-635, 1987. By permission of WB Saunders Company.)

disproportionately mild in comparison with the severity of the ventricular dysfunction. The coronary arteries are normal.

Histologic changes are nonspecific (Fig 19A-3). Indeed, in their end stage, idiopathic dilated cardiomyopathy and a host of specific heart muscle diseases have features that are morphologically indistinguishable. Myocardial fibers show a loss of myofibrils.[11] The nuclei show the changes of hypertrophy, consisting of pyknosis or vesicular changes that are attributed to attenuation of fibers. There is an increase in fibrous tissue due to interstitial collagen or to replacement of myocardial fibers.[11] The small vessels are usually normal except in areas of fibrosis, where there may be intimal thickening which is considered secondary to the surrounding fibrosis. There may be hypertrophy of the smooth muscle in the endocardium due to chamber dilatation.[12] Foci of a few inflammatory cells may be found, but, in contrast with myocarditis, the adjacent myocardial fibers are intact and have a smooth contour. Morphologic changes in familial cases are not distinctive. However, in families in which conduction system abnormalities are a major manifestation, abnormalities of the conduction system may dominate the histologic picture.[13] Histochemical analyses reveal nonspecific abnormalities.[14,15]

Electron microscopic findings include hypertrophy with an increase in mitochondria, ribosomes, and convolutions of nuclear membranes.[16,17] In addition, there is dilatation of the tubular system, and the Golgi apparatus is prominent. There are also foci of irregularly arranged myofibrils, including areas of abnormal crossover between fibers. An increase in nuclear pores has been reported, and it was speculated that this might indicate an increase in transport of materials for RNA-mediated protein synthesis.[18]

Etiology. By definition, the cause is unknown. Idiopathic dilated cardiomyopathy may represent a final common pathway of response to various causes. Etiologic studies have proceeded along several lines, including infectious, immunologic, toxic, nutritional/metabolic, vascular, and neurohumoral. It may be that an initial insult is followed by a considerable latent period, after which the disease becomes manifest. Risk factors such as genetic predisposition, infection, alcohol, pregnancy, hypertension, and smoking may, alone or in combination, lower the threshold for the development of dilated cardiomyopathy.[19,20] It is not known why the disease progresses over time in many patients, although neurohumoral factors could be important (see chapter 15).

Familial dilated cardiomyopathy is well known, but its frequency has probably been underestimated. Recent studies of patients with dilated cardiomyopathy in a referral population suggest that when family members are thoroughly screened, approximately one-fifth of cases are found to be familial[20] (see chapter 68).

Speculative interest has centered on the possibility of an immunologic cause.[21] It is possible that viral myocarditis may appear to resolve and then, after a latent period and perhaps in the presence of conditioning factors, an autoimmune process leads to dilated cardiomyopathy[8,21-24] (Fig 19A-4). Results of studies in murine models support this hypothesis.[25-27] Recent studies using molecular biology techniques have yielded evidence for persistent enteroviral presence in some patients with dilated cardiomyopathy.[28-30] Although such findings support the hypothesis that viral infection may result in dilated cardiomyopathy, causality has not been established and further studies are needed to confirm this mechanism of chronic myocardial injury.[31]

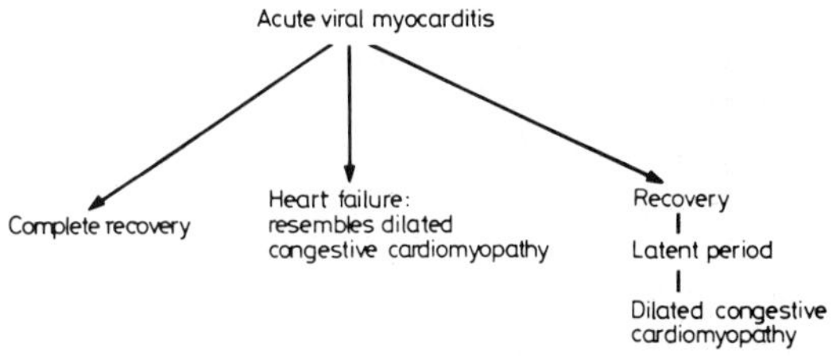

Fig 19A-4 Possible relationship between acute viral myocarditis and dilated cardiomyopathy. (From Goodwin JF: The frontiers of cardiomyopathy. *Br Heart J* 48:1-18, 1982. By permission.)

Other investigations have approached the question of an autoimmune mechanism by studying the immune system itself. During the 1980s, much evidence was obtained from patients with abnormalities in peripheral blood lymphocyte populations,[24,32-35] although the significance of these findings was controversial. More recent studies have reported that sera from patients with dilated cardiomyopathy contain autoantibodies to specific myocyte structures, including the adenine nucleotide translocator, myosin, and the β_1-adrenergic receptor.[36-40] Antibodies to these structures could have a direct effect on myocardial cellular energetics and contractility.[41]

Most patients are not hypertensive, and they do not have retinal or renal evidence of significant hypertension. Because peripheral vascular resistance is frequently increased in congestive cardiomyopathy, there may be transient hypertension, particularly diastolic, during periods of decompensation. Another potential cause involves myocardial ischemia resulting from abnormal regulation of the coronary microvasculature (loss of coronary vasodilatory function).[42,43] Neurohumoral abnormality[44-47] and defective parasympathetic function[48,49] also have been described, but they may be, in part, a consequence of the development of circulatory failure.

Clinical aspects. The clinical presentations of idiopathic dilated cardiomyopathy include cardiomegaly, arrhythmias and conduction disturbances, congestive heart failure, and sudden death. An asymptomatic stage in which cardiomegaly is the presenting feature has been well documented and may be the initial manifestation.

With low output, minimal symptoms such as fatigue and weakness may be early manifestations. With the development of congestive heart failure, patients have exertional dyspnea, orthopnea, paroxysmal nocturnal dyspnea, peripheral edema, or abdominal pain due to hepatic congestion. Chest pain typical of angina pectoris and atypical chest pains occur in approximately 10% of the patients.[50,51] The onset of symptoms may be gradual, with progression over a period of months or years. However, other cases present dramatically, sometimes in association with acute respiratory infection or flulike illness. Symptoms of pulmonary or systemic embolism are found in about 18% of cases.[7,52]

In as many as half the cases, arrhythmias are an early manifestation.[51] Ventricular arrhythmias and atrial fibrillation are especially common. Sudden cardiac death, presumably due to tachyarrhythmias or bradyarrhythmias, may occur early or at any time in the course of the illness.

Physical examination in the low-output stage may reveal cold, cyanotic extremities, a small-volume arterial pulse, and increased venous pressure. The systemic blood pressure may be normal or low, although sometimes the diastolic pressure is increased, which results in a small pulse pressure. Pulsus alternans denotes advanced left ventricular failure. Examination of the jugular venous pulse may confirm the increase in venous pressure but, in addition, may show prominent "a" wave or, in the presence of tricuspid insufficiency, a large cv wave.

On palpation, the precordial impulse tends to be diffuse. There may also be a left parasternal lift. Auscultation may reveal muffled heart sounds, paradoxic splitting of the second heart sound, or an accentuated pulmonic component of the second heart sound. Atrial gallop rhythm and early diastolic gallop rhythm are frequently heard, and at higher heart rates these may summate to simulate a diastolic murmur. Systolic murmurs of tricuspid or mitral regurgitation are heard when there is dilatation of the AV rings, and these may diminish or disappear with treatment. During decompression, rales or dullness, signifying pulmonary edema or effusion, may be present. There may be hepatomegaly, peripheral edema, or ascites.

Laboratory findings. The chest radiograph shows generalized cardiomegaly without calcification of valves or coronary arteries. If there is a large, globular silhouette, pericardial effusion may be suspected. The appearance of the pulmonary vasculature may suggest increased pulmonary venous pressure. There may be evidence of pulmonary edema, pleural effusion, or pulmonary infarction due to embolism.

The electrocardiogram (ECG) in symptomatic patients is almost always nonspecifically abnormal. There may be Q waves associated with patchy fibrosis, which may lead to a mistaken interpretation of myocardial infarction.[53] Significant left axis deviation is common. Almost any rhythm abnormality may be seen; atrial fibrillation is seen in 20% of patients.[54] Ventricular arrhythmias are also common, and ventricular tachycardia may be found in 50% to 60% of patients by ambulatory monitoring.[55-57] AV conduction abnormalities are frequently seen and sometimes are the presenting manifestation. Intraventricular conduction defects, especially left bundle-branch block,[58] are common. A high prevalence of H-Q prolongation on His bundle recordings has been reported in patients with dilated cardiomyopathy.[59]

Two-dimensional echocardiography is a valuable tool in the diagnosis and assessment of idiopathic dilated cardiomyopathy. It is helpful in differentiating this condition from hypertrophic cardiomyopathy, restrictive cardiomyopathy, and valvular or pericardial disease.

Radionuclide imaging reveals ventricular dilatation and generalized decreased contractility, especially of the left ventricle. Reversible perfusion defects are common in patients with idiopathic dilated cardiomyopathy and with ischemic ventricular dysfunction.[60]

Cardiac catheterization reveals hemodynamic and angiographic evidence of globular dilatation of the left ventricle, with generalized poor contraction, increased end-diastolic pressures, and increases in the pulmonary and right heart pressures.[61] Rarely, right-sided involvement may predominate. Left ventricular hypertrophy is common, which may or may not be appropriate to the degree of chamber dilatation.[10,62] Mitral regurgitation is often present and must be differentiated from regurgitation secondary to rheumatic or other primary valvular disease. Tricuspid regurgitation may be found. The coronary arteries are usually normal.

In early stages, hemodynamic parameters at rest may be normal or show only an increased left ventricular end-diastolic pressure; however, exercise or interventions to increase afterload[5,61] may uncover subtle abnormalities.

Endomyocardial biopsy is relatively safe, and specimens satisfactory for light and electron microscopy are obtained (see chapter 19B). However, challenges exist in interpretation, and the optimal application of this technique in the clinical setting remains to be fully realized.[14,50,63-65] It is sometimes useful in identifying specific heart muscle disease such as sarcoidosis or myocarditis.[65-69]

Differential diagnosis. In taking the history it is important to inquire about the use of alcohol or exposure to other toxic substances. In addition, one should inquire about infections, hypertension, and various systemic illnesses, including rheumatic fever, known to be associated with specific myocardial disease and to result in dilated cardiomyopathy.

Frequently the differential diagnosis is between idiopathic dilated cardiomyopathy and ischemic ventricular dysfunction. The issue is not academic, since the entity of "hibernating myocardium" with ischemic left ventricular dysfunction is probably more common than previously realized. The importance of identifying ischemic dysfunction lies in its potential for reversibility.[70,71] The history may be unrevealing because a significant number of myocardial infarctions are not clinically recognized, and in some patients this syndrome may evolve without chest pain. Conversely, chest pain may be a feature of idiopathic dilated cardiomyopathy. Clues may be derived from noninvasive studies, including radionuclide imaging.[60] However, coronary angiography may be indicated to resolve the issue.

Myocarditis should be considered in patients with a relatively short history, particularly if there was an antecedent febrile illness; in such cases, endomyocardial biopsy should be considered.[66-69,72]

Occasionally, long-standing valvular disease may result in myocardial failure which may or may not be reversible upon correction of the valvular fault. In severe aortic stenosis with very low cardiac output, the characteristic auscultatory features of aortic stenosis may be absent, so that the initial presentation may mimic cardiomyopathy.

When hypertrophic cardiomyopathy has progressed to

congestive heart failure, there may be symptoms suggestive of idiopathic dilated cardiomyopathy. Auscultatory features and an echocardiogram will usually resolve the issue. Restrictive/obliterative cardiomyopathy and pericardial disease also may be confused with dilated cardiomyopathy.

Selenium deficiency, described primarily in specific geographic areas of China where dietary selenium intake is low, can produce a dilated cardiomyopathy. Dietary supplementation can prevent this syndrome.[73,74] Selenium deficiency is rare in North America but has been reported during prolonged parenteral hyperalimentation.[75,76]

Natural history and prognosis. Idiopathic dilated cardiomyopathy most likely has a number of different causes; accordingly, the natural history is variable.[51] The stage in which diagnosis is made also is likely to affect the prognosis. Most reports derive from patients in congestive failure referred to tertiary medical centers, that is, patients in a relatively late stage of the disease. Although many of these patients have an initial favorable response to therapy—and in a few this is maintained—most have progression and die within a few years after diagnosis.

A "latent stage," in which cardiac enlargement precedes symptoms, may exist for many years. After symptoms have developed, the more severe the symptoms, the worse the prognosis generally is.[50,51,77]

In a long-term follow-up study of symptomatic patients with idiopathic dilated cardiomyopathy at the Mayo Clinic between 1960 and 1973,[52] 77% of patients had an accelerated course to death, with two-thirds of the deaths occurring within the first 2 years. Twenty-three percent of the patients had a normal survival, the great majority of them having clinical improvement and decreased or normal heart size. In 24 cases of idiopathic dilated cardiomyopathy in the young seen at the Mayo Clinic, 63% of the patients were alive at 1-year and 34% at 5-year follow-up.[78] Several other series have shown remarkably similar survival curves.[62,79-81] All of these studies took place in tertiary referral centers and suffer from potential referral bias in favor of sicker patients. A population-based cohort from Olmsted County, Minn., was studied to ascertain the magnitude of referral bias, and survival was found to be significantly better[82] (Fig 19A-5). The population-based cohort lacks the high early mortality, but the survival curve otherwise has a similar late downward slope. More recent follow-up of cohorts of referral patients at the Mayo Clinic suggests that patients seen in the 1980s may have a better survival than those seen in earlier eras.[83] This apparent change in prognosis could be related to better therapy, earlier diagnosis, or both.

Several prognostic features have particular importance in predicting poor outcome. Ejection fraction, increased pulmonary wedge pressure, increased right heart pressures, ventricular tachycardia, advanced age, and poor exercise capacity (as assessed by New York Heart Association [NYHA] class or by oxygen consumption) have all been shown to predict poor survival.[56,61,62,79,80,82,84-88] In addition, the failure to develop an appropriate degree of hypertrophy in the dilated ventricle indicates a poor prognosis.[10,62] Morphologic analysis of endomyocardial biopsy specimens has been performed in three studies, and its prognostic usefulness is controversial.[79,85,89]

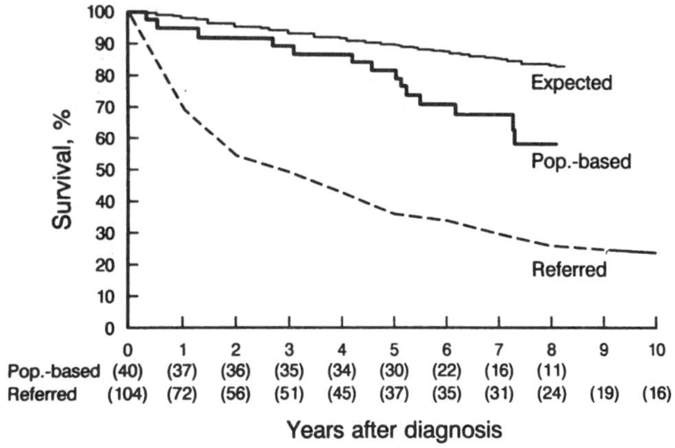

Fig 19A-5 Survival in population-based and referral cohorts. Survival after initial diagnosis of idiopathic dilated cardiomyopathy among residents of Olmsted County, Minn., 1975 to 1984 (*Pop.-based*), compared with survival after Mayo Clinic diagnosis of idiopathic dilated cardiomyopathy in a Mayo Clinic referral case series, 1960 to 1973 (*Referred*) and with survival of a 1980 Minnesota white cohort (*Expected*). (From Sugrue DD, Rodeheffer RJ, Codd MB, et al: The clinical course of idiopathic dilated cardiomyopathy: a population-based study. *Ann Intern Med* 117:117-123, 1992. By permission of American College of Physicians.)

The cause of death is most often progressive circulatory failure, but sudden death due to tachyarrhythmia or bradyarrhythmia may occur in up to 45% of cases.[7,77] A small number of patients die of embolic complications, either pulmonary or systemic.

Treatment. Management of patients with idiopathic dilated cardiomyopathy must take into consideration the duration and the severity of the illness, the presence of complications, possible contributing factors, the age of the patient, and response to previous therapeutic efforts. Aspects to be addressed include the patient's activities, diet, and exposure to potential toxins, pharmacologic interventions, and potential for surgical interventions. General measures include weight reduction when appropriate, restriction of sodium in the diet, abstinence from alcohol and tobacco, and correction of anemia, thyroid dysfunction, chronic tachyarrhythmia, or other deleterious conditions. Appropriate immunizations against influenza and pneumococcal pneumonia are recommended. A supervised exercise program is valuable in maintaining general fitness.

Pharmacotherapy includes vasodilators, diuretics, digoxin, anticoagulants, antiarrhythmics, and β-blockers. The quality of life can be improved and the occurrence of complications can be decreased by treatment (see chapter 17).

Because of the increased risk of pulmonary and systemic emboli, warfarin anticoagulation is recommended unless contraindications exist. This is particularly true if additional risk factors, such as age more than 60 years and atrial fibrillation, are also present.[90-94] The value of anticoagulation in mild dilated cardiomyopathy (ejection fraction >40%) and sinus rhythm is not known.

Atrial arrhythmias are common, particularly atrial fibrillation. Efforts should be made to achieve and maintain sinus rhythm, because doing so can improve cardiac output and exercise capacity and decrease the risks of embolic events. In addition, inadequately controlled atrial fibrillation rate may itself contribute to deterioration of ventricular function.[95] Although quinidine and procainamide have little negative inotropic risk and could be used, vigilance should be maintained because of their potential for precipitating ventricular arrhythmias. Nonsustained ventricular tachycardia is common in these patients, but controlled trials have not proven that antiarrhythmic drugs prevent sudden death in this population.[96] Nevertheless, intervention with antiarrhythmic agents may be warranted in patients who have had symptomatic sustained ventricular arrhythmias.

Corticosteroids used in a prospective, controlled clinical trial in a group of 102 patients resulted in a small, transient improvement in ejection fraction; almost half of the patients receiving steroids had notable treatment side effects.[97]

Patients with idiopathic dilated cardiomyopathy undergoing operation for mitral regurgitation have a high operative mortality,[98] and thus valvular surgery is not advisable in these patients. Mechanical circulatory-assist devices may be considered for judicious short-term use, particularly when a critically ill patient is being sustained for cardiac transplantation. Patients with severe idiopathic dilated cardiomyopathy undergoing cardiac transplantation have a significantly improved life expectancy. One-year survival for adults is approximately 85% and 5-year survival 70%[99] (see chapter 18).

Peripartum cardiomyopathy

Peripartum cardiomyopathy presents in the last month of gestation or the first several months post partum in patients with no previous heart disease or other cause for heart disease.[100,101] It is clinically indistinguishable from idiopathic dilated cardiomyopathy.[100,101] Although most cases probably represent the development of a new peripartal disease, it may not be possible to exclude the chance of a preexisting dilated cardiomyopathy exacerbated by the hemodynamic stress of pregnancy.

The incidence is estimated to be 1 in 1,300 to 4,000 deliveries in the United States.[100] In North America, the disease appears to be more common among black women.[102] The highest incidences have been reported in black African populations.[100,102,103] The risk is increased in multiparas, those who are lactating, those with hypertension, and those who have twins.[101,102]

Although the cause is unknown, a number of possibilities have been proposed. Lymphocytic myocarditis has been reported.[104] In a recent series, in which half the patients were black, myocarditis was found in 78% of patients in whom the endocardial biopsy specimen was obtained in the first few months after delivery.[105] In contrast, a series of predominantly white patients in whom biopsies were performed later in the course of disease showed a low incidence of myocarditis.[106] Myocardial inflammation could occur during the peripartum period because of altered sensitivity to viral infection, autoimmune dysregulation precipitated by exposure to fetal antigens, or unknown causes. The cause in high-incidence African populations may be unique for reasons of genetic predisposition or local customs of perinatal care.[100]

The usual treatment is that described above for idiopathic dilated cardiomyopathy. Corticosteroids have been associated with recovery in some patients with biopsy-proven myocarditis,[105] but given the potential for spontaneous recovery, the benefit of steroids cannot be considered proven.

The risk of recurrence during subsequent pregnancy appears to be related to the degree of recovery after the first occurrence. If cardiac function returns to normal, future pregnancies may be well tolerated.[107] The long-term prognosis appears also to be related to the degree of recovery of ventricular function.[101,106] In patients with ejection fractions of 35% or less, the 10-year actuarial survival rate has been estimated to be 42%.[106]

Right ventricular cardiomyopathy

Right ventricular cardiomyopathy (arrhythmogenic right ventricular dysplasia, Uhl's anomaly, parchment right ventricle) is a poorly understood condition that may become manifest at any age.[108-113] The right ventricle is often thinned, enlarged, and hypocontractile. There is replacement of myocardium by adipose and fibrous tissue. Arrhythmias, particularly of ventricular origin, are a prominent feature. In advanced cases, the left ventricle may also be enlarged and the clinical presentation may be that of dilated cardiomyopathy with refractory ventricular tachycardia. Indeed, in some reports of familial dilated cardiomyopathy, patients with dilated cardiomyopathy and patients with right ventricular cardiomyopathy have been found in the same kindred,[114] a suggestion that right ventricular cardiomyopathy is one form in which dilated cardiomyopathy may be expressed.

VIRAL MYOCARDITIS

Definitions

Infectious myocarditis is an inflammatory process of the myocardium due to viral infection. The inflammation may not be confined to the myocardium and sometimes involves the pericardium. Although a lymphocytic inflammatory reaction of the myocardium is often associated with known or presumed viral infection, histologically similar inflammatory reactions may follow a variety of insults, including exposure to drugs, chemicals, physical agents, bites and stings, and high levels of catecholamines.

Epidemiology

Geographic, socioeconomic, and demographic features exert a large influence on the incidence and prevalence of myocarditis, which, in turn, will influence the clinician's degree of alertness. In Europe and North America, viruses are believed to be the most common cause of infectious myocarditis. Although a variety of viral agents have been implicated as causes of myocarditis (Table 19A-1), the actual incidence of either viral infections or myocardial involvement is unknown because of difficulties in establishing the diagnosis. It has been estimated that 5% of all viral infections have some associated cardiac involvement,[25] but the prevalence of cardiac symptoms is only 0.5% to 5% in large series.[153,154] Coxsackie B appears to be the virus with the greatest cardiotropic potential in man.[153-155] The frequency of the disease is influenced by several factors including epidemic or sporadic outbreak, season, host age, pregnancy, and the sex of the patient. With current diagnostic criteria ("Dallas Criteria"; see below), the incidence of lymphocytic myocarditis in a large adult autopsy series, not all of which was viral in origin, was 1.06%.[156] However, when autopsy cases are selected for childhood and sudden death, myocarditis is found in 17% to 21%.[157] Familial clustering has been observed.[158]

During the first year of life, and especially in the neonatal period, there is a high incidence of myocarditis.[155] Then the frequency subsides in early childhood, only to increase again during late childhood and adolescence.[159]

Pregnancy may predispose a person to viral involvement of the heart. The incidence of severe poliomyelitis is increased during pregnancy and parturition, and there is

Table 19A-1 Viral myocarditis

Cause	Clinical features	Pathologic findings	Comments	References
Coxsackievirus	See text	See text	See text	25
Echovirus	See text	See text	See text	
Infuenza	Tachycardia, ECG abnormalities, dyspnea, anginal chest pain, congestive failure, complete heart block, and death	Myocarditis present in one-third of fatal cases; biventricular dilatation, subendocardial and subepicardial hemorrhage, and mononuclear perivascular inflammation	Treat type A with amantadine	115,116
Cytomegalovirus	Symptomatic disease rare; pericardial effusion occasionally present	Focal lymphocytic infiltration and fibrosis		117,118
Poliomyelitis	Often found in fatal cases; cardiovascular collapse, heart failure, and pulmonary edema		Immunization effective; maintain proper oxygenation and pulmonary function	119-121
Infectious mononucleosis	ECG changes common; cardiac symptoms unusual; rare congestive heart failure or death	Myocardial infiltrates of atypical lymphocytes and necrosis	Consider treatment with corticosteroids	122-125
Human immunodeficiency virus	Pericarditis, arrhythmias, ECG abnormalities, and dilated cardiomyopathy	Lymphocytic myocarditis, opportunistic myocardial infections, and ventricular dilatation	See text	126-130
Viral hepatitis	Usually transient; ECG abnormalities of bradycardia, ventricular premature complexes, ST-T changes; congestive failure and sudden death in severe cases	Focal necrosis and inflammation; petechial hemorrhage, including hemorrhage into conduction system		131,132
Mumps	Clinical and cardiac involvement uncommon; ST- and T-wave abnormalities more frequent	Cardiac dilatation and hypertrophy; mural thrombi; interstitial fibrosis and infiltration of mononuclear cells and focal necrosis; possible relationship of maternal mumps and fetal endocardial fibroelastosis		133-135

Continued.

Table 19A-1 Viral myocarditis—cont'd

Cause	Clinical features	Pathologic findings	Comments	References
Rubeola	Transient ECG abnormalities; rare congestive heart failure	Perivascular lymphocyte infiltrate		136, 137
Varicella	Rare bundle-branch block, conduction defects, heart failure, and sudden death; nonsustained ventricular tachycardia and fibrillation	Intranuclear inclusion bodies within myocardial cells, interstitial edema, cellular infiltrates, and myonecrosis		138-140
Variola and vaccinia	Myocarditis rare but may be fatal; myocarditis may follow vaccination by 2 weeks	Mononuclear infiltrate, interstitial edema, and necrosis	Variola now eradicated and immunization no longer recommended; myocarditis after vaccination has responded to steroids	141, 142
Arbovirus (chikungunya, dengue)	Myocarditis frequent; chest pain, dyspnea, palpitations, murmurs, gallops, and cardiomegaly; ST-T abnormalities, supraventricular and ventricular arrhythmias, and sudden death; chronicity	Embolization		143-145
Respiratory syncytial viruses	Rare congestive failure, complete heart block, and arrhythmias			146, 147
Herpes simplex virus		Chronic interstitial inflammation and fibrosis	Treat with adenine arabinoside or acyclovir, but effectiveness not proved	148, 149
Adenovirus	Myocarditis rare	Dilated right and left ventricles; mononuclear infiltrate		150
Yellow fever virus	Hepatitis, gastrointestinal bleeding, cardiovascular collapse, and bradycardia inappropriate to the fever	Pericardial petechial hemorrhages and myocyte degeneration		151
Rabies	Rare tachycardia, gallop rhythm, and hypotension	Diffuse interstitial infiltrate; myocardial necrosis		152

a higher incidence of myocarditis. Similar observations were made during an epidemic of Coxsackie B5 infection, during which the incidence of heart disease during pregnancy was greater than that of pleurodynia, in contrast with observations during the nonpregnant state.[160] The usual male-to-female proportion in viral heart disease associated with Coxsackie B infections is 2:1. However, during pregnancy the incidence in females increases.[25] Patients with peripartum cardiomyopathy have had biopsy evidence of acute myocarditis.[105]

Cardiac pathology

In acute viral myocarditis the heart is dilated, the papillary muscles and trabeculae carnae are flattened, and the myocardium is pale and often yellow-gray with yellow-brown streaks of minute hemorrhages. Microscopically, there may be serous effusion with only a few inflammatory cells, or there may be destruction and loss of muscle fibers, with polymorphonuclear leukocytes early and mononuclear cells later, including histiocytes and sometimes eosinophils (Fig 19A-3,F). Necrosis of myofibers occurs and may be either patchy or diffuse and may be found at any site, including the conduction system. Pericarditis may be found in association with myocarditis, and there may be serous effusion. Chronic and healed lesions show interstitial fibrosis and have evidence of loss of myofibers. After 7 to 10 days from the onset of symptoms, viruses can on rare occasions be cultured from the myocardium.[25]

Reports on myocarditis have been plagued by a lack of

uniform histologic criteria. In order to provide a common approach, the "Dallas Criteria" were published in 1987.[161] It is hoped that this histopathologic classification will improve our understanding of myocarditis and its therapy.

Pathogenesis

Evidence from animal experiments, chiefly in mice, indicates two possible mechanisms of injury to the heart. In viral myocarditis, direct invasion by the virus and replication are found early after the onset of infection and result in myocardial necrosis.[25] The infectious phase is usually 7 to 14 days, during which virus is recoverable from the heart, and this is usually followed by complete recovery. In this acute phase, a direct cytotoxic effect of the virus on the myocardium is postulated. Serum neutralizing antibody (IgM) develops within a week, and it is thought that this, together with mononuclear cell invasion, limits viral replication.[25] However, virus may persist in the myocardium for extended periods.[162] The susceptibility to infections and the severity of myocardial injury vary with the animal strain and with the viral strain.

The possibility that a similar pathogenesis occurs in human subjects has been based largely on epidemiologic evidence in the past (see above), since culture of virus from human myocardium has proven very difficult. However, newer molecular genetic techniques have provided important evidence for the presence of virus in the myocytes in human myocarditis.[29,30,163] Nevertheless, not all studies have supported the model of persistent viral presence and a chronic inflammatory response in human disease, and this hypothesis cannot be considered proven at this time.[30,31,164,165] Conflicting findings may be due to different patient populations, to obtaining data at different points in the course of the disease, and to use of different techniques to detect viral presence.

Other evidence suggests that immune mechanisms may be involved in myocyte injury or reversible myocyte dysfunction. Circulating heart-reactive antibodies are seen in myocarditis and dilated cardiomyopathy,[166,167] and myocarditis is characterized by induction of major histocompatibility antigens on the myocardium.[36,168] However, there is uncertainty about whether such antibodies are a primary mechanism for myocyte death or an epiphenomenon. A substantial body of evidence suggests that in some individuals, acute viral myocarditis may evolve into chronic dilated cardiomyopathy.[28-31,69,169-171] The mechanism may be a chronic immune-mediated injury initiated by an acute viral infection that alters the host myocyte antigenic profile in a way that produces persistent T-cell stimulation.[169,170,172,173]

In addition to the cell-mediated myocyte injury apparent on histopathologic examination,[69,161,172,173] there is evidence to support the concept of antibody-mediated and cytokine-mediated impairment of myocyte function;[36,173-175] this finding could help explain the discrepancy so often observed in myocarditis between a severe degree of ventricular dysfunction and a very mild cellular inflammatory infiltrate.

Experimental evidence in animals and circumstantial evidence in humans support the concept that myocardial injury from infection is a complex process. It has multiple causes, deriving from the convergence of several conditioning factors, one of which may be infection. Possible conditioning factors include familial predisposition, peripartum state, hypoxia, exercise, malnutrition, bacterial infection, ethanol intake, ionizing radiation, and exposure to heat or cold.[158,176]

Clinical aspects

As in other systemic illnesses, the generalized manifestations of infections may dominate the clinical picture. Fever, respiratory symptoms, gastrointestinal symptoms, headache, and myalgias are features common to a number of acute viral infections. Pleurodynia or rash may point to coxsackievirus syndromes.

Cardiac symptoms may be those of congestive failure, but unfortunately sudden death may be the initial presentation.[177] Occasionally, the presentation mimics acute myocardial infarction.[177]

Pericardial friction rubs commonly heard in patients with myocarditis and elevations of the ST segment are consistent with pericardial involvement. An S_3 gallop, cardiac palpatory asynergy, or pericardial rub may be present. Tachycardia disproportionate to the degree of fever is a frequent observation. A murmur of mitral regurgitation may be heard. Patients with overt heart failure may have elevated venous pressure, systemic hypotension with a narrowed pulse pressure, pulsus alternans, or peripheral edema. Other manifestations of Coxsackie B viral illness include pleurodynia, meningitis, hepatitis, orchitis, lymphadenopathy, and splenomegaly.[160] Patients with influenza syndromes may have evidence of pulmonary involvement. Patients with cytomegalovirus myocarditis may present with an infectious mononucleosis-like syndrome.

Evidence of myocarditis in adolescents and adults is most often apparent a week to 10 days after the onset of the acute systemic syndrome. In contrast, myocarditis in the neonate often appears early after the onset of the illness, and it tends to be more severe.

Laboratory findings

Radiologic examination of the chest may show a normal or an enlarged heart with evidence of pulmonary congestion. The cardiac silhouette may be enlarged by dilatation of the heart per se or by pericardial effusion. Pneumonia may sometimes be associated.

ECG abnormalities are common, occur more often than clinical syndromes of myocarditis, and may be transient. However, during an acute infection, ECG abnormalities may be found that are due not to the infection but rather to other factors, such as fever, tachycardia, ischemia, hypokalemia, and drugs. The most common changes are ST-segment and T-wave abnormalities; atrial and ventricular premature beats and arrhythmias may be seen, along with intraventricular conduction defects, and pathologic Q waves may rarely be present. Complete heart block may occur.

Serologic tests are important in incriminating a specific etiologic agent, but unfortunately they involve considerable delay; thus, they are often not helpful in the sporadic case. Frequently, the first serum sample has not been obtained before antibody formation, and thus an appropriate baseline titer is not available. A fourfold or more increase in the titer of a specific serum antibody supports the diagnosis. A positive culture of feces, urine, or sputum or from the pharynx is supporting, but by itself it is not conclusive proof of myocarditis due to that virus. Initially, the level of IgM antibody is increased and, later, IgG.[25] Leukocytosis of mild to moderate degree may be found, and during recovery some increase in eosinophils may be apparent. The erythrocyte sedimentation rate may be increased; if it is, this finding is helpful in following the clinical course. Intracellular cardiac enzymes will appear in the blood if there is sufficient myocardial necrosis.

Echocardiography may be useful in detecting dilatation and diminished cardiac function, excluding valvular disease, evaluating myocardial contraction abnormalities, and identifying pericardial thickening or effusion. The use of myocardial uptake of gallium for the identification of myocarditis has been reported[178] but has not proven to be sufficiently sensitive. Antimyosin antibody cardiac imaging may provide better sensitivity, and the predictive value of a normal scan appears to be high enough to be of clinical value.[179] Endomyocardial biopsy can demonstrate myocarditis, but sampling error contributes to a lack of sensitivity with this technique.[66,68,69,72,180-183] This variability in prevalence may be related to the nature of the patient population selected for study and the histopathologic criteria used.[184] Patients with a history of viral illness, severe heart failure, and a brief duration of illness are more likely to have myocarditis on biopsy.[69]

Treatment

When myocarditis is found in association with an acute systemic illness, bed rest in the hospital is warranted. Monitoring of the cardiac rhythm may be indicated. The diet should be restricted in salt, and alcohol should be forbidden. Temporary, and occasionally permanent, pacing may be indicated.

Congestive heart failure may necessitate use of digitalis, vasodilators, and diuretics. Anticoagulant therapy is indicated in patients with severe congestive failure unless there is prominent pericarditis or other contraindications exist. Antiarrhythmic agents may be required as well as intravenous inotropic support. Intra-aortic balloon pumps and ventricular-assist devices have been used for patients with cardiogenic shock, and cardiac transplantation may be indicated (see chapter 18).

The efficacy of immunosuppressive therapy for myocarditis has not been clearly defined. In the murine myocarditis model, administration of corticosteroids, ibuprofen, or cyclosporine during the early acute phase of illness exacerbates the extent of myocardial injury.[25,176,185,186] Likewise, cyclophosphamide has been shown to reduce inflammation but to increase mortality in the murine model.[187] Anti-T-cell antibodies have been shown to reduce inflammatory myocyte necrosis but to have a favorable effect on mortality only if all T-cell subsets are reduced.[188]

In human viral myocarditis, a substantial proportion of patients have spontaneous recovery with only supportive therapy,[69,182] so that reports of beneficial clinical response to immunosuppressive therapy are difficult to assess.[72,184,189,190] Prospective controlled clinical trials are under way to determine whether immunosuppression improves the rate of recovery from myocarditis in man.

Acquired immunodeficiency syndrome

There is a growing body of evidence for cardiac dysfunction in patients infected with the human immunodeficiency virus (HIV).[126,130] The prevalence of cardiac involvement may depend in part on the degree to which the disease has advanced in the population under study. Among the complications associated with HIV disease are pericarditis, myocarditis, ventricular tachycardia, endocarditis, cardiac malignancy (Kaposi's sarcoma, lymphoma), and dilated cardiomyopathy.[126-128] Although isolated echocardiographic and histologic abnormalities are common, symptomatic heart failure and tamponade occur infrequently.

In autopsy series, lymphocytic myocarditis is seen in 35% to 52% of cases,[129,191,192] and lymphocytic myocarditis has been associated with left ventricular dysfunction and ventricular tachycardia.[126] The cause of lymphocytic myocarditis is not known but could be related to opportunistic infection with viral, protozoan, bacterial, fungal, or mycobacterial pathogens.[126,192,193] It is not known whether HIV can itself infect or damage cardiac muscle. In addition, dilated cardiomyopathy in HIV-infected patients may be associated with zidovudine therapy.[194]

OTHER INFECTIOUS FORMS OF MYOCARDITIS

Rickettsial myocarditis

Table 19A-2 lists rickettsial myocarditides, with comments.

Bacterial myocarditis, *Mycoplasma pneumoniae*, and psittacosis

Table 19A-3 summarizes this topic.

Diphtheritic myocarditis. Myocardial involvement occurs in about a quarter of the cases of diphtheria and is the most common cause of death.[204,205] Signs of myocarditis may appear at about 1 week of illness and include cardiomegaly, congestive heart failure with gallop rhythm, and pulmonary congestion.[205] Sudden death may occur.

The ECG is useful for evaluating severity and following progress. ST- and T-wave abnormalities are common, but atrial and ventricular arrhythmias, bundle-branch block, and mild to high-grade AV block may occur. Abnormalities may be transient or permanent.

The exotoxin produced by diphtheria alters cellular respiration, affecting first tissue with high energy requirements such as nerve or heart. Myocardial carnitine is depleted[203] and the diphtheria toxin appears to interfere with cellular protein synthesis.[229,230] The cardiac conduction system appears to be particularly vulnerable to the

Table 19A-2 Rickettsial myocarditis

Cause	Clinical features	Pathologic findings	Comments	References
Scrub typhus *(R. tsutsugamushi)*	Myocarditis common, usually mild, and resolves without sequelae; occasional fatalities	Focal panvasculitis of small blood vessels with proliferative endothelial changes and perivascular round cell infiltrate	Antibiotic therapy	195-197
Rocky Mountain spotted fever *(R. rickettsii)*	Peripheral vascular collapse	Interstitial mononuclear myocarditis; immunofluorescent demonstration of rickettsia in myocardial capillaries, venules, and arterioles	Antibiotic therapy	198-200
Q fever *(R. burnetii)*	Endocarditis and pericarditis dominate picture; ECG ST and T changes and ventricular arrhythmias	Pericardial petechial hemorrhage; scattered necrosis and fibrosis of myocardium	Antibiotic therapy	201, 202

Table 19A-3 Bacterial myocarditis, *Mycoplasma pneumoniae,* and psittacosis

Cause	Clinical features	Pathologic findings	Comments	References
Diphtheria	See text	See text	See text	203-206
Enteric fever, typhoid fever (salmonella)	See text	See text	See text	207-212
Tuberculosis	See text	See text	See text	213-216
Streptococci	Acute myocarditis, distinct from rheumatic carditis; may accompany scarlet fever; conduction abnormalities and arrhythmia uncommon, and sudden death rare	Interstitial infiltrate of mononuclear cells and polymorphonuclear cells; bacteria sometimes detectable in the heart	Antibiotic therapy	217, 218
Meningococci	Myocardium commonly involved, especially in fatal cases; pericardial effusions, heart block, congestive heart failure, and death	Interstitial myocarditis and hemorrhagic myocardial lesions	Antibiotic therapy	219-221
Brucellosis	Endocarditis, conduction system disturbance	Tuberculoid granulomas	Antibiotic therapy	222
Clostridia		Gas bubbles in myocardium; organisms may be in tissues or intramural coronary arteries; myocardial abscess formation and purulent pericarditis	Antibiotic therapy	223, 224
Staphylococci	May be associated with endocarditis or overwhelming sepsis	Multiple abscesses; may complicate myocardial infarction; cardiac perforation	Antibiotic therapy	
Melioidosis	May mimic myocardial infarction	Abscess formation	Antibiotic therapy	225

Continued.

Table 19A-3 Bacterial myocarditis, *Mycoplasma pneumoniae,* and psittacosis—cont'd

Cause	Clinical features	Pathologic findings	Comments	References
Mycoplasma pneumoniae	Myalgias and ST-T abnormalities in up to one-third of patients; usually associated with pneumonia; may require intensive care; may result in permanent sequelae		Antibiotic therapy	226, 227
Psittacosis	Congestive heart failure; pericarditis; fever, chest pain, tachycardia, hypotension, and emboli	Inclusion bodies and plasma cells; subendocardial hemorrhage	Antibiotic therapy	228

toxin, and this accounts for the high frequency of conduction abnormalities.

Pathologically, gross examination reveals a dilated heart with fatty streaking of the myocardium. Histologically, there is fatty infiltration, interstitial inflammatory reaction, and hyaline necrosis of muscle fibers.[206]

Treatment consists of ensuring adequate ventilation and oxygenation. Adequate doses of diphtheria antitoxin should be administered promptly, and an antibiotic such as penicillin or erythromycin should be given. Rhythm should be monitored during the acute phase. Pacemaker insertion has been successfully employed in cases of advanced degrees of heart block. Treatment with corticosteroids has not proven useful,[231] but supplemental carnitine may be of benefit.[232]

Typhoid fever (enteric fever). Clinical evidence of myocarditis during *Salmonella typhi* infections is uncommon; however, ECG abnormalities are found in 11.9% to 80.8% of cases.[207-209] The availability of chloramphenicol therapy has not altered the frequency of ECG abnormalities.

Pathologically, fatal cases show biventricular dilatation, myocardial petechiae, hemorrhage, necrosis, and polymorphonuclear leukocyte infiltration. Coronary arteritis may be found, which may lead to thrombosis and infarction. There may be cloudy swelling or hyaline degeneration of myocardial fibers. In addition to myocarditis, shaggy fibrinous pericarditis may be seen, and endocarditis may occur. Myocardial abscess formation has been seen.[210]

Congestive heart failure is more likely to occur in severely ill children and is associated with significant mortality.[212] Bradycardia is frequent in typhoid fever, and therefore when tachycardia develops it may signal the onset of myocarditis. Hypotension and other evidence of circulatory failure are common in severe cases and do not necessarily reflect direct myocardial involvement.

ECG abnormalities most often appear in the second week and, in milder cases, resolve completely.[207,209] ST and T abnormalities are the most frequent abnormalities, followed by $Q\text{-}T_c$ prolongation. In addition, there may be conduction disturbances, and pathologic involvement of the conduction system has been shown.[210] Arrhythmias are not common, but when they do occur they indicate a poor prognosis. Cardiac enzyme levels are usually normal.[207,209]

Patients with typhoid fever require careful attention to fluid and electrolyte status. Appropriate antibiotic therapy should be instituted.

Tuberculosis. Tuberculosis of the myocardium was rare even before the availability of effective antituberculosis drugs. However, in an autopsy series of 100 fatal cases, a moderate to extensive degree of acute interstitial myocarditis was present in half the patients.[213] In miliary tuberculosis, the most frequent myocardial finding is miliary tuberculous infarctions, which tend to be seen most often in patients beyond the sixth decade of age.[213] Other cardiac lesions include nodule formation by tuberculomas and a diffuse infiltration. Nodules have a predilection for the right atrium but may be found elsewhere. Large tuberculomas have sometimes led to compression of chambers and obstruction of blood flow.[214] Complications include endocardial thrombosis with systemic embolization and aneurysm formation. Arrhythmias, including complete heart block, may result from myocardial tuberculosis.[215]

In advanced pulmonary tuberculosis, cardiac signs and symptoms may be overshadowed by the pulmonary disease. A tachycardia disproportionate to fever may be suggestive. Overt congestive heart failure is unusual. Treatment with appropriate antimicrobial agents is essential.

Rheumatic fever. Myocarditis is an integral part of acute rheumatic fever and is discussed in chapter 54.

Other bacterial infections. Other bacterial myocarditides are listed in Table 19A-3, with comments.

Spirochetal myocarditis

Lyme disease. Lyme disease was recognized in 1975 as a distinct disorder.[233] It has been shown to be a multisystem disease caused by the tick-borne spirochete *Borrelia burgdorferi.*[234,235] A characteristic rash, erythema chronicum migrans, may be associated with fever, lymph-

Table 19A-4 Spirochetal myocarditis

Cause	Clinical features	Pathologic findings	Comments	References
Syphilis	Arrhythmias and heart block	Myocarditis found in congenital syphilis; gummas may be found in myocardium, valves, and conduction system	Antibiotic therapy	244
Leptospirosis (Weil's disease)	ST and T abnormalities and arrhythmias with conduction defects; congestive heart failure rare	Interstitial inflammation and subepicardial hemorrhage	Antibiotic therapy	245-248
Relapsing fever (borrelia)	Tachyarrhythmias, AV conduction defects, hypotension, and heart failure	Petechiae and interstitial infiltrate	Antibiotic therapy	249
Lyme disease	Tick-borne; AV conduction defects; myocarditis; pericarditis	Thought to be immune mediated	Antibiotic therapy	233, 235, 237-240, 242, 243

adenopathy, myalgias, and arthralgias. Arthritis develops in most untreated patients; neurologic or cardiac complications may develop in a smaller proportion.[233] Myocarditis occurs in 4% to 10% of cases and is most commonly manifested by AV block.[236]

Recent reports of the isolation of organisms from endocardial biopsy specimens in patients with long-standing dilated cardiomyopathy have raised the possibility that Lyme disease may be a cause of dilated cardiomyopathy.[237-239] Laboratory studies in a hamster model of Lyme disease indicated that spirochetes perist in certain organs, particularly the heart, suggesting that the organism may have trophism for the myocardium.[240]

Serologic studies are useful to confirm the diagnosis, and the organisms may be found on endocardial biopsy.[241] Prompt antimicrobial treatment may prevent complications, but some patients require temporary or permanent pacemaker support.[242,243]

Other spirochetal infections. Myocarditides due to spirochetes are listed in Table 19A-4, with comments.

Fungal myocarditis

Candidiasis. Deep or systemic candidiasis, usually due to *Candida albicans,* is becoming more common with the use of antibiotics, immunosuppressive agents, and cancer chemotherapeutic drugs. Intravenous drug use and HIV infection have also contributed to the increased prevalence of *Candida* cardiac infections. Although endocarditis is the most common form of cardiac infection by *Candida* organisms, myocarditis and microabscesses occur often and may or may not be associated with endocarditis.[250,251] *Candida* was the most common fungal cardiac infection at the Johns Hopkins Hospital, constituting 34 of 51 cases recorded from 1889 through 1977. The fact that all occurred since 1954 suggests a relationship to the availability of antibiotics.[252]

Pathologically, microabscesses are found at random sites throughout the myocardium, including the cardiac conduction system. Pseudohyphae are found in the center of tubercles and are surrounded by yeast forms and, in the periphery, by polymorphonuclear leukocytes[252] (Fig 19A-6).

Clinically, hypotension and shock were frequent findings in one series. Sudden death may occur. The ECG commonly has shown T-wave abnormalities. Appearance of a new conduction disturbance is also common, and supraventricular arrhythmias and changes mimicking myocardial infarction may be observed. The diagnosis is often made at autopsy, but when it is diagnosed during life, antifungal therapy is indicated.

Other fungal infections. Other fungal myocarditides are listed in Table 19A-5, with comments.

Protozoal myocarditis

Chagas' disease. Chagas' disease is a chronic parasitosis caused by the protozoan *Trypanosoma cruzi.* The principal clinical manifestations are acute and chronic heart disease and achalasia of the esophagus or colon. It is a major health problem in Central and South America, where more than 7 million persons are estimated to be infected and nearly 20 million are at risk.[266,267] Genetic factors may influence susceptibility to cardiac damage.[268]

The natural vector of *T. cruzi* is the reduviid bug, an insect found in relatively warm and dry climates roughly between the 42nd parallel north in the United States and the 43rd parallel south in Argentina. At night the insect feeds on humans by puncturing the skin and sucking blood through a long proboscis. During feeding, they may defecate, and after the affected person scratches, the

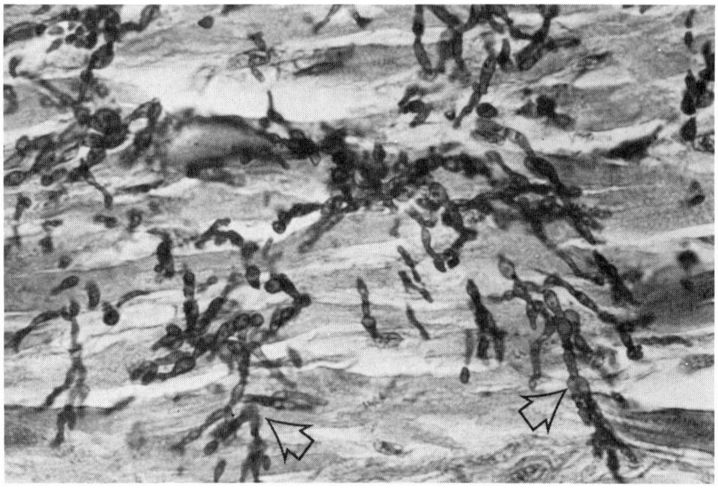

Fig 19A-6 Myocarditis due to *Candida* in case of acute myelocytic leukemia. Note pseudohyphae *(arrows)*. (Periodic acid-Schiff stain.) (Courtesy of William D. Edwards, M.D.)

Table 19A-5 Fungal myocarditis

Cause	Clinical features	Pathologic findings	Comments	References
Candidiasis	See text	See text	Antifungal therapy	250, 252
Aspergillosis	Compromised host	Endocarditis frequent; thrombosis of coronary vessels with infarction; invasion by fungus aided by elaboration of oxalic acid	Antifungal therapy	252-255
Cryptococcosis	Patients with malignancy; congestive heart failure and cardiomegaly; ventricular arrhythmias, first-degree AV block, and T-wave abnormalities	Cardiac dilatation; granuloma formation with giant cells and fibrosis	Antifungal therapy	256, 257
Histoplasmosis	Cardiac involvement rare; endocarditis and pericarditis; arrhythmias and T-wave abnormalities	Granulomas with *Histoplasma capsulatum* in phagocytes	Antifungal therapy	258, 259
Actinomycosis	Myocarditis rare; right and left heart failure	Extension of disease from thorax via pericardium or, less often, hematogenous spread; abscesses contain organism and are surrounded by granulation tissue	Antifungal therapy	260
Blastomycosis	Third and fourth decades of life; tachycardia, systolic murmur, dyspnea, cyanosis, and peripheral edema	Spreads from mediastinal lymph nodes, to pericardium, to myocardium, to endocardium, or by hematogenous miliary seeding; mural thrombi may form; caseation with tubercles and giant cells	Antifungal therapy	261, 262
Coccidioidomycosis	Pericarditis may be present	Myocarditis; focal interstitial and perivascular infiltrate; granulomas sometimes containing fungi	Antifungal therapy	263, 264
Mucormycosis	Cardiac involvement rare	Septic thrombosis; myocarditis; mycotic valvular thrombi	See Figure 19A-7 Antifungal therapy	265

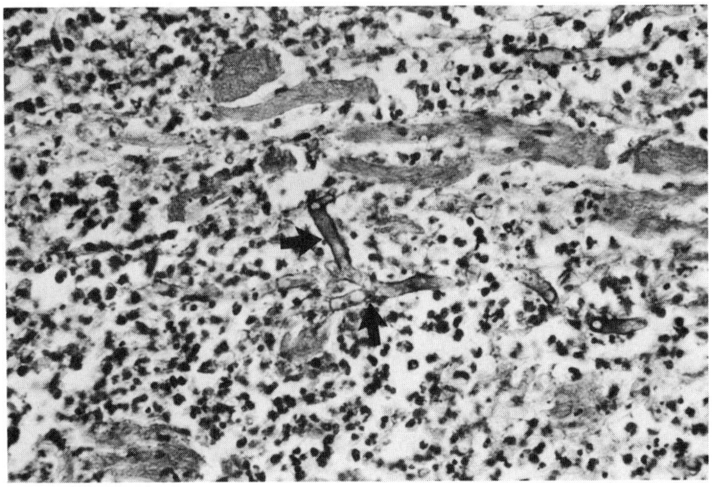

Fig 19A-7 *Mucor* myocarditis. Note hyphae *(arrows)* and intense inflammatory reaction. (Courtesy of William D. Edwards, M.D.)

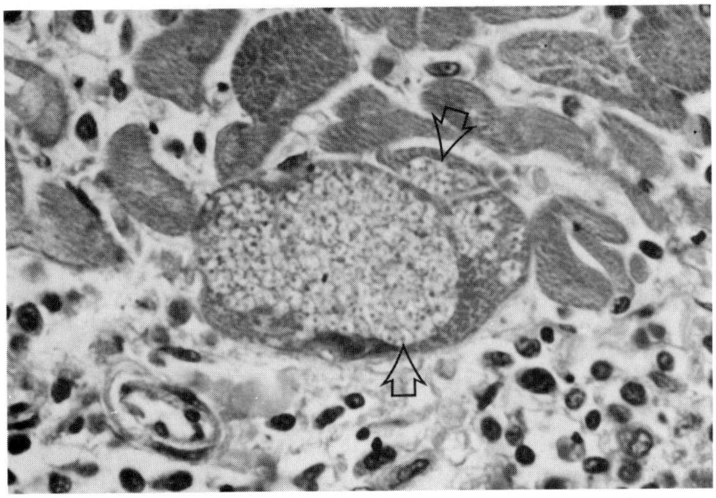

Fig 19A-8 Acute myocarditis of Chagas' disease. Note the many intracellular trypanosomes *(arrows).* (Courtesy of William D. Edwards, M.D.)

trypanosomes may enter the excoriated skin; they may also enter the intact conjunctiva. The organisms enter local tissues and cause an inflammatory reaction with edema. After transformation to a flagellate form, they enter the bloodstream and gain access to many tissues but have a predilection for myocardial cells, smooth muscle cells, and glia.

ACUTE CHAGAS' DISEASE. In most patients, acute Chagas' disease develops with little local or systemic reaction,[269] but some patients have generalized malaise, fever, sweats, muscular pain, irritability, anorexia, and sometimes vomiting and diarrhea. There may be generalized lymphadenopathy, hepatomegaly, and splenomegaly, together with signs and symptoms of acute myocarditis. Although most patients recover, in a very few cases there is a severe pancarditis and death.

Autopsy examination in acute Chagas' disease reveals a pronounced lymphocytic myocarditis associated with necrosis and contraction bands of myofibers and widely scattered parasitosis.[270] The parasite may be found within myocytes (Fig 19A-8), the pathologic findings in tissue are correlated with the presence of the parasite. There may be evidence of reactive lymphadenopathy, splenomegaly, and meningoencephalitis.[271]

Congestive heart failure is treated in the usual manner. Appropriate antiparasitic agents should be used. Because of significant developments in the treatment of parasitic diseases, the reader is advised to consult the Centers for Disease Control, Atlanta, or a comparable source for current treatment recommendations.

Patients who recover from acute Chagas' disease usually do so in 2 to 4 months. Sometimes there is residual lymphadenopathy, lymphocytosis, or elevated erythrocyte sedimentation rate, although such a finding may represent reinfection.[271]

CHRONIC CHAGAS' DISEASE. After the initial infection, there is a long latent period, during which parasitemia is found in a few patients, but all patients have positive complement-fixation tests or varying titers of hemagglutinins to *T. cruzi* antigens. Chronic chagasic myocarditis presents in three ways: congestive failure, arrhythmias and conduction disturbances, and sudden death. Insufficiency of tricuspid or mitral valves as a result of dilatation may be present. Gallop rhythms are frequent. Involvement of autonomic innervation may result in megaesophagus or megacolon.

The development of ECG abnormalities is associated with a poorer prognosis.[272] Right bundle-branch block is found in 30% to 60% of cases of chronic Chagas' myocarditis, with a high frequency of associated left anterior hemiblock. T-wave abnormalities are common, but left bundle-branch block is uncommon. Atrial fibrillation may develop in advanced stages of the disease. Patients commonly have multiform ventricular premature beats and ventricular tachycardia. Because of parasympathetic denervation, patients with Chagas' disease, in the absence of cardiac failure, may have a decreased heart rate response to exercise.[273]

Ventricular aneurysmectomy has been done for patients with malignant ventricular arrhythmias and ventricular aneurysms.[274] However, in a retrospective review of autopsy materials, no association was found between ventricular aneurysm and sudden death.[275] The presence of apical aneurysm predisposes to apical thrombus formation and to embolic complications.

CARDIAC PATHOLOGY. On gross pathologic examination, the heart in chronic Chagas' disease is enlarged and dilated, and there is hypertrophy of all chambers.[276] Left ventricular apical aneurysm and thrombosis are common. Right atrial thrombosis often occurs.

Histologically, there is evidence of focal lymphocytic infiltration with myocytolysis in some cases and with granulomatous lesions in rare cases. Extensive fibrosis is a prominent feature and may involve portions of the AV node, the right bundle branch, and anterior fascicles of the left bundle.[270] In chronic Chagas' disease, parasites are rarely seen. Ganglion neuronolysis may be seen in lesions of the parasympathetic nervous system.

PATHOGENESIS. Considerable interest has evolved in chronic Chagas' disease as a possible model of immune injury to the heart.[277] The paucity of intracellular parasites and the intense lymphocytic myocarditis are consistent with an allergic host reaction to a very immunogenic parasite. The fact that *T. cruzi*-sensitized lymphocytes have been shown to destroy allogeneic parasitized and nonparasitized heart cells in vitro suggests that a target antigen may reside in the sarcoplasmic reticulum of cardiac muscle.[278] Other evidence includes the presence of a circulating immunoglobulin (endotheliovascular interstitial antibody) that reacts with the endocardium, blood vessels, and the interstitium of the heart in patients with Chagas' cardiomyopathy.[279,280] The presence of antibodies that may involve the microvasculature supports the concept that the extensive myocardial fibrosis of Chagas' disease may be due in part to microvascular dysfunction and focal myocardial ischemia.[281] Evidence for a delayed hypersensitivity mechanism has been demonstrated in rabbits by the injection of a subcellular antigen that produces a disease similar to that seen after inoculation of the live organism. Eosinophil secretory products may also act as mediators of myocyte damage.[282] In addition to immune-mediated injury and microvascular disease, the autonomic nervous system dysfunction of chronic Chagas' disease may contribute to the cardiovascular manifestations of the disease.[281]

Toxoplasmosis. Toxoplasmosis is caused by the obligate intracellular parasite *Toxoplasma gondii.* It infects animals, including cats, cattle, sheep, and goats, around the world and is one of the more common causes of heart disease due to protozoa in North America.[283] Its role in idiopathic cardiomyopathy has not been fully defined; however, *Toxoplasma* was implicated in 28.6% of 70 cases of cardiomyopathy reported from Chile.[284]

The *Toxoplasma* parasite may be widespread in the body, with a miliary pattern of disease. In a glandular type of toxoplasmosis, only lymph nodes are involved, and there is a benign course resembling infectious mononucleosis. In a third type of toxoplasmosis, the parasites may be concentrated in one or two organs, including the heart, liver, eyes, muscles, kidneys, or brain and meninges. Congenital or acute miliary infection and acute myocarditis may be found in conjunction with myocardial necrosis and mononuclear cell infiltrates. In adults, viable cysts may be found throughout life.[285] The latent myocardial cysts may cause no injury, but cyst rupture can induce an immune response and diffuse interstitial fibrosis.[284]

Clinically, there may be no manifestations during the latent period, but with activation of the process, patients have precordial pain, arrhythmias, and cardiac failure.[283] Physical examination may reveal evidence of congestive heart failure. The ECG may show supraventricular or ventricular arrhythmias, bundle-branch block, or AV conduction abnormalities. Serologic tests indicating an increased *Toxoplasma* antibody titer suggest the diagnosis. Endocardial biopsy is useful in confirming the diagnosis.

Encouraging results have been reported with pyrimethamine and sulfadiazine therapy, but relapses may occur.[283]

Other protozoal infections. Other protozoal myocarditides are listed in Table 19A-6, with comments.

Helminthic myocarditis

Trichinosis. *Trichinella spiralis* infestation is a common human helminthic disease.[292] It is fatal in approximately 5% of cases, most often because of myocarditis. Encephalitis and pulmonary embolism due to venous thrombosis are other causes of death.

The parasite invades the heart but does not encyst there as it does in skeletal muscle. Pathologically, local infiltration of lymphocytes and eosinophils, interstitial edema, and scattered hemorrhages are found in a dilated and flabby heart. Pericardial effusion may be an associated finding. Serologic tests may support the diagnosis, but finding larvae or cysts by muscle biopsy during the third or fourth week of infection is specific proof of the disease. T-wave abnormalities are common, and there may be prolongation of the QRS complex or its voltage may be decreased. First- and second-degree AV block may be present, and arrhythmias may be seen. ECG abnormalities usually resolve over a period of weeks or months.

Clinically, as the systemic symptoms of trichinosis are diminishing, chest pain may appear in the second or third week, and congestive heart failure may ensue. Sudden death has been reported.[292,293] Recovery is generally expected with treatment. Eosinophilia is a prominent feature. Treatment with appropriate antiparasitic agents may be of value.

Echinococcosis (hydatid cyst). In sheep-raising areas of the world, echinococcosis is endemic. Hydatid disease occurs in fewer than 2% of cases of echinococcosis.[294] Ingestion of ova from contaminated dog feces infects

Table 19A-6 Protozoal myocarditis

Cause	Clinical features	Pathologic findings	Comments	References
Chagas' disease	See text	See text	*	256, 268-276, 278-282
Toxoplasmosis	See text	See text	*	283-285
African trypanosomiasis (*T. gambiense* and *T. rhodesiense*)	CNS (somnolence) dominates; Q-T prolongation and T-wave abnormalities common; cardiomegaly and congestive heart failure	Myocardial granulomas or diffuse interstitial infiltrates; primary arteritis and valvulitis	*	286, 287
Malaria	May have chest pain and rarely heart failure	Capillary thrombosis and occlusion by parasites; interstitial infiltrates and hemorrhage	*	288-290
Leishmaniasis (kala-azar)		Myocarditis and suppurative pericarditis; intracellular plasmatocytes with Leishman-Donovan bodies	*	288
Balantidiasis *(Balantidium coli)*		Subacute myocarditis, cardiac dilatation, and pericardial effusion; parasites within coronary vessels and myocardium	*	291
Sarcosporidiosis	Rare in humans	Sarcocysts in muscle fibers	*	288

CNS, central nervous system
*For current information regarding antiparasitic treatment, the reader is advised to consult the Centers for Disease Control, Atlanta, Georgia, or a comparable source.

human beings. Most parasites, on leaving the intestine, infest the lungs or liver, but a few develop in the heart, where they may grow larger than 10 cm.[295]

The most common site of cardiac cyst formation is the left ventricle, including the interventricular septum, but cysts may also be found in the right ventricle. They may reach such a large size that flow is obstructed. The cysts may degenerate and calcify, daughter cysts may develop, or cysts may rupture.[295] Rupture of the cysts is a dreaded complication resulting in an anaphylactic type of reaction. If rupture is into the pericardium, the result may be pericarditis with subsequent constriction. If rupture is into a cardiac chamber, the result may be systemic or pulmonic emboli.[296]

Clinically, the diagnosis may first be apparent on the chest radiograph because of a bulge in the cardiac silhouette, which may or may not be calcified. Another form of presentation is chest pain due to rupture of the cyst into the pericardium, or the pain may be due to compression of the myocardium.

The ECG may have nonspecific T-wave abnormalities or loss of QRS voltage, and AV conduction abnormalities may be seen.[297] Echocardiography may be used to identify these cysts. They may also be seen at angiography.[294,298] Surgical treatment is curative if it can be done without seeding of daughter cysts. However, late sudden death may occur in surgically treated cases, perhaps due to rupture of secondary pericardial cysts. Thus, a thorough exploration of the serosa is recommended, as well as extensive resection of the pericardium. Careful follow-up is recommended after surgery. Antiparasitic therapy may be of value.

Other helminthic infections. Other helminthic myocarditides are listed in Table 19A-7, with comments.

NONINFECTIOUS MYOCARDIAL DAMAGE

Alcoholic cardiomyopathy

Walshe[307] gave an early description of the adverse effects of alcohol on the heart in 1873. Subsequently, beriberi heart disease came to be linked with alcoholism, and this diverted attention from a pathogenetic role for alcohol. Then, several reports again focused attention on the effects of alcohol on the heart, pointing out features that differed from those of thiamine deficiency.[308] The complete pathogenesis has not yet been determined; nevertheless, there is now substantial evidence that alcohol is cardiotoxic. Inasmuch as an estimated two-thirds of adults in the Western world use alcohol, and approximately 10% or more are heavy users, its potential impact is apparent.[309] Whether alcoholic cardiomyopathy is a discrete entity or whether alcohol "unmasks" dilated cardiomyopathy in patients with other risk factors is unclear. What is far more important from a therapeutic standpoint is the realization that complete abstention may result in a

Table 19A-7 Helminthic myocarditis

Cause	Clinical features	Pathologic findings	Comments	References
Trichinosis	See text	See text	*	292, 293, 297
Echinococcosis	See text	See text	*	294-296, 298
Schistosomiasis	Cor pulmonale frequent; direct myocardial involvement infrequent	Ova in myocardium or coronary arteries with coronary thrombosis and myocardial infarction; inflammatory myocarditis and perivasculitis	Cardiac toxicity may also result from antimony derivatives used in treatment of schistosomiasis*	299, 300
Heterophyiasis	Chronic congestive heart failure; uncommonly, sudden death	Interstitial edema; capillary thrombosis; ova in myocardium; ova attached to mitral valve result in thickening and calcification	*	301
Cysticercosis	Cardiac involvement uncommon; ECG abnormalities; congestive heart failure occasionally	Intense tissue reaction resulting in cysts around degenerative larvae; cysts may calcify	*	302, 303
Visceral larva migrans *(Toxocara canis)*	Consider in young children with pica; congestive heart failure and death reported	Granulomas in myocardium	*	304, 305
Filariasis	Congestive heart failure; eosinophilia	Pericardial effusion; endocarditis	*	306

*For current information regarding antiparasitic treatment, the reader is advised to consult the Centers for Disease Control, Atlanta, Georgia, or a comparable source.

striking improvement in cardiac function.[310]

Pathogenesis. Among alcoholics, the extent of cardiac dysfunction correlates with the lifetime dose of ethanol.[311,312] Patients who consumed large quantities of alcohol and alcohol-fed animals that were subjected to additional interventions were found to have numerous biochemical, structural, and functional abnormalities that became manifest even before there was evidence of overt heart failure.[311,313-318] At autopsy, 43 alcoholics who were not clinically suspected of having cardiomyopathy were found to have a statistically significant increase in the ratio of mean heart weight to body weight and in mean absolute heart weight as well as microscopic cardiac pathologic changes consistent with alcoholic cardiomyopathy occurring in the absence of cardiomegaly.[319]

Cardiac dysfunction is demonstrable in normal persons who drink the quantities of alcohol commonly consumed in social drinking.[320-322] Ethyl alcohol and its metabolite acetaldehyde interfere with several cellular functions, including the transport and binding of calcium, mitochondrial respiration, myocardial lipid metabolism, myocardial protein synthesis, and myofibrillar ATPase. Among the possible mechanisms of myocardial injury are a coexisting dietary deficiency (e.g., thiamine) or the additive effects of other toxic agents. One well-publicized example of a cardiomyopathy occurring in heavy beer drinkers in the 1960s was shown to be a result, in part at least, of adding cobalt to beer.[323]

Pathologic aspects. The pathologic features of alcoholic cardiomyopathy are similar to those of idiopathic dilated cardiomyopathy. The heart has mild to moderate hypertrophy with dilatation of right and left ventricles. There are scattered small areas of myocytolysis and necrosis, and patchy fibrosis is evident (Fig 19A-9). There may be mural thrombi. Alcian-positive material accumulates in the interstitial tissues, and there are increased amounts of collagen. Electron microscopy reveals intracellular edema, lipid droplets, excessive glycogen, deranged elements of sarcoplasmic reticulum, and abnormal mitochondria.[315,324] Regan et al.[325] reported increased collagen fibers along the vascular system and periarterial fibrosis, raising the possibility of abnormal microvascular regulation.

Clinical aspects. Alcoholic cardiomyopathy is most often found in men in their third through fifth decades of life, among all socioeconomic classes. When obtained, the history is usually one of ingestion of six or more alcoholic drinks per day for 10 years or more, with sprees of drinking to intoxication.[310,326,327]

The symptom onset of alcoholic cardiomyopathy may be insidious or rather abrupt.

Palpitations, dyspnea on exertion, paroxysmal nocturnal dyspnea, orthopnea, edema, and nonspecific fatigue are early symptoms. Less common presentations are chest pain and cough.

On examination, many patients have edema and

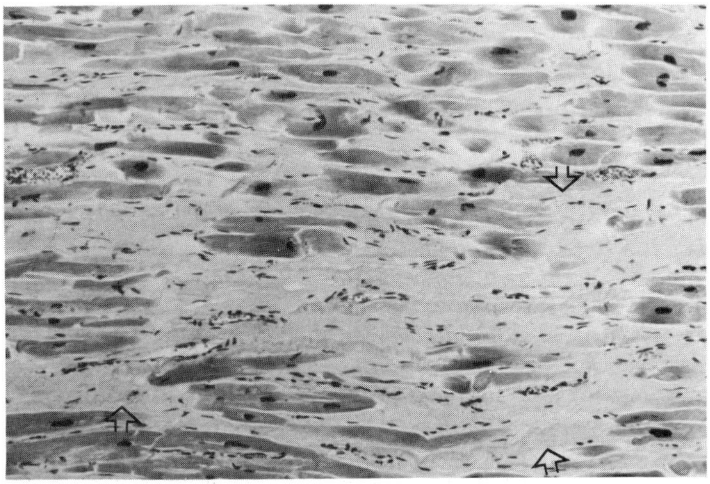

Fig 19A-9 Alcoholic cardiomyopathy in 39-year-old man. Note prominent interstitial fibrosis *(arrows)*. The sparse myocardial cells are hypertrophied. (Courtesy of William D. Edwards, M.D.)

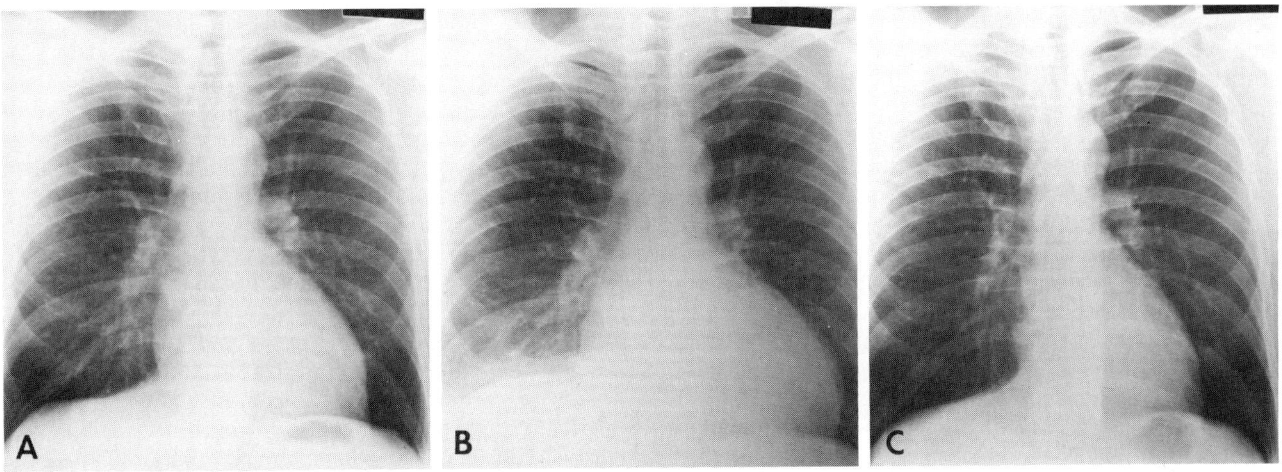

Fig 19A-10 Chest radiographs showing evolution and resolution of cardiomegaly in alcoholic cardiomyopathy. **A,** 4 months before hospitalization. **B,** at hospitalization, in congestive heart failure. **C,** 1 month after hospitalization.

hepatomegaly. Most patients have evidence of cardiomegaly and congestive heart failure. Cardiac rhythm is usually rapid and regular, but arrhythmias are common. Hypertension is common, especially diastolic hypertension. Neurologic and hepatic signs of alcohol toxicity are not always present.

The ECG in patients with heart failure from alcoholic cardiomyopathy displays a variety of abnormalities, but none of them is specific. Left ventricular hypertrophy with T-wave abnormalities is a frequent finding; however, the QRS voltage may be low or normal, and there may be nonspecific T-wave abnormalities. Atrial fibrillation,[328] ventricular arrhythmias,[329] or premature atrial beats may be seen, and a few patients have pathologic Q waves. Conduction disturbances include bundle-branch block and complete heart block. Electrophysiologic studies have shown P-R prolongation and intraventricular conduction defects in cases of alcoholic cardiomyopathy.[330]

An association has been found between excessive alcohol use and cardiac arrhythmias in the absence of overt cardiomyopathy and has been referred to as the "holiday heart."[331] Patients presented with atrial fibrillation after binge alcohol ingestion. Other arrhythmias have been observed.

Radiologic examination of the chest often shows cardiac enlargement and evidence of pulmonary venous congestion. Serial radiologic examinations may document a dramatic decrease in heart size with treatment, and this signals a good prognosis (Fig 19A-10). Macrocytosis or abnormalities of liver function tests found on examination of the blood, especially in conjunction with cardiomegaly, should alert the clinician to the possibility of heavy consumption of alcohol.

In patients with congestive heart failure, the echocardiogram shows findings similar to those of idiopathic dilated cardiomyopathy.[310,332] Hemodynamic study confirms low-output heart failure with poor ventricular contractile function, which is reflected in elevated end-diastolic pressure, low ejection fraction, and increased end-diastolic volume and tension.[333-335]

It would seem advantageous to detect any adverse effect of alcohol on the heart in the preclinical stage, before the development of overt heart disease. One means of accomplishing this may be the earlier diagnosis of alcoholism by the use of screening tests.[336] By echocardiography, 68% of chronic alcoholics without cardiac symptoms were found to have one or more of the following significant abnormalities: increased left ventricular mass, increased left ventricular dimensions, increased septal and left ventricular wall thickness, and increased left atrial dimension.[332] ECG in alcoholics who did not have overt cardiovascular disease was abnormal in 42.8% of cases studied.[337] The most frequent finding was a prolonged Q-T_c interval. Cardiomegaly was found on the chest radiograph in only 17.2%.

Treatment. Of utmost importance is perpetual abstinence from use of alcohol. Severe restriction of activities during the stage of decompensation is another essential part of treatment. Salt restriction and diuretics are used during the phase of congestive cardiopathy. Vasodilators, diuretics, and digitalis glycosides may be used as indicated for circulatory failure. Patients should receive a balanced diet, and any deficiencies should be corrected. Attention must be paid to electrolyte disturbances, including hypokalemia and hypomagnesemia. Arrhythmias are treated in the usual fashion. Inasmuch as thromboembolism is a significant risk in patients with severe chronic congestive cardiomyopathy, anticoagulant therapy is recommended for compliant patients.

Prognosis. Among patients with chronic circulatory failure who continue to use alcohol, the prognosis is poor, with a 3-year survival rate as low as 20%.[326] However, several reports document the reversibility of alcoholic cardiomyopathy in some cases.[338-340] Demakis et al.[326] found two factors to be associated with a favorable course: a short duration of symptoms before the initiation of therapy and abstention from alcohol. Of 15 patients who improved, 73% had abstained from alcohol. Unfortunately, more than 20% of patients who allegedly abstained continued to have a deteriorating course; this suggests that at some point the process becomes relentless and irreversible. In another study of 10 patients with alcoholic cardiomyopathy who abstained from alcohol throughout most of the follow-up period, there was a significantly more favorable prognosis than that in patients with nonalcoholic congestive cardiomyopathy.[340] Left ventricular function also has prognostic significance. Sudden unexpected death may occur in alcoholics.[341-346]

Since alcoholic cardiomyopathy is potentially reversible with abstinence, great emphasis should be placed on efforts to detect alcoholism and alcohol abuse and to rehabilitate the patient.

Tachycardia-induced cardiomyopathy

Sustained tachycardia itself has been suspected to predispose to the development of a dilated cardiomyopathy with congestive heart failure. Although the earliest observations were in patients with sustained atrial fibrillation, subsequent studies have demonstrated that other forms of incessant tachycardia may produce cardiac enlargement and circulatory failure.[347-350] In some patients, systolic dysfunction improves after correction of the tachycardia.[95,347-351] Depletion of intracellular energy stores may contribute to this form of cardiomyopathy.[352] The ability to use tachycardia to induce left ventricular dysfunction has provided a useful animal model of congestive heart failure.[352-354]

Cardiac toxicity due to drugs

Only a few of the many potential cardiotoxins have been shown to result in clinical heart disease. These are the antineoplastic agents, mood-altering drugs, anti-infective agents, antihypertensive drugs, and vaccines.

Some of these offenders have a direct toxic effect on the myocardium or the vasculature of the heart, or they may disturb primarily the functions of impulse formation and conduction. Some of them affect the heart indirectly by altering autonomic regulation of the heart. Disorders that are characterized by a direct toxic myocardial effect tend to reflect the intensity and duration of exposure.

In addition to agents that exert direct toxicity, there are drugs that have the potential to induce a generalized hypersensitivity reaction; the heart may become a target organ in such reactions and suffer significant inflammatory injury. The heart is caught up in a more generalized hypersensitivity reaction to a drug; an example of this is methyldopa.

In some instances, it is suspected that the interacion between environmental insults and host response results in cardiac toxicity. The multiplicity of potential insults, variable latent periods, and nonspecificity of cardiac responses all add to the difficulty of developing precise information about the pathogenesis of these diseases.

Antineoplastic drugs

DOXORUBICIN. Although the anthracycline drug doxorubicin (Adriamycin) is a valuable anticancer compound, its use is limited by its cardiac toxicity. A congestive cardiomyopathy may result at high doses, particularly if certain risk factors are present. Inasmuch as this cardiomyopathy is predictable, it may serve as a model of toxic cardiomyopathy and thereby have implications for pathogenesis, natural history, treatment, and prevention.

Pathology. Gross cardiac pathologic findings of doxorubicin toxicity are similar to those of other dilated cardiomyopathies.[355] Histologically, there is degeneration of myocytes with a loss of numbers of myocytes, interstitial edema, and, at certain stages, fibrosis (Fig 19A-11). Electron microscopy reveals vacuolated myocytes and dilated mitochondria. Lesions are disseminated mainly in the left ventricular free wall and the interventricular septum; the earliest lesions tend to occur in the subendocardium and ventricular trabeculae. Inflammatory infiltrates are not a feature of chronic anthracycline cardiotoxicity. A grading system has been devised to describe the extent of cell damage and the proportion of cells affected.[356] The cause of this myocardial injury has

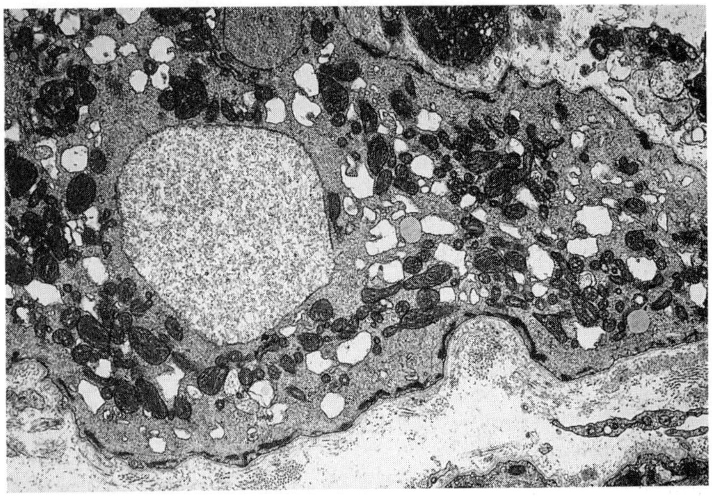

Fig 19A-11 Doxorubicin cardiomyopathy. Note vacuolization and myofibrillar degeneration. (Courtesy of William D. Edwards, M.D.)

not been proved but could be related to toxic metabolites of doxorubicin or free radical damage.[357,358]

Clinical Aspects. An acute cardiac effect, as judged by ECG changes, is seen in as many as 41% of patients receiving doxorubicin.[359] The most frequent change is nonspecific ST-T wave abnormalities; less common are sinus tachycardia, premature atrial and ventricular contractions, other cardiac arrhythmias, and low-voltage QRS complexes. With the possible exception of decreased QRS voltage, ECG abnormalities are reversible, do not correlate with the development of cardiomyopathy, and taken alone are not generally considered indications for discontinuation of treatment. In addition to acute effects, manifested primarily as ECG abnormalities, subacute effects of transient left ventricular dysfunction and a pericarditis-myocarditis syndrome may occur, but these are infrequently seen and are rarely of clinical importance.

Chronic cardiotoxicity of some degree will eventually develop in most patients given anthracyclines.[360] Several months pass before the full cytotoxic effect of a dose develops. Thus, if heart failure develops during the course of treatment, it will be several more weeks before the maximum degree of toxicity is seen. Therefore, patients in whom heart failure develops several months after the last dose can be expected to have a milder illness. At an early stage of the disease, either right or left ventricular dysfunction may predominate; in more advanced disease, there is biventricular failure with a low cardiac output and the usual clinical manifestations of congestive cardiomyopathy. Cardiomyopathy may occasionally be of a restrictive type with a normal heart size. This is particularly true if there was previous radiation-induced cardiac damage. With the development of cardiomyopathy, a mortality of up to 61% has been reported,[361] although the course may be more favorable in children.[362] Sudden cardiac death has been reported.[363] In some cases, cardiac toxicity is not manifest until years after therapy.[364]

Several factors have been identified which place patients at increased risk of doxorubicin toxicity. These are prior radiation therapy,[365] administration of cyclophosphamide,[365] old age,[360] and preexisting heart disease.

For treatment, patients should have rest and receive diuretics. Digitalis and vasodilators may be of benefit to some patients. Anticoagulant therapy is advised if left ventricular dysfunction is severe.

Efforts have been made to reduce cardiac toxicity by giving the drug on a weekly schedule,[360] and data suggest that administration by continuous infusion is less cardiotoxic than bolus injection.[366] A randomized trial has demonstrated a protective effect of the bispiperazinedione ICRF-187 when administered with doxorubicin.[368]

Several approaches have been taken for the early detection of cardiac toxicity before clinical manifestations. Decreased QRS voltage may appear with the onset of congestive heart failure but has not been useful in predicting clinical disease. Several investigators have determined the radionuclide ejection fraction at rest and, when feasible, with exercise,[369] and to date this appears to be a good, widely available noninvasive means of measuring cardiac performance.

Bristow et al.[356] described the dose effect and structure-function relationships in doxorubicin cardiomyopathy on the basis of which a strategy can be developed for cardiac monitoring in patients who receive anthracyclines. Patients are stratified for the presence or absence of risk factors. Those at low risk (young, no radiation, no heart disease, no increased potential for heart disease, including insulin-dependent diabetes) may be given cumulative doses of doxorubicin up to 450 mg/m^2. If higher doses are considered, the radionuclide ejection fraction, at rest and with exercise if feasible, should be determined before each additional 100 mg/m^2 is given. Patients who are at increased risk should undergo baseline ejection fraction measurement before treatment, after 350 mg/m^2 has been reached, and thereafter before every additional dose of 100 mg/m^2. An ejection fraction of less than 45% at rest, deterioration of more than 5% from baseline to a value less than 50% at rest, or failure to increase by at least 5% with exercise calls for discontinuation of the drug. However, if more doxorubicin is needed, right heart catheterization and endomyocardial biopsy should be performed at medical centers that are experienced in this technique and in histologic interpretation. On the basis of this information, a risk-benefit ratio can be estimated and a decision made whether to administer more of the drug. Routine monitoring of cardiac function can significantly reduce the incidence of congestive heart failure in these patients.[369]

DAUNOMYCIN. An anthracycline, daunomycin is used in the treatment of leukemia. It is similar to doxorubicin in that ECG abnormalities are common but are seldom clinically significant, but cardiomyopathy that is dose-related is a serious complication.[370] A mortality of 79% has been reported in patients with cardiomyopathy. A cumulative total dose of 600 mg/m^2 resulted in a 1.5% incidence of congestive heart failure, and a dose of 1,000 mg/m^2 resulted in an incidence of 12%.

The clinical presentation and management are the same as those for doxorubicin.

CYCLOPHOSPHAMIDES. Cyclophosphamides are alkylating agents. They may be used in massive doses in preparing patients for bone marrow transplantation. A retrospective analysis of 80 patients suggests that those receiving more than 6.2 g/m^2 have a greatly increased risk of fatal cardiotoxicity.[371] In a series of 32 patients who received 180 mg/kg over 4 days, left ventricular systolic function, as determined by echocardiogram, decreased substantially 5 to 16 days after the start of therapy.[372] Pericardial effusion was seen in 33% of patients, and ECG voltage decreased with or without pericardial effusion. Congestive heart failure was found in 28% of patients within 3 weeks of treatment, and 19% of patients died in heart failure. Pericardial tamponade occurred in 19%. Autopsy showed endothelial injury and hemorrhagic myopericarditis. Survivors of the toxic cardiomyopathy had a gradual recovery with a normal ECG and echocardiogram.

Antiparasitic drugs

EMETINE AND DEHYDROEMETINE. Emetine and dehydroemetine are used in the treatment of amebiasis and schistosomiasis. Emetine is also the principal component of ipecac, an emetic compound subject to abuse by some bulimic patients.[373] Emetine is believed to inhibit oxidative phosphorylation and thereby cause reversible damage to the mitochondria.[374] Myocardial lesions consisting of focal myocytolysis with interstitial and focal perivascular infiltration of lymphocytes have been seen in autopsies and in experimental animals.

ECG changes appear to be dose related and are almost always seen after a week of emetine therapy, or they may appear after completion of therapy.[375] T-wave abnormalities and Q-T prolongation are most often observed, and ventricular fibrillation has been seen. The T waves may gradually regress over a period of 1 or 2 months after drug therapy. Despite frequent ECG abnormalities, clinical evidence of myocardial disease is not common.[375] There may be elevations of the cardiac enzymes, and gallop rhythms may be audible. Adults seem to be more susceptible to toxicity than are children. Dehydroemetine is associated with similar ECG abnormalities, but they are generally less extensive and prolonged. Patients who are receiving parenteral treatment are more susceptible than those on oral administration.

Treatment consists of discontinuation of emetine or dehydroemetine therapy and bed rest. Administration of potassium under careful monitoring may be considered.

CHLOROQUINE. Chloroquine compounds are used in the prophylaxis and treatment of several parasitic diseases and for management of rheumatoid arthritis and systemic lupus erythematosus. Their cardiac toxicity is attributed to inhibition of cellular respiration by blocking of the Krebs cycle. Ultrastructural study reveals accumulation of lamellar bodies within myocytes (Fig 19A-12), a morphologic change suggesting that chloroquine toxicity is a drug-induced lipidosis.[376] ECG changes often occur and consist of T-wave abnormalities, ST-segment depression, and prolongation of the Q-T interval.

The diagnosis may be confirmed by endomyocardial biopsy.[376] Chloroquine has myocardial depressant action in large doses, but this is seldom apparent clinically. Toxicity from large doses of chloroquine has resulted in reduced cardiac output, bradycardia, arrhythmias, heart block, and death. Aggressive treatment of overdoses with mechanical ventilation, diazepam, and epinephrine may improve outcome.[377]

ANTIMONY. Sodium antimony tartrate and antimony dimercaptosuccinate have been used to treat schistosomiasis. Both drugs have a high incidence of associated ECG abnormalities, especially antimony tartrate.[378,379] Changes consist of abnormal T waves and prolonged Q-T interval. These changes disappear a few weeks after the conclusion of therapy.

Psychotropic drugs

PHENOTHIAZINES. Three commonly used mood-altering phenothiazine drugs are thioridazine (Mellaril), chlorpromazine (Thorazine), and trifluoperazine (Stelazine). Adverse cardiovascular effects include nonspecific ECG changes, abnormalities of conduction, myocardial irritability, hypotension, and cardiomyopathy.[380]

An estimated 50% to 70% of patients receiving long-term high-dose therapy have ECG changes. These include ST-segment depression, prolongation of the Q-T interval, T-wave inversion, appearance of U waves or increased U-wave amplitude, AV blocks, and ventricular irritability including ventricular fibrillation.[381] An increased incidence of sudden death in patients taking phenothiazines has been reported. These drugs have a quinidine-like effect; therefore, quinidine and procainamide are not advisable for treatment. Arrhythmias generally clear within 48 hours after discontinuation of the use of phenothiazines. Temporary cardiac pacing or administration of magnesium may shorten the Q-T interval and suppress ventricular arrhythmias.

Hypotension is a common side effect of phenothiazines and may be attributed either to an indirect effect due to depression of medullary vasopressor reflexes or to a direct effect on the heart and blood vessels because of α-adrenoceptor blocking properties. Hypotension is generally mild during oral administration but may be severe with parenteral administration. Hypotension may be treated with levarterenol or phenylephrine. Epinephrine may further lower the blood pressure and is therefore contraindicated.

A toxic cardiomyopathy due to phenothiazines has been reported.[382,383]

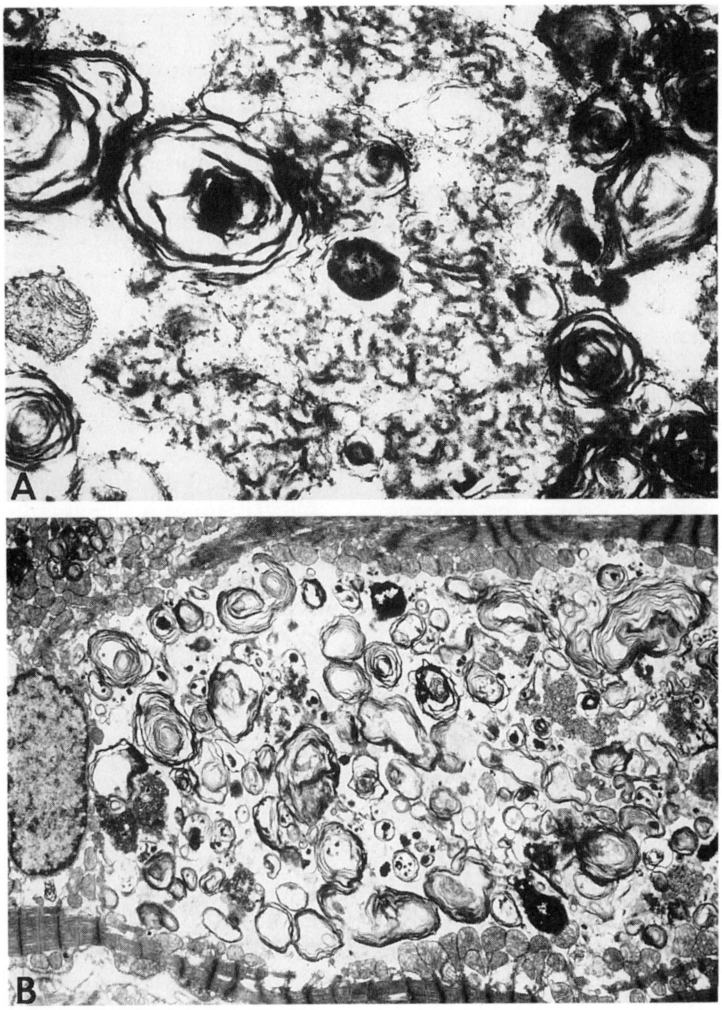

Fig 19A-12 Electron microscopic views of lamellar bodies characteristic of chloroquine toxicity. Original magnification: **A,** ×60,000; **B,** ×10,000.

TRICYCLIC ANTIDEPRESSANTS. ECG abnormalities have been reported in 20% of patients taking tricyclic antidepressant agents at therapeutic doses. Abnormalities include prolongation of the Q-T interval, ST-segment depression, T-wave abnormalities, intraventricular conduction defects, and AV conduction blocks.[384] Arrhythmias may be serious with overdosage, and they may persist several days because of the long half-life of the drugs and their affinity for cardiac tissue[385] and thus add to the difficulty of treatment.[386] In high doses, tricyclic antidepressants depress myocardial contractility, heart rate, and coronary blood flow. They may cause toxicity by direct myocardial depression, by their effect on adrenergic responses, or by anticholinergic activity. These arrhythmias should be treated with lidocaine, and hypotension should be treated with norepinephrine or dopamine.[386,387] Tricyclic antidepressants should be used with caution in patients with organic heart disease;[388] doxepin and maprotiline have been suggested by some investigators as preferable when one of these drugs is required.[389] Nevertheless, used in moderate dosage and with appropriate monitoring, tricyclic antidepressants cause relatively few side effects in cardiac patients.[390,391]

LITHIUM. ECG abnormalities are common in patients taking lithium at therapeutic levels. T-wave abnormalities are reported in 20% to 30% of patients. These generally revert to normal after lithium therapy is stopped and are thought to be benign.[392] Sinus node dysfunction or sinoatrial block has also been seen in patients taking therapeutic doses of lithium.[393] Ventricular irritability has been reported; it cleared on discontinuation of therapy and reappeared when therapy was reinstituted.[394] Myocardial irritability and ECG changes may be due to intracellular influx of lithium and its replacement of potassium. Exercise testing reveals no evidence of impairment of cardiovascular performance.[395] Myocarditis and heart failure have been reported in association with lithium therapy,[396,397] but these findings are controversial.[398,399]

Methysergide. Methysergide is an agonist of serotonin used primarily in the prevention of migraine headache. It can cause retroperitoneal, pleuropulmonary, and endocardial fibrosis. Its effect on the heart is somewhat similar to that in the carcinoid syndrome, but, in contrast with carcinoid syndrome, which largely affects the right side of the heart, methysergide affects primarily the left side.[400] Congestive heart failure, murmurs, and other findings of valvular stenosis and insufficiency have been reported, but fortunately they regressed when use of the drug was discontinued. Surgical therapy has been required for valvular lesions. Coronary ostial stenosis has been reported.[401] For the prevention of this complication, it is recommended that doses of more than 8 mg per day be avoided and that therapy be interrupted periodically.

Cocaine. Cocaine abuse has been associated with myocardial infarction (see chapter 30A), ventricular arrhythmias, myocarditis, and sudden death.[402] These cardiac events have been observed after intravenous and intranasal administration and may occur in the apparent absence of preexisting cardiac disease.[402,403] The mechanism is unknown but could be related to the intense sympathomimetic stimulation that occurs with cocaine use.

Hypersensitivity myocarditis. The myocardium may be damaged by hypersensitivity reactions. Clinical contexts include anaphylactic reactions, serum sickness, and reactions to vaccines and a number of drugs used therapeutically. For the most part, information on the incriminated drugs has appeared in case reports; however, hypersensitivity to the sulfonamides[404,406] and methyldopa[407-409] is well documented.

Histologically, the myocarditis of hypersensitivity is characterized by interstitial inflammatory infiltrate containing many eosinophils[410] (Fig 19A-13). In addition, foci of myocytolysis with sparse muscle cell necrosis, perivascular infiltrates, and absence of myocardial fibrosis or regeneration may be seen. The inflammatory lesions may be diffuse or focal in the myocardium.[409,411] These abnormalities are comparable to the lesions seen with delayed hypersensitivity drug reactions,[412] and it is suggested that these reactions may be similar to allergic reactions to penicillin, which are mediated immunologically. Fenoglio et al.[409] reported on autopsies of 24 patients with hypersensitivity myocarditis. Thirty-three percent of them were taking methyldopa, and some of these were also taking hydrochlorothiazide. Sulfonamides were taken by 21% and penicillin or ampicillin, by 17%. Hypersensitivity myocarditis was the presumed cause of death in 20 of 24 patients; the vast majority of deaths were sudden deaths, presumably from an arrhythmia.

Clinical criteria for drug hypersensitivity have been stated[405] and are as follows: (1) previous use of the drug without incident; (2) lack of relationship to dosage; (3) a reaction that is neither a pharmacologic nor a toxic effect of the drug: (4) classic allergic symptoms, symptoms of serum sickness, or a syndrome suggesting infectious disease; (5) immunologic confirmation; and (6) persistence of symptoms until the drug is withdrawn. The time from the initiation of drug therapy to symptoms or death is highly variable.

Symptoms have included dyspnea, chest pain, hypotension, syncope, and pain resembling that in myocardial infarction. Pericardial involvement with characteristic pain is sometimes associated. Palpitations or other indications of arrhythmias may be found. Examination may reveal tachycardia, fever, hypotension, and findings of biventricular heart failure or arrhythmias.

The ECG is frequently abnormal, with tachycardia or bradycardia, repolarization abnormalities, and conduction disturbances. There may be pathologic Q waves suggesting myocardial infarction. ECG observations may change often and abnormalities may correct themselves during clinical improvement.[406,409] Borderline increases in the levels of serum aspartate aminotransferase and lactic dehydrogenase may occur, consistent with myocarditis. The finding of jaundice or other evidence of hepatitis should raise one's suspicion. The observation that this process is uniformly found throughout the myocardium suggests that myocardial biopsy may be useful in making an early diagnosis.

When hypersensitivity myocarditis is suspected, use of the drug or drugs should be stopped immediately; myocardial biopsy should be considered. Corticosteroid therapy may be employed.[406]

Table 19A-8 lists drugs reported to cause hypersensitivity myocarditis, with comments.

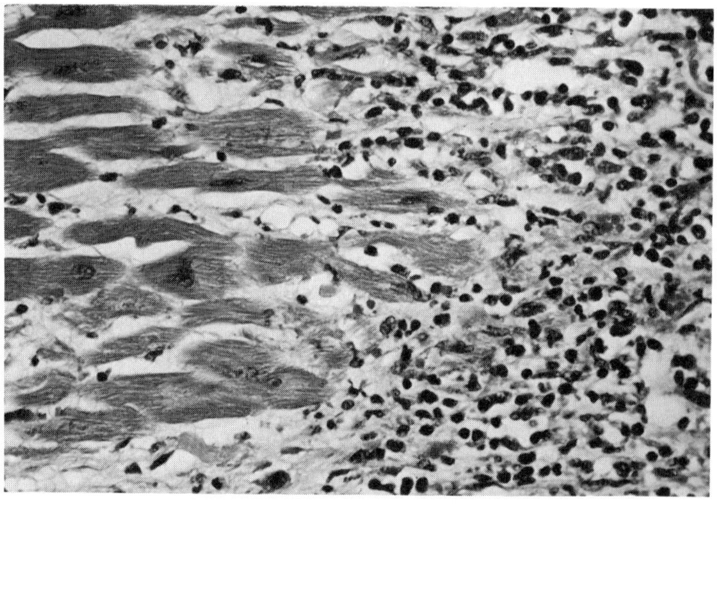

Fig 19A-13 Hypersensitivity myocarditis. Focal myocardial necrosis and inflammatory reaction. Mononuclear cells are most numerous, but many eosinophils also are present. (Courtesy of William D. Edwards, M.D.)

Table 19A-8 Hypersensitivity myocarditis

Drug	Symptoms	Mode of death	Pathology	References
Methyldopa	Shortness of breath, malaise, headache, fever, cerebrovascular accident	Sudden	Myocarditis, vasculitis, hepatitis	407-409
Sulfonamides (sulfadiazine, sulfisoxazole, sulfamethoxypyridazine, carbutamide)	Fever, shortness of breath	Sudden	Myocarditis, petechial hemorrhages, vasculitis, granulomas	406, 409
Penicillin, ampicillin	Rash, congestive heart failure	Sudden	Myocarditis, granulomas, pericarditis, myocardial infarction	409, 413
Phenylbutazone	Shortness of breath, fever, rash, chest pain, hypotension	Sudden	Myocarditis, hepatitis, myocardial giant cells, perivascular granulomas, fibrinoid degeneration, pericarditis	409, 414
Oxyphenbutazone	Congestive heart failure	Sudden	Myocarditis	409
Chlortetracycline	Fever, tachycardia		Interstitial and perivascular infiltrates	415
Chloramphenicol		Sudden	Myocarditis, hepatitis	409
Streptomycin	Chest pain, fever, rash	Sudden	Myocarditis, petechial hemorrhage, pericardial effusion	416
p-Aminosalicylic acid	Heart failure, hypotension, ventricular irritability			417
Phenytoin	Epistaxis	Sudden	Myocarditis	409, 410
Carbamazepine	Jaundice, fever, rash	Sudden	Myocarditis	409
Indomethacin	Cardiac arrest, fever	Brain damage	Myocarditis	409
Spironolactone with hydrochlorothiazide	Low back pain, fever	Sudden	Myocarditis	
Acetazolamide	Fever, rash	Uremia	Myocarditis, hepatitis	409
Amitriptyline		Sudden	Myocarditis	409
Phenindione			Myocarditis	409
Interleukin-2	Congestive heart failure; may occur within days of initiation of therapy		Myocarditis	418, 419

Table 19A-9 Cardiac toxicity due to chemicals

Chemical	Signs and symptoms	Mode of cardiac death	Cardiac pathology	References
Hydrocarbons	Congestive heart failure, arrhythmias, CNS depression, hepatic injury, dermatitis	Congestive heart failure, sudden	Myocytolysis	420-423
Carbon monoxide	Arrhythmias, angina	Congestive heart failure, sudden	Subendocardial infarction	424-427
Arsenic	Dyspnea, congestive heart failure, ECG changes of ischemia; chronic GI, CNS, hematologic, renal toxicity; arsine gas inhalation may be rapidly fatal	Congestive heart failure	Focal myocardial hemorrhages, pericardial effusion; arsine gas may cause myocardial necrosis	428, 429

CNS, central nervous system; GI, gastrointestinal.

Continued.

Table 19A-9 Cardiac toxicity due to chemicals—cont'd

Chemical	Signs and symptoms	Mode of cardiac death	Cardiac pathology	References
Lead	Chest pain, dyspnea, conduction system abnormalities, CNS and GI symptoms	Congestive heart failure	Myocardial inflammation and fibrosis	430, 431
Phosphorus	Pulmonary edema, arrhythmias	Congestive heart failure	Myocyte necrosis	432
Mercury	ST-T changes, QT prolongation			433
Cobalt	Congestive heart failure, arrhythmias	Congestive heart failure, sudden	Dilated cardiomyopathy	434, 435
Thallium	Cardiac and pulmonary toxicity, tachycardia, abdominal pain, ataxia, coma, alopecia, neuropathy	Death usually not attributable primarily to cardiac disturbance	Myocardial edema and inflammation	435

Table 19A-10 Cardiac toxicity due to physical agents

Agent	Signs and symptoms	Mode of cardiac death	Cardiac pathology	References
Radiation	Acute pericarditis, pericardial effusion, ventricular failure; late constrictive pericarditis, coronary disease, restrictive myocardial disease	Acute pericardial disease or congestive heart failure; late constriction, restriction, myocardial infarction	Pericarditis, myocytolysis, fibrosis, coronary disease	436-440
Heatstroke	ECG shows sinus tachycardia, ST-T changes, QT prolongation; central nervous system manifestations	Shock	Myocardial hemorrhage, right ventricular dilatation	441, 442
Hypothermia	ECG, ST-segment changes	Shock	Myocardial hemorrhage, chamber dilatation	443, 444

Table 19A-11 Cardiac toxicity due to bites and stings

Agent	Signs and symptoms	Mode of cardiac death	Cardiac pathology	Therapy	References
Scorpion venom	Tachycardia, mydriasis, sweating, pulmonary edema, priapism, ECG ST changes and conduction disturbances, neurotoxic symptoms	Sudden	Myocarditis, myocyte necrosis	? adrenergic blocking agents	445-447
Snake venom	ECG ST changes and QRS prolongation, dyspnea	Myocardial infarction, shock	Myocyte necrosis	Antivenom	448-451
Black widow spider venom	Arrhythmias, labile blood pressure	Shock		? β-blockers	452
Wasp venom	Cyanosis, pulmonary edema, chest pain	Shock	Myocardial hemorrhage		453
Tick paralysis	Congestive heart failure	Congestive heart failure	Cardiac dilatation		454

Other causes of cardiac toxicity

See Tables 19A-9, 19A-10, and 19A-11 for toxicities due to chemicals, physical agents, and bites and stings, respectively.

REFERENCES

1. Brandenburg RO, Chazov E, Cherian G, et al: Report of the WHO/ISFC Task Force on definition and classification of cardiomyopathies. *Circulation* 64:437A-438A, 1981
2. Torp A: Incidence of congestive cardiomyopathy. In *Congestive Cardiomyopathy.* Edited by JF Goodwin, Å Hjalmarson, EGJ Olsen. Mölndal, Sweden, AB Hässle, 1981, pp 18-22
3. Torp A: Incidence of congestive cardiomyopathy. *Postgrad Med J* 54:435-437, 1978
4. Codd MB, Sugrue DD, Gersh BJ, et al: Epidemiology of idiopathic dilated and hypertrophic cardiomyopathy: a population-based study in Olmsted County, Minnesota, 1975-1984. *Circulation* 80:564-572, 1989
5. Hamby RI: Primary myocardial disease: a prospective clinical and hemodynamic evaluation in 100 patients. *Medicine (Baltimore)* 49:55-78, 1970
6. Coughlin SS, Szklo M, Baughman K, et al: The epidemiology of idiopathic dilated cardiomyopathy in a biracial community. *Am J Epidemiol* 131:48-56, 1990
7. Johnson RA, Palacios I: Dilated cardiomyopathies of the adult. *N Engl J Med* 307:1051-1058; 1119-1126, 1982
8. Olsen EGJ: Pathology of congestive cardiomyopathy. In *Congestive Cardiomyopathy.* Edited by JF Goodwin, Å Hjalmarson, EGJ Olsen, Mölndal, Sweden, AB Hässle, 1981, pp 66-74
9. Roberts WC, Ferrans VJ: Pathologic anatomy of the cardiomyopathies: idiopathic dilated and hypertrophic types, infiltrative types, and endomyocardial disease with and without eosinophilia. *Hum Pathol* 6:287-342, 1975
10. Benjamin IJ, Schuster EH, Bulkley BH: Cardiac hypertrophy in idiopathic dilated congestive cardiomyopathy: a clinicopathologic study. *Circulation* 64:442-447, 1981
11. Schaper J, Froede R, Hein S, et al: Impairment of the myocardial ultrastructure and changes of the cytoskeleton in dilated cardiomyopathy. *Circulation* 83:504-514, 1991
12. Olsen EGJ: Pathological recognition of cardiomyopathy. *Postgrad Med J* 51:277-281, 1975
13. Schrader WH, Pankey GA, Davis RB, et al: Familial idiopathic cardiomegaly. *Circulation* 24:599-606, 1961
14. Olsen EGJ: Postmortem findings and histologic, histochemical, and electron microscopic findings of myocardial biopsies. In *Cardiomyopathy and Myocardial Biopsy.* Edited by M Kaltenbach, F Loogen, EGJ Olsen. Berlin, Springer-Verlag, 1978, pp 52-61
15. Rutenberg HL, Spann JF Jr: Alterations of cardiac sympathetic neurotransmitter activity in congestive heart failure. *Am J Cardiol* 32:472-480, 1973
16. Maron BJ, Ferrans VJ, Roberts WC: Ultrastructural features of degenerated cardiac muscle cells in patients with cardiac hypertrophy. *Am J Pathol* 79:387-434, 1975
17. Roberts WC, Ferrans VJ: Morphologic observations in the cardiomyopathies. In *Myocardial Disease.* Edited by NO Fowler. New York, Grune & Stratton, 1973, p 59
18. Goldstein MA: Nuclear pores in ventricular muscle cells from adult hypertrophied hearts. *J Mol Cell Cardiol* 6:227-235, 1974
19. Hartz AJ, Anderson AJ, Brooks HL, et al: The association of smoking with cardiomyopathy. *N Engl J Med* 311:1201-1206, 1984
20. Michels VV, Moll PP, Miller FA, et al: The frequency of familial dilated cardiomyopathy in a series of patients with idiopathic dilated cardiomyopathy. *N Engl J Med* 326:77-82, 1992
21. O'Connell JB: Evidence linking myocarditis to dilated cardiomyopathy in humans. In *Myocarditis: Precursor of Cardiomyopathy.* Edited by JA Robinson, JB O'Connell. Lexington, Massachusetts, The Collamore Press, 1983, pp 93-108
22. Abelmann WH, Miklozek CL, Modlin JF: The role of viruses in the etiology of congestive cardiomyopathy. In *Congestive Cardiomyopathy.* Edited by JF Goodwin, Å Hjalmarson, EGJ Olsen. Mölndal, Sweden, AB Hässle, 1981, pp 76-84
23. Das SK, Slein LD, Reynolds RT, et al: Immunologic studies in cardiomyopathy and pathophysiologic implications. In *Congestive Cardiomyopathy.* Edited by JF Goodwin, Å Hjalmarson, EGJ Olsen. Mölndal, Sweden, AB Hässle, 1981, pp 87-93
24. Anderson JL, Carlquist JF, Hammond EH: Deficient natural killer cell activity in patients with idiopathic dilated cardiomyopathy. *Lancet* 2:1124-1127, 1982
25. Woodruff JF: Viral myocarditis: a review. *Am J Pathol* 101:427-484, 1980
26. Matsumori A, Kawai C: An animal model of congestive (dilated) cardiomyopathy: dilatation and hypertrophy of the heart in the chronic stage in DBA/2 mice with myocarditis caused by encephalo-myocarditis virus. *Circulation* 66:355-360, 1982
27. Reyes MP, Ho K-L, Smith F, et al: A mouse model of dilated-type cardiomyopathy due to Coxsackievirus B3. *J Infect Dis* 144:232-236, 1981
28. Archard LC, Bowles NE, Cunningham L, et al: Molecular probes for detection of persisting enterovirus infection of human heart and their prognostic value. *Eur Heart J* 12 Suppl D:56-59, 1991
29. Jin O, Sole MJ, Butany JW, et al: Detection of enterovirus RNA in myocardial biopsies from patients with myocarditis and cardiomyopathy using gene amplification by polymerase chain reaction. *Circulation* 82:8-16, 1990
30. Ross RS, Chien KR: Of molecules and myocardium: PCR diagnosis of viral myocarditis in cardiac biopsies. *Circulation* 82:294-295, 1990
31. Tracy S, Wiegand V, McManus B, et al: Molecular approaches to enteroviral diagnosis in idiopathic cardiomyopathy and myocarditis. *J Am Coll Cardiol* 15:1688-1694, 1990
32. Eckstein R, Mempel W, Bolte H-D: Reduced suppressor cell activity in congestive cardiomyopathy and in myocarditis. *Circulation* 65:1224-1229, 1982
33. Anderson JL, Carlquist JF, Higashikuba R: Quantitation of lymphocyte subsets by immunofluorescence flow cytometry in idiopathic dilated cardiomyopathy. *Am J Cardiol* 55:1550-1554, 1985
34. Fowles RE, Bieber CP, Stinson EB: Defective in vitro suppressor cell function in idiopathic congestive cardiomyopathy. *Circulation* 59:483-491, 1979
35. Anderson JL, Carlquist JF, Hammond EH: Deficient natural killer cell activity in patients with idiopathic dilated cardiomyopathy. *Lancet* 2:1124-1127, 1982
36. Ansari AA, Wang YC, Danner DJ, et al: Abnormal expression of histocompatibility and mitochondrial antigens by cardiac tissue from patients with myocarditis and dilated cardiomyopathy. *Am J Pathol* 139:337-354, 1991
37. Caforio ALP, Bonifacio E, Stewart JT, et al: Novel organ-specific circulating cardiac autoantibodies in dilated cardiomyopathy. *J Am Coll Cardiol* 15:1527-1534, 1990
38. Goodwin JF: New serologic marker of cardiac autoimmunity in dilated cardiomyopathy. *J Am Coll Cardiol* 15:1535-1536, 1990
39. Magnusson Y, Marullo S, Hoyer S, et al: Mapping of a functional autoimmune epitope on the β_1-adrenergic receptor in patients with idiopathic dilated cardiomyopathy. *J Clin Invest* 86:1658-1663, 1990
40. Limas CJ, Limas C: Beta-adrenoceptor antibodies and genetics in dilated cardiomyopathy—an overview and review. *Eur Heart J* 12 Suppl D:175-177, 1991
41. Bristow MR, Anderson FL, Port D, et al: Differences in β-adrenergic neuroeffector mechanisms in ischemic versus idiopathic dilated cardiomyopathy. *Circulation* 84:1024-1039, 1991
42. Factor SM, Sonnenblick EH: Hypothesis: is congestive cardiomyopathy caused by a hyperreactive myocardial microcirculation (microvascular spasm)? *Am J Cardiol* 50:1149-1152, 1982
43. Treasure CB, Vita JA, Cox DA, et al: Endothelium-dependent dilation of the coronary microvasculature is impaired in dilated cardiomyopathy. *Circulation* 81:772-779, 1990
44. Dargie H, Amorin DS, Goodwin JF, et al: Sympathetic function in congestive cardiomyopathy. In *Congestive Cardiomyopathy.* Edited by JF Goodwin, Å Hjalmarson, EGJ Olsen. Mölndal, Sweden, AB Hässle, 1981, pp 166-170
45. Waldenström A, Hjalmarson Å: Biochemical basis for heart failure induced by catecholamines. In *Congestive Cardiomyopathy.* Edited by JF Goodwin, Å Hjalmarson, EGJ Olsen. Mölndal, Sweden, AB Hässle, 1981, pp 145-150
46. Kawai C, Yui Y, Hoshino T, et al: Myocardial catecholamines in hypertrophic and dilated (congestive) cardiomyopathy: a biopsy study. *J Am Coll Cardiol* 2:834-840, 1983
47. Yates JC, Beamish RE, Dhalla NS: Ventricular dysfunction and

necrosis produced by adrenochrome metabolite of epinephrine: relation to pathogenesis of catecholamine cardiomyopathy. *Am Heart J* 102:210-221, 1981

48. Amorin DS, Dargie HJ, Olsen EGJ, et al: Autonomic function in cardiomyopathies: heart rate and blood pressure responses. In *Congestive Cardiomyopathy.* Edited by JF Goodwin, Å Hjalmarson, EGJ Olsen. Mölndal, Sweden, AB Hässle, 1981, pp 174-191

49. Amorin DS, Dargie HJ, Heer K, et al: Is there autonomic impairment in congestive (dilated) cardiomyopathy? *Lancet* 1:525-527, 1981

50. Shirey EK, Proudfit WL, Hawk WA: Primary myocardial disease: correlation with clinical findings, angiographic and biopsy diagnosis; follow-up of 139 patients. *Am Heart J* 99:198-207, 1980

51. Hatle L, Örjavik O, Storstein O: Chronic myocardial disease. I. Clinical picture related to long-term prognosis. *Acta Med Scand* 199:399-405, 1976

52. Fuster V, Gersh BJ, Giuliani ER, et al: The natural history of idiopathic dilated cardiomyopathy. *Am J Cardiol* 47:525-531, 1981

53. Gau GT, Goodwin JF, Oakley CM, et al: Q waves and coronary arteriography in cardiomyopathy. *Br Heart J* 34:1034-1041, 1972

54. Mann B, Ray R, Goldberger AL, et al: Atrial fibrillation in congestive cardiomyopathy: echocardiographic and hemodynamic correlates. *Cathet Cardiovasc Diagn* 7:387-395, 1981

55. Huang SK, Messer JV, Denes P: Significance of ventricular tachycardia in idiopathic dilated cardiomyopathy: observations in 35 patients. *Am J Cardiol* 51:507-512, 1983

56. Holmes J, Kubo SH, Cody RJ, et al: Arrhythmias in ischemic and nonischemic dilated cardiomyopathy: prediction of mortality by ambulatory electrocardiography. *Am J Cardiol* 55:146-151, 1985

57. Meinertz T, Hofmann T, Kasper W, et al: Significance of ventricular arrhythmias in idiopathic dilated cardiomyopathy. *Am J Cardiol* 53:902-907, 1984

58. Kuhn H, Breithardt G, Knieriem H-J, et al: Prognosis and possible presymptomatic manifestations of congestive cardiomyopathy (COCM). *Postgrad Med J* 54:451-459, 1978

59. Probst P, Pachinger O, Murad AA, et al: The H-Q time in congestive cardiomyopathies. *Am Heart J* 97:436-441, 1979

60. Saltissi S, Hockings B, Croft DN, et al: Thallium-201 myocardial imaging in patients with dilated and ischaemic cardiomyopathy. *Br Heart J* 46:290-295, 1981

61. Hatle L, Stake G, Storstein O: Chronic myocardial disease. II. Haemodynamic findings related to long-term prognosis. *Acta Med Scand* 199:407-411, 1976

62. Feild BJ, Baxley WA, Russell RO Jr, et al: Left ventricular function and hypertrophy in cardiomyopathy with depressed ejection fraction. *Circulation* 47:1022-1031, 1973

63. Nippoldt TB, Edwards WD, Holmes DR Jr, et al: Right ventricular endomyocardial biopsy: clinicopathologic correlates in 100 consecutive patients. *Mayo Clin Proc* 57:407-418, 1982

64. Mason JW: Techniques for right and left ventricular endomyocardial biopsy. *Am J Cardiol* 41:887-892, 1978

65. O'Connell JB, Subramanian R, Robinson JA, et al: Endomyocardial biopsy: techniques and applications in heart disease of unknown cause. *Heart Transplant* 3:132-144, 1984

66. Edwards WD, Holmes DR Jr, Reeder GS: Diagnosis of active lymphocytic myocarditis by endomyocardial biopsy: quantitative criteria for light microscopy. *Mayo Clin Proc* 57:419-425, 1982

67. Parrillo JE, Aretz HT, Palacios I, et al: The results of transvenous endomyocardial biopsy can frequently be used to diagnose myocardial disease in patients with idiopathic heart failure: endomyocardial biopsies in 100 consecutive patients revealed a substantial incidence of myocarditis. *Circulation* 69:93-101, 1984

68. Fenoglio JJ Jr, Ursell PC, Kellogg CF, et al: Diagnosis and classification of myocarditis by endomyocardial biopsy. *N Engl J Med* 308:12-18, 1983

69. Dec GW Jr, Palacios IF, Fallon JT, et al: Active myocarditis in the spectrum of acute dilated cardiomyopathies: clinical features, histologic correlates, and clinical outcome. *N Engl J Med* 312:885-890, 1985

70. Rahimtoola SH: The hibernating myocardium. *Am Heart J* 117:211-221, 1989

71. Braunwald E, Rutherford JD: Reversible ischemic left ventricular dysfunction: evidence for the "hibernating myocardium." *J Am Coll Cardiol* 8:1467-1470, 1986

72. Mason JW, Billingham ME, Ricci DR: Treatment of acute inflammatory myocarditis assisted by endomyocardial biopsy. *Am J Cardiol* 45:1037-1044, 1980

73. Wei-Han Y: A study of nutritional and bio-geochemical factors in the occurrence and development of Keshan disease. *Jpn Circ J* 46:1201-1207, 1982

74. Lockitch G: Selenium: clinical significance and analytical concepts. *Crit Rev Clin Lab Sci* 27:483-541, 1989

75. Johnson RA, Baker SS, Fallon JT, et al: An occidental case of cardiomyopathy and selenium deficiency. *N Engl J Med* 304:1210-1212, 1981

76. Fleming CR, Lie JT, McCall JT, et al: Selenium deficiency and fatal cardiomyopathy in a patient on home parenteral nutrition. *Gastroenterology* 83:689-693, 1982

77. Franciosa JA, Wilen M, Ziesche S, et al: Survival in men with severe chronic left ventricular failure due to either coronary heart disease or idiopathic dilated cardiomyopathy. *Am J Cardiol* 51:831-836, 1983

78. Taliercio CP, Seward JB, Driscoll DJ, et al: Idiopathic dilated cardiomyopathy in the young: clinical profile and natural history. *J Am Coll Cardiol* 6:1126 1131, 1985

79. Schwarz F, Mall G, Zebe H, et al: Determinants of survival in patients with congestive cardiomyopathy: quantitative morphologic findings and left ventricular hemodynamics. *Circulation* 70:923-928, 1984

80. Diaz RA, Obasohan A, Oakley CM: Prediction of outcome in dilated cardiomyopathy. *Br Heart J* 58:393-399, 1987

81. Ikram H, Williamson HG, Won M, et al: The course of idiopathic dilated cardiomyopathy in New Zealand. *Br Heart J* 57:521-527, 1987

82. Sugrue DD, Rodeheffer RJ, Codd MB, et al: The clinical course of idiopathic dilated cardiomyopathy: a population-based study. *Ann Intern Med* 117:117-123, 1992

83. Redfield MM, Gersh BJ, Bailey KR, et al: Natural history of idiopathic dilated cardiomyopathy: effect of referral bias and secular trend. *J Am Coll Cardiol* 22:1921-1926, 1993

84. Keogh AM, Baron DW, Hickie JB: Prognostic guides in patients with idiopathic or ischemic dilated cardiomyopathy assessed for cardiac transplantation. *Am J Cardiol* 65:903-908, 1990

85. Unverferth DV, Magorien RD, Moeschberger ML, et al: Factors influencing the one-year mortality of dilated cardiomyopathy. *Am J Cardiol* 54:147-152, 1984

86. Romeo F, Pelliccia F, Cianfrocca C, et al: Predictors of sudden death in idiopathic dilated cardiomyopathy. *Am J Cardiol* 63:138-140, 1989

87. Mancini DM, Eisen H, Kussmaul W, et al: Value of peak exercise oxygen consumption for optimal timing of cardiac transplantation in ambulatory patients with heart failure. *Circulation* 83:778-786, 1991

88. Stewart RAH, McKenna WJ, Oakley CM: Good prognosis for dilated cardiomyopathy without severe heart failure or arrhythmia. *Q J Med* 74:309-318, 1990

89. Figulla HR, Rahlf G, Nieger M, et al: Spontaneous hemodynamic improvement or stabilization and associated biopsy findings in patients with congestive cardiomyopathy. *Circulation* 71:1095-1104, 1985

90. Stroke Prevention in Atrial Fibrillation investigators: Stroke Prevention in Atrial Fibrillation Study. *Circulation* 84:527-539, 1991

91. Boston Area Anticoagulation Trial for Atrial Fibrillation Investigators: The effect of low-dose warfarin on the risk of stroke in patients with nonrheumatic atrial fibrillation. *N Engl J Med* 323:1505-1511, 1990

92. Petersen P, Boysen G, Godtfredsen J, et al: Placebo-controlled, randomised trial of warfarin and aspirin for prevention of thromboembolic complications in chronic atrial fibrillation: the Copenhagen AFASAK study. *Lancet* 1:175-179, 1989

93. Stroke Prevention in Atrial Fibrillation Investigators: Predictors of thromboembolism in atrial fibrillation: I. Clinical features of patients at risk. *Ann Intern Med* 116:1-12, 1992

94. Ezekowitz MD, Bridgers SL, James KE, et al: Warfarin in the prevention of stroke associated with nonrheumatic atrial fibrillation. *N Engl J Med* 327:1406-1412, 1992

95. Grogan M, Smith HC, Gersh BJ, et al: Left ventricular dysfunction due to atrial fibrillation in patients initially believed to have idiopathic dilated cardiomyopathy. *Am J Cardiol* 69:1570-1573, 1992

96. Chatterjee K: Amiodarone in chronic heart failure. *J Am Coll Cardiol* 14:1775-1776, 1989

97. Parrillo JE, Cunnion RE, Epstein SE, et al: A prospective, randomized, controlled trial of prednisone for dilated cardiomyopathy. *N Engl J Med* 321:1061-1068, 1989

98. Phillips HR, Levine FH, Carter JE, et al: Mitral valve replacement for isolated mitral regurgitation: analysis of clinical course and late postoperative left ventricular ejection fraction. *Am J Cardiol* 48:647-654, 1981

99. The Registry of the International Society for Heart and Lung Transplantation: Ninth official report-1992. *J Heart Lung Transplant* 11:599-606, 1992
100. Homans DC: Peripartum cardiomyopathy. *N Engl J Med* 312:1432-1437, 1985
101. Demakis JG, Rahimtoola SH, Sutton GC, et al: Natural course of peripartum cardiomyopathy. *Circulation* 44:1053-1061, 1971
102. Julian DG, Szekely P: Peripartum cardiomyopathy. *Prog Cardiovasc Dis* 27:223-240, 1985
103. Adesanya CO, Anjorin FI, Adeoshun IO, et al: Peripartum cardiac failure: a ten year follow-up study. *Trop Geogr Med* 41:190-196, 1989
104. Melvin KR, Richardson PJ, Olsen EGJ, et al: Peripartum cardiomyopathy due to myocarditis. *N Engl J Med* 307:731-734, 1982
105. Midei MG, DeMent SH, Feldman AM, et al: Peripartum myocarditis and cardiomyopathy. *Circulation* 81:922-928, 1990
106. Davis MD, Murphy JG, Olson LJ, et al: Natural history and endomyocardial biopsy findings in peripartum cardiomyopathy (abstract). *Circulation* 86 Suppl 1:439, 1992
107. St. John Sutton M, Cole P, Saltzman D, et al: Risks of cardiac dysfunction in peripartum cardiomyopathy (PPCM) with subsequent pregnancy (abstract). *Circulation* 80 Suppl 2:320, 1989
108. Marcus FI, Fontaine GH, Guiraudon G, et al: Right ventricular dysplasia: a report of 24 adult cases. *Circulation* 65:384-398, 1982
109. Rossi P, Massumi A, Gillette P, et al: Arrhythmogenic right ventricular dysplasia: clinical features, diagnostic techniques, and current management. *Am Heart J* 103:415-420, 1982
110. Nava A, Scognamiglio R, Thiene G, et al: A polymorphic form of familial arrhythmogenic right ventricular dysplasia. *Am J Cardiol* 59:1405-1409, 1987
111. Ibsen HHW, Baandrup U, Simonsen EE: Familial right ventricular dilated cardiomyopathy. *Br Heart J* 54:156-159, 1985
112. Thiene G, Nava A, Corrado D, et al: Right ventricular cardiomyopathy and sudden death in young people. *N Engl J Med* 318:129-133, 1988
113. Maron BJ: Right ventricular cardiomyopathy: another cause of sudden death in the young (editorial). *N Engl J Med* 318:178-180, 1988
114. Mestroni L, Miani D, Di Lenarda A, et al: Clinical and pathologic study of familial dilated cardiomyopathy. *Am J Cardiol* 65:1449-1453, 1990
115. Verel D, Warrack AJN, Potter CW, et al: Observations of the A2 England influenza epidemic: a clinicopathological study. *Am Heart J* 92:290-296, 1976
116. Adams CW: Postviral myopericarditis associated with the influenza virus: report of eight cases. *Am J Cardiol* 4:56-67, 1959
117. Betts RF: Syndromes of cytomegalovirus infection. *Adv Intern Med* 26:447-466, 1980
118. Wilson RSE, Morris TH, Rees JR: Cytomegalovirus myocarditis. *Br Heart J* 34:865-868, 1972
119. Hildes JA, Schaberg A, Alcock AJW: Cardiovascular collapse in acute poliomyelitis. *Circulation* 12:986-993, 1955
120. Teloh HA: Myocarditis in poliomyelitis. *Arch Pathol* 55:408-411, 1953
121. Weinstein L, Shelokov A: Cardiovascular manifestations in acute poliomyelitis. *N Engl J Med* 244:281-285, 1951
122. Hudgins JM: Infectious mononucleosis complicated by myocarditis and pericarditis. *JAMA* 235:2626-2627, 1976
123. Frishman W, Kraus ME, Zabkar J, et al: Infectious mononucleosis and fatal myocarditis. *Chest* 72:535-538, 1977
124. Webster BH: Cardiac complications of infectious mononucleosis: a review of the literature and report of five cases. *Am J Med Sci* 234:62-69, 1957
125. Miller R, Ward C, Amsterdam E, et al: Focal mononucleosis myocarditis simulating myocardial infarction. *Chest* 63:102-105, 1973
126. Acierno LJ: Cardiac complications in acquired immunodeficiency syndrome (AIDS): a review. *J Am Coll Cardiol* 13:1144-1154, 1989
127. Steward JM, Kaul A, Gromisch DS, et al: Symptomatic cardiac dysfunction in children with human immunodeficiency virus infection. *Am Heart J* 117:140-144, 1989
128. Corallo S, Mutinelli MR, Moroni M, et al: Echocardiography detects myocardial damage in AIDS: prospective study in 102 patients. *Eur Heart J* 9:887-892, 1988
129. Reilly JM, Cunnion RE, Anderson DW, et al: Frequency of myocarditis, left ventricular dysfunction and ventricular tachycardia in the acquired immune deficiency syndrome. *Am J Cardiol* 62:789-793, 1988
130. Beschorner WE, Baughman K, Turnicky RP, et al: HIV-associated myocarditis. *Am J Pathol* 137:1365-1371, 1990
131. Bell H: Cardiac manifestations of viral hepatitis. *JAMA* 218:387-391, 1971
132. Nagaratnam N, de Silva DPKM, Gunawardene KRW: Myocardial involvement in infectious hepatitis. *Postgrad Med J* 47:785-788, 1971
133. Roberts WC, Fox SM III: Mumps of the heart: clinical and pathologic features. *Circulation* 32:342-345, 1965
134. Bengtsson E, Orndahl G: Complications of mumps with special reference to the incidence of myocarditis. *Acta Med Scand* 149:381-388, 1954
135. Brown NJ, Richmond SJ: Fatal mumps myocarditis in an 8-month-old child. *Br Med J* 281:356-357, 1980
136. Giustra FX, Nilsson DC: Myocarditis following measles: report of a case. *Am J Dis Child* 79:487-490, 1950
137. Goldfield M, Boyer NH, Weinstein L: Electrocardiographic changes during the course of measles. *J Pediatr* 46:30-35, 1955
138. Moore CM, Henry J, Benzing G III, et al: Varicella myocarditis. *Am J Dis Child* 118:899-902, 1969
139. Morales AR, Adelman S, Fine G: Varicella myocarditis: a case of sudden death. *Arch Pathol* 91:29-31, 1971
140. Fiddler GI, Campbell RWF, Pottage A, et al: Varicella myocarditis presenting with unusual ventricular arrhythmias. *Br Heart J* 39:1150-1153, 1977
141. Matthews AW, Griffiths ID: Post-vaccinial pericarditis and myocarditis. *Br Heart J* 36:1043-1045, 1974
142. Finlay-Jones LR: Fatal myocarditis after vaccination against smallpox: report of a case. *N Engl J Med* 270:41-42, 1964
143. Obeyesekere I, Hermon Y: Arbovirus heart disease: myocarditis and cardiomyopathy following dengue and chikungunya fever; a follow-up study. *Am Heart J* 85:186-194, 1973
144. Nagaratnam N, Siripala K, de Silva N: Arbovirus (dengue type) as a cause of acute myocarditis and pericarditis. *Br Heart J* 35:204-206, 1973
145. Obeyesekere I, Hermon Y: Myocarditis and cardiomyopathy after arbovirus infections (dengue and chikungunya fever). *Br Heart J* 34:821-827, 1972
146. Giles TD, Gohd RS: Respiratory syncytial virus and heart disease: a report of two cases. *JAMA* 236:1128-1130, 1976
147. Bairan AC, Cheery JD, Fagan LF, et al: Complete heart block and respiratory syncytial virus infection. *Am J Dis Child* 127:264-265, 1974
148. Ross CAC, Stevenson J: Herpes-simplex meningoencephalitis. *Lancet* 2:682-685, 1961
149. Bell RW, Murphy WM: Myocarditis in young military personnel: herpes simplex, trichinosis, meningococcemia, carbon tetrachloride, and idiopathic fibrous and giant cell types. *Am Heart J* 74:309-323, 1967
150. Henson D, Mufson MA: Myocarditis and pneumonitis with type 21 adenovirus infection: association with fatal myocarditis and pneumonitis. *Am J Dis Child* 121:334-336, 1971
151. Monath TP: Yellow fever virus. In *Principles and Practice of Infectious Diseases.* Second Edition. Edited by GL Mandell, RG Douglas Jr, JE Bennett. New York, John Wiley, 1985, pp 923-926
152. Cheetham HD, Hart J, Coghill NF, et al: Rabies with myocarditis: two cases in England. *Lancet* 1:921-922, 1970
153. Kitaura Y, Morita H: Secondary myocardial disease: virus myocarditis and cardiomyopathy. *Jpn Circ J* 43:1017-1031, 1979
154. Public Health Laboratory Service: Coxsackie B5 virus infections during 1965. *Br Med J* 4:575-577, 1967
155. Gravanis MB, Sternby NH: Incidence of myocarditis: a 10-year autopsy study from Mälmo, Sweden. *Arch Pathol Lab Med* 115:390-392, 1991
156. Bandt CM, Staley NA, Noren GR: Acute viral myocarditis: clinical and histologic changes. *Minn Med* 62:234-237, 1979
157. O'Connell JB, Fowles RE, Robinson JA, et al: Clinical and pathologic findings of myocarditis in two families with dilated cardiomyopathy. *Am Heart J* 107:127-135, 1984
158. Gear JHS, Measroch V: Coxsackievirus infections of the newborn. *Prog Med Virol* 15:42-62, 1973
159. Schmidt NJ, Magoffin RL, Lennette EH: Association of group B Coxsackieviruses with cases of pericarditis, myocarditis, or pleurodynia by demonstration of immunoglobulin M antibody. *Infect Immun* 8:341-348, 1973
160. Smith WG: Coxsackie B myopericarditis in adults. *Am Heart J* 80:34-46, 1970
161. Aretz HT, Billingham ME, Edwards WD, et al: Myocarditis: a

histopathologic definition and classification. *Am J Cardiovasc Pathol* 1:3-14, 1987

162. Cronin ME, Love LA, Miller FW, et al: The natural history of encephalomyocarditis virus-induced myositis and myocarditis in mice: viral persistence demonstrated by in situ hybridization. *J Exp Med* 168:1639-1648, 1988

163. Kandolf R, Ameis D, Kirschner P, et al: *In situ* detection of enteroviral genomes in myocardial cells by nucleic acid hybridization: an approach to the diagnosis of viral heart disease. *Proc Natl Acad Sci U S A* 84:6272-6276, 1987

164. Tracy S, Chapman NM, McManus BM, et al: A molecular and serologic evaluation of enteroviral involvement in human myocarditis. *J Mol Cell Cardiol* 22:403-414, 1990

165. Grasso M, Arbustini E, Silini E, et al: Search for coxsackievirus B3 RNA in idiopathic dilated cardiomyopathy using gene amplification by polymerase chain reaction. *Am J Cardiol* 69:658-664, 1992

166. Rose NR, Herskowitz A, Neumann DA, et al: Autoimmune myocarditis: a paradigm of post-infection autoimmune disease. *Immunol Today* 9:117-120, 1988

167. Neumann DA, Burek CL, Baughman KL, et al: Circulating heart-reactive antibodies in patients with myocarditis or cardiomyopathy. *J Am Coll Cardiol* 16:839-846, 1990

168. Herskowitz A, Ahmed-Ansari A, Neumann DA, et al: Induction of major histocompatibility complex antigens within the myocardium of patients with active myocarditis: a nonhistologic marker of myocarditis. *J Am Coll Cardiol* 15:624-632, 1990

169. Reyes MP, Lerner AM: Coxsackievirus myocarditis—with special reference to acute and chronic effects. *Prog Cardiovasc Dis* 27:373-394, 1985

170. Herzum M, Maisch B: Humoral and cellular immune response in human myocarditis and dilated cardiomyopathy. *Pathol Immunopathol Res* 7:240-250, 1988

171. Levi G, Scalvini S, Volterrani M, et al: Coxsackie virus heart disease: 15 years after. *Eur Heart J* 9:1303-1307, 1988

172. Deguchi H, Kitaura Y, Hayashi T, et al: Cell-mediated immune cardiocyte injury in viral myocarditis of mice and patients. *Jpn Circ J* 53:61-77, 1989

173. Lange LG, Schreiner GF: Immune mechanisms of cardiac disease. *N Engl J Med* 330:1129-1135, 1994

174. Drude L, Wiemers F, Maisch B: Impaired myocyte function in vitro incubated with sera from patients with myocarditis. *Eur Heart J* 12 Suppl D:36-38, 1991

175. Gulick T, Pieper SJ, Murphy MA, et al: A new method for assessment of cultured cardiac myocyte contractility detects immune factor-mediated inhibition of β-adrenergic responses. *Circulation* 84: 313-321, 1991

176. Kilbourne ED, Wilson CB, Perrier D: The induction of gross myocardial lesions by Coxsackie (pleurodynia) virus and cortisone. *J Clin Invest* 35:362-370, 1956

177. Wentworth P, Jentz LA, Croal AE: Analysis of sudden unexpected death in southern Ontario, with emphasis on myocarditis. *Can Med Assoc J* 120:676-680; 706, 1979

178. O'Connell JB, Henkin RE, Robinson JA, et al: Gallium-67 imaging in patients with dilated cardiomyopathy and biopsy-proven myocarditis. *Circulation* 70:58-62, 1984

179. Dec GW, Palacios I, Yasuda T, et al: Antimyosin antibody cardiac imaging: its role in the diagnosis of myocarditis. *J Am Coll Cardiol* 16:97-104, 1990

180. Hauck AJ, Kearney DL, Edwards WD: Evaluation of postmortem endomyocardial biopsy specimens from 38 patients with lymphocytic myocarditis: implications for role of sampling error. *Mayo Clin Proc* 64:1235-1245, 1989

181. Chow LH, Radio SJ, Sears TD, et al: Insensitivity of right ventricular endomyocardial biopsy in the diagnosis of myocarditis. *J Am Coll Cardiol* 14:915-920, 1989

182. Latham RD, Mulrow JP, Virmani R, et al: Recently diagnosed idiopathic dilated cardiomyopathy: incidence of myocarditis and efficacy of prednisone therapy. *Am Heart J* 117:876-882, 1989

183. Chow LC, Dittrich HC, Shabetai R: Endomyocardial biopsy in patients with unexplained congestive heart failure. *Ann Intern Med* 109:535-539, 1988

184. Lieberman EB, Hutchins GM, Herskowitz A, et al: Clinicopathologic description of myocarditis. *J Am Coll Cardiol* 18:1617-1626, 1991

185. Costanzo-Nordin MR, Reap EA, O'Connell JB, et al: A nonsteroid anti-inflammatory drug exacerbates coxsackie B3 murine myocarditis. *J Am Coll Cardiol* 6:1078-1082, 1985

186. O'Connell JB, Reap EA, Robinson JA: The effects of cyclosporine on acute murine Coxsackie B3 myocarditis. *Circulation* 73:353-359, 1986

187. Kishimoto C, Thorp KA, Abelmann WH: Immunosuppression with high doses of cyclophosphamide reduces the severity of myocarditis but increases the mortality in murine coxsackievirus B3 myocarditis. *Circulation* 82:982-989, 1990

188. Kishimoto C, Abelmann WH: Monoclonal antibody therapy for prevention of acute coxsackievirus B3 myocarditis in mice. *Circulation* 79:1300-1308, 1989

189. Daly K, Richardson PJ, Olsen EG, et al: Acute myocarditis: role of histological and virological examination in the diagnosis and assessment of immunosuppressive treatment. *Br Heart J* 51:30-35, 1984

190. Jones SR, Herskowitz A, Hutchins GM, et al: Effects of immunosuppressive therapy in biopsy-proved myocarditis and borderline myocarditis on left ventricular function. *Am J Cardiol* 68:370-376, 1991

191. Baroldi G, Corallo S, Moroni M, et al: Focal lymphocytic myocarditis in acquired immunodeficiency syndrome (AIDS): a correlative morphologic and clinical study in 26 consecutive fatal cases. *J Am Coll Cardiol* 12:463-469, 1988

192. Anderson DW, Virmani R, Reilly JM, et al: Prevalent myocarditis at necropsy in the acquired immunodeficiency syndrome. *J Am Coll Cardiol* 11:792-799, 1988

193. Roldan EO, Moskowitz L, Hensley GT: Pathology of the heart in acquired immunodeficiency syndrome. *Arch Pathol Lab Med* 111:943-946, 1987

194. Herskowitz A, Willoughby SB, Baughman KL, et al: Cardiomyopathy associated with antiretroviral therapy in patients with HIV infection: a report of six cases. *Ann Intern Med* 116:311-313, 1992

195. Levine HD: Pathologic study of thirty-one cases of scrub typhus fever with especial reference to the cardiovascular system. *Am Heart J* 31:314-328, 1946

196. Ognibene AJ, O'Leary DS, Czarnecki SW, et al: Myocarditis and disseminated intravascular coagulation in scrub typhus. *Am J Med Sci* 262:233-238, 1971

197. Woodward TE, McCrumb FR Jr, Carey TN, et al: Viral and rickettsial causes of cardiac disease, including the Coxsackie virus etiology of pericarditis and myocarditis. *Ann Intern Med* 53:1130-1150, 1960

198. Walker DH, Paletta CE, Cain BG: Pathogenesis of myocarditis in Rocky Mountain spotted fever. *Arch Pathol Lab Med* 104:171-174, 1980

199. Bradford WD, Hackel DB: Myocardial involvement in Rocky Mountain spotted fever. *Arch Pathol Lab Med* 102:357-359, 1978

200. Marin-Garcia J, Mirvis DM: Myocardial disease in Rocky Mountain spotted fever: clinical, functional, and pathologic findings. *Pediatr Cardiol* 5:149-154, 1984

201. Sheridan P, MacCraig JN, Hart RJC: Myocarditis complicating Q fever. *Br Med J* 2:155-156, 1974

202. Barraclough D, Popert AJ: Q fever presenting with paroxysmal ventricular tachycardia. *Br Med J* 2:423-424, 1975

203. Wittels B, Bressler R: Biochemical lesion of diphtheria toxin in the heart. *J Clin Invest* 43:630-637, 1964

204. Riley HD Jr, Weaver TS: Cardiovascular and nervous system complications of diphtheria. *Am Pract* 3:536-543, 1952

205. Tahernia AC: Electrocardiographic abnormalities and serum transaminase levels in diphtheritic myocarditis. *J Pediatr* 75:1008-1014, 1969

206. Morales AR, Vichitbandha P, Chandruang P, et al: Pathological features of cardiac conduction disturbances in diphtheritic myocarditis. *Arch Pathol* 91:1-7, 1971

207. Khosla SN: The heart in enteric (typhoid) fever. *J Trop Med Hyg* 84:125-131, 1981

208. Chowdhary S, Bhatnagar HNS, Singh SV: Myocarditis in enteric fever. *J Assoc Physicians India* 22:251-254, 1974

209. Thiruvengadam KV, Shetty MR, Mallick MA: Myocarditis in enteric fever. *J Indian Med Assoc* 48:115-119, 1967

210. Langaker OM, Svanes K: Myocardial abscess due to *Salmonella typhimurium*. *Br Heart J* 35:871-873, 1973

211. Kortleve JW, Düren DR, Becker AE: Cardiac aneurysm complicated by *Salmonella* abscess: a clinicopathologic correlation in two patients. *Am J Med* 68:395-400, 1980

212. Diem LV, Arnold K: Typhoid fever with myocarditis. *Am J Trop Med Hyg* 23:218-221, 1974

213. Roberts JE, Lisa JR: The heart in pulmonary tuberculosis: a

clinicopathological study of 100 autopsied patients. *Am Rev Tuberc* 47:253-262, 1943

214. Rawls WJ, Shuford WH, Logan WD, et al: Right ventricular outflow tract obstruction produced by a myocardial abscess in a patient with tuberculosis. *Am J Cardiol* 21:738-745, 1968

215. Kinare SG, Deshmukh MM: Complete atrioventricular block due to myocardial tuberculosis: report of a case. *Arch Pathol* 88:684-687, 1969

216. Wallis PJW, Branfoot AC, Emerson PA: Sudden death due to myocardial tuberculosis. *Thorax* 39:155-156, 1984

217. Gore I: Myocarditis in infectious diseases. *Am Pract* 1:292-298, 1947

218. Brody H, Smith LW: The visceral pathology in scarlet fever and related streptococcus infections. *Am J Pathol* 12:373-394, 1936

219. Robboy SJ: Atrioventricular-node inflammation: mechanism of sudden death in protracted meningococcemia. *N Engl J Med* 286:1091-1092, 1972

220. Hardman JM, Earle KM: Myocarditis in 200 fatal meningococcal infections. *Arch Pathol* 87:318-325, 1969

221. Denmark TC, Knight EL: Cardiovascular and coagulation complications of group C meningococcal disease. *Arch Intern Med* 127:238-240, 1971

222. Lubani M, Sharda D, Helin I: Cardiac manifestations in brucellosis. *Arch Dis Child* 61:569-572, 1986

223. Roberts WC, Berard CW: Gas gangrene of the heart in clostridial septicemia. *Am Heart J* 74:482-488, 1967

224. Guneratne F: Gas gangrene (abscess) of heart. *NY State J Med* 75:1766-1769, 1975

225. Sanford JP: *Pseudomonas* species (including melioidosis and glanders. In *Principles and Practice of Infectious Diseases.* Vol 2. Edited by GL Mandell, RG Douglas Jr, JE Bennett. New York, John Wiley & Sons, 1979, pp 1720-1726

226. Pönkä A: Carditis associated with *Mycoplasma pneumoniae* infection. *Acta Med Scand* 206:77-86, 1979

227. Sands MJ Jr, Satz JE, Turner WE Jr, et al: Pericarditis and perimyocarditis associated with active *Mycoplasma pneumoniae* infection. *Ann Intern Med* 86:544-548, 1977

228. Sutton GC, Morrissey RA, Tobin JR Jr, et al: Pericardial and myocardial disease associated with serological evidence of infection by agents of the psittacosis-lymphogranuloma venereum group (Chlamydiaceae). *Circulation* 36:830-838, 1967

229. Challoner DR, Prols HG: Free fatty acid oxidation and carnitine levels in diphtheritic guinea pig myocardium. *J Clin Invest* 51:2071-2076, 1972

230. Collier RJ, Pappenheimer AM Jr: Studies on the mode of action of diphtheria toxin. I. Phosphorylated intermediates in normal and intoxicated HeLa cells. *J Exp Med* 120:1007-1018, 1964

231. Thisyakorn U, Wongvanich J, Kumpeng V: Failure of corticosteroid therapy to prevent diphtheritic myocarditis or neuritis. *Pediatr Infect Dis J* 3:126-128, 1984

232. Ramos ACMF, Elias PRP, Barrucand L, et al: The protective effect of carnitine in human diphtheritic myocarditis. *Pediatr Res* 18:815-819, 1984

233. Steere AC, Taylor E, Wilson ML, et al: Longitudinal assessment of the clinical and epidemiological features of Lyme disease in a defined population. *J Infect Dis* 154:295-300, 1986

234. Steere AC, Grodzicki RL, Kornblatt AN, et al: The spirochetal etiology of Lyme disease. *N Engl J Med* 308:733-740, 1983

235. Burgdorfer W, Barbour AG, Hayes SF, et al: Lyme disease: a tick-borne spirochetosis? *Science* 216:1317-1319, 1982

236. Steere AC, Batsford WP, Weinberg M, et al: Lyme carditis: cardiac abnormalities of Lyme disease. *Ann Intern Med* 93:8-16, 1980

237. Stanek G, Klein J, Bittner R, et al: Isolation of *Borrelia burgdorferi* from the myocardium of a patient with longstanding cardiomyopathy. *N Engl J Med* 322:249-252, 1990

238. Vlay SC, Dervan JP, Elias J, et al: Ventricular tachycardia associated with Lyme carditis. *Am Heart J* 121:1558-1560, 1991

239. Klein J, Stanek G, Bittner R, et al: Lyme borreliosis as a cause of myocarditis and heart muscle disease. *Eur Heart J* 12 Suppl D:73-75, 1991

240. Goodman JL, Jurkovich P, Kodner C, et al: Persistent cardiac and urinary tract infections with *Borrelia burgdorferi* in experimentally infected Syrian hamsters. *J Clin Microbiol* 29:894-896, 1991

241. de Koning J, Hoogkamp-Korstanje JAA, van der Linde MR, et al: Demonstration of spirochetes in cardiac biopsies of patients with Lyme disease. *J Infect Dis* 160:150-153, 1989

242. Rahn DW, Malawista SE: Lyme disease: recommendations for diagnosis and treatment. *Ann Intern Med* 114:472-481, 1991

243. Steere AC: Medical progress: Lyme disease. *N Engl J Med* 321:586-596, 1989

244. Boss JH, Leffkowitz M, Freud M: Unusual manifestations of syphilitic cardiovascular disease. *Ann Intern Med* 55:824-831, 1961

245. Edwards GA, Domm BM: Human leptospirosis. *Medicine (Baltimore)* 39:117-156, 1960

246. Areán VM: Leptospiral myocarditis. *Lab Invest* 6:462-471, 1957

247. Sodeman WA, Killough JH: The cardiac manifestations of Weil's disease. *Am J Trop Med Hyg* 31:479-488, 1951

248. Usynowitz ML: Myocarditis and heart failure due to leptospira pomona. *Hawaii Med J* 23:41-44, 1963

249. Wengrower D, Knobler H, Gillis S, et al: Myocarditis in tick-borne relapsing fever. *J Infect Dis* 149:1033, 1984

250. Parker JC Jr: The potentially lethal problem of cardiac candidosis. *Am J Clin Pathol* 73:356-361, 1980

251. Atkinson JB, Connor DH, Robinowitz M, et al: Cardiac fungal infections: review of autopsy findings in 60 patients. *Hum Pathol* 15:935-942, 1984

252. Walsh TJ, Hutchins GM, Bulkley BH, et al: Fungal infections of the heart: analysis of 51 autopsy cases. *Am J Cardiol* 45:357-366, 1980

253. Williams AH: *Aspergillus* myocarditis. *Am J Clin Pathol* 61:247-256, 1974

254. Cade JF: Pulmonary aspergillosis with myocarditis. *Med J Aust* 1:581-584, 1966

255. Nime FA, Hutchins GM: Oxalosis caused by *Aspergillus* infection. *Johns Hopkins Med J* 113:183-194, 1973

256. Hutter RVP, Collins HS: The occurrence of opportunistic fungus infections in a cancer hospital. *Lab Invest* 11:1035-1045, 1962

257. Jones I, Nassau E, Smith P: Cryptococcosis of the heart. *Br Heart J* 27:462-464, 1965

258. Owen GE, Scherr SN, Segre EJ: Histoplasmosis involving the heart and great vessels. *Am J Med* 32:552-559, 1962

259. Prager RL, Burney P, Waterhouse G, et al: Pulmonary, mediastinal, and cardiac presentations of histoplasmosis. *Ann Thorac Surg* 30:385-390, 1980

260. Zoeckler SJ: Cardiac actinomycosis: a case report and survey of the literature. *Circulation* 3:854-858, 1951

261. Martin DS, Smith DT: Blastomycosis (American blastomycosis, Gilchrist's disease). I. A review of the literature. *Am Rev Tuberc* 39:275-304, 1939

262. Baker RD, Brian EW: Blastomycosis of the heart: report of two cases. *Am J Pathol* 13:139-147, 1937

263. Reingold IM: Myocardial lesions in disseminated coccidioidomycosis. *Am J Clin Pathol* 20:1044-1049, 1950

264. Larson R, Scherb RE: Coccidioidal pericarditis. *Circulation* 7:211-217, 1953

265. Virmani R, Connor DH, McAllister HA: Cardiac mucormycosis: a report of five patients and review of 14 previously reported cases. *Am J Clin Pathol* 78:42-47, 1982

266. Santos-Buch CA: American trypanosomiasis: Chagas' disease. *Int Rev Exp Pathol* 19:63-100, 1979

267. Rosenbaum MB: Chagasic myocardiopathy. *Prog Cardiovasc Dis* 7:199-225, 1964

268. Llop E, Rothhammer F, Acuña M, et al: HLA antigens in cardiomyopathic Chilean chagasics. *Am J Hum Genet* 43:770-773, 1988

269. Lima JAC, Szarfman A, Lima SD, et al: Absence of left ventricular dysfunction during acute chagasic myocarditis in the rhesus monkey. *Circulation* 73:172-179, 1986

270. Andrade ZA, Andrade SG, Oliveira GB, et al: Histopathology of the conducting tissue of the heart in Chagas' myocarditis. *Am Heart J* 95:316-324, 1978

271. Laranja FS, Dias E, Nobrega G, et al: Chagas' disease: a clinical, epidemiologic, and pathologic study. *Circulation* 14:1035-1060, 1956

272. Maguire JH, Hoff R, Sherlock I, et al: Cardiac morbidity and mortality due to Chagas' disease: prospective electrocardiographic study of a Brazilian community. *Circulation* 75:1140-1145, 1987

273. Gallo L Jr, Morelo Filho J, Maciel BC, et al: Functional evaluation of sympathetic and parasympathetic system in Chagas' disease using dynamic exercise. *Cardiovasc Res* 21:922-927, 1987

274. Castagnino HE, Jörg ME, Thompson AC: Ventricular aneurysms in chronic Chagas' cardiopathy. *J Cardiovasc Surg (Torino)* 23:28-33, 1982

275. Oliveira JSM, Mello de Oliveira JA, Frederigue U Jr, et al: Apical aneurysm of Chagas's heart disease. *Br Heart J* 46:432-437, 1981

276. Mott KE, Hagstrom JWC: The pathologic lesions of the cardiac autonomic nervous system in chronic Chagas' myocarditis. *Circulation* 31:273-286, 1965

277. Santos-Buch CA, Acosta AN: Chagas' disease. In *Immunology and Pathogenesis of Trypanosomiasis.* Edited by I Tizard. Boca Raton, Florida, CRC Press, 1985, pp 145-183

278. Santos-Buch CA, Teixeira ARL: The immunology of experimental Chagas' disease. III. Rejection of allogeneic heart cells in vitro. *J Exp Med* 140:38-53, 1974

279. Cossio PM, Laguens RP, Diez C, et al: Chagasic cardiopathy: antibodies reacting with plasma membrane of striated muscle and endothelial cells. *Circulation* 50:1252-1259, 1974

280. Cossio PM, Diez C, Szarfman A, et al: Chagasic cardiopathy: demonstration of a serum gamma globulin factor which reacts with endocardium and vascular structures. *Circulation* 49:13-21, 1974

281. Morris SA, Tanowitz HB, Wittner M, et al: Pathophysiological insights into the cardiomyopathy of Chagas' disease. *Circulation* 82:1900-1909, 1990

282. Molina HA, Kierszenbaum F: Immunohistochemical detection of deposits of eosinophil-derived neurotoxin and eosinophil peroxidase in the myocardium of patients with Chagas' disease. *Immunology* 64:725-731, 1988

283. Leak D, Meghji M: Toxoplasmic infection in cardiac disease. *Am J Cardiol* 43:841-849, 1979

284. Arribada A, Thiermann E: Contribution to diagnostic problem of cardiomyopathies produced by *Toxoplasma gondii. Recent Adv Stud Cardiac Struct Metab* 2:655-668, 1973

285. Feldman HA: Toxoplasmosis. *N Engl J Med* 279:1370-1375; 1431-1437, 1968

286. Poltera AA, Cox JN, Owor R: Pancarditis affecting the conducting system and all valves in human African trypanosomiasis. *Br Heart J* 38:827-837, 1976

287. Francis TI: Visceral complications of Gambian trypanosomiasis in a Nigerian. *Trans R Soc Trop Med Hyg* 66:140-144, 1972

288. Kean BH: Parasitic diseases of the heart. In *Pathology of the Heart and Blood Vessels.* Third edition. Edited by SE Gould. Springfield, Illinois, Charles C Thomas, Publisher, 1968, pp 812-833

289. Rojas RA, Deza D: Cardiac changes in malarial patients. *Am Heart J* 33:702-703, 1947

290. Simonson E, Keys A: Experimental malaria in man. III. The changes in the electrocardiogram. *J Clin Invest* 29:68-71, 1950

291. Sidorov P: Un cas de balantidiose chez l'homme suivi d'une myocardite granulomateuse. *Ann Anat Pathol (Paris)* 12:711-721, 1935

292. Barr R: Human trichinosis: report of four cases, with emphasis on central nervous system involvement, and a survey of 500 consecutive autopsies at the Ottawa Civic Hospital. *Can Med Assoc J* 95:912-917, 1966

293. Gray DF, Morse BS, Phillips WF: Trichinosis with neurologic and cardiac involvement: review of the literature and report of three cases. *Ann Intern Med* 57:230-244, 1962

294. Murphy TE, Kean BH, Venturini A, et al: Echinococcus cyst of the left ventricle: report of a case with review of the pertinent literature. *J Thorac Cardiovasc Surg* 61:443-450, 1971

295. Oliver JF, Sotillo JF, Domínguez FJ, et al: Two-dimensional echocardiographic features of echinococcosis of the heart and great blood vessels: clinical and surgical implications. *Circulation* 78:327-337, 1988

296. Chin DD, Rice JP, Lequesne DM: Hydatid cyst of the heart presenting as cerebral and cerebellar infarction. *Med J Aust* 2:556-557, 1981

297. Solarz SD: An electrocardiographic study of one hundred fourteen consecutive cases of trichinosis. *Am Heart J* 34:230-240, 1947

298. Leading Article: Medical treatment for hydatid disease? *Br Med J* 2:563, 1979

299. Wessel HU, Sommers HM, Cugell DW, et al: Variants of cardiopulmonary manifestations of Manson's schistosomiasis: report of two cases. *Ann Intern Med* 62:757-766, 1965

300. Al Zahawi S, Shukri N: Histopathology of fatal myocarditis due to ectopic schistosomiasis. *Trans R Soc Trop Med Hyg* 50:166-168, 1956

301. Kean BH, Breslau RC: *Parasites of the Human Heart.* New York, Grune & Stratton, 1964

302. Helimsky AM: Cysticercosis of the brain, heart and skeletal muscles. *Med Parazitol (Mosk)* 31:610-611, 1962

303. Ibarra-Pérez C, Fernández-Diez J, Rodriguez-Trujillo F: Myocardial cysticercosis: report of two cases with coexisting heart disease. *South Med J* 65:484-486, 1972

304. Schantz PM, Glickman LT: Toxocaral visceral larva migrans. *N Engl J Med* 298:436-439, 1978

305. Friedman S, Hervada AR: Severe myocarditis with recovery in a child with visceral larva migrans. *J Pediatr* 56:91-96, 1960

306. Tatibouet L, Eusen Y: Insuffisance cardiaque d'origine filarienne. *Sem Hop Paris* 37:3418-3420, 1961

307. Walshe WH: *The Practical Treatise on the Diseases of the Heart and Great Vessels, Including the Principles of Their Physical Diagnosis.* Fourth edition. London, Smith, Elder & Co, 1873

308. Burch GE, Walsh JJ: Cardiac insufficiency in chronic alcoholism. *Am J Cardiol* 6:864-874, 1960

309. Kaelber CT, Barboriak J (eds): Symposium on alcohol and cardiovascular diseases. *Circulation* 64 Suppl 3:1-84, 1981

310. Kopecky SL, Gersh BJ: Dilated cardiomyopathy and myocarditis: natural history, etiology, clinical manifestations, and management. *Curr Probl Cardiol* 12:569-647, 1987

311. Urbano-Marquez A, Estruch R, Navarro-Lopez F, et al: The effects of alcoholism on skeletal and cardiac muscle. *N Engl J Med* 320:409-415, 1989

312. Regan TJ: Alcohol and the cardiovascular system. *JAMA* 264:377-381, 1990

313. Segel LD, Rendig SV, Choquet Y, et al: Effects of chronic graded ethanol consumption on the metabolism, ultrastructure, and mechanical function of the rat heart. *Cardiovasc Res* 9:649-663, 1975

314. Pachinger O, Mao J, Fauvel J-M, et al: Mitochondrial function and excitation-contraction coupling in the development of alcoholic cardiomyopathy. *Recent Adv Stud Cardiac Struc Metab* 5:423-429, 1975

315. Klein H, Harmjanz D: Effect of ethanol infusion on the ultrastructure of human myocardium. *Postgrad Med J* 51:325-328, 1975

316. Segel LD, Rendig SV, Mason DT: Left ventricular dysfunction of isolated working rat hearts after chronic alcohol consumption. *Cardiovasc Res* 13:136-146, 1979

317. Horwitz LD, Atkins JM: Acute effects of ethanol on left ventricular performance. *Circulation* 49:124-128, 1974

318. Regan TJ: Alcoholic cardiomyopathy. *Prog Cardiovasc Dis* 27:141-152, 1984

319. Steinberg JD, Hayden MT: Prevalence of clinically occult cardiomyopathy in chronic alcoholism. *Am Heart J* 101:461-464, 1981

320. Friedman HS, Lieber CS: Cardiotoxicity of alcohol. *Cardiovasc Med* 2:111-112, 1977

321. Kelbaek H, Gjørup T, Brynjolf I, et al: Acute effects of alcohol on left ventricular function in healthy subjects at rest and during upright exercise. *Am J Cardiol* 55:164-167, 1985

322. Lang RM, Borow KM, Neumann A, et al: Adverse cardiac effects of acute alcohol ingestion in young adults. *Ann Intern Med* 102:742-747, 1985

323. Alexander CS: Cobalt-beer cardiomyopathy: a clinical and pathologic study of twenty-eight cases. *Am J Med* 53:395-417, 1972

324. Bing RJ, Tillmanns H: The effect of alcohol on the heart. In *Metabolic Aspects of Alcoholism.* Edited by CS Lieber. Lancaster, England, MTP Press Limited, 1977, pp 117-134

325. Regan TJ, Wu CF, Weisse AB, et al: Acute myocardial infarction in toxic cardiomyopathy without coronary obstruction. *Circulation* 51:453-461, 1975

326. Demakis JG, Proskey A, Rahimtoola SH, et al: The natural course of alcoholic cardiomyopathy. *Ann Intern Med* 80:293-297, 1974

327. Regan TJ, Ettinger PO, Lyons MM, et al: Ethyl alcohol as a cardiac risk factor. *Curr Probl Cardiol* 2:1-35, May 1977

328. Rich EC, Siebold C, Campion B: Alcohol-related acute atrial fibrillation: a case-control study and review of 40 patients. *Arch Intern Med* 145:830-833, 1985

329. Greenspon AJ, Stang JM, Lewis RP, et al: Provocation of ventricular tachycardia after consumption of alcohol. *N Engl J Med* 301:1049-1051, 1979

330. Luca C: Electrophysiological properties of right heart and atrioventricular conducting system in patients with alcoholic cardiomyopathy. *Br Heart J* 42:274-281, 1979

331. Ettinger PO, Wu CF, De La Cruz C Jr, et al: Arrhythmias and the "holiday heart": alcohol-associated cardiac rhythm disorders. *Am Heart J* 95:555-562, 1978

332. Mathews EC Jr, Gardin JM, Henry WL, et al: Echocardiographic abnormalities in chronic alcoholics with and without overt congestive heart failure. *Am J Cardiol* 47:570-578, 1981

333. Spodick DH, Pigott VM, Chirife R: Preclinical cardiac malfunction in chronic alcoholism: comparison with matched normal controls and with alcoholic cardiomyopathy. *N Engl J Med* 287:677-680, 1972

334. Gould L, Shariff M, Zahir M, et al: Cardiac hemodynamics in alcoholic patients with chronic liver disease and a presystolic gallop. *J Clin Invest* 48:860-868, 1969

335. Regan TJ, Levinson GE, Oldewurtel HA, et al: Ventricular function in noncardiacs with alcoholic fatty liver: role of ethanol in the production of cardiomyopathy. *J Clin Invest* 48:397-407, 1969

336. Hurt RD, Morse RM, Swenson WM: Diagnosis of alcoholism with a self-administered alcoholism screening test: results with 1,002 consecutive patients receiving general examinations. *Mayo Clin Proc* 55:365-370, 1980

337. Kino M, Imamitchi H, Morigutchi M, et al: Cardiovascular status in asymptomatic alcoholics, with reference to the level of ethanol consumption. *Br Heart J* 46:545-551, 1981

338. Schwartz L, Sample KA, Wigle ED: Severe alcoholic cardiomyopathy reversed with abstention from alcohol. *Am J Cardiol* 36:963-966, 1975

339. Baudet M, Rigaud M, Rocha P, et al: Reversibility of alcoholic cardiomyopathy with abstention from alcohol. *Cardiology* 64:317-324, 1979

340. Hung J, Harris PJ, Kelly DT, et al: Improvement of left ventricular function in alcoholic cardiomyopathy documented by serial gated cardiac pool scanning. *Aust NZ J Med* 9:420-422, 1979

341. Rosengren A, Wilhelmsen L, Pennert K, et al: Alcoholic intemperance, coronary heart disease and mortality in middle-aged Swedish men. *Acta Med Scand* 222:201-213, 1987

342. Rosengren A, Wilhelmsen L: Alcoholic registration and cardiovascular morbidity and mortality—a prospective study in middle aged Swedish men. *Acta Med Scand Suppl* 717:87-92, 1987

343. Rosengren A, Wilhelmsen L, Wedel H: Separate and combined effects of smoking and alcohol abuse in middle-aged men. *Acta Med Scand* 223:111-118, 1988

344. Lithell H, Åberg H, Selinus I, et al: Alcohol intemperance and sudden death. *Br Med J* 294:1456-1458, 1987

345. Suhonen O, Aromaa A, Reunanen A, et al: Alcohol consumption and sudden coronary death in middle-aged Finnish men. *Acta Med Scand* 221:335-341, 1987

346. Beard CM, Griffin MR, Offord KP, et al: Risk factors for sudden unexpected cardiac death in young women in Rochester, Minnesota, 1960 through 1974. *Mayo Clin Proc* 61:185-191, 1986

347. Phillips E, Levine SA: Auricular fibrillation without other evidence of heart disease: a cause of reversible heart failure. *Am J Med* 7:478-489, 1949

348. McLaran CJ, Gersh BJ, Sugrue DD, et al: Tachycardia induced myocardial dysfunction: a reversible phenomenon? *Br Heart J* 53:323-327, 1985

349. Gallagher JJ: Tachycardia and cardiomyopathy: the chicken-egg dilemma revisited. *J Am Coll Cardiol* 6:1172-1173, 1985

350. Packer DL, Bardy GH, Worley SJ, et al: Tachycardia-induced cardiomyopathy: a reversible form of left ventricular dysfunction. *Am J Cardiol* 57:563-570, 1986

351. Rabbani LE, Wang PJ, Couper GL, et al: Time course of improvement in ventricular function after ablation of incessant automatic atrial tachycardia. *Am Heart J* 121:816-819, 1991

352. Coleman HN III, Taylor RR, Pool PE, et al: Congestive heart failure following chronic tachycardia. *Am Heart J* 81:790-798, 1971

353. Redfield MM, Edwards BS, McGoon MD, et al: Failure of atrial natriuretic factor to increase with volume expansion in acute and chronic congestive heart failure in the dog. *Circulation* 80:651-657, 1989

354. Tomita M, Spinale FG, Crawford FA, et al: Changes in left ventricular volume, mass, and function during the development and regression of supraventricular tachycardia-induced cardiomyopathy: disparity between recovery of systolic versus diastolic function. *Circulation* 83:635-644, 1991

355. Kantrowitz NE, Bristow MR: Cardiotoxicity of antitumor agents. *Prog Cardiovasc Dis* 27:195-200, 1984

356. Bristow MR, Mason JW, Billingham ME, et al: Dose-effect and structure-function relationships in doxorubicin cardiomyopathy. *Am Heart J* 102:709-718, 1981

357. Olson RD, Mushlin PS, Brenner DE, et al: Doxorubicin cardiotoxicity may be caused by its metabolite, doxorubicinol. *Proc Natl Acad Sci U S A* 85:3585-3589, 1988

358. Singal PK, Deally CMR, Weinberg LE: Subcellular effects of Adriamycin in the heart: a concise review. *J Mol Cell Cardiol* 19:817-828, 1987

359. Praga C, Beretta G, Vigo PL, et al: Adriamycin cardiotoxicity: a survey of 1273 patients. *Cancer Treat Rep* 63:827-834, 1979

360. Bristow MR, Mason JW, Billingham ME, et al: Doxorubicin cardiomyopathy: evaluation by phonocardiography, endomyocardial biopsy, and cardiac catheterization. *Ann Intern Med* 88:168-175, 1978

361. Von Hoff DD, Layard MW, Basa P, et al: Risk factors for doxorubicin-induced congestive heart failure. *Ann Intern Med* 91:710-717, 1979

362. Goorin AM, Borow KM, Goldman A, et al: Congestive heart failure due to Adriamycin cardiotoxicity: its natural history in children. *Cancer* 47:2810-2816, 1981

363. Wortman JE, Lucas VS Jr, Schuster E, et al: Sudden death during doxorubicin administration. *Cancer* 44:1588-1591, 1979

364. Steinherz LJ, Steinherz PG, Tan CTC, et al: Cardiac toxicity 4 to 20 years after completing anthracycline therapy. *JAMA* 266:1672-1677, 1991

365. Chan PYM, Byfield JE, Lemkin SR, et al: Coincident Adriamycin (A) and x-ray therapy (XRT) in bronchogenic carcinoma (BC): response and cardiotoxicity (CT) (abstract). *Proc Am Assoc Cancer Res Am Soc Clin Oncol* 17:276, 1976

366. Weiss AJ, Metter GE, Fletcher WS, et al: Studies on Adriamycin using a weekly regimen demonstrating its clinical effectiveness and lack of cardiac toxicity. *Cancer Treat Rep* 60:813-822, 1976

367. Hortobagyi GN, Frye D, Buzdar AU, et al: Decreased cardiac toxicity of doxorubicin administered by continuous intravenous infusion in combination chemotherapy for metastatic breast carcinoma. *Cancer* 63:37-45, 1989

368. Speyer JL, Green MD, Kramer E, et al: Protective effect of the bispiperazinedione ICRF-187 against doxorubicin-induced cardiac toxicity in women with advanced breast cancer. *N Engl J Med* 319:745-752, 1988

369. Schwartz RG, McKenzie WB, Alexander J, et al: Congestive heart failure and left ventricular dysfunction complicating doxorubicin therapy: seven-year experience using serial radionuclide angiocardiography. *Am J Med* 82:1109-1118, 1987

370. Von Hoff DD, Rozencweig M, Layard M, et al: Daunomycin-induced cardiotoxicity in children and adults: a review of 110 cases. *Am J Med* 62:200-208, 1977

371. Goldberg MA, Antin JH, Guinan EC, et al: Cyclophosphamide cardiotoxicity: an analysis of dosing as a risk factor. *Blood* 68:1114-1118, 1986

372. Gottdiener JS, Appelbaum FR, Ferrans VJ, et al: Cardiotoxicity associated with high-dose cyclophosphamide therapy. *Arch Intern Med* 141:758-763, 1981

373. Schiff RJ, Wurzel CL, Brunson SC, et al: Death due to chronic syrup of ipecac use in a patient with bulimia. *Pediatrics* 78:412-416, 1986

374. Murphy ML, Bulloch RT, Pearce MB: The correlation of metabolic and ultrastructural changes in emetine myocardial toxicity. *Am Heart J* 87:105-108, 1974

375. Dempsey JJ, Salem HH: An enzymatic electrocardiographic study on toxicity of dehydroemetine. *Br Heart J* 28:505-511, 1966

376. Ratliff NB, Estes ML, Myles JL, et al: Diagnosis of chloroquine cardiomyopathy by endomyocardial biopsy. *N Engl J Med* 316:191-193, 1987

377. Riou B, Barriot P, Rimailho A, et al: Treatment of severe chloroquine poisoning. *N Engl J Med* 318:1-6, 1988

378. Honey M: The effects of sodium antimony tartrate on the myocardium. *Br Heart J* 22:601-616, 1960

379. Somers K, Rosanelli JD: Electrocardiographic effects of antimony dimercapto-succinate ("astiban"). *Br Heart J* 24:187-191, 1962

380. Elkayam U, Frishman W: Cardiovascular effects of phenothiazines. *Am Heart J* 100:397-401, 1980

381. Stimmel B: *Cardiovascular Effects of Mood-Altering Drugs.* New York, Raven Press, 1979

382. Alexander CS, Niño A: Cardiovascular complications in young patients taking psychotropic drugs: a preliminary report. *Am Heart J* 78:757-769, 1969

383. Deglin SM, Deglin JM, Chung EK: Drug-induced cardiovascular diseases. *Drugs* 14:29-40, 1977

384. Pinder RM, Brogden RN, Speight TM, et al: Doxepin up-to-date: a review of its pharmacological properties and therapeutic efficacy with particular reference to depression. *Drugs* 13:161-218, 1977

385. Pellinen TJ, Färkkilä M, Heikkilä J, et al: Electrocardiographic and clinical features of tricyclic antidepressant intoxication: a survey of 88 cases and outlines of therapy. *Ann Clin Res* 19:12-17, 1987

386. Pentel PR, Benowitz NL: Tricyclic antidepressant poisoning. Management of arrhythmias. *Med Toxicol* 1:101-121, 1986
387. Hayes JR, Born GF, Rosenbaum AH: Incidence of orthostatic hypotension in patients with primary effective disorders treated with tricyclic antidepressants. *Mayo Clin Proc* 52:509-512, 1977
388. Roose SP, Glassman AH, Giardina EGV, et al: Tricyclic antidepressants in depressed patients with cardiac conduction disease. *Arch Gen Psychiatry* 44:273-275, 1987
389. Richardson JW III, Richelson E: Antidepressants: a clinical update for medical practitioners. *Mayo Clin Proc* 59:330-337, 1984
390. Veith RC, Raskind MA, Caldwell JH, et al: Cardiovascular effects of tricyclic antidepressants in depressed patients with chronic heart disease. *N Engl J Med* 306:954-959, 1982
391. Georgotas A, McCue RE, Friedman E, et al: Electrocardiographic effects of nortriptyline, phenelzine, and placebo under optimal treatment conditions. *Am J Psychiatry* 144:798-801, 1987
392. Mitchell JE, Mackenzie TB: Cardiac effects of lithium therapy in man: a review. *J Clin Psychiatry* 43:47-51, 1982
393. Wilson JR, Kraus ES, Bailas MM, et al: Reversible sinus-node abnormalities due to lithium carbonate therapy. *N Engl J Med* 294:1223-1224, 1976
394. Tangedahl TN, Gau GT: Myocardial irritability associated with lithium carbonate therapy. *N Engl J Med* 287:867-869, 1972
395. Tilkian AG, Schroeder JS, Kao J, et al: Effect of lithium on cardiovascular performance: report on extended ambulatory monitoring and exercise testing before and during lithium therapy. *Am J Cardiol* 38:701-708, 1976
396. Swedberg K, Winblad B: Heart failure as complication of lithium treatment: preliminary report of a fatal case. *Acta Med Scand* 196:279-280, 1974
397. Tseng HL: Interstitial myocarditis probably related to lithium carbonate intoxication. *Arch Pathol* 92:444-448, 1971
398. Schou M: Lithium in heart muscle (letter to the editor). *Arch Pathol* 94:277, 1972
399. Singer I, Rotenberg D: Mechanisms of lithium action. *N Engl J Med* 289:254-260, 1973
400. Redfield MM, Nicholson WJ, Edwards WD, et al: Valve disease associated with ergot alkaloid use: echocardiographic and pathologic correlations. *Ann Intern Med* 117:50-52, 1992
401. Bana DS, MacNeal PS, LeCompte PM, et al: Cardiac murmurs and endocardial fibrosis associated with methysergide therapy. *Am Heart J* 88:640-655, 1974
402. Isner JM, Estes NAM III, Thompson PD, et al: Acute cardiac events temporally related to cocaine abuse. *N Engl J Med* 315:1438-1443, 1986
403. Mathias DW: Cocaine-associated myocardial ischemia: review of clinical and angiographic findings. *Am J Med* 81:675-678, 1986
404. French AJ, Weller CV: Interstitial myocarditis following the clinical and experimental use of sulfonamide drugs. *Am J Pathol* 18:109-121, 1942
405. Lilienfeld A, Hochstein E, Weiss W: Acute myocarditis with bundle branch block due to sulfonamide sensitivity. *Circulation* 1:1060-1064, 1950
406. MacSearraigh ETM, Patel KM: Cardiomyopathy as a complication of sulphonamide therapy. *Br Med J* 3:33, 1968
407. Bezahler GH: Fatal methyldopa-associated granulomatous hepatitis and myocarditis. *Am J Med Sci* 283:41-45, 1982
408. Seeverens H, de Bruin CD, Jordans JGM: Myocarditis and methyldopa. *Acta Med Scand* 211:233-235, 1982
409. Fenoglio JJ Jr, McAllister HA Jr, Mullick FG: Drug related myocarditis. I. Hypersensitivity myocarditis. *Hum Pathol* 12:900-907, 1981
410. Taliercio CP, Olney BA, Lie JT: Myocarditis related to drug hypersensitivity. *Mayo Clin Proc* 60:463-468, 1985
411. Burke AP, Saenger J, Mullick F, et al: Hypersensitivity myocarditis. *Arch Pathol Lab Med* 115:764-769, 1991
412. Mullick FG, McAllister HA Jr, Wagner BM, et al: Drug related vasculitis: clinicopathologic correlations in 30 patients. *Hum Pathol* 10:313-325, 1979
413. Schoenwetter AH, Silber EN: Penicillin hypersensitivity, acute pericarditis, and eosinophilia. *JAMA* 191:672-673, 1965
414. Hodge PR, Lawrence JR: Two cases of myocarditis associated with phenylbutazone therapy. *Med J Aust* 1:640-641, 1957
415. Kline IK, Kline TS, Saphir O: Myocarditis in senescence. *Am Heart J* 65:446-457, 1963
416. Chatterjee SS, Thakre MW: Fiedler's myocarditis: report of a fatal case following intramuscular injection of streptomycin. *Tubercle* 39:240-241, 1958
417. Barrett DA II, Dalldorf FG, Barnwell WH II, et al: Allergic giant cell myocarditis complicating tuberculosis chemotherapy. *Arch Pathol* 91:201-205, 1971
418. Schuchter LM, Hendricks CB, Holland KH, et al: Eosinophilic myocarditis associated with high-dose interleukin-2 therapy. *Am J Med* 88:439-440, 1990
419. Kragel AH, Travis WD, Steis RG, et al: Myocarditis or acute myocardial infarction associated with interleukin-2 therapy for cancer. *Cancer* 66:1513-1516, 1990
420. James FW, Kaplan S, Benzing G III: Cardiac complications following hydrocarbon ingestion. *Am J Dis Child* 121:431-433, 1971
421. Steiner MM: Syndromes of kerosene poisoning in children. *Am J Dis Child* 74:32-44, 1947
422. Zakhari S, Aviado DM: Cardiovascular toxicology of aerosol propellants, refrigerants, and related solvents. In *Cardiovascular Toxicology.* Edited by EW Van Stee. New York, Raven Press, 1982, pp 281-326
423. Aviado DM: Preclinical pharmacology and toxicology of halogenated solvents and propellants. In *Review of Inhalants: Euphoria to Dysfunction.* Edited by CW Sharp, ML Brehm. Washington, DC, US Department of Health, Education, and Welfare, 1977, pp 165-185
424. Anderson RF, Allensworth DC, deGroot WJ: Myocardial toxicity from carbon monoxide poisoning. *Ann Intern Med* 67:1172-1182, 1967
425. Stern FB, Halperin WE, Hornung RW, et al: Heart disease mortality among bridge and tunnel officers exposed to carbon monoxide. *Am J Epidemiol* 128:1276-1288, 1988
426. Corya BC, Black MJ, McHenry PL: Echocardiographic findings after acute carbon monoxide poisoning. *Br Heart J* 38:712-717, 1976
427. Orinius E: The late cardiac prognosis after acute carbon monoxide intoxication. *Acta Med Scand* 183:239-241, 1968
428. Glazener FS, Ellis JG, Johnson PK: Electrocardiographic findings with arsenic poisoning. *Calif Med* 109:158-162, August 1968
429. McKinstry WJ, Hickes JM: Emergency: arsine poisoning. *Arch Intern Med* 100:34-43, 1957
430. Kline TS: Myocardial changes in lead poisoning. *Am J Dis Child* 99:48-54, 1960
431. Freeman R: Reversible myocarditis due to chronic lead poisoning in childhood. *Arch Dis Child* 40:389-393, 1965
432. Talley RC, Linhart JW, Trevino AJ, et al: Acute elemental phosphorus poisoning in man: cardiovascular toxicity. *Am Heart J* 84:139-140, 1972
433. Dahhan SS, Orfaly H: Electrocardiographic changes in mercury poisoning. *Am J Cardiol* 14:178-183, 1964
434. Barborik M, Dusek J: Cardiomyopathy accompanying industrial cobalt exposure. *Br Heart J* 34:113-116, 1972
435. Roby DS, Fein AM, Bennett RH, et al: Cardiopulmonary effects of acute thallium poisoning. *Chest* 85:236-240, 1984
436. Karas JS, Stanbury JB: Fatal radiation syndrome from an accidental nuclear excursion. *N Engl J Med* 272:755-761, 1965
437. Stewart JR, Fajardo LF: Radiation-induced heart disease: an update. *Prog Cardiovasc Dis* 27:173-194, 1984
438. Kinsella TJ, Fraass BA, Glatstein E: Late effects of radiation therapy in the treatment of Hodgkin's disease. *Cancer Treat Rep* 66:991-1001, 1982
439. Applefeld MM, Slawson RG, Spicer KM, et al: Long-term cardiovascular evaluation of patients with Hodgkin's disease treated by thoracic mantle radiation therapy. *Cancer Treat Rep* 66:1003-1013, 1982
440. Gottdiener JS, Katin MJ, Borer JS, et al: Late cardiac effects of therapeutic mediastinal irradiation: assessment by echocardiography and radionuclide angiography. *N Engl J Med* 308:569-572, 1983
441. Kew MC, Tucker RBK, Bersohn I, et al: The heart in heatstroke. *Am Heart J* 77:324-335, 1969
442. Malamud N, Haymaker W, Custer RP: Heat stroke: a clinicopathologic study of 125 fatal cases. *Milit Surg* 99:397-449, 1946
443. Duguid H, Simpson RG, Stowers JM: Accidental hypothermia. *Lancet* 2:1213-1219, 1961
444. Read AE, Emslie-Smith D, Gouch KR, et al: Pancreatitis and accidental hypothermia. *Lancet* 2:1219-1221, 1961
445. Bawaskar HS: Diagnostic cardiac premonitory signs and symptoms of red scorpion sting. *Lancet* 1:552-554, 1982
446. Gueron M, Yaron R: Cardiovascular manifestations of severe scorpion sting: clinicopathologic correlations. *Chest* 57:156-162, 1970

447. Gueron M, Stern J, Cohen W: Severe myocardial damage and heart failure in scorpion sting: report of five cases. *Am J Cardiol* 19:719-726, 1967

448. Than-Than, Francis N, Tin-Nu-Swe, et al: Contribution of focal haemorrhage and microvascular fibrin deposition to fatal envenoming by Russell's viper (Vipera russeli siamensis) in Burma. *Acta Trop (Basel)* 46:23-38, 1989

449. Russell FE: Pharmacology of animal venoms. *Clin Pharmacol Ther* 8:849-873, 1967

450. Lefer AM, Curtis MT: Cardiotoxicity of naturally occurring animal peptides. In *Cardiovascular Toxicology.* Edited by EW Van Stee. New York, Raven Press, 1982, pp 221-258

451. Aravanis C, Ioannidis PJ, Ktenas J: Acute myocardial infarction and cerebrovascular accident in a young girl after viper bite. *Br Heart J* 47:500-503, 1982

452. Weitzman S, Margulis G, Lehmann E: Uncommon cardiovascular manifestations and high catecholamine levels due to "black widow" bite. *Am Heart J* 93:89-90, 1977

453. Levine HD: Acute myocardial infarction following wasp sting: report of two cases and critical survey of the literature. *Am Heart J* 91:365-374, 1976

454. Pearn JH: A case of tick paralysis with myocarditis. *Med J Aust* 1:629-630, 1966

CHAPTER

19

Cardiomyopathy and biopsy

B. Transvenous endomyocardial biopsy

William D. Edwards, M.D., and David R. Holmes, Jr., M.D.

ENDOMYOCARDIAL biopsy is a clinically safe procedure whereby a sample of cardiac muscle can be obtained nonsurgically from a living patient. It is useful for the diagnosis of acute cardiac transplant rejection and anthracycline cardiotoxicity and for the evaluation of myocarditis, unexplained arrhythmias, unexplained chest pain, cardiomyopathies, and secondary cardiac involvement by systemic diseases.[1,2] The biopsy tissue may be assessed by light or electron microscopy, immunofluorescent or immunoperoxidase studies, various histochemical and enzyme analyses, quantitative morphometric studies, or cultures for viruses, bacteria, or fungi.[1,2] The results of such studies may provide clinically useful information that is unobtainable by other conventional methods. Accordingly, endomyocardial biopsy may add a new dimension to the diagnosis and treatment of nonischemic myocardial diseases.

HISTORICAL BACKGROUND

The procurement of a sample of ventricular myocardium by transthoracic needle biopsy in the dog was described by Casten and Marsh[3] in 1953 and in human subjects, by Sutton and colleagues[4] in 1956. Shirey et al.[5] later published their experience with myocardial needle biopsies in 198 patients.

However, in 1962, Sakakibara and Konno[6] described a transvenous bioptome with which endomyocardial tissue could be obtained from the right ventricular apex. The bioptome has subsequently undergone several modifications in design.[7,8] Although this method of biopsy has been used extensively for the evaluation of acute cardiac transplant rejection, it has also gained acceptance for the evaluation of numerous primary and secondary myocardial diseases.

BIOPSY TECHNIQUE

Because of the stiffness of the bioptome, the pathway to the right ventricular apex should be short and relatively straight. Accordingly, the preferred entry site is the right internal jugular vein, as described in detail by Mason.[9] After the right side of the neck has been prepared and draped, the skin is locally anesthetized and the right internal jugular vein is entered with the use of standard percutaneous techniques. After placement of a venous sheath, the bioptome is advanced, under fluoroscopic visualization, across the tricuspid valve to the right ventricular apex.

Tissue is obtained from the septal surface to avoid perforation of the right ventricular free wall (Fig. 19B-1A). With each biopsy, the bioptome is removed and it is then reinserted for subsequent tissue procurement. After removal of the venous sheath and bioptome at the end of the procedure, local hemostasis is obtained by direct pressure and by elevation of the patient's head. Adequate hemostasis is essential to avoid hematomas; these may organize and form fibrous tissue, which would hinder future biopsies.

If the right internal jugular vein is not accessible, the right subclavian vein or the femoral veins may be used.[9] However, from these sites, the bioptome may be more difficult to manipulate and to orient properly in the right ventricle. In such circumstances, the left ventricle may be biopsied, as described by Mason[9] and by Brooksby et al.[10] After cannulation of the femoral artery, a long sheath is advanced retrogradely across the aortic valve and into the left ventricle; through this, the bioptome can be positioned within the ventricular chamber. Similarly, the brachial artery may be used if the femoral arteries are not accessible.[11] In addition, left ventricular biopsies may be performed via the femoral vein and an atrial transseptal approach.[11]

With either the right or the left ventricular approach, multiple biopsy specimens may be obtained. The biopsy may be performed as an independent procedure or it may be done at the time of cardiac catheterization or electrophysiologic study. It may also be performed as an outpatient procedure.

COMPLICATIONS

Endomyocardial biopsy of either ventricle is a very safe procedure. The incidence of complications was 1.7% in

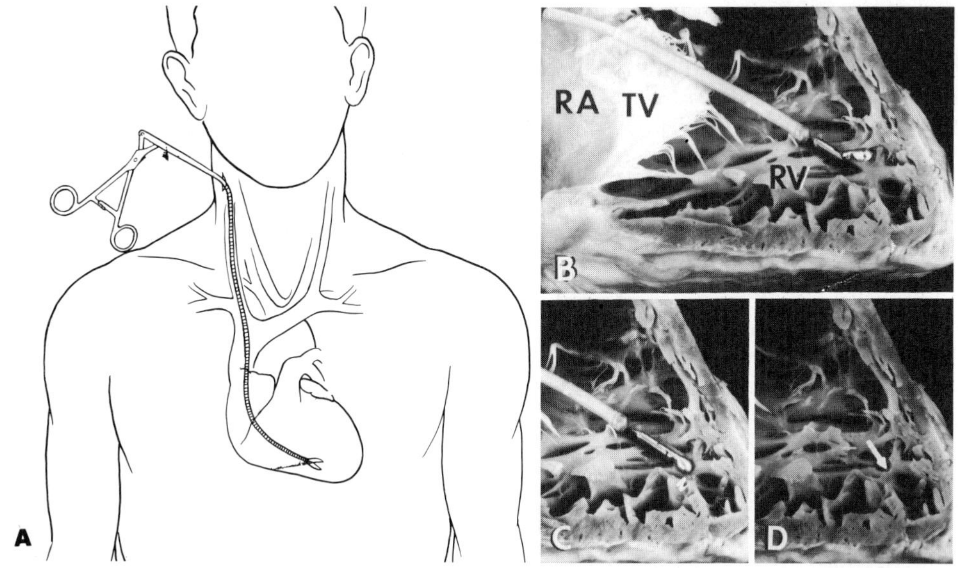

Fig 19B-1 Right ventricular endomyocardial biopsy. **A,** schematic diagram showing ease of access to right ventricular apex via right internal jugular vein. **B** to **D,** autopsy specimen used to simulate biopsy procurement, with bioptome jaws opened around a trabecula carnea **(B),** jaws closed **(C),** and appearance of biopsy site *(arrow)* **(D).** *RA,* right atrium; *RV,* right ventricle; *TV,* tricuspid valve. (From Nippoldt TB, Edwards WD, Holmes DR Jr, et al: Right ventricular endomyocardial biopsy: clinicopathologic correlates in 100 consecutive patients. *Mayo Clin Proc* 57:407-418, 1982. By permission, Mayo Foundation.)

2,337 biopsies reviewed by Richardson[12] and less than 1% in more than 4,000 biopsies performed at Stanford.[13] As one's experience increases, the morbidity from this procedure generally decreases. Deaths attributable to endomyocardial biopsy are extremely rare.

Cardiac biopsy, therefore, compares favorably with liver and renal biopsies. Liver biopsies have a reported morbidity of 5.9%[14] and a mortality of 0.015% to 0.17%.[15] Renal biopsies may have a morbidity of 8.1%[16] and a mortality of less than 0.1%.[17]

Among the potential complications of endomyocardial biopsy, perforation of the *right* ventricular free wall is uncommon. In 2,337 biopsies reviewed by Richardson,[12] it occurred in only nine (0.4%) but accounted for nearly one-quarter of the complications; operation was required in six of the nine to control the resultant hemopericardium. Right ventricular perforation during biopsy procedures occurs somewhat more frequently in children than in adults.[18] Although the left ventricle is thicker than the right, the true apex of the left ventricle is only 1 to 2 mm thick, even in hypertrophied hearts,[19] and perforation of the *left* ventricle by the bioptome potentially may occur.

Other complications of endomyocardial biopsy include right pneumothorax, vasovagal reaction, atrial or ventricular arrhythmias, infection, and transient nerve palsies.[1,2,9,12,19-21] Conceivably, friable intracavitary masses such as vegetations, mural thrombi, or neoplasms could become dislodged by the bioptome. Also, fresh thrombus may form on the instrument and become dislodged during the procedure; such embolization is a rare cause of systemic symptoms after left ventricular biopsy.[12] Meticulous attention to vessel entry, bioptome placement, specimen procurement, and adequate hemostasis will minimize these complications. Successful biopsy procedures are attainable in 95% to 100% of patients, including children.[18,22]

TISSUE PROCUREMENT AND PROCESSING

In the right ventricle, tissue is generally obtained from the trabeculae carneae rather than from the septum per se (see Fig 19B-1,B to D), whereas in the left ventricle actual septal myocardium is obtained. Since these 1- to 3-mm tissue specimens represent endocardium and subjacent myocardium, tissue more than 5 mm below the endocardial surface is generally not accessible to the bioptome.

As a result, sampling error may be significant, particularly in such cardiac disorders as hypertrophic cardiomyopathy, in which myocyte disarray tends to be limited to the core of the ventricular septum.[23] Similarly, sampling error may be difficult to avoid in such disorders as cardiac sarcoidosis, in which basal involvement is generally greater than apical.[24,25] Sampling error also may play an important role in the interpretation of processes such as lymphocytic myocarditis that are mild and focal in distribution or involve regions of the heart inaccessible to the bioptome.[26,27]

To increase the likelihood of a truly representative biopsy and to decrease the likelihood of sampling error, it is recommended that at least five specimens be obtained, particularly for the evaluation of possible lymphocytic myocarditis.[26,27] Since sampling error may still occur and may lead to false-negative diagnoses, only positive findings should be considered diagnostic; negative reports do not necessarily exclude the clinical diagnosis.

Right ventricular biopsies are generally preferred for the evaluation of diffuse myocardial disorders, such as idiopathic dilated cardiomyopathy, and for processes that affect primarily the right ventricle, such as carcinoid heart disease. Similarly, left ventricular biopsy is preferred for the assessment of disorders that involve primarily the left heart, such as endocardial fibroelastosis. Occasionally, biventricular biopsies may be useful. Finally, in the evaluation of a diffuse myocardial process, the presence of a second cardiac disorder in one chamber may necessitate biopsy of the other ventricle. The right ventricle is the proper chamber for biopsy when left ventricular mural thrombus is present, because of the possibility of biopsy-induced systemic embolization.

Biopsy specimens should be removed *gently* from the bioptome; rough handling by forceps may result in severe crush artifacts that render the tissue uninterpretable. For light microscopy, tissue should be fixed in 10% neutral buffered formalin and processed either for paraffin embedding and sectioning (4 to 5 μm in thickness) or for plastic embedding and sectioning (1 or 2 μm thick).[2]

Each glass slide should contain at least five sections of all specimens. Four slides should be prepared (two stained with hematoxylin and eosin, one stained for iron, and one stained for connective tissue (trichrome or sulfated Alcian blue).[2,9] If amyloid is suspected clinically, an additional battery of stains is recommended (sulfated Alcian blue, methyl violet, Congo red, and thioflavine T), since amyloid may stain quite variably.[2]

If special studies are indicated, additional biopsy specimens should be obtained. In certain storage diseases, extra specimens should be fixed in glutaraldehyde for transmission electron microscopy. Moreover, for the evaluation of anthracycline cardiotoxicity, *all* tissue should be processed for electron microscopy.[1] Although significant ultrastructural abnormalities are common in other cardiac disorders, they usually are not diagnostically specific.[2] In suspected myocarditis and some cases of dilated cardiomyopathy, viral cultures may seem appropriate; however, such cultures are rarely positive, even when positive stool cultures are obtained.[28,29] Furthermore, in suspected myocarditis, extra tissue may be frozen fresh for immunofluorescent studies, and some investigators have reported immunoglobulin deposition in cardiac biopsy material in this setting.[30]

Artifacts are commonly encountered in endomyocardial biopsy specimens and have been described in detail both for light microscopy[1,2] and for transmission electron microscopy.[31]

In the remainder of this chapter, the expected biopsy findings will be presented for various *clinical* diagnostic entities. Since response to injury in the heart is limited in scope, the morphological findings at biopsy are often common to several different clinical disorders and, therefore, may appear rather nonspecific.

BIOPSY FINDINGS IN VARIOUS CLINICAL DIAGNOSTIC ENTITIES

Cardiac allograft rejection

Right ventricular endomyocardial biopsy is the best method for evaluating episodic acute cardiac allograft rejection, particularly among patients receiving cyclosporine, in whom the clinical features of acute rejection are often masked.[1,32,33] The histologic alterations are diffuse, and there are no appreciable differences in severity between subendocardium and subepicardium, right ventricle and left ventricle, or septum and free wall.[32,33] Although four or more specimens are recommended, reliable results have been reported with only one or two biopsy specimens.[1,2]

Acute rejection is associated with an infiltration of T lymphocytes and may be graded histologically.[32,33] Although several classification systems have been proposed, the standardized working formulation published in 1990 is currently recommended[34-38] (Table 19B-1). According to this system, the first biopsy tissue obtained during an episode of acute rejection is designated as mild, moderate, or severe (grades 1-4), and subsequent specimens are interpreted as ongoing, resolving, or resolved rejection, by comparison with the most recent biopsy slides. For reviewing older slides that have been graded by another classification system, a comparison with the working formulation may be helpful (Table 19B-2).

The presence of a mononuclear inflammatory infiltrate, visible at low magnification, is the most reliable indicator of acute rejection,[39] and most diagnoses can be made by evaluating slides stained with hematoxylin and eosin alone (Fig 19B-2,A). Inflammation in an area of fibrosis, indicative of healing at a previous biopsy site, should not be misinterpreted as acute or resolving rejection[40,41] (Fig 19B-2,B). Although myocyte necrosis is emphasized as the important distinguishing feature between mild and moderate rejection,[34] other authors have found necrosis to be uncommon in biopsy specimens.[39,42]

Mild infiltrates behave unpredictably and may resolve spontaneously or progress to moderate rejection.[39,43] Although moderate rejection is reversible, severe cardiac allograft rejection is often difficult to control clinically. Like severe rejection, the presence of arteriolar vasculitis or occlusive endothelial proliferation correlates with a high risk for graft dysfunction or failure[44-46] (Fig 19B-2,C).

Among patients treated with cyclosporine, acute rejection develops and resolves more slowly than in those with other forms of immunosuppression.[47,48] Even in the absence of rejection episodes, sparse lymphocytic infiltrates and fine pericellular fibrosis may be observed in biopsy tissues.[1,49] A dense endocardial lymphoplasmacytic infiltrate has also been reported in cyclosporine-treated patients and is referred to as the Quilty effect, after the surname of the first patient in whom it was detected (Fig 19B-2,D). This should not be misinterpreted as acute rejection (if the myocardial interstitium is also free of infiltrates) or as lymphoma.

Infections in cardiac transplant recipients are common and are often pulmonary in nature.[50] However, the heart may also harbor organisms, and fungi, parasites, and viral

Table 19B-1 Standardized nomenclature for grading cardiac allograft rejection

Grade	Nomenclature	Microscopic features
0	No rejection	No evidence of rejection, or equivocal findings of rejection
1A	Focal mild rejection	Focal sparse perivascular or interstitial lymphocytic infiltrates without myocyte necrosis
1B	Diffuse mild rejection	Diffuse sparse perivascular or interstitial lymphocytic infiltrates without myocyte necrosis
2	Focal moderate rejection	Solitary circumscribed lymphocytic infiltrate (eosinophils optional) with myocyte damage
3A	Multifocal moderate rejection	Multifocal aggressive lymphocytic infiltrates (eosinophils optional) with myocyte damage
3B	Diffuse moderate rejection	Diffuse aggressive lymphocytic infiltrate with eosinophils and myocyte necrosis, without hemorrhage
4	Severe rejection	Diffuse aggressive infiltrate of lymphocytes, eosinophils, and neutrophils, with myocyte necrosis, vasculitis, edema, and hemorrhage
–	Humoral rejection	Positive immunofluorescence, vasculitis, or severe edema without cellular infiltrate
–	Ongoing rejection	Same grade as or higher grade than previous biopsy tissues
–	Resolving rejection	Lesser grade than previous biopsy tissues
0	Resolved rejection	Grade 0, after evidence of rejection in previous biopsy tissues

From Hauck AJ, Edwards WD: Histopathologic examination of tissues obtained by endomyocardial biopsy. In *Cardiac Biopsy.* Edited by RE Fowles. Mount Kisco, New York, Futura Publishing, 1992, pp 95-153. By permission.

Table 19B-2 Comparison of five classifications of acute cardiac allograft rejection

Classification	Designation of grade of severity			
Billingham[34]	None	Mild	Moderate	Severe
Rose and Uys[35]	0	0.5-2.0	2.5-4.0	4.5-15.0
McAllister et al.[36]	0	1-3	4-8	9-10
Kemnitz et al.[37]	A0	A1, A2	A3	A4
Billingham et al.[38]	0	1A, 1B	2, 3A, 3B	4

inclusions have each been reported in biopsy specimens.[1] Accordingly, the pathologist must evaluate such tissue not only for acute rejection but also for possible infections, such as toxoplasmosis and cytomegalovirus.

Myocarditis

Myocarditis represents a nonischemic inflammatory or immunologic disorder of the myocardium. It is characterized microscopically by an inflammatory infiltrate and by nonischemic injury or necrosis of adjacent myocytes, according to the Dallas criteria.[26,27] Primary forms are idiopathic, whereas secondary forms have an identifiable apparent cause such as coxsackievirus or drug hypersensitivity.

Studies utilizing endomyocardial biopsy findings have verified the diverse clinical presentations of myocarditis, including unexplained heart failure, life-threatening arrhythmias, and chest pain.[1,51] Furthermore, other myocardial disorders such as idiopathic dilated cardiomyopathy and acute myocardial infarction may have similar clinical presentations and thereby mimic myocarditis.[1,51,52] Consequently, false-positive and false-negative clinical diagnoses are expected and occur relatively commonly.

Moreover, biopsy interpretations also may be in error. False-positive histopathologic diagnoses may result from misinterpretation of noninflammatory interstitial cells as lymphocytes and from the pressure of strong clinical bias.[51] Sampling error appears to be the most common cause of false-negative tissue diagnoses. Although this may be minimized by procuring 5 to 10 biopsy specimens, false-negative results still occur in about 40% of patients.[53,54] Accordingly, only positive biopsy findings should be considered diagnostic; negative findings do not necessarily rule out the clinical diagnosis of myocarditis, due to the possibility of sampling error.

The aforementioned features indicate that discrepancies between clinical and biopsy tissue diagnosis are expected, and indeed this is documented in the literature. The clinical diagnosis of myocarditis has been substantiated by endomyocardial biopsy in only 17% to 29% of patients; in the remaining 71% to 83% of cases, the biopsy either was normal by light microscopy or, more commonly, had chronic features (hypertrophy and fibrosis) that suggested an evolving cardiomyopathy.[1,51] From another perspective, in one series,[55] only 11% of the biopsy diagnoses of myocarditis had been made in patients with a clinical diagnosis of myocarditis, and 89% had been

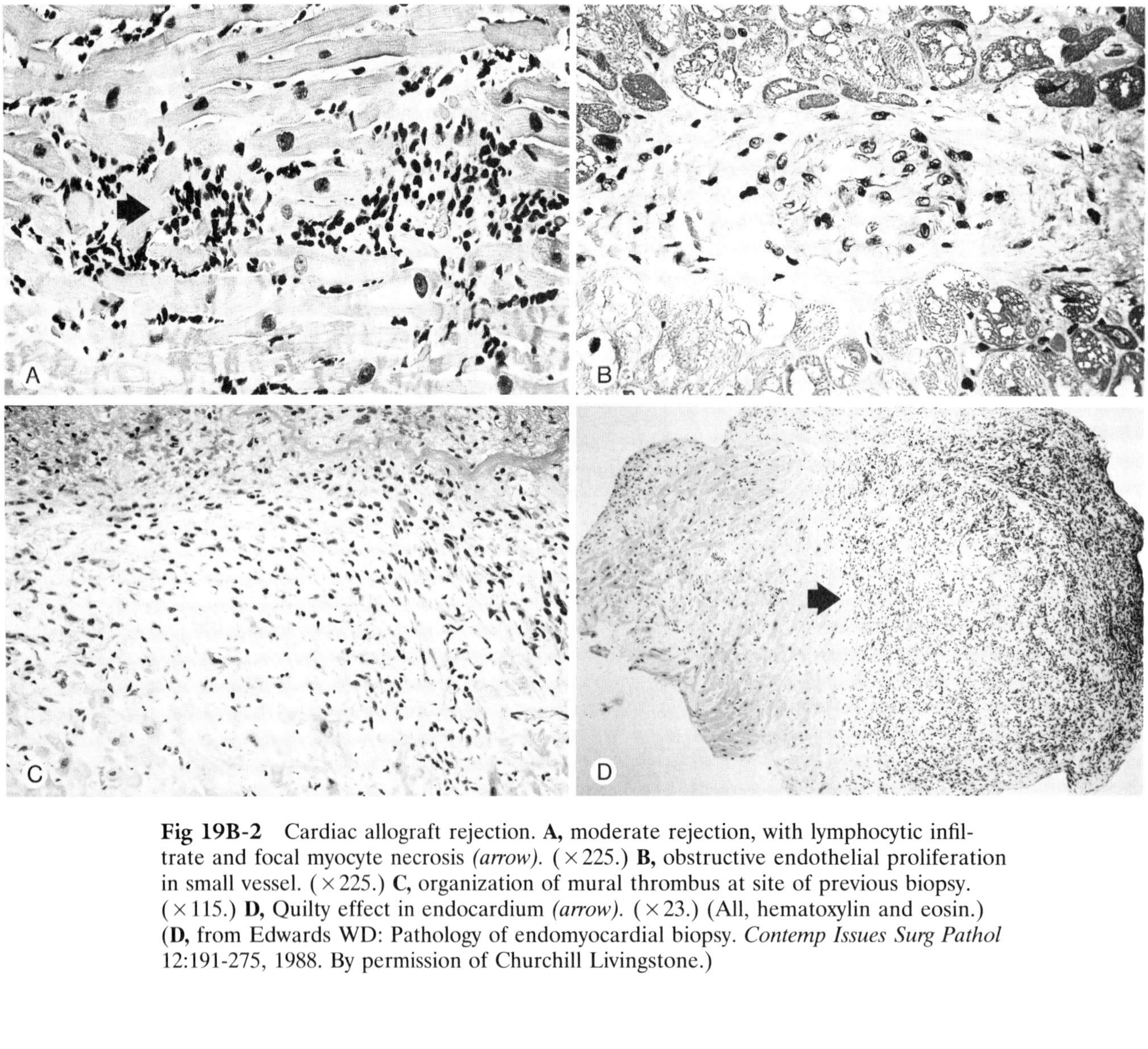

Fig 19B-2 Cardiac allograft rejection. **A,** moderate rejection, with lymphocytic infiltrate and focal myocyte necrosis *(arrow).* (×225.) **B,** obstructive endothelial proliferation in small vessel. (×225.) **C,** organization of mural thrombus at site of previous biopsy. (×115.) **D,** Quilty effect in endocardium *(arrow).* (×23.) (All, hematoxylin and eosin.) (**D,** from Edwards WD: Pathology of endomyocardial biopsy. *Contemp Issues Surg Pathol* 12:191-275, 1988. By permission of Churchill Livingstone.)

made in those without clinical suspicion of an inflammatory process.

By light microscopy, myocarditis is characterized by a leukocytic infiltrate, nonischemic myocardial cell injury, and, eventually, healing by resolution or by organization with fibrosis (Fig 19B-3).[26,27,51] The nature of the leukocytic infiltrate may shed light on the underlying cause (Table 19B-3), and the extent of injury (that is, myocyte damage and endocardial or interstitial fibrosis) may be important prognostically. Thus, in reports of endomyocardial biopsies, these histopathologic features should be described and designated as mild, moderate, or severe (Table 19B-4).[26,27,51] Because many drugs (see Table 19B-4) may be responsible for the different histopathologic types of myocarditis,[56-58] a thorough drug history should be recorded from all patients with biopsy-proved myocarditis.

In the past, without specific guidelines for evaluating myocarditis in biopsy tissues, a high rate of diagnostic disagreement occurred among pathologists.[59] Two separate sets of criteria were proposed—one based on lymphocyte counts[60] and another based on terminology for glomerulonephritis[61]—but neither was universally accepted.

In 1984, at the request of clinicians who were proposing a multicenter myocarditis trial,[62] eight pathologists convened in Dallas to formulate standardized guidelines for the biopsy diagnosis of myocarditis for use in the trial. The results of this and subsequent meetings culminated in publication of the so-called Dallas criteria,[26,27] and greater uniformity of diagnoses has now been achieved among pathologists using these guidelines in the multicenter myocarditis trial.[63] According to the Dallas criteria, myocarditis is defined microscopically by the presence of an inflammatory infiltrate *and* by nonischemic injury or necrosis of adjacent myocytes.[26,27]

Only three diagnostic categories exist for a patient's *first* biopsy: myocarditis, borderline myocarditis, and no myocarditis[26,27] (Table 19B-5). If an inflammatory infiltrate is present but is *not* associated with myocyte

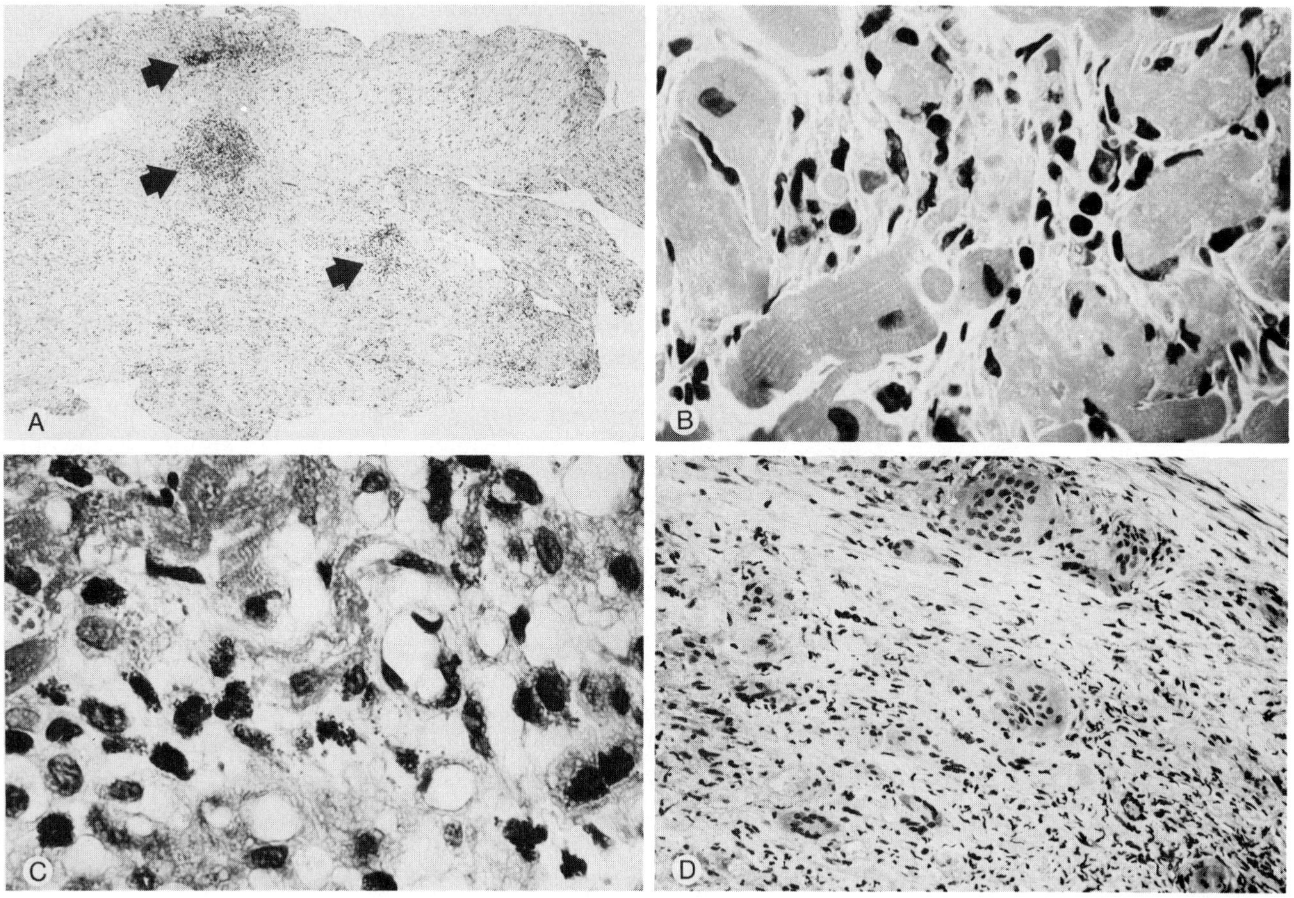

Fig 19B-3 Myocarditis. **A** and **B,** idiopathic lymphocytic myocarditis. Low-power view (**A,** *arrows*) shows focal nature of infiltrates. (×23.) High-power view (**B**) demonstrates myocyte injury and necrosis adjacent to lymphocytes. (×550.) **C,** eosinophilic myocarditis is associated with degranulation of eosinophils and myocyte necrosis. (×225.) **D,** giant cell myocarditis in a patient with cardiac sarcoidosis exhibits extensive replacement fibrosis in addition to inflammatory infiltrate. (×115.) (All, hematoxylin and eosin.) (**B,** from Edwards WD: Pathology of endomyocardial biopsy. *Contemp Issues Surg Pathol* 12:191-275, 1988. By permission of Churchill Livingstone. **C** and **D,** from Edwards WD, Wold LE: The cardiovascular system. In *Surgical Pathology.* Vol 1. Second edition. Edited by WF Coulson. Philadelphia, JB Lippincott Company, 1988, pp 462-505. By permission.)

injury, even after additional microscopic slides have been prepared and evaluated, borderline myocarditis is diagnosed, and rebiopsy may be considered. Use of adjectives with a temporal meaning (such as acute, subacute, chronic, ongoing, and resolving) is considered inappropriate because this implies that comparison has been made with previously obtained biopsy specimens.

In contrast, *subsequent* biopsy tissues should be evaluated relative to the most recently available previous tissues and compared with regard to severity. Three diagnoses are possible and include ongoing (or persistent), resolving (or healing), and resolved (or healed) myocarditis[26,27] (see Table 19B-5). Thus, the terminology of the Dallas criteria for myocarditis resembles that for the evaluation of cardiac allograft rejection (compare Tables 19B-1 and 19B-5).

However, despite similarities in terminology, myocarditis and rejection do not necessarily share the same patterns of intensity and distribution. For example, in contrast to acute rejection, lymphocytic myocarditis is usually mild, spotty, and uneven in its distribution.[53] Moreover, myocarditis may be limited to regions of the heart inaccessible to the bioptome, such as the subepicardium, ventricular free walls, and core of the ventricular septum. These features tend to maximize the likelihood of sampling error and false-negative results.[53,54]

With a false-negative rate that may be as high as 37% to 58%, based on the number of biopsy samples and the ventricle of origin,[53,54] one may question whether it is wise even to perform endomyocardial biopsy procedures in patients thought to have myocarditis clinically. This is particularly relevant for patients with lymphocytic myo-

Table 19B-3 Causes of various histopathologic forms of myocarditis in biopsy tissues

Lymphocytic	Eosinophilic
Idiopathic	Idiopathic
Viral syndrome	Hypereosinophilia
Polymyositis	Restrictive cardiomyopathy
Sarcoidosis	Asthmatic bronchitis
Lyme disease	Churg-Strauss syndrome
Kawasaki disease*	Parasitic infestations
AIDS†	Drug hypersensitivity
Mycoplasma pneumoniae	
Drug toxicity	
Neutrophilic or mixed	**Giant cell or granulomatous**
Idiopathic	Idiopathic
Infection	Sarcoidosis
Infarction	Infective
Drug toxicity	Rheumatoid
	Rheumatic
	Drug hypersensitivity

*Mucocutaneous lymph node syndrome.
†Acquired immunodeficiency syndrome.

carditis in whom the efficacy of immunosuppressive therapy is not yet known.

It is recognized, however, that patients with a clinical diagnosis of myocarditis may in fact have other illnesses that mimic the inflammatory state.[1,51,52] An evolving dilated cardiomyopathy is probably the most commonly encountered "look-alike," and its biopsy features (hypertrophy and fibrosis) allow differentiation not only from myocarditis but also from false-negative tissues in patients who actually do have myocarditis elsewhere in their hearts. Similarly, acute myocardial infarction was identified in biopsy tissues from one patient who had a clinical diagnosis of myocarditis.[51]

Thus, the rationale for endomyocardial biopsy in patients with clinically suspected myocarditis is not only to diagnose inflammatory disease but also to exclude other disorders that may mimic myocarditis. From this perspective, biopsy procedures are justified in this group of patients.

Another question that arises concerns the fate of patients who have a biopsy diagnosis of myocarditis. In some cases, inflammation remits and ventricular function returns to normal, whether or not the patient receives immunosuppressive therapy.[59] In others, however, the disease progresses to chronic heart failure and a state indistinguishable from dilated cardiomyopathy.[64] Among

Table 19B-4 Possible effects of various drugs on the heart*

Hypersensitivity myocarditis	Toxic myocarditis	Dilated cardiomyopathy
Acetazolamide	Amphetamines	Amphetamines
p-Aminosalicylic acid	Antihypertensives	Anthracyclines
Amitriptyline	Antimony	Chloroquine
Amphotericin B	Arsenicals	Cobalt
Carbamazepine	Barbiturates	Cocaine
Chloramphenicol	Caffeine	Ephedrine
Diphenylhydantoin	Catecholamines	Ethanol
Diphtheria toxin	Cocaine	Lithium
Horse serum	Cyclophosphamide	
Hydrochlorothiazide	Emetine	**Endocardial fibrosis**
Indomethacin	5-Fluorouracil	Anthracyclines
Isoniazid	Immunosuppressives	Busulfan
Methyldopa	Lithium	Ergotamine
Penicillins	Paraquat	Mercury
Phenindione	Phenothiazines	Methysergide
Phenylbutazone	Plasmocid	Serotonin
Smallpox vaccine	Quinidine	
Spironolactone	Rapeseed oil	**Myocardial fibrosis**
Streptomycin	Theophylline	Cyclosporine†
Sulfonamides		
Sulfonylureas		
Tetanus toxoid		
Tetracycline		

*Information from references 56, 57, and 58.
†In transplanted hearts only.

Table 19B-5 Diagnosis of myocarditis by endomyocardial biopsy

First biopsy

Myocarditis, with or without fibrosis
Borderline myocarditis (rebiopsy may be indicated)
No myocarditis

Subsequent biopsies

Ongoing (persistent) myocarditis, with or without fibrosis
Resolving (healing) myocarditis, with or without fibrosis
Resolved (healed) myocarditis, with or without fibrosis

Inflammation

Type: lymphocytic, eosinophilic, neutrophilic, giant cell, granulomatous, mixed
Distribution: focal, confluent, diffuse
Extent: mild, moderate, severe

Fibrosis

Type: perivascular, pericellular, replacement
Distribution: interstitial, endocardial
Extent: mild, moderate, severe

Modified from Aretz HT, Billingham ME, Edwards WD, Factor SM, Fallon JT, Fenoglio JJ Jr, Olsen EGJ, Schoen FJ: Myocarditis: a histopathologic definition and classification. *Am J Cardiovasc Pathol* 1:3-14, 1986

63 patients in three studies in whom a clinical diagnosis of acute heart failure and a biopsy diagnosis of myocarditis were made, severe chronic heart failure developed in 40% to 52%.[65-67] Thus, dilated cardiomyopathy develops in a substantial number of patients who have biopsy-proved myocarditis.

Unexplained arrhythmias

The sudden development of ventricular or supraventricular arrhythmias can represent the first clinical manifestation of an underlying disorder of the myocardium or cardiac conduction system. Such arrhythmias may present clinically as syncope or cardiac arrest (so-called resuscitated sudden death) and can remain unexplained even after cardiac catheterization and electrophysiologic studies. Hence, an endomyocardial biopsy may be indicated.

Most commonly, arrhythmias result from underlying myocardial disorders, such as ischemic heart disease, cardiomyopathy, and myocarditis, and are associated with an abnormal myocardium.[52,68] In other cases, arrhythmias are the cause of myocardial dysfunction (rather than the result), and successful treatment of the rhythm disturbance is attended by improved ventricular performance.[69-71] In still others, with conduction system disease or idiopathic arrhythmias, the myocardium remains normal in structure and function. Arrhythmias may also be associated with mitral valve prolapse or rare diseases, such as arrhythmogenic right ventricular dysplasia and histiocytoid cardiomyopathy.[55,72-75]

Consequently, endomyocardial biopsy findings are variable among patients with unexplained arrhythmias.[72,76-80] In some, the biopsy tissues appear normal. In others, the most commonly observed abnormalities are myocyte hypertrophy and interstitial fibrosis. Although these are chronic and nonspecific alterations, they may reflect an underlying cardiomyopathic state. Less commonly, biopsy specimens exhibit lymphocytic or giant cell myocarditis. For patients with arrhythmogenic right ventricular dysplasia, excessive interstitial adipose tissue has been reported, although hypertrophy and fibrosis also are usually present.[72,80]

Among 27 patients with unexplained arrhythmias reported from the Mayo Clinic, 55% had biopsy tissues that were either normal or nearly so, whereas 30% had chronic features suggestive of cardiomyopathy, and 15% had clinically unsuspected lymphocytic myocarditis.[55] The 27 patients included 7 with mitral valve prolapse, of whom 1 had myocarditis and 2 had changes consistent with cardiomyopathy.

Unexplained chest pain

In Western countries, chest pain due to cardiac disease is most commonly the result of obstructive coronary atherosclerosis. However, it may also occur in patients with aortic valve disease, myocarditis, pericarditis, and even the cardiomyopathies and infiltrative processes. When cardiac pain develops in patients with angiographically normal coronary arteries and no evidence of coronary artery spasm, endomyocardial biopsy tissues may be obtained and are often abnormal.[1,2,81,82]

Myocyte hypertrophy and interstitial fibrosis are the most commonly observed features.[81] These chronic and nonspecific alterations may be indicative of an evolving cardiomyopathy. Myocarditis is also frequently accompanied by chest pain[64] and may be detected in biopsy specimens, although the possibility of sampling error should be borne in mind.[53,54] Rarely, amyloid deposition in small intramural coronary vessels causes sufficient obstruction to produce myocardial ischemia and chest pain.[83,84]

Also, rarely, acute myocardial infarction may be misdiagnosed, usually as myocarditis, and the patients undergo endomyocardial biopsy.[51] In this situation, coagulative necrosis is likely to be observed, particularly if tissues are biopsied from the left ventricle. The endocardial defect caused by the biopsy procedure may allow tearing and eventual rupture of subjacent infarcted myocardium. Thus, before a left ventricular biopsy is performed in a patient with unexplained chest pain, the possibility of acute myocardial infarction must be ruled out.

Dilated cardiomyopathy

The most prevalent type of cardiomyopathy in the United States is the dilated form, accounting for 90% to 95% of cases.[52] In contrast, the hypertrophic form represents only 2% to 6%, and restrictive disease is the least common

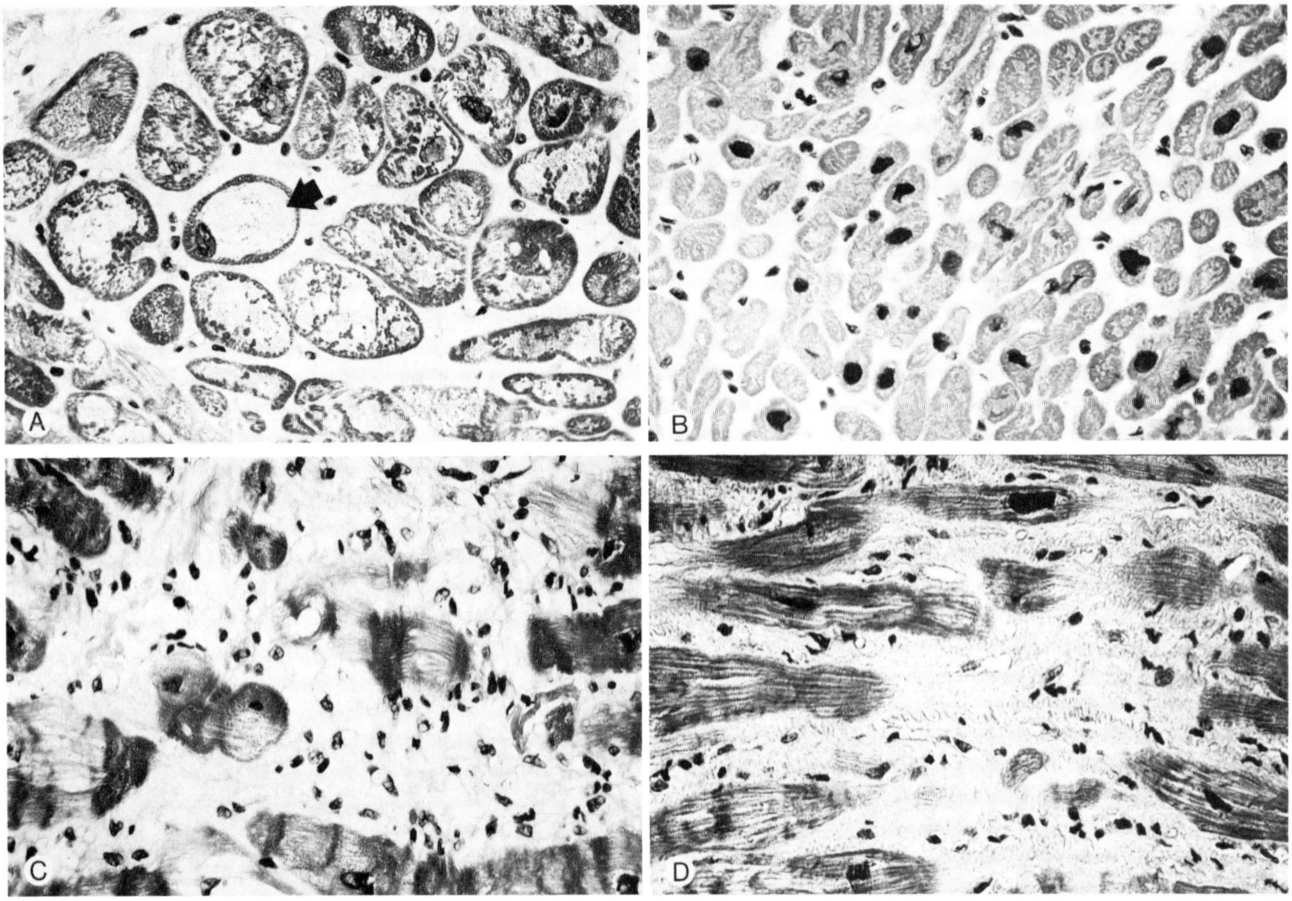

Fig 19B-4 Dilated cardiomyopathy. **A** and **B,** myocyte hypertrophy. Cells also exhibit focal loss of sarcoplasmic contractile elements (**A,** *arrow*) and attenuation, or stretching, due to cardiac dilatation (**B**). **C** and **D,** interstitial fibrosis. Biopsy tissues are involved by focal noninflammatory interstitial proliferation (**C**) and by patchy collagen deposition (**D**). (All, hematoxylin and eosin; ×225.) (**A** and **B,** from Edwards WD: Cardiomyopathies. *Hum Pathol* 18:625-635, 1987. By permission of WB Saunders Company. **C,** from Edwards WD, Wold LE: The cardiovascular system. In *Surgical Pathology.* Vol 1. Second edition. Edited by WF Coulson. Philadelphia, JB Lippincott Company, 1988, pp 462-505. By permission.)

form of all. Worldwide, however, these relative frequencies vary with geographic location, climate, and the prevalence of associated features, such as chronic alcoholism and peripheral eosinophilia. Although all three forms of cardiomyopathy represent distinct entities both clinically and in hearts at autopsy, their microscopic features in cardiac biopsy specimens are remarkably similar. This is true for children and adults.[19,52]

In idiopathic dilated cardiomyopathy, the light and electron microscopic findings are nonspecific and quite variable in severity.[1,2,52,55,85-89] Myocyte hypertrophy and interstitial fibrosis represent the most commonly observed lesions in biopsy tissues. Hypertrophy is often accompanied by cellular attenuation (or stretching), sarcoplasmic degenerative changes (vacuolization and loss of contractile elements), and nuclear alterations (enlargement, hyperchromicity, and irregularity in shape) (Fig 19B-4,A and B).

Interstitial fibrosis exhibits several patterns—pericellular, perivascular, and patchy or replacement types. Young fibrosis is characterized by proliferation of plump fibroblasts and other noninflammatory interstitial cells (not to be mistaken for myocarditis) and by deposition of more glycosaminoglycans than collagen (not to be mistaken for interstitial edema) (Fig 19B-4,C). In contrast, old fibrosis tends to be less cellular and to be associated with dense collagen and occasional small clusters of lymphocytes (Fig 19B-4,D). Pigmented macrophages in areas of fibrosis occur more often with ischemic heart disease than with the cardiomyopathies. In some patients, endocardial fibrosis may be prominent.

Some investigators have reported a good correlation between the severity of cardiac dysfunction and such biopsy abnormalities as hypertrophy and fibrosis,[90,91] whereas others have not.[81] Ultrastructurally, the extent to which myocyte contractile elements are lost, as determined by quantitative morphometry, appears to correlate well with prognosis.[92-95]

Table 19B-6 Frequency of lymphocytic myocarditis in endomyocardial biopsy tissue from 3,271 patients with unexplained heart failure or idiopathic dilated cardiomyopathy: summary of 30 reports

Reference	Year	Myocarditis	
		Number	%
Rose et al.[100]	1984	0/76	0
Baandrup et al.[81]	1981	0/68	0
Mason et al.[30]	1980	10/>400	2
Cassling et al.[105]	1985	2/80	3
Müller et al.[106]	1985	2/68	3
Dec et al.[67]	1988	20/637	3*
Bouhour et al.[112]	1988	4/91	4*
Chow et al.[113]	1988	4/90	4*
Popma et al.[114]	1989	3/61	5*
Noda[97]	1980	4/75	5
Edwards et al.[60]	1982	5/89	6
Kunkel et al.[96]	1978	4/66	6
Unverferth et al.[99]	1983	4/60	7
O'Connell et al.[101]	1984	5/68	7
Das et al.[98]	1981	1/12	8
Salvi et al.[115]	1989	38/420	9*
Obrador et al.[116]	1989	3/30	10*
Nippoldt et al.[55]	1982	4/34	12
Latham et al.[117]	1989	7/52	13*
Hosenpud et al.[107]	1985	6/38	16
Daly et al.[102]	1984	12/69	17
Ruzyllo and Rosnowski[108]	1985	12/69	17
Anderson et al.[111]	1987	14/79	18*
Mortensen et al.[109]	1985	12/65	18
Hobbs et al.[118]	1989	34/162	21
Fenoglio et al.[61]	1983	34/135	25
Parrillo et al.[103]	1984	19/74	26
Bolte and Ludwig[119]	1984	18/41	44†
Zee-Cheng et al.[104]	1984	22/35	63‡
Dec et al.[110]	1985	18/27	67§
Total		321/3,271	10

*Dallas criteria used for diagnosis; total: 93/1,460 = 6%.
†Represents only cases with suspected viral myocarditis.
‡Using Dallas criteria, probably 4 (12%) have myocarditis.
§Represents only cases of *acute* heart failure.
From Edwards WD: Endomyocardial biopsy and cardiomyopathy. *Cardiovasc Rev Rep* 11 no. 7:26-43, 1990.

Myocarditis, as defined by the Dallas criteria,[26,27] may be observed in endomyocardial biopsy tissue from some patients with idiopathic dilated cardiomyopathy. Among 30 studies in which the frequency of myocarditis was determined in biopsy tissues from 3,271 patients with unexplained heart failure or dilated cardiomyopathy, 321 patients (10%) had myocarditis[30,55,59,61,67,81,96-118] (Table 19B-6). Although the frequency ranged from 0 to 67% in these studies, this wide variance is misleading. In 24 of the 30, the frequency was less than 20%. Furthermore, in eight investigations in which the Dallas criteria were used, myocarditis cumulatively involved 93 (6%) of the 1,460 cases, and its prevalence ranged only from 3% to 18% (see Table 19B-6).

The three studies in which myocarditis occurred in more than 40% of the cases are readily explained. The report by Dec et al.[110] was limited exclusively to patients with *acute* heart failure, in whom a diagnosis of myocarditis is expected more often than among *chronic* cases. Similarly, the study by Bolte and Ludwig[119] involved patients thought to have viral myocarditis. In the study by Zee-Cheng et al.,[104] it is likely that only 4 patients, rather than 22, would have qualified as having myocarditis if the Dallas criteria (which were not available when the study was published) could now be applied.[52] Other investigators have also commented that myocarditis may have been appreciably overdiagnosed in this latter study.[120,121]

Thus, myocarditis is likely to be encountered in biopsy tissues in fewer than 10% (and certainly fewer than 20%) of patients with chronic idiopathic dilated cardiomyopathy. For comparison, 21% to 45% of patients with dilated cardiomyopathy have a history of chronic alcoholism.[122,123] From these data, one may conclude that other factors, such as chronic alcoholism, are more likely than myocarditis to play a role in the development of dilated cardiomyopathy.[52]

The biopsy features of idiopathic dilated cardiomyopathy are identical to those of alcoholic heart disease and overlap considerably with the biopsy findings in hypertrophic or restrictive cardiomyopathies.[1,2,52] Also, clinically significant ischemic, valvular, and hypertensive heart disease may have similar histopathologic findings. As a result, the diagnosis of dilated cardiomyopathy per se cannot be made by endomyocardial biopsy alone. However, the morphological diagnosis may be interpreted as consistent with dilated cardiomyopathy if the conditions that mimic this disorder can be excluded clinically.[1,2,52] Cardiac biopsy is justified in these patients to rule out myocarditis, hemochromatosis, storage diseases, and other disorders (Table 19B-7).

Hypertrophic cardiomyopathy

When seen in combination, three findings are highly specific and sensitive diagnostic hallmarks of hypertrophic cardiomyopathy: (1) asymmetric septal hypertrophy, (2) myocyte disarray, and (3) systolic anterior motion of the anterior mitral leaflet.[124-126] The cellular disarray may be quite patchy and variable in distribution, and it tends to be greatest deep within the core of the ventricular septum.[23,127] As a result, tissue with the typical histopathologic features of this disorder may be inaccessible to the transvenous bioptome, and the diagnosis of hypertrophic cardiomyopathy per se rarely will be possible by endomyocardial biopsy alone.[1,2,52] Although histologic criteria have been proposed to distinguish hypertrophic from dilated cardiomyopathies,[128-131] there is considerable overlap, and the criteria have not been widely accepted.

In biopsy tissue, the most common histologic features are myocardial cellular hypertrophy and interstitial fibro-

Table 19B-7 Differential diagnosis of the cardiomyopathies

Idiopathic dilated cardiomyopathy	Hypertrophic cardiomyopathy	Restrictive cardiomyopathy
Ischemic heart disease	Amyloidosis	Amyloidosis
Myocarditis	Chronic hypertension	Constrictive pericarditis
Hemochromatosis	Angled ventricular septum	Hypertrophic cardiomyopathy
Other disorders	Other disorders	Other disorders
Carnitine deficiency	Aortic valve stenosis	Anthracycline therapy
Fabry's disease	Congenital subaortic stenosis	Carcinoid heart disease
Hypereosinophilic syndrome	Fabry's disease	Cardiac lipomatosis
	Glycogen storage disease	Diabetes mellitus
	Hypercontractile states	Endocardial calcification
	Hypereosinophilic syndrome	Fabry's disease
	Infants of diabetic mothers	Glycogen storage disease
	Septal or pericardial hemorrhage	Hemochromatosis
		Metastatic disease
		Methysergide therapy
		Postoperative rheumatic heart disease
		Pseudoxanthoma elasticum
		Radiation therapy
		Sarcoidosis
		Scleroderma

Modified from Edwards WD: Cardiomyopathies. *Major Probl Pathol* 23:257-309, 1991.

sis, whereas classic myocyte disarray is rarely observed in subendocardial specimens.[1,2,52] Additionally, however, the biopsy may identify a pathologic process which mimics hypertrophic cardiomyopathy, particularly cardiac amyloid (see Table 19B-7). Herein lies the rationale for endomyocardial biopsy in patients with a clinical diagnosis of hypertrophic cardiomyopathy, especially the nonobstructive form.

Restrictive cardiomyopathy

According to the World Health Organization, restrictive cardiomyopathy encompasses eosinophilic endomyocardial diseases, including eosinophilic myocarditis, endomyocardial fibrosis, and the hypereosinophilic syndrome.[132] Generally, endomyocardial biopsy tissues show mural thrombus with or without eosinophils, endocardial granulation tissue or fibrosis, and subjacent myocardial interstitial fibrosis.[1,2,52] Some specimens also exhibit myocyte hypertrophy or eosinophilic myocarditis. Rarely, the tissues may appear histologically normal. The observed lesions depend, in part, on the stage of the disease (necrotic, thrombotic, or fibrotic).[52,133,134] If the endocardium is densely fibrotic, attainment of adequate biopsy specimens may be difficult or impossible.

In addition to the aforementioned patients with eosinophilic endomyocardial disease, there exists a group with *non*eosinophilic restrictive cardiomyopathy.[52,135-137] Biopsy features in these cases are characterized by interstitial fibrosis, with little evidence of myocyte hypertrophy or endocardial fibrosis and no evidence of mural thrombus or eosinophilic infiltrates.[138] Rarely, biopsy tissues may appear normal, even though the hemodynamic features are clearly due to myocardial rather than pericardial disease.[135]

Endomyocardial biopsy may also assist in the diagnosis of those disorders that mimic restrictive cardiomyopathy (see Table 19B-7). For example, cardiac amyloid can produce restrictive symptoms and is readily documented in biopsy tissue with special stains. When pericarditis causes significant constriction, myocytes generally will appear normal or atrophic,[139] in contrast to the features of restrictive disease.[140] Hypertrophic cardiomyopathy may mimic restrictive cardiomyopathy,[141] and the nonspecific biopsy findings may not allow histologic distinction between the two. Thus, endomyocardial biopsy is indicated not only to assess primary endomyocardial disease but also to rule out cardiac amyloid and, perhaps, constrictive pericarditis and other disorders.[1,2,52]

Cardiac amyloid

Endomyocardial biopsy is the diagnostic tool of choice for the tissue documentation of cardiac amyloid.[142] Although rectal biopsy was once the preferred biopsy procedure, neither the presence nor the absence of vascular amyloid in the rectum necessarily implies a similar status in the heart. Also, persistent bleeding from stiffened amyloid-filled vessels may render rectal biopsy more hazardous than heart biopsy.

Amyloid deposits can be identified easily in biopsy tissue (Fig 19B-5, A) and may encircle myocardial cells, form interstitial nodules, or involve blood vessels or endocardium.[142] The microscopic pattern of involvement tends to correspond to the type of amyloid encountered, although some overlap occurs. Thus, primary amyloidosis

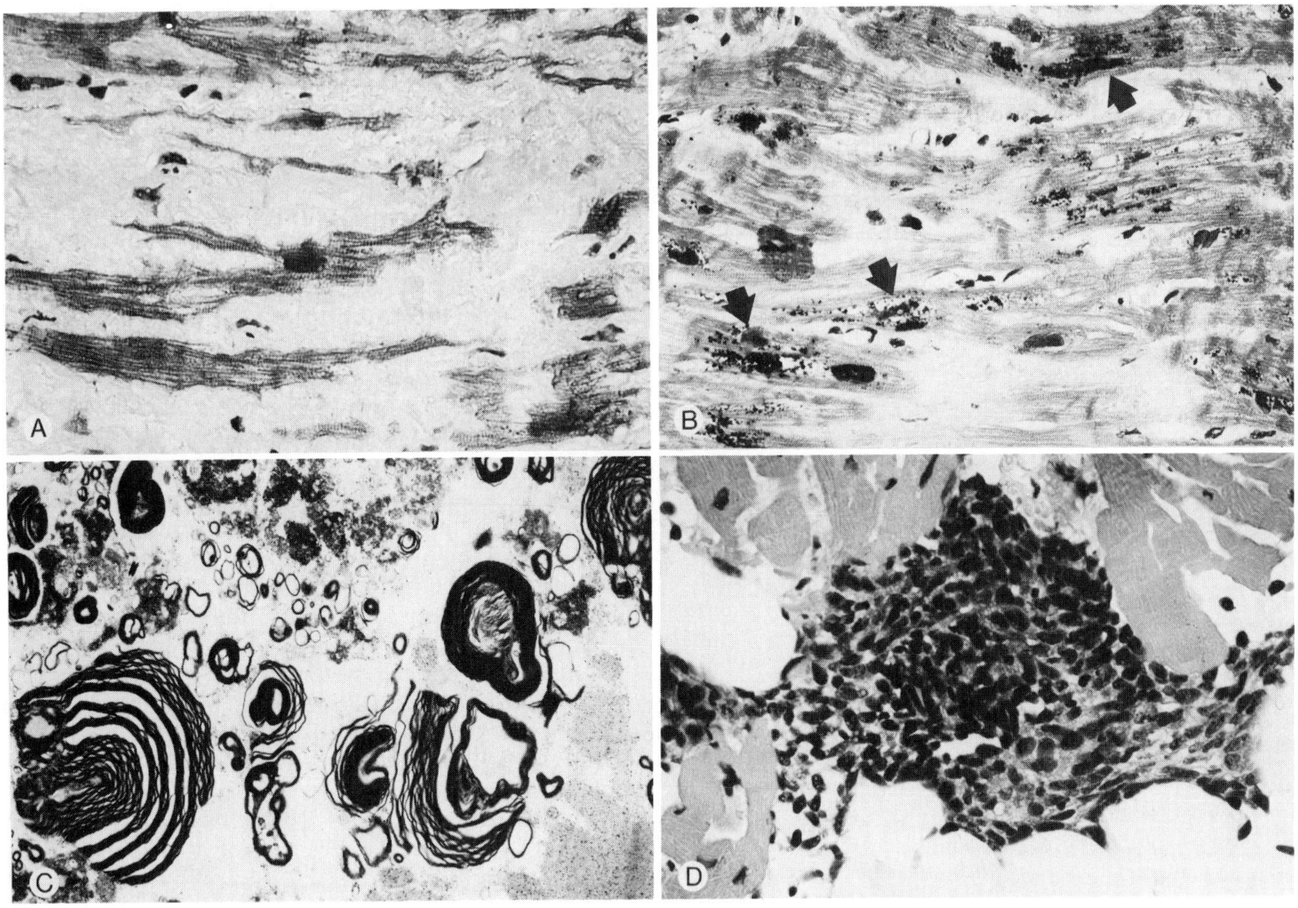

Fig 19B-5 Secondary myocardial disease. **A,** interstitium is extensively infiltrated by amyloid. (Hematoxylin and eosin; ×225.) **B,** myocytes contain abundant iron *(arrows)* in a patient with hemochromatosis and cardiac dysfunction. (Iron stain; ×225.) **C,** in Fabry's disease, myocytes are filled with glycolipid deposits that typically appear as membranous sacs and lamellar whorls by transmission electron microscopy. (Lead citrate and uranyl acetate; ×4,375.) **D,** metastatic malignant melanoma is present in endomyocardial biopsy tissue from patient with right ventricular outflow tract obstruction. (Hematoxylin and eosin; ×225.) (**A,** from Edwards WD: Cardiomyopathies. *Hum Pathol* 18:625-635, 1987. By permission of WB Saunders Company. **B** and **D,** from Edwards WD: Pathology of endomyocardial biopsy. *Contemp Issues Surg Pathol* 12:191-275, 1988. By permission of Churchill Livingstone. **C,** from Broadbent JC, Edwards WD, Gordon H, et al: Fabry cardiomyopathy in the female confirmed by endomyocardial biopsy. *Mayo Clin Proc* 56:623-628, 1981. By permission, Mayo Foundation.)

is usually associated with pericellular and vascular deposits, whereas senile cardiovascular amyloidosis generally produces nodular lesions without vascular involvement.[142-144]

Sulfated Alcian blue and methyl violet are the two favored amyloid stains at the Mayo Clinic. Congo red and, perhaps, thioflavine T stains may also be used, although satisfactory results may be difficult to achieve with Congo red. Immunohistochemical stains for κ and λ light chains and for transthyretin (prealbumin) are suggested for the evaluation of senile cardiovascular amyloidosis and, rarely, myeloma-associated light-chain disease[144,145] (Table 19B-8). Transmission electron microscopy may be necessary to document small amounts of amyloid.[1] In some cases, the initial clinical diagnosis will be hypertrophic or restrictive cardiomyopathy rather than amyloidosis (see Table 19B-7).

Anthracycline cardiotoxicity

Among the antineoplastic anthracycline antibiotics, doxorubicin (Adriamycin) is the most commonly used for a variety of solid and hematologic neoplasms in children and adults. However, its usefulness is limited by its cardiotoxicity, which is dose-related and is associated with 50% mortality once heart failure develops.[146] When functional cardiotoxicity develops, it usually occurs within 1 to 6 months after completion of therapy, although an

Table 19B-8 Types of amyloid involving the heart

Clinical classification	Chemical type of amyloid	Immunohistochemical staining
Primary	AL	κ or λ light chains
Myeloma-related	AL	κ or λ light chains
Secondary	AA	A-component
Senile	ASC1	Transthyretin (prealbumin)
Isolated atrial	ASC2	Atrial natriuretic factor

Table 19B-9 Histopathologic features of anthracycline cardiotoxicity: extent in relation to grade

Grade	Histopathologic features	Course of doxorubicin therapy
0	Normal biopsy tissue	Continue
1	Isolated myocytes (<5%) with early myofibrillar loss or sarcotubular dilatation	Continue
1.5	Small clusters of myocytes (5%-15%) with myofibrillar loss or sarcoplasmic vacuoles	Continue
2	Clustered myocytes (16%-25%) with marked myofibrillar loss or sarcoplasmic vacuoles	Continue cautiously, if hemodynamics are satisfactory
2.5	Large clusters of myocytes (26%-35%) with marked myofibrillar loss or coalescing sarcoplasmic vacuoles	Discontinue
3	Confluent or diffuse myocyte injury (>35%) with many severely damaged or necrotic cells	Discontinue

Modified from Billingham ME: The role of endomyocardial biopsy in the diagnosis and treatment of heart disease. In Cardiovascular Pathology. Edited by MD Silver. Vol 2. New York, Churchill Livingstone, 1983, pp 1205-1224, and Bristow MR: Toxic cardiomyopathy due to doxorubicin. *Hosp Pract* [Off] 17:101-111, 1982.

example 7 years after treatment has been reported.[147]

Although a cumulative dosage of more than 550 mg/m^2 generally results in a high incidence of cardiotoxic injury, there is considerable individual variation, and other factors (such as old age or prior irradiation) may lower the dosage at which toxicity develops.[146,148,149] On the other hand, some patients can tolerate much higher cumulative doses. Thus, in individual cases, the cumulative dosage is not always an accurate predictor of the likelihood for developing heart failure. However, serial endomyocardial biopsies provide a reliable and accurate method of evaluating doxorubicin cardiotoxicity *before* cardiac dilatation or heart failure supervenes.[1,150]

Several biopsy specimens should be obtained and processed for plastic embedding, sectioning at 1 μm thick, and staining with toluidine blue. At least 10 thick sections should be evaluated by light microscopy, and those with abnormalities should be examined by transmission electron microscopy.[1] Two lesions of cardiac muscle cells may be observed: (1) loss of contractile elements and (2) vacuolar degeneration due to sarcotubular dilatation; these may occur in separate cells or together in the same cell.[1,148,151,152] Mitochondria and nuclei are generally normal, although subtle nuclear alterations have been detected by electron microscopy.[153] In more advanced cases, necrotic myocardial cells are present and are characterized by nuclear pyknosis and mitochondrial degeneration.[1] There are no vascular lesions and no inflammatory cell infiltrates, but interstitial fibrosis may be observed.[1]

A histologic grading system based on the extent of damage both in individual cells and in the total population of myocardial cells has been established[151] (Table 19B-9). Although these changes are characteristic of anthracycline cardiotoxicity, they are not specific and may be observed in other disorders such as dilated cardiomyopathy.[1] For this reason, a reference biopsy is recommended before therapy is begun.

Other secondary myocardial diseases

In addition to amyloidosis and anthracycline cardiotoxicity, cardiac involvement by other secondary disorders can be documented by endomyocardial biopsy. The likelihood of a positive biopsy depends on the extent and distribution of lesions within the heart, the histologic specificity of the lesions, and the number of specimens obtained. The nature of the underlying disorder dictates how the tissue should be fixed, processed, and stained.

Hemochromatosis. Although stainable iron is not normally present in the myocardium, it accumulates within myocytes in both the primary and the secondary forms of hemochromatosis. Iron is uneven in its distribution and tends to involve sub*epi*cardial myocytes more extensively than the sub*endo*cardium.[154-156] However, if the disease is far enough advanced that systolic dysfunction is evident, iron accumulation throughout the heart will generally be sufficient for diagnosis, even in biopsy tissue from the subendocardium[157] (Fig 19B-5,B). Therefore, sampling error is not a limiting factor. Serial biopsies may be used to document a diminution in stainable iron in myocytes after treatment with phlebotomy or chelating agents.[158]

Generally, hemochromatosis produces a dilated and failing heart that mimics idiopathic dilated cardiomyopathy.[52] Occasionally, it is associated with restrictive or constrictive features or with arrhythmias. Because of the varied clinical presentations, it is recommended that iron staining be performed on all biopsy specimens from patients with chronic myocardial diseases of undetermined cause.

Sarcoidosis. The classic biopsy appearance of cardiac sarcoidosis is a giant cell or granulomatous myocarditis (see Fig 19B-3,D), and nonspecific patchy fibrosis is the typical feature of healed or inactive disease.[159] Biopsy specimens that include only the borders of inflammatory foci, however, may be free of giant cells and demonstrate lymphocytic myocarditis[160] (see Table 19B-3). Normal biopsy tissue should be interpreted with caution; it may be indicative of absence of cardiac involvement, inactive cardiac sarcoidosis, or sampling error in a patient with active lesions elsewhere in the heart. Because sarcoidosis tends to involve the base of the heart rather than the apex (where biopsy specimens are taken), sampling error is particularly likely.

Storage diseases. When storage diseases are suspected clinically, the processing of tissues often requires special considerations and should be discussed with a pathologist before the biopsy procedure is performed. For example, enzyme assays may be performed on fresh-frozen biopsy specimens in some cases.[161] Moreover, biopsy tissues should be fixed in absolute alcohol if aqueous-soluble substances are present, as in glycogen storage disease or Fabry's disease. Transmission electron microscopy is also recommended for the evaluation of most storage diseases, because specific ultrastructural alterations are generally present. Cardiac involvement has been documented by endomyocardial biopsy in glycogen storage disease, Fabry's disease, and Gaucher's disease[161-164] (Fig 19B-5,C).

Neoplastic diseases. Cardiac biopsy has also been used to demonstrate infiltration by benign and malignant primary cardiac neoplasms and by metastatic malignancies[165-170] (Fig 19B-5,D).

SUMMARY

Transvenous endomyocardial biopsy is a safe procedure that may provide clinically useful information in carefully selected patients with a variety of nonischemic cardiac disorders. It is the best procedure with which to diagnose acute cardiac allograft rejection, and it is a reliable and accurate method of evaluating anthracycline cardiotoxicity.[1,2,52]

In the clinical setting of myocarditis, unexplained life-threatening arrhythmias, or unexplained chest pain, the biopsy may document myocarditis or morphological changes suggestive of cardiomyopathy. However, sampling error is a problem.

In patients with idiopathic dilated cardiomyopathy, biopsy may be useful to rule out myocarditis, hemochromatosis, storage diseases, and other disorders. When hypertrophic cardiomyopathy, particularly the nonobstructive form, is diagnosed clinically, biopsy may be justified to rule out amyloid. Likewise, when restrictive cardiomyopathy is present, endomyocardial biopsy may be useful not only to evaluate eosinophilic endomyocardial disorders but also to rule out amyloid and, perhaps, constrictive pericarditis and other disorders (see Table 19B-7).

If cardiac amyloid is suspected clinically, cardiac biopsy is the best method for documentation. The biopsy also may be useful for the evaluation of cardiac involvement by other systemic diseases, such as hemochromatosis and sarcoidosis.

In general, a positive endomyocardial biopsy is diagnostic, but a negative biopsy does not necessarily exclude the clinical diagnosis, owing to possible sampling error. False-negative results are more commonly encountered with myocarditis than with amyloidosis or hemochromatosis.[53,54,142,157]

REFERENCES

1. Billingham ME: The role of endomyocardial biopsy in the diagnosis and treatment of heart disease. In *Cardiovascular Pathology.* Edited by MD Silver. New York, Churchill Livingstone, 1983, vol. 2, pp 1205-1224
2. Edwards WD: Pathology of endomyocardial biopsy. *Contemp Issues Surg Pathol* 12:191-275, 1988
3. Casten GG, Marsh JB: Metabolic studies on cardiac tissue obtained by needle biopsy in the intact unanesthetized dog. *Circ Res* 1:226-229, 1953
4. Sutton DC, Sutton GC, Kent G: Needle biopsy of human ventricular myocardium. *Q Bull Northwestern Univ Med Sch* 30:213-214, 1956
5. Shirey EK, Hawk WA, Mukerji D, et al: Percutaneous myocardial biopsy of the left ventricle: experience in 198 patients. *Circulation* 46:112-122, 1972
6. Sakakibara S, Konno S: Endomyocardial biopsy. *Jpn Heart J* 3:537-543, 1962
7. Caves PK, Schulz WP, Dong E Jr, et al: New instrument for transvenous cardiac biopsy. *Am J Cardiol* 33:264-267, 1974
8. Richardson PJ: King's endomyocardial bioptome. *Lancet* 1:660-661, 1974
9. Mason JW: Techniques for right and left ventricular endomyocardial biopsy. *Am J Cardiol* 41:887-892, 1978
10. Brooksby IAB, Jenkins BS, Davies MJ, et al: Left ventricular endomyocardial biopsy. I. Description and evaluation of the technique. *Cathet Cardiovasc Diagn* 3:115-121, 1977
11. Brooksby IAB, Coltart DJ, Webb-Peploe MM: Progress in endomyocardial biopsy. *Mod Concepts Cardiovasc Dis* 44:65-69, December 1975
12. Richardson PJ: Endomyocardial biopsy technique. In *Myocardial Biopsy: Diagnostic Significance.* Edited by H-D Bolte. Berlin, Springer-Verlag, 1980, pp 3-7
13. Fowles RE, Mason JW: Myocardial biopsy (editorial). *Mayo Clin Proc* 57:459-461, 1982
14. Perrault J, McGill DB, Ott BJ, et al: Liver biopsy: complications in 1000 inpatients and outpatients. *Gastroenterology* 74:103-106, 1978
15. Sherlock S: *Diseases of the Liver and Biliary System.* Sixth edition. Boston, Blackwell Scientific Publications, 1981, p 31
16. Diaz-Buxo JA, Donadio JV Jr: Complications of percutaneous renal biopsy: an analysis of 1,000 consecutive biopsies. *Clin Nephrol* 4:223-227, 1975
17. Zollinger HU, Mihatsch MJ: *Renal Pathology in Biopsy: Light, Electron and Immunofluorescent Microscopy and Clinical Aspects.* New York, Springer-Verlag, 1978, p 4
18. Yoshizato T, Edwards WD, Alboliras ET, et al: Safety and utility of endomyocardial biopsy in infants, children and adolescents: a review of 66 procedures in 53 patients. *J Am Coll Cardiol* 15:436-442, 1990
19. Bradfield JWB, Beck G, Vecht RJ: Left ventricular apical thin point. *Br Heart J* 39:806-809, 1977
20. Billingham ME, Bristow MR, Mason JW, et al: Endomyocardial biopsy. In *Congestive Heart Failure: Current Research and Clinical Applications.* Edited by E Braunwald, MB Mock, JT Watson. New York, Grune & Stratton, 1982, pp 237-251
21. Kober G, Kunkel B, Becker H-J, et al: Technical aspects, experiences, and complications of right and left ventricular endomyocardial biopsy. In *Cardiomyopathy and Myocardial Biopsy.* Edited by M Kaltenbach, F Loogen, EGJ Olsen. Berlin, Springer-Verlag, 1978, pp 40-47
22. Chandra RS: The role of endomyocardial biopsy, in the diagnosis

of cardiac disorders in infants and children. *Am J Cardiovasc Pathol* 1:157-172, 1987

23. Maron BJ, Roberts WC: Hypertrophic cardiomyopathy and cardiac muscle cell disorganization revisited: relation between the two and significance. *Am Heart J* 102:95-110, 1981

24. Roberts WC, McAllister HA Jr, Ferrans VJ: Sarcoidosis of the heart: a clinicopathologic study of 35 necropsy patients (group I) and review of 78 previously described necropsy patients (group II). *Am J Med* 63:86-108, 1977

25. Silverman KJ, Hutchins GM, Bulkley BH: Cardiac sarcoid: a clinicopathologic study of 84 unselected patients with systemic sarcoidosis. *Circulation* 58:1204-1211, 1978

26. Aretz HT, Billingham ME, Edwards WD, et al: Myocarditis: a histopathologic definition and classification. *Am J Cardiovasc Pathol* 1:3-14, 1987

27. Aretz HT: Myocarditis: the Dallas criteria. *Hum Pathol* 18:619-624, 1987

28. Cambridge G, MacArthur CGC, Waterson AP, et al: Antibodies to Coxsackie B viruses in congestive cardiomyopathy. *Br Heart J* 41:692-696, 1979

29. Waterson AP: Coxsackie viruses in acute and chronic cardiac disease. In *Myocardial Biopsy: Diagnostic Significance.* Edited by H-D Bolte. Berlin, Springer-Verlag, 1980, pp 116-118

30. Mason JW, Billingham ME, Ricci DR: Treatment of acute inflammatory myocarditis assisted by endomyocardial biopsy. *Am J Cardiol* 45:1037-1044, 1980

31. Olmesdahl PJ, Gregory MA, Cameron EWJ: Ultrastructural artefacts in biopsied normal myocardium and their relevance to myocardial biopsy in man. *Thorax* 34:82-90, 1979

32. Yacoub MH, Rose ML, Fraser AK, et al: T-cell phenotype characterization in human cardiac allografts. *Heart Transplant* 2:259-265, August 1983

33. Weintraub D, Masek M, Billingham ME: The lymphocyte subpopulations in cyclosporine-treated human heart rejection. *J Heart Transplant* 4:213-216, 1985

34. Billingham ME: Diagnosis of cardiac rejection by endomyocardial biopsy. *Heart Transplant* 1:25-30, 1981

35. Rose AG, Uys CJ: Pathology of acute rejection. In *Heart Transplantation: The Present Status of Orthotopic and Heterotopic Heart Transplantation.* Edited by DKC Cooper, RP Lanza. Lancaster, MTP Press, 1984, pp 157-176

36. McAllister HA Jr, Schnee MJM, Radovančević B, et al: A system for grading cardiac allograft rejection. *Tex Heart Inst J* 13:1-3, 1986

37. Kemnitz J, Cohnert T, Schäfers H-J, et al: A classification of cardiac allograft rejection: a modification of the classification by Billingham. *Am J Surg Pathol* 11:503-515, 1987

38. Billingham ME, Cary NRB, Hammond ME, et al: A working formulation for the standardization of nomenclature in the diagnosis of heart and lung rejection: Heart Rejection Study Group. *J Heart Transplant* 9:587-593, 1990

39. Sibley RK, Olivari M-T, Ring WS, et al: Endomyocardial biopsy in the cardiac allograft recipient: a review of 570 biopsies. *Ann Surg* 203:177-187, 1986

40. Rose AG, Novitzky D, Cooper DKC, et al: Endomyocardial biopsy site morphology: an experimental study in baboons. *Arch Pathol Lab Med* 110:622-625, 1986

41. Novitzky D, Rose AG, Cooper DKC, et al: Histopathologic changes at the site of endomyocardial biopsy: potential for confusion with acute rejection. *J Heart Transplant* 5:79-80, 1986

42. Myles JL, Ratliff NB, McMahon JT, et al: Reversibility of myocyte injury in moderate and severe acute rejection in cyclosporine-treated cardiac transplant patients. *Arch Pathol Lab Med* 111:947-952, 1987

43. Imakita M, Tazelaar HD, Billingham ME: Heart allograft rejection under varying immunosuppressive protocols as evaluated by endomyocardial biopsy. *J Heart Transplant* 5:279-285, 1986

44. Herskowitz A, Soule LM, Ueda K, et al: Arteriolar vasculitis on endomyocardial biopsy: a histologic predictor of poor outcome in cyclosporine-treated heart transplant recipients. *J Heart Transplant* 6:127-134, 1987

45. Smith SH, Kirklin JK, Geer JC, et al: Arteritis in cardiac rejection after transplantation. *Am J Cardiol* 59:1171-1173, 1987

46. Palmer DC, Tsai CC, Roodman ST, et al: Heart graft arteriosclerosis: an ominous finding on endomyocardial biopsy. *Transplantation* 39:385-388, 1985

47. Herskowitz A, Soule LM, Mellits ED, et al: Histologic predictors of acute cardiac rejection in human endomyocardial biopsies: a multivariate analysis. *J Am Coll Cardiol* 9:802-810, 1987

48. Carrier M, Paplanus SH, Graham AR, et al: Histopathology of acute myocardial necrosis: effects of immunosuppression therapy. *J Heart Transplant* 6:218-221, 1987

49. Stovin PGI, English TAH: Effects of cyclosporine on the transplanted human heart. *J Heart Transplant* 6:180-185, 1987

50. Hofflin JM, Potasman I, Baldwin JC, et al: Infectious complications in heart transplant recipients receiving cyclosporine and corticosteroids, *Ann Intern Med* 106:209-216, 1987

51. Edwards WD: Myocarditis and endomyocardial biopsy. *Cardiol Clin* 2:647-656, November 1984

52. Edwards WD: Cardiomyopathies. *Major Probl Pathol* 23:257-309, 1991

53. Hauck AJ, Kearney DL, Edwards WD: Evaluation of postmortem endomyocardial biopsy specimens from 38 patients with lymphocytic myocarditis: implications for role of sampling error. *Mayo Clin Proc* 64:1235 1245, 1989

54. Chow LH, Radio SJ, Sears TD, et al: Insensitivity of right ventricular endomyocardial biopsy in the diagnosis of myocarditis. *J Am Coll Cardiol* 14:915-920, 1989

55. Nippoldt TB, Edwards WD, Holmes DR Jr, et al: Right ventricular endomyocardial biopsy: clinicopathologic correlates in 100 consecutive patients. *Mayo Clin Proc* 57:407-418, 1982

56. Billingham ME: Morphologic changes in drug-induced heart disease. In *Drug-Induced Heart Disease.* Edited by MR Bristow. Amsterdam, Elsevier/North-Holland Biomedical Press, 1980, pp 127-149

57. McAllister HA Jr, Mullick FG: The cardiovascular system. In *Pathology of Drug-Induced and Toxic Diseases.* Edited by RH Riddell. New York, Churchill Livingstone, 1982, pp 201-228

58. Fenoglio JJ Jr: The effects of drugs on the cardiovascular system. In *Cardiovascular Pathology.* Vol 2. Edited by MD Silver. New York, Churchill Livingstone, 1983, pp 1085-1107

59. Shanes JG, Ghali J, Billingham ME, et al: Interobserver variability in the pathologic interpretation of endomyocardial biopsy results. *Circulation* 75:401-405, 1987

60. Edwards WD, Holmes DR Jr, Reeder GS: Diagnosis of active lymphocytic myocarditis by endomyocardial biopsy: quantitative criteria for light microscopy. *Mayo Clin Proc* 57:419-425, 1982

61. Fenoglio JJ Jr, Ursell PC, Kellogg CF, et al: Diagnosis and classification of myocarditis by endomyocardial biopsy. *N Engl J Med* 308:12-18, 1983

62. Mason JW: Endomyocardial biopsy: the balance of success and failure. *Circulation* 71:185-188, 1985

63. Billingham ME: Myocarditis and endomyocardial biopsy (letter to the editor). *Ann Intern Med* 100:165, 1989

64. Kereiakes DJ, Parmley WW: Myocarditis and cardiomyopathy. *Am Heart J* 108:1318-1326, 1984

65. Billingham ME, Tazelaar HD: The morphological progression of viral myocarditis. *Postgrad Med J* 62:581-584, 1986

66. Quigley PJ, Richardson PJ, Meany BT, et al: Long-term follow-up of acute myocarditis. Correlation of ventricular function and outcome. *Eur Heart J* 8 Suppl J:39-42, 1987

67. Dec GW Jr, Fallon JT, Southern JF, et al: Relation between histological findings on early repeat right ventricular biopsy and ventricular function in patients with myocarditis. *Br Heart J* 60:332-337, 1988

68. von Olshausen KV, Schäfer A, Mehmel HC, et al: Ventricular arrhythmias in idiopathic dilated cardiomyopathy. *Br Heart J* 51:195-201, 1984

69. McLaran CJ, Gersh BJ, Sugrue DD, et al: Tachycardia induced myocardial dysfunction: a reversible phenomenon? *Br Heart J* 53:323-327, 1985

70. Packer DL, Bardy GH, Worley SJ, et al: Tachycardia-induced cardiomyopathy: a reversible form of left ventricular dysfunction. *Am J Cardiol* 57:563-570, 1986

71. Fyfe DA, Gillette PC, Crawford FA Jr, et al: Resolution of dilated cardiomyopathy after surgical ablation of ventricular tachycardia in a child. *J Am Coll Cardiol* 9:231-234, 1987

72. Marcus FI, Fontaine GH, Guiraudon G, et al: Right ventricular dysplasia: a report of 24 adult cases. *Circulation* 65:384-398, 1982

73. Nava A, Thiene G, Canciani B, et al: Familial occurrence of right ventricular dysplasia: a study involving nine families. *J Am Coll Cardiol* 12:1222-1228, 1988

74. Saffitz JE, Ferrans VJ, Rodriguez ER, et al: Histocytoid cardio-

myopathy: a cause of sudden death in apparently healthy infants. *Am J Cardiol* 52:215-217, 1983

75. Kearney DL, Titus JL, Hawkins EP, et al: Pathologic features of myocardial hamartomas causing childhood tachyarrhythmias. *Circulation* 75:705-710, 1987

76. Strain JE, Grose RM, Factor SM, et al: Results of endomyocardial biopsy in patients with spontaneous ventricular tachycardia but without apparent structural heart disease. *Circulation* 68:1171-1181, 1983

77. Vignola PA, Aonuma K, Swaye PS, et al: Lymphocytic myocarditis presenting as unexplained ventricular arrhythmias: diagnosis with endomyocardial biopsy and response to immunosuppression. *J Am Coll Cardiol* 4:812-819, 1984

78. Sugrue DD, Holmes DR Jr, Gersh BJ, et al: Cardiac histologic findings in patients with life-threatening ventricular arrhythmias of unknown origin. *J Am Coll Cardiol* 4:952-957, 1984

79. Morgera T, Salvi A, Alberti E, et al: Morphological findings in apparently idiopathic ventricular tachycardia. An echocardiographic haemodynamic and histologic study. *Eur Heart J* 6:323-334, 1985

80. Sugrue DD, Edwards WD, Olney BA: Histologic abnormalities of the left ventricle in a patient with arrhythmogenic right ventricular dysplasia. *Heart Vessels* 1:179-181, 1985

81. Baandrup U, Florio RA, Rehahn M, et al: Critical analysis of endomyocardial biopsies from patients suspected of having cardiomyopathy. II. Comparison of histology and clinical/haemodynamic information. *Br Heart J* 45:487-493, 1981

82. Richardson PJ, Livesley B, Oram S, et al: Angina pectoris with normal coronary arteries: transvenous myocardial biopsy in diagnosis. *Lancet* 2:677-680, 1974

83. Smith RRL, Hutchins GM: Ischemic heart disease secondary to amyloidosis of intramyocardial arteries. *Am J Cardiol* 44:413-417, 1979

84. Saffitz JE, Sazama K, Roberts WC: Amyloidosis limited to small arteries causing angina pectoris and sudden death. *Am J Cardiol* 51:1234-1235, 1983

85. Baandrup U, Florio RA, Roters F, et al: Electron microscopic investigation of endomyocardial biopsy samples in hypertrophy and cardiomyopathy: a semiquantitative study in 48 patients. *Circulation* 63:1289-1298, 1981

86. Baandrup U, Olsen EGJ: Critical analysis of endomyocardial biopsies from patients suspected of having cardiomyopathy. I. Morphological and morphometric aspects. *Br Heart J* 45:475-486, 1981

87. Rose AG, Beck W: Dilated (congestive) cardiomyopathy: a syndrome of severe cardiac dysfunction with remarkably few morphological features of myocardial damage. *Histopathology* 9:367-379, 1985

88. Fast JH, Kubat K, van Haelst UJGM, et al: The usefulness of an endomyocardial biopsy in heart disease of unknown etiology. *Int J Cardiol* 11:317-328, 1986

89. O'Connell JB, Costanzo-Nordin MR, Subramanian R, et al: Dilated cardiomyopathy: emerging role of endomyocardial biopsy. *Curr Probl Cardiol* 11:445-507, 1986

90. Kunkel B, Lapp H, Kober G, et al: Correlations between clinical and morphologic findings and natural history in congestive cardiomyopathy. In *Cardiomyopathy and Myocardial Biopsy.* Edited by M Kaltenbach, F Loogen, EGJ Olsen. Berlin, Springer-Verlag, 1978, pp 271-283

91. Mall G, Schwarz F, Derks H: Clinicopathologic correlations in congestive cardiomyopathy: a study on endomyocardial biopsies. *Virchows Arch [A]* 397:67-82, 1982

92. Schwarz F, Mall G, Zebe H, et al: Quantitative morphologic findings of the myocardium in idiopathic dilated cardiomyopathy. *Am J Cardiol* 51:501-506, 1983

93. Schwarz F, Mall G, Zebe H, et al: Determinants of survival in patients with congestive cardiomyopathy: quantitative morphologic findings and left ventricular hemodynamics. *Circulation* 70:923-928, 1984

94. Figulla HR, Rahlf G, Nieger M, et al: Spontaneous hemodynamic improvement or stabilization and associated biopsy findings in patients with congestive cardiomyopathy. *Circulation* 71:1095-1104, 1985

95. Hammond EH, Menlove RL, Anderson JL: Predictive value of immunofluorescence and electron microscopic evaluation of endomyocardial biopsies in the diagnosis and prognosis of myocarditis and idiopathic dilated cardiomyopathy. *Am Heart J* 114:1055-1065, 1987

96. Kunkel B, Lapp H, Kober G, et al: Light-microscopic evaluation of myocardial biopsies. In *Cardiomyopathy and Myocardial Biopsy.* Edited by M Kaltenbach, F Loogen, EGJ Olsen. Berlin, Springer-Verlag, 1978, pp 62-70

97. Noda S: Histopathology of endomyocardial biopsies from patients with idiopathic cardiomyopathy: quantitative evaluation based on multivariate statistical analysis. *Jpn Circ J* 44:95-116, 1980

98. Das JP, Rath B, Das S, et al: Study of endomyocardial biopsies in cardiomyopathy. *Indian Heart J* 33:18-26, 1981

99. Unverferth DV, Fetters JK, Unverferth BJ, et al: Human myocardial histologic characteristics in congestive heart failure. *Circulation* 68:1194-1200, 1983

100. Rose AG, Fraser RC, Beck W: Absence of evidence of myocarditis in endomyocardial biopsy specimens from patients with dilated (congestive) cardiomyopathy. *S Afr Med J* 66:871-874, 1984

101. O'Connell JB, Henkin RE, Robinson JA, et al: Gallium-67 imaging in patients with dilated cardiomyopathy and biopsy-proven myocarditis. *Circulation* 70:58-62, 1984

102. Daly K, Richardson PJ, Olsen EGJ, et al: Acute myocarditis: role of histological and virological examination in the diagnosis and assessment of immunosuppressive treatment. *Br Heart J* 51:30-35, 1984

103. Parrillo JE, Aretz HT, Palacios I, et al: The results of transvenous endomyocardial biopsy can frequently be used to diagnose myocardial diseases in patients with idiopathic heart failure: endomyocardial biopsies in 100 consecutive patients revealed a substantial incidence of myocarditis. *Circulation* 69:93-101, 1984

104. Zee-Cheng C-S, Tsai CC, Palmer DC, et al: High incidence of myocarditis by endomyocardial biopsy in patients with idiopathic congestive cardiomyopathy. *J Am Coll Cardiol* 3:63-70, 1984

105. Cassling RS, Linder J, Sears TD, et al: Quantitative evaluation of inflammation in biopsy specimens from idiopathically failing or irritable hearts: experience in 80 pediatric and adult patients. *Am Heart J* 110:713-720, 1985

106. Müller S, Müller P, Meyer R, et al: Myocardial bioptic findings in correlation with TL-201 imaging and hemodynamic parameters in patients with latent cardiomyopathies suspected of having myocarditis. *Heart Vessels* 1 Suppl 1:111-115, 1985

107. Hosenpud JD, McAnulty JH, Niles NR: Lack of objective improvement in ventricular systolic function in patients with myocarditis treated with azathioprine and prednisone. *J Am Coll Cardiol* 6:797-801, 1985

108. Ruzyllo W, Rosnowski A: Endomyocardial biopsy study of cardiomyopathy in Poland. *Heart Vessels Suppl* 1:71-76, 1985

109. Mortensen SA, Baandrup U, Buch J, et al: Immunosuppressive therapy of biopsy proven myocarditis: experiences with corticosteroids and cyclosporin. *Int J Immunotherapy* 1:35-45, 1985

110. Dec GW Jr, Palacios IF, Fallon JT, et al: Active myocarditis in the spectrum of acute dilated cardiomyopathies: clinical features, histologic correlates, and clinical outcome. *N Engl J Med* 312:885-890, 1985

111. Anderson JL, Hammond EH, Menlove RL: Determining humoral and cellular-immune components in myocarditis: complementary diagnostic role of immunofluorescence microscopy in the evaluation of endomyocardial biopsy specimens. In *Cardiomyopathy Update 1: Pathogenesis of Myocarditis and Cardiomyopathy: Recent Experimental and Clinical Studies.* Edited by C Kawai, WH Abelmann. Tokyo, University of Tokyo Press, 1987, p 233

112. Bouhour JB, Helias J, de Lajartre AY, et al: Detection of myocarditis during the first year after discovery of a dilated cardiomyopathy by endomyocardial biopsy and gallium-67 myocardial scintigraphy: prospective multicentre French study of 91 patients. *Eur Heart J* 9:520-528, 1988

113. Chow LC, Dittrich HC, Shabetai R: Endomyocardial biopsy in patients with unexplained congestive heart failure. *Ann Intern Med* 109:535-539, 1988

114. Popma JJ, Cigarroa RG, Buja LM, et al: Diagnostic and prognostic utility of right-sided catheterization and endomyocardial biopsy in idiopathic dilated cardiomyopathy. *Am J Cardiol* 63:955-958, 1989

115. Salvi A, Di Lenarda A, Dreas L, et al: Immunosuppressive treatment in myocarditis. *Int J Cardiol* 22:329-338, 1989

116. Obrador D, Ballester M, Carrió I, et al: High prevalence of myocardial monoclonal antimyosin antibody uptake in patients with chronic idiopathic dilated cardiomyopathy. *J Am Coll Cardiol* 13:1289-1293, 1989

117. Latham RD, Mulrow JP, Virmani R, et al: Recently diagnosed idiopathic dilated cardiomyopathy: incidence of myocarditis and efficacy of prednisone therapy. *Am Heart J* 117:876-882, 1989

118. Hobbs RE, Pelegrin D, Ratliff NB, et al. Lymphocytic myocarditis and dilated cardiomyopathy: treatment with immunosuppressive agents. *Cleve Clin J Med* 56:628-635, 1989

119. Bolte H-D, Ludwig B: Viral myocarditis: symptomatology, clinical diagnostics and haemodynamics. In *Viral Heart Disease.* Edited by H-D Bolte. New York, Springer-Verlag, 1984, pp 177-186

120. Uretsky BF: Idiopathic "myocarditis"? (letter to the editor). *J Am Coll Cardiol* 4:1069, 1984

121. Tazelaar HD, Billingham ME: Leukocytic infiltrates in idiopathic dilated cardiomyopathy: a source of confusion with active myocarditis. *Am J Surg Pathol* 10:405-412, 1986

122. Fuster V, Gersh BJ, Giuliani ER, et al: The natural history of idiopathic dilated cardiomyopathy. *Am J Cardiol* 47:525-531, 1981

123. Roberts WC, Siegel RJ, McManus BM: Idiopathic dilated cardiomyopathy: analysis of 152 necropsy patients. *Am J Cardiol* 60:1340-1355, 1987

124. Maron BJ, Roberts WC: Quantitative analysis of cardiac muscle cell disorganization in the ventricular septum of patients with hypertrophic cardiomyopathy. *Circulation* 59:689-706, 1979

125. Maron BJ, Epstein SE: Hypertrophic cardiomyopathy. Recent observations regarding the specificity of three hallmarks of the disease: asymmetric septal hypertrophy, septal disorganization and systolic anterior motion of the anterior mitral leaflet. *Am J Cardiol* 45:141-154, 1980

126. Maron BJ, Bonow RO, Cannon RO III, et al: Hypertrophic cardiomyopathy: interrelations of clinical manifestations, pathophysiology, and therapy. *N Engl J Med* 316:780-789 (part 1); 844-852 (part 2), 1987

127. Tazelaar HD, Billingham ME: The surgical pathology of hypertrophic cardiomyopathy. *Arch Pathol Lab Med* 111:257-260, 1987

128. Van Noorden S, Olsen EGJ, Pearse AGE: Hypertrophic obstructive cardiomyopathy, a histological, histochemical, and ultrastructural study of biopsy material. *Cardiovasc Res* 5:118-131, 1971

129. Rose AG: Evaluation of pathological criteria for diagnosis of hypertrophic cardiomyopathy. *Histopathology* 8:395-406, 1984

130. Nunoda S, Genda A, Sekiguchi M, et al: Left ventricular endomyocardial biopsy findings in patients with essential hypertension and hypertrophic cardiomyopathy with special reference to the incidence of bizarre myocardial hypertrophy with disorganization and biopsy score. *Heart Vessels* 1:170-175, 1985

131. Sekiguchi M, Nunoda S, Hiroe M: The value of endomyocardial biopsy in diagnosing hypertrophic cardiomyopathy. In *Cardiomyopathy Update 2: Hypertrophic Cardiomyopathy.* Edited by H Toshima, BJ Maron. Tokyo, University of Tokyo Press, 1988, pp 59-69

132. Olsen EGJ (Chairman): Report of the WHO/ISFC task force on the definition and classification of cardiomyopathies. *Br Heart J* 44:672-673, 1980

133. Olsen EGJ: Pathological aspects of endomyocardial fibrosis. *Postgrad Med J* 59:135-139, 1983

134. Webb-Peploe MM: Obliterative and restrictive cardiomyopathies. *Eur Heart J* 9 Suppl G:159-167, 1988

135. Benotti JR, Grossman W, Cohn PF: Clinical profile of restrictive cardiomyopathy. *Circulation* 61:1206-1212, 1980

136. Siegel RJ, Shah PK, Fishbein MC: Idiopathic restrictive cardiomyopathy. *Circulation* 70:165-169, 1984

137. Child JS, Perloff JK: The restrictive cardiomyopathies. *Cardiol Clin* 6:289-316, 1988

138. Hosenpud JD, Niles NR: Clinical, hemodynamic and endomyocardial biopsy findings in idiopathic restrictive cardiomyopathy. *West J Med* 144:303-306, 1986

139. Dines DE, Edwards JE, Burchell HB: Myocardial atrophy in constrictive pericarditis. *Proc Staff Meet Mayo Clin* 33:93-99, 1958

140. Schoenfeld MH, Supple EW, Dec GW Jr, et al: Restrictive cardiomyopathy versus constrictive pericarditis: role of endomyocardial biopsy in avoiding unnecessary thoracotomy. *Circulation* 75:1012-1017, 1987

141. Maron BJ, Long L, Moller JH, et al: Cardiomyopathies characterized by evidence of resistance to left ventricular inflow. *Cathet Cardiovasc Diagn* 6:29-38, 1980

142. Pellikka PA, Holmes DR Jr, Edwards WD, et al: Endomyocardial biopsy in 30 patients with primary amyloidosis and suspected cardiac involvement. *Arch Intern Med* 148:662-666, 1988

143. Smith TJ, Kyle RA, Lie JT: Clinical significance of histopathologic patterns of cardiac amyloidosis. *Mayo Clin Proc* 59:547-555, 1984

144. Olson LJ, Gertz MA, Edwards WD, et al: Senile cardiac amyloidosis with myocardial dysfunction: diagnosis by endomyocardial biopsy and immunohistochemistry. *N Engl J Med* 317:738-742, 1987

145. McAllister HA Jr, Seger J, Bossart M, et al: Restrictive cardiomyopathy with κ light chain deposits in myocardium as a complication of multiple myeloma: histochemical and electron microscopic observations. *Arch Pathol Lab Med* 112:1151-1154, 1988

146. Bristow MR, Mason JW, Billingham ME, et al: Doxorubicin cardiomyopathy: evaluation by phonocardiography, endomyocardial biopsy, and cardiac catheterization. *Ann Intern Med* 88:168-175, 1978

147. Freter CE, Lee TC, Billingham ME, et al: Doxorubicin cardiac toxicity manifesting seven years after treatment: case report and review. *Am J Med* 80:482-485, 1986

148. Lefrak EA, Pitha J, Rosenheim S, et al: A clinicopathologic analysis of Adriamycin cardiotoxicity. *Cancer* 32:302-314, 1973

149. Billingham ME, Bristow MR, Glatstein E, et al: Adriamycin cardiotoxicity: endomyocardial biopsy evidence of enhancement by irradiation. *Am J Surg Pathol* 1:17-23, 1977

150. Mason JW, Bristow MR, Billingham ME, et al: Invasive and noninvasive methods of assessing Adriamycin cardiotoxic effects in man: superiority of histopathologic assessment using endomyocardial biopsy. *Cancer Treat Rep* 62:857-864, 1978

151. Billingham ME, Mason JW, Bristow MR, et al: Anthracycline cardiomyopathy monitored by morphologic changes. *Cancer Treat Rep* 62:865-872, 1978

152. Bristow MR, Mason JW, Billingham ME, et al: Dose-effect and structure-function relationships in doxorubicin cardiomyopathy. *Am Heart J* 102:709-718, 1981

153. Buja LM, Ferrans VJ, Mayer RJ, et al: Cardiac ultrastructural changes induced by daunorubicin therapy. *Cancer* 32:771-788, 1973

154. Buja LM, Roberts WC: Iron in the heart: etiology and clinical significance. *Am J Med* 51:209-221, 1971

155. Fitchett DH, Coltart DJ, Littler WA, et al: Cardiac involvement in secondary haemochromatosis: a catheter biopsy study and analysis of myocardium. *Cardiovasc Res* 14:719-724, 1980

156. Olson LJ, Edwards WD, McCall JT, et al: Cardiac iron deposition in idiopathic hemochromatosis: histologic and analytic assessment of 14 hearts from autopsy. *J Am Coll Caridol* 10:1239-1243, 1987

157. Olson LJ, Edwards WD, Holmes DR Jr, et al: Endomyocardial biopsy in hemochromatosis: clinicopathologic correlates in six cases. *J Am Coll Cardiol* 13:116-120, 1988

158. Short EM, Winkle RA, Billingham ME: Myocardial involvement in idiopathic hemochromatosis: morphologic and clinical improvement following venesection. *Am J Med* 70:1275-1279, 1981

159. Ratner SJ, Fenoglio JJ Jr, Ursell PC: Utility of endomyocardial biopsy in the diagnosis of cardiac sarcoidosis. *Chest* 90:528-533, 1986

160. Lemery R, McGoon MD, Edwards WD: Cardiac sarcoidosis: a potentially treatable form of myocarditis. *Mayo Clin Proc* 60:549-554, 1985

161. Olson LJ, Reeder GS, Noller KL, et al: Cardiac involvement in glycogen storage disease. III: Morphologic and biochemical characterization with endomyocardial biopsy. *Am J Cardiol* 53:980-981, 1984

162. Matsui S, Murakami E, Takekoshi N, et al: Cardiac manifestations of Fabry's disease: report of a case with pulmonary regurgitation diagnosed on the basis of endomyocardial biopsy findings. *Jpn Circ J* 41:1023-1036, 1977

163. Broadbent JC, Edwards WD, Gordon H, et al: Fabry cardiomyopathy in the female confirmed by endomyocardial biopsy. *Mayo Clin Proc* 56:623-628, 1981

164. Edwards WD, Hurd HP II, Partin JR: Cardiac involvement by Gaucher's disease documented by right ventricular endomyocardial biopsy. *Am J Cardiol* 52:654, 1983

165. Johnston IDA, Popple AW: Right ventricular outflow tract obstruction secondary to small intestinal lymphoma. *Br Heart J* 43:593-596, 1980

166. Hanley PC, Shub C, Seward JB, et al: Intracavitary cardiac melanoma diagnosed by endomyocardial left ventricular biopsy. *Chest* 84:195-198, 1983

167. Case records of the Massachusetts General Hospital (Case 29-1983). *N Engl J Med* 309:169-178, 1983

168. Hausheer FH, Josephson RA, Grochow LB, et al: Intracardiac sarcoma diagnosed by left ventricular endomyocardial biopsy. *Chest* 92:177-179, 1987

169. Adachi K, Tanaka H, Toshima H, et al: Right atrial angiosarcoma diagnosed by cardiac biopsy. *Am Heart J* 115:482-485, 1988

170. Flipse TR, Tazelaar HD, Holmes DR Jr: Diagnosis of malignant cardiac disease by endomyocardial biopsy. *Mayo Clin Proc* 65:1415-1422, 1990

CHAPTER

20

Hypertrophic cardiomyopathy

Rick A. Nishimura, M.D., Emilio R. Giuliani, M.D., Robert O. Brandenburg, M.D., and Gordon K. Danielson, M.D.

HYPERTROPHIC cardiomyopathy is a disease of the heart muscle of unknown etiology. Pathologically, it is characterized by a small left ventricular cavity and marked hypertrophy of the myocardium with myocardial fiber disarray. There may or may not be evidence of an associated intraventricular pressure gradient in one or both ventricles.

The first anatomic description of this entity was by Teare[1] in 1958, when he reported the pathologic findings in eight young patients, seven of whom died suddenly. There was massive hypertrophy of the ventricular septum and a small ventricular cavity. This gross picture was associated with microscopic evidence of myocardial disarray of the individual muscle fibers which was thought to be due to a benign tumor or hamartoma. Additionally, Brock[2] reported on several patients with functional subvalvular left ventricular outflow gradients confirmed by pressure recordings at catheterization. Many of his patients had accompanying aortic stenosis or hypertension, and the gradient was attributed by him to a secondary massive left ventricular hypertrophy developing from pressure overload. A specific disease process was suggested by Braunwald et al.[3] in 1960, when they described asymmetric septal hypertrophy with myocardial fiber disarray associated with a dynamic subvalvular pressure gradient. This was considered to be a primary process with no known cause. The possibility of genetic connection was suggested when a familial link was shown to be associated with this entity.[4] Recently, it was demonstrated that mutations in the cardiac myosin heavy chain genes are associated with hypertrophic cardiomyopathy in some families.[5,6]

This disease process has had a wide variety of names. It has been called "asymmetric septal hypertrophy," "idiopathic hypertrophic subaortic stenosis," "hypertrophic obstructive cardiomyopathy," and "muscular subaortic stenosis."[7] The World Health Organization has designated the term "hypertrophic cardiomyopathy" to describe this unique disease process.[8]

The diagnosis of hypertrophic cardiomyopathy (HCM) should be reserved for patients who have (1) significant hypertrophy of the myocardium in the absence of an underlying cause or (2) an inappropriate degree of hypertrophy in response to a known stimulus.[9] A dynamic left ventricular outflow gradient may or may not be present.[9] The epidemiology of HCM remains difficult to assess, because many patients do not have symptoms and the disease is undiagnosed. In Olmsted County, Minn., the age- and sex-adjusted incidence rate was found to be 2.5/100,000 person-years, with a prevalence rate of 19.7/100,000 population.[10] Although an impressive number of investigations have been generated concerning etiology, pathophysiology, natural history, and treatment, HCM remains a fascinating and often confusing disease entity.[11b]

ETIOLOGY

The characteristic pathologic and pathophysiologic features of HCM have intrigued many, and the result has been that a multitude of causes have been postulated for this disorder. A familial component has been demonstrated with the use of asymmetric septal hypertrophy as a marker. Clark et al.[4] showed that 46% of first-degree relatives of patients with HCM had asymmetric septal hypertrophy, and they concluded that this occurred on an autosomal dominant basis with a high degree of penetrance.

There has been an association of HCM with the human lymphocyte antigen HLA-DRw4 from several institutions,[12-14] consistent with a genetic component in susceptibility to HCM. Others have not found support for an association with the HLA antigens.[15] The high frequency of sporadic cases indicates that nongenetic causes may exist to produce phenotypically similar expressions of the disease.[11a]

Goodwin[7] postulated that HCM develops as a response to an increase in catecholamine stimulation. Animal experiments have shown that continuous exposure to a high level of catecholamines will result in asymmetric septal hypertrophy and an intraventricular pressure gradient.[16] Administration of a nerve growth factor in dogs produced an increase in sympathetic innervation of the heart, resulting in myocardial hypertrophy with histologic disarray of muscle fibers similar to that seen in patients with HCM.[17] Histochemical studies of resected portions of outflow tract muscles from patients with HCM revealed an increased sympathetic nerve supply[18,19] and possibly a higher norepinephrine content of the muscle.[18,19] The association of HCM with pheochromocytoma, multiple lentiginosis, and neurofibromatosis has raised the question of a neural crest disorder.[16,17,20,21]

A hereditary cardiomyopathy of Syrian hamsters has prompted some investigators to propose a calcium disorder as a cause of HCM.[22,23] These hamsters have increased myocardial calcium uptake and content; the cardiomyopathy may be prevented by the use of calcium-channel blocking agents.[22] In the Syrian hamster, there appears to be a defect in the calcium-channel antagonist binding site protein, resulting in 50% more calcium-channel binding sites. It was subsequently shown that the number of calcium antagonist receptors in the myocardium of patients with HCM is increased, presumably reflecting an increased density of voltage-sensitive calcium channels.[24] The increased density of the calcium channels and resultant increase in calcium entry into the myocardium have been the basis for implicating abnormal calcium kinetics in patients with HCM as a cause of the hyperdynamic contractility and delayed relaxation.[25]

In over half the patients, the disease is familial, with an autosomal dominance pattern of transmission with variable expression.[26] The remaining cases appear to be sporadic.[26] Up until recently, the genetics of this disorder were understood only in classic mendelian terms, but since 1989, investigation of the molecular biology of HCM has provided new insight into its causation.[5,6,27,28] Molecular genetics studies have demonstrated linkage of familial HCM to the cardiac myosin heavy-chain genes on chromosome 14 in some families.[5,29]

It has been shown that a missense mutation in the β myosin heavy-chain gene is the probable cause of HCM in a kindred.[30] Additional missense mutations have been identified in the β myosin heavy-chain gene in other families.[6] It is proposed that the mutated β myosin heavy-chain genes produce "poison polypeptides" that cause the formation of defective myofibrils in patients with HCM.[6] It is of great interest for future investigation that certain types of mutations may portend a poorer prognosis.[6] Transcripts of β myosin heavy-chain genes have been detected in blood lymphocytes and could potentially be used to screen for the mutations that cause HCM.[28]

PATHOLOGY

Gross examination of the heart in HCM reveals a small ventricular cavity with a flattened "S" shape from the pronounced septal thickening[31-34] (Fig 20-1). Measurements at autopsy of septal-to-free-wall ratio may not reflect asymmetric septal hypertrophy, even though this was present during life, because the postmortem heart usually has a systolic configuration that results in increased thickness of the free wall.[35] The mural endocardium is thickened by fibrous tissue, and there is often a plaque located on the upper septal area where the mitral valve has been apposed to the septum during diastole.[32] The mitral valve itself is usually intrinsically normal although distorted in shape from the myocardial hypertrophy.[31,32] In nearly all hearts, the left atrium is dilated at autopsy.[32]

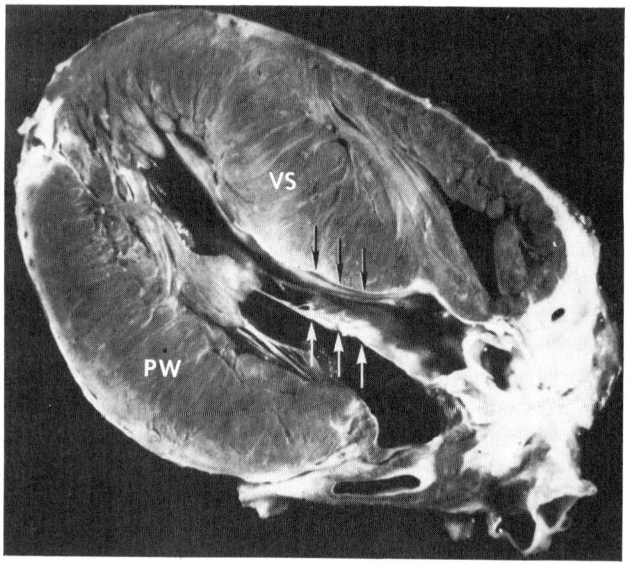

Fig 20-1 HCM from the long-axis view. Ventricular cavity is small and has pronounced septal and posterior wall thickening. *Arrows* indicate narrowing of the left ventricular outflow tract caused by the thickened ventricular septum and anterior leaflet of the mitral valve. *VS,* ventricular septum; *PW,* posterior wall of the left ventricle. (From Edwards WD, Zakheim R, Mattioli L: Asymmetric septal hypertrophy in childhood: unreliability of histologic criteria for differentiation of obstructive and nonobstructive forms. *Hum Pathol* 8:277-284, 1977. By permission of WB Saunders Company.)

The epicardial coronary arteries often are large in caliber without significant obstructive disease.[32] The incidence of significant obstructive coronary disease in patients with HCM is less than 25%, which is probably less than that in an age-matched normal population.[36] However, intramural coronary arterioles in the septum are abnormal, with thickening of the vessel wall and a decrease in lumen size.[32,37] The areas of myocardium supplied by these vessels are frequently associated with areas of myocardial fibrosis and may contribute to the myocardial ischemic manifestations found in patients with HCM.[37]

Teare,[1] in his original report, noted bizarre arrangements of muscle fibers separated by clefts lined with endothelium. The myocardial disarray consists of short runs of severely hypertrophied fibers interrupted by connective tissue; there are large, bizarre nuclei and fibrosis, degenerating muscle fibers, and disappearing muscle myofibrils. The disorganization results in a "whorling" of muscle fiber, which has been considered to be characteristic of HCM[31] (Fig 20-2). Myocardial disarray has been noted not only in the ventricular septum in patients with HCM but also in the left ventricular free wall and may be indicative of a more severe myopathic process when present in the free wall.[38] The myocardial disarray is not specific but can be seen in pressure-overloaded ventricles and even in normal hearts.[31,38,39] However, when quantitated, the disarray of HCM occupies a much larger proportion of myocardium than it does in the other

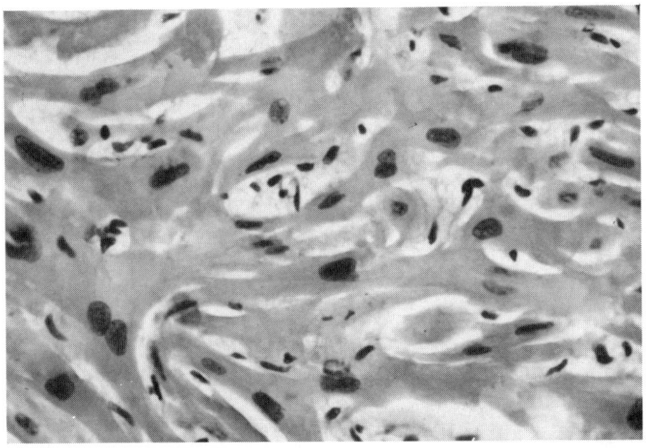

Fig 20-2 Photomicrograph of the myocardium in HCM. There is pronounced disarray and hypertrophy of the individual muscle fibers, resulting in a "whorling" appearance of the muscle fiber. (Hematoxylin and eosin; ×165.) (Photograph courtesy of William D. Edwards, M.D.)

entities.[40-42] It has been stated that even quantitative measurements of myocardial disarray are not diagnostic, because the plane of a section of tissue might profoundly influence the degree of disarray.[43] Histochemical studies have revealed increased glycogen stores in hearts of patients with HCM, but these are nonspecific findings, as is the disarray of myofibrils and myofilaments seen on electron microscopic studies.[41]

PATHOPHYSIOLOGY

Cardiac function in HCM is altered by a combination of structural and functional abnormalities—ventricular hypertrophy with supernormal systolic function, ventricular outflow gradients, abnormal diastolic relaxation and compliance, mitral regurgitation, myocardial ischemia, and cardiac arrhythmias.[44] The varying combination and varying degrees of these abnormalities account for the wide spectrum of presentation of HCM.[11b,45,46]

Diastolic function

Impaired diastolic filling of the heart is one of the major pathophysiologic mechanisms in patients with HCM.[11a,11b,47-50] Although decreased compliance of the left ventricle was first implicated in the early 1960s[51] as a cause for the symptoms in patients with HCM, only within the past decade has an understanding of the complex process of diastolic filling of the heart evolved.[52-54] Diastole is a complex series of multiple interrelated events, and its evaluation in the past has been difficult. With the advent of radionuclide angiography and Doppler echocardiography, a greater understanding of the diastolic filling process in patients with HCM has been possible.

Two processes during diastole are markedly changed in patients with HCM: relaxation is impaired, and chamber stiffness is increased.[49] Other factors, such as erectile coronary effect (coronary turgor), pericardial restraint, ventricular interaction, and viscoelastic forces, also probably contribute but are more difficult to assess.

Relaxation depends on load, inactivation, and nonuniformity,[52] all of which are abnormal in patients with HCM.[11a,49] The left ventricular outflow gradient poses a contraction load, and impaired coronary and ventricular filling impose a relaxation load.[47] Inactivation of the contractile elements is abnormal because of calcium overload.[52] Patients with HCM have a marked abnormality of nonuniformity of relaxation.[55,56] These factors all contribute to a marked impairment of relaxation. High-fidelity pressure measurements have demonstrated a slower rate of fall of left ventricular pressure that extends through early and mid diastole. This is manifested on radionuclide angiograms and Doppler mitral flow velocities as prolonged isovolumetric relaxation periods and decrease in peak filling rates. [55,57-63]

Compliance is also abnormal in HCM.[49] Compliance is the rise in pressure that occurs for a given increase in volume. Myocardial stiffness is increased, muscle mass is increased, and chamber volume is decreased, all of which decrease compliance.[47,49] Myocardial oxygen mismatch from the large myocardial muscle mass and from systolic compression of epicardial arteries leads to myocardial ischemia and further causes abnormalities of both relaxation and compliance.

The combination of relaxation and compliance abnormalities leads to increased diastolic pressures, which are reflected back to the pulmonary circulation and cause symptoms of dyspnea. The increased diastolic pressures also result in an increase in myocardial ischemia, because of a lower coronary perfusion gradient, and thus contribute to symptoms of angina pectoris. The abnormalities of diastolic filling of the heart may account for most symptoms in selected subgroups of patients with HCM.

Systolic function

The majority of patients with HCM have a normal to small left ventricular chamber size with normal to supernormal systolic function; development of a clinical picture dominated by congestive heart failure is rare.[45,46] Most patients have a normal to supernormal ejection fraction by angiography, with a pronounced increase in the speed and extent of ventricular emptying; this results in obliteration of the ventricular apex at end-systole.[3] The dp/dt during the ventricular ejection period is increased; 75% to 80% of the total stroke volume is ejected in the first half of systole.[3] Systolic function as measured by percentage shortening of the left ventricular cavity dimension, ejection fraction, and velocity of circumferential fiber shortening is normal or increased in patients with HCM.[64]

Left ventricular outflow pressure gradient

The original description by Brock[2] in 1957 emphasized functional subvalvular left ventricular outflow gradients at cardiac catheterization. The occurrence of catheter entrapment has been described in which the catheter tip lies in the obliterated left ventricular apex and causes an artificial increase in pressure.[65] An intraventricular gradient can also be produced in normal hearts in the absence of obstruction by isoproterenol infusion[65] or severe hypovolemia. Thus, the term "cavity obliteration" has been suggested,[65] in which an empty, contracted ventricular apex at end-systole can produce a higher systolic pressure than in the basal portion of the ventricle and form an intraventricular gradient. However, an outflow gradient may be demonstrated with the catheter tip placed within a nonobliterated portion of the left ventricle in patients with HCM—proving a true subaortic outflow gradient.[66]

The true significance of the intraventricular outflow gradient has been controversial.[67-70] It has been demonstrated that 80% of forward stroke output occurs during the first half of systole in patients with HCM compared with 57% in control subjects.[67] This results in a pronounced decrease in forward flow during the latter half of systole. It had been suggested that the intraventricular pressure gradient does not actually signify outflow obstruction but instead is a result of rapid and early emptying of a hyperdynamic ventricle.[68] Doppler echocardiographic studies have subsequently shown that true obstruction to outflow does exist, because forward flow continues throughout the entire systolic ejection period, which itself is prolonged.[47,49]

The outflow pressure gradients may be present at rest and may be labile or latent.[2,3,71-75] The reproducibility of the level of the gradient from day to day in an individual patient is poor;[73,75] this helps to explain why the magnitude of the outflow gradient as measured at catheterization does not correlate with symptoms or prognosis.[45,76]

Mitral regurgitation

Mitral regurgitation frequently occurs in patients with HCM, especially in those with left ventricular outflow obstruction.[71,77,78] As with the left ventricular outflow gradient, the severity of mitral regurgitation is dynamic. Mitral regurgitation decreases in severity as the degree of outflow obstruction decreases and vice versa. Most of the mitral regurgitation takes place late in systole after the onset of the obstruction, an occurrence supporting the concept that the regurgitation depends on distortion of the mitral valve apparatus caused by the obstruction.[47,78] The patients who have severe mitral regurgitation experience significant symptoms of dyspnea and are helped most by surgical myectomy to decrease the degree of regurgitation.

Myocardial ischemia

Chest pain is a common symptom in patients with HCM, even those with normal coronary arteries. It has been shown that regional myocardial ischemia does occur in these patients. Thallium-201 scintigraphy has demonstrated perfusion defects in most patients with HCM.[79] Positron emission tomography scanning has revealed both a decrease in myocardial blood flow and a decrease in myocardial glucose utilization in the septum of patients with HCM.[80] During atrial pacing, lactate production measured from the coronary sinus occurs, indicating that myocardial ischemia is present.[81]

The reason for myocardial ischemia is unclear, but it may be related to a number of factors. The increase of muscle mass and high left ventricular pressures from the outflow gradient serve to increase myocardial oxygen requirements.[11a,82] Coronary vascular resistance may be increased because of systolic compression of the large intramyocardial coronary arteries.[83] Inadequate coronary flow reserve and impaired oxygen extraction are present in patients with HCM.[82] Abnormalities of relaxation may have an adverse effect on coronary filling and myocardial ischemia.[49]

Abnormally small and thickened intramural coronary arteries have also been implicated in the production of myocardial ischemia.[37] Because these have been associated with areas of myocardial fibrosis, continued microinfarcts may be the mechanism for the left ventricular dysfunction and dilatation that occur in some patients.[37,84] This mechanism is further supported by thallium-201 studies, which show fixed defects in patients with reduced ejection fraction and thin walls and reversible defects in patients with supranormal ejection fractions and thick walls.[79]

Cardiac arrhythmias

Patients with HCM have a high incidence of both atrial and ventricular arrhythmias. These may be asymptomatic, may cause recurrent episodes of syncope, and are probably one of the major causes of sudden death that occurs in patients with HCM. Incidences of premature atrial contractions and supraventricular tachycardias have been shown to be high on Holter monitoring and treadmill exertion testing.[85,86] The rapid atrioventricular (AV) nodal conduction[87] and bypass tracts[88] associated with HCM may be the basis of hemodynamic deterioration that occurs when atrial fibrillation develops. The diseased myocardium[88] and abnormal refractory periods[89] in patients with HCM predispose them to ventricular arrhythmias, which have been documented in 20% to 40% of patients by Holter monitoring[86,90] and are the major cause for symptoms of syncope and sudden death.

Combination of pathophysiologic factors

It is very likely that some patients have pure diastolic dysfunction without outflow obstruction and other patients have pure outflow obstruction without diastolic abnormalities accounting for symptoms. Most patients most likely have a combination of both systolic and diastolic abnormalities to some degree. Myocardial ischemia and cardiac arrhythmias also contribute to the pathophysiology in these patients (Fig 20-3).

SYMPTOMS

The three major symptoms of HCM are dyspnea, angina, and syncope.[76,91-93] The variability in clinical presentation is wide. Symptoms may appear at all ages, but the majority of patients become symptomatic in the second or third decade. Two generalizations have consistently been found with respect to symptoms: (1) there has been a consistent lack of correlation of symptoms with the

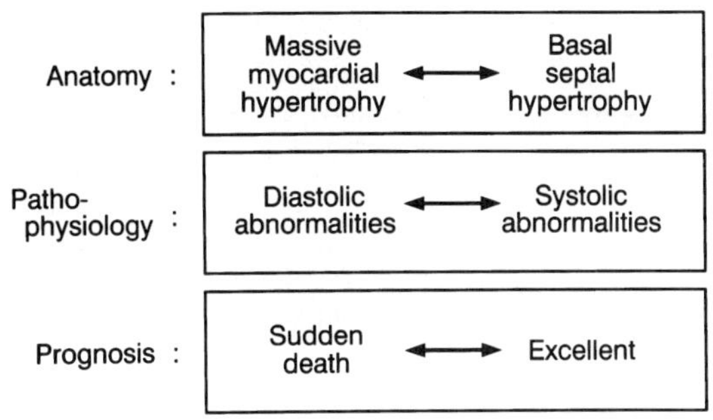

Fig 20-3 The wide spectrum of presentation of anatomy, pathophysiology, and prognosis in patients with hypertrophic cardiomyopathy.

outflow gradient,[45,91] and (2) the older patients tend to be more symptomatic.[45,93]

Dyspnea is a common symptom, occurring in up to 90% of all patients with HCM. The symptom of dyspnea has not been shown to correlate with any hemodynamic or echocardiographic measure of left ventricular outflow gradient or left ventricular systolic function. However, prolonged isovolumic relaxation as shown by echocardiography,[56,64,94] decreased rate of peak posterior wall thinning on angiography,[51] and decreased peak left ventricular filling rate on radionuclide studies[95,96] support the concept that abnormal diastolic function is the probable cause of symptoms of dyspnea.

Angina occurs in 70% to 80% of all patients with HCM,[36] and 15% of all patients at autopsy have associated myocardial infarction.[97] Approximately 25% of patients with HCM over 44 years old will have significant coronary artery disease noted on angiography,[36] but the remainder experience angina with normal extramural coronary arteries. The angina and myocardial infarction have a number of possible mechanisms: (1) small-artery narrowing as seen in some patients with normal extramural coronary arteries and myocardial infarction,[87,97] (2) intramyocardial compression of small arteries from massive muscular hypertrophy,[93] (3) abnormal diastolic filling resulting in an imbalance of oxygen supply-demand ratio because of the noncompliant, thickened ventricle,[64,98] and (4) coronary spasm.[99]

Syncope occurs in approximately 20% of patients with HCM, but 50% to 55% of all patients with this disorder will have presyncopal symptoms. An earlier suggested mechanism of syncope occurring immediately after exercise was a decrease in venous return with continued sympathetic stimulation to the heart, resulting in a critical increase in outflow gradient.[3,76,100,101] However, it has repeatedly been shown that syncopal symptoms do not correlate with outflow gradients, often occurring in those who have no or mild gradients at rest.[76,91,92] In most instances cardiac arrhythmia is the likely cause. Ambulatory monitoring of patients with HCM has shown frequent complex ventricular ectopy, with a 20% to 40% incidence of ventricular tachycardia.[85,90,102] Electrophysiologic studies have shown that the ventricular septum in these patients has different electrophysiologic properties, with abnormal refractory periods, which make them prone to ventricular reentry arrhythmias.[89] Rapid atrial arrhythmias are common, occurring in up to 50% of patients.[90,102] The frequently encountered rapid ventricular response and hemodynamic deterioration associated with atrial arrhythmias may be a result of an association of HCM with bypass tracts[76,88] or fetal dispersion of the AV node.[87] In other instances, it has been proposed that activation of left ventricular baroceptors could be the cause of exercise hypotention and hemodynamic collapse.[103-105] This hypothesis is based on the observation of syncope during sinus rhythm,[104] an abnormal response to exercise in one-third of patients,[105] and the frequent occurrence of hypotension during head-up tilt.[103] Hypotension suddenly occurring during head-up tilt is associated with bradycardia and a reduced cavity size, compatible with activation of a ventricular baroreflex.[103]

Deterioration to heart failure is uncommon,[45,100,101] occurring in fewer than 7% of patients with HCM. In the few patients in whom congestive failure develops, a decrease in intensity of the outflow murmur and a loss of outflow gradient have been noted.[45] Accompanying myocardial infarction may contribute to this mode of deterioration.[97]

PHYSICAL EXAMINATION

The classic physical findings in patients with HCM described below apply to patients who have left ventricular outflow gradients.[3,76,100,101] The subset of patients without outflow gradients will present only with features of left ventricular hypertrophy on physical examination.

Carotid pulse

The classic carotid impulse (Fig 20-4) is bisferiens and is characterized by a rapid rise ("percussion wave") followed by a midsystolic drop, which in turn is followed by a delayed slower wave ("tidal wave"). The drop in amplitude in early systole is associated with premature closure of the aortic valve and coincides with systolic anterior motion of the mitral valve.[71,106] The later peak is due to relief of the outflow gradient as the mitral leaflet returns to its original position.[107] This bifid contour is seen in approximately 60% to 70% of all patients who have gradients. Because of the supernormal systolic function, the upstroke time is much more rapid than normal; the pronounced hypertrophy causes a longer ejection time. The importance of recognizing the typical carotid pulsation is in the differential diagnosis of valvular aortic stenosis, in which there is both a decrease in rate of rise and a decrease in amplitude of the carotid pulsation. The pulse amplitude diminishes after a premature contraction in patients with HCM, as opposed to the increased amplitude seen in valvular outflow obstruction. This change is due to the postextrasystolic increase in ventricular contractility in HCM, which results in a greater outflow gradient and consequently a decrease in pulse amplitude.

Jugular venous pulse

The jugular venous pulsation is of little value in the diagnosis of HCM. An exception occurs when there is

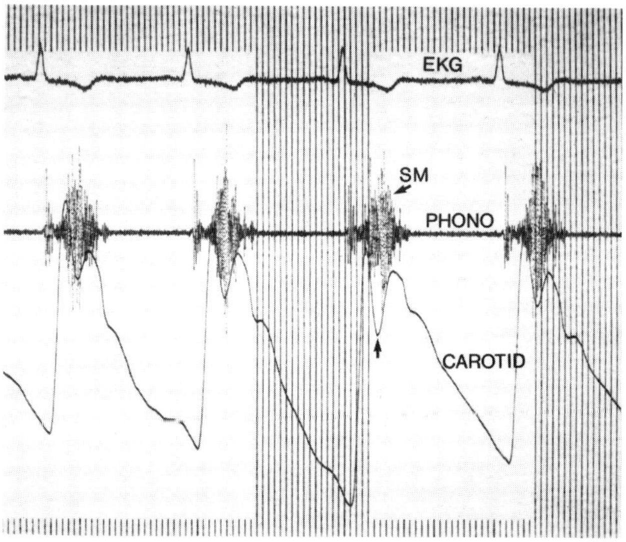

Fig 20-4 Carotid pulse tracing and phonocardiogram in HCM. Carotid pulsation is bisferiens; drop in amplitude in early systole coincides with the peak of the systolic murmur *(arrow). SM,* systolic murmur; *EKG,* electrocardiogram.

right ventricular involvement, in which case there will be a large "a" wave reflecting decreased compliance of the right ventricle.

Apical impulse

The apical impulse is a powerful systolic thrust, which is sustained throughout most of systole and is a reflection of left ventricular hypertrophy. There is often a bifid impulse due to a forceful atrial systole (palpable S_4) that distends a poorly compliant ventricle. About 20% to 25% of patients will have a triple impulse, the third component occurring near the end of the systole after relief of the outflow gradient.

A systolic thrill is palpable in approximately 40% of patients. Its location is lower in the chest than that for valvular aortic stenosis, usually between the lower left sternal border and the apex. The thrill has been associated with severe mitral regurgitation but is more common in the presence of a high outflow gradient.

Cardiac sounds

Auscultation reveals a normal first heart sound, usually preceded by a loud fourth heart sound, and sometimes a third heart sound is present because of the poorly compliant left ventricle. The presence of a systolic click should alert the clinician to an associated valvular abnormality. The second heart sound is usually split physiologically, yet 20% of patients have a paradoxic split, which has been associated with higher outflow gradients or left bundle-branch block.[76]

Murmurs

The outflow murmur is systolic in timing, crescendo-decrescendo in nature, and of mixed frequency or scratchy in quality; it is located at the left sternal border (see Fig 20-4). The intensity of the murmur is variable and is not related to the severity of the outflow gradient; however, a longer duration of the murmur does correlate with a higher gradient. In contrast to valvular aortic outflow murmurs, there is seldom radiation into the carotid arteries. Mitral regurgitation is present in 50% to 90% of patients with HCM and is the cause of an apical pansystolic murmur.

Various maneuvers differentiate the murmur of HCM from those of valvular aortic stenosis and mitral regurgitation (Fig 20-5). Maneuvers that decrease left ventricular volume, and hence the outflow tract diameter, such as the Valsalva maneuver, use of amyl nitrite, and assumption of the upright posture, will increase the amount of dynamic gradient and thus increase the intensity of the murmur. Maneuvers that increase left ventricular volume, such as squatting, leg raising in the supine position, or phenylephrine infusion, will decrease the dynamic gradient and result in a lower intensity of the murmur. The only other lesion that responds to volume changes in this manner is some instances of mitral valve prolapse, which should be distinguishable by the presence of nonejection systolic clicks and the location and quality of the murmur. As with any type of left ventricular outflow murmur, the response of the murmur of HCM after a premature ventricular contraction that increases the contractility of the postextrasystolic beat is an increase in intensity of the systolic murmur during the postpremature beat. The differentiation of the dynamic left ventricular outflow obstruction of HCM from other causes of left ventricular outflow obstruction can be made by palpation of the peripheral pulse after a premature contraction. In patients with HCM, the pulse amplitude following premature contraction is lower because of a marked increase in the degree of obstruction from increased contractility and decreased afterload. Exercise, amyl nitrite, and sympathetic drugs all increase contractility and will increase the intensity of the systolic murmur, as opposed to β-adrenergic blocking agents, which decrease contractility and decrease the intensity of the murmur.

The presence of an aortic diastolic decrescendo murmur should suggest another disease, such as aortic valvular disease or a subaortic fibromuscular diaphragm, that has caused a "jet" deformity of the aortic cusps. In the authors' experience, there are some patients, usually younger, with severe outflow gradients in whom a low-frequency apical diastolic rumble may be auscultated, probably reflecting transmitral flow into a thick, noncompliant ventricle.

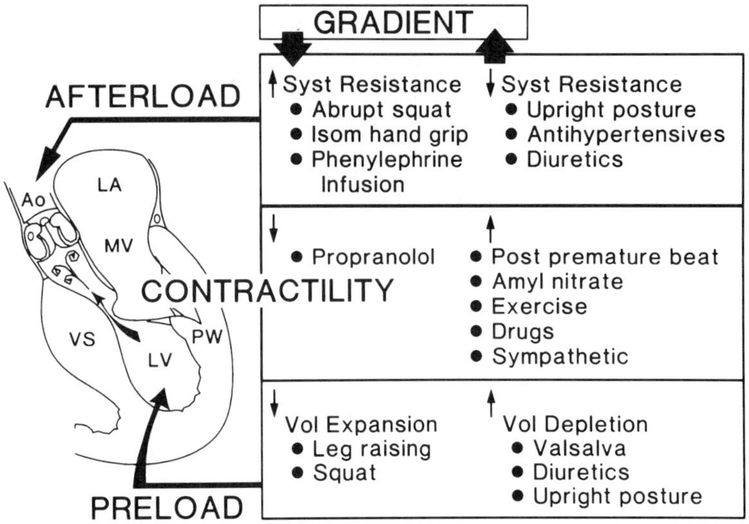

Fig 20-5 Interventions that change the outflow gradient, with resultant change in intensity of the systolic murmur in HCM. Outflow gradient is affected by changes in afterload, preload, and contractility. *Ao,* aorta; *LA,* left atrium; *MV,* mitral valve; *VS,* ventricular septum; *LV,* left ventricle; *PW,* posterior wall.

DIAGNOSTIC STUDIES

Electrocardiogram

The electrocardiogram (ECG) is abnormal in the majority of patients with HCM.[76] The basic rhythm is normal sinus rhythm, but ambulatory Holter recordings have shown a high incidence of supraventricular tachycardia (46%), multiform premature ventricular contractions (43%), and ventricular tachycardia (26%).[86] The onset of atrial fibrillation, which occurs in 10% of patients, is often associated with clinical deterioration.[108] Preexcitation has been associated with HCM,[76] and a rapid ventricular response with atrial fibrillation may further contribute to hemodynamic deterioration.

A normal axis is present in 60% of patients and a left axis in 30%. Approximately 70% to 80% of patients with HCM will demonstrate left ventricular hypertrophy on the ECG.[76] ECG findings of left ventricular hypertrophy occur more commonly in patients with extensive distribution of hypertrophy involving substantial portions of both the ventricular septum and the free wall.[109] The earlier report from Japan[110] suggesting that giant negative T wave had a high degree of specificity for apical HCM is not supported by the study of Alfonso et al.[111] In this study, giant negative T waves were present in 15%, and although associated with a greater degree of left ventricular hypertrophy, the T-wave abnormality was not limited to anatomic sites and the patients with the ECG feature did not differ from others in symptomatic status, ventricular function, evidence of ventricular arrhythmias, or outcome during follow-up. Although bundle-branch blocks and AV blocks are unusual, more than 80% of patients undergoing electrophysiologic studies demonstrated a prolonged H–V interval.[112] Abnormal Q waves simulating myocardial infarction are common (25%) and may appear in the limb leads, right precordial leads, or left precordial leads[109,113] (Fig 20-6). Vector analysis and electrophysiologic studies have shown that the Q waves are due to a disturbance of activation of the ventricular septum[89,114] and may disappear after septotomy.[115] A completely normal ECG is most commonly a manifestation of localized left ventricular hypertrophy.[109]

Chest radiograph

The chest radiograph depicts mild to moderate enlargement of the cardiac silhouette, with a rounded left ventricular contour consistent with concentric left ventricular hypertrophy.[76] The left atrium is often enlarged, but the right-sided chambers are usually not prominent.[76] The presence of aortic valvular calcification or a dilated ascending aorta should raise the question of aortic valvular disease. Cardiac fluoroscopy may demonstrate calcification of the mitral valve annulus.[116]

M-mode echocardiography

The advent of M-mode echocardiography heralded considerable advances in the knowledge of the pathophysiology and diagnosis of HCM.[35,64,94,107,117-146] The classic features of asymmetric septal hypertrophy, systolic anterior motion of the mitral valve, and early systolic closure of the aortic valve on M-mode echocardiography have allowed a reproducible noninvasive technique for the diagnosis of HCM. However, M-mode echocardiography as an isolated study may lead to erroneous diagnoses concerning HCM and is of historic interest only.

Asymmetric septal hypertrophy, defined as a septal-to-free-wall thickness ratio of more than 1.3, was at one time considered to be pathognomonic for HCM[117] (Fig 20-7). Subsequent studies by two-dimensional echocardiography have shown that HCM may involve concentric hypertrophy or areas of hypertrophy not visualized by an M-mode beam.[121,122] In addition, asymmetric septal hypertrophy occurs in a variety of situations that are not related to HCM.

Systolic anterior motion of the mitral valve was first described on angiography in 1966.[66] Subsequent reports of M-mode echocardiographic tracings confirmed the presence of systolic anterior motion in patients with

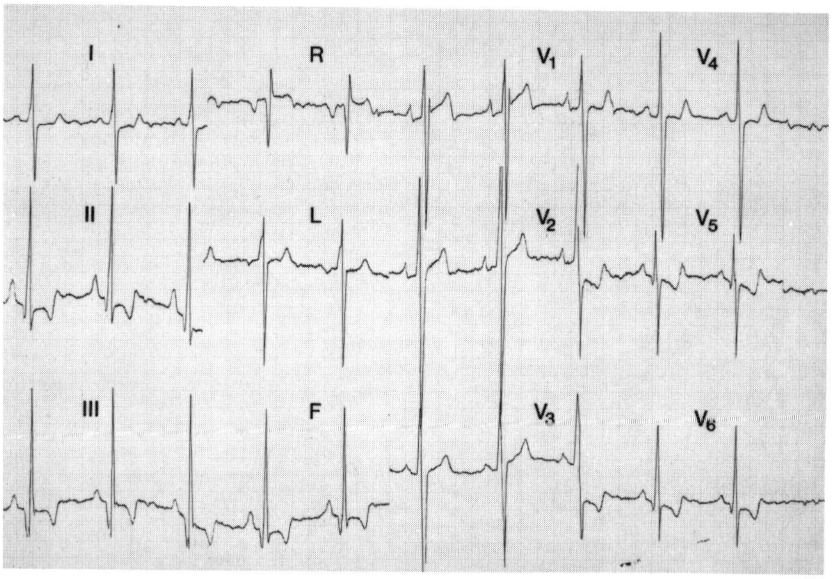

Fig 20-6 ECG tracing from a patient with HCM. There are pathologic Q waves in leads II, III, and aV_F *(F)* that simulate an inferior myocardial infarction. Voltage criteria for left ventricular hypertrophy are present.

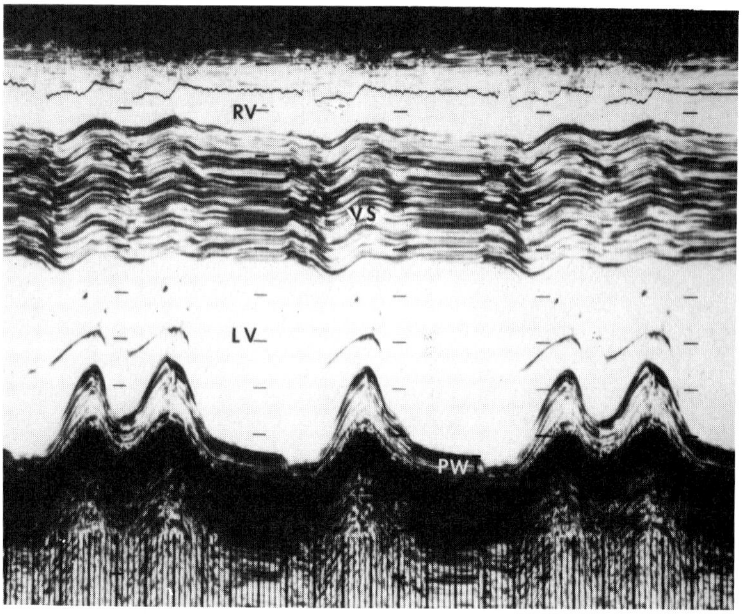

Fig 20-7 M-mode echocardiographic tracing at the level of the mid left ventricle in HCM. There a pronounced increase in ventricular septal *(VS)* thickness, whereas the posterior wall *(PW)* is of normal thickness. *LV,* left ventricle; *RV,* right ventricle.

HCM[107,135] (Fig 20-8). The left ventricular outflow gradient has been correlated with systolic anterior motion of the mitral valve.[71-76,107,132-136] Various mechanisms have been proposed as the cause of systolic anterior motion: (1) septal hypertrophy or forward position of the mitral valve at the onset of systole, causing a narrowed outflow tract and increased velocity of blood through the outflow tract, with a resulting Venturi effect, which pulls or sucks the anterior leaflet against the septum and brings it out of apposition to the posterior leaflet;[137,147] (2) abnormal papillary muscle contraction and abnormal rotation of the mitral valve, which then balloons into the outflow tract;[138,139] and (3) superior displacement of the papillary muscles, leading to chordal slackening with resultant anterior mitral motion.[148] The first explanation is the most plausible, but a combination of these factors may be involved.

Other characteristic M-mode features associated with HCM include early systolic aortic valve closure and decreased rate of septal thickening. The early systolic closure of the aortic valve was found to correlate with a resting gradient, and it disappeared after surgical relief of

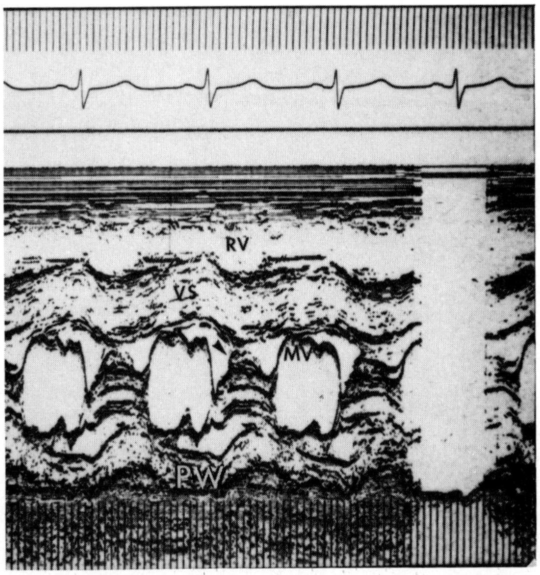

Fig 20-8 M-mode echocardiographic tracing at the level of the mitral valve in HCM. *Arrowhead* depicts systolic anterior motion of the mitral valve. *VS,* ventricular septum; *PW,* posterior wall; *MV,* mitral valve; *RV,* right ventricle.

the gradient;[142] however, it is nonspecific and has been seen in normal persons and in patients with ventricular septal defects, mitral regurgitation, double-outlet right ventricle, aortic root dissection, and congestive cardiomyopathy.[145] The decrease in excursion and in systolic thickening of the ventricular septum adds to the specificity of asymmetric septal hypertrophy in the diagnosis of HCM but will decrease its sensitivity.[131,136]

Two-dimensional echocardiography

By its ability to visualize all walls of the myocardium and valvular motion in real time, two-dimensional echocardiography has become the diagnostic tool of choice for patients in whom HCM is suspected. It is not only valuable for studying the dynamic pathology seen in patients with HCM but has also greatly expanded the concept of the diversity of anatomic variants of HCM.[149]

Three different sites of outflow tract narrowing have been demonstrated with two-dimensional echocardiography.[150,151] These are (1) classic narrowing between the basal septum and the mitral valve leaflet; (2) narrowing between the upper third of the ventricular septum and the distal free edge of the mitral valve; and (3) midventricular narrowing between the midseptum and the papillary muscle.

The classic two-dimensional echocardiographic features of a patient with HCM are shown in Figure 20-9. This demonstrates the pronounced thickening of the entire ventricular septum, extending from the base to the apex, out of proportion to the posterior wall. Systolic anterior motion of the mitral valve can be directly visualized in real time. By utilization of multiple views by two-dimensional echocardiography, all walls of the left ventricle can be visualized.

As seen by two-dimensional echocardiography, a wide spectrum of morphologic patterns is present in patients with HCM[47,77,121] (Fig 20-10). The septal hypertrophy can involve the entire septum or the anterior or posterior septum alone. Septal hypertrophy is not uniform from base to apex in all patients, for it may be localized to the base, middle, or apical third alone.[150,152,153] In most patients with HCM, the anterior and lateral free wall is also involved by the hypertrophic process.[47,77,119,121,150,152-154] Concentric hypertrophy may be present.[146]

The involvement by hypertrophy has been demonstrated to be related to the age of the patient.[155,156] In younger patients, hypertrophy is much more severe and is characterized by a crescent-shaped left ventricle and reversed septal curvature.[155,156] Older patients have less severe hypertrophy, including an ovoid contour of the left ventricle and normal septal curvature, but more distortion of the left ventricular outflow tract.[155,156]

The degree of hypertrophy found on two-dimensional echocardiography may have important implications. The extent of hypertrophy has been correlated with Doppler indices[157] and nuclear indices[158] of impaired relaxation and with the degree of left ventricular end-diastolic pressure elevation.[47] Thus, the more extensive the hypertrophy, the greater the abnormality of diastolic filling. This would explain why patients with the most widespread hypertrophy have the greatest functional limitation.[121] On Holter monitoring, the degree of hypertrophy has been shown to correlate with the occurrence of nonsustained ventricular tachycardia,[47,159,160] which itself is a marker for increased risk of sudden death. Most patients with no or mild symptoms who die suddenly have marked and diffuse left ventricular hypertrophy.[160,161] Sudden death is uncommon in the asymptomatic adult with relatively mild hypertrophy.[161]

Longitudinal echocardiographic studies have shown that the degree of hypertrophy may progress in children and adolescents.[162] This means that serial echocardiograms should be obtained until at least the end of puberty in all children thought to have HCM. Hypertrophy does not appear to progress in adults.[163]

Two-dimensional echocardiography has also depicted a unique subset of patients who have pronounced concentric hypertrophy localized to the left ventricular apex (apical hypertrophic cardiomyopathy).[143,164-166] This picture has been found with increased frequency in Japan, associated with giant negative T waves and high QRS voltage on the ECG.[143] A characteristic spade-like configuration of the left ventricle is seen in the right anterior oblique ventriculogram at end diastole as well as in the long-axis view on two-dimensional echocardiography. In the United States, apical HCM is less common, seen in 2% of all patients with HCM.[166] The appearance differs from the general description, for the hypertrophy is more diffuse and involves the middle and basal levels as well. The degree of T-wave inversion on the ECG is less. As in other patients with HCM, there is a positive family history and propensity toward sudden death.[166]

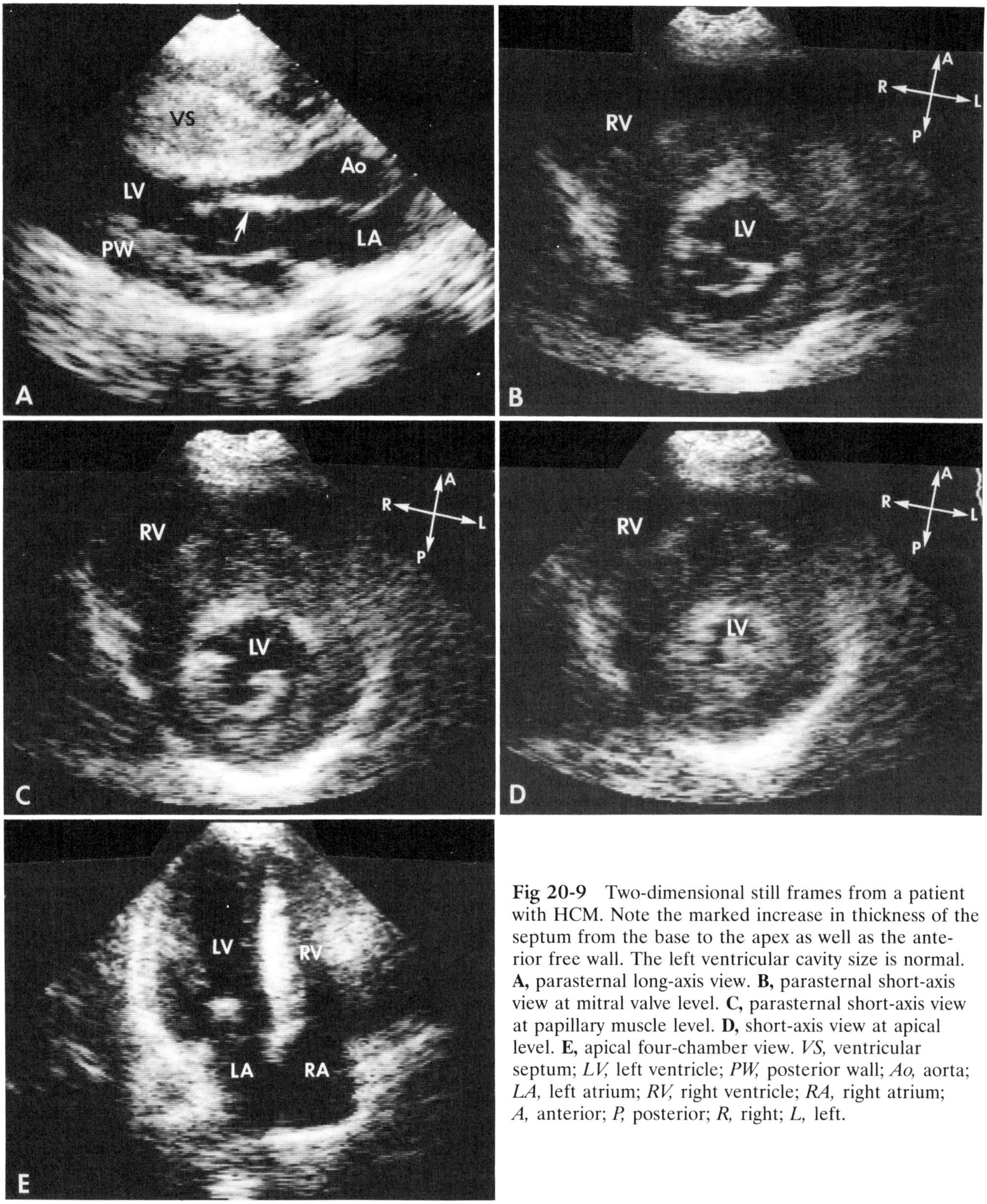

Fig 20-9 Two-dimensional still frames from a patient with HCM. Note the marked increase in thickness of the septum from the base to the apex as well as the anterior free wall. The left ventricular cavity size is normal. **A,** parasternal long-axis view. **B,** parasternal short-axis view at mitral valve level. **C,** parasternal short-axis view at papillary muscle level. **D,** short-axis view at apical level. **E,** apical four-chamber view. *VS,* ventricular septum; *LV,* left ventricle; *PW,* posterior wall; *Ao,* aorta; *LA,* left atrium; *RV,* right ventricle; *RA,* right atrium; *A,* anterior; *P,* posterior; *R,* right; *L,* left.

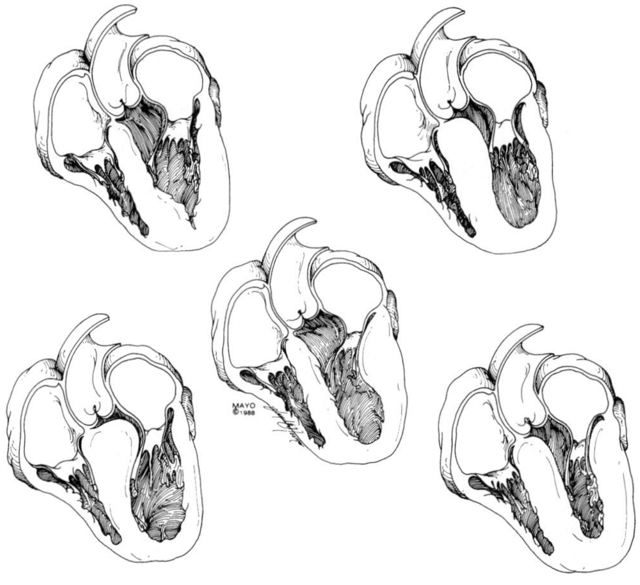

Fig 20-10 Variation in location of hypertrophy of the left ventricle in patients with HCM. (From Nishimura RA, Tajik AJ: Echocardiography. *Prog Cardiol* 2 No 2:135-156, 1989. By permission, Mayo Foundation.)

Two-dimensional echocardiography has also been useful in another variant of HCM—midventricular obstruction.[167] This may be associated with apical infarction, presumably due to increased oxygen demands from the high left ventricular apical pressures.[168]

Several other unique characteristics of HCM demonstrated by two-dimensional echocardiography have been described. An unusual ground-glass texture of the involved myocardium has been depicted by this method, which suggests closely spaced interfaces of different acoustic densities; it has been speculated that this finding correlates with the pathologic myofibril disarray seen in HCM.[154] This appearance, however, is not specific for HCM; it also is seen in cases of cardiac amyloid and in patients with chronic renal failure, and it can only be said to reflect an abnormal myocardial texture. Two-dimensional echocardiography has also demonstrated a pronounced deviation of the ventricular septum from the anterior aortic wall, resulting in an orientation of the left ventricle toward the left atrium rather than the aorta.[153] An intense endocardial echo located on the ventricular septum opposite the mitral valve leaflets has been described;[154] it most likely represents the echo correlate of the endocardial plaque seen at operation and autopsy and caused by apposition of the anterior mitral valve leaflet against the ventricular septum.

Several conditions have two-dimensional echocardiographic appearances similar to those in HCM yet are entirely different disease processes. These patients should not be diagnosed as having HCM on the basis of the echocardiogram alone. First, patients with severe ventricular hypertrophy as found in long-standing significant hypertension may have an echocardiographic appearance similar to that of HCM, with thickened walls (including disproportionate septal thickening) and even systolic anterior motion of the mitral chordal apparatus. The degree of thickness of the ventricular walls and septum should not approach that of HCM (it is usually less than 14 to 16 mm in thickness). The diagnosis of HCM in the presence of severe hypertension should be made with caution.

Second, there are patients with infiltrative diseases such as amyloidosis and hemochromatosis in whom markedly thickened ventricular walls develop that mimic HCM on two-dimensional echocardiography. These patients are usually distinguished from those with HCM on the basis of echocardiographic features of enlarged ventricular cavities, decreased systolic function, and accompanying pericardial effusion. In addition, low-voltage complexes will be seen on the ECG. However, some patients with amyloid heart disease have thick walls, hyperdynamic systolic function, and even dynamic left ventricular outflow obstruction and may be mistakenly thought to have HCM.

Patients with other disease entities, such as chronic renal failure requiring hemodialysis or Friedreich's ataxia, may show two-dimensional appearances that simulate HCM.

Doppler echocardiography

Doppler echocardiography has become a valuable adjunct to two-dimensional echocardiography in providing hemodynamic information as a complement to the anatomic images.[77,149,169-171] The severity of the left ventricular outflow tract gradient can be assessed by continuous-wave Doppler interrogation of the left ventricular outflow tract. This is typically a late-peaking, high-velocity signal[61,77,78] (Fig 20-11). The peak velocity can be converted to a pressure gradient by the modified Bernoulli equation ($P = 4V^2$) and accurately reflects the peak gradient between left ventricular apex and base.[172,173] The velocity signal, which reflects the dynamic nature of the gradient, varies under different loading conditions.

Mitral regurgitation frequently occurs in patients with HCM and can be evaluated by Doppler or flow imaging.[77,78] A semiquantitative estimate of its severity can be made from the extent of the jet into the left atrium. Since mitral regurgitation is visualized as a systolic flow away from the transducer from the apical position, these velocities may be mistaken for the left ventricular outflow tract velocity. Differentiation should be on the basis of velocity contour (symmetric in mitral regurgitation and dagger-shaped in outflow obstruction) and the timing of the onset of flow (at mitral valve closure in mitral regurgitation and after isovolumic contraction in outflow obstruction).

Aortic flow velocities measured by pulsed-wave Doppler echocardiography have shown continued flow throughout a prolonged ejection period, an indication that true obstruction to outflow does occur.[174] The different intracavitary velocities recorded during isovolumic relaxation and ventricular filling demonstrate the marked incoordination of relaxation present in patients with HCM.[165,175]

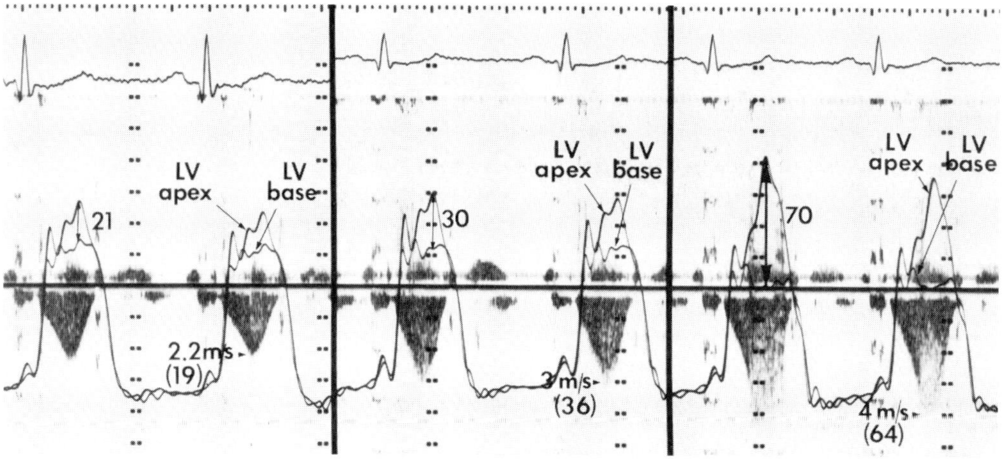

Fig 20-11 Simultaneous continuous-wave Doppler scan across the left ventricular outflow tract and cardiac catheterization pressures in the left ventricular apex and base. There is a correlation between the Doppler-derived pressure gradient and the catheter gradient between the base and the apex. **Left,** baseline. **Center,** low-dose isoproterenol. **Right,** high-dose isoproterenol. (From Nishimura RA, Tajik AJ: Echocardiography. *Prog Cardiol* 2/2:135-156, 1989. By permission, Mayo Foundation.)

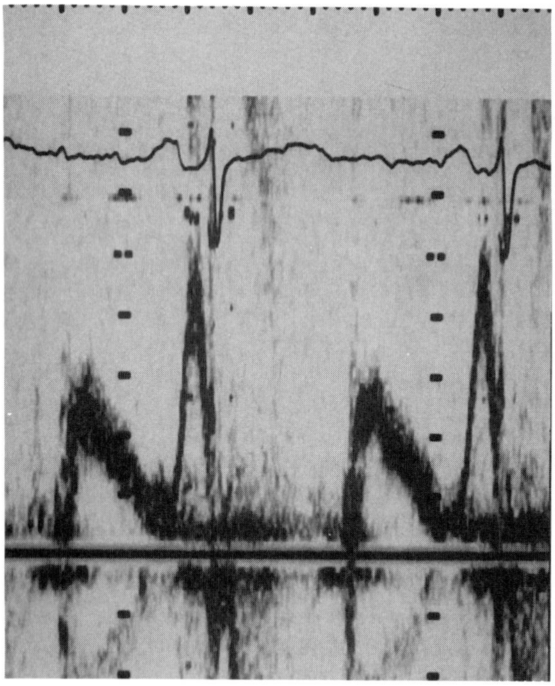

Fig 20-12 Mitral flow velocity curve demonstrating "abnormal relaxation," with a decrease in early initial velocity and an increase in velocity at atrial contraction.

Pulsed-wave Doppler examination of the mitral inflow velocities has been used to assess diastolic filling in patients with HCM.[60-63,77,171] In most patients, lower initial E velocity, prolongation of deceleration time, and lower E:A ratio reflect abnormal relaxation (Fig 20-12). However, these variables depend on several other factors, including loading conditions and coexistent valvular abnormalities.[176] Therefore, a normal-appearing mitral velocity curve may be present in a patient with abnormal relaxation but coexistent increased filling pressures or mitral regurgitation.[61,62] The pulmonary vein velocity curves are helpful in diagnosing this "pseudonormalization" of the mitral flow velocity curve by demonstrating a large reversal at atrial contraction[177] (Fig 20-13).

Radionuclide studies

Radionuclide imaging techniques add an important dimension in the evaluation of patients with HCM. The usefulness of gated blood-pool scanning as a diagnostic technique for HCM is limited, because with it one cannot directly visualize the ventricular walls or valve motion; however, it can be used to differentiate HCM from other cardiomyopathies (dilated and restrictive) by the evaluation of ventricular dimension, ventricular function, and septal abnormalities.[178] Evaluation of diastolic function in patients with HCM by gated blood-pool scanning has shown promise. Abnormalities in diastolic filling, as shown by a decrease in peak left ventricular filling rate and prolonged time to peak filling, have been demonstrated by radionuclide left ventricular time-activity curves.[55,57-59,95,96] Thallium-201 perfusion defects have been seen in patients with HCM and probably indicate myocardial ischemia, even when coronary arteries are normal.[79,179]

Holter and electrophysiologic studies

The findings of nonsustained ventricular tachycardia on 48- to 72-hour Holter monitoring have important impli-

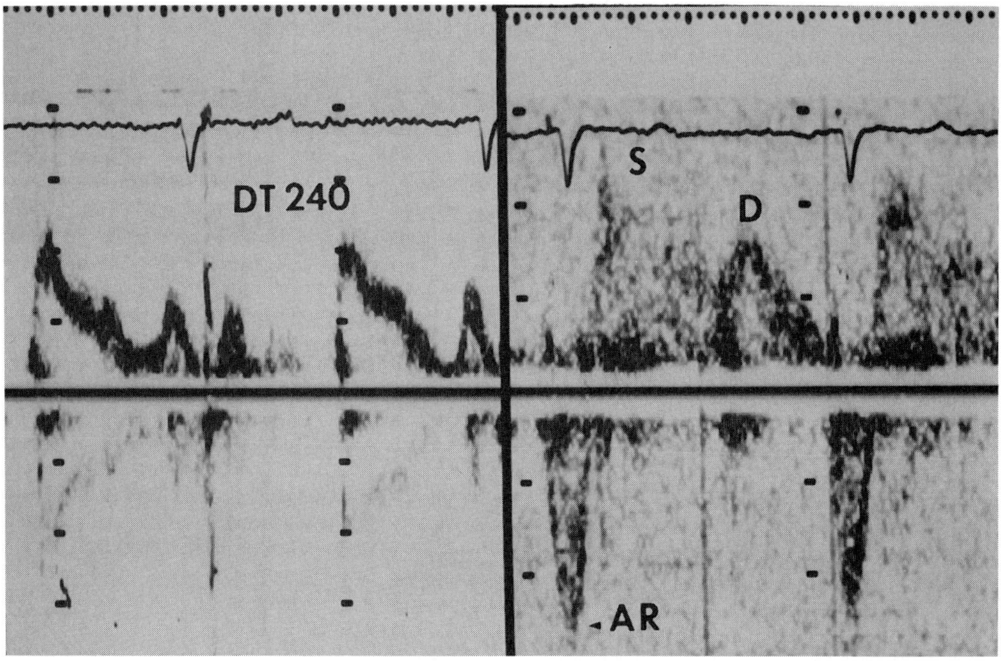

Fig 20-13 Mitral flow **(left)** and pulmonary vein **(right)** velocity curves in a patient with HCM. The mitral flow velocity curve shows a normal pattern with a deceleration time *(DT)* of 240 msec. In the pulmonary vein velocity curve, there is a decrease in the ratio of systolic *(S)* to diastolic *(D)* forward flow. The velocity at atrial contraction (atrial reversal *[AR]*) is significantly increased to 0.5 m/sec (normal, <0.2 m/sec), indicating a "pseudonormalization pattern" of the mitral flow velocity curve. The calibrations on the Doppler image are 0.2 m/sec.

cations for prognosis in patients with HCM. Of patients with nonsustained ventricular tachycardia, 25% die suddenly within 3 years, presumably because of ventricular arrhythmias.[90,102] Conversely, the incidence of arrhythmic events is very low (<5%) in patients without ventricular tachycardia on Holter monitoring. Thus, annual Holter monitoring is recommended for all patients receiving follow-up for the diagnosis of HCM. However, although these findings identify most adult patients with HCM who are at risk for sudden death, they may be relatively nonspecific for clinical decision-making, because 75% of patients with ventricular tachycardia do not experience clinical arrhythmias at 3-year follow-up. In addition, the association between ventricular tachycardia and sudden death does not exist in children.[180]

Other diagnostic modalities have been studied to try to further identify patients at risk for sudden death from electrical causes. Signal-averaged electrocardiography has been useful in predicting serious arrhythmias in patients with ischemic heart disease and has been investigated in patients with HCM.[181] An abnormal signal-averaged ECG is more common in patients with HCM than in controls (20% vs. 4%), and there is a significant association between nonsustained ventricular tachycardia on Holter monitoring and an abnormal signal-averaged ECG.[181] More extensive prospective follow-up studies are required to determine whether signal-averaged ECG is more useful for prognosis than Holter monitoring alone.

Electrophysiologic testing has been performed in selected patients with HCM at high risk for arrhythmic events (those with cardiac arrest, syncope, and asymptomatic ventricular tachycardia on Holter monitoring).[182,183] Electrophysiologic abnormalities were very common, occurring in 81% of patients. Abnormal sinus node function was present in 66% and His-Purkinje conduction abnormalities in 30%. An aggressive stimulation protocol induced nonsustained ventricular tachycardia in 14% and ventricular tachycardia in 43% of the patients. Occurrence of inducible ventricular tachycardia was highest in patients with previous cardiac arrest (77%) and second highest in those with syncope (49%), whereas the occurrence was only 10% in patients without previous clinical events or ventricular tachycardia on Holter monitoring.[182] Whether detection of these arrhythmias at electrophysiologic study will facilitate clinical decision-making remains to be investigated.

Cardiac catheterization initially contributed significantly to the diagnosis and pathophysiologic delineation of HCM.[2,3,72-75] Now, with the availability of newer noninvasive techniques, it is less often necessary. Selective left ventricular cineangiography demonstrates characteristic anatomic and functional features. Ventricular geometry is altered, the cavity assuming a sausage shape in the

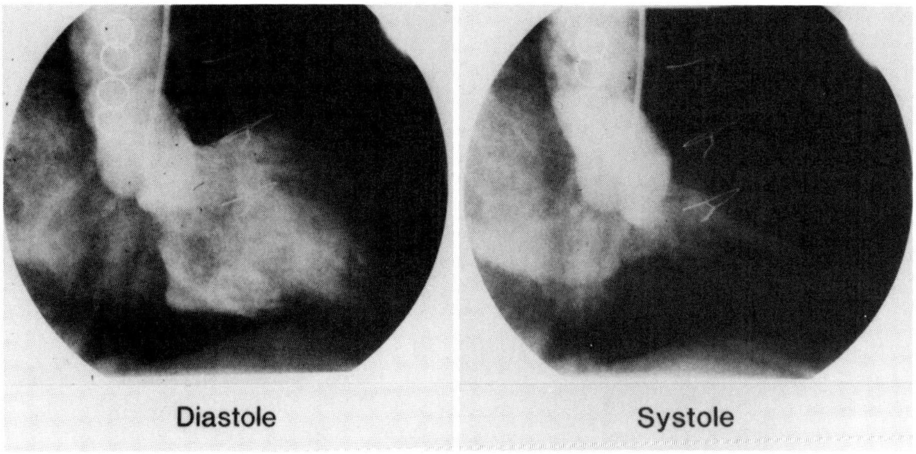

Fig 20-14 Left ventricular cineangiography in the right anterior oblique view during diastole and systole. Pronounced cavity obliteration is demonstrated during systole.

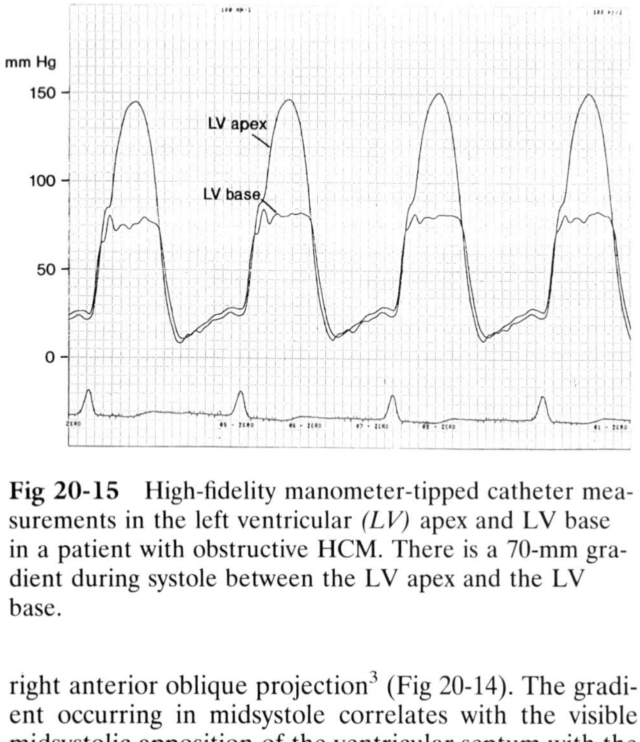

Fig 20-15 High-fidelity manometer-tipped catheter measurements in the left ventricular *(LV)* apex and LV base in a patient with obstructive HCM. There is a 70-mm gradient during systole between the LV apex and the LV base.

right anterior oblique projection[3] (Fig 20-14). The gradient occurring in midsystole correlates with the visible midsystolic apposition of the ventricular septum with the lower half of the anterior mitral valve.[71,74] Mitral regurgitation occurs in 50% to 90% of all patients studied by angiography.[71]

Measurement of the outflow gradient is an important part of the procedure for the diagnosis of HCM by cardiac catheterization: the classic pattern is a systolic gradient seen during catheter pull-back between the middle and basal regions of the left ventricle (Fig 20-15). Studies have documented the presence of midventricular gradients in a subset of patients.[151] The measurement of the outflow gradient by catheterization is prone to error, for the small hyperdynamic left ventricular cavity may cause "catheter entrapment." This occurs when the ventricular myocardium engulfs the catheter ports and leads to an erroneous false-positive gradient. This potential problem can be avoided by a transseptal technique in which the distal catheter is placed in the base or inflow portion of the left ventricle, where cavity obliteration does not occur.[47]

NATURAL HISTORY

The natural history of patients with HCM is highly variable.[45,76,91,92,184,185] Accompanying hypertension, coronary artery disease, and congenital heart disease may influence the prognosis. In the initial natural history studies, 50% to 75% of all patients presenting with HCM were shown to remain stable over a several-year follow-up, and 25% to 30% would die or show deterioration.[76,91,92] Deterioration was not correlated with outflow gradient, but some studies had shown that patients who had a higher left ventricular end-diastolic pressure had a less favorable course.[91] The onset of atrial fibrillation often heralded clinical deterioration. Approximately 10% of patients went on to experience congestive heart failure,[46] which was accompanied by a decrease in the intensity of the murmur and loss of the outflow gradient.[45] There was an annual reported mortality of 3% from HCM.[91,92]

However, these numbers cannot be applied to all patients with HCM, for there appears to be a wide spectrum of clinical presentations and natural history. Very young children have an extremely poor prognosis; during a 7-year follow-up in one series, 30% deteriorated and 30% experienced sudden death.[186] Young adults usually have a severe degree of hypertrophy and tend to have a hemodynamically stable course, but they are prone to sudden death.[76]

Elderly patients are usually asymptomatic or mildly symptomatic until the sixth or seventh decade, when they experience severe and sometimes intractable symptoms.[155,187] They have a different morphology: less hypertrophy but more distortion of the left ventricular outflow tract.[156] The entity of "hypertensive hypertrophic

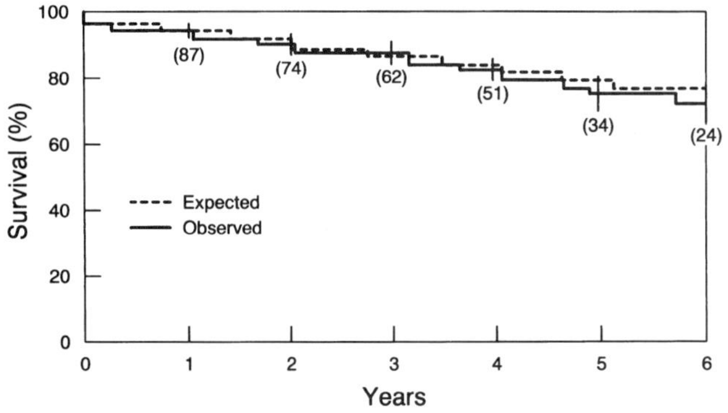

Fig 20-16 Survival rate in patients with HCM diagnosed after age 65 *(Observed)* compared with that in an age- and sex-matched control group *(Expected)*. Numbers in parentheses indicate number of patients at follow-up. (From Fay WP, Taliercio CP, Ilstrup DM, et al: Natural history of hypertrophic cardiomyopathy in the elderly. *J Am Coll Cardiol* 16:821-826, 1990. By permission of American College of Cardiology.)

cardiomyopathy," which is hypertrophy secondary to hypertension in older patients, may be encompassed within the overall spectrum of HCM.[188,189] Both groups have severe heart failure and angina secondary to outflow obstruction and diastolic dysfunction, with symptoms frequently exacerbated by therapy with afterload reducers and diuretics. The risk of sudden death does not seem to be high in these older patients.[190] The survival rate of patients in whom the diagnosis of HCM is made after age 65 has been shown to be similar to that in an age- and sex-matched control group[190] (Fig 20-16).

Much of the presented data originate from tertiary centers that are referral bases for patients with HCM. This consequence may introduce a bias, because these patients may have more symptoms and be at higher risk for events. A review of outpatients with HCM has demonstrated that the incidences of symptoms, clinical deterioration, and death are low.[187]

The reported cause of death varies, but 50% to 90% of all deaths will be sudden.[45,87,92] Sudden death may be the initial manifestation of the disease, as was seen in Teare's[1] original autopsy series of seven patients who died suddenly. HCM has been found to be associated with the majority of sudden deaths occurring in competitive athletes.[191] Sudden death appears to occur especially in younger males with a strong family history of sudden death[88,107]—the so-called malignant variety of HCM.[192,193] This subset has not been correlated with any hemodynamic abnormalities: it occurs in those with severe, mild, or no outflow gradient.[76,107] Pathologic and echocardiographic studies have shown that patients with no or mild symptoms who die suddenly have marked and diffuse left ventricular hypertrophy and that a relationship exists between the extent of hypertrophy and unexpected death.[161,192] A study of patients with HCM who have the "malignant" symptom of syncope often associated with sudden death disclosed three variables as significant independent predictors of syncope: age less than 30 years, left ventricular end-diastolic volume index less than 60 mL/m^2, and nonsustained ventricular tachycardia on 72-hour ambulatory ECG monitoring.[194] The identification of specific gene mutations in the β myosin heavy-chain gene may play a major role in the future for identification of patients at high risk.[5,6,29,30]

The mechanism of sudden death has not been well established. There have been cases of sudden death after severe exertion;[191,192] however, many will experience sudden death at rest.[76,87]

An electrical abnormality probably accounts for the majority of deaths. Death is usually sudden and unheralded by symptoms. The association of sudden death and the occurrence of ventricular tachycardia on Holter monitoring[90,102] has led to the conclusion that ventricular arrhythmias are the major cause of sudden death. The finding that sudden death is also associated with more marked and diffuse hypertrophy[161,192] further supports this concept, because the diseased, hypertrophied myocardium would predispose the patient to these ventricular arrhythmias.[159] Other electrical causes of sudden death have been documented, including asystole[195] and atrial fibrillation,[186,192] the latter associated with rapid AV conduction[87] or bypass tracts.[88]

Other complications of HCM include infective endocarditis, systemic embolism, congestive heart failure, and atrial fibrillation. Infective endocarditis occurs in 4% to 5% of patients with HCM.[76] The lesions are usually located at the point of apposition of the mitral valve against the septum but can involve the mitral valve and, less often, the aortic valve. Systemic embolism occurs in 10% of patients; this is usually associated with atrial fibrillation, and anticoagulation is advisable in patients in whom atrial fibrillation develops.

Progressive left ventricular systolic dysfunction may occur, causing a loss of the outflow gradient and congestive heart failure.[45,46,84,163,196] Myocardial fibrosis and wall thinning occur;[197] possibly they are related to continued myocardial ischemia.[37]

Atrial fibrillation itself is uncommon, occurring in approximately 10% of all patients. It indicates advanced disease[91,92] and is associated with clinical deterioration.[109,195] There are four reasons for deterioration with atrial fibrillation: (1) loss of atrial contribution to ventricular filling with a poorly compliant ventricle; (2) decreased rate of diastolic filling, leading to increased left ventricular outflow gradient from reduced diastolic filling time; (3) variable inotropic effects of varying cycle lengths, leading to intermittent outflow gradients; and (4) change in ventricular activation in some patients with bypass tracts, causing a lower stroke volume.[108] Acute atrial fibrillation should be regarded as a medical emergency, and immediate conversion to normal sinus rhythm may be indicated.

MANAGEMENT

The management of HCM is primarily medical, although there may be a need for surgical intervention. Medical management includes the selected use of β-adrenergic blocking drugs, calcium-channel blocking agents, antiarrhythmia agents, and prophylaxis for infective endocarditis. Operation has been proven to provide dramatic relief of symptoms in patients with severe symptoms despite maximal medical therapy. Preliminary studies have shown that there may be a role for dual-chamber pacing in relief of symptoms.

On the basis of findings of hyperdynamic ventricular function combined with gradient provocation by β-agonists, β-adrenergic blockade was employed in an attempt to improve hemodynamic abnormalities. Theoretic advantages of the use of β-blocking agents include (1) decreased heart rate response to exercise, (2) decreased outflow gradient, (3) relief of angina by a decrease in myocardial oxygen demand, (4) improved diastolic left ventricular filling, (5) antiarrhythmic effect, and (6) decreased left ventricular work with possible resultant halting of disease progression.[198] Acute hemodynamic studies show that β-blocking agents block the increase in gradient which occurs with isoproterenol and exercise but have no effect on the resting gradient.[91,199,200] Studies of the effect of long-term β-blockade demonstrate an initial improvement in angina,[201-203] exercise tolerance, and syncope[202-204] in 60% to 80% of patients; 40% of patients continue to have sustained improvement.[39,201,205] There is also a subset of patients whose condition deteriorates with increasing pulmonary congestion after β-blockade has been initiated, especially if the initial left ventricular end-diastolic pressure was high.[46,202]

The differentiation among patients with resting, labile, and latent gradients is not predictive of the clinical response to β-blockade.[39] There has been no proven reduction in the incidence of sudden death with β-blockade,[46,88] although there is some suggestion that large dosages of β-blocking drugs may prevent sudden death.[44] Although β-blockade should theoretically help decrease left ventricular compliance,[206] studies using propranolol have failed to show any improvement in diastolic ventricular function.[207] Nonetheless, when proper dosages are used (>320-mg equivalent of propranolol per day), β-blockade relieves symptoms in most patients to the point at which they can lead normally functioning lives.

The effects of calcium-channel blocking drugs suggest they may be of value in the treatment of HCM. Experimental work with calcium blockers as modifiers of ischemia-induced diastolic abnormalities[208] has prompted investigation of their use in HCM. By preventing calcium influx, they have the theoretic possibility of decreasing inotropy and chronotropy and improving diastolic compliance. Abnormal calcium metabolism has been postulated as a cause of HCM,[22,209] and this suggests that slow calcium-channel blockers might favorably affect the course of the disease. Clinical studies have shown a significant decrease in both basal and provoked gradients during acute drug intervention with verapamil.[210-212] Even patients who show no acute effect on outflow gradient with verapamil will have a decrease in gradient after long-term use.[205,212] There may be improvement in diastolic filling with verapamil as judged by radionuclide and angiographic studies.[51,212,213]

Long-term studies with verapamil have shown beneficial results. Both β-blockers and verapamil improve exercise tolerance by 20% to 30% in short-term follow-up.[214,215] Calcium-channel blockers have improved angina to a greater degree than β-blockers.[99] The beneficial effect on symptomatic improvement is sustained for several years.[214] Verapamil has been shown to decrease the Sokolov hypertrophy index of the ECG,[205,216] decrease cardiac size and volume,[99,205,216] and decrease coronary diameter,[205] which may reflect decreased muscle mass. The calcium blocker verapamil has been shown to diminish and, in some patients, prevent inducible silent ischemia in patients with HCM.[217]

There is, however, a subset of patients who will undergo hemodynamic deterioration with the calcium-channel blocking agents, specifically those with a large resting left ventricular outflow obstruction. If the systemic blood pressure is decreased by the vasodilatory effect of calcium-channel blockers, the outflow gradient and left ventricular end-diastolic pressure may actually increase with hemodynamic deterioration.[210] Death from pulmonary edema has been reported after therapy with verapamil.[212] It is for this reason that a calcium-channel blocking agent should be the second-line drug of choice only after β-blockers have failed to control symptoms. It should be used with extreme caution in patients with high left ventricular outflow gradients.

Disopyramide has been used as therapy in patients with HCM.[47,218] It has been found to decrease the outflow gradient, decrease the ejection time, and lower the left ventricular end-diastolic pressure without affecting cardiac output.[47,218] Because of the high incidence of anticholinergic side effects in the authors' experience, use of disopyramide has been limited to patients who are intolerant of β-blockers or calcium-channel blockers.

No drug has been shown to be of benefit in the prevention of sudden death. The current group I and group II antiarrhythmia drugs have not been shown to decrease the incidence of sudden death.[219] The antiarrhythmia agent amiodarone can completely abolish supraventricular and ventricular arrhythmias on Holter monitoring in patients with HCM.[214] Initial data suggested that high-risk patients with HCM and nonsustained ventricular tachycardia on Holter monitoring had very low mortality when treated with amiodarone.[220] Later studies, however, have shown that amiodarone causes conduction abnormalities in 20% of patients and actually facilitates electrophysiologically induced tachycardia in half of patients.[221] In addition, despite abolition of atrial and ventricular arrhythmias on Holter monitoring, empiric treatment with amiodarone did not prevent sudden death and may actually have resulted in a higher incidence of early sudden death after administration of amiodarone began.[222] Thus, there are conflicting data on the use of amiodarone in the empiric treatment of patients with HCM to prevent sudden death. Further long-term studies are required to determine the role of this antiarrhythmic drug in these high-risk patients.

Current medical therapy for patients with HCM continues to be controversial. However, a general approach, as outlined, based on symptoms and nondiagnostic testing

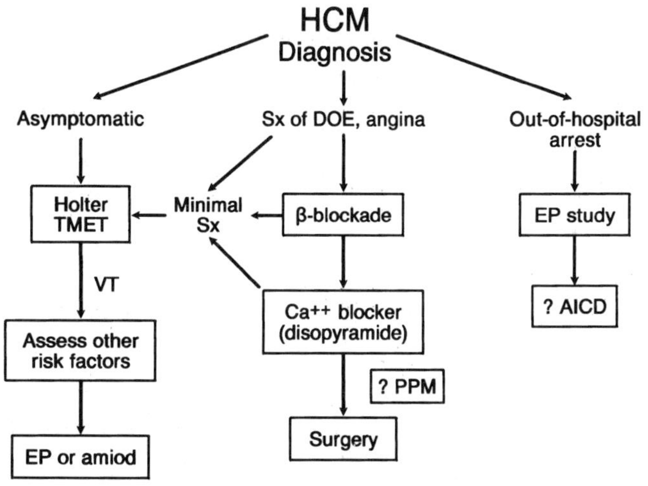

Fig 20-17 Evaluation of a patient with HCM. *AICD,* implantable cardioverter-defibrillator; *amiod,* amiodarone; *DOE,* dyspnea on exertion; *EP,* electrophysiologic; *PPM,* permanent pacemaker; *Sx,* symptoms; *TMET,* treadmill exertion testing; *VT,* ventricular tachycardia.

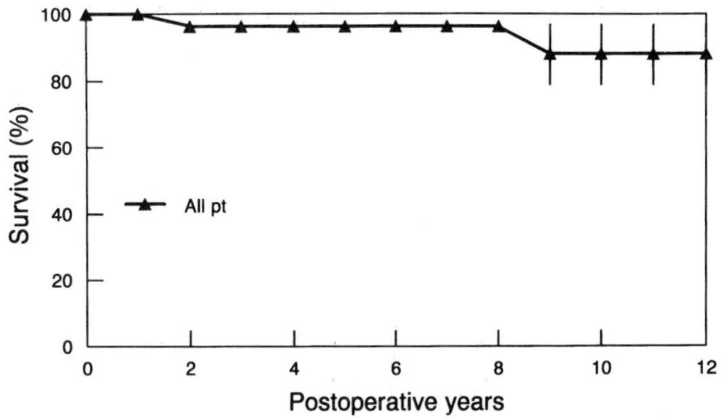

Fig 20-18 Actuarial survival curve after septal myectomy in patients younger than 65 years. (From Mohr R, Schaff HV, Puga FJ, et al: Results of operation for hypertrophic obstructive cardiomyopathy in children and adults less than 40 years of age. *Circulation* 80 Suppl 1:191-196, 1989. By permission of American Heart Association.)

(Fig 20-17) may be useful. Initial therapy for patients with limiting symptoms of dyspnea and angina should be with β-adrenergic blocking drugs. Large dosages are usually required, at times exceeding 320 mg of propranolol per day. The calcium-channel blockers are currently used for patients who do not respond or who are intolerant to β-adrenergic blocking drugs. Initial dosage with verapamil is 80 mg three times per day; this may be gradually increased to 240 mg three times per day as tolerated until relief of symptoms is obtained. The role of combined therapy with β-adrenergic blocking drugs and calcium-channel blockers requires further investigation. As stated previously, certain patients with HCM may show hemodynamic deterioration with the addition of calcium-channel blockers, so that they must be used with caution, especially with outflow obstruction at rest. Disopyramide may be used in patients who are intolerant of β-blockers and calcium-channel blockers.

In the patient who is asymptomatic or symptomatically improved after medical therapy, a 48- to 72-hour Holter monitor and treadmill exertion test is recommended to determine whether nonsustained ventricular tachycardia is present. If ventricular tachycardia is present, the patient should be assessed for other risk factors of sudden death, including a family history of sudden death, young age, male sex, and severe, diffuse hypertrophy. In patients with multiple risk factors, electrophysiology testing should be considered. If the risk is found to be very high, an automatic implantable defibrillator may be indicated.

The patient who has already experienced an out-of-hospital arrest is at high risk for recurrent events. In these patients, an electrophysiologic test is warranted, specifically to rule out causes for cardiac arrest other than ventricular tachycardia. These include atrial arrhythmias, accessory pathways, sinus node disease, and conduction disease, seen in approximately 30% of these patients.[183] If no other cause is identified, an automatic implantable cardiac defibrillator should be recommended.

Surgical therapy for HCM has been performed for longer than 2 decades.[223-229] Transaortic septal myectomy is the current operation of choice to relieve left ventricular outflow obstruction.[224,230] For preservation of the conduction system, relatively little tissue can be removed at the time of the operation. Therefore, the decrease in left ventricular outflow obstruction is accomplished not only by physical enlargement of the outflow tract but also by interruption of the pathophysiologic sequence of events that causes the outflow obstruction.

Replacement of the mitral valve with a low-profile mitral valve prosthesis has been proposed as an alternative to septal myectomy.[231] The major problem with this procedure is that one disease process is being replaced by another, that is, a prosthetic valve with all the problems of valve durability, infection, thromboembolization, and anticoagulation.[226,232] Because of these problems, mitral valve replacement should be considered only if primary mitral valve disease and significant mitral regurgitation are present or if the septum is not thought to be thick enough to undergo myectomy.[230]

Transaortic septal myectomy has a steep learning curve, and the procedure should be performed only at selected referral centers. The initial results of the operation included intraoperative mortality of 7% to 16% and late postoperative mortality of 7% to 10%.[223-225,230] Complications of the surgical procedure other than death included intraoperative complete heart block, late complete heart block, ventricular septal defect, left bundle-branch block, and septal aneurysms.[223,224,233] However, new advances in myocardial preservation techniques and anesthesia along with the key factor of surgical expertise have produced surgical results that are significantly different from those in the initial reports. In experienced centers, septal myectomy can now be performed with an overall mortality of 5.6%, reduced to 1.2% in patients younger than 65 years[234] (Fig 20-18) and even lower in children and young adults.[235] Relieving outflow obstruction has a proven benefit, with the average decrease in

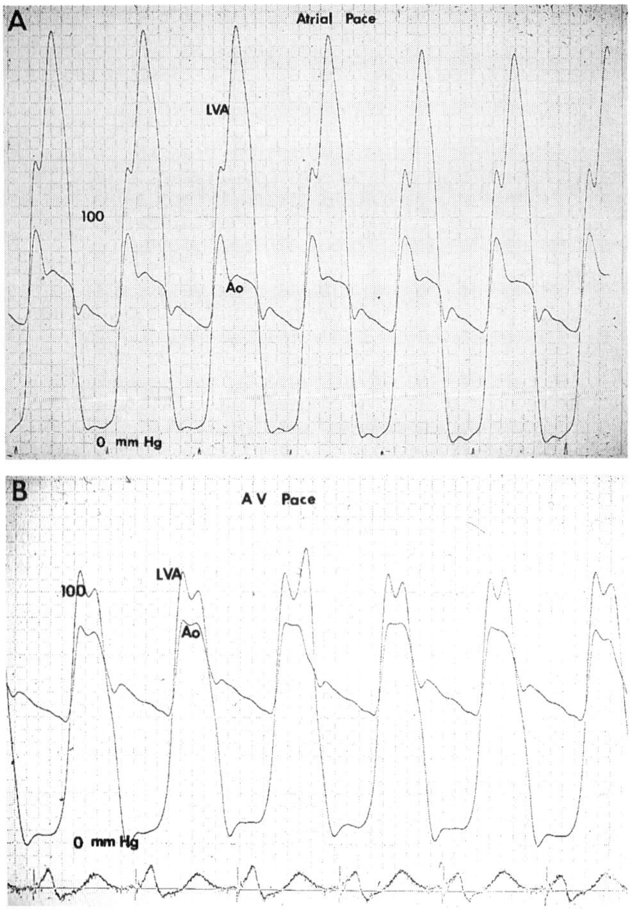

Fig 20-19 High-fidelity manometer pressures of the left ventricular apex *(LVA)* and aorta *(Ao)* in a patient with HCM. **A,** during atrial pacing, there is a severe gradient of over 100 mm Hg. **B,** during atrioventricular *(AV)* sequential pacing, there is a dramatic reduction in gradient to 15 mm Hg.

gradient from 70 ± 38 mm Hg to 9 ± 11 mm Hg. Frequently, mitral regurgitation, even when severe, is significantly improved after myectomy alone.[230,234] Studies have shown that myectomy favorably affects myocardial oxygen consumption and metabolism.[236] Left ventricular end-diastolic pressure is significantly decreased, an indication of overall improvement in diastolic filling of the heart.[21] Relief of symptoms is dramatic, with 90% of patients improving by at least one functional class and 73% being completely free of symptoms at long-term follow-up.[230,234,237] Although no randomized data compare myectomy with medical therapy for effect on survival, a 5-year survival rate of 93% has been reported for patients younger than 65 years[234] in whom annual mortality is known to be 3% to 4%.

Thus, operation with transaortic septal myectomy should be considered in patients with severe symptoms who have high left ventricular outflow tract gradients unresponsive to medical therapy. Mortality is relatively low, especially in patients younger than 65 years, if the procedure is done at experienced centers. The short- and long-term relief of symptoms is excellent.

Recently, use of dual-chamber pacing as an alternative to surgery has been reported in patients with HCM and left ventricular outflow tract obstruction who are intolerant of or not having a response to medical therapy[238-240] (Fig 20-19). An acute reduction in gradient of approximately 50% during AV pacing has been reported. Permanent pacing has resulted in abatement of symptoms over short-term follow-up. The mechanism is thought to be reduction in left ventricular outflow gradient from the abnormal septal motion caused by right ventricular pacing. There may also be a component of ventricular remodeling and even regression of hypertrophy after long-term pacing, as evidenced by ventricular dilatation at follow-up. In addition, some patients have had continued reduction of gradient, even after conversion to normal sinus rhythm, at follow-up. However, the experience with dual-chamber pacing in patients with HCM is early. The effect of dual-chamber pacing on other pathophysiologic mechanisms, such as diastolic abnormalities, coronary ischemia, mitral regurgitation, and arrhythmias, in patients with HCM is not known. Only short-term follow-up of a small number of patients is available, and it is not known whether these initial hemodynamic or symptomatic benefits will be sustained in long-term follow-up. Further studies are warranted to determine the optimal role of dual-chamber pacing in these patients.

SUMMARY AND CONCLUSIONS

HCM represents a broad spectrum of disease. It is a unique cardiac disease, characterized pathologically by a nondilated hypertrophied ventricle with microscopic findings of myofibrillar disarray. Recent molecular genetic studies have shown that a gene mutation is responsible for the occurrence of familial HCM in several kindreds. The major symptoms are dyspnea, angina, and syncope. HCM must be differentiated from other forms of left ventricular outflow obstruction, other cardiomyopathies, and other causes of ventricular hypertrophy. The introduction of two-dimensional and Doppler echocardiography has greatly contributed to the understanding of this disease process and its many variations. β-Adrenergic blockade has been the medical treatment of choice in the past; however, the introduction of calcium-channel blocking agents and the recognition of the frequency of arrhythmias as a cause of symptoms (syncope) and death enhance the opportunity for more effective treatment. Surgical therapy has resulted in improvement of a subset of patients with severe symptoms. Dual-chamber pacing is a promising but still investigational therapeutic modality. Further understanding of the cause, pathophysiology, prognosis, and treatment of this entity is required.

REFERENCES

1. Teare D: Asymmetrical hypertrophy of the heart in young adults. *Br Heart J* 20:1-8, 1958

2. Brock R: Functional obstruction of the left ventricle (acquired aortic subvalvar stenosis). *Guys Hosp Rep* 106:221-238, 1957

3. Braunwald E, Morrow AG, Cornell WP, et al: Idiopathic hypertrophic subaortic stenosis: clinical, hemodynamic and angiographic manifestations. *Am J Med* 29:924-945, 1960
4. Clark CE, Henry WL, Epstein SE: Familial prevalence and genetic transmission of idiopathic hypertrophic subaortic stenosis. *N Engl J Med* 289:709-714, 1973
5. Jarcho JA, McKenna W, Pare JAP, et al: Mapping a gene for familial hypertrophic cardiomyopathy to chromosome 14q1. *N Engl J Med* 321:1372-1378, 1989
6. Watkins H, Rosenzweig A, Hwang D-S, et al: Characteristics and prognostic implications of myosin missense mutations in familial hypertrophic cardiomyopathy. *N Engl J Med* 326:1108-1114, 1992
7. Goodwin JF: ? IHSS. ? HOCM. ? ASH: a plea for unity. *Am Heart J* 89:269-277, 1975
8. Brandenburg RO, Chazov E, Cherian G, et al: Report of the WHO/ISFC task force on definition and classification of cardiomyopathies. *Circulation* 64:437A–438A, 1981
9. Gersh BJ: Cardiomyopathies: editorial overview. *Curr Opin Cardiol* 4:377-378, 1989
10. Codd MB, Sugrue DD, Gersh BJ, et al: Epidemiology of idiopathic dilated and hypertrophic cardiomyopathy: a population-based study in Olmsted County, Minnesota, 1975-1984. *Circulation* 80:564-572, 1989
11. Maron BJ, Bonow RO, Cannon RO III, et al: Hypertrophic cardiomyopathy: interrelations of clinical manifestations, pathophysiology, and therapy. Parts 1 and 2. *N Engl J Med* 316:a, 780-789; b, 844-852, 1987
12. Matsumori A, Kawai C, Wakabayashi A, et al: HLA-DRW4 antigen linkage in patients with hypertrophic obstructive cardiomyopathy. *Am Heart J* 101:14-16, 1981
13. Zezulka A, MacKintosh P, Jobson S, et al: Human lymphocyte antigens in hypertrophic cardiomyopathy. *Int J Cardiol* 12:193-202, 1986
14. Firoito S, Autore C, Fragola PV, et al: HLA-DR3 antigen linkage in patients with hypertrophic obstructive cardiomyopathy. *Am Heart J* 111:91-94, 1986
15. Gardin JM, Gottdiener JS, Radvany R, et al: HLA linkage vs association in hypertrophic cardiomyopathy: evidence for the absence of an association in a heterogeneous Caucasian population. *Chest* 81:466-472, 1982
16. De Bono AH, Proctor E, Brock R: Dynamic obstruction of the left ventricle: its production and abolition by drugs in normal animals. *Guys Hosp Rep* 114:4-14, 1965
17. Kaye MP, Witzke DJ, Wells DJ, et al: Cardiac effects of nerve growth factor in dogs. In *Hypertrophic Cardiomyopathy: The Therapeutic Role of Calcium Antagonists.* Edited by M Kaltenbach, SE Epstein. Berlin, Springer-Verlag, 1982, pp 88-98
18. Pearse AGE: The histochemistry and electron microscopy of obstructive cardiomyopathy. In *CIBA Foundation Symposium on Cardiomyopathies.* Edited by GEW Wolstenholme, M O'Connor. Boston, Little, Brown & Company, 1964, pp 132-164
19. Van Noorden S, Olsen EGJ, Pearse AGE: Hypertrophic obstructive cardiomyopathy, a histological, histochemical, and ultrastructural study of biopsy material. *Cardiovasc Res* 5:118-131, 1971
20. Polani PE, Moynahan EJ: Progressive cardiomyopathic lentiginosis. *Q J Med* 41:205-225, 1972
21. St John Sutton MG, Tajik AJ, Giuliani ER, et al: Hypertrophic obstructive cardiomyopathy and lentiginosis: a little known neural ectodermal syndrome. *Am J Cardiol* 47:214-217, 1981
22. Dhalla NS: Involvement of membrane systems in heart failure due to intracellular calcium overload and deficiency (editorial). *J Mol Cell Cardiol* 8:661-667, 1976
23. Finkel MS, Marks ES, Patterson RE, et al: Increased cardiac calcium channels in hamster cardiomyopathy. *Am J Cardiol* 57:1205-1206, 1986
24. Wagner JA, Sax FL, Weisman HF, et al: Calcium-antagonist receptors in the atrial tissue of patients with hypertrophic cardiomyopathy. *N Engl J Med* 320:755-761, 1989
25. Braunwald E: Hypertrophic cardiomyopathy—continued progress (editorial). *N Engl J Med* 320:800-802, 1989
26. Maron BJ, Mulvihill JJ: The genetics of hypertrophic cardiomyopathy (editorial). *Ann Intern Med* 105:610-613, 1986
27. Curfman GD: Molecular insights into hypertrophic cardiomyopathy (editorial). *N Engl J Med* 326:1149-1151, 1992
28. Rosenzweig A, Watkins H, Hwang D-S, et al: Preclinical diagnosis of familial hypertrophic cardiomyopathy by genetic analysis of blood lymphocytes. *N Engl J Med* 325:1753-1760, 1991
29. Hejtmancik JF, Brink PA, Towbin J, et al: Localization of gene for familial hypertrophic cardiomyopathy to chromosome 14q1 in diverse US population. *Circulation* 83:1592-1597, 1991
30. Geisterfer-Lowrance AAT, Kass S, Tanigawa G, et al: A molecular basis for familial hypertrophic cardiomyopathy: a β cardiac myosin heavy chain gene missense mutation. *Cell* 62:999-1006, 1990
31. Olsen EGJ: The pathology of cardiomyopathies: a critical analysis. *Am Heart J* 98:385-392, 1979
32. Roberts WC: Valvular, subvalvular, and supravalvular aortic stenosis: morphologic features. *Cardiovasc Clin* 5 No 1:97-126, 1973
33. Davies MJ, Pomerance A, Teare RD: Pathological features of hypertrophic obstructive cardiomyopathy. *J Clin Pathol* 27:529-535, 1974
34. Roberts WC, Ferrans VJ: Pathologic anatomy of the cardiomyopathies: idiopathic dilated and hypertrophic types, infiltrative types, and endomyocardial disease with and without eosinophilia. *Hum Pathol* 6:287-342, 1975
35. Maron BJ, Henry WL, Roberts WC, et al: Comparison of echocardiographic and necropsy measurements of ventricular wall thicknesses in patients with and without disproportionate septal thickening. *Circulation* 55:341-346, 1977
36. Stewart S, Schreiner B: Coexisting idiopathic hypertrophic subaortic stenosis and coronary artery disease: clinical implication and operative management. *J Thorac Cardiovasc Surg* 82:278-280, 1981
37. Maron BJ, Wolfson JK, Epstein SE, et al: Intramural ("small vessel") coronary artery disease in hypertrophic cardiomyopathy. *J Am Coll Cardiol* 8:545-557, 1986
38. Maron BJ, Ferrans VT, Henry WL, et al: Differences in distribution of myocardial abnormalities in patients with obstructive and nonobstructive asymmetric septal hypertrophy (ASH): light and electron microscopic findings. *Circulation* 50:436-446, 1974
39. Stenson RE, Flamm MD Jr, Harrison DC, et al: Hypertrophic subaortic stenosis: clinical and hemodynamic effects of long-term propranolol therapy. *Am J Cardiol* 31:763-773, 1973
40. Maron BJ, Sato N, Roberts WC, et al: Quantitative analysis of cardiac muscle cell disorganization in the ventricular septum: comparison of fetuses and infants with and without congenital heart disease and patients with hypertrophic cardiomyopathy. *Circulation* 60:685-696, 1979
41. Maron BJ, Roberts WC: Quantitative analysis of cardiac muscle cell disorganization in the ventricular septum of patients with hypertrophic cardiomyopathy. *Circulation* 59:689-706, 1979
42. St John Sutton MG, Lie JT, Anderson KR, et al: Histopathological specificity of hypertrophic obstructive cardiomyopathy: myocardial fibre disarray and myocardial fibrosis. *Br Heart J* 44:433-443, 1980
43. Becker AE, Caruso G: Myocardial disarray: a critical review. *Br Heart J* 47:527-538, 1982
44. Canedo MI, Frank MJ: Therapy of hypertrophic cardiomyopathy: medical or surgical? Clinical and pathophysiologic considerations (editorial). *Am J Cardiol* 48:383-388, 1981
45. Shah PM, Adelman AG, Wigle ED, et al: The natural (and unnatural) history of hypertrophic obstructive cardiomyopathy: a multicenter study. *Circ Res* 35 Suppl 2:179-195, 1974
46. Swan DA, Bell B, Oakley CM, et al: Analysis of symptomatic course and prognosis and treatment of hypertrophic obstructive cardiomyopathy. *Br Heart J* 33:671-685, 1971
47. Wigle ED, Sasson Z, Henderson MA, et al: Hypertrophic cardiomyopathy. The importance of the site and the extent of hypertrophy. A review. *Prog Cardiovasc Dis* 28:1-83, 1985
48. Spirito P, Maron BJ, Chiarella F, et al: Diastolic abnormalities in patients with hypertrophic cardiomyopathy: relation to magnitude of left ventricular hypertrophy. *Circulation* 72:310-316, 1985
49. Wigle ED: Hypertrophic cardiomyopathy: a 1987 viewpoint (editorial). *Circulation* 75:311-322, 1987
50. Wigle ED, Heimbecker RO, Gunton RW: Idiopathic ventricular septal hypertrophy causing muscular subaortic stenosis. *Circulation* 26:325-340, 1962
51. Hanrath P, Mathey DG, Kremer P, et al: Effect of verapamil on left ventricular isovolumic relaxation time and regional left ventricular filling in hypertrophic cardiomyopathy. *Am J Cardiol* 45:1258-1264, 1980
52. Brutsaert DL, Rademakers FE, Sys SU: Triple control of relaxation: implications in cardiac disease (editorial). *Circulation* 69: 190-196, 1984
53. Gaasch WH, Levine HJ, Quinones MA, et al: Left ventricular compliance: mechanisms and clinical implications. *Am J Cardiol* 38:645-653, 1976

54. Nishimura RA, Housmans PR, Hatle LK, et al: Assessment of diastolic function of the heart: background and current applications of Doppler echocardiography. Part I. Physiologic and pathophysiologic features. *Mayo Clin Proc* 64:71-81, 1989
55. Bonow RO, Vitale DF, Maron BJ, et al: Regional left ventricular asynchrony and impaired global left ventricular filling in hypertrophic cardiomyopathy: effect of verapamil. *J Am Coll Cardiol* 9:1108-1116, 1987
56. Sanderson JE, Traill TA, St John Sutton MG, et al: Left ventricular relaxation and filling in hypertrophic cardiomyopathy: an echocardiographic study. *Br Heart J* 40:596-601, 1978
57. Chen Y-T, Chang K-C, Hu W-S, et al: Left ventricular diastolic function in hypertrophic cardiomyopathy: assessment by radionuclide angiography. *Int J Cardiol* 15:185-193, 1987
58. Betocchi S, Bonow RO, Bacharach SL, et al: Isovolumic relaxation period in hypertrophic cardiomyopathy: assessment by radionuclide angiography. *J Am Coll Cardiol* 7:74-81, 1986
59. Bonow RO, Frederick TM, Bacharach SL, et al: Atrial systole and left ventricular filling in hypertrophic cardiomyopathy: effect of verapamil. *Am J Cardiol* 51:1386-1391, 1983
60. Maron BJ, Spirito P, Green KJ, et al: Noninvasive assessment of left ventricular diastolic function by pulsed Doppler echocardiography in patients with hypertrophic cardiomyopathy. *J Am Coll Cardiol* 10:733-742, 1987
61. Bryg RJ, Pearson AC, Williams GA, et al: Left ventricular systolic and diastolic flow abnormalities determined by Doppler echocardiography in obstructive hypertrophic cardiomyopathy. *Am J Cardiol* 59:925-931, 1987
62. Takenaka K, Dabestani A, Gardin JM, et al: Left ventricular filling in hypertrophic cardiomyopathy: a pulsed Doppler echocardiographic study. *J Am Coll Cardiol* 7:1263-1271, 1986
63. Gidding SS, Snider AR, Rocchini AP, et al: Left ventricular diastolic filling in children with hypertrophic cardiomyopathy: assessment with pulsed Doppler echocardiography. *J Am Coll Cardiol* 8:310-316, 1986
64. St John Sutton MG, Tajik AJ, Gibson DG, et al: Echocardiographic assessment of left ventricular filling and septal and posterior wall dynamics in idiopathic hypertrophic subaortic stenosis. *Circulation* 57:512-520, 1978
65. Criley JM, Lewis KB, White RI Jr, et al: Pressure gradients without obstruction: a new concept of "hypertrophic subaortic stenosis." *Circulation* 32:881-887, 1965
66. Ross J Jr, Braunwald E, Gault JH, et al: The mechanism of the intraventricular pressure gradient in idiopathic hypertrophic subaortic stenosis. *Circulation* 34:558-578, 1966
67. Murgo JP, Alter BR, Dorethy JF, et al: Dynamics of left ventricular ejection in obstructive and nonobstructive hypertrophic cardiomyopathy. *J Clin Invest* 66:1369-1382, 1980
68. Murgo JP: Does outflow obstruction exist in hypertrophic cardiomyopathy? (Editorial). *N Engl J Med* 307:1008-1009, 1982
69. Pierce GE, Morrow AG, Braunwald E: Idiopathic hypertrophic subaortic stenosis. III. Intraoperative studies of the mechanism of obstruction and its hemodynamic consequences. *Circulation* 30 Suppl 4:152-206, 1964
70. Goodwin JF: The frontiers of cardiomyopathy. *Br Heart J* 48:1-18, 1982
71. Adelman AG, McLoughlin MJ, Marquis Y, et al: Left ventricular cineangiographic observations in muscular subaortic stenosis. *Am J Cardiol* 24:689-697, 1969
72. Braunwald E, Brockenbrough EC, Frye RL: Studies on digitalis. V. Comparison of the effects of ouabain on left ventricular dynamics in valvular aortic stenosis and hypertrophic subaortic stenosis. *Circulation* 26:166-173, 1962
73. Whalen RE, Cohen AI, Sumner RG, et al: Demonstration of the dynamic nature of idiopathic hypertrophic subaortic stenosis. *Am J Cardiol* 11:8-17, 1963
74. Simon AL, Ross J Jr, Gault JH: Angiographic anatomy of the left ventricle and mitral valve in idiopathic hypertrophic subaortic stenosis. *Circulation* 36:852-867, 1967
75. Braunwald E, Ebert PA: Hemodynamic alterations in idiopathic hypertrophic subaortic stenosis induced by sympathomimetic drugs. *Am J Cardiol* 10:489-495, 1962
76. Frank S, Braunwald E: Idiopathic hypertrophic subaortic stenosis: clinical analysis of 126 patients with emphasis on the natural history. *Circulation* 37:759-788, 1968
77. Rakowski H: Echocardiographic and Doppler assessment of hypertrophic cardiomyopathy. *J Am Soc Echocardiography* 1:31-47, 1988
78. Nishimura RA, Tajik AJ, Reeder GS, et al: Evaluation of hypertrophic cardiomyopathy by Doppler color flow imaging: initial observations. *Mayo Clin Proc* 61:631-639, 1986
79. O'Gara PT, Bonow RO, Maron BJ, et al: Myocardial perfusion abnormalities in patients with hypertrophic cardiomyopathy: assessment with thallium-201 emission computed tomography. *Circulation* 76:1214-1223, 1987
80. Grover-McKay M, Schwaiger M, Krivokapich J, et al: Regional myocardial blood flow and metabolism at rest in mildly symptomatic patients with hypertrophic cardiomyopathy. *J Am Coll Cardiol* 13:317-324, 1989
81. Ogata Y, Hiyamuta K, Terasawa M, et al: Relationship of exercise or pacing induced ST segment depression and myocardial lactate metabolism in patients with hypertrophic cardiomyopathy. *Jpn Heart J* 27:145-158, 1986
82. Cannon RO III, Schenke WH, Maron BJ, et al: Differences in coronary flow and myocardial metabolism at rest and during pacing between patients with obstructive and patients with nonobstructive hypertrophic cardiomyopathy. *J Am Coll Cardiol* 10:53-62, 1987
83. Pichard AD, Meller J, Teichholz LE, et al: Septal perforator compression (narrowing) in idiopathic hypertrophic subaortic stenosis. *Am J Cardiol* 40:310-314, 1977
84. Spirito P, Maron BJ, Bonow RO, et al: Severe functional limitation in patients with hypertrophic cardiomyopathy and only mild localized left ventricular hypertrophy. *J Am Coll Cardiol* 8:537-544, 1986
85. Ingham RE, Rossen RM, Goodman DJ, et al: Treadmill arrhythmias in patients with idiopathic hypertrophic subaortic stenosis. *Chest* 68:759-764, 1975
86. McKenna WJ, Chetty S, Oakley CM, et al: Arrhythmia in hypertrophic cardiomyopathy: exercise and 48 hour ambulatory electrocardiographic assessment with and without beta adrenergic blocking therapy. *Am J Cardiol* 45:1-5, 1980
87. James TN, Marshall TK: De subitaneis mortibus. XII. Asymmetrical hypertrophy of the heart. *Circulation* 51:1149-1166, 1975
88. Goodwin JF, Krikler DM: Arrhythmia as a cause of sudden death in hypertrophic cardiomyopathy. *Lancet* 2:937-940, 1976
89. Cosio FG, Moro C, Alonso M, et al: The Q waves of hypertrophic cardiomyopathy: an electrophysiologic study. *N Engl J Med* 302:96-99, 1980
90. McKenna WJ, England D, Doi YL, et al: Arrhythmia in hypertrophic cardiomyopathy. I. Influence on prognosis. *Br Heart J* 46:168-172, 1981
91. Adelman AG, Wigle ED, Ranganathan N, et al: The clinical course in muscular subaortic stenosis: a retrospective and prospective study of 60 hemodynamically proved cases. *Ann Intern Med* 77:515-525, 1972
92. Maron BJ, Epstein SE: Clinical course of patients with hypertrophic cardiomyopathy. *Cardiovasc Clin* 10 No 1:253-265, 1979
93. Shah PM: Newer concepts in hypertrophic obstructive cardiomyopathy II. *JAMA* 242:1771-1776, 1979
94. Hanrath P, Mathey DG, Siegert R, et al: Left ventricular relaxation and filling pattern in different forms of left ventricular hypertrophy: an echocardiographic study. *Am J Cardiol* 45:15-23, 1980
95. Bonow RO, Rosing DR, Bacharach SL, et al: Left ventricular systolic function and diastolic filling in patients with hypertrophic cardiomyopathy: effect of verapamil (abstract). *Circulation* 62 Suppl 3:317, 1980
96. Bonow RO, Rosing DR, Bacharach SL, et al: Long-term effects of verapamil on left ventricular diastolic filling in patients with hypertrophic cardiomyopathy (abstract). *Am J Cardiol* 47:409, 1981
97. Maron BJ, Epstein SE, Roberts WC: Hypertrophic cardiomyopathy and transmural myocardial infarction without significant atherosclerosis of the extramural coronary arteries. *Am J Cardiol* 43:1086-1102, 1979
98. Ten Cate FJ, Balakumaran K, McGhie J, et al: Angina pectoris in hypertrophic cardiomyopathy (HCM): cause or consequence of disturbed relaxation? (Abstract). *Circulation* 62 Suppl 3:317, 1980
99. Koide T, Kakihana M, Takabatake Y, et al: Long-term clinical effect of calcium inhibitors in hypertrophic cardiomyopathy compared to the effect of beta-blocking agents: a preliminary report with special reference to the beneficial effect of nifedipine on angina pectoris. *Jpn Heart J* 22:87-102, 1981

100. Epstein SE, Henry WL, Clark CE, et al: Asymmetric septal hypertrophy. *Ann Intern Med* 81:650-680, 1974

101. Braunwald E, Lambrew CT, Rockoff SD, et al: Idiopathic hypertrophic subaortic stenosis. I. A description of the disease based upon an analysis of 64 patients. *Circulation* 30 Suppl 4:3-119, 1964

102. Maron BJ, Savage DD, Wolfson JK, et al: Prognostic significance of 24 hour ambulatory electrocardiographic monitoring in patients with hypertrophic cardiomyopathy: a prospective study. *Am J Cardiol* 48:252-257, 1981

103. Gilligan DM, Nihoyannopoulos P, Chan WL, et al: Investigation of a hemodynamic basis for syncope in hypertrophic cardiomyopathy: use of a head-up tilt test. *Circulation* 85:2140-2148, 1992

104. McKenna W, Harris L, Deanfield J: Syncope in hypertrophic cardiomyopathy. *Br Heart J* 47:177-179, 1982

105. Frenneaux MP, Counihan PJ, Caforio ALP, et al: Abnormal blood pressure response during exercise in hypertrophic cardiomyopathy. *Circulation* 82:1995-2002, 1990

106. Wigle ED: The arterial pressure pulse in muscular subaortic stenosis. *Br Heart J* 25:97-105, 1963

107. Shah PM, Gramiak R, Kramer DH: Ultrasound localization of left ventricular outflow obstruction in hypertrophic obstructive cardiomyopathy. *Circulation* 40:3-11, 1969

108. Glancy DL, O'Brien KP, Gold HK, et al: Atrial fibrillation in patients with idiopathic hypertrophic subaortic stenosis. *Br Heart J* 32:652-659, 1970

109. Maron BJ, Wolfson JK, Ciró E, et al: Relation of electrocardiographic abnormalities and patterns of left ventricular hypertrophy identified by 2-dimensional echocardiography in patients with hypertrophic cardiomyopathy. *Am J Cardiol* 51:189-194, 1983

110. Sakamoto T, Tei C, Murayama M, et al: Giant T wave inversion as a manifestation of asymmetrical apical hypertrophy (AAH) of the left ventricle: echocardiographic and ultrasono-cardiotomographic study. *Jpn Heart J* 17:611-629, 1976

111. Alfonso F, Nihoyannopoulos P, Stewart J, et al: Clinical significance of giant negative T waves in hypertrophic cardiomyopathy. *J Am Coll Cardiol* 15:965-971, 1990

112. Ingham RE, Mason JW, Rossen RM, et al: Electrophysiologic findings in patients with idiopathic hypertrophic subaortic stenosis. *Am J Cardiol* 41:811-816, 1978

113. Prescott R, Quinn JS, Littmann D: Electrocardiographic changes in hypertrophic subaortic stenosis which simulate myocardial infarction. *Am Heart J* 66:42-48, 1963

114. Kariv I, Sherf L, Solomon M: Familial cardiomyopathy: with special consideration of electrocardiographic and vectorcardiographic findings. *Am J Cardiol* 13:734-749, 1964

115. Wigle ED, Baron RH: The electrocardiogram in muscular subaortic stenosis: effect of a left septal incision and right bundle-branch block. *Circulation* 34:585-594, 1966

116. Kronzon I, Glassman E: Mitral ring calcification in idiopathic hypertrophic subaortic stenosis. *Am J Cardiol* 42:60-66, 1978

117. Henry WL, Clark CE, Epstein SE: Asymmetric septal hypertrophy: echocardiographic identification of the pathognomonic anatomic abnormality of IHSS. *Circulation* 47:225-233, 1973

118. Mintz GS, Kotler MN, Segal BL, et al: Systolic anterior motion of the mitral valve in the absence of asymmetric septal hypertrophy. *Circulation* 57:256-263, 1978

119. Maron BJ, Gottdiener JS, Bonow RO, et al: Hypertrophic cardiomyopathy with unusual locations of left ventricular hypertrophy undetectable by M-mode echocardiography: identification by wide-angle two-dimensional echocardiography. *Circulation* 63:409-418, 1981

120. Larter WE, Allen HD, Sahn DJ, et al: The asymmetrically hypertrophied septum: further differentiation of its causes. *Circulation* 53:19-27, 1976

121. Maron BJ, Gottdiener JS, Epstein SE: Patterns and significance of distribution of left ventricular hypertrophy in hypertrophic cardiomyopathy: a wide angle, two dimensional echocardiographic study of 125 patients. *Am J Cardiol* 48:418-428, 1981

122. Maron BJ, Epstein SE: Hypertrophic cardiomyopathy: recent observations regarding the specificity of three hallmarks of the disease; asymmetric septal hypertrophy, septal disorganization and systolic anterior motion of the anterior mitral leaflet. *Am J Cardiol* 45:141-154, 1980

123. Kansal S, Roitman D, Sheffield LT: Interventricular septal thickness and left ventricular hypertrophy: an echocardiographic study. *Circulation* 60:1058-1065, 1979

124. Fowles RE, Martin RP, Popp RL: Erroneous diagnosis of asymmetric septal hypertrophy due to angled interventricular septum (abstract). *Am J Cardiol* 43:348, 1979

125. Goodman DJ, Harrison DC, Popp RL: Echocardiographic features of primary pulmonary hypertension. *Am J Cardiol* 33:438-443, 1974

126. Maron BJ, Verter J, Kapur S: Disproportionate ventricular septal thickening in the developing normal human heart. *Circulation* 57:520-526, 1978

127. Maron BJ, Edwards JE, Epstein SE: Disproportionate ventricular septal thickening in patients with systemic hypertension. *Chest* 73:466-470, 1978

128. Henning H, O'Rourke RA, Crawford MH, et al: Inferior myocardial infarction as a cause of asymmetric septal hypertrophy: an echocardiographic study. *Am J Cardiol* 41:817-822, 1978

129. Shah PM: Newer concepts in hypertrophic obstructive cardiomyopathy I. *JAMA* 242:1663-1665, 1979

130. Hamby RI, Roberts GS, Meron JM: Hypertension and hypertrophic subaortic stenosis. Am J Med 51:474-481, 1971

131. Rossen RM, Goodman DJ, Ingham RE, et al: Ventricular systolic septal thickening and excursion in idiopathic hypertrophic subaortic stenosis. *N Engl J Med* 291:1317-1319, 1974

132. Shah PM, Gramiak R, Adelman AG, et al: Echocardiographic assessment of the effects of surgery and propranolol on the dynamics of outflow obstruction in hypertrophic subaortic stenosis. *Circulation* 45:516-521, 1972

133. Abbasi A, MacAlpin RN, Eber LM, et al: Left ventricular hypertrophy diagnosed by echocardiography. *N Engl J Med* 289:118-121, 1973

134. Shah PM, Gramiak R, Adelman AG, et al: Role of echocardiography in diagnostic and hemodynamic assessment of hypertrophic subaortic stenosis. *Circulation* 44:891-898, 1971

135. Popp RL, Harrison DC: Ultrasound in the diagnosis and evaluation of therapy of idiopathic hypertrophic subaortic stenosis. *Circulation* 40:905-914, 1969

136. Tajik AJ, Giuliani ER: Echocardiographic observations in idiopathic hypertrophic subaortic stenosis. *Mayo Clin Proc* 49:89-97, 1974

137. Henry WL, Clark CE, Griffith JM, et al: Mechanism of left ventricular outflow obstruction in patients with obstructive asymmetric septal hypertrophy (idiopathic hypertrophic subaortic stenosis). *Am J Cardiol* 35:337-345, 1975

138. Björk VO, Hultquist G, Lodin H: Subaortic stenosis produced by an abnormally placed anterior mitral leaflet. *J Thorac Cardiovasc Surg* 41:659-669, 1961

139. Pridie RB, Oakley CM: Mechanism of mitral regurgitation of hypertrophic obstructive cardiomyopathy. *Br Heart J* 32:203-208, 1970

140. Gardin JM, Talano JV, Stephanides L, et al: Systolic anterior motion in the absence of asymmetric septal hypertrophy: a buckling phenomenon of the chordae tendineae. *Circulation* 63:181-188, 1981

141. Dinsmore RE, Sanders CA, Harthorne JW: Mitral regurgitation in idiopathic hypertrophic subaortic stenosis. *N Engl J Med* 275:1225-1228, 1966

142. Krajcer Z, Orzan F, Pechacek LW, et al: Early systolic closure of the aortic valve in patients with hypertrophic subaortic stenosis and discrete subaortic stenosis: correlation with preoperative and postoperative hemodynamics. *Am J Cardiol* 41:823-829, 1978

143. Yamaguchi H, Ishimura T, Nishiyama S, et al: Hypertrophic nonobstructive cardiomyopathy with giant negative T waves (apical hypertrophy): ventriculographic and echocardiographic features in 30 patients. *Am J Cardiol* 44:401-412, 1979

144. Henry WL, Clark CE, Roberts WC, et al: Differences in distribution of myocardial abnormalities in patients with obstructive and nonobstructive asymmetric septal hypertrophy (ASH): echocardiographic and gross anatomic findings. *Circulation* 50:447-455, 1974

145. Cotter L, Wong P: Aortic valve closure during early or middle systole. *Herz* 5:285-290, 1980

146. Maron BJ, Gottdiener JS, Roberts WC, et al: Left ventricular outflow tract obstruction due to systolic anterior motion of the anterior mitral leaflet in patients with concentric left ventricular hypertrophy. *Circulation* 57:527-533, 1978

147. Hoit BD, Penonen E, Dalton N, et al: Doppler color flow mapping studies of jet formation and spatial orientation in obstructive hypertrophic cardiomyopathy. *Am Heart J* 117:1119-1126, 1989

148. Rodger JC: Motion of mitral apparatus in hypertrophic cardiomyopathy with obstruction. *Br Heart J* 38:732-737, 1976

149. Nishimura RA, Tajik AJ: Echocardiography. *Prog Cardiol* 2 No 2:135-156, 1989

150. Tajik AJ, Seward JB, Hagler DJ: Detailed analysis of hypertrophic obstructive cardiomyopathy by wide-angle two-dimensional section echocardiography (abstract). *Am J Cardiol* 43:348, 1979

151. Falicov RE, Resnekov L, Bharati S, et al: Mid-ventricular obstruction: a variant of obstructive cardiomyopathy. *Am J Cardiol* 37:432-437, 1976

152. Rakowski H, Gilbert BW, Drobac M, et al: Anatomic variations in subgroups of hypertrophic cardiomyopathy as assessed by wide-angle two-dimensional echocardiography (abstract). *Am J Cardiol* 43:348, 1979

153. DeMaria AN, Bommer W, Lee G, et al: Value and limitations of two dimensional echocardiography in assessment of cardiomyopathy. *Am J Cardiol* 46:1224-1231, 1980

154. Martin RP, Rakowski H, French J, et al: Idiopathic hypertrophic subaortic stenosis viewed by wide-angle, phased-array echocardiography. *Circulation* 59:1206-1217, 1979

155. Lewis JF, Maron BJ: Elderly patients with hypertrophic cardiomyopathy: a subset with distinctive left ventricular morphology and progressive clinical course late in life. *J Am Coll Cardiol* 13:36-45, 1989

156. Lever HM, Karam RF, Currie PJ, et al: Hypertrophic cardiomyopathy in the elderly: distinctions from the young based on cardiac shape. *Circulation* 79:580-589, 1989

157. Utsunomiya T, Gardin JM, Henry WL: Relationship between the extent of muscular hypertrophy and diastolic function in patients with hypertrophic cardiomyopathy without left ventricular outflow gradients or mitral regurgitation (abstract). *J Am Coll Cardiol* 13 Suppl A:89, 1989

158. Liu P, Wilansky S, Poon P, et al: Myocardial mass quantitation by magnetic resonance imaging in hypertrophic cardiomyopathy (abstract). *Circulation* 74 Suppl 2:226, 1986

159. Spirito P, Watson RM, Maron BJ: Relation between extent of left ventricular hypertrophy and occurrence of ventricular tachycardia in hypertrophic cardiomyopathy. *Am J Cardiol* 60:1137-1142, 1987

160. Lazzeroni E, Domenicucci S, Finardi A, et al: Severity of arrhythmias and extent of hypertrophy in hypertrophic cardiomyopathy. *Am Heart J* 118:734-738, 1989

161. Spirito P, Maron BJ: Relation between extent of left ventricular hypertrophy and occurrence of sudden cardiac death in hypertrophic cardiomyopathy. *J Am Coll Cardiol* 15:1521-1526, 1990

162. Maron BJ, Spirito P, Wesley Y, et al: Development and progression of left ventricular hypertrophy in children with hypertrophic cardiomyopathy. *N Engl J Med* 315:610-614, 1986

163. Spirito P, Maron BJ: Absence of progression of left ventricular hypertrophy in adult patients with hypertrophic cardiomyopathy. *J Am Coll Cardiol* 9:1013-1017, 1987

164. Maron BJ, Bonow RO, Seshagiri TNR, et al: Hypertrophic cardiomyopathy with ventricular septal hypertrophy localized to the apical region of the left ventricle (apical hypertrophic cardiomyopathy). *Am J Cardiol* 49:1838-1848, 1982

165. Zoghbi WA, Haichin RN, Quinones MA: Mid-cavity obstruction in apical hypertrophy: Doppler evidence of diastolic intraventricular gradient with higher apical pressure. *Am Heart J* 116:1469-1474, 1988

166. Louie EK, Maron BJ: Apical hypertrophic cardiomyopathy: clinical and two-dimensional echocardiographic assessment. *Ann Intern Med* 106:663-670, 1987

167. Blazer D, Kotler MN, Parry WR, et al: Noninvasive evaluation of mid-left ventricular obstruction by two-dimensional and Doppler echocardiography and color flow Doppler echocardiography. *Am Heart J* 114:1162-1168, 1987

168. Gordon EP, Henderson MA, Rakowski H, et al: Midventricular obstruction with apical infarction and aneurysm formation (abstract). *Circulation* 70 Suppl 2:145, 1984

169. Hatle L, Angelsen B (eds): Doppler Ultrasound in Cardiology: Physical Principles and Clinical Applications. Philadelphia, Lea & Febiger, 1982

170. Nishimura RA, Miller FA Jr, Callahan MJ, et al: Doppler echocardiography: theory, instrumentation, technique, and application. *Mayo Clin Proc* 60:321-343, 1985

171. Pearson AC, Gudipati CV, Labovitz AJ: Systolic and diastolic flow abnormalities in elderly patients with hypertensive hypertrophic cardiomyopathy. *J Am Coll Cardiol* 12:989-995, 1988

172. Sasson Z, Yock PG, Hatle LK, et al: Doppler echocardiographic determination of the pressure gradient in hypertrophic cardiomyopathy. *J Am Coll Cardiol* 11:752-756, 1988

173. Stewart WJ, Schiavone WA, Salcedo EE, et al: Intraoperative Doppler echocardiography in hypertrophic cardiomyopathy: correlations with the obstructive gradient. *J Am Coll Cardiol* 10:327-335, 1987

174. Maron BJ, Gottdiener JS, Arce J, et al: Dynamic subaortic obstruction in hypertrophic cardiomyopathy: analysis by pulsed Doppler echocardiography. *J Am Coll Cardiol* 6:1-15, 1985

175. Sasson Z, Hatle L, Appleton CP, et al: Intraventricular flow during isovolumic relaxation: description and characterization by Doppler echocardiography. *J Am Coll Cardiol* 10:539-546, 1987

176. Nishimura RA, Abel MD, Hatle LK, et al: Assessment of diastolic function of the heart: background and current applications of Doppler echocardiography. Part II. Clinical studies. *Mayo Clin Proc* 64:181-204, 1989

177. Nishimura RA, Abel MD, Hatle LK, et al: Relation of pulmonary vein to mitral flow velocities by transesophageal Doppler echocardiography: effect of different loading conditions. *Circulation* 81:1488-1497, 1990

178. Goldman MR, Boucher CA: Value of radionuclide imaging techniques in assessing cardiomyopathy. *Am J Cardiol* 46:1232-1236, 1980

179. Pitcher D, Wainwright R, Maisey M, et al: Assessment of chest pain in hypertrophic cardiomyopathy using exercise thallium-201 myocardial scintigraphy. *Br Heart J* 44:650-656, 1980

180. McKenna WJ, Franklin RC, Nihoyannopoulos P, et al: Arrhythmia and prognosis in infants, children and adolescents with hypertrophic cardiomyopathy. *J Am Coll Cardiol* 11:147-153, 1988

181. Cripps TR, Counihan PJ, Frenneaux MP, et al: Signal-averaged electrocardiography in hypertrophic cardiomyopathy. *J Am Coll Cardiol* 15:956-961, 1990

182. Fananapazir L, Tracy CM, Leon MB, et al: Electrophysiologic abnormalities in patients with hypertrophic cardiomyopathy: a consecutive analysis in 155 patients. *Circulation* 80:1259-1268, 1989

183. Fananapazir L, Epstein SE: Hemodynamic and electrophysiologic evaluation of patients with hypertrophic cardiomyopathy surviving cardiac arrest. *Am J Cardiol* 67:280-287, 1991

184. Menges H Jr, Brandenburg RO, Brown AL Jr: The clinical, hemodynamic, and pathologic diagnosis of muscular subvalvular aortic stenosis. *Circulation* 24:1126-1136, 1961

185. Parker BM: The course in idiopathic hypertrophic muscular subaortic stenosis. *Ann Intern Med* 70:903-911, 1969

186. Maron BJ, Henry WL, Clark CE, et al: Asymmetric septal hypertrophy in childhood. *Circulation* 53:9-19, 1976

187. Spirito P, Chiarella F, Carratino L, et al: Clinical course and prognosis of hypertrophic cardiomyopathy in an outpatient population. *N Engl J Med* 320:749-755, 1989

188. Topol EJ, Traill TA, Fortuin NJ. Hypertensive hypertrophic cardiomyopathy of the elderly. *N Engl J Med* 312:277-283, 1985

189. Karam R, Lever HM, Healy BP: Hypertensive hypertrophic cardiomyopathy or hypertrophic cardiomyopathy with hypertension? A study of 78 patients. *J Am Coll Cardiol* 13:580-584, 1989

190. Fay WP, Taliercio CP, Ilstrup DM, et al: Natural history of hypertrophic cardiomyopathy in the elderly. *J Am Coll Cardiol* 16:821-826, 1990

191. Maron BJ, Roberts WC, McAllister HA, et al: Sudden death in young athletes. *Circulation* 62:218-229, 1980

192. Maron BJ, Roberts WC, Edwards JE, et al: Sudden death in patients with hypertrophic cardiomyopathy: characterization of 26 patients without functional limitation. *Am J Cardiol* 41:803-810, 1978

193. Maron BJ, Lipson LC, Roberts WC, et al: "Malignant" hypertrophic cardiomyopathy: identification of a subgroup of families with unusually frequent premature death. *Am J Cardiol* 41:1133-1140, 1978

194. Nienaber CA, Hiller S, Spielmann RP, et al: Syncope in hypertrophic cardiomyopathy: multivariate analysis of prognostic determinants. *J Am Coll Cardiol* 15:948-955, 1990

195. Hardarson T, de la Calzada CS, Curiel R, et al: Prognosis and mortality of hypertrophic obstructive cardiomyopathy. *Lancet* 2:1462-1467, 1973

196. Fighali S, Krajcer Z, Edelman S, et al: Progression of hypertrophic cardiomyopathy into a hypokinetic left ventricle: higher incidence in patients with midventricular obstruction. *J Am Coll Cardiol* 9:288-294, 1987

197. Bulkley BH, Weisfeldt ML, Hutchins GM: Isometric cardiac contraction: a possible cause of the disorganized myocardial pattern of idiopathic hypertrophic subaortic stenosis. *N Engl J Med* 296:135-139, 1977

198. Goodwin JF: Treatment of the cardiomyopathies. *Am J Cardiol* 32:341-351, 1973

199. Adelman AG, Shah PM, Gramiak R, et al: Long-term propranolol therapy in muscular subaortic stenosis. *Br Heart J* 32:804-811, 1970

200. Flamm MD, Harrison DC, Hancock EW: Muscular subaortic stenosis: prevention of outflow obstruction with propranolol. *Circulation* 38:846-858, 1968

201. Goodwin JF: The role of beta adrenergic stimulation in obstructive cardiomyopathy and its modification by blocking drugs and surgery. *UCLA Forum Med Sci* 13:161-172, 1970

202. Sloman G: Propranolol in management of muscular subaortic stenosis. *Br Heart J* 29:783-787, 1967

203. Cohen LS, Braunwald E: Amelioration of angina pectoris in idiopathic hypertrophic subaortic stenosis with beta-adrenergic blockade. *Circulation* 35:847-851, 1967

204. Cherian G, Brockington IF, Shah PM, et al: Beta-adrenergic blockade in hypertrophic obstructive cardiomyopathy. *Br Med J* 1:895-898, 1966

205. Kaltenbach M, Hopf R, Kober G, et al: Treatment of hypertrophic obstructive cardiomyopathy with verapamil. *Br Heart J* 42:35-42, 1979

206. Lewis BS, Mitha AS, Bakst A, et al: Haemodynamic effects of beta blockade in hypertrophic cardiomyopathy using Sectral (acebutolol; M & B 17803A). *Cardiovasc Res* 8:249-262, 1974

207. Speiser KW, Krayenbuehl HP: Reappraisal of the effect of acute beta-blockade on left ventricular filling dynamics in idiopathic hypertrophic subaortic stenosis (IHSS) (abstract). *Am J Cardiol* 43:380, 1979

208. Henry PD, Shuchleib R, Davis J, et al: Myocardial contracture and accumulation of mitochondrial calcium in ischemic rabbit heart. *Am J Physiol* 233:H677-H684, 1977

209. McFarland KF, Stefadouros MA, Abdulla AM, et al: Hypercalcemia and idiopathic hypertrophic subaortic stenosis. *Ann Intern Med* 88:57-58, 1978

210. Rosing DR, Kent KM, Borer JS, et al: Verapamil therapy: a new approach to the pharmacologic treatment of hypertrophic cardiomyopathy. I. Hemodynamic effects. *Circulation* 60:1201-1207, 1979

211. Rosing DR, Kent KM, Seides SF, et al: Hemodynamic effects of verapamil in patients with hypertrophic cardiomyopathy (abstract). *Am J Cardiol* 43:380, 1979

212. Raff GL, Brundage BH, Ports IA, et al: Dissociation between acute hemodynamic effects and clinical response to verapamil in hypertrophic cardiomyopathy (abstract). *Clin Res* 29:79A, 1981

213. Shaffer EM, Rocchini AP, Spicer RL, et al: Effects of verapamil on left ventricular diastolic filling in children with hypertrophic cardiomyopathy. *Am J Cardiol* 61:413-417, 1988

214. Rosing DR, Condit JR, Maron BJ, et al: Verapamil therapy: a new approach to the pharmacologic treatment of hypertrophic cardiomyopathy. III. Effects of long-term administration. *Am J Cardiol* 48:545-553, 1981

215. Rosing DR, Kent KM, Maron BJ, et al: Verapamil therapy: a new approach to the pharmacologic treatment of hypertrophic cardiomyopathy. II. Effects of exercise capacity and symptomatic status. *Circulation* 60:1208-1213, 1979

216. Lemke R, Hopf R, Kober G, et al: Echokardiographische Befunde unter calciumantagonistischer Therapie der hypertrophobstruktiven Myokardiopathie. *Z Kardiol* 69:661-668, 1980

217. Udelson JE, Bonow RO, O'Gara PT, et al: Verapamil prevents silent myocardial perfusion abnormalities during exercise in asymptomatic patients with hypertrophic cardiomyopathy. *Circulation* 79:1052-1060, 1989

218. Pollick C, Kimball B, Henderson M, et al: Disopyramide in hypertrophic cardiomyopathy. I. Hemodynamic assessment after intravenous administration. Am J Cardiol 62:1248-1251, 1988

219. McKenna WJ, Harris L, Perez G, et al: Hypertrophic cardiomyopathy: comparison of verapamil and amiodarone in treatment of arrhythmias (abstract). *Br Heart J* 45:354, 1981

220. McKenna WJ, Harris L, Rowland E, et al: Amiodarone for long-term management of patients with hypertrophic cardiomyopathy. *Am J Cardiol* 54:802-810, 1984

221. Fananapazir L, Epstein SE: Value of electrophysiologic studies in hypertrophic cardiomyopathy treated with amiodarone. *Am J Cardiol* 67:175-182, 1991

222. Fananapazir L, Leon MB, Bonow RO, et al: Sudden death during empiric amiodarone therapy in symptomatic hypertrophic cardiomyopathy. *Am J Cardiol* 67:169-174, 1991

223. Goodwin JF, Oakley CM: The cardiomyopathies (editorial). *Br Heart J* 34:545-552, 1972

224. Morrow AG, Reitz BA, Epstein SE, et al: Operative treatment in hypertrophic subaortic stenosis: techniques, and the results of pre and postoperative assessment in 83 patients. *Circulation* 52:88-102, 1975

225. Tajik AJ, Giuliani ER, Weidman WH, et al: Idiopathic hypertrophic subaortic stenosis: long-term surgical follow-up. *Am J Cardiol* 34:815-822, 1974

226. Roberts WC: Operative treatment of hypertrophic obstructive cardiomyopathy: the case against mitral valve replacement (editorial). *Am J Cardiol* 32:377-381, 1973

227. Cooley DA, Leachman RD, Wukasch DC: Diffuse muscular subaortic stenosis: surgical treatment. *Am J Cardiol* 31:1-6, 1973

228. Morrow AG, Fogarty TJ, Hannah H III, et al: Operative treatment in idiopathic hypertrophic subaortic stenosis: techniques, and the results of preoperative and postoperative clinical and hemodynamic assessments. *Circulation* 37:589-596, 1968

229. Maron BJ, Merrill WH, Freier PA, et al: Long-term clinical course and symptomatic status of patients after operation for hypertrophic subaortic stenosis. *Circulation* 57:1205-1213, 1978

230. McIntosh CL, Maron BJ: Current operative treatment of obstructive hypertrophic cardiomyopathy. *Circulation* 78:487-495, 1988

231. Cooley DA, Wukasch DC, Leachman RD: Mitral valve replacement for idiopathic hypertrophic subaortic stenosis: results in 27 patients. *J Cardiovasc Surg* 17:380-387, 1976

232. Krajcer Z, Leachman RD, Cooley DA, et al: Septal myotomy-myomectomy versus mitral valve replacement in hypertrophic cardiomyopathy: ten-year follow-up in 185 patients. *Circulation* 80 Suppl 1:57-64, 1989

233. Sasson Z, Prieur T, Skrobik Y, et al: Aortic regurgitation: a common complication after surgery for hypertrophic obstructive cardiomyopathy. *J Am Coll Cardiol* 13:63-67, 1989

234. Mohr R, Schaff HV, Danielson GK, et al: The outcome of surgical treatment of hypertrophic obstructive cardiomyopathy: experience over 15 years. *J Thorac Cardiovasc Surg* 97:666-673, 1989

235. Mohr R, Schaff HV, Puga FJ, et al: Results of operation for hypertrophic obstructive cardiomyopathy in children and adults less than 40 years of age. *Circulation* 80 Suppl 1:191-196, 1989

236. Cannon RO III, McIntosh CL, Schenke WH, et al: Effect of surgical reduction of left ventricular outflow obstruction on hemodynamics, coronary flow, and myocardial metabolism in hypertrophic cardiomyopathy. *Circulation* 79:766-775, 1989

237. Beahrs MM, Tajik AJ, Seward JB, et al: Hypertrophic obstructive cardiomyopathy: 10- to 21-year follow-up after partial septal myectomy. *Am J Cardiol* 51:1160-1166, 1983

238. Fananapazir L, Cannon RO III, Tripodi D, et al: Impact of dual-chamber permanent pacing in patients with obstructive hypertrophic cardiomyopathy with symptoms refractory to verapamil and β-adrenergic blocker therapy. *Circulation* 85:2149-2161, 1992

239. McDonald K, McWilliams E, O'Keeffe B, et al: Functional assessment of patients treated with permanent dual chamber pacing as a primary treatment for hypertrophic cardiomyopathy. *Eur Heart J* 9:893-898, 1988

240. Jeanrenaud X, Goy J-J, Kappenberger L: Effects of dual-chamber pacing in hypertrophic obstructive cardiomyopathy. *Lancet* 339:1318-1323, 1992

CHAPTER

21

Restrictive cardiomyopathy

Byron A. Olney, M.D.

HISTORICAL DEVELOPMENT AND DEFINITION

A precise and universally accepted definition of what constitutes a restrictive cardiomyopathy remains elusive. The identification of myocardial restriction as a functional category of cardiomyopathy evolved from bedside observations and right heart catheterization studies in patients presenting with findings "typical" for constrictive pericarditis but who proved not to have constricting pericardial structures.[1-4] Such patients have a relatively fixed limitation to ventricular volume expansion with an accentuated filling in early diastole that terminates abruptly at the end of the rapid filling phase and leads to a diastolic dip and plateau, or square-root sign, on pressure tracings. In restrictive cardiomyopathy, this hemodynamic profile is imposed by alterations in myocardial or endocardial tissues rather than, as in constrictive pericarditis, alterations in the pericardium. In this purest definition of restrictive cardiomyopathy, the myocardial or endocardial abnormality closely mimics constrictive pericarditis in its hemodynamic effects.

Cardiomyopathic conditions that are labeled "restrictive cardiomyopathy" often do not conform closely to this strict definition. The reason is related, in part, to the number and variety of pathologic conditions reported to be able to exhibit restrictive physiology. Further, the degree to which these diverse conditions simulate pericardial constriction may differ at different stages of the disease[5] and may also depend on a number of coexisting variables, such as intravascular volume, neuroendocrine status, valvular insufficiency, and unrelated cardiovascular disease. Moreover, with improved techniques for assessing diastolic function, diastolic filling abnormalities of the myocardium do not appear to be neatly segregated in an either/or manner; rather, they form a spectrum that includes both cases with the pure restrictive-constrictive defect and those with less distinct physiologic features and a more mixed pattern of diastolic filling abnormalities.[6,7] Thus, in daily practice, a broader definition of restrictive cardiomyopathy emerges that describes a condition of *decreased diastolic chamber compliance* with demonstrable impairment of ventricular filling without significant ventricular hypertrophy, systolic dysfunction, or pericardial disease. Conditions that meet this definition may or may not closely simulate constrictive pericarditis.

CLINICAL DIFFERENTIATION AND DIAGNOSIS

Comparison of constrictive and restrictive defects

Although an aggressive surgical approach is potentially curative in pericardial constriction, surgical exploration in restrictive cardiomyopathy carries potential for significant morbidity.[8,9] Thus, regardless of how one conceptualizes restrictive cardiomyopathy, its differentiation from pericardial constriction has major clinical importance. The advent of more sophisticated technology has greatly enhanced the ability to establish a clear diagnosis. Nonetheless, the unusual case remains in which uncertainty persists and surgical exploration may need to be considered.

Clinical profile and noninvasive evaluation

Patients with advanced pericardial constriction or myocardial restriction present with fatigue and dyspnea, jugular venous distention with a particularly prominent y descent, evidence of ascites and peripheral edema, and a relatively normal heart size. In these respects, the two conditions may be indistinguishable. Further compounding the diagnostic challenge is the fact that the two conditions may coexist in the same patient, for example, one who earlier received radiation therapy. However, certain features of the clinical history and examination may be helpful. Angina-like chest pain, a third heart sound, murmurs of mitral and tricuspid insufficiency, and the peripheral stigmata of a systemic disease known to cause myocardial infiltrates favor a diagnosis of restrictive cardiomyopathy. Conversely, a history of prior pericarditis or conditions known to cause chronic pericardial disease, auscultation of a pericardial knock, and calcification in the pericardium suggest constrictive pericarditis. The pericardial knock may be difficult to differentiate from a third heart sound, but it tends to occur slightly earlier and have a sharper sound quality. Major alterations in QRS morphology on electrocardiograms may be more characteristic of cardiomyopathy, but these and other electrocardiographic findings are nonspecific and rarely helpful.

Careful *Doppler echocardiographic* assessment of diastolic (transmitral) blood flow can help identify restriction to diastolic filling.[10-12] It has been proposed also as a

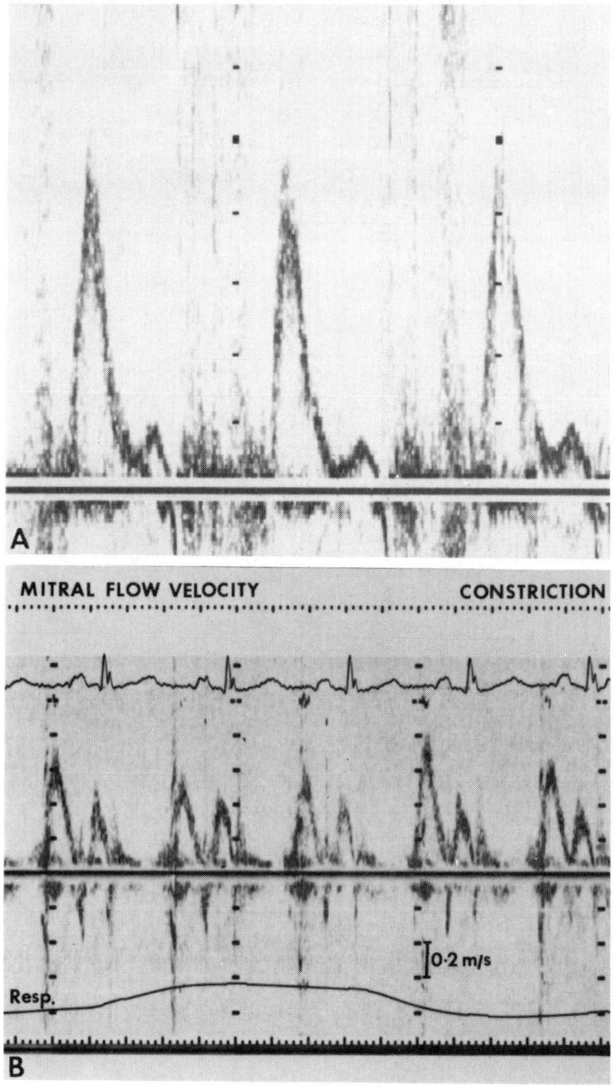

Fig 21-1 **A,** pulsed Doppler tracing illustrating the char acteristic transmitral diastolic flow pattern in a patient with myocardial restriction. Early filling is rapid, and deceleration time is shortened. Late filling is diminished, and the E:A ratio is increased. **B,** pulsed Doppler tracing from a patient with constrictive pericarditis illustrating the typical respiratory variation with diminished transmitral flow during inspiration. (From Seward JB: Restrictive cardiomyopathy: reassessment of definitions and diagnosis. *Curr Opin Cardiol* 3:391-395, 1988. By permission of Gower Academic Journals.)

means to differentiate restrictive myocardial disease from pericardial constriction,[13] although its sensitivity and specificity for this purpose have not been fully established.[14] Both phenomena exhibit accentuated early diastolic filling (E), shortened deceleration time, and diminished atrial filling (A), which result in an increased E:A ratio (Fig 21-1). However, when both ventricles are encased in a common constricting pericardial sac, an inspiratory increase in inflow into the right ventricle causes a reciprocal reduction in transmitral inflow into the left ventricle. Thus, a pattern of respiratory variation with diminished peak transmitral diastolic flow during inspiration is characteristic of pericardial constriction but not of myocardial restriction.[12,13]

Left ventricular peak filling rates can also be derived from time activity curves generated by *radionuclide angiography* and may be helpful in separating constrictive pericarditis from restrictive cardiomyopathy. Experience with this technique has been limited.[15,16]

Computed tomography and *magnetic resonance imaging* of the heart both allow visualization of the parietal pericardium, and these methods are the most accurate noninvasive means of demonstrating structural alterations of the pericardium.[17] In a small study in which thickened pericardium was used to differentiate constrictive pericarditis from nonpericardial causes of restrictive physiology, magnetic resonance imaging had a 93% accuracy in establishing a pericardial constrictive cause.[18] Such imaging modalities are therefore excellent means to screen for pericardial abnormalities. One must remember, however, that some exceptional patients with apparently normal pericardial thickness nevertheless have pericardial constriction and that others may have coexisting pericardial thickening and myocardial restrictive disease.

Cardiac catheterization

Cardiac catheterization often is used to attempt to differentiate constriction from restriction. The combination of increased right heart pressures, typical venous wave pattern, and the dip-plateau contour of the ventricular diastolic pressures (Fig 21-2) may be present in both pericardial and myocardial disorders. Thus, additional hemodynamic measurements have been sought and proposed to differentiate these two entities. The following criteria are said to favor a diagnosis of constrictive pericarditis: (1) equalization of left and right ventricular filling pressures, with a difference of no more than 5 mm Hg between the two sides;[19] (2) right ventricular end-diastolic pressure equal to or exceeding one-third of the level of the right ventricular systolic pressure;[20] (3) right ventricular systolic pressure of less than 50 mm Hg;[20] and (4) persistence of diastolic equalization of pressures under stress of exercise or fluid challenge.[19,21,22] In restrictive cardiomyopathy, variance between right and left ventricular diastolic pressures is more likely to be greater than 5 mm Hg, right ventricular end-diastolic pressure to be less than one-third the right ventricular systolic pressure, and right ventricular systolic pressure to be greater than 50 mm Hg.

A retrospective analysis of published experience with the first three of these hemodynamic diagnostic criteria indicates significant overlap between groups for any criterion. However, 91% (64 of 70) of these patients in whom all three criteria were satisfied proved to have constrictive pericarditis. Conversely, 94% (17 of 18) of those who had none or only one of these criteria had restrictive cardiomyopathy. Seventy-four percent of patients could be placed in one of these two categories, so that diagnosis was greater than 90% accurate. However,

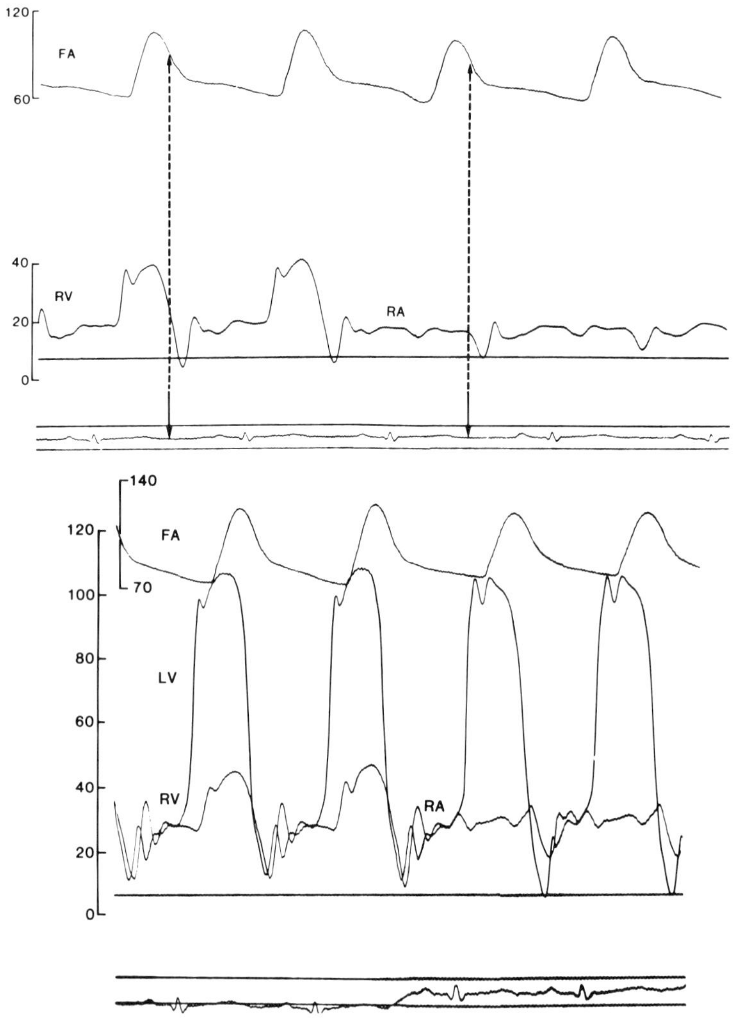

Fig 21-2 Intracardiac pressure tracings from a patient with an idiopathic primary restrictive cardiomyopathy. **Upper,** right ventricular *(RV)* and right atrial *(RA)* tracings with a typical diastolic square-root configuration in the right ventricular tracing and a prominent y descent in the early diastolic period of the right atrial tracing. *FA,* femoral artery. **Lower,** simultaneous left ventricular *(LV)*–right ventricular *(RV)* pressures and left ventricular–right atrial *(RA)* pressures, showing a square-root configuration in the left ventricular tracing and equalization of pressures during diastole in the three chambers. *FA,* femoral artery.

the other 26% of patients were in an intermediate category in which two of the criteria were satisfied, and this circumstance did not allow differentiation of constriction from restriction.

An increasingly frequent cause of constrictive pericarditis is the aftereffect of cardiac surgery, which may give rise to regional constriction or tamponade without equalization of filling pressures.

Endomyocardial biopsy

Percutaneous myocardial biopsy has proved to be very useful in certain cases in establishing whether endocardial or myocardial disease is present.[23] The biopsy sample may be taken from either the right or the left ventricle, and a growing experience with this technique indicates a high diagnostic yield in diseases that may appear with restrictive dynamics.[24] In cases in which the diagnosis remains in doubt after noninvasive studies and hemodynamic assessment, myocardial biopsy may be the most direct and definitive way of establishing a diagnosis of myocardial disease. This procedure is strongly advocated in such cases before exploratory surgery is done.[25]

Summary

Table 21-1 summarizes the clues to diagnostic differentiation of pericardial constriction from myocardial restriction. Figure 21-3 presents an algorithm for the evaluation of patients who present with restrictive or constrictive

Table 21-1 Clues to differentiation of pericardial constriction from myocardial restriction

Indices	Pericardial constriction	Myocardial restriction
Physical examination		
Peripheral	± Ascites, edema	± Ascites, edema; stigmata of systemic disease
Jugular venous pressure	Increased, with rapid y descent	Increased, with rapid y descent
Auscultation	Pericardial knock (40%)	± S_3, murmurs of mitral and tricuspid insufficiency
Noninvasive studies		
Chest radiograph	Heart size normal to increased; calcification of pericardium (40%)	Heart size normal to increased
Electrocardiogram	Nondiagnostic	Nondiagnostic
Echocardiogram/Doppler		
E	Increased	Increased
A	Decreased	Decreased
E:A	Increased	Increased
Deceleration time	Shortened	Shortened
Respiratory variation	Usually present*	Absent
CT or MRI	Thickened pericardium	Normal pericardium
Invasive studies		
Catheterization hemodynamics		
RV systolic pressure	≤50 mm Hg	≥50 mm Hg
RVEDP/RV systolic ratio	≥0.33	≤0.33
RVEDP/LVEDP equalization	≤5 mm Hg difference	>5 mm Hg difference
Cardiac biopsy	Normal myocardium	Abnormal myocardium, often diagnostic

A, atrial filling; CT, computed tomography; E, early diastolic filling; LVEDP, left ventricular end-diastolic pressure; MRI magnetic resonance imaging; RV, right ventricular; RVEDP, right ventricular end-diastolic pressure.
*May be absent, especially in cases of postoperative regionally circumscribed pericarditis.

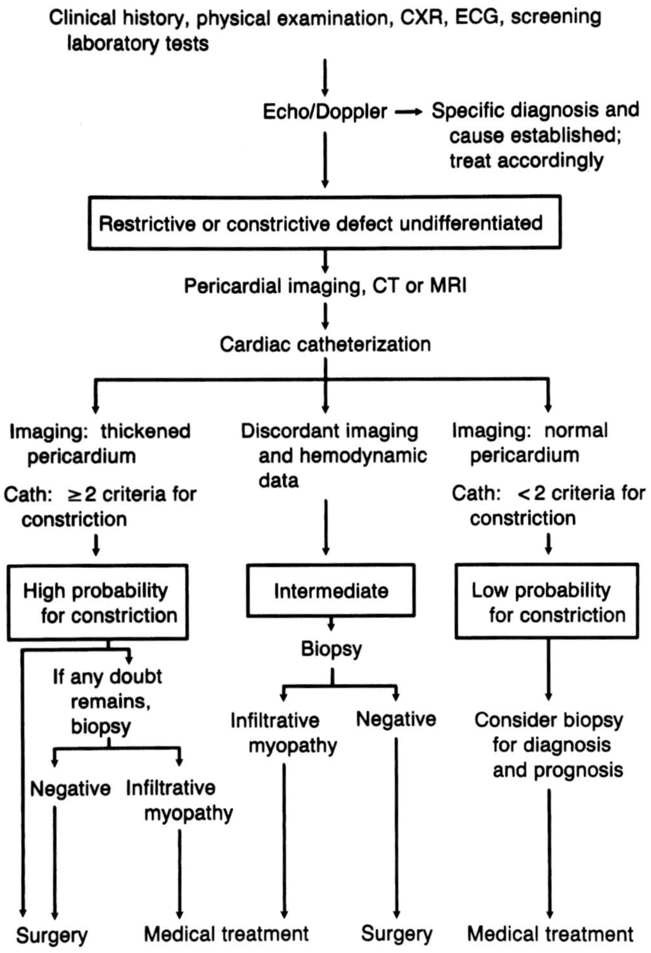

Fig 21-3 Algorithm for evaluation of patients with restrictive cardiomyopathy or constrictive pericarditis. *Cath*, cardiac catheterization; *CT*, computed tomography; *CXR*, chest radiograph; *ECG*, electrocardiogram; *Echo*, echocardiogram; *MRI*, magnetic resonance imaging. (Modified from Vaitkus PT, Kussmaul WG: Constrictive pericarditis versus restrictive cardiomyopathy: a reappraisal and update of diagnostic criteria. *Am Heart J* 122:1431-1441, 1991.)

disease. If such a scheme is used, the correct diagnosis can be established with few exceptions and inappropriate surgery avoided.

Differentiation from hypertrophic cardiomyopathy

A distinction should also be made between a restrictive abnormality of diastolic function and hypertrophic cardiomyopathy (see chapter 20). The latter may also be manifested by abnormalities of diastolic ventricular filling in a patient with relatively normal heart size. Unlike the occurrence in restrictive disorders, however, the ventricular filling in hypertrophic hearts is slow throughout diastole, without an early rapid-filling phase; this results from impaired diastolic relaxation. A longer period is required to complete the ventricular filling, and atrial contraction makes an important contribution at the end of diastole. Rapid heart rates and loss of atrial contractions are detrimental and may lead to rapid decompensation in hypertrophic cardiomyopathies. In contradistinction, in the true restrictive pattern, ventricular filling is rapid but abbreviated. Atrial contraction has little effect, and a moderate degree of tachycardia may be beneficial in compensating for a small, fixed stroke volume. In addition, the demonstration of pronounced ventricular hypertrophy, along with the characteristic systolic contractile abnormalities of hypertrophic cardiomyopathies, should automatically separate the hypertrophic from the restrictive category.

CLASSIFICATION OF RESTRICTIVE MYOCARDIAL DISEASES

The classification of cardiomyopathies formulated in 1980 by a World Health Organization task force[26] has served well as a general frame of reference to bring order to a broad and disparate area of cardiology. The definition of what constitutes a restrictive cardiomyopathy has evolved in the ensuing years, however, and the current concept is somewhat at variance with the original classification. Table 21-2 retains the broad distinction between the idiopathic cardiomyopathy and specific heart muscle disease that may be present with restrictive physiology. What now constitutes the idiopathic form was not recognized in the original classification, and endomyocardial fibrosis, which had been classified as idiopathic, is now listed as a specific disease entity.[27,28]

Primary restrictive cardiomyopathy

Numerous observers have noted a subset of patients with heart muscle disease of unknown cause manifested by heart failure and restrictive hemodynamics but without significant ventricular hypertrophy, endocardial thickening or fibrosis, associated eosinophilia, or other diagnostically distinct histopathologic features.[6,7,28-37] Such cases are labeled "primary restrictive cardiomyopathy," and reduced myocardial compliance is the physiologic common denominator, with myocardial fibrosis the most common histopathologic substrate (Fig 21-4).

Pathology. Although histologically lacking clear definition, these cases have a number of significant features in common. The decreased myocardial compliance cannot be accounted for by myocardial hypertrophy or the effects of coronary artery disease, and no specific infiltrative processes are evident. Pathologic examination shows normal-sized ventricular chambers without significant hypertrophy. The atria are usually enlarged, a reflection of the decreased compliance of the downstream chamber. The histologic features, as a rule, include interstitial fibrosis, which is minimal in some and extensive in others. The fibrosis is usually not severe, however, and the histologic picture is most accurately described as nonspecific.[31] As noted above, significant endocardial disease is not present.

Clinical profile. The symptoms generally consist of a combination of dyspnea, fatigue, and chest pain, although

Table 21-2 Restrictive myocardial disease

Restrictive cardiomyopathy	Specific heart muscle disease
Heart muscle disease of unknown cause presenting with findings of restriction to ventricular diastolic filling without ventricular hypertrophy or dilatation:	Heart muscle disease of specific cause or associated with more generalized underlying disease that often (+ + +), occasionally (+ +), or rarely (+) presents with restriction to ventricular diastolic filling:
Primary (idiopathic) restrictive cardiomyopathy	Eosinophilic endomyocardial disease (+ + +) Amyloid heart disease (+ + +) Hemochromatosis heart disease (+ +) Heart transplantation (+ +) Postradiation heart disease (+) Carcinoid heart disease (+) Doxorubicin and daunorubicin cardiotoxicity (+) Progressive systemic sclerosis (+) Pseudoxanthoma elasticum (+)

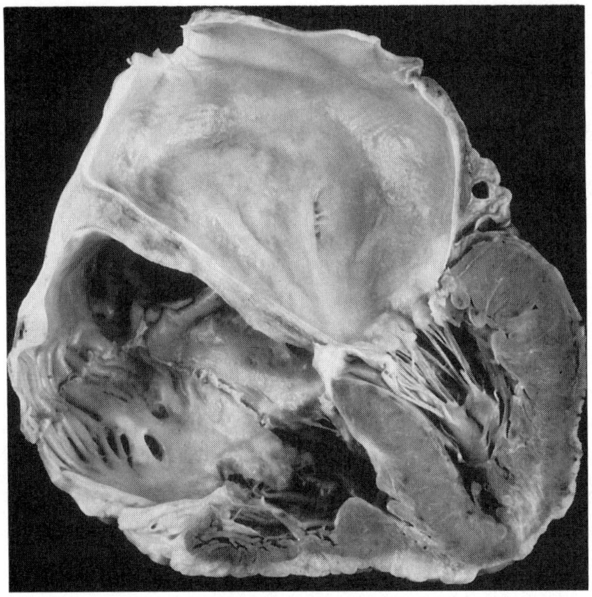

Fig 21-4 Long-axis section of the heart from a patient with primary restrictive cardiomyopathy. Note the relatively normal ventricular size and thickness with marked biatrial enlargement. There is no evident endocardial or pericardial disease. (From Edwards WD: Cardiomyopathies. *Hum Pathol* 18:625-635, 1987. By permission of WB Saunders Company.)

occasionally the patients may be virtually without symptoms.[31] The typical patient with symptoms has a heart of normal or near-normal size and experiences exertional dyspnea and fatigue far out of proportion to any demonstrable systolic dysfunction. The angina-like chest pain may be equally prominent, but coronary artery disease is absent. Males and females have been affected equally, and the disease has appeared throughout the pediatric and adult age ranges. A familial pattern has been noted in some cases of restrictive cardiomyopathy, and the possibility that it is an inherited disease has been advanced.[6,38] Systolic murmurs and S_3 gallops are common, and the murmurs may help to differentiate these cases from those of constrictive pericarditis. The jugular venous pressure is typically increased and has a rapid y descent. Mural thrombus and systemic emboli are not common in primary restrictive cardiomyopathy.

Diagnostic studies. Atrial fibrillation has been noted in 50% of patients and an increased cardiothoracic ratio on the chest radiograph in 70%. Echocardiographic studies have consistently shown normal ventricular dimensions without hypertrophy or dilatation. Indices of left ventricular systolic function may be normal or reduced. Biatrial enlargement is almost universal and may be quite striking in individual cases. This feature accounts for the radiographic appearance of cardiomegaly in most cases.[31]

Left ventriculography and hemodynamic assessment likewise show normal or near-normal global systolic function. The hemodynamic physiology corresponds with decreased ventricular compliance, which may be equally evident in both ventricles or may be predominantly on one side or the other. The classic diastolic dip and plateau is present in only about 50% of cases. When this pattern is present, the appearance may mimic constrictive pericarditis very closely[6,7] (see Fig 21-2).

Treatment and prognosis. No definitive or specific treatment has been developed for such restrictive cardiomyopathies, and most patients are treated symptomatically with standard inotropic agents, diuretics, and antiarrhythmic drugs. The clinical course and prognosis of this group vary, but at least some patients survive for several years with conventional therapy.[6,7,28] Others have a more relentless downhill course. The prognosis appears to be worse in children than in adults.[39] Children require relatively high filling pressures for maintenance of systolic output, and the therapeutic margin between volume depletion (leading to low output) and volume overload (leading to congestive heart failure) is narrowed. Limited experience suggests that morbidity and mortality are high in patients operated on for diagnosis or for mitral valve replacement when mitral regurgitation is present.[9,36]

Specific heart muscle disease with restrictive features

Eosinophilic endomyocardial disease. In 1936, Löffler[40] described two patients with a history of eosinophilia and heart failure due to a fibrous thickening of the endocardium. In 1948, Davies[41] reported on 36 cases of heart failure in Uganda, and these hearts also had fibrous thickening of the endocardium. The similarities in these separately described entities were noted early, and the possibility that they represented the same phenomenon was raised.[42] Meanwhile, other investigators[43-46] were identifying patients with a hypereosinophilic syndrome who also had a high incidence of cardiac lesions similar to those described by Löffler and Davies. Although eosinophilia has not been a consistent finding in Davies' tropical endomyocardial fibrosis, pathologic studies directly comparing these various entities[27,47,48] have supported the concept of a unified cause, with eosinophilia as the common denominator in the initiation of the disease. It has been proposed that Löffler's endocarditis, Davies' endomyocardial fibrosis, and the cardiac lesions associated with hypereosinophilic syndromes are all the same disease observed and described at different stages of development. Patients with isolated eosinophilia of whatever cause are at one end of the spectrum, and patients with advanced fibrosis of the endocardium and myocardium, most of whom no longer have eosinophilia, are at the other end. In between are patients with various degrees of eosinophilia associated with a progression of lesions from acute to chronic and from mild to severe.

It is now commonly acknowledged that the pathologic and clinical end results of Löffler's endocarditis and Davies' endomyocardial fibrosis are the same. However, acceptance of the unified eosinophilic etiologic theory is not universal, and numerous differences between the two entities have been noted[49-51] (Table 21-3). Eosinophilia is a consistent feature in Löffler's endocarditis, whereas its role in endomyocardial fibrosis is largely inferential.

Table 21-3 Comparison of Löffler's endocarditis with endomyocardial fibrosis

	Löffler's endocarditis	Endomyocardial fibrosis
Geographic distribution	Temperate zone	Tropical zone
Age	Adults	Children, young adults
Sex, M:F	3:1	1:1
Eosinophilia	Present	Uncommon
Organ involvement	Heart and other organs	Limited to the heart
Acuity	Both early acute and late chronic stages	Late chronic stage (acute form rarely identified)
Embolism	Frequent	Present but less frequent

There are relative differences in age and sex distribution, organ involvement, chronicity, and frequency of associated systemic embolism. An additional observation is that, even under favorable circumstances (e.g., presence of eosinophilia or habitation in tropical latitudes), the prevalence of disease expression varies widely. These discrepancies imply that other, non-eosinophilia-related factors must also contribute significantly to the clinical manifestations of the disease. Nonetheless, we believe it is valid to view these two entities as different expressions of a single disease process that has been designated "eosinophilic endomyocardial disease."[26]

THE EOSINOPHIL AND EOSINOPHILIA. An increased body of data implicates eosinophil granule proteins in the development of eosinophilic endomyocardial disease.[52] Typically, increased numbers of degranulated eosinophils in blood and tissues[53] imply a release of granules and their content.

Two eosinophil granule proteins in particular have been implicated—major basic protein and eosinophil cationic protein.[54] Both have demonstrated potential for cell damage or cell death, and both have been shown to be present in the cardiac tissue of patients with eosinophilic endomyocardial disease at all stages, acute and chronic.[55]

Eosinophilia may occur under a number of different circumstances. There are two broad categories: primary (idiopathic) and secondary (reactive). Associated with the primary group are the idiopathic hypereosinophilic syndrome and possibly a much smaller subgroup that meets the strict criteria for the diagnosis of eosinophilic leukemia. In the secondary, or reactive, group are the hypereosinophilias related to other disease processes, most notably allergic or hypersensitivity reactions and parasitic infestations. Endomyocardial fibrosis may occur in relation to either primary or secondary causes of eosinophilia. In tropical climates, parasitic infestations are the most common cause of eosinophilia, and filariasis, in particular, has often been associated with endomyocardial fibrosis.[56,57] In nontropical areas of the world, the largest number of cases of endomyocardial fibrosis have been reported in association with primary or idiopathic hypereosinophilia. In their review of reported cases on nontropical endomyocardial fibrosis (Löffler's endocarditis with and without eosinophilia), Brockington and Olsen[48] noted the following distribution of 112 cases: idiopathic primary hypereosinophilic syndrome, 65 (58%); reactive (secondary) hypereosinophilia, 25 (22%); and eosinophilia absent, 22 (20%).

There are no established boundaries for how severe eosinophilia need be or how long it must be present before heart disease appears. Furthermore, it seems clear that not all persons who have hypereosinophilia will experience heart disease. Nonetheless, in those in whom the hypereosinophilia is both severe and chronic, such as in the idiopathic hypereosinophilia syndrome, the incidence of associated heart disease of some degree is very high. It is estimated that 80% of patients with hypereosinophilia are found to have endomyocardial fibrosis within a 5-year follow-up period.[52]

PATHOLOGY. In his original description of African endomyocardial fibrosis, Davies[41] postulated the following pathologic natural history:

> For some reason, at present obscure, a myocardial infiltration with round cells and eosinophil cells takes place: either co-incidentally, or more probably subsequently, necrosis of the endocardium or the sub-endocardial myocardial fibers takes place: over the necrosed area a mural thrombus forms, . . . the mural thrombus is organised, dense fibrous tissue is laid down, and the inflammatory cells disappear so that the final result is a gross fibrosis of the endomyocardium manifested by congestive cardiac failure.

This general sequence of events has been supported by subsequent observers. The disease is thought to develop sequentially through the necrotic stage, the thrombotic stage, and the fibrotic stage, with much transitional overlap between stages. The necrotic stage is characterized by an intense myocarditis with eosinophils and an arteritis. The thrombotic stage shows some nonspecific thickening of the endocardium with overlying thrombus. The third, or final, stage is marked by a prominent layer of hyaline fibrous tissue in the thickened endocardium and fibrous septa penetrating the myocardium.[27]

Grossly, the fully developed case of endomyocardial fibrosis shows a pearly white thickening of the endocardium that affects the apices and the inflow tracts of one or both ventricles (Fig 21-5). The atria and the ventricular outflow tracts are relatively spared. Typically, the border between the affected and unaffected portions of the ventricles is clearly demarcated. In less advanced cases, intraventricular thrombus may be more prominent than fibrosis. The mural thrombosis (and subsequent fibrosis) often extends to involve the supporting structures of the atrioventricular (AV) valves, and this leads to mitral and tricuspid insufficiency (Fig 21-6 and 21-7). Mural thrombosis is present in most patients; it can occur in either ventricle and thus be a source of pulmonary or systemic emboli. At times the thrombus formation may be very extensive and, together with the thickened endocardium,

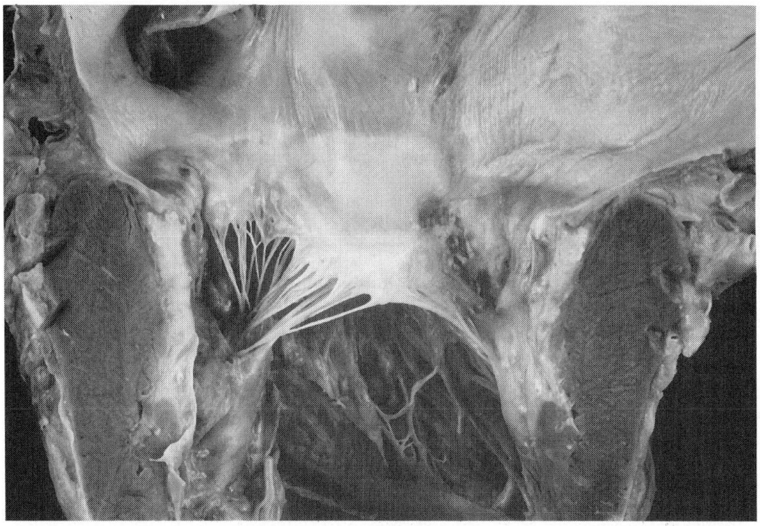

Fig 21-5 Long-axis section through the left ventricle in a case of eosinophilic endomyocardial disease. Note the pearly white endocardial thickening in the left ventricular inflow area, including the papillary muscles. (Courtesy of William D. Edwards, M.D.)

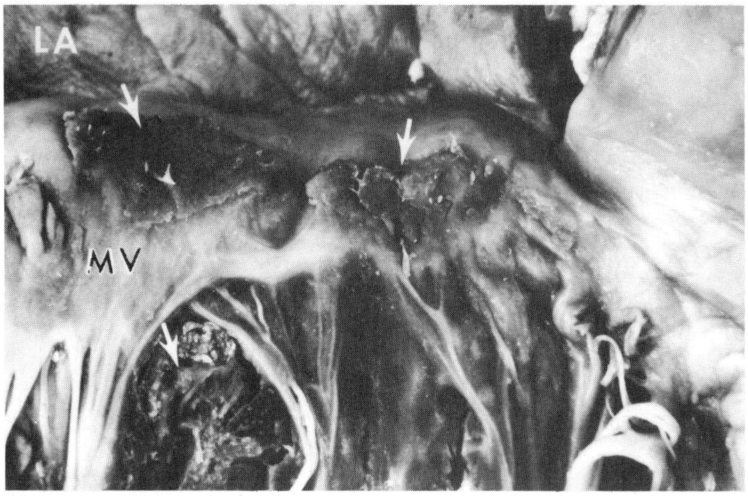

Fig 21-6 Close-up view of the mitral valve *(MV)* in a patient with hypereosinophilic endomyocardial disease, demonstrating accumulation of thrombus on and below the valve (*arrows*). *LA,* left atrium.

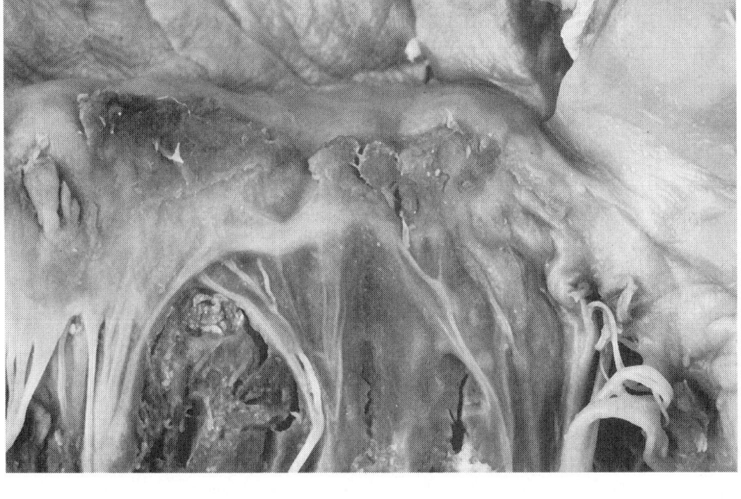

Fig 21-7 Close-up view of mitral valve from a patient with eosinophilic endomyocardial disease. Encroachment of thrombus under and on the mitral valve results in a clinical finding of mitral regurgitation. (From Edwards WD: Cardiomyopathies. *Hum Pathol* 18:625-635, 1987. By permission of WB Saunders Company.)

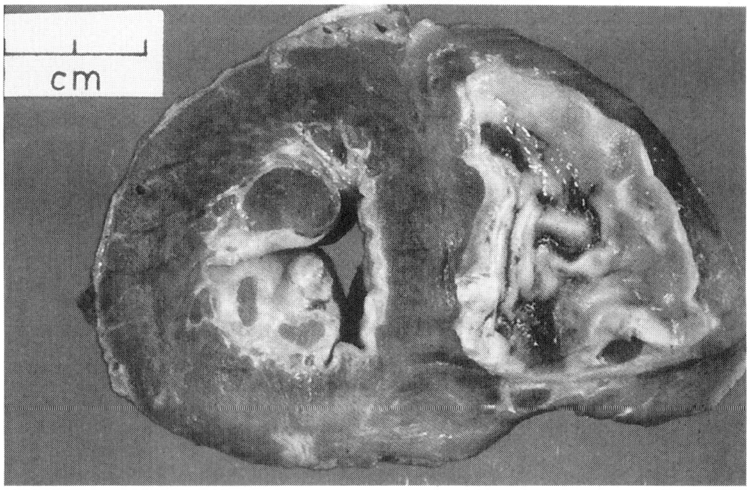

Fig 21-8 Transverse short-axis section through the ventricles at papillary muscle level in chronic nontropical endomyocardial fibrosis. A dense layer of fibrous tissue in both ventricles surrounds the papillary muscle. The apex of the right ventricle is obliterated. (From Davies MJ: *Colour Atlas of Cardiovascular Pathology*. New York, Oxford University Press, 1986, p 107. By permission of Harvey Miller Publishers.)

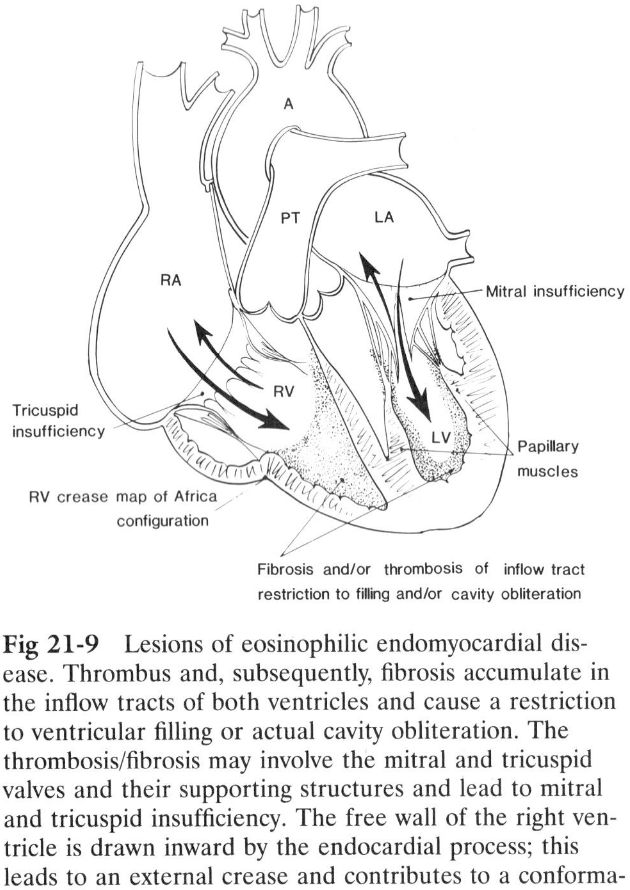

Fig 21-9 Lesions of eosinophilic endomyocardial disease. Thrombus and, subsequently, fibrosis accumulate in the inflow tracts of both ventricles and cause a restriction to ventricular filling or actual cavity obliteration. The thrombosis/fibrosis may involve the mitral and tricuspid valves and their supporting structures and lead to mitral and tricuspid insufficiency. The free wall of the right ventricle is drawn inward by the endocardial process; this leads to an external crease and contributes to a conformation likened to the "map of Africa." The atrial chambers are enlarged as a result of valvular insufficiency and resistance to ventricular filling. *A,* aorta; *PT,* pulmonary trunk; *RA,* right atrium; *LA,* left atrium; *RV,* right ventricle; *LV,* left ventricle.

can nearly fill the affected ventricular cavities, hence the term "obliterative cardiomyopathy" (Fig 21-8). This finding is more prevalent in the right ventricle than in the left. With such obliteration, drawing in of the anteroinferior wall of the right ventricle creates a deep crease or depression on the external surface.[58] Along with an outward bulging of the right ventricular outflow tract, this feature gives the right ventricle an external configuration likened to the "map of Africa."[59]

CLINICAL PROFILE. Most cases appear between the ages of 15 and 50 years, and there is no clear gender predominance. Heart failure and thromboembolism are the dominant cardiovascular manifestations of endomyocardial fibrosis. Other symptom complexes may range from none at all to sudden death. The heart failure may result from the restrictive effects of the endomyocardial disease, from obliteration of the ventricular cavities, from AV valve insufficiency, or from combinations of these (Fig 21-9). Intrinsic myocardial function, when assessed by a variety of different methods, is usually well preserved, and the heart failure is related to the structural and mechanical effects of the endomyocardial fibrosis. The clinical picture may be that of right or left ventricular failure or of biventricular failure, depending on the distribution of lesions. Atrial hypertension and dilatation are common, and with left ventricular involvement, pulmonary venous hypertension and pulmonary edema are usual. With right ventricular involvement, the findings are those of myocardial restriction-constriction, with increased jugular venous pressure and a rapid y descent. In advanced cases, the patient may present with ascites and peripheral edema; tricuspid insufficiency often obscures the restrictive venous wave pattern. Mitral insufficiency may dominate the cardiovascular picture in some cases,[60,61] and pulmonary hypertension may be important in others.[61,62]

DIAGNOSTIC STUDIES. The presence or absence of eosinophilia at the time of diagnosis is quite variable. It is relatively less common in far advanced cases and less common in tropical endomyocardial fibrosis than in the disease found in temperate zones.

The electrocardiogram most commonly shows nonspecific ST-T-wave changes and nondiagnostic changes in QRS morphology. Markers of left or right ventricular hypertrophy and atrial enlargement are relatively common electrocardiographic findings. Rhythm disorders and conduction disturbances that have been reported are atrial fibrillation, sick sinus syndrome, AV node block, and bundle-branch and fascicular blocks.[63]

The cardiac silhouette on the chest radiograph may be either normal or enlarged. Significant pulmonary congestion may be present despite a relatively normal heart size. When cardiomegaly is evident, it may be due to atrial enlargement rather than ventricular dilatation. Infrequently, endomyocardial calcification appears, once again confusing the distinction from pericarditis.

The echocardiogram has shown a variety of nonspecific abnormalities and has been useful for demonstrating early cardiac alterations in cases in which cardiac disease was not otherwise evident.[46] Common findings include increased left ventricular wall thickness and mass and left atrial enlargement. Pericardial effusion is present in one-third of cases; mural thrombus and cavity obliteration may be evident in the more advanced cases. Despite echocardiographic abnormalities in 82% of cases, global left ventricular function, as assessed by echocardiographic estimation of ejection fraction, was normal in all cases.[46]

Findings at cardiac catheterization depend on the distribution of involvement. The pathologic process can exhibit cardiac restriction and mimic the hemodynamic features of pericardial constriction more consistently than it can of any other specific myocardial problem. Increased right atrial pressure with rapid y descent, rapid early diastolic ventricular filling with a dip-plateau diastolic contour in either or both ventricles, and normal left ventricular size and systolic function may all be present. AV valve insufficiency is demonstrable in a high percentage of cases. Angiography typically shows a small, thick-walled ventricular cavity that may be significantly distorted by mural thrombus. The endocardial fibrosis gives the ventricular cavity outline a relatively smooth, featureless appearance.

Percutaneous ventricular endomyocardial biopsy can be very useful in helping to differentiate endomyocardial from pericardial disease and in demonstrating early cardiac involvement in cases of eosinophilia. Right ventricular biopsy studies have demonstrated characteristic histologic abnormalities in patients with hypereosinophilia, even in those without clinically evident cardiac disease.[46,64,65] Early changes include destructive changes in the endothelial cells of the endocardium and capillaries. More advanced cases demonstrate thrombus in various stages of organization, endocardial inflammation or thickening, myocardial cell damage, and myocardial fibrosis.

TREATMENT AND PROGNOSIS. The natural history of eosinophilic endomyocardial fibrosis usually features progressive cardiac dysfunction leading to death from end-stage heart failure. Sudden death has been reported in 9% of cases.[46] Overall survival at 10 years in these relatively young patients approximates 25%.[66] Features of the disease identified with a worsened prognosis are advanced functional class (New York Heart Association III or IV) at time of diagnosis, severe right ventricular involvement, mitral and tricuspid insufficiency, and embolic phenomena.[66,67] When the diagnosis is established early in the course of the illness, the prognosis appears more favorable, and survival to 24 years has been recorded.[65] The disease appears to be rapidly progressive in some patients and more static in others.[46,66,67] Whether this difference is related to a continuing myocardial destructive process in some or to a greater initial insult with more severe subsequent fibrosis is not clear.

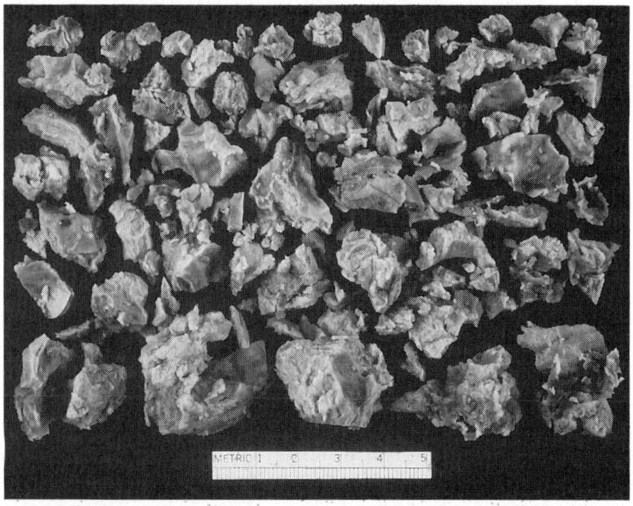

Fig 21-10 Surgically excised thrombus (42 g) from the right ventricle of a patient with eosinophilic endomyocardial disease. (From Wright RS, Simari RD, Orszulak TA, et al: Eosinophilic endomyocardial disease presenting as cyanosis, platypnea, and orthodeoxia. *Ann Intern Med* 117:482-483, 1992. By permission of American College of Physicians.)

Ideally, treatment is directed at both the cause and its consequences. In this disease, the eosinophil appears to be the offending agent, and mural thrombosis, thromboembolism, endocardial fibrosis with ventricular diastolic filling restriction, and AV valve incompetence are the secondary pathologic and functional consequences. Traditionally, use of digitalis preparations and diuretics has been the recommended approach, and these drugs continue to be commonly used. Newer drugs introduced for management of heart failure have also been tried, but there is no clear indication that they alter the natural progression of the disease.

More recently, it has been proposed that when eosinophilia is present, its suppression may be important in the control of progression of the disease. In cases of reactive (secondary) hypereosinophilia, such suppression may result from treatment of the underlying disease process. In hypereosinophilic syndrome, some reports have indicated that treatment with a combination of prednisone and hydroxyurea is effective in reducing the eosinophilia; patients thus treated are reported to have had significantly improved survival and prognosis in comparison with the outcome in untreated cases.[45,46,68,69] Anticoagulation should be strongly considered, especially when mural thrombus is known to be present or embolism has been part of the clinical description.

Experience with surgical treatment of endomyocardial fibrosis is growing.[59,66,70-74] Thrombectomy, endocardial stripping, and mitral or tricuspid valve replacement have all been used alone and in combination (Fig 21-10). Patients selected have generally had far advanced disease, and operative mortality has averaged 20%.[73]

Despite this high early operative mortality, continuing experience indicates that surgery can effect overall improvement in long-term survival and relief of symptoms by reversing otherwise intractable heart failure in these very ill patients. Survival, inclusive of operative mortality, approximates 60% at 5 years.[66,67,73] Significant improvement in functional class can be expected in 70% to 90% of survivors.[66,73] Recurrence of endomyocardial fibrosis after operation has not been observed.[72,74] Increased experience and improvements in surgical technique aimed at preserving the native mitral and tricuspid valves[74] offer a further promise for success in the surgical management of this problem.

Amyloidosis. Amyloidosis is characterized by intercellular accumulation of amyloid material in amounts sufficient to impair the function of the involved organs. Amyloid, in turn, is an amorphous ground substance containing a high concentration of characteristic protein fibrils. Precise knowledge of why or how amyloid is formed and deposited is very limited. There are four different varieties of amyloidosis: primary or myeloma-related amyloidosis, secondary amyloidosis, senile systemic amyloidosis, and familial amyloidosis. The amyloid protein composition is different in each of these varieties, and the degree and nature of the cardiac involvement are also different.

The cardiac involvement in primary amyloidosis is the form of the disease that is most commonly associated with restrictive physiology. Systemic senile amyloidosis may exhibit impaired diastolic filling properties but has other features more typical of a dilated cardiomyopathy.[75]

PATHOLOGY. The protein fibrils of primary amyloidosis are composed of immunoglobulin light chains. The amyloid material is distributed diffusely throughout the myocardium, giving it a firm and rubbery consistency, and typically the heart does not collapse when removed from the chest at autopsy (Fig 21-11).

PHYSIOLOGY. Diastolic filling abnormalities are a hallmark of cardiac amyloidosis, but the exact characteristics of these abnormalities appear to depend on the stage of the disease and severity of amyloid deposition.[5] In early cases with only modest increases in left ventricular wall thickness (greater than 12 mm but less than 15 mm), Doppler flow characteristics are most typical of impaired diastolic relaxation, with a diminished peak early velocity (E), accentuated late velocity (A), and decreased ratio of early to late velocity (E:A). In advanced cases (left ventricular wall thickness greater than 15 mm), the more typical restrictive filling pattern is seen with early peak velocity, diminished late filling, increased E:A ratio, and a short deceleration time. Thus, not all cases of cardiac amyloidosis display a typical restrictive physiology, but the more advanced the case, the more likely it is to do so.[5,76] A corollary of these observations is that restrictive diastolic dynamics strongly predict cardiac death in patients with amyloidosis.[77]

DIAGNOSIS. Differentiating amyloidosis from other forms of restriction or constriction is usually not difficult. Amyloid involvement of other organ systems, associated with typical urinary or serum protein abnormalities, and low QRS voltage despite the appearance of a thickened myocardium support the diagnosis. Myocardial biopsy is a reliable means of establishing the diagnosis if other means fail.[23]

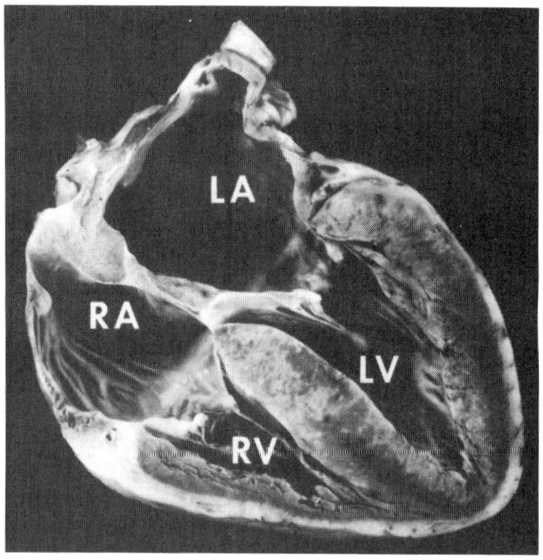

Fig 21-11 Amyloid-infiltrated heart. Amyloid material appears light-colored. There is transmural involvement at the base of the left ventricle *(LV)* and subendocardial involvement throughout; the papillary muscles also are involved. There is also diffuse thickening of the ventricular myocardium, but the ventricular chamber size and configuration have been maintained. The left atrium *(LA)* is dilated. Both the mitral and the tricuspid valves are thickened. *RA,* right atrium; *RV,* right ventricle. (From Edwards WD, Tajik AJ, Seward JB: Standardized nomenclature and anatomic basis for regional tomographic analysis of the heart. *Mayo Clin Proc* 56:479-497, 1981. By permission, Mayo Foundation.)

Hemochromatosis. In hemochromatosis, an iron-storage disease, a general increase in the body stores of iron is great enough to cause tissue damage and organ malfunction. Two forms of hemochromatosis are recognized: a primary (idiopathic) form characterized by a hereditary predisposition to absorb excessive amounts of iron from the gastrointestinal tract, and a secondary form related to chronic exogenous administration of iron, usually in the form of repeated blood transfusions for chronic anemia. Idiopathic hemochromatosis most commonly appears between the ages of 40 and 70 years and is very rare before age 20 years. Males predominate in a ratio of approximately 9:1.[78,79] Transfusion-related hemochromatosis occurs in either sex and in children as well as adults, the primary determinant being the number of transfusions received.[80] Regardless of these differences, the end result from a cardiac standpoint is similar.

PATHOLOGY. Microscopically, the cardiac iron deposition of hemochromatosis is predominantly intracellular and leads to cell destruction and replacement fibrosis. Overall, however, the amount of fibrosis is relatively modest, and the myocardial dysfunction is related to the large amounts of iron in the cells rather than to the number of cells destroyed or replaced by fibrosis.[81] The iron deposits are most heavily concentrated in the subepicardial layers of the ventricles, with significantly less in the subendocardium.[82] Grossly, the hearts usually are characterized by hypertrophy or dilatation (or both).

PHYSIOLOGY. Cardiac symptoms are evident in about 35% of untreated cases of idiopathic hemochromatosis,[78] and heart failure is the predominant presentation. The most typical pattern of heart failure is a dilated cardiomyopathy with significant systolic dysfunction. However, a restrictive pattern can also be seen in individual cases.[79,80,83-86] In one reported series of hemodynamically studied cases, one of eight had a restrictive pattern, four had objective evidence of predominantly systolic dysfunction, and three appeared to have features atypical for either congestive or restrictive cardiomyopathy.[79] Other investigators have estimated that 25% of cases of hemochromatosis will show findings of a restrictive disorder.[84]

DIAGNOSIS. The tetrad of diabetes mellitus, liver disease, increased skin pigmentation, and heart disease should be a clue to the diagnosis of hemochromatosis. Increases in serum iron concentration, percent saturation of total iron binding capacity, and serum ferritin level are strong markers of disease, and liver biopsy is diagnostic in virtually all cases.[78,79] Endomyocardial biopsy has been reported in a limited number of cases and proved to be a useful indicator of therapeutic response in one case.[87] The preferential localization of iron in the subepicardial layers may limit the sensitivity of this technique in some cases.[88]

Specific heart muscle disease infrequently associated with restrictive features

Certain other afflictions of the cardiac muscle are occasionally reported to have a clinical picture of restriction to diastolic filling (see Table 21-2). These will be described only briefly in this context because, for the most part, their presentation in this mode is atypical and infrequent. The list consists of conditions that may cause necrosis and fibrosis of the myocardium or conditions that may lead to thickening of the endocardium. Only a few such conditions are described below, but, in principle, any condition that can cause extensive myocardial fibrosis or endocardial thickening can result in restricted diastolic ventricular filling.

Heart transplantation. Follow-up studies on transplanted hearts have revealed that such hearts may develop restrictive physiology[89,90] that closely mimics constriction. This process is distinct from the changes of acute rejection and has necessitated retransplantation on occasion.[89,90] A hemodynamic survey of 64 heart transplant recipients 1 to 13 years after transplantation revealed that 10 patients (15%) had a "restrictive-constrictive" profile.[90] Donor heart characteristics and length of time since transplantation did not appear to have any causal association. The affected hearts tended to have more fibrosis on histologic examination and a history of more frequent previous episodes of rejection (six or more) than nonaffected hearts. Eight of the 10 patients had symptoms of heart failure.

Postirradiation fibrosis. Mediastinal radiation doses in excess of 40 Gy result in a high incidence of left ventricular dysfunction, and such doses also appear required for late appearance of significant myocardial

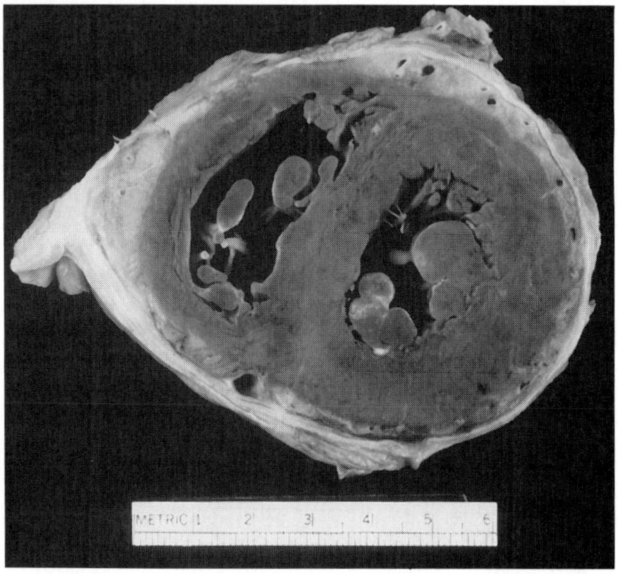

Fig 21-12 Transverse short-axis section through the ventricles of a patient with postradiation changes, including combined pericardial and myocardial fibrosis. (Courtesy of William D. Edwards, M.D.)

fibrosis and restriction. As with pericardial constriction, the myocardial fibrosis and restrictive pattern may first be evident several years after the irradiation. The differential diagnostic distinction between constriction and restriction may be particularly difficult in such patients, and the two commonly coexist[9,13] (Fig 21-12). In such cases, removal of a constricting pericardium does not necessarily eliminate the diastolic restriction. In addition, the surgical mortality both early and late is high.[9]

Carcinoid syndrome. The typical cardiac manifestations of the carcinoid syndrome, described elsewhere, usually feature right-sided valvular lesions most prominently. Endocardial plaque formation is also seen but is usually relatively limited. Valvular surgery may correct these problems and prolong the patient's survival. McGuire et al.[91] reported on one such patient, who, a year after valve surgery, acquired clinical and catheterization findings of a restrictive process presumed to be related to progressive development of more extensive carcinoid endocardial plaque. It is postulated that this complication may be representative of the extended natural history of the disease that may evolve after valve replacement.[91]

Doxorubicin and daunorubicin cardiotoxicity. The cardiotoxic effects of doxorubicin and of its closely related analogue daunorubicin are well known and include myofibril degeneration with myocardial fibrosis. Endocardial fibrosis and mural thrombi have been noted but usually are of minor degree.[92] Two cases with unusually extensive endocardial fibrosis closely resembling that described with hypereosinophilic endomyocardial disease have been recorded.[92,93] One case was associated with daunorubicin administration[93] and the other with doxorubicin.[92] In both, intractable heart failure resulted, and in one, mitral insufficiency developed.

Progressive systemic sclerosis (scleroderma). It is well documented that scleroderma may be accompanied by diffuse myocardial fibrosis with impaired cardiac function.[94] It has been demonstrated in such cases that despite overt signs of "congestive heart failure," ventricular contractile function remains normal.[95] Moreover, Todesco et al.[96] reported that of 13 patients with scleroderma and cardiac involvement in whom hemodynamic studies were done, 3 had a prominent diastolic dip-plateau pattern consistent with diastolic restriction.

Pseudoxanthoma elasticum. Cardiac involvement in pseudoxanthoma elasticum has only rarely been reported and has had little recognized clinical significance. Fibrous thickening of the endocardium has been described[97] and in one case[98] caused restriction to left ventricular filling, resulting in left atrial enlargement and "heart failure" with a normal left ventricular size. A dip-plateau pressure pattern was recorded at catheterization study, and at autopsy the left ventricular endocardium showed extensive thickening with fibrosis and layered elastic fiber proliferation.

Sarcoidosis. Sarcoid granulomas may be found in the heart in 20% to 30% of cases of systemic sarcoidosis; thus, cardiac sarcoidosis is categorized as a myocardial infiltrative disease. As such, it is commonly listed as a cause of myocardial restriction. However, hemodynamic evaluations of hearts affected by sarcoidosis have shown no consistent pattern.[99,100] Right-sided heart pressures and dynamics are dictated mainly by the extent of pulmonary sarcoid involvement, and some degree of pulmonary hypertension is a common finding.[99] Left-sided heart dynamics may be normal or consistent with systolic dysfunction.[99,100] Echocardiographic examination of patients with sarcoidosis showed evidence of cardiac impairment in 12 of 88 patients (13.6%). In each instance, the patient had a dilated cardiomyopathy with systolic contractile abnormalities.[101] A pattern typical of myocardial restriction has not been a characteristic feature of the hemodynamic profile of cardiac sarcoidosis.

REFERENCES

1. Goodwin JF, Gordon H, Hollman A, et al: Clinical aspects of cardiomyopathy. *Br Med J* 1:69-79, 1961
2. Couter WT, Reichert RE Jr: Primary systemic amyloidosis mimicking chronic constrictive pericardial disease. *Circulation* 2:441-444, 1950
3. Hetzel PS, Wood EH, Burchell HB: Pressure pulses in the right side of the heart in a case of amyloid disease and in a case of idiopathic heart failure simulating constrictive pericarditis. *Proc Staff Meet Mayo Clin* 28:107-112, 1953
4. Gunnar RM, Dillon RF, Wallyn RJ, et al: The physiologic and clinical similarity between primary amyloid of the heart and constrictive pericarditis. *Circulation* 12:827-832, 1955
5. Klein AL, Hatle LK, Burstow DJ, et al: Doppler characterization of left ventricular diastolic function in cardiac amyloidosis. *J Am Coll Cardiol* 13:1017-1026, 1989
6. Katritsis D, Wilmshurst PT, Wendon JA, et al: Primary restrictive cardiomyopathy: clinical and pathologic characteristics. *J Am Coll Cardiol* 18:1230-1235, 1991
7. Hirota Y, Shimizu G, Kita Y, et al: Spectrum of restrictive cardiomyopathy: report of the national survey in Japan. *Am Heart J* 120:188-194, 1990
8. Meaney E, Shabetai R, Bhargava V, et al: Cardiac amyloidosis, constrictive pericarditis and restrictive cardiomyopathy. *Am J Cardiol* 38:547-556, 1976
9. Seifert FC, Miller DC, Oesterle SN, et al: Surgical treatment of constrictive pericarditis: analysis of outcome and diagnostic error. *Circulation* 72 Suppl 2:264-273, 1985
10. Plotnick GD: Changes in diastolic function—difficult to measure, harder to interpret (editorial). *Am Heart J* 118:637-641, 1989
11. Nishimura RA, Housmans PR, Hatle LK, et al: Assessment of diastolic function of the heart: background and current applications of Doppler echocardiography. Part I. Physiologic and pathophysiologic features. *Mayo Clin Proc* 64:71-81, 1989
12. Nishimura RA, Abel MD, Hatle LK, et al: Assessment of diastolic function of the heart: background and current applications of Doppler echocardiography. Part II. Clinical studies. *Mayo Clin Proc* 64:181-204, 1989
13. Appleton CP, Hatle LK, Popp RL: Demonstration of restrictive ventricular physiology by Doppler echocardiography. *J Am Coll Cardiol* 11:757-768, 1988
14. DeMaria AN, Wisenbaugh TW, Smith MD, et al: Doppler echocardiographic evaluation of diastolic function. *Circulation* 84 Suppl 1:288-295, 1991
15. Aroney CN, Ruddy TD, Dighero H, et al: Differentiation of restrictive cardiomyopathy from pericardial constriction: assessment of diastolic function by radionuclide angiography. *J Am Coll Cardiol* 13:1007-1014, 1989
16. Gerson MC, Colthar MS, Fowler NO: Differentiation of constrictive pericarditis and restrictive cardiomyopathy by radionuclide ventriculography. *Am Heart J* 118:114-120, 1989
17. Sechtem U, Tscholakoff D, Higgins CB: MRI of the abnormal pericardium. *AJR* 147:245-252, 1986
18. Masui T, Finck S, Higgins CB: Constrictive pericarditis and restrictive cardiomyopathy: evaluation with MR imaging. *Radiology* 182:369-373, 1992
19. Wood P: Chronic constrictive pericarditis. *Am J Cardiol* 7:48-61, 1961
20. Yu PNG, Lovejoy FW Jr, Joos HA, et al: Right auricular and ventricular pressure patterns in constrictive pericarditis. *Circulation* 7:102-107, 1953
21. Benotti JR, Grossman W, Cohn PF: Clinical profile of restrictive cardiomyopathy. *Circulation* 61:1206-1212, 1980
22. Bush CA, Stang JM, Wooley CF, et al: Occult constrictive pericardial disease: diagnosis by rapid volume expansion and correction by pericardiectomy. *Circulation* 56:924-930, 1977
23. Schroeder JS, Billingham ME, Rider AK: Cardiac amyloidosis: diagnosis by transvenous endomyocardial biopsy. *Am J Med* 59:269-273, 1975
24. Mason JW, Billingham ME: Myocardial biopsy. *Prog Cardiol* 9:113-146, 1980
25. Schoenfeld MH, Supple EW, Dec GW Jr, et al: Restrictive cardiomyopathy versus constrictive pericarditis: role of endomyocardial biopsy in avoiding unnecessary thoracotomy. *Circulation* 75:1012-1017, 1987
26. Brandenburg RO, Chazov E, Cherian G, et al: Report of the WHO/ISFC task force on definition and classification of cardiomyopathies. *Circulation* 64:A-437-A-438, 1981
27. Olsen ECJ: Pathologic aspects of endomyocardial fibrosis. *Postgrad Med J* 59:135-139, 1983
28. Boffa GM, Thiene G, Nava A, et al: Cardiomyopathy: a necessary revision of the WHO classification. *Int J Cardiol* 30:1-7, 1991
29. Cortina Llosa A, González Camino F, Prieto Granda JA, et al: Miocardiopatías restrictivas. *Rev Lat Cardiol* 3:139-152, 1982
30. Lewis AB: Clinical profile and outcome of restrictive cardiomyopathy in children. *Am Heart J* 123:1589-1593, 1992
31. Patton JN, Tajik AJ, Reeder GS, et al: Echocardiographic nondilated, nonhypertrophic (restrictive) cardiomyopathy: clinical profile and natural history (abstract). *J Am Coll Cardiol* 1:738, 1983
32. Nye RE Jr, Lovejoy FW Jr, Yu PN: Clinical and hemodynamic studies of myocardial fibrosis. *Circulation* 16:332-338, 1957
33. Robin ED, Burwell CS: Hemodynamic aspects of diffuse myocardial fibrosis. *Circulation* 16:730-735, 1957
34. Arnold P, Brandt C, Reynert R, et al: Myocardiopathies primitives et syndrome hémodynamique d'adiastolie. *Coeur Med Interne* 11:35-52, 1972
35. Hansen AT, Eskildsen P, Götzsche H: Pressure curves from the right auricle and the right ventricle in chronic constrictive pericarditis. *Circulation* 3:881-888, 1951

36. Siegel RJ, Shah PK, Fishbein MC: Idiopathic restrictive cardiomyopathy. *Circulation* 70:165-169, 1984
37. Seward JB, Tajik AJ: Restrictive cardiomyopathy. *Curr Opin Cardiol* 2:499-501, 1987
38. Fitzpatrick AP, Shapiro LM, Rickards AF, et al: Familial restrictive cardiomyopathy with atrioventricular block and skeletal myopathy. *Br Heart J* 63:114-118, 1990
39. Rapezzi C, Ortolani P, Binetti G, et al: Idiopathic restrictive cardiomyopathy in the young: report of two cases. *Int J Cardiol* 29:121-126, 1990
40. Löffler W: Endocarditis parietalis fibroplastica mit Bluteosinophilie: Ein eigenartiges Krankheitsbild. *Schweiz Med Wochenschr* 66: 817-820, 1936
41. Davies JNP: Endocardial fibrosis in Africans. *East Afr Med J* 25:10-14, 1948
42. Gerbaux A, Ben Naceur M, de Brux J, et al: Contribution à l'étude de l'endocardite pariétale fibroplastique avec éosinophilie sanguine (endocardite de Löeffler). *Arch Mal Coeur* 49:689-715, 1956
43. Hardy WR, Anderson RE: The hypereosinophilic syndromes. *Ann Intern Med* 68:1220-1229, 1968
44. Chusid MJ, Dale DC, West BC, et al: The hypereosinophilic syndrome: analysis of fourteen cases with review of the literature. *Medicine (Baltimore)* 54:1-27, 1975
45. Parrillo JE, Borer JS, Henry WL, et al: The cardiovascular manifestations of the hypereosinophilic syndrome: prospective study of 26 patients, with review of the literature. *Am J Med* 67:572-582, 1979
46. Fauci AS, Harley JB, Roberts WC, et al: The idiopathic hypereosinophilic syndrome: clinical, pathophysiologic, and therapeutic considerations. *Ann Intern Med* 97:78-92, 1982
47. Roberts WC, Liegler DG, Carbone PP: Endomyocardial disease and eosinophilia: a clinical and pathologic spectrum. *Am J Med* 46:28-42, 1969
48. Brockington IF, Olsen EGJ: Löffler's endocarditis and Davies' endomyocardial fibrosis. *Am Heart J* 85:308-322, 1973
49. Littler WA: Restrictive cardiomyopathy. In *Diseases of the Heart.* Edited by DG Julian, AJ Camm, KM Fox, et al. London, Baillière Tindall, 1989, pp 925-927
50. Braunwald E: *Heart Disease: A Textbook of Cardiovascular Medicine*. Fourth edition. Philadelphia, WB Saunders Company, 1992, pp 1421-1423
51. Johnson RA, Fifer MA, Palacios IF: Dilated and restrictive cardiomyopathies. In *The Practice of Cardiology: The Medical and Surgical Cardiac Units at the Massachusetts General Hospital.* Vol 2. Second edition. Edited by KA Eagle, E Haber, RW DeSanctis, et al. Boston, Little, Brown and Company, 1989, pp 932-936
52. Spry CJF: The pathogenesis of endomyocardial fibrosis: the role of the eosinophil. *Springer Semin Immunopathol* 11:471-477, 1989
53. Spry CJF, Tai PC: Studies on blood eosinophils. II. Patients with Löffler's cardiomyopathy. *Clin Exp Immunol* 24:423-434, 1976
54. deMello DE, Liapis H, Jureidinri S, et al: Cardiac localization of eosinophil-granule major basic protein in acute necrotizing myocarditis. *N Engl J Med* 323:1542-1545, 1990
55. Tai P-C, Ackerman SJ, Spry CJF, et al: Deposits of eosinophil granule proteins in cardiac tissues of patients with eosinophilic endomyocardial disease. *Lancet* 1:643-647, 1987
56. Andy JJ, Bishara FF, Soyinka OO: Relation of severe eosinophilia and microfilariasis to chronic African endomyocardial fibrosis. *Br Heart J* 45:672-680, 1981
57. Ive FA, Willis AJP, Ikeme AC, et al: Endomyocardial fibrosis and filariasis. *Q J Med* 36:495-516, 1967
58. Davies JNP, Ball JD: The pathology of endomyocardial fibrosis in Uganda. *Br Heart J* 17:337-359, 1955
59. Graham JM, Lawrie GM, Feteih NM, et al: Management of endomyocardial fibrosis: successful surgical treatment of biventricular involvement and consideration of the superiority of operative intervention. *Am Heart J* 102:771-775, 1981
60. Bell JA, Jenkins BS, Webb-Peploe MM: Clinical, haemodynamic, and angiographic findings in Löffler's eosinophilic endocarditis. *Br Heart J* 38:541-548, 1976
61. D'Arbela PG, Mutazindwa T, Patel AK, et al: Survival after first presentation with endomyocardial fibrosis. *Br Heart J* 34:403-407, 1972
62. Solley GO, Maldonado JE, Gleich GJ, et al: Endomyocardiopathy with eosinophilia. *Mayo Clin Proc* 51:697-708, 1976
63. Raizner AE, Silverman ME, Waters WC III: Conduction disturbances and pacemaker failure in Löffler's endomyocarditis. *Am J Med* 53:343-347, 1972
64. Kim CH, Vlietstra RE, Edwards WD, et al: Steroid-responsive eosinophilic myocarditis: diagnosis by endomyocardial biopsy. *Am J Cardiol* 53:1472-1473, 1984
65. Take M, Sekiguchi M, Hiroe M, et al: Clinical spectrum and endomyocardial biopsy findings in eosinophilic heart disease. *Heart Vessels Suppl* 1:243-249, 1985
66. Gupta PN, Valiathan MS, Balakrishnan KG, et al: Clinical course of endomyocardial fibrosis. *Br Heart J* 62:450-454, 1989
67. Pereira Barretto AC, da Luz PL, de Oliveira SA, et al: Determinants of survival in endomyocardial fibrosis. *Circulation* 80 Suppl 1:177-182, 1989
68. Parrillo JE, Fauci AS, Wolff SM: Therapy of the hypereosinophilic syndrome. *Ann Intern Med* 89:167-172, 1978
69. Parrillo JE: Heart disease and the eosinophil (editorial). *N Engl J Med* 323:1560-1561, 1990
70. Dubost Ch, Maurice P, Gerbaux A, et al: The surgical treatment of constrictive fibrous endocarditis. *Ann Surg* 184:303-307, 1976
71. Davies J, Sapsford R, Brooksby I, et al: Successful surgical treatment of two patients with eosinophilic endomyocardial disease. *Br Heart J* 46:438-445, 1981
72. Metras D, Coulibaly AO, Ouattara K: The surgical treatment of endomyocardial fibrosis: results in 55 patients. *Circulation* 72 Suppl 2:274-279, 1985
73. da Costa FDA, Moraes CR, Rodriques JV, et al: Early surgical results in the treatment of endomyocardial fibrosis: a Brazilian cooperative study. *Eur J Cardiothorac Surg* 3:408-413, 1989
74. Oliveira SA, Pereira Barreto AC, Mady C, et al: Surgical treatment of endomyocardial fibrosis: a new approach. *J Am Coll Cardiol* 16:1246-1251, 1990
75. Olson LJ, Gertz MA, Edwards WD, et al: Senile cardiac amyloidosis with myocardial dysfunction: diagnosis by endomyocardial biopsy and immunohistochemistry. *N Engl J Med* 317:738-742, 1987
76. Klein AL, Hatle LK, Burstow DJ, et al: Comprehensive Doppler assessment of right ventricular diastolic function in cardiac amyloidosis. *J Am Coll Cardiol* 15:99-108, 1990
77. Klein AL, Hatle LK, Taliercio CP, et al: Prognostic significance of Doppler measures of diastolic function in cardiac amyloidosis: a Doppler echocardiography study. *Circulation* 83:808-816, 1991
78. Finch SC, Finch CA: Idiopathic hemochromatosis, an iron storage disease. *Medicine* 34:381-430, 1955
79. Mattheyses M, Hespel JP, Brissot P, et al: La myocardiopathie de l'hémochromatose idiopathique. *Arch Mal Coeur* 71:371-379, 1978
80. Faivre G, Gilgenkrantz JM, Cherrier F, et al: Hémochromatose et adiastolie: a propos d'une observation anatomo-clinique. *Arch Mal Coeur* 54:935-945, 1961
81. Arnett EN, Nienhuis AW, Henry WL, et al: Massive myocardial hemosiderosis: a structure-function conference at the National Heart and Lung Institute. *Am Heart J* 90:777-787, 1975
82. Buja LM, Roberts WC: Iron in the heart: etiology and clinical significance. *Am J Med* 51:209-221, 1971
83. Wasserman AJ, Richardson DW, Baird CL, et al: Cardiac hemochromatosis simulating constrictive pericarditis. *Am J Med* 32:316-323, 1962
84. Mathivat A, Catusse Ph, Normand JP, et al: Insuffisance cardiaque de type restrictif au cours de l'hémochromatose primitive. *Arch Mal Coeur* 67:911-923, 1974
85. Nody AC, Bruno MS, DePasquale NP, et al: Fulminating idiopathic hemochromatosis presenting as constrictive pericarditis (letter to the editor). *Ann Intern Med* 83:373-374, 1975
86. Cutler DJ, Isner JM, Bracey AW, et al: Hemochromatosis heart disease: an unemphasized cause of potentially reversible restrictive cardiomyopathy. *Am J Med* 69:923-928, 1980
87. Short EM, Winkle RA, Billingham ME: Myocardial involvement in idiopathic hemochromatosis: morphologic and clinical improvement following venesection. *Am J Med* 70:1275-1279, 1981
88. Fitchett DH, Coltart DJ, Littler WA, et al: Cardiac involvement in secondary haemochromatosis: a catheter biopsy study and analysis of myocardium. *Cardiovasc Res* 14:719-724, 1980
89. Valantine HA, Appleton CP, Hatle LK, et al: A hemodynamic and Doppler echocardiographic study of ventricular function in long-term cardiac allograft recipients: etiology and prognosis of restrictive-constrictive physiology. *Circulation* 79:66-75, 1989

90. Young JB, Leon CA, Short HD III, et al: Evolution of hemodynamics after orthotopic heart and heart-lung transplantation: early restrictive patterns persisting in occult fashion. *J Heart Transplant* 6:34-43, 1987

91. McGuire MR, Pugh DM, Dunn MI: Carcinoid heart disease: restrictive cadiomyopathy as a late complication. *J Kans Med Soc* 79:661-662; 665, 1978

92. Fitter W, deSa DJ, Pai KRM: Adriamycin cardiotoxicity: report of an unusual case with features resembling endomyocardial fibrosis. *J Clin Pathol* 34:602-605, 1981

93. Wilcox RG, James PD, Toghill PJ: Endomyocardial fibrosis associated with daunorubicin therapy. *Br Heart J* 38:860-863, 1976

94. Bulkley BH, Ridolfi RL, Salyer WR, et al: Myocardial lesions of progressive systemic sclerosis: a cause of cardiac dysfunction. *Circulation* 53:483-490, 1976

95. Siegel RJ, O'Connor B, Mena I, et al: Left ventricular function in scleroderma (abstract). *Circulation* 62 Suppl III:319, 1980

96. Todesco S, Gatta A, Glorioso S, et al: Cardiac involvement in progressive systemic sclerosis. *Acta Cardiol (Brux)* 34:311-322, 1979

97. Huang S, Kumar G, Steele HD, et al: Cardiac involvement in pseudoxanthoma elasticum: report of a case. *Am Heart J* 74:680-686, 1967

98. Navarro-Lopez F, Llorian A, Ferrer-Roca O, et al: Restrictive cardiomyopathy in pseudoxanthoma elasticum. *Chest* 78:113-115, 1980

99. Baughman RP, Gerson M, Bosken CH: Right and left ventricular function at rest and with exercise in patients with sarcoidosis. *Chest* 85:301-306, 1984

100. Thunell M, Bjerle P, Olofsson B-O, et al: Cardiopulmonary function in sarcoidosis. *Acta Med Scand* 215:215-220, 1984

101. Klein AL, Oh JK, Miller FA, et al: Two-dimensional and Doppler echocardiographic assessment of infiltrative cardiomyopathy. *J Am Soc Echocardiogr* 1:48-59, 1988

PART V *Arrhythmias and Conduction Abnormalities*

CHAPTER

22

Cardiac arrhythmias

A. Anatomic and pathophysiologic concepts

Win-Kuang Shen, M.D., David R. Holmes, Jr., M.D., and Douglas L. Packer, M.D.

SINUS NODE
Normal anatomy

The sinus node is a tapering cylindrical structure, approximately 15 by 3 by 2 mm, lying subepicardially in the sulcus terminalis on the anterolateral margin of the right atrium at its junction with the superior vena cava.[1-3] It develops as a unilateral structure from the right horn of the sinus venosus and can be identified early in life, at approximately 35 days of gestational age.[4,5] Rhythmic discharge has been detected early in fetal life in the sinoatrial portion of developing hearts even before the onset of visible contractions.[6]

The sinus node itself surrounds a central artery, which arises from the right coronary artery in 55% to 65% and from the left circumflex coronary artery in 35% to 45% of patients.[3,7,8] This artery may approach the sinus node from the posterior aspect of the superior vena cava, circling counterclockwise (viewed from the superior aspect of the heart), or from the anterior aspect of the superior vena cava, circling clockwise (Fig 22A-1). Occasionally, sinus node arteries approach from both directions and anastomose within the node itself.[1,9] The anatomic relationship between the sinoatrial node artery and the surrounding pacemaker tissue is rather intriguing and has stimulated many studies. A coupling mechanism has been postulated between changes in caliber of the sinus node artery and sinus node impulse formation.[10-12] The role this may play in the regulation of impulse formation in the intact heart remains unknown.[1]

Histologically, two major specialized types of cells are seen within the area of the sinoatrial node, both embedded in a connective tissue stroma of collagen. The round or ovoid P cell may be the site of impulse formation.[13-15] The myofibrils in these cells are short and sparse. The mitochondria, which are also sparse and small, have fewer cristae. The sarcoplasmic reticulum is scant, and there is no transverse tubular system. All these features are consistent with the idea that the contractile function of the P cell is small. The cells themselves are arranged in groups mainly in the central portions of the sinus node, where they form multiple junctions with one another and with transitional cells.[2,16] Although many nodal cells exist within the sinoatrial node, probably

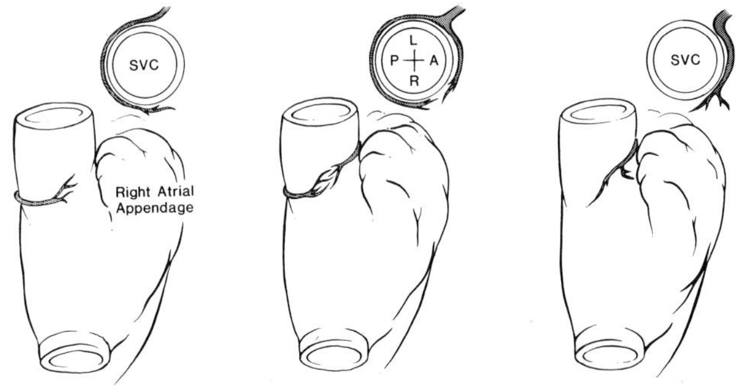

Fig 22A-1 Diagram of arterial supply to sinus node. The sinus node artery may approach the sinus node from the posterior aspect of the superior vena cava *(SVC) (left diagram)* or from the anterior aspect of the superior vena cava *(right diagram)*. Occasionally, there may be two sinus node arteries, which may anastomose within the node *(middle diagram)*. *L,* left; *R,* right; *P,* posterior; *A,* anterior. (Modified from Anderson RH, Becker AE: Gross anatomy and microscopy of the conducting system. In *Cardiac Arrhythmias: Their Mechanisms, Diagnosis, and Management.* Edited by WJ Mandel. Philadelphia, JB Lippincott Company, 1980, pp 12-54.)

only a few thousand serve as the primary pacemaker, the actual number of cells depending on specific membrane properties and distribution of intracellular connections. The functional implications of the sparsity of intracellular connections are currently under investigation. Using a two-dimensional model of electrically coupled cells, Michaels et al.[17] generated activation maps that demonstrated apparent wave front propagation from a leading pacemaker region to the rest of the matrix. Appropriate selection of pacemaker cycle lengths and intercellular resistances permitted accurate simulation of the activation sequence observed experimentally. With the aid of such a system, one can better understand the role of intercellular resistance in impulse propagation.

The second specialized cell type, the transitional cell, is seen in considerably larger numbers. These cells, which are the link between P cells and the rest of the heart, presumably facilitate impulse transmission from the P cells. Histologically, they form intercalated disks between P cells and the atrial myocardium.[2,15,16] In addition to these two major specialized cell types, myocytes are present along with a stroma of connective tissue fibers, predominantly collagen but also elastin.

The autonomic nervous system has a profound effect on impulse formation and propagation within the heart.[18-20] The detailed anatomic innervation varies substantially among species, and in many instances, distributions have not been correlated with the functional indices. In general, the sympathetic and vagal nerves on the right side influence the sinoatrial node more than the atrioventricular (AV) node and vice versa for the nerves on the left side. Numerous nerve endings have been documented within the sinus node, although ganglia have been found only along the margins.[21] At rest, parasympathetic tone, which is mediated by acetylcholine, is dominant. Sympathetic tone is mediated by norepinephrine. Changes in the balance between parasympathetic and sympathetic tone may result in actual shifts in the pacemaker site within the sinoatrial node.[22,23]

Pathologic anatomy

Many disease processes affect the sinus node by virtue of its subepicardial location, its central dominant artery, and its connective tissue stroma.[24] Its subepicardial location makes it susceptible to damage at the time of open heart operation, as can be seen in Figure 22A-2, which shows a suture that had inadvertently been placed around the sinus node artery. This has been a particularly important problem in patients undergoing corrective operations for transposition of the great vessels.[25-29] In these patients, postoperative arrhythmias due to trauma to the sinus node itself or to the atrial conduction pathways have been a significant clinical problem. Pericarditis can also affect the node by virtue of its location.[30] In addition, any inflammatory process involving the myocardium itself may also involve the sinus node; Figure 22A-3 shows intense inflammation of the sinus node in a child with myocarditis. Such inflammatory involvement may be asymptomatic or may result in a wide variety of supraventricular arrhythmias.

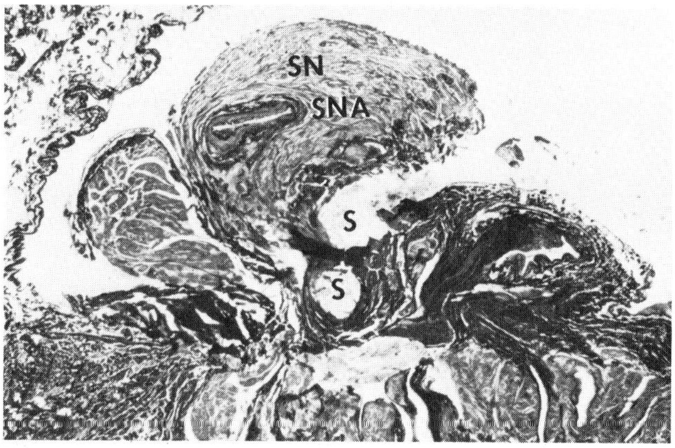

Fig 22A-2 Autopsy section from a 4-month-old infant who died after a Mustard procedure for transposition of the great arteries. There is acute necrosis of the sinus node *(SN)* and compression of the sinus node artery *(SNA)* as a result of snaring of the node by sutures *(S)*. Elastic-van Gieson; ×25. (From Edwards WD, Edwards JE: Pathology of the sinus node in d-transposition following the Mustard operation. *J Thorac Cardiovasc Surg* 75:213-218, 1978. By permission of Mosby-Year Book.)

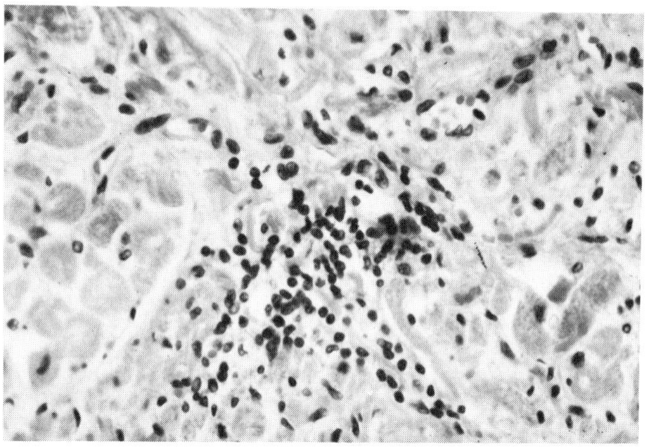

Fig 22A-3 Section taken near the sinus node of 16-year-old child who died of Coxsackie B_4 viral myocarditis, documenting intense round cell infiltrate. Hematoxylin-eosin; ×250. (Courtesy of Dr. W.D. Edwards.)

The connective tissue stroma may also be involved, as has been documented in patients with scleroderma and systemic lupus erythematosus.[31-35] During life, the total number of sinoatrial node cells and the fibrous stroma of the sinus node change. An increase in fibrous tissue occurs with aging[13,36] (Fig 22A-4). The general belief has been that the increase in quantity of the fibrous tissue is at the expense of sinoatrial node cells.[36-39] These changes may affect sinus node impulse formation and propagation and may be the anatomic substrate for sinus node dysfunction or the sick sinus syndrome.[38-42]

In a recent study, Shiraishi et al.[43] observed that the

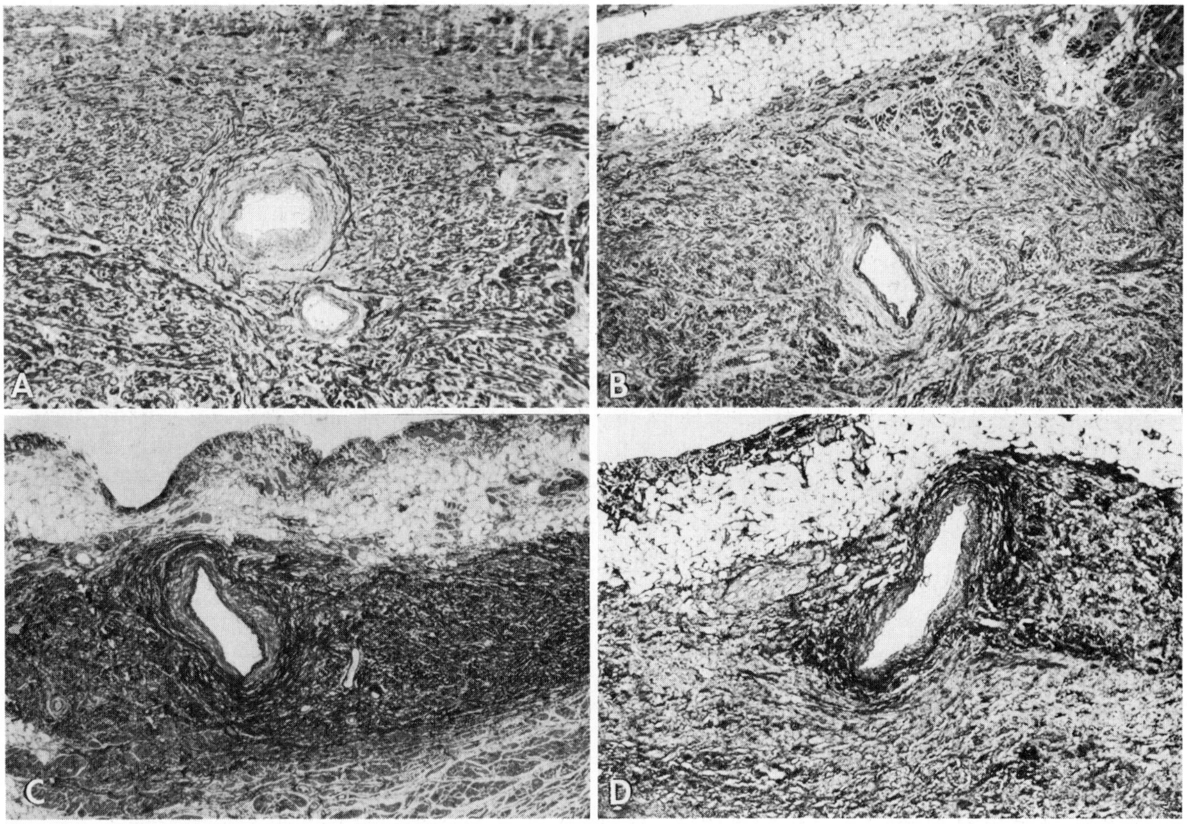

Fig 22A-4 **A,** normal sinus node in a 2-year-old girl. Gomori's trichrome; ×60. **B,** sinus node in a 20-year-old man showing increased fibrous tissue. Gomori's trichrome; ×25. **C,** sinus node in an 85-year-old man, showing significantly increased fibrous tissue in comparison with **A** and **B.** Elastic-van Gieson; ×25. **D,** excessive fibrosis in a 71-year-old man who had undergone previous mediastinal radiation therapy. Gomori's trichrome; ×25. (Courtesy of Dr. W.D. Edwards.)

actual volume of sinoatrial node cells increased during adolescence and young adulthood, although the volume percentage to the total sinoatrial node decreased because of the larger volume increase of the fibrous connective tissue. During aging, the volume of fibrous connective tissue remained unchanged, but the total volume and the volume percentage of the sinoatrial node cells significantly decreased.

Because of the central vascular supply of the sinoatrial node, arteriolar diseases may cause significant abnormalities of sinus node function.[31] Patients with vasculitis such as polyarteritis nodosa or systemic lupus erythematosus may have significant arrhythmias related to sinus node involvement.[44-46] Thrombotic occlusion has also been reported in patients with hematologic disorders, including thrombocytopenic thrombotic purpura.[47,48] Finally, atherosclerosis may result in ischemic injury or damage. Supraventricular arrhythmias, ranging from bradyarrhythmias such as sinus bradycardia to tachyarrhythmias including atrial flutter-fibrillation, are common in patients with acute myocardial infarction, occurring in up to 40% of such patients.[49-54] Some of these arrhythmias may be due to occlusion of the coronary artery that supplies the sinoatrial node. Some investigators have even maintained that the sick sinus syndrome is related in part to the consequences of chronic sick node ischemia.[55-57] This relationship requires continued evaluation, because sinus node dysfunction may occur in patients with normal sinoatrial node arteries.

DISTRIBUTION OF SINUS NODE IMPULSE AND ATRIAL CONDUCTION TISSUE

There has been continued controversy about the presence and function of specialized atrial tracts or bundles.[1,2,58-61] This controversy continues today and is in part dependent on the distinction between specialized anatomic pathways and specialized functional conduction pathways.

Normal anatomy

Several authors have described evidence for the preferential spread of atrial activation along three internodal pathways[59,60,62,63] (Fig 22A-5). These pathways allow sinus impulses to arrive with precise timing at the AV node and so facilitate optimal AV synchrony. The anterior

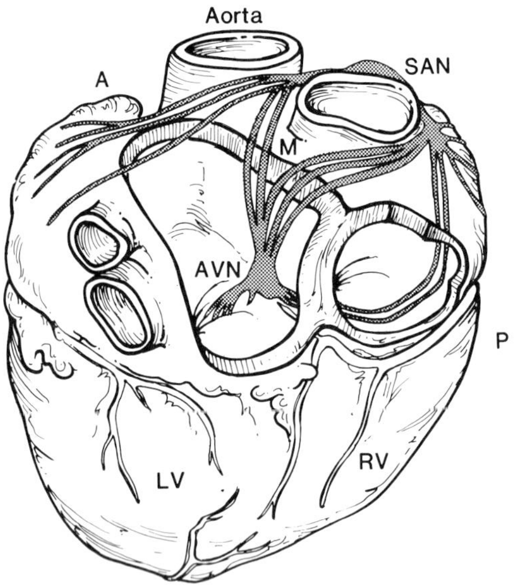

Fig 22A-5 Posterior schematic of the heart with internodal pathways connecting the sinus node *(SAN)* and atrioventricular node *(AVN)*. The anterior internodal tract *(A)* curves leftward and anteriorly around the superior vena cava. The middle internodal tract *(M)* crosses toward the interatrial system to join the anterior internodal tract. The posterior pathway *(P)* exits posteriorly and courses toward the inferior vena cava. *LV,* left ventricle; *RV,* right ventricle. See text for discussion.

internodal pathway curves leftward and anteriorly around the superior vena cava after leaving the sinoatrial node. It divides into two portions, one of which continues as Bachmann's bundle toward the left atrium, while the other descends in the interatrial septum to the crest of the AV node. The second pathway (middle internodal pathway, or Wenckebach's bundle) arises from the posterior aspect of the sinoatrial node and courses toward the interatrial septum, where it joins the anterior internodal pathway. The posterior internodal pathway exits posteriorly from the sinus node and runs within the crista terminalis toward the inferior vena cava. The terminal portion of this pathway passes over the coronary sinus ostium and enters the posterior margin of the AV node.

Morphologically, the concept of distinct atrial pathways remains unsettled. The internodal pathways are not anatomically separated from atrial myocardium by collagen sheaths.

Pathologic anatomy

Disease processes that affect the atrium may also affect the conduction of impulses from the sinus to the AV node. There is considerable redundancy in the intra-atrial and interatrial conduction systems, so that isolated focal lesions may have only minor effects on conduction. Widespread fibrosis has been identified in patients with unstable sinus rhythm and atrial arrhythmias, including atrial fibrillation.[16,64,65] Prolonged and fractionated right atrial electrograms during sinus rhythm in patients with paroxysmal atrial fibrillation and sick sinus syndrome have been reported and may reflect the anatomic abnormalities.[66]

In patients with atrial dilatation and abnormalities of the atrial septum, intra-atrial impulse transmission is often delayed.[67] In these patients, slowed conduction and dispersion of refractoriness may provide the substrate for the supraventricular arrhythmias that are seen in patients with atrial septal defect, mitral valvular disease, Ebstein's malformation, or AV canal defect.[68-72]

ATRIOVENTRICULAR NODE

Normal anatomy

The AV node is a small elliptical structure that lies in the subendocardium at the apex of Koch's triangle, which is formed by the ostium of the coronary sinus, the tendon of Todaro, and the septal attachment of the tricuspid valve. The AV node varies in size but is usually smaller than the sinoatrial node. In general, it is approximately 5 to 6 mm long, 2 to 3 mm wide, and 0.5 to 1 mm thick. Anderson and Becker[1] pointed out the discrepancies that have existed among the electrophysiologic, clinical, and morphologic definitions of the AV node. Some investigators have preferred the term "AV junctional area" to describe the part of the conduction system that extends from the base of the atrial septum through the central fibrous body to the ventricles.[73] Four different zones have been identified anatomically: (1) the transitional zone that intervenes between atrial myocardium and the discrete cells of the compact node; (2) the compact AV node (node of Tawara); (3) the penetrating AV bundle; and (4) the branching AV bundle.[73] Other authors, however, do not include the branching AV bundle in the AV node region.[74]

Embryologically, the AV junctional area develops from several sources, which include the sinoatrial ring, septum primum, AV ring, and primitive atrium.[75] In contrast to the sinoatrial node, the AV junctional area has a dual blood supply in most individuals.[8,73] The AV node artery arises at the crux of the heart and ascends to enter the AV junctional area. It is a branch of the right coronary artery in approximately 90% of patients, and it arises from the circumflex coronary artery in the remaining 10%.[8,73,76-78] The second major arterial supply is from the left anterior descending coronary artery via septal perforators (Fig 22A-6). There is significant variability in the blood supply to remaining regions of the AV junction and bundle branches. Occlusion of the arterial supply to a portion of the conduction system may have variable effects on the generation and conduction of the cardiac impulse. These effects depend on the location of the occlusion and the presence of alternative vascular sources via either a dual blood supply or collateral vessels. (See chapter 30 on myocardial infarction.)

Histologically, several cell types are seen within the AV junctional area, including atrial myocytes, slender transitional cells (which predominate), Purkinje's cells, P cells similar to those found in the sinoatrial node, and a connective tissue stroma.[73,79-83] At the level of the penetrating AV bundle, there is an actual connective tissue sheath formed in part by the fibrous tissue of the

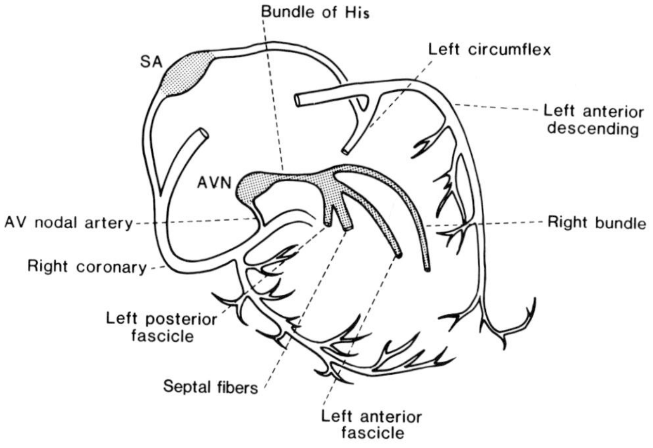

Fig 22A-6 Schematic of the vascular supply to the cardiac conduction system. The sinus node artery may arise from the right coronary artery (55% to 65%) or as a branch of the left circumflex (35% to 45%). The atrioventricular node *(AVN)* artery arises from the right coronary artery in 90% of patients. The right coronary artery also supplies the common His bundle and portions of the right bundle. The left anterior descending coronary artery also supplies blood to the His bundle via septal perforators and the "left anterior fascicle." The left posterior fascicle usually receives a blood supply from both the right coronary artery (posterior descending) and the left anterior descending artery. *SA,* sinoatrial node.

central body. The geometry of the fibers varies throughout the AV junction, from a transition zone at which the atrial myocardial cells form an interface with the compact node, to a longitudinally parallel orientation within the penetrating bundle, to a lattice-like network in the bundles.

Evidence for the rich autonomic innervation of the AV node has been documented by both functional and anatomic studies and also by studies in patients with cardiac homotransplantation.[21,80,84-89] In general, the sympathetic and vagal nerves on the left side predominantly influence the AV node. Stimulation of the left stellate ganglion consistently shortens the AV nodal conduction time and refractoriness, whereas stimulation of the left vagal nerve primarily slows AV nodal conduction and increases refractoriness. Experimentally, vagal stimulation may result in prolongation of AV node conduction with the development of first-degree and Mobitz type I and type II second-degree AV block.[90] Increased vagal tone in human subjects can be documented in the electrophysiology laboratory by the presence of abnormal AV node conduction and refractoriness, which can be reversed by atropine; such persons may be highly trained athletes, they may have asymptomatic bradycardia, or they may present with syncope or near syncope.[91-93]

Pathologic anatomy

As has previously been discussed for the sinoatrial node, vascular, infiltrative, inflammatory, and degenerative diseases all may affect the AV junctional area. The role of ischemia due to vascular occlusion in the genesis of conduction defects occurring during the course of acute myocardial infarction is well known and is discussed later in detail[94-102] (see chapter 30). Because of its size and location, the AV node artery may also be involved in patients who have polyarteritis nodosa.[46]

Disease processes also affect the connective tissue stroma, as is seen in patients with progressive systemic sclerosis in whom conduction disturbances are common.[33-35] In addition, in approximately 40% of patients with sick sinus syndrome, abnormalities of AV node function can also be documented electrophysiologically and are presumably due to increased fibrosis within the AV junctional area itself. In patients with a history of clinical AV conduction disturbances, histopathologic studies have revealed that the fibrotic lesions are usually diffuse. Consequently, clinical correlation of the location of the conduction disturbance (AV node or bundle of His) with histopathologic findings has been poor.

The AV junctional area enlarges during growth and development. Pediatric patients have more rapid AV node conduction and abbreviated AV node refractoriness. This may be related in part to the physical properties such as the size and shape of the AV junctional area. Retention of a "juvenile, small AV node" has been postulated as one mechanism for the rapid AV nodal conduction that can be seen in patients with accelerated or enhanced AV nodal conduction.[103-105]

Congenital complete heart block is of particular importance as it relates to the AV junctional area and may be seen in patients with or without associated congenital heart disease. In patients without associated congenital heart disease, two major types can be distinguished. In one there is discontinuity between atrial tissue and a hypoplastic nodal bundle axis, whereas in the second the AV node may be normal but there is discontinuity between the node and the ventricular conduction tissue.[106,107] Congenital complete heart block is also seen in association with structural congenital heart disease, perhaps most often with anomalies of great vessel development—for example, corrected transposition of the great arteries. It is also seen in a variety of other congenital heart disease patients, including those with univentricular heart and AV canal. In patients with corrected transposition of the great arteries, there is typically an anterior accessory AV node.[108-110] A penetrating bundle arises from this and follows a course along the superior aspect of the interventricular septum. This penetrating bundle may not connect with distal conduction tissue or may be damaged by fibrosis and hemorrhage, leading to the AV block.

SPECIALIZED VENTRICULAR CONDUCTION SYSTEM

Normal anatomy

In the normal heart the transmission of impulses arising in the sinoatrial node to the ventricle occurs exclusively via the AV node. As previously mentioned, the fibrous connective tissue sheath at the level of the penetrating bundle prevents the lateral spread of the wave front to

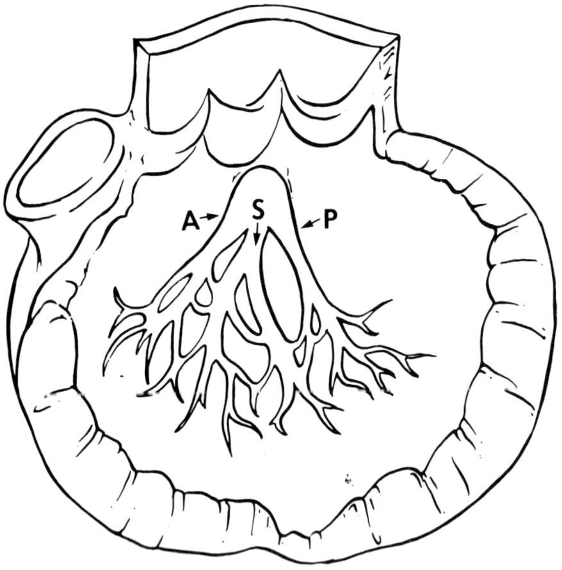

Fig 22A-7 Schematic of the left bundle branch viewed from the opened left ventricle, illustrating major divisions—anterior *(A)*, septal *(S)*, and posterior *(P)*—with numerous interconnections.

ventricular muscle and dictates antegrade impulse transmission only via the specialized ventricular conduction system, including the bundle branches and their peripheral ramifications and the Purkinje fiber/ventricular muscle junction.

The concepts of intraventricular conduction disturbances or, specifically, hemiblocks as popularized by Rosenbaum have facilitated the clinical management of conduction system disease.[111,112] As initially conceptualized, infra-His conduction defects could be categorized electrocardiographically as right bundle-branch block, left anterior hemiblock (or left anterior-superior fascicular block), and left posterior hemiblock (or left posterior-inferior fascicular block). The term "bifascicular block" was applied when there was electrocardiographic (ECG) evidence of block in two of the three fascicles. Although these concepts remain helpful clinically, from anatomic studies the bundle branches are considerably more complex.[1,113-118] Detailed studies in animals with the use of glycogen-staining techniques and serial sections in humans indicate that the left bundle branch has two or three major divisions (Fig 22A-7) and multiple peripheral anastomoses. Primarily, the left bundle branch divides into anterior and posterior fascicles. The posterior fascicle spreads as a broad band of fibers over the posterior and inferior endocardial surface of the left ventricle, and the anterior fascicle spreads out anteriorly and superiorly. In 33 of 49 human hearts (67%) studied by Demoulin and Kulbertus,[119] a third branch could easily be identified. This structure travels to the midseptal surface and emerges from either of the two fascicles on the left or directly from the bundle of His itself. The normal sequence of activation of the left ventricle via the left bundle has been identified.[120-127]

In contrast to the left bundle branch, the right bundle branch has aroused less controversy, mainly because it is structurally and functionally more isolated than the left bundle and its origin and distribution.[24,73,74,113] Activation of the right ventricle occurs initially at the right ventricular apex and spreads from there via peripheral branches to cover the interventricular septum and the right ventricular free wall.[128] There is a delay in the activation of the basal portion near the tricuspid valve ring. This delay is believed by some to be related to slow conduction through ventricular muscle because of the absence of specialized conduction fibers in that area.[127]

Histologically, the Purkinje cells in the bundle branches and peripheral branches are large (15 to 30 μm in diameter and 20 to 100 μm in length) and distinct from contracting ventricular myocardial cells. Compared with contracting ventricular muscle cells, there are no transverse tubules, the mitochondria are more loosely distributed, and there are fewer myofibrils. Well-developed intercalated disks are present, which facilitate diffusion of ions and transmission of impulses.[129,130]

Pathologic anatomy

Disease processes that involve the bundle-branch system may give rise to readily recognizable ECG abnormalities. After the widespread clinical acceptance of the hemiblock concept, attempts were made to find an exact pathologic basis to account for the characteristic ECG abnormalities. In addition, experimental models of selective destruction of portions of the bundle-branch system have been applied to the problem.[120,127,131] Some of these studies have yielded discordant results. Suffice it to say that with increasing age, fibrosis develops in the left-sided conduction system, and in patients with ECG conduction defects there are often widespread lesions throughout the left-sided conduction system.[24,118,132] In patients with right-sided conduction system disease, the pathology varies from central fibrosis to peripheral bundle-branch block seen in patients after right ventriculotomy. In patients with complete heart block, there is often extensive destruction of the His-Purkinje system.[24,133-135]

PREEXCITATION

Normal transmission of impulses from the atrium to the ventricle occurs only via the AV junction. In some patients alternative routes of transmission are available (Fig 22A-8). In these patients preexcitation exists—that is, ventricular muscle is activated by an atrial impulse earlier than expected in comparison with normal AV junctional transmission. In addition, in some of these patients, accessory pathways are present that can conduct only in a retrograde fashion (concealed bypass tracts). The importance of these alternative pathways lies in the clinical problems with which these patients present, including abnormal ECGs, reentrant tachycardia, atrial fibrillation, and the potential for sudden cardiac death.[136-154] Knowledge of the pathologic anatomy in these patients is important in understanding clinical problems and particularly important when catheter or surgical procedures, such

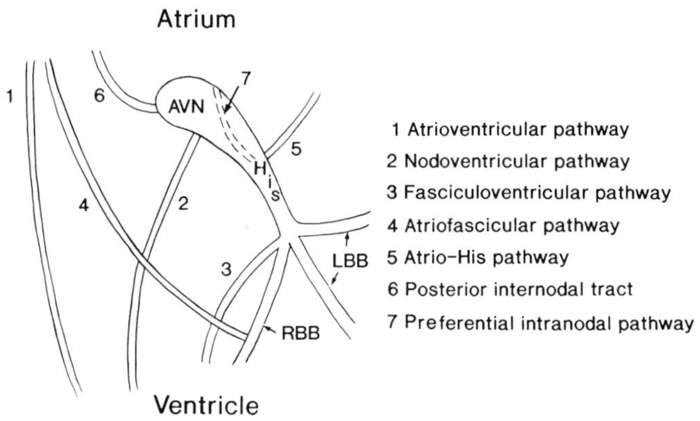

Fig 22A-8 Schematic of the anatomic substrates of preexcitation (see text for description). *AVN,* atrioventricular node; *LBB,* left bundle branch; *RBB,* right bundle branch. (Modified from Josephson ME, Seides SF: Preexcitation syndromes. In *Clinical Cardiac Electrophysiology: Techniques and Interpretations.* Philadelphia, Lea & Febiger, 1979, p 212. By permission.)

as ablation of the pathway, are contemplated.[1,155-169]

Multiple classifications of the anatomic substrate exist, some of which acknowledge and use the eponymous terms "Kent bundles," "James fibers," "Mahaim fibers," and "Brechenmacher fibers."[63,144,161,170-172] Part of the problem and confusion can be attributed to the fact that the anatomic substrates are multiple and varied and also that knowledge about the embryologic and anatomic substrates has lagged behind electrophysiologic description.[1,161,173] This lag is in turn related to the difficulties in pathologic study of the conduction system. The report by Lev et al.[174] in 1975 on a unique variety of ventricular preexcitation illustrates some of these difficulties; for analysis of the conduction system and AV rims in their study, 18,600 sections were taken.

A sound classification is important to our understanding and approach to patients with preexcitation, however. The European Study Group for Preexcitation recommended an anatomic classification for accessory pathways.[156] This classification suggested that "tract" be used to describe accessory pathways that insert into specialized conduction tissue and that "connection" be used when pathways terminate into contractile myocardium. A suggested division of the accessory pathways was as follows: (1) AV bypass connections, (2) nodoventricular connections, (3) fasciculoventricular connections, and (4) AV node bypass (atriofascicular) tracts. Subsequently, internodal bypass tracts were added to the classification.

Atrioventricular bypass connections

Atrioventricular bypass connections are the commonest cause of ventricular preexcitation (Wolff-Parkinson-White syndrome). The development and use of intraoperative mapping and ablation of accessory AV connections in patients with reentrant paroxysmal supraventricular tachycardia or atrial fibrillation and rapid antegrade bypass conduction has added a great deal to our knowledge of the anatomy of accessory AV conductions.[1,136,137,157-161,175,176] These pathways, previously referred to as Kent bundles, have been described both at autopsy and intraoperatively. On the left side they pass close to the epicardial aspect of the well-formed annulus fibrosis. This contrasts to right-sided pathways, which traverse the adipose tissue in the AV sulcus, sometimes at some distance from the less well formed annulus.

Nodofascicular/nodoventricular, fasciculoventricular, and atriofascicular pathways

Autopsy studies have documented the presence of conduction tissue in some hearts which links the compact node or the penetrating bundle with ventricular muscle.[1,156,174,177,178] This has been demonstrated postmortem in normal hearts and also in cases in which there had been symptomatic tachycardia. Nodofascicular or nodoventricular fibers, known as Mahaim fibers, may also function as the substrate for tachycardia by serving either as a component of a macroreentrant loop or as a bystander pathway during AV nodal reentrant tachycardia.[179] Studies have also demonstrated that some of these connections previously thought to originate in the AV node may, in fact, be atriofascicular bypass tracts with decremental properties.[180] Fasciculoventricular fibers originating in the bundle-branch system and inserting in myocardium have not been convincingly shown to be a critical component for the maintenance of any tachycardia.

Atrioventricular node bypass tracts

Several anatomic substrates have been postulated in patients with AV node bypass tracts.[63,103-105,156,171,181] These patients may present with abnormal ECGs (short P-R intervals but normal QRS complexes). Participation of AV node bypass tracts in supraventricular arrhythmias has not been clearly demonstrated. The presence of anatomic structures that could serve as bypass tracts remains controversial, but potentially they include atrial nodal or atrial His fibers, atrial His bundle tracts described by Brechenmacher, and posterior internodal tracts. Other possible mechanisms of rapid AV conduction as seen in these patients include the so-called juvenile AV node or preferential pathways of conduction within the AV node.

In addition to these classic anatomic explanations, the short P-R interval could be explained by rapid conduction properties, either intrinsic or resulting from alterations in autonomic tone.[104] "Enhanced AV nodal conduction" is a term that has been used to characterize short P-R intervals on the ECG and little or no prolongation of AV nodal conduction time in response to rapid atrial pacing. Jackman et al.[182] demonstrated that enhanced AV nodal conduction occurred in 11% of 160 consecutive patients, and this phenomenon represented one end of a continuous spectrum of normal AV nodal physiology.

IMPULSE FORMATION AND PROPAGATION

Although investigations of isolated perfused hearts demonstrated the importance of sodium and calcium in the maintenance of rhythmic electrical activity as early as 1880 to 1882, it was not until the development of the glass microelectrode that investigators were able to elucidate the mechanisms of impulse formation. With the application of microelectrode impalement techniques, it became apparent that action potentials recorded from different regions of the heart were distinct from one another (Fig 22A-9). (The action potential from cells in the sinoatrial node and certain portions of the AV junction differ from that in other cardiac tissue.) Most cells exhibited an initial rapid depolarization (phase 0), early limited rapid repolarization (phase 1), slow prolonged repolarization (phase 2), and terminal, more extensive rapid repolarization (phase 3) (Fig 22A-10). In addition, in spontaneously active cells, there was a phase of slow diastolic depolarization (phase 4), during which the action potential increased toward the threshold potential. Evidence for the underlying mechanisms responsible for the action potential dates back to the idea that electrical properties may reside in the cell membrane.[183] The additional application of voltage clamp techniques in studying the electrical properties of excitable cells and the use of pharmacologic agents have facilitated our understanding of the ionic currents in cardiac muscle.[184-187] Furthermore, the development of the single-cell voltage clamp, the single-channel patch-clamp, and lipid bilayer reconstitution techniques has greatly enhanced our understanding of the ionic basis for impulse formation and propagation. However, some areas remain controversial and are still under active investigation.

In normal cardiac muscle, microelectrode studies have documented that the resting transmembrane potential is approximately −90 mV (see Fig 22A-10). Maintenance of this voltage depends on active ionic exchange between the extracellular and intracellular fluids via the sodium-potassium pump and only transiently permeable membranes. The balance of chemical and electrical forces is particularly, but not exclusively, dependent on the potassium ion. At rest, the intracellular potassium concentration is approximately 35 times the extracellular potassium concentration. The cell membrane at rest is permeable to potassium ions, and thus they tend to diffuse outward along the existing concentration gradient. This outward movement of cations results in the formation of a net negative charge within the cell because the intracellular anions that are associated with intracellular proteins cannot pass through the intact cell membrane. In the situation in which the membrane is only permeable to potassium ions, they continue to diffuse outward along their concentration gradient until the development of a sufficient electrostatic negative intracellular charge. When these electrochemical forces balance each other, the outward movement of potassium stops. The Nernst equation describes the membrane potential at which the flux of potassium ions is zero.

$$E_K = \frac{RT}{F} \ln \frac{[K^+]_o}{[K^+]_i}$$

The equilibrium potential for potassium (E_K) is a function of the gas constant *(R)*, Faraday's constant *(F)*, the absolute temperature *(T)*, and the intracellular and extracellular potassium ion concentrations ($[K^+]_i$ and $[K^+]_o$).

This equation assumes a resting membrane that is permeable only to potassium. In fact, although the resting potential is determined mainly by potassium, the cell membrane is not exclusively permeable to potassium. There is in addition a small inward sodium current

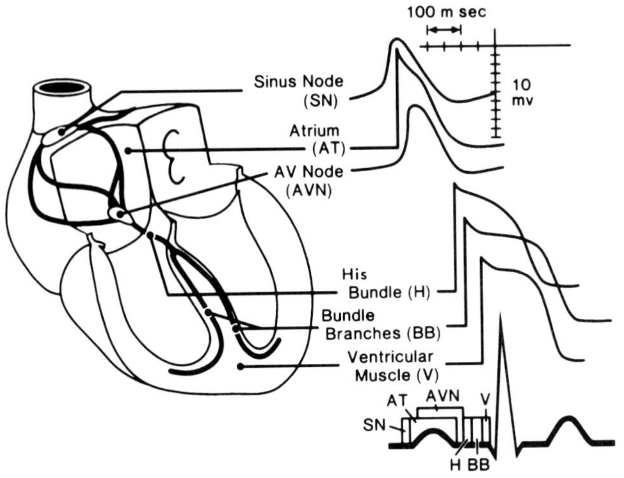

Fig 22A-9 Action potentials recorded from different regions of the heart. Action potentials from the sinus and certain cells in the AV node are similar and distinct from those from the rest of the heart.

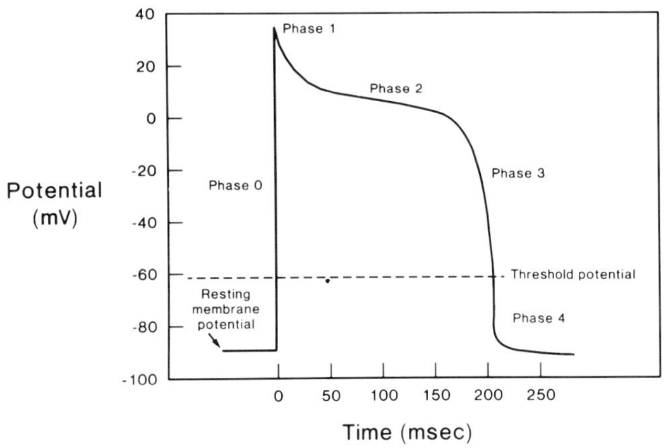

Fig 22A-10 Action potential with five phases. The resting membrane potential is −90 mV. In spontaneously active cells, there is slow diastolic depolarization during phase 4, which returns the fiber toward the threshold potential.

favored by both an electrical and a concentration gradient. Goldman[188] and Hodgkin and Katz[189] have described the resting membrane potential as it relates to a cell that is permeable to both sodium and potassium. The resting potential (V_r) is dependent on both intracellular and extracellular sodium and potassium concentrations ($[Na^+]_i$, $[Na^+]_o$, $[K^+]_i$, $[K^+]_o$) and on the ratio of the coefficients of sodium and potassium permeabilities (P_{Na}/P_K).

$$V_r = \frac{RT}{F}\ln\frac{[K^+]_o + (P_{Na}/P_K[Na^+]_o)}{[K^+]_i + (P_{Na}/P_K[Na^+]_i)}$$

The resting membrane potential may become less negative and move toward the threshold potential by a decrease in outward potassium current or an increase in a pacemaker or sodium-carried current.

Gadsby and Wit[190] simplified the equation, since the intracellular concentration of potassium is much greater than the intracellular concentration of sodium.

$$V_r = \frac{RT}{F}\ln\frac{[K^+]_o + 0.01\,[Na^+]_o}{[K^+]_i}$$

These equations are of practical significance. Changes in local ion concentrations due to drugs, ischemia, and other factors can result in changes in resting membrane potentials and affect both impulse formation and propagation. Furthermore, changes in sodium channel conductance resulting from local anesthetics, antiarrhythmic drugs, or other factors can also affect impulse propagation, given the apparent quadratic relationship between net membrane sodium currents and conduction velocity squared.[191,192]

THE ACTION POTENTIAL

The cardiac action potential has been studied intensively and has been the subject of numerous comprehensive reviews.[186,187,190,193-196] It has a characteristic time course, which depends on sequential changes in cell membrane permeability. These characteristic changes have been divided into five phases. The ionic occurrence responsible for the various phases of the action potential and their ionic mechanisms[197] are summarized in Table 22A-1.

Phase 0: rapid membrane depolarization. Phase 0 results from increased sodium permeability with a rapid

Table 22A-1 Cardiac action potential and underlying currents

Action potential	SA node	Atrial myocardium	AV node	Purkinje fiber	Ventricular myocardium
Phase 0					
Amplitude, mV	50-60	110-120	70-80	120	110-120
V_{max}, V/sec	1-10	100-200	5-15	500-700	100-200
Currents	i_{Ca} i_{Na}	i_{Na}	i_{Ca} i_{Na}	i_{Na}	i_{Na}
Phase 1					
Overshoot, mV	...	30	...	30	30
Currents	...	i_{to}	...	i_{to} i_{Cl}(?)	i_{to} i_{Cl}(?)
Phases 2 and 3					
Currents	i_{Ca} i_K	i_{Ca} i_K i_{K1}	i_{Ca} i_K	i_{Ca} i_K i_{K1}	i_{Ca} i_K i_{K1}
Action potential duration, msec	175-250	200-300	100-175	250-400	200-300
Propagation velocity, m/sec	<0.05	0.3-0.4	0.1	2-3	0.3-0.4
Phase 4					
Maximal diastolic potential, mV	−50 to −60	−80 to −90	−60 to −70	−90 to −95	−80 to −90
Spontaneous depolarization	+	−	+	+	−
Currents	i_{Ca} i_{f*}		i_{Ca} i_{f*}		

AV, atrioventricular; I_{Ca}, calcium current; i_{Cl}, chloride current; i_f, pacemaker current; i_K, delayed rectifier K current; i_{K1}, inward current; i_{Na}, sodium current; i_{to}, transient outward current; sa, sinoatrial.
*Presence or absence depends on maximal diastolic potential.

Table 22A-2 Distinguishing features of fast and slow inward currents of the action potential

Characteristic	Fast current	Slow current
Main ion	Na^+	Ca^{2+}
Rates of activation and inactivation	Rapid	Slow
Activation threshold, mV	−60 to −70	−30 to −40
Resting membrane potential, mV	−80 to −90	−40 to −70
Conduction velocity, m/sec	0.5 to 3.0	0.01 to 0.1
Action potential amplitude, mV	100 to 130	35 to 75
Recovery	Prompt	Delayed, outlasts full repolarization
Current decreased by	Tetrodotoxin Decreased resting membrane potential Local anesthetics	Manganese, verapamil, D600, nifedipine, diltiazem, perhexiline, acetylcholine
Current enhanced by	Veratridine	Catecholamines, cAMP
Role in nodal automaticity	Doubtful	Probable
Role in toxic or ischemic arrhythmias	?	Possible

inward sodium current. The concept of gated channels has been used to describe the transmembrane ionic fluxes.[196] According to this concept, the opening and closing of special sodium channels or gates control the changes in permeability. When a stimulus depolarizes the membrane, one three-component activation gate complex moves rapidly (within a fraction of a millisecond) to an open channel conformation. The other gate, an inactivation complex with a slower time course, closes the channel over many milliseconds. Several factors affect the rate of increase of phase 0, which is critically dependent on sodium conductance, including the absolute number of sodium channels ($\bar{g}_{Na}$), the fraction of channels in an activated state (m^3), the fraction of noninactivated channels (h), the size of the electrochemical potential sodium gradient ($E - E_{Na^+}$), and the absolute level of the threshold potential as shown:

$$g_{Na} = m^3 h\, \bar{g}_{Na}\, (E - E_{Na^+})$$

Phase 1: After the dominant action potential upstroke, there is a brief phase of repolarization, which temporarily returns the membrane potential toward normal. A transient outward current of potassium ions is now believed to be responsible for this rapid but brief repolarization.[198]

Phase 2: plateau phase. After phase 1 temporarily returns the action potential toward 0, the plateau phase is seen. This relatively prolonged phase results from a delicate balance of a small outward membrane current and, more importantly, a slow inward current, which is dependent mainly upon the movement of calcium ions. There has been increasing interest in this slow inward current.[195,199-206] These slow currents can be distinguished from fast inward currents by both electrophysiologic and pharmacologic features (Table 22A-2 and Fig 22A-11).

Cardiac cells can be classified with regard to the underlying dominant ionic mechanism of depolarization. Impulse formation and conduction in the sinoatrial and AV nodes is dependent upon the slow inward current. By

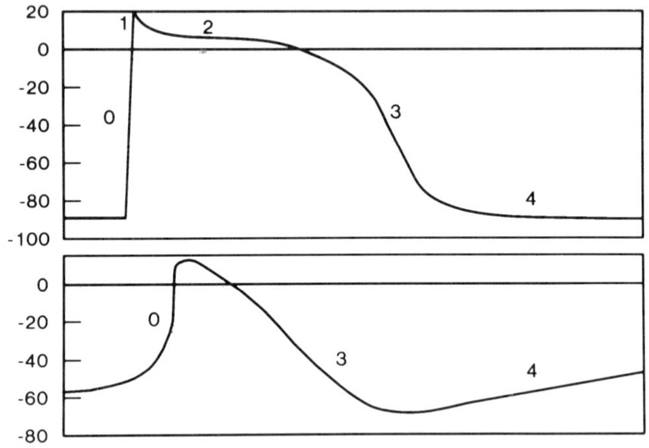

Fig 22A-11 Action potentials recorded by intracellular electrodes from two types of cardiac cells. **Top,** action potential recorded from a cell that is dependent mainly upon a rapid-current, fast-channel response. **Bottom,** action potential recorded from a sinus node cell that is dependent upon a slow inward current. The latter current is characterized by lower resting and activation potentials and slower conduction velocity. Numbers 0-4 refer to the phases shown in Figure 22A-10.

virtue of this, sinoatrial and AV node cells are characterized by lower resting and activation potentials and slower conduction velocities. Activation of most of the rest of the cardiac tissue is more dependent upon rapid-current fast-channel responses. In these fibers the slow inward calcium current can also be documented if the fast sodium channel is blocked. In these cells the slow inward current is responsible in part for the plateau phase of the action potential which occurs after inactivation of the rapid sodium current.

Increasing attention to the importance of the slow inward current in normal sinoatrial and AV node function, in the genesis of reentrant arrhythmias, and in the contractile-mechanical properties in cardiac and smooth muscle has led to the development and widespread use of calcium entry blocking drugs.

Phase 3: After the end of the plateau zone, repolarization takes place, during which time the membrane potential returns toward the resting level. This phase involves continued inactivation of the slow inward current and, more importantly, voltage-dependent changes in conductance with an efflux of potassium.[195,207,208]

Phase 4: The diastolic portion of the action potential is variable.[195,205,209-215] In normal cardiac muscle, no spontaneous diastolic depolarization occurs. During this time, there is active ionic movement with energy-dependent exchange of sodium and potassium. In other cardiac fibers (Purkinje's fibers, cells within the AV node, specialized atrial fibers, and, most prominently, the sinus node), spontaneous diastolic depolarization occurs, which forms the basis of automaticity. This phase depends on a reduction of outward current carried by potassium, leading to progressive membrane depolarization until the threshold potential has been reached. In addition, there is an inward component mediated by sodium.[209,210] The rate of diastolic depolarization is variable; it is highest in the sinoatrial node but is affected by local ion concentrations and catecholamines.

MECHANISMS OF ARRHYTHMIAS

Arrhythmias arise through three potential mechanisms: (1) disorders of impulse formation, (2) disorders of impulse conduction, and (3) mixed disorders.[190,193,195,216-221]

Disorders of impulse formation

Normal automaticity. Normal automaticity is defined as spontaneous diastolic depolarization (phase 4 action potential) occurring in cells with intrinsic automatic mechanisms. In addition to occurrence in the sinus node, intrinsic automaticity can be found in specialized atrial cells, in some regions of the AV junction, and in His-Purkinje fibers. These areas function as standby or subsidiary pacemakers; usually they are depolarized by propagated impulses from the sinus node before they reach threshold spontaneously. Atrial and ventricular cells normally do not exert automaticity.

Intrinsic automaticity is dependent upon three major factors: (1) the slope and rate of phase 4 depolarization which set the rate of impulse formation; (2) the threshold potential—the potential at which an action potential is initiated, and (3) the maximum diastolic potential—the potential from which phase 4 spontaneous depolarization begins. Any factors that slow the rate of phase 4 depolarization, make the threshold potential more positive, or make the maximum diastolic membrane potential more negative slow the rate of spontaneous pacemaker depolarization. The ionic mechanisms responsible for phase 4 depolarization have been previously discussed. The numerous factors capable of influencing the slope and rate of phase 4 depolarization include autonomic mediators, acid-base changes, hypoxia, temperature, extracellular and intracellular ion concentrations, cardioactive medications, and degree of tissue stretch.[193,195,216] These factors may act directly on the dominant pacemaker to slow or accelerate the heart rate or they may shift the dominant pacemaker either within the sinus node or to a subsidiary pacemaker. Boineau et al.[22,23] postulated a multicenter pacemaker complex with multiple subsidiary pacemakers, activated differently, in the region of the sinus node.

Abnormal automaticity. Abnormal automaticity can be defined as alteration of the normal automatic mechanisms (enhanced automaticity in cells with intrinsic automatic mechanisms) or as occurrence of abnormal automatic mechanisms in cells that do not have intrinsic automatic mechanisms.[193,195,216,222] Abnormal automaticity has been demonstrated in both ischemic and diseased cardiac tissues. Under experimental conditions, abnormal automaticity can occur by one of three mechanisms:[223,224] (1) depolarized resting membrane potential (less negative membrane potential), (2) increased slope of diastolic depolarization (phase 4 of action potential), and (3) more negative threshold membrane potential. Abnormal automaticity occurs most often when the resting membrane potential is partially depolarized, that is, in injured atrial or ventricular cells.

When atrial and ventricular resting membrane potentials are reduced to less than -60 mV, spontaneous depolarization may occur. At this membrane potential in partially depolarized fibers, the fast inward sodium current is inactivated whereas slow inward current mechanisms remain intact. In this setting, these slow inward current mechanisms may result in abnormal automaticity. These cellular observations may also explain why some automatic arrhythmias respond to calcium channel blockers and β-blockers. Singer et al.[216,225-227] demonstrated that approximately 90% of specimens of chronically diseased atrial tissue and 50% of ventricular myocardial specimens taken at the time of operation may have spontaneous activity. Clinically, it has been shown that some types of ectopic tachycardia are automatic. An example of atrial tachycardia is shown in Figure 22A-12.

Triggered activity and afterdepolarizations. An additional mechanism of arrhythmia generation that has received increasing attention is "triggered automaticity."[218-221,228,229] This general term is used to describe arrhythmias originating in afterdepolarizations, or oscillatory afterpotentials, the genesis of which is critically dependent on previous electrical activity of the heart.[230] These afterdepolarizations, or oscillatory afterpotentials, are referred to as "early afterdepolarizations" when they occur during phases 2 and 3 of the action potential[231-235] and as "delayed afterdepolarizations" when they occur after complete repolarization.[228,229,236-239] The characteristics of each type of afterdepolarization are substantially different from those of the other.

During the repolarization phases of action potential (phase 2 and phase 3), delayed rectifier (i_K) and inward rectifier (i_{K1}) are the major components of outward potassium currents. The inward currents are primarily the

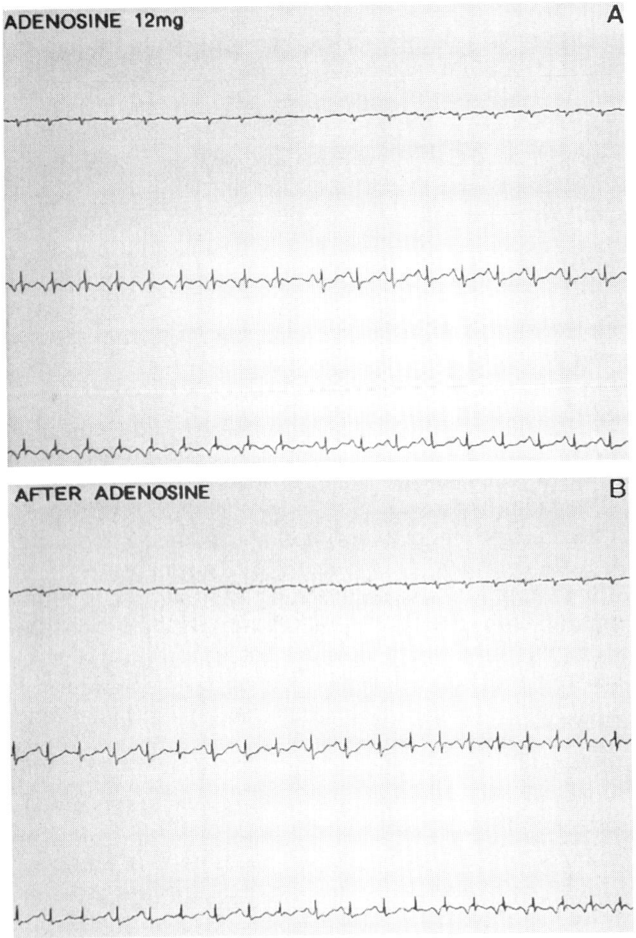

Fig 22A-12 Recordings from surface electrocardiogram leads I, II, and III. In **B,** the P-wave morphology in leads II and III suggests an ectopic atrial focus (inverted P wave). The response of the tachycardia to adenosine, i.e., transient suppression (**A** and **B**), is consistent with an automatic mechanism. (From Shen W-K, Kurachi Y: Mechanisms of adenosine-mediated actions on cellular and clinical cardiac electrophysiology. *Mayo Clin Proc* 70:274-291, 1995. By permission, Mayo Foundation.)

calcium (i_{Ca}) currents. Early afterdepolarization can theoretically occur when outward currents are inhibited or inward currents are enhanced.[230] During phase 2 of the action potential, because of the reduced membrane potential, the calcium current could be responsible for the early afterdepolarization. During phase 3 of the action potential, the membrane potential is more negative than in phase 2, and the sodium current could be responsible for early afterdepolarization. The sodium current most likely differs from the sodium current that is responsible for phase 0 of the action potential. The sodium current occurring during phase 3 of the action potential has been referred to as the "sodium window current."[206,240,241]

Because of these different mechanisms for early afterdepolarization, it is not surprising that pharmacologic response may vary for triggered arrhythmias caused by early afterdepolarization. Early afterdepolarization and

Table 22A-3 Factors that influence early afterdepolarization

	Increase	Decrease
Autonomic	↑ sympathetic tone ↑ catecholamines ↓ parasympathetic tone	↓ sympathetic tone ↓ catecholamines ↑ parasympathetic tone
Metabolic	↑ hypoxia ↑ acidosis	↑ O_2 ↓ acidosis
Electrolytes	C_s^+ Hypokalemia	K^+ Mg^{2+}
Drugs and metabolites	Sotalol *N*-acetylprocainamide Quinidine Aconitine Veratridine	Acetylcholine/adenosine Lidocaine Procainamide Ca^{2+} channel blockers β-Blockers Tetrodotoxin K^+ channel openers
Heart rate	Slow	Fast

triggered activity have been observed under the following conditions (Table 22A-3): hypokalemia,[234,235] membrane depolarization, hypoxia, acidosis (with or without catecholamines),[230] aconitine and veratridine (induced inward current),[242] cesium (inhibits i_K),[231-233] and antiarrhythmic agents, such as sotalol, *N*-acetylprocainamide, and quinidine.[235] Early afterdepolarization can be suppressed under the following conditions: increased potassium, acetylcholine (hyperpolarization of transmembrane potential), tetrodotoxin, magnesium, antiarrhythmic agents such as lidocaine and procainamide (suppressed sodium window current), calcium channel blockers and β-blockers (suppressed calcium currents), and potassium channel openers (enhanced potassium currents).

Delayed afterdepolarization and triggered activity have been observed with the following agents and conditions: faster heart rate,[243-245] cardiac glycosides,[237,246,247] hypokalemia,[248,249] hypercalcemia,[250] and catecholamines.[248,251,252] All these experimental conditions lead to a final common pathway, that is, increased intracellular concentration of calcium. The fluctuation of increased intracellular calcium concentration has been correlated to activation of an inward ionic current. This current has been named the "transient inward current."[253-255] The ionic channel responsible for the transient inward current is thought to be a nonselective monovalent cationic channel. This channel can conduct either sodium or potassium ions. Under physiologic conditions, this channel conducts sodium ions predominantly. The afterpotentials coupled to the oscillatory intracellular calcium concentration may eventually increase in amplitude, reach threshold, and produce a sustained arrhythmia (Fig

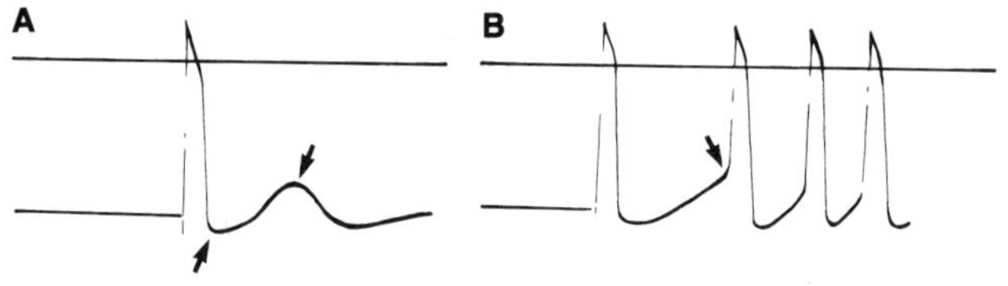

Fig 22A-13 Action potential from an atrial fiber. **A,** single stimulated action potential followed by an afterdepolarization *(arrows).* **B,** afterdepolarization reaches threshold potential *(arrow)* and results in triggered activity. (From Wit AL, Boyden PA, Gadsby DC, et al: Triggered activity as a cause of atrial arrhythmias. In *Cardiac Arrhythmias: Electrophysiology, Diagnosis, and Management.* Edited by OS Narula. Baltimore, Williams & Wilkins, 1979, pp 14-31. By permission.)

22A-13). In contrast to early afterdepolarizations, these oscillating afterpotentials are more likely precipitated by shorter pacing cycle lengths or coupling intervals, producing an increased amplitude of the afterdepolarizations and shortening of the coupling interval to the preceding action potential.[229,236,237]

The precise role of triggered activity in arrhythmogenesis is not completely established. Nevertheless, it has been proposed that early afterdepolarizations may be the mechanism underlying torsades de pointes.[233] In support of this hypothesis is the finding that these afterpotentials are generated by conditions or drugs commonly associated with clinical torsades de pointes. Furthermore, torsade has been reproduced in experimental animals by the administration of cesium, also shown to decrease outward potassium currents and produce early afterdepolarizations.[232,233]

Delayed afterdepolarization and triggered activity may be the underlying mechanism for arrhythmias occurring during digitalis toxicity, ischemia, enhanced catecholamines, hypokalemia, and hypercalcemia. The most convincing observation of clinical arrhythmias caused by delayed afterdepolarization is perhaps from the exercise-induced ventricular tachycardia in patients without any overt cardiac disease.[256,257] This tachycardia is catecholamine-dependent and calcium-sensitive. The exercise-induced ventricular tachycardia frequently responds to adenosine, calcium channel blockers, and β-blockers (Fig 22A-14). These pharmacologic agents decrease intracellular calcium concentration and therefore inhibit the transient inward current and suppress clinical tachycardia.

Arrhythmias related to abnormal impulse conduction

Arrhythmias related to reentry are more common than arrhythmias of abnormal automaticity.[177,187,193-195,216,221,222,259-261] Reentry involves three prerequisite conditions: (1) at least two functionally distinct conduction pathways, (2) unidirectional block in one pathway, and (3) slow conduction down the second pathway (Fig 22A-15).

Two or more functional pathways for conduction. During normal conditions, despite the fact that cross connections exist between fibers of the conduction system, the direction of impulse formation is uniform. Reentry requires an alteration in the uniform propagation of the impulse, so that two or more limbs are present that join proximally and distally to form final common pathways. The pathways may be anatomically distinct, as seen in patients with accessory AV connections, or they may be only functionally separate, as seen with dual AV node pathways and AV node reentry. Pathologic processes such as fibrosis or infarction may also result in distinct conduction pathways joining together to form a closed loop.

Unidirectional block in one pathway. For reentry to occur, there must be unidirectional block in one pathway. This allows an impulse that is being conducted antegradely down the second pathway to reenter the first pathway and excite it in a retrograde fashion. Unidirectional block may be due to structural conditions or it may be functional, depending on the disparity in refractoriness in the two limbs.

Slow conduction down the second pathway. The third prerequisite is slow conduction. Conduction velocity is dependent upon the threshold potential, the rate of increase of phase 0, the amplitude of the action potential, and the resistance. Slow conduction may be due to decremental conduction, in which the amplitude of the impulse decreases progressively during passage through the cardiac tissue. Such slow decremental conduction is seen in areas of the conduction system which are characterized by slow-fiber calcium currents such as the AV node. Slow decremental conduction can also be seen in fibers that normally are dependent upon fast-channel responses but that are exposed to ischemia or hypoxia. Slow conduction down one pathway allows recovery of the second pathway so that retrograde conduction and reentry can occur.

Reentry can occur at any level within the conduction system and can be macroreentrant with a large anatomic loop, such as is seen in patients with classic preexcitation with accessory AV pathways, or microreentrant[136,137,141,262-269] (Figs 22A-16 and 22A-17). Irrespective of the location and size of the pathway, the requisite requirements are the same. In Figure 22A-17, dual AV node pathways are depicted diagrammatically, with an α pathway characterized by slow conduction but rapid recovery and a β pathway with rapid conduction but slower recovery. Under normal conditions, all conduction is down the fast pathway, and this results in a normal P-R interval. An atrial premature contraction, however, finds the pathway unexcitable (unidirectional block), but it can be conducted, with delay, down the slow pathway, the result being P-R prolongation. Given the right circumstances, the impulse can then be conducted retrogradely up the fast pathway and give rise to an atrial echo. Sustained reentry results when critical timing exists to allow the impulse to return to the ventricle via the slow pathway.

Although reentry around an anatomic obstacle is undoubtedly the mechanism for many arrhythmias, in

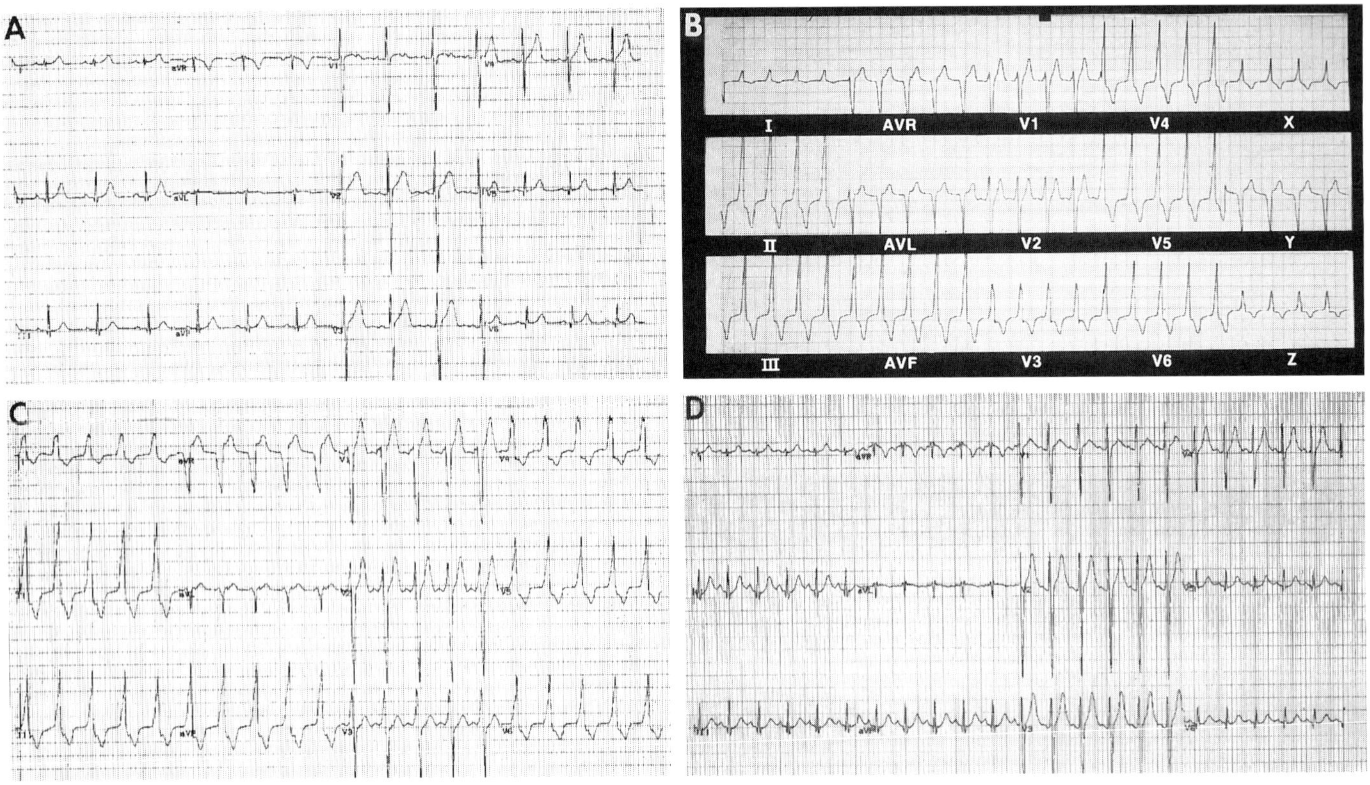

Fig 22A-14 Electrocardiograms from a 17-year-old boy with exercise-induced ventricular tachycardia and without any structural heart disease. **A,** baseline tracings show normal sinus rhythm. **B,** during treadmill exercise test, ventricular tachycardia was induced when the sinus rate reached 110 beats/min. Note the typical left bundle-branch block morphology and normal (inferior) axis, suggestive of a right ventricular outflow tract origin. **C,** at electrophysiologic testing, ventricular tachycardia became incessant during isoproterenol infusion. It was also inducible with programmed ventricular stimulation and with atrial and ventricular burst pacing (not shown). **D,** during infusion of isoproterenol, verapamil (10 mg intravenously) completely abolished spontaneous ventricular tachycardia. Tachycardia was also transiently terminated after injection of 6 mg of adenosine (not shown). Electrophysiologic and pharmacologic responses of this tachycardia are consistent with the triggered mechanism. See text and references 256, 257, and 258 for details.

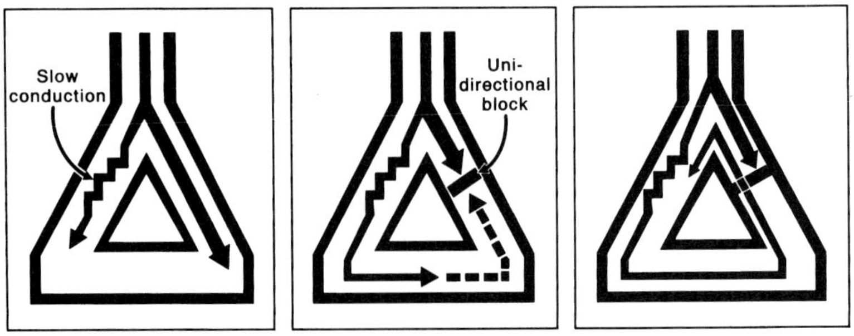

Fig 22A-15 Three conditions are necessary for reentry to occur: **left,** at least two functionally distinct conduction pathways in a continuous circuit; **middle,** unidirectional block in one pathway that permits conduction in only one direction; and **right,** slow conduction in the second pathway that allows the area proximal to the block in the first pathway to recover from the refractory state. Recovery allows the impulse to reenter and travel around the loop.

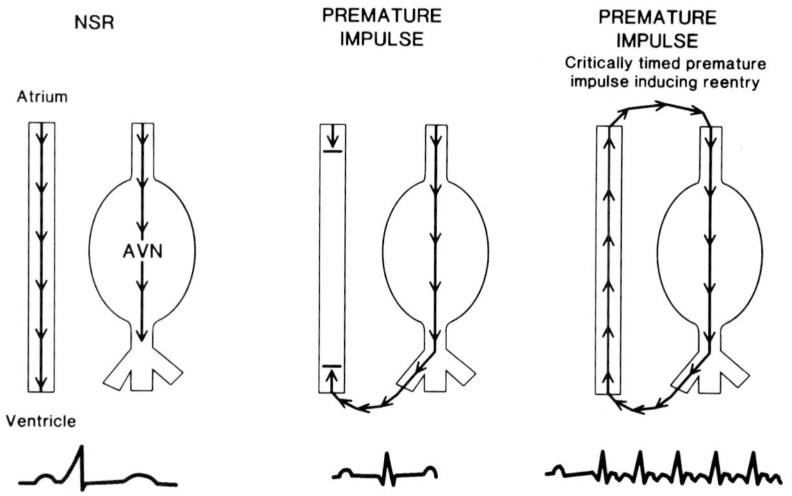

Fig 22A-16 Diagram of preexcitation and accessory AV pathways. **Left,** during normal sinus rhythm *(NSR),* the P-R interval is short; the slurred QRS complex is a result of fusion between ventricular activation via the accessory pathway and that from the AV node (AVN). **Middle,** a premature impulse finds the accessory pathway blocked but conducts normally through the AVN. The resultant ECG shows a normal P wave, P-R segment, and QRS. **Right,** a critically timed premature impulse finds the accessory pathway blocked in the antegrade direction. It is conducted normally through the AVN. On reaching the ventricle, it reenters the bypass in a retrograde fashion and initiates supraventricular tachycardia.

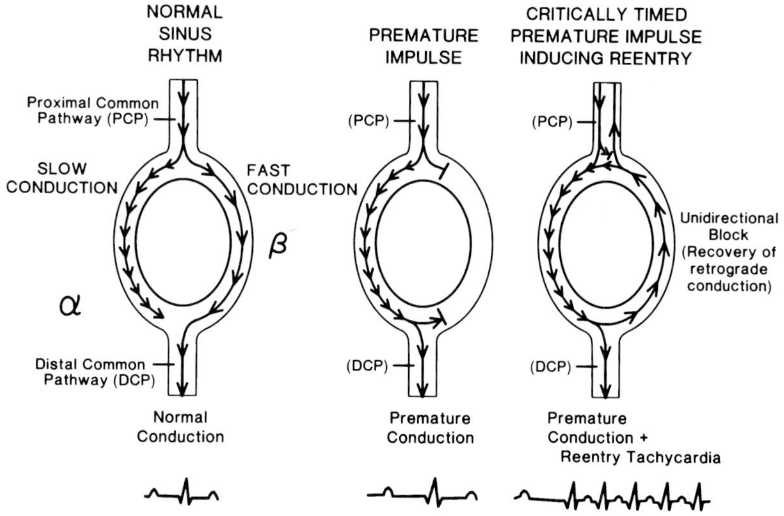

Fig 22A-17 Diagram of dual AV nodal pathways. There are a proximal and a distal common pathway and two functional limbs of a reentrant circuit. **Left,** during normal sinus rhythm, the impulse is conducted down the fast limb (β), and the result is a normal P-R interval. This limb has a longer refractory period than the slower-conducting (α) limb. **Middle,** a premature impulse finds the β pathway blocked but is conducted down the α pathway; a longer P-R interval results. **Right,** a critically timed premature impulse initiates tachycardia. It is conducted slowly down the α limb. When it reaches the distal common pathway, the β limb, which has recovered, conducts the impulse in a retrograde direction to produce either echo beats or sustained tachycardia.

other cases no fixed barrier may be present. In those cases, a reentrant arrhythmia may circle around an area of functional block that is disseminated in time and space. Such a mechanism has been demonstrated in rabbit atrial myocardium and other preparations in which, in the absence of a fixed inexcitable central obstacle, the center of a circus movement may be invaded by multiple centripetal wavelets converging on and producing block at the very center of the circuit. This mechanism, referred to as a "leading circle" concept, may likewise be responsible for clinically relevant rhythm disorders.[259]

Many important differences in characteristics of circuit movement reentry exist between an anatomically defined circuit and a functionally defined circuit. The reentry circuit of an anatomic obstacle usually has a defined length of the circuitry. A fully excitable gap is usually present between the head and the tail of the impulse. The revolution time is inversely reproportional to the conduction velocity. The revolution time does not depend on the refractory period, because the circuit length always exceeds the wavelength (conduction velocity times the refractory period) of the reentry pathway. The circuit length of the functional leading circle type is not fixed. It depends on the conduction velocity and the refractory period of the tissue involved. There is no fully excitable gap. The revolution time is directly proportional to the length of the refractory period.

Reentry can also be demonstrated over short distances and in isolated bundles of cardiac tissue. This has been called "reflection."[265-269] Experimentally,

> . . . an impulse arriving at a depressed area [of conduction] in an unbranched bundle of fibers undergoes marked delay. After that delay, an impulse may continue in the forward direction while an impulse is reflected back in the direction from which the original impulse came.[265] Reflection occurs in a one-dimensional structure in which the impulse is conducted to-and-fro from the same pathway. Reflection may be important in the generation of ventricular extrasystoles and of parasystolic pacemaker activity.[268]

Abnormal impulse formation and conduction

Abnormalities of impulse conduction and impulse formation can coexist and lead to clinical arrhythmias.[216,270-277] Parasystolic rhythms have attracted considerable clinical interest. They have been thought to result from a focus of myocardial cells that were undergoing cyclic diastolic depolarization at varying rates. These arrhythmias are characterized by abnormal conduction of the normal cardiac impulse into the focus (entrance block). They may also exhibit abnormal conduction of the impulse out of the focus (exit block). This abnormal conduction may be caused by localized changes in the diastolic potential in the myocardium surrounding the focus and in the focus itself. Some experimental parasystolic arrhythmias have been shown to have a high rate of discharge as a result of abnormal automaticity with rapid oscillatory afterpotentials, and this is then combined with abnormal conduction (exit block) out of the focus.

RELEVANCE OF ANATOMIC AND PATHOPHYSIOLOGIC MECHANISMS IN THE EVALUATION AND MANAGEMENT OF ARRHYTHMIAS

The body of information on mechanisms and management of arrhythmias has increased rapidly in recent years. This increase is related to the development of electrophysiology as a clinical tool and the introduction of new antiarrhythmia agents and new surgical and pacing techniques. The proper use of these new management approaches depends on knowledge of the underlying anatomic and pathophysiologic concepts. As growth continues in the evaluation of basic mechanisms of arrhythmias, there will be continued development of new drugs aimed at treating the underlying electrophysiologic abnormalities that are responsible for the arrhythmia. This in turn will permit more scientific and effective management of patients having a wide range of arrhythmias.

REFERENCES

1. Anderson RH, Becker AE: Gross anatomy and microscopy of the conducting system. In *Cardiac Arrhythmias: Their Mechanisms, Diagnosis, and Management.* Edited by WJ Mandel. Philadelphia, JB Lippincott Company, 1980, pp 12-54
2. Truex RC: The sinoatrial node and its connections with the atrial tissues. In *The Conduction System of the Heart: Structure, Function and Clinical Complications.* Edited by HJJ Wellens, KI Lie, MJ Janse. Philadelphia, Lea & Febiger, 1976, pp 209-226
3. James TN: Anatomy of the human sinus node. *Anat Rec* 141:109-139, 1961
4. Anderson RH, Ho SY, Becker AE, et al: The development of the sinus node. In *Workshop on Sinus Node.* Edited by FIM Bonke. The Hague, Boston, Martinus Nijhoff Medical Division, 1978
5. Walls EW: The development of the specialized conducting tissue of the human heart. *J Anat* 81:93-110, 1947
6. Van Mierop LHS: Location of pacemaker in chick embryo heart at the time of initiation of heartbeat. *Am J Physiol* 212:407-415, 1967
7. Kennel AJ, Titus JL: The vasculature of the human sinus node. *Mayo Clin Proc* 47:556-561, 1972
8. James TN: *Anatomy of the Coronary Arteries.* New York, Paul B Hoeber, Medical Division of Harper & Brothers, 1961
9. Anderson KR, Ho YS, Anderson RH: Location and vascular supply of sinus node in human heart. *Br Heart J* 41:28-32, 1979
10. James TN: The sinus node as a servomechanism. *Circ Res* 32:307-313, 1973
11. James TN, Nadeau RA: Sinus bradycardia during injections directly into the sinus node artery. *Am J Physiol* 204:9-15, 1963
12. James TN, Nadeau RA: Relation of retrograde pressure in the sinus node artery to sinus tachycardia from stellate stimulation. *J Lab Clin Med* 62:777-786, 1963
13. James TN: The sinus node. *Am J Cardiol* 40:965-986, 1977
14. Woods WT, Urthaler F, James TN: Spontaneous action potentials of cells in the canine sinus node. *Circ Res* 39:76-82, 1976
15. James TN, Sherf L, Fine G, et al: Comparative ultrastructure of the sinus node in man and dog. *Circulation* 34:139-163, 1966
16. James TN: Anatomy and pathology of the conduction system of the human heart. In *Fundamentals in Cardiac Pacing.* Vol. 3. Edited by HJT Thalen, CC Meere. The Hague, Boston, Martinus Nijhoff, 1979, pp 22-57
17. Michaels DC, Matyas EP, Jalife J: Mechanisms of sinoatrial pacemaker synchronization: a new hypothesis. *Circ Res* 61:704-714, 1987
18. Randall WC, Ardell JL: Nervous control of the heart: anatomy and pathophysiology. In *Cardiac Electrophysiology: From Cell to Bedside.* Edited by DP Zipes, J Jalife. Philadelphia, WB Saunders Company, 1990, pp 291-299
19. Zipes DP, Miyazaki T: The autonomic nervous system and the heart: basis for understanding interactions and effects on arrhythmia

development. In *Cardiac Electrophysiology: From Cell to Bedside.* Edited by DP Zipes, J Jalife. Philadelphia, WB Saunders Company, 1990, pp 312-330

20. Carlson MD, Geha AS, Hsu J, et al: Selective stimulation of parasympathetic nerve fibers to the human sinoatrial node. *Circulation* 85:1311-1317, 1992

21. James TN: Cardiac innervation: anatomic and pharmacologic relations. *Bull NY Acad Med* 43:1041-1086, 1967

22. Boineau JP, Schuessler RB, Mooney CR, et al: Multicentric origin of the atrial depolarization wave: the pacemaker complex. Relation to dynamics of atrial conduction, P-wave changes and heart rate control. *Circulation* 58:1036-1048, 1978

23. Boineau JP, Schuessler RB, Hackel DB, et al: Multicentric distribution and rate differentiation of the atrial pacemaker systems: pacemaker complex. In *Physiology of Atrial Pacemakers and Conductive Tissues.* Edited by RC Little. Mount Kisco, New York, Futura Publishing Company, 1980, pp 221-260

24. Davies MJ: *Pathology of Conducting Tissue of the Heart.* New York, Appleton-Century-Crofts; London, Butterworths, 1971, pp 16-20

25. El-Said G, Rosenberg HS, Mullins CE, et al: Dysrhythmias after Mustard's operation for transposition of the great arteries. *Am J Cardiol* 30:526-532, 1972

26. Lewis AB, Lindesmith GG, Takahashi M, et al: Cardiac rhythm following the Mustard procedure for transposition of the great vessels. *J Thorac Cardiovasc Surg* 73:919-926, 1977

27. Angelini P, Sandiford FM: Functional correction of transposition of the great arteries: a new approach to avoid postoperative arrhythmias. *J Thorac Cardiovasc Surg* 66:87-92, 1973

28. Issacson R, Titus JL, Merideth J, et al: Apparent interruption of atrial conduction pathways after surgical repair of transposition of great arteries. *Am J Cardiol* 30:533-535, 1972

29. Drago F, Turchetta A, Calzolari A, et al: Early identification of patients at risk for sinus node dysfunction after Mustard operation. *Int J Cardiol* 35:27-32, 1992

30. James TN: Pericarditis and the sinus node. *Arch Intern Med* 110:305-311, 1962

31. James TN, Rupe CE, Monto RW: Pathology of the cardiac conduction system in systemic lupus erythematosus. *Ann Intern Med* 63:402-410, 1965

32. James TN: De Subitaneis Mortibus. VIII. Coronary arteries and conduction system in the scleroderma heart disease. *Circulation* 50:844-856, 1974

33. Bulkley BH, Ridolfi RL, Salyer WR, et al: Myocardial lesions of progressive systemic sclerosis: a cause of cardiac dysfunction. *Circulation* 53:483-490, 1976

34. Bulkley BH: Progressive systemic sclerosis: cardiac involvement. *Clin Rheum Dis* 5:131-149, 1979

35. D'Angelo WA, Fries JF, Masi AT, et al: Pathologic observations in systemic sclerosis (scleroderma): a study of fifty-eight autopsy cases and fifty-eight matched controls. *Am J Med* 46:428-440, 1969

36. Davies MJ, Pomerance A: Quantitative study of ageing changes in the human sinoatrial node and internodal tracts. *Br Heart J* 34:150-152, 1972

37. Lev M: Aging changes in the human sinoatrial node. *J Gerontol* 9:1-9, 1954

38. Sims BA: Pathogenesis of atrial arrhythmias. *Br Heart J* 34:336-340, 1972

39. Thery C, Gosselin B, Lekieffre J, et al: Pathology of sinoatrial node: correlations with electrocardiographic findings in 111 patients. *Am Heart J* 93:735-740, 1977

40. Shaw DB: The etiology of sino-atrial disorder (sick sinus syndrome). *Am Heart J* 92:539-540, 1976

41. Ferrer MI: *The Sick Sinus Syndrome.* Mount Kisco, New York, Futura Publishing Company, 1974

42. Demoulin J-C, Kulbertus HE: Histopathological correlates of sinoatrial disease. *Br Heart J* 40:1384-1389, 1977

43. Shiraishi I, Takamatsu T, Minamikawa T, et al: Quantitative histological analysis of the human sinoatrial node during growth and aging. *Circulation* 85:2176-2184, 1992

44. James TN, Birk RE: Pathology of the cardiac conduction system in polyarteritis nodosa. *Arch Intern Med* 117:561-567, 1966

45. James TN: The George E. Brown Memorial Lecture: Small arteries of the heart. *Circulation* 56:2-14, 1977

46. Thiene G, Valente M, Rossi L: Involvement of the cardiac conducting system in panarteritis nodosa. *Am Heart J* 95:716-724, 1978

47. James TN, Monto RW: Pathology of the cardiac conduction system in thrombotic thrombocytopenic purpura. *Ann Intern Med* 65:37-43, 1966

48. James TN, Marshall ML, Craig MW: De Subitaneis Mortibus. VII. Disseminated intravascular coagulation and paroxysmal atrial tachycardia. *Circulation* 50:395-401, 1974

49. James TN: Myocardial infarction and atrial arrhythmias. *Circulation* 24:761-776, 1961

50. DeSanctis RW, Block P, Hutter AM Jr: Tachyarrhythmias in myocardial infarction. *Circulation* 45:681-702, 1972

51. Liberthson RR, Salisbury KW, Hutter AM Jr, et al: Atrial tachyarrhythmias in acute myocardial infarction. *Am J Med* 60:956-960, 1976

52. Klass M, Haywood LJ: Atrial fibrillation associated with acute myocardial infarction: a study of 34 cases. *Am Heart J* 79:752-760, 1970

53. Rotman M, Wagner GS, Wallace AG: Bradyarrhythmias in acute myocardial infarction. *Circulation* 45:703-722, 1972

54. Hindmann MC, Wagner GS: Arrhythmias during myocardial infarction: mechanisms, significance and therapy. In *Cardiac Arrhythmias: Mechanisms and Managements.* Edited by A. Castellanos Jr. Philadelphia, FA Davis Company, 1980, pp 81-103

55. Jordan J, Yamaguchi I, Mandel WJ: Characteristics of sinoatrial conduction in patients with coronary artery disease. *Circulation* 55:569-574, 1977

56. Scarpa WJ: The sick sinus syndrome. *Am Heart J* 92:648-660, 1976

57. Bharati S, Nordenberg A, Bauernfiend R, et al: The anatomic substrate for the sick sinus syndrome in adolescence. *Am J Cardiol* 46:163-172, 1980

58. Spach MS, Miller WT III, Barr RC, et al: Electrophysiology of the internodal pathways: determining the difference between anisotropic cardiac muscle and a specialized tract system. In *Physiology of Atrial Pacemakers and Conductive Tissues.* Edited by RC Little. Mount Kisco, New York, Futura Publishing Company, 1980, pp 367-380

59. Sherf L, James TN: Functional anatomy and ultrastructure of the internodal pathways. In *Physiology of the Atrial Pacemakers and Conductive Tissues.* Edited by RC Little. Mount Kisco, New York, Futura Publishing Company, 1980, pp 67-112

60. Merideth J, Titus JL: The anatomic atrial connections between sinus and A-V node. *Circulation* 37:566-579, 1968

61. Joyner RW, Ramón F, Moore JW: Stimulation of action potential propagation in an in homogeneous sheet of coupled excitable cells. *Circ Res* 36:654-661, 1975

62. James TN: The connecting pathways between the sinus node and A-V node and between the right and the left atrium in the human heart. *Am Heart J* 66:498-508, 1963

63. James TN: Morphology of the human atrioventricular node, with remarks pertinent to its electrophysiology. *Am Heart J* 62:756-771, 1961

64. Abildskov JA, Millar K, Burgess MJ: Atrial fibrillation. *Am J Cardiol* 28:263-267, 1971

65. Davies MJ, Pomerance A: Pathology of atrial fibrillation in man. *Br Heart J* 34:520-525, 1972

66. Tanigawa M, Fukatani M, Konoe A, et al: Prolonged and fractionated right atrial electrograms during sinus rhythm in patients with paroxysmal atrial fibrillation and sick sinus node syndrome. *J Am Coll Cardiol* 17:403-408, 1991

67. Leier CV, Meacham JA, Schaal SF: Prolonged atrial conduction: a major predisposing factor for the development of atrial flutter. *Circulation* 57:213-216, 1978

68. Brandenburg RO Jr, Holmes DR Jr, Brandenburg RO, et al: Clinical follow-up study of paroxysmal supraventricular tachyarrhythmias after operative repairs of a secundum type atrial septal defect in adults. *Am J Cardiol* 51:273-276, 1983

69. Anderson PAW, Rogers MC, Canent RV Jr, et al: Atrioventricular conduction in secundum atrial septal defects. *Circulation* 48:27-31, 1973

70. Roberts NK, Fink BW: Arrhythmias in the pediatric patient. In *Cardiac Arrhythmias.* Edited by WJ Mandel. Philadelphia, JB Lippincott Company, 1980, pp 454-469

71. Ng R, Somerville J, Ross D: Ebstein's anomaly: late results of surgical correction. *Eur J Cardiol* 9:39-52, 1979

72. Bialostozky D, Horwitz S, Espino-Vela J: Ebstein's malformation of the tricuspid valve: a review of 65 cases. *Am J Cardiol* 29:826-836, 1972

73. Becker AE, Anderson RH: Morphology of the human atrioventricular junctional area. In *The Conduction System of the Heart: Structure, Function and Clinical Implications.* Edited by HJJ Wellens, KI Lie, MJ Janse. Philadelphia, Lea & Febiger, 1976, pp 263-286

74. Hecht HH, Kossmann CE, Childers RW, et al: Atrioventricular and intraventricular conduction: revised nomenclature and concepts. *Am J Cardiol* 31:232-244, 1973

75. Anderson RH, Becker AE, Wenink ACG, et al: The development of the cardiac specialized tissue. In *The Conduction System of the Heart: Structure, Function and Clinical Implications.* Edited by HJJ Wellens, KI Lie, MJ Janse. Philadelphia, Lea & Febiger, 1976, pp 3-28

76. Frink RJ, James TN: Normal blood supply to the human His bundle and proximal bundle branches. *Circulation* 47:8-18, 1973

77. James TN: The coronary circulation and conduction system in acute myocardial infarction. *Prog Cardiovasc Dis* 10:410-449, 1968

78. James TN, Burch GE: Blood supply of the human interventricular septum. *Circulation* 17:391-396, 1958

79. James TN, Sherf L: Ultrastructure of the human atrioventricular node. *Circulation* 37:1049-1070, 1968

80. Tranum-Jensen J: The fine structure of the atrial and atrioventricular (AV) junctional specialized tissues of the rabbit heart. In *The Conduction System of the Heart: Structure, Function and Clinical Implications.* Edited by HJJ Wellens, KI Lie, MJ Janse. Philadelphia, Lea & Febiger, 1976, pp 55-81

81. James TN, Sherf L: Fine structure of the His bundle. *Circulation* 44:9-28, 1971

82. Truex RC, Smythe MQ: Reconstruction of the human atrioventricular node. *Anat Rec* 158:11-19, 1967

83. Lev M: The conduction system. In *Pathology of the Heart and Blood Vessels.* Third edition. Edited by SE Gould. Springfield, Illinois, Charles C Thomas, Publisher, 1968

84. Hirsch EF: Innervation of the human heart. III. The conductive system. *Arch Pathol* 74:427-439, 1962

85. Randall WC (ed): *Neural Regulation of the Heart.* New York, Oxford University Press, 1977

86. Levy MN, Martin PJ: Neural control of the heart. In *Handbook of Physiology. Section 2, The Cardiovascular System. Vol. I, The Heart,.* Edited by RM Berne, N Sperelakis, SR Geiger. Bethesda, Maryland, American Physiological Society, 1979, pp 581-620

87. Levitt B, Cagin N, Kleid J, et al: Role of the nervous system in the genesis of cardiac rhythm disorders. *Am J Cardiol* 37:1111-1113, 1976

88. Mason JW, Harrison DC: Electrophysiology and electropharmacology of the transplanted human heart. In *Cardiac Arrhythmia: Electrophysiology, Diagnosis and Management.* Edited by OS Narula. Baltimore, Williams & Wilkins Company, 1979, pp 66-81

89. Geis WP, Kaye MP, Randall WC: Major autonomic pathways to the atria and S-A and A-V nodes of the canine heart. *Am J Physiol* 224:202-208, 1973

90. Spear JF, Moore EN: Influence of brief vagal and stellate nerve stimulation on pacemaker activity and conduction within the atrioventricular conduction system of the dog. *Circ Res* 32:27-41, 1973

91. Meytles I, Kaplinsky E, Yahini JH, et al: Wenckebach A-V block: a frequent feature following heavy physical training. *Am Heart J* 90:426-430, 1975

92. DiMarco JP, Garan H, Harthorne JW, et al: Intracardiac electrophysiologic techniques in recurrent syncope of unknown cause. *Ann Intern Med* 95:542-548, 1981

93. Schlesinger Z, Barzilay J, Stryjer D, et al: Life-threatening "vagal reaction" to emotional stimuli. *Isr J Med Sci* 13:59-61, 1977

94. Lie KI, Durrer D: Acute and chronic aspects of conduction disturbances in acute myocardial infarction. In *Selected Topics in Cardiac Arrhythmias.* Edited by B Befeler, R Lazzara, BJ Scherlag. Mount Kisco, New York, Futura Publishing Company, 1980, pp 75-93

95. Sutton R, Davies M: The conduction system in acute myocardial infarction complicated by heart block. *Circulation* 38:987-992, 1968

96. Norris RM: Heart block in posterior and anterior myocardial infarction. *Br Heart J* 31:352-356, 1969

97. Davies MJ, Anderson RH, Becker AE: *The Conduction System of the Heart.* Boston, Butterworths, 1983, pp 9-94, 181-251, 281-300

98. Kostuk WJ, Beanlands DS: Complete heart block associated with acute myocardial infarction. *Am J Cardiol* 26:380-384, 1970

99. Brown RW, Hunt D, Sloman JG: The natural history of atrioventricular conduction defects in acute myocardial infarction. *Am Heart J* 78:460-466, 1969

100. Hunt D, Lie JT, Vohra J, et al: Histopathology of heart block complicating acute myocardial infarction: correlation with the His bundle electrogram. *Circulation* 48:1252-1261, 1973

101. Hackel DB, Estes EH Jr: Pathologic features of atrioventricular and intraventricular conduction disturbances in acute myocardial infarction. *Circulation* 43:977-979, 1971

102. Becker AE, Lie KI, Anderson RH: Bundle-branch block in the setting of acute anteroseptal myocardial infarction: clinicopathological correlation. *Br Heart J* 40:773-782, 1978

103. Childers R: The AV node: normal and abnormal physiology. *Prog Cardiovasc Dis* 19:361-364, 1977

104. Caracta AR, Damato AN, Gallagher JJ, et al: Electrophysiologic studies in the syndrome of short P-R interval, normal QRS complex. *Am J Cardiol* 31:245-253, 1973

105. Holmes DR Jr, Hartzler GO, Merideth J: The clinical and electrophysiologic characteristics of patients with accelerated atrioventricular nodal conduction. *Mayo Clin Proc* 57:339-344, 1982

106. Lev M, Silverman J, Fitzmaurice FM, et al: Lack of connection between the atria and the more peripheral conduction system in congenital atrioventricular block. *Am J Cardiol* 27:481-490, 1971

107. Lev M, Cuadros H, Paul MH: Interruption of the atrioventricular bundle with congenital atrioventricular block. *Circulation* 43:703-710, 1971

108. Anderson RH, Becker AE, Arnold R, et al: The conducting tissues in congenitally corrected transposition. *Circulation* 50:911-923, 1974

109. Kupersmith J, Krongrad E, Gersony WM, et al: Electrophysiologic identification of the specialized conduction system in corrected transposition of the great arteries. *Circulation* 50:795-800, 1974

110. Maloney JD, Ritter DG, McGoon DC, et al: Identification of the conduction system in corrected transposition and common ventricle at operation. *Mayo Clin Proc* 50:387-394, 1975

111. Rosenbaum MB, Elizari MV, Lazzari JO, et al: Intraventricular trifascicular blocks: review of the literature and classification. *Am Heart J* 78:450-459, 1969

112. Rosenbaum MB: The hemiblocks: diagnostic criteria and clinical significance. *Mod Concepts Cardiovasc Dis* 39:141-146, 1970

113. Massing GK, James TN: Anatomical configuration of the His bundle and bundle branches in the human heart. *Circulation* 53:609-621, 1976

114. Demoulin JC, Kulbertus HE: Histopathological examination of concept of left hemiblock. *Br Heart J* 34:807-814, 1972

115. Uhley HN: The quadrifascicular nature of the peripheral conduction system. In *Cardiac Arrhythmias.* Edited by LS Dreifus, W Liboff. New York, Grune & Stratton, 1973, pp 339-348

116. Uhley HN, Rivkin L: Peripheral distribution of the canine A-V conduction system: observations on gross morphology. *Am J Cardiol* 5:688-691, 1960

117. Uhley HN: Some controversy regarding the peripheral distribution of the conduction system (editorial). *Am J Cardiol* 30:919-920, 1972

118. Davies MJ, Anderson RH, Becker AE: *The Conduction System of the Heart.* Boston, Butterworths, 1983, pp 281-300

119. Demoulin JC, Kulbertus HE: Pathological basis of concept of left hemiblock. In *The Conduction System of the Heart: Structure, Function, and Clinical Implications.* Edited by HJJ Wellens, KI Lie, MJ Janse. Philadelphia, Lea & Febiger, 1976, pp 263-286

120. Myerburg RJ, Nilsson K, Gelband H: Physiology of the canine interventricular conduction system and endocardial excitation. *Circ Res* 30:217-243, 1972

121. Van Dam RTh: Ventricular activation in human and canine bundle branch block. In *The Conduction System of the Heart: Structure, Function and Clinical Implications.* Edited by HJJ Wellens, KI Lie, MJ Janse. Philadelphia, Lea & Febiger, 1976, pp 377-392

122. Roos JP, van Dam RTh, Durrer D: Epicardial and intramural excitation of normal heart in six patients 50 years of age and older. *Br Heart J* 30:630-637, 1968

123. Wyndham CB, Meeran MK, Smith T, et al: Epicardial activation of intact human heart without conduction defect. *Circulation* 59:161-168, 1979

124. Wiener I, Mindich B, Pitchon R, et al: Epicardial activation in patients with coronary artery disease: effects of regional contraction abnormalities. *Circulation* 65:154-160, 1982

125. Wyndham CRC, Smith T, Meeran MK, et al: Epicardial activation in patients with left bundle branch block. *Circulation* 61:696-703, 1980

126. Spielman SR, Untereker WJ, Horowitz LN, et al: Endocardial activation and refractoriness of the normal human left ventricle (abstract). *Am J Cardiol* 49:982, 1982

127. Myerburg RJ, Gelband H, Castellanos A Jr, et al: Electrophysiology of endocardial intraventricular conduction: the role and function of the specialized conducting system. In *The Conduction System of the Heart: Structure, Function and Clinical Implications.* Edited by HJJ Wellens, KI Lie, MJ Janse. Philadelphia, Lea & Febiger, 1976, pp 336-359

128. Nagao K, Toyama J, Kodama I, et al: Role of the conduction system in the endocardial excitation spread in the right ventricle. *Am J Cardiol* 48:864-870, 1981

129. Sommer JR, Johnson EA: Cardiac muscle: a comparative study of Purkinje fibers and ventricular fibers. *J Cell Biol* 36:497-526, 1968

130. Weidmann S: The diffusion of radiopotassium across intercalated disks of mammalian cardiac muscle. *J Physiol* 187:323-342, 1966

131. Watt TB Jr, Freud GE, Durrer D, et al: Left anterior arborization block combined with right bundle branch block in canine and primate hearts: an electrocardiographic study. *Circ Res* 22:57-63, 1968

132. Kulbertus HE, Demoulin JCI: Pathological basis of concept of left hemiblock. In *The Conduction System of the Heart: Structure, Function and Clinical Implications.* Edited by HJJ Wellens, KI Lie, MJ Janse. Philadelphia, Lea & Febiger, 1976, pp 287-295

133. Lenegre J: Etiology and pathology of bilateral bundle branch block in relation to complete heart block. *Prog Cardiovasc Dis* 6:409-444, 1964

134. Lev M: The pathology of complete atrioventricular block. *Prog Cardiovasc Dis* 6:317-326, 1964

135. Lev M: Anatomic basis for atrioventricular block. *Am J Med* 37:742-748, 1964

136. Gallagher JJ, Pritchett ELC, Sealy WC, et al: The preexcitation syndromes. *Prog Cardiovasc Dis* 20:285-327, 1978

137. Gallagher JJ, Gilbert M, Svenson RH, et al: Wolff-Parkinson-White syndrome: the problem, evaluation, and surgical correction. *Circulation* 51:767-785, 1975

138. Durrer D: Electrical aspects of human cardiac activity: a clinical-physiological approach to excitation and stimulation. *Cardiovasc Res* 2:1-18, 1968

139. Dreifus LS, Haiat R, Watanabe Y, et al: Ventricular fibrillation: a possible mechanism of sudden death in patients with Wolff-Parkinson-White syndrome. *Circulation* 43:520-527, 1971

140. Öhnell RF: Pre-excitation a cardiac abnormality: pathophysiological, patho-anatomical and clinical studies of an excitatory spread phenomenon bearing upon the problem of the WPW (Wolff, Parkinson and White) electrocardiogram and paroxysmal tachycardia. *Acta Med Scand [Suppl]* 152:1-167, 1944

141. Farshidi A, Josephson ME, Horowitz LN: Electrophysiologic characteristics of concealed bypass tracts: clinical and electrocardiographic correlates. *Am J Cardiol* 41:1052-1060, 1978

142. Gillette PC: Concealed anomalous cardiac conduction pathways: a frequent cause of supraventricular tachycardia. *Am J Cardiol* 40:848-852, 1977

143. Holmes DR Jr, Hartzler GO, Maloney JD: Concealed retrograde bypass tracts and enhanced atrioventricular nodal conduction: an unusual subset of patients with refractory paroxysmal supraventricular tachycardia. *Am J Cardiol* 45:1053-1060, 1980

144. Durrer D, Schuilenburg RM, Wellens HJJ: Pre-excitation revisited. *Am J Cardiol* 25:690-697, 1970

145. Benditt DG, Pritchett ELC, Gallagher JJ: Spectrum of regular tachycardias with wide QRS complexes in patients with accessory atrioventricular pathways. *Am J Cardiol* 42:828-838, 1978

146. Krahn AD, Manfreda J, Tate RB, et al: The natural history of electrocardiographic preexcitation in men: the Manitoba Follow-up Study. *Ann Intern Med* 116:456-460, 1992

147. Packer DL, Gallagher JJ, Prystowsky EN: Physiological substrate for antidromic reciprocating tachycardia: prerequisite characteristics of the accessory pathway and atrioventricular conduction system. *Circulation* 85:574-588, 1992

148. Chen P-S, Pressley JC, Tang ASL, et al: New observations on atrial fibrillation before and after surgical treatment in patients with the Wolff-Parkinson-White syndrome. *J Am Coll Cardiol* 19:974-981, 1992

149. Auricchio A, Klein H, Trappe HJ, et al: Lack of prognostic value of syncope in patients with Wolff-Parkinson-White syndrome. *J Am Coll Cardiol* 17:152-158, 1991

150. James TN: Syncope and sudden death in the Wolff-Parkinson-White syndrome. *J Am Coll Cardiol* 17:159-160, 1991

151. Fujimura O, Klein GJ, Yee R, et al: Mode of onset of atrial fibrillation in the Wolff-Parkinson-White syndrome: How important is the accessory pathway? *J Am Coll Cardiol* 15:1082-1086, 1990

152. Klein GJ, Bashore TM, Sellers TD, et al: Ventricular fibrillation in Wolff-Parkinson-White syndrome. *N Engl J Med* 301:1080-1085, 1979

153. Prystowsky EN, Fananapazir L, Packer DL, et al: Wolff-Parkinson-White syndrome and sudden cardiac death. *Cardiology* 74 Suppl 2:67-71, 1987

154. Sharma AD, Yee R, Guiraudon G, et al: Sensitivity and specificity of invasive and noninvasive testing for risk of sudden death in Wolff-Parkinson-White syndrome. *J Am Coll Cardiol* 10:373-381, 1987

155. Rossi L: Anatomic basis of pre-excitation. In *Selected Topics in Cardiac Arrhythmias.* Edited by B Befeler, R Lazzara, BJ Scherlag. Mount Kisco, New York, Futura Publishing Company, 1980, pp 261-275

156. Anderson RH, Becker AE, Brechenmacher C, et al: Ventricular preexcitation: a proposed nomenclature for its substrates. *Eur J Cardiol* 3:27-35, 1975

157. Sealy WC, Gallagher JJ: Surgical treatment of left free wall accessory pathways of atrioventricular conduction of the Kent type. *J Thorac Cardiovasc Surg* 81:698-706, 1981

158. Sealy WC, Gallagher JJ: Surgical problems with multiple accessory pathways of atrioventricular conduction. *J Thorac Cardiovasc Surg* 81:707-712, 1981

159. Sealy WC, Gallagher JJ: The surgical approach to the septal area of the heart based on experiences with 45 patients with Kent bundles. *J Thorac Cardiovasc Surg* 79:542-551, 1980

160. Becker AE, Anderson RH, Path MRC, et al: The anatomical substrates of Wolff-Parkinson-White syndrome: a clinicopathologic correlation in seven patients. *Circulation* 57:870-879, 1978

161. Anderson RH, Becker AE: Stanley Kent and accessory atrioventricular connection. *J Thorac Cardiovasc Surg* 81:649-658, 1981

162. Verduyn Lunel AA: Significance of annulus fibrosus of heart in relation to AV conduction and ventricular activation in cases of Wolff-Parkinson-White syndrome. *Br Heart J* 34:1263-1271, 1972

163. Fananapazir L, German LD, Gallagher JJ, et al: Importance of preexcited QRS morphology during induced atrial fibrillation to the diagnosis and localization of multiple accessory pathways. *Circulation* 81:578-585, 1990

164. Liebman J, Zeno JA, Olshansky B, et al: Electrocardiographic body surface potential mapping in the Wolff-Parkinson-White syndrome: noninvasive determination of the ventricular insertion sites of accessory atrioventricular connections. *Circulation* 83:886-901, 1991

165. Schlüter M, Geiger M, Siebels J, et al: Catheter ablation using radiofrequency current to cure symptomatic patients with tachyarrhythmias related to an accessory atrioventricular pathway. *Circulation* 84:1644-1661, 1991

166. Kuck K-H, Schlüter M: Single-catheter approach to radiofrequency current ablation of left-sided accessory pathways in patients with Wolff-Parkinson-White syndrome. *Circulation* 84:2366-2375, 1991

167. Schlüter M, Kuck K-H: Catheter ablation from right atrium of anteroseptal accessory pathways using radiofrequency current. *J Am Coll Cardiol* 19:663-670, 1992

168. Calkins H, Kim Y-N, Schmaltz S, et al: Electrogram criteria for identification of appropriate target sites for radiofrequency catheter ablation of accessory atrioventricular connections. *Circulation* 85:565-573, 1992

169. Calkins H, Langberg J, Sousa J, et al: Radiofrequency catheter ablation of accessory atrioventricular connections in 250 patients: abbreviated therapeutic approach to Wolff-Parkinson-White syndrome. *Circulation* 85:1337-1346, 1992

170. Anderson RH, Becker AE: Accessory atrioventricular connections (letter to the editor). *J Thorac Cardiovasc Surg* 78:310-311, 1979

171. Brechenmacher C: Atrio-His bundle tracts. *Br Heart J* 37:853-855, 1975

172. Ferrer MI: New concepts relating to the preexcitation syndrome. *JAMA* 201:1038-1039, 1967

173. Truex RC, Bishof JK, Hoffman EL: Accessory atrioventricular muscle bundles of the developing human heart. *Anat Rec* 131:45-59, 1958

174. Lev M, Fox SM III, Bharati S, et al: Mahaim fibers as a basis for a unique variety of preexcitation (abstract). *Am J Cardiol* 35:152, 1975

175. Sealy WC, Gallagher JJ, Pritchett ELC: The surgical anatomy of Kent bundles based on electrophysiological mapping and surgical exploration. *J Thorac Cardiovasc Surg* 76:804-814, 1978

176. Sealy WC, Gallagher JJ, Wallace AG: The surgical treatment of Wolff-Parkinson-White syndrome: evolution of improved methods for

identification and interruption of the Kent bundle. *Ann Thorac Surg* 22:443-457, 1976

177. Mahaim I: Kent's fibers and the A-V paraspecific conduction through the upper connections of the bundle of His-Tawara. *Am Heart J* 33:651-653, 1947

178. Gallagher JJ, Benditt D, Pritchett ELC, et al: Participation of Mahaim fibers in the genesis of cardiac dysrhythmias (abstract). *Circulation* 58 Suppl II:155, 1978

179. Gallagher JJ, Selle JG, Sealy WC, et al: Variants of preexcitation: update 1989. In *Cardiac Electrophysiology: From Cell to Bedside.* Edited by DP Zipes, J Jalife. Philadelphia, WB Saunders Company, 1990, pp 480-490

180. Tchou P, Lehmann MH, Jazayeri M, et al: Atriofascicular connection or a nodoventricular Mahaim fiber? Electrophysiologic elucidation of the pathway and associated reentrant circuit. *Circulation* 77:837-848, 1988

181. Lown B, Ganong WF, Levine SA: The syndrome of short P-R interval, normal QRS complex and paroxysmal rapid heart action. *Circulation* 5:693-706, 1952

182. Jackman WM, Prystowsky EN, Naccarelli GV, et al: Reevaluation of enhanced atrioventricular nodal conduction: evidence to suggest a continuum of normal atrioventricular nodal physiology. *Circulation* 67:441-448, 1983

183. Bernstein J: Untersuchungen zur Thermodynamik der bioelektrischen Ströme. *Arch Gesamte Physiol* 92:521-562, 1902

184. Cole KS, Marmont G: The effect of ionic environment upon the longitudinal impedance of the squid giant axon (abstract). *Fed Proc* 1:15-16, 1942

185. Hodgkin AL, Huxley AF: A quantitative description of membrane current and its application to conduction and excitation in nerve. *J Physiol* 117:500-544, 1952

186. Trautwein W: Membrane currents in cardiac muscle fibers. *Physiol Rev* 53:793-835, 1973

187. Cranefield PF: *The Conduction of the Cardiac Impulse.* Mount Kisco, New York, Futura Publishing Company, 1975

188. Goldman DE: Potential, impedance, and rectification in membranes. *J Gen Physiol* 27:37-60, 1943

189. Hodgkin AL, Katz B: The effect of sodium ions on the electrical activity of the giant axon of the squid. *J Physiol (Lond)* 108:37-77, 1949

190. Gadsby DC, Wit AL: Normal and abnormal electrophysiology of cardiac cells. In *Cardiac Arrhythmias: Their Mechanisms, Diagnosis, and Management.* Edited by WJ Mandel. Philadelphia, JB Lippincott Company, 1980, pp 55-82

191. Buchanan JW Jr, Saito T, Gettes LS: The effects of antiarrhythmic drugs, stimulation frequency, and potassium-induced resting membrane potential changes on conduction velocity and dV/dt_{max} in guinea pig myocardium. *Circ Res* 56:696-703, 1985

192. Packer DL, Grant AO, Strauss HC, et al: Characterization of concentration- and use-dependent effects of quinidine from conduction delay and declining conduction velocity in canine Purkinje fibers. *J Clin Invest* 83:2109-2119, 1989

193. Hoffman BF, Cranefield PF: The physiological basis of cardiac arrhythmias. *Am J Med* 37:670-684, 1964

194. Rosen MR, Wit AL, Hoffman BF: Electrophysiology and pharmacology of cardiac arrhythmias. I. Cellular electrophysiology of the mammalian heart. *Am Heart J* 88:380-385, 1974

195. Ten Eick RE, Baumgarten CM, Singer DH: Ventricular dysrhythmia: membrane basis of currents, channels, gates, and cables. *Prog Cardiovasc Dis* 24:157-188, 1981

196. Coraboeuf E: Ionic basis of electrical activity in cardiac tissues. *Am J Physiol* 234:H101-H116, 1978

197. Shen WK, Wharton JM, Strauss HC: Mechanisms of bradyarrhythmias and blocks. *Hosp Pract* 23 No. 7:93-110, 1988

198. Kenyon JL, Gibbons WR: Effects of low-chloride solutions on action potentials of sheep cardiac Purkinje fibers. *J Gen Physiol* 70:635-660, 1977

199. Fozzard HA: Cardiac muscle: excitability and passive electrical properties. *Prog Cardiovasc Dis* 19:343-359, 1977

200. Hauswirth O, Singh BN: Ionic mechanisms in heart muscle in relation to the genesis and the pharmacological control of cardiac arrhythmias. *Pharmacol Rev* 30:5-63, 1978

201. Reuter H: Divalent cations as charge carriers in excitable membranes. *Prog Biophys Mol Biol* 26:1-43, 1973

202. Zipes DP, Mendez C: Action of manganese ions and tetrodotoxin on atrioventricular nodal transmembrane potentials in isolated rabbit hearts. *Circ Res* 32:447-454, 1973

203. Zipes DP, Bailey JC, Elharrar V: *The Slow Inward Current and Cardiac Arrhythmias.* The Hague, Boston, Martinus Nijhoff, 1980

204. Reuter H: The dependence of slow inward current in Purkinje fibres on the extracellular calcium-concentration. *J Physiol (Lond)* 192:479-492, 1967

205. Noble D, Tsien RW: Outward membrane currents activated in the plateau range of potentials in cardiac Purkinje fibres. *J Physiol (Lond)* 200:205-231, 1969

206. Coraboeuf E, Deroubaix E, Coulombe A: Effects of tetrodotoxin on action potentials of the conducting system in the dog heart. *Am J Physiol* 236:H561-H567, 1979

207. Beeler GW, Reuter H: Reconstruction of the action potential of ventricular myocardial fibres. *J Physiol (Lond)* 268:177-210, 1977

208. McAllister RE, Noble D, Tsien RW: Reconstruction of the electrical activity of cardiac Purkinje fibres. *J Physiol (Lond)* 251:1-59, 1975

209. DiFrancesco D: A new interpretation of the pace-maker current in calf Purkinje fibers. *J Physiol (Lond)* 314:359-376, 1981

210. DiFrancesco D: A study of the ionic nature of the pace-maker current in calf Purkinje fibres. *J Physiol (Lond)* 314:377-393, 1981

211. Cleemann L, Morad M: Extracellular potassium accumulation and inward-going potassium rectification in voltage clamped ventricular muscle. *Science* 191:90-92, 1976

212. Tsien RW, Carpenter DO: Ionic mechanisms of pacemaker activity in cardiac Purkinje fibers. *Fed Proc* 37:2127-2131, 1978

213. Yanagihara K, Irisawa H: Inward current activated during hyperpolarization in the rabbit sinoatrial node cell. *Pflugers Arch* 385:11-19, 1980

214. Noma A, Irisawa H: A time- and voltage-dependent potassium current in the rabbit sinoatrial node cell. *Pflugers Arch* 366:251-258, 1976

215. Vassalle M: Analysis of cardiac pacemaker potential using a "voltage clamp" technique. *Am J Physiol* 210:1335-1341, 1966

216. Singer DH, Ten Eick RE: Chronic dysrhythmias: a new look at old questions. *Prog Cardiovasc Dis* 24:91-96, 1981

217. Wit AL, Rosen MR, Hoffman BF: Electrophysiology and pharmacology of cardiac arrhythmias. II. Relationship of normal and abnormal electrical activity of cardiac fibers to the genesis of arrhythmias. A. Automaticity. *Am Heart J* 88:515-524, 1974

218. Cranefield PF: Action potentials, afterpotentials, and arrhythmias. *Circ Res* 41:415-423, 1977

219. Wit AL, Cranefield PF: Triggered activity in cardiac muscle fibers of the simian mitral valve. *Circ Res* 38:85-98, 1976

220. Wit AL, Cranefield PF: Triggered and automatic activity in the canine coronary sinus. *Circ Res* 41:435-445, 1977

221. Wit AL, Rosen MR, Hoffman BF: Electrophysiology and pharmacology of cardiac arrhythmias. II. Relationship of normal and abnormal electrical activity of cardiac fibers to the genesis of arrhythmias. B. Re-entry. Section II. *Am Heart J* 88:798-806, 1974

222. Cranefield PF, Wit AL: Cardiac arrhythmias. *Annu Rev Physiol* 41:459-472, 1979

223. Hoffman BF: Experiments on abnormal automaticity. In *Frontiers of Cardiac Electrophysiology.* Edited by MB Rosenbaum, MV Elizari. The Hague, Martinus Nijhoff, 1983, pp 144-157

224. Noble D: The surprising heart: a review of recent progress in cardiac electrophysiology. *J Physiol (Lond)* 353:1-50, 1984

225. Singer DH, Ten Eick RE, DeBoer AA: Electrophysiologic correlates of human atrial tachyarrhythmias. In *Cardiac Arrhythmias.* Edited by LS Dreifus, W Likoff. New York, Grune & Stratton, 1973, pp 97-111

226. Ten Eick RE, Singer DH: Electrophysiological properties of diseased human atrium. I. Low diastolic potential and altered cellular response to potassium. *Circ Res* 44:545-557, 1979

227. Chua WT, Singer DH, Ten Eick RE: Ventricular dysrhythmia in man: cellular electrophysiologic aspects (abstract). *Clin Res* 29:181A, 1981

228. Wit AL, Boyden PA, Gadsby DC, et al: Triggered activity as a cause of atrial arrhythmias. In *Cardiac Arrhythmias: Electrophysiology, Diagnosis and Management.* Edited by OS Narula. Baltimore, Williams & Wilkins Company, 1979, pp 14-31

229. Rosen MR, Fisch C, Hoffman BF, et al: Can accelerated atrioventricular junctional escape rhythms be explained by delayed afterdepolarizations? *Am J Cardiol* 45:1272-1284, 1980

230. Rosen MR, Wit AL: Triggered activity. *Prog Cardiol* 1:39-46, 1988

231. Damiano BP, Rosen MR: Effects of pacing on triggered activity induced by early afterdepolarizations. *Circulation* 69:1013-1025, 1984

232. Levine JH, Spear JF, Guarnieri T, et al: Cesium chloride-induced long QT syndrome: demonstration of afterdepolarizations and triggered activity in vivo. *Circulation* 72:1092-1103, 1985

233. Brachmann J, Scherlag BJ, Rosenshtraukh LV, et al: Bradycardia-dependent triggered activity: relevance to drug-induced multiform ventricular tachycardia. *Circulation* 68:846-856, 1983

234. January CT, Riddle JM: Early afterdepolarizations: mechanism of induction and block: a role for L-type Ca^{2+} current. *Circ Res* 64:977-990, 1989

235. Davidenko JM, Cohen L, Goodrow R, et al: Quinidine-induced action potential prolongation, early afterdepolarizations, and triggered activity in canine Purkinje fibers: effects of stimulation rate, potassium, and magnesium. *Circulation* 79:674-686, 1989

236. Ferrier GR: Digitalis arrhythmias: role of oscillatory afterpotentials. *Prog Cardiovasc Dis* 19:459-474, 1977

237. Ferrier GR, Saunders JH, Mendez C: A cellular mechanism for the generation of ventricular arrhythmias by acetylstrophanthidin. *Circ Res* 32:600-609, 1973

238. Cranefield PF, Aronson RW: *Cardiac Arrhythmias: the Role of Triggered Activity and Other Mechanisms.* Mount Kisco, New York, Futura Publishing Company, 1988

239. January CT, Fozzard HA: Delayed afterdepolarizations in heart muscle: mechanisms and relevance. *Pharmacol Rev* 40:219-227, 1988

240. Attwell D, Cohen I, Eisner D, et al: The steady state TTX-sensitive ("window") sodium current in cardiac Purkinje fibres. *Pflugers Arch* 379:137-142, 1979

241. Coulombe A, Coraboeuf E, Malecot C, et al: Role of the Na window current and ionic currents in triggering early afterdepolarizations and resulting re-excitations in Purkinje fibers. In *Cardiac Electrophysiology and Arrhythmias.* Edited by DP Zipes, J Jalife. Orlando, Florida, Grune & Stratton, 1985, pp 43-49

242. Leichter DA, Danilo P, Rosen T, et al: Torsades de pointes induced by aconitine and quinidine in the canine heart (abstract). *Circulation* 74 Suppl 2:349, 1986

243. Aronson RS: Afterpotentials and triggered activity in hypertrophied myocardium from rats with renal hypertension. *Circ Res* 48:720-726, 1981

244. El-Sherif N, Gough WB, Zeiler RH, et al: Triggered ventricular rhythms in 1-day-old myocardial infarction in the dog. *Circ Res* 52:566-579, 1983

245. Nordin C, Gilat E, Aronson RS: Delayed afterdepolarizations and triggered activity in ventricular muscle from rats with streptozotocin-induced diabetes. *Circ Res* 57:28-34, 1985

246. Rosen MR, Gelband H, Merker C, et al: Mechanisms of digitalis toxicity: effect of ouabain of phase four of canine Purkinje fiber transmembrane potentials. *Circulation* 47:681-689, 1973

247. Hashimoto K, Moe GK: Transient depolarizations induced by acetylstrophanthidin in specialized tissue of dog atrium and ventricle. *Circ Res* 32:618-624, 1973

248. Henning B, Kline RP, Siegal MS, et al: Triggered activity in atrial fibres of canine coronary sinus: role of extracellular potassium accumulation and depletion. *J Physiol* 383:191-211, 1987

249. Eisner DA, Lederer WJ: Inotropic and arrhythmogenic effects of potassium-depleted solutions on mammalian cardiac muscle. *J Physiol* 294:255-277, 1979

250. Lipsius SL, Gibbons WR: Membrane currents, contractions, and aftercontractions in cardiac Purkinje fibers. *Am J Physiol* 243:H77-H86, 1982

251. Wit AL, Cranefield PF, Gadsby DC: Electrogenic sodium extrusion can stop triggered activity in the canine coronary sinus. *Circ Res* 49:1029-1042, 1981

252. Tseng G-N, Wit AL: Characteristics of a transient inward current that causes delayed afterdepolarizations in atrial cells of the canine coronary sinus. *J Molec Cell Cardiol* 19:1105-1119, 1987

253. Lederer WJ, Tsien RW: Transient inward current underlying arrhythmogenic effects of cardiogenic steroids in Purkinje fibres. *J Physiol* 263:73-100, 1976

254. Vassalle M, Mugelli A: An oscillatory current in sheep cardiac Purkinje fibers. *Circ Res* 48:618-631, 1981

255. Karagueuzian HS, Katzung BG: Voltage-clamp studies of transient inward current and mechanical oscillations induced by ouabain in ferret papillary muscle. *J Physiol* 327:255-271, 1982

256. Lerman BB, Belardinelli L, West GA, et al: Adenosine-sensitive ventricular tachycardia: evidence suggesting cyclic AMP-mediated triggered activity. *Circulation* 74:270-280, 1986

257. Lerman BB, Belardinelli L: Cardiac electrophysiology of adenosine: basic and clinical concepts. *Circulation* 83:1499-1509, 1991

258. Wit AL, Rosen MR: Afterdepolarizations and triggered activity: distinction from automaticity as in arrhythmogenic mechanism. In *The Heart and Cardiovascular System: Scientific Foundations.* Vol. 2. Second edition. Edited by HA Fozzard, E Haber, RB Jennings, et al. New York, Raven Press, 1993, pp 2113-2164

259. Allessie MA, Bonke FIM, Schopman FJG: Circus movement in rabbit atrial muscle as a mechanism of tachycardia. III. The "leading circle" concept: a new model of circus movement in cardiac tissue without the involvement of an anatomical obstacle. *Circ Res* 41:9-18, 1977

260. Allessie MA, Bonke FIM: Atrial arrhythmias: basic concepts. In *Cardiac Arrhythmias: Their Mechanisms, Diagnosis, and Management.* Edited by WJ Mandel. Philadelphia, JB Lippincott Company, 1980, pp 145-166

261. Binah O, Rosen MR: Mechanisms of ventricular arrhythmias. *Circulation* 85 Suppl 1:25-31, 1992

262. Moe GK, Mendez C: The physiologic basis of reciprocal rhythm. *Prog Cardiovasc Dis* 8:461-482, 1966

263. Moe GK, Preston JB, Burlington H: Physiologic evidence for a dual A-V transmission system. *Circ Res* 4:357-375, 1956

264. Josephson ME, Seides SF: *Clinical Cardiac Electrophysiology: Techniques and Interpretations.* Philadelphia, Lea & Febiger, 1979, pp 147-190

265. Wit AL, Hoffman BF, Cranefield PF: Slow conduction and reentry in the ventricular conduction system. I. Return extrasystole in canine Purkinje fibers. *Circ Res* 30:1-10, 1972

266. Cranefield PF, Klein HO, Hoffman BF: Conduction of the cardiac impulse. I. Delay, block, and one-way block in depressed Purkinje fibers. *Circ Res* 28:199-219, 1971

267. Wit AL, Cranefield PF, Hoffman BF: Slow conduction and reentry in the ventricular conduction system. II. Single and sustained circus movement in networks of canine and bovine Purkinje fibers. *Circ Res* 30:11-22, 1972

268. Antzelevitch C, Jalife J, Moe GK: Characteristics of reflection as a mechanism of reentrant arrhythmias and its relationship to parasystole. *Circulation* 61:182-191, 1980

269. Singer DH, Lazzara R, Hoffman BF: Interrelationships between automaticity and conduction in Purkinje fibers. *Circ Res* 21:537-558, 1967

270. Pick A: The electrophysiologic basis of parasystole and its variants. In *The Conduction System of the Heart: Structure, Function and Clinical Implications.* Edited by HJJ Wellens, KI Lie, MJ Janse. Philadelphia, Lea & Febiger, 1976, pp 143-162

271. Saunders JH, Ferrier GR, Moe GK: Conduction block associated with transient depolarizations induced by acetylstrophanthidin in isolated canine Purkinje fibers. *Circ Res* 32:610-617, 1973

272. El-Sherif N: The ventricular premature complex: mechanisms and significance. In *Cardiac Arrhythmias: Their Mechanisms, Diagnosis, and Management.* Edited by WJ Mandel. Philadelphia, JB Lippincott Company, 1980, pp 288-319

273. Lazzara R, El-Sherif N, Scherlag BJ: Electrophysiological properties of canine Purkinje cells in one-day-old myocardial infarction. *Circ Res* 33:722-734, 1973

274. Hoffman BF: The electrophysiology of heart muscle and the genesis of arrhythmias. In *Mechanisms and Therapy of Cardiac Arrhythmias.* Edited by LS Dreifus, W Likoff, JH Moyer. New York, Grune & Stratton, 1966, pp 27-34

275. Scherf D, Blumenfeld S, Yildiz M: Extrasystoles and parasystole. *Am Heart J* 64:357-363, 1962

276. Scherf D, Choi K-H, Bahadori A, et al: Parasystole. *Am J Cardiol* 12:527-538, 1963

277. Trautwein W: Mechanism of tachyarrhythmias and extrasystoles. In *Symposium on Cardiac Arrhythmias.* Edited by E Sandoe, E Flensted-Jensen, K Olesen. Sweden, Astra AB, 1970, p 53

CHAPTER

22

Cardiac arrhythmias

B. Supraventricular arrhythmias

Douglas L. Wood, M.D., Stephen C. Hammill, M.D., and Stephen L. Kopecky, M.D.

THE term "supraventricular arrhythmia" refers to a diverse group of abnormal rhythms ranging from chronic atrial fibrillation to paroxysmal sinus tachycardia due to reentry within the sinus node (Fig 22B-1). Although supraventricular tachycardia can be broadly defined as any tachycardia requiring the atrium or the atrioventricular (AV) node, either in whole or in part, for its perpetuation, more specific definitions will be provided for each of the common supraventricular arrhythmias. The atrial arrhythmias vary considerably in their rate and regularity, their clinical manifestations, and the setting in which they occur. These rhythms are characteristically abrupt in onset and termination and are often seen in patients who do not have evidence of organic heart disease. Although these disturbances in rhythm are generally benign, in patients with organic heart disease a rapid supraventricular rhythm may produce significant hemodynamic complications. In some patients with preexcitation syndromes and antegrade conduction down an accessory pathway, there is a distinct risk of sudden death.

Two major groups are included in the broad classification of supraventricular arrhythmia. The first is paroxysmal tachycardia and the second is atrial flutter-fibrillation. These two groups often have different anatomic and physiologic substrates, respond differently to therapeutic regimens, and often occur in different clinical settings. This chapter includes discussions of paroxysmal supraventricular tachycardia and of atrial flutter and fibrillation. The various types of tachycardia are defined in appropriate parts of the chapter. That component of supraventricular arrhythmias characterized by bradycardia is dealt with in the chapters on syncope, sudden death, and pacing (see chapters 23, 24A, and 25A, respectively).

PATHOPHYSIOLOGY OF SUPRAVENTRICULAR TACHYCARDIA

The systemic and cardiac diseases associated with supraventricular tachycardia are listed in Table 22B-1. Cardiac diseases include coronary artery disease,[1-4] congenital heart disease,[3,4] infectious and inflammatory diseases,[3,4] and cardiomyopathy and pericardial diseases.[3,4] Systemic disorders include pulmonary disease, neoplastic disease, metabolic disorders and electrolyte imbalance, and treatment with certain drugs.[3,4] In addition, a substantial number of patients with supraventricular tachycardia have no identifiable heart disease.

DIAGNOSIS OF SUPRAVENTRICULAR TACHYCARDIA

Definition of supraventricular tachycardia

Supraventricular tachycardia is defined electrocardiographically as a regular tachycardia of 140 to 240 beats/min, during which the QRS is of normal duration unless bundle-branch block is present. This tachycardia has been given many names, including paroxysmal supraventricular tachycardia, paroxysmal atrial tachycardia, and others (see Fig 22B-1). In this chapter, the term "supraventricular tachycardia" is used to describe any tachycardia that meets the electrocardiographic (ECG) definitions that have been mentioned. This does not include atrial flutter, which, although a regular tachycardia, is considered elsewhere in the chapter. In addition, this definition of supraventricular tachycardia excludes the irregularly irregular rhythm of atrial fibrillation, which is also discussed in another section. When P waves are identifiable, the P-wave morphology is often different from sinus P-wave morphology, and the P wave may precede, coincide with, or follow the QRS complex.

Clinically, supraventricular tachycardia is characterized by the sudden onset of a rapid, regular heart rate with termination that is equally abrupt, often after the performance of vagal maneuvers. Presyncope and syncope are other manifestations of supraventricular tachycardia. Symptoms reported by the patient or clinical signs that are present depend on associated clinical problems, specifically, the presence of associated cardiopulmonary disease.

Historical features

The historical details of the tachycardia or the details of symptoms of palpitations provided by the patient can

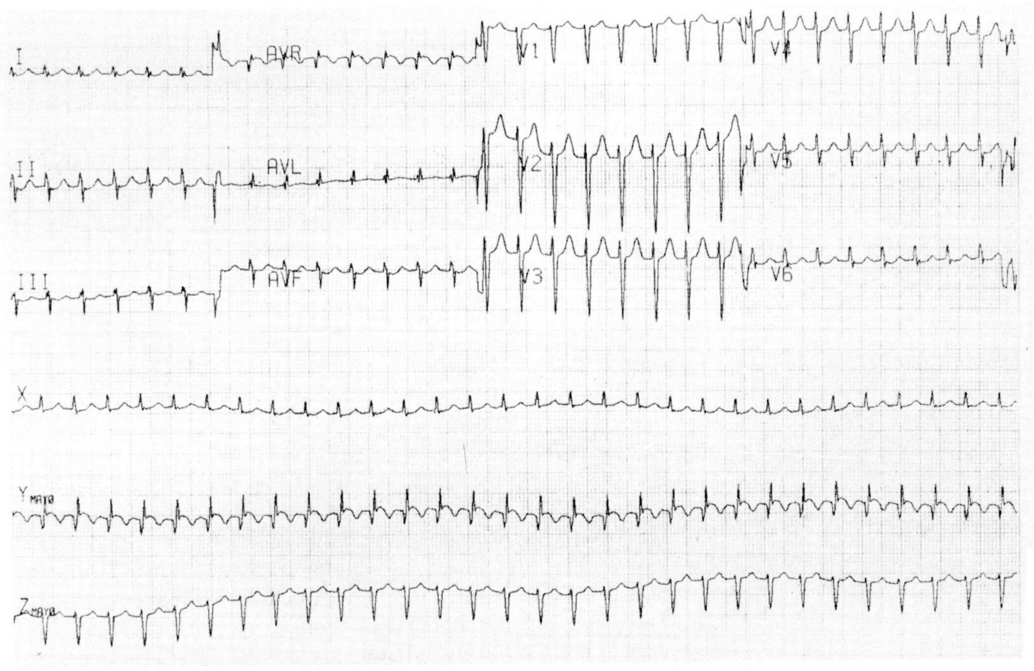

Fig 22B-1 Paroxysmal supraventricular tachycardia. ECG recording of supraventricular tachycardia also described as paroxysmal atrial tachycardia, atrial tachycardia, sinoatrial (SA node) reentry tachycardia, intra-atrial reentry tachycardia, AV node reentry tachycardia, reciprocating tachycardia, circus movement tachycardia, AV reentry tachycardia, and orthodromic AV reentry tachycardia.

Table 22B-1 Cardiac and systemic disorders that influence supraventricular tachycardias

Cardiac diseases

- Coronary artery disease
  - Angina (primary and secondary)
  - Acute myocardial infarction
- Congenital heart disease
  - Atrial septal defect
  - Ebstein's anomaly
  - Transposition of the great arteries
- Carditis
  - Viral myocarditis
  - Rheumatic carditis
  - Infective endocarditis
  - Collagen vascular disease
  - Sarcoid
- Cardiomyopathy
- Pericardial disease
- Mitral valve disease
- After cardiac surgery

Systemic disorders

- Chest trauma with myocardial contusion
- After thoracic or cardiac surgery
- Neoplasia
  - Leukemia
  - Lymphoma
  - Breast cancer
- Toxic exposure
  - Theophylline-like compounds
  - Catecholamines
  - Anticholinergic compounds
  - Digoxin
  - Stimulants, including alcohol, tobacco, and proprietary drugs
- Pulmonary diseases
  - Acute pneumonia
  - Chronic obstructive lung disease
- Metabolic and electrolyte disorders
  - Thyrotoxicosis
  - Pheochromocytoma
  - Hypokalemia

contribute greatly to the evaluation of patients with supraventricular tachycardia.

Objectives of the evaluation of supraventricular tachycardia are first to confirm the presence of and determine the mechanism for an arrhythmia and then to determine whether the arrhythmia is related to any precipitating factors that might be important in treatment. Another objective is to determine the functional consequences of the arrhythmia—specifically, its association with presyncope or syncope, fatigue, dyspnea, or chest pain. These aspects of the patient's clinical history will largely determine the extent and sequence of special diagnostic studies, including electrophysiologic studies. Finally, the frequency of the arrhythmia is important in deciding on the management of supraventricular tachycardias. Characteristically, these rhythms vary significantly over time, and these variations are critical to an understanding of the effects of therapy.

Electrocardiographic recording

Clearly the most important diagnostic test in the evaluation of patients with supraventricular tachycardia is an ECG recording during the tachycardia. These recordings can be obtained by ambulatory ECG, telephone transmitters, rhythm strips recorded in the office, or in-hospital ECG monitoring. For optimal rhythm analysis of ECGs, extreme care should be exercised to record distinct atrial and ventricular activity; also, a long, continuous rhythm strip made during an arrhythmia should be available for analysis. A 12-lead ECG should be recorded during tachycardia, and a long rhythm strip can be obtained by using the lead displaying the best atrial and ventricular activities.

Physiologic maneuvers used in association with an ECG recording can be very useful in the diagnosis of supraventricular tachycardia. The most common maneuver is carotid sinus massage. External pressure applied to the carotid artery with a gentle massaging motion will stimulate the baroreceptors of the carotid sinus and cause a significant increase in vagal tone. Increased vagal tone influences the AV node by prolonging AV nodal conduction and refractoriness, thereby facilitating the recognition of P waves that were not previously apparent. The most important application of carotid sinus massage is, in fact, to assist in the diagnosis of a rapid, regular tachycardia in which P waves are not easily seen.

Carotid sinus massage must be performed carefully, for it is not without significant risk, especially in elderly patients. Patients should be positioned supine with the neck relaxed. The head is then turned to the left for massage of the right carotid artery. If no response has been elicited after 10 to 20 seconds of very light massage, firmer pressure is exerted, but for no longer than 5 seconds. If no response is observed after several attempts on one side, the other side may be tried. One should never perform simultaneous massage of both carotid arteries.

Significant complications of carotid sinus massage include syncope, convulsions, stroke, prolonged asystole, ventricular tachyarrhythmias, and adverse hemodynamic reflexes.[5-7] Carotid sinus massage should therefore be avoided in patients with known cerebrovascular disease or with symptoms that suggest cerebrovascular disease, especially involving the external carotid arteries. Patients who have sick sinus syndrome may experience prolonged sinus arrest after the conversion of supraventricular tachycardia to sinus rhythm. Therefore, if the history suggests sick sinus syndrome, specifically with symptoms of syncope or presyncope, carotid sinus massage should be performed with extreme caution.

The general response of sinus tachycardia to carotid sinus massage is a gradual slowing of the rate before resumption of the premassage rate. Characteristically, supraventricular tachycardia due to reentry within the AV node or to utilization of an accessory pathway demonstrates an all-or-none effect, either terminating abruptly or changing little or not at all (Fig 22B-2). In atrial flutter, the degree of AV block is increased with carotid sinus massage, which allows better visualization of flutter waves.

Adenosine may be useful in differentiating atrial flutter with 2:1 AV conduction from supraventricular tachycardia and sinus tachycardia. Most supraventricular tachycardias in which the AV node is a critical part of the reentrant circuit are terminated by an intravenous injection of adenosine. Atrial flutter can be recognized when adenosine creates transient heart block and flutter waves become obvious. Adenosine may terminate other atrial arrhythmias, especially sinus node reentry tachycardia.[8]

Special procedures for detection of atrial activation

Since accurate analysis of the rhythm strip obtained from a patient with supraventricular tachycardia requires identification of atrial activity, any circumstance in which P waves are not easily identifiable from the surface tracing will make diagnosis virtually impossible. This is especially important when trying to differentiate supraventricular tachycardia with aberrant ventricular conduction from ventricular tachycardia. Therefore, concerted attempts must always be made to identify P waves. When standard ECG recording techniques fail to provide easily recognizable atrial activity, it may be necessary to place special electrodes. A common lead orientation used in this circumstance is the Lewis lead, in which the right and left arm leads are positioned in the second and fourth intercostal spaces, respectively, just to the right of the sternum. If this maneuver fails to identify distinct P waves, the right and left arm leads then may be moved empirically to the right and left of the sternum in an attempt to record adequate P waves. Then lead I is recorded, preferably in association with another lead that displays a clear QRS complex.

When surface recordings, including special lead orientations, fail to provide clear records of P-wave activity, esophageal recording of atrial activity should be considered. Bipolar electrodes can be placed in the lower esophagus so that they lie just behind the left atrium. A bipolar electrode or an appropriately filtered unipolar electrode so placed will detect a very prominent deflection during atrial depolarization. The development of newer

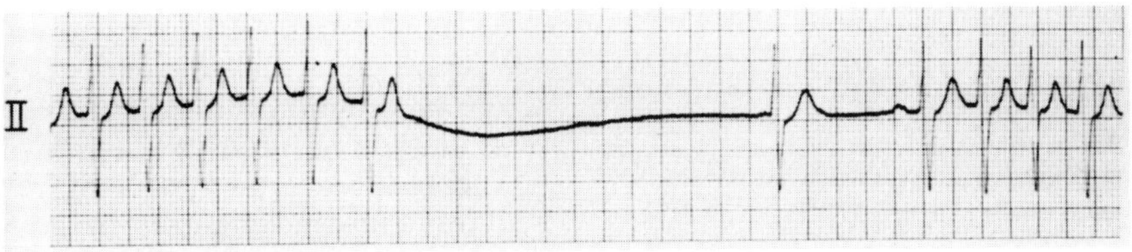

Fig 22B-2 Supraventricular tachycardia with a rate of approximately 165 beats/min is transiently terminated by carotid sinus massage.

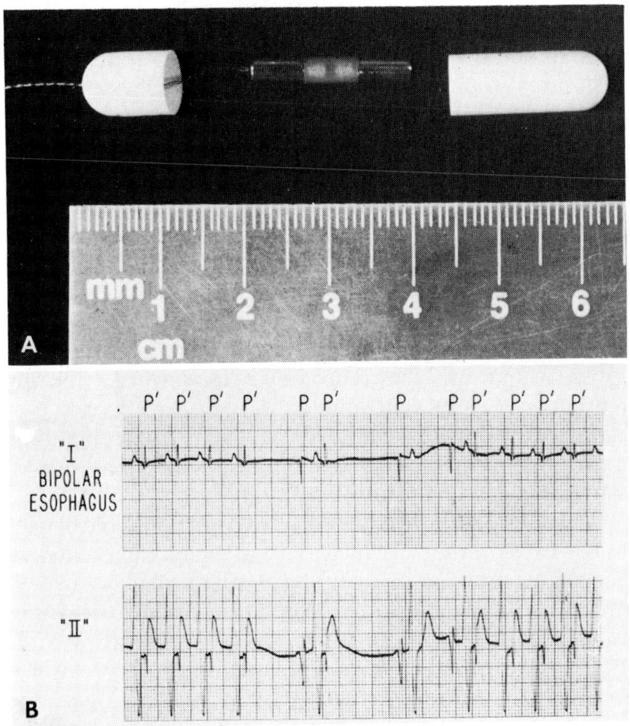

Fig 22B-3 Esophageal recording techniques. **A,** esophageal pill electrode originally described by Arzbaecher.[10] **B,** bipolar esophageal recording from a patient with paroxysmal AV tachycardia that utilizes a concealed accessory pathway. The bipolar esophageal lead recorded simultaneously with lead II during tachycardia clearly identifies retrograde P waves (P′) with a VA interval of approximately 150 msec. (From Hammill SC, Pritchett ELC: Dynamic electrocardiography in the investigation of supraventricular tachycardia and tachycardia associated with pre-excitation syndromes. In *Dynamic Electrocardiography.* Edited by R Campbell, A Murray. Edinburgh, Churchill Livingstone, 1985, pp 74-88. By permission.)

esophageal electrode recording techniques has made esophageal electrocardiography much easier[9] (Fig 22B-3). A convenient and readily available esophageal electrode is the permanent coronary sinus pacing electrode. This lead has an optimal interelectrode distance, is small and flexible, and has a small "leader" that facilitates passage intranasally. If esophageal electrode recordings fail to help in the diagnosis of supraventricular tachycardia, the use of more invasive ECG recording techniques will be necessary.

Table 22B-2 Indications for electrophysiologic testing in patients with supraventricular tachycardia

Narrow-complex tachycardia and significant associated symptoms with need for urgent effective therapy
Narrow-complex tachycardia refractory to standard therapy
Intractable tachycardia considered for antitachycardia pacing, catheter ablation, or surgical therapy
Preexcitation syndromes
Wide-complex tachycardia
Atrial flutter or fibrillation with rapid antegrade conduction down the accessory pathway

Atrial activity during supraventricular tachycardia can be recorded by passing an electrode catheter to the atrium from percutaneous entry into a vein in the antecubital fossa, the internal jugular vein, the subclavian vein, or a femoral vein. An electrode catheter positioned in the right atrium may also be used for programmed stimulation in the treatment of certain rhythm disorders.

Electrophysiologic study. The electrophysiologic evaluation of supraventricular tachycardia involves recording electrograms from the right atrium, right ventricle, region of the His bundle, and coronary sinus during programmed stimulation and during tachycardia (see chapter 22D). The goals of electrophysiologic study are to determine the mechanism of the tachycardia, its site of origin, the tissues used to sustain the tachycardia, and the potential benefit of alternative therapeutic approaches, including antiarrhythmia drugs, antitachycardia pacing systems, catheter ablation, and surgery.

Electrophysiologic investigations are indicated (Table 22B-2) for patients who have significant symptoms associated with supraventricular tachycardia, including presyncope and syncope; patients with preexcitation syndromes in whom atrial fibrillation with rapid ventricular response develops; patients who have tachycardia that has proved refractory to empiric therapy with antiarrhythmia drugs, to allow evaluation of further drug therapy or alternative therapeutic techniques; and patients with tachycardias who are considered candidates for catheter ablation or surgical treatment.

Table 22B-3 Treatment of supraventricular tachycardia

Arrhythmia	First-choice therapy	Alternative therapy
SA node reentry	β-Blockers	Calcium channel blockers
Intra-atrial reentry	Quinidine Disopyramide	Flecainide Propafenone Sotalol
	Procainamide	Radiofrequency ablation Electrosurgery
Automatic atrial	Quinidine Disopyramide	Flecainide Propafenone Sotalol
	Procainamide	Radiofrequency ablation
	Calcium blocker β-Blocker	Electrosurgery
AV node reentry	Radiofrequency ablation AV node blocking drugs	Flecainide Sotalol Electrosurgery
AV reentry	Radiofrequency ablation	Disopyramide
	AV node blocking drugs	Quinidine Procainamide Flecainide Propafenone Sotalol Amiodarone Electrosurgery
Atrial flutter*	Quinidine Procainamide Disopyramide	Flecainide Propafenone Amiodarone Electrosurgery Catheter ablation and pacing†
Atrial fibrillation*	Quinidine Procainamide	Flecainide Propafenone Sotalol
	Disopyramide	Amiodarone Electrosurgery Catheter ablation and pacing†

*The drugs listed are used to prevent paroxysms, and AV node blocking drugs are usually required in addition to control ventricular rate.
†Catheter ablation and permanent pacing are generally used only for control of ventricular rate. It may be possible to cure type I atrial flutter with catheter ablation.

GENERAL PRINCIPLES OF THE TREATMENT OF SUPRAVENTRICULAR TACHYCARDIA

Advances in the pharmacology of antiarrhythmia drugs and refinements in catheter ablation techniques have considerably altered our ability to treat arrhythmias. A large number of patients are treated without electrophysiologic studies, and in most of these circumstances treatment continues to be based on ECG rhythm strips. This method is successful in most patients.

Successful treatment of supraventricular tachycardias requires that the physician be knowledgeable regarding the mechanism and cause of the arrhythmia, the effect of the arrhythmia on the patient's cardiac function, the natural history of the arrhythmia, and the various forms of therapy that are available. Although some patients will be asymptomatic during the episodes of the arrhythmia, more often symptoms are present, and there may be significant potential for sudden death or severe deterioration in hemodynamic stability during these episodes. In most cases, then, the goal of treatment is to restore or maintain sinus rhythm while reducing the frequency of the tachycardia (Table 22B-3). If the tachycardia cannot be completely abolished, control of the ventricular rate during episodes of tachycardia becomes an important goal.

Treatment of cardiac arrhythmias depends first of all on careful diagnosis. Although many patients may complain of palpitations or rapid heart action, the physician must confirm whether a tachycardia is, in fact, present. This may be accomplished by recording a standard ECG during tachycardia, using an ambulatory ECG, recording a rhythm strip during tachycardia, using a transtelephonic monitoring system, or observing the patient in a hospital with continuous ECG monitoring.

A careful search should be made for the possible causes of an arrhythmia or factors that may aggravate it. Electrolyte imbalance, acid-base disturbances, hypoxemia, drug intoxication or other drug effect, coexistent diseases of the heart or lungs, or even central nervous system abnormalities should be sought and corrected if possible. In many of these circumstances, once the underlying cause of the arrhythmia has been corrected, long-term treatment of the arrhythmia is not needed. In some circumstances, particularly in elderly patients with thyrotoxicosis, a cardiac arrhythmia may be an early or the only manifestation of the underlying disorder. In this circumstance, treatment of the hyperthyroidism is clearly superior to attempts to suppress the atrial fibrillation with a rapid ventricular response with digoxin or propranolol.

The development of radiofrequency catheter ablation for supraventricular arrhythmias has changed the practice of cardiac electrophysiology. It is now feasible to consider a combined diagnostic and therapeutic electrophysiologic procedure rather than a staged approach with separate diagnostic studies followed by serial drug testing, antitachycardia pacing, or surgical therapy. Combined diagnostic and therapeutic procedures are safe and when used early cure tachycardia and eliminate the need for potentially risky lifelong antiarrhythmic drug treatment.[11] This approach also minimizes risk and expense to the patient.

SPECIFIC TREATMENT OF ACUTE NARROW-COMPLEX QRS TACHYCARDIA

Acute supraventricular tachycardia with a QRS complex of normal morphology is a common arrhythmia, which

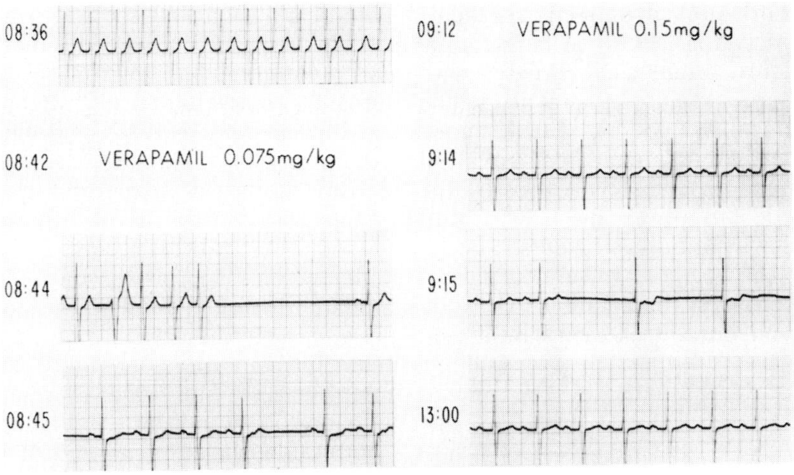

Fig 22B-4 Effect of verapamil in supraventricular tachycardia. Supraventricular tachycardia (rate, 150 beats/min) is treated with an initial verapamil dose of 0.075 mg/kg followed in 2 minutes by interruption of tachycardia. An additional dose of verapamil causes transient AV block.

usually causes symptoms even in normal patients. The goal of treatment is to terminate the rhythm or to slow the ventricular response. Vagal maneuvers, including carotid sinus massage or the Valsalva maneuver, can be attempted initially in the treatment of these arrhythmias. If these maneuvers fail, the acute treatment of narrow-complex supraventricular tachycardia involves intravenous administration of adenosine (6 mg given by rapid injection, followed in 5 to 10 minutes by a second dose) or verapamil (Fig 22B-4). The initial dose of verapamil, 0.075 mg/kg given intravenously over 2 minutes, may convert supraventricular tachycardia to sinus rhythm. When necessary, a subsequent dose of 0.15 mg/kg may be administered 20 minutes later. Verapamil, which inhibits calcium-dependent slow-channel responses in the SA node and also in the AV node, depresses conduction in both the fast and the slow pathways of patients with dual AV nodal pathways and interrupts AV nodal reentrant tachycardia. Verapamil also exerts a significant effect on the slow-conducting pathway in patients with intra-atrial reentrant tachycardia or reciprocating tachycardia that utilizes an accessory pathway. Use of verapamil acutely in the treatment of supraventricular tachycardia results in successful reversion to normal sinus rhythm in more than 80% of cases.[12,13]

Adenosine causes slowing and block in the AV node. The advantage of adenosine is that it has a very short plasma half-life (measured in seconds) and does not have the tendency to cause hypotension or have an adverse negative inotropic effect that verapamil might have in selected patients. In addition, its very short plasma half-life increases the level of safety for use in acute situations. It must be administered intravenously very rapidly (over 1 to 2 seconds) in an initial dose of 6 mg. Subsequent repeat doses of 12 mg may be administered on two separate occasions according to need.

Digoxin and propranolol also exert a significant effect on AV nodal conduction. Both digoxin and propranolol affect primarily the slow pathway, and they are generally effective in the treatment of AV nodal reentrant tachycardia because of their predominant effect on antegrade conduction of impulses down the slow pathway. In addition, both of these drugs may help terminate paroxysms of tachycardia by prolonging refractoriness in the fast pathway in which retrograde conduction occurs.

An alternative approach to the treatment of supraventricular tachycardia of acute onset is to induce a reflex increase in vagal tone by the use of edrophonium (10 mg intravenously) or neostigmine (0.5 to 2 mg subcutaneously, intramuscularly, or intravenously). It should be emphasized that verapamil is preferable to these drugs.

The long-term treatment of supraventricular tachycardia may include the use of class I antiarrhythmia agents, specifically procainamide, quinidine, or disopyramide, which may interrupt reentrant tachycardias by prolonging refractoriness in the fast (retrograde) pathway. These drugs may be useful in the treatment of tachycardias that utilize an accessory pathway. The class I antiarrhythmia drugs may be especially helpful in preventing repeated episodes of reentrant tachycardia by decreasing the number of atrial or ventricular premature beats that initiate such episodes. Propafenone, flecainide, sotalol, or amiodarone may be helpful for patients who are resistant to digoxin, β-adrenergic blocking agents, calcium channel blockers, or class I antiarrhythmia agents.

Patients with frequent or severely symptomatic tachycardias should be considered for electrophysiologic studies early. Patients who have been unsuccessfully treated with empiric antiarrhythmic drug therapy should be considered for invasive electrophysiologic studies and possible cure by catheter ablation techniques.

Catheter ablation should be considered for patients in whom therapy does not produce a response or electropharmacologic studies suggest failure of antiarrhythmic drugs. Radiofrequency ablation can be first-line therapy for AV reentrant tachycardia, AV node reentrant tachycardia, permanent reciprocating junctional tachycardia, and accessible intra-atrial reentrant tachycardias.[14]

Alternative surgical approaches to treatment include modification of AV conduction in patients with AV node reentrant tachycardia, surgical ablation of ectopic atrial arrhythmias, and ablation of accessory AV pathways. Patients with supraventricular tachycardia in whom an attempt at radiofrequency ablation has failed should be considered for surgical therapy. Electrosurgical procedures have effectively cured AV tachycardia, AV node reentrant tachycardia, and intra-atrial tachycardia (see chapter 26).

SPECIFIC SUPRAVENTRICULAR ARRHYTHMIAS AND THEIR TREATMENT

AV nodal reentry tachycardias

Supraventricular tachycardia is most often a result of reentry within the AV node. Almost half of patients with supraventricular tachycardia in the absence of preexcitation have this mechanism of tachycardia.

Clinical manifestations. These arrhythmias are characteristically abrupt in onset and termination and are variable in duration. Episodes may last from several minutes to hours or even days. Tachycardia may occur in patients without identifiable heart disease or in the setting of organic heart disease.[15] Patients with normal hearts may complain of a vague chest heaviness, palpitation or rapid heart beat, or presyncope. After prolonged bouts of this type, patients may be quite fatigued and unwell for several hours. However, patients with coexisting organic heart disease often complain of dyspnea, chest pain, or presyncope or syncope. Supraventricular tachycardia may be life threatening in some circumstances, especially when patients with organic heart disease have significant hemodynamic compromise as a consequence of the rapid rhythm.

Electrocardiographic characteristics. The ECG during supraventricular tachycardia related to AV nodal reentry shows a regular tachycardia with a rate of 150 to 230 beats/min and a narrow QRS complex unless bundle-branch block is present (see Fig 22B-1). The P waves occur before, simultaneously with, or shortly after the QRS complex. Long R-P intervals suggest an underlying AV reentrant tachycardia that utilizes an accessory pathway or permanent junctional reciprocating tachycardia.[9]

Electrophysiologic findings. Electrophysiologic studies permit a diagnosis to be made of the mechanism of supraventricular tachycardia in virtually all cases. Specifically, reentrant tachycardias can be differentiated from automatic ectopic tachycardias in that the former can be reliably initiated and terminated by programmed stimulation. In addition, the behavior of tachycardia involving an AV nodal reentrant mechanism differs from that involving AV tachycardia that utilizes an accessory pathway.

The concept of dual AV nodal pathways has come to be applied commonly in the description of patients with AV nodal reentrant tachycardia. The most common form of AV nodal reentrant tachycardia has been described earlier and has been called "slow-fast tachycardia." This form of tachycardia utilizes the slow pathway as the antegrade limb of the reentry circuit and the fast pathway as the retrograde limb of the reentry circuit (Fig 22B-5,A).

An unusual form of AV nodal reentrant tachycardia causes incessant tachycardia. It has variously been called "permanent junctional reciprocating tachycardia" and "fast-slow tachycardia."[16-18] The fast pathway has a short refractory period and serves as the antegrade limb of the tachycardia circuit, and the slow pathway has a long refractory period and serves as the retrograde limb of the circuit[16] (Fig 22B-5,B). This tachycardia involves an accessory AV connection capable of very slow retrograde

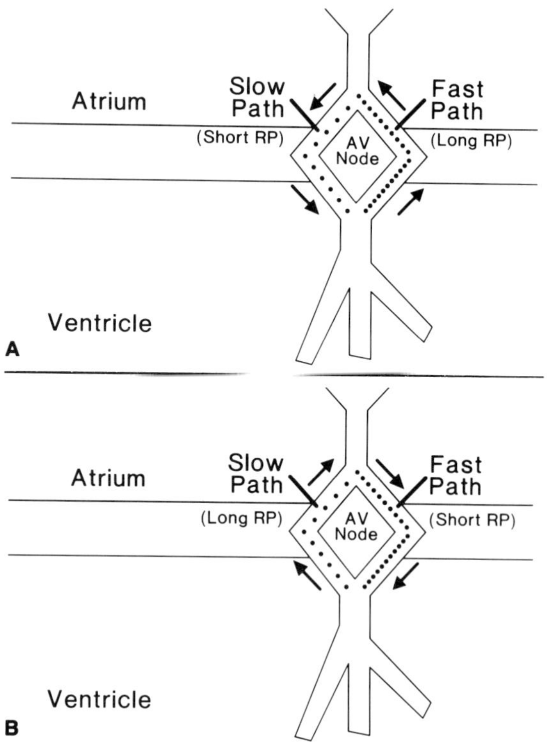

Fig 22B-5 Mechanisms of supraventricular tachycardia. **A,** slow-fast form. In this common form of AV nodal reentry tachycardia, a reentrant circuit is composed of a slow pathway with a short refractory period *(RP)* and a fast pathway with a long refractory period. A premature beat is required to initiate tachycardia, and the tachycardia utilizes the slow pathway for antegrade conduction and the fast pathway for retrograde conduction. **B,** fast-slow form. In this unusual form of AV nodal reentrant tachycardia, sometimes referred to as "incessant tachycardia," the slow pathway has a long refractory period and the fast pathway has a short refractory period. In contrast to the more common form of AV nodal reentrant tachycardia, a premature beat is not necessary to initiate tachycardia; a normally timed sinus beat may initiate tachycardia.

conduction but not antegrade conduction, and it takes a tortuous route through the septum. Endocardial mapping during tachycardia characteristically reveals eccentric atrial activation, with the earliest activation occurring in the region of the os of the coronary sinus. This type of supraventricular tachycardia is also unusual in that a critically timed premature beat is not necessary for its initiation. Instead, it may be triggered simply by a slight increase in sinus rate. Thus, autonomic changes may play an important role in the initiation, maintenance, termination, or even spontaneous cure of tachycardia in patients with this unusual form of tachycardia.

The differential diagnosis of supraventricular tachycardia with a long R-P interval and a short P-R interval includes four mechanisms: (1) intra-atrial tachycardia; (2) an unusual form of AV nodal tachycardia alluded to earlier in this chapter; (3) an accessory AV pathway (concealed bypass tract) with rapid retrograde conduction; and (4) an accessory pathway with slow retrograde conduction (thus, long R-P interval). Generally, patients with an accessory pathway have a P-R interval longer than the R-P interval and, for practical purposes, the major differential diagnosis lies between atrial tachycardia and tachycardia utilizing an accessory AV connection with slow conduction. This distinction can be made with the aid of a 12-lead ECG and carotid sinus massage.[19]

Most cases of supraventricular tachycardia due to AV nodal reentry can easily be reproduced in the electrophysiology laboratory by means of programmed stimulation. Critical to the initiation of tachycardia is a delay in conduction in the AV node.[20] Almost three-fourths of patients with AV nodal reentrant tachycardia are found to have AV dual nodal pathways during programmed atrial stimulation.[21-24] This circumstance is characterized by sudden lengthening of the A-H interval in response to premature atrial stimuli (Fig 22B-6). It is not uncommon for an electrophysiologic study to fail to demonstrate dual AV nodal pathways. This failure may be related to several factors, including similar refractory periods of the fast and slow pathways and a functional refractory period in the atrium which limits the prematurity with which atrial premature depolarizations can enter the AV node.[25]

Programmed ventricular stimulation may induce AV nodal supraventricular tachycardia in some circumstances, but ventricular premature extrastimuli will induce tachycardia less reliably than will atrial premature beats. Since ventriculoatrial (VA) conduction occurs over the fast pathway, the conduction delay between the ventricle and the atrium is inadequate to allow recovery of excitability in the slow pathway so that tachycardia can be initiated.

In some circumstances, however, ventricular premature beats or ventricular pacing may induce AV nodal reentrant tachycardia (Fig 22B-7). The most common is the occurrence of a ventricular premature beat followed by antegrade block in the rapid pathway with slow conduction in the slow pathway because of the concealed conduction of the ventricular premature depolarization in a retrograde fashion.

Another characteristic of supraventricular tachycardia involving reentry within the AV node is that neither the atria nor the ventricles are required to sustain the tachycardia. Maintenance of the tachycardia in the presence of AV block or AV dissociation suggests that little if any of the atrium is required to sustain the tachycardia[26-28] (Fig 22B-8). The development of Wenckebach behavior during the tachycardia is evidence that the ventricle is not required for the tachycardia to continue. The ability to depolarize the atrium with premature atrial beats during tachycardia without altering the tachycardia cycle length is further evidence that the atrium is not required.[28]

It has long been suggested that AV node reentry tachycardia occurs entirely within the AV node without involvement of perinodal tissue. The knowledge gained from the development of surgical modification of AV node function and radiofrequency catheter ablation has changed the concepts of the anatomic substrate for AV node reentry tachycardia. Electrophysiologic studies previously showed that AV node reentry could be sustained during dissociation of the atria and the ventricles from the tachycardia (see Fig 22B-8), suggesting that the substrate for this tachycardia was confined to the AV node proper and did not include perinodal tissue.[26-28] However, successful surgical cure of AV node reentry tachycardia demonstrated that atrial perinodal fibers are critical elements of the reentry circuit.[29,30]

Ablation of the fast pathway is associated with a high risk of heart block,[31] but a more posterior approach in which lesions are placed between the septal leaflet of the tricuspid valve and the coronary sinus os selectively ablates the slow pathway.[32,33] These findings suggest that the proximal common pathway for AV node reentrant tachycardia includes perinodal atrial tissue.

Mapping studies corroborate the conclusion that atrial tissue is, indeed, part of this reentrant circuit.[34] The combined information from these studies suggests that the atrial insertion of the slow pathway is at the base of the triangle of Koch near the coronary sinus os and that the atrial insertion of the fast pathway is near the apex of the triangle of Koch.

An important criterion of AV nodal reentrant tachycardia is the inability of a premature ventricular contraction to preexcite the atrium while the His-Purkinje system is refractory.

The sequence of retrograde atrial activation during AV nodal reentrant tachycardia is entirely normal, and the earliest site of retrograde activation recorded occurs in the His bundle electrogram or in the region of the os of the coronary sinus, as recorded from a quadripolar catheter positioned in the coronary sinus.[35,36] This is followed by depolarization of the low septal right atrium, as recorded from a His catheter, and then by the sequential depolarization of the remainder of the right and left atria (see Fig 22B-10,B).

Functional bundle-branch block may occur during supraventricular tachycardia, and because it is related to alterations in His-Purkinje conduction away from, and not part of, a reentrant circuit, it does not modify the reentrant process in the AV node. Functional bundle-branch block may prolong V-V intervals for a single cycle,

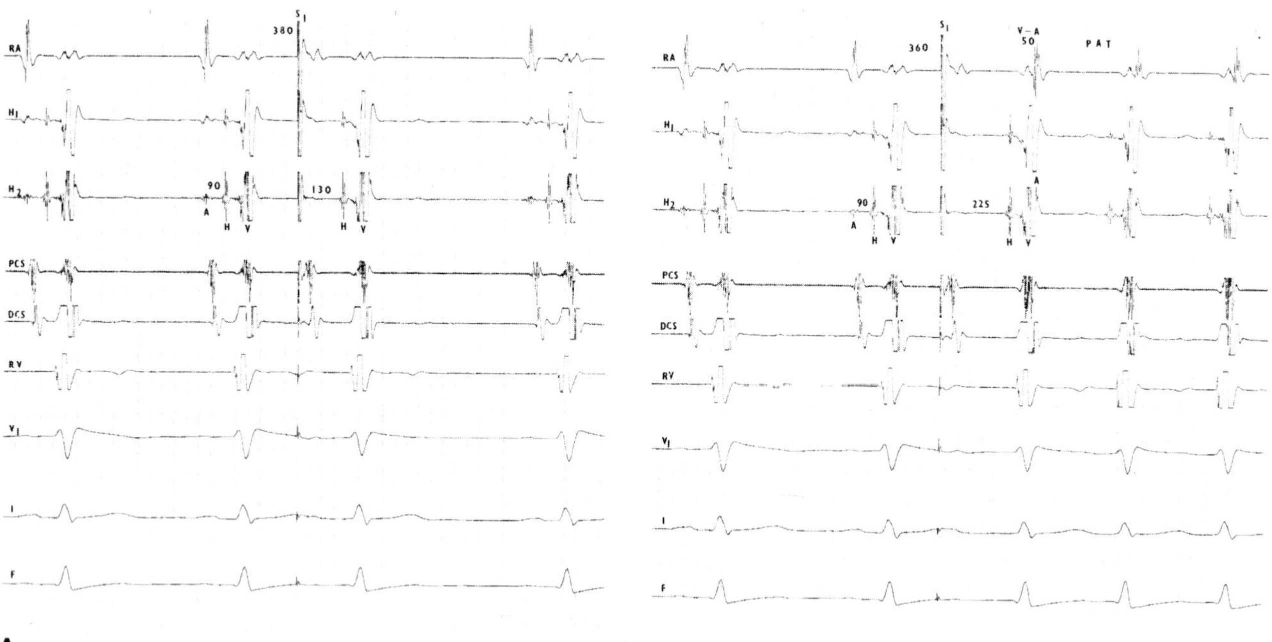

A

B

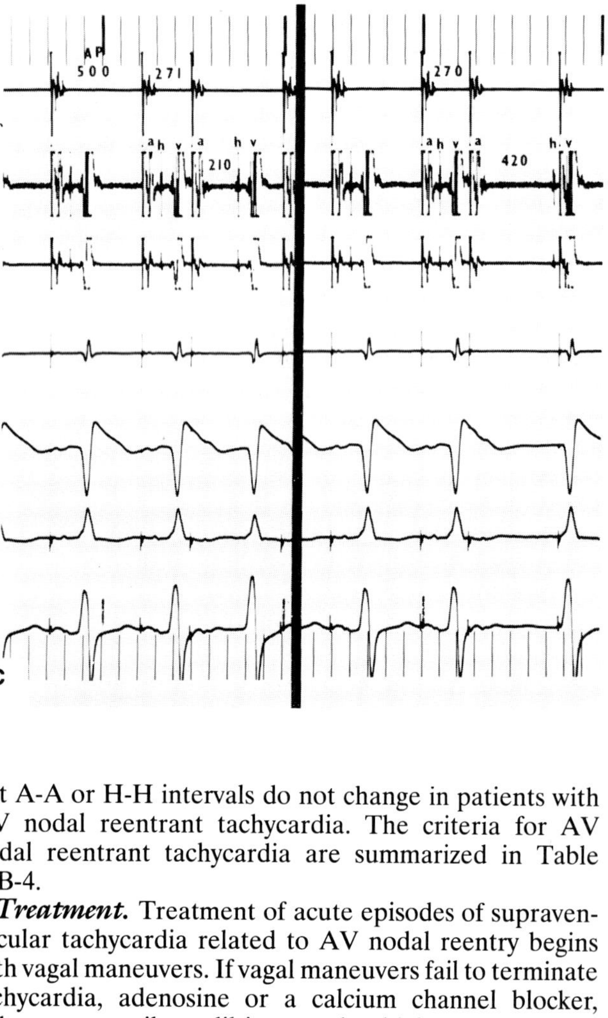

C

Fig 22B-6 Electrophysiologic diagnosis of dual AV nodal pathways. **A,** electrophysiologic recording obtained from a patient with dual AV nodal pathways. Recorded are electrograms from the high right atrium *(RA),* region of the His bundle (H_1 and H_2), coronary sinus (*PCS* and *DCS*), right ventricle *(RV),* and surface electrodes (V_1, *I, F*). In sinus rhythm, impulses are conducted down the fast pathway with a short H-V interval (A–H = 90 msec). When a premature impulse is introduced in the atrium (S_1 at a coupling interval of 380 msec after a sinus beat), the premature impulse is conducted with some delay down the fast pathway (A-H interval = 30 msec); supraventricular tachycardia is not induced. **B,** critically timed atrial premature impulse (S_1) is introduced at a coupling interval of 360 msec. This impulse is blocked in the fast pathway and travels down the slow pathway (A-H interval = 225 msec). It encounters excitable tissue in the distal limb of the fast pathway and is conducted in a retrograde fashion to the atrium, initiating supraventricular tachycardia. On occasion, the timing of a premature impulse needed to initiate tachycardia may be extremely critical. **C,** electrograms recorded from the high right atrium, His bundle, right ventricle, and surface, in that order. During atrial pacing *(AP)* at 120 beats/min (520-msec cycle length), a premature impulse is introduced at a coupling interval of 271 msec and is conducted down the fast pathway. A second premature impulse introduced at the coupling interval of 270 msec is blocked in the fast pathway but traverses the slow pathway. On this occasion, supraventricular tachycardia is not induced.

but A-A or H-H intervals do not change in patients with AV nodal reentrant tachycardia. The criteria for AV nodal reentrant tachycardia are summarized in Table 22B-4.

Treatment. Treatment of acute episodes of supraventricular tachycardia related to AV nodal reentry begins with vagal maneuvers. If vagal maneuvers fail to terminate tachycardia, adenosine or a calcium channel blocker, either verapamil or diltiazem, should be administered intravenously.

Long-term treatment of supraventricular tachycardia related to AV node reentry may include daily antiarrhythmia drug therapy, intermittent drug therapy, or catheter ablation.

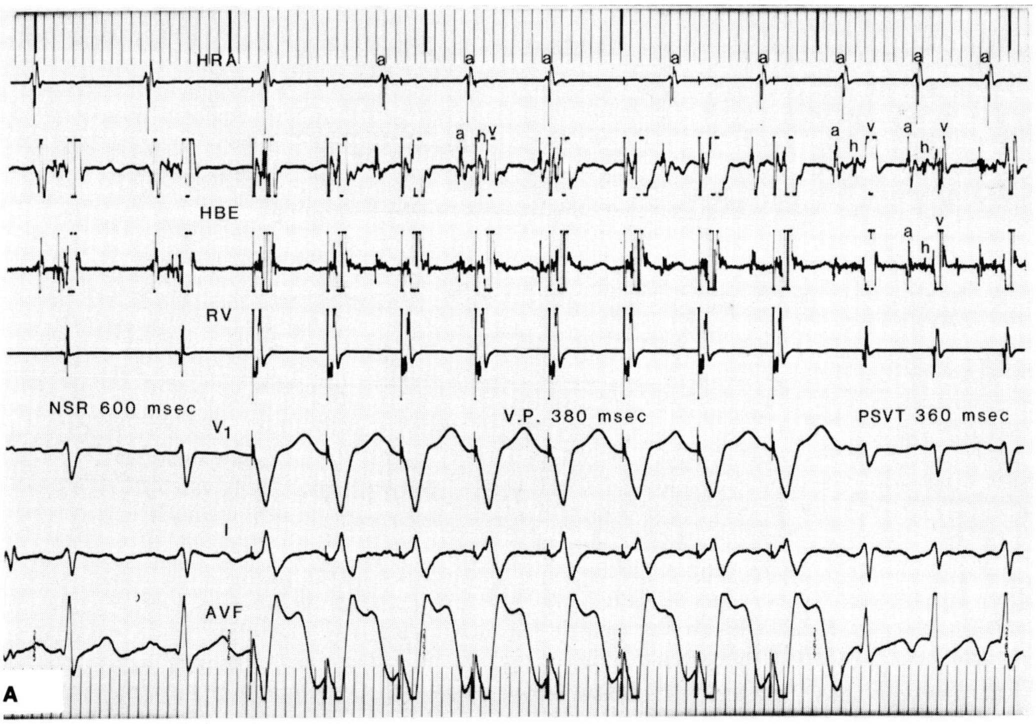

A

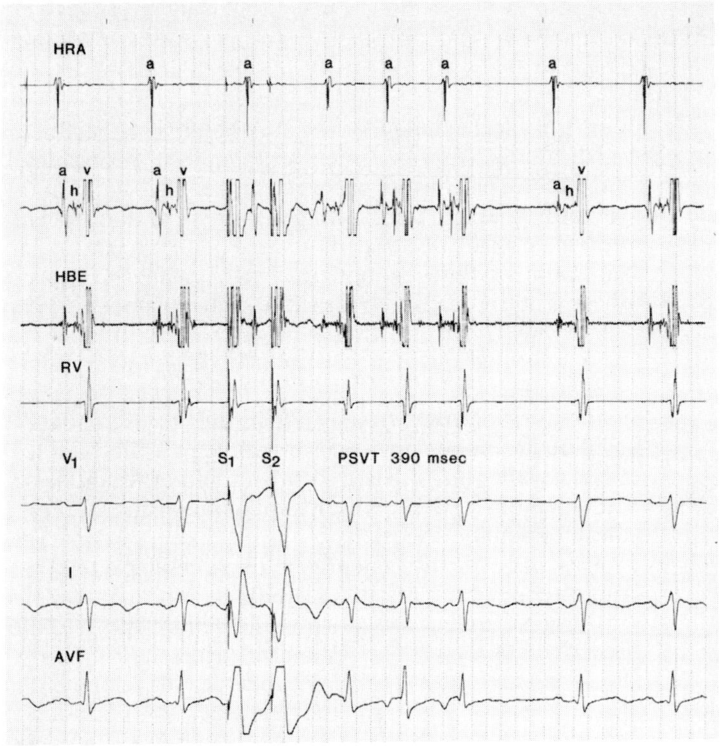

B

Fig 22B-7 Induction of supraventricular tachycardia by ventricular pacing or ventricular premature beats during electrophysiologic study. **A,** induction of supraventricular tachycardia by pacing. Recordings from the high right atrium *(HRA),* His bundle *(HBE),* right ventricle *(RV),* and surface leads, showing initiation of ventricular pacing *(V.P.)* at 380 msec (167 beats/min). VA Wenckebach behavior occurs, and supraventricular tachycardia *(PSVT)* is initiated. The cycle length of the tachycardia is 360 msec, and atrial activation is via the septal atrium. NSR, normal sinus rhythm. **B,** similar electrograms, but with two premature beats *(S_1, S_2)* delivered in the ventricle. The second premature impulse encounters a critical delay in its retrograde conduction to the atrium, which allows the initiation of a reentrant tachycardia with a cycle length of 390 msec.

AV node reentrant tachycardia is curable by radiofrequency ablation. The safety and efficacy of radiofrequency ablation make this intervention the treatment of choice in patients with bothersome symptoms. Alternative treatment options include antiarrhythmic drugs given daily or on an as-needed basis, antitachycardia pacing, and electrosurgery. The decision to proceed with radiofrequency ablation should be considered at the time that diagnostic electrophysiologic studies are discussed with the patient so that curative therapy can be applied when an appropriate substrate for supraventricular tachycardia is identified in the electrophysiology laboratory.

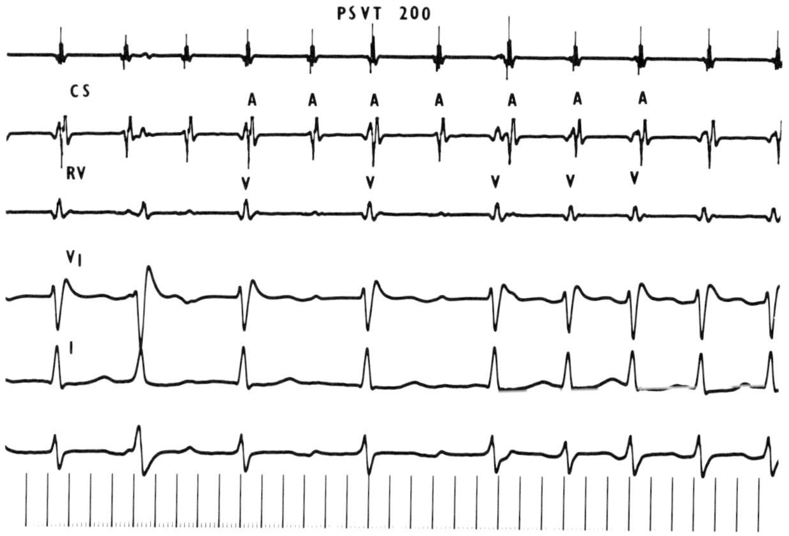

Fig 22B-8 Supraventricular tachycardia persisting in the face of AV block. Shown are electrograms recorded from the coronary sinus *(CS, top two channels),* right ventricle *(RV)* and surface leads V_1, *I,* and *aVF.* A supraventricular tachycardia *(PSVT)* at the rate of 200 beats/min is evident in the coronary sinus electrograms. However, the tachycardia persists in the face of AV block of the Wenckebach variety. This confirms that the ventricles are not a part of the reentry circuit.

Table 22B-4 Electrophysiologic criteria for AV nodal reentrant tachycardias

Initiation or termination of tachycardia by critically timed atrial or ventricular premature beats
Dual refractory curves during programmed atrial stimulation
Initiation of tachycardia dependent upon critical delay in conduction in the slow pathway
Normal retrograde atrial activation via the septum
Neither atrium nor ventricle required to maintain tachycardia
Supraventricular tachycardia slowed and abruptly terminated by carotid sinus massage
VA interval, ≤65 msec

It is preferable to ablate the slow pathway in AV node reentry to reduce the risk of heart block, since the slow pathway is remote from the His bundle. Care should be taken to evaluate the function of the fast pathway before ablation. If the fast pathway has a long antegrade refractory period, there is an increased likelihood of abnormal AV conduction after ablation of the slow pathway. In such patients, it may be preferable to selectively ablate the fast pathway to minimize the likelihood of heart block related to the procedure.

Patients who refuse radiofrequency ablation may be treated with a variety of interventions. If episodes of tachycardia are infrequent, patients should be taught to perform vagal maneuvers first and then to use short-acting medications (for example, verapamil or propranolol). Frequent episodes of tachycardia require daily antiarrhythmic therapy. Long-acting verapamil or diltiazem may be tried initially because of the ease of administration and low proarrhythmic potential. Tachycardia refractory to these simple drugs may be effectively treated with class IA or class IC drugs. Propafenone is quite effective and well tolerated, with a low proarrhythmic potential.[37,38] Flecainide has also been effective in treatment of patients with supraventricular tachycardia, but its use should be confined to patients without evidence of structural heart disease.[39,42] Sotalol has also proven effective and is safe provided that caution is used in patients with heart failure and pulmonary disease.[43-45]

Patients who have undergone unsuccessful attempts at radiofrequency ablation are candidates for curative electrosurgery. We have used a modification of the operation described by Cox et al.[29] and have successfully cured AV node reentry tachycardia without the development of heart block.[30] We have encountered no morbidity or mortality during cryosurgical modification of AV node conduction.

Reentry tachycardia utilizing a concealed accessory pathway

Supraventricular tachycardia may occur in patients with accessory pathways. These patients may have a variety of disturbances in rhythm associated with different functional characteristics of the accessory pathway. Tachycardia in these patients depends on the difference in

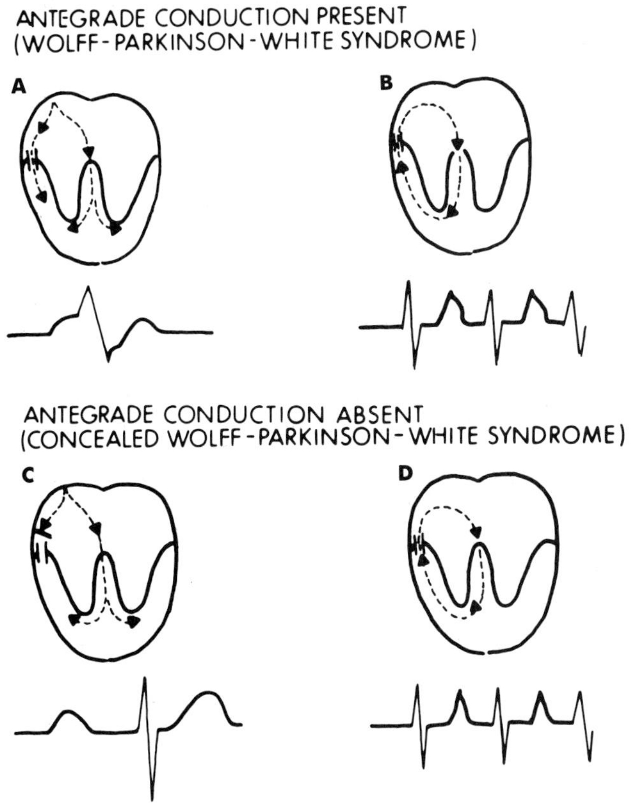

Fig 22B-9 Wolff-Parkinson-White syndrome with manifest (**A** and **B**) and concealed (**C** and **D**) conduction. When antegrade conduction is present down an accessory pathway, the QRS morphology is the product of fusion of input from the atria via the AV node and the accessory pathway producing the typical delta wave. When antegrade conduction down the accessory pathway is absent (**C**), activation of the ventricle proceeds in the normal fashion, and the QRS is normal (hence, concealed bypass tract). The mechanism of tachycardia in both cases is identical: antegrade conduction proceeds down the AV node, and retrograde conduction is via the bypass tract (**C** and **D**). (From Hammill SC, Pritchett ELC: Dynamic electrocardiography in the investigation of supraventricular tachycardia and tachycardia associated with pre-excitation syndromes. In *Dynamic Electrocardiography.* Edited by R Campbell, A Murray. Edinburgh, Churchill Livingstone, 1985, pp 74-88. By permission.)

conduction and refractoriness between the accessory pathway and the normal AV conduction system. Most commonly, the accessory pathway is capable of conduction in both an antegrade and a retrograde direction, although conduction may occur only in the antegrade[46] or retrograde direction. Antegrade conduction down an accessory pathway activates part of the ventricle earlier than would normally be expected and produces the commonly known delta wave in the ECG (Fig 22B-9,A and B). In certain patients the accessory pathway is not capable of antegrade conduction in sinus rhythm, and the ECG is normal; this situation has been described as one involving a "concealed" bypass tract (Fig 22B-9,C and D). Tachycardia that utilizes a concealed bypass tract constitutes almost one-third of cases of supraventricular tachycardia.[47-49]

Clinical manifestations. The symptoms experienced by patients who have tachycardia that utilizes an accessory pathway are similar to those described by patients with tachycardia due to reentry within the AV node. These patients usually are younger and have organic heart disease less often than do patients with AV nodal reentrant tachycardia.[15]

Electrocardiographic characteristics. The ECG manifestations of tachycardia that utilize a concealed accessory pathway are a rapid, regular tachycardia of 150 to 230 beats/min and a normal QRS morphology, unless functional bundle-branch block is present. P-wave morphology may be abnormal, and the R-P interval is lengthened to more than 65 msec. Functional bundle-branch block is more likely to be found in patients with supraventricular tachycardia that utilizes a concealed accessory pathway.

QRS alternans is not related to the mechanism of tachycardia. Rather, the phenomenon of QRS alternans is an expression of a form of aberrant conduction produced by oscillation of diastolic intervals.[50] The predictive accuracy of QRS alternans is greatly influenced by the rate of the tachycardia; at rates exceeding 180 beats/min, the positive predictive accuracy of QRS alternans for a diagnosis of orthodromic tachycardia using a concealed accessory pathway is slightly more than 80%.[51]

The location of a retrogradely conducting accessory pathway may be suggested by careful analysis of the P-wave morphology and axis during tachycardia. An inverted P wave in lead I during orthodromic tachycardia is common in left free-wall accessory pathways. An inverted P wave in lead I and all inferior leads (II, III, aVF) suggests a left posterior accessory pathway. A right-sided accessory pathway is suggested by a positive P wave in leads I, II, and aVL.

Electrophysiologic findings. The electrophysiologic behavior of tachycardia that utilizes a concealed bypass tract is different from that of tachycardia related to reentry within the AV node. Most episodes of tachycardia that utilizes a concealed bypass tract are initiated by atrial premature beats but, unlike AV nodal reentrant tachycardia, the initiation of tachycardia is not related to delay within the AV node, but to the total conduction time from the atrium to the ventricle. Ventricular stimulation can also induce tachycardia in patients with concealed bypass tracts, and commonly ventricular premature depolarizations will produce tachycardia more reliably in these patients (in as many as 50%) than in those with tachycardia related to AV nodal reentry.

In cases involving a concealed bypass tract, both the atria and the ventricles are obligatory parts of the reentrant circuit. Therefore, when a tachycardia exists in a patient with AV or VA block, a concealed bypass tract cannot be involved in the arrhythmia.

An important diagnostic point in the electrophysiologic evaluation of patients with supraventricular tachycardia is the analysis of retrograde atrial activation by means of right atrial electrograms and left atrial electro-

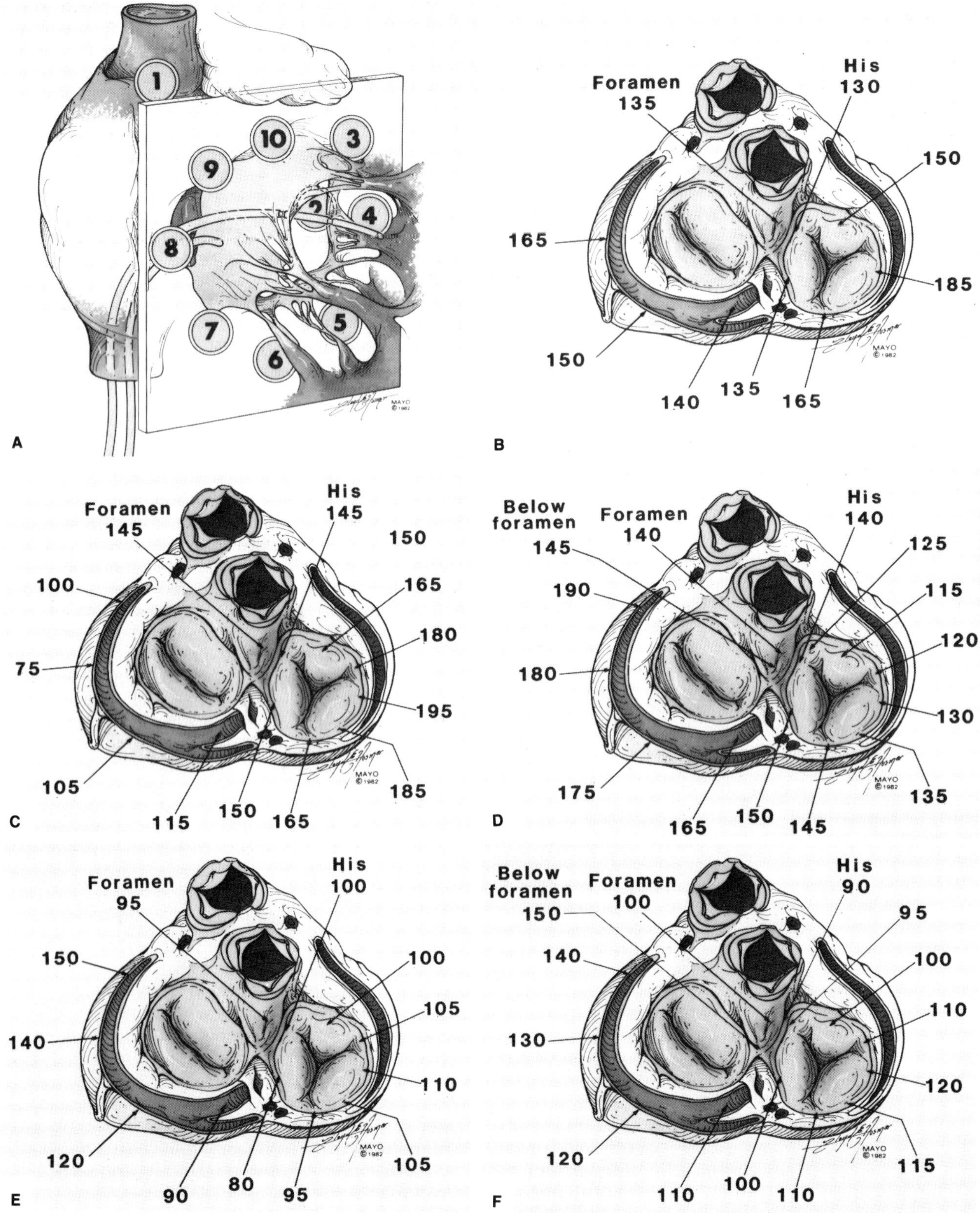
1
10
3
9
2
4
8
7
5
6
MAYO ©1982
A
Foramen 135
His 130
150
165
185
150
140
135
165
MAYO ©1982
B
Foramen 145
His 145
150
100
165
180
75
195
105
115
150
165
185
MAYO ©1982
C
Below foramen
145
Foramen 140
His 140
125
190
115
120
180
130
175
165
150
145
135
MAYO ©1982
D
Foramen 95
His 100
150
100
105
140
110
120
90
80
95
105
MAYO ©1982
E
Below foramen
150
Foramen 100
His 90
95
140
100
110
130
120
120
110
100
110
115
MAYO ©1982
F

Fig 22B-10 Electrophysiologic analysis of retrograde atrial activation during tachycardia. **A,** technique of analysis of atrial activation. Schematic representation of right atrium shows a tripolar catheter positioned across the tricuspid valve to record a His potential and a modified bipolar Brockenbrough catheter located proximally in the right atrium. During ventricular pacing and during tachycardia, the bipolar Brockenbrough catheter is moved in sequence to each of 10 different positions, and electrograms are recorded at each site. In this fashion, a map of atrial activation is constructed. **B,** normal pattern of retrograde activation of the atrium is recorded during ventricular pacing and may be recorded during AV nodal reentrant tachycardia. In this circumstance, the earliest area of activation is in the interatrial septum, followed by the proximal coronary sinus and then more lateral structures of the right and left atria. **C,** in the presence of a left lateral accessory pathway, the earliest activation is recorded in the left lateral AV groove, followed by activation of the intra-atrial septum. Activation of the right atrium occurs last. **D,** right anterior free wall accessory pathway causes earliest activation to occur in the high right atrium, followed by activation of the interatrial septum and finally the left atrium. **E,** accessory pathway located in the posteroseptal region activates the posterior interatrial septum first; activation then proceeds via septal structures, including the area around the foramen ovale and posterior atrial structures, before moving toward lateral atrial structures. **F,** anteroseptal accessory pathway causes earliest activation of anterior septal structures in the region of the His bundle during reciprocating tachycardia. Other septal structures are depolarized next, followed by a spread of the excitatory wave into other areas of the atria. (By permission, Mayo Foundation.)

grams. Detailed atrial mapping carried out during tachycardia and during ventricular pacing in patients with AV reentry tachycardia reveals that activation of the atria during tachycardia or rapid ventricular pacing is eccentric (Fig 22B-10) unless a septal accessory pathway is present.[48,49]

Because the ventricles are an obligatory part of AV tachycardia that utilizes a concealed bypass tract, the development of ipsilateral bundle-branch block will produce a slowing of the tachycardia (Fig 22B-11) because of lengthened VA conduction caused by prolongation of conduction through the ventricle.[48,49,52] Therefore, prolongation of the cycle length during tachycardia by more than 35 msec with the development of bundle-branch block is virtually diagnostic of an ipsilateral free-wall bypass tract if that lengthening is related to total VA prolongation.

Because the atrium is required to sustain AV reentrant tachycardia that utilizes an accessory pathway, it is difficult to depolarize the atria prematurely with atrial premature beats without affecting the cycle length of the tachycardia (Fig 22B-12). In addition, the introduction of critically timed ventricular premature beats while the His bundle is refractory may demonstrate that the atrium can be advanced with an atrial activation sequence that resembles the eccentric sequence recorded during reciprocating tachycardia[47-49,52] (see Fig 22B-12). This technique confirms the utilization of a concealed bypass tract for AV reentrant tachycardia, since the only pathway to the atrium which the ventricular premature contraction can use when the His bundle is refractory is an accessory connection. Supraventricular tachycardia that involves a concealed bypass tract usually is terminated by a ventricular premature depolarization that preexcites the atrium so that antegrade conduction down the AV node is impossible. Alternatively, a premature ventricular contraction may partially penetrate the AV node in a retrograde manner to produce block in the AV node (concealed conduction). The criteria for AV reentrant tachycardia that utilizes a concealed bypass tract are summarized in Table 22B-5.

Treatment. The principles of treatment of supraventricular tachycardia that utilizes a concealed bypass tract are the same as those for AV nodal reentrant tachycardia. Pharmacologic therapy of AV reentrant tachycardia that utilizes a concealed accessory pathway may be directed at either limb of the reentrant circuit—the accessory pathway or the AV node. On some occasions, the accessory pathway will be the weak link, but in other instances the AV node may be vulnerable to the appropriate antiarrhythmia drug.

Acute intervention may begin with vagal maneuvers, adenosine, or intravenously delivered verapamil or diltiazem.[53] The safety and efficacy of radiofrequency ablation also make this therapeutic intervention a first-line choice for orthodromic tachycardia using a concealed accessory pathway.[11,14] Patients in whom radiofrequency ablation fails should be considered for curative electrosurgery.

Patients who refuse curative therapy may be treated with antiarrhythmic drugs, including verapamil, propafenone, flecainide, sotalol, and amiodarone.

Sinus tachycardia

Clinical manifestations. Symptoms of sinus tachycardia are generally mild and are related to changing autonomic tone in response to physiologic and psychologic stress in the absence of fever, thyrotoxicosis, or other provocative factors. Characteristically, sinus tachycardia begins gradually and ends gradually, and it causes

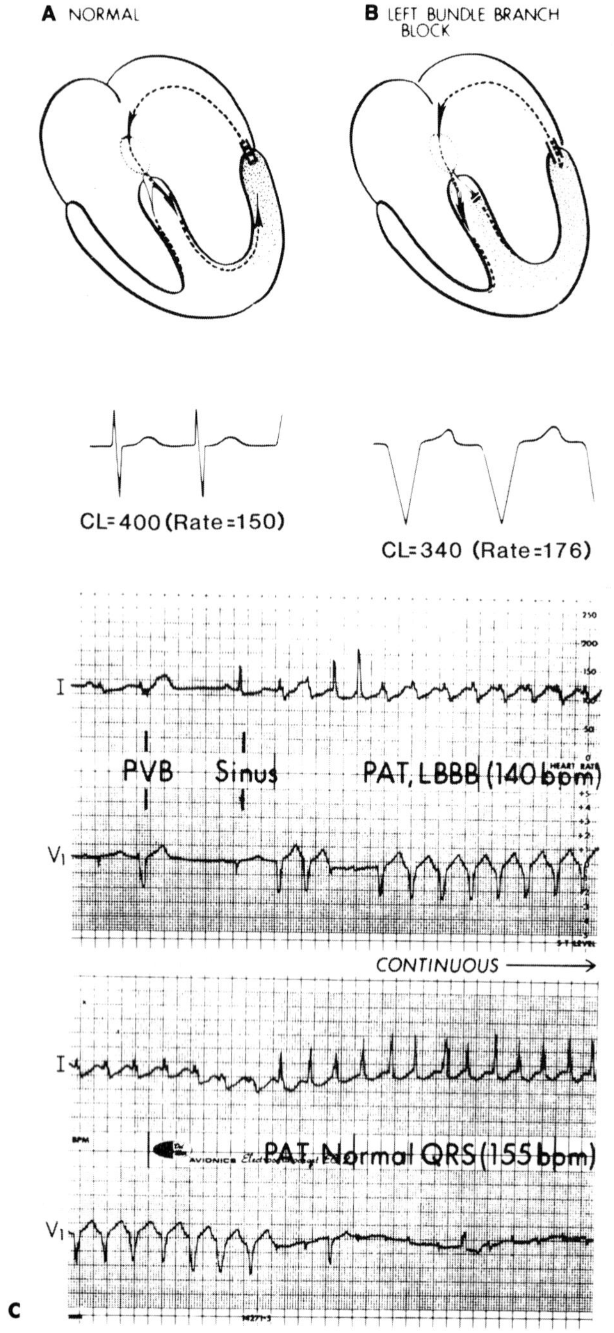

Fig 22B-11 Effect of bundle-branch block on circus movement tachycardia. **A**, usual conduction during reciprocating tachycardia in which antegrade conduction occurs down the AV node with retrograde conduction via the accessory pathway. **B**, with the development of left bundle-branch block, the cycle length of the tachycardia lengthens and the rate of the tachycardia slows with lengthening of the VA conduction time. **C**, ambulatory recording from a patient with a left ventricular free-wall accessory pathway. Paroxysmal atrial tachycardia *(PAT)* is initiated with a left bundle-branch block *(LBBB)* morphology. When the QRS normalizes, the tachycardia rate increases. *CL*, cycle length; *PVB*, premature ventricular beat. (**C** from Gallagher JJ, Pritchett ELC, Sealy WC, et al: The preexcitation syndromes. *Prog Cardiovasc Dis* 20:285-327, 1978. By permission of Grune & Stratton.)

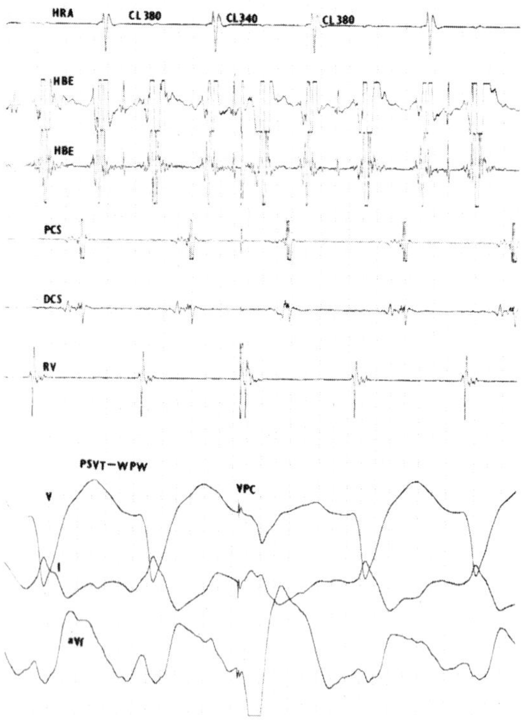

Fig 22B-12 Electrophysiologic study in Wolff-Parkinson-White (WPW) syndrome. Electrograms were recorded from the high right atrium *(HRA)*, His bundle region (*HBE*, channels 2 and 3), proximal coronary sinus *(PCS)*, distal coronary sinus *(DCS)*, right ventricle *(RV)*, and surface (*V, I,* and *aVF*) during reciprocating tachycardia. The cycle length *(CL)* of the tachycardia was 380 msec. During reciprocating tachycardia, a premature stimulus is introduced in the right ventricular apex, which then advances the response in the high right atrium by 40 msec. The only available route for an impulse to depolarize the atrium when the His bundle is refractory is an accessory pathway (see text). *PSVT,* paroxysmal supraventricular tachycardia; *VPC,* ventricular premature contraction.

Table 22B-5 Electrophysiologic criteria for AV reentrant tachycardia utilizing an accessory pathway

Tachycardia initiated or terminated by atrial or ventricular premature complexes with critical AV delay
Both atrium and ventricle required to maintain tachycardia
Eccentric atrial activation during tachycardia (except septal pathway)
Alteration of tachycardia cycle length with associated bundle-branch block (except septal pathway)
Ability to preexcite the atrium with a ventricular premature depolarization during tachycardia while the His bundle is refractory
Tachycardia slowed and abruptly terminated by carotid sinus massage
VA interval, ≥65 msec

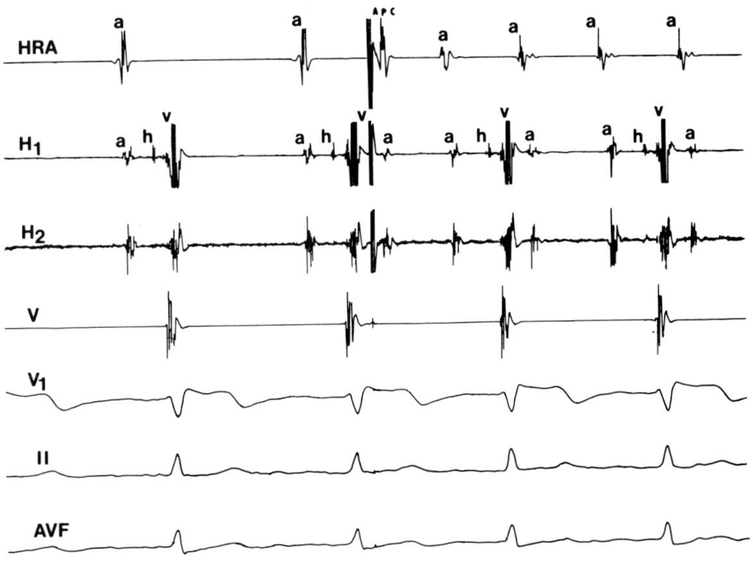

Fig 22B-13 SA node reentry tachycardia. Electrograms are recorded in order from the top: high right atrium *(HRA),* region of the His bundle (H_1 and H_2), right ventricle *(V)* and surface electrodes V_1, *II,* and *aVF*. In sinus rhythm, an atrial premature impulse *(APC)* is delivered in the high right atrium, and this initiates a reentrant tachycardia. The activation sequence of this tachycardia is from high to low. Specifically, the earliest activation is in the high right atrium, followed by activation of the septal right atrium as recorded from the His bundle electrodes.

symptoms of palpitations or rapid heart beat only when the heart rate exceeds 120 beats/min. Heart rates with sinus tachycardia generally range from 100 to 160 beats/min, although more rapid heart rates have been recorded. Usually, attacks of sinus tachycardia are short-lived. Heart disease is rare in patients with sinus tachycardia.

Electrocardiographic characteristics. The ECG in most patients with sinus tachycardia is entirely normal. During tachycardia, the P-wave morphology is normal, as are the QRS morphology and the P-R interval.

Electrophysiologic findings. Invasive electrophysiologic studies are not indicated for the diagnosis or management of supraventricular tachycardia of known sinus origin. If the cause of the tachycardia remains in question after a careful history has been taken in patients complaining of palpitations, the diagnosis can be made either by the use of ambulatory ECG or by means of a telephone transmitter.

Treatment. Rarely is any specific treatment necessary for sinus tachycardia. If reassurance fails to allay the symptoms, a small dose of a β-adrenergic blocking agent can be used. However, care should be taken to avoid side effects with this type of treatment.

Paroxysmal sinus tachycardia due to reentry within the SA node

Reentrant mechanisms are involved in the initiation and maintenance of paroxysmal sinus tachycardia.[54-58]

Clinical manifestations. The clinical manifestations of this type of tachycardia are the same as those of sinus tachycardia, except that the onset is typically more sudden and the termination is likewise sudden.

Electrocardiographic characteristics. The ECG reveals a normal P wave, but there may be slight prolongation of the P-R interval during the tachycardia.[59a] During ambulatory electrocardiography, short-lived episodes of sinus tachycardia of sudden onset and termination may be seen. Atrial premature beats are often quite rare in records obtained from patients with paroxysmal sinus tachycardia. The cycle length may be prolonged immediately before termination of the tachycardia.

Electrophysiologic findings. Invasive electrophysiologic studies are generally not needed for the diagnosis of paroxysmal sinus tachycardia due to reentry within the SA node (Figs 22B-13, 22B-14, and 22B-15). During tachycardia, the P-wave morphology is exactly like that observed during sinus rhythm, and the atrial activation sequence during tachycardia is normal. AV nodal block may exist without alteration of the tachycardia.

Treatment. The treatment of paroxysmal sinus tachycardia due to reentry within the SA node can often be accomplished with a minimum of intervention. Simple reassurance may be enough to dispel a patient's concern about episodes of sinus tachycardia, but if the symptoms are particularly bothersome, treatment with β-blockers may be undertaken. Alternative drugs are digoxin and verapamil. Class I antiarrhythmia agents have not been systematically studied in the treatment of this disorder but may be of benefit.

Supraventricular tachycardia due to true intra-atrial tachycardia

The term "paroxysmal atrial tachycardia" has been applied in general to describe a large number of supraventricular tachycardias, but true atrial tachycardia that involves either an automatic mechanism or reentry within the atrium itself independent of the SA or AV node is rare. *Automatic atrial tachycardias* may be related to the effects of certain drugs—specifically digoxin—or certain disease entities, as in the multifocal atrial tachycardia related to chronic obstructive lung disease.[60,61] *Tachycardias due to intra-atrial reentry* are rare in adults and constitute less than 5% of the supraventricular tachycardias. These tachycardias occur most commonly in younger adults and adolescents. In contrast, in the pediatric age group, intra-atrial reentrant tachycardias are a more common cause of supraventricular tachycardias.[61]

Clinical manifestations. Typically, atrial tachycardia begins suddenly and is marked by palpitations or rapid heartbeat. Spontaneous termination of attacks of atrial

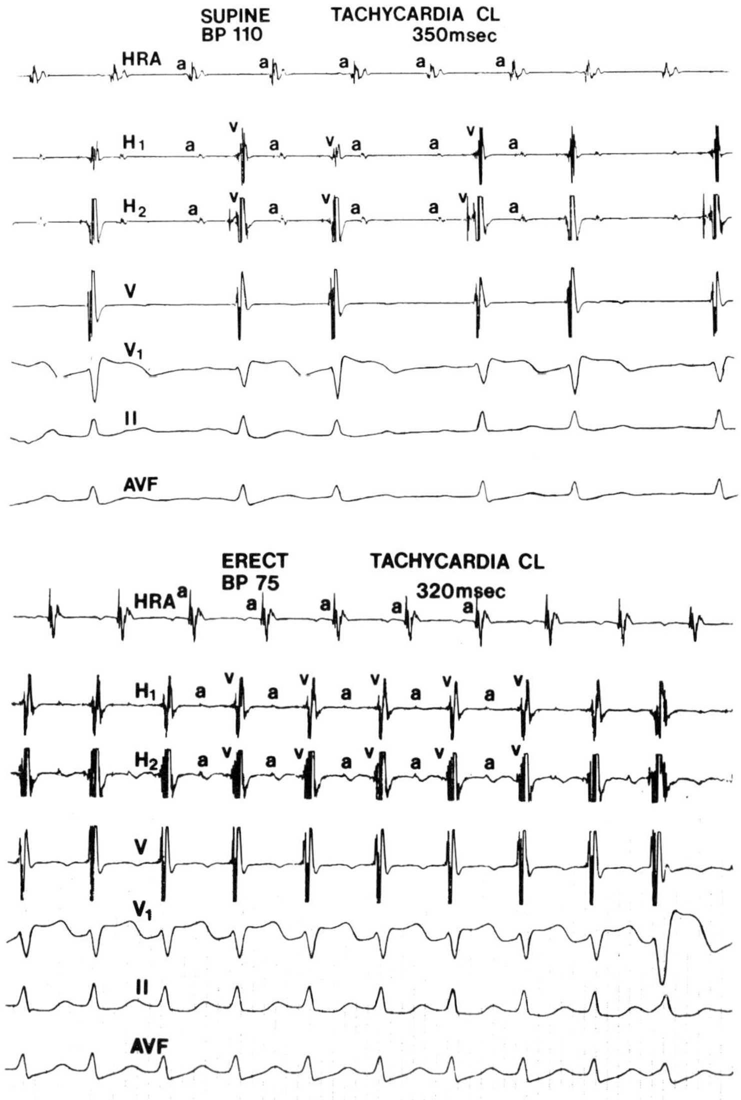

Fig 22B-14 Effect of posture on SA node reentry tachycardia. Electrograms recorded during electrophysiologic study of a patient with SA node reentry tachycardia. **A,** in supine position, tachycardia shows a cycle length *(CL)* of 350 msec and blood pressure *(BP)* is 110 mm Hg. **B,** patient is tipped into upright position. Cycle length of the tachycardia shortens to 320 msec, and the blood pressure falls to 75 mm Hg. This maneuver reproduced the patient's symptoms. *HRA,* high right atrium; H_1 and H_2, region of His bundle; *V,* right ventricle; V_1, *II,* and *aVF,* surface electrodes. (From Hammill SC, Holmes DR Jr, Wood DL, et al: Electrophysiologic testing in the upright position: improved evaluation of patients with rhythm disturbances using a tilt table. *J Am Coll Cardiol* 4:65-71, 1984. By permission of the American College of Cardiology.)

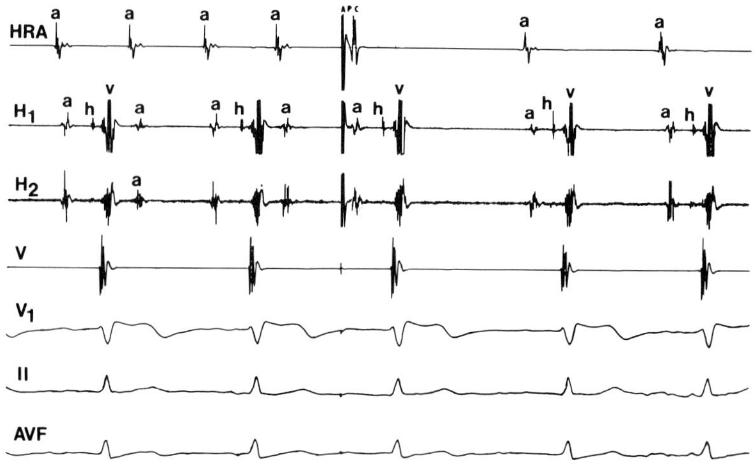

Fig 22B-15 Termination of SA node reentry tachycardia. Electrograms recorded during the electrophysiologic study of a patient with SA node reentry tachycardia as shown in Figures 22B-13 and 22B-14. Tachycardia that had been initiated with a single atrial premature contraction *(APC)* here has the characteristic activation from high to low with 2:1 AV nodal block present. The tachycardia is terminated by a single APC. *HRA,* high right atrium; H_1, and H_2, region of His bundle; *V,* right ventricle; V_1, *II,* and *aVF,* surface electrodes. (From Hammill SC, Holmes DR Jr, Wood DL, et al: Electrophysiologic testing in the upright position: improved evaluation of patients with rhythm disturbances using a tilt table. *J Am Coll Cardiol* 4:65-71, 1984. By permission of the American College of Cardiology.)

tachycardia is less common than in attacks of SA node or AV node reentry tachycardia. In addition, atrial tachycardia differs from tachycardia that utilizes dual AV nodal pathways or a concealed bypass tract in that it is relatively insensitive to vagal maneuvers, although AV nodal block may be produced. Patients with sustained intra-atrial reentrant tachycardia often have underlying structural heart disease with left atrial enlargement evident by echocardiographic examination. A history of atrial fibrillation or atrial flutter may be obtained in almost 70% of patients.[62]

Electrocardiographic characteristics. The heart rate during episodes of atrial tachycardia generally ranges from 140 to 200 beats/min. P-wave morphology during episodes of tachycardia is different from that during sinus rhythm, depending on the location of an automatic focus or reentrant circuit, and the P-R interval is also variable. A longer P-R interval may indicate an origin of tachycardia at some distance from the AV node, whereas a short P-R interval may indicate that the origin is near the AV node.[59b]

Electrophysiologic findings. The factors that suggest an automatic cause for intra-atrial tachycardia include a gradual acceleration of the tachycardia during atrial pacing or programmed atrial stimulation and alteration of the tachycardia under the influence of the autonomic nervous system.[60,61] In addition, the inability to initiate and terminate an atrial tachycardia with programmed stimulation routinely by means of a critically timed atrial premature beat suggests an automatic origin. Intra-atrial tachycardias that utilize reentrant mechanisms are easy to initiate and terminate with critically coupled atrial premature depolarizations. Atrial mapping (Fig 22B-16) during atrial tachycardia reveals that the atrial activation sequence differs from the activation sequence during sinus rhythm.[58,63]

It is possible that AV nodal block may exist without affecting supraventricular tachycardia due to intra-atrial reentry. Because vagal maneuvers may produce AV block without altering conduction within the atrium itself, these maneuvers often will not influence intra-atrial reentry tachycardia, although AV nodal block may be produced.

Treatment. The treatment of atrial tachycardia due to reentry or to an automatic focus is often empiric. The most effective treatment is to control the ventricular rate during tachycardia with digoxin, a β-blocker, or a calcium channel blocker.

Suppression of intra-atrial tachycardia is difficult to achieve with class IA drugs like procainamide and quinidine.[62] Amiodarone is particularly effective and can often be used in low doses, specifically maintenance doses of 200 mg/day, which are associated with a reduced likelihood of adverse effects. Propafenone and sotalol may also be effective. Although likely to be effective, flecainide should be used with caution because of the common finding of structural heart disease. Radiofrequency ablation may be curative when a single focus of tachycardia can be identified during diagnostic electrophysiologic studies. Surgical ablation may also be curative if other therapies fail. Lastly, if rate control alone is desired and drug therapy is ineffective or poorly tolerated, catheter ablation of AV conduction and permanent pacing can relieve symptoms.

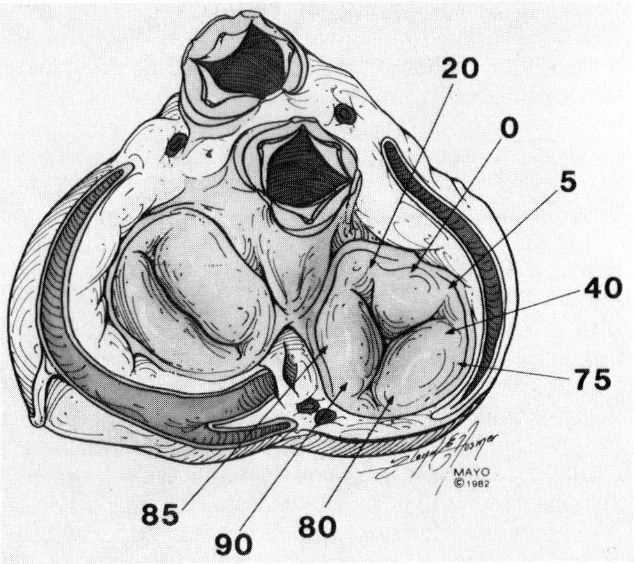

Fig 22B-16 Atrial activation during intra-atrial reentry tachycardia. At the time of electrophysiologic study, atrial activation during tachycardia was analyzed by mapping the right atrium with a modified Brockenbrough catheter (see Fig 22B-10). This figure shows the areas of the atrium that were mapped and the activation times measured against a reference electrogram recorded from the His catheter. The earliest activation is in the anterolateral right atrium followed by anterior and then lateral, posterior, and finally septal activation. This activation sequence was different from the activation sequence recorded during sinus rhythm. (By permission, Mayo Foundation.)

If there is a suspicion that digitalis intoxication is responsible for the atrial arrhythmia, the digitalis should be withdrawn for 48 hours while the rhythm is observed. If the rhythm improves, the digitalis should be reinstituted at a lower dose while the serum potassium level is checked; no other specific treatment is necessary. If patients are being treated concomitantly with verapamil or quinidine, usual doses of digoxin must be reduced. Because verapamil may not alter the serum digoxin concentration for 1 or 2 weeks after the drug has been administered, particular caution should be used in treating patients with supraventricular tachycardia who may have compromised renal function and who are at particular risk for digoxin intoxication during concomitant treatment with quinidine or verapamil.

Atrial flutter

Clinical manifestations. Atrial flutter may be a transitory acute disturbance in rhythm or it may be a chronic and recurrent disorder.[64] Atrial flutter commonly occurs in the setting of acute myocardial infarction,[65,66] after pneumonectomy, and after cardiac surgery in adults. It is an unusual rhythm disturbance in children.

Electrocardiographic characteristics. The typical ECG during atrial flutter shows a narrow QRS complex with a ventricular rate of approximately 150 beats/min. Atrial activity during atrial flutter causes a specific alteration in the surface ECG, giving the baseline a characteristic sawtooth appearance. When atrial activity is not readily evident, simultaneous recording of a rhythm strip during carotid sinus massage may allow recognition of P waves. The atrial rates in atrial flutter range from 250 to 350 beats/min, but they are remarkably close to 300 beats/min in most patients, with very little beat-to-beat variation (usually less than 20 msec).

The physiologic characteristics of the AV node require that AV block be present in virtually all cases of atrial flutter. The most common conduction ratio in patients with untreated atrial flutter is 2:1 AV block, which produces the typical ventricular rate of 150 beats/min. Higher grades of AV block in patients not treated with digitalis, β-blockers, or calcium channel blockers suggest the presence of AV nodal disease or enhanced vagal tone. Drugs that impair AV nodal conduction, specifically digitalis and verapamil, will also cause higher grades of AV block. In patients with accessory AV pathways, impulses may be conducted from the atrium to the ventricle without delay in the AV node. This rhythm is usually poorly tolerated and causes hemodynamic collapse. In children and adolescents with Wolff-Parkinson-White syndrome with 1:1 conduction from the atrium to the ventricle, hemodynamic instability is less common, and these patients may tolerate periods of extremely rapid tachycardia with only mild or moderate symptoms.

Electrophysiologic findings. The mechanism of atrial flutter is that of reentrant tachycardia.[67-71]

Atrial flutter has been divided into two types, one common and the other rare. This distinction depends on the morphology of the flutter waves.[72-74] The two types of atrial flutter differ in their electrophysiologic characteristics. Common atrial flutter, type I, generally has an atrial rate of 300 beats/min (range, 230 to 340), and atrial activation occurs in a counterclockwise sequence, producing negative P waves in leads I, II, III, and aVF. Type I atrial flutter is almost always amenable to treatment with rapid atrial pacing. The less common type of atrial flutter, type II, has a more rapid atrial rate (340 to 400 beats/min); atrial activation proceeds in a clockwise direction, and there are positive flutter waves in the inferior leads.

Regardless of the type of atrial flutter observed, electrophysiologic studies indicate that it is caused and maintained by reentrant mechanisms (Fig 22B-17). The electrophysiologic models that make use of an anatomic obstacle generally show an excitable gap between the beginning and the end of an impulse. In addition, there is an inverse relationship between the conduction velocity and the time required for an impulse to make a revolution about the circuit.

A peculiar characteristic of atrial flutter is the manner in which it can be terminated by atrial stimulation. Because atrial flutter is characterized by a very small excitable gap difficult to penetrate within the limits of atrial refractoriness, it is not commonly possible to interrupt atrial flutter with the introduction of critically timed single atrial premature beats. Rather, electrical interruption of atrial flutter generally requires sustained rapid pacing in the high right atrium or coronary sinus at very specific rates.[76,77]

Successful termination of atrial flutter in this manner is

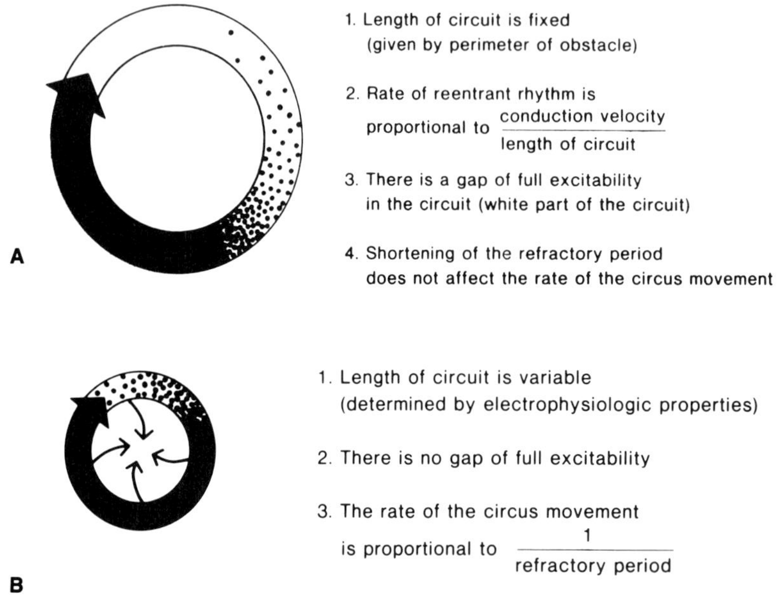

Fig 22B-17 Mechanism of atrial flutter. **A,** electrophysiologic characteristics of atrial flutter based on the theory of Mines.[75] **B,** electrophysiologic mechanism of atrial flutter proposed by Allessie et al.[69] (see text). (From Allessie MA, Bonke FIM: Atrial arrhythmias: basic concepts. In *Cardiac Arrhythmias: Their Mechanisms, Diagnosis, and Management.* Edited by WJ Mandel. Philadelphia, JB Lippincott Company, 1980, pp 145-166. By permission.)

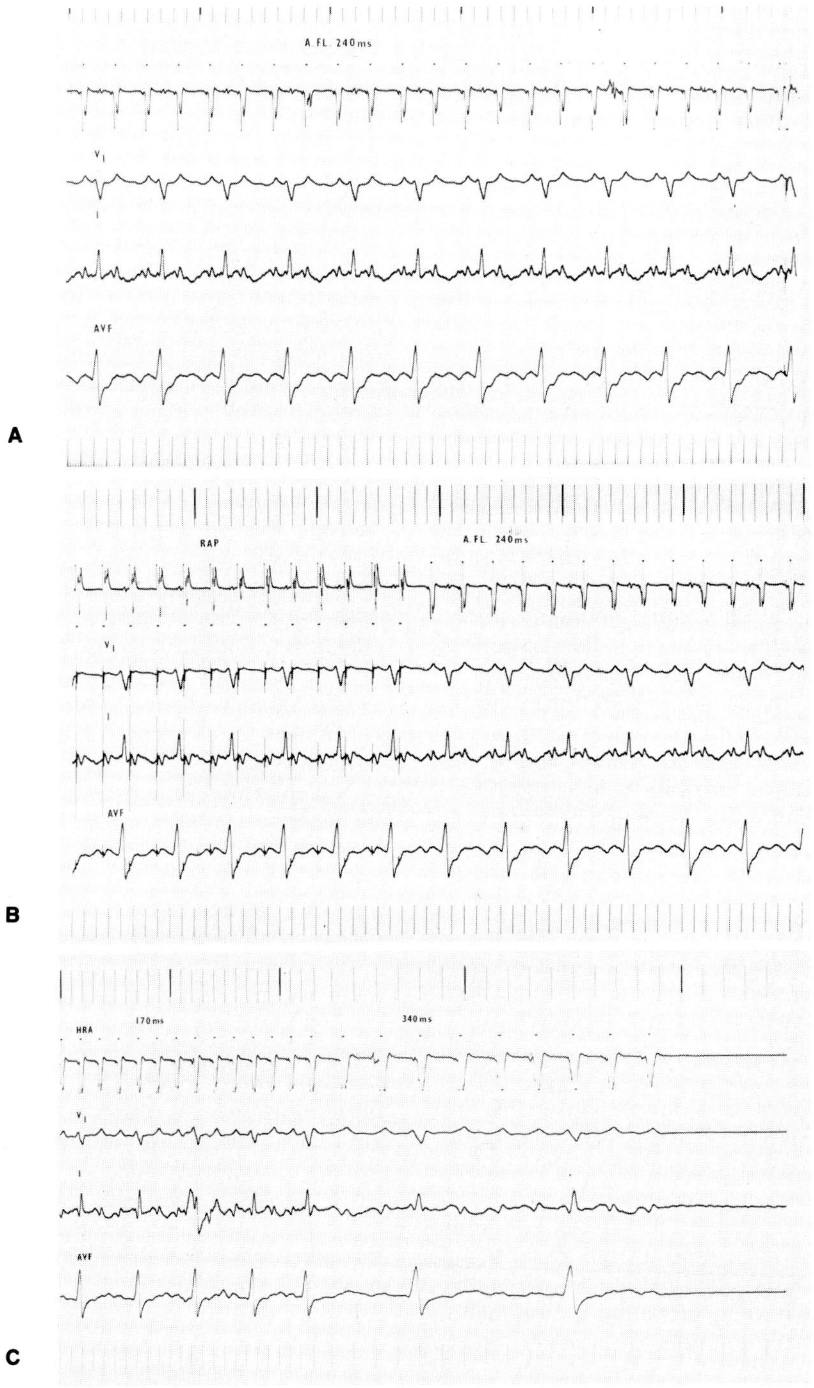

Fig 22B-18 Atrial flutter *(A. FL.)* and overdrive termination of atrial flutter. **A,** atrial electrogram *(HRA)* and three surface channels (V_1, *I,* and *aVF*) are recorded. Rate of atrial flutter was 250 beats/min (cycle length, 240 msec) with 2:1 AV block. **B,** rapid atrial pacing *(RAP)* captures the atrium. **C,** after pacing is abruptly discontinued, tachycardia terminates.

critically dependent upon the rate and duration of pacing. The critical rate at which flutter is terminated is approximately 125% of the basic flutter rate.[76] Pacing at more rapid rates causes atrial fibrillation, which is usually only transient before normal sinus rhythm returns. The technique of termination of atrial flutter with rapid pacing at cycle lengths that are shorter than the underlying flutter rate has been generally referred to as "entrainment" and is accompanied by an alteration in the morphology of the flutter waves in the inferior leads during pacing from a negative to a positive P wave (Fig 22B-18). The ability to terminate flutter by rapid atrial pacing is of importance for treatment and suggests that rapid pacing may be a preferred treatment for recurrent atrial flutter in patients who are recovering from surgery or from an acute myocardial infarction or those with digitalis toxicity.

Treatment. Atrial flutter occurs most often in the setting of organic heart disease and is not an uncommon consequence of acute myocardial infarction and cardiac or lung surgery. The goals of treatment of atrial flutter are to control the ventricular rate while attempting to restore sinus rhythm and prevent recurrences of atrial flutter. Emergency treatment of atrial flutter with a rapid ventricular response is best accomplished with direct-current cardioversion. Cardioversion should be undertaken in any circumstance in which the patient is hemodynamically compromised. If the hemodynamics are stable, however, urgent treatment of atrial flutter may be accomplished by the intravenous administration of propranolol or verapamil. When urgency is not required, oral digitalization will generally control the ventricular rate; if this is inadequate, propranolol or verapamil by mouth may provide the needed control.

Persistent atrial flutter can be treated by elective cardioversion. Atrial flutter has been terminated by the application of rapid atrial pacing.[76,77] This is, in fact, a quite convenient approach for patients in whom atrial flutter develops after cardiac surgery, who usually have temporary atrial pacing wires available. In most of these patients, the rhythm can be converted to sinus rhythm with little difficulty.

Prophylaxis for attacks of atrial flutter is probably best achieved with a combination of digoxin, a β-blocker or verapamil to control the ventricular rate, and a class I antiarrhythmia drug such as procainamide to provide prophylaxis by virtue of its membrane effects. Quinidine and disopyramide may also be used for this purpose, but neither of these drugs should be given until the patient has been adequately digitalized to prevent 1:1 conduction down the AV node during episodes of atrial flutter. In patients with repeated attacks of atrial flutter associated with atrial fibrillation and in those with a history of previous embolism during episodes of atrial flutter, anticoagulants should be utilized until the atrial rhythm abnormality has been controlled. When conventional drugs do not successfully control atrial flutter, use of amiodarone, flecainide, or propafenone may be necessary. The use of class IC drugs for the management of atrial fibrillation should be guided by caution, as was suggested earlier in this chapter for the use of these drugs in patients with supraventricular tachycardia. Patients with atrial flutter should always be evaluated with treadmill exercise testing once a stable antiarrhythmic drug dose is achieved and before hospital dismissal.

Atrial fibrillation

Atrial fibrillation is a common supraventricular arrhythmia and may occur in patients with and without organic heart disease. This rhythm disturbance is very common and coexists with many other arrhythmias and conduction defects. Although the atria are continuously depolarized and, therefore, not subject to other atrial arrhythmias, a combination of AV junctional arrhythmias and ventricular arrhythmias is common in patients who have atrial fibrillation. Some of these rhythms are related to the treatment of atrial fibrillation with drugs. Thus, one of the most common associated AV junctional rhythms is nonparoxysmal AV junctional tachycardia related to digitalis intoxication.[78]

Clinical manifestations. Paroxysmal atrial fibrillation is associated with the acute onset of a rapid, irregular rhythm. Patients with coexisting aortic or mitral valve disease, with hypertrophic cardiomyopathy, or who have had Fontan procedures usually will be acutely ill, with dyspnea or other signs of hemodynamic compromise. Atrial fibrillation may be an early manifestation of thyrotoxicosis in elderly patients.

In patients with atrial fibrillation and poorly controlled ventricular rates, heart failure may develop. This phenomenon was first described for patients with paroxysmal supraventricular tachycardia, but we have observed tachycardia-mediated heart failure and found that effective rate control can reverse ventricular dysfunction. It is not always necessary to restore normal sinus rhythm to improve ventricular function in patients with heart failure induced by atrial fibrillation.[79]

In general, patients with atrial fibrillation have an increased risk of stroke. However, patients with lone atrial fibrillation (defined as patients without identifiable heart disease or hypertension) are at low risk for stroke.[80] In patients with paroxysmal or chronic nonvalvular atrial fibrillation, there are significant clinical and echocardiographic predictors of thromboembolism that should be sought during evaluation.[81,82] The clinical predictors of stroke are recent congestive heart failure (within the last 3 months), history of hypertension, and previous arterial thromboemboli[81] (Table 22B-6). For a patient with none of these clinical predictors, the risk of thromboemboli is 2.5% per year; if one of the above-mentioned risk factors is present, the risk is approximately 7% per year; and if two or three of the clinical risk factors are present, the risk is almost 18% per year for a thromboembolic event. In echocardiographic examinations, the two strongest predictors of thromboembolism in atrial fibrillation from the Stroke Prevention in Atrial Fibrillation (SPAF) study were global left ventricular dysfunction and enlargement of the left atrium (M-mode measurement of greater than 2.4 cm/m^2 of body surface area or left atrial size greater than 4.7 cm).[82] Patients with nonvalvular atrial fibrillation without clinical or echocardiographic risk factors for thromboembolism have an extremely low risk for throm-

Table 22B-6 Clinical and echocardiographic predictors of risk of stroke in patients with atrial fibrillation

Predictor	Relative risk
History of hypertension	1.9
Recent congestive heart failure	2.0
Previous thromboembolism	1.9
Global left ventricular dysfunction	2.0
Left atrial size >2.4 cm/m^2, M-mode	1.6

boembolism (1.0% per year). However, more than one-third of patients without clinical risk factors were identified as being at moderate risk for thromboembolism (greater than 5.0% per year) when only one of the echocardiographic predictors was present.

Electrocardiographic characteristics. A typical ECG of atrial fibrillation shows a rapid irregular tachycardia in which recognizable P waves are absent. QRS complexes are generally normal, and the ventricular rate in patients with untreated atrial fibrillation generally ranges between 150 and 220 beats/min. However, in elderly patients, ventricular rates in untreated atrial fibrillation are typically slower. The ventricular rate may be accelerated in the presence of thyrotoxicosis, fever, catecholamines or catecholamine-like drugs, or conditions that enhance sympathetic tone. Although a cardinal feature of atrial fibrillation is irregularity of the R-R interval, at the most rapid ventricular rate this irregularity may be somewhat difficult to discern.

Electrophysiologic findings. The electrophysiologic mechanism of atrial fibrillation is not distinct. Multiple factors may be operative.[83-88] Atrial fibrillation is usually initiated by a premature atrial beat. Although an atrial premature depolarization may strike during a vulnerable period of atrial repolarization and cause atrial fibrillation as the initial rhythm, brief periods of rapid atrial tachycardia may precede the characteristic fibrillation.

Atrial fibrillation is a consequence of programmed atrial stimulation in 5% to 10% of normal patients.[89,90] In these circumstances the fibrillation is not sustained. Sustained atrial fibrillation provoked by programmed atrial stimulation generally correlates with the presence of spontaneously occurring atrial fibrillation. In patients with sustained atrial fibrillation, the mechanism is probably that of reentry tachycardia in which the heterogeneity of refractoriness of atrial tissue allows the development of intra-atrial conduction defects. In addition, sinus node dysfunction is more common in patients with sustained atrial fibrillation than in those who have nonsustained atrial fibrillation.[84]

Treatment. Acute atrial fibrillation may significantly impair hemodynamic stability in patients with acute myocardial infarction, valvular heart disease, or hypertrophic obstructive cardiomyopathy.[1] This circumstance dictates urgent treatment, which is best accomplished by direct-current cardioversion followed by the administration of digoxin to provide control of the ventricular rate in the event that atrial fibrillation recurs. If digoxin alone is inadequate in controlling the ventricular rate in these patients, either a β-blocker or a calcium channel blocker such as verapamil or diltiazem may be helpful. Intravenous administration of propranolol or verapamil should be used with caution in patients who have sustained acute myocardial infarction, because of the negative inotropic and dromotropic effects of these drugs. The use of the two together must be discouraged because of a propensity for causing complete heart block and heart failure. Other precipitating causes of atrial fibrillation should be sought and treated if found, including metabolic disorders, inflammatory processes, and drug intoxication.

The therapeutic goals in managing patients with atrial fibrillation are to maintain sinus rhythm or control ventricular rate (or both) and prevent stroke. Maintenance of sinus rhythm is difficult. The likelihood that quinidine will be effective in maintaining sinus rhythm for the long term is only 50%.[91] Flecainide,[92] propafenone,[93] and sotalol[94] may also be tried, but their long-term success in maintaining sinus rhythm is not substantially better than that of quinidine. Furthermore, there is an increased potential for proarrhythmia in patients with atrial fibrillation treated with class I drugs. Patients treated with class I drugs should undergo drug loading during ECG monitoring in the hospital and should have exercise testing before hospital dismissal to further evaluate the risk of proarrhythmia. Amiodarone is effective in maintaining sinus rhythm, especially in patients with atrial fibrillation that has been refractory to other antiarrhythmic drugs. When amiodarone is used to treat atrial fibrillation, maintenance doses can often be reduced to 200 mg/day. Low doses of amiodarone have fewer side effects than standard doses; the likelihood of pulmonary toxicity is low with daily maintenance doses of 200 mg, and proarrhythmia is far less than it is with other drugs.

When atrial fibrillation becomes established, control of the ventricular rate is the primary objective. The goal of therapy is to achieve resting ventricular rates of 70 to 80 beats/min and maximal exercise rates of less than 120 beats/min. Digoxin, calcium channel blockers, and β-blockers may be used to control ventricular rate. Amiodarone is also helpful in rate control. When satisfactory ventricular rate control cannot be achieved with drugs, catheter ablation of AV conduction and implantation of a permanent pacemaker are necessary.

A surgical approach to atrial fibrillation is also possible. This operation has been called "the maze procedure" because of the nature of the incisions made in the atrium to isolate the multiple reentrant circuits that characterize human atrial fibrillation. The maze operation appears to have the advantage of maintaining atrial kick, whereas previous surgical atrial isolation procedures failed to maintain a hemodynamic benefit. Early experience with the maze procedure is promising, but some patients have required pacing for sinus node dysfunction postoperatively. The discoveries made during the course of the development of the maze operation also hold promise for developing catheter ablation techniques for atrial flutter and fibrillation.

Stroke prevention in atrial fibrillation. Patients under age 60 with lone atrial fibrillation do not need long-term warfarin or aspirin therapy. Patients over age 60 with lone atrial fibrillation (defined as patients without identifiable heart disease or hypertension) are at a higher risk of transient ischemic attacks than those in an age- and sex-matched population and should be treated with long-term aspirin therapy (160 to 325 mg per day). If a transient ischemic attack occurs in an elderly person with lone atrial fibrillation, long-term warfarin therapy should be considered. The risks of major bleeding must also be weighed in the decision to treat older patients who have nonvalvular atrial fibrillation. In general, in patients less than 75 years of age who have no risk factors for bleeding (unstable gait, alcohol abuse, poor patient compliance, high-risk occupation, known bleeding disorder), the incidence of major bleeding is 1.0% to 1.5% per year with warfarin and 0.5% to 0.8% per year with aspirin.[95-98] However, major bleeding events (intracranial hemorrhage, bleeding causing death or requiring transfusion, surgery, or hospitalization) occur more frequently in patients aged 75 years and older. In this older age group, the incidence of major bleeding is 6% to 7% per year with warfarin and 1% to 1.5% per year with aspirin. The goal of warfarin therapy should be an international normalized ratio (INR) of 2.0 to 3.0.

Patients 75 years of age or younger who have nonvalvular atrial fibrillation without clinical or echocardiographic predictors of thromboemboli (approximately 25% of patients are in this group) are at low risk for stroke. This group could receive either aspirin (160 to 325 mg per day) or long-term warfarin therapy (INR, 2.0 to 3.0) if there are no contraindications. Patients 75 years old or younger who have one or more clinical or echocardiographic predictors of thromboemboli should receive long-term warfarin therapy if no bleeding contraindications exist. If there are bleeding contraindications, this age group should receive long-term aspirin therapy if possible. The treatment of patients older than 75 poses a complex problem. This age group, as noted above, has a higher incidence of major bleeding complications, but it has also been found that long-term aspirin therapy (up to 325 mg per day) does not significantly decrease this group's risk of thromboembolism. Therapy for this age group should be individualized on the basis of stroke and bleeding risk factors.

Preexcitation syndromes

Ventricular preexcitation[99] exists when any part of the ventricular myocardium is activated by an impulse originating in the atrium earlier than would be expected if the impulse reached the ventricles via the normal specialized conducting tissue. "Preexcitation" is a general term, however, and might be better defined as premature activation of any cardiac chamber by an impulse originating from the other chamber earlier than would be expected if the impulse were traveling through normal conducting tissue.[99] The clinical significance of the preexcitation syndrome is related to the high frequency of arrhythmias associated with the preexcitation.[100,101] In addition, preexcitation often gives rise to unusual ECG

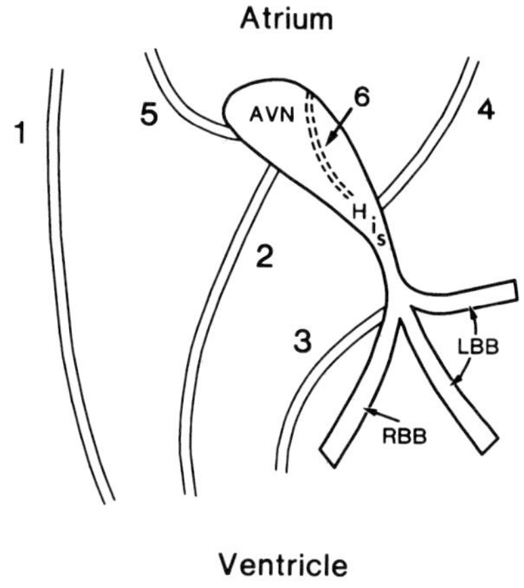

Fig 22B-19 Anatomic substrates of Wolff-Parkinson-White syndrome (see text). *1,* AV pathway; *2,* nodoventricular pathway; *3,* fasciculoventricular pathway; *4,* atrio-His pathway; *5,* posterior internodal tract; and *6,* preferential intranodal pathway. *AVN,* atrioventricular node; *LBB,* left bundle branch; *RBB,* right bundle branch.

tracings during tachycardia which can be a source of tremendous diagnostic difficulty. The delta wave patterns of preexcitation during sinus rhythm may be confused for myocardial infarction or other conditions. The most common clinical example of preexcitation is the Wolff-Parkinson-White syndrome.

The anatomic substrates for the preexcitation syndromes include several types of accessory AV connections[102,103] (Fig 22B-19). These connections include fibers that course directly from the atrium to the ventricle and are called "accessory AV pathways" (also called "Kent bundles"); fibers that connect the atria to the His bundle, called "atrio-Hisian fibers" (also called "James fibers"); fibers that course from the AV node to the ventricle, called "nodoventricular fibers" (also referred to as "Mahaim fibers"); and fibers that arise in the His bundle or bundle branches and course to the ventricular myocardium, called "fasciculoventricular fibers" and also "Mahaim fibers." Although the anatomic pathways may be present in any given heart, they may not be electrophysiologically active, and they may not explain the tachycardias in patients who have associated dual AV nodal pathways as potential substrates for their tachyarrhythmias.[101-105]

Electrocardiographic characteristics. The ECG in patients with the Wolff-Parkinson-White syndrome is noted for its characteristic delta wave and short P-R interval, described initially as bundle-branch block with a short P-R interval. Variance of this appearance is quite possible and reflects the fact that the ECG manifestations of preexcitation are determined by the location of the accessory pathway, the intra-atrial conduction time, the conduction time over the accessory pathway, and the AV nodal conduction time. The classic ECG occurs when the conduction time from the SA node to the ventricle via the accessory pathway is shorter than the conduction time over the normal AV conducting system; thus, the P-R interval is short, there is a delta wave, and associated

Table 22B-7 ECG localization of accessory pathways

Site of accessory connection	ECG criteria
Left free wall	Negative or isoelectric delta wave in any one of leads I, aVL, V_5, and V_6 RS in V_1 or V_2 Delta wave duration often <40 msec
Posteroseptal	Negative or isoelectric delta wave in any two of leads II, III, and aVF RS in V_1, V_2, or V_3 QR in V_1, V_2, or V_3 with Ebstein's anomaly
Right free wall	LBBB pattern, axis +30° to −60°
Right anteroseptal	LBBB pattern, axis +30° to +120°

LBBB, Left bundle-branch block.
Modified from Milstein S, Sharma AD, Guiraudon GM, et al: An algorithm for the electrocardiographic localization of accessory pathways in the Wolff-Parkinson-White syndrome. *PACE* 10:555-563, 1987.

alterations of the T wave reflect altered repolarization. However, in some circumstances the contribution of the accessory pathway may be minimal, so the P-R interval is normal and the QRS complex does not show the typical delta wave. Patients with left lateral accessory pathways and enhanced AV nodal conduction may have a normal QRS during sinus rhythm.

There has been some controversy about the usefulness of the 12-lead ECG in localizing the anatomic site of an accessory pathway in patients with Wolff-Parkinson-White syndrome. In our experience,[106] the 12-lead ECG is of limited use in the exact localization of the anatomic site of accessory pathways, especially when maximal preexcitation is absent. Milstein et al.[107] found that the surface ECG can effectively predict the site of an accessory pathway when a simplified system of localization is used that would place pathways in the left free wall, the posteroseptal region of the AV group, the right free wall, and the right anteroseptal region of the AV groove. Table 22B-7 summarizes the ECG criteria that may help in the localization of accessory pathways. The effective use of the 12-lead ECG in localizing accessory pathways may not require maximal preexcitation on the surface ECG. In fact, a minimal preexcitation pattern in an adult with Wolff-Parkinson-White syndrome is a useful first approximation to localizing the accessory pathway to the left lateral free wall.[108]

The development of radiofrequency ablation requires greater diagnostic precision in the localization of accessory pathways. Some patients with Wolff-Parkinson-White syndrome have multiple accessory pathways, and in these patients careful analysis of the surface ECG, especially during atrial fibrillation, is a critical part of the diagnostic evaluation and localization of pathways.

The ECG features that suggest multiple pathways are the occurrence of more than one preexcited QRS morphology and simultaneous preexcitation of the ventricles, creating a QRS pattern atypical for any single pathway.[109] It is important to record a 12-lead ECG with a long rhythm strip during all episodes of atrial fibrillation. In the electrophysiology laboratory, His bundle electrograms should be recorded during atrial fibrillation to minimize the confusion that can be created by premature ventricular beats or functional bundle-branch block. This maneuver helps avoid the conclusion that the altered QRS morphology related to such events is evidence of multiple pathways.

Other ECG findings that may suggest multiple accessory pathways are multiple P-wave configurations during orthodromic tachycardia, a spontaneous change from orthodromic to antidromic tachycardia or from one morphology of antidromic tachycardia to another, and a change in preexcitation noted after the administration of a drug.[110]

The incidence of the ECG pattern of preexcitation described as the Wolff-Parkinson-White syndrome has been reported to vary from 0.1 to 3 per 1,000, and there is no age predilection except that the incidence seems to decrease somewhat in elderly persons.[111] AV bypass tracts that are involved in tachycardia and are capable of antegrade conduction have been associated with certain heart diseases, specifically Ebstein's anomaly of the tricuspid valve, in which as many as 10% to 25% of patients will have preexcitation, usually involving an anatomically right-sided pathway.[112] A possible association has been reported between left-sided bypass tracts and mitral valve prolapse.[99] The Wolff-Parkinson-White syndrome has also been associated with various cardiomyopathies and congenital cardiac disorders.[99,111] In most patients, however, no heart disease is present even though preexcitation is found.

Arrhythmias associated with preexcitation. As indicated earlier, "preexcitation" is a general term that can be construed as indicating activation of the cardiac chamber earlier than would be expected. This general term has been used interchangeably with the eponymic description known to everyone, the Wolff-Parkinson-White syndrome. This is an occasional source of confusion, but an even greater source of confusion is the number of descriptions that are given of the tachycardias associated with preexcitation. They have been called "reciprocating tachycardia," "circus movement tachycardia," and "AV reentrant tachycardia." All of these terms imply that the tachycardia utilizes the accessory pathway for one limb of the tachycardia circuit. Although commonly the accessory pathway participates as the retrograde limb of the reentrant circuit, it may participate as the antegrade limb. Both mechanisms of tachycardia are described in detail below.

Most patients with AV pathways have arrhythmias, the most common of which is a reentrant tachycardia that uses the normal AV node and the His-Purkinje system as the antegrade limb of the reentry circuit and the bypass tract as the retrograde limb of the circuit (orthodromic tachycardia)[99,113] (Fig 22B-20,A). A typical attack of tachycardia results when a premature beat blocks an impulse in the accessory pathway and also conducts, with

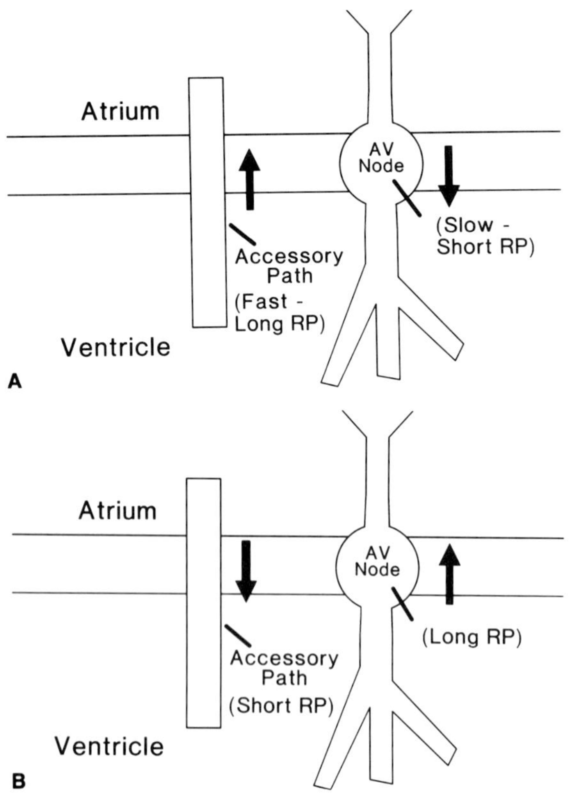

Fig 22B-20 Mechanisms of tachycardia in Wolff-Parkinson-White syndrome. **A,** reciprocating tachyardia (also called orthodromic tachycardia). This is the most common mechanism of tachycardia observed in Wolff-Parkinson-White syndrome. In this form, tachycardia is often initiated by a premature atrial beat that blocks in the accessory pathway and then is conducted antegrade down the AV node. The impulse then is conducted retrograde to the atrium over the accessory pathway and returns to the ventricle over the AV node. In this manner, a reciprocating tachycardia is sustained. Unless functional bundle-branch block is present, the QRS complex will be narrow, going to its antegrade conduction down normal AV conduction tissues. **B,** more unusual form of reciprocating tachycardia (sometimes called antidromic tachycardia) observed in Wolff-Parkinson-White syndrome in which the antegrade limb of the reentry circuit is the accessory pathway and the retrograde limb is the AV node. In this circumstance, the QRS complex is wide. RP, refractory period.

a physiologic delay, down the normal conducting tissue. The resulting QRS complex is of normal morphology because it has not been preexcited. The wave of excitability then spreads throughout the ventricle and finds the accessory pathway excitable; thus, conduction occurs in a retrograde direction across the pathway and allows reexcitation of the atrium. As a result, a reentrant circuit has been established and a tachycardia initiated. Detailed intra-atrial recordings during ventricular pacing and tachycardia will reveal an abnormal sequence of atrial activation and allow the localization of accessory pathways by mapping techniques in the electrophysiology laboratory.[99,114,115]

Occasionally in the electrophysiology laboratory, it may be difficult to catheterize the coronary sinus for the purpose of recording left atrial activation sequences during reciprocating tachycardia. Packer et al.[116] demonstrated the usefulness of the response to single and double ventricular premature beats introduced during reciprocating tachycardia in predicting the location of left free-wall accessory pathways. Retrograde preexcitation in response to a single ventricular extrastimulus during reciprocating tachycardia suggested a posterolateral location of the left free-wall pathway. Atrial preexcitation seen in response to paired ventricular extrastimuli during tachycardia suggested an intermediate location of the free-wall pathway, and failure of either single or paired ventricular extrastimuli during reciprocating tachycardia to preexcite the atrium suggested a location of accessory pathway beyond the lateral margin of the left ventricle or the very distal left AV groove.

Although the most common cause of a wide-QRS-complex tachycardia in patients with Wolff-Parkinson-White syndrome is orthodromic tachycardia with bundle-branch block, a less common type of reentrant tachycardia in patients with AV bypass tracts, "antidromic reciprocating tachycardia,"[99,114] also causes a wide QRS complex. In this circumstance, the AV bypass tract functions as the antegrade limb of the reentry circuit and the AV node constitutes the retrograde limb (Fig 22B-20,B). Since the impulse travels from the atrium to the ventricle down the accessory pathway, the ECG during tachycardia reveals the P wave just before the preexcited ventricular complex, which is wide. Thus, this type of tachycardia may often be confused with ventricular tachycardia. The ECG during normal sinus rhythm demonstrates the typical Wolff-Parkinson-White characteristics of a short P-R interval and a delta wave.

The remaining types of preexcitation syndromes are less common than the Wolff-Parkinson-White syndrome, which utilizes an accessory AV pathway.[99,115,117-119] Mahaim fibers originate either in the AV node (nodoventricular fibers) or in the bundle of His (fasciculoventricular fibers) and insert distally into the ventricle; thus, they bypass the distal AV conduction system. In most reported cases of supraventricular tachycardia involving a nodoventricular bypass tract and a wide-complex tachycardia, the bypass tract has been inserted into the right ventricle; this produces a QRS complex during tachycardia which has a left bundle-branch block morphology. Although Mahaim fibers are a common anatomic finding, supraventricular tachycardia that utilizes a fasciculoventricular pathway is rare.[99,120] Patients with Mahaim fibers have been found to have AV nodal reentrant tachycardias in which the Mahaim fibers are simply passive bystanders.[118,119,121] The presence of the delta wave in association with a normal P-R interval or a junctional premature beat that demonstrates ventricular preexcitation is a cardinal feature of the ECG which suggests the presence of Mahaim fibers.[118]

Accessory atrio-Hisian or atriofascicular connections have been described. Although such fibers have been considered to be the potential anatomic substrate of the

Lown-Ganong-Levine syndrome (short P-R interval and normal QRS morphology),[117] electrophysiologic studies in patients with this syndrome generally reveal enhanced AV node conduction. In these patients, conduction through the AV node is rapid at rest (A-H, <60 msec) but A-H intervals become longer with incremental atrial pacing, thereby excluding the involvement of accessory atrio-Hisian or atriofascicular connections in these patients.

It should be noted that the description of nodofascicular fibers as James fibers is imprecise. James[122] described a fiber present in normal hearts which passed from the eustachian ridge forward to insert into the junction of the AV node and bundle. The nodofascicular or atrio-Hisian connections are fibers that insert directly through the fibrous tissue collar and enter the penetrating AV bundle.[123]

Combinations of nodofascicular and fasciculoventricular fibers have been reported which give the ECG appearance of the Wolff-Parkinson-White syndrome. Physiologically, it appears that both nodofascicular and fasciculoventricular fibers are similar to normal AV conduction tissue.

Patients with multiple accessory pathways appear to have an increased risk for the development of ventricular fibrillation.[124] The reasons why patients with multiple pathways have this increased risk remain uncertain, but possible explanations are that a greater potential for complex wave fronts increases the risk of atrial fibrillation and, simply, that multiple pathways increase the likelihood that one pathway will have a short refractory period.

Atrial fibrillation in patients with bypass tracts. Patients with AV bypass tracts are susceptible to the development of very rapid ventricular rates during atrial fibrillation or flutter. During atrial fibrillation in a patient with an antegradely conducting AV bypass tract, the QRS complex will be wide as a result of ventricular preexcitation. However, the conduction down the AV node will result in a normal QRS complex or in fusion complexes. The ventricular rate and the morphology of the QRS complex depend on the refractory periods of the AV node and of the accessory pathway. Patients with AV bypass tracts or AV nodal bypass tracts can experience ventricular rates as rapid as 350 beats/min during atrial fibrillation or flutter, which may deteriorate to ventricular fibrillation and cause sudden death.[125,126] Patients with long effective refractory periods of the bypass tract have moderate ventricular responses during atrial fibrillation, but those with short refractory periods have more rapid ventricular responses. Patients with an effective refractory period of the accessory pathway of less than 220 msec are at the greatest risk for extremely rapid ventricular responses and ventricular fibrillation during atrial fibrillation.[127]

Given the risk of sudden death in patients with Wolff-Parkinson-White syndrome, there has been intense interest in the development of either invasive or noninvasive testing regimens that would predict with great accuracy which patients are at highest risk. Atrial fibrillation with a rapid ventricular rate may occur as the presenting arrhythmia in patients with Wolff-Parkinson-White syndrome. Investigators have confirmed the conclusion that invasive electrophysiologic studies are not useful in predicting the likelihood of sudden death in patients with Wolff-Parkinson-White syndrome.[128,129] Thus, invasive electrophysiologic studies should not be used as a routine screening test in asymptomatic patients with ventricular preexcitation.

Part of the explanation for low specificity includes the findings that atrial fibrillation is not a common arrhythmia and that the incidence of sudden death is low in patients with Wolff-Parkinson-White syndrome. Using noninvasive techniques to select patients for invasive studies has a limited value.[130] Infusion of procainamide has in the past been considered a possible noninvasive technique to identify patients who have Wolff-Parkinson-White syndrome or who are potentially at risk for sudden death, but the work of Fananapazir et al.[131] indicated a poor correlation between the use of procainamide infusion and the ability to risk-stratify patients with Wolff-Parkinson-White syndrome.

Thus, neither invasive electrophysiologic testing nor noninvasive techniques are useful in predicting risk of sudden death among asymptomatic patients with Wolff-Parkinson-White syndrome.

Treatment of tachyarrhythmias associated with preexcitation. Patients with the Wolff-Parkinson-White syndrome may seek medical attention because of a rapid tachycardia that is found to be atrial fibrillation or atrial flutter with 1:1 antegrade conduction down the accessory pathway. The most effective treatment in patients who are hemodynamically compromised is direct-current cardioversion. In the absence of such compromise, procainamide administered intravenously is especially useful in the acute therapy of atrial fibrillation with Wolff-Parkinson-White syndrome. Furthermore, procainamide and disopyramide are effective drugs for long-term prophylaxis of atrial fibrillation or flutter in Wolff-Parkinson-White syndrome. The use of lidocaine,[132-134] although controversial, may be successful in limiting the ventricular response in patients with atrial fibrillation and rapid antegrade conduction down an accessory pathway by virtue of its ability to produce antegrade block in the pathway. One should avoid using propranolol, which slows AV conduction but not conduction in the accessory pathway,[133,135] verapamil,[136,137] which decreases retrograde concealed conduction of the accessory pathway (Fig 22B-21), and digoxin,[138,139] which decreases the effective refractory period of the bypass tract. After the acute condition has been stabilized, the patient should be referred for invasive electrophysiologic testing.

Other patients with Wolff-Parkinson-White syndrome may experience periodic palpitations or episodes of tachycardia which are not as disabling as those associated with very rapid conduction down an accessory pathway. Since these patients may have a normal ECG between the episodes of tachycardia, the mechanisms of their tachycardia may not be evident to the examining physician. On other occasions, episodes of tachycardia may be sufficiently rare that invasive electrophysiologic study may not be warranted initially. In these circumstances, long-term antiarrhythmia therapy may be undertaken empirically. In such cases, a class I antiarrhythmia drug—disopyramide[140,141] (Fig 22B-22), quinidine,[142,143] or

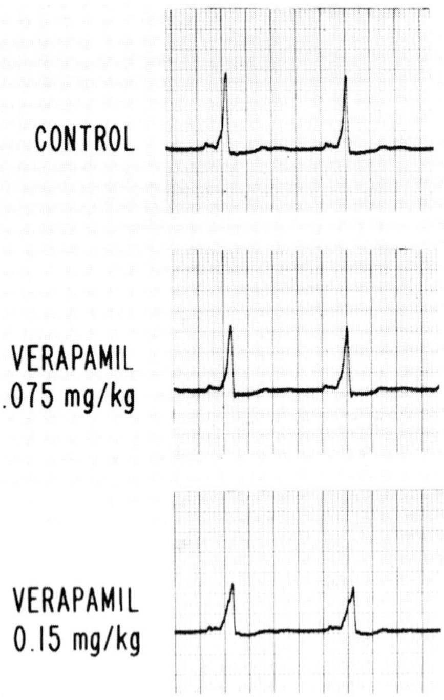

Fig 22B-21 Effect of verapamil in patients with Wolff-Parkinson-White syndrome. **Top panel,** two QRS complexes recorded from a patient with resting preexcitation. The P-R interval is short and the delta wave is evident. **Middle panel,** after administration of a small dose of verapamil, the delta wave is exaggerated, indicating preferential conduction down the accessory pathway. **Bottom panel,** as a higher dose of verapamil is given, conduction in the AV node is further slowed, and the ECG manifestation of preexcitation is exaggerated.

procainamide—all of which increase the effective refractory period of the accessory pathway,[142-144] may be effective. Flecainide, propafenone, and sotalol may also be effective in treating patients with Wolff-Parkinson-White syndrome so long as there is no underlying structural heart disease. If there is evidence of a long effective refractory period of the accessory pathway—specifically, if the delta wave disappears during increasing heart rates or if there is only intermittent accessory pathway function on routine ECGs—drugs such as propranolol, verapamil, and digoxin may be used. If empiric therapy fails to control the episodes of tachycardia or if there is a suggestion that the accessory pathway is capable of sustaining very rapid AV conduction, electrophysiologic studies must be performed.

The long-term treatment of patients with Wolff-Parkinson-White syndrome and reentrant reciprocating tachycardia is often guided by the results of invasive electrophysiologic testing. Catheter ablation of accessory connection is the best treatment for most patients with Wolff-Parkinson-White syndrome (see chapter 26).

Digitalis has an unpredictable effect on conduction and refractoriness in AV bypass tracts.[138,139] Therefore, a digitalis preparation should be administered with caution in patients with Wolff-Parkinson-White syndrome, especially when atrial fibrillation or flutter has occurred. Digitalis in these circumstances may cause the ventricular rate to increase to the point that ventricular fibrillation may ensue. If electrophysiologic testing demonstrates that digitalis does not shorten the refractory period of the AV accessory pathway, the drug may be quite useful in preventing episodes of reciprocating tachycardia by increasing AV nodal refractoriness and thereby disrupting the reentry circuit.

β-Adrenergic blocking agents have no direct effect on the AV bypass tract but, like digitalis, these drugs may be helpful in preventing orthodromic and antidromic tachycardia because of their effect on the AV node.[133,135]

Verapamil also behaves like digitalis in that it has no direct effect on the accessory pathway.[136] The salutary effect of verapamil in terminating a reciprocating tachycardia that utilizes an accessory pathway depends entirely on the effect of this drug on the AV node. Verapamil may paradoxically increase the ventricular rate during atrial fibrillation by altering retrograde conduction into the accessory pathway and increasing sympathetic tone as a result of peripheral vasodilation[137] (see Fig 22B-21).

Drugs that directly affect conduction and refractoriness of the accessory pathway are the mainstay of treatment of patients with the Wolff-Parkinson-White syndrome. Class I antiarrhythmia drugs—namely, procainamide, quinidine, and disopyramide[140,142-144]—lengthen refractoriness in the accessory pathway, the atrium, the ventricle, and the His-Purkinje system (see Fig 22B-22). Thus, these drugs may prolong conduction at virtually any point within the reentry circuit and thereby terminate episodes of reciprocating tachycardia. However, when the effective refractory period of the accessory pathway is short, usually less than 270 msec, these drugs are less likely to be beneficial.[145]

Amiodarone has been found to be effective in terminating and preventing episodes of circus movement tachycardia that utilizes accessory pathways.[146-148] Amiodarone prolongs the refractoriness of an accessory pathway as well as of the AV node. It may be especially helpful in preventing tachycardia in the Wolff-Parkinson-White syndrome by suppressing the number of atrial and ventricular premature beats that trigger reciprocating tachycardias. Evidence suggests that amiodarone may be ineffective at prolonging the refractoriness of accessory pathways of patients in whom the baseline effective refractory period of the accessory pathway is short.[149]

TREATMENT OF SUPRAVENTRICULAR TACHYCARDIA BY MEANS OF PACING SYSTEMS

Supraventricular tachycardia may be terminated by various forms of electrical stimulation, including single or paired stimuli delivered at a critical time during the cardiac cycle.[150,151] This can be achieved with an automatic scanning pacemaker,[150,152] or it can be done by competitive underdrive pacing[153-155] with the use of a demand pacemaker firing in the asynchronous mode or by bursts of stimuli delivered either by an automatic antitachycardia pacemaker[156] or a patient-activated radiofrequency pacemaker.[157-160]

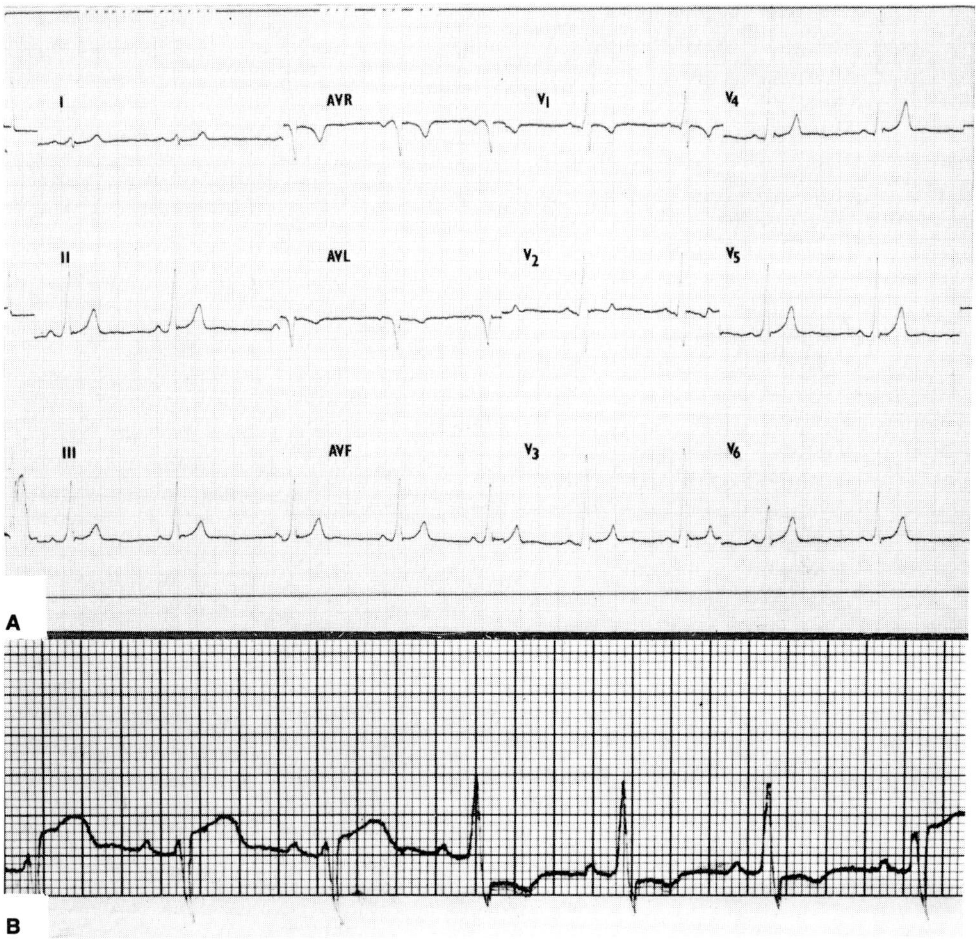

Fig 22B-22 Effect of disopyramide on accessory pathway conduction in a patient with Wolff-Parkinson-White syndrome. **A,** a 12-lead ECG recorded from a patient with a left lateral accessory pathway. Resting preexcitation is evident by virtue of short P-R interval and presence of a delta wave that is positive in leads II, III, *aVF,* and V_{1-6}. After an electrophysiologic study indicated that procainamide completely abolished conduction in an antegrade fashion down the accessory pathway, the patient was given disopyramide by mouth. **B,** after four doses of disopyramide, a rhythm strip showed intermittent evidence of preexcitation. The first three beats of this rhythm strip show normal AV conduction followed by three beats that were conducted down the accessory pathway followed again by conduction down the normal AV conduction system. After subsequent doses of disopyramide were administered, antegrade conduction down the pathway was abolished.

The treatment of supraventricular tachycardia by pacing techniques is based on the ability of an electrical stimulus to alter conduction in some portion of the reentry circuit so as to render an area of tissue unexcitable and thereby interrupt the recirculating wave front. All of the pacing modalities that may be applied to the treatment of supraventricular tachycardia have the propensity to initiate reentrant tachycardias or atrial fibrillation, and this is the chief limitation of antitachycardia pacing in the treatment of this tachycardia. In addition, significant problems are encountered in other aspects of pacemaker function in this unusual group of patients. A detailed description of the pacing techniques and associated problems for patients with supraventricular tachycardia is found in chapter 25B.

SURGICAL TREATMENT OF SUPRAVENTRICULAR TACHYCARDIA

The risks of long-term antiarrhythmic drug therapy and the safety and efficacy of radiofrequency catheter ablation in the treatment of patients with Wolff-Parkinson-White syndrome (see chapter 26), AV nodal reentrant tachycardia, and some intra-atrial tachycardias has changed the practice of electrosurgery. Catheter ablation techniques are rapidly replacing electrosurgery for treatment of symptomatic supraventricular tachycardia.

However, when radiofrequency ablation for supraventricular tachycardia fails to achieve the desired curative result, curative cardiac electrosurgery should still be considered.[161] The goal of surgical treatment is to excise an arrhythmogenic focus of tissue in the atrium,[162-165] to ablate an accessory pathway,[99,166,167] or to modify AV node function in patients with dual AV nodal pathways and supraventricular tachycardia.[29,30]

Certain patients may benefit from surgical treatment of the supraventricular tachycardia associated with the Wolff-Parkinson-White syndrome. A more detailed discussion of the surgical procedures used to divide accessory pathways is found in chapter 26. The selection of an optimal surgical candidate depends on an extensive preoperative evaluation, which includes invasive electrophysiologic testing. At the time of the preoperative electrophysiologic study, detailed right and left atrial mapping is undertaken to localize the bypass tract and to determine whether multiple bypass tracts are present. Another objective of a preoperative electrophysiologic study is to determine whether the accessory pathway is involved in the patient's reentry tachycardia. Factors that influence the decision for surgery include the nature of the patient's tachycardia, the hemodynamic consequences of the tachycardia, the risk for the development of ventricular fibrillation and sudden death, the response to other therapeutic modalities (including the need for long-term medical therapy), and the location and functional characteristics of the accessory pathway. Patients who are undergoing operation for congenital heart disease and have associated Wolff-Parkinson-White syndrome should undergo surgical division of the accessory pathway at the same operation.

CATHETER ABLATION IN THE MANAGEMENT OF SUPRAVENTRICULAR ARRHYTHMIAS

Closed chest ablation of the AV conduction system by means of a synchronized direct-current electrical discharge was originally described for treatment of refractory atrial fibrillation.[168-170] Improvements in catheter mapping techniques, better understanding of the mechanisms of reentrant arrhythmias in the AV junction, and the development of radiofrequency energy to replace direct current have broadened the indications for catheter ablation. Radiofrequency catheter ablation should be considered early in the treatment of paients with symptomatic AV node reentrant tachycardia[31-33,171,172] and AV reentrant tachycardia.[11,14,173-175] Patients with symptomatic intra-atrial tachycardia who are refractory to antiarrhythmic drugs should also be considered for catheter ablation.[62,176] A detailed description of catheter ablation techniques can be found in chapter 26.

REFERENCES

1. James TN: Arrhythmias and conduction disturbances in acute myocardial infarction. *Am Heart J* 64:416-426, 1962
2. Lippestad CT, Marton PF: Sinus arrest in proximal right coronary artery occlusion. *Am Heart J* 74:551-556, 1967
3. Davies MJ, Pomerance A: Pathology of atrial fibrillation in man. *Br Heart J* 34:520-525, 1972
4. Sims BA: Pathogenesis of atrial arrhythmias. *Br Heart J* 34:336-340, 1972
5. Greenwood RJ, Dupler DA: Death following carotid sinus pressure. *JAMA* 181:605-609, 1962
6. Porus RL, Marcus FI: Ventricular fibrillation during carotid-sinus stimulation. *N Engl J Med* 268:1338-1342, 1963
7. Alexander S, Ping WC: Fatal ventricular fibrillation during carotid sinus stimulation. *Am J Cardiol* 18:289-291, 1966
8. Griffith MJ, Garratt CJ, Ward DE, et al: The effects of adenosine on sinus node reentrant tachycardia. *Clin Cardiol* 12:409-411, 1989
9. Gallagher JJ, Smith WM, Kasell J, et al: Use of esophageal lead in the diagnosis of mechanisms of reciprocating supraventricular tachycardia. *PACE* 3:440-451, 1980
10. Arzbaecher R: A pill electrode for the study of cardiac arrhythmia. *Med Instrum* 12:277-281, 1978
11. Calkins H, Sousa J, el-Atassi R, et al: Diagnosis and cure of the Wolff-Parkinson-White syndrome or paroxysmal supraventricular tachycardias during a single electrophysiologic test. *N Engl J Med* 324:1612-1618, 1991
12. Schamroth L, Krikler DM, Garrett C: Immediate effects of intravenous verapamil in cardiac arrhythmias. *Br Med J* 1:660-662, 1972
13. Singh BN, Ellrodt G, Peter CT: Verapamil: a review of its pharmacological properties and therapeutic use. *Drugs* 15:169-197, 1978
14. Scheinman MM, Laks MM, DiMarco J, et al: Current role of catheter ablative procedures in patients with cardiac arrhythmias. A report for health professionals from the Subcommittee on Electrocardiography and Electrophysiology, American Heart Association. *Circulation* 83:2146-2153, 1991
15. Wu D, Denes P, Amat-y-Leon F, et al: Clinical, electrocardiographic and electrophysiologic observations in patients with paroxysmal supraventricular tachycardia. *Am J Cardiol* 41:1045-1051, 1978
16. Gallagher JJ, Sealy WC: The permanent form of junctional reciprocating tachycardia: further elucidation of the underlying mechanism. *Eur J Cardiol* 8:413-430, 1978
17. Brugada P, Vanagt EJ, Bär FWHM, et al: Incessant reciprocating atrioventricular tachycardia: factors playing a role in the mechanism of the arrhythmia. *PACE* 3:670-677, 1980
18. Coumel P: Junctional reciprocating tachycardias: the permanent and paroxysmal forms of A-V nodal reciprocating tachycardias. *J Electrocardiol* 8:79-90, 1975
19. Brugada P, Farré J, Green M, et al: Observations in patients with supraventricular tachycardia having a P-R interval: differentiation between atrial tachycardia and reciprocating atrioventricular tachycardia using an accessory pathway with long conduction times. *Am Heart J* 107:556-570, 1984
20. Goldreyer BN, Damato AN: The essential role of atrioventricular conduction delay in the initiation of paroxysmal supraventricular tachycardia. *Circulation* 43:679-687, 1971
21. Josephson ME, Kastor JA: Supraventricular tachycardia: mechanisms and management. *Ann Intern Med* 87:346-358, 1977
22. Wu D, Denes P: Mechanisms of paroxysmal supraventricular tachycardia. *Arch Intern Med* 135:437-442, 1975
23. Denes P, Wu D, Dhingra RC, et al: Demonstration of dual A-V nodal pathways in patients with paroxysmal supraventricular tachycardia. *Circulation* 48:549-555, 1973
24. Rosen KM, Mehta A, Miller RA: Demonstration of dual atrioventricular nodal pathways in man. *Am J Cardiol* 33:291-294, 1974
25. Josephson ME, Seides SF: *Clinical Cardiac Electrophysiology: Techniques and Interpretations.* Philadelphia, Lea & Febiger, 1979, p 152
26. Josephson ME, Kastor JA: Paroxysmal supraventricular tachycardia: is the atrium a necessary link? *Circulation* 54:430-435, 1976
27. Haft JI: Treatment of arrhythmias by intracardiac electrical stimulation. *Prog Cardiovasc Dis* 16:539-568, 1974
28. Wellens HJJ, Wesdorp JC, Düren DR, et al: Second degree block during reciprocal atrioventricular nodal tachycardia. *Circulation* 53:595-599, 1976
29. Cox JL, Holman WL, Cain ME: Cryosurgical treatment of atrioventricular node reentrant tachycardia. *Circulation* 76:1329-1336, 1987
30. Wood DL, Hammill SC, Porter CJ, et al: Cryosurgical modification of atrioventricular conduction for treatment of atrioventricular node reentrant tachycardia. *Mayo Clin Proc* 63:988-992, 1988

31. Lee MA, Morady F, Kadish A, et al: Catheter modification of the atrioventricular junction with radiofrequency energy for control of atrioventricular nodal reentry tachycardia. *Circulation* 83:827-835, 1991

32. Roman CA, Wang X, Friday KJ, et al: Catheter technique for selective ablation of slow pathway in AV nodal reentrant tachycardia (abstract). *PACE* 13:498, 1990

33. Haissaguerre M, Warin JF, Lemetayer P, et al: Closed-chest ablation of retrograde conduction in patients with atrioventricular nodal reentrant tachycardia. *N Engl J Med* 320:426-433, 1989

34. McGuire MA, Lau KC, Johnson DC, et al: Patients with two types of atrioventricular junctional (AV nodal) reentrant tachycardia. Evidence that a common pathway of nodal tissue is not present above the reentrant circuit. *Circulation* 83:1232-1246, 1991

35. Josephson ME, Scharf DL, Kastor JA, et al: Atrial endocardial activation in man: electrode catheter technique for endocardial mapping. *Am J Cardiol* 39:972-981, 1977

36. Amat-y-Leon F, Dhingra RC, Wu D, et al: Catheter mapping of retrograde atrial activation: observations during ventricular pacing and AV nodal re-entrant paroxysmal tachycardia. *Br Heart J* 38:355-362, 1976

37. Pritchett EL, McCarthy EA, Wilkinson WE: Propafenone treatment of symptomatic paroxysmal supraventricular arrhythmias. A randomized, placebo-controlled, crossover trial in patients tolerating oral therapy. *Ann Intern Med* 114:539-544, 1991

38. Hammill SC, McLaran CJ, Wood DL, et al: Double-blind study of intravenous propafenone for paroxysmal supraventricular reentrant tachycardia. *J Am Coll Cardiol* 9:1364-1368, 1987

39. Henthorn RW, Waldo AL, Anderson JL, et al: Flecainide acetate prevents recurrence of symptomatic paroxysmal supraventricular tachycardia. The Flecainide Supraventricular Tachycardia Study Group. *Circulation* 83:119-125, 1991

40. Pritchett EL, DaTorre SD, Platt ML, et al: Flecainide acetate treatment of paroxysmal supraventricular tachycardia and paroxysmal atrial fibrillation: dose-response studies. The Flecainide Supraventricular Tachycardia Study Group. *J Am Coll Cardiol* 17:297-303, 1991

41. Berns E, Rinkenberger RL, Jeang MK, et al: Efficacy and safety of flecainide acetate for atrial tachycardia or fibrillation. *Am J Cardiol* 59:1337-1341, 1987

42. Miles WM, Chang M-S, Heger JJ, et al: Electrophysiologic and antiarrhythmic effects of oral encainide in patients with atrioventricular nodal reentry or nodoventricular reentry. *Am Heart J* 114:26-33, 1987

43. Klein GJ, Yee R, Leitch JW: Pharmacological management of supraventricular tachycardia. *PACE* 13:1516-1524, 1990

44. Soyka LF, Wirtz C, Spangenberg RB: Clinical safety profile of sotalol in patients with arrhythmias. *Am J Cardiol* 65:74A-81A, 1990

45. Millar RNS: Efficacy of sotalol in controlling reentrant supraventricular tachycardias. *Cardiovasc Drugs Ther* 4 Suppl 3:625-629, 1990

46. Hammill SC, Pritchett ELC, Klein GJ, et al: Accessory atrioventricular pathways that conduct only in the antegrade direction. *Circulation* 62:1335-1340, 1980

47. Akhtar M, Damato AN, Ruskin JN, et al: Antegrade and retrograde conduction characteristics in three patterns of paroxysmal atrioventricular junctional reentrant tachycardia. *Am Heart J* 95:22-42, 1978

48. Farshidi A, Josephson ME, Horowitz LN: Electrophysiologic characteristics of concealed bypass tracts: clinical and electrocardiographic correlates. *Am J Cardiol* 41:1052-1060, 1978

49. Sung RJ, Gelband H, Castellanos A, et al: Clinical and electrophysiologic observations in patients with concealed accessory atrioventricular bypass tracts. *Am J Cardiol* 40:839, 1977

50. Morady F, DiCarlo LA Jr, Baerman JM, et al: Determinants of QRS alternans during narrow QRS tachycardia. *J Am Coll Cardiol* 9:489-499, 1987

51. Josephson ME, Wellens HJ: Differential diagnosis of supraventricular tachycardia. *Cardiol Clin* 8:411-412, 1990

52. Pritchett ELC, Tonkin AM, Dugan FA, et al: Ventriculoatrial conduction time during reciprocating tachycardia with intermittent bundle-branch block in Wolff-Parkinson-White syndrome. *Br Heart J* 38:1058-1064, 1976

53. Huycke EC, Sung RJ, Dias VC, et al: Intravenous diltiazem for termination of reentrant supraventricular tachycardia: a placebo-controlled, randomized, double-blind, multicenter study. *J Am Coll Cardiol* 13:538-544, 1989

54. Childers RW, Arnsdorf MF, de la Fuente DJ, et al: Sinus nodal echoes: clinical case report and canine studies. *Am J Cardiol* 31:220-231, 1973

55. Paulay KL, Weisfogel GM, Damato AN: Sinus nodal reentry: effect of quinidine. *Am J Cardiol* 33:617-622, 1974

56. Paulay KL, Varghese PJ, Damato AN: Atrial rhythms in response to an early atrial premature depolarization in man. *Am Heart J* 85:323-331, 1973

57. Weisfogel GM, Batsford WP, Paulay KL, et al: Sinus node reentrant tachycardia in man. *Am Heart J* 90:295-304, 1975

58. Wu D, Amat-y-Leon F, Denes P, et al: Demonstration of sustained sinus and atrial re-entry as a mechanism of paroxysmal supraventricular tachycardia. *Circulation* 51:234-243, 1975

59. Curry PVL, Shenasa M: Atrial arrhythmias: clinical concepts. In *Cardiac Arrhythmias: Their Mechanisms, Diagnosis, and Management.* Edited by WJ Mandel. Philadelphia, JB Lippincott Company, 1980, pp a, 175; b, 179

60. Goldreyer BN, Gallagher JJ, Damato AN: The electrophysiologic demonstration of atrial ectopic tachycardia in man. *Am Heart J* 85:205-215, 1973

61. Gillette PC, Garson A Jr: Electrophysiologic and pharmacologic characteristics of automatic ectopic atrial tachycardia. *Circulation* 56:571-575, 1977

62. Haines DE, DiMarco JP: Sustained intraatrial reentrant tachycardia: clinical, electrocardiographic and electrophysiologic characteristics and long-term follow-up. *J Am Coll Cardiol* 15:1345-1354, 1990

63. Paulay KL, Ruskin JN, Damato AN: Sinus and atrioventricular nodal reentrant tachycardia in the same patient. *Am J Cardiol* 36:810-816, 1975

64. Leier CV, Meacham JA, Schaal SF: Prolonged atrial conduction: a major predisposing factor for the development of atrial flutter. *Circulation* 57:213-216, 1978

65. Cristal N, Szwarcberg J (Shahar), Gueron M: Supraventricular arrhythmias in acute myocardial infarction. *Ann Intern Med* 82:35-39, 1975

66. Liberthson RR, Salisbury KW, Hutter AM Jr, et al: Atrial tachyarrhythmias in acute myocardial infarction. *Am J Med* 60:956-960, 1976

67. Rytand DA: The circus movement (entrapped circuit wave) hypothesis and atrial flutter. *Ann Intern Med* 65:125-157, 1966

68. Boineau JP, Schuessler RB, Mooney CR, et al: Natural and evoked atrial flutter due to circus movement in dogs: role of abnormal atrial pathways, slow conduction, nonuniform refractory period distribution and premature beats. *Am J Cardiol* 45:1167-1181, 1980

69. Allessie MA, Bonke FIM, Schopman FJG: Circus movement in rabbit atrial muscle as a mechanism of tachycardia. III. The "leading circle" concept: a new model of circus movement in cardiac tissue without the involvement of an anatomical obstacle. *Circ Res* 41:9-18, 1977

70. Rosenblueth A, Garcia Ramos J: Studies on flutter and fibrillation. II. The influence of artificial obstacles on experimental auricular flutter. *Am Heart J* 33:677-684, 1947

71. Watson RM, Josephson ME: Atrial flutter. I. Electrophysiologic substrates and modes of initiation and termination. *Am J Cardiol* 45:732-741, 1980

72. Prinzmetal M, Corday E, Brill IC, et al: *The Auricular Arrhythmias.* Springfield, Illinois, Charles C Thomas, Publisher, 1952

73. Kishon Y, Smith RE: Studies in human atrial flutter with the use of proximity electrodes. *Circulation* 40:513-525, 1969

74. Cohen SI, Koh D, Lau SH, et al: P loops during common and uncommon atrial flutter in man. *Br Heart J* 39:173-180, 1977

75. Mines GR: On dynamic equilibrium in the heart. *J Physiol (Lond)* 46:349-383, 1913

76. Waldo AL, MacLean WAH, Karp RB, et al: Entrainment and interruption of atrial flutter with atrial pacing: studies in man following open heart surgery. *Circulation* 56:737-745, 1977

77. MacLean WAH, Karp RB, Kouchoukos NT, et al: Uniformly successful interruption of atrial flutter with rapid atrial pacing in 100 patients (abstract). *Circulation* 54 Suppl 2:167, 1976

78. Kastor JA: Digitalis intoxication in patients with atrial fibrillation. *Circulation* 47:888-896, 1973

79. Grogan M, Smith HC, Gersh BJ, et al: Left ventricular dysfunction due to atrial fibrillation in patients initially believed to have idiopathic dilated cardiomyopathy. *Am J Cardiol* 69:1570-1573, 1992

80. Kopecky SL, Gersh BJ, McGoon MD, et al: The natural history of lone atrial fibrillation. A population-based study over three decades. *N Engl J Med* 317:669-674, 1987

81. The Stroke Prevention in Atrial Fibrillation Investigators: Predictors of thromboembolism in atrial fibrillation: I. Clinical features of patients at risk. *Ann Intern Med* 116:1-5, 1992

82. The Stroke Prevention in Atrial Fibrillation Investigators: Predictors of thromboembolism in atrial fibrillation: II. Echocardiographic features of patients at risk. *Ann Intern Med* 116:6-12, 1992

83. Loomis TA, Krop S: Auricular fibrillation induced and maintained in animals by acetylcholine or vagal stimulation. *Circ Res* 3:390-396, 1955

84. Kaplan BM, Langendorf R, Lev M, et al: Tachycardia-bradycardia syndrome (so-called "sick sinus syndrome"): pathology, mechanisms and treatment. *Am J Cardiol* 31:497-508, 1973

85. Engel TR, Luck JC, Leddy CL, et al: Diagnostic implications of atrial vulnerability. *PACE* 2:208-214, 1979

86. Anbe DT, Rubenfire M, Drake EH: Conversion of atrial flutter to atrial fibrillation with carotid sinus pressure. *J Electrocardiol* 2:377-380, 1969

87. Abildskov JA, Millar K, Burgess MJ: Atrial fibrillation. *Am J Cardiol* 28:263-267, 1971

88. Wells JL Jr, Karp RB, Kouchoukos NT, et al: Characterization of atrial fibrillation in man: studies following open heart surgery. *PACE* 1:426-438, 1978

89. Haft JI, Lau SH, Stein E, et al: Atrial fibrillation produced by atrial stimulation. *Circulation* 37:70-74, 1968

90. Josephson ME, Seides SF: *Clinical Cardiac Electrophysiology: Techniques and Interpretations.* Philadelphia, Lea & Febiger, 1979, p 206

91. Coplen SE, Antman EM, Berlin JA, et al: Efficacy and safety of quinidine therapy for maintenance of sinus rhythm after cardioversion. A meta-analysis of randomized control trials. *Circulation* 82:1106-1116, 1990

92. Anderson JL, Gilberg EM, Alpert BL, et al: Prevention of symptomatic recurrences of paroxysmal atrial fibrillation in patients initially tolerating antiarrhythmic therapy. A multicenter, double-blind, crossover study of flecainide and placebo with transtelephonic monitoring. Flecainide Supraventricular Tachycardia Study Group. *Circulation* 80:1557-1570, 1989

93. Hammill SC, Wood DL, Gersh BJ, et al: Propafenone for paroxysmal atrial fibrillation. *Am J Cardiol* 61:473-474, 1988

94. Reimold SC, Cantillon CO, Friedman PL, et al: Propafenone versus sotalol for suppression of recurrent symptomatic atrial fibrillation. *Am J Cardiol* 71:558-563, 1993

95. Stroke Prevention in Atrial Fibrillation Investigators: Stroke Prevention in Atrial Fibrillation Study. Final results. *Circulation* 84:527-539, 1991

96. Petersen P, Boysen G, Godtfredsen J, et al: Placebo-controlled, randomised trial of warfarin and aspirin for prevention of thromboembolic complications in chronic atrial fibrillation. The Copenhagen AFASAK study. *Lancet* 1:175-179, 1989

97. The Boston Area Anticoagulation Trial for Atrial Fibrillation Investigators: The effect of low-dose warfarin on the risk of stroke in patients with nonrheumatic atrial fibrillation. *N Engl J Med* 323:1505-1511, 1990

98. Connolly SJ, Laupacis A, Gent M, et al: Canadian Atrial Fibrillation Anticoagulation (CAFA) Study. *J Am Coll Cardiol* 18:349-355, 1991

99. Gallagher JJ, Pritchett ELC, Sealy WC, et al: The preexcitation syndromes. *Prog Cardiovasc Dis* 20:285-327, 1978

100. Bellet S: *Clinical Disorders of the Heart Beat.* Third edition, revised. Philadelphia, Lea & Febiger, 1971, p 506

101. Averill KH, Fosmoe RJ, Lamb LE: Electrocardiographic findings in 67,375 asymptomatic subjects. IV. Wolff-Parkinson-White syndrome. *Am J Cardiol* 6:108-129, 1960

102. Becker AE, Anderson RH, Durrer D, et al: The anatomical substrates of Wolff-Parkinson-White syndrome: a clinicopathologic correlation in seven patients. *Circulation* 57:870-879, 1978

103. Anderson RH, Becker AE, Brechenmacher C, et al: Ventricular preexcitation: a proposed nomenclature for its substrates. *Eur J Cardiol* 3:27-35, 1975

104. Wellens HJJ, Durrer D: The role of an accessory atrioventricular pathway in reciprocal tachycardia: observations in patients with and without the Wolff-Parkinson-White syndrome. *Circulation* 52:58-72, 1975

105. Pritchett ELC, Gallagher JJ, Wallace AG: Reentry within the atrioventricular node in man: a reassessment. *Eur J Cardiol* 6:437-447, 1978

106. Lemery R, Hammill SC, Wood DL, et al: Value of the resting 12 lead electrocardiogram and vectorcardiogram for locating the accessory pathway in patients with the Wolff-Parkinson-White syndrome. *Br Heart J* 58:324-332, 1987

107. Milstein S, Sharma AD, Guiraudon GM, et al: An algorithm for the electrocardiographic localization of accessory pathways in the Wolff-Parkinson-White syndrome. *PACE* 10:555-563, 1987

108. Teo WS, Klein GJ, Yee R, et al: Significance of minimal preexcitation in Wolff-Parkinson-White syndrome. *Am J Cardiol* 67:205-207, 1991

109. Fananapazir L, German LD, Gallagher JJ, et al: Importance of preexcited QRS morphology during induced atrial fibrillation to the diagnosis and localization of multiple accessory pathways. *Circulation* 81:578-585, 1990

110. Wellens HJ, Atie J, Smeets JL, et al: The electrocardiogram in patients with multiple accessory atrioventricular pathways. *J Am Coll Cardiol* 16:745-751, 1990

111. Mandel WJ, Laks MM, Fink B, et al: Comparative electrophysiologic features of the WPW syndrome in the pediatric and adult patient (abstract). *Am J Cardiol* 33:155, 1974

112. Wellens HJJ, Lubbers WJ, Losekoot TG: Preexcitation. In *Cardiac Arrhythmias in the Neonate, Infant, and Child.* Edited by NK Roberts, H Gelband. New York, Appleton-Century-Crofts, 1977, pp 231-263

113. Wellens HJJ: The Wolff-Parkinson-White and related syndromes. II. The value of cardiac pacing in study and treatment. In *Cardiac Arrhythmias: The Modern Electrophysiological Approach.* Edited by DM Krikler, JF Goodwin. Philadelphia, WB Saunders Company, 1975, pp 162-181

114. Wellens HJJ, Farré J, Bär FW: Wolff-Parkinson-White syndrome: value and limitations of programmed electrical stimulation. In *Cardiac Arrhythmias: Electrophysiology, Diagnosis and Management.* Edited by O Narula. Baltimore, Williams & Wilkins Company, 1979, pp 589-617

115. Gallagher JJ, Sealy WC, Kasell J, et al: Multiple accessory pathways in patients with the pre-excitation syndrome. *Circulation* 54:571-591, 1976

116. Packer DL, Ellenbogen KA, Colavita PG, et al: Utility of introducing ventricular premature complexes during reciprocating tachycardia in specifying the location of left free wall accessory pathways. *Am J Cardiol* 63:49-57, 1989

117. Benditt DG, Pritchett ELC, Smith WM, et al: Characteristics of atrioventricular conduction and the spectrum of arrhythmias in Lown-Ganong-Levine syndrome. *Circulation* 57:454-465, 1978

118. Gallagher JJ, Smith WM, Kasell JH, et al: Role of Mahaim fibers in cardiac arrhythmias in man. *Circulation* 64:176-189, 1981

119. Bharati S, Bauernfiend R, Scheinman M, et al: Congenital abnormalities in the conduction system of two patients with tachyarrhythmias. *Circulation* 59:593-606, 1979

120. Gallagher JJ, Benditt D, Pritchett ELC, et al: Participation of Mahaim fibers in the genesis of cardiac dysrhythmias (abstract). *Circulation* 58 Suppl 2:155, 1978

121. Castellanos A, Agha AS, Befeler B, et al: Double accessory pathways in Wolff-Parkinson-White syndrome. *Circulation* 51:1020-1025, 1975

122. James TN: Morphology of the human atrioventricular node, with remarks pertinent to its electrophysiology. *Am Heart J* 62:756-771, 1961

123. Brechenmacher C: Atrio-His bundle tracts. *Br Heart J* 37:853-855, 1975

124. Teo WS, Klein GJ, Guiraudon GM, et al: Multiple accessory pathways in the Wolff-Parkinson-White syndrome as a risk factor for ventricular fibrillation. *Am J Cardiol* 67:889-891, 1991

125. Dreifus LS, Haiat R, Watanabe Y, et al: Ventricular fibrillation: a possible mechanism of sudden death in patients with Wolff-Parkinson-White syndrome. *Circulation* 43:520-527, 1971

126. Bashore TM, Sellers TD, Gallagher JJ, et al: Ventricular fibrillation in the Wolff-Parkinson-White syndrome (abstract). *Circulation* 53 Suppl 2:187, 1976

127. Klein GJ, Bashore TM, Sellers TD, et al: Ventricular fibrillation in the Wolff-Parkinson-White syndrome. *N Engl J Med* 301:1080-1085, 1979

128. Leitch JW, Klein GJ, Yee R, et al: Prognostic value of electrophysiology testing in asymptomatic patients with Wolff-Parkinson-White pattern. *Circulation* 82:1718-1723, 1990

129. Beckman KJ, Gallastegui JL, Bauman JL, et al: The predictive value of electrophysiologic studies in untreated patients with Wolff-Parkinson-White syndrome. *J Am Coll Cardiol* 15:640-647, 1990

130. Sharma AD, Yee R, Guiraudon G, et al: Sensitivity and specificity of invasive and noninvasive testing for risk of sudden death in Wolff-Parkinson-White syndrome. *J Am Coll Cardiol* 10:373-381, 1987
131. Fananapazir L, Packer DL, German LD, et al: Procainamide infusion test: inability to identify patients with Wolff-Parkinson-White syndrome who are potentially at risk of sudden death. *Circulation* 77:1291-1296, 1988
132. Josephson ME, Kastor JA, Kitchen JG III: Lidocaine in Wolff-Parkinson-White syndrome with atrial flutter. *Ann Intern Med* 84:44-45, 1976
133. Rosen KM, Barwolf C, Ehsani A, et al: Effects of lidocaine and propranolol on the normal and anomalous pathways in patients with preexcitation. *Am J Cardiol* 30:801-809, 1972
134. Akhtar M, Gilbert CJ, Shenasa M: Effect of lidocaine on atrioventricular response via the accessory pathway in patients with Wolff-Parkinson-White syndrome. *Circulation* 63:435-441, 1981
135. Denes P, Cummings JM, Simpson R, et al: Effects of propranolol on anomalous pathway refractoriness and circus movement tachycardias in patients with preexcitation. *Am J Cardiol* 41:1061-1067, 1978
136. Spurrell RAJ, Krikler DM, Sowton E: Effects of verapamil on electrophysiological properties of anomalous atrioventricular connexion in Wolff-Parkinson-White syndrome. *Br Heart J* 36:256-264, 1974
137. Gulamhusein S, Ko P, Carruthers SG, et al: Acceleration of the ventricular response during atrial fibrillation in the Wolff-Parkinson-White syndrome after verapamil. *Circulation* 65:348-354, 1982
138. Wellens HJ, Durrer D: Effect of digitalis on atrioventricular conduction and circus-movement tachycardias in patients with Wolff-Parkinson-White syndrome. *Circulation* 47:1229-1233, 1973
139. Sellers TD Jr, Bashore TM, Gallagher JJ: Digitalis in the preexcitation syndrome: analysis during atrial fibrillation. *Circulation* 56:260-267, 1977
140. Spurrell RAJ, Thorburn CW, Camm J, et al: Effects of disopyramide on electrophysiological properties of specialized conduction system in man and on accessory atrioventricular pathway in Wolff-Parkinson-White syndrome. *Br Heart J* 37:861-867, 1975
141. Kerr CR, Prystowsky EN, Smith WN, et al: Electrophysiologic effects of disopyramide phosphate in patients with Wolff-Parkinson-White syndrome. *Circulation* 65:869-878, 1982
142. Sellers TD Jr, Campbell RWF, Bashore TM, et al: Effects of procainamide and quinidine sulfate in the Wolff-Parkinson-White syndrome. *Circulation* 55:15-22, 1977
143. Wellens HJJ, Durrer D: Effect of procaine amide, quinidine, and ajmaline in the Wolff-Parkinson-White syndrome. *Circulation* 50:114-120, 1974
144. Mandel WJ, Laks MM, Obayashi K, et al: The Wolff-Parkinson-White syndrome: pharmacologic effects of procaine amide. *Am Heart J* 90:744-754, 1975
145. Wellens HJ, Bär FW, Gorgels AP: Effect of drugs in WPW syndrome: importance of initial length of effective refractory period of accessory pathway (abstract). *Am J Cardiol* 41:372, 1978
146. Rosenbaum MB, Chiale PA, Ryba D, et al: Control of tachyarrhythmias associated with Wolff-Parkinson-White syndrome by amiodarone hydrochloride. *Am J Cardiol* 34:215-223, 1974
147. Wellens HJ, Lie KI, Bär FW, et al: Effect of amiodarone in the Wolff-Parkinson-White syndrome. *Am J Cardiol* 38:189-194, 1976
148. Rosenbaum MB, Chiale PA, Halpern MS, et al: Clinical efficacy of amiodarone as an antiarrhythmic agent. *Am J Cardiol* 38:934-944, 1976
149. Wellens HJ, Brugada P, Abdollah H: Effect of amiodarone in paroxysmal supraventricular tachycardia with or without Wolff-Parkinson-White syndrome. *Am Heart J* 106:876-879, 1983
150. Spurrell RAJ, Sowton E: Management of paroxysmal supraventricular tachycardia using a scanning pacing system (abstract). *Br Heart J* 38:536, 1976
151. Mandel WJ, Laks MM, Yamaguchi I, et al: Recurrent reciprocating tachycardias in the Wolff-Parkinson-White syndrome: control by the use of a scanning pacemaker. *Chest* 69:769-774, 1976
152. Spurrell RAJ, Nathan AW, Bexton RS, et al: Implantable automatic scanning pacemaker for termination of supraventricular tachycardia. *Am J Cardiol* 49:753-760, 1982
153. Ryan GF, Easley RM Jr, Zaroff LI, et al: Paradoxical use of a demand pacemaker in treatment of supraventricular tachycardia due to the Wolff-Parkinson-White syndrome: observation on termination of reciprocal rhythm. *Circulation* 38:1037-1043, 1968
154. Krikler D, Curry P, Buffet J: Dual-demand pacing for reciprocating atrioventricular tachycardia. *Br Med J* 1:1114-1116, 1976
155. Zipes DP, King RD, Duffin EG: Use of a new antiarrhythmic physiologic pacemaker in a patient with debilitating atrial tachyarrhythmia (abstract). *PACE* 2:A-80, 1979
156. Lister JW, Cohen LS, Bernstein WH, et al: Treatment of supraventricular tachycardias by rapid atrial stimulation. *Circulation* 38:1044-1059, 1968
157. Kahn A, Morris JJ, Citron P: Patient-initiated rapid atrial pacing to manage supraventricular tachycardia. *Am J Cardiol* 38:200-204, 1976
158. Fruehan CT, Meyer JA, Klie JH, et al: Refractory paroxysmal supraventricular tachycardia: treatment with patient controlled permanent radio frequency atrial pacemaker. *Am Heart J* 87:229-237, 1974
159. Vergara GS, Hildner FJ, Schoenfeld CB, et al: Conversion of supraventricular tachycardias with rapid atrial stimulation. *Circulation* 46:788-793, 1972
160. Waxman MB, Wald RW, Bonet JF, et al: Self-conversion of supraventricular tachycardia by rapid atrial pacing. *PACE* 1:35-48, 1978
161. Giannelli S Jr, Ayres SM, Gomprecht RF, et al: Therapeutic surgical division of the human conduction system. *JAMA* 199:155-160, 1967
162. Coumel P, Aigueperse J, Perrault M-A, et al: Repérage et tentative d'exérèse chirurgicale d'un foyer ectopique auriculaire gauche avec tachycardie rebelle. *Ann Cardiol Angeiol (Paris)* 22:189-199, 1973
163. Wyndham C, Smith T, Arnsdorf M, et al: Successful surgical excision of paroxysmal atrial tachycardia: in vivo and in vitro observation (abstract). *Clin Res* 27:442A, 1979
164. Anderson KP, Stinson EB, Mason JW: Surgical exclusion of focal paroxysmal atrial tachycardia. *Am J Cardiol* 49:869-874, 1982
165. Wood DL, Hammill SC, Danielson GK: Use of the cryoprobe to facilitate intraoperative electrophysiologic mapping by inhibiting sinus node function in automatic atrial tachycardia. *Am J Cardiol* 59:176, 1987
166. Holmes DR Jr, Osborn MJ, Gersh B, et al: The Wolff-Parkinson-White syndrome: a surgical approach. *Mayo Clin Proc* 57:345-350, 1982
167. Burchell HB: The surgical treatment of reentrant atrioventricular tachycardia (Wolff-Parkinson-White syndrome) (editorial). *Mayo Clin Proc* 57:387-389, 1982
168. Gallagher JJ, Svenson RH, Kasell JH, et al: Catheter technique for closed-chest ablation of the atrioventricular conduction system: a therapeutic alternative for the treatment of refractory supraventricular tachycardia. *N Engl J Med* 306:194-200, 1982
169. Scheinman MM, Morady F, Hess DS, et al: Catheter-induced ablation of the atrioventricular junction to control refractory supraventricular arrhythmias. *JAMA* 248:851-855, 1982
170. Wood DL, Hammill SC, Holmes DR Jr, et al: Catheter ablation of the atrioventricular conduction system in patients with supraventricular tachycardia. *Mayo Clin Proc* 58:791-796, 1983
171. Huang SK, Bharati S, Graham AR, et al: Closed chest catheter desiccation of the atrioventricular junction using radiofrequency energy – a new method of catheter ablation. *J Am Coll Cardiol* 9:349-358, 1987
172. Kunze K-P, Schlüter M, Geiger M, et al: Modulation of atrioventricular nodal conduction using radiofrequency current. *Am J Cardiol* 61:657-658, 1988
173. Warin J-F, Haissaguerre M, Lemetayer P, et al: Catheter ablation of accessory pathways with a direct approach: results in 35 patients. *Circulation* 78:800-815, 1988
174. Morady F, Scheinman MM, Kou WH, et al: Long-term results of catheter ablation of a posteroseptal accessory atrioventricular connection in 48 patients. *Circulation* 79:1160-1170, 1989
175. Bardy GH, Ivey TD, Coltorti F, et al: Developments, complications and limitations of catheter-mediated electrical ablation of posterior accessory atrioventricular pathways. *Am J Cardiol* 61:309-316, 1988
176. Evans GT Jr, Scheinman MM, Zipes DP, et al: The Percutaneous Cardiac Mapping and Ablation Registry: summary of results. *PACE* 10:1395-1399, 1987

CHAPTER

22

Cardiac arrhythmias

C. Ventricular arrhythmias

Win-Kuang Shen, M.D., and Stephen C. Hammill, M.D.

VENTRICULAR arrhythmias occur in a wide variety of patients, ranging from the asymptomatic patient with an occasional premature ventricular complex (PVC) to the patient with malignant ventricular tachycardia associated with severely compromised left ventricular function (ventricular fibrillation is discussed in a separate chapter dealing with sudden death—chapter 24). This variability among patients makes the treatment of ventricular arrhythmias challenging and, at times, frustrating. The physician must decide whether a patient's rhythm disturbance warrants treatment on the basis of the degree of symptoms and the relative risk the patient has of experiencing significant complications, including sudden death. If the physician concludes that a patient requires treatment, he or she has to decide what that treatment should be and the best way of determining whether it is effective. Since most antiarrhythmic drugs can actually worsen a ventricular arrhythmia—this occurs in 5% to 15% of cases[1-6]—the physician must also monitor the therapy closely to make certain that the patient has not been harmed by the treatment.

Ventricular arrhythmias in certain clinical situations are known to be associated with sudden death, and the suppression of such arrhythmias decreases the incidence of sudden death.[7-11] Knowledge of basic electrophysiology has improved our understanding of the mechanism of ventricular arrhythmias, and clinical electrophysiologic studies, including intracardiac recording and programmed stimulation, have aided in the diagnosis of ventricular arrhythmias and in directing appropriate therapy in patients with life-threatening ventricular tachycardia.[12-14] Advances in 24-hour ambulatory monitoring have permitted the detection and quantification of ventricular arrhythmias[15-17] and improved the physician's ability to confirm that antiarrhythmic drug therapy has in fact decreased the frequency of spontaneous ventricular arrhythmias. This chapter reviews the mechanisms of ventricular arrhythmias, including the PVC and ventricular tachycardia. It also discusses which patients require treatment, the various modalities of treatment available, and the different ways of monitoring therapy. Finally, cardiac abnormalities associated with ventricular arrhythmias are discussed.

MECHANISMS OF VENTRICULAR ARRHYTHMIAS

Reentry

The most common mechanism of formation of ventricular arrhythmias is reentry. The original model of reentry was proposed by Schmitt and Erlanger.[18] This model is depicted in Figure 22C-1 and includes three prerequisites for reentry: (1) two functionally distinct pathways, (2) a unidirectional block in one pathway, and (3) conduction over the second pathway. An electrical impulse encounters the reentrant circuit and, at critical intervals, finds one of the limbs refractory to conduction. The impulse then travels down the second limb, which conducts the impulse at a rate slow enough to allow the limb that was refractory to recover its ability to conduct. On reaching the distal end of the slowly conducting limb, the impulse is now able to return to the point of origin over the second limb, which has recovered its conductive ability. This forms a reentrant circuit, and if conditions are appropriate, the circuit can be maintained and a reentrant arrhythmia can develop. The amount of ventricular tissue needed to support a reentry circuit can vary from a macro reentry circuit that utilizes the specialized conduction system to a small reentry circuit that may be as short as 1.0 cm or less in pathologic conditions such as ischemia.[19-23]

The most common source for a reentrant PVC is found in the setting of myocardial ischemia.[24-26] In an ischemic myocardium, the impulse encounters myocardial fibers that are functionally dissociated with regard to their conductive characteristics. This gives rise to multiple potential reentrant circuits, as demonstrated in Figure 22C-2. In the ischemic zone, multiple irregular areas of severely depressed or unexcitable myocardium are interspersed with areas of less severely depressed myocardium. This allows slow conduction of an impulse to occur with the ability to excite myocardium that is no longer refractory and thus to initiate a reentrant arrhythmia.

Reentrant arrhythmias are variably affected by heart rate and may be absent at slower or faster heart rates.[24-26] Bradycardia is associated with ventricular ectopic rhythms in the setting of an acute myocardial infarction.[27,28] Several researchers[21,29,30] attributed this relationship to

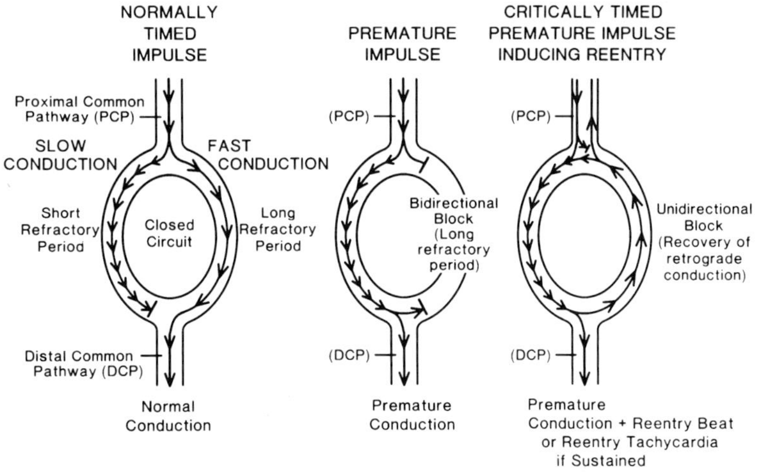

Fig 22C-1 Description of a reentrant circuit as a mechanism in initiating and sustaining tachycardia.

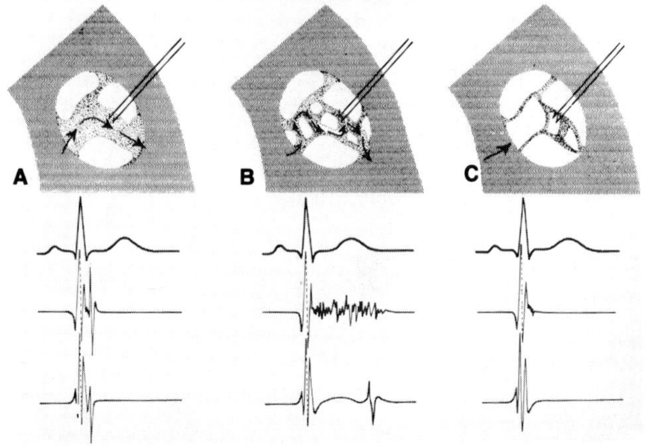

Fig 22C-2 Schematic representation of conduction in the infarction zone during three sinus beats. The *top tracing* is a standard ECG lead; the *middle tracing* was made from a composite electrode; the *bottom tracing* represents a close bipolar electrode. **A,** conduction of the sinus impulse through the infarction zone without significant delay. **B,** conduction of the sinus impulse through the infarction zone with conduction delay and persistent electrical activity as recorded by electrodes close to the infarction zone. This delay in conduction is the physiologic substrate necessary for reentrant arrhythmias to occur. **C,** conduction block into the infarction zone. (Modified from El-Sherif N, Scherlag BJ, Lazzara R, et al: Re-entrant ventricular arrhythmias in the late myocardial infarction period. 1. Conduction characteristics in the infarction zone. *Circulation* 55:686-702, 1977.)

the increased dispersion of refractoriness that is present in ischemic myocardium at slow rates and that would favor reentry by means of focal reexcitation. A second explanation is varying degrees of block at the area of reentrance.[24,25] At normal heart rates, reentrant pathways may exhibit complete or high-grade entrance block, whereas at slower heart rates there is less conduction block at the reentrant pathway, which would be more conducive to the establishment of a reentrant arrhythmia. Suppressing such mechanisms of arrhythmia in the setting of acute myocardial infarction has been accomplished by a technique known as "overdrive suppression," which is achieved either by pharmacologic methods such as with atropine or isoproterenol or by cardiac pacing.[31] Similarly, certain reentrant arrhythmias become worse with more rapid heart rates.[32-34] This change may be due to increased ischemia, which results in further slowing of conduction in the reentrant circuit and the establishment of a reentrant arrhythmia. The increased heart rate may also alter the refractoriness of both limbs of the reentrant circuit and cause enough disparity to foster reentry.

The only way to prove that an arrhythmia is of a reentry mechanism is to fulfill the criteria of Mines' original postulates, that is, to demonstrate unidirectional block, to map the complete reentrant pathway, and to terminate the arrhythmia interrupting the reentrant circuit.[35] Direct proof of a proposed reentrant mechanism is often difficult to obtain, even in animal experiments and isolated preparations. In human hearts, a reentrant mechanism is firmly established only in the accessory atrioventricular (AV) pathways. In the absence of direct proof, the strongest evidence to support the notion that reentry is the mechanism in most cases of clinical ventricular tachyarrhythmias is the response of the tachycardia to extrastimuli during programmed stimulation. Characteristics of the response of a reentrant ventricular tachycardia to extrastimuli have been established in electrophysiologic laboratories.[36]

Abnormal automaticity

Normal automaticity, such as that of the sinus pacemaker, is defined as spontaneous depolarizations arising from relatively high diastolic membrane potentials or resting membrane potentials that are normal for that tissue.

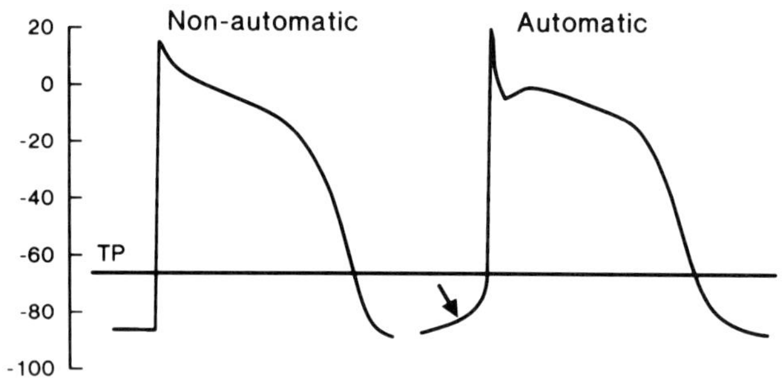

Fig 22C-3 Comparison of a schematic action potential from a nonautomatic and an automatic fiber. The automatic fiber demonstrates spontaneous phase 4 depolarization *(arrow),* which results in complete depolarization of the cell when the threshold potential *(TP)* is reached.

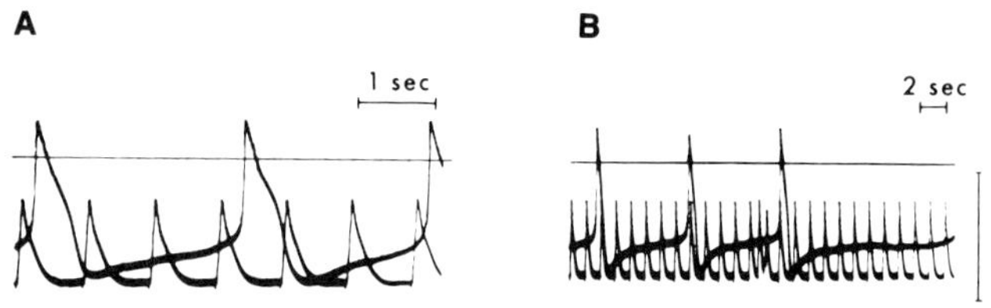

Fig 22C-4 Intracellular recordings from the infarction zone in a dog model of myocardial infarction. **A,** the large action potential represents a parasystolic pacemaker cell from within the infarction zone. The smaller action potential is obtained from a second recording site in the infarction zone which is following the drive stimulus at a cycle length of 1,000 msec (1 sec). The parasystolic pacemaker cell fails to follow the drive stimulus and thus demonstrates the presence of entrance block, a hallmark of a parasystolic focus. **B,** the long interval after the last recorded beat from the parasystolic cell is approximately twice the shorter parasystolic cycle length. This would be interpreted as being due to 2:1 exit block from the parasystolic focus as recorded by the surface ECG. However, this tracing demonstrates that the prolonged interval is due not to exit block but to pronounced spontaneous variation in the rate of the parasystolic focus. (From Lazzara R, El-Sherif N, Scherlag BJ: Electrophysiological properties of canine Purkinje cells in one-day-old myocardial infarction. *Circ Res* 33:722-734. 1973. By permission of American Heart Association.)

These rhythms can be suppressed by overdrive pacing.[37] Abnormal automaticity is the result of spontaneous depolarizations of tissue with low resting membrane potential. There is less tendency for overdrive pacing to result in suppression.[38] The onset of an abnormal automatic rhythm is often associated with a gradual increase in rate or a warm-up phenomenon.[39] Features suggesting an automatic mechanism are precipitation of ventricular tachyarrhythmias with catecholamine stimulation and inability to initiate or terminate ventricular tachycardia by ventricular programmed stimulation.

Abnormal automaticity in the ventricle occurs when a cell that is capable of spontaneous depolarization (Fig 22C-3) is no longer affected by the dominant cardiac rhythm as a consequence of entrance block or a rapid discharge rate. This cell then develops its own rhythm and at times can influence the basic rhythm. The abnormal automatic pacemaker is also termed a "parasystolic focus," because the focus is discharging along with the sinus pacemaker.

Several mechanisms that have been advanced to explain how the parasystolic focus is protected from being depolarized by the normal sinus pacemaker impulse include a zone of protective block surrounding the automatic focus,[40-42] lower excitability of an automatic center relative to the strength of the sinus impulse,[43] and slow diastolic depolarization of the pacemaker cell.[44,45] Studies on experimental parasystole suggest that the parasystolic center has a high inherent frequency of discharge that keeps the immediate tissue refractory to being discharged by the dominant rhythm[46] (Fig 22C-4).

Two major diagnostic criteria[47] for a parasystolic focus are the presence of pronounced variation of coupling of the ectopic beat to the normal beat and intervals between the ectopic beats that can be reduced to a single common denominator, implying a regular rate of the parasystolic focus with intermittent exit block. The majority of such rhythms also show fusion complexes. The rate of a parasystolic focus varies from 20 to 400 beats/min.[48] In general, the rates are slow and may have been present for several years.[49]

Ventricular parasystole is usually considered a rare disorder,[43] with a reported incidence of less than 1%, but these complexes were due to parasystole in 37 (46%) of 81 presumed healthy flying personnel with PVCs.[50] This suggests that the automatic rhythm is not rare in clinically healthy persons and that it is probably benign. Parasystolic rhythm occurs in association with myocardial infarction and in the postinfarction period in approximately 2% of such patients and is generally believed to be benign in this setting.[51]

Triggered activity

The phenomenon of triggered activity (Fig 22C-5) has been described in the basic electrophysiology laboratory,[52] but its relevance to clinical ventricular tachyarrhythmias has not been well established. Triggered activity results from oscillations in membrane potentials, known as afterdepolarizations.[53] Situations that predispose to increased triggered activity in the laboratory include fiber stretch, hypoxia, toxic dose of ouabain, and exposure of Purkinje fibers to high levels of epinephrine and potassium.[54,55] Afterdepolarizations have been divided into two types, early and delayed, on the basis of their timing relative to the repolarization of the preceding action potential. Early afterdepolarization occurs before the completion of repolarization. Recent studies suggest that early afterdepolarization may result in triggered activity and may be a mechanism for torsade de pointes in patients with prolonged QT syndrome.[56,57] Delayed afterdepolarization occurs after the completion of repolarization. Delayed afterdepolarization may result in inducement of triggered rhythms by digitalis, myocardial infarction, and

Fig 22C-5 The effect of ouabain on spontaneously firing diseased human atrial fibers. **A,** spontaneous cycle length of 2,100 msec in the control state. **B,** effects of superfusion with ouabain, resulting in delayed afterdepolarizations occurring during phase IV. **C,** a tachyarrhythmia occurs when the afterdepolarizations observed in **B** attain threshold potential. (From Hordof AJ, Spotnitz A, Mary-Rabine L, et al: The cellular electrophysiologic effects of digitalis on human atrial fibers. *Circulation* 57:223-229, 1978. By permission of American Heart Association.)

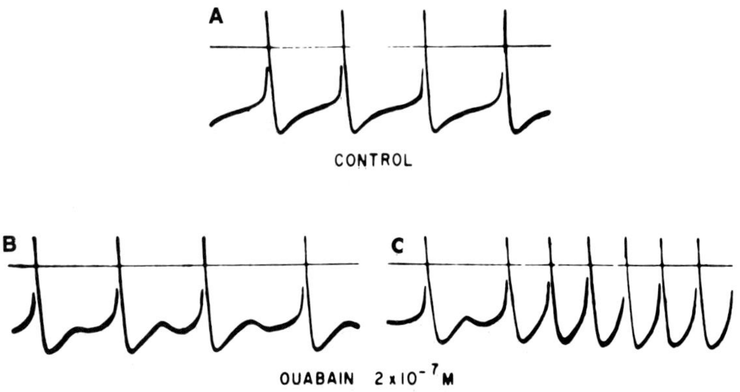

exercise.[58] A triggered mechanism underlying ventricular tachyarrhythmias can be invoked from the responses of the arrhythmia to various pharmacologic agents and programmed stimulation.[39,58]

SUDDEN CARDIAC DEATH

Sudden cardiac death is discussed in chapter 24. However, there is growing evidence that certain patients with PVCs and ventricular tachycardia are at an increased risk of sudden cardiac death.[59] This is a major group of patients who should be considered for antiarrhythmic therapy, and they form the basis of the discussion in this chapter. Sudden death is more formally defined in chapter 24, but, in general, patients who die soon after the onset of symptoms are said to have experienced sudden death, and this is almost always due to ventricular fibrillation, which is either primary or a result of ventricular tachycardia. It is generally believed that patients with simple ventricular ectopy and no associated heart disease are not at risk for sudden cardiac death,[60,61] whereas patients with more complex ventricular ectopy and associated heart disease are at risk for sudden cardiac death because of the presence of the ventricular arrhythmia.[62-64] Such patients often have coronary artery disease, and the sudden death may be associated with an acute ischemic event, including myocardial infarction or angina, but it may also occur in the absence of myocardial ischemia.

THE PREMATURE VENTRICULAR COMPLEX

Lown grading scale

Patients with recurrent episodes of ventricular tachycardia and syncope do not pose a difficult decision regarding treatment. Such patients require treatment, and the approach to evaluation and therapy are discussed later in this chapter. However, the decision is more difficult in the patient with only PVCs. In order to classify PVCs and to relate them to the risk of sudden cardiac death, Lown et al.[65,66] devised a grading scale (Table 22C-1) that attempts to correlate the complexity of a ventricular arrhythmia with the risk of sudden death. This scale has been criticized, specifically with regard to the high level of severity given to the so-called R-on-T phenomenon,[67-69] multiform PVCs, and PVCs in a bigeminal pattern. However, the grading system does provide a framework within which to evaluate patients' PVCs and to decide which patients require therapy.

Table 22C-1 Classification of premature ventricular complexes (PVCs)

Grade	Complexity of PVC
0	No PVCs
1	Fewer than 30 PVCs in 1 hr
1A	Fewer than 1 PVC in 1 min
1B	More than 1 PVC in 1 min
2	More than 1 PVC in 1 min and 30 in 1 hr
3	Multiform PVCs
4	Repetitive PVCs
4A	Couplets
4B	Salvos or ventricular tachycardia
5	Early PVCs (abutting or interrupting the T wave)

R-on-T

There is conflicting evidence regarding the importance of the so-called R-on-T phenomenon in the development of significant ventricular arrhythmias.[67,68,70-72] In the cardiac cycle, the middle third of the T wave corresponds to maximum dispersion of refractoriness within the ventricles. A PVC that falls in this period (hence, "R-on-T") has the potential to initiate repetitive ventricular activity, sustained ventricular tachycardia, or ventricular fibrillation[73,74] (Fig 22C-6). The ability of the PVC to generate such an abnormal ventricular rhythm is related to the development of reentry. As discussed previously, reentry depends on differing degrees of conduction and refractoriness within fibers that can complete a reentrant circuit. During the above-mentioned vulnerable period of the T wave, there is dispersion of refractoriness among the ventricular fibers which results from the various degrees of recovery during the process of repolarization. Because of this dispersion, some fibers are able to conduct slowly and

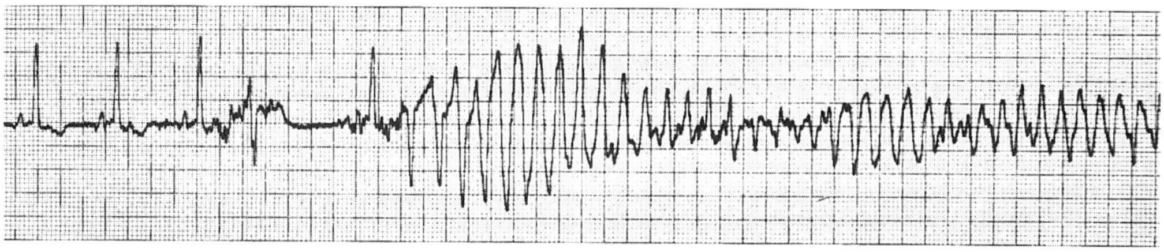

Fig 22C-6 R-on-T: rhythm strip from a patient with bradycardia shows frequent premature ventricular contractions. The second premature ventricular contraction occurred during repolarization (T wave) and triggered a run of polymorphic ventricular tachycardia.

other fibers are refractory and are not able to conduct. This creates an ideal environment for the establishment of a reentrant arrhythmia.

In a normal heart, the duration of the vulnerable period is short, and the magnitude of dispersion of recovery during repolarization in the ventricles is not great enough to allow reentry. In this environment, the risk that PVCs that fall on the T wave will result in a ventricular arrhythmia is low; however, in the diseased heart, the situation is quite different. The vulnerable period may be longer because repolarization can be prolonged, and this makes it more likely that a critically timed PVC can initiate a reentry arrhythmia.[75,76] The cardiac abnormalities that predispose to prolongation of the vulnerable period and heterogeneity of conduction and refractoriness include acute ischemia, myocardial infarction, volume overload or pressure overload of the ventricles, valvular heart disease, primary myocardial disease, and electrolyte or acid-base imbalance. Medications that result in a prolongation of repolarization are significant contributors to prolonging the vulnerable period and making reentrant ventricular arrhythmias more likely.

Simple PVCs

Simple PVCs have the following characteristics: (1) they occur beyond the T wave of the preceding QRS complex, (2) their morphology is uniform, (3) they occur in an isolated fashion and do not present as pairs or triplets, and (4) they generally exhibit constant coupling intervals with the preceding QRS complex. This type of PVC is frequent in the general population, occurring in 35% to 50% of healthy young adults during 24-hour ambulatory monitoring.[60,77] As persons increase in age, the frequency of such PVCs increases; approximately 70% of persons between the ages of 40 and 60 have simple PVCs, and they are seen in most individuals over the age of 60.[78,79]

Simple PVCs that occur in persons who do not have any type of cardiac disease do not require treatment. However, the physician must not overlook the fact that the majority of sudden deaths occur in persons who were previously believed to be healthy and normal. Therefore, when confronted with a patient with simple PVCs, the physician must rule out any associated cardiac or electrolyte abnormalities that may predispose the patient to sudden death. If the physician can be confident that there is no associated heart disease, then this type of PVC should not place the person at increased risk for sudden death.[16]

Complex PVCs

Complex ventricular ectopy can be defined as PVCs that (1) occur in pairs, triplets, or more prolonged runs of ventricular tachycardia; (2) fall in the vulnerable period of the cardiac cycle (R-on-T); and (3) have more than one morphology. A close correlation exists between the complexity of PVCs and the risk of developing ventricular tachycardia and fibrillation in patients with cardiac disease.[66,72,80] Patients who have complex ventricular ectopy without apparent cardiac disease only rarely experience life-threatening ventricular arrhythmias.[61,78]

Complex PVCs in association with myocardial infarction

The association between complex PVCs and ventricular fibrillation in patients with acute myocardial infarction is well known.[66,80] In the setting of acute myocardial infarction, ventricular fibrillation can occur as a result of critically timed simple and complex PVCs. Accordingly, ventricular ectopy is aggressively suppressed in the coronary care unit in an attempt to prevent ventricular fibrillation. Such treatment has resulted in a significant reduction in the frequency of in-hospital ventricular fibrillation, but has not reduced total mortality.[81,82] Ventricular fibrillation may occur in the absence of warning arrhythmias.

The physician must recognize that the frequency of PVCs during the acute phase of myocardial infarction as observed in the coronary care unit may be different from the frequency of PVCs that occur after the patient has been dismissed and begins rehabilitation.[83,84]

Several studies have indicated that ventricular arrhythmias are common after myocardial infarction and that the risk of sudden death can be associated with the frequent occurrence and complex forms of PVCs. The frequency and complexity of PVCs have a positive correlation with total mortality and with sudden death in patients after myocardial infarction[62-64,85-86] (Table 22C-2 and Fig 22C-7). Complex PVCs, especially nonsustained ventricular tachycardia (defined as three or more consecutive PVCs shorter than 30 seconds without associated loss of

Table 22C-2 Association of frequent and complex ventricular complexes with mortality and sudden death

Study	No. of patients	FU, mo	Total mortality, % With frequent PVCs†	Total mortality, % Without frequent PVCs†	Sudden cardiac death, % With frequent PVCs†	Sudden cardiac death, % Without frequent PVCs†	Sensitivity/specificity, %*	Positive predictive value*
Ruberman et al.[85]	1,739	24	27	13	15	5	54/76	15
Mukharji et al.[62]	533	18	29	9	13	4	34/87	13
Bigger et al.[63]	819	22	19	10	12	6	33/81	12
Kostis et al.[64]	1,640	25	20	9	9	4	25/88	9
Farrell et al.[86]	416	20	40	18	54‡	18‡	54/82	16
			With complex PVCs§	Without complex PVCs§	With complex PVCs§	Without complex PVCs§		
Ruberman et al.[72]	1,739	42	28	12	16	6	57/67	16
Moss et al.[87]	940	36	21	10	11	4	42/78	11
Bigger et al.[63]	819	22	20	9	13	5	48/73	13
Kostis et al.[64]	1,640	25	17	8	7	3	33/81	7

FU, follow-up; PVCs, premature ventricular complexes.
*Calculated for sudden death only.
†PVCs ≥ 10/hr.
‡Including sudden death and sustained ventricular tachycardia.
§R-on-T, pairs, multiform, bigeminy.
From Shen W-K, Hammill SC, Packer DL: Asymptomatic ventricular arrhythmias after MI: a therapeutic dilemma (Part 1). *CARDIO* 11:36-41, 50, 1994. By permission of the journal.

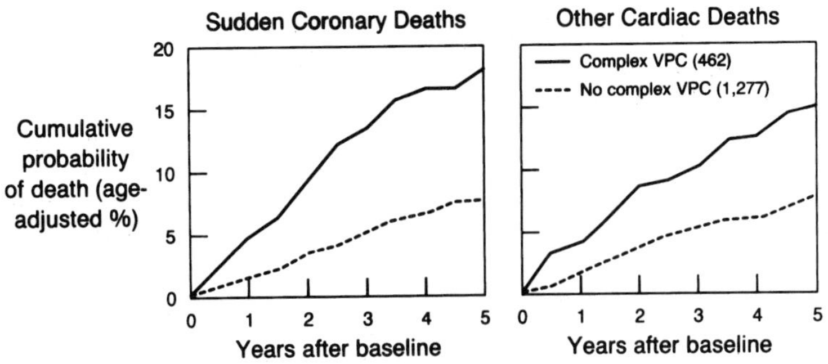

Fig 22C-7 Total cardiac mortality and sudden death are significantly higher in patients with complex ventricular premature contractions after myocardial infarction than in patients without complex ventricular premature contractions after myocardial infarction. (From Ruberman W, Weinblatt E, Goldberg JD, et al: Ventricular premature complexes and sudden death after myocardial infarction. *Circulation* 64:297-305, 1981. By permission of American Heart Association.)

consciousness) after myocardial infarction, also identify a group at increased risk for total mortality and for sudden cardiac death (Table 22C-3).[15,63,86,88,90] In a study of 430 patients after myocardial infarction who were evaluated with 24-hour ambulatory monitoring before dismissal from the hospital, it was determined that ventricular tachycardia was an independent risk factor for the development of sudden cardiac death.[15]

A review[72] of 1,739 survivors of myocardial infarction followed for 5 years who had complex ectopy on 1 hour of monitoring (R-on-T, pairs or longer runs, multiform types, bigeminy) demonstrated that complex PVC had the strongest influence on the risk of sudden cardiac death. This study did not specifically examine the relationship of the ejection fraction to the risk of sudden cardiac death, but it did evaluate the risk of conges-

Table 22C-3 Nonsustained ventricular tachycardia and mortality

Source	No. of patients	FU, mo	NSVT		Total mortality No NSVT	
			No	Yes	No.	%
Anderson et al.[88]	915	4-48	132†	66	11	8
Kleiger et al.[89]	289	12	201	88	14	7
Bigger et al.[15]	820	31	728	92‡	109	15
Bigger et al.[63]	430	36	380	50	44	12
Farrell et al.[86]	416	20	330	86	63	19

FU, follow-up; NSVT, nonsustained ventricular tachycardia; SCD, sudden cardiac death.
*Calculated for sudden cardiac death only.
†Number of control patients by matching to patients with nonsustained ventricular tachycardia.
‡Including two patients with sustained ventricular tachycardia.
Modified from Shen W-K, Hammill SC: Survivors of acute myocardial infarction: Who is at risk for sudden cardiac death? *Mayo Clin Proc* 66:950-962, 1991.

Table 22C-4 Relationship between ventricular arrhythmias and left ventricular (LV) dysfunction in predicting mortality

Source	No. of patients	Holter monitoring True interval from MI, wk	Duration, hr
Ruberman et al.[85]	1,739	12	1
Moss et al.[87]	940	2-3	6
Mukharji et al.[62]	533	1-2	24
Bigger et al.[63]	866	1-2	24
Kostis et al.[64]	1,640	1-3	24
Califf et al.[16]	1,293	Chronic	TMET
Califf et al.[103]	395	Chronic	24
Lichtlen et al.[104]	204	Chronic	20-24
Maisel et al.[105]	191*	1-3	24
	586†	1-3	24
Farrell et al.[86]	416	1	24
Richards et al.[95]	361	1-4	24

Angio, angiography; FU, follow-up; MI, myocardial infarction; RNV, radionuclide ventriculography; SCD, sudden cardiac death; TMET, treadmill exercise test; . . . , data not obtainable from report.
*Non-Q-wave myocardial infarction.
†Q-wave myocardial infarction.
‡Including SCD and sustained ventricular tachycardia.
Modified from Shen W-K, Hammill SC: Survivors of acute myocardial infarction: Who is at risk for sudden cardiac death? *Mayo Clin Proc* 66:950-962, 1991.

tive heart failure, diuretic use, and cardiomegaly and determined that the PVC had a stronger influence on the development of sudden cardiac death than any of these.

Electrophysiologic testing was proposed as a way of identifying patients at highest risk for sudden death after myocardial infarction but has subsequently proven to be disappointing.[91-95] An American Heart Association and American College of Cardiology consensus statement[96] concluded that (1) there were no indications for routine electrophysiologic studies in low-risk patients after myocardial infarction, (2) the indications at this time were uncertain for electrophysiologic studies in high-risk patients, and (3) electrophysiologic testing was beneficial in patients with sustained ventricular tachycardia or fibrillation after the first 24 hours of acute myocardial infarction.

Complex PVCs in patients without evidence of myocardial infarction

Persons who present with PVCs and appear to be normal by routine clinical and laboratory examinations may be found to have heart disease when studied more intensively. Several studies have identified subclinical abnormalities of left ventricular performance in apparently

Total mortality		SCD					
NSVT		No NSVT		NSVT			Positive
No.	%	No.	%	No.	%	Sensitivity/ specificity, %*	predictive value, %*
11	17	7	5	8	12	53/95	12
12	14	8	4	4	5	33/96	5
30	33	58	8	19	21	25/92	21
19	38	33	9	11	22	25/91	22
31	36	60	18	46	54‡	54/81	15

Assessment of LV function	FU, mo	Deaths, no.		Independence
		Total	SCD	
Clinical	24	208	85	Yes
Clinical	36	115	55	Yes
RNV	18	66	29	Yes
RNV	24	89	35	Yes
Clinical	25	163	76	Yes
Angio	36	...	...	No
Angio	36	60	35	No
Angio	18	...	19	No
RNV, angio	12	37	...	Yes
RNV, angio	12	46	...	No
RNV, angio	20	47	24‡	No
RNV	25	34	8	No

normal persons with asymptomatic PVCs.[97,98] It is essential to exclude any significant underlying heart disease in these patients. Several longitudinal studies have examined the prognostic significance of ventricular ectopy in apparently normal individuals.[61,99-102] For normal subjects with ventricular ectopy on a 12-lead electrocardiogram (ECG), the risk of death is not clearly increased; however, the risk of coronary artery disease developing seems to be increased, especially the risk of experiencing sudden death as a first manifestation of coronary heart disease.

Whether it is necessary to treat PVCs in patients who do not have evidence of myocardial ischemia or infarction is both a difficult and a common clinical question. Hinkle et al.[78,99] suggested that frequent PVCs and PVCs that fall in the vulnerable period of the cardiac cycle are associated with an increased risk of sudden cardiac death in middle-aged males who do not have active myocardial ischemia or a recent myocardial infarction. The PVC was an independent risk factor for sudden cardiac death in this study even when the patients exhibited the associated risk factors of coronary artery disease, heart failure, cardiac enlargement, hypertension, or chronic obstructive pulmonary disease. This study also indicated that the presence of frequent PVCs in patients who do not have other risk factors was rarely associated with subsequent sudden cardiac death.

Ventricular arrhythmia and ventricular dysfunction

The relationship of left ventricular function and PVCs to the subsequent development of sudden cardiac death remains controversial. The results of most studies show a strong relationship between PVCs and left ventricular dysfunction[16,62-64,85-87,95,103-105] (Table 22C-4). Total mortality and sudden cardiac death are significantly higher in patients with complex and frequent PVCs than in those without this finding. Left ventricular dysfunction also is a major predictor of total mortality and sudden cardiac death. The role of PVCs as an independent risk factor, however, remains uncertain. On the basis of early studies, which were handicapped by shorter monitoring periods and nonquantitative assessment of left ventricular function, investigators concluded that left ventricular dysfunction and ventricular arrhythmia were independent risk factors for sudden cardiac death.[85,87] Subsequently, other investigators found that ventricular arrhythmia was a marker of left ventricular dysfunction and did not contribute independently to the prediction of survival or certain cardiac death.[16,103,104]

A review of 655 patients undergoing cardiac catheterization and 24-hour ambulatory monitoring evaluated 395 patients with and 260 patients without significant coronary artery disease.[103] The arrhythmias were evaluated with the Lown grading system (see Table 22C-1). An increased risk of sudden cardiac death was found to be directly associated with an increased score on the Lown grading scale. However, these investigators also determined that ventricular arrhythmias were strongly correlated with left ventricular function and that if left ventricular function was known, the Lown score did not contribute independent prognostic information. This study concluded that left ventricular function, as reflected by the ejection fraction, was a better predictor of sudden death than complex ventricular ectopy. Ventricular ectopy was, however, a useful noninvasive marker for the relative risk of the occurrence of sudden cardiac death in patients with coronary artery disease. The risk of sudden cardiac death is extremely low in patients with asymptomatic complex ventricular ectopy and a left ventricular ejection fraction greater than 40%.[106]

Ventricular arrhythmias during exercise testing

The prognostic implications and clinical significance of ventricular arrhythmias that occur during exercise testing (Fig 22C-8) are currently under evaluation. Studies by Faris et al.[107] and Morris and McHenry[108] of clinically normal Indiana state policemen 22 to 54 years of age who were free of ventricular ectopy at rest identified a prevalence of exercise-induced ventricular arrhythmias of 30% during a single test, and the arrhythmias were not necessarily reproducible with subsequent exercise testing. This prevalence increased with age and was higher in patients suspected of having cardiovascular disease. The investigators concluded that ventricular arrhythmias occur commonly with exercise in clinically normal persons and that occurrence of these arrhythmias is not reproducible from one exercise test to another.

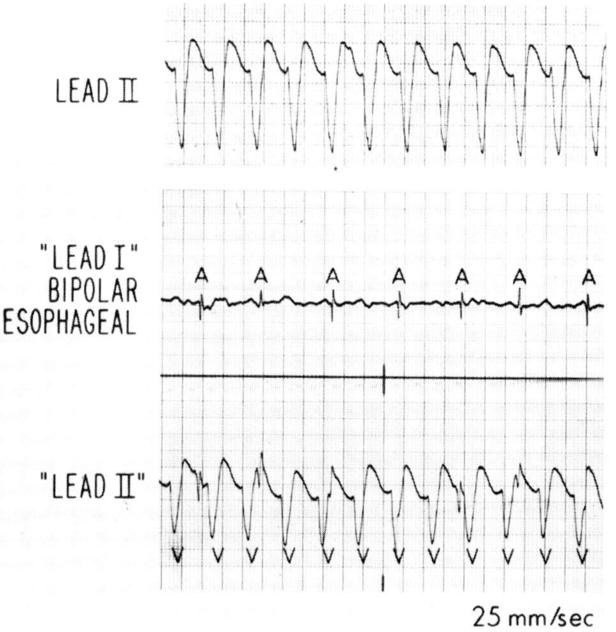

Fig 22C-8 Ventricular tachycardia during treadmill exercise stress testing. Lead II demonstrates a regular tachycardia of 150 beats/min with a wide QRS complex. The bipolar esophageal electrode records discrete atrial activity *(A)* that is dissociated from the ventricular activity *(V)* recorded simultaneously by "lead II." (From Hammill SC, Holmes DR Jr, Wood DL: Cardiac arrhythmias. In *Current Diagnosis 7.* Edited by RB Conn. Philadelphia, WB Saunders Company, 1985, pp 405-433. By permission.)

The frequency of PVCs appears to be highest in the early recovery period after the completion of exercise[109,110] and occurs more often during treadmill testing than with bicycle testing.[110] Unfortunately, neither of these observations helps to distinguish normal persons from those with coronary artery disease.[109] Patients whose ventricular arrhythmias are eliminated at high levels of exercise are not necessarily free from coronary artery disease, and this observation does not exclude patients with multiple-vessel coronary artery disease.

The presence of simple PVCs during exercise testing is of little diagnostic or prognostic importance; however, complex PVCs are more likely to occur in the presence of coronary artery disease; and if such arrhythmias occur at an exercise heart rate below 70% of predicted maximal heart rate in patients with coronary artery disease, there is a greater incidence of sudden cardiac death. Exercise ventricular ectopic activity after myocardial infarction is an important risk factor for subsequent sudden death.[111] Patients with exercise-induced sustained monomorphic ventricular tachycardia that is symptomatic can be treated by using the elimination of ventricular tachycardia during exercise as a therapeutic end point.[112]

Treating the patient with PVCs

The problem with using the PVC as a marker of ventricular instability and consequent need for antiarrhythmia therapy is, as we have seen, that the PVC has a widespread prevalence even among patients without obvious heart disease. The risk of sudden cardiac death is low in patients who have no underlying heart disease. In patients with heart disease, frequent and complex PVCs are associated with an increased risk of sudden cardiac death; however, the sensitivity and predicted value of these markers are poor[113] (see Tables 22C-2 and 22C-3). The sensitivity of complex PVCs as a marker for sudden cardiac death is approximately 25% to 50%. Thus, more than half of all cardiac patients who die suddenly would not have had complex PVCs on Holter monitoring. The positive predictive value of complex PVCs for sudden cardiac death is approximately 10% to 15%. This finding suggests that only 10% to 15% of all patients with complex PVCs will experience sudden cardiac death. If all patients with complex PVCs were treated with antiarrhythmic agents, more than 50% of patients dying suddenly would not have been treated, and 85% to 90% of all patients treated with antiarrhythmic agents would not have experienced sudden death if they had not been treated. Therefore, one can easily deduce that if frequent and complex PVCs are used as the sole indicator for treatment, a net benefit from antiarrhythmic treatment would not be attainable unless a nearly perfect antiarrhythmic agent existed, that is, one with no proarrhythmic effect and 100% efficacy.

In a recent review,[114] meta-analysis was performed on the results of antiarrhythmic therapy in 10 randomized, controlled trials between 1966 and 1989. These trials used a total of nine class I agents in patients after myocardial infarction; enrollments were within 60 days after myocardial infarction. Three studies showed a small beneficial effect of treatment,[115-117] two showed no difference,[118,119] and four showed a small adverse effect of treatment.[120-123] The alarming adverse effect can be best demonstrated by the recent Cardiac Arrhythmia Suppression Trial (CAST),[1,5,124,125] which assessed the effect of encainide and flecainide on subsequent mortality in patients with asymptomatic or mildly symptomatic complex ventricular ectopy after myocardial infarction (Fig 22C-9). Increased incidences of arrhythmic deaths, nonfatal cardiac arrests, and total mortality were significantly higher in the encainide and flecainide treatment group in all subsets of patients and resulted in discontinuation of the part of the trial involving these medications. The application of these data to patients without coronary disease is still under investigation. Nonetheless, this study highlights the danger of antiarrhythmic drugs producing a proarrhythmic effect and the subsequent risk of a worse survival in a low-risk population.

The issue of whether antiarrhythmia therapy that suppresses complex PVCs will result in a reduced incidence of sudden cardiac death has not been answered. However, Graboys et al.[65] presented their experience suggesting that the suppression of PVCs in patients who have a history of recurrent ventricular tachycardia or ventricular fibrillation protects against the recurrence or sudden cardiac death. They developed a drug-testing protocol that uses two phases. In the first phase, the patient is given a single large oral dose of antiarrhythmia medication and the ECG is monitored in the form of a programmed transcription that displays the time course of

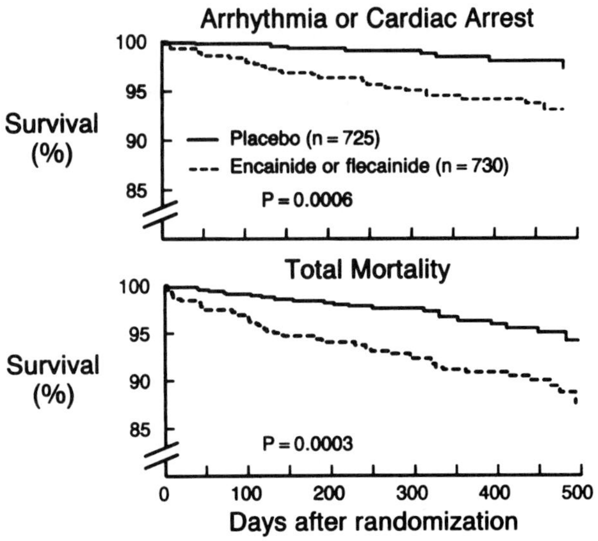

Fig 22C-9 Incidences of total mortality, ventricular tachycardia, and sudden death from the Cardiac Arrhythmia Suppression Trial. (From The Cardiac Arrhythmia Suppression Trial (CAST) Investigators: Preliminary report: effect of encainide and flecainide on mortality in a randomized trial of arrhythmia suppression after myocardial infarction. *N Engl J Med* 321:406-411, 1989. By permission of the journal.)

the action of the drug on the ventricular ectopy. Plasma levels of the drug are determined to allow correlation with the antiarrhythmia and toxic effects. These patients undergo exercise testing during this same period. A positive response to the acute phase of testing is elimination of grades 4B and 5 of complex PVCs (see Table 22C-1).

The second phase of drug testing consists of maintenance therapy for 48 to 96 hours with the drug that appeared to be most effective during phase-1 testing. During phase 2, drug efficacy is assessed with 24-hour ambulatory monitoring, maximal exercise stress testing, and psychologic stress testing. The end points of therapy during phase 2 include elimination of grades 4B and 5 PVCs, a reduction by 90% of grade 4A PVCs, and at least a 50% reduction of total PVCs.

Patients treated with this protocol are then given two antiarrhythmia drugs that exhibited effectiveness during phase-2 testing. Observations suggest that effective control of advanced grades of ventricular ectopy in patients with recurrent life-threatening arrhythmias is associated with a reduced incidence of sudden cardiac death.

Failure to prevent sudden cardiac death by suppressing asymptomatic PVCs may be due to spontaneous variability of PVCs,[126-128] suboptimal predictive value of the currently available diagnostic tools, and the lack of perfect pharmacologic therapy;[114,129-131] however, more fundamental issues, such as the mechanisms of sudden cardiac death, perhaps should be addressed. Does the ventricular ectopic activity trigger a sustained fatal ventricular arrhythmia? Do the frequent and complex PVCs degenerate or transform into a fatal sustained ventricular arrhythmia? Are spontaneous PVCs simply a reflection of more severe

Table 22C-5 Results of electrophysiologic studies after myocardial infarction

Study	No. of patients	Timing of EPS, mo	FU, mo	Inducibility, %
Greene et al.[132]	48	<3	18	40 (SVT, NSVT)
Hamer et al.[133]	70	<1	24	32
Richards et al.[134]	165	<1	8	23 (NSVT, SVT, VF)
Marchlinski et al.[135]	46	<2	18	22 (SVT, NSVT)
Roy et al.[91]	150	12 ± 2 days	10 ± 5	23 (VT, VF)
Denniss et al.[136]	403	<1	24	34 (VT, VF)
Bourke et al.[93]	1,209	7-10 days	32	6.2 (VT)
Richards et al.[95]	313	6-28 days	25	7.3 (VT)

EPS, electrophysiologic study; FU, follow-up; Ind, inducible; Neg, negative; Nonind, noninducible; NS, not significant; NSVT, nonsustained ventricular tachycardia; Pos, positive; SVT, sustained ventricular tachycardia; VF, ventricular fibrillation; VT, ventricular tachycardia.
Modified from Shen W-K, Hammill SC: Survivors of acute myocardial infarction: Who is at risk for sudden cardiac death? *Mayo Clin Proc* 66:950-962, 1991.

underlying heart disease? Suppression of PVCs should prevent sudden cardiac death if triggering or transformation is the underlying mechanism of sudden cardiac death. If, however, PVCs are simply markers of underlying heart disease, prevention of sudden cardiac death should be improved by optimizing treatment of the underlying heart disease and eliminating the source of the triggering and transforming events. If the triggering mechanisms for fatal arrhythmias cannot be prevented, alternative approaches, such as implantation of an automatic defibrillator (to abort the arrhythmia after it has been triggered), may be effective in preventing sudden death. At this time, we recommend treating patients with complex ectopy associated with significant symptoms. Asymptomatic patients should not be treated until additional information is available that therapy improves survival.

Electrophysiologic testing has been assessed as a method for determining the prognostic importance of asymptomatic nonsustained ventricular tachycardia and deciding who requires therapy (Table 22C-5). In a study of 110 patients with asymptomatic nonsustained ventricular tachycardia undergoing electrophysiologic testing, only the ejection fraction and congestive heart failure class were found to be independent predictors of outcome.[106] Of patients with asymptomatic nonsustained ventricular tachycardia and an ejection fraction of 40% or greater, 11% had sustained ventricular tachycardia induced and only two had arrhythmic events during follow-up (3.5%). This finding has been reported by others.[90,137] These patients did not benefit from electrophysiologic testing and do not appear to require antiarrhythmic therapy. Patients with coronary artery disease and an ejection fraction less than 40% had an inducibility rate of 40% to 50%,[106] which is consistent with those of other reports.[90,137-140] A negative study in this group did not confer a favorable prognosis, because 21% of patients died suddenly.[106] This finding is consistent with the reports of others,[138,140] whereas other investigators have found that a negative electrophysiology study confers a favorable prognosis.[90,137,139] Patients with a dilated cardiomyopathy and ejection fraction of less than 40% had a low incidence of inducibility (4%), had a high occurrence of ventricular tachycardia or cardiac arrest during follow-up (33%), and did not benefit from electrophysiologic testing,[106] results that confirm those of earlier investigations.[141-143]

VENTRICULAR TACHYCARDIA

Ventricular tachycardia (Fig 22C-10) is a difficult clinical problem for the physician.[145-147] The evaluation and treatment of such a rhythm disturbance are complicated by the fact that it often occurs in life-threatening situations that dictate rapid diagnosis and treatment. Ventricular tachycardia is due to abnormal impulses originating from areas of the specialized conduction system or ventricular myocardium that are distal to the bundle of His. It is defined as three or more consecutive ectopic complexes with a rate of 100 to 250 beats/min. The ability of patients to tolerate an episode of ventricular tachycardia generally depends on the rate of the tachycardia and the state of the patient's cardiovascular system. In patients with poor myocardial function and rapid tachycardia, there is often hemodynamic deterioration, resulting in diminished coronary artery perfusion and ventricular fibrillation. In contrast, patients with good myocardial function can often tolerate ventricular tachycardia for a prolonged period. This section discusses the electrophysiologic mechanisms of ventricular tachycardia, the clinical and ECG features, and the use of invasive electrophysiologic testing in the evaluation of patients with ventricular tachycardia.

As discussed previously, the three known electrophysiologic mechanisms involved in the initiation of ventricular tachycardia are enhanced automaticity, triggered activity, and reentry. The His-Purkinje system can depolarize spontaneously and function as an escape pacemaker. This serves an important role in the event that supraventricular impulses fail to reach the ventricles; however, under abnormal circumstances, the rate of automaticity in the His-Purkinje system can be enhanced and can result in ventricular tachycardia. Such circumstances include elec-

Mortality, %				Predictive value, %	
Ind	Nonind	*P*	Sensitivity/ specificity, %	Pos	Neg
79	14	<0.05	79/86	79	86
30	4	<0.05	78/75	32	96
32	2	<0.001	80/83	32	98
10	14	NS	7/78	10	86
3	3	NS	25/97	3	97
27	8	<0.01	64/71	27	92
25	2.9	<0.0005	47/95	19	98
30	2	<0.001	58/95	30	98

trolyte imbalance, catecholamine stimulation, and ischemia. Short runs of tachycardia which are observed during continuous monitoring and which cannot be initiated by programmed ventricular stimulation may be automatic in nature.[148,149] Ventricular tachycardia caused by a triggered mechanism has been observed under experimental conditions that resemble clinical circumstances, such as ischemia, digitalis toxicity, hypokalemia, hypercalcemia, and the influence of catecholamine.[58] Indirect observations also strongly suggest that exercise-induced ventricular tachycardia in young patients with normal hearts may be caused by a triggered mechanism.[150,151]

The more common mechanism for the initiation of ventricular tachycardia is reentry. Reentry can occur when there is inhomogeneous conduction and refractoriness such as is present in the ischemic myocardium. Ventricular tachycardia dependent upon a reentry mechanism is usually initiated by a critically timed premature impulse.[148,152,153] The initiating impulse may be a PVC, a supraventricular complex, or an artificial electrical impulse introduced during the electrophysiologic study or permanent pacing. The impulse can arrive during the vulnerable period to initiate episodes of tachycardia; however, late coupled PVCs are also able to initiate ventricular tachycardia.[68]

Ventricular tachycardia is often referred to as sustained or nonsustained. Sustained ventricular tachycardia refers to an episode of tachycardia that lasts at least 30 seconds and generally requires termination by antiarrhythmia drugs, antitachycardia pacing techniques, or electrical cardioversion. Nonsustained ventricular tachycardia suggests that the episodes are short (three beats or longer) and terminate spontaneously.

In general, ventricular tachycardia affects the diseased heart, although it has been described in patients with apparently normal hearts. Ventricular tachycardia is usually associated with coronary artery disease.[145-147] Patients who have ventricular tachycardia in the absence of coronary artery disease have other cardiac abnormalities, including cardiomyopathy, mitral valve prolapse, valvular heart disease, Q-T interval prolongation and an otherwise normal heart, and an abnormality described as primary electrical instability.[141] Other causes of ventricular tachycardia include sarcoidosis, beginning treatment in patients with myxedema, and drugs such as digitalis, sympathomimetic amines, and antiarrhythmia agents. Occasional runs of tachycardia are initiated by a change in posture, exercise, emotional excitement, or vagal stimulation.

Clinical features

Between episodes of tachycardia there generally is evidence of underlying heart disease. This may take the form of coronary artery disease and a history of ischemia or abnormal auscultation suggesting valvular heart disease or mitral valve prolapse. An episode of tachycardia is often associated with a falling blood pressure, angina, congestive heart failure, or pulmonary edema. The other physical findings depend on the relationship of the atrial rhythm to the ventricular tachycardia. In patients who demonstrate 1:1 retrograde conduction during tachycardia, a regular cannon "a" wave is present in the jugular venous pulse with each beat, and there is a constant intensity of the first heart sound. In patients with ventriculoatrial (VA) dissociation and a regular atrial rhythm, intermittent cannon "a" waves are present in the jugular pulse, and there is variation in the intensity of the first heart sound and beat-to-beat variation in the systolic blood pressure. Finally, in patients who have coexistent atrial fibrillation, no cannon "a" waves are present, and the first heart sound is constant.

Use of surface ECG to differentiate supraventricular tachycardia from ventricular tachycardia

It is critically important, yet often difficult, to differentiate supraventricular tachycardia with aberrancy from ventricular tachycardia. On the ECG these arrhythmias generally have similar rates, the rate of the ventricular tachycardia ranging from 100 to 250 beats/min.[152] Ven-

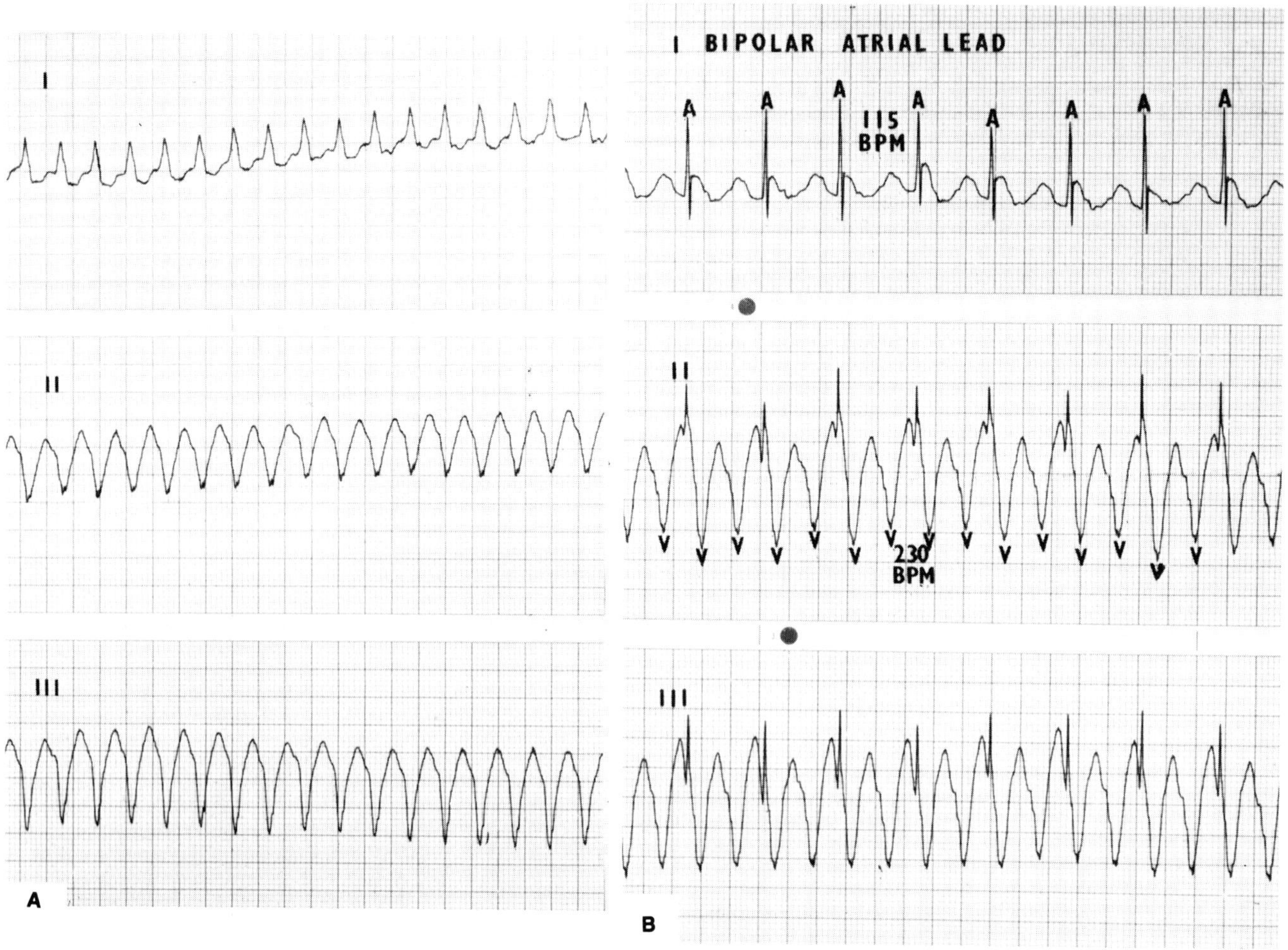

Fig 22C-10 **A,** tachycardia with a wide QRS morphology and a ventricular rate of 250 beats/min. **B,** use of a bipolar electrode that was placed percutaneously in the right atrium and is recorded simultaneously with surface leads II and III by means of a technique previously described.[144] The bipolar atrial lead records discrete atrial depolarization *(A)* (115 beats/min, BPM) and ventricular depolarization *(V)* (230 beats/min, BPM) is recorded in leads II and III. Retrograde ventriculoatrial conduction (2:1) is present. (**A** from Hammill SC, Holmes DR Jr, Wood DL: Cardiac arrhythmias. In *Current Diagnosis 7.* Edited by RB Conn. Philadelphia, WB Saunders Company, 1985, pp 405-433. By permission.)

Table 22C-6 Differentiation of supraventricular tachycardia with aberrancy (SVT) from ventricular tachycardia (VT) by means of the surface electrocardiogram*

Parameters	SVT, %	VT, %	Parameters	SVT, %	VT, %
Ventricular rate (beats/min)			Mean QRS axis, frontal plane		
100-130	1	13	−30° or less	7	69
130-170	27	47	Between −30° and +90°	47	11
170-200	60	21	More than +90°	43	17
>200	12	19	Undetermined	3	3
One-to-one atrial and ventricular relationship	100	33			
QRS width, msec					
<120	76	14			
120-140	24	19			
>140	0	67			

*Data from Wellens et al.[154] See text for morphological comparison.

WIDE QRS TACH - RBBB

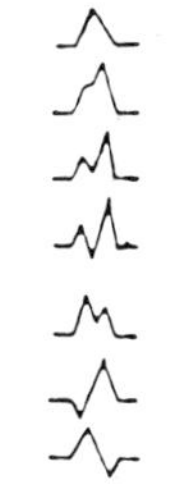

LEAD V1	ABERRATION	VT
		15
	11	17
	19	3
	38	3
		7
	1	16
		4

A

WIDE QRS TACH - LBBB

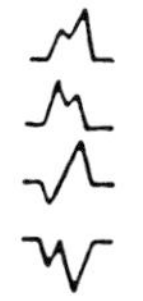

LEAD V6	ABERRATION	VT
	14	15
	17	14
		5
		1

B

Fig 22C-11 Differentiation of ventricular tachycardia *(VT)* from supraventricular tachycardia with aberrancy by QRS configuration in leads V_1 and V_6 during tachycardia *(TACH)*. **A,** configuration of right bundle-branch block *(RBBB)*-shaped QRS complexes in lead V_1 during tachycardia. **B,** configuration in leads V_6 in patients with left bundle-branch block *(LBBB)*-shaped QRS complex during ventricular tachycardia. (Modified from Wellens HJJ, Bär FWHM, Lie KI: The value of the electrocardiogram in the differential diagnosis of tachycardia with a widened QRS complex. *Am J Med* 64:27-33, 1978.)

tricular tachycardia is usually regular, although on occasion there may be a change in cycle length of 10 to 50 msec between two complexes during a sustained episode of ventricular tachycardia.[154] Both supraventricular and ventricular tachycardia may, in patients who have a QRS complex of normal width in sinus rhythm, be associated with QRS complexes wider than 120 msec; in contrast, ventricular tachycardia can show a QRS complex of 100 to 120 msec in duration.[154-156]

Wellens et al.[154] described the ECG characteristics of electrophysiologically documented ventricular tachycardia and compared these findings with the rhythms that were documented as supraventricular tachycardia with aberration. The following observations were observed more commonly during ventricular tachycardia (Table 22C-6 and Fig 22C-11): AV dissociation, superior QRS axis, QRS width exceeding 140 msec, monophasic or biphasic right bundle-branch block-shaped QRS complexes in V_1, and complexes with a QR or QS in V_6 with a left bundle-branch block morphology. Recording atrial activity with a bipolar recording lead placed in the esophagus (see Fig 22C-8) can often identify AV dissociation that was not apparent on the surface ECG.[144] The observation of fusion complexes also suggests a ventricular tachycardia.[154,157,158] The introduction of intracardiac recording of the His bundle has demonstrated that none of the surface ECG features is pathognomonic of ventricular tachycardia in the individual cases.[147]

Akhtar et al.[159] described the value and limitations of clinical and ECG criteria for separating supraventricular tachycardia with aberrancy from ventricular tachycardia. The standard ECG criteria for ventricular tachycardia had poor sensitivity and specificity individually but collectively allowed a correct diagnosis of ventricular tachycardia in 92% of patients with a clinical history of heart disease. Ventricular tachycardia was suggested by its association with structural heart disease, AV dissociation, positive QRS concordance and axis less than −90° to +180°, combination of left bundle-branch block and right axis deviation, QRS duration of greater than 140 msec with right bundle-branch block and greater than 160 msec with left bundle-branch block, and a QRS complex during tachycardia that differed from the baseline preexisting bundle-branch block. They concluded that ventricular tachycardia was the commonest underlying mechanism for a wide-QRS tachycardia and that a correct diagnosis can usually be made from clinical and surface ECG criteria.

In a recent study, Brugada et al.[160] prospectively analyzed 554 tachycardias (384 ventricular and 170 supraventricular) by using a four-step approach: (1) positive concordance in precordial leads, (2) at least one R-S interval greater than 100 msec, (3) AV dissociation, and (4) leads V_1 and V_6 both fulfilling classic criteria for ventricular tachycardia.[154,161,162] If the requirement is met at any step, a positive diagnosis of ventricular tachycardia is made. If the results of all four steps are negative, the diagnosis of supraventricular tachycardia with aberrancy is made by exclusion of ventricular tachycardia. The sensitivity of the four consecutive steps was 0.987, and the specificity was 0.965.

Use of intracardiac recordings to differentiate supraventricular tachycardia from ventricular tachycardia

An important application of electrophysiologic testing, including intracardiac recording and programmed stimulation, is to determine whether a tachycardia is supraventricular or ventricular in origin (Fig 22C-12). Despite the most careful scrutiny of a surface ECG, it is often difficult to determine the origin of a tachycardia. The use of intracardiac recordings has permitted the physician to identify more clearly the origin of a tachycardia. Electrophysiologic investigation has helped in determining the relative importance of the following in differentiating supraventricular from ventricular tachycardia: rate and regularity of the tachycardia, relationship of the ventricular and atrial activities during tachycardia, width of the QRS complex, morphology of the QRS complex, fusion beats during tachycardia, and the relationship of depolarization of the His bundle to depolarization of the ventricles.

Tachycardia rate. The ventricular rate during tachycardia does not help in distinguishing supraventricular tachycardia with aberrancy from ventricular tachycardia.

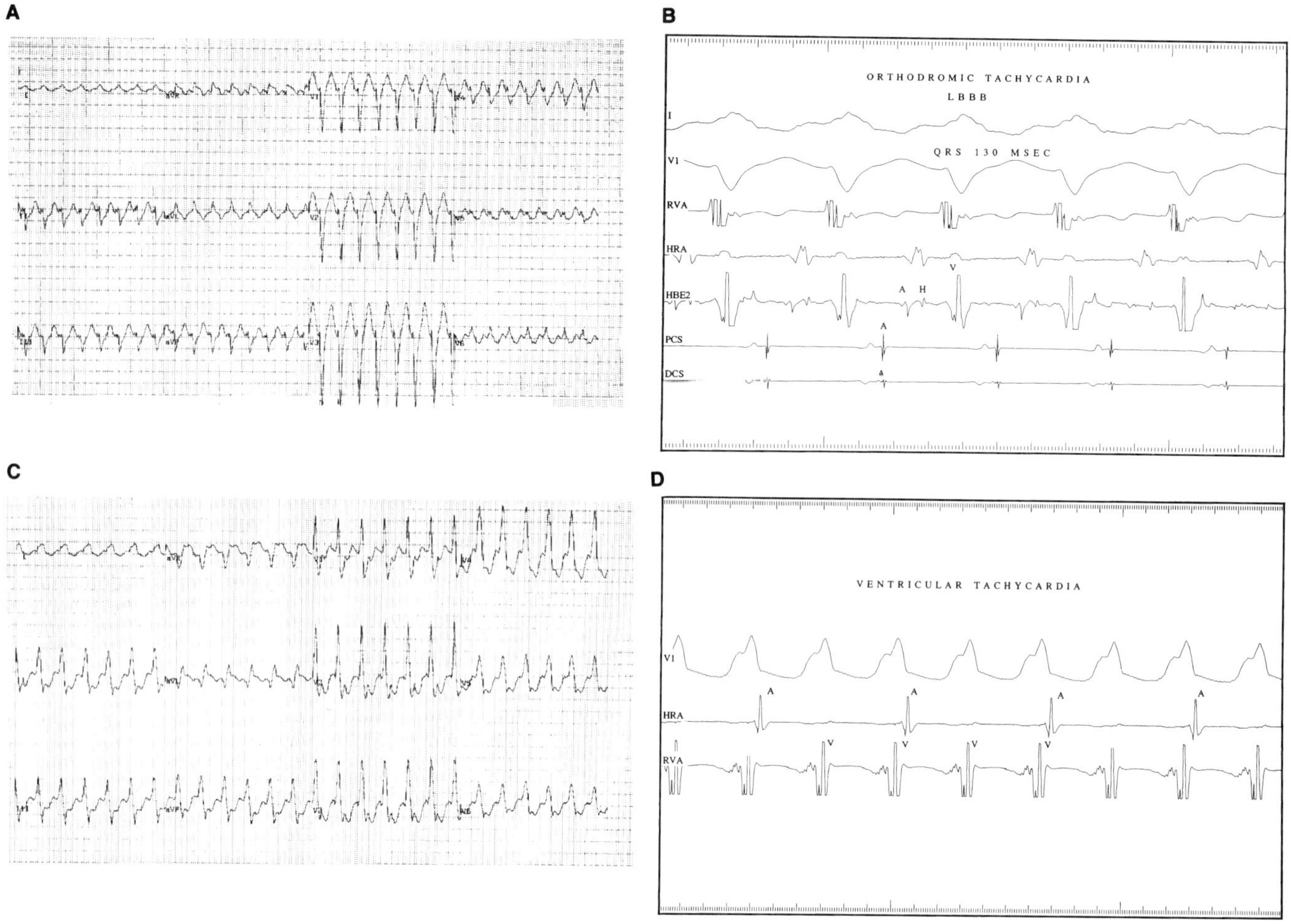

Fig 22C-12 Differentiation of wide complex tachycardia by electrophysiologic testing. **A,** a 12-lead ECG demonstrates a wide complex tachycardia of left bundle-branch block morphology. **B,** during electrophysiologic testing, it was confirmed that a concealed accessory pathway was located in the left posterior position. An orthodromic reentrance tachycardia with left bundle-branch block was induced. Surface leads I and V_1 are recorded. Intracardiac recordings from right ventricular apex *(RVA),* high right atrium *(HRA),* His bundle electrogram *(HBE2),* proximal coronary sinus *(PCS),* and distal coronary sinus *(DCS)* are recorded. *A* denotes intracardiac atrial signals, *H* denotes His bundle signal, and *V* denotes ventricular signal. **C,** a 12-lead ECG shows a wide complex tachycardia. **D,** during electrophysiologic testing, a ventricular tachycardia of a similar morphology was induced. Intracardiac recordings clearly demonstrated AV dissociation. This confirms the diagnosis of ventricular tachycardia.

Both supraventricular tachycardia and ventricular tachycardia are generally regular. Occasionally, ventricular tachycardia can vary from 10 to 50 msec between two ventricular complexes. Changes in regularity of more than 20 msec were observed in 21% of cases of ventricular tachycardia, compared with 6% of the cases of supraventricular tachycardia.[154]

Atrioventricular relationship. Electrophysiologic testing helps in evaluating the relationship of atrial and ventricular activity. The presence of AV dissociation (see Figs 22C-8 and 22C-10) has long been used as a clue in identifying ventricular tachycardia.[163] It has been well established that patients with ventricular tachycardia can have 1:1 AV relationships. In such cases the patients have retrograde VA conduction.[164,165] In general, electrophysiologic studies have demonstrated that VA conduction is often intact during ventricular tachycardia, and if block is present, it can occur at any portion of the conduction system between the ventricle and the atrium.[166] When patients with ventricular tachycardia are evaluated by means of the surface ECG, the patients may show a 1:1 AV relationship as a result of retrograde VA conduction. In such patients, the P waves will proceed from the low to the high portion of the atrium with an axis of −90°. Such P waves occur shortly after completion of the QRS complex and are similar to P waves associated with AV node reentrant tachycardia.[147]

During an episode of tachycardia with a wide QRS complex, the tachycardia is most likely ventricular in origin if the P waves that are seen are normal in

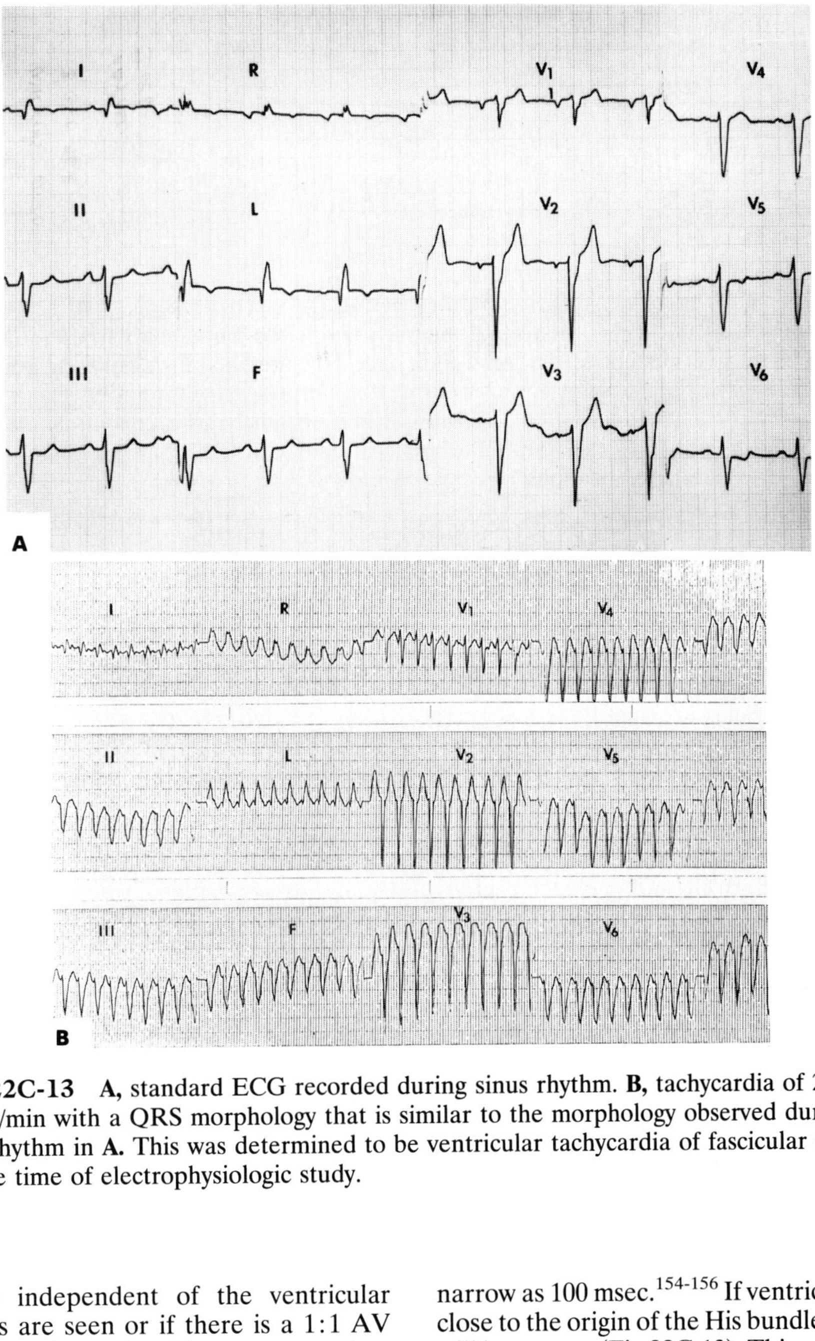

Fig 22C-13 **A,** standard ECG recorded during sinus rhythm. **B,** tachycardia of 250 beats/min with a QRS morphology that is similar to the morphology observed during sinus rhythm in **A.** This was determined to be ventricular tachycardia of fascicular origin at the time of electrophysiologic study.

morphology and are independent of the ventricular rhythm. If no P waves are seen or if there is a 1:1 AV relationship, the tachycardia can be either supraventricular or ventricular. Finally, if 2:1 VA conduction is observed, the diagnosis is ventricular tachycardia, because this relationship is only rarely produced by a rhythm other than ventricular tachycardia. On occasion, carotid sinus massage can help dissociate atrial activity from ventricular activity during ventricular tachycardia and establish the diagnosis.[147]

QRS width and morphology. The width of the QRS complex during tachycardia can help in identifying whether it is supraventricular or ventricular in origin. In general, a tachycardia with a QRS duration longer than 140 msec is ventricular tachycardia.[154] However, ventricular tachycardia may also be present with QRS complexes of less than 140 msec, and occasionally they can be as narrow as 100 msec.[154-156] If ventricular tachycardia arises close to the origin of the His bundle, the QRS morphology will be narrow (Fig 22C-13). This probably occurs because the ventricles are depolarized simultaneously from a focus that originates in the interventricular septum.[167] It is generally believed that a tachycardia with a right bundle-branch block morphology originates in the left ventricle and a tachycardia with a left bundle-branch morphology originates in the right ventricle. However, observations[168] during clinical electrophysiologic studies of 41 patients with ventricular tachycardia demonstrated that in 100% of the 22 patients with right bundle-branch morphology, the tachycardia originated in the left ventricle, and in 84% of the 19 patients with left bundle-branch morphology, the tachycardia originated in the left ventricle. All of these patients had coronary artery disease. In three (16%) of the patients with left bundle-

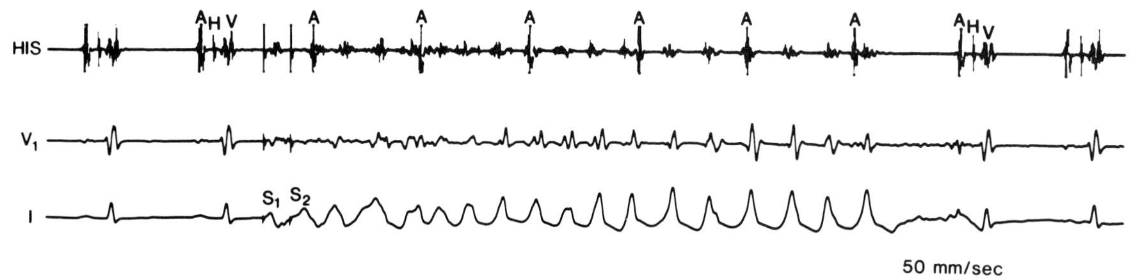

Fig 22C-14 Ventricular tachycardia recorded in the electrophysiology laboratory with surface leads V_1 and I recorded simultaneously with a His bundle electrode *(HIS)*. The patient is in sinus rhythm with normal A-H and H-V intervals. Two critically timed premature extrastimuli *(S_1S_2)* are introduced that initiate self-terminating ventricular tachycardia. A normal H-V interval is present in the sinus beats immediately preceding and upon termination of the ventricular tachycardia. Ventriculoatrial dissociation is also present. *A,* atrial depolarizations.

branch block morphology during tachycardia, the tachycardia originated in the right ventricle, and none of these patients had coronary artery disease.

Fusion beats. A fusion beat occurs during ventricular tachycardia when the ventricles are simultaneously activated by supraventricular and ventricular impulses. The fusion beat as recorded by the ECG combines the morphological features of the supraventricular beat and the beat occurring during ventricular tachycardia.[156,157] Fusion beats appear in approximately 12% of patients with ventricular tachycardia who undergo electrophysiologic testing,[154] and they are an important finding in differentiating supraventricular from ventricular tachycardia. During the electrophysiologic study, fusion beats demonstrate a short H-V interval. The His depolarization is a result of antegrade activation, whereas the onset of the QRS complex occurs early because of ventricular tachycardia. The presence of fusion beats on the surface ECG during tachycardia is good evidence that the tachycardia is ventricular in origin.

The H-V interval. The relationship of the His bundle depolarization to the onset of the QRS complex (H-V interval) is important in establishing the origin of a tachycardia[149,169] (Fig 22C-14). In the absence of preexcitation, supraventricular rhythms have a normal H-V interval. In contrast, during ventricular tachycardia, the His bundle deflection may not be observed because it is being activated retrogradely from the ventricles, and consequently the deflection is hidden in the ventricular deflection, or the His bundle may appear not to be related at all to the ventricular arrhythmia if there is ventricular atrial block at a level below the His bundle.[170] On occasion, ventricular tachycardia may be associated with a fixed H-V interval that is shorter than the H-V interval observed during sinus rhythm; this occurs when the tachycardia originates in the proximal portion of the ventricles. Such tachycardias are referred to as "fascicular" rhythms, and they begin in the specialized conduction system distal to the His bundle. These rhythms depolarize the ventricle in the antegrade direction and the His bundle in the retrograde direction; they thereby give rise to a fixed H-V interval shorter than that occurring when the patient is in sinus rhythm. The physician must make certain that a right bundle-branch potential is not being recorded during a supraventricular rhythm because this also will give rise to a short interval. When one attempts to identify whether a tachycardia is ventricular in origin by determining the relationship of the His bundle depolarization to the tachycardia, the His bundle deflection should be identified during sinus rhythm (see Fig 22C-13) or related to atrial depolarization during ventricular tachycardia to make certain that the His bundle catheter is in proper position.[170]

Electrophysiologic evaluation of patients with ventricular tachycardia

With the advent of programmed stimulation, it has become possible to induce and terminate tachycardias by pacing techniques. Such techniques have improved our understanding of ventricular tachycardia and have made the approach to therapy more rational. The technique of programmed stimulation to induce and terminate ventricular tachycardia can be performed with small risk to the patient in the controlled setting of the electrophysiology laboratory.[171] In patients who have sustained ventricular tachycardia that was documented before the electrophysiologic study, it will be possible to induce that tachycardia in the electrophysiology laboratory 90% of the time.[145,146,172-175] The induction of tachycardia depends on several factors, including the distance between the site of stimulation and the origin of the ventricular tachycardia, the conduction velocity between the two sites, and the refractoriness of the ventricle.[152,153]

The initiation of ventricular tachycardia by pacing can be performed by a variety of maneuvers. On occasion, ventricular tachycardia can be induced by a critically timed premature atrial complex. In general, however, ventricular stimulation is required for the initiation of ventricular tachycardia[176] (Figs 22C-15 and 22C-16). A common protocol for programmed stimulation includes the introduction of single and paired extrastimuli during

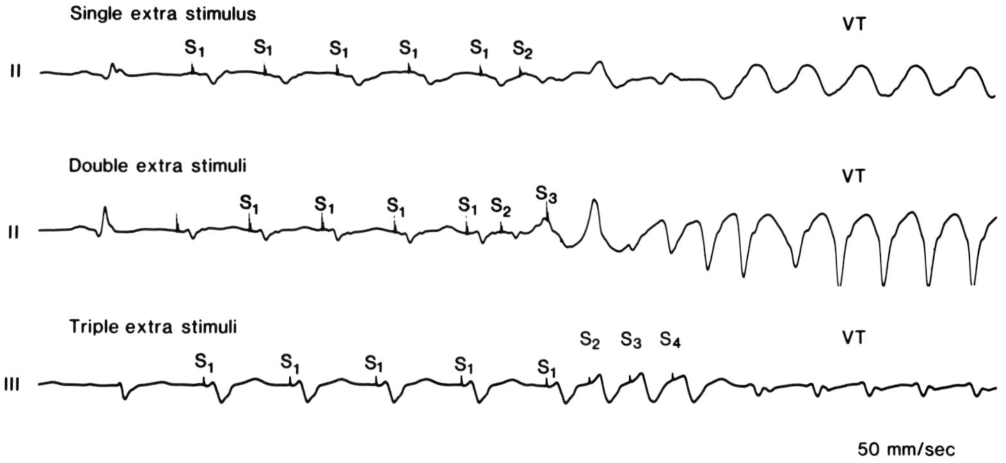

Fig 22C-15 Initiation of ventricular tachycardia *(VT)* in the electrophysiology laboratory with the use of single *(S_2)*, double *(S_2S_3)*, and triple *($S_2S_3S_4$)* extrastimuli introduced during ventricular pacing *(S_1)* at 120 beats/min.

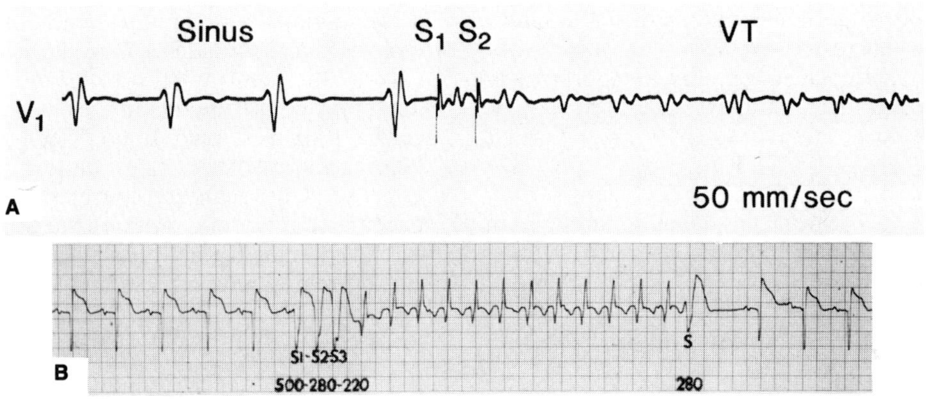

Fig 22C-16 **A,** initiation of ventricular tachycardia *(VT)* by critically timed paired premature extrastimuli *(S_1S_2)* introduced during sinus rhythm. **B,** initiation of tachycardia with the use of triple extrastimuli *($S_1S_2S_3$)*. Ventricular tachycardia is then terminated with a single *(S)* critically timed (280 msec) extrastimulus and sinus rhythm is restored.

ventricular pacing at cycle lengths of 600, 500, and 400 msec (100, 120, and 150 beats/min, respectively). Ventricular pacing is performed for eight beats, and then the extrastimulus is introduced. The stimuli are introduced at the end of diastole and brought progressively closer to the last QRS complex until refractoriness occurs. The impulse is then placed 20 msec later, and the second impulse is brought in during diastole. This scans diastole and attempts to alter the properties of the presumed reentrant circuit such that there will be block in one limb of the circuit with conduction through the slower pathway and formation of reentrant tachycardia. If single and paired extrastimuli fail to induce ventricular tachycardia, a third extrastimulus can be used. If ventricular tachycardia is not induced with this procedure, the catheter is generally repositioned in a different part of the right ventricle in an attempt to get closer to the presumed reentrant circuit.[152,153] The stimulation sequence is then repeated.

In general, the right ventricular apex and right ventricular outflow tract are the two most common areas used for stimulation. A small percentage of patients will require stimulation in the left ventricle to produce tachycardia that has previously been observed clinically.[177-179] In the evaluation of patients with previously observed sustained ventricular tachycardia, the tachycardia will be induced by a single premature beat in 15%, double premature beats in 45%, triple premature beats in 30%, and left ventricular stimulation in 6% to 10%.[180] The addition of a third premature beat to the stimulation protocol increases sensitivity from 60% to 90% and decreases specificity from 95% to 60%.[181]

In patients with ventricular tachycardia associated with exertion, it may be possible to induce the tachycardia at the time of electrophysiologic study only during the administration of a catecholamine such as isoproterenol.[176,178,182] On occasion, antiarrhythmia drugs such as procainamide[172,178,183] can facilitate the induction of ventricular tachycardia, presumably because they alter the properties of the reentrant circuit. Procainamide probably slows conduction in an asynchronous fashion in portions of the reentrant circuit and enhances the ability to induce tachycardia.

The ease of induction of ventricular tachycardia in the electrophysiology laboratory depends on several factors. Ventricular tachycardia is easier to induce in patients who have previously had sustained ventricular tachycardia and who have an associated cardiac abnormality such as coronary artery disease, ventricular aneurysms, or ischemic cardiomyopathy.[147,184] The electrophysiologic study is less likely to induce ventricular tachycardia in patients with nonsustained ventricular tachycardia, exercise-induced ventricular tachycardia, torsade de pointes, dilated cardiomyopathy, or mitral valve prolapse.[141,176,185] It is assumed that arrhythmias that are induced by pacing techniques are reentrant in nature and that arrhythmias that cannot be induced during the electrophysiologic study are due to automaticity. The demonstration of triggered activity in the research laboratory suggests that certain ventricular arrhythmias obtained in the clinical laboratory may be due to a triggered mechanism; however, most inducible arrhythmias in the clinical laboratory are believed to be reentrant in nature.

Termination of induced tachycardia

After ventricular tachycardia has been induced in the laboratory, the tachycardia must be terminated unless detailed mapping of its site of origin is to be undertaken. In terminating the tachycardia, attention is given to the patient's blood pressure and mental status. If the blood pressure deteriorates, termination of the tachycardia must be rapid, and this often requires electrical cardioversion. Sustained tachycardias that are hemodynamically stable can often be converted with pacing techniques[147,186] (Figs 22C-16, 22C-17, and 22C-18). These techniques include the introduction of single or double extrastimuli, pacing at a rate slower than the tachycardia (underdrive pacing), and pacing at a rate faster than the tachycardia (overdrive pacing). The most important factor that allows the technique of single or double ventricular extrastimuli to be used to terminate the tachycardia is the hemodynamic stability of the patient because of the length of time it takes to scan diastole during the tachycardia and determine the necessary coupling interval that is required for termination. If a tachycardia does not result in hemodynamic deterioration, single or double extrastimuli programmed into diastole will convert tachycardia in 80% to 90% of cases.[152,187,188] In general, this technique is more successful when the catheter tip is close to the origin of the tachycardia and the rate of the tachycardia is below 175 beats/min.[152]

Occasionally, the ventricle appears to be captured with a programmed extrastimulus without termination of the tachycardia.[189] In such cases, the extrastimulus has not entered the reentrant circuit because the excitable gap is anatomically or functionally too narrow; thus, the tachycardia is allowed to continue. When one is dealing with a tachycardia of slow rate, underdrive pacing can be effective. This technique converts the tachycardia when a paced beat randomly captures the ventricles at a coupling interval similar to the interval that was effective when a single programmed extrastimulus was able to convert the tachycardia.[152]

Often the only pacing technique that is effective in

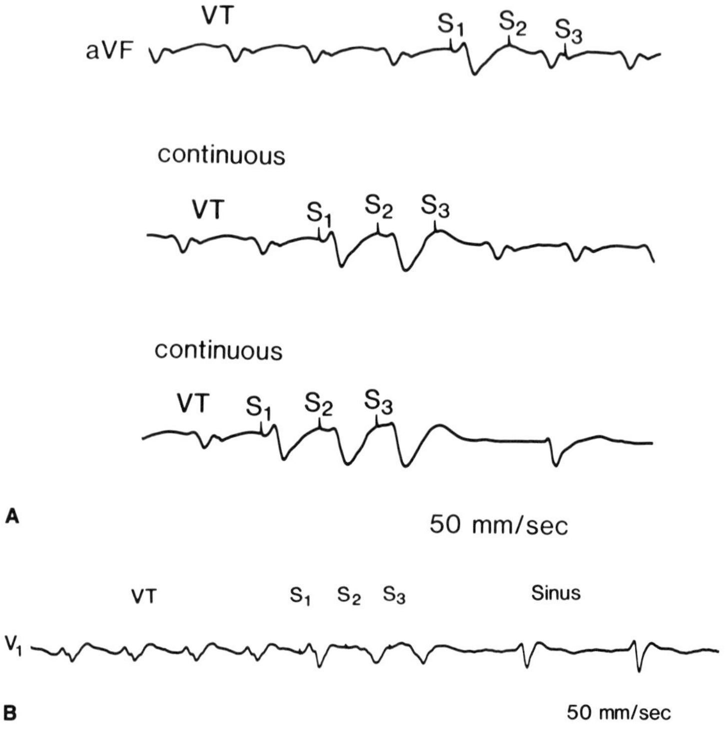

Fig 22C-17 Termination of ventricular tachycardia *(VT)* with critically timed premature extrastimuli. **A,** three extrastimuli *($S_1S_2S_3$)* are introduced during the tachycardia. S_1 captures the ventricle, but the tachycardia fails to terminate. Subsequently, S_1 and S_2 capture the ventricle, but again the tachycardia is not terminated. Finally, all three extrastimuli capture the ventricle and the tachycardia is terminated. **B,** termination of ventricular tachycardia with triple extrastimuli.

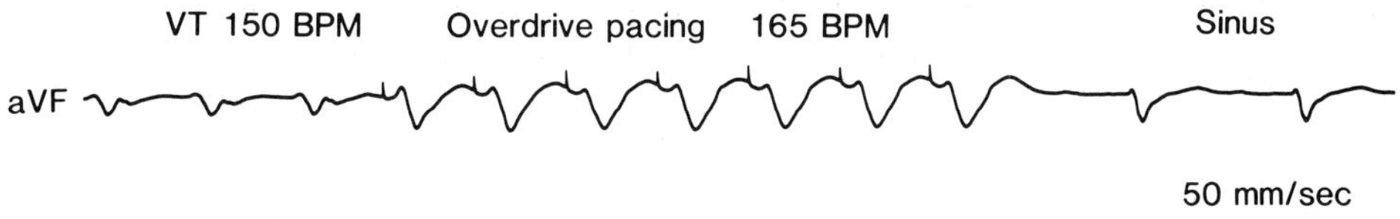

Fig 22C-18 Ventricular tachycardia *(VT)* at a rate of 150 beats/min is converted to sinus rhythm with overdrive pacing at 165 beats/min.

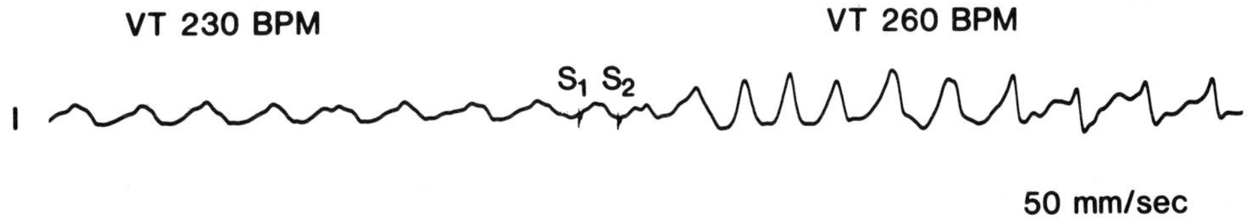

Fig 22C-19 Ventricular tachycardia *(VT)* at a rate of 230 beats/min is accelerated to a rate of 260 beats/min after two premature extrastimuli *(S_1S_2)*.

terminating a fast tachycardia is rapid overdrive pacing. Rapid overdrive pacing attempts to capture the entire ventricle and thus create a block in the reentrant circuit. This technique is less likely to succeed if the tachycardia is greater than 250 beats/min or the patient is in shock.[190] Overdrive pacing can result in acceleration of the tachycardia (Fig 22C-19) or the induction of ventricular fibrillation.[191,192]

Ventricular fibrillation may develop during an electrophysiologic study in the following situations: (1) when an attempt is made to induce a previously observed ventricular tachycardia; (2) when an electrophysiologic study is performed in patients who have been resuscitated from near sudden cardiac death or have had syncope; and (3) when an attempt is made to terminate ventricular tachycardia. If such a rhythm disturbance occurs, the patient is immediately treated with electrical cardioversion. The chance of producing cardiac or neurologic damage in such a situation is minimal.[171]

The repetitive ventricular response

There has been considerable controversy over the significance of the repetitive ventricular response. This phenomenon is defined as two to four ventricular depolarizations in response to a single induced ventricular extrastimulus. The repetitive ventricular response was initially believed to be predictive of patients who would experience ventricular tachycardia after recovery from a myocardial infarction.[132] However, subsequent studies have demonstrated that a repetitive ventricular response to a single ventricular extrastimulus introduced during normal sinus rhythm and atrial pacing is rare (although more commonly observed after a ventricular drive) and that it is not an accurate index of the susceptibility of the patient to serious ventricular arrhythmias and therefore not an adequate therapeutic end point.[193,194] A review of 100 patients with known ventricular tachycardia demonstrated that the repetitive ventricular response had a sensitivity of 92% and a specificity of 57%.[175] This response should not be used to predict which patients are susceptible to the development of ventricular tachycardia, and it is not an adequate model for the evaluation of antiarrhythmic therapy. It usually is possible in the electrophysiology laboratory to differentiate induced ventricular depolarizations due to a physiologic mechanism (pacer site reentry and bundle-branch reentry) from those due to a pathologic mechanism (reentry in or near scar tissue).

Sensitivity and specificity of the electrophysiologic study in patients with ventricular tachycardia

A review of 529 patients undergoing clinical electrophysiologic study determined the sensitivity and specificity of the procedure in patients with ventricular tachycardia.[174] Of 57 patients with sustained ventricular tachycardia before the electrophysiologic study, 54 patients had induction of sustained tachycardia in the electrophysiology laboratory. Of 29 patients with nonsustained ventricular tachycardia before the electrophysiologic study, 18 had ventricular tachycardia induced in the laboratory. Of 443 patients with no ventricular tachycardia before the study, only 3 (fewer than 1%) had ventricular tachycardia induced at the time of the electrophysiologic study. Of 454 patients who did not have ventricular tachycardia induced in the electrophysiology laboratory, only 14 (3%) had clinical ventricular tachycardia. Thus, in this group of patients the incidence of false-positive electrophysiologic studies was lower than 1% and that of false-negative studies was about 3%.

A review of 100 patients with known ventricular tachycardia before electrophysiologic testing determined that the electrophysiologic study was 65% sensitive and 98% specific with regard to induction of ventricular tachycardia in the laboratory.[175] This study concluded that ventricular tachycardia induced at the time of electrophysiologic evaluation is an excellent guide to the management of patients with ventricular tachycardia.

Electrophysiologic evaluation of patients with ventricular tachycardia in the absence of coronary artery disease

As confidence in the technique of intracardiac recording and programmed stimulation has increased, patients are being studied who present with sustained ventricular tachycardia without a history of coronary artery disease. Ventricular tachycardia in these patients is generally more difficult to induce in the laboratory. In an evaluation of 83 patients with ventricular tachycardia not due to coronary artery disease, programmed electrical stimulation in the electrophysiology laboratory induced ventricular tachycardia less often in patients whose tachycardia was not associated with coronary artery disease.[141] Also, there was less success in inducing tachycardia in the laboratory in patients with a history of nonsustained ventricular tachycardia than in those with a history of sustained ventricular tachycardia.

USE OF ELECTROPHYSIOLOGIC STUDY IN EVALUATING THE TREATMENT OF VENTRICULAR TACHYCARDIA

Pharmacologic therapy

Patients who have recurrent sustained ventricular tachycardia or have been resuscitated from cardiac arrest generally have a disturbance in rhythm that occurs sporadically, and empiric selection of therapy may not be effective in preventing recurrences.[195] A serious ventricular arrhythmia that occurs sporadically may not be observed during the initial phase when the patient starts taking a particular antiarrhythmia agent. If the antiarrhythmia drug chosen is not effective, a life-threatening arrhythmia may recur when the patient is not in a hospital setting where proper cardiac resuscitation is possible. There is also a risk that the antiarrhythmia agent chosen by empiric therapy will actually result in a faster ventricular arrhythmia and one that occurs more frequently[196] (Fig 22C-20). Therefore, electrophysiologic testing should be performed in patients who have serious, life-threatening ventricular arrhythmias because this form of evaluation provides an objective basis for the rational choice of therapy with an antiarrhythmia drug while the patient is in the hospital.[7,172,197,198] The patient is then dismissed on a therapeutic regimen that has been demonstrated to be effective in this setting. Initiation of the tachycardia is reproducible over a period of several days or months, and this provides an objective measure by which drugs can be evaluated.[176]

A typical protocol for assessment of the efficacy of various antiarrhythmia agents in preventing the induction of ventricular tachycardia or ventricular fibrillation is as follows. The patient undergoes a control study to determine whether the ventricular arrhythmia is inducible by programmed stimulation.

The patient is brought back on successive days until an effective antiarrhythmia agent is found. After an oral antiarrhythmia drug regimen has been started and adequate blood levels have been achieved, the patient returns to the electrophysiology laboratory to make certain that a tachycardia cannot be induced.

The response to intravenously administered procainamide in association with left ventricular ejection fraction has been reported in 106 patients to be predictive of identifying an effective drug regimen by serial drug testing[199] (Fig 22C-21). These results are provocative but require confirmation.

The use of programmed stimulation to evaluate to effect of antiarrhythmia drugs on known ventricular arrhythmias is based on two assumptions that have proved to be valid: (1) that the tachycardia produced in the electrophysiology laboratory is the same as the tachycardia occurring clinically[172,174,175] and (2) that the response to antiarrhythmia drugs in the setting of the

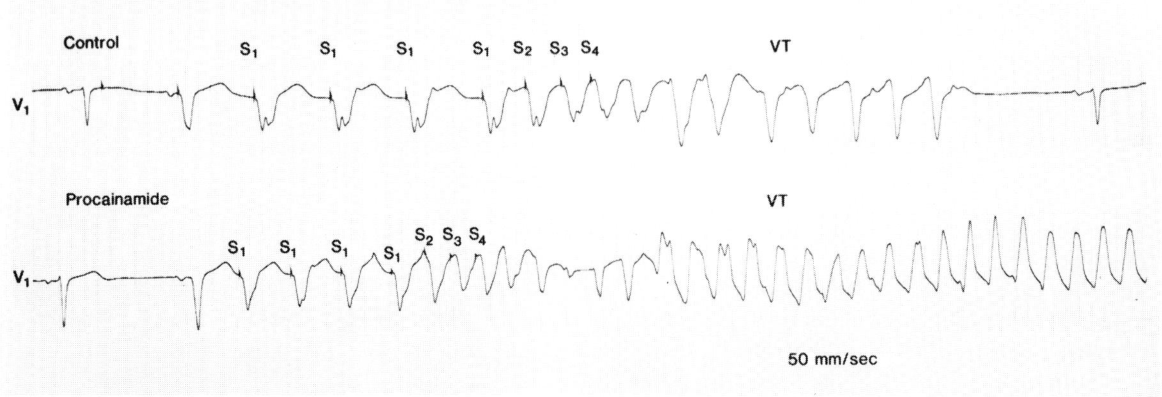

Fig 22C-20 Nonsustained ventricular tachycardia *(VT)* is induced during the control state with triple critically timed extrastimuli *($S_2S_3S_4$)* introduced during ventricular pacing *(S_1)*. After administration of procainamide, sustained ventricular tachycardia is induced.

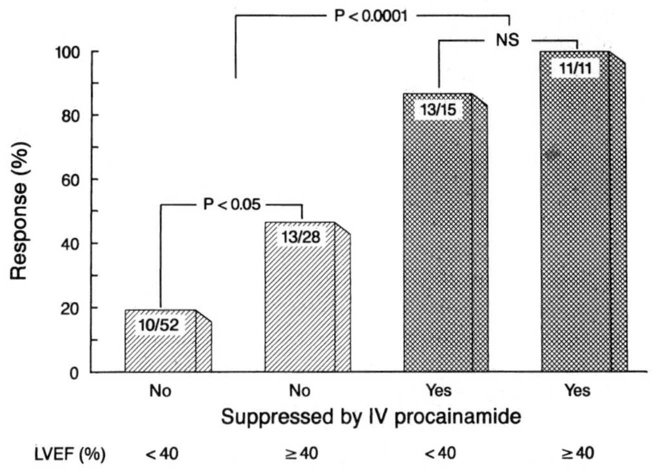

Fig 22C-21 Response to intravenously administered procainamide in association with left ventricular ejection fraction *(LVEF)* is predictive of identifying an effective drug regimen from serial drug testing. These results are provocative but require confirmation. Preliminary results from our institution suggest that left ventricular ejection fraction and clinical functional class are the two strongest predictors for drug response during serial drug testing. Response to intravenous *(IV)* administration of procainamide is not an independent predictor. *NS,* not significant. (From Kuchar DL, Rottman J, Berger E, et al: Prediction of successful suppression of sustained ventricular tachyarrhythmias by serial drug testing from data derived at the initial electrophysiologic study. *J Am Coll Cardiol* 12:982-988, 1988. By permission of American College of Cardiology.)

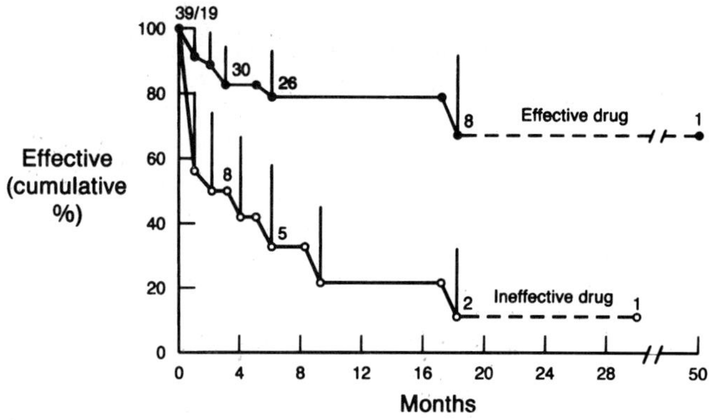

Fig 22C-22 The value of electrophysiologic testing and pharmacologic therapy guided by electrophysiologic testing in patients with sustained ventricular tachycardia. (From Mason JW, Winkle RA: Accuracy of the ventricular tachycardia-induction study for predicting long-term efficacy and inefficacy of antiarrhythmic drugs. *N Engl J Med* 303:1073-1077, 1980. By permission of the journal.)

electrophysiology laboratory can predict the clinical response.[7,145-147,173]

The antiarrhythmia drugs evaluated in the setting of electrophysiologic testing include procainamide, quinidine, disopyramide, tocainide, mexiletine, aprindine, encainide, flecainide, propafenone, amiodarone, and β-adrenoreceptor blockers. It is not possible to predict before electrophysiologic testing which drugs will be effective. The incidence of worsening the arrhythmia (easier to induce, a more rapid rate, or going from nonsustained to sustained tachycardia) is 5% to 25%, depending on the antiarrhythmia agent.[196]

If no antiarrhythmia drug or combination of drugs can be found that prevents the induction of ventricular tachycardia during electrophysiologic testing, the patient has a high probability of having a recurrence of the tachycardia after dismissal from the hospital[173] (Fig 22C-22). Thus, if a patient continues to have inducible ventricular tachycardia despite therapy with any of the available antiarrhythmia drugs, the likelihood of recurrence of the tachycardia is high. Even though electrophysiologic testing does not help in identifying a drug that prevents induction of tachycardia in such patients, the testing does allow identification of drugs that will make the arrhythmia more difficult to induce or reduces the tachycardia from sustained to nonsustained ventricular tachycardia, indicating a more favorable prognosis.[200] It is not unusual in the electrophysiology laboratory to administer antiarrhythmic drugs to patients and find their tachycardia becoming easier to induce, more sustained, more rapid, and less hemodynamically stable.

A pharmacologic regimen that prevents induction of tachycardia can be identified in 40% of patients who are resuscitated from cardiac arrest due to ventricular tachycardia or fibrillation.[7,201,202] These patients have a low incidence of recurrence of tachycardia when they are maintained on the long-term drug regimen that was selected during the electrophysiologic evaluation.

In assessing response to drug therapy in patients with sustained ventricular tachycardia or fibrillation, electrophysiologic testing has been demonstrated to be superior to noninvasive testing with use of Holter monitoring and treadmill exercise testing.[141,200]

Amiodarone (chapter 29C) is being used with increasing frequency in the treatment of patients with ventricular tachycardia.[203] The drug has given good results in this difficult group of patients, although up to 40% of patients with recurrent sustained ventricular tachycardia may experience a recurrence of their arrhythmia while taking amiodarone. In the majority of these patients, the tachycardia is slower and better tolerated. The usefulness of electrophysiologic testing in predicting the long-term antiarrhythmia efficacy of amiodarone is controversial—some investigators demonstrated that failure to induce ventricular tachycardia while the patient is taking amiodarone does predict long-term suppression of arrhythmia[204,205] and others found no such correlation.[206,207] More recent publications have indicated that electrophysiologic testing is helpful in predicting the long-term antiarrhythmia efficacy of amiodarone.

Pacemaker therapy for the control of ventricular tachycardia

Occasionally, patients are refractory to antiarrhythmia drugs and are not suitable candidates for surgical treatment of their ventricular tachycardia. Such patients were previously considered for antitachycardia pacing systems.[191,208-211] However, these systems did not have the capability of defibrillation, so that their use was significantly limited. The major complication with this form of therapy is acceleration of the ventricular arrhythmia.[209,212] On occasion, a critically timed premature beat occurring during an episode of ventricular tachycardia can either accelerate the tachycardia or cause degeneration of the tachycardia into ventricular flutter or fibrillation (see section below on the automatic implantable cardioverter-defibrillator).

Transvenous catheter ablation for treatment of patients with ventricular tachycardia

Transvenous catheter ablation has been used for the treatment of ventricular tachycardia refractory to medical therapy and unsuitable for antitachycardia pacing or surgical treatment.[213-223] The technique of ablation of ventricular tachycardia requires placement of an electrode catheter in the right or left ventricle close to the origin of the tachycardia. The sequence of ventricular endocardial activation is recorded during tachycardia to identify the point of earliest activation. This point is then assumed to be the site of the reentrant circuit, and ablation of this area is performed by using the electrode catheter. Electrical energy is transmitted through the electrode catheter to the electrode in contact with the endocardium in the area of the tachycardia focus. The electrical energy then returns to the cardioversion unit by way of a catheter on the other side of the interventricular septum or a back paddle.

Patients who undergo this technique have experienced frequent episodes of ventricular tachycardia that have been unresponsive to medical management. The tachycardia needs to be relatively hemodynamically stable to allow identification of the tachycardia focus. Most patients have ischemic heart disease and reduced ventricular function. In general, approximately one-third of patients have cure of their tachycardia, with no further recurrence and no requirement for medications. In another third of patients, the tachycardia circuit is modified such that antiarrhythmic drugs, although still required, are now effective. The technique is unsuccessful in the final third of patients, who require another form of therapy, which is usually endocardial resection or implantation of the automatic internal cardioverter-defibrillator.

Recently, there has been growing interest in using radiofrequency current as an alternative energy source for catheter ablation in patients with refractory ventricular tachycardia.[224-226] The limitations of direct current ablation and the potential advantages of radiofrequency current have been described and demonstrated in animal studies.[227,228] These studies show that radiofrequency current ablation causes insignificant left ventricular dysfunction and fewer ventricular arrhythmias. Histologically, radiofrequency current ablation induces more discrete and homogeneous necrosis with a smaller lesion size than that induced by direct current ablation. Although radiofrequency current ablation for ventricular tachycardia holds promise, only small subgroups of patients in whom radiofrequency current ablation may be particularly effective have been studied.[229,230] A broad application of radiofrequency current ablation for ventricular tachycardia awaits further evaluation.

Catheter ablation for ventricular tachycardia remains an investigational procedure and should be performed only by physicians who are experienced in electrophysiologic testing and intercardiac ablation procedures. The long-term sequelae of the ablation technique are unknown, and the duration of follow-up has been insufficient to ascertain whether any long-term complications ensue, such as arrhythmia arising from the area of scar induced by the ablation catheter.

Automatic implantable cardioverter-defibrillator

The automatic implantable cardioverter-defibrillator (AICD)[213,231-247] senses the onset of rapid ventricular tachycardia or ventricular fibrillation by analyzing the change in the baseline characteristics of the ECG or the rate of the arrhythmia (or both). When the arrhythmia criteria have been satisfied, the AICD can deliver a fixed high-energy shock at approximately 30 J (first-generation AICD), programmable low-energy cardioversion (second-generation AICD), or antitachycardia pacing (third-generation AICD) (Fig 22C-23). This device has reduced the 2-year mortality attributable to arrhythmia to 2%-5%.[231-233,241,248]

Currently, there are limitations to the use of the AICD. Although the perfect device is not yet available, several AICDs are under clinical investigation. Many of the desirable features of the "ideal device" related to sensing, pacing, cardioversion-defibrillation, and physical features have been discussed in detail in recent reviews.[249-251] Reliance on rate as the only detection criterion for ventricular tachycardia has high sensitivity but low specificity. Other rhythms, either physiologic (sinus tachycardia, for example) or pathologic (atrial fibrillation) can trigger device discharge, which leads to inappropriate therapy. Therefore, other criteria to improve the specificity of tachycardia recognition, such as stability of the R-R cycle length and the abruptness of the onset of tachycardia, have been incorporated into some devices, but with only mixed success.[252] One of the most important limitations of antitachycardia pacing for patients with ventricular tachycardia is the risk that the arrhythmia will accelerate to ventricular fibrillation. This event occurs in more than one-third of patients when pacing is used during electrophysiologic study to terminate ventricular tachycardia.[253] Availability of backup defibrillation in the same device eliminates sudden cardiac death from this change in rhythm but does not prevent syncope. A shock to the patient while awake is quite uncomfortable. Considerable physical constraints are also present in the currently approved AICDs. Thoracotomy is necessary for placement of the epicardial lead, and the pacemaker generator is large and cumbersome and must be implanted in the abdominal wall.

Pacemaker technology is evolving rapidly. New implant-

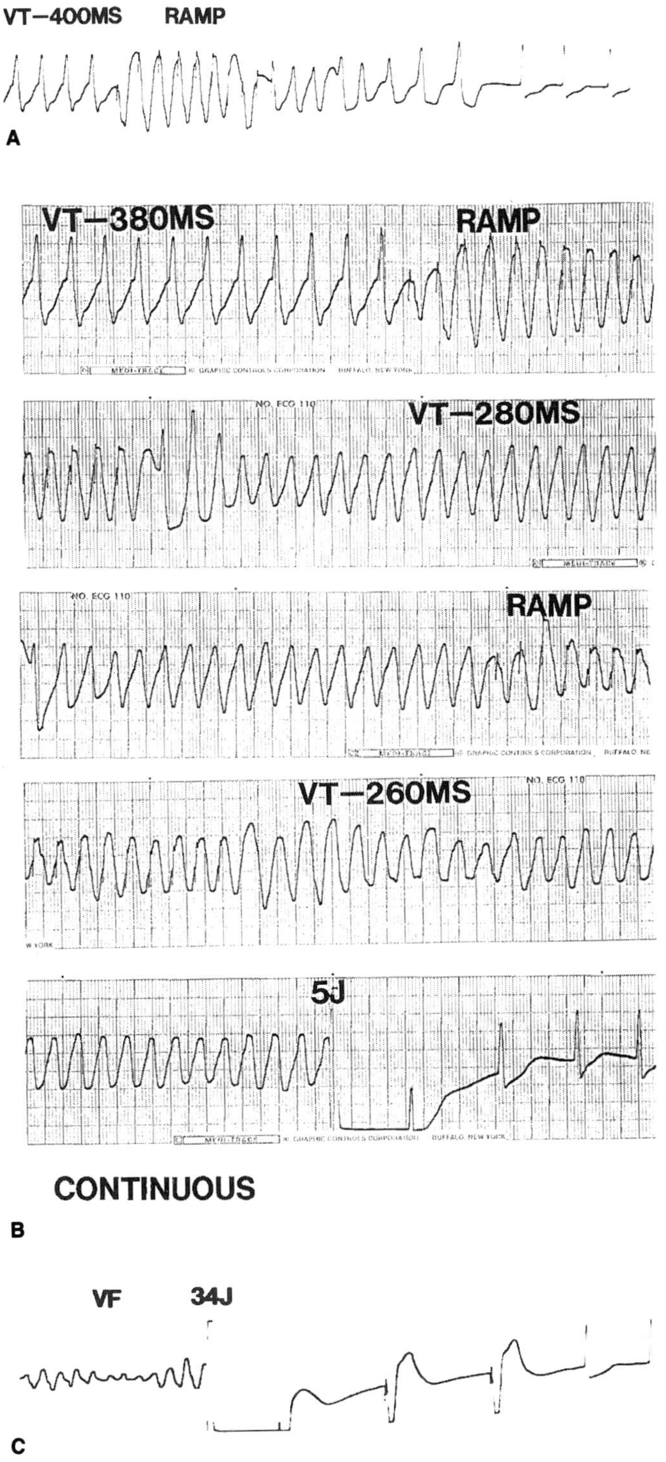

Fig 22C-23 Continuous recording from a patient with a third-generation implantable cardioverter and defibrillator. **A,** monomorphic ventricular tachycardia *(VT)* was terminated by decremental *(RAMP)* ventricular pacing. **B,** monomorphic ventricular tachycardia was accelerated by the second RAMP therapy. This rapid ventricular tachycardia was terminated by a low-energy shock of 5 J. **C,** ventricular fibrillation *(VF)* was terminated by a 34-J shock. Immediately after the termination of ventricular fibrillation, pacemaker activity was evident while the patient was experiencing bradycardia.

able devices are being investigated that will terminate ventricular tachycardia by using either pacing techniques or low-energy shock cardioversion, which is better tolerated by the patient. Reduction in defibrillator shocks with an implantable device combining antitachycardia pacing and shock therapy has been reported.[254] In instances in which the tachycardia cannot be terminated, the tachycardia is accelerated, or the initial tachycardia is ventricular fibrillation, defibrillation can be accomplished with high energy. In the newer devices, bradycardia pacing will also be available. Nonthoracotomy systems with a catheter alone or with a subcutaneous patch are under investigation.[255-259] Combinations of electrodes in the superior vena cava, coronary sinus, and right ventricular apex are being tested together with a chest wall electrode. In general, defibrillation thresholds of less than 18 J can be achieved in about 75% of patients with nonthoracotomy lead placement and sequential or simultaneous shock configurations. The capability to store ventricular electrograms before antitachycardia and shock therapy may also provide invaluable information in the diagnosis of arrhythmias precipitating electrical device shock therapy.[260] Major advances have been, and continue to be, made in antitachycardia devices. Newer devices with expanded capabilities, biphasic waveforms, and nonthoracotomy implantable features will provide better therapeutic options to patients with life-threatening ventricular arrhythmias.

Surgical treatment of patients with ventricular tachycardia

The past decade has seen improvement in various surgical techniques for use in approaching the problem of medically resistant ventricular tachycardia.[261,262] These techniques, discussed in chapter 26, include endocardial resection,[145,146] encircling endocardial ventriculotomy,[263] sympathectomy,[264,265] and cryoablation.[266,267] In such patients a detailed study in the electrophysiology laboratory is performed before the surgical procedure. The preoperative study establishes the nature of the tachycardia being considered for surgical treatment and the location of the reentrant circuit within either the right or the left ventricle.[145,146] Epicardial mapping at the time of surgery has limitations inasmuch as the site of origin of ventricular tachycardia on the endocardial surface may be quite distant from the site of epicardial breakthrough.[268] Consequently, endocardial mapping is performed at the time of surgery to localize the origin of the tachycardia.

When preoperative endocardial mapping of patients with ventricular tachycardia is performed in the electrophysiology laboratory, the technique is similar to that used in the routine electrophysiologic study. Most patients undergo coronary and left ventricular angiography before electrophysiologic study, to determine whether a ventricular aneurysm or an akinetic segment of the ventricle is present. Such abnormalities are known to be the sites of reentry circuits in patients with ventricular tachycardia.[269-273] The angiogram allows the electrophysiologist to determine whether structural abnormalities exist and to suggest the area of the ventricle that should be explored by the mapping catheter. During the electrophysiologic study, catheters are placed in the standard locations, including the right atrium, region of the His bundle, and right ventricular apex. A mapping catheter is then positioned in several locations of the right and left ventricles during tachycardia. The site as recorded by the exploring electrode catheter is compared with the reference catheter located in the right ventricular apex. The earliest site of activation generally precedes the onset of the QRS complex and identifies the origin of the recurrent circuit.[145,146]

Epicardial mapping at the time of surgery has been used to localize the site of origin of ventricular tachycardia with the use of techniques similar to those employed for surgical ablation of AV bypass tracts (see chapter 26B). During epicardial mapping,[274-277] electrograms from the epicardial surface are recorded by means of a hand-held probe or multielectrode computer-assisted mapping system. The timing of these electrograms is compared with timing of the surface electrograms and with reference electrograms obtained from fixed reference electrodes attached to the ventricle. Stimulating electrodes are also attached to the ventricle and the atrium in order to pace the patient into tachycardia. It has been demonstrated that ventricular tachycardia originates in the myocardium bordering aneurysms in patients with coronary artery disease.[269-272] The local activation times during intraoperative epicardial mapping have been demonstrated to be reproducible within the same patient.[278] The major limitation of epicardial mapping is that the epicardial breakthrough site may be several centimeters away from the site of origin of the tachycardia, which is located on the endocardial surface.[268,279,280] Consequently, endocardial mapping of the border of the aneurysm at the time of surgery is most productive, and such mapping generally agrees with the findings of the preoperative electrophysiologic study.

Aneurysmectomy or coronary artery bypass surgery that does not utilize electrophysiologic mapping for treatment of recurrent ventricular tachycardia has met with variable success.[281,282] Recurrent ventricular fibrillation due to reversible ischemia or associated with a recent myocardial infarction may respond favorably to coronary artery bypass grafting with associated infarctectomy.[261,283,284] However, recurrent sustained ventricular tachycardia is not optimally treated with coronary artery bypass grafting and myocardial resection and is better treated with electrophysiologically guided surgical techniques.[261] The introduction of electrophysiologic mapping of the site of origin of the tachycardia during surgery has improved the success rate in eliminating tachycardia.[145-147,269,285-292] In several published series, operative mortality rates varied between 5% and 17% (Table 22C-7). Operative risk has been shown to be primarily related to the residual left ventricular function after aneurysm resection.[294] From the University of Pennsylvania, risk analysis performed on 289 patients who had undergone endocardial resection showed that four risk factors were associated with early surgical mortality: (1) ejection fraction below 20%, (2) reoperation, (3) emergency operation, and (4) anterior and inferior aneurysms.[295] Postoperative reinducibility rates vary considerably, from 4% to 33% (see Table 22C-7). During long-term follow-up, sudden death is uncommon in both inducible and noninducible patient groups. Five-year actuarial survival has been approximately 60%, with the most common cause of death being heart failure.[287,288] Cryosurgery[296] and laser[297,298] ablation of the endocardial focus and transcoronary chemical ablation of the local myocardium have been reported to successfully treat patients with refractory ventricular tachycardia, although the series have been small.

General approach to the care of patients with spontaneous ventricular tachycardia

Patients with ventricular tachycardia should be evaluated to make certain that all reversible factors have been eliminated, such as electrolyte imbalance, ischemia, hypoxia, and drug effects, including those of antiarrhythmic drugs. When ventricular tachycardia is associated with hemodynamic compromise, it is imperative that a stable cardiac rhythm be restored. If the patient has impaired cerebral perfusion, hypotension, or coronary ischemia, the rhythm should be terminated by electrical cardioversion. Electrical cardioversion will abolish ventricular tachycardia and allow resumption of sinus rhythm in approximately 90% of patients. If time allows, the patient should be anesthetized with a short-acting barbiturate or with diazepam. In most patients the arrhythmia will convert with 50 J of energy; however, up to 200 J may be required for the conversion of ventricular tachycardia.

In patients who are hemodynamically stable and for whom urgent conversion to sinus rhythm is not required, pharmacologic agents can be tried. The drug usually tried first is lidocaine, and it may be administered to adults as a 75-mg intravenous (IV) bolus over 1 minute. If this is not effective, a 50-mg bolus can be given at 5 minutes, 10 minutes, and 15 minutes after the initial bolus. Once the arrhythmia has been controlled by lidocaine, a continuous IV infusion should be initiated at 1 to 5 mg/min, with evaluation for signs of toxicity and efficacy. Lidocaine is most useful for ventricular arrhythmias associated with myocardial ischemia. When lidocaine is not effective in terminating the ventricular tachycardia, procainamide is generally the second drug of choice and may be given IV in a dosage of 10 to 15 mg/kg by infusion at a rate of 50 mg/min. The patient has to be monitored for side effects, including QRS widening of more than 50% or significant hypotension. If the administration of procainamide is effective, it should be followed by institution of an IV infusion at 1 to 4 mg/min. In the unusual case in which lidocaine and procainamide are not effective, bretylium can be tried. Occasionally, patients will be able to terminate their ventricular tachycardia by performing the Valsalva maneuver.[150,299]

Once the acute episode of ventricular tachycardia has been terminated and no reversible causes have been identified, including myocardial ischemia, the patient should be evaluated for an oral antiarrhythmia drug regimen that is effective in preventing a recurrence of the tachycardia. The patient with a clinical model (sustained or nonsustained ventricular tachycardia) that is readily recorded by monitor can be treated by means of the technique developed by Lown et al.[300] This technique

Table 22C-7 Surgery for ventricular tachycardia with ischemic heart disease

Study	No. of patients	Operative mortality, %	Postoperative inducibility, %	Long-term mortality, %	SCD, %	FU, mo
Kehoe et al.[291]	79	13	23			
Swerdlow et al.[290]	98	17	32			
Kron et al.[289]	50	8	13			
Ostermeyer et al.[287]	93	5	19			
Hargrove et al.[288]	289	15	33			
Landymore et al.[293]	26	12	4	19	0	43
Garan et al.[294]	36	17	33	0	0	25

FU, follow-up; SCD, sudden cardiac death.

requires frequent spontaneous ventricular arrhythmias, and physicians who use this technique to treat patients must be aware of the presence of spontaneous day-to-day variation of ventricular arrhythmias.[127,128,301] The majority of patients with sustained ventricular tachycardia will benefit from electrophysiologic testing. Electrophysiologic testing offers the patient advantages over ambulatory electrocardiographic monitoring by providing a higher degree of accuracy in predicting the long-term clinical response to antiarrhythmia drugs.[200,302-304]

The patient with recurrent ventricular tachycardia who does not respond to antiarrhythmia drug therapy should be evaluated for an antitachycardia pacing and low-energy cardioversion system with defibrillation back-up, as described earlier. When an antitachycardia cardioverter-defibrillator system is not feasible, the patient should be considered for surgical therapy. Such patients undergo a preoperative evaluation that includes coronary angiography with left ventriculography. They then have a detailed electrophysiologic study for mapping of the left and right ventricles and determination of the site of origin of the ventricular tachycardia. When a patient has a tachycardia that is suitable for surgical intervention, endocardial electrophysiologic mapping is performed in the operating room at the time of the surgical procedure.

There are some unanswered questions with regard to the use of electrophysiologic testing in patients with ventricular arrhythmias, as follows.

1. In what fraction of normal patients and patients with coronary artery disease who are totally symptom free with regard to a rhythm disturbance can ventricular tachycardia be induced, and what is the long-term prognosis for this group of patients if they go untreated?
2. What are the end points of programmed stimulation? Are they the prevention of sustained ventricular tachycardia or nonsustained ventricular tachycardia or the altering of the tachycardia cycle length or mode of induction?
3. Should the patient with complex PVCs with associated heart disease who has never had ventricular tachycardia or fibrillation clinically but in whom one of these two rhythms is induced at the time of electrophysiologic testing be treated with long-term antiarrhythmia therapy, and if so, for how long?

These questions have not been totally answered; however, as experience with electrophysiologic testing in the setting of ventricular arrhythmias increases, it should become clearer which group of patients will benefit most from this technique.

Ventricular arrhythmias associated with mitral valve prolapse

In general, mitral valve prolapse is considered a benign condition; however, there is a low but significant incidence of sudden cardiac death in these patients.[305-310] In most such patients the cause of sudden cardiac death appears to be a ventricular arrhythmia.[306,311] During 24-hour ambulatory monitoring, the patient with mitral valve prolapse is found to have a higher incidence of ventricular arrhythmias than patients without this disorder.[312,313] The ventricular arrhythmias in patients with mitral valve prolapse range from isolated PVCs to frequent multiform types, PVCs occurring in the vulnerable period, and ventricular tachycardia.[60,314-316] The overall incidence of sudden cardiac death is not known, although a review of several series of patients with mitral valve prolapse noted a 1.4% incidence of sudden death.[308] These groups were probably biased because of symptoms and obvious cardiac signs; however, the condition of mitral valve prolapse may indeed be a relatively important cause of sudden death in patients who are otherwise young and healthy.

Patients with mitral valve prolapse and suspected ventricular arrhythmias should be evaluated with 24-hour ambulatory monitoring. This technique may identify potentially life-threatening arrhythmias; however, because it is merely a sample in time, it may not include arrhythmias that are the cause of the patient's symptoms of presyncope or syncope. If necessary, 24-hour ambulatory monitoring can be continued until arrhythmias are recorded. If a patient's episode of palpitation lasts long enough to allow the use of a telephone transmitter, this technique can be very helpful in identifying the cause of a patient's symptoms.[317] Patients with documented ventricular arrhythmias or episodes of syncope can benefit from electrophysiologic testing. A review of 18 patients with mitral valve prolapse demonstrated that in 5 patients who had a clinical history of sustained ventricular tachycardia, sustained ventricular tachycardia could be induced in 3 and nonsustained ventricular tachycardia in 2 in an electrophysiology laboratory; in contrast, in 5 of 13 patients with a history of syncope and nonsustained ventricular tachycardia, sustained ventricular tachycardia could not be induced.[141] Several other electrophysiologic studies of patients with mitral valve prolapse in association with cardiac arrest,[201,318,319] sustained ventricular tachycardia,[141] and complex ventricular ectopies with or without symptoms[137,141,184,318,319] have been reported. Because of the small number of patients involved, the inducibility of sustained ventricular tachycardia and reproducibility of electrophysiologic testing in patients with mitral valve prolapse have not been substantiated. The role of electrophysiologic testing in patients with mitral valve prolapse without associated syncope, cardiac arrest, or documented sustained arrhythmias has not been well defined. Some patients may have serious arrhythmias when they undergo exercise stress testing.[320,321] This is an appropriate initial evaluation in the attempt to induce arrhythmias in patients who have symptoms suggesting tachycardia. A normal exercise stress test does not exclude the possibility of sudden death at a later date, and the significance of ventricular ectopy in the absence of exercise-inducible ventricular tachycardia is not known.

Patients with mitral valve prolapse have abnormalities of the ECG. Unfortunately, little is known about the incidence of Q-T prolongation in a population of patients with mitral valve prolapse who have had no symptoms suggesting tachycardia. Similarly, there are few data regarding the overall incidence of ST-segment and T-wave changes in patients with mitral valve prolapse and an otherwise normal cardiac evaluation. In general, such changes on the ECG in patients with mitral valve prolapse should raise the suspicion of significant ventricular arrhythmias, and the patient should be evaluated further with 24-hour ambulatory monitoring and exercise stress testing.

No single drug is uniquely effective in controlling ventricular arrhythmias associated with mitral valve prolapse.[308] The drug of first choice is a β-blocking agent,[322,323] but successful management has been reported with other drugs, including procainamide, quinidine, disopyramide, and phenytoin. Delayed afterdepolarization and triggered activity have been observed in anterior mitral valve leaflets resected from patients with mitral valve prolapse.[324] This observation suggests that a triggering mechanism may be responsible for the arrhythmias occurring in patients with mitral valve prolapse. Theoretically, calcium channel blockers could be effective in this group of patients; however, no studies have been reported to date. Arrhythmias associated with mitral valve prolapse are difficult to control with antiarrhythmic medications.[323,325,326]

Ventricular arrhythmias in patients with hypertrophic cardiomyopathy

Patients with hypertrophic cardiomyopathy are known to have an increased incidence of sudden cardiac death compared with other patients without this disorder. It is generally believed that ventricular tachycardia and ventricular fibrillation are the usual causes; however, the triggering event is not always clear. Factors such as myocardial ischemia due to impaired coronary reserve and aggravation of hemodynamic abnormalities by supraventricular tachycardia or sympathetic activation may play an important role preceding the ventricular arrhythmias.

The use of electrophysiologic testing in patients with hypertrophic cardiomyopathy has been evaluated in subgroups of patients who experienced syncope or sudden death.[327-332] Most of these studies revealed a high prevalence of inducible polymorphic ventricular tachycardia. Induced polymorphic ventricular tachycardia is usually thought of as an artifact of extrastimulus testing; however, much higher inducibility of polymorphic ventricular tachycardia in patients with hypertrophic cardiomyopathy suggests that an arrhythmogenic substrate may be present.

The largest series to date reported the results of electrophysiologic testing in 155 patients at high risk.[332] Indications for electrophysiologic studies were cardiac arrest (14%), syncope (36%), presyncope (24%), nonsustained ventricular tachycardia (16%), palpitations (7%), and a strong family history of sudden death (5%). Electrophysiologic abnormalities were present in 124 (80%) patients. The authors concluded that electrophysiologic testing usually identifies abnormalities in selected patients with hypertrophic cardiomyopathy.

Induced polymorphic ventricular tachycardia, a nonspecific response in other clinical situations, remains problematic. Does this finding provide a marker of primary electrical instability or is it merely a nonspecific artifact of an aggressive stimulation protocol? The prognostic significance of these findings will be uncertain until the clinical outcome has been determined and compared with that in a large number of low-risk patients. The clinical relevance of inducible, sustained polymorphic ventricular tachycardia also depends on the reproducibility of the findings and ultimately on a prospective evaluation. Programmed ventricular stimulation may provide the measurements that will improve the predictive accuracy and identify those patients with episodes of nonsustained ventricular tachycardia during ECG monitoring who are at greatest risk and warrant more vigorous treatment. A broader application of programmed ventricular stimulation in adults with hypertrophic cardiomyopathy, however, does not seem warranted.[333,334]

Well-controlled clinical studies are not yet available to determine the exact role of β-blockers and calcium channel blockers in preventing sudden death. These drugs can relieve hemodynamic symptoms, but they do not substantially alter occurrence of ventricular tachycardia.[335,336] The efficacy of these drugs in preventing sudden death has not yet been determined. It is difficult to determine clinical variables that identify a subgroup of patients with hypertrophic cardiomyopathy who are at increased risk of sudden death. However, variables that may be of value in alerting physicians to patients at increased risk of sudden death are increased hypertrophy,[337] symptoms of syncope,[338] late potentials on signal-averaged electrocardiography,[339-341] a familial predilection for sudden premature death in families with known hypertrophic cardiomyopathy,[342] and asymptomatic ventricular tachycardia on 24-hour ambulatory monitoring.[343]

Ventricular tachycardia after repair of congenital heart disease

Advances in surgical techniques and improved postoperative care have increased the survival of patients undergoing correction of congenital cardiac defects. These patients are now approaching adulthood, and the long-term sequelae of these repairs are assuming more importance to the adult cardiologist. There are few data regarding the incidence of ventricular tachycardia in this group of patients, but information is becoming available with regard to certain subsets of patients, including those with repair of tetralogy of Fallot. The long-term electrophysiologic consequences of repair of tetralogy of Fallot include AV conduction defects, intraventricular conduction defects, ventricular arrhythmias, and sudden death.[344] A report of four patients with spontaneous episodes of sustained ventricular tachycardia after repair of tetralogy of Fallot indicated that the tachycardia could be reproducibly initiated and terminated by programmed electrical stimulation in the electrophysiology laboratory.[345] This study suggests that one cause of sustained ventricular tachycardia after repair of tetralogy of Fallot is reentry at the site of the previous operation in the right ventricular outflow tract. The development of significant ventricular arrhythmias in patients who have had total correction of tetralogy of Fallot is uncommon,[344] and it remains unclear why ventricular tachycardia will develop in certain patients. Patients with repair of tetralogy of Fallot who present with frequent and severe ventricular arrhythmias or have documented recurrent ventricular tachycardia should undergo electrophysiologic testing to characterize the rhythm disturbance and determine the most appropriate therapeutic approach. Ventricular arrhythmias also have been reported after surgical closure of isolated ventricular septal defect, and their prevalence is not statistically different from that in postoperative tetralogy of Fallot.[346] A high incidence of sudden cardiac death after surgical repair of more complex congenital heart disease, such as double-outlet right ventricle, has also been reported recently.[347]

Ventricular arrhythmias after aortic valve replacement

Sudden death is a complication of aortic valve disease even after successful aortic valve replacement has been performed, with improvement in the hemodynamic burden imposed by the aortic regurgitation and aortic stenosis.[348-350] Sudden death accounts for 15% to 20% of the late deaths in patients after aortic valve replacement and is most likely a consequence of ventricular arrhythmias.[348-354] A review of 45 patients who had aortic valve replacement an average of 3.3 years before they were evaluated with 48 hours of continuous ambulatory monitoring detected ventricular arrhythmias in 43 patients—multiform PVCs in 89%, bigeminy in 60%, couplets in 60%, and ventricular tachycardia in 36%.[355]

This study demonstrates that significant ventricular arrhythmias, including ventricular tachycardia, are commonly observed late after aortic valve replacement. This group of patients had not experienced significant symptoms suggesting prolonged episodes of tachycardia, and therefore the relationship of their ventricular arrhythmias to the occurrence of sudden death is not clear. The study suggests that the majority of patients who have had aortic valve replacement experience significant ventricular arrhythmias, and it implies a relationship between these ventricular arrhythmias and the occurrence of sudden cardiac death. However, it has not been demonstrated that the suppression of significant ventricular arrhythmias in patients who have had aortic valve replacement will decrease the incidence of sudden death. Patients with aortic valve replacement who have symptoms of presyncope or syncope suggesting prolonged episodes of tachycardia should be evaluated by 24-hour ambulatory monitoring or exercise stress testing and should be considered for electrophysiologic investigation.

Aggravation of ventricular arrhythmias by antiarrhythmia drugs

As we have seen, the use of ambulatory monitoring and exercise stress testing has enabled the physician to identify patients with significant ventricular arrhythmias who are at risk for sudden death. Once such a patient has been identified, treatment is instituted in an attempt to suppress the ventricular arrhythmia by the use of antiarrhythmia drugs. Yet often the drug therapy fails to control the arrhythmia even after "therapeutic" blood levels have been achieved.[356-360] Each antiarrhythmia drug has the potential of making the ventricular rhythm disturbance worse in a given patient[1,2,196] (see Fig 22C-20). This constitutes a significant threat to the patient being treated for ventricular arrhythmias and undoubtedly accounts for iatrogenic fatalities that could have been prevented had the physician been aware of this adverse reaction. Quinidine was the first drug to be associated with a paradoxic increase in ventricular arrhythmias.[361-363] In therapeutic doses, quinidine may induce ventricular tachycardia and ventricular fibrillation. It is now well appreciated that other antiarrhythmia drugs worsen ventricular arrhythmias[2,364,365] (Fig 22C-24).

In a retrospective analysis of antiarrhythmia drug action in 155 patients, 53 patients had a worsening of their ventricular arrhythmias.[196] This group of patients received a total of 722 antiarrhythmia drug trials, and 80 (11.1%) of the trials were associated with a significant worsening of ventricular arrhythmias. The evaluation was designed to eliminate the possibility that spontaneous variation in ventricular arrhythmia might be falsely interpreted as a worsening of an arrhythmia because of the antiarrhythmia drug itself. The design was such that an aggravation of arrhythmias was defined as the occurrence of a fourfold increase in frequency of ventricular prema-

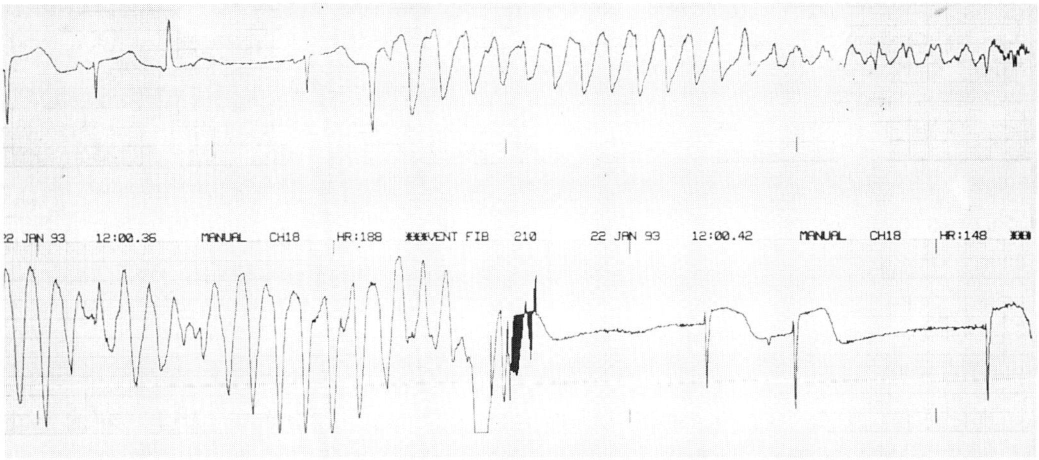

Fig 22C-24 Spontaneous polymorphic ventricular tachycardia occurring after treatment of atrial fibrillation with sotalol.[365]

ture complexes, a tenfold increase in repetitive forms, or the first emergence of sustained ventricular tachycardia coincident with the time course of action of the particular drug being studied. The aggravation of arrhythmias was noted with quinidine, procainamide, disopyramide, propranolol, metoprolol, aprindine, mexiletine, tocainide, and pindolol. The frequency of complications for each drug ranged from 5.9% to 15.8%; all plasma drug concentrations were in the therapeutic range. This study evaluated patients by means of continuous ECG monitoring.

Proarrhythmia and increased mortality have been demonstrated to occur with flecainide and encainide used to treat patients with complex ventricular ectopy after myocardial infarction,[1,6] and young patients with supraventricular and ventricular arrhythmias,[6] with class I antiarrhythmic agents in patients with complex ventricular ectopy after myocardial infarction,[4,114,366,367] with lidocaine during the first 24 to 48 hours after myocardial infarction,[368] and with quinidine for the treatment of paroxysmal atrial fibrillation.[3,369]

Similar observations have been made in the setting of the electrophysiology laboratory,[172,178,183,370] in which patients with nonsustained ventricular tachycardia induced at the time of electrophysiologic testing may acquire sustained ventricular tachycardia, often at an increased rate, after the tachycardia is reinduced while the patient is receiving an antiarrhythmia drug (see Fig 22C-20). It is critically important for the physician who is treating patients with significant ventricular arrhythmias to realize the potential that each antiarrhythmia drug has for worsening the ventricular arrhythmia. Thus, the physician must assess not only whether an antiarrhythmia drug is effective and has not resulted in toxicity but also whether the drug may have resulted in a paradoxic increase in the frequency of the patient's ventricular arrhythmias.

Arrhythmogenic right ventricular dysplasia

In 1952, Uhl[371] described a group of patients with right ventricular dysplasia in whom the right ventricle was paper thin, with apposition of the endocardium to the epicardium. Since this initial description, patients have been identified who have varying degrees of right ventricular dysplasia with right ventricular musculature that is partially or totally absent and has been replaced by fibrous and fatty tissue (Fig 22C-25). This abnormality primarily involves the right ventricle, and if the dysplasia is extensive, cardiomegaly will be detected on chest roentgenography, and congestive heart failure will occur in early childhood. Studies suggest that the left ventricle may be abnormal in patients with right ventricular dysplasia.[372] Patients may survive to adulthood and have asymptomatic cardiomegaly. The dysplasia may be limited to certain portions of the right ventricle and result in only minimal cardiac dysfunction. Such patients may present with ventricular tachycardia of right ventricular origin.[373-377]

A review of 22 patients with right ventricular dysplasia and recurrent ventricular tachycardia identified the following characteristics of this group of patients: (1) the male-to-female ratio was 2.7:1, with a mean age at the time of hospitalization of 39 years; (2) all the patients except one had ventricular tachycardia of left bundle-branch block configuration; (3) all patients had inverted T waves in the right precordial leads; (4) the heart generally showed cardiomegaly with normal pulmonary vasculature; and (5) right ventricular angiography demonstrated right ventricular enlargement in all but two patients, and both of these patients had either abnormalities of the right ventricle by M-mode echocardiography or systolic bulging of the right ventricular infundibulum by angiography.[373] Of the 22 patients, 10 were treated medically and 12 surgically. The medical treatment included amiodarone, aprindine, quinidine, procainamide, disopyramide, and propranolol. The surgical treatment consisted of one or more ventricular incisions in the right ventricle designed to disrupt the reentrant circuit. (This surgical approach has been used with limited success in patients with arrhythmogenic right ventricular dysplasia. Transvenous catheter ablation of the right ventricular focus has also been reported in a small number of patients.[215]) The most frequent areas of dysplasia and origin of ventricular

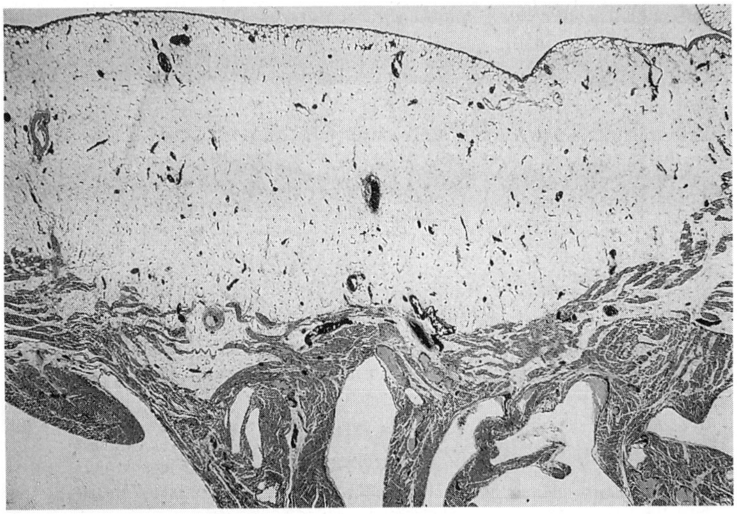

Fig 22C-25 Transmural section of right ventricular free wall from a patient with arrhythmogenic right ventricular dysplasia. At least 75% of the myocardium was replaced by adipose tissue. (Hematoxylin and eosin; original magnification, ×36.)

tachycardia were the anterior infundibulum, the right ventricular apex, and the inferior, or diaphragmatic, aspect of the right ventricle.

The clinical course of patients with arrhythmogenic right ventricular dysplasia treated either medically or surgically has not been well defined. Lemery et al.[378] reported the clinical course and long-term follow-up of 12 patients with arrhythmogenic right ventricular dysplasia and ventricular tachycardia. One patient underwent right ventricular disconnection and died of low cardiac output failure 1 week after the operation. The remaining 11 patients, all treated medically, were alive at a mean follow-up time of 7.9 years after the onset of symptoms. Of the 11 patients, 8 had recurrence of symptomatic and documented sustained monomorphic ventricular tachycardia. These results suggest that despite recurrence of ventricular tachycardia, patients with arrhythmogenic right ventricular dysplasia have a favorable outcome when treated medically. The diagnosis should be considered in patients who have ventricular tachycardia of unknown cause, especially if the tachycardia has a left bundle-branch block morphology on the surface ECG. A familial occurrence of arrhythmogenic right ventricular dysplasia has been reported.[379]

Ventricular arrhythmias associated with liquid protein diets

The protein-supplemented fast is recognized as an effective means of weight reduction; however, patients on the liquid protein diet have an increased incidence of sudden death.[380-382] Among 60 patients who died unexpectedly while on the diet, 12-lead ECGs were available in 11.[380] All 11 had ventricular tachycardia, and most had prolongation of the Q-T interval and decreased QRS voltage. At autopsy, the myocardium was atrophied in a manner similar to that observed with total starvation and cachexia. In a study designed to evaluate the liquid protein diet, the diet was administered to six patients, and their heart rhythm was monitored before and after the diet was initiated.[383] No abnormalities were found on 12-lead ECGs recorded before or after the diet was started. In three of the patients, no rhythm abnormality was detected by 24-hour monitoring during the control period or after institution of the diet; however, the remaining three patients had serious arrhythmias during the study period. These arrhythmias included an increased frequency of PVCs, sustained ventricular bigeminy, paired PVCs, and spontaneous ventricular tachycardia. Although other investigators[380] have reported low-voltage QRS complex and Q-T prolongation, this group of patients did not experience any abnormalities recorded on the 12-lead ECG.

Deficiencies of protein, electrolytes, trace elements, and micronutrients (such as essential fatty acids) may have a role in the development of significant ventricular arrhythmias; however, the exact cause remains unclear. This type of diet is not recommended. Patients who are on such diets should have 24-hour ambulatory monitoring and be warned of the increased risk of ventricular arrhythmias and sudden death. Routine chemical determination and metabolic balance studies have failed to identify patients who are at risk for the development of cardiac complications; thus, any sense of security based only on monitoring serum electrolytes would be a false one.

Torsade de pointes

Dessertenne[384] described a new ventricular arrhythmia in 1966 which he termed "torsade de pointes" ("twisting of points")[385-387] (Fig 22C-26). This arrhythmia may be misclassified as ventricular tachycardia or ventricular fibrillation; however, it is a distinct disturbance in rhythm. Torsade de pointes should be distinguished from ventricular fibrillation because of its unusual response to conventional treatment; antiarrhythmia drugs that prolong the Q-T interval may aggravate the frequency and duration of episodes of torsade de pointes. Such drugs include quinidine,[388,389] procainamide,[390] and disopyramide.[3,391]

The morphology of torsade de pointes is distinct, with cycles of alternating electrical polarity such that the peaks of the QRS complexes appear to twist around an isoelectric line. The alternating cycles may be seen to move in and out of episodes of rapid tachycardia with

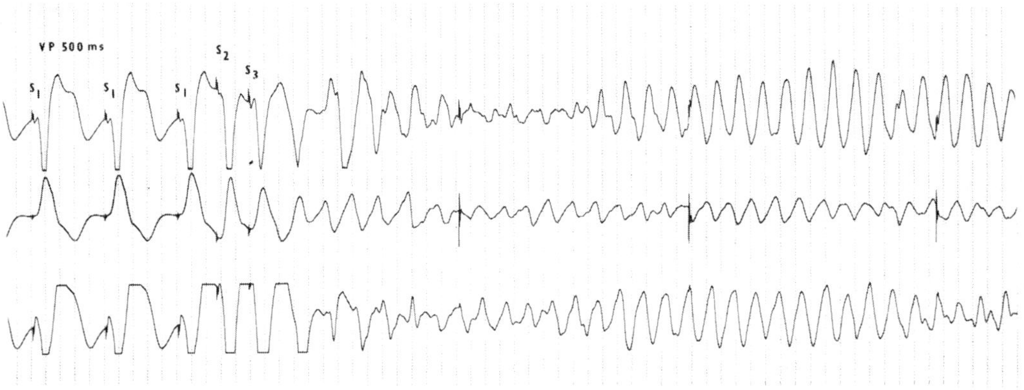

Fig 22C-26 Torsade de pointes induced at the time of electrophysiologic testing in a patient with congenital Q-T prolongation. A ventricular arrhythmia with a morphology consistent with torsade de pointes was induced after critically timed paired extrastimuli *(S_2S_3)* were introduced during ventricular pacing *(VP)* at a rate of 120 beats/min (cycle length equals 500 msec).

uniform morphology and polarity. The rhythm disturbance generally terminates spontaneously, but a fatal outcome is always possible. The rhythm has been reported to occur at all ages and often without evidence of associated heart disease. The rate of the tachycardia varies between 160 and 280 beats/min and is usually initiated by a PVC occurring late in diastole.[385] Torsade de pointes virtually always occurs in the setting of prolongation of the Q-T interval, and an enhanced U wave is often present.

The relationship among conventional ventricular tachycardia, torsade de pointes, and ventricular fibrillation remains unclear. Torsade de pointes appears to be a rhythm disturbance that is transitional between ventricular tachycardia and ventricular fibrillation. Any disturbance that results in Q-T prolongation can cause torsade de pointes. Such disturbances are listed in Table 22C-8. This rhythm disturbance is associated with syncope in patients with the syndrome of congenital Q-T prolongation, both with and without deafness.[385,392-394] The rhythm also occurs often in the setting of pronounced bradycardia or complete heart block, possibly because of a variation in sympathetic tone of the cardiac nerves and the consequent aggravation of the dispersion of repolarization which is already present at slow heart rates.[395] In patients who have syncope after starting quinidine therapy, torsade de pointes is the most likely cause. The incidence of Q-T prolongation with therapeutic levels of quinidine is 0.5% to 8.8%.[66,396] Procainamide,[390] disopyramide,[3,391] amiodarone,[397] and lidocaine[387] in high dosages have been associated with torsade de pointes. Other causes of torsade de pointes include organophosphate insecticide poisoning,[398,399] phenothiazines,[400-403] liquid protein diets,[380-382] and possibly tricyclic antidepressants[387,400] after overdosage. Hypokalemia[385,404] is an important cause of torsade de pointes, and cases of hypomagnesemia[405] in association with torsade de points have been reported. Although Q-T prolongation occurs with myocarditis, myocardial infarction, and variant angina, torsade de pointes is rare in these settings.

Table 22C-8 Conditions associated with torsade de pointes

I. Electrolyte abnormality
  A. Hypokalemia
  B. Hypomagnesemia
  C. Hypocalcemia (rare)
II. Drug-related
  A. Antiarrhythmia agents: quinidine, procainamide, disopyramide, amiodarone, lidocaine, aprindine
  B. Psychotropic agents: phenothiazines, tricyclic antidepressants
  C. Organophosphate poisoning
III. Liquid protein diets
IV. Cardiac disease
  A. Ischemia
  B. Myocarditis
  C. Bradycardia: sinus node disease, AV block with a slow escape rhythm
V. Central nervous system disease
  A. Intracranial trauma
  B. Subarachnoid hemorrhage
  C. Pneumoencephalography
VI. Congenital syndromes
  A. Romano-Ward
  B. Jervell and Lange-Nielsen

In a patient who has torsade de pointes, the treatment should be aimed at removing any predisposing causes and suppressing the arrhythmia until the Q-T interval returns to normal.[406] If the Q-T interval fails to return to normal after all possible predisposing causes have been eliminated, the diagnosis of congenital Q-T prolongation is then made (Romano-Ward syndrome and Jervell and Lange-Nielsen syndrome).

Prolonged episodes of torsade de pointes may require defibrillation; however, frequent recurrence of the tachy-

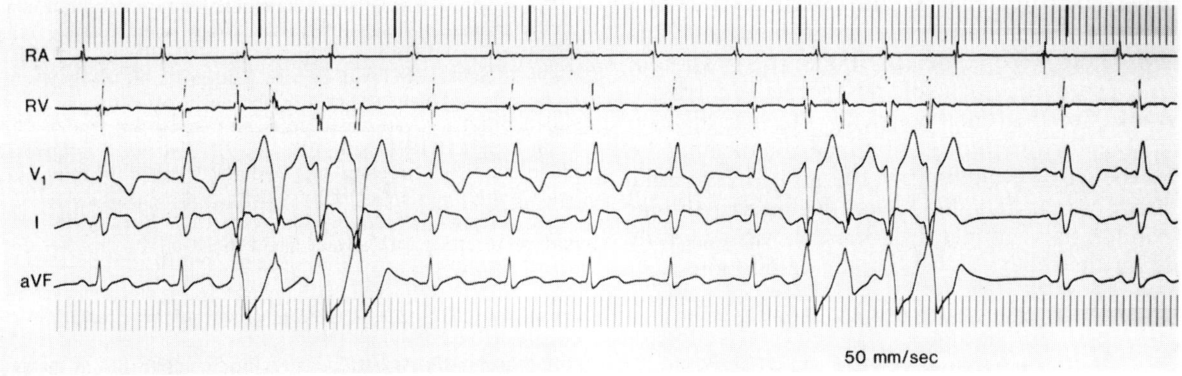

Fig 22C-27 Benign monomorphic ventricular tachycardia in an asymptomatic, otherwise healthy patient. Surface leads V_1, I, and aV_F are recorded simultaneously with electrograms from the right atrium *(RA)* and right ventricle *(RV)*. Four-beat runs of ventricular tachycardia are present during sinus rhythm.

cardia makes this technique less useful. Many antiarrhythmia drugs have been associated with torsade de pointes and result in prolongation of the Q-T interval. Lidocaine and propranolol have been associated with both success and failure in treating torsade de pointes, and bretylium has been reported to be successful.[385,406-409] The usual approach in the event that immediate control of the arrhythmia is necessary is the use of an isoproterenol infusion or overdrive pacing,[410-412] since both of these techniques reduce the dispersion of myocardial refractoriness. Initially, it may be necessary to use atrial pacing at 150 beats/min, but the pacing rate can usually be decreased subsequently. Intravenously administered magnesium has been reported to successfully control episodes of torsade de pointes.[57,413]

For the patient in whom Q-T prolongation is acquired, overdrive pacing can be discontinued when the predisposing causes have been eliminated. Prophylactic medication after a return of the Q-T interval to normal is not necessary. In the case of a patient who has a persistent prolongation of the Q-T interval, this usually indicates a congenital syndrome and requires treatment. Such patients generally respond to treatment with β-adrenergic blocking agents and refractory cases may require permanent cardiac pacing[414] or left stellate ganglion sympathectomy.[385,415] The fact that antiarrhythmia agents can aggravate preexisting ventricular arrhythmias has already been discussed. In the setting of torsade de pointes, this is exceedingly important. Such patients may have ventricular arrhythmias, experience Q-T prolongation with antiarrhythmia drugs, and then acquire torsade de pointes. Unless recognized, the torsade de pointes will be made worse if antiarrhythmia treatment is increased. The proper therapy is to discontinue use of the offending antiarrhythmia agent in such patients and substitute a new drug that does not result in Q-T prolongation but does suppress the initial ventricular arrhythmia. The role of electrophysiologic testing in patients with torsade de pointes is currently being evaluated.[156,416-419] Usually torsade de pointes is not inducible in the electrophysiology laboratory in patients who have had the rhythm clinically.

Repetitive monomorphic ("benign") ventricular tachycardia

Gallavardin[420] was the first physician to suggest that there may be a benign form of ventricular tachycardia. He described a ventricular arrhythmia characterized by single and double PVCs and brief episodes of ventricular tachycardia. The bursts of tachycardia were usually 3 to 10 complexes long, and all ectopic QRS complexes exhibited a uniform morphology. The intervening sinus complexes were normal, and the arrhythmia constantly occurred in alternation with normal sinus complexes (Fig 22C-27). This tachycardia has subsequently been called "benign ventricular tachycardia," "type II paroxysmal ventricular tachycardia," and "repetitive paroxysmal ventricular tachycardia."[421-423] The arrhythmia is usually associated with a good prognosis, but individual cases of sudden death have been reported[424-427] and may be examples of triggered activity.[428] The arrhythmia occurs in younger patients who do not demonstrate significant heart disease and it may persist for years, although spontaneous resolution has been reported. Occasionally, congestive heart failure will develop during the incessant ventricular tachycardia.[421] A review[102] of 18 patients who demonstrated repetitive ventricular tachycardia revealed the following clinical characteristics: (1) the mean age was 37 years; (2) in general, a long history of arrhythmia was present before evaluation; (3) only 2 patients had a history of syncope, and 6 were completely asymptomatic; (4) 14 patients had no evidence of underlying heart disease, whereas 3 patients had mitral valve prolapse and 1 patient had congestive cardiomyopathy; (5) 24-hour ambulatory monitoring demonstrated that the episodes of ventricular tachycardia tended to occur in clusters. Tachycardia could be induced in two of the nine patients who were studied in the electrophysiology laboratory, and the mechanism of the rhythm disturbance was believed to be due to automaticity. The patients were followed for a mean of 8 years (range, 1 to 18) after the arrhythmia was first recognized. There were no deaths and no progression of symptoms. Of six patients who did not receive antiarrhythmia therapy, five had no ventricular tachycardia on 24-hour ambulatory monitoring obtained at a mean of 3.6 years after the initial evaluation. In this group of patients, the incidence of mortality due to ventricular arrhythmias was low, and antiarrhythmia drug therapy was generally used only for the relief of symptomatic palpitations.

REFERENCES

1. The Cardiac Arrhythmia Suppression Trial (CAST) Investigators: Preliminary report: effect of encainide and flecainide on mortality in a randomized trial of arrhythmia suppression after myocardial infarction. *N Engl J Med* 321:406-411, 1989
2. Stanton MS, Prystowsky EN, Fineberg NS, et al: Arrhythmogenic effects of antiarrhythmic drugs: a study of 506 patients treated for ventricular tachycardia or fibrillation. *J Am Coll Cardiol* 14:209-215, 1989
3. Coplen SE, Antman EM, Berlin JA, et al: Efficacy and safety of quinidine therapy for maintenance of sinus rhythm after cardioversion: a meta-analysis of randomized control trials. *Circulation* 82:1106-1116, 1990
4. Morganroth J, Goin JE: Quinidine-related mortality in the short-to-medium-term treatment of ventricular arrhythmias: a meta-analysis. *Circulation* 84:1977-1983, 1991
5. Epstein AE, Bigger JT Jr, Wyse DG, et al: Events in the Cardiac Arrhythmia Suppression Trial (CAST): mortality in the entire population enrolled. *J Am Coll Cardiol* 18:14-19, 1991
6. Fish FA, Gillette PC, Benson DW Jr, et al: Proarrhythmia, cardiac arrest and death in young patients receiving encainide and flecainide. *J Am Coll Cardiol* 18:356-365, 1991
7. Ruskin JN, DiMarco JP, Garan H: Out-of-hospital cardiac arrest: electrophysiologic observations and selection of long-term antiarrhythmic therapy. *N Engl J Med* 303:607-613, 1980
8. Morady F, Scheinman MM, Hess DS, et al: Electrophysiologic testing in the management of survivors of out-of-hospital cardiac arrest. *Am J Cardiol* 51:85-89, 1983
9. Eldar M, Sauve MJ, Scheinman MM: Electrophysiologic testing and follow-up of patients with aborted sudden death. *J Am Coll Cardiol* 10:291-298, 1987
10. Wilber DJ, Garan H, Finkelstein D, et al: Out-of-hospital cardiac arrest: use of electrophysiologic testing in the prediction of long-term outcome. *N Engl J Med* 318:19-24, 1988
11. Waller TJ, Kay HR, Spielman SR, et al: Reduction in sudden death and total mortality by antiarrhythmic therapy evaluated by electrophysiologic drug testing: criteria of efficacy in patients with sustained ventricular tachyarrhythmia. *J Am Coll Cardiol* 10:83-89, 1987
12. Rosenbaum MS, Wilber DJ, Finkelstein D, et al: Immediate reproducibility of electrically induced sustained monomorphic ventricular tachycardia before and during antiarrhythmic therapy. *J Am Coll Cardiol* 17:133-138, 1991
13. Gomes JA, Winters SL, Ergin A, et al: Clinical and electrophysiologic determinants, treatment and survival of patients with sustained malignant ventricular tachyarrhythmias occurring late after myocardial infarction. *J Am Coll Cardiol* 17:320-326, 1991
14. Poole JE, Mathison TL, Kudenchuk PJ, et al: Long-term outcome in patients who survive out-of-hospital ventricular fibrillation and undergo electrophysiologic studies: evaluation by electrophysiologic subgroups. *J Am Coll Cardiol* 16:657-665, 1990
15. Bigger JT Jr, Weld FM, Rolnitzky LM: Prevalence, characteristics and significance of ventricular tachycardia (three or more complexes) detected with ambulatory electrocardiographic recording in the late hospital phase of acute myocardial infarction. *Am J Cardiol* 48:815-823, 1981
16. Califf RM, McKinnis RA, Burks J, et al: Prognostic implications of ventricular arrhythmias during 24 hour ambulatory monitoring in patients undergoing cardiac catheterization for coronary artery disease. *Am J Cardiol* 50:23-31, 1982
17. Schmidt G, Ulm K, Barthel P, et al: Evaluation of antiarrhythmic drug effects with simultaneous analysis of single ventricular premature contractions, couplets, and salvos. *J Am Coll Cardiol* 18:138-143, 1991
18. Schmitt FO, Erlanger J: Directional differences in the conduction of the impulse through heart muscle and their possible relation to extrasystolic and fibrillary contractions. *Am J Physiol* 87:326-347, 1928
19. de Bakker JMT, van Capelle FJL, Janse MJ, et al: Macroreentry in the infarcted human heart: the mechanism of ventricular tachycardias with a "focal" activation pattern. *J Am Coll Cardiol* 18:1005-1014, 1991
20. Henthorn RW, Rudy Y, Waldo AL: Evolving concepts regarding the role of tissue structure in arrhythmogenesis in the infarcted human heart. *J Am Coll Cardiol* 15:1608-1609, 1990
21. Bernstein RC, Frame LH: Ventricular reentry around a fixed barrier: resetting with advancement in an in vitro model. *Circulation* 81:267-280, 1990
22. Brugada J, Boersma L, Kirchof CJH, et al: Reentrant excitation around a fixed obstacle in uniform anisotropic ventricular myocardium. *Circulation* 84:1296-1306, 1991
23. Spach MS: Anisotropic structural complexities in the genesis of reentrant arrhythmias. *Circulation* 84:1447-1450, 1991
24. El-Sherif N, Scherlag BJ, Lazzara R, et al: Re-entrant ventricular arrhythmias in the late myocardial infarction period. 1. Conduction characteristics in the infarction zone. *Circulation* 55:686-702, 1977
25. El-Sherif N, Hope RR, Scherlag BJ, et al: Re-entrant ventricular arrhythmias in the late myocardial infarction period. 2. Patterns of initiation and termination of re-entry. *Circulation* 55:702-719, 1977
26. El-Sherif N, Lazzara R, Hope RR, et al: Re-entrant ventricular arrhythmias in the late myocardial infarction period. 3. Manifest and concealed extrasystolic grouping. *Circulation* 56:225-235, 1977
27. Han J, DeTraglia J, Millet D, et al: Incidence of ectopic beats as a function of basic rate in the ventricle. *Am Heart J* 72:632-639, 1966
28. Han J: Mechanisms of ventricular arrhythmias associated with myocardial infarction. *Am J Cardiol* 24:800-813, 1969
29. Han J, Millet D, Chizzonitti B, et al: Temporal dispersion of recovery of excitability in atrium and ventricle as a function of heart rate. *Am Heart J* 71:481-487, 1966
30. Gottlieb CD, Rosenthal ME, Stamato NJ, et al: A quantitative evaluation of refractoriness within a reentrant circuit during ventricular tachycardia: relation to termination. *Circulation* 82:1289-1295, 1990
31. Kastor JA, DeSanctis RW, Harthorne JW, et al: Transvenous atrial pacing in the treatment of refractory ventricular irritability. *Ann Intern Med* 66:939-945, 1967
32. Scherlag BJ, Helfant RH, Haft JI, et al: Electrophysiology underlying ventricular arrhythmias due to coronary ligation. *Am J Physiol* 219:1665-1671, 1970
33. Zipes DP, Knoebel SB: Rapid rate-dependent ventricular ectopy: adverse responses to atropine-induced rate increase. *Chest* 62:255-258, 1972
34. Kent KM, Smith ER, Redwood DR, et al: The deleterious electrophysiologic effects produced by increasing heart rate during experimental coronary occlusion (abstract). *Clin Res* 20:379, 1972
35. Mines GR: On dynamic equilibrium in the heart. *J Physiol (Lond)* 46:349-383, 1913
36. Janse MJ: Reentry arrhythmias. In *The Heart and Cardiovascular System: Scientific Foundations.* Vol. 2. Edited by HA Fozzard, E Haber, RB Jennings, et al. New York, Raven Press, 1992, pp 2055-2094
37. Jalife J, Antzelevitch C: Pacemaker annihilation: diagnostic and therapeutic implications. *Am Heart J* 100:128-130, 1980
38. Dangman KH, Hoffman BF: Studies on overdrive stimulation of canine cardiac Purkinje fibers: maximum diastolic potential as determinant of the response. *J Am Coll Cardiol* 2:1183-1190, 1983
39. Johnson NJ, Rosen MR: The distinction between triggered activity and other cardiac arrhythmias. In *Cardiac Arrhythmias: Where to Go From Here?* Edited by P Brugada, HJJ Wellens. Mount Kisco, New York, Futura Publishing Company, 1987, pp 129-145
40. Kaufmann R, Rothberger CJ: Beitrag zur Kenntnis der Entstehungsweise extrasystolischer Allorhythmien. *Z Ges Exp Med* 5:349-370, 1917
41. Kaufmann R, Rothberger CJ: Beiträge zur Entstehungsweise extrasystolischer Allorhythmien. *Z Ges Exp Med* 7:199-236, 1919
42. Kaufmann R, Rothberger CJ: Beiträge zur Entstehungsweise extrasystolischer Allorhythmien. 3. Die Wirkung der extrakardialen Herznerven. *Z Ges Exp Med* 9:104-122, 1919
43. Scherf D, Schott A: *Extrasystoles and Allied Arrhythmias.* New York, Grune & Stratton, 1953
44. Hoffman BF: The electrophysiology of heart muscle and the genesis of arrhythmias. In *Mechanisms and Therapy of Cardiac Arrhythmias.* Edited by LS Dreifus, W Likoff. New York, Grune & Stratton, 1966, pp 27-34

45. Lazzara R, El-Sherif N, Scherlag BJ: Electrophysiological properties of canine Purkinje cells in one-day-old myocardial infarction. *Circ Res* 33:722-734, 1973

46. Scherf D, Blumenfeld S, Yildiz M: Extrasystoles and parasystole. *Am Heart J* 64:357-363, 1962

47. Scherf D, Kyung-Hi-Choi, Bahadori A, et al: Parasystole. *Am J Cardiol* 12:527-538, 1963

48. Chung EKY: Parasystole. *Prog Cardiovasc Dis* 11:64-81, 1968

49. Watanabe Y: Reassessment of parasystole. *Am Heart J* 81:451-466, 1971

50. Myburgh DP, Lewis BS: Ventricular parasystole in healthy hearts. *Am Heart J* 82:307-311, 1971

51. Salazar J, McKendrick CS: Ventricular parasystole in acute myocardial infarction. *Br Heart J* 32:377-385, 1970

52. Wit AL, Cranefield PF: Triggered and automatic activity in the canine coronary sinus. *Circ Res* 41:435-445, 1977

53. Cranefield PF: Action potentials, afterpotentials, and arrhythmias. *Circ Res* 41:415-423, 1977

54. Rosen MR, Gelband H, Hoffman BF: Correlation between effects of ouabain on the canine electrocardiogram and transmembrane potentials of isolated Purkinje fibers. *Circulation* 47:65-72, 1973

55. Cranefield PF, Aronson RS: Initiation of sustained rhythmic activity by single propagated action potentials in canine cardiac Purkinje fibers exposed to sodium-free solution or to ouabain. *Circ Res* 34:477-481, 1974

56. Levine JH, Spear JF, Guarnieri T, et al: Cesium chloride-induced long QT syndrome: demonstration of afterdepolarizations and triggered activity in vivo. *Circulation* 72:1092-1103, 1985

57. Bailie DS, Inoue H, Kaseda S, et al: Magnesium suppression of early afterdepolarizations and ventricular tachyarrhythmias induced by cesium in dogs. *Circulation* 77:1395-1402, 1988

58. Wit AL, Rosen MR: Afterdepolarizations and triggered activity: distinction from automaticity as an arrhythmogenic mechanism. In *The Heart and Cardiovascular System: Scientific Foundations.* Edited by HA Fozzard, E Haber, RB Jennings, et al. Vol. 2. New York, Raven Press, 1992, pp 2113-2163

59. Shen W-K, Hammill SC: Survivors of acute myocardial infarction: Who is at risk for sudden cardiac death? *Mayo Clin Proc* 66:950-962, 1991

60. Brodsky M, Wu D, Denes P, et al: Arrhythmias documented by 24 hour continuous electrocardiographic monitoring in 50 male medical students without apparent heart disease. *Am J Cardiol* 39:390-395, 1977

61. Kennedy HL, Whitlock JA, Sprague MK, et al: Long-term follow-up of asymptomatic healthy subjects with frequent and complex ventricular ectopy. *N Engl J Med* 312:193-197, 1985

62. Mukharji J, Rude RE, Poole WK, et al: Risk factors for sudden death after acute myocardial infarction: two-year follow-up. *Am J Cardiol* 54:31-36, 1984

63. Bigger JT Jr, Fleiss JL, Kleiger R, et al: The relationships among ventricular arrhythmias, left ventricular dysfunction, and mortality in the 2 years after myocardial infarction. *Circulation* 69:250-258, 1984

64. Kostis JB, Byington R, Friedman LM, et al: Prognostic significance of ventricular ectopic activity in survivors of acute myocardial infarction. *J Am Coll Cardiol* 10:231-242, 1987

65. Graboys TB, Lown B, Podrid PJ, et al: Long-term survival of patients with malignant ventricular arrhythmia treated with antiarrhythmic drugs. *Am J Cardiol* 50:437-443, 1982

66. Lown B, Wolf M: Approaches to sudden death from coronary heart disease. *Circulation* 44:130-142, 1971

67. El-Sherif N, Myerburg RJ, Scherlag BJ, et al: Electrocardiographic antecedents of primary ventricular fibrillation: value of the R-on-T phenomenon in myocardial infarction. *Br Heart J* 38:415-422, 1976

68. De Soyza N, Bissett JK, Kane JJ, et al: Ectopic ventricular prematurity and its relationship to ventricular tachycardia in acute myocardial infarction in man. *Circulation* 50:529-533, 1974

69. Bigger JT Jr, Weld FM: Analysis of prognostic significance of ventricular arrhythmias after myocardial infarction: shortcomings of Lown grading system. *Br Heart J* 45:717-724, 1981

70. El-Sherif N, Scherlag BJ, Lazzara R: Electrode catheter recordings during malignant ventricular arrhythmia following experimental acute myocardial ischemia: evidence for re-entry due to conduction delay and block in ischemic myocardium. *Circulation* 51:1003-1014, 1975

71. Williams DO, Scherlag BJ, Hope RR, et al: The pathophysiology of malignant ventricular arrhythmias during acute myocardial ischemia. *Circulation* 50:1163-1172, 1974

72. Ruberman W, Weinblatt E, Goldberg JD, et al: Ventricular premature complexes and sudden death after myocardial infarction. *Circulation* 64:297-305, 1981

73. Kosowsky BD, Lown B, Whiting R, et al: Occurrence of ventricular arrhythmias with exercise as compared to monitoring. *Circulation* 44:826-832, 1971

74. Surawicz B: Dispersion of refractoriness in ventricular arrhythmias. In *Cardiac Electrophysiology: From Cell to Bedside.* Edited by DP Zipes, J Jalife. Philadelphia, WB Saunders Company, 1990, pp 377-385

75. Chardack WM, Ishikawa H, Fochler FJ, et al: Pacing and ventricular fibrillation. *Ann NY Acad Sci* 167:919-933, 1969

76. Garan H, Ruskin JN, Fallon JT: Heterogeneity of effective refractory periods within the infarct zone in dogs with chronic myocardial infarction (abstract). *Clin Res* 27:168A, 1979

77. Sobotka PA, Mayer JH, Bauernfeind RA, et al: Arrhythmias documented by 24-hour continuous ambulatory electrocardiographic monitoring in young women without apparent heart disease. *Am Heart J* 101:753-759, 1981

78. Hinkle LE Jr, Carver ST, Stevens M: The frequency of asymptomatic disturbances of cardiac rhythm and conduction in middle-aged men. *Am J Cardiol* 24:629-650, 1969

79. Bjerregaard P: Premature beats in healthy subjects 40-79 years of age. *Eur Heart J* 3:493-503, 1982

80. Lown B, Kosowsky BD, Klein MD: Pathogenesis, prevention, and treatment of arrhythmias in myocardial infarction. *Circulation* 40 Suppl 4:261-267, 1969

81. Koch-Weser J, Klein SW, Foo-Canto LL, et al: Antiarrhythmic prophylaxis with procainamide in acute myocardial infarction. *N Engl J Med* 281:1253-1260, 1969

82. Lie KI, Wellens HJ, van Capelle FJ, et al: Lidocaine in the prevention of primary ventricular fibrillation: a double-blind, randomized study of 212 consecutive patients. *N Engl J Med* 291:1324-1326, 1974

83. Vismara LA, DeMaria AN, Hughes JL, et al: Evaluation of arrhythmias in the late hospital phase of acute myocardial infarction compared to coronary care unit ectopy. *Br Heart J* 37:598-603, 1975

84. Schulze RA Jr, Rouleau J, Rigo P, et al: Ventricular arrhythmias in the late hospital phase of acute myocardial infarction: relation to left ventricular function detected by gated cardiac blood pool scanning. *Circulation* 52:1006-1011, 1975

85. Ruberman W, Weinblatt E, Goldberg JD, et al: Ventricular premature beats and mortality after myocardial infarction. *N Engl J Med* 297:750-757, 1977

86. Farrell TG, Bashir Y, Cripps T, et al: Risk stratification of arrhythmic events in postinfarction patients based on heart rate variability, ambulatory electrocardiographic variables and the signal-averaged electrocardiogram. *J Am Coll Cardiol* 18:687-697, 1991

87. Moss AJ, Davis HT, DeCamilla J, et al: Ventricular ectopic beats and their relation to sudden and nonsudden cardiac death after myocardial infarction. *Circulation* 60:998-1003, 1979

88. Anderson KP, DeCamilla J, Moss AJ: Clinical significance of ventricular tachycardia (3 beats or longer) detected during ambulatory monitoring after myocardial infarction. *Circulation* 57:890-897, 1978

89. Kleiger RE, Miller JP, Thanavaro S, et al: Relationship between clinical features of acute myocardial infarction and ventricular runs 2 weeks to 1 year after infarction. *Circulation* 63:64-70, 1981

90. Gomes JAC, Hariman RI, Kang PS, et al: Programmed electrical stimulation in patients with high-grade ventricular ectopy: electrophysiologic findings and prognosis for survival. *Circulation* 70:43-51, 1984

91. Roy D, Marchand E, Théroux P, et al: Programmed ventricular stimulation in survivors of an acute myocardial infarction. *Circulation* 72:487-494, 1985

92. Rahimtoola SH, Zipes DP, Akhtar M, et al: Consensus statement of the conference on the state of the art of electrophysiologic testing in the diagnosis and treatment of patients with cardiac arrhythmias. *Circulation* 75 Suppl 3:3-11, 1987

93. Bourke JP, Richards DAB, Ross DL, et al: Routine programmed electrical stimulation in survivors of acute myocardial infarction for prediction of spontaneous ventricular arrhythmias during follow-up: results, optimal stimulation protocol and cost-effective screening. *J Am Coll Cardiol* 18:780-788, 1991

94. Wilber DJ, Olshansky B, Moran JF, et al: Electrophysiological testing and nonsustained ventricular tachycardia: use and limitations in patients with coronary artery disease and impaired ventricular function. *Circulation* 82:350-358, 1990

95. Richards DAB, Byth K, Ross DL, et al: What is the best predictor

of spontaneous ventricular tachycardia and sudden death after myocardial infarction? *Circulation* 83:756-763, 1991

96. ACC/AHA Task Force Report: Guidelines for clinical intracardiac electrophysiologic studies: a report of the American College of Cardiology/American Heart Association Task Force on Assessment of Diagnostic and Therapeutic Cardiovascular Procedures (subcommittee to assess clinical intracardiac electrophysiologic studies). *J Am Coll Cardiol* 14:1827-1842, 1989

97. Kennedy HL, Pescarmona JE, Bouchard RJ, et al: Objective evidence of occult myocardial dysfunction in patients with frequent ventricular ectopy without clinically apparent heart disease. *Am Heart J* 104:57-65, 1982

98. Strain JE, Grose RM, Factor SM, et al: Results of endomyocardial biopsy in patients with spontaneous ventricular tachycardia but without apparent structural heart disease. *Circulation* 68:1171-1181, 1983

99. Hinkle LE, Carver ST, Argyros DC: The prognostic significance of ventricular premature contractions in healthy people and in people with coronary heart disease. *Acta Cardiol [Suppl] (Brux)* 18:5-32, 1974

100. Proudfit WL, Bruschke AVG, Sones FM Jr: Clinical course of patients with normal or slightly or moderately abnormal coronary arteriograms: 10-year follow-up of 521 patients. *Circulation* 62:712-717, 1980

101. Rabkin SW, Mathewson FA, Tate RB: Relationship of ventricular ectopy in men without apparent heart disease to occurrence of ischemic heart disease and sudden death. *Am Heart J* 101:135-142, 1981

102. Rahilly GT, Prystowsky EN, Zipes DP, et al: Clinical and electrophysiologic findings in patients with repetitive monomorphic ventricular tachycardia and otherwise normal electrocardiogram. *Am J Cardiol* 50:459-468, 1982

103. Califf RM, McKinnis RA, McNeer JF, et al: Prognostic value of ventricular arrhythmias associated with treadmill exercise testing in patients studied with cardiac catheterization for suspected ischemic heart disease. *J Am Coll Cardiol* 2:1060-1067, 1983

104. Lichtlen PR, Bethge K-P, Platiel H: Inzidenz des plötzlichen Herztodes bei Koronarpatienten in Abhängigkeit von Anatomie und Rhythmusprofil. *Z Kardiol* 69:639-648, 1980

105. Maisel AS, Scott N, Gilpin E, et al: Complex ventricular arrhythmias in patients with Q wave versus non-Q wave myocardial infarction. *Circulation* 72:963-970, 1985

106. Hammill SC, Trusty JM, Wood DL, et al: Influence of ventricular function and presence or absence of coronary artery disease on results of electrophysiologic testing for asymptomatic nonsustained ventricular tachycardia. *Am J Cardiol* 65:722-728, 1990

107. Faris JV, McHenry PL, Jordan JW, et al: Prevalence and reproducibility of exercise-induced ventricular arrhythmias during maximal exercise testing in normal men. *Am J Cardiol* 37:617-622, 1976

108. Morris SN, McHenry PL: Cardiac arrhythmias during exercise testing and exercise conditioning. *Cardiovasc Clin* 9 No 3:57-68, 1978

109. Goldschlager N, Cake D, Cohn K: Exercise-induced ventricular arrhythmias in patients with coronary artery disease: their relation to angiographic findings. *Am J Cardiol* 31:434-440, 1973

110. Jelinek MV, Lown B: Exercise stress testing for exposure of cardiac arrhythmia. *Prog Cardiovasc Dis* 16:497-522, 1974

111. Henry RL, Kennedy GT, Crawford MH: Prognostic value of exercise-induced ventricular ectopic activity for mortality after acute myocardial infarction. *Am J Cardiol* 59:1251-1255, 1987

112. Saini V, Graboys TB, Towne V, et al: Reproducibility of exercise-induced ventricular arrhythmia in patients undergoing evaluation for malignant ventricular arrhythmia. *Am J Cardiol* 63:697-701, 1989

113. Shen W-K, Hammill SC, Packer DL: Asymptomatic ventricular arrhythmias after MI: a therapeutic dilemma. Parts I and II. CARDIO (in press)

114. Hine LK, Laird NM, Hewitt P, et al: Meta-analyses of empirical long-term antiarrhythmic therapy after myocardial infarction. *JAMA* 262:3037-3040, 1989

115. Lovell RRH, Mitchell ME, Prineas RJ, et al: Phenytoin after recovery from myocardial infarction: controlled trial in 568 patients. *Lancet* 2:1055-1057, 1971

116. Gottlieb SH, Achuff SC, Mellits ED, et al: Prophylactic antiarrhythmic therapy of high-risk survivors of myocardial infarction: lower mortality at 1 month but not at 1 year. *Circulation* 75:792-799, 1987

117. Cardiac Arrhythmia Pilot Study (CAPS) Investigators: Effects of encainide, flecainide, imipramine and moricizine on ventricular arrhythmias during the year after acute myocardial infarction: the CAPS. *Am J Cardiol* 61:501-509, 1988

118. Nielsen BL, Clausen J, Nielsen JS: Can procainamide improve the prognosis of patients with ventricular arrhythmias after myocardial infarction? *Dan Med Bull* 25:121-125, 1978

119. Rydén L, Arnman K, Conradson T-B, et al: Prophylaxis of ventricular tachyarrhythmias with intravenous and oral tocainide in patients with and recovering from acute myocardial infarction. *Am Heart J* 100:1006-1012, 1980

120. Peter T, Ross D, Duffield A, et al: Effect on survival after myocardial infarction of long-term treatment with phenytoin. *Br Heart J* 40:1356-1360, 1978

121. Chamberlain DA, Jewitt DE, Julian DG, et al: Oral mexiletine in high-risk patients after myocardial infarction. *Lancet* 2:1324-1327, 1980

122. Bastian BC, Macfarlane PW, McLauchlan JH, et al: A prospective randomized trial of tocainide in patients following myocardial infarction. *Am Heart J* 100:1017-1022, 1980

123. IMPACT Research Group: International Mexiletine and Placebo Antiarrhythmic Coronary Trial. I. Report on arrhythmia and other findings. *J Am Coll Cardiol* 4:1148-1163, 1984

124. Wyse DG, Hallstrom A, McBride R, et al: Events in the Cardiac Arrhythmia Suppression Trial (CAST): mortality in patients surviving open label titration but not randomized to double-blind therapy. *J Am Coll Cardiol* 18:20-28, 1991

125. Capone RJ, Pawitan Y, El-Sherif N, et al: Events in the Cardiac Arrhythmia Suppression Trial (CAST): baseline predictors of mortality in placebo-treated patients. *J Am Coll Cardiol* 18:1434-1438, 1991

126. Anderson JL, Anastasiou-Nana MI, Menlove RL, et al: Spontaneous variability in ventricular ectopic activity during chronic antiarrhythmic therapy. *Circulation* 82:830-840, 1990

127. Pratt CM, Hallstrom A, Theroux P, et al: Avoiding interpretive pitfalls when assessing arrhythmia suppression after myocardial infarction: insights from the long-term observations of the placebo-treated patients in the Cardiac Arrhythmia Pilot Study (CAPS). *J Am Coll Cardiol* 17:1-8, 1991

128. Bigger JT Jr, Fleiss JL: The variability of spontaneous ventricular arrhythmias in the year after myocardial infarction. *J Am Coll Cardiol* 17:9-10, 1991

129. Furberg CD, Yusuf S: Antiarrhythmics and VPD suppression. *Circulation* 84:928-930, 1991

130. Cairns JA, Connolly SJ, Gent M, et al: Post-myocardial infarction mortality in patients with ventricular premature depolarizations: Canadian Amiodarone Myocardial Infarction Arrhythmia Trial Pilot Study. *Circulation* 84:550-557, 1991

131. Burkart F, Pfisterer M, Kiowski W, et al: Effect of antiarrhythmic therapy on mortality in survivors of myocardial infarction with asymptomatic complex ventricular arrhythmias. Basel Antiarrhythmic Study of Infarct Survival (BASIS). *J Am Coll Cardiol* 16:1711-1718, 1990

132. Greene HL, Reid PR, Schaeffer AH: The repetitive ventricular response in man: a predictor of sudden death. *N Engl J Med* 299:729-734, 1978

133. Hamer A, Vohra J, Hunt D, et al: Prediction of sudden death by electrophysiologic studies in high risk patients surviving acute myocardial infarction. *Am J Cardiol* 50:223-229, 1982

134. Richards DA, Cody DV, Denniss AR, et al: Ventricular electrical instability: a predictor of death after myocardial infarction. *Am J Cardiol* 51:75-80, 1983

135. Marchlinski FE, Buxton AE, Waxman HL, et al: Identifying patients at risk of sudden death after myocardial infarction: value of the response to programmed stimulation, degree of ventricular ectopic activity and severity of left ventricular dysfunction. *Am J Cardiol* 52:1190-1196, 1983

136. Denniss AR, Richards DA, Cody DV, et al: Prognostic significance of ventricular tachycardia and fibrillation induced at programmed stimulation and delayed potentials detected on the signal-averaged electrocardiograms of survivors of acute myocardial infarction. *Circulation* 74:731-745, 1986

137. Buxton AE, Waxman HL, Marchlinski FE, et al: Electrophysiologic studies in nonsustained ventricular tachycardia: relation to underlying heart disease. *Am J Cardiol* 52:985-991, 1983

138. Veltri EP, Platia EV, Griffith LSC, et al: Programmed electrical stimulation and long-term follow-up in asymptomatic, nonsustained ventricular tachycardia. *Am J Cardiol* 56:309-314, 1985

139. Klein RC, Machell C: Use of electrophysiologic testing in patients with nonsustained ventricular tachycardia: prognostic and therapeutic implications. *J Am Coll Cardiol* 14:155-161, 1989

140. Sulpizi AM, Friehling TD, Kowey PR: Value of electrophysiologic testing in patients with nonsustained ventricular tachycardia. *Am J Cardiol* 59:841-845, 1987

141. Naccarelli GV, Prystowsky EN, Jackman WM, et al: Role of electrophysiologic testing in managing patients who have ventricular tachycardia unrelated to coronary artery disease. *Am J Cardiol* 50:165-171, 1982

142. Meinertz T, Treese N, Kasper W, et al: Determinants of prognosis in idiopathic dilated cardiomyopathy as determined by programmed electrical stimulation. *Am J Cardiol* 56:337-341, 1985

143. Poll DS, Marchlinski FE, Buxton AE, et al: Sustained ventricular tachycardia in patients with idiopathic dilated cardiomyopathy: electrophysiologic testing and lack of response to antiarrhythmic drug therapy. *Circulation* 70:451-456, 1984

144. Hammill SC, Pritchett ELC: Simplified esophageal electrocardiography using bipolar recording leads. *Ann Intern Med* 95:14-18, 1981

145. Josephson ME, Horowitz LN: Recurrent ventricular tachycardia: an electrophysiologic approach. *Med Clin North Am* 63:53-71, January 1979

146. Josephson ME, Kastor JA, Horowitz LN: Electrophysiologic management of recurrent ventricular tachycardia in acute and chronic ischemic heart disease. *Cardiovasc Clin* 11 No 1:35-55, 1980

147. Kastor JA, Horowitz LN, Harken AH, et al: Clinical electrophysiology of ventricular tachycardia. *N Engl J Med* 304:1004-1020, 1981

148. Wellens HJJ: *Electrical Stimulation of the Heart in the Study and Treatment of Tachycardias.* Baltimore, University Park Press, 1971, pp 14-22

149. Gallagher JJ, Damato AN, Lau SH: Electrophysiologic studies during accelerated idioventricular rhythms. *Circulation* 44:671-677, 1971

150. Lerman BB, Belardinelli L, West GA, et al: Adenosine-sensitive ventricular tachycardia: evidence suggesting cyclic AMP-mediated triggered activity. *Circulation* 74:270-280, 1986

151. Lerman BB, Belardinelli L: Cardiac electrophysiology of adenosine: basic and clinical concepts. *Circulation* 83:1499-1509, 1991

152. Josephson ME, Horowitz LN, Farshidi A, et al: Recurrent sustained ventricular tachycardia. 1. Mechanisms. *Circulation* 57:431-440, 1978

153. Wellens HJJ, Düren DR, Lie KI: Observations on mechanisms of ventricular tachycardia in man. *Circulation* 54:237-244, 1976

154. Wellens HJJ, Bär FWHM, Lie KI: The value of the electrocardiogram in the differential diagnosis of tachycardia with a widened QRS complex. *Am J Med* 64:27-33, 1978

155. Ross DL, Vohra JK, Sloman JG: Similar QRS morphology in sinus rhythm and ventricular tachycardia. *PACE* 2:486-489, 1979

156. Wellens HJJ: Value and limitations of programmed electrical stimulation of the heart in the study and treatment of tachycardias. *Circulation* 57:845-853, 1978

157. Kastor JA, Goldreyer BN: Ventricular origin of bidirectional tachycardia: case report of a patient not toxic from digitalis. *Circulation* 48:897-903, 1973

158. Vermeulen A, Wellens HJ: Paroxysmal ventricular tachycardia showing fusion with reciprocal ventricular beats. *Br Heart J* 33:320-322, 1971

159. Akhtar M, Shenasa M, Jazayeri M, et al: Wide QRS complex tachycardia: reappraisal of a common clinical problem. *Ann Intern Med* 109:905-912, 1988

160. Brugada P, Brugada J, Mont L, et al: A new approach to the differential diagnosis of a regular tachycardia with a wide QRS complex. *Circulation* 83:1649-1659, 1991

161. Kindwall KE, Brown J, Josephson ME: Electrocardiographic criteria for ventricular tachycardia in wide complex left bundle branch block morphology tachycardias. *Am J Cardiol* 61:1279-1283, 1988

162. Akhtar M, Shenasa M, Tchou PJ, et al: Role of electrophysiologic studies in supraventricular tachycardia. In *Cardiac Arrhythmias: Where to Go From Here?* Edited by P Brugada, HJJ Wellens. Mount Kisco, New York, Futura Publishing Company, 1987, pp 232-242

163. Chapman JH, Schrank JP, Crampton RS: Idiopathic ventricular tachycardia: an intracardiac electrical, hemodynamic and angiographic assessment of six patients. *Am J Med* 59:470-480, 1975

164. Kistin AD, Tawakkol A, Massumi RA: Atrial rhythm in ventricular tachycardia occurring during cardiac catheterization. *Circulation* 35:10-14, 1967

165. Kistin AD: Retrograde conduction to the atria in ventricular tachycardia. *Circulation* 24:236-249, 1961

166. Josephson ME, Kastor JA: His-Purkinje conduction during retrograde stress. *J Clin Invest* 61:171-177, 1978

167. Josephson ME, Horowitz LN, Farshidi A, et al: Recurrent sustained ventricular tachycardia. 2. Endocardial mapping. *Circulation* 57:440-447, 1978

168. Josephson ME, Horowitz LN, Waxman HL, et al: Sustained ventricular tachycardia: role of the 12-lead electrocardiogram in localizing site of origin. *Circulation* 64:257-272, 1981

169. Castellanos A Jr, O'Brien H, Castillo CA, et al: Contribution of His bundle recordings to analysis of abnormal beats with right bundle-branch block—superior axis pattern. *Br Heart J* 34:795-799, 1972

170. Josephson ME, Seides SF: *Clinical Cardiac Electrophysiology: Techniques and Interpretations.* Philadelphia, Lea & Febiger, 1979, pp 5-21

171. DiMarco JP, Garan H, Ruskin JN: Complications in patients undergoing cardiac electrophysiologic procedures. *Ann Intern Med* 97:490-493, 1982

172. Horowitz LN, Josephson ME, Farshidi A, et al: Recurrent sustained ventricular tachycardia. 3. Role of the electrophysiologic study in selection of antiarrhythmic regimens. *Circulation* 58:986-997, 1978

173. Mason JW, Winkle RA: Accuracy of the ventricular tachycardia-induction study for predicting long-term efficacy and inefficacy of antiarrhythmic drugs. *N Engl J Med* 303:1073-1077, 1980

174. Vandepol CJ, Farshidi A, Spielman SR, et al: Incidence and clinical significance of induced ventricular tachycardia. *Am J Cardiol* 45:725-731, 1980

175. Livelli FD Jr, Bigger JT Jr, Reiffel JA, et al: Response to programmed ventricular stimulation: sensitivity, specificity and relation to heart disease. *Am J Cardiol* 50:452-458, 1982

176. Josephson ME, Seides SF: *Clinical Cardiac Electrophysiology: Techniques and Interpretations.* Philadelphia, Lea & Febiger, 1979, pp 247-280

177. Michelson EL, Spielman SR, Greenspan AM, et al: Electrophysiologic study of the left ventricle: indications and safety. *Chest* 75:592-596, 1979

178. Josephson ME, Horowitz LN: Electrophysiologic approach to therapy of recurrent sustained ventricular tachycardia. *Am J Cardiol* 43:631-642, 1979

179. Lin H-T, Mann DE, Luck JC, et al: Prospective comparison of right and left ventricular stimulation for induction of sustained ventricular tachycardia. *Am J Cardiol* 59:559-563, 1987

180. Robertson JF, Cain ME, Horowitz LN, et al: Anatomic and electrophysiologic correlates of ventricular tachycardia requiring left ventricular stimulation. *Am J Cardiol* 48:263-268, 1981

181. Morady F, DiCarlo L, Winston S, et al: A prospective comparison of triple extrastimuli and left ventricular stimulation in studies of ventricular tachycardia induction. *Circulation* 70:52-57, 1984

182. Reddy CP, Gettes LS: Use of isoproterenol as an aid to electric induction of chronic recurrent ventricular tachycardia. *Am J Cardiol* 44:705-713, 1979

183. Kang PS, Gomes JAC, El-Sherif N: Procainamide in the induction and perpetuation of ventricular tachycardia in man. *PACE* 5:311-322, 1982

184. Engel TR, Meister SG, Frankl WS: Ventricular extrastimulation in the mitral valve prolapse syndrome: evidence for ventricular reentry. *J Electrocardiol* 11:137-142, 1978

185. Wellens HJJ, Lie KI, Durrer D: Further observations on ventricular tachycardia as studied by electrical stimulation of the heart: chronic recurrent ventricular tachycardia and ventricular tachycardia during acute myocardial infarction. *Circulation* 49:647-653, 1974

186. Herre JM, Griffin JC, Nielsen AP, et al: Permanent triggered antitachycardia pacemakers in the management of recurrent sustained ventricular tachycardia. *J Am Coll Cardiol* 6:206-212, 1985

187. Wellens HJ, Schuilenburg RM, Durrer D: Electrical stimulation of the heart in patients with ventricular tachycardia. *Circulation* 46:216-226, 1972

188. Mason JW, Winkle RA: Electrode-catheter arrhythmia induction in the selection and assessment of antiarrhythmic drug therapy for recurrent ventricular tachycardia. *Circulation* 58:971-985, 1978

189. Josephson ME, Horowitz LN, Farshidi A, et al: Sustained ventricular tachycardia: evidence for protected localized reentry. *Am J Cardiol* 42:416-424, 1978

190. Fisher JD, Mehra R, Furman S: Termination of ventricular tachycardia with bursts of rapid ventricular pacing. *Am J Cardiol* 41:94-102, 1978

191. Ruskin JN, Garan H, Poulin F, et al: Permanent radiofrequency ventricular pacing for management of drug-resistant ventricular tachycardia. *Am J Cardiol* 46:317-321, 1980

192. Naccarelli GV, Zipes DP, Rahilly GT, et al: Influence of tachycardia cycle length and antiarrhythmic drugs on pacing termination and acceleration of ventricular tachycardia. *Am Heart J* 105:1-5, 1983

193. Ruskin JN, DiMarco JP, Garan H: Repetitive responses to single ventricular extrastimuli in patients with serious ventricular arrhythmias: incidence and clinical significance. *Circulation* 63:767-772, 1981

194. Mason JW: Repetitive beating after single ventricular extrastimuli: incidence and prognostic significance in patients with recurrent ventricular tachycardia. *Am J Cardiol* 45:1126-1131, 1980

195. Cobb LA, Baum RS, Alvarez H III, et al: Resuscitation from out-of-hospital ventricular fibrillation: 4 years follow-up. *Circulation* 52 Suppl 3:223-228, 1975

196. Velebit V, Podrid P, Lown B, et al: Aggravation and provocation of ventricular arrhythmias by antiarrhythmic drugs. *Circulation* 65:886-894, 1982

197. Hartzler GO, Maloney JD: Programmed ventricular stimulation in management of recurrent ventricular tachycardia. *Mayo Clin Proc* 52:731-741, 1977

198. Rae AP, Greenspan AM, Spielman SR, et al: Antiarrhythmic drug efficacy for ventricular tachyarrhythmias associated with coronary artery disease as assessed by electrophysiologic studies. *Am J Cardiol* 55:1494-1499, 1985

199. Kuchar DL, Rottman J, Berger E, et al: Prediction of successful suppression of sustained ventricular tachyarrhythmias by serial drug testing from data derived at the initial electrophysiologic study. *J Am Coll Cardiol* 12:982-988, 1988

200. Mitchell LB, Duff HJ, Manyari DE, et al: A randomized clinical trial of the noninvasive and invasive approaches to drug therapy of ventricular tachycardia. *N Engl J Med* 317:1681-1687, 1987

201. Roy D, Waxman HL, Kienzle MG, et al: Clinical characteristics and long-term follow-up in 119 survivors of cardiac arrest: relation to inducibility at electrophysiologic testing. *Am J Cardiol* 52:969-974, 1983

202. Benditt DG, Benson DW Jr, Klein GJ, et al: Prevention of recurrent sudden cardiac arrest: role of provocative electropharmacologic testing. *J Am Coll Cardiol* 2:418-425, 1983

203. Zipes DP, Prystowsky EN, Heger JJ: Amiodarone: electrophysiologic actions; pharmacokinetics and clinical effects. *J Am Coll Cardiol* 3:1059-1071, 1984

204. Naccarelli GV, Fineberg NS, Zipes DP, et al: Amiodarone: risk factors for recurrence of symptomatic ventricular tachycardia identified at electrophysiologic study. *J Am Coll Cardiol* 6:814-821, 1985

205. Horowitz LN, Greenspan AM, Spielman SR, et al: Usefulness of electrophysiologic testing in evaluation of amiodarone therapy for sustained ventricular tachyarrhythmias associated with coronary artery disease. *Am J Cardiol* 55:367-371, 1985

206. Waxman HL: The efficacy of amiodarone for ventricular arrhythmias cannot be predicted with clinical electrophysiological studies. *Int J Cardiol* 3:76-80, 1983

207. Hamer AW, Finerman WB Jr, Peter T, et al: Disparity between the clinical and electrophysiologic effects of amiodarone in the treatment of recurrent ventricular tachyarrhythmias. *Am Heart J* 102:992-1000, 1981

208. Fisher JD, Cohen HL, Mehra R, et al: Cardiac pacing and pacemakers. II. Serial electrophysiologic-pharmacologic testing for control of recurrent tachyarrhythmias. *Am Heart J* 93:658-668, 1977

209. Fisher JD, Kim SG, Furman S, et al: Role of implantable pacemakers in control of recurrent ventricular tachycardia. *Am J Cardiol* 49:194-206, 1982

210. Hartzler GO: Treatment of recurrent ventricular tachycardia by patient-activated radiofrequency ventricular stimulation. *Mayo Clin Proc* 54:75-82, 1979

211. Mirowski M, Reid PR, Mower MM, et al: Termination of malignant ventricular arrhythmias with an implanted automatic defibrillator in human beings. *N Engl J Med* 303:322-324, 1980

212. Brugada J, Brugada P, Boersma L, et al: On the mechanisms of ventricular tachycardia acceleration during programmed electrical stimulation. *Circulation* 83:1621-1629, 1991

213. Hammill SC, Sugrue DD, Gersh BJ, et al: Clinical intracardiac electrophysiologic testing: technique, diagnostic indications, and therapeutic uses. *Mayo Clin Proc* 61:478-503, 1986

214. Morady F, Frank R, Kou WH, et al: Identification and catheter ablation of a zone of slow conduction in the reentrant circuit of ventricular tachycardia in humans. *J Am Coll Cardiol* 11:775-782, 1988

215. Leclercq JF, Chouty F, Cauchemez B, et al: Results of electrical fulguration in arrhythmogenic right ventricular disease. *Am J Cardiol* 62:220-224, 1988

216. Fontaine G, Tonet JL, Frank R, et al: La fulguration endocavitaire. Une nouvelle méthode de traitement des troubles du rythme? *Ann Cardiol Angeiol (Paris)* 33:543-561, 1984

217. Belhassen B, Miller HI, Geller E, et al: Transcatheter electrical shock ablation of ventricular tachycardia. *J Am Coll Cardiol* 7:1347-1355, 1986

218. Morady F, Scheinman MM, Di Carlo LA Jr, et al: Catheter ablation of ventricular tachycardia with intracardiac shocks: results in 33 patients. *Circulation* 75:1037-1049, 1987

219. Hartzler GO: Electrode catheter ablation of refractory focal ventricular tachycardia. *J Am Coll Cardiol* 2:1107-1113, 1983

220. Stevenson WG, Weiss JN, Wiener I, et al: Slow conduction in the infarct scar: relevance to the occurrence, detection, and ablation of ventricular reentry circuits resulting from myocardial infarction. *Am Heart J* 117:452-467, 1989

221. Garan H, Kuchar D, Freeman C, et al: Early assessment of the effect of map-guided transcatheter intracardiac electric shock on sustained ventricular tachycardia secondary to coronary artery disease. *Am J Cardiol* 61:1018-1023, 1988

222. Borggrefe M, Breithardt G, Podczeck A, et al: Catheter ablation of ventricular tachycardia using defibrillator pulses: electrophysiological findings and long-term results. *Eur Heart J* 10:591-601, 1989

223. Morady F, Kadish A, Rosenheck S, et al: Concealed entrainment as a guide for catheter ablation of ventricular tachycardia in patients with prior myocardial infarction. *J Am Coll Cardiol* 17:678-689, 1991

224. Huang SKS, Graham AR, Wharton K: Radiofrequency catheter ablation of the left and right ventricles: anatomic and electrophysiologic observations. *PACE* 11:449-459, 1988

225. Davis MJE, Murdock C: Radiofrequency catheter ablation of refractory ventricular tachycardia. *PACE* 11:725-729, 1988

226. Cohen TJ, Chien WW, Lurie KG, et al: Radiofrequency catheter ablation for treatment of bundle branch reentry ventricular tachycardia: results and long-term follow-up. *J Am Coll Cardiol* 18:1767-1773, 1991

227. Jackman WM, Kuck K-H, Naccarelli GV, et al: Radiofrequency current directed across the mitral annulus with a bipolar epicardial-endocardial catheter electrode configuration in dogs. *Circulation* 78:1288-1298, 1988

228. Huang SKS, Graham AR, Lee MA, et al: Comparison of catheter ablation using radiofrequency versus direct current energy: biophysical, electrophysiologic and pathologic observations. *J Am Coll Cardiol* 18:1091-1097, 1991

229. Tchou P, Jazayeri M, Denker S, et al: Transcatheter electrical ablation of right bundle branch: a method of treating macroreentrant ventricular tachycardia attributed to bundle branch reentry. *Circulation* 78:246-257, 1988

230. Cowen TJ, Chien WW, Lurie KG, et al: Radiofrequency catheter ablation for treatment of bundle branch reentrant ventricular tachycardia: results and long-term follow-up. *J Am Coll Cardiol* 18:1767-1773, 1991

231. Tchou PJ, Kadri N, Anderson J, et al: Automatic implantable cardioverter defibrillators and survival of patients with left ventricular dysfunction and malignant ventricular arrhythmias. *Ann Intern Med* 109:529-534, 1988

232. Winkle RA, Mead RH, Ruder MA, et al: Long-term outcome with the automatic implantable cardioverter-defibrillator. *J Am Coll Cardiol* 13:1353-1361, 1989

233. Kelly PA, Cannom DS, Garan H, et al: The automatic implantable cardioverter-defibrillator: efficacy, complications and survival in patients with malignant ventricular arrhythmias. *J Am Coll Cardiol* 11:1278-1286, 1988

234. Guarnieri T, Levine JH, Veltri EP, et al: Success of chronic defibrillation and the role of antiarrhythmic drugs with the automatic implantable cardioverter/defibrillator. *Am J Cardiol* 60:1061-1064, 1987

235. Bardy GH, Ivey TD, Johnson G, et al: Prospective evaluation of initially ineffective defibrillation pulses on subsequent defibrillation success during ventricular fibrillation in survivors of cardiac arrest. *Am J Cardiol* 62:718-722, 1988

236. Winkle RA, Bach SM Jr, Mead RH, et al: Comparison of defibrillation efficacy in humans using a new catheter and superior vena cava spring–left ventricular patch electrodes. *J Am Coll Cardiol* 11:365-370, 1988

237. Chapman PD, Vetter JW, Souza JJ, et al: Comparative efficacy of monophasic and biphasic truncated exponential shocks for nontho-

racotomy internal defibrillation in dogs. *J Am Coll Cardiol* 12:739-745, 1988

238. Marchlinski FE, Flores B, Miller JM, et al: Relation of the intraoperative defibrillation threshold to successful postoperative defibrillation with an automatic implantable cardioverter defibrillator. *Am J Cardiol* 62:393-398, 1988

239. Bardy GH, Ivey TD, Allen MD, et al: Prospective comparison of sequential pulse and single pulse defibrillation with use of two different clinically available systems. *J Am Coll Cardiol* 14:165-171, 1989

240. Klein LS, Miles WM, Zipes DP: Antitachycardia devices: realities and promises. *J Am Coll Cardiol* 18:1349-1362, 1991

241. Fogoros RN, Elson JJ, Bonnet CA, et al: Efficacy of the automatic implantable cardioverter-defibrillator in prolonging survival in patients with severe underlying cardiac disease. *J Am Coll Cardiol* 16:381-386, 1990

242. Levine JH, Mellits ED, Baumgardner RA, et al: Predictors of first discharge and subsequent survival in patients with automatic implantable cardioverter-defibrillators. *Circulation* 84:558-566, 1991

243. Kim SG, Fisher JD, Furman S, et al: Benefits of implantable defibrillators are overestimated by sudden death rates and better represented by the total arrhythmic death rate. *J Am Coll Cardiol* 17:1587-1592, 1991

244. Henthorn RW, Waller TJ, Hiratzka LF: Are the benefits of the automatic implantable cardioverter-defibrillator (AICD) overestimated by sudden death rate? *J Am Coll Cardiol* 17:1593-1594, 1991

245. Troup PJ: Implantable cardioverters and defibrillators. *Curr Probl Cardiol* 14:675-843, 1989

246. Fogoros RN, Elson JJ, Bonnet CA, et al: Long-term outcome of survivors of cardiac arrest whose therapy is guided by electrophysiologic testing. *J Am Coll Cardiol* 19:780-788, 1992

247. Wyndham CRC: Implantable cardioverter defibrillators: Where do we go from here? *J Am Coll Cardiol* 19:789-791, 1992

248. Mirowski M: The automatic implantable cardioverter-defibrillator: an overview. *J Am Coll Cardiol* 6:461-466, 1985

249. de Belder MA, Camm AJ: Implantable cardioverter-defibrillators (ICDs) 1989: How close are we to the ideal device? *Clin Cardiol* 12:339-345, 1989

250. Saksena S, Poczobutt-Johanos M, Castle LW, et al: Long-term multicenter experience with a second-generation implantable pacemaker-defibrillator in patients with malignant ventricular tachyarrhythmias. *J Am Coll Cardiol* 19:490-499, 1992

251. Yee R, Klein GJ, Leitch JW, et al: A permanent transvenous lead system for an implantable pacemaker cardioverter-defibrillator: nonthoracotomy approach to implantation. *Circulation* 85:196-204, 1992

252. Ropella KM, Baerman JM, Sahakian AV, et al: Differentiation of ventricular tachyarrhythmias. *Circulation* 82:2035-2043, 1990

253. Roy D, Waxman HL, Buxton AE, et al: Termination of ventricular tachycardia: role of tachycardia cycle length. *Am J Cardiol* 50:1346-1350, 1982

254. Leitch JW, Gillis AM, Wyse G, et al: Reduction in defibrillator shocks with an implantable device combining antitachycardia pacing and shock therapy. *Am J Cardiol* 18:145-151, 1991

255. Bardy GH, Allen MD, Mehra R, et al: Transvenous defibrillation in humans via the coronary sinus. *Circulation* 81:1252-1259, 1990

256. Miles WM, Prystowski EN, Heger JJ, et al: The implantable transvenous cardioverter: long-term efficacy and reproducible induction of ventricular tachycardia. *Circulation* 74:518-524, 1986

257. Saksena S, Parsonnet V: Implantation of a cardioverter/defibrillator without thoracotomy using a triple electrode system. *JAMA* 259:69-72, 1988

258. McCowan R, Maloney J, Wilkoff B, et al: Automatic implantable cardioverter-defibrillator implantation without thoracotomy using an endocardial and submuscular patch system. *J Am Coll Cardiol* 17:415-421, 1991

259. Stanton MS, Hayes DL, Munger TM, et al: Consistent subcutaneous prepectoral implantation of a new implantable cardioverter defibrillator. *Mayo Clin Proc* 69:309-314, 1994

260. Hook BG, Marchlinski FE: Value of ventricular electrogram recordings in the diagnosis of arrhythmias precipitating electrical device shock therapy. *J Am Coll Cardiol* 17:985-990, 1991

261. Horowitz LN, Harken AH, Josephson ME, et al: Surgical treatment of ventricular arrhythmias in coronary artery disease. *Ann Intern Med* 95:88-97, 1981

262. Wellens HJJ, Bär FWHM, Vanagt EJDM, et al: Medical treatment of ventricular tachycardia: considerations in the selection of patients for surgical treatment. *Am J Cardiol* 49:186-193, 1982

263. Guiraudon G, Fontaine G, Frank R, et al: Encircling endocardial ventriculotomy: a new surgical treatment for life-threatening ventricular tachycardias resistant to medical treatment following myocardial infarction. *Ann Thorac Surg* 26:438-443, 1978

264. Moss AJ, McDonald J: Unilateral cervicothoracic sympathetic ganglionectomy for the treatment of long QT interval syndrome. *N Engl J Med* 285:903-904, 1971

265. Sealy WC, Oldham HN: Surgical treatment of malignant ventricular arrhythmias by sympathectomy, coronary artery grafts and heart wall resection. In *International Symposium on Clinical Electrophysiology*. Edited by DT Kelly. Lane Cove, NSW Australia, Telectronics Pty, 1978, pp 218-224

266. Camm J, Ward DE, Spurrell RAJ, et al: Cryothermal mapping and cryoablation in the treatment of refractory cardiac arrhythmias. *Circulation* 62:67-74, 1980

267. Gallagher JJ, Anderson RW, Kasell J, et al: Cryoablation of drug-resistant ventricular tachycardia in a patient with a variant of scleroderma. *Circulation* 57:190-197, 1978

268. Horowitz LN, Josephson ME, Harken AH: Epicardial and endocardial activation during sustained ventricular tachycardia in man. *Circulation* 61:1227-1238, 1980

269. Mason JW, Stinson EB, Winkle RA, et al: Surgery for ventricular tachycardia: efficacy of left ventricular aneurysm resection compared with operation guided by electrical activation mapping. *Circulation* 65:1148-1155, 1982

270. Friedman PL, Stewart JR, Wit AL: Spontaneous and induced cardiac arrhythmias in subendocardial Purkinje fibers surviving extensive myocardial infarction in dogs. *Circ Res* 33:612-626, 1973

271. Gallagher JJ, Oldham HN, Wallace AG, et al: Ventricular aneurysm with ventricular tachycardia: report of a case with epicardial mapping and successful resection. *Am J Cardiol* 35:696-700, 1975

272. Horowitz LN, Spear JF, Moore EN: Subendocardial origin of ventricular arrhythmias in 24-hour-old experimental myocardial infarction. *Circulation* 53:56-63, 1976

273. Josephson ME, Horowitz LN, Spielman SR, et al: Role of catheter mapping in the preoperative evaluation of ventricular tachycardia. *Am J Cardiol* 49:207-220, 1982

274. Gallagher JJ, Kasell JH, Cox JL, et al: Techniques of intraoperative electrophysiologic mapping. *Am J Cardiol* 49:221-240, 1982

275. Littmann L, Svenson RH, Gallagher JJ, et al: Functional role of the epicardium in postinfarction ventricular tachycardia: observations derived from computerized epicardial activation map, entrainment, and epicardial laser photoablation. *Circulation* 83:1577-1591, 1991

276. Svenson RH, Littmann L, Gallagher JJ, et al: Termination of ventricular tachycardia with epicardial laser photocoagulation: a clinical comparison with patients undergoing successful endocardial photocoagulation alone. *J Am Coll Cardiol* 15:163-170, 1990

277. Spielman SR: Activation mapping in ventricular tachycardia: role of the epicardium. *J Am Coll Cardiol* 15:171-173, 1990

278. Abendroth R-R, Ostermeyer J, Breithardt G, et al: Reproducibility of local activation times during intraoperative epicardial mapping. *Circulation* 62:75-79, 1980

279. Vaitkus PT, Kindwall KE, Marchlinski FE, et al: Differences in electrophysiological substrate in patients with coronary artery disease and cardiac arrest for ventricular tachycardia: insights from endocardial mapping and signal-averaged electrocardiography. *Circulation* 84:672-678, 1991

280. Kaltenbrunner W, Cardinal R, Dubuc M, et al: Epicardial and endocardial mapping of ventricular tachycardia in patients with myocardial infarction: Is the origin of the tachycardia always subendocardially localized? *Circulation* 84:1058-1071, 1991

281. Mason JW, Stinson EB, Winkle RA, et al: Relative efficacy of blind left ventricular aneurysm resection for the treatment of recurrent ventricular tachycardia. *Am J Cardiol* 49:241-248, 1982

282. Zee-Cheng C-S, Kouchoukos NT, Connors JP, et al: Treatment of life-threatening ventricular arrhythmias with nonguided surgery supported by electrophysiologic testing and drug therapy. *J Am Coll Cardiol* 13:153-162, 1989

283. Kelly P, Ruskin JN, Vlahakes GJ, et al: Surgical coronary revascularization in survivors of prehospital cardiac arrest: its effect on inducible ventricular arrhythmias and long-term survival. *J Am Coll Cardiol* 15:267-273, 1990

284. Kaiser GA, Thurer RJ: Surgical approaches to treatment of ventricular arrhythmias. *J Am Coll Cardiol* 15:274, 1990

285. Fontaine G, Guiraudon G, Frank R, et al: Surgical management of ventricular tachycardia unrelated to myocardial ischemia or infarction. *Am J Cardiol* 49:397-410, 1982

286. Boineau JP, Cox JL: Rationale for a direct surgical approach to control ventricular arrhythmias: relation of specific intraoperative techniques to mechanism and location of arrhythmic circuit. *Am J Cardiol* 49:381-396, 1982

287. Ostermeyer J, Borggrefe M, Breithardt G, et al: Direct operations for the management of life-threatening ischemic ventricular tachycardia. *J Thorac Cardiovasc Surg* 94:848-861, 1987

288. Hargrove WC III, Josephson ME, Marchlinski FE, et al: Surgical decisions in the management of sudden cardiac death: subendocardial resection, the automatic internal defibrillator, or both. *J Thorac Cardiovasc Surg* 97:923-928, 1989

289. Kron IL, Lerman BB, Nolan SP, et al: Sequential endocardial resection for the surgical treatment of refractory ventricular tachycardia. *J Thorac Cardiovasc Surg* 94:843-847, 1987

290. Swerdlow CD, Moran JW, Stinson EB, et al: Results of operations for ventricular tachycardia in 105 patients. *J Thorac Cardiovasc Surg* 92:105-113, 1986

291. Kehoe R, Zheutlin T, Finkelmeier B, et al: Visually directed endocardial resection for ventricular arrhythmia: long term outcome and functional status (abstract). *J Am Coll Cardiol* 5:497, 1985

292. Lawrie GM, Pacifico A, Kaushik R, et al: Factors predictive of results of direct ablative operations for drug-refractory ventricular tachycardia: analysis of 80 patients. *J Thorac Cardiovasc Surg* 101:44-55, 1991

293. Landymore RW, Gardner MA, McIntyre AJ, et al: Surgical intervention for drug-resistant ventricular tachycardia. *J Am Coll Cardiol* 16:37-41, 1990

294. Garan H, Nguyen K, McGovern B, et al: Perioperative and long-term results after electrophysiologically directed ventricular surgery for recurrent ventricular tachycardia. *J Am Coll Cardiol* 8:201-209, 1986

295. Miller JM, Gottlieb CD, Hargrove WC, et al: Factors influencing operative mortality in surgery for ventricular tachycardia (abstract). *Circulation* 78 Suppl 2:44, 1988

296. Caceres J, Werner P, Jazayeri M, et al: Efficacy of cryosurgery alone for refractory monomorphic sustained ventricular tachycardia due to inferior wall infarction. *J Am Coll Cardiol* 11:1254-1259, 1988

297. Svenson RH, Gallagher JJ, Selle JG, et al: Neodymium:YAG laser photocoagulation: a successful new map-guided technique for the intraoperative ablation of ventricular tachycardia. *Circulation* 76:1319-1328, 1987

298. Saksena S, Hussain M, Gielchinsky I, et al: Intraoperative mapping-guided argon laser ablation of malignant ventricular tachycardia. *Am J Cardiol* 59:78-83, 1987

299. Waxman MB, Wald RW, Finley JP, et al: Valsalva termination of ventricular tachycardia. *Circulation* 62:843-851, 1980

300. Lown B, Podrid PJ, DeSilva RA, et al: Sudden cardiac death: management of the patient at risk. *Curr Probl Cardiol* 4:1-62, March 1980

301. Michelson EL, Morganroth J: Spontaneous variability of complex ventricular arrhythmias detected by long-term electrocardiographic recording. *Circulation* 61:690-695, 1980

302. Platia EV, Reid PR: Comparison of programmed electrical stimulation and ambulatory electrocardiographic (Holter) monitoring in the management of ventricular tachycardia and ventricular fibrillation. *J Am Coll Cardiol* 4:493-500, 1984

303. Kim SG, Seiden SW, Matos JA, et al: Discordance between ambulatory monitoring and programmed stimulation in assessing efficacy of class IA antiarrhythmic agents in patients with ventricular tachycardia. *J Am Coll Cardiol* 6:539-544, 1985

304. Kim SG, Seiden SW, Felder SD, et al: Is programmed stimulation of value in predicting the long-term success of antiarrhythmic therapy for ventricular tachycardias? *N Engl J Med* 315:356-362, 1986

305. Campbell RWF: Arrhythmias in mitral valve prolapse. *Pract Cardiol* 8:124-135, 1982

306. Mills P, Rose J, Hollingsworth J, et al: Long-term prognosis of mitral-valve prolapse. *N Engl J Med* 297:13-18, 1977

307. Barlow JB, Bosman CK, Pocock WA, et al: Late systolic murmurs and non-ejection ("mid-late") systolic clicks: an analysis of 90 patients. *Br Heart J* 30:203-218, 1968

308. Swartz MH, Teichholz LE, Donoso E: Mitral valve prolapse: a review of associated arrhythmias. *Am J Med* 62:377-389, 1977

309. Dollar AL, Roberts WC: Morphologic comparison of patients with mitral valve prolapse who died suddenly with patients who died from severe valvular dysfunction or other conditions. *J Am Coll Cardiol* 17:921-931, 1991

310. Düren DR, Becker AE, Dunning AJ: Long-term follow-up of idiopathic mitral valve prolapse in 300 patients: a prospective study. *J Am Coll Cardiol* 11:42-47, 1988

311. Kostuk WJ, Boughner DR: Strokes: a complication of mitral-leaflet prolapse? *Lancet* 2:313-316, 1977

312. Darsee JR, Mikolich JR, Nicoloff NB, et al: Prevalence of mitral valve prolapse in presumably healthy young men. *Circulation* 59:619-622, 1979

313. Markiewicz W, Stoner J, London E, et al: Mitral valve prolapse in one hundred presumably healthy young females. *Circulation* 53:464-473, 1976

314. Campbell RWF, Godman MG, Fiddler GI, et al: Ventricular arrhythmias in syndrome of balloon deformity of mitral valve: definition of possible high risk group. *Br Heart J* 38:1053-1057, 1976

315. Ritchie JL, Hammermeister KE, Kennedy JW: Refractory ventricular tachycardia and fibrillation in a patient with the prolapsing mitral leaflet syndrome: successful control with overdrive pacing. *Am J Cardiol* 37:314-316, 1976

316. Jeresaty RM: Sudden death in the mitral valve prolapse-click syndrome. *Am J Cardiol* 37:317-318, 1976

317. Shen W-K, Holmes DR Jr, Hammill SC: Transtelephonic monitoring: documentation of transient cardiac rhythm disturbances. *Mayo Clin Proc* 62:109-112, 1987

318. Morady F, Shen E, Bhandari A, et al: Programmed ventricular stimulation in mitral valve prolapse: analysis of 36 patients. *Am J Cardiol* 53:135-138, 1984

319. Rosenthal ME, Hamer A, Gang ES, et al: The yield of programmed ventricular stimulation in mitral valve prolapse patients with ventricular arrhythmias. *Am Heart J* 110:970-976, 1985

320. Kavey RW, Sondheimer HM, Blackman MS: Detection of dysrhythmia in pediatric patients with mitral valve prolapse. *Circulation* 62:582-587, 1980

321. Sloman G, Wong M, Walker J: Arrhythmias on exercise in patients with abnormalities of the posterior leaflet of the mitral valve. *Am Heart J* 83:312-317, 1972

322. Winkle RA, Lopes MG, Goodman DJ, et al: Propranolol for patients with mitral valve prolapse. *Am Heart J* 93:422-427, 1977

323. Gooch AS, Vicencio F, Maranhao V, et al: Arrhythmias and left ventricular asynergy in the prolapsing mitral leaflet syndrome. *Am J Cardiol* 29:611-620, 1972

324. Wit AL, Fenoglio JJ Jr, Hordof AJ, et al: Ultrastructure and transmembrane potentials of cardiac muscle in the human anterior mitral valve leaflet. *Circulation* 59:1284-1292, 1979

325. Wei JY, Bulkley BH, Schaeffer AH, et al: Mitral-valve prolapse syndrome and recurrent ventricular tachyarrhythmias: a malignant variant refractory to conventional drug therapy. *Ann Intern Med* 89:6-9, 1978

326. Troup PJ, Zipes DP: Aprindine treatment of recurrent ventricular tachycardia in patients with mitral valve prolapse. *Am Heart J* 97:322-328, 1979

327. Anderson KP, Stinson EB, Derby GC, et al: Vulnerability of patients with obstructive hypertrophic cardiomyopathy to ventricular arrhythmia induction in the operating room: analysis of 17 patients. *Am J Cardiol* 51:811-816, 1983

328. Schiavone WA, Maloney JD, Lever HM, et al: Electrophysiologic studies of patients with hypertrophic cardiomyopathy presenting with syncope of undetermined etiology. *PACE* 9:476-481, 1986

329. Watson RM, Schwartz JL, Maron BJ, et al: Inducible polymorphic ventricular tachycardia and ventricular fibrillation in a subgroup of patients with hypertrophic cardiomyopathy at high risk for sudden death. *J Am Coll Cardiol* 10:761-774, 1987

330. Kuck K-H, Kunze K-P, Schlüter IM, et al: Programmed electrical stimulation in hypertrophic cardiomyopathy. Results in patients with and without cardiac arrest or syncope. *Eur Heart J* 9:177-185, 1988

331. Kowey PR, Eisenberg R, Engel TR: Sustained arrhythmias in hypertrophic obstructive cardiomyopathy. *N Engl J Med* 310:1566-1569, 1984

332. Fananapazir L, Tracy CM, Leon MB, et al: Electrophysiologic abnormalities in patients with hypertrophic cardiomyopathy: a consecutive analysis in 155 patients. *Circulation* 80:1259-1268, 1989

333. Maron BJ, Fananapazir L: Sudden cardiac death in hypertrophic cardiomyopathy. *Circulation* 85 Suppl 1:57-63, 1992

334. McKenna WJ, Camm AJ: Sudden death in hypertrophic cardiomyopathy: assessment of patients at high risk. *Circulation* 80:1489-1492, 1989

335. McKenna WJ, Harris L, Perez G, et al: Arrhythmia in hypertrophic cardiomyopathy. II: Comparison of amiodarone and verapamil in treatment. *Br Heart J* 46:173-178, 1981

336. McKenna WJ, Chetty S, Oakley CM, et al: Arrhythmia in hypertrophic cardiomyopathy: exercise and 48 hour ambulatory electrocardiographic assessment with and without beta adrenergic blocking therapy. *Am J Cardiol* 45:1-5, 1980

337. Spirito P, Watson RM, Maron BJ: Relation between extent of left ventricular hypertrophy and occurrence of ventricular tachycardia in hypertrophic cardiomyopathy. *Am J Cardiol* 60:1137-1142, 1987

338. Nienaber CA, Hiller S, Spielmann RP, et al: Syncope in hypertrophic cardiomyopathy: multivariate analysis of prognostic determinants. *J Am Coll Cardiol* 15:948-955, 1990

339. Cripps TR, Counihan PJ, Frenneaux MP, et al: Signal-averaged electrocardiography and hypertrophic cardiomyopathy. *J Am Coll Cardiol* 15:956-961, 1990

340. Brandenburg RO: Syncope and sudden death in hypertrophic cardiomyopathy. *J Am Coll Cardiol* 15:962-964, 1990

341. Fananapazir L, Barbour DJ, Winkler JB: Signal-averaged electrocardiographic identification of patients with inducible ventricular tachycardia with hypertrophic cardiomyopathy (abstract). *Circulation* 78 Suppl 2:51, 1988

342. Maron BJ, Lipson LC, Roberts WC, et al: "Malignant" hypertrophic cardiomyopathy: identification of a subgroup of families with unusually frequent premature death. *Am J Cardiol* 41:1133-1140, 1978

343. Maron BJ, Savage DD, Wolfson J, et al: Prognostic significance of 24 hour ambulatory electrocardiographic monitoring in patients with hypertrophic cardiomyopathy: a prospective study. *Am J Cardiol* 48:252-257, 1981

344. Wessel HU, Bastanier CK, Paul MH, et al: Prognostic significance of arrhythmia in tetralogy of Fallot after intracardiac repair. *Am J Cardiol* 46:843-848, 1980

345. Horowitz LN, Vetter VL, Harken AH, et al: Electrophysiologic characteristics of sustained ventricular tachycardia occurring after repair of tetralogy of Fallot. *Am J Cardiol* 46:446-452, 1980

346. Houyel L, Vaksmann G, Fournier NA, et al: Ventricular arrhythmias after correction of ventricular septal defects: importance of surgical approach. *J Am Coll Cardiol* 16:1224-1228, 1990

347. Shen W-K, Holmes DR Jr, Porter CJ, et al: Sudden death after repair of double-outlet right ventricle. *Circulation* 81:128-136, 1990

348. Ross J Jr, Braunwald E: Aortic stenosis. *Circulation* 38 Suppl 5:61-67, 1968

349. Samuels DA, Curfman GD, Friedlich AL, et al: Valve replacement for aortic regurgitation: long-term follow-up with factors influencing the results. *Circulation* 60:647-654, 1979

350. Rubin JW, Moore HV, Hillson RF, et al: Thirteen year experience with aortic valve replacement. *Am J Cardiol* 40:345-354, 1977

351. Starr A, Gurnkemeier GL, Lambert LE, et al: Aortic valve replacement: a ten-year follow-up of non-cloth-covered vs cloth-covered caged-ball prostheses. *Circulation* 56 Suppl 2:133-139, 1977

352. Duvoisin GE, Wallace RB, Ellis FH Jr, et al: Late results of cardiac-valve replacement. *Circulation* 37 Suppl 2:75-85, 1968

353. Barratt-Boyes BG, Roche AHG, Whitlock RML: Six year review of the results of freehand aortic valve replacement using an antibiotic sterilized homograft valve. *Circulation* 55:353-361, 1977

354. Lee SJK, Barr C, Callaghan JC, et al: Long-term survival after aortic valve replacement using Smeloff-Cutter prosthesis. *Circulation* 52:1132-1137, 1975

355. Gradman AH, Harbison MA, Berger HJ, et al: Ventricular arrhythmias late after aortic valve replacement and their relation to left ventricular performance. *Am J Cardiol* 48:824-831, 1981

356. Winkle RA, Alderman EL, Fitzgerald JW, et al: Treatment of recurrent symptomatic ventricular tachycardia. *Ann Intern Med* 85:1-7, 1976

357. Jelinek MV, Lohrbauer L, Lown B: Antiarrhythmic drug therapy for sporadic ventricular ectopic arrhythmias. *Circulation* 49:659-666, 1974

358. Myerburg RJ, Conde C, Sheps DS, et al: Antiarrhythmic drug therapy in survivors of prehospital cardiac arrest: comparison of effects on chronic ventricular arrhythmias and recurrent cardiac arrest. *Circulation* 59:855-863, 1979

359. Wellens HJJ, Bär FWHM, Lie KI, et al: Effects of procainamide, propranolol and verapamil on mechanism of tachycardia in patients with chronic recurrent ventricular tachycardia. *Am J Cardiol* 40:579-585, 1977

360. Schaffer WA, Cobb LA: Recurrent ventricular fibrillation and modes of death in survivors of out-of-hospital ventricular fibrillation. *N Engl J Med* 293:259-262, 1975

361. Koster RW, Wellens HJJ: Quinidine-induced ventricular flutter and fibrillation without digitalis therapy. *Am J Cardiol* 38:519-523, 1976

362. Selzer A, Wray HW: Quinidine syncope: paroxysmal ventricular fibrillation occurring during treatment of chronic atrial arrhythmias. *Circulation* 30:17-26, 1964

363. Jenzer HR, Hagemeijer F: Quinidine syncope: torsade de pointes with low quinidine plasma concentrations. *Eur J Cardiol* 4:447-451, 1976

364. Falk RH: Flecainide-induced ventricular tachycardia and fibrillation in patients treated for atrial fibrillation. *Ann Intern Med* 111:107-111, 1989

365. McKibbin JK, Pocock WA, Barlow JB, et al: Sotalol, hypokalaemia, syncope, and torsade de pointes. *Br Heart J* 51:157-162, 1984

366. Anderson JL: Reassessment of benefit-risk ratio and treatment algorithms for antiarrhythmic drug therapy after the Cardiac Arrhythmia Suppression Trial. *J Clin Pharmacol* 30:981-989, 1990

367. Salerno DM: Quinidine: Worse than adverse? *Circulation* 84:2196-2198, 1991

368. Hine LK, Laird N, Hewitt P, et al: Meta-analytic evidence against prophylactic use of lidocaine in acute myocardial infarction. *Arch Intern Med* 149:2694-2698, 1989

369. Pritchett ELC: Management of atrial fibrillation. *N Engl J Med* 326:1264-1271, 1992

370. Rae AP, Kay HR, Horowitz LN, et al: Proarrhythmic effects of antiarrhythmic drugs in patients with malignant ventricular arrhythmias evaluated by electrophysiologic testing. *J Am Coll Cardiol* 12:131-139, 1988

371. Uhl HS: A previously undescribed congenital malformation of the heart: almost total absence of the myocardium of the right ventricle. *Bull Johns Hopkins Hosp* 91:197-209, 1952

372. Manyari DE, Klein GJ, Gulamhusein S, et al: Arrhythmogenic right ventricular dysplasia: a generalized cardiomyopathy? *Circulation* 68:251-257, 1983

373. Marcus FI, Fontaine GH, Guiraudon G, et al: Right ventricular dysplasia: a report of 24 adult cases. *Circulation* 65:384-398, 1982

374. Fontaine G, Guiraudon G, Frank R: Mechanism of ventricular tachycardia with and without associated chronic myocardial ischemia: surgical management based on epicardial mapping. In *Cardiac Arrhythmias: Electrophysiology, Diagnosis and Management.* Edited by OS Narula. Baltimore, Williams & Wilkins Company, 1979, pp 516-545

375. Fontaine G, Frank R, Guiraudon G, et al: Relevant investigations in the diagnosis and treatment of resistant ventricular tachycardia in patients without coronary artery disease. In *International Symposium on Clinical Electrophysiology.* Edited by DT Kelly. Lane Cove, NSW Australia, Telectronics Pty, 1978, pp 184-203

376. Frank R, Fontaine G, Vedel J, et al: Electrocardiologie de quatre cas de dysplasie ventriculaire droite arythmogène. *Arch Mal Coeur* 71:963-972, 1978

377. Fontaine G, Guiraudon G, Frank R, et al: Stimulation studies and epicardial mapping in ventricular tachycardia: study of mechanisms and selection for surgery. In *Re-entrant Arrhythmias: Mechanisms and Treatment.* Edited by HE Kulbertus. Baltimore, University Park Press, 1976, pp 334-350

378. Lemery R, Brugada P, Janssen J, et al: Nonischemic sustained ventricular tachycardia: clinical outcome in 12 patients with arrhythmogenic right ventricular dysplasia. *J Am Coll Cardiol* 14:96-105, 1989

379. Nava A, Thiene G, Canciani B, et al: Familial occurrence of right ventricular dysplasia: a study involving nine families. *J Am Coll Cardiol* 12:1222-1228, 1988

380. Isner JM, Sours HE, Paris AL, et al: Sudden, unexpected death in avid dieters using the liquid-protein-modified-fast diet: observations in 17 patients and the role of the prolonged QT interval. *Circulation* 60:1401-1412, 1979

381. Singh BN, Gaarder TD, Kanegae T, et al: Liquid protein diets and *torsade de pointes. JAMA* 240:115-119, 1978

382. Brown JM, Yetter JF, Spicer MJ, et al: Cardiac complications of protein-sparing modified fasting. *JAMA* 240:120-122, 1978

383. Lantigua RA, Amatruda JM, Biddle TL, et al: Cardiac arrhythmias associated with a liquid protein diet for the treatment of obesity. *N Engl J Med* 303:735-738, 1980

384. Dessertenne F: La tachycardie ventriculaire à deux foyers opposés variables. *Arch Mal Coeur* 59:263-272, 1966

385. Smith WM, Gallagher JJ: "Les torsades de pointes": an unusual ventricular arrhythmia. *Ann Intern Med* 93:578-584, 1980

386. Soffer J, Dreifus LS, Michelson EL: Polymorphous ventricular tachycardia associated with normal and long Q-T intervals. *Am J Cardiol* 49:2021-2029, 1982

387. Krikler DM, Curry PVL: *Torsade de pointes,* an atypical ventricular tachycardia. *Br Heart J* 38:117-120, 1976

388. Binder MJ, Rosove L: Paroxysmal ventricular tachycardia and fibrillation due to quinidine. *Am J Med* 12:491-497, 1952

389. Oravetz J, Slodki SJ: Recurrent ventricular fibrillation precipitated by quinidine: report of a patient with recovery after 28 paroxysms. *Arch Intern Med* 122:63-65, 1968

390. Strasberg B, Sclarovsky S, Erdberg A, et al: Procainamide-induced polymorphous ventricular tachycardia. *Am J Cardiol* 47:1309-1314, 1981

391. Nicholson WJ, Martin CE, Gracey JG, et al: Disopyramide-induced ventricular fibrillation. *Am J Cardiol* 43:1053-1055, 1979

392. Schwartz PJ, Periti M, Malliani A: The long Q-T syndrome. *Am Heart J* 89:378-390, 1975

393. Weintraub RG, Gow RM, Wilkinson JL: The congenital long QT syndromes in childhood. *J Am Coll Cardiol* 16:674-680, 1990

394. Moss AJ, Robinson J: Clinical features of the idiopathic long QT syndrome. *Circulation* 85 Suppl 1:140-144, 1992

395. Fontaine GH, Frank R, Welti JJ, et al: Electrophysiology of torsades de pointes. In *Proceedings of the VI World Symposium on Cardiac Pacing.* Edited by C Meere. Montreal, Pacesym, 1979, chap 6

396. Radford MD, Evans DW: Long-term results of DC reversion of atrial fibrillation. *Br Heart J* 30:91-96, 1968

397. McComb JM, Logan KR, Khan MM, et al: Amiodarone induced ventricular fibrillation. *Eur J Cardiol* 11:381-385, 1980

398. Ludomirsky A, Klein HO, Sarelli P, et al: Q-T prolongation and polymorphous ("torsade de pointes") ventricular arrhythmias associated with organophosphorus insecticide poisoning. *Am J Cardiol* 49:1654-1658, 1982

399. Kiss Z, Fazekas T: Arrhythmias in organophosphate poisonings. *Acta Cardiol* 34:322-330, 1979

400. Fowler NO, McCall D, Chou T-C, et al: Electrocardiographic changes and cardiac arrhythmias in patients receiving psychotropic drugs. *Am J Cardiol* 37:223-230, 1976

401. Moore MT, Book MH: Sudden death in phenothiazine therapy (a clinicopathologic study of 12 cases). *Psychiatr Q* 44:389-402, 1970

402. Schoonmaker FW, Osteen RT, Greenfield JC Jr: Thioridazine (Mellaril®)-induced ventricular tachycardia controlled with an artificial pacemaker. *Ann Intern Med* 65:1076-1078, 1966

403. Giles TD, Modlin RK: Death associated with ventricular arrhythmia and thioridazine hydrochloride. *JAMA* 205:108-110, 1968

404. Curry P, Fitchett D, Stubbs W, et al: Ventricular arrhythmias and hypokalaemia. *Lancet* 2:231-233, 1976

405. Loeb HS, Pietras RJ, Gunnar RM, et al: Paroxysmal ventricular fibrillation in two patients with hypomagnesemia: treatment by transvenous pacing. *Circulation* 37:210-215, 1968

406. Khan MM, Logan KR, McComb JM, et al: Management of recurrent ventricular tachyarrhythmias associated with Q-T prolongation. *Am J Cardiol* 47:1301-1308, 1981

407. Kaplinsky E, Yahini JH, Barzilai J, et al: Quinidine syncope: report of a case successfully treated with lidocaine. *Chest* 62:764-766, 1972

408. VanderArk CR, Reynolds EW, Kahn DR, et al: Quinidine syncope: a report of successful treatment with bretylium tosylate. *J Thorac Cardiovasc Surg* 72:464-467, 1976

409. De Azevedo IM, Watanabe Y, Dreifus LS: Electrophysiologic antagonism of quinidine and bretylium tosylate. *Am J Cardiol* 33:633-638, 1974

410. Keren A, Tzivoni D, Gavish D, et al: Etiology, warning signs and therapy of torsade de pointes: a study of 10 patients. *Circulation* 64:1167-1174, 1981

411. DiSegni E, Klein HO, David D, et al: Overdrive pacing in quinidine syncope and other long QT-interval syndromes. *Arch Intern Med* 140:1036-1040, 1980

412. Anderson JL, Mason JW: Successful treatment by overdrive pacing of recurrent quinidine syncope due to ventricular tachycardia. *Am J Med* 64:715-718, 1978

413. Tzivoni D, Keren A, Cohen AM, et al: Magnesium therapy for torsades de pointes. *Am J Cardiol* 53:528-530, 1984

414. Eldar M, Griffin JC, Abbott JA, et al: Permanent cardiac pacing in patients with the long QT syndrome. *J Am Coll Cardiol* 10:600-607, 1987

415. Schwartz PJ, Locati EH, Moss AJ, et al: Left cardiac sympathetic denervation in the therapy of congenital long QT syndrome: a worldwide report. *Circulation* 84:503-511, 1991

416. Hartzler GO, Osborn MJ: Invasive electrophysiological study in the Jervell and Lange-Nielsen syndrome. *Br Heart J* 45:225-229, 1981

417. Hiejima K, Suzuki F, Satake S, et al: Electrophysiologic studies of Jervell, Lange-Nielsen syndrome. *Chest* 79:446-448, 1981

418. Evans TR, Curry PVL, Fitchett DH, et al: "Torsade de pointes" initiated by electrical ventricular stimulation. *J Electrocardiol* 9:255-258, 1976

419. Horowitz LN, Greenspan AM, Spielman SR, et al: Torsade de pointes: electrophysiologic studies in patients without transient pharmacologic or metabolic abnormalities. *Circulation* 63:1120-1128, 1981

420. Gallavardin L: Extra-systolie ventriculaire à paroxysmes tachycardiques prolongés. *Arch Mal Coeur* 15:298-306, 1922

421. Froment R, Gallavardin L, Cahen P: Paroxysmal ventricular tachycardia: a clinical classification. *Br Heart J* 15:172-178, 1953

422. Parkinson J, Papp C: Repetitive paroxysmal tachycardia. *Br Heart J* 9:241-262, 1947

423. Dimond EG, Hayes WL: Benign paroxysmal ventricular tachycardia: report of a case. *Ann Intern Med* 53:1255-1260, 1960

424. Maddox K: Intermittent ventricular tachycardia in youth: report of case with fatal termination (abstract). *Am Heart J* 33:739-740, 1947

425. Wilson FN, Wishart SW, Macleod AG, et al: A clinical type of paroxysmal tachycardia of ventricular origin in which paroxysms are induced by exertion. *Am Heart J* 8:155-169, 1932

426. Steffens TG, Pierce PL, Zegerius RJ: Multiple ventricular premature beats in five adolescents. *Eur J Cardiol* 8:177-184, 1978

427. Rally CR, Walters MB: Paroxysmal ventricular tachycardia without evident heart disease. *Can Med Assoc J* 86:268-273, 1962

428. Zimmermann M, Maisonblanche P, Cauchemez B, et al: Determinants of the spontaneous ectopic activity in repetitive monomorphic idiopathic ventricular tachycardia. *J Am Coll Cardiol* 7:1219-1227, 1986

CHAPTER

22

Cardiac arrhythmias

D. Clinical electrophysiologic assessment

Win-Kuang Shen, M.D., and David R. Holmes, Jr., M.D.

SINCE the 1950s, advances in catheter techniques, coupled with the development of programmed electrical stimulation, endocardial and epicardial mapping, and nonpharmacologic therapy, have resulted in the exceptionally rapid growth of clinical electrophysiology. Growth continues in this area as new mapping and stimulation techniques and effective antitachycardia devices are developed and applied in additional populations (e.g., ablation in patients with supraventricular[1-6] and ventricular[3,7-11] tachycardia [see chapter 26] and the implantable cardioverter-defibrillator[12-21] in patients with high risk of sudden cardiac death or sustained ventricular arrhythmias).

The objectives of clinical electrophysiologic assessment have continued to change since this approach was described in 1969.[22,23] At present the major aims[24] are for diagnosis or therapy.

1. Identification and analysis of the conduction system, including sinus node function and intra-atrial, AV node, and His-Purkinje conduction and refractoriness.
2. Evaluation of supraventricular and ventricular tachycardia with specific attention to the electrophysiologic anatomic substrate, mechanism, and site of tachycardia.
3. Identification of optimal treatment regimens by serial drug testing.
4. Evaluation of patients with suspected symptomatic bradyarrhythmias and those with syncope or near syncope of unknown cause.
5. Determination of cause in and optimal therapy for survivors of sudden cardiac arrest.
6. Risk stratification for therapeutic need in patients with increased risk for ventricular tachycardia or sudden cardiac arrest.
7. Assessment of patients for placement of an implantable cardioverter-defibrillator (ICD) (see chapter 25B).
8. Ablative therapy for patients with various types of supraventricular and ventricular tachyarrhythmias (see chapter 26).

The techniques used for evaluation of these areas of interest vary depending on the aim of the study. Assessment of these techniques involves knowledge of basic electrophysiologic terminology (Table 22D-1).[25]

TECHNICAL CONSIDERATIONS

Catheter selection and placement

Techniques, systems, and protocols for electrophysiologic testing vary from institution to institution. Catheter selection and placement depend on personal preference of the electrophysiologist, catheter availability, patient population studied (pediatric or adult), and clinical problem at hand. In our laboratory, woven polyester fiber (Dacron) catheters, sizes 5 to 7 French, are usually used during diagnostic studies. Smaller catheters are available and are useful in infants and small children. These catheters may be resterilized and reused if properly handled. Mapping and ablation catheters are discussed in chapter 26.

Electrode number, distance between electrodes, and configuration also vary widely (Fig 22D-1). Probably the most common type of diagnostic catheter has a 10-mm interelectrode distance in a sequential configuration. Selection of a specific catheter depends on the use for which it is intended. The number of electrodes per catheter varies from 2 to 12. The multiple-electrode catheters with more than four electrodes are used for recording from several sites simultaneously—e.g., during endocardial mapping. During a diagnostic study, tripolar and quadripolar catheters are used most often; the tripolar catheters are used for His bundle recording and the quadripolar for simultaneous stimulation and recording from the right atrium or right ventricle. An orthogonal catheter is best suited for coronary sinus pacing and recording. Other catheters are available with various electrode configurations or with special features, which include lumens for pressure monitoring and thermodilution sensors. In addition, an electrode catheter that fits over a modified transseptal stylet has been designed for atrial mapping in patients with atrial tachycardia or preexcitation syndromes.[26]

Placement of the catheters is also dictated by the

Table 22D-1 Definitions of electrophysiologic terms

Antegrade conduction: Conduction that proceeds from the atrium to the ventricle. The conduction can be over the normal AV conduction system or an accessory AV pathway
Automatic rhythm: Automatic rhythms can occur throughout the heart and result when cells undergo spontaneous diastolic (phase IV) depolarization and reach the threshold at a rate that is faster than the rate of the normal sinus rhythm
Concealed conduction: The effect of incomplete penetration of an impulse that can result in the following unexpected findings on an ECG: (1) a spontaneous pacemaker that demonstrates pauses; (2) failure of an impulse to propagate normally, resulting in high-grade block; and (3) prolongation of conduction, resulting in first-degree conduction block
Conduction intervals:
- *HV:* The time from the onset of depolarization of the His bundle to the onset of ventricular activity (usually recorded by an endocardial electrode). The range for the normal HV intervals is 35 to 55 msec
- *PP:* The time between two consecutive P waves
- *PR:* The time from the onset of the P wave to the onset of the QRS complex
- *QT:* The time from the onset of the Q wave to the termination of the T wave
- *RP:* The time from the onset of ventricular activity to the onset of atrial activity as manifested by the P wave. This interval is present when there is retrograde conduction from the ventricle to the atrium
- *VA:* The time from the onset of ventricular activity to the onset of atrial activity. This measurement is usually obtained by using intracardiac recordings or recordings of atrial activity from the esophagus

Escape complex: Any complex that occurs later than the time of the next expected complex
Mapping: The electrophysiologic procedure used to identify the anatomic location and conduction sequence of supraventricular or ventricular arrhythmias. The procedure is used before or at the time of catheter ablation (fulguration) or surgical procedures to treat tachycardia
Normal AV conduction system: The AV node, His bundle, and Purkinje fibers (also referred to as the "specialized conduction system")
Paroxysmal tachycardia: An arrhythmia that is present intermittently and has an abrupt onset and an abrupt termination
Programmed stimulation: The systematic introduction of single or multiple critically timed extrastimuli during a sensed or paced rhythm. Either the atrium or the ventricle is stimulated to stress the sinus node and AV conduction system or to induce supraventricular or ventricular tachycardia
Reentrant rhythm: Also referred to as a reciprocating rhythm, this rhythm abnormality can occur in multiple locations within the heart. A reentrant circuit consists of two functionally distinct pathways that join proximally and distally to create a closed conduction circuit. A critically timed impulse will encounter this circuit at a time when one of the limbs is refractory to conduction and the other limb is able to maintain conduction (unidirectional block). The conduction proceeds slowly down the unblocked pathway; thus, the previously blocked pathway is granted time to recover its ability to conduct the impulse. As the impulse reaches the distal end of the second pathway, it returns to the proximal common pathway and completes the reentrant circuit. If a single reentrant beat is produced, it is known as a reentrant, echo, or reciprocating beat. If the electrical impulse continues to move around the reentrant circuit, a reentrant tachycardia develops. Reentry may involve a microcircuit that includes a small area within the heart, such as the AV node or areas of ventricle associated with myocardial infarction, or a macrocircuit that encompasses larger areas of the heart, including the atria, ventricles, or His-Purkinje system
Refractory periods:
- *Effective:* The longest interval between two impulses that fail to be conducted through the tissue
- *Functional:* The shortest interval that can be obtained between two consecutively conducted impulses
- *Relative:* Prolongation of conduction of a premature impulse marking the end of the full recovery period

Retrograde conduction: Conduction that proceeds from the ventricle to the atrium. The conduction can be over the normal AV conduction system or an accessory AV pathway
Supraventricular impulses: Impulses that originate proximal to or within the His bundle
Ventricular impulses: Impulses that originate distal to the His bundle

From Hammill SC, Sugrue DD, Gersh BJ, et all: Clinical intracardiac electrophysiologic testing: technique, diagnostic indications, and therapeutic uses. *Mayo Clin Proc* 61:478-503, 1986. By permission, Mayo Foundation.

clinical problem and the available access to the circulation. In our laboratory, the catheters are introduced via the femoral veins with the use of local anesthesia and standard percutaneous techniques. Access via the right femoral vein is usually somewhat easier than that via the left femoral vein, although either can be used. Usually, three catheters are introduced through the same femoral vein: (1) a quadripolar catheter, the tip of which is placed in the right atrial appendage; (2) a tripolar catheter positioned across the tricuspid valve for His bundle recording; and (3) a quadripolar catheter, the tip of which is placed in the right ventricular apex. In patients with preexcitation or in those with suspected supraventricular tachycardia, a quadripolar or an orthogonal catheter is also placed in the coronary sinus to record left atrial and left ventricular depolarization (Fig 22D-2). This catheter

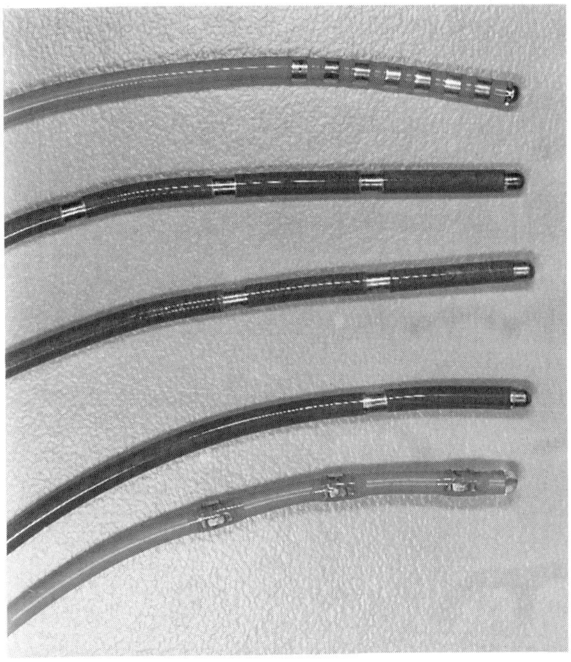

Fig 22D-1 Catheters used during electrophysiologic testing. From top to bottom: octopolar catheter, which may be used for atrial and ventricular stimulation or His bundle recording; quadripolar catheter for atrial and ventricular recording and stimulation; tripolar catheter for His bundle recording and pacing; bipolar catheter for either recording or stimulation; and orthogonal catheter, usually for coronary sinus recording and pacing.

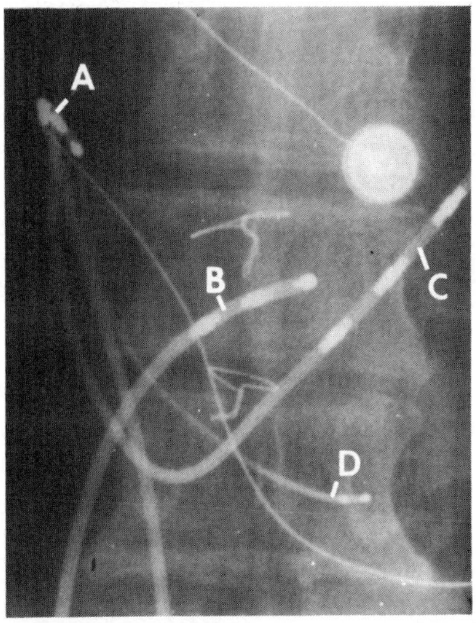

Fig 22D-2 Positioning of catheters in the heart: *A,* high right atrial quadripolar catheter for recording and stimulation, *B,* tripolar catheter for His bundle recording, *C,* coronary sinus catheter for recording and stimulation, and *D,* bipolar right ventricular catheter for recording or stimulation.

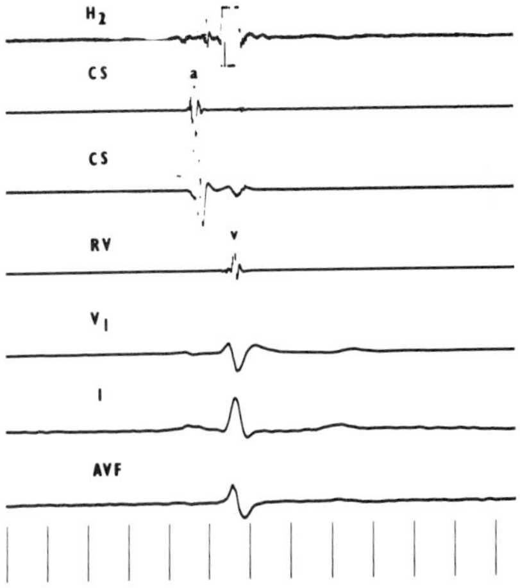

Fig 22D-3 Baseline recording from high right atrium *(HRA),* two His bundle channels *(H_1, H_2),* two coronary sinus recordings *(CS),* right ventricle *(RV),* and three surface ECG leads *(V_1, I,* and *aV_F). a,* atrial activation; *h,* His bundle potential; *v,* ventricular activation.

is usually introduced percutaneously from either the subclavian or the right internal jugular vein, although it may also be easily placed from the left arm. In patients in whom stimulation or recording of left ventricular events is required, this may be accomplished by placement of the catheter by a retrograde approach from the femoral or brachial arteries, via a patent foramen ovale, or by the transseptal technique.

Other placement techniques have been described and are used according to the specific patient and clinical problem.[27-29a] Placement of catheters for recording and stimulating the right atrium and left atrium and also the His bundle and right ventricle can be accomplished from brachial, subclavian, or jugular approaches. Stable positioning, however, particularly of the His bundle catheter, may be somewhat more difficult from the upper extremity approach.

Recording apparatus

Electrophysiologic studies may be performed and recorded in dedicated electrophysiology laboratories or in general catheterization laboratories. Commercially produced computerized recording and analysis units are available that combine filters, single or multiple oscilloscopes, monitors, and a paper recorder or a printer. In addition, tape recorders and storage oscilloscopes are incorporated in many laboratories. During a study, 4 to 16 intracardiac electrograms can be displayed simultaneously. These usually include recordings from the high right atrium, two His bundle channels, the right ventricular apex, and often the coronary sinus (Fig 22D-3). These channels require both high- and low-band-pass filters to record optimal signals (the usual setting is 40 to 400 mHz). In addition to the intracardiac electrograms, three surface electrocardiograms (ECGs) are usually recorded simultaneously to assess P-wave and QRS configuration, duration, and axis.

The recorder used must be able to generate high-quality records for both storage and analysis. Several commercial recorders are available. Some are ink-jet types; electrostatic recorders and laser printers are now more frequently used. High-fidelity, multichannel tape recorders are also used to record and store data from the entire study. An audiochannel for recording details during the procedure and correlating these with electrophysiologic findings is very useful.

Stimulation apparatus

The type of stimulator required depends on the aim of the electrophysiologic study. Evaluation of AV node conduction or sinus node recovery times by incremental atrial pacing can be performed with the temporary pacemakers commonly used in intensive care units. For most studies, the stimulator must be more complex. Several units are available commercially. These units allow for programmed intracardiac stimulation and are capable of pacing at variable cycle lengths; additionally, they can induce variably timed single and multiple extrastimuli as well as burst pace. These units can also be programmed to test the capability of pacemakers for termination of tachycardia.

TESTING PROCEDURES

Measurement of conduction intervals

Catheter positioning. Measurement of conduction intervals is an integral part of electrophysiologic testing. The lengths of intervals and refractory periods are expressed in milliseconds (msec). Heart rate and atrial and ventricular pacing rates may be expressed as cycle lengths in msec or in beats/min. To convert from cycle lengths to beats/min, the following formula is used:

$$\text{Beats/min} = \frac{60{,}000\ (\text{msec})}{\text{cycle length (msec)}}.$$

Conduction intervals are measured both at rest and during pacing. Proper placement of the catheters is essential for accurate and reproducible measurements. The high right atrial quadripolar catheter is placed in the atrial appendage whenever possible. This facilitates recording of adequate atrial electrograms close to the sinus node by means of the proximal pair of electrodes and a stable position for pacing with the distal pair. In patients who have undergone surgical procedures involving ligation of the right atrial appendage, stable positioning of the catheter can usually be obtained along the lateral right atrial wall.

Correct positioning of the catheter used for recording His bundle potentials is also vital. Optimal placement usually results in recording atrial and ventricular potentials that are relatively equal in amplitude (Fig 22D-4). If the catheter tip is positioned too far within the ventricle, small, poorly defined atrial potentials and a right bundle-branch potential may be recorded rather than the His bundle potential itself. Alternatively, if the catheter is distant from the His bundle, no potential may be identified. The finding of a large ventricular potential relative to the atrial potential usually indicates that the catheter is positioned too far in the right ventricle, and it should then be withdrawn while one applies clockwise rotation so as to bring the catheter tip against the interventricular septum. Although several authors have stressed the importance of validating the His bundle

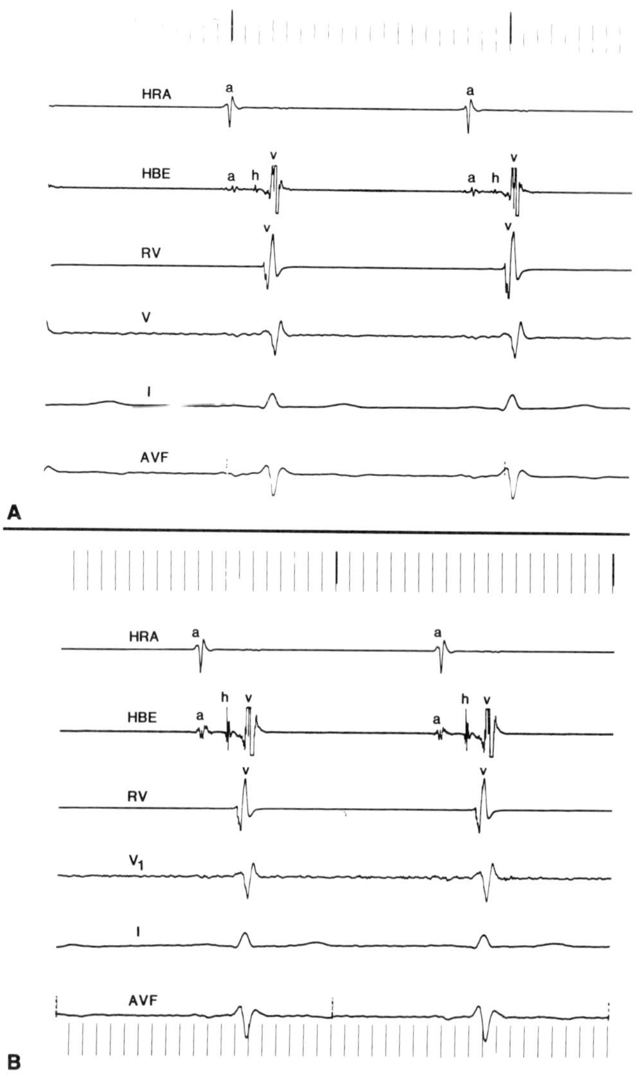

Fig 22D-4 Catheters positioned for recording from high right atrium *(HRA),* His bundle *(HBE),* right ventricle *(RV),* and three surface ECG leads. **A,** His bundle catheter is positioned remote from His bundle; it is too far within the right ventricle and this leads to small septal atrial activation *(a)* and small His potential *(h). v,* ventricular activation. **B,** withdrawal of catheter with clockwise rotation results in more optimal position and larger His potential *(h).*

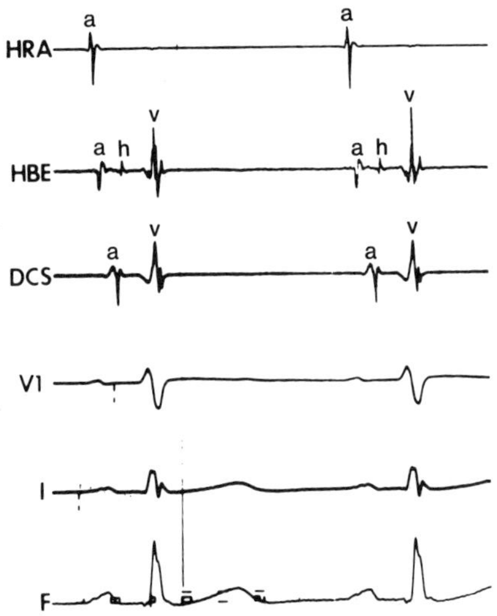

Fig 22D-5 Baseline recording from high right atrium *(HRA),* His bundle *(HBE),* distal coronary sinus *(DCS),* and three standard ECG leads. The P-A interval is measured from earliest onset of atrial activation either on surface ECG or HRA *(a)* to atrial activation *(a)* seen on HBE. The A-H interval is measured from atrial activation *(a)* on HBE to His depolarization *(h).* The H-V interval is measured from onset of *h* depolarization to earliest onset of ventricular activation *(v)* on either surface ECG or HBE. Normal atrial activation proceeds from high right atrium *(HRA,a)* to low septal right atrium *(HBE,a)* to left atrium *(DCS,a).*

potential by His bundle pacing,[30-33a] this may be difficult or not feasible and is usually not essential.

Placement of a catheter in the coronary sinus and one in the right ventricle allows recording of potentials from the left atrium and both the left and the right ventricles. In patients with atrial septal defects or with a patent foramen ovale, the left atrial electrogram can be measured directly, although the hazard exists that thrombus forming on the catheter could result in systemic thromboembolism. Left atrial potentials can also be recorded from the left pulmonary artery, although this is usually not necessary.

Resting intervals. The *P-A interval* is an approximation of the intra-atrial conduction time, although it more accurately reflects the conduction time between the area of the high right atrial recording electrodes and the low septal right atrium near the AV node (Fig 22D-5). In our laboratory, the P-A interval is measured from the earliest atrial activation, as seen either on the surface ECG or on the high right atrial electrogram, to the onset of atrial activation in the His bundle electrogram. Published reports of studies of normal values of this interval provide variable results (Table 22D-2). In our laboratory, the normal P-A interval ranges from 26 to 48 msec. Assessment of intra-atrial conduction also involves analysis of the atrial activation sequence (see Fig 22D-5). Usually, activation begins in the high right atrium and spreads to the low septal right atrium near the area of the AV node. In some patients, by means of endocardial mapping, atrial activation has been documented to begin in the midlateral right atrium.[38] Activation of the left atrium follows activation of the right atrium.

Table 22D-2 Range of normal electrophysiologic intervals

Source	Interval, msec P-A	A-H	H-V
Dhingra et al.[34]	9-45	54-130	31-55
Bekheit et al.[35]	10-50	50-125	35-45
Gallagher and Damato[36]	24-45	60-140	30-55
Fisher[30]	10-45	55-130	30-55
Josephson and Seides[29b]		60-125	35-55
Narula et al.[33a,37]	25-60	50-120	35-45
Present authors	26-48	54-130	35-55

The *A-H interval* is a reflection of the conduction time through the AV node and is the time for the depolarization wave front to pass through the AV node and reach the His bundle. It is measured from the onset of the right atrial potential on the His bundle electrogram (low septal activation) to the onset of the His bundle potential itself (see Fig 22D-5). The normal A-H interval in our laboratory ranges from 54 to 130 msec (see Table 22D-2). This wide range reflects not only the pronounced influence of the autonomic nervous system and the resting heart rate on AV node function but also the spectrum of AV node function in the population studied. A patient who is adequately sedated and relaxed during the electrophysiologic testing may have a different AV node function, including a different A-H interval, than the same patient would have if he or she were anxious and had a pronounced increase in sympathetic tone.

The *H-V interval* is a measure of His-Purkinje conduction. It is measured from the onset of the His potential to the earliest reproducible onset of ventricular depolarization, whether it be on the surface ECG or on the intracardiac electrogram (see Fig 22D-5). The normal range, 35 to 55 msec in our laboratory (see Table 22D-2), is considerably narrower than that seen with AV node conduction, in part because His-Purkinje conduction generally is not affected by changes in autonomic tone. The normal His potential is discrete and has a duration of less than 20 msec.[33a] The finding of a broad, fragmented potential may be due to filtering problems with the recording equipment or may be related to conduction delay within the His-Purkinje system.[39]

Programmed stimulation

Pacing. Pacing techniques play an integral role in electrophysiologic assessment. Pacing at various cycle lengths and from various sites is used to assess the function of the conduction system.

Atrial pacing permits assessment of sinus node function and AV node function. For these purposes, pacing is usually performed from the high right atrium with the use of the atrial appendage if possible because of the stability

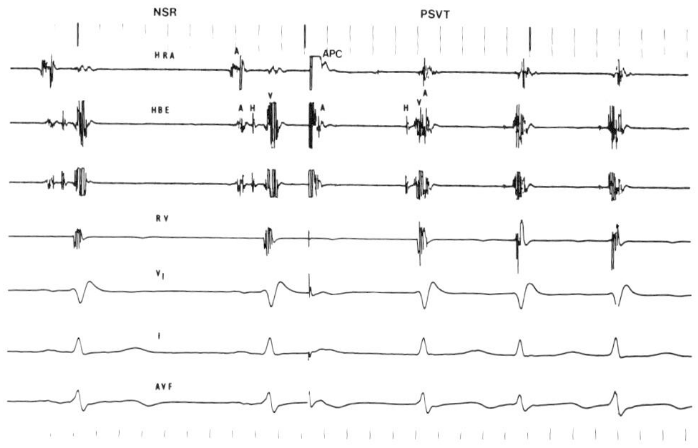

Fig 22D-6 Introduction of a critically timed atrial premature contraction *(APC)* results in induction of AV node reentry tachycardia. Left portion of figure shows recording from high right atrium *(HRA),* His bundle *(HBE),* right ventricle *(RV),* and three surface ECG leads during normal sinus rhythm *(NSR).* A critically timed atrial premature contraction results in prolongation of A-H interval as well as induction of typical AV node reentry tachycardia *(PSVT).* Other abbreviations as before.

of this position. On some occasions, however, pacing from other sites, such as the coronary sinus, is used to evaluate the effect of differential or selective input into the AV node.[40-43] Pacing from the coronary sinus usually results in a shorter A-H interval and may reflect more rapid AV node conduction.

For the assessment of sinus node recovery time, pacing is initiated at a cycle length 50 to 100 msec shorter than the spontaneous cycle length of the patient at rest. Progressively shorter cycle lengths are used, at least down to a cycle length of 300 msec (200 beats/min). A typical sequence would include pacing at cycle lengths of 600, 550, 500, 450, 400, 380, 360, 340, 320, and 300 msec. The duration of each pacing rate should be at least 15 seconds to allow for adequate sinus node suppression.[44]

Shortest 1:1 conduction and AV node Wenckebach period are determined by decremental atrial pacing. Pacing is initiated at a cycle length 50 to 100 msec shorter than the spontaneous sinus cycle length and continuously decremented by 20 msec until AV block is observed. The longest pacing cycle length at which AV block first occurs is defined as the AV node Wenckebach period. The shortest pacing cycle length immediately preceding the AV node Wenckebach period defines AV node shortest 1:1 conduction.

Atrial stimulation is also performed with single impulses or short bursts of rapid atrial pacing in an attempt to initiate or terminate paroxysmal supraventricular tachycardia, atrial fibrillation, or atrial flutter (Fig 22D-6). This may be accomplished by a "ramp technique," in which pacing is initiated at a slow rate, which is then incrementally increased until the desired rate is reached, tachycardia is initiated or terminated, or atrial capture is lost.

Ventricular pacing is also an essential component of electrophysiologic assessment. With ventricular pacing at cycle lengths ranging from 600 to 300 msec, ventriculoatrial (VA) conduction can be assessed. This is particularly important in patients in whom permanent pacing devices are contemplated. The presence of intact VA conduction in these persons may predispose them to supraventricular reentrant tachycardia or the pacemaker syndrome.[45] Pacing at shorter cycle lengths, ranging from 300 to 240 msec, for shorter durations (approximately 5 seconds) at a time to initiate tachycardia is useful in patients suspected of having ventricular arrhythmias. Ventricular pacing is usually performed at the right ventricular apex. In patients undergoing assessment for ventricular arrhythmias, however, pacing may be performed from the right ventricular apex, right ventricular outflow tract, and left ventricle.[29c,30,46-49]

Coupled extrastimulation. The technique of programmed electrical stimulation also involves the delivery of timed coupled extrastimuli in atrial or ventricular diastole and is usually performed both in sinus rhythm and during a paced rhythm. Extrastimuli are introduced usually every fourth beat during sinus rhythm and every eighth beat during paced rhythm. This technique is used to assess sinus node function and to evaluate the refractory periods of the atrium, AV node, and His-Purkinje system. It is essential in the induction and termination of supraventricular and ventricular arrhythmias.

Although each electrophysiologic study must be individualized, depending on the specific problem presented by the patient, it is important that standardized techniques be used. The extrastimuli should be given at a constant stimulus strength, which is usually twice the stimulation threshold. Alterations in current strength or stimulation duration may change refractoriness and may also affect the ability to initiate and terminate tachycardia.[50,51] Atrial extrastimuli are usually introduced during sinus rhythm or with atrial pacing at 100 and 150 beats/min. The extrastimuli are timed during the cardiac cycle so as to scan diastole; at first they are placed late in diastole, and then they are repeated at progressively earlier intervals in diastole until the stimulus fails to capture the atrium. This determines the effective refractory period of the atrium. By convention, the stimulation artifact and the atrial, His bundle, and ventricular electrograms during either sinus or paced rhythm are represented by S_1, A_1, H_1, and V_1, respectively. The stimulation artifact, atrial His bundle, and ventricular electrograms of the programmed extrastimuli are represented by S_2, A_2, H_2, and V_2 (Fig 22D-7). During attempts at arrhythmia induction, single, paired, and even triple extrastimuli may be placed (see Fig 22D-6).

Single ventricular extrastimuli are introduced both during unpaced rhythm and during ventricular pacing at 100, 120, and 150 beats/min. The ventricular stimuli are also timed so as to scan diastole; they are begun late in the cycle and are then repeated progressively earlier in diastole until the stimulus fails to capture the ventricle. This defines the effective refractory period of the ventricle. In patients in whom ventricular arrhythmias are suspected, a second and a third consecutive ventricular extrastimulus may be introduced to facilitate induction of arrhythmia.

In addition to induction of arrhythmia, programmed

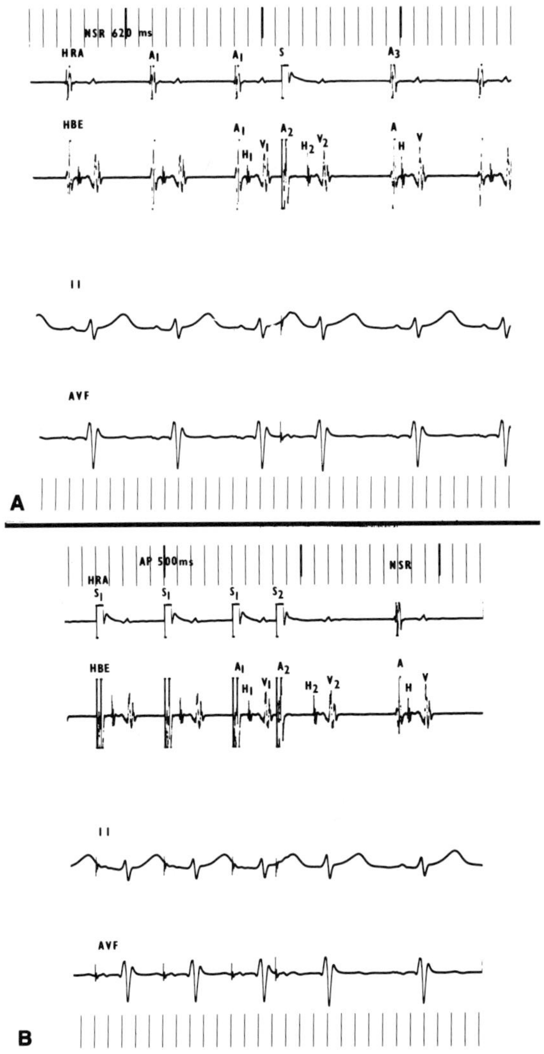

Fig 22D-7 **A,** recording during sinus rhythm *(NSR, 620 msec)* from high right atrium *(HRA),* His bundle *(HBE),* and two surface ECG leads. Atrial, His bundle, and ventricular potentials of the sinus beats are A_1, H_1, and V_1, respectively. *S,* premature atrial beat is delivered. Atrial, His bundle, and ventricular potentials of the premature stimulated beat are A_2, H_2, and V_2, respectively. **B,** recording during atrial-paced rhythm *(AP, 500 msec).* Stimulation artifact, and atrial, His bundle, and ventricular potentials of the paced rhythm are S_1, A_1, H_1, and V_1, respectively. S_2, premature atrial beat is delivered. Atrial, His bundle, and ventricular potentials of the premature stimulated beat are A_2, H_2, and V_2, respectively.

atrial and programmed ventricular stimulation are the methods used to evaluate refractoriness. Refractoriness is a measure of the ability of cardiac tissue to recover its excitability after depolarization. Atrial, AV node, His-Purkinje, and ventricular refractoriness all are assessed. In addition, in patients with preexcitation, the refractory period of the accessory pathway is also assessed. Because refractoriness is dependent on cycle length, it is usually assessed during sinus rhythm and during paced rhythm at multiple pacing rates.[52-55]

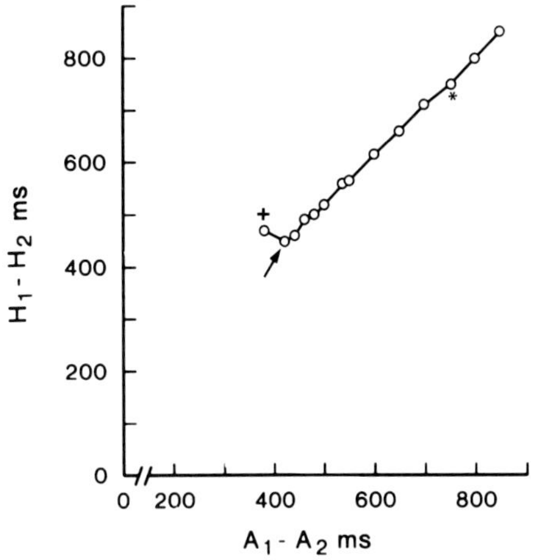

Fig 22D-8 Graphic display of AV node refractoriness. Functional refractory period of the AV node is the shortest H_1-H_2 obtained in response to atrial extrastimuli *(arrow).* Effective refractory period of the AV node is the longest A_1-A_2 interval that fails to result in conduction to the His bundle (+). Relative refractory period is the longest A_1-A_2 at which the H_1-H_2 interval exceeds the A_1-A_2 interval (*). See text for details.

Refractoriness is defined in three ways: (1) The *effective refractory period* is the longest coupling interval of a premature impulse that fails to capture the portion of the conduction system under study. This measurement is made just proximal to the refractory tissue. For example, the effective refractory period of the AV node is expressed as the longest A_1-A_2 interval that fails to result in conduction to the His bundle (Fig 22D-8). (2) The *functional refractory period* is the shortest interval between two consecutively conducted impulses. For example, at the level of the AV node, the functional refractory period is the shortest H_1-H_2 interval that is obtained in response to atrial extrastimuli. (3) The *relative refractory period* identifies full recovery of the cardiac tissue under study. It is the longest coupling interval of a premature stimulus that is conducted with some delay in relation to the drive cycle. For example, the relative refractory period of the AV node is the longest A_1-A_2 interval at which the H_1-H_2 interval exceeds the A_1-A_2 interval.

The refractory periods of the atrium, AV node, His-Purkinje system, and ventricles are shown in Table 22D-3.[53-55,58] The response of the refractory periods of the atrium, His-Purkinje system, and ventricles to changes in pacing rates differs from that of the AV node. Atrial functional and both atrial and ventricular effective refractory periods shorten with decreasing cycle length. AV node functional refractory periods shorten slightly with decreased cycle length; however, the effective refractory period of the AV node increases with decreasing cycle length.[53-55] This difference is probably related to the fact that the recovery of excitability of the AV node exceeds the action potential duration.[59,60]

Table 22D-3 Range of adult normal refractory periods

		Refractory period, msec					
	Cycle length,	In atrium		In AV node		In His-Purkinje	In ventricle
Source	msec	FRP	ERP	FRP	ERP	ERP	ERP
Denes et al.[54,56]	600-850	190-390	150-360	350-495	250-365	. . .	. . .
Akhtar et al.[57]*	500-1,000		230-330	320-680	280-430	340-430	190-290
Josephson and Seides[29b]			170-300	330-525	230-425	330-450	170-290
Present authors		235-375	144-300	338-502	186-374	. . .	170-290

FRP, functional refractory period; ERP, effective refractory period.
*Includes only patients with normal resting conduction intervals.

Interventions

Physiologic and pharmacologic interventions are used during electrophysiologic assessment to stress the conduction system, reproduce symptoms, and initiate tachycardia.

Physiologic intervention. Carotid sinus massage is a particularly useful adjunct to the evaluation of the autonomic tone on the conduction system.[61-71] Carotid sinus massage is carried out with firm pressure placed over the carotid sinus for 5 seconds. This is then performed on the contralateral side. Obviously, care must be taken to avoid massage in patients with carotid artery disease. During carotid sinus massage in patients with symptoms, the blood pressure should be monitored to assess the cardioinhibitory and vasodepressor effects of the maneuver. In some persons, carotid sinus massage may cause a decrease in blood pressure (vasodepressor effect) without significant change in heart rate.

The effect of changes in posture on the response to carotid sinus massage and on the ease of induction and termination of tachycardia can be assessed with the use of a tilt table.[72] This maneuver may be important in the attempt to reproduce a patient's symptoms. For example, in patients with supraventricular tachycardia and syncope, the successful induction of tachycardia in the supine position may cause only palpitations. When the patient is tilted to the full upright position, however, syncope may ensue and thus reproduce the patient's symptoms entirely (Fig 22D-9). The tilt table has also been used with increasing frequency in the evaluation of patients presenting with recurrent unexplained syncope. The degree and duration of tilt vary depending on the specific protocol.[70,73-83] Fitzpatrick and Sutton[74] used a maximum tilt of 60° for up to 45 minutes to reproduce symptoms. Other authors have used more extreme degrees of tilt, up to 80°, for a shorter time, up to 10 minutes.[73] This has also been combined with isoproterenol infusion in an attempt to reproduce neurally mediated syncope.[73,77-80]

Pharmacologic intervention. The type of pharmacologic intervention selected depends on the specific problem being studied. Some interventions are designed to stress the conduction system and thus expose latent abnormalities; others facilitate the induction of tachycardia. Some drugs are used to estimate resting autonomic tone. Finally, some medications are given to assess optimal therapeutic regimens to be prescribed for patients having symptomatic tachycardia.

1. Drugs that stress the conduction system. Intravenous (IV) atropine, 0.04 mg/kg, is the drug used most often to stress the conduction system. It improves conduction through the AV node and thus facilitates the entry of premature beats into the His-Purkinje system.[84-86] Intra- or infra-His conduction defects may be seen only after atropine administration when the usual conduction delay through the AV node has been reduced. In addition, in the evaluation of sinus node function, atropine may abolish sinoatrial entrance block and thus permit more consistent depolarization of the sinus node during atrial pacing and therefore more accurate assessment of sinus node function.[87-93]

Procainamide, 50 to 100 mg/min for a total dose of 10 to 15 mg/kg, is also often used to expose latent His-Purkinje conduction system disease.[94-96] Other drugs have also been used to stress the conduction system, including lidocaine and ajmaline.[97-99] Each of these three drugs may produce high-grade AV block necessitating temporary pacing.

2. Drugs that facilitate induction of tachycardia. Atropine is used most commonly in patients with a history of supraventricular tachycardia during attempts to induce this arrhythmia.[100,101] In patients with dual AV node pathways, atropine enhances antegrade slow-pathway conduction and retrograde fast-pathway conduction and may facilitate the induction and maintenance of sustained paroxysmal supraventricular tachycardia.[102,103] In patients with accessory pathways, atropine may have differing actions on the potential limbs of the reentrant circuit and also facilitate macroreentrant tachycardia.

Isoproterenol, 0.02 to 0.08 μg/kg, may also be useful in the induction of either supraventricular or ventricular tachycardia, particularly in patients with a history of exercise- or catecholamine-induced arrhythmia.[25,104-115] Successful induction of tachycardia by isoproterenol may depend on drug-induced changes in refractoriness or conduction or the initiation of abnormal automaticity.[29c] Isoproterenol has also been used to provoke or reproduce

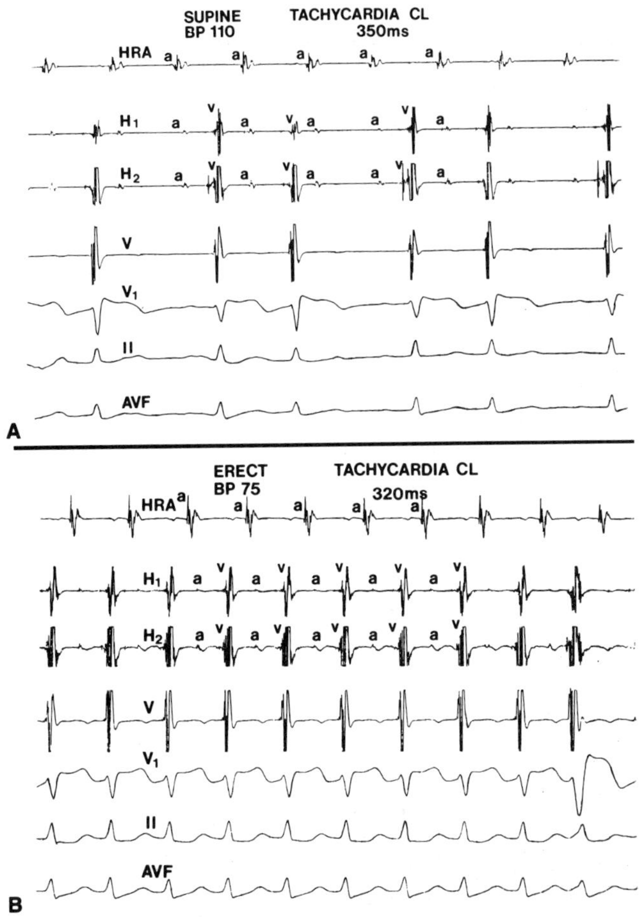

Fig 22D-9 Electrophysiologic study in a 72-year-old woman with paroxysmal tachycardia and near-syncope. Recordings are from high right atrium *(HRA),* two His bundle channels *(H_1, H_2),* right ventricle *(V),* and three surface ECG leads. **A,** in supine position, patient complained of palpitations only. Sinoatrial nodal reentry tachycardia is present with an atrial rate of 171 beats/min and 3:2 AV block; blood pressure *(BP)* was 110 mm Hg systolic. **B,** in upright position, patient's symptoms were reproduced with near-syncope, pronounced weakness, and dizziness. Sinoatrial node reentry tachycardia is present with an atrial rate of 187 beats/min, 1:1 AV conduction, and BP of 75 mm Hg. *CL,* cycle length; other abbreviations as before.

neurally mediated syncope.[73,77-80] The rationale for this use rests on the finding of increased levels of circulating catecholamines preceding syncope.[116,117] It is possible that catecholamine excess and the resultant increase in the force of cardiac contraction may enhance the susceptibility to syncope by stimulation of intracardiac mechanoreceptors. In the setting in which this has been a postulated mechanism, electrophysiologic testing has been performed on a tilt table to reduce central volume and been combined with an isoproterenol infusion. Isoproterenol can also be used to predict recurrence of paroxysmal supraventricular tachycardia in patients with preexcitation syndromes.[109] After drug or ablation therapy and before dismissal, electrophysiologic testing may be repeated in these patients during isoproterenol infusion.[109,118-123] If tachycardia cannot be reinduced, the chances of it recurring spontaneously may be decreased. Finally, in some patients, IV procainamide paradoxically may result in sustained ventricular tachycardia.[124]

3. Drugs used to assess or affect autonomic tone. Variation in autonomic tone and balance often plays a significant role in the genesis of rhythm disturbances and cardiac symptoms, and manipulation of this factor is useful in studying patients. This is particularly important in patients who have carotid sinus hypersensitivity, hypervagotonia, or sinus node dysfunction. Atropine is most commonly used.[61,62,87,125,126] There has been increased interest in the usefulness of combined parasympathetic and sympathetic blockade in the evaluation of patients with sinus node dysfunction. Combined blockade allows assessment of the electrophysiologic properties of the sinus node itself without the confounding variables of sympathetic and parasympathetic tones, both of which can influence impulse formation and conduction. The most common agents used are atropine, 0.04 mg/kg, and propranolol, 0.1 to 0.2 mg/kg, in combination.[127-130]

Assessment of therapy. (See subsequent section on drug testing.) Serial drug intervention for the purpose of identifying optimal therapeutic regimens has become widely used in the management of tachycardia. The drugs tested vary greatly with the laboratory and the availability of investigational agents. Procainamide and lidocaine are most commonly used in patients with ventricular tachycardia, although acute administration of quinidine is also useful. In patients with supraventricular tachycardia, digoxin, propranolol, verapamil, and procainamide are most often used.

APPLICATIONS OF ELECTROPHYSIOLOGIC TESTING

Assessment of sinus node function

The assessment of sinus node function has received considerable attention. This interest arises from the recognition of sinus node dysfunction as a common cause of symptoms, including syncope and near-syncope, the frequency with which drugs may adversely affect sinus node function, and pacing systems that depend on normal sinus node function. Evaluation includes the assessment of automaticity, conduction, and refractoriness, for abnormalities of any one of these may result in symptomatic arrhythmias.[25,44,87,131-142] Although direct recordings of sinus node automaticity and conduction have been documented in humans, indirect assessment is still the rule.[143-145]

Automaticity. The suppression of the normal pacemaker of the heart by pacing the heart at a faster rate (overdrive pacing) is the basis of the assessment of sinus node automaticity. The mechanism of overdrive suppression may be related to the release of autonomic neurotransmitters—for example, acetylcholine—or hyperpolarization of membrane potential due to activation of the Na^+/K^+ pump leading to the disruption of the intrinsic

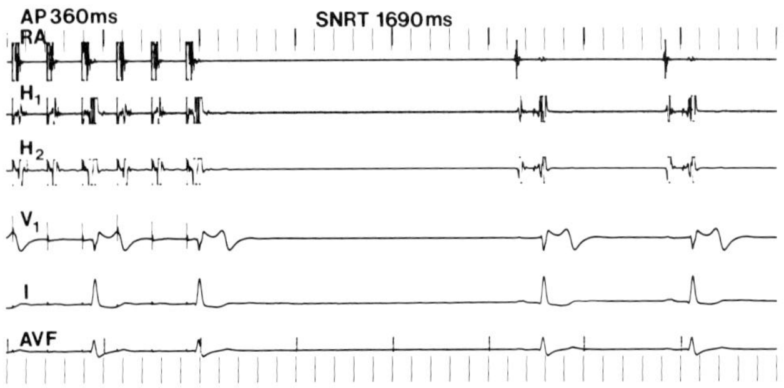

Fig 22D-10 Measurement of sinus node recovery time *(SNRT)*. Rapid atrial pacing *(AP)* at 166 beats/min *(360 msec)* is abruptly terminated. SNRT (measured at the time interval from the last paced atrial beat to the spontaneous sinus beat) is prolonged at 1,690 msec. *RA*, high right atrium; other abbreviations as before.

Table 22D-4 Sinus node function: range of normal values

Source	Time, msec SNRT	CSNRT	SACT
Rosen et al.[154]	<1,400		
Breithardt et al.[131]	<1,480	<508	<120
Narula et al.[150]		<525	
Mandel et al.[44]	1,040 ± 56		
Jordan et al.[155]		<450	
Josephson and Seides[29d]	<1.3 (SCL) + 101	<550	
Present authors	<1,500	<525	<125

SNRT, sinus node recovery time; CSNRT, corrected sinus node recovery time; SACT, sinoatrial conduction time; SCL, sinus cycle length.

control of automaticity.[146-148] The critical variable is the time it takes the sinus node to depolarize spontaneously after a period of atrial overdrive pacing. The sinus node recovery time is measured as the time interval from the last paced atrial depolarization to the first spontaneous sinus node beat (Fig 22D-10). This recovery time is a function of the automaticity of the sinus node but is subject to modification by other factors, which include the proximity of the pacing site to the sinus node, the conduction time into and out of the sinus node, and the duration of atrial pacing.[29d,44,136,149-152]

The normal sinus node is suppressed by pacing for at least 15 to 30 seconds.[44,150] For studies in our laboratory, pacing is continued for 30 seconds and then abruptly terminated. It is initiated at rates just exceeding the sinus rate, followed by a stepwise increase in rates up to 200 beats/min – usually 100, 120, 133, 150, 156, 166, 176, 187, and 200 beats/min. The importance of pacing at increasing rates (decreasing cycle lengths) derives from the fact that sinus node recovery time depends in part on the length of the paced cycle.[44] At faster pacing rates, there may be sinus node entrance block, and not all paced atrial beats enter the sinus node and depolarize it. Pacing at rapid rates may thus lead to spuriously short estimates of sinus node recovery time as a result of this entrance block.[149,153]

Normal sinus node recovery time varies in published studies up to 1,500 msec (Table 22D-4). After the termination of pacing, the cycle length should return to baseline within seven beats. Long secondary pauses, more than 1.5 seconds, occurring during this time are abnormal and may indicate sinus node dysfunction, reflecting either suppression of automaticity or a shift in the pacemaker site[156] (Fig 22D-11). The sinus node recovery time is in part dependent upon the length of the resting cycle. For this reason, sinus node recovery time is commonly given as a corrected sinus node recovery time (sinus node recovery time minus the cycle length of the spontaneous rhythm). Other corrections for sinus node recovery time involve regression equations, which are less often used.[29d,44,132] Because sinus node function may be profoundly influenced by changes in autonomic tone, sinus node recovery time should routinely be assessed before and after atropine. After atropine, 0.04 mg/kg, the sinus rate should increase to more than 90 beats/min or more than 25% to 50% above the resting baseline.[29d,135,157-160] Atropine usually results in a decrease in sinus node recovery time and corrected sinus node recovery time, although, as previously noted, abolition of entrance block into the sinus node may cause a paradoxic increase in sinus node recovery time.[87-89]

After analysis of the effect of atropine, IV propranolol, 0.1 to 0.2 mg/kg, may be given. The combined use of these drugs eliminates the influence of the autonomic nervous system. After autonomic blockade, the resultant heart rate, called the "intrinsic" heart rate, is measured. This is believed by some authors to be an excellent test of sinus node function.[29d,127,130,136] Evaluation of the effect of other drugs, such as IV isoproterenol at 1 to 3 μg/min, which should increase the sinus rate in normals by more than 25%, is also recommended by some authors but is not used as widely.[132,135,160,161]

Conduction. In addition to abnormalities of sinus node automaticity, abnormal sinus node conduction with exit block from the sinus node may cause symptomatic bradycardia. Conduction of impulses into and out of the sinus node is evaluated by assessment of sinoatrial conduction times. There are two major methods, both of which are indirect. The most common method involves the introduction of programmed atrial extrastimuli at progressively earlier intervals during diastole.[131,132,137,162-164] Four responses are seen. If the premature atrial extrastimulus is introduced during the last 20% to 30% of diastole, the wave front of the atrial premature depolarization collides with the spontaneous sinus impulse but does not penetrate and reset the sinus node. The cycle length of the next spontaneous sinus impulse is unchanged (zone of non-reset). With the introduction of progressively earlier premature impulses, the sinus node is reset (zone II). This zone occupies up to 50% of middiastole, during which time the return cycle or pause remains relatively constant. With increasingly premature beats, two or more zones may be seen: zone III, the zone of interpolation, and zone IV, the zone of reentry (Fig 22D-12).

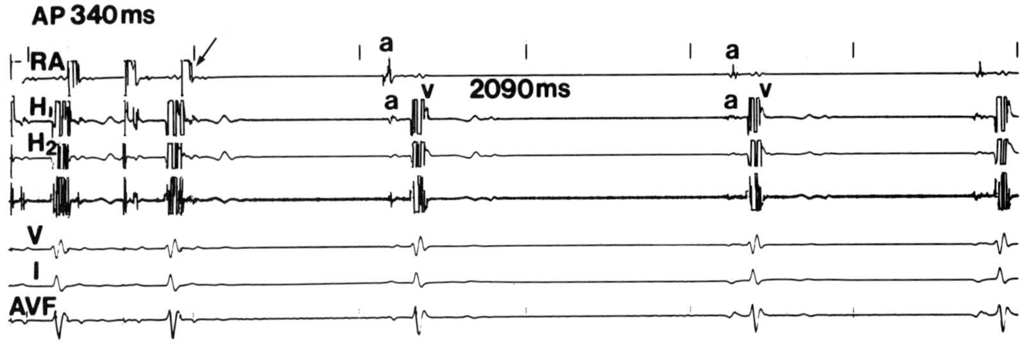

Fig 22D-11 Atrial pacing *(AP)* at 176 beats/min *(340 msec)* is abruptly terminated *(arrow).* Return of first sinus beat is normal but is followed by a long secondary pause (2,090 msec), indicating sinus node dysfunction. Abbreviations as before.

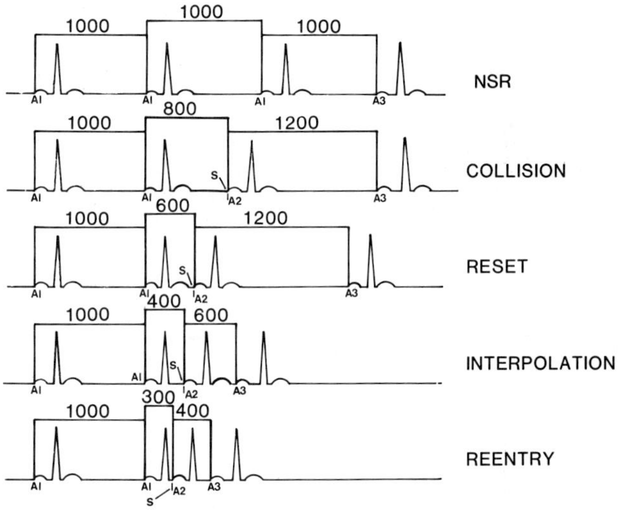

Fig 22D-12 Sinus node responses to programmed atrial extrastimuli. *Normal sinus rhythm (NSR):* A_1-A_1 cycle length is 1,000 msec. *Zone of collision:* Atrial premature contraction (APC) (A_2) introduced at 800-msec coupling interval *(S)* collides with emerging sinus node impulse but does not enter and reset sinus node pacemaker. Return cycle (A_2-A_3) is 1,200 msec. Sum of A_1-A_2 and A_2-A_3 is equal to A_1-$A_1 \times 2$. *Zone of reset:* APC (A_2) introduced at 600 msec is conducted and it enters and resets sinus node pacemaker. Return cycle A_2-A_3 is 1,200 msec. Sum of A_1-A_2 and A_2-A_3 is less than A_1-$A_1 \times 2$. *Zone of interpolation:* APC (A_2) introduced at 400 msec fails to enter sinus node and, in addition, fails to inhibit transmission of subsequent sinus node impulse. Return cycle is early. A_1-A_2 + A_2-A_3 may be equal to A_1-A_1 as pictured here. *Zone of reentry:* APC (A_2) introduced at 200 msec results in earlier return cycle as a result of sinus node reentry. A_1-A_2 + A_2-A_3 is less than A_1-A_1. (Adapted from Jordan JL, Mandel WJ: Disorders of sinus function. In *Cardiac Arrhythmias: Their Mechanisms, Diagnosis, and Management.* Edited by WJ Mandel. Philadelphia, JB Lippincott Company, 1980, p 125.)

Zone II is used to calculate the sinoatrial conduction time (Fig 22D-13). Calculation of the sinoatrial conduction time is based in part on several assumptions, including (1) that the conduction times into and out of the sinoatrial node are equal and (2) that isolated atrial premature contractions cause no shift in the pacemaker site and no change in automaticity of the sinus node.[29d,133,136,162,165] These assumptions have not been proved to be valid experimentally. Depression of automaticity by an atrial premature contraction has been documented experimentally.[166-168] Also, antegrade and retrograde conduction times are not equal.[169] Despite this, assessment of sinoatrial conduction time by atrial premature contractions is still often performed and is useful in the electrophysiologic evaluation of sinus node function.[170] Published normal ranges are variable, depending in part upon the patient population studied (see Table 22D-4). Some authors express the sinoatrial conduction

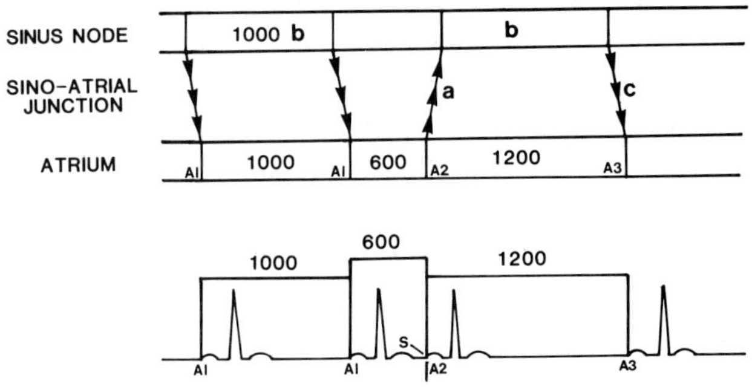

Fig 22D-13 Calculation of sinoatrial conduction time. An atrial premature contraction (A_2) delivered at 600 msec *(S)* penetrates and resets the sinus node pacemaker. Return cycle is 1,200 msec. This return cycle is made up of conduction time of the premature impulse into the sinus node *(a),* underlying cycle length of the pacemaker *(b),* and conduction time out of the sinus node *(c).* Assuming that a = c, sinoatrial conduction time is calculated as $\frac{1}{2}[(A_2\text{-}A_3) - (A_1\text{-}A_1)]$.

time as the total of antegrade and retrograde conduction, while others assume equal antegrade and retrograde conduction and express the value as half of the total sinoatrial conduction time.[133,157,165,171]

A second method of estimating sinoatrial conduction time—by the use of atrial pacing—has been introduced.[172] With this method, atrial pacing is performed slightly in excess of the sinus rate (less than 10 beats/min greater than the sinus rate) for eight beats. The sinoatrial conduction time is again calculated on the first cycle length after the end of pacing. The return interval (A_2-A_3) minus the basic cycle length (A_1-A_1) equals conduction into and out of the sinus node. This again assumes no change in automaticity and no shift in the pacemaker and also assumes equal conduction into and out of the sinus node. Continued evaluation of this approach to sinus node testing will establish its usefulness.[173]

The role of invasive electrophysiologic testing in the evaluation of sinus node function and dysfunction continues to generate considerable debate.[87,134,137,152,174-178] Controversy exists because of the large range of normal values, the variable percentage of positive and negative tests in patients with sinus node dysfunction, and the actual definition of sinus node dysfunction itself. In general, sinus node recovery time is a more sensitive indicator of sinus node dysfunction, although sensitivity varies widely, whereas sinoatrial conduction time may be more specific.[133,170,171,174] The optimal diagnosis of symptomatic sinus node dysfunction is made by ECG monitoring during a typical symptomatic episode.

Refractoriness. Direct measurement of antegrade sinus node refractoriness during electrophysiologic testing has not been developed, because it requires direct extrastimulus testing of the sinus node and downstream atrial recording. Determination of retrograde sinus node refractoriness is theoretically possible and is based on the observation that prolonged refractoriness of the sinoatrial node underlies disturbances of conduction elsewhere in the heart and may cause sinoatrial exit block and affect sinus node recovery time and sinoatrial conduction time.[91,139,151,152,179,180] The effective refractory period of the sinoatrial node corresponds to the coupling interval of an induced premature atrial contraction that marks the transition from an interpolated premature contraction to a reset response. It has been proposed that interpolation occurs as the entering atrial impulse encroaches on the refractory period of the preceding sinus beat. Determination of sinus node refractoriness during atrial pacing also has been established to ensure regulation of conduction times and activation patterns. The effective refractory period of the sinus node has been reported to be 325 ± 39 msec in normal persons and 522 ± 20 msec in patients with sinus node dysfunction. Although measurement of sinus node refractoriness has not been a standard part of sinoatrial nodal evaluation, it may provide an additional sensitive index of sinus node function.

Assessment of intra-atrial conduction

After impulse formation in the sinus node, the impulse spreads to the AV node. The functional-anatomic substrate for impulse transmission remains a subject of considerable controversy; some authors favor the presence of discrete internodal pathways and others support the concept of preferential conduction through the atrial wall without histologically specialized internodal tracts being present.[181-183] Conventionally, intra-atrial conduction is assessed by measuring the P-A interval as previously discussed. Normal atrial activation is seen in Figure 22D-5, in which the high right atrium is depolarized first, with the impulse spreading to the low right atrium and low septal right atrium and later to the left atrium. For more detailed studies of intra-atrial conduction both during normal rhythm and during tachycardia, multiple recording sites are necessary.[29b,38,184] Atrial conduction and refractoriness are also assessed during rapid atrial pacing and programmed atrial stimulation, respectively. The finding of prolonged atrial conduction and abnormal atrial refractoriness is of some value, for it identifies the electrophysiologic substrate for the development of atrial flutter and atrial fibrillation.[29e,185-189]

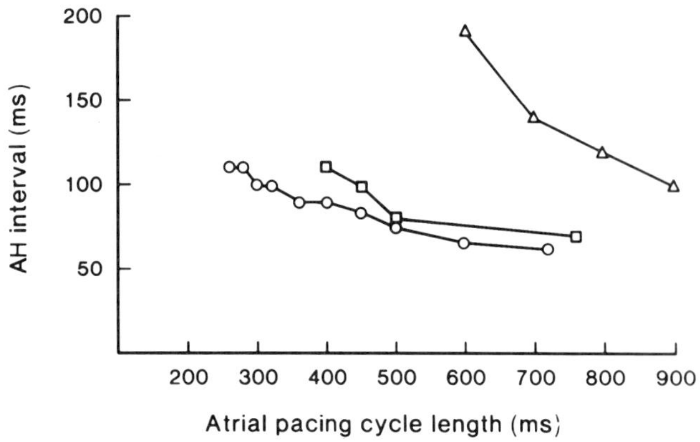

Fig 22D-14 Response of AV node to atrial pacing. Most common response is a gradual increase in the A-H interval and then AV node block at less than 200 beats/min. This is seen in patient □, in whom the resting A-H is 70 msec at 80 beats/min and increases to 110 msec at 150 beats/min and then AV node Wenckebach periodicity. Patient ○ had accelerated AV node conduction with an initial A-H of 60 msec, which increased to 110 msec with atrial pacing at 250 beats/min (240 msec). Patient △ had abnormal AV node conduction and an initial A-H of 100 msec, which increased to 190 msec with pacing at 100 beats/min (600 msec). AV node Wenckebach periodicity then developed.

Assessment of AV node function

AV node function is assessed both in the resting state and with rapid atrial pacing and programmed atrial stimulation. During incremental rapid atrial pacing, the AV node conduction time, which is measured as the A-H interval, normally lengthens.[30,34,190] The most common response is gradual prolongation of the A-H interval and then AV node Wenckebach periodicity. The AV node Wenckebach periodicity occurs with atrial pacing between 120 and 190 beats/min in most adults (Fig 22D-14). Patients with abnormally accelerated AV node conduction have been described in whom atrial pacing at more than 200 beats/min results in 1:1 AV conduction.[191-194] The underlying electrophysiologic mechanism in these patients varies. Some may have unrecognized augmentation of sympathetic tone. Others may have a juvenile or a small AV node or a partial bypass of the AV node.[195-198] At the other end of the spectrum is the appearance of Wenckebach periodicity occurring at less than 120 beats/min. This may occur as a result of intrinsic AV node disease or, often, as a consequence of increased vagal tone. Increased vagal tone may be seen in symptom-free, well-trained athletes or in patients who have experienced syncope or near-syncope.[199-202] Although type II second-degree AV block has been reported in the AV node, it is rare and its documentation has been questioned.[203,204] Congenital AV block is usually at the level of the AV node and typically is associated with an escape rhythm originating in the AV junction which is characterized by a narrow QRS complex on the ECG. Congenital AV block has also been documented at lower levels within the conduction system.[205-207]

As is true for the assessment of sinoatrial node function, repeat testing of AV node function after pharmacologic intervention is often of significant benefit. Commonly, atropine is administered, particularly in patients who have Wenckebach periodicity at low atrial pacing rates. In patients with enhanced vagal tone, atropine normalizes AV node conduction and refractoriness in comparison with patients with intrinsic AV node disease, in whom atropine does not change the abnormal AV node function. At the same time that sinoatrial node and atrial refractoriness are being assessed with programmed atrial stimulation, AV node refractoriness is also evaluated. In general, abnormalities in AV node conduction are usually associated with abnormalities in AV node refractoriness. On occasion, however, after atropine is given, one of these variables improves while the other remains abnormal. These persons may have a combination of abnormally enhanced vagal tone and intrinsic AV node disease.

Assessment of His-Purkinje conduction

The His-Purkinje system is assessed by measuring conduction from the His bundle to the ventricle both during sinus rhythm and during ventricular pacing and programmed atrial and ventricular stimulation (Fig 22D-15). At rest, the H-V interval in our laboratory is between 35 and 55 msec. During atrial pacing, the H-V interval usually remains constant. However, with rapid atrial pacing or very premature programmed atrial extrasystoles, there may be functional His-Purkinje delays with prolonged H-V interval or block distal to the bundle of His.[29b,f,208-210] The occurrence of block distal to the His bundle or a pronounced increase in the H-V interval associated with premature atrial extrastimuli introduced with a coupling interval of more than 360 to 400 msec or atrial pacing at rates of less than 150 beats/min should raise concern about disease of the His-Purkinje conduction system. Both type I and type II second-degree AV block have been documented in the His-Purkinje system, although the latter is, of course, more common[29g,33b,211-213] (Fig 22D-16).

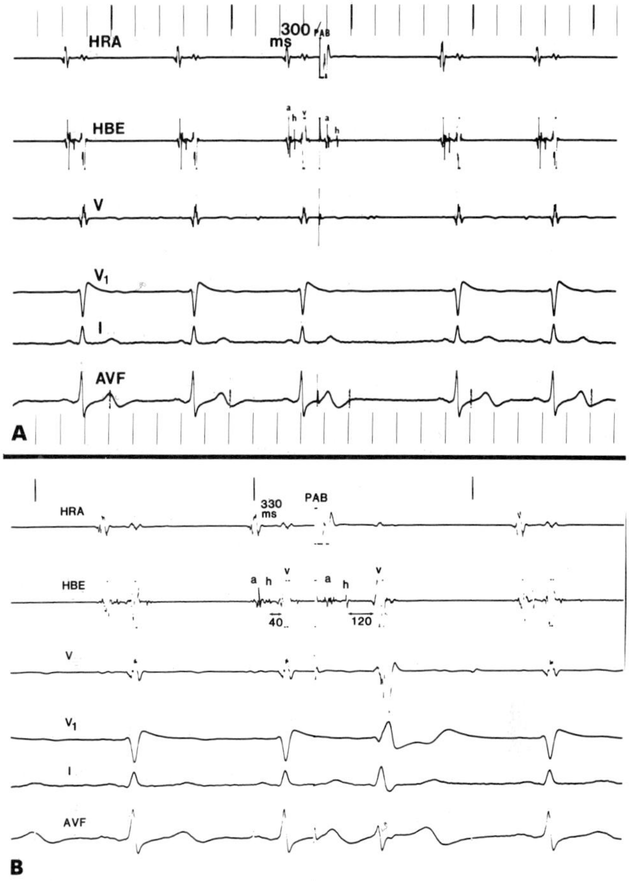

Fig 22D-15 Response of His-Purkinje system to premature atrial extrastimuli. **A,** electrophysiologic study with high right atrial *(HRA),* His bundle *(HBE),* and right ventricular *(V)* electrograms and three surface ECGs. Premature atrial beat *(PAB)* placed at a coupling interval of 300 msec results in block distal to the His bundle potential. Other abbreviations are as before. **B,** in same patient, PAB later in diastole with a coupling interval of 330 msec results in conduction to the ventricle but with delay and prolongation of H-V interval from 40 to 120 msec.

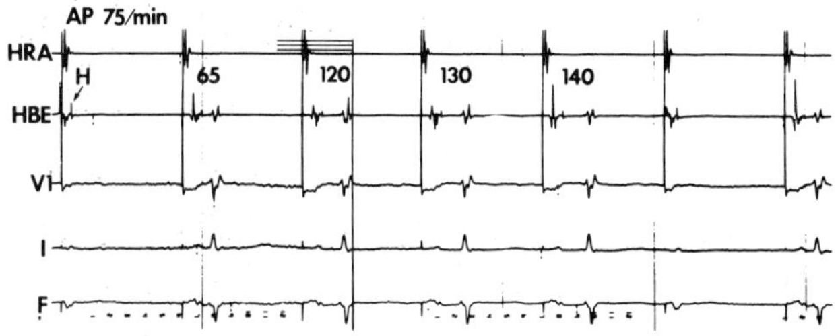

Fig 22D-16 Recordings from high right atrium *(HRA),* His bundle *(HBE),* and three surface ECG leads during atrial pacing *(AP)* at 75 beats/min. During atrial pacing there is gradual prolongation of the H-V interval from 65 to 140 msec and then block distal to His bundle *(H).*

The significance of prolonged His-Purkinje conduction continues to generate considerable clinical interest. Prolonged H-V intervals may occur in the setting of conduction defects on the surface ECG or with a normal surface QRS complex. The finding of significant H-V prolongation in patients with syncope in whom no other abnormality is found suggests that intermittent high-grade AV block may be the cause of the syncope.[30,33b,214-218] In addition, the finding of significantly prolonged H-V intervals (> 100 msec) in patients with bifascicular block may be predictive of the development of cardiogenic syncope.[29g,215-217] In these groups of patients, permanent pacing will often successfully alleviate recurrent symptoms of syncope or near-syncope. It is important to remember, however, that syncope in these patients may be due to other cardiovascular mechanisms, including sinus node dysfunction and ventricular arrhythmias.[218,219]

Repeat measurements of the H-V interval both at rest and with atrial pacing and programmed atrial stimulation are usually made after the administration of atropine and procainamide. In addition, other medications have been used to stress the His-Purkinje system. As previously discussed, the goal with the use of atropine is to increase conduction through the AV node and thus expose the His-Purkinje system to premature stimuli and rapid atrial pacing rates. Procainamide in and of itself causes an increase in the H-V interval and may result in infra-His block.[94,95] This finding in patients who will need class I antiarrhythmia agents is of vital importance because it indicates the need for prophylactic ventricular pacing. Other medications, including lidocaine and ajmaline, have been used for the assessment of His-Purkinje conduction, although less often.[97-99] It remains important to remember that these drugs may result in high-grade AV block requiring temporary pacing.

Evaluation of tachycardia

A major application of electrophysiologic testing is in the evaluation of tachycardia. The goal of testing is to (1) reproduce and characterize the tachycardia, (2) identify the anatomic and physiologic substrate of the tachycardia, (3) identify potential therapeutic modalities including pacing techniques and antiarrhythmia drugs, and (4) identify patients in whom electrophysiologically guided ablation or surgical therapy may be useful (see chapter 26). The techniques for this evaluation are the same as those used for assessment of sinoatrial node, atrial, and AV node function—i.e., rapid pacing and programmed extrastimuli with and without pharmacologic intervention and carotid sinus massage.

Electrophysiologic testing has allowed identification of the three major mechanisms of arrhythmias—reentry, abnormal automaticity, and triggered activity (see chapter 22A). The ability to initiate and terminate tachycardia reliably by programmed stimulation has been considered the hallmark of the reentrant mechanism. Although there are some known exceptions to this, in general these criteria are still accepted as working definitions.[29h,30,220,221]

Supraventricular tachycardia. The development of electrophysiologic testing has revolutionalized the classification of supraventricular tachycardia. From the anatomic locations, supraventricular tachycardia can originate in the sinoatrial node, atrial myocardium, or AV junction. Reentrant tachyarrhythmias in patients with Wolff-Parkinson-White syndrome utilize the accessory pathway, AV node, and atrial and ventricular myocardium as the obligatory components of the tachycardia circuit. Responses to programmed stimulation and pharmacologic intervention during electrophysiologic testing further allow a differentiation of the underlying electrophysiologic mechanisms: reentry, abnormal automaticity, and triggered activity. The most common specific type of paroxysmal supraventricular tachycardia among patients studied in most series is tachycardia secondary to dual AV node pathways.[29h,220,222-224] Josephson and Wellens,[225] in a review of 708 consecutive patients presenting with supraventricular tachycardia, found that 50% had AV nodal reentrant tachycardia, 35% had AV reentrant tachycardia utilizing an accessory pathway, and 15% had other forms of atrial tachycardia. Reentry is the most common mechanism of paroxysmal supraventricular tachycardia in patients undergoing electrophysiologic testing.

The evaluation of the anatomic-electrophysiologic substrate of supraventricular tachycardia is based on analysis of specific events during induction and termination of the the tachycardia and events during the tachycardia itself.[226-229] Essential features are (1) the mode of initiation and termination of paroxysmal supraventricular tachycardia, (2) the timing of the atrial activation sequence and of VA conduction during tachycardia, and (3) the participation of and requirement for atrial and ventricular excitation and depolarization during tachycardia. Analysis of these events, in addition to the assessment of AV conduction as previously described, will allow identification of the anatomic and electrophysiologic substrates, such as dual AV node pathways, anomalous AV connections and participation of these pathways in tachycardia (see chapter 22B), and atrial (sinus node or ectopic focus) tachycardia. Finally, specific information is sought concerning the effects of drug intervention and pacing on the paroxysmal supraventricular tachycardia.

In the case of atrial flutter/atrial fibrillation, electrophysiologic studies have also resulted in a new classification.[30,230-235] With atrial flutter, two types have been identified by some investigators: (1) a more common type, type I, with counterclockwise atrial activation in the frontal plane, a flutter rate of 230 to 340 beats/min, and negative deflection of the flutter waves in the inferior ECG leads; and (2) a less common type of flutter, type II, with somewhat faster flutter rates (340 to 430 beats/min) and clockwise atrial activation with small positive deflections of the flutter waves in the inferior ECG leads. Although there is considerable overlap, this classification may have potential clinical value because some investigators have found that the response to specific therapeutic modalities such as rapid atrial pacing is related to the type of flutter. Improved mapping techniques also led to the recent advancement in ablation therapy for atrial fibrillation and atrial flutter.[4,236-239] Electrophysiologic testing in patients with atrial flutter or atrial fibrillation is valuable in the following ways: (1) to evaluate the electrophysiologic substrate, i.e., conduction delay or dispersion of refractoriness,[185,186] (2) to assess AV conduction and ventricular rate during atrial fibrillation or atrial flutter, (3) to map and ablate the reentry circuit in patients with classic type I atrial flutter,[240] and (4) to map and ablate or modify the AV node in patients with atrial fibrillation and rapid ventricular rate.[241,242]

Ventricular arrhythmias. The application of electrophysiologic studies to the evaluation of patients with ventricular arrhythmias and out-of-hospital cardiac arrest has been well established[29c,104,106-108,243-270] (see chapters 22C and 24A). This is related in part to the life-threatening nature of the arrhythmia, to its frequency as a major cause of morbidity and mortality, and to the efficacy of the technique in determining arrhythmogenic substrate and appropriate therapy.[104,243,271-275] There are several goals of electrophysiologic testing for ventricular arrhythmias. One is confirmation of the diagnosis. Although published criteria for the surface ECG diagnosis are available, widely used, and often helpful, accurate diagnosis may remain a problem.[276-279] Other goals are induction and identification of the mechanism of the ventricular tachycardia, localization of the site of tachycardia by endocardial mapping of both the right and the left ventricles, and assessment of pharmacologic, ablation, or device treatment.

Protocols for this assessment vary from laboratory to laboratory and depend on the aim of the study. If the goal is identification of patients for electrophysiologically directed operation or ablation, detailed electrophysiologic mapping of the right and left ventricles during tachycardia is essential. On the other hand, if the goal is assessment of drug or ICD therapy, detailed mapping is not necessary. Although atrial pacing and programmed atrial extrastimulation may induce ventricular tachycardia, in most instances ventricular stimulation is necessary.[280-282] For induction of tachycardia, we routinely use single, paired, and triple ventricular premature contractions during sinus rhythm and during ventricular pacing at two or more ventricular-paced cycle lengths—i.e., usually 600, 500, and 400 msec (Fig 22D-17). In addition, short bursts of ventricular pacing of up to 250 beats/min for 15 beats are also used. Initial stimulation is usually performed at the right ventricular apex; however, if no tachycardia is induced, repeat stimulation is performed at another right ventricular site (usually the right ventricular outflow tract) or the left ventricle.[46-48]

The specific protocol used is of considerable importance, as is the clinical setting in which it is used.[108,248,257-260,262,264-266] The aim is to reproduce a clinical arrhythmia with a high degree of specificity and sensitivity. In patients with known sustained ventricular tachycardia documented electrocardiographically so that the morphology is known, electrophysiologic testing is useful to assess the inducibility and reproducibility of the clinical arrhythmia and thereby to guide therapy. In patients with syncope without documented ventricular arrhythmia, a consistent stimulation protocol is critical to

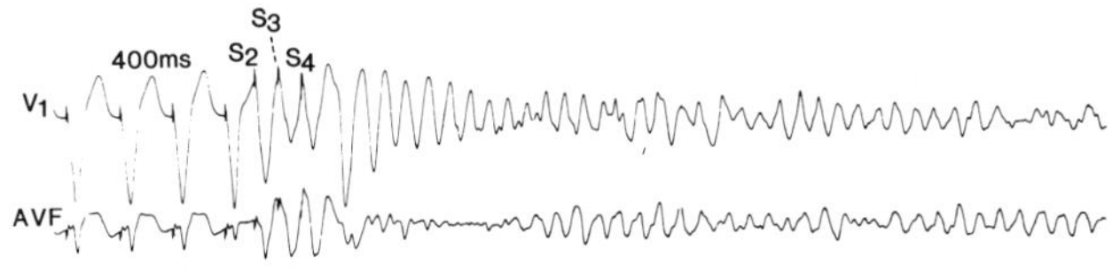

Fig 22D-17 Induction of ventricular fibrillation by ventricular pacing at 150 beats/min (400 msec) and adding three ventricular premature contractions *(S_2, S_3, S_4)*.

avoid obtaining a false-positive result. In the latter patients, ventricular flutter or ventricular fibrillation may be a false-positive finding. Initiation of ventricular tachycardia usually requires two ventricular extrastimuli. Adding another extrastimulus, for example, either a third or a fourth, increases the sensitivity but decreases the specificity of the test.[257,258,264-268] The nature of the induced arrhythmia, however, is important in this regard. Induction of ventricular flutter or ventricular fibrillation in a patient with a history of syncope and no known cardiac disease, although uncommon, would most likely be considered a false-positive result. On the other hand, induction of sustained monomorphic ventricular tachycardia is rarely a false-positive finding.

In patients with previously documented ventricular tachycardia in whom stimulation from two right ventricular sites does not induce ventricular tachycardia, repeat programmed ventricular stimulation with an infusion of isoproterenol may be of benefit.[104-107,110-112,249,266,283,284] In this situation, it may facilitate induction of arrhythmia. In reported series, details of administration have varied considerably, so that evaluation of the specific usefulness of this approach is difficult. If isoproterenol facilitates induction of tachycardia, β-blockers may then be used as specific treatment, although this protocol needs further evaluation and testing.

Left ventricular stimulation is also used, although incorporating three extrastimuli from two right ventricular sites has decreased the need for this approach.[107,249,265] Reported series have documented a small increase in sensitivity of electrophysiologic testing in patients with sustained ventricular tachycardia when left ventricular stimulation is used (3% to 7% increase). In patients with a history of sudden cardiac arrest, the increase in sensitivity is somewhat higher.

In addition to details of the protocol used, specific patient characteristics, including type and extent of cardiac disease and the specific clinical arrhythmia, affect outcome of ventricular stimulation. Arrhythmia induction rates are higher in patients with coronary artery disease than in patients with cardiomyopathy or primary electrical disorders.[251,255,259,266] This is particularly true in patients with a history of cardiac arrest or nonsustained ventricular tachycardia. The extent of disease also plays a role. In patients with more severe left ventricular dysfunction, arrhythmia induction rates tend to be higher, particularly in those undergoing evaluation of nonsustained ventricular tachycardia.

The specific clinical arrhythmia plays an even more important role in the outcome of testing.[106,249,250,257,259,266] Patients with a history of sustained ventricular tachycardia, particularly if they have coronary artery disease, have the highest induction rates. The arrhythmia can be repeatedly induced, often by identical stimulation protocols. Also, it can often be repeatedly terminated by identical stimulation protocols. In these patients, electrophysiologic testing can be useful to document the arrhythmia, to identify drug regimens that can be predicted to have a high likelihood of success in preventing recurrence, and to identify pacing modalities that can terminate tachycardia.

Nonsustained ventricular tachycardia has proven to be a more heterogeneous and difficult arrhythmia.[248,255,262,266,285,286] (see chapter 22C). Of the patients afflicted, some have had syncope, some have had palpitations, and some are asymptomatic. In patients with syncope and documented nonsustained ventricular tachycardia, the goal of the study is to identify a causal relationship between the two. In patients with asymptomatic nonsustained ventricular tachycardia, the goals have been to identify those at high risk for the development of sustained ventricular tachycardia or ventricular fibrillation and to identify those who might benefit from antiarrhythmia therapy. Although this latter group of patients has been repeatedly evaluated, overall conclusions have been difficult to draw because of variability in patient selection and differences in ventricular stimulation protocols and treatment algorithms. Many of the reports have been descriptions of clinical practice rather than scientific studies of specific problems. A further confounding variable has been the lack of any documentation that drug treatment of a large group of these patients reliably improves outcome.

Electrophysiologic results in these patients have depended on the type and severity of cardiac disease. In patients with coronary artery disease and depressed left ventricular function, induction rates are higher than in patients with cardiomyopathy and well-preserved left ventricular function. In the former group of patients, subsequent event rates are higher. Electrophysiologic testing may help to identify a high-risk group as well as help to select optimal therapy.

Currently, a randomized trial is testing the hypothesis that by treating patients with antiarrhythmia therapy guided by electrophysiologic studies, the risk of sustained ventricular tachycardia or sudden death can be reduced in patients with coronary artery disease, decreased left ventricular function, and asymptomatic or mildly symptomatic nonsustained ventricular tachycardia. In these patients, signal-averaged electrocardiograms may also play an important role in selecting which patients need either electrophysiologic study or treatment or need both.[287]

At present in our *clinical* practice, because patients with asymptomatic nonsustained ventricular tachycardia and an ejection fraction ≥40% have a low rate of inducibility as well as a good outcome, we do not perform electrophysiologic studies nor do we recommend routine antiarrhythmia therapy.[255] In patients with nonsustained ventricular tachycardia, coronary artery disease, and an ejection fraction of <40%, inducible rates of approximately 40% to 50% are seen; in these patients, electrophysiologically guided therapy may be helpful in decreasing arrhythmic events during follow-up. Finally, in patients with nonsustained ventricular tachycardia, a dilated cardiomyopathy, and an ejection fraction of <40%, the ability to induce an arrhythmia at electrophysiologic study is low and event rates remain high. These patients may not benefit from electrophysiologic testing. Benefit from antiarrhythmia therapy based on noninvasive monitoring has not been confirmed.

Patients with a history of cardiac arrest not associated with acute infarction should undergo electrophysiologic testing,[25,249,251,266] usually preceded by coronary angiography. These patients have a high rate of follow-up events. Electrophysiologic testing is aimed at reproducing the arrhythmia and identifying a drug therapy regimen effective in preventing recurrences. In these patients, electrophysiologic testing is also essential in evaluating the role of an ICD[253,256,288-290] (see chapter 25B). As was true for sustained ventricular tachycardia, inducibility rates in patients with a history of cardiac arrest are higher in those with coronary artery disease than in those with cardiomyopathy.

Evaluation of pacing. Attempts at termination of tachycardia by electrical stimulation are an integral part of electrophysiologic assessment. Termination of tachycardia by pacing is dependent upon several factors. These include the rate of the tachycardia, the characteristics and location of the reentry circuit, the site of stimulation and speed of conduction of the impulse to the site of the reentry circuit, and the mode of stimulation used.[29c,h,291,292] The importance of this evaluation was underscored by the development of implantable antitachycardia pacing devices in the mid-1980s. However, the high effectiveness of catheter ablation for patients with supraventricular tachycardia and ICD therapy for patients with ventricular tachycardia have made the evaluation of pacing for termination of tachycardia less critical for therapeutic purposes. For diagnostic purposes, response to pacing during tachycardia provides invaluable information in the differential diagnosis of the specific types and mechanisms of tachyarrhythmias as well as tachycardia localization.

In 1971, Wellens[292] distinguished five different modes of stimulation of the heart in the treatment of the various types of tachycardia: (1) a single premature stimulus delivered in either the atrium or the ventricle,[29c,291,293,294] (2) paired premature stimuli,[295,296] (3) simultaneous stimulation of the atrium and ventricle,[297-301] (4) overdrive pacing, and (5) pacing at regular rates to prevent tachycardia. These five different modes continue to be used in the electrophysiologic laboratory for the treatment and diagnosis of induced tachycardia. In ICDs recently approved by the Food and Drug Administration, overdrive pacing is the preferred initial therapy for monomorphic ventricular tachycardia in most patients.

Single or *paired extrastimuli* may be delivered in either the atrium or the ventricle during tachycardia[29c,h,291,293,294] (Figs 22D-18, 22D-19, and 22D-20). A single stimulus is introduced during each cycle at progressively more premature coupling intervals until either termination of the tachycardia or failure to capture at the stimulation site. The ability of a single premature beat to terminate tachycardia is particularly dependent upon the

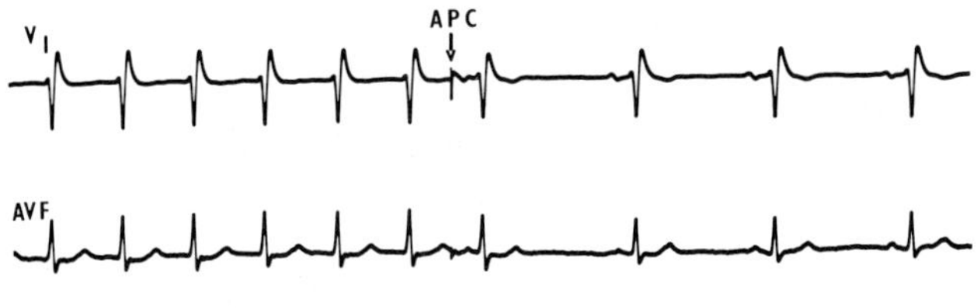

Fig 22D-18 AV node reentry tachycardia terminated by the introduction of a critically timed atrial premature contraction *(APC)*.

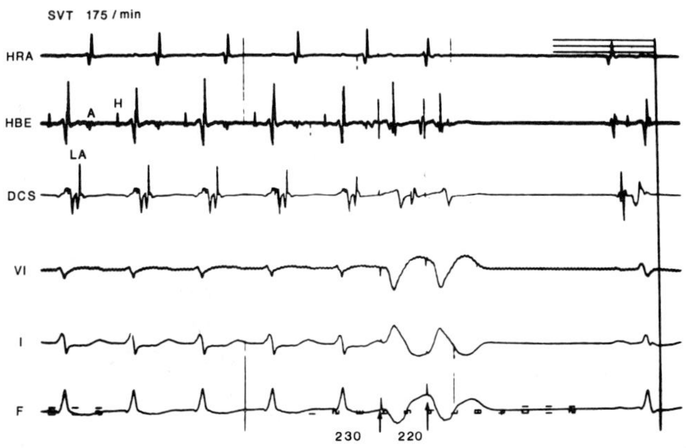

Fig 22D-19 Electrophysiologic study with recording from right atrium *(HRA)*, His bundle *(HBE)*, coronary sinus *(DCS)*, and three surface ECG leads. Supraventricular tachycardia *(SVT)* at 175 beats/min in a patient with preexcitation was interrupted by two critically timed ventricular premature beats at 230 and 220 msec. *LA,* left atrium; other abbreviations as before.

location of the stimulation site relative to the reentrant circuit, the conduction of the impulse to the reentry circuit, and the rate of tachycardia.[29c,h,291] Rapid paroxysmal AV node supraventricular tachycardia at rates of more than 175 beats/min may not be terminated by a single atrial premature beat; it often requires the introduction of paired stimuli or the use of pacing plus programmed extrastimuli. This technique is useful in altering refractoriness of cardiac tissue between the stimulation site and the reentrant circuit and thus allowing programmed extrastimuli to reach and interrupt the reentrant circuit.[29c,h,293,294,302] In our experience, the use of single and paired stimuli is not as effective in terminating ventricular tachycardia, because the ventricular tachycardia is often quite rapid and is not well tolerated. However, in patients with slow, stable ventricular tachycardia, single and paired ventricular premature extrastimuli may also be used to disrupt the reentry circuit and terminate the tachycardia (see Fig 22D-20).

Overdrive pacing (burst and ramp pacing) is often used to terminate tachycardia in the electrophysiologic laboratory, in the postoperative period with temporary pacing wires, and in patients with permanent pacemakers and ICDs.[231,233,293,303-307] This method is useful for both supraventricular and ventricular tachycardias (Figs 22D-21 and 22D-22). Depending on the specific rhythm, overdrive pacing may capture and change conduction and refractoriness in one limb of the reentrant circuit, result in suppression of an ectopic focus, or induce unstable atrial fibrillation followed by return to sinus rhythm. In the electrophysiologic laboratory, evaluation of overdrive pacing involves the following.

1. Determination of the optimal stimulation rate and its duration. Excessively rapid stimulation in the atrium during paroxysmal supraventricular tachycardia may result in undesirable atrial fibrillation, whereas rapid

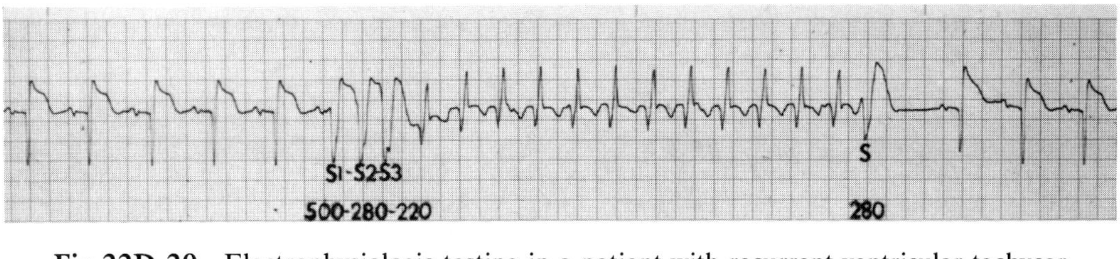

Fig 22D-20 Electrophysiologic testing in a patient with recurrent ventricular tachycardia. Ventricular tachycardia was induced with three ventricular beats *(S_1, S_2, S_3)* from the right ventricular apex. Termination of the ventricular tachycardia was then achieved with a single critically timed ventricular premature contraction at 280 msec *(S)*.

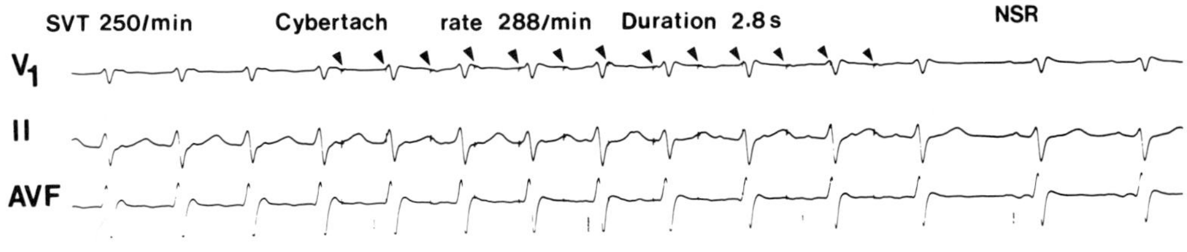

Fig 22D-21 Rhythm strip from patient with supraventricular tachycardia *(SVT)* at a rate of 250 beats/min. Automatic-burst atrial pacemaker (Cybertach) sensed the tachycardia and delivered a train of rapid atrial beats at 288 beats/min for 2.8 msec, and this resulted in return to normal sinus rhythm *(NSR)*.

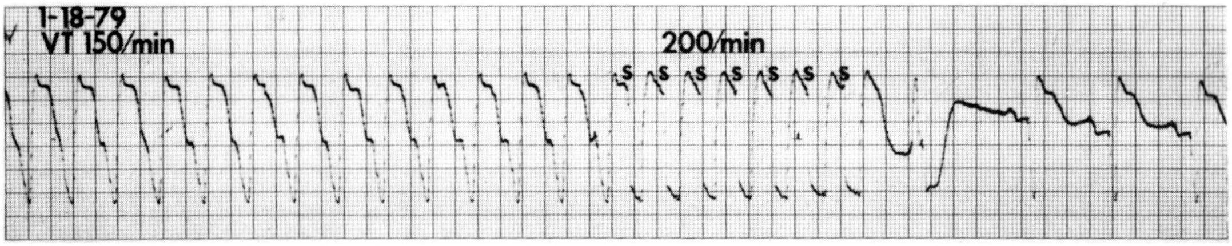

Fig 22D-22 Rhythm strip in a patient with ventricular tachycardia *(VT)* at 150 beats/min. Rapid ventricular pacing at 200 beats/min *(S)* then returned patient to normal sinus rhythm.

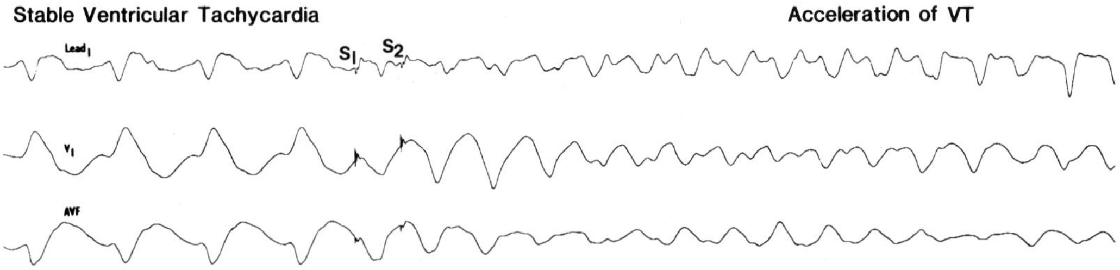

Fig 22D-23 Stable ventricular tachycardia induced during electrophysiologic testing. Two ventricular premature beats were introduced *(S_1, S_2,)* and the result was acceleration of the ventricular tachycardia *(VT)* and hemodynamic collapse.

stimulation in the ventricle may be poorly tolerated hemodynamically or result in an actual increase in the spontaneous rate of the tachycardia, with adverse consequences. Identification of the proper duration of such stimulation is important, since continued pacing after the cessation of tachycardia may reinduce the tachycardia it had terminated.

2. Determination of the optimal stimulation site. As is true with single extrastimuli, the closer the stimulation site to the reentry circuit, the easier, in general, is the termination.

3. Identification of potentially adverse sequelae of overdrive pacing. The most common complication of overdrive pacing is acceleration of the tachycardia, with its adverse hemodynamic consequences. In addition, overdrive pacing may convert one arrhythmia to another. Rapid atrial pacing may convert atrial flutter to atrial fibrillation; this often reverts spontaneously to normal sinus rhythm.[230,233,293] In patients with ventricular tachycardia, acceleration of the tachycardia or conversion to a different arrhythmia may cause a more serious problem (Fig 22D-23), as when rapid pacing results in conversion to ventricular flutter or fibrillation.[104,308]

In addition to its use in the termination of tachycardia induced during electrophysiologic testing, overdrive permanent pacing is useful for the treatment of tachycardia in carefully selected patients.[293,303-307] Permanent pacing for treatment of supraventricular tachycardia is no longer recommended because of the recent success of ablation therapy. Pacing as monotherapy for ventricular tachycardia without backup cardioversion or defibrillation poses significant risk for patients because of the possibility of tachycardia acceleration associated with hemodynamic collapse.

Evaluation of drug testing.[104,243,244,271,272,309-313] The utility of electrophysiologically guided pharmacologic therapy has been under increasing debate as nonpharmacologic therapy continues to improve and expand. Drug testing is based on four major assumptions: (1) that clinically symptomatic episodic tachycardia can be reproduced in the electrophysiologic laboratory; (2) that inducible sustained tachycardia can be induced usually only in patients having a clinical history compatible with episodic tachycardia; (3) that the effect of drugs administered during serial drug testing in the laboratory accurately reflects the clinical response to the chronic use of the same drugs; and (4) that in patients with inducible arrhythmia, induction is reproducible from day to day. The accuracy of these assumptions depends on the underlying arrhythmogenic substrate. Inducibility and reproducibility of serial drug testing are most reliable in patients with a fixed substrate for reentrant tachyarrhythmias. In 80% to 95% of patients with coronary artery disease who have had documented episodes of sustained ventricular tachycardia, the tachycardia can be induced in the laboratory. For patients with cardiomyopathy, inducibility rates are lower. Up to 90% of patients with documented paroxysmal supraventricular tachycardia have inducible tachycardia. The underlying assumption that the effect of drugs administered acutely reflects the long-term clinical response is dependent on four factors: (1) that the blood levels of the drug obtained over the long term are similar to those shown to be effective after the acute IV administration of the drug; (2) that the auto-

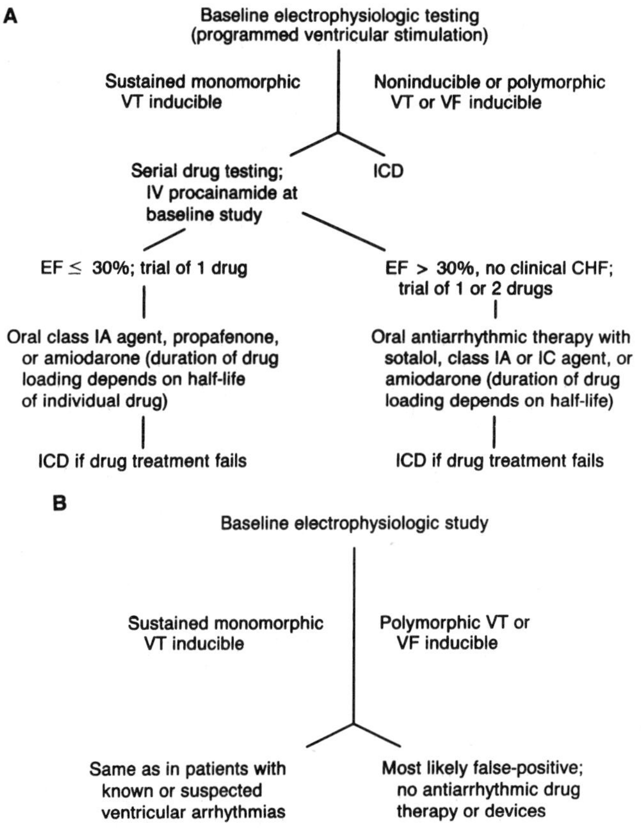

Fig 22D-24 General guidelines for electrophysiologic testing and electrophysiologically guided therapy **(A)** in patients with known or suspected (survivors of sudden cardiac arrest) ventricular arrhythmias and **(B)** in patients with coronary artery disease who have syncope or minimally symptomatic or asymptomatic nonsustained ventricular tachycardia *(VT)*. *CHF,* congestive heart failure; *EF,* ejection fraction; *ICD,* implantable cardioverter-defibrillator; *IV,* intravenous; *VF,* ventricular fibrillation.

nomic effects of IV and oral drugs used are similar; (3) that the oral drug does not depend on active metabolites of it; and (4), most importantly, that arrhythmogenic substrate does not change with time. Considerable variability in tachycardia induction rates and results of long-term treatment has been reported between different laboratories. These differences are probably related to different patient populations studied, differences in protocol design, different medications assessed, and the time-dependent change in substrate.

The details of the study protocol used vary from patient to patient, depending upon the type of arrhythmia, associated clinical problems, and previous drug therapy. With the techniques discussed above, an attempt is first made to induce the tachycardia and evaluate its electrophysiologic basis and mechanism. In addition, the reproducibility with which the arrhythmia can be initiated and maintained is evaluated. This baseline study is performed if possible after all antiarrhythmia medications have been discontinued for five half-lives of each drug. Once tachycardia has been induced and characterized, antiarrhythmia agents are administered sequentially. The order of administration and selection of drugs depend on the clinical setting. After administration of a drug, attempts are made to reinduce the tachycardia. If reinduction is achieved, another single drug may then be tested. It is important to determine the blood level of the drug at the time of testing. If a drug prevents initiation of tachycardia at a given blood level after acute administration and if a similar blood level can be achieved with oral administration, this usually is predictive of a good response. Depending on the outcome of the initial testing, other drugs may be tested on subsequent days (Fig 22D-24).

Variations in the technique include the following.

1. The medications studied. Some laboratories test a large battery of drugs irrespective of the response, whereas other laboratories discontinue the testing of drugs after an effective regimen has been identified.

2. Definition of success.[30,104,243,314,315] The best criterion of success is the inability to initiate tachycardia. In some laboratories, the ease of induction is considered to be a measure of success. In addition, in some laboratories a change from sustained to nonsustained tachycardia is believed to represent a successful result. These less stringent definitions of success may give rise to less than optimal results with a given therapeutic regimen and are probably a less reliable predictor of a good clinical outcome. This has important implications, particularly for patients receiving treatment with amiodarone.[254,266] In these patients, suppression of inducible ventricular tachycardia is the goal because it predicts an excellent outcome. However, with amiodarone, failure of the drug to suppress induction of ventricular tachycardia does not necessarily preclude a good outcome. In these patients, even if tachycardia can be reinduced, if it is more stable with a longer cycle length or requires a more aggressive ventricular stimulation protocol for induction, the long-term outcome is still often favorable. If, however, ventricular tachycardia in the patient receiving amiodarone remains easily inducible or is hemodynamically unstable, other therapeutic strategies should be strongly considered.

3. Restudy of the same drug after several days of oral administration. In some institutions, such as ours, repeat programmed stimulation is often performed to confirm drug efficacy before the patient is dismissed from the hospital.

4. Drug testing to evaluate proarrhythmic effects of drugs.[263] Proarrhythmic effects have been documented with all antiarrhythmia drugs, although with some the incidence is considerably higher. Proarrhythmic events or adverse drug-related events may include easier induction of tachycardia, more sustained tachycardia (e.g., converting nonsustained ventricular tachycardia to sustained ventricular tachycardia), more rapid tachycardia rates, or more unstable tachycardia either hemodynamically or electrically. Documentation of such events mandates evaluation of other therapies. Proarrhythmic events are modulated by underlying patient factors such as ventricular function. In patients with poor left ventricular function, for example, proarrhythmic effects are more com-

mon and more serious with some drug classes, such as class IC antiarrhythmia agents.

5. In patients with paroxysmal supraventricular tachycardia, drug testing to guide therapy.[109] This may be particularly valuable in patients with preexcitation syndromes. Drug effects in these patients may be reversed by increased levels of catecholamines. This result may have implications for predicting long-term drug efficacy, particularly when class IC antiarrhythmia drugs are used. In some patients, isoproterenol may be used to assess the potential for tachycardia recurrence in this setting.

Testing in patients with syncope

Electrophysiologic testing for the evaluation of syncope has gone through several cycles.[73,74,77,199,262,316-322] Patients with syncope present a formidable diagnostic and therapeutic challenge, particularly when routine testing, including 12-lead electrocardiography, 12-hour Holter monitoring, neurologic evaluation, and exercise testing, fails to identify the cause.[318,323] In these patients, recurrence may be common and mortality, particularly when the syncope is related to a cardiovascular cause, is increased. Early studies documented that in approximately two-thirds of patients, electrophysiologic testing could identify a presumptive mechanism.[199,316] In these patients, treatment was usually successful in abolishing recurrence. Subsequent to that, the importance of baseline characteristics of the patients undergoing electrophysiologic testing was emphasized; in patients without evidence of organic heart disease, the results of routine electrophysiologic testing are quite limited. Enthusiasm for testing in this situation subsequently declined. More recently, however, new electrophysiologic techniques have been used.[73,76,77] Increased concentration of circulating catecholamines has been documented prior to syncopal spells.[116,117,324,325] This increase could potentially enhance susceptibility of patients in the upright position to bradycardia and hypotension. Electrophysiologic testing using 60° tilt alone or in combination with isoproterenol has been evaluated as a means to identify susceptibility to neurally mediated recurrent syncope. This approach has been found to increase the yield of electrophysiologic testing and has fostered development of alternative therapeutic strategies in these patients, such as low-dose administration of cardioselective β_1-adrenergic receptor blockers.

Evaluation of ICD

Electrophysiologic assessment is required for consideration and use of ICD devices (see chapter 25B). Baseline assessment to document the ventricular arrhythmia, the patient's hemodynamic response to it, and the effect of drugs on it is essential.[256] During implantation, electrophysiologic testing to determine the optimal configuration of the device for tachycardia termination and to document its effectiveness is required. Finally, before dismissal, postoperative testing with tachycardia induction to document the integrity and usefulness of the system is mandatory.

RISKS AND COMPLICATIONS

Any intravascular catheterization has the potential for adverse consequences, particularly when performed in high-risk patients such as those with coronary artery disease and recurrent unstable ventricular tachycardia or cardiac arrest. With invasive electrophysiologic testing, there are two major potential types of complications. The first may arise from the intravascular catheterization itself and includes bleeding from the site of venous or arterial entry, thrombus formation and potential embolization, phlebitis, and myocardial perforation. These complications are similar to those seen after other catheterization procedures.[29a,326,327] As is true with all such procedures, careful and meticulous attention to detail markedly reduces morbidity.

The second major category of potential complications is related to the electrophysiologic techniques themselves. These include (1) adverse hemodynamic consequences of rapid pacing or rapid arrhythmias, and (2) adverse hemodynamic consequences of induced bradycardia. In patients with angina pectoris or cerebrovascular disease, rapid rates produced by either pacing or tachycardia may result in angina or altered consciousness. This is particularly important in patients undergoing evaluation for ventricular arrhythmias. In these patients, programmed ventricular stimulation may result in ventricular fibrillation or unstable ventricular tachycardia or it may accelerate stable ventricular tachycardia and result in hemodynamic collapse. In our laboratory, anesthesia coverage is available as needed for each study. Careful monitoring of the patient's symptoms and clinical condition and the capability for prompt reversal of unstable ventricular tachycardia or ventricular fibrillation by defibrillation are essential parts of any electrophysiologic evaluation.

PATIENT SELECTION

Electrophysiology remains a demanding discipline.[328,329] Knowledge and application of catheterization techniques, theoretic concepts, and clinical pharmacology are required. Also important, however, is proper patient selection, for the test is invasive, time-consuming, and costly. Proper patient selection enhances the yield from the procedure. Criteria for patient selection vary from institution to institution. In Table 22D-5 are listed the criteria for patient selection in our institution. In these patients, electrophysiologic testing plays a valuable role in both clinical assessment and management. As techniques improve and new patient subsets are delineated, the role of electrophysiologic testing can be expected to evolve and increase.

SUMMARY

Invasive electrophysiologic testing plays an important role in modern cardiology.[30,292,330] It has substantiated many theoretic concepts that were based on deductive reasoning and analysis of surface ECGs. Use of the techniques described (Table 22D-6) has also helped the clinician to document and understand the mechanisms, types, and natural histories of conduction defects. Application of

Table 22D-5 Clinical uses of invasive electrophysiologic testing

Problem	Objective of study
Arrhythmia that cannot be diagnosed from the body surface ECG	To ascertain the diagnosis, mechanism, prognosis, and appropriate treatment of the arrhythmia
Syncope or near-syncope without apparent neurologic or metabolic cause	To evaluate sinus node function and AV conduction; to detect covert atrial or ventricular tachyarrhythmias; to assess neural, hemodynamic, and physiologic causes
Recurrent palpitations with normal Holter ECG recording	To search for inducible atrial fibrillation, paroxysmal supraventricular tachycardia, or ventricular tachycardia
Suspected sinus node dysfunction (sick sinus syndrome)	To ascertain the mechanism and magnitude of dysfunction; to assess the need for pacemaker therapy; to evaluate the efficacy or safety of drug therapy
AV conduction defect	To ascertain the site and extent of block, the prognosis, and the need for pacemaker therapy
Recurrent, sustained supraventricular tachycardia or ventricular tachycardia	To induce the arrhythmia, evaluate its mechanism, and determine effective therapy (medical, ablation device, or surgical)
Survival after cardiac arrest	To ascertain whether inducible ventricular tachycardia or fibrillation is present and to find effective treatment
Wolff-Parkinson-White syndrome	To induce atrial fibrillation or supraventricular tachycardia and ascertain the ventricular rate; to ascertain number and location of anomalous AV connections; to guide medical, ablation, and surgical therapy
Mitral valve prolapse, idiopathic subaortic stenosis, or long QT syndrome, with palpitations or near-syncope	To search for supraventricular tachycardia, anomalous AV connections, and inducible ventricular tachycardia and to find effective treatment
Asymptomatic, self-limited nonsustained ventricular tachycardia in patients with coronary artery disease and poor left ventricular function (EF <40%)	To search for inducible, sustained ventricular tachycardia and, if present, find effective, safe drug therapy
Uncertain safety of cardioactive drugs (digitalis or antiarrhythmic, tricyclic antidepressant or antihypertensive drugs) in patients with sinus node or AV conduction system disease	To search for potential adverse effects on cardiac automaticity and conduction in a controlled environment (acute drug testing for safety)

Modified from the Medical Knowledge Self-Assessment Program (MKSAP) VI Syllabus.

Table 22D-6 Electrophysiologic assessment

Function assessed	Parameters evaluated*	Techniques
Sinus node	SNRT	Atrial pacing
	SACT	Programmed atrial stimulation
	Intrinsic heart rate	Pharmacologic assessment
AV node	AV node conduction	Atrial pacing
	AV node refractoriness	Programmed atrial stimulation
	VA conduction	Ventricular pacing
His-Purkinje system	His-Purkinje conduction	Resting intervals
		Atrial pacing
	His-Purkinje refractoriness	Programmed atrial stimulation
		Pharmacologic challenge
Tachycardia		
Supraventricular	Initiation and maintenance of tachycardia	Atrial and ventricular pacing
	Electrophysiologic substrate	Programmed atrial and ventricular stimulation
		Atrial mapping
	Potential treatment regimens	Drug testing, ablation
Ventricular	Initiation and maintenance of tachycardia	Ventricular pacing
		Atrial pacing
	Electrophysiologic substrate	Programmed ventricular stimulation
		Ventricular mapping
	Potential treatment regimens	Drug testing, ablation, ICD, surgery

*SNRT, sinus node recovery time; SACT, sinoatrial conduction time; VA, ventriculoatrial; ICD, implantable cardioverter-defibrillator.

these techniques in patients with supraventricular or ventricular tachycardia has been particularly rewarding. In these patients, testing has delineated the anatomic-pathophysiologic substrates for the initiation, maintenance, and termination of the tachycardia. This information has been essential to the development of new devices and to the successful application of electrophysiologically guided ablation and surgical treatment. Because of the effectiveness of ablation in the treatment of supraventricular tachycardia and devices (ICDs) in the treatment of ventricular tachycardia, the role of electrophysiologically guided serial drug testing is currently undergoing reevaluation. Improved patient care and survival, in addition to expanded therapeutic options, particularly in patients with tachycardia, have resulted from this growth of invasive electrophysiologic testing.

REFERENCES

1. Kugler JD, Danford DA, Deal BJ, et al: Radiofrequency catheter ablation for tachyarrhythmias in children and adolescents. The Pediatric Electrophysiology Society. *N Engl J Med* 330:1481-1487, 1994
2. Chang AC, McAreavey D, Tripodi D, et al: Radiofrequency catheter atrioventricular node ablation in patients with permanent cardiac pacing systems. *PACE* 17:65-69, 1994
3. Hindricks G: The Multicentre European Radiofrequency Survey (MERFS):complications of radiofrequency catheter ablation of arrhythmias. The Mulitcentre European Radiofrequency Sruvey (MERFS) investigators of the Working Group on Arrhythmias of the European Society of Cardiology. *Eur Heart J* 14:1644-1653, 1993
4. Lesh MD, Van Hare GF, Epstein LM, et al: Radiofrequency catheter ablation of atrial arrhythmias. Results and mechanisms. *Circulation* 89:1074-1089, 1994
5. Chen SA, Chiang CE, Yang CJ, et al: Accessory pathway and atrioventricular node reentrant tachycardia in elderly patients: clinical features, electrophysiologic characteristics and results of radiofrequency ablation. *J Am Coll Cardiol* 23:702-708, 1994
6. Morady F, Calkins H, Langberg JJ, et al: A prospective randomized comparison of direct current and radiofrequency ablation of the atrioventricular junction. *J Am Coll Cardiol* 21:102-109, 1993
7. Blanck Z, Dhala A, Deshpande S, et al: Catheter ablation of ventricular tachycardia. *Am Heart J* 127:1126-1133, 1994
8. Wen MS, Yeh SJ, Wang CC, et al: Radiofrequency ablation therapy in idiopathic left ventricular tachycardia with no obvious structural heart disease. *Circulation* 89:1690-1696, 1994
9. Kim YH, Sosa-Suarez G, Trouton TG, et al: Treatment of ventricular tachycardia by transcatheter radiofrequency ablation in patients with ischemic heart disease. *Circulation* 89:1094-1102, 1994
10. Morady F, Kadish A, Rosenheck S, et al: Concealed entrainment as a guide for catheter ablation of ventricular tachycardia in patients with prior myocardial infarction. *J Am Coll Cardiol* 17:678-689, 1991
11. Garan H, Kuchar D, Freeman C, et al: Early assessment of the effect of map-guided transcatheter intracardiac electric shock on sustained ventricular tachycardia secondary to coronary artery disease. *Am J Cardiol* 61:1018-1023, 1988
12. Kolettis TM, Saksena S: Prophylactic implantable cardioverter defibrillator therapy in high-risk patients with coronary artery disease. *Am Heart J* 127:1164-1170, 1994
13. Borggrefe M, Chen X, Martinez-Rubio A, et al: The role of implantable cardioverter defibrillators in dilated cardiomyopathy. *Am Heart J* 127:1145-1150, 1994
14. Sweeney MO, Ruskin JN: Mortality benefits and the implantable cardioverter-defibrillator. *Circulation* 89:1851-1858, 1994
15. Manolis AS: Transvenous endocardial cardioverter defibrillator systems. Is the future here? *Arch Intern Med* 154:617-622, 1994
16. Callans DJ, Josephson ME: Future developments in implantable cardioverter defibrillators: the optimal device. *Prog Cardiovasc Dis* 36:227-244, 1993
17. Moss AJ: Influence of the implantable cardioverter defibrillator on survival: retrospective studies and prospective trials. *Prog Cardiovasc Dis* 36:85-88, 1993
18. Akhtar M, Jazayeri M, Sra J, et al: Implantable cardioverter defibrillator for prevention of sudden cardiac death in patients with ventricular tachycardia and ventricular fibrillation: ICD therapy in sudden cardiac death. *PACE* 16:511-518, 1993
19. Fogoros RN: The effect of the implantable cardioverter defibrillator on sudden death and on total survival. *PACE* 16:506-510, 1993
20. Troup PJ: Implantable cardioverters and defibrillators. *Curr Probl Cardiol* 14:673-843, 1989
21. Fogoros RN, Elson JJ, Bonnet CA, et al: Efficacy of the automatic implantable cardioverter-defibrillator in prolonging survival in patients with severe underlying cardiac disease. *J Am Coll Cardiol* 16:381-386, 1990
22. Scherlag BJ, Lau SH, Helfant RH, et al: Catheter technique for recording His bundle activity in man. *Circulation* 39:13-18, 1969
23. Damato AN, Lau SH, Helfant RH, et al: Study of atrioventricular conduction in man using electrode catheter recordings of His bundle activity. *Circulation* 39:287-296, 1969
24. Zipes DP (Chairman): Guidelines for clinical intracardiac electrophysiologic studies. A report of the American College of Cardiology/American Heart Association Task Force on Assessment of Diagnostic and Therapeutic Cardiovascular Procedures (Subcommittee to Assess Clinical Intracardiac Electrophysiologic Studies). *J Am Coll Cardiol* 14:1827-1842, 1989
25. Hammill SC, Sugrue DD, Gersh BJ, et al: Clinical intracardiac electrophysiologic testing: technique, diagnostic indications, and therapeutic uses. *Mayo Clin Proc* 61:478-503, 1986
26. Gallagher JJ, Sealy WC, Wallace AG, et al: Correlation between catheter electrophysiological studies and findings on mapping of ventricular excitation in the W.P.W. syndrome. In *The Conduction System of the Heart: Structure, Function and Clinical Implications.* Edited by HJJ Wellens, KI Lie, MJ Janse, Philadelphia, Lea & Febiger, 1976, pp 588-612
27. Gallagher JJ, Damato AN, Lau SH, et al: Antecubital vein approach for recording His bundle activity in man. *Am Heart J* 85:199-204, 1973
28. Narula OS, Runge M, Samet P: A new catheter technique for His bundle recordings via the arm veins. *Br Heart J* 35:1226-1233, 1973
29. Josephson ME, Seides SF: *Clinical Cardiac Electrophysiology: Techniques and Interpretations.* Philadelphia, Lea & Febiger, 1979, a, pp 5-21; b, pp 23-59; c, pp 247-280; d, pp 61-78; e, pp 191-210; f, pp 103-118; g, pp 79-101; h, pp 147-190
30. Fisher JD: Role of electrophysiologic testing in the diagnosis and treatment of patients with known and suspected bradycardias and tachycardias. *Prog Cardiovasc Dis* 24:25-90, 1981
31. Narula OS (ed): *His Bundle Electrocardiography and Clinical Electrophysiology.* Philadelphia, FA Davis Company, 1975, pp 65-93
32. Narula OS, Scherlag BJ, Samet P: Pervenous pacing of the specialized conducting system in man: His bundle and A-V nodal stimulation. *Circulation* 41:77-87, 1970
33. Narula OS (ed): *Cardiac Arrhythmias: Electrophysiology, Diagnosis and Management.* Baltimore, Williams & Wilkins Company, 1979, a, pp 57-65; b, pp 85-113
34. Dhingra RC, Rosen KM, Rahimtoola SH: Normal conduction intervals and responses in sixty-one patients using His bundle recording and atrial pacing. *Chest* 64:55-59, 1973
35. Bekheit S, Murtagh JG, Morton P, et al: Measurements of sinus impulse conduction from electrogram of bundle of His. *Br Heart J* 33:719-724, 1971
36. Gallagher JJ, Damato AN: Technique of recording His bundle activity in man. In *Cardiac Catheterization and Angiography.* Second edition. Edited by W Grossman. Philadelphia, Lea & Febiger, 1980, pp 283-301
37. Narula OS, Cohen LS, Samet P, et al: Localization of A-V conduction defects in man by recording of the His bundle electrogram. *Am J Cardiol* 25:228-237, 1970
38. Josephson ME, Scharf DL, Kastor JA, et al: Atrial endocardial activation in man: electrode catheter technique for endocardial mapping. *Am J Cardiol* 39:972-981, 1977
39. Varghese PJ, Elizari MV, Lau SH, et al: His bundle electrograms of dog: correlation with intracellular recordings. *Circulation* 48:753-760, 1973
40. Aranda J, Castellanos A, Moleiro F, et al: Effects of the pacing site on A-H conduction and refractoriness in patients with short P-R intervals. *Circulation* 53:33-39, 1976

41. Batsford WP, Akhtar M, Caracta AR, et al: Effect of atrial stimulation site on the electrophysiological properties of the atrioventricular node in man. *Circulation* 50:283-292, 1974

42. Janse MJ: Influence of the direction of the atrial wave front on A-V nodal transmission in isolated hearts of rabbits. *Circ Res* 25:439-449, 1969

43. Ross DL, Brugada P, Bar FWHM, et al: Comparison of right and left atrial stimulation in demonstration of dual atrioventricular nodal pathways and induction of intranodal reentry. *Circulation* 64:1051-1058, 1981

44. Mandel W, Hayakawa H, Danzig R, et al: Evaluation of sinoatrial node function in man by overdrive suppression. *Circulation* 44:59-66, 1971

45. Nishimura RA, Gersh BJ, Vliestra RE, et al: Hemodynamic and symptomatic consequences of ventricular pacing. *PACE* 5:903-910, 1982

46. Robertson JF, Cain ME, Horowitz LN, et al: Anatomic and electrophysiologic correlates of ventricular tachycardia requiring left ventricular stimulation. *Am J Cardiol* 48:263-268, 1981

47. Michelson EL, Spielman SR, Greenspan AM, et al: Electrophysiologic study of the left ventricle: indications and safety. *Chest* 75:592-596, 1979

48. Prystowsky EN, Naccarelli GV, Rahilly GT, et al: Electrophysiologic and anatomic characteristics associated with ventricular tachycardia induced at the right ventricular outflow tract but not at the apex (abstract). *Am J Cardiol* 49:959, 1982

49. Wellens HJJ, Düren DR, Lie KI: Observations on mechanisms of ventricular tachycardia in man. *Circulation* 54:237-244, 1976

50. Waxman HL, Cain ME, Greenspan AM, et al: Termination of ventricular tachycardia with ventricular stimulation: salutary effect of increased current strength. *Circulation* 65:800-804, 1982

51. Mercer AB, Simpson RJ Jr, Gettes LS, et al: Strength-interval testing to enhance ventricular tachycardia induction during clinical electrophysiologic study (abstract). *Am J Cardiol* 49:958, 1982

52. DuBrow IW, Fisher EA, Amat-y-Leon F, et al: Comparison of cardiac refractory periods in children and adults. *Circulation* 51:485-491, 1975

53. Cagin NA, Kunstadt D, Wolfish P, et al: The influence of heart rate on the refractory period of the atrium and A-V conducting system. *Am Heart J* 85:358-366, 1973

54. Denes P, Wu D, Dhingra R, et al: The effects of cycle length on cardiac refractory periods in man. *Circulation* 49:32-41, 1974

55. Wiener I, Kunkes S, Rubin D, et al: Effects of sudden change in cycle length on human atrial, atrioventricular nodal and ventricular refractory periods. *Circulation* 64:245-248, 1981

56. Wu D, Denes P, Rosen KM: Refractoriness of atrioventricular conduction. In *His Bundle Electrocardiography and Clinical Electrophysiology.* Edited by OS Narula. Philadelphia, FA Davis Company, 1975, pp 95-103

57. Akhtar M, Damato AN, Batsford WP, et al: A comparative analysis of antegrade and retrograde conduction patterns in man. *Circulation* 52:766-778, 1975

58. Guss SB, Kastor JA, Josephson ME, et al: Human ventricular refractoriness: effects of cycle length, pacing site and atropine. *Circulation* 53:450-455, 1976

59. Simson MB, Spear JF, Moore EN: Electrophysiologic studies on atrioventricular nodal Wenckebach cycles. *Am J Cardiol* 41:244-258, 1978

60. Merideth J, Mendez C, Mueller WJ, et al: Electrical excitability of atrioventricular nodal cells. *Circ Res* 23:69-85, 1968

61. Hartzler GO, Maloney JD: Cardioinhibitory carotid sinus hypersensitivity: intracardiac recordings and clinical assessment. *Arch Intern Med* 137:727-731, 1977

62. Walter PF, Crawley IS, Dorney ER: Carotid sinus hypersensitivity and syncope. *Am J Cardiol* 42:396-403, 1978

63. Davies AB, Stephens MR, Davies AG: Carotid sinus hypersensitivity in patients presenting with syncope. *Br Heart J* 42:583-586, 1979

64. Sigler LH: The cardioinhibitory carotid sinus reflex: its importance as a vagocardiosensitivity test. *Am J Cardiol* 12:175-183, 1963

65. McIntosh SJ, Lawson J, Kenny RA: Clinical characteristics of vasodepressor, cardioinhibitory, and mixed carotid sinus syndrome in the elderly. *Am J Med* 95:203-208, 1993

66. Hopson JR, Rea RF, Kienzle MG: Alterations in reflex function contributing to syncope: orthostatic hypotension, carotid sinus hypersensitivity and drug-induced dysfunction. *Herz* 18:164-174, 1993

67. Kenny RA, Allen JA, Wallace WF: Autonomic reflexes in patients with cardioinhibitory carotid sinus syncope. *Clin Auton Res* 3:101-105, 1993

68. Brignole M, Menozzi C, Gianfranchi L, et al: Carotid sinus massage, eyeball compression, and head-up tilt test in patients with syncope of uncertain origin and in healthy control subjects. *Am Heart J* 122:1644-1651, 1991

69. Brignole M, Menozzi C, Gianfranchi L, et al: Neurally mediated syncope detected by carotid sinus massage and head-up tilt test in sick sinus syndrome. *Am J Cardiol* 68:1032-1036, 1991

70. Almquist A, Gornick C, Benson DW Jr, et al: Carotid sinus hypersensitivity: evaluation of the vasodepressor component. *Circulation* 71:927-936, 1985

71. Schweitzer P, Teicholz LE: Carotid sinus massage. Its diagnostic and therapeutic value in arrhythmias. *Am J Med* 78:645-654, 1985

72. Waxman MB, Bonet JF, Finley JP, et al: Effects of respiration and posture on paroxysmal supraventricular tachycardia. *Circulation* 62: 1011-1020, 1980

73. Almquist A, Goldenberg IF, Milstein S, et al: Provocation of bradycardia and hypotension by isoproterenol and upright posture in patients with unexplained syncope. *N Engl J Med* 320:346-351, 1989

74. Fitzpatrick A, Sutton R: Tilting towards a diagnosis in recurrent unexplained syncope. *Lancet* 1:658, 660, 1989

75. Kenny RA, Ingram A, Bayliss J, et al: Head-up tilt: a useful test for investigating unexplained syncope. *Lancet* 1:1352-1355, 1986

76. Abi-Samra F, Maloney JD, Fouad-Tarazi FM, et al: The usefulness of head-up tilt testing and hemodynamic investigations in the workup of syncope of unknown origin. *PACE* 11:1202-1214, 1988

77. Waxman MB, Yao L, Cameron DA, et al: Isoproterenol induction of vasodepressor-type reaction in vasodepressor-prone persons. *Am J Cardiol* 63:58-65, 1989

78. Sheldon R, Splawinski J, Killam S: Reproducibility of isoproterenol tilt-table tests in patients with syncope. *Am J Cardiol* 69:1300-1305, 1992

79. Sheldon R, Killam S: Methodology of isoproterenol-tilt table testing in patients with syncope. *J Am Coll Cardiol* 19:773-779, 1992

80. Kapoor WN, Brant N: Evaluation of syncope by upright tilt testing with isoproterenol. A nonspecific test. *Ann Intern Med* 116:358-363, 1992

81. Raviele A, Gasparini G, Di Pede F, et al: Usefulness of head-up tilt test in evaluating patients with syncope of unknown origin and negative electrophysiologic study. *Am J Cardiol* 65:1322-1327, 1990

82. Grubb BP, Temesy-Armos P, Hahn H, et al: Utility of upright tilt-table testing in the evaluation and management of syncope of unknown origin. *Am J Med* 90:6-10, 1991

83. Grubb BP, Temesy-Armos P, Moore J, et al: Head-upright tilt-table testing in evaluation and management of the malignant vasovagal syndrome. *Am J Cardiol* 69:904-908, 1992

84. Markel ML, Miles WM, Zipes DP, et al: Parasympathetic and sympathetic alterations of Mobitz type II heart block. *J Am Coll Cardiol* 11:271-275, 1988

85. Sadr-Ameli MA, Shenasa M, Lacombe P, et al: Effect of autonomic nervous system modulation on retrograde atrioventricular nodal conduction in the human heart. *Cardiovasc Res* 21:45-54, 1987

86. Paraskos JA: Cardiovascular pharmacology. III: Atropine, calcium, calcium blockers, and beta-blockers. *Circulation* 74 Suppl 4:86-89, 1986

87. Gupta PK, Lichstein E, Chadda KD, et al: Appraisal of sinus nodal recovery time in patients with sick sinus syndrome. *Am J Cardiol* 34:265-270, 1974

88. Bashour T, Hemb R, Wickramesekaran R: An unusual effect of atropine on overdrive suppression (letter to the editor). *Circulation* 48:911-912, 1973

89. Reiffel JA, Bigger JT, Giardina E-GV: "Paradoxical" prolongation of sinus nodal recovery time after atropine in the sick sinus syndrome. *Am J Cardiol* 36:98-104, 1975

90. Marcus B, Gillette PC, Garson A Jr: Electrophysiologic evaluation of sinus node dysfunction in postoperative children and young adults utilizing combined autonomic blockade. *Clin Cardiol* 14:33-40, 1991

91. Kerr CR: Effect of pacing cycle length and autonomic blockade on sinus node refractoriness. *Am J Cardiol* 62:1192-1196, 1988

92. Kuga K, Yamaguchi I, Sugishita Y, et al: Assessment by autonomic blockade of age-related changes of the sinus node function and autonomic regulation in sick sinus syndrome. *Am J Cardiol* 61:361-366, 1988

93. Cappato R, Alboni P, Paparella N, et al: Bedside evaluation of sinus bradycardia: usefulness of atropine test in discriminating organic from autonomic involvement of sinus automaticity. *Am Heart J* 114:1384-1388, 1987

94. Josephson ME, Caracta AR, Ricciutti MA, et al: Electrophysiologic properties of procainamide in man. *Am J Cardiol* 33:596-603, 1974

95. Scheinman MM, Weiss AN, Shafton E, et al: Electrophysiologic effects of procaine amide in patients with intraventricular conduction delay. *Circulation* 49:522-529, 1974

96. Twidale N, Heddle WF, Tonkin AM: Procainamide administration during electrophysiology study—utility as a provocative test for intermittent atrioventricular block. *PACE* 11:1388-1397, 1988

97. Gupta PK, Lichstein E, Chadda KD: Lidocaine-induced heart block in patients with bundle branch block. *Am J Cardiol* 33:487-492, 1974

98. McKenna WJ, Rowland E, Davies J, et al: Failure to predict development of atrioventricular block with electrophysiological testing supplemented by ajmaline. *PACE* 3:666-669, 1980

99. Chiale PA, Przybylski J, Laiño RA, et al: Usefulness of the ajmaline test in patients with latent bundle branch block. *Am J Cardiol* 49:21-26, 1982

100. Kim YH, Leitch JW, Klein GJ, et al: Effect of atropine and isoproterenol on tachycardia induction in asymptomatic patients with Wolff-Parkinson-White electrocardiographic pattern. *Can J Cardiol* 8:716-720, 1992

101. Toda I, Kawahara T, Murakawa Y, et al: Electrophysiological study of young patients with exercise related paroxysms of palpitation: role of atropine and isoprenaline for initiation of supraventricular tachycardia. *Br Heart J* 61:268-273, 1989

102. Wu D, Denes P, Bauernfeind R, et al: Effects of atropine on induction and maintenance of atrioventricular nodal reentrant tachycardia. *Circulation* 59:779-788, 1979

103. Akhtar M, Damato AN, Batsford WP, et al: Induction of atrioventricular nodal reentrant tachycardia after atropine: report of five cases. *Am J Cardiol* 36:286-291, 1975

104. Mason JW, Winkle RA: Electrode-catheter arrhythmia induction in the selection and assessment of antiarrhythmic drug therapy for recurrent ventricular tachycardia. *Circulation* 58:971-985, 1978

105. Reddy CP, Gettes LS: Use of isoproterenol as an aid to electric induction of chronic recurrent ventricular tachycardia. *Am J Cardiol* 44:705-713, 1979

106. Freedman RA, Swerdlow CD, Echt DS, et al: Facilitation of ventricular tachyarrhythmia induction by isoproterenol. *Am J Cardiol* 54:765-770, 1984

107. Morady F, Hess D, Scheinman MM: Electrophysiologic drug testing in patients with malignant ventricular arrhythmias: importance of stimulation at more than one ventricular site. *Am J Cardiol* 50:1055-1060, 1982

108. Morady F, DiCarlo L, Winston S, et al: A prospective comparison of triple extrastimuli and left ventricular stimulation in studies of ventricular tachycardia induction. *Circulation* 70:52-57, 1984

109. Niazi I, Naccarelli G, Dougherty A, et al: Treatment of atrioventricular node reentrant tachycardia with encainide: reversal of drug effect with isoproterenol. *J Am Coll Cardiol* 13:904-910, 1989

110. Wesley RC Jr, Taylor R, Nadamanee K: Catecholamine-sensitive right ventricular tachycardia in the absence of structural heart disease: a mechanism of exercise-induced cardiac arrest. *Cardiology* 79:237-243, 1991

111. Shimizu W, Ohe T, Kurita T, et al: Early afterdepolarizations induced by isoproterenol in patients with congenital long QT syndrome. *Circulation* 84:1915-1923, 1991

112. Haissaguerre M, Le Metayer P, D'Ivernois C, et al: Distinctive response of arrhythmogenic right ventricular disease to high dose isoproterenol. *PACE* 13:2119-2126, 1990

113. Szabo TS, Klein GJ, Sharma AD, et al: Usefulness of isoproterenol during atrial fibrillation in evaluation of asymptomatic Wolff-Parkinson-White pattern. *Am J Cardiol* 63:187-192, 1989

114. Huycke EC, Lai WT, Nguyen NX, et al: Role of intravenous isoproterenol in the electrophysiologic induction of atrioventricular node reentrant tachycardia in patients with dual atrioventricular node pathways. *Am J Cardiol* 64:1131-1137, 1989

115. Brembilla-Perrot B, Terrier de la Chaise A, Pichene M, et al: Isoprenaline as an aid to the induction of catecholamine dependent supraventricular tachycardias during programmed stimulation. *Br Heart J* 61:348-355, 1989

116. Chosy JJ, Graham DT: Catecholamines in vasovagal fainting. *J Psychosom Res* 9:189-194, 1965

117. Vingerhoets AJJM: Biochemical changes in two subjects succumbing to syncope. *Psychosom Med* 46:95-103, 1984

118. Markel ML, Miles WM, Luck JC, et al: Differential effects of isoproterenol on sustained ventricular tachycardia before and during procainamide and quinidine antiarrhythmic drug therapy. *Circulation* 87:783-792, 1993

119. Manolis AS, Katsaros C, Cokkinos DV: Electrophysiological and electropharmacological studies in pre-excitation syndromes: results with propafenone therapy and isoproterenol infusion testing. *Eur Heart J* 13:1489-1495, 1992

120. Helmy I, Scheinman MM, Herre JM, et al: Electrophysiologic effects of isoproterenol in patients with atrioventricular reentrant tachycardia treated with flecainide. *J Am Coll Cardiol* 16:1649-1655, 1990

121. DiCarlo LA Jr, Susser F, Winston SA: The role of beta-blockade therapy for ventricular tachycardia induced with isoproterenol: a prospective analysis. *Am Heart J* 120:1347-1355, 1990

122. Jazayeri MR, Van Wyhe G, Avitall B, et al: Isoproterenol reversal of antiarrhythmic effects in patients with inducible sustained ventricular tachyarrhythmias. *J Am Coll Cardiol* 14:705-711, 1989

123. Manolis AS, Estes NA III: Reversal of electrophysiologic effects of flecainide on the accessory pathway by isoproterenol in the Wolff-Parkinson-White syndrome. *Am J Cardiol* 64:194-198, 1989

124. Strasberg B, Sclarovsky S, Erdberg A, et al: Procainamide-induced polymorphous ventricular tachycardia. *Am J Cardiol* 47:1309-1314, 1981

125. Dhingra RC, Amat-y-Leon F, Wyndham C, et al: Electrophysiologic effects of atropine on sinus node and atrium in patients with sinus nodal dysfunction. *Am J Cardiol* 38:848-855, 1976

126. Breithardt G, Seipel L, Both A, et al: The effect of atropine on calculated sinoatrial conduction time in man. *Eur J Cardiol* 4:49-57, 1976

127. Kang PS, Gomes JAC, El-Sherif N: Differential effects of functional autonomic blockade on the variables of sinus nodal automaticity in sick sinus syndrome. *Am J Cardiol* 49:273-282, 1982

128. Kang PS, Gomes JA, Kelen G, et al: Role of autonomic regulatory mechanisms in sinoatrial conduction and sinus node automaticity in sick sinus syndrome. *Circulation* 64:832-838, 1981

129. Jose AD: Effect of combined sympathetic and parasympathetic blockade on heart rate and cardiac function in man. *Am J Cardiol* 18:476-478, 1966

130. Desai JM, Scheinmann MM, Strauss HC, et al: Electrophysiologic effects of combined autonomic blockade in patients with sinus node disease. *Circulation* 63:953-960, 1981

131. Breithardt G, Seipel L, Loogen F: Sinus node recovery time and calculated sinoatrial conduction time in normal subjects and patients with sinus node dysfunction. *Circulation* 56:43-50, 1977

132. Strauss HC, Bigger JT Jr, Saroff AL, et al: Electrophysiologic evaluation of sinus node function in patients with sinus node dysfunction. *Circulation* 53:763-776, 1976

133. Steinbeck G, Lderitz B: Comparative study of sinoatrial conduction time and sinus node recovery time. *Br Heart J* 37:956-962, 1975

134. Reiffel JA, Bigger JT Jr, Cramer M, et al: Ability of Holter electrocardiographic recording and atrial stimulation to detect sinus nodal dysfunction in symptomatic and asymptomatic patients with sinus bradycardia. *Am J Cardiol* 40:189-194, 1977

135. Mandel WJ, Laks MM, Obayashi K: Sinus node function: evaluation in patients with and without sinus node disease. *Arch Intern Med* 135:388-394, 1975

136. Jordan JL, Mandel WJ: Disorders of sinus function. In *Cardiac Arrhythmias: Their Mechanisms, Diagnosis, and Management.* Edited by WJ Mandel. Philadelphia, JB Lippincott Company, 1980, pp 107-144.

137. Strauss HC, Grant AO, Scheinman MM, et al: The use of cardiac stimulation techniques to evaluate sinus node dysfunction. In *Physiology of Atrial Pacemakers and Conductive Tissues.* Edited by RC Little. Mount Kisco, New York, Futura Publishing Company, 1980, pp 339-365

138. Jordan JL, Yamaguchi I, Mandel WJ: Studies on the mechanism of sinus node dysfunction in the sick sinus syndrome. *Circulation* 57:217-223, 1978

139. Kerr CR, Strauss HC: The measurement of sinus node refractoriness in man. *Circulation* 68:1231-1237, 1983

140. Wu DL, Yeh SJ, Lin FC, et al: Sinus automaticity and sinoatrial conduction in severe symptomatic sick sinus syndrome. *J Am Coll Cardiol* 19:355-364, 1992

141. Reiffel JA, Ferrick K, Zimmerman J, et al: Electrophysiologic

studies of the sinus node and atria. *Cardiovasc Clin* 16:37-59, 1985

142. Tonkin AM, Heddle WF: Electrophysiological testing of sinus node function. *PACE* 7:735-748, 1984

143. Reiffel JA, Gang E, Gliklich J, et al: The human sinus node electrogram: a transvenous catheter technique and a comparison of directly measured and indirectly estimated sinoatrial conduction time in adults. *Circulation* 62:1324-1334, 1980

144. Hariman RJ, Krongrad E, Boxer RA, et al: Methods for recording electrograms of the sinoatrial node during cardiac surgery in man. *Circulation* 61:1024-1029, 1980

145. Hariman RJ, Krongrad E, Boxer RA, et al: A method for recording of extracellular sinoatrial electrograms during cardiac surgery in man (abstract). *Am J Cardiol* 41:375, 1978

146. Lange G: Action of driving stimuli from intrinsic and extrinsic sources on in situ cardiac pacemaker tissues. *Circ Res* 17:449-459, 1965

147. Lu H-H, Lange G, Brooks CM: Factors controlling pacemaker action in cells of the sinoatrial node. *Circ Res* 17:460-471, 1965

148. Furchgott RF, de Gubareff T, Grossman A: Release of autonomic mediators in cardiac tissue by suprathreshold stimulation. *Science* 129:328-329, 1959

149. Goldreyer BN, Damato AN: Sinoatrial-node entrance block. *Circulation* 44:789-802, 1971

150. Narula OS, Samet P, Javier RP: Significance of the sinus-node recovery time. *Circulation* 45:140-158, 1972

151. Yee R, Strauss HC: Electrophysiologic mechanisms: sinus node dysfunction. *Circulation* 75 Suppl 3:12-18, 1987

152. Benditt DG, Gornick CC, Dunbar D, et al: Indications for electrophysiologic testing in the diagnosis and assessment of sinus node dysfunction. *Circulation* 75 Suppl 3:93-102, 1987

153. Kulbertus HE, de Leval-Rutten F, Mary L, et al: Sinus node recovery time in the elderly. *Br Heart J* 37:420-425, 1975

154. Rosen KM, Loeb HS, Sinno MZ, et al: Cardiac conduction in patients with symptomatic sinus node disease. *Circulation* 43:836-844, 1971

155. Jordan JL, Yamaguchi I, Mandel WJ: The sick sinus syndrome: pathophysiology, significance, and treatment. *Cardiol Dig* 12:11-22, 1977

156. Benditt DG, Strauss HC, Sheinman MM, et al: Analysis of secondary pauses following termination of rapid atrial pacing in man. *Circulation* 54:436-441, 1976

157. Narula OS, Shantha N, Narula LK, et al: Clinical and electrophysiological evaluation of sinus node function. In *Cardiac Arrhythmias: Electrophysiology, Diagnosis and Management.* Edited by OS Narula. Baltimore, Williams & Wilkins Company, 1979, pp 176-206

158. Eckberg DL, Drabinsky M, Braunwald E: Defective cardiac parasympathetic control in patients with heart disease. *N Engl J Med* 285:877-883, 1971

159. Morton HJV, Thomas ET: Effect of atropine on the heart-rate. *Lancet* 2:1313-1315, 1958

160. Mandel WJ, Hayakawa H, Allen HN, et al: Assessment of sinus node function in patients with the sick sinus syndrome. *Circulation* 46:761-769, 1972

161. Cleaveland CR, Rangno RE, Shand DG: A standardized isoproterenol sensitivity test: the effects of sinus arrhythmia, atropine, and propranolol. *Arch Intern Med* 130:47-52, 1972

162. Strauss HC, Saroff AL, Bigger JT Jr, et al: Premature atrial stimulation as a key to the understanding of sinoatrial conduction in man: presentation of data and critical review of the literature. *Circulation* 47:86-93, 1973

163. Breithardt G, Seipel L: The effect of premature atrial depolarization on sinus node automaticity in man. *Circulation* 53:920-925, 1976

164. Dhingra RC, Wyndham C, Amat-y-Leon F, et al: Sinus nodal responses to atrial extrastimuli in patients without apparent sinus node disease. *Am J Cardiol* 36:445-452, 1975

165. Masini G, Dianda R, Graziina A: Analysis of sino-atrial conduction in man using premature atrial stimulation. *Cardiovasc Res* 9:498-508, 1975

166. Bonke FIM, Bouman LN, Schopman FJG: Effect of an early atrial premature beat on activity of the sinoatrial node and atrial rhythm in the rabbit. *Circ Res* 29:704-715, 1971

167. Bonke FIM, Bouman LN, van Rijn HE: Change of cardiac rhythm in the rabbit after an atrial premature beat. *Cir Res* 24:533-544, 1969

168. Steinbeck G, Lüderitz B: Sinoatrial pacemaker shift following atrial stimulation in man. *Circulation* 56:402-409, 1977

169. Miller HC, Strauss HC: Measurement of sinoatrial conduction time by premature atrial stimulation in the rabbit. *Circ Res* 35:935-947, 1974

170. Jordan J, Yamaguchi I, Mandel WJ: Characteristics of sinoatrial conduction in patients with coronary artery disease. *Circulation* 55:569-574, 1977

171. Scheinman MM, Strauss HC, Abbott JA, et al: Electrophysiologic testing in patients with sinus pauses and/or sinoatrial exit block. *Eur J Cardiol* 8:51-60, 1978

172. Narula OS, Shantha N, Vasquez M, et al: A new method for measurement of sinoatrial conduction time. *Circulation* 58:706-714, 1978

173. Breithardt G, Seipel L: Comparative study of two methods of estimating sinoatrial conduction time in man. *Am J Cardiol* 42:965-972, 1978

174. Evans TR, Callowhill EA, Kirkler DM: Clinical value of tests of sino-atrial function. *PACE* 1:2-7, 1978

175. Lüderitz B, Steinbeck G, d'Alnoncourt CN, et al: Relevance of diagnostic stimulation for pacemaker treatment in sinoatrial disease. In *The Sinus Node: Structure, Function, and Clinical Relevance.* Edited by FIM Bonke. The Hague, Martinus Nijhoff, 1978, pp 77-88

176. Schweitzer P, Mark H: The values and limitations of deductive analysis and electrophysiological testing in patients with sinoatrial arrhythmias. *PACE* 7:403-420, 1984

177. Cain ME: Electrophysiologic assessment of sinus node function: discussion. *Circulation* 75 Suppl 3:100-102, 1987

178. Rahimtoola SH, Zipes DP, Akhtar M, et al: Consensus statement of the Conference on the State of the Art of Electrophysiologic Testing in the Diagnosis and Treatment of Patients with Cardiac Arrhythmias. *Circulation* 75 Suppl 3:3-11, 1987

179. Kerr CR, Prystowsky EN, Browning DJ, et al: Characterization of refractoriness in the sinus node of the rabbit. *Circ Res* 47:742-756, 1980

180. Kerr CR, Strauss HC, Aiama N: Effect of basic pacing cycle length on sinus node refractoriness in the rabbit. *Am J Cardiol* 56:162-167, 1985

181. Anderson RH, Becker AE: Gross anatomy and microscopy of the conducting system. In *Cardiac Arrhythmias: Their Mechanisms, Diagnosis, and Management.* Edited by WJ Mandel. Philadelphia, JB Lippincott Company, 1980, pp 12-54

182. Spach MS, Miller WT III, Barr RC, et al: Electrophysiology of the internodal pathways: determining the difference between anisotropic cardiac muscle and a specialized tract system. In *Physiology of Atrial Pacemakers and Conductive Tissues.* Edited by RC Little. Mount Kisco, New York, Futura Publishing Company, 1980, pp 367-380

183. Sherf L, James TN: Functional anatomy and ultrastructure of the internodal pathways. In *Physiology of Atrial Pacemakers and Conductive Tissues.* Edited by RC Little. Mount Kisco, New York, Futura Publishing Company, 1980, pp 67-112

184. Amat-y-Leon F, Dhingra RC, Wu D, et al: Catheter mapping of retrograde atrial activation: observations during ventricular pacing and AV nodal re-entrant paroxysmal tachycardia. *Br Heart J* 38:355-362, 1976

185. Watson RM, Josephson ME: Atrial flutter. I. Electrophysiologic substrates and modes of initiation and termination. *Am J Cardiol* 45:732-741, 1980

186. Leier CV, Meacham JA, Schaal SF: Prolonged atrial conduction: a major predisposing factor for the development of atrial flutter. *Circulation* 57:213-216, 1978

187. Allessie MA, Bonke FIM: Atrial arrhythmias: basic concepts. In *Cardiac Arrhythmias: Their Mechanisms, Diagnosis, and Management.* Edited by WJ Mandel, Philadelphia, JB Lippincott Company, 1980, pp 145-166

188. Misier AR, Opthof T, van Hemel NM, et al: Increased dispersion of "refractoriness" in patients with idiopathic paroxysmal atrial fibrillation. *J Am Coll Cardiol* 19:1531-1535, 1992

189. Kumagai K, Akimitsu S, Kawahira K, et al: Electrophysiological properties in chronic lone atrial fibrillation. *Circulation* 84:1662-1668, 1991

190. Wit AL, Weiss MB, Berkowitz WD, et al: Patterns of atrioventricular conduction in the human heart. *Circ Res* 27:345-359, 1970

191. Benditt DG, Epstein ML, Arentzen CE, et al: Enhanced atrioventricular conduction in patients without preexcitation syndrome: relation to heart rate in paroxysmal reciprocating tachycardia. *Circulation* 65:1474-1479, 1982

192. Holmes DR Jr, Hartzler GO, Merideth J: The clinical and electrophysiologic characteristics of patients with accelerated atrioventricular nodal conduction. *Mayo Clin Proc* 57:339-344, 1982

193. Holmes DR Jr, Hartzler GO, Maloney JD: Concealed retrograde bypass tracts and enhanced atrioventricular nodal conduction: an unusual subset of patients with refractory paroxysmal supraventricular tachycardia. *Am J Cardiol* 45:1053-1060, 1980
194. Benditt DG, Pritchett ELC, Smith WM, et al: Characteristics of atrioventricular conduction and the spectrum of arrhythmias in Lown-Ganong-Levine syndrome. *Circulation* 57:454-465, 1978
195. Caracta AR, Damato AN, Gallagher JJ, et al: Electrophysiologic studies in the syndrome of short P-R interval, normal QRS complex. *Am J Cardiol* 31:245-253, 1973
196. Childers R: The AV node: normal and abnormal physiology. *Prog Cardiovas Dis* 19:361-384, 1977
197. Gallagher JJ, Sealy WC, Kasell J, et al: Multiple accessory pathways in patients with the pre-excitation syndrome. *Circulation* 54:571-591, 1976
198. Brechenmacher C: Atrio-His bundle tracts. *Br Heart J* 37:853-855, 1975
199. DiMarco JD, Garan H, Harthorne JW, et al: Intracardiac electrophysiologic techniques in recurrent syncope of unknown cause. *Ann Intern Med* 95:542-548, 1981
200. Meytes I, Kaplinsky E, Yahini JH, et al: Wenckebach A-V block: a frequent feature following heavy physical training. *Am Heart J* 90:426-430, 1975
201. Schlesinger Z, Barzilay J, Stryjer D, et al: Life-threatening "vagal reaction" to emotional stimuli. *Isr J Med Sci* 13:59-61, 1977
202. Cullen KJ, Collin R: Daily running causing Wenckebach heart-block. *Lancet* 2:729-730, 1964
203. Rosen KM, Loeb HS, Gunnar RM, et al: Mobitz type II block without bundle-branch block. *Circulation* 44:1111-1119, 1971
204. Yeh BK, Tao P, deGuzman N: Mobitz type II A-V block as a manifestation of digitalis toxicity. *J Electrocardiol* 5:74-77, 1972
205. Pinsky WW: Diagnosis and management of congenital complete atrioventricular block. In *Pediatric Cardiac Dysrhythmias.* Edited by PC Gillette, A Garson Jr. New York, Grune & Stratton, 1981, pp 383-396
206. Rosen KM, Mehta A, Rahimtoola SH, et al: Sites of congenital and surgical heart block as defined by His bundle electrocardiography. *Circulation* 44:833-841, 1971
207. Anderson RH, Wenick ACG, Losekoot TG, et al: Congenitally complete heart block: developmental aspects. *Circulation* 56:90-101, 1977
208. Damato AN, Varghese PJ, Caracta AR, et al: Functional 2:1 A-V block within the His-Purkinje system: stimulation of type II second-degree A-V block. *Circulation* 47:534-542, 1973
209. Dhingra RC, Wyndham C, Bauernfeind R, et al: Significance of block distal to the His bundle induced by atrial pacing in patients with chronic bifascicular block. *Circulation* 60:1455-1464, 1979
210. Reddy CP, Damato AN, Akhtar M, et al: Study of the temporal effects on conduction and refractoriness of the His-Purkinje system in man. *Am Heart J* 96:316-325, 1978
211. Narula OS, Samet P: Wenckebach and Mobitz type II A-V block due to block within the His bundle and bundle branches. *Circulation* 41:947-965, 1970
212. Peuch P, Grolleau R, Giumond C: Incidence of different types of A-V block and their localization by His bundle recordings. In *The Conduction System of the Heart: Structure, Function and Clinical Implications.* Edited by HJJ Wellens, KI Lie, MJ Janse. Philadelphia, Lea & Febiger, pp 467-484
213. Narula OS, Shantha N: Atrioventricular block: clinical concepts and His bundle electrocardiography. In *Cardiac Arrhythmias: Their Mechanisms, Diagnosis, and Management.* Edited by WJ Mandel. Philadelphia, JB Lippincott Company, 1980, pp 437-453
214. Altschuler H, Fisher JD, Furman S: Significance of isolated H-V interval prolongation in symptomatic patients without documented heart block. *Am Heart J* 97:19-26, 1979
215. Scheinman M, Weiss A, Kunkel F: His bundle recordings in patients with bundle branch block and transient neurologic symptoms. *Circulation* 48:322-330, 1973
216. Rosen KM, Dhingra RC, Wyndham CRC, et al: Significance of H-V interval in 515 patients with chronic bifascicular block (abstract). *Am J Cardiol* 45:405, 1980
217. Vera Z, Mason DT, Fletcher RD, et al: Prolonged His-Q interval in chronic bifascicular block: relation to impending complete heart block. *Circulation* 53:46-55, 1976
218. Dhingra RC, Denes P, Wu D, et al: Syncope in patients with chronic bifascicular block: significance, causative mechanisms, and clinical implications. *Ann Intern Med* 81:302-306, 1974
219. Click RL, Gersh BJ, Sugrue DD, et al: Role of invasive electrophysiologic testing in patients with symptomatic bundle branch block. *Am J Cardiol* 59:817-823, 1987
220. Bauernfeind RA, Wyndham C, Dhingra RC, et al: Paroxysmal supraventricular tachycardia. In *Cardiac Arrhythmias: Their Mechanisms, Diagnosis, and Management.* Edited by WJ Mandel. Philadelphia, JB Lippincott Company, 1980, pp 193-204
221. Wit AL, Rosen MR: Afterdepolarizations and triggered activity: distinction from automaticity as an arrhythmogenic mechanism. In *The Heart and the Cardiovascular System.* Second edition. Edited by HA Fozzard, RE Haber, RB Jennings, et al. New York, Raven Press, 1991, pp 2113-2163
222. Josephson ME: Paroxysmal supraventricular tachycardia: an electrophysiologic approach (editorial). *Am J Cardiol* 41:1123-1126, 1978
223. Wu D, Denes P, Amat-y-Leon F, et al: Clinical, electrocardiographic and electrophysiologic observations in patients with paroxysmal supraventricular tachycardia. *Am J Cardiol* 41:1045-1051, 1978
224. Josephson ME, Kastor JA: Supraventricular tachycardia: mechanisms and management. *Ann Intern Med* 87:346-358, 1977
225. Josephson ME, Wellens HJ: Differential diagnosis of supraventricular tachycardia. *Cardiol Clin* 8:411-442, 1990
226. Akhtar M, Jazayeri MR, Sra J, et al: Atrioventricular nodal reentry. Clinical, electrophysiological, and therapeutic considerations. *Circulation* 88:282-295, 1993
227. Jazayeri MR, Sra JS, Akhtar M: Atrioventricular nodal reentrant tachycardia. Electrophysiologic characteristics, therapeutic interventions, and specific reference to anatomic boundary of the reentrant circuit. *Cardiol Clin* 11:151-181, 1993
228. Wathen MS, Klein GJ, Yee R, et al: Classification and terminology of supraventricular tachycardia. Diagnosis and management of the atrial tachycardias. *Cardiol Clin* 11:109-120, 1993
229. Oren JW IV, Beckman KJ, McClelland JH, et al: A functional approach to the preexcitation syndromes. *Cardiol Clin* 11:121-149, 1993
230. Waldo AL, MacLean WAH, Karp RB, et al: Entrainment and interruption of atrial flutter with atrial pacing: studies in man following open heart surgery. *Circulation* 56:737-745, 1977
231. Waldo AL, Wells JL Jr, Plumb VJ, et al: Characterization of atrial flutter: studies in patients following open heart surgery. In *Cardiac Arrhythmias: Electrophysiology, Diagnosis and Management.* Edited by OS Narula. Baltimore, Williams & Wilkins Company, 1979, pp 256-271
232. Wells JL Jr, MacLean WAH, James TN, et al: Characterization of atrial flutter: studies in man after open heart surgery using fixed atrial electrodes. *Circulation* 60:665-673, 1979
233. Waldo AL, MacLean WAH: Diagnosis and treatment of arrhythmias following open-heart surgery. In *Cardiac Arrhythmias: Their Mechanisms, Diagnosis, and Management.* Edited by WJ Mandel. Philadelphia, JB Lippincott Company, 1980, pp 514-533
234. Simpson RJ Jr: Clinical electrophysiology of the normal and diseased human atria. In *Atrial Fibrillation: Mechanisms and Management.* Edited by RH Falk, PJ Podrid. New York, Raven Press, 1992, pp 321-332
235. Waldo AL: Mechanisms of atrial fibrillation, atrial flutter, and ectopic atrial tachycardia—a brief review. *Circulation* 75 Suppl 3:37-40, 1987
236. Calkins H, Leon AR, Deam AG, et al: Catheter ablation of atrial flutter using radiofrequency energy. *Am J Cardiol* 73:353-356, 1994
237. Rodriguez LM, Smeets JL, Xie B, et al: Improvement in left ventricular function by ablation of atrioventricular nodal conduction in selected patients with lone atrial fibrillation. *Am J Cardiol* 72:1137-1141, 1993
238. Cosio FG, Goicolea A, Lopez-Gil M, et al: Catheter ablation of atrial flutter circuits. *PACE* 16:637-642, 1993
239. Cosio FG, Lopez-Gil M, Goicolea A, et al: Radiofrequency ablation of the inferior vena cava-tricuspid valve isthmus in common atrial flutter. *Am J Cardiol* 71:705-709, 1993
240. Feld GK, Fleck RP, Chen PS, et al: Radiofrequency catheter ablation for the treatment of human type 1 atrial flutter. Identification of a critical zone in the reentrant circuit by endocardial mapping techniques. *Circulation* 86:1233-1240, 1992
241. Wood DL, Hammill SC, Holmes DR Jr, et al: Catheter ablation of the atrioventricular conduction system in patients with supraventricular tachycardia. *Mayo Clin Proc* 58:791-796, 1983
242. Williamson BD, Man KC, Daoud E, et al: Radiofrequency catheter modification of atrioventricular conduction to control the ventricular rate during atrial fibrillation. *N Engl J Med* 331:910-917, 1994
243. Horowitz LN, Josephson ME, Kastor JA: Intracardiac electro-

physiologic studies as a method for the optimization of drug therapy in chronic ventricular arrhythmia. *Prog Cardiovasc Dis* 23:81-98, 1980

244. Hartzler GO, Maloney JD: Programmed ventricular stimulation in management of recurrent ventricular tachycardia. *Mayo Clin Proc* 52:731-741, 1977

245. Josephson ME, Horowitz LN: Electrophysiologic approach to therapy of recurrent sustained ventricular tachycardia. *Am J Cardiol* 43:631-642, 1979

246. Myerburg RJ, Conde CA, Sung RJ, et al: Clinical, electrophysiologic and hemodynamic profile of patients resuscitated from prehospital cardiac arrest. *Am J Med* 68:568-576, 1980

247. Josephson ME, Horowitz LN, Spielman SR, et al: Electrophysiologic and hemodynamic studies in patients resuscitated from cardiac arrest. *Am J Cardiol* 46:948-955, 1980

248. Gomes JAC, Hariman RI, Kang PS, et al: Programmed electrical stimulation in patients with high-grade ventricular ectopy: electrophysiologic findings and prognosis for survival. *Circulation* 70:43-51, 1984

249. Morady F. Scheinman MM, Hess DS, et al: Electrophysiologic testing in the management of survivors of out-of-hospital cardiac arrest. *Am J Cardiol* 51:85-89, 1983

250. Platia EV, Reid PR: Comparison of programmed electrical stimulation and ambulatory electrocardiographic (Holter) monitoring in the management of ventricular tachycardia and ventricular fibrillation. *J Am Coll Cardiol* 4:493-500, 1984

251. Morady F, DiCarlo L, Winston S, et al: Clinical features and prognosis of patients with out of hospital cardiac arrest and a normal electrophysiologic study. *J Am Coll Cardiol* 4:39-44, 1984

252. Horowitz LN, Greenspan AM, Spielman SR, et al: Usefulness of electrophysiologic testing in evaluation of amiodarone therapy for sustained ventricular tacharrhythmias associated with coronary heart disease. *Am J Cardiol* 55:367-371, 1985

253. Mirowski M: The automatic implantable cardioverter-defibrillator: an overview. *J Am Coll Cardiol* 6:461-466, 1985

254. DiCarlo LA Jr, Morady F, Sauve MJ, et al: Cardiac arrest and sudden death in patients treated with amiodarone for sustained ventricular tachycardia or ventricular fibrillation: risk stratification based on clinical variables. *Am J Cardiol* 55:372-374, 1985

255. Hammill SC, Trusty JM, Wood DL, et al: Influence of ventricular function and presence or absence of coronary artery disease on results of electrophysiologic testing for asymptomatic nonsustained ventricular tachycardia. *Am J Cardiol* 65:722-728, 1990

256. Holmes DR Jr: Automatic implantable cardioverter defibrillator. In *A Practice of Cardiac Pacing.* Second edition. Edited by S Furman, DL Hayes, DR Holmes Jr. Mount Kisco, New York, Futura Publishing Company, 1989, pp 427-455

257. Brugada P, Wellens HJJ: Comparison in the same patient of two programmed ventricular stimulation protocols to induce ventricular tachycardia. *Am J Cardiol* 55:380-383, 1985

258. Mann DE, Luck JC, Griffin JC, et al: Induction of clinical ventricular tachycardia using programmed stimulation: value of third and fourth extrastimuli. *Am J Cardiol* 52:501-506, 1983

259. Doherty JU, Kienzle MG, Waxman HL, et al: Programmed ventricular stimulation at a second right ventricular site: an analysis of 100 patients, with special reference to sensitivity, specificity and characteristics of patients with induced ventricular tachycardia. *Am J Cardiol* 52:1184-1189, 1983

260. Schoenfeld MH, McGovern B, Garan H, et al: Long-term reproducibility of responses to programmed cardiac stimulation in spontaneous ventricular tachyarrhythmias. *Am J Cardiol* 54:564-568, 1984

261. Veltri EP, Platia EV, Griffith LSC, et al: Programmed electrical stimulation and long-term follow-up in asymptomatic, nonsustained ventricular tachycardia. *Am J Cardiol* 56:309-314, 1985

262. Sulpizi AM, Friehling TD, Kowey PR: Value of electrophysiologic testing in patients with nonsustained ventricular tachycardia. *Am J Cardiol* 59:841-845, 1987

263. Poser RF, Podrid PJ, Lombardi F, et al: Aggravation of arrhythmia induced with antiarrhythmic drugs during electrophysiologic testing. *Am Heart J* 110:9-16, 1985

264. Brugada P, Green M, Abdollah H, et al: Significance of ventricular arrhythmias initiated by programmed ventricular stimulation: the importance of the type of ventricular arrhythmia induced and the number of premature stimuli required. *Circulation* 69:87-92, 1984

265. Buxton AE, Waxman HL, Marchlinski FE, et al: Role of triple extrastimuli during electrophysiologic study of patients with documented sustained ventricular tachyarrhythmias. *Circulation* 69:532-540, 1984

266. Prystowsky EN: Electrophysiologic-electropharmacologic testing in patients with ventricular arrhythmias. *PACE* 11:225-251, 1988

267. Roy D, Waxman HL, Kienzle MG, et al: Clinical characteristics and long-term follow-up in 119 survivors of cardiac arrest: relation to inducibility at electrophysiologic testing. *Am J Cardiol* 52:969-974, 1983

268. DiMarco JP: Work-up and management of sudden cardiac death survivors. *Cardiol Clin* 11:11-19, 1993

269. Hsia HH, Buxton AE: Work-up and management of patients with sustained and nonsustained monomorphic ventricular tachycardias. *Cardiol Clin* 11:21-37, 1993

270. Grogin HR, Scheinman M: Evaluation and management of patients with polymorphic ventricular tachycardia. *Cardiol Clin* 11:39-54, 1993

271. Mason JW, Winkle RA: Accuracy of the ventricular tachycardia-induction study for predicting long-term efficacy and inefficacy of antiarrhythmic drugs. *N Engl J Med* 303:1073-1077, 1980

272. Ruskin JN, DiMarco JP, Garan H: Out-of-hospital cardiac arrest: electrophysiologic observations and selection of long-term antiarrhythmic therapy. *N Engl J Med* 303:607-613, 1980

273. Wyse DG: Pharmacologic therapy in patients with ventricular tachyarrhythmias. *Cardiol Clin* 11:65-83, 1993

274. Kim YH, O'Nunain S, Ruskin JN, et al: Nonpharmacologic therapies in patients with ventricular tachyarrhythmias. Catheter ablation and ventricular tachycardia surgery. *Cardiol Clin* 11:85-96, 1993

275. Akhtar M, Jazayeri MR, Sra JS, et al: Implantable cardioverter-defibrillator therapy for prevention of sudden cardiac death. *Cardiol Clin* 11:97-108, 1993

276. Schamroth L: *The Disorders of Cardiac Rhythm.* Oxford, Blackwell Scientific Publications, 1971, pp 124-126

277. Sandler IA, Marriott HJL: The differential morphology of anomalous ventricular complexes of RBBB-type in lead V_1: ventricular ectopy versus aberration. *Circulation* 31:551-556, 1965

278. Krikler D: Ventricular tachycardia and ventricular fibrillation. In *Cardiac Arrhythmias: Their Mechanism, Diagnosis, and Management.* Edited by WJ Mandel. Philadelphia, JB Lippincott Company, 1980, pp 320-341

279. Wellens HJJ, Bär FWHM, Lie KI: The value of the electrocardiogram in the differential diagnosis of a tachycardia with a widened QRS complex. *Am J Med* 64:27-33, 1978

280. Wellens HJJ Bär FW, Farré J, et al: Initiation and termination of ventricular tachycardia by supraventricular stimuli: incidence and electrophysiologic determinants as observed during programmed stimulation of the heart. *Am J Cardiol* 46:576-582, 1980

281. Zipes DP, Foster PR, Troup PJ, et al: Atrial induction of ventricular tachycardia: reentry versus triggered automaticity. *Am J Cardiol* 44:1-8, 1979

282. Berman ND: Ventricular tachycardia initiated by both normally and aberrantly conducted atrial premature beats. *PACE* 3:519-525, 1980

283. DeLacey WA, Nath S, Haines DE, et al: Adenosine and verapamil-sensitive ventricular tachycardia originating from the left ventricle: radiofrequency catheter ablation. *PACE* 15:2240-2244, 1992

284. Lerman BB: Response of nonreentrant catecholamine-mediated ventricular tachycardia to endogenous adenosine and acetylcholine. Evidence for myocardial receptor-mediated effects. *Circulation* 87:382-390, 1993

285. Shen W-K, Hammill SC, Packer DL: Asymptomatic ventricular arrhythmias after MI: a therapeutic dilemma (part 1). *CARDIO* 11:36-41;50, 1994

286. Farrell TG, Bashir Y, Cripps T, et al: Risk stratification for arrhythmic events in postinfarction patients based on heart rate variability, ambulatory electrocardiographic variables and the signal-averaged electrocardiogram. *J Am Coll Cardiol* 18:687-697, 1991

287. Kuchar DL, Thorburn CW, Sammel NL: Prediction of serious arrhythmic events after myocardial infarction: signal-averaged electrocardiogram, Holter monitoring and radionuclide ventriculography. *J Am Coll Cardiol* 9:531-538, 1987

288. Akhtar M, Avitall B, Jazayeri M, et al: Role of implantable cardioverter defibrillator therapy in the management of high-risk patients. *Circulation* 85 Suppl 1:131-139, 1992

289. Akhtar M, Garan H, Lehmann MH, et al: Sudden cardiac death: management of high-risk patients. *Ann Intern Med* 114:499-512, 1991

290. Winkle RA, Mead RH, Ruder MA, et al: Long-term outcome with the automatic implantable cardioverter-defibrillator. *J Am Coll Cardiol* 13:1353-1361, 1989

291. Wellens HJJ: Value and limitations of programmed electrical stimulation of the heart in the study and treatment of tachycardias. *Circulation* 57:845-853, 1978

292. Wellens HJJ: *Electrical Stimulation of the Heart in the Study and Treatment of Tachycardias.* Baltimore, University Park Press, 1971, pp 122-127

293. Foster PR, Zipes DP: Pacing and cardiac arrhythmias. In *Cardiac Arrhythmias: Their Mechanisms, Diagnosis, and Management.* Edited by WJ Mandel. Philadelphia, JB Lippincott Company, 1980, pp 605-624

294. Ward DE, Camm AJ, Spurrell RAJ: The response of regular re-entrant supraventricular tachycardia to right heart stimulation. *PACE* 2:586-595, 1979

295. Spurrell RAJ, Nathan AW, Bexton RS, et al: Implantable automatic scanning pacemaker for termination of supraventricular tachycardia. *Am J Cardiol* 49:753-760, 1982

296. Critelli G, Grassi G, Chiariello M, et al: Automatic "scanning" by radiofrequency in the long-term electrical treatment of arrhythmias. *PACE* 2:289-296, 1979

297. Krikler D, Curry P, Buffet J: Dual-demand pacing for reciprocating atrioventricular tachycardia. *Br Med J* 1:1114-1116, 1976

298. Sung RJ, Styperek JL, Castellanos A: Complete abolition of the reentrant supraventricular tachycardia zone using a new modality of cardiac pacing with simultaneous atrioventricular stimulation. *Am J Cardiol* 45:72-78, 1980

299. Dreifus LS, Berkovits BV, Kimibiris D, et al: Use of atrial and bifocal cardiac pacemakers for treating resistant dysrhythmias. *Eur J Cardiol* 3:257-266, 1975

300. Spurrell RAJ, Sowton E: Pacing techniques in the management of supraventricular tachycardias. Part 2. An implanted atrial synchronous pacemaker with a short atrioventricular delay for the prevention of paroxysmal supraventricular tachycardias. *J Electrocardiol* 9:89-96, 1976

301. Curry PVL, Rowland E, Krikler DM: Dual-demand pacing for refractory atrioventricular re-entry tachycardia. *PACE* 2:137-151, 1979

302. Wellens HJJ, Durrer D: The role of an accessory atrioventricular pathway in reciprocal tachycardia: observations in patients with and without the Wolff-Parkinson-White syndrome. *Circulation* 52:58-72, 1975

303. Fisher JD, Kim SG, Furman S, et al: Role of implantable pacemakers in control of recurrent ventricular tachycardia. *Am J Cardiol* 49:194-206, 1982

304. Ruskin JN, Garan H, Poulin F, et al: Permanent radiofrequency ventricular pacing for management of drug-resistant ventricular tachycardia. *Am J Cardiol* 46:317-321, 1980

305. Kahn A, Morris JJ, Citron P: Patient-initiated rapid atrial pacing to manage supraventricular tachycardia. *Am J Cardiol* 38:200-204, 1976

306. Cooper TB, MacLean WAH, Waldo AL: Overdrive pacing for supraventricular tachycardia: a review of theoretical implications and therapeutic techniques. *PACE* 1:196-221, 1978

307. Hartzler GO, Holmes DR Jr, Osborn MJ: Patient-activated transvenous cardiac stimulation for the treatment of supraventricular and ventricular tachycardia. *Am J Cardiol* 47:903-909, 1981

308. Fisher JD, Mehra R, Furman S: Termination of ventricular tachycardia with bursts of rapid ventricular pacing. *Am J Cardiol* 41:94-102, 1978

309. Wu D, Amat-y-Leon F, Simpson RJ Jr, et al: Electrophysiological studies with multiple drugs in patients with atrioventricular reentrant tachycardias utilizing an extranodal pathway. *Circulation* 56:727-736, 1977

310. Bauernfeind RA, Wyndham CR, Dhingra RC, et al: Serial electrophysiologic testing of multiple drugs in patients with atrioventricular nodal reentrant paroxysmal tachycardia. *Circulation* 62:1341-1349, 1980

311. Wu D, Wyndham CR, Denes P, et al: Chronic electrophysiological study in patients with recurrent paroxysmal tachycardia: a new method for developing successful oral antiarrhythmic therapy. In *Re-Entrant Arrhythmias: Mechanisms and Treatment.* Edited by HE Kulbertus. Baltimore, University Park Press, 1977, pp 294-311

312. Fisher JD: Nonsurgical treatment of ventricular tachycardia: the value of serial provocative testing. In *Cardiac Arrhythmias: Electrophysiology, Diagnosis and Management.* Edited by OS Narula. Baltimore, Williams & Wilkins Company, 1979, pp 494-515

313. Klein GJ, Gulamhusein S, Prystowsky EN, et al: Comparison of the electrophysiologic effects of intravenous and oral verapamil in patients with paroxysmal supraventricular tachycardia. *Am J Cardiol* 49:117-124, 1982

314. Fisher JD, Cohen HL, Mehra R, et al: Cardiac pacing and pacemakers. II. Serial electrophysiologic-pharmacologic testing for control of recurrent tachyarrhythmias. *Am Heart J* 93:658-668, 1977

315. Horowitz LN, Josephson ME, Farshidi A, et al: Recurrent sustained ventricular tachycardia. 3. Role of the electrophysiologic study in selection of antiarrhythmic regimens. *Circulation* 58:986-997, 1978

316. Brandenburg RO Jr, Holmes DR Jr, Hartzler GO: The electrophysiologic assessment of patients with syncope (abstract). *Am J Cardiol* 47:433, 1981

317. Morady F, Shen E, Schwartz A, et al: Long-term follow-up of patients with recurrent unexplained syncope evaluated by electrophysiologic testing. *J Am Coll Cardiol* 2:1053-1059, 1983

318. Kapoor W, Karpf M, Levey GS: Issues in evaluating patients with syncope (editorial). *Ann Intern Med* 100:755-757, 1984

319. Gulamhusein S, Naccarelli GV, Ko PT, et al: Value and limitations of clinical electrophysiologic study in assessment of patients with unexplained syncope. *Am J Med* 73:700-705, 1982

320. Sugrue DD, Gersh BJ, Holmes DR Jr, et al: Symptomatic "isolated" carotid sinus hypersensitivity: natural history and results of treatment with anticholinergic drugs or pacemaker. *J Am Coll Cardiol* 7:158-162, 1986

321. McLaran CJ, Gersh BJ, Osborn MJ, et al: Increased vagal tone as an isolated finding in patients undergoing electrophysiological testing for recurrent syncope: response to long term anticholingeric agents. *Br Heart J* 55:53-57, 1986

322. Shen W-K, Gersh BJ: Syncope: mechanisms, approach, and management. In *Clinical Autonomic Disorders: Evaluation and Management.* Edited by PA Low. Boston, Little, Brown and Company, 1993, pp 605-640

323. Kapoor WN, Karpf M, Wieand S, et al: A prospective evaluation and follow-up of patients with syncope. *N Engl J Med* 309:197-204, 1983

324. Goldstein DS, Spanarkel M, Pitterman A, et al: Circulatory control mechanisms in vasodepressor syncope. *Am Heart J* 104:1071-1075, 1982

325. Engel GL: Psychologic stress, vasodepressor (vasovagal) syncope, and sudden death. *Ann Intern Med* 89:403-412, 1978

326. DiMarco JP, Garan H, Ruskin JN: Morbidity associated with electrophysiologic procedures (abstract). *Am J Cardiol* 49:959, 1982

327. Horowitz LN: Safety of electrophysiologic studies. *Circulation* 73 Suppl 2:28-31, 1986

328. Surawicz B: Intracardiac extrastimulation studies: how to? Where? By whom? (editorial) *Circulation* 65:428-431, 1982

329. Ross DL, Farre J, Bar FWHM, et al: Comprehensive clinical electrophysiologic studies in the investigation of documented or suspected tachycardias: time, staff, problems and costs. *Circulation* 61:1010-1016, 1980

330. Wiener I: Current applications of clinical electrophysiologic study in the diagnosis and treatment of cardiac arrhythmias. *Am J Cardiol* 49:1287-1292, 1982

CHAPTER

23

Syncopal disorders

Stephen C. Hammill, M.D., and Juergen E. Thomas, M.D.

A brief disturbance in normal consciousness is one of the commoner casual ailments. When it is an isolated occurrence with an adequate explanation, the physician is seldom consulted. However, if the disturbance recurs, it may become a matter of concern and may require that the physician weigh such episodes as possible evidence of an underlying disease and distinguish—often on the basis of history alone—among syncope, epilepsy, vertigo, hyperventilation, and a host of other conditions.

The terms "syncope" and "faint"—which will henceforth be used interchangeably—refer to a transient, rapid, or even abrupt disturbance of consciousness associated with an inability to maintain postural tone and often accompanied by autonomic manifestations. Its basic mechanism is a global impairment in cerebral perfusion.

Syncope accounts for 1% of hospital admissions and approximately 3% of emergency room visits. Three percent of the general population will experience syncope during long-term observation.[1,2] The most common cause of syncope is vasovagal in approximately 60% of patients. Patients with syncope of unknown cause have a 6% 1-year mortality and a 4% incidence of sudden death; and patients with a cardiac cause of syncope have an 18% to 33% 1-year mortality and a 24% incidence of sudden death.[3,4] One-third of patients presenting with syncope will experience a repeat episode during 30 months of follow-up regardless of the cause.

Many attempts have been made at classifying syncopal disorders, and all have fulfilled a purpose to the classifier. From the clinical point of view, we believe that a complicated classification does not outrank a simple listing of the major etiologic categories as illustrated in Table 23-1. We shall proceed along this line in our subsequent discussion.

Table 23-1 Major clinical types of syncopal disorders

Vasodepressor or vasovagal syncope
Orthostatic syncope
Poor autonomic adjustment to upright posture
Orthostatic hypotension
Cardiac syncope
Cardiac arrhythmias
Sick sinus syndrome
Paroxysmal supraventricular tachyarrhythmias
AV dissociation
Paroxysmal ventricular tachyarrhythmias
Ischemic heart disease
Valvular heart disease
Congenital heart disease
Syncope due to primary pulmonary hypertension
Carotid sinus syncope
Hyperactive carotid sinus reflex
Carotid sinus syndrome
Cardioinhibitory type
Vasodepressor type
Glossopharyngeal-vagal syncope
Cerebrovascular syncope
Micturition syncope
Pressor-postpressor syncope

Modified from Hammill SC, Holmes DR Jr, Wood DL: Cardiac arrhythmias. In *Current Diagnosis 7.* Edited by RB Conn. Philadelphia, WB Saunders Company, 1985, pp 405-433.

VASODEPRESSOR OR VASOVAGAL SYNCOPE

This is the classic benign faint. Among its predisposing factors are unaccustomed physical and mental exhaustion, chronic debility, a hot, stuffy environment, anxiety, head trauma, and pregnancy. The precipitating events vary widely and include emotional shocks, somatic or visceral pain, loss of blood, dehydration, and prolonged motionless standing. Vasodepressor syncope does not spare any age, but it particularly affects young persons and is reported to occur in 16% of patients referred for evaluation of syncope.[5]

The clinical picture is remarkably uniform regardless of cause. The patient is usually standing but may be sitting at the onset of the attack. He or she first notices a sense of weakness and apprehension. This is followed by nausea, pallor, cold perspiration, and perhaps epigastric distress. Within seconds or minutes, lightheadedness and blurring of vision set in, and, unless protective measures are taken, the patient slumps to the floor, unconscious. In the recumbent position, consciousness is quickly restored.

Although anoxic convulsion is more likely to occur in cardiac and pressor-postpressor syncope, even a vasovagal faint can cause such a convulsion if loss of consciousness is sufficiently abrupt and prolonged.[6] This consists of extensor rigidity of the body, with clenching of the fists, often followed or sometimes preceded by several clonic jerks. If the bladder happens to be full, urinary incontinence may be observed. "Malignant vasovagal syncope" describes abrupt loss of consciousness from asystole due to a neurogenic vasodepressor mechanism.

Physiologic studies suggest that the essential element in syncope is a profound decrease in total peripheral vascular resistance unaccompanied by an increase in cardiac output. This alteration causes compromise of cerebral perfusion and unconsciousness; peripheral venodilatation is no longer thought to be a contributing factor.

The treatment of vasodepressor syncope is well known. The immediate management consists of placing the patient in a flat position, preferably with the legs elevated, loosening tight clothing, and leaving him or her recumbent until strength has been regained. The patient should rise slowly and sit for a minute or two before going on his or her way. Repeat fainters should try to eliminate or avoid factors that they know tend to predispose them to or precipitate an attack.

Patients with a clinical history of syncope consistent with a vasodepressor mechanism and a normal cardiac and neurologic evaluation, including electrophysiologic testing and carotid sinus massage, may have their clinical syndrome reproduced by β-adrenergic receptor stimulation with isoproterenol in association with upright tilting.[7-10] This response is believed to be due to stimulation of C fibers in the left ventricle during vigorous contraction of a relatively volume-depleted chamber and is the postulated mechanism of vasodepressor syncope. Suggested treatments have been β-adrenergic receptor blockade with propranolol or metoprolol,[11] decreased contractility with disopyramide,[12] adenosine receptor blockade with theophylline,[13] and dual-chamber pacing.[14] Long-term success rates of the different therapies are being evaluated.

ORTHOSTATIC SYNCOPE

Physiologic studies[15] have delineated the adaptive cardiovascular changes that normally swing into action on assumption of the erect position. These include (1) reflex arteriolar constriction mediated through pressor receptors in the carotid sinus and aortic arch, (2) reflex venous constriction and reflex augmentation of respiration to resist pooling of blood and to facilitate venous return to the heart, (3) reflex acceleration of heart rate to maintain cardiac output, (4) increase in muscle tone and tissue pressure in the legs and in abdominal muscles, and (5) immediate increase in plasma catecholamines and, later, activation of the renin-angiotensin-aldosterone system.

The postural changes in blood pressure and cardiac rate as modified by the above adaptive mechanisms normally result in a transient decrease in systolic arterial pressure of up to 25 mm Hg and either no change or an increase in diastolic pressure of smaller magnitude. These changes are accompanied by an acceleration in heart rate of 5 to 25 beats/min.

Insufficiency of postural blood pressure adaptation can be divided into (1) poor autonomic adjustment to the upright posture and (2) orthostatic hypotension. Both conditions can be associated with syncope.

Poor autonomic adjustment to upright posture

This postural problem is an affliction especially of young persons of tall, asthenic habitus who have poorly developed musculature but are healthy otherwise. It also occurs among the elderly whose postural reflexes are slowed by physiologic aging. Other conditions that favor the development of poor postural adjustment through impedance of venous return to the heart and stasis of blood in the dependent body parts include physical exhaustion, prolonged recumbency, hot weather, pregnancy, and gastrectomy.

The cardiovascular alterations that occur in poor adjustment to upright posture consist of an exaggerated pooling of blood in the distended capillary beds of the splanchnic and subpapillary skin plexuses, leading to a decrease in effective blood volume, an inadequate cardiac venous return, and an increase in peripheral vascular resistance. The net result is an abnormal decrease in systolic pressure, an abnormal increase in diastolic pressure, and an excessive acceleration in heart rate.

On assuming the upright position or after prolonged standing, persons with poor autonomic adjustment may complain of lightheadedness, faintness, blurred vision, cold perspiration, yawning, and apprehension. These symptoms may culminate in fleeting loss of consciousness. Lying down provides prompt relief of all symptoms. Poor autonomic adjustment to upright posture is usually a harmless condition, and it responds to supportive therapy and removal of precipitating and aggravating factors.

Orthostatic hypotension

In orthostatic hypotension, postural regulation is severely and often persistently impaired because the cardiovascular system, even in the absence of stress, is no longer able to activate its compensatory mechanisms in response to the body's upright position or peripheral vasodilatation during and after exercise. Reflex arteriolar constriction fails, cardiac output lessens, and peripheral vascular resistance may decrease. The result is a pronounced postural fall in systolic and diastolic pressures. If the orthostatic hypotension is secondary to autonomic dysfunction, nausea, pallor, and sweating are often absent, and a concomitant increase in heart rate may be lacking because of inactivation of the cardioaccelerator nerves. Conversely, in orthostatic hypotension due to volume depletion—with autonomic function intact—standing up induces pronounced tachycardia through a compensatory increase in sympathetic activity.

We believe that a clinical diagnosis of orthostatic hypotension can be considered established when, on standing, a patient shows a consistent and persistent decrease of 30 mm Hg or more in systolic and a decrease of 15 mm Hg or more in diastolic pressure, provided that assumption of the upright position or exercise also induces clinical symptoms. We do not determine blood pressure

Table 23-2 Classification of disorders of postural blood pressure regulation

Poor autonomic adjustment to upright posture
Young persons with tall, asthenic habitus
Advanced age
Physical exhaustion
Prolonged recumbency
Pregnancy
Gastrectomy
Orthostatic hypotension
Secondary orthostatic hypotension
Endocrinologic-metabolic disorders
Diabetes mellitus
Primary amyloidosis
Primary and secondary adrenal insufficiency
Pheochromocytoma
Primary aldosteronism with pronounced hypokalemia
Porphyria
Central and peripheral nervous system disorders
Intracranial tumors
Idiopathic Parkinson's disease
Wernicke's encephalopathy
Multiple cerebral infarcts
Brain stem lesions
Tabes dorsalis
Syringomyelia
Traumatic, inflammatory myelopathies
Guillain-Barré syndrome
Chronic inflammatory polyradiculoneuropathy
Peripheral neuropathies
Familial dysautonomia (Riley-Day syndrome)
Miscellaneous disorders
Hypovolemia
Hypochromic anemia
Electrolyte disturbance
Psychotropic and antihypertensive drug use
Extensive surgical sympathectomy
Chronic hemodialysis
Anorexia nervosa
Hyperbradykininism
Primary or idiopathic orthostatic hypotension
Idiopathic orthostatic hypotension
Idiopathic orthostatic hypotension with somatic neurologic deficit (Shy-Drager syndrome)

responses to passive tilting but prefer to measure blood pressure and pulse rate while the patient is supine and standing. With the patient standing up, the blood pressure is recorded at intervals of 1 to 2 minutes for 10 minutes, if this is tolerated. If necessary, this procedure is supplemented by measurement of the blood pressure immediately after exercise, such as walking for a few minutes or after a standard treadmill test.

On assuming the erect position, patients with orthostatic hypotension may complain of lightheadedness, faintness, blurring or even loss of vision, a sense of profound weakness, tightness in neck and shoulders, and imbalance. The postural symptoms are often worse in the morning and are aggravated by heat, humidity, a heavy meal, and exercise. The patient may lose consciousness at the height of the decrease in postural blood pressure. Usually, syncope lasts no longer than seconds, but on rare occasions it has been observed to last as long as a minute or two, particularly if the patient is prevented from lying down.

It is customary to divide orthostatic hypotension into the secondary and the primary or idiopathic varieties.

Disorders that cause secondary orthostatic hypotension can be placed into three categories: endocrinologic-metabolic disorders, primary diseases of the central or peripheral nervous system, and a group of miscellaneous conditions. Table 23-2 provides a classification of the various causes.

Primary or idiopathic orthostatic hypotension is a separate entity with a characteristic evolution of symptoms and signs. Since it represents a disease of the autonomic nervous system—as do many cases of secondary orthostatic hypotension—other autonomic dysfunction, such as impairment of sweating, impotence, or bowel-bladder dysregulation, is a frequent accompaniment.

An as yet unknown number of patients eventually suffer somatic neurologic manifestations in addition to the autonomic deficit (Shy-Drager syndrome), consisting most prominently of involvement of central motor tracts. Affected are the corticobulbar-corticospinal, extrapyramidal, and cerebellar systems. In some patients, only one motor system is affected; in others, all are involved. Sensory systems are almost uniformly spared, and the intellect is not usually impaired. The prognosis is invariably poor. Details regarding the quality spectrum and the natural history of the neurologic syndrome can be found in other publications.[16]

Treatment modalities to be considered in patients with orthostatic hypotension are summarized in Table 23-3.

SYNCOPE ASSOCIATED WITH CARDIAC DYSFUNCTION

Syncope due to cardiac dysfunction is caused by a transiently diminished cardiac output as a result of a cardiac arrhythmia or reduced stroke volume. The major cardiac abnormalities that result in syncope include cardiac arrhythmias, ischemic heart disease, valvular heart disease, and congenital anomalies of the heart.

The onset of cardiac syncope is usually more rapid than the onset of other types of fainting. In fact, it may be so sudden that there seem to be no premonitory symptoms at all. If symptoms do occur, they consist of varying degrees of lightheadedness, nausea, blurring of vision, a sense of rapid heart action, or other cardiac distress. The recovery from a syncopal spell due to cardiac dysfunction may be equally rapid. In general, the patient is not left with lingering postsyncopal discomfort. Patients with cardiac syncope may exhibit anoxic convulsions during the spell. A distinguishing characteristic of cardiac syncope is that

Table 23-3 Treatment modalities for orthostatic hypotension

Disease-specific modalities

- Eliminate conditions that favor pooling of blood and impede venous return
- Correct electrolyte disturbance and volume depletion; discontinue hypotension-inducing drugs; treat adrenal insufficiency, hypothyroidism, anemia, and other treatable diseases

Other modalities

- Mechanical measures
  - Head-up position of bed
  - Elasticized body garment
  - Mild exercise if tolerated
- Plasma and extracellular fluid volume expanders
  - High-salt diet
  - 9α-Fluorohydrocortisone
- Vasoconstrictor drugs
  - Ephedrine
  - Vasopressin
  - Amphetamine
  - Methylphenidate
  - Monoamine oxidase inhibitors with amphetamine
- Other drugs
  - Indomethacin
  - Propranolol
  - Midodrine (investigational)
  - Dihydroergotamine (investigational)

Table 23-4 Disturbances in cardiac rhythm associated with syncope

Sick sinus syndrome

- Sinoatrial conduction block
- Tachycardia-bradycardia syndrome

Paroxysmal supraventricular tachyarrhythmias

- Atrial fibrillation
- Atrial flutter
- Atrial tachycardia
- Anomalies resulting in enhanced AV conduction during paroxysmal supraventricular tachyarrhythmias
  - Wolff-Parkinson-White syndrome
  - Lown-Ganong-Levine syndrome
  - Enhanced AV node conduction

AV dissociation

- Type I AV block (hypervagotonia)
- Type II AV block (His-Purkinje disease)
- Complete heart block
  - Congenital heart block
  - Drug toxicity (digitalis, verapamil, quinidine, lidocaine, phenytoin)
  - Electrolyte disturbances
  - Valvular heart disease
  - Myocarditis (viral, rheumatic fever, toxoplasmosis, syphilis, mumps, diphtheria)
  - Coronary artery disease
  - Infiltrative cardiomyopathy (amyloidosis, sarcoidosis, hemochromatosis)
  - Collagen vascular disease
  - Cardiac tumors (primary, metastatic)
  - Degenerative disease (Lenegre's disease, Lev's disease)
  - Neuromuscular diseases (Duchenne's and myotonic dystrophy, Friedreich's ataxia)

Paroxysmal ventricular tachyarrhythmias

- Ventricular tachycardia
- Ventricular fibrillation
- Prolonged Q-T syndrome
  - Primary (Jervell and Lange-Nielsen syndrome, Romano-Ward syndrome)
  - Secondary (quinidine, procainamide, disopyramide; hypokalemia, hypocalcemia, hypomagnesemia; cerebral contusion, stroke)

Modified from Hammill SC, Holmes DR Jr, Wood DL: Cardiac arrhythmias. In *Current Diagnosis 7.* Edited by RB Conn. Philadelphia, WB Saunders Company, 1985, pp 405-433.

it may occur when the patient is in either the recumbent or the upright position.

Cardiac arrhythmias

In this group belong the excessively slow and fast heart rates that may result in syncope from severely reduced cardiac output. Any of these disturbances in rhythm may be transitory and not necessarily found at a subsequent examination. Disturbances in cardiac rhythm associated with syncope include the sick sinus syndrome, paroxysmal supraventricular tachycardia, high-degree atrioventricular (AV) block, paroxysmal ventricular tachycardia or fibrillation, and asystole with failure of subsidiary pacemakers to maintain an adequate cardiac output (Table 23-4).

Sick sinus syndrome. Sinus node dysfunction is an important cause of syncope.[17] The "sick sinus syndrome" is a general term used to describe disorders of sinus node function that result in failure of the sinus node impulse to activate the atrium (sinoatrial conduction block) or failure of the sinus node to perform its pacemaking function adequately. A major subset of the sick sinus syndrome is the tachycardia-bradycardia syndrome, which is characterized by episodes of paroxysmal supraventricular tachycardia and sinus bradycardia. At the termination of supraventricular tachycardia, there is often prolonged delay before sinus rhythm returns. Patients may experience syncope during this transition phase from paroxysmal tachycardia to sinus rhythm. Generally, sinus node dysfunction is found in association with abnormalities of the subsidiary pacemakers in the AV node and His-Purkinje system such that they do not maintain adequate cardiac rhythm during the absence of sinus node activity. Treatment of patients with symptomatic tachycardia requires medications to slow conduction through the AV node (digoxin, calcium antagonists, β-adrenoreceptor blocker) and to prevent paroxysms (class IA, IC, and III antiarrhythmic drugs). Pacing is used to treat patients with symptomatic bradycardia.[18]

Paroxysmal supraventricular tachycardia. Patients with paroxysmal episodes of atrial fibrillation, atrial flutter, or atrial tachycardia may have a history of syncope.[19] In general, syncope during these arrhythmias is due to a rapid ventricular rate and subsequent inability of the heart to maintain an adequate cardiac output—which may further aggravate myocardial ischemia in patients with coronary artery disease. Heart rates in excess of 180 to 200 beats/min will generally be necessary before consciousness becomes clouded or lost. However, most patients can tolerate such accelerated heart rates without significant alteration in consciousness. Accelerated AV conduction resulting in a rapid ventricular rate and syncope during episodes of paroxysmal supraventricular tachycardia can occur in patients with a preexcitation syndrome[20] (Wolff-Parkinson-White syndrome, Lown-Ganong-Levine syndrome) and patients with enhanced AV nodal conduction[21] (chapter 22B).

Atrioventricular block. Syncope in patients with AV block can result from superimposed tachyarrhythmias[22] or a failure of subsidiary pacemakers to maintain cardiac rhythm.[23,24] The causes of AV block, including complete heart block, are included in Table 23-4.

Paroxysmal ventricular tachyarrhythmias. Paroxysmal ventricular tachycardia or ventricular fibrillation can occur not only in patients with ischemic heart disease but also in those who appear to have otherwise normal cardiac function.[25,26] As with paroxysmal supraventricular tachycardia, patients with paroxysmal ventricular tachycardia and otherwise normal cardiac function generally do not experience syncope; however, syncope may be experienced by patients whose ventricular tachycardia results in a rapid ventricular rate or who have an associated cardiac disease (ischemic, myopathic, valvular, or congenital heart disease).

The long Q-T syndrome[27] is associated with rapid paroxysmal ventricular arrhythmias and syncope. Patients with a prolonged Q-T interval, congenital deafness, and the association of syncope and sudden death are classified as having the Jervell and Lange-Nielsen syndrome. Patients with a similar syndrome excluding deafness are classified as having the Romano-Ward syndrome. Both syndromes are familial. The long Q-T syndrome can also result from use of drugs, including quinidine, procainamide, disopyramide, and the phenothiazines, and from electrolyte imbalance, including hypokalemia, hypomagnesemia, and hypocalcemia. This syndrome is discussed in further detail in chapter 22C.

Asystole. Asystole can develop in the presence of complete heart block when the subsidiary pacemakers fail to pace the heart. In addition, asystole can result from atrial standstill with a failure of subsidiary pacemakers to maintain cardiac rhythm, as in patients with the sick sinus syndrome.

Ischemic heart disease

During cardiac ischemia,[28] syncope can result from ventricular arrhythmias or conduction disturbances, increased parasympathetic activity with consequent bradycardia and hypotension, and severely impaired left ventricular function. The syncopal event is generally preceded by dyspnea and anginal pain, and myocardial infarction should always be suspected in a patient in whom low blood pressure, weak pulse, pallor, and sweating persist after syncope.

Valvular heart disease and hypertrophic cardiomyopathy

Patients who have valvular heart disease that results in a relatively fixed cardiac output (aortic and pulmonary stenosis) can experience syncope.[29,30] Characteristically, their syncope is in association with exertion and does not occur at rest. Syncope during exertion results from increased peripheral vasodilatation with a failure to increase cardiac output commensurately. The cause of the inadequate cardiac output is believed to lie either in an inability to increase cardiac output with exertion (fixed cardiac output) or in a reflex increase in parasympathetic tone elicited by pressure changes in the left ventricle.[31] The most common valvular abnormality associated with syncope is aortic stenosis. Syncope occurs in 10% to 25% of cases and is almost always induced by physical activity. The syncopal spell can be ushered in by dyspnea, weakness, dizziness, and angina pectoris. Rarely, mitral stenosis gives rise to syncope because of a markedly decreased cardiac output after exercise or a ball-valve type of thrombus. Myxomas can also result in syncope as a result of ball-valve obstruction of cardiac outflow.[32] Patients with prosthetic cardiac valves who have syncope should be treated aggressively because the syncope may be secondary to mechanical malfunction or obstruction caused by damage to the valve or by formation of thrombus on the valve structures.[33] Finally, syncope may be associated with dynamic left ventricular outflow obstruction as seen in hypertrophic cardiomyopathy.[34] In hypertrophic cardiomyopathy, syncope is associated with events that result in decreased systolic left ventricular cavity diameter, such as increased contractility, or decreased afterload and thus decreased left ventricular distending pressure. This may occur during exertion or after the administration of drugs that have a positive inotropic effect, such as digitalis or isoproterenol, or drugs that result in peripheral vasodilatation. Also, arrhythmia due to valvular heart disease (or ischemic or congenital heart disease) may cause syncope.

Congenital heart disease

Transient loss of consciousness in patients with congenital heart disease has been most commonly observed with tetralogy of Fallot but also occurs in truncus arteriosus, Eisenmenger's complex, aortic stenosis, pulmonary stenosis, transposition of the great vessels, and ventricular septal defects.[35] Syncope usually becomes manifest in early childhood and is precipitated by physical activity. The syncope may be secondary to a decrease in cardiac output, cardiac arrhythmias, or arterial oxygen desaturation. In patients with tetralogy of Fallot, syncope can result from an increase in the right-to-left shunting, such as that occurring with peripheral vasodilatation during exercise. This increase in shunting results in a decrease in arterial oxygen saturation. The patient quickly learns that certain positions, such as squatting, help abort an episode of syncope; they do so by increasing systemic pressure and thus decreasing the right-to-left intracardiac shunt and improving arterial oxygenation.

SYNCOPE ASSOCIATED WITH PRIMARY PULMONARY HYPERTENSION

Syncope due to primary pulmonary hypertension is also characteristically an effort syncope.[36] Dresdale et al.[36] found that it occurred in 20% of their patients with this disease. It is often preceded by dizziness, epigastric distress, and faintness and may be followed by nausea, vomiting, and abdominal cramps. The episodes last from a few seconds to several minutes. Effort syncope is highly suggestive of primary pulmonary hypertension if the patient is found to have dilatation of the pulmonary artery, accentuation of the pulmonary second sound, or right ventricular hypertrophy. The cause of the faint seems to lie in the impaired ability to raise cardiac output during the vasodilatation of exercise and thus an inability to maintain sufficient arterial pressure. Again, arrhythmia secondary to severe right ventricular hypertrophy and hypertension can occur and precipitate syncope.

CAROTID SINUS SYNCOPE

The recognition that the carotid sinus reflex has not only physiologic but pathologic implications as well is as old as the discovery of the reflex itself. Numerous accounts have appeared in the medical literature of instances of syncope and even convulsions in response to mechanical manipulation of the carotid sinus in man. Persons so afflicted were said to have a "hyperactive carotid sinus reflex." As a logical extension of this observation, the sinus reflex was studied as a possible cause of spontaneously occurring syncope, and a relationship was shown to exist in some patients. Spontaneously occurring carotid sinus symptoms with or without syncope were referred to as the carotid sinus syndrome.

Hyperactive carotid sinus reflex

This term applies when digital stimulation of the carotid sinus results in pronounced slowing of cardiac rate or in cardiac asystole accompanied by a decrease in systemic blood pressure. In some cases, only the blood pressure decreases and cardiac rhythm remains unaffected. Franke,[37] who studied the carotid sinus reflex extensively, considered cardiac asystole of 3 seconds or more and a decrease in systolic blood pressure of 50 mm Hg or more as clearly abnormal, and a slowing of heart rate by 30% to 40%, cardiac asystole lasting 2 seconds, and a decrease of 30 mm Hg in systolic blood pressure as constituting a borderline response.

The hyperactive sinus reflex, as defined above, almost never occurs in the first 2 decades of life,[37] whereas in men more than 50 years old the frequency has been estimated to be 25% to 30%.[38] Males are affected twice as often as females. The reflex may be evoked more easily from the right than the left sinus and it may be present bilaterally.

Carotid sinus stimulation test. The test begins with a check for satisfactory pulsation of the carotid and temporal arteries and auscultation of the carotid vessels for bruits. Patients with obvious cerebrovascular disease are tested by carotid sinus stimulation under strict indications only.

The patient is placed in the supine position, significant head rotation is avoided, and the head is kept in a neutral position between flexion and extension. The examiner's fingers feel gently for the fusiform carotid sinus or the area of greatest arterial pulsation lying in front of the sternomastoid muscle at the upper border of the thyroid cartilage. The carotid sinus is pressed for 5 to 10 seconds while the examiner monitors heart rate and blood pressure. The right carotid sinus is stimulated first, followed by the left several minutes later. Never are both sinuses stimulated together. The sinus stimulation test should ideally be carried out under electrocardiographic (ECG) control.

The carotid sinus stimulation test is not without hazard. Complications have ranged from visual disturbances to hemiplegia to sudden death, the last-named mostly in seriously ill patients or during anesthesia or operation.

Clinical manifestations. A variety of symptoms and signs occur during the stimulation test in persons with a hyperactive carotid sinus reflex. The ease of induction, intensity, and duration of these manifestations are influenced by the position of the body, the age of the person, the status of the cerebral circulation, and the psychologic makeup of the patient.

Among the subjective manifestations, lightheadedness is the most common and is often the initial symptom. Other frequent manifestations are faintness, blurring of vision, a feeling of general weakness, and pressure or fullness in the head. Also, tinnitus, paresthesias in the hands, dyspnea, headache, nausea, and sweating have been reported. These symptoms are not specific and can be part of any other type of syncope as well.

In some cases of hyperactive carotid sinus reflex, the above symptoms culminate in loss of consciousness, usually of sudden onset. This is immediately preceded or accompanied by pallor of the face, coldness of the skin, and deep respiration. During the faint, the patient is usually motionless and limp; but occasionally, when cardiac asystole is prolonged, a tonic spasm of the body and a few clonic jerks of limbs and face can be seen. A fleeting, intense facial flush may accompany the convulsive movements.

Unconsciousness is brief, lasting from seconds to a minute or two at the longest. The sensorium is quickly restored, and the person feels well again. After a prolonged spell, there may be short-lasting drowsiness or lassitude. To be productive of syncope, cardiac asystole must last anywhere from 5 to 15 seconds. The occurrence of syncope is an indication for immediate cessation of the stimulation test.

The cardiovascular response on digital stimulation of the carotid sinus was divided by Weiss and Baker[39] into three types: (1) the cardioinhibitory type with bradycardia or asystole with or without systemic hypotension, (2) the vasodepressor type not associated with cardiac slowing, and (3) a primary cerebral type not accompanied by either systemic hypotension or bradycardia.

The cardioinhibitory type is by far the most common variety of the hyperactive carotid sinus reflex. Its incidence has been estimated to vary from 34% to 78% among persons with carotid sinus hypersensitivity. The pure vasodepressor type is rare, making up only 10% to 15% of cases.

Whether the so-called primary cerebral type exists is highly debatable. Undoubtedly, many of the cases that had previously been regarded as "cerebral" were in fact a result of mechanical compromise of carotid blood flow during the stimulation test when there was occlusive disease involving the opposite carotid, the anterior cerebral, or the vertebral-basilar arterial system. If the cerebral form of the carotid sinus hypersensitivity exists, it must be exceedingly rare.

In the cardioinhibitory type, the cardiac manifestations depend largely on the reflex responsiveness of the heart at the time of the test. Cardiac asystole may last from 2 to 15 seconds. Electrocardiographic abnormalities include sinoatrial slowing, atrial conduction defects, prolongation of the P-R interval, AV block, sinoatrial arrest, nodal escape, complete asystole, and ventricular ectopic beats.

As noted above, the vasodepressor type of carotid sinus hypersensitivity is rare. The symptoms it causes are the same as those in the cardioinhibitory type, except that syncope probably never occurs in the recumbent position. The symptoms tend to follow a more protracted course because the blood pressure may not recover its normal level for minutes. However, symptoms and signs commence just as quickly as in the cardiac form—namely, within the first 15 to 20 seconds of sinus stimulation.

Carotid sinus syndrome (carotid sinus syncope)

Although the hyperactive carotid sinus reflex has limited clinical significance and does not give rise to spontaneous symptoms, the carotid sinus syndrome (also called spontaneous carotid sinus syncope) is clinically significant and should be considered separately because in this condition symptoms occur spontaneously. Most patients who exhibit abnormal sinus sensitivity on manual testing do not suffer spontaneous carotid syncope. Conversely, patients with spontaneous sinus syncope usually do have a hyperactive reflex. The two may be closely related, differing perhaps only in severity. By definition, the diagnosis of spontaneous carotid sinus syndrome is said to be established if spontaneously occurring symptoms of dizziness, blurring of vision, faintness, or fainting can be reproduced by stimulation of one or both carotid sinuses, provided that carotid blood flow is preserved during the test.

Carotid sinus syncope is a rare condition. Some 5% to 20% of persons with a hyperactive reflex are said to have it. As in the hyperactive reflex, carotid sinus syncope occurs more often in men than in women and is commoner in the older age groups.

Clinical manifestations. The symptoms occurring in the spontaneous syndrome are the same as those that occur as a result of the hyperactive reflex. The attacks occur for the most part in the sitting or standing position and tend to follow a similar course in the individual patient, but changes in symptom content and in severity from one attack to the next are known to occur. Frequencies of several episodes a day to one every few months have been reported.

The spontaneous syndrome, like the hyperactive reflex, has been divided into the cardioinhibitory, vasodepressor, and cerebral types. This division is nearly always made on the basis of the patient's response to the sinus stimulation test because one is rarely able to study the patient during one of his or her spontaneous attacks.

Precipitating and predisposing factors. In most patients suffering from spontaneous carotid sinus syncope, no obvious cause for the spells can be identified. However, when there are trigger mechanisms, these may be of extravascular or intravascular origin.

Among the extravascular factors, forced head turning when backing a car, hyperextension of the neck, working overhead, and the like are said to have been responsible for the syncope. Other local triggering factors have included pressure of constricting neckwear, stretching of the skin over the neck when shaving, and carrying heavy shoulder loads.

Pathologic changes adjacent to the carotid sinus, such as thyroid tumor, carotid body tumor, and inflammatory and malignant lymph nodes, are other extravascular conditions that are believed to have precipitated the spontaneous syndrome, just as they are blamed for some cases of hyperactive carotid sinus reflex.[40]

Diagnosis. The diagnosis of carotid sinus syndrome is made on the basis of (1) spontaneously occurring episodes of syncope, often preceded by dizziness, weakness, and faintness, and (2) the reproduction of the same symptom complex on digital stimulation of the carotid sinus but not on pressure on the carotid artery elsewhere.

Arriving at a diagnosis in this fashion is unsatisfactory. First, there is nothing unique about the symptom quality of the carotid sinus syndrome. The presyncopal discomfort is as nonspecific as the syncope itself. Although the abrupt onset of symptoms will alert the physician to a possible reflex nature of the syncope, the carotid sinus is just one of several sites from which reflex syncope may arise.

Second, to regard the reproduction of symptoms on digital sinus stimulation as diagnostic confirmation of the carotid sinus etiology is highly speculative. The hyperactive carotid sinus reflex occurs much more often than the spontaneous syndrome, and the presence of an overactive reflex in a patient with spontaneous faints may therefore be coincidental. A history of repeated syncope clearly related to maneuvers that press or stretch the sinus in a patient who also has a positive reaction on carotid stimulation is diagnostically helpful. However, most patients do not furnish such a history. If spontaneous syncope and hyperactive sinus reflex coexist and therapeutic measures directed at the carotid sinus abolish both, a common etiologic bond may be assumed to have been present.

In the patient with presumed carotid sinus syncope, electrophysiologic testing can be used to exclude other cardiogenic causes for syncope, such as intermittent complete heart block and ventricular tachycardia. Carotid sinus massage can then be performed in the electrophysiology laboratory with the patient in the upright position to help separate the cardioinhibitory from the vasodepressor components. If the patient exhibits asystole and hypotension during carotid sinus massage, AV pacing is performed and carotid sinus massage repeated to determine if a vasodepressor component persists despite maintenance of normal heart rate.[41] Patients with mixed carotid sinus hypersensitivity should be forewarned that pacing may not entirely relieve their near-syncope or syncope.

Treatment. Since there are no spontaneous symptoms, a hyperactive carotid sinus reflex requires no treatment.

In patients with spontaneous but infrequent carotid sinus syncope, an explanation of the problem and reassurance are sufficient. When the frequency of occurrence is significant, a careful search for remediable precipitating factors should be undertaken. Focal lesions about the carotid sinus should be removed and trigger mechanisms (for example, tight neckwear) avoided.

Patients with cardioinhibitory carotid sinus hypersensitivity can be treated with anticholinergic therapy or permanent pacing. Anticholinergic therapy is achieved with propantheline bromide in doses ranging from 7.5 mg three times daily to 15 mg four times daily. Anticholinergic therapy may be limited by side effects, which include blurred vision, constipation, dry mouth, and urinary difficulties. This form of therapy is contraindicated in patients known to have glaucoma. Permanent pacing is the other standard form of treatment for patients with cardioinhibitory carotid sinus hypersensitivity, with AV pacing being used most commonly. The vasodepressor component of carotid sinus hypersensitivity can be treated with elastic stockings that go to the thigh or waist, fluid expansion with a high-salt diet or fluorohydrocortisone, or a vasoconstrictor medication such as ephedrine.[42]

Severe carotid sinus syncope requires energetic treatment measures. Radiation therapy[43] and surgical denervation of the carotid sinus[44] have given inconsistent results in such cases. The cardioinhibitory type of carotid sinus syncope has been treated with placement of a transvenous demand pacemaker.[45]

GLOSSOPHARYNGEAL-VAGAL SYNCOPE

An interesting type of syncope is that associated with glossopharyngeal neuralgia. Fainting occurs concomitantly with pain that affects the pharynx, tonsillar area, base of the tongue, and ear. An ECG recorded during a syncopal spell discloses bradycardia or asystole. Complete relief of pain is usually obtained by sectioning of the glossopharyngeal nerve. Anticholinergic agents may reverse the cardiovascular changes. Also, phenytoin or carbamazepine may be of benefit. It has been suggested that the cardiovascular effects of the syndrome are attributable to excitation of the dorsal motor nucleus of the vagus by way of secondary afferent collaterals from the nucleus solitarius.[46]

Other types of reflexly induced syncope, mediated through the vagal system (vagovagal syncope), have occasionally been described in pharyngeal, esophageal, laryngeal, bronchial, and mediastinal lesions, during bronchoscopy and esophagoscopy, with "needling" of body cavities, following ocular pressure, and in digitalis intoxication. Also, pleural and pulmonary processes such as pulmonary embolism may be associated with syncope, and the rare cases of swallow syncope likewise arise on the basis of a vagovagal reflex. Loss of consciousness is usually abrupt and of short duration. In clinical practice, these forms of fainting are rare.

CEREBROVASCULAR SYNCOPE

In cerebrovascular diseases as a group, fainting is an uncommon clinical manifestation.[47,48] When it occurs, there is usually partial and sometimes complete occlusion of one or more of the large arteries in the neck.[49] The more severely these vessels are affected, the more likely will syncope be part of the clinical picture. This general rule is best exemplified in the "aortic arch syndrome" (pulseless disease) in which occlusive processes involve the aortic arch and markedly narrow the ostia of its main branches, including the innominate, subclavian, and common carotid arteries. Syncope occurs in as many as 40% of these cases and is characteristically induced by physical activity. It is often preceded by lightheadedness, blurring of vision, and confusion.

Stenosis or occlusion of the vertebral arteries has been held responsible for those syncopal attacks that occur in relation to certain positions of the head, especially hyperextension and lateral rotation.

Disturbance of consciousness on exercise of an upper extremity may be part of the "subclavian steal syndrome," which is caused by occlusive disease of the subclavian artery, usually the left, proximal to the origin of the vertebral vessel. Because of the reduction in pressure in that artery and the resultant reversal of the pressure gradient between its proximal and distal portions, blood is shunted from the vertebral artery via the distal subclavian artery into the arm. Exercise of the arm may evoke symptoms of cerebrovascular insufficiency, including syncope. The presence of a subclavian steal syndrome is suggested by (1) a difference in brachial pressure of at least 20 mm Hg, (2) a bruit audible in the area of the subclavian-vertebral junction, and (3) a delay in pulse arrival time on the involved side. Arch aortography provides more specific information.

MICTURITION SYNCOPE

Micturition syncope can occur during or right after urination in the upright position, and the person so affected has almost always been recumbent for some time. Micturition syncope is probably caused by a circulatory collapse that occurs when the postural adaptive mechanisms, impaired by recumbency in a warm bed and perhaps alcohol consumption the night before, are not allowed their usual period of adjustment. Visceral afferent stimulation from a full bladder has been thought to play a contributing part, and a similar type of syncope has been seen after drainage of a distended bladder. Consciousness is usually lost abruptly, sometimes after symptoms such as dizziness, weakness, or nausea or after injuries have been sustained. Recovery is usually rapid and complete. Whether micturition syncope constitutes a truly separate entity is doubtful. More likely, it represents a simple postural faint accentuated by the Valsalva maneuver.

PRESSOR-POSTPRESSOR SYNCOPE

Symptoms such as lightheadedness and blurring of vision are seen in some persons during strenuous activities such as laughing, coughing, straining at stool, vomiting, sneezing, and lifting. Occasionally, these symptoms may culminate in syncope. Best known is "tussive syncope," the faint accompanying an attack of coughing. This almost exclusively affects men more than 40 years old who are of a pyknic or athletic habitus and are capable of considerable muscular effort. Chronic bronchopulmonary disease may be a predisposing factor. The attack is ushered in by a series of strenuous expiratory coughs without inspiratory relief and is not necessarily prolonged. The patient's face becomes congested, his eyes tear, he seems to be dazed, and at the height of the coughing attack or at its cessation he slumps to the floor unconscious and may display an anoxic convulsion. Recovery is prompt. The attacks can occur when the patient is in the erect or recumbent position. The cause of tussive syncope and other pressor symptoms is believed to lie in the greatly increased intrathoracic pressure, which results in decreased venous return to the heart, diminution in cardiac output, and peripheral vasodilatation following the cough. Other factors include an increase in cerebrovascular resistance by the hypocapnia of coughing, an increase in spinal fluid pressure, and perhaps a concussive effect caused by the sudden increase in intracranial pressure transmitted via the cerebrospinal fluid from the thorax and abdomen.[50,51]

EVALUATION OF THE PATIENT WITH SYNCOPE

The cause of syncope is apparent in the majority of patients after a thorough history and physical examination. The history should be obtained with emphasis on the description of the syncopal episode, including the presence or absence of any premonitory symptoms and the relationship of the disorder to such activities as postural changes of the body, eating, coughing, micturition, defecation, or movements of the neck that might irritate the carotid sinus. It is important to elucidate the associated symptoms, including gastrointestinal distress and symptoms suggesting cardiac disease, and also the relation of the syncope to the occurrence of pain, prolonged standing, use of medications, or diseases that might otherwise predispose the patient to fainting spells.

The physical examination should emphasize a thorough neurologic and cardiovascular workup for the presence of orthostatic hypotension, cerebrovascular disease, congenital or acquired cardiac conditions, and carotid sinus hypersensitivity.

Specialized laboratory tests that may be considered in selected patients with syncope include plasma aldosterone and mineralocorticoid determinations in cases of suspected adrenocortical insufficiency; supine and standing plasma catecholamine levels in patients suspected of having idiopathic orthostatic hypotension or diabetic autonomic neuropathy, in which the recumbent values may be low and the postural response blunted or absent, or pheochromocytoma, in which the values for plasma catecholamines, fractionated urinary catecholamines, and urinary 4-hydroxy-3-methoxymandelic acid are elevated; ophthalmodynamometry, oculopneumoplethysmography, or other tests designed to evaluate cerebral blood pressure; glucose tolerance test to check for functional hypoglycemia or insulin-secreting tumor; and electroencephalography awake and asleep to test for seizure disorder.[52]

A significant number of patients in whom the syncope is suspected to be of cardiac origin will have an otherwise normal history, physical examination, and laboratory evaluation. In such cases, the exact mechanism of the suspected rhythm disturbance should be determined in order to administer appropriate treatment. The study of disturbances in cardiac rhythm in patients with syncope has become easier with the introduction of the telephone transmitter, 24-hour ambulatory monitoring, and electrophysiologic testing. The telephone transmitter is a device that allows transmission of an ECG over the telephone. This device is not useful in patients who have syncope in the absence of premonitory symptoms. Twenty-four-hour ambulatory monitoring of the ECG has proved to be helpful in determining the cause of syncope in patients who are suspected of having disorders of cardiac rhythm.[53,54] It is not usually possible to record the cardiac rhythm during a faint because of its infrequent, paroxysmal occurrence. However, brief disturbances in rhythm can be recorded which, if prolonged, could potentially induce syncope and hence suggest a cardiac etiology. Event recorders and newer devices allow long-term monitoring that is convenient for the patient and are useful for recording the rhythm during symptomatic episodes of brief duration.[55,56]

An abnormal ECG is found in approximately 50% of patients with syncope, but in most patients it is not diagnostic. The ECG can identify potential cause of syncope in 2% to 11% of patients. Twenty-four-hour ambulatory monitoring will identify a potential arrhythmia as the cause for syncope in 10% to 64% of patients, although concurrently symptomatic arrhythmias occur in only 2% to 3% of patients.[57,58]

The electrophysiologic test (chapter 22D) is helpful when the diagnosis of syncope remains obscure despite the history, physical examination, laboratory tests, electroencephalogram, and use of 24-hour ambulatory monitoring.

Abnormal findings at the time of electrophysiologic testing in patients with syncope include sinus node recovery time of 3 seconds or longer, pacing-induced block in the His-Purkinje system, an H-V interval longer than 100 msec, paroxysmal supraventricular tachycardia with symptomatic hypotension, and sustained monomorphic ventricular tachycardia.[1,59] Predictors of a negative electrophysiologic study in patients with syncope include an absence of heart disease, normal ECG and 24-hour ambulatory monitoring, an ejection fraction greater than 40%, an absence of injury during syncope, and multiple or

Table 23-5 Results of electrophysiologic testing in patients with syncope of uncertain etiology

Study	Pt (n = 809)	Abn ET, %	ET abnormality* SVT, %	VT, %	Conduction,† %	Other,‡ %
Di Marco[66]	25	68	6	53	18	24
Gulamhusein[67]	34	18	50	0	50	0
Hess[68]	32	56	61	6	33	0
Akhtar[69]	30	53	0	68	32	0
Olshansky[70]	105	50	18	56	22	10
Doherty[71]	119	66	29	40	11	19
Denes[72]	50	74	12	8	60	24
Sugrue[73]	175	71	12	30	45	12
Teichman[74]	150	75	11	22	54	12
Denes[75]	89	71	15	15	41	0
Mean %		60	21	30	37	10

*Patients have more than one abnormality. †Includes abnormal sinus node, atrioventricular node, or His-Purkinje function. ‡Includes hypervagotonia, carotid sinus hypersensitivity. §Excludes data from Denes. Abn, abnormal; ET, electrophysiologic testing; Nl, normal; SVT, supraventricular tachycardia; VT, ventricular tachycardia.

From Kapoor WN, Hammill SC, Gersh BJ: Diagnosis and natural history of syncope and the role of invasive electrophysiologic testing. *Am J Cardiol* 63:730-734, 1989. By permission of Cahners Publishing Company, a Division of Reed Publishing USA.

prolonged (more than 5 minutes) episodes of syncope.[59] Several authors[60-65] have reported their findings from electrophysiologic evaluation of patients with syncope of unknown cause (Table 23-5). In these studies, a mean of 60% of patients had abnormalities at the time of electrophysiologic testing that were assumed to be the cause of syncope; ventricular tachycardia and conduction disturbances were the most frequently identified abnormalities. Patients with abnormalities identified at electrophysiologic testing who were treated had a mean recurrence rate of syncope of 15%, a mortality rate of 7%, and a higher incidence of heart disease. In contrast, patients with normal results at electrophysiologic testing had a recurrence rate of 35%, cardiac mortality of 3%, and a lower incidence of heart disease. The use of the tilt table[5-10,76] helps to identify patients with vasodepressor syncope and vasodepressor carotid sinus hypersensitivity and to correlate the symptoms during the electrophysiologically induced rhythm abnormality with the patient's clinical presentation.

Diurnal blood pressure variations can be more accurately assessed and correlated with cardiac rhythm and the patient's symptoms by simultaneous automatic blood pressure monitoring and 24- to 48-hour ambulatory ECG recording. The results of such testing are then compared with a detailed symptom diary provided by the patient for the same span of time.

DIFFERENTIAL DIAGNOSIS

Conditions with clinical features that can be confused with syncope include epilepsy, vertigo, hyperventilation, migraine, and hysteria. Narcoleptic cataplexy, hypoglycemia, and tetany are sometimes mentioned in the differential diagnosis of syncope, but in almost every instance a careful history will reveal obvious points of distinction.

Epilepsy

In the evaluation of passing-out spells, the most frequent uncertainty is related to a distinction between epilepsy and syncope, and there are times when the history alone does not permit a clear choice. For the most part, the differentiation can be made with the following points in mind.

Rapidity of onset. Most syncopal attacks feature a period of warning before consciousness is lost—a fading or graying of vision, squeamishness in the stomach, cold perspiration, nausea, and weakness. One must distinguish these complaints from the aura of an epileptic state, and one of the most obvious differences is the favorable influence of recumbency on syncope. Many convulsive episodes begin abruptly, without warning of any kind. Even when there is an aura, it is usually a repetitive chain of events, more often sensory than motor and having little in common with presyncopal symptoms. However, an abrupt onset without warning does not exclude the diagnosis of syncope, for cardiac and occasionally orthostatic faints may manifest themselves in just this way. Nonetheless, the great majority of such episodes prove to be epileptic in nature.

Consistency of pattern. A consistent pattern is a characteristic of epilepsy but not of syncope. Once the chain of events has been triggered in epilepsy, it tends to run an identical course each time. A syncopal spell, on the other hand, may be modified by prompt remedial measures (especially recumbency), and its course is variable in duration, severity, and manifestations. Consciousness is rarely lost as abruptly as in epilepsy, and the fall tends to be less forceful. In the epileptic seizure, breathing is labored after the apneic phase has subsided, whereas in a faint, respiration is mostly shallow.

Postural influences. Except for cardiac syncope, which can occur when the patient is in any position, syncopal

Mean follow-up, mo	Recurrent syncope		Cardiac mortality	
	Abn ET, %	Nl ET, %	Abn ET, %	Nl ET, %
18	18	50	6	0
15	0	39	0	0
21	11	29	11	0
17	13	80	0	0
26	28	20	6	0
27	32	24	13	4
23	5	8	14	8
17	14	36	—	—
31	15	47	5	14
47	11	13	41*	9*
24	15	35	7§	3§

episodes happen when the patient is upright, usually standing but sometimes sitting. A clinical history of spells occurring often during recumbency or sleep favors a diagnosis of epilepsy over that of syncope.

Motor phenomena. Convulsive movements are not confined to the epileptic seizure. In fact, stiffening of the body—at times severe—and brief twitching of face and arms are not rare in syncope. As a rule, the more suddenly consciousness is lost and the longer the patient remains unconscious, the more likely it is that such motor phenomena will occur in syncope. Although these motor discharges have been called "anoxic convulsions," they are unlike epilepsy clinically and electrophysiologically. They usually last no longer than 10 to 20 seconds and do not follow the orderly sequence of an epileptic grand mal seizure. Occasionally, though, syncopal convulsions lasting 1 to 2 minutes can be observed. When convulsive movements precede loss of consciousness, the spell is almost always epileptic.

Skin changes. Changes in the skin may be helpful in the differential diagnosis, because syncope usually features pronounced pallor accompanied by cold perspiration. Occasionally, a patient in an akinetic epileptic state may also appear pale, but flushing or cyanosis with warm perspiration is much more in keeping with an epileptic attack. Although most types of faints are accompanied by autonomic hyperactivity, orthostatic syncope due to failure of the autonomic nervous system may conspicuously lack such symptoms as nausea, pallor, and cold perspiration.

Incontinence and tongue biting. Urinary incontinence is not pathognomonic of epilepsy. It may occur in fainting spells when loss of consciousness is sudden and the bladder happens to be full. Bowel incontinence, on the other hand, is highly atypical in syncope. Tongue biting likewise distinctly suggests epilepsy, but it is possible for a patient to faint so abruptly that the tongue is injured in the fall.

Recovery. After a generalized epileptic seizure there is transient depression of cerebral function. Consciousness returns gradually, and the patient may remain confused for several minutes. He or she will then often sleep for an hour or longer and on awakening may not remember the seizure and may complain of headache. After a faint, the patient is rarely confused, and he or she has no amnesia. In fact, sometimes the spell is vividly recalled, even including audible events that occurred after the patient seemed to have lost consciousness. Physical weakness, however, often persists, and dizziness, nausea, and sometimes postsyncopal oliguria may linger for some time. If the patient rises too soon, he or she may be overcome by another faint.

In spite of these distinguishing features, spells will occur about which a definite decision cannot be made. In these instances an electroencephalogram may be helpful. However, a normal interictal record does not exclude epilepsy any more than a moderate dysrhythmia in the electroencephalogram excludes syncope.

Vertigo

Vertigo will seldom be confused with syncope if the patient can describe precisely what is being experienced. In vertigo there is a sense of motion, either of the environment or of the patient. Falling may be abrupt and violent, but consciousness is not usually lost. Nausea is frequent, and the associated pallor and cold sweat may suggest a faint to the unwary observer. The increased distress with head movements is characteristic of vertigo and is seldom seen in syncope. Vertigo as an epileptic phenomenon (tornado epilepsy) is very rare.

Hyperventilation

Several clinical states, including syncope itself, may be complicated by hyperventilation. It is usually a manifestation of an emotional disturbance, but when it occurs repetitively it can pose a diagnostic problem. The sensation of air hunger, with resultant deep and rapid breathing, may not be described spontaneously by the patient and may have to be described spontaneously by the patient and may have to be inquired after specifically. Symptoms of faintness, lightheadedness, and paresthesias of the fingers and face, usually bilateral, should stimulate such an inquiry. Hyperventilation spells may themselves constitute the entire problem, or they may be a reaction that is secondary to a true syncopal attack. These two conditions are not mutually exclusive.

Migraine

Attacks of migraine ordinarily have no syncopal features, but Selby and Lance[77] and later Bickerstaff[78] drew attention to a rare situation in which the basilar arterial system may be involved in addition to or instead of the more commonly affected carotid system. In these patients, usually adolescent girls, the premonitory aura of a migrainous episode terminates in deep unconsciousness of several minutes' duration, followed by a severe headache, typically occipital in location.

Hysteria

Hysteria can often be distinguished from syncope by the calm detachment with which the patient describes the symptoms; the vagueness of description; the absence of pallor, sweating, and cardiovascular changes during an attack; the often prolonged duration; and the almost invariable presence of an audience. These episodes are not dependent on the upright position and do not respond as promptly to recumbency. Hyperventilation may be part of the picture. The patient is often either a naive, unsophisticated young person or an older one in whom a previous conversion tendency can be established. One should always be skeptical, however, of "hysteria" that appears unheralded in middle age or later. It may prove to be something else.

REFERENCES

1. Kapoor WN, Hammill SC, Gersh BJ: Diagnosis and natural history of syncope and the role of invasive electrophysiologic testing (editorial). *Am J Cardiol* 63:730-734, 1989
2. Kapoor WN: Diagnostic evaluation of syncope. *Am J Med* 90:91-106, 1991
3. Kapoor WN, Karpf M, Wieand S, et al: A prospective evaluation and follow-up of patients with syncope. *N Engl J Med* 309:197-204, 1983
4. Eagle KA, Black HR, Cook EF, et al: Evaluation of prognostic classifications for patients with syncope. *Am J Med* 79:455-460, 1985
5. Fitzpatrick A, Theodorakis G, Vardas P, et al: The incidence of malignant vasovagal syndrome in patients with recurrent syncope. *Eur Heart J* 12:389-394, 1991
6. Grubb BP, Gerard G, Roush K, et al: Cerebral vasoconstriction during head-upright tilt-induced vasovagal syncope: a paradoxic and unexpected response. *Circulation* 84:1157-1164, 1991
7. Waxman MB, Yao L, Cameron DA, et al: Isoproterenol induction of vasodepressor-type reaction in vasodepressor-prone persons. *Am J Cardiol* 63:58-65, 1989
8. Fitzpatrick AP, Theodorakis G, Vardas P, et al: Methodology of head-up tilt testing in patients with unexplained syncope. *J Am Coll Cardiol* 17:125-130, 1991
9. Chen XC, Chen MY, Remole S, et al: Reproducibility of head-up tilt-table testing for eliciting susceptibility to neurally mediated syncope in patients without structural heart disease. *Am J Cardiol* 69:755-760, 1992
10. Kapoor WN, Brant N: Evaluation of syncope by upright tilt testing with isoproterenol: a nonspecific test. *Ann Intern Med* 116:358-363, 1992
11. Sra JS, Murthy VS, Jazayeri MR, et al: Use of intravenous esmolol to predict efficacy of oral beta-adrenergic blocker therapy in patients with neurocardiogenic syncope. *J Am Coll Cardiol* 19:402-408, 1992
12. Milstein S, Buetikofer J, Dunnigan A, et al: Usefulness of disopyramide for prevention of upright tilt-induced hypotension-bradycardia. *Am J Cardiol* 65:1339-1344, 1990
13. Nelson SD, Stanley M, Love CJ, et al: The autonomic and hemodynamic effects of oral theophylline in patients with vasodepressor syncope. *Arch Intern Med* 151:2425-2429, 1991
14. Fitzpatrick A, Theodorakis G, Ahmed R, et al: Dual chamber pacing aborts vasovagal syncope induced by head-up 60° tilt. *PACE* 14:13-19, 1991
15. Page EB, Hickam JB, Sieker HO, et al: Reflex venomotor activity in normal persons and in patients with postural hypotension. *Circulation* 11:262-270, 1955
16. Thomas JE, Schirger A: Idiopathic orthostatic hypotension: a study of its natural history in 57 neurologically affected patients. *Arch Neurol* 22:289-293, 1970
17. Strauss HC, Bigger JT Jr, Saroff AL, et al: Electrophysiologic evaluation of sinus node function in patients with sinus node dysfunction. *Circulation* 53:763-776, 1976
18. Brignole M, Menozzi C, Lolli G, et al: Pacing for carotid sinus syndrome and sick sinus syndrome. *PACE* 13:2071-2075, 1990
19. Leitch JW, Klein GJ, Yee R, et al: Syncope associated with supraventricular tachycardia: an expression of tachycardia rate or vasomotor response? *Circulation* 85:1064-1071, 1992
20. Paul T, Guccione P, Garson A Jr: Relation of syncope in young patients with Wolff-Parkinson-White syndrome to rapid ventricular response during atrial fibrillation. *Am J Cardiol* 65:318-321, 1990
21. Benditt DG, Pritchett ELC, Smith WM, et al: Characteristics of atrioventricular conduction and the spectrum of arrhythmias in Lown-Ganong-Levine syndrome. *Circulation* 57:454-465, 1978
22. Jensen G, Sigurd B, Sandoe E: Adams-Stokes seizures due to ventricular tachydysrhythmias in patients with heart block: prevalence and problems of management. *Chest* 67:43-48, 1975
23. Kastor JA: Atrioventricular block. *N Engl J Med* 292:462-465, 1975
24. Karpawich PP, Gillette PC, Garson A Jr, et al: Congenital complete atrioventricular block: clinical and electrophysiologic predictors of need for pacemaker insertion. *Am J Cardiol* 48:1098-1102, 1981
25. Shen W-K, Hammill SC: Survivors of acute myocardial infarction: Who is at risk for sudden cardiac death? *Mayo Clin Proc* 66:950-962, 1991
26. Wellens HJJ, Lemery R, Smeets JL, et al: Sudden arrhythmic death without overt heart disease. *Circulation* 85 Suppl 1:92-97, 1992
27. Moss AJ, Robinson J: Clinical features of the idiopathic long QT syndrome. *Circulation* 85 Suppl 1:140-144, 1992
28. Igarashi Y, Yamazoe M, Suzuki K, et al: Possible role of coronary artery spasm in unexplained syncope. *Am J Cardiol* 65:713-717, 1990
29. Danielsen R, Nordrehaug JE, Vik-Mo H: Clinical and haemodynamic features in relation to severity of aortic stenosis in adults. *Eur Heart J* 12:791-795, 1991
30. Johnson LW, Grossman W, Dalen JE, et al: Pulmonic stenosis in the adult: long-term follow-up results. *N Engl J Med* 287:1159-1163, 1972
31. Mark AL, Abboud FM, Schmid PG, et al: Reflex vascular responses to left ventricular outflow obstruction and activation of ventricular baroreceptors in dogs. *J Clin Invest* 52:1147-1153, 1973
32. Bulkley BH, Hutchins GM: Atrial myxomas: a fifty year review. *Am Heart J* 97:639-643, 1979
33. Copans H, Lakier JB, Kinsley RH, et al: Thrombosed Björk-Shiley mitral prostheses. *Circulation* 61:169-174, 1980
34. Nienaber CA, Hiller S, Spielmann RP, et al: Syncope in hypertrophic cardiomyopathy: multivariate analysis of prognostic determinants. *J Am Coll Cardiol* 15:948-955, 1990
35. Garson A Jr, Gillette PC, McNamara DG: *A Guide to Cardiac Dysrhythmias in Children.* New York, Grune & Stratton, 1980
36. Dresdale DT, Schultz M, Michtom RJ: Primary pulmonary hypertension. I. Clinical and hemodynamic study. *Am J Med* 11:686-705, 1951

37. Franke H: *Über das Karotissinus-Syndrom und den sogenannten hyperaktiven Karotissinus-Reflex.* Stuttgart, FK Schattauer Verlag, 1963

38. Volkmann H, Schnerch B, Kühnert H: Diagnostic value of carotid sinus hypersensitivity. *PACE* 13:2065-2070, 1990

39. Weiss S, Baker JP: The carotid sinus reflex in health and disease: its rôle in the causation of fainting and convulsions. *Medicine (Baltimore)* 12:297-354, 1933

40. Papay FA, Roberts JK, Wegryn TL, et al: Evaluation of syncope from head and neck cancer. *Laryngoscope* 99:382-388, 1989

41. Hammill SC, Gersh BJ: Hypersensitive carotid sinus syndrome. In *Current Management of Arrhythmias.* Edited by LN Horowitz. Philadelphia, Brian C. Decker, 1991, pp. 232-235

42. Sugrue DD, Gersh BJ, Holmes DR Jr, et al: Symptomatic "isolated" carotid sinus hypersensitivity: natural history and results of treatment with anticholinergic drugs or pacemaker. *J Am Coll Cardiol* 7:158-162, 1986

43. Greeley HP, Smedal MI, Most W: The treatment of the carotid-sinus syndrome by irradiation. *N Engl J Med* 252:91-94, 1955

44. Simpson RK Jr, Pool JL, Grossman RG, et al: Neurosurgical management of carotid sinus hypersensitivity: report of three cases. *J Neurosurg* 67:757-759, 1987

45. Keating EC, Burks JM, Calder JR Jr: Mixed carotid sinus hypersensitivity: successful therapy with pacing, ephedrine, and propranolol. *PACE* 8:356-359, 1985

46. Adams RD, Braunwald E: Faintness, syncope, and episodic weakness. In *Harrison's Principles of Internal Medicine.* Ninth edition. Edited by KJ Isselbacher, RD Adams, E Braunwald, et al. New York, McGraw-Hill Book Company, 1980, pp 77-82

47. Davidson E, Rotenberg Z, Fuchs J, et al: Transient ischemic attack-related syncope. *Clin Cardiol* 14:141-144, 1991

48. Constantin L, Martins JB, Fincham RW, et al: Bradycardia and syncope as manifestations of partial epilepsy. *J Am Coll Cardiol* 15:900-905, 1990

49. Yanagihara T, Klass DW, Piepgras DG, et al: Brief loss of consciousness in bilateral carotid occlusive disease. *Arch Neurol* 46:858-861, 1989

50. Sharpey-Schafer EP: The mechanism of syncope after coughing. *Br Med J* 2:860-863, 1953

51. McIntosh HD, Estes EH, Warren JV: The mechanism of cough syncope. *Am Heart J* 52:70-82, 1956

52. Davis TL, Freemon FR: Electroencephalography should not be routine in the evaluation of syncope in adults. *Arch Intern Med* 150:2027-2029, 1990

53. Luxon LM, Crowther A, Harrison MJG, et al: Controlled study of 24-hour ambulatory electrocardiographic monitoring in patients with transient neurological symptoms. *J Neurol Neurosurg Psychiatry* 43:37-41, 1980

54. Bass EB, Curtiss EI, Arena VC, et al: The duration of Holter monitoring in patients with syncope: Is 24 hours enough? *Arch Intern Med* 150:1073-1078, 1990

55. Linzer M, Pritchett ELC, Pontinen M, et al: Incremental diagnostic yield of loop electrocardiographic recorders in unexplained syncope. *Am J Cardiol* 66:214-219, 1990

56. Murdock CJ, Klein GJ, Yee R, et al: Feasibility of long-term electrocardiographic monitoring with an implanted device for syncope diagnosis. *PACE* 13:1374-1378, 1990

57. Gibson TC, Heitzman MR: Diagnostic efficacy of 24-hour electrocardiographic monitoring for syncope. *Am J Cardiol* 53:1013-1017, 1984

58. Kapoor WN, Cha R, Peterson JR, et al: Prolonged electrocardiographic monitoring in patients with syncope: importance of frequent or repetitive ventricular ectopy. *Am J Med* 82:20-28, 1987

59. Krol RB, Morady F, Flaker GC, et al: Electrophysiologic testing in patients with unexplained syncope: clinical noninvasive predictors of outcome. *J Am Coll Cardiol* 10:358-363, 1987

60. Moazez F, Peter T, Simonson J, et al: Syncope of unknown origin: clinical, noninvasive, and electrophysiologic determinants of arrhythmia induction and symptom recurrence during long-term follow-up. *Am Heart J* 121:81-88, 1991

61. Sra JS, Anderson AJ, Sheikh SH, et al: Unexplained syncope evaluated by electrophysiologic studies and head-up tilt testing. *Ann Intern Med* 114:1013-1019, 1991

62. Muller T, Roy D, Talajic M, et al: Electrophysiologic evaluation and outcome of patients with syncope of unknown origin. *Eur Heart J* 12:139-143, 1991

63. Seliem MA, Benson DW Jr, Strasburger JF, et al: Complex ventricular ectopic activity in patients < 20 years of age with or without syncope, and the role of ventricular extrastimulus testing. *Am J Cardiol* 68:745-750, 1991

64. Manolis AS, Linzer M, Salem D, et al: Syncope: current diagnostic evaluation and management. *Ann Intern Med* 112:850-863, 1990

65. Fujimura O, Yee R, Klein GJ, et al: The diagnostic sensitivity of electrophysiologic testing in patients with syncope caused by transient bradycardia. *N Engl J Med* 321:1703-1707, 1989

66. DiMarco JP, Garan H, Harthorne JW, et al: Intracardiac electrophysiologic techniques in recurrent syncope of unknown cause. *Ann Intern Med* 95:542-548, 1981

67. Gulamhusein S, Naccarelli GV, Ko PT, et al: Value and limitations of clinical electrophysiologic study in assessment of patients with unexplained syncope. *Am J Med* 73:700-705, 1982

68. Hess DS, Morady F, Scheinman MM: Electrophysiologic testing in the evaluation of patients with syncope of undetermined origin. *Am J Cardiol* 50:1309-1315, 1982

69. Akhtar M, Shenasa M, Denker S, et al: Role of cardiac electrophysiologic studies in patients with unexplained recurrent syncope. *PACE* 6:192-201, 1983

70. Olshansky B, Mazuz M, Martins JB: Significance of inducible tachycardia in patients with syncope of unknown origin: a long-term follow-up. *J Am Coll Cardiol* 5:216-223, 1985

71. Doherty JU, Pembrook-Rogers D, Grogan EW, et al: Electrophysiologic evaluation and follow-up characteristics of patients with recurrent unexplained syncope and presyncope. *Am J Cardiol* 55:703-708, 1985

72. Denes P, Uretz E, Ezri MD, et al: Clinical predictors of electrophysiologic findings in patients with syncope of unknown origin. *Arch Intern Med* 148:1922-1928, 1988

73. Sugrue D, Holmes D, Hammill S, et al: Intracardiac electrophysiological studies (EPS) in patients with unexplained syncope (abstract). *Chest* 88 Suppl 1:24, 1985

74. Teichman SL, Felder SD, Matos JA, et al: The value of electrophysiologic studies in syncope of undetermined origin: report of 150 cases. *Am Heart J* 110:469-479, 1985

75. Denes P, Ezri MD: The role of electrophysiologic studies in the management of patients with unexplained syncope. *PACE* 8:424-435, 1985

76. Hammill SC, Holmes DR Jr, Wood DL, et al: Electrophysiologic testing in the upright position: improved evaluation of patients with rhythm disturbances using a tilt table. *J Am Coll Cardiol* 4:65-71, 1984

77. Selby G, Lance JW: Observations on 500 cases of migraine and allied vascular headache. *J Neurol Neurosurg Psychiatry* 23:23-32, 1960

78. Bickerstaff ER: Impairment of consciousness in migraine. *Lancet* 2:1057-1059, 1961

CHAPTER

24

Sudden cardiac death

A. Mechanisms, incidence, and prevention of sudden cardiac death

Michael J. Osborn, M.D.

Sudden cardiac death represents one of the major public health problems in the world. In the industrially developed countries, it is the leading cause of death. It represents approximately 30% of all nontraumatic and 50% of all coronary artery-related deaths.[1,2] In the United States, 1,200 to 1,400 persons die suddenly and unexpectedly each day (approximately 400,000 persons yearly).[3-7] At least one-third of these persons are under the age of 65 years, and sudden death is the leading cause of death among men of age 20 to 64 years, accounting for 32% of the total deaths in this age group, during the most productive time of life.[8,9]

The incidence of sudden death increases with age. In young people, the incidence is less than 1 per 1,000 population per year, but it doubles with each decade of life after 45 years of age.[10-12] Sudden death occurs more frequently in men than in women. On the average, the incidence is three times higher in men, and although the rate increases in women with increasing age, they lag behind men by 20 years.[11-13]

There has been a reduction in the total number of patients dying suddenly in this country each year (from more than 600,000 annually in 1971 to the present rate of approximately 400,000 per year).[14,15] This decline may be primarily a result of the development of emergency response teams of highly trained paramedical personnel, the training of the general population in principles and techniques of cardiopulmonary resuscitation, the control of cardiac risk factors, the development of cardiac intensive care units with an aggressive approach to treatment and prophylaxis in acute cardiac events, and more vigorous treatment of ischemic heart disease. Much attention and effort have been given the identification of subgroups of patients at increased risk of sudden death. The use of prophylactic therapy in these patients *may* also have contributed to the overall reduction in the rate of sudden death.

DEFINITION OF SUDDEN DEATH

There is no generally accepted definition for sudden death. In addition to the problem of inclusion of patients who do not die, no consensus exists concerning the appropriate duration of time from the onset of symptoms to death. As a result, there seem to be as many criteria for sudden death as there are investigators interested in the problem. The definitions have ranged from death within minutes of the onset of symptoms to death within 24 hours of the onset of symptoms.[16-23] Thus, classifications such as instantaneous death (within minutes of the onset of symptoms), very sudden death (less than 1 hour after the onset of symptoms), sudden death (1 to 24 hours after the onset of symptoms), and nonsudden death (more than 24 hours after the onset of symptoms) have also been developed.[24,25]

The lack of a precise definition of sudden death poses significant problems. Attempts to define populations of patients who are at risk of sudden death, to determine the pathophysiology of sudden death, to assess the significance of different types of underlying cardiac disease, and to compare programs of prophylaxis against recurrence of sudden death may prove very difficult when patients who die instantaneously are grouped with patients who die within 24 hours, or when witnessed and unwitnessed deaths are grouped together.

Some studies attempt to differentiate "instant" and "sudden" death, but most have grouped these potentially heterogeneous patients together. The potential problem related to this approach is the difficulty in determining the true incidence of acute myocardial infarction or acute coronary arterial thrombotic occlusion in cases of sudden death. It is quite possible that the incidence of associated acute myocardial infarction (both in survivors and in nonsurvivors of cardiac arrest) and of acute coronary thrombosis in nonsurvivors would increase if the duration of time from the onset of symptoms to death was relatively long.[26,27] Romo,[28] in a series of 1,267 cases of acute myocardial infarction, found that of the patients who died suddenly, only 50% died less than 1 hour after the onset of symptoms. Corday[8] found that the incidence of acute thrombosis at autopsy was 4% when death occurred within 30 seconds of the onset of symptoms and increased to 33% when death occurred within 1 hour of the onset of symptoms. These differences might affect the design of programs aimed at preventing sudden death.

The proportion of sudden deaths that are unwitnessed is variable but significant in many population studies. In a large metropolitan area, approximately 20% of 100 consecutive deaths classified as sudden (by World Health Organization criteria) occurred in patients who had been found dead without any information about the manifestations or duration of the attack.[29] Kuller et al.[30] estimated that up to one-third of all sudden deaths are unwitnessed. These are most likely to occur in women, in persons who live alone, or in patients whose episode occurs at home. The inability to determine such factors as the duration of time between the onset of symptoms and death and the nature of the episode quite obviously compromises any population studies, which include a large percentage of unwitnessed sudden deaths.

The study of these patients would be made less difficult by the adoption of a clear definition of sudden death. It should eliminate any potentially noncardiac deaths, unwitnessed deaths, and deaths with a relatively long period from the onset of symptoms to the time of death.[15] A definition proposed by Myerburg[31] seems to be the most reasonable:

> natural death due to cardiac causes, occurring either instantaneously or up to one hour after the onset of symptoms in a patient who may or may not have known pre-existing heart disease but in whom the time and mode of death occur unexpectedly.

A definition such as this has generally been accepted for use by clinical trials attempting to define methods of prophylactic therapy for prevention of arrhythmic death. However, a strictly time-based criterion of 1 hour or less after the onset of symptoms has resulted in errors of up to 27% in classification of arrhythmic deaths (that is, some deaths secondary to arrhythmia have a duration of symptoms greater than 1 hour and many nonarrhythmic deaths have a very short period from symptom onset to death).[32]

CAUSES OF SUDDEN DEATH

Associated cardiac arrhythmias

In general, it can be stated that sudden death usually results from severe disturbances of cardiac impulse generation or conduction which cause cardiac output to fall to levels that cannot sustain cerebral or cardiac function.

Since 1889, when McWilliam[33] suggested that sudden death in man was due to "fibrillar contraction" of the ventricular wall, it had been assumed that most (if not all) cases of sudden death were caused by ventricular fibrillation. With the development of rapid-response mobile emergency units, the disturbances in rhythm associated with sudden death have been documented. The majority of cases are indeed related to ventricular tachyarrhythmias, but a significant percentage are associated with profound bradyarrhythmias.[14,34-41] In a series of 352 consecutive episodes of witnessed out-of-hospital cardiac arrest that were attended by paramedics within 4 minutes of the onset of symptoms, 62% were found to involve ventricular fibrillation, 7% ventricular tachycardia, and 31% bradyarrhythmias as the first rhythm recorded.[42] A study of 133 patients with spontaneous out-of-hospital cardiac arrest attended by paramedics within 10 minutes after the onset of symptoms found that 75% had ventricular fibrillation and 25% had extreme bradycardia or asystole. The bradyarrhythmias documented were sinus arrest or profound sinus bradycardia in 90% and complete atrioventricular (AV) block with absent or markedly retarded escape rhythms in 10%.[39,43] Similar results were found in 87 patients attended within 4 minutes of the onset of symptoms. Eighty-four percent had ventricular fibrillation, and 16% had cardiac standstill (asystole). However, the finding by the same investigators that patients who were not monitored until more than 4 minutes after the onset of symptoms had a significantly greater incidence of asystole (80%) suggested that the asystole documented in some patients may not have been the mechanism of arrest but rather a result of sustained myocardial anoxia.[44]

In a series of patients with recurrent out-of-hospital cardiac arrest, 77% had ventricular fibrillation and 23% had asystole when first monitored. In this group of patients, those with asystole usually had unwitnessed episodes (70%), whereas those with ventricular fibrillation usually had witnessed episodes (76%); this again suggested the possibility that asystole in some of these patients may not have been the initial rhythm disturbance.[20] Regardless of the exact percentages, it is obvious that not all episodes of cardiac arrest (sudden death) are related to ventricular tachyarrhythmias.

Several studies have reported the fortuitous occurrence of cardiac arrest during ambulatory electrocardiographic (ECG) monitoring. Once again, the majority of episodes were due to ventricular tachyarrhythmias, but profound bradycardia or asystole occurred in 16% to 26%.[39-41,45-48] Sudden collapse and death was also rarely seen despite the persistence of a regular cardiac rhythm (electromechanical dissociation).[49,50]

Ventricular fibrillation is the most common terminal tachyarrhythmia but in most instances begins as a monomorphic or polymorphic ventricular tachycardia that degenerates to fibrillation.[39,41,51,52] Torsade de pointes type of fibrillation occurs infrequently with Q-T interval prolongation and usually is related to antiarrhythmic drug therapy and electrolyte abnormalities.[39,53]

In addition to confirming the nature of terminal arrhythmias, Holter monitoring during cardiac arrest has allowed observation of the rhythms that lead up to ventricular tachycardia and fibrillation. An increase in heart rate ($\geq 20\%$) and in the frequency and complexity of ventricular arrhythmias in the hour before sudden death has frequently been observed[15,41,52,54] and may reflect a significant increase in sympathetic tone preceding these tachycardia events.[55] The precipitating ventricular premature complexes do not consistently occur close to the preceding T wave (the so-called R-on-T phenomenon) and in some series are most frequently seen late in the cardiac cycle.[41,51]

Other potential causes of sudden cardiac death include supraventricular tachycardias resulting in very rapid ventricular rates[54] (for example, atrial fibrillation associated with the Wolff-Parkinson-White syndrome), cardiac rupture in the setting of acute myocardial infarction,[56] pericardial effusion with associated cardiac tamponade, rupture of an abdominal aortic aneurysm, and rupture of a dissecting aortic aneurysm. These are, of course, very uncommon causes of sudden death.

Factors predisposing patients to "malignant" arrhythmias

Mechanism of sudden death. From the observation that a variety of arrhythmias (tachycardia as well as bradycardia) are associated with sudden death, it is obvious that no uniform or predictable pathophysiologic process applies to all episodes or all patients. Ventricular fibrillation and ventricular tachycardia appear to be the most common arrhythmias, and hence an understanding of the factors that lead to their occurrence is important if we hope to identify populations at risk and formulate approaches to prevention.

In general, three factors are involved in the initiation and perpetuation of a ventricular tachyarrhythmia: triggers, a pathophysiologic substrate for arrhythmia, and modulating factors. Ordinarily, these must act in concert to result in sustained arrhythmias. The triggers are almost invariably ventricular premature beats. The pathophysiologic substrate may be acute (myocardial infarction or ischemia) or chronic (healed myocardial infarction, cardiomyopathy, ventricular hypertrophy), and the modulating factors could include changes in autonomic tone, hemodynamic abnormalities, myocardial ischemia, electrolyte imbalance, or drugs. Each of the functional modifiers may interact with one or more of the structural abnormalities to generate specific responses that serve as an initiating event for a fatal arrhythmia. If the functional factor alone is of sufficient severity or intensity, it *may* itself initiate a fatal arrhythmia in the absence of structural disease.[57]

Ventricular fibrillation is favored by any inhomogeneity of myocardial excitability and refractoriness.[58,59] The triggering of ventricular fibrillation requires the operation of transient changes that momentarily alter cardiac refractoriness and conduction.[60] A ventricle that is totally uniform electrically will not fibrillate. Ventricular fibrillation may occur after stimulation during the so-called vulnerable period of the cardiac cycle, which occurs within a 30-msec interval preceding the apex of the T wave. During this vulnerable period, maximum asynchrony of the action potential duration and refractoriness would be expected. Stimulation at that time causes the depolarization wave front to encounter some cells that are fully repolarized, others that are partially repolarized, and still others that are absolutely refractory. Thus, the wave front becomes fractionated into areas of normal conduction, slowed conduction, and block – providing an electrophysiologic substrate for reentry.[61]

The threshold for ventricular fibrillation is altered in patients with diseased ventricular myocardium such as in coronary artery disease. Diseased ventricular myocardium should be more vulnerable to ventricular fibrillation because reentrant activity and fractionation of wave fronts of excitation are more likely to occur in the presence of localized areas of depressed excitability and conduction as a result of myocardial damage.[62]

Electrical stimulation of the ventricle during the vulnerable period has resulted in ventricular tachycardia/fibrillation in experimental animals. In animals without underlying heart disease, multiple repetitive electrical stimuli or single stimuli at very high levels of electrical energy have been required to produce arrhythmia.[63] The repetitive extrasystole threshold has been used as a measure of ventricular vulnerability to fibrillation in these animals.[64] This threshold of ventricular vulnerability or fibrillation threshold can be altered experimentally by the creation of coronary artery stenoses (with resultant myocardial ischemia or infarction),[64] reinstitution of coronary blood flow after coronary occlusion (that is, coronary reperfusion after balloon occlusion of a coronary artery),[65] central nervous system stimulation,[66] and psychologic stress.[67] These alterations in the electrical milieu of the ventricle seem to be required for the initiation of ventricular fibrillation by ventricular stimuli. Such experimental situations have obvious clinical correlations in man.

Myocardial infarction. Comparisons of infarcted and noninfarcted regions by catheter technique in patients with acute myocardial infarction have revealed an increased threshold of excitability and prolongation of refractory periods at infarction sites; these findings confirm the existence of considerable electrophysiologic disparity between infarcted and noninfarcted myocardium.[68] These changes in myocardial conduction and refractoriness resulting from muscle necrosis or ischemia create the anatomic and physiologic substrate for malignant ventricular tachyarrhythmias. Most patients who die acutely in the setting of myocardial infarction do so as a result of such a malignant arrhythmia. It is conceivable that infarction or severe ischemia localized to the sinoatrial node, AV node, or other parts of the conduction system could result in profound bradyarrhythmias which could result in sudden death[38] directly (asystole) or indirectly (bradycardia causing hemodynamic deterioration that leads to ventricular tachycardia/fibrillation).

However, most patients who die suddenly do not have associated myocardial infarction. In a large number of studies the incidence of acute myocardial infarction associated with sudden cardiac death ranged from 0% to 39%.[7,20-22,42,56,69-78] Once again, this is somewhat dependent upon the definition of sudden death. The longer the period from the onset of symptoms to the time of death, the greater is the likelihood of finding myocardial necrosis at postmortem examination. Studies comparing autopsy findings in patients who died within 30 seconds, 1 hour, and 24 hours after the onset of symptoms have found that acute coronary lesions are present in 0% to 4% of patients dying instantaneously (less than 30 seconds), in 33% of those dying within 1 hour, and in 82% of those dying within 24 hours.[4,79]

Myocardial ischemia. There is reasonable circumstantial evidence to implicate myocardial ischemia – clinically manifest or silent – as a major pathogenetic mechanism in sudden death.[14]

Histologically, there are two basic categories of myocardial cell injury or necrosis: myocardial infarction and myofibrillar degeneration.[80] This myofibrillar degeneration (distortion or loss of the normal linear arrangement and regularly spaced cross striations of individual muscle fibers and the presence of contraction bands alternating with lightly staining granular cytoplasm) is one of the three histologic criteria for myocardial ischemia. The two others are sinuous (wavy) fiber distortion and positive staining with hematoxylin basic fuchsin-picric acid.[4]

Whereas myocardial infarction occurs relatively infrequently, myofibrillar degeneration or the other histologic changes of myocardial ischemia are seen in the majority of patients who die suddenly. In 120 patients who died less than 6 hours after the onset of symptoms, 52% had all three of the histologic findings and 81% had at least one of the three.[4] In 54 cases of sudden death, Alexandru and Dobrescu[81] identified positive hematoxylin basic fuchsin-picric acid staining in 46%.

In a study of 50 consecutive patients who died within 2 hours of the onset of symptoms, myofibrillar degeneration was identified in 88%. The number of cells that exhibited this change varied considerably, not only from patient to patient but also at different locations within the same heart. In addition, electron microscopic evaluation of these same patients identified abnormal but not necrotic myocardial cells, which could not be differentiated from normal by the usual techniques of light microscopy.[80] Any or all of these abnormal cells or groups of cells could function as the anatomic or physiologic substrate of a ventricular arrhythmia.

Experimentally, myofibrillar degeneration has been produced by situations other than permanent vascular obstruction. These include transient myocardial ischemia, catecholamines, hypokalemia, central nervous system stimulation, and electrical discharge.[80] These experimental data suggest that a variety of clinical situations could lead to an abnormal electrical milieu of the myocardium and thus to lethal ventricular tachyarrhythmias.

Transient myocardial ischemia is a result of an imbalance between myocardial oxygen demands and myocardial blood flow. It can be precipitated in a setting of stable coronary artery disease by excessive physical activity or profound emotional stress. Although most patients who die suddenly do so during normal activity or at rest, 7% to 25% of these persons die during vigorous activity or under emotional stress,[20,22,56,82] probably as a result of a severe imbalance in oxygen supply and demand. This is especially true in middle-aged (or older) adults, the overwhelming majority of whom have significant coronary artery disease.[83-86]

In addition, transient myocardial ischemia can be caused by coronary artery spasm. ST-segment alternans (on the surface ECG) has been observed in a significant percentage of patients during an episode of coronary artery spasm with associated transmural myocardial ischemia.[87] ST-segment alternans is a sign on the surface ECG of a disequilibrium of conduction and refractoriness during ischemia that can predispose the heart to reentrant arrhythmias.[87-89]

During episodes of coronary artery spasm associated with ST-segment electrical alternans on the surface ECG, ventricular arrhythmias occur almost invariably. Ventricular tachycardia has been observed in up to 63% of these episodes and ventricular fibrillation in 33%. When coronary artery spasm occurs in the absence of ST-segment alternans, complex ventricular ectopy is not observed.[88,90] It is conceivable that a significant proportion of victims of sudden death (without explicable cause) had sustained reversible ischemia on the basis of coronary artery spasm which initiated a lethal ventricular arrhythmia.[91]

Coronary artery spasm could result in malignant ventricular tachyarrhythmias during the release phase with subsequent coronary reperfusion.[61,88,92] Ventricular fibrillation has been produced experimentally by the reinstitution of flow in a previously occluded coronary artery.[93-95] Bulkley et al.[96] found contraction band myocardial necrosis, which suggested reperfusion of focally nonperfused myocardium, in several patients who died suddenly. All had normal intramural and extramural coronary arteries.

Another potential cause of focal myocardial ischemia is focal obliteration of the small intramyocardial arteries by microemboli or microthrombi. These microemboli and microthrombi could be made up of aggregates of platelets. In experimental animals, intracoronary or intraventricular infusion of adenosine diphosphate, which induces platelet aggregation, led to focal ischemic myocardial necrosis, myocardial infarction, and sudden cardiac death. Prior induction of thrombocytopenia in these animals prevented these changes in response to adenosine disphosphate infusion.[97] On this basis, it has been postulated that platelet microthrombi or microemboli can result in permanent focal or extensive myocardial ischemia and lethal arrhythmia. Platelet aggregation has been found in large and small coronary blood vessels in up to 30% of patients with sudden death; therefore, this appears to be more than just a theoretical cause of cardiac arrest.[98,99] Since catecholamines have been shown to cause myocardial injury, this effect may be not only a direct effect but also related to catecholamine-induced platelet aggregation.[72]

A number of studies have found that there appears to be a diurnal variation in the incidence of sudden cardiac death. Most of these events occur in the midmorning hours, a time when the tendency to platelet aggregation is also maximal.[100-103] In the Beta-Blocker Heart Attack Trial, 38% of all sudden deaths occurred between the hours of 5 and 11 a.m., whereas in the β-blocker treatment group, only 24% of patients died during that time. This result suggests that β-blockade is protective during the morning hours, when a surge of sympathetic activity may increase the risk of sudden death.[104]

Other contributing factors. Experimental evidence indicates that environmental stress of diverse types can injure the heart, lower the threshold of cardiac vulnerability to ventricular fibrillation, and, in animals with coronary artery occlusion, produce potentially malignant ventricular arrhythmias.[67]

Psychologic stresses have also been shown to precipitate arrhythmias in man.[105] The provocative emotional patterns include startle, fright, anger, helplessness, excitement, and even joy.[60] It would appear that these psychologic (or emotional) factors may be mediated by the sympathetic nervous system or be a manifestation of a withdrawal or disruption of central neural inhibitory influences on cardiac activity.[106] Evidence in support of this thesis has been derived from animal studies in which stimulation of hypothalamic and reticular activating systems resulted in ventricular fibrillation in animals with associated coronary artery occlusive lesions.[107,108]

Autonomic nervous system activity during acute myocardial infarction may also be a major determinant in the occurrence of ventricular fibrillation. Sympathetic activation can trigger malignant arrhythmias, whereas vagal activity may exert a protective effect. The antifibrillatory effect of vagal activation has also been shown to prevent ventricular fibrillation during acute ischemia in animal studies.[109] Studies in man have demonstrated that alterations in autonomic tone after acute myocardial infarction may be highly predictive of subsequent sudden death.[110,111]

Not all episodes of sudden death occur in association with acute myocardial infarction or ischemia, as can be ascertained on clinical grounds and by pathologic studies. A significant number of patients have no symptoms to suggest ischemia before an episode.[112,113] Silent ischemia is absent by Holter criteria in approximately 90% of episodes of spontaneous ventricular tachycardia or ventricular fibrillation, and ECG evidence of myocardial ischemia during exercise testing is absent in most survivors of out-of-hospital cardiac arrest.[39] Many episodes of sudden death are secondary to sustained ventricular tachycardia (or ventricular tachycardia that degenerates to ventricular fibrillation), and this arrhythmia is an uncommon manifestation of acute ischemia or infarction.[40,41,52,114]

Ventricular tachycardia encompasses a clinical spectrum with various symptom presentations, including hemodynamic collapse and death. This clinical spectrum depends on a variety of factors, including rate, ventricular systolic and diastolic function, and lack of AV synchrony. Hemodynamic collapse can lead to myocardial ischemia, which in turn causes degeneration of arrhythmia to ventricular fibrillation. Some ventricular tachycardias are poorly tolerated, and victims of cardiac arrest may be experiencing their first episode and thus not have a history of recurrent ventricular tachycardia.[115] These arrhythmias arise from myocardial regions electrophysiologically altered by remote infarction (or other underlying disease processes).[116,117] Most victims of sudden death have healed myocardial infarction or scar, which commonly serves as an anatomic substrate for reentrant ventricular arrhythmias, and approximately one-third have left ventricular aneurysms.[118] Furthermore, ventricular arrhythmias are inducible in more than three-fourths of patients with coronary artery disease who survive cardiac arrest unrelated to acute infarction. The inducibility of these arrhythmias does not depend on ischemia, as evidenced by the absence of symptoms or ECG changes during programmed ventricular stimulation. One study suggested that nearly 50% of survivors of out-of-hospital cardiac arrest had ischemia (determined by myocardial lactate production) during induction of ventricular tachycardia.[119] In another study, however, the elimination of metabolic evidence of ischemia by the administration of a calcium-channel blocker did not affect the ability to induce ventricular tachycardia.[120]

Additionally, it must be remembered that not all episodes of sudden death are related to ventricular fibrillation or tachycardia, and while it is conceivable that acute infarction or ischemia could result in profound bradycardia, most episodes of bradyarrhythmic cardiac arrest or electromechanical dissociation occur in patients with significant congestive heart failure.[41] In a series of 21 patients with severe heart failure who suffered monitored cardiac arrest, only 38% of the episodes were secondary to tachyarrhythmia. Bradycardia or electromechanical dissociation was the terminal event in all patients with dilated cardiomyopathy but in only 36% of those with heart failure secondary to coronary artery disease.[121] This finding suggests that these deaths are secondary to a hemodynamic derangement rather than an electrical one.[78]

UNDERLYING CARDIAC DISEASE ASSOCIATED WITH SUDDEN DEATH (TABLE 24A-1)

The majority of patients who die suddenly have associated coronary artery disease. The incidence (again depending on study design) has varied from 75% to 100%. This association is not unexpected when one considers the high prevalence of coronary artery disease and its propensity to produce the conditions of myocardial ischemia and injury conducive to fatal arrhythmia.[20,38,69,73,122-125]

Other cardiac pathologic conditions commonly associated with sudden death include cardiomyopathy (dilated, hypertrophic, or restrictive), valvular heart disease (aortic stenosis and mitral valve prolapse primarily), and hypertensive cardiac disease. Of interest is that from 5% to 20% of patients who die suddenly have no evidence of underlying cardiac disease, either by gross autopsy examination or by cardiac catheterization.[38,122-124,126]

There remain a large number of additional potential causes of sudden cardiac death which either have been definitely implicated in isolated cases or theoretically provide anatomic or physiologic substrates for these events. Diseases of the coronary arteries other than atherosclerosis that have been associated with significant myocardial ischemia and sudden death are anomalous origin of the right or left coronary artery;[127-129] dissecting aneurysms of the coronary arteries (especially in the Marfan syndrome or during pregnancy);[130,131] coronary artery embolism, primarily in the presence of bacterial endocarditis or prosthetic valves;[132] a coronary artery ostial lesion related to syphilis (now rare)[133] or atheromatous disease;[134] and generalized inflammatory polyarthritis with associated involvement of the coronary arteries.[135]

All forms of myocarditis are complicated by a wide spectrum of atrial and ventricular arrhythmias and conduction defects. It is not surprising, therefore, that sudden death is an associated feature. Among the types of myocarditis most likely to be associated with sudden death are sarcoidosis,[136] viral myocarditis, other forms of

Table 24A-1 Cardiovascular disease states associated with sudden death

- Coronary artery disease
  - Atherosclerosis
  - Infectious disease (syphilis)
  - Inflammatory disorder (rheumatic vasculitis)
  - Congenital anomaly
  - Coronary artery embolism
  - Coronary artery aneurysm
- Valvular heart disease
  - Mitral valve prolapse
  - Aortic stenosis
- Cardiomyopathy or myocarditis
  - Idiopathic disorder
  - Hypertrophic cardiomyopathy
  - Infectious disease
  - Sarcoidosis
  - Amyloidosis
  - Muscular dystrophy
  - Arrhythmogenic ventricular dysplasia
- Prolonged Q-T interval
  - Idiopathic disorder
  - Congenital anomaly
  - Medication-related disorder
  - Liquid protein diet
- Metabolic abnormalities
  - Hyperkalemia or hypokalemia
  - Hypercalcemia or hypocalcemia
  - Hypomagnesemia
  - Increased levels of catecholamines
- Congenital heart disease
  - Primary pulmonary hypertension
  - Tetralogy of Fallot
  - Congenital heart block
  - Ebstein's anomaly of the heart
- Medication
  - Antiarrhythmic agents
  - Antidepressant drugs
  - Major tranquilizers
- Intracardiac tumor
  - Primary
  - Metastatic
- Cardiac ganglionitis
- Wolff-Parkinson-White syndrome
- No apparent underlying cardiac disease

infectious myocarditis,[137] and amyloidosis (but usually only in the presence of heavy ventricular muscle involvement and particularly if the bundle branches are infiltrated).[138]

Acute hypokalemia, hyperkalemia, hypocalcemia, hypercalcemia, and hypomagnesemia all are associated with sudden cardiac arrest. These biochemical changes may lead to pronounced ECG changes in the absence of morphological abnormalities of the myocardium.[139,140] Production of catecholamines by pheochromocytoma will produce focal myocardial injury and is therefore associated with a tendency to ventricular fibrillation and sudden death.[141]

The use of certain types of drugs (both in the usual therapeutic dosage and in toxic amounts) has led to fatal cardiac arrhythmias. Most of the antiarrhythmic agents used to treat both ventricular and supraventricular arrhythmias have resulted in ventricular fibrillation or hemodynamically unstable ventricular tachycardia.[140] This has been well documented for class IA (quinidine), class IC (flecainide or encainide), and class III (amiodarone) antiarrhythmic agents.[142,143] Flecainide and encainide have been associated with the greatest degree of proarrhythmia and sudden death. When proarrhythmia was defined as the occurrence of a new form of ventricular tachycardia, temporally associated with the initiation of drug therapy or an increase in drug dosage, the incidences were 4% and 11% in patients with ventricular tachycardia treated with flecainide and encainide, respectively.[144] In a study of more than 550 patients using either drug for control of supraventricular tachycardia or ventricular tachycardia, the rate of sudden death was 2.3% in those taking flecainide and 7.5% in those taking encainide. Cardiac arrest occurred predominantly in patients with underlying heart disease but also in patients with normal hearts being treated for supraventricular tachycardia.[145] The tricyclic antidepressants[146,147] and phenothiazine-type major tranquilizers[140] are other commonly implicated drugs. They appear to alter myocardial repolarization with resultant prolongation of the Q-T interval, which may lead to arrhythmic generation.

Some forms of congenital heart disease are associated with sudden cardiac death, especially primary pulmonary hypertension, in which syncope and sudden death are common initial symptoms.[148] Some patients with congenital heart block are at risk for sudden death. Identification of this subset of patients has been difficult. The only finding that has been shown to correlate with risk of sudden death is a resting heart rate of fewer than 50 beats/min.[129,149] After the successful complete surgical repair of tetralogy of Fallot, the reported incidence of late sudden death is as high as 4.6%. Ventricular arrhythmias (especially ventricular fibrillation) are the most likely cause of sudden death in this group of patients, although complete heart block has been observed.[150-153] Other congenital heart lesions that are associated with sudden death are Eisenmenger's complex, transposition of the great arteries (especially after surgical repair), Ebstein's anomaly, and cyanotic congenital lesions with pulmonary stenosis or atresia.[126,129,154]

In patients younger than 40 years, the spectrum of cardiac disease accompanying sudden death is different from that in the older age groups. Most have some form of underlying cardiac disease, but 10% to 40% have structurally normal hearts. In patients younger than 20 years, acute myocarditis, cardiomyopathy (especially hypertrophic cardiomyopathy), and primary electrical disease of the heart are the most common causes, and coronary artery disease occurs only in patients with congenital anomalies of these vessels. In patients between 20 and 40 years of age, however, atherosclerotic coronary artery disease becomes the most prominent form of underlying cardiac disease.[155-159] In young people, episodes of cardiac arrest not infrequently occur during or shortly after strenuous exercise, and in these patients, conditions such as hypertrophic cardiomyopathy and arrhythmogenic right ventricular dysplasia are more likely to be present than in age- and sex-matched patients with nonexertional sudden cardiac death.[158,159] In this age group, sudden death secondary to toxic exposures, especially to cocaine, is becoming increasingly more frequent. Cocaine-related sudden death occurs primarily in young men or users of intravenous drugs. Accelerated coronary atherosclerosis and vasospasm are two common abnormalities noted in these patients.[160,161]

Coronary artery disease

As stated previously, most patients who die suddenly have associated coronary artery disease. This is expected in light of the fact that the physiologic milieu for sudden death is frequently some type of myocardial injury or necrosis. It is also clear that the type of coronary artery disease present in these patients can be fixed atheromatous disease (with or without complete coronary artery occlusion) or coronary artery spasm, or a combination of the two.

Not only do most of these patients have coronary artery disease, but it is distributed extensively throughout the coronary artery tree.[20,23,80] The minimum degree of coronary artery disease which can reasonably be associated with sudden death is one area of 85% stenosis, and most patients have multiple areas with this degree of stenosis.[138,162] In angiographic studies of survivors of out-of-hospital cardiac arrest, the majority had 70% or more stenosis of two or more coronary arteries, and one-half had significant triple-vessel disease.[16,38,69,124,163] Although obviously some patients have significant stenosis of only a single coronary artery, this degree of disease without associated stenosis (50% to 75%) of other coronary arteries is extremely uncommon.[23,164] These findings are not limited to middle-aged or elderly patients. The vast majority of patients between the ages of 24 and 44 years who die suddenly have extensive advanced atherosclerotic coronary disease.[13,165,166]

Autopsy studies have confirmed the findings of angiography. In 31 patients with sudden death due to coronary artery disease, 36% of 5-mm segments of the coronary arteries had 75% to 100% luminal narrowing, whereas only 7% of these segments had 25% or less narrowing.[167] In that study, the distribution of disease proximally and distally within a single vessel and in the three major vessels was the same. This is also the case in the angiographic studies, although it has been noted that involvement of the left anterior descending coronary artery is almost universal.[69]

The extent of coronary artery disease in patients who die suddenly is significantly greater than that in patients with coronary artery disease alone (manifested by angina or old infarction) or in those who die from other causes (but are matched for age and sex). In patients with coronary artery disease manifested by angina pectoris, approximately 25% will have more than 50% stenosis of the three major vessels, whereas in the sudden death group, more than 50% will have disease of that severity.[163] Autopsy studies comparing victims of sudden death with "matched controls" revealed incidences of significant two- and three-vessel disease of 60% to 80% in the former and 8% to 25% in the latter.[23,82] When the coronary arteries were sectioned in 5-mm segments, 70% revealed more than 50% narrowing in the sudden death group as opposed to 25% in matched controls.[167] In addition, patients who have a cardiac arrest with an associated myocardial infarction have less severe and less extensive coronary artery disease than those who have the arrest unassociated with an infarction.[69]

In addition to fixed and chronic coronary artery stenosis, many postmortem studies have demonstrated complicating acute coronary lesions—plaque fissure, plaque rupture, and thrombosis formation. The reported incidence of these acute events varies greatly (18% to 74%) and may reflect the length of time between symptoms and death (the frequency of thrombus formation increases with the duration of time between symptoms and death), the nature of the associated arrhythmias (a larger percentage of acute thrombosis occurs in patients with bradycardiac arrest), or associated acute myocardial infarction.[75,168,169]

A postmortem study demonstrated a difference in the types of acute coronary lesions in patients with sudden death and those with acute myocardial infarction. In the acute infarction group, the characteristic lesions were occlusive fibrin thrombi overlying areas of plaque rupture and hemorrhage. In the sudden death group, the incidence of plaque rupture was very low and thrombus, if present, was nonocclusive and composed almost entirely of platelets.[170] The incidences of acute myocardial infarction and ischemia have been discussed earlier. Healed myocardial infarction is also present in a significant number (38% to 91%) of patients who die suddenly, and ventricular aneurysm has been found in 18% to 56%.[22,23,69,116,171-173] There is no difference in the severity of coronary disease in patients who survive a cardiac arrest and in those who die as a result; however, whether overt cardiac disease is present before the cardiac arrest does have a bearing on the prognosis. A greater incidence of old myocardial infarction and symptomatic heart disease was found in patients who did not survive the event than in those who did.[74]

Sudden death can be the first manifestation of disease of the coronary arteries. It has been estimated that between 25% and 33% of patients who die suddenly in a setting of coronary artery disease have not had symptoms suggestive of cardiac disease for which they sought a physician's advice.[20-23,38,163] This may be particularly true of men between the ages of 25 and 44 years. In this age group, 87% of the deaths related to cardiac disease are sudden.[165] Among patients who have evidence of coronary artery disease before cardiac arrest, the manifestations are usually either angina pectoris (stable or unstable) or a history of prior myocardial infarction. If angina pectoris is present before a cardiac event, it is usually stable. Tresch et al.[69] reported that approximately 50% of a group of patients who survived sudden death had angina pectoris before the event. Only 10% of this group had accelerated or unstable symptoms at the time of or before the cardiac event.

Valvular heart disease

Aortic stenosis. Sudden death is a well-recognized complication of severe aortic stenosis and is the first manifestation of the disease in adults in approximately 5%. In adult patients who have symptoms related to aortic stenosis (angina, heart failure, syncope), the incidence increases to 15% to 20%.[174] In children, the incidence of sudden death, even in the absence of symptoms, is higher than in adults, ranging from 1% to 18% and averaging 7.5%. The mechanism of sudden death in this group of patients is not totally clear, but it is most likely related to an arrhythmia (either bradycardia or tachycardia). In patients with monitored sudden death (in the setting of critical aortic stenosis—that is, a valve area of 0.6 cm^2 or smaller), a variety of arrhythmias have been documented, including ventricular fibrillation, ventricular tachycardia, sinus arrest with a slow junctional rhythm, and heart block with an idioventricular escape rhythm.[175] The cause of the tachyarrhythmias (and perhaps the bradyarrhythmias as well) is probably myocardial ischemia. Many patients with aortic stenosis have been shown to have subendocardial necrosis resulting from the failure of adequate subendocardial perfusion via the coronary arteries in a setting of elevated left ventricular diastolic intercavitary pressure.[176] Bradyarrhythmia may result from heart block caused by encroachment of calcium on the conduction system as it passes adjacent to the aortic valve in the intraventricular septum.[177,178] Bradyarrhythmias may also be reflexly triggered by activation of left ventricular baroreceptors.[179] The evaluation of treatment of aortic valvular disease and its complications is discussed in chapters 32 and 33.

Mitral valve prolapse. Myxomatous degeneration of the mitral valve apparatus with associated systolic prolapse is a common cardiac abnormality, affecting approximately 5% to 10% of the population.[180,181] The condition is benign in most patients, but there is a distinct risk of sudden death in this group, as demonstrated by the fact that most series of consecutive sudden deaths list mitral valve prolapse as the probable underlying cause in 4% to 7%.[20,123,124,159] The risk of sudden death is relatively small, however, averaging 1 to 2 per 100 patients with documented prolapse.[182-184]

The mechanism of sudden death is speculative but is probably related to ventricular tachyarrhythmias in the majority of cases.[6,182,185,186] A variety of ventricular arrhythmias have been reported in somewhat more than 50% of patients with mitral valve prolapse at rest, during ambulatory monitoring, or during treadmill exercise tests.[174,182,187] Complex ventricular ectopy (defined as multiform premature ventricular beats, pairs, and salvos of three or more consecutive beats) has been demonstrated in as many as one-third of these patients.[184] Ventricular tachycardia has been seen in approximately 5% of patients at rest or during normal daily activity and in a larger percentage (approximately 15%) during formal exercise testing.[183,184] In addition, prolongation of the $Q\text{-}T_c$ interval occurs in these patients, and this also may predispose them to ventricular tachyarrhythmias.[174,184]

The majority of patients with mitral valve prolapse and associated ventricular arrhythmias are women.[123] As expected in the reported cases of sudden death in the setting of mitral valve prolapse, the majority (approximately 75%) also are women. Most of these patients have had a history of presyncope/syncope and have had abnormal ECGs.

The mechanism of the ventricular tachyarrhythmias in these patients is unclear. The explanations include a myopathic process of the left ventricle (with associated changes in refractoriness and conduction in the myocardium), abnormality of the left circumflex coronary artery, coronary artery spasm occurring as a reflex response to prolapse of the mitral leaflet, or tension of the papillary muscles with resultant ischemia,[138,188] but these are clearly only speculative.

Cardiomyopathy

The general category of cardiomyopathy includes various hemodynamic entities (that is, dilated, restrictive, and obstructive) and underlying pathologic conditions. In most series of consecutive cases of sudden death, cardiomyopathies have a prominent place as the associated cardiac condition. The incidence ranges from 1 to 30 cases of cardiomyopathy (of all types) per 100 consecutive cases of sudden cardiac death.[20,38,42,73,109,122-124] The types of cardiomyopathy found in these patients include dilated cardiomyopathy, infiltrative cardiomyopathy (scleroderma, sarcoid, and so on), myocarditis (viral, bacterial, and the like), hypertrophic cardiomyopathy, and arrhythmogenic right ventricular dysplasia.[96,136,137,189-192] The relationship among hypertrophic cardiomyopathy, arrhythmogenic right ventricular dysplasia, and sudden death will be discussed in greater detail.

Sudden death is a recognized complication of hypertrophic cardiomyopathy, particularly in children (older than 10 years) and young adults.[193-195] Two separate studies followed large numbers of patients for 5 years. The most common kind of death was sudden death, which occurred in 14% to 16% of the patients during that period.[196,197] It is quite commonly the first manifestation of cardiac disease, especially in young patients.[198] Of 21 patients in whom sudden death was the first symptom associated with hypertrophic cardiomyopathy, 67% were younger than 18 years and 90% were younger than 25 years.[199,200]

The occurrence of sudden death has been reported among many members of the same family. In a study of eight families with hypertrophic cardiomyopathy and premature cardiac death, it was found that of the 41 patients in the study, 56% died suddenly during the period of observation. Again, the patients were commonly children and young adults, and in this study they were often asymptomatic before the episode.[198] In a retrospective study of 26 patients who died suddenly as the first manifestation of cardiac disease, 33% had a positive family history of sudden death in a first-degree relative.[199] Thus, a positive family history of sudden death appears to be a very poor prognostic sign in this group of patients.

It has been stated by some authors that sudden death

is seen primarily in symptomatic patients or in those with very severe disease, especially associated with pronounced elevation in left ventricular end-diastolic pressure.[193,201] However, as indicated above, sudden death is often the first manifestation of disease, and therefore it is seen also in asymptomatic patients.[195] In addition, 12 asymptomatic patients who died suddenly had had cardiac catheterizations performed a short time before the event. Half of the patients had had either no or only a small gradient across the left ventricular outflow tract, and half had had a gradient of 50 mm Hg or more. There had been modest elevation of the left ventricular end-diastolic pressure in 75% of the group, and they all had significant septal thickening.[199]

The mechanism of sudden death in this group of patients is probably ventricular tachycardia or fibrillation. Of 26 patients who died suddenly, 20% had documented ventricular fibrillation after sudden collapse, 5% had complex ventricular ectopy on a resting ECG, and 5% had ventricular tachycardia induced during a treadmill exercise test.[199] More than 20% of these patients show ventricular tachycardia on long-term ambulatory monitoring.[202] In a study of 86 consecutive patients, 24- to 48-hour periods of ambulatory ECG monitoring demonstrated nonsustained ventricular tachycardia in 28%. During a follow-up period of 3 years, 21% of this group of patients died suddenly.[203]

The possible mechanisms of ventricular fibrillation are many, and they all are potentially additive in any patient. Left ventricular outflow obstruction of a mild or severe degree can be aggravated by inotropic stimulation (that is, emotion, exercise, or some other factor), which could lead to complete obstruction and result in ventricular fibrillation. The fact that a significant percentage (about 40%) of the sudden deaths in these patients occurred during or immediately after physical activity supports this mechanism. The reduction and impairment of ventricular filling present in this condition can also be aggravated by inotropic stimulation. This stimulation alone can further hinder diastolic filling, and the resulting tachycardia will decrease the diastolic period. The onset of atrial fibrillation in these patients will cause a sudden loss of atrial "kick" and a decreased duration of diastolic filling time, which could result in precipitous drops in cardiac output and cause ventricular fibrillation. Acute myocardial ischemia as a result of compression of subendocardial and intramural coronary arteries could also result in arrhythmia. Finally, the disordered hypertrophic myocardium may cause temporal dispersion of depolarization and repolarization, leading to primary ventricular tachyarrhythmias.[122]

The presence of accessory conduction pathways (with antegrade conduction in the Wolff-Parkinson-White syndrome or concealed retrograde conduction alone) has been demonstrated in patients with hypertrophic cardiomyopathy.[204] A supraventricular tachycardia with accessory pathway conduction (especially with atrial fibrillation and rapid antegrade conduction) could also cause a significant reduction in cardiac output and result in sudden death. In patients in whom arrhythmias have been recorded before or immediately after collapse, about 10% had atrial tachycardias, and this suggests that in some patients the event may be due to supraventricular arrhythmias.[200]

Attempts to determine the clinical characteristics that might identify the subgroup of patients who are at risk for sudden death have met with variable success. There appear to be no hemodynamic parameters that are predictive of sudden death.[200] The presence or absence of symptoms is also of no predictive value. However, studies comparing patients with and without a history of cardiac arrest have demonstrated a relationship between the magnitude of left ventricular hypertrophy and the risk of sudden death. Extremely marked and diffuse hypertrophy was eight times more common in the sudden death group.[205] In addition, in patients who died suddenly, two factors were virtually constant: All had significant asymmetrical septal hypertrophy, and all had abnormal ECGs.

No entirely characteristic abnormality was seen, but the most common findings were left ventricular hypertrophy, ST-T changes, and deep, wide Q waves, especially in the precordial leads.[199,200] The presence of spontaneous nonsustained ventricular tachycardia during monitoring also identifies patients at increased risk.[194,203,206] In 86 patients with nonsustained ventricular tachycardia documented during periods of monitoring, the rate of sudden death was 21% in 3 years. In patients with the same clinical and hemodynamic variables without nonsustained ventricular tachycardia, only 3% died suddenly during the same follow-up period.[203]

The use of amiodarone in patients with spontaneous ventricular tachycardia or syncope (or both) has resulted in significant reduction in the rate of sudden death.[194] Eighty-two patients were screened by ambulatory ECG monitoring, and nonsustained ventricular tachycardia was demonstrated in 25%. These patients were then treated with amiodarone (average dose, 300 mg daily). During the period of follow-up, none of these patients experienced an arrhythmic event.[203]

This beneficial effect of amiodarone has not been found in all studies. In 50 patients with hypertrophic cardiomyopathy treated with amiodarone for relief of symptoms, the rate of sudden death was 14% in 2 years, most deaths (83%) occurring within the first 6 months of therapy. A history of syncope and the presence of nonsustained ventricular tachycardia on monitoring before the initiation of therapy were common in the group of patients with sudden death.[207] Electrophysiologic evaluation of patients with hypertrophic cardiomyopathy has demonstrated the frequent correlation of inducible supraventricular tachycardia, ventricular tachycardia, and severe conduction system disease in those with antecedent symptoms.[208] These studies question the validity of empirical use of amiodarone in all patients with hypertrophic cardiomyopathy and nonsustained ventricular tachycardia, especially if these disorders are accompanied by unexplained syncope.

Another type of cardiomyopathy causing sudden death in young patients is arrhythmogenic right ventricular dysplasia.[209] This disorder is characterized by fibrofatty transformation of the ventricular myocardium. The most commonly affected regions are the right ventricular inflow tract, the right ventricular outflow tract, and the right ventricular free wall in the inferoapical region. The ventricular free wall in the inferoapical region. The transformation may lead to generalized right ventricular enlargement or discrete aneurysmal deformities in the affected areas. The process affects the right ventricle predominantly but may also affect the left ventricle and become a generalized condition. Spontaneous ventricular arrhythmias causing palpitations, syncope, or sudden death are the most common presenting complaints, and because these symptoms typically occur at a younger age, the disease is an important cause of sudden death in juveniles and young adults. Patients with arrhythmogenic right ventricular dysplasia commonly have evidence of right ventricular enlargement by radiography or nonspecific ST-T changes on the ECG, but they may be otherwise asymptomatic, with normal cardiac examinations, ECGs, and chest radiographs. Careful echocardiographic or angiographic examination of the right ventricle is required for diagnosis. Sudden death has commonly occurred during exercise, and exercise testing has been useful in precipitating ventricular tachycardia in many patients.[191,192]

These patients frequently have a family history of ventricular tachycardia, syncope, or sudden death, and right ventricular dysplasia has been documented in the members of many families with such a history.[179] The mode of inheritance in these studies is thought to be autosomal dominant with incomplete penetrance.[210]

Thus, in young people with a family history of sudden death, a careful search for right ventricular dysplasia should be made with echocardiography (and perhaps angiography), because identification of this abnormality should lead to further diagnostic testing (especially exercise testing) to define a population of patients at increased risk of sudden death.

Aside from these two specific types of cardiomyopathy, most other pathophysiologic processes that result in global reduction of ventricular function are grouped under the heading of dilated cardiomyopathy. This disease entity carries with it a significant risk of sudden death.[205,211-213] In the Framingham study, the biannual age-adjusted sudden death rate was 31.4 per 1,000 men and 9.9 per 1,000 women with heart failure, compared with rates of 5.7 and 1.8 per 1,000 for men and women without heart failure.[214,215] Of the 400,000 patients with heart failure who die yearly, from 35% to 45% die suddenly, presumably as a consequence of malignant tachyarrhythmia. As the clinical condition of patients worsens, the rate of sudden death increases. Sudden death occurs in 8% to 10% of patients in New York Heart Association (NYHA) class I and in 20% of those in classes II through IV.[212,216]

Many potential mechanisms for sudden death are related to arrhythmia in these patients. Ventricular myocardial fibrosis, scarring, and hypertrophy could be associated with heterogeneity of depolarization and repolarization, creating an ideal setting for the occurrence of ventricular arrhythmias. The frequent use of diuretics could result in metabolic abnormalities that favor initiation of arrhythmia. As most of these patients have concomitant coronary artery disease, regional myocardial ischemia may occur, precipitating lethal arrhythmias.[216,217]

Prolonged Q-T interval syndromes

A relation between prolongation of the Q-T interval on the resting ECG and an increased risk of sudden cardiac death has been recognized since 1957, when Jervell and Lange-Nielsen[218] described a Norwegian family with a history of syncope and sudden death among siblings. Four of the six children experienced syncope in the first year of life, and three of those affected died suddenly at ages 4, 5, and 9 years, respectively. Further investigation of these (and similar) patients demonstrated an associated severe bilateral high-frequency loss of hearing. In this disorder—the Jervell and Lange-Nielsen syndrome—the inheritance is autosomal recessive. Heterozygotes are clinically normal but may have slight prolongation of the Q-T interval.[219]

In 1963, Romano et al.[220] and Ward[221] separately described patients with prolongation of the Q-T interval, syncope, and sudden death, with normal hearing. The mode of inheritance in these patients proved to be autosomal dominant. It was documented that ventricular arrhythmias coincided with the syncopal episodes in these patients, and it was assumed that sudden death resulted from ventricular fibrillation.

Since the identification of these two groups of patients, many more syndromes of prolonged Q-T interval (more than 440 to 460 msec when corrected for heart rate[222]) have been described, most associated with syncope and sudden death. Patients with prolonged Q-T intervals can be divided into two groups: (1) primary or idiopathic forms with or without heritable features and (2) acquired forms. Among the many causes of acquired Q-T interval prolongation are medications (antiarrhythmic agents, hypnotic agents, and major tranquilizers), electrolyte imbalance, hypothermia, cerebrovascular accidents, and liquid protein diets.[222-224]

Idiopathic syndromes of prolonged Q-T interval. Evidence suggests that prolongation of the Q-T interval or the appearance of giant U waves (Q-TU-interval prolongation) is directly related to the episodes of syncope and sudden death in all syndromes. For example, in the Romano-Ward syndrome, the Q-T interval is consistently prolonged at the time of unconsciousness, whereas it may be normal at other times.[225] Also, the Q-T interval has been noted to become normal synchronously with the spontaneous termination of ventricular tachycardia or fibrillation. If the Q-T interval remains normal in these patients, the ventricular arrhythmias do not recur.[223]

Prolongation of the Q-T interval is caused by delayed ventricular repolarization and usually represents an increase in refractoriness of myocardial and cardiac conduction tissue with an associated temporal dispersion of tissue recovery. Such dispersion leads to prolongation of the vulnerable period and may thereby enhance susceptibility to ventricular tachyarrhythmias.

Although there is a clear association between prolongation of the Q-T interval and episodic syncope or sudden death in some patients, it can be an incidental ECG finding in otherwise normal patients who are not at risk for sudden death. In addition, certain patients with idiopathic Q-T prolongation have a wide variability in the Q-T interval duration, depending on sympathetic tone and other nervous system influences at the time of the ECG recording. In these patients, the Q-T interval may, in fact, be normal most of the time and markedly prolonged at other times, such as during maximal exercise testing.[91]

The pathogenesis of the abnormal ventricular repolarization leading to Q-T interval prolongation is unknown, but most studies suggest that abnormalities of the cardiac sympathetic nervous system are the cause.[51] A number of facts tend to support this hypothesis. Syncope in this syndrome is commonly triggered by events (exercise, startle, anxiety, fear, and the like) that are known to increase sympathetic activity.[107,226,227] In addition to prolongation of the Q-T interval, patients with syncope commonly demonstrate T-wave alternans before or after an episode of ventricular fibrillation. These two ECG signs can be produced by asymmetrical alterations in sympathetic tone,[227] and, as pointed out earlier, stimulation of the central nervous system and the sympathetic nervous system in particular has resulted in a lowering of ventricular fibrillation threshold and has precipitated ventricular tachyarrhythmias.[107,228] Thus, the ventricular fibrillation and sudden death that occur in these patients are at least in some cases probably a result of an inhomogeneity of ventricular recovery times and a decrease in fibrillation thresholds resulting from imbalances in sympathetic tone.[219]

In addition, postmortem examination by James et al.[226] of patients with Q-T interval prolongation and sudden death has demonstrated focal neuritis and neural degeneration of unknown cause within the sinoatrial node, AV node, His bundle, and ventricular myocardium. This degeneration was present equally in males and females and was independent of age at the time of death and of duration of symptoms. It was speculated by these authors that many of the degenerating nerves in the ventricular myocardium must be sympathetic and that their focal destruction would explain the abnormal myocardial repolarization seen as Q-T interval prolongation and T-wave distortion. The apparently progressive nature of the neural disease could explain the waxing and waning of the electrophysiologic abnormalities, since different nerves would be involved at different times and thereby vary the asymmetrical neural influence randomly.[226]

About 30% of patients with long Q-T syndrome are identified during clinical evaluation of unexplained syncope or aborted sudden death. Approximately 60% are identified when family members of a patient with symptoms are screened by ECG. The remaining 10% are identified in a variety of ways but usually when unexpected prolongation of the Q-T interval is noted on routine examination.[229] The three hallmarks of the long Q-T syndrome are unequivocal Q-T prolongation, syncope, and family members with Q-T interval prolongation associated with syncope or premature sudden death. Once ECG and clinical diagnoses are established, all living relatives should be screened with ECG and a family pedigree developed, with special attention to symptoms. Treadmill exercise can also be used as a screening test. Exaggerated Q-T prolongation and T-wave enlargement can be elicited during and after exercise in these patients.[230,231]

Recently, linkage analysis performed on a family predisposed to sudden death from cardiac arrhythmias and a long Q-T syndrome confirmed the genetic basis of the trait. The gene associated with this abnormality was localized on the short arm of chromosome 11. The existence of genetic markers will greatly improve our ability to identify families and family members who are at the greatest risk of sudden death.[232]

Patients who do not have a family history of sudden death or symptoms of recurrent syncope or arrhythmia do not require therapy. Treatment is recommended, however, for patients with Q-T-interval prolongation associated with symptoms (syncope, arrhythmia, sudden death) or those who have no symptoms but who have a family history of sudden death or who have associated complex ventricular arrhythmias.[233] In untreated patients with syncope, the rate of recurrent events is 5% to 9% per year.[230,233]

β-Adrenergic blocking agents serve as the foundation for treatment. Therapy has to be individualized, and the dose of β-blockers should be maximized to ensure adequate competitive blockade of the myocardial β-adrenergic receptors. Dosage should be assessed by observation of a resting bradycardia, especially a blunted heart rate response to exercise. When treatment is used in this way, many studies have demonstrated a significant reduction in syncope recurrence and sudden deaths.[146,222,227,234] Pacing therapy is indicated only if therapy with β-blockers results in profound bradycardia or symptomatic pauses.[229,230,235] Despite adequate β-blockade, some patients continue to have syncope or cardiac arrest.

In this group of patients, left cervical sympathectomy and stellate ganglionectomy have been recommended.[236] In experimental animals, ablation of the right stellate ganglion or stimulation of the left has produced prolongation of the Q-T interval, decreased threshold for ventricular fibrillation, increased ventricular excitability, and ventricular arrhythmias.[222,237,238] In man, T-wave alternans and ventricular arrhythmias have been produced by stimulation of the left stellate ganglion or blockade of the right stellate ganglion, and they have been abolished by blockade of the left stellate ganglion.[222,239] Removal of the left stellate ganglion and the first three or four thoracic cervical ganglia (cervicothoracic sympathetic ganglionectomy) has been performed for treatment of refractory arrhythmias in an attempt to prevent sudden death.[229] The results have been encouraging but not uniformly successful, and at least 5% of these patients have had symptomatic recurrences.[226,227] In this group of patients, an implantable defibrillator has been used successfully.[229] Antiarrhythmic therapy has not been shown to be of benefit and may have a deleterious effect.

Acquired Q-T prolongation due to medication. Prolongation of the Q-T interval and sudden cardiac death have been reported in association with the use of a wide variety of drugs. Chief among these are the antiarrhythmic agents (quinidine, procainamide, disopyramide), phenothiazine tranquilizers, and tricyclic antidepressants.[138,140,146,222,223]

Antiarrhythmic agents such as quinidine, disopyramide, procainamide, and amiodarone all lengthen the Q-T interval when given in therapeutic doses. Quinidine syncope (the prototype of the medication-induced prolonged Q-T syndromes) is characterized by short paroxysms of ventricular tachycardia/fibrillation which may result in sudden death. In most cases, syncope has occurred when quinidine was administered for treatment of nonsustained ventricular tachycardia or atrial flutter-fibrillation.[240] In 20% of the cases, syncope or sudden death was seen within the first 24 hours of therapy, and 75% of the patients had received less than 1.0 g of medication.[223]

Most patients have a period of hours to days during which all episodes of tachycardia are brief and relatively well tolerated. When an episode of sustained ventricular tachycardia or fibrillation occurs, however, frequent recurrences are common. In general, arrhythmias in patients receiving class IA agents occur when drug levels are low or in the therapeutic range. Fifty percent of all episodes occur in the first 4 days of therapy, the rest occurring weeks to years later. The episodes are commonly linked to change in drug dose (increase or decrease), change in drug preparation, addition of other drugs, reinitiation of therapy after a brief discontinuation, concomitant electrolyte imbalance, bradycardias, and conversion of atrial fibrillation to sinus rhythm.[99,144,223,240-244]

Patients who have experienced syncope as a result of therapy with a class IA agent are likely to have similar occurrences when other antiarrhythmic agents (with similar electrophysiologic properties) are given.[242] Eleven patients who had ventricular fibrillation (torsades) while receiving a class IA agent were treated with another class IA or a class III agent, and 81% had recurrent episodes. The time to symptoms varied, and several days of monitoring would not have protected all patients.[32,245]

The phenothiazine tranquilizers, the tricyclic antidepressants, and lithium carbonate have electrophysiologic properties that are similar to those of quinidine. Q-T interval prolongation, life-threatening ventricular arrhythmias, and sudden death have been reported with these agents, even in usual therapeutic dosage.[242,246,247]

Acquired Q-T prolongation due to metabolic abnormalities. Various metabolic abnormalities have been associated with prolongation of the Q-T interval, syncope, and sudden death. As noted before, many electrolyte imbalances involving potassium and magnesium result in Q-T prolongation and its accompanying disturbances in rhythm.[139,140,222] Abnormalities in serum calcium (that is, hypocalcemia) result in prolongation of the Q-T interval. However, hypocalcemia does not affect phase 3 of the action potential and does not result in prolongation of T-wave or U-wave formation; consequently, there is no associated risk of ventricular fibrillation in this situation.[248,249]

Therapy for the group of patients with acquired prolongation of the Q-T interval and associated complications should be aimed at correcting the underlying causes, such as discontinuing use of all possible offending drugs and correcting any metabolic abnormalities. Because patients remain at risk while the primary problem is being treated, additional measures aimed at shortening the repolarization period should be employed. The treatment of choice at present appears to be overdrive pacing from the atrium or ventricle, although ventricular pacing, even in the absence of AV block, may be the more effective of the two methods.[140,227] Pacing rates of 90 to 110 beats/min have been shown to be most effective. If pacing is not possible, increasing the heart rate to this level by an infusion of isoproterenol may be beneficial.[248,249] Magnesium sulfate (1 to 2 mg intravenously) may suppress episodes even if the serum magnesium concentration is normal, and this agent is a reasonable adjunct to any therapy in this situation.[249,250]

MORTALITY

Sudden cardiac death usually occurs in out-of-hospital settings. The chances of surviving such an event depend on a number of factors, including the nature of the rhythmic disturbance (bradycardia or tachycardia), whether the episode is witnessed or unwitnessed, and the ability of paramedical personnel or nonmedical bystanders to respond quickly and in an appropriate manner.[251]

In 1974, Liberthson et al.[22] described 301 patients, all of whom had out-of-hospital cardiac arrest due to ventricular fibrillation. In this group, 66% were successfully defibrillated, but 49% of these patients died en route to the hospital. Therefore, only about 33% of the patients could be resuscitated and brought to the hospital for further care[22] (Table 24A-2). Similar findings were reported in several other studies.[20,122]

The rhythm disturbance related to the episode of cardiac arrest has a significant influence on the likelihood of initial resuscitation. In 352 consecutive episodes of prehospital cardiac arrest, when the rhythm disturbance was ventricular tachycardia, 88% of patients were successfully resuscitated; when it was ventricular fibrillation, 40% were resuscitated; and when it was bradyarrhythmia, only 9% were resuscitated.[42] In two other series of 195 patients, bradyarrhythmia and asystole were documented in 44 patients, of whom only 1 (2.3%) was successfully resuscitated.[43,54]

In addition to the large number of patients who die either at the scene of a cardiac arrest or en route to the hospital, the in-hospital mortality is very high. In the early experience with management, only 4% to 25% of patients who had an episode of cardiac arrest recovered to be dismissed from the hospital.[21,22,42,122,252-255] Studies in which early cardiopulmonary resuscitation and rapid defibrillation were emphasized demonstrated a significant improvement, although only 30% to 40% of patients survived to hospital dismissal.[34,255,256]

Although more than 50% of the patients successfully admitted to the hospital have recurrent ventricular tachycardia or fibrillation (usually within the first 24 hours),[22] only about 10% of in-hospital mortality is related to these disturbances in rhythm. The rest of the deaths are related to low cardiac output states, severe anoxic encephalopathy, or sepsis resulting from the required respiratory support.[42] Not only is the number of these patients who survive small, but only about 60% of patients dismissed from the hospital return to functional NYHA class I or II status or achieve their prehospital status.[22,122] This means that for every 100 patients with out-of-hospital cardiac arrest, only about 10 ever achieve their prehospital status.

Table 24A-2 Results after out-of-hospital cardiac arrest*

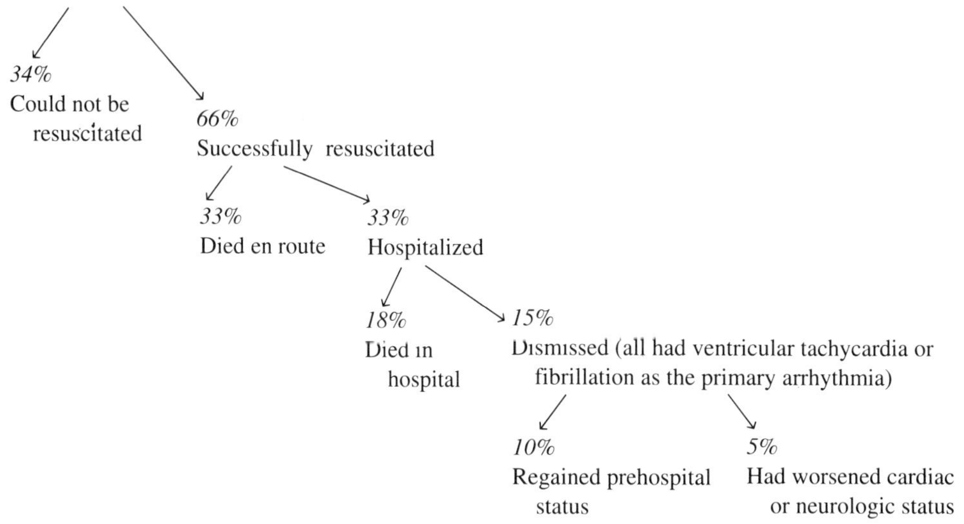

*Modified from Liberthson RR, Nagel EL, Hirschman JC, et al: Prehospital ventricular fibrillation: prognosis and follow-up course. *N Engl J Med* 291:317-321, 1974.

The specific rhythm disturbance involved is an important factor in long-term as well as short-term survival after a cardiac arrest. When ventricular fibrillation was the underlying arrhythmia, more than 20% of these patients survived to be dismissed from the hospital, whereas in all reported series, when the underlying arrhythmia was cardiac asystole (or other profound bradyarrhythmia), none lived to be dismissed from the hospital.[20,34,42,43,257]

The postresuscitation heart rate and rhythm appeared to have some predictive value for prehospital and in-hospital mortality. Postresuscitation bradycardia predicts a very poor prognosis (90% prehospital and in-hospital mortality), whereas a heart rate greater than 100 beats/min is associated with a significantly greater chance of ultimate hospital dismissal.[258] Likewise, if the post-resuscitation rhythm is sinus, paced, or atrial fibrillation, chances of survival are improved.[255]

The availability of rapidly responding, highly trained emergency paramedical teams has clearly reduced the short- and long-term mortality associated with an episode of cardiac arrest. The education of the nonmedical population in the techniques of cardiopulmonary resuscitation has also contributed to the reduction in mortality. In a study of 316 patients with cardiac arrest (all due to ventricular fibrillation), the effect of bystander-initiated cardiopulmonary resuscitation was evaluated. Of the patients in whom cardiopulmonary resuscitation was initiated by a trained bystander, 43% survived the event and were dismissed from the hospital. On the other hand, only 22% of patients who were not given cardiopulmonary resuscitation at the scene survived and left the hospital.[259] In a review of nine studies involving 608 patients, 30% of those who did, but only 9% of those who did not, receive bystander cardiopulmonary resuscitation survived to hospital dismissal.[260] It also appears that early defibrillation is very important in ultimate patient survival. There is a significant improvement in the success of resuscitation and subsequent hospital dismissal in patients in whom defibrillation is implemented immediately, compared with those given cardiopulmonary resuscitation for any length of time before defibrillation[215,261,262] (Table 24A-3).

Table 24A-3 Survival in patients with out-of-hospital cardiac arrest

Chances of survival are increased if:
- Initial rhythm is ventricular tachycardia or fibrillation rather than brady-asystole
- Cardiopulmonary resuscitation is initiated quickly
- Defibrillation is implemented immediately
- Heart rate after initial defibrillation is more than 100 beats/min
- Postresuscitation rhythm is sinus, paced, or atrial fibrillation

Even if patients survive these episodes of cardiac arrest and are dismissed from the hospital functionally unimpaired, they are at risk of recurrent episodes. Schaffer and Cobb[20] in 1975 reported that 27% of patients resuscitated and dismissed from the hospital had a subsequent cardiac arrest within a median of 20 weeks between the two episodes. One-third of these patients had their arrest within 3 months after hospital dismissal. Liberthson and associates[22] noted that 28% of patients had recurrent episodes of cardiac arrest after dismissal, and Weaver et al.[163] reported that 22% had recurrent episodes in a mean follow-up of 20 months. Thus, persons who have survived an episode of cardiac arrest are at very high risk of recurrent episodes. One-third of these episodes occur within 3 months after hospital dismissal, and one-half occur within the first year. However, the risk of recurrence of cardiac arrest continues up to 5 years after the initial event.[20,263] In a study of 139 survivors of cardiac arrest, the rate of recurrence at 1 year after the event was 12% and at 5 years had increased to 27%.[264]

Not unexpectedly, the prehospital and in-hospital mortality for subsequent episodes is almost identical to that of the first episode. In a series of 45 patients with recurrent cardiac arrest, the overall mortality was 83% (that is, 17% could be dismissed from the hospital). However, in this group of patients, more than 80% had ventricular fibrillation as the arrhythmia leading to arrest. Thus, the overall survival is somewhat less than would be expected in a comparable group of patients suffering their initial episode.[20]

The 2-year mortality after hospital dismissal is very different for patients whose cardiac arrest is associated with an acute myocardial infarction or myocardial necrosis (demonstrated by elevated levels of cardiac enzymes) compared with those who do not have evidence of myocardial damage. In 146 patients dismissed from the hospital after successful resuscitation, the *overall* mortality was 26% at 1 year and 38% at 2 years. For patients who had an associated myocardial infarction, the mortality was 0% at 1 year and 14% at 2 years. Without associated infarction, the mortality was 32% and 43%, respectively. Most of the deaths in this 2-year period were sudden.[21] Cobb et al.[71] compared survivors of cardiac arrest with and without associated myocardial infarction and found a sudden death recurrence rate of 31% in the group without infarction and 5% in those with infarction.

It is apparent, therefore, that the patients who are at highest risk for sudden cardiac death are those who have survived a previous cardiac arrest that was not associated with acute myocardial infarction.

PREVENTION OF SUDDEN DEATH

Prodromal symptoms

It would seem logical that, if a symptom complex that precedes episodes of sudden death could be identified, the recognition of these symptoms might allow us to intervene with specific or prophylactic therapy in a population that is at risk for sudden death.

Although, in general, patients with coronary artery disease have prodromal symptoms much more frequently than do patients without coronary artery disease,[265] its presence is not suspected in a large percentage of these patients and sudden death is the first manifestation of coronary artery disease in about one-third of them.

Sudden death appears to be truly unexpected both in patients with and in those without antecedent symptoms of cardiac disease. In a study of 301 patients with out-of-hospital cardiac arrest, about 30% of them had seen a physician within a few weeks before the event. Although about 28% had either new or changing symptoms of chest pain or dyspnea within about 4 weeks of the cardiac arrest, only 12% saw their physicians because of the new complaint.[22] In similar studies, it was found that between 8% and 25% of patients with unexpected sudden death had seen a physician within a week before their demise.[82,138] Either the majority of patients have no warning of the event or they ignore or misinterpret symptoms that might identify them as persons who are at risk.

Not only do patients not have a change in symptoms days to weeks before an event, but also the majority do not have symptoms suggesting a change in health status immediately preceding the event. In the large study by Liberthson et al.,[22] 17% of patients had chest pain or dyspnea within 4 hours of the event, 19% had chest pain or dyspnea preceding the cardiac arrest by 1 to 30 minutes, and 65% had either no symptoms or symptoms within 1 minute of the attack. However, other studies have demonstrated that in patients with clinically apparent coronary artery disease, antecedent chest pain or dyspnea may occur in up to 50%.[113,266]

In addition, the level of activity of most persons at the time of a cardiac arrest also suggests an absence of preceding symptoms. Most patients have their attacks during rest or normal daily activity, and a significant percentage die during sleep.[20,22,54] Young patients, who are more likely to have cardiac arrest during or after exertion, have reported prodromal symptoms more frequently than populations of older patients. In these patients, presyncope and syncope are the most common symptoms and may reflect the fact that sudden death in many of these patients is unrelated to coronary artery disease.[155,157,159]

The presence of prodromal symptoms appears to be more common in patients who have an associated myocardial infarction than in those who do not. In this group of patients, the symptoms seem to precede the event by a significant time. Of a group of patients in whom ventricular fibrillation developed after the arrival of medical aid, 87% had prodromal symptoms and 50% had an associated acute myocardial infarction, whereas in patients in whom ventricular fibrillation was present when the emergency medical team arrived, only 20% had prodromal symptoms and 10% had associated myocardial infarction.[21] In patients in whom intracoronary thrombus or platelet aggregates are found at postmortem examination, the incidence of any prodromal symptoms or unstable angina is significantly greater than in patients in whom no acute coronary lesions are noted.[98,168]

Thus, it appears that prodromal symptoms are uncommon either minutes or weeks before an episode of sudden death and are particularly unusual in patients with primary sudden death (not associated with acute infarction). Although attempts to identify patients at risk by identification of prodromal symptoms is clearly important, it may not be helpful in most cases.

Identification of populations at risk

Because ventricular tachyarrhythmias have been shown to be the cause of most episodes of sudden death and because ventricular ectopy is the trigger for these episodes, most of the studies attempting to define high-risk groups of patients and to assess treatment programs have focused on the relationship of ventricular arrhythmias to sudden death and on the benefits of arrhythmia control. As will become obvious, many questions remain unanswered.

General population. In the healthy general population, the risk of sudden death is less than 1% per year.[267,268] On the other hand, the frequency of ventricular ectopy of all types, including complex ventricular ectopy, is quite high.[269-272] Definitions vary, but the term "complex ventricular ectopy" usually implies multiform ventricular premature beats, couplets, and salvos of three or more consecutive ventricular premature beats (nonsustained ventricular tachycardia). Frequent ventricular premature beats are not uniformly included in this definition. Random 6-hour Holter monitoring in healthy men revealed ventricular ectopy in 62% of the group, and in about 20% complex ventricular ectopy was noted.[271] Complex ventricular ectopy has been detected by routine ECGs in 0.03%, during continuous monitoring in 8%, and during maximum exercise in 3% of healthy normal adults.[3] Twenty-four-hour Holter monitoring before angiography documented complex ventricular ectopy (multiform ventricular premature complexes and repetitive beating) in 25% of the patients in whom the subsequent catheterization results were normal.[273]

Two large studies have attempted to determine the significance of ventricular ectopy in the population in general. In both, the resting or ambulatory ECG recordings were obtained randomly, and in both approximately 50% of the patients had ischemic heart disease (by history of angina, infarction, or other evidence) and 50% did not. In the Tecumseh[2] study of 5,129 patients, it was found that 6% of the patients with ventricular ectopy died suddenly during the period of observation, whereas only 1% of the patients without ventricular ectopy did so (again, less than 1% per year in both groups). Similar results were found in a different study of 888 patients who had 24-hour Holter monitoring for a wide variety of reasons. In a follow-up period of 2 to 5 years, 4% of the patients with and 1% of those without ventricular ectopy died suddenly. In patients who were identified as having ischemic heart disease, the incidence of sudden death was 6% in those with and 2% in those without associated ectopy. There was no difference in death rates in the presence of simple as compared with complex ventricular ectopy.[274] This study also demonstrated that patients without ischemic heart disease had a very low risk of sudden death in the presence of ventricular ectopy. Several other authors have also shown that the presence of ventricular ectopy (including nonsustained ventricular tachycardia) in the absence of overt ischemic heart disease has no prognostic significance with respect to sudden death.[3,270,275-278]

In patients without a substrate that permits initiation of ventricular tachycardia or ventricular fibrillation, sudden death is unlikely to result from ventricular ectopy irrespective of its frequency or complexity. Therefore, its presence is prognostically irrelevant and its suppression would be necessary only for troublesome symptoms.[279]

Patients with ventricular dysfunction. The Framingham study demonstrated that in asymptomatic patients, the risk of sudden death varied over a wide range of risk factors, such as blood pressure, serum cholesterol, smoking, and resting ECG. However, when overt coronary artery disease was present, these risk factors had much less influence on the risk of sudden death, which became determined chiefly by indicators of intrinsic myocardial damage, especially reduced ventricular function.[280] Since complex ventricular ectopy and sudden death are common in patients with depressed ventricular function and heart failure, physicians have assumed that ventricular arrhythmias are the most important cause of sudden death.

Follansbee et al.[281] identified 37 patients (of 518 consecutive patients referred for ambulatory ECG monitoring for a wide variety of reasons) who had asymptomatic nonsustained ventricular tachycardia, defined as three or more ventricular premature complexes in a row. The majority of patients had ventricular tachycardia of only three consecutive beats, but about 10% had runs of more than five beats in a row. These investigators found that 27% of these patients died during the follow-up period (14 to 24 months). Of the patients who died, 90% had a history of congestive heart failure or an associated dilated cardiomyopathy at the time of the Holter monitoring. Only 5% of the group with nonsustained ventricular tachycardia without evidence of ventricular dysfunction died suddenly.

Several other studies used ambulatory monitoring to evaluate patients with reduced left ventricular function. The incidence of nonsustained ventricular tachycardia was very high in these patients (42% to 60%) regardless of the cause of left ventricular dysfunction, and total mortality and rate of sudden death also were high.[214,282] Some of these studies found that the combination of left ventricular dysfunction (ejection fraction of $<40\%$) and nonsustained ventricular tachycardia identified patients at a considerably increased risk of sudden death. In these studies, most patients had coronary artery disease with associated left ventricular dysfunction.[279,283,284] In studies in patients with dilated cardiomyopathy, however, the rate of sudden death was quite variable, and most results indicated that although the frequency of nonsustained ventricular tachycardia was high, monitoring was of little help in the identification of patients at increased risk of sudden death.[285-287] In severe heart failure (NYHA class III-IV), even though nonsustained ventricular tachycardia becomes even more prevalent, the rate of sudden death no longer increases despite a marked increase in total mortality.[158,216] Among 88 patients with idiopathic dilated cardiomyopathy and moderate heart failure, progressive ventricular dysfunction developed more frequently in those with nonsustained ventricular tachycardia than in those without ectopy. This finding suggests that in this group of patients, nonsustained ventricular tachycardia may be a marker more for hemodynamic and clinical instability than for sudden death.[288]

Electrophysiologic testing would seem to be of potential benefit in this group of patients for a variety of reasons:

1. Patchy scarring of the myocardium (especially in patients with coronary artery disease) may allow the development of conduction block and delayed conduction in parts of the myocardium.
2. Spontaneous ventricular ectopy (if appropriately timed) may result in reentrant arrhythmias.
3. These arrhythmias are the cause of a significant number of sudden deaths.
4. Programmed electrical stimulation commonly causes ventricular tachycardia in susceptible patients.

5. Identification of patients at high risk might justify aggressive therapeutic intervention.
6. Identification of patients at no risk would greatly enhance patient management.[289]

Several studies have attempted to evaluate the utility of this procedure in risk stratification in this group of patients. The majority had *coronary artery disease,* and all had asymptomatic complex ventricular ectopy, including nonsustained ventricular tachycardia. Sustained ventricular tachycardia was induced in 17% to 45% of this group despite the absence of a spontaneous arrhythmia. The cardiac event rate (sudden death or spontaneous ventricular tachycardia) in patients in whom the arrhythmias were not treated was between 50% and 100%. The event rate was 0 to 4% in those without an inducible arrhythmia.[290-296] When left ventricular function was correlated with inducibility in a group of patients with coronary artery disease, it was found that all the patients had left ventricular ejection fractions of less than 40%.[291] The conclusions drawn from these studies were that (1) patients with no inducible arrhythmias and those with left ventricular ejection fractions greater than 40% have a low probability of sudden death and do not require therapy and (2) patients with inducible ventricular tachycardias are at a significantly increased risk of sudden death.[291,294,297]

The utility of programmed ventricular stimulation and overall patient management has been evaluated in patients with *dilated cardiomyopathy* and nonsustained ventricular tachycardia. In this situation, the technique has proved to be of little value. The rates of arrhythmia inducibility are low, and there is no predictive value from either a positive or a negative test.[298-304]

The predictive value of the signal-averaged ECG has been evaluated in two studies involving patients with heart failure. Among patients with coronary artery disease and reduced left ventricular function, the probability of sudden death was higher in those with abnormal late potentials. However, if the cause of heart failure was idiopathic dilated cardiomyopathy or if heart failure (whatever the cause) was severe, the signal-averaged ECG was of no predictive value. Late potentials are poor predictors of the risk of sudden death when congestive heart failure is advanced, possibly because the causes of sudden death in this group are heterogeneous and ventricular tachyarrhythmia is only one of many possible mechanisms.[212,213]

It is clear that patients with nonsustained ventricular tachycardia who have concomitant heart disease with abnormal ventricular function are at an increased risk of sudden death. In patients with coronary artery disease, there appears to be a correlation between the two entities, and electrophysiologic testing further defines a population at significantly increased risk. In patients with dilated cardiomyopathy, the correlation is less clear, and no test clearly identifies subpopulations that could be selected for therapy.

The approach to therapy in these patients is discussed later in this chapter.

Survivors of acute myocardial infarction. Patients who survive hospitalization for acute myocardial infarction have a significant yearly mortality which to a large degree is due to sudden cardiac death. The average rate of sudden death at 1 year after hospital dismissal is 10%, and most of these patients die within the first 6 to 7 months.[6,16,70,171,289,305-312] In the Multicenter Investigation of the Limitations of Infarct Size (MILIS) study, 79% of all sudden deaths occurred in the first 7 months and the overall sudden death rate was low after these first few months.[313] However, long-term studies have demonstrated that the sudden death rate continues to increase slowly with time. In studies of patients from 9 to 12 years after infarction, the cumulative sudden death rate was 25% to 27%.[314,315] These figures are significantly greater than those for the population as a whole,[82,307] for whom the rate of sudden death is far less than 1% per year. As a result, many attempts have been made to more carefully define subgroups of patients at increased risk.

PRESENCE OF VENTRICULAR ECTOPY. When cardiac monitoring was first used in the management of patients during acute myocardial infarction, it was noted that a large percentage of them had ventricular ectopy of all types. Early studies suggested that as many as 80% had complex ventricular ectopy and that there was a correlation between complex ventricular ectopy and subsequent sudden death mortality.[316]

After these early observations, many studies involving some type of ECG monitoring of patients in the *late* hospital recovery phase (several days after the acute event) demonstrated a similar prevalence of ventricular ectopy,[306] with about 30% to 50% of instances considered to be complex ventricular ectopy.[171,305,309,317,318]

The predictive value of these complex ventricular arrhythmias in the identification of a population at risk for sudden death is controversial, although most studies support this concept.[19,76,319-322] As an example, in a study of 1,739 survivors of acute myocardial infarction who were followed for 5 years, the rate of sudden death was 2.6 times higher in patients who had complex ventricular ectopy during 1 hour of in-hospital ECG monitoring at rest than in those with no ventricular ectopy or with simple ventricular ectopy (single unifocal ventricular premature beats) regardless of frequency. When these studies were adjusted for the age of the patient, the presence of complex ventricular ectopy increased the rate of sudden death by three or four times.[16,70]

Although complex ventricular ectopy is associated with other factors (for example, left ventricular dysfunction) suggesting severe myocardial damage, a number of studies have demonstrated that complex ventricular ectopy is an independent risk factor for sudden death in this group of patients.[16,70,319,320,323] In the Beta-Blocker Heart Attack Trial involving 1,640 patients, complex ventricular ectopy was found to be an independent predictor of mortality. In addition, complex ventricular ectopy increased the risk of all other predictive factors.[324]

The same correlation between the presence of complex ventricular ectopy and the risk of sudden death was found in patients who were monitored in the posthospital period. In a study of 85 patients, it was found that if complex ventricular ectopy was demonstrated on three or more Holter recordings in the first 4 weeks after hospital dismissal, the incidence of sudden death in the first year was 22%. Thus, the persistence or appearance of complex ventricular premature contractions early after hospital dismissal may be a marker for continued myocardial electrical instability and for an increased risk of sudden death.[309,310]

Not all studies have found a correlation between the risk of sudden death and complex ventricular ectopy alone. Some have found that the risk is increased in patients with any type of ventricular ectopy, whether complex or noncomplex, frequent or infrequent.[305,325] The Coronary Drug Project Research Group[326] suggested that there was an increased risk of sudden death in patients with complex or frequent forms but also demonstrated a significantly increased risk for patients with infrequent uniform ventricular premature beats. Still other studies have shown only that complex ventricular ectopy has been associated with an increased rate of cardiac death without distinguishing between sudden and nonsudden death.[327] In a study of 978 patients followed over 3 years, no clinical variables, including complex ventricular ectopy, recorded on 24-hour Holter monitoring distinguished between sudden and nonsudden death, although patients with complex ectopy constituted one of the groups who were at higher risk for sudden death.[6]

The optimal duration of monitoring after myocardial infarction and the timing (in the hospital or after dismissal) of the monitoring are unknown. It would appear that the longer a patient is monitored, the greater is the frequency of detection of all forms of ectopy.[17,305] However, it may be that ventricular ectopy is predictive of sudden death only when it is frequent enough to be easily detected by less thorough methods of arrhythmia detection or shorter periods of monitoring.[328] In a study of 160 patients who had four resting ECGs and 12-hour Holter monitoring after infarction, it was found that only about one-third of those who had ventricular ectopy detected by Holter monitoring also had it detected on a resting ECG. Of interest is that 70% of the episodes of sudden death in this group occurred in patients in whom ectopy was detected by the resting ECG.[316]

Taylor et al.[17] studied 61 patients with myocardial infarction by means of 24-hour monitoring during and after hospitalization. They found complex ventricular ectopy in 32% of the patients in the hospital and in another 36% of the patients during the period after dismissal. In their opinion, a normal 24-hour ECG in the late hospital phase of recovery from myocardial infarction provides little assurance that a patient will not have more serious arrhythmias after dismissal. However, complex ventricular ectopy appears to have predictive value for a relatively short time after an acute infarction. In 160 patients who had 12-hour ambulatory monitoring 3 months after infarction, complex ventricular ectopy still identified patients at increased risk.[316] Moss et al.,[19,76] however, found that monitoring at 5 months was of no value.

It is also well known that the frequency and complexity of ventricular ectopy vary considerably, from hour to hour and from day to day.[329,330] This variability adds increasing problems for the use of any kind of ECG monitoring to identify subsets of patients who are at increased risk for sudden death.

The finding of complex ventricular ectopy seems to identify patients at increased risk of sudden death after myocardial infarction. However, because the specificity and predictive accuracy of this method are very poor, it clearly cannot be used alone to select patients for therapy with antiarrhythmic agents.

VENTRICULAR DYSFUNCTION. Because left ventricular dysfunction is a reflection of the extent of myocardial damage secondary to necrosis and ischemia, it is reasonable to assume that there is a correlation between left ventricular dysfunction and postinfarction mortality (both total and sudden death mortality). A number of studies have confirmed that left ventricular dysfunction is indeed an independent risk factor for sudden death after infarction.[171,308,331-334] A left ventricular ejection fraction of less than 40% (determined by an imaging technique, although usually by radionuclide angiography) is the value usually selected to reflect left ventricular dysfunction of significance. When more severe reductions in left ventricular ejection fraction are used as a marker for left ventricular dysfunction, the predictive value appears to increase.[284] As in the case of left ventricular dysfunction secondary to stable coronary artery disease or dilated cardiomyopathy, marked reduction in ejection fraction seems to be a more sensitive predictor of total mortality (although sudden death is a significant component). Patients with an ejection fraction of less than 20% have been found to have a 1-year mortality of 45%, compared with 4% if the ejection fraction is greater than or equal to 40%.[252]

Although ventricular ectopy and ventricular dysfunction are thought to be independent risk factors, they have greater predictive value when combined to assess risk. For patients with "complicated" ventricular ectopy (frequent ventricular premature contractions, multiform ventricular premature contractions, pairs, and ventricular tachycardia) and left ventricular dysfunction (left ventricular ejection fraction of $<40\%$), the 1-year mortality was 30% to 40%, compared with 2% when neither risk factor was present.[309,335] In the MILIS study, the sudden death rate was 18% in patients with both frequent ventricular premature contractions and left ventricular dysfunction but only 1.6% in the absence of either abnormality.[313]

SIGNAL-AVERAGED ELECTROCARDIOGRAPHY. Signal-averaged ECG is a noninvasive technique used to detect and measure microvolt-level signals (late potentials) that are contiguous with the terminal portion of the QRS complex.[336] These late potentials have been correlated with occurrence of spontaneous ventricular tachycardia.[337] They have also been used in an attempt to stratify risk of sudden death after acute myocardial infarction.

Studies performed in large numbers of patients after infarction (more than 1,600 patients combined) have demonstrated that the signal-averaged ECG is positive in 21% to 44% of patients. In these patients, between 8% and 29% had a cardiac arrhythmia event (ventricular tachycardia, ventricular fibrillation, or sudden death) in 12 to 24 months of follow-up. In patients with negative signal-averaged ECGs, the event rate was 1% to 4%.[331,338-342]

The timing of a signal-averaged ECG in relation to an

acute myocardial infarction appears to have prognostic significance. In a study of 190 patients evaluated by signal-averaged ECG within the first 3 days, at 2 weeks, and 6 months after a *first* myocardial infarction, only the results obtained within the first 3 days after infarction were predictive of episodes of ventricular tachycardia or ventricular fibrillation.[333]

These results appear to be independent of left ventricular dysfunction and ventricular arrhythmias, but they have even greater predictive value when combined with them. Patients with an abnormal signal-averaged ECG and left ventricular dysfunction (left ventricular ejection fraction of $<40\%$) have an arrhythmia event rate of 34% to 36% in 1 year. If left ventricular function and the signal-averaged ECG are normal, the event rate is 0 to 4%.[171,338,343] More than 50% of patients with complex ventricular ectopy, left ventricular dysfunction, and an abnormal signal-averaged ECG had ventricular tachycardia, ventricular fibrillation, or sudden death within 12 months, whereas in the absence of all three risk factors, no patients had a cardiac event.[171,338]

The signal-averaged ECG may also be of benefit in the selection of patients for electrophysiologic study, because there is a significant correlation between a positive test and the ability to induce ventricular tachycardia.[338,344]

RESPONSE TO PROGRAMMED ELECTRICAL STIMULATION. Two of the initial studies suggested that programmed electrical stimulation had significant predictive value. In 235 patients with complicated and uncomplicated transmural myocardial infarctions, repetitive ventricular beating (more than 6 to 10 repetitive beats) could be induced in approximately 20% by aggressive stimulation. This was associated with a risk of sudden death of 33% to 35% in a follow-up period of 1 year. The inability to initiate abnormal ventricular beating suggested a significantly better prognosis (sudden death rate, 0 to 8%).[289,312]

Following these initial studies, a number of similar studies demonstrated significant variability in the rates of inducibility and risk of sudden death or ventricular tachycardia in groups with and without inducible arrhythmias.[262,289,312,323,345-351] In patients with uncomplicated myocardial infarction (without spontaneous ventricular tachycardia, major conduction abnormalities, or heart failure), the cardiac arrhythmia event rate varies from 0 to 15% in those with inducible arrhythmias and is not significantly different from the event rate (0 to 11%) in patients in whom a sustained arrhythmia cannot be induced.[308,339,347-351] In a series of 50 patients with acute myocardial infarction complicated by new major conduction disturbances, heart failure, or spontaneous ventricular tachycardia, programmed electrical stimulation identified two groups of patients (group 1, inducible sustained or nonsustained ventricular tachycardia, and group 2, no inducible arrhythmias). Sudden death or ventricular tachycardia was seen in 41% of those in group 1 but was not seen in group 2 patients.[345]

As a result of these studies, it appeared that programmed electrical stimulation was not indicated in patients with uncomplicated acute myocardial infarction who appear to be at low risk for subsequent arrhythmia events but *might* be indicated in patients with complicated acute myocardial infarction, especially because the predictive accuracy of a negative test is quite high, an indication that in most patients without inducible arrhythmias, tachycardia does not subsequently develop.[289]

These studies were extremely difficult to interpret and compare because of significant variability in (1) patient selection (uncomplicated versus complicated acute myocardial infarction), (2) stimulation protocols, (3) definition of an abnormal response, (4) influence of anti-ischemic or β-blocker therapy, (5) concomitant revascularization procedures, and (6) the end point of follow-up.[352]

Recently, several studies again suggested that arrhythmia inducibility during electrophysiologic testing is an independent predictor of subsequent sudden death or arrhythmic events.[353] Two of the studies established sustained monomorphic ventricular tachycardia as the only indicator of an abnormal response to programmed stimulation. The rate of inducibility was low (11% to 19%), but 47% to 75% of these patients had recurrent arrhythmic events, whereas 0 to 2% of patients had events after a negative study.[334,354] In a study involving 1,206 patients with uncomplicated infarction, sustained monomorphic ventricular tachycardia was inducible in 6%. Arrhythmia events (ventricular tachycardia or sudden death) occurred in only 3% of the entire patient population but were significantly more frequent in the group with inducible arrhythmias (19%) than in the noninducible group (2%).[355] In this study, it was pointed out that more than 1,200 patients would have required electrophysiologic study to identify 14 patients with a possible risk of sudden death and that only 0.4% of the total group had a fatal outcome.[352] Thus, although refinements in technique, patient selection, and end points are being made, the issue of the use of electrophysiologic testing in survivors of acute myocardial infarction has yet to be resolved.

Evaluation of ventricular ectopy has not been of benefit in patient selection in these studies, whereas in some (though not all), decreased left ventricular function has identified patients more likely to have an inducible arrhythmia.[312,349-351] Despite the evidence to suggest that a positive signal-averaged ECG is predictive of arrhythmia inducibility, it has not been proven to be of benefit in patient selection in these studies.[353,354]

OTHER FACTORS OF PREDICTIVE VALUE. The heart receives a rich neural supply of both sympathetic and parasympathetic fibers, and the electrical stability of the myocardium depends on a synergism between the two components. Parasympathetic discharge has a protective effect on ventricular fibrillation thresholds, whereas increased sympathetic tone may have a deleterious effect. Areas of selective sympathetic or parasympathetic denervation may occur in the region of infarction and may lead to uncoupling of autonomic modulation, inappropriate sympathetic tone, or loss of protective vagal influences.[356,357] Studies have demonstrated a temporal dispersion of parasympathetic activity in the weeks immediately following acute infarction, coincident with the period during which the risk of arrhythmia events is highest.[358,359]

Two tests that have been used to evaluate autonomic function are heart rate variability (the standard deviation of R-R intervals during normal cardiac cycles obtained over a 24-hour period) and baroreceptor sensitivity (correlation of R-R interval changes with increasing blood pressure in response to phenylephrine administration). Heart rate variability is suppressed in the first 2 weeks after infarction and returns to normal within 6 months, so that the reduction in risk of sudden death in the 6 to 12 months after infarction appears to correlate with the progressive resumption of vagal activity and normalization of autonomic balance.[109,111]

Studies in patients after infarction have demonstrated a correlation between reduction in heart rate variability or baroreceptor sensitivity and the incidence of subsequent total mortality and sudden death. When these tests are combined with reduction in left ventricular function, positive signal-averaged ECGs, or arrhythmia inducibility at electrophysiologic study, the predictive accuracy improves.[110,342,360] Further verification of the utility of these techniques in risk stratification is required before they receive more widespread acceptance and use.

Other factors are also associated with an increased risk of sudden death, although not to the extent of those discussed above. Abnormalities such as cardiomegaly, a history of angina or prior myocardial infarction, left ventricular aneurysm, treatment with diuretics, conduction defects, persistent ST segment depression, and resting sinus tachycardia have all been shown to be associated with a slightly increased incidence of sudden death when controlled for ventricular ectopy.[16,17,70,326,327,352,361] When some of these factors are present in association with complex ventricular ectopy and ventricular dysfunction, the risk of sudden death increases even more.[324] For example, the combination of persistent ST depression and complex ectopy was associated with a risk of sudden death three to four times greater than that in patients with only one of these variables.[325]

In patients with acute myocardial infarction, studies have strongly suggested that residual myocardial ischemia adversely affects short- and long-term survival.[362,363] The evaluation and treatment of myocardial ischemia in this and other clinical settings are discussed in chapter 29.

Survivors of out-of-hospital cardiac arrest. Survivors of out-of-hospital cardiac arrest represent the group of patients who are at greatest risk for sudden death. All studies involving these patients have reported a significant rate of recurrent episodes. Weaver et al.[163] reported a 22% rate of recurrence in a mean follow-up of 2 years. Among a group of 301 survivors of out-of-hospital cardiac arrest, Liberthson et al.[22] noted recurrences in 28% in approximately the same period of follow-up. Another large study documented 30% recurrence of sudden death at 1 year and 45% at 2 years. Within the first year, the repeat events took place in a median time of 20 weeks, and one-third occurred within the first 3 months.[20] As noted before, however, the risk of recurrence persists for several years after the initial event.[164,263,264,279]

Within this total group, the patients can be separated into those at very high risk and those at relatively low risk. In the absence of acute myocardial infarction at the time of the cardiac arrest, the recurrence rate has been reported as 18% in 15 months by one group and 31% at 1 year by another. In these same studies, the risks for those with an associated acute myocardial infarction for the same period of follow-up were 0 and 5%, respectively.[20,38] Baum et al.[21] compared the 1- and 2-year mortality in patients who survived cardiac arrest with or without associated myocardial infarction and found similar results. In those with associated infarction, the 1- and 2-year mortality rates were 0 and 14%, respectively, whereas in those without infarction they were 32% and 43%, respectively. The vast majority of these deaths were sudden.

Other factors appear to separate patients who are at high risk for recurrence from those who are at a lesser risk. Comparing patients who had recurrence of sudden death with those who did not showed that the recurrence group had a greater incidence of congestive heart failure, three-vessel coronary artery disease (64% vs. 22%), and abnormal left ventricular ejection fractions (mean, 0.39 vs. 0.51) and more severe left ventricular contraction abnormalities than the nonrecurrence group.[116,117,163,263] This finding implies that patients with more severe myocardial disease or dysfunction are at greater risk for recurrent cardiac arrest.

The presence of complex ventricular ectopy is almost universal in this group of patients. Among 146 survivors of out-of-hospital cardiac arrest, a 24-hour Holter monitor evaluation detected complex ventricular ectopy (frequent ventricular premature contractions, pairs, salvos, bigeminy, ventricular tachycardia) in 84%.[21] Because ventricular ectopy of a complex nature is present in so many of these patients, it does not appear to separate high-risk from low-risk groups. However, in some studies the presence of complex ventricular ectopy was thought to be of predictive value for subsequent death.[266,364] It should be noted that complex ventricular arrhythmias in these patients correlate with left ventricular dysfunction and wall motion abnormalities and so may not be an independent predictor of increased risk.[263]

In survivors of out-of-hospital cardiac arrest, the use of signal-averaged ECG has demonstrated that correlation with arrhythmia inducibility is poor. This result is primarily related to inducible ventricular fibrillation and may represent a significant limitation of this technique in identification of patients at risk of sudden death.[335]

Electrophysiologic studies and their use in the determination of effective drug regimens in patients with recurrent ventricular tachyarrhythmias are discussed in detail in chapter 22D. They have also been used in an attempt to stratify the survivors of cardiac arrest in groups at high or low risk of recurrence.

Between 60% and 80% of patients with out-of-hospital cardiac arrest secondary to ventricular tachycardia or ventricular fibrillation have these arrhythmias reproducibly induced by programmed electrical stimulation. As discussed in the section on therapy, the successful identification of drug suppression of arrhythmia inducibility significantly reduces the risk of rhythm recurrence.[116,171,172,365-372] Early experience suggested that patients in whom no arrhythmia could be induced at the time of initial electrophysiologic study were at significantly lower risk than other patients. In these studies, the risk of recurrence was 0 to 6% in patients without inducible arrhythmias but 30% to 31% in patients with inducible arrhythmias in whom no successful therapy could be identified.[172,203,365,370-372] However, a number of subsequent studies could not confirm these findings and demonstrated an arrhythmia recurrence or sudden death rate of 3% to 32% in patients with normal electrophysiologic studies. These studies did identify a *small* group of patients with well-preserved left ventricular function and normal electrophysiologic studies in whom the long-term prognosis was excellent without specific antiarrhythmia drug therapy.[116,171,366,368,373-375]

Patients with inducible arrhythmias are more likely to have remote infarction, a history of heart failure, an ejection fraction of less than 40%, a left ventricular aneurysm, or a history of cardiac arrest. Those without an inducible arrhythmia are more likely to have structurally and functionally normal hearts, left ventricle segments in ischemic jeopardy (stenoses in proximal coronary artery segments supplying contracting and presumably normal myocardium), and factors suggesting ischemia at the time of the arrhythmia (cardiac arrest with activity or stress or clear spontaneous angina).[116,298,301,366,376,377]

In two studies involving 35 patients with a normal electrophysiologic test result who had no recurrence of arrhythmia events, 91% had coronary artery disease and were treated with surgery, percutaneous transluminal coronary angioplasty, or medication.[373,376] This result suggested that prognosis is good when therapy is directed at identifiable underlying heart disease. Another group of 19 survivors of out-of-hospital cardiac arrest underwent electrophysiologic testing before and during exercise testing. If there was no evidence of ischemia, ventricular tachycardia or ventricular fibrillation could be induced before and after exercise. However, if there was evidence of ischemia (by coronary sinus lactate analysis), 83% of these patients had ventricular tachycardia or ventricular fibrillation induced only during exercise but not at rest when there was no evidence of ischemia.[119] These studies suggest that myocardial ischemia may be a requirement for the spontaneous or stimulation-provoked occurrence of ventricular tachycardia or fibrillation in some patients with coronary artery disease who survive out-of-hospital cardiac arrest and might explain the excellent prognosis in some of these patients without specific antiarrhythmic drug therapy.

Clearly, patients who have survived one or more episodes of cardiac arrest, especially in the absence of associated myocardial infarction, are at great risk for recurrent events and deserve some form of therapeutic intervention.

THERAPY FOR PATIENTS AT INCREASED RISK FOR SUDDEN DEATH

Pharmacologic

If a decision has been made that a given patient should be treated with medication in an attempt to prevent sudden death, the next step is the choice of the appropriate agent or agents from the array of drugs that are currently available. Since ventricular fibrillation is the most common cause of sudden death, drugs that might be capable of decreasing the incidence of sudden death would be either antiarrhythmic agents or other agents that influence the pathophysiologic processes that lead to sudden death. Protection from sudden death might be achieved by drugs in one of several ways: (1) by preventing ventricular arrhythmias (antiarrhythmic agents or β-adrenergic receptor blocking agents), (2) by preventing degeneration of ventricular tachycardia to ventricular fibrillation (antifibrillatory agents, such as amiodarone, or β-blockers), (3) by preventing or reducing myocardial ischemia (nitrates, calcium channel blockers), (4) by affecting platelet function to reduce platelet aggregation (platelet-active agents), and (5) by improving ventricular mechanical function (vasodilators or positive inotropic agents).

Prevention of ventricular tachyarrhythmias. Three basic approaches to drug therapy with antiarrhythmic agents can be taken. The first is empiric therapy—that is, treating a patient with an antiarrhythmic agent without determining, by direct monitoring, its effect on the arrhythmia. The second is treatment with an antiarrhythmic agent in an attempt to reduce or eliminate ventricular ectopy noted on the ECG (either resting or ambulatory monitoring). The third is treatment based on some type of provocative testing (either treadmill exercise testing or electrophysiologic studies). The use of calcium channel blockers, β-blockers, vasodilators, or antiplatelet agents is on an empiric basis only.

EMPIRIC ANTIARRHYTHMIC THERAPY. In patients with ventricular ectopy, the empiric approach to antiarrhythmic therapy is commonly used. Unfortunately, most studies suggest that it is the least successful in the prevention of sudden cardiac death.

Virtually all of the early studies of patients who had recurrent episodes of cardiac arrest revealed that most of these patients were receiving antiarrhythmic therapy on an empiric basis.[19,22,305,317] In Baum and associates' series[21] of 143 survivors of sudden death, 58% of those with recurrent cardiac arrest were receiving antiarrhythmic agents. Schaffer and Cobb[20] described 64 patients with recurrent cardiac arrest, 73% of whom were receiving empiric antiarrhythmic therapy at the time of recurrence.

The same experience has also been described in patients who died suddenly after an acute myocardial infarction.[294,323] In a group of 64 patients followed for 2 years after an infarction, 18% died suddenly. All of the patients had ventricular ectopy late in the recovery phase, and two-thirds of them were receiving empiric antiarrhythmic therapy.[305] In a review of patients who had survived myocardial infarction, it was found that 12% of those receiving and 7% of those not receiving antiarrhythmic agents had died suddenly. A number of large single and multicenter trials have been undertaken to determine if the empiric use of antiarrhythmic agents (including procainamide, disopyramide, aprindine, tocainide, mexiletine, and dilantin) can reduce the rate of sudden death (and overall mortality) in the post-myocardial-infarction period. In these studies, most of the patients were free of complex arrhythmias and no attempt was made to modify the frequency of any ectopy that was present. None of these trials demonstrated any benefit from treatment, and several of them found that the sudden death rate was higher in patients in the treatment groups.[378-382]

Three studies have been reported comparing the empiric use of class IA or IB antiarrhythmic agents (in therapeutic amounts) with placebo in patients with complex ventricular ectopy and associated poor ventricular function. None of the studies found any difference in the rates of sudden death between the patients treated with antiarrhythmic drugs and those not treated.[147,279,339] One of these studies was not originally designed to involve the use of a placebo but ended that way because about 50% of the patients could not tolerate antiarrhythmic agents.[147]

The only antiarrhythmic agent with demonstrated benefit when used empirically is class III amiodarone. In studies involving patients with nonsustained ventricular tachycardia in a variety of clinical situations, including hypertrophic cardiomyopathy, dilated cardiomyopathy, and coronary artery disease (after myocardial infarction), use of amiodarone in a low dose has been associated with a lower rate of sudden death than that in patients receiving no therapy or other antiarrhythmic agents.[194,383,384] This observation has not been universal, however, and it should not lead to the conclusion that amiodarone should be routinely used in patients with nonsustained ventricular tachycardia who are at increased risk of sudden death.

The lack of success in the prevention of sudden death by the empiric use of antiarrhythmic agents is most likely a result of one or more of the following factors: incorrect choice of antiarrhythmic agent, inadequate dosage of the antiarrhythmic agent, poor patient compliance, and an adverse effect directly related to drug use. The potentially hazardous effects of drug use include impaired intracardiac conduction, depression of myocardial contractility, and proarrhythmia.[385,386] Additionally, because not all episodes of sudden death are primary electrical events, antiarrhythmic therapy (even if appropriately selected) will not have a beneficial effect in all cases.

Another form of empiric therapy involves the prophylactic use of β-adrenergic blocking agents after acute myocardial infarction in an attempt to reduce the rate of sudden death. The rationale for these studies is based on observations suggesting that sympathetic tone should be tempered for protection against sudden death. These observations include evidence of transient ischemia preceding some arrhythmias, increased heart rate occurring before some lethal arrhythmias, arrhythmias associated exclusively with exercise or inducible during isoproterenol infusion, and increased risk of sudden death in patients with reduced vagal influence.[387,388] In addition, β-blockers may have a primary antiarrhythmic effect, increase the fibrillation threshold in experimental animals,[389] and have an antiplatelet effect.[390]

In 1974, a study comparing alprenolol with placebo given to patients after myocardial infarction demonstrated a reduction in the short-term rate of sudden death after hospital dismissal.[391] These results were confirmed in a study of 230 patients (half treated with placebo, the other half with alprenolol) in which the rate of sudden death with placebo was 10% and that with alprenolol was 3%. The difference in the rate of sudden death was particularly striking in patients with electromechanical (ectopy, AV block, left ventricular dysfunction) cardiac damage.[392] In subsequent years a similar study comparing practolol with placebo demonstrated a 35% reduction in the group treated with this β-blocking agent. However, the degree of significant side effects related to practolol made the use of this drug unreasonable.[393]

The Norwegian Multicenter Study Group[394] evaluated the effects of timolol (a noncardiac selective β-adrenergic blocking agent without intrinsic sympathomimetic activity) in patients with recent myocardial infarction. The use of timolol resulted in a 44% reduction in the rate of sudden death and a 39% reduction in total mortality. The fact that this difference in death rate increased throughout the entire study period indicates that the protective effect of the drug persisted through the period of treatment. Similar results were obtained during the Beta-Blocker Heart Attack Trial in this country. In this trial, which compared propranolol with placebo given 5 to 21 days after acute myocardial infarction, a 28% reduction in the rate of sudden death was noted in the propranolol-treated group. This effect also persisted over the 27 months of the trial.[395]

To date, approximately 18,000 patients who survived acute myocardial infarction have been evaluated in a variety of trials with β-blocker therapy. The average reduction in sudden death mortality has been 30% regardless of age, sex, race, site of infarction, severity of underlying coronary artery disease or infarction, or comparative risk profiles.[394,396,397] Patients with complex ventricular ectopy continue to have a higher rate of sudden death than those without ectopy, but the rate is much reduced from that in patients not treated with β-blockers.[398] These trials have demonstrated that the only effective β-blockers are those that reduce the resting heart rate. Those that have no effect on heart rate (that is, those with intrinsic sympathomimetic activity) have not exhibited any benefit or have resulted in an increased frequency of sudden death.[388]

There is no consensus for use of β-blockers in the postinfarction period. Most would favor their use in patients with a myocardial infarction complicated by electrical instability, labile ischemia, or mild left ventricular dysfunction in the absence of prohibitive contraindications or unacceptable side effects.[386,399]

THERAPY TO SUPPRESS VENTRICULAR ECTOPY. In heart disease complicated by ventricular ectopic beats of all varieties, antiarrhythmic agents are often used to suppress the ectopy on the assumption that this will lead to a decreased risk of sudden death. This approach is based on two postulates: first, that suppression of these risk factors will alter the risk of sudden death; and second, that suppression of ectopy is, in fact, feasible. Conversely, it is often assumed that failure to suppress chronic ventricular ectopy may indicate an ominous prognosis.

However, many authors have suggested that the correlation between suppression of asymptomatic ventricular ectopy and prevention of sudden death is unclear. In many cases, sudden death appeared to be prevented by drugs without much reduction in the frequency or complexity of the ectopy.[73,327,400] Studies have shown that background ventricular ectopy in patients with a propensity to ventricular tachycardia responds differently to varying levels of antiarrhythmic agents than do the episodes of tachycardia themselves. In a study that evaluated the effects of procainamide on ventricular ectopy and ventricular tachycardia, the average percentage suppression of ventricular ectopy was only 36% at levels that prevented recurrence of the tachycardia.[401] In a series of patients who had survived an out-of-hospital cardiac arrest in whom stable therapeutic levels of antiarrhythmic agents reduced the rate of sudden death, there was little change in the frequency of complex ectopy.[122] In these patients, the use of antiarrhythmic agents may be altering refractoriness or conduction in a reentry circuit without altering the frequency of ventricular ectopy.[46] Conversely, life-threatening arrhythmias may occur in the absence of a significant number of ectopic beats; thus, the pronounced reduction of ventricular ectopy does not necessarily protect patients from recurrent cardiac arrest.[46,400,401]

In addition to this apparent lack of correlation between suppression of ventricular ectopy and prevention of ventricular tachyarrhythmias, other problems are inherent in this therapeutic approach.

Variation in the frequency of ventricular ectopy can be so great without any therapeutic intervention that it might be very difficult to distinguish between spontaneous variation and the effect of antiarrhythmic drugs.[402] Two studies in which healthy patients were monitored for various periods found significant spontaneous variation in the frequency of ventricular ectopy. It was noted in these studies that patients with infrequent ventricular ectopy might show even more variability.[330,403]

A significant reduction in the total frequency of ventricular ectopy does not uniformly reflect the absence of periods of advanced ectopic activity. In Myerburg and associates' series,[73] 47% of the tapes with infrequent ventricular premature beats had episodes of complex ventricular ectopy. Because it appears that the risk of sudden death in most groups correlates with associated complex ectopy, even significant drug-related reduction in the frequency of ectopy may not be the desired result.

It should be noted that much less rigorous definitions of reasonable drug efficacy are used in practice. It is commonly recommended that antiarrhythmic therapy used to control spontaneously occurring ventricular arrhythmias result in a 50% or greater reduction in ectopy frequency, a 90% or greater reduction in multiform ventricular premature contractions, and elimination of all repetitive forms in two successive 24-hour periods.[123,382]

In survivors of acute myocardial infarction complicated by complex ventricular ectopy (including nonsustained ventricular tachycardia), two large multicenter trials were initiated to test the premise that arrhythmia suppression would reduce the risk of sudden death. The Cardiac Arrhythmia Pilot Study (CAPS) trial demonstrated that suppression of complex ventricular ectopy was feasible. The use of class IC antiarrhythmic agents resulted in an 80% reduction in frequency of ventricular premature contractions and a greater than 90% suppression in nonsustained ventricular tachycardia.[32] This study was followed by the Cardiac Arrhythmia Suppression Trial (CAST), which used these antiarrhythmic agents (primarily flecainide and encainide) in a double-blind, placebo-controlled fashion. The total mortality and sudden death mortality rates were 3.6 times higher in the treatment group than in the placebo group.[382,388,404]

In another study, involving 312 postinfarction patients, the use of drugs that significantly reduced ectopy frequency and eliminated complex forms (by the criteria established above) was nevertheless associated with a rate of sudden death similar to that with no antiarrhythmia therapy.[405]

These studies have thrown a shadow on the theory that suppression of ventricular premature contractions protects against sudden death in patients in whom complex ventricular ectopy has been associated with an increased risk of sudden death. On the basis of all available data from drug trials in patients with complex ventricular ectopy in the period after myocardial infarction, it seems clear that drug therapy (at least with class I antiarrhythmic agents) does not improve survival and, consequently, cannot be recommended.

Patients with aborted sudden death or sustained ventricular arrhythmias have been managed by suppression of ectopy and elimination of repetitive ventricular premature contractions documented by serial periods of in-hospital or ambulatory monitoring. Lown et al.[65] reported success with rigorous monitoring during normal activity and exercise. The program of management of their patients required use of at least two drugs that were successful in reducing ectopy frequency by 50% over baseline and eliminating all repetitive forms during these monitoring periods. In patients who fulfilled management criteria, the yearly mortality was 3%, whereas in those who did not, the mortality was approximately 50% per year.[406]

A number of other studies have compared the noninvasive (ectopy suppression by monitor) with the invasive (electrophysiologic testing) approach to drug therapy for ventricular tachycardia. Although drug regimens predicted to be effective could commonly be identified by the noninvasive approach, the actuarial rate of arrhythmia event recurrence has been reported to be between 20% and 67% in 2 years. The consensus has been that drug therapy directed by ambulatory monitoring does not accurately predict a clinical response.[368,407,408] These studies have been criticized, however, for lack of randomization.

One randomized trial involved 57 patients with a history of spontaneous ventricular tachycardia or ventricular fibrillation. Noninvasive therapy required fewer days in the hospital and few drug trials, but although therapy predicted to be effective in 100% of patients was identified, the arrhythmia recurrence rate was 50% at 2 years. For the group managed by electrophysiologic testing, the recurrence rate was 20% during the same period.[409]

A large multicenter trial (Electrophysiologic Study Versus Electrocardiographic Monitoring) in progress for several years in an attempt to determine whether electrophysiologic testing or Holter monitoring more accurately predicts drug efficacy in patients with aborted sudden death or sustained ventricular tachycardia unfortunately has not resolved this controversy.[388]

THERAPY BASED ON PROVOCATIVE TESTING. Treadmill exercise testing has been suggested for the identification of subgroups of patients who are at increased risk for sudden death, but the method has not been used extensively to identify therapeutic interventions (other than those which alleviate myocardial ischemia) that will prevent death in these patients. Exercise testing appears to suffer from the same problems of spontaneous variation that make resting and ambulatory ECG monitoring difficult to use in attempts to identify efficacious antiarrhythmic agents. The prevalence of exercise-induced arrhythmias is quite high in patients with and without heart disease, and it increases with age. It has been demonstrated in 20% to 30% of males 25 to 35 years of age and in 40% to 50% of patients more than 50 years old.[271,272] More importantly, the reproducibility of induction of these arrhythmias is only about 50% to 60% in repeated tests, which is only slightly more than the reproducibility by chance alone.[271,272] This obviously would make any assessment of drug effectiveness very difficult.

Electrophysiologic testing has been used very effectively in patients with spontaneous ventricular tachycardia or ventricular fibrillation for patient evaluation and the selection of therapy.

Josephson et al.[410] published the first experience with programmed electrical stimulation in patients resuscitated from cardiac arrest. Of these 52 patients, 63% had arrhythmias that could be induced in the electrophysiology laboratory. Forty-three percent of patients in whom ventricular fibrillation was the first arrhythmia recorded at the time of cardiac arrest had inducible arrhythmias, whereas 90% of patients with ventricular tachycardia as the initial rhythm had inducible arrhythmia. In general, between 60% and 80% of survivors of cardiac arrest have inducible ventricular arrhythmias (ventricular tachycardia, ventricular fibrillation, or nonsustained ventricular tachycardia).[70,171,172,365-369,373,411,412] The variability in rates of arrhythmia induction is secondary to differences in stimulation protocol, in arrhythmia end points, in types of underlying heart disease, and in the presenting arrhythmia. At present, a sustained ventricular tachyarrhythmia is considered an appropriate arrhythmia end point.

In another early study, Ruskin et al.[370] evaluated 31 patients resuscitated from out-of-hospital cardiac arrest. A ventricular tachyarrhythmia was induced in the laboratory in 25 (81%), and an acutely effective drug regimen was identified by serial drug testing in 19 patients (76%), all of whom were free of symptoms during a 15-month period of observation. Of the six patients in whom no effective drug regimen could be identified and hence in whom only empiric therapy could be initiated, 50% died suddenly within six months (Table 24A-4).

Many other studies have demonstrated that effective drug regimens (those that prevent inducibility of arrhythmia) can be identified in 20% to 50% of patients through serial drug testing. Patients treated with acutely effective drugs generally do well, with a cardiac arrest recurrence rate of 0 to 6% at 1 year and 9% to 15% at 4 years in most studies. Those in whom effective drug regimens cannot be identified have a high rate of arrhythmia recurrence and sudden death (20% to 100%) when treated with drugs alone.[116,117,376] Clearly, this group requires some form of alternative therapy—either endocardial resection or, much more commonly, implantation of an automatic cardioverter-defibrillator.[413]

Table 24A-4 Out-of-hospital cardiac arrest: electrophysiologic studies*

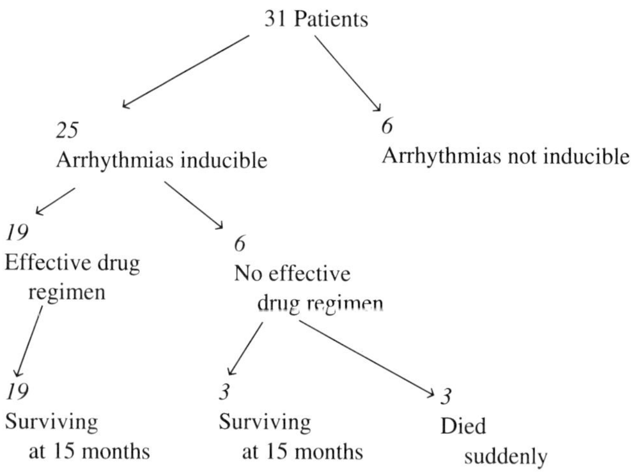

*Modified from Ruskin JN, DiMarco JP, Garan H: Out-of-hospital cardiac arrest: electrophysiologic observations and selection of long-term antiarrhythmic therapy. *N Engl J Med* 303:607-613, 1981.

As pointed out earlier, a significant number of survivors of cardiac arrest do not have inducible arrhythmias and hence are not candidates for serial drug testing. Early studies[368] suggested that these patients had a benign prognosis, but it is now apparent that 20% to 30% are at risk of recurrent cardiac arrest without therapy,[116,172,304,366,367,370,413] especially those with reduced left ventricular function or no demonstrable myocardial ischemia. Patients in whom no sustained arrhythmias are provoked by electrophysiologic testing should be evaluated for the presence or absence of myocardial ischemia and ventricular dysfunction. In patients with normal left ventricular function and evidence of myocardial ischemia, aggressive anti-ischemic management with drugs or revascularization is associated with an excellent prognosis.[116,373,413] In patients with decreased left ventricular function or normal left ventricular function without demonstrable ischemia, the risk of sudden death remains high and the absence of an inducible arrhythmia should not be routinely interpreted as a prognostically favorable finding.[116,171,172,366,367] These patients should be managed with implantation of an automatic cardioverter-defibrillator.

The use of electrophysiologic studies to determine programs of treatment is clearly indicated in all patients who have survived an episode of cardiac arrest. In patients with coronary artery disease, programmed electrical stimulation may identify patients at *risk* of sudden death, and drug testing may prove beneficial in reducing this risk. Several studies have demonstrated that patients whose inducible arrhythmias could be effectively suppressed by serial drug testing had an excellent prognosis, with rates of arrhythmia events and sudden death of 0 to 8%, whereas if no drugs were effective, the rates of sudden death were very high.[295,414] In a study of 52 patients, rates of sudden death (0 to 3%) in those treated with electrophysiologically directed antiarrhythmic therapy were comparable with rates in those without inducible arrhythmia.[296] All of these studies suggested either that electrophysiologic studies were not predictive of arrhythmia recurrence or that electrophysiologically guided drug therapy significantly reduced the risk of sudden death. At present, a multicenter study (Multicenter Unsustained Tachycardia Trial) is attempting to answer this question.

In patients with dilated cardiomyopathy, electrophysiologic testing has not proved to be of benefit in selecting therapy for those at an increased risk of sudden death. The inducibility rates are low in these patients, and identification of antiarrhythmic agents that prevent reinitiation of arrhythmia has not changed the rate of sudden death.

Other forms of pharmacologic therapy. As stated before, it is not known whether ventricular arrhythmias are always a primary electrical event or whether other mechanisms trigger the fatal arrhythmias as a secondary phenomenon. This is especially in question because the CAST and other trials of ventricular premature contraction suppression in survivors of acute myocardial infarction have demonstrated no benefit from antiarrhythmic agents (with the exception of amiodarone) given empirically or to suppress ectopy.

β-Adrenergic blocking agents have demonstrated a significant benefit in this group of patients. β-Blockers and calcium-channel blockers have approximately equally potent anti-ischemic effects in patients with coronary artery disease. Therefore, if the net effect on myocardial ischemia were the predominant mechanism of β-blockers to account for the decrease in sudden death mortality, calcium-channel blockers should be as effective. However, pooled data from short- and long-term trials with a variety of calcium-channel antagonists indicate either no benefit or a slight increase in the risk of sudden death in comparison with placebo control results.[388,415,416]

Because acute ischemia and infarction can lead to ventricular arrhythmias, recurrent thrombosis perhaps is a factor in triggering arrhythmias in some of these patients. If this is the case, antithrombotic therapy may be effective.[417-419] In the Persantine-Aspirin Reinfarction Study, Part II, antithrombotic therapy was successful in reducing sudden death mortality. However, this result was derived from a small group of asymptomatic patients with non-Q-wave infarction and no previous infarction who were receiving concomitant β-blocker therapy. This supports the idea (already discussed) that sudden death may be thrombotic or ischemic in nature in patients with well-preserved ventricular function.[115]

In patients with heart failure, sudden death is common, but as the severity increases, total mortality increases without a concomitant rise in the rate of sudden death.[216] Thus, it appears that the major cause of death in severe congestive heart failure is progressive deterioration in left ventricular function. It is not surprising, therefore, that antiarrhythmic therapy alone has not demonstrated significant reduction in mortality in these patients.

Vasodilator therapy of all types—with nitrates, α-receptor antagonists, and angiotensin converting enzyme inhibitors—has demonstrated significant improvement in total mortality without demonstrating any benefit in sudden death mortality.[420,421] The use of phosphodiesterase inhibitors has also not shown a beneficial effect and may actually increase the frequency of serious arrhythmia.[383] Because these data suggest that therapy directed at ameliorating the hemodynamic and neuroendocrine abnormalities of chronic heart failure does not favorably influence the incidence of sudden death, concomitant use of antiarrhythmic agents may be required to decrease the occurrence of lethal arrhythmias in these patients. To date, studies have not demonstrated this benefit, probably because the proarrhythmic and negative inotropic effects of these drugs may offset their potential benefits.[421,422]

Surgery

Three kinds of surgical procedures have been performed in an attempt to prevent sudden death. One, left stellate ganglionectomy, was discussed earlier in this chapter. Another, ventricular aneurysmectomy, with or without intraoperative electrophysiologic mapping, is discussed in the section on surgery for arrhythmias (chapter 26B). The third, coronary artery revascularization, is discussed here.

As in virtually all other areas of the problem of sudden death, there is controversy about the role of saphenous vein bypass graft surgery in the prevention of sudden death. It is clear that in certain patients with precarious coronary artery anatomy (that is, high-grade left main coronary artery stenosis or high proximal three-vessel disease), mortality is reduced in surgically treated patients as compared with those treated medically, and some of this reduction has been due to a reduction in the rate of sudden death. However, even though some studies suggest a significant reduction in sudden death in surgically treated patients, it must be remembered that although some but not all were randomized studies, they were not controlled for other forms of therapy, in particular antiarrhythmic agents.[423-426] Additionally, the greatest reduction in sudden death rate in surgically treated patients was in those with three-vessel coronary artery disease.[427] In patients with coronary artery disease (with or without a prior myocardial infarction), it is not reasonable at this time to recommend coronary artery revascularization in an attempt to prevent sudden death, in the absence of the aforementioned critical coronary artery stenoses.

As indicated above, coronary revascularization is the treatment of choice in survivors of cardiac arrest who have demonstrable ischemia, significant coronary artery disease, normal left ventricular function, and no inducible ventricular arrhythmias.[413] However, although coronary artery bypass graft surgery may be indicated for the alleviation of ischemia, it will not modify the electrophysiologic milieu for ventricular tachyarrhythmias in most patients.

In a study that evaluated patients who had survived out-of-hospital cardiac arrest before and after coronary artery bypass graft surgery, 65% of those who had inducible ventricular tachycardia preoperatively had the same arrhythmia inducible postoperatively.[428] In patients with significant coronary artery disease and ischemia, we recommend electrophysiologic evaluation before and after revascularization. If ventricular arrhythmias are induced preoperatively, serial drug testing should be carried out postoperatively. If no arrhythmias are inducible, the need for additional therapy is based on whether left ventricular dysfunction is present. If it is present, we recommend implantation of an automatic cardioverter-defibrillator at the time of revascularization.

It would appear, then, that coronary artery revascularization should be offered to patients in this group for the same reason that it is offered to patients with coronary artery disease in general—namely, for relief of symptoms and reduction of mortality risk in patients with precarious coronary artery anatomy. Only in the very small group of patients with normal left ventricular function and no inducible arrhythmias is it offered to prevent recurrence of cardiac arrest.

Automatic implantable cardioverter-defibrillator

The use of implanted defibrillators has been a very important adjunct in the management of patients at risk for sudden death, especially those resuscitated from an episode of cardiac arrest. A more detailed description of the use of these devices is found in chapter 25B.

In 1983, the initial clinical experience from Johns Hopkins University was reported. The automatic internal defibrillator was used in 52 patients who had survived out-of-hospital cardiac arrest. In 33% of these patients, the device discharged 62 episodes of ventricular tachycardia or ventricular fibrillation and resuscitated the patient. The mortality (one-year) was 23%, and the sudden death rate was 8.5%. When the first defibrillator discharge was used as an indicator of sudden death, the mortality rate (without the use of the defibrillator) was estimated to be 48%. Thus, the use of the device was associated with a 52% reduction in overall mortality.[429]

Since then, more than 12,000 patients have received implantable defibrillators of all types.[430,431] On the basis of pooled data from more than 10,000 patients, the rate of sudden death in these patients was 1.6% at 1 year, 3% at 3 years, and 4.5% at 5 years, compared with a sudden death rate of 25% at 1 year and 40% at 5 years in the absence of treatment.[432-434]

The defibrillator would appear to be of greatest use for patients in whom no effective drug regimens can be found at the time of electrophysiologic testing. However, it can also be used as an adjunct to other forms of therapy. As an example, in 23 patients who had survived out-of-hospital cardiac arrest, the device was used in combination with surgical revascularization. Thirty-five percent of the group had automatic implantable cardioverter-defibrillator resuscitative discharges during a period of two years. The use of the device reduced the two-year mortality to 9%.[385] The device has been used with equal success in combination with ventricular aneurysmectomy and subendocardial resection.

REFERENCES

1. Kuller L, Cooper M, Perper J: Epidemiology of sudden death. *Arch Intern Med* 129:714-719, 1972
2. Chiang BN, Perlman LV, Fulton M, et al: Predisposing factors in sudden cardiac death in Tecumseh, Michigan: a prospective study. *Circulation* 41:31-37, 1970
3. Peter T, Hamamoto H, Jordon J, et al: Indications for antiarrhythmic therapy as prophylaxis against sudden death. *Cardiovasc Clin* 11 No 1:249-266, 1980
4. Lie JT, Titus JL: Pathology of the myocardium and the conduction system in sudden coronary death. *Circulation* 52 Suppl 3:41-52, 1975
5. Lie JT: Histopathology of the conduction system in sudden death from coronary heart disease. *Circulation* 51:446-452, 1975
6. Moss AJ: Prediction and prevention of sudden cardiac death. *Annu Rev Med* 31:1-14, 1980
7. Mazur NA, Zhukov VN: Sudden death of acute coronary insufficiency. *Kardiologiia* 16:27-31, 1976
8. Corday E: Symposium on identification and management of the candidate for sudden cardiac death: introduction. *Am J Cardiol* 39:813-815, 1977
9. Lown B: Sudden cardiac death: the major challenge confronting contemporary cardiology. *Am J Cardiol* 43:313-328, 1979
10. Madsen JK: Ischaemic heart disease and prodromes of sudden cardiac death: is it possible to identify high risk groups for sudden cardiac death? *Br Heart J* 54:27-32, 1985
11. Kannel WB, Schatzkin A: Sudden death: lessons from subsets in population studies. *J Am Coll Cardiol* 5 Suppl B:141-149, 1985
12. Schatzkin A, Cupples LA, Heeren T, et al: Sudden death in the Framingham Heart Study: differences in incidence and risk factors by sex and coronary disease status. *Am J Epidemiol* 120:888-899, 1984
13. Särkioja T, Hirvonen J: Causes of sudden unexpected deaths in young and middle-aged persons. *Forensic Sci Int* 24:247-261, 1984
14. Meissner MD, Morganroth J: Silent myocardial ischemia as a mechanism of sudden cardiac death. *Cardiol Clin* 4:593-605, 1986
15. Myerburg RJ: Epidemiology of ventricular tachycardia/ventricular fibrillation and sudden cardiac death. *PACE* 9:1334-1338, 1986
16. Ruberman W, Weinblatt E, Goldberg JD, et al: Ventricular premature complexes and sudden death after myocardial infarction. *Circulation* 64:297-305, 1981
17. Taylor GJ Jr, Humphries JO, Pitt B, et al: Complex ventricular arrhythmias after myocardial infarction during convalescence and follow-up: a harbinger of multi-vessel coronary disease, left ventricular dysfunction and sudden death. *Johns Hopkins Med J* 149:1-5, 1981
18. Oberman A, Ray M, Turner ME, et al: Sudden death in patients evaluated for ischemic heart disease. *Circulation* 52 Suppl 3:170-172, 1975
19. Moss AJ, DeCamilla J, Davis H: Cardiac death in the first six months after myocardial infarction: potential for mortality reduction in the early posthospital period. *Am J Cardiol* 39:816-820, 1977
20. Schaffer WA, Cobb LA: Recurrent ventricular fibrillation and modes of death in survivors of out-of-hospital ventricular fibrillation. *N Engl J Med* 293:259-262, 1975
21. Baum RS, Alvarez H III, Cobb LA: Survival after resuscitation from out-of-hospital ventricular fibrillation. *Circulation* 50:1231-1235, 1974
22. Liberthson RR, Nagel EL, Hirschman JC, et al: Prehospital ventricular fibrillation: prognosis and follow-up course. *N Engl J Med* 291:317-321, 1974
23. Perper JA, Kuller LH, Cooper M: Arteriosclerosis of coronary arteries in sudden, unexpected deaths. *Circulation* 52 Suppl 3:27-33, 1975
24. Bruce RA, DeRouen TA: Exercise testing as a predictor of heart disease and sudden death. *Hosp Pract* 13:69-75, September 1978
25. Bruce RA, DeRouen T, Peterson DR, et al: Noninvasive predictors of sudden cardiac death in men with coronary artery disease: predictive value of maximal stress testing. *Am J Cardiol* 39:833-840, 1977
26. Spain DM, Bradess VA: Sudden death from coronary heart disease: survival time, frequency of thrombi, and cigarette smoking. *Chest* 58:107-110, 1970
27. Roberts WC, Buja LM: The frequency and significance of coronary arterial thrombi and other observations in fatal acute myocardial infarction: a study of 107 necropsy patients. *Am J Med* 52:425-443, 1972
28. Romo M: Factors related to sudden death in acute ischaemic

heart disease: a community study in Helsinki. *Acta Med Scand [Suppl]* 547:1-92, 1972

29. Najem GR, Najem AJ, Najem NH, et al: Diagnosis on death certificates of sudden death due to ischemic heart disease. *South Med J* 73:1597-1598, 1980

30. Kuller LH, Perper JA, Cooper MC: Sudden and unexpected death due to arteriosclerotic heart diseases. *Mod Trends Cardiol* 3:292-332, 1975

31. Myerburg RJ: Sudden death. *Cont Educ Cardiol* 13:15-29, 1978

32. Shah A, Schwartz H: Mexiletine for treatment of torsade de pointes. *Am Heart J* 107:589-591, 1984

33. McWilliam JA: Cardiac failure and sudden death. *Br Med J* 1:6-8, 1889

34. Greene HL: Sudden arrhythmic cardiac death—mechanisms, resuscitation and classification: the Seattle perspective. *Am J Cardiol* 65:4B-12B, 1990

35. Cobb LA, Conn RD, Samson WE, et al: Early experiences in the management of sudden death with a mobile intensive/coronary care unit (abstract). *Circulation* 42 Suppl 3:144, 1970

36. Adgey AAJ, Geddis JS, Mulholland HC, et al: Incidence, significance, and management of early bradyarrhythmia complicating acute myocardial infarction. *Lancet* 2:1097-1101, 1968

37. Adgey AAJ, Pantridge JF: The prehospital phase of treatment for myocardial infarction. *Geriatrics* 27:102-110, May 1972

38. Bonchek LI, Olinger GN, Keelan MH Jr, et al: Management of sudden coronary death. *Ann Thorac Surg* 24:337-344, 1977

39. Bayés de Luna A, Coumel P, Leclercq JF: Ambulatory sudden cardiac death: mechanisms of production of fatal arrhythmia on the basis of data from 157 cases. *Am Heart J* 117:151-159, 1989

40. Panidis IP, Morganroth J: Sudden death in hospitalized patients: cardiac rhythm disturbances detected by ambulatory electrocardiographic monitoring. *J Am Coll Cardiol* 2:798-805, 1983

41. Kempf FC Jr, Josephson ME: Cardiac arrest recorded on ambulatory electrocardiograms. *Am J Cardiol* 53:1577-1582, 1984

42. Myerburg RJ, Kessler KM, Zaman L, et al: Survivors of prehospital cardiac arrest. *JAMA* 247:1485-1490, 1982

43. Iseri LT, Humphrey SB, Siner EJ: Prehospital brady-asystolic cardiac arrest. *Ann Intern Med* 88:741-745, 1978

44. Pantridge JF: Mobile coronary care. *Chest* 58:229-234, 1970

45. Pool J, Kunst K, van Wermeskerken JL: Two monitored cases of sudden death outside hospital. *Br Heart J* 40:627-629, 1978

46. Lahiri A, Balasubramanian V, Raftery EB: Sudden death during ambulatory monitoring. *Br Med J* 1:1676-1678, 1979

47. Medina-Ravell V, Rodriguez-Salas L, Castellanos A, et al: Death due to paroxysmal atrioventricular block during ambulatory electrocardiographic monitoring. *PACE* 12:65-69, 1989

48. Bayés de Luna A, Guindo J: Sudden death in ischemic heart disease. *Rev Port Cardiol* 9:473-479, 1990

49. Raizes G, Wagner GS, Hackel DB: Instantaneous nonarrhythmic cardiac death in acute myocardial infarction. *Am J Cardiol* 39:1-6, 1977

50. Roelandt J, Klootwijke P, Lubsen J, et al: Sudden death during longterm ambulatory monitoring. *Eur Heart J* 5:7-20, 1984

51. Martin GJ, Magid NM, Myers G, et al: Heart rate variability and sudden death secondary to coronary artery disease during ambulatory electrocardiographic monitoring. *Am J Cardiol* 60:86-89, 1987

52. Milner PG, Platia EV, Reid PR, et al: Ambulatory electrocardiographic recordings at the time of fatal cardiac arrest. *Am J Cardiol* 56:588-592, 1985

53. Rettig G, Sen S: Sudden cardiac death during ambulatory Holter monitoring: report on 3 documented cases. *Jpn Heart J* 25:639-649, 1984

54. Olshausen KV, Witt T, Pop T, et al: Sudden cardiac death while wearing a Holter monitor. *Am J Cardiol* 67:381-386, 1991

55. Coumel P, Leclercq J-F, Leenhardt A: Arrhythmias as predictors of sudden death. *Am Heart J* 114:929-937, 1987

56. Lovegrove T: Sudden death from ischaemic heart disease: a review of five hundred consecutive cases. *Med J Aust* 1:128-129, 1977

57. Myerburg RJ, Kessler KM, Castellanos A: Pathophysiology of sudden cardiac death. *PACE* 14:935-943, 1991

58. Han J, Moe GK: Nonuniform recovery of excitability in ventricular muscle. *Circ Res* 14:44-60, 1964

59. Moe GK, Harris AS, Wiggers CJ: Analysis of the initiation of fibrillation by electrographic studies. *Am J Physiol* 134:473-492, 1941

60. Lown B, Temte JV, Reich P, et al: Basis for recurring ventricular fibrillation in the absence of coronary heart disease and its management. *N Engl J Med* 294:623-629, 1976

61. Zipes DP: Electrophysiological mechanisms involved in ventricular fibrillation. *Circulation* 52 Suppl 3:120-130, 1975

62. Han J: Mechanisms of ventricular arrhythmias associated with myocardial infarction. *Am J Cardiol* 24:800-813, 1969

63. Lown B, Wolf M: Approaches to sudden death from coronary heart disease. *Circulation* 44:130-142, 1971

64. DeSilva RA, Verrier RL, Lown B: Effects of psychologic stress and morphine sulfate upon ventricular electrical instability in the conscious dog (abstract). *Am J Cardiol* 39:276, 1977

65. Lown B: Sudden cardiac death—1978. *Circulation* 60:1593-1599, 1979

66. Verrier RL, Calvert A, Lown B: Effect of posterior hypothalamic stimulation on ventricular fibrillation threshold. *Am J Physiol* 228:923-927, 1975

67. Lown B, Verrier RL, Rabinowitz SH: Neural and psychologic mechanisms and the problem of sudden cardiac death. *Am J Cardiol* 39:890-902, 1977

68. Kienzle MG, Doherty JU, Cassidy D, et al: Electrophysiologic sequelae of chronic myocardial infarction: local refractoriness and electrographic characteristics of the left ventricle. *Am J Cardiol* 58:63-69, 1986

69. Tresch DD, Grove R, Siegal R, et al: Survivals of prehospitalization sudden death: characteristic clinical and angiographic features. *Arch Intern Med* 141:1154-1157, 1981

70. Ruberman W, Weinblatt E, Goldberg JD, et al: Ventricular premature beats and mortality after myocardial infarction. *N Engl J Med* 297:750-757, 1977

71. Cobb LA, Baum RS, Alvarez H III, et al: Resuscitation from out-of-hospital ventricular fibrillation: 4 years follow-up. *Circulation* 52 Suppl 3:223-228, 1975

72. Warren JV: Recurrent "sudden death." *N Engl J Med* 293:298-299, 1975

73. Myerburg RJ, Conde C, Sheps DS, et al: Antiarrhythmic drug therapy in survivors of prehospital cardiac arrest: comparison of effects on chronic ventricular arrhythmias and recurrent cardiac arrest. *Circulation* 59:855-863, 1979

74. Reichenbach DD, Moss NS, Meyer E: Pathology of the heart in sudden cardiac death. *Am J Cardiol* 39:865-872, 1977

75. Fawal MAEL, Berg GA, Wheatley DJ, et al: Sudden coronary death in Glasgow: nature and frequency of acute coronary lesions. *Br Heart J* 57:329-335, 1987

76. Moss AJ, DeCamilla J, Mietlowski W, et al: Prognostic grading and significance of ventricular premature beats after recovery from myocardial infarction. *Circulation* 52 Suppl 3:204-210, 1975

77. Greene HL, Richardson DW, Barker AH, et al: Classification of deaths after myocardial infarction as arrhythmic or nonarrhythmic (the Cardiac Arrhythmia Pilot Study). *Am J Cardiol* 63:1-6, 1989

78. Packer M: Lack of relation between ventricular arrhythmias and sudden death in patients with chronic heart failure. *Circulation* 85 Suppl 1:50-56, 1992

79. Eliot RS, Salhany EA: Sudden death and acute myocardial infarction: clues to differences in pathophysiology. *Postgrad Med* 64:52-58, October 1978

80. Reichenbach DD, Moss NS: Myocardial cell necrosis and sudden death in humans. *Circulation* 52 Suppl 3:60-62, 1975

81. Alexandru E, Dobrescu G: Histochemical and histoenzymic researches in coronary sudden death. *Morphol Embryol (Bucur)* 24:229-232, 1978

82. Friedman M, Manwaring JH, Rosenman RH, et al: Instantaneous and sudden deaths: clinical and pathological differentiation in coronary artery disease. *JAMA* 225:1319-1328, 1973

83. Waller BF: Exercise-related sudden death: what autopsy findings reveal about its causes in conditioned persons over age 30 years. *Postgrad Med* 83:273-282, 1988

84. Epstein SE, Maron BJ: Sudden death and the competitive athlete: perspectives on preparticipation screening studies. *J Am Coll Cardiol* 7:220-230, 1986

85. Cobb LA, Weaver WD: Exercise: at risk for sudden death in patients with coronary heart disease. *J Am Coll Cardiol* 7:215-219, 1986

86. Maron BJ, Epstein SE, Roberts WC: Causes of sudden death in competitive athletes. *J Am Coll Cardiol* 7:204-214, 1986

87. Rozanski JJ, Meller J, Kleinfeld M, et al: Nonmechanical ST-segment alternans in Prinzmetal's angina. *Ann Intern Med* 89:76-77, 1978

88. Kleinfeld MJ, Rozanski JJ: Alternans of the ST segment in Prinzmetal's angina. *Circulation* 55:574-577, 1977

89. Rozanski JJ, Kleinfeld M: ST segment alternans in Prinzmetal's angina and associated ventricular arrhythmias (abstract). *Circulation* 54 Suppl 2:77, 1976

90. Rozanski JJ, El-Sherif N, Kleinfeld M, et al: ST segment alternans and ventricular arrhythmias in Prinzmetal's angina (abstract). *Circulation* 58 Suppl 2:239, 1978

91. Rozanski JJ, Castellanos A, Myerburg RJ: Ventricular ectopy and sudden death. *Cardiovasc Clin* 11 No 1:127-142, 1980

92. Hillis LD, Braunwald E: Coronary-artery spasm. *N Engl J Med* 299:695-702, 1978

93. Tennant R, Wiggers CJ: The effect of coronary occlusion on myocardial contraction. *Am J Physiol* 112:351-361, 1935

94. Harris AS, Guevara Rojas A: The initiation of ventricular fibrillation due to coronary occlusion. *Exp Med Surg* 1:105-122, 1943

95. Sommers HM, Jennings RB: Ventricular fibrillation and myocardial necrosis after transient ischemia: effect of treatment with oxygen, procainamide, reserpine, and propranolol. *Arch Intern Med* 129:780-789, 1972

96. Bulkley BH, Klacsmann PG, Hutchins GM: Angina pectoris, myocardial infarction and sudden cardiac death with normal coronary arteries: a clinicopathologic study of 9 patients with progressive systemic sclerosis. *Am Heart J* 95:563-569, 1978

97. Jørgensen L, Rowsell HC, Hovig T, et al: Adenosine diphosphate-induced platelet aggregation and myocardial infarction in swine. *Lab Invest* 17:616-644, 1967

98. Davies MJ, Thomas AC, Knapman PA, et al: Intramyocardial platelet aggregation in patients with unstable angina suffering sudden ischemic cardiac death. *Circulation* 73:418-427, 1986

99. Keren A, Tzivoni D, Gavish D, et al: Etiology, warning signs and therapy of torsade de pointes: a study of 10 patients. *Circulation* 64:1167-1174, 1981

100. Muller JE, Tofler GH, Willich SN, et al: Circadian variation of cardiovascular disease and sympathetic activity. *J Cardiovasc Pharmacol* 10 Suppl 2:S104-S109, 1987

101. Willich SN, Levy D, Rocco MB, et al: Circadian variation in the incidence of sudden cardiac death in the Framingham Heart Study population. *Am J Cardiol* 60:801-806, 1987

102. Tofler GH, Brezinski D, Schafer AI, et al: Concurrent morning increase in platelet aggregability and the risk of myocardial infarction and sudden cardiac death. *N Engl J Med* 316:1514-1518, 1987

103. Willich SN: Epidemiologic studies demonstrating increased morning incidence of sudden cardiac death. *Am J Cardiol* 66:15G-17G, 1990

104. Peters RW: Propranolol and the morning increase in sudden cardiac death (the Beta-Blocker Heart Attack Trial experience). *Am J Cardiol* 66:57G-59G, 1990

105. Eliot RS, Clayton FC, Pieper GM, et al: Influence of environmental stress on pathogenesis of sudden cardiac death. *Fed Proc* 36:1719-1724, 1977

106. Wolf S (ed): *Advances in Experimental Medicine and Biology. Vol. 16B. The Artery and the Process of Arteriosclerosis: Measurement and Modification.* New York, Plenum Press, 1972, pp 213-275

107. Mauck HP Jr, Hockman CH: Central nervous system mechanisms mediating cardiac rate and rhythm. *Am Heart J* 74:96-109, 1967

108. Satinsky J, Kosowsky B, Lown B, et al: Ventricular fibrillation induced by hypothalamic stimulation during coronary artery occlusion (abstract). *Circulation* 44 Suppl 2:60, 1971

109. Schwartz PJ, La Rovere MT, Vanoli E: Autonomic nervous system and sudden cardiac death: experimental basis and clinical observations for post-myocardial infarction risk stratification. *Circulation* 85 Suppl 1:77-91, 1992

110. La Rovere MT, Specchia G, Mortara A, et al: Baroreflex sensitivity, clinical correlates, and cardiovascular mortality among patients with a first myocardial infarction: a prospective study. *Circulation* 78:816-824, 1988

111. Lombardi F, Sandrone G, Pernpruner S, et al: Heart rate variability as an index of sympathovagal interaction after acute myocardial infarction. *Am J Cardiol* 60:1239-1245, 1987

112. Marcus FI, Cobb LA, Edwards JE, et al: Mechanism of death and prevalence of myocardial ischemic symptoms in the terminal event after acute myocardial infarction. *Am J Cardiol* 61:8-15, 1988

113. Goldstein S, Vanderburg Medendorp S, Landis JR, et al: Analysis of cardiac symptoms preceding cardiac arrest. *Am J Cardiol* 58:1195-1198, 1986

114. Miller DD, Waters DD, Szlachcic J, et al: Clinical characteristics associated with sudden death in patients with variant angina. *Circulation* 66:588-592, 1982

115. Meissner MD, Akhtar M, Lehmann MH: Nonischemic sudden tachyarrhythmic death in atherosclerotic heart disease. *Circulation* 84:905-912, 1991

116. Wilber DJ, Garan H, Finkelstein D, et al: Out-of-hospital cardiac arrest: use of electrophysiologic testing in the prediction of long-term outcome. *N Engl J Med* 318:19-24, 1988

117. Furukawa T, Rozanski JJ, Nogami A, et al: Time-dependent risk of and predictors for cardiac arrest recurrence in survivors of out-of-hospital cardiac arrest with chronic coronary artery disease. *Circulation* 80:599-608, 1989

118. McLaran CJ, Gersh BJ, Sugrue DD, et al: Out-of-hospital cardiac arrest in patients without clinically significant coronary artery disease: comparison of clinical, electrophysiological, and survival characteristics with those in similar patients who have clinically significant coronary artery disease. *Br Heart J* 58:583-591, 1987

119. Morady F, DiCarlo LA Jr, Krol RB, et al: Role of myocardial ischemia during programmed stimulation in survivors of cardiac arrest with coronary artery disease. *J Am Coll Cardiol* 9:1004-1012, 1987

120. Orlow SW, Peters TF, Holmes EW, et al: Myocardial ischemia during programmed stimulation: modification by nifedipine (abstract). *Circulation* 80 Suppl 2:224, 1989

121. Luu M, Stevenson WG, Stevenson LW, et al: Diverse mechanisms of unexpected cardiac arrest in advanced heart failure. *Circulation* 80:1675-1680, 1989

122. Myerburg RJ, Briese FW, Conde C, et al: Long-term antiarrhythmic therapy in survivors of prehospital cardiac arrest: initial 18 months' experience. *JAMA* 238:2621-2624, 1977

123. Lown B, Graboys TB: Management of patients with malignant ventricular arrhythmias. *Am J Cardiol* 39:910-918, 1977

124. Myerburg RJ, Sung RJ, Conde C, et al: Intracardiac electrophysiologic studies in patients resuscitated from unexpected cardiac arrest outside the hospital (abstract). *Am J Cardiol* 39:275, 1977

125. Goldstein S: The epidemiology of tachyfibrillation in sudden death. *PACE* 9:1339-1342, 1986

126. Vetter VL: Sudden death in infants, children, and adolescents. *Cardiovasc Clin* 15 No 3:301-313, 1985

127. Lauridson JR: Sudden death and anomalous origin of the coronary arteries from the aorta. A case report and review. *Am J Forensic Med Pathol* 9:236-240, 1988

128. Isner JM, Shen EM, Martin ET, et al: Sudden unexpected death as a result of anomalous origin of the right coronary artery from the left sinus of Valsalva. *Am J Med* 76:155-158, 1984

129. Neuspiel DR, Kuller LH: Sudden and unexpected natural death in childhood and adolescence. *JAMA* 254:1321-1325, 1985

130. Shaver PJ, Carrig TF, Baker WP: Postpartum coronary artery dissection. *Br Heart J* 40:83-86, 1978

131. Claudon DG, Claudon DB, Edwards JE: Primary dissecting aneurysm of coronary artery: a cause of acute myocardial ischemia. *Circulation* 45:259-266, 1972

132. Wenger NK, Bauer S: Coronary embolism: review of the literature and presentation of fifteen cases. *Am J Med* 25:549-557, 1958

133. Heggtveit HA: Syphilitic aortitis: a clinicopathologic autopsy study of 100 cases, 1950 to 1960. *Circulation* 29:346-355, 1964

134. Rissanen V: Occurrence of coronary ostial stenosis in a necropsy series of myocardial infarction, sudden death, and violent death. *Br Heart J* 37:182-191, 1975

135. Thiene G, Valente M, Rossi L: Involvement of the cardiac conducting system in panarteritis nodosa. *Am Heart J* 95:716-724, 1978

136. James TN: De subitaneis mortibus. XXV. Sarcoid heart disease. *Circulation* 56:320-326, 1977

137. Wentworth P, Jentz LA, Croal AE: Analysis of sudden unexpected death in southern Ontario, with emphasis on myocarditis. *Can Med Assoc J* 120:676-680; 706, 1979

138. Davies MJ, Popple A: Sudden unexpected cardiac death: a practical approach to the forensic problem. *Histopathology* 3:255-277, 1979

139. Cohen HC, Rosen KM, Pick A: Disorders of impulse conduction and impulse formation caused by hyperkalemia in man. *Am Heart J* 89:501-509, 1975

140. Krikler DM, Curry PVL: *Torsades de pointes,* an atypical ventricular tachycardia. *Br Heart J* 38:117-120, 1976
141. Kline IK: Myocardial alterations associated with pheochromocytomas. *Am J Pathol* 38:539-551, 1961
142. Zipes DP: Proarrhythmic events. *Am J Cardiol* 61:70A-76A, 1988
143. Kuck KH, Kunze KP, Roewer N, et al: Sotalol-induced torsade de pointes. *Am Heart J* 107:179-180, 1984
144. Keren A, Tzivoni D, Gottlieb S, et al: Atypical ventricular tachycardia (torsade de pointes) induced by amiodarone: arrhythmia previously induced by quinidine and disopyramide. *Chest* 81:384-386, 1982
145. Fish FA, Gillette PC, Benson DW Jr: Proarrhythmia, cardiac arrest and death in young patients receiving encainide and flecainide. *J Am Coll Cardiol* 18:356-365, 1991
146. Moir DC, Crooks J, Sawyer P, et al: Cardiotoxicity of tricyclic antidepressants. *Br J Pharmacol* 44:371P-372P, 1972
147. Aronow WS, Mercando AD, Epstein S, et al: Effect of quinidine or procainamide versus no antiarrhythmic drug on sudden cardiac death, total cardiac death, and total death in elderly patients with heart disease and complex ventricular arrhythmias. *Am J Cardiol* 66:423-428, 1990
148. James TN: On the cause of syncope and sudden death in primary pulmonary hypertension. *Ann Intern Med* 56:252-264, 1962
149. Karpawich PP, Gillette PC, Garson A Jr, et al: Congenital complete atrioventricular block: clinical and electrophysiologic predictors of need for pacemaker insertion. *Am J Cardiol* 48:1098-1102, 1981
150. Fuster V, McGoon DC, Kennedy MA, et al: Long-term evaluation (12 to 22 years) of open heart surgery for tetralogy of Fallot. *Am J Cardiol* 46:635-642, 1980
151. Katz NM, Blackstone EH, Kirklin JW, et al: Late survival and symptoms after repair of tetralogy of Fallot. *Circulation* 65:403-410, 1982
152. Garson A Jr, Porter CJ, Gillette PC, et al: Induction of ventricular tachycardia during electrophysiologic study after repair of tetralogy of Fallot. *J Am Coll Cardiol* 1:1493-1502, 1983
153. Chandar JS, Wolff GS, Garson A Jr, et al: Ventricular arrhythmias in postoperative tetralogy of Fallot. *Am J Cardiol* 65:655-661, 1990
154. Maron BJ, Epstein SE, Roberts WC: Hypertrophic cardiomyopathy: a common cause of sudden death in the young competitive athlete. *Eur Heart J* 4 Suppl F:135-143, 1983
155. Drory Y, Turetz Y, Hiss Y, et al: Sudden unexpected death in persons < 40 years of age. *Am J Cardiol* 68:1388-1392, 1991
156. Kron J, Oliver RP, Norsted S, et al: The automatic implantable cardioverter-defibrillator in young patients. *J Am Coll Cardiol* 16:896-902, 1990
157. Drory Y, Kramer MR, Lev B: Exertional sudden death in soldiers. *Med Sci Sports Exerc* 23:147-151, 1991
158. Burke AP, Farb A, Virmani R, et al: Sports-related and non-sports-related sudden cardiac death in young adults. *Am Heart J* 121:568-575, 1991
159. Corrado D, Thiene G, Nava A, et al: Sudden death in young competitive athletes: clinicopathologic correlations in 22 cases. *Am J Med* 89:588-596, 1990
160. Kolodgie FD, Virmani R, Cornhill JF, et al: Increase in atherosclerosis and adventitial mast cells in cocaine abusers: an alternative mechanism to cocaine-associated coronary vasospasm and thrombosis. *J Am Coll Cardiol* 17:1553-1560, 1991
161. McKelway R, Vieweg V, Westerman P: Sudden death from acute cocaine intoxication in Virginia in 1988. *Am J Psychiatry* 147:1667-1669, 1990
162. Davies MJ: Pathological view of sudden cardiac death. *Br Heart J* 45:88-96, 1981
163. Weaver WD, Lorch GS, Alvarez HA, et al: Angiographic findings and prognostic indicators in patients resuscitated from sudden cardiac death. *Circulation* 54:895-900, 1976
164. Fawal MAEL, Berg GA, Wheatley DJ, et al: Sudden coronary death in Glasgow: the severity and distribution of chronic coronary atherosclerotic stenoses. *Br Heart J* 57:420-426, 1987
165. Johnson WD, Strong JP, Oalmann MC, et al: Sudden death from coronary heart disease in young men: pathologic findings. *Arch Pathol Lab Med* 105:227-323, 1981
166. Warnes CA, Roberts WC: Comparison at necropsy by age group of amount and distribution of narrowing by atherosclerotic plaque in 2995 five-mm long segments of 240 major coronary arteries in 60 men aged 31 to 70 years with sudden coronary death. *Am Heart J* 108:431-435, 1984
167. Roberts WC, Jones AA: Quantitation of coronary arterial narrowing at necropsy in sudden coronary death: analysis of 31 patients and comparison with 25 control subjects. *Am J Cardiol* 44:39-45, 1979
168. Davies MJ, Thomas A: Thrombosis and acute coronary-artery lesions in sudden cardiac ischemic death. *N Engl J Med* 310:1137-1140, 1984
169. Warnes CA, Roberts WC: Sudden coronary death: comparison of patients with to those without coronary thrombus at necropsy. *Am J Cardiol* 54:1206-1211, 1984
170. Kragel AH, Gertz SD, Roberts WC: Morphologic comparison of frequency and types of acute lesions in the major epicardial coronary arteries in unstable angina pectoris, sudden coronary death and acute myocardial infarction. *J Am Coll Cardiol* 18:801-808, 1991
171. Eldar M, Sauve MJ, Scheinman MM: Electrophysiologic testing and follow-up of patients with aborted sudden death. *J Am Coll Cardiol* 10:291-298, 1987
172. Morady F, Scheinman MM, Hess DS: Electrophysiologic testing in the management of survivors of out-of-hospital cardiac arrest. *Am J Cardiol* 51:85-89, 1983
173. Alderman EL, Bourassa MG, Cohen LS, et al: Ten-year follow-up of survival and myocardial infarction in the randomized Coronary Artery Surgery Study. *Circulation* 82:1629-1646, 1990
174. Ross J Jr, Braunwald E: Aortic stenosis. *Circulation* 38 Suppl 5:61-67, 1968
175. Iskandrian AS, Segal BL, Wasserman L, et al: Sudden death in severe aortic stenosis following cardiac catheterization. *Cathet Cardiovasc Diagn* 4:419-425, 1978
176. Davies MJ: The pathology of myocardial ischaemia. *J Clin Pathol* 30 Suppl 11:45-52, 1977
177. Thompson R, Mitchell A, Ahmed M, et al: Conduction defects in aortic valve disease. *Am Heart J* 98:3-10, 1979
178. Dhingra RC, Amat-y-Leon F, Pietras RJ, et al: Sites of conduction disease in aortic stenosis: significance of valve gradient and calcification. *Ann Intern Med* 87:275-280, 1977
179. Cohle SD, Graham MA, Dowling G, et al: Sudden death and left ventricular outflow disease. *Pathol Annu* 23:97-124, 1988
180. Procacci PM, Savran SV, Schreiter SL, et al: Prevalence of clinical mitral-valve prolapse in 1169 young women. *N Engl J Med* 294:1086-1088, 1976
181. Darsee JR, Mikolich JR, Nicoloff NB, et al: Prevalence of mitral valve prolapse in presumably healthy young men. *Circulation* 59:619-622, 1979
182. Swartz MH, Teichholz LE, Donoso E: Mitral valve prolapse: a review of associated arrhythmias. *Am J Med* 62:377-389, 1977
183. Jeresaty RM: Sudden death in the mitral valve prolapse-click syndrome (editorial). *Am J Cardiol* 37:317-318, 1976
184. Gooch AS, Vicencio F, Maranhao V, et al: Arrhythmias and left ventricular asynergy in the prolapsing mitral leaflet syndrome. *Am J Cardiol* 29:611-620, 1972
185. Ritchie JL, Hammermeister KE, Kennedy JW: Refractory ventricular tachycardia and fibrillation in a patient with the prolapsing mitral leaflet syndrome: successful control with overdrive pacing. *Am J Cardiol* 37:314-316, 1976
186. Jeresaty RM: Mitral valve prolapse-click syndrome. *Prog Cardiovasc Dis* 15:623-652, 1973
187. DeMaria AN, Amsterdam EA, Vismara LA, et al: Arrhythmias in the mitral valve prolapse syndrome: prevalence, nature, and frequency. *Ann Intern Med* 84:656-660, 1976
188. Nakhjavan FK, Natarajan G, Seshachary P, et al: The relationship between prolapsing mitral leaflet syndrome and angina and normal coronary arteriograms. *Chest* 70:706-710, 1976
189. Simonsen J, Falk E: A case of sudden cardiac death in connection with *Salmonella typhimurium* infection. *Forensic Sci Int* 16:283-287, 1980
190. Di Bello R: Cardiac echinococcosis: late sudden death after surgical treatment. *Chest* 79:110-111, 1981
191. Nava A, Canciani B, Daliento L, et al: Juvenile sudden death and effort ventricular tachycardias in a family with right ventricular cardiomyopathy. *Int J Cardiol* 21:111-123, 1988
192. Thiene G, Nava A, Corrado D, et al: Right ventricular cardiomyopathy and sudden death in young people. *N Engl J Med* 318:129-133, 1988
193. Swan DA, Bell B, Oakley CM, et al: Analysis of symptomatic course and prognosis and treatment of hypertrophic obstructive cardiomyopathy. *Br Heart J* 33:671-685, 1971

194. McKenna WJ, Franklin RC, Nihoyannopoulos P, et al: Arrhythmia and prognosis in infants, children and adolescents with hypertrophic cardiomyopathy. *J Am Coll Cardiol* 11:147-153, 1988
195. McKenna WJ, Deanfield JE: Hypertrophic cardiomyopathy; an important cause of sudden death. *Arch Dis Child* 59:971-975, 1984
196. Hardarson T, de la Calzada CS, Curiel R, et al: Prognosis and mortality of hypertrophic obstructive cardiomyopathy. *Lancet* 2:1462-1467, 1973
197. Shah PM, Adelman AG, Wigle ED, et al: The natural (and unnatural) history of hypertrophic obstructive cardiomyopathy: a multicenter study. *Circ Res* 35 Suppl 2:179-195, 1974
198. Maron BJ, Lipson LC, Roberts WC, et al: "Malignant" hypertrophic cardiomyopathy: identification of a subgroup of families with unusually frequent premature death. *Am J Cardiol* 41:1133-1140, 1978
199. Maron BJ, Roberts WC, Edwards JE, et al: Sudden death in patients with hypertrophic cardiomyopathy: characterization of 26 patients without functional limitation. *Am J Cardiol* 41:803-810, 1978
200. Maron BJ, Roberts WC, Edwards JE, et al: Sudden death in previously asymptomatic patients with asymmetric septal hypertrophy (abstract). *Am J Cardiol* 39:270, 1977
201. Goodwin JF, Krikler DM: Arrhythmia as a cause of sudden death in hypertrophic cardiomyopathy. *Lancet* 2:937-940, 1976
202. McKenna WJ, Chetty S, Oakley CM, et al: Arrhythmia in hypertrophic cardiomyopathy: exercise and 48 hour ambulatory electrocardiographic assessment with and without beta adrenergic blocking therapy. *Am J Cardiol* 45:1-5, 1980
203. McKenna WJ, Oakley CM, Krikler DM, et al: Improved survival with amiodarone in patients with hypertrophic cardiomyopathy and ventricular tachycardia. *Br Heart J* 53:412-416, 1985
204. Krikler DM, Davies MJ, Rowland E, et al: Sudden death in hypertrophic cardiomyopathy: associated accessory atrioventricular pathways. *Br Heart J* 43:245-251, 1980
205. Spirito P, Maron BJ: Relation between extent of left ventricular hypertrophy and occurrence of sudden cardiac death in hypertrophic cardiomyopathy. *J Am Coll Cardiol* 15:1521-1526, 1990
206. Watson RM, Schwartz JL, Maron BJ, et al: Inducible polymorphic ventricular tachycardia and ventricular fibrillation in a subgroup of patients with hypertrophic cardiomyopathy at high risk for sudden death. *J Am Coll Cardiol* 10:761-774, 1987
207. Fananapazir L, Leon MB, Bonow RO, et al: Sudden death during empiric amiodarone therapy in symptomatic hypertrophic cardiomyopathy. *Am J Cardiol* 67:169-174, 1991
208. Fananapazir L, Tracy CM, Leon MB, et al: Electrophysiologic abnormalities in patients with hypertrophic cardiomyopathy: a consecutive analysis in 155 patients. *Circulation* 80:1259-1268, 1989
209. Blomstrom-Lundqvist C, Sabel KG, Olsson SB: A long term follow up of 15 patients with arrhythmogenic right ventricular dysplasia. *Br Heart J* 58:477-488, 1987
210. Buja GF, Nava A, Martini B, et al: Right ventricular dysplasia: a familial cardiomyopathy? *Eur Heart J* 10 Suppl D:13-15, 1989
211. Middlekauff HR, Stevenson WG, Stevenson LW: Prognostic significance of atrial fibrillation in advanced heart failure: a study of 390 patients. *Circulation* 84:40-48, 1991
212. Middlekauff HR, Stevenson WG, Woo MA, et al: Comparison of frequency of late potentials in idiopathic dilated cardiomyopathy and ischemic cardiomyopathy with advanced congestive heart failure and their usefulness in predicting sudden death. *Am J Cardiol* 66:1113-1117, 1990
213. Ohnishi Y, Inoue T, Fukuzaki H: Value of the signal-averaged electrocardiogram and a predictor of sudden death in myocardial infarction and dilated cardiomyopathy. *Jpn Circ J* 54:127-136, 1990
214. Kannel WB, Plehn JF, Cupples LA: Cardiac failure and sudden death in the Framingham Study. *Am Heart J* 115:869-875, 1988
215. Hessen SE, Nydegger CC, Kutalek SP: Use of programmed stimulation in identifying patients at high risk for sudden cardiac death. *Cardiology* 77:230-239, 1990
216. Kjekshus J: Arrhythmias and mortality in congestive heart failure. *Am J Cardiol* 65:42I-48I, 1990
217. Goldstein S: Toward a new understanding of the mechanism and prevention of sudden death in coronary artery heart disease. *Circulation* 82:284-288, 1990
218. Jervell A, Lange-Nielsen F: Congenital deaf-mutism, functional heart disease with prolongation of the Q-T interval, and sudden death. *Am Heart J* 54:59-68, 1957
219. Vincent GM, Abildskov JA, Burgess MJ: Q-T interval syndromes. *Prog Cardiovasc Dis* 16:523-530, 1974
220. Romano C, Gemme G, Pongiglione R: Aritmie cardiache rare dell'eta' pediatrica. II. Accessi sincopali per fibrillazione ventricolare parossistica. *Clin Pediatr (Bologna)* 45:656-683, 1963
221. Ward OC: *Report Council Royal Academy of Medicine in Ireland,* 1963
222. Moss AJ, Schwartz PJ: Sudden death and the idiopathic long Q-T syndrome. *Am J Med* 66:6-7, 1979
223. Reynolds EW, Vander Ark CR: Quinidine syncope and the delayed repolarization syndromes. *Mod Concepts Cardiovasc Dis* 45:117-122, 1976
224. Siegel RJ, Cabeen WR Jr, Roberts WC: Prolonged QT interval-ventricular tachycardia syndrome from massive rapid weight loss utilizing the liquid-protein-modified-fast diet: sudden death with sinus node ganglionitis and neuritis. *Am Heart J* 102:121-124, 1981
225. Levine SA, Woodworth CR: Congenital deaf-mutism, prolonged QT interval, syncopal attacks and sudden death. *N Engl J Med* 259:412-417, 1958
226. James TN, Froggatt P, Atkinson WJ Jr, et al: De subitaneis mortibus. XXX. Observations on the pathophysiology of the long QT syndromes with special reference to the neuropathology of the heart. *Circulation* 57:1221-1231, 1978
227. Schwartz PJ, Periti M, Malliani A: The long Q-T syndrome. *Am Heart J* 89:378-390, 1975
228. Kliks BR, Burgess MJ, Abildskov JA: The influence of sympathetic tone on ventricular fibrillation threshold during experimental coronary occlusion (abstract). *Circulation* 46 Suppl 2:115, 1972
229. Moss AJ, Robinson J: Clinical features of the idiopathic long QT syndrome. *Circulation* 85 Suppl 1:140-144, 1992
230. Jackman WM, Friday KJ, Anderson JL, et al: The long QT syndromes: a critical review, new clinical observations and a unifying hypothesis. *Prog Cardiovasc Dis* 31:115-172, 1988
231. Benhorin J, Hewitt D, Moss AJ: Relationship between repolarization duration and cycle length during exercise testing in normals and long QT syndrome patients (abstract). *J Am Coll Cardiol* 17 Suppl A:60, 1991
232. Keating M, Atkinson D, Dunn C, et al: Linkage of a cardiac arrhythmia, the long QT syndrome, and the Harvey *ras*-1 gene. *Science* 252:704-706, 1991
233. Moss AJ, Schwartz PJ, Crampton RS, et al: The long QT syndrome: prospective longitudinal study of 328 families. *Circulation* 84:1136-1144, 1991
234. Olley PM, Fowler RS: The surdo-cardiac syndrome and therapeutic observations. *Br Heart J* 32:467-471, 1970
235. Abdalla ISH, Prineas RJ, Neaton JD, et al: Relation between ventricular premature complexes and sudden cardiac death in apparently healthy men. *Am J Cardiol* 60:1036-1042, 1987
236. Schwartz PJ, Randall WC, Anderson EA, et al: Task Force 4: sudden cardiac death; nonpharmacologic interventions. *Circulation* 76 Suppl 1:215-219, 1987
237. Schwartz PJ, Stone HL, Brown AM: Effects of unilateral stellate ganglion blockade on the arrhythmias associated with coronary occlusion. *Am Heart J* 92:589-599, 1976
238. Schwartz PJ, Stone HL: Role of right stellate ganglion during exercise (abstract). *Eur J Clin Invest* 6:328, 1976
239. Moss AJ, McDonald J: Unilateral cervicothoracic sympathetic ganglionectomy for the treatment of long QT interval syndrome. *N Engl J Med* 285:903-904, 1971
240. Roden DM, Woosley RL, Primm RK: Incidence and clinical features of the quinidine-associated long QT syndrome: implications for patient care. *Am Heart J* 111:1088-1093, 1986
241. Tzivoni D, Keren A, Stern S, et al: Disopyramide-induced *torsade de pointes. Arch Intern Med* 141:946-947, 1981
242. Wald RW, Waxman MB, Colman JM: Torsade de pointes ventricular tachycardia: a complication of disopyramide shared with quinidine. *J Electrocardiol* 14:301-307, 1981
243. Jackman WM, Clark M, Friday KJ, et al: Ventricular tachyarrhythmias in the long QT syndromes. *Med Clin North Am* 68:1079-1109, September 1984
244. Nguyen PT, Scheinman MM, Seger J: Polymorphous ventricular tachycardia: clinical characterization, therapy, and the QT interval. *Circulation* 74:340-349, 1986

245. Maloney JD, Nissen RG, McColgan JM: Open clinical studies at a referral center: chronic maintenance tocainide therapy in patients with recurrent sustained ventricular tachycardia refractory to conventional antiarrhythmic agents. *Am Heart J* 100:1023-1030, 1980

246. Burda CD: Electrocardiographic abnormalities induced by thioridazine (Mellaril). *Am Heart J* 76:153-156, 1968

247. Moss AJ: Prolonged QT-interval syndromes. *JAMA* 256:2985-2987, 1986

248. Khan MM, Logan KR, McComb JM, et al: Management of recurrent ventricular tachyarrhythmias associated with Q-T prolongation. *Am J Cardiol* 47:1301-1308, 1981

249. Bonatti V, Rolli A, Botti G: Monophasic action potential studies in human subjects with prolonged ventricular repolarization and long QT syndromes. *Eur Heart J* 6 Suppl D:131-143, 1985

250. Stern S, Keren A, Tzivoni D: Torsade de pointes: definitions, causative factors, and therapy: experience with sixteen patients. *Ann NY Acad Sci* 427:234-240, 1984

251. Hearne TR, Cummins RO: Improved survival from cardiac arrest in the community. *PACE* 11:1968-1973, 1988

252. Amey BD, Harrison EE, Straub EJ: Sudden cardiac death: a retrospective and prospective study. *JACEP* 5:429-433, 1976

253. Sharma B, Wyeth RP: Six-year survival of patients with and without painless myocardial ischemia and out-of-hospital ventricular fibrillation. *Am J Cardiol* 61:9F-12F, 1988

254. Agnew TM, Lauder IM, Fisher CA, et al: Sudden cardiac death: results of resuscitation begun outside hospital. *N Z Med J* 96:465-467, 1983

255. Dunn HM, McComb JM, MacKenzie G, et al: Survival to leave hospital from ventricular fibrillation. *Am Heart J* 112:745-751, 1986

256. Roth R, Stewart RD, Rogers K, et al: Out-of-hospital cardiac arrest: factors associated with survival. *Ann Emerg Med* 13:237-243, April 1984

257. Ng AY, Clinton JE, Peterson G: Nontraumatic prehospital cardiac arrest ages 1 to 39 years. *Am J Emerg Med* 8:87-91, 1990

258. Nagel EL, Liberthson RR, Hirschman JC, et al: Emergency care. *Circulation* 52 Suppl 3:216-218, 1975

259. Thompson RG, Hallstrom AP, Cobb LA: Bystander-initiated cardiopulmonary resuscitation in the management of ventricular fibrillation. *Ann Intern Med* 90:737-740, 1979

260. Cummins RO, Eisenberg MS: Prehospital cardiopulmonary resuscitation: is it effective? *JAMA* 253:2408-2412, 1985

261. Eisenberg MS, Copass MK, Hallstrom AP, et al: Treatment of out-of-hospital cardiac arrests with rapid defibrillation by emergency medical technicians. *N Engl J Med* 302:1379-1383, 1980

262. Weaver WD, Cobb LA, Hallstrom AP, et al: Factors influencing survival after out-of-hospital cardiac arrest. *J Am Coll Cardiol* 7:752-757, 1986

263. Ritchie JL, Hallstrom AP, Troubaugh GB, et al: Out-of-hospital sudden coronary death: rest and exercise radionuclide left ventricular function in survivors. *Am J Cardiol* 55:645-651, 1985

264. Tresch DD, Keelan MH Jr, Siegel R, et al: Long-term survival after prehospital sudden cardiac death. *Am Heart J* 108:1-5, 1984

265. Kannel WB, McGee DL: Epidemiology of sudden death: insights from the Framingham Study. *Cardiovasc Clin* 15 No 3:93-105, 1985

266. Goldstein S, Landis JR, Leighton R, et al: Predictive survival models for resuscitated victims of out-of-hospital cardiac arrest with coronary heart disease. *Circulation* 71:873-880, 1985

267. Rabkin SW: Electrocardiographic abnormalities in apparently healthy men and the risk of sudden death. *Drugs* 28 Suppl 1:28-43, 1984

268. Kannel WB, McGee DL, Schatzkin A: An epidemiological prospective of sudden death: 26-year follow-up in the Framingham Study. *Drugs* 28 Suppl 1:1-14, 1984

269. Kennedy HL, Underhill SJ: Frequent or complex ventricular ectopy in apparently healthy subjects: a clinical study of 25 patients. *Am J Cardiol* 38:141-148, 1976

270. Hinkle LE Jr, Carver ST, Stevens M: The frequency of asymptomatic disturbances of cardiac rhythm and conduction in middle-aged men. *Am J Cardiol* 24:629-650, 1969

271. Faris JV, McHenry PL, Jordan JW, et al: Prevalence and reproducibility of exercise-induced ventricular arrhythmias during maximal exercise testing in normal men. *Am J Cardiol* 37:617-622, 1976

272. Ekblom B, Hartley LH, Day WC: Occurrence and reproducibility of exercise-induced ventricular ectopy in normal subjects. *Am J Cardiol* 43:35-40, 1979

273. Calvert A, Lown B, Gorlin R: Ventricular premature beats and anatomically defined coronary heart disease. *Am J Cardiol* 39:627-634, 1977

274. Stern Z, Tzivoni D, Keren A, et al: Relationship between ventricular arrhythmias detected by ambulatory ECG monitoring and subsequent sudden cardiac death. *Cardiology* 67:90-102, 1981

275. Rodstein M, Wolloch L, Gubner RS: Mortality study of the significance of extrasystoles in an insured population. *Circulation* 44:617-625, 1971

276. Alexander S, Desai DC, Hershberg PI: Clinical significance of ventricular premature beats in an outpatient population (abstract). *Am J Cardiol* 29:250, 1972

277. Kluger J, Hinkle LE: Factors affecting prognosis of men with ventricular premature complexes (abstract). *Circulation* 54 Suppl 2:9, 1976

278. Kennedy HL, Whitlock JA, Sprague MK, et al: Long-term follow-up of asymptomatic healthy subjects with frequent and complex ventricular ectopy. *N Engl J Med* 312:193-197, 1985

279. Chakko CS, Gheorghiade M: Ventricular arrhythmias in severe heart failure: incidence, significance, and effectiveness of antiarrhythmic therapy. *Am Heart J* 109:497-504, 1985

280. Kannel WB, Gagnon DR, Cupples LA: Epidemiology of sudden coronary death: population at risk. *Can J Cardiol* 6:439-444, 1990

281. Follansbee WP, Michelson EL, Morganroth J: Nonsustained ventricular tachycardia in ambulatory patients: characteristics and association with sudden cardiac death. *Ann Intern Med* 92:741-747, 1980

282. Packer M, Gottlieb SS, Blum MA: Immediate and long-term pathophysiologic mechanisms underlying the genesis of sudden cardiac death in patients with congestive heart failure. *Am J Med* 82 Suppl 3A:4-10, 1987

283. Holmes J, Kubo SH, Coty RJ, et al: Arrhythmias in ischemic and nonischemic dilated cardiomyopathy: prediction of mortality by ambulatory electrocardiography. *Am J Cardiol* 55:146-151, 1985

284. Bigger JT Jr, Fleiss JL, Kleiger R, et al: The relationships among ventricular arrhythmias, left ventricular dysfunction, and mortality in the 2 years after myocardial infarction. *Circulation* 69:250-258, 1984

285. Ikegawa T, Chino M, Hasegawa H, et al: Prognostic significance of 24-hour ambulatory electrocardiographic monitoring in patients with dilative cardiomyopathy: a prospective study. *Clin Cardiol* 10:78-82, 1987

286. von Olshausen K, Schäfer A, Mehmel HC, et al: Ventricular arrhythmias in idiopathic dilated cardiomyopathy. *Br Heart J* 51:195-201, 1984

287. Olshausen KV, Stienen U, Schwarz F, et al: Long-term prognostic significance of ventricular arrhythmias in idiopathic dilated cardiomyopathy. *Am J Cardiol* 61:146-151, 1988

288. Packer M: Asymptomatic ventricular tachycardia identifies patients with heart failure at risk of clinical progression rather than sudden death (abstract). *Circulation* 80 Suppl 2:120, 1989

289. Richards DA, Cody DV, Denniss AR, et al: Ventricular electrical instability: a predictor of death after myocardial infarction. *Am J Cardiol* 51:75-80, 1983

290. Kharsa MH, Gold RL, Moore H, et al: Long-term outcome following programmed electrical stimulation in patients with high-grade ventricular ectopy. *PACE* 11:603-609, 1988

291. Gomes JAC, Hariman RI, Kang PS, et al: Programmed electrical stimulation in patients with high-grade ventricular ectopy: electrophysiologic findings and prognosis for survival. *Circulation* 70:43-51, 1984

292. Schoenfeld MH, McGovern B, Garan H, et al: Determinants of the outcome of electrophysiologic study in patients with ventricular tachyarrhythmias. *J Am Coll Cardiol* 6:298-306, 1985

293. Zheutlin TA, Roth H, Chua W, et al: Programmed electrical stimulation to determine the need for antiarrhythmic therapy in patients with complex ventricular ectopic activity. *Am Heart J* 111:860-867, 1986

294. Buxton AE, Marchlinski FE, Flores BT, et al: Nonsustained ventricular tachycardia in patients with coronary artery disease: role of electrophysiologic study. *Circulation* 75:1178-1185, 1987

295. Wilber DJ, Olshansky B, Moran JF, et al: Electrophysiological testing and nonsustained ventricular tachycardia: use and limitations in patients with coronary artery disease and impaired ventricular function. *Circulation* 82:350-358, 1990

296. Manolis AS, Estes NAM III: Value of programmed ventricular stimulation in the evaluation and management of patients with nonsustained ventricular tachycardia associated with coronary artery disease. *Am J Cardiol* 65:201-205, 1990

297. Zimmerman M, Adamec R, Simonin P, et al: Prognostic significance of ventricular late potentials in coronary artery disease. *Am Heart J* 109:725-732, 1985

298. Poll DS, Marchlinski FE, Buxton AE, et al: Sustained ventricular tachycardia in patients with idiopathic dilated cardiomyopathy: electrophysiologic testing and lack of response to antiarrhythmic drug therapy. *Circulation* 70:451-456, 1984

299. Stamato NJ, O'Connell JB, Murdock DK, et al: The response of patients with complex ventricular arrhythmias secondary to dilated cardiomyopathy to programmed electrical stimulation. *Am Heart J* 112:505-508, 1986

300. Poll DS, Marchlinski FE, Buxton AE, et al: Usefulness of programmed stimulation in idiopathic dilated cardiomyopathy. *Am J Cardiol* 58:992-997, 1986

301. Das SK, Morady F, DiCarlo L Jr, et al: Prognostic usefulness of programmed ventricular stimulation in idiopathic dilated cardiomyopathy without symptomatic ventricular arrhythmias. *Am J Cardiol* 58:998-1000, 1986

302. Meinertz T, Treese N, Kasper W, et al: Determinants of prognosis in idiopathic dilated cardiomyopathy as determined by programmed electrical stimulation. *Am J Cardiol* 56:337-341, 1985

303. Brembilla-Perrot B, Donetti J, de la Chaise AT: Diagnostic value of ventricular stimulation in patients with idiopathic dilated cardiomyopathy. *Am Heart J* 121:1124-1131, 1991

304. Stevenson WG, Stevenson LW, Weiss J, et al: Inducible ventricular arrhythmias in sudden death during vasodilator therapy of severe heart failure. *Am Heart J* 116:1447-1454, 1988

305. Vismara LA, Amsterdam EA, Mason DT: Relation of ventricular arrhythmias in the late hospital phase of acute myocardial infarction to sudden death after hospital discharge. *Am J Med* 59:6-12, 1975

306. Oxman HA, Connolly DC, Nobrega FT, et al: Identification of the patients at highest risk for sudden death within five years following their first myocardial infarction (abstract). *Am J Cardiol* 31:150, 1973

307. Schwartz PJ, Wolf S: QT interval prolongation as predictor of sudden death in patients with myocardial infarction. *Circulation* 57:1074-1077, 1978

308. Marchlinski FE, Buxton AE, Waxman HL, et al: Identifying patients at risk of sudden death after myocardial infarction: value of the response to programmed stimulation, degree of ventricular ectopic activity and severity of left ventricular dysfunction. *Am J Cardiol* 52:1190-1196, 1983

309. Olson HG, Lyons KP, Troop P, et al: The high-risk acute myocardial infarction patient at 1-year follow-up: identification at hospital discharge by ambulatory electrocardiography and radionuclide ventriculography. *Am Heart J* 107:358-366, 1984

310. Olson HG, Lyons KP, Troop P, et al: Prognostic implications of complicated ventricular arrhythmias early after hospital discharge in acute myocardial infarction: a serial ambulatory electrocardiography study. *Am Heart J* 108:1221-1228, 1984

311. Denniss AR, Baaijens H, Cody DV, et al: Value of programmed stimulation and exercise testing in predicting one-year mortality after acute myocardial infarction. *Am J Cardiol* 56:213-220, 1985

312. Hamer A, Vohra J, Hunt D, et al: Prediction of sudden death by electrophysiologic studies in high risk patients surviving acute myocardial infarction. *Am J Cardiol* 50:223-229, 1982

313. Mukharji J, Rude RE, Poole WK, et al: Risk factors for sudden death after acute myocardial infarction: two-year follow-up. *Am J Cardiol* 54:31-36, 1984

314. Daly LE, Hickey N, Graham IM, et al: Predictors of sudden death up to 18 years after a first attack of unstable angina or myocardial infarction. *Br Heart J* 58:567-571, 1987

315. Luria MH, Debanne SM, Osman MI: Long-term follow-up after recovery from acute myocardial infarction: observations on survival, ventricular arrhythmias, and sudden death. *Arch Intern Med* 145:1592-1595, 1985

316. Kotler MN, Tabatznik B, Mower MM, et al: Prognostic significance of ventricular ectopic beats with respect to sudden death in the late postinfarction period. *Circulation* 47:959-966, 1973

317. Vismara LA, Vera Z, Foerster JM, et al: Identification of sudden death risk factors in acute and chronic coronary artery disease. *Am J Cardiol* 39:821-828, 1977

318. Federman J, Whitford JA, Anderson ST, et al: Incidence of ventricular arrhythmias in first year after myocardial infarction. *Br Heart J* 40:1243-1250, 1978

319. Bigger JT Jr: Methodology for clinical trials with antiarrhythmic drugs to prevent cardiac death: US experience. *Cardiology* 74 Suppl 2:40-56, 1987

320. Coronary Drug Project Research Group: The Coronary Drug Project: design, methods, and baseline results. *Circulation* 47 Suppl 1:1-50, 1973

321. Locksley R, Moss AJ, DeCamilla J, et al: Prognostic grading and significance of VPBs after myocardial infarction (abstract). *Circulation* 50 Suppl 3:121, 1974

322. Oliver GC, Nolle FM, Tiefenbrunn AJ, et al: Ventricular arrhythmias associated with sudden death in survivors of acute myocardial infarction (abstract). *Am J Cardiol* 33:160, 1974

323. Schulze RA Jr, Strauss HW, Pitt B: Sudden death in the year following myocardial infarction: relation to ventricular premature contractions in the late hospital phase and left ventricular ejection fraction. *Am J Med* 62:192-199, 1977

324. Kostis JB, Byington R, Friedman LM, et al: Prognostic significance of ventricular ectopic activity in survivors of acute myocardial infarction. *J Am Coll Cardiol* 10:231-242, 1987

325. Ruberman W, Weinblatt E, Goldberg JD, et al: Ventricular premature complexes in prognosis of angina. *Circulation* 61:1172-1178, 1980

326. Coronary Drug Project Research Group: Prognostic importance of premature beats following myocardial infarction: experience in the Coronary Drug Project. *JAMA* 223:1116-1124, 1973

327. Moss AJ, Davis HT, DeCamilla J, et al: Ventricular ectopic beats and their relation to sudden and nonsudden cardiac death after myocardial infarction. *Circulation* 60:998-1003, 1979

328. Winkle RA: Ambulatory electrocardiography and the diagnosis, evaluation, and treatment of chronic ventricular arrhythmias. *Prog Cardiovasc Dis* 23:99-128, 1980

329. Oliver GC, Miller JP, Kleiger RE, et al: Ventricular arrhythmias in the early post hospital phase of myocardial infarction (abstract). *Circulation* 52 Suppl 2:223, 1975

330. Morganroth J, Michelson EL, Horowitz LN, et al: Limitations of routine long-term electrocardiographic monitoring to assess ventricular ectopic frequency. *Circulation* 58:408-414, 1978

331. Verzoni A, Romano S, Pozzoni L, et al: Prognostic significance and evolution of late ventricular potentials in the first year after myocardial infarction: a prospective study. *PACE* 12:41-51, 1989

332. Norris RM, Barnaby PF, Brandt PWT, et al: Prognosis after recovery from first acute myocardial infarction: determinants of reinfarction and sudden death. *Am J Cardiol* 53:408-413, 1984

333. Rodriguez LM, Krijne R, van den Dool A, et al: Time course and prognostic significance of serial signal-averaged electrocardiograms after a first acute myocardial infarction. *Am J Cardiol* 66:1199-1202, 1990

334. Iesaka Y, Nogami A, Aonuma K, et al: Prognostic significance of sustained monomorphic ventricular tachycardia induced by programmed ventricular stimulation using up to triple extrastimuli in survivors of acute myocardial infarction. *Am J Cardiol* 65:1057-1063, 1990

335. Dolack GL, Callahan DB, Bardy GH, et al: Signal-averaged electrocardiographic late potentials in resuscitated survivors of out-of-hospital ventricular fibrillation. *Am J Cardiol* 65:1102-1104, 1990

336. Vatterott PJ, Hammill SC, Bailey KR, et al: Signal-averaged electrocardiography: a new noninvasive test to identify patients at risk for ventricular arrhythmias. *Mayo Clin Proc* 63:931-942, 1989

337. Simson MB: Use of signals in the terminal QRS complex to identify patients with ventricular tachycardia after myocardial infarction. *Circulation* 64:235-242, 1981

338. Gomes JA, Winters SL, Stewart D, et al: A new noninvasive index to predict sustained ventricular tachycardia and sudden death in the first year after myocardial infarction: based on signal-averaged electrocardiogram, radionuclide ejection fraction and Holter monitoring. *J Am Coll Cardiol* 10:349-357, 1987

339. Denniss AR, Richards DA, Cody DV, et al: Prognostic significance of ventricular tachycardia and fibrillation induced at programmed stimulation and delayed potentials detected on the signal-averaged electrocardiograms of survivors of acute myocardial infarction. *Circulation* 74:731-745, 1986

340. Kuchar DL, Thorburn CW, Sammel NL: Late potentials detected after myocardial infarction: natural history and prognostic significance. *Circulation* 74:1280-1289, 1986

341. Ozawa Y, Yakubo S, Hatano M: Prospective study of late potentials to predict cardiac sudden death and ventricular tachycardias

in patients with myocardial infarction surviving over 4 weeks. *Jpn Circ J* 54:1304-1314, 1990

342. Farrell TG, Bashir Y, Cripps T, et al: Risk stratification for arrhythmic events in postinfarction patients based on heart rate variability, ambulatory electrocardiographic variables and the signal-averaged electrocardiogram. *J Am Coll Cardiol* 18:687-697, 1991

343. Kuchar DL, Thorburn CW, Sammel NL: Predictor of serious arrhythmic events after myocardial infarction: signal-averaged electrocardiogram, Holter monitoring and radionuclide ventriculography. *J Am Coll Cardiol* 9:531-538, 1987

344. Simson MB: Clinical application of signal averaging. *Cardiol Clin* 1 no 1:109-119, 1983

345. Waspe LE, Seinfeld D, Ferrick A, et al: Prediction of sudden death and spontaneous ventricular tachycardia in survivors of complicated myocardial infarction: value of the response to programmed stimulation using a maximum of three ventricular extrastimuli. *J Am Coll Cardiol* 5:1292-1301, 1985

346. Roy D, Marchand E, Théroux P, et al: Programmed ventricular stimulation in survivors of an acute myocardial infarction. *Circulation* 72:487-494, 1985

347. Santarelli P, Bellocci F, Loperfido F, et al: Ventricular arrhythmia induced by programmed ventricular stimulation after acute myocardial infarction. *Am J Cardiol* 55:391-394, 1985

348. Bhandari AK, Rose JS, Kotlewski A, et al: Frequency and significance of induced sustained ventricular tachycardia or fibrillation two weeks after acute myocardial infarction. *Am J Cardiol* 56:737-742, 1985

349. Bhandari AK, Au PK, Rose JS, et al: Decline in inducibility of sustained ventricular tachycardia from two to twenty weeks after acute myocardial infarction. *Am J Cardiol* 59:284-290, 1987

350. Roy D, Marchand E, Théroux P, et al: Long-term reproducibility and significance of provokable ventricular arrhythmias after myocardial infarction. *J Am Coll Cardiol* 8:32-39, 1986

351. Kuck K-H, Costard A, Schlüter M, et al: Significance of timing programmed electrical stimulation after acute myocardial infarction. *J Am Coll Cardiol* 8:1279-1288, 1986

352. Dhingra RC: Electrophysiologic studies during acute myocardial infarction: Do they prognosticate? *J Am Coll Cardiol* 18:789-791, 1991

353. Richards DAB, Byth K, Ross DL, et al: What is the best predictor of spontaneous ventricular tachycardia and sudden death after myocardial infarction? *Circulation* 83:756-763, 1991

354. Cripps T, Bennett ED, Camm AJ, et al: Inducibility of sustained monomorphic ventricular tachycardia as a prognostic indicator in survivors of recent myocardial infarction: a prospective evaluation in relation to other prognostic variables. *J Am Coll Cardiol* 14:289-296, 1989

355. Bourke JP, Richards DAB, Ross DL, et al: Routine programmed electrical stimulation in survivors of acute myocardial infarction for prediction of spontaneous ventricular tachyarrhythmias during follow-up: results, optimal stimulation protocol and cost-effective screening. *J Am Coll Cardiol* 18:780-788, 1991

356. Barber MJ, Mueller TM, Davies BG, et al: Interruption of sympathetic and vagal-mediated afferent responses by transmural myocardial infarction. *Circulation* 72:623-631, 1985

357. Minisi AJ, Thames MD: Effect of chronic myocardial infarction on vagal cardiopulmonary baroreflex. *Circ Res* 65:396-405, 1989

358. Rothschild M, Rothschild A, Pfeifer M: Temporary decrease in cardiac parasympathetic tone after acute myocardial infarction. *Am J Cardiol* 62:637-639, 1988

359. Schwartz PJ, Zaza A, Pala M, et al: Baroreflex sensitivity and its evolution during the first year after myocardial infarction. *J Am Coll Cardiol* 12:629-636, 1988

360. Kleiger RE, Miller JP, Bigger JT Jr, et al: Decreased heart rate variability and its association with increased mortality after acute myocardial infarction. *Am J Cardiol* 59:256-262, 1987

361. Hassapoyannes CA, Stuck LM, Hornung CA, et al: Effect of left ventricular aneurysm on risk of sudden and nonsudden cardiac death. *Am J Cardiol* 67:454-459, 1991

362. The Multicenter Postinfarction Research Group: Risk stratification and survival after myocardial infarction. *N Engl J Med* 309:331-336, 1983

363. Théroux P, Waters DD, Halphen C, et al: Prognostic value of exercise testing soon after myocardial infarction. *N Engl J Med* 301:341-345, 1979

364. Weaver WD, Cobb LA, Hallstrom AP, et al: Significance of ventricular dysrhythmias during ambulatory monitoring in patients resuscitated from the sudden death syndrome (abstract). *Circulation* 54 Suppl 2:172, 1976

365. Kehoe RP, Maron JM, Zheutlin T, et al: Electrophysiological study to direct therapy in survivors of pre-hospital ventricular fibrillation (abstract). *Am J Cardiol* 49:928, 1982

366. Roy D, Waxman HL, Kienzle MG, et al: Clinical characteristics and long-term follow-up in 119 survivors of cardiac arrest: relation to inducibility at electrophysiologic testing. *Am J Cardiol* 52:969-974, 1983

367. Benditt DG, Benson DW Jr, Klein GJ, et al: Prevention of recurrent sudden cardiac arrest: role of provocative electropharmacologic testing. *J Am Coll Cardiol* 2:418-425, 1983

368. Skale BT, Miles WM, Heger JJ, et al: Survivors of cardiac arrest; prevention of recurrence by drug therapy as predicted by electrophysiologic testing or electrocardiographic monitoring. *Am J Cardiol* 57:113-119, 1986

369. Wilber DJ, Garan H, Kelly E, et al: Out-of-hospital cardiac arrest: role of electrophysiologic testing in prediction of long-term outcome (abstract). *Circulation* 74 Suppl 2:482, 1986

370. Ruskin JN, DiMarco JP, Garan H: Out-of-hospital cardiac arrest: electrophysiologic observations and selection of long-term antiarrhythmic therapy. *N Engl J Med* 303:607-613, 1980

371. Benson DW Jr, Hession WT, Zavoral JH, et al: Sudden cardiac arrest in young adults: clinical and electrophysiological findings (abstract). *Am J Cardiol* 49:928, 1982

372. Ruskin JN, Garan H, DiMarco JP, et al: Electrophysiologic testing in survivors of prehospital cardiac arrest: therapy and long-term follow-up (abstract). *Am J Cardiol* 49:958, 1982

373. Morady F, DiCarlo L, Winston S, et al: Clinical features and prognosis of patients with out of hospital cardiac arrest and a normal electrophysiologic study. *J Am Coll Cardiol* 4:39-44, 1984

374. Zheutlin T, Steinman R, Summers C, et al: Long-term outcome in survivors of cardiac arrest with non-inducible ventricular tachycardia during programmed stimulation (abstract). *Circulation* 70 Suppl 2:399, 1984

375. Wellens HJJ, Brugada P, Stevenson WG: Programmed electrical stimulation of the heart in patients with life-threatening ventricular arrhythmias: What is the significance of induced arrhythmias and what is the correct stimulation protocol? *Circulation* 72:1-7, 1985

376. Kehoe R, Tommaso C, Zheutlin T, et al: Factors determining programmed stimulation responses and long-term arrhythmic outcome in survivors of ventricular fibrillation with ischemic heart disease. *Am Heart J* 116:355-363, 1988

377. Meinertz T, Hofmann T, Kasper W, et al: Significance of ventricular arrhythmias in idiopathic dilated cardiomyopathy. *Am J Cardiol* 53:902-907, 1984

378. Peter T, Ross D, Duffield A, et al: Effect on survival after myocardial infarction of long-term treatment with phenytoin. *Br Heart J* 40:1356-1360, 1978

379. Kosowsky BD, Taylor J, Lown B, et al: Long-term use of procaine amide following acute myocardial infarction. *Circulation* 47:1204-1210, 1973

380. Hugenholtz PA, Hagemeijer F, Lubsen J, et al: One year follow-up in patients with persistent ventricular dysrhythmias after myocardial infarction treated with aprindine or placebo. Excerpta Medica International Congress Series No 458, 1978, pp 572-577

381. UK Rythmodan Multicentre Study Group: Oral disopyramide after admission to hospital with suspected acute myocardial infarction. *Postgrad Med* 60:98-107, 1984

382. The CAPS Investigators: The Cardiac Arrhythmia Pilot Study. *Am J Cardiol* 57:91-95, 1986

383. Simonton CA, Daly PA, Kereiakes D, et al: Survival in severe left ventricular failure treated with the new nonglycosidic, nonsympathomimetic oral inotropic agents. *Chest* 92:118-123, 1987

384. Dargie HJ, Cleland JGF, Leckie BJ, et al: Relation of arrhythmias and electrolyte abnormalities to survival in patients with severe chronic heart failure. *Circulation* 75 Suppl 4:98-107, 1987

385. Fonger JD, Guarnieri T, Griffith LSC, et al: Impending sudden cardiac death: treatment with myocardial infarction revascularization and the automatic implantable cardioverter defibrillator. *Ann Thorac Surg* 46:13-16, 1988

386. Chamberlain DA: Overview of completed sudden death trials: European experience. *Cardiology* 74 Suppl 2:10-23, 1987

387. Coumel P, Leclercq J-F, Zimmerman M: The clinical use of

beta-blockers in the prevention of sudden death. *Eur Heart J* 7 Suppl A:187-201, 1986

388. Singh BN: When is drug therapy warranted to prevent sudden cardiac death? *Drugs* 41 Suppl 2:24-46, 1991

389. Furberg CD: Overview of completed sudden death trials: US experience. *Cardiology* 74 Suppl 2:24-31, 1987

390. Weksler BB, Gillick M, Pink J: Effect of propranolol on platelet function. *Blood* 49:185-196, 1977

391. Ahlmark G, Saetre H, Korsgren M: Reduction of sudden deaths after myocardial infarction (letter to the editor). *Lancet* 2:1563, 1974

392. Wilhelmsson C, Vedin JA, Wilhelmsen L, et al: Reduction of sudden deaths after myocardial infarction by treatment with alprenolol: preliminary results: *Lancet* 2:1157-1160, 1974

393. Barber JM, Boyle DMcC, Chaturvedi NC, et al: Practolol in acute myocardial infarction. *Acta Med Scand [Suppl]* 587:213-216, 1976

394. Norwegian Multicenter Study Group: Timolol-induced reduction in mortality and reinfarction in patients surviving acute myocardial infarction. *N Engl J Med* 304:801-807, 1981

395. β-Blocker Heart Attack Study Group: The β-blocker heart attack trial. *JAMA* 246:2073-2074, 1981

396. Editorial: Beta-blockers after myocardial infarction. *Lancet* 1:873-874, 1981

397. Yusuf S, Peto R, Lewis J, et al: Beta blockage during and after myocardial infarction: an overview of the randomized trials. *Prog Cardiovasc Dis* 27:335-371, 1985

398. Kostis JB, Wilson AC, Sanders MR, et al: Prognostic significance of ventricular ectopic activity in survivors of acute myocardial infarction who receive propranolol. *Am J Cardiol* 61:975-978, 1988

399. Chamberlain D, Campbell S: Which patients for secondary prevention with beta-blocking drugs? *Eur Heart J* 7 Suppl B:53-58, 1986

400. Winkle RA: Measuring antiarrhythmic drug efficacy by suppression of asymptomatic ventricular arrhythmias (editorial). *Ann Intern Med* 91:480-482, 1979

401. Myerburg RJ, Kessler KM, Kiem I, et al: Relationship between plasma levels of procainamide, suppression of premature ventricular complexes and prevention of recurrent ventricular tachycardia. *Circulation* 64:280-290, 1981

402. Winkle RA, Gradman AH, Fitzgerald JW: Antiarrhythmic drug effect assessed from ventricular arrhythmia reduction in the ambulatory electrocardiogram and treadmill test: comparison of propranolol, procainamide and quinidine. *Am J Cardiol* 42:473-480, 1978

403. Winkle RA, Antiarrhythmic drug effect mimicked by spontaneous variability of ventricular ectopy. *Circulation* 57:1116-1121, 1978

404. The Cardiac Arrhythmia Suppression Trial (CAST) Investigators: Preliminary report: effect of encainide and flecainide on mortality in a randomized trial of arrhythmia suppression after myocardial infarction. *N Engl J Med* 321:406-412, 1989

405. Burkart F, Pfisterer M, Kiowski W, et al: Effect of antiarrhythmic therapy on mortality in survivors of myocardial infarction with asymptomatic complex ventricular arrhythmias: Basel Antiarrhythmic Study of Infarct Survival (BASIS). *J Am Coll Cardiol* 16:1711-1718, 1990

406. Podrid PJ, Blatt CM: Sudden cardiac death: an approach to management of the patient at risk. *Herz* 9:65-76, 1984

407. Platia EV, Reid PR: Comparison of programmed electrical stimulation and ambulatory electrocardiographic (Holter) monitoring in the management of ventricular tachycardia and ventricular fibrillation. *J Am Coll Cardiol* 4:493-500, 1984

408. Ezri MD, Huang SK, Denes P: The role of Holter monitoring in patients with recurrent sustained ventricular tachycardia: an electrophysiologic correlation. *Am Heart J* 108:1229-1236, 1984

409. Mitchell LB, Duff HJ, Manyari DE, et al: A randomized clinical trial of the noninvasive and invasive approaches to drug therapy of ventricular tachycardia. *N Engl J Med* 317:1681-1687, 1987

410. Josephson ME, Horowitz LN, Spielman SR, et al: Electrophysiologic and hemodynamic studies in patients resuscitated from cardiac arrest. *Am J Cardiol* 46:948-955, 1980

411. Myerburg RJ, Conde CA, Sung RJ, et al: Clinical, electrophysiologic and hemodynamic profile of patients resuscitated from prehospital cardiac arrest. *Am J Med* 68:568-576, 1980

412. Rae AP, Spielman SR, Kutalek SP, et al: Electrophysiologic assessment of antiarrhythmic drug efficacy for ventricular tachyarrhythmias associated with dilated cardiomyopathy. *Am J Cardiol* 59:291-295, 1987

413. Ruskin JN: Role of invasive electrophysiological testing in the evaluation and treatment of patients at high risk for sudden cardiac death. *Circulation* 85 Suppl 1:152-159, 1992

414. Kowey PR, Waxman HL, Greenspon A, et al: Value of electrophysiologic testing in patients with previous myocardial infarction and nonsustained ventricular tachycardia. *Am J Cardiol* 65:594-598, 1990

415. Bigger JT Jr, Coromilas J, Rolnitzky LM, et al: Effect of diltiazem on cardiac rate and rhythm after myocardial infarction. *Am J Cardiol* 65:539-546, 1990

416. Yusuf S, Furberg CD: Effects of calcium channel blockers on survival after myocardial infarction. *Cardiovasc Drugs Ther* 1:343-344, 1987

417. Verheugt FWA, van der Laarse A, Funke-Küpper AJ, et al: Effects of early intervention with low-dose aspirin (100 mg) on infarct size, reinfarction and mortality in anterior wall acute myocardial infarction. *Am J Cardiol* 66:267-270, 1990

418. Smith P, Arnesen H, Holme I: The effect of warfarin on mortality and reinfarction after myocardial infarction. *N Engl J Med* 323:147-152, 1990

419. Verheugt FWA, Brugada P: Sudden death after acute myocardial infarction: the forgotten thrombotic view. *Am J Cardiol* 67:1130-1134, 1991

420. The CONSENSUS Trial Study Group: Effects of enalapril on mortality in severe congestive heart failure: results of the Cooperative North Scandinavian Enalapril Survival Study (CONSENSUS). *N Engl J Med* 316:1429-1435, 1987

421. Francis GS: Should asymptomatic ventricular arrhythmias in patients with congestive heart failure be treated with antiarrhythmic drugs? *J Am Coll Cardiol* 12:274-283, 1988

422. Chatterjee K: Protagonist's viewpoint. *J Am Coll Cardiol* 12:276-280, 1988

423. Hammermeister KE, DeRouen TA, Murray JA, et al: Effect of aortocoronary saphenous vein bypass grafting on death and sudden death: comparison of nonrandomized medically and surgically treated cohorts with comparable coronary disease and left ventricular function. *Am J Cardiol* 39:925-934, 1977

424. Vismara LA, Miller RR, Price JE, et al: Improved longevity due to reduction of sudden death by aortocoronary bypass in coronary atherosclerosis: prospective evaluation of medical versus surgical therapy in matched patients with multivessel disease. *Am J Cardiol* 39:919-924, 1977

425. Hammermeister KE, DeRouen TA, Murray JA, et al: Comparison of late survival and incidence of sudden cardiac death in similar medically and surgically treated coronary disease patients (abstract). *Am J Cardiol* 39:286, 1977

426. Holmes DR Jr, Davis K, Gersh BJ, et al: Risk factor profiles of patients with sudden cardiac death and death from other cardiac causes: a report from the Coronary Artery Surgery Study (CASS). *J Am Coll Cardiol* 13:524-530, 1989

427. Holmes DR Jr, Davis KB, Mock MB, et al: The effect of medical and surgical treatment on subsequent sudden cardiac death in patients with coronary artery disease: a report from the Coronary Artery Surgery Study. *Circulation* 73:1254-1263, 1986

428. Garan H, Ruskin JN, DiMarco JP, et al: Electrophysiologic studies before and after myocardial revascularization in patients with life-threatening ventricular arrhythmias. *Am J Cardiol* 51:519-524, 1983

429. Mirowski M, Reid PR, Winkle RA, et al: Mortality in patients with implanted automatic defibrillators. *Ann Intern Med* 98:585-588, 1983

430. Grubb BP, Mancini M, Temesy-Armos P, et al: Resolution of high initial epicardial patch defibrillation thresholds following chronic implantation. *PACE* 14:149-151, 1990

431. Fisher JD, Kim SG, Furman S, et al: Role of implantable pacemakers in control of recurrent ventricular tachycardia. *Am J Cardiol* 49:194-206, 1982

432. Palatianos GM, Thurer RJ, Cooper DK, et al: The implantable cardioverter-defibrillator: clinical results. *PACE* 14:297-301, 1991

433. Nisam S, Mower M, Moser S: ICD clinical update: first decade, initial 10,000 patients. *PACE* 14:255-262, 1991

434. Singer I, Austin E, Nash W, et al: The initial clinical experience with an implantable cardioverter defibrillator/antibody cardiac pacemaker. *PACE* 14:1119-1128, 1991

CHAPTER

24

Sudden cardiac death

B. Out-of-hospital intervention in sudden cardiac death

Roger D. White, M.D.

SUDDEN cardiac death remains a major health problem, claiming 350,000 to 400,000 persons annually in the United States.[1] Most of these deaths occur outside the hospital, and ventricular fibrillation (VF) is the most commonly observed initial arrhythmia upon arrival of emergency rescue personnel, although monomorphic or pleomorphic ventricular tachycardia (VT) that degenerates into VF is a frequent initiating sequence.[2] In an effort to reduce this mortality, prehospital emergency medical services systems have been developed nationwide, with a major focus on rapid intervention in patients experiencing out-of-hospital cardiac arrest. Because of the frequency of VF as the presenting rhythm in such patients, recent emphasis has been directed toward making defibrillation available as rapidly as possible by use of various non-advanced-life-support systems to reach patients in VF with defibrillators. This chapter describes the spectrum of intervention employed in the management of patients experiencing sudden cardiac arrest, beginning with basic life support and extending to the full array of advanced life support procedures often needed to restore spontaneous circulation.

CARDIOPULMONARY RESUSCITATION: PERFORMANCE AND RATIONALE

The timely application of properly performed cardiopulmonary resuscitation (CPR) is frequently the major determinant of the success of all other maneuvers to save the patient who has cardiac arrest. A detailed description of the procedures employed in CPR is available in the document that defines national guidelines for CPR and emergency cardiac care.[3] CPR can be learned best by hands-on supervised practice on manikins. Certainly all physicians should be thoroughly acquainted with currently recommended techniques and the physiologic rationale for their use. A brief description of these techniques follows. The most recent guidelines should be reviewed for further information pertaining to current recommendations for CPR and emergency cardiac care.[3]

Techniques of CPR

Having confirmed that a person who has collapsed is indeed unresponsive, the rescuer calls the Emergency Medical Services (EMS) system to initiate an advanced life support response and then immediately opens the airway. The head tilt-chin lift method is used, or, alternatively, the jaw thrust maneuver can be used to restore a patent airway. The rescuer then confirms that the patient is apneic by observing the chest for appropriate motion, listening for air movement, and feeling over the nose and mouth for the flow of expired air. This can be accomplished in 5 seconds. The rescuer then applies two mouth-to-mouth ventilations, each with sufficient volume to effect rise and fall of the chest. Compact masks with one-way valves are available as an alternative to mouth-to-mouth ventilation. The carotid pulse is palpated to confirm the absence of spontaneous circulation. The location of the carotid artery makes it an immediately accessible site for confirming pulselessness, although the femoral artery is an equally acceptable alternative. If no pulse is present, the diagnosis of cardiac arrest is confirmed.

External chest compressions are then begun. The lower half of the sternum is quickly located by identifying with the fingers of one hand the notch where the ribs unite with the sternum just above the xiphoid. The heel of the other hand is then placed just above this notch. The chest is compressed smoothly and rhythmically, with equal lengths of time for downstroke and upstroke. The chest is compressed 4 to 5 cm with each downstroke, and pressure is released during the upstroke to permit the chest wall to return to its resting position. When only one rescuer is present, the chest is compressed 15 times at a rate of 80 to 100 per minute, and then the lungs are ventilated twice in succession, so that the ratio of compressions to ventilation during one-rescuer CPR is 15:2. This compression rate allows an adequate number of compressions to be applied per minute, given the interruptions needed to ventilate the lungs. When two rescuers are present, the compression rate remains 80 to 100 per minute, and the second rescuer can deliver a ventilation after every fifth

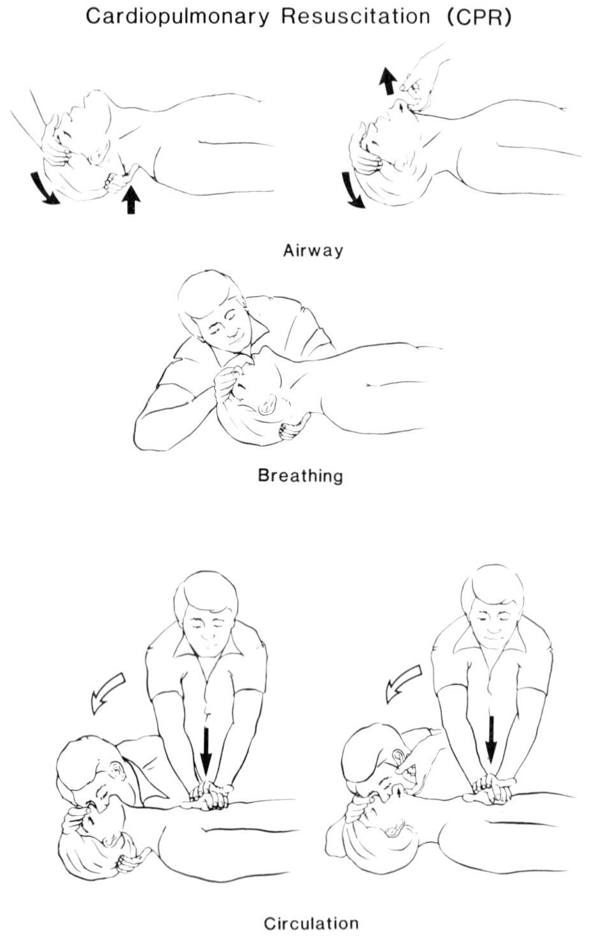

Fig 24B-1 The ABCs of CPR. The airway is opened, preferably by the head tilt-chin lift maneuver *(Airway),* and mouth-to-mouth ventilation is performed *(Breathing).* External chest compression *(Circulation)* is then combined with breathing to become cardiopulmonary resuscitation. The previously used head tilt-neck lift method is also illustrated here. Because the chin lift is easier to learn and may be more effective, it is recommended as the preferred technique.

compression. The lungs are ventilated during a brief pause at the end of every fifth chest compression. During ventilation, inspiratory time should approximate 2 seconds in an attempt to provide more effective lung inflation and to minimize high upper airway pressures that can promote gastric distention. Thus, the ratio of compressions to ventilation is 5:1. This 5:1 compression-to-ventilation ratio seems to maintain adequate flow and pressure, allows cardiac refilling, avoids rapid fatigue of the rescuer, and facilitates coordination of ventilation with compression.

The sequential steps of opening the airway (head tilt-chin lift), performing mouth-to-mouth ventilation, and applying external chest compression are illustrated in Figure 24B-1.

Physiologic considerations

The mechanisms of blood flow and ventilation during cardiopulmonary arrest continue to be the subject of both experimental and clinical investigations. It has been assumed since the early 1960s, when CPR became a widespread clinical technique, that blood is propelled forward as a direct result of actual compression of the heart between the sternum and the vertebral column. This effect is now commonly referred to as the "cardiac pump mechanism." During experimental porcine CPR, echocardiographic and hemodynamic measurements demonstrated that both mitral and tricuspid valves opened during the upstroke phase of external compression and closed during the downstroke. A reduction in left ventricular area was observed during the downstroke.[4] These observations support direct cardiac compression as the mechanism providing forward blood flow during CPR. Transesophageal echocardiography in humans with cardiac arrest provides an opportunity to assess changes in cardiac dimensions and valve positions during chest compressions and in directional blood flow. This method of assessment has confirmed that, at least in some patients, direct cardiac compression is the predominant mechanism of blood flow during external chest compressions.[5,6] Right and left ventricular compression, mitral valve closure during the downstroke of the compression phase, and opening of the mitral valve during the upstroke, or relaxation phase, are all consistent with direct cardiac compression, or the cardiac pump mechanism[5,6] (Fig 24B-2).

Because repeated, forceful coughing (cough CPR) can sustain consciousness during VF for as long as 100 seconds, mechanisms other than direct compression of the heart may account for forward blood flow during cardiac arrest in some circumstances.[7] Indeed, vigorous coughing has been shown to produce an arterial pressure pulse associated with forward blood flow and to cause opening of the aortic valve during pressure and flow generation.[8] These findings support the proposal that increases in intrathoracic pressure generate forward blood flow.[9] This is commonly referred to as the "thoracic pump mechanism" for movement of blood. The increasing intrathoracic pressure during chest compression equalizes intravascular pressures within the thorax. On the venous side, valves and venous collapse at the thoracic inlet limit transmission of retrograde pressure or flow. The arterial system, which is relatively resistant to collapse, transmits pressure and flow into the extrathoracic arterial tree. A peripheral arteriovenous pressure difference is thus established that permits blood to flow forward in the extrathoracic vascular system. Some studies suggest that during compression or vigorous coughing, the left side of the heart acts as a passive conduit for the transfer of pulmonary venous blood out into the peripheral arterial circulation. During compression, blood flows from the lungs through the left ventricle and toward the periphery. The pulmonary valve is closed and the mitral and aortic valves are open during periods of high intrathoracic pressure when the chest is compressed.[10]

Cyclic increases in intrathoracic pressure (the thoracic

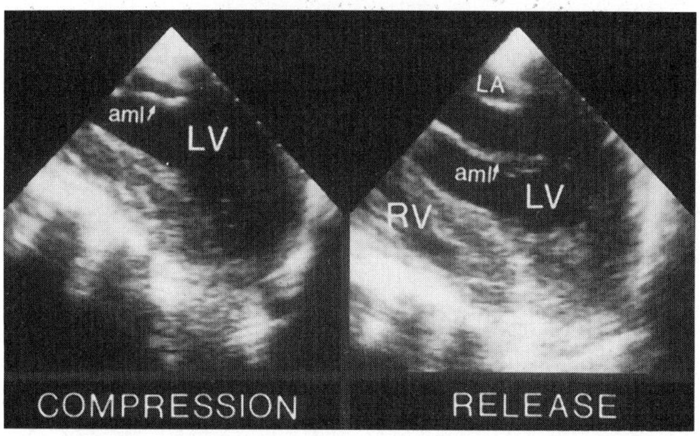

Fig 24B-2 Transesophageal echocardiographic images obtained during external chest compression in a human with cardiac arrest. During the downstroke (compression), the right ventricle *(RV)* is obliterated, the left ventricle *(LV)* is compressed, and the mitral valve closes. During the upstroke (release), the mitral valve opens and left ventricular filling occurs. *aml,* anterior mitral leaflet; *LA,* left atrium. (From Higano ST, Oh JK, Ewy GA, et al: The mechanism of blood flow during closed chest cardiac massage in humans: transesophageal echocardiographic observations. *Mayo Clin Proc* 65:1432-1440, 1990. By permission, Mayo Foundation for Medical Education and Research.)

pump) have been applied in patients in cardiac arrest by means of circumferential compression of the thorax with a pneumatic vest. In a preliminary study, "vest CPR" increased aortic and coronary perfusion pressures more than manual CPR, but neither restoration of spontaneous circulation nor survival was significantly improved.[11]

Another mechanism of "direct" cardiac compression during CPR—referred to as "high-impulse CPR"—has been proposed. The physical and physiologic mechanisms in support of this proposal have been described in detail.[12] The underlying principle is that manual chest compressions delivered in a high-impulse (brief duration, high velocity) manner induce direct cardiac compression rather than increases in intrathoracic pressure. Supporting this hypothesis is experimental evidence that the left ventricle is indeed deformed by chest compression, an indication that the heart experiences direct compressive force.[13]

Interposed abdominal counterpulsation is a form of CPR in which the abdomen is compressed during the upstroke of the chest compression phase in an attempt to sustain aortic diastolic pressure and thus improve coronary perfusion pressure, a critical determinant of successful restoration of spontaneous circulation. There is experimental evidence that carotid blood flow[14] and end-diastolic arteriovenous pressure difference,[15] an index of coronary perfusion pressure, are increased with this form of CPR. A recent randomized controlled trial of interposed abdominal counterpulsation CPR in cardiac arrest in humans provides suggestive preliminary evidence that survival to hospital dismissal is improved with this form of CPR.[16] Additional clinical trials will be needed to confirm the benefit of this technique.

The most recent addition to the varieties of techniques and devices intended to improve blood flow during CPR is active compression-decompression (ACD) CPR.[17-21] This procedure accomplishes compression and active decompression of the thorax by means of a device containing a suction header, bellows, and compression area within the bellows. Preliminary data from a comparison of ACD CPR with standard CPR in humans with cardiac arrest provided evidence of hemodynamic benefit, with higher systolic arterial pressure and end-tidal carbon dioxide concentrations and echocardiographic demonstration of increased velocity time integral, an analogue of cardiac output.[17] Transesophageal echocardiographic imaging during ACD CPR disclosed increased transmitral flow and stroke volume with ACD resuscitation.[18]

Studies in patients undergoing frequent periods of induction of VF during surgical implantation of cardioverter-defibrillators have confirmed increased arterial and coronary perfusion pressures with ACD CPR compared with standard CPR, along with increased minute ventilation and negative inspiratory pressure.[20] After in-hospital cardiac arrest, ACD CPR, in a comparison with standard CPR, was shown to improve the rate of initial resuscitation and survival and neurologic condition at 24 hours,[19] but neither this study nor two studies of ACD CPR during out-of-hospital cardiac arrest[21] were able to demonstrate a statistically significant improvement in dismissal survival. It is evident that larger studies are needed to assess the impact of this form of CPR on the ultimate determinant of benefit—neurologically intact survival after cardiac arrest.

Until the clinical relevance of any of these observations is established, standard CPR techniques as described and illustrated above are recommended. What is certain is that CPR, regardless of mechanism of blood flow and technique, is only a temporizing procedure and requires rapid supplementation with advanced cardiac life support, most critically rapid defibrillation of the fibrillating heart.

OUT-OF-HOSPITAL EMERGENCY MEDICAL SERVICES

The feasibility of mobile advanced life support (ALS) emerged from experience with mobile coronary care described by Pantridge and Adgey in Belfast in the late 1960s.[22] Their approach to sudden cardiac death used physicians as participants in the mobile coronary care response team. Furthermore, this effort was directed specifically and almost exclusively at acute cardiac events. The lack of availability of physicians for this function and the obvious advantages of a system capable of responding to all causes of life-threatening events, not only cardiac, led to the development and implementation of mobile ALS systems capable of rapid response to a variety of life-threatening emergencies. These systems became functional in the early 1970s in several metropolitan areas of the United States. In Rochester, Minn., this form of prehospital emergency care became established in mid-1973 and was first described in 1974.[23]

Functional components of an EMS system

Sudden cardiac death imposes the greatest challenge to the functional capability of an EMS system, because the sequence and timing of responses are critical to a successful outcome. It begins with prompt recognition of collapse and cardiopulmonary arrest and institution of CPR. The EMS system must be activated quickly, and mobile ALS must be brought to and applied at the scene within minutes of the collapse. A breakdown in any one of these responses rapidly diminishes the chances for survival of the victim of sudden cardiac arrest. The decisive role of bystanders in prompt initiation of CPR has been documented.[24,25] It is clear that bystander-initiated CPR before the arrival of rescue personnel is a major determinant of outcome. Unfortunately, in most EMS systems, this remains a major limitation of the effectiveness of mobile ALS. No matter how promptly and aggressively this support is applied at the scene of collapse, if CPR is not begun within a few minutes of arrest, the chance of the patient's survival without neurologic deficit is very low unless defibrillation and restoration of spontaneous circulation can be executed within a few minutes after collapse.

The critical role of rapid defibrillation in improving survival from out-of-hospital cardiac arrest (OHCA) has been well documented.[26-31] The American Heart Association has promulgated nationwide implementation of early defibrillation as an essential component of a chain of survival for victims of OHCA.[32-34] The American Heart Association has also developed an early defibrillation training program to promote and incorporate this intervention in prehospital emergency cardiac care. The advent of the automated external defibrillator (AED) that contains microprocessor-based cardiac rhythm detection circuitry has already expedited the introduction of rapid defibrillation into EMS systems.[35-37] This device is attached to the patient's chest by means of two adhesive monitor-defibrillation electrode pads. Once activated, the AED analyzes the surface ECG through a series of filters that assess such variables as waveform amplitude, slope, regularity, isoelectric content, rate, and QRS complex width. Impedance measurements and noise filters restrict analysis to an acceptable electrocardiographic (ECG) signal. If sufficient criteria for VF or VT in a pulseless and apneic patient are fulfilled, the AED "advises," by means of a visual display or voice synthesizer (or both), the delivery of a shock. This semiautomated cycle of analyze, advise, and shock can be executed and repeated rapidly. All events are preserved on a dual-channel cassette tape that records all voice and ECG data from the moment the device is turned on. In addition, most AEDs have an additional documentation system, such as a solid-state memory module, that stores priority ECG segments and times for subsequent review and printout. An example of an AED is shown in Figure 24B-3, and a printed record from a memory module from an actual event is reproduced in Figure 24B-4.

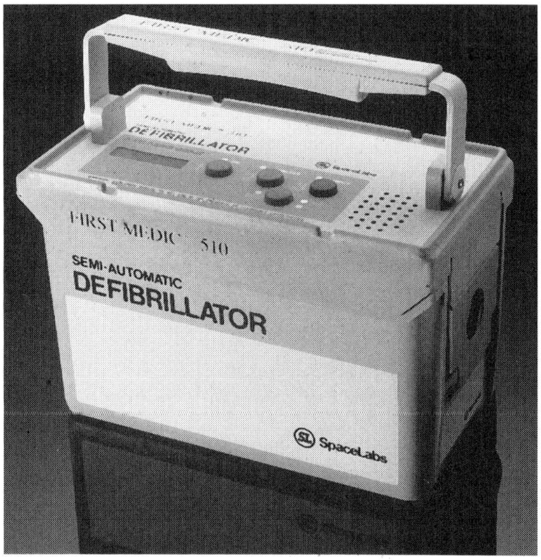

Fig 24B-3 Example of a semiautomated external defibrillator. Visual prompts, displayed on the screen to the left of the controls, and voice messages from the speaker on the right side guide the user in operation. (Courtesy of SpaceLabs, Inc., Redmond, Washington.)

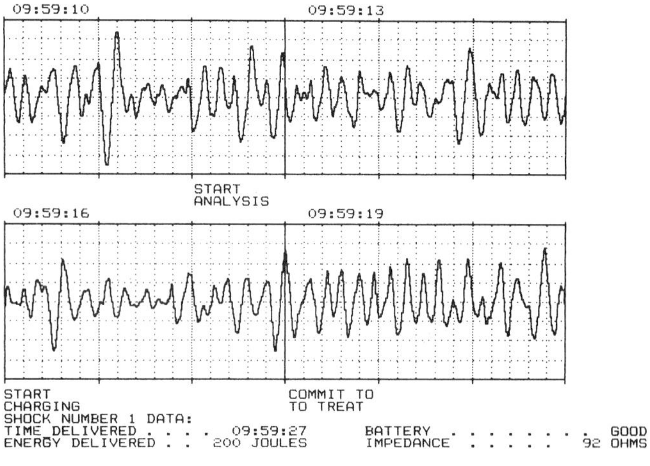

Fig 24B-4 Recording of events during defibrillation with a semiautomated defibrillator. A 200-J shock was delivered 15 seconds after automated analysis of the rhythm was begun. The rhythm depicted in the bottom panel, recorded 44 seconds after shock delivery, was accompanied by strong peripheral pulses.

Early and rapid defibrillation, more than any other intervention, improves survival from OHCA. To effect this improvement, AEDs must be readily available. Basic life support ambulances staffed by basic (nonparamedic)

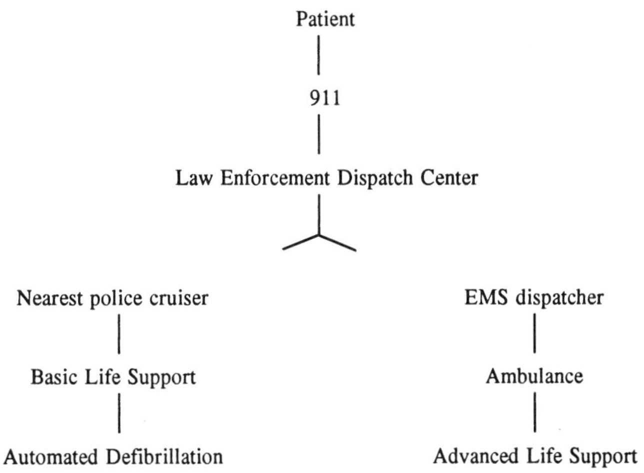

Fig 24B-5 Emergency Medical Services (EMS) system response network. Components and function are described in the text.

emergency medical technicians should be equipped with AEDs unless long response times and small population bases preclude the likelihood of benefit from early defibrillation. Likewise, first responders such as police officers and fire personnel can be trained to operate AEDs and deliver shocks before arrival of an ambulance in many situations.

A critical issue surrounding widespread implementation of early defibrillation is proper operation and maintenance of AEDs. The Food and Drug Administration has documented major deficiencies in this area.[38] In fact, potentially life-threatening problems caused by improper operation and maintenance exist wherever defibrillators are located, whether in ambulances or in the hospital. The Food and Drug Administration has developed checklists for both manual and automated defibrillators that are intended to reduce substantially the incidence and magnitude of such problems and thus permit early defibrillation to confer maximal benefit on survival from OHCA.[39]

In our community, mobile ALS is provided by an ambulance service serving a population base of approximately 90,000 persons in a geographical area of about 660 square miles. The area serviced utilizes the universal emergency telephone number 911 for access. The mechanisms of system entry and response to an emergency are illustrated in Figure 24B-5. The 911 call for help is received in the county law enforcement dispatch center. The nearest police car is dispatched to the scene of the emergency, and at the same time an EMS dispatcher receives the call via a telephone hot line. An ambulance with ALS capability is dispatched immediately on reception of the 911 call. Within the city, the average response time for the police car is 2.6 minutes from the time of receipt of the call. The ambulance response time averages 4.5 minutes. Although these times in themselves are favorable, they do not include whatever time may be lost between the moment of the victim's collapse and the activation of the EMS system via the 911 call. All city police and county sheriff's officers are trained in CPR and therefore act as the first medical responders in the event of cardiac arrest. They are a vital component of the EMS system for that reason. As part of a continuing pilot project, several city police cars carry AEDs and all officers have been trained to operate the devices. These compact and rugged AEDs (see Fig 24B-3) are carried in the car beside the officer, immediately available in the event of a 911 call indicative of an OHCA.

Our initial experience with police defibrillation was recently reported.[40] Of 14 patients in VF initially treated by police with one to three shocks before ambulance arrival, 7 regained pulses with police shocks only. The remaining seven required additional ALS care. Ten of the 14 patients in VF initially treated by police survived to leave the hospital.

The responding ALS ambulance team consists of two ALS emergency medical technician (EMT)-paramedics. All are registered with the National Registry of Emergency Medical Technicians, the national certifying agency for EMTs, and are required to fulfill the stringent entry and reregistration requirements of the Registry to be a part of our system. In the event of a cardiac arrest, backup EMT-paramedics are immediately dispatched to assist the primary team.

Emergency cardiac care as part of ALS

One of the major thrusts of ALS in cardiac emergencies is to provide medical intervention before cardiac arrest takes place. Prompt recognition of warning signs of an acute cardiac event by the patient or the patient's family, followed by activation of the EMS system, facilitates this level of intervention. Emergency care in these situations includes the administration of oxygen, ECG monitoring, placement of an intravenous infusion line, and administration of drugs, if necessary. Drug therapy may consist of nitroglycerin sublingually or morphine intravenously for the control of pain and the injection of such drugs as lidocaine, atropine, verapamil,[41] and adenosine[42] for suppression of arrhythmias. Much of this care is accomplished by means of standing orders in a protocol for ALS (Table 24B-1) for the initiation of therapy in potentially life-threatening circumstances. Further treatment requires radio or telephone consultation with a physician. Ambulance-to-hospital ECG telemetry was used for several years in our system but has been discontinued. Technical problems with telemetry equipment and ECG transmission, our satisfaction with the technicians' ability to interpret life-threatening arrhythmias, and the prompt and continuous availability of radio or telephone consultation with a physician all were factors in our decision to discontinue ECG telemetry. Incorporation of national standards and guidelines for emergency cardiac care into our ALS protocols has facilitated the immediate application of appropriate care by EMT-paramedics in acute cardiac emergencies.

Prehospital emergency cardiac care encompasses assessment and management of patients with a variety of cardiac arrhythmias. Examples include multifocal atrial tachycardia as the presenting rhythm in patients experi-

Table 24B-1 Emergency cardiac care procedures in patients **not** in cardiac arrest

I. Standard Cardiac Care Protocol
  A. Oxygen by mask or cannula at 5-8 L/min. If patient has emphysema, do not exceed 2 L/min.
  B. Have patient sit in a comfortable position.
  C. Evaluate cardiac rhythm.
  D. Start IV infusion with D5W.
  E. Check vital signs every 5 min and record significant changes.
  F. Give nitroglycerin, 0.4 mg (1 tablet) sublingually, for chest pain if systolic pressure is ≥100 mm Hg. May be *repeated* once or twice at intervals of 4-5 min.
  G. Give further pain medication or sedation on M.D. order as follows:
    Morphine—not to exceed 4 mg at one time, by IV push SLOWLY.
    Diazepam (Valium)—not to exceed 5 mg at one time, by IV push SLOWLY.
  H. Transport as soon as possible.

II. Sinus Bradycardia
  A. Standard cardiac care.
  B. Observe to determine whether
    Patient alert.
    Skin warm and dry.
    Blood pressure stable.
  C. If blood pressure is low (≤90 mm Hg systolic) or premature ventricular complexes or clinical signs of impaired perfusion (confusion, disorientation, diaphoresis) are present:
    Give atropine, 0.5-1.0 mg, by IV push. Consult M.D. for further therapy.
    Atropine may be given in additional increments up to 3 mg. Transcutaneous pacing (TCP) can be used in atropine-refractory patients or as first treatment for severe bradycardia on M.D. order.

III. Supraventricular Tachycardia
  A. For general treatment purposes, this includes paroxysmal supraventricular tachycardia and atrial flutter or atrial fibrillation with rapid ventricular response.
  B. Standard cardiac care.
  C. Observe to determine whether
    Patient alert and blood pressure stable.
  D. Valsalva maneuver with patient supine.
  E. On order of M.D., inject adenosine, 6 mg IV through antecubital venous catheter. Repeat in 2-3 min with 12 mg if needed. Verapamil, 5 mg, can be used on M.D. order.
  F. On order of M.D., be prepared to use synchronized cardioversion at 50-75 J. Diazepam, 5 mg IV, may be ordered before shock if patient responsive.
  G. On occasion, M.D. may order lidocaine bolus, 50-100 mg IV.
  H. Transport as soon as possible.

IV. First-Degree Heart Block
  A. Standard cardiac care.
  B. Observe for progression of heart block to higher degrees.

V. Second-Degree Heart Block
  A. Standard cardiac care.
  B. Observe to determine whether
    Patient alert.
    Skin warm and dry.
    Blood pressure stable.
  C. If blood pressure is ≤90 mm Hg systolic or premature ventricular complexes or clinical signs of impaired perfusion are present:
    Give atropine, 0.5-1.0 mg, by IV push. Consult M.D. Be prepared, on order, to repeat atropine or go to D.
  D. TCP on M.D. order. This is the preferred intervention for Mobitz type II block or wide-QRS complete heart block in symptomatic patients.
  E. Monitor for significant changes.

VI. Complete Heart Block
  A. Standard cardiac care.
  B. Observe to determine whether
    Patient alert.
    Skin warm and dry.
    Blood pressure stable.

CPR, cardiopulmonary resuscitation; D5W, 5% dextrose in water; IV, intravenous(ly).

Table 24B-1 Emergency cardiac care procedures in patients **not** in cardiac arrest—cont'd

- C. If blood pressure is ≤90 mm Hg systolic or clinical signs of impaired perfusion are present:
  Give atropine, 0.5-1.0 mg, by IV push. Consult M.D. Be prepared, on order, to repeat atropine or go to D.
- D. TCP on M.D. order. TCP is treatment of choice in symptomatic complete heart block with wide QRS complexes.
- E. If patient loses consciousness, initiate CPR.

VII. Ventricular Ectopy (Premature Ventricular Complexes)
- A. Standard cardiac care.
- B. Give lidocaine, 1.0-1.5 mg/kg, by IV bolus. Consult M.D.
- C. On M.D. order, give repeat 0.5-1.5 mg/kg every 5-10 min to 3 mg/kg.
- D. On M.D. order, give lidocaine, 1.0 g in 250 mL of D5W, with minidrip infusion set. Infuse at 1-4 mg/min, 15-60 minidrops/min. (Dilution is 4 mg/mL.)
- E. Observe patient for confusion, seizure activity, or decreasing level of response during administration of lidocaine. Watch for early signs of toxicity, e.g., slurred speech, paresthesias, muscle twitching.

VIII. Wide-Complex Tachycardia
- A. Standard cardiac care.
- B. Give lidocaine, 1.0-1.5 mg/kg, by IV bolus. Consult M.D.
- C. Repeat lidocaine, 0.5-0.75 mg/kg, every 5-10 min to 3 mg/kg.
- D. If tachycardia persists, consult M.D. about adenosine.
- E. If cardioversion ordered for persistent or severely symptomatic tachycardia:
  Give diazepam, 5 mg IV, on order. Use synchronized shock at 100 J. Consult M.D. if tachycardia persists.
- F. If patient is initially unresponsive, use 200-J shock immediately.

encing acute myocardial infarction (AMI)[43] (Fig 24B-6), paroxysmal supraventricular tachycardia (Fig 24B-7), pleomorphic ventricular tachycardia[44] (Fig 24B-8), and monomorphic ventricular tachycardia (Fig 24B-9). In all circumstances such as these, the need for therapeutic intervention is based on assessment of the patient's condition and the decision of the consulting on-line medical control physician. If a potentially life-threatening, hemodynamically unstable arrhythmia is present, EMT-paramedics are authorized to institute treatment immediately using standing orders and then consult a physician for further direction.

The role of thrombolytic intervention in prehospital emergency cardiac care is not yet established.[45-47] Only 4.2%[48] to 18%[49] of patients whose chief symptom is nontraumatic chest pain during prehospital care by EMS services are shown subsequently to have experienced an AMI. Of those patients with AMI, 24%[49] to 54%[50,51] have prehospital 12-lead ECGs diagnostic of AMI. Finally, only 4% to 5% of patients attended by EMS systems who have chest pain as the chief symptom are considered candidates for thrombolytic therapy.[48,51,52] A randomized European study demonstrated the feasibility and safety of prehospital thrombolytic therapy but did not confirm a definite reduction in overall mortality.[53] Likewise in the United States, a randomized, controlled trial of prehospital-initiated thrombolytic therapy compared with hospital-initiated treatment demonstrated no improvement in outcome after initiation of treatment outside the hospital.[54] In EMS systems with short transport times from the site of the emergency to the hospital, such as is the case in our system, deriving a cost-effective benefit from prehospital thrombolytic therapy is very unlikely. However, it is possible to obtain historical and ECG data at the scene and during transportation that will expedite delivery of thrombolytic therapy on arrival at the hospital.[49,54,55] The accuracy of on-scene computer-interpreted 12-lead ECGs,[56] without need for ambulance-to-hospital ECG transmission, has potential prehospital cost-effective application in EMS systems with relatively long times before arrival at a hospital. When this is not the case, emphasis should be placed on shortening the time between arrival at the emergency department and initiation of thrombolytic treatment ("door-to-drug" time interval).

As noted earlier, out-of-hospital sudden cardiac death imposes the greatest demands on a mobile ALS system. Experience has shown that unless the patient can be resuscitated and stabilized at the scene by aggressive emergency cardiac care, the likelihood of survival is very low indeed.[25,57] In fact, if spontaneous circulation cannot be restored during prehospital care, little or no benefit is gained by transporting the patient in arrest to the hospital.[58-61] Therefore, the immediate end point of out-of-hospital resuscitation from cardiac arrest is restoration of a functional circulation before transportation. To this end, standing orders in ALS protocols are deliberately designed to permit EMT-paramedics to execute treatment as quickly as possible and in a rapidly moving series of steps appropriate for the specific form of cardiac arrest (Table 24B-2). Protocols for cardiorespiratory arrest are based on the national guidelines for emergency cardiac care.[3] These guidelines are further developed in the American Heart Association's *Textbook of Advanced Cardiac Life Support*[62] and in the text *Advanced Emergency Care for Paramedic Practice.*[63] A description of a typical response to out-of-hospital cardiac arrest follows.

When a 911 emergency call is received at the dispatch center, the nearest police car is dispatched to the scene.

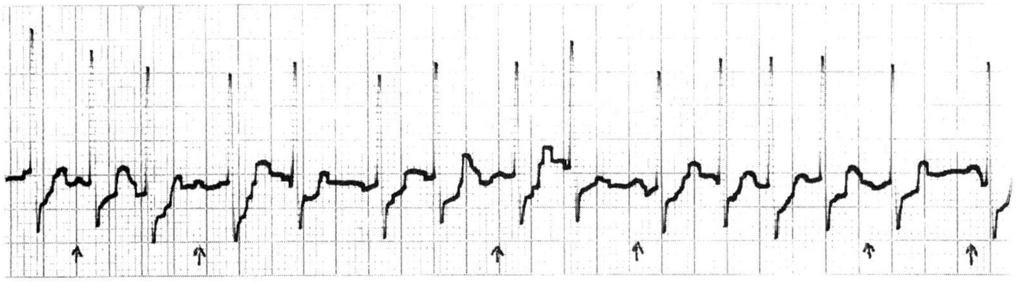

Fig 24B-6 Multifocal atrial tachycardia as the initial rhythm during prehospital care in a patient experiencing an acute myocardial infarction. *Arrows* mark P waves with varying morphology and polarity. (From White RD: Prehospital recognition of multifocal atrial tachycardia: association with acute myocardial infarction. *Ann Emerg Med* 21:753-756, 1992. By permission of American College of Emergency Physicians.)

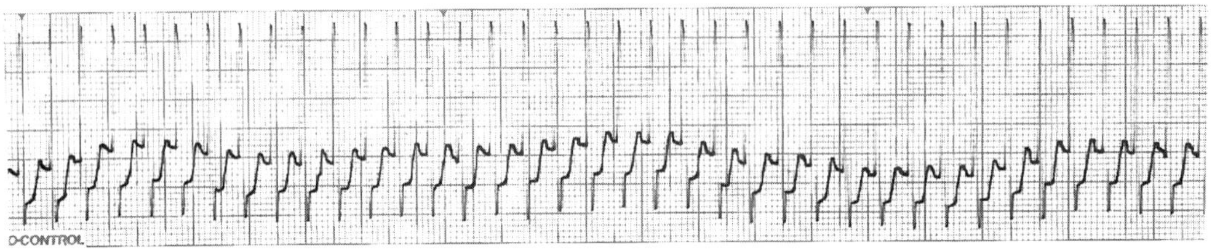

Fig 24B-7 Paroxysmal supraventricular tachycardia during prehospital care. Adenosine and verapamil are both available for treatment of this arrhythmia.

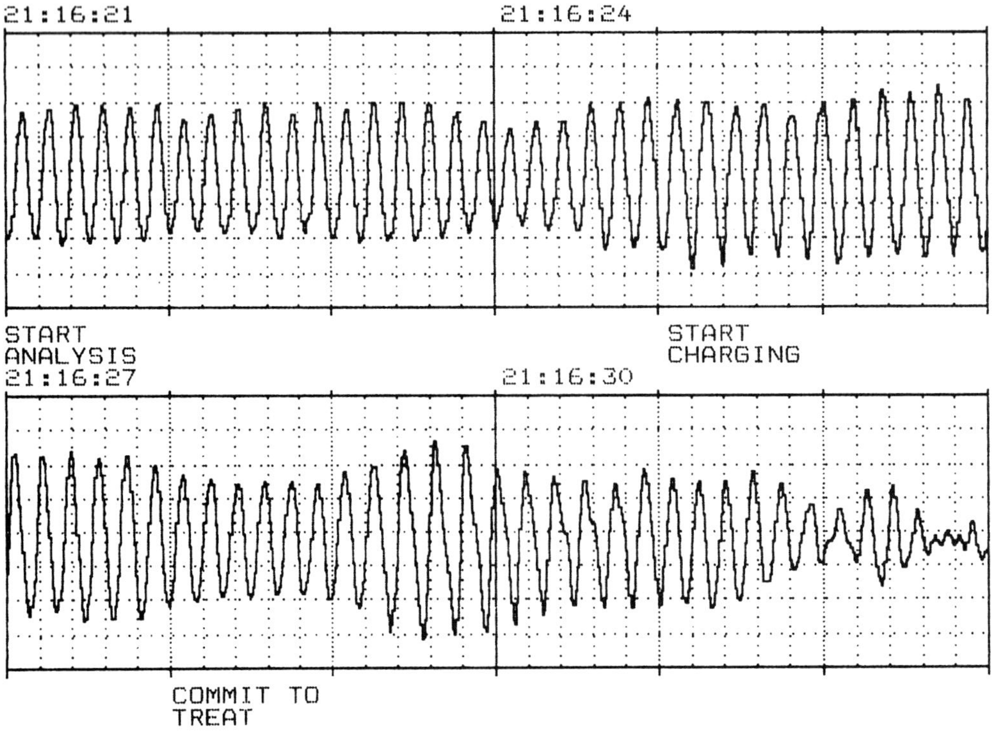

Fig 24B-8 Pleomorphic ventricular tachycardia occurring during the course of resuscitation. A semiautomated defibrillator analyzed, charged, and defibrillated this tachycardia. (From White RD, Wood DL: Prehospital polymorphic ventricular tachycardia [reply]. *Ann Emerg Med* 22:1368-1369, 1993. By permission of American College of Emergency Physicians.)

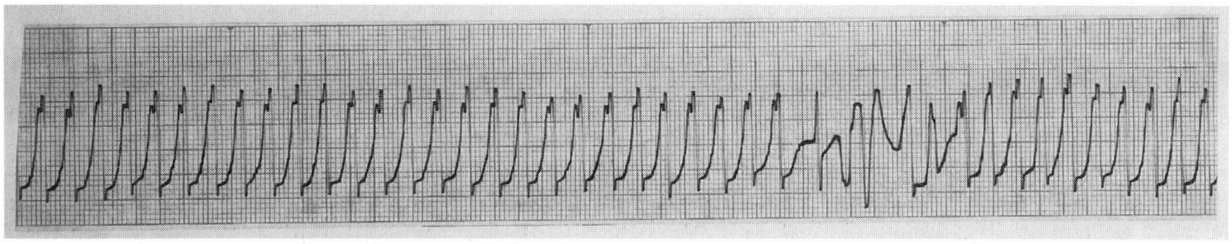

Fig 24B-9 Monomorphic ventricular tachycardia with fusion complexes observed by emergency medical technician-paramedics as the presenting rhythm.

Table 24B-2 Protocol for therapy in patients with cardiopulmonary arrest

I. Ventricular Fibrillation (VF) and Pulseless Ventricular Tachycardia (VT)
   A. Initiate or continue CPR.
   B. Confirm VF.
   C. Deliver 200-J shock; if VF still present, shock at 300 J and then at 360 J.
   D. If arrest persists, resume CPR, intubate trachea, connect automatic transport ventilator (ATV) and capnograph, and ventilate 10-12/min with VT 800-1,000 mL.
   E. Start IV infusion and inject 1 mg of epinephrine. Thereafter, either standard dose (1 mg) or alternative dose* of epinephrine can be ordered by M.D. *All doses are given every 3-5 min.*
   F. Deliver 360-J shock.
   G. For persistent VF, give lidocaine, 1.5 mg/kg, and follow with 360-J shock. Repeat lidocaine, 1.5 mg/kg, in 3-5 min if needed. Defibrillate after each dose of each drug throughout resuscitation for persistent VF.
   H. After lidocaine dose has reached 3 mg/kg, switch to bretylium, 5 mg/kg, and shock at 360 J. Repeat bretylium in 5 min at 10 mg/kg, and repeat 10 mg/kg dose again to 35 mg/kg maximum.
   I. Sodium bicarbonate, 1 mEq/kg, on M.D. order. This can be used earlier in resuscitation on order and repeated at 0.5 mEq/kg every 10 min.
   J. For refractory VF, consult M.D. about magnesium sulfate ($MgSO_4$), 1-2 g over 2 min; potassium chloride, 10 mEq over 10-15 min; or procainamide, 30 mg/min to 17 mg/kg. If pleomorphic VT ("torsade" appearance) at any point in resuscitation, consult M.D. for immediate $MgSO_4$ order.

II. Pulseless Electrical Activity
   A. Initiate or continue CPR.
   B. Intubate, connect ATV and capnograph, and start IV infusion.
   C. Consider possible causes and inform M.D. of findings for specific therapy.
   D. Epinephrine in doses in VF/VT protocol.
   E. If bradycardia present, atropine, 1 mg, and repeat in 3-5 min to 3 mg. Transcutaneous pacing may be ordered by M.D. if patient atropine-refractory.
   F. Sodium bicarbonate as in VF/VT protocol.

III. Asystole
   A. Initiate or continue CPR.
   B. Intubate, connect ATV and capnograph, and start IV infusion.
   C. Immediate transcutaneous pacing if witnessed arrest.
   D. Epinephrine in doses in VF/VT protocol.
   E. Atropine, 1 mg. Repeat in 3-5 min to 3 mg.
   F. Sodium bicarbonate as in VF/VT protocol.
   G. Consult M.D. regarding cessation of resuscitation.

CPR, cardiopulmonary resuscitation; IV, intravenous.
*Standard dose, 1 mg; intermediate dose, 2-5 mg; escalating dose, 1 mg, 3 mg, 5 mg; high dose, 0.1 mg/kg.

If cardiac arrest is confirmed, CPR is begun by the police officer. If the police defibrillator arrives before the ambulance, it is attached immediately and the rhythm analyzed. If indicated, shocks are delivered by the officer. An example of a police-officer-delivered shock that restored spontaneous circulation is depicted in Figure 24B-4.

When the first ambulance arrives, CPR is continued, if necessary, by police officers while one EMT-paramedic prepares to ventilate with 100% oxygen and then to intubate the trachea. The other attaches an AED with an oscilloscope and defines further treatment according to the observed rhythm and the dictates of the standing orders (see Table 24B-2). Backup EMT-paramedics are

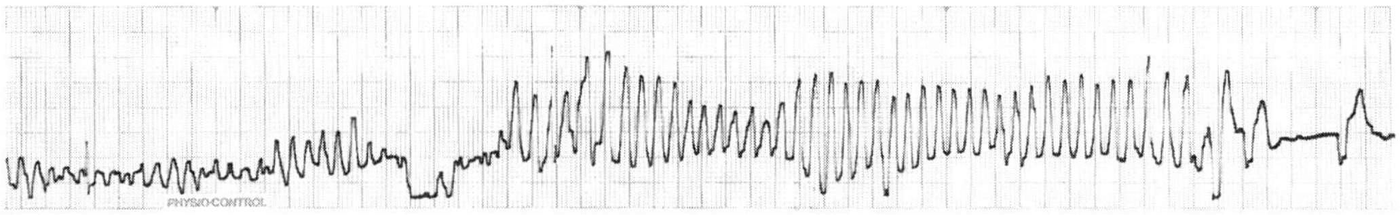

Fig 24B-10 Pleomorphic ventricular tachycardia as the initial rhythm on arrival of the emergency medical technician-paramedics. A precordial thump converted the rhythm. (From White RD, Wood DL: Out-of-hospital pleomorphic ventricular tachycardia and resuscitation: association with acute myocardial ischemia and infarction. *Ann Emerg Med* 21:1282-1287, 1992. By permission of American College of Emergency Physicians.)

also dispatched to the scene as soon as cardiac arrest is confirmed. In most instances (70% to 75% in our experience), VF is the presenting rhythm. Pleomorphic VT has also been observed as the rhythm at presentation or during the course of prehospital resuscitation[44] (Fig 24B-8 and 24B-10). Up to three initial defibrillatory shocks are used for VF. If VF persists after three shocks (delivered by a police officer or an EMT-paramedic, or both), an intravenous infusion is begun and pharmacologic therapy instituted as outlined in the protocol.

Epinephrine is the major pharmacologic agent used to improve cerebral and myocardial blood flow during cardiac arrest.[64] High-dose therapy with epinephrine (0.2 mg/kg) has been shown to increase coronary perfusion pressure.[65] However, there is no evidence that high doses of epinephrine in adult cardiac arrest improve hospital dismissal rates or the neurologic condition of patients dismissed.[66-69] Until a survival benefit from high-dose therapy is determined, our policy is to begin with 1 mg of epinephrine and then at the physician's option permit use of alternative doses, including high doses, thereafter.

For persistent or recurrent VF or VT, lidocaine and bretylium remain the prehospital antiarrhythmic drugs of choice. The protocol shown in Table 24B-2 describes their use.

The role of sodium bicarbonate therapy in the treatment of the metabolic acidosis of cardiac arrest remains unresolved, although the weight of evidence indicates that it probably is not beneficial and may be detrimental. A decrease in coronary perfusion pressure that occurred during experimental cardiac arrest in which sodium bicarbonate was used was attributed to its hypertonicity.[70] Because it is a potent generator of carbon dioxide, it may worsen mixed-venous and tissue acidosis.[71] There is evidence that sodium bicarbonate is incapable of reversing intramyocardial acidosis during arrest,[72] and alternatives to sodium bicarbonate, such as an equimolar mixture of sodium bicarbonate and sodium carbonate (Carbicarb), have been shown experimentally also to be ineffective in ameliorating this acidosis.[73] Currently, sodium bicarbonate is usually used only after other interventions defined in the protocols have been used.

Monitoring the effectiveness of a resuscitative effort has been difficult and subjective, with reliance on skin color, palpable pulses, and pupil size. All of these assessments have inherent limitations. The pressure of carbon dioxide in end-expired gas ($P_{ET}CO_2$) is an objective index of pulmonary blood flow, provided that minute ventilation is controlled and physiologic carbon dioxide production assumed to be constant.[74,75] There is growing evidence that $P_{ET}CO_2$ can be used during cardiac arrest and resuscitation as an indication of pulmonary blood flow and, therefore, cardiac output during chest compressions.[76,77] It may also be useful in predicting the likelihood of restoration of spontaneous circulation and the outcome of resuscitation.[78-80] For accurate interpretation of $P_{ET}CO_2$ measurements, minute ventilation during resuscitation must be kept controlled and constant.[74] Control is now possible with time-cycled, constant-flow automatic ventilators, which we use routinely in all patients with cardiac arrest. Semiquantitative colorimetric $P_{ET}CO_2$ indicators are available for confirming correct endotracheal tube placement, but in the low-flow state of cardiac arrest and CPR, these devices lack sensitivity in making this determination.[81,82] Nevertheless, the color changes observed with these indicators during resuscitation provide an index of pulmonary blood flow and prognosis for survival to hospital admission.[83]

What is needed to fully apply the potential benefit of $P_{ET}CO_2$ measurement during OHCA is a portable, battery-powered capnometer that displays the capnographic waveform in real time on a breath-to-breath basis. Such a device, coupled with a time-cycled automatic ventilator, would confer a significant advance in the assessment of the patient with OHCA undergoing resuscitation. Capnometers with these capabilities are now becoming available. Our preliminary experience with quantitative capnography during OHCA and CPR has confirmed the feasibility of this noninvasive procedure and has demonstrated that changes in $P_{ET}CO_2$ track changes in pulmonary blood flow during CPR or during spontaneous circulation.[84] Our observations also indicate that $P_{ET}CO_2$ measurements during the first few minutes of CPR are prognostic for restoration of spontaneous circulation during OHCA.[85] Further development of these findings may enable quantitative capnography to be used early in resuscitation to identify when efforts should cease rather than persist in futile attempts to restore the circulation.

Asystole or bradysystole is the presenting disorder in 25% to 30% of cases of OHCA. Mortality in this circumstance approaches 100% despite vigorous treatment in the field. In most instances, this is an end-stage, irreversible derangement for which currently available interventions are ineffectual. External transthoracic pacing has not been shown to improve survival in these patients,[86] although there is a subset of patients with symptomatic bradycardia refractory to atropine for whom external pacing may be beneficial.

Electromechanical dissociation (EMD), an organized electrical rhythm that does not generate pressure, presents a problem in differential diagnosis. Although it may reflect acute power failure from extensive AMI, other causes need to be considered in preparation for treatment and the decision to transport the patient rapidly to the hospital. Possible causes of this disorder are hypovolemia (for example, from a ruptured abdominal aortic aneurysm), massive pulmonary embolism, anaphylaxis, cardiac tamponade, tension pneumothorax, and AMI. The initial assessment of the patient, the history, and the circumstances surrounding the collapse all dictate the course of treatment. If hypovolemia is suspected, a fluid challenge is used. If hypovolemia is tentatively confirmed by the response to this fluid challenge, the patient is immediately transported so that definitive hospital care can be instituted. Unfortunately, the cause of this disorder is commonly found at autopsy to be severe coronary atherosclerosis with acute and irreversible pump failure or cardiac tamponade from left ventricular rupture following AMI.

Every attempt is made to achieve circulatory stabilization before movement of the patient and transportation. As indicated earlier, failure to accomplish this at the scene is almost invariably followed by failure to resuscitate at the hospital. This outcome underscores the need for vigorous attempts to achieve return of spontaneous circulation before movement and transportation are begun.

Experience with out-of-hospital emergency cardiac care

Extensive experience has been gained across the country since the advent of mobile ALS systems. Most studies report results as percentage of patients with OHCA who are ultimately dismissed from the hospital. Survival varies widely among EMS systems, depending in large measure on the prompt availability of bystander CPR, early defibrillation, and early, definitive, on-scene ALS.[24] Improved outcome is invariable when the arrest is witnessed, bystander CPR is started, the presenting rhythm is VF, and prompt defibrillation is applied.[25,33] The most recent data indicate that the highest dismissal survival rates in ALS EMS systems are in the range of 15% to 26% when VF is the initial rhythm.[87-90] However, in one large metropolitan ALS EMS system, a very low dismissal survival rate from VF (3%) was observed.[91] This disproportionately low rate of survival was attributed primarily to a long interval between collapse and defibrillation (mean of 16 minutes). This result underscores the critical role of rapid defibrillation in improving survival from OHCA caused by VF.

When asystole or various forms of pulseless electrical activity are the initial rhythms, survival from OHCA is uniformly low in all studies (<6%), most likely because these arrhythmias often represent long intervals between collapse and initiation of treatment and because in other instances they accompany irreversible cardiac insults. Exceptions may be EMD and pseudo-EMD, forms of pulseless electrical activity that may be more amenable to treatment if high priority is given to the possible correctable causes.

Our experience in a relatively small population base compares favorably with results in most large metropolitan EMS systems. The first full year of operation of our prehospital ALS system was 1974. From 1974 through 1994, 591 patients with OHCA and VF as the presenting rhythm were treated. Of these, 144 (24%) survived to be dismissed without significant neurologic impairment. In the first half of this 18-year period (1974 through 1982), 303 patients with VF were treated and 56 (18.5%) survived to be dismissed to home. In the latter half (1983 through 1993), 288 patients with VF were treated and 87 (30%) were dismissed to home. Any patients with neurologic impairment requiring prolonged nursing home care were excluded from the dismissal figures. In the 5-year period between 1983 and 1988, the Seattle group[92] reported that 24% of 1,132 patients with OHCA and VF were dismissed to home. Our overall survival data are quite comparable with the much larger experience observed in Seattle during a similar period. On the basis of the 18-year experience in Seattle with 5,120 patients who had OHCA and VF as the initial rhythm, Cobb et al.[92] proposed that there may be an upper limit for survival rates from OHCA and VF, perhaps at a level of approximately 30%. Whether widespread community implementation of rapid automated defibrillation within an already existing well-organized and rapidly responding ALS EMS system can increase this upper limit has not yet been established.

REFERENCES

1. Brooks R, McGovern BA, Garan H, et al: Current treatment of patients surviving out-of-hospital cardiac arrest. *JAMA* 265:762-768, 1991

2. Bayés de Luna A, Coumel P, Leclercq JF: Ambulatory sudden cardiac death: mechanisms of production of fatal arrhythmia on the basis of data from 157 cases. *Am Heart J* 117:151-159, 1989

3. Emergency Cardiac Care Committee and Subcommittees, American Heart Association: Guidelines for cardiopulmonary resuscitation and emergency cardiac care. *JAMA* 268:2171-2302, 1992

4. Deshmukh HG, Weil MH, Gudipati CV, et al: Mechanism of blood flow generated by precordial compression during CPR. I. Studies on closed chest precordial compression. *Chest* 95:1092-1099, 1989

5. Higano ST, Oh JK, Ewy GA, et al: The mechanism of blood flow during closed chest cardiac massage in humans: transesophageal echocardiographic observations. *Mayo Clin Proc* 65:1432-1440, 1990

6. Kühn C, Juchems R, Frese W: Evidence for the 'Cardiac Pump Theory' in cardiopulmonary resuscitation in man by transesophageal echocardiography. *Resuscitation* 22:275-282, 1991

7. Harada Y, Fuseno H, Ohtomo T, et al: Self-administered hyperventilation cardiopulmonary resuscitation for 100 s of cardiac arrest during Holter monitoring. *Chest* 99:1310-1312, 1991

8. Criley JM, Niemann JT, Rosborough JP, et al: Modifications of cardiopulmonary resuscitation based on the cough. *Circulation* 74 Suppl 4:42-50, 1986

9. Halperin HR, Weisfeldt ML: Movement of blood by intrathoracic pressure fluctuations during cardiopulmonary resuscitation. In *Acute Coronary Care in the Thrombolytic Era.* Edited by RM Califf, DB Mark, GS Wagner. Chicago, Year Book Medical Publishers, 1988, pp 114-126

10. Cohen JM, Chandra N, Alderson PO, et al: Timing of pulmonary and systemic blood flow during intermittent high intrathoracic pressure

cardiopulmonary resuscitation in the dog. *Am J Cardiol* 49:1883-1889, 1982

11. Halperin HR, Tsitlik JE, Gelfand M, et al: A preliminary study of cardiopulmonary resuscitation by circumferential compression of the chest with use of a pneumatic vest. *N Engl J Med* 329:762-768, 1993
12. Feneley MP, Maier GW, Rankin JS: Mechanisms of blood flow during cardiopulmonary resuscitation: analysis of recent experimental observations on the importance of the chest compression technique. In *Acute Coronary Care in the Thrombolytic Era.* Edited by RM Califf, DB Mark, GS Wagner. Chicago, Year Book Medical Publishers, 1988, pp 127-148
13. Feneley MP, Maier GW, Gaynor JW, et al: Sequence of mitral valve motion and transmitral blood flow during manual cardiopulmonary resuscitation in dogs. *Circulation* 76:363-375, 1987
14. Einagle V, Bertrand F, Wise RA, et al: Interposed abdominal compressions and carotid blood flow during cardiopulmonary resuscitation: support for a thoracoabdominal unit. *Chest* 93:1206-1212, 1988
15. Lindner KH, Ahnefeld FW, Bowdler IM: Cardiopulmonary resuscitation with interposed abdominal compression after asphyxial or fibrillatory cardiac arrest in pigs. *Anesthesiology* 72:675-681, 1990
16. Sack JB, Kesselbrenner MB, Bregman D: Survival from in-hospital cardiac arrest with interposed abdominal counterpulsation during cardiopulmonary resuscitation. *JAMA* 267:379-385, 1992
17. Cohen TJ, Tucker KJ, Lurie KG, et al: Active compression-decompression: a new method of cardiopulmonary resuscitation. *JAMA* 267:2916-2923, 1992
18. Tucker KJ, Redberg RF, Schiller NB, et al: Active compression-decompression resuscitation: analysis of transmitral flow and left ventricular volume by transesophageal echocardiography in humans. *J Am Coll Cardiol* 22:1485-1493, 1993
19. Cohen TJ, Goldner BG, Maccaro PC, et al: A comparison of active compression-decompression cardiopulmonary resuscitation with standard cardiopulmonary resuscitation for cardiac arrests occurring in the hospital. *N Engl J Med* 329:1918-1921, 1993
20. Shultz JJ, Coffeen P, Sweeney M, et al: Evaluation of standard and active compression-decompression CPR in an acute human model of ventricular fibrillation. *Circulation* 89:684-693, 1994
21. Schwab TM, Callaham ML, Madsen CD, et al: A randomized clinical trial of active compression-decompression CPR vs standard CPR in out-of-hospital cardiac arrest in two cities. *JAMA* 273:1261-1268, 1995
22. Pantridge JF, Adgey AAJ: Pre-hospital coronary care: the mobile coronary care unit. *Am J Cardiol* 24:666-673, 1969
23. White RD, O'Donovan TPB: Prehospital life-support systems in traumatic and cardiac emergencies. *Anesth Analg* 53:734-743, 1974
24. Eisenberg MS, Horwood BT, Cummins RO, et al: Cardiac arrest and resuscitation: a tale of 29 cities. *Ann Emerg Med* 19:179-186, 1990
25. Spaite DW, Hanlon T, Criss EA, et al: Prehospital cardiac arrest: the impact of witnessed collapse and bystander CPR in a metropolitan EMS system with short response times. *Ann Emerg Med* 19:1264-1269, 1990
26. Eisenberg MS, Copass MK, Hallstrom AP, et al: Treatment of out-of-hospital cardiac arrests with rapid defibrillation by emergency medical technicians. *N Engl J Med* 302:1379-1383, 1980
27. Stults KR, Brown DD, Schug VL, et al: Prehospital defibrillation performed by emergency medical technicians in rural communities. *N Engl J Med* 310:219-223, 1984
28. Weaver WD, Cobb LA, Hallstrom AP, et al: Factors influencing survival after out-of-hospital cardiac arrest. *J Am Coll Cardiol* 7:752-757, 1986
29. Weaver WD, Copass MK, Bufi D, et al: Improved neurologic recovery and survival after early defibrillation. *Circulation* 69:943-948, 1984
30. Weaver WD, Hill D, Fahrenbruch CE, et al: Use of the automatic external defibrillator in the management of out-of-hospital cardiac arrest. *N Engl J Med* 319:661-666, 1988
31. Haynes BE, Mendoza A, McNeil M, et al: A statewide early defibrillation initiative including laypersons and outcome reporting. *JAMA* 266:545-547, 1991
32. Cummins RO, Thies W: Encouraging early defibrillation: the American Heart Association and automated external defibrillators. *Ann Emerg Med* 19:1245-1248, 1990
33. Cummins RO, Ornato JP, Thies WH, et al: Improving survival from sudden cardiac arrest: the "Chain of Survival" concept: a Statement for Health Professionals from the Advanced Cardiac Life Support Subcommittee and the Emergency Cardiac Care Committee, American Heart Association. *Circulation* 83:1832-1847, 1991
34. Kerber RE: Statement on early defibrillation: from the Emergency Cardiac Care Committee, American Heart Association. *Circulation* 83:2233, 1991
35. Stults KR, Brown DD, Kerber RE: Efficacy of an automated external defibrillator in the management of out-of-hospital cardiac arrest: validation of the diagnostic algorithm and initial clinical experience in a rural environment. *Circulation* 73:701-709, 1986
36. Cummins RO, Eisenberg MS, Stults KR: Automatic external defibrillators: clinical issues for cardiology. *Circulation* 73:381-385, 1986
37. Cummins RO, Austin D Jr, Graves JR, et al: An innovative approach to medical control: semiautomatic defibrillators with solid-state memory modules for recording cardiac arrest events. *Ann Emerg Med* 17:818-824, 1988
38. Cummins RO, Chesemore K, White RD, et al: Defibrillator failures: causes of problems and recommendations for improvement. *JAMA* 264:1019-1025, 1990
39. White RD: Maintenance of defibrillators in a state of readiness. *Ann Emerg Med* 22:302-306, 1993
40. White RD, Vukov LF, Bugliosi TF: Early defibrillation by police—initial experience with measurement of critical time intervals and patient outcome. *Ann Emerg Med* 23:1009-1013, 1994
41. O'Toole KS, Heller MB, Menegazzi JJ, et al: Intravenous verapamil in the prehospital treatment of paroxysmal supraventricular tachycardia. *Ann Emerg Med* 19:291-294, 1990
42. McCabe JL, Adhar GC, Menegazzi JJ, et al: Intravenous adenosine in the prehospital treatment of paroxysmal supraventricular tachycardia. *Ann Emerg Med* 21:358-361, 1992
43. White RD: Prehospital recognition of multifocal atrial tachycardia: association with acute myocardial infarction. *Ann Emerg Med* 21:753-756, 1992
44. White RD, Wood DL: Out-of-hospital pleomorphic ventricular tachycardia and resuscitation: association with acute myocardial ischemia and infarction. *Ann Emerg Med* 21:1282-1287, 1992
45. Gokli AR, Kovar JL, Kowalenko T, et al: Prehospital care of acute myocardial infarction: a review. *Henry Ford Hosp Med J* 39:170-175, 1991
46. Kereiakes DJ, Weaver WD, Anderson JL, et al: Time delays in the diagnosis and treatment of acute myocardial infarction: a tale of eight cities: report from the Pre-Hospital Study Group and the Cincinnati Heart Project. *Am Heart J* 120:773-780, 1990
47. Kowalenko T, Kereiakes DJ, Gibler WB: Prehospital diagnosis and treatment of acute myocardial infarction: a critical review. *Am Heart J* 123:181-190, 1992
48. Gibler WB, Kereiakes DJ, Dean EN, et al: Prehospital diagnosis and treatment of acute myocardial infarction: a North-South perspective. *Am Heart J* 121:1-11, 1991
49. Weaver WD, Eisenberg MS, Martin JS, et al: Myocardial infarction triage and intervention project—Phase I: Patient characteristics and feasibility of prehospital initiation of thrombolytic therapy. *J Am Coll Cardiol* 15:925-931, 1990
50. Aufderheide TP, Hendley GE, Thakur RK, et al: The diagnostic impact of prehospital 12-lead electrocardiography. *Ann Emerg Med* 19:1280-1287, 1990
51. Aufderheide TP, Haselow WC, Hendley GE, et al: Feasibility of prehospital r-TPA therapy in chest pain patients. *Ann Emerg Med* 21:379-383, 1992
52. Grim PS, Feldman T, Childers RW: Evaluation of patients for the need of thrombolytic therapy in the prehospital setting. *Ann Emerg Med* 18:483-488, 1989
53. The European Myocardial Infarction Project Group: Prehospital thrombolytic therapy in patients with suspected acute myocardial infarction. *N Engl J Med* 329:383-389, 1993
54. Weaver WD, Cerqueira M, Hallstrom AP, et al: Prehospital-initiated vs hospital-initiated thrombolytic therapy. The Myocardial Infarction Triage and Intervention Trial. *JAMA* 270:1211-1216, 1993
55. Karagounis L, Ipsen SK, Jessop MR, et al: Impact of field-transmitted electrocardiography on time to in-hospital thrombolytic therapy in acute myocardial infarction. *Am J Cardiol* 66:786-791, 1990
56. Kudenchuk PJ, Ho MT, Weaver WD, et al: Accuracy of computer-interpreted electrocardiography in selecting patients for thrombolytic therapy. *J Am Coll Cardiol* 17:1486-1491, 1991
57. Lewis LM, Ruoff B, Rush C, et al: Is emergency department

resuscitation of out-of-hospital cardiac arrest victims who arrive pulseless worthwhile? *Am J Emerg Med* 8:118-120, 1990

58. Kellermann AL, Staves DR, Hackman BB: In-hospital resuscitation following unsuccessful prehospital advanced cardiac life support: 'Heroic Efforts' or an exercise in futility? *Ann Emerg Med* 17:589-594, 1988

59. Gray WA, Capone RJ, Most AS: Unsuccessful emergency medical resuscitation—are continued efforts in the emergency department justified? *N Engl J Med* 325:1393-1398, 1991

60. Bonnin MJ, Pepe PE, Kimball KT, et al: Distinct criteria for termination of resuscitation in the out-of-hospital setting. *JAMA* 270:1457-1462, 1993

61. Kellermann AL, Hackman BB, Somes G: Predicting the outcome of unsuccessful prehospital advanced cardiac life support. *JAMA* 270:1433-1436, 1993

62. Cummins RO (ed): *Textbook of Advanced Cardiac Life Support.* Dallas, American Heart Association, 1994, pp 1-24

63. Breiter M: Cardiovascular emergencies. In *Advanced Emergency Care for Paramedic Practice.* Edited by SA Jones, A Weigel, RD White, et al. Philadelphia, JB Lippincott Company, 1991, pp. 405-520

64. Ornato JP: Use of adrenergic agonists during CPR in adults. *Ann Emerg Med* 22:411-416, 1993

65. Paradis NA, Martin GB, Rosenberg J, et al: The effect of standard- and high-dose epinephrine on coronary perfusion pressure during prolonged cardiopulmonary resuscitation. *JAMA* 265:1139-1144, 1991

66. Callaham M, Barton CW, Kayser S: Potential complications of high-dose epinephrine therapy in patients resuscitated from cardiac arrest. *JAMA* 265:1117-1122, 1991

67. Stiell IG, Hebert PC, Weitzman BN, et al: High-dose epinephrine in adult cardiac arrest. *N Engl J Med* 327:1045-1050, 1992

68. Brown CG, Martin DR, Pepe PE, et al: A comparison of standard-dose and high-dose epinephrine in cardiac arrest outside the hospital. *N Engl J Med* 327:1051-1055, 1992

69. Callaham M, Madsen CD, Barton CW, et al: A randomized clinical trial of high-dose epinephrine and norepinephrine vs standard-dose epinephrine in prehospital cardiac arrest. *JAMA* 268:2667-2672, 1992

70. Kette F, Weil MH, Gazmuri RJ: Buffer solutions may compromise cardiac resuscitation by reducing coronary perfusion pressure. *JAMA* 266:2121-2126, 1991

71. Hindman BJ: Sodium bicarbonate in the treatment of subtypes of acute lactic acidosis: physiologic considerations. *Anesthesiology* 72:1064-1076, 1990

72. Kette F, Weil MH, von Planta M, et al: Buffer agents do not reverse intramyocardial acidosis during cardiac resuscitation. *Circulation* 81:1660-1666, 1990

73. Gazmuri RJ, von Planta M, Weil MH, et al: Cardiac effects of carbon dioxide-consuming and carbon dioxide-generating buffers during cardiopulmonary resuscitation. *J Am Coll Cardiol* 15:482-490, 1990

74. Isserles SA, Breen PH: Can changes in end-tidal P_{CO_2} measure changes in cardiac output? *Anesth Analg* 73:808-814, 1991

75. Ornato JP, Garnett AR, Glauser FL: Relationship between cardiac output and the end-tidal carbon dioxide tension. *Ann Emerg Med* 19:1104-1106, 1990

76. Falk JL, Rackow EC, Weil MH: End-tidal carbon dioxide concentration during cardiopulmonary resuscitation. *N Engl J Med* 318:607-611, 1988

77. Gudipati CV, Weil MH, Bisera J, et al: Expired carbon dioxide: a noninvasive monitor of cardiopulmonary resuscitation. *Circulation* 77:234-239, 1988

78. Kern KB, Sanders AB, Voorhees WD, et al: Changes in expired end-tidal carbon dioxide during cardiopulmonary resuscitation in dogs: a prognostic guide for resuscitation efforts. *J Am Coll Cardiol* 13:1184-1189, 1989

79. Sanders AB, Kern KB, Otto CW, et al: End-tidal carbon dioxide monitoring during cardiopulmonary resuscitation: a prognostic indicator for survival. *JAMA* 262:1347-1351, 1989

80. Callaham M, Barton C: Prediction of outcome of cardiopulmonary resuscitation from end-tidal carbon dioxide concentration. *Crit Care Med* 18:358-362, 1990

81. Ping STS, Mehta MP, Symreng T: Accuracy of the EEF CO_2 detector in the assessment of endotracheal tube placement. *Anesth Analg* 74:415-419, 1992

82. Varon AJ, Morrina J, Civetta JM: Clinical utility of a colorimetric end-tidal CO_2 detector in cardiopulmonary resuscitation and emergency intubation. *J Clin Monit* 7:289-293, 1991

83. Ornato JP, Shipley JB, Racht EM, et al: Multicenter study of a portable, hand-size, colorimetric end-tidal carbon dioxide detection device. *Ann Emerg Med* 21:518-523, 1992

84. White RD, Asplin BR: Out-of-hospital quantitative monitoring of end-tidal carbon dioxide pressure during CPR. *Ann Emerg Med* 23:25-30, 1994

85. Asplin BR, White RD: Prognostic value of end-tidal carbon dioxide pressures during out-of-hospital cardiac arrest. *Ann Emerg Med* 25:756-761, 1995

86. Cummins RO, Graves JR, Eisenberg MS, et al: Early transcutaneous pacing (TCP) for out-of-hospital cardiac arrest: no benefit when performed by emergency medical technicians (EMTs) or paramedics (abstract). *Circulation* 84 Suppl 2:417, 1991

87. Valenzuela TD, Spaite DW, Meislin HW, et al: Case and survival definitions in out-of-hospital cardiac arrest: effect on survival rate calculation. *JAMA* 267:272-274, 1992

88. Longstreth WT Jr, Cobb LA, Fahrenbruch CE, et al: Does age affect outcomes of out-of-hospital cardiopulmonary resuscitation? *JAMA* 264:2109-2110, 1990

89. Greene HL: Sudden arrhythmic cardiac death—mechanisms, resuscitation and classification: the Seattle perspective. *Am J Cardiol* 65:4B-12B, 1990

90. Eisenberg MS, Cummins RO, Damon S, et al: Survival rates from out-of-hospital cardiac arrest: recommendations for uniform definitions and data to report. *Ann Emerg Med* 19:1249-1259, 1990

91. Becker LB, Ostrander MP, Barrett J, et al: Outcome of CPR in a large metropolitan area—where are the survivors? *Ann Emerg Med* 20:355-361, 1991

92. Cobb LA, Weaver WD, Fahrenbruch CE, et al: Community-based interventions for sudden cardiac death: impact, limitations, and changes. *Circulation* 85 Suppl 1:98-102, 1992

CHAPTER

25

Pacing

A. Antibradycardia devices

David L. Hayes, M.D., and Michael J. Osborn, M.D.

Few areas in clinical medicine are more dependent upon, and have been affected more by, advances in engineering technology than cardiac pacing. In the more than 30 years since the first implantation of a pacing system, there has been a significant change not only in pulse generators (power sources, circuitry) and leads but also in the indications for pacing, pacing modalities, implantation techniques, and follow-up of patients with implanted pacing devices. These changes are largely a direct result of engineering improvements in the implantable devices and the external systems used to monitor and to modify pacemaker function.

Initially, pacemaker therapy was used to prevent death and to prolong the life of patients with bradyarrhythmias. In this regard it has been highly successful. There has been a significant reduction in the mortality rate of patients with atrioventricular (AV) block (those paced compared to those not paced). The survival rates for patients given pacemakers for all types of conduction abnormalities are decreased slightly for each decade of life (compared to actuarial life tables), but even in the ninth decade there is an acceptable prognosis.

In addition to the prolongation of life by prevention of life-threatening bradyarrhythmias, the proliferation of "physiologic" pacing devices has allowed us to improve the quality of life for selected patients and has given us more therapeutic options in the management of bradyarrhythmias.

HISTORICAL BACKGROUND

In the early 1930s the first artificial device used to stimulate the heart was developed and introduced into clinical medicine by Albert Hyman.[1] The generator was large, weighing more than 6.8 kg (15 lb) and mechanically driven by a spring motor. He applied a stimulus from the pacemaker to the right atrium by passing a long needle (electrode) through the chest wall into the atrial myocardium. It was successful in 14 of 43 cases.

By using the electrode in the esophagus and another electrode over the precordium in a dog, Paul Zoll[2] demonstrated that electrical stimuli could cause atrial or ventricular electrical responses and effective myocardial contractions. He subsequently found that use of two surface electrodes, one on each side of the precordium, was just as effective as the combination of a precordial and an esophageal electrode. Large amounts of current (30-150 V or 50-200 mA) were required to stimulate the heart effectively, but the use of short pulse widths (2 to 3 msec) reduced the danger of initiating ventricular tachyarrhythmias.

In 1952 this technique was expanded to human use in two patients with symptomatic and complete heart block. The intensity of the current (130 V) necessary to produce ventricular beats in one of the patients caused "slight contraction of the thoracic muscles, but was not disturbing to the patient." The heart was kept beating for 25 minutes in one patient and for 5 days in the other. The first patient died of cardiac tamponade. In the second, the myocardium ultimately recovered spontaneously, with depolarization resulting in an idioventricular rhythm.[3]

Although helpful in some patients on a temporary basis, this technique was not an acceptable system for long-term pacing. It was clear that direct stimulation of the myocardium would be required. In 1957 a temporary stainless steel cathodal lead was sutured to the myocardium at the time of thoracotomy and attached to an external pulse generator for the purpose of temporary pacing in patients with Stokes-Adams attacks.[4] Stimulation failed uniformly within about 7 weeks because of increasing thresholds for myocardial capture secondary to a foreign body tissue reaction to sterile contaminants in the electrode surface.[2]

In 1958 the first totally implantable pacing system (pulse generator and lead) was utilized by Senning.[5] The patient was a 43-year-old man who suffered from Stokes-Adams attacks. Two myocardial electrodes were sutured into the left ventricle and connected to a nickel/cadmium battery-powered rechargeable pulse generator placed into the abdominal wall beneath the rectus fascia. The first generator failed after 3 hours; the second failed after 8 days. The patient was not treated by pacing again until 3 years later, when he was given a mercury battery-powered pulse generator.

The first clinical application of right heart catheterization to stimulate the ventricular endocardium via venous catheter was made by Furman and Schwedel[6] in 1958. The catheter was introduced into the venous system via the median basilic vein (antecubital cutdown) and guided into the right ventricle under fluoroscopic observation. The first patient had complete heart block with associated syncope and was paced temporarily during a gastrointestinal operation; he died due to an episode of asystole shortly after discontinuation of pacing. The second patient had atrial fibrillation with complete AV dissociation and Stokes-Adams attack. Attempts to manage his rhythm disturbance by pharmacologic intervention and the use of an external pacemaker were unsuccessful. Therefore, an endocardial pacing catheter was positioned in the right ventricle, and temporary pacing was instituted and continued for approximately 6 weeks, until he again developed atrial fibrillation with AV conduction. He had been confined to a bed or bedside chair; with his temporary pacing device placed on a small table and use of a 50-ft extension cord, he was able to walk for short distances. With resumption of a conducted rhythm, ambulation was allowed. The catheter was finally withdrawn 96 days after the initiation of endocardial pacing.

The demonstration that the heart could be stimulated by using either myocardial or endocardial pacing electrodes and the development of a fully implantable battery-powered pacing system with reliable transistors[7] led to the increased use of this therapeutic modality in the treatment of AV block. A battery-powered, hand-held atrial synchronous pacemaker that detected atrial depolarization and amplified the signal sufficiently to produce ventricular stimulation was described in 1957.[8] Two years later, a P-synchronous system that detected the atrial electrogram and stimulated the ventricle after a preset delay was developed and implanted. However, widespread clinical use of this type of pacing modality lagged by almost 20 years. The same can be said for AV sequential type pacing devices, which were first introduced in the late 1950s.[9]

The sensing requirements of the atrial synchronous units led to the development of sophisticated sensing circuits and the introduction of single-chamber demand pacing systems in 1963.[10]

In the early 1970s two further developments occurred that have had a profound effect on the field of cardiac pacing. These were the use of lithium batteries as a power source for implantable pulse generators and the introduction of programmability based on complementary metal oxide semiconductor technology.[11] In the 1980s, pacemakers capable of rate adaptation were introduced. Rate-adaptive pacemakers allowed the paced rate to be increased through a sensor incorporated into the pacemaker that monitored some physiologic variable. By the late 1980s, rate-adaptive pacemakers were used frequently.

INDICATIONS

The precise criteria for the implantation of a permanent pacemaker vary from institution to institution. However, there are certain conditions that are generally accepted to be definite indications for permanent pacing and certain conduction disturbances in which it is generally agreed that a permanent pacemaker is not necessary. Because of changes in diagnosis and therapy as well as continued research and development, there seems to be some degree of constant change in absolute indications for permanent pacing. Difficulties arise in attempting to list rigid indications for permanent pacemaker insertion. A joint committee of the American College of Cardiology and the American Heart Association has developed guidelines for permanent pacemaker implantation. This statement is an excellent guide for clinical decision-making in determining the need for permanent pacing.[12]

The decision for implantation of a permanent pacemaker must be arrived at by adherence to a fundamental principle of clinical medicine—careful, thoughtful analysis of each patient by the responsible physician. This includes giving attention to the general medical status of the patient as well as the specifics of the cardiac rhythm disturbance.

The indication for permanent pacing must meet generally accepted clinical guidelines, such as those set forth by the American College of Cardiology and American Heart Association. The need for the pacemaker and supporting evidence, such as electrocardiographic (ECG) tracings, must be clearly documented in the patient's medical record. Clear documentation is required to assure reimbursement by Medicare or third-party payers.

The literature abounds with articles dealing with indications for cardiac pacing.[13] Pacing is appropriate for the control of any symptomatic bradyarrhythmia, particularly bradyarrhythmias not responsive to medical management. The continued expansion of pacemaker technology also increased the indications for permanent pacing. Nevertheless, many times it is not clear when a permanent pacemaker should be utilized. Areas in which controversy still exists regarding the use of permanent pacemakers include bifascicular and trifascicular block,[14] new-onset bundle-branch block in the setting of an acute myocardial infarction,[15,16] and treatment of low cardiac output syndromes in the presence of bradycardia (specifically, to aid in the treatment of chronic congestive heart failure or renal failure).

Acquired AV block, AV block occurring with myocardial infarction, bifascicular and trifascicular block (chronic), sinus node dysfunction and sinus bradycardia, and carotid hypersensitivity will be discussed in terms of whether indications for permanent pacemakers are definite, probable, or lacking. Indications for antitachycardia pacing are dealt with in chapter 25B.

Acquired AV block

AV block is defined as an impairment of conduction from the atrium to and within the specialized conducting tissue of the ventricular septum resulting in a complex variety of clinical and ECG findings. AV block is further classified traditionally into first-degree, second-degree, or third-degree (or complete) heart block. It can be defined anatomically as occurring at a supra-Hisian, intra-Hisian,

Table 25A-1 Indications for permanent pacemaker in acquired AV block

Necessary	Probably necessary	Probably not necessary
Symptomatic complete heart block, intermittent or permanent Second-degree AV block of any type or site associated with symptoms due to bradycardia	Asymptomatic complete heart block at any anatomic site, permanent or intermittent Asymptomatic, type II, second-degree AV block at the intra-Hisian or infra-Hisian level Congenital complete heart block	First-degree AV block Asymptomatic, type I, second-degree AV block at the AV node level

or infra-Hisian location. More specifically, if the patient has a wide QRS complex, there is a greater probability that the conduction disturbance is infra-Hisian.

Patients with abnormalities of AV conduction may be asymptomatic or may experience severe symptoms related to profound bradycardia or ventricular arrhythmias. Decisions regarding the need for an implanted pacemaker in the presence of impaired AV conduction are influenced by a number of factors, but most importantly by the presence or absence of symptoms that may be attributable directly to the arrhythmia (Table 25A-1). Patients who have complete heart block associated with syncope survive longer with permanent pacing. However, there is no evidence to suggest that survival is enhanced by pacemaker therapy in patients with isolated first-degree AV block, and the prognosis in type I second-degree AV block (Wenckebach), when it is due to AV nodal delay, is usually benign as well. However, in patients who have type II second-degree heart block, either intra- or infra-Hisian, the symptoms are frequent and the prognosis is compromised because progression to complete heart block is common.[17]

Acquired AV block is most commonly idiopathic and related to aging, but there are many potential causes (Table 25A-2).

AV block with myocardial infarction

Patients with myocardial infarction may experience a variety of chronic or permanent conduction disturbances related largely to the site of infarction.[19] Indications for permanent pacing after myocardial infarction in patients experiencing AV block are related in large measure to the presence of intraventricular conduction defects (Table 25A-3). Patients may also develop chronic sinus node dysfunction after myocardial infarction or drug-resistant tachyarrhythmia.

The requirement for temporary pacing in acute myocardial infarctions does not necessarily constitute an indication for permanent pacing. The long-term prognosis in survivors of acute myocardial infarction who have had AV block is related primarily to the extent of myocardial injury rather than to the AV block per se.[20] The need for permanent pacing in patients with myocardial infarction and AV block does not necessarily depend on the presence of symptoms.

Permanent pacing for persistent tachycardia-brady-

Table 25A-2 Causes of acquired AV block

- Idiopathic (senescent) AV block
- Coronary artery disease
- Calcific valvular disease
- Postoperative or traumatic condition
- AV node ablation[18]
- Therapeutic irradiation of the chest
- Infectious
  - Syphilis
  - Diphtheria
  - Chagas' disease
  - Tuberculosis
  - Toxoplasmosis
  - Lyme disease*
  - Viral myocarditis (Epstein-Barr, varicella, etc.)
  - Infective endocarditis
- Collagen-vascular
  - Rheumatoid arthritis
  - Scleroderma
  - Dermatomyositis
  - Ankylosing spondylitis
  - Polyarteritis nodosa
  - Systemic lupus erythematosus
  - Marfan's syndrome
- Infiltrative
  - Sarcoidosis
  - Amyloidosis
  - Hemochromatosis
  - Malignant disease (lymphomatous or solid tumor)
- Neuromuscular
  - Progressive external ophthalmoplegia (Kearns-Sayre syndrome)
  - Myotonic muscular dystrophy
  - Peroneal muscular atrophy (Charcot-Marie-Tooth disease)
  - Scapuloperoneal syndrome
  - Limb-girdle dystrophy
- Drug effect
  - Digoxin
  - β-Blocking agents
  - Calcium-blocking agents
  - Amiodarone
  - Procainamide
  - Class 1C agents: propafenone, encainide, flecainide

*AV block secondary to Lyme disease does not require permanent pacing.

Table 25A-3 Indications for permanent pacemaker in AV block with myocardial infarction

Necessary	Probably necessary	Probably not necessary
Mobitz type II or complete AV block (symptomatic or asymptomatic) Bilateral bundle-branch block Symptomatic bradyarrhythmias of any origin or mechanism	New right bundle-branch block with new left axis deviation Left anterior or left posterior hemiblock alone Transient bifascicular block Tachycardia/bradycardia syndrome	First-degree AV block Asymptomatic Wenckebach AV block in inferior myocardial infarction Asymptomatic or transient sinus or AV junctional (nodal) delay New asymptomatic bradyarrhythmias Right bundle-branch block

Table 25A-4 Indications for permanent pacemaker in sinus node dysfunction

Necessary	Probably necessary	Probably not necessary
Sinus node dysfunction with documented symptomatic bradycardia Symptomatic sinus bradycardia due to long-term drug therapy for which there is no acceptable alternative	Sinus node dysfunction with documented rates less than 45 beats/min without clear-cut association between significant symptoms consistent with bradycardia	Sinus node dysfunction in asymptomatic patients Sinus bradycardia (less than 45 beats/min) in asymptomatic patients

cardia or sinus node dysfunction after myocardial infarction is reserved for patients who have symptoms. If drug therapy results in symptomatic bradycardia, criteria for permanent pacing should follow the guidelines given for sinus node dysfunction (Table 25A-4).

Bifascicular and trifascicular block (chronic)

Trifascicular heart block causing symptoms is associated with a high mortality and a significant incidence of sudden death.[21]

Syncope is uncommon in patients with bifascicular block. It usually is not recurrent, nor is it associated with increased incidence of sudden death.[22] However, in the presence of complete heart block, either permanent or transient, syncope is associated with an increased incidence of sudden death.[22] Thus, being unable to define the cause of syncope in the presence of bifascicular or trifascicular block, it appears reasonable to assume that the syncope may be due to transient complete heart block and therefore prophylactic permanent pacing is indicated.

The evidence is impressive that the rate of progression of bifascicular block to complete heart block is low. Furthermore, no single clinical or laboratory variable including bifascicular block identifies patients at high risk of death from a future bradyarrhythmia due to a fascicular block.[14] Therefore, as noted in Table 25A-5, pacing is probably not necessary for asymptomatic bifascicular or trifascicular block.

Of the many laboratory variables, the P-R and H-V intervals have been singled out as possible predictors of complete heart block and sudden death. Evidence indicates that P-R prolongation is common in patients with bifascicular block; however, the prolongation is most often at the level of the AV node. Furthermore, there is no correlation between the P-R and H-V intervals nor between the length of the P-R interval and progression to complete heart block and death.[23-25]

In the symptomatic patient, i.e., with syncope or near-syncope, an H-V interval of 100 msec or greater is generally an accepted indication for permanent pacing. If the patient is to receive cardioactive drugs, e.g., procainamide, that may further prolong the H-V interval, some would consider permanent pacing for an H-V interval of 70 msec or greater.

Sinus node dysfunction

Sinus node dysfunction or "sick sinus syndrome" includes various cardiac arrhythmias that have been classified in many ways. Sinoatrial disturbances associated with sinus node dysfunction include symptomatic sinus bradycardia, sinus arrest, sinoatrial block, and paroxysmal supraventricular tachycardia alternating with periods of bradycardia or even asystole. The definition of bradycardia varies from institution to institution, but it generally includes a rate, during waking hours, less than 40 to 50 beats/min. There is disagreement as to the absolute cycle length at which treatment should be required. It is known that during sleep some people have sinus pauses as long as 4 seconds.[26] Therefore, during ambulatory monitoring of the awake patient, the interval between sinus depolariza-

Table 25A-5 Indications for permanent pacemaker in bifascicular and trifascicular block

Necessary	Probably necessary	Probably not necessary
Bifascicular block with intermittent complete heart block associated with symptomatic bradyarrhythmias Bifascicular block with intermittent Mobitz type II heart block with symptoms attributable to the heart block	Bifascicular or trifascicular block with intermittent Mobitz type II AV block without symptoms Bifascicular or trifascicular block with syncope thought to be due to bradyarrhythmia	Fascicular blocks without AV block or symptoms Fascicular blocks with first-degree AV block without symptoms

tions generally is considered to be abnormal if it is greater than 3 seconds (the absolute value depends on the specific local definition of this abnormality).

In sinus node dysfunction, symptoms should be correlated with the specific arrhythmia. Pacing should be considered for any recurrent symptomatic sinus bradycardia.[27-31] Many patients who have episodes of both tachycardia and bradycardia are asymptomatic. Others are symptomatic until medication required for treatment of the tachycardia is given, which then exacerbates the tendency toward bradycardia. The treatment of tachycardia episodes therefore leads to the need for permanent pacing for the bradycardia (see Table 25A-4).

Neurocardiogenic syncope

Permanent pacing may be indicated for some of the several types of neurally mediated syncope. The terminology used for the various disorders is unnecessarily confusing. The disorders are asymptomatic carotid sinus hypersensitivity, carotid sinus syndrome, benign vasovagal syncope, and malignant vasovagal syncope.

Understanding the physiology involved is crucial to understanding the clinical manifestations. The carotid sinus reflex is the physiologic response to pressure exerted on the carotid sinus. Stimulation results in activation of baroreceptors within the wall of the carotid sinus. Vagal efferents then result in cardiac slowing. Although this reflex is physiologic, some persons have an exaggerated or even pathologic response. This reflex has two components, a cardioinhibitory response and a vasodepressor response. A cardioinhibitory response results from increased parasympathetic tone and may be manifested by any or all of the following: sinus bradycardia, P-R prolongation, and advanced AV block. The vasodepressor response is due to decreased sympathetic activity and secondary hypotension. Although a pure cardioinhibitory or pure vasodepressor response may occur, a mixed response is most common.

The definitions of normal and abnormal responses are somewhat arbitrary. Ventricular asystole of 3 seconds or a substantial decrease in blood pressure (30 to 50 mm Hg), or both, is abnormal. An abnormal response to carotid sinus massage occurs in 25% to 30% of patients over 50 years of age. Men are affected approximately twice as frequently as women, and the right carotid sinus usually is more sensitive than the left. Although most of these patients are asymptomatic during carotid sinus massage and have no clinical history of syncope, others may have had recurrent syncope. Patients with syncope may have a typical history related to a tight collar or neck extension but more commonly have not identified any definite provocative maneuvers. If carotid sinus massage reproduces the patient's symptoms and is associated with significant cardioinhibition or vasodepression, a diagnosis of carotid sinus syndrome can be made and treatment could be initiated. If carotid sinus massage has a positive result but does not reproduce the patient's symptoms, a hypersensitive carotid reflex that may not be of clinical significance has been demonstrated, and other causes for syncope should be investigated. If the result of carotid sinus massage is negative, however, tilt testing may be indicated.

Tilt testing can provide the physiologic environment to reproduce malignant vasovagal syncope.[32,33] With head-up tilt, susceptible patients have decreased venous return and subsequent decrease in left ventricular filling, which may result in efferent vagal discharge. Stimulation of baroreceptors and adrenergic discharge may also result in efferent vagal discharge. Vasodilatation and hypotension as well as cardiac slowing may result from efferent vagal discharge. It is important to document whether the predominant cause of symptoms is cardioinhibitory or vasodepressor in origin because therapy differs. Tilt-table testing is often helpful in determining the predominant cause. In the patient with significant cardioinhibition, permanent pacing is appropriate and should eliminate most, if not all, of the patient's symptoms. In the patient with pure vasodepression, however, other measures, such as drugs and compressive stockings, are best for treatment. In the patient with a mixed response but a significant vasodepressor response, dual-chamber permanent pacing helps to blunt the vasodepressor-related symptoms.[34-36] In this situation, the ideal dual-chamber pacemaker would have the capability of hysteresis. The device would be programmed to a hysteresis rate (40 to 50 ppm) that would allow the patient to remain in normal sinus rhythm most of the time, with a pacing rate of 80 to 100 ppm. Therefore, when an episode of cardioinhibition and vasodepression occurs and the patient's intrinsic heart rate slows to less than the hysteresis rate, the pacemaker begins pacing at the programmed rate of 80 to 100 ppm. Ideally, to allow restoration of the patient's intrinsic rhythm, the pacemaker should be capable of "search hysteresis," whereby the pacemaker intermittently, at programmed intervals, suspends pacing to determine if the patient's intrinsic rate is once again greater than the hysteresis rate.

Benign vasovagal syncope, or a "simple faint," usually does not require therapy. Associated rhythms are usually prolonged sinus arrest without nodal or ventricular escape and may be associated with dramatic symptoms, including syncope, often undiagnosed for prolonged periods. Syncope has been reported during many activities such as swallowing, coitus, cough, micturition, and respiration. Pacemaker implantation may be an effective means of preventing syncope, but whether these patients should receive permanent pacing is somewhat controversial. The argument against pacing is that such vagally mediated events do not usually result in significant reduction in mortality. However, the events may occur during situations such as operation of a motor vehicle or heavy machinery that predispose the patient or bystanders to danger.

Permanent pacing for cardiomyopathic states

Hypertrophic obstructive cardiomyopathy. Dual-chamber pacing has been proposed as a therapeutic modality for patients with severe, symptomatic hypertrophic obstructive cardiomyopathy.[37,38] Initial reports have shown a significant reduction in the left ventricular tract gradient and symptomatic improvement in patients with hypertrophic obstructive cardiomyopathy in whom dual-chamber pacemakers have been implanted. The mechanism of action of dual-chamber pacing on patients with hypertrophic obstructive cardiomyopathy remains uncertain. It is hypothesized that the altered septal activation caused by right ventricular pacing may result in less narrowing of the left ventricular outflow tract and a subsequent decrease in the Venturi effect, causing systolic anterior motion of the mitral valve. On the basis of the initial studies, it has been proposed that dual-chamber pacing be instituted in all patients with symptomatic hypertrophic obstructive cardiomyopathy who would otherwise be surgical candidates.[38]

It has been recognized that AV timing is critical if optimal hemodynamic improvement is to be achieved. Although some patients with hypertrophic obstructive cardiomyopathy have optimal improvement with a very short AV interval, others may have hemodynamic deterioration if the AV interval is too short. Further investigation is necessary to determine the best method for programming the AV interval. It has also been recognized that depolarization of the ventricle must occur via the pacemaker. Some investigators have advocated AV nodal ablation to assure paced ventricular depolarization if rapid intrinsic AV nodal conduction prevents total ventricular depolarization via the pacing stimulus.

Permanent pacing in patients with hypertrophic cardiomyopathy may possibly result in a long-term remodeling effect of the left ventricle. Additional studies will be necessary to determine if remodeling does occur.

The optimal role of pacing for treatment of hypertrophic cardiomyopathy remains to be defined. Although it may improve symptoms in some patients, it has been ineffective in others, and the long-term outcome is not yet clear.

Dilated cardiomyopathy. Dual-chamber pacing has been reported to be effective in the treatment of patients with idiopathic dilated cardiomyopathy. Four papers on the use of DDD pacing in this disorder, including long-term follow-up experience, have been published since 1990. A small number of abstracts and some unpublished, anecdotal, and largely undocumented reports also exist.

Treatment of idiopathic dilated cardiomyopathy with short AV interval DDD pacing was first reported by Hochleitner et al.[39] They treated 16 patients with idiopathic dilated cardiomyopathy refractory to pharmacologic therapy (digitalis, vasodilators, angiotensin-converting enzyme inhibitors). All were in New York Heart Association functional class III or IV. All were critically ill and either awaiting heart transplant (40%) or had no hope of transplant (60%). Eight were in cardiogenic shock. Hochleitner et al. reported dramatic improvement in New York Heart Association functional class and a reduction in mortality over that expected at 1 year. Hemodynamic findings included an increase in left ventricular ejection fraction and blood pressure and normalization of heart rate.

Kataoka[40] reported results of studies performed in one patient in an attempt to replicate the Hochleitner et al. results. Although this report of a single case must be interpreted cautiously, it consistently supports the conclusions of Hochleitner et al. with similar hemodynamic findings.

Brecker et al.[41] presented evidence that patients with dilated cardiomyopathy have reduced ventricular filling time associated with loss of atrial-ventricular synchrony and mitral-tricuspid valve regurgitation. In their study, 12 patients treated with temporary or permanent short AV interval DDD pacing had improvement in ventricular filling and a reduction in regurgitant flow. These patients showed improvements in hemodynamic indices and increases in exercise time.

Hochleitner et al.[42] subsequently published 5-year follow-up results for their original patient cohort. Excluding four patients who received transplants, median survival in this critically ill population was 22 months. Improvements in hemodynamic function continued throughout the five cases with known cause; except for one death due to cancer, all deaths were due to embolic events. None resulted from continued deterioration in ventricular function. No patient needed rehospitalization due to a worsening of heart failure after pacemaker implantation.

Not all patients with dilated cardiomyopathy respond to permanent pacing. The mechanisms by which permanent pacing may result in improvement remain uncertain, but improvement probably is due to optimization of AV synchrony. Further work is needed to identify those who will have a response to permanent pacing.

Pacing for the prevention of atrial fibrillation

It is theorized that atrial fibrillation occurs when dispersion of refractoriness is present within the atria and that this leads to regions of functional block and zones of slow conduction when spontaneous premature atrial impulses occur. It is possible that reducing this dispersion of refractoriness may prevent atrial premature complexes from causing fibrillation. One method to decrease the dispersion of refractoriness may be to pace the atrium from dual sites.

Daubert et al.[43] reported on five patients with paroxysmal atrial rhythm disturbances who were paced from the right atrium and the coronary sinus simultaneously. During a short follow-up period, 2 to 8 months, none of the patients had recurrent atrial rhythm disturbances with dual-site atrial pacing. Other centers are currently investigating this potential application for pacing.

PACEMAKER LEADS

The evolution through several generations of transvenous leads, from bare tips of wires inserted in the myocardium to stainless steel pins protruding from a silicone rubber pad placed in a myocardial stab wound, has been rewarding.

As transvenous leads evolved, it became obvious that they were easier and less traumatic to implant than those requiring a transthoracic approach. However, although the transvenous approach rapidly became more popular than the transthoracic, the results of the former method were not as reliable in the early years. Problems with the early transvenous systems included dislodgment, perforation, and other complications that required reoperation.

The flange, or wedge-tip, transvenous lead was one of the first designed to provide a nondislodging connection. This design has changed extensively in recent years, and there now are various "positive fixation" or "self-anchoring" mechanisms. They operate by active or passive means. Passive fixation refers to leads that do not invade the myocardium but achieve permanent fixation by special positioning features, entrapment among the trabeculae, or tissue ingrowth. Active fixation leads are those that actually penetrate the myocardium. A number of such leads have been tested. These range from the most popular "screw-in" mechanism to barbs, darts, grips, and pincers.

Tined electrodes remain the most widely used of the passive variety; screw-in leads are the most popular active-fixation device. It has not been clearly established that one type is superior, each having its own advantages.

Conductor

Various conductor configurations have been utilized, including multistrand unipolar conductor, tightly wound unipolar conductor, space-wound unifilar unipolar conductor, parallel bipolar conductors, coaxial bipolar conductor, four-filar single-strand tinsel wire, six-filar multistranded tinsel wire, and multifilar close-wound unipolar conductors. Current widely used conductor types include single-filar coils, multifilar coils, and multifilar coils composed of superalloys.

Classically, platinum/iridium alloy has been used because platinum is a good electrical conductor in biologic fluids as a consequence of modulation of oxygen adsorption on its surface. Activated pyrolytic carbon tip also displays catalytic behavior at the electrode/myocardium interface, but because of higher polarization potentials, it results in lower chronic thresholds of stimulation, which means energy saving and greater pacemaker longevity for the patient.

Electrode tip design may be either solid or porous. Porous surface and solid electrodes have about the same acute threshold performance, but porous surface electrodes have somewhat lower chronic thresholds.[44] Many designs have now been introduced to achieve low chronic thresholds.[45]

The steroid-eluting electrode tip is capable of gradually eluting dexamethasone from a steroid-silicone rubber compound core in an attempt to minimize fibrous encapsulation and, in turn, to lower the chronic stimulation threshold. These leads produce a dramatic reduction in pacing threshold and largely abolish the transient threshold increase seen with conventional leads.[46,47] Other steroid-eluting designs, such as a porcelain collar positioned near the tip, are also being investigated in the United States and are clinically available in other countries.

Insulation

Silicone rubber and polyurethane are commonly used insulation materials. There has been concern about the long-term performance of the polyurethane lead because of the unacceptable failure rate of several specific polyurethane leads.[48-50] In these specific leads, difficulties in manufacturing were identified that appear to have been limited to those leads and were not indicative of overall polyurethane experience.

Epicardial leads

Epicardial electrodes are used in only a small percentage of patients receiving permanent pacemakers. This type generally is used only when the patient has undergone cardiac surgery; epicardial leads are placed at the time of operation because of an anticipated need for permanent pacing or when the transvenous approach is abandoned because of technical difficulties. Epicardial pacing has been largely abandoned not only because of the lower morbidity and mortality associated with transvenous techniques but also because epicardial pacing usually results in higher chronic stimulation thresholds and a higher incidence of exit block as well as a greater fracture rate and lack of a good atrial epicardial lead.

Porous, platinized-platinum epicardial electrode design with or without steroid elution appears, in early experience, to significantly lower chronic epicardial pacing thresholds.[51] For patients in whom transvenous pacing is not appropriate, epicardial leads with improved chronic pacing thresholds will be very important.

Table 25A-6 Compatibility of pacemaker headers and pacing leads

Header	Lead
VS-1/IS-1	Accepts only VS-1/IS-1 leads
VS-1A/IS-1A	Accepts VS-1/IS-1 leads and Cordis-style 3.2-mm in-line leads (incorporates a longer connector pin)
VS-1B/IS-1B	Accepts VS-1/IS-1 leads and 3.2-mm in-line leads of Cordis, Medtronic, CPI, and Telectronics styles (incorporates a longer connector pin and sealing rings) (see Fig 25A-1)

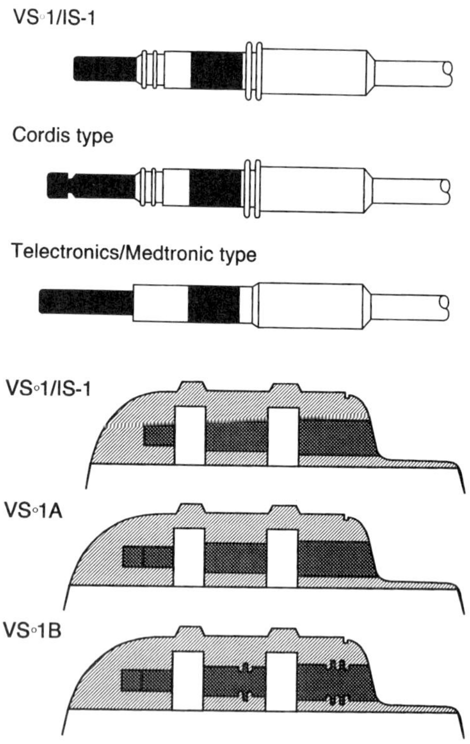

Fig 25A-1 The VS-1/IS-1 connectors are intended to restore universal interconnection of all leads and pulse generators via the newly standardized 3.2-mm connectors. The pin is connected to the negative output, and the ring is connected to the positive terminal in the pulse generator header. Unipolar leads of similar configuration exist but without a positive terminal; they are of the same size and are interchangeable with a bipolar receptacle. The four ridges represent the sealing rings, which prevent the ingress of fluid into the header. Leads designated VS-1A accept VS-1 leads and Cordis-style 3.2-mm in-line leads (incorporating a longer pin). Leads designated VS-1B accept Cordis, Medtronic, CPI, and Telectronics styles of 3.2-mm in-line leads (incorporating a longer pin and sealing rings). (From A short course on VS-1/IS-1. Teleceptor™ Vol. 3, no 5, September 1989. By permission of Teletronics Pacing Systems.)

Lead connectors

A confusing issue for many years has been that of pacemaker-lead compatibility. Pacemakers from different manufacturers have had different-sized receptacles. Representatives of major pacemaker lead manufacturers developed ad hoc specifications for a "voluntary standard," or VS-1, design to standardize all connectors, unipolar and in-line bipolar, to a single size, i.e., 3.2 mm.[52] A formal, international pacing connector standard, the "international standard," or IS-1, design, was then jointly endorsed by the International Standards Organization (ISO) and International Electrotechnical Commission (IEC) after the addition of performance requirements to the VS-1 standards.[53]

VS-1/IS-1 pacing leads are 3.2 mm in diameter, have sealing rings on the lead, and have a short (0.508 cm) terminal pin. VS-1/IS-1 pacing leads fit all 3.2-mm pacemakers. VS-1/IS-1 pacemaker headers are 3.2 mm in diameter, have *no* sealing rings, have a short (5.08 cm) receptacle for the lead terminal, and accept only VS-1/IS-1 pacing leads. Table 25A-6 provides an abbreviated compatibility guide for various pacing leads and pacemaker headers. Pacemaker headers with the designation VS-1A and VS-1B still exist as a point of confusion. Pacemakers designated VS-1A are 3.2 mm in diameter, have no sealing rings, and have a long (0.851 cm) receptacle for the lead terminal. Pacemakers with the VS-1B designation have sealing rings in the header but are otherwise like the VS-1A designation (Fig 25A-1). This terminology need not be confusing. Dimensions are the same for both unipolar and bipolar VS-1/IS-1 leads and pacemakers. There is only one configuration for VS-1 and IS-1 lead connectors. The VS-1 and IS-1 designs have provisions within the pacemaker connector for three functional options (see Table 25A-6).

PACEMAKER IMPLANTATION TECHNIQUES

Epicardial pacing systems

Epicardial lead types. Although the choice of epicardial lead design is expanding, it is still rather limited in comparison with the endocardial variety.

One of the earlier epicardial lead designs has been called the "cobra-head" design because of its appearance (Fig 25A-2). The lead is attached directly to the myocardium by sutures after a hole for the electrode is made by a surgical blade.

One of the most commonly used designs for years was the corkscrew design. The electrode screws directly into the myocardium and does not require suturing. It is available in a two-turn model and a three-turn model (Fig 25A-3).

A third design is the "fish-hook" or "barbed" configuration (Fig 25A-4). The hook is placed into the myocardium and the lead sutured to the myocardium.

Surgical procedures. Several surgical procedures allow implantation of epicardial pacing electrodes. The two most commonly used are lateral thoracotomy for implan-

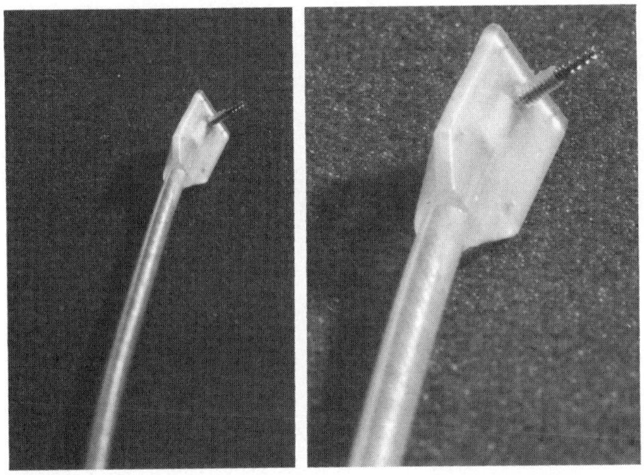

Fig 25A-2 "Cobra-head" epicardial lead. The lead is attached directly to the myocardium by sutures passed through holes in each of four corners of distal lead.

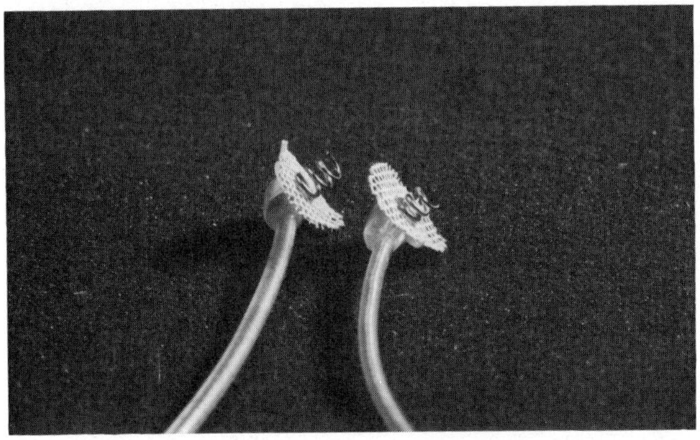

Fig 25A-3 Epicardial (corkscrew) electrodes: three-turn model **(left)** and two-turn model **(right)**.

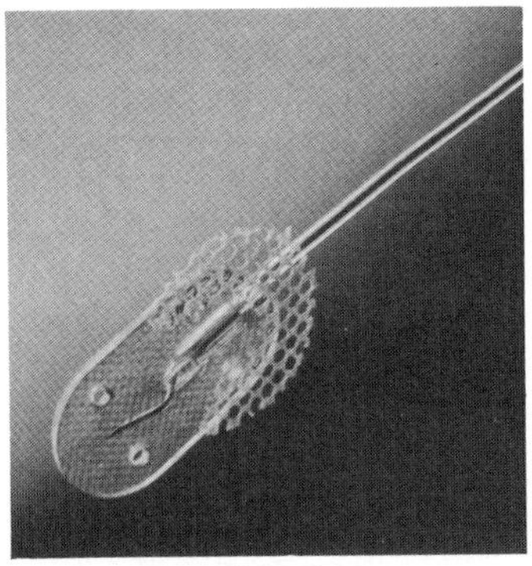

Fig 25A-4 Epicardial electrode of the "fish-hook" or "barbed" configuration. The barbed electrode is placed in the myocardium and the lead is fixed to the epicardium by nonabsorbable suture.

tation of electrodes on the left ventricular free wall, and subxiphoid or left subcostal approach for implantation of the sutureless electrodes on the left or right ventricle. In addition, various other techniques have been developed, including mediastinal implantation of atrial sensing electrodes, extrapleural thoracotomy, and intrapleural implantation of lead impulse generator.

Endocardial pacing systems

The vast majority of the patients who require pacing at our institution receive endocardial pacing systems. The leads and generators are implanted by cardiologists in a specially designed and equipped operating suite in a cardiac catheterization laboratory. A permanent C-arm fluoroscope enables us to guide the pacing catheters and to determine the adequacy of the final position in both the anteroposterior and lateral projections. The equipment necessary for appropriate patient monitoring, defibrillation, and resuscitation is always available in the room. The implanting physician is assisted by a scrub nurse (or technician), a circulating nurse (or technician), and a nurse who continuously monitors the ECG, measures lead and pulse generator parameters, records and measures intracardiac electrograms, and records all this information in the patient's permanent file. An anesthesia technician is also in attendance for airway management and in the event that IV medication is required either to control arrhythmia or for the patient's comfort.

The procedures are generally performed with local anesthesia (1% lidocaine), and the patients are given small amounts of sedatives or analgesics or both for additional relief of pain or anxiety. We ordinarily use general anesthesia only for patients unable to cooperate during the procedure because of age or confused mental status.

Venous access

SUBCLAVIAN VEIN. Subclavian venipuncture became increasingly popular after the reports by McNeill and Taylor[54] and by Littleford et al.[55] of the successful use of this technique in large clinical trials in Great Britain and in the United States, respectively. This approach has been used almost exclusively at our institution since 1978.[56]

An incision about two fingerbreadths below and parallel to the clavicle is made and carried down to the prepectoral fascia. A subcutaneous pocket is then created for the pulse generator as outlined above. The pocket is enlarged superiorly toward the clavicle (and subclavian vein) by blunt dissection. This additional space makes it easier to cannulate the subclavian vein and to fix the leads to the prepectoral fascia.

The subclavian vein is cannulated with a thin-walled 18-gauge needle. The needle is passed under the clavicle at the junction of its middle and lateral thirds and aimed toward the suprasternal notch (Fig 25A-5,A). When venous blood is freely aspirated, a J-tipped guide wire is advanced through the needle into the superior vena cava or right atrium, and the position is confirmed fluoroscopically (Fig 25A-5,B). The needle is then removed, leaving only the guide wire in the venous system. We have found that in most patients the subclavian vein can be cannu-

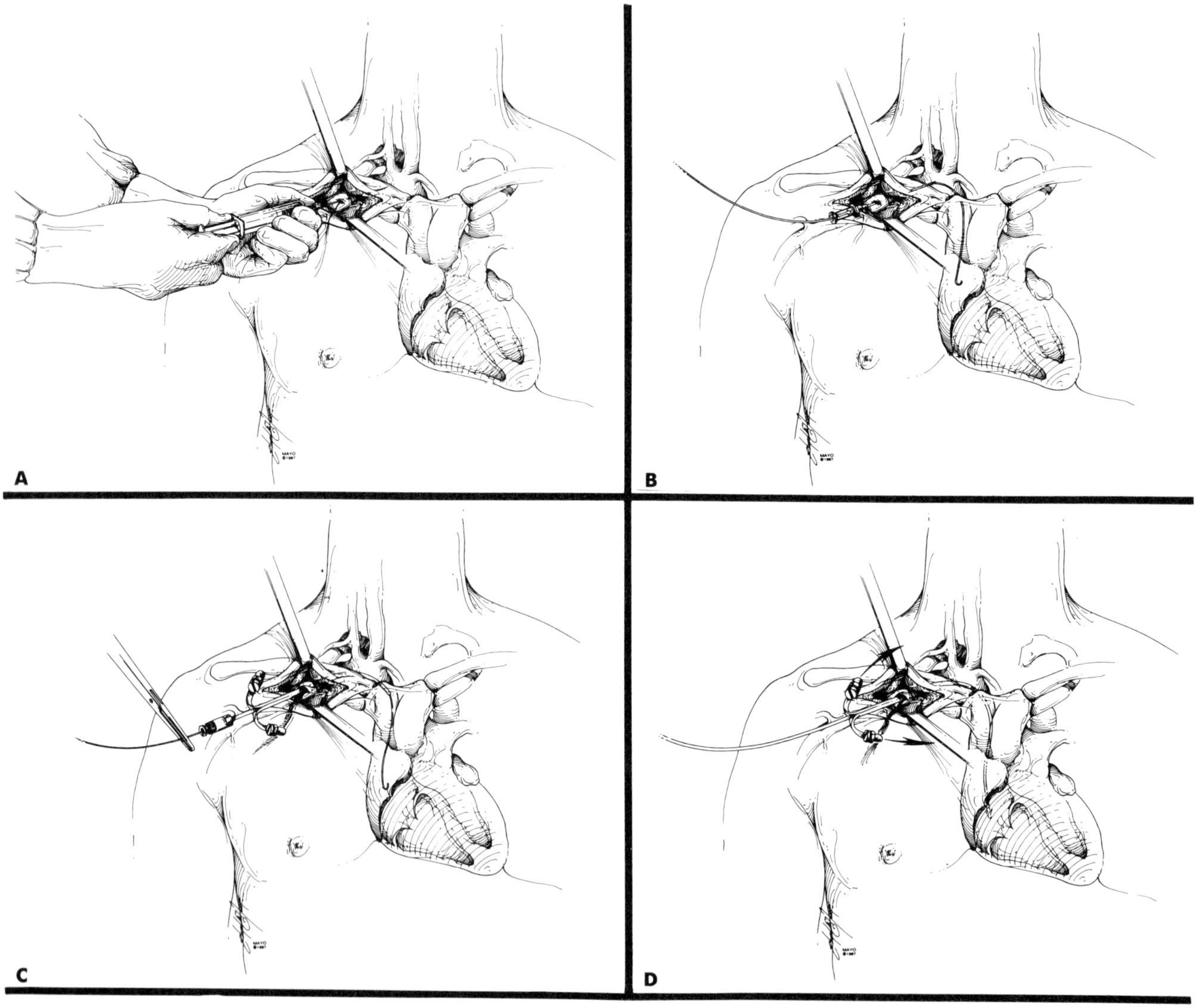

Fig 25A-5 Subclavian vein can be used for single- or dual-lead placement. **A,** initial step involves puncturing the vein with an 18-gauge needle. Blood is aspirated to ensure proper positioning in venous structure. **B,** syringe is removed and flexible guide wire is passed through needle until proximal end is in region of right atrium. **C,** with guide wire in place, needle is pulled back and off the wire. Dilator and peel-away sheath are then placed over guide wire and passed into subclavian vein. Sizes of dilator and peel-away sheath depend on size of lead or leads to be used. As dilator and sheath are being passed into vein, hemostat is placed on guide wire to prevent wire from being lost into the venous circulation. **D,** guide wire and dilator are removed from sheath, and pacing lead is quickly passed through sheath into right side of heart. *Arrows* indicate pulling the peel-away introducer away from the lead. If a second lead is to be used, a second subclavian puncture can be performed parallel to the already placed pacing lead. Care should be taken to avoid puncturing the indwelling lead.

lated in this manner with the patient lying flat. The operating table is usually placed in the Trendelenburg position during subclavian puncture.

The vein dilator and surrounding peel-away sheath are then passed over the guide wire into the superior vena cava (Fig 25A-5,C). The size of the sheath is determined by the size of the lead or leads to be inserted into the heart. For most leads, a 10F sheath is used. A few leads require a 12F sheath. If two leads are to be inserted via a single sheath, a 12F sheath is commonly used. The insertion of sheath and dilator is also monitored by fluoroscopy to ensure that they pass easily into the superior vena cava.

Once the sheath is in place, the dilator and guide wire are removed and the open end of the sheath is obstructed with a finger or by squeezing the sheath firmly to prevent

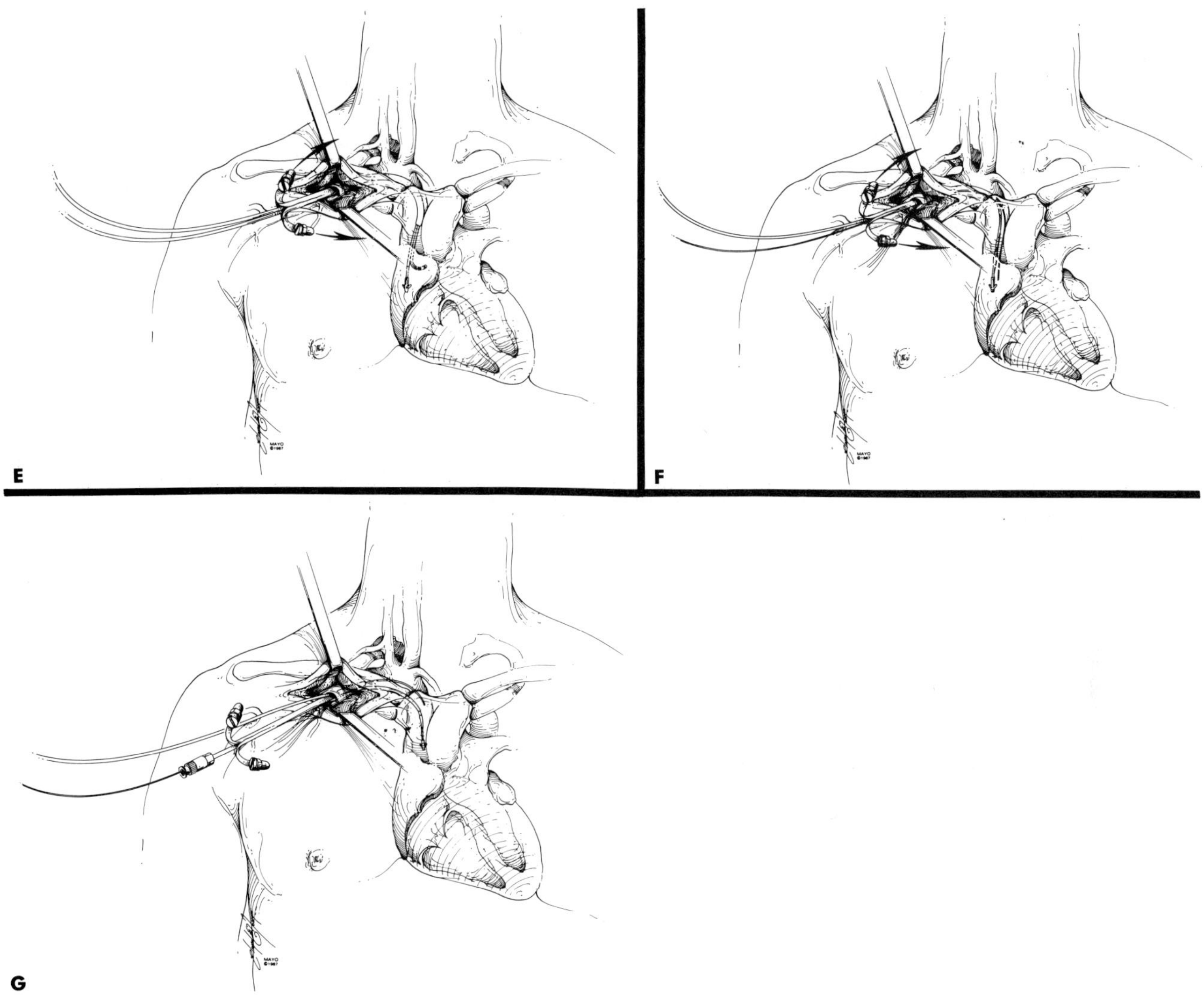

Fig 25A-5, cont'd. **E,** if two pacing leads are necessary, both leads can be inserted simultaneously if a peel-away introducer large enough to accommodate both leads is used. With straight stylets in place, one lead is staggered 1 to 2 cm behind the other, they are passed simultaneously into the right side of the heart, and the introducer is peeled away. **F,** two leads can be placed without a second subclavian puncture and without simultaneously passing the leads. As dilator and guide wire are removed and the initial pacing lead is passed into the right side of the heart, the guide wire is reinserted through a peel-away introducer alongside the pacing lead. The introducer is then peeled away, and pacing lead and guide wire are left in place. **G,** a second introducer is then placed over the guide wire. (From Holmes DR, Hayes DL, Furman S: Permanent pacemaker implantation. In *A Practice of Cardiac Pacing.* Second edition. Edited by S Furman, DL Hayes, DR Holmes Jr. Mount Kisco, New York, Futura Publishing Company, 1989, pp 239-287. By permission.)

bleeding or the aspiration of air. We perform this maneuver while the patient is holding his or her breath to decrease further the chance of air embolism. This should not be done after a deep inspiration, which will reduce intrathoracic pressure; rather, the patient is instructed to cease breathing without inhaling. Other authors have suggested placing the patient in the Trendelenburg position to increase venous pressure or, if this is not possible, raising the patient's legs to accomplish this same purpose.

Finally, the lead is passed through the sheath into the right atrium (Fig 25A-5,D). When the catheter position has been verified by fluoroscopy, the sheath is withdrawn from the vein and peeled off the catheter (see Fig

25A-5,D). The lead should be advanced as this sheath is withdrawn to prevent accidental withdrawal of the lead from the vein.

If the pacing system to be implanted requires the use of two leads, then a modification of the procedure is required. Either two venipunctures are performed and each lead is advanced through a separate sheath, or a single venipuncture is performed and both leads are advanced through a single sheath.

If two separate venipunctures are performed, we cannulate the vein twice and insert both guide wires into it. The first cannulation of the vein is done slightly medial to our usual position. The second cannulation is then performed lateral to the first. The lateral guide wire is clipped to the surgical drapes, and the ventricular lead is inserted into the heart through a 10-F sheath. When the ventricular lead is in an acceptable position in the right ventricular apex, the atrial lead is inserted and positioned. Movement of both catheters is very easy, with minimal interaction between the two. There have been no problems with bleeding related to the two separate venipunctures, nor have we encountered an increased incidence of other complications, primarily pneumothorax.

If only one venipuncture is performed, both leads can be inserted simultaneously via a larger dilator and sheath than would ordinarily be required. The atrial and ventricular leads are prepared for implantation by inserting straight stylets into both leads. The atrial electrode tip is placed 1 to 2 cm behind the ventricular electrode tip, and both are inserted with one motion immediately after removal of the dilator (Fig 25A-5,E). The passage of the leads may be facilitated by the use of a small amount of lubricant. Because both leads are entering the same opening, friction between the two may produce motion of both leads when either is moved. When positioning one lead, firmly grasping the other reduces this problem and permits independent manipulation of each lead.

A modification of the single-venipuncture technique has been occasionally used when the decision about the need for a dual-chamber pacing device is to be made intraoperatively. The vein is cannulated once and, through the usual peel-away sheath, the ventricular lead and a guide wire are advanced into the right heart (Fig 25A-5,F). If it is elected to insert two leads, the guide wire is in place and may be used; if not, it can be simply removed and a single lead system implanted (Fig 25A-5,G).

Various complications have been described as a consequence of subclavian venipuncture, including septic thrombosis, pneumothorax, AV fistula, and air embolism. The three major concerns that physicians have had about the use of the subclavian approach for lead implant include two of these complications (pneumothorax and air embolism) and concern about leakage around the venipuncture site with resultant hematoma formation.

A more medial subclavian puncture technique has been described that should minimize complications of subclavian vein puncture.[57] More medial placement of the lead may, however, increase the likelihood of crush injury to the lead between the clavicle and the first rib. Cadaver studies have indicated that subclavian crush injury may actually be caused by pressure from the subclavius muscle and not directly from bony injury.[58-60]

Subclavian puncture may also be facilitated and complications minimized by the use of contrast venography.[61] With contrast medium in the vein, the venipuncture needle can be positioned directly into the subclavian vein with fluoroscopic guidance.

The subclavian artery can be accidentally punctured, especially if the needle is aimed too far cephalad during venipuncture; usually this is without any significant ill effects. Firm pressure over the puncture site should control the bleeding without difficulty.

There have been some fatal complications related to this technique, including the cannulation of the pulmonary artery and superior vena cava with resultant prolonged and significant bleeding and massive air embolism.

The advantages of the technique are many and in our experience far outweigh the potential complications. These advantages include reduction in the time required for pacemaker implantation, ease of implantation of dual-chamber systems, and reduction in the requirement for intraoperative manipulations, which decreases the amount of surgical expertise required.

CEPHALIC VEIN. Before the development and utilization of the subclavian vein approach for lead insertion, the cephalic vein was the preferred route for endocardial lead insertion. The vein is exposed in the deltopectoral groove via an overlying incision and looped proximally and distally by nonabsorbable suture (Fig 25A-6). The proximal suture is tied and placed under slight tension. A small venotomy is performed with small iris scissors, and with a lead introducer, the lead is inserted into the venous system.

The cephalic vein approach has been widely used because of the ease with which the vein can be exposed and because of the minimal vascular and pulmonary complications that occur with cephalic use. Because the vein is not blindly approached as it is in the subclavian puncture, the complication rate is lower if the operator is comfortable with the cephalic technique[62] (see Fig 25A-6). The introducer technique can be used with the cephalic vein.[63] In most cases, two leads can be placed via the cephalic vein to accommodate dual-chamber pacing.[64]

JUGULAR VEINS. The internal and external jugular veins have been used as alternative approaches, primarily when the subclavian or cephalic vein could not be used (Fig 25A-7).

The external jugular vein can be exposed by making an incision over the sternocleidomastoid muscle and extending it laterally. The vein is controlled proximally and distally in a manner similar to that used for the cephalic vein. Alternatively, the external jugular vein can be exposed by using a large subclavicular incision, raising a subcutaneous flap over the clavicle in the area of the vein, and freeing it beneath the platysma.[65]

If the external jugular vein cannot be used, the sternocleidomastoid muscle is split between its sternal and clavicular heads and the internal jugular vein is exposed. The vein is again controlled proximally and distally and is entered via an anterolateral venotomy. Usually a purse-string suture is placed around the port of

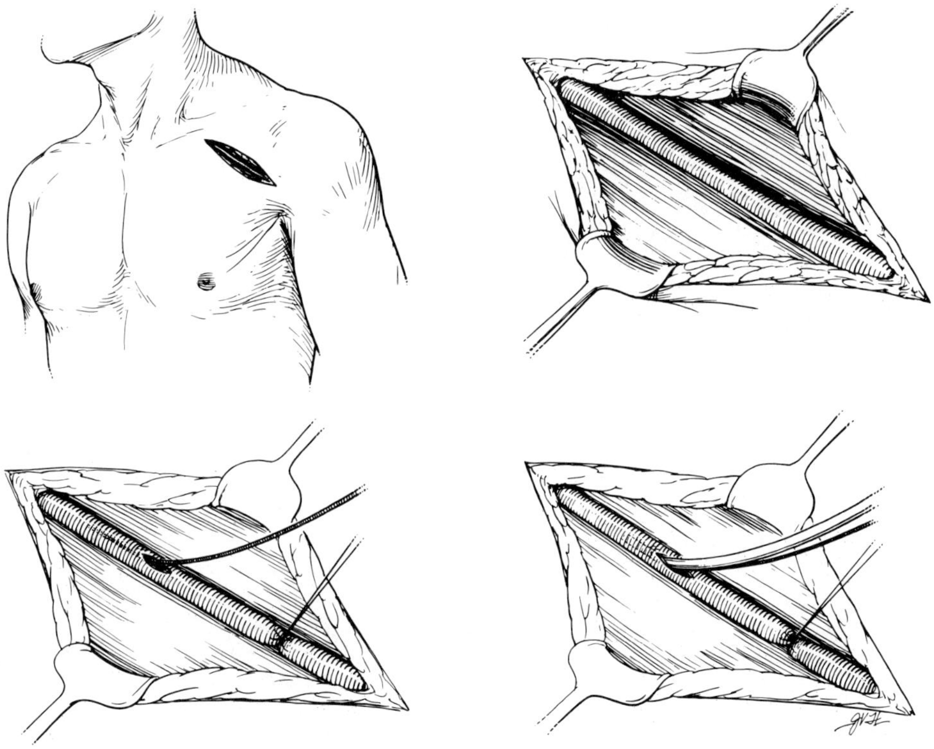

Fig 25A-6 A partial cephalic cutdown, introducer technique involves exposure of the cephalic vein in the deltopectoral groove **(upper left, upper right).** If the vein is too small to accept a lead, a guide wire is placed **(lower left)** and an introducer over it. The guide wire may be reintroduced to facilitate placement of a second lead **(lower right).** (From Holmes DR, Hayes DL, Furman S: Permanent pacemaker implantation. In *A Practice of Cardiac Pacing.* Second edition. Edited by S Furman, DL Hayes, DR Holmes Jr. Mount Kisco, New York, Futura Publishing Company, 1989, pp 239-287. By permission.)

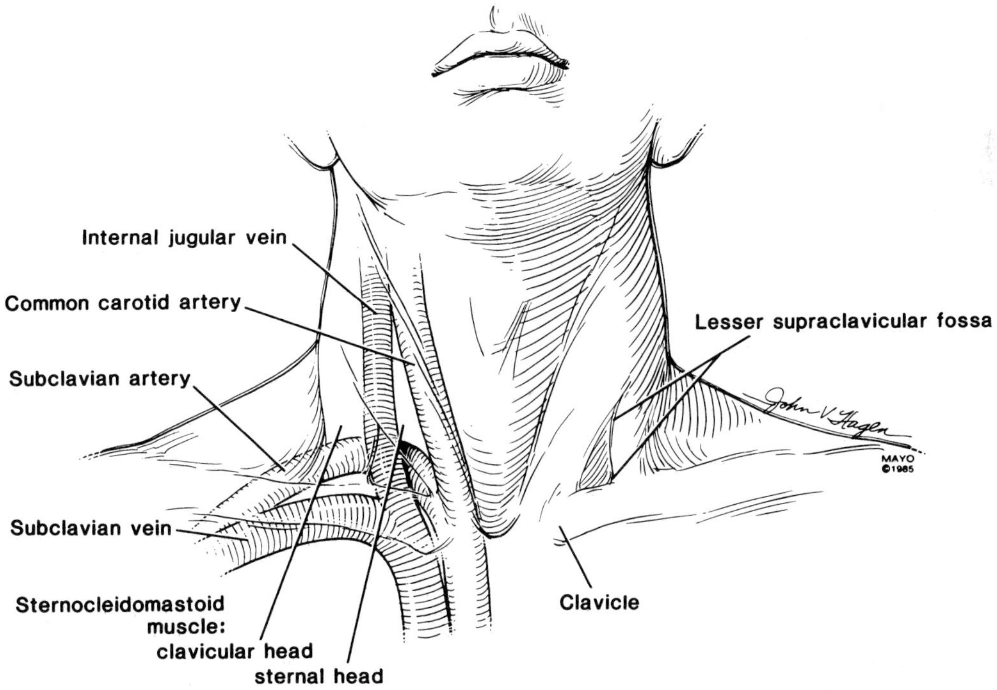

Fig 25A-7 Relationship of jugular vein to carotid artery and sternocleidomastoid muscle. (From Hayes DL, Holmes DR Jr, Furman S: Permanent pacemaker implantation. In *A Practice of Cardiac Pacing.* Third edition. Edited by S Furman, DL Hayes, DR Holmes Jr. Mount Kisco, New York, Futura Publishing Company, 1993, pp 261-307. By permission, Mayo Foundation.)

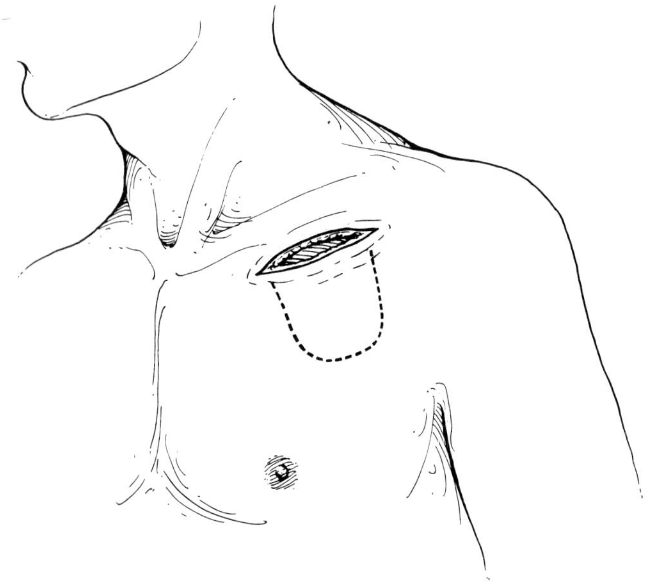

Fig 25A-8 Location of subcutaneous pacemaker pocket in upper left aspect of chest. Note that incision is made parallel to and several centimeters below lower clavicular margin. (From Hayes DL, Holmes DR Jr, Furman S: Permanent pacemaker implantation. In *A Practice of Cardiac Pacing.* Third edition. Edited by S Furman, DL Hayes, DR Holmes Jr. Mount Kisco, New York, Futura Publishing Company, 1993, pp 261-307. By permission.)

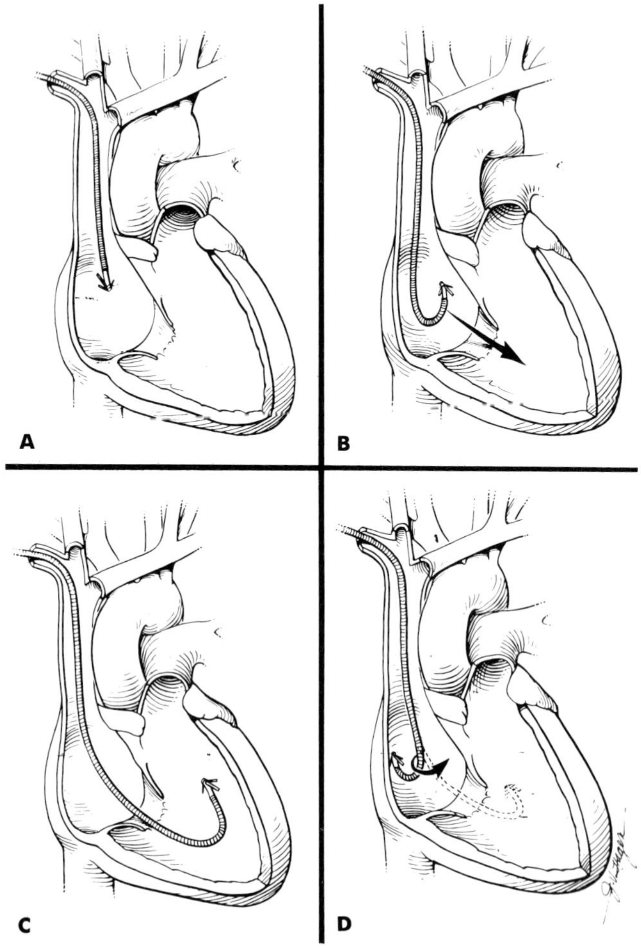

Fig 25A-9 **A,** lead in middle of right atrium with straight stylet in place. **B,** mid-atrial position with curved stylet in place. **C,** conventional (or straight pass) approach to cross tricuspid valve. **D,** lead rotation approach to cross tricuspid valve.

entry of the lead to secure it, but, if necessary, the vein can be totally ligated without untoward effects. The lead (or leads) is then tunnelled either over or beneath the clavicle to join the infraclavicular incision.

The disadvantages of the use of the jugular veins are the need for two separate incisions, the requirement for an increased amount of surgical expertise, increased difficulty with lead repositioning, and increased frequency of lead complications.

Pacemaker pocket formation. Regardless of the site or method of venous access, a pocket is fashioned in the upper thoracic region (left or right) for the pulse generator. The pocket is made in the plane between the subcutaneous tissue and the underlying pectoralis major muscle. If the pocket is made in the subcutaneous fat rather than deep to it, the blood supply of the subcutaneous tissues and the overlying skin may be compromised, increasing the chances of early or late erosion. When the appropriate tissue plane has been identified, a pocket is created by blunt finger dissection, minimizing the amount of bleeding. The pocket is then packed with neomycin-soaked sponges (one or two) to maintain wound sterility and to aid in hemostasis while the leads are positioned (Fig 25A-8).

Endocardial ventricular lead positioning. The lead is inserted into the vein and advanced to the level of the mid-right atrium with a straight stylet in place. This stylet is then replaced by one in which a gentle curve has been fashioned. The lead is then advanced to cross the tricuspid valve into the right ventricle. It is usually possible to accomplish this by a direct "forward pass" approach, but occasionally the lead tip must be flipped across the valve by lead rotation (Fig 25A-9).

There may be problems advancing the lead in patients with enlarged right atria or with any degree of tricuspid regurgitation. In these patients it is sometimes necessary to cross the valve with the body of the lead preceding the tip. With the stylet withdrawn into the body of the vein, the tip electrode is placed against the lateral atrial wall and a soft loop is made in the atrium. The stylet is then advanced carefully across the valve (without advancing it into the lead). When the stylet and body of the lead are in the right ventricular cavity, the lead is pulled back over the stylet (maintaining the stylet position in the right ventricle) until the tip is free in the right ventricular cavity (Fig 25A-10).

Once the tip of the electrode is in the right ventricular

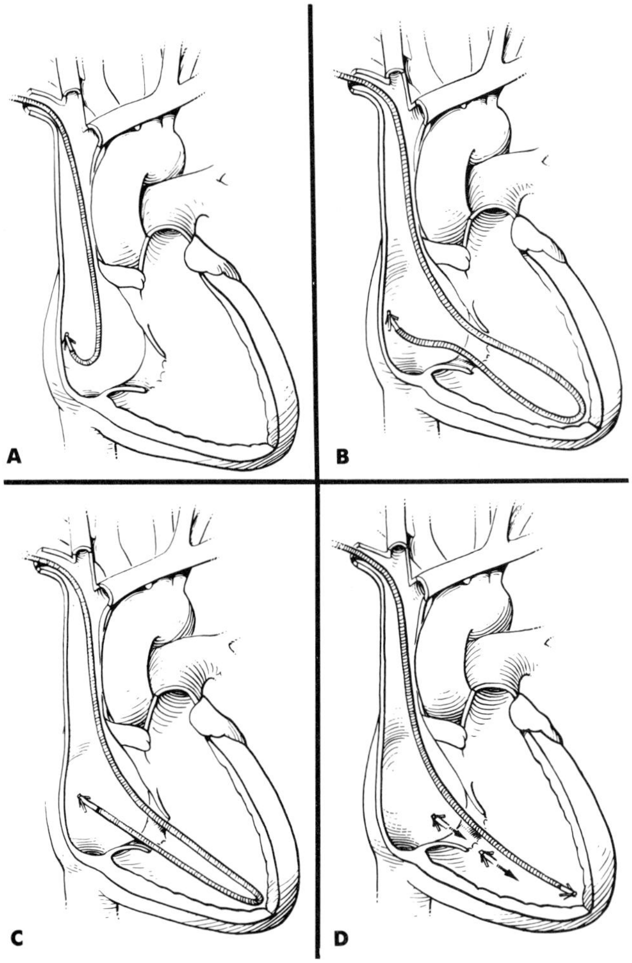

Fig 25A-10 **A,** reverse loop in right atrium with curved stylet in place. **B,** stylet partially removed and loop advanced across tricuspid valve. **C,** straight stylet inserted to region of right ventricular apex. **D,** lead "pulled over" the stylet to right ventricular apex position.

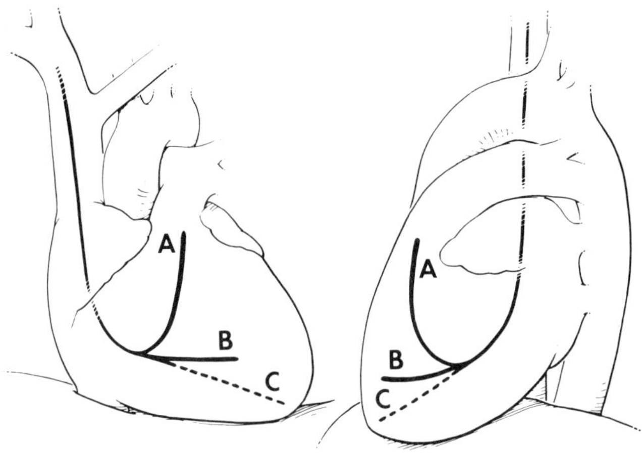

Fig 25A-11 A, advancement of pacemaker lead into pulmonary outflow tract. B, lead is withdrawn until it is free in right ventricular cavity. C, lead is then advanced to right ventricular apex.

cavity, it should be advanced into the right or left pulmonary artery. This serves two purposes: (1) to establish that the lead is clearly in the right ventricle and not in the coronary sinus, and (2) to orient the tip electrode for maneuvering into the right ventricular apex. (If the technique described in Figure 25A-10 is used, it may not be necessary to pass the lead into the pulmonary outflow tract.)

With the distal electrode in the pulmonary artery, the curved stylet is removed and replaced with a straight one. The lead is then slowly withdrawn as a straight stylet is advanced until the tip falls free in the right ventricular cavity. The lead is then slowly and carefully advanced until a stable position is achieved in the right ventricular apex. The stylet is withdrawn for about 5 cm, and the lead again is advanced to achieve a final position. The stylet is then withdrawn to the level of the superior vena cava. A gentle loop in the catheter is then formed in the right atrium. The final curvature in the loop should be determined during held deep inspiration to allow adequate lead redundancy (to minimize the chances of lead dislodgment) (Fig 25A-11).

The fluoroscopic appearance of the distal electrode catheter should be carefully checked. Ideally, the terminal portion of the lead should be relatively stationary except for slight longitudinal motion synchronous with systole. The position should be checked during cough and deep inspiration to ensure the absence of tip motion. If lateral fluoroscopy is available, it should be used to confirm the anterior position of the electrode in the right ventricular apex.

If a ventricular screw-in electrode is used, it should be secured to the ventricular endocardium in a manner that will be discussed later.

Endocardial atrial lead positioning. Most commonly, atrial lead placement is performed as part of dual-chamber pacing, and single-chamber atrial pacing is used relatively uncommonly in the United States. The right atrial appendage is the most common position for the atrial lead (Fig 25A-12), although satisfactory pacing can be achieved from various right atrial sites. Active or passive fixation leads, with or without preformed J configuration, may be used. An active fixation (screw-in) lead can potentially allow a greater variety of pacing positions. Once the lead is in the superior vena cava, it is advanced with a straight stylet in place into the middle portion of the right atrium (Fig 25A-13, A).

If a preformed J lead is used, the stylet is then withdrawn and the lead returns to its J shape (Fig 25A-13, B). After this, the entire lead is withdrawn with medial rotation into the right atrial appendage (Fig 25A-13, C). Placement of the lead in the right atrial appendage can be recognized by the to-and-fro lateral motion of the catheter during atrial systole (Fig 25A-13, D). A stable position is essential and should be checked by noting the effects of torque and deep breathing. During inspiration, the two limbs of the J widen toward an L shape, but the angle

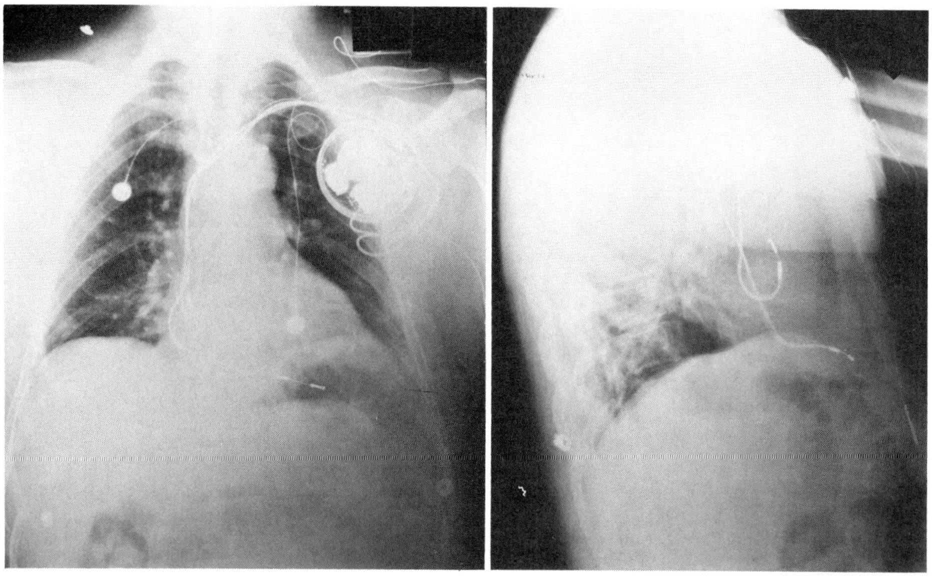

Fig 25A-12 Chest radiographs showing typical position of pacing catheter in right atrial appendage. Note anterior position of lead tip on lateral view **(right).**

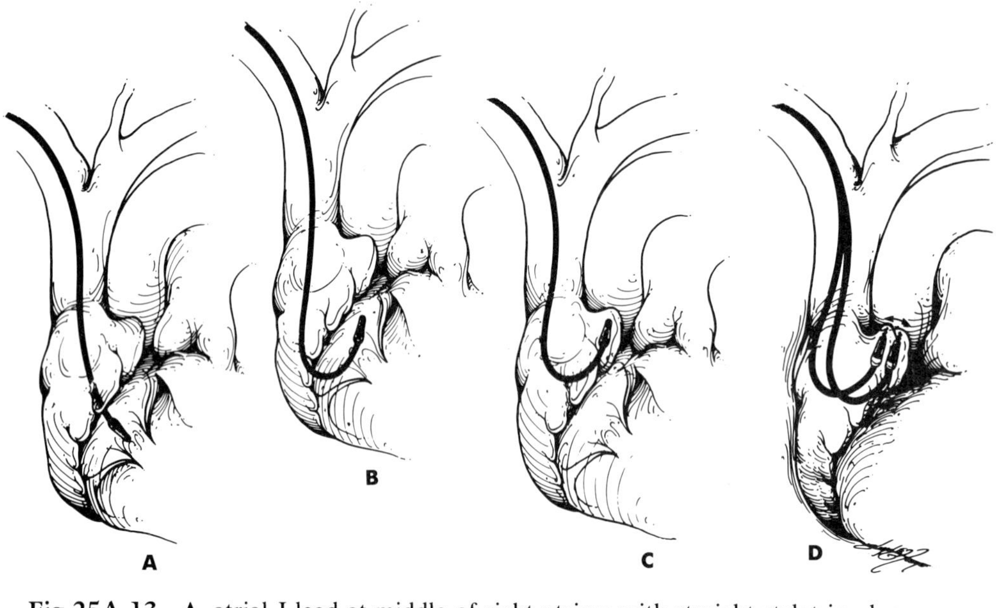

Fig 25A-13 **A,** atrial J lead at middle of right atrium with straight stylet in place. **B,** straight stylet is removed; removal allows catheter to assume the preformed J configuration. **C,** entire lead is pulled back and tip of electrode is allowed to enter right atrial appendage. **D,** characteristic to-and-fro motion of lead when positioned in right atrial appendage. (From Holmes DR, Hayes DL, Furman S: Permanent pacemaker implantation. In *A Practice of Cardiac Pacing.* Second edition. Edited by S Furman, DL Hayes, DR Holmes Jr. Mount Kisco, New York, Futura Publishing Company, 1989, pp 239-287. By permission, Mayo Foundation.)

should not exceed approximately 80°. During expiration, the two limbs should form an acute angle.

If a straight (nonpreformed J) lead is used, the same procedure is followed except that a curved or J stylet is introduced after the lead is passed into the midportion of the right atrium. With the stylet in place, the lead is directed toward the desired position in the atrium. If an active fixation lead is used, the lead can then be fixed and the stylet removed. Enough slack is left in the lead to allow the J shape and angulation described. Many implanters prefer a straight lead because of increased ease in manipulating it to sites other than the atrial appendage. In pediatric patients and certain adults, the atrium may be too small to accommodate preformed J leads.

The atrial appendage may not be suitable for lead placement because of amputation or ligation from a previous cardiac operation or because of poor sensing or pacing thresholds in this location. In such cases, other locations in the right atrium should be used, and lateral fluoroscopy is helpful for exploring the right atrium. Any atrial position that allows adequate pacing and sensing thresholds can be used so long as no extracardiac stimulation occurs with pacing.

Intraoperative measurements

After adequate anatomic lead position is achieved, whether the procedure is performed via the transvenous route under fluoroscopic control or through the epicardial route under direct visualization, it must be established that this position will result in adequate and reliable myocardial stimulation and sensing of intrinsic cardiac electrical activity.

Stimulation threshold. The threshold for cardiac pacing may be defined as the smallest amount of electrical activity that produces consistent myocardial capture outside the refractory period of the heart.[66] The threshold may vary according to a number of factors, including the duration of the stimulus (pulse width), the type of electrode and its age, and the site of stimulation. It also may be influenced by electrolyte or acid-base imbalance, drug administration, the state of the myocardium, and the type of measuring equipment used.

The acute threshold is determined at the time of implantation and is usually expressed in terms of the voltage or current (milliamperes) requirements for myocardial capture. This threshold will increase shortly after implantation. After the initial increase, the threshold falls again and usually reaches its stable value after 4 to 6 weeks.[67] This increase seems to be the result of the growth of fibrous tissue about the electrode, which increases the effective size of the interface between the electrode and the myocardium.[68] (With steroid-eluting leads, little if any acute threshold rise occurs.)

One should remember that although the threshold for stimulation is described in terms of voltage or current, it is equally important that the pulse duration (the amount of time a given amount of energy is delivered to the heart) is also known. The shortest duration of an electrical impulse that produces consistent capture (at a constant pulse amplitude—current or voltage) represents the threshold of stimulation as a function of the pulse duration. Comparison of stimulation thresholds at various pulse widths (durations) allows determination of the strength-duration curve. This measurement is particularly important in the evaluation of leads because the proper adjustment of pulse duration and output voltage will allow long-term pacing with maximal conservation of energy (Fig 25A-14).

The thresholds for capture should be measured in both volts and milliamperes at the pulse duration to be utilized.

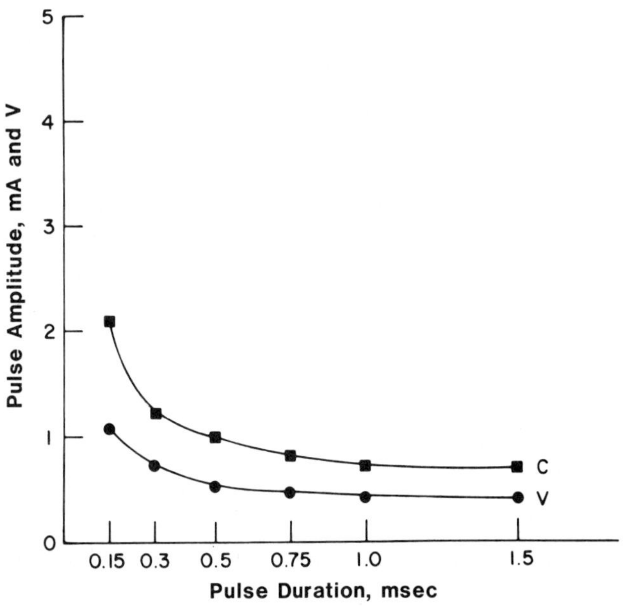

Fig 25A-14 Acute strength-duration curves for voltage (●) and current (■). As the pulse duration decreases, the energy requirements to maintain myocardial stimulation (capture) increase. Initial implant data from 25 patients.

For bipolar leads the positive and negative test cables are attached to the positive and negative poles of the lead. For unipolar systems, the positive test cable has to be connected to a ground placed in the pacemaker pocket. Two thresholds should be measured—the stimulation threshold and the pacing threshold. The output of the pacing systems analyzer is set at 5 V (10 mA) and slowly decreased until myocardial capture is lost (stimulation threshold); then the output is slowly increased until consistent capture is maintained (pacing threshold). The pacing threshold is ordinarily slightly higher than the stimulation threshold, and it is this value that should be accepted and recorded.

The acceptable values for ventricular pacing thresholds should be 1.0 V or less at a pulse width of 0.5 msec.

The acceptable values for atrial pacing thresholds should be 1.5 V or less at a pulse width of 0.5 msec, although we search for thresholds less than 1.0 V whenever possible. Great care should be taken to find the lowest possible pacing threshold in each patient.

Intracardiac electrogram measurement. For any pulse generator to be triggered or inhibited by intrinsic cardiac activity, the intracardiac electrograms generated by that activity must be of sufficient magnitude to be sensed by the generator.

There are three important components of any acute intracardiac electrogram (either R wave or P wave): the amplitude (millivolts), the slew rate, and the magnitude of the current of injury (ST-T change). The amplitude and slew rate are determined from that part of the electrogram called the "intrinsic deflection." It is the rapid biphasic portion of the electrogram that occurs as the muscle adjacent to the electrode becomes electronegative with the passing depolarization wave.[69] The current of injury appears as an elevation immediately following the intrinsic deflection and is believed to be due to a small area of damaged endocardium caused by irritation from the electrode (Fig 25A-15).

The electrogram evolves from acute to chronic, demonstrating the following changes: (1) voltage amplitude is decreased by an average of 15% (ventricle) to 18% (atrium);[70] (2) slew rates are reduced by 59% (average); and (3) current of injury pattern is no longer present[71] (Fig 25A-16).

Ordinarily there are no significant differences in the intracardiac electrograms obtained by using unipolar or bipolar catheter electrodes. However, because the bipolar signal is a result of the potential difference between two intracardiac poles, if the axis of the bipole is at a right angle to the depolarization pathway the resultant signal may be very small and unacceptable for pulse generator sensing.

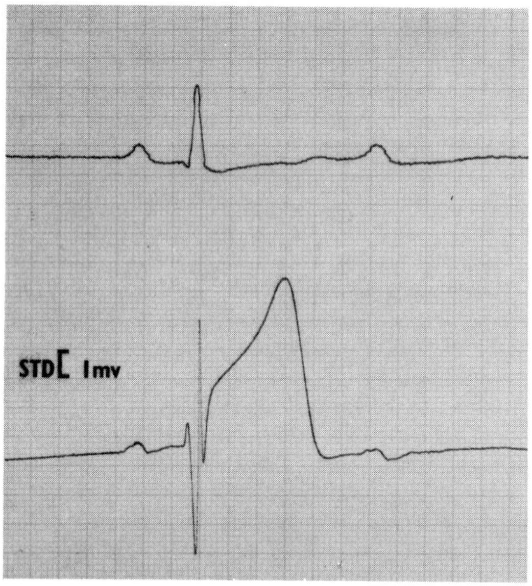

Fig 25A-15 Acute ventricular electrogram demonstrating amplitude of 8 mV, rapid slew rate, and typical current of injury (ST-segment elevation).

Because of the relative lack of muscle mass, the average P waves generated in the atrium are of a lesser magnitude than the R waves generated in the ventricle. P waves may vary in amplitude from approximately 2.0 to 5.9 mV. We attempt to locate a site in the atrium that yields a P wave of 2.0 to 2.5 mV or greater if any P-wave sensing pacing system is to be used. P-wave amplitude will vary with atrial lead position.

If a lead position is found where the stimulation threshold is acceptable and the R wave or P wave is of adequate amplitude, measurement of the slew rate and recording of intracardiac electrograms usually are not necessary. They are most helpful if the measured R wave or P wave is lower than desired and a better position cannot be found. Recording the slew rate and appropriate intracardiac electrogram more accurately determines whether adequate sensing will be possible from that position. Several pacing system analyzers now have the capability of telemetering intracardiac electrograms and measuring slew rates.

Lead impedance. The lead impedance, or resistance to current flow is determined by Ohm's law: $E = IR$, in which E is voltage, I is current in milliamperes, and R is resistance in ohms. By simultaneously measuring voltage and the resultant current, the resistance can be easily calculated by transposing the equation: $R = E/I$. We measure impedance routinely by pacing the heart at a constant output of 5 V and recording the resultant current. The presently accepted range of normal lead impedance is approximately 300 to 1,000 ohms. Average impedance tends to fall slightly after initial implantation of the lead, and then stabilizes.[67] In the absence of lead

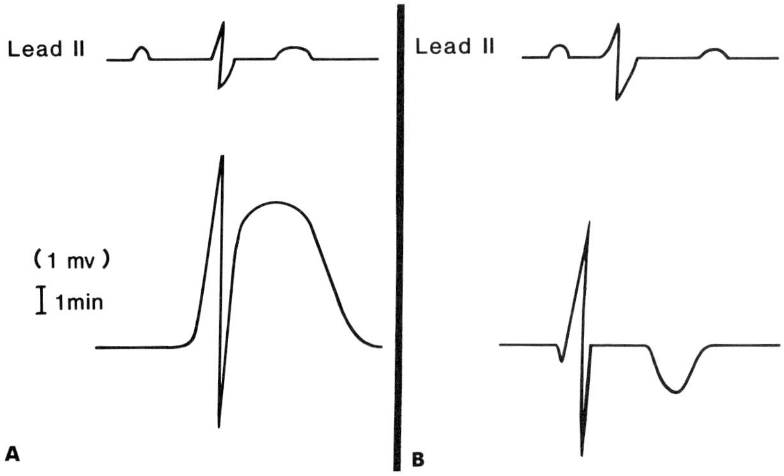

Fig 25A-16 **A,** acute ventricular electrogram, exhibiting adequate sensing amplitude and ST elevation reflecting the current of injury. **B,** chronic ventricular electrogram, exhibiting loss of the current of injury pattern and T-wave inversion.

complications or myocardial abnormalities, the long-term values for impedance tend to remain constant and do not differ significantly from the original value.

Measurement of lead impedance is especially important at the time of elective replacement of a pulse generator or during intraoperative pacemaker troubleshooting because it offers the best information concerning the integrity of the catheter electrode.

It should be stressed that establishing the adequacy of lead position is done by using all of the information available at the time of lead implantation—appropriate position by anteroposterior and lateral fluoroscopy, low stimulation thresholds, electrograms of adequate amplitude and slew rate with evidence of myocardial contact by ST-segment shift, and the consistency of these measurements during forced inspiration and cough.

Diaphragmatic stimulation testing. Once an adequate position of the lead electrode has been obtained, stimulation through the lead at twice the output of the implantable pulse generator (i.e., 10 V) should be done to check for the possibility of diaphragmatic stimulation. If this occurs, it necessitates lead repositioning.

Final steps of implantation

The lead or leads should be secured to the prepectoral fascia. Leads are equipped with sliding silicone rubber sleeves (Fig 25A-17). The sleeve is moved to the appropriate point on the extravascular portion of the lead and is secured by an encircling suture. (Sutures should not be placed directly on the lead, because the insulation may be damaged. This is especially true of polyurethane-insulated leads but may also occur with silicone rubber-insulated leads.) Although the sleeve is used to protect the lead, very tight encircling sutures may compress the insulation. Actual insulation damage is unlikely when the sleeve is used, but extremely tight ligatures around the sleeve could potentially damage the insulation. If a sleeve is not part of the lead design, silicone "butterfly" sleeves can be used (see Fig 25A-17).

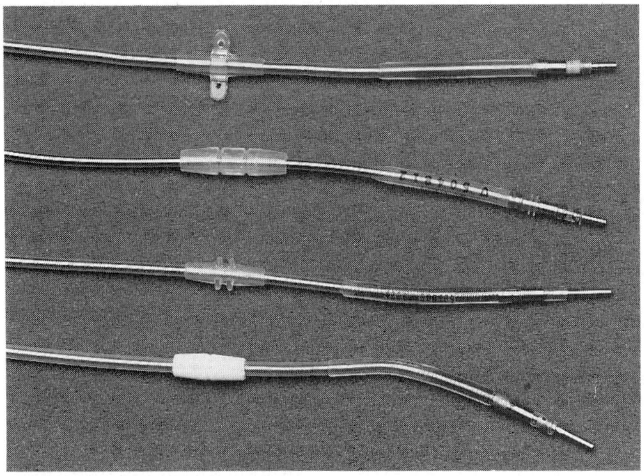

Fig 25A-17 Several different types of sleeves are used to fix the lead to adjacent tissue. The sleeve protects the lead from damage that could be induced by placing the ligature directly on the lead. (From Hayes DL, Holmes DR Jr, Furman S: Permanent pacemaker implantation. In *A Practice of Cardiac Pacing.* Third edition. Edited by S Furman, DL Hayes, DR Holmes Jr. Mount Kisco, New York, Futura Publishing Company, 1993, pp 261-307. By permission.)

The lead is then connected to the pulse generator and the function of the system is assessed. Appropriate myocardial capture (pacing) and sensing (inhibition of pacemaker activity during normal cardiac function) should be noted. If no pacemaker function is evident because of a normal cardiac rhythm, then a magnet should be applied to convert the system to the asynchronous mode so that pacing can be seen.

The pacemaker pocket should be irrigated with a dilute antibacterial solution, such as 0.25% neomycin. The pulse generator should then be positioned in the preformed pocket with the redundant lead coiled under it to avoid the possibility of damage at the time of reoperation. Care should be taken to position the pulse generator properly in the pacemaker pouch. Unipolar systems are coated with plastic to prevent stimulation of surrounding tissues with each pacing impulse. Only a small area is left uncoated to act as the cathode. This area should be facing away from the pectoral muscles to avoid muscle stimulation. We perform the closure in three layers. The deep subcutaneous and subcutaneous layers are closed in a continuous fashion with an absorbable 2-0 suture; the skin is closed with a continuous subcuticular absorbable 4-0 suture.

The length of time the patient should be kept in the hospital after pacemaker implantation is controversial and varies significantly among institutions. In our practice, patients who are not pacemaker-dependent are allowed to walk the evening of the procedure and are dismissed the following morning.[72] The patient is monitored during the overnight stay. Before dismissal, thresholds are documented and the pacemaker is programmed to its final settings. If a rate-adaptive pacemaker has been implanted, informal exercise is performed the morning after implantation and the rate-responsive parameters are adjusted to fit the needs of the patient. Pacemaker-dependent patients may be kept in the hospital for 1 or 2 nights, but the practice is moving toward a single night stay. When the patient's pulse generator reaches battery depletion indicators, replacement is performed as an outpatient procedure.

A number of implanting physicians now perform initial pacemaker implantation as an outpatient procedure. Some physicians do outpatient implantation only in non-pacemaker-dependent patients, whereas others perform outpatient procedures regardless of dependency status. The results are encouraging, and it is possible that ambulatory pacemaker implantation with outpatient follow-up the next day may become the norm.

The day after the procedure is used for teaching the patient about the pacemaker and transtelephonic monitoring. Chest radiographs (posteroanterior and lateral) are also obtained at this time.

We have traditionally given antibiotics parenterally immediately before the procedure and for 24 hours after the procedure and orally for 3 days thereafter. However, there is little information to support intravenous or oral antibiotic administration. The best deterrent to infection is careful sterile technique and irrigation of the pocket with an antibiotic solution.[73]

PROGRAMMABILITY

"Programmability" is a property of a pacemaker system that permits stable, but reversible, changes in function to be made noninvasively. The pacemaker contains a set of circuits from which one feature or function or several can be selected for variation within a restricted range. By using a programmer, one can select among the desired functions but cannot produce a completely new program.

Initially, "programmability" referred mainly to noninvasive adjustment of rate or pulse width. Currently, pacemaker programmability varies widely depending on the capabilities of the individual pulse generator. The most significant variable is whether or not the pacemaker is pacing one or two chambers. Optimal programming with any pacemaker can have a profound effect on pacemaker longevity, patient well-being, and avoidance of further invasive procedures.[74,75]

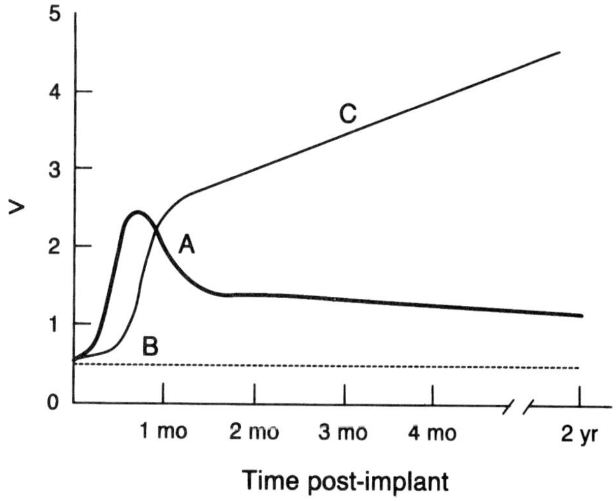

Fig 25A-18 Schematic representation of potential acute and chronic pacing threshold variations. Voltage (V) is shown on the abscissa and time after implantation on the ordinate. *A*, typical threshold course with early rise in threshold and subsequent decrease and plateau; *B*, chronic rise in threshold, i.e., exit-block; *C*, flat or nearly flat threshold response typical of steroid-eluting pacing leads.

Programming of rate

Rate is the most frequently used programmable feature. The major use of rate programming is to allow a patient to remain in sinus rhythm rather than in paced rhythm when sinus bradycardia with intermittent sinus arrest or intermittent AV block exists. Programming the rate to 60 ppm, or even as low as 40 to 50 ppm, might allow the patient's intrinsic rhythm to exist most of the time. Slower pacing rates allow dominance of the patient's intrinsic rhythm when the bradyarrhythmia is intermittent.

Faster pacing rates—i.e., greater than 70 ppm—are most commonly utilized in pediatric patients. An occasional patient will require and tolerate rapid pacing for prolonged periods. Sometimes, faster pacing rates can be useful to increase cardiac output for any reason, transiently or permanently, and may occasionally be used to prevent other rhythm disturbances (overdrive pacing).

A newer feature for lower rate limit control is that of Circadian Response (Intermedics, Inc.).[76] This feature allows a lower rate to be programmed for the approximate time the patient is sleeping. A separate, potentially faster lower rate limit may then be programmed for waking hours. (For example, the lower rate limit during waking hours may be programmed to 70 ppm and the lower rate limit during sleeping hours may be programmed to 50 ppm.)

Programming of energy (pulse width and voltage amplitude)

For any given patient, early and long-term threshold behavior cannot be predicted from the threshold value obtained at implantation (Fig 25A-18). The importance of output programmability in maintaining the widest margin of patient safety becomes evident.

The output function that should be programmed to provide the most effective control of threshold increases is still uncertain. Of the options available, it is likely that voltage programming coupled with pulse duration programming over a narrow range—e.g., 0.05 to 1.0 msec—is the most effective. It has been shown that programming to a pulse width greater than 1 msec on a long-term basis probably does not provide any additional pacing margin of safety and may lead to high current and energy drain without producing ventricular capture.[77] Indications for increasing the output of the pulse generator might include maintaining cardiac pacing in a patient with poor electrode position or microdislodgment prior to lead revision and controlling temporary high threshold evolution. It should be pointed out that at no time should output programmability be used as a substitute for proper lead placement.

Reduction of energy output is safe for many patients and translates into prolonged longevity of the pulse generator.[71,78] By programming of the output to an efficient but safe level, the projected battery life can theoretically be increased by as much as 50%. A decrease in energy output can be used not only to increase pulse generator longevity but also to eliminate phrenic or diaphragmatic stimulation[79] and to eliminate local pectoral muscle stimulation.

The feasibility of automatic output regulation has been explored since the early 1970s. Despite the desirability of such a feature, automatic output regulation has never been made available in a clinically released pacemaker. Such a feature would automatically determine capture threshold and adjust output accordingly.[80] Because output adjustment is so critical for both extremes, i.e., maintaining an adequate safety margin and prolonging

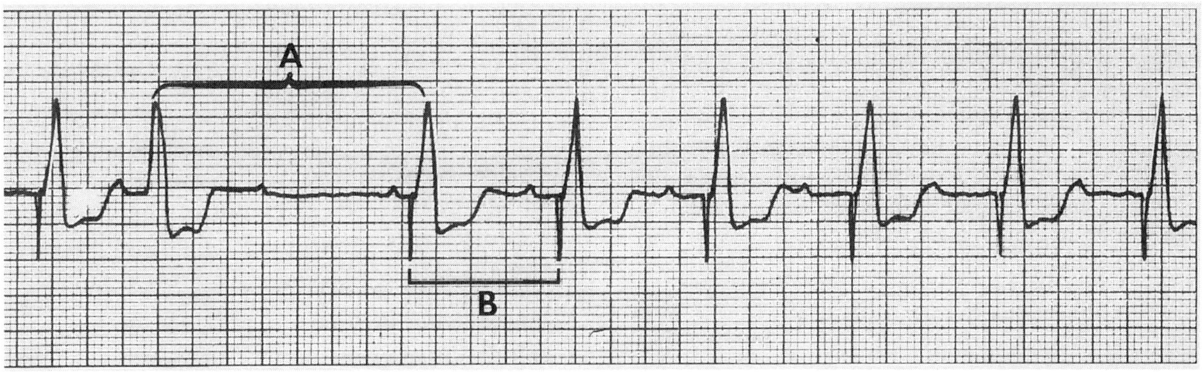

Fig 25A-19 Ventricular demand (VVI) pacing at a programmed rate of 72 ppm (833 msec, interval B). The preceding interval (interval A) is approximately 1,550 msec in duration and represents normal VVI pacing with hysteresis. The prolonged cycle following a sensed ventricular event allows a longer period for the patient's intrinsic conduction system to escape before pacing begins at the programmed rate. (From Hayes DL: Pacemaker electrocardiography. In *A Practice of Cardiac Pacing.* Third edition. Edited by S Furman, DL Hayes, DR Holmes Jr. Mount Kisco, New York, Futura Publishing Company, 1993, pp 309-359. By permission.)

battery longevity, automatic output regulation most certainly will become a standard feature of future pacemakers.

Programming of sensitivity

All noncompetitive pulse generators contain a sensing circuit that amplifies and filters the intracardiac electrogram delivered through the lead electrode. For ventricular sensing, the R wave must have a minimal amplitude and slew rate for proper sensing to occur. The sensitivity of the pulse generator is the lowest amplitude of R wave that the unit will recognize as ventricular depolarization (QRS complex). For nonprogrammable models, the sensitivity is usually preset at 1.2 to 2.5 mV, and sensing malfunction will develop if the amplitude of the intracardiac R wave is below the programmed sensitivity. The amplitude of the intracardiac R wave may decrease for various reasons, including metabolic or drug effects, lead dislodgment, and organic disease. In addition, ventricular extrasystoles or supraventricular beats conducted with aberrancy may not be sensed if they do not meet the required amplitude and slew rate criteria.

If the pacemaker is being used in the atrial position, the P wave must have a minimum amplitude and slew rate for proper sensing to occur, as described above for ventricular pacing.

Sensitivity programming can be accomplished by increasing the sensitivity of the amplifier—e.g., by decreasing the amplitude of the signal required to trigger the unit—but maintaining the same frequency spectrum. Because poor QRS and P waves contain a predominance of low-frequency signals, a program shift to lower frequencies as well as an increase in gain can be useful and may obviate additional operative procedures. Programming the pacemaker to a less sensitive setting is useful in eliminating oversensing of nonphysiologic electromagnetic interference signals or such physiologic signals as pectoral muscle artifacts.

Programming of hysteresis

Programming of hysteresis permits prolongation of the first escape interval of the pacemaker (Fig 25A-19). For example, the pacemaker programmed at a cycle of 1,000 msec (i.e., a rate of 60 ppm) and at a hysteresis of 50/ ppm (or +200 msec) will discharge a pulse escape at 1,200 msec after the last QRS complex. Unless another QRS complex is recognized, the pacemaker will then revert to the programmed rate of 60 ppm (1,000-msec cycling). The advantages of hysteresis reside in the ability to maintain the intrinsic rhythm as long as possible.

In addition, in most patients with symptomatic ventriculoatrial (VA) conduction, hysteresis may allow less frequent pacing and, therefore, relieve symptoms secondary to the intact VA conduction or "pacemaker syndrome."[81]

Programming of refractory periods

Programming in single-chamber pacemakers. Refractory period programming in single-chamber pacing can be advantageous in two situations. The first is in a pacemaker the refractory period of which is so long that it is prevented from sensing some ventricular electrograms. Should this occur, the subsequent pacemaker stimulus could fall on the T wave on the unsensed beat. Conversely, a refractory period too short can allow sensing of the T wave and inappropriate inhibition of the pulse generator. In the second situation, less commonly seen, some older pulse generators have sensed the afterpotential following a stimulus. The problem can be corrected by prolongation of the refractory period or reduction of the pulse duration if an adequate pacing margin of safety still exists. If a single-chamber, unipolar generator is used for atrial pacing, a longer refractory period is desirable to avoid sensing the QRS electrogram.

Programming in dual-chamber pacemakers. Refractory periods in dual-chamber, dual-sensing pacemakers are much more complex than in single-chamber pacemakers because the events and timing cycles in one channel affect those in the other.

AV interval

To properly program the AV interval, one must first understand the components of a normal AV interval (Fig 25A-20).

Ventricular safety pacing. Crosstalk is the sensing of the output of one pacemaker channel in the other. (Other "noise" sensed on the ventricular lead could also result in the appearance of crosstalk.) The major concern is the sensing of an atrial stimulus in the ventricular channel. To prevent ventricular inhibition by crosstalk, a blanking period begins in the ventricular channel simultaneously with the atrial stimulus. During this period, the sensing circuits are insensitive. This interval is most commonly of 12 to 50 msec, depending on the pulse generator, and is programmable in many pulse generators. If the blanking period is too long, a spontaneous R wave, occurring soon after the atrial stimulus, will not be sensed and a competitive ventricular stimulus will be emitted. This situation is of greater concern with longer blanking periods. Any blanking period in excess of 100 msec has greater potential of competing with a ventricular premature contraction and exaggerating ventricular competition if episodic atrial undersensing is present. If the blanking period is too short, the possibility exists that crosstalk and ventricular inhibition may result. Crosstalk occurs more frequently as the voltage output of the atrial stimulus increases or, less commonly, as pulse duration increases. The potential for crosstalk should be carefully evaluated and the blanking period appropriately lengthened.

In an effort to create the safest situation possible while retaining a relatively short blanking period, this period is followed in many pacemakers by another portion of the AV interval, during which activity sensed in the ventricular channel results in ventricular pacing (see Fig 25A-20). This occurrence has been referred to as "ventricular safety pacing" or the "nonphysiologic AV delay." Both terms are descriptive, because the paced interval is often shorter than the programmed AV interval and is present to assure ventricular pacing when crosstalk or other "noise" is sensed early in the AV interval. Since the "safety" stimulus occurs at a fixed delay after the beginning of the "safety pacing" interval, the total AV interval is likely to be abbreviated. Because several early pulse generators had a ventricular safety pacing interval of 110 msec, the designation "110-msec phenomenon" has also been used.

Differential AV interval. An option of a differential AV interval is an attempt to provide a P-R interval, i.e., the hemodynamic interval, of equal duration whether the atrial contraction is paced or sensed.[82] The AV interval following a sensed atrial event is shorter than that following a paced atrial event (Fig 25A-21). In some pacemakers the differential is programmable, and in

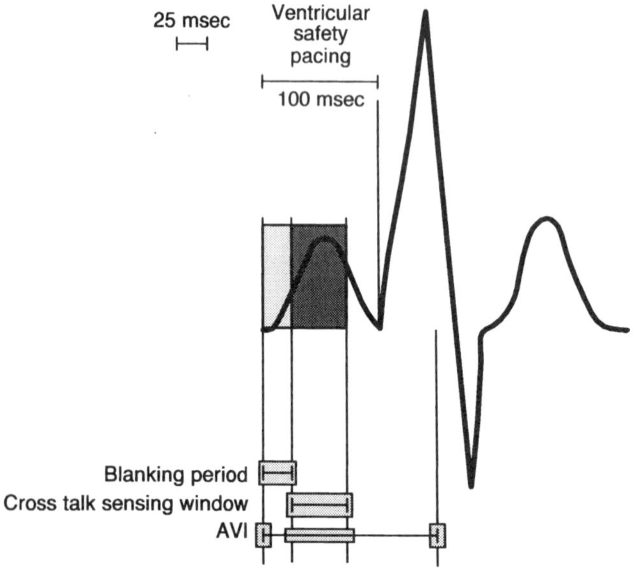

Fig 25A-20 The AV interval (AVI) should be considered a single interval with two subportions. The entire AVI corresponds to the programmed value. The initial portion of the AVI is the blanking period *(lighter shading)*. This interval is followed by the cross-talk sensing window *(darker shading)*. (From Hayes DL, Levine PA: Pacemaker timing cycles. In *Cardiac Pacing.* Edited by KA Ellenbogen. Boston, Blackwell Scientific Publications, 1992, pp 263-308. By permission.)

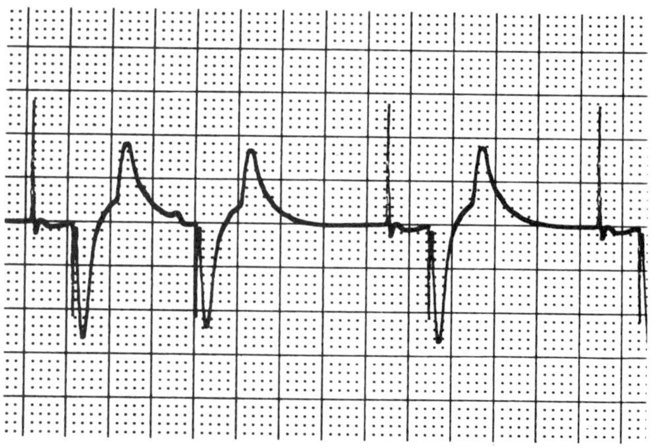

Fig 25A-21 ECG recording from a patient with a DDD pacemaker with differential AV interval. The AV interval following the paced atrial artifacts is 200 msec. The AV interval following the sensed atrial event is 150 msec. (Modified from Hayes DL: Pacemaker electrocardiography. In *A Practice of Cardiac Pacing.* Third edition. Edited by S Furman, DL Hayes, DR Holmes Jr. Mount Kisco, New York, Futura Publishing Company, 1993, pp 309-359.)

others a preset differential is used when the differential AV interval is programmed "on."

Rate-variable or rate-adaptive AV interval. Some DDDR pacemakers have the capability of shortening the AV interval during AV sequential sensor-driven pacing.[83] Rate-adaptive or rate-variable AV interval is intended to optimize the cardiac output by mimicking the normal physiologic decrease in P-R interval that occurs in the normal heart as the atrial rate increases. The rate-related shortening of the AV interval may also improve atrial sensing by shortening the total atrial refractory period and thereby giving more time for the atrial sensing window. Alternatively, the atrial sensing window could be maintained if the PVARP were automatically shortened as the ventricular rate increased.[84]

Polarity programmability

Polarity programmability allows programming from unipolar to bipolar functions.[85] This appears to be most helpful in patients who have myopotential or electromagnetic inhibition in the unipolar mode but not in the bipolar mode. Unipolar and bipolar electrograms may have distinctly different characteristics, and programming from one polarity to the other may result in superior sensing of an electrogram or the elimination of the sensing of an unwanted electrogram or an interfering signal.[86-89]

Some generators allow several variations of polarity programmability,[90] so that one can selectively program the polarity for sensing and pacing. In most dual-chamber pacemakers with polarity programmability as an option, the same polarity must be programmed in both channels. However, in some pacemakers, it is possible to program unipolar programmability in one channel and bipolar in the other.

Phantom programming

Several categories of phantom or spurious programming have been defined. Included are misprogramming that can occur from faulty program emission signals, dysprogramming from anomalous sources, and phantom physician programming.[91] Despite the fact that telemetry capability continues to improve, programming problems persist. One of the largest problems at this time is that each pacemaker is programmed by an individual programmer, and the programmers continue to become more and more complex. There has been some interest in the pacemaker industry to create a "universal" programmer. Whether or not such a universal programmer will ever exist remains to be seen. However, for the present, the physician should become familiar with each individual programmer and sequence of programming for a particular event and remember to verify the patient's programmed sequence after each program change has been completed.

CLINICAL APPLICATION OF PACING MODALITIES

As a result of the constant improvement in pacemaker technology, many types of pacing modalities are available to practicing physicians. Once the decision has been made to use pacing in an individual patient, the most appropriate mode of pacing must be selected.

Pacemaker code system

Because of the proliferation of pacing systems with many different types of function, a code system was developed, and then revised, so that the precise function of each unit would be clear for all who intended to use them.

A three-letter code was introduced in 1974,[92] and in 1981 the pacemaker study group revised the code system to allow the code to contain information about the programmable function and antitachycardia function of any given pulse generator.[93] In 1987, the North American Society of Pacing and Electrophysiology (NASPE) in conjunction with the British Pacing and Electrophysiology Group (BPEG) revised the code for permanent pacemakers.[94] The current code ("NBG" designating the combined American and British organizations) is shown in Table 25A-7.

With this code system, a ventricular-demand pacemaker capable of rate modulation would be designated "VVIR." A dual-chamber, non-rate-modulated pacemaker with telemetric capability would be designated "DDDC."

Pulse generator mode selection

The pacing mode utilized should be one that optimizes cardiac output and exercise capacity, prevents symptomatic VA conduction (pacemaker syndrome), reduces the incidence of paroxysmal tachycardia, and reduces the chances of systemic or pulmonary thromboembolism.[95]

Pacemaker influence on cardiac output. Many elements contribute to the ultimate effect of any pacing system on cardiac output. In general, these have been thought to include the site from which the heart is paced,[96] the status of myocardial function (or the presence or absence of underlying cardiac disease), the rate at which the heart is paced, the AV interval, and the sequence of ventricular activation.

Each element will be discussed separately, but it is obvious that there is significant interaction among all factors.

SITE OF CARDIAC PACING. The heart can be paced from the ventricle, the atrium, or both chambers. A major factor underlying the importance of the pacing site is the presence or absence of AV synchrony.

The contraction of the atrium aids in transport of blood to the ventricle. It increases ventricular end-diastolic pressure without concomitant increase in atrial pressure.[97,98] This reduction in preload (without effect on venous pressure) facilitates venous return and prevents systemic and pulmonary venous congestion. The enhancement of ventricular filling (end-diastolic volume) results in an increase in fiber length which enhances the force of myocardial contraction,[99-101] which in turn leads to an increase in stroke volume and cardiac output.

The increase in ventricular pressure resulting from atrial systole is sufficient during early atrial diastole to

Table 25A-7 The NBG* generic pacemaker code

Position†	**I**	**II**	**III**	**IV**	**V**
Category‡	**Chamber(s) paced**	**Chamber(s) sensed**	**Response to sensing**	**Programmability, rate modulation**	**Antitachy-arrhythmia function(s)**
	O = None A = Atrium V = Ventricle D = Dual (A + V)	O = None A = Atrium V = Ventricle D = Dual (A + V)	O = None T = Triggered I = Inhibited D = Dual (T + I)	O = None P = Simple programmable M = Multiprogrammable C = Communicating R = Rate modulation	O = None P = Pacing (antitachyarrhythmia) S = Shock D = Dual (P + S)
Manufacturer's designation only	S = single (A or V)	S = single (A or V)			

*The North American Society of Pacing and Electrophysiology and the British Pacing and Electrophysiology Group.
†Positions I through III are used exclusively for antibradyarrhythmia function.
‡Pacing modes are currently designated with a 3- to 5-letter code. For example, DDDR denotes a pacing function with atrial and ventricular pacing and sensing, with a dual mode of response, and with rate modulation.
From Bernstein AD, Camm AJ, Fletcher RD, et al: The NASPE/BPEG generic pacemaker code for antibradyarrhythmia and adaptive-rate pacing and antitachyarrhythmia devices. *PACE* 10:794-799, 1987. By permission of Futura Publishing Company.

reverse the AV pressure gradient, thus placing the AV valve leaflets in approximation before or at the onset of ventricular systole.[102]

Conversely, when the atria and ventricles contract at or about the same time rather than separately and sequentially, the ventricles are deprived of the atrial contribution to ventricular filling, mean atrial pressure increases in relation to the ventricular end-diastolic pressure, the end-diastolic pressure is lower, and the ventricles produce less external work.

The magnitude of the decrease in cardiac output, stroke volume, etc., has been shown in many studies that have compared atrial (intact AV conduction) with ventricular pacing or compared sinus rhythm with rhythms not having consistent atrial contraction (atrial fibrillation or ventricular pacing).

When AV dissociation is artificially created by ventricular pacing (with retrograde VA block), there is a reduction in cardiac output and stroke volume (15% to 20%) when ventricular systole is not preceded by atrial systole.

In studies in patients with undefined degrees of cardiac disease (many normal patients), comparison of atrial to ventricular pacing at the same heart rate demonstrated increases, of 15% to 50%,[100,103,104] in cardiac output with atrial pacing.

Mitral regurgitation may occur in the absence of AV synchrony and may also be contributing to the decrease in cardiac output and ventricular performance. The increase in left ventricular pressure resulting from the atrial contraction can close the AV valve; however, when the ventricle contracts without a preceding atrial systole, the valve swings closed from the open position and regurgitation into the atrium during this interval results. The presence of AV valve regurgitation during ventricular pacing would be expected to reduce ventricular volume at the moment of ventricular excitation and therefore reduce forward stroke volume.

The magnitude of mitral regurgitation is variable, and the lack of a properly timed atrial contraction probably does not induce AV valve incompetence of clinical importance in the majority of patients.[97] However, in some patients the degree of acute mitral regurgitation may be severe. It is thought by some authors that, in the presence of preexisting AV valve regurgitation (especially mitral regurgitation), ventricular pacing significantly accentuates the degree of insufficiency, and cardiac output may fall.[105]

When this has been shown to be a significant problem, restoration of AV synchrony has minimized the valvular regurgitation.

FUNCTIONAL STATUS OF THE MYOCARDIUM. The effect of AV synchrony on cardiac output and other measures of cardiac performance may be of particular importance in patients with myocardial disease and resultant resistance to myocardial filling due to changes in ventricular compliance.[106]

Some questions have been raised about the benefits of atrial synchrony in patients with severe ventricular dysfunction.[107] In a comparison of patients with congenital heart block with and without associated myocardial disease, it was found that AV synchrony was less effective in augmenting right ventricular stroke volume in symptomatic patients (13% increase) than in patients without myocardial disease (40% increase), even though there were increases in both groups.[108]

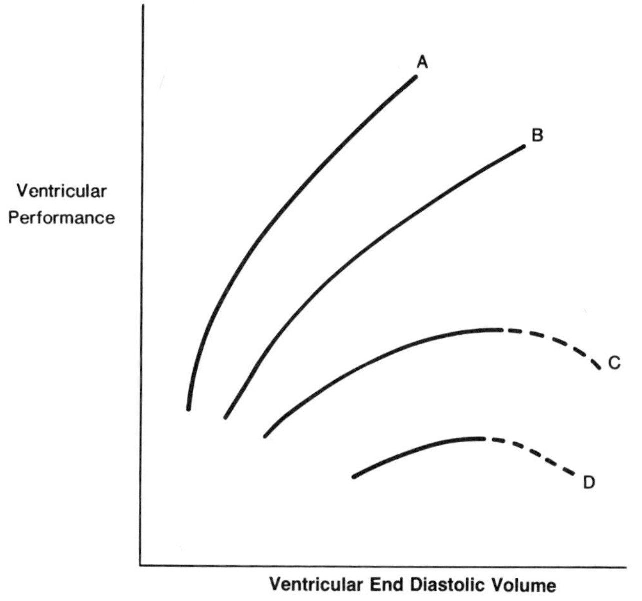

Fig 25A-22 Starling's law (curve) of the heart. A-D reflect progressively worsening ventricular function. As ventricular performance worsens, increases in end-diastolic volume have less beneficial effects and may actually result in a deterioration in ventricular function.

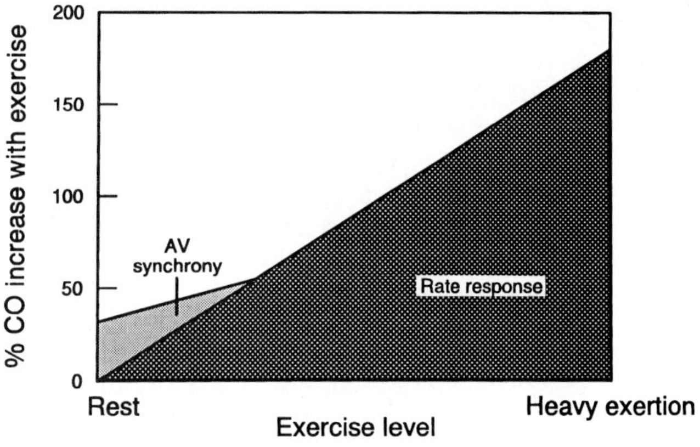

Fig 25A-23 Schematic representation of relative contribution of AV synchrony and rate response with increasing levels of exercise. At high levels of exercise, rate response is largely responsible for the increase in cardiac output. AV synchrony is more important at rest and lower levels of activity. This difference should not be underestimated, because most older persons with pacemakers are at rest or low levels of exercise most of the time. (Courtesy of D. Benditt, M.D., University of Minnesota.)

Greenberg et al.[109] have pointed out that the level of end-diastolic pressure would be expected to influence contribution to cardiac output. When the end-diastolic pressure is in the normal range, the left ventricular function curve is steepest and the atrial contraction should increase stroke volume maximally (Fig 25A-22). When the end-diastolic pressure is increased, further increments in pressure would be expected to have progressively less effect in augmenting stroke volume. In a series of patients (all with abnormal resting ejection fractions), the authors found that the stroke volume index was higher (by an average of 25%) with atrial pacing.

However, there was a significant decrease in the atrial contribution to stroke volume with increased pulmonary capillary wedge pressure or with overt heart failure. This would suggest that patients with severe myocardial dysfunction might not achieve the hemodynamic improvement hoped for by maintaining AV synchrony.[109]

Even modest increases in cardiac output may be of benefit to patients with myocardial dysfunction, and the decreases in hemodynamic parameters that have been seen as a result of ventricular pacing could result in further decompensation in some patients.[99]

All the studies cited have pointed out that there is a considerable variability among patients in the hemodynamic response to maintenance of AV synchrony. In some patients with or without severe cardiac dysfunction, the loss of atrial systole is compensated for (partially or completely) by other adaptive mechanisms. The factors that contribute to the ability of effective atrial contraction to augment integrated cardiac performance are still poorly defined.[110] It seems clear that the decision to use a pacing system that maintains AV synchrony should be based (at least in part) on some assessment of the patient's potential for hemodynamic benefit.

Cardiac output is the product of stroke volume times heart rate. Thus, cardiac output is closely dependent on heart rate, especially at rates below which stroke volume is maximal (Fig 25A-23). The increased metabolic demands of the body in response to routine activity and exercise are met through an increase in cardiac output and oxygen delivery. Patients who lack rate responsiveness must rely solely on an increased stroke volume to provide the necessary adjustments in cardiac output, which may limit their ability to exercise.[111] This may be true especially in some patients with myocardial dysfunction who are unable to increase stroke volume with exercise. In some, stroke volume tended to decrease even during mild exertion.

Questions have been raised about the relative roles of AV synchrony and increased heart rate in the maintenance of optimal cardiac output. Karlöf[97] compared atrial synchronous pacing and fixed ventricular pacing. When a ventricular rate fixed at 70 beats/min was compared to a rate-response system, there was a 27% average increase in cardiac output during exercise, when the ventricular rate was allowed to increase by atrial synchrony. But, when the fixed ventricular rate was adjusted to coincide with the maximal atrial rate achieved during exercise, there was only an 8% increase in cardiac output with atrial synchronous pacing.[97] Fananapazir et al.[112] demonstrated that there was a similar increase in work capacity (compared to fixed-rate pacing) in patients with rate-responsive pacemakers maintaining AV synchrony or with pacemakers triggered by chest wall stimulation at a rate slightly faster than the atrial rate, thus eliminating AV synchrony. This suggests that the rate response, not the maintenance of AV synchrony, is the major determinant in improvement of cardiac performance.[112]

Regardless of the controversy over the relative importances of AV synchrony and rate in the maintenance of optimal exercise capacity, two things are clear from all of the above studies. First, rate is an important factor in determination of cardiac output, and second, the combination of the two is clearly a very effective means of allowing rate responsiveness in pacing. As will be discussed later, these two factors have been very successfully combined in many atrial synchronous pacing systems.

AV INTERVAL. If preservation of AV synchrony is important in optimizing cardiac output, it would seem obvious that the timing of atrial and ventricular contractions also is of importance.

If the AV interval is excessively long, the atria may contract against closed AV valves during the preceding ventricular systole and therefore make no contribution to, or actually decrease, stroke volume. In addition, if atrial contraction occurs very early in ventricular diastole during the rapid ventricular filling phase, atrial contraction may not significantly augment ventricular filling.[108] An inappropriately short AV interval may not enhance cardiac output because of the lack of adequate time for antegrade atrial emptying before ventricular systole. There is marked variability of the optimal AV intervals from patient to patient, with wide ranges over which cardiac output and stroke volume are maintained. This is true for patients with normal or abnormal myocardial function.

It is known from several studies that the most effective P-R interval is related to the heart rate—i.e., short P-R intervals are more effective as the heart rate increases[113-118] (Fig 25A-24). These data indicate the importance of properly timed atrial systole in determining stroke volume, especially at rapid heart rates. Thus, this capability should be incorporated into the adjustments of programmable rate-responsive pulse generators.

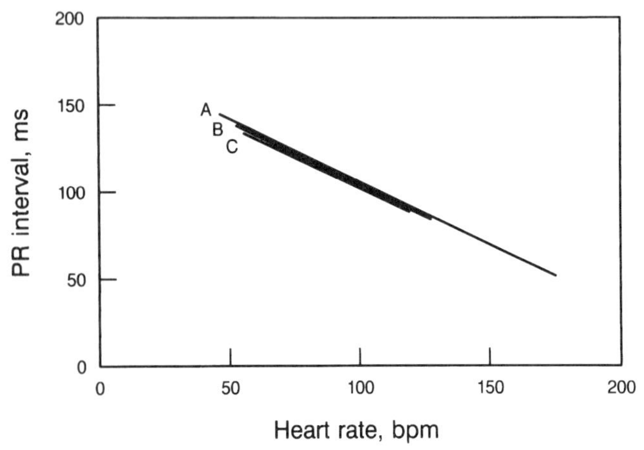

Fig 25A-24 Linear regression of P-R interval (milliseconds) and heart rate (beats per minute) from electrocardiograms in young healthy subjects (group A), older healthy subjects (group B), and subjects after myocardial infarction (group C). (From Rees M, Haennel RG, Black WR, et al: Effect of rate-adapting atrioventricular delay on stroke volume and cardiac output during atrial synchronous pacing. *Can J Cardiol* 6:445-452, 1990. By permission of the journal.)

VA conduction

INCIDENCE. VA conduction implies conduction of cardiac impulses in a retrograde fashion from ventricles to the atria via the normal conduction pathways or via an accessory conduction pathway.

The incidence of VA conduction is quite variable and is dependent upon the presence of disease in other areas of the conduction system. VA conduction will be present in 64% to 68%[119-121] of those with normal antegrade conduction (by resting ECG). A similar percentage of patients with fascicular block (bundle-branch block with or without hemiblock) will also have intact VA conduction.[119] In patients with second-degree AV block, the incidence of VA conduction ranges from 20% (with AV node level block) to 36% (with intra-Hisian or infra-Hisian level block).[119] If complete AV block is present, VA conduction is still possible, depending on the level of the block. If the block is in the AV node, virtually no patients exhibit VA conduction. But if the level is below the AV node, VA conduction can be expected to occur in 15% to 20%.[119-121]

In patients with sinus node dysfunction there is a variable incidence of associated AV nodal conduction system disease.[122] It is important to note that VA conduction is present in about 50% of all patients requiring implantation of a permanent pacing system. When AV conduction is intact, the VA interval is variable and has ranged from 120 to 420 msec (mean, about 230 msec).[123]

It has been shown that atrial natriuretic peptide levels rise significantly above normal levels with ventricular pacing and intact VA conduction[124] (Fig 25A-25). This finding suggests that VA conduction results in a significant increase in atrial wall tension. With DDD pacing, the

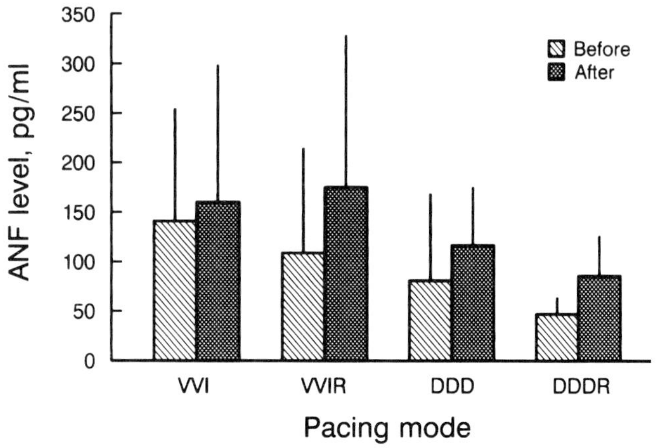

Fig 25A-25 Effect of various pacing modes on levels of atrial natriuretic peptide *(ANF)* before and immediately after exercise. DDDR pacing resulted in the least increase in ANF levels, both at rest and after exercise.

atrial natriuretic peptide levels at rest are usually near normal.[125]

It should be remembered that the VA conduction may be modified by autonomic tone and drugs, and it may be absent during ventricular pacing (at the lowest possible rates) if the spontaneous sinus rate is fast, only to return when this rate slows.[126]

CONSEQUENCES. The presence of VA conduction has the potential for causing two significant problems: pacemaker syndrome and the initiation of tachyarrhythmias.[125,127] Embolic phenomena have also been shown to occur more commonly in VVI than in DDD pacing modes in patients with intact VA conduction.[128]

The term "pacemaker syndrome" is used to describe a symptom complex that develops as a result of or worsens during ventricular pacing.[122,129-133] Potential symptoms are listed in Table 25A-8. The decrease in cerebral blood flow is a result of a decrease in cardiac output that may occur secondary to the loss of AV synchrony[97] and may be aggravated by abnormal timing of AV valve closure, resulting in AV valve regurgitation. However, the hallmark of the pacemaker syndrome appears to be retrograde VA conduction, which leads to persistent contraction of the atrium against the closed mitral and tricuspid valves.[97,122,134]

The decrease in cardiac output caused by this persistent contraction of the atria against closed AV valves is likely to be more profound than that caused by the intermittent variation in AV synchrony resulting from AV disassociation with ventricular pacing because the loss of atrial contribution to cardiac output is maximal when VA synchrony is 1:1.[135]

If persistent, this could lead to a profound decrease in cardiac output and hypotension in some patients[101] (Fig 25A-26).

Hemodynamic studies in patients with atrial pacing or ventricular pacing in the presence of persistent VA conduction have demonstrated not only a significant reduction in cardiac output and ventricular end-diastolic pressure but also persistent changes in pulmonary artery wedge pressure tracings, suggesting or simulating acute severe mitral regurgitation and concomitant increases in pulmonary venous pressure.

In addition to the marked reduction in cardiac output resulting from VA conduction, the triggering of atrial stretch reflexes by persistent atrial dilatation in susceptible patients may lead to inappropriate peripheral vasodilatation or a reduction in the normal compensatory mechanism (in the face of systemic hypotension), which would aggravate a maldistribution of systemic blood flow and lead to decreased cerebral perfusion.[101]

The absence of an atrial contribution to cardiac output may be perpetuated in the presence of VA conduction. By capturing the atrium on a consistent basis, VA conduction may prevent the emergence of sinus rhythm and the establishment of normal AV synchrony.

In a series of nine patients, we found that symptoms of presyncope and syncope that occurred during ventricular pacing were associated with significant decreases in systolic blood pressure (greater than 20 mm Hg).[135] These symptoms accompanied intact VA conduction and were alleviated in most patients by reestablishment of AV synchrony by use of AV pacing. In those patients who

Table 25A-8 Potential symptoms of pacemaker syndrome

- Weakness
- Near-syncope
- Syncope
- Fatigue
- Lassitude
- Cough
- Apprehension
- Chest pain
- Hypotension
- Congestive heart failure
- Dyspnea
- Jugular venous pulsations
- Abdominal pulsations

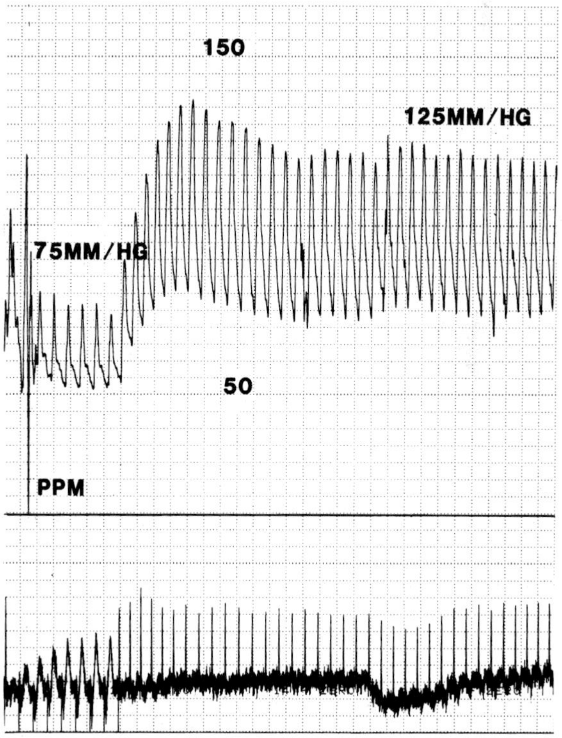

Fig 25A-26 Arterial pressure changes with and without ventricular pacing. Ventricular pacing of the first seven beats results in a systolic arterial pressure of approximately 75 mm Hg. Subsequent intrinsic rhythm results in a systolic arterial pressure of approximately 125 mm Hg. (From Hayes DL, Holmes DR Jr: Hemodynamics of cardiac pacing. In *A Practice of Cardiac Pacing.* Third edition. Edited by S Furman, DL Hayes, DR Holmes Jr. Mount Kisco, New York, Futura Publishing Company, 1993, pp 195-218. By permission.)

Table 25A-9 Studies assessing atrial fibrillation and mortality with mode of permanent pacing

First author	Patients, no.	Follow-up, mo	AF, %	Deaths, %	Difference in survival of $P \leq 0.05$?*	Only patients with SND analyzed?†	Comment
Alpert[30]							
DDD or DVI	49	1-18 yr	NA	16	NA	Yes	
VVI	79	1-18 yr	NA	27			
Bianconi[138]							
AAI/DDD	153	44	18	14	No	Yes	Abstract
VVI	150	59	39	31	0.08		
Feuer[139]							
DDD or DDI	110	40	8	7	NR‡	NR	
VVI	110	48	18	15			
Grimm[140]							
DDD	41	32	2	NA	NA	No	
VVI	203	69	32				
Hayes[141]							
DDD or DVI	172	1-13 yr	NR	29	Yes	No	Abstract
VVI	389	1-13 yr	NR	43			
Hesselson[142]							
DVI/DDD	58/308	2-14 yr	5/8	33/20	Yes	No	
VVI	193	2-14 yr	26	47			
Kosakai[143]							
AAI/AV-sequential	87/57	NR	16/23	NA	NA	No	
VVI	51	NR	57	NA			
Langenfeld[127]							
DDD	43	63	2	NA	NA	No	
CCI	203	63	31	NA			
Markewitz[144]							
AAI/DDI	67/69	51/13	14/3	NA	NA	Yes	
VVI	87	32	27	NA			
Nürnberg[145]							
AAI/DDD	15/22	41	13/18	27/23	Yes	No	Abstract
VVI	93	41	38	47			
Pieper[146]							
DDD/DVI	78/98	62	NR	NA	Yes§	Yes	
VVI	457	62	NR	NA			
Rosenqvist[29]							
AAI	89	44	7	8	Yes	Yes	
VVI	79	47	47	23			
Santini[147]							
AAI/DDD	135/79	60	4/12	13/16	Yes	Yes	
VVI	125	60	44	30			
Santomauro[148]							
DDD	186	51	NR	17	Yes	No	Abstract
VVI	204	51	NR	28			
Sasaki[149]							
AAI/DDD	17/24	39	0	13	Yes	Yes	
VVI	34	62	36	24			

NA, not available; NR, not reported; SND, sinus node dysfunction.
*Study included patients with other rhythm disturbances, but data in this table reflect the sinus node dysfunction subset only.
†Difference in survival statistically significant when AAI or dual-chamber pacing mode is compared with VVI mode.
‡No *P* value reported, but results suggest a significant difference in survival.
§Survival differences by Kaplan-Meier method.
Modified from Hesselson AB, Parsonnet V, Bernstein AD, et al: Deleterious effects of long-term single-chamber ventricular pacing in patients with sick sinus syndrome: the hidden benefits of dual-chamber pacing. *J Am Coll Cardiol* 19:1542-1549, 1992.

Table 25A-9 Studies assessing atrial fibrillation and mortality with mode of permanent pacing—cont'd

First author	Patients, no.	Follow-up, mo	AF, %	Deaths, %	Difference in survival of $P \leq 0.05$?*	Only patients with SND analyzed?†	Comment
Sethi[150]							
AAI	40	47	3	10	No	Yes	
VVI	47	50	21	15			
Stangl[151]							
AAI	110	40	6	17	Yes	Yes	
VVI	112	33	19	27			
Sutton[152]							
AAI	410	33	4	NA	NA	Yes	
VVI	651	39	22	NA			
van Erckelens[153]							
DDD	44	99	2	NA	Yes	No	
VVI	163	99	14	NA			
Witte[154]							
AAI/DDD	1,092/152	NR	NA	11	Yes	Yes	
VVI	3,440	NR	NA	23			
Zanini[155]							
AAI	53	45	4	9	Yes	Yes	
VVI	57	40	18	18			

continued to have symptoms, vasodepressor carotid sinus hypersensitivity (a decrease in blood pressure in response to carotid sinus massage despite normal atrial or AV pacing) was identified as a likely cause.

The incidence of pacemaker syndrome is difficult to determine and depends on how one defines pacemaker syndrome. If the definition is limited to patients with clinical limitations during any pacing mode that results in AV dissociation, the incidence is probably in the range of 7% to 10% of patients with VVI pacing, as estimated in a review by Ausbubel and Furman.[136] In a study by Heldman et al.,[137] patients with DDD pacemakers who were randomized to DDD or VVI pacing mode for 1 week and subsequently programmed to the alternate mode completed questionnaires comparing 16 symptoms during each pacing mode. With this approach, some degree of pacemaker syndrome was thought to be present in 83% of those studied. The most common symptoms reported were shortness of breath, dizziness, fatigue, pulsations in the neck or abdomen, cough, and apprehension. It can be concluded from this study that if patients with VVI pacing have some basis for comparison, they may be more aware of symptoms with VVI pacing.

The key to therapy in this situation appears to be *avoidance* of VA conduction. Our approach is to use intraoperative testing: recording the intra-atrial electrogram to assess VA conduction in both the supine and semi-erect positions (using a tilt table) and measuring supine and erect blood pressure changes during ventricular pacing. If VA conduction and/or a significant (greater than 20 mm Hg) decrease in blood pressure are confirmed, dual-chamber pacing is implemented.

Effect of pacing mode on morbidity and mortality. An early prospective study by Rosenqvist et al.[29] initiated much of the initial interest in the effect of pacing mode on survival. Although this study was not without criticism (patients were not randomized to the AAI and VVI pacing modes and there was a question of selection bias in the criteria allowing patients to be in the AAI group), the 4-year analysis of the data was, and remains, impressive. At 4 years of follow-up, atrial fibrillation had occurred in 47% of the VVI group versus 7% of the AAI group ($P < 0.0005$) and congestive heart failure in 37% of the VVI group versus 15% of the AAI group ($P < 0.005$); mortality was 23% in the VVI group versus 8% in the AAI group ($P < 0.025$).

RETROSPECTIVE ANALYSES. The Rosenqvist et al. study prompted many other investigators to perform retrospective reviews to assess the effect of pacing mode on mortality[30,127,138-156] (Table 25A-9). Some studies considered mortality as the only end point, whereas others assessed the incidence of thromboembolic disease or atrial fibrillation, or both.

The study by Hesselson et al.[142] merits discussion. The authors performed long-term follow-up of 950 patients with sinus node dysfunction and various pacing modes. Results were analyzed by presence or absence of sinus node dysfunction and pacing mode. Modes considered were DDD, DVI, and VVI. At 7 years of follow-up in patients with sinus node dysfunction, atrial fibrillation had developed in 5% of the DDD group, 9% of the DVI group, and 26% of the VVI group. Mortality in the group with sinus node dysfunction at 7 years of follow-up was 20% in DDD, 33% in DVI, and 47% in VVI. Interestingly, in the cohort without sinus node dysfunction, atrial fibrillation developed in 2% of the DDD group, 8% of the DVI group, and 5% of the VVI group.

In a recent study, Lamas et al.[157] reported survival in a large population (n = 20,948) of patients with sinus node dysfunction. The population was a random sample of the complete United States cohort of Medicare patients with pacing for sinus node dysfunction in 1988 through 1990. DDD/DDDR pacing mode was an independent correlate of survival (odds ratio, 0.80; 95% confidence interval, 0.73 to 0.88).

The issue of paroxysmal atrial fibrillation has also been addressed in the retrospective studies. It is an issue of importance because there have been anecdotal reports of less frequent paroxysmal atrial fibrillation in patients with pacing in a dual-chamber or AAI pacing mode than in those with VVI pacing. In a recent study, Santomauro et al.[148] demonstrated better survival with dual-chamber pacing than with ventricular single-chamber pacing in a group of 390 patients and analyzed survival by whether patients had atrial fibrillation or paroxysmal atrial fibrillation. At 5 years, survival was 72% with VVI pacing and 83% with DDD (P < 0.01); survival without atrial fibrillation was 74% in VVI-paced patients and 86% in DDD-paced patients (P < 0.001). However, in patients with paroxysmal atrial fibrillation, the difference was less marked: survival was 70% with VVI pacing and 72% with DDD pacing (not significant).

In assessing Table 25A-9, despite the retrospective nature of all the studies, with the exception of Rosenqvist et al.,[29] and all the inherent weaknesses of retrospective analyses, it is difficult to dismiss the similar outcomes among all the studies. Nonetheless, these studies lack definitive answers that could be provided by a prospective outcome-based study.

PROSPECTIVE ANALYSES. In a 1992 review and critique of the retrospective literature on the effect of pacing mode on the development of atrial fibrillation and survival, Lamas et al.[158] called for a prospective randomized, controlled trial. The authors stated that "the current retrospective data support the need for a randomized trial, but do not allow a definitive recommendation to be made regarding atrial pacing to prevent atrial fibrillation in patients with sick sinus syndrome." They proposed implantation of a DDD pacemaker with randomization to DDD or VVI in patients with sinus node dysfunction and thought that such a study would require approximately 1,000 patients and follow-up of 3 years to allow detection of a 30% reduction in the incidence of atrial fibrillation.

Lamas et al. then proceeded with a prospective randomized trial. Pacing Mode and Survival in the Elderly (PASE) began enrolling patients in January 1993.[159] This multicenter trial will compare quality of life as a primary end point in patients with pacemakers programmed to DDDR and VVIR modes. Secondary end points include all causes of mortality, hospitalization for congestive heart failure or cerebrovascular accidents, and atrial fibrillation. A total of 400 patients, 65 years of age or older, will be enrolled. Patient enrollment is expected to be completed in 1994 and follow-up in all patients to extend at least 1 year after enrollment.

Andersen et al.[160] published the first prospective data on pacing mode and survival. They randomized 225 patients with sinus node dysfunction to AAI or VVI pacing. The data were analyzed and presented in "intermediate status," that is, final follow-up was to have been accomplished 1 year later. They found that mortality was 10.9% in the AAI group and 13% in the VVI group; atrial fibrillation occurred in 9.7% of the AAI group and 19% of the VVI group and cerebrovascular disease in 3.8% of the AAI group and 9.3% of the VVI group. Even though the difference in mortality between the two groups was not significant at the time the data were analyzed, it is a distinct possibility that mortality could reach significance

Table 25A-10 Prospective trials of pacing modes and survival

Trial	Modes	Patients, no.	Rhythm disturbance	Date of inception	Anticipated date of enrollment completion	End points (primary & secondary)
Andersen et al.[160]	VVI vs. AAI	225	SND	1988	1991	Mortality, AF, CVA, CHF
PASE*	VVIR vs. DDDR	400	All conduction system abnormalities	1993	1994	Quality of life, all causes of mortality, CHF, CVA, AF
CTOPP†	VVIR vs. AIR or DDDR	2,500	SND or AVB or both	1993	1995	Mortality, CVA, cardiac death, CHF, AF
U.K.-PACE‡	VVI vs. DDD	NA	2nd- or 3rd-degree AVB	1994	NA	NA

AF, atrial fibrillation; AVB, atrioventricular block; CHF, congestive heart failure; CVA, cerebrovascular accident; NA, information not available; SND, sinus node dysfunction.
*Pacing Mode Selection in the Elderly; Lamas GA: Personal communication, June 1994.
†Canadian Trial of Physiologic Pacing; Kerr CA: Personal communication, June 1994.
‡Camm AJ: Personal communication.

at later follow-up given the higher incidences of atrial fibrillation and cerebrovascular disease in the VVI group.

Other trials are under way or proposed (Table 25A-10). The Canadian Trial of Physiologic Pacing (CTOPP) was initiated in 1993. This prospective, randomized study will compare VVIR with AAIR or DDDR.[161] Patients with sinus node dysfunction or AV block (or both) as an indication for pacing are eligible, with the exception of AV block secondary to AV nodal ablation. To date, approximately 800 patients have been enrolled, and the goal is 2,500 patients.[162] Expected completion date for enrollment is 1995, with initial follow-up results available 1 year after enrollment is completed. Primary end points for the study are overall mortality and cerebrovascular accidents. Secondary end points are atrial fibrillation, hospitalizations for congestive heart failure, and death due to cardiac cause.

A prospective, randomized British trial, U.K.-PACE, recently begun, will compare DDD and VVI pacing modes in patients 70 years of age and older requiring permanent pacing for second- or third-degree AV block.[163]

Pacemaker modes

Selection of the pacing modality is dependent upon factors other than the ability to control bradyarrhythmias, although this is still the primary indication for use of a pacing device. In this section we review each of the types of pacing modalities commercially available and discuss the functional characteristics of each device, the indications or contraindications for use, the problems that can arise from the use of these devices, and clinical experience to date with them (when it is applicable).

Atrial or ventricular asynchronous (AOO, VOO) pacing

FUNCTION. Asynchronous pacing systems, whether they pace in the atrium or ventricle, are designed to provide a train of stimuli at a fixed rate regardless of any intrinsic cardiac activity (Fig 25A-27). They are the simplest pulse generators because they consist of only an output circuit with no sensing circuits present. These generators (especially the ventricular) were the first types of pacemakers to be used clinically.

There is really no indication for implanting a device with the intention of pacing in an asynchronous mode. An asynchronous mode may occasionally be used in an attempt to eliminate inappropriate bradycardia secondary to oversensing T waves, myopotentials, and so forth.

The major contraindication to asynchronous pacing is potential competition with the intrinsic rhythm. Competitive pacing could potentially lead to induction of unfavorable rhythm disturbances; for example, VOO pacing could potentially induce ventricular fibrillation if a ventricular stimulus occurred during the ventricular vulnerable period.

Ventricular demand (VVI) or ventricular triggered (VVT) pacing

FUNCTION. Demand pacing systems differ from asynchronous systems in that they have a sensing circuit in the pulse generator. The pacing rate of this type of system is determined by the preset or programmable escape interval—for example, for a rate of 70 beats/min the escape interval (or stimulus interval) is 857 msec.

Intracardiac activity detected by the sensing circuit modifies the escape interval in one of two ways. In inhibited systems, intracardiac activity (atrial or ventricular electrograms) occurring and detected during the intrastimulus interval (before the escape interval has elapsed) resets the pulse generator, so that the next

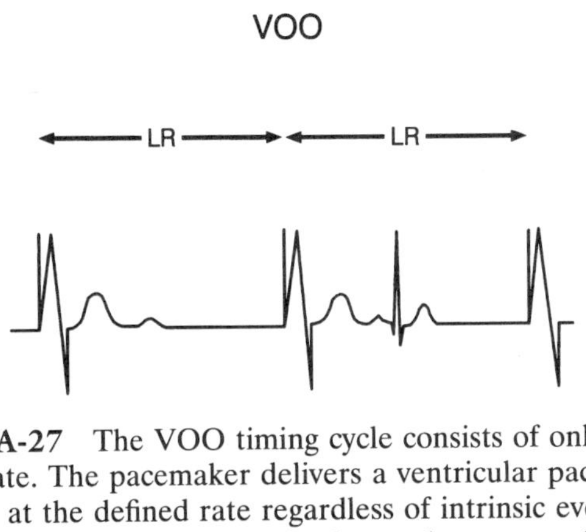

Fig 25A-27 The VOO timing cycle consists of only a defined rate. The pacemaker delivers a ventricular pacing artifact at the defined rate regardless of intrinsic events. In this example, an intrinsic QRS complex occurs after the second paced complex, but because there is no sensing in the VOO mode, the interval between the second and the third paced complex remains stable. *LR,* lower rate limit. (From Hayes DL, Levine PA: Pacemaker timing cycles. In *Cardiac Pacing.* Edited by KA Ellenbogen. Boston, Blackwell Scientific Publications, 1992, pp 263-308. By permission.)

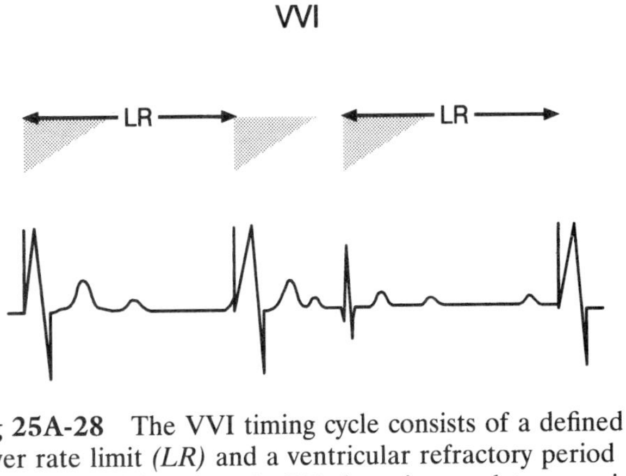

Fig 25A-28 The VVI timing cycle consists of a defined lower rate limit *(LR)* and a ventricular refractory period *(shaded triangle)*. When the LR timer is complete, a pacing artifact is delivered in the absence of a sensed intrinsic ventricular event. If an intrinsic QRS occurs, the LR timer is started from that point. A ventricular refractory period begins with any sensed or paced ventricular activity. (From Hayes DL, Levine PA: Pacemaker timing cycles. In *Cardiac Pacing.* Edited by KA Ellenbogen. Boston, Blackwell Scientific Publications, 1992, pp 263-308. By permission.)

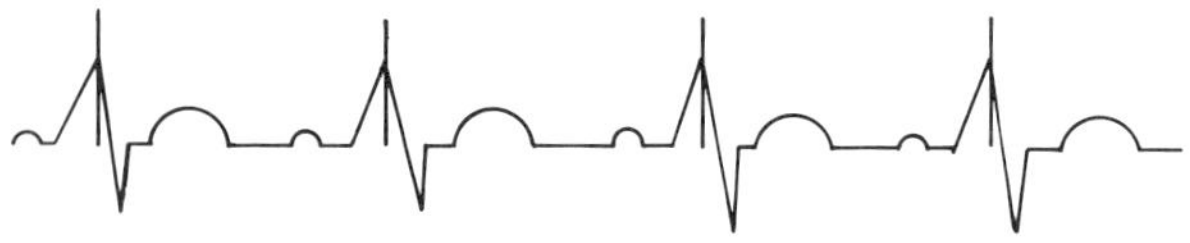

Fig 25A-29 Ventricular triggered pacing. When cardiac activity is sensed, a pacing stimulus is delivered at a time when ventricular stimulation cannot occur (during the ventricular refractory period).

stimulus occurs at the preset escape interval after the intrinsic activity (Fig 25A-28). In triggered systems, if the rate of spontaneous cardiac activity is faster than the preset pacemaker rate, an output stimulus occurs within the spontaneous electrogram during the absolute refractory period of the atrium or ventricle (to avoid initiation of repetitive beating) (Fig 25A-29).

ADVANTAGES AND DISADVANTAGES. The main advantage of the ventricular demand systems is their simplicity. The disadvantages are more numerous, including loss of AV synchrony with associated deterioration in hemodynamics, potential for retrograde VA conduction with its attendant problems, and lack of rate responsiveness to allow maximal exercise performance.

INDICATIONS AND CONTRAINDICATIONS. Indications for VVI pacing have declined (Table 25A-11). Some practices continue to use VVI pacing for a significant number of patients. Others now reserve VVI for patients in whom the atrium cannot be paced (i.e., atrial fibrillation) and in whom there is little potential for chronotropic incompetence developing. Because this is obviously hard to predict, others advocate implanting only ventricular demand systems that have the capability of rate modulation (VVIR) should the need arise in the future. VVI pacing may also remain appropriate for patients with very rare bradycardia (i.e., as a backup system) and in patients with associated terminal illness in whom it is thought that pacing is appropriate despite the associated illness.

VVI is specifically contraindicated if hemodynamic deterioration is noted during ventricular pacing, due either to loss of AV synchrony or to persistent VA conduction.

Atrial demand (AAI) or atrial triggered (AAT) pacing

FUNCTION. The atrial demand system is exactly like the ventricular demand system except that it functions by sensing atrial electrical activity and responding accordingly (Fig 25A-30).

ADVANTAGES AND DISADVANTAGES. The advantages of atrial pacing include preservation of AV synchrony, thereby optimizing cardiac output and other hemodynamic parameters; reduction of myocardial oxygen consumption; prevention of VA conduction; and control of atrial and ventricular arrhythmias by improvement in hemodynamics and elimination of atrial and ventricular bradycardia.[105,164,165] Several studies have shown a lower incidence of atrial fibrillation in patients with sinus node dysfunction who are paced AAI rather than VVI. A lower incidence of thromboembolic phenomena has also been demonstrated.[128]

There are two specific disadvantages of atrial demand pacing systems. The first is the lack of protection in the event of ventricular bradycardia. Therefore, atrial pacing systems are contraindicated in patients with AV nodal dysfunction. The second is that if the patient is being paced for sinus node dysfunction and has chronotropic incompetence, an atrial demand pacing system will not restore rate responsiveness. For most patients receiving an atrial demand pacing system for sinus node dysfunction, an AAIR pacemaker is most appropriate.

INDICATIONS AND CONTRAINDICATIONS. The clinical indication for atrial demand pacing systems would be sinus node dysfunction without evidence of AV conduction system disease in an attempt to give patients all the benefits of AV synchrony and eliminate the problems of VA conduction (Table 25A-12). A significant number of patients who either are chronotropically incompetent or will become chronotropically incompetent have clinical evidence of sinus node dysfunction. This has led to less use of AAI systems and a greater utilization of pacemakers with rate-modulated (AAIR) capability.

AAI pacing is contraindicated in the presence of AV node or His-Purkinje conduction system disease (because there is no protection against ventricular bradycardia), atrial flutter or fibrillation (because of the inability to

Table 25A-11 Ventricular demand pacing system

Indications:
Atrial fibrillation with complete heart block or slow ventricular response but without chronotropic incompetence
Rare episodes of bradycardia requiring "backup" pacing capability
Contraindications:
Hemodynamic deterioration secondary to
Loss of AV synchrony
VA conduction

Table 25A-12 Atrial demand pacing system

Indications:
Sinus node dysfunction with normal AV conduction
To optimize cardiac output
To prevent atrial tachyarrhythmia
To prevent VA conduction
To decrease the incidence of thromboembolism
Contraindications:
AV node or His-Purkinje conduction system disease
Chronic atrial flutter or fibrillation
Carotid sinus hypersensitivity

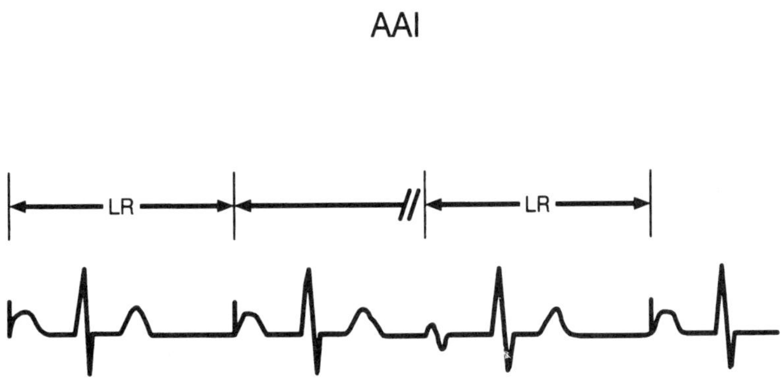

Fig 25A-30 Atrial demand (AAI) pacing. The interval from one atrial pacing artifact to the next is the lower rate *(LR)* interval. If an intrinsic atrial event occurs, the timing cycle is reset. (From Hayes DL, Levine PA: Pacemaker timing cycles. In *Cardiac Pacing.* Edited by KA Ellenbogen. Boston, Blackwell Scientific Publications, 1992, pp 263-308. By permission.)

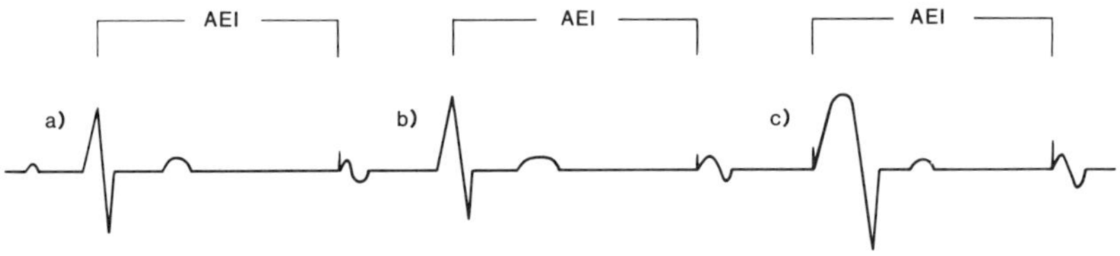

Fig 25A-31 AV sequential (DVI) pacing, demonstrating the atrial escape interval (*AEI;* VA interval), which is the period of ventricular sensing from a spontaneous or paced ventricular event to the initiation of atrial pacing. **a,** spontaneous atrial and ventricular activity; **b,** atrial pacing followed by spontaneous ventricular activity; **c,** atrial and ventricular pacing.

cause atrial stimulation), carotid sinus hypersensitivity (because of the potential for associated AV node block in addition to profound sinus bradycardia), and atrial disease resulting in poor P-wave generation (because of inherent problems in sensing with potential for competitive atrial rhythms).

Some form of electrophysiologic testing is required to determine if atrial demand pacing can be used safely in the presence of sinus node dysfunction. The incidence of associated AV node or His-Purkinje conduction system disease has been documented (or estimated) at between 36% and 67%.[122,166] These values have been based on the presence of conduction abnormalities on surface ECGs and include first-degree AV block, fascicular disease, bundle-branch block, and second-degree and third-degree AV block. The number of patients who actually go on to have AV block is much smaller and has been shown to be very low.[167,168]

Many authors have been satisfied to use the response to intraoperative atrial pacing as a guide to the safety of this system for pacing, without the benefits of a full electrophysiologic study. Others have stated that if 1:1 AV conduction is maintained at atrial pacing rates of 120 beats/min or greater, long-term atrial pacing could be carried out safely.

AV sequential (DVI) pacing

FUNCTION. This form of pacing involves the use of pacing electrode catheters in both the atrium and the ventricle but sensing only ventricular intracardiac activity. A new atrial escape interval begins with each sensed intraventricular electrogram (whether paced or occurring spontaneously).[169] If no ventricular activity is seen before the atrial escape interval has been completed, the atrium is stimulated by the pulse generator (Fig 25A-31).

Dual-chamber pacemakers capable of DVI pacing only are no longer implanted in the United States. However, many available dual-chamber pacemakers offer the DVI pacing mode as a programmable option. Therefore, an understanding of DVI function is important.

DVI pacing systems have been described as being committed or noncommitted. In the *noncommitted variety* (see Fig 25A-31), if no ventricular activity occurs before the first sensing cycle has expired, atrial pacing occurs. If ventricular activity occurs between the two sensing cycles (which is the preset AV interval), the pulse generator is inhibited and resets the atrial and ventricular escape intervals. If no ventricular activity is sensed during the AV interval, the ventricle and the atrium are paced.[170]

In the uncommonly seen *committed variety,* an atrial pacing stimulus is always followed by a ventricular pacing stimulus, whether or not a spontaneous ventricular event occurs within the pacemaker AV interval (Fig 25A-32).

In the DVI pacing mode, there is a real potential for competitive atrial beating and initiation of atrial tachyarrhythmias, particularly atrial fibrillation, because there is no atrial sensing.[171]

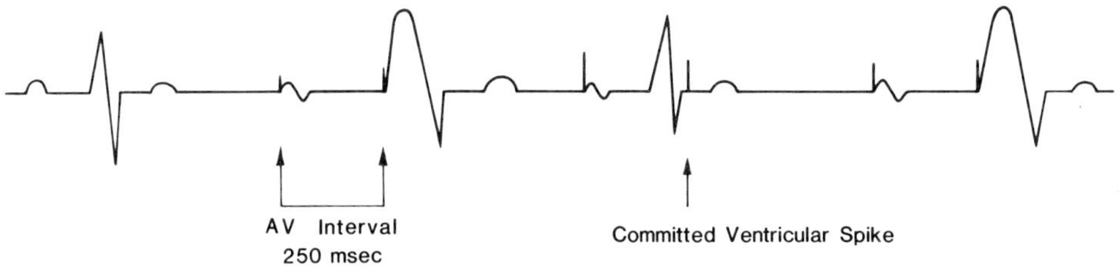

Fig 25A-32 Committed DVI (AV sequential) function. A ventricular stimulus always follows an atrial stimulus, despite normal AV conduction.

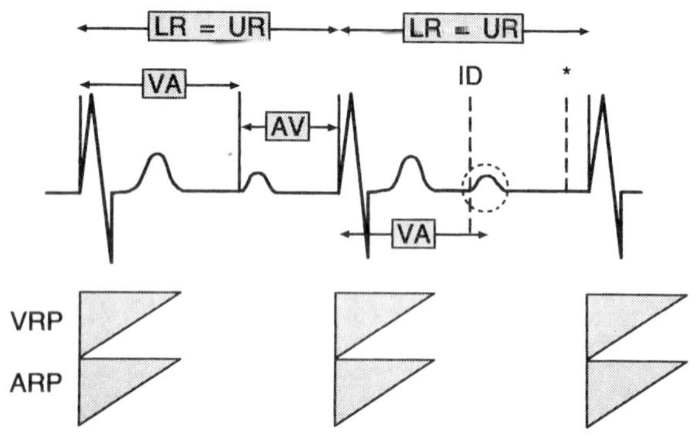

Fig 25A-33 The DDI timing cycle consists of a lower rate limit *(LR),* an AV interval, a ventricular refractory period *(VRP),* and an atrial refractory period *(ARP).* Paced or sensed ventricular activity initiates a VRP and a postventricular ARP. The LR cannot be violated, even if the sinus rate is faster. In this example, the first paced ventricular complex begins the ventriculoatrial *(VA)* interval. At the completion of the VA interval and in the absence of an intrinsic P wave, paced atrial activity occurs and is followed by paced ventricular activity at the completion of the AV interval. During the subsequent VA interval, an intrinsic P wave occurs *(broken circle;* sensed at *broken line ID).* However, the next ventricular pacing artifact cannot be delivered until the LR interval is complete. The dashed line with asterisk indicates the length of the programmed AV interval. *ID,* intrinsic deflection, *UR,* upper rate limit. (From Hayes DL: Timing cycles of permanent pacemakers. *Cardiol Clin* 10:593-608, 1992. By permission of WB Saunders Company.)

DDI pacing. DDI pacing can be viewed as DDD without P-wave tracking or DVI with atrial sensing. The advantage over DVI is that it eliminates competitive atrial pacing, and the obvious disadvantage over DDD is the inability to track normal sinus rhythm (Fig 25A-33). In the past, DDI was used for patients requiring dual-chamber pacing with associated paroxysmal supraventricular arrhythmias.[172] Such patients would probably be better served with DDDR pacing programmed in one of the several ways described in the subsequent section on DDDR pacing. The other option available in some pacemakers is DDD with mode-switching (see DDDR).

Atrial synchronous (VDD) pacing

FUNCTION. Atrial synchronous pacing systems function primarily by atrial sensing and ventricular pacing after a preset AV interval (Fig 25A-34).

Two timing circuits are incorporated in the generator to establish upper and lower rate limits (Fig 25A-35). If the intrinsic atrial (sinus) rhythm falls below the preset low rate limit, the pulse generator will revert to the ventricular demand mode at the programmed lower rate. When the atrial rate exceeds the lower rate limit, the ventricle will be paced in a 1:1 fashion (in the absence of spontaneous ventricular activity) until the preset upper rate limit is reached. When the atrial rate exceeds the programmed upper rate limit, pseudo-Wenckebach behavior is usually seen. With pseudo-Wenckebach behavior, there is a progressive increase in interval between the sensed atrial P wave and the pacer stimulus until the P wave occurs in the pacemaker atrial refractory period. This P wave is not sensed and therefore a ventricular stimulus is not delivered and the cycle then begins to repeat itself.

INDICATIONS. The dedicated VDD pacemaker had largely been supplanted by DDD pacemakers, although the mode was a programmable option in many DDD pacemakers. However, the VDD pacing mode as a single-lead pacing system has gained renewed interest. Single-lead VDD pacing systems are clinically available in the United States, and investigational work is continuing with VDDR pacemakers (a single-lead VDD system with VVIR capability as well).

With the single-lead VDD system, atrial sensing electrodes are incorporated in the pacing lead in the portion of the lead that resides in the atrial cavity (Fig 25A-36). Atrial sensing is bipolar, and ventricular pacing is unipolar. Single-lead VDD pacing systems have functioned very well, with excellent long-term atrial sensing.[173,174]

DDD pacing

FUNCTION. The DDD pacing system combines the functions of ventricular, atrial, AV sequential, and atrial synchronous. Pacing and sensing occur in both atrium and ventricle. The atrium is stimulated if sinus (atrial) bradycardia exists. Both atrium and ventricle are stimulated if bradycardia exists independently in both chambers; if heart block exists with normal sinus function the ventricle will be paced in synchrony with the atrium, and if sinus rhythm exists the pacemaker will be totally inhibited. Therefore, there are four different rhythms that can be seen as a result of normal pacemaker function: (1)

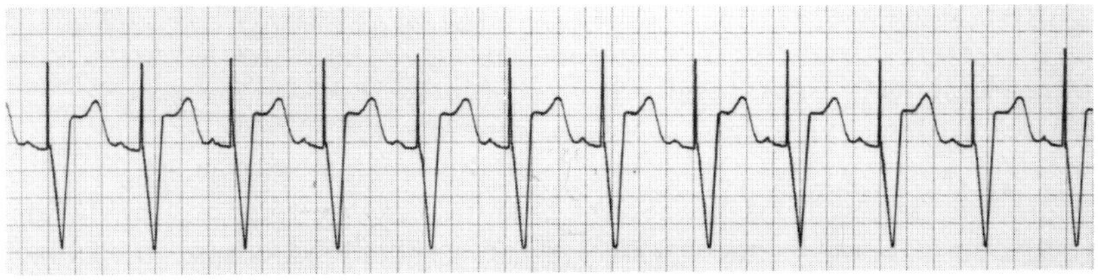

Fig 25A-34 Atrial synchronous (VDD) pacing. Normal spontaneous atrial activity followed by 1:1 ventricular pacing after AV interval of 175 msec.

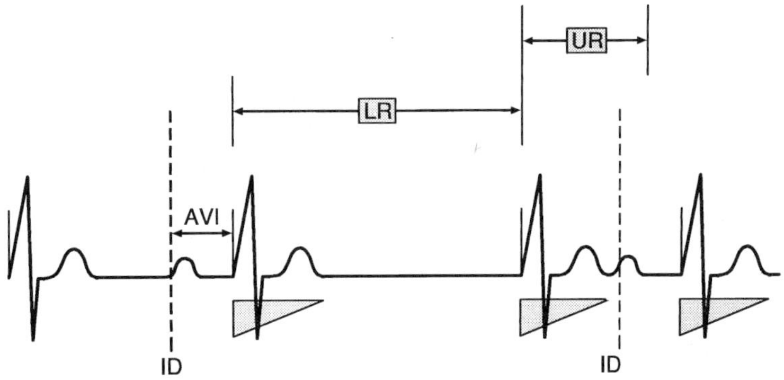

Fig 25A-35 The VDD timing cycle consists of a lower rate limit *(LR),* and AV interval *(AVI),* a ventricular refractory period, a postventricular atrial refractory period (PVARP), and an upper rate limit *(UR).* A sensed P wave initiates the AVI (during the AVI, the atrial sensing channel is refractory). At the end of the AVI, a ventricular pacing artifact is delivered if no intrinsic ventricular activity has been sensed, that is, P-wave tracking. Ventricular activity, paced or sensed, initiates the PVARP and the ventriculoatrial interval (the LR interval minus the AVI). If no P-wave activity occurs, the pacemaker escapes with a ventricular pacing artifact at the LR. *Shaded triangles* represent the duration of the PVARP. *ID,* intrinsic deflection. (From Hayes DL: Timing cycles of permanent pacemakers. *Cardiol Clin* 10:593-608, 1992. By permission of WB Saunders Company.)

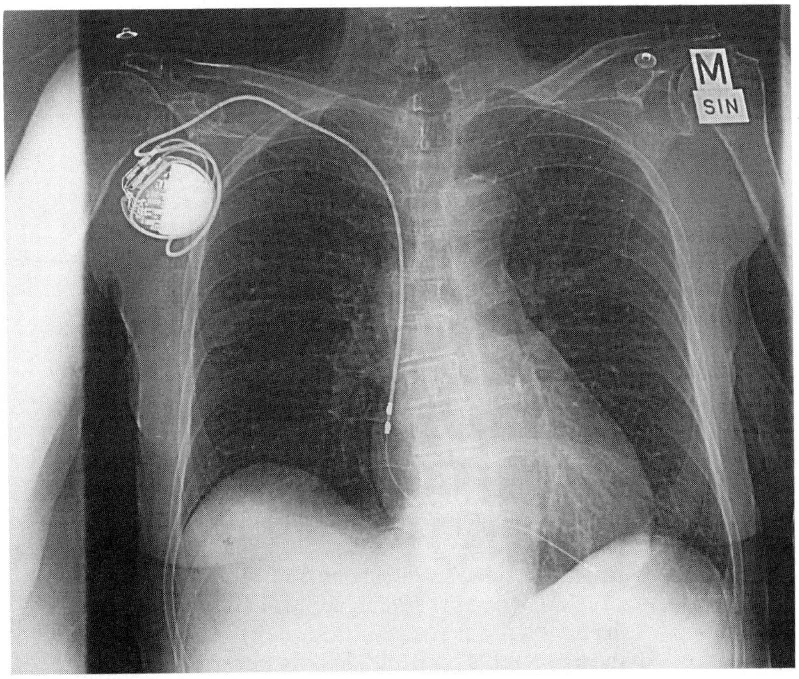

Fig 25A-36 Chest radiograph from a patient with a single-lead VDD pacing system. In the portion of the lead that lies within the atrium, two electrodes can be seen. These electrodes provide bipolar sensing of atrial activity. At the tip of the lead, right ventricular apex, another electrode provides unipolar ventricular pacing and sensing. (Courtesy of Intermedics, Inc.)

normal sinus rhythm; (2) atrial pacing (sinus bradycardia with intact AV conduction); (3) AV sequential pacing (atrial and ventricular bradycardia); and (4) atrial synchronous pacing (heart block with normal sinus activity)[175] (Fig 25A-37).

As with other atrial synchronous type systems, the atrial tracking function occurs between two preset limits. If the atrial rate falls below the lower rate limit, AV sequential pacing will occur. If the atrial rate exceeds the upper limit, some form of pacemaker-induced heart block will occur. This pacemaker-induced heart block could be 2:1 or pacemaker Wenckebach behavior, or it could take the form of ventricular fall-back. In ventricular fall-back, the ventricular rate will slowly decrease to a preset level (Fig 25A-38).

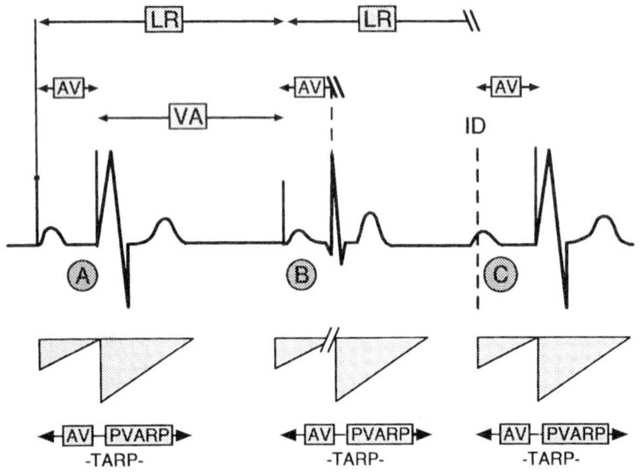

Fig 25A-37 Potential pacing combinations that can occur in the DDD pacing mode. Portions of the timing cycle induce a lower rate limit *(LR),* an AV interval, a ventricular refractory period, a postventricular atrial refractory period *(PVARP),* and an upper rate limit. (The AV interval and PVARP form the total atrial refractory period [*TARP*].) If intrinsic activity in both the atrium and the ventricle occurs before the LR times out, both channels are inhibited and no pacing occurs. *A,* if no intrinsic ventricular activity occurs before the termination of the AV interval, a ventricular pacing artifact is delivered: AV sequential pacing. (The intrinsic P wave is sensed during the early portion of the P wave. The AV interval is initiated at the point of the intrinsic deflection [*ID*] of atrial activity, as seen on the atrial electrogram.) *B,* if no atrial activity is sensed before the ventriculoatrial interval *(VA)* is completed, an atrial pacing artifact is delivered and initiates the AV interval. If intrinsic ventricular activity occurs before the termination of the AV interval, ventricular output from the pacemaker is inhibited: atrial pacing. *C,* if a P wave is sensed before the VA interval is completed (the LR minus the AV interval), output from the atrial channel is inhibited. The AV interval is initiated, and if no ventricular activity is sensed before the AV interval terminates, a ventricular pacing artifact is delivered: P-synchronous pacing. (From Hayes DL: Timing cycles of permanent pacemakers. *Cardiol Clin* 10:593-608, 1992. By permission of WB Saunders Company.)

ADVANTAGES AND DISADVANTAGES. The primary advantage of any type of atrial synchronous system is the ability to increase the ventricular rate to match the atrial rate in a 1:1 fashion as dictated by the physiologic needs of the body. With this system, there is an inherent ability to increase cardiac output during exercise secondary to the associated increase in cardiac rate, and thus there is no need for excessive increases in stroke volume or ventricular filling pressure. This system combines the benefits of AV synchrony and rate responsiveness in the chronotropically competent patient.

The main disadvantage of DDD pacing is the lack of rate responsiveness in patients with sinus node dysfunction, i.e., chronotropic incompetence.

INDICATIONS AND CONTRAINDICATIONS. The DDD pacing mode has traditionally been used for patients with normal sinus node function and AV block. In patients with sinus node dysfunction and AV block, DDDR pacing would be more appropriate if there were associated chronotropic incompetence. DDD or DDDR pacing is considered to be the mode of choice in neurocardiogenic syncope when there is significant vasodepression in addition to cardioinhibition.

DDD pacing is contraindicated in patients with chronic atrial flutter or fibrillation or with a paralyzed or inexcitable atrium.

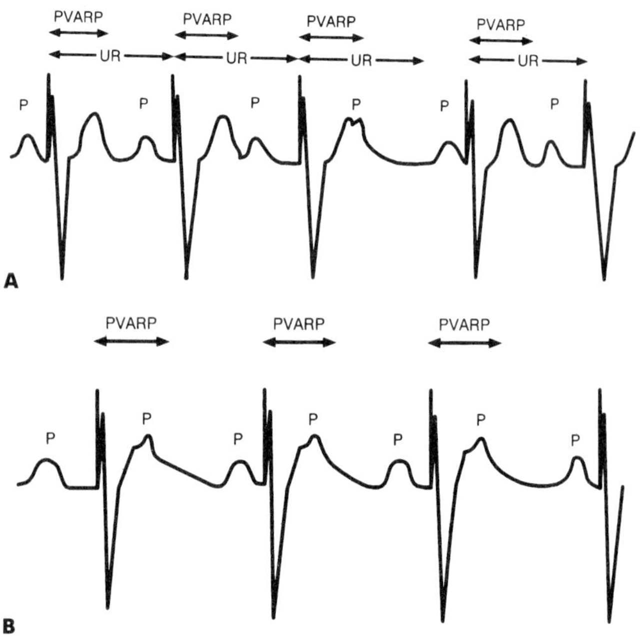

Fig 25A-38 **A,** the sinus rate exceeds the programmed upper rate limit *(UR),* resulting in pseudo-Wenckebach behavior. The fourth P wave falls in the postventricular atrial refractory period *(PVARP)* and is not sensed.
B, as the sinus rate becomes even faster, every other P wave falls in the PVARP, resulting in 2:1 block and a significantly slower ventricular rate. (From Hayes DL, Levine PA: Pacemaker timing cycles. In *Cardiac Pacing.* Edited by KA Ellenbogen. Boston, Blackwell Scientific Publications, 1992, pp 263-308. By permission.)

COMPLICATIONS. A potential problem with the use of all systems that have the capability of atrial synchronous pacing is pacemaker mediation of a reciprocating tachycardia. The term "endless-loop tachycardia" has been used in the literature to describe this type of arrhythmia. The anatomic and functional components of this tachycardia are the pacemaker itself (the antegrade limb) and normal conduction tissue (the retrograde limb). The requirements for the tachycardia are intact retrograde VA conduction, the artificial AV conduction (provided by the pacemaker), and a retrograde VA conduction time that exceeds the atrial (pacemaker) refractory period (measured after a sensed or paced ventricular event)[176] (Fig 25A-39).

The precipitating event may be (1) a ventricular ectopic beat with retrograde atrial conduction; (2) intermittent sensing of intrinsic atrial electrical activity (which will force the pulse generator to function in the low-rate mode, which, for a VDD system, is ventricular pacing); (3) escape to ventricular pacing during sinus bradycardia or pause (VDD); and (4) a ventricular ectopic beat that causes the AV disable mechanism to function (if the next beat is a ventricular paced beat, VA conduction could then ensue) (Fig 25A-40).

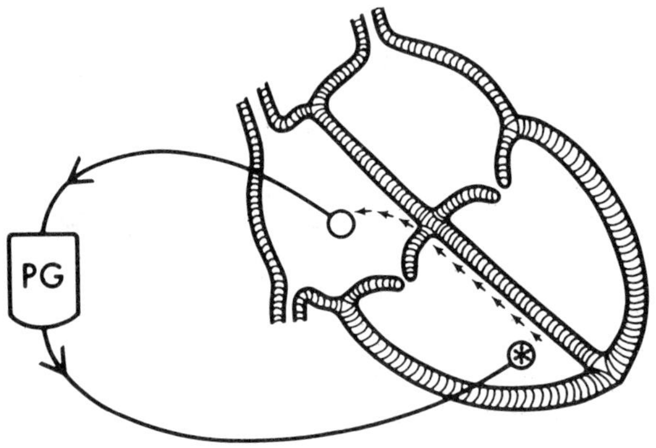

Fig 25A-39 Schematic representation of the components of an endless-loop tachycardia circuit: pulse generator *(PG)* to ventricular pacing lead to retrograde AV node conduction to atrial sensing lead.

The retrograde activity that results from any of these precipitating events will stimulate the atrium. Because the pulse generator cannot distinguish retrograde from antegrade atrial activation, it would synchronize with the atrial event. After an AV delay, the ventricle will be stimulated, which will result in VA conduction, atrial activation, pulse generator synchronization, ventricular pacing, etc.[177]

Several methods have been used to prevent endless-loop tachycardia. Programmable postventricular atrial refractory periods have had the greatest impact in preventing endless-loop tachycardia.[121,178] Unfortunately, lengthening this period may significantly limit the upper rate limit. Some tachycardia-terminating algorithms have been very successful at limiting the length of endless-loop tachycardia.[179] Discriminant atrial sensing, that is, distinguishing between antegrade and retrograde P waves, could potentially solve the problem of endless-loop tachycardia.[180,181]

If the refractory period of the pacemaker exceeds the retrograde VA conduction time, then no tracking of retrograde atrial activity can occur and therefore no tachycardia can be mediated by the pacemaker. Many pulse generators have great flexibility in refractory period programmability but it must be remembered that any increase in the pacemaker refractory period will limit the upper rate characteristics of the system. During the AV interval and the PVARP, atrial activity is not sensed. (The sum of the AV interval and the PVARP is the total atrial refractory period, or TARP.) If every other atrial beat falls within the TARP, 2:1 heart block will occur. Thus, if exercise capacity is the desired goal of atrial synchronous pacing, care must be taken to preset the shortest AV interval and pacemaker refractory period possible.

DDDR pacing overcomes the problem of upper rate limitation in patients who require a longer TARP because of endless-loop tachycardia. Even if the ability to track the intrinsic atrial rate is limited by a long TARP, the patient can achieve desired AV sequential pacing at rapid rates via sensor activation.

LIMITATIONS OF DUAL-CHAMBER PACING DEVICES. As discussed above, the greatest limitation of DDD pacing is in the patient with chronotropic incompetence who, despite the capability of P-wave tracking, lacks rate responsiveness.

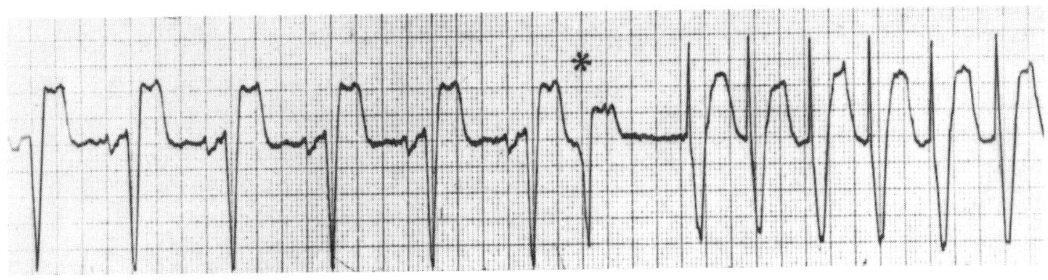

Fig 25A-40 AV disable mechanism. The ventricular premature beat (*) results in two consecutive ventricular events without intervening atrial activity. This causes atrial tracking to be disabled followed by a ventricular paced escape beat. In this case, a pacemaker-mediated tachycardia results.

Rate-adaptive pacemakers. Whenever possible, there should be some preimplantation assessment of the patient's chronotropic competence.[182,183] This information is helpful to assess the need for a rate-adaptive pacemaker. Some have advocated routinely using only pacemakers with rate-adaptive capability in the event chronotropic incompetence develops in the future. Such advocates have contended that it is difficult to predict in whom chronotropic incompetence will develop. The rate-adaptive antagonists have advocated using such a device only when chronotropic incompetence can be demonstrated and have noted that the current cost difference between rate-adaptive and non-rate-adaptive pacemakers cannot justify use of the rate-adaptive device in all pacemaker recipients.

Since the introduction of the first rate-adaptive pacemaker for general clinical use in the United States in 1986, rapid technologic advances have been made, and rate-adaptive pacemakers have rapidly been accepted as beneficial pacing modes. Multiple sensors are currently undergoing either laboratory or clinical investigation.

TERMINOLOGY. Multiple terms have been used to describe pacemakers with the ability to increase the pacing rate with activity or metabolic demand, but no single term has been universally accepted. In this chapter, the term "rate-adaptive pacing" will be used. Other terms are "rate-responsive pacing," "rate-modulated pacing," and "sensor-driven pacing."

In an effort to classify sensors on the basis of their response to physiologic variables, Rossi[184] divided sensors into five orders (Table 25A-13).

Table 25A-13 Classification of sensors by response to physiologic variables

Order	Physiologic variable
First – A sensor that directly measures O_2 consumption or energy expenditure	Oxygen uptake
Second – A sensor with a linear relationship to sensors of the first order	Cardiac output, minute ventilation,* atrioventricular O_2 difference
Third – A sensor with a linear relationship to sensors of the second order	Heart rate,* stroke volume,† mixed O_2 saturation,† respiratory rate,* tidal volume
Fourth – A sensor that relies on changes in sympathetic activity and circulating catecholamines	QT interval,* right ventricular dp/dt,† preejection interval,† ventricular depolarization gradient†
Fifth – A sensor that responds to physiologic feedback mechanisms in terms of metabolic activity or receptor reflexes	Central venous pH, central venous temperature,* right atrial pressure,† mixed venous lactate and bicarbonate levels

*Available clinically in the United States or Europe.
†Under investigation.
Data from Rossi P: Rate-responsive pacing: biosensor reliability and physiological sensitivity. *PACE* 10:454-466, 1987.

AVAILABLE RATE-ADAPTIVE SENSORS. At this writing, three types of sensors (activity, temperature, and minute volume) are available in the United States for general clinical use. Other sensors are available outside the United States, and multiple sensors are currently undergoing laboratory or clinical investigation.

Although few generalizations can be made about rate-adaptive systems, one can be made about the pacing lead. It is generally thought to be advantageous if a standard pacing lead can be used. If the rate-adaptive system requires that the sensor or part of the sensing apparatus be incorporated in the pacing lead, the pacing lead is less likely to be compatible with any other pacemaker in the event a change in pulse generator is required. Whether pacing leads that incorporate a special sensing apparatus will have an increased rate of failure remains to be seen.

Activity-detecting sensors. The first sensor to be introduced in the United States was an activity, or motion, sensor. A piezoelectric crystal glued to the inside of the pacemaker can sense body movement, which deforms the crystal. This mechanical energy is transformed into electrical energy. The electrical signal is filtered and fed into the pacemaker circuitry and results in a response from the rate-response algorithm. Other activity-detecting rate-adaptive pacing systems have incorporated an accelerometer. This works in much the same way as a piezoelectric crystal-based system but has the advantage of sensing anterior and posterior motion.[185-189] Although there may be a slight clinical advantage of an accelerometer over a piezoelectric crystal-based rate-adaptive pacing system in some patients, both types of activity sensors have performed very well clinically.

To determine the pacemaker's response to activity, one must program threshold and rate response. The threshold determines the level of activity sensed. For example, a low threshold setting would filter out very few activity signals and would allow the pacemaker to respond to low-level activity. A high threshold is less sensitive and would filter out everything but high-level activities. When the programmed threshold is exceeded, the rate response, or slope, can be programmed to allow the rate increment most appropriate for the individual patient.[190]

The major disadvantage of an activity sensor is that it does not respond to an indicator of metabolic demands. It is difficult to place the activity sensor in any one of Rossi's five categories.[184] Activity-sensing devices could result in unexpected or inappropriate increases in pacing rate. For example, the rate may increase in response to riding in a vehicle on rough terrain or from tapping on the pacemaker. The rate response to climbing stairs from an activity-sensing pacemaker is opposite to that of normal physiology. An activity-sensing pacemaker almost always produces a lesser rate response for walking up stairs than for walking down stairs.

Despite these limitations, the activity-sensing pacemakers have been quite successful and are reliable for long-term use. Activity-driven pacemakers use a standard pacing lead, so that an existing pacing system can be upgraded to VVIR/AAIR or DDDR if needed without placing new leads in the patient.

Minute volume. Minute volume (respiratory rate times tidal volume) has an excellent correlation with metabolic demand.[191-193] Measurement of minute volume is accomplished by emitting a small charge of known current (1 mA every 15 msec) from the pulse generator every 50 msec and measuring the resulting voltage at the lead tip.[194] When both current and voltage are known, transthoracic impedance can be measured between the ring electrode and the pulse generator can. Because transthoracic impedance varies with respiration and its amplitude varies with tidal volume, the impedance measurement can be used to determine respiratory rate and tidal volume. A pacing algorithm uses the minute volume measurements to alter pacing rate.

After initial programming to a rate-adaptive pacing mode, the pacemaker accrues data on the patient's respiration characteristics and makes a determination of the appropriate rate response parameter setting, referred to as the "rate-response factor." After programming to the rate-adaptive mode and the suggested rate-response factor, the patient should be exercised to determine if the rate-response factor does indeed result in appropriate rate-adaptation for the patient. For example, if the rate response is inadequate, a higher rate-response factor can be programmed and the patient re-exercised. If the rate response at the initial setting is too fast, a lower rate-response factor can be programmed and the patient re-exercised.

Long-term reliability of the minute volume sensor has been excellent.[195] Rate-adaptive pacing systems with minute volume sensing are clinically available in single- and dual-chamber pacemakers.[196]

Central venous temperature. Central venous temperature increases with exercise as heat is generated by skeletal muscles. This rise in temperature can be measured by a thermistor contained within the right ventricular portion of the pacing lead.[197,198] With the onset of exercise, central venous temperature decreases as cooler peripheral blood returns to the right ventricle. After this initial dip, the temperature increases as a function of absolute workload. Available thermistors are capable of an accuracy of 0.01°C change in temperature.

Although central venous temperature is an excellent correlate of metabolic demand at high workloads, response is less adequate at low workloads because of the relatively slow response of central venous temperature. One temperature-sensing pacemaker has demonstrated sensor reliability in a 1- to 14-month follow-up study.[199]

SENSORS NOT CLINICALLY AVAILABLE. Several other sensors have been or are being evaluated for their appropriateness in rate-adaptive pacing. Sensors that have undergone clinical investigation include dp/dt, stroke volume, preejection interval, oxygen saturation, and paced depolarization integral. Stimulus-T or QT sensing rate-adaptive pacing systems have been available in Europe and other countries for many years.

The *preejection interval* is measured by an impedance catheter in the right ventricle.[200] The preejection interval is the systolic time interval from the onset of electrical ventricular depolarization to the onset of ventricular ejection. In terms of ventricular pacing, the preejection interval is the interval between a right ventricular pacing stimulus and the onset of contraction determined by an impedance catheter.[201] The preejection interval shortens as exercise workload increases and can be used as a signal to increase the pacing rate. An increase in heart rate does not appreciably affect the preejection interval; that is, no significant positive feedback occurs.

Stroke volume, also measured by an impedance catheter in the right ventricle, can be used for rate-adaptive pacing by incorporation of a pacing algorithm that alters the pacing rate to keep the right ventricular stroke volume relatively constant and within physiologic values.

Change in right ventricular pressure, *dp/dt,* is measured by incorporating a pressure transducer in the right ventricular portion of the pacing lead.[202] In clinical investigations and in follow-up, the sensor has performed very well.[203]

Mixed venous oxygen saturation varies with physical activity, and the change begins rapidly with the onset of exercise. Oxygen saturation is measured with hemoreflectance oximetry. For a rate-adaptive pacing system, the oximeter is incorporated in the right ventricular portion of the pacing lead. The greatest challenge has been to find a stable sensor. Initial studies in animals and humans are encouraging.[204]

Paced depolarization integral is a less well known physiologic sensor that has been investigated as a single-sensor system but never market-released.[205] The concept of paced depolarization integral is somewhat complex and refers to the vector integral of the paced QRS, or ventricular depolarization gradient.[206] Lau[207] explained the clinical response of this gradient as follows. During fixed-rate ventricular pacing, exercise and the effect of circulating catecholamines decrease the ventricular depolarization gradient. An increase in pacing rate increases the gradient. Therefore, in a normal heart the ventricular depolarization gradient should remain relatively unchanged during exercise and other forms of stress and represents a "closed loop" rate-adaptive pacing system.

The paced depolarization integral responds relatively rapidly, similar to the rate response of an activity sensor. The disadvantage of this sensor has been the potential for rate response to decrease after the initial rate response despite an increase in the workload. In addition, a paradoxical response to posture has been seen, resulting in a lower pacing rate when the patient is upright during a head-up tilt.[207]

The interval from the onset of a paced QRS complex to the end of the T wave has been used for rate adaptation. This *stimulus-T interval* is affected by autonomic activity and heart rate. This relationship allows measurement of the stimulus-T interval to be used for rate adaptation.[208,209] The QT-sensing rate-adaptive pacing system has been very successful clinically but has not yet been introduced in the United States.

Right atrial pressure has been investigated as a measurement for rate adaptation but does not appear promising at present. Although mean right atrial pressure has the advantage of being a rapidly responding variable with a nearly constant sensitivity, the problem lies in the high sensitivity that would be necessary for detection of the relatively small pressure changes that occur in the right atrium. A sensitive enough to reliably detect such small pressure changes would probably be susceptible to many extraneous disturbances.

Central venous pH was the first metabolic parameter to be used for rate adaptation.[210] The pH change is an excellent indicator of metabolic demand, but long-term sensor reliability has been a problem. Because of sensor instability, pH is unlikely to be useful for rate adaptation in a permanent pacemaker.

DUAL-SENSOR COMBINATIONS. The overall performance of market-approved single-sensor rate-adaptive systems has been excellent. However, the perfect sensor would mimic the response of the normal sinus node. This includes appropriate response to all levels of activity, such as acceleration and deceleration of heart rate and emotional stress.

Clinical problems with available rate-adaptive pacing systems have been minimal. Both activity-sensing and minute-ventilation devices may respond to nonphysiologic stimuli. For example, with activity-sensing systems, rate acceleration may occur when the pulse generator is tapped or the patient rolls over on the pacemaker. A paradoxical rate response has also been shown; for example, sensor-driven rate response is often faster during descent of stairs than during ascent.[211] Minute-ventilation rate response may be interrupted if the patient is talking during exercise, and arm movement may result in a rate increase even if minute ventilation remains unchanged. These changes occur because minute ventilation is an impedance-based measurement and may be affected by any movement that alters thoracic impedance. Although response to nonphysiologic stimuli represents less-than-perfect specificity of the sensor response, both activity sensing and minute ventilation have served patients very well.

The perfect sensor would be resistant to these nonphysiologic stimuli. Although some "closed-loop" physiologic sensors could potentially be at or near 100% specificity, none are available clinically. A multisensor rate-adaptive pacing system could improve specificity by having one sensor verify or cross-check the other. For example, a dual-sensor pacemaker could be designed so that if sensor one reacted to a stimulus with a rate response but sensor two indicated that a rate increase was inappropriate, no rate increase would occur. Both sensors would have to indicate a rate increase before it would be allowed.

Several basic concerns had to be addressed in developing a dual-sensor pacemaker, including sensor interaction and programming. Sensor interaction could potentially be designed in several ways (Table 25A-14). The method of programming the rate-adaptive response and sensor interaction was also critical. Early concerns were raised about the potential complexity of programming two or more sensors, especially if programming of the sensors was done independently of one another.

Dual-sensor systems undergoing clinical investigation in humans. The first VVIR dual-sensor pacemaker began clinical investigation in August 1991 and was clinically released in Europe in January 1992. This device combines activity and Q-T interval sensing. Sensor combinations that are market-released in Europe or Asia or are in clinical investigation in the United States or elsewhere are shown in Table 25A-15.

Problems with a multi-sensor rate-adaptive pacemaker. Lau[212] lists several potential concerns with dual-sensor pacing systems, including more complex programming and greater battery consumption because two or more

Table 25A-14 Potential sensor interactions

Pacemaker rate responds only to
- Rate of change of sensor one and absolute value of sensor two
- Sensor one to a certain level of exertion and thereafter sensor two
- Sensor one when sensor two also indicates a rate change
- Sensor one when sensor two is above or below a certain value

Data from Nappholz T: Personal communication, 1989.

Table 25A-15 Sensor combinations undergoing clinical investigation in the United States

Sensors	Company	Model	Single or dual chamber	Status in U.S.
Minute ventilation & activity*	Medtronic	Legend Plus	Single	CI
Q-T interval & activity*	Vitatron	Topaz	Single	NA
Q-T interval & activity*	Vitatron	Diamond	Dual	NA
Q-T interval & activity	Vitatron	Ruby	Dual	NA
Q-T interval & activity*	Vitatron	Sapphire	VDD/VDDR; single-pass lead system	NA
PDI & minute ventilation	Telectronics	Sentri	Single	CI

CI, clinical investigation; NA, not available at the time of manuscript preparation; PDI, paced depolarization integral.
*Activity sensory is piezoelectric crystal.

sensors are monitored and activated. However, given the limited experience with multisensor systems, most concerns are hypothetical and follow-up data are too limited to allow long-term assessment of dual-sensor reliability.

Taborsky et al.[213] attempted to compare time and technologic components necessary for follow-up of a dual-sensor system. In a limited assessment of 10 patients, they concluded that the dual-sensor system did not prolong the time required for regular follow-up of single-sensor pacemakers, in part because of the "automatic" features available on the dual-sensor pacemaker.

Proving the clinical benefit of two or more sensors. During initial clinical evaluation of single-sensor rate-adaptive pacemakers, the clinical advantages of rate adaptation over fixed-rate pacing in the chronotropically incompetent patient were easily and repeatedly demonstrated. It may be more difficult to demonstrate objective clinical gains with a dual-sensor rate-adaptive pacemaker over a single-sensor device.

From the initial studies with dual-sensor pacemakers, the advantage of one sensor verifying the rate response of the other sensor and preventing a response to a nonphysiologic event seems evident. What has not yet clearly emerged is whether dual sensors will impart any improvement in exercise tolerance either objectively or subjectively.

Other potential dual-sensor benefits. Another potential application of sensors is for the detection of tachyarrhythmias. Cohen and Liem[214] designed a dual-sensor algorithm using mean right atrial pressure and mixed venous oxygen saturation as the sensors. With this combination of sensors, detection of tachyarrhythmias had 100% sensitivity and 73% specificity.

Combining multiple physiologic sensors could theoretically provide clinical information helpful in managing various cardiopulmonary disorders.

MECHANISMS AND INDICATIONS FOR RATE-ADAPTIVE PACEMAKERS. Current indications for rate-adaptive pacemakers are listed in Table 25A-16.

Table 25A-16 Indications for rate-responsive pacemakers

VVIR	AAIR	DDDR
Atrial fibrillation with symptomatic slow ventricular response Paralyzed or inexcitable atrium with symptomatic slow ventricular response	Sinus node dysfunction with associated chronotropic incompetence and normal AV node function*	Combined sinus node and AV node dysfunction

AV, atrioventricular.
*See text.

The timing cycle of VVIR pacing is relatively simple. After lower and upper rate limits are defined, the cycle length varies between these limitations, depending on sensor activation (Fig 25A-41).

The primary indication for VVIR pacing is atrial fibrillation with a slow ventricular response. VVIR is contraindicated if ventricular pacing results in retrograde (VA) conduction or a decrease in blood pressure. This response to ventricular pacing suggests potential pacemaker syndrome. VVIR pacing should not be used as an excuse to forgo attempts at placing an atrial lead in a patient who is undergoing pacemaker implantation, has normal sinus node function, and would benefit from rate-adaptive pacing.[215,216] If the sinus node is intact, P-synchronous pacing should still be considered the optimal rate-adaptive parameter and be used when possible.

AAIR pacing follows the same timing cycle as that described for VVIR, with the obvious exception of stimulation occurring in the atrium (Fig 25A-42). AAIR pacing can be considered in the patient with sinus node dysfunction and normal AV node function. If AAIR pacing is contemplated, normal AV node conduction must first be determined as described earlier for AAI pacing.

DDDR pacing is designed to restore rate responsiveness while maintaining AV synchrony for the paced patient. DDDR can be thought of as a hybrid of DDD and SSIR technology. DDDR by definition indicates that there are pacing and sensing in both the atrial and the ventricular chambers, that the response to sensing includes both triggered pacing and inhibition by intrinsic

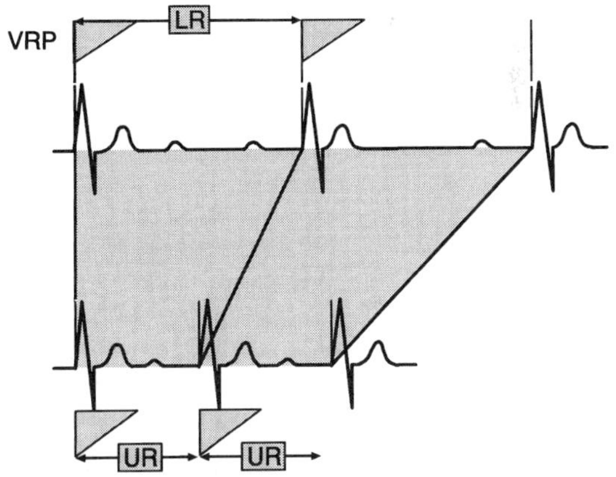

Fig 25A-41 The VVIR timing cycle consists of a lower rate limit *(LR),* upper rate limit *(UR),* and a ventricular refractory period *(VRP; shaded triangles).* As indicated by sensor activity, the VV cycle length will shorten accordingly. (The *shaded area* represents the range of sensor-driven VV cycle lengths.) In most VVIR pacemakers, the VRP remains fixed despite the changing VV cycle length. In newer VVIR pacemakers, the VRP may have the capability of shortening as the cycle length shortens. (From Hayes DL: Timing cycles of permanent pacemakers. *Cardiol Clin* 10:593-608, 1992. By permission of WB Saunders Company.)

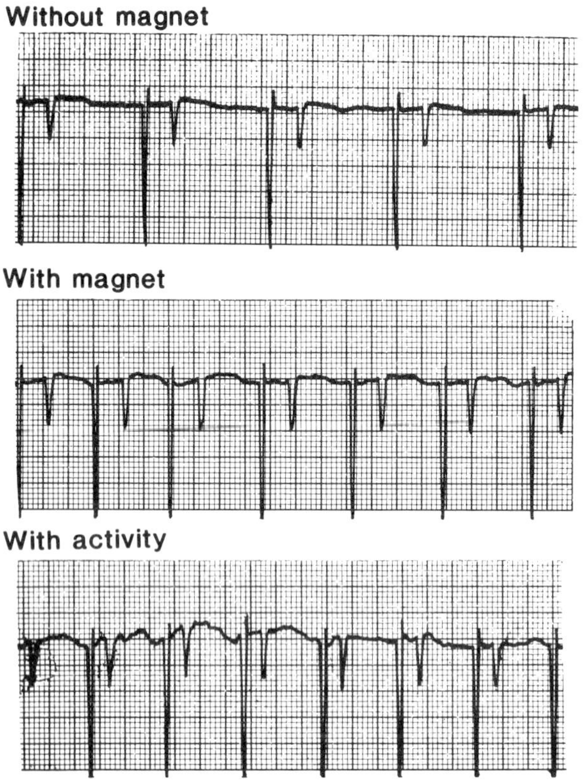

Fig 25A-42 Transtelephonically obtained ECGs from a patient with an activity-sensing AAIR pacemaker (Medtronic Activitrax model 8403). The upper panel demonstrates atrial pacing at the programmed base rate of 60 ppm. The middle panel is obtained after magnet application, which results in three initial beats at 100 ppm followed by a rate of 85 ppm. The lower panel is obtained after the patient has exercised in place. With exercise, the paced atrial rate increases to approximately 96 ppm.

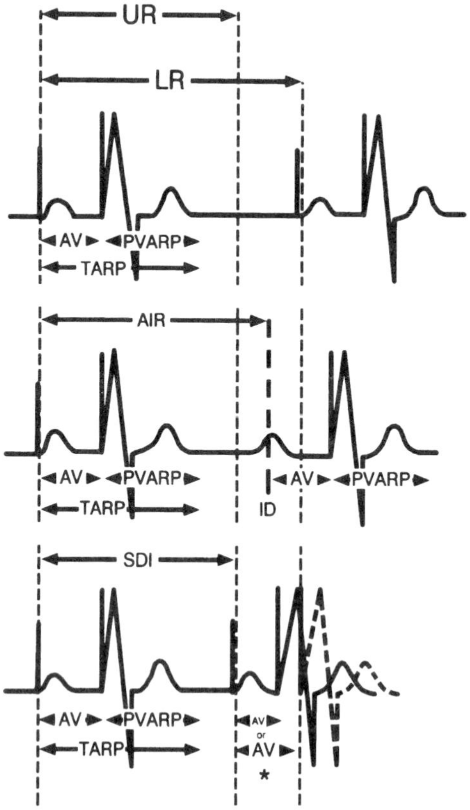

Fig 25A-43 DDDR pacemakers are capable of all pacing variations previously described for DDD pacemakers. **Top,** AV sequential pacing occurs at the lower rate limit *(LR).* **Middle,** AV sequential pacing is followed by P-synchronous pacing. **Bottom,** sensor-driven AV sequential pacing occurs at the upper rate limit *(UR).* The *asterisk* denotes a variable AV interval that can occur if the pacemaker is capable of a rate-adaptive AV interval. If the AV interval shortens at faster pacing rates, the shorter AV interval shown by the *continuous line* occurs. If the AV interval does not vary with rate, that is, is fixed, the timing of the paced ventricular complex is indicated by the *broken line. AIR,* atrial-indicated rate; *ID,* intrinsic deflection; *PVARP,* postventricular atrial refractory period; *SDI,* sensor-driven interval; *TARP,* total atrial refractory period. (Modified from Hayes DL, Levine PA: Pacemaker timing cycles. In *Cardiac Pacing.* Edited by KA Ellenbogen. Boston, Blackwell Scientific Publications, 1992, pp 263-308.)

activity in each chamber, and that the device has rate-adaptive capability (Fig 25A-43). As with any DDD pacemaker, a DDDR pacemaker must have a programmed lower rate as well as an upper rate limit or maximum P-tracking limit. In DDDR, however, the maximum pacing rate may be determined by sensor activity. Sensor function and programmability of the sensor depend on the type of sensor incorporated in the pacemaker. Despite a closer mimicking of normal physiology, the paced DDDR ECG may be more difficult to interpret. As with any paced ECG, correct interpretation depends on adequate familiarity with the pacemaker and knowledge of all the programmed variables. Telemetric functions, such as intracardiac electrograms and surface electrocardiograms with markers, can be very valuable.

A significant difference in the timing cycle of DDD pacing from that of DDDR pacing is the ability to pace the atrium during the PVARP in the DDDR mode (Fig 25A-44). The DDD mode does not have this ability because paced atrial activity does not occur until the lower rate limit has timed out, a point, by definition, that must be after the PVARP. In the DDDR mode, however, even though the atrial sensing channel is refractory during the PVARP, sensor-driven atrial output can still occur.

DDDR pacing mode further increases the complexity of the upper rate behavior because the pacemaker can be driven by either intrinsic atrial activity to cause PV pacing or a sensor whose input signal is not identifiable on the ECG to result in AV or AR (atrial paced event followed by intrinsic R wave) pacing. The eventual upper rate also depends on the type of sensor incorporated in the pacemaker and how the sensor is programmed. Between

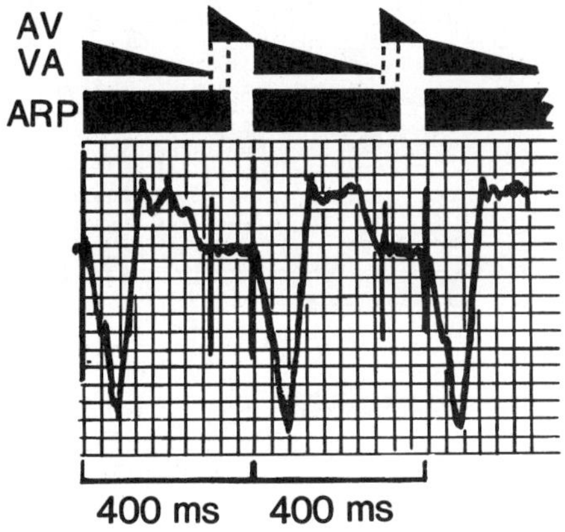

Fig 25A-44 In this ECG example from a DDDR pacemaker, the maximum sensor rate is 150 ppm (400 msec), the atrial refractory period *(ARP)* is 350 msec, and the AV interval is 100 msec. The block diagrams above the ECG illustrate the two sensor-driven atrial pacing artifacts that occur during the terminal portion of the postventricular atrial refractory period (PVARP). Although no atrial sensing can occur during the PVARP (as indicated in this example by the intrinsic P wave that occurs immediately after the first-paced ventricular depolarization), a sensor-driven atrial pacing artifact is not prevented by the PVARP. Whether a sensor-driven atrial pacing artifact is delivered depends on the sensor-indicated rate at that time, not the PVARP. (From Hayes DL, Higano ST: DDDR pacing: follow-up and complications. In *New Perspectives in Cardiac Pacing.* Second edition. Edited by SS Barold, J Mugica. Mount Kisco, New York, Futura Publishing Company, 1991, pp 473-491. By permission.)

the programmed lower rate limit and the programmed upper rate limit there may be stable P-wave synchronous pacing, P-wave synchronous pacing alternating with AV sequential pacing, or stable AV sequential pacing at rates that exceed the base rate (Fig 25A-45). AV sequential pacing rates may increase as high as the programmed maximum sensor rate (MSR).

Although the MSR and maximum tracking rate (MTR) are closely related, they are not identical. The tracking rate refers to the rate when the pacemaker is sensing and tracking endogenous atrial activity. The MTR is the maximum ventricular paced rate that is allowed in response to sensed atrial rhythms. This may result in the fixed block, Wenckebach, fallback, or rate smoothing response, depending on the design of the system. The sensor-controlled rate is the rate of the pacemaker that is determined by the sensor-input signal. The MSR is the maximum rate that the pacemaker is allowed to achieve under sensor control. In some units in which the MTR and MSR can be independently programmed, the ventricular paced rate under sensor drive might exceed that attained when endogenous atrial activity is being tracked.

Whether at the MTR or during rate acceleration below the MTR, the rhythm that results may be in part sensor-driven and in part sinus-driven (P-wave tracking) and not purely one or the other. Which of these mechanisms predominates depends on the integrity of the sinus node and the sensor and how it is programmed. DDDR pacing can result in a type of rate smoothing we have designated as "sensor-driven rate smoothing" (Fig 25A-46). If the sensor is optimally programmed, as the atrial rate exceeds the maximum tracking rate, the PR interval displays minimal variation between sinus-driven and sensor-driven pacing. In the DDDR mode, the RR interval is allowed to lengthen only as much as the

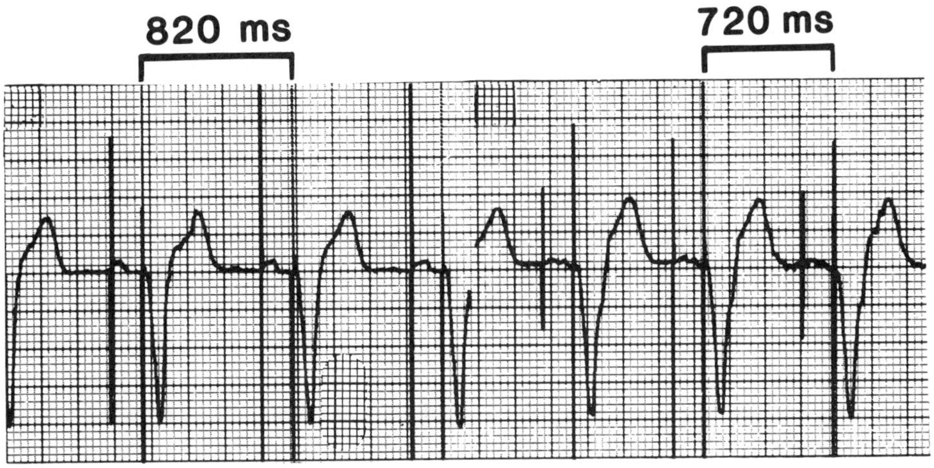

Fig 25A-45 ECG from a patient with a DDDR pacemaker. This tracing was obtained during exercise at 1.5 mph on a 6% grade. The paced RR cycle length is 820 msec at the beginning of the tracing; at the end, it has shortened to 720 msec. (From Hayes DL, Higano ST, Eisinger G: Electrocardiographic manifestations of a dual-chamber, rate-modulated (DDDR) pacemaker. PACE 12:555-562, 1989. By permission of Futura Publishing Company.)

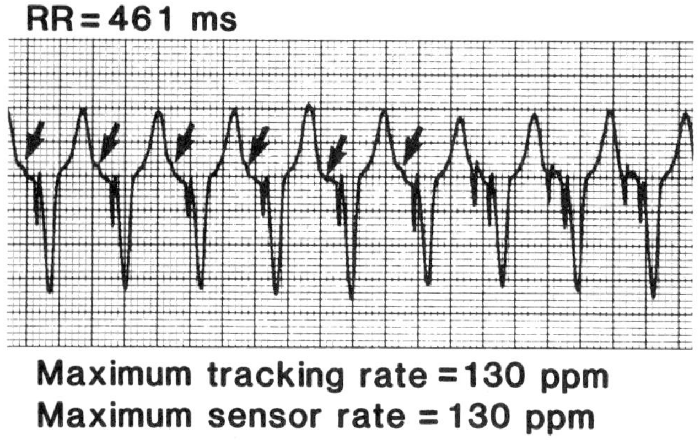

Fig 25A-46 ECG from a patient with a DDDR pacemaker shows P-synchronous pacing at 130 ppm with intermittent sensor-driven AV sequential pacing at the same rate. *Arrows* indicate P waves. (From Hayes DL, Higano ST, Eisinger G: Electrocardiographic manifestations of a dual-chamber, rate-modulated (DDDR) pacemaker. *PACE* 12:555-562, 1989. By permission of Futura Publishing Company.)

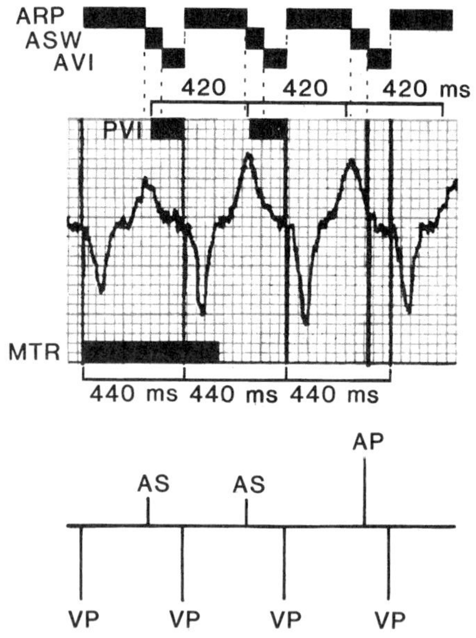

Fig 25A-47 Diagram showing the relationship between the postventricular atrial refractory period (noted in this figure as *ARP*), atrial sensing window *(ASW),* and AV interval *(AVI).* Increasing the ARP and the AVI shortens the ASW. At rapid pacing rates, the ASW may become very short or disappear. In this diagram, the ASW is 65 msec and the AVI is 100 msec. The intrinsic atrial rate is 143 bpm (420 msec). The sensor rate is 136 ppm (440 msec). At the bottom, a diagram in Marker-Channel (Medtronic, Inc., Minneapolis, MN) fashion demonstrates the ECG findings. *AP,* atrial paced event; *AS,* atrial sensed event; *MTR,* maximum tracking rate; *PVI,* postventricular interval; *VP,* ventricular paced event. (From Higano ST, Hayes DL: P wave tracking above the maximum tracking rate in a DDDR pacemaker. *PACE* 12:1044-1048, 1989. By permission of Futura Publishing Company.

difference between the MTR and the activity sensor rate interval. For example, if a device is programmed to a P-wave tracking limit of 120 ppm and the patient's atrial rate exceeds this, the pacemaker operates in a Wenckebach-type block. If the sensor-indicated rate at this time is 100 ppm, the paced rate drops from 120 ppm (500 msec) to an AV sequential paced rate of 100 ppm (600 msec) for the Wenckebach cycle and then returns to P-wave tracking at a rate of 120 ppm. This behavior usually shortens the DDD Wenckebach interval, but this interval depends on the atrial rate and the programmed values for the MTR and the TARP.

Maximal sensor-driven rate smoothing requires optimal programming of the sensor parameter. If the rate-responsive circuitry is programmed to mimic the native atrial rate, the paced ventricular rate does not demonstrate the 2:1, or Wenckebach-type, behavior. Conversely, if the rate-responsive circuitry is programmed to very low levels of sensor-driven pacing, little or no rate smoothing takes place.

Another aspect of DDDR timing cycles is the atrial sensing window (ASW) (Fig 25A-47). The portion of the RR cycle that is not part of the PVARP or the AV interval (AVI) is the period during which the atrial sensing channel is alert, the ASW. If the PVARP or the AVI is extended, there may effectively be no ASW, and even a DDD pacemaker will function as a DVI system. Conversely, if a DDDR pacemaker has exceeded the programmed MTR and is pacing at faster rates based on sensor activation, an appropriately timed intrinsic P wave can still inhibit sensor-driven atrial pacing artifact and give the appearance of P-wave tracking at rates greater than the MTR. Although the MTR is programmed to a single value in DDDR pacing, it behaves as if it were variable and equal to the sensor-driven rate when the sensor-driven rate exceeds the programmed MTR if a P-wave occurs during the ASW to inhibit output of an atrial pacing artifact.

EFFECT OF VENTRICULAR-BASED AND ATRIAL-BASED TIMING SYSTEMS ON DDDR TIMING CYCLES. In a ventricular-based timing system, the effective atrial paced rate could theoretically be significantly higher than the programmed MSR if AR conduction were present. (Fig 25A-48,A). If it is assumed that the maximum sensor-controlled rate is 150 ppm (a cycle length of 400 msec), with a programmed AVI of 200 msec, the atrial escape interval (AEI) would also be 200 msec. If AV conduction were intact so that the AR interval (ARI) was 150 msec, the actual pacing interval would be the ARI + AEI or 150 msec + 200 msec or 350 msec. A cycle length of 350 msec is equal to 171 ppm, which is significantly higher than the programmed MSR of 150 ppm. Although this potentially achievable faster rate may not be troublesome or even advantageous for some patients, it could create problems for other patients. If the MTR and the MSR are independently programmable, such rate acceleration can be avoided. If the MSR is programmed lower than the

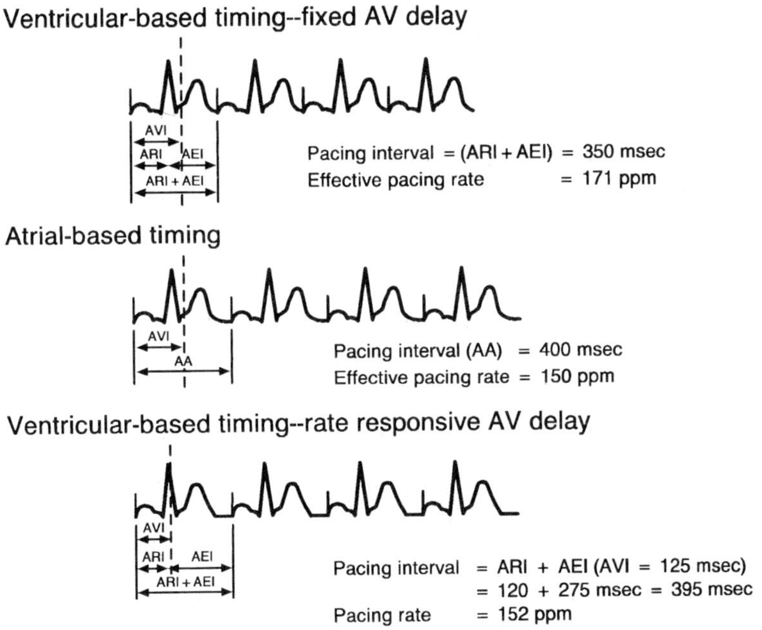

Fig 25A-48 Effect of different timing systems on maximum sensor rate with intact, stable AV nodal conduction (AR [atrial paced event followed by intrinsic R wave] pacing). **Top,** in a ventricular-based timing system, there is a significant theoretical increase in the paced atrial rate, exceeding that programmed. Although the maximum sensor rate programmed is 150 ppm (400 msec), the effective pacing rate achieved is 171 ppm, because the effective pacing rate is a function of the AR interval *(ARI)* and the atrial escape interval *(AEI);* that is, 140 + 200 = 350 msec (171 ppm). **Middle,** in a theoretical pure atrial-based DDDR system, the R wave sensed during the AV interval *(AVI)* does not alter the basic timing during stable AR pacing and results in atrial pacing at the sensor-indicated rate. **Bottom,** the addition of rate-adaptive AVI to a ventricular-based timing system minimizes the increase in the paced atrial rate above the programmed sensor-indicated rate. Other mechanisms for correcting any rate increase above the programmed sensor-indicated rate are available and are often pacemaker-specific. (From Hayes DL: Pacemaker electrocardiography. In *A Practice of Cardiac Pacing.* Third edition. Edited by S Furman, DL Hayes, DR Holmes Jr. Mount Kisco, New York, Futura Publishing Company, 1993, pp 309-359. By permission.)

MTR, the absolute rate achievable can be defined by the programmed MTR. In atrial-based timing systems, sensor-driven pacing does not exceed the programmed maximum pacing rate because the AA interval is maintained (Fig 25A-48,B).

Rate acceleration can also be minimized in a ventricular-based timing system by a variety of mechanisms. One of the first mechanisms for controlling this behavior was by incorporation of a rate-responsive AV delay (RRAVD) (Fig 25A-48,C). As the sinus or sensor-driven rate progressively increases, RRAVD causes the AVI to progressively shorten. Shortening the AVI with RRAVD results in a shorter TARP (shorter AVI + PVARP). This increases the intrinsic atrial rate that can be sensed, reducing the likelihood of both a fixed block upper rate response and functional atrial undersensing. It also minimizes the chance of an inappropriately long AVI at the higher rate, as may occur with a fixed AV delay that is programmed appropriately for lower rate behavior. In this case, the AV delay may be too long at higher rates. In a DDDR system, when the AVI shortens, the ventricular rate drive is held to that governed by the sensor, causing the time subtracted from the AVI to be added to the AEI. Thus, at a rate of 150 ppm and pacing interval of 400 msec, if the RRAVD caused the AVI to shorten by 75 msec from an initally programmed AVI of 200 msec, the AVI would shorten to 125 msec. Since the overall ventricular timing is held constant, the 75 msec subtracted from the AVI is added to the AEI, increasing it to 275 msec.

The RRAVD serves both to provide a more physiologic AVI at the faster rate and to minimize the degree of rate increase over the programmed MSR if AR conduction is intact. If it is assumed that the rate is 150 ppm and the initial AVI is 200 msec, the RRAVD is 125 msec, resulting in AV sequential pacing at the sensor programmed rate when the ARI is 140 msec. If intact AV conduction is present at 120 msec, the overall shortening of the pacing interval is only 5 msec above that at 150 ppm, a rate of 152 ppm.

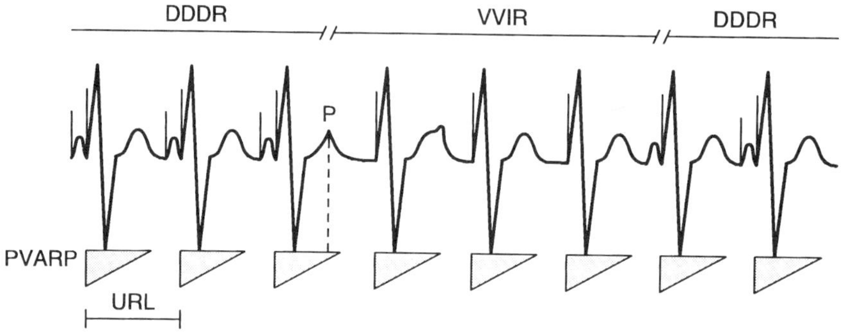

Fig 25A-49 ECG illustration of automatic mode switching. The first three cycles are sensor-driven AV sequential pacing at the upper rate limit *(URL)*. An intrinsic P wave occurs at the dashed line, within the postventricular atrial refractory period *(PVARP; triangles)*. The P wave occurring in the PVARP results in a mode change to VVIR. This continues until a P wave is sensed outside the PVARP, at which time DDDR pacing resumes. (From Hayes DL: Timing cycles of permanent pacemakers. *Cardiol Clin* 10:593-608, 1992. By permission of WB Saunders Company.)

The ideal patient for DDDR pacing has combined sinus node and AV nodal dysfunction. DDDR pacing is appropriate for the patient with pure sinus node dysfunction if the implanting physician is uncomfortable with AAIR pacing. DDDR pacing is also appropriate for the patient with associated paroxysmal supraventricular tachycardia who requires pacing. In the past, DDD pacing was relatively contraindicated in a patient with paroxysmal supraventricular tachycardias because the pacemaker would potentially track the tachycardia, resulting in rapid paced ventricular rates. With DDDR pacemakers, several options are available. If automatic mode switching is a programmable option, the pacemaker has the capability of reprogramming from DDDR to VVIR if the pacemaker detects an atrial rhythm that meets the pacemaker's criteria for being pathologic. When a physiologic atrial rhythm returns, the pacemaker automatically is reprogrammed to DDDR (Fig 25A-49). (This feature is now an option in the DDD pacing mode in some pacemakers. Detection of a pathologic atrial rhythm would result in reprogramming to the VVI pacing mode.)

DDIR pacing is another option for patients with paroxysmal supraventricular rhythm disturbances. This pacing mode, by definition, does not allow tracking of any atrial rhythm, pathologic or physiologic. Although DDIR pacing has been used successfully in many patients, the lack of P-synchronous pacing in a patient who is predominantly in sinus rhythm is a definite disadvantage.

A third option for this group of patients is discrepant MSRs and MTRs. Even if the pacemaker does not allow independent programming of these variables, discrepant rates can be achieved by programming the TARP to the desired MTR and allowing a faster upper rate limit to be reached via the sensor.

If a patient previously paced with a DDD pacemaker has had symptoms with normal DDD upper rate behavior, that is, symptomatic pseudo-Wenckebach or 2:1 pacing, it is reasonable to change to DDDR pacing at the time of pulse generator replacement. Sensor-driven rate smooth-

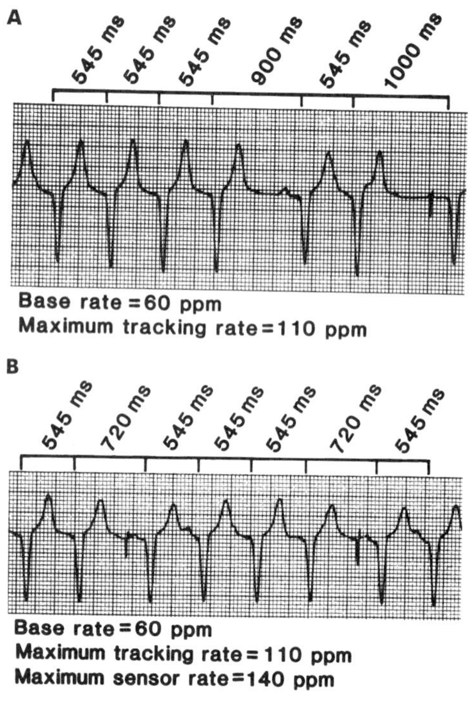

Fig 25A-50 **A,** ECG showing DDD pacing (sensor is programmed "passive") with Wenckebach-type block at the maximum tracking rate of 110 ppm. RR cycle length varies from 545 to 1,000 msec. **B,** ECG showing DDDR pacing in the same patient with the same maximum tracking rate (110 ppm) and a maximum sensor rate of 140 ppm. With the sensor "on," there is less variation in cycle length, 545 to 720 msec. (From Hayes DL, Higano ST, Eisinger G: Electrocardiographic manifestations of a dual-chamber, rate-modulated (DDDR) pacemaker. *PACE* 12:555-562, 1989. By permission of Futura Publishing Company.)

ing avoids the marked variations in paced ventricular cycle length and should avoid symptomatic upper rate behavior if the sensor is optimally programmed (Fig 25A-50).

DDDR pacing is contraindicated in patients with chronic atrial fibrillation.

PACEMAKER COMPLICATIONS

Complications can occur as a direct result of the implantation technique or because of failure of a component of the pacing system.[217] Many complications are directly related to the experience of the implanter. One study demonstrated a significantly higher incidence of complications when implanters performed fewer than 12 implantations per year.[218]

Abnormalities of pacemaker function

Failure of the pacing stimulus to capture the myocardium (failure to pace). In general, there are three potential causes for failure to pace: abnormalities of pulse generator function, abnormalities in the pulse generator-lead circuit, and abnormalities of the myocardium.[219] These abnormalities can result in a complete or intermittent failure to capture the myocardium (Fig 25A-51).

PULSE GENERATOR ABNORMALITIES. These include power source failure (either accelerated or expected end of battery life), random component failure in the timing or output circuit, loss of adequate hermetic sealing of the pulse generator case, allowing tissue fluid to come in contact with the components of the pulse generator, and improper pulse generator output programming (pulse width or voltage below threshold requirements).

Premature power source failure is infrequent with lithium batteries. The characteristic changes that occur at end of battery life include a decrease in voltage output, a decrease in pacing rate, and an increase in pulse width. These are predictable but vary from manufacturer to manufacturer and are best demonstrated during asynchronous pacing with magnet application. These changes are gradual and allow for elective pulse generator change long before a dangerous reduction in energy occurs.

PULSE GENERATOR-LEAD CIRCUIT ABNORMALITIES. Included in this group of abnormalities are complete or intermittent electrode wire fracture, current leakage secondary to a break in lead insulation, discontinuity between the pulse generator and the lead (secondary to poor set-screw connection), and improper lead position (occurring at the time of initial implantation or secondary to subsequent lead dislodgment or myocardial perforation).

A. Conductor coil fracture. The most common manifestation of a conductor coil fracture is total pacing failure without a demonstrable pacemaker stimulus artifact.[219,220] This may be intermittent if the fractured ends are opposed and are interrupted only by intermittent catheter movement. It also may be manifested as a changing of the amplitude and spatial orientation (vector) of a stimulus artifact with or without associated demonstration of failure to capture the myocardium.

The usual sites of fracture are at the junction of the pacing lead and pulse generator, at sites where there is an acute angulation of a catheter (e.g., sites where the catheter curves over the clavicle if the internal or external jugular vein is used for venous access), or at the point where the lead passes under the clavicle when the subclavian vein has been used if the space between the first rib and the clavicle is narrow.[221] Wire fracture may occur spontaneously or be secondary to trauma. Fracture can also be seen at a site where a suture is placed directly around the lead. This practice is no longer acceptable. Leads are equipped with a sleeve around which ligatures can be placed to secure the lead to the underlying tissue and obviate placing a ligature directly on the lead.

Correction of this problem requires surgical intervention with repair (if the area of fracture is accessible) or replacement of the electrode catheter (if repair is impossible or the area of fracture is within the venous system). There are multiple descriptions of lead repair in the literature, but repair of a fractured lead should be attempted only by someone with experience. The lead should otherwise be replaced.

B. Insulation break. A break in the electrode catheter insulation allows some of the current from the electrode to escape into the surrounding tissues. If the degree of current leakage is sufficient, complete or intermittent failure of myocardial capture will result. Insulation breaks may occur at the point where a lead passes between the clavicle and the first rib if subclavian placement has been used. Insulation breaks could also be caused by placing a suture directly around the lead (see above) and occasionally occur at the site where a ligature has been appropriately placed around the sleeve. As in the case of wire fracture, resolution of this problem usually requires surgical replacement of the pacing lead.

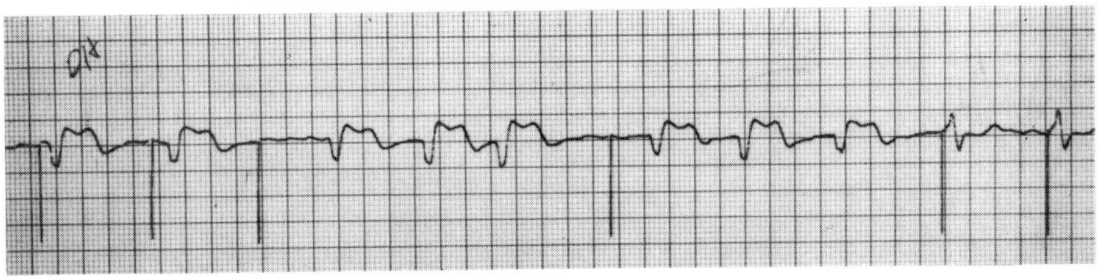

Fig 25A-51 Ventricular demand pacing system exhibiting intermittent failure to pace with normal sensing.

MYOCARDIAL ABNORMALITIES. Complete or intermittent failure to capture may occur as a result of expected or accelerated changes in threshold requirements for myocardial capture that occur with time or as a result of electrolyte imbalance or concomitant drug therapy (or drug toxicity).[222] The most common electrolyte abnormality to interfere with pacemaker function is hyperkalemia. Hyperkalemia may result in failure to capture and failure to sense. The most common cardioactive drugs to interfere with pacemaker function are the class C antiarrhythmic agents.[223,224] Flecainide, encainide, and propafenone have all been reported to raise pacing thresholds. Sensing abnormalities have also been reported with some class C agents.

These abnormalities might be overcome by noninvasively increasing the pulse generator output (either increasing pulse width or increasing stimulation voltage) and additionally by correcting any reversible metabolic or drug-related abnormalities. In some cases of chronic progressive increases in threshold requirements, lead replacement is required.

PSEUDOMALFUNCTION. Apparent failure to pace will be noted if a pacemaker stimulus occurs during the refractory period of a spontaneous beat. This is referred to as "functional noncapture" (Fig 25A-52).

Sensing abnormalities. These can be broken down into the true abnormalities undersensing (a lack of recognition of normal intrinsic cardiac activity) and oversensing (unexpected sensing of an intrinsic or extrinsic electrical signal) and pseudomalfunction, which mimics both oversensing and undersensing.

UNDERSENSING. The inappropriate lack of sensing of intrinsic cardiac activity is a relatively common abnormality which results in a pacemaker output that is undesirably competitive (Fig 25A-53). Once again, true malfunctions may be the result of abnormalities of the pulse generator, the catheter electrode, or myocardial function. In addition, apparent malfunctions (pseudomalfunctions) may occur despite, or as a result of, normal pacemaker function and must be differentiated from pathologic conditions.

A. Pulse generator abnormalities. Pulse generator abnormalities result in undersensing despite proper lead position and function and despite delivery of an adequate intracardiac electrogram to the pulse generator. This may be the result of impending power source failure, a random component failure in the sensing circuit, abnormal reedswitch function, or, most commonly, inappropriate pulse generator programming (decreased sensitivity or prolonged pulse generator refractory period).[225]

The reedswitch is made of metal strips that are separated from one another—"open"—when the pulse generator is functioning in the demand mode. When a magnet (or programmer head that incorporates a magnet) is placed over the pulse generator, the strips become magnetized and come into contact with one another—"closed." This converts a demand to an asynchronous (fixed-rate) pacing system. Mechanical failure of the reedswitch, which is now rare, may cause pacemaker malfunction by allowing it to remain in the open or closed position regardless of the presence or absence of an external magnetic field. If a reedswitch remains in a closed position (a "sticky" reedswitch), the system will exhibit consistent asynchronous pacing without myocardial sensing.[225]

Pulse generator failure or abnormal reedswitch function requires replacement of the pulse generator. Abnormal pulse generator programming can be corrected easily and noninvasively in most situations.

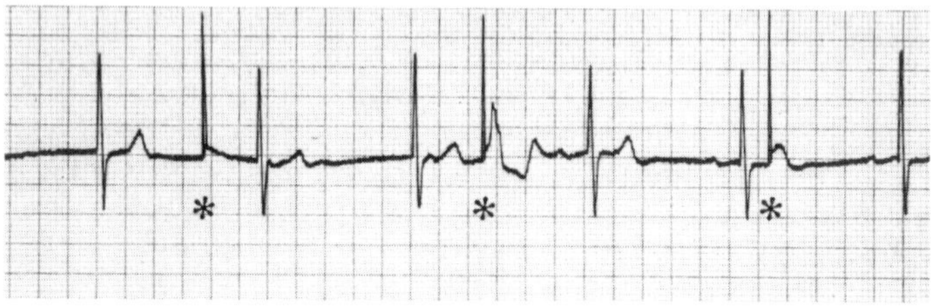

Fig 25A-52 VVI pacing with failure to capture *(first asterisk),* normal capture *(second asterisk),* and functional noncapture *(third asterisk)* because pacing artifact occurs during ventricular refractoriness.

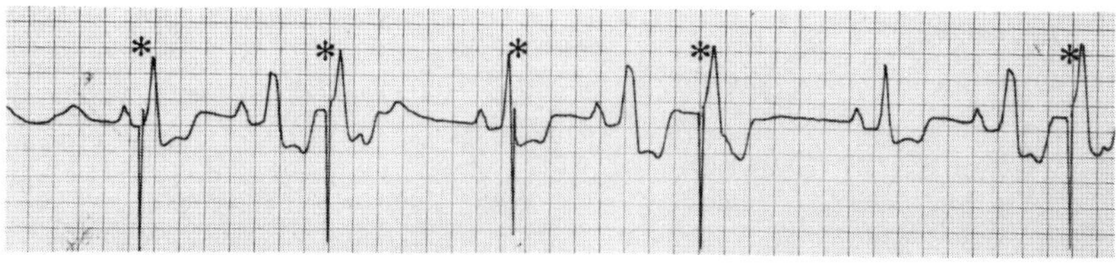

Fig 25A-53 VVI pacing with undersensing, which results in potentially undesirable competitive ventricular stimulation *(first and fourth asterisks).*

B. Catheter electrode abnormalities. Undersensing may be due to problems with the pacemaker lead. This is most commonly the result of poor lead position either at the time of initial implantation or as a result of early or late lead dislodgment[222] (Fig 25A-54). In addition, sensing abnormalities may be seen as a result of a loss of lead insulation.

C. Myocardial abnormalities. Most commonly undersensing is a result of delivery of a poor cardiac electrical signal to a normally functioning pulse generator lead system. In elderly patients with atherosclerotic or degenerative cardiac disease, in the setting of myocardial infarction (either acutely or chronically as a result of myocardial scar formation), as a consequence of progressive fibrosis and thrombus organization at the electrode myocardial junction or with electrolyte imbalance or drug toxicity, the myocardium may not be able to generate electrical activity of sufficient magnitude to be properly sensed.[222,226] In these situations an R or P wave that was acceptable initially may be diminished to a level that cannot be sensed by the pulse generator.

A normally functioning pacing system will at times fail to detect atrial or ventricular extrasystoles because the voltage generated is not sufficient to be sensed. This cannot always be anticipated unless extrasystoles of the same morphology occur during implantation and can be measured.

D. Pseudomalfunctions. The occurrence of fusion and pseudofusion beats is a result of superimposition of an ineffective pacemaker spike on a spontaneously occurring P wave or QRS complex. It usually is the consequence of pacemaker discharge during the refractory period of atrial or ventricular activity before sufficient intracardiac voltage is generated to activate the sensing circuit. This would be expected to occur when the pacing rate and the intrinsic heart rate are very similar (Fig 25A-55). Pseudofusion beats also may be the result of a delayed arrival of ventricular activity (in a ventricular demand system) due to intraventricular conduction abnormalities at the site of the sensing electrodes. Right ventricular apical activation may be delayed up to 65 msec after the beginning of the surface QRS complex by right bundle-branch block (and even more by ectopic beats originating in the left ventricle).[227] Therefore, it is not surprising that, in this

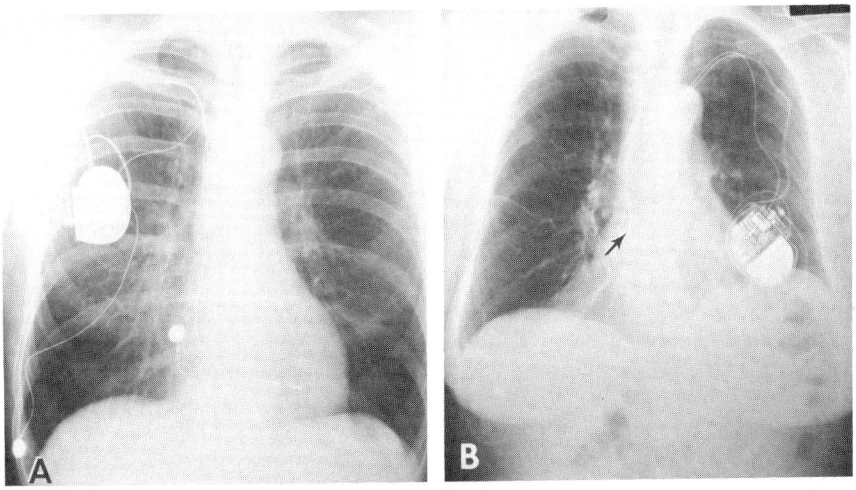

Fig 25A-54 **A,** chest radiograph showing acceptable position of a ventricular pacing catheter in the right ventricular apex. **B,** gross dislodgment of the ventricular pacing lead *(arrow)* with retraction of the lead from the usual apical position.

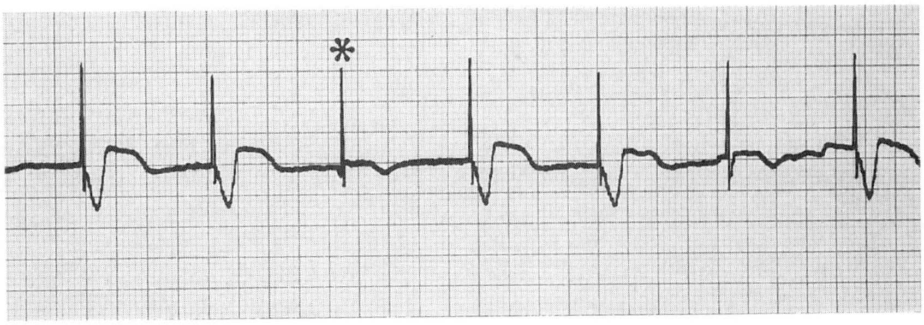

Fig 25A-55 Rhythm strip demonstrates pseudofusion beat *(asterisk)* and fusion beat (sixth pacing stimulus).

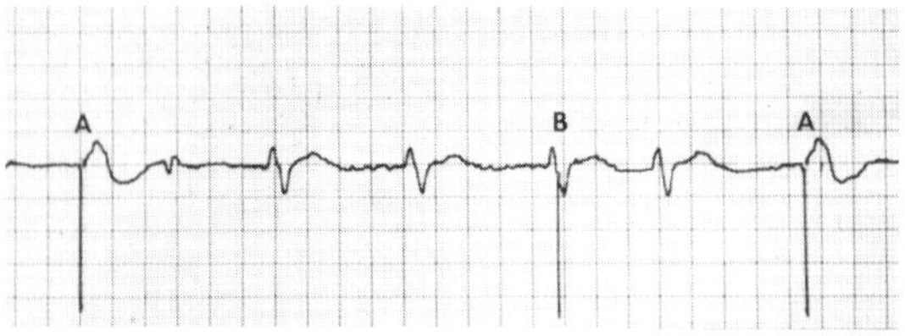

Fig 25A-56 Intermittent pacing in a patient whose native QRS complex exhibits an intraventricular conduction delay. A delay in right ventricular activation could result in an apparent failure to sense (B). *A,* paced ventricular depolarization; *B,* pseudofusion beat.

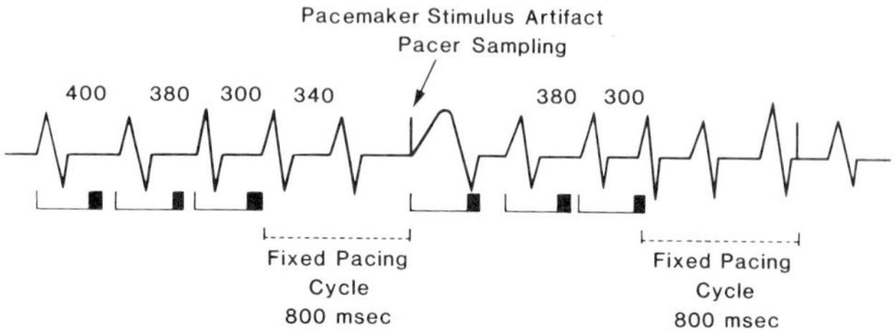

Fig 25A-57 During atrial fibrillation, QRS complexes that fall within the noise sampling cycle of the pulse generator will cause single-cycle fixed-rate pacing, resulting in random undersensing. Note that the second pacing artifact or stimulus fails to capture because it falls within the refractory period of the preceding QRS.

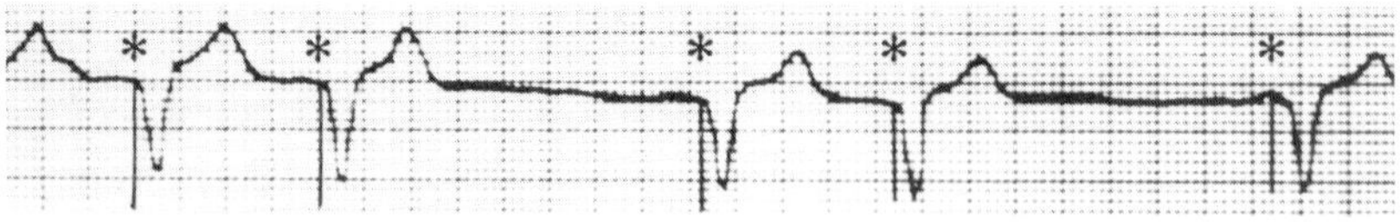

Fig 25A-58 Oversensing, resulting in an inappropriate, irregular pacemaker bradycardia. It is impossible to tell what is being oversensed in this ECG tracing.

situation, there may be pacemaker discharge into the QRS, mimicking pacemaker malfunction. This phenomenon also has been seen in the presence of left bundle-branch block with a left ventricular epicardial pacing system[228] (Fig 25A-56).

Electromagnetic interference (electrical noise) during the last portion of the refractory period of a pulse generator—termed the "noise-sampling period"—will disable the demand function of the pacemaker and cause reversion to its fixed-rate mode for one timing cycle (or automatic pacing interval), thus creating the impression of an undersensing malfunction. In the presence of short R-to-R intervals (i.e., during tachycardia), a very early QRS may fall within the noise-sampling period and be interpreted as electrical interference, which could lead to apparent random undersensing. If this occurs, each random fixed-rate cycle should include two QRS complexes: the first in the noise-sampling period and resulting in asynchronous function for one cycle, and the second during this asynchronous cycle and not sensed. This is most commonly seen when the pulse generator refractory period is long and can be solved by shortening the refractory period (Fig 25A-57).

The rhythm strip of a pacemaker functioning normally in the atrial- or ventricular-triggered mode (AAT or VVT) could be mistakenly interpreted as undersensing if the physician is not completely familiar with the patient and the pacing system. Some QRS-inhibited pulse generators will exhibit partial recycling after a ventricular premature beat. If this occurs, the escape interval after the premature beat will be shorter than the automatic interval because of partial saturation of the sensing amplifier. This shortened escape interval will give the impression of intermittent undersensing.

OVERSENSING. Oversensing is associated with the unexpected sensing of an intracardiac or extracardiac signal. It may be intermittent, resulting in irregularly delayed pacemaker stimulation, or it may be permanent, leading to a markedly decreased pacing rate or total inhibition of synchronous (demand) output (Fig 25A-58). Electrical signals that are commonly the cause of oversensing include T waves, myopotential interference, afterpotential delay, P waves, and isoelectric extrasystoles. Oversensing can frequently be corrected by reprogramming the sensitivity or at times by reprogramming the refractory period.

A. Intracardiac signals. Abnormal sensing of P waves by a ventricular lead is usually secondary to lead malposition. This could occur if a right ventricular catheter became displaced near the tricuspid valve or if an epicardial electrode was placed near the AV groove. In these situations, if retrograde VA conduction follows ventricular pacing, the P waves might be sensed if the retrograde conduction time exceeded the duration of the pacemaker refractory period.

Sensing of T waves occurs in the presence of prominent T waves with a high rate of rise or fall of electrical potential (Fig 25A-59). It is often intermittent and can be eliminated by extending the refractory period of the pulse generator to incorporate the T wave.

During atrial demand pacing, the R wave that results from normal AV conduction may be of sufficient magnitude to be sensed by the atrial lead, which would lead to an inappropriately slowed atrial pacing rhythm. This can be eliminated by extension of the refractory period.

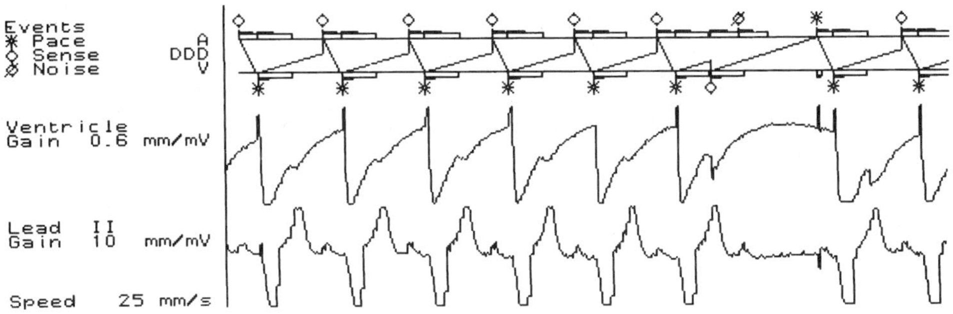

Fig 25A-59 Simultaneous ECG tracings from a patient with a DDD pacemaker. In the initial portion of the tracing, P-synchronous pacing occurs with a ventricular paced beat at the programmed AV interval of 200 msec after the P wave. The last four ventricular depolarizations are intrinsic QRS complexes that are preceded by a P wave at an AV interval of approximately 300 msec, not at the programmed AV interval of 200 msec. This is not atrial undersensing. Intermittently, a T wave of a paced ventricular depolarization is sensed by the ventricular lead. Having sensed what are interpreted as two consecutive ventricular events, the paced ventricular beat and the T wave, without an intervening atrial event, the pacemaker presumes that a premature ventricular event has occurred and the postventricular atrial refractory period (PVARP) is extended. In this example, the PVARP is extended from the programmed value of 300 msec to 480 msec. When the next true ventricular event occurs, the first of the four intrinsic QRS complexes, the pacemaker has still not sensed an atrial event, so that the PVARP is extended again. This process will continue until the cycle is once again interrupted by a P wave occurring outside the extended PVARP.

An uncommon cause of oversensing is afterpotential sensing. After pacemaker discharge, the current is transferred from the electrode tissue interface, through the catheter, back to the pulse generator. This usually is not sensed but, under certain circumstances, it can be. Sensing may occur when pacing is achieved at relatively high levels of energy. This oversensing is related to a modification in the normal current wave form caused by the high current density.[229] Afterpotential oversensing should always be considered when there is intermittent irregular prolongation of the stimulus-to-stimulus interval of less than twice the automatic interval. However, it may be difficult to differentiate after-potential oversensing from T-wave oversensing.[230]

Hysteresis may suggest oversensing. If hysteresis is a feature of the pacing system, the escape interval will be longer than the pacing interval. This feature is used primarily to allow maintenance of sinus rhythm in patients with intermittent bradycardia, but it may lead to problems in interpretation of the ECG (see Fig 25A-19).

Ventricular extrasystoles may result in very small QRS deflections (which may be inapparent), depending on the orientation of a depolarization pathway to the recording electrodes.[231] The diagnosis can be made by changing the position of the recording electrodes, which makes the extrasystoles more apparent.

B. Extracardiac causes

1. Skeletal muscle myopotentials. Significant biogalvanic electrical myopotentials can be generated by a contracting muscle mass.[232] Myopotentials of up to 2 to 3 mV generated by the pectoral muscles have been recorded[233] and these are well within the sensing capabilities of most modern pulse generators.

Myopotential interference is a problem primarily with unipolar systems (although bipolar systems have been implicated infrequently as well).[234] Unipolar pacing represents an open electrical circuit that is closed by the tissues between the tip of the electrode in the atrium or ventricle and the indifferent electrode which commonly consists of a large part of the metallic casing of the pulse generator. Because myopotential inhibition is most likely to occur with a large anodal area in contact with a large muscle mass, especially if the anode and catheter are on opposite sides of the contracting muscle, it is not surprising that it happens frequently during unipolar pacing.[235] Inhibition of pacemaker output by myopotentials has been documented in as many as 70% to 85% of patients with unipolar pacing systems.[236] Among these patients, approximately 20% reported transient symptoms (lightheadedness, dizziness, presyncope, and syncope) related to the transient sensation of pacemaker activity[236] (Fig 25A-60).

Pacemakers that are unipolar and bipolar pacemakers capable of unipolar pacing are coated with a plastic material on the side of the pacemaker that is to be placed in contact with the underlying pectoral muscle. Avoiding direct contact of metal and muscle is of help in minimizing myopotential inhibition.

If symptomatic myopotential inhibition occurs, there are some steps that can be taken to lessen or eliminate the problem. A unipolar system can be replaced with a bipolar system. The pulse generator can be reprogrammed to the

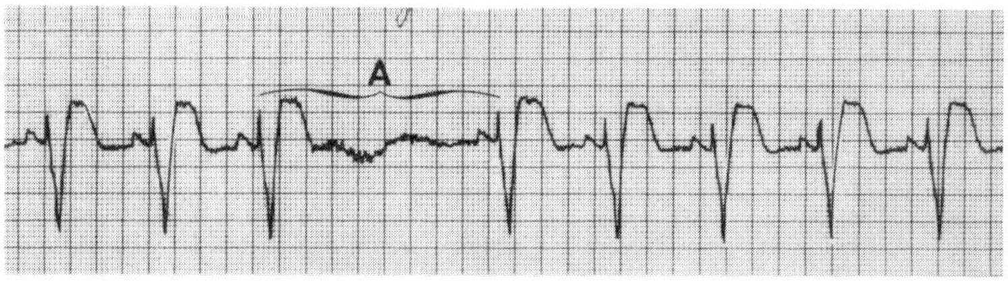

Fig 25A-60 During P-synchronous pacing, oversensing of myopotentials results in an irregular prolongation of the R-R interval.

bipolar mode if the pulse generator is polarity programmable and a bipolar lead is in place, or the sensitivity can be reprogrammed to a less sensitive value (although this can lead to inadequate sensing of normal intracardiac electrograms).

2. Electromagnetic interference. A disadvantage of any demand pacing system is its potential susceptibility to external electromagnetic interference which, depending on its frequency, may enter the pulse generator directly or via the lead that acts as an antenna. Although many improvements have been made (especially encapsulation of the pulse generator in metal) that have decreased the number of potentially hazardous electromagnetic or radiofrequency signals, there may be instances in which patients are subjected to uncomfortable or life-threatening symptoms.[237]

Protection from high-frequency signals is achieved by metallic shielding or filtering measures, and protection from low-frequency signals is provided by circuitry that converts demand into fixed-rate pacing if a *continuous uniform* signal reaches the pulse generator.[237] However, demand pacemakers still remain sensitive to bursts or pulsed fields of energy.

Electromagnetic energy sources such as microwave ovens and airport security magnetometers produce high-frequency interference that is easily rejected by current pulse generators. However, devices such as electrocautery or electrocoagulation units, therapeutic diathermy, and electrical or arc welding machines can inhibit pacemaker function.[219,237,238] Transcutaneous nerve stimulation may rarely inhibit a pacemaker[239] but is generally thought to be safe.[240] In addition, the use of surgical (electrocautery) or physiotherapeutic diathermy can lead to pulse generator damage due to local heat production, myocardial burning, or ventricular fibrillation when used intraoperatively. Transient, very rapid pacing rates[237] and ventricular fibrillation have been produced by electrocautery used 8 to 25 cm away from a catheter electrode and 16 to 33 cm from pulse generators. However, the most common problem after subjecting a pacemaker to any of these sources of electromagnetic interference is reprogramming of the pacemaker, most commonly to its backup parameters.

Patients with permanent pacemakers are usually prohibited from undergoing magnetic resonance imaging. The magnet results in asynchronous operation of the pacemaker, which usually would not cause any untoward effects. In animal studies, it has been shown that the pacemaker can pace rapidly at the frequency cycle of the magnetic resonance (e.g., if the magnetic resonance imaging frequency is at 200 msec, the output of the pacemaker will be 300 ppm).[241] This is not a predictable phenomenon. If magnetic resonance imaging is the only diagnostic modality that can provide the necessary information for a paced patient, methods have been used to allow the non-pacemaker-dependent patient to undergo imaging. Uncomplicated magnetic resonance imaging has been reported in patients with a stable underlying rhythm when the pacemaker could be programmed in such a way that the stimulus delivered in the ventricle was subthreshold, i.e., failed to depolarize the ventricle. Therefore, even if rapid pacing occurs, it is ineffectual. If this method is used, the patient should be monitored in some way to assure adequate heart rate and blood pressure throughout the test.

Precautions must also be taken when pacemaker patients are subjected to extracorporeal shock wave lithotripsy.[242] Dual-chamber pacemakers should be programmed to the ventricular demand mode during the procedure if the patient paces in the atrium. If such a patient is left in a dual-chamber mode of operation, the lithotripsy can be triggered by the atrial paced event and induce ventricular inhibition. Activity-sensing pulse generators should be reprogrammed to a non-rate-adaptive mode, because action by the lithotriptor could result in sensor activation with inappropriately high pacing rates. An effort should be made to avoid placing any pacemaker at the focal point of the lithotriptor, especially an activity-sensing, rate-adaptive pacemaker that incorporates a piezoelectric crystal. The action of the lithotriptor could shatter the piezoelectric crystal.[243]

3. Spurious electrical discharges. Spurious electrical potentials can be recorded as a result of intimate contact between two endocardial electrodes when one is active and the other is inactive. The electrical activity has been demonstrated to cause inhibition of a demand pacemaker and stimulation of a synchronous unit. It is relatively unlikely that this would result in a clinically significant problem and usually would not warrant removal of a noninfected abandoned lead.

Other situations that are associated with the generation of electrical discharges include current leakage from a pulse generator, loose connection between lead and pulse generator, and insulation break in the catheter electrode.[244,245]

C. Therapy. The need for an aggressive therapeutic approach to sensing abnormalities depends upon the frequency of the sensing malfunction and the problems that occur as a result. Untreated bradycardia requires surgical revision if it cannot be corrected by reprogramming. Occasional and asymptomatic episodic sensing abnormalities can be treated safely by observation alone.[246]

Defibrillation. Because of the large amount of energy discharged during defibrillation, this procedure may result in various problems for patients with implanted permanent pacing systems.

A shunting circuit, known as a Zener diode, has been incorporated in all pulse generators to protect them against electrical damage during defibrillation. The diode may be considered to be a switch that is open during normal pacemaker function but closes when defibrillation voltage is detected, protecting the pulse generator's integrated circuits. However, damage is still possible if the defibrillation signal has a rapid rise time that prevents switch closure or the amount of energy transmitted is greater than the protective device can control. In addition, the characteristics of the diode are such that a low-resistance pathway may exist between the pulse generator and the electrode tip if sufficient voltage is applied externally, and therefore injury can result independently of pulse generator damage.

The complications that have resulted from the use of defibrillation in patients with implanted pacing systems include electrical damage to the pulse generator, which may be permanent or transient and which may be delayed in onset for several days; myocardial thermal damage secondary to transmission of electrical discharge to the heart via the leads (resulting in myocardial infarction or ventricular fibrillation or both); and inappropriate programming of programmable pulse generators.

To prevent these complications, defibrillation paddles should be placed at least 7.5 cm from the pulse generator or subcutaneous lead. Ideally, the paddles should be oriented perpendicularly to the line joining the pulse generator to the electrode tip to reduce the quantity of energy passing through the pacemaker sensing circuit. This can best be accomplished by using an anterior-posterior position of the defibrillation paddles, which will orient the defibrillation vector in a more perpendicular fashion than will an anterior-anterior (cross chest) position of the paddles.[247]

Because of the potential for complications, the pacing system should be checked after any defibrillation discharge.

Runaway pacemaker. This term refers to an increasing pacing rate beyond 150 beats/min with sufficient output to capture the heart. With lithium batteries, hermetic sealing, and reliable electronic circuits with runaway protection, the incidence has decreased significantly, although isolated instances still occur.[248,249] At the present time, when runaway does occur, it is secondary to random electronic component failure or therapeutic radiation resulting in component failure.

Because of the rapid pacing rates, hemodynamic embarrassment can occur, and the development of pacemaker runaway should be considered a medical emergency requiring immediate disconnection of the patient from the offending unit. This can be accomplished rapidly by local infiltration of anesthetic in the area of the pulse generator lead connection followed by incision into the area to isolate and cut the wires. If the patient is pacemaker dependent, a temporary pacemaker can be connected to the exposed wires to protect the patient from bradycardia-related symptoms.[248]

HISTORY. If symptoms have developed after implantation of the pacing system, they need to be assessed carefully. A return of the patient's preimplantation symptoms (especially syncope or presyncope) suggests complete or intermittent pacemaker failure. The development of new symptoms suggestive of hypotension (presyncope or episodic lightheadedness) in patients with ventricular demand systems may indicate the need for restoration of AV synchrony. Palpitations may indicate undersensing with initiation of competitive pacemaker rhythms.

INTRAOPERATIVE EVALUATION. Intraoperative pacemaker system evaluation is indicated in patients with documented complete or intermittent failure to capture, complete or symptomatic intermittent sensing abnormalities, or symptoms suggestive of serious pacemaker malfunction in whom a diagnosis cannot be made by noninvasive evaluation.

The pulse generator should be removed and inspected, and its function should be tested (output, pacing rate, pulse width, sensing capability, etc.) by use of a pacing system analyzer. Prior to disconnection of the pulse generator from the lead, the adequacy of that connection should be checked. The leads should be mobilized and also inspected for wire fracture or insulation break.

The voltage and current thresholds for myocardial capture should be checked, and lead impedance should be calculated during pacing at 5 V. For a bipolar lead, this testing should be accomplished in both a bipolar and a unipolar configuration.

These parameters aid in the assessment not only of

Table 25A-17 Intraoperative evaluation of pacing system

Defect	Voltage threshold	Current threshold	Lead impedance	Electrogram
Wire fracture	High	High, normal, or low	High	Variable
Insulation break	Low	High	Low	Variable
Lead dislodgment	High	High	Normal	Low
Exit block	High	High	Normal	Normal

patients with sensing abnormalities but also of patients with complete or intermittent failure to capture (Table 25A-17). With fracture of the electrode catheter wire, the voltage requirement for capture will be high, the resultant current requirement will be high, normal, or low, the lead impedance will be high, and the electrogram will be variable. If an insulation break is present, the voltage will be low, the current high, the impedance low, and the electrogram variable. Lead dislodgment will result in increased voltage and current thresholds, normal lead impedance, and a poor (low) electrogram. With exit block (abnormalities of myocardium-lead interface secondary to fibrosis), voltage and current thresholds will be high, the impedance will be normal, and in many cases the electrogram will also be normal.

When all this information has been collected, a reasoned decision can be made concerning which of the elements of the pacing system is malfunctioning and should be repaired or replaced.

Pathologic changes that may occur in the cardiovascular system secondary to transvenous electrode implantation

Intracardiac fibrosis. Transvenous electrodes are quickly incorporated into the right ventricular endocardium by the development of fibrous rings around various portions of the lead, resulting in firm attachment to the ventricular musculature and other cardiac and venous structures.[68,250,251] This retention, secondary to fibrosis, is particularly true with silicone rubber or polyethylene catheters that are known to encourage a fairly prominent endothelial reaction. Electrodes of polyurethane-coated woven polyester fibers provoke much less reaction, even though they remain in the heart for long periods.[252]

Postmortem examinations of patients bearing transvenous electrodes reveal that the catheters are endothelialized to varying degrees, depending on the length of time the catheter has been in the heart. The process begins within 12 hours of implantation,[253] and by 4 to 5 days there is a marked thrombosis along the catheter and at the point of attachment of the catheter to the myocardium. A gradual process of endothelialization then begins and is completed by about 7 months. A fibrin sheath surrounds the electrode catheter with multiple points of attachment of the sheath to the endocardium. Between 33% and 60% of all catheters evaluated at necropsy were firmly attached to the chordae tendineae or tricuspid valve without other evidence of tricuspid valve dysfunction.[254,255] However, there are reports of murmurs of tricuspid valve origin developing after catheter implantation and disappearing when the lead is repositioned,[256] and an isolated case of supravalvular, valvular, and infravalvular tricuspid stenosis secondary to a transvenous catheter has also been reported.[257] In addition, about 45% of all catheters exhibit thrombosis or fibrous organization, or both, in the region of the sinoatrial node.[254]

Because of these fibrous attachments, attempted lead removal in the event of lead malfunction has the potential for cardiac damage. Various complications of forceful traction have been reported, including arrhythmia with hypotension secondary to invagination of the right ventricle into the tricuspid valve, ventricular tachycardia, ventricular fibrillation, intracardiac lead rupture, hemopericardium secondary to a tear in the right ventricular myocardium, and tricuspid valve damage. In the absence of infection, a retained lead rarely causes a problem, and most authors would favor removal only if the lead could be explanted without forceful traction.[252]

One of the problems that has been associated with a retained lead is migration. This has occurred primarily when the lead was severed at the vein level and then sutured to the vein or other tissue. The migration usually has been to the lower part of the body (i.e., the inferior vena cava or hepatic venous system); however, on occasion the retained lead may migrate to the pulmonary circuit. Regardless of location, migration has been associated with serious complications, including thrombosis with embolism, sepsis, and death. For this reason, if migration occurs the catheter should be removed—transvenously if possible, but if this is not successful, then by a direct surgical approach. To prevent the problem of migration, the lead should not be severed close to the level of venous access and should be anchored securely to surrounding tissue.

Thrombosis, stenosis, and embolism secondary to transvenous electrode placement

INTRACARDIAC THROMBOSIS. The development of a clinically significant thrombus in the right atrium around a permanent transvenous catheter is rare. It may be manifested by recurrent pulmonary embolism or right heart inflow obstruction.[258] In the cases reported in the literature, the mortality rate associated with this complication has been very high. In the patient with symptoms, surgical evacuation of the thrombus may rarely be necessary. Heparin therapy can be considered, as can thrombolytic therapy unless the thrombus occurs in the early postimplantation period. Asymptomatic pulmonary embolism in the absence of an identified right atrial thrombus has been said to occur in as many as 15% of patients with new pacemaker implants.[259]

A pacing catheter that is malpositioned in the left ventricle (septal perforation or via an atrial or ventricular septal defect) may serve as a source of arterial thromboembolism and should be removed and repositioned in the right ventricle.

VENOUS THROMBOSIS OR STENOSIS. Superior vena caval obstruction is a rare complication usually secondary to thrombus formation, particularly in the region of a fractured catheter electrode,[260] but it also has been reported secondary to stenosis of the superior vena cava at the site of the proximal cut end of a retained endocardial electrode or of fibrosis encircling the catheter at the right atrium–superior vena cava junction. The usual therapy includes anticoagulation and the use of diuretics to reduce the edema until collateral venous channels develop.

Symptomatic subclavian vein obstruction may occur in patients with uncomplicated endocardial pacing systems, in an incidence varying from 1.2% to 12%.[261] The symptoms usually are confined to painless, unilateral, upper extremity edema or prominence of the venous pattern in the arm, chest, or neck.[261] Acute subclavian or axillary thrombophlebitis and resultant pulmonary embolism are rarely encountered.

Although the incidence of symptomatic venous obstruction is quite low, contrast venography performed on asymptomatic patients has produced abnormal venograms in 30% to 45%, with total obstruction of the subclavian vein in 13% to 20%.[262] Conversely, a study of paced pediatric patients revealed no significant venous thrombosis in any of the patients studied. Isotope venographic studies have demonstrated similar abnormalities and suggest that the incidence may be higher in patients with multiple electrodes. Some studies have indicated that the incidence of thrombosis around severed retained leads left unsecured intraluminally may be extremely high.

The discrepancy between the incidence of venous obstruction and the lack of associated symptoms would suggest that subclavian obstruction occurs gradually, allowing an adequate collateral circulation to develop and so prevent the development of edema.

Because of the low risk of symptomatic thrombosis, prophylactic anticoagulation to prevent this complication is not indicated. However, if symptoms do result from thrombotic subclavian obstruction, therapy with heparin, elevation, and elastic support will allow collateralization to occur with resolution of symptoms. Anticoagulation with warfarin probably should be continued for several weeks after the resolution of acute symptoms.

We have reported on percutaneous balloon venoplasty to enable placement of an additional pacing lead through a stenotic subclavian vein.[263] This procedure is rarely necessary, but in patients with limited venous access and the need for an additional pacing lead, it may be considered.

Pacemaker infections

Pacemaker implantation, like all surgical procedures, entails the risk of infection. The incidence of infection after pacemaker surgery has been reported to vary from 0.3% to 6.0%.[264] More recent experience, including our own, indicates that at present the annual incidence is between 0% and 3%.[265] The fact that the pacing system is an implanted foreign body enhances the significance of infection and may impair the ability to eradicate the infection by antibiotic therapy alone.

The various clinical manifestations of pacemaker infections include erosion of part of the pacing system through the skin with secondary infection, inflammation or abscess of the pulse generator pocket, septicemia in a patient with an implanted pacemaker without another identifiable source, and infective endocarditis. These manifestations may occur alone or in various combinations.

Clinical manifestations

EROSION. Erosion of part of the pacing system through the skin with infection occurring at that site has been the sole clinical manifestation of infection in about 20% of the patients referred to our institution for pacing system infection.[265] It appears to result primarily from pressure necrosis of the skin caused by the pulse generator.

As expected, it is a late complication, occurring (on the average) 16 months after pacemaker implantation. In our series, skin necrosis occurred in 83% of the patients whose infections occurred more than 24 months after implantation; only 10% of patients whose infections occurred less than 24 months after implantation had skin necrosis.[266] Erosion is also more likely to occur in patients whose most recent surgical procedure was pulse generator replacement rather than implantation of a new pacing system.

Actual erosion of the skin by part of the pacing system may be preceded by "pre-erosion," which is manifested by an area of thin, tight, reddened skin over the generator or lead. Pre-erosion may also result in localized pain in the absence of predisposing factors (such as trauma). As long as the skin is intact, it will be a barrier to infection, but because of the potential for skin breakdown with resultant infection, the pacemaker pocket should be revised immediately.

PULSE GENERATOR INFLAMMATION OR ABSCESS. Inflammation or abscess formation within the pulse generator pocket is the most common manifestation of pacemaker infection, occurring in about 40% of all cases as the only manifestation and in more than 70% in combination with erosion or sepsis.[265,266]

This complication usually presents as erythema, tenderness, and swelling over the pulse generator, with or without skin necrosis. It may occur soon after a pacemaker surgical procedure or be delayed by weeks or months.[267] In our experience, virtually all the acute pacemaker infections (i.e., those occurring less than 2 weeks after a surgical procedure) presented as pulse generator pocket abscesses.[265,266]

SEPSIS AND ENDOCARDITIS. Fever (with or without chills) associated with positive blood cultures in the absence of another focus of infection in any patient with an implanted pacemaker should be considered to be a manifestation of a potentially fatal pacemaker infection.

Sepsis is the least common primary clinical manifestation of a pacemaker infection, occurring in about 15% to 20% of patients.[265] When it occurs as a sole manifestation of infection, the length of time between the most recent surgical procedure and the onset of infection is usually short.

Endocarditis may accompany septicemia and should be considered to exist when there is a sustained bacteremia.[268,269] There are rarely any systemic manifestations of endocarditis, and in the past it was thought that this was an extremely rare occurrence. However, studies have demonstrated an associated mural endocarditis of the right atrial wall surrounding the electrode in patients with sepsis.

Bacteremia also may be documented in the absence of septicemia. In a series of 46 patients, only 66% of the patients with bacteremia had clinical manifestations of sepsis. Although blood cultures were not obtained in all cases, when they were they were positive in 30%,[266] which might imply that the incidence of bacteremia in an apparently uncomplicated pacemaker infection is much higher than anticipated.

Microbiology. In all reported series, the majority of pacemaker infections are caused by a *Staphylococcus* sp.—*S. aureus* or *S. epidermidis.* Many other organisms

Table 25A-18 Organisms documented in pacing system infections

Frequently identified
Staphylococcus epidermidis
Staphylococcus aureus
Less frequently identified
Klebsiella pneumoniae
Enterobacter cloacae
Pseudomonas aeruginosa
Escherichia coli
Proteus mirabilis
Alcaligenes faecalis
Serratia marcescens
Peptostreptococcus
Micrococcus
α-Hemolytic streptococcus
β-Hemolytic streptococcus
Flavobacterium
Propionibacterium
Isolated reports
Candida albicans
Petriellidium boydii
Mycobacterium avium
Haemophilus parainfluenzae
Actinobacillus actinomycetemcomitans
Aspergillus flavus

(alone or as a mixed infection) also have been implicated as the cause of a pacing system infection (Table 25A-18).

The infecting organism tends to vary according to the clinical manifestation of infection. Septicemia and infections that occur shortly after operation are most frequently caused by *S. aureus,* whereas *S. epidermidis* is more frequently associated with pulse generator pocket infections or infections of a more indolent nature.[265]

The diagnosis of infection must be confirmed and the proper selection of antibiotic therapy must be guided by identification of the infecting organism by culture. Positive cultures have been obtained from the pulse generator pocket, catheter electrode, blood, pericardium, and pleura. In our experience, cultures were positive in 94% from the pulse generator pocket, in 88% from the electrode, and in 30% from blood.[266] In most reported series the diagnosis of infection depended on obtaining positive cultures. In a 12-year review of infections, Lemire et al.[270] found that in 15% of obviously infected systems the cultures were sterile. The reasons for this were not given but could include concomitant antibiotic therapy and inadequate culture technique.

Predisposing factors. Various factors have been identified as appearing to increase the chances of infection after pacemaker implantation. These include multiple pacemaker-related surgical procedures, the need to reposition the catheter electrode acutely, drain placement, postoperative hematoma formation (especially if associated with attempted needle aspiration), chest wall trauma, diabetes mellitus, presence of an underlying malignancy, and concomitant steroid or anticoagulant therapy.[265] There does not seem to be a difference in the rate of infection if the surgical procedure is performed in a catheterization laboratory as opposed to an operating suite.

Few data support the routine use of parenteral or oral antibiotic therapy before, during, or after pacemaker implantation. Some data support the use of an antibiotic solution to irrigate the pacemaker pocket at the time of the procedure. This practice, coupled with good sterile technique, is the best deterrent to infection.[73,271]

Therapy. Many therapeutic approaches to the eradication of a pacemaker infection have been proposed.[272,273] For skin erosion (especially if not grossly infected), it has been suggested that the creation of a new pocket adjacent to the area of erosion combined with local irrigation with antibiotic solution (the same generator and lead are used) or creation of a new pulse generator pocket (the old catheter is used but the generator is replaced) may be successful in some patients.

In the case of pulse generator pocket inflammation or abscess, success with a combination of local debridement, systemic antibiotic therapy, and continuous irrigation with an antiseptic solution without removal of the pacing system has been reported when the infecting organism was *S. epidermidis.* However, in our experience, therapy that has not included removal of all pacing hardware has been almost uniformly unsuccessful in eradication of the infectious process.[273] In nine patients with epicardial systems with pulse generator pocket infections (78% *S. epidermidis*), conservative nonsurgical therapy failed in 100% and lead transection with partial lead removal failed in 57%. When the system was totally removed, all patients were cured.[273]

If sepsis (or positive blood cultures without systemic symptoms) occurs, there is uniform agreement that treatment should include local pocket irrigation, systemic antibiotic therapy, and removal of the pulse generator and catheter electrode, even if thoracotomy is required.

When the infected system is removed, the timing of implantation of the new generator and lead is a disputed matter. Many authors have suggested that after the infected system is removed, implantation of a new system at a fresh site (either the contralateral side of chest or abdomen) should be carried out either shortly after removal in the case of localized infections or after an interval of temporary pacing and systemic antibiotic therapy if bacteremia is present. We have used both this two-stage procedure and a one-stage procedure in all types of infections (including sepsis) with equal success.

The one-stage procedure involves isolation of the infected site from the one to be used and then implantation of the new system followed by removal of the infected system. This one-stage procedure has decreased patient morbidity related to temporary pacing and has decreased the average length of hospital stay significantly. It has also been suggested that there is inherent danger associated with the long-term breach of skin required during

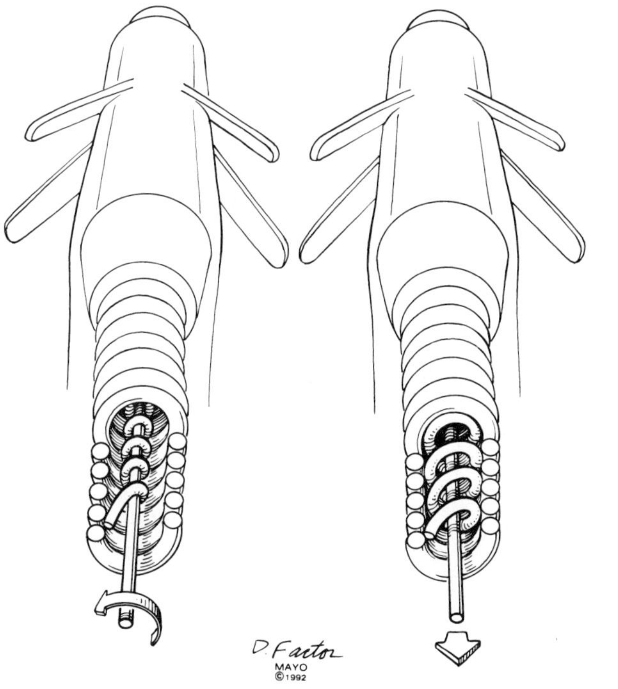

Fig 25A-61 The locking stylet technique is based on the ability to grasp the inner coil of a bipolar lead with a locking guide wire so that inflexible traction can be applied to the tip of the lead. **Left,** the locking guide is inserted and rotated counterclockwise. The locking stylet is insinuated and grasps the coil. **Right,** the rotation can then be relaxed and traction applied. (From Furman S: Troubleshooting. In *A Practice of Cardiac Pacing.* Third edition. Edited by S Furman, DL Hayes, DR Holmes Jr. Mount Kisco, New York, Futura Publishing Company, 1993, pp 685-723. By permission, Mayo Foundation.)

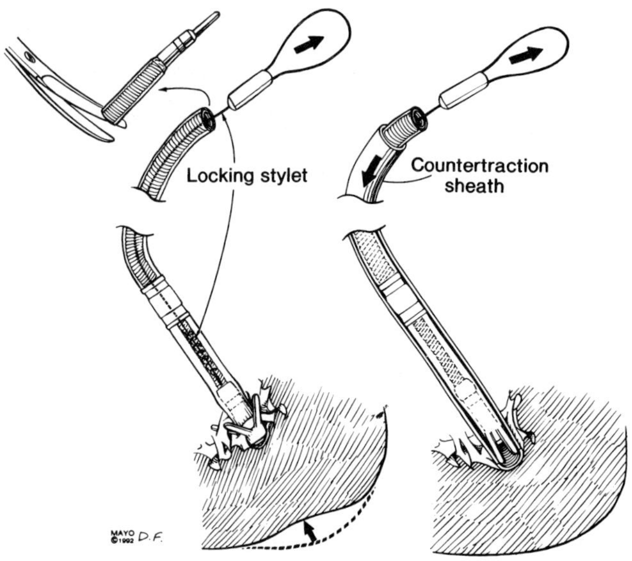

Fig 25A-62 The entire locking stylet process is described as follows: **Left,** the connector is cut from the lead. The locking stylet is then insinuated into the lead (see Fig 25A-61). Traction is applied to the lead, which may pull it from the heart. **Right,** if the preceding maneuvers are not successful in removing the lead, a series of plastic sheaths is placed over the lead and advanced to the endocardial surface. The sheath is then pushed against the endocardial surface to provide countertraction while the locking guide pulls on the lead. (From Furman S: Troubleshooting. In *A Practice of Cardiac Pacing.* Third edition. Edited by S Furman, DL Hayes, DR Holmes Jr. Mount Kisco, New York, Futura Publishing Company, 1993, pp 685-723. By permission, Mayo Foundation.)

long-term temporary pacing, and this is eliminated by the one-stage procedure.[274]

The recommended duration of systemic antibiotic therapy also varies with the type of infection encountered. For localized infections, antibiotic therapy usually is continued for 2 to 4 weeks, whereas when sepsis is present therapy for at least 4 weeks is usually indicated.

Pacemaker lead extraction

When a decision is made to remove a chronically implanted lead, the lead must be carefully mobilized and a stylet introduced into it. If the lead has an active fixation mechanism, it should be withdrawn from the endocardium if possible. Traction should be used as the initial method of lead retraction. Traction under fluoroscopy should be exerted while the lead is watched. Cardiac rhythm should also be monitored during traction. Traction on a ventricular lead usually results in premature ventricular contractions, and more malignant rhythm disturbances are possible. If the lead is successfully dislodged from the endocardial surface, traction should be continued as the lead is pulled into the superior vena cava and remaining venous structures. It is possible that the lead could be dislodged from the endocardial surface but be adherent within the venous structures, so that retraction would be impossible.

When traction is not successful for removal of chronically implanted leads, other techniques are available. Special lead extractors have been developed. The most commonly used is the Cook extractor, which is applied in the Byrd extraction technique, named after the primary developer, Dr. Charles Byrd. With this technique, after the lead connector is transected, a special "locking stylet" is sized to the lead and inserted (Fig 25A-61). Once the stylet is locked into the lead, pulling the stylet places traction at the tip of the lead and not throughout the entire lead, which could result in the lead stretching or insulation separating from the lead. If traction on the locking stylet fails to remove the lead, a series of sleeves is placed over the lead and passed along the exterior of the lead to break up fibrous adhesions. The sleeves or dilators are passed all the way to the attachment of the electrode to the myocardium if necessary. Traction on the locking stylet with counterpressure on the sleeve usually allows lead extraction while preventing invagination of the right ventricle (Fig 25A-62).

Experienced persons have achieved excellent results

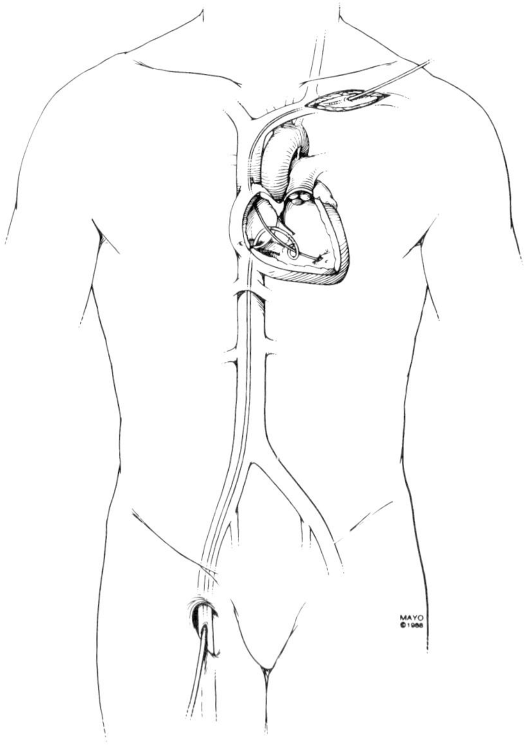

Fig 25A-63 A pigtail catheter is passed through the right femoral vein into the right ventricle. The pigtail portion of the catheter is positioned around the permanent pacing lead as close to the tip of the lead as possible. (From Furman S: Troubleshooting. In *A Practice of Cardiac Pacing.* Second revised and enlarged edition. Edited by S Furman, DL Hayes, DR Holmes Jr. Mount Kisco, New York, Futura Publishing Company, 1989, pp 611-650. By permission, Mayo Foundation.)

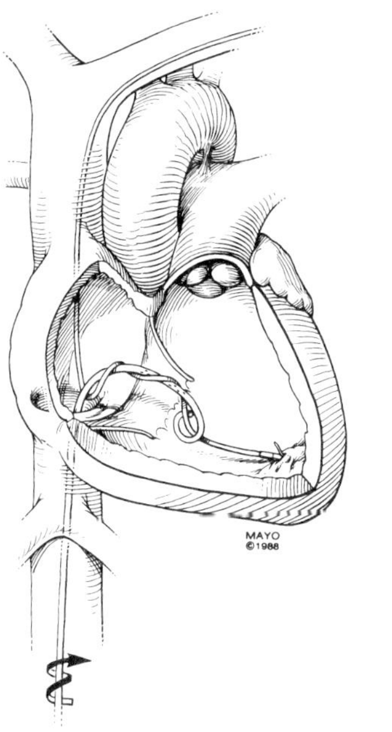

Fig 25A-64 The pigtail catheter is twisted clockwise. This movement effectively entwines the pigtail catheter and the permanent pacing lead. (From Furman S: Troubleshooting. In *A Practice of Cardiac Pacing.* Second revised and enlarged edition. Edited by S Furman, DL Hayes, DR Holmes Jr. Mount Kisco, New York, Futura Publishing Company, 1989, pp 611-650. By permission, Mayo Foundation.)

with this technique. In a reported series of attempted removal of 829 leads by this extraction technique, 85% were completely removed, 8% were partially removed, and 7% were not removed. Success with this technique is higher with active fixation leads and bipolar leads and is obviously also related to physician experience and the length of time the lead has been in place.

This technique is not without potential complications. Nonlethal complications that have been reported include avulsion of myocardium, hemothorax, and pulmonary embolism. The need for emergency thoracotomy has been reported.

Another technique used at the Mayo Clinic is as follows: If the tip of the lead cannot be removed by traction, a pigtail catheter is passed into the heart via the femoral vein. The pigtail portion of the catheter is positioned around the permanent pacing lead, as close to the tip as possible (Fig 25A-63). Twisting the pigtail catheter several times in a clockwise direction entwines the pacing lead in the catheter (Fig 25A-64). Traction is then applied to the pigtail catheter. Frequently, traction to the pacing lead near its point of endocardial attachment frees the lead (Fig 25A-65,A). If the lead tip is dislodged from the endocardial surface, traction is continued on the pigtail catheter, and the lead is pulled into the inferior vena cava. Because the entwined pacing lead and pigtail catheter are bulky and because with traction the catheter may now slip off the free end of the pacing lead, the pigtail catheter is removed by twisting it in a counterclockwise direction (Fig 25A-65,B). Once the pigtail catheter is removed, a Dotter retriever is passed into the inferior vena cava through the femoral vein. The Dotter retriever consists of a retractable wire basket passed within a sheath. When the wire basket is extended beyond the sheath, the basket opens, and the operator attempts to catch a portion of the pacing lead in the wire basket. When the retractor is pulled back, the pacing lead is firmly entrapped in the Dotter retriever. Applying traction on the retriever extracts the lead via the femoral vein. Before extraction is attempted, the connector portion at the proximal end of the pacing lead must be transected (Fig 25A-65,C).

If initial traction on the entwined pigtail catheter does not dislodge the tip of the pacing lead, any redundancy in the lead is pulled into the inferior vena cava in an effort to form a small loop of pacing lead that can subsequently be grasped by the Dotter retriever (Fig 25A-66,A). Again, turning the pigtail catheter in a counterclockwise direction frees it from the pacing lead, and the catheter is removed. The Dotter retriever is passed into the inferior vena cava, and with the basket extended, an attempt is

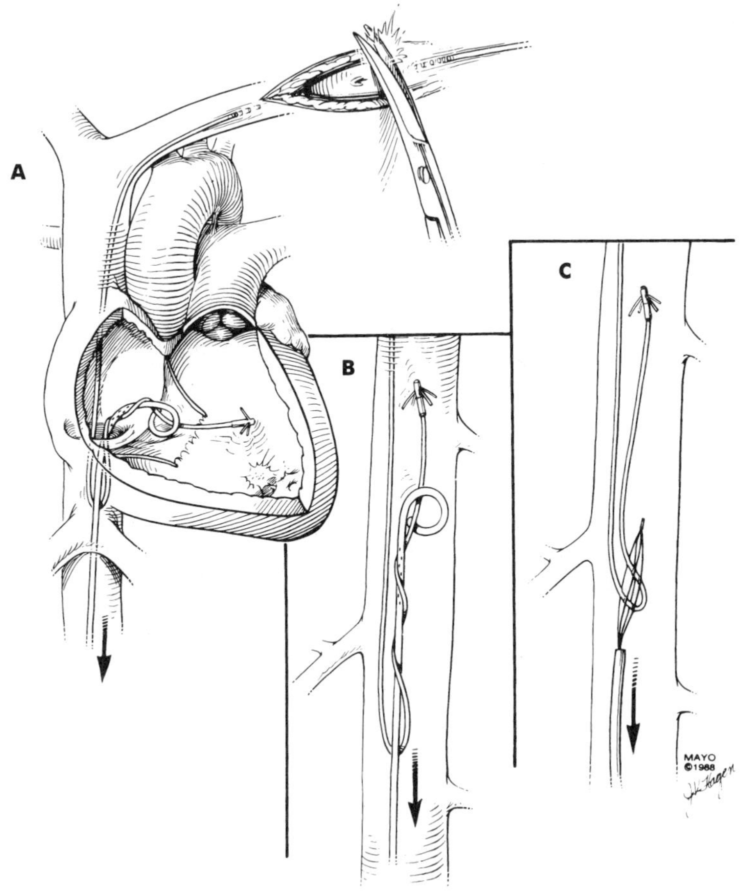

Fig 25A-65 **A,** with the pigtail catheter and the permanent pacing lead firmly entwined, traction is applied on the catheter in an attempt to free the lead tip from the endocardial surface. **B,** if traction is successful in freeing the tip of the lead, the lead is pulled into the inferior vena cava. The pigtail catheter is rotated in a counterclockwise direction to free it from the lead and is then removed via the femoral vein. **C,** the pigtail catheter is replaced with a Dotter retriever. The wire basket is extended and under fluoroscopy is positioned so that a portion of the pacing lead is within the wire basket. The wire basket is then retracted around a portion of the pacing lead so that the lead is firmly caught in the Dotter retriever. Traction is then applied to the Dotter retriever in an attempt to extract the whole lead via the femoral vein. The most proximal portion of the pacing lead (the lead connector) should be transected before extraction. (From Furman S: Troubleshooting. In *A Practice of Cardiac Pacing.* Second revised and enlarged edition. Edited by S Furman, DL Hayes, DR Holmes Jr. Mount Kisco, New York, Futura Publishing Company, 1989, pp 611-650. By permission, Mayo Foundation.)

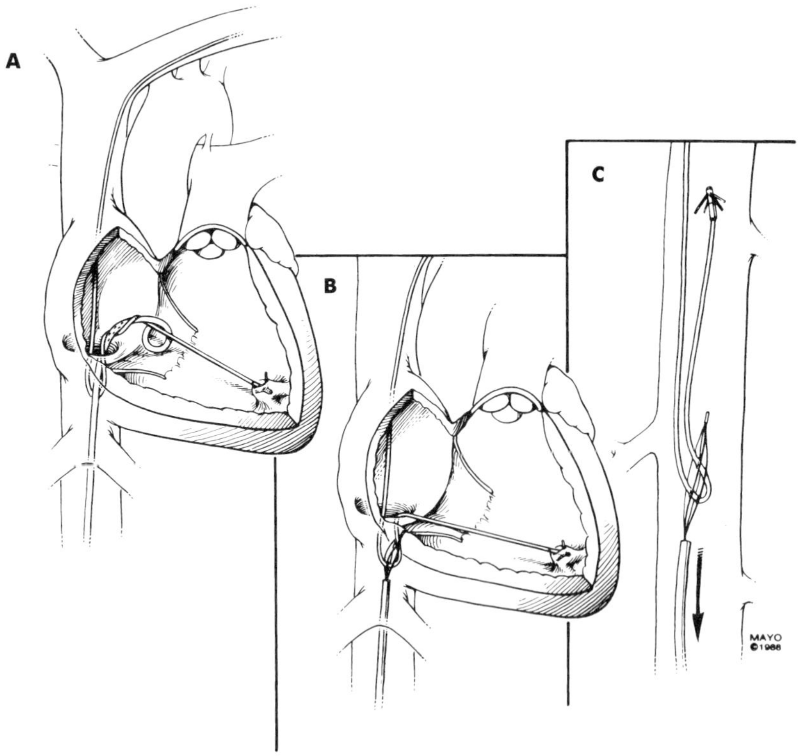

Fig 25A-66 **A,** with the pigtail catheter firmly entwined with the permanent pacing lead, traction is applied, but the lead tip cannot be dislodged from the endocardial surface. Traction is applied on the pigtail catheter and the still attached lead to position a small loop of the pacing catheter within the inferior vena cava. The pigtail catheter is then rotated in a counterclockwise direction to separate the catheter from the pacing lead. The pigtail catheter is removed. **B,** the Dotter retriever is passed into the inferior vena cava. With the Dotter retriever extended, an attempt is made to snare the loop of the pacing lead in the retriever. Once this is accomplished, the basket portion of the Dotter retriever is retracted, firmly securing a portion of the pacing lead in the retriever. Traction is then applied on the Dotter retriever to free the tip of the pacing lead from the endocardial surface. **C,** if the tip of the pacing lead is successfully dislodged from the endocardial surface, the lead is extracted via the femoral vein. (From Furman S: Troubleshooting. In *A Practice of Cardiac Pacing.* Second revised and enlarged edition. Edited by S Furman, DL Hayes, DR Holmes Jr. Mount Kisco, New York, Futura Publishing Company, 1989, pp 611-650. By permission, Mayo Foundation.)

made to capture the loop of pacing lead. Once the pacing lead has been entrapped in the wire basket, the retractor is pulled back. With the pacing lead firmly snared, traction is placed on the Dotter retriever in an effort to dislodge the tip of the lead (Fig 25A-66,B). The Dotter retriever sometimes can dislodge the lead tip when the pigtail catheter has failed, because better traction can be applied with the pacing lead securely snared in the retriever. If the lead tip is successfully dislodged, traction is continued on the Dotter retriever, and the lead is extracted via the femoral vein (Fig 25A-66,C). Extracting the lead through the femoral vein while it is still entangled in the Dotter retriever has the potential to damage the femoral vein because of the bulk of the catheters being extracted. In our experience, significant hematomas have not resulted from the extraction and venous repair has never been required. A pressure dressing should be placed over the puncture site, and the site must be carefully observed.

Although time-consuming and technically difficult, this procedure may obviate thoracotomy.

Myocardial perforation

Penetration and perforation of the myocardium by a pacing catheter electrode is infrequent. Cardiac perforation may present clinically as intermittent (or complete) failure to pace, diaphragmatic stimulation, or hemopericardium with or without tamponade. In addition, the diagnosis can be suggested by the development of friction rub on examination, a change in the ECG, or a change in

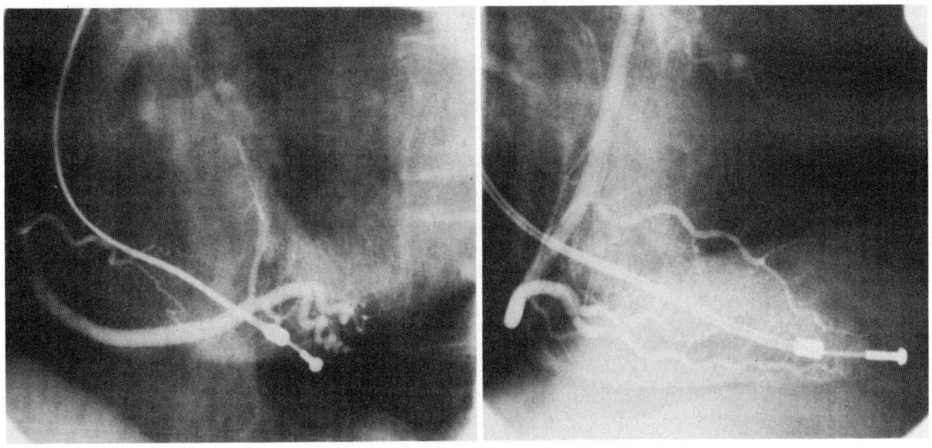

Fig 25A-67 Still frame from a cineangiogram reveals cardiac perforation by the permanent pacing lead. Note that the lead tip extends beyond the border of the ventricle as determined by the position of the coronary arteries.

lead position apparent on a chest roentgenogram (Fig 25A-67). The diagnosis should always be entertained for a patient who exhibits failure to pace (complete or intermittent) with normal sensing if the stimulus artifact is still present on the ECG and no lead dislodgment is apparent by x-ray examination. This would be reinforced if other abnormalities suggesting perforation (e.g., friction rub, diaphragmatic stimulation) were also present.

Even though pacemaker malfunction or tamponade may result from perforation, it is likely that the majority of patients do not exhibit these abnormalities clinically.

Various ECG changes (including a change in bundle-branch block pattern during pacing, deep T-wave inversion, or a change in the vector of the pacemaker stimulus artifact) have been reported to occur as a result of perforation. However, there is no absolute diagnostic pattern, which limits the value of the surface ECG in this situation. When possible, the intracardiac electrogram may be helpful, particularly if a change in the QRS morphology and vector and the development of a current of injury pattern (consistent with normal endocardial pacing) occur during careful withdrawal of the pacing electrode.

If lead perforation occurs, the lead should be repositioned. This should be done under fluoroscopic control, and the signs of cardiac tamponade should be watched for carefully.

Twiddler's syndrome

This term refers to dislodgment or fracture of a transvenous pacing electrode by repeated manipulation and turning of the pulse generator in the subcutaneous pocket. This can result in retraction of the electrode into the right atrium or superior vena cava. This is a very uncommon cause of lead dislodgment. The vast majority of these patients are elderly women with large, loose pulse generator pockets, and virtually all patients deny manipulation of the pulse generator. The location of the pulse generator (chest or abdomen) or the catheter (endocardial or epicardial) has no bearing on the occurrence of the complication.

This syndrome may be prevented by avoiding the creation of excessively large pulse generator pockets, fixation of the pulse generator by an anchoring suture (especially if the pocket is larger than necessary at the time of pulse generator replacement), or anchoring the lead to the prepectoral fascia by a butterfly or sleeve.

Miscellaneous

Skeletal muscle stimulation. Pectoral or abdominal muscles may be stimulated by the indifferent plate of a unipolar system or as a result of an electrical current leak from the lead (insulation break) or pulse generator. Most unipolar pulse generators are covered with a plastic coating, an area of metal being left bare to act as the anode plate. The non-coated surface (bare metal) should be placed facing subcutaneous tissue, not muscle.

Phantom programming. Inappropriate modification of the programmable functions of a pulse generator can occur after defibrillation, after electrocautery, after application of a magnet, or occasionally after exposure to a strong electromagnetic field. The function of a pulse generator should be carefully checked in any of these circumstances.

Allergy. This is an extremely rare complication of pacemaker implantation. If patients are sensitive to nickel or chromium, they may be sensitive to a pulse generator coated with stainless steel. Most generators are coated with titanium, which has been considered to be nonallergenic. However, titanium allergy with recurrent inflammation around the pulse generator has been documented.[275]

FOLLOW-UP OF THE PACED PATIENT

When a pacemaker is implanted, the physician who performed the operation or the institution at which it was done should assume responsibility for follow-up of the patient. The physician may elect to do this at his or her own institution, through any number of commercial pacemaker follow-up centers, or through the company that manufactured the pacemaker.

The most important reason for careful pacemaker follow-up still is to identify pacemaker failure before it occurs.[276-278] The incidence of catastrophic pacemaker failure continues to decline with advances in pacemaker technology. Other problems, such as programming difficulties or other inherent circuitry problems, also must be watched for.

We have adopted a standard pacemaker surveillance program for our patients as follows.

1. All patients who are to be followed at our institution (approximately 96% of those receiving implants at our institution) are given educational material and instruction by a nurse trained in pacemaker care and surveillance prior to dismissal from the hospital after the implantation procedure. The topics include care of the wound in the immediate postoperative period, general principles of cardiac pacing, how to check the peripheral pulse, specific capabilities of the patient's pacemaker, myths and realities of electromagnetic interference, technique of transtelephonic monitoring, and discussion of activities for the pacemaker patient. At that time the patient is given an appointment for the first transtelephonic pacemaker check.

2. For all new pacemaker implants, other than those under clinical investigation, the telephone schedule is as follows: weekly transmission for 1 month; transmission every 3 months thereafter until the first indication of battery depletion; transmission every month after indications of battery depletion until battery end-of-life indicators are reached.

ECG strips, obtained via telephone and recorded with and without a magnet placed over the pulse generator, are analyzed and kept as part of the permanent record. Some pacemaker centers have the capability of digitizing the ECG tracings to allow a permanent ECG record to be stored in the computer.

3. For those patients who return for a battery pack change only, they are checked transtelephonically 1 week after the implantation and then they resume their usual schedule.

4. Follow-up of patients bearing "clinical investigation units" is based on the follow-up requirements of the pacemaker manufacturer.

5. All patients are requested to return for an office visit at 3 months after the implantation procedure. At the time of that visit the patient should be interviewed, and certain specific questions should be asked. Has the pacemaker caused you any discomfort? Have you resumed normal activities? Have those symptoms that initially prompted the medical attention that resulted in implantation of the permanent pacemaker now resolved. Rhythm strips with and without magnet application are obtained. If the pacemaker is programmed to a rate-adaptive pacing mode, the patient is exercised to determine appropriateness of rate response. (Exercise is usually accomplished informally; that is, the patient walks at a casual or brisk pace in the clinic or hospital corridor while heart rate is monitored.) If the patient has a pacemaker capable of rate adaptation but it is not programmed to a rate-adaptive pacing mode, the patient's rate response should be assessed to determine whether benefit might be derived from a rate-adaptive pacing mode.

During the physical examination, special attention is given to the incision and pulse generator pocket.

6. A full programming routine is carried out prior to hospital dismissal, again at 3 months, and thereafter annually. Full programming would allow *(a)* a decrease in pulse width or amplitude in those patients who display a safe pacing margin of safety at the lower energy output; *(b)* an increase in pulse width to ensure an adequate pacing margin of safety in those patients with increasing thresholds in the early postimplantation period; *(c)* a decrease in rate in patients who may display normal conduction during the majority of their activities; *(d)* change in any number of programming combinations that may need changing in the patient with a rate variable pacemaker—i.e., lower rate, upper rate, AV delay, or rate-adaptive parameters; and *(e)* display of all telemetered values available.

Many pacemaker centers, like ours, are now computerized. This allows the nurse or technician who receives the calls or sees the patient in the pacemaker clinic to retrieve data concerning last follow-up: most recent measured pacing parameters, appropriate magnet response of the patient's pulse generator, age of the unit and lead, programmed settings, most recent programmings, etc. This will minimize paperwork and errors from trying to remember failure modes and magnet response for each pulse generator.

REFERENCES

1. Hyman AS: Resuscitation of the stopped heart by intracardiac therapy. *Arch Intern Med* 46:553-568, 1930
2. Zoll PM: Historical development of cardiac pacemakers. *Prog Cardiovasc Dis* 14:421-429, 1972
3. Zoll PM: Resuscitation of the heart in ventricular standstill by external electric stimulation. *N Engl J Med* 247:768-771, 1952
4. Weirich WL, Gott VL, Lillehei CW: The treatment of complete heart block by the combined use of a myocardial electrode and an artificial pacemaker. *Surg Forum* 8:360-363, 1957
5. Senning A: Cited by Irnich W, Parsonnet V, Myers GH[11]
6. Furman S, Schwedel JB: An intracardiac pacemaker for Stokes-Adams seizures. *N Engl J Med* 261:943-948, 1959
7. Greatbatch W, Chardack WM: A transistorized implantable pacemaker for the long-term correction of complete A-V block. *J Med Elec* 48:643, 1959
8. Folkman MJ, Watkins E: An artificial conduction system for the management of experimental complete heart block. *Surg Forum* 8:331-334, 1957
9. Stephenson SE Jr, Edwards WH, Jolly PC, et al: Physiologic P-wave cardiac stimulator. *J Thorac Cardiovasc Surg* 38:604-609, 1959
10. Nathan DA, Center S, Wu C-Y, et al: An implantable, synchro-

nous pacemaker for the long-term correction of complete heart block. *Circulation* 27:682-685, 1963

11. Irnich W, Parsonnet V, Myers GH: Introduction and historical review. *PACE* 1:371-374, 1978
12. A Report of the Joint American College of Cardiology/American Heart Association Task Force on Assessment of Cardiovascular Procedures (Subcommittee on Pacemaker Implantation): Guidelines for permanent cardiac pacemaker implantation, May 1984. *J Am Coll Cardiol* 4:434-442, 1984
13. Goldschlager N: Permanent cardiac pacing for bradyarrhythmia. *Postgrad Med* 83:156-174, 1988
14. McAnulty JH, Rahimtoola SH, Murphy E, et al: Natural history of "high-risk" bundle branch block: final report of a prospective study. *N Engl J Med* 307:137-143, 1982
15. Hindman MC, Wagner GS, JaRo M, et al: The clinical significance of bundle branch block complicating acute myocardial infarction. 1. Clinical characteristics, hospital mortality, and one-year follow-up. *Circulation* 58:679-688, 1978
16. Kones RJ, Phillips JH: Bundle branch block in acute myocardial infarction: current concepts and indications. *Acta Cardiol (Brux)* 35:469-478, 1980
17. Norris RM, Mercer CJ, Croxson MS: Conduction disturbances due to anteroseptal myocardial infarction and their treatment by endocardial pacing. *Am Heart J* 84:560-566, 1972
18. Bru P, Lévy S, Metge M, et al: Remote occurrence of high degree heart block following failure of transcatheter AV junctional ablation: incidence and clinical significance. *PACE* 10:937-942, 1987
19. Nicod P, Gilpin E, Dittrich H, et al: Long-term outcome in patients with inferior myocardial infarction and complete atrioventricular block. *J Am Coll Cardiol* 12:589-594, 1988
20. Hindman MC, Wagner GS, JaRo M, et al: The clinical significance of bundle branch block complicating acute myocardial infarction. 2. Indications for temporary and permanent pacemaker insertion. *Circulation* 58:689-699, 1978
21. Edhag O, Swahn Å: Prognosis of patients with complete heart block or arrhythmic syncope who were not treated with artificial pacemakers: a long-term follow-up study of 101 patients. *Acta Med Scand* 200:457-463, 1976
22. Fisch GR, Zipes DP, Fisch C: Bundle branch block and sudden death. *Prog Cardiovasc Dis* 23:187-224, 1980
23. Scheinman MM, Peters RW, Modin G, et al: Prognostic value of infranodal conduction time in patients with chronic bundle branch block. *Circulation* 56:240-244, 1977
24. McAnulty JH, Kauffman S, Murphy E, et al: Survival in patients with intraventricular conduction defects. *Arch Intern Med* 138:30-35, 1978
25. Denes P, Dhingra RC, Wu D, et al: Sudden death in patients with chronic bifascicular block. *Arch Intern Med* 137:1005-1010, 1977
26. Hayes DL: Indications for permanent pacing. In *A Practice of Cardiac Pacing*. Third edition. Edited by S Furman, DL Hayes, DR Holmes Jr. Mount Kisco, New York, Futura Publishing Company, 1993, pp 1-28
27. Vintila M, Fagarasanu R, Luca R: Pacemaker therapy in a group of 132 patients with sick sinus syndrome—indications and results. *Med Interne* 26:305-309, 1988
28. Sasaki Y, Shimotori M, Akahane K, et al: Long-term follow-up of patients with sick sinus syndrome: a comparison of clinical aspects among unpaced, ventricular inhibited paced, and physiologically paced groups. *PACE* 11:1575-1583, 1988
29. Rosenqvist M, Brandt J, Schüller H: Long-term pacing in sinus node disease: effects of stimulation mode on cardiovascular morbidity and mortality. *Am Heart J* 116:16-22, 1988
30. Alpert MA, Curtis JJ, Sanfelippo JF, et al: Comparative survival following permanent ventricular and dual-chamber pacing for patients with chronic symptomatic sinus node dysfunction with and without congestive heart failure. *Am Heart J* 113:958-965, 1987
31. Alt E, Völker R, Wirtzfeld A, et al: Survival and follow-up after pacemaker implantation: a comparison of patients with sick sinus syndrome, complete heart block, and atrial fibrillation. *PACE* 8:849-855, 1985
32. Abi-Samra F, Maloney JD, Fouad-Tarazi FM, et al: The usefulness of head-up tilt testing and hemodynamic investigations in the workup of syncope of unknown origin. *PACE* 11:1202-1214, 1988
33. Almquist A, Goldenberg IF, Milstein S, et al: Provocation of bradycardia and hypotension by isoproterenol and upright posture in patients with unexplained syncope. *N Engl J Med* 320:346-351, 1989
34. Brignole M, Menozzi C, Lolli G, et al: Pacing for carotid sinus syndrome and sick sinus syndrome. *PACE* 13:2071-2075, 1990
35. Fitzpatrick A, Theodorakis G, Ahmed R, et al: Dual chamber pacing aborts vasovagal syncope induced by head-up 60° tilt. *PACE* 14:13-19, 1991
36. Sutton R: Pacing in patients with carotid sinus and vasovagal syndromes (abstract). *PACE* 12:1260-1263, 1989
37. Jeanrenaud X, Goy JJ, Kappenberger L: Effects of dual-chamber pacing in hypertrophic obstructive cardiomyopathy. *Lancet* 339:1318-1323, 1992
38. Fananapazir L, Cannon RO III, Tripodi D, et al: Impact of dual-chamber permanent pacing in patients with obstructive hypertrophic cardiomyopathy with symptoms refractory to verapamil and β-adrenergic blocker therapy. *Circulation* 85:2149-2161, 1992
39. Hochleitner M, Hörtnagl H, Ng C-K, et al: Usefulness of physiologic dual-chamber pacing in drug-resistant idiopathic dilated cardiomyopathy. *Am J Cardiol* 66:198-202, 1990
40. Kataoka H: Hemodynamic effect of physiological dual chamber pacing in a patient with end-stage dilated cardiomyopathy: a case report. *PACE* 14:1330-1335, 1991
41. Brecker SJ, Xiao HB, Sparrow J, et al: Effects of dual-chamber pacing with short atrioventricular delay in dilated cardiomyopathy. *Lancet* 340:1308-1312, 1992
42. Hochleitner M, Hortnagl H, Hortnagl H, et al: Long-term efficacy of physiologic dual-chamber pacing in the treatment of end-stage idiopathic dilated cardiomyopathy. *Am J Cardiol* 70:1320-1325, 1992
43. Daubert C, Cazeau S, Limousin M, et al: Atrial resynchronization: a new algorithm in DDD pacing (abstract). *Eur J Card Pacing Electrophysiol* 4:41, 1994
44. Gould L, Patel C, Becker W: Long-term threshold stability with porous tip electrodes. *PACE* 9:1202-1205, 1986
45. Djordjevic M, Stojanov P, Velimirovic D, et al: Target lead—low threshold electrode. *PACE* 9:1206-1210, 1986
46. Kruse IM: Long-term performance of endocardial leads with steroid-eluting electrodes. *PACE* 9:1217-1219, 1986
47. Mond H, Stokes K, Helland J, et al: The porous titanium steroid eluting electrode: a double blind study assessing the stimulation threshold effects of steroid. *PACE* 11:214-219, 1988
48. Phillips R, Frey M, Martin RO: Long-term performance of polyurethane pacing leads: mechanisms of design-related failures. *PACE* 9:1166-1172, 1986
49. Hayes DL, Holmes DR Jr, Merideth J, et al: Bipolar tined polyurethane ventricular lead: a four-year experience. *PACE* 8:192-196, 1985
50. Hayes DL, Graham KJ, Irwin M, et al: A multicenter experience with a bipolar tined polyurethane ventricular lead. *PACE* 15:1033-1039, 1992
51. Karpawich PP, Hakimi M, Arciniegas E, et al: Improved chronic epicardial pacing in children: steroid contribution to porous platinized electrodes. *PACE* 15:1151-1157, 1992
52. Calfee RV, Saulson SH: A voluntary standard for 3.2 mm unipolar and bipolar pacemaker leads and connectors. *PACE* 9:1181-1185, 1986
53. Draft International Standards (ISO/DIS 5841-3)
54. McNeill GP, Taylor NC: Use of subclavian vein for permanent cardiac pacing. *Br Heart J* 40:114-116, 1978
55. Littleford PO, Parsonnet V, Spector SD: Method for the rapid and atraumatic insertion of permanent endocardial pacemaker electrodes through the subclavian vein. *Am J Cardiol* 43:980-982, 1979
56. Miller FA Jr, Holmes DR Jr, Gersh BJ, et al: Permanent transvenous pacemaker implantation via the subclavian vein. *Mayo Clin Proc* 55:309-314, 1980
57. Belott PH, Byrd CL: Recent developments in pacemaker implantation and lead retrieval. In *New Perspectives in Cardiac Pacing. 2.* Edited by SS Barold, J Mugica. Mount Kisco, New York, Futura Publishing Company, 1991, pp 105-131
58. Jacobs DM, Fink AS, Miller RP, et al: Anatomical and morphological evaluation of pacemaker lead compression. *PACE* 16:434-444, 1993
59. Magney JE, Flynn DM, Parsons JA, et al: Anatomical mechanisms explaining damage to pacemaker leads, defibrillator leads, and failure of

central venous catheters adjacent to the sternoclavicular joint. *PACE* 16:445-457, 1993

60. Magney JE, Staplin DH, Flynn DM, et al: A new approach to percutaneous subclavian venipuncture to avoid lead fracture or central venous catheter occlusion. *PACE* 16:2133-2142, 1993

61. Higano ST, Hayes DL, Spittell PC: Facilitation of the subclavian-introducer technique with contrast venography. *PACE* 13:681-684, 1990

62. Furman S: Subclavian puncture for pacemaker lead placement (letter from the editor). *PACE* 9:467, 1986

63. Goren CC: Ease of insertion of exposed helical coil tip and tined silicone leads through single cephalic vein. *PACE* 10:949-950, 1987

64. Ong LS, Barold SS, Lederman M, et al: Cephalic vein guide wire technique for implantation of permanent pacemakers. *Am Heart J* 114:753-756, 1987

65. Kemler RL: A simple method for exposing the external jugular vein for placement of a permanent transvenous pacing catheter electrode. *Ann Thorac Surg* 26:266-268, 1978

66. Furman S: Basic concepts. In *A Practice of Cardiac Pacing.* Second edition. Edited by S Furman, DL Hayes, DR Holmes Jr. Mount Kisco, New York, Futura Publishing Company, 1989, pp 23-78

67. Platia EV, Brinker JA: Time course of transvenous pacemaker stimulation impedance, capture threshold, and electrogram amplitude. *PACE* 9:620-625, 1986

68. Beyersdorf F, Schneider M, Kreuzer J, et al: Studies of the tissue reaction induced by transvenous pacemaker electrodes. I. Microscopic examination of the extent of connective tissue around the electrode tip in the human right ventricle. *PACE* 11:1753-1759, 1988

69. Furman S, Hurzeler P, DeCaprio V: Cardiac pacing and pacemakers. III. Sensing the cardiac electrogram. *Am Heart J* 93:794-801, 1977

70. Perrins EJ, Sutton R, Kalebic B, et al: Modern atrial and ventricular leads for permanent cardiac pacing. *Br Heart J* 46:196-201, 1981

71. Furman S, Hurzeler P, DeCaprio V: The ventricular endocardial electrogram and pacemaker sensing. *J Thorac Cardiovasc Surg* 73:258-266, 1977

72. Hayes DL, Vlietstra RE, Trusty JM, et al: A shorter hospital stay after cardiac pacemaker implantation. *Mayo Clin Proc* 63:236-240, 1988

73. Ramsdale DR, Charles RG, Rowlands DB, et al: Antibiotic prophylaxis for pacemaker implantation: a prospective randomized trial. *PACE* 7:844-849, 1984

74. Pless P, Simonsen E, Arnsbo P, et al: Superiority of multiprogrammable to nonprogrammable VVI pacing: a comparative study with special reference to management of pacing system malfunctions. *PACE* 9:739-744, 1986

75. Jung W, Manz M, Lüderitz B: Which programmable pacemaker features are available and what is their clinical relevance? *Herz* 16:158-170, 1991

76. Lee MT, Baker R: Circadian rate variation in rate-adaptive pacing systems. *PACE* 13:1797-1801, 1990

77. Hynes JK, Holmes DR Jr, Merideth J, et al: An evaluation of long-term stimulation thresholds by measurement of chronic strength duration curves. *PACE* 4:376-379, 1981

78. Hill WE, Murray A, Bourke JP, et al: Minimum energy for cardiac pacing. *Clin Phys Physiol Meas* 9:41-46, 1988

79. Furman S, Escher D, Fisher J: Seven year experience with programmable pulse generators (abstract). *PACE* 2:A-60, 1979

80. Feld GK, Love CJ, Camerlo J, et al: A new pacemaker algorithm for continuous capture verification and automatic threshold determination: elimination of pacemaker afterpotential utilizing a triphasic charge balancing system. *PACE* 15:171-178, 1992

81. Rosenqvist M, Vallin HO, Edhag KO: Rate hysteresis pacing: How valuable is it? A comparison of the stimulation rates of 70 and 50 beats per minute and rate hysteresis in patients with sinus node disease. *PACE* 7:332-340, 1984

82. Janosik DL, Pearson AC, Buckingham TA, et al: The hemodynamic benefit of differential atrioventricular delay intervals for sensed and paced atrial events during physiologic pacing. *J Am Coll Cardiol* 14:499-507, 1989

83. Sulke AN, Chambers JB, Sowton E: The effect of atrio-ventricular delay programming in patients with DDDR pacemakers. *Eur Heart J* 13:464-472, 1992

84. Begemann MJS, Boute WIM: Automatic refractory period. *PACE* 11:1684-1686, 1988

85. Mond HG: Unipolar versus bipolar pacing—poles apart. *PACE* 14:1411-1424, 1991

86. McAlister HF, Klementowicz PT, Calderon EM, et al: Atrial electrogram analysis: antegrade versus retrograde. *PACE* 11:1703-1707, 1988

87. Gabry MD, Behrens M, Andrews C, et al: Comparison of myopotential interference in unipolar-bipolar programmable DDD pacemakers. *PACE* 10:1322-1330, 1987

88. Klementowicz PT, Furman S: Stability of atrial sensing and pacing after dual chamber pulse generator implantation. *J Am Coll Cardiol* 6:1338-1341, 1985

89. Jochheim R, Lutzmann A, Bisler H, et al: Comparison of sensing behaviour of unipolar and bipolar electrodes. *Herz Kreislauf* 23:113-118, 1991

90. de Boer H, Kofflard M, Scholtes T, et al: Differential bipolar sensing of a dual chamber pacemaker. *PACE* 11:158-165, 1988

91. Fieldman A, Dobrow RJ: Phantom pacemaker programming. *PACE* 1:166-171, 1978

92. Parsonnet V (Chairman), Furman S, Smyth NPD: Implantable cardiac pacemakers. Status report and resource guideline: pacemaker study group. *Circulation* 50:A-21-A-35, 1974

93. Parsonnet V, Furman S, Smyth NPD: A revised code for pacemaker identification: pacemaker study group. *Circulation* 64:60A-62A, 1981

94. Bernstein AD, Camm AJ, Fletcher RD, et al: The NASPE/BPEG generic pacemaker code for antibradyarrhythmia and adaptive-rate pacing and antitachyarrhythmia devices. *PACE* 10:794-799, 1987

95. Baig MW, Perrins EJ: The hemodynamics of cardiac pacing: clinical and physiological aspects. *Prog Cardiovasc Dis* 33:283-298, 1991

96. Nordlander R, Hedman A, Pehrsson SK: Rate responsive pacing and exercise capacity—a comment. *PACE* 12:749-751, 1989

97. Karlöf I: Haemodynamic effect of atrial triggered versus fixed rate pacing at rest and during exercise in complete heart block. *Acta Med Scand* 197:195-206, 1975

98. Samet P, Castillo C, Bernstein WH, et al: Hemodynamic results of right atrial pacing in cardiac subjects. *Dis Chest* 53:133-137, 1968

99. Benchimol A, Ellis JG, Dimond EG: Hemodynamic consequences of atrial and ventricular pacing in patients with normal and abnormal hearts: effect of exercise at a fixed atrial and ventricular rate. *Am J Med* 39:911-922, 1965

100. Samet P, Castillo C, Bernstein WH: Hemodynamic consequences of sequential atrioventricular pacing: subjects with normal hearts. *Am J Cardiol* 21:207-212, 1968

101. Ogawa S, Dreifus LS, Shenoy PN, et al: Hemodynamic consequences of atrioventricular and ventriculoatrial pacing. *PACE* 1:8-15, 1978

102. Little RC: Effect of atrial systole on ventricular pressure and closure of the A-V valves. *Am J Physiol* 166:289-295, 1951

103. Samet P, Bernstein WH, Nathan DA, et al: Atrial contribution to cardiac output in complete heart block. *Am J Cardiol* 16:1-10, 1965

104. Curtis JJ, Madigan NP, Whiting RB, et al: Clinical experience with permanent atrioventricular sequential pacing. *Ann Thorac Surg* 32:179-185, 1981

105. Furman S: Therapeutic uses of atrial pacing. *Am Heart J* 86:835-840, 1973

106. Miller M, Fox S, Jenkins R, et al: Non-invasive evaluation of cerebral blood flow during ventricular and A-V sequential pacing (abstract). *Am J Cardiol* 47:435, 1981

107. Mukharji J, Rehr RB, Hastillo A, et al: Comparison of atrial contribution to cardiac hemodynamics in patients with normal and severely compromised cardiac function. *Clin Cardiol* 13:639-643, 1990

108. Gillespie WJ, Greene DG, Karatzas NB, et al: Effect of atrial systole on right ventricular stroke output in complete heart block. *Br Med J* 1:75-79, 1967

109. Greenberg B, Chatterjee K, Parmley WW, et al: The influence of left ventricular filling pressure on atrial contribution to cardiac output. *Am Heart J* 98:742-751, 1979

110. Kroetz FW, Leonard JJ, Shaver JA, et al: The effect of atrial contraction on left ventricular performance in valvular aortic stenosis. *Circulation* 35:852-867, 1967

111. Shapland JE, MacCarter D, Tockman B, et al: Physiologic benefits of rate responsiveness. *PACE* 6:329-332, 1983

112. Fananapazir L, Bennett DH, Monks P: Atrial synchronized

ventricular pacing: contribution of the chronotropic response to improved exercise performance. *PACE* 6:601-608, 1983

113. Barbieri D, Percoco GF, Toselli T, et al: AV delay and exercise stress tests: behavior in normal subjects. *PACE* 13:1724-1727, 1990

114. Daubert C, Ritter P, Mabo P, et al: Rate modulation of the AV delay in DDD pacing. In *Progress in Clinical Pacing.* Edited by M Santini, M Pistolese, A Alliegro. New York, Elsevier Science Publishing Company, 1990, pp 415-430

115. Haskell RJ, French WJ: Optimum AV interval in dual chamber pacemakers. *PACE* 9:670-675, 1986

116. Luceri RM, Brownstein SL, Vardeman L, et al: PR interval behavior during exercise: implications for physiological pacemakers. *PACE* 13:1719-1723, 1990

117. Rees M, Haennel RG, Black WR, et al: Effect of rate-adapting atrioventricular delay on stroke volume and cardiac output during atrial synchronous pacing. *Can J Cardiol* 6:445-452, 1990

118. Ritter P, Daubert C, Mabo P, et al: Haemodynamic benefit of a rate-adapted A-V delay in dual chamber pacing. *Eur Heart J* 10:636-646, 1989

119. Schuilenburg RM: Patterns of V-A conduction in the human heart in the presence of normal and abnormal A-V conduction. In *The Conduction System of the Heart: Structure, Function and Clinical Implications.* Edited by HJJ Wellens, KI Lie, MJ Janse. Philadelphia, Lea & Febiger, 1976, pp 485-503

120. Akhtar M: Retrograde conduction in man. *PACE* 4:548-562, 1981

121. Hayes DL, Furman S: Atrio-ventricular and ventriculo-atrial conduction times in patients undergoing pacemaker implant. *PACE* 6:38-46, 1983

122. Van Mechelen R, Hagemeijer F, de Boer H, et al: Atrioventricular and ventriculo-atrial conduction in patients with symptomatic sinus node dysfunction. *PACE* 6:13-21, 1983

123. Hartzler GO, Maloney JD, Curtis JJ, et al: Hemodynamic benefits of atrioventricular sequential pacing after cardiac surgery. *Am J Cardiol* 40:232-236, 1977

124. Clemo HF, Baumgarten CM, Stambler BS, et al: Atrial natriuretic factor: implications for cardiac pacing and electrophysiology. *PACE* 17:70-91, 1994

125. Stangl K, Weil J, Seitz K, et al: Influence of AV synchrony on the plasma levels of atrial natriuretic peptide (ANP) in patients with total AV block. *PACE* 11:1176-1181, 1988

126. Lévy S, Corbelli J-L, Labrunie P, et al: Retrograde (ventriculoatrial) conduction. *PACE* 6:364-371, 1983

127. Langenfeld H, Grimm W, Maisch B, et al: Atrial fibrillation and embolic complications in paced patients. *PACE* 11:1667-1672, 1988

128. Ebagosti A, Gueunoun M, Saadjian A, et al: Long-term follow-up of patients treated with VVI pacing and sequential pacing with special reference to VA retrograde conduction. *PACE* 11:1929-1934, 1988

129. Patel AK, Yap VU, Thomsen JH: Adverse effects of right ventricular pacing in a patient with aortic stenosis: hemodynamic documentation management. *Chest* 72:103-105, 1977

130. Witte J, Bondke H, Müller S: The pacemaker syndrome: a haemodynamic complication of ventricular pacing. *Cor Vasa* 30:393-399, 1988

131. Schüller H, Brandt J: The pacemaker syndrome: old and new causes. *Clin Cardiol* 14:336-340, 1991

132. Travill CM, Sutton R: Pacemaker syndrome: an iatrogenic condition. *Br Heart J* 68:163-166, 1992

133. Ellenbogen KA, Stambler BS: Pacemaker syndrome. In *Clinical Cardiac Pacing.* Edited by KA Ellenbogen, GN Kay, BL Wilkoff. Philadelphia, WB Saunders Company, 1995, pp 419-431

134. El Gamal MIH, Van Gelder LM: Chronic ventricular pacing with ventriculo-atrial conduction versus atrial pacing in three patients with symptomatic sinus bradycardia. *PACE* 4:100-105, 1981

135. Nishimura RA, Gersh BJ, Holmes DR Jr, et al: Outcome of dual-chamber pacing for the pacemaker syndrome. *Mayo Clin Proc* 58:452-456, 1983

136. Ausbubel K, Furman S: The pacemaker syndrome. *Ann Intern Med* 103:420-429, 1985

137. Heldman D, Mulvihill D, Nguyen H, et al: True incidence of pacemaker syndrome. *PACE* 13:1742-1750, 1990

138. Bianconi L, Boccadamo R, Di Florio A, et al: Atrial versus ventricular stimulation in sick sinus syndrome: effects on morbidity and mortality (abstract). *PACE* 12:1236, 1989

139. Feuer JM, Shandling AH, Messenger JC: Influence of cardiac pacing mode on the long-term development of atrial fibrillation. *Am J Cardiol* 64:1376-1379, 1989

140. Grimm W, Langenfeld H, Maisch B, et al: Symptoms, cardiovascular risk profile and spontaneous ECG in paced patients: a five-year follow-up study. *PACE* 13:2086-2090, 1990

141. Hayes DL, Espinosa RE, Neubauer SA, et al: Association of atrial fibrillation, pacing mode, and survival following pacemaker implantation (abstract). *PACE* 16:919, 1993

142. Hesselson AB, Parsonnet V, Bernstein AD, et al: Deleterious effects of long-term single-chamber ventricular pacing in patients with sick sinus syndrome: the hidden benefits of dual-chamber pacing. *J Am Coll Cardiol* 19:1542-1549, 1992

143. Kosakai Y, Ohe T, Kamakura S, et al: Long term follow-up of incidence of embolism in sick sinus syndrome after pacing (abstract). *PACE* 14:680, 1991

144. Markewitz A, Schad N, Hemmer W, et al: What is the most appropriate stimulation mode in patients with sinus node dysfunction? *PACE* 9:1115-1120, 1986

145. Nürnberg M, Frohner K, Podczeck A, et al: Is VVI pacing more dangerous than AV-sequential pacing in patients with sick sinus node syndrome? (Abstract.) *PACE* 14:674, 1991

146. Pieper S, Shen W, Hammill S, et al: Survival advantage of DDD pacing (abstract). *Eur J Card Pacing Electrophysiol* 4:35, 1994

147. Santini M, Alexidou G, Ansalone G, et al: Relation of prognosis in sick sinus syndrome to age, conduction defects and modes of permanent cardiac pacing. *Am J Cardiol* 65:729-735, 1990

148. Santomauro M, Pappone C, Damiano M, et al: Effects of different pacing modes on patients survival (abstract). *Eur J Card Pacing Electrophysiol* 4:34, 1994

149. Sasaki Y, Furihata A, Suyama K, et al: Comparison between ventricular inhibited pacing and physiologic pacing in sick sinus syndrome. *Am J Cardiol* 67:771-774, 1991

150. Sethi KK, Bajaj V, Mohan JC, et al: Comparison of atrial and VVI pacing modes in symptomatic sinus node dysfunction without associated tachyarrhythmias. *Indian Heart J* 42:143-147, 1990

151. Stangl K, Seitz K, Wirtzfeld A, et al: Differences between atrial single chamber pacing (AAI) and ventricular single chamber pacing (VVI) with respect to prognosis and antiarrhythmic effect in patients with sick sinus syndrome. *PACE* 13:2080-2085, 1990

152. Sutton R, Kenny RA: The natural history of sick sinus syndrome. *PACE* 9:1110-1114, 1986

153. van Erckelens F, Sigmund M, Lambertz H, et al: Atrial fibrillation in rate responsive-, DDD- and VVI-pacing: incidence, time of onset, influencing factors (abstract). *PACE* 13:1194, 1990

154. Witte J, v. Knorre GH, Volkmann H-J, et al: Survival rate in sick-sinus-syndrome patients: AAI/DDD versus VVI-pacing (abstract). *PACE* 16:1149, 1993

155. Zanini R, Facchinetti A, Gallo G, et al: Morbidity and mortality of patients with sinus node disease: comparative effects of atrial and ventricular pacing. *PACE* 13:2076-2079, 1990

156. Barold SS, Santini M: Natural history of sick sinus syndrome after pacemaker implantation. In *New Perspectives in Cardiac Pacing. 3.* Edited by SS Barold, J Mugica. Mount Kisco, New York, Futura Publishing Company, 1993, pp 169-211

157. Lamas GA, Pashos C, Normand S-L, et al: Natural history of sick sinus syndrome (SSS) following pacemaker implantation (abstract). *Eur J Card Pacing Electrophysiol* 4:34, 1994

158. Lamas GA, Estes NM III, Schneller S, et al: Does dual chamber or atrial pacing prevent atrial fibrillation? The need for a randomized controlled trial. *PACE* 15:1109-1113, 1992

159. Lamas GA: Personal communication

160. Andersen HR, Thuesen L, Bagger JP, et al: Prospective randomised trial of atrial versus ventricular pacing in sick-sinus syndrome. *Lancet* 344:1523-1528, 1994

161. Kerr CA, Connolly S: Pacemaker mode selection. *ACC Current Journal Rev* 2:29-32, 1993

162. Kerr CA: Personal communication

163. Camm AJ: Personal communication

164. Chamberlain DA, Leinbach RC, Vassaux CE, et al: Sequential atrioventricular pacing in heart block complicating acute myocardial infarction. *N Engl J Med* 282:577-582, 1970

165. DeSanctis RW: Diagnostic and therapeutic uses of atrial pacing. *Circulation* 43:748-761, 1971

166. Narula OS: Atrioventricular conduction defects in patients with sinus bradycardia: analysis by His bundle recordings. *Circulation* 44:1096-1110, 1971

167. Hayes DL, Furman S: Stability of AV conduction in sick sinus node syndrome patients with implanted atrial pacemakers. *Am Heart J* 107:644-647, 1984

168. Hayes DL, Holmes DR Jr: Atrial pacing: A viable pacing mode for the 1980s? *Clin Prog Pacing Electrophysiol* 2 No 4:339-348, 1984

169. Barold SS, Falkoff MD, Ong LS, et al: Characterization of pacemaker arrhythmias due to normally functioning AV demand (DVI) pulse generators. *PACE* 3:712-723, 1980

170. Luceri RM, Ramirez AV, Castellanos A, et al: Ventricular tachycardia produced by a normally functioning AV sequential demand (DVI) pacemaker with "committed" ventricular stimulation. *J Am Coll Cardiol* 1:1177-1179, 1983

171. Calfee RV: Dual-chamber committed mode pacing. *PACE* 6:387-391, 1983

172. Irwin M, Harris L, Cameron D, et al: DDI pacing: indications, expectations, and follow-up. *PACE* 17:274-279, 1994

173. Antonioli GE, Ansani L, Barbieri D, et al: Single-lead VDD pacing. In *New Perspectives in Cardiac Pacing. 3.* Edited by SS Barold, J Mugica. Mount Kisco, New York, Futura Publishing Company, 1993, pp 359-381

174. Antonioli GE, Ansani L, Barbieri D, et al: Italian multicenter study on a single lead VDD pacing system using a narrow atrial dipole spacing. *PACE* 15:1890-1893, 1992

175. Funke HD, Neumann G, Herpers L, et al: Performance of physiological pacing by DDD stimulation—two years of experience (abstract). *PACE* 3:371, 1980

176. Furman S, Fisher JD: Endless loop tachycardia in an AV universal (DDD) pacemaker. *PACE* 5:486-489, 1982

177. Messenger JC, Greenberg PS, Warren J, et al: Atrial synchronous ventricular inhibited pacing (VDD): an underutilized mode of pacing. *PACE* 6:392-398, 1983

178. Klementowicz P, Ausubel K, Furman S: The dynamic nature of ventriculoatrial conduction. *PACE* 9:1050-1054, 1986

179. Nitzsché R, Gueunoun M, Lamaison D, et al: Endless-loop tachycardias: description and first clinical results of a new fully automatic protection algorithm. *PACE* 13:1711-1718, 1990

180. Timmis GC, Westveer DC, Bakalyar DM, et al: Discrimination of anterograde from retrograde atrial electrograms for physiologic pacing. *PACE* 11:130-140, 1988

181. Hayes DL: Endless-loop tachycardia: The problem has been solved? In *New Perspectives in Cardiac Pacing.* Edited by SS Barold, J Mugica. Mount Kisco, New York, Futura Publishing Company, 1988, pp 375-386

182. Benditt DG, Mianulli M, Fetter J, et al: An office-based exercise protocol for predicting chronotropic response of activity-triggered, rate-variable pacemakers. *Am J Cardiol* 64:27-32, 1989

183. Wilkoff BL, Corey J, Blackburn G, et al: Techniques in the definition of chronotropic incompetence (abstract). *PACE* 13:501, 1990

184. Rossi P: Rate-responsive pacing: biosensor reliability and physiological sensitivity. *PACE* 10:454-466, 1987

185. Bacharach DW, Hilden TS, Millerhagen JO, et al: Activity-based pacing: comparison of a device using an accelerometer versus a piezoelectric crystal. *PACE* 15:188-196, 1992

186. Lau C-P, Tai Y-T, Fong P-C, et al: Clinical experience with an activity sensing DDDR pacemaker using an accelerometer sensor. *PACE* 15:334-343, 1992

187. Perrins EJ, Astridge PS: Clinical trials and experience. In *Clinical Cardiac Pacing.* Edited by KA Ellenbogen, GN Kay, BL Wilkoff. Philadelphia, WB Saunders Company, 1995, pp 399-418

188. Alt E, Millerhagen JO, Heemels J-P. Accelerometers. In *Clinical Cardiac Pacing.* Edited by KA Ellenbogen, GN Kay, BL Wilkoff. Philadelphia, WB Saunders Company, 1995, pp 267-276

189. Benditt DG, Duncan JL: Activity-sensing, rate-adaptive pacemakers. In *Clinical Cardiac Pacing.* Edited by KA Ellenbogen, GN Kay, BL Wilkoff. Philadelphia, WB Saunders Company, 1995, pp 167-186

190. Hayes DL, Christiansen JR, Vliestra RE, et al: Follow-up of an activity-sensing, rate-modulated pacing device, including transtelephonic exercise assessment. *Mayo Clin Proc* 64:503-508, 1989

191. McElroy PA, Janicki JS, Weber KT. Physiologic correlates of the heart rate response to upright isotonic exercise: relevance to rate-responsive pacemakers. *J Am Coll Cardiol* 11:94-99, 1988

192. Vai F, Bonnet JL, Ritter PH, et al: Relationship between heart rate and minute ventilation, tidal volume and respiratory rate during brief and low level exercise. *PACE* 11:1860-1865, 1988

193. Mond H, Strathmore N, Kertes P, et al: Rate responsive pacing using a minute ventilation sensor. *PACE* 11:1866-1874, 1988

194. Nappholtz T, Valenta H, Maloney J, et al: Electrode configurations for a respiratory impedance measurement suitable for rate responsive pacing. *PACE* 9:960-964, 1986

195. Li H, Neubauer SA, Hayes DL: Long-term performance of a rate-adaptive pacemaker using a minute volume sensor (abstract). *Eur J Card Pacing Electrophysiol* 2 No 2:49, 1992

196. Vanerio G, Patel S, Ching E, et al: Early clinical experience with a minute ventilation sensor DDDR pacemaker. *PACE* 14:1815-1820, 1991

197. Jolgren D, Fearnot N, Geddes L: A rate-responsive pacemaker controlled by right ventricular blood temperature. *PACE* 7:794-801, 1984

198. Alt E, Hirgstetter C, Heinz M, et al: Measurement of right ventricular blood temperature during exercise as a means of rate control in physiological pacemakers. *PACE* 9:970-977, 1986

199. Sellers TD, Fearnot N, Kelvin 500 Investigator Group: A multicenter experience with a temperature based rate modulating pacemaker (Kelvin 500) (abstract). *PACE* 11:486, 1988

200. Salo R, O'Donoghue S, Platia EV: The use of intracardiac impedance-based indicators to optimize pacing rate. In *Clinical Cardiac Pacing.* Edited by KA Ellenbogen, GN Kay, BL Wilkoff. Philadelphia, WB Saunders Company, 1995, pp 234-249

201. Chirife R: Physiological principles of a new method for rate responsive pacing using the pre-ejection interval. *PACE* 11:1545-1554, 1988

202. Bennett TD, Olson WH, Bornzin GA, et al: Rate-responsive pacing: alternative modes for physiological cardiac pacing. Proceedings of AAMI 20th Annual Meeting, Boston, MA, 1985, p 12

203. Yee R, Bennett TD: Rate-adaptive pacing controlled by dynamic right ventricular pressure (dP/dtmax). In *Clinical Cardiac Pacing.* Edited by KA Ellenbogen, GN Kay, BL Wilkoff. Philadelphia, WB Saunders Company, 1995, pp 212-218

204. Kay GN, Bornzin GA: Rate-modulated pacing controlled by mixed venous oxygen saturation. In *Clinical Cardiac Pacing.* Edited by KA Ellenbogen, GN Kay, BL Wilkoff. Philadelphia, WB Saunders Company, 1995, pp 187-200

205. Singer I, Callaghan FJ: Evoked potentials as a sensor for rate-adaptive pacing. In *Clinical Cardiac Pacing.* Edited by KA Ellenbogen, GN Kay, BL Wilkoff. Philadelphia, WB Saunders Company, 1995, pp 258-266

206. Callaghan F, Vollmann W, Livingston A, et al: The ventricular depolarization gradient: effects of exercise, pacing rate, epinephrine, and intrinsic heart rate control on the right ventricular evoked response. *PACE* 12:1115-1130, 1990

207. Lau CP: Ventricular depolarization gradient and output pulse parameters. In *Rate Adaptive Cardiac Pacing: Single and Dual Chamber.* Edited by CP Lau. New York, Futura Publishing Company, 1993, pp 137-146

208. Donaldson RM, Rickards AF: The ventricular endocardial paced evoked response. *PACE* 6:253-259, 1983

209. Connelly DT, Rickards AF: The evoked QT interval. In *Clinical Cardiac Pacing.* Edited by KA Ellenbogen, GN Kay, BL Wilkoff. Philadelphia, WB Saunders Company, 1995, pp 250-257

210. Cammilli L, Alcidi L, Papeschi G, et al: Preliminary experience with the pH-triggered pacemaker. *PACE* 1:448-457, 1978

211. Soberman J, McAlister H, Klementowicz P, et al: Paradoxical responses in activity-sensing pacemakers (abstract). *PACE* 11:507, 1988

212. Lau CP: The combination of sensors and algorithms. In *Rate Adaptive Cardiac Pacing: Single and Dual Chamber.* Edited by CP Lau. New York, Futura Publishing Company, 1993, pp 213-227

213. Taborsky M, Neuzil P, Vopalka R: Follow-up of patients with dual sensor pacemakers place more demand on time and technology? (Abstract.) *PACE* 16:1205, 1993

214. Cohen TJ, Liem LB: A combined oxygen-pressure sensing algorithm improves tachyarrhythmia detection (abstract). *PACE* 16:857, 1993

215. Linde-Edelstam C, Hjemdahl P, Pehrsson SK, et al: Is DDD pacing superior to VVI,R? A study on cardiac sympathetic nerve activity and myocardial oxygen consumption at rest and during exercise. *PACE* 15:425-434, 1992
216. Oldroyd KG, Rae AP, Carter R, et al: Double blind crossover comparison of the effects of dual chamber pacing (DDD) and ventricular rate adaptive (VVIR) pacing on neuroendocrine variables, exercise performance, and symptoms in complete heart block. *Br Heart J* 65:188-193, 1991
217. Love CJ, Hayes DL: Evaluation of pacemaker malfunction. In *Clinical Cardiac Pacing.* Edited by KA Ellenbogen, GN Kay, BL Wilkoff. Philadelphia, WB Saunders Company, 1995, pp 656-683
218. Parsonnet V, Bernstein AD, Lindsay B: Pacemaker-implantation complication rates: an analysis of some contributing factors. *J Am Coll Cardiol* 13:917-921, 1989
219. Hayes DL: Pacemaker complications. In *A Practice of Cardiac Pacing.* Second edition. Edited by S Furman, DL Hayes, DR Holmes Jr. Mount Kisco, New York, Futura Publishing Company, 1989, pp 485-507
220. Alt E, Völker R, Blömer H: Lead fracture in pacemaker patients. *Thorac Cardiovasc Surg* 35:101-104, 1987
221. Fyke FE III: Simultaneous insulation deterioration associated with side-by-side subclavian placement of two polyurethane leads. *PACE* 11:1571-1574, 1988
222. Hayes DL: Pacemaker electrocardiography. In *A Practice of Cardiac Pacing.* Second edition. Edited by S Furman, DL Hayes, DR Holmes Jr. Mount Kisco, New York, Futura Publishing Company, 1989, pp 289-321
223. Bianconi L, Boccadamo R, Toscano S, et al: Effects of oral propafenone therapy on chronic myocardial pacing threshold. *PACE* 15:148-154, 1992
224. Hayes DL: Effects of drugs and devices on permanent pacemakers. *CARDIO* 1:70-75, 1991
225. Driller J, Barold SS, Parsonnet V: Normal and abnormal function of the pacemaker magnetic reed switch. *J Electrocardiol* 9:283-292, 1976
226. Nordlander R, Pehrsson SK: Incidence and management of pacemaker-related complications during dual-chamber pacing. *Acta Med Scand* 218:293-298, 1985
227. Castellanos A Jr, Agha AS, Befeller B, et al: A study of arrival of excitation at selected ventricular sites during human bundle branch block using close bipolar catheter electrodes. *Chest* 63:208-213, 1973
228. Vera Z, Mason DT, Swan NA, et al: Lack of sensing by demand pacemakers due to intraventricular conduction defects. *Circulation* 51:815-822, 1975
229. Barold SS, Gaidula JJ: Evaluation of normal and abnormal sensing functions of demand pacemakers. *Am J Cardiol* 28:201-210, 1971
230. Cheng TO, Chaithiraphan S, Baltazar A, et al: Supression by a prominent T-wave: an unusual case of malfunction of a transvenous demand pacemaker. *Chest* 60:502-504, 1971
231. Massumi RA, Mason DT, Amsterdam EA, et al: Apparent malfunction of demand pacemaker caused by nonpropagated (concealed) ventricular extrasystoles. *Chest* 61:426-431, 1972
232. Irnich W: Muscle noise and interference behavior in pacemakers: a comparative study. *PACE* 10:125-132, 1987
233. Ohm O-J, Bruland H, Pedersen OM, et al: Interference effect of myopotentials on function of unipolar demand pacemakers. *Br Heart J* 36:77-84, 1974
234. Barold SS, Ong LS, Falkoff MD, et al: Inhibition of bipolar demand pacemaker by diaphragmatic myopotentials. *Circulation* 56:679-683, 1977
235. Berger R, Jacobs W: Myopotential inhibition of demand pacemakers: etiologic, diagnostic, and therapeutic considerations. *PACE* 2:596-602, 1979
236. Anderson ST, Davis BB: Interference with function of unipolar pacemaker due to muscle potentials. *J Thorac Cardiovasc Surg* 71:698-703, 1976
237. Irnich W, de Bakker JMT, Bisping H-J: Electromagnetic interference in implantable pacemakers. *PACE* 1:52-61, 1978
238. Levine PA, Balady GJ, Lazar HL, et al: Electrocautery and pacemakers: management of the paced patient subject to electrocautery. *Ann Thorac Surg* 41:313-317, 1986
239. Chen D, Philip M, Philip PA, et al: Cardiac pacemaker inhibition by transcutaneous electrical nerve stimulation. *Arch Phys Med Rehabil* 71:27-30, 1990. (Published erratum appears in *Arch Phys Med Rehabil* 71:388, 1990.)
240. Rasmussen MJ, Hayes DL, Vlietstra RE, et al: Can transcutaneous electrical nerve stimulation be safely used in patients with permanent cardiac pacemakers? *Mayo Clin Proc* 63:443-445, 1988
241. Hayes DL, Holmes DR Jr, Gray JE: Effect of 1.5 tesla nuclear magnetic resonance imaging scanner on implanted permanent pacemakers. *J Am Coll Cardiol* 10:782-786, 1987
242. Fetter J, Patterson D, Aram G, et al: Effects of extracorporeal shock wave lithotripsy on single chamber rate response and dual chamber pacemakers. *PACE* 12:1494-1501, 1989
243. Cooper D, Wilkoff B, Masterson M, et al: Effects of extracorporeal shock wave lithotripsy on cardiac pacemakers and its safety in patients with implanted cardiac pacemakers. *PACE* 11:1607-1616, 1988
244. Waxman MB, Berman ND, Sanz G, et al: Demand pacemaker malfunction due to abnormal sensing: report of two cases. *Circulation* 50:389-394, 1974
245. Pickers BA, Goldberg MJ: Inhibition of a demand pacemaker and interference with monitoring equipment by radio-frequency transmissions. *Br Med J* 2:504-506, 1969
246. Furman S: Cardiac pacing and pacemakers VI. Analysis of pacemaker malfunction. *Am Heart J* 94:378-386, 1977
247. Gould L, Patel S, Gomes GI, et al: Pacemaker failure following external defibrillation. *PACE* 4:575-577, 1981
248. Mickley H, Andersen C, Nielsen LH: Runaway pacemaker: a still existing complication and therapeutic guidelines. *Clin Cardiol* 12:412-414, 1989
249. Rodriguez F, Filimonov A, Henning A, et al: Radiation-induced effects in multiprogrammable pacemakers and implantable defibrillators. *PACE* 14:2143-2153, 1991
250. Bilgutay AM, Jensen NK, Schmidt WR, et al: Incarceration of transvenous pacemaker electrode: removal by traction. *Am Heart J* 77:377-379, 1969
251. Imparato AM, Kim GE: The trapped endocardial electrode: removal by prolonged graded skin traction. *Ann Thorac Surg* 14:605-608, 1972
252. Furman S, Behrens M, Andrews C, et al: Retained pacemaker leads. *J Thorac Cardiovasc Surg* 94:770-772, 1987
253. Lagergren H, Dahlgren S, Nordenstam H: Cardiovascular tissue response to intracardiac pacemaking. *Acta Chir Scand* 132:696-704, 1966
254. Huang T-Y, Baba N: Cardiac pathology of transvenous pacemakers. *Am Heart J* 83:469-474, 1972
255. Robboy SJ, Harthorne JW, Leinbach RC, et al: Autopsy findings with permanent pervenous pacemakers. *Circulation* 39:495-501, 1969
256. Gibson TC, Davidson RC, DeSilvey DL: Presumptive tricuspid valve malfunction induced by a pacemaker lead: a case report and review of the literature. *PACE* 3:88-95, 1980
257. Lee ME, Chaux A: Unusual complications of endocardial pacing. *J Thorac Cardiovasc Surg* 80:934-940, 1980
258. Nicolosi GL, Charmet PA, Zanuttini D: Large right atrial thrombosis: rare complication during permanent transvenous endocardial pacing. *Br Heart J* 43:199-201, 1980
259. Seeger W, Scherer K: Asymptomatic pulmonary embolism following pacemaker implantation. *PACE* 9:196-199, 1986
260. Krug H, Zerbe F: Major venous thrombosis: a complication of transvenous pacemaker electrodes. *Br Heart J* 44:158-161, 1980
261. Stoney WS, Addlestone RB, Alford WC Jr, et al: The incidence of venous thrombosis following long-term transvenous pacing. *Ann Thorac Surg* 22:166-170, 1976
262. Spittell PC, Hayes DL: Venous complications after insertion of a transvenous pacemaker. *Mayo Clin Proc* 67:258-265, 1992
263. Spittell PC, Vlietstra RE, Hayes DL, et al: Venous obstruction due to permanent transvenous pacemaker electrodes: treatment with percutaneous transluminal balloon venoplasty. *PACE* 13:271-274, 1990
264. Goldman BS, MacGregor DC: Management of infected pacemaker systems. *Clin Prog Pacing Electrophysiol* 2:220-235, 1984
265. Lewis AB, Hayes DL, Holmes DR Jr, et al: Update on infections involving permanent pacemakers. Characterization and management. *J Thorac Cardiovasc Surg* 89:758-763, 1985
266. Choo MH, Holmes DR Jr, Gersh BJ, et al: Permanent pacemaker infections: characterization and management. *Am J Cardiol* 48:559-564, 1981
267. Wohl B, Peters RW, Carliner N, et al: Late unheralded

pacemaker pocket infection due to *Staphylococcus epidermidis:* a new clinical entity. *PACE* 5:190-195, 1982

268. Schwartz IS, Pervez N: Bacterial endocarditis associated with a permanent transvenous cardiac pacemaker. *JAMA* 218:736-737, 1971

269. Bryan CS, Sutton JP, Saunders DE Jr, et al: Endocarditis related to transvenous pacemakers: syndromes and surgical implications. *J Thorac Cardiovasc Surg* 75:758-762, 1978

270. Lemire GG, Morin JE, Dobell ARC: Pacemaker infections: a 12-year review. *Can J Surg* 18:181-184, 1975

271. Hartstein AI, Jackson J, Gilbert DN: Prophylactic antibiotics and the insertion of permanent transvenous cardiac pacemakers. *J Thorac Cardiovasc Surg* 75:219-223, 1978

272. Harjula A, Järvinen A, Virtanen KS, et al: Pacemaker infections—treatment with total or partial pacemaker system removal. *Thorac Cardiovasc Surg* 33:218-220, 1985

273. Choo MH, Holmes DR Jr, Gersh BJ, et al: Infected epicardial pacemaker systems: partial versus total removal. *J Thorac Cardiovasc Surg* 82:794-796, 1981

274. Townsend ER, Parker DJ, Siddons AHM, et al: The management of surgical complications of permanent transvenous pacing (abstract). *PACE* 2:A-34, 1979

275. Peters MS, Schroeter AL, van Hale HM, et al: Pacemaker contact sensitivity. *Contact Dermatitis* 11:214-218, 1984

276. Byrd CL, Schwartz SJ, Gonzales M, et al: Pacemaker clinic evaluations: key to early identification of surgical problems. *PACE* 9:1259-1264, 1986

277. Dreifus LS, Zinberg A, Hurzeler P, et al: Transtelephonic monitoring of 25,919 implanted pacemakers. *PACE* 9:371-378, 1986

278. Luceri RM, Hayes DL: Follow-up of DDD pacemakers. *PACE* 7:1187-1194, 1984

CHAPTER

25

Pacing

B. Antitachycardia devices

Michael J. Osborn, M.D.

PACEMAKER THERAPY FOR TACHYARRHYTHMIAS

There are basically three ways in which pacing may be used to treat tachycardia: to prevent the initiation of tachyarrhythmia, to terminate it once it has been initiated, and, rarely, to alter the rate of the tachycardia, or the associated hemodynamic status, without actually terminating it.

Table 25B-1 Prevention of tachycardia

Elimination of bradycardia
Elimination of VA conduction
Suppression of ectopy
Creation of homogeneous depolarization
AV synchronous pacing

Prevention of tachycardia

Some tachycardias can be prevented by improving a patient's hemodynamic status, preventing ventriculoatrial (VA) conduction, maintaining basic atrial or ventricular rate support, using overdrive suppression of ectopy, increasing heart rate to create a homogeneous process of myocardial repolarization, or maintaining artificial atrioventricular (AV) synchrony with a short AV interval by simultaneous or sequential AV stimulation[1-5] (Table 25B-1).

Elimination of bradycardia. In some patients with sinus node dysfunction associated with paroxysms of tachycardia in addition to profound bradycardia, the occurrence of tachycardia can be suppressed or prevented simply by increasing the heart rate by pacing.[1] The same can be said for complete heart block because the ventricular arrhythmias that commonly occur can be suppressed by ventricular pacing at physiologic rates.[6-8]

Pacing therapy aimed at the prevention of tachycardia is probably most useful against rhythms caused by enhanced automaticity.[9,10] Because bradyarrhythmias allow a greater opportunity for an ectopic pacemaker focus to discharge, shortening diastole by increasing the pacing rate provides less opportunity for ectopic activity to arise.[6,11] Other mechanisms by which the prevention of bradycardia may be useful in preventing tachycardia include reduced diastolic ventricular volume, decreased Purkinje fiber stretch, and increased cardiac output, with increased coronary artery flow reducing the likelihood of myocardial ischemia.[5,12] In addition, however, rate control may be a factor in prevention of some reentrant arrhythmias. These tachycardias may be prevented by shortening the time interval during which the reentrant circuit is able to respond to an initiating stimulus, eliminating long cycle lengths that predispose to reciprocating conduction by premature beats, and suppressing the ectopic premature depolarizations that may initiate tachycardias.[3,5,13-17]

In two studies involving 21 patients with a variety of supraventricular and ventricular arrhythmias, prevention of bradycardia by pacing (AAI, DDD, or VVI) was associated with a significant decrease in the frequency of both supraventricular and ventricular tachyarrhythmias.[18,19]

Elimination of VA conduction. In the patient with intact VA conduction, ventricular pacing has the potential for initiating tachycardia.[20] Various supraventricular arrhythmias, including atrial fibrillation, atrial flutter, AV nodal reentry, and AV reentry by accessory pathways, have been described as a result of ventricular pacing.[13,21-23] The artificial maintenance of AV synchrony prevents VA conduction and eliminates the potential for tachycardia.

Overdrive suppression of ectopy. This pacing technique has been successful in the management of supraventricular tachycardias but is most frequently used for control of ventricular ectopy and ventricular tachyarrhythmias.[15] Some of the other clinical settings in which

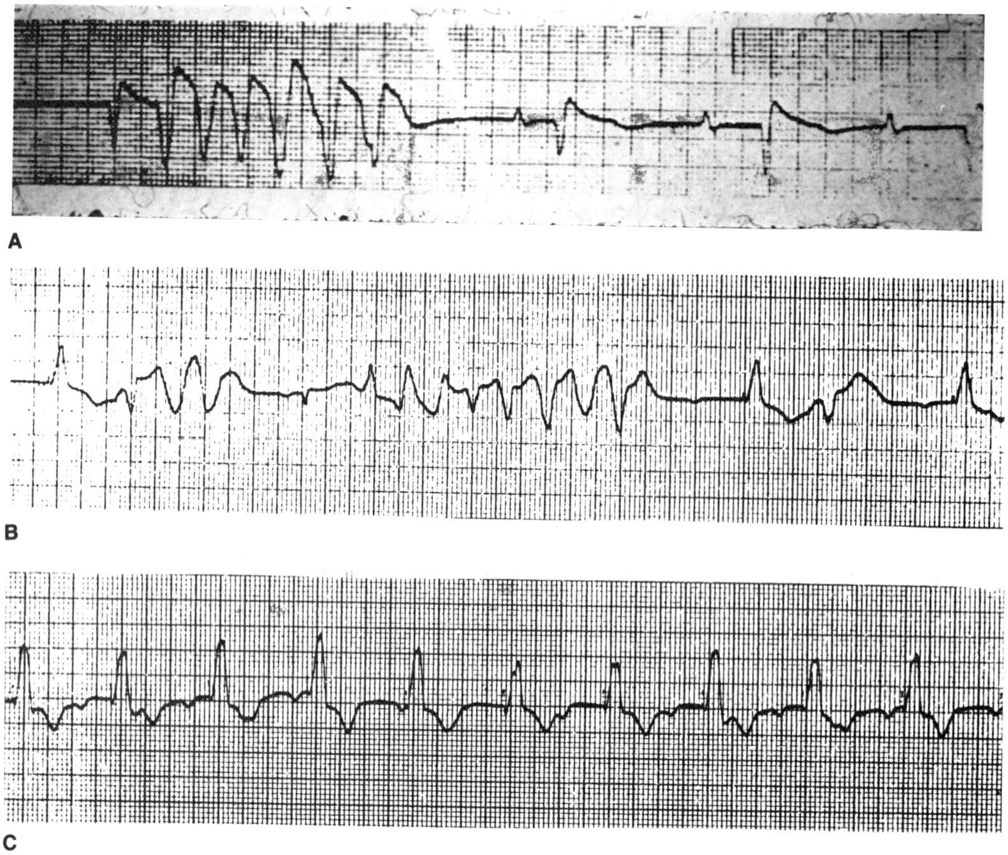

Fig 25B-1 Overdrive suppression. Episodic heart block with a slow ventricular escape focus associated with nonsustained ventricular tachycardia. Ventricular pacing led to suppression of ectopy. **A,** heart block with nonsustained rapid ventricular tachycardia. **B,** ventricular pacing at 60 beats/min did not control the tachycardia episodes. **C,** ventricular pacing at 75 beats/min resulted in complete elimination of both bradycardia and tachycardia.

overdrive pacing (especially on a temporary basis)[1] has been effective in controlling ventricular arrhythmia include acute myocardial infarction,[24] the period after cardiac surgery,[25] and situations of transient electrical instability secondary to metabolic disturbances[26] or digitalis toxicity.[16,27] In some patients, permanent overdrive pacing can be used to prevent refractory paroxysmal supraventricular tachycardia or paroxysmal ventricular tachycardia by suppression of atrial or ventricular extra beats.[15,28] It must be remembered that overdrive pacing is not always successful in preventing tachycardias because there is not always a direct relationship between the presence of premature beats and the development of tachycardia. A permanent pacemaker should be implanted only if temporary pacing proves effective.[6,28-30]

If overdrive pacing is used to control arrhythmia, two important factors must be taken into consideration: the rate at which the heart is paced, and the pacing site. The pacing rates that have proved to be successful in a number of studies are quite variable (range, 75 to 140 beats/min), and there is no clear consensus concerning ideal rates.[16,30-36] Quite clearly, the rate must be determined for each patient individually. The simplest approach is to increase the pacing rate until the arrhythmia is eliminated, allow the patient to stabilize, and then slowly reduce the rate to the lowest level that prevents recurrence[37] (Fig 25B-1). Care must be taken in patients with ischemic heart disease because increasing the heart rate may increase myocardial oxygen demand and ischemia and may worsen the arrhythmia.[38]

Suppression of arrhythmias depends not only on reaching a critical heart rate but sometimes also on the pattern of cardiac activation after the paced impulse. Therefore, in some situations atrial (or AV sequential) pacing may be far more effective than ventricular pacing, and in other situations the opposite may be true.[6,12,13,39] Once again, the site of pacing must be determined for each patient by comparisons of the effectiveness of pacing therapy in different atrial and ventricular locations.

Creation of homogeneous myocardial repolarization. A commonly occurring ECG abnormality associated with recurrent ventricular tachycardia is prolongation of the Q-T interval. This abnormality is produced by an increase in the amount of time that is required for ventricular repolarization and could possibly indicate a temporal dispersion of the repolarization of ventricular myocardial fibers. Any therapy that decreases this degree of temporal dispersion may be beneficial, and because there is an inverse relationship between the heart rate and the speed of ventricular repolarization (and, therefore, the Q-T interval), this decrease can be accomplished by increasing the heart rate.[5,31,37]

A number of clinical studies have documented the utility of overdrive pacing in the control and prevention of recurrent ventricular tachycardia or fibrillation in association with prolonged Q-T interval from various causes (usually secondary to the use of drugs, specifically antiarrhythmic or antidepressant agents).[7,31-33,37] When the underlying problem is drug toxicity, overdrive pacing can be carried out for short periods until the effects of the offending agent have disappeared. However, permanent overdrive pacing can be used for patients in whom the repolarization abnormality is chronic—for example, patients with congenital or idiopathic Q-T interval prolongation.[13,28,31] Once again, the pacing rate and location must be individualized.

AV synchronous pacing

A very specialized pacing approach to prevent refractory paroxysmal supraventricular tachycardias, due either to AV nodal reentry or to AV reentry utilizing accessory pathways, is the use of dual-chamber pacing devices that are either atrial or atrial and ventricular synchronous. The initiation of a reentrant arrhythmia requires that the tissue in the reentrant circuit be excitable to allow propagation of a premature impulse. If the reentrant pathway ahead of a premature stimulus is made refractory, the reentry loop cannot be completed, and tachycardia will not be initiated or sustained. By synchronization of ventricular depolarization to atrial activation, a premature complex previously able to initiate reentry is now followed by ventricular activation that retrogradely invades the opposite end of the reentry circuit and thus prevents the arrhythmia[4,39] (Fig 25B-2).

Coumel[40] demonstrated that incessant paroxysmal supraventricular tachycardia could be prevented by simultaneous (rather than sequential) stimulation of both the atrium and ventricle in two patients with intractable tachycardia. It was postulated that both AV nodal pathways were invaded simultaneously by the atrial and ventricular stimuli, consequently preventing reentry as long as stimulation was continued (Fig 25B-3). This technique was used successfully in six of seven patients with AV nodal or AV reentry tachycardia. It was shown that simultaneous pacing resulted in a marked alteration in AV nodal refractoriness that prevented the achievement of any necessary critical delays through the AV node.[31,41]

A further extension of this pacing technique was the development of a dual-chamber system capable of sensing either atrial or ventricular signals and, in turn, triggering simultaneous AV stimulation (DDT pacing).[42] This has been used successfully in patients with refractory supraventricular tachycardia secondary to AV nodal reentry. All atrial and ventricular premature stimuli elicited simultaneous AV stimulation with resultant impulse

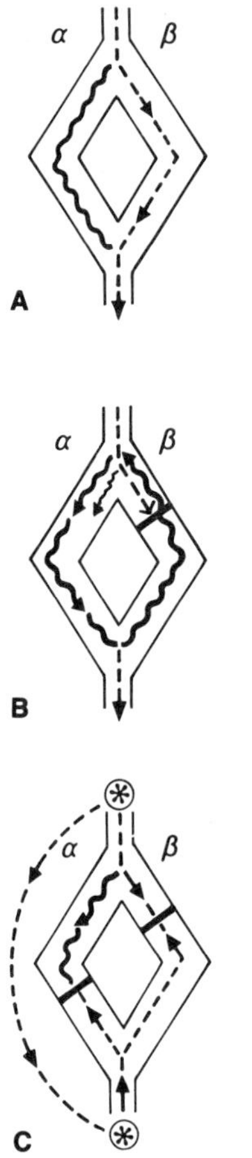

Fig 25B-2 **A,** reentrant circuit. More rapid conduction in the β pathway allows preferential antegrade conduction. Slower conduction in the α pathway finds the distal common pathway refractory to antegrade conduction. **B,** a premature beat may cause block in one pathway (β) while allowing conduction via the other pathway (α). Because of slowed conduction (α), the impulse may find the β pathway totally excitable and hence result in a reentrant arrhythmia. **C,** an atrial synchronous ventricular paced beat might enter the pathway, causing refractoriness in the α pathway at the same time as the β pathway is rendered refractory by the antegrade atrial impulse, thereby preventing reentry.

collision in the AV junction, consequently abolishing the initiation of the tachycardia (Fig 25B-4).

Although these devices have been successful in isolated cases, there are some clear limitations to their use. If very premature, the atrial premature beat that initiates the tachycardia may fall within the refractory period of the pacemaker and therefore not be sensed. The reentrant circuit associated with AV nodal reentry is anatomically small; therefore, the paced ventricular stimulus may not be able to penetrate the circuit (especially with rapid tachycardia rates). There may be distinct differences in the antegrade and retrograde conduction properties of the tachycardia circuit, limiting the ability of the system to prevent tachycardia and possibly even resulting in initiation of tachycardia.[6,28,42]

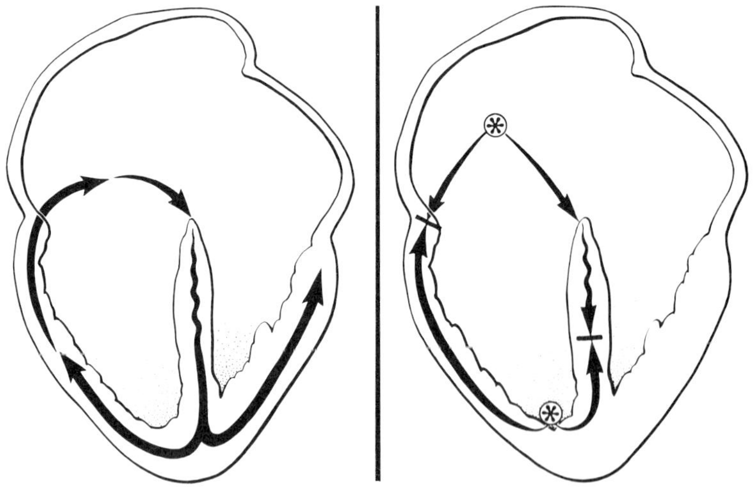

Fig 25B-3 **Left,** reentrant circuit of an incessant AV reentry tachycardia utilizing a right-sided accessory pathway. **Right,** DOO pacing with simultaneous atrial and ventricular depolarization, causing refractoriness/block in all parts of the reentrant circuit.

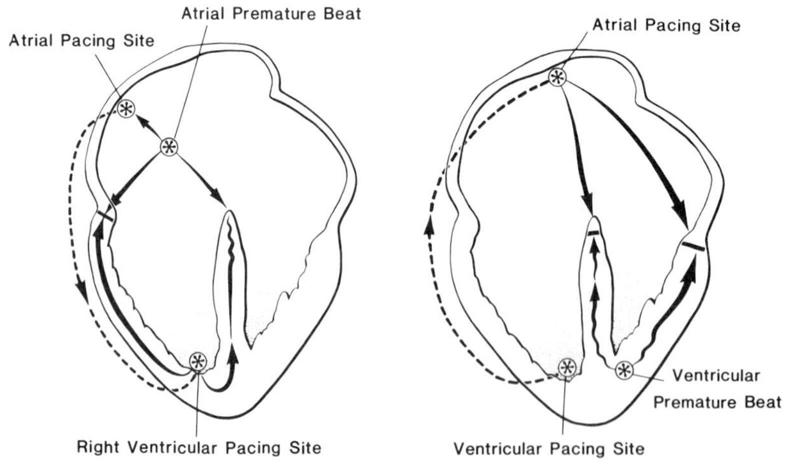

Fig 25B-4 **Left,** DDT pacing. Atrial premature beats sensed by the atrial catheter will result in ventricular pacing, causing refractoriness and block in a conduction pathway. **Right,** DDT pacing. Ventricular premature beats sensed by the ventricular pacing catheter will result in atrial pacing, causing refractoriness/block in the conduction pathways.

Alteration of tachycardia rate or associated hemodynamic status

Pacing techniques that attempt to improve the hemodynamic status during an episode of tachycardia without actually terminating the arrhythmia have been used very infrequently and almost exclusively on a temporary basis (Table 25B-2).

Paired or coupled pacing. The concept of paired pacing was developed to increase cardiac output in patients with decreased ventricular function by potentiating the effects of myocardial contractility.[43] It was noted that the effective heart rate could be slowed considerably by this technique. During spontaneous tachycardia (coupled pacing), or at a paced rate slightly faster than the tachycardia (paired pacing), premature beats are introduced that are so closely coupled to the preceding beat that they have no hemodynamic effects but do render the heart refractory to the next beat of the arrhythmia.[44] The

Table 25B-2 Tachycardia modification
Paired or coupled pacing
Ventricular synchronous atrial pacing
Rapid atrial pacing

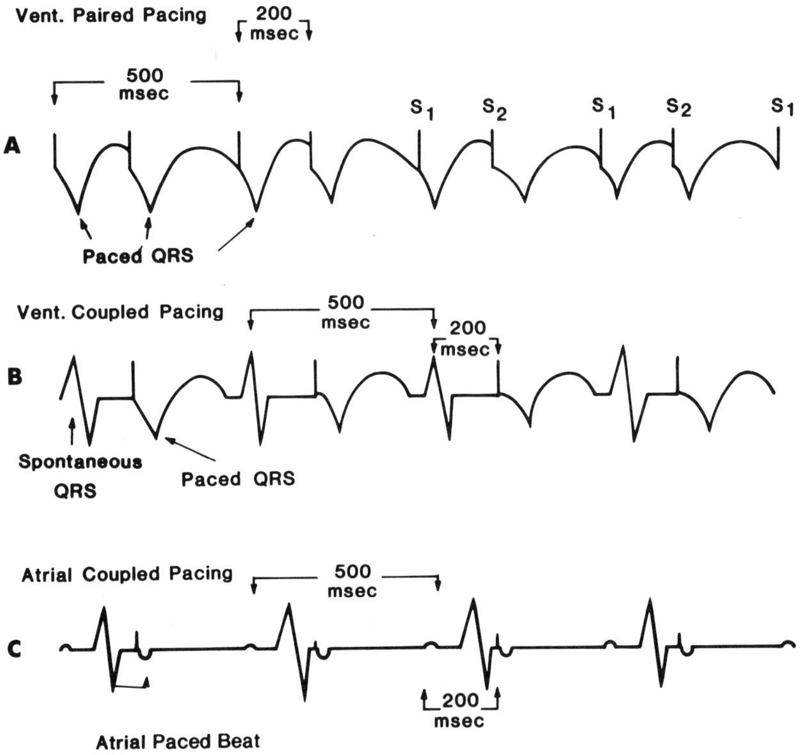

Fig 25B-5 **A,** during ventricular paired pacing, all ventricular beats are paced. The S_1-S_2 interval (200 msec) is shorter than the S_2-S_1 interval (300 msec). The S_1-S_2 interval is short enough to allow an electrical event without a significant ventricular contraction. **B,** during ventricular coupled pacing, a paced ventricular event follows each spontaneous QRS. **C,** during atrial coupled pacing, the atrium is stimulated *after* the atrial refractory period to allow atrial capture but *during* the AV node refractory period to ensure AV node block.

paired, or coupled, stimulus is timed to produce an electrical but not a mechanical response, and therefore the mechanical pulse rate may be halved while the electrical pulse rate remains the same, leading to hemodynamic improvement[30] (Fig 25B-5).

Both atrial[44] and ventricular[45] paired stimulation have been used to control the heart rate in patients with intractable, very rapid atrial tachycardias (associated with hemodynamic embarrassment). This also may be an effective therapeutic option in some patients with intractable tachycardia and resultant ventricular dysfunction, because heart rate reduction can improve cardiac function.[46,47]

Ventricular synchronous atrial pacing. A pacing technique that results in the restoration of AV synchrony during ventricular tachycardia may improve hemodynamics during that arrhythmia. In this pacing mode (AVT—ventricular synchronous atrial pacing), the atrium is paced at selected intervals after ventricular sensing. Although this is exclusively a temporary pacing technique, it may help to stabilize patients while all diagnostic and therapeutic approaches are being evaluated[30] (Fig 25B-6). It has also been used successfully to manage patients with hemodynamically significant tachycardias immediately after cardiopulmonary bypass surgery.[48]

Rapid atrial pacing. Finally, rapid atrial pacing can be used to slow the ventricular rate during supraventricular tachycardia by causing increased degrees of AV nodal block. This technique was introduced in 1968 by Wiener and Dwyer,[49] who used it in a patient with intractable supraventricular tachycardia. Rapid atrial pacing led to the induction of atrial fibrillation with a significant reduction of ventricular rate and improvement in hemodynamics. Since that time, several other reports have confirmed the utility of rapid atrial pacing to cause atrial fibrillation or atrial tachycardia with 2:1 (or higher degrees) AV block in patients with intractable and hemodynamically compromising atrial tachycardias.[50,51] This technique appears to have its greatest benefit as a temporary measure, although a permanently implanted radiofrequency unit has been successfully used chronically in at least one patient.[52]

Termination of tachyarrhythmias

Mechanisms of tachycardia termination. In general, tachyarrhythmias are divided into those based on abnormal automaticity and those resulting from an impulse circulating in an anatomically or functionally defined pathway (reentrant or reciprocating rhythms).[53]

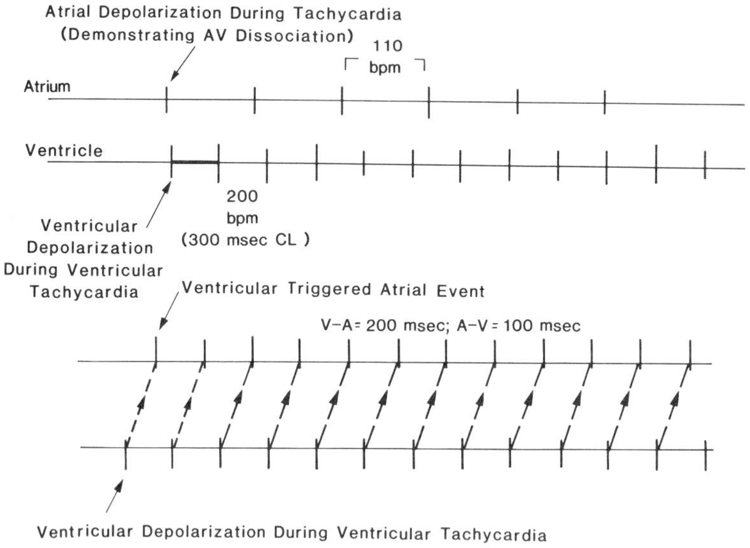

Fig 25B-6 **Upper,** AV dissociation during ventricular tachycardia eliminates the potential benefits of atrial contraction. **Lower,** artificial maintenance of AV synchrony (1:1 AV conduction with a 100-msec AV interval) by ventricular triggered atrial pacing may improve cardiac output during ventricular tachycardia. *CL,* cycle length.

The initiation and, more importantly, the termination of tachyarrhythmias by premature stimuli given within well-defined timing intervals or by rapid overdrive pacing suggests that they are reentrant in type.[54-56] By the same token, the inability to demonstrate termination by either premature electrical stimulation or overdrive pacing has been accepted as suggestive of abnormal automatic behavior.[8,39,57] Another potential electrophysiologic mechanism of arrhythmogenesis has been described as "triggered focal activity" (or triggered automaticity) and also may be terminated by pacing techniques.[58]

These definitions may be artificial, but they are useful for several reasons.[59] The mere fact that the classification of arrhythmias as reentrant requires that they be terminated by programmed stimulation or pacing makes them potentially amenable to pacing therapy. The use of the reentry model allows for a firmer understanding of the means by which pacing devices are effective and improves our ability to select a pacing device to fit the patient's needs. Therefore, electrophysiologic testing can be used to identify potential pacing candidates and to determine the optimal pacing systems for them.

The arrhythmias that are considered to be reentrant include atrial flutter, AV nodal reentry, sinoatrial node reentry, AV reentry utilizing accessory conduction pathways as one of the reentrant limbs, intra-atrial reentry, and ventricular tachycardia.[57,60-64] Consequently, for the majority of rhythm disturbances seen clinically, various pacing techniques may be attractive therapeutic options.

In a reentrant tachycardia, the circulation of the impulse will stop when refractory tissue is encountered in the reentrant pathway.[7] An appropriately timed atrial or ventricular paced beat may enter the reentry pathway and render the circuit refractory to further reciprocation, thus terminating the tachycardia.[29,65-67] This could be accomplished by random premature stimulation[68] or by rapid overdrive pacing.[69,70]

The factors that are important in determining the ability of a pacing stimulus to enter the tachycardia circuit include the location of the conduction pathways of the reentrant circuit; the distance between the site or sites of stimulation and the reentry circuit; the electrophysiologic properties of the tissues between the site or sites of stimulation and the tachycardia circuit; the size of the tachycardia circuit; and the rate of the tachycardia.[27-29,38,57,71,72]

In general, the effectiveness of programmed stimulation in termination of paroxysmal tachycardia is inversely related to the rate of the arrhythmias.[14,15] During episodes of tachycardia at rapid rates, the site and size of the reentry circuit and the distance between the circuit and the stimulation site become increasingly important factors in the determination of the ability of a given mode of pacing (underdrive, overdrive, scanning, etc.) to terminate an arrhythmia.[39] A single stimulus given close to a large, well-defined pathway with a slow rate of reciprocation will easily enter the circuit and terminate the arrhythmia. However, a single stimulus given far away from a small circuit with a rapid tachycardia rate may not terminate the arrhythmia as easily.[57]

With rapid tachycardias, multiple premature stimuli or trains of rapid pacing stimuli may be required to terminate the arrhythmias.[15,39,73,74] The site of stimulation will also affect the ability of any type of stimulation protocol (single stimuli, multiple stimuli, or rapid pacing) to terminate an arrhythmia. If stimulation can be performed near the tachycardia circuit, the chances of success increase and the numbers of stimuli required commonly decrease.

Patient selection. The basic therapeutic approaches in the management of recurrent tachyarrhythmias include administration of antiarrhythmia drugs, surgical interruption or removal of reentrant circuits, catheter ablation of conduction pathways, and implantable devices for tachycardia termination (pacemakers and defibrillators).

Although in most situations drug therapy remains the treatment of choice,[42] antiarrhythmia drugs do not always safely and reliably terminate arrhythmias. Also, in many cases, drug selection involves a prolonged hospital stay in a monitored area and repeat invasive electrophysiologic studies. Even after a drug has been carefully chosen in this fashion, the chances of long-term success are by no means absolute. Additionally, there is a potential for the development of significant cardiac or noncardiac toxicity.[75] Patients should be considered for pacing when commercially available and investigational drugs are ineffective or when the use of such drugs is contraindicated because of toxicity, allergy, or poor patient compliance.[13] In young women, freedom from the use of potentially teratogenic antiarrhythmia agents may also be very important.

In some patients, especially those with Wolff-Parkinson-White syndrome (or concealed retrogradely conducting accessory pathways), conditions exist that make them ideal candidates for catheter ablation or surgery.[76] Patients being considered for pacing therapy should not be ablation or surgical candidates or they should have refused this option.[30,77]

The magnitude of the patient's problems related to the episodes of tachycardia should have a strong bearing on patient selection. Pacing may represent an effective and safe therapeutic modality in patients with a long history of paroxysmal tachycardia, especially if the episodes are frequent, of long duration, characterized by rapid tachycardia rates, associated with significant symptoms (e.g., syncope, angina, dyspnea, lightheadedness), and cannot be self-terminated (e.g., by vagal maneuvers) and therefore require emergency room visits or hospitalization for termination.[30,77] In patients with frequent episodes, the ability to terminate them promptly must be weighed against the potential for rapid battery depletion and the need for frequent efforts to terminate tachycardia with patient-activated devices. As a result, patients being considered for pacing therapy should have relatively infrequent (fewer than one per week) episodes of tachycardia[72] (Table 25B-3).

In addition to the obvious symptoms that may be associated with these episodes, more insidious problems can arise as a result of paroxysmal tachycardias. Daily activities may be restricted by the patient for fear of inducing the tachycardia. There may be significant psychologic repercussions, including an unwanted change in lifestyle and dependence on the availability of medical assistance. In these situations, a strong search for alternatives to routine medical therapy is clearly warranted.[78] A group that is frequently overlooked are those patients with episodic tachycardias who also have conduction system disease requiring the use of a permanent pacemaker for control of bradycardia. If a device were available that could maintain basic rate support and function to terminate an episode of tachycardia, this use would be an ideal therapeutic option.[79] The use of automatic internal cardioverter-defibrillators for treatment of ventricular fibrillation and tachycardia is becoming more widespread. Concomitant use of antitachycardia pacemakers would aid in the management of patients with more stable forms of ventricular tachycardia, allowing burst or scanning arrhythmia termination while providing backup defibrillation in the event of tachycardia acceleration or degeneration to ventricular fibrillation.[80,81]

Table 25B-3 Situations in which pacing therapy should be considered

Tachycardias unsuitable for surgical therapy
Tachycardias refractory to pharmacologic therapy
Tachycardias associated with significant symptoms
Tachycardias requiring hospitalization for termination
Tachycardias of long duration
Tachycardias associated with alterations of lifestyle or significant psychologic repercussions
Concomitant conduction system disease requiring pacing for control of bradycardia
Concomitant use of an implantable defibrillator

Table 25B-4 Patient evaluation

Evaluation of spontaneous arrhythmias
Evaluation of the range of the intrinsic heart rate
Electrophysiologic evaluation
Confirm tachycardia mechanism
Determine most effective pacing mode
Consistent termination
Absence of arrhythmia acceleration
Repeat testing of pacing mode
Different days, different postures, different autonomic tone
With exercise
With concomitant drug therapy
Postimplantation evaluation of the pacing system

Patient evaluation. Selection of a safe and reliable method of pacing depends on an accurate diagnosis of the arrhythmia, a clear understanding of the electrophysiologic properties of the arrhythmia, and a careful evaluation of pacing techniques.[54,62]

The basic approach to patient evaluation should include the following: careful determination of the need for treatment by a permanent pacing device; evaluation of the spontaneous characteristics of the arrhythmia and any accompanying conduction or rhythm abnormalities; comparison of the sinus rate response to exercise with spontaneous tachycardia rates; assessment of the potential benefits of AV synchrony; and detailed electrophysiologic evaluation[78,82-84] (Table 25B-4).

Careful electrophysiologic evaluation of each patient is the most important element in patient management. The results are used to determine the most successful type of pacing, defined as the one that terminates the greatest percentage of tachycardia episodes with the least number of complications.[83] During evaluation, the tachycardia must be initiated to determine its mechanism, rate, and hemodynamic consequences and to confirm the inherent stability of the arrhythmia. The antegrade and retrograde properties of all AV connections (both the normal connections and any existing accessory pathways) should be determined. Each potential method of termination of the arrhythmia should be tested from many different pacing sites to determine its effectiveness, the stability of the *atrium or ventricle* with maximal stimulation protocols, and the presence or absence of complicating arrhythmias. The ability of the patient or the implanted pacemaker to sense the tachycardia appropriately should be assessed, as should the potential for post-termination bradycardia. Antiarrhythmia drugs should be given and their effect on the tachycardia evaluated.[72,78,83,85-87]

Termination by the most effective pacing method should then be carried out multiple times to assess the efficacy and safety of the technique. The absence of pacemaker-induced tachycardia acceleration, induction of other arrhythmias (particularly atrial or ventricular fibrillation), and rapid AV conduction via a functioning extranodal conduction pathway are prerequisites for the selection of any pacing method.[74,77,88]

The initial study commonly identifies patients who definitely are *not* pacing candidates. In a study of patients with ventricular tachycardia, 26% of all induced episodes of ventricular tachycardia and 39% of the patients required immediate countershock because of hemodynamic instability.[83,89] In electrophysiologic studies evaluating supraventricular tachycardia, from 6% to 37% of patients had problems with pacing-induced atrial fibrillation or ventricular tachycardia, precluding the use of certain pacing techniques.[72,90]

It is very important to remember that the stimulation protocol required to terminate an arrhythmia may vary at different times. This may be related to many factors, including the concomitant use of drugs that will affect the electrophysiologic properties of the tachycardia circuit and surrounding tissue,[74] spontaneous day-to-day variability in the excitable gaps, associated exercise, changes in position, and changes in autonomic tone during spontaneous episodes of tachycardia.[69,78,90-92] During the evaluation the patient should be taking the drugs that are likely to be prescribed for use after dismissal from the hospital.[6,9,82] Also, the reliability of tachycardia termination by any pacing mode should be tested while the patient is supine, in the semiupright position (by tilt table), or exercising to assess the effects of changing autonomic tone and posture.[69,85,87,91,93]

Ten patients with supraventricular tachycardia were managed by an automatic antitachycardia pacing device with the capacity for Holter monitoring and telemetry and the ability to allow noninvasive electrophysiologic testing. Only four of these patients had tachycardias that could be initiated in the supine, sitting, and standing positions. Changing position varied the rate of tachycardia as well as the timing of initiation of termination sequences.[94] Thus, failure of a pacing system to terminate an arrhythmia may be the result of incomplete electrophysiologic evaluation.

It has been recommended that before pacemaker implantation, at least 100 consecutive episodes of tachycardia (with a temporary catheter in the pacing site to be used) should be successfully terminated in various positions and during exercise without pacing-induced acceleration or degeneration of the arrhythmia.[38,93,95-97] Ideally, this should be accomplished with a pulse generator similar to the one to be implanted.[88] Only after these stringent criteria have been met should a pacemaker be implanted. In a study involving 16 patients with supraventricular tachycardia or ventricular tachycardia who had a minimum of only 50 tachycardia conversions with a success rate of only 85% before implantation of the device, 50% of the devices failed to terminate the tachycardia during long-term follow-up.[93]

Clearly, if these stringent criteria are required, a significant number of patients will not qualify for antitachycardia pacing. For example, 37 patients with supraventricular tachycardia or ventricular tachycardia were identified by careful electrophysiologic evaluation as potential candidates for pacing. After a more prolonged evaluation, only 52% of the patients with supraventricular tachycardia and 25% of the patients with ventricular tachycardia met the criteria for pacemaker insertion.[93] It has also been suggested that the ability of the implanted system to terminate tachycardia should be evaluated during the immediate postimplantation period to ensure that the stimulation protocol programmed into the system will continue to be effective.[85,92,98,99] Unfortunately, even extensive, successful in-hospital evaluations do not always predict uniform success with long-term use of these devices.[81] Hence, careful postdismissal follow-up and periodic testing of the device are necessary.

An evaluation of this magnitude is quite time-consuming and potentially very expensive; hence, it may not be feasible in most patients. The use of adaptive pacing modes (which adapt the pacing therapy to changing physiologic conditions and tachycardia rates by automatically adjusting the pacing cycle) shortens the time required for testing and the tailoring of therapy and allows many more patients to be candidates for pacing therapy. In addition, the increased use of devices with defibrillator backup expands the number of potential pacing candidates.[100]

Because of the exhaustive preimplantation and postimplantation evaluations required and because of the potential need for periodic checking of pacemaker detection and therapy algorithms, pacing systems have the capability for noninvasive electrophysiologic testing.[84,101] This can be accomplished in various ways, including magnet application, chest wall stimulation, or programmed stimulation through the pulse generator itself.[91,102,103] The implantation of such a device may obviate maintenance of a temporary electrode for long-term study, placement of a temporary electrode for subsequent study, and, in some cases, hospitalization during follow-up studies.[102] These devices could also be used to carry out serial drug testing in patients with ventricular tachycardia and again eliminate the need for insertion of a temporary catheter.[92,104]

Table 25B-5 Advantages and disadvantages of automatic antitachycardia pacing devices

Advantages:
Rapid response to tachycardia
Rapid pacing termination after arrhythmia conversion
Patient interaction not required
Programmable functions
Disadvantages:
Accurate intracardiac sensing required
Tachycardia criteria not uniformly accurate
May initiate serious arrhythmia (without medical personnel available)

Automatic and patient-activated pacing devices

Regardless of the pacing modality used, the implanted pacing systems must be able to respond to the tachycardia when it occurs spontaneously. A pulse generator may possess a sensing circuit that is capable of detecting increases in heart rate above a predetermined (programmable) rate and then initiating a pacing response.[87,105,106] The device may require patient activation either by the application of a magnet (creating asynchronous pacing)[76,95] or, in the case of radiofrequency-type devices, by the transmission of impulses from an external source to an implanted receiver.[10]

Automatic pacing devices (Table 25B-5). These units offer automatic tachycardia recognition and response without delay and without requiring any patient interaction.[82] This means that the device will respond even in the presence of profound symptoms (e.g., syncope),[9] or if the tachycardia is not detected by the patient, it will respond before hemodynamic deterioration occurs.[30] In the case of underdrive pacing devices, the absence of delay in pacemaker response to tachycardia ensures use of this system at a time when the chances for tachycardia termination are the greatest and increases the likelihood that tachycardia episodes will be short, thereby reducing the possibility of associated symptoms.[69,84,93] Immediate inhibition of pacemaker antitachycardia function after conversion decreases the potential for reinitiation of arrhythmia by competitive pacing during sinus rhythm.[69]

Until recently, tachycardia rate and duration have been the only diagnostic measures for detection of tachycardia. With these criteria only, a pacemaker cannot differentiate among sinus tachycardia, rapidly conducting atrial fibrillation, paroxysmal supraventricular tachycardia, and ventricular tachycardia.[92] In addition, if the tachycardia criteria are limited, the generator may respond inappropriately to sinus tachycardia brought about by such stimuli as exercise.[87] This response was reported in up to 36% of patients with devices implanted for treatment of supraventricular tachycardia in which rate was the only criterion for tachycardia detection.[107] Therefore, patients are subject to therapy for the wrong rhythm.

Other sensing algorithms have been developed and are available in current antitachycardia devices. These are high rate, sudden onset, rate stability, sustained high rate, and combinations of them. "High rate" defines the rate cutoff for identification of any tachycardia. It is identical to the detection criterion used in earlier pacing devices. The sudden-onset criterion is fulfilled if the comparison of the first high-rate interval with the preceding three intervals satisfies a programmable value (20 to 100 msec) indicating an abrupt change in rate (Fig 25B-7). Rate stability involves the determination of the P-P (or R-R) interval changes on a beat-to-beat basis. The number of intervals required and the allowable variability are also programmable functions (Fig 25B-8). The sustained-high-rate function allows detection of a tachycardia that has satisfied the high-rate criterion but has not fulfilled the sudden-onset or rate-stability criterion. This is accomplished by allowing an extended number of intervals to expire (up to 250), after which the arrhythmia is identified as pathologic and a device response is triggered.[108,109]

The sudden-onset criterion should differentiate sinus tachycardia from pathologic arrhythmias.[60,98,110,111] Rate stability may differentiate atrial fibrillation from other arrhythmias.[107] Sustained high rate could be useful in the management of patients with frequent episodes of nonsustained arrhythmias.

As with any therapeutic modality, there are disadvantages and limitations. Because these systems automatically respond to tachycardias, the ability to sense intra-atrial or ventricular electrograms accurately during an episode is crucial. Oversensing and undersensing can occur in automatic antitachycardia devices just as they can in any pacing system. Undersensing most commonly occurs in the atrium as a result of small-amplitude P waves (sinus or atrial premature complexes). If undersensing occurs, a generator does not respond appropriately to a spontaneously occurring arrhythmia or the tachycardia may be induced by competitive atrial or ventricular beating during sinus rhythm.[88,112,113] Oversensing has been reported secondary to electrical mechanical interference and myopotentials. This has led to inappropriate pacing during sinus rhythm and initiation of tachvcardia[91,113] (see Table 25B-5).

If an automatic device is being used for treatment of ventricular tachycardia, the risk of initiation of ventricular fibrillation by competitive ventricular beating is always a possibility. This could occur during a normal pacemaker response to ventricular tachycardia or during a response to rapid ventricular rate developed as a result of supraventricular tachyarrhythmia.[61,88]

Patient-activated pacing devices. There are two types of patient-activated devices: one with an implanted power source and one with a source supplied by an external electromagnetically coupled unit.[99,103] The most common types of patient-activated systems are the so-called radiofrequency units. These consist of a small implanted receiver and an external (usually handheld) portable transmitter which sends out signals that are transformed into 2-msec pulses by the receiver. The pulsing frequency is adjustable from approximately 50 to 400 pulses/min. To provide stimulation, the antenna of the transmitter is

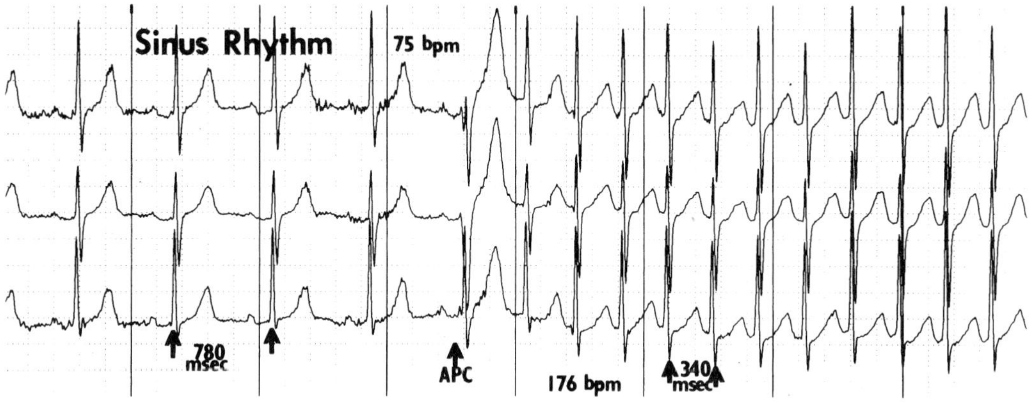

Fig 25B-7 Sudden onset: spontaneous episode of supraventricular tachycardia initiated by an aberrantly conducted atrial premature contraction *(APC)*. The resting heart rate is 75 beats/min (780 msec), and the tachycardia rate is 176 beats/min (340 msec). The abrupt change in heart rate easily satisfies a sudden-onset criterion of 100 msec.

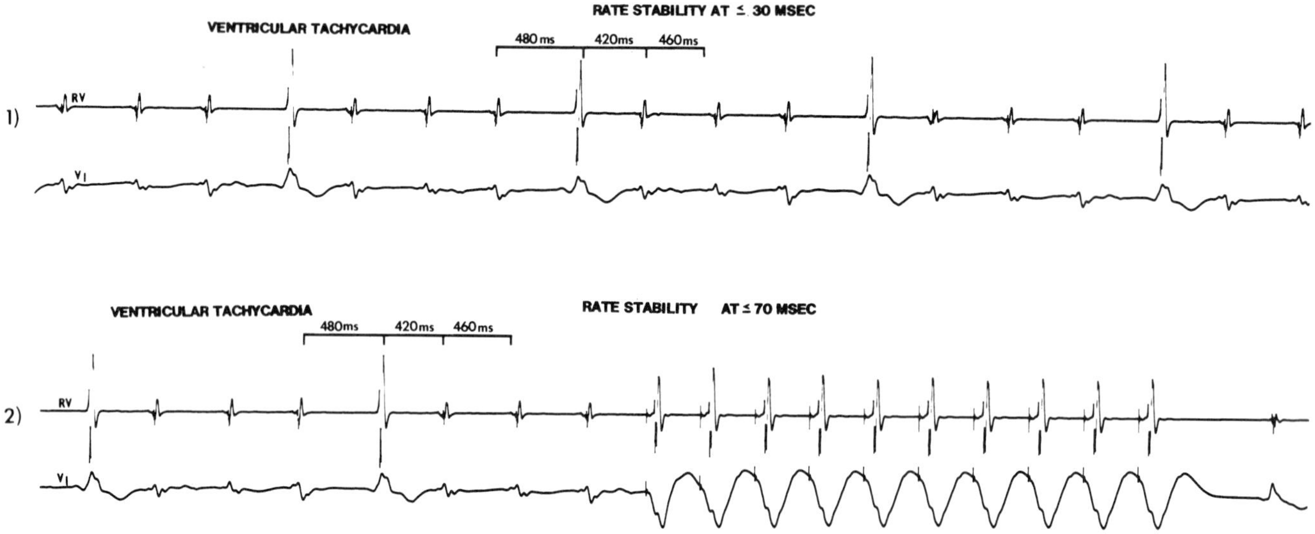

Fig 25B-8 Rate stability: spontaneous episode of ventricular tachycardia with significant variability in cycle length. (1) With rate stability ≤ 30 msec, the arrhythmia is not detected. (2) Adjusting the rate stability to ≤ 70 msec allows tachycardia detection and antitachycardia pacing. (From Osborn MJ: Antitachycardia pacing. In *Interventional Cardiology*. Edited by DR Holmes Jr, RE Vlietstra. Philadelphia, FA Davis Company, 1989, pp 266-296. By permission, Mayo Foundation.)

placed over the receiver and the "on/off" button is depressed. As long as the button is depressed, stimulus signals are transmitted to the receiver.[10,78] To utilize the pacing system properly, the patient must be able to recognize that a rhythm disturbance is occurring, to initiate stimulation, to maintain stimulation for a preset period, and to recognize the successful termination of the arrhythmia.[70]

The major advantage to this system is the external power source (Table 25B-6). This has significantly reduced the size of the implantable generator and has made frequent surgical procedures for battery change unnecessary.[9] This system does not require internal sensing and therefore the characteristics of intracardiac electrograms (in sinus rhythm or tachycardia) are not important for overdrive or underdrive systems.[68] However, because many scanning devices require triggering from intracardiac electrograms in these systems, adequate sensing will still be necessary.

The use of pacing devices to terminate arrhythmias is always associated with the risk of conversion of stable to unstable arrhythmias. Patients who use radiofrequency units can go to a hospital emergency room before activating the device, thereby ensuring that resuscitation

Table 25B-6 Advantages and disadvantages of patient-activated antitachycardia pacing devices

Advantages:
External power source
Intracardiac sensing not required in most systems
Tachycardia can be terminated in the presence of medical personnel
Disadvantages:
Patient initiation required
No bradycardia protection
High-energy output
External device must be constantly available

equipment will be available should a life-threatening arrhythmia be initiated.[30,114]

There are several potential disadvantages to the use of patient-activated devices. The patient must be able to perceive the presence of tachycardia correctly; the system will not be effective if the patient is rapidly disabled and it may leave residual symptoms if the period required to perceive and to respond to the tachycardia is prolonged.[9,30,82,105] Just as important, the patient must be able to perceive the absence of tachycardia. If this is difficult, then the unit may be used inappropriately during sinus rhythm or sinus tachycardia, or the arrhythmia may be reinitiated if there is a delay in deactivating the system after a successful conversion to sinus rhythm.[69,70,78,103]

In some radiofrequency devices, there is no bradycardia protection. Therefore, the patients are at risk of asystole after conversion of the tachycardia.[69,70] The transmitter may deliver large amounts of pacing energy to the myocardium (greater than 8 V) and this fact, in addition to the nonuniform (and potentially long) burst durations, may increase the chance of initiation of ventricular or atrial fibrillation.[10,105]

The external controlling device must be constantly available to the patient. Each termination requires patient interaction; therefore, hemodynamic and psychologic stability are required. Significant time may elapse from the onset of the tachycardia to its termination—time to perceive the tachycardia, locate the activating device, and terminate the arrhythmia. This lapse may make termination more difficult because of changes in cardiovascular reflex and autonomic tone. These factors all limit the use of any patient-activated device.[38,72,84,93,103,115]

Antitachycardia pacing methods

Although temporary pacing is commonly effective for the termination of tachycardias,[96,116] the use of implantable units has been limited. The limiting factors have included the lack of reliable response to the programmed pacing technique, the dangers of rhythm acceleration or degeneration, the difficulty in differentiating pathologic from physiologic tachycardias, the paucity of clinically available antitachycardia pacing techniques, and the lack of adaptive pacing methods.[117,118]

Table 25B-7 Antitachycardia pacing methods

Underdrive pacing
Single chamber
Dual chamber
Extrastimulus pacing
Fixed
Adaptive
Cycle-length scanning
Fixed
Adaptive
Rapid overdrive (burst) pacing
Combination of scanning and burst pacing
Autodecremental
Shifting (adaptive) burst
Scanning burst

At present, an increasing number of pacing techniques are commercially available. These include the use of underdrive pacing (single- or dual-chamber), extrastimulus pacing (fixed or adaptive), tachycardia cycle length scanning (fixed or adaptive), rapid (burst) overdrive pacing, combinations of scanning and burst pacing techniques or rapid burst (train stimulation). Rapid overdrive (burst pacing) and combinations of scanning and burst pacing techniques (especially ramp and autodecremental pacing) are being coupled with the use of automatic cardioverter-defibrillators in the treatment of all forms of ventricular tachyarrhythmias (Table 25B-7).

Underdrive pacing. Simply stated, underdrive pacing represents asynchronous atrial, ventricular, or AV pacing during an episode of tachycardia at a rate slower than the rate of the tachycardia.

SINGLE-CHAMBER. Competitive fixed-rate pacing at a slower rate will stimulate the atrium, ventricle, AV node, or accessory pathways randomly during various portions of the tachycardia cycle until one of these impulses is fortuitously delivered at a critical time within the termination zone of the reentry circuit to cause termination of the tachyarrhythmia[9,27,68] (Fig 25B-9).

The single-chamber underdrive devices have limited utility. For this type of system to be effective, the tachycardia rate must be slow (fewer than 160 beats/min for most arrhythmias), a wide tachycardia termination zone must be present, pacing must be initiated quickly to ensure the greatest chance of termination, pacing should be performed as close to the tachycardia circuit as possible (i.e., on the same side as an accessory pathway or in the same ventricle as the origin of ventricular tachycardia), and the tachycardia must respond consistently to a single stimulus during extensive electrophysiologic testing[15,39,60,71,87,103,118,119] (Table 25B-8). Additionally, the tachycardia must be well tolerated because of the length of time that might be required for its termination.[95]

This type of pacing is most likely to be effective for the termination of AV reentry (utilizing accessory pathways)

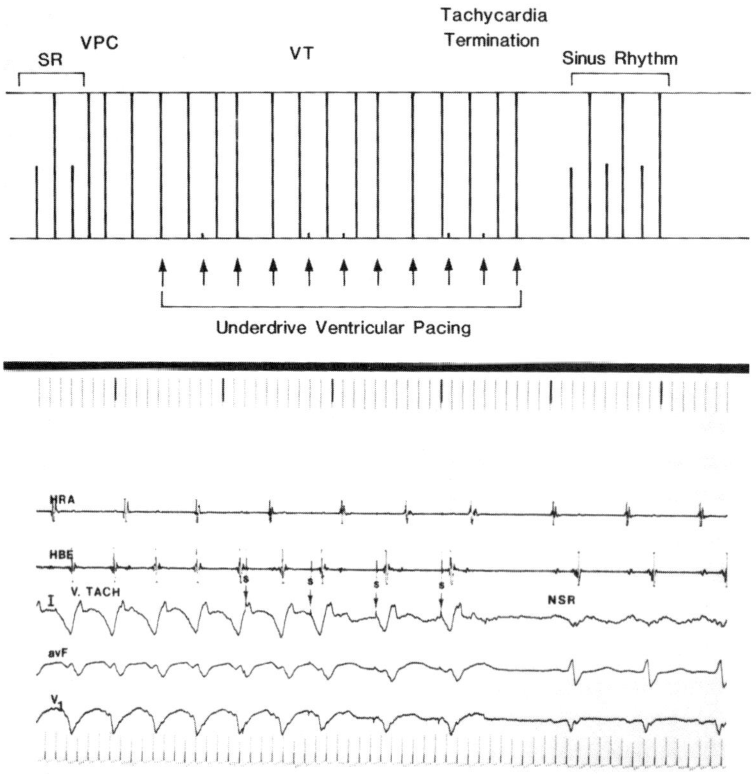

Fig 25B-9 **Upper,** underdrive pacing, With the onset of tachycardia *(VT),* underdrive pacing begins. Note that the third and seventh beats result in ventricular capture but not tachycardia termination. The last pacing stimulus captures the ventricle and invades the tachycardia circuit, terminating the arrhythmia. **Lower,** single-chamber underdrive termination of ventricular tachycardia. Four consecutive stimuli *(S)* are delivered during tachycardia, the last two of which interrupt the tachycardia circuit and restore sinus rhythm *(NSR). HBE,* His bundle electrogram; *HRA,* high right atrium; *SR,* sinus rhythm; *VPC,* ventricular premature contraction.

Table 25B-8 Criteria for use of an underdrive pacing device

Tachycardia rate < 160 beats/min
Wide termination zone
Rapid initiation of pacing
Site of pacing close to reentry circuit
Well-tolerated tachycardia

or slow ventricular tachycardia. In a series of patients with AV reentry studied by programmed stimulation, the tachycardia could be terminated by a single ventricular premature contraction in 43%, and it was speculated that the technique may be effective during tachycardias of up to 200 beats/min if stimulation were on the same side of the heart as the pathway.[9,70] In a similar study, underdrive pacing had a similar pattern of success (i.e., during supraventricular tachycardia at slow rates) but was less effective than a single timed extrastimulus.[119] In studies of patients with ventricular tachycardia, 37% to 57% had a response to a single right ventricular stimulus, and the greatest success occurred during episodes of slow ventricular tachycardia.[7,118,120] However, although a significant percentage of tachycardia episodes were terminated, only 5% of the patients had reliable termination with a single extrastimulus over several days of study.[118] Reports of success in patients with other types of tachycardias (AV nodal reentry or atrial flutter) are rare because these arrhythmias almost always require more than a single premature stimulus to bring about the termination.[39,87] In a large series[30] evaluating all types of arrhythmias, underdrive pacing did not prove useful in any patient.

Antiarrhythmia drugs often prove to be very useful when they are combined with underdrive pacing devices. They may slow the tachycardia rate and allow termination of the arrhythmia by a single stimulus and therefore increase the potential usefulness of these devices.[10,57,95,121]

DUAL-CHAMBER. Dual-chamber underdrive pacing can terminate supraventricular tachycardia when the relationship between atrial and ventricular depolarization is such that the ventricular paced impulse arrives at the tachycardia circuit early enough to collide with the impulse

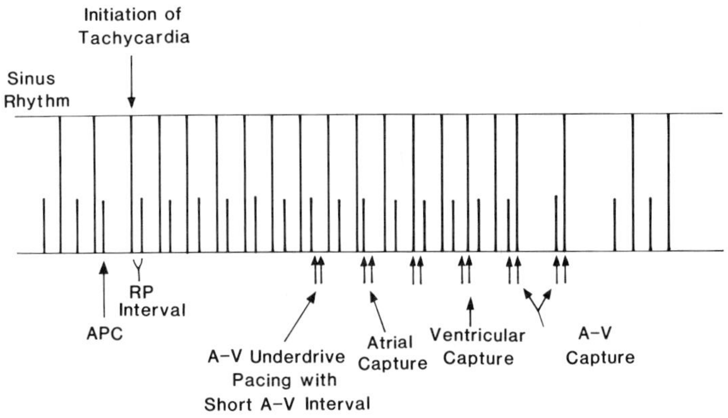

Fig 25B-10 An atrial premature beat (APC) initiates AV reentry with a long R-P interval. Dual-chamber underdrive pacing results in intermittent atrial or ventricular capture without tachycardia termination. Atrial and ventricular capture terminates the tachycardia.

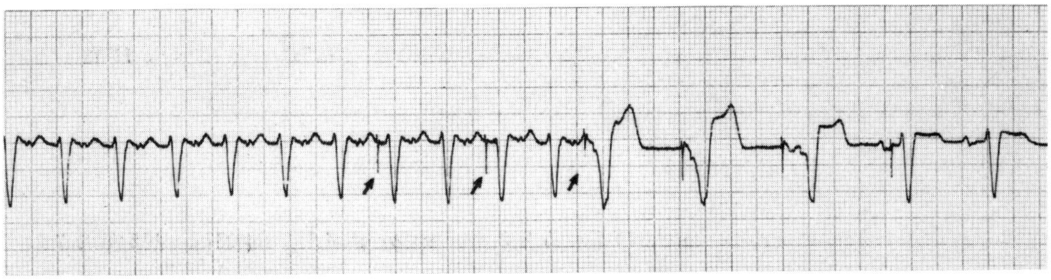

Fig 25B-11 During supraventricular tachycardia, underdrive AV pacing with a short P-R interval results in AV capture and interruption of tachycardia. (From Holmes DR: Pacing for tachycardia. In *A Practice of Cardiac Pacing.* Edited by S Furman, DL Hayes, DR Holmes Jr. Mount Kisco, New York, Futura Publishing Company, 1986, pp 413-431. By permission, Mayo Foundation.)

traveling from the atrium in the antegrade pathway and reaches the pathway used for retrograde conduction (i.e., accessory pathway or AV node) when it is refractory in order to prevent reinitiation of the tachycardia[15,122] (Fig 25B-10). Stimulation should be as close to the reentrant circuit as possible to increase the likelihood of tachycardia termination, because an impulse initiated at a distance from the circuit may not have enough time to traverse the intervening tissue and arrive at the circuit at the moment required to interrupt the reciprocating mechanism.[19,122]

The advantages of this type of pacing device over a single-chamber underdrive system include stimulation in both atrium and ventricle, which may improve the chances of tachycardia termination,[123] and protection against bradycardia in patients with spontaneous or drug-induced sinus bradycardia or AV block[6] with the potential benefit of reduction of the frequency of tachycardia episodes by maintenance of AV synchrony and atrial and ventricular rate support[2] (Fig 25B-11).

Dual-chamber underdrive pacing has been successfully utilized clinically in patients with various supraventricular arrhythmias, including classic AV node reentry (slow antegrade pathway–rapid retrograde pathway), atypical or incessant AV node reentry (rapid antegrade pathway), atypical or incessant AV node reentry (rapid antegrade pathway–slow retrograde pathway), AV reentry, and other extranodal reentrant tachycardias, including intra-atrial reentry.[3,13,15,122,123]

In the largest clinical series in the literature, involving 23 patients with various supraventricular tachycardias, no episodes of sustained tachycardia were noted and many short episodes were easily terminated. Of interest is the fact that arrhythmia occurrence was prevented in more than 50% of the patients despite discontinuation of antiarrhythmia therapy in 90%.[13] A report on the performance of a second-generation device indicates the same benefit in carefully selected patients.[75]

Extrastimulus pacing. If a single extrastimulus does not successfully terminate tachycardia, multiple extrastimuli may be effective. Extrastimulus pacing involves the sensing of atrial or ventricular electrograms during tachycardia with the introduction of two or more premature stimuli at a coupling interval following a sensed activity[38] (Fig 25B-12).

The coupling intervals may be fixed or adaptive. In the fixed mode, the interval from the last-sensed spontaneous

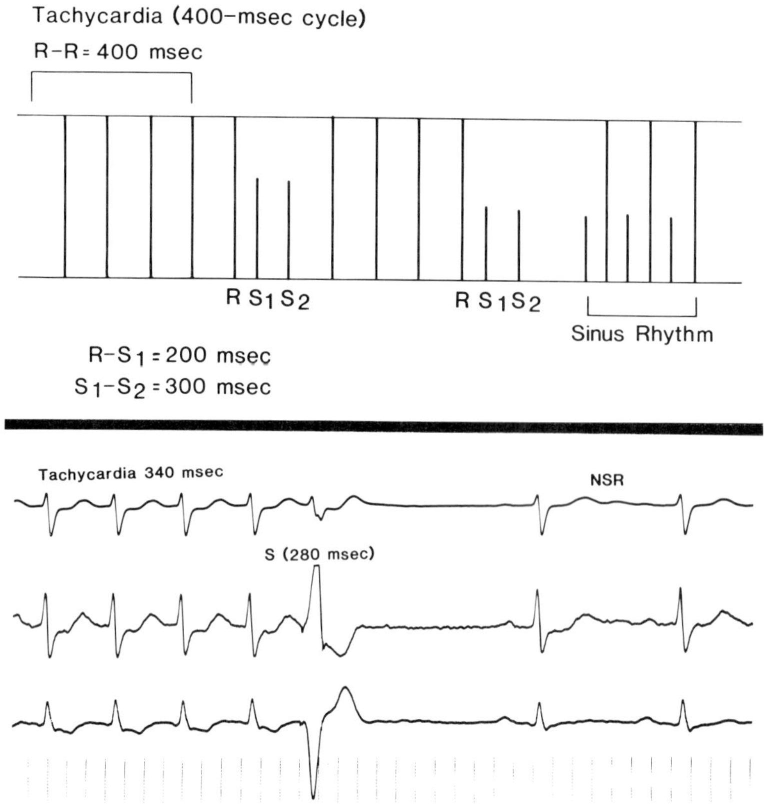

Fig 25B-12 **Upper,** during tachycardia, coupled premature stimuli at fixed intervals (R-S_1 and S_1-S_2) result in tachycardia termination. **Lower,** rhythm strip demonstrating the use of a single fixed stimulus *(S)* to interrupt a tachycardia and convert it to sinus rhythm *(NSR).*

beat and the intervals between each of the stimuli remain fixed during each subsequent pacing therapy. In the adaptive mode, coupling intervals are programmed to be some percentage of the tachycardia cycle length and, therefore, potentially adjust to changes in, for example, tachycardia rate, autonomic tone, position, and drug effects.[99] The number of stimuli to be used can also be fixed or increased to a preset value if an antitachycardia therapy is unsuccessful.[103]

Because fixed, programmed extrastimuli are commonly used in an attempt to terminate arrhythmias in the electrophysiologic laboratory, a rather large experience has developed with the technique. For all varieties of supraventricular tachycardia, two or more atrial extrastimuli are effective in more than 70% and two or more ventricular extrastimuli are effective in at least 75%.[72,124] In patients with ventricular tachycardia, the effectiveness is somewhat lower, ranging from 43% to 63%.[72,89,90,96,114,116,125,126] The rate of arrhythmia acceleration or the initiation of an unstable arrhythmia is increased significantly over that with a single extrastimulus. The overall rate of arrhythmia initiation (primarily atrial fibrillation) has been reported to be as high as 20% for two extrastimuli and 22% for three extrastimuli (atrial or ventricular).[90,125] When ventricular extrastimuli were used to terminate supraventricular tachycardia, ventricular tachycardia or ventricular fibrillation was initiated in 3%.[72]

Success increases with increasing tachycardia cycle lengths (slower rate). A tachycardia cycle length of 300 msec (200 beats/min) tends to separate tachycardias that require rapid pacing or direct current shock from those amenable to extrastimulus therapy.[96,110,116] The risk of tachycardia acceleration with two stimuli ranges from 8% to 20%, regardless of the tachycardia rate.[60,62,72,89,96] When more than two extrastimuli are used, the rate of acceleration is lightly increased.[62] With the use of multiple adaptive stimuli (up to six stimuli), the success rate is improved but the risk of acceleration still exists.[38]

Clinical experience with implanted devices using either fixed or adaptive extrastimuli has been limited, but the published results with the device in the adaptive mode for treatment of supraventricular tachycardia and ventricular tachycardia have been excellent: more than 90% of the tachycardia episodes have been successfully terminated with an arrhythmia acceleration rate of less than 1%.[99,103] It should be noted that in the clinical and electrophysiologic experience with this pacing method, three to five attempts were required (on an average) for termination of tachycardia and the mean time requirement was up to 15 seconds (depending on the type of adaptive mode used).[99] This potentially lengthy time requirement for termination of tachycardia has been noted with other adaptive modes as well; therefore, the technique may be inappropriate for patients with rapid hemodynamic deterioration.[85]

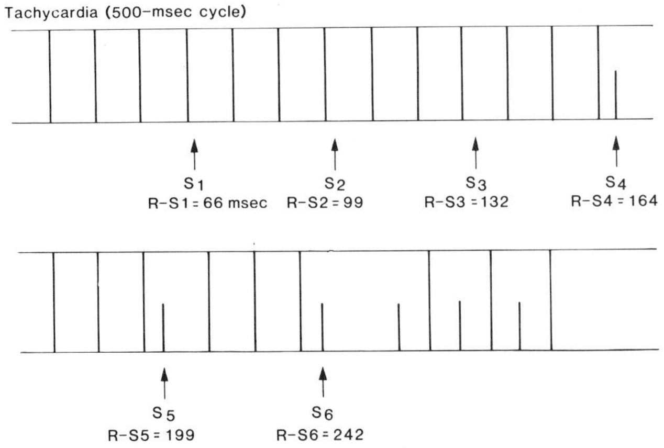

Fig 25B-13 During tachycardia, the cycle length is spanned by premature stimuli with increasingly longer coupling intervals. The first three stimuli fall within the refractory period and do not result in myocardial capture. The final (critically timed) premature stimulus terminates the arrhythmia.

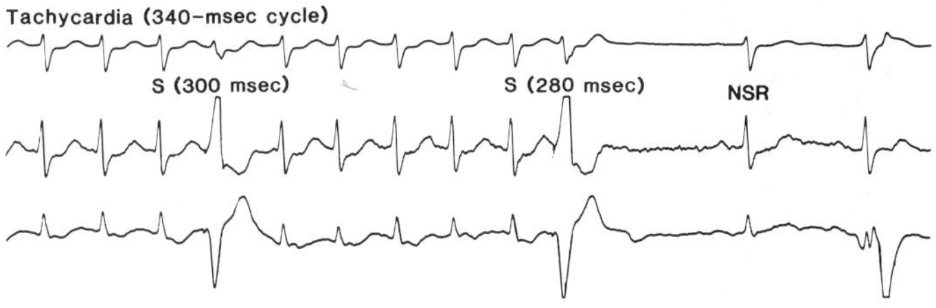

Fig 25B-14 Supraventricular tachycardia terminated by ventricular premature stimuli *(S)* that span the tachycardia at progressively shorter coupling intervals. *NSR,* normal sinus rhythm.

Tachycardia cycle length scanning. In addition to the adaptive pacing techniques, several other pacing methods have been developed to deal with the problem of a variable tachycardia termination zone. These include incremental or decremental sequential tachycardia cycle length scanning, an automatic increase in the number of stimuli given during a pacing treatment (which can be part of extrastimulus scanning or burst pacing techniques), and high-frequency (train) stimuli that begin in the refractory period.[103,104,127-129]

The theoretical advantages to the scanning technique, in addition to its inherently adaptive function, are that a very small number of stimuli are required for termination of tachycardia, the coupling intervals are programmable or adaptive, and the scanning stimuli are triggered off sensed cardiac events; thus, the chance of stimulation during the vulnerable period is decreased.[93,130,131]

Many methods have been devised for scanning of R-R cycle lengths. The simplest of these methods involves either incremental or decremental sequential scanning. In incremental scanning, the initial stimulus is delivered just beyond the refractory period, and the R-R interval is scanned by extrastimuli that follow a predetermined number of spontaneous tachycardia beats at progressive delays of 6 to 40 msec (Fig 25B-13). In decremental scanning, the initial extrastimulus is delivered at a preset delay that is slightly longer than the tachycardia cycle length, and the R-R interval is scanned by extrastimuli with progressively shorter coupling intervals. If a single stimulus is ineffective in either form, two stimuli can be used. The interval between the two stimuli is constant in incremental scanning but may be varied in decremental scanning[106,129,132] (Fig 25B-14).

In a reported series of patients with supraventricular and ventricular tachycardias treated with decremental scanning, total success (i.e., totally asymptomatic patients with rapid termination of tachycardia) was reported in 50%. Another 30% had short-lived episodes of tachycardia with eventual termination. In 20%, there was failure to terminate at least one episode of tachycardia, acceleration of tachycardia (atrial fibrillation), or incapacitating symptoms at the onset of tachycardia. There was no acceleration of ventricular tachycardia or initiation of ventricular fibrillation in any of the patients with ventricular stimulation for ventricular tachycardia or supraventricular tachycardia. Similar results were reported in other clinical experiences. However, reprogramming after dismissal from the hospital was required in up to 66% of patients, usually because of a change in the tachycardia rate or the need to modify the scanning program.[93,131-134]

Electrophysiologic testing using this technique for supraventricular and ventricular tachycardias demonstrated efficacy rates of 90% and 80%, respectively, with arrhythmia acceleration in 20% of patients with ventricular tachycardia. However, the mean duration of pacing for termination of tachycardia was 80.7 seconds in supraventricular tachycardia and 62.5 seconds in ventricular tachycardia.[99]

Very sophisticated forms of scanning are incorporated into some of the newer antitachycardia pacing systems. In the "self-searching" mode, the intervals of the extrastimuli are adjusted automatically by the generator, depending on their effect on the tachycardia. If the delivered stimulus produces tachycardia reset (alteration in tachycardia cycle lengths), the coupling intervals are too long and will be decreased at the next attempt. If no reset occurs, the intervals will be increased.

In adaptive "table scanning," a table of the five most successful stimulus intervals is compiled by the pacemaker. When the tachycardia occurs, these are tried first. If they are unsuccessful, a search is started.[91,98,135]

In short-term studies using these two scanning techniques in patients with supraventricular tachycardia, both were totally successful without acceleration of tachycardia.[98] In long-term follow-up, 90% of the patients had complete control of recurrent tachycardia by the device alone. Because of its adaptive nature, this pacing system was able to terminate new supraventricular tachycardias (not seen at initial electrophysiologic study) that developed during the period of follow-up.[94]

Rapid overdrive (burst) pacing. The most successful pacing technique for conversion of a tachycardia to sinus rhythm regardless of the mechanism of the arrhythmia is rapid overdrive pacing.[136,137] The technique was initially applied in 1967 for treatment of atrial flutter and in 1971

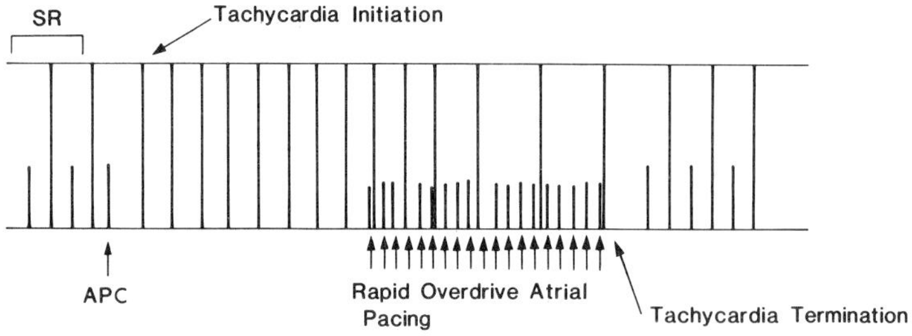

Fig 25B-15 An atrial premature beat *(APC)* results in the initiation of tachycardia. Rapid overdrive atrial pacing leads to progressive AV node block, resulting in tachycardia termination. *SR,* sinus rhythm.

was used for the treatment of ventricular tachycardia.[56,59]

If the rate of the tachycardia is rapid, if the reentry circuit or focus is distant from the site of stimulation, and if the circuit is small, the chances of termination of the arrhythmias by single or coupled stimuli are significantly reduced.[9,39,59,138] Brief bursts of pacing may decrease the refractoriness in the tissues near the pacing site and the tachycardia circuit or its site of origin and thereby facilitate penetration of the pathway by one or more stimuli, resulting in the interruption of a tachycardia.[74,139] In addition, the faster rates result in shorter coupling intervals for the pacing-induced depolarizations, allowing impulses to arrive at the site of the circuit earlier and thus facilitating invasion into the area.[39] The goal is not to have each impulse capture the heart but rather to increase the statistical probability of one impulse falling within the termination zone of the tachycardia circuit[27] (Fig 25B-15).

Rapid atrial pacing may terminate many different types of supraventricular tachycardia effectively, including atrial flutter, AV node reentry, AV reentry, intra-atrial or sinoatrial reentry, and junctional tachycardias.[1] The mechanisms by which this can occur include interruption of a reentry tachycardia circuit by depolarizing atrial, AV (accessory pathway), or AV nodal portions of the pathway;[1,29,67] conversion of the stable rhythm to an unstable one, which then reverts to sinus rhythm (i.e., paroxysmal supraventricular tachycardia → atrial fibrillation → sinus rhythm);[50,66] and, *possibly,* overdrive suppression of an atrial ectopic focus that allows the sinus mechanism to supervene[59,70,140] (Fig 25B-16).

The same potential modes of tachycardia termination would be expected as a result of rapid ventricular pacing during ventricular tachycardia.[141] The responses to ventricular pacing in this situation are immediate tachycardia termination, increased ventricular rate with or without spontaneous conversion to sinus rhythm, slowing of the rate of tachycardia to more acceptable levels, or no response with or without ventricular capture[95] (Fig 25B-17).

For successful termination of tachycardia by overdrive pacing, three important variables must be taken into consideration – site, rate, and duration of pacing. There is an inverse relationship between the pacing rate and the duration of pacing required to terminate tachycardias.[78] The rate necessary to terminate an episode of tachycardia is generally 10 or more beats/min faster than the tachycardia when pacing is applied for 1 to 15 seconds.[38] However, pacing at rates only slightly faster than the tachycardia rate is likely to result in entrainment (increased tachycardia rate by fusion with paced beats) without termination, which may lead to hemodynamic compromise.[141,142] Hence, it is more appropriate to consider effective burst pacing to be at rates at least 30 or more beats/min faster than the tachycardia for 4 to 15 extrastimuli (5 to 10 captured beats).[30,78,95] The more rapid the pacing rate, the greater the chance of inducing atrial or ventricular fibrillation; therefore, if rapid rates are required, they should be maintained for the shortest period of time possible.[78]

In patients with supraventricular tachycardia, burst pacing in the atrium or ventricle can be successful, although atrial pacing is much safer. For ventricular tachycardia, ventricular pacing is virtually always required, although atrial burst pacing has been reported to be successful when the tachycardia rate is slow.[27,143,144] The mechanism of termination of ventricular tachycardia by atrial pacing involves either conduction of the atrial stimuli to the reentrant circuit via the AV node or an overdrive suppressive effect of atrial pacing.[143]

The major advantages of burst pacing are its predictable effectiveness for virtually all types of tachycardias and the very brief period of time required for tachycardia termination.[9,15,59,60,65,95,145] The disadvantages relate primarily to the possibility of increasing the heart rate during tachycardia or initiating life-threatening arrhythmias.

In the electrophysiologic laboratory, *supraventricular tachycardia* can be terminated by burst pacing in 92% to 100% of episodes regardless of the nature of the arrhythmia or the tachycardia rate. The incidence of arrhythmia acceleration or initiation of atrial fibrillation varies from 0% to 20%.[72,98,99,112,119,146] In most cases, atrial fibrillation is transient and sinus rhythm is eventually resumed.[119] The frequency of initiation of atrial fibrillation is increased when burst pacing is used to terminate tachycardias with a rate of more than 175 beats/min, a suggestion that more rapid pacing rates increase the chance of acceleration.[90] The risk of initiation of atrial fibrillation can be decreased significantly by keeping the burst to fewer than 250 beats/min.[27,139]

Another potential consequence of rapid atrial pacing is 1:1 AV conduction to the ventricle via intranodal or extranodal pathways, with the potential for hemodynamic instability secondary to rapid ventricular rates or the

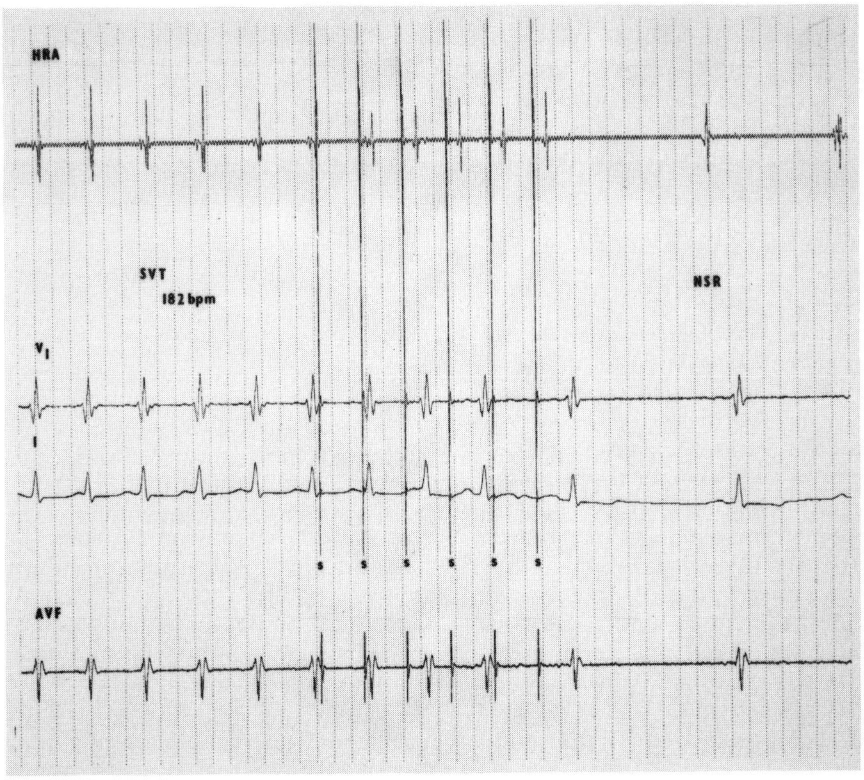

Fig 25B-16 A short burst of pacing in the right atrium terminates supraventricular tachycardia *(SVT)*, restoring sinus rhythm *(NSR)*.

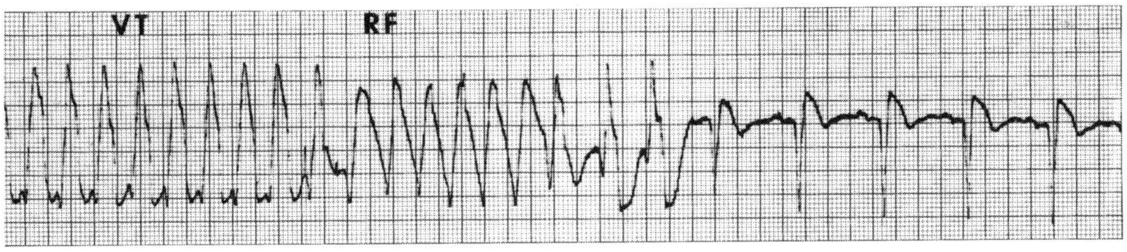

Fig 25B-17 A short burst of rapid ventricular pacing (utilizing a patient-activated radiofrequency *[RF]* device) results in termination of ventricular tachycardia *(VT)*.

initiation of ventricular arrhythmias.[39,49,78,105,147,148] As a rule, atrial stimulation at a rate of more than 200 beats/min should not have the potential for 1:1 conduction to the ventricle.[149]

Rapid ventricular pacing for control of *ventricular tachycardia* in the electrophysiologic laboratory results in termination of tachycardia in 62% to 89% of tachycardia episodes.[60,72,95,96,116,145-150] The percentage of episodes terminated is significantly higher at slower tachycardia rates than at faster rates (e.g., 83% of tachycardia episodes are terminated when the tachycardia rate is 250 beats/min or slower, whereas only 50% are terminated when the tachycardia rate is 220 beats/min or faster).[151] When the tachycardia rate exceeds 200 beats/min, burst pacing is commonly the only pacing technique that will convert the arrhythmia.[72,96,116] Burst pacing may be successful when all other methods of termination fail, regardless of the tachycardia rate.[89] Because it is the most effective means of terminating tachycardia, requiring less time than other forms of pacing therapy, it is a potential benefit in patients who are rapidly symptomatic.[150]

The hazards of ventricular pacing include acceleration of the rate of ventricular tachycardia, induction of ventricular fibrillation, initiation of ventricular tachycardia if pacing occurs inappropriately during a sinus rhythm, and hemodynamic compromise during sustained rapid ventricular pacing.[10,30,71,74,95,152] Most of the information on acceleration of ventricular tachycardia and induction of ventricular fibrillation comes from experience in the electrophysiology laboratory. The incidence of acceleration of ventricular tachycardia or initiation of ventricular fibrillation has been reported to be between 3% and 50% of tachycardia episodes, and occurrence is at least once in 32% to 50% of patients.[72,91,95,96,116,145,150,152,153]

Some studies have suggested that acceleration is most likely to occur with very aggressive pacing techniques at very rapid pacing rates.[10,72,153] Other studies have shown no statistical difference in the incidence of acceleration regardless of the pacing rate.[96] The incidence can possibly be reduced by reducing the burst rate and duration to the lowest effective level and by the concomitant use of antiarrhythmia agents to slow the tachycardia rate and hence the rate and duration requirements for termination of tachycardia.[8,10,30,74,95]

CLINICAL EXPERIENCE

A. Supraventricular tachycardia. Despite the potential problems with the use of rapid pacing, burst pacing is very effective in the management of refractory paroxysmal supraventricular tachycardia. Regardless of the type of tachycardia, more than 70% of cases will respond clinically to overdrive pacing.[1,15,147] In a consecutive series of 150 patients with paroxysmal supraventricular tachycardia, it was found that 5 (3%) were candidates for overdrive pacing on the basis of strict clinical and electrophysiologic criteria. All of these patients frequently successfully converted episodes of tachycardia to sinus rhythm without the induction of a complicating arrhythmia. Each noted a dramatic improvement in quality of life and was able to return to a normal lifestyle because of the knowledge that the pacing system would successfully and reliably terminate all episodes.[78]

In another series of 12 patients with refractory paroxysmal supraventricular tachycardia, during a mean follow-up period of 26 months more than 6,000 episodes of tachycardia were successfully terminated with only one transient failure.[70] Many of the reports of short-term clinical experience have demonstrated that the implanted devices are being used by more than 80% of patients, in whom more than 80% of tachycardia episodes were promptly terminated, with a very low rate of tachycardia acceleration.[70,84,104,116,149,154-157]

Recently, the long-term follow-up experience with antitachycardia pacing (primarily burst pacing) in patients with supraventricular tachycardia has been evaluated. In patients who had exhibited consistent short-term termination of tachycardia, continued pacing efficacy varied from 36% to 78%, and in a significant number, concomitant drug therapy was required.[93,97,107,158,159] These studies suggest that the major impediments to successful long-term therapy are changes in the electrophysiologic properties of the reentrant circuits and the inability to adequately sense chronic atrial electrograms in sinus rhythm and during tachycardia.[107,159]

B. Ventricular tachycardia. The clinical use of implanted devices is less extensive for ventricular tachycardia than for supraventricular tachycardia because of the potential for the initiation of life-threatening arrhythmias.[160] Most studies indicate that about 60% of patients continue to use implanted devices reliably after a mean follow-up of 13 to 17 months. In a series of 20 patients with antitachycardia pacing therapy of ventricular tachycardia, the actuarial efficacy of the devices was 78% at 1 year and 55% at 5 years.[97] The rate of arrhythmia acceleration ranges from 0% to 33% and the rate of sudden death from 7% to 34% in multiple clinical studies. Although most sudden deaths have no relationship to the use of the pacemaker, some episodes could have been secondary to pacemaker-induced ventricular fibrillation.[10,30,74,84,93,95,104,116,119,161,162]

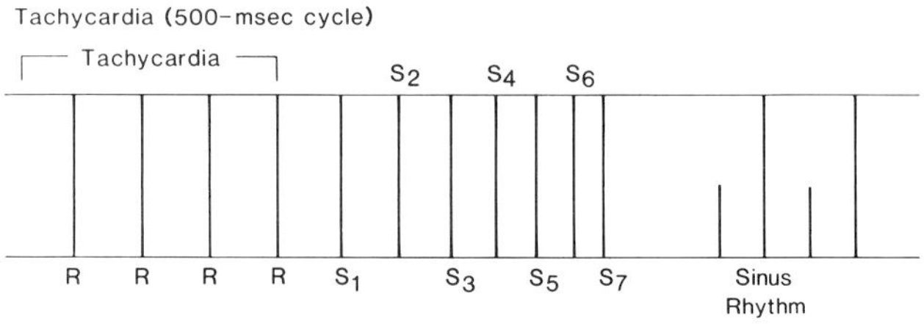

Fig 25B-18 During tachycardia, autodecremental pacing results in tachycardia termination. The first extrastimulus is delivered at a coupling interval equal to the tachycardia cycle length (R-R) minus a preset value, D (40 msec in this example). Each subsequent stimulus-to-stimulus coupling interval is reduced by D: R-S_1 = 460 msec; S_1-S_2 = 420 msec; S_2-S_3 = 380 msec; S_3-S_4 = 340 msec; S_4-S_5 = 300 msec; S_5-S_6 = 260 msec; S_6-S_7 = 220 msec.

Because of this potential for the initiation of lethal arrhythmias, the use of this and other pacing techniques for ventricular tachycardia has been greatly curtailed in the absence of defibrillator backup.[163] Antitachycardia pacing and automatic internal cardioverter-defibrillators have been used successfully in concert,[135] and implantable defibrillators that combine the two treatment modalities are now available.

Combination of scanning and burst pacing techniques. As a means to combine the effectiveness of rapid stimulation with adaptive pacing techniques, to minimize the risks of close-coupled stimulation, and to avoid the hemodynamic consequences associated with long bursts of pacing, the principles of both burst overdrive and scanning extrastimulus pacing have been combined in several pacing methods, including autodecremental pacing, shifting (adaptive) burst pacing, and scanning burst (concertina) pacing.[85,134]

AUTODECREMENTAL, OR RAMP, PACING. This is a rate-related accelerating overdrive method of pacing. On detection of tachycardia, the first pacing cycle interval is equal to the tachycardia cycle length minus a preset decrement value, D (e.g., 40 msec). Each subsequent pacing stimulus is reduced by the same value, gradually accelerating the pacing rate until a plateau of 100 beats/min faster than the tachycardia is reached[86] (Fig 25B-18).

This system has the theoretical advantages of being synchronous (to avoid stimulation within the vulnerable period), adaptive, and potentially less arrhythmogenic than competitive constant rate pacing. Scanning various pacing rates in a progressive and beat-to-beat manner allows the refractoriness of the myocardium to be peeled back incrementally after penetration of the tachycardia circuit.[72,110,134,146]

In a series of patients with ventricular tachycardia with a cycle length of more than 280 msec in which an adaptive decremental value of 3.5% of the tachycardia cycle length was used, 92% of all episodes in 95% of patients were terminated without acceleration of tachycardia. The termination rate and acceleration rate compared very well

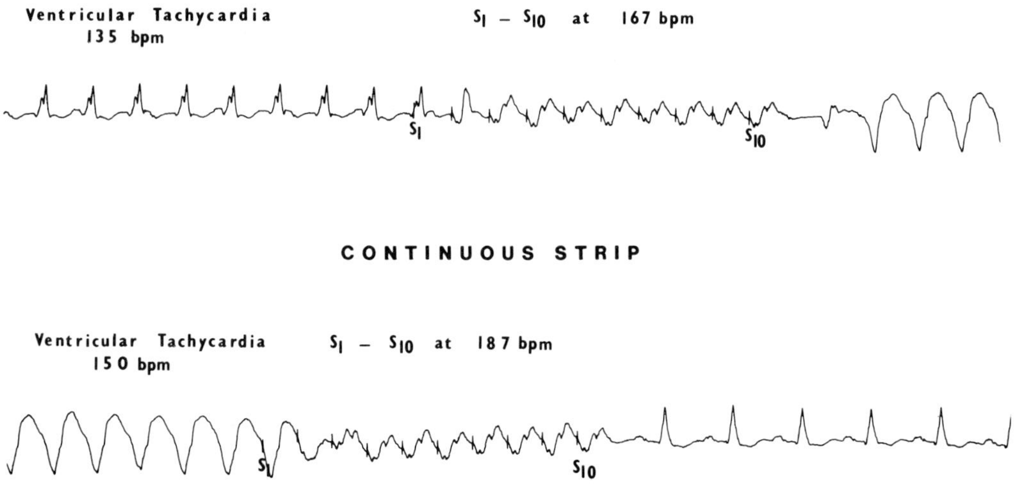

Fig 25B-19 Shifting (adaptive) burst pacing. Ventricular tachycardia at 135 beats/min (450 msec cycle length) triggers a sequence of burst pacing at 80% of the tachycardia cycle length (167 beats/min, or 360 msec). This results in a faster tachycardia that responds to another adaptive burst of pacing.

with those of burst pacing when the two methods were evaluated in the same patients.[110] However, in another study, although the system was successful, termination took a considerable amount of time, with long pacing bursts, which may have adverse hemodynamic consequences.[134] As with all stimulation techniques, the potential for acceleration of arrhythmia exists with autodecremental pacing.

SHIFTING (ADAPTIVE) BURST PACING. In this pacing technique, the first stimulus is synchronized to the last-sensed tachycardia beat and is delivered at a preset percentage of the tachycardia cycle length. The stimuli that follow may be delivered at the same interval or at a shorter interval but, unlike autodecremental pacing, remain fixed. The interval from the last tachycardia beat to the initiation of the burst can also remain fixed or be made decremental (shortened), a trait that allows some scan of the tachycardia cycle length in addition to burst pacing[139] (Fig 25B-19).

In a series of 14 patients, temporary adaptive burst pacing was used with a burst cycle length equal to 7% of the spontaneous tachycardia rate. With this protocol, 88% of ventricular tachycardia episodes were terminated and ventricular tachycardia was accelerated in 7%.[124]

SCANNING BURST, OR "CONCERTINA," PACING. In response to tachycardia, several premature beats are generated, the first of which occurs at a specified delay from the last detected tachycardia beat. If more than one stimulus is used, subsequent pacing intervals are the same as the initial coupling interval (the same principle as that of the adaptive burst mode). However, if tachycardia persists, the pacemaker automatically reduces the coupling interval. Reduction may be repeated up to 15 times; thus, short bursts may be generated that, if unsuccessful, are repeated at faster rates during subsequent events while scanning the tachycardia cycle length (Fig 25B-20).[85,134]

CLINICAL EXPERIENCE. The antitachycardia pacing devices in common use at present are capable of multiple pacing therapies, including extrastimuli, burst pacing (fixed or adaptive), and autodecremental pacing. The number of pacing stimuli within a sequence, the number of pacing attempts, and the sequence of pacing therapies are programmable. The device can be programmed to use a single pacing therapy (e.g., adaptive burst) or multiple therapies in sequence (e.g., adaptive burst pacing followed by autodecremental pacing) if tachycardia persists.[109] The tachycardia detection criteria include heart rate, sudden onset, rate stability, sustained high rate, and any combination of these.[164]

A. Supraventricular tachycardia. In the treatment of supraventricular tachycardia, adaptive burst and autodecremental pacing are the therapies most commonly used. With these pacing modes, the ability to control supraventricular arrhythmias has been excellent. Multiple studies have reported both short- and long-term success in tachycardia termination in 80% to 99% of patients.[94,100,108,164-166] The need for hospitalization of these patients has also been significantly reduced.[100,109] In a study of 22 patients, the average number of hospitalizations was 3.6 per year before and 0.1 per year after pacemaker implantation.[164] However, development of atrial fibrillation secondary to pacing therapy remains a problem, even with adaptive pacing modes. The incidence of sustained atrial fibrillations with adaptive pacing for treatment of supraventricular tachycardia has been reported to be 0 to 7%.[87,108,164,166] The flexibility these devices provide, because of their programmable tachycardia detection and therapy features, and the adaptiveness of the pacing therapies are the major reasons for their success in the management of a wide variety of supraventricular tachycardias, including atrial flutter, AV nodal reentry, and AV reentry. Their utility may be diminished by the advent of ablation procedures, which have the potential for complete eradication of an arrhythmia, but they remain an effective therapeutic option for supraventricular tachycardia.

B. Ventricular tachycardia. The development of adap-

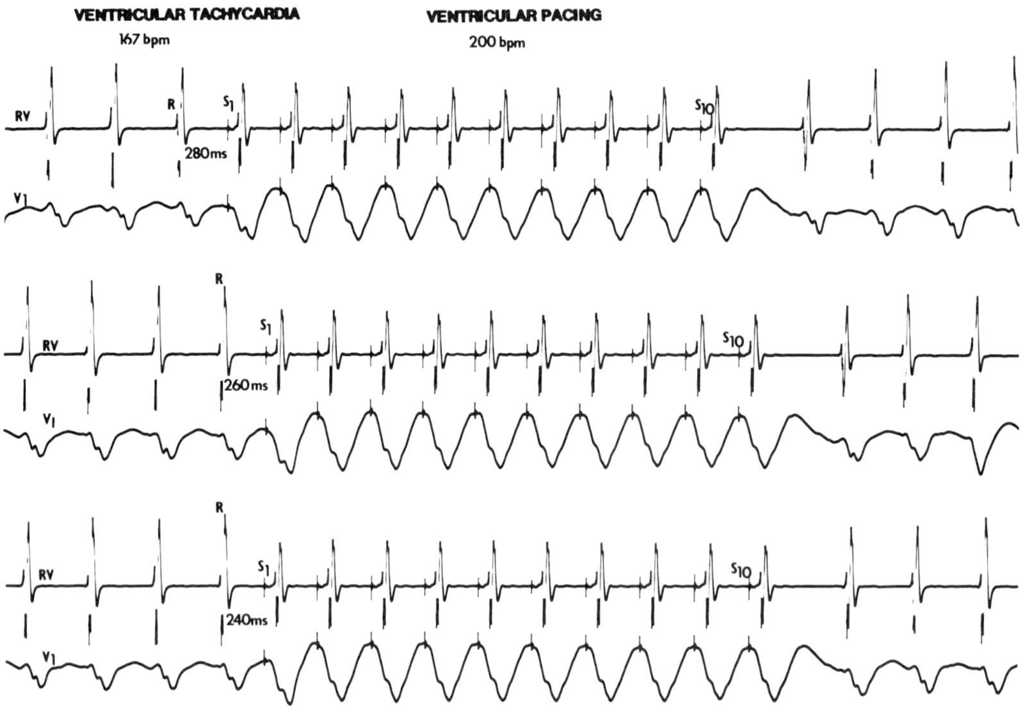

Fig 25B-20 Scanning burst pacing. Continuous tracing—three synchronous 10-beat bursts of ventricular pacing (S_1-S_{10}). Note progressive shortening of coupling interval between last beat of tachycardia and first extrastimulus as tachycardia cycle length is scanned. *bpm,* beats per minute; *RV,* right ventricular electrogram; V_1, electrocardiographic lead. (From Osborn MJ: Antitachycardia pacing. In *Interventional Cardiology.* Edited by DR Holmes Jr, RE Vlietstra. FA Davis Company, Philadelphia, 1989, pp 266-296. By permission, Mayo Foundation.)

tive burst, scanning burst, and autodecremental pacing therapies and their incorporation in antitachycardia pacemakers occurred at about the same time as implantable defibrillators began to be used in the management of ventricular tachyarrhythmias. Before devices with combined antitachycardia pacing and defibrillation capacity became available, some patients were treated by implantation of two separate devices. In a study of 10 such patients (who were very highly selected), antitachycardia pacing therapy (autodecremental or adaptive burst) terminated 89% of all ventricular tachycardia episodes. The rate of arrhythmia acceleration was less than 1%. However, the implanted defibrillator was activated at least once in all patients, primarily for spontaneous rapid ventricular tachycardia or ventricular fibrillation.[167] Despite the success of the pacing devices, it was still apparent that even in patients with stable ventricular tachycardia, automatic antitachycardia pacing devices should be implanted only with concomitant defibrillator backup.

These pacing therapies have been incorporated into the newest generation of implantable defibrillators, and most of the clinical experience has been derived from patients with these devices. From 51% to 93% of ventricular tachycardias terminated, and arrhythmia acceleration occurred in 0 to 29%. Therapeutic efficacy is enhanced and the rate of acceleration is much less when autodecremental rather than burst pacing therapies are selected and when they are used in relatively slow and stable arrhythmias.[168-172] It is quite likely that in some cases the evaluation of pacing therapy is less rigorous than suggested because of the ability to use shock therapy, which clearly affects the rate of arrhythmia conversion and acceleration.

In properly selected patients, pacing therapy is an extremely useful treatment option, and it will enhance our ability to use implantable devices in the management of patients with all types of arrhythmias.

Concomitant antiarrhythmia drug therapy

Because pharmacologic therapy is the accepted standard approach to management of arrhythmias, virtually all patients in whom pacing therapy is used will be taking antiarrhythmia drugs. Ideally, pacing therapy can be used in lieu of drug therapy, but not infrequently (especially in the case of ventricular tachycardia), the two must be used in concert.[93,103,118,133,158] This has been shown to be the case regardless of the type of antitachycardia pacing technique used.

Drugs have been used concomitantly with pacing for various reasons: (1) to slow the rate of sinus tachycardia to avoid inappropriate pacemaker discharge; (2) to decrease the incidence of tachycardia; (3) to slow the rate of tachycardia; (4) to decrease the incidence and significance of pacing-induced arrhythmias; (5) to modify shrinking or disappearing tachycardia termination windows that occur with changes in, for example, position and autonomic tone; (6) to facilitate termination of tachycardia; (7) to decrease the frequency of atrial or ventricular ectopy; (8) to modify the electrophysiologic characteristics of accessory pathways; (9) to eliminate nonsustained arrhythmias; and (10) to prevent competing arrhythmias (e.g., atrial fibrillation in patients with ventricular tachycardia).[72,83,97-99,103,109,113,164,173,174]

A reduction in tachycardia rate can be of benefit for two reasons: (1) to improve hemodynamic stability and so allow the use of pacing techniques (e.g., scanning) that may require more time but are inherently safer[10,39,95,121] and (2) to facilitate termination of tachycardia by any pacing method.[89,96]

Changes in the electrophysiologic properties of the reentrant circuit may also make termination of tachycardia more difficult.[83,116] If drugs are used with pacing, their effects must be carefully evaluated.

Temporary pacing

Temporary pacing may be useful for any situation in which recurrent tachycardia is posing a therapeutic problem. Transvenous or transesophageal placement of a pacing electrode may provide a safe and effective method for controlling recurrent arrhythmias.[38,175-179] It has several advantages for direct-current cardioversion: general anesthesia is not required; asystole that may occur in patients with sinus node dysfunction is avoided by pacing; during supraventricular tachycardia secondary to digitalis intoxication, the chance of ventricular instability is reduced because the ventricle is not stimulated; and the technique can be used diagnostically by recording atrial and ventricular electrograms.[9,180,181]

The technique is of particular importance in the postoperative period because temporary wire electrodes can be placed on the epicardial surface of the atrium and ventricle during the operation, brought out through the anterior chest wall, and used to assist in the diagnosis and treatment of postoperative arrhythmias. In addition, they can be used in noninvasive electrophysiologic studies after surgery for ventricular tachycardia or the Wolff-Parkinson-White syndrome.[182,183]

The most common rhythm disturbance in the postoperative period is atrial flutter. Rapid atrial pacing has proved very useful in controlling this arrhythmia. The standard approach to termination of atrial flutter is atrial pacing at 10 beats/min faster than the atrial flutter rate during monitoring of the ECG. When the atrial rate has increased to the pacing rate, the latter rate is increased until the P waves change shape. Pacing is then abruptly terminated, or the rate is quickly slowed. A constant-rate technique can also be used. The atrium is paced at 120% to 130% of the spontaneous rate for 30 seconds, and then pacing is stopped abruptly or quickly slowed. If this maneuver is unsuccessful, the pacing rate is increased by 5 to 10 beats/min until termination occurs.[138,184]

Temporary noninvasive pacing may also be used to terminate tachycardia. Standard transcutaneous pacemakers have been shown to be effective in patients with supraventricular (AV nodal or AV reentry) and ventricular tachycardias.[125,185-188] The thresholds for atrial and ventricular capture are high, and although the technique is reportedly well tolerated, in at least one study severe or intolerable discomfort was noted in approximately one-half of the patients.[125] A number of implantable permanent (bradycardia) pacemakers can respond to external stimulation in a triggered mode to allow noninvasive electrophysiologic studies. Chest wall stimulation has also been used to trigger rapid ventricular pacing in DDD systems (atrial sensing of the chest wall stimulation), with successful termination of ventricular tachycardia.[189]

AUTOMATIC IMPLANTABLE CARDIOVERTER-DEFIBRILLATOR

Antitachycardia pacing is not suitable for the management of all patients with ventricular tachyarrhythmias because it does not prevent or terminate every tachycardia episode, it carries the risk of arrhythmia acceleration or conversion to ventricular fibrillation, and it is ineffective in patients with ventricular fibrillation. As a result, other forms of electrical therapy for tachycardia termination (cardioversion and defibrillation) have been developed, and all these technologies have been merged in the newest generation of implantable devices.

History

The impetus for the development of an automatic implantable cardioverter-defibrillator (AICD) has been the problem of sudden cardiac death. More than 300,000 episodes of sudden death occur yearly, most of which are secondary to ventricular fibrillation.[136,190-193] Once the arrhythmia has started, the only reliable form of therapy is prompt defibrillation.

The two major stumbling blocks to the development of an AICD have been pulse generator size and ability to detect ventricular fibrillation (or tachycardia) and reliably differentiate these arrhythmias from other cardiac rhythms.

A cardioverter-defibrillator must contain a power source, a sensing system, a switching mechanism, and a means of energy delivery.[194] The primary space elements of the power source are batteries and capacitors. The capacitors are indispensible because batteries are not able to deliver cardioversion or defibrillation energy instantaneously. Therefore, the size of the pulse generator is a function of the capacitor, which in turn is directly related to the amount of energy delivered.

Transthoracic defibrillation requires a large amount of energy (200 to 400 J), much of which is dissipated in extracardiac tissue.[195] Internal defibrillation using low energy was first suggested in 1954 by Hopps and Bigelow.[196] Testing of a variety of implantable lead systems resulted in the development of an endocardial catheter that allowed successful and consistent defibrillation at 5 to 20 J in animals.[197,198] The first human defibrillation with a similar endocardial system was accomplished by Mirowski et al.[199] in 1972. In a series of patients undergoing cardiac surgery, defibrillation after cardioplegic arrest was accomplished with 5- to 15-J shocks. These studies demonstrated the feasibility of low-energy intracardiac catheter defibrillation in man.

This accomplishment, together with the observations of Garrey[200] (who had demonstrated that ventricular fibrillation could be consistently maintained in large animal hearts but not in small hearts), Mower et al.[201] (who found three distinct patters of defibrillation, only one of which was characterized by instantaneous conversion of ventricular fibrillation to normal sinus rhythm), and Zipes et al.[202] (who were able to terminate ventricular fibrillation by depolarizing limited amounts of myocardium by localized electrical shocks or potassium infusion) led to the formulation of the concept of critical mass. This stated that ventricular defibrillation can be accomplished without simultaneous and complete depolarization of the ventricular myocardium and may occur when the amount of fibrillating myocardium required for maintenance of the fibrillatory process is reduced below a critical level.[201]

The next problem that required solving was the ability of the pulse generator (cardioverter-defibrillator) to monitor the heart and sense ventricular fibrillation (or ventricular tachycardia). Initially, attempts were made to monitor right ventricular pressure. A marked reduction in pressure and abolition of its phasic nature served as an indication of ventricular fibrillation.[203,204] This sensing system proved impractical, and therefore a system that recognized ventricular fibrillation by the electrical characteristic of the arrhythmia itself was developed. This involved a concept of probability density function, which is a measure of the amount of time an electrical signal spends at different amplitude levels (see "Sensing function," below).[205]

The implantation of the automatic internal defibrillator (AID) in humans was first performed in 1980;[206] the device relied on the probability density function as the only tachycardia indicator. An endocardial spring coil electrode was placed at the junction of the superior vena cava with the right atrium, and a left ventricular patch electrode allowed stable lead positioning and adequate defibrillation thresholds. In 1982, R-wave synchronization and a second criterion for tachycardia detection (rate counting with a standard ventricular bipolarplacing catheter) were added, giving the system the capability for cardioversion as well as defibrillation (AICD).[151,194] In October 1985, the AID and AICD devices, which had been limited to a few investigating centers, were released for general (noninvestigational) use by the Food and Drug Administration.[207] Since then, fully integrated circuitry has been added to streamline the manufacturing process, improve generator reliability,[207] and increase availability of the device.[208] Second-generation devices, which allow modification of sensing parameters and defibrillation energy by external programming, were first implanted in 1988 and are now also commercially available. Third-generation devices, which incorporate antitachycardia pacing therapies with those of cardioversion and defibrillation, are currently under investigation, as are systems that can be implanted without the requirement for thoracotomy.[209]

General configuration and function

Defibrillator generator. The defibrillator generator is a large (200 to 240 g) device that consists of sensing circuits, batteries, and energy storage capacitors encased in titanium and hermetically sealed.[210,211] Because the power source must have both low standby power for a long rhythm-monitoring life and a rapidly induced peak output for defibrillation, special lithium batteries characterized by low internal resistance and high-energy density are used. These batteries are capable of charging two capacitors to approximately 700 V in 7 to 9 seconds.[182] With this power source, the implanted defibrillator can generate truncated exponential pulses, which require a lower peak voltage and peak current than other wave forms, in a very short time after the onset of ventricular fibrillation.[212] Second- and third-generation devices also incorporate circuitry for bradycardia pacing backup and antitachycardia pacing.

Lead system. The leads have four basic functions: tachycardia sensing, antitachycardia pacing, shock delivery, and bradycardia pacing. Most currently available (and investigational) systems have two standard epicardial pacing leads and two or three patch electrodes. The leads are used for bradycardia pacing, antitachycardia pacing, and tachycardia sensing, and the patches are used for tachycardia detection and shock delivery.[171]

The patch electrodes have a surface area of 10 to 60 cm^2 and consist of a titanium mesh with a silicone rubber coating.[171,210,213] The shape of the patch varies, although most are either hexagonal or oval.[172] A variety of designs are being investigated, including large, contoured asymmetrical patches that may reduce defibrillation energy requirements. The patch is placed on the epicardial surface either intrapericardially or extrapericardially.[171,209,214] The outer surface of the patch is insulated to enhance current distribution[194] (Fig 25B-21).

In an attempt to eliminate the need for thoracotomy or sternotomy, nonthoracotomy lead systems have been developed and are being investigated. One to three endocardial leads are used for tachycardia detection, bradycardia pacing, antitachycardia pacing, and shock delivery, and a subcutaneous epicostal patch is used for shock delivery.[171,215] Endocardial leads have one or two spring coil electrodes for shock delivery. The subcutaneous patch is structurally identical to the epicardial patches but has a larger surface area[216] (Fig 25B-22).

Sensing function. Two sensing circuits utilize separate sensing algorithms in most implantable defibrillators. The spring coil or patch electrodes are used in some devices to detect QRS morphology as well as to deliver shocks. The morphology-detection channel examines the shape of the differentiated and filtered electrogram. The filtering process eliminates the P- and T-wave electrogram signals and allows primary interrogation of the QRS complex. The morphology-detection criteria are based on the probability density function (PDF). Simply stated, the PDF reflects the amount of time during the cardiac cycle that the ventricular electrogram signals spend near (or, conversely, away from) the zero potential or isoelectric baseline assigned to the P-QRS-T amplitude level. In sinus rhythm and arrhythmias other than ventricular fibrillation, the QRS wave form spends most of its time on the isoelectric segment. In ventricular fibrillation (or coarse ventricular tachycardia), the wave form is away from the baseline a high percentage of time and produces

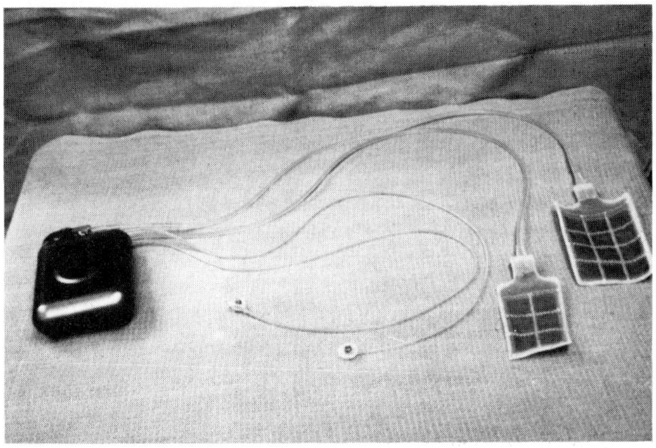

Fig 25B-21 A commercially available implantable cardioverter-defibrillator with defibrillating (patch) electrodes and rate-sensing (standard epicardial pacing) electrodes attached.

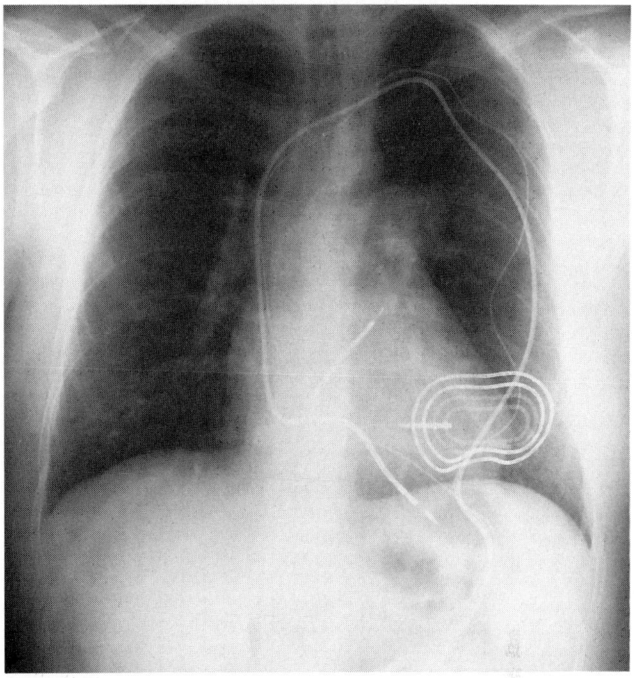

Fig 25B-22 Chest radiograph after implantation of a nonthoracotomy automatic cardioverter-defibrillator system. The system consists of two endocardial leads—one in the right ventricular apex and the other in the coronary sinus—and a subcutaneous patch placed in the anterior axillary line.

a sinusoidal waveform. This satisfies the morphology-sensing criteria that the defibrillator requires to identify a pathologic ventricular arrhythmia[182,203,212,213,217,218] (Fig 25B-23).

Because many persons with ventricular tachycardia have baseline QRS widening secondary to bundle-branch block or intraventricular conduction delays, supraventricular tachycardia may inappropriately satisfy the PDF criteria. In addition, rapid supraventricular tachycardias may also result in QRS widening secondary to aberrant conduction.[210,219] Therefore PDF morphology sensing does not eliminate the possibility of shock delivery during rhythms other than ventricular fibrillation or ventricular tachycardia. Use of the PDF criteria could also prevent the appropriate detection of ventricular tachycardia with a relatively narrow QRS complex and might increase the time required for arrhythmia detection.[208] Consequently, this form of tachycardia detection has largely been abandoned in favor of tiered detection criteria.

A bipolar electrode pair senses ventricular electrograms to determine heart rate and to allow for R-wave synchronization of the generator discharge. The first- and second-generation devices have a single preset or programmable rate criterion that must be exceeded to allow delivery of defibrillatory shocks. The combination of antitachycardia pacing with low- and high-energy cardioversion has expanded the number of clinical situations in which such a device can be used. Thus, third-generation devices make use of a variety of tachycardia detection criteria based on rate, including multiple rate levels (to allow differentiation of slow ventricular tachycardia from rapid ventricular tachycardia or ventricular fibrillation), rate onset, rate stability, and sustained high rate.

The desired goal in the development of implantable antitachycardia devices has been graded or tiered therapy for ventricular tachyarrhythmias. Ideally, a device capable of graded or tiered therapy would treat hemodynamically stable arrhythmias with pacing therapy and reserve shock therapy for tachycardias that are either unresponsive to pacing or hemodynamically unstable.

Tachycardias can be classified into three or more zones defined by two or more preset intervals. Sinus rhythm is defined by any heart rate below a tachycardia detection interval. Ventricular fibrillation (or any rhythm expected to be hemodynamically unstable) can be defined by any heart rate above the fibrillation detection interval. Arrhythmias with heart rates between these two intervals are considered to represent ventricular tachycardia. In addition, the ventricular tachycardia zone can be subdivided by other rate detection levels. Therapies can then be determined for each zone[168,170,171,220] (Fig 25B-24).

Therapy function. Devices that are commercially available have the capacity for low- and high-energy shock delivery. In the future, devices that have concomitant antitachycardia pacing will also be commercially available and will supplant the use of devices with more limited capability.

ANTITACHYCARDIA PACING. The pacing therapies utilized are scanning burst, adaptive burst, and autodecremental (ramp) pacing.[170-172,214,220] Each device has two pacing therapies available, although all make use of autodecremental pacing. Each of the therapies is adaptive and can be tailored to each tachycardia by a variety of programmable features, including the number of sequences per therapy, the number of impulses per sequence, and the degree of interval scanning with each therapy sequence. For example, autodecremental or fixed-interval burst pacing could be used with four total sequences of 10 impulses during each sequence, with each successive sequence of pulse intervals decreasing by a

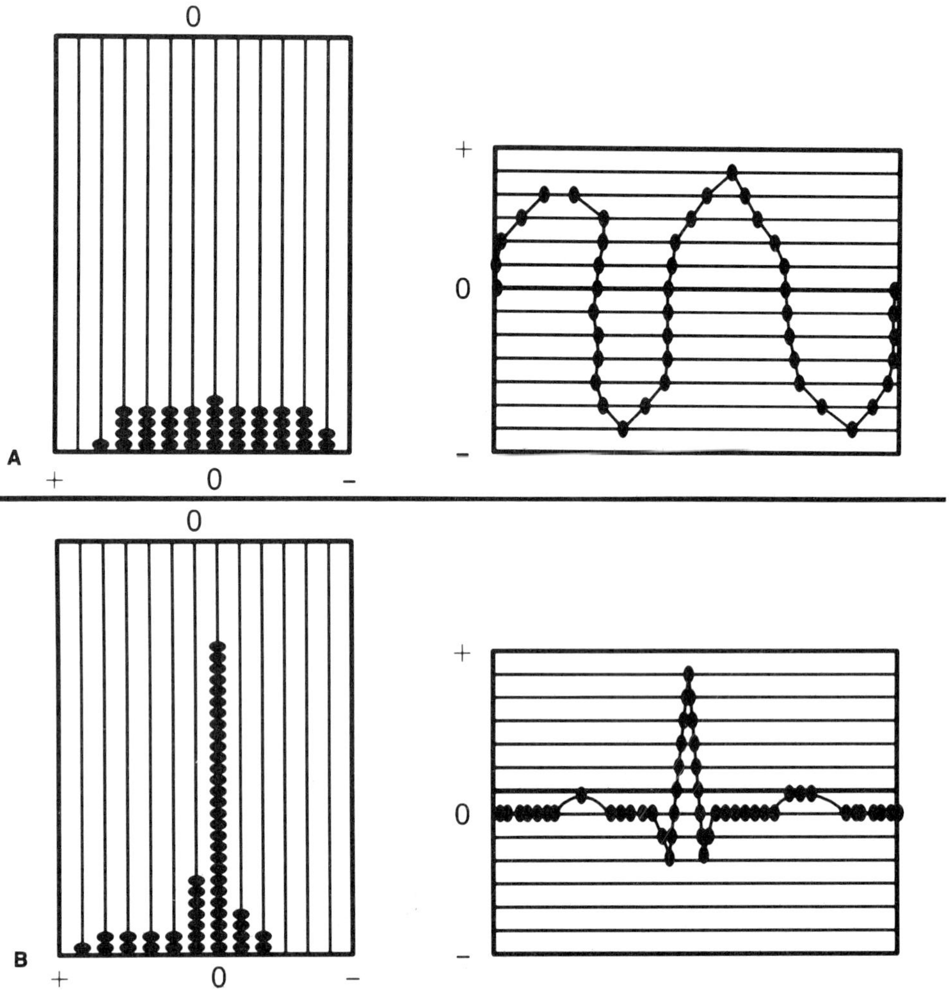

Fig 25B-23 **A,** probability density function of ventricular fibrillation. Left panel, graphic representation of the frequency of the electrogram signals demonstrates that most of the signals do not have zero potential or occur on the isoelectric line. Right panel, electrograms recorded during ventricular fibrillation. **B,** probability density function of a normal ECG. Left panel, change in the orientation of the graph demonstrates the frequency with which signals of different magnitudes occur. During sinus rhythm, most of the electrical signals have zero potential or occur at or near the isoelectric line. Right panel, electrograms recorded during sinus rhythm. Each dot represents a unit of time (ordinate). The abscissa is a measure of the magnitude of the electrical current (positive or negative) with respect to a zero potential or isoelectric line.

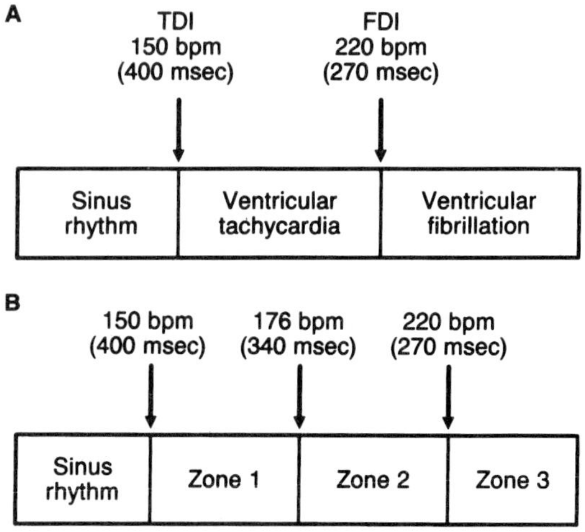

Fig 25B-24 Tachycardia-sensing algorithms. **A,** two rate detection intervals. The TDI (tachycardia detection interval) determines the rate criterion for a pathologic arrhythmia to which the device will respond. The FDI (fibrillation detection interval) can be used to differentiate stable from potentially unstable arrhythmias and results in more aggressive therapies. **B,** three rate detection intervals. Each zone is defined by predetermined rate limits and has its own set of treatment options. This may allow more flexibility in treatment, especially for patients who have multiple ventricular tachyarrhythmias of different rates and hemodynamic stability.

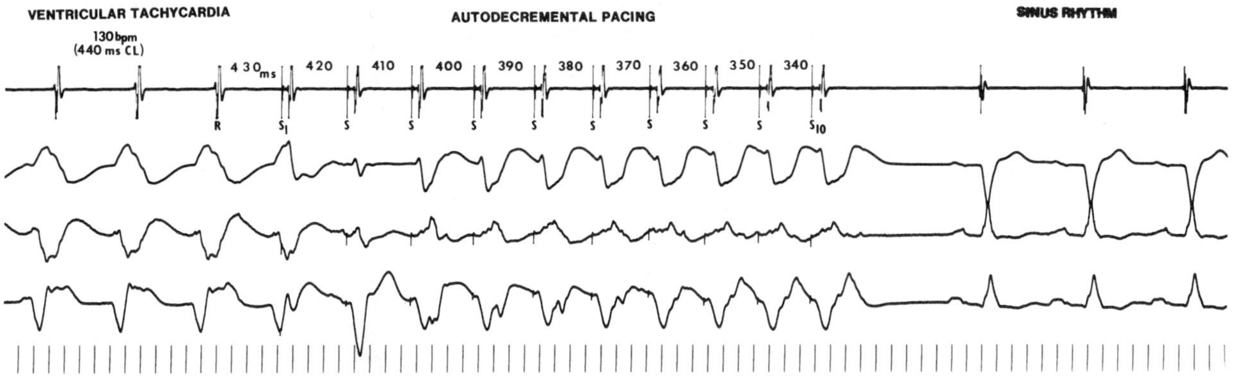

Fig 25B-25 Autodecremental (ramp) pacing: spontaneous ventricular tachycardia at 130 beats/min (440 msec cycle length). Autodecremental pacing therapy is successful. The initial impulse *(S_1)* is delivered at 97% of the tachycardia cycle length, with 10-msec decrements between successive impulses. (From Osborn MJ: Antitachycardia pacing. In *Interventional Cardiology.* Edited by DR Holmes Jr, RE Vlietstra. Philadelphia, FA Davis Company, 1989, pp 266-296. By permission, Mayo Foundation.)

programmed value, e.g., 10 msec, and thereby increasing the pacing rate (Fig 25B-25).

SHOCK THERAPY. The shock energy is delivered as a monophasic or biphasic truncated exponential waveform of 0.2 to 37 J. The energy delivery is programmable to low-energy (cardioversion) or high-energy (defibrillation) levels.

CARDIOVERSION. Any attempt to apply device therapy to all patients with ventricular arrhythmias must deal with the group of patients in whom antitachycardia pacing is ineffective and defibrillation is inappropriate because of hemodynamic stability during the arrhythmia. Low-energy cardioversion may fulfill this purpose.

The use of a transvenous catheter capable of cardioversion and defibrillation was first described in 1981 by Wibel et al.[204,221-223] Initial studies using the catheter coupled with the external defibrillator demonstrated that monomorphic ventricular tachycardia could be converted to sinus rhythm in 62% to 95% of ventricular tachycardia episodes at shock energies of 0.01 to 0.10 J with an associated rate of tachycardia acceleration of 0% to 14%.[222,224-226] The rate of acceleration was very low if the shock could be consistently synchronized to the R wave but much more frequent if it discharged during the ST-T segment.[224] With the same catheter-defibrillator combination, the conversion rate for rapid tachycardias (more than 300 beats/min) and ventricular fibrillation was very low (20% to 39%), even with the use of high energy.

In 1984, the first series of implantations with a fully programmable automatic cardioverter with bradycardia backup was reported. The generator (because of size limitations) could deliver a maximum discharge of 2.0 J. In seven patients with monomorphic ventricular tachycardia, the device successfully terminated most episodes. Complications, reported in 28%, included inappropriate discharge during atrial fibrillation and acceleration of ventricular tachycardia necessitating rescue transthoracic cardioversion. Shocks of 0.5 J were well tolerated by conscious patients.[227] Another study involving a fully implanted system demonstrated consistent success in 82% of patients with use of discharges of 0.2 to 2.0 J. There was no change in sensing capabilities and a modest increase in energy requirement for successful cardioversion noted over a 15-month period of follow-up.[228]

More recent studies have demonstrated similar rates of successful cardioversion (50% to 80% of slow ventricular tachycardia episodes), with acceleration to more unstable arrhythmias in 7.5% to 23% of ventricular tachycardia episodes at discharge energies of 0.5 to 3.0 J with use of transvenous endocardial electrodes (with or without an epicardial or submuscular patch)[150,214,216,222,223,229-231] (Fig 25B-26). The use of epicardial patches for shock delivery may prove to be more efficacious, because in a study of seven patients with slow ventricular tachycardia, all arrhythmia episodes were terminated with 5 J or less when delivery was through two large epicardial patches.[172]

All studies demonstrated that low-energy shock therapy was infrequently successful in converting polymorphic ventricular tachycardia or ventricular fibrillation to sinus rhythm. They also indicated that (1) discharges of greater than 2.5 J were not well tolerated by patients, (2) conversion was successful primarily in patients with relatively slow tachycardias, (3) the success rate for rapid overdrive pacing was similar to that of cardioversion, and (4) low-energy cardioversion resulted in a significant incidence of atrial fibrillation, a phenomenon not seen with antitachycardia pacing.

DEFIBRILLATION. When the rate criterion for ventricular fibrillation or rapid ventricular tachycardia has been satisfied, the defibrillator delivers an electrical shock through the patch or spring coil electrodes in an attempt to restore an effective cardiac rhythm. The device usually requires several seconds to sense the arrhythmia and 5 to 15 seconds to charge the storage capacitors before it delivers a defibrillatory shock of 18 to 37 J. The total elapsed time between onset of arrhythmia and delivery of the first electrical countershock is typically 10 to 35 seconds. If the arrhythmia persists, up to six additional

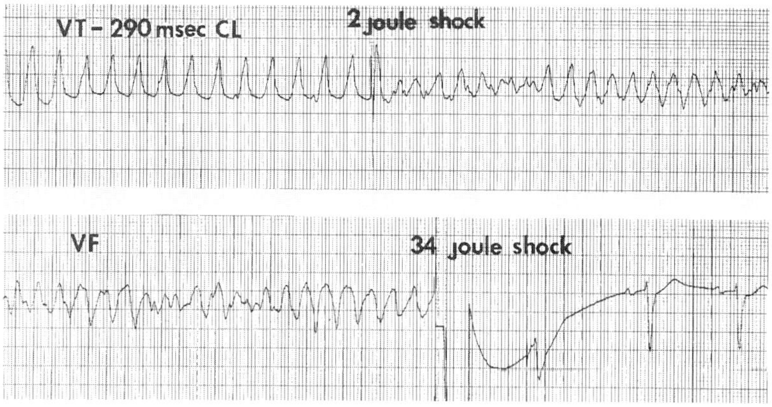

Fig 25B-26 Ventricular tachycardia shock therapy: spontaneous ventricular tachycardia *(VT)* at 290-msec cycle length *(CL)*. The first ventricular tachycardia therapy was a low-energy (2-J) shock that in this case accelerated the arrhythmia to ventricular fibrillation *(VF)*. Ventricular fibrillation therapies one through five were 34-J discharges. The first discharge terminated the arrhythmia.

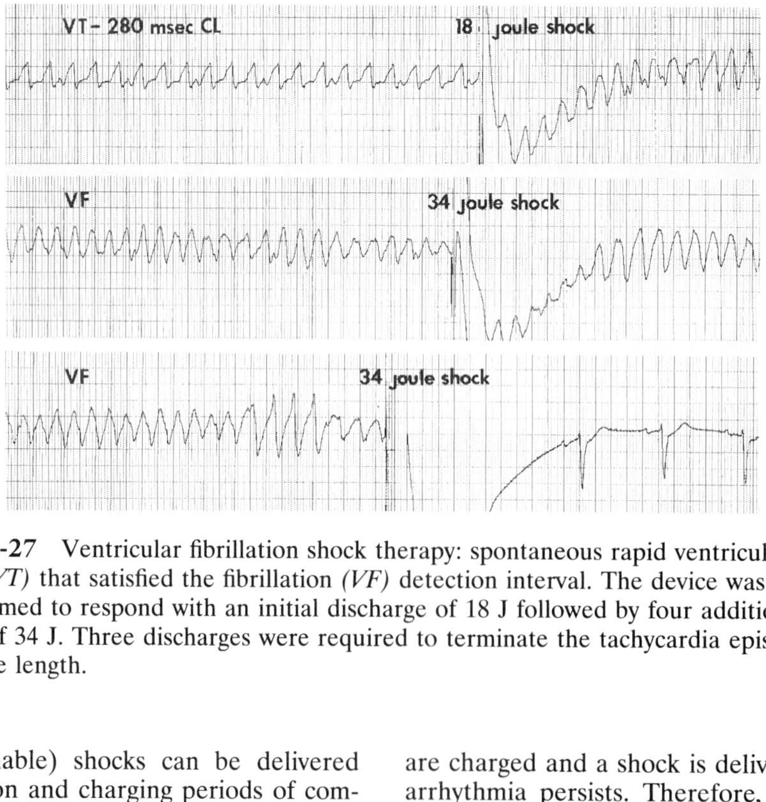

Fig 25B-27 Ventricular fibrillation shock therapy: spontaneous rapid ventricular tachycardia *(VT)* that satisfied the fibrillation *(VF)* detection interval. The device was programmed to respond with an initial discharge of 18 J followed by four additional shocks of 34 J. Three discharges were required to terminate the tachycardia episode. *CL,* cycle length.

high-energy (programmable) shocks can be delivered after additional detection and charging periods of comparable length (Fig 25B-27). After the final discharge, the device remains quiescent despite persistence of arrhythmia. However, after 35 seconds of a rhythm other than the one to which the sensing circuits responded, the pulse generator resets and is then capable of another sequence of high-energy shocks. Rhythms such as heart block, asystole, slower tachycardias, and paced rhythms in addition to sinus rhythm satisfy the 35-second reset.[34,168,170,171,182,212,213,217,220]

Most of the devices respond to ventricular fibrillation in a committed fashion. That is, once an arrhythmia meets the fibrillation detection criterion, the device capacitors are charged and a shock is delivered whether or not the arrhythmia persists. Therefore, these devices have the potential to respond to nonsustained arrhythmias with shock therapy. Some devices are noncommitted. Sensing continues through the period of capacitor charging and for a short time thereafter. No shock is delivered unless the tachycardia persists.[170,214,220]

Devices that use two defibrillating electrodes (patch or spring coil) deliver single shocks from the cathode (negative pole) to the anode (positive pole). Many devices use three defibrillating electrodes (epicardial, endocardial, and epicostal) for energy delivery. In an attempt to reduce the energy requirement for defibrillation, increase pulse generator longevity, and reduce the size of im-

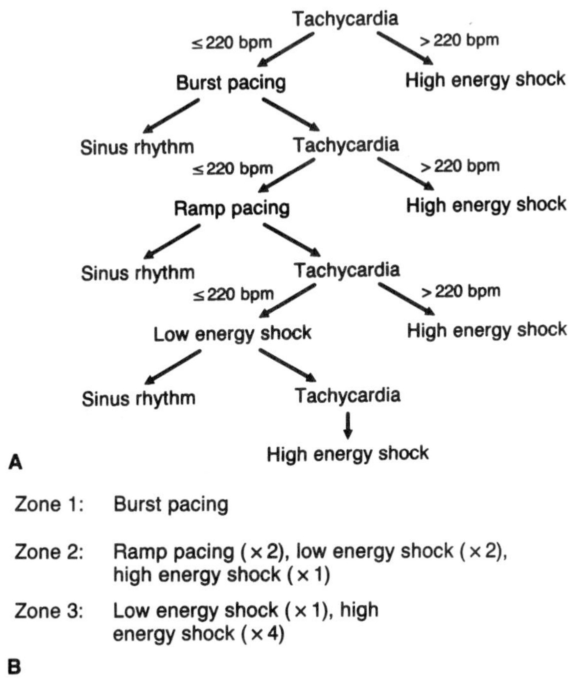

Fig 25B-28 Tachycardia treatment algorithms. **A,** an example of the response to a spontaneous episode of tachycardia by a device with two rate detection criteria (i.e., tachycardia detection interval of 150 beats/min and fibrillation detection interval of 280 beats/min). This device is programmed to respond to tachycardias with rates between 150 and 220 beats/min by a series of therapies—burst pacing followed by ramp pacing and then low- and high-energy shock delivery. Tachycardia episodes exceeding 220 beats/min are treated with high-energy shock delivery. After each delivered therapy, a period of sensing occurs. If the heart rate is < 150 beats/min, no further therapy is delivered. If the rate remains between 150 and 200 beats/min, the next programmed therapy is delivered. If the rate exceeds 220 beats/min, a high-energy shock is delivered. This process continues until the arrhythmia is terminated or all treatment options have been exhausted. **B,** in a device with multiple detection zones, a variety of treatment options are possible. For slow tachycardia (zone 1), therapy can be limited to antitachycardia pacing. For more rapid arrhythmias (with the potential for hemodynamic instability), low- and high-energy shock therapy can be provided in addition to antitachycardia pacing. For very rapid (and likely hemodynamically unstable) tachycardias, very aggressive therapy can be used exclusively.

planted devices, the use of bidirectional discharges (through three electrodes) rather than unidirectional discharges has been carefully investigated. Bidirectional pulses result in less myocardial energy dispersion because their total energy is divided between the pulses, so that the peak current and voltage for each pulse are reduced.[232] The use of two current pathways is likely to increase the volume of myocardium receiving high-current density and thereby facilitate defibrillation[233] and reduce the defibrillation energy requirement.[234]

The two defibrillatory shocks can be delivered simultaneously or sequentially. In a simultaneous discharge, the two shocks are delivered concomitantly over two current pathways by a single common cathode and dual anodes. Sequential pulse defibrillation involves the delivery of pulses of energies over each current pathway temporarily separated by an intershock interval of 0.2 msec.[171,232,235]

A number of studies in animals and humans comparing single and bidirectional shocks demonstrated reductions in energy requirements for defibrillation when the shock was delivered over two pathways.[183,199,233-239] When simultaneous and sequential shocks were compared, there was significant interpatient variability; therefore, the type of energy delivery must be individually tailored.[171] It seems important, however, that the defibrillation energy pass from cathode to anode through the intraventricular septum, because all pathways incorporating the septum have lower defibrillation energy requirements than those that do not.[240]

STAGED OR TIERED THERAPY. A device that allows flexibility in tachycardia detection and offers a variety of tachycardia therapies has a potential for the automatic delivery of tiered therapy based on an individually described therapeutic hierarchy. Antitachycardia pacing could be used for slow and hemodynamically well-tolerated ventricular tachycardia, cardioversion could be used as a therapeutic alternative for ventricular tachycardias that do not respond well to antitachycardia pacing, and defibrillation could be provided as primary therapy for ventricular fibrillation and as a backup for arrhythmia accelerated by pacing or low-energy shock therapy (Fig 25B-28).

Implantation procedure

Lead implantation

ENDOCARDIAL LEADS. Many devices, especially nonthoracotomy lead systems (see below), require implantation of one or more endocardial leads. Standard techniques of subclavian venipuncture and fluoroscopic monitoring of lead positioning, similar to those for pacemaker implantation, are used.

EPICARDIAL LEADS. Three surgical approaches are used for implantation of epicardial or pericardial leads: subxiphoid, left anterolateral thoracotomy, and median sternotomy.

The subxiphoid approach is usually employed in patients without previous cardiac surgery in whom simultaneous heart surgery for other reasons is not contemplated.[168,241-243]

The left anterolateral thoracotomy approach can be used for implantation of a single patch, epicardial leads and a single patch, or a complete epicardial system (i.e., two or three epicardial patches and an epicardial sensing lead).[236,244]

The median sternotomy approach is most commonly used when a defibrillator implantation is combined with cardiac surgery or when two patches are placed.[242] Regardless of the surgical approach, the patch electrodes are placed over the epicardial surface in positions that result in optimal defibrillation thresholds.

MORBIDITY AND COMPLICATIONS. The ultimate decision about the lead system and configuration (Fig 25B-29)

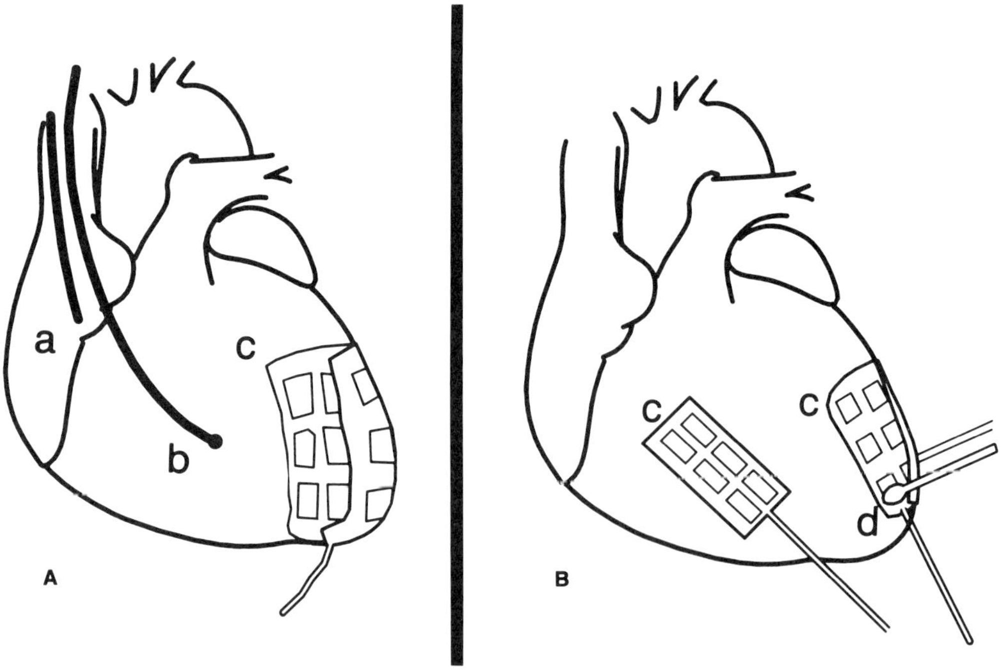

Fig 25B-29 Potential lead configuration for AICD. **A,** superior vena cava spring electrode *(a),* apical patch electrode *(c),* and intravascular bipolar sensing catheter (b). **B,** two epicardial patch electrodes *(c)* and rate-sensing provided by two sutureless screw-in electrodes *(d).* (From Mower MM, Reid PR, Watkins L Jr, et al: Automatic implantable cardioverter-defibrillator structural characteristics. *PACE* 7:1331-1337, 1984. By permission of Futura Publishing Company.)

depends on the adequacy of defibrillation thresholds (see below). However, issues of operative morbidity and system complications related to the type of procedure may have a bearing on patient management. For example, the incidence of pulmonary complications (pneumonia and pleural effusion) and localized wound sepsis is much higher with thoracotomy and median sternotomy than with a subxiphoid approach.[245,246] Pericarditis (acute and chronic) is more common when two patches are used.[247] Problems such as venous thrombosis, lead migration, and lead dislodgment are seen almost exclusively in systems utilizing endocardial leads.[171,182,246,248]

Generator implantation. Because of the large size of the generator and the necessity for placement of at least one lead on the surface of the heart, the pulse generator is implanted in the abdomen. A subcutaneous or submuscular pocket is developed in the left periumbilical region, and electrodes are tunneled subcutaneously into the pocket and connected to the generator.[242] Our practice is to tunnel the endocardial leads from the chest incision to the generator in the same fashion.

Intraoperative testing

Defibrillation threshold. The most important aspect of defibrillator implantation is determination that the system will respond to the patient's arrhythmia and convert it to sinus rhythm. This is accomplished by evaluation of the defibrillation threshold (DFT).

Defibrillation is related to the delivery of current density (for a sufficient period) adequate to depolarize a critical mass of the myocardium.[202] The DFT is defined as the minimum energy required to defibrillate the heart to sinus rhythm.[182,229]

The technique for determining DFT involves induction of ventricular fibrillation (and ventricular tachycardia if clinically indicated) and measurement of the amount of energy delivered through the defibrillation electrodes to terminate the arrhythmia. A major factor in achieving an acceptable DFT is the output delivery capacity of the generator. A generator whose capacity is exceeded by the DFT will not successfully defibrillate if it is implanted.[206]

A study of 33 patients attempted to determine the relation between intraoperative DFT and successful termination of postoperative inducible ventricular fibrillation.[249] In 55% of this group, the intraoperative DFT was 15 J or lower, and in the postoperative period, ventricular fibrillation was successfully terminated by the implanted defibrillator in all cases. However, in patients with an acute DFT of 20 J or higher, the rate of successful defibrillation was only 73%. In all patients without successful defibrillation, the difference between the DFT and the AICD energy output was 10 J or less.[249] This and similar observations have led to the recommendation that a DFT of 18 J or lower is optimal and acceptable without lead modification.[168,171,172,236] DFTs higher than 18 J would be considered acceptable by some if 25 J was always successful, 20 J was nearly uniformly successful, and 15 J was effective 50% of the time.[246,250] Others have stated that a safety margin of at least 10 J between the DFT and defibrillator output is required.[251]

If the initial DFT is not acceptable, some modification in the system will be required. Factors that should be taken into consideration when DFTs are unacceptable include left ventricular mass,[252] cardiomegaly (associated with increased thresholds),[229,253] lead configuration and orientation,[203,254] and concomitant drug therapy.[251,253] A comparison of the acute DFTs in patients with a spring coil and left ventricular patch configuration and in those with two ventricular patches demonstrated a mean DFT of 19 J in the former group and 9 J in the latter.[253] Thus, in patients with a spring coil and patch lead configuration in whom acute DFTs are unacceptable, a switch to a two-patch system (especially two large patches) often results in acceptable DFTs.[210,213,250,254]

Several options are available if DFTs remain high: changing the polarity of the defibrillating electrodes, repositioning endocardial or epicardial leads, adding a third electrode (usually an epicardial patch electrode), and implanting the lead system that gives the best DFTs (without generator implantation) and then reevaluating with threshold testing 7 to 15 days after surgery.[172,210,213,236,250,255] One study reported experience with six patients in whom no DFT less than 40 J could be obtained at initial implantation with any patch configuration. Half the patients had concomitant cardiopulmonary bypass procedures, and prolonged testing was precluded in all the patients because of hemodynamic compromise. All patches were placed in an anterior (right ventricular) and posterior (left ventricular) configuration arbitrarily. After 10 to 15 days, the DFTs were checked through the patches, and in all patients adequate DFTs were obtained (mean, 18 J).[256]

The concomitant use of antiarrhythmic agents, especially amiodarone,[243,253] can significantly alter acute DFTs. In a group of 42 patients, the DFTs were significantly higher in those taking amiodarone. In another group of 97 patients, 5% had an acute DFT greater than 25 J. All these patients were taking amiodarone, and 75% of those in whom administration of the drug was discontinued had acceptable DFTs on repeat testing within 6 to 10 weeks.[236] In other studies, however, no difference in DFTs was found between patients receiving amiodarone and those not receiving the drug.[257] If acceptable acute defibrillation thresholds cannot be achieved in patients receiving amiodarone, leads should be implanted without generator implantation and DFT tests repeated several weeks after discontinuation of the drug.[213]

Because of the time required for arrhythmia detection and capacitor charging before the defibrillation shock is delivered, questions have been raised about the effect of the duration of ventricular fibrillation on defibrillation efficacy. Animal studies suggest that there is an increase in acute DFT with increasing arrhythmia duration.[258] In a study of 10 survivors of out-of-hospital cardiac arrest, however, there was no statistical difference in DFT between ventricular fibrillation of 10 seconds' and that of 20 seconds' duration.[259] It is recommended that at least 10 to 15 seconds elapse between the onset of ventricular tachycardia or fibrillation and any attempted defibrillation because of the delays in response adherent in AICD function.[229,260,261] In a study of 11 patients in whom the AICD functioned to terminate spontaneous or induced ventricular tachycardia or fibrillation, the average time from arrhythmia onset to defibrillation was 18 seconds (range, 14 to 22 seconds), confirming the appropriateness of this time delay.[262]

Serial DFTs obtained over 25 months increased from 12.3 J to 16.9 J in one study, but the increase was significant only in patients receiving amiodarone (10.9 J to 20 J). In patients who were not taking amiodarone, the mean DFT decreased with time.[253] In a study comparing DFTs at implantation with those at elective replacement of the pulse generator, there was no change in the majority, reduction in some, and an increase of no more than 5 J in the rest.[229] In the large experience at Stanford University, fewer than 1% of 270 patients had late increases in DFTs.[250] This result is very reassuring but does not imply that careful evaluation of the lead system at pulse generator replacement is unnecessary.

A margin of safety also should be provided for the rate-detection criterion. If the ability to sense R waves during tachycardia is inadequate, lead revision may be required. Additionally, the rate of any inducible ventricular tachyarrhythmias must exceed the generator rate criterion. For polymorphic ventricular tachycardia, the rate should be at least 30 beats/min faster than the rate criterion, and for monomorphic ventricular tachycardia, at least 10 beats/min faster.[213]

Equipment and technique. The implantation of an AICD requires the cooperative effort of surgeons, a cardiac electrophysiologist, and experienced technical staff. The equipment required for implantation includes ECG monitoring leads (placed in such a way as not to interfere with external defibrillation), high-energy external defibrillation capacity (for use if internal defibrillation fails), an electrophysiologic recorder and stimulator, the AICD generator and appropriate leads, special cables for all the connections, and the proper device programmer for defibrillation threshold determination and generator evaluation.

After implantation, the leads are connected to the programmer. Ventricular tachycardia or ventricular fibrillation is induced by programmed ventricular stimulation or ventricular ramp (rapid accelerating) pacing. If this is not successful, ventricular fibrillation is induced by a standard AC fibrillator.[246,263] After 15 to 20 seconds, a shock is delivered by the programmer through the implanted leads in an attempt to convert the arrhythmia to sinus rhythm (Table 25B-9).

The programmer delivers a truncated exponential shock wave identical to the AICD waveform and has adjustable outputs from 0.5 to 40 J.[253] Usually, the initial energy delivered is 18 J, and if this is successful, the arrhythmia is reinduced and the shock therapy is maintained or decreased. Three successful defibrillations at an energy delivery of 18 J or less are required before a lead configuration is accepted. If an attempt is not success-

Table 25B-9 Determination of defibrillation threshold

Defibrillation and placement of sensing electrodes
Initiation of clinical tachycardia (and ventricular fibrillation)
Defibrillation attempted at 18 J
  If successful, repeat at same or decreased energy
  If not successful, rescue at 40 J
Defibrillation thresholds acceptable if ≤ 18 J
If not acceptable
  Lead modification
  No AICD implant

ful, it should be followed by a high-energy rescue shock delivered through the patches or by external defibrillation.[171,172,221,229]

Determining the defibrillation threshold in all patients is important, even if the clinical arrhythmia is ventricular tachycardia, because of the potential for acceleration or degeneration of ventricular tachycardia by discharges of any energy level.[210,229] Ventricular tachycardia cardioversion thresholds can also be determined if testing is clinically indicated.[171,172]

After DFT with an adequate margin of safety has been identified, a generator is connected to the implanted leads. Inactive when shipped from the manufacturer, the generator should be activated by programmer application and tested with the use of the programmer.[264,265] It should then be deactivated before attachment to the leads. After lead attachment and placement of the generator into the subcutaneous pocket, it is placed in a standby mode to allow reinitiation of ventricular fibrillation by programmed ventricular stimulation or an AC fibrillator. The arrhythmia is then reinduced, and the AICD is allowed (by programming) to automatically sense and terminate the arrhythmia (Fig 25B-30). If the AICD successfully terminates the arrhythmia, it is again deactivated and the operation completed. We routinely wait until the day after surgery (or until any postoperative arrhythmias are controlled) before reactivating the device.

Clinical experience

In 1985 (before Food and Drug Administration release of defibrillators for noninvestigational use), 400 devices had been implanted worldwide.[208] By 1988, approximately 4,000 devices had been implanted, and as of June 1990, more than 12,000 patients had received implantable defibrillators of all types.[190,209]

Worldwide experience confirms the profound effect that the implantable defibrillator has had on sudden death and total mortality in patients at very high risk. Individual studies report the rate of sudden death in patients with implantable devices to be 0 to 2% at 1 year, 3% to 10% at 3 years, and 3% to 20% at 5 years. Pooled data from more than 10,000 patients yield a sudden death rate of 1.6% at 1 year, 3% at 3 years, and 4.5% at 5 years. The extrapolated rate of sudden death without a device (assuming that the first defibrillation implies that sudden death would have occurred) is approximately 25% at 1 year and 40% at 3 and 5 years. The reported overall rate of defibrillator discharges is 44% to 70%, with most occurring in response to ventricular tachycardia or ventricular fibrillation. The vast majority of patients who receive shocks experience their first shock within the first year after implantation.[48] The total mortality in this group of patients remains high despite defibrillator implantation, varying from 5% to 20% at 1 year to 22% to 47% at 5 years, but it is significantly improved over anticipated rates.[236,243,246,266-272] Most deaths are cardiac in origin, but most are not sudden and are secondary to heart failure or electromechanical dissociation.[136,250]

The benefits of the implanted defibrillator are applied to the elderly as well as young patients and to patients with significant reductions in left ventricular function. In a study of 133 patients, 40% of whom were older than 65, there was no difference in the survival rates at 1 year and 3 years at any age.[273] Three studies evaluated the benefits of defibrillator implantation in patients with left ventricular ejection fractions of less than 30%. The projected mortality in these patients was 70%, 79%, and 90% at 1, 2, and 3 years, respectively, whereas the actual mortality was 23%, 28%, and 35%, an indication that defibrillator implantation can have a major impact on the survival of patients with poor left ventricular function.[274-276]

The clinical experience with third-generation devices (i.e., those with the capability of treating a variety of ventricular arrhythmias with antitachycardia pacing, low-energy cardioversion, and high-energy defibrillation) has also been excellent. The overall success in the management of ventricular tachycardia and ventricular fibrillation episodes has been 97% to 100%.[170,214] When antitachycardia pacing was the first therapy (in a tiered hierarchy of therapies), the success rate was 51% to 93%. Likewise, when cardioversion was used in a similar fashion, 70% to 100% of ventricular tachycardia episodes were terminated. Ventricular tachycardia accelerated by antitachycardia pacing or cardioversion, rapid primary ventricular tachycardia, and primary ventricular fibrillation episodes were successfully terminated by high-energy shock therapy in all cases.[168-172,214] Rates of total mortality and sudden death mortality are comparable to those reported for pure defibrillators.

Not only does device implantation influence mortality but also it allows most patients to resume a fairly normal lifestyle and prevents (or reduces) hospital intensive care readmission.[254,277] Thus, the device has clearly proved itself an extremely effective therapeutic tool in the management of patients at risk of sudden death.

Indications and contraindications

At present, the indications for implantation of an AICD (with or without antitachycardia capability) include patients with spontaneous ventricular tachycardia or ventricular fibrillation in whom (1) no other therapy is successful by virtue of drug inefficacy or patient intolerance or noncompliance, (2) surgical or ablation therapy is

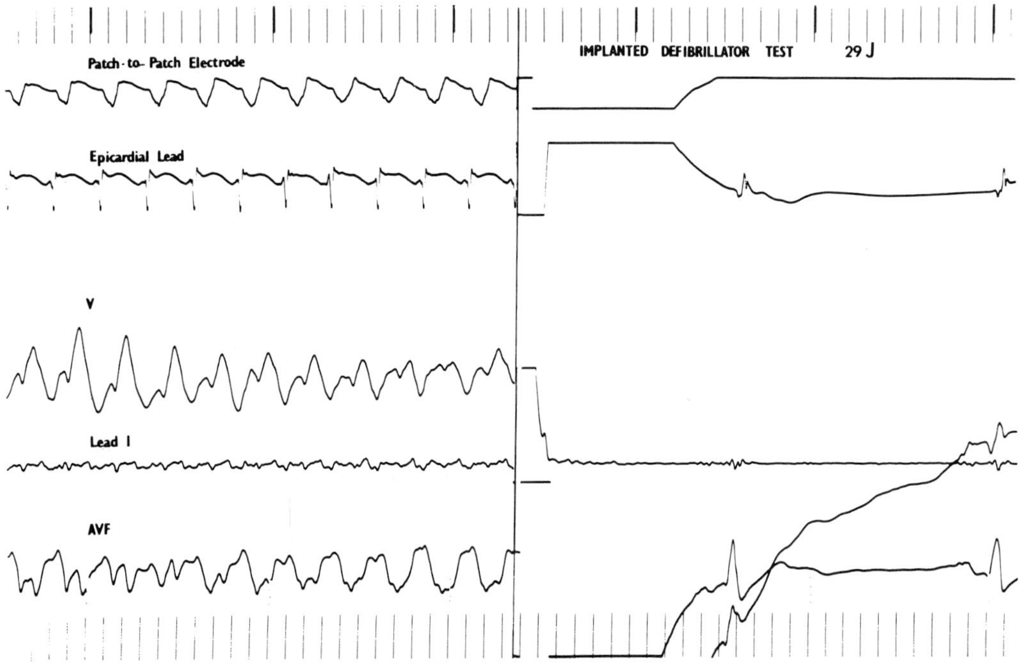

Fig 25B-30 Termination of ventricular fibrillation in the operating room by the AICD. This is the final stage in the process of intraoperative evaluation of defibrillation thresholds.

contraindicated or ineffective, or (3) no satisfactory end point exists to judge therapeutic efficacy (e.g., out-of-hospital cardiac arrest in a patient who has no arrhythmia inducible by electrophysiologic testing).[182,213,254,278,279] In the third group of patients, the use of implantable defibrillators has been associated with appropriate device discharges in response to life-threatening arrhythmia in 15%.[280]

Device implantation is a treatment option in patients with syncope of unknown origin who have clinically relevant ventricular tachycardia or ventricular fibrillation induced at electrophysiologic study and in whom antiarrhythmic therapy is limited by drug inefficacy, intolerance, or noncompliance.[279] These devices can be used as adjuncts to other forms of therapy, especially in patients who have had out-of-hospital cardiac arrest and are undergoing coronary artery bypass graft surgery or subendocardial resection, or both.[281] Of 23 patients with out-of-hospital cardiac arrest who had combined coronary artery bypass graft surgery and AICD implantation, 35% had a defibrillator resuscitation in a mean follow-up period of 24 months.[191]

Despite undergoing subendocardial resection, some patients do not have adequate arrhythmia control, even with drug therapy.[127,281] In patients with multiple infarct scars, multiple tachycardia morphologies, and multifocal or very rapid tachycardia, the chances of recurrent arrhythmias are as high as 25% to 38%.[282-284] AICDs implanted at the time of subendocardial resection have been successful in a small but significant population[282,284,285] (Table 25B-10). Device implantation has been used very successfully in patients with a history of ventricular tachycardia or ventricular fibrillation who are awaiting cardiac transplantation. In this group, the incidence of recurrent arrhythmias is exceedingly high in the short term, and AICD implantation represents a very efficacious means of aborting sudden death and serving as a bridge to transplantation.[286]

Table 25B-10 Candidates for AICD implantation

- Patients resuscitated from one or more episodes of cardiac arrest in whom
  - No effective drug therapy can be identified by serial drug testing
  - No arrhythmias can be induced at initial electrophysiologic testing
  - Drug therapy is not efficacious because of intolerance or noncompliance
- Patients with hemodynamically unstable ventricular tachycardia in whom drug therapy is ineffective
- Patients with syncope of unknown origin and inducible ventricular arrhythmias in whom drug therapy is ineffective

Instead of implantation of a complete AICD system, defibrillator patches can be placed at the time of cardiac surgery in patients at risk for postoperative arrhythmia (i.e., patients who survive out-of-hospital cardiac arrest and who have coronary artery bypass graft surgery

Table 25B-11 Complications of AICD use

Related to surgical procedure
Operative and perioperative mortality
Pneumonia
Pleural effusion
Infection
Postoperative arrhythmia
Related to leads
Dislodgment
Migration
Fracture
Insulation defect
Coronary artery erosion
Thrombosis formation
Pericarditis
Related to generator
Component failure
Premature battery depletion
Capacitor deformation
Related to defibrillation
Myocardial fibrosis or necrosis
Inappropriate discharges

performed before formal drug testing directed by electrophysiologic testing is done).[281] Although prophylactic patch implantation has the theoretical advantage of avoidance of a second major surgical procedure, it must be weighed against the possibility of complication (infection, primarily) and therefore should not be done routinely.

Absolute contraindications to AICD implantation are recent acute myocardial infarction; severe heart failure or other diseases in patients whose lives would not be significantly prolonged by AICD implantation; ventricular arrhythmias secondary to electrolyte imbalance, drug toxicity, electrocution, or drowning; and emotional or psychiatric disorders that might be aggravated by AICD implantation or discharges.[213,254] Relative contraindications to defibrillator implantation might include frequent episodes of ventricular tachycardia, which lead to frequent triggering of the device and rapid battery depletion, and episodes of supraventricular tachycardia or nonsustained ventricular tachycardia, which place the patient at the risk of defibrillator discharge while awake. However, with the capacity for antitachycardia pacing and cardioversion therapies for ventricular tachycardia as well as improved arrhythmia detection algorithms, these clinical situations are less a problem now than in the past.

Complications

The use of implantable defibrillators is associated with a variety of potential problems. The reported total complication rates vary from 12% to 51%.[246,261,267] Many complications reflect the fact that this is a new and rapidly evolving therapeutic technology that until relatively recently was purely investigational (Table 25B-11).

Surgical complications. The operative and perioperative mortality related to device implantation is approximately 3% in the worldwide experience.[168,182,190,236,243,246,250,267,270,272,284,285,287-290] If AICD implantation is combined with coronary artery bypass graft surgery or subendocardial resection, the mortality increases to 10% to 14%.[271,281,282,285]

The most common complications related to the surgical procedures are pulmonary (pneumonia or symptomatic pleural effusion); these occur in 20% to 30% of cases and are most common with a left anterior thoracotomy approach.[236,246] Symptomatic acute pericarditis occurs in about 3% of patients.[236] Constrictive pericarditis secondary to marked fibrosis around the patch electrodes is very uncommon but has required pericardial stripping in isolated cases.[247,262] Infection is a serious problem, although the incidence has been very low (0 to 2% worldwide). Onset may be delayed and insidious, and management requires explantation of the entire system.[182,190,213,236,246,250,260,291] Since early postoperative arrhythmias, such as atrial fibrillation and ventricular tachycardia, are observed in about 20% of patients and may result in defibrillator discharge,[236] AICDs should not be activated until after the early postoperative period.

Lead problems. Complications related to the leads are similar to those experienced with pacemakers. Lead dislodgment, migration, fracture, and insulation defects are the most common abnormalities (Fig 25B-31). The reported incidence varies from 1.5% to 33%[182,190,213,246,250,260,261] and is significantly higher for the endocardial defibrillating electrodes than for the patch or rate-sensing electrode.[215,246,250,260] Epicardial patches have rarely caused coronary artery erosion, atrial laceration, or local pericarditis,[246,281] and in the vast majority of cases, there have been no documented significant alterations of global or regional left ventricular function related to the use of the patches.[288]

Generator problems. The most common complications related to the implanted generator are electronic component failure, premature battery depletion, and capacitor deformation. The incidence of these complications (especially of premature battery depletion) was quite high with first- and second-generation devices (13% to 26%),[136,190,267,292] but with generators currently available for clinical use, the incidence is less than 1%.[190]

In addition to the complications noted above, some generator features are considered to be major limitations of AICD use, including large size, limited battery longevity, absence of reliable end-of-life indicators, and expense.[280,291,293,294]

Pathologic changes secondary to device use. Histopathologic evaluation of the heart, lungs, and great vessels of humans and animals in whom defibrillators have been implanted demonstrates a variety of abnormalities. Localized pericarditis and fibrosis surrounding implanted patches occur in all patients. Thrombus formation is associated with the spring-coil electrodes in 17% and to a much lesser extent with the rate-sensing electrodes.

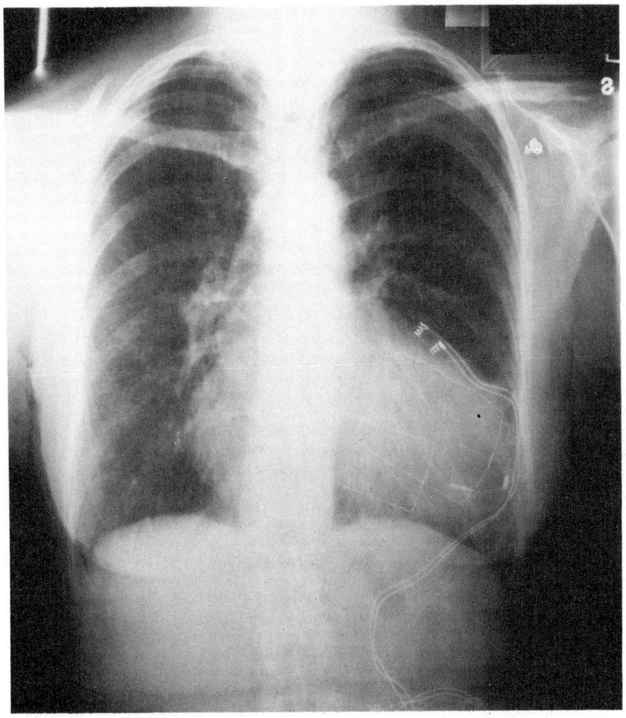

Fig 25B-31 Complete disruption of the defibrillator leads secondary to trauma.

Table 25B-12 Causes of inappropriate defibrillation discharges

Supraventricular tachycardia
Paroxysmal supraventricular tachycardia
Sinus tachycardia
Atrial fibrillation-flutter
Nonsustained ventricular tachycardia
Sensing lead fracture
Lead migration
Pacemaker action
Oversensing of cardiac or extracardiac electrical activity
Misdirected test discharge
Pulse generator abnormalities
Unknown

Asymptomatic pulmonary embolism has been noted in 8% of necropsies.[295,296]

Abnormalities related to defibrillation consist primarily of mild contraction band necrosis, fibrosis, and loss of myocytes in the myocardium under the patch electrode or adjacent to the implanted catheter electrodes.[248,296] Clinically, defibrillation testing and spontaneous device discharge are not associated with evidence of myocardial damage (creatine kinase release or pyrophosphate scanning) unless multiple discharges occur in very rapid succession.[222] Transient nonspecific ST-T changes have been demonstrated in 43% of patients in response to device testing or spontaneous discharges.[214,297]

Inappropriate defibrillator discharge. An inappropriate (also called "spurious" or "problematic") discharge is one that is documented as such by monitor or one that is not associated with a clinical event. The occurrence of these inappropriate shocks is a major clinical problem because of the discomfort associated with the discharge and the potential for triggering a lethal arrhythmia[182,260,298] (Table 25B-12).

Inappropriate discharges are frequent, accounting for 8% to 42% of all generator discharges.[182,236,246,250,292,295] The most common causes of inappropriate defibrillator discharge are supraventricular tachycardia (including sinus tachycardia and atrial fibrillation) that exceeds the tachycardia rate criterion of the defibrillator, nonsustained ventricular tachycardia, and clinical situations in which a shock is delivered for unclear reasons while the patient is awake and asymptomatic.[137,236,246,250,299,300]

Nonsustained ventricular tachycardia can present an especially difficult problem. Spontaneous complex ventricular ectopy (including nonsustained ventricular tachycardia) is common in patients who survive out-of-hospital cardiac arrest. If the episodes are long enough to be sensed by the generator but are self-terminating and not associated with hemodynamic collapse, they can result in unpleasant defibrillator discharges. This is a problem primarily in systems with committed cardioversion or defibrillator function, or both. Sensing algorithms that are noncommitted require arrhythmia reconfirmation before any therapy is delivered.[279]

Other, less common, causes of inappropriate discharges are afterpotential sensing caused by lead fracture, lead migration, interaction with pacemakers (especially double counting of a pacemaker stimulus and the evoked QRS complex), T-wave oversensing (sensing of both the QRS and the T-wave signals may exceed the rate cutoff),[301] pulse generator abnormalities, and misdirection of test shocks to the patient rather than to the internal resistor.[137,190,236,246,250,302,303]

Before implantation of the defibrillator, extensive monitoring during rest, normal ambulation, and formal exercise testing should be carried out to evaluate each patient for the possibility of inappropriate triggering of the AICD. Frequent episodes of supraventricular tachycardia, atrial fibrillation, or nonsustained ventricular tachycardia may exclude a patient as a candidate for defibrillator therapy and can certainly identify patients who will require concomitant antiarrhythmic drug therapy. Excessive exercise heart rate may require exercise limitations or the addition of β-blockade.

It is often very difficult to ascertain whether a given device discharge was appropriate and in response to sustained ventricular tachycardia or fibrillation. The hemodynamic status of the patient does not always differentiate between supraventricular tachycardia and ventricular tachycardia, since a significant percentage of patients do not experience syncope before an appropriate discharge.[304] The pattern of shock therapy may be helpful, because a single discharge is usually in response to ventricular tachycardia, whereas multiple discharges or grouped discharges as a result of device recycling often occur in response to atrial fibrillation or other supraventricular tachycardias.[305]

```
TELEMETRY
---------
 PERM TELEMETRY ENABLE          OFF HRS
 TELEMETRY TYPE                 MRKR


DATA
----
 DEVICE STATUS:
  MEMORY RETENTION OK
  CHARGE CIRCUIT                 OK
  LAST CHARGE TIME              0.24 SEC
  BATTERY VOLTAGE               6.26 V
  BATTERY OK

 VT ONSET COUNTER               2410

 VT EPISODE AND THERAPY DATA:
  EPISODE COUNT                   7
  VT THERAPY #1 SUCCESS COUNT     7
  VT THERAPY #2 SUCCESS COUNT     0
  VT THERAPY #3 SUCCESS COUNT     0
  VT THERAPY #4 SUCCESS COUNT     0
  # OF VT'S INEFFECTIVE           0
  DEVICE EFFICACIOUS ON LAST VT YES
  LAST THERAPY USED              #1
  #SEQ IN LAST PACE THERAPY       2
  R-R AVG FOR LAST PACE THRPY   430 MS


 VF EPISODE AND THERAPY DATA:
  EPISODE COUNT                   0
  VF THERAPY #1 SUCCESS COUNT     0
  VF THERAPY #2 SUCCESS COUNT     0
  VF THERAPY #3 SUCCESS COUNT     0
  VF THERAPY #4 SUCCESS COUNT     0
  # OF VF'S INEFFECTIVE           0
  DEVICE EFFICACIOUS ON LAST VF ---
  LAST THERAPY USED             NONE
```

```
LAST EPISODE DETECTION SEQUENCE:
 -19. R-R INTERVAL- 440 MS
 -18. R-R INTERVAL- 430 MS
 -17. R-R INTERVAL- 430 MS
 -16. R-R INTERVAL- 430 MS
 -15. R-R INTERVAL- 440 MS
 -14. R-R INTERVAL- 430 MS
 -13. R-R INTERVAL- 420 MS
 -12. R-R INTERVAL- 430 MS
 -11. R-R INTERVAL- 430 MS
 -10. R-R INTERVAL- 430 MS
  -9. R-R INTERVAL- 430 MS
  -8. R-R INTERVAL- 430 MS
  -7. R-R INTERVAL- 430 MS
  -6. R-R INTERVAL- 430 MS
  -5. R-R INTERVAL- 440 MS
  -4. R-R INTERVAL- 430 MS
  -3. R-R INTERVAL- 420 MS
  -2. R-R INTERVAL- 430 MS
  -1. R-R INTERVAL- 430 MS
  -0. R-R INTERVAL- 440 MS
  -0. VT DETECTED


EVENTS AFTER LAST THERAPY:
  +0. VT THERAPY #1 DELIVERED
  +1. R-R INTERVAL- 1000 MS
  +2. R-R INTERVAL- 860 MS
  +3. R-R INTERVAL- 860 MS
  +4. R-R INTERVAL- 860 MS
  +5. R-R INTERVAL- 800 MS
  +6. R-R INTERVAL- 860 MS
  +7. R-R INTERVAL- 860 MS
  +8. R-R INTERVAL- 860 MS
  +9. R-R INTERVAL- 860 MS
 +10. R-R INTERVAL- 760 MS
 +10. THERAPY WAS SUCCESSFUL
```

Fig 25B-32 Follow-up evaluation of a patient with an implanted cardioverter-defibrillator for treatment of recurrent ventricular tachycardia. The device was capable of two levels of therapy: zone 1, or ventricular tachycardia (480 to 330 msec, 125 to 200 beats/min), and zone 2, or ventricular fibrillation ($<$300 msec, $<$200 beats/min). The patient reported seven episodes of near-syncope, confirmed as ventricular tachycardia *(VT)* by the device. Ventricular tachycardia therapy #1 (in this case, ramp pacing) was successful in all episodes. There were no episodes of ventricular fibrillation *(VF)* or tachycardias with rates $<$200 beats/min during the period of observation. The last episode of tachycardia to which the device responded was a stable arrhythmia at a cycle length of 420 to 430 msec. Immediately after therapy was delivered, the rate slowed and therapy was interpreted as successful.

Patient evaluation is mandatory when the cause of device discharge is unclear. Third-generation devices have memory and telemetry function of different levels of sophistication. All provide a log of the number of tachycardia events detected, the therapies delivered, and the response of the arrhythmia to those therapies (success or failure). Some provide more detailed information about the last therapy detected by indicating the heart rate immediately before, during, and after the tachycardia episode. From this information, the mechanism of the arrhythmia can be inferred by rate, regularity, and type of therapy given (Fig 25B-32). Other devices provide electrograms from every tachycardia episode along with a record of therapy and results.[168,170,171,219,220] This capability obviously makes patient evaluation easier, but in many instances the mechanism of tachycardias leading to device therapy remains unclear. In these situations, electrophysiologic assessment may be required.[172]

Interaction with pacemakers. Some patients who need an AICD also require cardiac pacing to treat symptomatic bradycardia, to prevent bradycardia that occurs after defibrillation, to provide a rate floor to reduce the frequency of bradycardia-related ventricular arrhythmias, or to terminate arrhythmias by antitachycardia pacing.[71,72] The problems that can result from the concomitant use of defibrillators and pacemakers are shown in Table 25B-13.

During ventricular fibrillation, pacemaker undersensing may occur, resulting in inappropriate pacing function. The defibrillator may in turn sense the pacemaker spikes, ignore ventricular fibrillation, and fail to deliver defibrillatory shocks.[182] Inappropriate oversensing of pacemaker

Table 25B-13 Pacemaker and AICD interactions

Pacemaker undersensing of ventricular fibrillation, resulting in inappropriate pacemaker function
Double counting of pacemaker stimuli and extracardiac electrograms
Postdefibrillation changes in pacing or sensing variables
Defibrillation discharge during pacemaker magnet or programmer application
Pacemaker malfunction after defibrillation

Table 25B-14 Drug effects that may alter AICD function

Alteration of QRS morphology
Alteration of tachycardia cycle length
Conversion of sustained ventricular tachycardia to nonsustained ventricular tachycardia
Alterations in defibrillation threshold

spikes, especially in dual-chamber pacing systems, may lead to device discharge.[213] Because these complications are most likely to occur with unipolar pacing systems, they should not be implanted in patients with defibrillators.[182,246] In patients who require concomitant pacing, the potential for inappropriate pacemaker-device interaction should be evaluated at the time of device implantation.[182,213,301]

Pacemaker noncapture has been reported after spontaneous high-energy defibrillation discharges.[301,306] In addition, total pacemaker system failure has been reported after defibrillation in a patient with an endocardial defibrillating catheter placed in close proximity to a preexisting pacemaker lead.[215] The potential for postshock bradycardia (reported in up to 20% of patients) and the ability of an implanted pacemaker to reliably capture during this period should be evaluated.[220,279,301]

Because of the frequent requirement for pacing in these patients and the problems associated with pacemaker-device interactions, the capability for bradycardia pacing is incorporated in the newest devices. To date, very few problems have been reported as a result of the use of these devices.[307]

Drug interactions. Antiarrhythmia agents are commonly used in conjunction with AICDs for a variety of reasons: to reduce the frequency of spontaneous ventricular tachycardia, to eliminate or reduce the frequency of episodes of nonsustained ventricular tachycardia, and to prevent atrial fibrillation and other supraventricular tachycardias.[236,250] Potential drug-device interactions that can adversely affect defibrillator function are listed in Table 25B-14.

Antiarrhythmic therapy may result in a change in defibrillation thresholds and is, therefore, a potentially significant problem if initiated after device implantation. Classes IA and IB antiarrhythmic agents (e.g., procainamide, quinidine, and mexiletine) have little if any effect, whereas classes IC and III agents (e.g., propafenone, flecainide, and amiodarone) may result in elevation of the energy requirements for defibrillation.[251,253,308-311] Classes IA, IC, and III antiarrhythmic agents produce slowing in conduction that can slow the tachycardia cycle length and result in a failure to satisfy the tachycardia rate criterion.[312] These effects on conduction may also lead to an increase in QRS duration during exercise or supraventricular tachycardia, which could lead to fulfillment of the PDF criterion in devices that incorporate it for tachycardia detection.[297] As a result, careful electrophysiologic evaluation, including a determination of the efficacy of tachycardia and defibrillation therapies, is required when antiarrhythmic therapy is modified after device implantation.

Postoperative patient management

After defibrillator implantation, the patient is carefully monitored at rest and during ambulation to confirm adequate control of supraventricular arrhythmias and nonsustained ventricular tachycardia. An exercise test is performed to reassess the heart rate response to exercise and to exclude exercise-induced arrhythmias. For the first 12 to 24 hours after implantation, the device is inactive, after which it is activated by external programming.

After all necessary adjustments in antiarrhythmia therapy have been made, an electrophysiologic test is repeated to assess defibrillator function. With the AICD in the electrophysiologic test mode, the patient's clinical arrhythmia is induced, and in the case of ventricular tachycardia, antitachycardia pacing and cardioversion therapy are tested and tiered therapy is programmed into the device. If tachycardia termination is successful, ventricular fibrillation is induced (if it is not the clinical arrhythmia), and the ability of the defibrillator to terminate it is confirmed. We perform this testing with the patient fully anesthetized to minimize the morbidity associated with arrhythmia initiation and termination. During this procedure, any adjustments in the AICD (e.g., tachycardia criteria, pacing, therapy, shock output) that are required for consistent arrhythmia termination should be made.

In the postimplantation period at our institution, a specially trained nurse reviews defibrillator function, follow-up requirements, activity restrictions, instructions for contacting medical personnel, and basic life support (cardiopulmonary resuscitation) with the patient and members of the patient's family. The patient is instructed to contact a physician in the event of any defibrillator discharge, change in cardiovascular status, or development of symptoms suggesting a surgical complication (e.g., fever). The patient is advised to modify activity to avoid excessive heart rates during exercise, to avoid electromagnetic interference, and to avoid situations in which a spontaneous arrhythmia could result in serious injury (e.g., the patient is told *not* to drive under any circumstances). The patient must realize that the purpose of the

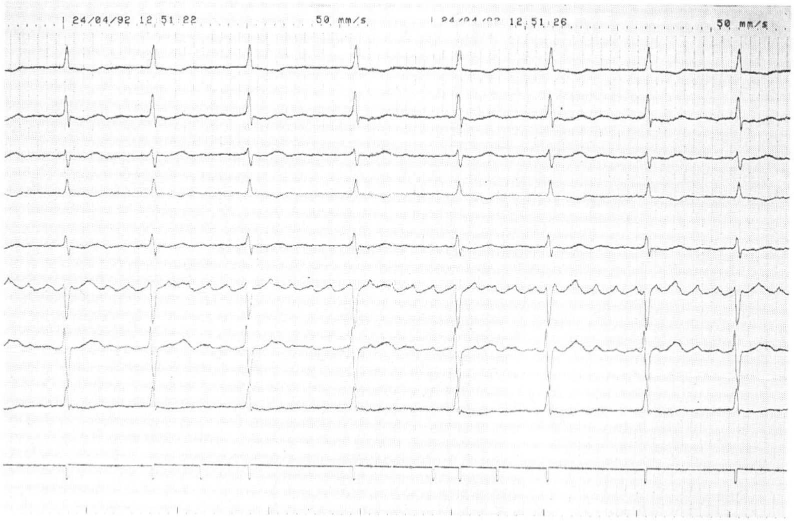

Fig 25B-33 Electrocardiographic tracings and marker channel recordings (bottom channel) obtained during follow-up evaluation of an implantable cardioverter-defibrillator. The marker channel indicates that in addition to each QRS, some extracardiac signals are also being sensed. Further evaluation demonstrated a fracture of the rate-sensing electrode.

defibrillator is to prevent *death,* not loss of consciousness.

Patients are seen in the outpatient department on a routine basis every 3 months or after tachycardia episodes if they occur frequently or if there is a possibility of inappropriate therapy (e.g., discharges without symptoms).

During these outpatient visits, an interim history is obtained and an examination is performed. The only routine laboratory evaluation is x-ray evaluation of lead integrity every 6 to 12 months.

During each visit, the device is interrogated to determine battery status, number of spontaneous tachycardia episodes, number and types of treatments delivered, and rate of therapeutic success. Depending on the device, information on all tachycardia episodes or the most recent one is also obtained. Pacing thresholds are determined, R waves are evaluated by telemetry, and marker channels are reviewed for oversensing or undersensing by the device (Fig 25B-33). The capacitors are reformed by a 34-J internal discharge, and a charge time is obtained by telemetry. Noninvasive electrophysiologic testing is done only when a patient's history requires verification of tachycardia detection and therapy or if antitachycardia drug therapy has been modified.[277,300,308]

Future of implantable device therapy

Many deficiencies in implantable devices have been eliminated by the addition of bradycardia pacing, antitachycardia pacing, low-energy cardioversion, tiered therapy based on more flexible detection algorithms, memory and telemetry, noninvasive electrophysiologic testing capability, and programmability of all functions. However, the ideal implantable antitachycardia device does not yet exist. The need for a major surgical procedure to accomplish device implantation and the delivery of shock therapy to asymptomatic patients are still major limitations. It is hoped that the former will be eliminated by the use of nonthoracotomy lead systems and the latter by incorporation of hemodynamic sensors into the sensing algorithms.

Nonthoracotomy lead systems. The use of nonthoracotomy lead systems could significantly reduce the mortality and morbidity associated with the implantation of epicardial lead systems. They may be especially useful in patients who have had cardiovascular surgery.

The systems currently being evaluated use either a single tripolar endocardial lead and an epicostal patch or multiple endocardial electrodes (right ventricular, right atrial, and coronary sinus) and an epicostal patch for sensing, pacing, and shock delivery. The endocardial lead or leads are implanted by the standard approach through the subclavian vein. The subcutaneous (epicostal) patch is positioned in the submuscular plane deep to the latissimus dorsi muscle and overlying the serratus anterior. It is commonly placed in the region of the fifth intercostal space in the midaxillary line, although a more precise location can be found by the use of a temporary patch during determination of the defibrillation threshold.[215,216]

The initial studies with bielectrode transvenous catheters demonstrated limited usefulness because the defibrillation energy requirements were too high; hence, three-electrode systems capable of bidirectional shock delivery are being evaluated at present.[172,313] A DFT of 18 J or less is required for defibrillator implantation, and this has been achieved in approximately 75% of patients. It seems likely that improvements in electrode design and energy waveforms will increase this figure.[168,214]

Multiple configurations using electrodes in the right

ventricle or atrium and the coronary sinus and the epicostal patch should be tried until a satisfactory DFT is achieved. If inadequate thresholds are obtained, the endocardial lead or leads should be repositioned. Movement of the epicostal patch does not seem to improve thresholds.[216] Most studies have demonstrated that the most favorable lead configuration for termination of ventricular fibrillation is to have the right ventricular electrode as cathode and the right atrial electrode and epicostal patch as anodes.[171,216,314]

The early experience with these leads has demonstrated a high rate of lead malfunction in both the endocardial leads and the epicostal patch. All failures appear to be related to disruption of the connector coil by fracture or electrical arcing between the coils after insulation breakdown. Apparently, the size of the single endocardial catheter (12F) causes crimping at the junction of the clavicle and the first rib. The use of multiple endocardial leads has apparently eliminated this problem. The epicostal patches may be traumatized by the stress of physical activity along the lead as it courses through the subcutaneous tissue. Improved lead design will be required for long-term use of these electrodes.[215]

Hemodynamic sensors. Hemodynamic variables could be combined with electrogram analysis by use of microprocessors. Stable tachyarrhythmias could be treated with less aggressive methods (e.g., pacing), and unstable arrhythmias could be treated by more aggressive measures (cardioversion followed by defibrillation). In addition, zoned rate detection could be combined with hemodynamic criteria to select treatment (tiered therapy). Extremely rapid rhythms could be defibrillated (without consideration of hemodynamic state), and less rapid tachycardias could be evaluated by both hemodynamic and rate criteria to select the most appropriate termination therapy.[211,219] Hemodynamic variables such as myocardial oxygen consumption, right ventricular pressure, and right atrial pressure have been combined with heart rate in sensing algorithms. Compared with heart rate alone, improvement in specificity was significant without any change in sensitivity in all cases.[315-317]

Although this concept has great potential, there are many unanswered questions, and the application of these sensors in chronically implanted systems requires further research and development.

REFERENCES

1. DeSanctis RW: Diagnostic and therapeutic uses of atrial pacing. *Circulation* 43:748-761, 1971

2. Maloney JD, Holmes DR Jr, Gersh B, et al: Control, conversion, and prevention of resistant dysrhythmias with demand and double-demand atrioventricular sequential pacing (abstract). *PACE* 3:379, 1980

3. Berkovits B, Castellanos A, Dreifus LS, et al: Double demand sequential pacing for treatment of paroxysmal reentry tachyarrhythmias (abstract). *PACE* 3:364, 1980

4. Spurrell RAJ, Sowton E: Pacing techniques in the management of supraventricular tachycardias. Part 2. An implanted atrial synchronous pacemaker with a short atrioventricular delay for the prevention of paroxysmal supraventricular tachycardias. *J Electrocardiol* 9:89-96, 1976

5. Han J, Millet D, Chizzonitti B, et al: Temporal dispersion of recovery of excitability in atrium and ventricle as a function of heart rate. *Am Heart J* 71:481-487, 1966

6. Dreifus LS, Berkovits BV, Kimibiris D, et al: Use of atrial and bifocal cardiac pacemakers for treating resistant dysrhythmias. *Eur J Cardiol* 3:257-266, 1975

7. Sowton E, Leatham A, Carson P: The suppression of arrhythmias by artificial pacemaking. *Lancet* 2:1098-1100, 1964

8. Fisher JD, Cohen HL, Mehra R, et al: Cardiac pacing and pacemakers II. Serial electrophysiologic-pharmacologic testing for control of recurrent tachyarrhythmias. *Am Heart J* 93:658-668, 1977

9. Wiener I: Pacing techniques in the treatment of tachycardias. *Ann Intern Med* 93:326-329, 1980

10. Hartzler GO: Treatment of recurrent ventricular tachycardia by patient-activated radiofrequency ventricular stimulation. *Mayo Clin Proc* 54:75-82, 1979

11. Han J, DeTraglia J, Millet D, et al: Incidence of ectopic beats as a function of basic rate in the ventricle. *Am Heart J* 72:632-639, 1966

12. DeSanctis RW, Kastor JA: Rapid intracardiac pacing for treatment of recurrent ventricular tachyarrhythmias in the absence of heart block. *Am Heart J* 76:168-172, 1968

13. Medina-Ravell V, Castellanos A, Portillo-Acosta B, et al: Management of tachyarrhythmias with dual-chamber pacemakers. *PACE* 6:333-345, 1983

14. Coumel P: Different modes of pacemaking in management of paroxysmal tachycardia. In *Symposium on Cardiac Arrhythmias.* Edited by E Sandøe, E Flensted-Jensen, KH Olesen. Södertälje, Sweden, Astra, 1972, p 783

15. Wellens HJJ: *Electrical Stimulation of the Heart in the Study and Treatment of Tachycardias.* Baltimore, University Park Press, 1971, p 122

16. Lew HT, March HW: Control of recurrent ventricular fibrillation by transvenous pacing in the absence of heart block. *Am Heart J* 73:794-797, 1967

17. Han J, Moe GK: Nonuniform recovery of excitability in ventricular muscle. *Circ Res* 14:44-60, 1964

18. Silka MJ, Manwill JR, Kron J, et al: Bradycardia-mediated tachyarrhythmias in congenital heart disease and responses to chronic pacing and physiologic rates. *Am J Cardiol* 65:488-493, 1990

19. Murphy P, O'Keefe DB: Effect of atrial pacing on the frequency of tachycardia in patients with recurrent junctional tachycardia. *PACE* 14:404-409, 1991

20. Burchell HB: Analogy of electronic pacemaker and ventricular parasystole with observations on refractory period, supernormal phase, and synchronization. *Circulation* 27:878-889, 1963

21. Waxman MB, Wald RW: Recurrent paroxysmal supraventricular tachycardia: a complication of ventricular pacing in a patient with occult Wolff-Parkinson-White syndrome. *J Electrocardiol* 10:291-298, 1977

22. Kastor JA, DeSanctis RW: Reciprocal beating from artificial ventricular pacemaker: report of a case. *Circulation* 35:1170-1173, 1967

23. Moss AJ, Rivers RJ Jr: Atrial pacing from the coronary vein: ten-year experience in 50 patients with implanted pervenous pacemakers. *Circulation* 57:103-106, 1978

24. Bennett MA, Pentecost BL: Suppression of ventricular tachyarrhythmias by transvenous intracardiac pacing after acute myocardial infarction. *Br Med J* 4:468-470, 1970

25. Eraklis AJ, Green WT Jr, Watson CG: Recurrent paroxysms or ventricular tachycardia following mitral valvuloplasty: case report. *Ann Surg* 161:63-66, 1965

26. Lichstein E, Chadda K, Fenig S: Atrial pacing in the treatment of refractory ventricular tachycardia associated with hypokalemia. *Am J Cardiol* 30:550-553, 1972

27. Wirtzfeld A, Schmidt G, Klein G, et al: External electrical stimulation in the management of acute tachyarrhythmias. *PACE* 4:679-691, 1981

28. Johnson RA, Hutter AM Jr, DeSanctis RW, et al: Chronic overdrive pacing in the control of refractory ventricular arrhythmias. *Ann Intern Med* 80:380-383, 1974

29. Moss AJ, Rivers RJ Jr: Termination and inhibition of recurrent tachycardias by implanted pervenous pacemakers. *Circulation* 50:942-947, 1974

30. Fisher JD, Kim SG, Furman S, et al: Role of implantable pacemakers in control of recurrent ventricular tachycardia. *Am J Cardiol* 49:194-206, 1982

31. DiSegni E, Klein HO, David D, et al: Overdrive pacing in quinidine syncope and other long QT-interval syndromes. *Arch Intern Med* 140:1036-1040, 1980

32. Sclarovsky S, Strasberg B, Lewin RF, et al: Polymorphous

ventricular tachycardia: clinical features and treatment. *Am J Cardiol* 44:339-344, 1979

33. Schoonmaker FW, Osteen RT, Greenfield JC Jr: Thioridazine (Mellaril)-induced ventricular tachycardia controlled with an artificial pacemaker. *Ann Intern Med* 65:1076-1078, 1966
34. Kastor JA, DeSanctis RW, Harthorne JW, et al: Transvenous atrial pacing in the treatment of refractory ventricular irritability. *Ann Intern Med* 66:939-945, 1967
35. Moss AJ, Rivers RJ Jr, Griffith LSC, et al: Transvenous left atrial pacing for the control of recurrent ventricular fibrillation. *N Engl J Med* 278:928-931, 1968
36. Sowton E, Balcon R, Preston T, et al: Long-term control of intractable supraventricular tachycardia by ventricular pacing. *Br Heart J* 31:700-706, 1969
37. Keren A, Tzivoni D, Golhman JM, et al. Ventricular pacing in atypical ventricular tachycardia. *J Electrocardiol* 14:201-205, 1981
38. Kerr CR, Klein GJ, Cooper JA, et al: Use of electrical pacemakers in the treatment of ventricular tachycardia and ventricular fibrillation. *Cardiovasc Clin* 16:215-237, 1985
39. Wellens HJJ, Bär FW, Gorgels AP, et al: Electrical management of arrhythmias with emphasis on the tachycardias. *Am J Cardiol* 41:1025-1034, 1978
40. Coumel P: Junctional reciprocating tachycardias: the permanent and paroxysmal forms of A-V nodal reciprocating tachycardias. *J Electrocardiol* 8:79-90, 1975
41. Akhtar M, Gilbert CJ, Al-Nouri M, et al: Electrophysiologic mechanisms for modification and abolition of atrioventricular junctional tachycardia with simultaneous and sequential atrial and ventricular pacing. *Circulation* 60:1443-1454, 1979
42. Sung RJ, Styperek JL, Castellanos A: Complete abolition of the reentrant supraventricular tachycardia zone using a new modality of cardiac pacing with simultaneous atrioventricular stimulation. *Am J Cardiol* 45:72-78, 1980
43. Braunwald E, Ross J Jr, Frommer PL, et al: Clinical observations on paired electrical stimulation of the heart: effects on ventricular performance and heart rate. *Am J Med* 37:700-711, 1964
44. Arbel ER, Cohen HC, Langendorf R, et al: Successful treatment of drug-resistant atrial tachycardia and intractable congestive heart failure with permanent coupled atrial pacing. *Am J Cardiol* 41:336-340, 1978
45. Waldo AL, Krongrad E, Kupersmith J, et al: Ventricular paired pacing to control rapid ventricular heart rate following open heart surgery: observations on ectopic automaticity; report of a case in a four-month-old patient. *Circulation* 53:176-181, 1976
46. Fruehan CT, Meyer JA, Klie JH, et al: Refractory paroxysmal supraventricular tachycardia: treatment with patient controlled permanent radio frequency atrial pacemaker. *Am Heart J* 87:229-237, 1974
47. Engel TR, Bush CA, Schaal SF: Tachycardia-aggravated heart disease. *Ann Intern Med* 80:384-388, 1974
48. Till JA, Rowland E: Atrial pacing as an adjunct to the management of post-surgical His bundle tachycardia. *Br Heart J* 66:225-229, 1991
49. Wiener L, Dwyer EM Jr: Electrical induction of atrial fibrillation: an approach to intractable atrial tachycardia. *Am J Cardiol* 21:731-734, 1968
50. Furman S: Therapeutic uses of atrial pacing. *Am Heart J* 86:835-840, 1973
51. Davidson RM, Wallace AG, Sealy WC, et al: Electrically induced atrial tachycardia with block: a therapeutic application of permanent radiofrequency atrial pacing. *Circulation* 44:1014-1021, 1971
52. Preston TA, Haynes RE, Gavin WA, et al: Permanent rapid atrial pacing to control supraventricular tachycardia. *PACE* 2:331-334, 1979
53. Cranefield PF: *The Conduction of the Cardiac Impulse: The Slow Response and Cardiac Arrhythmias.* Mount Kisco, New York, Futura Publishing Company, 1975
54. Wellens HJJ, Lie KI, Durrer D: Further observations on ventricular tachycardia as studied by electrical stimulation of the heart: chronic recurrent ventricular tachycardia and ventricular tachycardia during acute myocardial infarction. *Circulation* 49:647-653, 1974
55. Bigger JT Jr, Goldreyer BN: The mechanism of supraventricular tachycardia. *Circulation* 42:673-688, 1970
56. Bennett MA, Pentecost BL: Reversion of ventricular tachycardia by pacemaker stimulation. *Br Heart J* 33:922-927, 1971
57. Wellens HJJ: Value and limitations of programmed electrical stimulation of the heart in the study and treatment of tachycardias. *Circulation* 57:845-853, 1978
58. Cranefield PF: Action potentials, afterpotentials, and arrhythmias. *Circ Res* 41:415-423, 1977
59. Haft JI, Kosowsky BD, Lau SH, et al: Termination of atrial flutter by rapid electrical pacing of the atrium. *Am J Cardiol* 20:239-244, 1967
60. Josephson ME, Horowitz LN, Farshidi A, et al: Recurrent sustained ventricular tachycardia. 1. Mechanisms. *Circulation* 57:431-440, 1978
61. Wellens HJ, Overdijk AD, Durrer D: Traitement d'une tachycardie ventriculaire itérative chronique par l'implantation d'un pacemaker. *Coeur Med Interne* 13:683-685, 1974
62. Wellens HJJ, Duren DR, Lie KI: Observations on mechanisms of ventricular tachycardia in man. *Circulation* 54:237-244, 1976
63. Janse MJ, van Capelle FJL, Anderson RH, et al: Electrophysiology and structure of the atrioventricular node of the isolated rabbit heart. In *The Conduction System of the Heart: Structure, Function and Clinical Implications.* Edited by HJJ Wellens, KI Lie, MJ Janse. Philadelphia, Lea & Febiger, 1976, pp 296-335
64. Wellens HJ, Schuilenburg RM, Durrer D: Electrical stimulation of the heart in patients with ventricular tachycardia. *Circulation* 46:216-226, 1972
65. Massumi RA, Kistin AD, Tawakkol AA: Termination of reciprocating tachycardia by atrial stimulation. *Circulation* 36:637-643, 1967
66. Pittman DE, Makar JS, Kooros KS, et al: Rapid atrial stimulation: successful method of conversion of atrial flutter and atrial tachycardia. *Am J Cardiol* 32:700-706, 1973
67. Scheinman MM: The treatment of paroxysmal supraventricular tachycardia. *Ration Drug Ther* 10:1-6, 1976
68. Williams DO, Davison PH: Long-term treatment of refractory supraventricular tachycardia by patient-controlled inductive atrial pacing. *Br Heart J* 36:336-340, 1974
69. Curry PVL, Rowland E, Fox KM, et al: The relationship between posture, blood pressure and electrophysiological properties in patients with paroxysmal supraventricular tachycardia. *Arch Mal Coeur* 71:293-299, 1978
70. Kahn A, Morris JJ, Citron P: Patient-initiated rapid atrial pacing to manage supraventricular tachycardia. *Am J Cardiol* 38:200-204, 1976
71. Josephson ME, Horowitz LN: Electrophysiologic approach to therapy of recurrent sustained ventricular tachycardia. *Am J Cardiol* 43:631-642, 1979
72. German LD, Strauss HC: Electrical termination of tachyarrhythmias by discrete pulses. *PACE* 7:514-521, 1984
73. Barold SS, Linhart JW: Recent advances in the treatment of ectopic tachycardias by electrical pacing. *Am J Cardiol* 25:698-706, 1970
74. Ruskin JN, Garan H, Poulin F, et al: Permanent radiofrequency ventricular pacing for management of drug-resistant ventricular tachycardia. *Am J Cardiol* 46:317-321, 1980
75. Zipes DP, Prystowsky EN, Miles WM, et al: Initial experience with Symbios Model 7008 pacemaker. *PACE* 7:1301-1305, 1984
76. Gallagher JJ, Svenson RH, Sealy WC, et al: The Wolff-Parkinson-White syndrome and the preexcitation dysrhythmias: medical and surgical management. *Med Clin North Am* 60:101-123, January 1976
77. Griffin JC, Mason JW, Ross DL, et al: The treatment of ventricular tachycardia using an automatic tachycardia terminating pacemaker. *PACE* 4:582-588, 1981
78. Waxman MB, Wald RW, Bonet JF, et al: Self-conversion of supraventricular tachycardia by rapid atrial pacing. *PACE* 1:35-48, 1978
79. Osborn MJ, Holmes DR Jr: Antitachycardia pacing. *Clin Prog Pacing Electrophysiol* 3:239-267, 1985
80. Furman S, Mercando AD: Antitachycardia pacing and implantable cardioverter defibrillators. *Ann Rev Med* 40:123-136, 1989
81. Fromer M, Kus T, Page P, et al: Termination of sustained ventricular tachycardia with a new antitachycardia pacemaker: role of the nonautomatic mode to follow pacemaker function. *Can J Cardiol* 5:42-46, 1989
82. Castellanos A, Waxman HL, Berkovits BV, et al: Implantable pacemakers for cardiac tachyarrhythmias. *Cardiovasc Clin* 11 No 1:159-173, 1980
83. Brugada P, den Dulk D, Waldecker B, et al: Role of programmed electrical stimulation of the heart in the selection and design of implantable units for the treatment of recurrent tachycardia. *Eur Heart J* 7:728-734, 1986
84. Griffin JC, Sweeney M: The management of paroxysmal tachycardias using the Cybertach-60. *PACE* 7:1291-1295, 1984
85. Spurrell RAJ, Nathan AW, Camm AJ: Clinical experience with implantable scanning tachycardia reversion pacemakers. *PACE* 7:1296-1300, 1984

86. Ward DE, Camm AJ, Gainsborough J, et al: Autodecremental pacing: a microprocessor based modality for the termination of paroxysmal tachycardias. *PACE* 3:178-191, 1980

87. Curry PVL, Rowland E, Krikler DM: Dual-demand pacing for refractory atrioventricular re-entry tachycardia. *PACE* 2:137-151, 1979

88. Barold SS, Sweeney M, Falkoff MD, et al: Clinical utility of an implantable multiprogrammable automatic antitachycardia pulse generator as an external device. *PACE* 4:571-574, 1981

89. Waldecker B, Brugada P, Zehender M, et al: Importance of modes of electrical termination of ventricular tachycardia for the selection of implantable antitachycardia devices. *Am J Cardiol* 57:150-155, 1986

90. Spurrell RAJ: Artificial cardiac pacemakers. In *Cardiac Arrhythmias: The Modern Electrophysiological Approach.* Edited by DM Krikler, JF Goodwin. Philadelphia, WB Saunders Company, 1975, pp 238-258

91. Sowton E: Clinical results with the tachylog antitachycardia pacemaker. *PACE* 7:1313-1317, 1984

92. Fåhraeus T, Lassvik C, Sonnhag C: Tachycardias initiated by automatic antitachycardia pacemakers. *PACE* 7:1049-1054, 1984

93. Peters RW, Scheinman MM, Morady F, et al: Long-term management of recurrent paroxysmal tachycardia by cardiac burst pacing. *PACE* 8:35-44, 1985

94. Sulke AN, Bucknall CA, Sowton E: Supraventricular tachycardia control with Tachylog II: long-term follow-up. *PACE* 13:1960-1966, 1990

95. Fisher JD, Mehra R, Furman S: Termination of ventricular tachycardia with bursts of rapid ventricular pacing. *Am J Cardiol* 41:94-102, 1978

96. Naccarelli GV, Zipes DP, Rahilly GT, et al: Influence of tachycardia cycle length and antiarrhythmic drugs on pacing termination and acceleration of ventricular tachycardia. *Am Heart J* 105:1-5, 1983

97. Fisher JD, Johnston DR, Furman S, et al: Long-term efficacy of antitachycardia pacing for supraventricular and ventricular tachycardias. *Am J Cardiol* 60:1311-1316, 1987

98. Holt P, Crick JCP, Sowton E: Antitachycardia pacing: a comparison of burst overdrive, self-searching and adaptive table scanning programs. *PACE* 9:490-497, 1986

99. den Dulk K, Kersschot IE, Brugada P, et al: Is there a universal antiarrhythmia pacing mode? *Am J Cardiol* 57:950-955, 1986

100. den Dulk K, Brugada P, Sweets JL, et al: Long-term antitachycardia pacing experience for supraventricular tachycardia. *PACE* 13:1020-1030, 1990

101. Barold SS, Falkoff MD, Ong LS, et al: Clinical usefulness of chest wall stimulation in patients with automatic tachycardia-terminating pacemakers. *PACE* 9:634-643, 1986

102. Herre JM, Griffin JC, Nielsen AP, et al: Permanent triggered antitachycardia pacemakers in the management of recurrent sustained ventricular tachycardia. *J Am Coll Cardiol* 6:206-212, 1985

103. den Dulk K, Bertholet M, Brugada P, et al: Clinical experience with implantable devices for control of tachyarrhythmias. *PACE* 7:548-556, 1984

104. Saksena S, Pantopoulos D, Parsonnet V, et al: Usefulness of an implantable antitachycardia pacemaker system for supraventricular or ventricular tachycardia. *Am J Cardiol* 58:70-74, 1986

105. Griffin JC, Mason JW, Calfee RV: Clinical use of an implantable automatic tachycardia-terminating pacemaker. *Am Heart J* 100:1093-1096, 1980

106. Janssen M, Spurrell RAJ: The P.A.S.A.R. (Programmable Automatic Scanning Arrhythmia Revision) system: a new automatic scanning tachycardia terminating pacemaker. In *The Third Decade of Cardiac Pacing: Advances in Technology and Clinical Applications.* Edited by SS Barold, J Mugica. Mount Kisco, New York, Futura Publishing Company, 1982, pp 275-292

107. Schnittger I, Lee JT, Hargis JT, et al: Long-term results of antitachycardia pacing in patients with supraventricular tachycardia. *PACE* 12:936-941, 1989

108. Shandling AH, Curtis KL, Thomas L: Sustained effectiveness of an atrial antitachycardia pacemaker during follow-up. *PACE* 13:833-838, 1990

109. Fukushige J, Porter CJ, Hayes DL, et al: Antitachycardia pacemaker treatment of postoperative arrhythmias in pediatric patients. *PACE* 14:546-556, 1991

110. Charos GS, Haffajee CI, Gold RL, et al: A theoretically and practically more effective method for interruption of ventricular tachycardia: self-adapting autodecremental overdrive pacing. *Circulation* 73:309-315, 1986

111. Fisher JD, Goldstein M, Ostrow E, et al: Maximal rate of tachycardia development: sinus tachycardia with sudden exercise vs. spontaneous ventricular tachycardia. *PACE* 6:221-228, 1983

112. Echt DS: Potential hazards of implanted devices for the electrical control of tachyarrhythmias. *PACE* 7:580-587, 1984

113. Lerman BB, Waxman HL, Buxton AE, et al: Tachyarrhythmias associated with programmable automatic atrial antitachycardia pacemakers. *Am Heart J* 106:1029-1035, 1983

114. Greene HL, Gross BW, Preston TA, et al: Termination of ventricular tachycardia by programmed extrastimuli from an externally-activated permanent pacemaker. *PACE* 5:434-439, 1982

115. den Dulk K, Bertholet M, Brugada P, et al: A versatile pacemaker system for termination of tachycardias. *Am J Cardiol* 52:731-738, 1983

116. Roy D, Waxman HL, Buxton AE, et al. Termination of ventricular tachycardia: role of tachycardia cycle length. *Am J Cardiol* 50:1346-1350, 1982

117. Fisher JD, Kim SG, Matos JA et al: Pacing for ventricular tachycardia. *PACE* 7:1278-1290, 1984

118. Fisher JD, Kim SG, Matos JA, et al: Comparative effectiveness of pacing techniques for termination of well-tolerated sustained ventricular tachycardia. *PACE* 6:915-922, 1983

119. Ward DE, Camm AJ, Spurrell RAJ: The response of regular re-entrant supraventricular tachycardia to right heart stimulation. *PACE* 2:586-595, 1979

120. Josephson ME, Horowitz LN: Electrophysiologic approach to therapy of recurrent sustained ventricular tachycardia. *Am J Cardiol* 43:631-642, 1979

121. Wellens HJJ, Bär FWHM, Lie KI, et al: Effect of procainamide, propranolol and verapamil on mechanism of tachycardia in patients with chronic recurrent ventricular tachycardia. *Am J Cardiol* 40:579-585, 1977

122. Castellanos A, Waxman HL, Moleiro F, et al: Preliminary studies with an implantable multimodal A-V pacemaker for reciprocating atrioventricular tachycardias. *PACE* 3:257-265, 1980

123. Leclercq JF, Rosengarten MD, Delcourt P, et al: Prevention of intra-atrial reentry by chronic atrial pacing. *PACE* 3:162-170, 1980

124. Luck JC, Grubb BP, Artman SE, et al: Termination of sustained ventricular tachycardia by external noninvasive pacing. *Am J Cardiol* 61:574-577, 1988

125. Estes NAM III, Deering TF, Manolis AS, et al: External cardiac programmed stimulation in noninvasive termination of sustained supraventricular and ventricular tachycardia. *Am J Cardiol* 63:177-183, 1989

126. Rosenthal ME, Stamato NJ, Almendral JM, et al: Coupling intervals of ventricular extrastimuli causing resetting of sustained ventricular tachycardia secondary to coronary artery disease: relation to subsequent termination. *Am J Cardiol* 61:770-774, 1988

127. Hammon JW Jr, Echt DS, Merrill WH, et al: Indications for different modes of surgical therapy in medically refractory ventricular arrhythmias. *Ann Surg* 203:679-683, 1986

128. Chapman PD, Troup P: The automatic implantable cardioverter-defibrillator: evaluating suspected inappropriate shocks. *J Am Coll Cardiol* 7:1075-1078, 1986

129. Critelli G, Grassi G, Chiariello M, et al: Automatic "scanning" by radiofrequency in the long-term electrical treatment of arrhythmias. *PACE* 2:289-296, 1979

130. Spurrell RAJ, Nathan AW, Bexton RS, et al: Implantable automatic scanning pacemaker for termination of supraventricular tachycardia. *Am J Cardiol* 49:753-760, 1982

131. Reddy CP, Todd EP, Kuo CS, et al: Treatment of ventricular tachycardia using an automatic scanning extrastimulus pacemaker. *J Am Coll Cardiol* 3:225-230, 1984

132. Spurrell RAJ, Sowton E: The management of paroxysmal supraventricular tachycardia using a scanning pacemaker system. *Excerpta Medica International Congress Series* No 395, 1976, pp 187-189

133. Palakurthy PR, Slater D: Automatic implantable scanning burst pacemakers for recurrent tachyarrhythmias. *PACE* 11:185-192, 1988

134. Nathan AW, Spurrell RAJ, Camm AJ: Steps towards the development of a safe and effective tachycardia terminating pacemaker. *Eur Heart J* 5:993-1003, 1984

135. Manz M, Gerckens U, Funke HD, et al: Combination of antitachycardia pacemaker and automatic implantable cardioverter/defibrillator for ventricular tachycardia. *PACE* 9:676-684, 1986

136. Luceri RM, Habal SM, Castellanos A, et al: Mechanism of death in patients with the automatic implantable cardioverter defibrillator. *PACE* 11:2015-2022, 1988

137. Chapman PD, Veseth-Rogers JL, Duguette SE, et al: The implantable defibrillator and the emergency physician. *Ann Emerg Med* 18:579-585, 1989

138. Waldo AL, MacLean WAH, Karp RB, et al: Entrainment and interruption of atrial flutter with atrial pacing: studies in man following open heart surgery. *Circulation* 56:737-745, 1977

139. Batchelder JE, Zipes DP: Treatment of tachyarrhythmias by pacing. *Arch Intern Med* 135:1115-1124, 1975

140. Lange G: Action of driving stimuli from intrinsic and extrinsic sources on in situ cardiac pacemaker tissues. *Circ Res* 17:449-459, 1965

141. MacLean WAH, Plumb VJ, Waldo AL: Transient entrainment and interruption of ventricular tachycardia. *PACE* 4:358-366, 1981

142. Hoffman BF, Cranefield PF: *Electrophysiology of the Heart.* New York, McGraw-Hill Book Company, 1960

143. Tanabe A, Ikeda H, Fujiyama M, et al: Termination of ventricular tachycardia by an implantable atrial pacemaker and external pacemaker activator. *PACE* 8:532-538, 1985

144. Waxman MB, Bonet JF, Wald RW: Self-conversion of drug resistant ventricular tachycardia by rapid atrial pacing. *PACE* 6:900-907, 1983

145. Mason JW, Winkle RA: Electrode-catheter arrhythmia induction in the selection and assessment of antiarrhythmic drug therapy for recurrent ventricular tachycardia. *Circulation* 58:971-985, 1978

146. Nathan A, Hellestrand K, Ward D, et al: Rate-related accelerating (autodecremental) atrial pacing for reversion of paroxysmal supraventricular tachycardia. *J Electrocardiol* 15:77-84, 1982

147. Lister JW, Gosselin AJ, Nathan DA, et al: Rapid atrial stimulation in the treatment of supraventricular tachycardia. *Chest* 63:995-1001, 1973

148. Dreifus LS, Haiat R, Watanabe Y, et al: Ventricular fibrillation: a possible mechanism of sudden death in patients with Wolff-Parkinson-White syndrome. *Circulation* 43:520-527, 1971

149. Solti F, Szabó Z, Czakó E, et al: Refractory supraventricular reentry tachycardia treated by radiofrequency atrial pacemaker. *PACE* 5:275-277, 1982

150. Saksena S, Chandran P, Shah Y, et al: Comparative efficacy of transvenous cardioversion and pacing in patients with sustained ventricular tachycardia: a prospective, randomized, crossover study. *Circulation* 72:153-160, 1985

151. Winkle RA, Bach SM Jr, Echt DS, et al: The automatic implantable defibrillator: local ventricular bipolar sensing to detect ventricular tachycardia and fibrillation. *Am J Cardiol* 52:265-270, 1983

152. Spielman SR, Farshidi A, Horowitz LN, et al: Ventricular fibrillation during programmed ventricular stimulation: incidence and clinical implications. *Am J Cardiol* 42:913-918, 1978

153. Gardner MJ, Waxman HL, Buxton AE, et al: Termination of ventricular tachycardia: evaluation of a new pacing method. *Am J Cardiol* 50:1338-1345, 1982

154. Vohra J, Hamer A, Mond H, et al: Patient initiated implantable pacemakers for paroxysmal supraventricular tachycardia. *Aust NZ J Med* 11:27-34, 1981

155. Peters RW, Shafton E, Frank S, et al: Radiofrequency-triggered pacemakers: uses and limitations. *Ann Intern Med* 88:17-22, 1978

156. Griffin JC, Rothman MT, Echt DS, et al: Long-term follow-up of patients with an automatic tachycardia terminating burst pacemaker (abstract). *PACE* 6:142, 1983

157. Peters RW, Shafton E, Frank S, et al: Radiofrequency-triggered pacemakers: uses and limitations; a long-term study. *Ann Intern Med* 88:17-22, 1978

158. Kappenberger L, Valin H, Sowton E: Multicenter long-term results of antitachycardia pacing for supraventricular tachycardias. *Am J Cardiol* 64:191-193, 1989

159. Pfitzner P, Gerckens U, Funke HD, et al: Supraventrikuläre tachykardie: therapie mit variablem antitachykardem stimulationsmodus. *Z Kardiol* 77:366-372, 1988

160. Zipes DP: Pacing 1980. *PACE* 4:182-192, 1981

161. Higgins JR: Automatic burst extrastimulus pacemaker to treat recurrent ventricular tachycardia in a patient with mitral valve prolapse: more than 2,000 documented successful tachycardia terminations. *J Am Coll Cardiol* 8:446-450, 1986

162. Hartzler GO, Holmes DR Jr, Osborn MJ: Patient-activated transvenous cardiac stimulation for the treatment of supraventricular and ventricular tachycardia. *Am J Cardiol* 47:903-909, 1981

163. Saksena S, Camm AJ (Co-Chairman): Clinical investigation of implantable antitachycardia devices: report of the policy conference of the North American Society of Pacing and Electrophysiology. *J Am Coll Cardiol* 10:225-229, 1987

164. McComb JM, Jameson S, Bexton RS: Atrial antitachycardia pacing in patients with supraventricular tachycardia: clinical experience with the Intertach pacemaker. *PACE* 13:1948-1954, 1990

165. Fisher JD, Kim SJ, Mercando AD: Electrical devices for treatment of arrhythmias. *Am J Cardiol* 61:45A-57A, 1988

166. Fromer M, Gloor H, Kus T, et al: Clinical experience with the Intertach 262-12 pulse generator in patients with recurrent supraventricular tachycardia and ventricular tachycardia. *PACE* 13:1955-1959, 1990

167. Masterson M, Pinski SL, Wilkoff B, et al: Pacemaker and defibrillator combination therapy for recurrent ventricular tachycardia. *Cleve Clin J Med* 57:330-338, 1990

168. Leitch JW, Gillis AM, Wyse G, et al: Reduction in defibrillator shocks with an implantable device combining antitachycardia pacing and shock therapy. *J Am Coll Cardiol* 18:145-151, 1991

169. Yee R, Klein GJ, Murdock C, et al: Efficacy of antitachycardia pacing in cardioversion with the pacemaker-cardioverter-defibrillator (abstract). *J Am Coll Cardiol* 15 Suppl A:60, 1990

170. Winkle RA: The implantable defibrillator: progression from first- to third-generation devices. In *Cardiac Electrophysiology: From Cell to Bedside.* Edited by DP Zipes, J Jalife. Philadelphia, WB Saunders Company, 1990, pp 963-969

171. Saksena S, Mehta D, Krol RB, et al: Experience with a third-generation implantable cardioverter-defibrillator. *Am J Cardiol* 67:1375-1384, 1991

172. Fromer M, Schläpfer J, Fischer A, et al: Experience with a new implantable pacer-cardioverter-defibrillator for the therapy of recurrent sustained ventricular tachyarrhythmias: a step toward a universal ventricular tachyarrhythmia control device. *PACE* 14:1288-1298, 1991

173. Fromer M, Schlaepfer J, Goy J-J, et al: Initial experience with a new tachyarrhythmia control device (abstract). *J Am Coll Cardiol* 15:68, 1990

174. Gering LE, Miles WM, Klein LS, et al: Experience with a new pacemaker/cardioverter/defibrillator (abstract). *J Am Coll Cardiol* 17 Suppl A:129, 1991

175. Das G, Anand KM, Ankineedu K, et al: Atrial pacing for cardioversion of atrial flutter in digitalized patients. *Am J Cardiol* 41:308-312, 1978

176. Kerr CR, Cooper J, Chung DC, et al: Termination of sustained ventricular tachycardia by transesophageal atrial pacing. *Am J Cardiol* 61:463-464, 1988

177. Harte MT, Teo KK, Horgan JH: The diagnosis and management of supraventricular tachycardia by transesophageal cardiac stimulation and recording. *Chest* 93:339-344, 1988

178. Dick M II, Scott WA, Serwer GS, et al: Acute termination of supraventricular tachyarrhythmias in children by transesophageal atrial pacing. *Am J Cardiol* 61:925-927, 1988

179. Smith MS, Lindsay WC, Flowers NC: Treatment of torsades de pointes with esophageal atrial pacing. *Am J Med* 83:971-972, 1987

180. Radford DJ, Julian DG: Sick sinus syndrome: experience of a cardiac pacemaker clinic. *Br Med J* 3:504-507, 1974

181. MacLean WAH, Cooper TB, Waldo AL: Use of cardiac electrodes in diagnosis and treatment of tachyarrhythmias. *Cardiovasc Med* 3:965-980, 1978

182. Thurer RJ, Luceri RM, Bolooki H: Automatic implantable cardioverter-defibrillator: techniques of implantation and results. *Ann Thorac Surg* 42:143-147, 1986

183. Bourland JD, Tacker WA Jr, Wessale JL, et al: Sequential pulse defibrillation for implantable defibrillators. *Med Instrum* 20:138-142, 1986

184. Radford DJ, Julian DG: Sick sinus syndrome: experience of a cardiac pacemaker clinic. *Br Med J* 3:504-507, 1974

185. Altamura G, Bianconi L, Boccadamo R, et al: Treatment of ventricular and supraventricular tachyarrhythmias by transcutaneous cardiac pacing. *PACE* 12:331-338, 1989

186. Luck JC, Davis D: Termination of sustained tachycardia by external noninvasive pacing. *PACE* 10:1125-1129, 1987

187. Altamura G, Bianconi L, Toscono S, et al: Transcutaneous cardiac pacing for termination of tachyarrhythmias. *PACE* 13:2026-2030, 1990

188. Grubb BP, Temesy-Armos P, Hahn H, et al: The clinical use of external noninvasive pacing in the termination of sustained ventricular tachycardia. *PACE* 13:1092-1095, 1990

189. Barold SS, Falkoff MD, Ong LS, et al: Termination of ventricular tachycardia by chest wall stimulation during DDD pacing: a report of two cases. *Am J Med* 84:549-554, 1988

190. Thomas AC, Moser SA, Smutka ML, et al: Implantable defibrillation: eight years clinical experience. *PACE* 11:2053-2058, 1988

191. Fonger JD, Guarnieri T, Griffith LSC, et al: Impending sudden cardiac death: treatment with myocardial revascularization and the automatic implantable cardioverter defibrillator. *Ann Thorac Surg* 46:13-16, 1988

192. Mirowski M, Reid PR, Winkle RA, et al: Mortality in patients with implanted automatic defibrillators. *Ann Intern Med* 98:585-588, 1983

193. Kalbfleisch KR, Lehmann MH, Steinman RT, et al: Reemployment following implantation of the automatic cardioverter defibrillator. *Am J Cardiol* 64:199-202, 1989

194. Mirowski M, Mower MM, Reid PR, et al: The automatic implantable defibrillator: new modality for treatment of life-threatening ventricular arrhythmias. *PACE* 5:384-401, 1982

195. Frame LH: The effect of chronic oral and acute intravenous amiodarone administration on ventricular defibrillation threshold using implantable electrodes in dogs. *PACE* 12:339-346, 1989

196. Hopps JA, Bigelow WG: Electrical treatment of cardiac arrest: a cardiac stimulator-defibrillator. *Surgery* 36:833-849, 1954

197. Schuder JC, Stoeckle H, Gold JH, et al: Experimental ventricular defibrillation with an automatic and completely implanted system. *Trans Am Soc Artif Intern Organs* 16:207-212, 1970

198. Mower MM, Mirowski M, Denniston RH: Intraventricular defibrillation in dogs with impaired coronary circulation (abstract). *Clin Res* 20:388, 1972

199. Mirowski M, Mower MM, Gott VL, et al: Transvenous automatic defibrillator—preliminary clinical tests of its defibrillating subsystem. *Trans Am Soc Artif Intern Organs* 18:520-525, 1972

200. Garrey WE: The nature of fibrillatory contraction of the heart. Its relation to tissue mass and form. *Am J Physiol* 33:397-414, 1914

201. Mower MM, Mirowski M, Spear JF, et al: Patterns of ventricular activity during catheter defibrillation. *Circulation* 49:858-861, 1974

202. Zipes DP, Fischer J, King RM, et al: Termination of ventricular fibrillation in dogs by depolarizing a critical amount of myocardium. *Am J Cardiol* 36:37-44, 1975

203. Mirowski M, Mower MM, Staewen WS, et al: Standby automatic defibrillator: an approach to prevention of sudden coronary death. *Arch Intern Med* 126:158-161, 1970

204. Wibel FH, Kallok MJ, Schollmeyer MP, et al: Impedance mechanogram and electrogram for detection of ventricular fibrillation in dogs (abstract). *Med Instrum* 15:328, 1981

205. Langer A, Heilman MS, Mower MM, et al: Considerations in the development of the automatic implantable defibrillator. *Med Instrum* 10:163-167, 1976

206. Mirowski M, Reid PR, Mower MM, et al: Termination of malignant ventricular arrhythmias with an implanted automatic defibrillator in human beings. *N Engl J Med* 303:322-324, 1980

207. Mower MM, Nisam S: AICD indications (patient selection): past, present and future. *PACE* 11:2064-2070, 1988

208. Mirowski M: The automatic implantable cardioverter-defibrillator: an overview. *J Am Coll Cardiol* 6:461-466, 1985

209. Nisam S, Mower M, Moser S: ICD clinical update: first decade, initial 10,000 patients. *PACE* 14:255-263, 1991

210. Winkle RA, Stinson EB, Echt DS, et al: Practical aspects of automatic cardioverter/defibrillator implantation. *Am Heart J* 108:1335-1346, 1984

211. Cohen TJ, Liem LB: Biosensor applications to antitachycardia devices. *PACE* 14:322-328, 1991

212. Winkle RA: The implantable defibrillator in ventricular arrhythmias. *Hosp Pract [Off]* 18:149-165, March 1983

213. Cannom DS, Winkle RA: Implantation of the automatic implantable cardioverter defibrillator AICD: practical aspects. *PACE* 9:793-809, 1986

214. Klein LS, Miles WM, Zipes DP: Antitachycardia devices: realities and promises. *J Am Coll Cardiol* 18:1349-1362, 1991

215. Tullo NG, Saksena S, Krol RB, et al: Management of complications associated with a first-generation endocardial defibrillation lead system for implantable cardioverter-defibrillators. *Am J Cardiol* 66:411-415, 1990

216. McCowan R, Maloney J, Wilkoff B, et al: Automatic implantable cardioverter-defibrillator implantation without thorocotomy using an endocardial and submuscular patch system. *J Am Coll Cardiol* 17:415-421, 1991

217. Mirowski M, Mower MM, Langer A, et al: A chronically implanted system for automatic defibrillation in active conscious dogs: experimental model for treatment of sudden death from ventricular fibrillation. *Circulation* 58:90-94, 1978

218. Mower MM, Reid PR, Watkins L Jr, et al: Automatic implantable cardioverter-defibrillator: structural characteristics. *PACE* 7:1331-1337, 1984

219. Johnson NJ, Marchlinski FE: Arrhythmias induced by device antitachycardia therapy due to diagnostic nonspecificity. *J Am Coll Cardiol* 18:1418-1425, 1991

220. Singer I, Austin E, Nash W, et al: The initial clinical experience with an implantable cardioverter defibrillator/antitachycardia pacemaker. *PACE* 14:1119-1128, 1991

221. Nathan AW, Bexton RS, Spurrell RAJ, et al: Internal transvenous low energy cardioversion for the treatment of cardiac arrhythmias. *Br Heart J* 52:377-384, 1984

222. Waspe LE, Kim SG, Matos JA, et al: Role of a catheter lead system for transvenous countershock and pacing during electrophysiologic tests: an assessment of the usefulness of catheter shocks for terminating ventricular tachyarrhythmias. *Am J Cardiol* 52:477-484, 1983

223. Ciccone JM, Saksena S, Shah Y, et al: A prospective randomized study of the clinical efficacy and safety of transvenous cardioversion for termination of ventricular tachycardia. *Circulation* 71:571-578, 1985

224. Jackman WM, Zipes DP: Low-energy synchronous cardioversion of ventricular tachycardia using a catheter electrode in a canine model of subacute myocardial infarction. *Circulation* 66:187-195, 1982

225. Zipes DP, Jackman WM, Heger JJ, et al: Clinical transvenous cardioversion of recurrent life-threatening ventricular tachyarrhythmias: low energy synchronized cardioversion of ventricular tachycardia and termination of ventricular fibrillation in patients using a catheter electrode. *Am Heart J* 103:789-794, 1982

226. Yee R, Zipes DP, Gulamhusein S, et al: Low energy countershock using an intravascular catheter in an acute cardiac care setting. *Am J Cardiol* 50:1124-1129, 1982

227. Zipes DP, Heger JJ, Miles WM, et al: Early experience with an implantable cardioverter. *N Engl J Med* 311:485-490, 1984

228. Miles WM, Prystowsky EN, Heger JJ, et al: The implantable transvenous cardioverter: long-term efficacy and reproducible induction of ventricular tachycardia. *Circulation* 74:518-524, 1986

229. Winkle RA, Stinson EB, Bach SM Jr, et al: Measurement of cardioversion/defibrillation thresholds in man by a truncated exponential waveform and an apical patch-superior vena cava spring electrode configuration. *Circulation* 69:766-771, 1984

230. Lindsay BD, Saksena S, Rothbart ST, et al: Prospective evaluation of a sequential pacing and high-energy bidirectional shock algorithm for transvenous cardioversion in patients with ventricular tachycardia. *Circulation* 76:601-609, 1987

231. Saksena S, An H: Clinical efficacy of dual electrode systems for endocardial cardioversion of ventricular tachycardia: a prospective randomized crossover trial. *Am Heart J* 119:15-22, 1990

232. Jones DL, Sohla A, Bourland JD, et al: Internal ventricular defibrillation with sequential pulse countershock in pigs: comparison with single pulses and effects of pulse separation. *PACE* 10:497-502, 1987

233. Jones DL, Klein GJ, Guiraudon GM, et al: Internal cardiac defibrillation in man: pronounced improvement with sequential pulse delivery to two different lead orientations. *Circulation* 73:484-491, 1986

234. Wetherbee JN, Chapman PD, Klopfenstein HS, et al: Nonthoracotomy internal defibrillation in dogs: threshold reduction using a subcutaneous chest wall electrode with a transvenous catheter electrode. *J Am Coll Cardiol* 10:406-411, 1987

235. Bardy GH, Stewart RB, Ivey TD, et al: Intraoperative comparison of sequential-pulse and single-pulse defibrillation in candidates for automatic implantable defibrillators. *Am J Cardiol* 60:618-624, 1987

236. Kelly PA, Cannom DS, Garan HS, et al: The automatic implantable cardioverter-defibrillator: efficacy, complications and survival in patients with malignant ventricular arrhythmias. *J Am Coll Cardiol* 11:1278-1286, 1988

237. Hannekum A, Dalichau H, Kochs M, et al: Sequential or single pulse defibrillation? Investigations towards energy reduction in experimental animals. *Thorac Cardiovasc Surg* 35:270-276, 1987

238. Saksena S, Parsonnet V: Implantation of a cardioverter/defibrillator without thoracotomy using a triple electrode system. *JAMA* 259:69-72, 1988

239. Montenero AS, Bombardieri G, Barilaro C, et al: Comparison between two versus three patches single pulse shock defibrillation in pigs. *PACE* 14:362-365, 1991

240. Chang M-S, Inoue H, Kallok MJ, et al: Double and triple sequential shocks reduce the ventricular defibrillation thresholds in dogs with and without myocardial infarction. *J Am Coll Cardiol* 8:1393-1405, 1986

241. Watkins L Jr, Mirowski M, Mower MM, et al: Implantation of the automatic defibrillator: the subxiphoid approach. *Ann Thorac Surg* 34:575, 1982

242. Watkins L Jr, Mower MM, Reid PR, et al: Surgical techniques for implanting the automatic implantable defibrillator. *PACE* 7:1357-1362, 1984

243. O'Neill PG, Lawrie GM, Kaushik RR, et al: Late results of the left subcostal approach for automatic implantable cardioverter defibrillator implantation. *Am J Cardiol* 67:387-390, 1991

244. Watkins L Jr, Mirowski M, Mower MM, et al: Automatic defibrillation in man: the initial surgical experience. *J Thorac Cardiovasc Surg* 82:492-500, 1981

245. Leclercq JF, Menasché P, Laborde F, et al: Clinical use of automatic implantable defibrillators. *Eur Heart J* 8 Suppl D:143-147, 1987

246. Marchlinski FE, Flores BT, Buxton AE, et al: The automatic implantable cardioverter-defibrillator: efficacy, complications, and device failures. *Ann Intern Med* 104:481-488, 1986

247. Almassi GH, Chapman PD, Troup PJ, et al: Constrictive pericarditis associated with patch electrodes of the automatic implantable cardioverter-defibrillator. *Chest* 92:369-371, 1987

248. Singer I, Hutchins GM, Mirowski M, et al: Pathologic findings related to the lead system and repeated defibrillations in patients with the automatic implantable cardioverter-defibrillator. *J Am Coll Cardiol* 10:382-388, 1987

249. Marchlinski FE, Flores B, Miller JM, et al: Relation of the intraoperative defibrillation threshold to successful postoperative defibrillation with an automatic implantable cardioverter defibrillator. *Am J Cardiol* 62:393-398, 1988

250. Winkle RA, Mead RH, Ruder MA, et al: Long-term outcome with the automatic implantable cardioverter-defibrillator. *J Am Coll Cardiol* 13:1353-1361, 1989

251. Troup PJ, Chapman PD, Olinger GN, et al: The implanted defibrillator: relation of defibrillating lead configuration and clinical variables to defibrillation threshold. *J Am Coll Cardiol* 6:1315-1321, 1985

252. Chapman PD, Sagar KB, Wetherbee JN, et al: Relationship of left ventricular mass to defibrillation threshold for the implantable defibrillator: a combined clinical and animal study. *Am Heart J* 114:274-278, 1987

253. Guarnieri T, Levine JH, Veltri EP, et al: Success of chronic defibrillation and the role of antiarrhythmic drugs with the automatic implantable cardioverter/defibrillator. *Am J Cardiol* 60:1061-1064, 1987

254. Vlay SC: The automatic internal cardioverter-defibrillator: comprehensive clinical follow-up, economic and social impact—the Stony Brook experience. *Am Heart J* 112:189-194, 1986

255. O'Neill PG, Boahene KA, Lawrie GM, et al: The automatic implantable cardioverter-defibrillator: effect of patch polarity on defibrillation threshold. *J Am Coll Cardiol* 17:707-711, 1991

256. Grubb BP, Mancini M, Temesy-Armos P, et al: Resolution of high initial epicardial patch defibrillation thresholds following chronic implantation. *PACE* 14:149-151, 1990

257. Huang SKS, Tan de Guzman WL, Chenarides JG, et al: Effects of long-term amiodarone therapy on the defibrillation threshold and the rate of shocks of the implantable cardioverter-defibrillator. *Am Heart J* 122:720-727, 1991

258. Echt DS, Barbey JT, Black JN: Influence of ventricular fibrillation duration on defibrillation energy in dogs using bidirectional pulse discharges. *PACE* 11:1315-1323, 1988

259. Bardy GH, Ivey TD, Allen M, et al: A prospective, randomized evaluation of effect of ventricular fibrillation duration on defibrillation thresholds in humans. *J Am Coll Cardiol* 13:1362-1366, 1989

260. Echt DS, Armstrong K, Schmidt P, et al: Clinical experience, complications, and survival in 70 patients with the automatic implantable cardioverter/defibrillator. *Circulation* 71:289-296, 1985

261. Luceri RM, Thurer RJ, Palatianos GM, et al: The automatic implantable cardioverter-defibrillator: results, observations, and comments. *PACE* 9:1343-1348, 1986

262. Reid PR, Mirowski M, Mower MM, et al: Clinical evaluation of the internal automatic cardioverter-defibrillator in survivors of sudden cardiac death. *Am J Cardiol* 51:1608-1613, 1983

263. Grubb BP, Mancini M: A technique for intraoperative arrhythmia induction during automatic implantable defibrillator placement. *PACE* 13:958-960, 1990

264. Physicians manual for the CPI, AICD: St. Paul, Cardiac Pacemaker, Inc., 1985

265. Physicians manual for CPI AICD Ventak model generation. St. Paul, Cardiac Pacemaker, Inc., 1986

266. Mercando AD, Furman S, Johnston D, et al: Survival of patients with the automatic implantable cardioverter defibrillator. *PACE* 11: 2059-2063, 1988

267. Paull DL, Fellows CL, Guyton SW, et al: Early experience with the automatic implantable cardioverter defibrillator in sudden death survivors. *Am J Surg* 157:516-518, 1989

268. Tchou PJ, Kadri N, Anderson J, et al: Automatic implantable cardioverter defibrillators and survival of patients with left ventricular dysfunction and malignant ventricular arrhythmias. *Ann Intern Med* 109:529-534, 1988

269. Palatianos GM, Thurer RJ, Cooper DK, et al: The implantable cardioverter-defibrillator: clinical results. *PACE* 14:297-301, 1991

270. Porterfield JG, Porterfield LM, Bray L: Long-term community hospital experience with internal defibrillator. *PACE* 14:263-266, 1991

271. Kron J, Oliver RP, Norsted S, et al: The automatic implantable cardioverter-defibrillator in young patients. *J Am Coll Cardiol* 16:896-902, 1990

272. Kim SG, Fisher JD, Furman S, et al: Benefits of implantable defibrillators are overestimated by sudden death rates and better represented by total arrhythmic death rate. *J Am Coll Cardiol* 17:1587-1592, 1991

273. Tresch DD, Troup PJ, Thakur RK, et al: Comparison of efficacy of automatic implantable cardioverter defibrillator in patients older and younger than 65 years of age. *Am J Med* 90:717-724, 1991

274. Fogoros RN, Elson JJ, Bonnet CA, et al: Efficacy of the automatic implantable cardioverter-defibrillator in prolonging survival in patients with severe underlying cardiac disease. *J Am Coll Cardiol* 16:381-386, 1990

275. Axtell K, Tchou P, Akhtar M: Survival in patients with depressed left ventricular function treated by implantable cardioverter defibrillator. *PACE* 14:291-296, 1991

276. de Marchena E, Chakko S, Fernandez P, et al: Usefulness of the automatic implantable cardioverter defibrillator in improving survival of patients with severely depressed left ventricular function associated with coronary artery disease. *Am J Cardiol* 67:812-816, 1991

277. Fain ES, Lee JT, Winkle RA: Effects of acute intravenous and chronic oral amiodarone on defibrillator energy requirements. *Am Heart J* 114:8-17, 1987

278. Handelsman H: Implantation of the automatic cardioverter-defibrillator. *Health Technol Assess Rep* No 10:1-9, 1990

279. Lehmann MH, Saksena S: Implantable cardioverter defibrillators in cardiovascular practice: report of the Policy Conference of the North American Society of Pacing and Electrophysiology. *Pacing Clin Electrophysiol* 14:969-979, 1991

280. Epstein AE, Shepard RB, Kirklin JK, et al: Failure of elective replacement indicator to predict end-of-life of the automatic implantable cardioverter-defibrillator. *PACE* 11:569-574, 1988

281. Manolis AS, Rastegar H, Estes NAM III: Prophylactic automatic implantable cardioverter-defibrillator patches in patients at high risk for postoperative ventricular tachyarrhythmias. *J Am Coll Cardiol* 13:1367-1373, 1989

282. Platia EV, Griffith LSC, Watkins L Jr, et al: Treatment of malignant ventricular arrhythmias with endocardial resection and implantation of the automatic cardioverter-defibrillator. *N Engl J Med* 314:213-216, 1986

283. Winkle RA, Bach SM Jr, Mead RH, et al: Comparison of defibrillation efficacy in humans using a new catheter and superior vena cava spring–left ventricular patch electrodes. *J Am Coll Cardiol* 11:365-370, 1988

284. Watkins L Jr, Platia EV, Mower MM, et al: The treatment of malignant ventricular arrhythmias with combined endocardial resection and implantation of the automatic defibrillator: preliminary report. *Ann Thorac Surg* 37:60-65, 1984

285. Watkins L Jr, Mower MM, Reid PR, et al: Trials of the automatic implantable defibrillator in man: a three-year program report. *J Thorac Cardiovasc Surg* 86:381-387, 1983

286. Bolling SF, Deeb GM, Morady F, et al: Automatic internal cardioverter defibrillator: a bridge to heart transplantation. *J Heart Lung Transplant* 10:562-566, 1991

287. Slater AD, Singer I, Stavens CS, et al: Treatment of malignant ventricular arrhythmias with the automatic implantable cardioverter defibrillator. *Ann Surg* 209:635-641, 1989

288. Trappe H-J, Daniel WG, Klein H, et al: Evaluation of global and regional left ventricular function using two-dimensional and M-mode echocardiography in patients with an automatic implantable cardioverter defibrillator. *PACE* 11:1070-1076, 1988

289. Kron IL, Haines DE, Tribble CG, et al: Operative risks of the implantable defibrillator *versus* endocardial resection. *Ann Surg* 211:600-603, 1990

290. Edel TB, Castle LW, Morant VA, et al: Effect of combined cardiac surgery during implantable defibrillator placement on operative mortality and morbidity, late mortality and shock analysis (abstract). *PACE* 13:529, 1990

291. Rosenthal ME, Josephson ME: Current status of antitachycardia devices. *Circulation* 82:1889-1899, 1990

292. Brodman R, Fisher JD, Furman S, et al: Implantation of automatic cardioverter-defibrillators via median sternotomy. *PACE* 7:1363-1369, 1984

293. Rosenfeld LE: Device therapy of ventricular tachyarrhythmias. *Cardiol Clin* 6:437-448, 1988

294. Department of Health and Human Services. Health Care Financing Administration. Implantation of automatic defibrillators. Section 35-95, 1986

295. Gabry MD, Brodman R, Johnston D, et al: Automatic implantable cardioverter-defibrillator: patient survival, battery longevity and shock delivery analysis. *J Am Coll Cardiol* 9:1349-1356, 1987

296. Van Vleet JF, Tacker AW Jr, Bourland JD, et al: Cardiac damage in dogs with chronically implanted automatic defibrillator electrode catheters and given four episodes of multiple shocks. *Am Heart J* 106:300-307, 1983

297. Gottlieb CD, Horowitz LN: Potential interactions between antiarrhythmic medication and the automatic implantable cardioverter defibrillator. *PACE* 14:898-904, 1991

298. Echt DS, Winkle RA: Management of patients with the AICD. *Clin Prog EP Pacing* 3:4, 1985

299. Schuger CD, Jackson K, Steinman RT, et al: Atrial sensing to augment ventricular tachycardia detection by the automatic implantable cardioverter defibrillator: a utility study. *PACE* 11:1456-1464, 1988

300. Maloney J, Masterson M, Khoury D, et al: Clinical performance of the implantable cardioverter defibrillator: electrocardiographic documentation of 101 spontaneous discharges. *PACE* 14:280-285, 1991

301. Singer I, Guarnieri T, Kupersmith J: Implanted automatic defibrillators: effects of drugs and pacemakers. *PACE* 11:2250-2262, 1988

302. Singer I, deBorde R, Veltri EP, et al: The automatic implantable cardioverter defibrillator: T wave sensing in the newest generation. *PACE* 11:1584-1591, 1988

303. Gottlieb C, Miller JM, Rosenthal ME, et al: Automatic implantable defibrillator discharge resulting from routine pacemaker programming. *PACE* 11:336-338, 1988

304. Axtell KA, Akhtar M: Incidence of syncope prior to implantable cardioverter defibrillator discharges (abstract). *Circulation* 82 Suppl 3:211, 1990

305. Fogoros RN, Elson JJ, Bonnet CA: Actuarial incidence and pattern of occurrence of shocks following implantation of the automatic implantable cardioverter defibrillator. *PACE* 12:1465-1473, 1989

306. Khastgir T, Aarons D, Veltri E: Sudden bradyarrhythmic death in patients with the implantable cardioverter-defibrillator: report of two cases. *PACE* 14:395-398, 1991

307. Callans DJ, Hook BG, Marchlinski FE: Paced beats following single nonsensed complexes in a "codependent" cardioverter defibrillator and bradycardia pacing system: potential for ventricular tachycardia induction. *PACE* 14:1281-1287, 1991

308. Fain ES, Dorian P, Davy J-M, et al: Effects of encainide and its metabolites on energy requirements for defibrillation. *Circulation* 73:1334-1341, 1986

309. Reiffel JA, Coromilas J, Zimmerman JM, et al: Drug-device interactions: clinical considerations. *PACE* 8:369-373, 1985

310. Dawson AK, Steinberg MI, Shapland JE, et al: Effect of class I and class III drugs on current and energy required for internal defibrillation (abstract). *Circulation* 72 Suppl 3:384, 1985

311. Deeb GM, Hardesty RL, Griffith BP, et al: The effects of cardiovascular drugs on the defibrillation threshold and the pathological effects on the heart using an automatic implantable defibrillator. *Ann Thorac Surg* 35:361-366, 1983

312. Vaitkus PT, Buxton AE, Josephsen ME, et al: Cycle-length response of ventricular tachycardia associated with coronary artery disease to procainamide and amiodarone. *Am J Cardiol* 66:710-714, 1990

313. Jones DL, Klein GJ, Rattes MF, et al: Internal cardiac defibrillation: single and sequential pulses and a variety of lead orientations. *PACE* 11:583-591, 1988

314. Bach SM Jr, Barstad J, Harper N, et al: Initial clinical experience: Endotak—implantable transvenous defibrillator system (abstract). *J Am Coll Cardiol* 13 Suppl A:65, 1989

315. Cohen TJ, Liem LB: Mixed venous oxygen saturation for differentiating stable from unstable tachycardias. *Am Heart J* 122:733-740, 1991

316. Cohen TJ, Liem LB: A hemodynamically responsive antitachycardia system: development and basis for design in humans. *Circulation* 82:394-406, 1990

317. Sharma AD, Bennett TD, Erickson M, et al: Right ventricular pressure during ventricular arrhythmias in humans: potential implications for implantable antitachycardia devices. *J Am Coll Cardiol* 15:648-655, 1990

CHAPTER

26

Ablative therapy for cardiac arrhythmias

Douglas L. Packer, M.D.

For more than 20 years, antiarrhythmic drug therapy has been the mainstay of treatment for patients with supraventricular or ventricular tachycardias. Although many patients have derived substantial benefit from this therapy, inefficacy, significant side effects, and proarrhythmia have prevented optimal outcome in others. These problems have provided the incentive for the development of innovative alternative forms of therapy for patients with arrhythmias. When Dr. Will Sealy and associates in 1968 were successful in surgically interrupting an accessory pathway in a North Carolina fisherman with Wolff-Parkinson-White syndrome, a new era of nonpharmacologic therapy for a wide variety of arrhythmias was ushered in.[1] Subsequent improvements in electrophysiologic mapping and operative techniques enabled successful interruption of accessory pathways for permanent cure of arrhythmias related to accessory pathways in more than 1,000 patients.[2,3] On the basis of this progress, surgical techniques have also been developed for the treatment of other arrhythmias, including atrioventricular (AV) nodal reentrant,[4-6] ectopic atrial,[7] and more life-threatening ventricular tachycardias.[8-11]

CATHETER ABLATION OF THE AV CONDUCTION SYSTEM

Despite impressive rates of success, the potential morbidity and mortality of these surgical procedures made the development of less invasive catheter-based techniques for the elimination of arrhythmias desirable. The first progress toward that end came in the early 1980s when several groups demonstrated that 200 to 300 J of direct current energy could be delivered from an external defibrillator through a catheter to successfully interrupt the normal AV conduction system.[12,13] Typically, this technique was applied in patients with atrial fibrillation and a rapid ventricular response rate that could not be controlled adequately with antiarrhythmic medication. Enthusiasm for this technique was tempered, however, by the requirement of permanent pacemaker implantation after the procedure and the risk of sudden cardiac death that accompanied scar formation at the ablation site.[14] In addition, this approach could not be used in patients with the Wolff-Parkinson-White syndrome because of the propensity for rapid anterograde conduction during atrial fibrillation. In such patients, interruption of the normal AV conduction system does not deal with the underlying risk of sudden cardiac death and may even aggravate that risk by eliminating retrograde concealed conduction into the accessory pathway. Attention was, therefore, turned toward primary ablation of the accessory pathway in these patients.

ACCESSORY PATHWAY ABLATION

Although ablation of an accessory connection held theoretical promise, early applications of direct current to the pathway produced disappointing results. Brodman and Fisher[15] found that 35- to 45-J shocks delivered in the canine coronary sinus produced extensive fibrosis of the AV groove, coronary sinus occlusion, and intimal hyperplasia of the accompanying circumflex coronary artery. Subsequently, a patient who received 100- and 150-J shocks experienced coronary sinus rupture requiring emergency operation,[16] a further demonstration that the risk of applying this technique to ablate left-sided accessory pathways outweighed potential benefit. Furthermore, early investigators demonstrated that standard delivery of direct current energy via the coronary sinus was unlikely to interrupt accessory pathway conduction.[16]

Despite this disappointing initial experience with left free-wall connections, posteroseptal accessory pathways were found to be more amenable to delivery of direct current energy. After an initial report demonstrating incidental elimination of the posteroseptal accessory pathway in a patient undergoing direct current ablation of the normal AV conduction system,[13] others achieved success rates of 60% to 75% in patients with pathways in this location.[17-19] Although these rates provided cause for optimism, at least three patients undergoing this technique sustained coronary sinus rupture with accompanying cardiac tamponade.[19,20] Right coronary artery spasm following ablation to a right free-wall pathway after delivery of direct current energy was also reported.[21]

Subsequently, several important developments improved the success rate and substantially decreased the risk accompanying pathway ablation. First, Warin et al.[22] conclusively demonstrated that reduced-output direct current energy shocks from an endocardial approach were sufficient for ablation of accessory pathways, including those on the left side of the heart. These investigators found that a series of 160-J shocks successfully eliminated accessory pathway conduction in 91% of patients without producing significant complications. Others provided similar documentation of the safety and efficacy of low-energy direct current deliveries.[23] Another advancement was the development of flexible, steerable catheters that enabled more precise mapping of both the tricuspid and the mitral valve annuli. These catheters could also be more readily retroflexed beneath the respective valve leaflets to record discrete potentials from accessory pathways[24] and thus enable more precise localization of those connections.

Creation of lesions with radiofrequency energy

An additional step forward came when radiofrequency energy sources were developed for the ablation of cardiac tissue. During radiofrequency ablation, a 300- to 500-kHz oscillating sine wave signal applied to cardiac tissue via catheters heats the tissue at the catheter-tissue interface.[25-28] With sufficient heat generation, irreversible tissue desiccation occurs, and discrete, well-circumscribed lesions are created. This lesion production is a function of several factors. Hoyt et al.[27] found irreversible myocardial damage with energy delivery above a threshold of 20 J. In addition, they found that the volume and depth of lesions correlated with the absolute energy delivered. These investigators also determined that the diameter and depth of lesions paralleled increments in catheter contact pressure. Others[26] showed that lesion size was related to catheter or electrode radius. In other work, Haines and Verow[28] found that lesion size was proportional to peak temperature and that temperature was more predictive of lesion size than power, current, or energy characteristics.[25] Similar findings were reported by others.[29] In this regard, several groups showed that irreversible tissue desiccation occurred at a threshold temperature of 48° to 67°C.[25,29] Because of this relationship, thermistor-tipped catheters were developed to allow temperature monitoring to guide radiofrequency catheter ablation.[30] In addition, heating of the catheter-tissue interface to temperatures near 100°C produces coagulum formation on the catheter tip and tissue charring, manifested electrically as an abrupt increase in measured impedance.[28] In vitro and in vivo studies[28,31] documented that this impedance rise is accompanied by the explosive generation of microcavitation produced by boiling at that catheter-tissue interface. Boiling appears to be a function of energy delivered, duration of energy delivery,[31] and tissue contact pressure in excess of 80 g.[32] The incorporation of temperature-sensing thermistors was also proposed as a means to monitor and avoid these excessive increases in temperature. From information acquired in animal testing, radiofrequency energy was then directed toward ablation of accessory pathways.

Results and risks of ablation

Left free-wall accessory pathways. During the past 4 years, progress has been rapid and more than 5,000 patients have successfully undergone closed-chest elimination of their accessory pathways, resulting in cure of their symptomatic arrhythmias. Because of this progress, the need for cardiac surgery for this purpose has largely been eliminated.

In most series, 50% to 60% of all accessory pathways are located in the left free-wall position.[33-37] Several different methods have been developed to obtain access to these pathways, including transaortic[33,34] and transseptal approaches.[36,38-40] In both cases, the location of the accessory pathway is initially identified with the aid of a catheter positioned in the coronary sinus. In the retrograde aortic approach, an ablation catheter, typically with a 4-mm tip, is introduced percutaneously into a femoral artery, advanced via the aorta, and retroflexed across the aortic valve. Both catheter torque and flexion-extension of the distal catheter segment are used to position the tip beneath the mitral valve leaflet near the AV groove (Fig 26-1) in a position corresponding to the pathway location identified with the aid of the coronary sinus catheter. In this position, ablation-guiding atrial and ventricular deflections on intracardiac electrograms can be recorded.

The electrogram markers of pathway location include (1) an accessory pathway potential originating in the bypass tract, (2) the shortest local AV interval in patients in whom the pathway is identified during normal sinus rhythm or during atrial pacing, and (3) the point of earliest local ventricular activation at the ventricular insertion of the accessory pathway, as referenced to the onset of the surface QRS complex.[33-35,41] Each of these findings is illustrated in Figure 26-2,A, in which an accessory pathway potential is seen immediately before the earliest local ventricular activation that preceded the onset of the surface QRS complex on the electrocardiogram (ECG) by 20 msec. In addition, when mapping is performed during orthodromic reciprocating tachycardia or ventricular pacing, the pathway location may be indicated by the shortest local ventriculoatrial interval observed. In the optimal catheter position, the amplitude of the atrial electrogram is maximized and local AV conduction times are between 20 and 35 msec.[33,36] No one observation appears to be preferential to others in identifying the pathway location. Rather, combinations of these findings allow the direction of the catheter to the most appropriate ablation site. Energy delivered at the accessory pathway location identified in Figure 26-2,A eliminated the pathway, as shown in Figure 26-2,B.

An additional approach for the elimination of left free-wall pathways is a transseptal route.[36,38,40] Standard transseptal needle techniques are used to position a transseptal sheath across the interatrial septum. An ablation catheter is then introduced through the sheath to a position on the mitral valve annulus (Fig 26-3) where electrograms with more nearly equal atrial and ventricular

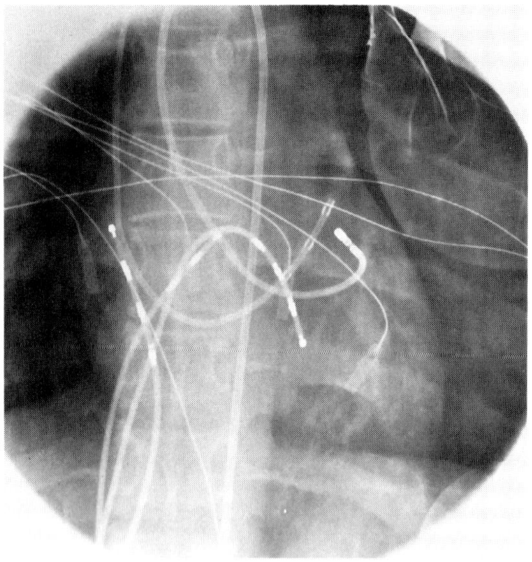

Fig 26-1 Anteroposterior chest radiograph showing transaortic catheter positioning for ablation of a left free-wall accessory pathway. Multipolar electrode catheters were introduced percutaneously and positioned in the high right atrium, right ventricle, region of the His bundle, and coronary sinus to localize the accessory pathway. As shown, the ablation catheter is advanced through the aortic valve and positioned beneath the mitral valve leaflet near the accessory connection.

deflections are seen. This approach offers the theoretical advantage of permitting catheter manipulation without interference from papillary muscle or other valvular support structures.[36,40] Similarly, the transseptal approach avoids the use of an arterial access site, which may be complicated by development of an arterial pseudoaneurysm or other vascular damage. In addition, damage to the aortic valve is possible with the transaortic approach.[42] In contrast, catheter stability in the region of the annulus may be less easily obtained with the transseptal approach. Figure 26-4 shows recordings before and after ablation in a patient in whom a left free-wall pathway was eliminated within 2.3 seconds of energy delivery by this approach. Here, the atrial and ventricular deflections recorded on the ablation catheter (RFDIST) are nearly fused, indicating the precise pathway location.

After mapping, radiofrequency energy is delivered between the catheter tip and an indifferent skin patch electrode positioned on the back near the scapula. Radiofrequency voltages between 40 and 70 V, yielding ablation powers of 25 to 40 W, are routinely used.[33-37] Available information suggests that disappearance of accessory pathway function within 4 seconds after the initiation of energy delivery predicts long-term success in elimination of the pathway, provided that energy application can be continued for at least 12 seconds.[43] Comparable success rates are possible with both the transaortic and the transseptal routes.[38-40] Energy delivery with either approach is relatively pain-free, allowing ablation without

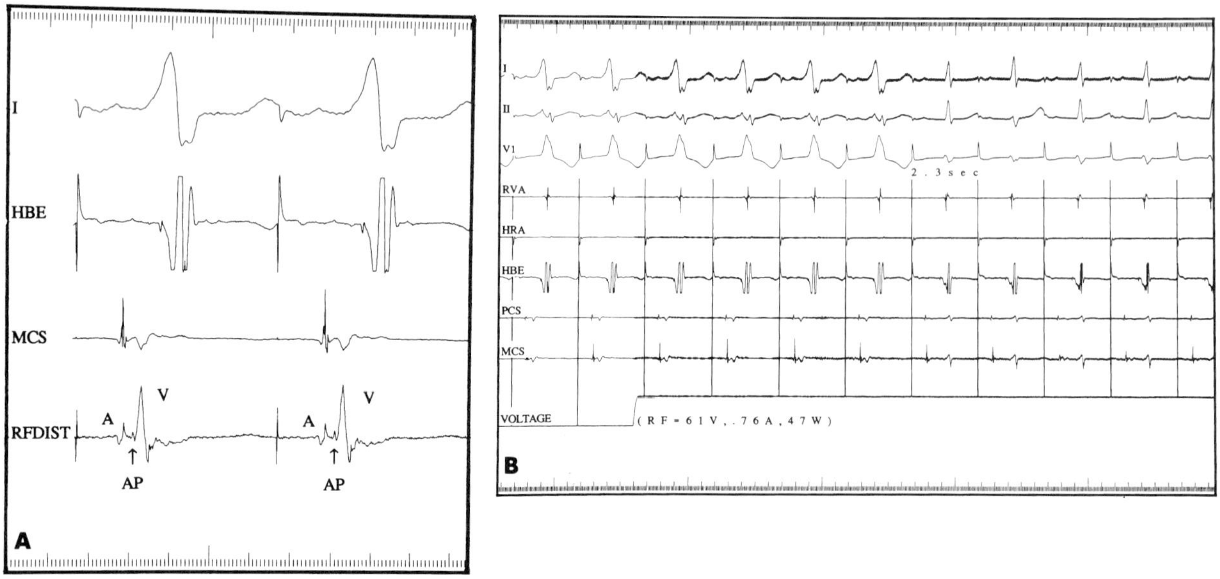

Fig 26-2 Recordings from a 10-year-old patient with a left lateral free-wall accessory pathway. **A**, shown are preablation tracings, including surface ECG lead I and intracardiac leads from the His bundle electrogram (*HBE*), the mid-coronary sinus position (*MCS*), and the distal tip of the ablation tip (*RFDIST*). Atrial (*A*) and ventricular (*V*) deflections and a discrete deflection from the accessory pathway (*AP*) were recorded from a catheter tip position below the mitral valve leaflet. The 25-msec AV interval and the accessory pathway potential indicated the precise location of the accessory pathway. **B**, energy delivery at this site resulted in successful elimination of the accessory pathway in 2.3 seconds, as indicated by the loss of preexcitation with prolongation of the AV interval recorded from both the PCS and the MCS positions. *HRA*, high right atrium; *PCS*, proximal coronary sinus; *RF*, radiofrequency; *RVA*, right ventricular apex.

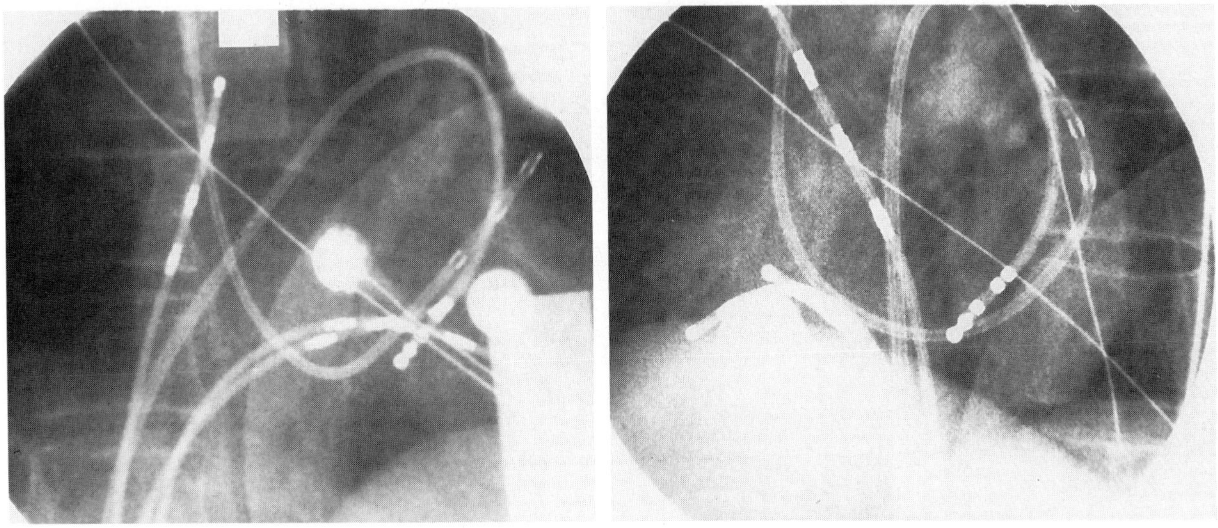

Fig 26-3 Shallow left anterior oblique (**A**) and right anterior oblique (**B**) fluoroscopic images obtained during ablation of a left paraseptal accessory pathway using a transseptal technique. Here, a Brockenbrough needle technique was used to advance the ablation catheter across the interatrial septum and position it on the mitral valve annulus in the region of the pathway. The right anterior oblique projection shows the ablation catheter looped back toward the septum on a course parallel to the coronary sinus catheter. The left anterior oblique projection shows a similar relationship between the ablation and the coronary sinus catheters as well as the proximity of the distal ablation catheter electrode and the septum, marked by the His bundle and right ventricular catheters.

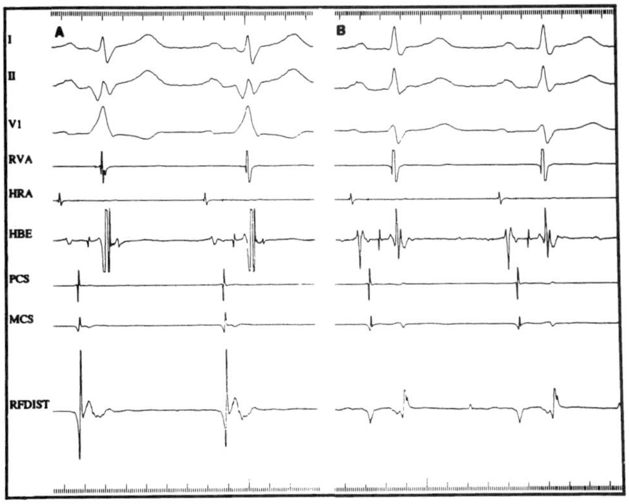

Fig 26-4 Preablation (**A**) and postablation (**B**) recordings from a 47-year-old patient with a left lateral free-wall accessory pathway. Shown are surface leads I, II, and V_1 and intracardiac recordings from the right ventricular apex (*RVA*), high right atrium (*HRA*), His bundle region (*HBE*), and proximal (*PCS*) and middle (*MCS*) coronary sinus positions and from the distal recording pair of the ablation catheter (*RFDIST*). **A**, preexcitation with a short His-ventricular interval recorded during normal sinus rhythm. The ablation catheter was positioned transseptally to an annular recording site. The RFDIST electrogram also shows the temporal relationship between atrial (sharp deflection) and ventricular (broad deflection) activation proceeding anterogradely across the accessory pathway. The two components of the RFDIST electrograms are nearly fused, indicating the location of the accessory pathway. **B**, recordings made during normal sinus rhythm after ablation. Note the absence of preexcitation, the normalization of the PR segment and the His-ventricular interval on the HBE electrogram, and the prolongation of the local AV interval recorded on the RFDIST catheter, all indicating successful interruption of the accessory pathway.

general anesthesia. Excellent rates of success have also been reported with low direct current energy delivery by the transseptal route,[22,23] although general anesthesia is required.

Posteroseptal pathway ablation. Ablation of posteroseptal accessory pathways, observed in 15% to 30% of patients with the Wolff-Parkinson-White syndrome, is complicated by the complexity of the posterior pyramidal space. As a result, these pathways are not a homogeneous group. In approximately 25% of patients, the posteroseptal pathway must be approached from the left side of the septum. An additional 25% of pathways may be immediately posterior to the normal AV conduction system in an intermedial septal position. Most pathways, however, are located in the posterior aspect of the triangle of Koch in

A

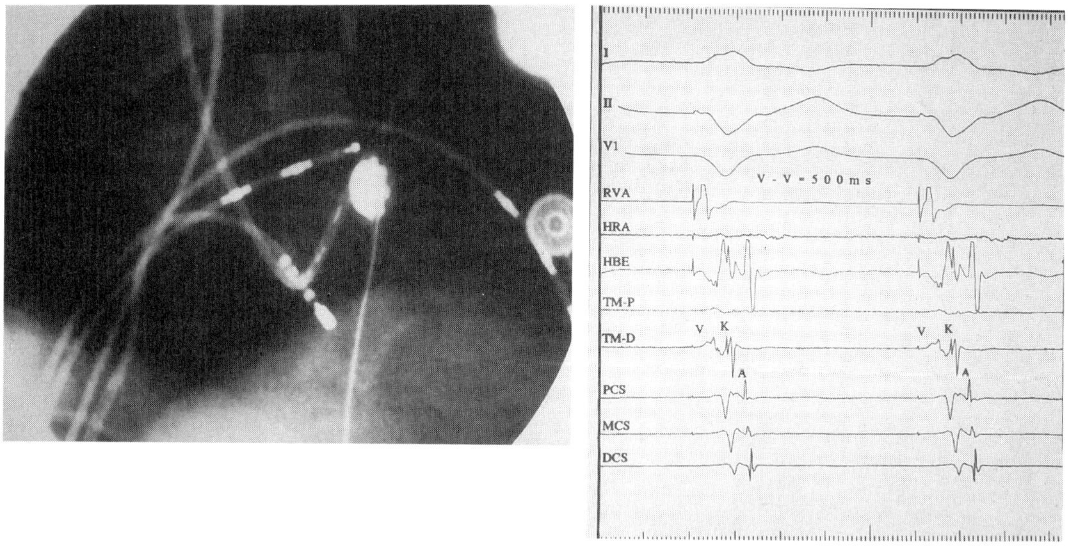

B

Fig 26-5 Fluoroscopic and intracardiac recordings during ablation of a posteroseptal accessory pathway. **A**, right anterior oblique x-ray image showing a large-tipped ablation catheter in the posterior aspect of the triangle of Koch. Other catheters are positioned in the His bundle region, right ventricular apex, and coronary sinus (going away from the plane of view). **B**, preablation tracings obtained during right ventricular pacing at a cycle length of 500 msec. Shown are surface leads I, II, and V_1 along with intracardiac leads from the right ventricular apex (*RVA*), high right atrium (*HRA*), His bundle region (*HBE*), proximal (*TM-P*) and distal (*TM-D*) poles of the tricuspid annulus mapping catheter, and proximal (*PCS*), middle (*MCS*), and distal (*DCS*) coronary sinus positions. The discrete deflection or pathway potential (*K*) is between the ventricular (*V*) and atrial (*A*) potentials originating in the pathway. The local ventriculoatrial interval of 25 msec also indicates the proximity of the distal catheter pole to the pathway. Ablation at this site successfully eliminated the pathway.

a region bounded by the coronary sinus orifice, the tendon of Todaro, and the posterior aspect of the tricuspid valve annulus (Fig 26-5,A). In Figure 26-5,A, the pathway location is also reflected by the pathway potential and the short ventriculoatrial interval seen on the recording from the distal pole of the tricuspid annulus mapping catheter (TM-D). Energy delivery at this site ablated the pathway. With the highly flexible catheters now available, each of these pathway locations is readily accessible, although success rates for the elimination of posteroseptal accessory pathways are slightly lower than those with the left free-wall variety. Figure 26-6 shows elimination of the posteroseptal pathway and cure of supraventricular tachycardia. In some cases, elimination of these pathways requires the delivery of lower energies inside the middle cardiac vein or in the mouth of the coronary sinus orifice. With these deliveries, voltages are usually decreased to the 15- to 30-V range. The risk of perforation appears to be substantially lower with delivery of radiofrequency energy in these locations than with delivery of direct current energy, in part because of the absence of barotrauma accompanying the radiofrequency energy delivery. Initial success rates of 70% to 95% have been reported, and recurrence rates of accessory pathway conduction may be 3% to 9%.[33-35,37]

Right free-wall pathway ablation. From 15% to 20% of pathways are located in the right free-wall position. With either the superior or the inferior vena cava as an access route, these pathways are approachable but are somewhat more difficult to localize and eliminate than pathways in other locations. Because there is no vein analogous to the coronary sinus, the catheter positioning is guided predominantly by fluoroscopy, and the pathway location is identified by an electrogram marker similar to that used for left free-wall pathways.[33,44] Exploring the right coronary artery with a 2F mapping catheter may provide information analogous to that obtainable with a coronary sinus catheter in patients with left free-wall pathways.[35,36] Whether this mapping technique will result in more frequent acute or chronic coronary artery damage is not clear. In many cases, the ablation catheter is positioned on the tricuspid valve annulus, where equal-sized atrial and ventricular recordings are obtainable, or is positioned underneath the tricuspid valve leaflets.[33] With energy delivery using these approaches, success rates of 80% to 98% have been possible.[33-37]

Anteroseptal accessory pathway ablation. Like the posteroseptal accessory pathways, those located in the anteroseptal position (5% to 10% of cases) pose a challenge to the electrophysiologist. Although the specific location of the pathway may be readily identified, the risk of heart block is significantly increased because of inadvertent delivery of energy to the AV conduction system. If the energy is delivered on the ventricular side

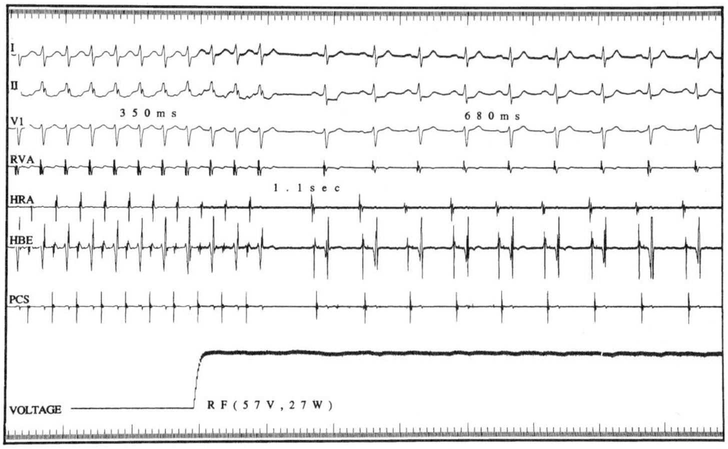

Fig 26-6 Elimination of a posteroseptal accessory pathway with radiofrequency (*RF*) energy delivery. Shown are surface leads I, II, and V_1 and intracardiac recordings from the right ventricular apex (*RVA*), high right atrium (*HRA*), His bundle region (*HBE*), and proximal coronary sinus (*PCS*). Also shown is a tracing of the delivered voltage. The left side of the figure shows supraventricular tachycardia with a cycle length of 350 msec. At 1.1 seconds after the onset of radiofrequency energy delivery, the pathway was permanently interrupted. Subsequently, normal sinus rhythm with conduction via the normal AV conduction system was present.

Table 26-1 Outcome of ablation of accessory pathways

Site	Patients, no.	Success No.	Success %	Accessory pathways, no.	Success No.	Success %	Accessory pathway return No.	Accessory pathway return %	Second procedure No.	Second procedure %
Oklahoma City[33]	164	166	99	177	175	99	15	9	17	10
Ann Arbor[34]	250	235	94	267	252	94	17	7	39	16
San Francisco[35]	100	89	89	109	98	90	9	9	17	17
Hamburg[37]	92	79	86	96	79	82	4	4	16	17
Washington, D.C.[36]	114	108	95	122	116	95	10	9	16	14
Rochester, Minn. (Mayo)	140	132	94	154	146	95	12	9	20	14

of the annulus, however, this risk may be diminished. As in other right-sided pathway locations, the success rates of 85% to 90% may be less than those with left free-wall accessory pathway ablation.[33-37]

Overall, an accessory pathway is permanently eliminated by a first procedure in 80% to 95% of cases.[33-36] In 7% to 11% of cases, accessory pathway function may return, typically within the first 2 months after the ablation procedure.[33-36] Including patients successfully treated with a second procedure, the largest available series indicate that 90% to 98% of patients can be cured of their accessory pathway-related arrhythmias (Table 26-1). Despite favorable results in early studies, additional improvements will further increase rates of success in the future. For example, continuous temperature monitoring during radiofrequency catheter ablation has already facilitated an improvement in ablation success.[30] With on-line temperature readings, energy output can be increased as necessary to produce catheter-tissue interface temperatures in a region, enabling complete and permanent pathway interruption, or decreased to avoid the impedance rise accompanying excessive temperature generation.

Risk of pathway ablation. Radiofrequency energy can eliminate pathways in all locations with relatively low risk to the patient. The relative technical difficulty and risk of pathway ablation in each location are summarized in Figure 26-7. Damage to an aortic valve due to catheter trauma[42] and untoward damage to a mitral valve related to the ablation of left free-wall pathways have occurred, although these complications affect fewer than 0.5% of patients. Although possible, tricuspid valve damage also appears to be rare, as judged by echocardiographic evaluations. Unlike delivery of direct current energy in the coronary sinus, there appears to be no evidence of untoward damage to coronary arteries when radiofrequency energy is delivered inside the heart.[45] Prolonged catheter manipulation on the left side of the heart may

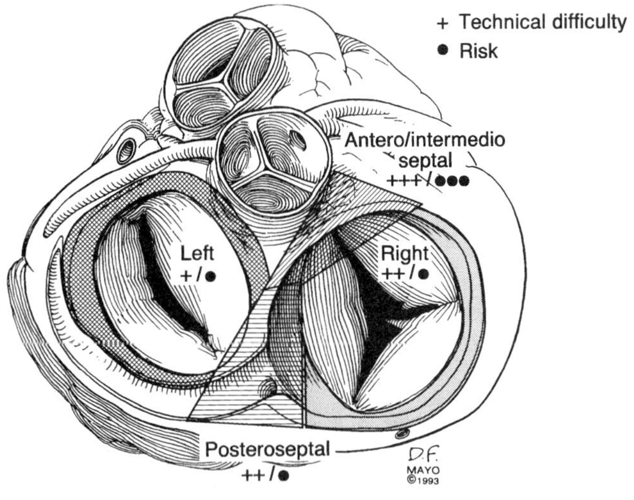

Fig 26-7 Summary of the technical difficulty and complication risk encountered in the ablation of accessory pathways. Ablation of right and left free-wall pathways is less demanding technically, unless Ebstein's malformation of the tricuspid valve is present, which increases the difficulty of ablation. The risk of a complication is similarly lower with free-wall pathways. The interruption of intermedioseptal and anteroseptal pathways in the region of the normal AV conduction system is accompanied by a greater risk of inadvertent complete heart block. (By permission, Mayo Foundation.)

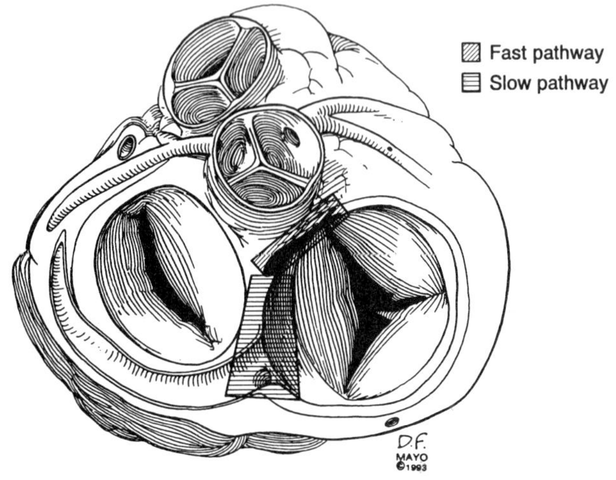

Fig 26-8 Typical locations of the fast and slow pathways participating in AV nodal reentrant tachycardia. The fast pathway is located anteriorly in the apex of the triangle of Koch. In contrast, the slow pathway, which may give rise to discrete potentials, is typically located in the posterior aspect of the triangle closer to the coronary sinus orifice. As a result, the risk of complete heart block with energy delivery in the slow pathway region is less than that with ablation of the fast pathway. (By permission, Mayo Foundation.)

also predispose to transient ischemic attacks or strokes, although with adequate anticoagulation during the procedure, the risk of this occurrence appears to be about 0.5%.[33,34] Thus, the risk of left free-wall pathway ablation appears to be low and less than the expected risk accompanying open heart surgical procedures for pathway elimination.

Ablation of septal pathways neighboring the normal AV conduction system may be accompanied by the risk of complete heart block.[33,34,36] Thus, the risk of potentially serious complications is approximately 2%, and the risk of a vascular complication is 1% to 3%. Fortunately, these untoward sequelae can usually be successfully managed without long-term consequences. Nevertheless, the decline in complication rates with additional experience suggests that radiofrequency ablation of accessory pathways should be performed only by experienced operators.

In addition to these possibilities, the development of a malignant lesion or blood dyscrasia related to fluoroscopy exposure is a theoretical risk. Calculations based on fluoroscopy times of 45 to 70 minutes suggest that this risk is about 0.1%.[36,46] Obviously, as catheter design and the experience of the operator improve, overall catheter ablation and fluoroscopy times can be reduced. Nevertheless, this eventuality has encouraged the development of alternative means of imaging radiofrequency procedures to decrease the duration of required x-ray exposure.

Indications for catheter ablation

In the past, surgical therapy for the elimination of an accessory pathway was reserved for patients with the Wolff-Parkinson-White syndrome who were at risk of sudden cardiac death. In these patients, a rapid ventricular response rate during atrial fibrillation, as indicated by the shortest R-R interval between two consecutively preexcited complexes of 250 msec or less, was used as a predictor of subsequent development of ventricular fibrillation. In addition, patients with arrhythmias refractory to medical therapy were considered to be candidates for surgery. With the further development of surgical techniques and improved myocardial protection, open pathway ablation was also offered to patients who otherwise faced a lifetime of medical therapy.[2,3]

Each of these indications may also be applied to patients in whom radiofrequency ablation is contemplated. Given the lower risk of the catheter approach, however, the indications have been expanded to include patients without adequate readily accessible health care to deal with any episodic tachycardia that might occur, patients with higher risk professions or the desire to participate in competitive sports, and patients with a family history of sudden cardiac death. In many cases, radiofrequency ablation is now being offered as first-line therapy for patients with symptoms.

Although catheter ablation has supplanted surgery for treatment of accessory pathways, operation may still be required for patients in whom radiofrequency ablation is unsuccessful and for patients with associated cardiac diseases requiring operation, such as Ebstein's anomaly.

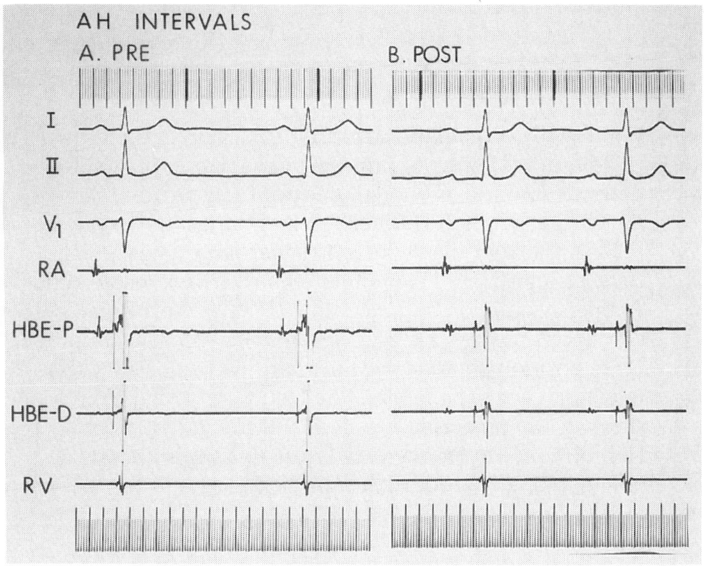

Fig 26-9 Preablation (**A**) and postablation (**B**) recordings in a patient undergoing elimination of the fast AV nodal pathway. Shown are surface ECG leads I, II, and V_1 and endocardial recordings from the high right atrium (*RA*), proximal (*HBE-P*) and distal (*HBE-D*) regions of the His bundle, and the right ventricle (*RV*). **A**, the atrio-His interval was 60 msec before ablation, reflecting AV conduction down the fast AV nodal pathway. **B**, the A-H interval has lengthened to 200 msec after the ablation of the fast connection, and AV conduction proceeds via the slower pathway. The P-R interval is also prolonged.

ATRIOVENTRICULAR NODAL REENTRANT TACHYCARDIA

Experience with the ablation of other supraventricular tachycardias is also accumulating. An additional common supraventricular arrhythmia that may be approached with catheter techniques is AV nodal reentrant tachycardia. Unlike the reentrant arrhythmias observed with the Wolff-Parkinson-White syndrome, in which the accessory pathway may be far removed from the normal AV conduction system, with AV nodal reentrant tachycardia both anterograde and retrograde components of the reentrant circuit are confined to the AV nodal or perinodal regions.

In the mid-1980s, nonpharmacologic surgical treatment for this type of arrhythmia consisted of either sharp dissection[5,6] or cryosurgical modification[4,47] of perinodal atrial tissue. In previously published reports, either technique could eliminate AV nodal reentrant tachycardia in more than 90% of patients. This success provided the impetus for development of catheter ablation techniques to produce similar modification of the AV node. In the earliest experience with such techniques, 160- to 240-J direct current shocks were delivered from the distal pole of a catheter positioned in perinodal tissue slightly posterior to the expected body of the AV node. In a series of 21 patients so treated, Haissaguerre et al.[48] demonstrated that tachycardia could not be induced in 14 of the patients during follow-up electrophysiology studies. In 16 of the patients, the procedure also abolished the clinical arrhythmia over a mean follow-up period of 14 ± 8 months without a requirement for pacemaker or subsequent drug therapy. Two other patients, however, sustained complete heart block requiring pacemaker implantation. In this series, retrograde conduction was eliminated in 15 patients. P-R prolongation after ablation was also noted, suggesting that the "fast" retrograde and anterograde AV nodal pathway was interrupted and the slow pathway was left for AV conduction.

Substantial progress in the ablation of this arrhythmia has also been made since the development of radiofrequency energy delivery methods. Energy delivery has been focused in two regions of the septum. For elimination of the fast pathway, the tip of the ablation catheter is positioned slightly anterior and superior to the AV node.[49-51] in the general region shown in Figure 26-8. Here, atrial electrogram amplitude is maximized, leaving small residual His bundle and ventricular deflections. Radiofrequency energy delivery of 20 to 60 V at this site successfully eliminated tachycardia in 95% to 98% of patients in most large series,[50] although lower success rates (70%) were also reported.[51] Since retrograde ventriculoatrial conduction is usually via the "fast" pathway, total retrograde block may occur in up to 63% of patients.[49] The P-R and atrio-His intervals also increase significantly as anterograde conduction after ablation shifts to the "slow" pathway (Fig 26-9). Because of the proximity of the ablation site to the AV node, the risk of complete heart block is appreciable, and rates between 7% and 25% have been reported.[49,51]

An additional approach for the elimination of AV nodal reentrant tachycardia is ablation of the slow pathway. The elimination of tachycardia with ablation in the more posterior aspect of the triangle of Koch (see Fig 26-8) suggests that the atrial insertion of this pathway may be confined to perinodal or extranodal tissue.[49,52,53] In many respects, elimination of this pathway is similar to ablation of more typical posteroseptal accessory pathways approachable from a posterior tricuspid annular position. In addition, as with mapping of posteroseptal pathways, discrete "slow pathway" potentials have been recorded (Fig 26-10) that are highly useful in guiding energy delivery. With this approach, success rates of 90% to 98% are possible.[51-54] In 1% to 10% of the cases, tachycardia may recur, requiring a second procedure.[49,51,53] In 40% to 65% of cases, although tachycardia is eliminated, dual AV nodal physiology persists, a result suggesting that modification of perinodal tissue or the entrance of an electrical impulse into the AV node may be critical in eliminating tachycardia.[49,52,53] After ablation, single AV nodal reen-

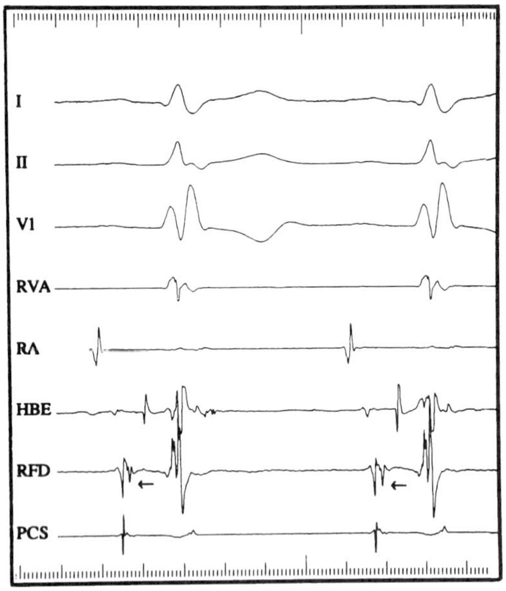

Fig 26-10 Preablation recordings during normal sinus rhythm in a 15-year-old undergoing ablation of the slow pathway to cure AV nodal reentrant tachycardia. Shown are surface leads I, II, and V_1 along with intracardiac recordings from the right ventricular apex (*RVA*), high right atrium (*RA*), His bundle region (*HBE*), distal radiofrequency ablation catheter tip (*RFD*), and proximal coronary sinus (*PCS*). The electrogram recorded from the RFD position shows a second sharp deflection (*arrows*) immediately after the atrial deflection recorded from a position in the posterior aspect of the triangle of Koch. Radiofrequency energy delivery at this site successfully eliminated AV nodal reentrant tachycardia in this patient.

A **B**

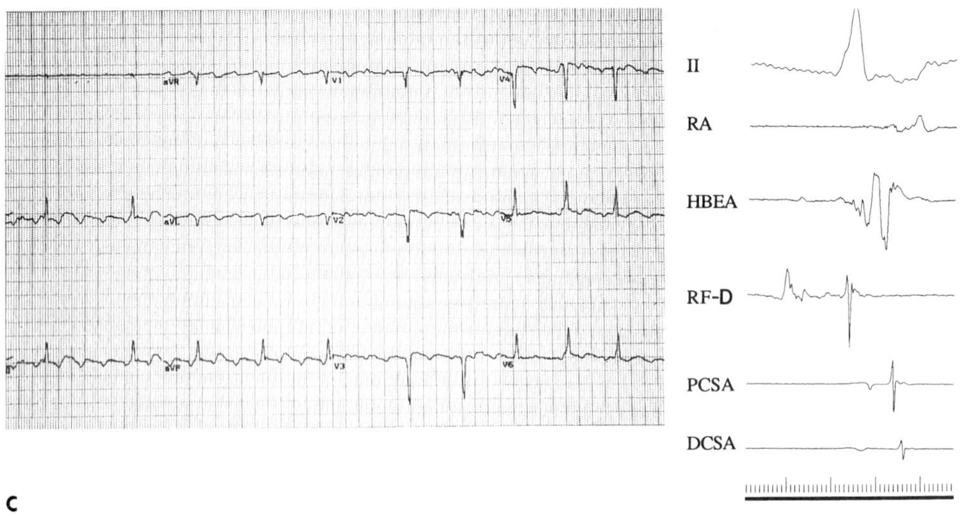

C

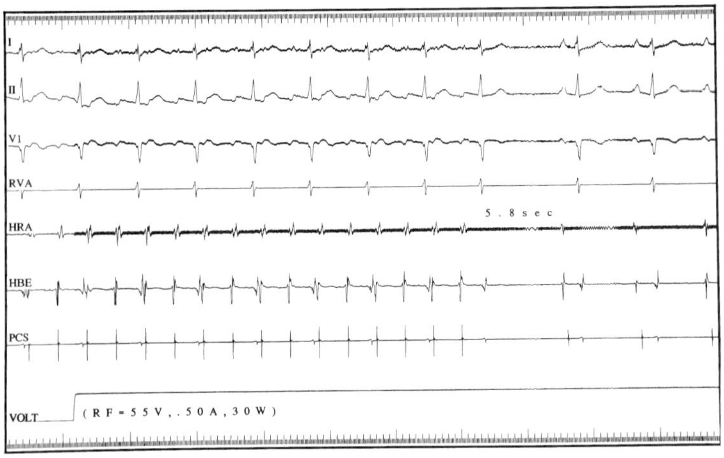

Fig 26-11 Recordings obtained during ablation of atrial flutter in a 57-year-old patient. **A**, ECG with classic (type I) atrial flutter with a saw-toothed P-wave pattern in leads II, III, and aVF. Here, the atrial activation sequence proceeded from the low posteroseptal region to the high right atrium, a reflection of a classic flutter circuit in which the reentrant impulse passes in a counterclockwise direction between the opening of the inferior vena cava and the posterior aspect of the tricuspid valve annulus. **B**, local atrial electrogram recorded from this isthmus region. Note the double atrial deflections, which were thought to indicate the remarkably slow conduction or local block observed in this region. **C**, energy delivery during atrial flutter at this site resulted in successful elimination of the arrhythmia after 5.8 seconds of 30-W radiofrequency (*RF*) energy. *DCSA*, distal coronary sinus; *HBE*, *HBEA*, His bundle region; *HRA, RA*, high right atrium; *PCS*, *PCSA*, proximal coronary sinus; *RF-D*, distal radiofrequency ablation catheter; *RVA*, right ventricular apex.

trant echo beats occur in 34% to 54% of patients, although this phenomenon does not appear to predict recurrent tachycardia.[49,53,54] Because the slow pathway location is farther posterior, the incidence of complete heart block complicating energy delivery at this site decreases to 1% to 3%.[49,51,53] This slow pathway ablation approach is, therefore, preferable to fast pathway elimination.

ATRIAL FLUTTER

Catheter and operative mapping studies[55] have indicated that in many cases the reentrant impulse responsible for classic saw-toothed atrial flutter (Fig 26-11,A) proceeds down the lateral aspect of the right atrium near the crista terminalis and passes along the isthmus of tissue between the tricuspid valve annulus and the atrial mouth of the inferior vena cava before returning back through the atria by a septal route.[56-58] This posterior annular location has also been identified as a site of relatively slow conduction in the flutter circuit,[59,60] as indicated by electrogram fractionation (Fig 26-11,B), prolonged duration of stimulus spike to local electrogram conduction times, and entrainment of the reentrant circuit with pacing immediately proximal to this inferior vena cava–tricuspid annular site.[56,60,61] In patients with such slow conduction and a classic saw-toothed flutter pattern of negative P waves in surface ECG leads II, III, and aVF, delivery of radiofrequency energy in this region has been successful in eliminating the arrhythmia. Feld et al.[56] eliminated atrial flutter in 9 of 12 patients studied. Others have reported 75% to 85% success rates in curing atrial flutter.[57,58] Figure 26-11,C shows the elimination of classic atrial flutter in a 57-year-old patient. In other patients, atypical atrial flutter with variable P-wave morphology may be present. In some cases, the flutter circuit passes in a reverse, or clockwise, direction through the isthmus of tissue between the tricuspid valve annulus and the inferior vena cava. In these patients, the P waves may appear to be upright in ECG leads II, III, and aVF. Although ablation in this region may eliminate this kind of atypical atrial flutter, circuits localized to other regions of the right or left atria may be less amenable to catheter elimination. Although relatively few patients have undergone ablation for the various types of atrial flutter, initial results are promising and suggest that this may be an additional atrial arrhythmia approachable by nonpharmacologic ablation techniques.

ECTOPIC ATRIAL TACHYCARDIAS

Catheter ablation techniques have been increasingly applied to patients with ectopic atrial tachycardias. In these patients, an ectopic focus of an automatic, triggered, or reentrant mechanism may arise in regions of the atria other than the sinus node. The origin of these ectopic foci has been localized to the right atrial free wall in approximately 68% of cases, to the intra-atrial septum in 6%, and within the left atrium in approximately 25%.[7] Most of these are also associated with the cristae terminalis of the right atrium.[62] Previously, patients with this kind of arrhythmia required open heart surgery for nonpharmacologic treatment.[7] Recently, catheter techniques have been applied to patients with this kind of arrhythmia, including those with left atrial foci.[63-65] An early report described the use of closed-chest catheter techniques with delivery of direct current energy in four patients with ectopic atrial tachycardias, two of which were located in the right atrial appendage.[63] These tachycardias were ablated with 50 or 100 J of direct current energy. In a more recent report, Kay et al.,[63] using radiofrequency energy, successfully eliminated an atrial focus of tachycardia in 13 of 15 (87%) patients. Overall, subsequent radiofrequency ablation studies show success rates of 75% to 92%.[63-66] Although concern has been raised about the possibility of perforation with energy delivery in thin-walled atrial structures, this does not appear to be a substantial problem to date. Additional experience is required to more carefully chronicle the success rates and potential complications that might be expected with the ablation of ectopic atrial tachycardias.

ATRIAL FIBRILLATION

Atrial fibrillation not only is the most common atrial arrhythmia but also may be the most difficult to treat, given the goal of maintaining normal sinus rhythm when possible or controlling the ventricular response rate if sinus rhythm is not readily restored. In the latter case, nonpharmacologic measures may be required to eliminate AV conduction if a patient has persistently rapid ventricular response rates at rest or during exercise despite therapy. Early in 1981, the original closed-chest direct current catheter technique for the ablation of the AV conduction system was developed, largely for this group of patients.[12,13] Since that time, hundreds of patients have undergone the catheter creation of complete heart block and have had significant relief of symptoms. In a study comparing catheter and open surgical procedures, the 88% success rate with the creation of complete heart block by the catheter approach was equivalent to that in patients treated with open surgical division of the AV conduction system.[67] The catheter approach, however, offers a decrease in recovery time and short-term periprocedure complications.

The quality of life in these patients after successful catheter ablation has also been excellent.[68] Although successful elimination of the normal AV conduction system is realized in 80% to 90%, approximately 9% of patients have resumption of conduction after attempted ablation but may have sufficiently modified AV conduction systems to relieve or eliminate symptoms without antiarrhythmic drugs.[14] An additional 10% to 12% of patients may become asymptomatic with antiarrhythmic agents that were ineffective before ablation.[14] In some cases, the AV conduction system can also be approached from within the left ventricle.

The application of radiofrequency energy has benefited these patients as well, and success rates in excess of 90% have been possible.[69] In addition, the risk of late sudden cardiac death appears to be lower than with delivery of direct current energy, the underlying escape rhythms

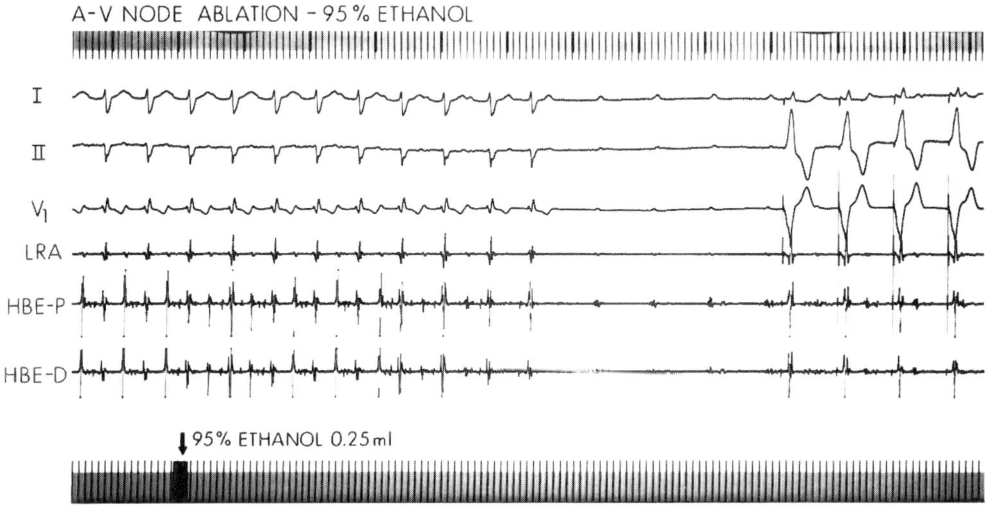

Fig 26-12 Creation of complete heart block with the injection of 95% ethanol into the AV nodal artery. A 50:50 combination of contrast material and 95% ethanol was injected into the region of the AV node through a 2F perfusion catheter introduced via the right coronary artery into the AV nodal artery. Complete block was observed in approximately 5 seconds. Subsequently, ventricular pacing was initiated, as noted in the right portion of the figure. *HBE-D*, distal region of the His bundle; *HBE-P*, proximal region of the His bundle; *LRA*, low right atrium.

appear to be more stable, and the radiofrequency approach does not require the use of general anesthesia. With successful control of the ventricular response rate, an improvement in ejection fraction may be possible in patients with a tachycardia-induced cardiomyopathy.[70,71] Preliminary studies have also suggested that in some patients, radiofrequency energy directed at the posterior septal region may sufficiently modify the ventricular response rate during atrial fibrillation to obviate complete elimination of the AV conduction system and subsequent pacemaker implantation.[72,73] Additional studies are required to determine the utility of such an approach.

Another recent development has been the evolution of techniques for ethanol ablation of the AV conduction system.[74,75] With this approach, a perfusion catheter is advanced via the dominant coronary artery into the AV nodal artery. A mixture of 0.95% alcohol and contrast material is injected to eliminate normal AV conduction (Fig 26-12). Although success rates in excess of 80% have been reported, the long-term consequences of this approach are less well defined. The greatest limitation for this approach is the requirement of a patent coronary artery leading to an identifiable AV nodal artery. Nevertheless, this may be an effective addition to the armamentarium for the elimination of the AV conduction system when other ablative attempts fail.

Although catheter treatment of atrial fibrillation and atrial flutter aims to interrupt AV conduction, techniques for surgical therapy of these atrial arrhythmias have been designed to restore sinus rhythm, prevent reentrant atrial arrhythmias, and allow normal atrial transport function. The maze procedure, described by Cox et al.,[76,77] is a series of incisions in the right and left atria that prevent reentrant tachycardia. The operation is performed with the aid of cardiopulmonary bypass and has been used in the management of patients who have symptomatic atrial fibrillation refractory to pharmacologic therapy and in patients who have atrial fibrillation and are undergoing another operative procedure, such as mitral valve repair or replacement, closure of an atrial septal defect, or septal myectomy.[78-82] The maze procedure appears to be highly effective, with success rates of 75% to 95%, with a 1% to 3% operative risk, depending on whether the patients have associated cardiac diseases.[83,84] At present, there is insufficient follow-up to know the long-term outcome of surgical treatment of atrial arrhythmias, but the approach appears to have promise, especially for younger patients with symptomatic atrial fibrillation and for selected patients who require concomitant cardiac surgical procedures.

ABLATION OF VENTRICULAR TACHYCARDIA

Attention has also been turned toward the development of similar closed-chest catheter techniques for the ablation of ventricular tachycardia (VT). In the earliest studies, direct current energy was delivered from a catheter tip positioned at the earliest site of tachycardia emergence, indicated by the point at which the local endocardial electrogram preceded the onset of the surface QRS by the greatest margin of time. Early studies, limited by small numbers of patients, indicated that the primary success rates for catheter ablation at this site were between 12% and 45%.[85-88] The Percutaneous Cardiac Mapping and Ablation Registry provided additional information on the efficacy of this direct current approach.[89] Of 88 patients who underwent closed-chest

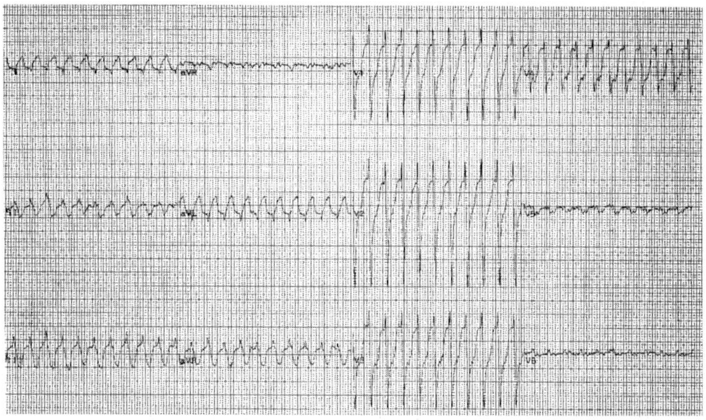

Fig 26-13 Twelve-lead surface ECG in a 62-year-old patient with coronary artery disease shows characteristic left bundle-branch block, left-axis deviation ventricular tachycardia due to a bundle-branch reentrant mechanism.

catheter ablation for a focus of VT, 29 (33%) were asymptomatic without medication on long-term postablation follow-up. An additional 33 (38%) were asymptomatic with antiarrhythmic medication administered because of persistently inducible arrhythmia. Finally, ablation failed completely in 26 (29%) of the patients. This limited success was accomplished at unacceptably high complication rates, including procedure-related deaths due to electromechanical dissociation or perforation and late sudden deaths possibly related to the ablation scars.[88,89] Such "proarrhythmia" has also occurred in animal models after direct current ablation.[90,91] On the basis of this information, the initial conclusion was that catheter ablation of VT was a procedure of last resort with marginal results.

Subsequent investigators, however, identified factors that could be exploited to improve the results of VT ablation. Additional studies showed that ventricular arrhythmias could be eliminated by ablation at the area of slow conduction within the tachycardia circuit.[92-94] Preliminary observations were validated by Fitzgerald et al.[92] in a series of 10 patients with 14 monomorphic VTs. VT in all seven patients with ablation at such an area of slow conduction, indicated by isolated mid-diastolic potentials, was successfully eliminated, although one patient required a second attempt. Two patients had persistently inducible, morphologically distinct VTs that had not been observed clinically. With these patients included, the success rate of VT ablation was 71%. The use of the earliest local ventricular activation site as a target for ablation in other patients was significantly less successful, with tachycardia elimination in only 3 of 12 (25%) energy deliveries. In similar studies, the delivery of energy at the region of slow conduction, whether from direct current or radiofrequency energy sources, significantly improved success rates to 60% to 70% of tachycardias.[93-95] The identification of the area of slow conduction, however, requires meticulous mapping, including resetting and entrainment studies, in which conduction times in various regions of the apparent VT circuit are exploited for use as a guide to energy delivery.[93-95] The use of radiofrequency energy for VT ablation may be a second factor in improving outcome of patients undergoing ablation. Although the success rate with this form of energy is no better than that with direct current energy, the risks of perforation, electromechanical dissociation, and proarrhythmia appear to be less than with direct current energy.

The catheter approach to the ablation of VTs remains limited by several factors. First, for successful ablation of a tachycardia focus, the arrhythmia must be inducible and sufficiently well tolerated hemodynamically to permit adequate mapping studies. This requirement eliminates many candidates for the procedure. Second, although patients with a single form of VT are most suited to catheter ablation techniques, it is not uncommon for patients with ventricular arrhythmias to have multiple VT morphologies. Successful treatment requires elimination of each VT. Therefore, the success rate in these patients may be less than that in patients with only one VT type. Third, VT originating from the high basal intraventricular septum may be more difficult to ablate because of difficulties with catheter access to the VT site. In some patients, the VT focus may also originate in a more epicardial location, which increases the difficulty of catheter ablation attempts. Obviously, many patients do not meet these criteria. In these patients, implantation of a device with both antitachycardia pacing and defibrillation capabilities may be more appropriate.

Several subtypes of VT may be more easily treated with an ablation technique. The first is bundle-branch reentrant VT. Typically, these tachycardias produce a left bundle-branch block, left-axis deviation, and QRS morphology (Fig 26-13) and are most commonly (but not exclusively) observed in patients with dilated cardiomyopathy.[96,97] Since the circuit for these tachycardias typically proceeds down the right bundle, crosses the intraventricular septum, and returns by the left bundle branch, ablation of the proximal right bundle branch may be highly successful in eliminating the tachycardia (Fig 26-14). Several groups have achieved success rates of nearly 100% in eliminating this VT variant by use of either direct current or radiofrequency energy.[96-99] Because this

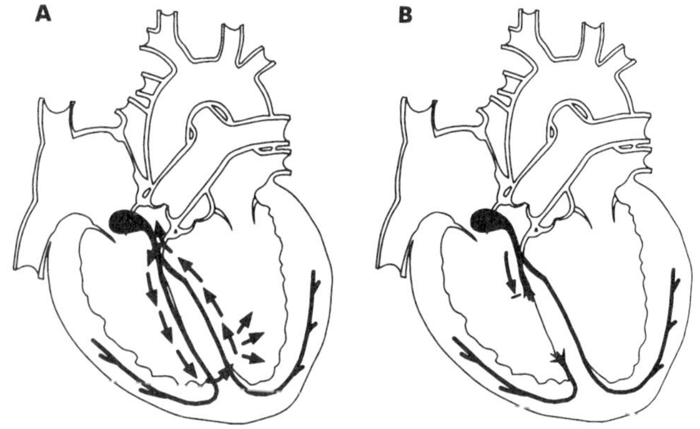

Fig 26-14 Ablation of the right bundle branch for the elimination of bundle-branch reentrant ventricular tachycardia. **A**, ventricular activation proceeds from the right bundle branch, producing a left bundle-branch block, left-axis deviation QRS morphology. The circuit subsequently proceeds across the interventricular septum and retrogradely up the left bundle branch. **B**, with interruption of the right bundle branch, the bundle-branch reentrant tachycardia circuit is interrupted.

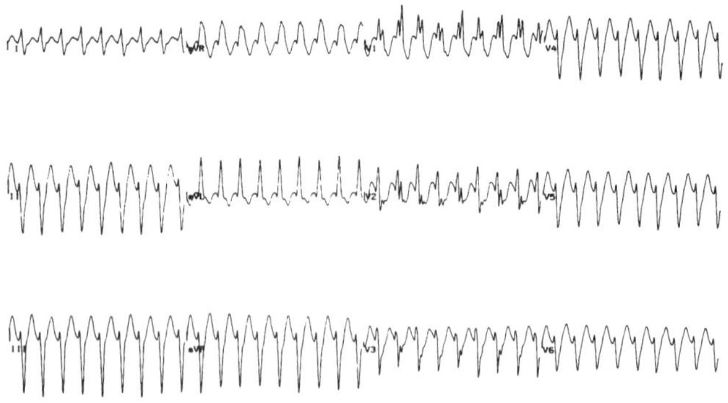

Fig 26-15 Surface 12-lead ECG showing classic right bundle-branch block, left-axis deviation ventricular tachycardia typically occurring in the absence of other organic heart disease. The earliest site of origin of this tachycardia is usually the posterior aspect of the left ventricular septum.

tachycardia is highly amenable to ablative techniques, VT studies should be performed with a His catheter in position to allow careful recording of His bundle deflections during VT. Nevertheless, these patients may have other foci of VT and are still subject to morbidity and mortality from their underlying disease.[97,98]

Two other "idiopathic" forms of VT occurring without other heart disease may be similarly amenable to ablation. Foci of tachycardia originating in the right ventricular outflow tract typically produce a left bundle, inferior axis morphology and may respond well to energy delivery.[100,101] Twelve-lead surface ECG criteria have been developed to aid localization of these foci of tachycardia.[100,102] In patients with a negative QRS complex in leads I and aVL, the focus of tachycardia is more likely to be near the septal side of the outflow tract, whereas in those with positive deflections in those leads, the earliest focus of tachycardia usually appears closer to the tricuspid valve. Delivery of energy at the earliest site of ventricular activation may successfully eliminate the tachycardia in 90% to 95% of cases. This likelihood of success also applies to patients with repetitive nonsustained monomorphic VT arising in this location, which is accompanied by marked clinical symptoms.[101] Similarly, a small fraction of patients with ventricular arrhythmias and structurally normal hearts may demonstrate a right bundle, left-axis deviation morphology during VT ablation (Fig 26-15). Entrainment of this arrhythmia from the right ventricular outflow tract suggests that these arrhythmias are likewise of a reentrant mechanism. In these patients, careful mapping of the VT circuit demonstrates prepotentials of small amplitude occurring immediately before the local ventricular activation at a posterior septal location in the middle to apical region of the left ventricle.[103] These deflections, when appropriately validated, appear to be markers of a successful ablation site. Success rates in excess of 90% have also been realized with energy delivery at this location. With both of these forms of "idiopathic" VT, this nonpharmacologic approach eliminates the need for subsequent drug therapy. Although experience with the elimination of these kinds of tachycardia has been recent, early results suggest that the indications for catheter ablation as first-line therapy may soon be expanded to include patients with these forms of ventricular arrhythmias.

The role of surgery in the treatment of ventricular arrhythmias has undergone a radical transformation, not only because of the availability of catheter ablation but also because of the effectiveness and sophistication of implantable cardioverter-defibrillators. Operation may still be preferred, however, for patients who have serious ventricular arrhythmias coupled with symptomatic coronary artery disease. In these patients, left ventricular aneurysmectomy and endocardial resection can prevent tachycardia in 80% to 85%, and the operative risk in properly selected patients is approximately 6% to 15%.[104,105] The advantage of endocardial resection combined with revascularization is that arrhythmias may be cured, and the patient will not be subjected to repeated cardioversion. Also, surgical treatment may reduce the risk of ischemic events in the future when revascularization is combined with left ventricular aneurysmectomy and endocardial excision.

SUMMARY

Over the past 10 years, catheter ablation techniques for both atrial and ventricular arrhythmias have developed rapidly and have achieved a position of preference in the nonpharmacologic elimination of arrhythmias. In general, these offer the patient permanent cure of the arrhythmia and a decrease in the risk of therapy. Available catheter technology also permits a more focused creation of a therapeutic lesion. Undoubtedly, with the development of new energy sources, such as microwave and ultrasound, along with expected improvement in catheter design, these techniques should be more readily applicable to patients with serious arrhythmias. Judging from the development of techniques over the past 5 years, substantial further improvement in these treatment modalities can be expected in the near future. This kind of progress should, in turn, result in a decrease in morbidity and mortality from serious ventricular arrhythmias as well as improve the quality of life in patients with supraventricular tachycardias.

REFERENCES

1. Cobb FR, Blumenschein SD, Sealy WL, et al: Successful surgical interruption of the bundle of Kent in a patient with Wolff-Parkinson-White syndrome. *Circulation* 38:1018-1029, 1968
2. Gallagher JJ, Sealy WC, Cox JL, et al: Results of surgery for preexcitation caused by accessory atrioventricular pathways in 267 consecutive cases. In *Tachycardias: Mechanisms, Diagnosis, Treatment*. Edited by ME Josephson, HJJ Wellens. Philadelphia, Lea & Febiger, 1984, pp 259-269
3. Packer DL, Prystowsky EN: Wolff-Parkinson-White syndrome: further progress in evaluation and treatment. *Prog Cardiol* 1/1:147-187, 1988
4. Cox JL, Holman WL, Cain ME: Cryosurgical treatment of atrioventricular node reentrant tachycardia. *Circulation* 76:1329-1336, 1987
5. Ross DL, Johnson DC, Denniss AR, et al: Curative surgery for atrioventricular junctional ("AV nodal") reentrant tachycardia. *J Am Coll Cardiol* 6:1383-1392, 1985
6. Ross DL, Johnson DC, Koo CC, et al: Surgical treatment of supraventricular tachycardia without the WPW syndrome: current indications, techniques, and results. In *Cardiac Arrhythmias: Where To Go From Here*? Edited by P Brugada, HJJ Wellens. Mt. Kisco, New York, Futura Publishing Company, 1987, pp 591-603
7. Lowe JE, Hendry PJ, Packer DL, et al: Surgical management of chronic ectopic atrial tachycardia. *Semin Thorac Cardiovasc Surg* 1:58-66, 1989
8. Harken AH, Horowitz LN, Josephson ME: Comparison of standard aneurysmectomy and aneurysmectomy with directed endocardial resection for the treatment of recurrent sustained ventricular tachycardia. *J Thorac Cardiovasc Surg* 80:527-534, 1980
9. Borggrefe M, Podczeck A, Ostermeyer J, et al: Long-term results of electrophysiologically guided antitachycardia surgery in ventricular tachyarrhythmias: a collaborative report on 665 patients. In *Nonpharmacological Therapy of Tachyarrhythmias*. Edited by G Breithardt, M Borggrefe, DP Zipes. Mount Kisco, New York: Futura Publishing Company, 1987, pp 109-132
10. Swerdlow CD, Mason JW, Stinson EB, et al: Results of operations for ventricular tachycardia in 105 patients. *J Thorac Cardiovasc Surg* 92:105-113, 1986
11. Horowitz LN, Harken AH, Kastor JA, et al: Ventricular resection guided by epicardial and endocardial mapping for treatment of recurrent ventricular tachycardia. *N Engl J Med* 302:589-593, 1980
12. Scheinman MM, Morady F, Hess DS, et al: Catheter-induced ablation of the atrioventricular junction to control refractory supraventricular arrhythmias. *JAMA* 248:851-855, 1982
13. Gallagher JJ, Svenson RH, Kasell JH, et al: Catheter technique for closed-chest ablation of the atrioventricular conduction system: a therapeutic alternative for the treatment of refractory supraventricular tachycardia. *N Engl J Med* 306:194-200, 1982
14. Evans GT Jr, Scheinman MM, Zipes DP, et al.: The Percutaneous Cardiac Mapping and Ablation Registry: final summary of results. *PACE* 11:1621-1626, 1988
15. Brodman R, Fisher JD: Evaluation of a catheter technique for ablation of accessory pathways near the coronary sinus using a canine model. *Circulation* 67:923-929, 1983
16. Fisher JD, Brodman R, Kim SG, et al: Attempted nonsurgical electrical ablation of accessory pathways via the coronary sinus in the Wolff-Parkinson-White syndrome. *J Am Coll Cardiol* 4:685-694, 1984
17. Morady F, Scheinman MM, Kou WH, et al: Long-term results of catheter ablation of a posteroseptal accessory atrioventricular connection in 48 patients. *Circulation* 79:1160-1170, 1989
18. Ruder MA, Mead RH, Gaudiani V, et al: Experience with catheter ablation of accessory pathways (abstract). *J Am Coll Cardiol* 9:251A, 1987
19. Bardy GH, Ivey TD, Coltorti F, et al: Developments, complications and limitations of catheter-mediated electrical ablation of posterior accessory atrioventricular pathways. *Am J Cardiol* 61:309-316, 1988
20. Linker NJ, Ward DE, Davies MJ, et al: Fatal coronary sinus rupture following attempted catheter ablation of an accessory pathway. *J Electrophysiol* 3:2-6, 1989
21. Hartzler GO, Giorgi LV, Diehl AM, et al: Right coronary spasm complicating electrode catheter ablation of a right lateral accessory pathway. *J Am Coll Cardiol* 6:250-253, 1985
22. Warin J-F, Haissaguerre M, Lemetayer P, et al: Catheter ablation of accessory pathways with a direct approach: results in 35 patients. *Circulation* 78:800-815, 1988
23. Lemery R, Talajic M, Roy D, et al: Success, safety, and late electrophysiological outcome of low-energy direct-current ablation in patients with the Wolff-Parkinson-White syndrome. *Circulation* 85:957-962, 1992
24. Jackman WM, Friday KJ, Fitzgerald DM, et al: Localization of left free-wall and posteroseptal accessory atrioventricular pathways by direct recording of accessory pathway activation. *PACE* 12:204-214, 1989.
25. Haines DE, Watson DD: Tissue heating during radiofrequency catheter ablation: a thermodynamic model and observations in isolated perfused and superfused canine right ventricular free wall. *PACE* 12:962-976, 1989
26. Haines DE, Watson DD, Verow AF: Electrode radius predicts lesion radius during radiofrequency energy heating: validation of a proposed thermodynamic model. *Circ Res* 67:124-129, 1990
27. Hoyt RH, Huang SK, Marcus FI, et al: Factors influencing trans-catheter radiofrequency ablation of the myocardium. *J Appl Cardiol* 1:469-486, 1986
28. Haines DE, Verow AF: Observations on electrode-tissue interface temperature and effect on electrical impedance during radiofrequency ablation of ventricular myocardium. *Circulation* 82:1034-1038, 1990
29. Hindricks G, Haverkamp W, Gülker H, et al: Radiofrequency coagulation of ventricular myocardium: improved prediction of lesion size by monitoring catheter tip temperature. *Eur Heart J* 10:972-984, 1989
30. Langberg JJ, Calkins H, El-Atassi R, et al: Temperature monitoring during radiofrequency catheter ablation of accessory pathways. *Circulation* 86:1469-1474, 1992
31. Packer DL, Kappler JH, Hammill SC, et al: Characterization of the pathophysiologic sequelae of the impedance rise during radiofrequency ablation of accessory pathways (abstract). *Circulation* 84 Suppl 2:709, 1991
32. Ring ME, Huang SKS, Gorman G, et al: Determinants of impedance rise during catheter ablation of bovine myocardium with radiofrequency energy. *PACE* 12:1502-1513, 1989
33. Jackman WM, Wang X, Friday KJ, et al: Catheter ablation of accessory atrioventricular pathways (Wolff-Parkinson-White syndrome) by radiofrequency current. *N Engl J Med* 324:1605-1611, 1991
34. Calkins H, Langberg J, Sousa J, et al: Radiofrequency catheter ablation of accessory atrioventricular connections in 250 patients: abbreviated therapeutic approach to Wolff-Parkinson-White syndrome. *Circulation* 85:1337-1346, 1992
35. Lesh MD, Van Hare GF, Schamp KJ, et al: Curative percutaneous catheter ablation using radiofrequency energy for accessory pathways in all locations: results in 100 consecutive patients. *J Am Coll Cardiol* 19:1303-1309, 1992
36. Swartz JF, Tracy CM, Fletcher RD: Radiofrequency endocardial catheter ablation of accessory atrioventricular pathway atrial insertion sites. *Circulation* 87:487-499, 1993
37. Schlüter M, Geiger M, Siebels J, et al: Catheter ablation using radiofrequency current to cure symptomatic patients with tachyarrhythmias related to an accessory atrioventricular pathway. *Circulation* 84:1644-1661, 1991
38. Packer DL, Hammill SC, Holmes DR: Comparison of transaortic and transseptal approaches for the ablation of left-sided accessory pathways (abstract). *Circulation* 86 Suppl 1:783, 1992
39. Lesh MD, Van Hare GF, Scheinman MM, et al: What is the best

approach to radiofrequency ablation of left-sided accessory pathways: retrograde or transseptal? (Abstract.) *PACE* 15:535, 1992

40. Natale A, Wathen M, Yee R, et al: Atrial and ventricular approaches for radiofrequency catheter ablation of left-sided accessory pathways. *Am J Cardiol* 70:114-116, 1992

41. Chen X, Borggrefe M, Shenasa M, et al: Characteristics of local electrogram predicting successful transcatheter radiofrequency ablation of left-sided accessory pathways. *J Am Coll Cardiol* 20:656-665, 1992

42. Seifert MJ, Morady F, Calkins HG, et al: Aortic leaflet perforation during radiofrequency ablation. *PACE* 14:1582-1585, 1991

43. Twidale N, Wang X, Beckman KJ, et al: Factors associated with recurrence of accessory pathway conduction after radiofrequency catheter ablation. *PACE* 14:2042-2048, 1991

44. Calkins H, Kim Y-N, Schmaltz S, et al: Electrogram criteria for identification of appropriate target sites for radiofrequency catheter ablation of accessory atrioventricular connections. *Circulation* 85:565-573, 1992

45. Calkins H, Niklason L, Sousa J, et al: Radiation exposure during radiofrequency catheter ablation of accessory atrioventricular connections. *Circulation* 84:2376-2382, 1991

46. Solomon AJ, Tracy CM, Swartz JF, et al: Effect on coronary artery anatomy of radiofrequency catheter ablation of atrial insertion sites of accessory pathways. *J Am Coll Cardiol* 21:1440-1444, 1993

47. Wood DL, Hammill SC, Porter CJ, et al: Cryosurgical modification of atrioventricular conduction for treatment of atrioventricular node reentrant tachycardia. *Mayo Clin Proc* 63:988-992, 1988

48. Haissaguerre M, Warin JF, Lemetayer P, et al: Closed-chest ablation of retrograde conduction in patients with atrioventricular nodal reentrant tachycardia. *N Engl J Med* 320:426-433, 1989

49. Jazayeri MR, Hempe SL, Sra JS, et al: Selective transcatheter ablation of the fast and slow pathways using radiofrequency energy in patients with atrioventricular nodal reentrant tachycardia. *Circulation* 85:1318-1328, 1992

50. Lee MA, Morady F, Kadish A, et al: Catheter modification of the atrioventricular junction with radiofrequency energy for control of atrioventricular nodal reentry tachycardia. *Circulation* 83:827-835, 1991

51. Mitrani RD, Klein LS, Hackett FK, et al: Radiofrequency ablation for atrioventricular node reentrant tachycardia: comparison between fast (anterior) and slow (posterior) pathway ablation. *J Am Coll Cardiol* 21:432-441, 1993

52. Kay GN, Epstein AE, Dailey SM, et al: Selective radiofrequency ablation of the slow pathway for the treatment of atrioventricular nodal reentrant tachycardia: evidence for involvement of perinodal myocardium within the reentrant circuit. *Circulation* 85:1675-1688, 1992

53. Jackman WM, Beckman KJ, McClelland JH, et al: Treatment of supraventricular tachycardia due to atrioventricular nodal reentry by radiofrequency catheter ablation of slow-pathway conduction. *N Engl J Med* 327:313-318, 1992

54. Haissaguerre M, Gaita F, Fischer B, et al: Elimination of atrioventricular nodal reentrant tachycardia using discrete slow potentials to guide application of radiofrequency energy. *Circulation* 85:2162-2175, 1992

55. Klein GJ, Guiraudon GM, Sharma AD, et al: Demonstration of macroreentry and feasibility of operative therapy in the common type of atrial flutter. *Am J Cardiol* 57:587-591, 1986

56. Feld GK, Fleck RP, Chen P-S, et al: Radiofrequency catheter ablation for the treatment of human type 1 atrial flutter: identification of critical zone in the reentrant circuit by endocardial mapping techniques. *Circulation* 86:1233-1240, 1992

57. Saoudi N, Atallah G, Kirkorian G, et al: Catheter ablation of the atrial myocardium in human type I atrial flutter. *Circulation* 81:762-771, 1990

58. Lesh MD, Van Hare GF, Kwasman JA, et al: Curative radiofrequency (RF) catheter ablation of atrial tachycardia and flutter (abstract). *J Am Coll Cardiol* 21 Suppl A:374, 1993

59. Kirkorian G, Canu G, Atallah G, et al: Radiofrequency ablation: a promising approach to the treatment of atrial flutter (abstract). *J Am Coll Cardiol* 21 Suppl A:374, 1993

60. Olshansky B, Okumura K, Hess PG, et al: Demonstration of an area of slow conduction in human atrial flutter. *J Am Coll Cardiol* 16:1639-1648, 1990

61. Cosio FG, Arribas F, Palacios J, et al: Fragmented electrograms and continuous electrical activity in atrial flutter. *Am J Cardiol* 57:1309-1314, 1986

62. Shenasa H, Merrill JJ, Hamer ME, et al: Distribution of ectopic atrial tachycardia along the crista terminalia. *Circulation* 88 Suppl 1:1-29, 1993

63. Kay GN, Chong F, Epstein AE, et al: Expanding the spectrum of arrhythmias curable with radiofrequency catheter ablation: experience with primary atrial tachycardias (abstract). *J Am Coll Cardiol* 19 Suppl A:184, 1992

64. Tracy CM, Swartz JF, Hoops HG, et al: Radiofrequency catheter ablation of ectopic atrial tachycardia using activation pace mapping (abstract). *J Am Coll Cardiol* 19 Suppl A:184, 1992

65. Gillette PC, Wampler DG, Garson A Jr, et al: Treatment of atrial automatic tachycardia by ablation procedures. *J Am Coll Cardiol* 6:405-409, 1985

66. Walsh EP, Saul JP, Hulse JE, et al: Transcatheter ablation of ectopic atrial tachycardia in young patients using radiofrequency current. *Circulation* 86:1138-1146, 1992

67. Marchese AC, Pressley JC, Sintetos AL, et al: Cryosurgical versus catheter ablation of the atrioventricular junction. *Am J Cardiol* 59:870-873, 1987

68. Kay GN, Bubien RS, Epstein AE, et al: Effect of catheter ablation of the atrioventricular junction on quality of life and exercise tolerance in paroxysmal atrial fibrillation. *Am J Cardiol* 62:741-744, 1988

69. Yeung-Lai-Wah JA, Alison JF, Lonergan L, et al: High success rate of atrioventricular node ablation with radiofrequency energy. *J Am Coll Cardiol* 18:1753-1758, 1991

70. Packer DL, Bardy GH, Worley SJ, et al: Tachycardia-induced cardiomyopathy: a reversible form of left ventricular dysfunction. *Am J Cardiol* 57:563-570, 1986

71. Grogan M, Smith HC, Gersh BJ, et al: Left ventricular dysfunction due to atrial fibrillation in patients initially believed to have idiopathic dilated cardiomyopathy. *Am J Cardiol* 69:1570-1573, 1992

72. Feld GK, Prothro DL, Fujimura O, et al: Radiofrequency catheter ablation of human type I atrial flutter--acute and chronic followup (abstract). *Circulation* 88 Suppl 1:584, 1993

73. Blanck Z, Dhala A, Krum D, et al: Dramatic reduction in ventricular response during atrial fibrillation by ablating the atrioventricular nodal slow pathway: electrophysiologic and clinical implications (abstract). *Circulation* 88 Suppl 1:584, 1993

74. Wang PJ, Sosa-Suarez G, Friedman PL: A-V nodal ablation by selective A-V nodal artery infusion of ethanol (abstract). *Circulation* 80 Suppl 2:324, 1989

75. de Swart H, Brugada P, Smeets J, et al: Transcoronary chemical ablation of atrioventricular conduction (abstract). *J Am Coll Cardiol* 15 Suppl A:103, 1990

76. Cox JL: The surgical treatment of atrial fibrillation. IV. Surgical technique. *J Thorac Cardiovasc Surg* 101:584-592, 1991

77. Cox JL, Schuessler RB, D'Agostino HJ Jr, et al: The surgical treatment of atrial fibrillation. III. Development of a definitive surgical procedure. *J Thorac Cardiovasc Surg* 101:569-583, 1991

78. Cox JL: Evolving applications of the maze procedure for atrial fibrillation. *Ann Thorac Surg* 55:578-580, 1993

79. McCarthy PM, Castle LW, Maloney JD, et al: Initial experience with the maze procedure for atrial fibrillation. *J Thorac Cardiovasc Surg* 105:1077-1087, 1993

80. Bonchek LI, Burlingame MW, Worley SJ, et al: Cox/maze procedure for atrial septal defect with atrial fibrillation: management strategies. *Ann Thorac Surg* 55:607-610, 1993

81. Blitz A, McLoughlin D, Gross J, et al: Combined maze procedure and septal myectomy in a septuagenarian. *Ann Thorac Surg* 54:364-365, 1992

82. Chua YL, Schaff HV, Orszulak TA, et al: Outcome of mitral valve repair in patients with preoperative atrial fibrillation: Should the maze procedure be combined with mitral valvuloplasty? *J Thorac Cardiovasc Surg* 107:408-415, 1994

83. Guiraudon GM: Surgical treatment of atrial fibrillation. *Herz* 18:51-59, 1993

84. Cox JL, Boineau JP, Schuessler RB, et al: Five-year experience with the maze procedure for atrial fibrillation. *Ann Thorac Surg* 56:814-823, 1993

85. Tonet JL, Fontaine G, Frank R, et al: Treatment of ventricular tachycardias by endocardial catheter fulguration: further experience and long-term follow-up (abstract). *Circulation* 78 Suppl 2:306, 1988

86. Garan H, Kuchar D, Freeman C, et al: Early assessment of the effect of map-guided transcatheter intracardiac electric shock on

sustained ventricular tachycardia secondary to coronary artery disease. *Am J Cardiol* 61:1018-1023, 1988

87. Morady F, Scheinman MM, Di Carlo LA Jr, et al: Catheter ablation of ventricular tachycardia with intracardiac shocks: results in 33 patients. *Circulation* 75:1037-1049, 1987

88. Borggrefe M, Breithardt G, Podczeck A, et al: Catheter ablation of ventricular tachycardia using defibrillator pulses: electrophysiological findings and long-term results. *Eur Heart J* 10:591-601, 1989

89. Evans GT Jr, Scheinman MM, Zipes DP, et al: Catheter ablation for control of ventricular tachycardia: a report of the Percutaneous Cardiac Mapping and Ablation Registry. *PACE* 9:1391-1395, 1986

90. Hauer RNW, de Medina EOR, Borst C: Proarrhythmic effects of ventricular electrical catheter ablation in dogs. *J Am Coll Cardiol* 10:1350-1356, 1987

91. Lerman BB, Weiss JL, Bulkley BH, et al: Myocardial injury and induction of arrhythmia by direct current shock delivered via endocardial catheters in dogs. *Circulation* 69:1006-1012, 1984

92. Fitzgerald DM, Friday KJ, Yeung Lai Wah JA, et al: Electrogram patterns predicting successful catheter ablation of ventricular tachycardia. *Circulation* 77:806-814, 1988

93. Morady F, Frank R, Kou WH, et al: Identification and catheter ablation of a zone of slow conduction in the reentrant circuit of ventricular tachycardia in humans. *J Am Coll Cardiol* 11:775-782, 1988

94. Morady F, Kadish A, Rosenheck S, et al: Concealed entrainment as a guide for catheter ablation of ventricular tachycardia in patients with prior myocardial infarction. *J Am Coll Cardiol* 17:678-689, 1991

95. Stevenson WG, Weiss JN, Wiener I, et al: Slow conduction in the infarct scar: relevance to the occurrence, detection, and ablation of ventricular reentry circuits resulting from myocardial infarction. *Am Heart J* 117:452-467, 1989

96. Caceres J, Jazayeri M, McKinnie J, et al: Sustained bundle branch reentry as a mechanism of clinical tachycardia. *Circulation* 79:256-270, 1989

97. Tchou P, Jazayeri M, Denker S, et al: Transcatheter electrical ablation of right bundle branch: a method of treating macroreentrant ventricular tachycardia attributed to bundle branch reentry. *Circulation* 78:246-257, 1988

98. Cohen TJ, Chien WW, Lurie KG, et al: Radiofrequency catheter ablation for treatment of bundle branch reentrant ventricular tachycardia: results and long-term follow-up. *J Am Coll Cardiol* 18:1767-1773, 1991

99. Touboul P, Kirkorian G, Atallah G, et al: Bundle branch reentrant tachycardia treated by electrical ablation of the right bundle branch. *J Am Coll Cardiol* 7:1404-1409, 1986

100. Wilber DJ, Baerman J, Olshansky B, et al: Adenosine-sensitive ventricular tachycardia: clinical characteristics and response to catheter ablation. *Circulation* 87:126-134, 1993

101. Klein LS, Shih H-T, Hackett FK, et al: Radiofrequency catheter ablation of ventricular tachycardia in patients without structural heart disease. *Circulation* 85:1666-1674, 1992

102. Lee RJ, Kwasman MA, Grogin HR, et al: Surface electrocardiographic localization of right ventricular outflow tract tachycardia (abstract). *J Am Coll Cardiol* 21 Suppl A:403, 1993

103. Nakagawa H, Beckman K, McClelland J, et al: Radiofrequency ablation of idiopathic left ventricular tachycardia guided by a Purkinje potential (abstract). *PACE* 16:890, 1993

104. Ostermeyer J, Kirklin JK, Borggrefe M, et al: Ten years electrophysiologically guided direct operations for malignant ischemic ventricular tachycardia--results. *Thorac Cardiovasc Surg* 37:20-27, 1989

105. Kron IL, Kern JA, Theodore P, et al: Does a posterior aneurysm increase the risk of endocardial resection? *Ann Thorac Surg* 54:617-620, 1992

CHAPTER

27

Coronary circulation

A. Pathophysiology of myocardial ischemia and reperfusion

Kirk N. Garratt, M.D., and James P. Morgan, M.D., Ph.D.

Ischemia may be defined as the pathophysiologic state produced when blood flow to a tissue bed is reduced below a level adequate to supply oxygen and nutrients commensurate with the metabolic needs of the tissue. Ischemic tissues are characterized by at least three consistent physiologic abnormalities: (1) hypoxia, that is, an insufficient supply of oxygen to support oxidative metabolism; (2) the accumulation of toxic metabolites, many of which reflect a shift from aerobic to anaerobic metabolism; and (3) the development of acidosis, or the accumulation of hydrogen ions produced by catabolic reactions in the absence of a suitable electron acceptor. Reperfusion, or the restoration of adequate blood flow, alleviates the physiologic abnormalities of ischemia but may be associated with biochemical events that adversely affect subsequent cellular function. This chapter examines the metabolic, cellular, physiologic, electrical, and structural abnormalities produced when ischemic conditions are imposed upon myocardial tissue and on the consequences of reperfusion after a period of ischemia.

EFFECTS OF ISCHEMIA ON INTERMEDIARY METABOLISM

Normal cardiac function depends on an adequate supply of high-energy phosphate compounds, in particular adenosine triphosphate (ATP). Under aerobic conditions, ATP is produced from adenosine diphosphate (ADP), chiefly in mitochondria, through the process of oxidative phosphorylation. The importance of this process to myocyte metabolism is evidenced by the fact that mitochondria account for more than 30% of the intracellular volume of the myocytes.[1] When hypoxia occurs, oxidative phosphorylation is inhibited and the intracellular stores of ATP decline dramatically. The myocyte is capable of producing limited amounts of ATP under hypoxic conditions; however, the reduced perfusion that characterizes ischemia leads to the accumulation of metabolites that have inhibitory effects on anaerobic energy production. Ischemia has profound effects on lipid, carbohydrate, and protein metabolism in the heart; this chapter summarizes these effects.

Carbohydrate metabolism

Glucose enters the cell by combining with a carrier protein in the cell membrane, a process that is facilitated by insulin. Once inside the cell, glucose is phosphorylated to glucose-6-phosphate by the enzyme hexokinase, which prevents glucose from diffusing back out of the cell. Glucose-6-phosphate then either is converted to its storage form, glycogen, or passes down the glycolytic pathway, where it is catabolized to pyruvate, with the net formation of two moles of pyruvate and two moles of ATP for every mole of glucose consumed. Under aerobic conditions, pyruvate is converted to acetylcoenzyme A (acetyl-CoA), which is further oxidized via the tricarboxylic acid cycle to yield carbon dioxide and water. Two moles of guanine triphosphate per mole of glucose consumed are directly generated from the tricarboxylic acid cycle. Also, hydrogen ions produced by glycolysis and the tricarboxylic acid cycle are bound by oxidized cofactors, principally nicotinamide adenine dinucleotide (NAD^+) and flavoprotein carriers, which transport this cytosolic "reducing power" into the mitochondria to fuel the process of oxidative phosphorylation, which yields another 34 moles of ATP. As the final hydrogen ion acceptor in the oxidative phosphorylation process, oxygen is converted to water. Therefore, a net total of 36 moles of high-energy ATP is generated by aerobic metabolism of 1 mole of glucose.[2] Additional high-energy phosphate compounds may be formed by the conversion of lactate to pyruvate (a reaction that produces additional reduced cofactors), which then enters the tricarboxylic acid cycle, and by the generation of guanine triphosphate by the enzyme succinylcoenzyme A synthetase within the tricarboxylic acid cycle.

Under hypoxic conditions, oxygen is not available to receive hydrogen ions, and the pool of reduced cofactors, especially reduced nicotinamide adenine dinucleotide (NADH), builds up. This excess of reduced cofactors inhibits oxidation of acetyl-CoA; pyruvate cannot enter the tricarboxylic acid cycle and is instead converted to lactate by the enzyme lactate dehydrogenase. This reaction produces enough oxidized cofactor to support glycolysis. Pyruvate may also bind ammonia moieties (NH_3), generated by the breakdown of adenine nucleotides under anaerobic conditions, via a transaminase reaction to form alanine. Although alanine is significantly less toxic than free NH_3, lactate may have direct toxic effects on cytosolic and mitochondrial functions.[3] Under hypoxic conditions, then, only the 2 moles of ATP netted from glycolysis of

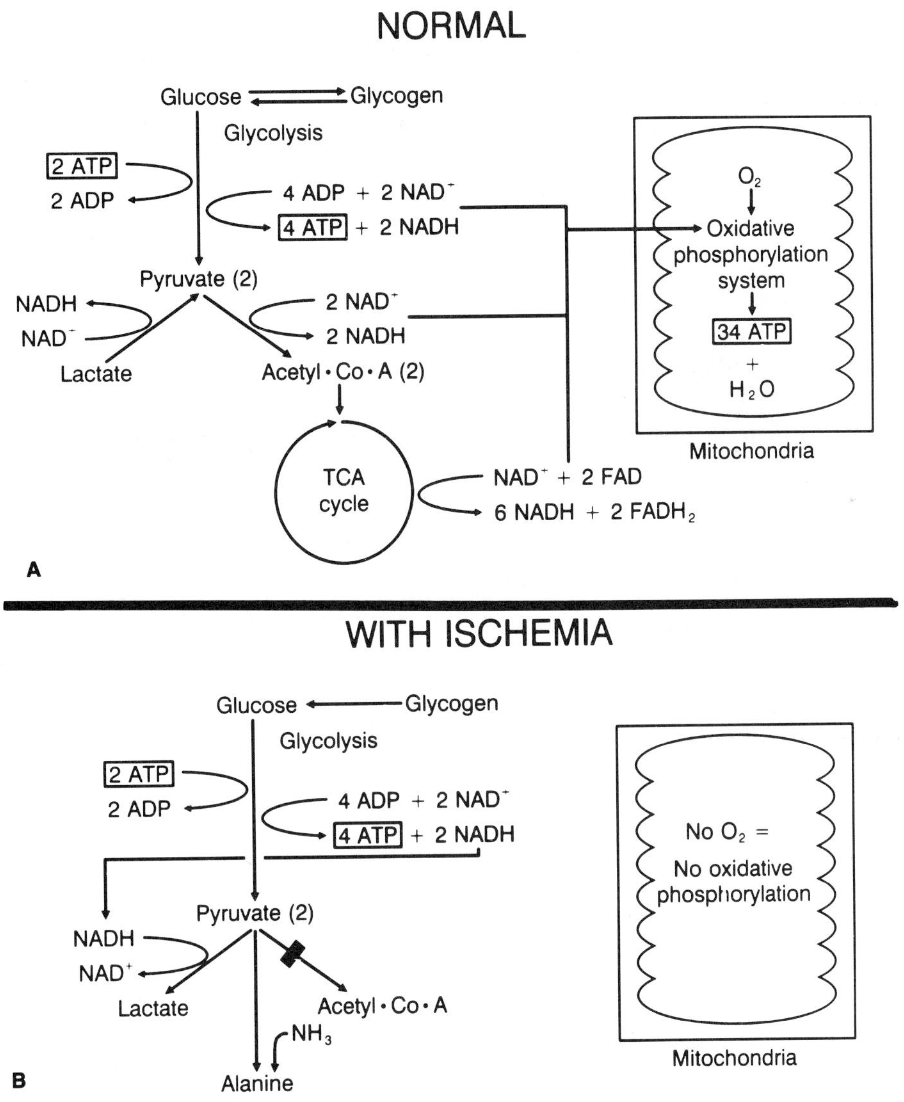

Fig 27A-1 Normal and ischemic glucose metabolism. **A,** net production of 36 moles of adenosine triphosphate *(ATP)* results from the aerobic catabolism of 1 mole of glucose and utilization of the reduced cofactors nicotinamide adenine dinucleotide *(NADH)* and flavin adenine dinucleotide *($FADH_2$)* in the mitochondrial process of oxidative phosphorylation. **B,** when oxygen is not available, NADH and $FADH_2$ levels rise and shut off the tricarboxylic acid *(TCA)* cycle. Pyruvate is converted to lactate, which leaks from the myocyte. Pyruvate also binds ammonia *(NH_3)* to form the less toxic compound alanine. Net production of just 2 moles of ATP results from the anaerobic catabolism of 1 mole of glucose. *ADP,* adenosine diphosphate.

glucose to pyruvate, rather than 36 moles, are generated from each mole of glucose consumed. Maximal anaerobic glycolysis can produce only about 7% of the usual high-energy phosphate needs of the myocardial cell.[3]

When additional amounts of glucose are required for energy production in the cell, glycogen is broken down by the enzyme phosphorylase to glucose-1-phosphate, which is converted to glucose-6-phosphate and enters the glycolytic pathway. Phosphorylase can exist in an active *(a)* and a less active *(b)* form. The enzyme phosphorylase kinase mediates the rapid conversion of phosphorylase *b* to phosphorylase *a* and is activated directly by calcium. Cyclic adenosine monophosphate (cyclic AMP) levels in the heart indirectly regulate the activity of phosphorylase kinase through their effects on a protein kinase (phosphorylase kinase kinase), which catalyzes the conversion of phosphorylase kinase to its active form, so that as cyclic AMP levels rise, the activity of phosphorylase kinase increases.[2] It is by these mechanisms that glycogenolysis appears to be regulated, providing an appropriate amount of glucose for passage down the glycolytic pathway.

The primary metabolic disturbance in the ischemic or hypoxic myocardium is the blockade of aerobic synthesis of high-energy phosphate compounds and a shift to anaerobic metabolism.[4-8] Ischemia increases the release of catecholamines from stores localized within the heart, and they stimulate phosphorylase kinase activity. Metabolic breakdown products, including citrate, ADP, AMP, and inorganic phosphate, accumulate in the sarcoplasm and stimulate the activity of phosphofructokinase, the primary enzyme controlling glycolysis, as well as other enzymes. Glycogen is rapidly consumed because glucose is needed to support the relatively inefficient anaerobic production of ATP. Instead of extracting lactic acid from arterial blood, hypoxic myocardium produces lactic acid as an end product of anaerobic metabolism. The accumulation of lactic and other organic acids results in a falling intracellular pH; if severe enough, this acidosis inhibits even anaerobic metabolism at several enzymatic steps,[9] and the initial burst of glycolytic activity induced by hypoxia is reversed as the production of high-energy phosphate compounds ceases altogether. The differences

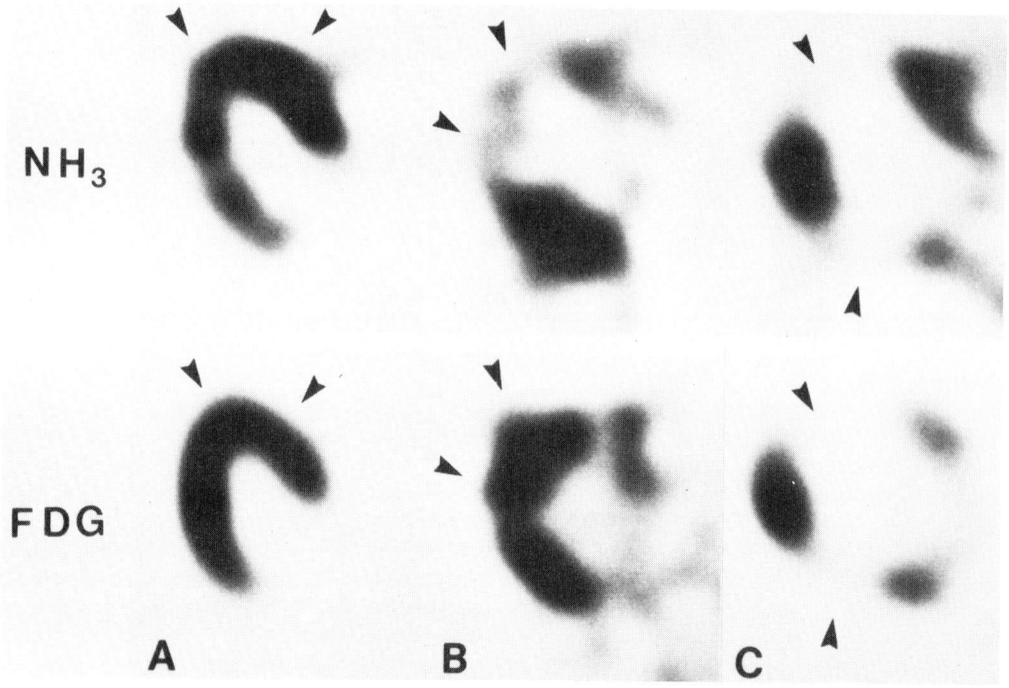

Fig 27A-2 Cross-sectional positron emission tomography images from the left ventricles of three patients. By isotope ventriculography, all three patients displayed contraction abnormalities (region between arrowheads). Positron-emitting ammonia ($^{13}NH_3$) uptake reflects blood flow, and labeled fluorodeoxyglucose (^{18}FDG) uptake reflects active carbohydrate metabolism. **A,** normal $^{13}NH_3$ and ^{18}FDG uptake in anteroseptal and apical regions, consistent with adequate blood flow to prevent ischemia. **B,** reduced uptake of $^{13}NH_3$ in anterolateral and apical regions with continued uptake of ^{18}FDG, consistent with continued carbohydrate metabolism in regions of abnormal blood flow (ischemia). **C,** concordant decrease in uptake of $^{13}NH_3$ and ^{18}FDG in apical and posterior regions, consistent with reduced blood flow and diminished metabolism after myocardial infarction. (From Tillisch J, Brunken R, Marshall R, et al: Reversibility of cardiac wall-motion abnormalities predicted by positron tomography. *N Engl J Med* 314:884-888, 1986. By permission of the journal.)

in aerobic and anaerobic glucose metabolism are illustrated in Figure 27A-1.

Positron emission tomography (PET) has made imaging areas of ischemic myocardium possible by exploiting differences in the way ischemic and nonischemic tissues metabolize glucose and other energy substrates.[10-12] Regional rates of utilization of glucose analogues labeled with positron-emitting isotopes can be assessed noninvasively. Impaired utilization of ^{18}F-2-fluoro-deoxyglucose is characteristic of severely ischemic myocardium; serial studies permit the differentiation of regions of reversible ischemia from irreversibly injured myocardium (Fig 27A-2).

Lipid metabolism

Under aerobic conditions, approximately two-thirds of the energy requirement of cardiac muscle cells is obtained from the oxidation of fatty acids. Fatty acids are derived from the hydrolysis of neutral fats or triglycerides to fatty acids and glycerol, a process that occurs principally in the liver and to a limited extent within the myocardial cells. After uptake or formation in the myocardium, fatty acids are metabolized to molecules of acylcoenzyme A (acyl-CoA) by the process of β-oxidation. After transport across the inner mitochondrial membrane via the carnitine acyl transferase system, acyl-CoA is converted to acetyl-CoA, which enters the tricarboxylic acid cycle to produce water, carbon dioxide, and high-energy phosphate compounds. Carnitine is an essential cofactor for the transport of long-chain fatty acids into the mitochondria. A deficiency of carnitine may lead to decreased oxidation of fatty acids in the mitochondria and increased cytosolic accumulation of lipids. Interestingly, carnitine deficiency has been reported as a cause of reversible cardiomyopathy.[13] Catabolism of fatty acids regulates glucose utilization by inhibiting glucose uptake and glycolysis.

As described above, hypoxic conditions result in an accumulation of NADH and other reduced cofactors. NADH inhibits β-oxidation and the acyl carnitine transferase system. Consequently, acyl-CoA accumulates in the cytosol and combines with glycerol (produced from accelerated glycolysis); the result is increased quantities of triglycerides in the ischemic cell. High levels of acyl-CoA inhibit the formation of esters of fatty acids, so that fatty acids are lost from the ischemic cell. The increased acyl-CoA levels also inhibit the translocase responsible for transporting ATP synthesized in the mitochondria to the cytosol,[14-16] further impairing the normal functioning of energy-requiring cytosolic metabolic processes.

Just as PET scanning can measure utilization of glucose analogues in ischemic tissues, it can also measure uptake and catabolism of lipids in ischemic myocardium.[17-19] Positron-emitting ^{11}C is used to label fatty acids. Diminished uptake of fatty acids in ischemic zones can then be imaged by PET. A particularly useful fatty acid analogue is [^{11}C]palmitate. The uptake of [^{11}C]palmitate is not diminished with a reduction in blood flow alone, since its extraction fraction will increase;[20] however, if oxidative phosphorylation is impaired, a region of decreased [^{11}C]palmitate uptake is detectable by PET.[18,19]

Table 27A-1 Major effects of ischemia on intermediary metabolism

Accumulation of reduced cofactors nicotinamide adenine dinucleotide and flavin adenine dinucleotide
Blockade of the tricarboxylic acid cycle
Inhibition of β-oxidation of fatty acids
Diminished translocation of ATP from mitochondria to cytoplasm
Dependence on ATP produced by glycolysis

Protein metabolism

Before they can be used for energy, amino acids must be transformed to tricarboxylic acid cycle substrates by deamination, that is, removal of the amino moieties. Although amino acids are not a major source of energy for myocardial cells, deamination of amino acids under ischemic conditions can result in toxic levels of intracellular ammonia. Pyruvate may scavenge these ammonia moieties to form alanine; an increase in the concentration of alanine in the coronary sinus effluent is a marker of myocardial ischemia.[21]

The major effects of ischemia on intermediary metabolism are summarized in Table 27A-1.

DETERMINANTS OF MYOCARDIAL OXYGEN CONSUMPTION

Normal myocardium uses 8 to 10 mL of oxygen per 100 g of muscle per minute in resting subjects; even when the normothermic heart is arrested with cardioplegic solution, about 7% of basal oxygen needs is still required.[22] With exercise, the oxygen consumption of the heart may increase 200% to 300%. The mechanical efficiency (that is, work divided by the energy equivalent of oxygen consumed) of the human heart estimated from levels of oxygen utilization is 17.8% in the normal subject at rest, 20.6% in the normal subject during heavy exercise, 32.9% in the trained athlete during heavy exercise, and 11.4% in the patient with heart failure.[23] The three most important determinants of myocardial oxygen demand are heart rate, wall tension, and contractility.

Heart rate

An increase in heart rate increases myocardial oxygen consumption by increasing the frequency of cardiac contractions per unit of time. In addition, an increase in heart rate leads to an increase in contractility, probably due to enhanced availability of intracellular Ca^{2+} for activation of the myofilaments.[24]

Wall tension

Tension in the myocardial wall is an important determinant of cardiac energy expenditure and, subsequently, myocardial oxygen consumption. According to the

Laplace relationship, wall tension is directly proportional to the ventricular pressure and the ventricular radius and inversely proportional to the ventricular wall thickness. As ventricular pressure, radius, and wall thickness vary throughout the cardiac cycle, wall tension varies from diastole to systole. Oxygen consumption must increase under conditions that increase systolic pressure or radius, such as hypertension and aortic stenosis, and conditions that increase diastolic pressure or radius, such as aortic regurgitation and heart failure.

Contractility

Myocardial contractility is a complex concept that expresses both the number and the rate of cross-bridge cyclings by actin and myosin during a cardiac cycle. Factors that increase contractility, such as the clinically useful inotropic agents dopamine and dobutamine, also increase the rate of oxygen consumption. Unfortunately, no completely satisfactory index of contractility is available. The rate of increase of pressure during isovolumic contraction, dp/dt, has been the most widely used index of contractility in the clinical setting. The inverse of the negative pressure differential (1/[−dp/dt], or tau) is equally useful as a measure of relaxation during the isovolumic phase of diastole. Although less well studied, an increase in tau also reflects an alteration in myocardial wall tension and contractile dynamics and may also contribute to an increase in myocardial oxygen consumption.[25]

Energy expenditure by the heart is approximately proportional to the degree of tension developed times the duration that tension is maintained (tension-time index). A less precise index that can easily be measured at the bedside is the systolic blood pressure times the heart rate (the double product); this index parallels oxygen consumption over a wide range of changing conditions. Because the double product is related to oxygen consumption, energy expenditure may also be expressed in terms of metabolic units (1 MET = oxygen consumption of 3.5 mL O_2/[kg · min]); this convenient unit is commonly used during cardiac stress testing.

EFFECTS OF ISCHEMIA ON ELECTRICAL ACTIVITY

Electrophysiologic study of normal and ischemic myocardial tissue has revealed important differences in electrical properties. Early in ischemia, the resting potential of the myocyte membrane is reduced, and the amplitude, velocity, and duration of the action potential are reduced.[26-28] After this early phase, the action potential duration tends to be prolonged. In some regions of the ischemic zone, postrepolarization refractoriness develops in which the refractory period is longer than the full repolarization period.[29] Abnormal repolarization times and nonuniformity of repolarization through the ischemic area predispose the ischemic zone to unidirectional block and the establishment of reentrant dysrhythmias.[26-29]

Abnormalities in electrochemical gradients produced by potassium,[30,31] magnesium,[30] sodium,[32] and calcium[33] all appear to contribute to ischemic arrhythmogenesis, and indeed interrelationships of fluxes of these ions may be critical to the development of ventricular arrhythmias.[32] Calcium fluxes appear to play a key role in arrhythmias related to reperfusion (see below). Adrenergic receptor stimulation[34] and pathologic catabolites of membrane phospholipids[29,35] may facilitate some arrhythmias. The major mechanisms whereby these disturbances contribute to arrhythmias are listed in Table 27A-2. The clinical recognition and management of ischemia-related arrhythmias are discussed in chapter 29.

Table 27A-2 Major electrophysiologic effects of acute ischemia

Heterogeneous rates of action potential conduction (unidirectional block)
Heterogeneous rates of myocyte repolarization (unidirectional block)
Increased delayed afterpotentials (increased automaticity)
Increased α_1-adrenergic receptor activity (increased automaticity)

EFFECTS OF ACUTE ISCHEMIA ON CONTRACTILE FUNCTION

When coronary blood flow to a portion of the heart is interrupted, the contractile function of the ischemic regions decreases almost immediately. The ischemic regions begin to bulge outward during systole because they are unable to overcome the intraventricular pressure generated by the normally perfused myocardium. Electron microscopy studies demonstrate significant overstretching of sarcomeres in the ischemic zone.[36] This paradoxic "dyskinetic" motion of ischemic myocardium is readily detected by echocardiography or radionuclide imaging.

Since the mechanical function of ischemic myocardium deteriorates in the same manner as acutely anoxic myocardium, lack of oxygen must play a key role in contractile dysfunction. As described above, hypoxia brings about a shift from aerobic to anaerobic metabolism, with a decrease in the production of the high-energy phosphate compounds needed for contraction. However, myocardial stores of high-energy phosphates do not appear to be significantly depleted during very early ischemia, when contractile function is significantly depressed;[37,38] furthermore, noninfarcted myocardium that is reperfused after an ischemic period may have a normal or higher than normal oxygen consumption[38-40] with adequate ATP production[41] and yet may have a persisting contraction abnormality. These observations suggest that depletion of ATP is not the sole explanation for the observed contractile dysfunction.

Calcium is required during muscular excitation-contraction coupling. Calcium is normally sequestered in the sarcoplasmic reticulum until an electrical impulse triggers its release. Transport of calcium requires an

Table 27A-3 Major subcellular events contributing to decreased contractility during the early phases of ischemia

Decreased Ca^{2+} entry during the plateau phase of the action potential
Impaired uptake and release of Ca^{2+} by sarcoplasmic reticulum
Decreased sensitivity of myofilaments to Ca^{2+}

ATP-dependent transport protein. Reduced activity levels of this transport protein under ischemic conditions have been observed;[42] the resulting decrease in cytosolic calcium may account, in part, for the contractile abnormalities observed under ischemic conditions (Table 27A-3). Also, acidosis impairs the ability of sarcoplasmic reticulum to accept and release calcium and decreases the sensitivity of contractile proteins to the calcium ion.[43-45]

Mechanical activity accounts for utilization of 75% or more of the energy produced by the myocyte under normal conditions.[30] Therefore, a reduction in contractility may have certain advantages to ischemic myocardium. If energy expenditures on contractility are reduced, more high-energy phosphate compounds are presumably available for maintaining homeostasis and repairing damages incurred during the ischemic episode, so that the development of cellular necrosis is delayed. Indeed, reperfused, reversibly injured myocardium appears to generate and utilize large quantities of high-energy phosphates without substantial improvement in contractility over that in the acutely ischemic state; thus, it appears that energy usually reserved for mechanical work is being used to restore normalcy in the postischemic myocyte.[40,41]

EFFECTS OF ACUTE ISCHEMIA ON DIASTOLIC FUNCTION

Gross diastolic abnormalities have long been recognized in patients with failing hearts, but the subtler forms of diastolic dysfunction among patients with myocardial ischemia are just now becoming clear.[46,47] Abnormal diastolic function occurs as the result of left ventricular wall thickness (pathologic myocardial hypertrophy), an increase in interstitial collagen content (as occurs, for instance, after myocardial ischemic injury), or abnormal intrinsic relaxation properties (as measured by tau). A change in tau is the earliest measurable cardiac abnormality during transient ischemia;[48] this may reflect the fact that the energy-requiring step in excitation-contraction coupling (release of calcium from its binding site on troponin C, allowing the actin-myosin cross-bridges to dissociate) occurs during diastole.[49] Impaired relaxation shifts the left ventricular diastolic pressure-volume relation upward (reflecting increased pressure relative to volume), which may result in congestive symptoms. Pathologic left ventricular hypertrophy is associated with a decrease in ventricular wall compliance, that is, increased wall stiffness. This may reflect an increase in the content of interstitial collagen[50] or abnormalities in calcium sequestration,[51] or both. Certainly, interstitial fibrosis, such as that seen after infarction or even prolonged ischemia, reduces ventricular compliance and impairs diastolic function. Since diastole and systole are intricately linked and since most patients with ischemic heart disease have some degree of both systolic and diastolic dysfunction, it is difficult to be certain of the relative contributions of each to clinical symptoms.

Successful therapy of diastolic dysfunction must be directed toward the likely cause of the dysfunction. Relief of ischemia is fundamental to functional improvement. Calcium antagonist drugs are usually of benefit, because they reduce afterload and attenuate calcium release from sarcoplasmic reticulum. Reducing ventricular dimensions (relative to ventricular wall dimensions) lowers wall tension and improves diastolic properties; β-blocking drugs and angiotensin converting enzyme inhibitors, in addition to calcium antagonists, can accomplish this. Fibrosis after prolonged ischemia or infarction is irreversible, but inhibition of the angiotensin converting enzyme system appears to limit fibrosis after myocardial injury.[50]

IRREVERSIBLE ISCHEMIC INJURY

The metabolic, electrical, and functional abnormalities accompanying acute myocardial ischemia are reversible if the duration of ischemia is brief. Irreversible injury, that is, injury that results in myocyte necrosis even if the ischemia is relieved, occurs if ischemia is prolonged. The pioneering work of Reimer et al.[52-54] demonstrated that prolonged ischemia first causes irreversible injury of the subendocardial layer, where wall stress is highest and oxygen needs are greatest; necrosis then proceeds in an endocardial-to-epicardial wave front, eventually becoming transmural. Irrversible injury of subendocardial cells begins within 40 to 60 minutes of total myocardial ischemia, with transmural infarction becoming complete in 3 to 6 hours.[30,53,54] The key event differentiating reversible from irreversible cell injury appears to be loss of the integrity of the cellular membrane.[30] Presumably, depletion of ATP and accumulation of toxic metabolites disrupt key membrane ionic pumps, causing the cell to lose its ability to maintain essential biochemical and electrochemical gradients.[55-57] The appearance of cytoplasmic contents, such as creatine kinase, lactate dehydrogenase, myoglobin, and aspartate aminotransferase, in the bloodstream is indicative of membrane disruption and ischemic cell death. Although most metabolic and ultrastructural abnormalities begin early in the reversible stage of ischemic cell injury and persist into the irreversible stage, the development of amorphous mitochondrial matrix densities and of small areas of plasmalemmal disruption is unique to the irreversibly injured cell.[55,56]

Although early ischemia is characterized by a decrease in Ca^{2+} entry, irreversibly injured myocytes have a greatly increased cytosolic Ca^{2+} concentration. This arises in part from impaired Ca^{2+} sequestration by the sarcoplasmic reticulum, because accelerated phospholipid degeneration prevents partitioning of intracellular Ca^{2+} stores,[58,59] and from increased permeability to extracellular Ca^{2+} sources. Intracellular complexes of Ca^{2+} form. This feature of irreversibly injured cells has been put to diagnostic use through ^{99m}Tc-stannous pyrophosphate scans, which depend on an increased intracellular Ca^{2+} concentration for accumulation of the radiolabeled tracer.[60]

CHRONICALLY ISCHEMIC MYOCARDIUM: HIBERNATING MYOCARDIUM

Coronary obstruction from atherosclerosis typically develops over a long period, with symptoms of ischemia in the distal tissue bed developing only when blood flow is significantly impaired. Although hyperemic coronary flow may be slightly impaired at lesser degrees of obstruction, a 50% reduction of hyperemic flow beyond an obstruction does not occur until the epicardial artery involved is stenosed to less than 30% of its original luminal diameter, and resting flow is not impaired until the lesion reduces the arterial lumen to 20% of its original diameter.[61] Chronic but reversible contraction abnormalities may occur if ischemia is prolonged but not severe enough to cause tissue necrosis. This chronic regional depression of contraction, termed "hibernating myocardium," may represent a protective mechanism whereby myocytes reduce their oxygen demand when the supply of oxygen is reduced.[62] The precise mechanism for this contraction abnormality is unclear, but abnormal calcium handling probably is involved and perhaps also impaired energy production or utilization.[63] If the abnormality is very prolonged, microfocal subendocardial fibrosis, myocyte vacuolar change, and microvascular variceal transformation occur;[64,65] even some of these dramatic changes may be reversible with relief of ischemia.[66]

Medical therapies are often effective in alleviating clinical symptoms of chronic ischemia (see chapter 29B) and may be effective in improving contractile function by improving flow to the ischemic bed or by reducing oxygen demand. Direct revascularization by bypass surgery or percutaneous techniques, such as angioplasty, is associated with improved regional wall motion.[67,68]

POSTISCHEMIC CONTRACTILE DYSFUNCTION: STUNNED MYOCARDIUM

Acute myocardial ischemia is most commonly the result of acute thrombus development over an atherosclerotic plaque with a disrupted surface.[69-71] Intervention by administration of a thrombolytic drug or direct recanalization of the occluded artery with balloon angioplasty has resulted in salvage of jeopardized myocardium.[72-74] However, contractile function does not return immediately but rather is delayed, sometimes for several weeks.[63,75,76] Although this phenomenon was described 20 years ago,[77] the pathophysiology underlying *myocardial stunning* is still not completely understood.

Several mechanisms may participate in myocardial stunning (Fig 27A-3). Since ATP levels may be reduced during ischemia and recover with a time course that parallels the recovery of contractile function, an early hypothesis suggested that mitochondrial ATP production was the principal factor accounting for myocardial stunning.[78] However, a consistent relationship between ATP content and contractile function has not been observed, and artificially increasing myocardial ATP levels in experimental preparations does not augment contractile function.[41,79] Furthermore, mitochondrial function can be supranormal in stunned myocardium.[79] Since inotropic stimulation can increase contractility in stunned myocardium, it is unlikely that limited availability or utilization of ATP[79,80] is a major factor in postischemic contractile dysfunction.

Cytosolic calcium increases during ischemia, probably as a result of impaired sequestration by the sarcoplasmic reticulum and an increase in the activity of the Na^+-Ca^{2+} exchange channel.*[81,82] Excess cytosolic calcium can activate degradative enzymes such as membrane phospholipases[83] and can trigger xanthine oxidase-mediated oxygen radical formation.[84] Since less calcium is stored in the sarcoplasmic reticulum, the calcium flux during excitation is reduced; hence, attenuated calcium release during systole may explain excitation-contraction uncoupling during stunning.[42,81] Some animal studies suggest that myofilaments may also have decreased sensitivity to intracellular calcium during stunning.[43] The role of calcium overload in myocardial stunning is currently under intense investigation.

Oxygen-derived free radicals, chiefly superoxide anion ($\cdot O_2-$), hydrogen peroxide (H_2O_2), and the hydroxyl radical ($\cdot OH$), are generated during ischemia.[85,86] Iron has also been implicated in myocardial stunning and may contribute by catalyzing the formation of $\cdot OH$.[87] Attenuation of myocardial stunning has been reported in animals treated with compounds that scavenge these reactive oxygen species, such as superoxide dismutase, catalase, and *N*-2-mercaptopropionyl glycine, and by compounds that chelate iron, such as desferrioxamine.[88] These and perhaps other mechanisms are likely to be operative simultaneously during myocardial stunning. Figure 27A-3 illustrates the potentially complex relationship between reversible ischemia and mechanical dysfunction. A significant question has been raised about the triggering event for myocardial stunning: Is it a consequence of the ischemic event or of injury that occurs at the moment of tissue reperfusion following ischemia, that is, reperfusion injury?

LETHAL REPERFUSION INJURY

After a prolonged period of severe ischemia, reperfusion of a myocardial bed with unmodified whole blood can,

*Intracellular Na^+ increases during ischemia because of a decrease in the activity of the Na^+-K^+-ATPase membrane enzyme, which expels intracellular Na^+ against an electrochemical gradient under normal conditions. Also, an increase in intracellular pH results in more H^+ ions being available to the Na^+-H^+ exchange protein complex, which exchanges an intracellular H^+ ion for an extracellular Na^+ ion.

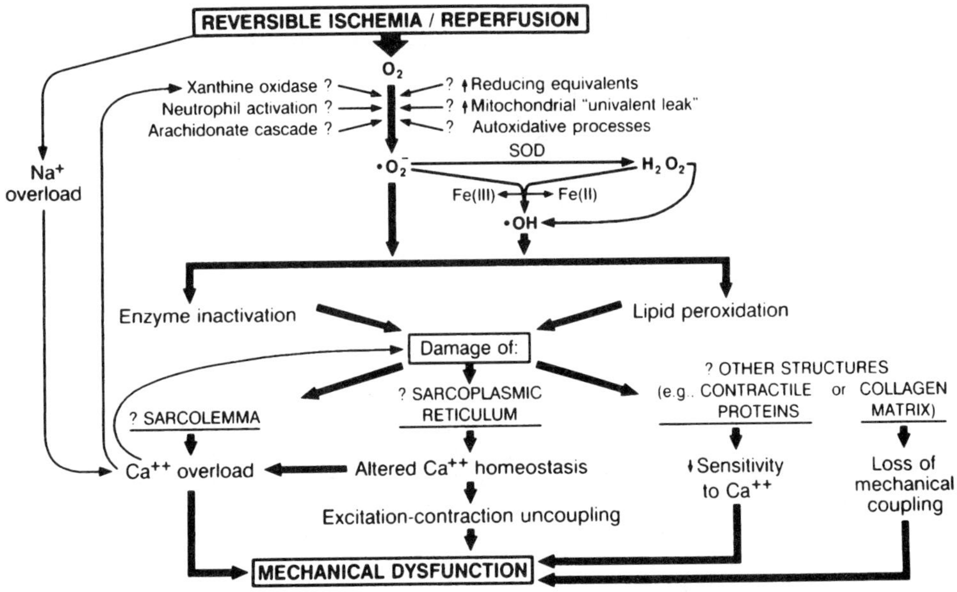

Fig 27A-3 Proposed mechanisms of postischemic myocardial dysfunction. Ischemia followed by reperfusion results in formation of superoxide radicals ($\cdot O_2^-$). Several mechanisms are proposed that may contribute to $\cdot O_2^-$ production. Through the action of superoxide dismutase *(SOD)* and catalytic iron *(Fe)*, $\cdot O_2^-$ may be converted to hydrogen peroxide *(H_2O_2)* and hydroxyl radicals ($\cdot OH$), respectively. These species damage lipid membranes and enzymatic proteins. Damage to sarcolemma and sarcoplasmic reticulum may result in deranged calcium *(Ca^{++})* homeostasis, whereas damage to contractile proteins or other structural cellular elements (e.g., collagen) may lead to excitation-contraction uncoupling and, consequently, mechanical dysfunction. Inhibition of Na^+-K^+-ATPase activity and enhanced activity of the Na^+-H^+ exchange system during acidosis lead to intracellular Na^+ overload. Excess intracellular Na^+ could activate the Na^+-Ca^{++} exchange system, which would lead to additional intracellular Ca^{++}. Increased intracellular Ca^{++} activates damaging phospholipases and other degradative enzymes and promotes oxygen radical formation by activating formation of xanthine oxidase. (From Bolli R: Mechanism of myocardial "stunning." *Circulation* 82:723-738, 1990. By permission of American Heart Association.)

paradoxically, be deleterious. This effect was first recognized as an "oxygen paradox."[89] Rosenkranz and Buckberg[90] refined the concept as applied to coronary perfusion and reperfusion during coronary bypass surgery; modifying cardioplegic solutions to increase the buffering capacity and osmolality, decrease ionized calcium, and provide glutamate or a similar substrate to support phosphorylation in the ischemic tissue improved postoperative cardiac performance.[91,92] Myocardial stunning is a form of reversible reperfusion injury, but *irreversible (lethal) reperfusion injury* may also occur. Several mechanisms may be operational in this phenomenon (Table 27A-4).

A favored hypothesis to explain lethal reperfusion injury contends that the fundamental cellular injury is lipid peroxidation by oxygen-derived free radicals. Although some authors have argued that during ischemia little free oxygen is available and intrinsic free-radical scavengers are abundant,[30] a wealth of indirect evidence, as well as direct evidence of oxygen radical formation and probable binding to lipids demonstrated by electron paramagnetic resonance spectroscopy,[85,93] indicates that radical species are operative during the postischemic phase. These oxygen radicals may be metabolic byproducts of the ischemic-postischemic cell or may be derived from neutrophils, which accumulate along the borders of the ischemic area after reperfusion.[94,95] Although treatment with drugs to block free-radical generation or scavenge generated radicals generally results in attenuated reperfusion injury,[86] granulocyte depletion does not prevent oxygen radical formation or reperfusion injury, perhaps because mast cells resident in the heart participate in the pathologic process.[96] Neutrophil adhesion to endothelial cells after ischemia is associated with endothelial damage and edema,[97] and activation of leukocytes causes them to stiffen and lose their conformability; these factors may contribute to leukocyte plugging of capillaries in an ischemic zone,[98] which has been implicated in the phenomenon of "no reflow" after reperfusion.[99]

The calcium ion plays a central role in the ultrastructural, metabolic, and electrical abnormalities that accompany reperfusion injury.[88] Sudden reperfusion with whole blood after prolonged ischemia results in a massive rise in intracellular Ca^{2+}, particularly within the mitochondria,

Table 27A-4 Possible mechanisms and consequences of reperfusion injury

Mechanism	Consequence
Cytosolic oscillatory Ca^{2+} overload	Early ventricular arrhythmias
Sustained Ca^{2+} overload	Stunning
	Accelerated necrosis
	Lethal reperfusion injury
Oxygen-derived free radicals	Lipid peroxidation
	Ventricular arrhythmias
	Stunning
	Lethal reperfusion injury
Neutrophil activation	Endothelial injury
	Late stunning
	Oxygen-derived free radicals
	Capillary plugging
	"No reflow"

Modified from Opie LH: Where do we stand with respect to reperfusion in the 1990s? Clinical and experimental perspectives. In *Myocardial Protection: the Pathophysiology of Reperfusion and Reperfusion Injury.* Edited by DM Yellon, RB Jennings. New York, Raven Press, 1992, pp 197-208.

Table 27A-5 Major mediators of reperfusion injury

Lipid peroxidation by oxygen-derived free radicals
Intracellular and intramitochondrial calcium overload
Phospholipid degradation due to insufficient ATP stores
Thromboxane and other cytotoxic arachidonate derivatives
Neutrophil-related endothelial injury and microvascular plugging

accompanied by cellular edema and myofibrillar disruption.[29,30] The functional abnormalities that characterize stunned myocardium can be ablated with calcium antagonists or chelators.[100-102]

During ischemia, production of high-energy phosphate compounds is reduced. ATP degrades to adenosine and inorganic phosphate, and adenine nucleotide purine metabolites diffuse out of the cell.[41,103] Magnesium, the bulk of which is normally bound to high-energy phosphates in the cell, also diffuses out of the myocyte.[104] These substrate shortages may limit ATP production once the ischemia is relieved; in fact, perfusion of ischemic tissue beds with solutions rich in ATP precursor compounds or energy precursors (e.g., glucose-insulin-potassium mixtures with or without magnesium[104,105]) limits postischemic injury or contractile dysfunction. Reduced high-energy phosphate levels result in degradation of phospholipid membranes, causing a further increase in permeability, loss of intracellular compartmentalization ability, and increased levels of arachidonic acid.[106] Although the role of arachidonate derivatives in ischemia is not fully understood, inhibition of thromboxane production appears to limit reperfusion injury, perhaps through endoperoxidase shunting with increased prostaglandin E_1 production. Prostaglandin E_1 may limit postischemic injury by reducing afterload pressure, by inhibiting superoxide production by neutrophils, or through cellular membrane stabilizing and cytoprotective mechanisms[107] (Table 27A-5).

In animal models, ventricular arrhythmias have been observed in conjunction with reperfusion of acutely ischemic myocardium.[108,109] Dispersion of refractoriness with heterogeneous rates of action potential conduction through the ischemic zone most likely underlies reentrant arrhythmias; heterogeneity of electrical properties appears to be maximal at 20 to 30 minutes after reperfusion, a time that correlates with the period of greatest incidence of malignant arrhythmias.[109] Also, increased cytosolic Ca^{2+} concentration, especially when accompanied by elevated cyclic AMP, catecholamine, and lysophosphoglyceride levels, can cause spontaneous calcium-induced calcium release with the generation of delayed afterpotentials, which may result in triggered arrhythmias.[27,29,33,110]

Despite all that is known about lethal reperfusion injury, its existence is still controversial. Demonstration of lethal reperfusion injury in animal experiments is not straightforward, since it is very difficult to know with certainty that the cells that are dead after reperfusion were not already dead before reperfusion: the accelerated appearance of structural abnormalities (sarcolemmal disruption, cellular edema, contracture of and damage to the microvasculature) after reperfusion may simply reflect a change in the time course or pattern of necrosis development among cells that are fatally injured before reperfusion. However, several lines of experimental evidence (summarized by Jennings and Yellon[92]) implicate the act of reperfusion with unmodified whole blood as a mediator of additional injury to viable ischemic myocytes. If reperfusion injury does exist, the potential clinical relevance of therapies that reduce lethal myocyte injury during treatment of acute myocardial infarction is enormous. Such therapies could potentially enhance early recovery of pump function, reduce ventricular arrhythmias, reduce the occurrence of ventricular rupture and aneurysm development, and facilitate more nearly complete and favorable postinfarction ventricular remodeling.

Of the many agents known to limit reperfusion injury in animals (Table 27A-6), adenosine is a particularly promising compound. Adenosine is a purine nucleoside produced endogenously through the decomposition of ATP.[111] Endogenous adenosine may be of benefit during ischemia because it can (1) reduce myocardial oxygen demand by its negative inotropic and chronotropic effects and its antiadrenergic effects; (2) augment energy stores by enhancing anaerobic glycolysis; and (3) inhibit the activation and aggregation of platelets and neutrophilic leukocytes.[112] Exogenous adenosine administered during the perireperfusion period reduces the structural and

Table 27A-6 Agents demonstrated to reduce lethal reperfusion injury in animals and their probable mechanisms of action

Agent	Probable mechanisms of action
Vasodilators	Enhance collateral blood flow Reduce leukocyte plugging
Calcium-channel antagonists	Limit cytosolic calcium overload Vasorelaxation ? Inhibition of endothelin
Xanthine oxidase inhibitors	Reduce oxygen-derived free radicals
Superoxide dismutase	Reduces oxygen-derived free radicals
N-2-mercaptopriopionyl glycine	Reduces oxygen-derived free radicals
Desferrioxamine	Reduces oxygen-derived free radicals
Na^+-channel blockers	Limit cytosolic calcium overload
Thromboxane synthetase inhibitors	Limit platelet adhesion
Thromboxane receptor antagonists	Limit platelet adhesion
Adenosine	All of the above

functional adverse consequences of unmodified reperfusion;[112-116] concomitant lidocaine may also be beneficial.[117] Both adenosine and lidocaine are available for intravenous infusion and are familiar to cardiologists. We are currently studying the effects of lidocaine and adenosine given intravenously to patients with acute myocardial infarction who undergo direct balloon angioplasty; myocardial salvage is measured by sestamibi radionuclide imaging.[118] Preliminary findings on safety are good,[119] but data pertaining to myocardial salvage are not yet available.

PRECONDITIONING

In the mid-1980s, animal experiments were conducted that allowed intermittent release of arterial occlusion during an ischemic period so that washout of toxic metabolites could take place. The investigators expected to isolate the effects of ATP depletion from the effects of toxic metabolite accumulation. They were surprised to find that such an experimental design did not produce myocardium that was deficient in ATP.[120] Furthermore, sustained ischemia after these brief ischemic episodes produced significantly less myocyte necrosis than expected.[121] The ability of one or more sublethal ischemic episodes to improve myocardial tolerance to subsequent prolonged ischemia has been termed *preconditioning.* The mechanisms operational in preconditioning are not clear, but reduced consumption of ATP is involved; this slows the depletion of high-energy phosphate stores, preserves creatine phosphate, limits the production of toxic catabolites, and maintains normal intracellular pH, all of which should prolong cell viability.[120-123] Excitation-contraction uncoupling may partially explain the reduced consumption of ATP.[124] Preconditioning does not appear to be the result of enhanced collateral blood flow.[123] The transcription of new mRNA with the production of myoprotective stress proteins may contribute to preconditioning,[125] although the rapid development and disappearance of preconditioning argues against this mechanism. Some recent evidence links endogenous adenosine production to preconditioning, at least in some animal species.[126] Activation of adenosine A1 receptors during ischemia stimulates anaerobic glycolysis, which helps to preserve ATP stores[126] and also limits intracellular calcium overload by stimulation of the ATP-regulated K^+ channel.[127] Further studies are needed to define the biologic basis and potential therapeutic implications of preconditioning.

REFERENCES

1. Page E, McCallister LP: Quantitative electron microscopic description of heart muscle cells: application to normal, hypertrophied and thyroxin-stimulated hearts. *Am J Cardiol* 31:172-181, 1973

2. Katz AM: *Physiology of the Heart.* New York, Raven Press, 1977, pp 35-50

3. Kobayashi K, Neely JR: Control of maximum rates of glycolysis in rat cardiac muscle. *Circ Res* 44:166-175, 1979

4. Opie LH: Myocardial ischemia – metabolic pathways and implications of increased glycolysis. *Cardiovasc Drugs Ther* 4 Suppl 4:777-790, 1990

5. Das DK, Engelman RM, Rousou JA, et al: Aerobic vs anaerobic metabolism during ischemia in heart muscle. *Ann Chir Gynaecol* 76:68-76, 1987

6. Näveri L, Näveri H, Härkönen M: Myocardial energy metabolism. *Ann Chir Gynaecol* 76:3-11, 1987

7. McDaniel HG, Jenkins RL, Digerness SB, et al: Myocardial fuel and energy balance, acute ischemia and diabetes. *Am J Med Sci* 295:207-211, 1988

8. Schwaiger M, Neese RA, Araujo L, et al: Sustained nonoxidative glucose utilization and depletion of glycogen in reperfused canine myocardium. *J Am Coll Cardiol* 13:745-754, 1989

9. Liedtke AJ: Alterations of carbohydrate and lipid metabolism in the acutely ischemic heart. *Prog Cardiovasc Dis* 23:321-336, 1981

10. Schelbert HR, Buxton D: Insights into coronary artery disease gained from metabolic imaging. *Circulation* 78:496-505, 1988

11. Schelbert HR, Phelps ME, Hoffman E, et al: Regional myocardial blood flow, metabolism and function assessed noninvasively with positron emission tomography. *Am J Cardiol* 46:1269-1277, 1980

12. Camici P, Ferrannini E, Opie LH: Myocardial metabolism in ischemic heart disease: basic principles and application to imaging by positron emission tomography. *Prog Cardiovasc Dis* 32:217-238, 1989

13. Tripp ME, Katcher ML, Peters HA, et al: Systemic carnitine deficiency presenting as familial endocardial fibroelastosis: a treatable cardiomyopathy. *N Engl J Med* 305:385-390, 1981

14. Vrobel TR, Jorgensen CR, Bache RJ: Myocardial lactate and adenosine metabolite production as indicators of exercise-induced myocardial ischemia in the dog. *Circulation* 66:555-561, 1982

15. Shrago E, Shug A, Elson C: Regulation of cell metabolism by mitochondrial transport systems. In *Gluconeogenesis: Its Regulation in Mammalian Species.* Edited by RW Hanson, MA Mehlman. New York, John Wiley & Sons, 1976, pp 221-238

16. Shrago E, Sul HS: Adenine nucleotide translocase activity during myocardial ischemia. In *Pathophysiology and Therapeutics of Myocardial*

Ischemia. Edited by AM Lefer, GJ Kelliher, MJ Rovetto. New York, Spectrum Publications, 1977, pp 239-255

17. Vanoverschelde J-L, Wijns W, Kolanowski J, et al: Competition between palmitate and ketone bodies as fuels for the heart: study with positron emission tomography. *Am J Physiol* 264:H701-H707, 1993

18. Tamaki N, Kawamoto M, Takahashi N, et al: Assessment of myocardial fatty acid metabolism with positron emission tomography at rest and during dobutamine infusion in patients with coronary artery disease. *Am Heart J* 125:702-710, 1993

19. Beanlands R, Schwaiger M: Cardiac applications of positron-emission tomography. *Curr Opin Radiol* 3:817-827, 1991

20. Goldstein RA, Klein MS, Sobel BE: Distribution of exogenous labeled palmitate in ischemic myocardium: implications for positron emission transaxial tomography. *Adv Cardiol* 27:71-82, 1980

21. Chazov E, Smirnov VN, Mazaev AV, et al: Myocardial ammonia metabolism in patients with heart disease as revealed by coronary sinus catheterization study. *Circulation* 47:1327-1334, 1973

22. Engelman RM, Rousou JH: Methods for assessing preservation techniques – a metabolic approach. In *A Textbook of Clinical Cardioplegia.* Edited by RM Engelman, S Levitsky. Mount Kisco, New York, Futura Publishing Company, 1982, pp 81-88

23. Gibbs CL, Chapman JB: Cardiac energetics. In *Handbook of Physiology. Section 2: The Cardiovascular System. Vol. 1. The Heart.* Edited by RM Berne, N Sperelakis, SR Geiger. Bethesda, Maryland, American Physiological Society, 1979, pp 775-804

24. Westerhof N, Elzinga G: Heart rate and cardiac energetics. *Cardioscience* 2:217-219, 1991

25. Thomas JD, Flachskampf FA, Chen C, et al: Isovolumic relaxation time varies predictably with its time constant and aortic and left atrial pressures: implications for the noninvasive evaluation of ventricular relaxation. *Am Heart J* 124:1305-1313, 1992

26. Corr PB, Sobel BE: The role of biochemical factors in ventricular dysrhythmia accompanying ischemia. *Adv Cardiol* 27:346-360, 1980

27. Singer DH, Baumgarten CM, Ten Eick RE: Cellular electrophysiology of ventricular and other dysrhythmias: studies on diseased and ischemic heart. *Prog Cardiovasc Dis* 24:97-156, 1981

28. Gettes LS: Effect of ischemia on cardiac electrophysiology. In *The Heart and Cardiovascular System: Scientific Foundations.* Vol. 2. Edited by HA Fozzard, E Haber, RB Jennings, et al. New York, Raven Press, 1986, pp 1317-1341

29. Corr PB, Pogwizd SM: Mechanisms contributing to arrhythmogenesis during early myocardial ischemia, subsequent reperfusion, and chronic infarction. *Angiology* 39:684-699, 1988

30. Reimer KA, Jennings RB: Myocardial ischemia, hypoxia, and infarction. In *The Heart and Cardiovascular System: Scientific Foundations.* Vol. 2. Edited by HA Fozzard, E Haber, RB Jennings, et al. New York, Raven Press, 1986, pp 1133-1201

31. Downar E, Janse MJ, Durrer D: The effect of "ischemic" blood on transmembrane potentials of normal porcine ventricular myocardium. *Circulation* 55:455-462, 1977

32. Fozzard HA, Makielski JC: The electrophysiology of acute myocardial ischemia. *Ann Rev Med* 36:275-284, 1985

33. Fabiato A: Calcium-induced release of calcium from the cardiac sarcoplasmic reticulum. *Am J Physiol* 245:C1-C14, 1983

34. Sheridan DJ, Penkoske PA, Sobel BE, et al: Alpha adrenergic contributions to dysrhythmia during myocardial ischemia and reperfusion in cats. *J Clin Invest* 65:161-171, 1980

35. Heathers GP, Yamada KA, Kanter EM, et al: Long-chain acylcarnitines mediate the hypoxia-induced increase in α_1-adrenergic receptors on adult canine myocytes. *Circ Res* 61:735-746, 1987

36. Crozatier B, Ashraf M, Franklin D, et al: Sarcomere length in experimental myocardial infarction: evidence for sarcomere overstretch in dyskinetic ventricular regions. *J Moll Cell Cardiol* 9:785-797, 1977

37. Katz AM: Effects of interrupted coronary flow upon myocardial metabolism and contractility. *Prog Cardiovasc Dis* 10:450-465, 1968

38. Neely JR, Grotyohann LW: Role of glycolytic products in damage to ischemic myocardium: dissociation of adenosine triphosphate levels and recovery of function of reperfused ischemic hearts. *Circ Res* 55:816-824, 1984

39. Laxson DD, Homans DC, Dai X-Z, et al: Oxygen consumption and coronary reactivity in postischemic myocardium. *Circ Res* 64:9-20, 1989

40. Stahl LD, Weiss HR, Becker LC: Myocardial oxygen consumption, oxygen supply/demand heterogeneity, and microvascular patency in regionally stunned myocardium. *Circulation* 77:865-872, 1988

41. Ambrosio G, Jacobus WE, Mitchell MC, et al: Effects of ATP precursors on ATP and free ADP content and functional recovery of postischemic hearts. *Am J Physiol* 256:H560-H566, 1989

42. Krause SM, Jacobus WE, Becker LC: Alterations in cardiac sarcoplasmic reticulum calcium transport in the postischemic "stunned" myocardium. *Circ Res* 65:526-530, 1989

43. Kusuoka H, Koretsune Y, Chacko VP, et al: Excitation-contraction coupling in postischemic myocardium: Does failure of activator Ca^{2+} transients underlie stunning? *Circ Res* 66:1268-1276, 1990

44. Blinks JR, Wier WG, Morgan JP, et al: Regulation of intracellular Ca^{++} by cardiotonic drugs. In *Advances in Pharmacology and Therapeutics II. Vol. 3. Cardio-renal and Cell Pharmacology.* Edited by H Yoshida, Y Hagihara, S Ebashi. New York, Pergamon Press, 1982, p 205

45. Nakamaru Y, Schwartz A: Possible control of intracellular calcium metabolism by [H^+]: sarcoplasmic reticulum of skeletal and cardiac muscle. *Biochem Biophys Res Commun* 41:830-836, 1970

46. Nishimura RA, Abel MD, Hatle LK, et al: Assessment of diastolic function of the heart: background and current applications of Doppler echocardiography. Part II. Clinical studies. *Mayo Clin Proc* 64:181-204, 1989

47. Litwin SE, Grossman W: Diastolic dysfunction as a cause of heart failure. *J Am Coll Cardiol* 22 Suppl A:49-55, 1993

48. Simari RD, Bell MR, Schwartz RS, et al: Ventricular relaxation and myocardial ischemia: a comparison of different models of tau during coronary angioplasty. *Cathet Cardiovasc Diagn* 25:278-284, 1992

49. Katz AM: *Physiology of the Heart.* Second edition. New York, Raven Press, 1992, pp 219-273

50. Weber KT, Brilla CG: Pathological hypertrophy and cardiac interstitium: fibrosis and renin-angiotensin-aldosterone system. *Circulation* 83:1849-1865, 1991

51. Morgan JP: Abnormal intracellular modulation of calcium as a major cause of cardiac contractile dysfunction. *N Engl J Med* 325:625-632, 1991

52. Reimer KA, Jennings RB: The "wavefront phenomenon" of myocardial ischemic cell death. II. Transmural progression of necrosis within the framework of ischemic bed size (myocardium at risk) and collateral flow. *Lab Invest* 40:633-644, 1979

53. Reimer KA, Lowe JE, Rasmussen MM, et al: The wavefront phenomenon of ischemic cell death. 1. Myocardial infarct size vs duration of coronary occlusion in dogs. *Circulation* 56:786-794, 1977

54. Reimer KA, Jennings RB, Tatum AH: Pathobiology of acute myocardial ischemia: metabolic, functional and ultrastructural studies. *Am J Cardiol* 52:72A-81A, 1983

55. Jennings RB, Reimer KA: Lethal myocardial ischemic injury. *Am J Pathol* 102:241-255, 1981

56. Farber JL, Chien KR, Mittnacht S Jr: The pathogenesis of irreversible cell injury in ischemia. *Am J Pathol* 102:271-281, 1981

57. Chien KR, Abrams J, Serroni A, et al: Accelerated phospholipid degradation and associated membrane dysfunction in irreversible, ischemic liver cell injury. *J Biol Chem* 253:4809-4817, 1978

58. Jennings RB, Ganote CE: Structural changes in myocardium during acute ischemia. *Circ Res* 35 Suppl 3:156-168, 1974

59. Chien KR, Pfau RD, Farber JL: Ischemic myocardial cell injury: prevention by chlorpromazine of an accelerated phospholipid degradation and associated membrane dysfunction. *Am J Pathol* 97:505-539, 1979

60. Holman BL, Wynne J: Infarct avid (hot spot) myocardial scintigraphy. *Radiol Clin North Am* 18:487-499, December 1980

61. Gould KL, Hamilton GW, Lipscomb K, et al: Method for assessing stress-induced regional malperfusion during coronary arteriography: experimental validation and clinical application. *Am J Cardiol* 34:557-564, 1974

62. Rahimtoola SH: The hibernating myocardium (editorial). *Am Heart J* 117:211-221, 1989

63. Kloner RA, Przyklenk K, Patel B: Altered myocardial states. The stunned and hibernating myocardium. *Am J Med* 86:14-22, 1989

64. Geer JC, Crago CA, Little WC, et al: Subendocardial ischemic myocardial lesions associated with severe coronary atherosclerosis. *Am J Pathol* 98:663-680, 1980

65. Hoyt JC, Hutchins GM: Variceal transformation of the subendocardial microvasculature in regions of chronic myocardial ischemia. *Am Heart J* 117:830-836, 1989

66. Pirolo JS, Hutchins GM, Moore GW: Myocyte vacuolization in infarct border zones is reversible. *Am J Pathol* 121:444-450, 1985

67. Hamouratidis ND, Handler CE, Pipilis A, et al: Effects of coronary artery surgery on left ventricular performance, segmental wall movement, and exertional ischaemia. *Br Heart J* 60:23-29, 1988

68. Presti CF, Gentile R, Armstrong WF, et al: Improvement in regional wall motion after percutaneous transluminal coronary angioplasty during acute myocardial infarction: utility of two-dimensional echocardiography. *Am Heart J* 115:1149-1155, 1988

69. Holmes DR Jr, Hartzler GO, Smith HC, et al: Coronary artery thrombosis in patients with unstable angina. *Br Heart J* 45:411-416, 1981

70. Falk E: Unstable angina with fatal outcome: dynamic coronary thrombosis leading to infarction and/or sudden death: autopsy evidence of recurrent mural thrombosis with peripheral embolization culminating in total vascular occlusion. *Circulation* 71:699-708, 1985

71. Davies MJ, Thomas AC: Plaque fissuring—the cause of acute myocardial infarction, sudden ischaemic death, and crescendo angina. *Br Heart J* 53:363-373, 1985

72. Simoons ML, Serruys PW, van den Brand M, et al: Early thrombolysis in acute myocardial infarction: limitation of infarct size and improved survival. *J Am Coll Cardiol* 7:717-728, 1986

73. Stack RS, O'Connor CM, Mark DB, et al: Coronary perfusion during acute myocardial infarction with a combined therapy of coronary angioplasty and high-dose intravenous streptokinase. *Circulation* 77:151-161, 1988

74. Gibbons RJ, Holmes DR, Reeder GS, et al: Immediate angioplasty compared with the administration of a thrombolytic agent followed by conservative treatment for myocardial infarction. *N Engl J Med* 328:685-691, 1993

75. Bolli R, Patel BS, Hartley CJ, et al: Nonuniform transmural recovery of contractile function in the stunned myocardium. *Am J Physiol* 257:H375-H385, 1989

76. Braunwald E, Kloner RA: The stunned myocardium: prolonged, postischemic ventricular dysfunction. *Circulation* 66:1146-1149, 1982

77. Heyndrickx GR, Millard RW, McRitchie RJ, et al: Regional myocardial functional and electrophysiological alterations after brief coronary artery occlusion in conscious dogs. *J Clin Invest* 56:978-985, 1975

78. Reimer KA, Hill ML, Jennings RB: Prolonged depletion of ATP and of the adenine nucleotide pool due to delayed resynthesis of adenine nucleotides following reversible myocardial ischemic injury in dogs. *J Mol Cell Cardiol* 13:229-239, 1981

79. Taegtmeyer H, Roberts AFC, Raine AEG: Energy metabolism in reperfused heart muscle: metabolic correlates to return of function. *J Am Coll Cardiol* 6:864-870, 1985

80. Greenfield RA, Swain JL: Disruption of myofibrillar energy use: dual mechanisms that may contribute to postischemic dysfunction in stunned myocardium. *Circ Res* 60:283-289, 1987

81. Krause S, Hess ML: Characterization of cardiac sarcoplasmic reticulum dysfunction during short-term, normothermic, global ischemia. *Circ Res* 55:176-184, 1984

82. Lazdunski M, Frelin C, Vigue P: The sodium/hydrogen exchange system in cardiac cells: its biochemical and pharmacological properties and its role in regulating internal concentrations of sodium and internal pH. *J Mol Cell Cardiol* 17:1029-1042, 1985

83. Opie LH: Reperfusion injury and its pharmacologic modification. *Circulation* 80:1049-1062, 1989

84. McCord JM: Oxygen-derived free radicals in postischemic tissue injury. *N Engl J Med* 312:159-163, 1985

85. Bolli R, Patel BS, Jeroudi MO, et al: Demonstration of free radical generation in "stunned" myocardium of intact dogs with the use of the spin trap α-phenyl N-*tert*-butyl nitrone. *J Clin Invest* 82:476-485, 1988

86. Bolli R: Oxygen-derived free radicals and postischemic myocardial dysfunction ("stunned myocardium"). *J Am Coll Cardiol* 12:239-249, 1988

87. Halliwell B, Gutteridge JMC: Oxygen toxicity, oxygen radicals, transition metals and disease. *Biochem J* 219:1-14, 1984

88. Bolli R: Postischemic myocardial "stunning": pathogenesis, pathophysiology, and clinical relevance. In *Myocardial Protection: the Pathophysiology of Reperfusion and Reperfusion Injury.* Edited by DM Yellon, RB Jennings. New York, Raven Press, 1992, pp 105-150

89. Hearse DJ: Reperfusion of the ischemic myocardium (editorial). *J Mol Cell Cardiol* 9:605-616, 1977

90. Rosenkranz ER, Buckberg GD: Myocardial protection during surgical coronary reperfusion. *J Am Coll Cardiol* 1:1235-1246, 1983

91. Follette DM, Fey K, Buckberg GD, et al: Reducing postischemic damage by temporary modification of reperfusate calcium, potassium, pH, and osmolarity. *J Thorac Cardiovasc Surg* 82:221-238, 1981

92. Jennings RB, Yellon DM: Reperfusion injury: definitions and historical background. In *Myocardial Protection: the Pathophysiology of Reperfusion and Reperfusion Injury.* Edited by DM Yellon, RB Jennings. New York, Raven Press, 1992, pp 1-11

93. Bolli R, McCay PB: Use of spin traps in intact animals undergoing myocardial ischemia/reperfusion: a new approach to assessing the role of oxygen radicals in myocardial "stunning." *Free Radic Res Commun* 9:169-180, 1990

94. Tada M, Kuzuya T, Hoshida S, et al: Arachidonate metabolism in myocardial ischemia and reperfusion. *J Mol Cell Cardiol* 20 Suppl 2:135-143, 1988

95. Dreyer WJ, Michael LH, West MS, et al: Neutrophil accumulation in ischemic canine myocardium: insights into the time course, distribution, and mechanism of localization during early reperfusion. *Circulation* 84:400-411, 1991

96. Keller AM, Clancy RM, Barr ML, et al: Acute reoxygenation injury in the isolated rat heart: role of resident cardiac mast cells. *Circ Res* 63:1044-1052, 1988

97. Kloner RA, Ganote CE, Jennings RB: The "no-reflow" phenomenon after temporary coronary occlusion in the dog. *J Clin Invest* 54:1496-1508, 1974

98. Engler RL, Dahlgren MD, Peterson MA, et al: Accumulation of polymorphonuclear leukocytes during 3-h experimental myocardial ischemia. *Am J Physiol* 251:H93-H100, 1986

99. Ambrosio G, Weisman HF, Mannisi JA, et al: Progressive impairment of regional myocardial perfusion after initial restoration of postischemic blood flow. *Circulation* 80:1846-1861, 1989

100. Przyklenk K, Kloner RA: Effect of verapamil on postischemic "stunned" myocardium: importance of the timing of treatment. *J Am Coll Cardiol* 11:614-623, 1988

101. Klein HH, Pich S, Lindert S, et al: Treatment of reperfusion injury with intracoronary calcium channel antagonists and reduced coronary free calcium concentration in regionally ischemic, reperfused porcine hearts. *J Am Coll Cardiol* 13:1395-1401, 1989

102. Przyklenk K, Ghafari GB, Eitzman DT, et al: Nifedipine administered after reperfusion ablates systolic contractile dysfunction of postischemic "stunned" myocardium. *J Am Coll Cardiol* 13:1176-1183, 1989

103. Pasque MK, Wechsler AS: Metabolic intervention to affect myocardial recovery following ischemia. *Ann Surg* 200:1-12, 1984

104. Shattock MJ, Hearse DJ, Fry CH: The ionic basis of the anti-ischemic and anti-arrhythmic properties of magnesium in the heart. *J Am Coll Nutr* 6:27-33, 1987

105. Maroko PR, Libby P, Sobel BE, et al: Effect of glucose-insulin-potassium infusion on myocardial infarction following experimental coronary artery occlusion. *Circulation* 45:1160-1175, 1972

106. Fiedler VB: Role of arachidonic acid metabolites in cardiac ischemia and reperfusion injury. *Pharmacotherapy* 8:158-168, 1988

107. Farber NE, Gross GJ: Prostaglandin E_1 attenuates postischemic contractile dysfunction after brief coronary occlusion and reperfusion. *Am Heart J* 118:17-24, 1989

108. Manning AS, Hearse DJ: Reperfusion-induced arrhythmias: mechanisms and prevention. *J Mol Cell Cardiol* 16:497-518, 1984

109. Corr PB, Witkowski FX: Arrhythmias associated with reperfusion: basic insights and clinical relevance. *J Cardiovasc Pharmacol* 6 Suppl 6:S903-S909, 1984

110. Wit AL, Rosen MR: Afterdepolarizations and triggered activity. In *The Heart and Cardiovascular System: Scientific Foundations.* Vol. 2. Edited by HA Fozzard, E Haber, RB Jennings, et al. New York, Raven Press, 1986, pp 1449-1490

111. Berne RM: The role of adenosine in the regulation of coronary blood flow. *Circ Res* 47:807-813, 1980

112. Forman MB, Velasco CE, Jackson EK: Adenosine attenuates reperfusion injury following regional myocardial ischemia. *Cardiovasc Res* 27:9-17, 1993

113. Olafsson B, Forman MB, Puett DW, et al: Reduction of reperfusion injury in the canine preparation by intracoronary adenosine: importance of the endothelium and the no-reflow phenomenon. *Circulation* 76:1135-1145, 1987

114. Babbitt DG, Virmani R, Forman MB: Intracoronary adenosine administered after reperfusion limits vascular injury after prolonged ischemia in the canine model. *Circulation* 80:1388-1399, 1989

115. Pitrays CJ II, Virmani R, Vildibill HD Jr, et al: Reduction of myocardial reperfusion injury by intravenous adenosine administered during the early reperfusion period. *Circulation* 83:237-247, 1991

116. Forman MB, Velasco CE: Role of adenosine in the treatment of myocardial stunning. *Cardiovasc Drugs Ther* 5:901-908, 1991

117. Homeister JW, Hoff PT, Fletcher DD, et al: Combined adenosine and lidocaine administration limits myocardial reperfusion injury. *Circulation* 82:595-608, 1990

118. Gibbons RJ, Verani MS, Behrenbeck T, et al: Feasibility of tomographic ^{99m}Tc-hexakis-2-methoxy-2-methylpropyl-isonitrile imaging for the assessment of myocardial area at risk and the effect of treatment in acute myocardial infarction. *Circulation* 80:1277-1286, 1989

119. Garratt KN, Gibbons RJ, Reeder GS, et al: Intravenous adenosine and lidocaine in the limitation of infarct size: preliminary safety data. In: *Adenosine and Adenine Nucleotides: From Molecular Biology to Integrative Physiology*. Edited by L Bellardinelli: A Pelleg. Boston, Kluver Academic Publishers, 1995, pp 447-460

120. Reimer KA, Murry CE, Yamasawa I, et al: Four brief periods of myocardial ischemia cause no cumulative ATP loss or necrosis. *Am J Physiol* 251:H1306-H1315, 1986

121. Murry CE, Jennings RB, Reimer KA: Preconditioning with ischemia: a delay of lethal cell injury in ischemic myocardium. *Circulation* 74:1124-1136, 1986

122. Kida M, Fujiwara H, Ishida M, et al: Ischemic preconditioning preserves creatine phosphate and intracellular pH. *Circulation* 84:2495-2503, 1991

123. Li GC, Vasquez JA, Gallagher KP, et al: Myocardial protection with preconditioning. *Circulation* 82:609-619, 1990

124. Murry CE, Richard VJ, Jennings RB, et al: Myocardial protection is lost before contractile function recovers from ischemic preconditioning. *Am J Physiol* 260:H796-H804, 1991

125. Fleischmann KE, Brand T, Sharma HS, et al: Gene expression in a preconditioning model (abstract). *Circulation* 82 Suppl 3:464, 1990

126. Omar B, Hanson A, Bose S, et al: Reperfusion with pyruvate eliminates ischemic preconditioning: an apparent role for enhanced glycolysis (abstract). *FASEB J* 5:A1257, 1991

127. Auchampach JA, Gross GJ: Myocardial preconditioning is mediated by the activation of the ATP-regulated potassium channel (abstract). *FASEB J* 5:A1103, 1991

CHAPTER

27

Coronary circulation

B. Intravascular ultrasonography

Stuart T. Higano, M.D., and Rick A. Nishimura, M.D.

INTRAVASCULAR ultrasonography is an exciting new technique in which a tiny ultrasound transducer mounted on the tip of a catheter is inserted directly into an artery to provide high-resolution images of lumen size and arterial structure. Although still in its early stage of development, intravascular ultrasonography has great potential for use in the diagnosis and treatment of atherosclerotic cardiovascular disease.

HISTORY

Initial research in intraluminal ultrasound techniques began in the mid-1950s when Cieszynski[1] used a single-element ultrasound crystal mounted perpendicularly on a catheter tip to measure the inner walls of the ventricle and pulmonary arteries on an "A-mode scan." Technical progress developed slowly until 1969 when Bom et al.[2] first introduced a catheter incorporating 32 transducer elements in a cylindrical phased array that could provide real-time tomographic images.

Nearly 2 decades passed before interest was generated in the use of intravascular ultrasonography in the United States. In the late 1980s, several commercially available intravascular ultrasound instruments were introduced in the United States and generated a high level of interest and enthusiasm. Industry responded to this enthusiasm with significant advances in catheter technology and image quality during the next few years.

CURRENT CATHETER TECHNOLOGY

The first catheters used for intravascular ultrasonography were relatively large (8F or 9F) and inflexible, and the images produced were of poor quality. Recent technologic advances have resulted in much smaller and more flexible catheters, some of which are now 3F to 5F (1.0 to 1.5 mm in diameter). Image resolution is now of high quality, and consistently reliable images are obtainable in most instances.

Imaging an arterial structure from within the lumen requires a mechanism to allow for rotation of the ultrasound beam around the circumference of the vessel. Two basic imaging systems have been incorporated into intravascular ultrasound catheters—the mechanical and the dynamic aperture array.

The mechanical scanning systems incorporate a mechanism for mechanically rotating the ultrasound beam, and several methods have been developed. The simplest device has a transducer element attached to a rotating central core. Another type has a fixed ultrasound transducer at the tip of the catheter. The ultrasound beam is directed proximally along the axis of the catheter and is then reflected off a rotating mirror angled at 45°, so that it emanates perpendicular to the catheter. A third type of mechanical system has both the ultrasound transducer and the angled mirror mounted on a rotating core (Fig 27B-1). In all current mechanical systems, the rotating portion revolves at 1,500 to 3,000 rpm and produces a tomographic image perpendicular to the catheter. The proximal end of the catheter is attached to a drive motor that provides torque to the central core. For accurate image reconstruction, the central core must provide a one-to-one correspondence in rotation between the drive

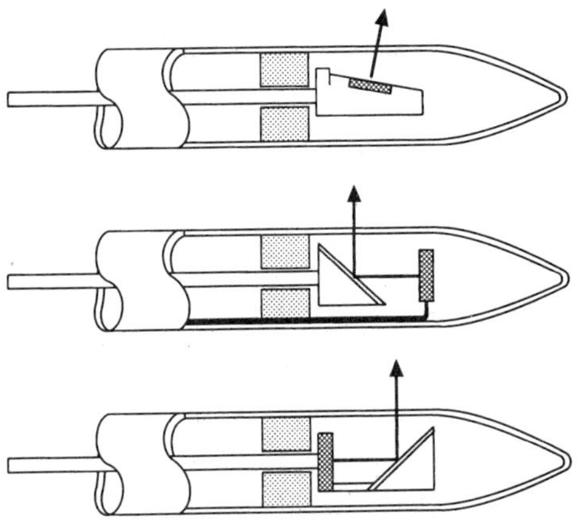

Fig 27B-1 Three types of mechanical catheters: **top**, rotating transducer; **middle**, rotating mirror; **bottom**, rotating mirror and transducer (see text for details).

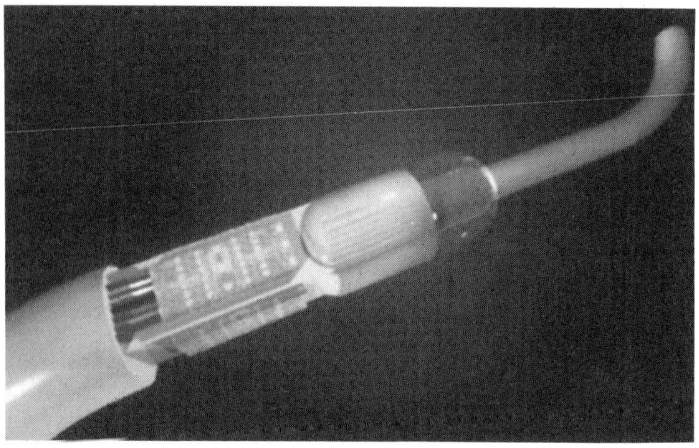

Fig 27B-2 Artist's representation of the dynamic aperture-array catheter. The cylindrically arranged ultrasound crystals are controlled by miniaturized integrated circuits (see text for details). (Courtesy of Endosonics, Inc., Pleasanton, California.)

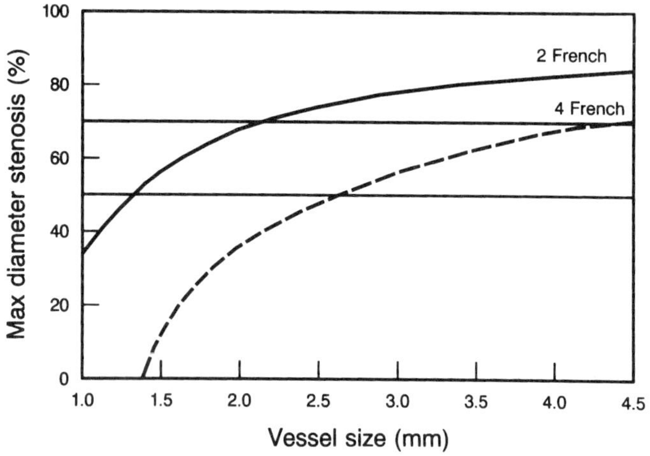

Fig 27B-3 Maximal percent diameter stenosis plotted against vessel size for 2F and 4F ultrasound catheters; circular dimensions are assumed. For example, a 4F catheter in a 2.5-mm vessel would not fit in a stenosis >50% without plaque stretching or disruption. The horizontal lines indicate the 50% and 70% stenosis levels. Decreasing the catheter size to 2F improves the ability to image stenoses.

motor and the tip of the catheter. Deviation from this one-to-one rotation results in image distortion.

The dynamic aperture array system incorporates a principle similar to that of the phased-array transducers on a transthoracic echocardiographic system. Multiple transducer elements (32 to 64) are located in a circular configuration around the catheter tip. The transducer elements on the wave-front side of the catheter are activated electronically. Appropriate timing of each transducer element allows a uniform ultrasound beam to be emitted perpendicular to the catheter. The beam sweeps electronically around the catheter, creating a 360° image. The ultrasound images are controlled by a microprocessor on the catheter tip, immediately proximal to the crystals (Fig 27B-2).

The size of the catheter varies with the manufacturer but is usually 6F to 8F for peripheral vascular imaging and 3F to 5F for coronary imaging. The ultrasound frequency for intravascular imaging is much higher than that used in transthoracic imaging; the resulting higher image resolution is at the expense of lower tissue penetration. Peripheral vascular imaging catheters usually operate at frequencies of 15 to 20 MHz and image to depths of 1 to 2 cm. Coronary imaging catheters usually have frequencies of 20 to 40 MHz and imaging depths of 3 to 5 mm.

Intravascular ultrasound catheters are delivered to the vascular system by the same type of technology used in interventional therapeutic procedures. For intracoronary imaging, the ultrasound catheter is delivered through a regular angioplasty-guided catheter. Most of the catheters are delivered to the arterial tree with an angioplasty guide wire. Many of the catheters incorporate a "monorail" design. Peripheral vascular systems are often placed through an arterial access sheath without either an over-the-wire system or a fixed wire at the catheter tip. The ultrasound catheters are usually placed under fluoroscopic guidance. Arterial structure is visually analyzed from the real-time ultrasound image, and videotape recording is available for off-line quantitation.

Significant advances in catheter technology remain to be accomplished, especially for imaging the coronary circulation. The major limitation at present for the mechanical scanners is the relatively large and bulky size of the catheters. Optimal imaging of a vessel requires a surrounding column of blood between the transducer and the arterial wall, because the ultrasound image depends on acoustic interfaces. Thus, an artery lumen must be at least 20% greater in diameter than the diameter of the catheter if an image of adequate quality is to be obtained. Since a transducer element (or mirror) is rotated at high speeds at the distal end of a catheter, the catheter shaft must be large enough to accommodate both the transducer wires and the motor driveshaft. With current technology, interrogation by mechanical transducers is limited to moderate stenoses in large vessels or after catheter-based interventions (Fig 27B-3). Although the dynamic aperture array models can be smaller and more flexible, image resolution may be poorer than that with the mechanical transducers. Technologic advances to allow smaller-sized catheters may consist of the development of miniaturized motor drives that can propel the transducers directly at the top of the catheters.

IMAGE INTERPRETATION

An intravascular ultrasound image represents a tomographic cross section of a vessel (Fig 27B-4). The catheter itself, which is located within the lumen of the vessel, appears as a black circle. The arterial lumen can be outlined, and it has been well documented that intravascular ultrasonography provides a highly accurate and reproducible measurement of luminal area. This result has been shown in both in vitro models and comparative

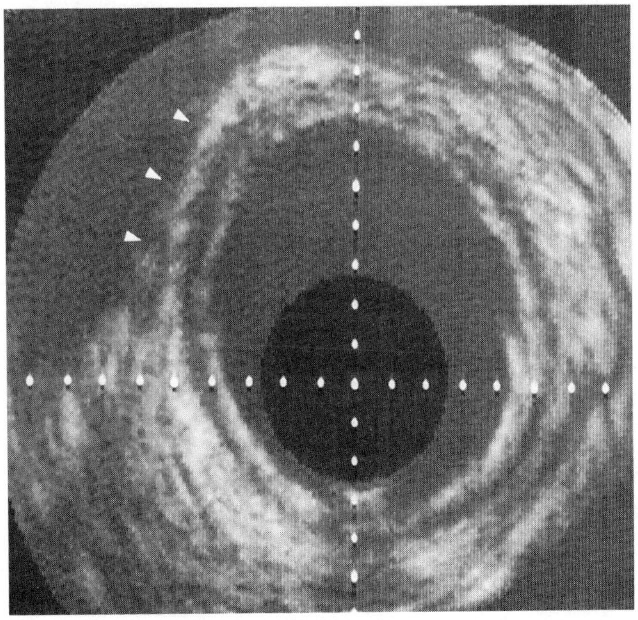

Fig 27B-4 Intravascular ultrasound image of a normal coronary artery. Three mural layers are readily apparent. The black hole in the lumen represents the catheter. (From Nishimura RA, Edwards WD, Warnes CA, et al: Intravascular ultrasound imaging: in vitro validation and pathologic correlation. *J Am Coll Cardiol* 16:145-154, 1990. By permission of American College of Cardiology.)

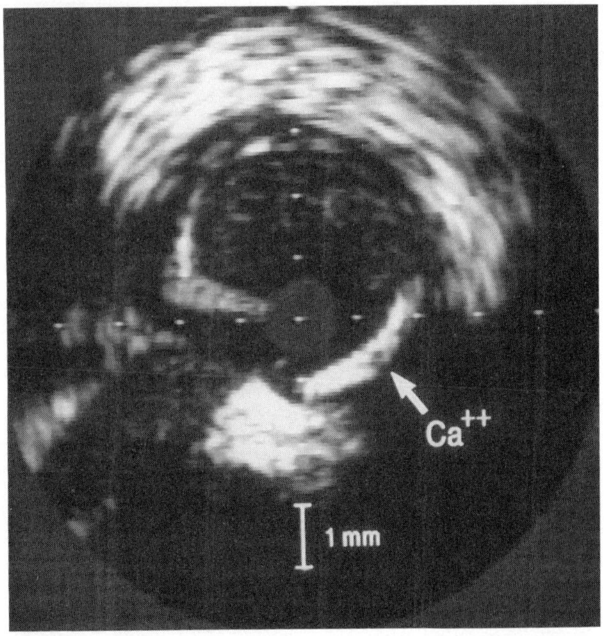

Fig 27B-5 Intravascular ultrasound image of a calcified atherosclerotic plaque adjacent to a septal perforator branch. Calcium (Ca^{++}) is echogenic (bright) and shadows the far field.

histopathologic studies.[3-8] An accurate measurement of luminal area assumes that the catheter is parallel to the long axis of the vessel, because any deviation from this long axis distorts the luminal area. Fortunately, the deviation that occurs during in vivo imaging is negligible and does not significantly affect the measured vessel area.[9]

The normal artery was initially thought to have a "trilayer appearance" consisting of an inner bright layer, a middle sonolucent area, and an outer dense layer. These layers were at first believed to represent the intima, media, and adventitia, respectively. Subsequent studies showed that this three-layered appearance is not always present.[4,10] In young patients with completely normal coronary arteries on histopathologic examination, the inner bright layer is absent. This inner layer is seen only in older patients who have an intimal thickness of at least 178 μm.[11] This inner bright layer most likely represents differences in acoustic impedance among blood-tissue interface, thickened intima, and ultrasound reflections from the internal elastic membrane.

In the normal artery, a middle sonolucent area may be present, most likely representing the media, with the adventitia represented by a dense outer layer. However, not all arteries have this distinct ultrasound appearance of the two layers. Whether these two layers are present depends on the type of artery (muscular or elastic), the composition of each layer, and the type of instrument used.[12] Instruments with different dynamic ranges and different levels of gray scale may result in different appearances of the multiple layers.

In atherosclerotic disease, the thickness of the inner layer is increased on intravascular ultrasound images. Intravascular ultrasonography is clearly able to diagnose early and diffuse atherosclerosis, which may not be evident on angiographic examination.

The ultrasound features have been used to characterize the composition of an atherosclerotic plaque[5] (Fig 27B-5). Plaque calcium has a high reflectivity and can be recognized on the intravascular ultrasound image as a bright echodensity with acoustic far-field shadowing. Lipid zones, or "lipid lakes," are seen as sonolucent regions that are visibly separate from the underlying media. Fibrous plaque typically has an intermediate ultrasound texture and frequently blends in with the underlying media. Intra-arterial thrombus has a granular or speckled heterogeneous appearance.[13,14]

CLINICAL UTILITY

Peripheral circulation

Intravascular ultrasonography of the peripheral circulation is a safe and accurate method to determine severity of stenosis in patients with arteriosclerosis obliterans. A peripheral vascular imaging catheter may be inserted through the femoral artery and placed under fluoroscopic guidance at the level of the descending thoracic aorta. Slowly withdrawing the catheter provides multiple tomographic images of the arterial circulation (Fig 27B-6). Because of the relatively large size of these arteries, high-resolution images are consistently obtained. The

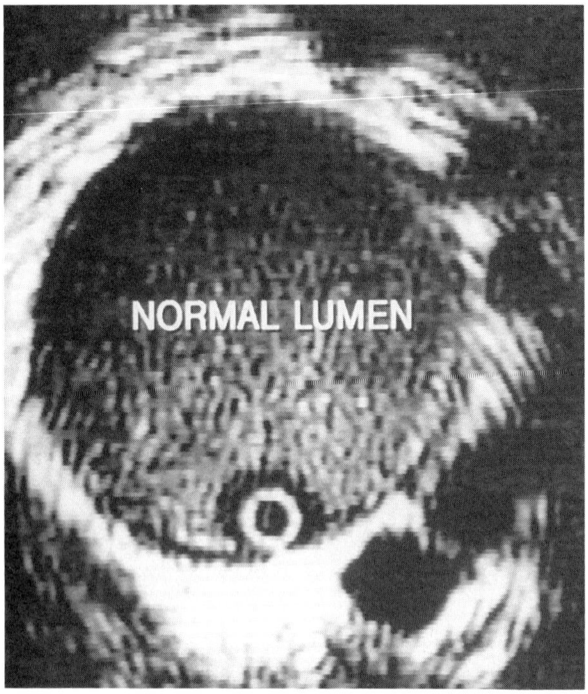

Fig 27B-6 Intravascular ultrasound image of the descending aorta. The catheter (black hole) is adjacent to the intimal surface.

multiple tomographic cross-sectional images allow three-dimensional reconstruction (Fig 27B-7).

As experience is gained with intravascular ultrasound imaging of the peripheral circulation and advances in computer technology allow on-line three-dimensional reconstruction, intravascular ultrasonography may become the imaging modality of choice in the evaluation of a patient with arteriosclerosis obliterans.

Intravascular ultrasound imaging has also been used for the evaluation of suspected aortic dissection,[15-18] because it gives extremely high resolution of arterial structure and can easily detect whether an intimal flap is present (Fig 27B-8). A scan of the aorta can define the extent of the dissection flap, its relationship to branch vessels, and the exact location of entry and exit points. Studies are under way comparing the utility of intravascular ultrasonography with that of other modalities, such as computed tomographic scanning and magnetic resonance imaging, for the diagnosis of aortic dissection. Since the intravascular ultrasound machine can easily be brought to a patient's bedside, its diagnostic accuracy and portability may in the future make this imaging modality the best one to use for patients with suspected dissection.

Coronary arteries

Coronary angiography has many limitations in defining the extent and severity of atherosclerotic disease. Coronary angiography produces a two-dimensional view of luminal area and thus may significantly underestimate the severity of stenoses in patients with eccentric lesions and

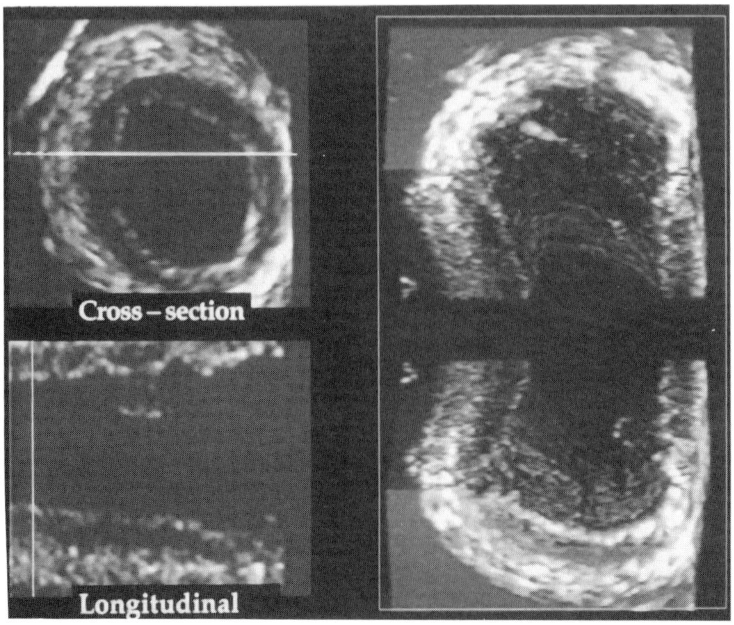

Fig 27B-7 Three-dimensional images of a coronary artery produced by sequential pull-back imaging. Both longitudinal and "clamshell" (*right*) methods of display are shown above with a representative cross section. (Courtesy of Cardiovascular Imaging Systems, Inc., Sunnyvale, California.)

overlapping vessels. Histopathologic studies have shown that coronary angiography cannot define severe narrowing of the coronary arteries if diffuse, concentric atherosclerosis is present[19-21] (Fig 27B-9). Intracoronary ultrasonography overcomes these inherent problems of coronary angiography by providing multiple tomographic cross sections of arterial structure.

The relatively large size of the catheters, however, limits current clinical application of diagnostic intracoronary ultrasonography to evaluation of indeterminate stenoses in the larger proximal vessels. Even with modern, sophisticated equipment in the cardiac catheterization laboratory, a coronary lesion may be angiographically indeterminate because of tortuosity or overlapping segments of

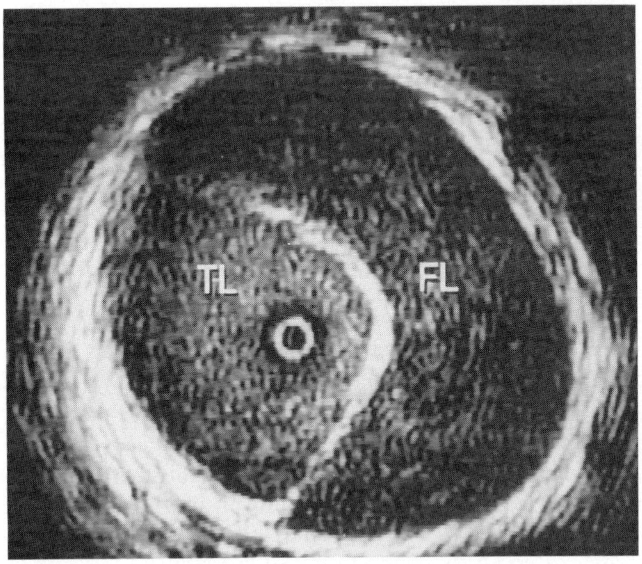

Fig 27B-8 Intravascular ultrasound image of an aortic dissection. The catheter (black hole) is in the true lumen (*TL*). *FL*, false lumen.

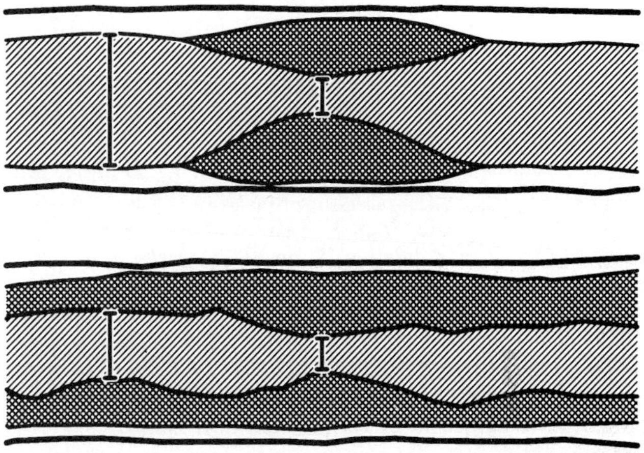

Fig 27B-9 Diagram of the difficulty in quantitating diffuse atherosclerosis by angiography. Both upper and lower vessels have similar luminal diameters at the tightest stenosis. However, the diffuse disease in the lower causes an underestimation of the lesion by percent diameter stenosis.

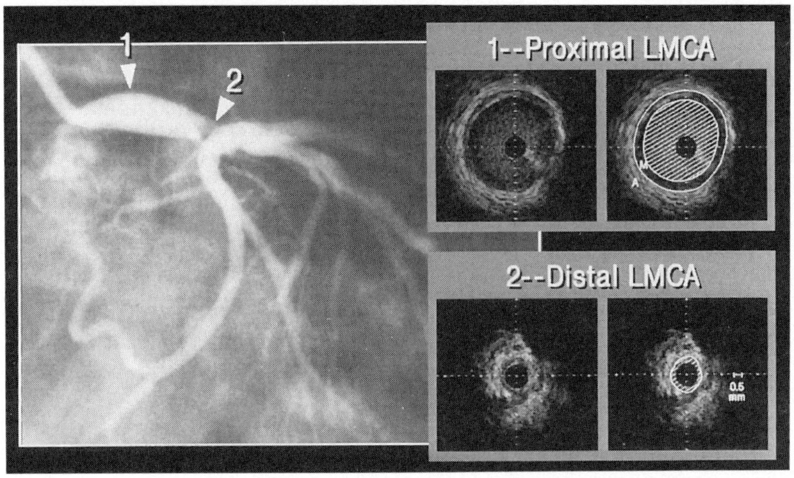

Fig 27B-10 Coronary angiogram and left main coronary artery (*LMCA*) intravascular sonograms. **Left**, right anterior oblique view of an indeterminate lesion in the distal LMCA. **Right**, intravascular ultrasound images from the proximal (*1*) and distal (*2*) LMCA. The distal LMCA has an 80% area stenosis. Hatched area represents the luminal area. The internal and external elastic membranes are outlined. *A*, adventitia; *M*, media. (From Nishimura RA, Higano ST, Holmes DR Jr: Utility of intracoronary ultrasound imaging for assessing left main coronary artery disease. *Mayo Clin Proc* 68:134-140, 1993. By permission, Mayo Foundation for Medical Education and Research.)

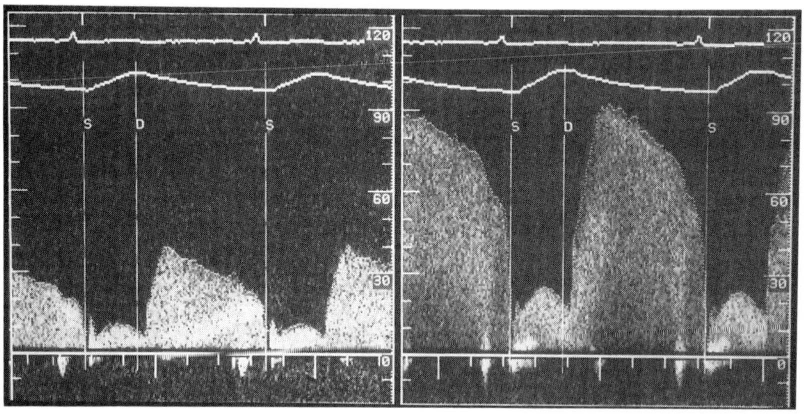

Fig 27B-11 Intracoronary Doppler study shows the measurement of coronary flow reserve. Tracings are from the left anterior descending coronary artery before (*left*) and after (*right*) 18 μg of adenosine was delivered by intracoronary administration. *D*, onset of diastole; *S*, onset of systole.

the arteries. Ultrasound imaging has been used in patients with indeterminate lesions in the left main coronary artery (Fig 27B-10) and the proximal right coronary artery. It is hoped that future developments in intracoronary ultrasound catheters will allow placement of these catheters in more severe stenoses in middle and distal coronary vessels. In addition, the Doppler guide wire now provides a method for measuring flow, which adds physiologic information to the anatomic information provided by intracoronary ultrasonography (Fig 27B-11). Since intravascular ultrasound imaging is the most sensitive method for detecting early atherosclerosis, it may become the ideal modality in the future for quantitating changes in the severity of atherosclerosis in trials examining progression and regression of coronary artery disease by different drugs and interventions.

Guiding therapy

One of the major expectations of intravascular ultrasonography has been for guidance of catheter-based interventions. Currently, percutaneous transluminal coronary angioplasty, atherectomy, laser angioplasty, and intracoronary stents are being used in the treatment of patients with coronary artery disease. However, a chance for acute complications and a high rate of restenosis remain after all these catheter-based therapies. It has been postulated that intracoronary ultrasound imaging may help in decreasing both acute complications and restenosis. However, benefits of this technique are speculative, and large multicenter trials are under way to determine its ultimate role in interventional cardiology.

Percutaneous transluminal coronary angioplasty is the most commonly used method for treatment of stenotic coronary artery lesions. The mechanism of successful balloon angioplasty is usually disruption of atherosclerotic plaque. An acute increase in cross-sectional area may also result from stretching of the noninvolved arterial wall, that is, "elastic recoil." If elastic recoil is the primary mechanism for acute enlargement in luminal area, "early restenosis" will occur as the expanded arterial wall returns to its normal size after several days. It has been proposed that when ultrasound imaging demonstrates that plaque has not fractured, a bulk removal method, such as directional atherectomy, be selected.[22]

In a selected subgroup of patients, extensive dissection may occur, causing abrupt closure of an artery. Clinical and angiographic methods have failed to accurately predict the occurrence of large flow-limiting dissections.[23] Dissections have been shown to occur in areas of calcification in the arterial wall detected by intracoronary ultrasound imaging, because nonuniform stress is placed on the plaque by an inflated balloon.[24,25] In the future, intravascular ultrasonography may be useful in identifying patients at high risk for large dissection with conventional percutaneous transluminal coronary angioplasty.

Restenosis remains a large problem after percutaneous transluminal coronary angioplasty, approaching 50% to 55% at 6 months. Restenosis is thought to occur from several mechanisms, including the problems associated with elastic recoil or medial injury with stimulation of atherogenesis. One of the major causes of apparent "restenosis" is an inadequate initial result. The multiple dissection channels and cleavages after angioplasty may cause "haziness" on coronary angiography, precluding accurate assessment of the final acute result. Intracoronary ultrasound imaging should provide a much better method for assessing the final luminal area after angioplasty, so that decisions on proceeding with larger balloon sizes or other interventional devices can be made.

Other catheter-based therapies used to treat coronary arterial lesions, such as directional atherectomy, rotational atherectomy, laser angioplasty, and stent placement, have had high initial success rates. However, the restenosis rate with each of these modalities remains high. It is hoped that intracoronary ultrasound imaging will prevent further recurrence by enhancing the results of the different therapies, that is, ensuring removal of the optimal amount of tissue in atherectomy, guiding laser ablation, and optimizing stent placement. For directional atherectomy, the ultrasound appearance of the plaque may influence the rate of restenosis. The restenosis rate appears to be significantly higher in the echolucent plaques than in the echodense plaques.[26,27] Intravascular ultrasonography may be of great utility in assuring complete apposition and expansion of intracoronary stents. Stent placement guided by intravascular ultrasonography may eliminate the need for anticoagulation.[28]

SUMMARY

Intravascular ultrasonography is an exciting new technique providing high-resolution images of arterial structure. Before it can be applied to daily clinical practice, however, significant advances must be made in catheter technology and prognostic and therapeutic benefits must be proved. Future technologic advances will include miniaturization of catheters, forward-looking catheters, and combination catheters (ultrasound-Doppler, ultrasound-angioplasty, and ultrasound-atherectomy). On-line three-dimensional reconstruction should prove to be particularly useful for assessment of the results of catheter-based therapy.

REFERENCES

1. Cieszynski T: Intracardial method for the investigation of structure of the heart with the aid of ultrasonics. *Arch Immun Ter Dosw* 8:551-557, 1960
2. Bom N, Lancée CT, van Egmond FC: An ultrasonic intracardiac scanner. *Ultrasonics* 10:72-76, 1972
3. Wenguang L, Gussenhoven WJ, Zhong Y, et al: Validation of quantitative analysis of intravascular ultrasound images. *Int J Card Imaging* 6:247-253, 1991
4. Nishimura RA, Edwards WD, Warnes CA, et al: Intravascular ultrasound imaging: in vitro validation and pathologic correlation. *J Am Coll Cardiol* 16:145-154, 1990
5. Potkin BN, Bartorelli AL, Gessert JM, et al: Coronary artery imaging with intravascular high-frequency ultrasound. *Circulation* 81: 1575-1585, 1990
6. Tobis JM, Mallery JA, Gessert J, et al: Intravascular ultrasound cross-sectional arterial imaging before and after balloon angioplasty in vitro. *Circulation* 80:873-882, 1989
7. Pandian NG, Kreis A, O'Donnell T: Intravascular ultrasound estimation of arterial stenosis. *J Am Soc Echocardiogr* 2:390-397, 1989
8. Hodgson JMcB, Graham SP, Savakus AD, et al: Clinical percutaneous imaging of coronary anatomy using an over-the-wire ultrasound catheter system. *Int J Card Imaging* 4:187-193, 1989
9. St. Goar FG, Pinto FJ, Alderman EL, et al: Intravascular ultrasound imaging of angiographically normal coronary arteries: an in vivo comparison with quantitative angiography. *J Am Coll Cardiol* 18:952-958, 1991
10. Nissen SE, Gurley JC, Grines CL, et al: Intravascular ultrasound assessment of lumen size and wall morphology in normal subjects and patients with coronary artery disease. *Circulation* 84:1087-1099, 1991
11. Fitzgerald PJ, St. Goar FG, Connolly AJ, et al: Intravascular ultrasound imaging of coronary arteries. Is three layers the norm? *Circulation* 86:154-158, 1992
12. Nishimura RA, Kennedy KD, Warnes CA, et al: Intravascular ultrasonography: image interpretation and limitations. *Echocardiography* 7:469-474, 1990
13. Pandian NG, Kreis A, Brockway B: Detection of intraarterial thrombus by intravascular high frequency two-dimensional ultrasound imaging: in vitro and in vivo studies. *Am J Cardiol* 65:1280-1283, 1990
14. Jain A, Ramee SR, Mesa J, et al: Intracoronary thrombus: chronic urokinase infusion and evaluation with intravascular ultrasound. *Cathet Cardiovasc Diagn* 26:212-214, 1992
15. Cavaye DM, French WJ, White RA, et al: Intravascular ultrasound imaging of an acute dissection aortic aneurysm: a case report. *J Vasc Surg* 13:510-512, 1991
16. Pande A, Meier B, Fleisch M, et al: Intravascular ultrasound for diagnosis of aortic dissection. *Am J Cardiol* 67:662-663, 1991
17. Weintraub AR, Schwartz SL, Pandian NG, et al: Evaluation of acute aortic dissection by intravascular ultrasonography (letter to the editor). *N Engl J Med* 323:1566-1567, 1990
18. Chandrasekaran K, Quinn V, Ross JJ Jr, et al: Diagnostic utility and clinical applicability of intravascular ultrasonography in the evaluation of aortic disorders: initial experience in 48 patients (abstract). *Circulation* 86 Suppl 1:364, 1992
19. Arnett EN, Isner JM, Redwood DR, et al: Coronary artery narrowing in coronary heart disease: comparison by cineangiographic and necropsy findings. *Ann Intern Med* 91:350-356, 1979
20. Grondin CM, Dyrda I, Pasternac A, et al: Discrepancies between cineangiographic and postmortem findings in patients with coronary artery disease and recent myocardial revascularization. *Circulation* 49:703-708, 1974
21. Schwartz JN, Kong Y, Hackel DB, et al: Comparison of angiographic and postmortem findings in patients with coronary artery disease. *Am J Cardiol* 36:174-178, 1975
22. Honye J, Mahon DJ, Jain A, et al: Morphological effects of coronary balloon angioplasty in vivo assessed by intravascular ultrasound imaging. *Circulation* 85:1012-1025, 1992
23. Waller BF, Orr CM, Pinkerton CA, et al: Coronary balloon angioplasty dissections: "the good, the bad, and the ugly." *J Am Coll Cardiol* 20:701-706, 1992
24. Fitzgerald PJ, Ports TA, Yock PG: Contribution of localized calcium deposits to dissection after angioplasty: an observational study using intravascular ultrasound. *Circulation* 86:64-70, 1992
25. Potkin BN, Keren G, Mintz GS, et al: Arterial responses to balloon coronary angioplasty: an intravascular ultrasound study. *J Am Coll Cardiol* 20:942-951, 1992
26. Yock PG, Fitzgerald PJ, Sykes C, et al: Morphologic features of successful coronary atherectomy determined by intravascular ultrasound imaging (abstract). *Circulation* 82 Suppl 3:676, 1990
27. Súarez de Lezo J, Romero M, Medina A, et al: Intracoronary ultrasound assessment of directional coronary atherectomy: immediate and follow-up findings. *J Am Coll Cardiol* 21:298-307, 1993
28. Colombo A, Hall P, Nakamura S, et al: Intracoronary stenting without anticoagulation accomplished with intravascular ultrasound guidance. *Circulation* 91:1676-1688, 1995

CHAPTER

28A

Atherosclerosis

A. Pathogenesis: initiation, progression, acute coronary syndromes, and regression

Valentin Fuster, M.D., Ph.D., and James H. Chesebro, M.D.

DEFINITION

Arteries normally undergo an aging process characterized by thickening of the intima, loss of elasticity, increase in calcium content, and increase in diameter. These changes are thought to occur generally throughout the major arterial system;[1] they were first referred to as "arteriosclerosis" by Lobstein.[2] In contrast to this natural process, atherosclerosis is a focal pathologic phenomenon affecting the large arteries, mainly the aorta and the coronary, carotid, iliac, and femoral arteries. In 1958, a study group of the World Health Organization[3] defined atherosclerosis as a "variable combination of changes of the intima of arteries (as distinguished from arterioles) consisting of the focal accumulation of lipids, complex carbohydrates, blood and blood products, fibrous tissue and calcium deposits, and associated with medial changes." During the past 3 decades, significant advances have been made in our understanding of this pathologic phenomenon.

Atherosclerotic disease primarily affects arteries ranging in size from the aorta down to the tertiary branches of coronary arteries (1 mm diameter). Atherosclerosis is characterized by atherosis (soft "gruel") and sclerosis (hard, collagenous). Most patients have plaques containing variable amounts of both hard and soft components.[4] The connection, if any, between the hard collagenous and the soft atheromatous components is uncertain, and most attempts to reconstruct a dynamic sequence in the evolution of atherosclerotic plaques on the basis of morphology and composition of advanced lesions have been disappointing. Some observers believe that plaques soften with time: the older the individual[5,6] and the larger the plaque,[7,8] the more gruel. It has been suggested, however, that softening of the inner part of the plaque occurs early during the evolution of fibrous plaques[9] and that hard lesions could represent the late, sclerotic phase of the disease,[10] with softening then being more localized at the base of the plaque.[9]

Portions of this manuscript are modified from Fuster et al.[4,9]

INITIATION AND LOCALIZATION OF ATHEROSCLEROSIS

Identification of the earliest events in lesion development is important if we are to understand the critical pathogenic mechanisms that become obscure as the lesions progress (Fig 28A-1 and 28A-2). In the 19th century, two major hypotheses explained the pathogenesis of atherosclerosis: the encrustation hypothesis and the lipid hypothesis. The encrustation theory, proposed by Rokitansky in 1851,[11] suggested that intimal thickening resulted from fibrin deposition, with subsequent organization by fibroblast and secondary lipid accumulation. The lipid theory, proposed by Virchow in 1856,[12] suggested that blood lipids transudate into the arterial wall, interact with proteoglycans, and promote intimal proliferation.

Vascular response to injury hypothesis

The prevalent view of atherogenesis proposed by Ross integrates both theories into a more complex "response to injury" hypothesis,[13] in which atherosclerosis is considered a healing response of the arterial wall to various injurious stimuli. For easier understanding of the pathogenesis of the disease and better formulation of therapeutic strategies, we have proposed a pathophysiologic classification of vascular injury or damage into three categories representing stages of increasing severity[14] (Fig 28A-3). Type I injury consists of functional alterations of endothelial cells without substantial morphologic changes, as it occurs in the initial stage of atherosclerosis; type II injury is characterized by endothelial denudation, as it may occur in relatively earlier stages of atherosclerosis (see below) or in the latest stages when plaques are very stenotic; and type III injury is characterized by endothelial denudation with damage to the intima and the media, as it occurs in plaque fissuring and rupture in later stages of atherosclerosis.

Hypercholesterolemia and other systemic risk factors somehow lead to endothelial dysfunction (type I injury) (Table 28A-1), but not necessarily to endothelial denu-

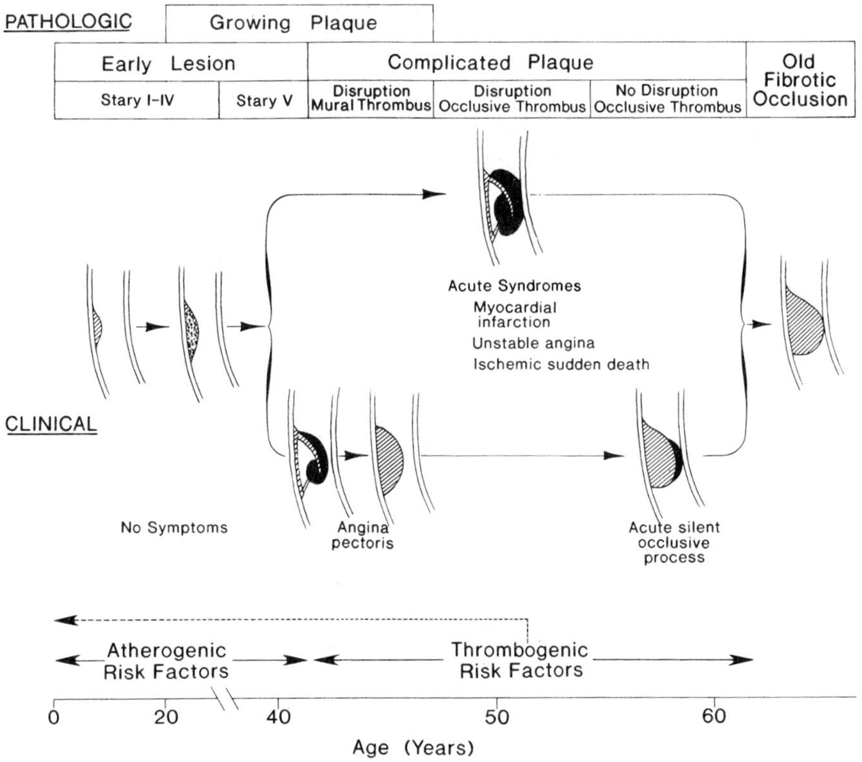

Fig 28A-1 Typical early evolution and progression of coronary atherosclerosis according to the pathologic and clinical findings. (From Fuster V, Badimon L, Badimon JJ, et al: The pathogenesis of coronary artery disease and the acute coronary syndromes. *N Engl J Med* 326:242-250; 310-318, 1992. By permission of journal.)

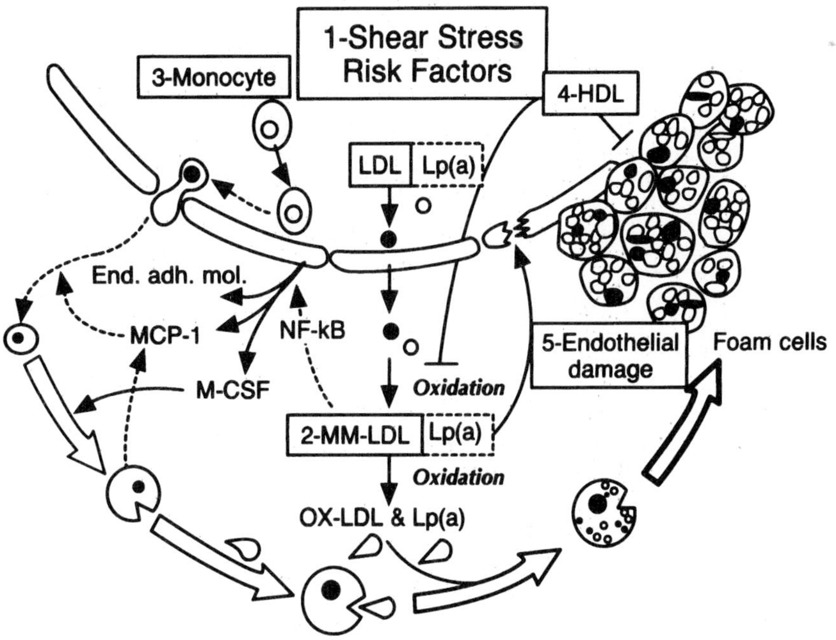

Fig 28A-2 Biologic factors involved in the initiation of atherosclerosis. See text for details. *end. adh. mol.,* endothelial adhesion molecule; *HDL,* high-density lipoprotein; *LDL,* low-density lipoprotein; *LP(a),* lipoprotein a; *MCP-1,* monocyte chemotactic protein-1; *M-CSF,* modified colony-stimulating factor; *MM-LDL,* minimally modified low-density lipoprotein; *OX-LDL,* oxidized low-density lipoprotein. (Modified from Steinberg D: Antioxidants and atherosclerosis. A current assessment [editorial]. *Circulation* 84:1420-1425, 1991.)

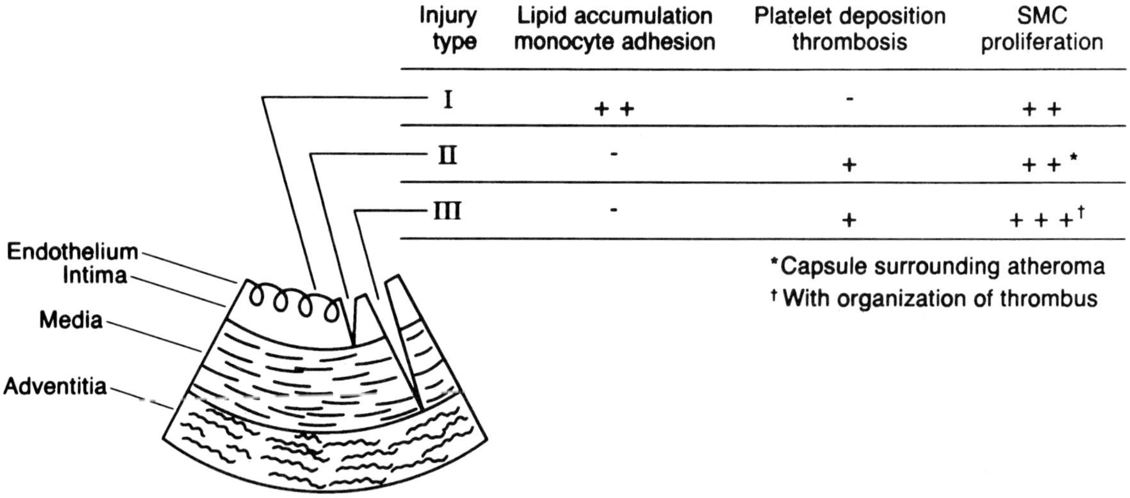

Fig 28A-3 Classification of vascular injury or damage and vascular response. See text for details. *SMC,* smooth muscle cell.

Table 28A-1 Atherogenesis: influence of risk factors

Biology	Dyslipoproteinemia	Hypertension	Smoking	Genetics	Diabetes*
Endothelial injury (type I injury)	+	+	+	−	+
Lipoprotein—monocytes	+ +	−	−	+ +	+ +
Platelet deposition (over type II injury)	+	−	+ +	−	+
SMC—collagen	+	+	−	+ +	+ +
Plaque disruption (type III injury)	+ +	+	−	+ +	−
Thrombosis	+	−	+ +	+	+ +
Microvasculature	+	+ +	+	−	+ +†

SMC, smooth muscle cell. +, slight influence; + +, significant influence; −, no influence.
*Glycemia: advanced glycosylation end product (more so in insulin-dependent than in non-insulin-dependent diabetes mellitus).
†Insulin resistance (non-insulin-dependent diabetes mellitus): increased triglycerides, decreased high-density lipoprotein, hypertension.

dation. Dysfunctional endothelium is characterized by increased permeability to lipoproteins and the expression of specific adhesive glycoproteins on its surface. Numerous studies have suggested that modified (oxidized) low-density lipoprotein (LDL), presumably accumulated within the arterial wall (often related to dissolution or cytolysis of saturated foam cells), may also be a key component in type II endothelial injury with cell necrosis.[15-17] Endothelial cells have the ability to oxidize lipoproteins as they are transported into the artery wall.[13,18] In vitro, smooth muscle cells and macrophages have also shown the ability to oxidize native LDL.[19-21]

Despite exposure to the same lipoprotein concentration, spontaneous atherosclerotic lesions develop only in certain locations. Therefore, in addition to systemic factors, local factors must have a role in determining the location and possibly the rate of atherosclerosis progression.[22] The preferred sites of atherogenesis are regions of low shear stress with complex secondary flow patterns, zones of standing recirculation, and regions of oscillatory hemodynamic changes occurring mostly at bending points and bifurcations.[22-24] Several hypotheses have been advanced to explain the mechanism by which low shear stress to vessel walls might promote the development of atherosclerotic lesions. Endothelial cells undergo morphologic alterations in response to changes in the degree and orientation of shear stress; elongated endothelial cells are located in regions of high shear stress, whereas polygonal endothelial cells are located in regions of low shear stress.[25] These alterations may be responsible for changes in endothelial cell permeability to atherogenic lipoprotein particles.[23] It has also been hypothesized that in regions of low shear stress, reduction or stagnation in the velocity of blood flow permits increased uptake of atherogenic particles as a result of increased residence time or prolonged contact with the endothelium, which would allow concentration-induced endocytosis.[15]

Besides local shear forces, probably enhanced in hypertension, and atherogenic lipoproteins, forms of injury such as those that can be induced by advanced glycosylated end products in diabetes, chemical irritants in tobacco smoke, circulating vasoactive amines, immunocomplexes, and infection all may lead to type I chronic endothelial injury favoring accumulation of lipids in the intima[9,14] (see Table 28A-1). Because T lymphocytes are present with macrophages in early lesions, an immunologic reaction may occur during the early process of atherogenesis and may be related to specific antigens.[13,26] No such antigen has been identified, although autoantibodies to oxidized LDL have been found.[13]

Clinical studies have shown that dysfunctional endothelium is present in very early stages of atherosclerosis.[27] High-resolution ultrasonography performed in femoral and brachial arteries of symptom-free children and young adults with risk factors for atherosclerosis demonstrated impairment in endothelium-dependent vasodilatation even before anatomic evidence of plaque formation.

Lipid entry into the arterial wall

Clinical and experimental studies have firmly established that high levels of LDL are associated with atherosclerosis.[26,27] Lipids deposited in the atherosclerotic lesions are mostly derived from plasma LDL. The internalization and intravascular accumulation of cholesterol and its esters depend on two mechanisms: one is active and dependent on specific receptors located in the wall membrane, and the other is passive and receptor-independent. Whether endothelial type I injury tends to increase the active one or, through the direct interaction of plasma LDL with glycosaminoglycans into the vessel wall,[26] the passive one is open to debate.

A specific LDL receptor in the liver is responsible for the metabolization and elimination of plasma cholesterol.[28] The number of these LDL receptors seems to be, in part, genetically determined, and this observation helps explain why a family history of hypercholesterolemia may be a risk factor for coronary artery disease. Among various receptors expressed by cultured macrophages, the β-VLDL (very-low-density lipoprotein) and the acetyl-LDL, or scavenger, receptors are poorly regulated by the intracellular cholesterol levels in contrast to the classic LDL receptor.[29] Monocytes and macrophages take up LDL via the LDL receptor at a very low rate without formation of cholesterol deposits, but chemically modified (oxidized) LDL is taken up much more rapidly via the acetyl-LDL, or scavenger, receptor.[30] Since the macrophage receptors for modified LDL are not regulated, excessive intracellular accumulation of this lipoprotein may lead to the destruction of the cell and subsequent release of oxidized LDL and free radicals, which can cause cytoxicity and further damage to the endothelium or deendothelialization or type II injury.

Monocyte-macrophage recruitment into the arterial wall

Monocyte-macrophages are present throughout all stages of plaque pathogenesis. From the initial events in atherogenesis (increased vascular permeability, increased monocyte adherence, and intimal recruitment) to the established disease (monocyte-macrophage-derived foam cells and formation of lipid core), macrophages may act as an antigen-presenting cell to T lymphocytes, as a scavenger cell to remove noxious materials, and as a source of growth-regulating molecules and cytokines.

Table 28A-2 Endothelial adhesion molecules

EC adhesion protein	Structure	Ligand cell type
E-selectin (ELAM-1)	Selectin	PMN, monocyte
P-selectin (PADGEM/GMP-140)	Selectin	PMN, monocyte
VCAM-1	Ig	Lymphocyte, monocyte
ICAM-1	Ig	Lymphocyte, monocyte, PMN
ICAM-2	Ig	Lymphocyte, monocyte, PMN
Athero-ELAM (rabbit)	Ig	Monocyte

EC, endothelial cell; ELAM, endothelial-leukocyte adhesion molecule; GMP, granule membrane protein; ICAM, intracellular adhesion molecule; PADGEM, platelet activation-dependent granule external membrane protein; PMN, polymorphonuclear neutrophilic leukocyte; VCAM, vascular cell adhesion molecule.
Modified from Bevilacqua MP, Nelson RM: Selectins. *J Clin Invest* 91:379-387, 1993, and Kim JA, Territo MC, Wayner E, et al: Partial characterization of leukocyte binding molecules on endothelial cells induced by minimally oxidized LDL. *Arterioscler Thromb* 14:427-433, 1994.

Focal accumulation of monocyte-macrophages in atherogenesis appears to involve the local expression of specific adhesive glycoproteins on the endothelial surface and the generation of chemotactic factors by altered endothelium, its adherent leukocytes, and, possibly, underlying smooth muscle cells. Oxidized LDL may have an initial role in monocyte recruitment by inducing the expression of adhesive cell-surface glycoproteins in the endothelium (Table 28A-2), the most important being vascular cell adhesion molecule-1 (athero-endothelial-leukocyte adhesion molecule).[13] Later, several specific molecules may be relevant in attracting and modifying monocytes within the subendothelial space, such as a specific chemotactic protein (monocyte chemotactic protein-1 [MCP-1]) synthesized by vascular cells,[31,32] colony-stimulating factors (CSFs),[33] and transforming growth factor-β (TGF-β).[34] In more advanced stages, during which there has been significant connective tissue production and tissue necrosis, peptide fragments from fibrin, fibronectin, elastin, collagen degradation,[35-37] and thrombin[38] may be the predominant monocyte chemoattractants elaborated.

Intimal hyperplasia versus areas prone to atherosclerosis

When atherosclerosis develops, advanced lesions form first in some regions with adaptive intimal thickening.[39,40] These intimal regions, coincident with locations at which advanced atherosclerotic lesions develop later, have been called the atherosclerosis-prone areas of arteries. Whether eccentric intimal thickening should be considered atherosclerotic has been much debated. The evidence available indicates that the specific mechanical stress, previously described, in locations of the arterial tree with adaptive intimal thickening causes the thickening whether or not high concentrations of atherogenic lipoproteins are present. When atherogenic lipoproteins exceed certain critical levels, the same mechanical forces may enhance lipoprotein deposition in the same regions, leading to transformation into atheromatous lesions. However, in severely hypercholesterolemic humans and in several species of animals subjected to severe hypercholesterolemia, nearly all regions of the aorta and many arteries may ultimately be the sites of advanced lesions. Thus, advanced lesions may not be confined to regions with adaptive intimal thickening. In answer to this question, the Committee on Vascular Lesions of the Council on Arteriosclerosis of the American Heart Association[40] in 1992 stated that the regions of intimal thickening simply mark locations where, under the influence of atherogenic stimuli, lesions form earlier and more rapidly than elsewhere.

PROGRESSION OF ATHEROSCLEROSIS

The progression of atherosclerotic lesions (see Fig 28A-1) to clinically manifest, enlarging atherosclerotic plaques, such as those causing exertional angina, is often more rapid in persons with coronary risk factors and in those whose lesions have certain topographic characteristics.[9,41] Proximal or midvessel location of lesions and complex lesion morphology were identified as predictors of angiographic progression in the Coronary Artery Surgery Study (CASS).[41] In most early lesions, progression is slow and probably a continuation of the complex biologic process initiated by chronic types I and II endothelial injury. In more advanced lesions, however, progression is probably rapid, suggesting recurrent minor fissures of the most fatty or atheromatous plaques, the so-called type III injury, with subsequent thrombus formation and fibrotic organization.[9]

Slow, early progression of atherosclerosis

Morphologic features. The morphologic studies by Stary[39,42] have provided many answers about plaque evolution (Fig 28A-4, 28A-5, and 28A-6). Detailed studies were made of the arteries in young subjects, ranging in age from infancy to over 30 years, who died suddenly from noncardiac causes.

The first observation made by Stary was that in all human infants, focal thickening of the intima develops because of smooth muscle cell proliferation. Initial atherosclerotic lesions (Stary type I) are only microscopically and chemically perceivable, consisting of isolated groups of macrophages filled with lipid droplets. Macrophages without lipid droplets in this type of lesion are twice the number normally present in intima. Such minimal alterations were found in the coronary arteries of

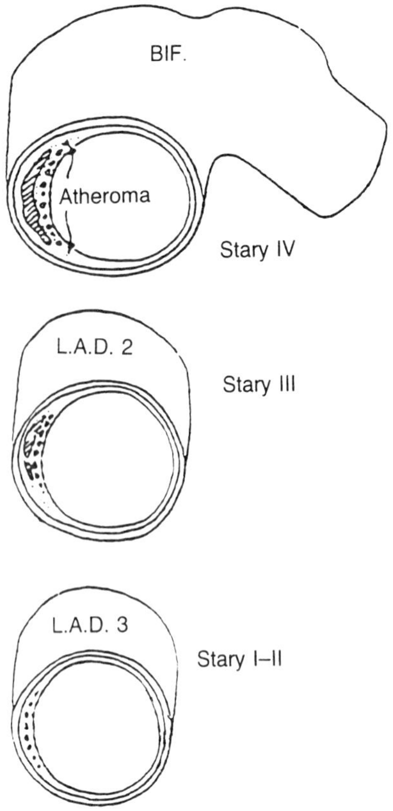

Fig 28A-4 Early evolution of spontaneous atherosclerosis according to the classification of Stary.[39] See text for details. *BIF,* bifurcation; *L.A.D.,* left anterior descending artery.

45% of infants in the first 8 months of life, located in areas of adaptative eccentric intimal thickening, where more advanced lesions usually develop in older children and adults.[42] Type II lesions, or fatty streaks, are composed of more lipid-laden cells than initial lesions. Microscopically, they appear as fatty dots or streaks barely raised above the intimal surface. Each lesion is made up of one or more layers of lipid-filled foam cells within the intima. Although most of the lipids visible by electron microscopy are within cells, some smaller lipid particles are extracellular. Usually, no smooth muscle cell proliferation is evident in fatty streaks, and the endothelium probably is intact.[43] There is some evidence that such streaks are precursors of larger plaques. Pathologic studies show that transitional forms exist between fatty streaks and advanced plaques and that advanced plaques develop in the sites where fatty streaks are more frequent. However, not all fatty streaks progress.[44]

The cohort studies by Stary show that progression beyond the fatty streak stage is associated with a sequence of changes starting with the appearance of extracellular lipid, which begins to form a lesion that is more elevated (Stary type III). Extracellular lipids accumulate deep in the elastin-rich part of the intima, just below the layers of foam cells, and replace intercellular matrix proteoglycans

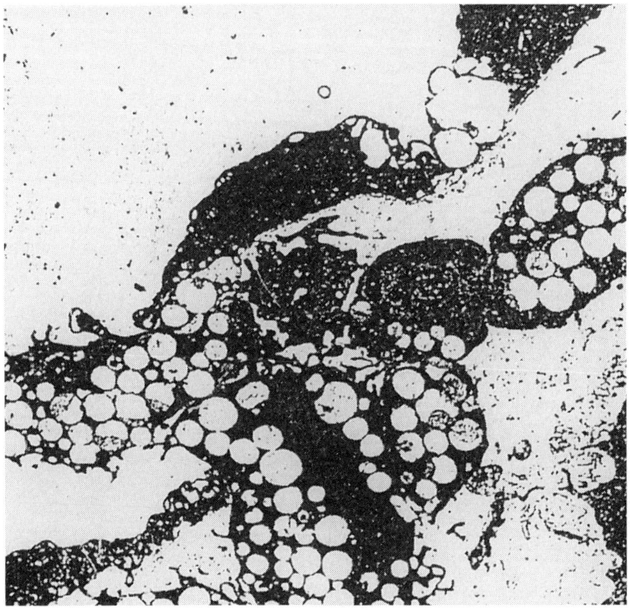

Fig 28A-5 Photomicrograph of macrophages with abundant cytoplasmic lipid inclusions (foam cells) in the vessel intima. The specimen was obtained from atherosclerotic porcine aorta. (x5,000.)

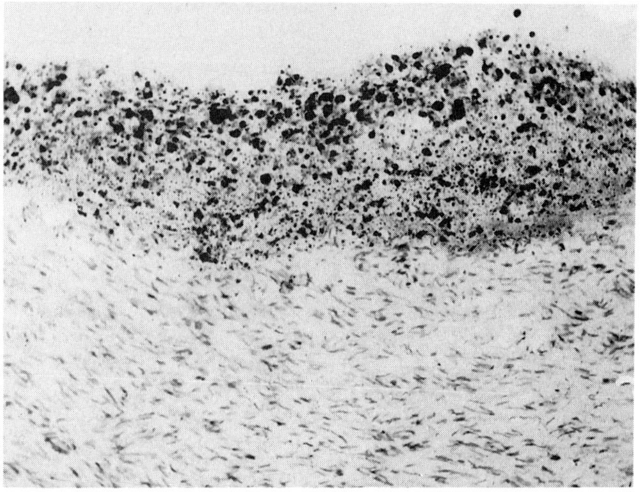

Fig 28A-6 Early atherosclerotic lesions in the pig model. Intracellular fat and extracellular fat are identified as regions staining with Sudan IV. (x350.)

and fibers, driving smooth muscle cells apart. Multiple scattered pools of extracellular lipid may progress to a massive, confluent accumulation of extracellular lipid—the lipid core characteristic of Stary type IV lesions. The core of an atheroma precedes the smooth muscle cell proliferation and collagen deposition that eventually may thicken the region above the lipid core, forming the fibrotic cap of the lesion. In Stary type IV lesions, most of the tissue above the lipid core represents the upper (proteoglycan) part of the preexisting adaptive thickening. In Stary type V lesions (fibroatheroma) or fibrolipid lesions, smooth muscle cells migrate into and proliferate within the plaque, forming a layer over the luminal side of the lipid core.[39,45] More and more collagen is produced, and plaque size increases. The process culminates in what is known as a raised fibrolipid, or advanced, plaque. In the aorta, such plaques may be 1 cm or more in length. Raised fibrolipid plaques have a very characteristic microanatomy, with a core of extracellular lipid separated from the media by smooth muscle cells and insulated from the lumen by a thick cap of collagen-rich fibrous tissue containing smooth muscle cells. Surrounding the lipid core are lipid-filled foam cells. The lipid-rich core is avascular and usually almost totally acellular, consisting of pultaceous debris with abundant cholesterol crystals.[7] Part of the core lipid is thought to be derived from the death of lipid-containing macrophage foam cells and the release of their intracytoplasmatic content. Some of the lipid core bordering foam cells appears disintegrated (dead), and cell constituents may be found extracellularly within the core, indicating that cell necrosis has contributed to its growth.[46]

Lesions with visible thrombotic deposits or marked hemorrhage in addition to lipid and collagen are Stary type VI lesions (complicated fibroatheroma, or complicated lesions). The term "calcific lesion" (Stary type VII lesion) may be applied to some advanced, largely mineralized lesions, particularly after the fourth decade. Calcium deposits replace the accumulated remnants of dead cells and extracellular lipid. Finally, some atherosclerotic lesions, possibly more often in arteries of the lower extremities, may consist entirely or almost entirely of scar collagen. Lipid may have regressed, or it may never have been in the lesion. The term "fibrotic lesions" (Stary type VIII lesions) is best reserved for lesions with this morphology.

The aorta and coronary arteries of adults show all stages of plaque development, implying that new lesions are generated throughout adult life. Even in the same individual there are major plaque-to-plaque variations in the relative proportions of extracellular lipid and collagen that are present. The work by Stary indicates that a plaque can take from 10 to 15 years to fully develop.

Biologic mechanisms. The progression of atherosclerotic lesions from one morphologic type to another is believed to depend on the balance between positive and negative feedback loops generated by their cellular components[9] (Fig 28A-7). Through a network of cellular interactions, the release of one molecule (growth factors, cytokines, and other chemicals) can lead to expression of a second molecule in a target cell that can then either stimulate its neighbors in a paracrine way or stimulate itself in an autocrine way. The underlying biologic events that follow the initial endothelial injury, lipid entry, and monocyte recruitment now are related to a similar but chronic early progression phenomenon up to Stary type V lesions and include (1) monocyte-macrophage-foam cell accumulation and activity, with a significant contribution by lipoproteins and immunomechanisms (related to types

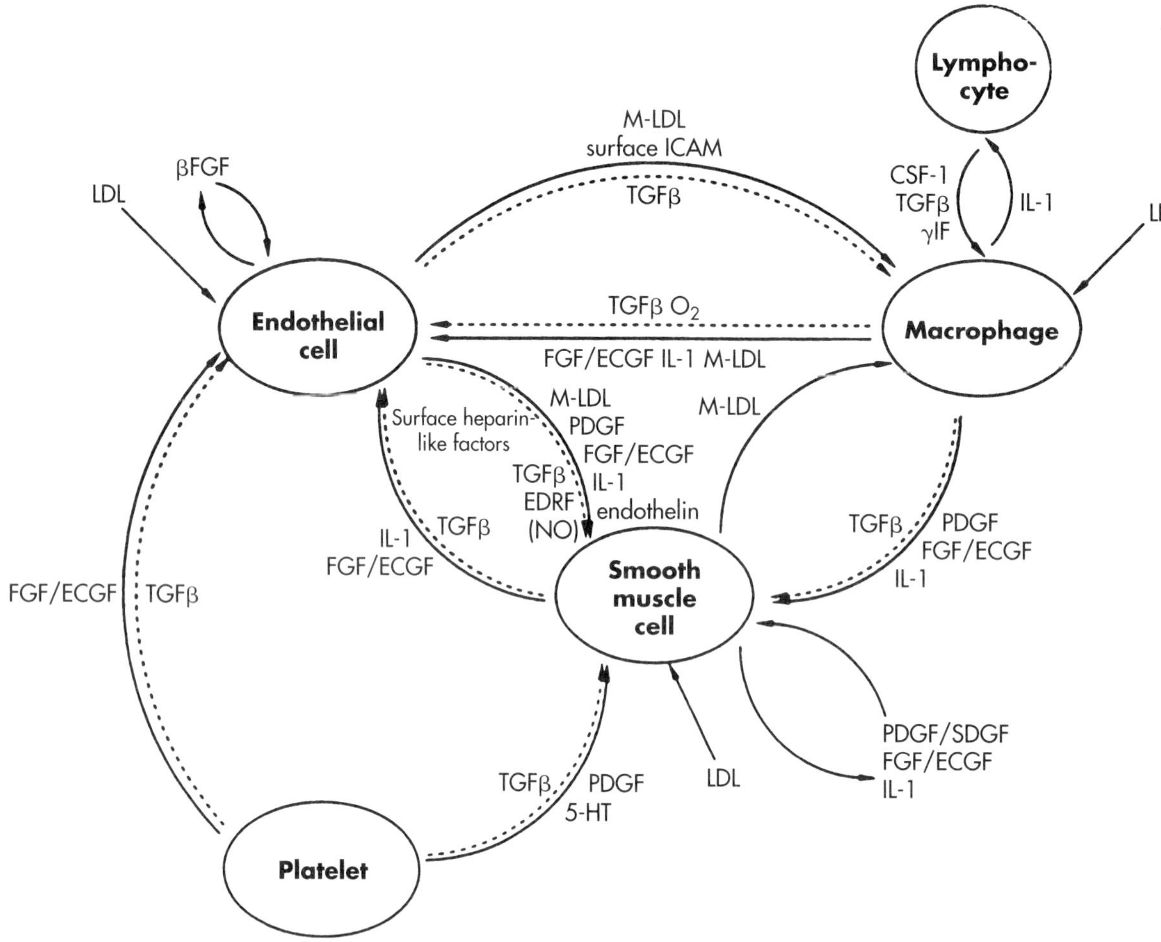

Fig 28A-7 Early evolution of spontaneous atherosclerosis. Shown are some of the complex interactions between and among the cells of major importance in atheroma formation. Molecules with a predominantly stimulatory function (described more completely in Table 28A-4) in growth, contraction, adhesion, secretion, or gene expression are depicted with solid lines. Molecules that inhibit any of the functions above are depicted with broken lines. *CSF-1,* colony-stimulating factor-1; *ECGF,* endothelial-cell growth factor; *EDRF,* endothelium-derived relaxing factor; *FGF,* fibroblast growth factor; *βFGF,* β-fibroblast growth factor; *5-HT,* serotonin; *ICAM,* intracellular adhesion molecules; *γIF,* interferon gamma; *IL-1,* interleukin-1; *LDL,* low-density lipoprotein cholesterol; *M-LDL,* modified low-density lipoprotein cholesterol; *NO,* nitrous oxide; *O_2,* oxygen; *PDGF,* platelet-derived growth factor; *SDGF,* smooth muscle cell-derived growth factor; *TGFβ,* transformation growth factor-β. (From Fuster V, Badimon L, Badimon JJ, et al: The pathogenesis of coronary artery disease and the acute coronary syndromes. *N Engl J Med* 326:242-250; 310-318, 1992. By permission of journal.)

I and II endothelial injury), (2) smooth muscle cell migration and proliferation (mainly as a result of types II and III endothelial injury), and (3) subsequent synthesis of extracellular matrix.

MONOCYTE-MACROPHAGE-FOAM CELL ACTIVITY AND THE ROLES OF LIPOPROTEINS AND IMMUNE MECHANISMS: RELATION TO TYPES I AND II ENDOTHELIAL INJURY (SEE FIG 28A-2)

Monocyte-macrophage-foam cell accumulation and activity. More than 3 decades ago, Poole and Florey[47] presented evidence for the possible role of monocytes in the development of atherosclerotic lesions. Two decades later, Gerrity et al.[48] reported that monocytic accumulation in subendothelial space was responsible for the formation of fatty streak in early lesions of atherosclerosis in cholesterol-fed swine (see Fig 28A-5). Subsequently, Ross[13] confirmed that monocyte invasion of the intima was the earliest cellular event in the evolution of an atherosclerotic lesion in monkeys and rabbits on an atherogenic diet. There is an indication that foam cells in human fatty streaks are also predominantly monocytes that by accumulating fat become macrophages;[39] to a lesser degree, smooth muscle cells with a content of fat can also contribute to foam cells. Overall, lipid uptake in the form of macrophages or foam cells represents the major mechanism of lipid accumulation in the formation of fatty streak and early atheroma formation.[39,49,50] These monocytes, macrophages, or foam cells are functionally very active in a number of ways.

First, the molecular mechanism underlying monocytic attachment to the vessel wall is unknown, but it appears to depend on the interaction between a series of glycoproteins present on the monocyte surface and the monocyte binding sites on the dysfunctional endothelial surface[51,52] (see Table 28A-2), this occurring as a result of the type I injury already described. The possible mechanisms of increased monocyte adhesion to endothelium may involve the regulation of the expression of these receptor sites by the oxidized LDL within the vessel wall (discussed earlier) and various atherogenic stimuli.[51] Second, after accumulation in the subendothelial space, monocytes have a high uptake of modified (oxidized) cholesterol, becoming macrophages and foam cells (this process is discussed in more detail in the next section on lipoproteins). And third, macrophages or foam cells before or after rupture can liberate a large number of products that can participate in the evolution of the atherosclerotic lesion. Thus, products such as interleukins, complement factor fragments, and tumor necrosis factors can enhance monocyte adhesiveness and chemotaxis and so form an amplification mechanism for recruitment of further monocytes into the lesion.[52] In addition, monocytes and macrophages can release enzymes, oxidized cholesterol, and oxygen-derived free radicals that may promote further endothelial injury and cytolysis and, most importantly, plaque rupture; furthermore, macrophages can synthesize tissue factor, also contributing with plaque rupture to subsequent thrombus formation leading to the rapid progression of the atherosclerotic plaque or to an acute coronary syndrome. Finally, released mitogens, such as macrophage-derived growth factor, may have a key role in smooth muscle cell migration and subsequent proliferation.[52]

Role of lipoproteins. One of the major features of atherosclerosis is the intracellular and extracellular accumulation of lipids (see Fig 28A-6), specifically cholesterol esters. Whereas cholesterol linoleate is the major cholesterol ester of plasma, cholesterol oleate is the major ester that accumulates in atherosclerotic plaques.[53] Characteristically, cholesterol esters are water insoluble and form an oil-lipid crystalline phase; however, at later stages of plaque development, the additional accumulation of free cholesterol results in the formation of cholesterol monohydrate crystals.[54]

The three basic cell types that participate in lipid accumulation in the arterial wall are endothelial cells, smooth muscle cells, and macrophages. Endothelial cells form a continuous monolayer lining of the arterial inner wall and normally act as a barrier to the migration of lipoprotein particles into the wall. Minimal damage of the endothelial cell barrier, or type I injury, predisposes to entry of lipoprotein particles from the plasma. Some studies in experimental animals given high cholesterol diets suggest that circulating plasma cholesterol in high levels may itself contribute to endothelial injury at the initial stages of atherosclerosis.[9,13]

Smooth muscle cells, especially those migrating to the arterial intima under the influence of three growth factors[13] (see later section), are thought to play a role, through specific and self-regulated membrane receptors,[53] in LDL uptake and accumulation; it is possible that such intracellular accumulation of cholesterol also may be secondarily mitogenic by favoring cell membrane formation.[13]

The potential role of the macrophages (derived from circulating monocytes) in lipid accumulation has aroused considerable interest in recent years. In general terms, the sources of cholesterol entering the cells include LDLs[53] and remnant particles[55] that result from the peripheral hydrolysis of VLDL and chylomicrons by lipoprotein lipase[56] and, most importantly, modified LDLs (oxidative modifications).[53] The uptake of these particles by the cells of the vessel wall requires their interaction with a variety of specific membrane receptors in fibroblasts and smooth muscle cells[53] and, most importantly, results from poorly defined non-receptor-regulated uptake by monocytes and macrophages.[52,57,58] After the lipoprotein particles have been taken up, they undergo hydrolysis by lysosomal hydrolases and proteases, and the resulting free cholesterol is reesterified with oleic rather than linoleic acid by the microsomal enzyme acyl-cholesterol acyltransferase. This results in accumulation of cholesterol oleate.[53,55] Extracellular accumulation of cholesterol appears to be mainly due to rupture of macrophages or to accumulated debris resulting from cell death.

Oxidative modification of LDLs and their nonregulated uptake by monocytes and macrophages may play a key role in the formation of the fatty streaks and early atheromatous lesions.[57,59] First, oxidized LDL rather than native LDL is recognized by the non-down-regulating scavenger receptors of macrophages and thus could promote foam cell formation; second, modified LDL may be atherogenic by being chemotactic for monocytes, thereby potentially serving to recruit monocytes into the subendothelial space; and third, oxidized LDL (often related to dissolution or cytolysis of saturated foam cells) is cytotoxic and may provide a potential mechanism for endothelial injury and necrosis, or type II injury.

The mechanisms responsible for "reverse cholesterol transport," or removal mechanisms, are essentially the same for macrophages and smooth muscle cells. These mechanisms involve the hydrolysis of cholesterol esters by a neutral supernatant cholesterol ester hydrolase, transfer of free cholesterol across the cell membrane, binding of free cholesterol to apolipoprotein A-I and phospholipids, resynthesis of cholesterol esters (mostly cholesterol linoleate) by the enzyme lecithin-cholesterol acyltransferase, transfer of cholesterol esters to other lipoproteins through the action of apolipoprotein D, and, finally, transport of high-density lipoprotein (HDL) particles to the liver for disposal.[60] The lipid accumulation occurs when cellular cholesterol input exceeds the capacity of "reverse cholesterol transport." Studies in our laboratory suggest that a defect in reverse cholesterol transport may be the most common lipoprotein abnormality associated with angiographically significant coronary artery disease and coronary artery disease progression.[61,62] Such studies support the epidemiologic data indicating a consistent correlation between low concentration of HDL cholesterol and increased incidence of coronary disease.[63]

The possible ultrastructural and biochemical role of lipids in atherosclerotic plaque formation may be summarized as follows: 1. It is probable that high serum levels of LDL contribute to the process of type I endothelial injury; in addition, oxidized LDL within the vessel wall may favor type I endothelial injury. 2. Oxidized LDL accumulated within the arterial wall may lead to type II endothelial injury with cell necrosis. 3. According to studies with smooth muscle cell cultures, lipoproteins may be secondarily mitogenic, perhaps by contributing to cell membrane formation; however, this mitogenic role is not yet established. 4. The space-occupying intracellular (macrophages) and extracellular accumulation of cholesterol and cholesterol esters, as described above, may significantly contribute to the growth of the atherosclerotic plaque. 5. It has been suggested that factors, such as low HDL cholesterol, that impair the process of removal of cholesterol from the arterial wall may favor its accumulation and thus progession of the disease; indeed, recent data have established a consistent correlation between low concentration of HDL cholesterol and apolipoprotein A-I in plasma and an increased incidence and progression of atherosclerotic disease. 6. The regions of the atherosclerotic plaques with a high content of fat are soft and vulnerable to rupture, or type III injury, with subsequent thrombus formation leading to the rapid progression of the plaque or to an acute coronary syndrome (see later section); the liberation of products from macrophages, including enzymes, favors such a process of rupture. 7. There is evidence that lipoproteins enhance platelet reactivity[64,65] and may alter the production of prostaglandins.[66] This, together with the above-mentioned predisposition of fatty plaque to rupture and enhance thrombosis and the recent evidence that a lipoprotein fraction, Lp(a), may chemically compete with plasminogen activator and impair natural fibrinolysis,[67] establishes a link between lipoproteins and thrombosis in atherogenesis and thrombogenesis.

Immune mechanisms in atherogenesis (Table 28A-3). Substantial amounts of T lymphocytes are present in both early fatty lesions and advanced fibrous lesions in humans.[68] In addition, T lymphocytes in the intima are frequently associated with monocytes and macrophages.[13] Although the precise role of T lymphocytes in atherogenesis is still unknown and is highly speculative, this close association with monocytes and macrophages is not surprising in view of the well-known regulatory interactions of these two cell types.[13] For example, the secretion of monocyte chemotactic factor can enhance the adhesion and migration of circulating monocytes, and the release of lymphokines and interleukins from activated T lymphocytes can regulate the lipoprotein uptake by the macrophage and thus may influence foam cell formation. In addition, the complex regulatory roles of these cytokines on the expression of growth factor receptors and smooth muscle cell growth further raise the possibility that the T lymphocytes have a pivotal role in atherogenesis.[13]

Other components of the immune system, such as immunoglobulins and various activated complement factors, have also been identified in the human atherosclerotic plaque.[13,65] Although their presence does not necessarily imply a cause-and-effect relationship, it may indicate a continuing immune response in the process of atherosclerosis. In this context, Seifert et al.[69] demonstrated the deposition of complement C5b,9 complex in the endothelial layer and intima in rabbits as early as 2 weeks after a high-fat diet began. Monocyte accumulation and foam cell formation at the same sites of complement deposition were noted at 6 weeks. On the other hand, monocytes and macrophages were not detected in locations devoid of complement activation products. In this regard, some complement peptides have been shown to be chemotactic for monocytes.[69] In addition, studies of C3-binding proteins in human plaques demonstrated that the smooth muscle cells of the atherosclerotic lesion (but not of the normal artery) express a decay-accelerating factor that protects the cells from complement-mediated lysis by inhibiting C3 and C5 convertase formation.[70] This

Table 28A-3 Cytokines secreted by atheroma-associated cells

	Endothelial cell	Smooth muscle cell	Monocyte	T cell
IL-1	+	+	+ + +	−
TNF	−	+	+ + +	+
LT	−	−	−	+ + +
IL-2	−	−	−	+ + +
IL-6	+	+ + +	+ + +	
IL-8	+	?	+ +	−
MCP-1	+	+	+	
IFN-γ	−	−	−	+ + +

+, slight secretion; + +, significant secretion; + + +, very significant secretion; −, no secretion. IFN, interferon; IL, interleukin; LT, leukotriene; MCP-1, monocyte chemotactic protein-1; TNF, tumor necrosis factor.

Data from Hansson GK: Immune and inflammatory mechanisms in the development of atherosclerosis. *Br Heart J* 69 Suppl:38-41, 1993; and Hansson GK, Holm J, Jonasson L: Detection of activated T lymphocytes in the human atherosclerotic plaque. *Am J Pathol* 135:169-175, 1989.

result shows that the phenotypic changes of smooth muscle cells during atherogenesis may involve the induction of complement-regulatory molecules.

These provocative findings are just a few examples in a rapidly growing body of data on the role of immune mechanisms in atherogenesis. The interplay of these cellular components provides numerous potential mechanisms for mediating the inflammatory, reparative, and proliferative changes in atherosclerotic lesions.

SMOOTH MUSCLE CELL MIGRATION AND PROLIFERATION MAINLY AS A RESULT OF TYPES II AND III ENDOTHELIAL INJURY. Proliferation of smooth muscle cells is a key prerequisite process leading to vascular occlusion in both spontaneous and accelerated atherosclerosis (see Fig 28A-7). Animal models of vascular injury, designed for the study of the "response to injury" hypothesis, have suggested that migration of the smooth muscle cells and subsequent proliferation of the cells depend on the milieu created by the interactions of the blood-borne cells with types II and III endothelial injury or necrosis. Elimination of the growth inhibitory effect of intact endothelium and the release of growth factors from activated platelets, monocytes, injured endothelial cells, and smooth muscle cells, coupled with thrombosis and thrombus organization, provide the mitogenic stimuli for smooth muscle cell growth.

Migration of smooth muscle cells: phenotypic change of the cell from "contractile" to "synthetic" mode. Vascular smooth muscle cells can express different phenotypes.[71] In young, developing arteries, smooth muscle cells have the ability to proliferate and produce large amounts of collagen, elastin, and proteoglycans. In the adult artery, their main function is to regulate wall tension, but they may modulate back into a "synthetic" phenotype and participate in tissue repair of atherogenesis. In forming atherosclerotic lesions, smooth muscle cells appear to regain the phenotypic characteristics of smooth muscle cells in young and developing arteries.[71]

Campbell and Campbell,[71] in a study of the phenotypic changes of smooth muscle cells in primary culture, demonstrated that when smooth muscle cells from the aortic media of young adult rabbits were dispersed into single cells in such a way that a confluent monolayer was present, the cells attained the "contractile" state characterized by fusiform shape with abundant bundles of myofilaments in the cytoplasm, and they could respond to mechanical and electrical stimuli by slow contraction. If the isolated cells were sparsely seeded, they spontaneously underwent a change of phenotype to the "synthetic" state, with a loss of the thick myosin-containing filaments and an increase of synthetic matrix. These cells also became broader and flatter and lost their contractility. However, modulation into this "synthetic" state in vitro was inhibited if smooth muscle cells were grown on a confluent layer of endothelial cells.

Similar phenotypic changes of medial smooth muscle cells from a "contractile" to a "synthetic" mode have been demonstrated in various models of vascular injury.[72] After massive endothelial loss from an artery, smooth muscle cells proliferate first in the media and later in the intima. In the balloon-injured rat carotid artery, about 30% of the medial smooth muscle cell population participated in the immediate proliferative response, reaching a maximum at 48 hours. These cells were ultrastructurally similar to the "synthetic-state" cells in culture, with large amounts of rough endoplasmic reticulum, free ribosomes, and mitochondria and fewer myofilaments. These changes could persist up to 3 weeks after type II endothelial injury. Smooth muscle cells then began to migrate into the intima at 4 days, and proliferation was maximum in the intima at 7 days.[72,73] Increase in intimal thickening continued into the eighth week after vascular injury and appeared to be due mainly to synthesis and accumulation of extracellular matrix and connective tissue. By further analysis of smooth muscle cell types with tritiated thymidine, it was demonstrated that about 50% of the cells that migrated into the intima never divided, and they accounted for approximately 10% of the intimal cell population.[74] Thus, migration alone without proliferation could make up a significant part of the accumulation of intimal smooth muscle cells.

Individual smooth muscle cells are believed to possess different degrees of migrating and proliferative ability.[75] Thus, some populations of migrating smooth muscle cells lack the ability to divide. Whether this heterogeneity in the proliferative potential of smooth muscle cells helps determine the degree of intimal hyperplasia after vascular injury remains to be established.

Proliferation of smooth muscle cells. Proliferation of intimal smooth muscle cells (Table 28A-4) has been established as a key event in the evolution of atherosclerosis.[9,13] One of the principal issues in atherosclerosis is the determination of the biochemical signal or signals that underlie smooth muscle cell proliferation. In the normal quiescent state, smooth muscle cells proliferate at a very low rate. Experimental evidence[76] suggests that intact endothelium plays the central role in maintaining the low proliferative state of smooth muscle cells under normal vascular conditions. In types II and III vascular injury, either induced experimentally or in humans after coronary angioplasty, the platelets, injured endothelial cells, and smooth muscle cells can release platelet-derived growth factor and other mitogens necessary for growth of smooth muscle cells. To a much lesser extent, it is possible that in type I injury, as in hypercholesterolemia, adherent monocytes and platelets and possibly endothelial cells and smooth muscle cells may also secrete mitogens that can cause proliferation of smooth muscle cells.

Inhibitory effect of endothelial cells with intact function. Findings from in vivo experimental models of vascular injury and smooth muscle cell proliferation suggest that intact endothelium is a potent inhibitor of smooth muscle cell growth. Smooth muscle cell proliferation ceases when a mechanically denuded area is reendothelialized. As previously described, using an air-dry model for injury in the rat carotid artery, Fishman et al.[76] demonstrated that maximal myointimal thickening occurred in areas with minimal reendothelialization. Similarly, reendothelialization was much faster after superficial nylon-induced injury than after balloon injury and appeared to correlate with the lack of smooth muscle cell proliferation.[77,78] The mechanism of apparent inhibition of smooth muscle cell

Table 28A-4 Regulatory substances of mitogenic and other cell functions

Stimulators	
Platelet-derived growth factor	
Endothelial cell growth factor	
Fibroblast growth factor	
Smooth muscle cell-derived growth factor	
Interleukin-1	
Interleukin-6	
Transforming growth factor-β	
Low-density lipoproteins	
Vasoactive substances	
	Angiotensin II
	Epinephrine
	Norepinephrine
	Serotonin
	Neuropeptide substances P and K
	Endothelin
Thrombin	
Leukotriene B_4, C_4, D_4	
Prostaglandin E_2, prostacyclin	
Inhibitors	
Transforming growth factor-β	
Heparin-like factors	
Vasorelaxant substances	
	Endothelium-derived relaxing factor
Prostaglandin E, E_2; prostacyclin	
Interferon gamma	

growth by endothelial cells is not entirely clear. However, it has been shown that cultured endothelial cells could produce a heparin-like substance that inhibits smooth muscle cell proliferation in vivo.

In contrast to the inhibitory effect of functionally intact endothelial cells, platelet-derived growth factors and other similar mitogens have been found to enhance modulation of smooth muscle cells into the "synthetic" state.[79-81] Sources of these growth factors include endothelial cells, platelets, macrophages, and smooth muscle cells.

Stimulatory effect by platelets. Platelets are excellent candidates for the initiators of intimal plaque formation after types II and III injury. In almost all in vivo experimental models studied, immediate platelet adhesion and degranulation were followed by proliferation of smooth muscle cells within 48 hours of denudation.[82,83] Mitotic activity declines considerably thereafter as platelets disappear. The fact that intimal thickening induced by moderate balloon injury is significantly inhibited in severely thrombocytopenic rabbits[84] lends additional support to the notion that platelet-derived growth factor may contribute to the induction of proliferative response after vascular injury. In a model of endothelial injury induced by homocysteinemia, Harker et al.[85] demonstrated desquamation of endothelial cells followed by platelet adhesion, thrombus formation, smooth muscle cell migration from the media to the intima, and subsequent proliferation leading to intimal thickening; antiplatelet therapy with sulfinpyrazone inhibited this process. In humans, it is highly likely that platelets are involved in early lesion formation in catheter-induced injury, in perianastomotic lesions of vascular grafts, and in other traumatic vascular injury. The role of platelets after type I injury is less certain, as indicated by several experimental atherosclerosis models in which proliferation of smooth muscle cells and intimal thickening occurred without obvious platelet participation.[86-89] However, Fuster et al.[90-92] demonstrated that extensive proliferative atheromatous lesions developed in normal swine given a normal or mildly hypercholesterolemic diet, whereas less proliferative lesions developed in swine homozygous for von Willebrand's disease and thus lacking factor VIII and defective in platelet-vessel wall interaction. Similarly, Cohen and McCombs[93] showed that thrombocytopenia could reduce atherosclerostic lesions in rabbits. Indeed, as discussed later, although platelets may not be essential in the initiation of atherosclerosis related to minimal (type I) injury, they may contribute to the subsequent progression of the disease.[9]

Platelet-derived growth factor (PDGF) is a major mitogen for smooth muscle cells. It is a basic protein consisting of two disulfide-linked polypeptide chains (A and B) and is one of the primary constituents of the platelet α granule.[94] One or both of its chains can also be synthesized by several other cells, including endothelial cells, macrophages, and even smooth muscle cells. The early response to activation of the PDGF receptor on smooth muscle cells includes a tyrosine-specific autophosphorylation of the receptor in intracellular calcium and active exclusion of protons via Na/K exchanger. The end result is an activation of several PDGF-responsive genes and production of their specific proteins.[94] These proteins probably are essential in such processes as smooth muscle cell proliferation and migration.

Stimulating effect by damaged endothelial cells. Endothelial cells from every source tested, including bovine, monkey, and pig aorta, rat heart, and human umbilical vein, possess growth-promoting activity for cultured smooth muscle cells and fibroblasts.[95] The mitogenic activity is due to the secretion of at least two major mitogens, which are separable by biochemical and immunologic methods. One of these mitogens is closely related to, if not identical to, PDGF. The mechanism by which growth factor production is regulated in endothelial cells is not known. The amount of growth factor produced by cultured endothelial cells can be greatly increased by raising the pH or by lethally injuring the endothelial cells with such agents as endotoxin.[95] A mathematical model applied to these cell injury experiments suggests that a dying endothelial cell produces in less than 3 days as much growth factor as a healthy cell produces over a 19-day period.[95] These data support the modified version of the "response to injury" hypothesis, in which focal lethal damage to the endothelium could lead to high local mitogenic activity that can attract and stimulate neighboring smooth muscle cells. On the other hand, as previously mentioned, endothelial cells with intact function may exert an inhibitory effect on neighboring smooth muscle cells.

Stimulating effect by monocytes and macrophages. The relevance of monocytes in atherogenesis,[96] besides the accumulation of lipid, appears to be related to their ability to stimulate growth of smooth muscle cells. The role of monocytes and macrophages in fibroplasia was first investigated by Leibovich and Ross[97] in studies of wound repair in monocytopenic guinea pigs and subsequently in tissue culture studies. Fibroblast proliferation was inhibited when the availability of monocytes was diminished. It has been reported[98] that at least part of the macrophage-derived mitogenic activity is due to production of a growth factor similar to, if not identical to, PDGF.

Self-stimulating effect of smooth muscle cells. Adult arterial smooth muscle cells in primary culture can spontaneously modulate from a "contractile" to a "synthetic" phenotype. This transition is followed by rapid growth partly independent of exogenous mitogens and accompanied by endogenous production of a PDGF-like protein.[99] The ability to grow in serum-free medium ceases as the cells reach confluence but reappears if a wound is produced in the culture. Libby et al.[100] demonstrated that smooth muscle cells isolated from human atheroma could secrete mitogenic proteins, some of which resembled PDGF. This capacity to produce endogenous, potentially self-stimulating growth factors may help to explain how replication of smooth muscle cells can begin early in atherogenesis even while the endothelial barrier remains morphologically intact. On the other hand, it can also explain why replication of smooth muscle cells can continue after aggregation of blood cells (platelets and monocytes) has ceased a few weeks after vascular injury.

Many additional growth factors present in platelets and atheroma cells are mitogenic toward vascular smooth muscle cells and also lead to other contractile and metabolic changes. These include interleukin-1, α- and β-fibroblast growth factors, serotonin, and thrombospondin.[13] Various neurotransmitters and hormones, such as catecholamines and angiotensin II, are likewise implicated in growth regulation of smooth muscle cells.[13]

SYNTHESIS OF EXTRACELLULAR MATRIX. The formation of fibrous tissue in the arteries contributes significantly to the initiation of the atherosclerotic plaque[13,101] and, most importantly, to its progression, as discussed later. The formation of fibrous tissue is regulated by the fibroblasts and smooth muscle cells when they are stimulated by the growth factors. Aside from plaque components (e.g., LDL, fibrinogen), the principal elements that make up this fibrous tissue are collagen, proteoglycans, elastin, and glycoproteins.

Collagen formation (Table 28A-5) is the major contributor to the growth of the atherosclerotic plaque; several excellent reviews have summarized the biochemical events of this collagen deposition.[13,101] Of the various types of collagen, type I is the primary component of the plaque (70% of the total collagen), followed by collagen type III and much less prominent collagens IV, V, and VI.[101] The various types of collagen are synthesized by

Table 28A-5 Atherosclerosis: extracellular matrix

Collagens (I, III, IV, V, VI): structural
Elastin: structural
Proteoglycans: transport and regulation (cells, molecules)
Plasma components (low-density lipoprotein, fibrinogen, etc.)

	Collagen type				
Structure	**I**	**III**	**IV**	**V**	**VI**
Normal intima	−	−	+	−	−
Fibrous plaque	+ +	+ +	+ +	+	+
Atheromatous plaque, fibrous cap	+ + +	+ + +	+ + +	+ +	+ +

+, slight content; + +, significant content; + + +, very significant content; −, no content.

arterial smooth muscle cells[13,40] when they are stimulated by the growth factors (see later discussion).

Extracellular proteoglycans, mainly chondroitin sulfate, because of their large physical size, concentration, and ionic properties, function in arterial permeability, ion exchange, transport, and deposition of plasma materials, such as LDL. Small-sized extracellular proteoglycans, such as dermatan sulfate, may function to regulate collagen fibrillogenesis but also may regulate ionically complex LDL.[101] Proteoglycans are also synthesized by the arterial smooth muscle cells, under the influence of the growth factors, and by the endothelial cells, specifically the heparan sulfate-like proteoglycans.[40]

The concentration of elastin in atherosclerotic plaques is low in comparison with that in normal arteries;[13] however, it has been suggested that the atherosclerotic arterial wall has an abnormal elastin, and this appears to be synthesized by the arterial smooth muscle cells.[13] Elastin fibers appear to be important in the binding of lipid to the arterial wall;[40,101] in addition, they contribute significantly to the process of calcification of the atherosclerotic plaque.[101] Regardless of the mechanisms involved, calcium is clearly a very common but highly variable component in advanced atherosclerotic lesions. Unfortunately, as is true of fibrous proteins, very little is known about the factors controlling the quantity of calcium in the lesions. These important and often dominant components justify more intensive study.[101]

Both chemical and mechanical factors stimulate smooth muscle cells to make connective tissue. One of the most widespread and potent chemical factors potentially involved in matrix formation is TGF-β.[34,102] TGF-β is not only a potent inhibitor of mitogenesis but also the most potent stimulator of connective tissue formation known. It can induce gene expression for fibronectin, collagen types I, III, IV, and V, and numerous glycosaminoglycan and elastic fiber proteins. In most circumstances, TGF-β is in a latent form that requires exposure to acidic conditions or specific enzymes, such as plasmin or trypsin-like proteases, to release the active form.[34,102] TGF-β seems to inhibit cell proliferation by suppression of transcription of the proto-oncogene *c-myc* and by increased deposition of connective tissue around the cells.[34,103] In addition, it appears that chronic pulsatile distention in the arterial region favors the synthesis of collagen by the smooth muscle cells[104,105] and, thus, the slow progression of the atherosclerotic plaque.

Rapid thrombus-mediated progression of atherosclerosis

Angiographic studies show that the progression of coronary artery disease in humans is neither linear nor predictable. New high-grade lesions often appear in segments of artery that were normal at previous angiographic examination.[106] Two-thirds of the lesions presumably responsible for acute ischemic events (unstable angina or myocardial infarction) have been previously only mildly to moderately stenotic.[106,107] This unpredictable and espisodic progression can be explained by the occurrence of plaque rupture with subsequent thrombosis and changes in plaque geometry and local rheologic factors leading to intermittent plaque growth[14] (Fig 28A-1 and 28A-8).

Fibrolipid lesions (Stary type V) surrounded by a thin fibrous capsule can be easily disrupted, an event leading to type III injury with thrombus formation.[108] Plaque rupture occurs when the strain within the fibrous cap exceeds the deformability of its component material.[109] Marked oscillations in shear stress, acute changes in coronary pressure or tone, and bending and twisting of an artery during each heart contraction could contribute to plaque rupture.[108] For artery walls with heterogeneous composition, like those in atherosclerotic lesions, focal concentrations of circumferential stress may occur that might well lead to plaque fissuring.[109] Areas with decreased load-bearing capabilities, such as a lipid pool, result in increased stress elsewhere in the vessel wall. An extracellular lipid pool in a plaque exceeding about 45% of the vessel circumference increases stress at the lateral edge of the plaque, a frequent site of plaque rupture.[109] However, because plaque rupture does not always occur at the regions of highest stress, local variations in plaque material properties may also contribute to plaque rupture.[110] Thrombi after rupture may be clinically silent, be lysed, or become organized, contributing to the growth of the atherosclerotic plaque.[9,39,43,111,112] When thrombi are large and occlusive, they can contribute to acute coronary syndromes such as unstable angina, myocardial infarction, and sudden ischemic death.[108,111] Ultimately, they can be partially lysed or become organized into a chronic fibrotic occlusion.

Morphologic features. Pathologic studies have revealed that atherosclerotic plaques prone to rupture are commonly composed of a crescentic mass of soft lipids, with abundant cholesterol crystals, separated from the

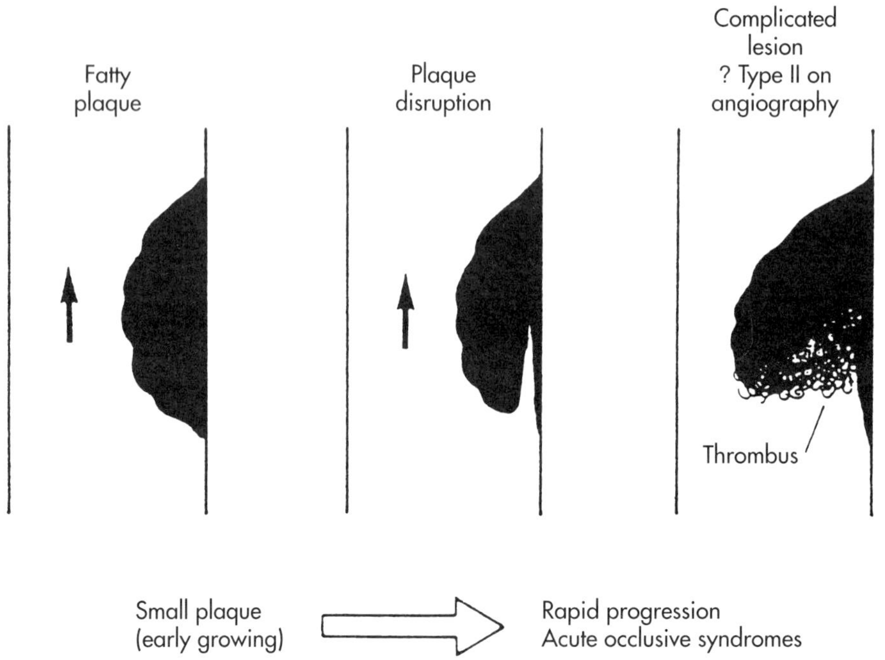

Fig 28A-8 Evolution of the coronary lesion from a stable fatty plaque (asymptomatic or stable angina phase) to plaque disruption with or without superimposed thrombus formation, leading to rapid progression of the plaque or to an acute occlusion syndrome (unstable angina, acute myocardial infarction, or sudden ischemic death). Angiographic type II lesion represents an eccentric stenosis with scalloped or overhanging edges, frequently seen in unstable angina and non-Q-wave infarct (see text).

vessel lumen by a fibrous cap (Stary type V lesions)[109] (see Fig 28A-8 and 28A-9). Ruptured plaques contain more extracellular lipid and less collagen, fewer smooth muscle cells, and less calcium than intact plaques. Fissures tend to occur at the margins of plaques, where caps are necrotic, very thin, and extensively infiltrated by macrophages.[109,113] Plaques in which the extracellular lipid core makes up more than 40% of the overall plaque volume are particularly susceptible.[114] It is likely that many variables determine whether an unstable plaque proceeds rapidly to an occlusive thrombus with the potential for acute infarction or persists at an intermediate stage as a mural nonocclusive thrombus. Local factors such as quantity (fissure size) and quality (plaque composition) of thrombogenic substrate exposed after plaque rupture, as well as rheologic status of blood flow at the site of rupture, are the major local determinants of thrombotic response after plaque rupture.[115] Systemic factors such as fibrinolytic system, catecholamines, and lipoprotein(a) also modulate thrombosis, but it is unknown whether they are less influential than substrate thrombogenicity and rheology.[9] Lp(a) contains apolipoprotein(a), which has considerable amino acid sequence homology with plasminogen, but because of a crucial substitution of serine or arginine, Lp(a) has no enzymatic activity.[116] Therefore, Lp(a) may compete with serum plasminogen for binding sites and inhibit the activation of plasminogen by t-plasminogen activator (t-PA), thus serving as a procoagulant.

Plaque fissuring comes in various shapes and sizes. The tear may be small, 100 to 200 μm across. Such tears allow blood to enter and expand the plaque but may not result in thrombus formation in the arterial lumen. Plaque expansion produces acute changes in plaque geometry with subsequent alternations in local rheology that may further stimulate lesion progression.[22] The healing organization process of intraplaque thrombi may also contribute to subclinical progression of the lesions.[9] Indeed, analysis of the coronary tree in patients who died of ischemic heart disease[117] showed a morphologic appearance consistent with previously healed fissures at different stages of thrombosis and thrombus organization. Furthermore, studies in which monoclonal antibodies were used to identify fibrin, fibrinogen, and their degradation products have also supported the evidence for thrombosis and thrombus incorporation as part of plaque progression.[118] In advanced and fibrous plaques, fibrin and fibrin-related products were detected in the intima, in the neointima, and even in the deeper medial layer, particularly around areas with thrombus incorporation (smaller quantities of these fibrin and fibrin-related products were also found in early lesions and in normal arteries). In addition, the results of a 5-year trial of platelet inhibitor therapy in the angiographic progression of coronary disease[115] indicate that antiplatelet agents may be helpful in preventing the angiographic progression of coronary disease, supporting the hypothesis that recurrent thrombotic events are important contributors to the progression of atherosclerosis.

The tear may be large, and thrombus formed within the lumen may occlude the vessel. Lastly, it may either be removed by lysis or become replaced in the process of organization by the ubiquitous vascular repair response (smooth muscle cell proliferation and collagen production). Of interest, acute occlusive thrombus may be invaded by several neovascular channels and appears partially open at angiography.[117]

Biologic mechanisms. Before rupture, macrophages may be a key factor in determining plaque susceptibility to

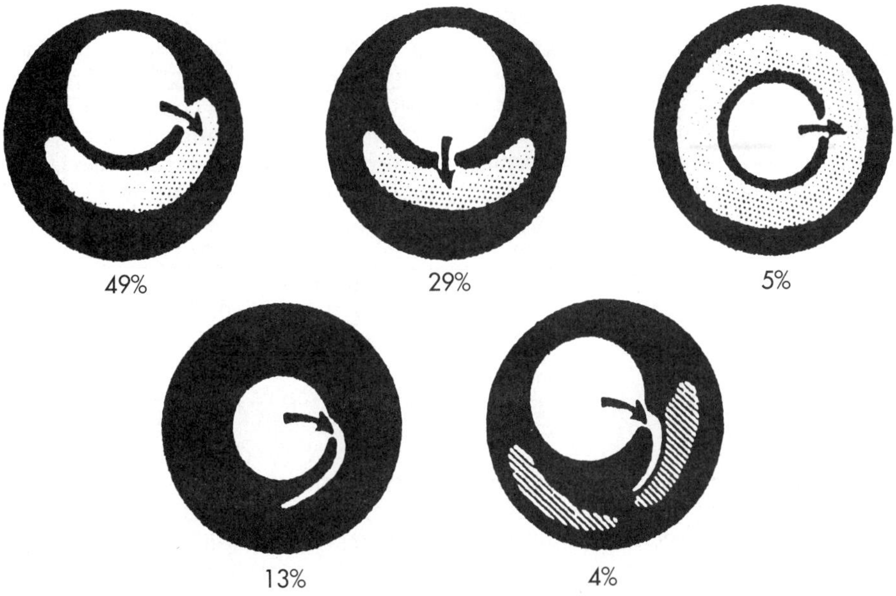

Fig 28A-9 Types of coronary plaque (seen in cross section) undergoing intimal tearing and sites of tearing (*arrows*). Percentages indicate proportion of plaques with various morphologies. *Stippling,* lipid; *cross-hatching,* calcification; *black,* fibrous tissue.

rupture, whereas after rupture, platelets, thrombin, fibrin, and fibrinogen may be the main promoters of lesion progression.

MACROPHAGES. As mentioned earlier, macrophages are involved in the development of fatty streaks and advanced atherosclerotic plaques. Moreover, macrophages may reduce the strength of collagen, elastin, and other structural proteins by releasing proteases.[117,119,120] These proteases may lead to erosion of the fibrous cap overlying a lipid pool, increasing the concentration of wall stress while reducing the ability of the cap to resist deformation. Although ruptured plaques contain a higher concentration of macrophages,[114,119] comparative quantification of protease activity in ruptured and stable plaques has not been performed.

PLATELETS. Emerging evidence suggests that platelet aggregation and thrombosis after types II and III injury have a key role in the progression of the disease. Platelets may induce the migration and proliferation of smooth muscle cells by secreting PDGF.[13,121] Other mitogenetic factors, such as TGF-β, acidic and basic fibroblast growth factor (FGF), and platelet-derived endothelial cell growth factor (PD-ECGF), may also contribute to thrombosis and subsequent myofibrotic response of atherosclerosis.[13,122]

THROMBIN. After vascular damage, as a result of vessel wall tissue factor activator, the enzymatically active thrombin is produced and is incorporated into the thrombus and into the extracellular matrix.[123,124] Subsequently, it may be released gradually in active form during spontaneous fibrinolysis or during thrombus organization. Surface-bound fibrin, in particular, may act as a reservoir for enzymatically active thrombin.[124] Several studies have demonstrated that thrombin is a potent mitogen for mesenchyme-derived cells,[125,126] and it is chemotactic for monocytes.[127] In addition, through the activation of platelets and the elaboration of fibrin polymers and fibrinopeptide A and B fragments, thrombin may also bear direct, adverse atherogenic consequences in the vascular milieu.

FIBRIN, FIBRINOGEN, AND THEIR DEGRADATION PRODUCTS. Fibrin and fibrinogen are believed to contribute to atherogenesis through several mechanisms. These include the stimulation of migration and proliferation of smooth muscle cells.[128] Fibrin and fibrinogen degradation products released from fibrin and fibrinogen by the action of plasmin (and thrombin) may also contribute to atherogenesis by their ability to stimulate vascular cell proliferation.[128,129]

Risk factors and their role in the progression of atherosclerosis

Among the most important risk factors are cigarette smoking, genetic factors or family history of atherosclerotic disease, dyslipoproteinemia, hypertension, and diabetes mellitus. Such risk factors increase the primary incidence rate of atherosclerotic disease,[130-132] promote manifestation of the disease at an earlier age,[133] and, once the disorder is clinically apparent, accelerate its progression.[131,134]

Cigarette smoking. The statement issued by the Public Health Service in 1964 warning about the hazards of smoking is a milestone in primary prevention.[135] Increasingly forthright statements have been produced over the past few years,[136,137] and it is logical to conclude that the recent declines in the death rates from coronary heart disease and lung cancer in men in the United States are in major part a reflection of these preventive efforts.[137,138]

How does cigarette smoking play an important role in atherogenesis? First, it is now widely recognized that cigarette smoking enhances platelet reactivity and that it may alter prostaglandin production—mechanisms that may promote the development of atherosclerosis.[139,140] This effect on thrombogenicity appears to be the most important one, since after discontinuation of smoking, there is a sharp decrease in acute thrombotic events.[138] Second, smoking enhances the process of atherosclerotic disease by its direct effect on the vessel wall. Thus, the carbon monoxide in tobacco smoke results in arterial tissue hypoxia;[141-143] nicotine leads to the mobilization of catecholamines, which may increase platelet reactivity and cause injury to the arterial wall;[144] and a tobacco glycoprotein may lead to a hypersensitivity reaction affecting the arterial wall.[145] Third, smoking may decrease the serum levels of HDL apoproteins.[146]

Genetic factors. Excluding patients with familial hyperlipoproteinemia, familial low HDL cholesterol (see later), and familial hypertension, there is strong evidence that genetic factors are important in the development of atherosclerosis, particularly at a young age.[132,137,147] However, even though the familial tendency may be influenced by genetic transmission, it is not completely clear to what extent the genetic elements act in combination with nutritional, socioeconomic, and other environmental risk factors.[132,137,147,148]

In our experience, it is uncommon to see a patient 50 years of age or younger with coronary atherosclerotic disease who does not have a strong family history of coronary atherosclerotic disease at a young age and cigarette smoking habits.[149] It is more common to see older patients with coronary atherosclerotic disease who do not have any of the known risk factors; possibly in such patients some genetic predisposition or environmental factors alone have contributed to the development of the disease.

Genetic factors may contribute to a hyperactive response by the arterial wall to the endothelial injury; that is, the injury might induce exaggerated proliferation of smooth muscle cells or fibroblasts or excessive production of collagen beginning before or just after birth. Compatible with this hypothesis is the increase in smooth muscle cell proliferation or intimal thickening observed at a young age in populations genetically disposed to the development of atherosclerotic plaques in focal areas of intimal thickening (intimal cushions). Dock[150] pointed out that male infants begin life with about three times the amount of focal intimal thickening found in female infants; he proposed that these differences in intimal thickening were responsible for the differences in the incidence of coronary atherosclerotic disease between men and women. Pesonen[151] measured intimal thickening in the coronary arteries of Finnish infants under 1 year of age who died of noninfectious causes. Besides an increased degree of intimal thickening in boys, he also noted that children whose parents, and especially whose grandparents, were born in eastern Finland had a greater degree of intimal thickening than did children whose parents or grandparents were born in western Finland. From the genetic standpoint, this finding is of interest, because it has been known for many years that the incidence of coronary artery disease is much higher in eastern Finland than in the western portion of the country.

In regard to some genetic disposition of the disease, it is possible that in vivo the smooth muscle cell that proliferates after endothelial injury is a mutation of an arterial smooth muscle cell that replicates and gives rise to a monoclonal proliferative thickening of the intima. Indeed, cell cultures of atherosclerotic plaques often consist of cells of just one type.[13] Nevertheless, the response to in vivo injury appears to be hyperplastic rather than neoplastic,[152] but some types of cell selection must be considered.

Finally, apart from familial hyperlipoproteinemia, a rare but well-defined genetic abnormality that has been associated with a high incidence of atherosclerosis is homocystinuria.[153,154] Harker et al.[155] suggested that the vascular disease is related to endothelial damage produced by homocystinemia.

Dyslipoproteinemia. Evidence in general suggests that hyperlipoproteinemia, particularly hypercholesterolemia at a young age, increases the incidence and progression of atherosclerotic disease.[131,137,156] Indeed, familial hypercholesterolemia related to an increased uptake of cholesterol by the arterial wall is the most classic and convincing risk factor for atherosclerotic disease.[156]

As discussed above in more detail, there are several mechanisms by which an alteration effects the atherosclerotic process. Briefly, hypercholesterolemia possibly favors endothelial injury and initiation of the atherosclerotic plaque.[9,13] It may be that lipoproteins promote the proliferation of smooth muscle cells by favoring formation of smooth muscle cell membrane.[9,13] Accumulation of fat in the arterial wall contributes to growth of atherosclerotic plaque.[39] The regions of the atherosclerotic plaques with a high content of fat are soft, vulnerable, and prone to rupture; subsequent thrombus formation leads to the rapid progression of the plaque or to an acute coronary syndrome.[105,157] There is evidence that lipoproteins enhance platelet reactivity[64,65] and may alter production of prostaglandins.[66] As mentioned in a previous section, this increase in platelet reactivity, the predisposition of fatty plaques to rupture and thrombosis, and the recent evidence that a lipoprotein fraction—Lp(a)—may impair natural fibrinolysis[67] all establish a link between lipoproteins and thrombosis in atherogenesis and thrombogenesis.

Importantly, a decrease in the plasma concentration of HDL cholesterol without associated hyperlipoproteinemia is common in patients with a strong family history of atherosclerotic disease.[158] Such a decrease is perhaps the crucial metabolic abnormality in some patients with a strong family history of atherosclerotic disease in whom no other specific risk factors of atherosclerosis can be detected.[158] In addition, a low concentration of HDL cholesterol associated with an increased risk of atherosclerosis has been observed in uremic patients;[159] conversely, a high concentration of HDL cholesterol, perhaps associated with a decreased risk of atherosclerosis, has been observed in persons who exercise regularly[160] and in those who use alcohol moderately.[161]

Hypertension. Although hypertension may increase the incidence of atherosclerotic disease,[132,134,137,162] it is better known as a secondary risk factor that worsens the prognosis in patients already known to have the clinical manifestations of atherosclerotic disease.[134,163]

Hypertension and arterial pulsatile distention may lead to smooth muscle cell proliferation with medial thickening and to an increase in the arterial wall content of elastin, collagen, and glycosaminoglycans,[13,161] all of which contribute to the growth of the atherosclerotic plaque. Also, a key role of hypertension in the development and progression of atherosclerosis might be the triggering of acute plaque rupture caused by the effect of shear stress on the arterial wall.[108,164,165] Furthermore, it has been proposed that in hypertension, the chronic effect of shear stress produces an increased permeability of the endothelium that allows increased uptake of cholesterol,[166] increased platelet and monocyte interaction with the vessel wall, and subsequent liberation of growth factors known to promote proliferation of smooth muscle cells.

Diabetes mellitus. Accelerated atherosclerosis is a major complication of juvenile-onset insulin-dependent diabetes mellitus (IDDM)[167,168] and, to a lesser extent, of non-insulin-dependent diabetes mellitus (NIDDM). The vascular effects of IDDM may be a result of advanced glycosylation end products (AGEs), which can contribute to the various stage-by-stage mechanisms of atherosclerotic plaque progression[169-173] (see Table 28A-1). On the other hand, insulin resistance—typical of NIDDM, which is often associated with hypertension and obesity—may also enhance the process of atherogenesis through enhanced lipolysis, high triglycerides, low HDL, or associated risk factors[173] (see Table 28A-1). Conventional risk factors for coronary artery disease (e.g., hypertension, hyperlipidemia, smoking), which may damage the endothelium of the epicardial arteries and also cause vasoconstriction, may also affect the endothelium of the microcirculation, leading to vasoconstriction dependent on endothelin I during coronary thrombotic occlusion.[9] To a lesser extent, such effect on the microcirculation has also been described in IDDM through high AGEs[173] (see Table 28A-1). Experimentally, aortic atherosclerosis induced by a high cholesterol diet in monkeys was strikingly aggravated by the induction of diabetes mellitus.[174]

There is evidence that platelet reactivity is enhanced in diabetes mellitus[175] and that a plasma factor,[176] perhaps an increase in plasma von Willebrand's factor, an alteration of the free cholesterol content of platelet membranes secondary to the changes of plasma lipoproteins, or an alteration in the control of platelet production of prostaglandins, may be responsible for platelet activation. Consistent with the enhancement in platelet reactivity,

Table 28A-6 Comparison between spontaneous atherosclerosis and accelerated atherosclerosis

	Atherosclerosis	
	Spontaneous	Accelerated
Endothelial injury	Type I	Types II and III
Early platelet involvement	−	+
Early monocyte involvement	+ +*	+
Sources of growth factors	Endothelium, monocyte, SMC	Endothelium, platelet, SMC
Pathology	Intimal SMC proliferation; lipid, fibrosis; late thrombosis	Intimal SMC proliferation; lipid, fibrosis; early or late thrombosis (or both)
Duration of process	Decades	3 months to 2 years

SMC, smooth muscle cell; −, absent; +, present; + +, very much present.
*If hyperlipidemic.

substantial platelet microthrombi have been observed in diabetic microangiopathy.[177,178]

Estrogens. Several large observational epidemiologic studies have reported a reduction of up to 50% in the rate of cardiovascular mortality in postmenopausal women treated with replacement estrogens.[179-181] This powerful protective effect may be due in part to the 15% increase in HDL cholesterol, 15% decrease in LDL cholesterol, and inhibition of cholesterol deposition in vascular endothelium due to estrogens.[182] However, since reduced mortality has been observed in estrogen-treated women without alteration in lipids, these favorable alterations in lipid metabolism are not likely to account for all the effects of estrogen.[183]

Compelling lines of evidence argue for direct anti-ischemic effects of estrogen. First, estrogens have favorable systemic hemodynamic effects in pregnant sheep, resulting in increased cardiac output, decreased systemic vascular resistance and blood pressure, and increased myocardial perfusion.[184] In humans, estrogens decrease the carotid artery "pulsatility" index;[185] stabilize vulvar, forearm, and thenar eminence blood flow in elderly women;[186] and increase blood flow through affected intracranial vessels during migraine attacks.[187] Second, estrogens appear to be direct coronary artery vasodilators.[188] Endothelium-dependent, endothelium-independent, and possible calcium-antagonist mechanisms have been proposed. In cynomolgus monkeys with diet-induced coronary disease, estrogens reverse acetylcholine-induced coronary artery vasoconstriction.[189] Estrogens may be direct coronary artery vasodilators in humans as well.

Acquired syndromes of accelerated atherosclerosis secondary to intervention

The process of plaque formation in accelerated atherosclerosis resembles that of spontaneous atherosclerosis.[14] However, because the vascular injury is more acute and severe, the platelet and thrombotic phenomena as well as the smooth muscle cell proliferation response are more predominant than the chronic lipid deposition (Tables 28A-6 and 28A-7). Specifically, in contrast to spontaneous

Table 28A-7 Biologic factors in the pathogenesis of the syndromes of accelerated atherosclerosis

	Transplant atherosclerosis	Vein graft atherosclerosis	PTCA restenosis
Vascular injury	I-II	II-III	III
Platelets, thrombosis	+	+ +	+ +
Hyperlipidemia	+ +	+ +	+/−
Immunologic	+	+/−	−

PTCA, percutaneous transluminal coronary angioplasty; −, no effect; +, mild; + +, moderate.

atherosclerosis, in accelerated atherosclerosis types II and III vascular injuries appear to be the critical initiating events that lead to platelet aggregation, thrombosis and thrombus organization, very apparent smooth muscle cell proliferation, and lesion formation. Type II vascular injury has been found in patients after heart transplantation[190] and coronary vein graft bypass[191] (although type I appears to be most frequent in transplantation), and type III vascular injury invariably occurs in patients after coronary angioplasty.[192-195] In accelerated atherosclerosis, unlike in spontaneous atherosclerosis, platelet aggregation and thrombosis can be found early in the formation of atherosclerotic lesions in these three clinical situations.[190-195] Processes of lipoprotein modification and monocyte accumulation probably are as important in the late progression of the early lesions in heart transplantation and vein graft atherosclerosis as they are in spontaneous atherosclerosis.

ACUTE CORONARY SYNDROMES: PLAQUE DISRUPTION AND THROMBOSIS

Rupture of an atherosclerotic plaque in the coronary arteries is fundamental in the development of the acute

Table 28A-8 Thrombosis frequency in plaque rupture

Disease entity	Rupture, %	With thrombosis, %
Noncardiac death[112]		
No risk factors	9	. . .
Risk factors	22	5
Cardiac death		
Cause	90	80[4]
Associated[196]	2.5 per patient	

Data from Davies MJ, Bland JM, Hangartner JR, et al: Factors influencing the presence or absence of acute coronary artery thrombi in sudden ischaemic death. *Eur Heart J* 10:203-208, 1989; Davies MJ, Thomas A: Thrombosis and acute coronary-artery lesions in sudden cardiac ischemic death. *N Engl J Med* 310:1137-1140, 1984; Davies MJ: A macro and micro view of coronary vascular insult in ischemic heart disease. *Circulation* 82 Suppl 2:38-46, 1990; and Falk E: Plaque rupture with severe pre-existing stenosis precipitating coronary thrombosis. Characteristics of coronary atherosclerotic plaques underlying fatal occlusive thrombi. *Br Heart J* 50:127-134, 1983.

Table 28A-9 Angiographic evolution of acute coronary syndromes

Syndrome	Initial stenosis		
	<50%	50%-70%	>70%
Unstable angina, %			
n = 25[206]	72	16	12
Myocardial infarction, %			
n = 23[106]	48	30	22
n = 41[107]	66	31	3
n = 92[207]	78	9	13
n = 39[208]	59	15	26
Mean, %	65	20	15

ischemic syndromes (Table 28A-8), as clearly shown in pathologic studies of patients who died suddenly or shortly after an episode of unstable angina or myocardial infarction.[117,196] Disrupted atherosclerotic plaques are commonly associated with formation of mural or occlusive thrombi, usually anchored to fissures in the ruptured or ulcerated plaque. In addition, as already discussed, emerging evidence suggests that small plaque rupture or fissuring thrombosis and fibrous organization of the thrombus are much more frequent, having an important part in the progression of atherosclerosis in patients without symptoms and in those with stable angina (see Table 28A-8).

Plaque disruption

The process of atherosclerotic plaque disruption leading to thrombus formation has been known for many years.[197-200] More recent angiographic, angioscopic, and pathologic studies have clearly established an association between plaque fissuring or ulceration and the development of unstable angina, acute myocardial infarction, and sudden ischemic death.[111,117,196-204] The anatomic and physiologic characteristics of ruptured plaques, the ability to identify and predict which lesions are prone to rupture, and measures aimed at reversal of this pathologic process are subjects currently being explored by many investigators around the world. Four aspects will be analyzed here: (1) rupture of small atherosclerotic plaques, (2) lipid-rich plaques, (3) role of macrophages, and (4) effects of stress on plaque rupture.

Rupture of plaques not severely stenotic. The severity of coronary artery stenosis and the number of diseased vessels are known to be markers for future cardiac morbidity and mortality.[205] Only within the past few years has it become apparent that coronary lesions with less severe angiographic disease are associated with significant progression to severe stenosis or total occlusion and that these lesions may account for up to two-thirds of patients in whom unstable angina or acute myocardial infarction develops.[106,206] Originally, a study from our laboratory in patients with unstable angina who underwent two sequential angiograms revealed that 72% of the lesions that showed progression had less than 50% stenosis on the first angiogram[206] (Table 28A-9). Morphologic analysis of coronary lesions that progressed to less than total occlusion revealed type II, or eccentric, lesions with a narrow neck and overhanging edges or scalloped borders in 71% of cases (Fig 28A-10). Lesions with this particular structure are thought to represent plaque disruption with or without a partially occlusive thrombus.[206] Indeed, postmortem angiographic studies[204] have shown that eccentric lesions with irregular borders commonly represent plaque rupture or hemorrhage or superimposed partially occluding or recanalized thrombus.

Four studies[106,107,207,208] have addressed the issue of angiographic progression of coronary disease in patients with myocardial infarction (see Table 28A-9). When these studies are analyzed together, it is apparent that lesions presumably responsible for the acute ischemic event (unstable angina or myocardial infarction) have only mild to moderate stenosis in a substantial number of patients at the time of the first evaluation. In a separate study, Brown et al.,[209] using highly magnified angiographic images of coronary arteries during streptokinase infusion for acute myocardial infarction, found that the original lesions responsible for the infarction had less than 60% stenosis in two-thirds of patients.

Two important issues need to be considered in the evaluation of patients with coronary disease. First, angiography is helpful as a marker of severity of coronary disease but cannot accurately predict the site of future coronary occlusion, since acute ischemic events result from disruption of only mild-to-moderate stenotic lesions in a substantial proportion of patients. Second, angiography may underestimate the extent and severity of atherosclerotic involvement of coronary arteries.

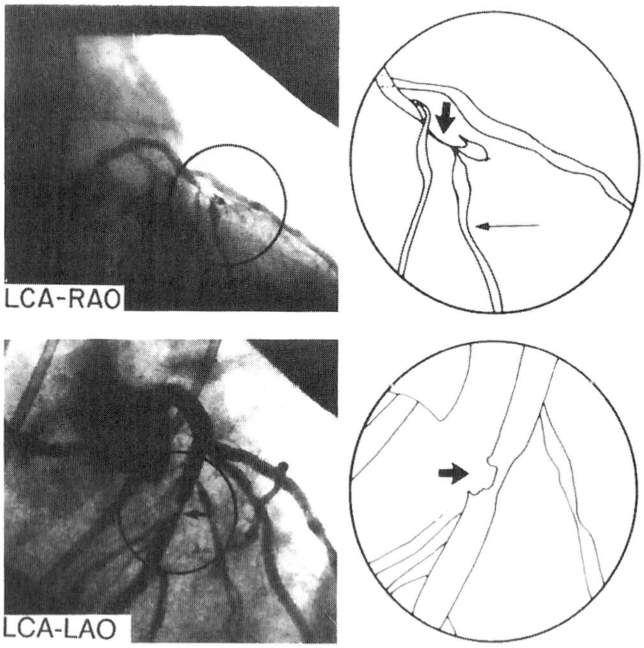

Fig 28A-10 Left coronary angiograms *(LCA)* and diagrams of left anterior descending arteries in two patients with unstable angina. The *thick arrows* indicate the lesions, characterized by narrow neck and irregular or "overhanging" edges, which represent plaque rupture or partially occlusive thrombi. The *thin arrow* indicates the distal vessel. Projections: *RAO,* right anterior oblique; *LAO,* left anterior oblique.

Lipid-rich plaques (see Fig 28A-10). Pathologic studies have revealed that atherosclerotic plaques prone to rupture are commonly composed of a crescentic mass of lipids separated from the vessel lumen by a fibrous cap.[109] Indeed, plaques that undergo disruption tend to be relatively soft and have a high concentration of cholesterol and its esters; thinning of the fibrous cap overlying the lipid core probably precedes its rupture.[109] In addition, a particular configuration of the plaque, in which the lipid pool is situated eccentrically, is most commonly associated with fissuring.[109]

Increased shear rate in the area of stenosis, acute changes in coronary pressure or tone, and bending and twisting of an artery during each heart contraction perhaps contribute to plaque rupture, particularly when plaques are soft and fatty. In this context, when aortas of pigs with spontaneous or diet-induced atherosclerosis were analyzed,[90,91] we observed extensive plaque formation and ulceration in areas of lipid accumulation, as assessed by Evans blue dye staining.

Noninvasive imaging of plaques with a high content of lipid is emerging as an important research tool, given the susceptibility of these plaques to rupture. It may soon be possible to detect fatty plaques within the vascular system by several techniques, including magnetic resonance imaging with spectroscopy, ultrafast computed tomography, and intravascular echocardiography. Experiments using labeling with technetium 99m[210,211] have shown the feasibility of noninvasive imaging of LDLs, which would facilitate studies of their biodistribution and catabolism in several disease states, including atherosclerosis, and the effect of drugs or diet.

Role of macrophages (see Figs 28A-2 and 28A-5). As previously discussed, macrophages can release proteases (elastase and collagenase)[120] that, together with the generation of toxic products (free radicals, products of lipid oxidation), may facilitate vessel wall damage or plaque rupture. Histologic specimens of ruptured plaques leading to thrombosis have disclosed macrophages infiltrating the cap of atherosclerotic plaques.[109]

Effects of local stress on plaque rupture. Using computer modeling for analysis of tensile stress across the vessel wall, Richardson et al.[109] found high concentrations of stress on the plaque cap overlying an area of lipid pool. In this area, the plaque cap lacks underlying collagen support, so that perhaps it is more susceptible to rupture. They suggested that the risk of fissuring can be predetermined by the plaque configuration and the biochemical and structural properties of the cap components.[109]

Although the experimental model above is helpful in understanding the distribution of stress in plaques that protrude into the vessel lumen, it does not clearly explain why rupture or ulceration occurs in plaques that are relatively flat and do not encroach on the lumen. A possible explanation for the latter process is that stress produced by turbulent blood flow in areas of stenosis or at branching points contributes to tearing of the plaque, particularly in the thinner portion of the fibrous cap. Therefore, not only intrinsic characteristics of the atherosclerotic lesion but also forces external to the plaque itself, such as turbulence[165] or marked oscillations in shear stress,[164] may contribute to the development of plaque growth and, perhaps, rupture. At this juncture, these are only speculations.

Thrombus formation

Having discussed the participation of thrombus formation in the progression of atherosclerosis and in the acute coronary syndromes, as recently reviewed by us,[9] we now examine the local and systemic factors present at the time of coronary plaque disruption that may influence the degree and the duration of thrombus deposition and account for the various pathologic and clinical manifestations (Table 28A-10).

Degree of plaque disruption. Badimon et al.[212-214] developed a computer-assisted nuclear-scintigraphic method with an extracorporeal perfusion system to study the pattern of platelet deposition in various degrees of vascular injury (types II and III) and on different components of the exposed vessel. The exposure of superficially damaged vessel wall (mimicking type II, mild vascular damage) to blood at high shear rates (mimicking a stenosed coronary artery) induced within minutes platelet adhesion and aggregation to the exposed vessel. However, because the thrombus could be partially dislodged from the substrate by the flowing blood, the thrombus might be labile. The exposure of fibrillar

Table 28A-10 Evolving local and systemic risk factors for thrombogenesis

Factor or condition	Degree of risk
Local factor	
Degree of plaque disruption (collagen, tissue factor)	. . .
Degree of stenosis (change in geometry)	. . .
Surface of residual thrombus (thrombin)	. . .
Systemic factor	
Epinephrine levels (stress, circadian variation, smoking)	. . .
Cholesterol levels	. . .
Lipoprotein(a) and plasminogen activator inhibitor type I (impaired fibrinolysis)	. . .
Fibrinogen and factor VII levels	. . .
Clinicopathologic condition	
Mural thrombus, progressive disease, angina	Low
Labile occlusive thrombus, unstable angina, non-Q-wave infarction	Medium
Fixed occlusive thrombus, Q-wave infarction	High

collagen (mimicking type III, deep injury) to blood produced a dense platelet thrombus that could not be dislodged. In addition to the fibrillar collagen, exposed tissue factor[46,215] may be macrophage-dependent and probably also contributes to the high thrombogenicity of deep or severe injury by activating the clotting system.

In unstable angina, aside from the angiographic and angioscopic data showing mural or transient thrombosis close to the time of chest pain in patients at rest,[202,216] Hirsh et al.[217] showed that a temporal relation between chest pain and increases in the transcardiac concentration of thromboxane A_2 by platelets or other local cells[218,219] is associated with transient or labile platelet aggregation in patients with unstable angina. In addition, another product of platelet secretion, serotonin, is increased in some patients with frequent angina and complex coronary artery lesions.[220] These observations do not suggest that transient platelet activation and secretion occur in unstable coronary syndromes. Furthermore, increases in thromboxane A_2 and serotonin concentrations at sites of plaque disruption probably increase the level of platelet aggregation, promote vasoconstriction, and contribute to neointimal proliferative response.[221]

When only the surface of the atherosclerotic plaque is disrupted, the thrombogenic stimulus is relatively limited, resulting either in mural thrombosis with subsequent growth of the plaque or in a thrombotic occlusion that is transient, as in unstable angina. Conversely, deep plaque disruption or ulceration exposes the lipid core with macrophages and tissue factor, leading to relatively persistent thrombotic occlusion and myocardial infarction.[4,222]

Degree of stenosis. Experimentally, Badimon et al.[212,213] found that platelet deposition increased significantly with increased stenosis, indicating shear-induced platelet activation. In addition, analysis of the axial distribution of platelet deposition indicated that the apex was the segment of greatest platelet accumulation, whereas the flow recirculation zone distal to the apex is most prone to fibrinogen deposition.[223] These data suggest that the acute platelet response to plaque disruption depends in part on the sudden geometric changes or degree of stenosis following the disruption—that is, after plaque disruption, a small geometric change with only mild stenosis may result in a small mural thrombus, whereas a larger geometric change or severe stenosis may result in a transient or persistent platelet-rich thrombotic occlusion, causing an acute coronary syndrome. Furthermore, the disruption of a plaque at the apex may result in a thrombus that is richer in platelets[212,213] and therefore less amenable to fibrinolytic agents[224] than a thrombus formed in a zone distal to the apex.[212,213,223]

Residual thrombus. Pharmacologic or spontaneous lysis of thrombi appears to play a part in unstable angina[108,220] as well as in acute myocardial infarction.[225,226] A residual mural thrombus predisposes patients with unstable angina or acute myocardial infarction and those undergoing pharmacologic lysis to residual stenosis[209,227] and to recurrent thrombotic vessel occlusion.[227-229]

Several factors that contribute to rethrombosis have been identified. First, the residual mural thrombus may encroach on the vessel lumen, resulting in increased stenosis with an increased shear rate, which facilitates the activation and deposition of platelets.[213,214,223] Second, Fitzgerald and Fitzgerald[230] reported that reocclusion of a recanalized artery in a dog model of coronary thrombolysis was mainly related to the high local thrombin activity on the surface of the fragment thrombus, a concept previously suggested by others[231] and recently confirmed.[232] Thus, after lysis of a thrombus, thrombin bound to fibrin may become exposed to the circulating blood, leading to platelet and clotting activation and further thrombosis. Unlike heparin molecules, molecules of hirudin and other specific antithrombins are at least 10 times smaller than the heparin-antithrombin III complex and have no natural inhibitors, and unlike antithrombin III receptors of fibrin-bound thrombin, thrombin receptors to direct antithrombins are not masked by fibrin bound to thrombin.[233] Finally, studies have suggested that the enhancement of platelet and thrombin activity by the thrombolytic agents themselves contributes to rethrombosis.[232-235]

Systemic thrombogenic risk factors. Recent evidence, experimental and clinical, suggests that a primary hypercoagulable or thrombogenic state of circulation can favor focal thrombosis. Thus, platelet aggregation and the generation of thrombin may be activated by circulating catecholamines.[236] This mechanism and catecholamine-dependent vasoconstriction may be of major importance in humans, because they may link emotional stress,[237,238] circadian variation,[239-241] catecholamine effects,[238-240] and the development of arterial thrombosis and vasoconstriction. Of particular importance is the growing evidence of enhanced platelet reactivity in cigarette smokers,[139] which also may be related to the release of catecholamines.[242] Indeed, the sharp decrease in the incidence of acute thrombotic events after the discontinuation of smoking[137,243] supports the thrombogenic role of cigarette smoking.

Also of significance is the increasing evidence of hypercoagulability[244] and enhanced platelet reactivity at sites of vascular damage in patients with hypercholesterolemia.[245] Enhanced platelet reactivity has also been documented in young patients with a strong family history of coronary disease, whether or not the coronary disease is related to hyperlipidemia.[139]

Other metabolic abnormalities, such as high plasma levels of homocysteine and Lp(a), have also been identified as powerful risk factors in young patients with coronary disease. Heterozygous homocystinuria or homocystinemia is now considered to be a possible risk factor for atherosclerotic disease in young people with a strong family history of vascular disease.[153,246] However, since endothelial damage with a subsequent proliferative response has been observed in experimental homocystinemia,[155] this metabolic condition may be an atherogenic rather than a thrombogenic risk factor.

Lp(a) is very similar to LDL cholesterol in its molecular configuration and is an important risk factor for ischemic heart disease and presumably for thrombotic occlusion,[247] particularly in familial hypercholesterolemia.[248,249] Apolipoprotein(a) is a glycoprotein present in Lp(a) that has close structural homology with plasminogen,[250] and both genes are clearly linked on the long arm of chromosome 6.[251] Evidence suggests that the close homology of Lp(a) with plasminogen results in competitive inhibition of the fibrinolytic properties of plasminogen,[252] thus predisposing patients to thrombotic complications.

The above discussion of metabolic abnormalities, specifically the role of Lp(a) in coronary disease, supports the concept that defective fibrinolysis is a thrombogenic risk factor in patients with coronary disease. However, since available methods for studying fibrinolysis are neither sensitive nor specific, this concept has yet to be proved. One of the components of the fibrinolytic system now being examined is plasminogen activator inhibitor; although some studies suggest that high levels of this inhibitor are a risk factor for ischemic heart disease[253] and myocardial infarction,[253-255] the results of other studies are less convincing.[153,155,244-256] Finally, other hemostatic proteins, specifically fibrinogen and factor VII, have also been implicated as thrombogenic risk factors. For example, several prospective studies have shown that high plasma fibrinogen concentrations are independent risk factors for coronary artery disease[257,258] and are specifically associated with myocardial infarction.[257,259] It is noteworthy that fibrinogen levels are increased in relation to age and the degree of obesity, hyperlipidemia, diabetes, smoking, and emotional stress.[259,260] High levels of factor VII coagulant activity are also associated with an increased risk of coronary events[257,259] and with the risk factors associated with fibrinogen, as well as with menopause and oophorectomy[261] – two factors known to increase the risk of coronary artery disease. Thus, fibrinogen and factor VII activity may be considered thrombogenic risk factors for coronary events, and their classification as such may also explain some of the other risk factors associated with the disease.

Role of vasoconstriction

Although many episodes of unstable angina and acute myocardial infarction are caused by the fissuring or disruption of plaque with superimposed thrombosis, other mechanisms that alter the balance between myocardial oxygen supply and demand must be considered. Studies by Maseri et al.[262] that used hemodynamic, electrocardiographic, and angiographic monitoring suggested that coronary vasoconstriction has an important role in the pathogenesis of ischemic heart disease. Indeed, vasospasm was found to be an important contributor to intermittent coronary occlusion in patients with acute myocardial infarction treated with intracoronary streptokinase.[227]

In the acute coronary syndromes, vasoconstriction either may be a response to deep arterial damage or plaque disruption or may occur as a response to a mildly dysfunctional endothelium (Fig 28A-11).

Plaque disruption or deep arterial damage (type III) and vasoconstriction. Several recent studies have aimed at elucidating the pathophysiology of vasoconstriction in coronary disease. Platelet-dependent vasoconstriction, mediated by serotonin and thromboxane A_2,[118,220,263,264] and thrombin-dependent vasoconstriction[264] occur if the endothelium has been injured or removed (type II or III injury), an event suggesting that these substances directly interact with the vascular smooth muscle cells. This information, along with recent data obtained in humans after percutaneous transluminal coronary angioplasty,[265,266] supports the angiographic observation that transient vasoconstriction accompanies plaque disruption or fissuring and thrombosis in the acute coronary syndromes.[227]

Physiologically, focal thrombus formation and vasoconstriction probably serve as defense mechanisms to prevent bleeding when microvascular – arteriolar and capillary – damage occurs. Such protective processes do not distinguish between this type of damage and that occurring in the major arteries (plaque disruption or fissuring), so that the response may be detrimental and contribute to the acute coronary syndromes. If the endothelium is intact, however, the platelet-dependent vascular response is relaxation[264] and the active platelet products are serotonin and adenine nucleotides. Hence, although focal arterial damage and thrombosis are detrimental, if the products of thrombosis reach the downstream vascular bed protected by endothelium, distal relaxation and blood flow may increase and thus limit ischemia.[267]

Normal or dysfunctional (type I) endothelium and vasoconstriction. The endothelium can profoundly affect vascular tone by releasing relaxing factors such as

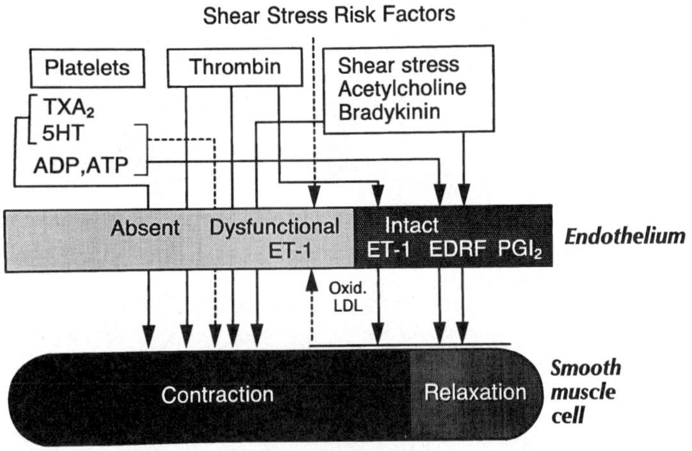

Fig 28A-11 The effects of shear stress, acetylcholine, and bradykinin lead intact endothelium to generate and release endothelium-derived relaxing factor (*EDRF*) and prostacyclin (*PGI_2*), which cause relaxation of the smooth muscle. The effect of thrombin leads the intact endothelium to generate endothelin-1 (*ET-1*), which causes vasoconstriction of a smooth muscle. After type I injury or damage, dysfunctional endothelium may not generate relaxing substances; in this circumstance, all the above-mentioned stimulants exert a vasoconstrictive effect, either through the enhancement of endothelium-derived contracting factors or directly. As a result of type II or III injury or damage, in areas of deendothelialization (*Absent*), thrombin and the platelet products thromboxane A_2 (*TXA_2*) and serotonin (*5HT*) induce direct vasoconstriction of the smooth muscle. *ADP,* adenosine diphosphate; *ATP,* adenosine triphosphate; *Oxid. LDL,* oxidized low-density lipoprotein. (Modified from Fuster V, Badimon L, Badimon JJ, et al: The pathogenesis of coronary artery disease and the acute coronary syndromes. *N Engl J Med* 326:242-250; 310-318, 1992.)

prostacyclin and endothelium-derived relaxing factor (nitric oxide), which also prevent platelet deposition, and contracting factors such as endothelin-1.[268] Under physiologic conditions, endothelium-derived relaxing factor seems to predominate. However, an alteration in the endothelium, such as that occurring in type I injury, may cause endothelial cells to generate more mediators that enhance constriction and fewer mediators that enhance dilation. Evidence suggests that atherosclerotic arteries have increased vascular tone, perhaps related to a deficiency in the production or release of endothelium-derived relaxing factor. For example, a paradoxical vasoconstrictor response to acetylcholine has been demonstrated in atherosclerotic coronary arteries in humans[238,269] and in various animal species,[270-272] and this response has been attributed to endothelial dysfunction. Recent coronary arteriographic studies in humans suggested that there is a progressive impairment of endothelial vasoactive function, beginning with a selective endothelial dysfunction in angiographically normal arteries in patients with hypercholesterolemia and progressing to vasoconstriction in response to several agonists in atherosclerotic coronary arteries.[273] Indeed, local secretion of endothelium-derived relaxing factor seems to be diminished in atherosclerotic human coronary arteries.[9]

On the basis of these observations, it appears that in acute coronary syndromes there is a predisposition for platelet-dependent and thrombin-dependent transient vasoconstriction at the site of plaque disruption and thrombosis. Chronic atherosclerosis is associated with abnormal vasodilatation or an exaggerated vasoconstrictor response, perhaps due to endothelial dysfunction with loss or impaired diffusion of endothelium-derived relaxing factor through the altered vascular wall. Similarly, atherogenic risk factors such as hypercholesterolemia may increase the likelihood of vasoconstriction.

INTEGRATED PATHOGENESIS OF THE CORONARY SYNDROMES

In patients with stable coronary artery disease, angina commonly results from an increase in myocardial oxygen demand that outstrips the ability of stenosed coronary arteries to increase its delivery (Fig 28A-12). In contrast, unstable angina, non-Q-wave myocardial infarction, and Q-wave infarction are a continuum of the disease process and are usually characterized by an abrupt reduction in coronary flow. Thus, local and systemic thrombogenic risk factors present at the time of plaque disruption may modify the extent and duration of thrombus deposition and account for the various pathologic and acute clinical manifestations (see Table 28A-10).

In unstable angina, a relatively small fissuring or disruption of an atherosclerotic plaque may lead to an acute change in plaque structure and a reduction in coronary blood flow, resulting in exacerbation of angina. Transient

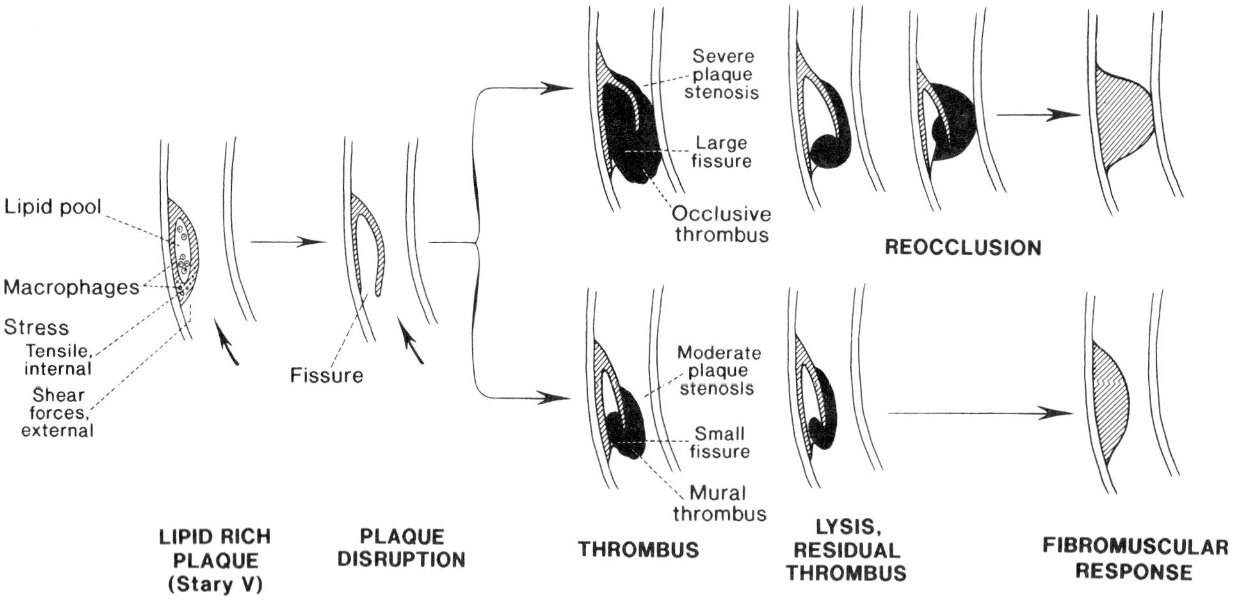

Fig 28A-12 Typical dynamic evolution of the complicated disrupted plaque shown in Figure 28A-1. See text for details. (From Fuster V, Badimon L, Badimon JJ, et al: The pathogenesis of coronary artery disease and the acute coronary syndromes. *N Engl J Med* 326:242-250; 310-318, 1992. By permission of journal.)

episodes of thrombotic vessel occlusion at the site of plaque injury may occur, leading to angina at rest.[108,274,275] This thrombus is usually labile and results in temporary vascular occlusion, perhaps lasting only 10 to 20 minutes.[108] In addition, release of vasoactive substances by platelets and vasoconstriction secondary to endothelial vasodilator dysfunction may contribute to a reduction in coronary flow. Alterations in perfusion and myocardial oxygen supply probably account for two-thirds of episodes of unstable angina; the rest may be caused by transient increases in myocardial oxygen demand.[276]

In non-Q-wave infarction, more severe plaque damage results in more persistent thrombotic occlusion, perhaps lasting up to 1 hour. About one-fourth of patients with non-Q-wave infarction may have an infarct-related vessel occluded for more than 1 hour, but the distal myocardial territory is usually supplied by collaterals.[277] ST-segment elevation in the electrocardiogram, an early peak in plasma creatine kinase concentration, and a high rate of angiographic patency of the involved vessel in early angiograms support these speculations. Resolution of vasospasm may also be pathogenically important in non-Q-wave infarction.[278,279] Therefore, spontaneous thrombolysis, spasm resolution, and collateral circulation are important in preventing the formation of Q-wave infarction by limiting the duration of myocardial ischemia.

In Q-wave infarction, larger plaque fissures may result in the formation of a fixed and persistent thrombus. This leads to abrupt cessation of myocardial perfusion for more than 1 hour, resulting in transmural necrosis of the involved myocardium. Because the coronary lesion responsible for the infarction is frequently only mildly to moderately stenotic, plaque rupture with superimposed thrombus rather than the severity of the underlying lesion may be the primary determinant of acute occlusion.[106,107] It is conceivable that in patients with severe coronary stenosis, well-developed collaterals prevent or reduce the extent of infarction.[109] In perhaps one-fourth of patients, coronary thrombosis results from superficial intimal injury or blood stasis in areas of high-grade stenosis.[112] Additionally, myocardial infarction may be promoted by alterations in hemostasis, such as increased activation of the coagulation system, increased platelet aggregability, increased fibrinogen and factor VII activity, and deficient fibrinolytic mechanisms.

Sudden coronary death probably involves a rapidly progressive coronary lesion in which plaque rupture and resultant thrombosis lead to ischemia and fatal ventricular arrhythmias.[111] Absence of collateral flow to the myocardium distal to the occlusion or platelet microemboli[280] perhaps contribute to the development of sudden ischemic death.

THE CORONARY MICROCIRCULATION AND COLLATERALS

Diseases of the coronary arteries have generally been considered from the vantage point of the epicardial coronary vessels because of the widespread use of coronary angiography as the standard means for the diagnosis of coronary artery disease. In the past decade, advances in the ability to assess the microcirculatory compartment of the human coronary circulation have led

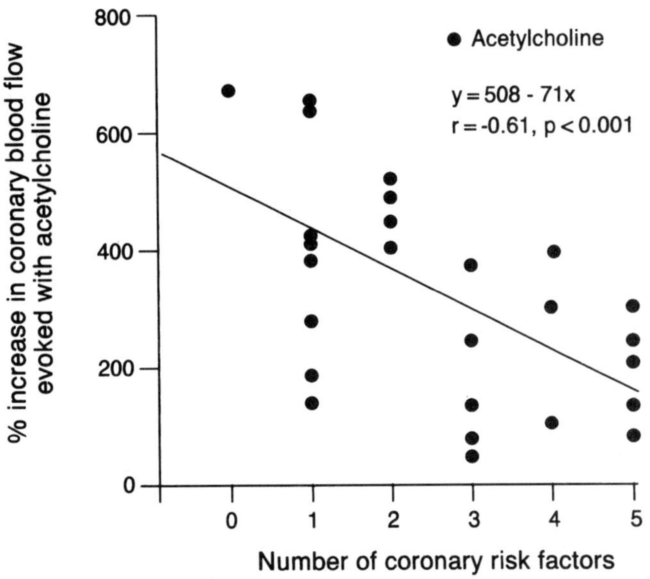

Fig 28A-13 Coronary blood flow evoked by acetylcholine. Decrease is proportional to number of risk factors. (Modified from Egashira K, Inou T, Hirooka Y, et al: Impaired coronary blood flow response to acetylcholine in patients with coronary risk factors and proximal atherosclerotic lesions. *J Clin Invest* 91:29-37, 1993.)

to new concepts in coronary artery disease.[281] Recent work has revealed that the cardiovascular risk factors known to affect the epicardial coronary arteries also affect coronary microcirculatory function[282] (Fig 28A-13). These factors include atherosclerosis, cardiomyopathy, and postangioplasty and post-myocardial infarction syndromes. There are also diseases that may exclusively involve the microvasculature (subsets of the so-called syndrome X).

The lesion common to all these entities is possibly a defect in endothelium-mediated vasomotor regulation, which is assessed clinically by measurement of the vasomotor regulation, which in turn is assessed clinically by measurement of the vasodilator reserve. For the clinician, data suggest that control of cardiovascular risk factors, such as hypercholesterolemia and hypertension, may be of greater benefit than previously appreciated, with evidence that they can independently and reversibly[54] alter vasomotor responses in the microcirculation.[282]

An important anatomic factor of the microcirculation that may modify the hemodynamic effects of an atherosclerotic obstruction is collateral circulation. Collaterals are anastomotic connections without an intervening capillary bed between portions of the same artery or between different arteries. In human hearts, the distribution and extent of collateral vessels are quite variable. Under physiologic conditions, collateral vessels are generally less than 40 μm in diameter and appear to have little or no function. However, when myocardial perfusion is compromised by obstructions affecting major vessels, these collateral vessels enlarge and blood flow through them increases.[283-286] Collaterals become angiographically visible only when coronary occlusion is complete or virtually so. Collaterals may equal perfusion through a vessel with 90% stenosis of the luminal diameter,[285,286] providing just enough perfusion to maintain myocardial viability and prevent myocardial infarction. There is very little information about the ways in which coronary collateral circulation can be stimulated. Exercise[287,288] and gradual rather than abrupt coronary occlusion[286] appear to enhance the development of collaterals. Advances in our knowledge of vascular biology, particularly the critical roles played by the vascular endothelium in regulating vascular tone, in hemostasis, and in controlling the growth of the microvessels (angiogenesis), lead to opportunities for new strategies in coronary artery disease.

STABILIZATION OR REGRESSION OF THE ATHEROSCLEROTIC PLAQUE

Risk factor modification: lipid-modifying trials

Approaches that have been taken toward retardation or even reversibility of atherosclerotic lesions in humans include better control of risk factors, especially by reducing plasma cholesterol levels; enhancement of lipid-removal pathways from the vessel wall, particularly by increasing plasma HDL levels (successful experimentally);[289,290] and reduction of LDL oxidation by use of antioxidant agents, such as probucol, which has been associated with regression of atherosclerosis in animal models to a greater degree than that expected by its lipid-lowering action alone.[58] Each of these approaches, by acting on the lipid-rich plaque more prone to rupture, might prevent progression and even induce removal of fat and regression of atherosclerotic plaque.

However, numerous trials have shown only slight regression of atherosclerotic lesions despite substantial reduction in the incidence of acute cardiac events[291-300] (Table 28A-11 and Fig 28A-14). It is possible that removal of lipids from the relatively small lipid-rich layers, not necessarily angiographically visible,[301] and increased relative collagen content of the plaque, together with the production of heavily cross-linked collagen, may account for increasing plaque stability without significant reduction in plaque size.[302] It is striking that the greatest reduction of events occurs within the first 6 months of treatment.[303] Also of great interest is the substantial reduction in angina in several trials despite minimal or no regression of atherosclerotic lesions. Indeed, according to the previously discussed detrimental effect of dyslipoproteinemia and other risk factors on microvascular flow, lipid modification might reverse such phenomena and thus the degree of angina.

Angiotensin-converting enzyme inhibitors and β-blockers

Recent evidence from trials of angiotensin-converting enzyme inhibitors in patients with ischemic heart disease

Table 28A-11 Progression and regression of coronary disease

Study	Progression (P) (control), %	Regression (R) (treated), %	Event reduction* (treated), %
NHLBI II	...	...	33
CLAS I II	...	...	34
POSCH	...	...	62
Lifestyle	3.4	2.2	...
FATS	2.1	0.8	75
UC-SCOR	0.8	1.5	...
STARS	5.8	1.5	79
SCRIP	...	...	50
CCAIT	...	...	47
Average	3.0(P)	1.4(R)	54

*Death, myocardial infarction, unstable angina (revascularization).

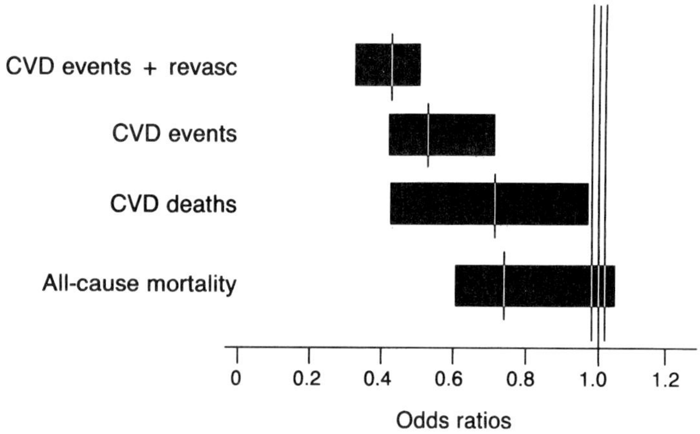

Fig 28A-14 Coronary events in the regression trials. *CVD,* cardiovascular disease. (From Blankenhorn DH, Hodis HN: Arterial imaging and atherosclerosis reversal. *Arterioscler Thromb* 14:177-192, 1994. By permission of American Heart Association.)

points to a reduction of 14% to 28% in the incidence of ischemic cardiac events.[304,305] The mechanism of any possible reduction in the incidence of plaque rupture by angiotensin-converting enzyme inhibitors is uncertain. The effect may be due to a reduction in arterial wall stress caused by lower blood pressure or reduced levels of neurohumoral activation[306] or their effect on protein synthesis influencing plaque composition so that the likelihood of plaque rupture is reduced. Meta-analysis of secondary prevention trials with β-blockers has shown a 20% reduction in cardiac mortality, an additional 25% reduction in the incidence of reinfarction, and a 30% reduction in the incidence of sudden death.[307] Treatment with β-blockers reduces the circumferential plaque stress by reducing blood pressure and blunting hypertensive pressure surges.[308] β-Blockers may also prevent plaque rupture by increasing the ability of the fibrous cap of the plaque to withstand stress. Because plaque stiffness increases with heart rate, β-blockers may increase plaque tensile strength by reducing heart rate.[309]

Antithrombotic approaches to prevention

Since thrombus formation seems to be an important factor in the progression of coronary artery disease and in the conversion of chronic to acute events after plaque disruption, a promising approach is to prevent these processes with antithrombotic therapy. Preliminary information indicates that antiplatelet agents may offer some promise in preventing the progression of small coronary atherosclerotic plaques.[115] Otherwise, the most beneficial effect of antiplatelet and anticoagulant agents has been observed in the prevention of acute coronary events.[310-315]

The best-suited, least toxic, and most widely used antithrombotic agent in acute chronic coronary artery disease is aspirin. It has been shown to be effective in unstable angina and acute myocardial infarction during and after coronary revascularization, in the secondary prevention of chronic coronary and cerebrovascular disease, and in primary prevention, particularly in persons at high risk.[310] Aspirin interferes with only one of the three pathways of platelet activation—the one dependent on thromboxane A_2. The other two pathways, one dependent on adenosine diphosphate and collagen and the other on thrombin, remain unaffected, and so does the coagulation system. On the other hand, anticoagulant agents interfere only partially with the coagulation system and are ineffective in platelet activation. It is not surprising, therefore, that aspirin, heparin, and oral anticoagulants cannot completely prevent thrombotic events.

It is noteworthy that in coronary artery disease, the overall antithrombotic effectiveness of aspirin or anticoagulant agents is clinically similar.[316] Combination therapy with low doses of aspirin and anticoagulant agents may have an additive effect. The rationale behind this combination is to block to some extent both platelet activation and the generation of thrombin by the intrinsic and extrinsic coagulation systems. The hope is to achieve this objective without enhancing bleeding; thus far, such therapy is being considered only for the short term (<1 week to 3 months) in patients at high risk for thrombotic events, such as those with unstable angina or acute myocardial infarction, and in patients who have had coronary thrombolysis or revascularization[317] (Table 28A-12). In addition, low doses of aspirin and oral anticoagulants are being tested in chronic coronary disease (see Table 28A-12).

Table 28A-13 outlines some of the newer antithrombotic approaches under active investigation, either blocking of the early stage of platelet activation with the specific antithrombins hirudin[318,319] and hirulog[323] or direct blocking of the platelet-membrane receptor glycoprotein IIb/IIIa.[326]

Table 28A-12 Antithrombotic therapy in coronary artery disease

Syndrome	Risk	ASA	AC	AC + ASA < 1 wk	AC + ASA ≥ 1 wk
Unstable angina	High	+	+	+*	±†
MI (acute), no lysis	High	+	±	?*	?‡
MI (acute), lysis	High	+	±	±*	?‡
MI (acute), LV anterior	Medium	−	+	−	−
PTCA	High	+	+	+	−
SVBG	High	+	±	?†	?†
MI (> 1 mo-3 yr)	Medium	±	+		?‡
Chronic or stable CAD	Medium	+	+		?†
Primary prevention	Low	±†	?		−

AC, anticoagulant; ASA, aspirin; CAD, coronary artery disease; LV, left ventricular; MI, myocardial infarction; PTCA, percutaneous transluminal coronary angioplasty; SVBG, saphenous vein bypass graft.
**GUSTO* II (hirudin).
†Evolving approach in high risk: need for trials.
‡*CARS* (AC + ASA low dose and fixed).

Table 28A-13 New antithrombotic approaches for coronary artery disease: Clinical experience, 1993-1994

	Unstable angina	Myocardial infarction	PTCA occlusion
Hirudin	GUSTO pilot[318] GUSTO II OASIS	TIMI-5 pilot (rt-PA)[319] TIMI-6 pilot (SK) TIMI-9 GUSTO-II OASIS	Rotterdam pilot[320] GUSTO II HELVETICA
Hirulog	Montreal pilot[321] TIMI-7 pilot[323] TIMI-8	Montreal pilot (SK)[321] ISIS-5 HERO (SK)	Topol et al.[322]
IIb/IIIa receptor block	ECSG pilot[324] Hopkins pilot[327] CAPTURE	TAMI-8[325] IMPACT MI	EPIC[326] IMPACT PTCA[328]

MI, myocardial infarction; PTCA; percutaneous transluminal coronary angioplasty; rt-PA, recombinant tissue-type plasminogen activator; SK, streptokinase.

REFERENCES

1. Restrepo C, Strong JP, Guzman MA, et al: Geographic comparisons of diffuse intimal thickening of the aorta. *Atherosclerosis* 32:177-193, 1979
2. Lobstein JF: Cited by Li P-L: Adaptation in veins to increased intravenous pressure, with special reference to the portal system and inferior vena cava. *J Pathol Bacteriol* 50:121-136, 1940
3. Classification of atherosclerotic lesions: report of a study group. *WHO Tech Rep Ser* 143:1-20, 1958
4. Fuster V: Lewis A. Conner Memorial Lecture. Mechanisms leading to myocardial infarction: insights from studies of vascular biology. *Circulation* 90:2126-2146, 1994
5. Tracy RE, Kissling GE: Comparisons of human populations for histologic features of atherosclerosis. A summary of questions and methods for geographic studies. *Arch Pathol Lab Med* 112:1056-1065, 1988
6. Angelini A, Thiene G, Frescura C, et al: Coronary arterial wall and atherosclerosis in youth (1-20 years): a histological study in a northern Italian population. *Int J Cardiol* 28:361-370, 1990
7. Dollar AL, Kragel AH, Fernicola DJ, et al: Composition of atherosclerotic plaques in coronary arteries in women less than 40 years of age with fatal coronary artery disease and implications for plaque reversibility. *Am J Cardiol* 67:1223-1227, 1991
8. Baroldi G, Silver MD, Mariani F, et al: Correlation of morphological variables in the coronary atherosclerotic plaque with clinical patterns of ischemic heart disease. *Am J Cardiovasc Pathol* 2:159-172, 1988
9. Fuster V, Badimon L, Badimon JJ, et al: The pathogenesis of coronary artery disease and the acute coronary syndromes. *N Engl J Med* 326:242-250; 310-318, 1992
10. Cliff WJ, Heathcote CR, Moss NS, et al: The coronary arteries in cases of cardiac and noncardiac sudden death. *Am J Pathol* 132:319-329, 1988
11. Rokitansky C: *A Manual of Pathological Anatomy.* Vol. 4 (Translated from German by GE Day). London, Sydenham Society, 1852, pp 271-273
12. Virchow R: *Gesammelte Abhandlungen zur wissenschaftlichen Medicin.* Frankfurt, Meidinger Sohn Company, 1856, p 458

13. Ross R: The pathogenesis of atherosclerosis: a perspective for the 1990s. *Nature* 362:801-809, 1993
14. Ip JH, Fuster V, Badimon L, et al: Syndromes of accelerated atherosclerosis: role of vascular injury and smooth muscle cell proliferation. *J Am Coll Cardiol* 15:1667-1687, 1990
15. Rosenfeld ME, Palinski W, Yla-Herttuala S, et al: Macrophages, endothelial cells, and lipoprotein oxidation in the pathogenesis of atherosclerosis. *Toxicol Pathol* 18:560-571, 1990
16. Steinbrecher UP, Zhang HF, Lougheed M: Role of oxidatively modified LDL in atherosclerosis. *Free Rad Biol Med* 9:155-168, 1990
17. Steinberg D: Antioxidants and atherosclerosis. A current assessment (editorial). *Circulation* 84:1420-1425, 1991
18. Henriksen T, Mahoney EM, Steinberg D: Interactions of plasma lipoproteins with endothelial cells. *Ann N Y Acad Sci* 401:102-116, 1982
19. Heinecke JW, Rosen H, Chait A: Iron and copper promote modification of low density lipoprotein by human arterial smooth muscle cells in culture. *J Clin Invest* 74:1890-1894, 1984
20. Morel DW, DiCorleto PE, Chisolm GM: Endothelial and smooth muscle cells alter low density lipoprotein in vitro by free radical oxidation. *Arteriosclerosis* 4:357-364, 1984
21. Fogelman AM, Schechter I, Seager J, et al: Malondialdehyde alteration of low density lipoproteins leads to cholesteryl ester accumulation in human monocyte-macrophages. *Proc Natl Acad Sci U S A* 77:2214-2218, 1980
22. Gibson CM, Diaz L, Kandarpa K, et al: Relation of vessel wall shear stress to atherosclerosis progression in human coronary arteries. *Arterioscler Thromb* 13:310-315, 1993
23. Asakura T, Karino T: Flow patterns and spatial distribution of atherosclerotic lesions in human coronary arteries. *Circ Res* 66:1045-1066, 1990
24. MacIsaac AI, Thomas JD, Topol EJ: Toward the quiescent coronary plaque. *J Am Coll Cardiol* 22:1228-1241, 1993
25. Levesque MJ, Liepsch D, Moravec S, et al: Correlation of endothelial cell shape and wall shear stress in a stenosed dog aorta. *Arteriosclerosis* 6:220-229, 1986
26. Badimon JJ, Fuster V, Chesebro JH, et al: Coronary atherosclerosis. A multifactorial disease. *Circulation* 87 Suppl 2:3-16, 1993
27. Celermajer DS, Sorensen KE, Gooch VM, et al: Non-invasive detection of endothelial dysfunction in children and adults at risk of atherosclerosis. *Lancet* 340:1111-1115, 1992
28. Brown MS, Kovanen PT, Goldstein JL: Regulation of plasma cholesterol by lipoprotein receptors. *Science* 212:628-635, 1981
29. Shepherd J, Packard CJ: Lipoprotein receptors and atherosclerosis. *Clin Sci* 70:1-6, 1986
30. Goldstein JL, Ho YK, Basu SK, et al: Binding site on macrophages that mediates uptake and degradation of acetylated low density lipoprotein, producing massive cholesterol deposition. *Proc Natl Acad Sci U S A* 76:333-337, 1979
31. Valente AJ, Rozek MM, Sprague EA, et al: Mechanisms in intimal monocyte-macrophage recruitment. A special role for monocyte chemotactic protein-1. *Circulation* 86 Suppl 3:20-25, 1992
32. Berliner JA, Territo M, Almada L, et al: Monocyte chemotactic factor produced by large vessel endothelial cells in vitro. *Arteriosclerosis* 6:254-258, 1986
33. Stanley ER: The macrophage colony-stimulating factor, CSF-1. *Methods Enzymol* 116:564-587, 1985
34. Sporn MB, Roberts AB, Wakefield LM, et al: Some recent advances in the chemistry and biology of transforming growth factor-beta. *J Cell Biol* 105:1039-1045, 1987
35. Norris DA, Clark RA, Swigart LM, et al: Fibronectin fragment(s) are chemotactic for human peripheral blood monocytes. *J Immunol* 129:1612-1618, 1982
36. Hunninghake GW, Davidson JM, Rennard S, et al: Elastin fragments attract macrophage precursors to diseased sites in pulmonary emphysema. *Science* 212:925-927, 1981
37. Postlethwaite AE, Kang AH: Collagen- and collagen peptide-induced chemotaxis of human blood monocytes. *J Exp Med* 143:1299-1307, 1976
38. Bar-Shavit R, Kahn A, Fenton JW II, et al: Chemotactic response of monocytes to thrombin. *J Cell Biol* 96:282-285, 1983
39. Stary HC: Evolution and progression of atherosclerotic lesions in coronary arteries of children and young adults. *Arteriosclerosis* 9 Suppl 1:19-32, 1989
40. Stary HC, Blankenhorn DH, Chandler AB, et al: A definition of the intima of human arteries and of its atherosclerosis-prone regions. A report from the Committee on Vascular Lesions of the Council on Arteriosclerosis, American Heart Association. *Circulation* 85:391-405, 1992
41. Alderman EL, Corley SD, Fisher LD, et al: Five-year angiographic follow-up of factors associated with progression of coronary artery disease in the Coronary Artery Surgery Study (CASS). CASS Participating Investigators and Staff. *J Am Coll Cardiol* 22:1141-1154, 1993
42. Stary HC: Composition and classification of human atherosclerotic lesions. *Virchows Arch A Pathol Anat Histopathol* 421:277-290, 1992
43. Davies MJ, Woolf N, Rowles PM, et al: Morphology of the endothelium over atherosclerotic plaques in human coronary arteries. *Br Heart J* 60:459-464, 1988
44. Restrepo C, Tracy RE: Variations in human aortic fatty streaks among geographic locations. *Atherosclerosis* 21:179-193, 1975
45. Falk E: Why do plaques rupture? *Circulation* 86 Suppl 3:30-42, 1992
46. Wilcox JN, Smith KM, Schwartz SM, et al: Localization of tissue factor in the normal vessel wall and in the atherosclerotic plaque. *Proc Natl Acad Sci U S A* 86:2839-2843, 1989
47. Poole JCF, Florey HW: Changes in the endothelium of the aorta and the behaviour of macrophages in experimental atheroma of rabbits. *J Pathol Bacteriol* 75:245-252, 1958
48. Gerrity RG, Naito HK, Richardson M, et al: Dietary induced atherogenesis in swine. Morphology of the intima in prelesion stages. *Am J Pathol* 95:775-792, 1979
49. Schwartz CJ, Kelley JL, Nerem RM, et al: Pathophysiology of the atherogenic process. *Am J Cardiol* 64:23G-30G, 1989
50. Mitchinson MJ, Ball RY: Macrophages and atherogenesis. *Lancet* 2:146-148, 1987
51. Patarroyo M, Prieto J, Beatty PG, et al: Adhesion-mediating molecules of human monocytes. *Cell Immunol* 113:278-289, 1988
52. Prieto J, Beatty PG, Clark EA, et al: Molecules mediating adhesion of T and B cells, monocytes and granulocytes to vascular endothelial cells. *Immunology* 63:631-637, 1988
53. Brown MS, Goldstein JL: A receptor-mediated pathway for cholesterol homeostasis. *Science* 232:34-47, 1986
54. Small DM, Shipley GG: Physical-chemical basis of lipid deposition in atherosclerosis. *Science* 185:222-229, 1974
55. Fielding CJ: The endothelium, triglyceride-rich lipoproteins, and atherosclerosis: insights from cell biology and lipid metabolism. *Diabetes* 30 Suppl 2:19-23, 1981
56. Sherrill BC, Dietschy JM: Characterization of the sinusoidal transport process responsible for uptake of chylomicrons by the liver. *J Biol Chem* 253:1859-1867, 1978
57. Steinberg D, Parthasarathy S, Carew TE, et al: Beyond cholesterol. Modifications of low-density lipoprotein that increase its atherogenicity. *N Engl J Med* 320:915-924, 1989
58. Carew TE, Schwenke DC, Steinberg D: Antiatherogenic effect of probucol unrelated to its hypocholesterolemic effect: evidence that antioxidants in vivo can selectively inhibit low density lipoprotein degradation in macrophage-rich fatty streaks and slow the progression of atherosclerosis in the Watanabe heritable hyperlipidemic rabbit. *Proc Natl Acad Sci U S A* 84:7725-7729, 1987
59. Palinski W, Rosenfeld ME, Yla-Herttuala S, et al: Low density lipoprotein undergoes oxidative modification in vivo. *Proc Natl Acad Sci U S A* 86:1372-1376, 1989
60. Gordon DJ, Rifkind BM: High-density lipoprotein—the clinical implications of recent studies. *N Engl J Med* 321:1311-1316, 1989
61. Maciejko JJ, Holmes DR, Kottke BA, et al: Apolipoprotein A-I as a marker of angiographically assessed coronary-artery disease. *N Engl J Med* 309:385-389, 1983
62. Webster MWI, Chesebro JH, Kottke BA, et al: Apolipoprotein AI and coronary disease progression: a 5-year angiographic study (abstract). *J Am Coll Cardiol* 15 Suppl A:114, 1990
63. Gordon DJ, Probstfield JL, Garrison RJ, et al: High-density lipoprotein cholesterol and cardiovascular disease. Four prospective American studies. *Circulation* 79:8-15, 1989
64. Shattil SJ, Bennett JS, Colman RW, et al: Abnormalities of cholesterol-phospholipid composition in platelets and low-density lipoproteins of human hyperbetalipoproteinemia. *J Lab Clin Med* 89:341-353, 1977
65. Harker LA, Hazzard W: Platelet kinetic studies in patients with hyperlipoproteinemia: effects of clofibrate therapy. *Circulation* 60:492-496, 1979

66. Stuart MJ, Gerrard JM, White JG: Effect of cholesterol in production of thromboxane β_2 by platelets in vitro. *N Engl J Med* 302:6-10, 1980

67. Scott J: Lipoprotein(a). Thrombogenesis linked to atherogenesis at last? *Nature* 341:22-23, 1989

68. van der Wal AC, Das PK, Bentz van de Berg D, et al: Atherosclerotic lesions in humans. In situ immunophenotypic analysis suggesting an immune mediated response. *Lab Invest* 61:166-170, 1989

69. Seifert PS, Hugo F, Hansson GK, et al: Prelesional complement activation in experimental atherosclerosis. Terminal C5b-9 complement deposition coincides with cholesterol accumulation in the aortic intima of hypercholesterolemic rabbits. *Lab Invest* 60:747-754, 1989

70. Seifert PS, Hansson GK: Decay-accelerating factor is expressed on vascular smooth muscle cells in human atherosclerotic lesions. *J Clin Invest* 84:597-604, 1989

71. Campbell GR, Campbell JH: Smooth muscle phenotypic changes in arterial wall homeostasis: implications for the pathogenesis of atherosclerosis. *Exp Mol Pathol* 42:139-162, 1985

72. Manderson JA, Mosse PR, Safstrom JA, et al: Balloon catheter injury to rabbit carotid artery. I. Changes in smooth muscle phenotype. *Arteriosclerosis* 9:289-298, 1989

73. Clowes AW, Clowes MM, Reidy MA: Kinetics of cellular proliferation after arterial injury. III. Endothelial and smooth muscle growth in chronically denuded vessels. *Lab Invest* 54:295-303, 1986

74. Clowes AW, Schwartz SM: Significance of quiescent smooth muscle migration in the injured rat carotid artery. *Circ Res* 56:139-145, 1985

75. Haudenschild CC, Grunwald J: Proliferative heterogeneity of vascular smooth muscle cells and its alteration by injury. *Exp Cell Res* 157:364-370, 1985

76. Fishman JA, Ryan GB, Karnovsky MJ: Endothelial regeneration in the rat carotid artery and the significance of endothelial denudation in the pathogenesis of myointimal thickening. *Lab Invest* 32:339-351, 1975

77. Reidy MA, Clowes AW, Schwartz SM: Endothelial regeneration. V. Inhibition of endothelial regrowth in arteries of rat and rabbit. *Lab Invest* 49:569-575, 1983

78. Walker LN, Ramsay MM, Bowyer DE: Endothelial healing following defined injury to rabbit aorta. Depth of injury and mode of repair. *Atherosclerosis* 47:123-130, 1983

79. Thyberg J, Palmberg L, Nilsson J, et al: Phenotype modulation in primary cultures of arterial smooth muscle cells. On the role of platelet-derived growth factor. *Differentiation* 25:156-167, 1983

80. Libby P, Warner SJ, Friedman GB: Interleukin 1: a mitogen for human vascular smooth muscle cells that induces the release of growth-inhibitory prostanoids. *J Clin Invest* 81:487-498, 1988

81. Winkles JA, Friesel R, Burgess WH, et al: Human vascular smooth muscle cells both express and respond to heparin-binding growth factor I (endothelial cell growth factor). *Proc Natl Acad Sci U S A* 84:7124-7128, 1987

82. Stemerman MB, Spaet TH, Pitlick F, et al: Intimal healing. The pattern of reendothelialization and intimal thickening. *Am J Pathol* 87:125-142, 1977

83. Reidy MA: A reassessment of endothelial injury and arterial lesion formation. *Lab Invest* 53:513-520, 1985

84. Friedman RJ, Stemerman MB, Wenz B, et al: The effect of thrombocytopenia on experimental arteriosclerotic lesion formation in rabbits. Smooth muscle cell proliferation and re-endothelialization. *J Clin Invest* 60:1191-1201, 1977

85. Harker LA, Harlan JM, Ross R: Effect of sulfinpyrazone on homocysteine-induced endothelial injury and arteriosclerosis in baboons. *Circ Res* 53:731-739, 1983

86. Faggiotto A, Ross R, Harker L: Studies of hypercholesterolemia in the nonhuman primate. I. Changes that lead to fatty streak formation. *Arteriosclerosis* 4:323-340, 1984

87. Faggiotto A, Ross R: Studies of hypercholesterolemia in the nonhuman primate. II. Fatty streak conversion to fibrous plaque. *Arteriosclerosis* 4:341-356, 1984

88. Seddon AM, Woolf N, La Ville A, et al: Hereditary hyperlipidemia and atherosclerosis in the rabbit due to overproduction of lipoproteins. II. Preliminary report of arterial pathology. *Arteriosclerosis* 7:113-124, 1987

89. Davies PF, Reidy MA, Goode TB, et al: Scanning electron microscopy in the evaluation of endothelial integrity of the fatty lesion in atherosclerosis. *Atherosclerosis* 25:125-130, 1976

90. Fuster W, Bowie EJ, Lewis JC, et al: Resistance to arteriosclerosis in pigs with von Willebrand's disease. Spontaneous and high cholesterol diet-induced arteriosclerosis. *J Clin Invest* 61:722-730, 1978

91. Fuster V, Fass DN, Kaye MP, et al: Arteriosclerosis in normal and von Willebrand pigs: long-term prospective study and aortic transplantation study. *Circ Res* 51:587-593, 1982

92. Fuster V, Griggs TR: Porcine von Willebrand disease: implications for the pathophysiology of atherosclerosis and thrombosis. *Prog Hemost Thromb* 8:159-183, 1986

93. Cohen P, McCombs HL: Platelets and atherogenesis. 2. Amelioration of cholesterol atherogenesis in rabbits with reduced platelet counts as the result of ^{32}P administration. *J Atheroscler Res* 8:389-398, 1968

94. Ross R, Raines EW, Bowen-Pope DF: The biology of platelet-derived growth factor. *Cell* 46:155-169, 1986

95. Fox PL, DiCorleto PE: Regulation of production of a platelet-derived growth factor-like protein by cultured bovine aortic endothelial cells. *J Cell Physiol* 121:298-308, 1984

96. Bylock AL, Gerrity RG: Visualization of monocyte recruitment into atherosclerotic arteries using fluorescent labelling. *Atherosclerosis* 71:17-25, 1988

97. Leibovich SJ, Ross R: The role of the macrophage in wound repair. A study with hydrocortisone and antimacrophage serum. *Am J Pathol* 78:71-100, 1975

98. Bonner JC, Hoffman M, Brody AR: A platelet-derived growth factor homolog secreted by alveolar macrophages is complexed to an alpha-macroglobulin. *Transplant Proc* 21:3704-3705, 1989

99. Majesky MW, Benditt EP, Schwartz SM: Expression and developmental control of platelet-derived growth factor A-chain and B-chain/Sis genes in rat aortic smooth muscle cells. *Proc Natl Acad Sci U S A* 85:1524-1528, 1988

100. Libby P, Warner SJ, Salomon RN, et al: Production of platelet-derived growth factor-like mitogen by smooth-muscle cells from human atheroma. *N Engl J Med* 318:1493-1498, 1988

101. Stary HC, Chandler AB, Dinsmore RE, et al: A definition of advanced atherosclerotic lesions and a classification of atherosclerosis. *Circulation* (in press), 1995

102. Roberts AB, Sporn MB: The transforming growth factor-βs. In *Handbook of Experimental Pharmacology: Peptide Growth Factors and Their Receptors I.* Edited by MB Sporn, AB Roberts. Berlin, Springer-Verlag, 1990, pp 419-472

103. Moses HL, Yang EY, Pietenpol JA: TGF-beta stimulation and inhibition of cell proliferation: new mechanistic insights. *Cell* 63:245-247, 1990

104. Leung DY, Glagov S, Mathews MB: Cyclic stretching stimulates synthesis of matrix components by arterial smooth muscle cells in vitro. *Science* 191:475-477, 1976

105. Iwatsuki K, Cardinale GJ, Spector S, et al: Hypertension: increase of collagen biosynthesis in arteries but not in veins. *Science* 198:403-405, 1977

106. Ambrose JA, Tannenbaum MA, Alexopoulos D, et al: Angiographic progression of coronary artery disease and the development of myocardial infarction. *J Am Coll Cardiol* 12:56-62, 1988

107. Little WC, Constantinescu M, Applegate RJ, et al: Can coronary angiography predict the site of a subsequent myocardial infarction in patients with mild-to-moderate coronary artery disease? *Circulation* 78:1157-1166, 1988

108. Fuster V, Badimon L, Cohen M, et al: Insights into the pathogenesis of acute ischemic syndromes. *Circulation* 77:1213-1220, 1988

109. Richardson PD, Davies MJ, Born GV: Influence of plaque configuration and stress distribution on fissuring of coronary atherosclerotic plaques. *Lancet* 2:941-944, 1989

110. Cheng GC, Loree HM, Kamm RD, et al: Distribution of circumferential stress in ruptured and stable atherosclerotic lesions. A structural analysis with histopathological correlation. *Circulation* 87: 1179-1187, 1993

111. Falk E: Unstable angina with fatal outcome: dynamic coronary thrombosis leading to infarction and/or sudden death. Autopsy evidence of recurrent mural thrombosis with peripheral embolization culminating in total vascular occlusion. *Circulation* 71:699-708, 1985

112. Davies MJ, Bland JM, Hangartner JR, et al: Factors influencing the presence or absence of acute coronary artery thrombi in sudden ischaemic death. *Eur Heart J* 10:203-208, 1989

113. Constantinides P: Cause of thrombosis in human atherosclerotic arteries. *Am J Cardiol* 66:37G-40G, 1990
114. Davies MJ, Richardson PD, Woolf N, et al: Risk of thrombosis in human atherosclerotic plaques: role of extracellular lipid, macrophage, and smooth muscle cell content. *Br Heart J* 69:377-381, 1993
115. Chesebro JH, Webster MW, Zoldhelyi P, et al: Antithrombotic therapy and progression of coronary artery disease. Antiplatelet versus antithrombins. *Circulation* 86 Suppl 3:100-110, 1992
116. Moliterno DJ, Lange RA, Meidell RS, et al: Relation of plasma lipoprotein(a) to infarct artery patency in survivors of myocardial infarction. *Circulation* 88:935-940, 1993
117. Davies MJ: Thrombosis and coronary atherosclerosis. In *Thrombolysis in Cardiovascular Disease.* Edited by DG Julian, W Kubler, RM Norris, et al. New York, Marcel Dekker, 1989, pp 25-43
118. Bini A, Fenoglio JJ Jr, Mesa-Tejada R, et al: Identification and distribution of fibrinogen, fibrin, and fibrin(ogen) degradation products in atherosclerosis. Use of monoclonal antibodies. *Arteriosclerosis* 9:109-121, 1989
119. Woolf N, Davies MJ: Interrelationship between atherosclerosis and thrombosis. In *Thrombosis in Cardiovascular Disorders.* Edited by V Fuster, M Verstraete. Philadelphia, WB Saunders Company, 1992, pp 41-77
120. Shah PK, Falk E, Badimon J, et al: Human monocyte-derived macrophages express collagenase and induce collagen breakdown in atherosclerotic fibrous caps: implications for plaque rupture (abstract). *Circulation* 88 Suppl 1:254, 1993
121. Ferns GA, Raines EW, Sprugel KH, et al: Inhibition of neointimal smooth muscle accumulation after angioplasty by an antibody to PDGF. *Science* 253:1129-1132, 1991
122. Loscalzo J: The relation between atherosclerosis and thrombosis. *Circulation* 86 Suppl 3:95-99, 1992
123. Bar-Shavit R, Eldor A, Vlodavsky I: Binding of thrombin to subendothelial extracellular matrix. Protection and expression of functional properties. *J Clin Invest* 84:1096-1104, 1989
124. Weitz JI, Hudoba M, Massel D, et al: Clot-bound thrombin is protected from inhibition by heparin-antithrombin III but is susceptible to inactivation by antithrombin III-independent inhibitors. *J Clin Invest* 86:385-391, 1990
125. Bar-Shavit R, Benezra M, Eldor A, et al: Thrombin immobilized to extracellular matrix is a potent mitogen for vascular smooth muscle cells: nonenzymatic mode of action. *Cell Regulation* 1:453-463, 1990
126. Berk BC, Taubman MB, Griendling KK, et al: Thrombin-stimulated events in cultured vascular smooth-muscle cells. *Biochem J* 274:799-805, 1991
127. Jones A, Geczy CL: Thrombin and factor Xa enhance the production of interleukin-1. *Immunology* 71:236-241, 1990
128. Naito M, Hayashi T, Kuzuya M, et al: Effects of fibrinogen and fibrin on the migration of vascular smooth muscle cells in vitro. *Atherosclerosis* 83:9-14, 1990
129. Kaplan KL, Mather T, DeMarco L, et al: Effect of fibrin on endothelial cell production of prostacyclin and tissue plasminogen activator. *Arteriosclerosis* 9:43-49, 1989
130. Paul O: Background of the prevention of cardiovascular disease. II. Arteriosclerosis, hypertension, and selected risk factors. *Circulation* 80:206-214, 1989
131. The Expert Panel: Report of the National Cholesterol Education Program Expert Panel on Detection, Evaluation, and Treatment of High Blood Cholesterol in Adults. *Arch Intern Med* 148:36-69, 1988
132. Devereux RB, Alderman MH: Role of preclinical cardiovascular disease in the evolution from risk factor exposure to development of morbid events. *Circulation* 88:1444-1455, 1993
133. Fuster V, Frye RL, Connolly DC, et al: Arteriographic patterns early in the onset of the coronary syndromes. *Br Heart J* 37:1250-1255, 1975
134. The 1988 report of the Joint National Committee on Detection, Evaluation, and Treatment of High Blood Pressure. *Arch Intern Med* 148:1023-1038, 1988
135. Smoking and Health: A Report of the Surgeon General (NIH Publication No 79-50066). US Department of Health, Education, and Welfare. Washington DC, US Public Health Service, 1964
136. Gunby P: Surgeon General emphasizes nicotine addiction in annual report on tobacco use, consequences. *JAMA* 259:2811, 1988
137. Cullen JW, McKenna JW, Massey MM: International control of smoking and the US experience. *Chest* 89 Suppl:206S-218S, 1986
138. Strong WB, Deckelbaum RJ, Gidding SS, et al: Integrated cardiovascular health promotion in childhood. A statement for health professionals from the Subcommittee on Atherosclerosis and Hypertension in Childhood of the Council on Cardiovascular Disease in the Young, American Heart Association. *Circulation* 85:1638-1650, 1992
139. Fuster V, Chesebro JH, Frye RL, et al: Platelet survival and the development of coronary artery disease in the young adult: effects of cigarette smoking, strong family history and medical therapy. *Circulation* 63:546-551, 1981
140. Bierenbaum ML, Fleischman AI, Stier A, et al: Effect of cigarette smoking upon in vivo platelet function in man. *Thromb Res* 12:1051-1057, 1978
141. Astrup P: Some physiological and pathological effects of moderate carbon monoxide exposure. *Br Med J* 4:447-452, 1972
142. Davies RF, Topping DL, Turner DM: The effect of intermittent carbon monoxide exposure on experimental atherosclerosis in the rabbit. *Atherosclerosis* 24:527-536, 1976
143. Becker CG, Dubin T, Wiedemann HP: Hypersensitivity to tobacco antigen. *Proc Natl Acad Sci U S A* 73:1712-1716, 1976
144. Koch A, Hoffmann K, Steck W, et al: Acute cardiovascular reactions after cigarette smoking. *Atherosclerosis* 35:67-75, 1980
145. Becker CG, Dubin T: Activation of factor XII by tobacco glycoprotein. *J Exp Med* 146:457-467, 1977
146. Berg K, Borresen AL, Dahlen G: Effect of smoking on serum levels of HDL apoproteins. *Atherosclerosis* 34:339-343, 1979
147. Grech ED, Ramsdale DR, Bray CL, et al: Family history as an independent risk factor of coronary artery disease. *Eur Heart J* 13:1311-1315, 1992
148. Lindpaintner K: Blood pressure and heredity. Is it all in the genes, or not? (Editorial.) *Hypertension* 22:147-149, 1993
149. Chesebro JH, Fuster V, Elveback LR, et al: Strong family history and cigarette smoking as risk factors of coronary artery disease in young adults. *Br Heart J* 47:78-83, 1982
150. Dock W: The predilection of atherosclerosis for the coronary arteries. *JAMA* 131:875-878, 1946
151. Pesonen E: Coronary wall thickening in children. An analysis of the factors associated with the growth of arterial layers. *Atherosclerosis* 20:173-187, 1974
152. Lee KT, Thomas WA, Florentin RA, et al: Evidence for a polyclonal origin and proliferative heterogeneity of atherosclerotic lesions induced by dietary cholesterol in young swine. *Ann N Y Acad Sci* 275:336-347, 1976
153. Boers GH, Smals AG, Trijbels FJ, et al: Heterozygosity for homocystinuria in premature peripheral and cerebral occlusive arterial disease. *N Engl J Med* 313:709-715, 1985
154. Murphy-Chutorian DR, Wexman MP, Grieco AJ, et al: Methionine intolerance: a possible risk factor for coronary artery disease. *J Am Coll Cardiol* 6:725-730, 1985
155. Harker LA, Ross R, Slichter SJ, et al: Homocystine-induced arteriosclerosis. The role of endothelial cell injury and platelet response in its genesis. *J Clin Invest* 58:731-741, 1976
156. Gotto AM Jr: Status report: plasma lipids, lipoproteins, and coronary artery disease. *Atheroscler Rev* 4:17-28, 1979
157. Stehbens WE: Vascular complications in experimental atherosclerosis. *Prog Cardiovasc Dis* 29:221-237, 1986
158. Brunzell JD, Sniderman AD, Albers JJ, et al: Apoproteins B and A-I and coronary artery disease in humans. *Arteriosclerosis* 4:79-83, 1984
159. Mordasini R, Frey F, Flury W, et al: Selective deficiency of hepatic triglyceride lipase in uremic patients. *N Engl J Med* 297:1362-1366, 1977
160. Tall AR, Small DM: Plasma high-density lipoproteins. *N Engl J Med* 299:1232-1236, 1978
161. Wilson DE, Schreibman PH, Brewster AC, et al: The enhancement of alimentary lipemia by ethanol in man. *J Lab Clin Med* 75:264-274, 1970
162. Dannenberg AL, Drizd T, Horan MJ, et al: Progress in the battle against hypertension. Changes in blood pressure levels in the United States from 1960 to 1980. *Hypertension* 10:226-233, 1987
163. Moss AJ, DeCamilla J, Davis H, et al: The early posthospital phase of myocardial infarction. Prognostic stratification. *Circulation* 54:58-64, 1976
164. Ku DN, Giddens DP, Zarins CK, et al: Pulsatile flow and atherosclerosis in the human carotid bifurcation. Positive correlation between plaque location and low oscillating shear stress. *Arteriosclerosis* 5:293-302, 1985

165. Weinberger J, Ramos L, Ambrose JA, et al: Morphologic and dynamic changes of atherosclerotic plaque at the carotid artery bifurcation: sequential imaging by real time B-mode ultrasonography. *J Am Coll Cardiol* 12:1515-1521, 1988

166. Wolinsky H: Effects of hypertension and its reversal on the thoracic aorta of male and female rats. Morphological and chemical studies. *Circ Res* 28:622-637, 1971

167. Getz GS: Report on the workshop on diabetes and mechanisms of atherogenesis. September 17th and 18th, 1992, Bethesda, Maryland. *Arterioscler Thromb* 13:459-464, 1993

168. The Diabetes Control and Complications Trial Research Group: The effect of intensive treatment of diabetes on the development and progression of long-term complications in insulin-dependent diabetes mellitus. *N Engl J Med* 329:977-986, 1993

169. Jacoby RM, Nesto RW: Acute myocardial infarction in the diabetic patient: pathophysiology, clinical course and prognosis. *J Am Coll Cardiol* 20:736-744, 1992

170. Reichard P, Nilsson BY, Rosenqvist U: The effect of long-term intensified insulin treatment on the development of microvascular complications of diabetes mellitus. *N Engl J Med* 329:304-309, 1993

171. Savage PJ, Soad MF: Insulin and atherosclerosis: villain, accomplice, or innocent bystander? (Editorial.) *Br Heart J* 69:473-475, 1993

172. DeFronzo RA: Insulin resistance, hyperinsulinemia, and coronary artery disease: a complex metabolic web. *Coron Artery Dis* 3:11-25, 1992

173. Schwartz CJ, Valente AJ, Sprague EA, et al: Pathogenesis of the atherosclerotic lesion. Implications for diabetes mellitus. *Diabetes Care* 15:1156-1167, 1992

174. Lehner ND, Clarkson TB, Lofland HB: The effect of insulin deficiency, hypothyroidism, and hypertension on atherosclerosis in the squirrel monkey. *Exp Mol Pathol* 15:230-244, 1971

175. Schneider DJ, Sobel BE: Effect of diabetes on the coagulation and fibrinolytic systems and its implications for atherogenesis. *Coron Artery Dis* 3:26-32, 1992

176. Colwell JA, Sagel J, Crook L, et al: Correlation of platelet aggregation, plasma factor activity, and megathrombocytes in diabetic subjects with and without vascular disease. *Metabolism* 26:279-285, 1977

177. Bloodworth JMB Jr, Molitor DL: Ultrastructural aspects of human and canine diabetic retinopathy. *Invest Ophthalmol* 4:1037-1048, 1965

178. Timperley WR, Preston FE, Ward JD: Cerebral intravascular coagulation in diabetic ketoacidosis. *Lancet* 1:952-956, 1974

179. Stampfer MJ, Colditz GA, Willett WC, et al: Postmenopausal estrogen therapy and cardiovascular disease. Ten-year follow-up from the Nurses' Health Study. *N Engl J Med* 325:756-762, 1991

180. Colditz GA, Willett WC, Stampfer MJ, et al: Menopause and the risk of coronary heart disease in women. *N Engl J Med* 316:1105-1110, 1987

181. Nabulsi AA, Folsom AR, White A, et al: Association of hormone-replacement therapy with various cardiovascular risk factors in postmenopausal women. The Atherosclerosis Risk in Communities Study Investigators. *N Engl J Med* 328:1069-1075, 1993

182. Grady D, Rubin SM, Petitti DB, et al: Hormone therapy to prevent disease and prolong life in postmenopausal women. *Ann Intern Med* 117:1016-1037, 1992

183. Rosano GM, Sarrel PM, Poole-Wilson PA, et al: Beneficial effect of oestrogen on exercise-induced myocardial ischaemia in women with coronary artery disease. *Lancet* 342:133-136, 1993

184. Magness RR, Rosenfeld CR: Local and systemic estradiol-17 beta: effects on uterine and systemic vasodilation. *Am J Physiol* 256:E536-E542, 1989

185. Gangar KF, Vyas S, Whitehead M et al: Pulsatility index in internal carotid artery in relation to transdermal oestradiol and time since menopause. *Lancet* 338:839-842, 1991

186. Ginsburg J, Hardiman P, O'Reilly B: Peripheral blood flow in menopausal women who have hot flushes and in those who do not. *BMJ* 298:1488-1490, 1989

187. Brass LM, Kisiel D, Sarrel PM: A correlation between estrogen and middle cerebral artery blood velocity at different times in the menstrual cycle in women with catamenial migraines. *J Cardiovasc Technol* 9:68, 1990

188. Collins P, Rosano GM, Jiang C, et al: Cardiovascular protection by oestrogen—a calcium antagonist effect? *Lancet* 341:1264-1265, 1993

189. Williams JK, Adams MR, Herrington DM, et al: Short-term administration of estrogen and vascular responses of atherosclerotic coronary arteries. *J Am Coll Cardiol* 20:452-457, 1992

190. Kushwaha SS, Bustami M, Lythall DA, et al: Coronary endothelial function in cardiac transplant recipients with accelerated coronary disease. *Coron Artery Dis* 5:147-154, 1994

191. Fuster V, Chesebro JH: Role of platelets and platelet inhibitors in aortocoronary artery vein-graft disease. *Circulation* 73:227-232, 1986

192. Landau C, Lange RA, Hillis LD: Percutaneous transluminal coronary angioplasty. *N Engl J Med* 330:981-993, 1994

193. Lange RA, Willard JE, Hillis LD: Southwestern internal medicine conference: restenosis: the Achilles heel of coronary angioplasty. *Am J Med Sci* 306:265-275, 1993

194. Libby P, Schwartz D, Brogi E, et al: A cascade model for restenosis. A special case of atherosclerosis progression. *Circulation* 86 Suppl 3:47-52, 1992

195. Haudenschild CC: Pathobiology of restenosis after angioplasty. *Am J Med* 94:40S-44S, 1993

196. Falk E: Plaque rupture with severe pre-existing stenosis precipitating coronary thrombosis. Characteristics of coronary atherosclerotic plaques underlying fatal occlusive thrombi. *Br Heart J* 50:127-134, 1983

197. Benson RL: Present status of coronary arterial disease. *Arch Pathol* 2:876-916, 1926

198. Constantinides P: Plaque fissures in human coronary thrombosis. *J Atheroscler Res* 6:1-17, 1966

199. Chandler AB: Mechanisms and frequency of thrombosis in the coronary circulation. *Thromb Res* 4 Suppl 1:3-23, 1974

200. Fulton WFM: Thrombosis and atherosclerosis: an essay on the genesis and microanatomy of atherosclerosis of the coronary arteries. In *The Coronary Arteries: Arteriography, Microanatomy, and Pathogenesis of Obliterative Coronary Artery Disease.* Springfield, Illinois, Charles C Thomas, 1965, pp 230-302

201. Ambrose JA, Winters SL, Stern A, et al: Angiographic morphology and the pathogenesis of unstable angina pectoris. *J Am Coll Cardiol* 5:609-616, 1985

202. Sherman CT, Litvack F, Grundfest W, et al: Coronary angioscopy in patients with unstable angina pectoris. *N Engl J Med* 315:913-919, 1986

203. Ambrose JA, Hjemdahl-Monsen CE, Borrico S, et al: Angiographic demonstration of a common link between unstable angina pectoris and non-Q-wave acute myocardial infarction. *Am J Cardiol* 61:244-247, 1988

204. Levin DC, Fallon JT: Significance of the angiographic morphology of localized coronary stenoses: histopathologic correlations. *Circulation* 66:316-320, 1982

205. Moise A, Lesperance J, Theroux P, et al: Clinical and angiographic predictors of new total coronary occlusion in coronary artery disease: analysis of 313 nonoperated patients. *Am J Cardiol* 54:1176-1181, 1984

206. Ambrose JA, Winters SL, Arora RR, et al: Angiographic evolution of coronary artery morphology in unstable angina. *J Am Coll Cardiol* 7:472-478, 1986

207. Giroud D, Li JM, Urban P, et al: Relation of the site of acute myocardial infarction to the most severe coronary arterial stenosis at prior angiography. *Am J Cardiol* 69:729-732, 1992

208. Nobuyoshi M, Tanaka M, Nosaka H, et al: Progression of coronary atherosclerosis: is coronary spasm related to progression? *J Am Coll Cardiol* 18:904-910, 1991

209. Brown BG, Gallery CA, Badger RS, et al: Incomplete lysis of thrombus in the moderate underlying atherosclerotic lesion during intracoronary infusion of streptokinase for acute myocardial infarction: quantitative angiographic observations. *Circulation* 73:653-661, 1986

210. Vallabhajosula S, Paidi M, Badimon JJ, et al: Radiotracers for low density lipoprotein biodistribution studies in vivo: technetium-99m low density lipoprotein versus radioiodinated low density lipoprotein preparations. *J Nucl Med* 29:1237-1245, 1988

211. Lees AM, Lees RS, Schoen FJ, et al: Imaging human atherosclerosis with ^{99m}Tc-labeled low density lipoproteins. *Arteriosclerosis* 8:461-470, 1988

212. Badimon L, Badimon JJ, Turitto VT, et al: Platelet thrombus formation on collagen type I. A model of deep vessel injury. Influence of blood rheology, von Willebrand factor, and blood coagulation. *Circulation* 78:1431-1442, 1988

213. Badimon L, Badimon JJ: Mechanisms of arterial thrombosis in nonparallel streamlines: platelet thrombi grow on the apex of stenotic severely injured vessel wall. Experimental study in the pig model. *J Clin Invest* 84:1134-1144, 1989

214. Lassila R, Badimon JJ, Vallabhajosula S, et al: Dynamic monitoring of platelet deposition on severely damaged vessel wall in flowing blood. Effects of different stenoses on thrombus growth. *Arteriosclerosis* 10:306-315, 1990

215. Drake TA, Morrissey JH, Edgington TS: Selective cellular expression of tissue factor in human tissues. Implications for disorders of hemostasis and thrombosis. *Am J Pathol* 134:1087-1097, 1989

216. Capone G, Wolf NM, Meyer B, et al: Frequency of intracoronary filling defects by angiography in angina pectoris at rest. *Am J Cardiol* 56:403-406, 1985

217. Hirsh PD, Hillis LD, Campbell WB, et al: Release of prostaglandins and thromboxane into the coronary circulation in patients with ischemic heart disease. *N Engl J Med* 304:685-691, 1981

218. Fitzgerald DJ, Roy L, Catella F, et al: Platelet activation in unstable coronary disease. *N Engl J Med* 315:983-989, 1986

219. van den Berg EK, Schmitz JM, Benedict CR, et al: Transcardiac serotonin concentration is increased in selected patients with limiting angina and complex coronary lesion morphology. *Circulation* 79:116-124, 1989

220. Willerson JT, Golino P, Eidt J, et al: Specific platelet mediators and unstable coronary artery lesions. Experimental evidence and potential clinical implications. *Circulation* 80:198-205, 1989

221. Willerson JT, Yao SK, McNatt J, et al: Frequency and severity of cyclic flow alternations and platelet aggregation predict the severity of neointimal proliferation following experimental coronary stenosis and endothelial injury. *Proc Natl Acad Sci U S A* 88:10624-10628, 1991

222. Fernandez-Ortiz A, Badimon JJ, Falk E, et al: Characterization of the relative thrombogenicity of atherosclerotic plaque components: implications for consequences of plaque rupture. *J Am Coll Cardiol* 23:1562-1569, 1994

223. Mailhac A, Badimon JJ, Fallon JT, et al: Effect of an eccentric severe stenosis on fibrin(ogen) deposition on severely damaged vessel wall in arterial thrombosis. Relative contribution of fibrin(ogen) and platelets. *Circulation* 90:988-996, 1994

224. Davies SW, Marchant B, Lyons JP, et al: Coronary lesion morphology in acute myocardial infarction: demonstration of early remodeling after streptokinase treatment. *J Am Coll Cardiol* 16:1079-1086, 1990

225. Rentrop KP, Feit F, Sherman W, et al: Serial angiographic assessment of coronary artery obstruction and collateral flow in acute myocardial infarction. Report from the second Mount Sinai-New York University Reperfusion Trial. *Circulation* 80:1166-1175, 1989

226. Van Lierde J, De Geest H, Verstraete M, et al: Angiographic assessment of the infarct-related residual coronary stenosis after spontaneous or therapeutic thrombolysis. *J Am Coll Cardiol* 16:1545-1549, 1990

227. Hackett D, Davies G, Chierchia S, et al: Intermittent coronary occlusion in acute myocardial infarction. Value of combined thrombolytic and vasodilator therapy. *N Engl J Med* 317:1055-1059, 1987

228. Davies SW, Marchant B, Lyons JP, et al: Irregular coronary lesion morphology after thrombolysis predicts early clinical instability. *J Am Coll Cardiol* 18:669-674, 1991

229. Badimon L, Badimon JJ, Lassila R, et al: Re-thrombosis on an evolving thrombus is mediated by thrombus-bound thrombin that is not inhibited by systemic heparin (abstract). *Thromb Haemost* 65 Suppl:321, 1991

230. Fitzgerald DJ, Fitzgerald GA: Role of thrombin and thromboxane A_2 in reocclusion following coronary thrombolysis with tissue-type plasminogen activator. *Proc Natl Acad Sci U S A* 86:7585-7589, 1989

231. Francis CW, Markham RE Jr, Barlow GH, et al: Thrombin activity of fibrin thrombi and soluble plasmic derivatives. *J Lab Clin Med* 102:220-230, 1983

232. Meyer BJ, Badimon JJ, Mailhac A, et al: Inhibition of growth of thrombus on fresh mural thrombus. Targeting optimal therapy. *Circulation* 90:2432-2438, 1994

233. Weitz JI, Hudoba M: Mechanism by which clot-bound thrombin is protected from inactivation by fluid-phase inhibitors (abstract). *Circulation* 86 Suppl 1:413, 1992

234. Fitzgerald DJ, Catella F, Roy L, et al: Marked platelet activation in vivo after intravenous streptokinase in patients with acute myocardial infarction. *Circulation* 77:142-150, 1988

235. Eisenberg PR, Sherman LA, Jaffe AS: Paradoxic elevation of fibrinopeptide A after streptokinase: evidence for continued thrombosis despite intense fibrinolysis. *J Am Coll Cardiol* 10:527-529, 1987

236. Badimon L, Lassila R, Badimon J, et al: An acute surge of epinephrine stimulates platelet deposition to severely damaged vascular wall (abstract). *J Am Coll Cardiol* 15 Suppl A:181, 1990

237. Grignani G, Soffiantino F, Zucchella M, et al: Platelet activation by emotional stress in patients with coronary artery disease. *Circulation* 83 Suppl 2:128-136, 1991

238. Yeung AC, Vekshtein VI, Krantz DS, et al: The effect of atherosclerosis on the vasomotor response of coronary arteries to mental stress. *N Engl J Med* 325:1551-1556, 1991

239. Muller JE, Stone PH, Turi ZG, et al: Circadian variation in the frequency of onset of acute myocardial infarction. *N Engl J Med* 313:1315-1322, 1985

240. Tofler GH, Brezinski D, Schafer AI, et al: Concurrent morning increase in platelet aggregability and the risk of myocardial infarction and sudden cardiac death. *N Engl J Med* 316:1514-1518, 1987

241. Willich SN, Linderer T, Wegscheider K, et al: Increased morning incidence of myocardial infarction in the ISAM Study: absence with prior beta-adrenergic blockade. *Circulation* 80:853-858, 1989

242. Winniford MD, Wheelan KR, Kremers MS, et al: Smoking-induced coronary vasoconstriction in patients with atherosclerotic coronary artery disease: evidence for adrenergically mediated alterations in coronary artery tone. *Circulation* 73:662-667, 1986

243. Buhler FR, Vesanen K, Watters JT, et al: Impact of smoking on heart attacks, strokes, blood pressure control, drug dose, and quality of life aspects in the International Prospective Primary Prevention Study in Hypertension. *Am Heart J* 115:282-288, 1988

244. Hunt BJ: The relation between abnormal hemostatic function and the progression of coronary disease. *Curr Opin Cardiol* 5:758-765, 1990

245. Badimon JJ, Badimon L, Turitto VT, et al: Platelet deposition at high shear rates is enhanced by high plasma cholesterol levels. In vivo study in the rabbit model. *Arterioscler Thromb* 11:395-402, 1991

246. Genest JJ Jr, McNamara JR, Upson B, et al: Prevalence of familial hyperhomocyst (e) inemia in men with premature coronary artery disease. *Arterioscler Thromb* 11:1129-1136, 1991

247. Rosengren A, Wilhelmsen L, Eriksson E, et al: Lipoprotein (a) and coronary heart disease: a prospective case-control study in a general population sample of middle aged men. *BMJ* 301:1248-1251, 1990

248. Dahlen GH, Guyton JR, Attar M, et al: Association of levels of lipoprotein Lp(a), plasma lipids, and other lipoproteins with coronary artery disease documented by angiography. *Circulation* 74:758-765, 1986

249. Seed M, Hoppichler F, Reaveley D, et al: Relation of serum lipoprotein(a) concentration and apolipoprotein(a) phenotype to coronary heart disease in patients with familial hypercholesterolemia. *N Engl J Med* 322:1494-1499, 1990

250. McLean JW, Tomlinson JE, Kuang WJ, et al: cDNA sequence of human apolipoprotein(a) is homologous to plasminogen. *Nature* 330: 132-137, 1987

251. Frank SL, Klisak I, Sparkes RS, et al: The apolipoprotein(a) gene resides on human chromosome 6q26-27, in close proximity to the homologous gene for plasminogen. *Hum Genet* 79:352-356, 1988

252. Loscalzo J: Lipoprotein(a). A unique risk factor for atherothrombotic disease. *Arteriosclerosis* 10:672-679, 1990

253. Olofsson BO, Dahlen G, Nilsson TK: Evidence for increased levels of plasminogen activator inhibitor and tissue plasminogen activator in plasma of patients with angiographically verified coronary artery disease. *Eur Heart J* 10:77-82, 1989

254. Hamsten A, de Faire U, Walldius G, et al: Plasminogen activator inhibitor in plasma: risk factor for recurrent myocardial infarction. *Lancet* 2:3-9, 1987

255. Aznar J, Estelles A, Tormo G, et al: Plasminogen activator inhibitor activity and other fibrinolytic variables in patients with coronary artery disease. *Br Heart J* 59:535-541, 1988

256. Oseroff A, Krishnamurti C, Hassett A, et al: Plasminogen activator and plasminogen activator inhibitor activities in men with coronary artery disease. *J Lab Clin Med* 113:88-93, 1990

257. Meade TW, North WR, Chakrabarti R, et al: Haemostatic function and cardiovascular death: early results of a prospective study. *Lancet* 1:1050-1054, 1980

258. Kannel WB, D'Agostino RB, Belanger AJ: Fibrinogen, cigarette smoking, and risk of cardiovascular disease: insights from the Framingham Study. *Am Heart J* 113:1006-1010, 1987

259. McGill DA, Ardlie NG: The relationship between blood fibrinogen level and coronary artery disease. *Coron Artery Dis* 1:557-565, 1990

260. Rosengren A, Wilhelmsen L, Welin L, et al: Social influences and cardiovascular risk factors as determinants of plasma fibrinogen concentration in a general population sample of middle aged men. *BMJ* 300:634-638, 1990

261. Scarabin PY, Bonithon-Kopp C, Bara L, et al: Factor VII activation and menopausal status. *Thromb Res* 57:227-234, 1990

262. Maseri A, L'Abbate A, Baroldi G, et al: Coronary vasospasm as a possible cause of myocardial infarction. A conclusion derived from the study of "preinfarction" angina. *N Engl J Med* 299:1271-1277, 1978

263. Lam JY, Chesebro JH, Steele PM, et al: Is vasospasm related to platelet deposition? Relationship in a porcine preparation of arterial injury in vivo. *Circulation* 75:243-248, 1987

264. Vanhoutte PM, Shimokawa H: Endothelium-derived relaxing factor and coronary vasospasm. *Circulation* 80:1-9, 1989

265. Fischell TA, Derby G, Tse TM, et al: Coronary artery vasoconstriction routinely occurs after percutaneous transluminal coronary angioplasty. A quantitative arteriographic analysis. *Circulation* 78:1323-1334, 1988

266. el-Tamimi H, Davies GJ, Hackett D, et al: Abnormal vasomotor changes early after coronary angioplasty. A quantitative arteriographic study of their time course. *Circulation* 84:1198-1202, 1991

267. Araki H, Nishi K, Jougasaki M: Effects of thrombosis on vascular tone in rat mesenteric arteries with endothelium in vivo. *Circ Res* 67:312-318, 1990

268. Lerman A, Webster MW, Chesebro JH, et al: Circulating and tissue endothelin immunoreactivity in hypercholesterolemic pigs. *Circulation* 88:2923-2928, 1993

269. McLenachan JM, Vita J, Fish DR, et al: Early evidence of endothelial vasodilator dysfunction at coronary branch points. *Circulation* 82:1169-1173, 1990

270. Cohen RA, Zitnay KM, Haudenschild CC, et al: Loss of selective endothelial cell vasoactive functions caused by hypercholesterolemia in pig coronary arteries. *Circ Res* 63:903-910, 1988

271. Osborne JA, Lento PH, Siegfried MR, et al: Cardiovascular effects of acute hypercholesterolemia in rabbits. Reversal with lovastatin treatment. *J Clin Invest* 83:465-473, 1989

272. McLenachan JM, Williams JK, Fish RD, et al: Loss of flow-mediated endothelium-dependent dilation occurs early in the development of atherosclerosis. *Circulation* 84:1273-1278, 1991

273. Zeiher AM, Drexler H, Wollschlager H, et al: Modulation of coronary vasomotor tone in humans. Progressive endothelial dysfunction with different early stages of coronary atherosclerosis. *Circulation* 83:391-401, 1991

274. Willerson JT, Hillis LD, Winniford M, et al: Speculation regarding mechanisms responsible for acute ischemic heart disease syndromes. *J Am Coll Cardiol* 8:245-250, 1986

275. Braunwald E: Unstable angina. A classification. *Circulation* 80:410-414, 1989

276. Gotoh K, Minamino T, Katoh O, et al: The role of intracoronary thrombus in unstable angina: angiographic assessment and thrombolytic therapy during ongoing anginal attacks. *Circulation* 77:526-534, 1988

277. DeWood MA, Stifter WF, Simpson CS, et al: Coronary arteriographic findings soon after non-Q-wave myocardial infarction. *N Engl J Med* 315:417-423, 1986

278. Gibson RS, Beller GA, Gheorghiade M, et al: The prevalence and clinical significance of residual myocardial ischemia 2 weeks after uncomplicated non-Q wave infarction: a prospective natural history study. *Circulation* 73:1186-1198, 1986

279. Timmis AD, Griffin B, Crick JC, et al: The effects of early coronary patency on the evolution of myocardial infarction: a prospective arteriographic study. *Br Heart J* 58:345-351, 1987

280. Fuster V, Stein B, Ambrose JA, et al: Atherosclerotic plaque rupture and thrombosis. Evolving concepts. *Circulation* 82 Suppl 2:47-59, 1990

281. Maseri A, Crea F, Cianflone D: Myocardial ischemia caused by distal coronary vasoconstriction (editorial). *Am J Cardiol* 70:1602-1605, 1992

282. Egashira K, Inou T, Hirooka Y, et al: Impaired coronary blood flow response to acetylcholine in patients with coronary risk factors and proximal atherosclerotic lesions. *J Clin Invest* 91:29-37, 1993

283. Fuster V, Frye RL, Kennedy MA, et al: The role of collateral circulation in the various coronary syndromes. *Circulation* 59:1137-1144, 1979

284. Habib GB, Heibig J, Forman SA, et al: Influence of coronary collateral vessels on myocardial infarct size in humans. Results of phase I Thrombolysis in Myocardial Infarction (TIMI) trial. The TIMI Investigators. *Circulation* 83:739-746, 1991

285. Cohen M, Sherman W, Rentrop KP, et al: Determinants of collateral filling observed during sudden controlled coronary artery occlusion in human subjects. *J Am Coll Cardiol* 13:297-303, 1989

286. Patterson RE, Jones-Collins BA, Aamodt R, et al: Differences in collateral myocardial blood flow following gradual vs abrupt coronary occlusion. *Cardiovasc Res* 17:207-213, 1983

287. Cohen MV, Yipintsoi T, Scheuer J: Coronary collateral stimulation by exercise in dogs with stenotic coronary arteries. *J Appl Physiol* 52:664-671, 1982

288. Bloor CM, White FC, Sanders TM: Effects of exercise on collateral development in myocardial ischemia in pigs. *J Appl Physiol* 56:656-665, 1984

289. Badimon JJ, Badimon L, Galvez A, et al: High density lipoprotein plasma fractions inhibit aortic fatty streaks in cholesterol-fed rabbits. *Lab Invest* 60:455-461, 1989

290. Badimon JJ, Badimon L, Fuster V: Regression of atherosclerotic lesions by high density lipoprotein plasma fraction in the cholesterol-fed rabbit. *J Clin Invest* 85:1234-1241, 1990

291. Brown G, Albers JJ, Fisher LD, et al: Regression of coronary artery disease as a result of intensive lipid-lowering therapy in men with high levels of apolipoprotein B. *N Engl J Med* 323:1289-1298, 1990

292. Ornish D, Brown SE, Scherwitz LW, et al: Can lifestyle changes reverse coronary heart disease? The Lifestyle Heart Trial. *Lancet* 336:129-133, 1990

293. Blankenhorn DH, Nessim SA, Johnson RL, et al: Beneficial effects of combined colestipol-niacin therapy on coronary atherosclerosis and coronary venous bypass grafts. *JAMA* 257:3233-3240, 1987

294. Brensike JF, Levy RI, Kelsey SF, et al: Effects of therapy with cholestyramine on progression of coronary arteriosclerosis: results of the NHLBI Type II Coronary Intervention Study. *Circulation* 69:313-324, 1984

295. Cashin-Hemphill L, Mack WJ, Pogoda JM, et al: Beneficial effects of colestipol-niacin on coronary atherosclerosis. A 4-year follow-up. *JAMA* 264:3013-3017, 1990

296. Buchwald H, Varco RL, Matts JP, et al: Effect of partial ileal bypass surgery on mortality and morbidity from coronary heart disease in patients with hypercholesterolemia. Report of the Program on the Surgical Control of the Hyperlipidemias (POSCH). *N Engl J Med* 323:946-955, 1990

297. Watts GF, Lewis B, Brunt JN, et al: Effects on coronary artery disease of lipid-lowering diet, or diet plus cholestyramine, in the St Thomas' Atherosclerosis Regression Study (STARS). *Lancet* 339:563-569, 1992

298. Vogel RA: Comparative clinical consequences of aggressive lipid management, coronary angioplasty and bypass surgery in coronary artery disease (editorial). *Am J Cardiol* 69:1229-1233, 1992

299. Haskell WL, Alderman EL, Fair JM, et al: Effects of intensive multiple risk factor reduction on coronary atherosclerosis and clinical cardiac events in men and women with coronary artery disease. The Stanford Coronary Risk Intervention Project (SCRIP). *Circulation* 89:975-990, 1994

300. Waters D, Higginson L, Gladstone P, et al: Effects of monotherapy with an HMG-CoA reductase inhibitor on the progression of coronary atherosclerosis as assessed by serial quantitative arteriography. The Canadian Coronary Atherosclerosis Intervention Trial. *Circulation* 89:959-968, 1994

301. Brown BG, Zhao XQ, Sacco DE, et al: Lipid lowering and plaque regression. New insights into prevention of plaque disruption and clinical events in coronary disease. *Circulation* 87:1781-1791, 1993

302. Loree HM, Tobias BJ, Gibson LJ, et al: Mechanical properties of model atherosclerotic lesion lipid pools. *Arterioscler Thromb* 14:230-234, 1994

303. Pearson TA, Marx HJ: The rapid reduction in cardiac events with lipid-lowering therapy: mechanisms and implications (editorial). *Am J Cardiol* 72:1072-1073, 1993

304. Pfeffer MA, Braunwald E, Moye LA, et al: Effect of captopril on mortality and morbidity in patients with left ventricular dysfunction after myocardial infarction. Results of the Survival and Ventricular Enlargement trial. *N Engl J Med* 327:669-677, 1992

305. The SOLVD Investigators: Effect of enalapril on mortality and the development of heart failure in asymptomatic patients with reduced left ventricular ejection fractions. *N Engl J Med* 327:685-691, 1992

306. Francis GS: Neuroendocrine activity in congestive heart failure. *Am J Cardiol* 66:33D-38D, 1990

307. Yusuf S, Peto R, Lewis J, et al: Beta blockade during and after myocardial infarction: an overview of the randomized trials. *Prog Cardiovasc Dis* 27:335-371, 1985

308. Frishman WH, Lazar EJ: Reduction of mortality, sudden death and non-fatal reinfarction with beta-adrenergic blockers in survivors of acute myocardial infarction: a new hypothesis regarding the cardioprotective action of beta-adrenergic blockade. *Am J Cardiol* 66:66G-70G, 1990

309. Loree HM, Kamm RD, Stringfellow RG, et al: Effects of fibrous cap thickness on peak circumferential stress in model atherosclerotic vessels. *Circ Res* 71:850-858, 1992

310. Fuster V, Dyken ML, Vokonas PS, et al: Aspirin as a therapeutic agent in cardiovascular disease. *Circulation* 87:659-675, 1993

311. Hirsh J, Fuster V: Guide to anticoagulant therapy. 1. Heparin. *Circulation* 89:1449-1468, 1994

312. Hirsh J, Fuster V: Guide to anticoagulant therapy. 2. Oral anticoagulants. *Circulation* 89:1469-1480, 1994

313. Antiplatelet Trialists' Collaboration: Collaborative overview of randomised trials of antiplatelet therapy—I: prevention of death, myocardial infarction, and stroke by prolonged antiplatelet therapy in various categories of patients. *BMJ* 308:81-106, 1994

314. Antiplatelet Trialists' Collaboration: Collaborative overview of randomised trials of antiplatelet therapy—II: maintenance of vascular graft or arterial patency by antiplatelet therapy. *BMJ* 308:159-168, 1994

315. ISIS-2 (Second International Study of Infarct Survival) Collaborative Group: Randomised trial of intravenous streptokinase, oral aspirin, both, or neither among 17,187 cases of suspected acute myocardial infarction: ISIS-2. *Lancet* 2:349-360, 1988

316. Smith P: Antithrombotic therapy in the chronic phase of myocardial infarction. In *Thrombosis in Cardiovascular Disorders.* Edited by V Fuster, M Verstraete. Philadelphia, WB Saunders Company, 1992, pp 343-362

317. Cohen M, Adams PC, Parry G, et al: Combination antithrombotic therapy in unstable rest angina and non-Q-wave infarction in nonprior aspirin users. Primary end points analysis from the ATACS trial. *Circulation* 89:81-88, 1994

318. Topol EJ, Fuster V, Harrington RA, et al: Recombinant hirudin for unstable angina pectoris. A multicenter, randomized angiographic trial. *Circulation* 89:1557-1566, 1994

319. Cannon CP, McCabe CH, Henry TD, et al: A pilot trial of recombinant desulfatohirudin compared with heparin in conjunction with tissue-type plasminogen activator and aspirin for acute myocardial infarction: results of the Thrombolysis in Myocardial Infarction (TIMI) 5 trial. *J Am Coll Cardiol* 23:993-1003, 1994

320. van den Bos AA, Deckers JW, Heyndrickx GR, et al: PTCA with hirudin associated with less acute cardiac complications than with heparin (abstract). *Circulation* 86 Suppl 1:372, 1992

321. Lidon RM, Theroux P, Lesperance J, et al: A pilot, early angiographic patency study using a direct thrombin inhibitor as adjunctive therapy to streptokinase in acute myocardial infarction. *Circulation* 89:1567-1572, 1994

322. Topol EJ, Bonan R, Jewitt D, et al: Use of a direct antithrombin, hirulog, in place of heparin during coronary angioplasty. *Circulation* 87:1622-1629, 1993

323. Fuchs J, McCabe CH, Antman EM, et al: Hirulog in the treatment of unstable angina: results of the TIMI 7 trial (abstract). *J Am Coll Cardiol* 23 Suppl A:56, 1994

324. Simoons ML, de Boer MJ, van den Brand MJ, et al: Randomized trial of a GPIIb/IIIa platelet receptor blocker in refractory unstable angina. *Circulation* 89:596-603, 1994

325. Kleiman NS, Ohman EM, Califf RM, et al: Profound inhibition of platelet aggregation with monoclonal antibody 7E3 Fab after thrombolytic therapy. Results of the Thrombolysis and Angioplasty in Myocardial Infarction (TAMI) 8 Pilot Study. *J Am Coll Cardiol* 22:381-389, 1993

326. Califf RM, Shadoff N, Valett N, et al: Use of a monoclonal antibody directed against the platelet glycoprotein IIB/IIIA receptor in high-risk coronary angioplasty. *N Engl J Med* 330:956-961, 1994

327. Schulman SP, Goldschmidt-Clermont PJ, Navetta FI, et al: Integrelin in unstable angina: a double-blind randomized trial (abstract). *Circulation* 88 Suppl 1:608, 1993

328. Tcheng JE, Kleiman NS, Harrington RA, et al: Outcome of patients treated with the GPIIb/IIIa inhibitor integrelin during coronary angioplasty: results of the IMPACT study (abstract). *Circulation* 88 Suppl 1:595, 1993

CHAPTER

28

Atherosclerosis

B. Antithrombotic agents in cardiac disease: platelet inhibitors, anticoagulants, and thrombolytic agents

Valentin Fuster, M.D., William P. Fay, M.D., and James H. Chesebro, M.D.

HEMOSTASIS is a major body defense mechanism. This process is activated to prevent the loss of blood after vascular injury and depends on complex interactions among the dynamics of blood flow, components of the vessel wall, blood platelets, and plasma proteins. A thrombus can be considered as the product of an unregulated or inappropriate form of hemostasis and is composed of a mass of cellular material held together by a fibrous network. The relative proportion of cells to fibrin may vary considerably, depending on other conditions that cause formation of the thrombus and on its age.[1a]

The primary condition affecting the composition of a thrombus is the nature of blood flow.[2] Under conditions of relatively slow flow, as in a vein or within the chambers of the heart, thrombi resemble blood clots formed in vitro; the cellular elements are uniformly distributed, and the fibrin lattice is a major component of such "red" thrombi. Conventional anticoagulants, such as heparin and warfarin sodium (Coumadin), are usually effective in the management of these thrombi because they interfere with the process of fibrin formation.[3]

Thrombi that develop in areas of rapid flow, such as systemic arteries, have a different pathogenesis and different morphologic features. Formation of such thrombi is primarily related to interaction of an abnormal vascular surface with elements of blood, particularly platelets.[2] An example is development of thrombus on an ulcerated atherosclerotic plaque of a coronary artery. Such thrombi consist of a predominant platelet-rich component near the interface with the damaged vascular wall (with some fibrin formation to maintain the stability of the platelet thrombus) and of a predominant fibrin component with erythrocytes and leukocytes more distally.[3] The proximal concentration of platelets may give the "head" of the thrombi a white appearance.[1a] Thus, platelets play a major role in thrombus formation and embolization, especially in the arterial system. In addition, platelet deposition and thrombus formation can contribute to the growth and progression of atherosclerotic plaques. For these reasons, considerable attention has been focused recently on the question of whether drugs that inhibit certain platelet functions can prevent or modify the course of arterial thromboembolic disease and atherosclerotic disease in humans.[1b,1c]

This chapter addresses the following issues: (1) the role of platelet activation and fibrin formation in thrombogenesis, (2) clinicopathologic presentation and fate of the thrombus, (3) pathogenesis of thrombosis and embolism in coronary arteries, cardiac chambers, and prosthetic valves, (4) pharmacology of the antithrombotic agents, and (5) the role of antithrombotic therapy in cardiac disease.

Some sections of this chapter are a modification of Ip JH, Fuster V, Fay WP, et al: Antithrombotic therapy in cardiac disease. In *Cardiology: An Illustrated Text/Reference.* Vol. 1: Physiology, Pharmacology, Diagnosis. Philadelphia, JB Lippincott Company, 1991, pp 2.143-2.171.

ROLE OF PLATELET ACTIVATION AND FIBRIN FORMATION IN THROMBOGENESIS

An arterial thrombus appears to develop in three phases (Fig 28B-1): platelet adhesion, platelet aggregation, and activation of the clotting mechanisms. In addition, endogenous inhibitors tend to limit thrombus formation or extension.

Platelet adhesion: role of collagen fibers and von Willebrand's factor

The term "platelet adhesion" refers to the attachment of platelets to a surface other than another platelet. Platelets tend to adhere to damaged or disrupted endothelial

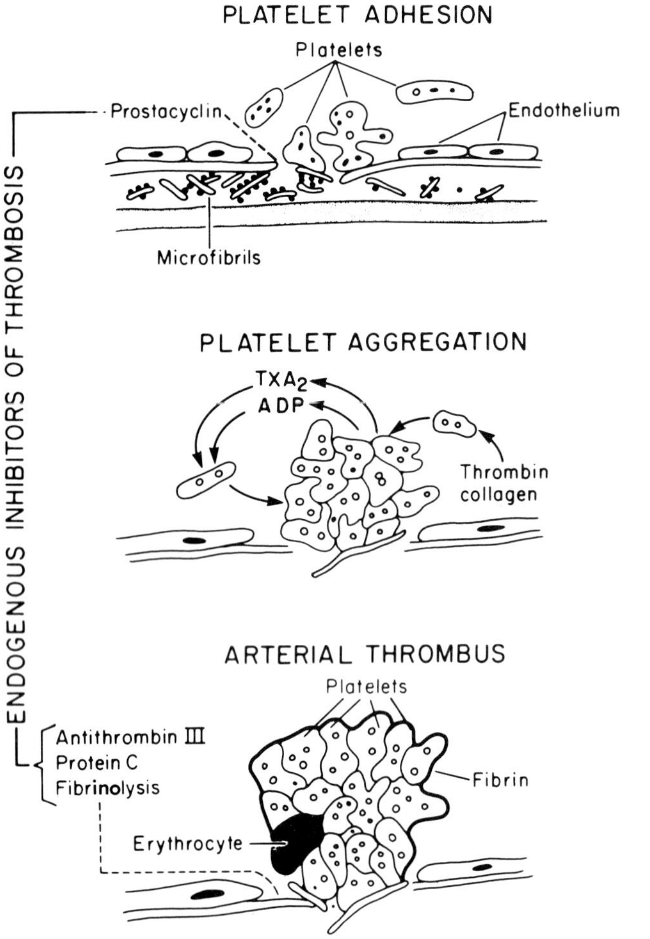

Fig 28B-1 Microscopic phases of arterial thrombus formation: platelet adhesion and spreading, platelet aggregation, activation of the coagulation system and thrombus formation, and activation of the endogenous inhibitors of thrombosis. *Dashed line* denotes an inhibitory reaction. *ADP,* adenosine diphosphate; *TXA*$_2$, thromboxane A_2 (From Stein B, Fuster V, Israel DH, et al: Platelet inhibitor agents in cardiovascular disease: an update. *J Am Coll Cardiol* 14:813-836, 1989. By permission of the American College of Cardiology.)

surfaces, such as an ulcerated atherosclerotic plaque, or to an artificial surface, such as a prosthetic heart valve, a Scribner arteriovenous shunt for hemodialysis, or a peripheral vascular prosthetic graft. Circulating platelets do not adhere to intact endothelium. After removal of the endothelial lining of a normal blood vessel by a mild or superficial injury, the subendothelium becomes coated by a layer of adherent platelets.[4] Adhesion depends on the interaction of platelet membrane glycoproteins with several components of the subendothelial matrix[4] (Fig 28B-2). Glycoprotein Ib appears to be important for initial contact of platelets with von Willebrand's factor on the subendothelial surface. Glycoprotein Ia, which binds to exposed subendothelial collagen, may also be important. The glycoprotein IIb-IIIa complex binds von Willebrand's factor, fibronectin, and fibrinogen.

In the clinical context, subtle injury of the endothelial cell layer—for example, that produced by flowing blood at arterial branch points or through stenoses—may trigger platelet adhesion. The release of platelet and endothelial cell growth factors may contribute to the early process of atherogenesis. In the acute coronary syndromes, severe vascular injury (plaque disruption) exposes components of the arterial media, particularly smooth muscle cells (contain prothrombin and provide lipid [cell] membrane for formation of prothrombin activator complex, which markedly accelerates thrombin generation) and fibrillar collagen (with type I being more prevalent in diseased vessels and type III in normal vessels), which in addition to other mediators discussed later, induces platelet adhesion, aggregation, and thrombus formation.[4-8] In addition, the atheromatous fatty core, which is associated with and exposed after disruption of the plaque, is the most thrombogenic component of human atherosclerotic plaques. Platelet deposition is fourfold to sixfold greater on atheromatous core than on other plaque components, such as collagen.[9]

Platelet adhesion is determined not only by the degree of vascular injury as described above but also by transportation to the injured area. Transportation is determined by the wall shear rate, which is a measure of the difference in blood velocity between the center of the vessel and along the wall. At higher wall shear rates, characteristic of medium-sized stenotic arteries, the initial platelet deposition rate and maximum extent of deposition are significantly higher.[10,11]

On artificial surfaces, the process of platelet adhesion is less understood. A film of adsorbed plasma proteins forms immediately after exposure of the surface to blood, and apparently different surfaces become coated with different proteins that, by means of their surface charge, react differently with platelets.[12] Among the adsorbed plasma proteins that have been studied are fibrinogen, which tends to increase platelet adherence, and albumin, which tends to have the opposite effect.

Platelet aggregation and release: role of collagen, thrombin, thromboxane A_2, adenosine diphosphate, and serotonin

In this second stage, platelets adhere to each other and the platelet mass builds (see Fig 28B-1). Platelet aggregation appears to depend primarily on an increase in cytoplasmic calcium, which is mediated by three pathways. First, concomitant with the process of platelet adhesion, there is an activation of platelets by extrinsic stimuli, specifically collagen and thrombin; second, during such platelet activation, there is the release of platelet intracytoplasmic granule constituents, particularly adenosine diphosphate (ADP), which further activate neighboring platelets and cause aggregation; and third, also during platelet activation, there are synthesis and release of the platelet prostanoid thromboxane A_2 (TXA_2), which also causes platelet aggregation.

The primary and pivotal role of thrombin in the in vivo

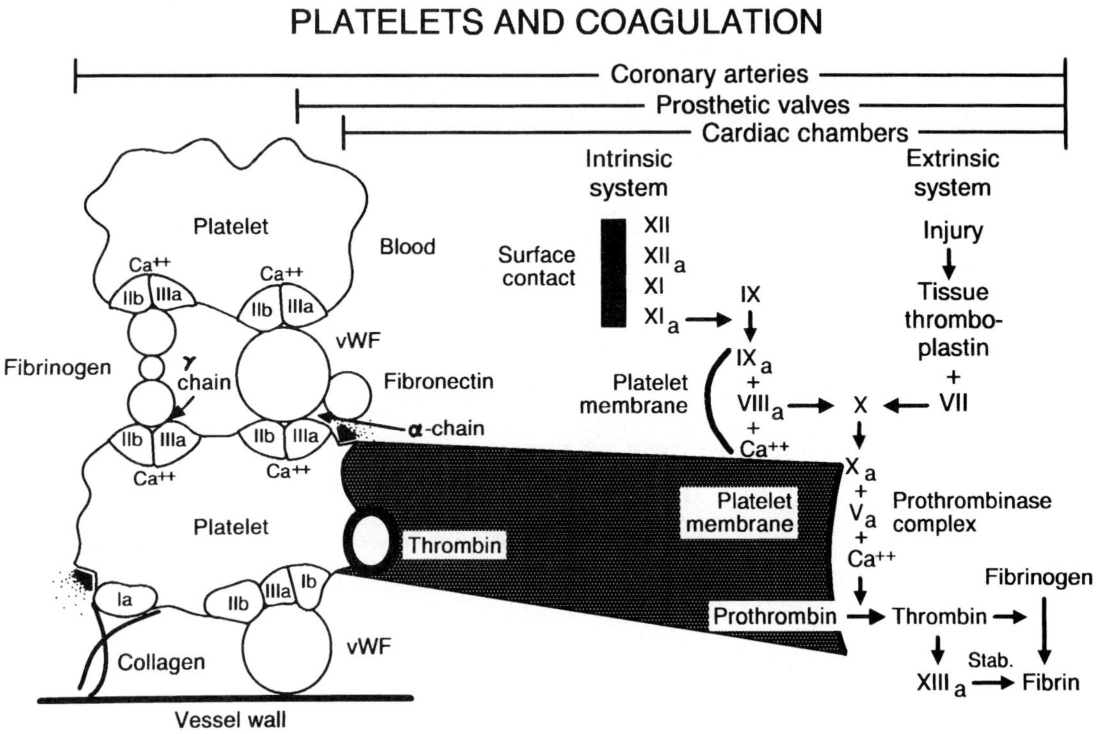

Fig 28B-2 **Left,** interactions among platelet membrane receptors (glycoproteins Ia, Ib, and IIb/IIIa), adhesive macromolecules, and the disrupted vessel wall. **Right,** the intrinsic and extrinsic systems of the coagulation cascade. Note the interaction between clotting factors and the platelet membrane. *Ca,* calcium; *Stab.,* stabilization; *vWF,* von Willebrand's factor. (Modified from Stein B, Fuster V, Halperin JL, et al: Antithrombotic therapy in cardiac disease: an emerging approach based on pathogenesis and risk. *Circulation* 80:1501-1513, 1989.)

aggregation of platelets and maintenance of the platelet thrombus by thrombin is documented by the action of the direct and specific thrombin inhibitor hirudin. After deep arterial injury, hirudin blocks platelet thrombus formation and limits platelet deposition to a single layer or less.[13] In addition, administration of hirudin 30 minutes after the formation of arterial thrombus leads to deaggregation of in vivo arterial thrombus by 90% over the next hour.[14] This finding shows that maintenance of platelet-rich arterial thrombus also depends on continued thrombin activity.

The first pathway. As discussed above, in certain pathologic situations, such as when an atherosclerotic plaque disrupts, extrinsic factors may be very potent in triggering calcium release and platelet aggregation. Specifically, exposed collagen, smooth muscle cells, and lipid core or gruel initiates thrombin generation from activation of the extrinsic and intrinsic clotting systems (Figs 28B-2 and 28B-3). Through the actions of these extrinsic activators, calcium is then released from the platelet-dense tubular system into the cytoplasm, which, in turn, is associated with the activation of the actin-myosin system. These reactions in the adherent platelets and in the circulating neighboring platelets cause platelet contraction and the release of ADP and serotonin (see second pathway). In addition, TXA_2 is synthesized and released[4,15] (see third pathway). Collagen and thrombin may have a direct effect on platelets, possibly through a platelet-activating factor (see Fig 28B-3) that may expose the platelet membrane glycoprotein IIb-IIIa complex to fibrinogen and von Willebrand's factor and thus promote aggregation[4, 15-17] (see Figs 28B-2 and 28B-3). For the purpose of this discussion, these reactions, which depend on collagen and thrombin, constitute the first pathway of platelet activation and aggregation. Both collagen and thrombin are strong agonists (cause secretion of platelet α granules and dense bodies regardless of aggregation, do not require TXA_2 for aggregation, and are not blocked by aspirin).[17] The primary role of thrombin in comparison with TXA_2 in the continuous growth of thrombus on fresh thrombus is documented by the total inhibition of thrombus growth by the specific thrombin inhibitor hirudin and no effect by aspirin.

The second pathway. After the adherent platelets and circulating neighboring platelets have been exposed to collagen and thrombin, the second pathway may be activated. This pathway is mediated by ADP and serotonin, which are weak agonists (cause aggregation only when TXA_2 is produced; platelet secretion depends on aggregation)[17] released from platelet-dense granules after contraction (see Figs 28B-2 and 28B-3). ADP is a potent

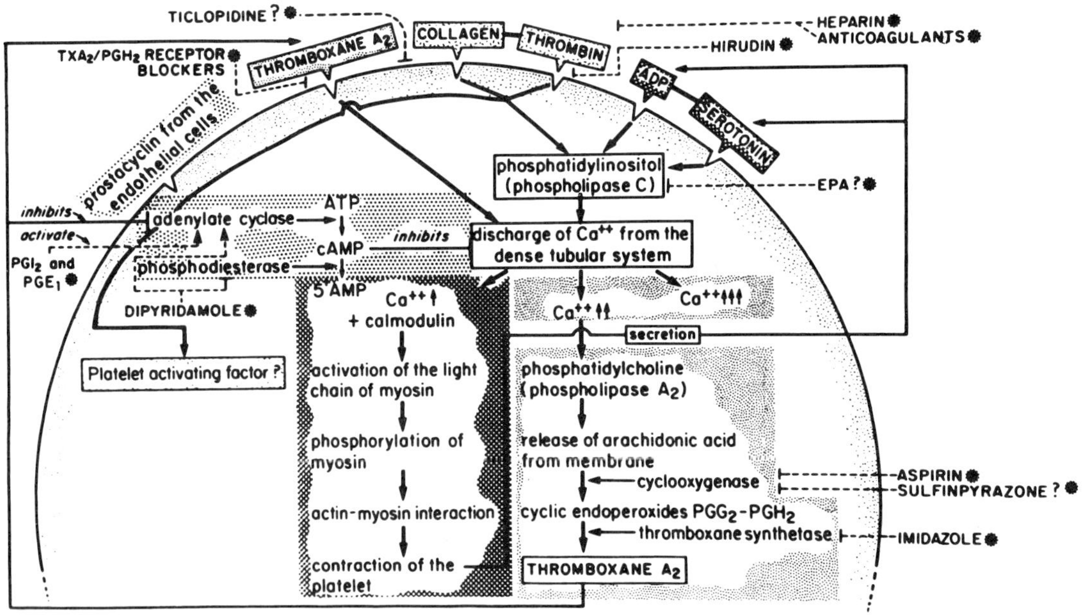

Fig 28B-3 Mechanisms of platelet activation and presumed sites of action of various platelet inhibitor agents. Platelet agonists lead to the mobilization of calcium *(Ca^{++})*, which functions as a mediator of platelet activation through metabolic pathways dependent on adenosine diphosphate *(ADP)*, thromboxane A_2 *(TXA_2)*, thrombin, and collagen. Cyclic adenosine monophosphate *(cAMP)* inhibits calcium mobilization from the dense tubular system. Note that thrombin and collagen may independently activate platelets by means of platelet-activating factor. *Asterisk* (*) indicates a platelet inhibitor. *Dashed line* indicates a presumed site of drug action. *ATP,* adenosine triphosphate; *EPA,* eicosapentaenoic acid; *PGE_1,* prostaglandin E_1; *PGG_2,* prostaglandin G_2; *PGH_2,* prostaglandin H_2; *PGI_2,* prostaglandin I_2. (From Stein B, Fuster V, Israel DH, et al: Platelet inhibitor agents in cardiovascular disease: an update. *J Am Coll Cardiol* 14:813-836, 1989. By permission of the American College of Cardiology.)

inducer of platelet aggregation in the presence of calcium and fibrinogen. It stimulates neighboring platelets and, most importantly, exposes the platelet membrane glycoprotein IIb-IIIa complex,[4,15,16,18,19] thus promoting aggregation (see Figs 28B-2 and 28B-3). Furthermore, the turbulence present in stenotic areas and at branching points within the arterial tree promotes erythrocyte lysis, with the subsequent release of ADP, which activates platelets and promotes their aggregation.

The third pathway. After the adherent platelets have been exposed to collagen and thrombin, a third pathway of TXA_2 synthesis may be activated (see Figs 28B-2 and 28B-3). This pathway is mediated by arachidonic acid, which is released from the platelet membrane by the action of phospholipase A_2 on phosphatidylcholine.[20] Cyclooxygenase converts arachidonic acid into proaggregatory prostaglandin endoperoxide intermediates (prostaglandins G_2 and H_2); TXA_2 is formed by the action of thromboxane synthetase, particularly on prostaglandin H_2. TXA_2 is both a potent platelet-aggregating agent and a vasoconstrictor. It stimulates platelet aggregation by promoting the mobilization of intracellular calcium, which causes a conformational change in the glycoprotein IIb-IIIa complex. This results in exposure of previously occult binding sites for fibrinogen and von Willebrand's factor and, thus, promotion of aggregation[4,15,16,18,19] (see Figs 28B-2 and 28B-3). In addition, short interaction between a-thrombin and platelets triggers long-lasting exposure of glycoprotein IIb-IIIa receptors. Prostacyclin induces rapid closure of glycoprotein IIb-IIIa binding sites on platelets. However, thrombin-treated platelets cannot close glycoprotein IIb-IIIa binding sites, which remain open as long as thrombin remains bound to platelets.[21]

In summary, collagen, fatty gruel, thrombin, and products of platelet secretion such as ADP and TXA_2 enhance the thrombotic process by stimulating platelets and causing the exposure of platelet membrane glycoprotein receptors to fibrinogen and von Willebrand's factor. These reactions promote further platelet aggregation and thrombus growth. The pivotal role of thrombin is documented by its specific inhibition with hirudin for the prevention of thrombosis[13] and thrombus growth[22] and the maintenance of platelet thrombi.[14]

Activation of the clotting mechanism: role of thrombin and fibrin formation

During platelet adhesion and aggregation, the clotting mechanism is activated and thrombin is generated (see Figs 28B-1 and 28B-2); this further promotes platelet aggregation and leads to the formation and polymerization of fibrin, which maintains the stability of the platelet-rich arterial thrombus.

The coagulation cascade is composed of a series of proenzyme activations that allows amplification of the initial thrombotic stimulus.[23] Historically, the coagulation system has been divided into intrinsic and extrinsic pathways[24] (see Fig 28B-2). In the intrinsic pathway, all necessary factors are present in the circulating blood (hence the name), and the initial reaction is triggered by contact of the blood with a negatively charged (e.g., subendothelial collagen) or foreign (e.g., the glass wall of a test tube) surface. In the extrinsic activation pathway, tissue fluid, not a plasma component, initiates the blood coagulation process; after vessel damage, this tissue factor, called "tissue thromboplastin," mixes with blood and starts coagulation. After activation of factor X, the two pathways merge into one. In addition, both appear to be equally necessary to ensure normal hemostasis. More specifically, and as outlined in Figure 28B-2, in the intrinsic system, coagulation is initiated by the adsorption of factor XII onto a foreign surface or collagen. Both kallikrein and high-molecular-weight kininogen are required for the rapid surface activation of factor XII. Also, high-molecular-weight kininogen increases the reactivity of factor XIIa in the conversion of factor XI to XIa. Factor XIa converts factor IX to activated protease factor IXa, whereupon factors VIII and IXa form a complex, activating factor X. Both platelet phospholipid, made available by aggregated platelets, and calcium (Ca^{2+}) are essential for maximal activation of factor X.

The prothrombinase activator complex is the assembly of factors Va, Xa, prothrombin (factor II), and calcium on a phospholipid membrane (platelets or smooth muscle cells). This activator complex accelerates thrombin generation by 278,000 times and protects activated factors from inhibition by antithrombin III. Thrombin cleaves fibrinogen to fibrin; activates factor V, which is essential for thrombin generation; activates factor XIII, which cross-links fibrin; and induces platelet secretion and aggregation.[17]

Platelet aggregation may be activated by circulating catecholamines. This may be of major importance because it may be a link between conditions of stress and the development of arterial thrombosis. Of no less importance is the increasing evidence of an enhanced thrombogenicity in cigarette smokers and in patients with a strong family history of coronary disease,[1a,25] with hyperlipidemia,[26] and with diabetes mellitus.[1a]

Endogenous inhibitors of thrombosis: role of prostacyclin, protein C, fibrinolysis, and antithrombin III

During platelet activation and fibrin formation, endogenous mechanisms tend to limit thrombus formation. The most important are prostacyclin, antithrombin III, protein C, and the fibrinolytic system (see Fig 28B-1).

Prostacyclin (PGI_2), discovered by Moncada and colleagues,[27] appears to be the principal prostaglandin metabolite in vascular tissue. It is most highly concentrated on the intimal surface, particularly the endothelium, and progressively decreasing in activity toward the adventitial surface. PGI_2 is a potent systemic vasodilator and a potent inhibitor of platelet aggregation. The platelet-inhibitory action of PGI_2 seems to be related to an activation of platelet membrane adenylate cyclase enzyme, which leads to an increase in platelet adenosine 3′,5′-cyclic monophosphate (cAMP). Presumably, similar to the synthesis of the prostanoid TXA_2 by platelets, the vessel wall synthesizes PGI_2 from its own precursors (see Fig 28B-3).

It has been claimed that PGI_2 can be produced by the cells of the vessel wall in response to stimulation by endothelial injury or thrombin; most importantly, platelets adhering to sites of vascular damage not only release TXA_2, which promotes aggregation of other platelets, but also concomitantly release endoperoxides, which potentiate PGI_2 synthesis by the arterial wall. Thus, the process of platelet aggregation and thrombosis may tend to be limited or prevented. In this context, Greenland Eskimos, who have a bleeding tendency but in whom thrombosis or atherosclerosis does not develop, seem to have little platelet TXA_2 (or rather a biologically low active TXA_3) and a substantial amount of a prostacyclin-type substance (prostaglandin I_3, the synthesis of which is not inhibited by aspirin), all of these factors presumably related to diet.[28,29] Indeed, it has been suggested that an imbalance between platelet proaggregating and disaggregating activity of both prostaglandin systems (TXA_2 and PGI_2) may be an important factor leading to thrombosis and vascular disease.[20] Thus, it has been suggested that certain of the so-called risk factors of atherosclerosis and thrombosis may promote vascular disease by altering this TXA_2-PGI_2 equilibrium system.[1a]

Antithrombin III, a critical endogenous anticoagulant, is enhanced by heparin and inhibits thrombin and activated factors IX, X, XI, and XII.[17] The actions of antithrombin III and heparin cofactor II are blocked by binding of thrombin to fibrin or arterial wall matrix. Natural inhibitors block secretion of platelet factor 4 and conversion of fibrinogen to fibrin monomer II.[17,30] A deficiency of antithrombin III is associated with thrombosis.[31]

Protein C is activated by the thrombin:thrombomodulin complex (Fig 28B-4). In addition to being a potent anticoagulant, activated protein C may promote fibrinolysis, in part by complexing with plasminogen activator inhibitor.[32] Certain findings underscore the importance of the fibrinolytic system in maintaining normal hemostasis and suggest that the balance between plasminogen activators and inhibitors[33,34] may be important in both arterial and venous thrombotic disorders. Indeed, patients who are congenitally deficient in protein C and persons who have low fibrinolytic response or have thrombolysis blocked by aprotinin are prone to recurrent thrombosis.[35-37]

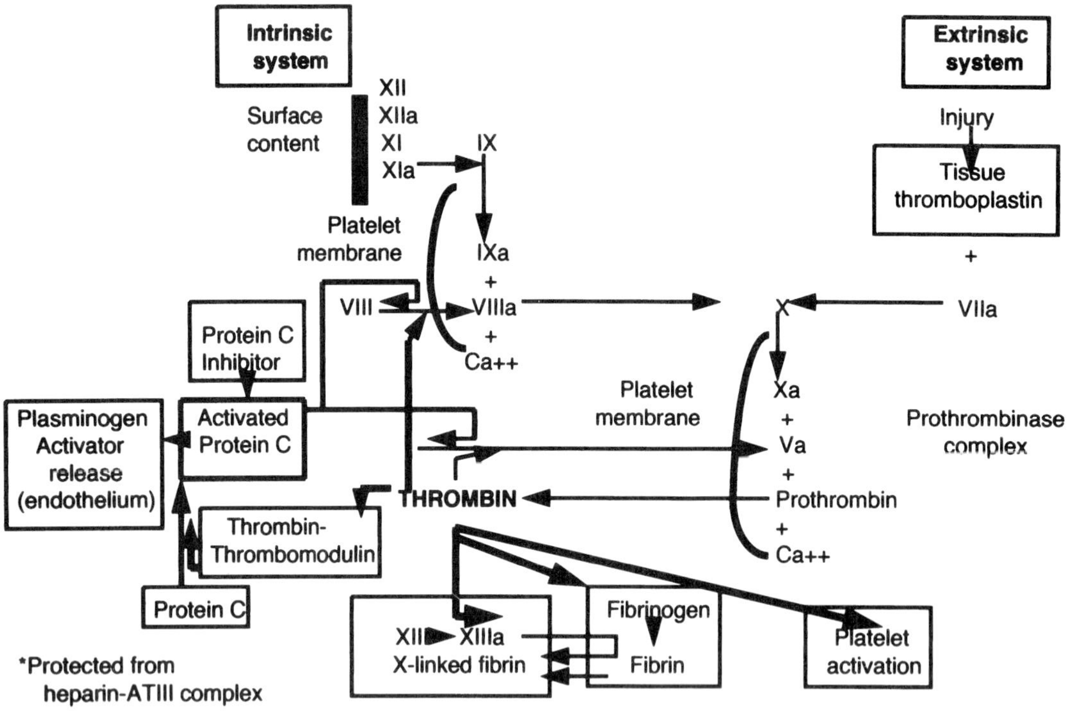

Fig 28B-4 Thrombin generation (with amplification by activator complexes) and activity and relationship to actions of activated protein C and fibrinolysis as initiated by tissue plasminogen activator, which converts plasminogen to plasmin. The intrinsic and extrinsic coagulation systems are illustrated, with the final common pathway being thrombin generation. The three major actions of thrombin are shown below: platelet activation, conversion of fibrinogen to fibrin, and cross-linking of fibrin by activation of factor XIII. In addition, thrombin binds to thrombomodulin on endothelium, which is necessary for the activation of protein C. Activated protein C decreases thrombin generation by inactivating factors VIIIa and Va and enhances thrombolysis by binding to plasminogen activator inhibitor and stimulating the release of tissue plasminogen activator from endothelium for the conversion of plasminogen to plasmin. In addition, plasmin activates factor V to Va. Activated factors are shown by attached "a."

CLINICOPATHOLOGIC PRESENTATION AND FATE OF THROMBUS

Platelet activation appears to be associated with the initiation and growth of the atherosclerotic plaque by the release of platelet-derived growth factors. In some instances, platelet adhesion tends to progress to platelet aggregation and thrombus formation. From the clinicopathologic standpoint, the arterial thrombus thus formed usually has one of the following three outcomes (Fig 28B-5).

Subclinical mural thrombi

Subclinical mural thrombi are probably the most common and consist of a partial thrombotic obstruction of the vascular lumen insufficient to cause clinical symptoms. Such thrombi tend to occur over an ulcerated atherosclerotic plaque, such as in the coronary or carotid system, or on an artificial surface, such as a prosthetic heart valve. Although such thrombi can totally or partially disappear in situ by lysis or embolization,[1a] they may persist and eventually undergo phagocytosis, endothelialization, or atherogenic transformation.[38] Such atherogenic transformation of arterial thrombi may contribute to accelerated atherosclerosis in some patients.

Clinically acute or subacute thrombotic occlusion

At the time of arterial plaque disruption, local and systemic factors influence the degree and duration of thrombus formation and account for a variety of pathologic and clinical manifestations. Three local factors greatly influence the degree of thrombus formation. First, the degree of plaque disruption in terms of depth of injury (and thus substrates exposed to flowing blood, with lipid gruel, smooth muscle cells, and types I and III collagen being very thrombogenic), surface area, and configuration

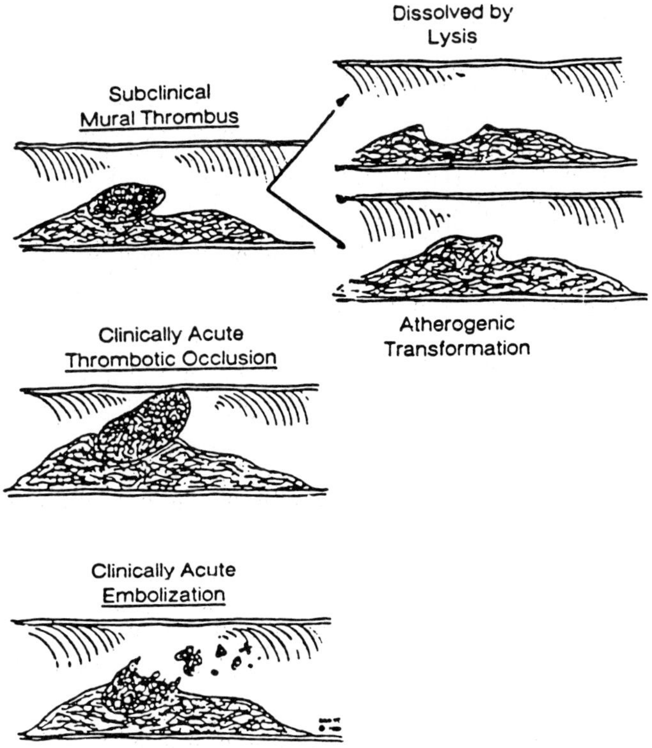

Fig 28B-5 Clinicopathologic presentation and fate of an arterial thrombus that develops over an atherosclerotic plaque. (From Fuster V, Chesebro JH: Antithrombotic therapy: role of platelet-inhibitor drugs. I. Current concepts of thrombogenesis: role of platelets. *Mayo Clin Proc* 56:102-112, 1981. By permission, Mayo Foundation.)

of injury is a major contributor. In approximately one-fourth of cases, there is only superficial injury (thrombus easily dispersed) in a branch or distal artery with high-grade stenosis. Second, the degree of stenosis and arterial size influence blood flow velocity (directly related to platelet deposition) and luminal radius (platelet deposition inversely related to the third power of luminal radius). Third, residual thrombus is extremely thrombogenic and influences blood rheology, shear force, and, thus, platelet deposition.[22,38,39] Systemic risk factors, such as epinephrine, high low-density lipoprotein and low high-density lipoprotein cholesterol, high Lp(a) lipoprotein, and elevated coagulation factors, such as factor VII and fibrinogen, also influence thrombosis.[39] Many of the factors above also influence vasoconstriction.

Vasoconstriction may be platelet-dependent (and thus related to the degree of arterial injury and platelet deposition), endothelium-dependent (presence of, absence of, or dysfunctional), thrombin-dependent (thrombin releases the potent vasoconstrictor endothelin), and lipid- or cholesterol-dependent (cholesterol feeding is associated with vascular wall production of endothelin-1). Normal endothelium protects against vasoconstriction because it produces the vasodilators prostacyclin and endothelium-derived relaxing factor (nitric oxide—synthesized from arginine), which are both vasodilatory and antithrombotic, probably because they increase platelet cAMP and cyclic guanosine monophosphate (cGMP), respectively.[39-43] Contributors to arterial vasoconstriction are summarized in Figure 28B-6.

Acute embolization

A thrombus at a site in the arterial system, particularly the subclinical mural or partially obstructive type, can dislodge and embolize to a distal artery or arteries. The acute embolization can result from forces of blood flow dislodging large masses of thrombi (macroembolism) and can lead to an acute cerebrovascular accident or an occlusion of a limb artery, typically in patients with ulcerated thromboatherosclerotic carotid arteries, ulcerated plaques in the aortic arch, or ulcerated abdominal aorta or in patients with prosthetic heart valves.[1a,44]

Ulcerated plaques in the aortic arch are common in patients with stroke, and the frequency increases with age and heart weight (index of hypertension) (Table 28B-1).[44] The prevalence of ulcerative plaques was 61% among the 28 patients with no known cause of cerebral infarction compared with 22% among the 135 patients with a known cause of cerebral infarction ($P < 0.001$). Because ulcerated plaques in the aortic arch were not correlated with extracranial internal carotid artery stenosis, these lesions may be two independent risk factors for stroke.[44]

Acute embolization can also result from digestion of fibrin in the thrombus by the fibrinolytic enzymatic system, causing small platelet masses to embolize (microembolism); this process can be clinically apparent if the site of the embolus is vitally important, such as in transient cerebral ischemic attacks in patients with carotid atherosclerotic disease[45,46] (see Table 28B-1).

Embolization of thrombotic or calcified atherosclerotic material in the coronary microcirculation has been proposed as one of the causes of ventricular fibrillation and sudden death.[6,47,48] Nevertheless, although mural thrombi or calcified atherosclerotic material of diseased coronary arteries most likely may embolize and obstruct the microcirculation of the heart, determining how frequently this occurs in relationship to other mechanisms that lead to ventricular fibrillation and sudden death is difficult.

Development of thromboembolism and its detection by laboratory tests

From the clinical standpoint, arterial thromboembolic disease usually becomes manifest acutely or subacutely. Nevertheless, whether the thromboembolic episode is subclinical or clinically apparent, increasing evidence has indicated that a continuous process of dynamic thrombus formation and lysis frequently persists in the region of arterial thrombus formation both before and after the thromboembolic event. This evidence probably explains why, in many patients with a clinically acute thromboembolic episode, a persistent increase in platelet consumption or turnover, as measured by the rate of disappearance of autologous platelets labeled with chromium 51 (^{51}Cr)

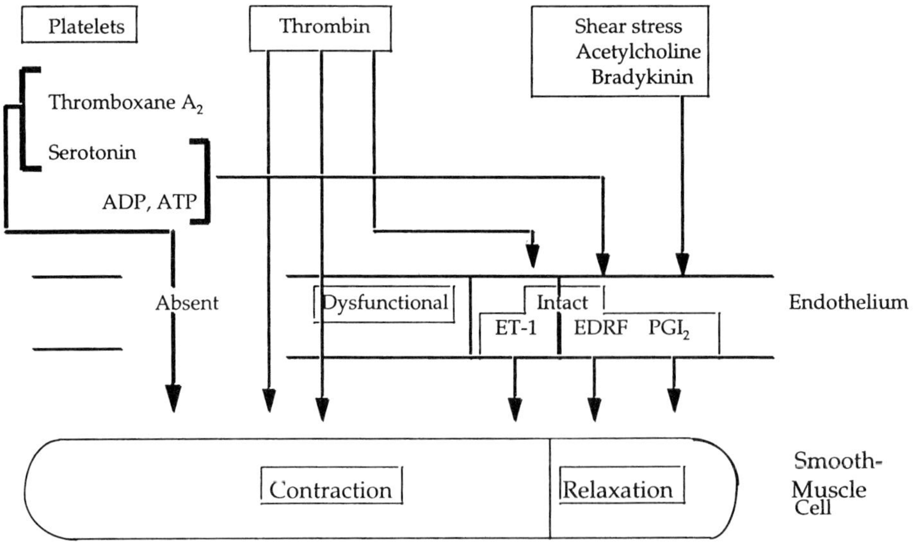

Fig 28B-6 The effects of shear stress, acetylcholine, and bradykinin lead intact endothelium to generate and release endothelium-derived relaxing factor *(EDRF)* and prostacyclin *(PGI_2)*, which in turn cause relaxation of the smooth muscle. The effect of thrombin leads the intact endothelium to generate endothelin-1 *(ET-1)*, which causes vasoconstriction of the smooth muscle. After type I injury or damage, dysfunctional endothelium may not generate relaxing substances; in these circumstances, all the stimulants mentioned above exert a vasoconstrictive effect, either through the enhancement of endothelium-derived contracting factors or directly. As a result of type II or III injury or damage in areas of deendothelialization *(Absent)*, thrombin and the platelet products thromboxane A_2 and serotonin induce direct vasoconstriction of the smooth muscle cell. *ADP,* adenosine diphosphate; *ATP,* adenosine triphosphate. (From Fuster V, Badimon L, Badimon JJ, et al: The pathogenesis of coronary artery disease and the acute coronary syndromes [part 2]. *N Engl J Med* 326:310-318, 1992. By permission of the journal.)

Table 28B-1 Prevalence of ulcerated plaques in the aortic arch according to age group and diagnosis

	Cerebral infarction (n = 183)			Other neurologic diseases (n = 261)			
		Pt with ulcerated plaques			Pt with ulcerated plaques		
Age, yr	**No. of pt**	**No.**	**%**	**No. of pt**	**No.**	**%**	***P****
<40	2	0	0	28	0	0	–
40-49	4	0	0	25	0	0	–
50-59	14	0	0	54	0	0	–
60-69	28	6	21	59	3	5	0.019
70-79	71	22	31	69	5	7	0.001
80-89	58	20	34	23	4	17	0.128
≥90	6	3	50	3	1	33	0.63

*For the comparison between the patients with cerebral infarction and those with other neurologic diseases.
From Amarenco P, Duyckaerts C, Tzourio C, et al: The prevalence of ulcerated plaques in the aortic arch in patients with stroke. *N Engl J Med* 326:221-225, 1992. By permission of the journal.

Table 28B-2 Biochemical markers of thrombosis and thrombolysis

Reaction coagulation	Marker	$t_{1/2}$
$FX \rightarrow Xa$	FX activation peptide[51]	30 min
Prothrombin → thrombin (thrombin generation)	Prothrombin activation fragment 1.2[52-57]	90 min
	Thrombin-antithrombin III[58]	15 min
	Hirudin-thrombin complex[59-61]	3-4 hr
Fibrinogen → fibrin (thrombin activity)	Fibrinopeptide A (FPA)[62]	3-5 min
Activation of protein C	Protein C activation peptide[63]	5 min
	APC-protein C inhibitor[64,65]	40 min
	APC-1_1 antitrypsin complex[66]	140 min
	APC-1_2 macroglobulin complex[67]	–
Platelet secretion of		
Thromboxane A_2	Thromboxane A_2[68,69]	30 sec
	Thromboxane B_2[68,69]	5-7 min
	2,3-Dinor-thromboxane B_2*[68,69]	15 min
	11-Dehydro-thromboxane B_2*[68,69]	1 hr
	Platelet factor 4[70]	2.1 (fast), 70 min (slow component)
	β-Thromboglobulin[70]	8.4 (fast), 63 min (slow component)
Thrombolysis by plasmin on		
Cross-linked fibrin	D-D dimer[71,72]	8 hr
Fibrin II	B-b 15-42 fragment	–
Fibrin I/fibrinogen	B-b 1-42 fragment	–

*Not subject to artifactual formation during sampling.

or indium 111 (^{111}In), can be detected weeks or months after, or even before, the clinical event.[49]

Several in vitro methods are available for evaluation of platelet reactivity. Although these tests provide important information on platelet function and metabolism in some bleeding disorders, they have been of lesser value in the evaluation of thromboembolism.[1a] However, spontaneous platelet aggregation in vitro, an index of platelet hyperreactivity, has been associated with increased mortality and coronary events in survivors of myocardial infarction.[50] Several methods for in vivo assessment of platelet function and ex vivo measurement of coagulation (Table 28B-2) are of use in the evaluation of thromboembolic disease. These include (1) evaluation of platelet survival time, (2) assessment of platelet deposition with external radioisotopic imaging, (3) detection of platelet-specific proteins (i.e., platelet factor 4 and β-thromboglobulin), (4) measurement of thrombin generation using prothrombin fragment 1.2 or inhibitors bound to thrombin and activity using fibrin-dependent products (e.g., fibrinopeptide A) released into the plasma during platelet activation and fibrin formation, and (5) measurement of plasma and urine metabolites of TXA_2 (see Table 28B-2).

Platelet survival time. Until recently, platelet survival time was measured by the rate of disappearance, during an 8-day period, of autologous platelets labeled with ^{51}Cr. The platelet survival time has been found to be abnormally shortened in patients with thrombotic and atherosclerotic disease.[49,73] Indeed, evidence suggests that measurement of platelet survival may detect some patients in whom atherosclerotic or thrombotic disease is developing but who are still asymptomatic.[25] After experience with more than 2,000 patients, we believe that the measurement of platelet survival time is a reasonably sensitive and specific hematologic procedure for the assessment of arterial thromboembolism and of the therapeutic effects of platelet-inhibitor drugs.[49,74] Unfortunately, this procedure is very specialized, and currently we view it primarily as a research tool.[49]

A more recent radioisotopic technique uses ^{111}In-labeled platelets.[75] Survival data are comparable to those obtained with ^{51}Cr-labeled platelets; unlike ^{51}Cr, ^{111}In has a high labeling efficiency and a high γ-ray emission. These features permit, respectively, the use of a small volume of blood for the labeling procedure and the capability to define, by external imaging, the site of platelet deposition in some clinical and experimental conditions.[76]

In vivo imaging. The capability of external imaging in humans with in vivo quantitation by use of ^{111}In-labeled platelets is providing meaningful information for the visualization of thrombi, particularly in the left ventricle[77] and in prosthetic materials.[78] In addition, this permits assessment of different antithrombotic regimens for the prevention of thrombosis as evaluated in animals[79] and in humans.[80] Regional injection of ^{111}In-labeled platelets, use of ^{111}In-labeled monoclonal antibody to platelet surface receptors, or use of platelets labeled with technetium Tc 99m hexamethyl propylenamine oxime (^{99m}Tc HMPAO) in conjunction with dynamic computerized imaging may have a more promising future for the in vivo detection of thrombi than currently used techniques.[81,82] New solid state local isotope surface detectors, 2 cm in length, consisting of cadmium-tellurium crystals with tungsten shielding and collimation, that are connected to a portable personal computer and modified into a gamma spectrometer with a storage base for data are being developed and evaluated for simultaneous double or triple isotope detection with individual data points for each isotope every 1 or 2 minutes. This simultaneous continuous monitoring of platelets and fibrin may potentially revolutionize the in vivo and ex vivo evaluation of antithrombotic therapy and dose-activity responses before a major clinical trial.

Platelet-specific proteins (platelet factor 4 and β-thromboglobulin) released into plasma. Increasing evidence has suggested that platelets can be activated and even degranulated and yet can continue to circulate. For this reason, measurement of platelet-specific proteins released into the plasma during platelet activation and degranulation may be a more sensitive marker of platelet activation than platelet survival time. Platelet factor 4 and β-thromboglobulin are two platelet-specific proteins liberated from the platelet α granules during platelet activation. The specificity and clinical value of measurements of these proteins in systemic or regional circulation remain controversial, in part because artifacts are increased and β-thromboglobulin is metabolized in the kidneys and increased in renal insufficiency.[70,83]

Thrombin generation and activity. Figure 28B-6 shows the formation of biochemical markers of thrombin generation and activity. As with any plasma marker, great care must be taken in blood drawing, which should be into tubes containing multiple blockers of coagulation and fibrinolysis (ethylenediaminetetraacetic acid, chlormethyl ketone [P-PACK], and aprotinin) to avoid artifactual coagulation changes.[54,55]

Prothrombin fragment 1.2, a marker of thrombin generation, is released in the conversion of prothrombin to thrombin, has a plasma half-life of 90 minutes, is increased in patients with unstable angina or myocardial infarction, and remains elevated 6 months later for unexplained reasons.[55] Fibrinopeptide A is specific for the cleavage of fibrinogen by thrombin (see Fig 28B-6), has a half-life of 3 to 5 minutes, is largely (70%) degraded by peptidases, and is filtered (30%) by the kidney (which then catabolizes most of this), and only about 0.5% is excreted in the urine.[52,53] Thus, fibrinopeptide A is a marker of thrombin activity, may be artifactually increased by a suboptimal blood drawing technique (>6.0 nmol/L in normal persons), is increased in patients with unstable angina or acute myocardial infarction, and decreases to the upper limit of normal 6 months later in these patients.[55] Fibrinopeptide A may decrease during heparin or other antithrombin therapy during continuing arterial thrombosis, both experimentally in pigs (Heras M, Chesebro JH: Unpublished data) and in patients with reocclusion of the infarct-related artery after thrombolysis.[56] Thus, decreased fibrinopeptide A appears necessary but is not specific for protection against arterial thrombosis by antithrombin therapy. This may occur during heparin therapy, which is effective in reducing heart fibrin formation but has a weak effect against platelets,[13] in part because of the difficulty in inhibiting thrombin bound to platelets, fibrin, or arterial wall matrix. Likewise, low doses of thrombin-inhibiting agents may inhibit fibrin formation but not platelet-rich macroscopic thrombus.[13]

Increased thrombin generation increases thrombin bound to thrombomodulin and thus increases activation of protein C, which causes release of tissue plasminogen activator and, thus, fibrinolysis, with release of fibrinogen-fibrin degradation products, including D-dimer (see Fig 28B-4 and 28B-6).[62,84]

Another marker of thrombin generation is the formation of the natural inhibitor complex whereby thrombin is bound irreversibly by antithrombin III. This complex has a plasma half-life of 15 minutes and is accelerated 3 to 4 times in its formation by heparin.[58,85,86]

Thrombin/antithrombin III complex (TAT) increases during hemodialysis despite heparin therapy and increases during cardiopulmonary bypass operation but decreases with low-molecular-weight heparin therapy.[86] In experimental disseminated intravascular coagulation, the antithrombin/heparin complex inhibits thrombin activity (formation of fibrin and disappearance of fibrinogen) but not thrombin generation (prothrombin consumption).[87] These studies suggest that an antithrombin inhibits thrombin activity but not its generation.

The newest method of measuring thrombin generation uses very-low-dose hirudin, the specific, rapid, and nearly irreversible inhibitor of thrombin, which, unlike antithrombin III, binds free and bound thrombin rapidly and selectively by 1:1 stoichiometry.[59] Even therapeutic anticoagulation with hirudin does not decrease prothrombin fragment 1.2 but does decrease TAT plasma levels, because hirudin binds thrombin more rapidly than antithrombin III.[60] The hirudin-thrombin complex is inactive, has a circulating half-life of 3 to 4 hours, can be measured during therapeutic or subtherapeutic anticoagulation with hirudin, and documents persistent thrombin generation in patients with stable coronary disease or unstable angina during therapeutic anticoagulation with hirudin.[59-61]

Plasma and urine thromboxane levels. TXA_2 is a prostanoid product of platelet arachidonic acid metabolism that is synthesized during platelet activation.[20,88] The substance is highly unstable, with a half-life of only 30 seconds, but it has stable metabolites of thromboxane B_2 in urine (2,3 dinor thromboxane B_2) and plasma (II dehydrothromboxane B_2), which are not subject to artifactual formation during sampling and for which radioimmunoassays are available.[68,69,89] (see Table 28B-2). In patients with unstable angina, 84% of episodes of spontaneous ischemia at rest were associated with elevation of urinary 2,3 dinor thromboxane B_2 or plasma 2 dehydrothromboxane B_2.[68] Similar elevations were observed in patients with persistent unstable angina or postinfarction angina and were frequently associated with angiographic evidence of thrombus formation.[69] Today, with at least 50% to 80% of patients presenting with acute coronary syndromes taking aspirin, thromboxane synthesis is blocked, and measurement of these metabolites as a measure of thrombosis is not valid.

PATHOGENESIS OF THROMBOSIS AND EMBOLISM IN CORONARY ARTERIES, CARDIAC CHAMBERS, AND PROSTHETIC VALVES

Coronary arteries—platelets and fibrin

The concept of vascular injury—platelets and fibrin. Vascular injury and thrombus formation are the key events in the progression of atherosclerosis and in the pathogenesis of acute coronary syndromes. We previously proposed a pathologic classification of vascular injury and its pathophysiologic cellular responses in an attempt to aid understanding of the pathogenesis of various vascular diseases and formulate therapeutic strategies in the prevention of these diseases.[38,90] We proposed that vascular injury be classified into three types: type I, functional alterations of endothelial cells without significant morphologic changes; type II, endothelial denudation and intimal injury but intact internal elastic lamina and media; and type III, endothelial denudation with damage of intima and media.

In type I endothelial injury, monocyte rather than platelet deposition or thrombus formation can be demonstrated (in part because of lipid infiltration) and can contribute, by the release of growth factors, to some intimal hyperplasia; this may be the basis of the initiation of the atherosclerotic process. In contrast, with type II injury, an obvious monolayer of a few layers of platelets with or without thrombus formation can be seen; the release of platelet growth factors may contribute to an accelerated intimal hyperplasia, such as that occurring in the coronary vein graft within the first postoperative year.

In type III injury with exposure of components of the medial layer, particularly type I collagen, marked platelet aggregation with mural thrombus formation follows. Vascular injury of this magnitude also stimulates thrombin formation through both the intrinsic (surface-activated) and extrinsic (tissue factor-dependent) coagulation pathways, in which the platelet and smooth muscle cell membranes facilitate interaction between clotting factors (see Fig 28B-2). Platelets, smooth muscle cells, and the coagulation system are therefore clearly interrelated in the genesis of arterial thrombosis after deep, type III, injury, such as that seen in the acute coronary syndromes or after coronary angioplasty.

Labile compared with fixed thrombus. Delivery and activation of platelets at the site of vascular injury are dependent on both shear rate, which is a measure of the difference in blood velocity between the center and the periphery of the vessel,[91] and the degree of vessel injury (type II or type III). In areas of luminal stenosis, high shear rate promotes contact between blood elements and the vessel wall[11] and favors platelet activation. Most importantly, the influence of the severity of vascular injury on thrombus formation has been demonstrated in perfusion chamber experiments[9,10] in which different tissue substrates were exposed to blood at various shear rates. With type II vascular injury, platelet deposition and thrombus formation may occur, but the phenomenon is usually transient; with type III injury, platelet aggregation is considerably increased, leading to fixation of thrombus and persistent vascular occlusion.

Clinical correlations of vascular injury and thrombosis. These concepts of vascular injury and thrombosis are important in the understanding of the pathogenesis of various vascular diseases, including the initiation and progression of atherosclerosis, the acute coronary syndromes, vein graft disease, and restenosis after coronary angioplasty.

INITIATION AND PROGRESSION OF ATHEROSCLEROSIS. The process of type I vascular injury followed by intermittent deposition of monocytes, lipid accumulation, smooth muscle cell proliferation, and resultant plaque formation represents the prevalent view of the initiation of spontaneous atherogenesis.[92] However, the precise nature of the injury remains unknown; that is, whether the turbulence of blood flow injures the endothelium or toxic lipids (oxidized cholesterol) cause injury from inside the vessel wall is controversial.

Accumulating evidence suggests that repetitive fissures of soft fatty plaques (see "Acute Coronary Syndromes," below) with thrombus formation is a major mechanism for the progression of atherosclerosis.[38,93] In an autopsy study of coronary arteries of 129 patients with atheromatous disease who died of noncardiac causes, Davies et al.[47] found that 16% of patients studied had fissures in atherosclerotic plaque (type II injury) and, in some cases, overlying thrombi. This degree of frequency of plaque fissure (type II injury) in a static pathologic evaluation suggests that a single plaque may undergo many fissures, with subsequent thrombus formation and organization, during the evolution and progression into an advanced lesion. Indeed, analysis of coronary trees in patients dying of ischemic heart disease showed that morphologic appearance consistent with previously healed fissures and various stages of thrombus incorporation and organization was almost ubiquitous and suggested that most fissures probably reseal and incorporate overlying thrombus without manifestation of clinical symptoms.[6,93]

Further evidence for supporting thrombosis and thrombus incorporation as part of plaque progression is provided by a study using monoclonal antibodies to identify fibrin, fibrinogen, and fibrinogen degradation products.[94] In advanced fibrous plaque, fibrin and fibrin-related products were detected in the intima, neointima, subintima, and even the deeper medial layer, especially around thrombus, collagen, and smooth muscle cells; on the other hand, these fibrin and related products were found in small quantities in early lesions and normal arteries. Although it is as yet unknown how prevalent this process is, its clinical significance is potentially enormous because mural thrombi in the region of fissures may be prevented by platelet inhibitors or anticoagulant agents.

ACUTE CORONARY SYNDROMES. Pathologic,[6,48] angioscopic,[95] and angiographic[96,97] data have firmly established that type III vascular injury—major plaque and plaque rupture—with formation of mural or occlusive thrombus is a common mechanism leading to the acute coronary syndromes, namely, unstable angina, acute myocardial infarction, and sudden death. In addition, accumulating evidence indicates that the process of type III injury and the resulting intraluminal thrombotic process are dynamic and repetitive; it has been suggested that this dynamic process provides a physiologic link between these clinical syndromes.[5,98] Indeed, pathologic studies by Falk[48] in patients with unstable angina leading to infarction or sudden death revealed layers of thrombi of different ages in most cases, suggesting that recurrent episodes of mural thrombosis and organization rather than a single abrupt thrombotic event occurred in the transition between these syndromes.

Similarly, studies[97,99] in patients with unstable angina have demonstrated both rapid progression of stenosis angiographically and clinical deterioration to myocardial infarction in a significant percentage of patients. This finding reflects the dynamic process of intraluminal thrombosis and organization in these clinical syndromes. In addition, the coronary lesion responsible for unstable angina and acute myocardial infarction is frequently only mildly to moderately stenotic. For example, Ambrose and co-workers[97,99,100] demonstrated that more than 70% of the lesions responsible for unstable angina have a prior stenosis of less than 50% and that about one-half of the lesions leading to acute myocardial infarction have nonsignificant narrowing. These findings strongly support the conclusion that type III injury of a small plaque with superimposed thrombosis, rather than the severity of the underlying lesion, is the primary determinant of acute occlusion in a significant proportion of patients with acute coronary syndromes. Similar pathogenic mechanisms of sudden death can also be inferred from the pathologic data. For example, Davies et al.[47] reported that more than 70% of sudden cardiac death cases have evidence of recent mural or occlusive intraluminal thrombus overlying the sites of plaque fissure and rupture at autopsy.

Thus, type III vascular injury—plaque rupture—with thrombus formation appears to be the major mechanism leading to the acute coronary syndromes. In a proportion of patients with unstable angina, type III vascular injury in the form of fissure may lead to transient vessel occlusion and ischemia by labile thrombus; in some of these patients, a more permanent occlusion may lead to infarction or sudden death. Indeed, myocardial infarction may result from type III vascular injury in the form of an ulcer and thus be associated with more persistent and fixed thrombotic coronary occlusion in the face of inadequate collateral flow. In addition, spontaneous or pharmacologic lysis of thrombus occurs in some patients, placing them at high risk for reocclusion.[5,98] Why rupture of a plaque occurs and then leads to growth of the atherosclerotic plaque or acute coronary syndromes is under investigation. It appears that small plaques that rupture have a high fat content (vulnerable plaques); in addition, they contain numerous macrophages that favor the formation of an abscess.[5,38,39,101]

VEIN GRAFT DISEASE. Vascular injury also appears to be the critical initiating event in coronary vein graft disease. Vein grafts are subject to mechanical injury that may occur when the veins are harvested and by handling during the operation, resulting in a transient, predominantly type III injury that may lead to acute thrombotic occlusion; in most cases, however, the vessel wall heals quickly.[102,103] The exposure of the vein grafts to relatively high-pressure flow and the presence of biologic risk factors, such as hypercholesterolemia and smoking, may induce and perpetuate type II injury and hinder the process of reendothelialization that might otherwise occur under normal conditions. During the first postoperative year, the most notable and consistent histologic change in the vein graft is marked intimal thickening, characterized by proliferation of smooth muscle cells and an increase in hyaline matrix.[103]

Lie et al.[104] reported that even within 3 weeks after the operation, smooth muscle cells appear in the subendothelial portion of the intima, followed by proliferation and fibrointimal thickening. Beyond the first year after operation, there is further connective tissue synthesis from smooth muscle cells and fibroblasts, followed by incorporation of lipid into the lesions. If various biologic risk factors are present, this process can be accelerated and enhanced, leading to vascular occlusion. Few changes occur during the second and third years after operation. Beyond the third year, lipid incorporation becomes evident with formation of complex atherosclerotic lesions, often with a lipid core: a mixture of fibrous plaque with intimal hyperplasia, ulceration, cholesterol clefts, foam cells, and, in some areas, calcification with disruption of the medial layer.[105] In addition, because of the predisposition of fatty plaques to rupture (type III injury), occlusive or nonocclusive thrombus formation may also occur during this late stage of graft disease, as documented in surgical specimens and autopsy studies.[104,105] In one report, two-thirds of the vein grafts removed during a second coronary artery bypass operation showed evidence of mural or occlusive thrombus.[106]

POSTANGIOPLASTY RESTENOSIS. Type III vascular injury associated with intense platelet aggregation and mural thrombi formation also results in the release of various cellular growth factors and in a significant hyperplastic response; this appears to be the pathogenic mechanism for coronary restenosis after percutaneous transluminal coronary angioplasty.[90] In a study of restenosis in pigs, type III injury was induced, with marked platelet aggregation and mural thrombus formation, immediately after balloon injury to the carotid arteries.[107] Necrosis of the medial smooth muscle cells was evident at 24 hours, and the process of progressive intimal proliferation of smooth muscle cells and reorganization and incorporation of thrombi finally led to partial or total occlusion of the lumen.

Type III changes in the vessel wall seen in patients who died several days after angioplasty included denudation of the endothelium, intimal necrosis, medial tear, adventitial hemorrhage, and thrombosis.[108-110] Coronary angioscopy studies[111,112] also described mural thrombi, intimal flaps, dissection, and ruptured atheroma as common findings. In contrast to these acute morphologic features, specimens obtained weeks to months after successful angioplasty showed marked circumferential fibrointimal thickening and organized thrombi at sites of chronic restenosis.[108-110] Similarly, tissues removed from restenotic segments via atherectomy were composed mainly of smooth muscle cells and collagen, with some thrombus present in two-thirds of restenotic lesions.[113] The mitogenic stimuli appear to be due to the release of growth factors from aggregating platelets and also from endothelial cells and smooth muscle cells via paracrine and autocrine mechanisms.[110]

Cardiac chambers – predominance of fibrin component

Intracavitary mural thrombi develop frequently in patients with acute myocardial infarction, chronic left ventricular aneurysm, dilated cardiomyopathy, and atrial fibrillation. The pathogenesis of thrombosis may be outlined along the lines established more than a century ago by the pathologist Rudolf Virchow, who defined a triad of precipitating factors: endothelial injury, a zone of circulatory stasis, and a hypercoagulable state.[114] In addition to these factors, the clinical significance derives from the risk of systemic embolism, which depends on dynamic forces of the circulation and the underlying disease.

Endothelial injury. In the first few days after acute myocardial infarction, leukocyte infiltration separates endothelial cells from their basal lamina.[115] The resulting exposure of subendothelial tissue to blood serves as the nidus for thrombus development. Specific endocardial abnormalities have also been identified histologically in surgical and postmortem specimens from patients with left ventricular aneurysms[116] and at necropsy in patients with idiopathic dilated cardiomyopathy.[117]

Blood stasis. Both experimental[118] and clinical[119,120] studies have emphasized the importance of wall motion abnormalities in the development of left ventricular thrombi, and it seems clear that stasis of blood in regions of akinesis or dyskinesis is the essential factor. Similarly, stasis is important in the development of atrial thrombi[121] when effective mechanical atrial activity is impaired, as occurs in atrial fibrillation, atrial enlargement, mitral stenosis, and cardiac failure. Stasis is paramount to conditions of low shear rate, in which activation of coagulation factors rather than of platelets leads to fibrin formation and constitutes the predominant pathogenic mechanism in the development of intracavitary thrombi (see Fig 28B-2).

Hypercoagulable state. One study of patients with acute myocardial infarction found a significantly greater incidence of thromboembolism in cases of increased serum fibrinogen levels,[122] suggesting a hypercoagulable tendency in this condition. A systemic procoagulant state is present during acute myocardial infarction (increased thrombin generation and activity)[55] and probably predisposes to thrombotic events. More relevant is experimental evidence that the surface of a fresh thrombus is itself highly thrombogenic because of increased thrombin generation, producing at least a local, if not a systemic, hypercoagulable state.[5]

Underlying disease. Risk of thromboembolism varies with (1) the underlying disease (myocardial infarction or type of valvular heart disease), (2) severity of underlying disease (size of anterior myocardial infarction), (3) timing after onset and development of disease (two-thirds of left ventricular thrombi formed within 48 hours of onset of anterior myocardial infarction), (4) presence or absence of risk factors for thromboembolism (clinical risks of hypertension, recent heart failure, or previous thromboembolism in patients with atrial fibrillation), and (5) pathogenesis of underlying disease (acute disruption of fatty plaque with ulceration causes anchored major thrombi with embolic potential in coronary arteries in three-fourths of patients with acute coronary syndromes; endothelial denudation within a severe stenosis causes a small labile thrombus; if coronary collateral circulation has developed, few or no symptoms result).

Dynamic forces of the circulation. The problems of thromboembolism originating from the cardiac chambers prompt consideration of the balance between the effects of regional injury, stasis, and procoagulant factors, which favor thrombus formation, and dynamic forces of the circulation, which are responsible for the migration of thrombotic material into the systemic circulation. Even though stasis favors thrombus formation within the sac of a left ventricular aneurysm, isolation from dynamic circulatory forces protects against embolic migration.[123,124] In diffusely dilated cardiomyopathy, on the other hand, mural thrombus is not isolated from the circulation, and the embolic risk is higher. Thus, factors leading to thrombus formation are not the same as those that produce systemic embolism, and this paradox must not be neglected in the selection of therapeutic options.

Prosthetic valves – fibrin and platelets

Mechanical prosthesis. The pathologic events leading to thromboembolism begin during surgery. The damaged perivalvular tissue and prosthetic materials activate platelets as soon as blood starts flowing across the valve, and immediate platelet deposition results.[125,126] A Dacron sewing ring is common to all prosthetic valves, both mechanical and bioprosthetic. Platelet deposition on this ring can be demonstrated by use of ^{111}I-labeled platelets within the first 24 hours after operation when either a mechanical or a bioprosthetic valve is placed.[125,126] More importantly, prosthetic materials can activate the intrinsic clotting system,[127] with subsequent fibrin formation. In addition, the abnormal hemodynamic characteristics of prosthetic devices promote mainly fibrin generation and, less importantly, platelet activation (see Fig 28B-2). Finally, the process of fibrin thrombus formation can be facilitated in areas with stasis and decreased blood flow, such as in the left atrium during atrial fibrillation and in the left ventricle during low cardiac output state secondary to left ventricular dysfunction.

Biologic prosthesis. Bioprosthetic valves are considerably less thrombogenic,[128] mainly because of the biologic properties of the material used in their construction and also because of characteristic axial flow profile and leaflet pliability.[129]

PHARMACOLOGY OF ANTITHROMBOTIC AGENTS

This section reviews the pharmacology of platelet inhibitors, heparin, oral anticoagulants, and thrombolytic agents.

Platelet inhibitors

There has been continuous interest in the mechanism of action of drugs that interfere with platelet function in atherosclerosis, thrombosis, and embolism (see Fig 28B-3). Platelet inhibitors may exert their effects through several mechanisms, including inhibition of the arachidonic acid pathway, increase in platelet cAMP and cGMP levels, inhibition of platelet glycoprotein membrane receptors (IIb-IIIa), and inhibition of thrombin generation and activity.

Inhibitors of the arachidonic acid pathway

INHIBITORS OF PLATELET CYCLOOXYGENASE: ASPIRIN

Mechanism of action. Aspirin (Fig 28B-7) and other nonsteroidal anti-inflammatory drugs acetylate the platelet enzyme cyclooxygenase and thus inhibit the formation of TXA_2. Aspirin only partially inhibits platelet aggregation induced by ADP, collagen, or thrombin (at low concentrations). The adherence of the initial layer of platelets to the subendothelium and the release of granule contents are not inhibited by aspirin.[130] Consequently, the effects of platelet-derived growth factor and other mitogens on smooth muscle cell proliferation may still occur in the presence of cyclooxygenase inhibitors.[131] In contrast, these drugs inhibit platelet aggregation on the layer of adherent platelets, presumably by blocking TXA_2 synthesis.

The acetylation of platelet cyclooxygenase is permanent,[132] so that the effects of the drug persist for the life of the platelets. The long-term administration of aspirin, 1 mg/kg per day, effectively inhibits platelet cyclooxygenase and TXA_2 formation. In contrast, aspirin may only temporarily reduce vascular endothelial cyclooxygenase activity, because these cells are capable of synthesizing new enzymes within several hours. Contrary to earlier suggestive findings, platelet cyclooxygenase is not more sensitive than arterial wall cyclooxygenase to low-dose aspirin. Slow-release low-dose aspirin (within the enterohepatic circulation) avoids inhibition of vascular wall cyclooxygenase[133] but has not been clinically valuable (see below).

Ideal dose. Beneficial effects of aspirin on cyclooxygenase-dependent platelet aggregation may be approximately equivalent over a dose range of at least 75 to 1,500 mg daily. Numerous clinical studies have demonstrated the protective effects of aspirin in this dose range in patients with unstable angina or acute myocardial infarction and in primary and secondary prevention of cardiovascular disease.[134-138] For example, three randomized clinical trials[134,135] using aspirin in doses of 75 to 325 mg and 1,300 mg daily in patients with unstable angina showed similar reduction in mortality and nonfatal myocardial infarction. Similarly, in a recent overview of 145 clinical trials[138] using antiplatelet agents in the secondary prevention of cardiovascular disease, aspirin used in doses ranging from 75 to 1,500 mg per day reduced vascular mortality by 17%, nonfatal myocardial infarction by 34%, nonfatal stroke by 35%, and all important vascular events by 25%. There was no evidence that doses of 900 to 1,500 mg of aspirin daily were any more effective in avoiding cardiovascular events than a lower dose of 75 to 325 mg, or one standard aspirin tablet, per day. This observation is pharmacologically plausible, because doses lower than 300 mg/day would have been sufficient to produce virtually complete inhibition of cyclooxygenase-dependent platelet aggregation. Reductions in vascular events were statistically significant in middle and old age,

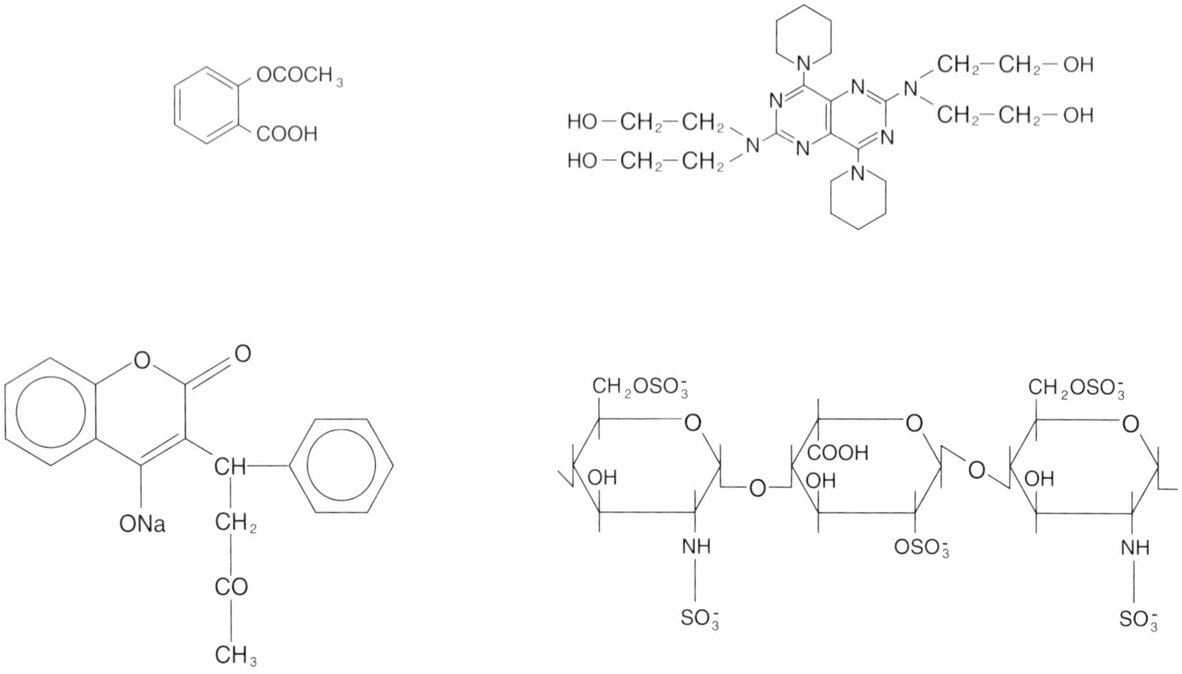

Fig 28B-7 Chemical structure of the antithrombotic agents most commonly used in the United States: *(clockwise from upper left)* acetylsalicylic acid (aspirin), dipyridamole (Persantine), heparin, and warfarin sodium.

in men and women, in hypertensive and normotensive patients, and in diabetic and nondiabetic patients. In pooling all high-risk cardiovascular patients together, there were reductions of about one-third in nonfatal myocardial infarction, one-third in nonfatal stroke, and one-sixth in vascular death (all highly significant).[138] At present, the best studied, most inexpensive, and least toxic dose range is 75 to 325 mg per day.

Side effects. Aspirin side effects are mainly gastrointestinal (GI).[139] Aspirin rarely causes significant generalized bleeding unless it is combined with anticoagulant therapy. There is evidence that aspirin affects the gastric mucosa by inhibiting synthesis of prostaglandins.[140] The effect of aspirin on gastric mucosa is reduced by treatment with cimetidine or antacid and by the use of enteric-coated aspirin.[141]

Most of the side effects of aspirin are dose-related. The United Kingdom Transient Ischaemic Attack Trial compared two daily doses of aspirin with placebo among 2,345 patients with a history of transient ischemic attacks or mild ischemic stroke.[142] It was, therefore, possible to compare the frequencies of side effects reported at 300 mg/day and at 1,200 mg/day. Symptoms, including indigestion, nausea, heartburn, and constipation as well as GI bleeding, were lowest in the placebo group, somewhat higher in the group receiving 300 mg/day, and highest among those receiving 1,200 mg/day. Since there is no evidence that higher doses are more effective than lower doses, an aspirin dose of 75 to 325 mg/day for the prevention of thromboembolic disease is currently recommended.

Other inhibitors of platelet cyclooxygenase. Although nonsteroidal anti-inflammatory drugs reversibly inhibit cyclooxygenase, the antithrombotic activity of these compounds has not been properly tested in large randomized trials; therefore, their use cannot be recommended.[143] Furthermore, one of the nonsteroidal anti-inflammatory agents, indomethacin, has been found to increase coronary vascular resistance and exacerbate ischemic attacks in patients with coronary disease.[144]

DRUGS THAT ALTER PLATELET MEMBRANE PHOSPHOLIPIDS (OMEGA-3 FATTY ACIDS). Both eicosapentaenoic acid and docosahexaenoic acid are present in high concentration in most salt-water fish and may account for the lower incidence of coronary heart disease in Greenland Eskimos and populations that consume large amounts of fish.[29,145] Eicosapentaenoic acid competes with arachidonic acid for platelet cyclooxygenase. This leads to the formation of two endoperoxidases (prostaglandins G_3 and H_3) and thromboxane A_3, which have minimal biologic activity.[146] Furthermore, eicosapentaenoic acid does not inhibit endothelial cell prostacyclin production and stimulates the formation of prostaglandin I_3, which has antiplatelet activity. The net result is a shift in the hemostatic balance toward an antiaggregative and vasodilative state. Docosahexaenoic acid also has platelet inhibitory effects and undergoes retroconversion to eicosapentaenoic acid.[147] Feeding cod liver oil to pigs before balloon-induced deep arterial injury caused a mild increase in the eicosapentaenoic acid-arachidonic acid ratio to >0.5, which was associated with a modest but significant reduction in postinjury platelet deposition and vasoconstriction.[148] Although fish consumption may decrease the incidence of coronary artery disease, fish oils are associated with some potentially adverse events, such as increased bleeding diathesis and reduced inflammatory and immune responses.[147] Before fish oils are recommended for the prevention of atherosclerosis, more properly designed and controlled human trials are necessary.[146] The role of fish oils in the prevention of restenosis after coronary angioplasty is reviewed later.

INHIBITORS OF THROMBOXANE SYNTHETASE. Imidazole analogue thromboxane synthetase inhibitors (see Fig 28B-3) have been developed with the expectation of not only suppressing TXA_2 biosynthesis but also sparing or even enhancing the formation of prostacyclin by the vascular endothelium.[149] The rationale behind this hypothesis is that in the presence of a thromboxane synthetase inhibitor, platelet-derived prostaglandin G_2 would be transferred to the endothelial cells and used in the production of prostacyclin. Although thromboxane synthetase inhibitors have shown some benefits in experimental models,[150] their effects in clinical trials[151,152] of coronary artery disease have been disappointing. This may be a result of two factors: (1) TXA_2 may not be completely suppressed by the available compounds and (2) the prostaglandin endoperoxide intermediates that result from thromboxane synthetase inhibition have themselves significant proaggregating effects.

BLOCKERS OF THROMBOXANE AND PROSTAGLANDIN ENDOPEROXIDE RECEPTORS. Specific inhibition of proaggregating and vasoconstrictive TXA_2 by blocking its synthase and combining prostaglandin endoperoxide receptor blockade (to reduce platelet-activating effects of accumulating endoperoxides) to reduce TXA_2 and increase prostacyclin (so as to increase platelet cAMP) is theoretically appealing (see Fig 28B-3). Ridogrel, a potent inhibitor of TXA_2 synthase activity at low concentrations (1×10^{-8} mol/L) and a comparatively weak and competitive TXA_2-prostaglandin endoperoxide receptor blocker at substantially higher concentrations (1×10^{-5} mol/L), can be administered in doses achieving dual activity. However, despite inhibiting TXA_2 and enhancing prostacyclin production, ridogrel was not superior to aspirin in enhancing fibrinolytic efficacy of streptokinase or in maintaining patency of the infarct-related coronary artery after thrombolysis with streptokinase in patients who did not receive any heparin.[153] Similarly, using a prostacyclin-sparing slow-release aspirin offers no clinical benefit over conventional aspirin in patients with unstable angina who also receive heparin followed by warfarin.[154]

Drugs that increase platelet cyclic adenosine monophosphate levels

DIPYRIDAMOLE. Dipyridamole (see Figs 28B-3 and 28B-7) increases platelet cAMP by three mechanisms: 1. It blocks its breakdown by inhibiting phosphodiesterase. 2. It activates adenylate cyclase by a prostacyclin-mediated effect on the platelet membrane.[155] 3. It increases the levels of plasma adenosine by inhibiting its uptake by vascular endothelium and erythrocytes.[156,157] Adenosine, in turn, enhances platelet adenylate cyclase activity. In addition, the vasodilative effects of dipyridamole appear to be related to the increase in plasma adenosine levels. Although in vitro data support dipyridamole's mechanisms of action on the platelet, no firm clinical evidence exists that such mechanisms contribute to a significant antithrombotic effect in humans.[157]

In contrast to aspirin, dipyridamole has antithrombotic effects that are more evident on prosthetic materials (artificial heart valves[158,159] and arteriovenous cannulas[73]) than on biologic surfaces. Although one study[74] showed that aspirin potentiates the efficacy of dipyridamole in experimental thromboembolism on prosthetic surfaces, other studies[157] yielded conflicting results on the pharmacologic interaction of these two agents. Furthermore, aspirin alone was as effective as the combination of aspirin and dipyridamole in several antithrombotic trials[160-164] in myocardial infarction, saphenous vein graft disease, and stroke. On the basis of these findings, there is little evidence to support the use of dipyridamole as an antithrombotic agent except in combination with warfarin in high-risk patients with a mechanical prosthesis[165-169] and perhaps in the period preceding coronary artery bypass surgery[170,171] to prevent platelet activation by the extracorporeal pump; however, the latter indication has not been properly tested.

PROSTAGLANDIN E_1 AND PROSTACYCLIN (PGI_2). These prostaglandins are powerful systemic vasodilators and inhibitors of platelet aggregation by virtue of their ability to increase platelet cAMP. Intravenous infusions of prostaglandin E_1 are commonly used in neonates with congenital heart disease who are dependent on the persistence of a patent ductus arteriosus until surgical correction is done. These agents have also been used to improve myocardial function in patients with acute myocardial infarction and to treat peripheral vascular disease.[172]

Prostacyclin is a potent platelet inhibitor synthesized by normal endothelium and adjacent subendothelial cells. Its clinical use has been limited by its instability at neutral pH and its propensity to cause significant systemic hypotension at the doses required for platelet inhibition. Its duration of action is very short, and the pharmacologic effects disappear in 30 minutes. Infusion of prostacyclin strongly limits platelet interaction with artificial surfaces and preserves platelet number and function during cardiopulmonary bypass.[173,174] The effects of prostacyclin in patients with ischemic heart disease and peripheral vascular insufficiency are controversial.[172]

PROSTACYCLIN ANALOGUES. Iloprost, a synthetized prostacyclin analogue, is chemically stable at neutral pH. In an in vitro comparison with equimolar concentrations of prostaglandin E_1 and prostacyclin, iloprost was found to be more potent in increasing the levels of cAMP and inhibiting platelet aggregation by various agonists, particularly thrombin.[175] However, in vivo studies in animals and humans with acute myocardial infarction did not show any benefit when iloprost was combined with a thrombolytic agent.[176,177] Another prostacyclin analogue, ciprostene, was found to reduce the rate of ischemic events in patients after coronary angioplasty but did not reduce the incidence of restenosis.[178] Thus, chemically stable analogues of prostacyclin may have antiplatelet activity, but they do not appear sufficiently potent at doses for safe administration without hypotension.

Other platelet inhibitors

TICLOPIDINE. Ticlopidine (see Fig 28B-3) is chemically unrelated to other antiplatelet drugs; its mechanism of action is not completely understood. It may act on the platelet membrane to alter its reactivity, perhaps by blocking the interaction of von Willebrand's factor and fibrinogen with platelets.[179] It inhibits platelet aggregation induced by adenosine diphosphate and low concentrations of thrombin, collagen, and TXA_2 (but high concentrations may overcome this effect); prolongs bleeding time; and normalizes shortened platelet survival.[180] Optimal efficacy is reached only after 3 days of administration, and its effects last for several days after administration has been stopped.

Clinical evaluation of ticlopidine is now under way. An Italian multicenter trial[181] suggests that ticlopidine is effective in patients with unstable angina for the prevention of myocardial infarction and cardiovascular death. Two studies in patients undergoing coronary angioplasty showed reduced incidences of acute occlusion and ischemic events after angioplasty, but the rate of restenosis was not reduced.[182,183] In addition, this agent was found to be effective in reducing vein graft closure in patients after aortocoronary bypass surgery.[184] Recently published data[185,186] suggest that ticlopidine reduces cardiovascular morbidity and mortality in patients with stroke and is more effective than aspirin in patients with transient ischemic attacks. However, ticlopidine is associated with occasional side effects, including rash and neutropenia. A sister compound, clopidogrel, has reduced side effects and is being evaluated in comparison with aspirin in patients with recent myocardial infarction, stroke, or peripheral vascular disease (Clopidogrel versus Aspirin in Patients at Risk of Ischemic Events – CAPRIE study).

SULFINPYRAZONE. Sulfinpyrazone (see Fig 28B-3) is structurally related to phenylbutazone but has minimal anti-inflammatory activity. In contrast to aspirin, sulfinpyrazone is a competitive inhibitor of platelet cyclooxygenase, but the exact mechanism of its antithrombotic activity is not well understood.[74] It inhibits the formation of thrombus on the subendothelium and protects the endothelium from chemical injury in vitro and possibly in vivo. In addition, sulfinpyrazone produces a dose-dependent inhibition of experimental thromboembolism in artificial cannulas,[74] reduces the rate of thrombotic events in patients with arteriovenous cannulas,[187] and normalizes platelet survival in patients with artificial heart valves.[188] Overall, beneficial effects have been more consistent on prosthetic than on biologic surfaces. Sulfinpyrazone did not reduce platelet deposition after deep arterial injury in pigs.[189] Thus, despite a beneficial trend in decreasing vascular events after myocardial infarction[190] and reducing the occlusion rates in saphenous vein coronary grafts,[164,191] sulfinpyrazone was found to have no additional benefit in unstable angina[135] and stroke.[192] Side effects of sulfinpyrazone include increased sensitivity to warfarin, hypoglycemia when combined with sulfonylureas, exacerbation of peptic ulcer, and precipitation of uric acid stones or transient renal insufficiency.

DEXTRAN. Dextran of molecular weight 65,000 to 80,000 daltons prolongs the bleeding time. Its mechanism of action is unclear. It may involve some alteration of platelet membrane function[193] or interference with factor VIII-von Willebrand's factor complex.[194] Although some experimental studies[195] have shown an antithrombotic effect of dextran, no effect was found in a randomized trial[196] in patients undergoing coronary angioplasty. Furthermore, dextran has been associated with a low but disturbing incidence (0.6%) of anaphylactoid reactions.[197] Data supporting the role of dextran as an antithrombotic agent on foreign materials (i.e., arterial stents and vascular grafts) are lacking.

Inhibition of platelet membrane adhesive glycoproteins. The final common pathway of platelet aggregation is mediated through binding of platelet membrane adhesive glycoproteins (see Fig 28B-2), such as the von Willebrand factor and fibrinogen, to platelet glycoprotein IIb-IIIa. This interaction may be blocked by short peptides containing the amino acid sequence Arg-Gly-Asp (RGD), by arginine mimetics, and by monoclonal antibodies against glycoprotein IIb-IIIa. Thus, short-term complete inhibition of platelet aggregation may be achieved with peptides or antibodies that block either the platelet membrane receptor (glycoprotein IIb-IIIa) or adhesive macromolecules, such as von Willebrand's factor.[198,199] Thus, these agents may inhibit the platelet membrane receptors necessary for platelet adhesion, may be useful for short-term therapy, and may cause an exceptionally high risk of bleeding. However, such therapy requires concomitant use of a thrombin inhibitor, such as heparin, to prevent fibrin formation and thrombin-mediated platelet aggregation.[200] In addition, glycoprotein IIb-IIIa receptor inhibitors appear to be effective experimentally at high shear with less effect at low shear; this poses a disadvantage for arterial injury in a larger coronary artery without a severe stenosis or after a stenosis is reduced by angioplasty.

Thrombin inhibitors. Thrombin inhibitors may inhibit platelet deposition weakly (heparin dose to an activated partial thromboplastin time [aPTT] of two times control), modestly (high-dose heparin, as in the cardiac catheterization laboratory, to activated coagulation time of more than 300 seconds), markedly (direct thrombin inhibition with hirudin to an aPTT of two to three times control), or poorly (direct thrombin inhibition with intravenously delivered argatroban to an aPTT of 3.8 times control).[13,14,22,201-203]

Direct thrombin inhibition by peptides. The direct and specific thrombin inhibitor hirudin is now made recombinantly, is derived from the anticoagulant in leech saliva *(Hirudo medicinalis)*, and is the prototype and most potent direct, specific thrombin inhibitor. Hirudin blocks the conversion of fibrinogen to fibrin at lower doses and at higher doses blocks platelet activation, aggregation, and deposition on deeply injured arterial wall.[13,202,204] Since platelets are exquisitely sensitive to tiny amounts of thrombin,[205] there is a sharp definition of the dose-activity response of hirudin for preventing mural thrombus on deeply injured arterial wall (thrombus occurred at an aPTT of 1.7 times control but not at more than two times control).[13] More thrombin appears to be generated after deep arterial injury (and more hirudin is required to prevent thrombosis) than after subendothelial injury, intravascular coagulation, or venous thrombosis. The half-life of hirudin in patients with coronary artery disease is 2 to 3 hours, and the aPTT is the best laboratory test for monitoring therapy.[206,207]

Because thrombosis and thrombolysis are dynamic and simultaneous in vivo processes, the most potent antithrombotic therapy will best accelerate thrombolysis and promote endogenous thrombolysis. Hirudin blocks thrombus growth, accelerates thrombolysis, and promotes dethrombosis and endogenous thrombolysis in animals and patients.[14,22,208] Hirudin appears promising for patients with unstable angina, acute myocardial infarction, and recent arterial occlusions.[207-209] Ongoing clinical trials are testing hirudin in acute coronary syndromes, including myocardial infarction with and without thrombolysis (GUSTO II) and thrombolysis for acute myocardial infarction (TIMI 9).

Heparin

Mechanisms of action. Heparin (see also chapter 30B) is a highly sulfated glycosaminoglycan (see Fig 28B-7) that is derived from porcine intestinal mucosa or bovine lung. The effect of heparin as an anticoagulant is essentially direct and immediate and depends on its ability to accelerate the action of the naturally occurring protease inhibitor antithrombin III; indeed, the absence or near absence of antithrombin III renders heparin useless for antithrombotic therapy. Antithrombin III inhibits thrombin and several other proteases of the coagulation cascade by the formation of covalent protease-inhibitor complexes. The interaction of heparin with antithrombin III leads to a conformational change in the inhibitor that greatly accelerates its interaction with coagulation proteases, particularly thrombin and factor Xa.[210,211]

Heparin can be fractionated on the basis of either molecular weight or affinity for antithrombin III. Low-molecular-weight heparin (molecular weight of 5,000 to 7,000) effectively catalyzes the inactivation of factor Xa by antithrombin III but does not prolong the aPTT (i.e., less antithrombin effect) or interact with platelets to the extent that high-molecular-weight heparin does.[212,213] The antithrombin effect of heparin appears more important than the anti-Xa effect for prevention of platelet deposition and arterial thrombosis.[214] Therefore, it has been suggested that low-molecular-weight heparin may be an effective antithrombotic agent with a relatively low risk of hemorrhagic side effects[215] for patients with venous thrombosis but less satisfactory for arterial thrombosis unless used at a higher dose with a measurable aPTT.[214]

Dose, administration, and control of therapy. The major aim of heparin administration is to prevent both the formation and the extension of thrombi while minimizing the risk of bleeding. Heparin is not absorbed by the GI mucosa and must be given intravenously or subcutaneously. Absorption from sites of intramuscular injection is erratic and frequently results in hematoma formation; hence, this route of delivery should be avoided. Both calcium and sodium salts of heparin seem to be equally safe and effective. Heparin is distributed mainly in the intravascular space, because it binds to several plasma proteins, including platelet factor IV, which is released by platelet activation. This protein binding contributes to the reduced bioavailability at low concentrations, to the variable anticoagulant response to fixed-dose administrations in patients with thrombotic disorders, and to the laboratory phenomenon of heparin resistance. Heparin also binds to endothelial cells and macrophages. The saturable phase of heparin clearance is due to the binding of heparin to the cells, where it is internalized and metabolized. The slower nonsaturable clearance is mainly renal. At therapeutic doses, most heparin is cleared via the rapid saturable, dose-dependent mechanism. This causes a nonlinear, ever-increasing anticoagulant response in intensity and duration with increasing dose. Thus, the biologic half-life of intravenously administered heparin increases from 30 minutes with a bolus of 25 U/kg to 60 minutes with a bolus of 100 U/kg to 150 minutes with a bolus of 400 U/kg. Patients with massive thrombosis (such as deep venous thrombosis pulmonary embolism) usually require higher dosages early in the treatment course.[216]

At present, no test is completely satisfactory for monitoring heparin effect. The most commonly used test is the aPTT,[211,216-218] which measures the effect of heparin on the intrinsic and common coagulation pathways (see Fig 28B-2). The protamine sulfate neutralization assay, which measures the amount of protamine sulfate (a heparin inactivator) necessary to normalize the thrombin clotting time, can also be used.[211,216,219,220] Anticoagulation with heparin should be maintained at a level equal to 0.2 to 0.5 U of heparin per million (using the protamine sulfate titration standard curve), which corresponds to an aPTT of 1.5 to 2.5 times control. Unfortunately, no international standard is available for the different procoagulants and reagents used in the aPTT system.[216] When larger doses of heparin are needed, such as during cardiopulmonary bypass and percutaneous transluminal coronary angioplasty in the catheterization laboratory, the activated clotting time, which measures the effect of heparin on whole blood clotting stimulated by diatomaceous earth, allows rapid determination of the anticoagulant effect of heparin, although it is less sensitive at lower heparin levels.[221,222]

Treatment of patients with active thrombosis should be initiated by an intravenous bolus to immediately saturate heparin binding sites and be followed by administration by one of the two preferred routes, intravenous infusion or subcutaneous injection, to prolong coagulation within a predefined range. Patients at higher risk of bleeding may receive intravenous infusion to allow more rapid adjustment of anticoagulation. Patients with massive thrombosis require a larger initial bolus (such as 10,000 U for those with massive venous thrombosis pulmonary embolism). Higher average doses are required for maintenance by subcutaneous injection (average of 35,000 U/24 hr from five studies) than by continuous intravenous infusion (30,000 U/24 hr). Average therapeutic doses may range between 25,000 and 50,000 U/24 hr (Table 28B-3). Intermittent intravenous injections at 4-hour intervals in full therapeutic doses are seldom used because of the greater difficulty in monitoring, greater risks of supertherapeutic or subtherapeutic levels, and potentially greater risk of bleeding (or greater risk of thrombosis if the daily doses of heparin are similar to doses used during continuous intravenous infusion). Subtherapeutic levels of heparin achieved by injecting a low dose subcutaneously are effective for routine prevention of venous thrombosis (during and after elective general surgery), because heparin affects multiple levels of the coagulation

Table 28B-3 Heparin regimens

Dosage (U/24 hr)	Route	Clinical indications	Therapeutic range (aPTT ratio)
Low (10,000-15,000)	Subcutaneous (continuous IV)	Elective general surgery (not including major orthopedic procedures)	
Intermediate (18,000)	Subcutaneous* (continuous IV)	Orthopedic procedures	1.1-1.2
Intermediate (24,000-30,000)	Subcutaneous* (continuous IV)	Acute myocardial infarction, heart failure, and immobilization	1.5-2.0
		After acute venous thromboembolism	1.5-2.0
Average, or "therapeutic" (25,000-50,000)	IV (continuous or intermittent) or subcutaneous	Acute thromboembolism	1.5-2.0
High (40,000-60,000)	IV (continuous or intermittent)	Massive acute venous thromboembolism	2.0-2.5

aPTT, activated partial thromboplastin time; IV, intravenous.
*Starting with subcutaneous dosing every 12 hours without IV bolus may prolong achievement of therapeutic aPTTs for 36 to 48 hours.[223]

cascade, is administered before the appearance of thrombus and amplification of the coagulation cascade, and is not administered for higher risk situations of local injury (as in major orthopedic procedures or acute myocardial infarction).

CONTINUOUS INFUSION. Continuous infusion of heparin (Fig 28B-8 and Table 28B-3) is used in patients with acute coronary syndromes, cardiac chamber thrombosis, and venous thrombosis or pulmonary embolism. Heparin is administered as an initial bolus (5,000 U routinely or 10,000 U for massive thrombosis), which is followed by maintenance doses with an automatic infusion pump.[211,216] The laboratory test for monitoring anticoagulation (usually aPTT) is performed approximately 6 hours after therapy begins and at least once more during the first 24 hours (assuming each test result is in target range). Twice daily monitoring is continued until anticoagulation is stabilized in the target range.

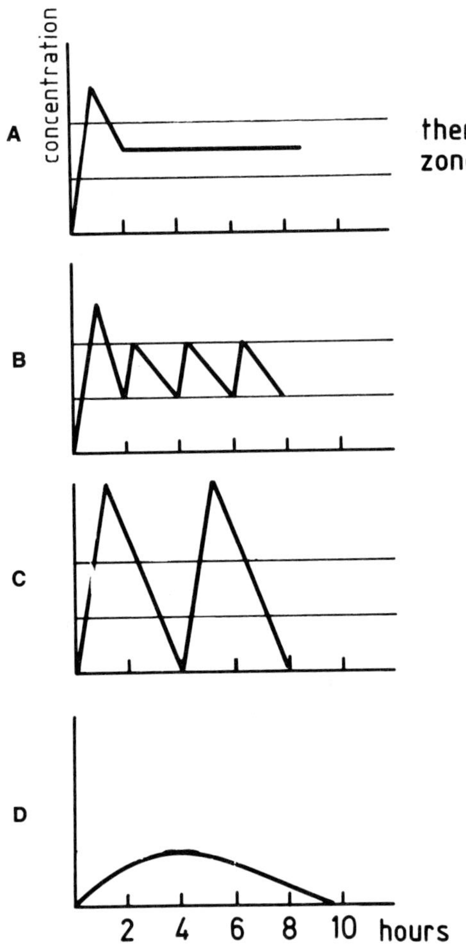

Fig 28B-8 Blood concentration of heparin after (**A**) bolus injection followed by continuous IV infusion (**B** and **C**), intermittent IV injections, and (**D**) subcutaneous injection. The risk of bleeding is higher when high-dose intermittent IV injection (**C**) is used and lower with subcutaneous injection (**D**). (From Verstraete M, Vermylen J: *Thrombosis.* Oxford, Pergamon Press, 1984, pp 76-112. By permission.)

The average maintenance infusion is 30,000 U/24 hr. This dose is adjusted according to the result of the test for monitoring anticoagulation. Protamine sulfate titration equivalent to 0.3 to 0.4 U/mL of heparin corresponds to an aPTT of 1.5 to 2.0 times control (approximately 60 to 85 seconds) and is the heparin concentration that prevents the extension of experimental thrombi.[216] The level is adjusted slightly higher for patients with pulmonary embolism (0.4 to 0.5 U/mL of heparin, corresponding to an aPTT of 2.0 to 2.5 times control); in some patients, this may require an infusion of nearly 50,000 U/24 hr. An algorithm for adjusting heparin dosage is given in Table 28B-4. During the first 2 or 3 days, dosage requirements may change, but thereafter the dose response for a given patient is usually stable.

Patients in the early postoperative period or with a hemostatic defect may be treated with lower doses of heparin. An initial bolus of 2,000 U is followed by maintenance dosage of 15,000 to 20,000 U/24 hr, with an anticoagulation effect of heparin monitored more frequently than usual to maintain the heparin level between 0.1 and 0.2 U/mL, corresponding to an aPTT of 1.25 to 1.5 times control (aPTT approximately 45 to 59 seconds).[211,216]

INTERMITTENT INTRAVENOUS INJECTION. Intermittent intravenous injections of heparin, used extensively in the past,[224,225] are no longer routinely recommended, because intravenous infusion or subcutaneous administration is more easily monitored, avoids peaks that may produce bleeding and nadirs that may produce thrombosis, and overall may require higher doses to avoid drifting to subtherapeutic levels. However, this appears to increase the risk of bleeding.[224-226] Intermittent intravenous heparin therapy certainly would not be recommended for patients at increased hemorrhagic risk, especially the elderly and those receiving thrombolysis.[216,226]

SUBCUTANEOUS INJECTION. Heparin can be given subcutaneously in low, intermediate, or full therapeutic doses[227] (see Fig 28B-8 and Table 28B-3). When heparin is used prophylactically in patients undergoing elective abdominal or thoracic surgery, it is usually given by subcutaneous injection in doses of 5,000 U every 8 or 12 hours.[228-230] The first subcutaneous dose is given 2 hours before operation, and administration continues thereafter every 8 or 12 hours for the first 7 days, preferably until 2 days after complete mobilization. For this administration, 0.2 mL of concentrated heparin containing 5,000 U is used. Monitoring of the aPTT is usually not required.

An intermediate heparin regimen of about 10,000 U given every 12 hours is of prophylactic value in patients at very high risk for venous thromboembolism and can also be used for the secondary prevention of venous thrombosis after a 7- to 10-day course of full-dose heparin.[230] A dose of 10,000 to 15,000 U given every 12 hours has been successful in acute myocardial infarction for the prevention of recurrence[231] and for prevention of left ventricular thrombi.[223] The dose is adjusted so that the aPTT 6 hours after injection is about 1½ times control (heparin level, 0.2 to 0.3 U/mL).[211,216,230-232]

Table 28B-4 Intravenous heparin: monitoring and dosage adjustment*

aPTT, sec†	Infusion change, mL/hr	Dose change, U/24 hr	Additional action	Next aPTT
≤45	+6	+5,760	Rebolus with 5,000 U	4-6 hr
46-54	+3	+2,880	None	4-6 hr
55-59	+2	+1,920	None	4-6 hr
60-85‡	0	0	None	Next morning§
86-110	−3	−2,880	Stop infusion 1 hr	4-6 hr after restart
>110	−6	−5,760	Stop infusion 1 hr	4-6 hr after restart

aPTT, activated partial thromboplastin time.
*A starting bolus of 5,000 U (thrombolysis) to 10,000 U (massive venous thrombosis or pulmonary embolism) intravenously followed by intravenous infusion of 1,000 U/hr (thrombolysis) or 1,200 U/hr (acute coronary syndromes without thrombolysis or venous thrombosis) or 1,300 U/hr (pulmonary embolism); heparin, 20,000 U in 500 mL D5W and 25 mL/hr for 1,000 U/hr, 30 mL/hr for 1,200 U/hr, or 33 mL/hr for 1,300 U/hr. The concentration of heparin is 40 U/mL. When aPTT is checked at 6 hours or longer, steady-state kinetics can be assumed. Dosage adjustments are made as in table above.
†Normal aPTT with Dade-Actin FS reagent of 27 to 35 seconds.
‡Therapeutic range of 60 to 80 seconds is approximately equivalent to a plasma heparin concentration of 0.2 to 0.4 U/mL by protamine titration or to 0.35 to 0.7 U/mL by inhibition of factor Xa. The therapeutic range varies with different aPTT reagents and coagulation machines.
§During the first 24 hours, repeat aPTT in 4 to 6 hours. Thereafter, monitor aPTT daily unless it is subtherapeutic.
Modified from Hyers TM, Hull RD, Weg JG: Antithrombotic therapy for venous thromboembolic disease. *Chest* 102 Suppl 4:408S-425S, 1992.

Side effects and neutralization of heparin. Side effects of heparin and the relative frequency are listed in Table 28B-5. Intracranial bleeding is the most serious and is related to the use of thrombolytic agents, level of anticoagulation (especially aPTTs over 100 seconds), increased age, lower body weight, female gender, and systolic blood pressure exceeding 150 mm Hg (based on results from pooling of all patients treated in the International Study of Infarct Survival trials).[233,234] Major bleeding was more prominent during the first 24 hours (approximately 40% of episodes) after the beginning of therapy, perhaps reflecting the greater anticoagulation after the initial bolus, than during the subsequent plateau level of anticoagulation (see Fig 28B-8). Bleeding related to early increased anticoagulation was especially evident with the direct antithrombin hirudin, which also was associated with increased bleeding in patients with diminished renal function, which increases anticoagulation because of the renal dependence of hirudin excretion. These two studies emphasize the narrow therapeutic window for administration of heparin (and direct antithrombins) with thrombolytic therapy. Bleeding with heparin was greater in the GUSTO IIa trial than in GUSTO I with only slight increases in dosage administration (increased infusion rates of 1,100 to 1,300 U/hr by weight, and the upper target range of aPTT increased from 85 to 90 seconds). Increased bleeding was evident with both streptokinase and recombinant tissue-type plasminogen activator therapies, resulting in increases in hemorrhagic stroke to as high as 2% to 3% with streptokinase plus heparin.[233,234]

Risk factors for bleeding for all patients receiving heparin (with or without thrombolytic therapy) include competence of hemostasis prior to heparin therapy, invasive procedures (especially arterial punctures with large-bore devices), aspirin therapy, trauma, and surgery (recent or during therapy). Generally, therapy with heparin should not be used in patients with hemorrhagic diatheses, persistent hypertension (>180/105 mm Hg), major trauma, cerebrovascular hemorrhage, acute ulceration, or overt bleeding from the respiratory, gastrointestinal, or genitourinary tracts. Bleeding risks appear to increase with heparin dose. Heparin administered alone in patients with coronary artery disease is not associated with an increased bleeding risk in the absence of the above risk factors.[226]

With continuous heparin infusion, the anticoagulant effect disappears within hours of discontinuing administration; this eliminates the threat of minor bleeding. When heparin is administrated as a bolus, the duration of anticoagulation depends on dose (3 to 4 hours after 4,000 to 5,000 U, and 6 hours after 15,000 U). Heparin maintained by subcutaneous therapy is sustained for up to 12 hours or more. If bleeding is severe, protamine sulfate (1% solution) is the drug of choice for neutralizing heparin. The protamines are low-molecular-weight proteins that are rich in arginine and thus strongly basic. They bind quickly to heparin, forming salts devoid of anticoagulant activity. One milligram of protamine sulfate neutralizes about 100 U of heparin. Only 50% of the calculated protamine sulfate dose should be administered, and only 25% of the calculated dose should be administered if 2 hours have elapsed since heparin administration. No more than 50 mg of protamine sulfate should be administered in any 10-minute interval. Because severe toxic reactions, including hypotension and anaphylaxis, may occur, epinephrine and corticosteroids should be available when protamine is used (especially if use was recent or multiple).

Heparin may cause thrombocytopenia (platelet count of $<100{,}000/mm^3$) in 3% to 10% of patients.[211,216,232,235,236] Thrombocytopenia appears to be

Table 28B-5 Side effects of heparin

Effect	Frequency
Bleeding	Common
Thrombocytopenia	Uncommon
Thrombocytopenia and thrombosis	Uncommon
Osteoporosis	Uncommon
Painful nodules at subcutaneous injection sites	Uncommon
Anaphylactic reaction	Rare
Alopecia	Rare
Elevation of hepatic transaminases	Rare
Skin necrosis	Rare
Urticaria (local)	Rare
Hypoaldosteronism	Rare

immune-mediated and typically occurs from 6 to 12 days after heparin therapy begins. This is unique among drug-induced thrombocytopenias, since it can be complicated by arterial thromboembolism. The diagnosis of heparin-induced thrombocytopenia is confirmed by a rapid normalization of the platelet count after discontinuation of heparin. It is not prevented by substituting low-molecular-weight heparin.

Transition from heparin to warfarin. The overlap of heparin with warfarin appears critical in patients with acute thromboembolism or a high likelihood of thrombosis to prevent enhancement of thrombosis in the absence of therapeutic heparin or reactivation of thrombotic events when heparin administration is stopped. Starting warfarin therapy alone without simultaneous heparin administration when stimuli for newly formed thrombus are present (e.g., in patients with anterior transmural myocardial infarction) increases the incidence of thrombus (e.g., in the left ventricle).[237] Overlap is not necessary when warfarin is administered as prophylaxis in the absence of a recent thrombotic event.

In addition, acute withdrawal of heparin alone after a mean of 6 days of treatment in patients with unstable angina causes reactivation of coronary events in 13% of patients within 96 hours (median, 9.5 hours). Reactivation of coronary events is reduced to 5.1% within 96 hours when withdrawal is from heparin plus aspirin, aspirin alone, or placebo alone.[238] Reactivation of thrombosis appears to be from residual mural thrombus overlying the disrupted atherosclerotic plaque of the culprit coronary artery. This thrombus is rich in thrombin and thrombin-generating activator complexes.[205,239] Heparin reduces the activity of thrombin but not its generation.[87] Thus, cessation of heparin alone may unmask the activity of thrombin when thrombin generation goes unchecked. For this reason, it appears critical to overlap heparin with warfarin for at least 24 hours after a therapeutic prothrombin time has been achieved so that rethrombosis can be prevented in patients with a recent thrombotic event, since they have a high likelihood of residual thrombus.

The overlap of heparin for 24 hours after a therapeutic prothrombin time has been achieved is necessary because the antithrombotic effect of warfarin is delayed relative to its anticoagulant effect on the prothrombin time.[240] The reason is that the early anticoagulant effect is caused by replacement of the normal factor VII, with a half-life of 6 to 7 hours, by the decarboxylated species, but the full antithrombotic effect is delayed for 72 to 96 hours because the half-lives of the other three vitamin K-dependent clotting factors (II, IX, X) are considerably longer. In addition, the half-life of protein C, the endogenous vitamin K-dependent anticoagulant and antithrombotic, is short and similar to that of factor VII. A course of heparin therapy also transiently depresses antithrombin III levels. Thus, a relative prothrombotic state due to the early decrease of protein C and decreased antithrombin III could be created by discontinuing administration of heparin as soon as the prothrombin time enters the therapeutic range. If the goal is a therapeutic international normalized ratio (INR) of 2.0 to 3.0, an INR in the upper portion of the range (e.g., 2.6 to 3.0) would be advised, because heparin may contribute to INR prolongation. After heparin administration is stopped, a therapeutic INR from warfarin alone is needed.[240]

Table 28B-6 Transition from intravenous (IV) heparin to warfarin bridging with outpatient subcutaneous (SC) heparin to reduce hospitalization

- Start SC heparin, 15,000 U; 12 hours later start 17,000 U every 12 hours*
- During continuous IV infusion of heparin, continue infusion for 2 hours after initial SC dose
- Obtain aPTTs at baseline, 6, 12, and 20 hours (8 hours after initial SC heparin)
- Give warfarin, 5 to 10 mg (double the anticipated maintenance dose) every day for 2 days and 3 to 5 mg every day thereafter
- Teach self-administration (or by spouse or visiting nurse) of SC heparin
- Obtain aPTTs daily during SC heparin administration (6 to 10 hours after SC dose)
- Determine prothrombin times daily for 5 days (starting on day 2), next at 1, 2, and 3 weeks, and then every 3 or 4 weeks
- Stop SC heparin when international normalized ratio reaches upper part of target range (e.g., 2.6 to 3.0 for target range of 2.0 to 3.0)

*Average of five reported studies.[211]

Transition from intravenously delivered heparin to warfarin with heparin overlap of 4 to 5 days or more can be initiated in the hospital and the patient dismissed in 24 hours if a switch is made from intravenous to subcutaneous administration of heparin, as outlined in Table 28B-6. This transition, using subcutaneous administration of heparin, serves the patient for approximately 4 hospital days. It requires a coordinated effort between physician and nursing personnel, which is most efficiently carried out at a large medical institution by means of an anticoagulation clinic.

Oral anticoagulants

Mechanism of action. During the hot summer of 1931, a few Canadian farmers in the province of Alberta were alarmed by the death of several cattle from hemorrhage. A peculiar intense smell of spoiled sweet clover, which these animals had been given to eat, was also noticed. The heat had favored the exuberant growth of molds, from which K. P. Link eventually isolated bishydroxycoumarin, or dicumarol, a potent anticoagulant. Since then, hundreds of congeneric substances of dicumarol have been synthesized, the most important of which is warfarin sodium (see Fig 28B-7) (see also chapter 30B).

Coagulation factors II, VII, IX, and X, protein C, and protein S are vitamin K-dependent proteins that are synthesized in hepatocytes. Post-translational modification of these proteins is necessary to yield biologically active molecules and involves the γ-carboxylation of glutamic acid residues. Coumarin anticoagulants inhibit vitamin K 2,3-epoxide reductase within hepatic microsomes and thus prevent recycling of vitamin K, which is necessary for the synthesis of γ-carboxyglutamic acid residues.[240] The carboxylation of coagulation factors is necessary for calcium binding and binding onto phospholipid surfaces, where biochemical reactions of the coagulation cascade are markedly accelerated by 200,000 to 300,000 times.

Circulating coagulation factors in plasma are normally in a state of dynamic but steady equilibrium. With an oral dose of anticoagulant (e.g., warfarin) large enough to block hepatic synthesis, each vitamin K-dependent coagulation factor decreases at a rate depending on its biologic half-life. When oral anticoagulation is discontinued, the coagulation factors return to normal at a rate depending on their intrinsic synthetic rates. After a latent period specific for each oral anticoagulant, the prothrombin time becomes prolonged, mainly from the effect of lowering the plasma level of factor VII, the vitamin K-dependent factor with the shortest half-life (6 to 7 hours). Plasma concentrations of the other vitamin K-dependent coagulation factors decrease more slowly because their half-lives are longer (20 to 60 hours for factors IX and X, and 80 to 100 hours for prothrombin). After 3 to 5 days of coumarin treatment, the lowered blood levels of the affected coagulation factors become virtually uniform. For effective treatment of thrombosis, the levels of factors II, VII, IX, and X should remain at approximately 25% of normal.

In North America, warfarin sodium is preferred among the coumarin drugs. The indanedione drugs are seldom used for oral anticoagulant therapy because they are more prone to side effects and more difficult to control. Although the various coumarin congeners differ in speed of induction of effect and in their individual metabolism, they all induce quantitatively similar effects on the clotting mechanism. Warfarin is extremely soluble in an aqueous medium and is completely absorbed from the GI tract and reaches maximal plasma concentrations in normal persons in 90 minutes. It is almost totally bound to plasma proteins, which may be partially responsible for its long plasma half-life. The biologic half-life of warfarin ranges from 36 to 42 hours and is independent of dose.[216] Warfarin is metabolized by hepatic microsomal enzymes. It can cross the placental barrier, but there is no firm evidence that the drug appears in breast milk in significant amounts. In one study involving mothers and infants, no warfarin was found either in the mother's milk or in the plasma of the breast-fed infant.[241]

Dose, administration, and control of therapy. Treatment with warfarin is usually begun by the oral route. O'Reilly and Aggeler[242] were the first to suggest that the danger of hemorrhage in sensitive patients is reduced by avoiding large loading doses.[240,242] A simple protocol for predicting early dosage adjustments has been devised for warfarin: A dose of 10 mg on the first day of treatment is followed for the next 3 days by daily adjustments on the basis of the prothrombin time determined 16 hours later.[243] Half to one-third of the initial dose may be considered if the patient is now nursed, is older than 75 to 80 years, has liver disease, or is receiving medication, which can significantly potentiate the effect of warfarin. If the INR on day 2 (16 hours after the initial dose) is less than 1.5, another 10 mg of warfarin is administered. If the INR is more than 1.5, the dose is decreased to less than 10 mg. If the INR on day 3 (16 hours after the second dose of warfarin) is less than 1.5, a greater than average maintenance dose (>5 mg) is suggested. If the INR is 1.5 to 2.0, an average dose of 4.5 mg per day is suggested. If the INR exceeds 2.0, a lower than average maintenance dose (<4.5 mg) is suggested. Data from the Stroke Prevention in Atrial Fibrillation Study targeting an INR of 2.0 to 3.0 suggest the following average warfarin dose for stabilized patients: under age 60, 5 mg/day; 60 to 70, 4 mg/day; 70 to 80, 3.5 mg/day; and over 80, 3 mg/day. To establish the optimal regimen for each patient, the prothrombin time should be monitored two or three times a week for the first few weeks of therapy. As a stable dosing regimen is established, this interval may be increased to 1 to 2 weeks and then eventually to 3 to 4 weeks. It is inadvisable to obtain prothrombin times at intervals of more than 1 month.

Oral anticoagulants are contraindicated in patients with a hemorrhagic diathesis, poorly controlled hypertension, cerebrovascular hemorrhage, major trauma, active peptic ulcer disease, unsteady gait with high risk of frequent falling, or overt bleeding from the GI, genitourinary, or respiratory tracts. Inadequate laboratory facilities and unsatisfactory patient cooperation should also be considered contraindications. Relative contraindications to oral anticoagulation include concomitant use of aspirin in a dose causing gastric erosion (over 325 mg/day), vasculitis, bacterial endocarditis, pericarditis complicating acute myocardial infarction, renal or liver disease, and thyrotoxicosis treated with radioactive iodine (because of the possibility of gland hemorrhage). Adequate treatment of concomitant disease before administration of oral anticoagulants may reduce the hazard of bleeding and disorders such as steatorrhea, sprue, ulcerative colitis, and pancreatitis. In diabetic patients, who may require long-term warfarin therapy, the risk of thromboembolism must be weighed against the risk of vitreous or retinal hemorrhage with anticoagulation.[244] Advanced age has been considered a relative contraindication to long-term oral anticoagulation because of potentially lethal side effects and the frequent use of other drugs that may interact with warfarin.[244,245] Nevertheless, clear evidence on the risk-benefit ratio of oral anticoagulation in elderly patients is not available, and age alone should not proscribe the use of warfarin in patients at high risk of thromboembolism.[246-248]

Numerous medications interact with warfarin. Therefore, it is vital to instruct all patients receiving warfarin to report promptly when any drug is deleted from or added to their therapeutic regimen, including nonprescription compounds. Frequent prothrombin time determinations permit dose adjustments that can prevent either under- or over-anticoagulation. Similarly, any major change in diet (e.g., leafy vegetables, green beans, and liver contain large amounts of vitamin K) should be reported so that drug dosage can be adjusted by more frequent determinations of the prothrombin time. Drugs that interact with warfarin can do so by altering warfarin absorption, plasma protein binding, and metabolism, causing significant potentiation or inhibition of the drug's anticoagulant effect. A list of the most important interactions is presented in Table 28B-7.

Prothrombin time is the test most frequently used to monitor warfarin therapy. It is performed by adding calcium and thromboplastin to citrated plasma and then measuring the time to fibrin formation. Thromboplastin is an extract of brain, lung, or placenta that contains tissue factor and phospholipid, which are necessary for the activation of factor X by factor VII.[249] Thromboplastins extracted from different organs or species can vary significantly in their sensitivity to reductions in levels of vitamin K-dependent factors. Thus, a single plasma sample from a patient receiving coumarin could yield significantly different prothrombin times if assayed in two different laboratories that used different commercial thromboplastins. In addition, the results of the prothrombin time also depend on the instrument used for measurement of coagulation.

Table 28B-7 Drugs affecting the anticoagulant activity of warfarin

Enhanced effect	Decreased effect
Chloramphenicol	Vitamin K
Cimetidine	Oral contraceptives
Anabolic steroids	Rifampin
D-Thyroxine	Griseofulvin
Clofibrate	Glutethimide
Metronidazole	Cholestyramine
Phenylbutazone	Barbiturates
Sulfinpyrazone	Phenytoin
Quinidine	
Disulfiram	
Sulfonamides	
Chloral hydrate	
Alcohol (abuse only)	
Allopurinol	
Amiodarone	
Antibiotics	
Methyldopa	
Aspirin (in high doses)	

The prothrombin time can be standardized either by comparing a given thromboplastin through a standard thromboplastin or by using standard plasmas from normal persons and patients with a known anticoagulation status. The INR system uses the former method and compares the local thromboplastin with a World Health Organization (WHO) standard. The INR is the prothrombin time ratio that would have been obtained if the WHO primary standard for thromboplastin had been used.

Any prothrombin time system (i.e., a combination of the thromboplastin and the clotting instrument) can be related to the INR scale by calibration of the thromboplastin. The calibration is performed by measuring the prothrombin time of normal persons in patients receiving anticoagulant therapy with both the local thromboplastin and the WHO standard. Usually, 20 normal persons and 60 patients are required for the comparison. The prothrombin times are plotted on double logarithmic scales and an international sensitivity index (ISI) is calculated by orthogonal regression analysis. The INR is an exponential function that is calculated as follows: INR = (patients' prothrombin time/mean normal prothrombin time for laboratory)^{ISI}. The prothrombin times are expressed in seconds. Note that the mean normal for the laboratory is used in this calculation, not the control for the day.

In summary, the INR is calculated from the prothrombin time ratio, which is a simple calculation, and the ISI, which is the exponent applied to the ratio. The ISI is calculated by the manufacturer of thromboplastin, by the laboratory performing the test, or by both. The ISI of the WHO standard is by definition 1.0. Recombinant tissue factor is now being manufactured with an ISI of 1.0. This will simplify laboratory reporting of the prothrombin time and INR, since the prothrombin time ratio is the same as the INR when the ISI is 1.0.

The INR offers several advantages: 1. Smooth regulation of anticoagulant therapy. 2. Benefit to patients who travel or use different laboratories for monitoring. The INR provides consistency among laboratories using different types of thromboplastin. This is critical for avoiding both thrombosis due to low prothrombin times and bleeding due to excessive prothrombin times. 3. Standardization of anticoagulant therapy in clinical trials and scientific publications. The INR is applied only to patients receiving long-term anticoagulant therapy or whose conditions are stable.[240,249]

The intensity of oral anticoagulation necessary to properly treat or prevent intravascular thrombosis varies depending on the clinical situation. The American College of Chest Physicians Conference on Antithrombotic Therapy offered the following recommendations for oral anticoagulant therapy:[240]

A. A less intense degree of oral anticoagulation

(INR = 2.0 to 3.0) should be used in the following clinical situations:

1. Prevention of venous thromboembolism in high-risk patients.
2. Treatment of venous thrombosis and pulmonary embolism (after an initial course of heparin).
3. Prevention of systemic embolism in patients with tissue cardiac valve prostheses, nonvalvular atrial fibrillation with risk factors, valvular heart disease and atrial fibrillation, acute transmural anterior wall myocardial infarction, or dilated cardiomyopathy.

B. A more intense degree of oral anticoagulation (INR = 2.5 to 3.5) should be used in patients with mechanical cardiac valve prostheses, recurrent systemic thromboembolism, or recent arterial thrombosis (Table 28B-8).

Side effects. The most important side effect of oral anticoagulation is bleeding. The risk of bleeding varies from patient to patient, depending on the intensity of anticoagulation, the indication for its use, and the presence of comorbid conditions. Hull et al.[250] showed that in patients with venous thrombosis, those randomized to more intense anticoagulant therapy (INR, 2.5 to 4.5) have a more than fivefold greater risk of bleeding (22% compared with 4%) than those randomized to less intense anticoagulation (INR, 2.0). Levine et al.[226,232,251] pooled data from 171 studies dealing with rates of bleeding in patients receiving long-term oral anticoagulant therapy. The risk of major bleeding (intracranial or retroperitoneal bleeding or bleeding leading directly to death, hospitalization, or transfusion) was 8.1% in venous thromboembolism, 7% in ischemic cerebrovascular disease, 4.7% in ischemic heart disease, and 2.4% with prosthetic cardiac valves. The incidence of major bleeding is best expressed as rate per 100 patient-years of therapy and is from 2 to 22 per 100 patient-years in ischemic cerebrovascular disease, 0 to 7.7 per 100 patient-years in myocardial infarction, and 0.8 per 100 patient-years in patients with prosthetic cardiac valves. Levine et al. concluded that the reason for the relatively high incidence of bleeding complications in patients with ischemic cerebrovascular disease and venous thromboembolism is the frequent presence of comorbid conditions, such as hypertension, malignancy, and recent surgery.

Bleeding in patients receiving oral anticoagulants may occur at unusual sites. Hemorrhage into the bowel lumen, the intestinal wall, the mesentery, the rectus muscle, or the corpus luteum may simulate an acute abdominal crisis. Similarly, genitourinary bleeding may mimic a renal tumor. Hematomas may cause carpal tunnel compression, and, rarely, there may be pericardial, adrenal, or retro-

Table 28B-8 Antithrombotic approach to cardiovascular disease based on pathogenesis and thromboembolic risk

	Thromboembolic risk		
Pathogenesis	**High (>6%/yr)**	**Medium (2%-6%/yr)**	**Low (<2%/yr)**
Arterial system	Unstable angina Acute MI After thrombolysis PTCA, early phase SVBG, early phase	Chronic stable angina Chronic phase after MI PTCA, chronic phase SVBG, chronic phase	Primary prevention of coronary disease
Platelets and fibrin	Platelet inhibitors plus anticoagulants*	Platelet inhibitors or anticoagulants (INR, 2.0-3.0)†	Platelet inhibitors‡
Cardiac chambers	AF, prior embolism AF, mitral stenosis	AF, other forms of organic heart disease Early phase after anterior MI Dilated cardiomyopathy	Idiopathic AF Chronic LV aneurysm
Fibrin	Anticoagulants (INR, 2.5-3.5 in prior embolism or 2.0-3.0 in mitral stenosis)	Anticoagulants (INR, 2.0-3.0)	Usually no need for therapy
Prosthetic valves	Old mechanical prostheses Mechanical prostheses, prior embolism	Recent mechanical prostheses Bioprostheses, AF	Bioprostheses, normal rhythm
Fibrin and platelets	Anticoagulants (INR, 2.5-3.5) plus platelet inhibitors *or* Anticoagulants (INR, 3.0-4.0)	Anticoagulants (INR, 2.5-3.5 in mechanical prostheses or 2.0-3.0 in bioprostheses)	Usually no need for therapy

AF, atrial fibrillation; INR, international normalized ratio of prothrombin suppression; LV, left ventricular; MI, myocardial infarction; PTCA, percutaneous transluminal coronary angioplasty; SVBG, saphenous vein bypass graft.
*Heparin may be used in the acute phase (aPTT, 60-85 sec, 1.5-2.0 times control).
†Although both are beneficial, platelet inhibitor therapy is recommended because of lower toxicity, ease of administration, and cost.
‡Recommended for persons at high risk for coronary disease.

peritoneal hemorrhage. Whether to search for the cause of an episode of spontaneous bleeding, such as from the genitourinary or GI tract, can best be decided if the prothrombin time is obtained within 24 hours of hemorrhage. Experience has shown that when the INR is in the range of 2.0 to 3.5, the likelihood of finding a localized lesion is greater than if the INR is in excess of 4.5. In the former situation, further efforts to identify the bleeding source should be undertaken promptly.

Minor bleeding in patients with prolonged prothrombin times can be treated by withholding warfarin temporarily. Major bleeding may additionally require the administration of vitamin K_1 or blood products. The dose of vitamin K_1 depends not only on the end point desired but also on the intensity of the warfarin effect. A common mistake is the administration of a high dose of vitamin K_1 in an effort to return the prothrombin time to normal more rapidly. Larger doses of vitamin K_1 do not increase the rate of synthesis of the individual vitamin K-dependent clotting factors; rather, vitamin K_1 restores extrinsic synthesis rates for a period that is dose-dependent. The route of vitamin K_1 administration may be intravenous, subcutaneous, or oral, depending on the nature and urgency of the clinical situation. Some correction of the prothrombin time is noted within 6 hours, and full correction occurs within 24 hours. If the patient is to continue receiving warfarin, the dose of vitamin K_1 should be 0.5 to 1.0 mg. Higher amounts, up to 10 mg, may be indicated if therapy is not to be maintained after the hemorrhage is controlled. Large doses of vitamin K_1 may make the patient resistant to warfarin for many days, preventing effective anticoagulant therapy for that period. An immediate reversal of the clotting defect can be achieved by transfusion of blood, plasma, or plasma concentrates rich in the vitamin K-dependent clotting factors. Because these factors are relatively stable, they remain fully potent in ordinary banked blood or banked or lyophilized plasma. Three units of blood or plasma or 15 mL/kg should suffice for an initial effect, providing time for concomitant vitamin K_1 administration to exert its action. In patients with limited cardiac reserve, the recommended volumes of blood or plasma may precipitate pulmonary edema unless significant blood loss has occurred or patients are receiving diuretic therapy. Plasma concentrates rich in factors II, VII, IX, and X avoid the hazard of hypervolemia but carry with them the risk of thrombosis, hepatitis, and acquired immunodeficiency syndrome.

Nonhemorrhagic side effects of warfarin include coumarin embryopathy and coumarin-induced skin necrosis. Coumarin readily crosses the placenta and has been found to be teratogenic, particularly during the first trimester of pregnancy.[252] Fetal bone and cartilage development appears sensitive to warfarin, as evidenced by the best-described abnormalities of coumarin embryopathy, nasal deformity, and stippling of the bony epiphyses. This effect may be mediated by deficiency of osteocalcin, a vitamin K-dependent protein.[253] An increased incidence of fetal wastage and central nervous system defects has also been observed with exposure to warfarin during pregnancy.[254] For this reason, most experts advise substitution of subcutaneously administered heparin (e.g., approximately 12,500 to 17,000 units subcutaneously every 12 hours, with target aPTT of 1½ to 2 times control) for coumarin, at least during the first trimester of pregnancy and for several weeks before delivery.[255] Indeed, high doses of heparin given subcutaneously throughout the pregnancy have been advocated by many.[252,253] Therefore, fertile women receiving warfarin must be warned of the risks of teratogenicity and should be advised to notify their physicians at the earliest suspicion of pregnancy.

Coumarin-induced necrosis of the skin and subcutaneous tissues is a rare but striking complication of warfarin therapy that has been associated with hereditary protein C deficiency.[256] The lesion appears within 3 to 10 days of drug administration, usually in the lower half of the body. It occurs particularly in women and in areas of abundant subcutaneous fat, such as the buttocks, breasts, thighs, and abdomen. The initial manifestation of coumarin-induced skin necrosis is an erythematous patch. Frank hemorrhagic necrosis may develop within 24 hours. Coumarin necrosis should not be confused with purple toe syndrome,[257] in which pain and bluish discoloration develop in the toes, often accompanied by livedo reticularis to the knees or to the iliac crest; this is believed to represent atheromatous embolization to the extremities, perhaps accentuated by warfarin.[258] When coumarin-induced necrosis occurs, warfarin administration should be discontinued. If further anticoagulation is indicated, heparin therapy should be initiated.

Thrombolytic agents

The acute coronary syndromes, including acute myocardial infarction, unstable angina, and sudden death, are caused by thrombotic occlusion of critically situated blood vessels. Timely pharmacologic dissolution of blood clots therefore aborts the evolution of these syndromes, preserves the myocardium, and reduces mortality. Dissolution can be achieved with intravenous infusion of plasminogen activators[259,260] (see also chapter 30B), which convert plasminogen, the inactive proenzyme of the fibrinolytic system, to the proteolytic enzyme plasmin (see Fig 28B-4). Plasmin is a serine protease that digests fibrin to soluble degradation products. Natural inhibition of the fibrinolytic system occurs both at the level of the plasminogen and at the level of the plasmin. Plasminogen is a single-chain glycoprotein consisting of 790 amino acids; it is converted to plasmin by cleavage of the Arg560-Val561 peptide bond by plasminogen activators, which are serine proteases with a high specificity for plasminogen. The plasminogen molecule contains structures called "kringles" that mediate its binding to fibrin and accelerate the interactions of plasmin with its physiologic inhibitor α_2-antiplasmin.

Currently, five thrombolytic agents are either approved for clinical use or under clinical investigation in patients with acute myocardial infarction: streptokinase, recombinant tissue-type plasminogen activator (rt-PA), acylated plasminogen streptokinase activator complex (APSAC), urokinase, and single-chain urokinase-type plasminogen activator (scu-PA, or prourokinase).[259-262] This section presents a brief overview of the current status of thrombolysis, a field in which progress is rapid.

Streptokinase

MECHANISM OF ACTION. Streptokinase is produced by Lancefield group C strains of β-hemolytic streptococci. It is a nonenzymatic antigenic protein that forms a 1:1 stoichiometric complex with plasminogen. This complexing exposes the active site of the light chain of plasminogen. The complex is then converted spontaneously to streptokinase-plasmin complex, which is a potent activator of plasminogen. Streptokinase complexes consist of both circulating and fibrin-bound plasminogen for conversion to plasmin. Initially, circulating plasmin is neutralized by α-antiplasmin, which is consumed, and the result is that plasmin exerts its proteolytic effect on plasma coagulation proteins, including fibrinogen and factors V and VIII. This consumption of fibrinogen and coagulation factor contributes to the bleeding risk of streptokinase, especially when it is combined with heparin or other antithrombins to an aPTT of more than 100 seconds. The half-life of circulating streptokinase is approximately 30 minutes.[233,234,259]

REPERFUSION. Many factors influence the success of thrombolytic therapy. Some are related to the occlusion, such as the age, location, and concentration of plasminogen and plasmin inhibitors on the thrombus. Others are related to the therapeutic regimen, such as the dosage of the agent used, the duration of the therapy, and the speed with which treatment is begun.[259-262a,b] Because of the dynamic and simultaneous processes of thrombosis and thrombolysis and the critical role of thrombin in thrombosis, adjunctive therapy with a direct thrombin inhibitor accelerates reperfusion both experimentally and now clinically.[263,264] The direct thrombin inhibitor hirulog increased coronary artery patency at 90 minutes from 47% with heparin to 77% with hirulog.[264] Rentrop et al.[265] pioneered the intracoronary use of streptokinase in patients with acute myocardial infarction. The enthusiasm stemmed in part from the anticipated greater incidence of thrombolysis when the drug was delivered directly to the vicinity of the clot, the potential for efficacy with a lower dose, and the advantage of confirmation of an occlusive thrombus before treatment and angiographic assessment of its response to lytic therapy. Although these advantages are real, the delay associated with intracoronary administration and the relatively limited immediate availability of cardiac catheterization facilities for most patients presenting with acute infarction have led to virtual abandonment of the intracoronary route as the primary or sole approach for most patients. The collective experience from numerous earlier studies of intracoronary delivery of streptokinase with a dose of 250,000 units in patients with acute myocardial infarction indicates that thrombolysis with reperfusion occurs in about 85% of patients.[266-268]

The reported patency rate of intravenously administered streptokinase in patients with acute myocardial infarction is much lower than that achieved with intracoronary streptokinase. The cumulative database from 13 angiographic studies indicated that the infarct vessel patency rate at 60 to 120 minutes was approximately 48% with the use of 1.5 million units infused over 1 hour.[269-281] However, a definite "catch-up" phenomenon for streptokinase was recently documented by serial angiography performed up to 24 hours after the onset of symptoms. By the time of late follow-up cardiac catheterization, the patency rate of arteries treated with streptokinase approached 80%.[281] However, it is the reperfusion to normal or Thrombolysis in Myocardial Infarction (TIMI) grade 3 flow at 90 minutes that predicts subsequent mortality and left ventricular function (salvage).[282]

COMPLICATIONS. The complications of intracoronary administration of streptokinase are related to the catheterization and angiographic procedures, the thrombolytic agent, the adverse effects of reperfusion, and the consequences of reocclusion. The major risk of streptokinase is hemorrhage.[283] A systemic lytic state with fibrinogenolysis is induced even when subtherapeutic or low doses of intracoronary streptokinase are administered. Bleeding occurs most frequently at the site of vascular puncture. However, systemic hemorrhage, including cerebral, GI, mediastinal, and urinary tract, may be encountered, particularly when occult predisposing causes are present. The reported prevalence of hemorrhage requiring transfusion after intracoronary or intravenous administration of streptokinase has ranged from 1.3% to 18%, but most studies report an incidence of 10% or less. Fortunately, intracerebral bleeding is rare, occurring in fewer than 1% of patients.[259-262a,b,283,284] Also, transient episodes of hypotension have been reported in approximately 9% and 17% of patients, respectively, after intracoronary and intravenous administration of streptokinase.[283] However, hypotension has generally responded to transient interruption of the infusion of streptokinase and to administration of fluids or atropine. Another side effect of streptokinase is related to its antigenicity. Overt allergic reactions are not common. Frank anaphylaxis is extremely rare, and skin rash, swollen lips, and urticaria occur in less than 2% of patients.[283]

Recombinant tissue-type plasminogen activators

MECHANISM OF ACTION. Wild-type tissue-type plasminogen activator (t-PA) is a trypsin-like serine protease composed of 527 amino acids and is produced by recombinant DNA technology.[259-262] Because of limited plasmin action on the fibrin surface, wild-type t-PA is rapidly converted to the two-chain form, which has comparable fibrinolytic activity (but different amidolytic activity in vitro). The heavy, or A, chain of this molecule contains two regions that share a high degree of homology with the five kringles of plasminogen, and the catalytic site is located on the light, or B, chain.

In the absence of fibrin, t-PA is a poor plasminogen activator. In the presence of fibrin, however, t-PA activates plasminogen several hundredfold more rapidly. The underlying principle of this phenomenon is that both plasminogen and t-PA bind to fibrin and form a ternary complex. Thus, fibrin serves as a cofactor for plasminogen activation by lowering the K_m of t-PA for plasminogen. As a consequence of these kinetic characteristics, plasmin is predominantly generated on the fibrin surface.[259-262] This in turn results in a relative sparing of circulating fibrinogen and other plasma proteins to plasmin-mediated degradation. Recombinant tissue-type plasminogen activator (rt-PA) is mainly single-chain t-PA and the only one currently on the market for clinical use.

REPERFUSION. Accelerated administration of rt-PA (intravenous bolus of 15 mg followed by an infusion of 0.75

mg/kg over 30 minutes [maximum, 50 mg] and then an infusion of 0.5 mg/kg over a 60-minute period [maximum, 35 mg], along with aspirin and intravenous heparin) maximizes coronary artery patency at 90 minutes and reduces mortality and left ventricular dysfunction relative to streptokinase.[281,282,284] This accelerated-dose rt-PA and heparin administration resulted in coronary artery patency with normal flow at 90 minutes in 54% of patients, compared with 29% to 32% of patients in the streptokinase groups.[282] Double-bolus rt-PA therapy (two bolus injections of 50 mg of rt-PA separated by 30 minutes) resulted in normal or TIMI grade 3 flow in 86% of patients at 60 minutes and 88% of patients at 90 minutes.[285] Reocclusion after administration of either rt-PA or streptokinase was minimized at 5 to 7 days after thrombolysis with the use of combined antithrombotic therapy with heparin plus aspirin; reocclusion rates were very low in all groups, ranging from 4.9% to 6.4%.[282]

COMPLICATIONS. Speculation has ranged from a prediction that rt-PA would be associated with less bleeding because of the absence of a systemic lytic state[286,287] to fear that it would result in an increased risk of bleeding secondary to augmented fibrinolytic potency.[262a,288] Direct comparative trial data with streptokinase showed little difference in extracranial bleeding complications. The incidence of intracranial hemorrhage was 0.5% in 2,742 patients treated with 100 mg[289] and 0.72% in 10,396 patients treated with front-loaded rt-PA.[284] However, the overall combined end point of death and stroke from all causes was significantly lower in patients treated with front-loaded rt-PA than in those treated with streptokinase. Contrary to protocols in other large mortality trials,[290-293] this overall low frequency was established with detailed data collection and routine computed tomographic scanning for any new neurologic deficit. In contrast to streptokinase, rt-PA is nonantigenic and lacks hypotensive effects.

Acylated plasminogen streptokinase activator complex

MECHANISM OF ACTION. Acylated plasminogen streptokinase activator complex (APSAC) is a complex of streptokinase and human lys-plasminogen.[259-262,294,295] Its catalytic center is acetylated, which renders the molecule inactive. The acyl group is hydrolyzed after intravenous injection, with a deacylation half-life of 40 minutes, thus exposing the active center. This transient blocking of the active center theoretically allows time for APSAC to bind to fibrin via the kringles of plasminogen before becoming active (without being inactivated by α_2-antiplasmin), resulting in fibrin-specific plasminogen activation. In fact, however, when the drug is administered intravenously in a therapeutic dose (30 U), systemic fibrinogenolysis is constant. The half-life of APSAC is 90 minutes, compared with 23 minutes for streptokinase. This prolonged half-life results in long-lasting thrombolytic effects. Because the intravenous injection of the complex does not cause profound hemodynamic effects, the drug can be administered in a bolus injection.[259-262,295,296]

REPERFUSION. Results of several clinical studies indicate that the patency rate for infarct-related arteries at 90 minutes after intravenously administered APSAC (30 U) is approximately 69%. Comparison of intravenously administered APSAC and streptokinase in a French randomized, open-designed, multicenter study demonstrated a slightly higher patency rate in patients receiving APSAC than in those given streptokinase (72% compared with 55%).[297]

COMPLICATIONS. The bleeding complication rate produced by APSAC is remarkably similar to that of other thrombolytic agents with or without fibrin specificity. In a French multicenter trial involving 231 patients, hemorrhage was observed in 6.5% of the APSAC-treated patients, and only half these patients required blood transfusion.[297]

Urokinase and single-chain urokinase-type plasminogen activator

MECHANISM OF ACTION. Urokinase is a double-chain glycoprotein and a trypsin-like serine protease that occurs in two molecular forms – S1 (32 kd) and S2 (54 kd) – the former being a proteolytic degradation product of the latter.[259-261] Urokinase isolated from human urine or cultured embryonic kidney cells is nonantigenic. It directly activates plasminogen and generates plasmin by cleaving the Arg560-Val561 bond of the plasminogen molecule. Urokinase is not specific for fibrin and activates fibrin-bound as well as circulating plasminogen. Thus, it also includes a systemic activation of the fibrinolytic system as soon as the α_2-antiplasmin level is reduced. The half-life of urokinase is about 10 minutes, so that the persistence of thrombolysis may be less than that with streptokinase. Single-chain urokinase-type plasminogen activator (scu-PA), or prourokinase, is a single-chain glycoprotein containing 411 amino acids; it is converted to urokinase by plasmin-mediated hydrolysis of the Lys158-Ile159 peptide bond. Although scu-PA has very little activity toward synthetic substrates, it has intrinsic plasminogen-activating potential, with a catalytic efficiency that is two orders of magnitude lower than that of urokinase. The half-life of scu-PA is about 8 minutes.[259-261]

REPERFUSION. Two reports[298,299] showed that the patency rate at 60 minutes in patients with acute myocardial infarction given urokinase by either intracoronary or intravenous administration is about 60%. This moderately fibrin-selective thrombolytic agent can be given intravenously with a reduced systemic lytic state and predictably lower bleeding risk than intravenously administered streptokinase. The recanalization rate of scu-PA in patients with acute myocardial infarction is about 78%, as reported by Van de Werf et al.,[300] with use of 70 mg of scu-PA infused over 1 hour. The potential value of these two agents is that they may provide synergistic effects on clot lysis and reperfusion when combined with other thrombolytic agents. Topol et al.[301] demonstrated that although the patency rate in patients with acute myocardial infarction given the combination of t-PA and urokinase was not significantly higher than that achieved by t-PA alone, the reocclusion rate was substantially lower. Similarly, some beneficial effects on bleeding complications and reocclusion were observed when the combination of t-PA and scu-PA was used.[302] Other combinations, such as t-PA and streptokinase, are currently being evaluated. These synergistic combinations of thrombolytic agents may offer better cost-benefit and risk-benefit ratios than those obtainable with single-agent therapy. However, if valid conclusions are to be drawn, continued investigation of synergism needs to be done with appropriate procedures of experimental design and data analysis and requires combined investigation between pharmaceutical companies, which has previously been difficult.

ROLE OF ANTITHROMBOTIC THERAPY IN CARDIAC DISEASE

In the foregoing sections, we established the importance of pathogenesis at the site of thrombosis: platelet and fibrin components in arterial disease, predominance of fibrin in cardiac chambers, and predominance of fibrin over platelet component in prosthetic valves. We can also classify the various clinical cardiac syndromes according to absolute and relative risk of thromboembolic events developing[303] (Table 28B-8). We shall discuss three general risk categories derived from the number of episodes per 100 patients per year: (1) highest risk, more than six, (2) medium risk, two to six, and (3) lower risk, fewer than two. Persons without overt evidence of heart disease have a comparable annual event rate below 1%. Pathogenesis and risk stratification are conducive to the therapeutic role and intensity of the various antithrombotic strategies in preventing thromboembolism in coronary arteries, cardiac chambers, and prosthetic heart valves (see Table 28B-8).

Coronary arteries

Acute coronary syndromes. As discussed earlier, type III vascular injury with recurrent thrombosis is the major mechanism linking the acute coronary syndromes. During the early phase of the acute coronary syndromes of unstable angina and acute myocardial infarction, the risk of thrombotic occlusion (or reocclusion after vessel reperfusion) developing is substantial, varying between 5% and 20%.[303] This high risk of thrombotic occlusion or reocclusion makes antithrombotic therapy mandatory in patients with unstable angina and myocardial infarction.

UNSTABLE ANGINA

Platelet inhibitors. The results of four randomized trials support administration of aspirin as a platelet inhibitor to patients with unstable angina and no previous use of aspirin. A Veterans Administration cooperative study[134] found a 51% collective reduction in mortality and nonfatal myocardial infarction with a daily dose of 324 mg during a period of 12 weeks, and benefit was still detected after a full year. A Canadian multicenter trial[135] corroborated these findings using a higher aspirin dosage (1,300 mg daily) for a mean of 18 months; an identical 51% reduction in myocardial infarction and death was found; sulfinpyrazone conferred no added benefit. The effects of aspirin or heparin, or both, were compared in a short-term (6-day) randomized trial conducted in two Montreal hospitals;[304] aspirin (325 mg twice daily) reduced the combined rate of fatal and nonfatal myocardial infarction by 72% in a placebo comparison. In a Swedish study,[305] 75 mg of aspirin daily reduced the continued incidence of cardiac death and nonfatal myocardial infarctions by 63%. The Italian multicenter trial[181] of ticlopidine (250 mg twice a day) in patients with unstable angina revealed that this potent platelet inhibitor significantly reduced the combined incidence of cardiac death and nonfatal myocardial infarction by 46% (13.6% in controls to 7.3% in the treated group).

Unfortunately, at least half the patients treated with aspirin have further ischemic events. In addition, up to 50% to 80% of patients presenting with unstable angina to hospitals today in the United States are already taking aspirin regularly. These previous users of aspirin appear to be at greater risk of early cardiac events than those without prior aspirin use.[306] Thus, additional therapy with anticoagulation added to aspirin appears to be warranted in these patients.

ANTICOAGULANTS (WITH AND WITHOUT ASPIRIN). An earlier study of unstable angina suggested that intravenously administered heparin reduced the incidence of myocardial infarction by as much as 80%, but deficiencies in patient recruitment left the conclusions of this trial less credible.[307] In the Montreal study[304] mentioned above, the 240 patients treated with heparin, with or without aspirin, had an 89% reduction in the rate of infarction compared with placebo results. Because there was a trend favoring heparin over aspirin, the study was extended in the heparin only and aspirin only groups. Myocardial infarction occurred in only 0.8% (2 of 240 patients) randomized to heparin and 3.7% (9 of 244 patients) randomized to aspirin alone ($P = 0.035$). This study documents that heparin alone prevents myocardial infarction better than aspirin alone during the acute phase of unstable angina.[308]

Combined anticoagulation plus aspirin in patients with unstable rest angina and non-Q-wave infarction significantly reduces recurrent ischemic events in the early phase (days and weeks) of unstable angina in patients without previous use of aspirin.[309] Pooled analysis of three trials comparing aspirin plus heparin with aspirin alone showed that myocardial infarction or death was significantly reduced during the first 5 days of this treatment for unstable angina. In one of these trials, Antithrombotic Therapy in Acute Coronary Syndromes (ATACS), heparin was replaced by warfarin, and administration was continued for 3 months. In this study, 214 patients were randomized to either aspirin alone (162.5 mg/day) or aspirin and anticoagulation with heparin (aPTT, 1.5 to 2 times control) followed by warfarin to an INR of 2 to 3 for 3 months. There was a significant reduction in primary ischemic events with combined therapy in the first 14 days (10.5% versus 27%, $P = 0.004$) with a trend toward beneficial effects at 90 days (13% versus 25%, $P = 0.06$) (Fig 28B-9). In patients with unstable angina, reaction events (refractory angina, myocardial infarction, or death) were associated with cessation of heparin alone (13% incidence over 96 hours; median time for reactivation event was 9.5 hours) and were lower in patients treated with heparin plus aspirin (5% incidence over 96 hours, with no early clustering of reactivation events).[238]

Because 3 to 6 months may be required for a disrupted plaque to heal,[5] the risk of early reactivation of events with heparin alone and the reduced event rate with combined therapy (especially when heparin is replaced by warfarin) suggest that combined anticoagulation plus aspirin is the most efficacious treatment for patients presenting with

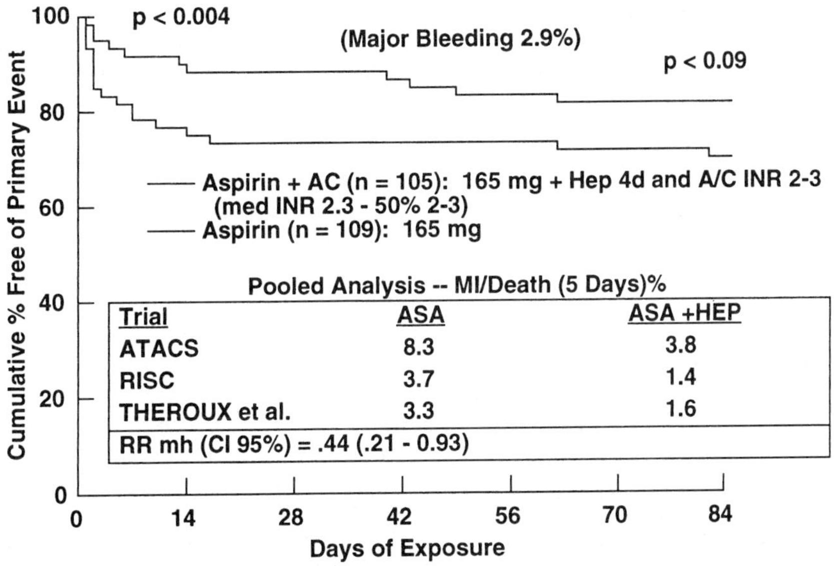

Fig 28B-9 The Unstable Angina in Non-Q-Wave Infarction (ATACS) trial comparing anticoagulation (starting with heparin and switching to warfarin) plus aspirin versus aspirin alone, showing the incidence of ischemic events over the first 3 months for each group. *Boxed data,* antithrombotic therapy in unstable angina comparing heparin (HEP) plus aspirin (ASA) versus ASA alone in a pooled analysis for the end point of myocardial infarction or death from three randomized controlled trials after 5 days of therapy. (Modified from Cohen M, Adams PC, Parry G, et al: Combination antithrombotic therapy in unstable rest angina and non-Q-wave infarction in nonprior aspirin users. Primary end points analysis from the ATACS trial. *Circulation* 89:81-88,1994.)

unstable angina. At hospital admission, heparin should be administered intravenously in a bolus of 5,000 U. This dose is followed by intravenous infusion of heparin at 1,000 U/hr if the patient's weight is less than 60 kg, 1,200 U/hr if weight is 60 to 80 kg, and 1,300 U/hr if weight is over 80 kg (with aPTT monitoring to 1.5 to 2 times control, or between 60 and 85 seconds). Aspirin administration should begin simultaneously with heparin at a loading dose of 160 mg on admission to the hospital and be continued at 80 mg/day. For patients being referred for coronary angiography and possible coronary angioplasty, combined antithrombotic therapy should continue for at least 3 days to minimize the risk of thrombotic events, including acute coronary occlusion after angioplasty. For patients being treated medically, conversion of heparin to warfarin and continuation of low-dose aspirin for at least 3 months (and then clinically aspirin alone) appear to minimize the risk of future ischemic events.

Direct thrombin inhibitors (the prototype is hirudin) would probably be superior to heparin in blocking the growth of thrombus and encouraging endogenous lysis and thus would have the potential for reducing the need for coronary revascularization procedures.[207,208,310] The GUSTO II trial is currently comparing hirudin with heparin in patients with unstable angina who are also taking aspirin.

Thrombolytic therapy. As predicted,[311] thrombolytic therapy in patients with unstable angina was of no benefit or worsened the outcome in 19 smaller trials.[312-330] In the largest trial (1,473 patients), the incidence of fatal and nonfatal acute myocardial infarction was increased within 42 days in rt-PA-treated patients from 4.9% in the placebo group to 7.4% in the treated group (P = 0.04).[331] These findings are consistent with the lack of survival benefit in the large GISSI-I and ISIS-II trials in the subgroups of patients with myocardial infarction who had ST-segment depression at presention; with streptokinase treatment, no survival benefit was observed over that with placebo.[332]

In addition, significant differences between coronary substrates leading to unstable angina and those leading to acute myocardial infarction probably explain why the success of thrombolytic therapy in myocardial infarction cannot be duplicated in unstable angina.[311] First, of patients presenting with an acute myocardial infarction with ST-segment elevation, 70% to 90% have total occlusion of the infarct-related artery on angiography. In unstable angina, the frequency of total occlusion of the ischemia-related artery is significantly less and as low as 8%.[99] Second, the thrombus formation in unstable angina develops slowly after type III injury, and much of the thrombus in these lesions may be partially organized by the time of clinical presentation. This partial organization may explain the pathologic finding by Falk,[48] who found layering of thrombus in most patients who died after an episode of unstable angina. Therefore, in such patients, only small amounts of thrombus would be present and amenable to thrombolysis. In addition, thrombus formation in patients with unstable angina may occur not within the lumen but beneath the fibrous cap of the plaque. Moreover, after type III injury, there may be a geometric change in the shape of the plaque without significant intraluminal thrombus formation. In both situations, little thrombus would be available for thrombolysis.[311] The extent of type III injury in unstable angina is probably less than in acute myocardial infarction and may thus result in a smaller amount of intraluminal thrombus formation.[311]

Finally, the extent of thrombin generation and formation within thrombus is greater adjacent to deep arterial injury, increasing platelet-rich thrombus and fibrin deposition with increased cross-linking of the fibrin, all of which make the thrombus more resistant to thrombolysis.[205]

Thus, thrombolysis is not indicated in patients with unstable angina, since it results in no benefit and appears to increase the risk of myocardial infarction and probably intracranial bleeding. Rather, combination antithrombotic therapy with anticoagulation plus aspirin appears indicated at present. Newer antithrombotic therapy with direct antithrombins or platelet membrane receptor inhibitors, or both, appears especially promising and is being tested in randomized trials.

ACUTE MYOCARDIAL INFARCTION. As in unstable angina, type III vascular injury and superimposed thrombotic occlusion play major roles in the development of acute myocardial infarction.[6] In some patients, particularly those with non-Q-wave infarction, spontaneous reperfusion occurs as a result of thrombolysis or resolution of vasospasm, limiting myocardial necrosis[333,334] but setting the stage for subsequent ischemic events. The more extensive necrosis that occurs in Q-wave infarction probably results from persistent thrombotic coronary occlusion with inadequate collateral flow. In addition, because spontaneous vessel recanalization seems to occur in both non-Q- and Q-wave infarction, an aggressive antithrombotic approach, including thrombolytic agents for Q-wave infarction, is beginning to emerge for achieving successful lysis, continuing endogenous lysis, and preventing thrombotic reocclusion by reducing residual thrombus and blocking thrombus regrowth.

Thrombolytic therapy and rethrombosis. The use of thrombolytic therapy in acute myocardial infarction is discussed in chapter 30B. We therefore will concentrate on one of the major problems encountered in patients after successful thrombolytic therapy—rethrombosis.

Reocclusion after successful recanalization is a frequent problem that precludes improvement in left ventricular function, increases mortality, and reduces the benefits of early reperfusion.[29,335,336] Serial coronary angiography is necessary before, during, and after therapy to assess reperfusion. Consequently, few studies have systematically determined the incidence of reocclusion. Some studies have defined nonangiographic clinical reperfusion and reocclusion, but the definition is unreliable because of spasm or silent reocclusion with or without collaterals. In this context, early reocclusion is defined as the angiographic closure of a reperfused or patent artery within the first 24 hours of thrombolytic therapy and late occlusion as angiographic closure usually assessed just before hospital dismissal. The rate of early reocclusion is quite variable;[291,335] it ranges from 0% to 45% and usually is 4% to 18%. Late reocclusion ranges from 5% to 30%. Both processes are due to rethrombosis, which in turn appears to depend on two main factors:[335] (1) the pathologic substrate, namely, type III vascular injury, with exposure of lipid gruel and collagen and the thrombogenic surface of the residual thrombus on the atherosclerotic plaque, and (2) the rheologic factors, or the increase in shear rate and turbulent flow created by the residual stenosis.[5,10-12,22,335]

Type III vascular injury with the exposure of various thrombotic elements creates a strong stimulus for thrombosis (see above). Furthermore, during lysis (endogenous or exogenous), there is release of active thrombin from within the dissolving thrombus and activation of platelets by the active surface of the thrombus. There is now evidence that combined therapy with heparin plus aspirin minimizes the incidence of reocclusion.[282,335] Prevention of reocclusion, therefore, requires inhibition of mechanisms involved in rethrombosis and includes two basic principles: thorough lysis and antithrombotic therapy.

Antiplatelet therapy. The value of aspirin in patients with acute myocardial infarction is demonstrated in the large Second International Study of Infarct Survival (ISIS-2).[136] Patients with suspected myocardial infarction treated within 24 hours had a 23% greater reduction in 5-week vascular mortality than those given placebo. This striking benefit was possibly related to prevention of reinfarction in patients with spontaneous vessel recanalization. Indeed, aspirin reduced the rate of nonfatal reinfarction by almost half.[136]

As discussed previously, patients with acute myocardial infarction treated with thrombolytic agents are at high risk for early reocclusion, which approaches 5% to 30%.[282,291,292] The importance of concomitant platelet inhibitor therapy in patients undergoing thrombolysis was emphasized by the results of the ISIS-2 trial,[136] in which streptokinase alone decreased early cardiovascular mortality by 25% and the combination of aspirin and streptokinase decreased the death rate by 42%. The benefits of these agents appeared independent of one another, and the addition of aspirin to streptokinase reduced the clinical reinfarction rate by 50%. A meta-analysis of studies from the literature on the use of aspirin versus no aspirin (in all but a few studies, the patients were also receiving heparin infusion) after thrombolysis showed a reduction in reocclusion from 25% without aspirin to 11% with aspirin.[337] The lowest rates of reocclusion were achieved in the GUSTO angiographic study, in which heparin plus aspirin reduced reocclusion to 4.9% to 6.3% in all groups.[282] Thus, we advocate aspirin (160 mg loading dose and then 80 to 160 mg daily) as early as possible in the treatment of acute myocardial infarction, whether or not thrombolytic agents are given. Daily use of aspirin should be continued after dismissal.

Anticoagulant therapy. The issue of short-term anticoagulation in acute myocardial infarction, aimed at reducing the incidence of death, infarct extension, or reinfarction, is still not settled. Despite a large number of studies published during the past 40 years, only three randomized, controlled trials[338-340] were large enough to establish a significant reduction in mortality with anticoagulants. Of these, only one[339] found a statistically significant decrease in mortality; the other two[338,340] showed a beneficial trend. In addition, all three revealed a trend toward lower reinfarction rate. When the results of the only six published randomized trials were pooled,[341] a significant 21% reduction in mortality in treated patients emerged. Despite the limitation inherent in retrospective meta-analysis of heterogeneous trials, short-term anticoagulation in acute myocardial infarction appears to provide a modest reduction in early mortality. Because of the high risk of reinfarction, however, the combination of aspirin and an anticoagulant appears promising[303] and is being tested in the Coumadin-Aspirin Reinfarction Study (CARS) and in the CHAMPS study.

As expected from the pharmacokinetics of heparin, low to medium doses of heparin administered subcutaneously twice daily beginning 4 to 12 hours after thrombolytic therapy in patients with acute myocardial infarction showed no clinical benefit in reducing mortality in two large trials.[290,293] However, three angiographic trials provided solid evidence for improved infarct-related arterial patency with heparin administration,[342-344] but the relationship of these outcomes to mortality is uncertain. Heparin with adequate aPTTs (compared with heparin and inadequate aPTTs) has been shown to improve the patency of the infarct-related artery and the minimal lumen diameter by angiography after 3 weeks of administration in patients receiving streptokinase as thrombolytic therapy.[345] Thus, it is recommended that every patient who receives thrombolytic therapy be considered for adjuvant anticoagulant therapy lasting at least 48 hours, followed by continuing anticoagulant therapy. This recommendation is based on clinical interpretation of trials from the prethrombolysis era and the results of angiographic evaluations of heparin therapy in conjunction with thrombolysis.[291] The GUSTO trial documents the efficacy and safety of the initial heparin therapy in decreasing the reocclusion rates for streptokinase and rt-PA to the lowest so far reported in the medical literature in a large prospective trial (4.9% to 6.3% after 5 to 7 days). The heparin regimen in GUSTO that was associated with a lower incidence of bleeding was 5,000 U in an intravenous bolus followed by 1,000 U/hr, with maintenance of the aPTT at 1.5 to 2 times control (60 to 85 seconds). In the APRICOT study, infarct-related artery patency at 3 to 6 months after myocardial infarction was low (60%) when warfarin was not administered[346] or when suboptimal doses of heparin (20,000 U/24 hours as a fixed intravenous infusion) were used during hospitalization before therapy with warfarin.[347]

Chronic phase after myocardial infarction. Survivors of acute myocardial infarction are at medium risk for recurrent infarction or cardiac death.[348] Because cardiac morbidity and mortality during the period may be related to a number of factors, including left ventricular dysfunction, ventricular arrhythmias, and recurrent myocardial infarction, proving that antithrombotic therapy is beneficial in these patients has been difficult and has generated controversy for several decades.[303]

PLATELET INHIBITORS. Since 1974, there have been no fewer than 10 randomized trials involving platelet inhibitors in patients with prior myocardial infarction, and an extensive meta-analysis[138] of these studies has been published. Despite the inherent problems of pooled data, this overview concluded that among survivors of myocardial infarction, platelet inhibitors reduced vascular mortality by 22% (from 11.7% to 9.3%), nonfatal reinfarction by 54% (from 2.2% to 1.0%), nonfatal stroke by 40% (from 0.6% to 0.4%), and all important vascular events by 29% (from 14.4% to 10.6%).[138] Aspirin alone was at least as effective as the combination of aspirin and dipyridamole and more effective than sulfinpyrazone. Available data do not justify the additional cost and frequency of administration of platelet inhibitors other than aspirin in this group of patients.[138]

ANTICOAGULANTS. Although controversy has existed about the effect of oral anticoagulants on postinfarction morbidity and mortality,[349,350] the results of several well-designed clinical trials indicate that there is a beneficial effect. The Veterans Administration Cooperative Study demonstrated a significant reduction in mortality for the first 3 years after myocardial infarction in patients treated with oral anticoagulants.[351] The Warfarin Reinfarction Study[352] demonstrated a 24% reduction in mortality, a 34% reduction in reinfarction, and a 55% reduction in stroke with warfarin therapy in postinfarction patients, compared with placebo. In this study, the incidence of serious bleeding in warfarin-treated patients was 0.6 per 100 patient-years.

Considering the above data, either aspirin or warfarin can be used for the secondary prevention of cardiac events. However, at a daily dose of 325 mg, aspirin offers several advantages over long-term anticoagulation in cost, ease of administration, and side effects. Thus, to survivors of myocardial infarction, daily use of aspirin is recommended. Studies evaluating combined low-dose warfarin and aspirin after myocardial infarction are in progress (CARS and CHAMPS).

Chronic stable coronary artery disease. Patients with a remote history of myocardial infarction (beyond 2 years) and those with chronic stable angina are at medium risk of coronary ischemic events, which vary between 2.5% and 5% per year.[348] In patients with remote myocardial infarction, recurrent thrombotic events are probably the main cause of mortality. Most studies of platelet inhibitors in survivors of myocardial infarction showed a beneficial trend toward lower mortality and reinfarction, which became significant only when the data derived from all available trials were pooled.[138]

In the Sixty Plus Reinfarction Study Research Group,[353] patients older than 60 who were treated with warfarin for a median of 6 years after myocardial infarction were randomly assigned to continue taking the anticoagulant or to take a placebo instead. The design was double-blind, and anticoagulant dosage was tightly controlled for 2 more years, at which point the anticoagulated group had a 26% lower mortality ($P = 0.07$) and 55% lower incidence of reinfarction ($P = 0.0005$) than the placebo group. It appears, therefore, that both aspirin and anticoagulants are effective in preventing reinfarction and reducing mortality in asymptomatic patients after remote myocardial infarction, but the former is associated with lower cost and risk.

Although no randomized trial of antithrombotic therapy in chronic stable angina has been published, the sustained beneficial effects of aspirin after initial therapy for patients with unstable angina and after coronary angiography (5-year follow-up in patients receiving aspirin and dipyridamole compared with those receiving placebo) suggest a role for aspirin in stable coronary disease.[134,135,138,205] A dose of 160 to 325 mg daily is associated with minimal GI toxicity and should be considered in these patients. As suggested from a 5-year follow-up angiographic study in patients with stable coronary disease randomized to platelet inhibitor therapy or placebo, significant thrombi may be prevented or reduced in some patients, and this definitely reduces the incidence of acute myocardial infarction and may reduce new lesion progression.[205]

Primary prevention of coronary events. In the final report from the U.S. Physicians' Health Study,[137] which included 22,071 male physicians followed up for 4.8 years, aspirin (325 mg every other day) significantly reduced the incidence of myocardial infarction by 44%, from about 0.4% to 0.2% per year. The incidence of cardiovascular death was identical in the aspirin and placebo groups, but aspirin was associated with a slight increase in the number of hemorrhagic strokes (although this did not attain statistical significance). In a British primary prevention trial[354] involving 5,139 male physicians, two-thirds were randomly assigned to take aspirin (500 mg daily) and one-third were instructed to avoid it (no placebo was given). After 6 years, no difference in the incidence of myocardial infarction or cardiovascular mortality was detected. Although the number of enrolled subjects was smaller than in the American trial, cardiovascular event rates were 5 to 10 times higher. When both studies are considered together, there appears to be a reduction in coronary events with aspirin but at the price of an increased risk of hemorrhagic stroke. The long-term effects of aspirin on the prostaglandin system in various tissues, especially the brain, are unknown. Aspirin is recommended for primary prevention only in individuals at high risk for coronary artery disease for whom the benefits of therapy outweigh the risk. Additional analysis of the U.S. Physicians' Health Study suggests that aspirin exerts a much greater effect on patients at higher risk for coronary events, mainly those with cardiovascular risk factors or evidence of cerebral or peripheral vascular disease.[355]

Coronary interventions

VEIN GRAFT DISEASE AFTER BYPASS SURGERY. Coronary vein graft disease contributes to significant morbidity and mortality after coronary artery surgery. Vein graft occlusion rates are 8% to 10% at 1 to 2 weeks, 8% to 18% of distal anastomoses at 1 month, and 6% to 16% of distal anastomoses at 1 year after operation.[102,103] The occlusion rate is then 2% to 4% per year in grafts still patent at 1 year. At the end of 5 years, up to 35% of vein grafts are occluded. Vein graft disease can be divided into two main stages: an early postoperative stage of thrombotic occlusion related to type III injury and a late stage of accelerated atherosclerotic process secondary to repetitive type II injury, which begins within the first year and is due to lipid accumulation, fibrointimal proliferation, and thrombus organization resembling spontaneous atherosclerosis and the final stages of atheroma formation.[102,103]

Early graft occlusion. As discussed in previous sections, early occlusion seems to be related to a type III vascular injury caused by surgical manipulation and exposure of the graft to high rates of arterial blood flow.[102] This process is mainly thrombotic in origin, and platelets play a major pathogenic role. Antithrombotic therapy is most effective in reducing the rate of early postoperative thrombotic occlusion.

Several trials of *platelet inhibitors*[102,163,164,170,184,356,357] have documented that aspirin, with or without dipyridamole, or ticlopidine reduces the incidence of early vein graft occlusion. Antiplatelet therapy should be instituted preoperatively or in the immediate postoperative period, because the benefit is lost if therapy is initiated more than 3 days after surgery. Because administration of aspirin before surgery carries the risk of increased postoperative bleeding,[164] we begin giving aspirin alone down the nasogastric tube within 1 hour after surgery.[356] Whether the addition of dipyridamole preoperatively offers any real value over aspirin alone postoperatively is unknown. Because extracorporeal circulation activates the coagulation system and platelets, the routine use of heparin intraoperatively may be important in the prevention of thrombus formation and early graft occlusion. Thus, the combination of heparin intraoperatively and platelet inhibitor drugs perioperatively effectively reduces the incidence of graft occlusion in this high-risk population. Aspirin is advised within an hour of operation.[356]

Two studies of *anticoagulants*[358,359] have addressed the effect of anticoagulation on vein graft patency. In one,[358] there was a trend toward a higher patency rate with warfarin given for 3 to 4 days postoperatively. In another,[359] this drug offered no advantage over a placebo. These studies were compromised by incomplete angiographic follow-up, small sample size, or late implementation of antithrombotic therapy. Although no comparative studies have been published, it is difficult to advocate the use of anticoagulants alone because of the impressive success of aspirin after saphenous vein graft surgery. One option is to begin administration of platelet inhibitor and heparin after the operation and then convert to oral anticoagulation, which is continued long term to prevent vein graft occlusion, as done in an earlier trial.[360] This may be useful for patients with vein grafts and a prosthetic valve.

Late graft occlusion. The beneficial effect of antiplatelet therapy is less apparent, however, in late graft occlusion, because a different pathologic process supervenes. This process includes smooth muscle cell proliferation, lipid accumulation, and recurrent thrombus formation and organization, a process similar to that of spontaneous atherosclerosis.[102] Although the beneficial effects of antiplatelet agents in reducing late occlusion are less striking, the risk of thrombotic and ischemic events developing is moderate, and long-term aspirin therapy appears sensible.

CORONARY ANGIOPLASTY. Coronary angioplasty has gained worldwide acceptance as the procedure of choice in many patients with coronary disease since its first clinical application by Andreas Grüntzig in 1977.[361] Despite improvement in equipment and technique, acute reocclusion after successful angioplasty occurs in about 5% of patients and late restenosis, generally within 3 to 6 months, occurs in 25% to 35% of patients.[90,362,363] As discussed in previous sections, acute occlusion appears to be secondary to a type III vascular injury with resultant intraluminal thrombus formation and the process of late restenosis to be due to intimal proliferation and thrombus organization.

Acute occlusion. Several studies[182,364-366] have clearly shown that pretreatment of patients with aspirin, aspirin and dipyridamole, or ticlopidine (all in association with heparin) significantly reduces the rate of acute thrombotic complications after angioplasty. The role of heparin alone in prevention of acute vessel occlusion during angioplasty has not been properly tested clinically, but there is experimental evidence that suggests an inverse relation between the dose of heparin and both platelet deposition and mural thrombosis.[202,367] In addition, uncontrolled preliminary studies in patients with unstable angina have demonstrated that pretreatment with heparin for 1 to 8 days reduces the incidence of acute thrombotic occlusion during and after angioplasty.[368-370] Therefore, heparin in high doses is widely used during this intervention. Given the substantial risk of acute thrombotic complications associated with angioplasty, pretreatment with aspirin combined with adequate heparinization throughout the procedure is strongly recommended. The angiographic appearance of intraluminal thrombus or vessel dissection usually dictates the duration of heparin therapy on completion of the procedure. The addition of a thrombolytic agent to heparin and aspirin has increased rather than decreased thrombus formation and its complications.[371] However, ischemic complications of coronary angioplasty and atherectomy were reduced from 12.8% to 8.3% within 30 days of the procedure in high-risk patients (all received aspirin plus heparin bolus and a 12-hour heparin infusion) given the chimeric monoclonal antibody Fab fragment (c7E3 Fab) directed against the platelet glycoprotein IIb-IIIa receptor (versus placebo), although the risk of major bleeding was substantially increased (from 7% to 14% of patients).[372]

Late restenosis.[357,362,363] The effects of antithrombotic therapy on late restenosis have been disappointing. Clinical trials[182,365,366] using different platelet-inhibiting regimens have shown no impact on the restenosis rate. Similarly, anticoagulation with heparin[373] or coumadin[374] was of no benefit when compared with aspirin therapy. However, long-term aspirin therapy is recommended for these patients on the basis of favorable experience in chronic coronary artery disease for secondary prevention of ischemic complications.[303]

Cardiac chambers

Atrial fibrillation. Systemic embolism is a common and potentially devastating complication of atrial fibrillation associated with both mitral valve disease and certain other forms of organic heart disease. Blood stasis appears to play a predominant pathogenic role in thrombus formation in patients with atrial fibrillation. Patients at highest risk are those with a history of systemic embolism in the previous 2 years; in this group, the embolic risk approaches 10% to 20% in the first 1 or 2 years.[303] Although no prospective randomized trials of anticoagulants are available, the current recommendation is for long-term anticoagulant therapy aimed at prolonging the prothrombin time to an INR of 2.5 to 3.5 in these patients.[303,375]

Patients at somewhat lower but nevertheless substantial risk of embolism (which approaches 6% per year) are those with atrial fibrillation associated with mitral stenosis. Data from numerous nonrandomized and uncontrolled trials have suggested that anticoagulation reduces by 25% the rates of embolism and death in patients with rheumatic valvular disease.[376] On the basis of known embolic risk and the results of clinical trials, chronic anticoagulation to prolong the prothrombin time to an INR of 2.0 to 3.0 is recommended for these patients. In addition, patients who have atrial fibrillation associated with uncontrolled hyperthyroidism or heart failure appear to be at increased risk of embolism.[376] Although anticoagulation in these patients has not been evaluated by prospective randomized trials, this therapy is recommended until the patient becomes euthyroid and reversion to sinus rhythm has been achieved.

At the lower end of the spectrum of embolic risk in atrial fibrillation are patients without evidence of associated organic heart disease. The natural history of lone atrial fibrillation was addressed by the Framingham investigators,[377] who observed 30 of these patients for more than 10 years and found a fourfold increase in the incidence of stroke in comparison with that in matched controls. Aside from the small sample size, other limitations of the analysis were the relatively advanced age of the subjects (mean, 70 years) and the inclusion of patients with hypertension (now known to be a marker of increased risk for thromboembolism in patients with nonvalvular atrial fibrillation).[378] In another study,[379] 97 normotensive patients younger than 60 years with lone atrial fibrillation were followed up for a mean of 17 years at the Mayo Clinic. Anticoagulants were used in just a few subjects. Only eight embolic events were identified, an overall incidence well below 1% per year. Very low rates were also found for stroke in those over age 60.[380] However, the total vascular risk is high for fatal and nonfatal myocardial infarction and stroke (4.6% per year), and chronic atrial fibrillation, a higher incidence of extracranial vascular disease, and an increasing prevalence of disrupted plaques in the ascending aorta and arch develop in two-thirds of patients.[44,380-383] These data suggest that in the absence of heart disease and clinical risks for thromboembolism, the major risk is atherosclerotic vascular disease and one aspirin a day (325 mg) is rational.

A large group of patients with nonvalvular atrial fibrillation associated with various forms of cardiovascular disease have an intermediate risk for thromboembolism and account for nearly half of all thromboembolic events of cardiac origin. Nonvalvular atrial fibrillation appears at a mean age of 64 years, is present in more than 1 million persons in the U.S., imparts a risk of stroke of 5% to 8% per year (about 35% in a lifetime), is associated with more than 75,000 strokes per year in the U.S., and is the single most important risk marker for stroke in women older than 70.[383] A population-based study of persons under age 60 with no cardiopulmonary or vascular disease or hypertension evaluated the effect of atrial fibrillation in a "normal" population and documented that the incidence of stroke is no greater than in the normal population.[379] Thus, atrial fibrillation appears to be a risk marker rather than a risk factor for stroke.[383]

Mechanisms for stroke in patients with nonvalvular atrial fibrillation are multiple, may be difficult to assess in the individual patient, and include stasis of blood in cardiac chambers (left ventricle and atrium), structural abnormalities on valves or their apparatus, and vascular disease of the ascending aorta and arch and carotid and vertebral arteries. Since plaque disruption or ulceration more often involves arteries with minor stenoses, may involve more than half of patients over age 60, and increases with age, a vascular source may be difficult to localize. It has been estimated that as many as 25% to 40% of patients older than 60 with atrial fibrillation may have stroke on a vascular basis. Thus, it is understandable why many of these patients may have a response to aspirin.[44,375,383]

A retrospective study of warfarin compared with control predicted the prospective success of warfarin.[384] Five randomized trials of patients with nonvalvular atrial fibrillation have shown that warfarin (INR range, 1.5 to 4.5) significantly reduces the incidence of stroke compared with placebo or no anticoagulation (Table 28B-9). The risk of intracranial bleeding is low (0.3% per year, including intracerebral bleeding, 0.2% per year; control, 0.1% per year). Aspirin, 325 mg per day, was also effective in patients under age 75 (see Table 28B-9) and especially in those without clinical risk factors of hypertension, previous stroke, and recent heart failure. Patients without clinical risk factors for stroke, including men of all ages and women under age 75 who were taking aspirin (325 mg per day), had a risk of stroke of 0.5% per year (no greater than that in the general population) and did not appear to require warfarin therapy.[387,391]

Two prospective studies have sufficient numbers of patients and stroke events for reliable multivariate analysis for risk stratification.[378,392] Clinical and echocardiographic risk factors for stroke and the risk in low-risk and high-risk cohorts acquired from prospective data analysis are shown in Table 28B-10. Other studies show a direct relation of stroke in atrial fibrillation to underlying heart disease, hypertension, female sex (probably), and especially age and absence of anticoagulation (Table 28B-11). About half of strokes related to atrial fibrillation occur in patients older than 75.[387,395] Predictors of stroke in patients receiving aspirin are shown in Table 28B-12.[391] Thus, it is not surprising that patients with previous thromboembolism have a poor response to aspirin.[396] Guidelines for antithrombotic therapy are shown in Table 28B-13. Patients with chronic or paroxysmal atrial fibrillation appear to have a similar risk for thromboembolic stroke.[387,391]

Patients under age 60 with lone atrial fibrillation (no associated cardiopulmonary disease or systemic hypertension, normal left atrial size) have a very low risk of embolic events (<0.5% per year) and do not require anticoagulation.[379,380,386] Those older than 60 should receive one aspirin a day because of the total vascular high risk of 4.6% per year for nonfatal and fatal stroke and myocardial infarction.[380]

Cardioversion for atrial fibrillation. Anticoagulation with warfarin (INR, 2.0 to 3.0) should be given for 3 weeks before elective cardioversion and for at least 4 weeks after cardioversion. In patients who have not received anticoagulation for 3 weeks, the use of transesophageal echocardiography enables cardioversion to be done immediately if left atrial (and, of course, left ventricular) thrombus is excluded, allows longer anticoagulation before cardioversion if thrombus is present, but does not obviate anticoagulation during and after cardioversion, when left atrial thrombus may form because of stunning of left atrial contraction with a delay in the return of normal left atrial function for as long as 1 month. The duration of left atrial stunning after cardioversion

Table 28B-9 Anticoagulants and aspirin in patients with atrial fibrillation

Study	No. of pt	INR	Stroke rate, control, %/yr	Stroke risk reduction on warfarin, %	Stroke rate on ASA, %/yr	Major bleeding rate, %/yr
AFSAK[385]	1,007	2.8-4.2	5.5	53	4.7	0.5
SPAF[386,387]	1,330	2.0-4.5†	7.4	67	3.6	1.5
BAATAF[388]	420	1.5-2.7†	3.0	86	—	0.8
CAFA[389]	383	2.0-3.0	5.2	35	—	2.1
SPINAF[390]	538	1.4-2.8†	4.3	74	—	1.1
Aggregate			4.5	69 (1.4%/yr)		1.2

ASA, aspirin; INR, international normalized ratio.
*Requiring hospitalization, blood transfusion, or surgery.
†Estimated from prothrombin time ratio.

Table 28B-10 Independent predictors of thromboembolic risk in atrial fibrillation

	SPAF-1 placebo[378]	AFI pooled analysis[392]	SPAF echo analysis[393]
No. of patients	568	1,236	568
No. of events	46	81	46
High-risk variables	Hx of hypertension Prior stroke or TIA Diabetes Recent heart failure	Hx of hypertension Prior stroke or TIA Diabetes Age >65 yr	Hx of hypertension Prior stroke or TIA Recent heart failure LA >2.5 cm/m² LV dysfunction
Thromboembolic rate (95% CI)			
No risk factor	1.4%/yr (0.05-3.7)	1.0%/yr (0.3-3.1)	1.0%/yr (0.2-4.0)
One high-risk variable	>7%/yr	5%/yr	>6%/yr
More than one high-risk variable	18%		
Percent at low risk	38%	15%	26%

AFI, Atrial Fibrillation Investigators; CI, confidence interval; Hx, history; LA, left atrial size by M-mode echocardiography; LV, left ventricular dysfunction by two-dimensional echocardiography; SPAF, Stroke Prevention in Atrial Fibrillation study; TIA, transient ischemic attack.
The SPAF-1 placebo data set[378] is included in the pooled analysis of clinical trials by the Atrial Fibrillation Investigators.[392]

Table 28B-11 Atrial fibrillation, age, stroke, and anticoagulation (AC)[394]

Age, yr	Stroke with AC, %/yr	Stroke without AC, %/yr
40-50	0.0	0.0
50-60	2.8	6.7
60-70	2.1	8.1
70-80	4.9	21.3
80-90	7.1	36.2
	3.8 (3.0-6.3)[385-390]	14.7* (70,000/yr U.S.)

*10% to 38% withdraw from AC (based on references 385-390).

Table 28B-12 Predictors of stroke in patients taking aspirin

	% of cohort	Stroke risk, %/yr
LV dysfunction	20	6.2
Systolic BP >160 mm Hg	17	8.1
Female >75 yr old	9	6.9
Prior thromboembolism	4	5.8
One or more	46	6.3
None	54	1.8

BP, blood pressure; LV, left ventricular.

appears to be directly related to the duration of atrial fibrillation before cardioversion, with less than a week of atrial fibrillation causing less than a 24-hour return to function but more than 6 weeks of atrial fibrillation leading to up to 1 month before return of left atrial function. It also appears that transesophageal echocardiography during the initial hospitalization for atrial fibrillation may not only guide the timing of cardioversion but also, when used without previous transthoracic echocardiography, be the least expensive and most effective procedure for hospitalized patients with atrial fibrillation. After 4 weeks of warfarin treatment, patients who have had only one or two episodes of atrial fibrillation, have no left atrial enlargement or risk factors for stroke with nonvalvular atrial fibrillation, and are expected to remain in normal sinus rhythm may have warfarin administration discontinued after a short 4 weeks of therapy. All patients

Table 28B-13 Guidelines for selection of antithrombotic therapy in atrial fibrillation

Age	No risk factors*	With risk factors
<60	No treatment	Warfarin
60-75	Aspirin	Warfarin
>75†	Warfarin	Warfarin

*No history of stroke, transient ischemic attack, hypertension, diabetes, coronary artery disease, or congestive heart failure.
†Risk of intracerebral hemorrhage may be increased; monitor carefully and keep international normalized ratio <2.5.
Data from Albers GW: Atrial fibrillation and stroke: three new studies, three remaining questions. *Arch Intern Med* 154:1443-1448, 1994.

expected to have recurrent paroxysmal atrial fibrillation (most patients who have had more than one short bout of atrial fibrillation) probably need indefinite anticoagulation with warfarin to prevent stroke and thromboembolism. On the average, antiarrhythmic therapy intended to maintain normal sinus rhythm is successful in accomplishing this in only about half of patients who are rechecked 6 to 12 months after cardioversion.[396-398]

Acute myocardial infarction. In approximately one-third of patients with acute anterior myocardial infarction and in less than 5% of those with inferior infarction, left ventricular mural thrombi develop.[399] These thrombi tend to occur in the first week and particularly in the first 2 days. Thrombi are more likely to form if infarcts are large (peak serum creatine kinase, >2,000 units/L). Systemic embolism, which occurs in about 10% of cases in which left ventricular thrombi are echocardiographically apparent, is the most important complication, affecting 2% to 5% of victims of myocardial infarction.[303,399] Echocardiographically, thrombi that protrude into the left ventricular cavity and have increased mobility are more likely to embolize than those without these characteristics.[399]

Because the incidence of embolism is highest in the first 1 to 3 months after myocardial infarction and short-term anticoagulation has been demonstrated to reduce the embolic rate by 25% to 75%,[338-340] the following approach is recommended: Patients with increased embolic risk, namely, those with large anterior infarcts, congestive heart failure, or atrial fibrillation, should receive heparin on admission (aimed at prolonging the aPTT to 1.5 to 2.0 times control, 55 to 85 seconds).[303] A study by Turpie et al.[223] demonstrated that when compared with low doses of heparin (5,000 units twice daily), high doses of heparin (12,500 units every 12 hours) given subcutaneously significantly reduced the incidence of mural thrombosis in patients with anterior infarcts. Heparin therapy may be followed by warfarin to prolong the prothrombin time to an INR of 2.0 to 3.0 in patients with echocardiographic evidence of mural thrombi, a large akinetic region at the time of hospital dismissal, or a Q-wave anterior myocardial infarction (in those without echocardiography).

Warfarin administration may be stopped after 1 to 3 months unless heart failure or impaired left ventricular function is still present.[303] The optimal duration of anticoagulation in this group has not been determined. Patients with anterior Q-wave myocardial infarction receiving anticoagulation with warfarin during and after hospitalization should continue to receive therapeutic heparin (aPTT, 55 to 85 seconds) for at least 3 to 5 days of overlap with warfarin therapy until the INR reaches 2.0 to 3.0, because starting warfarin therapy in patients not receiving heparin or receiving a subtherapeutic dose of heparin was associated with an increased prevalence of left ventricular thrombus.[237]

Chronic left ventricular aneurysm. In contrast to the prevalence of thromboembolism in acute myocardial infarction, the incidence of embolism in chronic left ventricular aneurysm is significantly lower (0.35% per year).[400] The reason for this difference is probably twofold. First, thrombi formed after acute myocardial infarction are usually mobile and friable and protrude into the ventricular cavity, whereas thrombi in chronic aneurysms are laminated and more adherent to the endocardium.[116,399] Second, thrombi located within an aneurysmal sac, which is devoid of contractile fibers, are less prone to propulsion into the left ventricular outflow tract.[124] Although some investigators have found a persistent risk of embolism in postinfarction patients, the mobility and protrusion of thrombus rather than the presence of an aneurysm predicted embolic events. On the basis of available data, patients with remote infarction and chronic left ventricular aneurysm are at low risk of embolism and need not receive anticoagulants. Whether these drugs should be given to patients with echocardiographic evidence of mobile and protruding thrombi, however, remains to be established.

Dilated cardiomyopathy. Postmortem studies[117] have found a high prevalence of right and left ventricular mural thrombi in patients with idiopathic dilated cardiomyopathy. Blood stasis and low shear rate in a dilated, hypocontractile ventricle lead to activation of coagulation processes. Because the mural thrombus is not mechanically isolated, as in a ventricular aneurysm, embolism of thrombotic materials may occur. In a retrospective study,[401] patients treated with anticoagulants had no evidence of systemic embolism, whereas those not anticoagulated had an embolic rate of 3.5% per year. Although any prospective trial of antithrombotic therapy in these patients at medium risk for embolism is lacking, this evidence supports long-term administration of warfarin,[401] particularly in patients with overt heart failure or atrial fibrillation and in patients with global left ventricular dysfunction and an ejection fraction of <30%.

Prosthetic valves

Mechanical prostheses. Prosthetic surfaces are thrombogenic by virtue of their ability to activate both the intrinsic coagulation system and platelets. Increased shear rate, blood stasis (particularly in high-profile prosthetic devices), and associated disturbances of the cardiac chambers predispose to thromboembolism.[127] Patients with a history of embolism and a valve manufactured before the mid-1970s are at highest risk, which exceeds six events per 100 patients per year.[128,129] Atrial fibrillation and left ventricular thrombus contribute additional risk. Patients with newer mechanical valves have a risk of thromboembolism that ranges between 1% and 5% per year despite anticoagulants.

ANTICOAGULANTS. Warfarin, at a dose sufficient to prolong the prothrombin time to an INR of 2.5 to 4.0, is the most important agent for prevention of thromboembolism.[128,402] Studies in patients with mechanical prostheses have consistently shown that anticoagulation significantly reduces the incidence of valvular thrombosis and embolism.[129,402] In fact, inadequate anticoagulation increases the thromboembolic risk twofold to sixfold,[128,129] whereas excessive anticoagulation (prothrombin time more than 2.5 times control) increases the risk of bleeding complications fourfold to eightfold.

ANTICOAGULANTS AND PLATELET INHIBITORS. Platelet inhibitors alone have not been found to confer protection against embolism in patients with mechanical prostheses. Indeed, studies of aspirin with dipyridamole in these patients have shown an incidence of thromboembolism as high as 10% per year.[403,404] Patients with mechanical valves treated with warfarin had significantly fewer thromboembolic events than those treated with aspirin combined with either dipyridamole or pentoxifylline.[404] It seems clear, therefore, that patients with mechanical prostheses should receive anticoagulant therapy indefinitely, aimed at a prothrombin time INR of 2.5 to 3.5.[128,402] However, the addition of a platelet inhibitor, such as dipyridamole (300 to 400 mg daily), to warfarin may reduce the thromboembolic risk below that of warfarin alone. Indeed, the antithrombotic effects of dipyridamole are more evident on prosthetic materials such as artificial heart valves than on biologic surfaces.[303] In patients with mechanical prostheses, the combination of warfarin (INR, 2.5 to 3.5) and low-dose aspirin (100 mg/day) has recently been shown to benefit patients with mechanical prosthetic heart valves who are at high risk of thromboembolism (especially those with associated vascular disease) without increasing the risk of bleeding.[405] Certainly, the risk of GI bleeding increases as the dose of aspirin is increased with warfarin, especially when it reaches 500 mg or more per day.[127]

Biologic prostheses. Although bioprosthetic valves are less thrombogenic than mechanical valves, thromboembolism may occur in 2 or 3 per 100 patients per year, particularly in the first 3 months after surgery, and more often in patients with mitral rather than aortic prostheses and in those with atrial fibrillation or previous embolism.[128,129,402] The thromboembolic rate is particularly high during the first 3 months after operation, especially after mitral valve replacement. Risk factors for thromboembolism include lack of anticoagulation, mitral valve location, and increasing age in addition to those noted above.[406] Patients with mitral bioprostheses should receive warfarin postoperatively, with a target INR of 3.0 for the first 3 months, at which time warfarin administration can be stopped unless there is an enlarged left atrium, left ventricular dysfunction, prior history of thromboembolism, or persistent atrial fibrillation, in which case warfarin should be used indefinitely.[128,402] Since 50% to 70% of prothrombin times are low in the early postoperative period, intravenous use of heparin should be seriously considered for particularly high-risk patients while administration of warfarin is beginning. Although aortic bioprostheses are associated with a lower incidence of embolism, concomitant atrial fibrillation may warrant long-term warfarin therapy in these patients as well.

Patients in whom normal sinus rhythm is maintained postoperatively without left ventricular dysfunction or previous embolism are at low risk. In these patients, sustained anticoagulant therapy may not be needed. This is particularly true for patients with aortic bioprostheses, in whom even a platelet inhibitor may be unnecessary.[128,402] No randomized, controlled studies of platelet inhibitors in patients with bioprostheses have been reported. In an uncontrolled trial, long-term administration of aspirin was associated with a low incidence of embolism in these patients.

Special situations. Four specific situations should be considered in prescribing anticoagulant therapy for patients with prosthetic heart valves.[128]

1. For patients undergoing a noncardiac operation, it appears safe to discontinue anticoagulation for 7 to 10 days. However, we recommend the use of a therapeutic dose of heparin (aPTT, 55 to 85 seconds) and dipyridamole (300 to 400 mg/day) until 4 to 5 hours before the operation and low doses of heparin (5,000 U subcutaneously every 12 hours) during and early after the operation. Warfarin administration should begin again about 1 to 2 days after the operation.
2. For pregnant patients with prosthetic heart valves, the use of heparin and oral anticoagulants is problematic, because neither the safety of oral anticoagulant therapy during pregnancy nor the efficacy of heparin therapy for prophylaxis of systemic embolism is established. Nevertheless, it is highly likely that full doses of heparin are effective in preventing thromboembolism. Two approaches have been recommended. The first is to use heparin throughout pregnancy, administered every 12 hours by subcutaneous injection in doses adjusted to keep the aPTT at least 1½ times the control value (aPTT, 55 to 85 seconds). The second approach is to use heparin until the 13th week, change to warfarin until the middle of the third trimester, and return to heparin therapy until delivery. Although the latter approach might avoid warfarin embryopathy, other fetopathic effects (e.g., central nervous system abnormalities) are still possible. Therefore, before this approach is recommended, the potential risks should be explained to the patient. A further potential problem with the use of anticoagulants during pregnancy arises from the clear statement in the manufacturer's package insert that coumadin is contraindicated during pregnancy. This statement thus carries significant medicolegal implications.
3. For patients sustaining a cerebral event caused by an embolus originating from the heart, it is recommended that anticoagulation be continued in those who are nonhypertensive, who have had small to moderate-sized embolic strokes, and in whom a computed tomography scan done 24 hours or longer after the stroke has excluded hemorrhagic transformations. Anticoagulant therapy should be postponed several days in patients with large embolic strokes or severe hypertension (who are prone to late hemorrhagic transformation). In patients with hemorrhagic complications, anticoagulant therapy should be postponed for 8 to 10 days.
4. For patients with prosthetic valve endocarditis, it is recommended that anticoagulation be continued unless there are specific contraindications. However, the risk of intracranial hemorrhage is substantial. It is strongly recommended that anticoagulant therapy not be given to patients with normal sinus rhythm and uncomplicated infective endocarditis involving a native valve or a bioprosthetic valve. The reasons for this recommendation are the increased incidence of hemorrhage in these patients and the lack of demonstrated efficacy of anticoagulation in this setting. In these patients, the role of aspirin is being investigated.

Conclusions

An approach to antithrombotic therapy in various cardiovascular diseases has emerged based on the evolving concept of vascular injury and thrombosis, a knowledge of pathophysiology, and an appreciation of different clinical features determining morbid risk. The essential elements of this approach form the framework of Table 28B-8.

In the arterial circulation, types II and III injury leads to both platelet activation and production of thrombin and fibrin, so that the therapeutic approach suggested is with a platelet inhibitor, an anticoagulant, or a combination of both (acutely and short-term). The propensity to thrombosis determines the intensity of antithrombotic therapy. High-risk patients with unstable angina and evolving acute myocardial infarction should be treated aggressively with a platelet inhibitor and acutely with an anticoagulant as well. Patients undergoing coronary angioplasty or saphenous vein bypass surgery should receive platelet inhibitors (and adequate anticoagulation during the procedure). Patients with coronary disease are at more moderate risk in the chronic phase of stable angina, past myocardial infarction, angioplasty, or bypass surgery; at this time, such patients are best managed with a platelet inhibitor rather than an anticoagulant for reasons of convenience, safety, and economy. In low-risk patients in whom prevention of complications of atherosclerosis is desired, aspirin may be prescribed to those with certain risk factors such as diabetes, family history, tobacco exposure, and hypercholesterolemia that cannot be fully modified. However, because long-term administration of aspirin may be associated with an escalated chance of intracerebral hemorrhage, aspirin should not be used indiscriminately; furthermore, the long-term effects (benefits or risks) of aspirin therapy are unknown.

Within the cardiac chambers, stasis of blood flow causes coagulation to predominate over platelet activation as the principal mechanism of thrombus formation, and anticoagulant therapy alone seems most appropriate in management of these patients. At highest risk are patients with atrial fibrillation and previous embolism; at somewhat lower but yet substantial risk are patients with atrial fibrillation associated with mitral stenosis or uncontrolled hyperthyroidism. In all such patients at high risk, high-intensity anticoagulation is recommended. Patients at medium risk are those in the period immediately after large anterior myocardial infarction and uncompensated dilated cardiomyopathy; for these patients, there is sufficient evidence to indicate moderately intense long-term anticoagulation. Some patients with nonvalvulopathic atrial fibrillation associated with other forms of cardiac disease benefit from warfarin therapy, but subgroups in this population have not yet been sufficiently identified. At lowest risk are younger patients with atrial fibrillation without overt heart disease and those with chronic left ventricular aneurysm; they do not require anticoagulants.

The thrombogenicity of prosthetic heart valves involves both fibrin formation and, to a lesser extent, platelet activation and is considerably greater for mechanical than for biologic devices. Patients at highest risk—those with older mechanical prostheses or previous embolism—should be treated with a combination of an anticoagulant and a platelet inhibitor; although either dipyridamole or, to a lesser extent, aspirin may be beneficial, dipyridamole has the advantage of not potentiating bleeding. At medium risk are patients with modern mechanical valves and those with bioprostheses who have atrial fibrillation; they can be successfully managed with an anticoagulant alone. In patients with bioprostheses and normal sinus rhythm, the embolic risk is low enough that antithrombotic therapy may not be needed.

REFERENCES

1. Fuster V, Chesebro JH: Antithrombotic therapy: role of platelet-inhibitor drugs. I. Current concepts of thrombogenesis: role of platelets. II. Pharmacologic effects of platelet-inhibitor drugs. III. Management of arterial thromboembolic and atherosclerotic disease. *Mayo Clin Proc* 56:a, 102-112 (part I); b, 185-195 (part II); c, 265-273 (part III), 1981
2. Baumgartner HR: The role of blood flow in platelet adhesion, fibrin deposition, and formation of mural thrombi. *Microvasc Res* 5:167-179, 1973
3. Davies MJ, Thomas T: The pathological basis and microanatomy of occlusive thrombus formation in human coronary arteries. *Philos Trans R Soc Lond [Biol]* 294:225-228, 1981
4. Hawiger J: Formation and regulation of platelet and fibrin hemostatic plug. *Hum Pathol* 18:111-122, 1987
5. Fuster V: Lewis A. Conner Memorial Lecture. Mechanisms leading to myocardial infarction: insights from studies of vascular biology. *Circulation* 90:2126-2146, 1994
6. Davies MJ, Thomas AC: Plaque fissuring—the cause of acute myocardial infarction, sudden ischaemic death, and crescendo angina. *Br Heart J* 53:363-373, 1985
7. Miller RS, Hassinger NL, McBane RD, et al: Tissue prothrombin (abstract). *Thromb Haemost* 69:1210, 1993
8. Mann KG, Nesheim ME, Church WR, et al: Surface-dependent reactions of the vitamin K-dependent enzyme complexes. *Blood* 76:1-16, 1990
9. Fernandez-Ortiz A, Badimon JJ, Falk E, et al: Characterization of the relative thrombogenicity of atherosclerotic plaque components: implications for consequences of plaque rupture. *J Am Coll Cardiol* 23:1562-1569, 1994
10. Badimon L, Badimon J-J, Galvez A, et al: Influence of arterial damage and wall shear rate on platelet deposition: ex vivo study in a swine model. *Arteriosclerosis* 6:312-320, 1986
11. Badimon L, Badimon JJ: Mechanisms of arterial thrombosis in nonparallel streamlines: platelet thrombi grow on the apex of stenotic severely injured vessel wall; experimental study in the pig model. *J Clin Invest* 84:1134-1144, 1989
12. Lindon JN, Collins RE, Coe NP, et al: In vivo assessment in sheep of thromboresistant materials by determination of platelet survival. *Circ Res* 46:84-90, 1980
13. Heras M, Chesebro JH, Webster MW, et al: Hirudin, heparin,and placebo during deep arterial injury in the pig. The in vivo role of thrombin in platelet-mediated thrombosis. *Circulation* 82:1476-1484, 1990
14. Wysokinski WE, McBane RD, Hassinger NL, et al: "Dethrombosis": effect of thrombin inhibition on thrombus propagation and maintenance (abstract). *Thromb Haemost* 69:692, 1993
15. Stein B, Fuster V, Israel DH, et al: Platelet inhibitor agents in cardiovascular disease: an update. *J Am Coll Cardiol* 14:813-836, 1989
16. Coller BS: Activation affects access to the platelet receptor for adhesive glycoproteins. *J Cell Biol* 103:451-456, 1986
17. Mruk JS, Chesebro JH, Webster MWI: Platelet aggregation and interaction with the coagulation system: implications for antithrombotic therapy in arterial thrombosis. *Coronary Artery Dis* 1:149-158, 1990
18. Peerschke EIB: The platelet fibrinogen receptor. *Semin Hematol* 22:241-259, 1985
19. Shattil SJ, Brass LF: Induction of the fibrinogen receptor on human platelets by intracellular mediators. *J Biol Chem* 262:992-1000, 1987
20. Moncada S, Vane JR: Arachidonic acid metabolites and the interactions between platelets and blood-vessel walls. *N Engl J Med* 300:1142-1147, 1979

21. van Willigen G, Akkerman JW: Regulation of glycoprotein IIB/IIIA exposure on platelets stimulated with alpha-thrombin. *Blood* 79:82-90, 1992

22. Meyer BJ, Badimon JJ, Mailhac A, et al: Inhibition of growth of thrombus on fresh mural thrombus. Targeting optimal therapy. *Circulation* 90:2432-2438, 1994

23. Nemerson Y: The tissue factor pathway of blood coagulation. In *Hemostasis and Thrombosis: Basic Principles and Clinical Practice.* Third edition. Edited by RW Coleman, J Hirsh, VJ Marder, et al. Philadelphia, JB Lippincott Company, 1994, pp 81-93

24. DeLa Cadena RA, Wachtfogel YT, Coleman RW: Contact activation pathway: inflammation and coagulation. In *Hemostasis and Thrombosis: Basic Principles and Clinical Practice.* Third edition. Edited by RW Coleman, J Hirsh, VJ Marder, et al. Philadelphia, JB Lippincott Company, 1994, pp 219-240

25. Fuster V, Chesebro JH, Frye RL, et al: Platelet survival and the development of coronary artery disease in the young adult: effects of cigarette smoking, strong family history and medical therapy. *Circulation* 63:546-551, 1981

26. Badimon JJ, Badimon L: Platelet deposition in areas of stenosis is stimulated by high plasma cholesterol levels (abstract). *J Am Coll Cardiol* 13 Suppl A:145, 1989

27. Moncada S, Gryglewski R, Bunting S, et al: An enzyme isolated from arteries transforms prostaglandin endoperoxides to an unstable substance that inhibits platelet aggregation. *Nature* 263:663-665, 1976

28. Dyerberg J, Bang HO, Stoffersen E, et al: Eicosapentaenoic acid and prevention of thrombosis and atherosclerosis? *Lancet* 2:117-119, 1978

29. Kromhout D, Bosschieter EB, Coulander CDL: The inverse relation between fish consumption and 20-year mortality from coronary heart disease. *N Engl J Med* 312:1205-1209, 1985

30. Weitz JI, Hudoba M, Massel D, et al: Clot-bound thrombin is protected from inhibition by heparin-antithrombin III but is susceptible to inactivation by antithrombin III-independent inhibitors. *J Clin Invest* 86:385-391, 1990

31. Egeberg O: Inherited antithrombin deficiency causing thrombophilia. *Thromb Diath Haemorrh* 13:516-530, 1965

32. Krishnamurti C, Young GD, Barr CF, et al: Enhancement of tissue plasminogen activator-induced fibrinolysis by activated protein C in endotoxin-treated rabbits. *J Lab Clin Med* 118:523-530, 1991

33. Erickson LA, Ginsberg MH, Loskutoff DJ: Detection and partial characterization of an inhibitor of plasminogen activator in human platelets. *J Clin Invest* 74:1465-1472, 1984

34. Fay WP, Owen WG: Platelet plasminogen activator inhibitor: purification and characterization of interaction with plasminogen activators and activated protein C. *Biochemistry* 28:5773-5778, 1989

35. Griffin JH, Evatt B, Zimmerman TS, et al: Deficiency of protein C in congenital thrombotic disease. *J Clin Invest* 68:1370-1373, 1981

36. Dreyer NA, Pizzo SV: Blood coagulation and idiopathic thromboembolism among fertile women. *Contraception* 22:123-135, 1980

37. Cosgrove DM III, Heric B, Lytle BW, et al: Aprotinin therapy for reoperative myocardial revascularization: a placebo-controlled study. *Ann Thorac Surg* 54:1031-1036, 1992

38. Fuster V, Badimon L, Badimon JJ, et al: The pathogenesis of coronary artery disease and the acute coronary syndromes (part 1). *N Engl J Med* 326:242-250, 1992

39. Fuster V, Badimon L, Badimon JJ, et al: The pathogenesis of coronary artery disease and the acute coronary syndromes (part 2). *N Engl J Med* 326:310-318, 1992

40. Lam JYT, Chesebro JH, Steele PM, et al: Is vasospasm related to platelet deposition? Relationship in a porcine preparation of arterial injury in vivo. *Circulation* 75:243-248, 1987

41. Ludmer PL, Selwyn AP, Shook TL, et al: Paradoxical vasoconstriction induced by acetylcholine in atherosclerotic coronary arteries. *N Engl J Med* 315:1046-1051, 1986

42. Lerman A, Webster MW, Chesebro JH, et al: Circulating and tissue endothelin immunoreactivity in hypercholesterolemic pigs. *Circulation* 88:2923-2928, 1993

43. Davies MJ, Woolf N, Rowles PM, et al: Morphology of the endothelium over atherosclerotic plaques in human coronary arteries. *Br Heart J* 60:459-464, 1988

44. Amarenco P, Duyckaerts C, Tzourio C, et al: The prevalence of ulcerated plaques in the aortic arch in patients with stroke. *N Engl J Med* 326:221-225, 1992

45. Gunning AJ, Pickering GW, Robb-Smith AHT, et al: Mural thrombosis of the internal carotid artery and subsequent embolism. *Q J Med* 33:155-195, 1964

46. Barnett HJM: Pathogenesis of transient ischemic attacks. *Cerebrovascular Dis* 10:1-21, 1976

47. Davies MJ, Bland JM, Hangartner JRW, et al: Factors influencing the presence or absence of acute coronary artery thrombi in sudden ischaemic death. *Eur Heart J* 10:203-208, 1989

48. Falk E: Unstable angina with fatal outcome: dynamic coronary thrombosis leading to infarction and/or sudden death; autopsy evidence of recurrent mural thrombosis with peripheral embolization culminating in total vascular occlusion. *Circulation* 71:699-708, 1985

49. Fuster V, Chesebro JH, Badimon L, et al: Platelet survival. *Methods Hematol* 8:189-215, 1983

50. Trip MD, Cats VM, van Capelle FJL, et al: Platelet hyperreactivity and prognosis in survivors of myocardial infarction. *N Engl J Med* 322:1549-1554, 1990

51. Bauer KA, Kass BL, ten Cate H, et al: Detection of factor X activation in humans. *Blood* 74:2007-2015, 1989

52. Nossel HL, Yudelman I, Canfield RE, et al: Measurement of fibrinopeptide A in human blood. *J Clin Invest* 54:43-53, 1974

53. Alkjaersig N, Fletcher AP: Catabolism and excretion of fibrinopeptide-A. *Blood* 60:148-156, 1982

54. Bauer KA, Weiss LM, Sparrow D, et al: Aging-associated changes in indices of thrombin generation and protein C activation in humans. Normative Aging Study. *J Clin Invest* 80:1527-1534, 1987

55. Merlini PA, Bauer KA, Oltrona L, et al: Persistent activation of coagulation mechanism in unstable angina and myocardial infarction. *Circulation* 90:61-68, 1994

56. Rapold HJ, de Bono D, Arnold AE, et al: Plasma fibrinopeptide A levels in patients with acute myocardial infarction treated with alteplase. Correlation with concomitant heparin, coronary artery patency, and recurrent ischemia. The European Cooperative Study Group. *Circulation* 85:928-934, 1992

57. Bauer KA, Barzegar S, Rosenberg RD: Influence of anticoagulants used for blood collection on plasma prothrombin fragment F1 + 2 measurements. *Thromb Res* 63:617-628, 1991

58. Collen D, de Cock F, Verstraete M: Quantitation of thrombin-antithrombin III complexes in human blood. *Eur J Clin Invest* 7:407-411, 1977

59. Zoldhelyi P, Chesebro JH, Owen WG: Hirudin as a molecular probe for thrombin in vitro and during systemic coagulation in the pig. *Proc Natl Acad Sci U S A* 90:1819-1823, 1993

60. Zoldhelyi P, Bichler J, Owen WG, et al: Persistent thrombin generation in humans during specific thrombin inhibition with hirudin. *Circulation* 90:2671-2678, 1994

61. Zoldhelyi P, Bichler J, Owen WG, et al: Measurement of thrombin-hirudin complex documents persistent thrombin formation in patients with unstable angina during anticoagulation with recombinant hirudin (abstract). *Circulation* 88 Suppl 1:319, 1993

62. Kruskal JB, Commerford PJ, Franks JJ, et al: Fibrin and fibrinogen-related antigens in patients with stable and unstable coronary artery disease. *N Engl J Med* 317:1361-1365, 1987

63. Bauer KA, Kass BL, Beeler DL, et al: Detection of protein C activation in humans. *J Clin Invest* 74:2033-2041, 1984

64. Espana F, Griffin JH: Determination of functional and antigenic protein C inhibitor and its complexes with activated protein C in plasma by ELISA's. *Thromb Res* 55:671-682, 1989

65. Espana F, Gruber A, Heeb MJ, et al: In vivo and in vitro complexes of activated protein C with two inhibitors in baboons. *Blood* 77:1754-1760, 1991

66. Espana F, Vicente V, Tabernero D, et al: Determination of plasma protein C inhibitor and of two activated protein C-inhibitor complexes in normals and in patients with intravascular coagulation and thrombotic disease. *Thromb Res* 59:593-608, 1990

67. Toh CH, Hoogendoorn H, Scully MF, et al: Quantification of activated protein C (APC) in complex with α_2-macroglobulin (α_2M) by ELISA in patients with disseminated intravascular coagulation (DIC) (abstract). *Blood* 78 Suppl 1:74a, 1991

68. Fitzgerald DJ, Roy L, Catella F, et al: Platelet activation in unstable coronary disease. *N Engl J Med* 315:983-989, 1986

69. Lawson JA, Patrono C, Ciabattoni G, et al: Long-lived enzymatic metabolites of thromboxane B_2 in the human circulation. *Anal Biochem* 155:198-205, 1986

70. Niewiarowski S, Holt JC, Cook JJ: Biochemistry and physiology of secreted platelet proteins. In *Hemostasis and Thrombosis: Basic Principles*

and Clinical Practice. Third edition. Edited by RW Coleman, J Hirsh, VJ Marder, et al. Philadelphia, JB Lippincott Company, 1994, pp 546-556

71. Whitaker AN, Elms MJ, Masci PP, et al: Measurement of cross linked fibrin derivatives in plasma: an immunoassay using monoclonal antibodies. *J Clin Pathol* 37:882-887, 1984

72. Eisenberg PR, Jaffe AS, Stump DC, et al: Validity of enzyme-linked immunosorbent assays of cross-linked fibrin degradation products as a measure of clot lysis. *Circulation* 82:1159-1168, 1990

73. Harker LA: Platelet survival time: its measurements and use. *Prog Hemost Thromb* 4:321-347, 1978

74. Hanson SR, Harker LA, Bjornsson TD: Effects of platelet-modifying drugs on arterial thromboembolism in baboons: aspirin potentiates the antithrombotic actions of dipyridamole and sulfinpyrazone by mechanism(s) independent of platelet cyclooxygenase inhibition. *J Clin Invest* 75:1591-1599, 1985

75. Wahner HW, Dunn WL, Dewanjee MK, et al: Survival time and organ distribution of ^{111}In-oxine-labeled human platelets in normal subjects. In *World Congress of Nuclear Medicine.* Vol 1. Edited by C Raynaud. New York, Pergamon Press, 1983, pp 918-921

76. du P Heyns A, Lötter MG, Badenhorst PN: Platelet imaging. *Methods Hematol* 8:216-234, 1983

77. Ezekowitz MD, Wilson DA, Smith EO, et al: Comparison of indium-111 platelet scintigraphy and two-dimensional echocardiography in the diagnosis of left ventricular thrombi. *N Engl J Med* 306:1509-1513, 1982

78. Pumphrey CW, Chesebro JH, Dewanjee MK, et al: In vivo quantitation of platelet deposition on human peripheral arterial bypass grafts using indium-111-labeled platelets: effect of dipyridamole and aspirin. *Am J Cardiol* 51:796-801, 1983

79. Steele PM, Chesebro JH, Fuster V: The natural history of arterial balloon angioplasty in pigs and intervention with platelet-inhibitor therapy: implications for clinical trials (abstract). *Clin Res* 32:209A, 1984

80. Stratton JR, Ritchie JL: The effects of antithrombotic drugs in patients with left ventricular thrombi: assessment with indium-111 platelet imaging and two-dimensional echocardiography. *Circulation* 69:561-568, 1984

81. Peters AM, Lavender JP, Needham SG, et al: Imaging thrombus with radiolabelled monoclonal antibody to platelets. *Br Med J [Clin Res]* 293:1525-1527, 1986

82. Becker W, Börner W, Borst U, et al: Tc-99m-HMPAO: a new platelet labelling compound? (Letter to the editor.) *Eur J Nucl Med* 13:267-268, 1987

83. Kaplan KL, Owen F: Radioimmunoassays of platelet alpha-granule proteins. *Methods Hematol* 8:115-125, 1983

84. Soria C, Soria J, Mirshahi M, et al: Dynamic coronary fibrinolysis evaluation in patients with myocardial infarction and unstable angina by specific plasma fibrin degradation product determination. *Thromb Res* 45:383-392, 1987

85. Shifman MA, Pizzo SV: The in vivo metabolism of antithrombin III and antithrombin III complexes. *J Biol Chem* 257:3243-3248, 1982

86. Deguchi K, Noguchi M, Yuwasaki E, et al: Dynamic fluctuations in blood of thrombin/antithrombin III complex (TAT). *Am J Hematol* 38:86-89, 1991

87. Spannagl M, Hoffmann H, Siebeck M, et al: A purified antithrombin III-heparin complex as a potent inhibitor of thrombin in porcine endotoxin shock. *Thromb Res* 61:1-10, 1991

88. Hamberg M, Svensson J, Samuelsson B: Thromboxanes: a new group of biologically active compounds derived from prostaglandin endoperoxides. *Proc Natl Acad Sci U S A* 72:2994-2998, 1975

89. Hamm CW, Lorenz RL, Bleifeld W, et al: Biochemical evidence of platelet activation in patients with persistent unstable angina. *J Am Coll Cardiol* 10:998-1006, 1987

90. Ip JH, Fuster V, Badimon L, et al: Syndromes of accelerated atherosclerosis: role of vascular injury and smooth muscle cell proliferation. *J Am Coll Cardiol* 15:1667-1687, 1990

91. Goldsmith HL, Turitto VT: Rheological aspects of thrombosis and haemostasis: basic principles and implications; ICTH-report-Subcommittee on Rheology of the International Committee on Thrombosis and Haemostasis. *Thromb Haemost* 55:415-435, 1986

92. Ross R: The pathogenesis of atherosclerosis: a perspective for the 1990s. *Nature* 362:801-809, 1993

93. Woolf N, Davies MJ: Interrelationship between atherosclerosis and thrombosis. In *Thrombosis in Cardiovascular Disorders.* Edited by V Fuster, M Verstraete. Philadelphia, WB Saunders Company, 1992, pp 41-77

94. Bini A, Fenoglio JJ Jr, Mesa-Tejada R, et al: Identification and distribution of fibrinogen, fibrin, and fibrin(ogen) degradation products in atherosclerosis. Use of monoclonal antibodies. *Arteriosclerosis* 9:109-121, 1989

95. Sherman CT, Litvack F, Grundfest W, et al: Coronary angioscopy in patients with unstable angina pectoris. *N Engl J Med* 315:913-919, 1986

96. Levin DC, Fallon JT: Significance of the angiographic morphology of localized coronary stenoses: histopathologic correlations. *Circulation* 66:316-320, 1982

97. Ambrose JA, Winters SL, Stern A, et al: Angiographic morphology and the pathogenesis of unstable angina pectoris. *J Am Coll Cardiol* 5:609-616, 1985

98. Gorlin R, Fuster V, Ambrose JA: Anatomic-physiologic links between acute coronary syndromes (editorial). *Circulation* 74:6-9, 1986

99. Ambrose JA, Tennenbaum MA, Alexopoulos D, et al: Angiographic progression of coronary artery disease and the development of myocardial infarction. *J Am Coll Cardiol* 12:56-62, 1988

100. Ambrose JA, Hjemdahl-Monson CE, Borrico S, et al: Angiographic demonstration of a common link between unstable angina pectoris and non-Q wave acute infarction. *Am J Cardiol* 61:244-247, 1988

101. Richardson PD, Davies MJ, Born GVR: Influence of plaque configuration and stress distribution on fissuring of coronary atherosclerotic plaques. *Lancet* 2:941-944, 1989

102. Chesebro JH, Goldman S: Coronary artery bypass surgery: antithrombotic therapy. In *Thrombosis in Cardiovascular Disorders.* Edited by V Fuster, M Verstraete. Philadelphia, WB Saunders Company, 1992, pp 375-388

103. Ip JH, Fuster V, Badimon L, et al: Interactions between blood and coronary arterial wall. *Curr Opin Cardiol* 4:772-777, 1989

104. Lie JT, Lawrie GM, Morris GC Jr: Aortocoronary bypass saphenous vein graft atherosclerosis. Anatomic study of 99 vein grafts from normal and hyperlipoproteinemic patients up to 75 months postoperatively. *Am J Cardiol* 40:906-914, 1977

105. Atkinson JB, Forman MB, Vaughn WK, et al: Morphologic changes in long-term saphenous vein bypass grafts. *Chest* 88:341-348, 1985

106. Solymoss BC, Nadeau P, Millette D, et al: Late thrombosis of saphenous vein coronary bypass grafts related to risk factors. *Circulation* 78 Suppl 1:140-143, 1988

107. Steele PM, Chesebro JH, Stanson AW, et al: Balloon angioplasty: natural history of the pathophysiological responses to injury in a pig model. *Circ Res* 57:105-112, 1985

108. Waller BF, Gorfinkel HJ, Rogers FJ, et al: Early and late morphologic changes in major epicardial coronary arteries after percutaneous transluminal coronary angioplasty. *Am J Cardiol* 53 Suppl:42C-47C, 1984

109. Waller BF: "Crackers, breakers, stretchers, drillers, scrapers, shavers, burners, welders, and melters"—the future treatment of atherosclerotic coronary artery disease? A clinical-morphologic assessment. *J Am Coll Cardiol* 13:969-987, 1989

110. Ip JH, Fuster V, Israel D, et al: The role of platelets, thrombin and hyperplasia in restenosis after coronary angioplasty. *J Am Coll Cardiol* 17 Suppl B:77-88, 1991

111. Uchida Y, Hasegawa K, Kawamura K, et al: Angioscopic observation of the coronary luminal changes induced by percutaneous transluminal coronary angioplasty. *Am Heart J* 117:769-776, 1989

112. Mizuno K, Miyamoto A, Shibuya T, et al: Changes of angioscopic macromorphology following coronary angioplasty (PTCA) (abstract). *Circulation* 78 Suppl 2:289, 1988

113. Johnson DE, Hinohara T, Selmon MR, et al: Primary peripheral arterial stenoses and restenoses excised by transluminal atherectomy: a histopathologic study. *J Am Coll Cardiol* 15:419-425, 1990

114. Virchow RLK: *Gesammelte Abhandlungen zur wissenschaftlichen Medicin.* Frankfurt, Medinger Sohn & Company, 1856, pp 219-732

115. Johnson RC, Crissman RS, DiDio LJA: Endocardial alterations in myocardial infarction. *Lab Invest* 40:183-193, 1979

116. Hochman JS, Platia EB, Bulkley BH: Endocardial abnormalities in left ventricular aneurysms: a clinicopathologic study. *Ann Intern Med* 100:29-35, 1984

117. Roberts WC, Siegel RJ, McManus BM: Idiopathic dilated cardiomyopathy: analysis of 152 necropsy patients. *Am J Cardiol* 60:1340-1355, 1987

118. Mikell FL, Asinger RW, Elsperger KJ, et al: Regional stasis of blood in the dysfunctional left ventricle: echocardiographic detection and differentiation from early thrombosis. *Circulation* 66:755-763, 1982

119. Asinger RW, Mikell FL, Elsperger J, et al: Incidence of

left-ventricular thrombosis after acute transmural myocardial infarction: serial evaluation by two-dimensional echocardiography. *N Engl J Med* 305:297-302, 1981

120. Weinreich DJ, Burke JF, Pauletto FJ: Left ventricular mural thrombi complicating acute myocardial infarction: long-term follow-up with serial echocardiography. *Ann Intern Med* 100:789-794, 1984

121. Shrestha NK, Moreno FL, Narciso FV, et al: Two-dimensional echocardiographic diagnosis of left atrial thrombus in rheumatic heart disease: a clinicopathologic study. *Circulation* 67:341-347, 1983

122. Fulton RM, Duckett K: Plasma-fibrinogen and thromboemboli after myocardial infarction. *Lancet* 2:1161-1164, 1976

123. Fuster V, Halperin JL: Left ventricular thrombi and cerebral embolism (editorial). *N Engl J Med* 320:392-394, 1989

124. Cabin HS, Roberts WC: Left ventricular aneurysm, intraaneurysmal thrombus and systemic embolus in coronary heart disease. *Chest* 77:586-590, 1980

125. Dewanjee MK, Fuster V, Rao SA, et al: Noninvasive radioisotopic technique for detection of platelet deposition in mitral valve prostheses and quantification of visceral microembolism in dogs. *Mayo Clin Proc* 58:307-314, 1983

126. Acar J, Vahanian A, Fauchet M, et al: Detection of prosthetic valve thrombosis using Indium 111 platelet imaging (abstract). *Eur Heart J* 10 Suppl:261, 1989

127. Chesebro JH, Adams PC, Fuster V: Antithrombotic therapy in patients with valvular heart disease and prosthetic heart valves. *J Am Coll Cardiol* 8 Suppl B:41-56, 1986

128. Fuster V, Badimon L, Badimon JJ, et al: Prevention of thromboembolism induced by prosthetic heart valves. *Semin Thromb Hemost* 14:50-58, 1988

129. Edmunds LH Jr: Thrombotic and bleeding complications of prosthetic heart valves. *Ann Thorac Surg* 44:430-445, 1987

130. Tschopp TB: Aspirin inhibits platelet aggregation, but not adhesion to, collagen fibrils: an assessment of platelet adhesion and deposited platelet mass by morphometry and ^{51}Cr-labeling. *Thromb Res* 11:619-632, 1977

131. Clowes AW, Karnovsky MJ: Failure of certain antiplatelet drugs to affect myointimal thickening following arterial endothelial injury in the rat. *Lab Invest* 36:452-464, 1977

132. Roth GJ, Majerus PW: The mechanism of the effect of aspirin on human platelets. I. Acetylation of a particulate fraction protein. *J Clin Invest* 56:624-632, 1975

133. Clarke RJ, Mayo G, Price P, et al: Suppression of thromboxane A_2 but not of systemic prostacyclin by controlled-release aspirin. *N Engl J Med* 325:1137-1141, 1991

134. Lewis HD Jr, Davis JW, Archibald DG, et al: Protective effects of aspirin against acute myocardial infarction and death in men with unstable angina: results of a Veterans Administration Cooperative Study. *N Engl J Med* 309:396-403, 1983

135. Cairns JA, Gent M, Singer J, et al: Aspirin, sulfinpyrazone, or both in unstable angina: results of a Canadian Multicenter Trial. *N Engl J Med* 313:1369-1375, 1985

136. ISIS-2 (Second International Study of Infarct Survival) Collaborative Group: Randomised trial of intravenous streptokinase, oral aspirin, both or neither among 17,187 cases of suspected acute myocardial infarction: ISIS-2. *Lancet* 2:349-360, 1988

137. Steering Committee of the Physicians' Health Study Research Group: Final report on the aspirin component of the ongoing Physicians' Health Study. *N Engl J Med* 321:129-135, 1989

138. Antiplatelet Trialists' Collaboration: Collaborative overview of randomised trials of antiplatelet therapy—I: Prevention of death, myocardial infarction, and stroke by prolonged antiplatelet therapy in various categories of patients. *BMJ* 308:81-106, 1994

139. Graham DY, Smith JL: Aspirin and the stomach. *Ann Intern Med* 104:390-398, 1986

140. Ali M, Zamecnik J, Cerskus AL, et al: Synthesis of thromboxane B_2 and prostaglandins by bovine gastric mucosal microsomes. *Prostaglandins* 14:819-827, 1977

141. MacKercher PA, Ivey KJ, Baskin WN, et al: Protective effect of cimetidine on aspirin-induced gastric mucosal damage. *Ann Intern Med* 87:676-679, 1977

142. Farrell B, Godwin J, Richards S, et al: The United Kingdom transient ischaemic attack (UK-TIA) aspirin trial: final results. *J Neurol Neurosurg Psychiatry* 54:1044-1054, 1991

143. Neri Serneri GG, Castellani S: Platelet and vascular prostaglandins: pharmacological and clinical implication. In *Antiplatelet Therapy; Twenty Years' Experience: Proceedings of a European Conference.* Edited by GVR Born, GG Neri Serneri. Amsterdam, Elsevier Science Publishers, 1987, pp 37-51

144. Friedman PL, Brown EJ Jr, Gunther S, et al: Coronary vasoconstrictor effect of indomethacin in patients with coronary-artery disease. *N Engl J Med* 305:1171-1175, 1981

145. Shekelle RB, Missel L, Paul O, et al: Fish consumption and mortality from coronary heart disease (letter to the editor). *N Engl J Med* 313:820, 1985

146. Von Schacky C: Prophylaxis of atherosclerosis with marine omega-3 fatty acids: a comprehensive strategy. *Ann Intern Med* 107:890-899, 1987

147. Leaf A, Weber PC: Cardiovascular effects of n-3 fatty acids. *N Engl J Med* 318:549-557, 1988

148. Lam JY, Badimon JJ, Ellefson RD, et al: Cod liver oil alters platelet-arterial wall response to injury in pigs. *Circ Res* 71:769-775, 1992

149. FitzGerald GA, Reilly IAG, Pedersen AK: The biochemical pharmacology of thromboxane synthase inhibition in man. *Circulation* 72:1194-1201, 1985

150. Mullane KM, Fornabaio D: Thromboxane synthetase inhibitors reduce infarct size by a platelet-dependent, aspirin-sensitive mechanism. *Circ Res* 62:668-678, 1988

151. Reuben SR, Kuan P, Cairns J, et al: Effects of dazoxiben on exercise performance in chronic stable angina. *Br J Clin Pharmacol* 15 Suppl:83S-86S, 1983

152. Thaulow E, Dale J, Myhre E: Effects of a selective thromboxane synthetase inhibitor, dazoxiben, and of acetylsalicylic acid on myocardial ischemia in patients with coronary artery disease. *Am J Cardiol* 53:1255-1258, 1984

153. The Ridogrel Versus Aspirin Patency Trial (RAPT): Randomized trial of ridogrel, a combined thromboxane A_2 synthase inhibitor and thromboxane A_2/prostaglandin endoperoxide receptor antagonist, versus aspirin as adjunct to thrombolysis in patients with acute myocardial infarction. *Circulation* 89:588-595, 1994

154. Cohen M, Parry G, Xiong J, et al: Double blind randomized trial of a prostacyclin sparing aspirin formulation in rest angina and non-Q wave infarction. *J Am Coll Cardiol* 21 Suppl A:269, 1993

155. Moncada S, Korbut R: Dipyridamole and other phosphodiesterase inhibitors act as antithrombotic agents by potentiating endogenous prostacyclin. *Lancet* 1:1286-1289, 1978

156. Crutchley DJ, Ryan US, Ryan JW: Effects of aspirin and dipyridamole on the degradation of adenosine diphosphate by cultured cells derived from bovine pulmonary artery. *J Clin Invest* 66:29-35, 1980

157. FitzGerald GA: Dipyridamole. *N Engl J Med* 316:1247-1257, 1987

158. Harker LA, Slichter SJ: Studies of platelet and fibrinogen kinetics in patients with prosthetic heart valves. *N Engl J Med* 283:1302-1305, 1970

159. Weily HS, Steele PP, Davies H, et al: Platelet survival in patients with substitute heart valves. *N Engl J Med* 290:534-537, 1974

160. The Persantine-Aspirin Reinfarction Study Research Group: Persantine and aspirin in coronary heart disease. *Circulation* 62:449-461, 1980

161. Bousser MG, Eschwege E, Haguenau M, et al: "AICLA" controlled trial of aspirin and dipyridamole in the secondary prevention of athero-thrombotic cerebral ischemia. *Stroke* 14:5-14, 1983

162. The American-Canadian Co-Operative Study Group: Persantine aspirin trial in cerebral ischemia. Part II: Endpoint results. *Stroke* 16:406-415, 1985

163. Brown BG, Cukingnan RA, DeRouen T, et al: Improved graft patency in patients treated with platelet-inhibiting therapy after coronary bypass surgery. *Circulation* 72:138-146, 1985

164. Goldman S, Copeland J, Moritz T, et al: Improvement in early saphenous vein graft patency after coronary artery bypass surgery with antiplatelet therapy: results of a Veterans Administration Cooperative Study. *Circulation* 77:1324-1332, 1988

165. Sullivan JM, Harken DE, Gorlin R: Pharmacologic control of thromboembolic complications of cardiac-valve replacement. *N Engl J Med* 284:1391-1394, 1971

166. Kasahara T: Clinical effect of dipyridamole ingestion after prosthetic heart valve replacement—especially on the blood coagulation system. *Nippon Kyobu Geka Gakkai Zasshi* 25:1007-1021, 1977

167. Groupe de Recherche PACTE: Prevention des accidents thromboemboliques systemiques chez les porteurs de prosthesis valvulaires artificielles: essai cooperatif controle du dipyridamole. *Coeur* 9:915-969, 1978

168. Rajah SM, Sreeharan N, Joseph A, et al: A prospective trial of

dipyridamole and warfarin in heart valve patients (abstract). *Acta Therapeutic* 6 Suppl 93:54, 1980

169. Chesebro JH, Fuster V, Elveback LR, et al: Trial of combined warfarin plus dipyridamole or aspirin therapy in prosthetic heart valve replacement: danger of aspirin compared with dipyridamole. *Am J Cardiol* 51:1537-1541, 1983

170. Chesebro JH, Clements IP, Fuster V, et al: A platelet-inhibitor-drug trial in coronary-artery bypass operations: benefit of perioperative dipyridamole and aspirin therapy on early postoperative vein-graft patency. *N Engl J Med* 307:73-78, 1982

171. Chesebro JH, Fuster V, Elveback LR, et al: Effect of dipyridamole and aspirin in late vein-graft patency after coronary bypass operations. *N Engl J Med* 310:209-214, 1984

172. Weksler BB: Prostaglandins and vascular function. *Circulation* 70 Suppl 3:63-71, 1984

173. Coppe D, Sobel M, Seamans L, et al: Preservation of platelet function and number by prostacyclin during cardiopulmonary bypass. *J Thorac Cardiovasc Surg* 81:274-278, 1981

174. Smith MC, Danviriyasup K, Crow JW, et al: Prostacyclin substitution for heparin in long-term hemodialysis. *Am J Med* 73:669-678, 1982

175. Fisher CA, Kappa JR, Sinha AK, et al: Comparison of equimolar concentrations of iloprost, prostacyclin, and prostaglandin E_1 on human platelet function. *J Lab Clin Med* 109:184-190, 1987

176. Nicolini FA, Mehta JL, Nichols WW, et al: Prostacyclin analogue iloprost decreases thrombolytic potential of tissue-type plasminogen activator in canine coronary thrombosis. *Circulation* 81:1115-1122, 1990

177. Topol EJ, Ellis SG, Califf RM, et al: Combined tissue-type plasminogen activator and prostacyclin therapy for acute myocardial infarction. Thrombolysis and Angioplasty in Myocardial Infarction (TAMI) 4 Study Group. *J Am Coll Cardiol* 14:877-884, 1989

178. Raizner A, Hollman J, Demke D, et al: Beneficial effects of Ciprostene in PTCA: a multicenter, randomized, controlled trial (abstract). *Circulation* 78 Suppl 2:290, 1988

179. Defreyn G, Bernat A, Delebassee D, et al: Pharmacology of ticlopidine: a review. *Semin Thromb Hemost* 15:159-166, 1989

180. McTavish D, Faulds D, Goa KL: Ticlopidine. An updated review of its pharmacology and therapeutic use in platelet-dependent disorders. *Drugs* 40:238-259, 1990

181. Balsano F, Rizzon P, Violi F, et al: Antiplatelet treatment with ticlopidine in unstable angina: a controlled multicenter clinical trial. *Circulation* 82:17-26, 1990

182. White CW, Chaitman B, Lassar TA, et al: Antiplatelet agents are effective in reducing the immediate complications of PTCA: results from the Ticlopidine Multicenter Trial (abstract). *Circulation* 76 Suppl 4:400, 1987

183. Bertrand ME, Allain H, Lablanche JM: Results of a randomized trial of ticlopidine versus placebo for prevention of acute closure and restenosis after coronary angioplasty (PTCA). The TACT Study (abstract). *Circulation* 82 Suppl 3:190, 1990

184. Limet R, David J-L, Magotteaux P, et al: Prevention of aorta-coronary bypass graft occlusion: beneficial effect of ticlopidine on early and late patency rates of venous coronary bypass grafts: a double-blind study. *J Thorac Cardiovasc Surg* 94:773-783, 1987

185. Gent M, Blakeley JA, Easton JD, et al: The Canadian American Ticlopidine Study (CATS) in thromboembolic stroke. *Lancet* 1:1215-1220, 1989

186. Hass WK, Easton JD, Adams HP Jr, et al: A randomized trial comparing ticlopidine hydrochloride with aspirin for the prevention of stroke in high-risk patients. Ticlopidine Aspirin Stroke Study Group. *N Engl J Med* 321:501-507, 1989

187. Kaegi A, Pineo GF, Shimizu A, et al: Arteriovenous-shunt thrombosis: prevention by sulfinpyrazone. *N Engl J Med* 290:304-306, 1974

188. Steele P, Rainwater J, Vogel R: Platelet suppressant therapy in patients with prosthetic cardiac valves: relationship of clinical effectiveness to alteration of platelet survival time. *Circulation* 60:910-913, 1979

189. Lam JY, Chesebro JH, Steele PM, et al: Antithrombotic therapy for deep arterial injury by angioplasty. Efficacy of common platelet inhibition compared with thrombin inhibition in pigs. *Circulation* 84:814-820, 1991

190. Report from the Anturan Reinfarction Italian Study: Sulphinpyrazone in post-myocardial infarction. *Lancet* 1:237-242, 1982

191. Baur HR, VanTassel RA, Pierach CA, et al: Effects of sulfinpyrazone on early graft closure after myocardial revascularization. *Am J Cardiol* 49:420-424, 1982

192. The Canadian Cooperative Study Group: A randomized trial of aspirin and sulfinpyrazone in threatened stroke. *N Engl J Med* 299:53-59, 1978

193. Harker LA, Fuster V: Pharmacology of platelet inhibitors. *J Am Coll Cardiol* 8 Suppl B:21-32, 1986

194. Åberg M, Hedner U, Bergentz S-E: Effect of dextran 70 on factor VIII and platelet function in von Willebrand's disease. *Thromb Res* 12:629-634, 1978

195. Weiss HJ: The effect of clinical dextran on platelet aggregation, adhesion, and ADP release in man: in vivo and in vitro studies. *J Lab Clin Med* 69:37-46, 1967

196. Swanson KT, Vlietstra RE, Holmes DR Jr, et al: Efficacy of adjunctive dextran during percutaneous transluminal coronary angioplasty. *Am J Cardiol* 54:447-448, 1984

197. Brown RI, Aldridge HE, Schwartz L, et al: The use of dextran-40 during percutaneous transluminal coronary angioplasty: a report of three cases of anaphylactoid reactions—one near fatal. *Cathet Cardiovasc Diagn* 11:591-595, 1985

198. Coller BS: A new murine monoclonal antibody reports an activation-dependent change in the conformation and/or microenvironment of the platelet glycoprotein IIb/IIIa complex. *J Clin Invest* 76:101-108, 1985

199. Mousa SA, Bozarth JM, Forsythe MS, et al: Antiplatelet and antithrombotic efficacy of DMP 728, a novel platelet GPIIb/IIIa receptor antagonist. *Circulation* 89:3-12, 1994

200. Frelinger AL III, Roncinske RA, Adelman B, et al: RGD and anti-GPIIb/IIIa insensitive thrombin induced platelet aggregation (abstract). *Circulation* 86 Suppl 1:684, 1992

201. Hanson SR, Harker LA: Interruption of acute platelet-dependent thrombosis by the synthetic antithrombin D-phenylalanyl-L-prolyl-L-arginylcholomethyl ketone. *Proc Natl Acad Sci U S A* 85:3184-3188, 1988

202. Heras M, Chesebro JH, Penny WJ, et al: Effects of thrombin inhibition on the development of acute platelet-thrombus deposition during angioplasty in pigs: heparin versus recombinant hirudin, a specific thrombin inhibitor. *Circulation* 79:657-665, 1989

203. Hassinger NL, McBane RD, Mruk JS, et al: All thrombin inhibitors are not created equal: the paradox of anticoagulant versus antithrombotic efficacy (abstract). *Thromb Haemost* 69:888, 1993

204. Markwardt F, Kaiser B, Nowak G: Studies on antithrombotic effects of recombinant hirudin. *Thromb Res* 54:377-388, 1989

205. Chesebro JH, Webster MW, Zoldhelyi P, et al: Antithrombotic therapy and progression of coronary artery disease. Antiplatelet versus antithrombins. *Circulation* 86 Suppl 6:100-110, 1992

206. Zoldhelyi P, Webster MW, Fuster V, et al: Recombinant hirudin in patients with chronic, stable coronary artery disease. Safety, half-life, and effect on coagulation parameters. *Circulation* 88:2015-2022, 1993

207. Topol EJ, Fuster V, Harrington RA, et al: Recombinant hirudin for unstable angina pectoris. A multicenter, randomized angiographic trial. *Circulation* 89:1557-1566, 1994

208. Chesebro JH, Rao AK, Schwartz D, et al: Endogenous thrombolysis and recanalization of occluded aortocoronary vein grafts with recombinant hirudin in patients with unstable angina (abstract). *Circulation* 90 Suppl 1:568, 1994

209. Cannon CP, McCabe CH, Henry TD, et al: A pilot trial of recombinant desulfatohirudin compared with heparin in conjunction with tissue-type plasminogen activator and aspirin for acute myocardial infarction: results of the Thrombolysis in Myocardial Infarction (TIMI) 5 trial. *J Am Coll Cardiol* 23:993-1003, 1994

210. Rosenberg RD: Biochemistry of heparin antithrombin interactions, and the physiologic role of this natural anticoagulant mechanism. *Am J Med* 87 Suppl 3B:2S-9S, 1989

211. Hirsh J: Heparin. *N Engl J Med* 324:1565-1574, 1991

212. Carter CJ, Kelton JG, Hirsh J, et al: The relationship between the hemorrhagic and antithrombotic properties of low molecular weight heparin in rabbits. *Blood* 59:1239-1245, 1982

213. Salzman EW, Rosenberg RD, Smith MH, et al: Effect of heparin and heparin fractions on platelet aggregation. *J Clin Invest* 65:64-73, 1980

214. Heras M, Chesebro JH, Webster MW, et al: Antithrombotic efficacy of low-molecular-weight heparin in deep arterial injury. *Arterioscler Thromb* 12:250-255, 1992

215. Samama M, Boissel JP, Combe-Tamzali S, et al: Clinical studies with low molecular weight heparins in the prevention and treatment of venous thromboembolism. *Ann N Y Acad Sci* 556:386-405, 1989

216. Hirsh J, Dalen JE, Deykin D, et al: Heparin: mechanism of

action, pharmacokinetics, dosing considerations, monitoring, efficacy, and safety. *Chest* 102 Suppl 4:337S-351S, 1992

217. Basu D, Gallus A, Hirsh J, et al: A prospective study of the value of monitoring heparin treatment with the activated partial thromboplastin time. *N Engl J Med* 287:324-327, 1972

218. Schriever HG, Epstein SE, Mintz MD: Statistical correlation and heparin sensitivity of activated partial thromboplastin time, whole blood coagulation time, and an automated coagulation time. *Am J Clin Pathol* 60:323-329, 1973

219. Perkins HA, Osborn JJ, Hurt R, et al: Neutralization of heparin in vivo with protamine; a simple method of estimating the required dose. *J Lab Clin Med* 48:223-226, 1956

220. Chiu HM, Hirsh J, Yung WL, et al: Relationship between the anticoagulant and antithrombotic effects of heparin in experimental venous thrombosis. *Blood* 49:171-184, 1977

221. Esposito RA, Culliford AT, Colvin SB, et al: The role of the activated clotting time in heparin administration and neutralization for cardiopulmonary bypass. *J Thorac Cardiovasc Surg* 85:174-185, 1983

222. Ogilby JD, Kopelman HA, Klein LW, et al: Adequate heparinization during PTCA: assessment using activated clotting time (abstract). *J Am Coll Cardiol* 11 Suppl A:237, 1988

223. Turpie AGG, Robinson JG, Doyle DJ, et al: Comparison of high-dose with low-dose subcutaneous heparin to prevent left ventricular mural thrombosis in patients with acute transmural anterior myocardial infarction. *N Engl J Med* 320:352-357, 1989

224. Salzman EW, Deykin D, Shapiro RM, et al: Management of heparin therapy: controlled prospective trial. *N Engl J Med* 292:1046-1050, 1975

225. Glazier RL, Crowell EB: Randomized prospective trial of continuous vs intermittent heparin therapy. *JAMA* 236:1365-1367, 1976

226. Levine MN, Hirsh J, Landefeld S, et al: Hemorrhagic complications of anticoagulant treatment. *Chest* 102 Suppl 4:352S-363S, 1992

227. Hyers TM, Hull RD, Weg JG: Antithrombotic therapy for venous thromboembolic disease. *Chest* 102 Suppl 4:408S-425S, 1992

228. Salzman EW: Heparin for prophylaxis of venous thromboembolism. *Ann N Y Acad Sci* 556:371-377, 1989

229. Kakkar VV: Current recommendations in prevention of thrombosis in surgery. *Blood Rev* 1:237-244, 1987

230. Gold EW: Prophylaxis of deep venous thromboembolism: literature review. *Orthopedics* 11:1197-1201, 1988

231. The SCATI (Studio Sulla Calciparina Nell'Angina e Nella Trombosi Ventricolare Nell'Infartol) Group: Randomised controlled trial of subcutaneous calcium-heparin in acute myocardial infarction. *Lancet* 2:182-186, 1989

232. Levine MN, Hirsh J, Salzman EW: Side effects of antithrombotic therapy. In *Hemostasis and Thrombosis, Basic Principles and Clinical Practice.* Third edition. Edited by RW Coleman, J Hirsh, VJ Marder, et al. Philadelphia, JB Lippincott Company, 1994, pp 936-955

233. The Global Use of Strategies to Open Occluded Coronary Arteries (GUSTO) IIa Investigators: Randomized trial of intravenous heparin versus recombinant hirudin for acute coronary syndromes. *Circulation* 90:1631-1637, 1994

234. Antman EM: Hirudin in acute myocardial infarction. Safety report from the Thrombolysis and Thrombin Inhibition in Myocardial Infarction (TIMI) 9A Trial. *Circulation* 90:1624-1630, 1994

235. Miller ML: Heparin-induced thrombocytopenia. *Cleve Clin J Med* 56:483-490, 1989

236. Warkentin TE, Kelton JG: Heparin-induced thrombocytopenia. *Annu Rev Med* 40:31-44, 1989

237. Kontny F, Dale J, Abildgaard U, et al: Adverse effect of warfarin in acute myocardial infarction: increased left ventricular thrombus formation in patients not treated with high-dose heparin. *Eur Heart J* 14:1040-1043, 1993

238. Theroux P, Waters D, Lam J, et al: Reactivation of unstable angina after the discontinuation of heparin. *N Engl J Med* 327:141-145, 1992

239. Chesebro JH, Fuster V: Thrombosis in unstable angina (editorial). *N Engl J Med* 327:192-194, 1992

240. Hirsh J, Dalen JE, Deykin D, et al: Oral anticoagulants. Mechanism of action, clinical effectiveness, and optimal therapeutic range. *Chest* 102 Suppl 4:312S-326S, 1992

241. Baty JD, Breckenridge A, Lewis PJ, et al: May mothers taking warfarin breast feed their infants? (Letter to the editor.) *Br J Clin Pharmacol* 3:969, 1976

242. O'Reilly RA, Aggeler PM: Studies on coumarin anticoagulant drugs: initiation of warfarin therapy without a loading dose. *Circulation* 38:169-177, 1968

243. Fennerty A, Dolben J, Thomas P, et al: Flexible induction dose regimen for warfarin and prediction of maintenance dose. *Br Med J* 288:1268-1270, 1984

244. Scott PJW: Anticoagulant drugs in the elderly: the risks usually outweigh the benefits. *BMJ* 297:1261; 1263, 1988

245. Wintzen AR, de Jonge H, Loeliger EA, et al: The risk of intracerebral hemorrhage during oral anticoagulant treatment: a population study. *Ann Neurol* 16:553-558, 1984

246. Second Report of the Sixty Plus Reinfarction Study Research Group: Risks of long-term oral anticoagulant therapy in elderly patients after myocardial infarction. *Lancet* 1:64-68, 1982

247. Joglekar M, Mohanaruban K, Bayer AJ, et al: Can old people on oral anticoagulants be safely managed as out-patients? *Postgrad Med J* 64:775-777, 1988

248. Lowe GDO: Anticoagulant drugs in the elderly: valuable in selected patients. *BMJ* 297:1260; 1262, 1988

249. Poller L, Hirsh JL: Optimal therapeutic ranges for oral anticoagulation. In *Thrombosis in Cardiovascular Disorders.* Edited by V Fuster, M Verstraete. Philadelphia, WB Saunders Company, 1992, pp 161-174

250. Hull R, Hirsh J, Jay R, et al: Different intensities of oral anticoagulant therapy in the treatment of proximal-vein thrombosis. *N Engl J Med* 307:1676-1681, 1982

251. Levine MN, Raskob G, Hirsh J: Hemorrhagic complications of long-term anticoagulant therapy. *Chest* 95:26S-36S, 1989

252. Ginsberg JS, Hirsh J: Anticoagulants during pregnancy. In *Thrombosis in Cardiovascular Disorders.* Edited by V Fuster, M Verstraete. Philadelphia, WB Saunders Company, 1992, pp 485-489

253. Ginsberg JS, Hirsh J: Use of antithrombotic agents during pregnancy. *Chest* 102 Suppl 4:385S-390S, 1992

254. Sareli P, England MJ, Berk MR, et al: Maternal and fetal sequelae of anticoagulation during pregnancy in patients with mechanical heart valve prostheses. *Am J Cardiol* 63:1462-1465, 1989

255. Howie PW: Anticoagulants in pregnancy. *Clin Obstet Gynecol* 13:349-363, 1986

256. McGehee WG, Klotz TA, Epstein DJ, et al: Coumarin necrosis associated with hereditary protein C deficiency. *Ann Intern Med* 101:59-60, 1984

257. Feder W, Auerbach R: "Purple toes": an uncommon sequela of oral coumarin drug therapy. *Ann Intern Med* 55:911-917, 1961

258. Kazmier FJ, Sheps SG, Bernatz PE, et al: Livedo reticularis and digital infarcts: a syndrome due to cholesterol emboli arising from atheromatous abdominal aortic aneurysms. *Vasc Dis* 3:12-24, 1966

259. Verstraete M, Collen D: Thrombolytic agents. In *Thrombosis in Cardiovascular Disorders.* Edited by V Fuster, M Verstraete. Philadelphia, WB Saunders Company, 1992, pp 175-189

260. Collen D, Gold HK: Fibrin specific thrombolytic agents and new approaches to coronary arterial thrombolysis. In *Thrombolysis in Cardiovascular Disease.* Edited by DG Julian, W Kubler, RM Norris, et al. New York, M Dekker, 1989, pp 45-67

261. Collen D, Stump DC, Gold HK: Thrombolytic therapy. *Annu Rev Med* 39:405-423, 1988

262. Marder VJ, Sherry S: Thrombolytic therapy: current status. *N Engl J Med* 318: a, 1512-1520 (part 1); b, 1585-1595 (part 2), 1988

263. Chesebro JH, Fuster V: Dynamic thrombosis and thrombolysis. Role of antithrombins (editorial). *Circulation* 83:1815-1817, 1991

264. Lidon RM, Theroux P, Lesperance J, et al: A pilot, early angiographic patency study using a direct thrombin inhibitor as adjunctive therapy to streptokinase in acute myocardial infarction. *Circulation* 89:1567-1572, 1994

265. Rentrop KP, Feit F, Blanke H, et al: Effects of intracoronary streptokinase and intracoronary nitroglycerin infusion on coronary angiographic patterns and mortality in patients with acute myocardial infarction. *N Engl J Med* 311:1457-1463, 1984

266. Kennedy JW, Ritchie JL, Davis KB, et al: Western Washington randomized trial of intracoronary streptokinase in acute myocardial infarction. *N Engl J Med* 309:1477-1482, 1983

267. Simoons ML, Serruys PW, Brand Mv/d, et al: Improved survival after early thrombolysis in acute myocardial infarction: a randomized trial by the Interuniversity Cardiology Institute in the Netherlands. *Lancet* 2:578-581, 1985

268. Rentrop KP: Thrombolytic therapy in patients with acute myocardial infarction. *Circulation* 71:627-631, 1985

269. Verstraete M, Bernard R, Bory M, et al: Randomised trial of

intravenous recombinant tissue-type plasminogen activator versus intravenous streptokinase in acute myocardial infarction: report from the European Cooperative Study Group for recombinant tissue-type plasminogen activator. *Lancet* 1:842-847, 1985

270. Verstraete M, Bleifeld W, Brower RW, et al: Double-blind randomised trial of intravenous tissue-type plasminogen activator versus placebo in acute myocardial infarction. *Lancet* 2:965-969, 1985

271. Verstraete M, Arnold AER, Brower RW, et al: Acute coronary thrombolysis with recombinant human tissue-type plasminogen activator: initial patency and influence of maintained infusion on reocclusion rate. *Am J Cardiol* 60:231-237, 1987

272. Simoons ML, Arnold AER, Betriu A, et al: Thrombolysis with tissue plasminogen activator in acute myocardial infarction: no additional benefit from immediate percutaneous coronary angioplasty. *Lancet* 1:197-203, 1988

273. Topol EJ, Morris DC, Smalling RW, et al: A multicenter, randomized, placebo-controlled trial of a new form of intravenous recombinant tissue-type plasminogen activator (Activase) in acute myocardial infarction. *J Am Coll Cardiol* 9:1205-1213, 1987

274. Topol EJ, Califf RM, George BS, et al: A randomized trial of immediate versus delayed elective angioplasty after intravenous tissue plasminogen activator in acute myocardial infarction. *N Engl J Med* 317:581-588, 1987

275. Topol EJ, George BS, Kereiakes DJ, et al: A randomized controlled trial of intravenous tissue plasminogen activator and early intravenous heparin in acute myocardial infarction. *Circulation* 79:281-286, 1989

276. Gold HK, Leinbach RC, Garabedian HD, et al: Acute coronary reocclusion after thrombolysis with recombinant human tissue-type plasminogen activator: prevention by a maintenance infusion. *Circulation* 73:347-352, 1986

277. The TIMI Research Group: Immediate vs delayed catheterization and angioplasty following thrombolytic therapy for acute myocardial infarction: TIMI II A results. *JAMA* 260:2849-2858, 1988

278. Johns JA, Gold HK, Leinbach RC, et al: Prevention of coronary artery reocclusion and reduction in late coronary artery stenosis after thrombolytic therapy in patients with acute myocardial infarction: a randomized study of maintenance infusion of recombinant human tissue-type plasminogen activator. *Circulation* 78:546-556, 1988

279. Stack RS, O'Connor CM, Mark DB, et al: Coronary perfusion during acute myocardial infarction with a combined therapy of coronary angioplasty and high-dose intravenous streptokinase. *Circulation* 77:151-161, 1988

280. Brochier ML, Quilliet L, Kulbertus H, et al: Intravenous anisoylated plasminogen streptokinase activator complex versus intravenous streptokinase in evolving myocardial infarction. Preliminary data from a randomised multicentre study. *Drugs* 33 Suppl 3:140-145, 1987

281. Neuhaus KL, von Essen R, Tebbe U, et al: Improved thrombolysis in acute myocardial infarction with front-loaded administration of alteplase: results of the rt-PA-APSAC Patency Study (TAPS). *J Am Coll Cardiol* 19:885-891, 1992

282. The GUSTO Angiographic Investigators: The effects of tissue plasminogen activator, streptokinase, or both on coronary-artery patency, ventricular function, and survival after acute myocardial infarction. *N Engl J Med* 329:1615-1622, 1993

283. Bono DD: Problems in thrombolysis. In *Thrombolysis in Cardiovascular Disease.* Edited by DG Julian, W Kubler, RM Norris, et al. New York. M. Dekker, 1989, pp 279-292

284. The GUSTO Investigators: An international randomized trial comparing four thrombolytic strategies for acute myocardial infarction. *N Engl J Med* 329:673-682, 1993

285. Purvis JA, McNeill AJ, Siddequi RA, et al: Angiographic assessment of efficacy of double bolus alteplase in acute myocardial infarction (abstract). *Circulation* 88 Suppl 1:292, 1993

286. Collen D, Topol EJ, Tiefenbrunn AJ, et al: Coronary thrombolysis with recombinant human tissue-type plasminogen activator: a prospective, randomized, placebo-controlled trial. *Circulation* 70:1012-1017, 1984

287. Collen D: Human tissue-type plasminogen activator: from the laboratory to the bedside (editorial). *Circulation* 72:18-20, 1985

288. Pitt B: Clot-specific thrombolytic agents: Is there an advantage? (Editorial.) *J Am Coll Cardiol* 12:588, 1988

289. The TIMI Study Group: Comparison of invasive and conservative strategies after treatment with intravenous tissue plasminogen activator in acute myocardial infarction: results of the Thrombolysis in Myocardial Infarction (TIMI) phase II trial. *N Engl J Med* 320:618-627, 1989

290. Gruppo Italiano per lo Studio della Sopravvivenza nell'Infarto Miocardico: GISSI-2: a factorial randomised trial of alteplase versus streptokinase and heparin versus no heparin among 12,490 patients with acute myocardial infarction. *Lancet* 336:65-71, 1990

291. Cairns JA, Fuster V, Kennedy JW: Coronary thrombolysis. *Chest* 102 Suppl 4:482S-507S, 1992

292. Sobel BE: Thrombolysis in the treatment of acute myocardial infarction. In *Thrombosis in Cardiovascular Disorders.* Edited by V Fuster, M Verstraete. Philadelphia, WB Saunders Company, 1992, pp 289-326

293. ISIS-3 (Third International Study of Infarct Survival) Collaborative Group: ISIS-3: a randomised comparison of streptokinase vs tissue plasminogen activator vs anistreplase and of aspirin plus heparin vs aspirin alone among 41,299 cases of suspected acute myocardial infarction. *Lancet* 339:753-770, 1992

294. AIMS Trial Study Group: Effect of intravenous APSAC on mortality after acute myocardial infarction: preliminary report of a placebo-controlled clinical trial. *Lancet* 1:545-549, 1988

295. Monk JP, Heel RC: Anisoylated plasminogen streptokinase activator complex (APSAC): a review of its mechanism of action, clinical pharmacology and therapeutic use in acute myocardial infarction. *Drugs* 34:25-49, 1987

296. Anderson JL, Rothbard RL, Hackworthy RA, et al: Multicenter reperfusion trial of intravenous anisoylated plasminogen streptokinase activator complex (APSAC) in acute myocardial infarction: controlled comparison with intracoronary streptokinase. *J Am Coll Cardiol* 11:1153-1163, 1988

297. Bassand JP, Machecourt J, Cassagnes J, et al: Multicenter trial of intravenous anisoylated plasminogen streptokinase activator complex (APSAC) in acute myocardial infarction: effects on infarct size and left ventricular function. *J Am Coll Cardiol* 13:988-997, 1989

298. Mathey DG, Schofer J, Sheehan FH, et al: Intravenous urokinase in acute myocardial infarction. *Am J Cardiol* 55:878-882, 1985

299. Tennant SN, Dixon J, Venable TC, et al: Intracoronary thrombolysis in patients with acute myocardial infarction: comparison of the efficacy of urokinase with streptokinase. *Circulation* 69:756-760, 1984

300. Van de Werf F, Vanhaecke J, de Geest H, et al: Coronary thrombolysis with recombinant single-chain urokinase-type plasminogen activator in patients with acute myocardial infarction. *Circulation* 74:1066-1070, 1986

301. Topol EJ, Califf RM, George BS, et al: Coronary arterial thrombolysis with combined infusion of recombinant tissue-type plasminogen activator and urokinase in patients with acute myocardial infarction. *Circulation* 77:1100-1107, 1988

302. Collen D, Van de Werf F: Coronary arterial thrombolysis with low-dose synergistic combinations of recombinant tissue-type plasminogen activator (rt-PA) and recombinant single-chain urokinase-type plasminogen activator (rscu-PA) for acute myocardial infarction. *Am J Cardiol* 60:431-434, 1987

303. Stein B, Fuster V, Halperin JL, et al: Antithrombotic therapy in cardiac disease: an emerging approach based on pathogenesis and risk. *Circulation* 80:1501-1513, 1989

304. Théroux P, Ouimet H, McCans J, et al: Aspirin, heparin, or both to treat acute unstable angina. *N Engl J Med* 319:1105-1111, 1988

305. The RISC Group: Risk of myocardial infarction and death during treatment with low dose aspirin and intravenous heparin in men with unstable coronary artery disease. *Lancet* 336:827-830, 1990

306. Haghani K, Shah PK, Cercek B: Unstable angina developing in patients on chronic aspirin therapy is associated with an increased risk of early adverse cardiac events (abstract). *J Am Coll Cardiol* 21 Suppl A:270, 1993

307. Telford AM, Wilson C: Trial of heparin versus atenolol in prevention of myocardial infarction in intermediate coronary syndrome. *Lancet* 1:1225-1228, 1981

308. Théroux P, Waters D, Qiu S, et al: Aspirin versus heparin to prevent myocardial infarction during the acute phase of unstable angina. *Circulation* 88:2045-2048, 1993

309. Cohen M, Adams PC, Parry G, et al: Combination antithrombotic therapy in unstable rest angina and non-Q-wave infarction in nonprior aspirin users. Primary end points analysis from the ATACS trial. *Circulation* 89:81-88, 1994

310. Lidon RM, Theroux P, Juneau M, et al: Initial experience with a direct antithrombin, Hirulog, in unstable angina. Anticoagulant, antithrombotic, and clinical effects. *Circulation* 88:1495-1501, 1993

311. Waters D, Lam JY: Is thrombolytic therapy striking out in unstable angina? (Editorial.) *Circulation* 86:1642-1644, 1992

312. Lawrence JR, Shepherd JT, Bone I, et al: Fibrinolytic therapy in unstable angina pectoris: a controlled clinical trial. *Thromb Res* 17:767-777, 1980

313. Rentrop P, Blanke H, Karsch KR, et al: Selective intracoronary thrombolysis in acute myocardial infarction and unstable angina pectoris. *Circulation* 63:307-317, 1981

314. Vetrovec GW, Leinbach RC, Gold HK, et al: Intracoronary thrombolysis in syndromes of unstable ischemia: angiographic and clinical results. *Am Heart J* 104:946-952, 1982

315. Mandelkorn JB, Wolf NM, Singh S, et al: Intracoronary thrombus in nontransmural myocardial infarction and in unstable angina pectoris. *Am J Cardiol* 52:1-6, 1983

316. Ambrose JA, Hjemdahl-Monsen C, Borrico S, et al: Quantitative and qualitative effects of intracoronary streptokinase in unstable angina and non-Q wave infarction. *J Am Coll Cardiol* 9:1156-1165, 1987

317. Gold HK, Johns JA, Leinbach RC, et al: A randomized, blinded, placebo-controlled trial of recombinant human tissue-type plasminogen activator in patients with unstable angina pectoris. *Circulation* 75:1192-1199, 1987

318. Gotoh K, Minamino T, Katoh O, et al: The role of intracoronary thrombus in unstable angina: angiographic assessment and thrombolytic therapy during ongoing angina attacks. *Circulation* 77:526-534, 1988

319. de Zwaan C, Bar FW, Janssen JHA, et al: Effects of thrombolytic therapy in unstable angina: clinical and angiographic results. *J Am Coll Cardiol* 12:301-309, 1988

320. Topol EJ, Nicklas JM, Kander NH, et al: Coronary revascularization after intravenous tissue plasminogen activator for unstable angina pectoris: results of a randomized, double-blind, placebo-controlled trial. *Am J Cardiol* 62:368-371, 1988

321. Williams DO, Topol EJ, Califf RM, et al: Intravenous recombinant tissue-type plasminogen activator in patients with unstable angina pectoris. *Circulation* 82:376-383, 1990

322. Chaudhary H, Crozier I, Hamer A, et al: Tissue plasminogen activator using a rapid-infusion low-dose regimen for unstable angina. *Am J Cardiol* 69:173-175, 1992

323. Bar FW, Verheugt FW, Col J, et al: Thrombolysis in patients with unstable angina improves the angiographic but not the clinical outcome. Results of UNASEM, a multicenter, randomized, placebo-controlled, clinical trial with anistreplase. *Circulation* 86:131-137, 1992.

324. Freeman MR, Langer A, Wilson RF, et al: Thrombolysis in unstable angina. Randomized double-blind trial of t-PA and placebo. *Circulation* 85:150-157, 1992

325. Schreiber TL, Rizik D, White C, et al: Randomized trial of thrombolysis versus heparin in unstable angina. *Circulation* 86:1407-1414, 1992

326. Saran RK, Bhandari K, Narain VS, et al: Intravenous streptokinase in the management of a subset of patients with unstable angina: a randomized controlled trial. *Int J Cardiol* 28:209-213, 1990

327. Neri Serneri GG, Gensini GF, Poggesi L, et al: Effect of heparin, aspirin, or alteplase in reduction of myocardial ischaemia in refractory unstable angina. *Lancet* 335:615-618, 1990

328. Steffenino G, DiLeo M, Bergerone S, et al: No clinical benefit from early intracoronary streptokinase in unstable angina: a prospective, randomized study (abstract). *Eur Heart J* 11 Suppl:387, 1990

329. Nicklas JM, Topol EJ, Kander N, et al: Randomized, double-blind, placebo-controlled trial of tissue plasminogen activator in unstable angina. *J Am Coll Cardiol* 13:434-441, 1989

330. Mont L, Betriu A, Azqueta M, et al: Early angiography and thrombolysis in patients with unstable angina (abstract). *Circulation* 78 Suppl 2:420, 1988

331. The TIMI IIIB Investigators: Effects of tissue plasminogen activator and a comparison of early invasive and conservative strategies in unstable angina and non-Q-wave myocardial infarction. Results of the TIMI IIIB Trial. *Circulation* 89:1545-1556, 1994

332. Gruppo Italiano per lo Studio della Streptochinasi nell'Infarto Miocardico (GISSI): Effectiveness of intravenous thrombolytic treatment in acute myocardial infarction. *Lancet* 1:397-402, 1986

333. Gibson RS, Beller GA, Gheorghiade M, et al: The prevalence and clinical significance of residual myocardial ischemia 2 weeks after uncomplicated non-Q wave infarction: a prospective natural history study. *Circulation* 73:1186-1198, 1986

334. Timmis AD, Griffin B, Crick JCP, et al: The effects of early coronary patency on the evolution of myocardial infarction: a prospective arteriographic study. *Br Heart J* 58:345-351, 1987

335. Chesebro JH, Badimon JJ, Ortiz AF, et al: Conjunctive antithrombotic therapy for thrombolysis in myocardial infarction. *Am J Cardiol* 72:66G-74G, 1993

336. Braunwald E: The open-artery theory is alive and well—again (editorial). *N Engl J Med* 329:1650-1652, 1993

337. Roux S, Christeller S, Ludin E: Effects of aspirin on coronary reocclusion and recurrent ischemia after thrombolysis: a meta-analysis. *J Am Coll Cardiol* 19:671-677, 1992

338. Report of the Working Party on Anticoagulant Therapy in Coronary Thrombosis to the Medical Research Council: Assessment of short-term anticoagulant administration after cardiac infarction. *Br Med J [Clin Res]* 1:335-342, 1969

339. Drapkin A, Merskey C: Anticoagulant therapy after acute myocardial infarction: relation of therapeutic benefit to patient's age, sex, and severity of infarction. *JAMA* 222:541-548, 1972

340. Veterans Administration Hospital Investigators: Anticoagulants in acute myocardial infarction: results of a cooperative clinical trial. *JAMA* 225:724-729, 1973

341. Chalmers TC, Matta RJ, Smith H Jr, et al: Evidence favoring the use of anticoagulants in the hospital phase of acute myocardial infarction. *N Engl J Med* 297:1091-1096, 1977

342. Bleich SD, Nichols TC, Schumacher RR, et al: Effect of heparin on coronary arterial patency after thrombolysis with tissue plasminogen activator in acute myocardial infarction. *Am J Cardiol* 66:1412-1417, 1990

343. Hsia J, Hamilton WP, Kleiman N, et al: A comparison between heparin and low-dose aspirin as adjunctive therapy with tissue plasminogen activator for acute myocardial infarction. Heparin-Aspirin Reperfusion Trial (HART) Investigators. *N Engl J Med* 323:1433-1437, 1990

344. de Bono DP, Simoons ML, Tijssen J, et al: Effect of early intravenous heparin on coronary patency, infarct size, and bleeding complications after alteplase thrombolysis: results of a randomised double blind European Cooperative Study Group trial. *Br Heart J* 67:122-128, 1992

345. Cuccia C, Volterrani M, Volpini M, et al: Relationship between anticoagulation level, ischemic events and angiographic characteristics of infarct-related artery following streptokinase in patients with acute myocardial infarction. *J Am Coll Cardiol* 19 Suppl A:92, 1992

346. Topol EJ, Califf RM, Vandormael M, et al: A randomized trial of late reperfusion therapy for acute myocardial infarction. Thrombolysis and Angioplasty in Myocardial Infarction-6 Study Group. *Circulation* 85:2090-2099, 1992

347. Meijer A, Verheugt FW, Werter CJ, et al: Aspirin versus coumadin in the prevention of reocclusion and recurrent ischemia after successful thrombolysis:a prospective placebo-controlled angiographic study. Results of the APRICOT Study. *Circulation* 87:1524-1530, 1993

348. Kannel WB, Wolf PA, Garrison RJ: Survival following initial cardiovascular events. Framingham study. Section 35. United States Department of Health and Human Services, National Institute of Health. United States Department of Commerce. Publication No. PB 88-204049, 1988

349. Breddin K, Loew D, Lechner K, et al: The German-Austrian Aspirin Trial: a comparison of acetylsalicylic acid, placebo and phenprocoumon in secondary prevention of myocardial infarction. *Circulation* 62 Suppl 5:63-72, 1980

350. An International Anticoagulant Review Group: Collaborative analysis of long-term anticoagulant administration after acute myocardial infarction. *Lancet* 1:203-209, 1970

351. Ebert RV, Borden CW, Hipp HR, et al: Long-term anticoagulant therapy after myocardial infarction: final report of the Veterans Administration Cooperative Study. *JAMA* 207:2263-2267, 1969

352. Smith P, Arnesen H, Holme I: The effect of warfarin on mortality and reinfarction after myocardial infarction. *N Engl J Med* 323:147-152, 1990

353. Report of the Sixty Plus Reinfarction Study Research Group: A double-blind trial to assess long-term oral anticoagulation therapy in elderly patients after myocardial infarction. *Lancet* 2:989-994, 1980

354. Peto R, Gray R, Collins R, et al: Randomised trial of prophylactic daily aspirin in British male doctors. *Br Med J [Clin Res]* 296:313-316, 1988

355. Fuster V, Cohen M, Halperin J: Aspirin in the prevention of coronary disease. *N Engl J Med* 321:129-135, 1989

356. Gavagham TP, Gebski V, Baron DW: Immediate postoperative aspirin improves vein graft patency early and late after coronary artery bypass graft surgery. A placebo-controlled, randomized study. *Circulation* 83:1526-1533, 1991

357. Stein PD, Dalen JE, Goldman S, et al: Antithrombotic therapy in patients with saphenous vein and internal mammary artery bypass grafts following percutaneous transluminal coronary angioplasty. *Chest* 102 Suppl 4:508S-515S, 1992

358. McEnany MT, Salzman EW, Mundth ED, et al: The effect of antithrombotic therapy on patency rates of saphenous vein coronary artery bypass grafts. *J Thorac Cardiovasc Surg* 83:81-89, 1982
359. Pantely GA, Goodnight SH Jr, Rahimtoola SH, et al: Failure of antiplatelet and anticoagulant therapy to improve patency of grafts after coronary-artery bypass: a controlled, randomized study. *N Engl J Med* 301:962-966, 1979
360. Gohlke H, Gohlke-Barwolf C, Sturzenhofecker P, et al: Improved graft patency with anticoagulant therapy after aortocoronary bypass surgery: a prospective, randomized study. *Circulation* 64 Suppl 2:22-27, 1981
361. Grüntzig AR, Senning Å, Siegenthaler WE: Nonoperative dilatation of coronary-artery stenosis: percutaneous transluminal coronary angioplasty. *N Engl J Med* 301:61-68, 1979
362. Landau C, Lange RA, Hillis LD: Percutaneous transluminal coronary angioplasty. *N Engl J Med* 330:981-993, 1994
363. Chesebro JH, Badimon JJ, Badimon L, et al: Arterial angioplasty: injury, mural thrombus, and restenosis. In *The Practice of Interventional Cardiology.* Second edition. Edited by JHK Vogel, SB King III. St. Louis, Mosby Year Book, 1993, pp 509-520
364. Barnathan ES, Schwartz JS, Taylor L, et al: Aspirin and dipyridamole in the prevention of acute coronary thrombosis complicating coronary angioplasty. *Circulation* 76:125-134, 1987
365. Schwartz L, Bourassa MG, Lesperance J, et al: Aspirin and dipyridamole in the prevention of restenosis after percutaneous transluminal coronary angioplasty. *N Engl J Med* 318:1714-1719, 1988
366. White CW, Knudson M, Schmidt D, et al: Neither ticlopidine nor aspirin-dipyridamole prevents restenosis post PTCA: results from a randomized placebo-controlled multicenter trial (abstract). *Circulation* 76 Suppl 4:213, 1987
367. Heras M, Chesebro JH, Penny WJ, et al: Importance of adequate heparin dosage in arterial angioplasty in a porcine model. *Circulation* 78:654-660, 1988
368. Lukas MA, Deutsch E, Laskey WK: Beneficial effect of heparin therapy on PTCA outcome in unstable angina (abstract). *J Am Coll Cardiol* 11 Suppl A:132, 1988
369. Douglas JS Jr, Lutz JF, Clements SD, et al: Therapy of large intracoronary thrombi in candidates for percutaneous transluminal coronary angioplasty (abstract). *J Am Coll Cardiol* 11 Suppl A:238, 1988
370. Pow TK, Varricchione TR, Jacobs AK, et al: Does pretreatment with heparin prevent abrupt closure following PTCA? (Abstract.) *J Am Coll Cardiol* 11 Suppl A:238, 1988
371. Ambrose JA, Almeida OD, Sharma SK, et al: Adjunctive thrombolytic therapy during angioplasty for ischemic rest angina: results of the TAUSA Trial. *Circulation* 90:69-77, 1994
372. The EPIC Investigation: Use of a monoclonal antibody directed against the platelet glycoprotein IIb/IIIa receptor in high-risk coronary angioplasty. *N Engl J Med* 330:956-961, 1994
373. Ellis SG, Roubin GS, Wilentz J, et al: Results of a randomized trial of heparin and aspirin vs. aspirin alone for prevention of acute closure (AC) and restenosis (R) after angioplasty (PTCA) (abstract). *Circulation* 76 Suppl 4:213, 1987
374. Thornton MA, Gruentzig AR, Hollman J, et al: Coumadin and aspirin in prevention of recurrence after transluminal coronary angioplasty: a randomized study. *Circulation* 69:721-727, 1984
375. Halperin JL, Hart RG: Atrial fibrillation and stroke: new ideas, persisting dilemmas. *Stroke* 19:937-941, 1988
376. Laupacis A, Albers G, Dunn M, et al: Antithrombotic therapy in atrial fibrillation. *Chest* 102 Suppl 4:426S-433S, 1992
377. Brand FN, Abbott RD, Kannel WB, et al: Characteristics and prognosis of lone atrial fibrillation: 30-year follow-up in the Framingham Study. *JAMA* 254:3449-3453, 1985
378. The Stroke Prevention in Atrial Fibrillation Investigators: Predictors of thromboembolism in atrial fibrillation: I. Clinical features of patients at risk. *Ann Intern Med* 116:1-5, 1992
379. Kopecky SL, Gersh BJ, McGoon MD, et al: The natural history of lone atrial fibrillation: a population-based study over three decades. *N Engl J Med* 317:669-674, 1987
380. Kopecky SL, Gersh BJ, McGoon MD, et al: Lone atrial fibrillation in the elderly: a population-based long-term study (abstract). *Circulation* 80 Suppl 2:409, 1989
381. Weinberger J, Rothlauf E, Materese E, et al: Noninvasive evaluation of the extracranial carotid arteries in patients with cerebrovascular events and atrial fibrillations. *Arch Intern Med* 148:1785-1788, 1988
382. Fisher CM, Gore I, Okabe N, et al: Atherosclerosis of the carotid and vertebral arteries--extracranial and intracranial. *J Neuropathol Exp Neurol* 24:455-476, 1965
383. Chesebro JH, Fuster V, Halperin JL: Atrial fibrillation—risk marker for stroke (editorial). *N Engl J Med* 323:1556-1558, 1990
384. Roy D, Marchand E, Gagné P, et al: Usefulness of anticoagulant therapy in the prevention of embolic complications of atrial fibrillation. *Am Heart J* 112:1039-1043, 1986
385. Peterson P, Godtfredsen J, Boysen G, et al: Placebo-controlled, randomised trial of warfarin and aspirin for prevention of thromboembolic complications in chronic atrial fibrillation: the Copenhagen AFASAK study. *Lancet* 1:175-179, 1989
386. Stroke Prevention in Atrial Fibrillation Study Group Investigators: Preliminary report of the Stroke Prevention in Atrial Fibrillation Study. *N Engl J Med* 322:863-868, 1990
387. Stroke Prevention in Atrial Fibrillation Investigators: Stroke Prevention in Atrial Fibrillation Study: final results. *Circulation* 84:527-539, 1991
388. The Boston Area Anticoagulation Trial for Atrial Fibrillation Investigators: The effect of low-dose warfarin on the risk of stroke in patients with nonrheumatic atrial fibrillation. *N Engl J Med* 323:1505-1511, 1990
389. Connolly SJ, Laupacis A, Gent M, et al: Canadian Atrial Fibrillation Anticoagulation (CAFA) Study. *J Am Coll Cardiol* 18:349-355, 1991
390. Ezekowitz MD, Bridgers SL, James KE, et al: Warfarin in the prevention of stroke associated with nonrheumatic atrial fibrillation. Veterans Affairs Stroke Prevention in Nonrheumatic Atrial Fibrillation Investigators. *N Engl J Med* 327:1406-1412, 1992
391. Stroke Prevention in Atrial Fibrillation Investigators: Warfarin versus aspirin for prevention of thromboembolism in atrial fibrillation: Stroke Prevention in Atrial Fibrillation II Study. *Lancet* 343:687-691, 1994
392. Atrial Fibrillation Investigators: Risk factors for stroke and efficacy of antithrombotic therapy in atrial fibrillation. Analysis of pooled data from five randomized controlled trials. *Arch Intern Med* 154:1449-1457, 1994
393. The Stroke Prevention in Atrial Fibrillation Investigators: Predictors of thromboembolism in atrial fibrillation: II. Echocardiographic features of patients at risk. *Ann Intern Med* 116:6-12, 1992
394. Wolf PA, Abbott RD, Kannel WB: Atrial fibrillation: a major contributor to stroke in the elderly. The Framingham Study. *Arch Intern Med* 147:1561-1564, 1987
395. Wolf PA, Abbott RD, Kannel WB: Atrial fibrillation as an independent risk factor for stroke: The Framingham Study. *Stroke* 22:983-988, 1991
396. EAFT (European Atrial Fibrillation Trial) Study Group: Secondary prevention in non-rheumatic atrial fibrillation after transient ischaemic attack or minor stroke. *Lancet* 342:1255-1262, 1993
397. Grimm RA, Stewart WJ, Black IW, et al: Should all patients undergo transesophageal echocardiography before electrical cardioversion of atrial fibrillation? *J Am Coll Cardiol* 23:533-541, 1994
398. Fatkin D, Kuchar DL, Thorburn CW, et al: Transesophageal echocardiography before and during direct current cardioversion of atrial fibrillation: evidence for "atrial stunning" as a mechanism of thromboembolic complications. *J Am Coll Cardiol* 23:307-316, 1994
399. Meltzer RS, Visser CA, Fuster V: Intracardiac thrombi and systemic embolization. *Ann Intern Med* 104:689-698, 1986
400. Lapeyre AC III, Steele PM, Kazmier FJ, et al: Systemic embolism in chronic left ventricular aneurysm: incidence and the role of anticoagulation. *J Am Coll Cardiol* 6:534-538, 1985
401. Fuster V, Gersh BJ, Giuliani ER, et al: The natural history of idiopathic dilated cardiomyopathy. *Am J Cardiol* 47:525-531, 1981
402. Stein PD, Alpert JS, Copeland J, et al: Antithrombotic therapy in patients with mechanical and biological prosthetic heart valves. *Chest* 102 Suppl 4:445S-455S, 1992
403. Myers ML, Lawrie GM, Crawford ES, et al: The St. Jude valve prosthesis: analysis of the clinical results in 815 implants and the need for systemic anticoagulation. *J Am Coll Cardiol* 13:57-62, 1989
404. Mok CK, Boey J, Wang R, et al: Warfarin versus dipyridamole-aspirin and pentoxifylline-aspirin for the prevention of prosthetic heart valve thromboembolism: a prospective randomized clinical trial. *Circulation* 72:1059-1063, 1985
405. Turpie AG, Gent M, Laupacis A, et al: A comparison of aspirin with placebo in patients treated with warfarin after heart-valve replacement. *N Engl J Med* 329:524-529, 1993
406. Heras M, Chesebro JH, Fuster V, et al: High risk of thromboemboli early after bioprosthetic cardiac valve replacement. *J Am Coll Cardiol* 25:1111-1119, 1995

CHAPTER

29

Myocardial ischemia clinical syndromes

A. Silent myocardial ischemia

Joseph L. Blackshear, M.D., and Robert E. Safford, M.D., Ph.D.

RENEWED interest in the totality of myocardial ischemia beyond symptoms has followed the rapid development of new or modified techniques for detection of ischemia. Although the many contributions to the literature on the subject suggest clinical relevance, the conclusions of recent American Heart Association, American College of Cardiology, and American College of Physicians task forces have not favored the widespread application of techniques for detection of silent ischemia.[1,2] These recommendations were issued before publication of a large body of data suggesting that silent myocardial ischemia potentially has independent prognostic importance. After reviewing silent ischemia in general, we discuss the data on prognosis in some detail and address the usefulness of various techniques in clinical management.

DEFINITION

Silent myocardial ischemia is transient or persistent, but reversible, dysfunction of the myocardium evidenced by electrocardiographic (ECG) abnormalities, myocardial perfusion or metabolic abnormalities, increase in filling pressures, or development of wall motion abnormalities without associated angina-equivalent syndromes in patients with known coronary artery disease or coronary artery spasm.[3] Without symptoms, identification of ischemia relies entirely on methods of detection interpreted with full knowledge of the pathophysiologic mechanisms that produce ischemia and affect pain perception.

MYOCARDIAL ISCHEMIA

Myocardial ischemia results when the supply of myocardial oxygen is less than the demand. It is accompanied by reduced clearance of metabolites from tissue due to decreased perfusion.[4] Decades of animal studies and clinical observations have documented that numerous factors have the potential to influence this supply-demand ratio (Fig 29A-1) (see chapter 27A).

Fixed luminal obstruction of epicardial coronary arteries may increase resistance to coronary arterial flow in such a way that when maximal autoregulatory dilatation of a coronary artery beyond a stenosis has occurred, further reduction of perfusion pressure or worsening of obstruction reduces coronary blood flow. In addition, dynamic changes in resistance to coronary artery flow may occur due to spasm or thrombosis. Increases in left ventricular end-diastolic pressure may be transmitted to the subendocardial vessels. The pressure difference (gradient) between the aorta and the myocardial capillaries is thereby lessened and the flow of nutrients reduced. Increases in heart rate, systolic blood pressure, left ventricular wall tension, and contractility all increase the demand for myocardial oxygen. Tachycardia, by shortening diastolic perfusion time, reduces coronary blood flow relative to increased demands from a higher heart rate.

The ischemic cascade

It is now well established that a predictable cascade of events follows occlusion of a coronary artery. As illustrated in Figure 29A-2, abnormal myocardial relaxation occurs within a few seconds after balloon inflation during coronary angioplasty in man. This is followed relatively quickly by abnormalities of contraction, then by measurable increases in diastolic pressure, only later by ECG changes (ST segment depression or elevation), and ultimately by angina pectoris in some but not all instances.[5] It seems reasonable to propose, therefore, that many episodes of ischemia, especially those that are brief or not particularly severe, might terminate at some point along the ischemic cascade before angina pectoris develops.

Another, perhaps more physiologic, illustration of the ischemic cascade is the spontaneous exercise-induced or

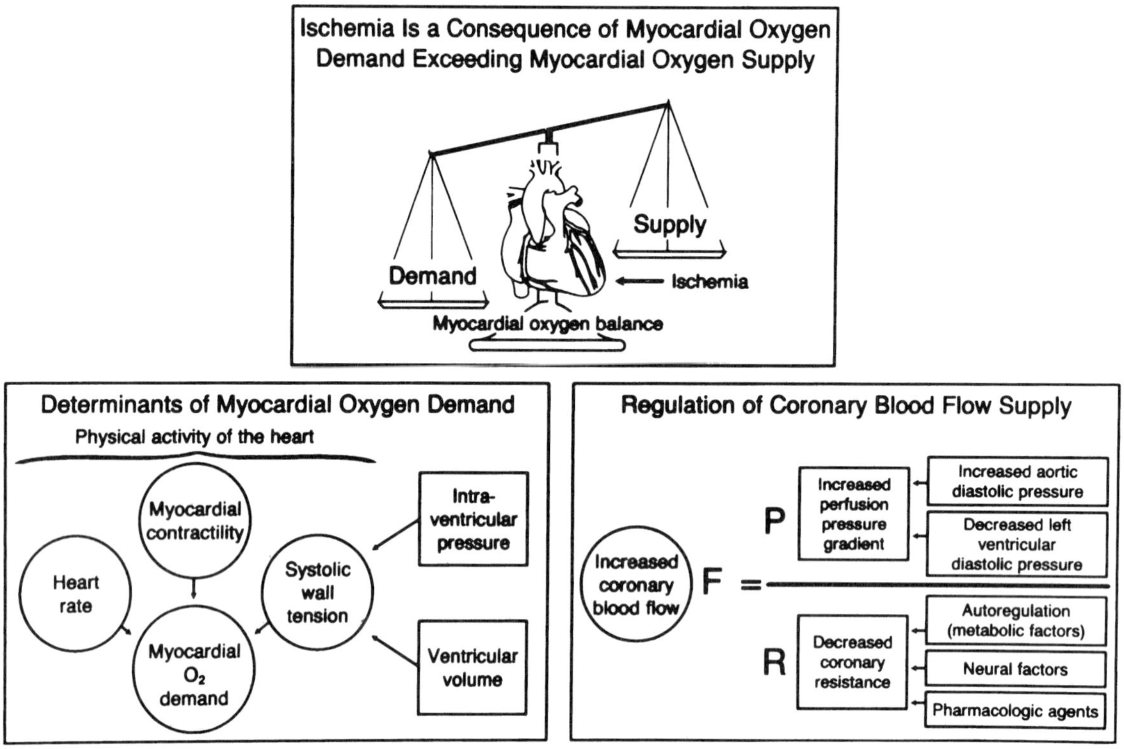

Fig 29A-1. Factors affecting the balance of myocardial oxygen demand and supply. (Modified from Topics in Cardiovascular Disease: Angina. ICI Americas, Wilmington, Delaware, 1984, pp 13-15.)

ergonovine-induced spasm of one or more coronary arteries. Figure 29A-3 is a reproduction of the ST-segment shifts that developed during exercise in a patient with variant angina superimposed on moderate fixed stenosis of the left anterior descending coronary artery. The onset of ST-segment elevation preceded the development of anginal pain by 1 1/2 minutes, during which time the heart rate progressively increased and further ST elevation occurred in multiple leads. New anteroapical akinesis was documented by echocardiography immediately after exercise, and the patient later had spontaneous near-total occlusion of the middle left anterior descending artery with chest pain during coronary angiography. This example illustrates the occurrence of ST-segment shifts before symptoms in a patient with coronary artery spasm. However, a variety of studies summarized by Cohn[6] have shown that silent ischemic episodes are not necessarily briefer or associated with less impressive wall motion or scintigraphic perfusion abnormalities than are symptomatic episodes.

Abnormalities of pain perception

Since the patient's awareness of any symptom requires an intact peripheral nervous system for sensation to occur and an intact central nervous system to allow the sensation to be perceived, neurologic abnormalities may cause myocardial ischemia to be symptomless in some patients, whereas in other patients the same degree of ischemia produces symptoms. Droste and Roskamm[7] and Glazier et al.[8] concluded that many patients with silent ischemia have defective perception of painful stimuli, because they documented increased pain thresholds in these subjects. It was speculated that increased levels of endorphins might be the cause of defective pain perception in these patients,[9] but normal endorphin levels were found in three studies,[9-11] and infusions of naloxone, an opioid-receptor blocking agent, did not produce anginal pain during exercise in patients known to have silent ischemia on previous treadmill tests.[12]

The higher prevalence of silent myocardial infarction in diabetic patients than in nondiabetic patients[13,14] is speculated to be the result of sensory neuropathy.[15] Abnormalities of the cardiac parasympathetic and sympathetic nerves have been found in patients with diabetes,[16] and age itself may contribute to decreased perception of ischemic cardiac pain.[17] The absence of symptoms due to myocardial ischemia after cardiac transplantation is common and is attributed to surgical denervation. Although precise definition of the mechanisms is unclear, it is generally accepted that many patients with myocardial ischemia have a "defective anginal warning system," a term coined by Cohn[18] in 1980.

Coronary artery vasoconstriction

The notion that coronary vasospasm may precipitate silent myocardial ischemia was first suggested by ambulatory

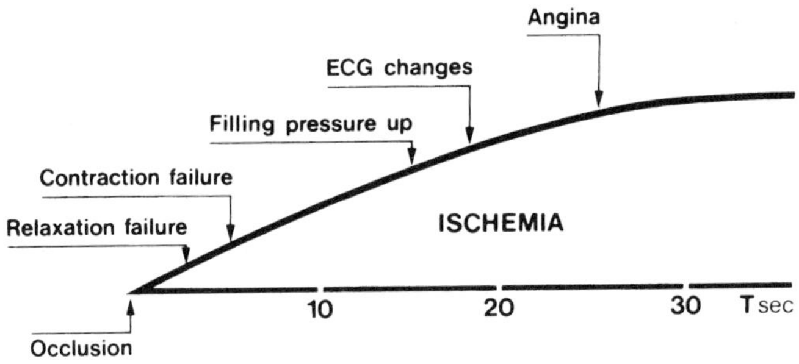

Fig 29A-2. The ischemia cascade. (From Sigwart U, Grbic M, Payot M, et al: Ischemic events during coronary artery balloon obstruction. In *Silent Myocardial Ischemia.* Edited by W Rutishauser, H Roskamm. Berlin, Springer-Verlag, 1984, pp 29-36. By permission.)

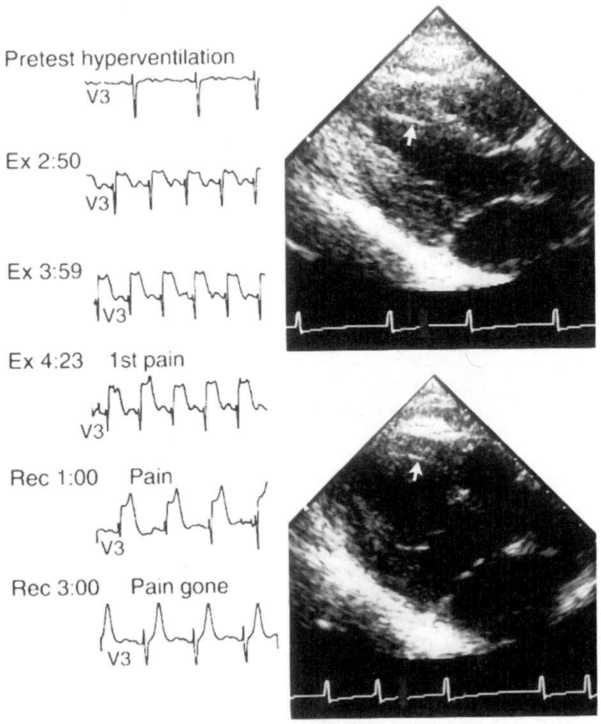

Fig 29A-3. Painless ST-segment elevation during treadmill exercise in a 53-year-old woman. Parasternal long-axis echocardiogram shows normal anteroseptal end-systolic thickness with patient at rest and anteroapical bulging and failure to thicken immediately after exercise (*arrows*). Coronary angiography showed moderate atherosclerotic left anterior descending stenosis with superimposed spontaneous spasm.

ECG studies in which heart rate during exercise testing in the same patient was usually lower at the onset of silent episodes than during painful episodes of ischemia.[18] Reduced rubidium 82 uptake in the myocardium during silent ST-segment changes, documented by Deanfield et al.,[19] provided strong evidence that the ECG changes indeed reflected ischemia. Later, it was shown that mental arithmetic and cigarette smoking also produced silent ST-segment depression, corresponding transient perfusion defects, and regional wall motion abnormalities in many patients with coronary artery disease.[20-23] Similar events occur during cocaine withdrawal.[24] Thus, transient reductions in myocardial oxygen supply on the basis of coronary vasoconstriction are believed to be a cause of silent ischemia when significant increases in myocardial oxygen demand are lacking (Fig 29A-4).

At the cellular level, understanding of the biochemistry and pharmacology of arterial endothelium has been advanced with the discovery of an endothelium-derived relaxant factor, nitric oxide.[25-27] It is now known that in atherosclerotic coronary arteries, concentrations of nitric oxide are reduced in the endothelium adjacent to plaque.[28] Consequently, local vasodilatory response is reduced and coronary vasomotor tone increased at these sites,[29] particularly in coronary arteries with eccentric stenoses.[30] This effect may be particularly prominent at times when circulating catecholamine levels are increased; consequent α-adrenergic-mediated coronary vasoconstriction may reduce the myocardial oxygen supply and result in ischemia at levels of myocardial oxygen demand lower than those normally occurring with exercise.[31] Since conventional vasodilators (nitrates, calcium-channel entry blockers) may remain effective at these sites in the coronary arteries, it is not surprising that they have been found effective in the treatment of silent myocardial ischemia.[32]

Platelet aggregation on the surfaces of atherosclerotic plaques may also cause transient reductions of coronary flow or episodic coronary occlusion, as shown by Folts et al.[33] and Davies et al.[34] Nicotine is also known to cause platelet aggregation and may contribute to silent ischemia via thrombosis in addition to direct coronary vasoconstriction.[35] A large body of data suggests that the pathophysiology of ischemia, silent or symptomatic, in unstable angina differs from that in stable angina because of intracoronary thrombus.[36,37] Clot formation, propagation, and dissolution; local release of vasoactive mediators with different effects on normal and abnormal areas of coronary endothelial surface; fluctuating myocardial oxygen demand; and abnormalities of pain perception, either endogenous or analgesia-induced, are currently perceived to be dynamic mechanisms underlying silent ischemia in patients with unstable angina.[37,38]

Myocardial oxygen demand and circadian periodicity

Careful studies have established that statistically significant increases in heart rate and systolic blood pressure frequently precede the onset of silent ischemic episodes during routine daily activities[39-41] (Fig 29A-5). The duration of increased heart rate influences the threshold of ischemia.[42] Prolonged (30 minutes) modest increases in heart rate may lower the ischemic threshold, in part explaining why silent ischemia during daily life may occur at a lower heart rate than ischemia during exercise testing.

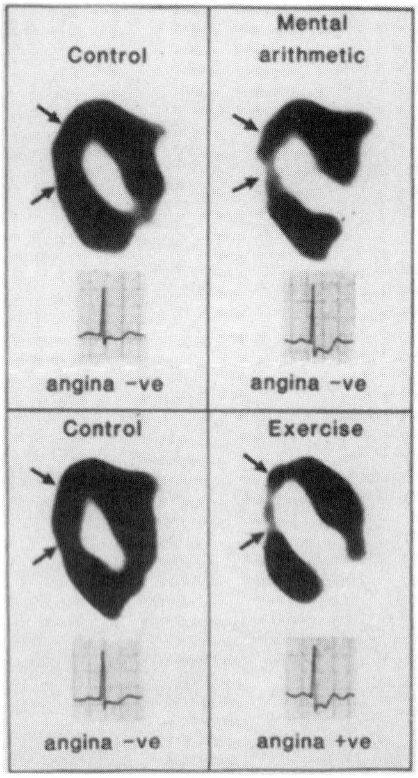

Fig 29A-4. Regional myocardial uptake of rubidium 82 before and after mental arithmetic and exercise correlated with electrocardiogram and symptoms. Scans demonstrate diminished apical-lateral perfusion (*arrows*), indicating silent myocardial ischemia induced by mental stress. *+ve*, angina present; *-ve*, angina absent. (From Deanfield JE, Shea M, Kensett M, et al: Silent myocardial ischaemia due to mental stress. *Lancet* 2:1001-1005, 1984. By permission of the journal.)

There is a striking circadian variation in serum catecholamine levels,[43] platelet aggregation,[44] heart rate, forearm vascular resistance, and systolic blood pressure in both healthy individuals and those with hypertension[41,45] (Fig 29A-6). The peak levels of these variables all occur within the first 4 hours after awakening and correlate with clinical events, because the maximal likelihoods of acute myocardial infarction,[46] sudden cardiac death,[47] coronary artery spasm,[48] and silent ST depression[40] all have the same time course. Interestingly, fibrinolytic activity follows a circadian pattern, with minimal activity occurring in the first few hours after awakening.[49] The combination of coronary vasospasm and increased platelet aggregation predisposes to coronary thrombosis.

Early after acute myocardial infarction, the circadian pattern of silent ischemia changes to a pattern of maximal activity in the evening (6 p.m. to midnight).[50] By a month after infarction, the pattern has reverted to that of patients with chronic stable angina, that is, the morning peak of silent ischemia has returned.[51]

Silent myocardial ischemia is but one of many ischemic syndromes that are related to the complex interaction of autonomic, endocrine, endothelial, hematologic, and environmental factors in patients with coronary artery disease.

METHODS OF DETECTION OF SILENT MYOCARDIAL ISCHEMIA

Clinically silent myocardial ischemia manifested by ST-segment depression during exercise was first described 60 years ago (see Epstein et al.[52]). More than 30 years ago, Holter,[53] in a paper describing the development of a prototype ambulatory ECG monitor, illustrated cases of myocardial ischemia during daily life. Subsequently, ex-

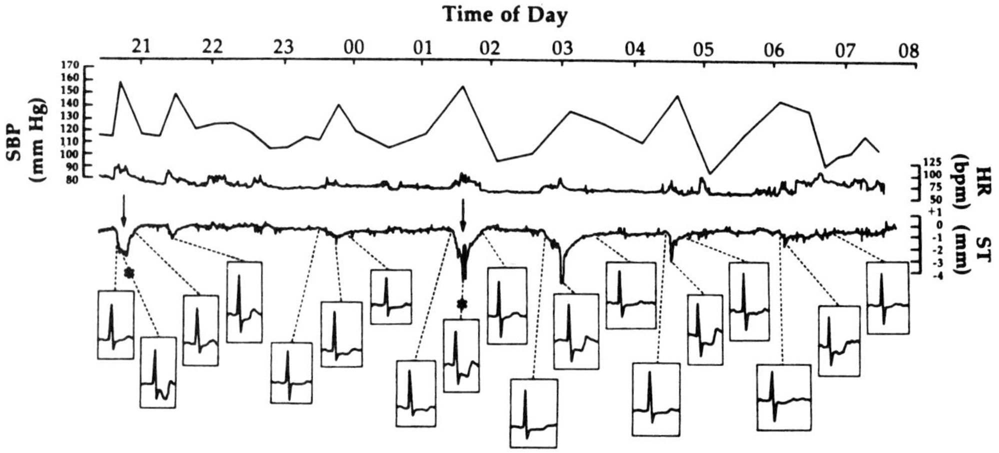

Fig 29A-5. Simultaneous ambulatory electrocardiogram and blood pressure monitoring data in a man with coronary artery disease. Data show an increase in heart rate (*HR*) and blood pressure preceding and during ischemic periods, most of which were asymptomatic. *Arrows* indicate angina. *ST*, ST segment. (From Deedwania PC, Nelson JR: Pathophysiology of silent myocardial ischemia during daily life: hemodynamic evaluation by simultaneous electrocardiographic and blood pressure monitoring. *Circulation* 82:1296-1304, 1990. By permission of American Heart Association.)

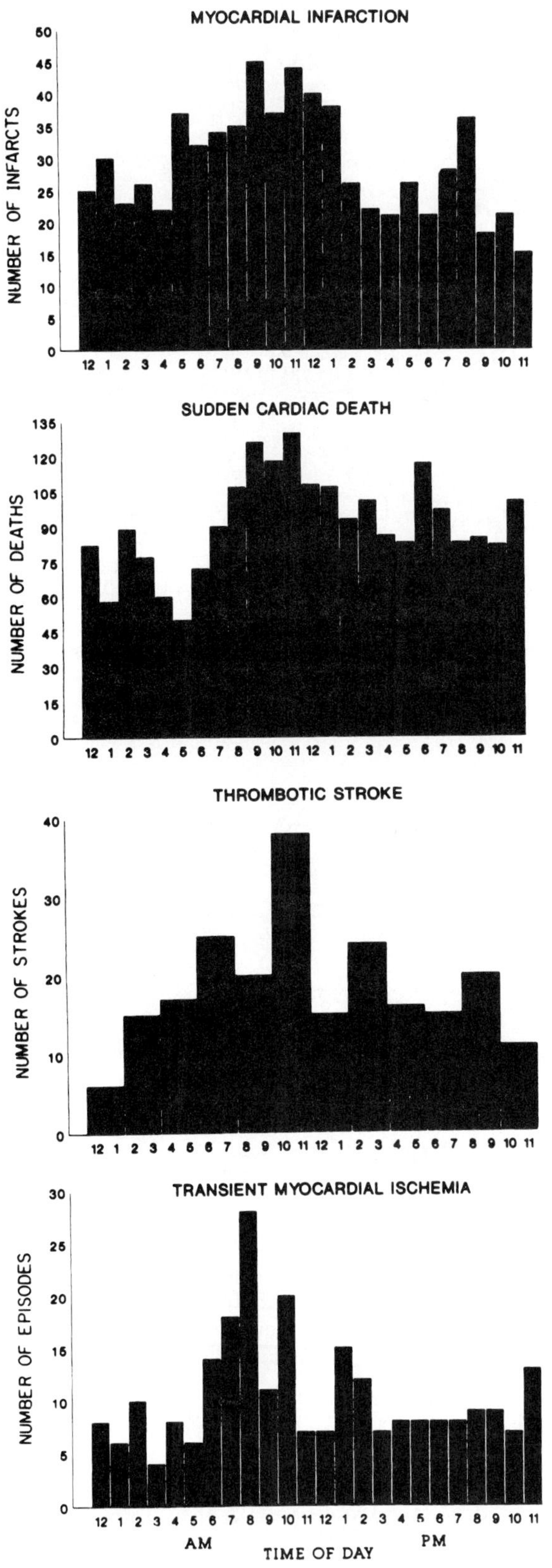

Fig 29A-6. Circadian variation of time of onset of myocardial infarction, sudden cardiac death, thrombotic stroke, and transient myocardial ischemia. Each illness occurs with greatest frequency between 6:00 a.m. and noon. (From Muller JE, Tofler GH, Stone PH: Circadian variation and triggers of onset of acute cardiovascular disease. *Circulation* 79:733-743, 1989. By permission of American Heart Association.)

ercise stress testing and ambulatory ECG monitoring ("Holter monitoring") became the most widely used methods for detecting silent myocardial ischemia. However, as shown in Table 29A-1, myocardial ischemia is detected by many other methods and in various clinical situations, such as ECG ST-segment changes in the operating room, perfusion defects on nuclear scans, wall motion abnormalities detected by a wide variety of techniques, and directly measured hemodynamic changes.[54]

Exercise electrocardiography

The rationale, technique, accuracy, limitations, and pitfalls of exercise stress testing are described in chapter 3B.

Traditionally, the ECG criterion for ischemia is 0.1 mV (1 mm with usual standardization) of horizontal or downsloping ST-segment depression at 80 msec from the J-point lasting from 30 to 60 seconds.[55,56] Even if one is

Table 29A-1 Methods of detection and clinical settings in silent myocardial ischemia

Example	Detected by
Ambulatory painless ST depression or elevation during normal activity with known CAD	Ambulatory ST monitoring
Painless ST depression during exercise testing with known CAD	Exercise ECG
Painless ST depression or elevation on balloon inflation during PTCA	ECG
ST depression in the operating room under anesthesia with known CAD	ECG
Painless ST depression or elevation recurring after thrombolysis or PTCA	ECG
Thallium or rubidium perfusion defects during exercise, smoking, or spontaneous activity	Thallium scintigraphy, positron-emission tomography
Increased LVEDP during spontaneous painless ST depression	ECG and pulmonary artery catheter measurements
Painless ventricular wall motion abnormalities with mental stress	Radionuclide or contrast ventriculography, echocardiography

CAD, coronary artery disease; ECG, electrocardiography; LVEDP, left ventricular end-diastolic pressure; PTCA, percutaneous transluminal coronary angioplasty.

From Blackshear JL: Ambulatory monitoring of silent myocardial ischemia: What is its utility? *South Med J* 85:293-298, 1992. By permission of Southern Medical Association.

careful to exclude conditions known to cause false-positive ECG responses, including left ventricular hypertrophy, ventricular conduction defects, Wolff-Parkinson-White syndrome, mitral valve prolapse, hypokalemia, and digitalis therapy, false-positive findings nevertheless exist, particularly when the patient population includes those at low risk for coronary artery disease. The accuracy of exercise ECG is therefore predictably low in asymptomatic subjects. In a study of more than 7,000 patients with minimal risk factors for coronary artery disease who underwent treadmill exercise testing and had ST-segment depression, the true-positive rate for the test was 21%. Approximately four of every five patients identified by such a program would have false-positive results and require further evaluation.[57] On the other hand, in a study of 269 patients with angiographically proven coronary artery disease and 141 normal subjects, the specificity of treadmill exercise testing was 93% and the sensitivity 64%, results indicating the usefulness of the test when the prevalence of coronary artery disease is high.[58] Patients with severe coronary artery disease and positive findings on treadmill exercise tolerance tests at a low workload have a poor prognosis, regardless of whether they do or do not have symptoms, and should be considered for revascularization.[52] Thus, ECG techniques are most reliable and helpful in the evaluation of high-risk populations or patients with known coronary artery disease.

Ambulatory ECG monitoring

Although ambulatory ECG monitoring has most often been used for the diagnosis and evaluation of arrhythmias, the technique has been known since Holter's first work to have the potential for detection of ST-segment shifts indicative of myocardial ischemia[53] (Fig 29A-7). Unfortunately, the technical aspects of accurate detection of ST-segment shifts are considerably different from those required for the accurate detection of arrhythmias. Consequently, an extensive literature describes the technologic development of such devices, the advantages and disadvantages of one type of device over another, and other factors.[59-61] An American College of Cardiology and American Heart Association task force report on guidelines for ambulatory electrocardiography[1] and a directory of suitable monitoring equipment[62] have been published.

Frequency modulation recorders have been the standard against which all other ambulatory monitors have been compared for the assessment of myocardial ischemia because of their extended low-frequency response and low incidence of phase shifts,[60] but newer amplitude modulation systems have been shown to be equally reliable.[59] The newest type of recording device has a very-high-density semiconductor memory into which digitized signals can be stored, and the recorder is smaller because of elimination of mechanical parts, including the magnetic tape recorder.[63] Although these solid-state devices have many advantages over traditional tape-based amplitude modulation and frequency modulation systems, including better signal-to-noise ratio, they have the disadvantage of interpretation that is based solely on the digitized, stored ECG waveforms, and in some models no recall of the original data is possible should the ordering physician doubt the accuracy of the interpretation.[64]

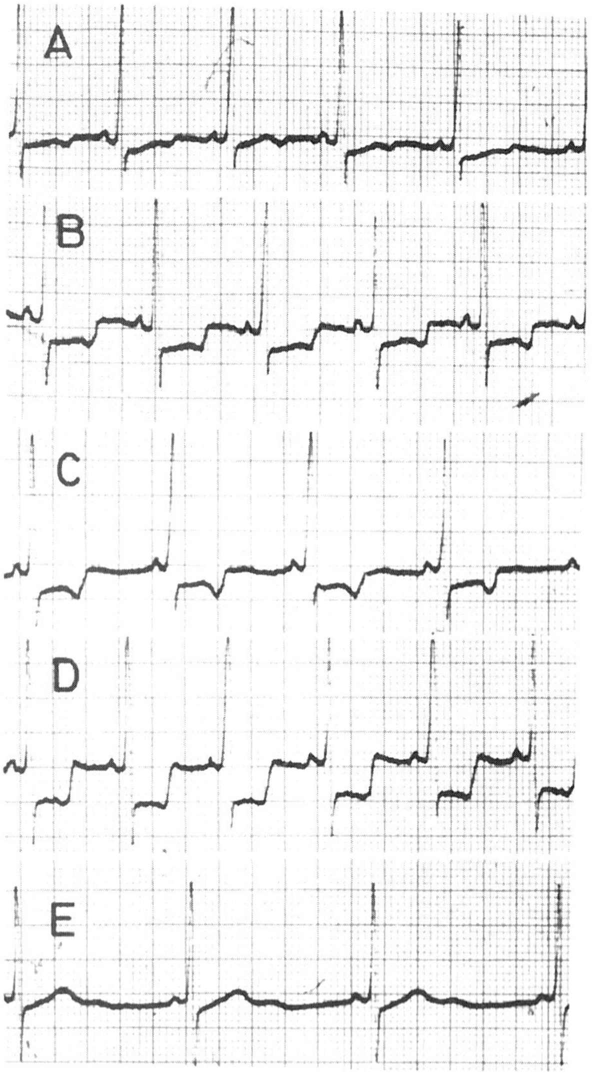

Fig 29A-7. Ambulatory electrocardiogram showing silent and symptomatic ischemia in a 56-year-old man. **A**, baseline. **B**, slight asymptomatic ST depression after meals. **C**, silent ischemia at rest; note more marked ST depression. **D**, patient walking with angina. **E**, during sleep. (From Stern S, Tzivoni D: The dynamic nature of the ST-T segment in ischemic heart disease. *Am Heart J* 91:820-822, 1976. By permission of Mosby-Year Book.)

Meticulous technique is required with ambulatory ECG monitoring for the detection of myocardial ischemia. In addition to selection of proper equipment and suitable patients, the technician must properly prepare the skin to minimize skin-electrode impedance, properly apply the electrodes, and then test the patient for ST-segment changes during hyperventilation or with changes of position. Patients who have ST-segment deviation during postural changes are not thought to be suitable candidates

Table 29A-2 Advantages and disadvantages of ambulatory electrocardiographic monitoring

Advantages:
Is the only practical method
May allow detection of triggers of ischemia
Is relatively inexpensive
May allow assessment of anti-ischemic therapy
Disadvantages:
Is subject to the day-to-day variability of ischemia
Requires much equipment and highly trained personnel
Lacks established therapeutic end points

for ambulatory monitoring because of the significant risk of false-positive responses. The leads selected should be those most likely to show the greatest ST-segment depression with ischemia. Usually, II, V_1, and V_5 are chosen. If exercise testing has been performed, it can be used to help select the proper leads. The patient should be instructed to keep a detailed diary listing all activities and symptoms.[65]

Although nonspecific ST-segment changes, such as upsloping ST-segment depression or T-wave changes, are common in normal persons,[66] horizontal or downsloping ST-segment depression is exceedingly rare in normal individuals. Stern and Tzivoni[67] and Tzivoni et al.[68] found no flat or downsloping ST-segment depression in 33 ambulatory and 42 sleeping normal subjects in one study and in 78 of 80 normal volunteers in another study during ambulatory ECG monitoring. Thus, with accurate equipment in properly selected patients, the specificity of ST-segment shifts during ambulatory monitoring for myocardial ischemia is good. Hammill,[69] comparing ambulatory ECG monitoring with treadmill exercise testing in 143 patients at the Mayo Clinic, found the sensitivity of the Holter system to be 89%, the specificity 96%, and the positive predictive accuracy 91%.

The number and duration of ischemic events vary from one 24-hour period to another.[70] In one study, day-to-day variability of ST-segment depression was 36% for number of episodes and 51% for duration of ST-segment depression in individual patients.[71] Consequently, although a 24-hour period of monitoring has been recommended by most authors,[72] others have thought that ambulatory monitoring should be continued for at least 48 hours, especially when a response to therapy is being assessed. Detry et al.[73] developed an algorithm to calculate the integral of total ST-segment elevation or depression over time from ambulatory ECG data, an approach that may help day-to-day comparisons.

With these caveats, the advantages of ambulatory ECG monitoring (Table 29A-2) are that it is the only practical method for diagnosing silent ischemia in the ambulatory state, that in individual patients it may be helpful in identifying the triggers of ischemia, and that it is relatively inexpensive. In selected patients, ambulatory monitoring may be helpful in the evaluation of anti-ischemic drug therapies. This capability may be particularly important in the future if the continuing randomized studies of silent ischemia indicate conclusively that eradication of silent ischemia improves prognosis.

The disadvantages of ambulatory ECG monitoring are the day-to-day variability of ischemia, which may require prolonged periods of monitoring; the considerable equipment and the technical expertise required to properly obtain and process the data; and the lack of established guidelines for a therapeutic end point should silent ischemia be detected.

ECG monitoring in the intensive care unit and operating room

Continuous monitoring of a single-lead ECG in the hospital has long been a standard practice in patients admitted with suspected or proven acute myocardial infarction, arrhythmias, new-onset heart failure, unstable angina, pulmonary embolism, severe obstructive lung disease when bronchodilator therapy is to be initiated, drug overdoses, and a host of other clinical situations. Initially, this was done for the detection of cardiac arrhythmias, but in recent years it has been advocated for the detection of silent myocardial ischemia as well. There has been significant interest in the monitoring of high-risk surgical patients, because preoperative ischemia has been found to be common,[74,75] prognostically important,[76-81] and amenable to intervention.[82-84]

Recently, a portable, programmable, microprocessor-driven, real-time, 12-lead ECG monitoring device was developed and approved for clinical use. It appears to address some of the limitations of conventional telemetric ECG monitoring and has been shown to be helpful in detecting reperfusion by thrombolytic therapy or coronary angioplasty during acute myocardial infarction and coronary reocclusion after these procedures[85,86] (Fig 29A-8). The device has an automatic monitoring system, so that ischemic ECG changes beyond a preset level of severity or duration trigger an alarm. The device is now being tested for its sensitivity, specificity, and clinical usefulness in patients with unstable coronary syndromes and for intraoperative and postoperative monitoring.

Myocardial perfusion, metabolism, and wall motion studies

Beller[87] reviewed the use of myocardial perfusion imaging for detection of silent myocardial ischemia. Maseri et al.[88,89] first demonstrated transient regional reductions of myocardial perfusion in patients having chest pain at rest due to coronary artery spasm. Since then, thallium 201 has been used to detect silent myocardial ischemia during exercise or during drug-induced stress, such as that produced by infusion of vasodilators (dipyridamole or adenosine) or catecholamines.[90-96]

Deanfield et al.[20,21,97] pioneered the use of myocardial perfusion imaging using rubidium 82 and positron-emission tomography to detect silent myocardial ischemia

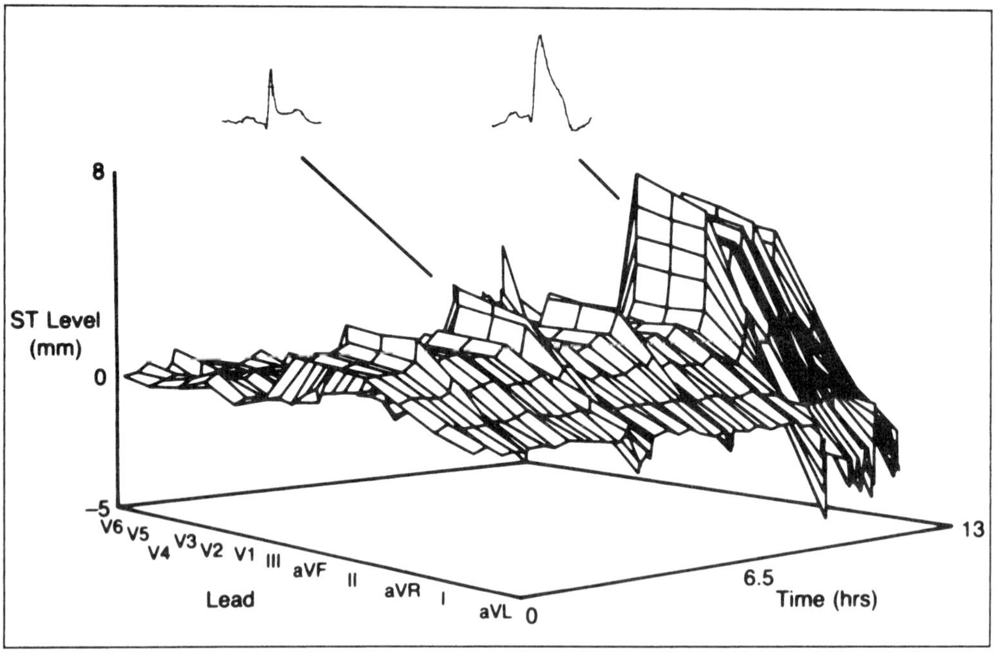

Fig 29A-8. Asymptomatic reocclusion of right coronary artery after thrombolytic therapy of acute inferior wall myocardial infarction detected by microprocessor-driven, real-time, 12-lead electrocardiographic monitor. (From Krucoff MW, Wagner NB, Pope JE, et al: The portable programmable microprocessor-driven real-time 12-lead electrocardiographic monitor: a preliminary report of a new device for the noninvasive detection of successful reperfusion or silent coronary reocclusion. *Am J Cardiol* 65:143-148, 1990. By permission of Excerpta Medica.)

in patients in the basal state, during exercise, during cold pressor stress, with mental stress, and during cigarette smoking (see Fig 29A-4). Furthermore, when positron-emission tomography was used to simultaneously assess perfusion and glucose metabolism, regions of ischemic myocardium could be differentiated from scar.[98] Magnetic resonance imaging also has the potential to be useful for the assessment of myocardial metabolism with patients at rest, because it can identify abnormalities of the high-energy phosphates.[99]

Left ventricular regional wall motion abnormalities are early manifestations of myocardial ischemia. Radionuclide ventriculography can be used to detect transient wall motion abnormalities with or without simultaneous ECG changes.[100-105] The examination can be done with the patient at rest, during exercise, during vasodilator stress or catecholamine infusions, or during atrial or ventricular pacing. An ambulatory nuclear monitoring device ("cardiac vest") may also prove to be useful.[106]

Echocardiography with exercise- or drug-induced stress[107,108] provides similar data but also allows simultaneous evaluation of the cardiac valves and detection of any thrombi, pericardial effusion, or septal defects. Assessment of global and regional function by echocardiography is extremely useful in patients who have congestive heart failure of unknown cause. Many such patients restudied after revascularization procedures have improved systolic function, a suggestion that the initial left ventricular dysfunction was the result of silent ischemia. Thus, there is much to be said for echocardiography in patients with coronary artery disease, and its use is increasing. Gated magnetic resonance imaging, if the images can be obtained more quickly and if the cost can be mitigated, may have a similar role in the future.[109]

Hemodynamic monitoring

Hemodynamic monitoring of patients with pulmonary artery flotation catheters in the intensive care unit has shown that transient episodes of myocardial ischemia, whether asymptomatic or associated with angina, correlate with simultaneous increases in pulmonary artery diastolic and pulmonary capillary wedge pressures[110-112] (Fig 29A-9). Similarly, Hirzel et al.[113] showed that silent ischemia during exercise was correlated not only with ECG changes, a decrease in the left ventricular ejection fraction, and new regional wall motion abnormalities but also with transient elevation of the left ventricular end-diastolic pressure. Therefore, in the intensive care unit, the operating room, and the catheterization laboratory, transient elevation of filling pressures on the left side of the heart can in the right circumstances indicate silent myocardial ischemia. However, changes in Swan-Ganz catheter pressures appear to be relatively insensitive for the detection of ischemia in comparison with intraoperative transesophageal echocardiographic wall motion anal-

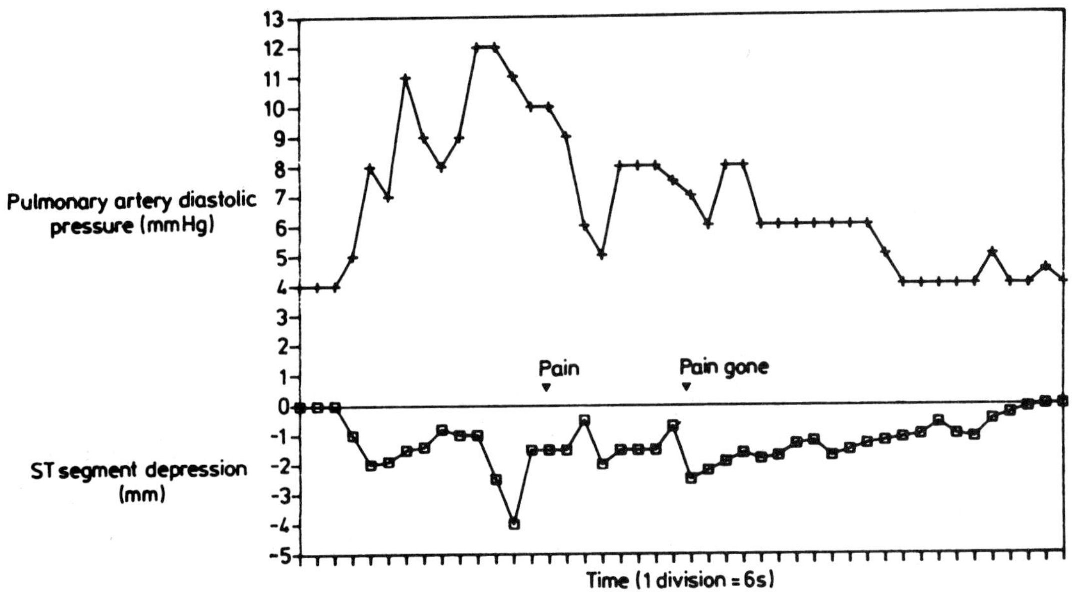

Fig 29A-9. Simultaneous measurement of changes in pulmonary artery diastolic pressure and ST-segment level from baseline values in an ambulatory patient with coronary artery disease. Note that the maximum increase in pulmonary artery diastolic pressure corresponded to the maximum degree of ST-segment depression and that the evidence of ischemia and left ventricular dysfunction preceded the onset of angina. (From Levy RD, Shapiro LM, Wright C, et al: The haemodynamic significance of asymptomatic ST segment depression assessed by ambulatory pulmonary artery pressure monitoring. *Br Heart J* 56:526-530, 1986. By permission of the journal.)

ysis. This finding suggests that changes in central pressures may detect only relatively severe ischemia.[114]

Summary

Stress testing, usually with treadmill exercise, remains the most widely used technique for the detection of silent myocardial ischemia. Exclusion of patients with resting ECGs in which the ST-segment tracings are not normal and interpretation of the results in the light of the pretest probability of coronary artery disease are vital to the accurate application of this technique. Assessment of myocardial perfusion by nuclear techniques and assessment of wall motion abnormalities by nuclear or echocardiographic techniques improve the sensitivity and specificity for the detection of myocardial ischemia and may allow detection of some episodes of ischemia in which no ECG changes occur. Ambulatory ECG monitoring may yield information on triggers of ischemia and the presence of ischemia in patients unable to exercise, in those with a mixed anginal pattern, in those thought to have Prinzmetal's variant angina, and preoperatively in high-risk patients. Careful patient selection and attention to technical factors are critical. Hemodynamic monitoring with pulmonary artery catheters and intraoperative transesophageal echocardiography may allow detection of transient myocardial ischemia in some circumstances.

PREVALENCE AND PROGNOSIS

Asymptomatic subjects

Estimates of the incidence and prevalence of silent myocardial ischemia in asymptomatic individuals are questionable but may be derived from ambulatory ECG monitoring, exercise ECG, and exercise perfusion imaging. As discussed in detail above and in other chapters, the sensitivity and specificity of all ECG methods for detection of ischemia vary with the prevalence of disease in the population being studied. In a review of studies of ambulatory ECG monitoring in asymptomatic subjects, the frequency of ST-segment shifts of 1 mm or more lasting 30 seconds varied from one study to another by 0 to 30%. Spontaneous ST elevation and T-wave inversion were also relatively frequent in asymptomatic individuals and often were related to postural change or hyperventilation.[115] Ambulatory ST-segment monitoring was performed in 394 Swedish men aged 60 or older who had no definite history of coronary heart disease. Of these subjects, 23% had ST-segment depression on ambulatory monitoring. Because this estimate incorporates false-positive ECG evidence of ischemia and true silent ischemia, it is probably an overestimation of true prevalence. Because of their age and sex, however, a significant number of these persons probably had true silent ischemia.[116]

Subjects with painless ST-segment depression on the

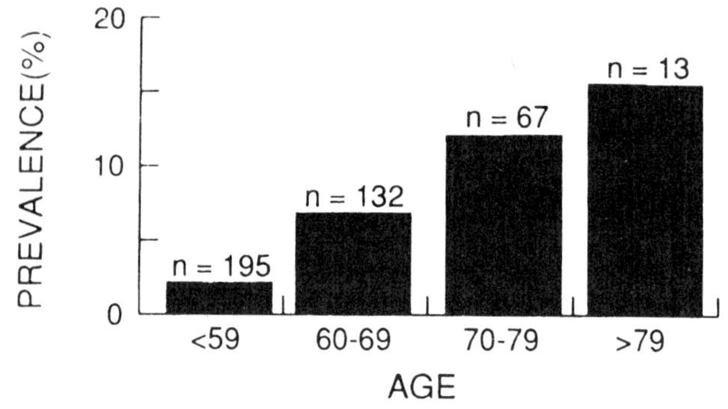

Fig 29A-10. Prevalence of exercise electrocardiographic and thallium scintigraphic positivity in asymptomatic persons as a function of age. (From Fleg JL, Gerstenblith G, Zonderman AB, et al: Prevalence and prognostic significance of exercise-induced silent myocardial ischemia detected by thallium scintigraphy and electrocardiography in asymptomatic volunteers. *Circulation* 81:428-436, 1990. By permission of American Heart Association.)

treadmill also include those with true ischemia and false-positive ST-segment depression. Rozanski and Berman[31,117] reviewed exercise ECG evidence of ischemia in asymptomatic individuals. Ischemic ECG changes occurred in approximately 13%. However, slightly more than one-fourth of a similar group of individuals, all of whom had cardiac catheterization, had normal coronary arteries.

Because it required both thallium perfusion defects and ECG evidence of ischemia, the study of Fleg et al.[118] from the Baltimore Longitudinal Study on Aging probably gives the best available conservative estimate (6%) for the prevalence of silent myocardial ischemia in asymptomatic individuals (Fig 29A-10). Moreover, the prevalence of 2% to 6% is similar to estimates of significant coronary disease in asymptomatic individuals subjected to coronary angiography.[119] However, approximately one-third of patients with angina and angiographically documented coronary disease have negative exercise ECGs, perhaps because of disease in posterior vessels remote from chest or inferior ECG leads. Thus, the requirement of ECG and thallium scintigraphic positivity in the study of Fleg et al.[118] probably resulted in an underestimation of the prevalence of ischemia. For example, a thallium perfusion abnormality was identified in 14% of patients. On the other hand, men outnumbered women by 2.8 to 1 in the study and the prevalence (both thallium and ECG results positive) was 6.2% in men and 2.2% in women overall. This factor suggests an overestimation of prevalence in comparison with that in an evenly distributed population of men and women.

Silent ischemia increased the risk of death, myocardial infarction, or development of angina by 3.6 times in the Fleg et al. study. A fourfold increased risk of cardiac events was noted in the Swedish study of ambulatory ST-segment monitoring in men older than 60.[116] Of 50 asymptomatic Norwegian men who had painless ECG positivity and subsequent positive angiographic findings, cardiac events increased fourfold to fivefold.[120]

As a group, asymptomatic subjects with treadmill exercise positivity have a threefold to fivefold greater risk of cardiac events than do those without exercise-induced ST-segment depression.[121-123] McHenry et al.[124] used serial exercise ECGs for follow-up in 916 asymptomatic men during a 13-year period. One-third of these patients with positive exercise ECG results had a cardiac event during this interval. However, 32 of 36 subjects who died or had a myocardial infarction had never had a positive exercise ECG result during initial or follow-up studies.

Data on the evaluation of asymptomatic persons support the following conclusions:[66,121,124-126]

1. If significant cardiac risk factors or symptoms are absent, most positive exercise ECG results or instances of ambulatory ST-segment depression falsely suggest ischemia.
2. True ischemia identified in asymptomatic persons has an important negative effect on prognosis.
3. Most adverse events in large asymptomatic populations during follow-up occur in patients with negative screening test results.
4. Because most asymptomatic patients have an excellent prognosis, any program designed to exhaustively discern true-positive from false-positive study results is unlikely to prolong life more by early revascularization than by symptom-directed follow-up.

Chronic stable angina pectoris

Among patients with angiographically proven significant coronary artery disease and a history of angina, data from the Duke data bank and the Coronary Artery Surgery Study (CASS) registry suggest that ST-segment depression develops in approximately 50% of patients during treadmill exercise, one-third of whom do not have angina.[127] This finding is in contrast to an approximate silent-to-symptomatic ratio of 2:1 when evaluation is by ambulatory ECG, a suggestion that symptoms are more likely to occur on the treadmill than during ordinary activity.[128]

Most studies of ambulatory ST-segment depression in patients with chronic stable angina are biased by requirements that exercise ECG positivity (usually prior to Bruce stage III) be present before ambulatory monitoring. Among such patients, ST-segment depression during ambulation is present 40% to 50% of the time. Three-fourths of episodes occur without anginal pain.[129] Four groups of investigators studied ambulatory ischemia and ischemia induced by treadmill exercise in patients with chronic stable angina documented by coronary angiography *without* the prestudy requirement of exercise ECG positivity. Mulcahy et al.[130] found that exercise ECG results were positive in 67% of patients. Of all episodes of ambulatory ST-segment depression in this angiographically defined group, 92% occurred in those who also had positive findings on exercise ECG. The only patient who had a negative result with exercise testing had documented coronary artery spasm. Ambulatory ST-segment depression occurred in 33% of patients. In a separate group of 172 patients with stable angina by history (no angiographic or exercise ECG criteria), the prevalence of ambulatory ST-segment depression was 42%.[131] Kawanishi et al.[132] and Mody et al.[133] suggested prevalences of ambulatory silent ischemia of 19% and 33%, respectively, in patients with angiographically defined significant coronary artery disease. Aronow et al.[134] found ambulatory ST evidence of ischemia in 33% of elderly nondiabetic patients and 38% of elderly diabetic patients in whom significant coronary disease was defined as a history of or ECG evidence of previous myocardial infarction or a history of typical angina. These and other data suggest that of patients with chronic stable angina, from one-fifth to one-third have ambulatory ST-segment depression, one-half to two-thirds have exercise ECG ST depression, and 90% have positive exercise thallium scans[135] (Figs 29A-11 and 29A-12).

Quyyumi et al.[136] performed gated exercise radionuclide angiography and ambulatory monitoring in 155 patients with angiographically documented coronary artery disease. Among patients with ambulatory ST-segment depression, 94% had radionuclide angiographic evidence of exercise-induced ischemia. However, among those with a positive radionuclide response, only 55% had ambulatory ST-segment depression. Most disturbing was the absence of ambulatory ST-segment depression in patients with radionuclide ischemia who had preexisting left ventricular dysfunction. This finding suggests that sensitivity is low in the highest risk subgroup of patients with coronary artery disease.

Both Weiner et al.[128] from a study of 2,982 CASS registry patients and Mark et al.[127] from a study of 1,698 Duke patients demonstrated that asymptomatic treadmill-induced ST-segment depression in patients with documented coronary artery disease was a significant adverse prognostic factor. The CASS investigators found that angina did not convey additional prognostic information. In contrast, the Duke investigators found that a history of exercise-limiting angina provided unique prognostic information in addition to the ST-segment deviation.

In patients who have angina and documented exercise ECG evidence of ischemia, occurrence of silent ischemia during ambulatory monitoring is associated with an increased risk of death or nonfatal infarction (Fig 29A-13). In general, a twofold to fourfold increase in risk has been observed. In the study by Rocco et al.[137] of 86 patients with stable angina and positive exercise ECGs, ambulatory ECG monitoring was performed after administration of antianginal medication was stopped. Fifty-seven percent of these patients had evidence of silent ischemia, and most adverse events occurred in the group with ambulatory ischemia. Of 107 patients who continued to take antianginal medication in a study by Deedwania and Carbajal,[138] 44% had silent ischemia, which was associated with an increased risk of death. Aronow et al.[134] and Tzivoni et al.[139] noted similar results. In contrast, Mulcahy et al.[140] found that during 2 years of follow-up in 172 patients with stable angina, only two of the nine cardiac deaths or nonfatal infarctions occurred in the 72 patients with an ambulatory episode of ST-segment depression.

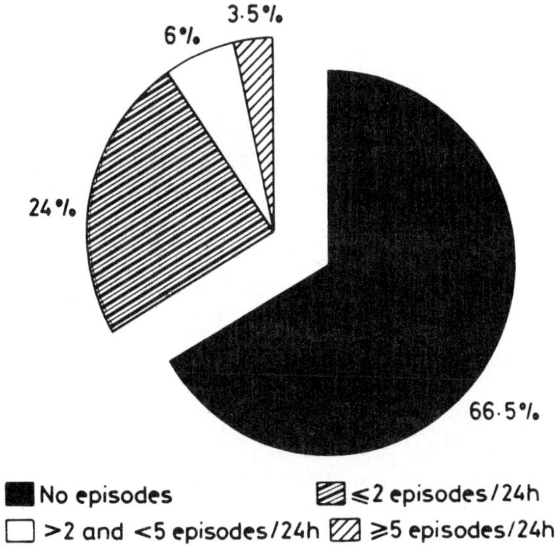

Fig 29A-11. Frequency of silent ischemia detected by ambulatory ST-segment monitoring in 114 patients with angina and angiographically proven coronary artery disease but without the requirement of positive treadmill exercise tests. (From Mulcahy D, Keegan J, Lindsay D, et al: Silent myocardial ischaemia in patients referred for coronary bypass surgery because of angina: a comparison with patients whose symptoms were well controlled on medical treatment. *Br Heart J* 61:496-501, 1989. By permission of the journal.)

Comparing the prognostic value of treadmill exercise data and ambulatory ST-segment depression data is difficult. The studies of Rocco et al.[137] and Deedwania and Carbajal[138] suggested that superior prognostic information was provided by ambulatory ST-segment data above and beyond treadmill data. In both studies, however, patients who had ambulatory silent ischemia had evidence of treadmill-induced ischemia earlier than those without ambulatory silent ischemia. It is possible, therefore, that all data obtained during treadmill exercise ECG were underutilized. Mark et al.[141] have proposed a scoring system for increasing the prognostic yield of treadmill data. The scoring system uses treadmill exercise time on a Bruce protocol, the presence or absence of exercise-limiting angina, and maximal ST-segment depression during the test. This method incorporates multiple treadmill variables while still identifying adverse prognostic risk in patients without anginal pain (but with ST depression at a low workload) or without ST depression (but with angina at a low workload). Comparative studies of the prognostic value of this treadmill ECG scoring system and ambulatory ST-segment depression have not been done.

A significant limitation of treadmill exercise testing and ambulatory ST-segment monitoring is the absence of ECG changes, which can occur in one-third of patients with significant coronary artery disease and angina.[142] The inability to detect residual ischemia in patients with preexisting left ventricular dysfunction also limits the

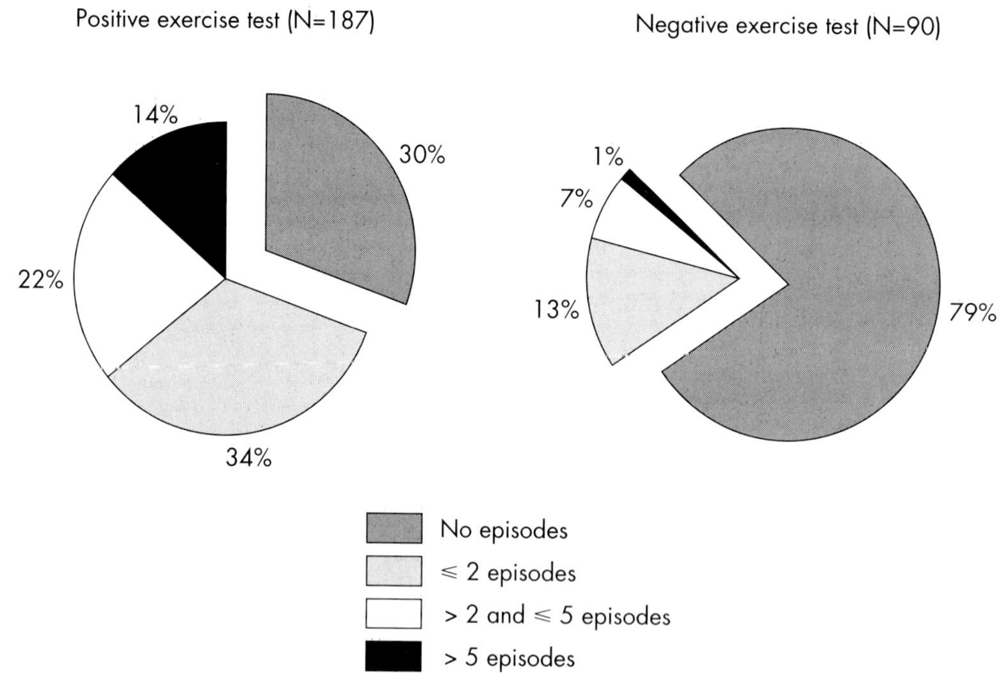

Fig 29A-12. Frequency of treadmill exercise positivity (187 of 277 patients, or 68%) and the relationship of ambulatory ST-segment depression to results of treadmill testing in 277 patients with angiographically documented coronary artery disease. The data indicate that a positive treadmill electrocardiogram identifies most patients who will have ambulatory ischemia. (From Mulcahy D, Keegan J, Sparrow J, et al: Ischemia in the ambulatory setting—the total ischemic burden: relation to exercise testing and investigative and therapeutic implications. *J Am Coll Cardiol* 14:1166-1172, 1989. By permission of American College of Cardiology.)

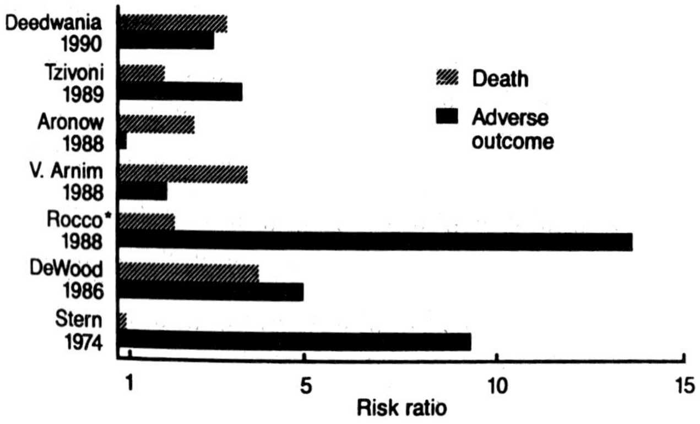

Fig 29A-13. Impact of ambulatory ST-segment evidence of ischemia on death or adverse outcomes in patients with stable angina or stable coronary disease. The range of follow-up is 6 to 36 months. (*Antianginal medications had been discontinued.) (From Pepine CJ: Is silent ischemia a treatable risk factor in patients with angina pectoris? *Circulation* 82 Suppl 2:135-142, 1990. By permission of American Heart Association.)

clinical utility of ambulatory monitoring.[136] The data suggest little justification for the use of ambulatory ST-segment monitoring in patients with negative exercise ECGs unless coronary artery spasm is suspected.[140]

Prinzmetal's variant angina

Nademanee et al.[143] studied the incidence of silent ST-segment shifts in patients with variant angina and documented angiographically normal coronary arteries. Eighty percent of episodes showed ST elevation, and up to 90% of episodes were painless. The number of episodes was threefold to fourfold greater per 24-hour period than in a comparison group of patients with chronic stable angina. The peak occurrence of episodes was in the hours between midnight and 6 a.m. Araki et al.[144] documented that 79% of episodes of ST-segment elevation were asymptomatic in 26 patients with variant angina. The same diurnal variation occurred. In this group of patients, criteria for a diagnosis of variant angina included ST-segment elevation on a 12-lead ECG during pain. All patients had at least one episode. However, occurrence varied from 1 to 68 episodes a day, with most patients having 1 to 5 episodes. Ventricular tachycardia occurred in only three patients. Morikami and Yasue[145] studied 14 patients with recurrent spontaneous angina associated with ST-segment elevation and angiographically docu-

Table 29A-3 Ischemia detected by ambulatory monitoring and risk of future events in patients with unstable angina

Source	No. of patients	Follow-up, mo	Patients with detectable ischemia, %	Risk ratio	
				Adverse outcome*	Death
Langer et al.[152]	135	In-hospital	66	2.5	3.7
Pozzati et al.[153]	88	12	55	2.1	2.7
Arnim et al.[154]	38	1	42	2.0	3.4
Nademanee et al.[155]	49	6	59	13.8	3.4
Gottlieb et al.[156]	70	24	53	3.2	9.0
Johnson et al.[157]	72	3	17	3.4	2.7
Total, ranges	452	In-hospital to 24	17-66	2.0-13.8	2.7-9.0

*Includes death and nonfatal myocardial infarction.
From Pepine CJ: Is silent ischemia a treatable risk factor in patients with angina pectoris? *Circulation* 82 Suppl 2:135-142, 1990. By permission of American Heart Association.

mented coronary spasm. As in the other studies, the peak occurrence of episodes was between midnight and 9 a.m. Significant suppression of the number and duration of attacks was associated with nifedipine therapy.

Between 10% and 30% of patients with Prinzmetal's angina have angina and ST elevation during exercise testing. Exercise ST elevation is more prevalent in patients with Prinzmetal's angina who have a high daily frequency of painful attacks and is associated with fixed coronary lesions and superimposed spasm.[146,147] The prevalence of symptomless ST deviation with exercise or during ambulatory monitoring in this subgroup of patients is not known.

Although a number of studies discuss prognosis in patients with variant angina, no data thus far have specifically evaluated the contribution of the results of ambulatory monitoring to prognosis. The recurring important prognostic variables are the extent of fixed coronary obstructive disease and indices of recent disease activity. For example, patients with evidence of spasm only with ergonovine provocation have an excellent prognosis, whereas those with multiple daily spontaneous attacks who are hospitalized have an incidence of infarction of approximately 25% within 3 months.[148-151] Because of the nine to one preponderance of silent over symptomatic episodes in patients with Prinzmetal's angina, it seems likely that ambulatory ST-segment data will provide prognostic information related to the activity of the disease.

Unstable angina

Pepine[129] reviewed the prevalence and prognostic significance of ambulatory ST-segment shifts in unstable angina (Table 29A-3). ST-segment deviation occurs in from 40% to 70% of these patients during in-hospital Holter monitoring. Important differences in entry criteria, time of initiation of monitoring, and exclusion criteria hampered comparison of individual studies. Langer et al.[152] reported the results of two-lead 24-hour ECG monitoring in 135 patients in whom the qualifying event was destabilization of anginal pain without enzyme evidence of infarction. No entry 12-lead ECG criteria were used, and monitoring was begun 6.5 hours after the qualifying episodes of pain. This study documented ST-segment shifts earlier in an unstable angina episode than did any other study. Two-thirds of the patients had significant ST-segment deviation lasting at least 60 seconds, and one-fifth had transient ST elevation. Sixty-eight percent of the patients had ECG changes without any symptoms, and 6% had ECG changes exclusively with anginal pain. Overall, 92% of the episodes of ST-segment deviation in this study occurred without symptoms.

Gottlieb et al.[38] required significant 12-lead ECG ST-segment depression as an entry criterion and monitored ST-segment shifts during the first 2 days of medical stabilization for unstable angina. Time from the last qualifying episode of chest pain or 12-lead ECG with ischemia was not published. Fifty-three percent of patients had ST-segment shifts during monitoring, and more than 90% of episodes occurred without symptoms.

Nyman et al.[158] studied 740 patients with predismissal exercise ECG after an episode of unstable angina or non-Q-wave myocardial infarction. Approximately 30% of the patients had neither angina nor ST-segment shifts during exercise testing, and an additional 30% had both. Approximately 20% had painless ST-segment depression on the treadmill, and an additional 20% had angina without ECG changes.

In patients with unstable angina, silent ischemia or total ischemia time, especially when it exceeds 60 minutes during a 24-hour period, has been associated with a fivefold increased risk of in-hospital death[152] and a twofold to ninefold increased risk of death within 2 to 6 years.[38,155,159] In addition, silent ischemia correlates with angiographically defined left main and multivessel coronary disease. When angiographic results were excluded from a multiple regression model, the duration of ST-segment deviation on Holter monitoring was the best predictor of unfavorable outcome.[152] Pepine[129] tabulated prognostic data on silent ischemia in unstable angina from multiple studies.

In summary, silent ischemia predominates over symptomatic ischemia by approximately nine to one in patients with unstable angina, in contrast to a three-to-one ratio in those with stable angina. Its presence identifies a subset of patients in both classes of angina at greater risk for death and nonfatal infarction. These data support the potential use of Holter ST-segment monitoring in these patients to more precisely define the severity of ischemia and identify patients at high risk.

Prior myocardial infarction

After myocardial infarction, residual ischemia, the extent of myocardial damage, the degree of left ventricular dilatation, and the presence of ventricular arrhythmias are major prognostic factors (see chapter 30). Ischemia detection is uncertain because of baseline ST-segment abnormalities and alteration in anginal pain perception. A large body of data has accumulated from exercise ECG, ambulatory ST-segment monitoring, and exercise perfusion studies.

In studies of predismissal exercise ECG after infarction, 18% to 45% of patients had exercise-induced ST-segment depression, with one-third to two-thirds of episodes not accompanied by anginal pain[41,43] (Table 29A-4). Transient ST elevation during predismissal exercise testing strongly predicts residual peri-infarction ischemia, as assessed by thallium imaging. T-wave pseudonormalization is less helpful (50% predictive).[167]

Petretta et al.[168] studied ambulatory monitoring in a large group of consecutive patients with myocardial infarction. Of 441 patients, 392 survived; 122 were excluded because of advanced age, early angina during hospitalization, and resting ST-segment abnormalities or ventricular arrhythmias. Of the remaining 270 patients, including some with resting ST-segment depression, 24% had spontaneous episodes of an additional 0.1 mV (1 mm) of ST-segment change lasting 60 seconds or longer. Monitoring was performed an average of 13 days after admission for infarction. In the studies of Gottlieb et al.,[169] Tzivoni et al.,[170] and Ouyang et al.,[171] the prevalence varied between 29% and 46%. Restrictive selection criteria were used in these studies. Thus, the consecutive series of patients in the Petretta et al. study is probably more representative of postinfarction patients in general. In all four studies cited in this paragraph, ambulatory ST depression after infarction suggested an increased risk of cardiac death or reinfarction of 2.5-fold to fourfold.

Bolognese et al.[108] used dipyridamole echocardiography in the evaluation of 217 consecutive patients recovering from a first myocardial infarction. During dipyridamole echocardiography, more than half the patients had new wall motion abnormalities suggestive of residual ischemia. Three-fourths of the patients had no symptoms during dipyridamole-induced ischemia. There was no difference in the outcome, angiographic severity, or extent of wall motion abnormalities between those with and those without symptoms.

Most, but not all, studies support the notion that ST-segment depression induced by treadmill exercise after myocardial infarction portends an adverse prognosis, as do limited exercise capacity, exercise-induced ventricular arrhythmia, and abnormal blood pressure response to exercise. The independent importance of angina varies significantly from study to study. No increase or up to an eightfold increase in mortality during the first postinfarction year has been predicted.[160,161,172,173] Recent infarction (less than 2 weeks) and treadmill-associated ST-segment depression suggested a poor prognosis in the large exercise ECG series of Callaham et al.[142]

After infarction, exercise perfusion or radionuclide wall motion studies or echocardiography may be more useful than ECG methods to overcome the problems of baseline ECG abnormalities and altered pain perception and to provide data on left ventricular function. These studies require the stress of exercise or pharmacologic intervention, as described in detail in other chapters. Nonetheless, a substantial percentage of patients with previous myocardial infarction have transient exercise- or dipyridamole-induced scintigraphic abnormalities.[92] Thallium scintigraphy provides extremely powerful prognostic information in this group of patients.[174]

In summary, in patients with negative results of exercise tests after myocardial infarction, ambulatory ECG probably does not provide additional information. In those with positive exercise ECG results, additional adverse prognostic information is suggested by spontaneous ST-segment depression on ambulatory monitoring. Scintigraphic data with exercise or wall motion studies may provide even greater accuracy for the detection of residual ischemia and important prognostic information about left ventricular function or perfusion defects in multiple vascular territories. These factors are extremely important because many patients with significant left ventricular

Table 29A-4 Prevalence of exercise-induced myocardial ischemia in patients recovering from acute myocardial infarction

Source	No. of patients	≥1 mm ST, %	Angina, %
Krone et al.[160]	667	25	17
Waters et al.[161]	225	31	. . .
Jespersen et al.[162]	126	37	9
Théroux et al.[163]	210	34	20
Starling et al.[164]	130	32	27
Davidson and DeBusk[165]	195	22	15
Markiewicz et al.[166]	46	45	. . .

From Deedwania PC: Transient myocardial ischemia in survivors of acute myocardial infarction. In *Silent Myocardial Ischemia and Angina: Prevalence, Prognostic, and Therapeutic Significance.* Edited by BN Singh. New York, Pergamon Press, 1988, pp 157-173. By permission of McGraw-Hill.

dysfunction and significant ischemia may be completely free of angina. Patients with preexisting left ventricular dysfunction and inducible ischemia have the greatest benefit from surgical therapy.[175,176] In determining whether to recommend surgery for a given patient, it is thus extremely important to attempt to differentiate the extent of infarction from residual ischemia, as schematized by Rahimtoola[177] (Fig 29A-14).

After bypass surgery or angioplasty

Droste et al.[178] and Mulcahy et al.[179] studied patients before and after coronary bypass grafting with ambulatory ST-segment monitoring and found a preoperative prevalence of ST depression between 28% and 55%, depending on whether medications were continued or withdrawn. Three weeks after surgery, the interpretation of ST segments was restricted by baseline abnormalities. At 6 months after surgery, 22% to 29% of patients continued to have episodes of ambulatory silent ST depression, a frequency similar to that documented by Kennedy et al.[180] 12 months postoperatively. Similar data for treadmill exercise ECG positivity 6 months postoperatively were reported by Dubach et al.[181] and Weiner et al.[182] Although this high prevalence of ECG-designated ischemia may suggest incomplete revascularization or early graft failure, previous studies have shown a poor correlation of exercise ST-segment changes with graft patency. The addition of perfusion imaging may improve accuracy. Huikuri et al.[183] studied consecutive patients 3 months after coronary artery bypass grafting with exercise thallium scintigraphy and cardiac catheterization. Twenty-two patients had no symptoms occurring spontaneously or induced by bicycle ergometry. In the totally asymptomatic group, thallium scintigraphy accurately predicted graft patency in 17 of 22 patients. Exercise ECG with thallium predicted the graft status of all but 1 of 22 patients. A higher cumulative cardiac event rate in patients with than in those without ambulatory ST-segment depression after coronary artery bypass grafting has been reported.[184]

A reproducible pattern of ischemic change in 12-lead ECG occurs during balloon angioplasty occlusion of a coronary artery in approximately 90% of patients. Abrupt reocclusion occurs in about 8% of patients within the first 24 hours after coronary angioplasty, whereas many other patients have chest pain after angioplasty but do not have coronary reocclusion.[185,186] In patients with chest pain due to coronary reocclusion in the first 24 hours after angioplasty, a similar pattern of ischemic change was observed. Patients with chest pain but without angiographic evidence of reocclusion did not show similar ECG changes. If additional larger studies confirm these findings, continuous 12-lead ECG monitoring with an alarm system has the potential to replace early repeat coronary angiography after angioplasty in patients who have chest pain after the procedure and to detect silent reocclusion. The utility of this approach in patients with single-vessel disease appears relatively straightforward. Whether it will be reliable in patients with multivessel disease and incomplete revascularization is problematic.[187]

The application of ambulatory or exercise ST-segment analysis after hospital dismissal for percutaneous transluminal coronary angioplasty may be questionable. Mulcahy et al.[179] documented ambulatory ST-segment depression in only 13 of 40 patients before and 6 of 40 patients after angioplasty. Of the 40 patients, 20 had exercise ECG positivity before angioplasty and 13 after. Studies by Laarman et al.,[188] Kaul et al.,[187] and Deligonul et al.[189] also found evidence of painless ST-segment depression on the treadmill in approximately 20% of patients with recent angioplasty. The sensitivity of ECG data was only 24% when compared with that of

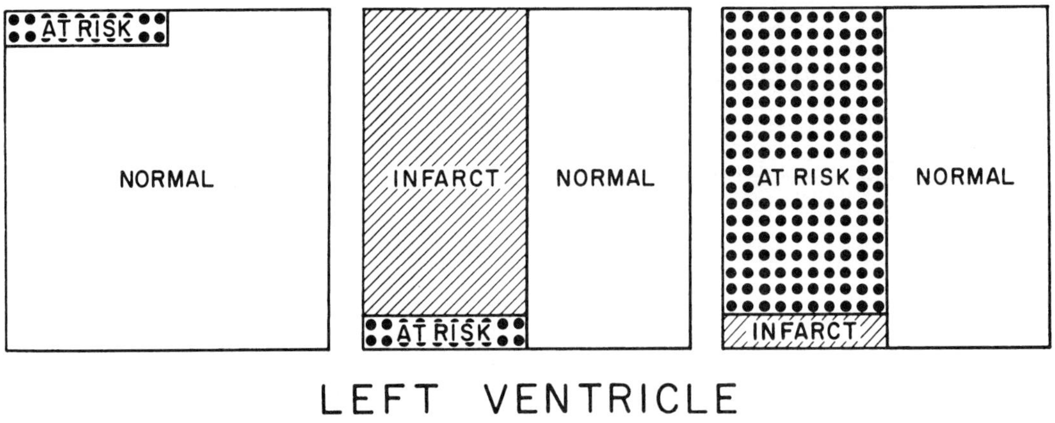

Fig 29A-14. Schematic representation of a spectrum of normal myocardium (**left panel**), largely infarcted myocardium (**middle panel**), and minimally infarcted myocardium with large residual risk area (**right panel**). Accurate identification of these areas is the goal of testing for ischemia after myocardial infarction. (From Rahimtoola SH: Clinical overview of management of chronic ischemic heart disease. *Circulation* 84 Suppl 1:81-84, 1991. By permission of American Heart Association.)

quantitative coronary angiography[188] and 40% when compared with that of thallium single-photon-emission computed tomography in asymptomatic subjects after angioplasty. In contrast, thallium single-photon-emission computed tomography was 90% sensitive and had a predictive accuracy of 89% in asymptomatic patients after angioplasty.[190]

For patients who have undergone previous revascularization procedures in whom a question of recurrent ischemia is important, exercise and ambulatory ECG do not provide a high degree of accuracy, partly because of a low prevalence of positive findings before revascularization. Important information on exercise capacity and symptom threshold is obtainable from treadmill exercise independent of ST-segment behavior. If accurate detection and quantification of ischemia are important clinically, stress or pharmacologic wall motion or perfusion imaging studies are required.

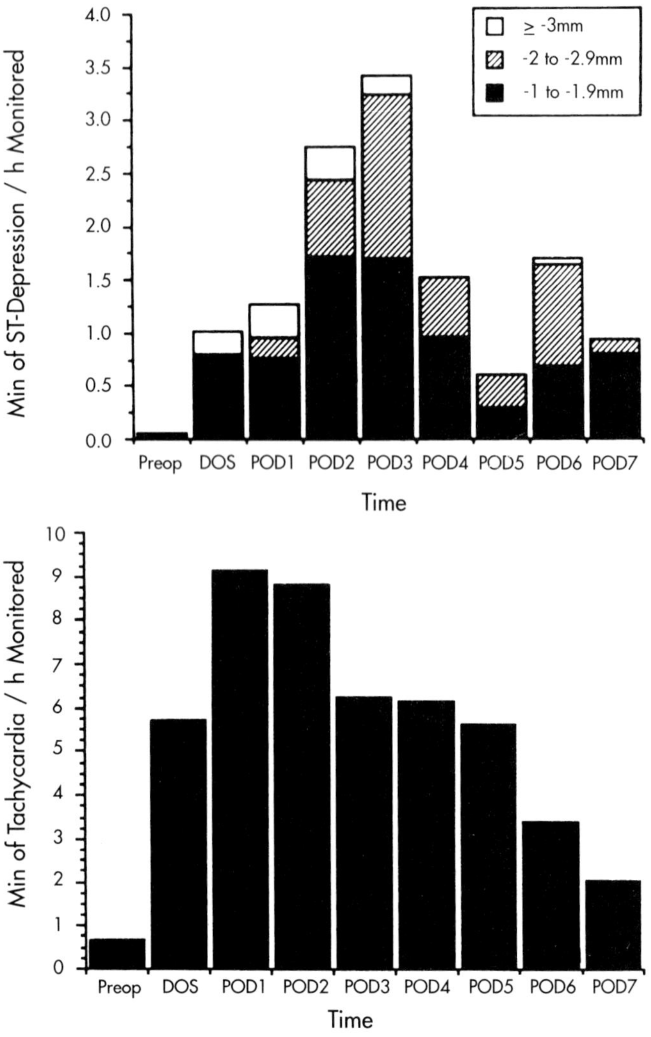

Fig 29A-15. Incidence and severity of perioperative ischemia and tachycardia. *DOS*, day of surgery; *POD*, postoperative day. (From Mangano DT, Wong MG, London MJ, et al: Perioperative myocardial ischemia in patients undergoing noncardiac surgery—II: Incidence and severity during the 1st week after surgery. *J Am Coll Cardiol* 17:851-857, 1991. By permission of American College of Cardiology.)

Noncardiac surgery

Preoperative screening for ischemia is extensively discussed in chapter 67. Continuous ST-segment monitoring, because of its unobtrusiveness, full-disclosure capability, and portability, has become an accepted research tool for the assessment of perioperative ischemia. Of 474 consecutive men with known coronary disease or significant risk factors for coronary artery disease studied by Mangano et al.,[81] 407 had acceptable continuous two-lead tracings. Forty-one percent of the patients had postoperative episodes of ST depression, and 20% to 25% had preoperative and intraoperative episodes. ST depression occurred without symptoms in 97% of patients. The optimal leads for detection of ischemia, in descending order of preference, were V_5, V_4, and II, and the sensitivity of all three leads combined was 96%.[191] Postoperative ischemia was significantly related to increased heart rate[192] (Fig 29A-15). Raby et al.[77] documented that preoperative ST-segment depression detected by continuous ECG monitoring of an inferior ECG lead and a lateral one occurred in 18% of patients undergoing peripheral vascular surgery. Both Mangano et al. and Raby et al. used ST-segment monitoring without concurrent nuclear, echocardiographic, or catheterization studies to verify that coronary disease was present. However, approximately half the patients in the Mangano et al. series had coronary disease documented by history or had significant risk factors, including the need for peripheral vascular surgery. Thus, ST-segment depression in this very-high-risk group probably represented ischemia most of the time. There were undoubtedly some false-positive results due to left ventricular hypertrophy not manifest on the ECG.

In the series of Mangano et al.,[81] perioperative ST-segment depression increased the risk of cardiac death, myocardial infarction, or unstable angina by a factor of nine. A substantially increased risk was also detected by Raby et al.[77,80] in patients undergoing peripheral vascular operations. Importantly, freedom from adverse events was predicted by the absence of preoperative ischemia in the Raby et al. study. Perioperative ST depression predicted increased risk of cardiac events in the first 2 postoperative years in both studies.

These important early results should pave the way for the more widespread use of this relatively inexpensive monitoring technology in the perioperative assessment of patients at moderate or high risk. Moreover, Mangano et al.[83] recently reported the efficacy of intensive analgesia in reducing the magnitude, duration, and severity of ischemia in patients undergoing coronary artery bypass surgery. Similar investigations should continue to demonstrate the therapeutic efficacy of anti-ischemic and adjunctive perioperative therapies.[84]

Sudden death

Data from animal studies and clinical experience with acute myocardial infarction and coronary artery spasm support an association of myocardial ischemia with life-threatening ventricular arrhythmias.[193] Furthermore, Sharma et al.[194] documented exercise-induced silent ischemia in survivors of sudden cardiac arrest. However, Gomes et al.,[195] in a study of survivors of out-of-hospital cardiac arrest with both electrophysiologic testing and ambulatory ST-segment monitoring, suggested that electrophysiologic inducibility of ventricular arrhythmia was of greater importance than ambulatory ischemia in the genesis of survivable cardiac arrest. Hausmann et al.[196] studied the relationship of spontaneous ST-segment shifts and ventricular arrhythmia in 97 patients who had documented coronary artery disease. Arrhythmia was rarely associated with ischemia. Because criteria for entry into these studies included surviving cardiac arrest in the first place, the results may not be representative of sudden death overall.

Perhaps the most pertinent study is that of Pepine et al.,[197] who retrospectively analyzed data on 35 patients who died during ambulatory ST-segment monitoring (Fig 29A-16). One-third of the tracings were uninterpretable for ischemia because of technical abnormalities or resting ST-segment changes. Of the patients with interpretable tracings, one-half had evidence of ischemia or infarction preceding death, and most of these patients had multiple episodes. The terminal events were either bradycardia-asystole or ventricular tachycardia-fibrillation. Data on symptoms were not available. This study supports a significant contribution of ischemia to sudden cardiac death.

THERAPEUTIC ISSUES

The use of medical antianginal therapy, the selection of patients for revascularization in stable and unstable angina, and the pharmacology of specific agents and combinations of agents are delineated in other chapters of this text. This section focuses on the therapeutic implications of ambulatory ST-segment monitoring in patients with known coronary artery disease.

When silent ischemia is identified by ambulatory ST-segment monitoring in patients with chronic stable angina, β-adrenergic blockers, calcium entry blockers, and nitrates all reduce the frequency of ischemia.[198] However, three studies have suggested that control of anginal symptoms with medical therapy does not result in total control of ischemic episodes.

Cohn et al.[199] reported the results of the multicenter Nifedipine-Total Ischemia Awareness Program study of patients with mild to moderate angina. In this study, a positive exercise ECG was an entry criterion for the great majority of patients, explaining the higher than expected prevalence (44%) of silent ischemic episodes in patients undergoing medical therapy with nitrates and β-blockers at study entry. In addition, monitoring was continued for 48 hours and resulted in a high relative rate of detection. Forty percent of this group had residual angina, and approximately one-fourth of the patients with a history of angina had residual ischemia that was totally silent during medical therapy. Deedwania and Carbajal[138] studied 118 consecutive patients with stable angina who were receiving medical therapy and whose symptoms were controlled. ECG criteria were not required for entry. Monitoring was done for 24 hours. Of the 107 patients who had analyzable ST segments on ambulatory monitoring during medical therapy, one-third had ST-segment depression and none had anginal symptoms. Mulcahy et al.[131] found that a similar fraction of patients had residual silent ischemia. These studies suggest that one-fourth to one-third of patients with angina have residual totally silent myocardial ischemia during medical treatment. Thus, reliance on control of symptoms leaves a large portion of patients with angina untreated for silent ischemic episodes.

Heart rate is important as a precipitant of silent ischemic episodes. In comparative therapeutic studies, atenolol was superior to nifedipine in reducing the frequency and duration of ischemic episodes.[32] Long-acting propranolol was compared with sustained-release diltiazem and nifedipine in patients with stable angina undergoing ambulatory ST-segment monitoring for 48 hours. Only propranolol significantly reduced the frequency and duration of ischemic events.[200] Similar data were obtained in a comparison of continuous-release metoprolol with sustained-action nifedipine.[201] These studies suggest that β-blockers are superior to calcium entry blockers for maximal suppression of ischemia and emphasize the importance of control of heart rate in the therapy of ischemia, both silent and symptomatic.

Whether to eliminate or only to diminish ischemia remains an extremely controversial issue. This is an important question because excessive therapy that has no effect on symptoms may produce unwanted side effects. Furthermore, excessive therapy may negatively affect prognosis, as shown in the Cardiac Arrhythmia Suppression Trial study of antiarrhythmic drug suppression of premature ventricular beats in patients with prior infarction.[202] Finally, total control of ischemia may require unwanted lifestyle restrictions that may not be necessary to optimize prognosis. In one study, patients with angiographically documented coronary disease who had painless exercise-induced radionuclide angiographic abnormalities benefited prognostically from medical therapy that eradicated the ischemic response.[136] This result can also be interpreted to suggest that patients have a poorer prognosis with medically refractory silent ischemia than with medically responsive silent ischemia.

It is clear that frequent episodes of silent ischemia suggest a poor prognosis and that medical treatment can reduce ischemia, but proof of the impact of therapeutic suppression of ischemic episodes cannot yet be assumed. Furthermore, optimal guided therapy for ischemia without symptoms is also undefined. Four trials addressing the effect of anti-ischemic therapy on ischemia frequency, cardiovascular events, and quality of life in patients with asymptomatic or minimally symptomatic ischemia are under way: the Atenolol Silent Ischemia Trial, the Canadian Amlodipine Silent Ischemia Study, the National

Heart, Lung, and Blood Institute's Asymptomatic Cardiac Ischemia Pilot, and the Total Ischemic Burden European Trial.[129,203-206]

CURRENT RECOMMENDATIONS, FUTURE DIRECTIONS

In 1989, a combined American College of Cardiology and American Heart Association subcommittee on ambulatory electrocardiography recommended ambulatory Holter monitoring only in patients thought to have Prinzmetal's variant angina.[1] The American College of Physicians, in 1990, suggested that ambulatory ST-segment monitoring be used only when coronary artery disease status is known.[2] A cautious interpretation of data obtained since then suggests that these indications may be reinterpreted and broadened somewhat. Because of problems with sensitivity and specificity, totally asymptomatic individuals who have ST-segment depression during ambulatory monitoring for assessment of arrhythmia pose a particular problem. Our current recommendations are to review the patient's history of cardiac risk factors, physical examination record, resting ECG, and chest radiograph and to follow those at low clinical risk

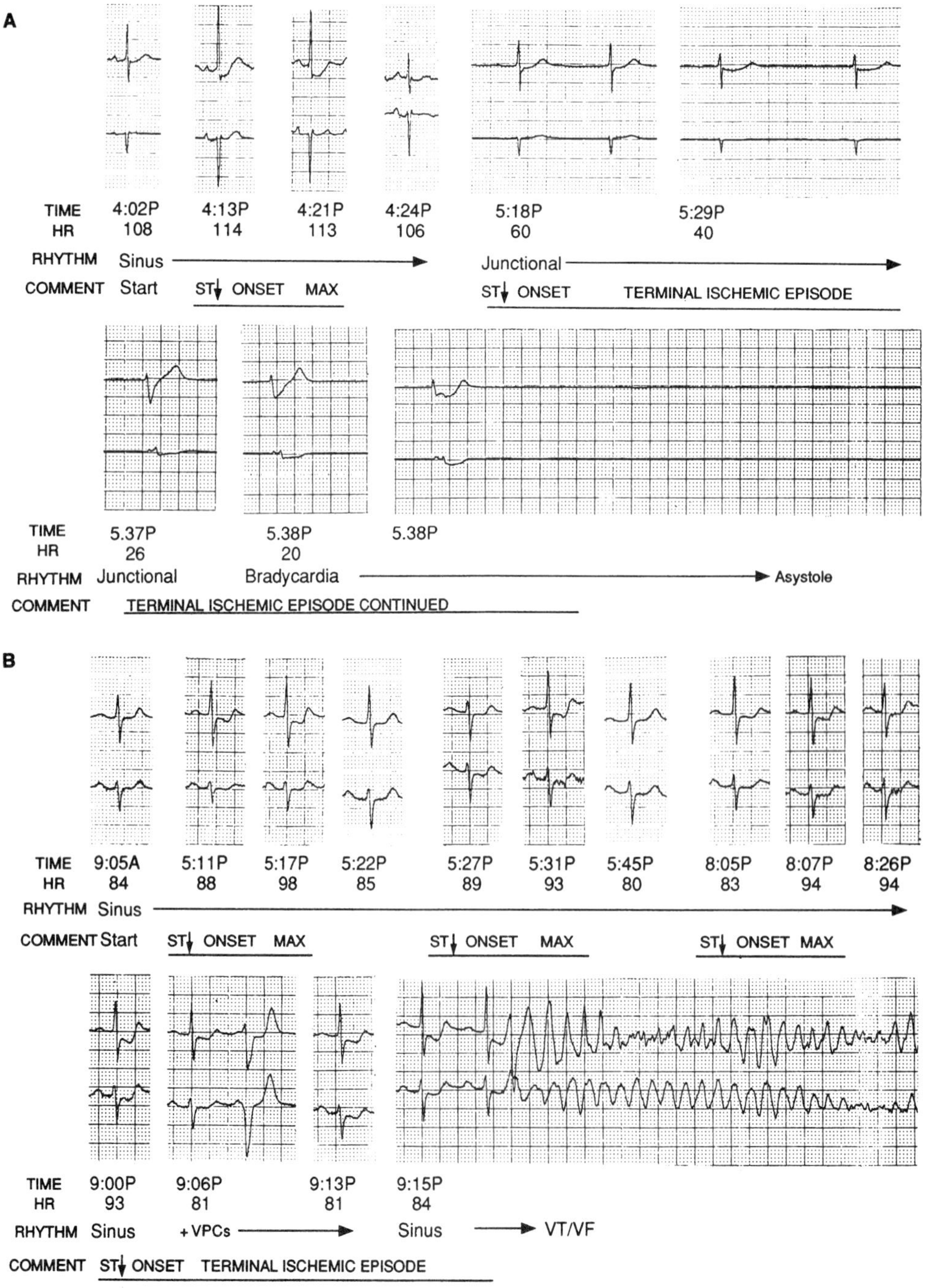

Table 29A-5 Suggested indications for ambulatory ST-segment monitoring

Inability to exercise or inadequate exercise workload. Does ST-segment depression occur? (vs. pharmacologic stress testing)
Negative exercise electrocardiogram but symptoms compatible with coronary spasm (nocturnal angina) (vs. cardiac catheterization and ergonovine)
After acute infarction or unstable angina. Is active ischemia relieved? (vs. exercise testing)
Effects of medical therapy or assessment of prognosis in patients with chronic severe disease (48 hr) (vs. exercise testing)
Postoperative period after noncardiac surgery in high-risk patients

From Blackshear JL: Ambulatory monitoring of silent myocardial ischemia: What is its utility? *South Med J* 85:293-298, 1992. By permission of Southern Medical Association.

Table 29A-6 Ischemic responses associated with high risk

ETT criteria*
Failure to complete ≥6.5 METS or attain HR ≥ 120
≥2 mm ST ↓
Postexercise ST ↓ >6 min
ST ↓ in multiple leads
Flat or declining SBP response
Exercise-induced VT
^{201}Tl criteria
New defect at low workload
Increased lung uptake
Multiple defects
Enlargement of cardiac pool
ECHO/MUGA criteria
EF ≤ 40%
Exercise-induced EF ↓ >5%
Multiple new defects
AEM criteria
≥2 mm ST ↓
≥60 min/24 hr
>6 episodes/24 hr

AEM, ambulatory electrocardiographic monitoring; ECHO, echocardiogram; EF, ejection fraction; ETT, exercise tolerance test; HR, heart rate; METS, metabolic equivalents; MUGA, multiuniform gated acquisition (scan); SBP, systolic blood pressure; ST ↓, ST-segment depression; VT, ventricular tachycardia.
*A patient meeting ETT criteria for high-risk ischemia may be tested further with thallium 201 (^{201}Tl), echocardiography and multigated image acquisition, and ambulatory electrocardiography. High-risk markers on these tests indicate the necessity for coronary angiography.
From Pepine CJ, Kern MJ, Boden WE: Advisory group reports on silent myocardial ischemia, acute intervention after myocardial infarction, and postinfarction management. *Am J Cardiol* 69:41B-46B, 1992. By permission of Excerpta Medica.

Fig 29A-16. Two examples of fatal events recorded by ambulatory ST-segment monitoring. **A**, patient with ischemia-related bradycardia/asystole. The ambulatory electrocardiographic recorder was applied at 4 p.m. when the ST segment was isoelectric and the patient in sinus rhythm. Approximately 11 minutes later, an ischemic episode was detected as 1.0 mm of ST-segment depression in lead V_5 (*top tracing*) and reached a maximum (*MAX*) of 2.5 mm after 8 minutes. This episode slowly subsided, but at 5:18 p.m. a junctional rhythm developed in association with 1.0 mm ST-segment depression. Eleven minutes later, the junctional rhythm slowed to 40 beats/min as ST-segment depression increased and R-wave amplitude diminished. The rate slowed progressively, and asystole occurred. *HR*, heart rate. **B**, patient with multiple ischemic episodes terminating in ventricular tachycardia (*VT*)/fibrillation (*VF*). The ambulatory electrocardiographic recorder was applied at 9:05 a.m. when the patient was in sinus rhythm. The ST segment remained isoelectric until 5:11 p.m. and reached a maximum (*MAX*) of 2.0 mm 6 minutes later in lead V_5 (*top tracing*) as R-wave amplitude and heart rate (*HR*) increased. This initial ischemic episode subsided slowly over the next 5 minutes. A second ischemic episode was recorded at 5:27 p.m. with a similar pattern of increasing R-wave amplitude and ST-segment depression. Another ischemic episode was recorded at 8:05 p.m., and a fourth and terminal ischemic episode was recorded at 9 p.m. During this episode, ST-segment depression reached 2.0 mm and at 9:06 p.m. was associated with ventricular premature contractions *(VPCs)* occurring late in the cycle. At 9:15 p.m., a ventricular premature contraction occurred during the T wave and was followed by ventricular tachycardia/fibrillation. (From Pepine CJ, Morganroth J, McDonald JT, et al: Sudden death during ambulatory electrocardiographic monitoring. *Am J Cardiol* 68:785-788, 1991. By permission of Excerpta Medica.)

without further testing. In patients with cardiac risk factors, exercise testing with perfusion or wall motion imaging is used in an attempt to demonstrate the presence and extent of ischemia and to place patients in high- or low-risk strata.

For patients with known coronary artery disease or with suspected coronary spasm, we have suggested some revised indications[54] (Table 29A-5). Use of ambulatory ST-segment monitoring for these indications presupposes knowledge of the prognostic import of the findings that may be obtained. Stratification of risk in patients with known stable and unstable angina may be improved with the knowledge that frequent silent ischemic episodes are present. Because ST-segment depression may be less likely to occur in patients with preexisting left ventricular dysfunction,[136] ambulatory monitoring should supplement but not replace exercise or pharmacologic wall motion or perfusion risk assessment in such patients.

Perioperative assessment of ST-segment behavior in patients with known coronary disease or risk factors is an extremely promising approach. The number of perioperative events in high-risk patients suggests that effective medical regimens should yield significant differences in patient outcomes. The study of different analgesic regimens related to the incidence of perioperative ischemia by Mangano et al.[83] is a notable example. An additional important question is whether extensive preoperative testing, the current conventional approach to patients with known or suspected disease, guides appropriate perioperative medical management decisions. Future studies will also evaluate the use of the on-line alarm-driven systems for interactive detection and treatment of ischemia. This should be extremely useful in patients under anesthesia or sedation or with unstable or Prinzmetal's angina in whom the preponderant ischemic episodes are silent.

Results of trials of optimal ischemia-guided therapeutics in patients with chronic stable angina may be available in the next few years. Meanwhile, we routinely prescribe aspirin, 160 to 325 mg/day, to prevent thrombotic episodes and have patients carry a sublingual nitroglycerin product. In addition, the impact of thrombolytic therapy on mortality in myocardial infarction is discussed, and each patient is admonished to urgently seek medical care within minutes of the onset of chest discomfort unresponsive to sublingual nitrate therapy. Our current approach to antianginal therapy is to suppress symptoms with the fewest drugs and lowest doses possible. This is done in concert with knowledge of overall risk, including left ventricular function and the ischemia threshold determined by an exercise test when feasible. For patients with documented coronary artery disease and no symptoms or ambiguous symptoms, an approach to therapy based on objective assessment of ischemia and low- or high-risk stratification seems most appropriate. Criteria for high risk (Table 29A-6) and a treatment algorithm (Fig 29A-17) have been proposed by the Council for Myocardial Ischemia and Infarction.[205] It has been suggested that low-risk patients receive aspirin and modify risk factors, with consideration of medical anti-ischemic therapy and with scheduled follow-up. Pending results from the clinical trials, which are continuing, the recom-

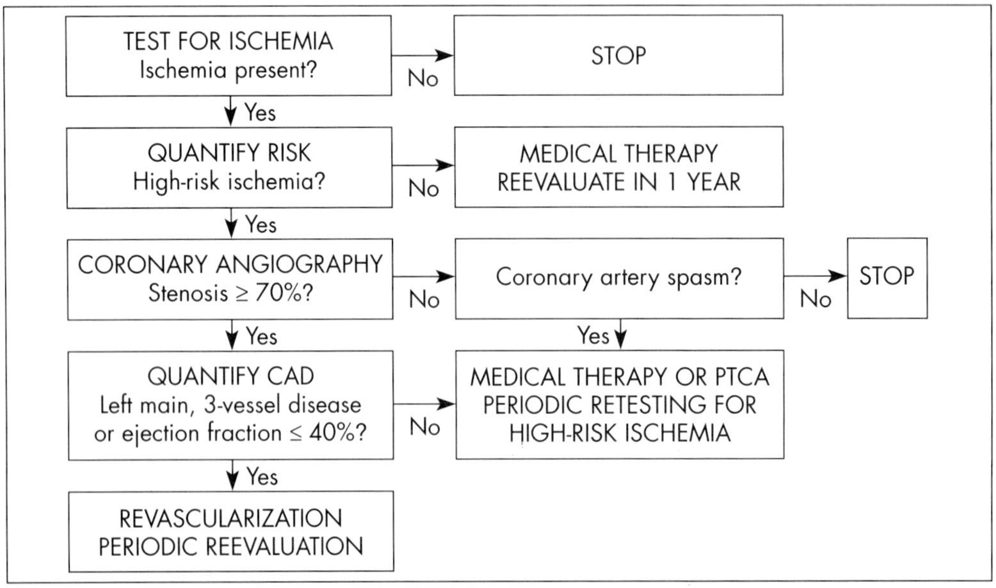

Fig 29A-17. Proposed algorithm based on tests of ischemia for management of patients at ischemic risk. *CAD*, coronary artery disease; *PTCA*, percutaneous transluminal coronary angioplasty. (From Pepine CJ, Kern MJ, Boden WE: Advisory group reports on silent myocardial ischemia, acute intervention after myocardial infarction, and postinfarction management. *Am J Cardiol* 69:41B-46B, 1992. By permission of Excerpta Medica.)

mendation is that high-risk patients receive sufficient medical treatment to convert high-risk ischemic test responses to low-risk responses or be considered for revascularization.[206]

REFERENCES

1. ACC-AHA Task Force: Guidelines for ambulatory electrocardiography: a report of the American College of Cardiology/American Heart Association Task Force on Assessment of Diagnostic and Therapeutic Cardiovascular Procedures (subcommittee on ambulatory electrocardiography). *J Am Coll Cardiol* 13:249-258, 1989
2. Dimarco JP, Philbrick JT: Ambulatory electrocardiographic (Holter) monitoring. *Ann Intern Med* 113:77-79, 1990
3. Pepine CJ: Silent myocardial ischemia: definition, magnitude, and scope of the problem. *Cardiol Clin* 4:577-581, 1986
4. Braunwald E, Sobel BE: Coronary blood flow and myocardial ischemia. In *Heart Disease: a Textbook of Cardiovascular Medicine*. Vol. 2. Edited by E Braunwald. Philadelphia, WB Saunders Company, 1980, pp 1279-1308
5. Sigwart U, Grbic M, Payot M, et al: Ischemic events during coronary artery balloon obstruction. In *Silent Myocardial Ischemia*. Edited by W Rutishauser, H Roskamm. Berlin, Springer-Verlag, 1984, pp 29-36
6. Cohn PF: Silent myocardial ischemia. *Ann Intern Med* 109:312-317, 1988
7. Droste C, Roskamm H: Experimental pain measurement in patients with asymptomatic myocardial ischemia. *J Am Coll Cardiol* 1:940-945, 1983
8. Glazier JJ, Chierchia S, Brown MJ, et al: Importance of generalized defective perception of painful stimuli as a cause of silent myocardial ischemia in chronic stable angina pectoris. *Am J Cardiol* 58:667-672, 1986
9. Sheps DS, Adams KF, Hinderliter A, et al: Endorphins are related to pain perception in coronary artery disease. *Am J Cardiol* 59:523-527, 1987
10. Weidinger F, Hammerle A, Sochor H, et al: Role of beta-endorphins in silent myocardial ischemia. *Am J Cardiol* 58:428-430, 1986
11. Heller GV, Garber CE, Connolly MJ, et al: Plasma beta-endorphin levels in silent myocardial ischemia induced by exercise. *Am J Cardiol* 59:735-739, 1987
12. Ellestad MH, Kuan P: Naloxone and asymptomatic ischemia: failure to induce angina during exercise testing. *Am J Cardiol* 54:982-984, 1984
13. Bradley RF, Schonfeld A: Diminished pain in diabetic patients with myocardial infarction. *Geriatrics* 17:322-326, 1962
14. Cabin HS, Roberts WC: Quantitative comparison of extent of coronary narrowing and size and healed myocardial infarct in 33 necropsy patients with clinically recognized and in 28 with clinically unrecognized ("silent") previous acute myocardial infarction. *Am J Cardiol* 50:677-681, 1982
15. Langer A, Freeman MR, Josse RG, et al: Detection of silent myocardial ischemia in diabetes mellitus. *Am J Cardiol* 67:1073-1078, 1991
16. Faerman I, Faccio E, Milei J, et al: Autonomic neuropathy and painless myocardial infarction in diabetic patients: histologic evidence of their relationship. *Diabetes* 26:1147-1153, 1977
17. Miller PF, Sheps DS, Bragdon EE, et al: Aging and pain perception in ischemic heart disease. *Am Heart J* 120:22-30, 1990
18. Cohn P: Silent myocardial ischemia in patients with a defective anginal warning system. *Am J Cardiol* 45:697-702, 1980
19. Deanfield JE, Maseri A, Selwyn AP, et al: Myocardial ischaemia during daily life in patients with stable angina: its relation to symptoms and heart rate changes. *Lancet* 2:753-758, 1983
20. Deanfield JE, Shea M, Kensett M, et al: Silent myocardial ischaemia due to mental stress. *Lancet* 2:1001-1005, 1984
21. Deanfield JE, Shea MJ, Wilson RA, et al: Direct effects of smoking on the heart: silent ischemic disturbances of coronary flow. *Am J Cardiol* 57:1005-1009, 1986
22. Bairey CN, Krantz DS, Rozanski A: Mental stress as an acute trigger of ischemic left ventricular dysfunction and blood pressure elevation in coronary artery disease. *Am J Cardiol* 66:28G-31G, 1990
23. Agati L, Penco M, Sciomer S, et al: Painless versus painful myocardial ischemia: different left ventricular dysfunction detected by echocardiography. *Int J Cardiol* 22:321-327, 1989
24. Nademanee K, Gorelick DA, Josephson MA, et al: Myocardial ischemia during cocaine withdrawal. *Ann Intern Med* 111:876-880, 1989
25. Cherry PD, Furchgott RF, Zawadzki JV, et al: Role of endothelial cells in relaxation of isolated arteries by bradykinin. *Proc Natl Acad Sci U S A* 79:2106-2110, 1982
26. Griffith TM, Edwards DH, Lewis MJ, et al: The nature of endothelium-derived vascular relaxant factor. *Nature* 308:645-647, 1984
27. Furchgott RF, Vanhoutte PM: Endothelium-derived relaxing and contracting factors. *FASEB J* 3:2007-2018, 1989
28. Ganz P, Alexander RW: New insights into the cellular mechanisms of vasospasm. *Am J Cardiol* 56:11E-15E, 1985
29. Okumura K, Yasue H, Matsuyama K, et al: Effect of acetylcholine on the highly stenotic coronary artery: difference between the constrictor response of the infarct-related coronary artery and that of the noninfarct-related artery. *J Am Coll Cardiol* 19:752-758, 1992
30. Freudenberg H, Lichtlen PR: The normal wall segment in coronary stenoses: a postmortal study. *Z Kardiol* 70:863-869, 1981
31. Rozanski A, Berman DS: Silent myocardial ischemia. I. Pathophysiology, frequency of occurrence, and approaches toward detection. *Am Heart J* 114:615-626, 1987
32. Deedwania PC, Carbajal EV, Nelson JR, et al: Anti-ischemic effects of atenolol versus nifedipine in patients with coronary artery disease and ambulatory silent ischemia. *J Am Coll Cardiol* 17:963-969, 1991
33. Folts JD, Crowell EB Jr, Rowe GG: Platelet aggregation in partially obstructed vessels and its elimination with aspirin. *Circulation* 54:365-370, 1976
34. Davies MJ, Thomas AC, Knapman PA, et al: Intramyocardial platelet aggregation in patients with unstable angina suffering sudden ischemic cardiac death. *Circulation* 73:418-427, 1986
35. Maouad J, Fernandez F, Barrillon A, et al: Diffuse or segmental narrowing (spasm) of the coronary arteries during smoking demonstrated on angiography. *Am J Cardiol* 53:354-355, 1984
36. Lewis HD Jr, Davis JW, Archibald DG, et al: Protective effects of aspirin against acute myocardial infarction and death in men with unstable angina: results of a Veterans Administration cooperative study. *N Engl J Med* 309:396-403, 1983
37. Shah PK, Forrester JS: Pathophysiology of acute coronary syndromes. *Am J Cardiol* 68:16C-23C, 1991
38. Gottlieb SO, Weisfeldt ML, Ouyang P, et al: Silent ischemia as a marker for early unfavorable outcomes in patients with unstable angina. *N Engl J Med* 314:1214-1219, 1986
39. Quyyumi AA, Wright CA, Mockus LJ, et al: Mechanisms of nocturnal angina pectoris: importance of increased myocardial oxygen demand in patients with severe coronary artery disease. *Lancet* 1:1207-1209, 1984
40. Deedwania PC, Nelson JR: Pathophysiology of silent myocardial ischemia during daily life: hemodynamic evaluation by simultaneous electrocardiographic and blood pressure monitoring. *Circulation* 82: 1296-1304, 1990
41. Deedwania PC, Carbajal EV: Silent myocardial ischemia: a clinical perspective. *Arch Intern Med* 151:2373-2382, 1991
42. McLenachan JM, Weidinger FF, Barry J, et al: Relations between heart rate, ischemia, and drug therapy during daily life in patients with coronary artery disease. *Circulation* 83:1263-1270, 1991
43. Cohn PF: *Silent Myocardial Ischemia and Infarction*. Second edition. New York, Marcel Dekker, 1989
44. Tofler GH, Brezinski D, Schafer AI, et al: Concurrent morning increase in platelet aggregability and the risk of myocardial infarction and sudden cardiac death. *N Engl J Med* 316:1514-1518, 1987
45. Millar-Craig MW, Bishop CN, Raftery EB: Circadian variation of blood pressure. *Lancet* 1:795-797, 1978
46. Muller JE, Stone PH, Turi ZG, et al: Circadian variation in the frequency of onset of acute myocardial infarction. *N Engl J Med* 313:1315-1322, 1985
47. Muller JE, Lundmer PL, Willich SN, et al: Circadian variation in the frequency of sudden cardiac death. *Circulation* 75:131-138, 1987
48. Yasue H, Omote S, Takizawa A, et al: Circadian variation of exercise capacity in patients with Prinzmetal's variant angina: role of exercise-induced coronary arterial spasm. *Circulation* 59:938-948, 1979
49. Rosing DR, Brakman P, Redwood DR, et al: Blood fibrinolytic activity in man: diurnal variation and the response to varying intensities of exercise. *Circ Res* 27:171-184, 1970
50. Mickley H, Pless P, Nielsen JR, et al: Circadian variation of transient myocardial ischemia in the early out-of-hospital period after first acute myocardial infarction. *Am J Cardiol* 67:927-932, 1991

51. Currie P, Saltissi S: Transient myocardial ischaemia after acute myocardial infarction. *Br Heart J* 64:299-303, 1990

52. Epstein SE, Quyyumi AA, Bonow RO: Myocardial ischemia—silent or symptomatic. *N Engl J Med* 318:1038-1043, 1988

53. Holter NJ: New method for heart studies: continuous electrocardiography of active subjects over long periods is now practical. *Science* 134:1214-1220, 1961

54. Blackshear JL: Ambulatory monitoring of silent myocardial ischemia: What is its utility? *South Med J* 85:293-298, 1992

55. Cohn PF, Kannel WB: Recognition, pathogenesis, and management options in silent coronary artery disease: summary. *Circulation* 75 Suppl 2:54, 1987

56. Hammill SC, Khandheria BK: Silent myocardial ischemia. *Mayo Clin Proc* 65:374-383, 1990

57. Josephson RA, Fleg JL: The role of exercise stress tests in screening asymptomatic patients for silent ischemia. *Prim Cardiol* 17:50-61, March 1991

58. Goldschlager N, Selzer A, Cohn K: Treadmill stress tests as indicators of presence and severity of coronary artery disease. *Ann Intern Med* 85:277-286, 1976

59. Shook TL, Balke CW, Kotilainen PW, et al: Comparison of amplitude-modulated (direct) and frequency-modulated ambulatory techniques for recording ischemic electrocardiographic changes. *Am J Cardiol* 60:895-900, 1987

60. Hinderliter A, Bragdon E, Herbst M, et al: A comparison of amplitude-modulated and frequency-modulated ambulatory monitoring systems. *Am J Cardiol* 64:76-80, 1989

61. Sheffield LT, Berson A, Bragg-Remschel D, et al: Recommendations for standards of instrumentation and practice in the use of ambulatory electrocardiography: the Task Force of the Committee on Electrocardiography and Cardiac Electrophysiology of the Council on Clinical Cardiology. *Circulation* 71:A-626-A-636, 1985

62. Benhorin J, Tzivoni D: A directory of ambulatory ECG monitoring equipment. *J Myocardial Ischemia* 3:1527, 1991

63. Kennedy HL, Wiens RD: Ambulatory (Holter) electrocardiography using real-time analysis. *Am J Cardiol* 59:1190-1195, 1987

64. Silber S, Bajaj RK, Kirk KA, et al: Accuracy of digital Holter monitoring of extent and duration of ischemic episodes compared to analog recording. *Am J Cardiol* 65:383-388, 1990

65. Deedwania PC, Carbajal EV: Ambulatory ECG monitoring for myocardial ischemia—state-of-the-art. *J Myocardial Ischemia* 4:52-71, 1992

66. Deanfield JE, Ribiero P, Oakley K, et al: Analysis of ST-segment changes in normal subjects: implications for ambulatory monitoring in angina pectoris. *Am J Cardiol* 54:1321-1325, 1984

67. Stern Z, Tzivoni D: Dynamic changes in the ST-T segment during sleep in ischemic heart disease. *Am J Cardiol* 32:17-20, 1973

68. Tzivoni D, Stern Z, Keren A, et al: Electrocardiographic characteristics of neurocirculatory asthenia during every day activities. *Br Heart J* 44:426-432, 1980

69. Hammill SC: Evaluation of a Holter system to record ST-segment changes. *J Electrocardiol* 20 Suppl:12-15, 1987

70. Nabel EG, Barry J, Rocco MB, et al: Variability of transient myocardial ischemia in ambulatory patients with coronary artery disease. *Circulation* 78:60-67, 1988

71. Tzivoni D, Gavish A, Benhorin J, et al: Day-to-day variability of myocardial ischemic episodes in coronary artery disease. *Am J Cardiol* 60:1003-1005, 1987

72. Khurmi NS, Raftery EB: Reproducibility and validity of ambulatory ST segment monitoring in patients with chronic stable angina pectoris. *Am Heart J* 113:1091-1096, 1987

73. Detry J-M, Fesler R, Berckmans T, et al: A new semiautomated algorithm to quantify Holter-detected myocardial ischemia: preliminary experiences with the Trimetazidine European Multicenter Trial (TEMS). *Cardiovasc Drugs Ther* 4 Suppl 4:841-846, 1990

74. Slogoff S, Keats AS: Does perioperative myocardial ischemia lead to postoperative myocardial infarction? *Anesthesiology* 62:107-114, 1985

75. Knight AA, Hollenberg M, London MJ, et al: Myocardial ischemia in patients awaiting coronary artery bypass grafting. *Am Heart J* 117:1189-1195, 1989

76. Coriat P, Harari A, Daloz M, et al: Clinical predictors of intraoperative myocardial ischemia in patients with coronary artery disease undergoing non-cardiac surgery. *Acta Anaesth Scand* 26:287-290, 1982

77. Raby KE, Goldman L, Creager MA, et al: Correlation between preoperative ischemia and major cardiac events after peripheral vascular surgery. *N Engl J Med* 321:1296-1300, 1989

78. Pasternack PF, Grossi EA, Baumann FG, et al: The value of silent myocardial ischemia monitoring in the prediction of perioperative myocardial infarction in patients undergoing peripheral vascular surgery. *J Vasc Surg* 10:617-625, 1989

79. Shah KB, Kleinman BS, Rao TLK, et al: Angina and other risk factors in patients with cardiac diseases undergoing noncardiac operations. *Anesth Analg* 70:240-247, 1990

80. Raby KE, Goldman L, Cook EF, et al: Long-term prognosis of myocardial ischemia detected by Holter monitoring in peripheral vascular disease. *Am J Cardiol* 66:1309-1313, 1990

81. Mangano DT, Browner WS, Hollenberg M, et al: Association of perioperative myocardial ischemia with cardiac morbidity and mortality in men undergoing noncardiac surgery. *N Engl J Med* 323:1781-1788, 1990

82. Mangano DT, Hollenberg M, Fegert G, et al: Perioperative myocardial ischemia in patients undergoing noncardiac surgery. I: Incidence and severity during the 4 day perioperative period. *J Am Coll Cardiol* 17:843-850, 1991

83. Mangano DT, Siliciano D, Hollenberg M, et al: Postoperative myocardial ischemia: therapeutic trials using intensive analgesia following surgery. *Anesthesiology* 76:342-353, 1992

84. Goldman L: Perioperative myocardial ischemia: to everything there is a season. *Anesthesiology* 76:331-333, 1992

85. Krucoff MW, Parente AR, Bottner RK, et al: Stability of multilead ST-segment "fingerprints" over time after percutaneous coronary angioplasty and its usefulness in detecting reocclusion. *Am J Cardiol* 61:1232-1237, 1988

86. Krucoff MW, Wagner NB, Pope JE, et al: The portable programmable microprocessor-driven real-time 12-lead electrocardiographic monitor: a preliminary report of a new device for the noninvasive detection of successful reperfusion or silent coronary reocclusion. *Am J Cardiol* 65:143-148, 1990

87. Beller GA: Myocardial perfusion imaging for detection of silent myocardial ischemia. *Am J Cardiol* 61:22F-26F, 1988

88. Maseri A, Mimmo R, Chierchia S, et al: Coronary artery spasm as a cause of acute myocardial ischemia in man. *Chest* 68:625-633, 1975

89. Maseri A, Parodi O, Severi S, et al: Transient transmural reduction of myocardial blood flow demonstrated by thallium-201 scintigraphy as a cause of variant angina. *Circulation* 54:280-288, 1976

90. Hecht HS, Shaw RE, Bruce T, et al: Silent ischemia: evaluation by exercise and redistribution tomographic thallium-201 myocardial imaging. *J Am Coll Cardiol* 14:895-900, 1989

91. Heller LI, Tresgallo M, Sciacca RR, et al: Prognostic significance of silent myocardial ischemia on a thallium stress test. *Am J Cardiol* 65:718-721, 1990

92. Gasperetti CM, Burwell LR, Beller GA: Prevalence and variables associated with silent myocardial ischemia on exercise thallium-201 stress testing. *J Am Coll Cardiol* 16:115-123, 1990

93. Leppo J, Boucher CA, Okada RD, et al: Serial thallium-201 myocardial imaging after dipyridamole infusion: diagnostic utility in detecting coronary stenoses and relationship to regional wall motion. *Circulation* 66:649-657, 1982

94. Boucher CA, Brewster DC, Darling RC, et al: Determination of cardiac risk by dipyridamole-thallium imaging before peripheral vascular surgery. *N Engl J Med* 312:389-394, 1985

95. Levinson JR, Boucher CA, Coley CM, et al: Usefulness of semiquantitative analysis of dipyridamole-thallium-201 redistribution for improving risk stratification before vascular surgery. *Am J Cardiol* 66:406-410, 1990

96. Younis LT, Byers S, Shaw L, et al: Prognostic importance of silent myocardial ischemia detected by intravenous dipyridamole thallium myocardial imaging in asymptomatic patients with coronary artery disease. *J Am Coll Cardiol* 14:1635-1641, 1989

97. Deanfield JE, Shea M, Ribiero P, et al: Transient ST-segment depression as a marker of myocardial ischemia during daily life. *Am J Cardiol* 54:1195-1200, 1984

98. Marshall RC, Tillisch JH, Phelps ME, et al: Identification and differentiation of resting myocardial ischemia and infarction in a man with positron computed tomography. ^{18}F-labeled fluorodeoxyglucose and N-13 ammonia. *Circulation* 67:766-778, 1983

99. Carbajal EV, Deedwania PC: Silent myocardial ischemia: mechanisms, diagnosis, prevalence. *Prim Cardiol* 17:30-37, October 1991

100. Borer JS, Kent KM, Bacharach SL, et al: Sensitivity, specificity and predictive accuracy of radionuclide cineangiography during exercise in patients with coronary artery disease: comparison with exercise electrocardiography. *Circulation* 60:572-580, 1979

101. Gibson RS, Beller GA: Should exercise electrocardiographic testing be replaced by radioisotope methods? *Cardiovasc Clin* 13 No 1:1-33, 1983

102. Cohn PF, Brown EJ, Wynne J, et al: Global and regional left ventricular ejection fraction abnormalities during exercise in patients with silent myocardial ischemia. *J Am Coll Cardiol* 1:931-933, 1983

103. Bonow RO, Bacharach SL, Green MV, et al: Prognostic implications of symptomatic versus asymptomatic (silent) myocardial ischemia induced by exercise in mildly symptomatic and in asymptomatic patients with angiographically documented coronary artery disease. *Am J Cardiol* 60:778-783, 1987

104. Berman DS, Rozanski A, Knoebel SB: The detection of silent ischemia: cautions and precautions. *Circulation* 75:101-105, 1987

105. Breitenbücher A, Pfisterer M, Hoffmann A, et al: Long-term follow-up of patients with silent ischemia during exercise radionuclide angiography. *J Am Coll Cardiol* 15:999-1003, 1990

106. Kayden DS, Remetz MS, Cabin HS, et al: Validation of continuous radionuclide left ventricular function monitoring in detecting silent myocardial ischemia during balloon angioplasty of the left anterior descending coronary artery. *Am J Cardiol* 67:1339-1343, 1991

107. Ryan T, Armstrong WF, O'Donnell JA, et al: Risk stratification after myocardial infarction by means of exercise two-dimensional echocardiography. *Am Heart J* 114:1305-1316, 1987

108. Bolognese L, Rossi L, Sarasso G, et al: Silent versus symptomatic dipyridamole-induced ischemia after myocardial infarction: clinical and prognostic significance. *J Am Coll Cardiol* 19:953-959, 1992

109. Pettigrew RI: Dynamic magnetic resonance imaging in acquired heart disease. *Semin Ultrasound CT MR* 12:61-91, 1991

110. Chierchia S, Lazzari M, Freedman B, et al: Impairment of myocardial perfusion and function during painless myocardial ischemia. *J Am Coll Cardiol* 1:924-930, 1983

111. Singh BN, Nademanee K, Figueras J, et al: Hemodynamic and electrocardiographic correlates of symptomatic and silent myocardial ischemia: pathophysiologic and therapeutic implications. *Am J Cardiol* 58:3B-10B, 1986

112. Levy RD, Shapiro LM, Wright C, et al: The haemodynamic significance of asymptomatic ST segment depression assessed by ambulatory pulmonary artery pressure monitoring. *Br Heart J* 56:526-530, 1986

113. Hirzel HO, Leutwyler R, Krayenbuehl HP: Silent myocardial ischemia: hemodynamic changes during dynamic exercise in patients with proven coronary artery disease despite absence of angina pectoris. *J Am Coll Cardiol* 6:275-284, 1985

114. van Daele ME, Sutherland GR, Mitchell MM, et al: Do changes in pulmonary capillary wedge pressure adequately reflect myocardial ischemia during anesthesia? A correlative preoperative hemodynamic, electrocardiographic, and transesophageal echocardiographic study. *Circulation* 81:865-871, 1990

115. Feldman T, Resnekov L: Ambulatory ECG recording for detecting silent myocardial ischemia. *Cardiovasc Clin* 18 No 3:23-41, 1988

116. Hedblad B, Juul-Möller S, Svensson K, et al: Increased mortality in men with ST segment depression during 24 h ambulatory long-term ECG recording. *Eur Heart J* 10:149-158, 1989

117. Rozanski A, Berman D: The frequency, pathophysiology and prognosis of exercise-induced silent ischemia. In *Silent Ischemia. Current Concepts and Management*. Edited by TV Arnim, A Maseri. New York, Springer-Verlag, 1987, pp 96-106

118. Fleg JL, Gerstenblith G, Zonderman AB, et al: Prevalence and prognostic significance of exercise-induced silent myocardial ischemia detected by thallium scintigraphy and electrocardiography in asymptomatic volunteers. *Circulation* 81:428-436, 1990

119. Erikssen J, Thaulow E: Follow-up of patients with asymptomatic myocardial ischemia. In *Silent Myocardial Ischemia*. Edited by W Rutishauser, H Roskamm. Berlin, Springer-Verlag, 1984, pp 156-164

120. Erikssen J: Prognostic importance of silent ischemia during long-term follow-up of patients with coronary artery disease. *Herz* 12:359-368, 1987

121. Hlatky MA: Exercise stress testing to screen for coronary artery disease in asymptomatic persons. *J Occup Med* 28:1020-1025, 1986

122. Multiple Risk Factor Intervention Trial Research Group: Exercise electrocardiogram and coronary heart disease mortality in the Multiple Risk Factor Intervention Trial. *Am J Cardiol* 55:16-24, 1985

123. Gordon DJ, Ekelund L-G, Karon JM, et al: Predictive value of the exercise tolerance test for mortality in North American men: the Lipid Research Clinics Mortality Follow-up Study. *Circulation* 74:252-261, 1986

124. McHenry PL, O'Donnell J, Morris SN, et al: The abnormal exercise electrocardiogram in apparently healthy men: a predictor of angina pectoris as an initial coronary event during long-term follow-up. *Circulation* 70:547-551, 1984

125. Cohn PF: Clinical importance of silent myocardial ischemia in asymptomatic subjects. *Circulation* 81:691-693, 1990

126. Yusuf S: Design of studies to critically evaluate if detection of asymptomatic ST-segment deviation (silent ischemia) is of medical or public health importance. In *Silent Myocardial Ischemia and Angina*. Edited by BN Singh. New York, Pergamon Press, 1988, pp 206-219

127. Mark DB, Hlatky MA, Califf RM, et al: Painless exercise ST deviation on the treadmill: long-term prognosis. *J Am Coll Cardiol* 14:885-892, 1989

128. Weiner DA, Ryan TJ, McCabe CH, et al: Significance of silent myocardial ischemia during exercise testing in patients with coronary artery disease. *Am J Cardiol* 59:725-729, 1987

129. Pepine CJ: Is silent ischemia a treatable risk factor in patients with angina pectoris? *Circulation* 82 Suppl 2:135-142, 1990

130. Mulcahy D, Keegan J, Sparrow J, et al: Ischemia in the ambulatory setting—the total ischemic burden: relation to exercise testing and investigative and therapeutic implications. *J Am Coll Cardiol* 14:1166-1172, 1989

131. Mulcahy D, Keegan J, Lindsay D, et al: Silent myocardial ischaemia in patients referred for coronary bypass surgery because of angina: a comparison with patients whose symptoms were well controlled on medical treatment. *Br Heart J* 61:496-501, 1989

132. Kawanishi DT, Reid CL, Morrison EC, et al: Response of angina and ischemia to long-term treatment in patients with chronic stable angina: a double-blind randomized individualized dosing trial of nifedipine, propranolol and their combination. *J Am Coll Cardiol* 19:409-417, 1992

133. Mody FV, Nademanee K, Intarachot V, et al: Severity of silent myocardial ischemia on ambulatory electrocardiographic monitoring in patients with stable angina pectoris: relation to prognostic determinants during exercise stress testing and coronary angiography. *J Am Coll Cardiol* 12:1169-1176, 1988

134. Aronow WS, Mercando AD, Epstein S: Prevalence of silent myocardial ischemia detected by 24-hour ambulatory electrocardiography, and its association with new coronary events at 40-month follow-up in elderly diabetic and nondiabetic patients with coronary artery disease. *Am J Cardiol* 69:555-556, 1992

135. Mahmarian JJ, Pratt CM, Cocanougher MK, et al: Altered myocardial perfusion in patients with angina pectoris or silent ischemia during exercise as assessed by quantitative thallium-201 single-photon emission computed tomography. *Circulation* 82:1305-1315, 1990

136. Quyyumi AA, Panza JA, Diodati JG, et al: Relation between left ventricular function at rest and with exercise and silent myocardial ischemia. *J Am Coll Cardiol* 19:962-967, 1992

137. Rocco MB, Nabel EG, Campbell S, et al: Prognostic importance of myocardial ischemia detected by ambulatory monitoring in patients with stable coronary artery disease. *Circulation* 78:877-884, 1988

138. Deedwania PC, Carbajal EV: Silent ischemia during daily life is an independent predictor of mortality in stable angina. *Circulation* 81:748-756, 1990

139. Tzivoni D, Weisz G, Gavish A, et al: Comparison of mortality and myocardial infarction rates in stable angina pectoris with and without ischemic episodes during daily activities. *Am J Cardiol* 63:273-276, 1989

140. Mulcahy D, Parameshwar J, Holdright D, et al: Value of ambulatory ST segment monitoring in patients with chronic stable angina: Does measurement of the "total ischaemic burden" assist with management? *Br Heart J* 67:47-52, 1992

141. Mark DB, Shaw L, Harrell FE Jr, et al: Prognostic value of a treadmill exercise score in outpatients with suspected coronary artery disease. *N Engl J Med* 325:849-853, 1991

142. Callaham PR, Froelicher VF, Klein J, et al: Exercise-induced silent ischemia: age, diabetes mellitus, previous myocardial infarction and prognosis. *J Am Coll Cardiol* 14:1175-1180, 1989

143. Nademanee K, Intarachot V, Josephson MA, et al: Circadian variation in occurrence of transient overt and silent myocardial ischemia

and chronic stable angina and comparison with Prinzmetal angina in men. *Am J Cardiol* 60:494-498, 1987

144. Araki H, Koiwaya Y, Nakagaki O, et al: Diurnal distribution of ST-segment elevation and related arrhythmias in patients with variant angina: a study by ambulatory ECG monitoring. *Circulation* 67:995-1000, 1983

145. Morikami Y, Yasue H: Efficacy of slow-released nifedipine on myocardial ischemic episodes in variant angina pectoris. *Am J Cardiol* 68:580-584, 1991

146. Castello R, Alegria E, Merino A, et al: The value of exercise testing in patients with coronary artery spasm. *Am Heart J* 119:259-263, 1990

147. Chaitman BR, Waters DD, Theroux P, et al: S-T segment elevation and coronary spasm in response to exercise. *Am J Cardiol* 47:1350-1358, 1981

148. Mark DB, Califf RM, Morris KG, et al: Clinical characteristics and long-term survival of patients with variant angina. *Circulation* 69:880-888, 1984

149. Yasue H, Takizawa A, Nagao M, et al: Long-term prognosis for patients with variant angina and influential factors. *Circulation* 78:1-9, 1988

150. Nakamura M, Takeshita A, Nose Y: Clinical characteristics associated with myocardial infarction, arrhythmias, and sudden death in patients with vasospastic angina. *Circulation* 75:1110-1116, 1987

151. Walling A, Waters DD, Miller DD, et al: Long-term prognosis of patients with variant angina. *Circulation* 76:990-997, 1987

152. Langer A, Freeman MR, Armstrong PW: ST segment shift in unstable angina: pathophysiology and association with coronary anatomy and hospital outcome. *J Am Coll Cardiol* 13:1495-1502, 1989

153. Pozzati A, Bugiardini R, Borghi A, et al: Prognostic significance of myocardial ischemia refractory to maximal medical therapy in unstable angina (abstract). *Circulation* 78 Suppl 2:421, 1988

154. Arnim Th v, Gerbig HW, Krawietz W, et al: Prognostic implications of transient—predominantly silent—ischaemia in patients with unstable angina pectoris. *Eur Heart J* 9:435-440, 1988

155. Nademanee K, Intarachot V, Josephson MA, et al: Prognostic significance of silent myocardial ischemia in patients with unstable angina. *J Am Coll Cardiol* 10:1-9, 1987

156. Gottlieb SO, Weisfeldt ML, Ouyang P, et al: Silent ischemia predicts infarction and death during 2 year follow-up of unstable angina. *J Am Coll Cardiol* 10:756-760, 1987

157. Johnson SM, Mauritson DR, Winniford MD, et al: Continuous electrocardiographic monitoring in patients with unstable angina pectoris: identification of high-risk subgroup with severe coronary disease, variant angina, and/or impaired early prognosis. *Am Heart J* 103:4-12, 1982

158. Nyman I, Larsson H, Areskog M, et al: The predictive value of silent ischemia at an exercise test before discharge after an episode of unstable coronary artery disease. *Am Heart J* 123:324-331, 1992

159. Romeo F, Rosano GMC, Martuscelli E, et al: Unstable angina: role of silent ischemia and total ischemic time (silent plus painful ischemia), a 6-year follow-up. *J Am Coll Cardiol* 19:1173-1179, 1992

160. Krone RJ, Gillespie JA, Weld FM, et al: Low-level exercise testing after myocardial infarction: usefulness in enhancing clinical risk stratification. *Circulation* 71:80-89, 1985

161. Waters DD, Bosch X, Bouchard A, et al: Comparison of clinical variables and variables derived from a limited predischarge exercise test as predictors of early and late mortality after myocardial infarction. *J Am Coll Cardiol* 5:1-8, 1985

162. Jespersen CM, Kassis E, Edeling C-J, et al: The prognostic value of maximal exercise testing soon after first myocardial infarction. *Eur Heart J* 6:769-772, 1985

163. Théroux P, Waters DD, Halphen C, et al: Prognostic value of exercise testing soon after myocardial infarction. *N Engl J Med* 301:341-345, 1979

164. Starling MR, Crawford MH, Kennedy GT, et al: Exercise testing early after myocardial infarction: predictive value for subsequent unstable angina and death. *Am J Cardiol* 46:909-914, 1980

165. Davidson DM, DeBusk RF: Prognostic value of a single exercise test 3 weeks after uncomplicated myocardial infarction. *Circulation* 61:236-242, 1980

166. Markiewicz W, Houston N, DeBusk RF: Exercise testing soon after myocardial infarction. *Circulation* 56:26-31, 1977

167. Margonato A, Ballarotto C, Bonetti F, et al: Assessment of residual tissue viability by exercise testing in recent myocardial infarction: comparison of the electrocardiogram and myocardial perfusion scintigraphy. *J Am Coll Cardiol* 19:948-952, 1992

168. Petretta M, Bonaduce D, Bianchi V, et al: Characterization and prognostic significance of silent myocardial ischemia on predischarge electrocardiographic monitoring in unselected patients with myocardial infarction. *Am J Cardiol* 69:579-583, 1992

169. Gottlieb SO, Gottlieb SH, Achuff SC, et al: Silent ischemia on Holter monitoring predicts mortality in high-risk postinfarction patients. *JAMA* 259:1030-1035, 1988

170. Tzivoni D, Gavish A, Zin D, et al: Prognostic significance of ischemic episodes in patients with previous myocardial infarction. *Am J Cardiol* 62:661-664, 1988

171. Ouyang P, Shapiro EP, Chandra NC, et al: An angiographic and functional comparison of patients with silent and symptomatic treadmill ischemia early after myocardial infarction. *Am J Cardiol* 59:730-734, 1987

172. Froelicher VF, Perdue ST, Atwood JE, et al: Exercise testing of patients recovering from myocardial infarction. *Curr Probl Cardiol* 11:370-444, 1986

173. Mark DB, Hlatky MA, Pryor DB: The exercise treadmill test in patients recovering from an acute myocardial infarction. In *Acute Coronary Care in the Thrombolytic Era*. Edited by RM Califf, DB Mark, GS Wagner. Chicago, Year Book Medical Publishers, 1988, pp 573-591

174. Brown KA: Prognostic value of thallium-201 myocardial perfusion imaging: a diagnostic tool comes of age. *Circulation* 83:363-381, 1991

175. Akins CW, Pohost GM, DeSanctis RW, et al: Selection of angina-free patients with severe left ventricular dysfunction for myocardial revascularization. *Am J Cardiol* 46:695-700, 1980

176. Bounous EP, Mark DB, Pollock BG, et al: Surgical survival benefits for coronary disease patients with left ventricular dysfunction. *Circulation* 78 Suppl 1:151-157, 1988

177. Rahimtoola SH: Clinical overview of management of chronic ischemic heart disease. *Circulation* 84 Suppl 1:81-84, 1991

178. Droste C, Lemmen S, Nitsche R, et al: ST segment monitoring before, three weeks and six months after aortocoronary bypass surgery. *Eur Heart J* 9 Suppl N:169-175, 1988

179. Mulcahy D, Keegan J, Phadke K, et al: Effects of coronary artery bypass surgery and angioplasty on the total ischemic burden: a study of exercise testing and ambulatory ST segment monitoring. *Am Heart J* 123:597-603, 1992

180. Kennedy HL, Seiler SM, Sprague MK, et al: Relation of silent myocardial ischemia after coronary artery bypass grafting to angiographic completeness of revascularization and long-term prognosis. *Am J Cardiol* 65:14-22, 1990

181. Dubach P, Froelicher V, Klein J, et al: Use of the exercise test to predict prognosis after coronary artery bypass grafting. *Am J Cardiol* 63:530-533, 1989

182. Weiner DA, Ryan TJ, Parsons L, et al: Prevalence and prognostic significance of silent and symptomatic ischemia after coronary bypass surgery: a report from the Coronary Artery Surgery Study (CASS) randomized population. *J Am Coll Cardiol* 18:343-348, 1991

183. Huikuri HV, Ikäheimo MJ, Korhonen UR, et al: Thallium scintigraphy in prediction of occlusion of bypass grafts in asymptomatic and symptomatic patients. *Acta Med Scand* 222:311-318, 1987

184. Egstrup K: Asymptomatic myocardial ischemia as a predictor of cardiac events after coronary artery bypass grafting for stable angina pectoris. *Am J Cardiol* 61:248-252, 1988

185. Stäblein A, von Pölnitz A, Reuschel-Janetschek E, et al: Multiple lead monitoring during and after PTCA. *Eur Heart J* 10 Suppl G:9-12, 1989

186. Bush HS, Ferguson JJ III, Angelini P, et al: Twelve-lead electrocardiographic evaluation of ischemia during percutaneous coronary angioplasty and its correlation with acute reocclusion. *Am Heart J* 121:1591-1599, 1991

187. Kaul U, De V, Manchanda SC, et al: Silent myocardial ischemia after percutaneous transluminal coronary angioplasty and its prognostic significance. *Clin Cardiol* 14:563-566, 1991

188. Laarman G, Luijten HE, van Zeyl LGPM, et al: Assessment of "silent" restenosis and long-term follow-up after successful angioplasty in single vessel coronary artery disease: the value of quantitative exercise electrocardiography and quantitative coronary angiography. *J Am Coll Cardiol* 16:578-585, 1990

189. Deligonul U, Vandormael MG, Younis LT, et al: Prognostic significance of silent myocardial ischemia detected by early treadmill exercise after coronary angioplasty. *Am J Cardiol* 64:1-5, 1989

190. Hecht HS, Shaw RE, Chin HL, et al: Silent ischemia after coronary angioplasty: evaluation of restenosis and extent of ischemia in asymptomatic patients by tomographic thallium-201 exercise imaging and comparison with symptomatic patients. *J Am Coll Cardiol* 17:670-677, 1991
191. London MJ, Hollenberg M, Wong MG, et al: Intraoperative myocardial ischemia: localization by continuous 12-lead electrocardiography. *Anesthesiology* 69:232-241, 1988
192. Mangano DT, Wong MG, London MJ, et al: Perioperative myocardial ischemia in patients undergoing noncardiac surgery—II: Incidence and severity during the 1st week after surgery. *J Am Coll Cardiol* 17:851-857, 1991
193. Podrid PJ: Silent ischemia, ventricular arrhythmia and sudden cardiac death. *J Am Coll Cardiol* 16:55-56, 1990
194. Sharma B, Asinger R, Francis GS, et al: Demonstration of exercise-induced painless myocardial ischemia in survivors of out-of-hospital ventricular fibrillation. *Am J Cardiol* 59:740-745, 1987
195. Gomes JA, Alexopoulos D, Winters SL, et al: The role of silent ischemia, the arrhythmic substrate and the short-long sequence in the genesis of sudden cardiac death. *J Am Coll Cardiol* 14:1618-1625, 1989
196. Hausmann D, Nikutta P, Trappe H-J, et al: Incidence of ventricular arrhythmias during transient myocardial ischemia in patients with stable coronary artery disease. *J Am Coll Cardiol* 16:49-54, 1990
197. Pepine CJ, Morganroth J, McDonald JT, et al: Sudden death during ambulatory electrocardiographic monitoring. *Am J Cardiol* 68:785-788, 1991
198. Cohn PF: *Silent Myocardial Ischemia and Infarction*. Second edition. New York, Marcel Dekker, 1989, pp 203-215
199. Cohn PF, Vetrovec GW, Nesto R, et al: The Nifedipine-Total Ischemia Awareness Program: a national survey of painful and painless myocardial ischemia including results of antiischemic therapy. *Am J Cardiol* 63:534-539, 1989
200. Stone PH, Gibson RS, Glasser SP, et al: Comparison of propranolol, diltiazem, and nifedipine in the treatment of ambulatory ischemia in patients with stable angina: differential effects on ambulatory ischemia, exercise performance, and anginal symptoms. *Circulation* 82:1962-1972, 1990
201. Ardissino D, Savonitto S, Egstrup K, et al: Transient myocardial ischemia during daily life in rest and exertional angina pectoris and comparison of effectiveness of metoprolol versus nifedipine. *Am J Cardiol* 67:946-952, 1991
202. Task Force of the Working Group on Arrhythmias of the European Society of Cardiology: CAST and beyond: implications of the Cardiac Arrhythmia Suppression Trial. *Circulation* 81:1123-1127, 1990
203. Pepine CJ, Cohn PF, Deedwania PC, et al: The prognostic and economic implications of a strategy to detect and treat asymptomatic ischemia. The Atenolol Silent Ischemia Trial (ASIST) protocol. *Clin Cardiol* 14:457-462, 1991
204. Fox KM, Mulcahy DA: Therapeutic rationale for the management of silent ischemia. *Circulation* 82 Suppl 2:155-160, 1990
205. Pepine CJ, Kern MJ, Boden WE: Advisory group reports on silent myocardial ischemia, acute intervention after myocardial infarction, and postinfarction management. *Am J Cardiol* 69:41B-46B, 1992
206. Stern S, Cohn PF, Pepine CJ: Silent myocardial ischemia. *Curr Probl Cardiol* 18:301-359, 1993

CHAPTER

29

Myocardial ischemia clinical syndromes

B. Angina pectoris and coronary heart disease

Clarence Shub, M.D., Roger L. Click, M.D., Ph.D., and Michael D. McGoon, M.D.

INTRODUCTION

Definitions

Angina pectoris refers to a symptom complex that reflects transient inadequacy of myocardial blood flow. Myocardial ischemia may occur because of decreased myocardial blood supply or increased myocardial oxygen demand or, often, both. The anginal syndrome may be divided into several forms: (1) classic angina, (2) atypical angina, (3) angina equivalent, (4) variant or Prinzmetal's angina (coronary vasospasm), and (5) unstable angina. *Classic angina* consists of a transient discomfort or distressing sensation occurring in the precordium, typically provoked by exertion (in addition to other factors) and relieved promptly by rest and the use of nitrates. *Atypical angina* refers to a similar symptom complex but one that is different (atypical) in the usual provoking or alleviating factors, duration, or location of discomfort.

Angina equivalent refers to the sensation of dyspnea or, less commonly, fatigue or weakness as the sole or major manifestation of cardiac ischemia. This may be a frequent manifestation in the older patient. Some physicians also refer to an isolated pain referral pattern—for example, jaw or localized arm pain—as representing an anginal equivalent. *Variant* or *Prinzmetal's angina* refers to angina pectoris that occurs at rest, is usually prolonged, and often presents with certain stereotyped patterns such as nocturnal symptoms or symptoms that occur only after exercise. Variant angina is thought to be caused by coronary artery spasm (a transient narrowing of a major epicardial branch of a coronary artery) (see "Coronary artery spasm," below).

The features of classic angina are compared with those of variant angina in Table 29B-1. *Unstable angina* is a syndrome that is intermediate in severity between chronic stable angina and myocardial infarction. Its main feature and most common manifestation is angina at rest, but recent onset or changing pattern of angina also should be considered unstable.

Angina, by definition, is a transient clinical event and is not associated with clinically detectable myocardial necrosis. When angina pectoris is prolonged, however (that is, more than 30 to 60 minutes), as in some cases of unstable angina, small foci of myocardial necrosis may result yet remain unrecognized by standard clinical techniques. The prolonged anginal syndrome may then merge imperceptibly with the syndrome of acute myocardial infarction. Angina pectoris is usually related to coronary artery disease and may be associated with varying degrees of coronary narrowing, ranging from

Table 29B-1 Comparison of classic and variant angina

Factor	Classic angina	Variant angina
Onset of symptoms	Exertional	Rest
Time of day	Variable	Usually nocturnal
ECG	ST depression	ST elevation*
Subsequent myocardial infarction	Common	Rare
Exercise stress test	Provokes pain and ECG abnormalities	Usually no pain, rare ECG abnormalities†
Treatment	Nitrates, β-blockers, calcium antagonists	Nitrates, calcium antagonists (β-blockers may worsen symptoms)

*ST depression may also occur in some patients with variant angina.
†On occasion, ECG abnormalities such as ventricular tachycardia and ST elevation or depression may occur late in the postexercise recovery period.

single-vessel disease to severe, extensive, and diffuse disease.

PATHOPHYSIOLOGY OF ANGINA PECTORIS

Although the terms "myocardial ischemia" and "angina" are not synonymous (that is, a patient may have ischemia without angina), it is generally accepted that angina pectoris is due to myocardial ischemia. The ischemia, in turn, results from an imbalance between the energy supply and demand in the heart. Because of the aerobic nature of myocardial metabolism and the ability of the heart to extract more oxygen from the blood than any other organ, oxygen supply is dependent primarily on coronary blood flow rather than on increasing oxygen extraction. Myocardial ischemia therefore occurs because of decreased myocardial blood flow or increased myocardial oxygen demand (in the presence of either "fixed" coronary stenosis or an increase in coronary vascular tone)[1-4] or, as in many patients, a combination of these factors (Table 29B-2).

Exertional angina is primarily related to an increased myocardial oxygen demand. During spontaneous attacks of angina, the rate-pressure product* is variable.[6] Thus, angina may occur at levels of workload well tolerated at other times. Ambulatory electrocardiographic (ECG) recordings in patients with chronic stable angina show that the heart rate at the onset of ischemic episodes during routine daily activities frequently varies by 20 beats/min or more.[5,7] Factors that modulate the ischemic threshold in such patients are shown in Table 29B-3. Furthermore, a vasospastic mechanism of rest angina has been demonstrated in these patients.[14] Patients with coronary heart disease may have limited coronary vasodilatory reserve, and superimposed coronary vasoconstriction may contribute to myocardial ischemia.[1,15]

Coronary spasm has been implicated in attacks of rest angina associated with ST depression[16] and, less commonly, in exertional angina as well.[17,18] The variable interplay of both mechanisms has been referred to as "mixed angina."[19]

Cardiac pain has been assumed to be transmitted primarily via afferent cardiac sympathetic nerves. In the spinal cord, these cardiac nerves join somatic cervical thoracic nerves in the same ascending spinal pathways, and this probably accounts for the phenomenon of referred pain (Fig 29B-1). Experimentally, cardiac afferent fibers, which appear to arise from the coronary arteries, can be excited by various mechanical (for example, coronary occlusion) and chemical (for example, bradykinin) stimuli.

Not infrequently, hypertension and tachycardia, presumably of reflex sympathetic origin, can appear simultaneously with ECG signs of ischemia and can precede (or follow) chest pain.[20]

Myocardial ischemia is a complex process. Possibilities exist for a variety of potential interconnecting "vicious cycles" to occur (Fig 29B-2).

Myocardial ischemia can cause ventricular systolic dysfunction ("pump failure"), diastolic dysfunction (decreased ventricular compliance and impaired filling), or both. Increased left ventricular filling pressure may aggravate ischemia by reducing the coronary perfusion gradient. Myocardial ischemia can also cause ventricular ectopy or sustained tachyarrhythmias, and the tachyarrhythmias, in turn, can worsen the ischemia.

*The product of heart rate times systolic blood pressure, referred to either as "double product" or more properly as "rate-pressure product," reflects myocardial oxygen demand. For a given patient, it tends to reach a constant level at the onset of angina,[5] unless there is superimposed coronary spasm or progression of coronary artery disease. Thus, the type of exercise may differ, but one may still characterize the imposed oxygen demand by using this simple calculation.

Table 29B-2 Determinants of myocardial oxygen supply and demand

Parameter	Determinant
Coronary blood flow	Coronary resistance
	Fixed stenosis
	Dynamic vascular tone
	Left ventricular wall stress
	Coronary perfusion pressure
	Duration of diastole
Myocardial oxygen consumption	Left ventricular wall tension*
	Preload
	Afterload
	Contractile state
	Heart rate

*Tension = transmural pressure x radius.

NATURAL HISTORY OF CORONARY HEART DISEASE

Coronary heart disease is prevalent throughout North America, Western Europe, and other industrialized countries (except Japan).

Table 29B-3 Factors that modulate the ischemia threshold

"Dynamic" coronary stenoses[2,8]
Vasomotor changes in distal coronary vessels (including arteriolar "resistance" vessels)[3]
Transmural distribution of myocardial perfusion[9]
- Adenosine-mediated coronary artery dilatation of nonischemic regions[10]
- β_2-Adrenergic subepicardial coronary artery dilatation[11]
- α_2-Adrenergic subendocardial vasoconstriction[12]
- Changes in prearteriolar coronary vessels[13]

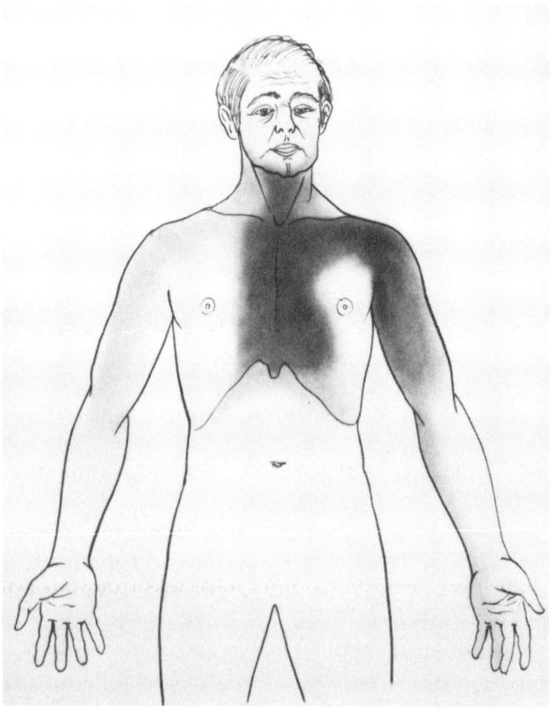

Fig 29B-1 Patterns of referred pain in the anginal syndrome. Only the anterior surface of the chest and volar surfaces of the arm are shown. Pain occurs more often in the heavily shaded than the lightly shaded zones. Pain can also occur in the upper back and the posterolateral surfaces of the arms. See text.

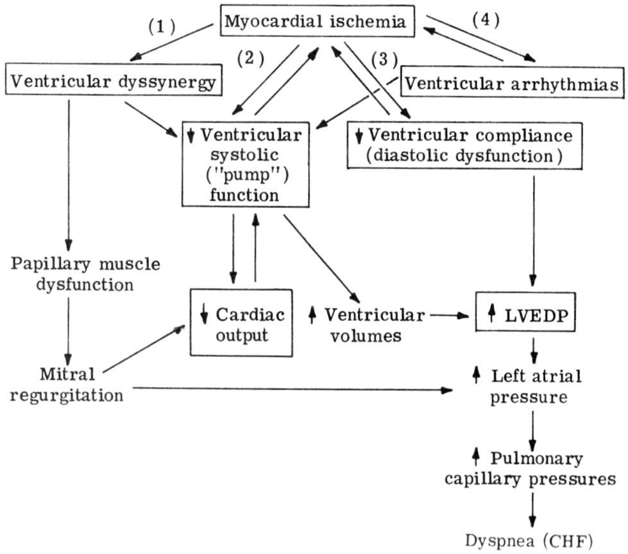

Fig 29B-2 Potential pathophysiologic consequences of myocardial ischemia. *LVEDP,* left ventricular end-diastolic pressure. Numbers in parentheses indicate the following: (1) ischemia-induced ventricular dyssynergy may cause papillary muscle dysfunction and mitral regurgitation or decreased systolic function; (2) ischemia-induced left ventricular "pump" failure may further aggravate ischemia if LVEDP increases or cardiac output decreases, which in turn may lead to further decrease in coronary flow; (3) ischemia-induced decreases in left ventricular compliance may cause increased LVEDP, which in turn may aggravate subendocardial ischemia; (4) ischemia may cause ventricular arrhythmias, which, by decreasing cardiac output, may in turn worsen ischemia.

In the Framingham study,[21] angina was the presenting symptom of coronary heart disease in 61% of the women and 38% of the men. Eight years later, 50% of the men with angina over the age of 45 years had evidence of myocardial infarction. The mortality for patients with angina was 4% per year (44% of these deaths were sudden). Mortality has been shown to be increased for men and patients who have risk factors such as hypertension, previous myocardial infarction, and abnormal ECGs.[22] Previous studies of patients with angina showed an annual mortality of 7% for men and 5% for women over the predicted death rate.[23]

More recent studies have shown that in patients with coronary heart disease who have not undergone coronary artery bypass surgery, the annual mortality has decreased somewhat to approximately 3% to 4%. Survival has improved for medically treated patients, especially those with mild coronary heart disease and low risk. Patients at high risk benefit from coronary revascularization.[24]

Among patients with coronary heart disease, prognosis for survival depends on several factors (Table 29B-4).

Interestingly, the severity and duration of symptoms in patients with coronary heart disease are not related to prognosis. The absence of symptoms does not exclude severe coronary heart disease; conversely, the presence of severe angina may be associated with one-, two-, or three-vessel coronary artery disease.[27,28]

THE SYNDROME OF ANGINA PECTORIS

Clinical description[29]

The symptom complex of angina pectoris can be quite variable. In any given patient, however, fairly predictable and consistent patterns may occur.

Anatomic location of anginal symptoms (patterns of referred pain). The various patterns of referred cardiac pain may make the diagnosis of angina pectoris very challenging. Possible areas of referred pain are shown in Figure 29B-1. Discomfort occurs in certain zones more commonly than in others. For example, substernal and left arm distress are more common than isolated shoulder, jaw, or right arm discomfort. As a general rule, left-sided chest discomfort is more common than right-sided discomfort. Isolated left precordial pain is less common than centrally located (substernal) pain. Not infrequently, the patient will describe a diffuse anterior chest pain coursing between the breasts. Jaw pain, when it occurs, is most often central and mandibular rather than maxillary. Angina only very rarely causes pain referable to the temporomandibular joints or forehead. Exceptions occur and can be dramatic—for example, unilateral pain referred to the jaw,[30] which can be misdiagnosed as tooth pain from dental caries and result in repeated dental examinations and even extractions.

Quality and duration of anginal symptoms. The original use of the term "angina" was applied more to a sensation of strangling or constriction than to actual pain. Like its other characteristics, the quality and duration of angina pectoris may vary considerably from patient to patient and within the same patient. At times, the patient may refuse to call the symptoms "painful," finding it difficult and even frustrating to describe the exact nature of the discomfort. Any of the following descriptive terms may be elicited from the patient, either alone or in combination: "pressure," "heaviness," "fullness," "a feeling like a weight," "squeezing," "burning," "ache," "just a pain," or "gas." Some patients clench a fist over the sternum in trying to describe the sensation. It is usually reported to be a "dull" (implying visceral etiology) rather than a "sharp" sensation. Angina is not influenced by respiration. Brief, sharp, stabbing precordial sensations that last only a few seconds and are unrelated to exertion are unlikely to be anginal.

Some patients experience dyspnea as the primary complaint (angina equivalent), and some are unable to differentiate dyspnea from chest discomfort. At times, both dyspnea and angina may occur. Dyspnea, in this circumstance, may reflect transient left ventricular dysfunction induced by ischemia. Dyspnea as an angina equivalent should be similar to typical angina in the manner in which it can be provoked and relieved.

Table 29B-4 Factors determining prognosis in patients with coronary heart disease

Extent and severity of coronary disease
Left ventricular function[25]
Left ventricular wall motion score*
Presence of ventricular ectopy
Ischemia on stress testing[26]

*Wall motion score is a regional assessment of left ventricular function determined by ventriculography or echocardiography.

A change in quality and severity of symptoms, especially if it is preceded by a stable symptom complex, may suggest increasing ischemia. For example, a patient who has had stable exertion-related chest "pressure" who suddenly gets "crushing" precordial pain occurring at rest, especially if prolonged and severe, is most likely experiencing a more severe ischemic episode and possibly is in the early phases of myocardial infarction.

Severity. The severity of anginal discomfort varies widely from slight distress to disabling pain. Most patients with chronic, stable angina do not have exquisite pain (like that of biliary or renal colic). Many patients can stop their provoking activity (such as exertion) and rest momentarily or take nitroglycerin and thereby obtain prompt relief from their symptoms. In some patients the discomfort may be severe enough to hamper normal activities, cause unacceptable work disability, and also render them unable to pursue other normal lifestyle activities (disabling angina).

Frequency. Some patients with angina pectoris have daily symptoms, whereas others have less frequent symptoms, perhaps less than once a week. Some have varying frequency of symptoms and so may find it difficult to characterize the exact number of attacks.

If possible, it is useful to classify the severity of the angina. Two simple classifications, which are applicable primarily for classic, effort-related angina and are quite similar, are shown in Tables 29B-5 and 29B-6. The limitations of this classification include the inability to classify patients who are not accurate observers, the overlap between classes, and the inapplicability of this system for the patient who does not have typical exertion-related angina.

An increase in the frequency of angina is an important clinical observation, which generally implies more severe ischemia. One method of gauging the frequency of angina is to ask the patient about the pattern of nitroglycerin consumption. An increase in the "tempo" of the angina pattern, nocturnal or rest angina, and ST-T wave abnormalities are predictive of future adverse cardiac events.[31] Uncommonly, the frequency of angina may decrease spontaneously (without a change in provocative factors). The reason for this phenomenon is unclear. Some possibilities include development of collateral circulation,

Table 29B-5 Functional classification of angina pectoris*

Functional class	Occurrence of symptoms	Exercise tolerance (METs)†	Functional impairment
I	With unusual activity	7-8 (or more)	Minimal or none
II	With prolonged or slightly more than usual activity	5-6	Mild (can do light and general industrial work)
III	With usual activity of daily living	3-4	Moderate (may be able to do desk job)
IV	At rest	1-2	Severe (incapacitated)

*Modified from Hackett TP, Cassem NH: Psychologic aspects of rehabilitation following myocardial infarction. In *Rehabilitation of the Coronary Patient.* Edited by NK Wenger, HK Hellerstein. New York, John Wiley & Sons, 1978, pp 243-253.
†One metabolic equivalent (MET) = Vo_2 of 3.5 mL O_2/(kg · min) while patient is sitting.

Table 29B-6 Canadian Cardiovascular Society classification for angina pectoris

Class I	*Ordinary physical activity* (such as walking or climbing stairs) *does not cause angina.* Angina may occur with strenuous, rapid, or prolonged exertion (work or recreation).
Class II	There is *slight limitation of ordinary activity.* Angina may occur with walking or climbing stairs rapidly; walking uphill; walking or stair climbing after meals or in the cold, in the wind, or under emotional stress; walking more than two blocks on the level and climbing one flight of stairs at a normal pace under normal conditions.
Class III	There is *marked limitation of ordinary physical activity.* Angina may occur after walking one or two blocks on the level or climbing one flight of stairs in normal conditions at a normal pace.
Class IV	There is *inability to carry on any physical activity without discomfort; angina* may be present *at rest.*

unrecognized infarction of an ischemic zone, or the training effect of an exercise program.

Provocative factors

Factors that either decrease coronary blood flow or increase myocardial oxygen demand (see Tables 29B-2 and 29B-3) and thus cause angina are referred to as "provocative" factors. Commonly recognized provocative factors are shown in Table 29B-7.

Exertion. Exertion-provoked angina can be caused by two general categories of exercise: (1) dynamic (or isotonic) exercise and (2) static (or isometric) exercise. An example of the former is walking; an example of the latter is lifting heavy objects. Physical work may involve varying degrees of both types of activity. The myocardial oxygen demands during isometric exercise[33] generally exceed those during isotonic exercise. This difference is presumably due to the excess sympathetic nervous system response and the elevated blood pressure associated with isometric activity. Both types of exercise may occur together and interact so as to influence the "ischemic threshold" (Fig 29B-3) for the combined activity. For example, a patient with angina may be able to walk (dynamic exercise) for several city blocks before symptoms occur. However, if he or she carries heavy luggage at the same time (additional isometric load), angina, at an equivalent heart rate, may occur at a much shorter walking distance (lower workload) (see Fig 29B-3).

Ischemic threshold (see Fig 29B-3), tension-time index,[34] and rate-pressure product provide useful, objective

Table 29B-7 Provocative factors for angina

Exertion
Emotion, excitement
Mental stress
Eating
Cold, heat, humidity
Sexual intercourse
Nicotine*
Carbon monoxide
Thyrotoxicosis
Fever
Tachycardia
Anemia (hemoglobin <9-10 g/dL)

*The nicotine effect of cigarette smoking increases heart rate and systemic blood pressure and leads to reduced exercise capacity.[32]

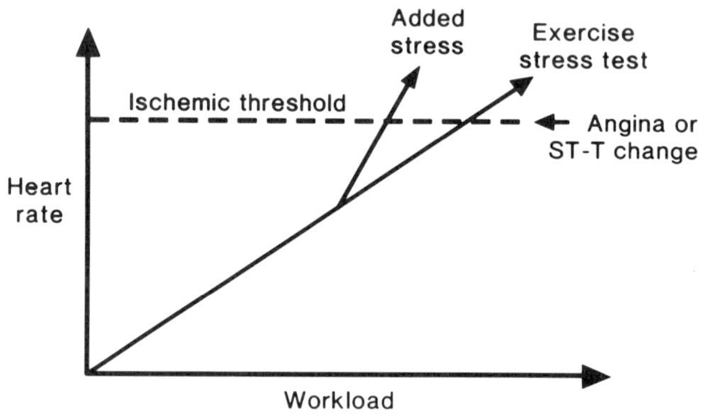

Fig 29B-3 Concept of ischemic threshold.

information regarding physical activities that provoke angina. Other things being equal, each physical activity causes a reproducible effect on the cardiovascular system in terms of myocardial oxygen demand. The level of physical activity which causes oxygen demand to exceed supply and thus causes myocardial ischemia is referred to as the anginal (if symptoms are produced) or ischemic threshold for that activity.

The concept of work-dependent anginal threshold, although useful, is limited by the observation that at times this threshold may vary. For example, a patient may report that at certain times of the day he or she may walk one block at the usual pace and experience angina and at other times may be able to walk several blocks before angina occurs. Differences in central autonomic neural output or other factors influencing coronary vasomotor tone (see Table 29B-2) may be responsible for this observation. The so-called second-wind phenomenon, in which a patient may be able to participate in a physical activity that just a short time before could not be undertaken, may also be an example of this.

At times, angina is provoked by physical activity involving only the upper extremities, such as hammering, painting, carpentry, and the like.

A cardinal feature of exercise-induced angina is the prompt abatement of symptoms, usually within a few minutes, when the physical activity ceases. Sublingual nitroglycerin taken on cessation of physical activity often hastens recovery, or sublingual nitroglycerin taken before an activity may prevent symptoms.

Emotions. Certain emotional reactions may provoke angina. The pathophysiologic mechanism for emotion-induced angina is an increase in myocardial oxygen demand due to increased heart rate and systemic blood pressure, which are themselves caused by enhanced sympathetic activity.[35] Autonomic-mediated increases in coronary vasomotor tone may also play a role.

In comparison with exertion-related angina, which usually abates promptly at the cessation of activity, emotion-related angina often persists for longer periods because the stimulus and response cannot be terminated as quickly.

Cold, heat, and humidity. Cold air may provoke angina at rest in as many as 50% of patients with coronary heart disease and even more often when exercise is combined with the exposure to cold. Cooling of the skin causes an increase in cardiac work which results from an increase in peripheral resistance.[36,37] Skin cooling seems to be a more important mechanism than inhaling moderately cold air (−10°C). Inhaling very cold air (−35°C), however, does cause changes in work capacity.[38] Exposing the face to cold air or immersing the hand in ice water provokes changes in peripheral vascular resistance, whereas cold air exposure limited to the abdomen does not.[39] The exact mechanism for cold-induced angina remains unclear.[40] Possibilities include an exaggerated arterial pressure and heart rate response to cold[41] and a cold-induced increase in coronary vasomotor tone.

Exercising in a hot, humid environment leads to a greater acceleration in heart rate for any given level of exercise.[42] Extreme degrees of humidity, regardless of temperature, may also provoke angina.[43]

Meals. Eating-induced angina usually occurs after a heavy meal and is often aggravated by exercise in the immediate postprandial period. The mechanism for eating-induced angina may be related to (1) a physiologic shift of blood flow to the vessels of the gastrointestinal tract, (2) a transient change in blood clotting and viscosity which occurs in response to postprandial hyperlipidemia,[44,45] (3) the effect of increased free-fatty acid levels on release of thromboxane and platelet aggregation,[46] and (4) a relatively greater than normal increase in heart rate and cardiac output with postprandial exercise.[47,48] Autonomic-mediated increases in coronary vasomotor tone may also play a role.

Sexual intercourse. The physiologic responses to sexual activity in coronary patients are the same as those in age-matched normals. An increase in rate-pressure product invariably occurs, but the spectrum of response is quite broad. The hemodynamic changes that occur during coitus are the net result of a moderate physical stress and an autonomic discharge of variable degree.

During coitus, there is in men an average heart rate of 101 beats/min (range, 90 to 144), or approximately 60% of maximal oxygen uptake as previously determined in the same patients by a bicycle exercise test.[49,50] Peak blood pressure and heart rate occur at orgasm,[51] but both rapidly decrease during the resolution phase. Hellerstein and Friedman[49] calculated that a maximum of 5 metabolic equivalents (METs) of activity was expended for less than 30 seconds, and an average of 3.7 METs was expended in the periods before and after orgasm. Thus, most patients with functional class II impairment (see Tables 29B-5 and 29B-6) can generally perform sexual intercourse without difficulty. Some class III patients, with proper treatment, may also be able to engage in sexual activities.

Sexual intercourse-induced angina generally occurs in either the orgasmic phase or, more commonly, immediately after orgasm in the resolution phase (that is, at or immediately after the occurrence of peak rate-pressure product). Hyperventilation-induced respiratory alkalosis that occurs during arousal and orgasm may cause coronary artery spasm or may adversely affect hemoglobin oxygen release. The actual incidence of coitus-induced angina in patients with coronary heart disease remains unknown; reported rates vary from approximately 20%[49,52] to as high as 65%.[53] Although deaths occur during coitus, they are apparently very rare.[54]

The use of nitrates before intercourse may prevent angina. Many of these patients will be taking either long-acting nitrates or other agents. β-Adrenergic blocking drugs may be useful under these circumstances but may cause impotence.

Characteristics of relief

When sublingual nitrates are effective, they almost always act promptly—within a few minutes—in accord with their rapid pharmacologic effect (see chapter 29C). Sometimes a second tablet is required for relief, however. The time within which relief occurs is of diagnostic value. Relief of symptoms which occurs only after 20 to 30 minutes or longer after use of sublingual nitrates suggests that the symptoms are not due to ischemia. Unfortunately, there are exceptions to this rule, and one cannot exclude a diagnosis of angina on this basis alone.

Carotid sinus pressure, by increasing vagal tone and slowing the heart rate, can bring about relief of pain in some patients and, if effective, is a useful bedside diagnostic maneuver. It must be applied cautiously, however, especially in patients with carotid or cerebrovascular disease and in the elderly, in whom a hypersensitive carotid sinus response may occur.

There is increasing evidence that the endogenous opiate system mediates the extent of pain sensation and relief. It is generally accepted that plasma endorphins act as natural analgesics and that different levels explain not only symptomatic (angina) and asymptomatic (silent) ischemia but also various degrees of exercise tolerance and individual relief of pain.[55]

Angina decubitus and nocturnal angina

Nocturnal angina may have more than one mechanism. Angina occurring within the first few hours of sleep appears to be similar to paroxysmal nocturnal dyspnea in its pathophysiology. Both symptoms are related to the increased cardiopulmonary blood volume of recumbency. Such patients often complain of dyspnea as well as angina, and they get relief by assuming the upright position in addition to taking nitroglycerin. Chest pain that occurs immediately after lying down is rarely due to ischemia.

A second type of nocturnal angina occurs during the later phases of sleep, especially in the early morning hours, and is associated with rapid eye movements and dreaming. This phase of sleep is characterized by pronounced fluctuations in heart rate and systemic blood pressure, presumably mediated by autonomic mechanisms.

DIFFERENTIAL DIAGNOSIS OF ANGINA

Noncardiovascular causes of chest pain (Table 29B-8)

Gastrointestinal. *Esophageal disorders,* especially if associated with esophageal spasm, may mimic angina pectoris.[56,57] Both diseases, which may coexist in about 20% of patients, may cause epigastric and substernal symptoms, be relieved by nitroglycerin, and cause radiation of pain to the neck, jaw, or arms. Whereas stooping or bending may provoke symptoms as a result of esophageal reflux, other types of physical exertion, such as walking or climbing stairs, usually do not. Symptoms due to esophageal reflux are more likely to occur soon after assuming the recumbent position and especially after eating a heavy meal or certain foods, whereas recumbent angina (angina decubitus) usually occurs a few hours after reclining or falling asleep. Esophageal reflux symptoms are often relieved by antacids; angina is not. An esophageal acid perfusion test, if it reproduces the patient's symptoms, may be helpful diagnostically. Similarly, *peptic ulcer disease* and *gastritis* can be differentiated from angina by their lack of relationship to exertion and by their response to antacids and specific foods.

Cholecystitis, especially if chronic, can be difficult to differentiate from atypical angina. Recurrent nocturnal attacks of epigastric pain, especially if the patient paces in an agitated manner, suggest gallbladder disease. The patient with nocturnal angina prefers to sit up and take nitroglycerin but only rarely prefers to pace back and forth. The diagnostic difficulty is increased if the patient has simultaneous cholelithiasis and coronary heart disease, especially since attacks of cholecystitis may precipitate angina. At times, it is impossible to separate the symptoms of atypical angina from chronic, recurrent attacks of cholecystitis, and elective cholecystectomy is then indicated.

Neuromusculoskeletal. Although classic *Tietze's syndrome* (painful swelling of the left costochondral junctions) is rare, *nonspecific chest wall pain* is common. Chest wall pain is often vaguely described, long in duration (lasting for hours or days), and usually not exertion related. Certain types of movement—for example, abduction or extension of the arms—may aggravate symptoms. Also, nonspecific chest wall pain is often aggravated by motion of the thorax, such as twisting or deep breathing; and variable tenderness, sometimes reproducing the symptoms, may be elicited by manual compression of the sternum or left anterior rib region. Nitroglycerin does not relieve these symptoms in any predictable manner. A therapeutic trial of heat, physical therapy, salicylates, or nonsteroidal anti-inflammatory agents may be helpful in both the diagnosis and the treatment of these conditions.

In comparison with the pain pattern of angina, *radiculopathic pain* is typically constant, and there may be associated abnormal neurologic signs. Similarly, *shoulder arthropathies* such as bursitis, tendinitis, and degenerative joint disease can cause continuous symptoms, and motion of the involved shoulder will typically aggravate them. In certain conditions, such as bicipital tendinitis, a localized zone of tenderness may be found, and local injection of anesthetic or steroid may aid in the diagnosis and provide relief.

Thoracic-respiratory. *Pneumothorax, mediastinitis,* and *pleuritis* present with sufficiently distinct clinical patterns that only rarely will there be diagnostic difficulty. The chronic chest pain of *intrathoracic malignancy* is usually continuous and does not have the precipitating or relief characteristics of angina.

Psychologic. Psychosomatization, conversion reactions, or malingering may cause diagnostic difficulty. The symptoms in these conditions are not as reproducible in terms of provocative or relief characteristics and can be quite bizarre. The patient with both coronary heart disease and psychologic difficulties can be difficult to manage. Exercise stress testing may help identify which of the patient's various symptoms are due to ischemia. Some of these patients will improve if enrolled in an exercise program.

Table 29B-8 Differential diagnosis of chest pain syndromes

- Cardiovascular
- Gastrointestinal
  - Esophageal disorders (esophagitis, esophageal spasm, hiatal hernia)
  - Peptic ulcer disease
  - Gastritis
  - Cholecystitis
- Neuromusculoskeletal
  - Costochondritis (Tietze's syndrome)
  - Chest wall pain
  - Cervical or thoracic radiculopathy
  - Shoulder arthropathies
- Thoracic-respiratory
  - Pneumothorax
  - Mediastinitis
  - Pleuritis
  - Intrathoracic malignancy
- Psychologic

Cardiovascular causes of chest pain other than coronary heart disease (Table 29B-9)

Angina occurs in approximately 50% to 60% of cases of *aortic stenosis,*[58] is usually exertional, and is indistinguishable from that due to coronary artery disease. It too is a result of excessive myocardial oxygen demand for the available supply. Angina due to coronary heart disease is more common with aortic valve disease than with mitral valve disease.[59] Angina is less common in *aortic regurgitation* than in aortic stenosis and is more often atypical. Angina in these patients can occur with or without concomitant coronary artery disease. Angina in *hypertrophic cardiomyopathy* may be related to subendocardial ischemia with or without coexisting coronary artery disease. The frequency of coronary artery disease in hypertrophic cardiomyopathy is as high as 25% in patients over the age of 40 years but is uncommon in young females.[60] Angina is relatively uncommon (approximately 10%) in patients with *idiopathic dilated cardiomyopathy,* and its mechanism is unclear. End-stage ischemic heart disease with dilated ventricles may at times be indistinguishable from idiopathic dilated cardiomyopathy on clinical grounds alone.

The chest pain of *pericarditis* is typically affected by certain positions and by respiration. Fever and a pericardial rub may be found, and there are usually diffuse and characteristic ECG abnormalities. The pain of *aortic dissection* is severe, excruciating, and abrupt in onset, rather than slowly waxing and waning in intensity as in angina. It may migrate after a short time to the back or abdomen. A younger patient may have a marfanoid habitus, and an older patient will usually be hypertensive. Although the chest pain of aortic dissection is typically abrupt in onset and severe, the patient may present with subacute, atypical chest pain. A high degree of clinical suspicion is warranted, especially in a hypertensive patient. Careful evaluation of the aortic shadow on chest radiographs is important, especially before exercise testing, because such testing can be hazardous in patients with aortic dissection.

The acute chest pain of *pulmonary embolus* often occurs in a specific clinical setting, such as after prolonged immobilization or after hip surgery. Although the clinical findings of acute pulmonary embolus may be quite variable, the patient is often severely ill with dyspnea, tachypnea, and cyanosis, in which case the differential diagnosis might include acute myocardial infarction.

Patients with *pulmonary hypertension,* either primary or secondary, may have symptoms that are interpreted as representing angina. The clinical, ECG, chest x-ray, and echocardiographic findings are helpful in the evaluation.

There is a subset of patients who have *angina pectoris and normal coronary anatomy* (as assessed by coronary arteriography) without spontaneous or ergonovine-induced epicardial coronary spasm. Terms such as "syndrome X,"[61] "microvascular angina,"[62] and "impaired coronary reserve" have been used to describe the condition in these patients. These patients, many of whom are female, have a good prognosis.[63] In long-term follow-up, the incidence of myocardial infarction is very low (<2%). Nearly half the patients have diminished chest pain. Symptoms are unchanged in one-fourth and worse in 29%. Patients with a "slow flow" phenomenon on coronary angiography are more likely to have constant or worse chest pain at follow-up.[64]

Approximately 20% of these patients have ST-T wave abnormalities during exercise testing and may have abnormal left ventricular function responses to exercise as assessed by radionuclide angiography.[65] The cause of the angina is unknown. "Small vessel disease" of the myocardium, hemoglobin-oxygen dissociation defects, coronary adrenergic hyperactivity,[66] a variant of the hyperdynamic heart syndrome, altered pain sensation,[67,68] and endothelial dysfunction[69] are some of the mechanisms that have been proposed. Intravenous administration of dipyridamole may precipitate angina in these patients. An inadequate coronary vasodilator response to pacing and a failure of coronary vessels to dilate normally after dipyridamole administration have been described. Some of these patients respond to calcium-entry blocker therapy,[70] others to tricyclic antidepressant agents or β-blockers.[71]

Table 29B-9 Cardiovascular causes of chest pain

Coronary artery disease (atherosclerotic and nonatherosclerotic)
Aortic valve disease (aortic stenosis or insufficiency)
Cardiomyopathy
Hypertrophic obstructive
Dilated
Pericarditis
Aortic dissection and aneurysm
Pulmonary embolism
Pulmonary hypertension

PHYSICAL EXAMINATION

General physical examination

The results of a general physical examination may provide important diagnostic insights in a patient with angina. For example, the presence of xanthomas or xanthelasma, especially in a young patient, should raise the possibility of familial hypercholesterolemia. Similarly, arcus cornealis, especially in white patients younger than 50 years old, is a stigma of hyperlipidemia. The finding of arcus cornealis has much less specificity in blacks and in the elderly.

Evidence of peripheral vascular occlusive disease—carotid or femoral bruits or a history of claudication—suggests that diffuse arteriosclerosis obliterans may be present and thus increases the possibility that simultaneous obstructive coronary artery disease is present.

A deep, husky voice with slowed speech in an overweight patient who has dry skin and thinning of the eyebrows laterally should suggest hypothyroidism. The presence of hypothyroidism increases the possibility of coronary heart disease and also has therapeutic implications. Similarly, the presence of systemic hypertension has important diagnostic and therapeutic implications, since increased blood pressure accelerates atherosclerosis and lowering of blood pressure may, by itself, significantly decrease the frequency of angina. Anemia, which may be suspected from the general clinical examination (appearance of the skin, conjunctivae, and so on), may exacerbate angina because of the associated decrease in myocardial oxygen delivery.

Physical findings on cardiac examination (Table 29B-10)

Palpation of the precordium. In the supine position, precordial palpation permits an estimate of cardiac size. Even more information is gained by palpating the apical impulse with the patient in the left lateral decubitus position. The apical impulse reflects the motion of the anteroapical left ventricular wall as it strikes the thoracic wall during contraction. Using this simple palpation technique at the bedside, one may assess the width and contour of the apical impulse. For example, a widened apical impulse implies left ventricular enlargement, and a presystolic impulse ("a" wave) suggests the presence of a vigorous atrial contraction into a poorly compliant left ventricle. A sustained impulse may reflect a large akinetic or dyskinetic left ventricular segment or left ventricular hypertrophy. In some patients, a delayed systolic outward bulge (signifying a dyskinetic segment) may be found only during an attack of angina pectoris. A triple impulse consisting of a prominent "a" wave and a bifid ventricular systolic wave should lead one to suspect hypertrophic obstructive cardiomyopathy. Less commonly in patients with coronary heart disease, a left parasternal (right ventricular) lift may be detected when secondary pulmonary hypertension is present. The frequency with which these abnormalities are detected (and they may be quite subtle) varies with the experience, skill, and diligence of the examiner.

Table 29B-10 Cardiac abnormalities detected on physical examination in patients with angina pectoris*

Finding	May be present on routine examination†	May be present during angina only†
Palpation		
Prominent "a" wave	+ +	+
Sustained apical impulse	+	±
Double impulse (late systolic bulge)‡	+	+
Widened impulse	+	±
Rapid filling wave	+	±
Auscultation		
Decreased intensity of S_1§	±	±
Paradoxic split S_2	+	+
Increased P_2	+	±
S_4	+ +	+
S_3‖	+	+
Systolic murmur (mitral regurgitation)	+	+
Diastolic murmur (CAVF)¶	±	−

*Frequency of these abnormalities is increased when special recording devices are used such as phonocardiography and apex cardiography.
†+ +, common; +, occasional; ±, rare; −, usually does not occur.
‡A double impulse, if subtle, may seem to the examiner like a sustained left ventricular impulse; both imply dyskinetic contraction of the left ventricle.
§Decreased S_1 may be better appreciated during serial examinations of the same patient.
‖Presence of S_3 implies severe left ventricular dysfunction.
¶CAVF, coronary arteriovenous fistula (in the absence of mitral stenosis or aortic regurgitation).

Auscultation. Although a softening of the mitral component of S_1 may occur with ischemic left ventricular dysfunction, it is only rarely detected at the bedside. A paradoxically split S_2 (in the absence of left bundle-branch block) is uncommon and generally reflects left ventricular asynergy with global left ventricular dysfunction. A paradoxically split S_2 may be heard only during an anginal episode, in which case, like the transient murmur of papillary muscle dysfunction (see below), it may prove of diagnostic value. S_4, which is generally best heard at the site of maximal apical impulse, is very common in patients with coronary heart disease and presumably reflects decreased left ventricular compliance and an elevated left ventricular end-diastolic pressure. It can also be found in some adults who have no known coronary heart disease, and it increases in frequency in the elderly. If, however, by precordial palpation, a prominent apical "a" wave is also found, this suggests that the audible S_4 is pathologically significant, regardless of the patient's age.

In contrast to the frequent finding of S_4 in patients with coronary heart disease, an audible S_3 at rest is less commonly heard (in the absence of overt congestive heart failure or significant mitral or aortic regurgitation). The S_3 is associated with increased middiastolic in addition to end-diastolic pressure.[72] This finding has clinical relevance, since the S_3 implies left ventricular failure. The presence of left ventricular failure due to ischemia suggests severe coronary heart disease with reduced left ventricular ejection fraction and implies a poor prognosis. Rarely, both S_4 and S_3 may be heard at the same time, or S_3 may be found without concomitant S_4. After medical treatment (for example, with nitrates or diuretics), the S_3 may decrease or disappear, only to return during subsequent bouts of cardiac decompensation. S_4 usually persists despite therapy, although its intensity may vary.

A systolic nonejection click (at times followed by a late systolic murmur) may be heard and represents a form of secondary mitral valve prolapse associated with papillary muscle dysfunction.[72] In this situation, myxomatous degeneration of the mitral valve, the pathologic substrate for primary mitral valve prolapse, is not present. However, the latter condition also may be found in patients with coronary heart disease.

If carefully sought, an apical systolic murmur, indicating mitral regurgitation, can be found. It may be due to (1) papillary muscle dysfunction (most often), (2) dilatation of the mitral valve annulus in cases of dilated left ventricles, or (3) other, nonrelated, abnormalities of the mitral valve apparatus, such as calcified mitral annulus (especially in the elderly). The apical systolic murmur of mitral regurgitation in coronary heart disease may be quite localized and soft. It can be missed on initial examination, only to be heard later, perhaps after an exercise test or during an episode of angina. Patients with severe left ventricular failure and low cardiac output may have concomitant ischemia-related mitral regurgitation (resulting from papillary muscle dysfunction), which may be underestimated or even undetected ("silent" mitral regurgitation). At times, the mitral regurgitation murmur may be misinterpreted as an aortic outflow murmur, especially in the elderly.

The presence of a systolic and diastolic murmur, especially in a young patient with angina, should raise the possibility of aortic regurgitation or coronary arteriovenous fistula. A localized diastolic murmur (in the absence of aortic regurgitation), although very rare, has been described and presumably represents turbulent blood flow across a severely stenotic coronary artery.

STANDARD DIAGNOSTIC TESTS[73]

Electrocardiogram

The ECG remains an important and relatively inexpensive standard diagnostic test for patients with angina. Possible abnormal findings include (1) prior myocardial infarction (pathologic Q waves), (2) presence of resting ischemia (ST-T abnormalities), and (3) disorders of atrioventricular or intraventricular conduction (P-R interval, atrioventricular block, QRS frontal plane axis deviation, bundle-branch block, and others).

These findings are not specific for coronary heart disease. Pseudoinfarction patterns can be seen with other disease states, such as amyloid heart disease or hypertrophic cardiomyopathy. ST-T abnormalities may be found in cases of mitral valve prolapse, left ventricular hypertrophy, dilated cardiomyopathy, myocarditis, hypokalemia, and other disorders. In the elderly, conduction disorders occur more commonly in primary (sclerodegenerative) disorders of the conduction system.

The resting ECG may be normal in patients with angina due to coronary heart disease (one-, two-, or three-vessel coronary involvement). Even patients with a history of severe angina may show ST-T abnormalities only during chest pain. Patients with significant left ventricular asynergy, however, only rarely have an entirely normal ECG.[74]

The most common ECG finding in patients with coronary heart disease is nonspecific repolarization (ST-T-wave) abnormality. Left axis deviation, left ventricular conduction delay, and ventricular ectopic beats can also be seen. Abnormal Q waves, indicating prior myocardial infarction, may be found, but Q waves may attenuate or even disappear over time.[75]

It has been suggested that in patients with coronary heart disease, the presence of left ventricular hypertrophy on the ECG is uncommon, and if left ventricular hypertrophy is found, one should consider the possibility of another disease process, such as aortic stenosis, hypertrophic obstructive cardiomyopathy, or hypertension. In a group of patients with end-stage ischemic heart disease (so-called ischemic cardiomyopathy), we have found ECG evidence of left ventricular hypertrophy, sometimes in combination with left ventricular conduction delay (unpublished observations). These findings may reflect increased left ventricular mass.

Certain ventricular conduction abnormalities occur in association with ECG evidence of prior myocardial infarction (postinfarction intraventricular conduction delay), especially anterior infarction. Left axis deviation is the most common ventricular conduction abnormality. Left bundle-branch block due to ischemic heart disease is also common and has been correlated with an increased incidence of congestive heart failure and cardiomegaly.[75] The presence of ventricular conduction defects—for example, left bundle-branch block—in addition to abnormal Q waves and resting ischemic ST-T-wave abnormalities has been associated with a poor prognosis.

Notches of the QRS complex may represent myocardial fibrosis and thus be relics of prior infarction. This depolarization abnormality is nonspecific, however, and may be seen in other cardiac diseases (myocardial fibrosis, left ventricular hypertrophy, cardiomyopathy, and others). Left atrial enlargement has also been described in patients with coronary heart disease.[76]

Obtaining an ECG during chest pain and finding new ST-T-wave abnormalities can be extremely helpful from a diagnostic standpoint in patients with angina due either to coronary heart disease or to coronary spasm. Resting U-wave inversion has been reported to be predictive of significant left anterior descending or left main coronary artery disease.[77] New T-wave inversions in the anterior precordial leads found during angina suggest left anterior descending coronary artery disease. The ECG may show only nonspecific abnormalities or even remain normal if the ischemia is due to left circumflex coronary artery disease.[78]

The presence of ECG evidence of prior myocardial infarction has been correlated with both the severity and the extent of coronary artery disease. Also, the localization of an infarct by ECG (anterior vs. inferior) correlates well with localization of lesions in a particular coronary artery (left anterior descending vs. right coronary artery). The absence of ECG evidence of myocardial infarction does not imply absence of extensive coronary artery disease.

Chest x-ray findings

Although the chest x-ray film is usually normal in patients with coronary heart disease, cardiomegaly (with or without evidence of pulmonary congestion) may be found in as many as 15% of patients.[75] Cardiomegaly in such patients is usually related to a history of congestive heart failure and prior myocardial infarction and is associated with an adverse prognosis. In a group of patients with end-stage ischemic heart disease (unpublished observations), we found that an increased cardiothoracic ratio on a chest x-ray film was a powerful predictor of increased mortality.

Occasionally, mild to moderate cardiac enlargement on the chest x-ray film may occur without a history of congestive heart failure.[75] Many such patients will have evidence of prior myocardial infarction. The cardiac enlargement is due primarily to left ventricular dilatation, but left or even right atrial enlargement may contribute to the enlarged cardiac silhouette on the posteroanterior view. Left ventricular hypertrophy or associated valvular abnormalities (mitral regurgitation, for example) may also contribute to cardiac enlargement in some patients. Valve calcification or an abnormality of left ventricular contour suggesting left ventricular aneurysm can sometimes be found on the routine chest radiograph.

SPECIAL DIAGNOSTIC TESTS

Stress testing

Stress testing plays a critical role in the diagnosis of patients with coronary heart disease (see also chapter 3B). In most cases, the diagnostic aim of stress testing is to increase cardiac workload. This can be accomplished by physiologic stress testing, for example, treadmill or bicycle stress tests, or pharmacologic stress testing, for example, intravenous infusion of dipyridamole, adenosine, or dobutamine. Under controlled circumstances, the clinical response and ECG changes are observed. In addition, cardiac imaging with echocardiography or radionuclide techniques can be used to determine coronary flow reserve. The ultimate goal is to differentiate a normal response from an ischemic one. For patients with ischemia, classification into high-, intermediate-, and low-risk subsets is helpful. For patients with a high-risk response, coronary angiography testing may be indicated. The results must be interpreted in the overall context of each patient's symptoms, expectations, prognosis, and risks.

Exercise ECG stress testing. If an adequate workload is achieved, the sensitivity of exercise ECG stress testing for the diagnosis of coronary artery disease ranges from 62% to 80% (average, about 65%) and the specificity from 77% to 96% (average, about 85%).[79-81]

Variables assessed and end points include workload and duration of exercise, ST-segment and T-wave changes, blood pressure and heart rate response, and symptoms (chest pain or dyspnea). Exercise-induced downsloping ST-segment depression indicates two- or three-vessel coronary artery disease more often than does horizontal or upsloping ST-segment depression.[82] Exercise-induced ST-segment elevation may indicate (1) severe transmural myocardial ischemia, (2) worsening segmental wall motion abnormality in an area of previous myocardial infarction, or (3) exercise-induced coronary spasm. In the general population, the ST-segment re-

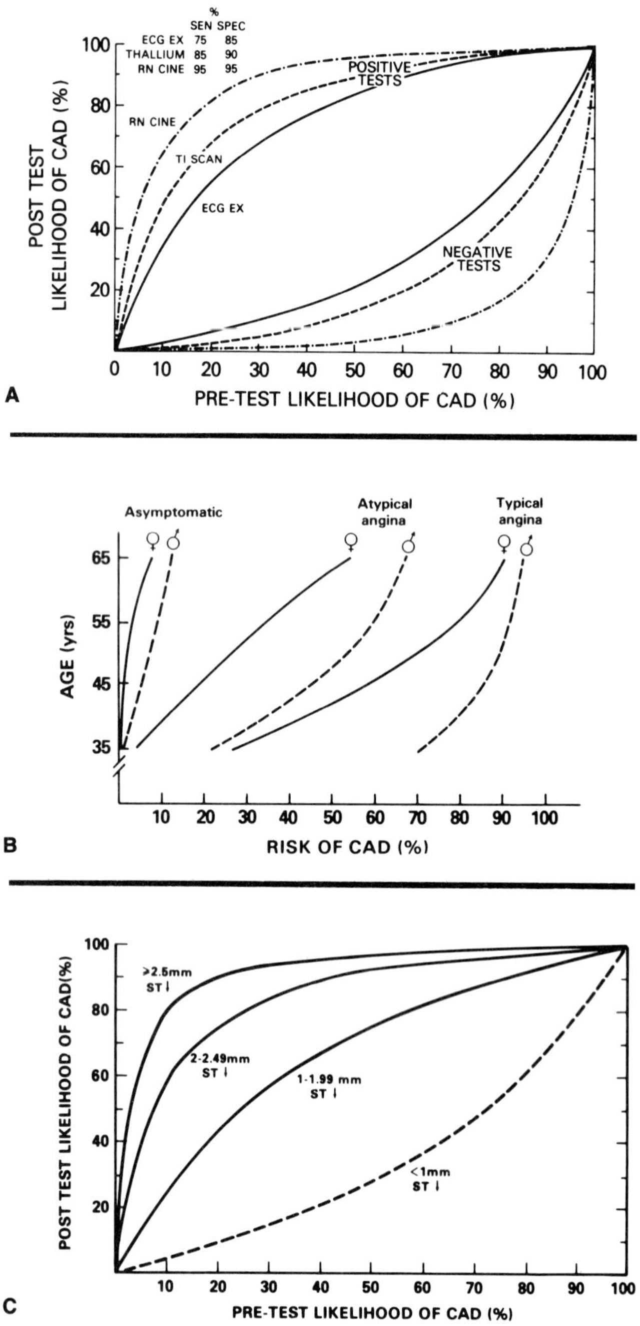

Fig 29B-4 Assessing the likelihood of coronary artery disease *(CAD).* **A,** effect of combining the exercise electrocardiogram *(ECG EX),* thallium scanning *(Tl scan),* and radionuclide angiography *(RN CINE)* on the pretest and posttest likelihood of coronary artery disease. **B,** interactive influence of age, symptoms, and sex on the risk of coronary artery disease. **C,** effect of the degree of ST-segment abnormality induced on exercise stress testing on the likelihood of coronary artery disease. (From Epstein SE: Implications of probability analysis on the strategy used for noninvasive detection of coronary artery disease: role of single or combined use of exercise electrocardiographic testing, radionuclide cineangiography and myocardial perfusion imaging. *Am J Cardiol* 46:491-499, 1980. By permission of Technical Publishing Company.)

sponse is of greater predictive value than the duration of exercise, and the degree of ST-segment depression influences the likelihood of severe coronary artery disease (Fig 29B-4,C), whereas in patients with known coronary artery disease, the duration of exercise is of greater prognostic value.[83]

ECG or clinical signs suggesting significant ischemia induced by exercise are shown in Table 29B-11. The presence of these signs implies one or more of the following entities: multivessel coronary artery disease, left main coronary artery disease, and left ventricular dysfunction. An early positive ECG ischemic response (i.e., in the first stage of exercise) is predictive of future adverse cardiac events.[84,85] Patients with an abnormal early exercise response are more likely to have severe coronary artery disease and should be considered candidates for coronary angiography. The amount of exercise performed correlates with functional class and the degree of functional impairment.

Patients who are able to achieve stage IV of an exercise test without significant ST-T abnormalities have a low prevalence (23%) of three-vessel coronary artery disease and are very unlikely (1%) to have significant left main coronary artery disease. In addition, patients who are able to reach stage IV or a maximal heart rate of more than 160 beats/min have an excellent (94%) 4-year survival rate.[86]

Exercise-induced ventricular arrhythmias may occur during the test and prevent its completion. Simple ventricular ectopy during exercise testing is common and nonspecific and may even disappear during the test. However, in high-risk populations, it has a negative prognostic implication, especially if associated with ischemic ST-T wave abnormalities on the exercise ECG.[87] Exercise testing should be stopped if ischemic ST-segment changes and increasing or complex ventricular ectopy occur.

Observation of the patient by the physician during the exercise stress test has many advantages. In addition to assessing the ECG response, the physician can correlate the symptoms observed during the test with the patient's usual symptoms. This may clarify a diagnosis of atypical angina. Because of the wide variation (both emotional and physical) of human reactions to disease, patients differ in their willingness and ability to perform exercise. Some will go beyond their perceived limits, perhaps to please the physician or to "prove" themselves. Others may wish to stop prematurely and may need encouragement. The blood pressure response (cuff method) is monitored; a decrease in blood pressure usually indicates an inappropriately low cardiac output response to exercise and is an indication to stop the procedure. Although a decrease in systolic blood pressure during stress testing occurs most often in patients with severe coronary artery disease and ischemia-induced left ventricular dysfunction, it has also been noted in patients with cardiomyopathy, in those taking various drugs, e.g., calcium antagonists, in those during prolonged strenuous exercise, and even in some patients without coronary artery disease. A decrease in systolic blood pressure below the preexercise value was found to be associated with an adverse prognosis, whereas lesser degrees of exercise-induced hypotension had no predictive value.[88]

False-positive ECG responses can occur when the resting tracing is abnormal. They are most common when repolarization abnormalities due to digitalis, left ventricular hypertrophy, or bundle-branch block (especially left bundle-branch block) or an electrolyte abnormality such as hypokalemia is present. When the resting ECG is abnormal, an added imaging modality, either echocardiography or a radionuclide procedure, is generally preferable.

A level of exercise sufficient to induce ischemia must be achieved; otherwise, the test must be considered "inadequate" rather than "negative." Ordinarily, 85% to 90% of predicted maximal heart rate for age, sex, and level of conditioning should be achieved for a test result to be considered negative.

The use of β-adrenergic blockers (by blunting the exercise heart rate and blood pressure response) may confound the test results. Calcium-entry blockers and long-acting nitrates also may delay or mask the appearance of ischemic changes during exercise ECG testing. When the diagnosis is unclear, it is ideal, but not always practical, to taper or discontinue the use of cardiac drugs before exercise testing.

For patients unable to use their legs, dynamic arm exercise testing (arm-cycle ergometer) may be used as an alternative, but it seems to be less sensitive than leg exercise testing.[89] (Alternative methods of stress testing with pharmacologic agents for patients who cannot exercise are discussed in the next sections.)

Finally, once angina has been diagnosed, the exercise stress test can be used to assess functional capacity or to assess the adequacy of drug treatment.

Radionuclide procedures. The methods, indications, and uses of radionuclide procedures in the diagnosis of angina pectoris are discussed in chapter 6. To assist in the diagnosis of coronary heart disease, one can use currently available radionuclide tests, including technetium-labeled erythrocyte cardiac scintigraphy (either by gated blood-pool scanning or by the first-pass technique), also referred to as "radionuclide angiography," and thallium-201 or sestamibi myocardial perfusion scanning. There are advantages and disadvantages of each technique in the diagnosis of angina.

The resting radionuclide angiogram provides useful

Table 29B-11 Abnormal exercise electrocardiographic stress test results indicating severe ischemia

Greater than 2 mm of ST depression (flat or downsloping)
ST depression at low workloads
Persistent ST depression after discontinuing exercise
Exercise-induced hypotension
Low heart rate response ("chronotropic incompetence")
Exercise-induced S_3 gallop

information with regard to global (ejection fraction) and regional (assessment of regional wall motion abnormalities) left ventricular function. Ejection fractions obtained are reproducible and compare favorably with results of contrast angiography.

As with contrast ventriculography, the assessment of regional wall motion is subjective and is prone to variation both for technical reasons and because of interobserver differences in interpretation. The presence of regional wall motion abnormalities is not specific for coronary heart disease; regional variation in contractility can occur with other disease states such as cardiomyopathy and cardiac amyloid.

When coronary angiography is indicated and left ventricular contrast angiography is believed to represent an increased risk, as in cases of severe renal insufficiency or a failing left ventricle, alternative assessment of left ventricular systolic function can be made with radionuclide angiography or echocardiography.

For the diagnosis of angina, additional information is obtained when an exercise radionuclide study is performed (Fig 29B-5). (This may be especially important when there is an abnormal resting ECG, such as with left bundle-branch block, which might limit the diagnostic value of an exercise ECG stress test.) The induction by exercise of new regional wall motion abnormalities or an abnormal ejection fraction response increases diagnostic sensitivity. The sensitivity of radionuclide angiography for the detection of coronary artery disease is in the 85% to 90% range, higher than that of treadmill ECG testing alone. The diagnostic specificity is approximately 75%. It is important to emphasize, however, that if sufficient exercise cannot be performed, as in patients with arthritis or other disabilities that might limit exercise performance, this test will be of limited diagnostic value and may not be cost-effective. Also, an abnormal ejection fraction response is not specific and can be seen in other disease states, including cardiomyopathy and valvular heart disease.

Although experience varies, the sensitivity (87%) and specificity (85% to 90%) of *quantitative* thallium scintigraphy have been reported to be greater than those of the standard exercise ECG test. The specificity of *qualitative* thallium imaging (75% to 80%) is lower, especially if artifacts, for example, diaphragmatic or breast attenuation, are misinterpreted. The appearance of thallium perfusion defects in two or three separate left ventricular segmental regions identifies approximately 75% of patients with multivessel coronary artery disease. Approximately 95% of patients with three-vessel coronary artery disease have abnormal scans.[90] Thallium stress testing seems to be more useful than standard exercise ECG testing in women with suspected coronary artery disease, since both sensitivity and specificity are improved signifi-

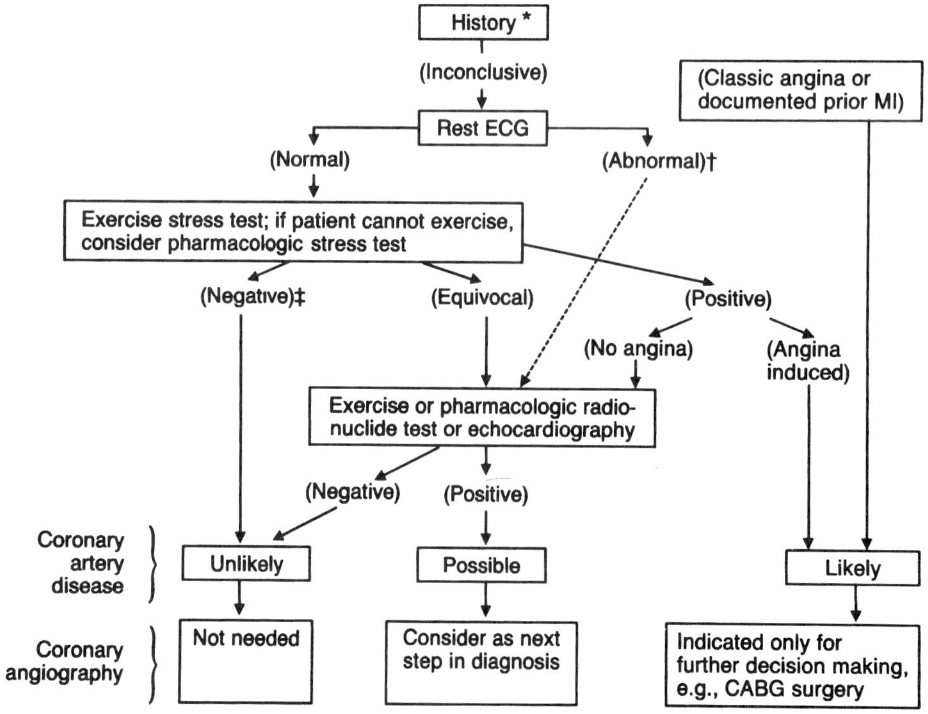

Fig 29B-5 Clinical strategies in the diagnosis of coronary heart disease. *Includes assessment of risk factors, age, and sex. †Examples of abnormal ECG include left bundle-branch block and repolarization abnormality. ‡Negative stress test assumes (1) that there are no cardiac symptoms or significant ECG changes and (2) that adequate workload has been achieved on a standard graded-exercise protocol. *CABG,* coronary artery bypass graft; *MI,* myocardial infarction.

cantly.[91] In terms of specificity, diseases other than coronary artery disease, such as aortic stenosis, cardiomyopathy, and mitral valve prolapse, can also produce perfusion defects.[92] Dipyridamole thallium or adenosine thallium scintigraphy has been shown to be useful in patients who are unable to exercise[93-97] and in patients with left bundle-branch block. Intravenous administration of these agents may cause ECG ST-T wave abnormalities or chest pain, but severe ischemic responses seem to be relatively rare. The effects are reversible by intravenous administration of aminophylline. In patients with asthma, dipyridamole or adenosine intravenously may cause bronchospasm. Patients at highest risk can be screened by pulmonary function testing with a methylcholine challenge.

A normal result of thallium exercise testing implies an excellent prognosis, even when coronary artery disease is present.[98] Conversely, the extent of perfusion defects (number of myocardial regions with redistribution defects) and severity of hypoperfusion have prognostic implications for future coronary events, especially if an adequate workload is achieved.[94,99] The exercise thallium stress test has been shown to be comparable to cardiac catheterization for determining long-term prognosis.[100] Increased lung uptake of thallium during exercise testing, a phenomenon related to increased pulmonary capillary wedge pressures, is correlated with the number of diseased vessels as well as with ventricular function and is also predictive of future cardiac events.[101] Thallium exercise testing has been used in patients unable to exercise completely (but who can still achieve a moderate workload) or who have inconclusive results of treadmill ECG tests. In these patients, thallium testing has a sensitivity of 70% and a specificity of 95% for detecting coronary artery disease.[102] Other patients in whom thallium exercise testing may be useful are selected asymptomatic patients with abnormal results of ECG testing, men with typical angina who have "negative" results of treadmill exercise testing, and women with typical angina who have equivocal results of ECG stress testing.

Abnormal thallium perfusion images have been reported in patients with angiographically normal coronary arteries.[103] Whether such patients have abnormalities of coronary microperfusion or significant coronary lesions that were not detected on standard coronary angiography or had false-positive results is unclear.

Radionuclide tests are expensive and require a high level of technical sophistication to perform and interpret properly. Thallium exercise testing is preferable (1) in patients with atrial fibrillation or frequent ventricular ectopy (which can cause ECG "gating" problems with radionuclide angiography), (2) when exercise-induced left ventricular dysfunction may be caused by a concomitant cardiac condition (such as valvular heart disease), or (3) when it is already known that the resting ejection fraction is markedly depressed. However, if left ventricular systolic function must be determined for clinical purposes, radionuclide angiography is preferred.

Pharmacologic stress testing. In patients unable to exercise, pharmacologic stress testing offers an alternative to evaluate for suspected coronary artery disease. Radionuclide testing includes the use of dipyridamole, adenosine, and dobutamine along with thallium or sestamibi scanning.[104,105] In echocardiographic pharmacologic stress testing, the primary agent to provoke ischemia has been dobutamine,[106-108] although dipyridamole and adenosine have also been used.[109,110] The tests have some differences in cost and convenience, but sensitivities and specificities generally are similar. The primary factor determining the choice of test is the expertise in performing it at each center. Details of these tests are found in chapters 5C and 6.

Use of echocardiography in coronary heart disease

The two-dimensional echocardiogram provides a safe, noninvasive method of evaluating the heart in patients with angina pectoris. Adequate images of the heart can be obtained in most patients, and the two-dimensional echocardiogram is thus a very useful alternative to radionuclide cardiac imaging. The major indication for echocardiography in patients with coronary heart disease is to evaluate regional and global left ventricular function, although other information, such as assessment of cardiac valves, pericardium, ventricular wall thickness, and the presence of left ventricular aneurysms and thrombi, can be obtained simultaneously. Exercise echocardiography is useful in patients with coronary artery disease in whom adequate images can be obtained and compares favorably with radionuclide testing.[111-116]

Echocardiographic estimates of ejection fraction have been limited because of difficulties with assumptions regarding the geometry of the left ventricle. Technologic advances have improved the accuracy of this calculation, however.[117]

The addition of the two-dimensional echocardiographic technique has permitted visualization of regions of the heart (such as the cardiac apex) that previously were inaccessible for imaging. Newer tomographic views have improved the assessment of regional wall motion. Using this technique, one can conceptually divide the left ventricle into different wall segments, and each segment can be analyzed separately. By qualitative visual analysis (similar to analysis of a left ventricular angiogram), specific abnormalities of systolic wall motion and appearance can be described, including hypokinesis, akinesis, dyskinesis, and abnormal wall thinning. The extent of left ventricular dysfunction can be expressed as the percentage of abnormally contracting segments (wall motion score). This derived index of left ventricular function is of prognostic value in patients with ischemic heart disease.[118] A distortion of diastolic contour, along with localized wall thinning and akinetic or dyskinetic regional motion, identifies a left ventricular aneurysm (see chapter 5C).

Other noninvasive procedures

Newer cardiac imaging techniques, including positron emission tomography (see chapter 9), magnetic resonance imaging (see chapter 7), and contrast echocardiography (see chapter 5), are potentially useful in assessing regional and global left ventricular function, perfusion, myocardial metabolism, and coronary anatomy in patients with coronary heart disease, but their clinical roles are not yet certain. In addition, ultrafast computed tomography scanning to detect coronary artery calcification may prove to be a useful screening tool (see chapter 8).

Coronary angiography

The decision to proceed with coronary arteriography (see also chapter 10A) is made after the clinician has decided that the patient would be a potential candidate for revascularization.

In general, coronary arteriography should be considered[119] under the following circumstances.

1. When revascularization or recanalization is being contemplated as a possible therapeutic modality. Examples include the following clinical circumstances: disabling angina unresponsive to standard medical therapy, unstable angina, postinfarction angina, a strongly positive treadmill test that suggests the presence of either left main coronary disease or severe three-vessel coronary disease, and selected postcoronary surgical bypass patients in whom angina redevelops.

2. For further assessment of complications after myocardial infarction. This includes recurrent, severe ventricular tachyarrhythmias, suspicion of left ventricular aneurysm, ruptured septum, and papillary muscle dysfunction or rupture.

3. To confirm or exclude the diagnosis of coronary heart disease when the clinical examination and noninvasive tests are equivocal or discordant (see Fig 29B-5) or in patients who are in positions of responsibility for the lives of others, such as airline pilots, when the clinical data indicate suspicion but not diagnosis of coronary heart disease.

It is controversial whether *routine* coronary angiography should be performed in adults with valvular heart disease or atrial septal defect without angina who will be undergoing corrective cardiac surgery.

Routine coronary angiography is not indicated in patients with minimal likelihood of coronary heart disease, such as a young woman with atypical chest pain (see Fig 29B-4,B), especially if noninvasive tests can be used instead to substantiate the diagnosis (see Fig 29B-5).

If coronary angiography is performed, however, valuable clinical and prognostic information may be obtained. Abnormally elevated left ventricular end-diastolic volume and decreased resting ejection fraction correlate with a history of congestive heart failure and cardiomegaly. The absence of cardiomegaly on the chest radiograph does not exclude left ventricular dysfunction because a decreased ejection fraction has been found in about one-third of patients with normal heart size on the radiograph.[75]

Increased left ventricular end-diastolic volume and reduced ejection fraction are found more often in patients with prior anterior myocardial infarction on the ECG than in patients with inferior myocardial infarction or a normal QRS. These ventriculographic abnormalities also seem to be more often associated with left bundle-branch block on the ECG than either isolated left axis deviation or right bundle-branch block. Patients with a normal resting ECG usually have a normal left ventricular ejection fraction. The correlation of the extent of coronary artery disease with left ventricular function is complex. Some patients with severe coronary artery disease may have normal or near-normal left ventricular function, whereas patients with single-vessel disease, especially if the proximal left anterior descending coronary artery is involved, may have abnormal left ventricular function.

Coronary heart disease is often accompanied by regional wall motion abnormalities (hypokinesis, akinesis, dyskinesis) on left ventriculography,[120] and these abnormalities, if extensive, are associated with congestive heart failure. In a study by Hamby,[75] 69% of 510 patients had abnormalities of left ventricular contractility, including a small number with diffuse hypokinesis. All patients with congestive heart failure had regional wall motion abnormalities, especially in the anterior and apical regions. Also, the presence of radiographic evidence of cardiomegaly was associated with regional wall motion abnormalities of the anterior wall.

Although ECG evidence of prior myocardial infarction is often accompanied by regional wall motion abnormalities, a significant number (50%) of patients without known prior myocardial infarction also can have regional wall motion abnormalities. Ventricular asynergy may thus reflect either prior myocardial damage or a functional disturbance due to ischemia. The location of regional wall motion abnormalities can be related to the ECG site of infarction, and the frequency of asynergy has been related to both the severity and the extent of coronary artery disease.

It is the extent and severity of coronary artery disease on angiography and, most important, the status of left ventricular function,[25] in addition to other factors such as history of congestive heart failure and prior myocardial infarction, that influence survival.[27,121]

In the study by Bruschke et al.,[27,121] patients with single-vessel disease had a 5-year mortality of 14% compared with a 5-year mortality of 37% and 53%, respectively, in patients with double- and triple-vessel disease.

Significant left main coronary artery disease is also associated with a high mortality. Older patients generally have more severe disease than younger patients, especially at the extremes of old age. In the cooperative Coronary Artery Surgery Study (CASS), the mere presence of angina among middle-aged men identified 43% of patients with three-vessel or left main coronary artery disease.[122] The 10-year follow-up survival rates in CASS confirmed early reports on medical compared with surgical management in patients with coronary artery disease. In patients with an ejection fraction of less than 0.50, survival was better with initial surgical treatment (medical, 61%; surgical, 79%). In patients with a normal ejection fraction (greater than 0.50), long-term survival remained the same (medical, 84%; surgical, 83%).[123] These findings have important implications for the management of patients with mild, stable angina who are tolerating medical therapy.

CLINICAL STRATEGIES IN THE DIAGNOSIS OF ANGINA

Figure 29B-5 is an algorithm for the clinical diagnosis of angina. The history and clinical examination are foremost in this scheme, and in some cases no further diagnostic testing is required. The exercise stress test plays a central role in this approach, especially because it can provide additional prognostic information.

In view of the pronounced variability of symptoms in patients with coronary heart disease, and the fact that no single noninvasive test provides 100% diagnostic accuracy, diagnostic strategies differ among different institutions and clinicians. Although there are always exceptions to generalizations in clinical medicine, the physician can be guided by a Bayesian approach to the diagnosis of coronary heart disease (estimating the pretest likelihood of disease in an individual patient in a given population). Figure 29B-4,B shows the influence of age, sex, and symptoms on the pretest likelihood of finding significant coronary heart disease. For example, in a young female patient without symptoms, a positive ECG response to exercise would be expected to be associated with a low probability of coronary heart disease. However, a markedly positive response, such as an ST depression of 2.5 mm, would override the low pretest probability. Conversely, even minor exercise-induced ECG changes (for example, ST depression of 0.5 mm) in a middle-aged male with a history of angina indicates a high probability of coronary disease (Fig 29B-4,C). In the former case – low probability, markedly positive response – if indicated, a second noninvasive test, such as a radionuclide or echocardiographic exercise procedure, can be performed, and if it is normal (as it often is), the patient can be reassured. This may obviate coronary angiography. In the latter example – minor exercise-induced changes but positive history in a middle-aged male – since coronary heart disease is strongly suspected, further *noninvasive* testing may not be necessary for diagnostic purposes only. If revascularization or recanalization is being contemplated as a therapeutic possibility (see Fig 29B-5) – e.g., severe typical angina in a middle-aged man – one can then proceed directly to coronary angiography. If the patient is unable to exercise, pharmacologic testing can be performed (see Fig 29B-5).

Risk stratification

Because coronary artery bypass graft surgery has been demonstrated to prolong life in certain high-risk subgroups of patients with coronary artery disease (left main or three-vessel coronary artery disease), the noninvasive identification of such patients assumes increasing importance. Low- and high-risk subgroups can be differentiated. Variables shown to be independently predictive of left main or three-vessel coronary artery disease include (in decreasing order of importance): (1) magnitude of exercise-induced ST-segment depression, (2) exercise ejection fraction, (3) exercise rate-pressure product, (4) sex of patient, (5) exercise end-systolic volume, (6) ratio of exercise systolic blood pressure to end-systolic volume, and (7) the number of METs achieved during exercise. The number of high-risk patients when the ST-segment depression is less than 1 mm is relatively small, regardless of exercise ejection fraction or rate-pressure product. Conversely, with 2 mm of ST-segment depression, the percentage of high-risk patients is large despite a satisfactory exercise ejection fraction and adequate workload.[124]

Use of the four most important variables for predicting high and low risk in patients (Fig 29B-6) emphasizes the importance of incorporating clinical variables, exercise ECG and hemodynamic response, and left ventricular function into a composite assessment of risk. However, using noninvasive tests for risk stratification may give misleading information as well.[125] Noninvasive tests are designed to detect physiologically significant coronary stenosis or ischemia with the implication that even asymptomatic patients are at increased risk for cardiac death and myocardial infarction. However, previous data suggest that a significant number of morbid events result from rapid progression of disease in segments of the coronary artery that initially had only minimal obstruction.[126-128] In such patients, it is anticipated that results of stress tests designed to provoke ischemia may be negative. In addition, patient selection is important. For example, the low prevalence of cardiac events in patients who are able to exercise results in a poor positive predictive value. Finally, from a therapeutic standpoint, only cardiac catheterization has been shown in randomized trials to predict which patients are candidates for revascularization. Thus, although a variety of noninvasive stress testing techniques are currently in use, questions have been raised about their ability to identify the high-risk patient.

Coronary artery disease in women

There has been increasing concern over the past several years that diagnostic and management decisions on coronary heart disease are influenced by the sex of the patient.[129,130] Coronary heart disease is the leading cause of death in women, and more women die of coronary heart disease than of all neoplastic diseases combined[131] (see chapter 65). Physicians tend to attribute chest pain in women to noncardiac causes rather than to angina,[132] and if angina is suspected, physicians tend to believe a woman is less likely than a man to have a serious cardiovascular event.[133] Women are less likely to be referred for cardiac catheterization, even when a noninvasive test indicates coronary artery disease.[132,134]

In women hospitalized for coronary heart disease, fewer diagnostic and therapeutic procedures are performed.[130] Finally, women tend to be referred to bypass surgery later in the course of disease, when they have more advanced disease, have more symptoms, are less stable, and are at greater risk, which may in part explain the higher mortality for bypass surgery in women.[134] Further studies are needed to determine long-term outcomes and whether the differences in rates of procedures reflect appropriate clinical practice or compromised care of women.

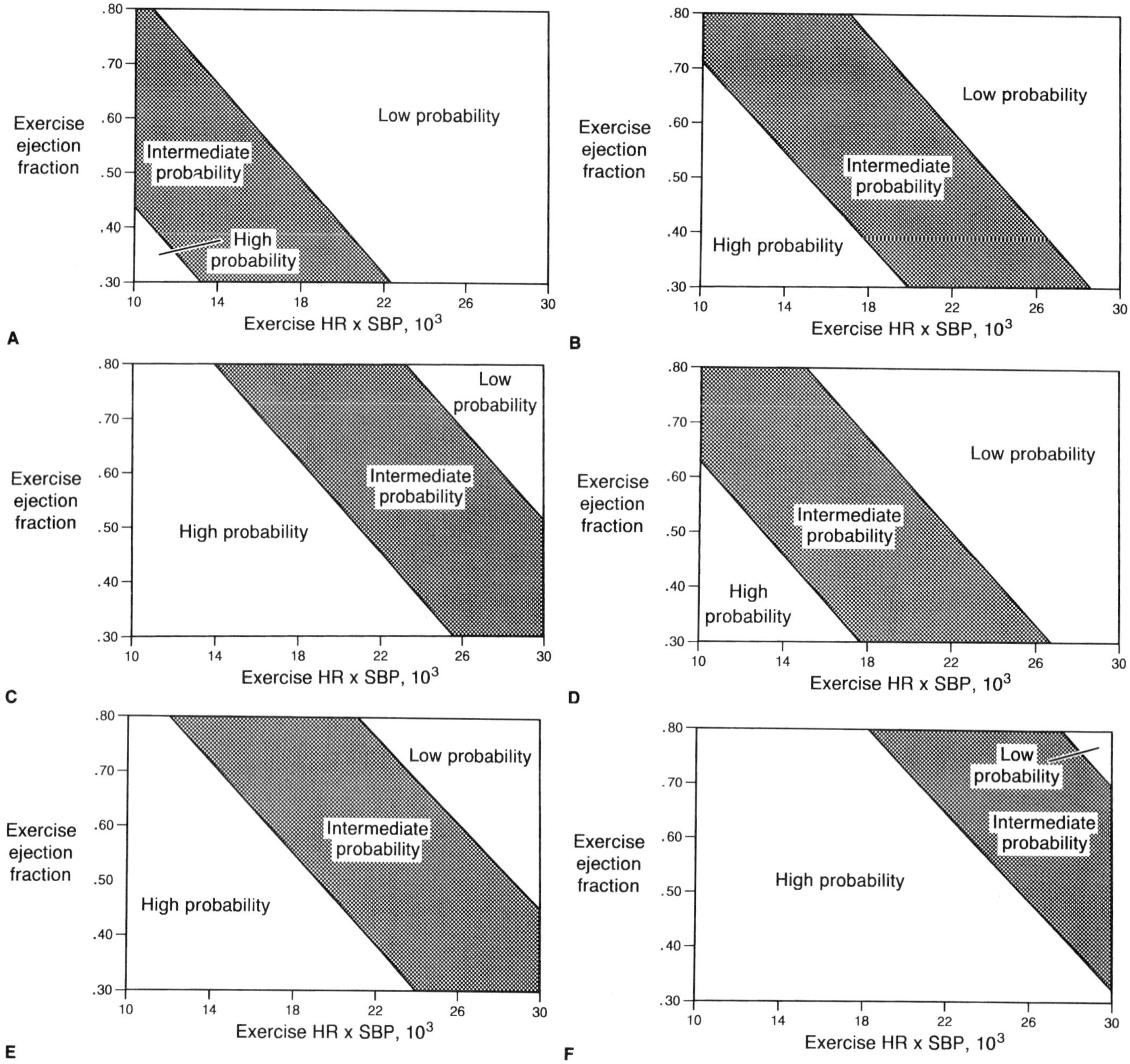

Fig 29B-6 Risk assessment for predicting presence of left main or triple-vessel coronary artery disease from four variables: (1) exercise ejection fraction (vertical axis), (2) rate-pressure product (horizontal axis), (3) degree of exercise-induced ST-segment depression, and (4) sex. **A, B,** and **C,** risk in female subjects with ST-segment depression of less than 1 mm (**A**), 1 mm (**B**), or 2 mm (**C**). **D, E,** and **F,** risk in male subjects with ST-segment depression of less than 1 mm (**D**), 1 mm (**E**), or 2 mm (**F**). *HR,* heart rate; *SBP,* systolic blood pressure. (From Gibbons RJ, Fyke FE III, Clements IP, et al: Noninvasive identification of severe coronary artery disease using exercise radionuclide angiography. *J Am Coll Cardiol* 11:28-34, 1988. By permission of American College of Cardiology.)

NONATHEROSCLEROTIC CORONARY ARTERY DISEASE

Even though coronary atherosclerosis is overwhelmingly the predominant underlying pathologic lesion in patients with angina due to coronary heart disease, rarely other pathologic processes involving the coronary arteries can cause angina (Table 29B-12).[135] Depending on the nature of the specific disease process—for example, vasculitis or vasospasm—large (epicardial) or small (myocardial) coronary arteries (or both) can be involved.

In 1959, Prinzmetal et al.[136] described a group of patients who had a variant of angina pectoris with features distinguishing it from classic exertional (Heberden's) angina, and they suggested that the syndrome was related to temporary alterations of vessel wall tone.

Pathophysiology. The term "coronary vasospasm" as used in this chapter refers to transient active increases in epicardial coronary artery smooth muscle tone which result in diminished luminal cross-sectional area, decreased coronary artery flow, and myocardial ischemia. Changes in tone of more distal precapillary resistance arterioles contribute to the autoregulation of coronary artery flow, and, although vasospasm may involve these vessels, a definite pathophysiologic role has not been documented.

Hemodynamic and symptomatic consequences of vasospasm (or change in vascular smooth muscle tension) depend not only on its intensity but also on the baseline caliber of the vessel. Vasospasm that produces ischemia in an otherwise normal coronary artery must be more intense than that superimposed on a site with a preexisting atherosclerotic lesion obstructing 75% of the luminal diameter.

Table 29B-12 Nonatherosclerotic coronary artery diseases that can cause angina*

Acquired disorders of the coronary arteries
Coronary artery embolism
Aortic dissection (involving the coronary ostia)
Syphilitic aortitis
Collagen-vascular and other systemic diseases
Polyarteritis nodosa
Rheumatoid arthritis
Systemic lupus erythematosus
Amyloid
Tumor infiltration
Miscellaneous
Mediastinal irradiation
Nitrate withdrawal
Hereditary connective tissue disorders
Pseudoxanthoma elasticum
Homocystinuria
Gargoylism
Cystic medial necrosis
Congenital disorders of the coronary arteries
Anomalous origin of a coronary artery from the pulmonary artery, aorta, or another coronary artery
Coronary arteriovenous fistula
Coronary artery aneurysm

*Modified from Hillis LD, Cohn PF: Nonatherosclerotic coronary artery disease. In *Diagnosis and Therapy of Coronary Artery Disease.* Edited by PF Cohn. Boston, Little, Brown & Company, 1979, pp 481-494.

Variant angina results from reduced coronary blood flow and not from increased myocardial oxygen demand. The initial evidence that ischemia may be the result of decreased flow was based on the absence of a concurrent increase in myocardial oxygen demand. Heart rate and blood pressure seldom change significantly before or at the onset of an episode of variant angina. Conversely, indices of left ventricular function, such as left ventricular filling pressure and left ventricular rate of increase of pressure during isovolumetric contraction (dp/dt), often become markedly abnormal at the onset of an attack, and this suggests the presence of inadequate myocardial perfusion. Angiographic observations of transient vessel narrowing during spontaneous or provoked episodes of variant angina have provided further evidence of directly compromised coronary artery flow. There is further angiographic evidence that patients with coronary vasospasm have a diffuse defect in coronary artery tone reflected by a generalized reduction of the diameter of coronary arteries other than those with discrete vasospasm after administration of ergonovine.[137] Assessment of coronary artery flow by means of radionuclide techniques has confirmed that regional myocardial perfusion is diminished during episodes of variant angina,[138] as shown by a relative decrease in regional left ventricular uptake of thallium 201 during spontaneous or provoked symptoms. In addition, measurements of coronary artery blood flow in patients during spontaneous variant angina have demonstrated that flow is diminished in the region that shows ECG changes of ischemia[138,139] (Fig 29B-7) or angiographically documented vessel narrowing.

Cause and mechanism of coronary arterial spasm. A number of hypotheses have been advanced to explain the occurrence of abnormal coronary vascular smooth muscle spasm, although all remain unproved.

LOCAL PHENOMENA. Discrete areas of vasospasm suggest that a local abnormality of the blood vessel wall leads to an exaggerated response to vasoconstrictor stimuli. Such an abnormality may permit a hypercontractile response of an otherwise normal-appearing vessel to either neurogenic or humoral stimuli. In regions of associated atherosclerotic disease, the abnormal response may be related to (1) hydrodynamic phenomena in which a partial stenosis is increased during periods of low perfusion pressure, low coronary arterial resistance distal to the stenosis, or superimposed vasoconstrictor stimuli;[140] (2) geometric considerations in which normal variations in resting vasomobility are amplified at stenotic sites as a result of proportionately greater encroachment on the already narrowed lumen,[141] and the fact that resistance, according to Poiseuille's law,* is inversely

*$R = \frac{8\mu L}{\pi r^4}$, in which R = resistance, μ = blood viscosity, L = length of the obstructing lesion, and r = radius of the vessel at the stenosis.

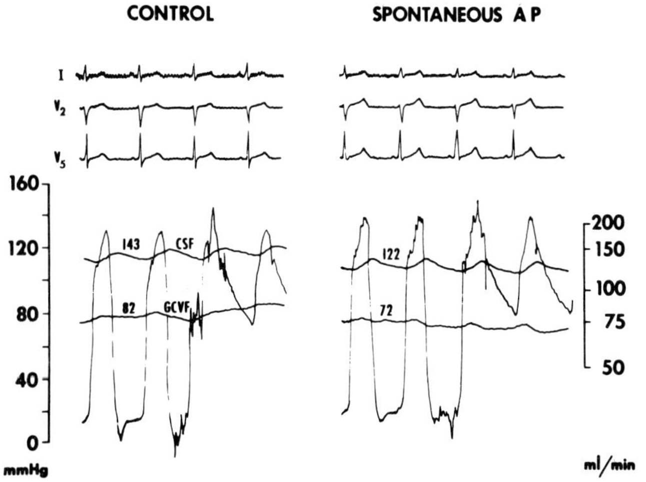

Fig 29B-7 Hemodynamic measurements in patient during a control period and spontaneous angina pectoris *(AP)*. Coronary sinus flow *(CSF)* and great cardiac vein flow *(GCVF)* decreased during angina, whereas aortic and left ventricular pressures changed little. (From Feldman RL, Pepine CJ, Whittle JL, et al: Coronary hemodynamic findings during spontaneous angina in patients with variant angina. *Circulation* 64:76-83, 1981. By permission of American Heart Association.)

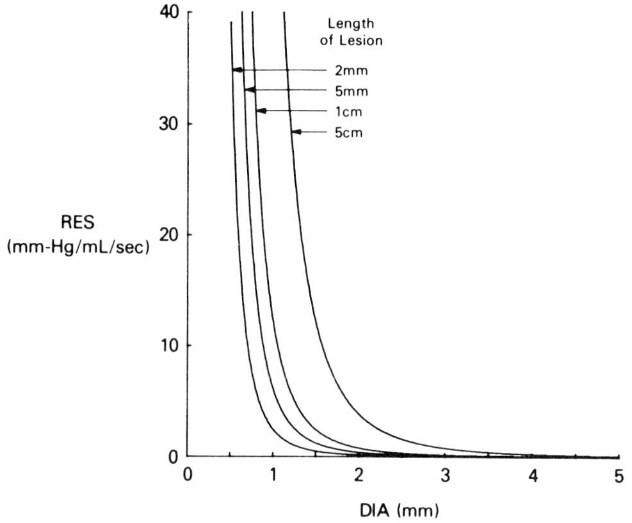

Fig 29B-8 Relation between coronary arterial diameter *(DIA)* and resistance *(RES)* to flow. Obstructive lesions of various lengths are represented by the four curves. Since resistance is proportional to the fourth power of vessel diameter, the diameter has the preponderant influence on resistance. (From Epstein SE, Talbot TL: Dynamic coronary tone in precipitation, exacerbation and relief of angina pectoris. *Am J Cardiol* 48:797-803, 1981. By permission of Technical Publishing Company, a Division of Dun-Donnelly Publishing Corporation.)

proportional to the fourth power of the vessel's radius[142](Fig 29B-8); or (3) a true focal or general[137] hypersensitivity to vasoconstrictor influences,[143,144] which may, in part, be due to abnormalities of the endothelium and its products.[145-148]

NEUROGENIC FACTORS. α-Adrenergic receptor stimulation may be involved in the pathogenesis of coronary vasospasm. This conclusion is supported by observations that α-adrenergic blockade with phenoxybenzamine or phentolamine can block vasospasm, symptoms of variant angina, and ECG abnormalities after ergonovine administration.[149,150] The administration of selective α_1-adrenergic blockers has yielded conflicting results.[151,152]

Parasympathetic activity has been proposed as having a role in coronary vasospasm. Intracoronary injection of the parasympathetic neurotransmitter acetylcholine causes spasm of epicardial arteries in most patients with variant angina[153,154] and in some patients with coronary atherosclerosis and effort angina.[155] Even in patients who exhibit acetylcholine-induced epicardial artery vasoconstriction, the arteriolar resistance vessels dilate, resulting in an overall increase in coronary flow measured in the coronary sinus.[156] Atropine blocks spasm induced by acetylcholine in patients with variant angina.[153]

HUMORAL MECHANISMS. Circulating endogenous epinephrine may hypothetically induce vasospasm in susceptible patients (in the same manner as exogenously administered epinephrine) by α-adrenergic stimulation, although presumably norepinephrine released from nerve endings in the vessel wall is the predominant adrenergic transmitter involved.

Pharmacologic evidence suggests that serotonin receptors may mediate vasoconstriction in canine coronary artery smooth muscle,[157-160] though attempts to block ergonovine-induced coronary spasm in patients by pretreatment with ketanserin, a selective serotonin$_2$-inhibitor, have been unsuccessful.[161] Since in patients with variant angina the administration of serotonin induces severe epicardial coronary arterial spasm[162] that is not reversed by ketanserin, serotonin$_1$-receptor subtypes may be implicated in mediating the vasospastic response.[163]

Thromboxane A_2, which is produced by aggregating platelets, is a potent platelet-activating agent and vasoconstrictor; prostaglandin I_2 (prostacyclin), which is synthesized in endothelial cells, is an inhibitor of platelet aggregation and a potent vasodilator. The opposing effects of these agents led to the hypothesis that they may be involved in the maintenance of normal platelet function, preventing aggregation in areas of normal endothelium by appropriately balanced proaggregatory and antiaggregatory influences. Endothelial damage, on the other hand, might tend to favor platelet aggregation due to inadequate prostacyclin production, which in turn would initiate release of thromboxane A_2 and other vasoconstrictors, such as serotonin, thereby promoting further aggregation and vasoconstriction. Such a mechanism would have physiologic importance in the regulation of the hemostatic function of platelets and vessels after loss of vessel wall integrity, but it could also provoke inappropriate coronary spasm in areas of deficient prostacyclin production or accelerated release of thromboxane A_2. It has been noted that sites of atherosclerotic disease are relatively defective in prostacyclin generation.[164,165]

Clinical manifestations of coronary artery spasm

HISTORY. Patients with variant angina characteristically experience symptoms of angina at rest and often nocturnally, although various degrees of exertional angina often occur intercurrently. Exertional symptoms in this setting may be due to either the simultaneous presence of atherosclerotic disease or exercise-induced vasospasm.

Symptoms at rest in variant angina may occur in a cyclic pattern; patients often note that they are awakened by pain at about the same time each night. The pain is often described as more severe and longer than that of typical exertional angina. Symptoms may wax and wane with time, so that remissions or asymptomatic interludes independent of therapy are not unusual.

Approximately 50% of patients with documented coronary vasospasm experience arrhythmias during an attack. Therefore, a history of syncopal episodes during chest pain should suggest that the angina may be related to coronary vasospasm. Occasionally, patients give a history of migraine headaches, Raynaud's disease, or symptomatic venospasm, suggesting a generalized vasospastic disorder.

ELECTROCARDIOGRAPHIC MANIFESTATIONS. Transient ST-segment elevation during chest pain is considered the ECG sine qua non of variant angina. However, not every episode of chest pain is necessarily associated with ST-segment elevation; conversely, prolonged monitoring has revealed frequent episodes of *asymptomatic* ST-segment elevation in patients with variant angina.[166] The occurrence of ST-segment elevation, which is often quite pronounced, reflects the temporary acute transmural myocardial ischemia caused by sudden occlusion of a proximal coronary artery. Reversible ST-segment elevation may occur in up to one-third of patients with significant fixed obstructive coronary artery disease and unstable angina. ST-segment depression also may occur in patients with variant angina.

Other ECG abnormalities associated with symptomatic episodes of coronary vasospasm include ventricular arrhythmias, second-degree and complete atrioventricular block, asystole, abnormally tall and broad R waves, ST-segment alternans, pseudonormalization of inverted T waves, and transient Q-wave development.

Exercise ECG in patients with variant angina shows variable results. More than 50% of patients with variant angina exhibit abnormalities of the exercise ECG. Approximately one-third of patients experience ST-segment elevation, one-third have ST-segment depression, and one-third show no change.[167,168] The occurrence of ST-segment depression in these patients has been associated with more significant fixed obstruction and may identify patients who are more likely to benefit from aortocoronary bypass grafting.[168] The development of ST-segment *elevation* with exercise appears to occur more often in patients with active disease (in terms of symptom frequency) than in those with relatively quiescent disease.[167]

ANGIOGRAPHY AND PROVOCATIVE TESTING. Coronary angiography of patients with clinically suspected variant angina may show any degree of severity of atherosclerotic coronary artery disease; approximately 10% have normal coronary arteries.[169] The angiographic diagnosis of ischemia depends on the fortuitous observation of spontaneous vessel spasm or a positive provocative test. Several general types of provocative testing have been employed: pharmacologic, cold pressor, hyperventilation, and exercise. Of these, only pharmacologic provocative testing has been systematically used during angiographic investigation.

Pharmacologic agents used for provocative testing have included ergonovine, methylergonovine maleate, acetylcholine, and methylcholine. Although the experience with ergonovine has generated the most clinical data in the United States, this agent is no longer manufactured. The clinical utility of methylergonovine appears to be clinically equivalent to ergonovine, and cardiac catheterization laboratories are converting to its use.[170]

Response to ergonovine administration was a sensitive and specific indicator of pathologic coronary vasospasm, with a true-positive rate of 93% to 99% and a false-positive rate of 0% to 5%.[171-174] A positive ergonovine test consisted of the production of focal coronary artery narrowing accompanied by other evidence of myocardial ischemia—that is, ST-segment elevation or symptoms. The occurrence of diffuse narrowing was not considered pathologic, and pain as the only symptom is unreliable, because it may occur in up to 20% of patients without coronary artery spasm or ischemia. Of 1,089 unselected consecutive patients undergoing coronary artery catheterization (except those with documented spontaneous spasm, left main disease, or severe three-vessel disease) who were given methylergonovine, 12% demonstrated focal spasm. Thirty-eight percent of patients with rest angina experienced spasm, compared with 14% with effort and rest angina, 4% with exertional angina, and 1% with atypical chest pain. Spasm was superimposed on fixed atherosclerotic lesions in 60% of these patients.[175] Acetylcholine provokes coronary spasm in 95% of patients with variant angina and in 10% of patients without clinical coronary artery disease.[176]

Major arrhythmias were reported in 10% to 20% of patients in the course of a positive ergonovine test or spontaneous spasm during angiography,[177] but were effectively managed by the reversal of vasospasm with nitroglycerin. Although rare, cases of ergonovine-induced coronary vasospasm were reported which were refractory to sublingual and intravenous nitroglycerin and resulted in death or myocardial infarction.[178,179] Intracoronary nitroglycerin (100 to 600 μg), however, may be more efficacious in the treatment of otherwise irreversible vasospasm.[178]

Provocative testing for coronary spasm is most likely to yield clinically useful information in patients who have a normal or near-normal coronary angiogram and (1) ST-segment depression or T-wave changes during chest pain, (2) major arrhythmias or syncope during chest pain, (3) a normal ECG during chest pain suggestive of angina, (4) left bundle-branch block or pacemaker rhythm and chest pain at rest, or (5) chest pain at rest but without the possibility of simultaneous ECG monitoring.[177] A provocative study may also be useful in a patient with severe fixed obstruction in one vessel but ECG changes of ischemia in a region supplied by a normal-appearing vessel. In patients with ST-segment elevation during pain and a normal coronary angiogram, the diagnosis of variant angina is virtually certain, and further testing is not warranted. In addition, patients with a typical history and ST-segment elevation on 12-lead or ambulatory ECG during a spontaneous episode of symptoms do not require provocative testing to establish the diagnosis of variant angina.

Provocative testing is best avoided in patients with (1) a recent myocardial infarction, (2) cerebrovascular disease, (3) multiple severe fixed coronary artery lesions or left main coronary artery disease, (4) severe hypertension, (5) uncontrolled chest pain or ventricular arrhythmias, (6) severe left ventricular failure, or (7) severe aortic stenosis.

SPECIFIC TREATMENT ISSUES. The mainstay of management of patients with variant angina consists of pharmacologic therapy with vasodilators. Nitrates are effective for terminating most acute episodes, whether spontaneous or provoked.

Calcium-entry blocking agents have become the primary mode of prophylactic therapy. Nifedipine, verapamil, and diltiazem all have demonstrated efficacy in reducing symptoms and evidence of ischemia in patients with variant angina. β-Adrenergic blocking drugs, which are useful in classic exertional angina as a result of their ability to limit myocardial oxygen demands, may exacerbate symptoms in variant angina, perhaps by unmasking α-adrenergic vasoconstriction.[180] Serotoninergic blockers have failed to demonstrate clinical benefit in the treatment of variant angina.[181] Intravenously administered magnesium sulfate may alleviate exercise-related angina in these patients, perhaps by inhibiting coronary vascular smooth muscle contraction.[182]

Coronary artery bypass surgery may be effective in reducing symptoms when vasospasm is superimposed on significant atherosclerotic obstructive disease. In general, however, the results of surgery are unsatisfactory in patients with insignificant or no obstructive lesions, and symptoms tend to recur.[183] Although percutaneous transluminal coronary angioplasty is technically feasible in patients with variant angina and associated obstructive lesions, symptoms of coronary artery spasm usually persist or recur,[184] and a high rate of restenosis has been observed.[185]

PROGNOSIS. The survival of patients with variant angina is largely dependent on associated factors, especially the extent and severity of concomitant fixed obstructive coronary artery disease.[169,186-189] Long-term survival ranges from as low as 77% at 5 years to as high as 93% at 10 years among patients treated medically (Fig 29B-9). The presence of atherosclerotic coronary artery disease demonstrably decreases longevity in these patients (Fig 29B-10). The risk of myocardial infarction also varies among studies (Fig 29B-11) and is predominantly a function, again, of obstructive coronary artery disease (Fig 29B-12). Perhaps because of the contribution by fixed obstructive disease to mortality and infarction, patients who undergo revascularization exhibit improved survival.[188] Among medically treated patients, the use of calcium-entry blockers has been shown to correlate with improved longevity[186,189] or to reduce the risk of myocardial infarction.[187] Apparent remission of the disease has been noted in a significant number of patients, particularly those in whom the only documentation of coronary spasm had been during provocative testing.[190] Although most patients without significant concomitant coronary artery atherosclerosis have a good prognosis, it may be difficult to predict which patients will have a poor outcome.[191]

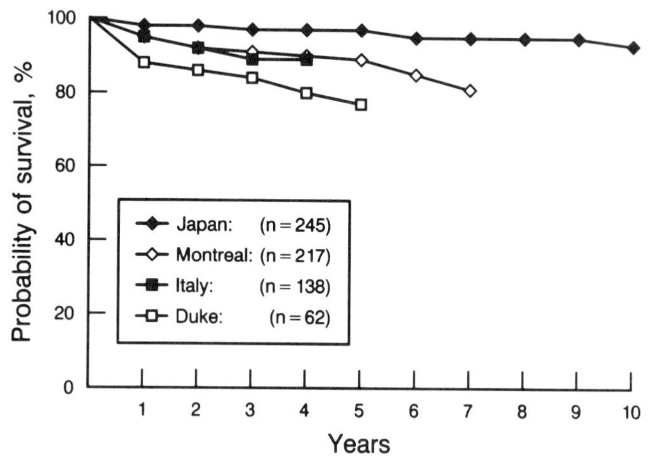

Fig 29B-9 Survival of patients with variant angina as reported in four large series from Japan,[186] Montreal,[187] Italy,[169] and Duke University.[188]

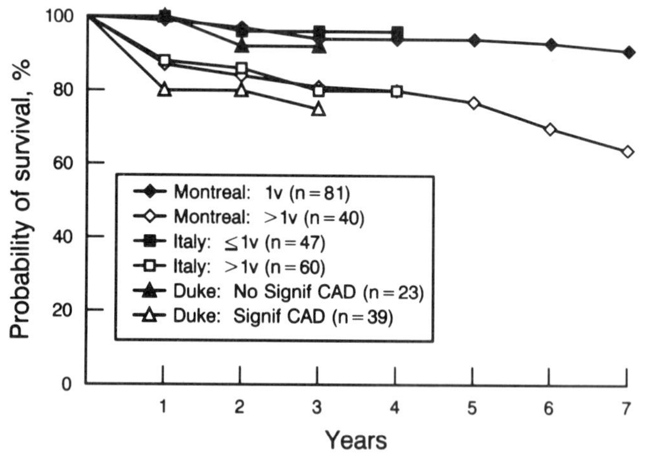

Fig 29B-10 Survival of subgroups of patients with variant angina and differing severity of coronary artery disease *(CAD). v,* vessels involved with obstructive *CAD.* References as in legend for Fig 29B-9.

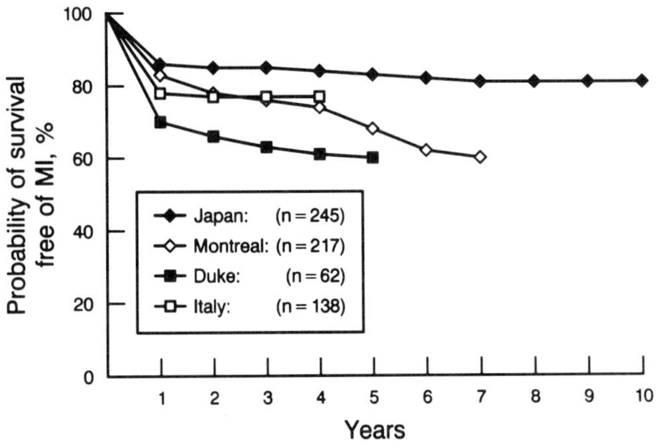

Fig 29B-11 Survival free of myocardial infarction *(MI)* in patients with variant angina as reported in four large series. References as in legend for Fig 29B-9.

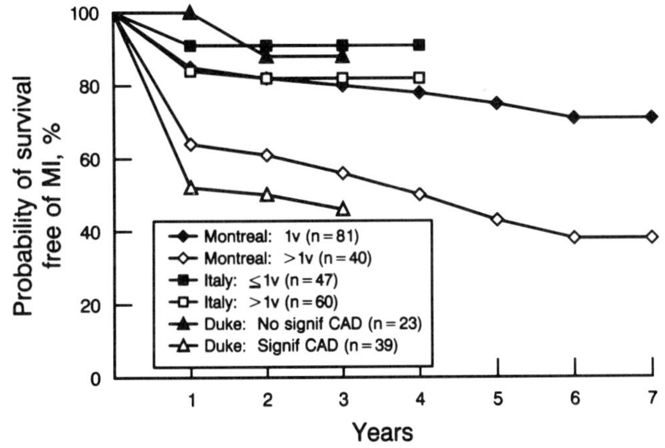

Fig 29B-12 Survival free of myocardial infarction *(MI)* in subgroups of patients with variant angina and differing severity of coronary artery disease *(CAD)*. *V,* vessels involved with CAD. References as in legend for Fig 29B-9.

Other manifestations of coronary artery spasm

EXERTIONAL ANGINA. Symptoms of exertional angina in some patients have been ascribed to exercise-induced vasospasm. Although patients with exertional angina experience symptoms due to increased myocardial oxygen demands associated with obstructive lesions, a component of the underlying pathophysiologic state may be attributable to dynamic coronary artery tone superimposed on obstructive lesions. Furthermore, coronary spasm may contribute to progression of coronary atherosclerotic disease, with resulting symptoms or myocardial infarction.[192] However, in patients with reproducible coronary spasm at the same sites documented over a period of approximately 2 years, progression of atherosclerotic stenoses appears to be no faster or more common at sites with spasm than in arterial segments without spasm.[193]

MYOCARDIAL INFARCTION. Patients with variant angina or angina with normal coronary arteries may sustain myocardial infarction.[194] Although spasm may be a component of the constellation of events leading to myocardial infarction, the results of acute angiography during evolving myocardial infarctions and the pattern of thrombolytic efficacy suggest that the main causative factor is intracoronary thrombosis in most patients.

SUDDEN DEATH. Coronary vasospasm is associated with a high incidence of major arrhythmias and has led to the hypothesis that some cases of unexplained sudden death may represent the first manifestation of ischemic heart disease or spasm.[189] Among patients with documented coronary vasospasm, the incidence of sudden death is 2% to 16%.[189] Patients with sudden death or serious arrhythmias appear to differ from others in that, during monitored spontaneous episodes of chest pain, maximal ST-segment elevation is higher, a finding that presumably reflects greater ischemia. Experimental animal studies suggest that the risk of ventricular fibrillation immediately after spasm and during reperfusion is higher in the *absence* of associated fixed obstruction. This corresponds to the observation that, in patients with variant angina, serious arrhythmias are more often detected in those with normal coronary angiograms.

Acquired disorders of the coronary arteries

Syphilitic involvement of the coronary arteries may produce angina by two mechanisms: (1) coronary ostial stenosis (most commonly) due to aortitis and usually associated with aortic regurgitation, and (2) syphilitic coronary arteritis involving the proximal coronary arteries (very rarely). If indicated, antibiotic therapy is warranted to eliminate smoldering spirochetal infection. Both coronary arteriotomy and bypass surgery have been successfully employed to treat ischemic symptoms.

Although *cardiac amyloid* is usually associated with diffuse myocardial infiltrates, large amyloid deposits can obstruct the coronary artery lumen and cause angina. *Metastatic cancer* can rarely encroach (externally) on a coronary artery and cause angina or myocardial infarction.

Periarteritis nodosa is a generalized form of periarteritis with multisystem involvement. The epicardial coronary arteries are involved with a necrotizing, obliterative vasculitis in 60% to 70% of adults with periarteritis nodosa. Despite this, clinical ischemic symptoms seem to be rare. In some cases, nodular coronary artery aneurysms form, which may eventually rupture or thrombose. A vasculitis of the small (myocardial) coronary arteries can also occur. Steroids have been used with varying degrees of success.

Some patients with *rheumatoid arthritis* have, as part of a diffuse systemic involvement, a coronary arteritis that most commonly involves the smaller (myocardial) arterioles. *Systemic lupus erythematosus* can cause a vasculitis of the large coronary arteries with symptoms of myocardial ischemia. Also, in some younger patients with lupus, early, severe coronary atherosclerosis has been found and has raised the possibility that steroid therapy may be responsible for accelerating atherosclerosis.

High-dose x-irradiation of the coronary arteries can cause coronary luminal narrowing that results in angina. In experimental animals, therapeutic doses of radiation accelerate the atherosclerotic process by an unknown mechanism, although hypercholesterolemia may contribute to this.[195]

Withdrawal from chronic nitroglycerin exposure (as in workers in nitrate factories) can induce angina and even myocardial infarction in patients without underlying coronary atherosclerosis.[196] Typically, anginal symptoms begin within 48 hours after nitroglycerin withdrawal. Presumably, this is due to reflex coronary vasoconstriction. The symptoms can be relieved by nitroglycerin.

Hereditary connective tissue disorders

Patients with *pseudoxanthoma elasticum* experience a diffuse degeneration of the arterial system at a relatively young age and present with any combination of angina, claudication, and hypertension. Although in *Marfan's syndrome* aortic dissection is more common, dissection of the coronary arteries themselves can also occur.

Congenital disorders of the coronary arteries

Anomalous origin of a coronary artery from the pulmonary artery is a rare disorder; 80% of infants with this anomaly die during the first year of life. This anomaly most often involves the left coronary artery, but involvement of the right coronary or of both vessels can occur. Patients with extensive collaterals may survive into adulthood and present with angina and a continuous precordial murmur caused by constant blood flow through the intracoronary anastomoses. Definitive diagnosis is by coronary angiography, and surgical treatment is required in most of these patients. Postoperative survival for as long as 8 years has been reported.[197]

An *aberrant coronary artery*—for example, the left circumflex arising from the right sinus of Valsalva or from the proximal right coronary artery—will cause symptoms only if its anatomic course is abnormal and it fails to provide blood flow to its usual myocardial territory.[198] There have been reports of sudden death in patients with an aberrant left coronary artery arising from the right coronary sinus and following a proximal course between the aorta and the pulmonary trunk.[198] In the CASS registry, the incidence of coronary artery anomalies (origin from opposite cusp, noncoronary cusp, or opposite artery) was 0.3%. The most common anomaly involved the circumflex coronary artery arising from a separate ostium in the right coronary sinus. Anomalous circumflex coronary arteries had a significantly greater degree of stenosis than nonanomalous arteries but were not associated with a difference in long-term survival.[199]

In patients with *coronary arteriovenous fistula,* a coronary artery may communicate with the right atrium, coronary sinus, right ventricle, or pulmonary artery. Most commonly, the right coronary artery drains into the right ventricle. The hemodynamic significance is based primarily on the degree of left-to-right shunt present, and symptoms are usually due to congestive heart failure if a large shunt is present. Occasionally, however, angina may also occur and is probably due to diversion of coronary blood flow away from its normal myocardial territory (a "macro" coronary "steal" phenomenon). On physical examination, there is evidence of a hyperdynamic precordium consistent with intracardiac shunting and a variably located continuous murmur heard over the precordium.

THERAPY OF ANGINA PECTORIS*

General principles

Proper medical management of the patient with angina due to coronary heart disease should take into account the effects of the disease on the whole person (including physical, psychosocial, and economic aspects). The physician should ascertain the impact of the disease process on both the patient and his or her family. Contributory conditions, both physical (such as anemia) and emotional (such as severe personal stress), should be sought and treated if possible.

An adjustment in lifestyle is warranted in most patients with angina. This includes an exercise training program (if possible), dietary education, weight reduction (if indicated), cessation of cigarette smoking, and avoidance of isometric exercise or exercising in the cold or immediately after a meal. Compliance is often limited, and some patients either cannot or will not change their specific lifestyle or habits. Some patients initially alter their patterns of behavior, but recidivism is common. Even if the patient is to undergo coronary surgery, continued attention to risk factors remains important in long-term care.

Every attempt should be made to have the patient continue to work and remain active and productive. Unfortunately, some types of work, especially those requiring heavy labor, cannot be done by the patient with angina. By means of an exercise test, an assessment of functional capacity (see Tables 29B-5 and 29B-6) can help classify these patients in terms of their job disability.

Medical therapy, which includes altering risk factors and treating associated diseases, as well as the use of antianginal drugs (see chapter 29C), improves angina in most (80% to 90%) patients with chronic stable angina. Patients who do not respond to this approach can be considered "treatment failures," and coronary revascularization should be considered.

All patients should be carefully instructed in the proper use of nitroglycerin. The patient should be trained to recognize symptoms of worsening ischemia and instructed to seek prompt medical assistance if indicated—for example, prolonged chest pain at rest unrelieved by nitroglycerin.

---

*See chapter 29C for a discussion of the pharmacologic treatment of angina, chapter 10B for catheter-based intervention, and chapter 31 for issues related to coronary revascularization.

The role of exercise training in the treatment of angina pectoris

Exercise programs that progressively increase physical endurance and reduce the heart rate, and thus reduce total cardiac work,[200,201] at any given level of physical activity lead to improvement in cardiac performance and prolong exercise time before angina occurs. Indeed, it has been shown[202] that as many as three-fourths of patients with angina will show an improved treadmill time after a daily walking program. Some patients may even experience complete elimination of angina after a prolonged, vigorous rehabilitation program.[203] In a small group of patients with stable coronary artery disease, stress-induced myocardial ischemia (as assessed by thallium 201 scintigraphy) was significantly decreased after a 1-year program of supervised exercise and low-cholesterol diet.[204]

A word of caution is necessary, however, especially in the untrained individual. Excessive physical activity in patients with coronary heart disease may worsen cardiac function and also unpredictably provoke ventricular fibrillation. Most of these patients, however, fall into a high-risk subgroup that can be identified beforehand because they have significant ST-wave depression on treadmill exercise examination.[205] Thus, an individual program should be outlined for each patient only after an exercise stress test has been completed.

Although data from some animal experiments suggest that training can improve collateral blood flow to the ischemic myocardium,[206,207] this has not been shown to occur in humans with coronary heart disease.[208]

Trained patients with angina also show a slight reduction in resting systolic blood pressure and a slightly lower systolic blood pressure at any given level of physical activity.[209] Although the increase in cardiac output is slightly less at equivalent workloads, there is also a significant peripheral effect resulting from increased enzyme activity in skeletal muscle and alterations in oxygen uptake.[209]

Although swimming can improve a patient's oxygen transport ability, this type of exercise (depending on its intensity) can exact large oxygen demands and should not be undertaken by angina patients who are deconditioned or who possess limited physical skills. In one study of patients with coronary disease, swimming was found to result in ST-wave depression that was similar to that from bicycling, implying that bicycle exercise testing might prove useful in predicting the safety of this type of cardiac rehabilitation.[210]

A walking program is both easy and inexpensive (if not limited by climate and weather conditions). A progressively increasing exercise program can be advised according to individual patient needs and capacities.[211] Other types of exercise can vary according to individual patient needs and desires and these include jogging, swimming (see above), and bicycling. A recommended exercise protocol[211] involves a warm-up phase (about 5 minutes), a workout (approximately 20 to 30 minutes), and a cool-down period (approximately 5 minutes) to allow for circulatory adjustments to exercise. Three to five exercise periods per week are generally recommended to achieve appropriate cardiovascular conditioning.

CONCOMITANT DISEASES AND SPECIAL DIAGNOSTIC AND THERAPEUTIC PROBLEMS IN THE TREATMENT OF ANGINA

Angina in the elderly[212]

A history of classic angina is often difficult to obtain in the elderly (defined as more than 65 years old). Nevertheless, angina pectoris is the presenting symptom in over 80% of elderly patients with symptomatic coronary artery disease.[213] The elderly have limited physical activity and are less likely to have typical exertional symptoms. However, bending, stooping, and use of the arms may provoke angina. The difficulty in obtaining an adequate history in these patients may be compounded by receptive or expressive speech difficulties due to prior cerebrovascular accident, auditory deficit (presbycusis), and memory impairment due to aging or other neurologic processes.

The elderly patient may complain of dyspnea rather than actual anginal pain. Exertional dyspnea (angina equivalent) may be erroneously attributed to chronic obstructive pulmonary disease, deconditioning, or congestive heart failure. Exertional syncope, coughing during emotional stress, palpitations, and sweating with exertion are commonly observed.[213,214] Angina at rest, prolonged angina, and nocturnal angina have the same significance as in younger patients and usually are associated with severe three-vessel coronary disease. In the CASS registry, the elderly were found to have more multivessel coronary artery disease, left main coronary artery disease, and left ventricular dysfunction than younger patients.[215]

Since as many as 50% of persons older than 65 will have an abnormal ECG (left axis deviation, left bundle-branch block, left ventricular hypertrophy, or the like), the ECG is even less specific in this age group than in younger patients.[216]

Similarly, the exercise stress test is of limited usefulness because of the frequently abnormal baseline ECG and physical limitations due to peripheral vascular disease, arthritis, or other disorders. Effort fatigue is usually the limiting factor during an exercise stress test. In elderly patients able to perform even moderate levels of exertion, rest and exercise thallium testing may be helpful in diagnosing ischemia.[213,214]

Data from the nonrandomized CASS registry show that in patients older than 65 years who are at "low risk" (mild angina, preserved left ventricular function, and no left main coronary artery disease), medical therapy is as effective as surgical therapy in regard to survival.[217]

The patient with indeterminate chest pain at rest

Occasionally, the clinician is confronted with a patient who has recurrent chest pain of undetermined cause at rest. If ischemia seems unlikely (see Fig 29B-4,B), one may proceed according to the plan outlined in Figure 29B-5 (see "Clinical Strategies in the Diagnosis of Angina," above). However, if ischemia is a strong possibility, as in a middle-aged male with several risk factors, and if symptoms are of recent onset, the patient should be hospitalized for close observation and monitoring. He should be examined during the time he is experiencing his symptoms (see "General Physical Examination," above), and, if possible, an ECG should be obtained during the symptoms. Any response to nitroglycerin should be recorded. Rarely, rest pain continues and the diagnosis still remains unclear. Echocardiography during and after pain may demonstrate reversible regional wall motion abnormalities. Likewise, sestamibi injection during pain with scanning soon afterward compared with reinjection and rescanning when pain-free may reveal perfusion defects. Finally, hemodynamic monitoring (Swan-Ganz catheter) should be considered. A transient increase in pulmonary wedge (occlusion) pressure coincident with the patient's symptoms suggests that the symptoms are ischemic in origin.

UNSTABLE ANGINA

Unstable angina is a syndrome that is intermediate in severity between chronic stable angina and myocardial infarction.[218,219] Synonyms applied to this syndrome include coronary insufficiency, intermediate coronary syndrome, and preinfarction angina.

Definitions and pathophysiology

Although definitions vary, the syndrome of unstable angina usually includes ischemic ST-T-wave abnormalities on ECG, along with any of the following clinical patterns: (1) new onset of exertional angina of moderate to severe degree, especially if accompanied by rest symptoms; (2) acceleration of previous stable angina pectoris (increasing frequency, intensity, or duration of symptoms), usually including rest or nocturnal symptoms and less responsive to medical therapy; and (3) prolonged rest angina (longer than 15 minutes) unrelieved by nitroglycerin.[220,221] Adding the requirement of ischemic ECG repolarization abnormalities to the definition of unstable angina increases diagnostic specificity. Even so, approximately 10% of patients with normal coronary arteries[222,223] will generally be found in any large series of patients with unstable angina who undergo diagnostic cardiac catheterization. In the majority of properly selected patients with unstable angina, the extent of coronary artery involvement is similar to that in patients with stable angina, except for a slightly increased frequency of left main coronary artery lesions.[222]

The pathophysiology of unstable angina has been clarified over the past several years. Unstable angina usually results from rupture of an atherosclerotic plaque and subsequent formation of thrombus and partial occlusion or transient total occlusion of flow.[224-227] The concept of acute coronary syndrome to describe this clinical entity includes unstable angina, acute myocardial infarction, and sudden cardiac death.[224,228,229]

Specific treatment issues

Management of patients with unstable angina consists of hospitalization, preferably in a monitored setting such as a coronary care unit, bed rest, and correction of reversible precipitating factors, such as anemia, hypoxia, and hypertension. The mainstays of medical management are nitrates and heparin. The initial goals of medical therapy are to stabilize the patient and to gain control of the angina. Initially, sublingual nitroglycerin should be used until nitroglycerin can be administered intravenously. In most patients, faster and more complete control of the angina is obtained with intravenous administration.[230] The dose can easily be titrated upward to control angina or downward if the patient becomes hypotensive. Abrupt discontinuation of intravenous administration of nitroglycerin may cause rebound ischemia.[231] All patients should be fully heparinized and given aspirin.[232-235] Angina may recur when heparin administration is stopped.[236]

β-Adrenergic blockers have proven to be effective in reducing the number of anginal episodes and progression to myocardial infarction.[236-240] β-Blockers should be used in patients with unstable angina unless contraindicated (poor left ventricular function, asthma, atrioventricular block, bradycardia, or previously demonstrated coronary spasm).

Although controversial,[241] calcium antagonists are potentially useful in unstable angina. Verapamil has been shown to decrease the frequency of ST deviation[242] and to be superior to propranolol alone in treating unstable angina.[243] When diltiazem was compared with propranolol, both agents decreased the number of episodes of chest pain but no difference in outcome was seen during follow-up.[244] Nifedipine has been found to be of benefit in a trial comparing it with placebo, especially in patients with ST-segment elevation,[245] and is equal to nitrates in relieving spasm.[246] However, in a large multicenter trial (Holland Interuniversity Nifedipine/Metoprolol Trial), nifedipine was beneficial only when combined with a β-blocker.[247] In general, calcium antagonists are believed to be more successful when combined with other drugs than when given as monotherapy,[248] and they should be added[249] to a regimen of nitroglycerin (given intravenously), heparin, and aspirin if this drug combination does not control symptoms. More than 75% of patients with unstable angina will respond to initial medical management with heparin, aspirin, nitroglycerin (intravenously), β-blockers, and calcium antagonist if needed.[250]

Thrombolytic therapy in unstable angina theoretically should be beneficial because of the underlying pathophysiology (ruptured plaque with thrombus formation). Early studies showed improved outcome with thrombolytic therapy.[251,252] Subsequent studies have shown resolution of intracoronary thrombus with lytic therapy but no clear-cut clinical benefit over standard anticoagulation and antiplatelet treatments.[253-255] In some patients, combined medical therapy fails to control symptoms (medically refractory group) and urgent coronary angiography should be considered,[256,257] especially in those with ST depression. Revascularization is required in many of these patients, even though the risk appears to be increased.[250] Some patients with a response to medical therapy can continue with conservative treatment, but others require subsequent revascularization as well. Continued evidence of ischemia (despite optimal medical treatment) and advanced age portend a poor prognosis. Independent predictors of long-term prognosis are left main coronary artery disease, multivessel coronary artery disease, and increased left ventricular end-diastolic pressure.[258]

Recognition of clinical markers of an early unfavorable course may be of value in defining management strategies. Recurrence of chest pain within 48 hours of admission and ECG changes on admission appear to be relevant markers for patients with a poorer prognosis.[259]

If the patient becomes asymptomatic with medical therapy, some physicians would not order coronary angiography as the next diagnostic step, especially in the elderly or in other patients who would be at high risk in relation to coronary artery bypass graft surgery. Instead, they would gradually mobilize the patient and consider low-level exercise testing under closely supervised conditions or continuous ST-segment analysis using ambulatory ECG monitoring. If the patient has any further evidence of ischemia, angiography would be recommended. However, in view of the significant incidence of left main and three-vessel coronary artery disease in a significant number of these patients, and especially men older than 50, a convincing argument can be made to perform elective coronary angiography in most of these patients.

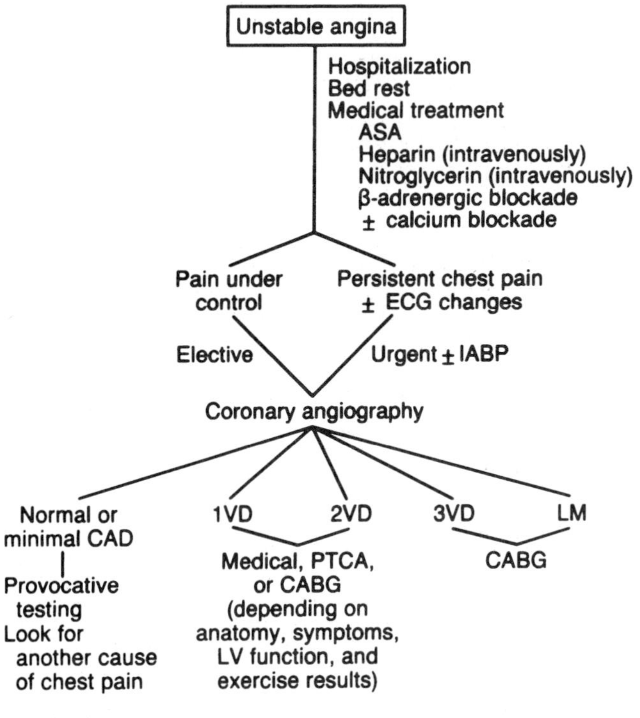

Fig 29B-13 General management strategy for unstable angina. *ASA,* acetylsalicylic acid; *CABG,* coronary artery bypass grafting procedure; *CAD,* coronary artery disease; *ECG,* electrocardiographic; *IABP,* intra-aortic balloon pulsation; *LM,* left main coronary artery involvement; *LV,* left ventricular; *PTCA,* percutaneous transluminal coronary angioplasty; *1VD, 2VD,* and *3VD:* one-vessel, two-vessel, and three-vessel disease. (From Munger TM, Oh JK: Unstable angina. *Mayo Clin Proc* 65:384-406, 1990. By permission, Mayo Foundation for Medical Education and Research.)

For the subgroup of patients who are unresponsive to this initial medical approach and have continued chest pain, intraaortic balloon pumping can be considered, followed by early angiography. However, only physicians who are skilled and experienced with the technique should perform this procedure because of the high incidence of vascular complications. Figure 29B-13 outlines the approach to management of unstable angina.

REFERENCES

1. Gunther S, Green L, Muller JE, et al: Inappropriate coronary vasoconstriction in patients with coronary artery disease: a role for nifedipine? *Am J Cardiol* 44:793-797, 1979

2. Gage JE, Hess OM, Murakami T, et al: Vasoconstriction of stenotic coronary arteries during dynamic exercise in patients with classic angina pectoris: reversibility by nitroglycerin. *Circulation*73:865-876, 1986

3. Cannon RO III, Watson RM, Rosing DR, et al: Angina caused by reduced vasodilator reserve of the small coronary arteries. *J Am Coll Cardiol* 1:1359-1373, 1983

4. Ellis AK, Klocke FJ: Effects of preload on the transmural distribution of perfusion and pressure-flow relationships in the canine coronary vascular bed. *Circ Res* 46:68-77, 1980

5. Deanfield JE, Maseri A, Selwyn AP, et al: Myocardial ischaemia during daily life in patients with stable angina: its relation to symptoms and heart rate changes. *Lancet* 2:753-758, 1983

6. Chierchia S, Muiesan L, Davies A, et al: Role of the sympathetic nervous system in the pathogenesis of chronic stable angina: implications for the mechanism of action of β-blockers. *Circulation* 82 Suppl 2:71-81, 1990

7. Chierchia S, Gallino A, Smith G, et al: Role of heart rate in the pathophysiology of chronic stable angina. *Lancet* 2:1353-1357, 1984

8. Epstein SE, Talbot TL: Dynamic coronary tone in precipitation, exacerbation and relief of angina pectoris. *Am J Cardiol* 48:797-803, 1981

9. Hoffman JIE, Spaan JAE: Pressure-flow relations in coronary circulation. *Physiol Rev* 70:331-390, 1990

10. Crea F, Pupita G, Galassi AR, et al: Effect of theophylline on exercise-induced myocardial ischaemia. *Lancet* 1:683-686, 1989

11. Domenech RJ, MacLellan PR: Transmural ventricular distribution of coronary blood flow during coronary beta 2-adrenergic receptor activation in dogs. *Circ Res* 46:29-36, 1980

12. Heusch G, Deussen A, Schipka J, et al: α_1- and α_2-adrenoceptor-mediated vasoconstriction of large and small canine coronary arteries *in vivo. J Cardiovasc Pharmacol* 6:961-968, 1984

13. Maseri A, Crea F, Kaski JC, et al: Mechanisms of angina pectoris in syndrome X. *J Am Coll Cardiol* 17:499-506, 1991

14. Maseri A, L'Abbate A, Baroldi G, et al: Coronary vasospasm as a possible cause of myocardial infarction: a conclusion derived from the study of "preinfarction" angina. *N Engl J Med* 299:1271-1277, 1978

15. Mudge GH Jr, Goldberg S, Gunther S, et al: Comparison of metabolic and vasoconstrictor stimuli on coronary vascular resistance in man. *Circulation* 59:544-550, 1979

16. Maseri A, Severi S, De Nes M, et al: "Variant" angina: one aspect of a continuous spectrum of vasospastic myocardial ischemia; pathogenetic mechanisms, estimated incidence and clinical and coronary arteriographic findings in 138 patients. *Am J Cardiol* 42:1019-1035, 1978

17. Specchia G, de Servi S, Falcone C, et al: Coronary arterial spasm as a cause of exercise-induced ST-segment elevation in patients with variant angina. *Circulation* 59:948-954, 1979

18. Yasue H, Omote S, Takizawa A, et al: Circadian variation of exercise capacity in patients with Prinzmetal's variant angina: role of exercise-induced coronary arterial spasm. *Circulation* 59:938-948, 1979

19. Maseri A, Chiechia S, Kaski JC: Mixed angina pectoris. *Am J Cardiol* 56:30E-33E, 1985

20. Remme WJ, de Leeuw PW, Bootsma M, et al: Systemic neurohumoral activation and vasoconstriction during pacing-induced acute myocardial ischemia in patients with stable angina pectoris. *Am J Cardiol* 68:181-186, 1991

21. Kannel WB, Feinleib M: Natural history of angina pectoris in the Framingham study: prognosis and survival. *Am J Cardiol* 29:154-163, 1972
22. Hilton TC, Chaitman BR: The prognosis in stable and unstable angina. *Cardiol Clin* 9:27-38, 1991
23. Richards DW, Bland EF, White PD: A completed twenty-five-year follow-up study of 456 patients with angina pectoris. *J Chronic Dis* 4:423-433, 1956
24. Pryor DB, Harrell FE Jr, Rankin JS, et al: The changing survival benefits of coronary revascularization over time. *Circulation* 76 Suppl 5:13-21, 1987
25. Vlietstra RE, Assad-Morell JL, Frye RL, et al: Survival predictors in coronary artery disease: medical and surgical comparisons. *Mayo Clin Proc* 52:85-90, 1977
26. Bonow RO, Kent KM, Rosing DR, et al: Exercise-induced ischemia in mildly symptomatic patients with coronary-artery disease and preserved left ventricular function: identification of subgroups at risk of death during medical therapy. *N Engl J Med* 311:1339 1345, 1984
27. Bruschke AVG, Proudfit WL, Sones FM Jr: Progress study of 590 consecutive nonsurgical cases of coronary disease followed 5-9 years. I. Arteriographic correlations. *Circulation* 47:1147-1153, 1973
28. Webster JS, Moberg C, Rincon G: Natural history of severe proximal coronary artery disease as documented by coronary cineangiography. *Am J Cardiol* 33:195-200, 1974
29. Shub C: Stable angina pectoris: 1. Clinical patterns. *Mayo Clin Proc* 65:233-242, 1990
30. Natkin E, Harrington GW, Mandel MA: Anginal pain referred to the teeth: report of a case. *Oral Surg* 40:678-680, 1975
31. Califf RM, Mark DB, Harrell FE Jr, et al: Importance of clinical measures of ischemia in the prognosis of patients with documented coronary artery disease. *J Am Coll Cardiol* 11:20-26, 1988
32. Aronow WS, Kaplan MA, Jacob D: Tobacco: a precipitating factor in angina pectoris. *Ann Intern Med* 69:529-536, 1968
33. Quarry VM, Spodick DH: Cardiac responses to isometric exercise: comparative effects with different postures and levels of exertion. *Circulation* 49:905-920, 1974
34. Sarnoff SJ, Braunwald E, Welch GH Jr, et al: Hemodynamic determinants of oxygen consumption of the heart with special reference to the tension-time index. *Am J Physiol* 192:148-156, 1958
35. Lane FM: Mental mechanisms and the pain of angina pectoris. *Am Heart J* 85:563-568, 1973
36. Neill WA, Duncan DA, Kloster F, et al: Response of coronary circulation to cutaneous cold. *Am J Med* 56:471-476, 1974
37. Epstein SE, Stampfer M, Beiser GD, et al: Effects of a reduction in environmental temperature on the circulatory response to exercise in man: implications concerning angina pectoris. *N Engl J Med* 280:7-11, 1969
38. Lassvik C, Areskog N-H: Angina pectoris during inhalation of cold air: reactions to exercise. *Br Heart J* 43:661-667, 1980
39. Hayward JM, Holmes WF, Gooden BA: Cardiovascular responses in man to a stream of cold air. *Cardiovasc Res* 10:691-696, 1976
40. Hattenhauer M, Neill WA: The effect of cold air inhalation on angina pectoris and myocardial oxygen supply. *Circulation* 51:1053-1058, 1975
41. Lassvik CT, Areskog N-H: Angina in cold environment: reactions to exercise. *Br Heart J* 42:396-401, 1979
42. Ansari A, Burch GE: Influence of hot environments on cardiovascular system: a clinical study of 23 cardiac patients at rest. *Arch Intern Med* 123:371-378, 1969
43. Sohar E, Shoenfeld Y, Shapiro Y, et al: Effects of exposure to Finnish sauna. *Isr J Med Sci* 12:1275-1282, 1976
44. Williams AV, Higginbotham AC, Knisely MH: Increased blood cell agglutination following ingestion of fat, a factor contributing to cardiac ischemia, coronary insufficiency, and anginal pain: a contribution to the biophysics of disease. *Angiology* 8:29-40, 1957
45. Regan TJ, Binak K, Gordon S, et al: Myocardial blood flow and oxygen consumption during postprandial lipemia and heparin-induced lipolysis. *Circulation* 23:55-63, 1961
46. Lewy RI: Effect of elevated plasma-free fatty acids on thromboxane release in patients with coronary artery disease. *Haemostasis* 9:134-140, 1980
47. Goldstein RE, Redwood DR, Rosing DR, et al: Alterations in the circulatory response to exercise following a meal and their relationship to postprandial angina pectoris. *Circulation* 44:90-100, 1971
48. Cowley AJ, Fullwood LJ, Stainer K, et al: Post-prandial worsening of angina: All due to changes in cardiac output? *Br Heart J* 66:147-150, 1991
49. Hellerstein HK, Friedman EH: Sexual activity and the postcoronary patient. *Arch Intern Med* 125:987-999, 1970
50. Nemec ED, Mansfield L, Kennedy JW: Heart rate and blood pressure responses during sexual activity in normal males. *Am Heart J* 92:274-277, 1976
51. Littler WA, Honour AJ, Sleight P: Direct arterial pressure, heart rate and electrocardiogram during human coitus. *J Reprod Fertil* 40:321-331, 1974
52. Datey KK: Sex and heart disease. *J Assoc Physicians India* 25:647-652, 1977
53. Jackson G: Sexual intercourse and angina pectoris. *Br Med J* 2:16, 1978
54. Ueno M: The so-called coition death. *Jpn J Leg Med* 17:330-340, 1963
55. Droste C: Influence of opiate systems in pain transmission during angina pectoris. *Z Kardiol* 79 Suppl 3:31-43, 1990
56. Benjamin SB: The relationship between esophageal motility disorders and microvascular angina. *Med Clin North Am* 75:1135-1142, 1991
57. Garrin Pulido J, Patel PH, Hunter WC, et al: Esophageal contribution to chest pain in patients with coronary artery disease. *Chest* 98:806-810, 1990
58. Basta LL, Raines D, Najjar S, et al: Clinical, haemodynamic, and coronary angiographic correlates of angina pectoris in patients with severe aortic valve disease. *Br Heart J* 37:150-157, 1975
59. Baxter RH, Reid JM, McGuiness JB, et al: Relation of angina to coronary artery disease in mitral and in aortic valve disease. *Br Heart J* 40:918-922, 1978
60. Lardani H, Serrano JA, Villamil RJ: Hemodynamics and coronary angiography in idiopathic hypertrophic subaortic stenosis. *Am J Cardiol* 41:476-481, 1978
61. Cannon RO III, Camici PG, Epstein SE: Pathophysiological dilemma of syndrome X. *Circulation* 85:883-892, 1992
62. Epstein SE, Cannon RO III, Bonow RO: Exercise testing in patients with microvascular angina. *Circulation* 83 Suppl 3:73-76, 1991
63. Bemiller CR, Pepine CJ, Rogers AK: Long-term observations in patients with angina and normal coronary arteriograms. *Circulation* 47:36-43, 1973
64. Voelker W, Euchner U, Dittmann H, et al: Long-term clinical course of patients with angina and angiographically normal coronary arteries. *Clin Cardiol* 14:307-311, 1991
65. Cannon RO III, Bonow RO, Bacharach SL, et al: Left ventricular dysfunction in patients with angina pectoris, normal epicardial coronary arteries, and abnormal vasodilator reserve. *Circulation* 71:218-226, 1985
66. Montorsi P, Fabbiocchi F, Loaldi A, et al: Coronary adrenergic hyperreactivity in patients with syndrome X and abnormal electrocardiogram at rest. *Am J Cardiol* 68:1698-1703, 1991
67. Cannon RO III: Microvascular angina: cardiovascular investigations regarding pathophysiology and management. *Med Clin North Am* 75:1097-1118, 1991
68. Shapiro LM, Crake T, Poole-Wilson PA: Is altered cardiac sensation responsible for chest pain in patients with normal coronary arteries? Clinical observation during cardiac catheterisation. *BMJ* 296:170-171, 1988
69. Motz W, Vogt M, Rabenau O, et al: Evidence of endothelial dysfunction in coronary resistance vessels in patients with angina pectoris and normal coronary angiograms. *Am J Cardiol* 68:996-1003, 1991
70. Cannon RO, Watson RM, Rosing DR, et al: Efficacy of calcium channel blocker therapy for angina pectoris resulting from small-vessel coronary artery disease and abnormal vasodilator reserve. *Am J Cardiol* 56:242-246, 1985
71. Bugiardini R, Borghi A, Biagetti L, et al: Comparison of verapamil versus propranolol in syndrome X. *Am J Cardiol* 63:286-290, 1989
72. Steelman RB, White RS, Hill JC, et al: Midsystolic clicks in arteriosclerotic heart disease: a new facet in the clinical syndrome of papillary muscle dysfunction. *Circulation* 44:503-515, 1971
73. Shub C: Stable angina pectoris: 2. Cardiac evaluation and diagnostic testing. *Mayo Clin Proc* 65:243-255, 1990
74. Swartz MH, Pichard AD, Meller J, et al: The normal electrocardiogram as a predictor of left ventricular function in patients with coronary artery disease. *Br Heart J* 39:208-211, 1977

75. Hamby RI: Angina pectoris: a clinical-electrocardiographic-angiographic correlative study in 510 patients. *Cardiovasc Clin* 8 No 3:79-109, 1977

76. Shettigar UR, Barry WH, Hultgren HN: P wave analysis in ischaemic heart disease: an echocardiographic, haemodynamic, and angiographic assessment. *Br Heart J* 39:894-899, 1977

77. Gerson MC, McHenry PL: Resting U wave inversion as a marker of stenosis of the left anterior descending coronary artery. *Am J Med* 69:545-550, 1980

78. Haines DE, Raabe DS, Gundel WD, et al: Anatomic and prognostic significance of new T-wave inversion in unstable angina. *Am J Cardiol* 52:14-18, 1983

79. Goldschlager N, Selzer A, Cohn K: Treadmill stress tests as indicators of presence and severity of coronary artery disease. *Ann Intern Med* 85:277-286, 1976

80. Martin CM, McConahay DR: Maximal treadmill exercise electrocardiography: correlations with coronary arteriography and cardiac hemodynamics. *Circulation* 46:956-962, 1972

81. Gianrossi R, Detrano R, Mulvihill D, et al: Exercise-induced ST depression in the diagnosis of coronary artery disease: a meta-analysis. *Circulation* 80:87-98, 1989

82. Goldschlager N: Use of the treadmill test in the diagnosis of coronary artery disease in patients with chest pain. *Ann Intern Med* 97:383-388, 1982

83. Podrid PJ, Graboys TB, Lown B: Prognosis of medically treated patients with coronary-artery disease with profound ST-segment depression during exercise testing. *N Engl J Med* 305:1111-1116, 1981

84. Mukharji J, Kremers M, Lipscomb K, et al: Early positive exercise test and extensive coronary disease: effect of antianginal therapy. *Am J Cardiol* 55:267-270, 1985

85. Ellestad MH, Wan MKC: Predictive implications of stress testing: follow-up of 2700 subjects after maximal treadmill stress testing. *Circulation* 51:363-369, 1975

86. McNeer JF, Margolis JR, Lee KL, et al: The role of the exercise test in the evaluation of patients for ischemic heart disease. *Circulation* 57:64-70, 1978

87. Udall JA, Ellestad MH: Predictive implications of ventricular premature contractions associated with treadmill stress testing. *Circulation* 56:985-989, 1977

88. Dubach P, Klein J, Froelicher VF: Which definition of exertional hypotension should be used to identify patients at increased risk? (Abstract.) *Circulation* 78 Suppl 2:109, 1988

89. Balady GJ, Weiner DA, McCabe CH, et al: Value of arm exercise testing in detecting coronary artery disease. *Am J Cardiol* 55:37-39, 1985

90. Gibson RS, Taylor GJ, Watson DD, et al: Predicting the extent and location of coronary artery disease during the early postinfarction period by quantitative thallium-201 scintigraphy. *Am J Cardiol* 47:1010-1019, 1981

91. Friedman TD, Greene AC, Iskandrian AS, et al: Exercise thallium-201 myocardial scintigraphy in women: correlation with coronary arteriography. *Am J Cardiol* 49:1632-1637, 1982

92. Bodenheimer MM, Banka VS, Helfant RH: Nuclear cardiology. II. The role of myocardial perfusion imaging using thallium-201 in diagnosis of coronary heart disease. *Am J Cardiol* 45:674-684, 1980

93. Boucher CA, Brewster DC, Darling RC, et al: Determination of cardiac risk by dipyridamole-thallium imaging before peripheral vascular surgery. *N Engl J Med* 312:389-394, 1985

94. Detrano R, Janosi A, Lyons KP, et al: Factors affecting sensitivity and specificity of a diagnostic test: the exercise thallium scintigram. *Am J Med* 84:699-710, 1988

95. Robertson WS, Feigenbaum H, Armstrong WF, et al: Exercise echocardiography: a clinically practical addition in the evaluation of coronary artery disease. *J Am Coll Cardiol* 2:1085-1091, 1983

96. Wackers FJT: Adenosine-thallium imaging: Faster and better? (Editorial.) *J Am Coll Cardiol* 16:1384-1386, 1990

97. Parodi O, Marcassa C, Casucci R, et al: Accuracy and safety of technetium-99m hexakis 2-methoxy-2-isobutyl isonitrile (sestamibi) myocardial scintigraphy with high dose dipyridamole test in patients with effort angina pectoris: a multicenter study. *J Am Coll Cardiol* 18:1439-1444, 1992

98. Pamelia FX, Gibson RS, Watson DD, et al: Prognosis with chest pain and normal thallium-201 exercise scintigrams. *Am J Cardiol* 55:920-926, 1985

99. Ladenheim ML, Kotler TS, Pollock BH, et al: Incremental prognostic power of clinical history, exercise electrocardiography and myocardial perfusion scintigraphy in suspected coronary artery disease. *Am J Cardiol* 59:270-277, 1987

100. Kaul S, Lilly DR, Gascho JA, et al: Prognostic utility of the exercise thallium-201 test in ambulatory patients with chest pain: comparison with cardiac catheterization. *Circulation* 77:745-758, 1988

101. Gill JB, Ruddy TD, Newell JB, et al: Prognostic importance of thallium uptake by the lungs during exercise in coronary artery disease. *N Engl J Med* 317:1485-1489, 1987

102. Iskandrian AS, Wasserman LA, Anderson GS, et al: Merits of stress thallium-201 myocardial perfusion imaging in patients with inconclusive exercise electrocardiograms: correlation with coronary arteriograms. *Am J Cardiol* 46:553-558, 1980

103. Berger BC, Abramowitz R, Park CH, et al: Abnormal thallium-201 scans in patients with chest pain and angiographically normal coronary arteries. *Am J Cardiol* 52:365-370, 1983

104. Gupta NC, Esterbrooks DJ, Hilleman DE, et al: Comparison of adenosine and exercise thallium-201 single-photon emission computed tomography (SPECT) myocardial infusion imaging. *J Am Coll Cardiol* 19:248-257, 1992

105. Pennell DJ, Underwood SR, Swanton RH, et al: Dobutamine thallium myocardial perfusion tomography. *J Am Coll Cardiol* 18:1471-1479, 1991

106. Mazeika PK, Nardazdin A, Oakley CM: Dobutamine stress echocardiography for detection and assessment of coronary artery disease. *J Am Coll Cardiol* 19:1203-1211, 1992

107. Segar DS, Brown SE, Sawada SG, et al: Dobutamine stress echocardiography: correlation with coronary lesion severity as determined by quantitative angiography. *J Am Coll Cardiol* 19:1197-1202, 1992

108. Sawada SG, Segar DS, Ryan T, et al: Echocardiographic detection of coronary artery disease during dobutamine infusion. *Circulation* 83:1605-1614, 1991

109. Martin TW, Seaworth JF, Johns JP, et al: Comparison of adenosine, dipyridamole, and dobutamine in stress echocardiography. *Ann Intern Med* 116:190-196, 1992

110. Zoghbi WA, Cheirif J, Kleiman NS, et al: Diagnosis of ischemic heart disease with adenosine echocardiography. *J Am Coll Cardiol* 18:1271-1279, 1991

111. Lam JYT, Chaitman BR, Glaenzer M, et al: Safety and diagnostic accuracy of dipyridamole-thallium imaging in the elderly. *J Am Coll Cardiol* 11:585-589, 1988

112. Armstrong WF, O'Donnell J, Dillon JC, et al: Complementary value of two-dimensional exercise echocardiography to routine treadmill exercise testing. *Ann Intern Med* 105:829-835, 1986

113. Limacher MC, Quinones MA, Lawrence LR, et al: Detection of coronary artery disease with exercise two-dimensional echocardiography: description of a clinically applicable method and comparison with radionuclide ventriculography. *Circulation* 67:1211-1218, 1983

114. Marwick TH, Nemec JJ, Pashkow FJ, et al: Accuracy and limitations of exercise echocardiography in a routine clinical setting. *J Am Coll Cardiol* 19:74-81, 1992

115. Ryan T, Vasey CG, Presti CF, et al: Exercise echocardiography: detection of coronary artery disease in patients with normal left ventricular wall motion at rest. *J Am Coll Cardiol* 11:993-999, 1988

116. Quiñones MA, Verani MS, Haichin RM, et al: Exercise echocardiography versus ^{201}Tl single-photon emission computed tomography in evaluation of coronary artery disease: analysis of 292 patients. *Circulation* 85:1026-1031, 1992

117. Quinones MA, Waggoner AD, Reduto LA, et al: A new, simplified and accurate method for determining ejection fraction with two-dimensional echocardiography. *Circulation* 64:744-753, 1981

118. Nishimura RA, Tajik AJ, Shub C, et al: Role of two-dimensional echocardiography in the prediction of in-hospital complications after acute myocardial infarction. *J Am Coll Cardiol* 4:1080-1087, 1984

119. Brandenburg RO, Fuster V, Giuliani ER: Indications for cardiac catheterization and coronary arteriography in the adult. *Cardiovasc Clin* 10 No 3:83-88, 1980

120. Herman MV, Heinle RA, Klein MD, et al: Localized disorders in myocardial contraction: asynergy and its role in congestive heart failure. *N Engl J Med* 277:222-232, 1967

121. Bruschke AVG, Proudfit WL, Sones FM Jr: Progress study of 590 consecutive nonsurgical cases of coronary disease followed 5-9 years. II. Ventriculographic and other correlations. *Circulation* 47:1154-1163, 1973

122. Chaitman BR, Bourassa MG, Davis K, et al: Angiographic prevalence of high-risk coronary artery disease in patient subsets (CASS). *Circulation* 64:360-367, 1981
123. Alderman EL, Bourassa MG, Cohen LS, et al: Ten-year follow-up of survival and myocardial infarction in the randomized Coronary Artery Surgery Study. *Circulation* 82:1629-1646, 1990
124. Gibbons RJ, Fyke FE III, Clements IP, et al: Noninvasive identification of severe coronary artery disease using exercise radionuclide angiography. *J Am Coll Cardiol* 11:28-34, 1988
125. Bodenheimer MM: Risk stratification in coronary disease: a contrary viewpoint. *Ann Intern Med* 116:927-936, 1992
126. Brensike JF, Levy RI, Kelsey SF, et al: Effects of therapy with cholestyramine on progression of coronary arteriosclerosis: results of the NHLBI Type II Coronary Intervention Study. *Circulation* 69:313-324, 1984
127. Lichtlen PR, Hugenholtz PG, Rafflenbeul W, et al: Retardation of angiographic progression of coronary artery disease by nifedipine: results of the International Nifedipine Trial on Antiatherosclerotic Therapy (INTACT). *Lancet* 335:1109-1113, 1990
128. Ambrose JA, Winters SL, Arora RR, et al: Angiographic evolution of coronary artery morphology in unstable angina. *J Am Coll Cardiol* 7:472-478, 1986
129. Steingart RM, Packer M, Hamm P, et al: Sex differences in the management of coronary artery disease. *N Engl J Med* 325:226-230, 1991
130. Ayanian JZ, Epstein AM: Differences in the use of procedures between women and men hospitalized for coronary heart disease. *N Engl J Med* 325:221-225, 1991
131. Eaker ED, Packard B, Thom TJ: Epidemiology and risk factors for coronary heart disease in women. *Cardiovasc Clin* 19 No. 3:129-145, 1989
132. Tobin JN, Wassertheil-Smoller S, Wexler JP, et al: Sex bias in considering coronary bypass surgery. *Ann Intern Med* 107:19-25, 1987
133. Wenger NK: Gender, coronary artery disease, and coronary bypass surgery (editorial). *Ann Intern Med* 112:557-558, 1990
134. Khan SS, Nessim S, Gray R, et al: Increased mortality of women in coronary artery bypass surgery: evidence for referral bias. *Ann Intern Med* 112:561-567, 1990
135. Hillis LD, Cohn PF: Nonatherosclerotic coronary artery disease. In *Diagnosis and Therapy of Coronary Artery Disease.* Edited by PF Cohn. Boston, Little, Brown & Company, 1979, pp 481-494
136. Prinzmetal M, Kennamer R, Merliss R, et al: Angina pectoris. I. A variant form of angina pectoris: preliminary report. *Am J Med* 27:375-388, 1959
137. Hoshio A, Kotake H, Mashiba H: Significance of coronary artery tone in patients with vasospastic angina. *J Am Coll Cardiol* 14:604-609, 1989
138. Feldman RL, Pepine CJ, Whittle JL, et al: Coronary hemodynamic findings during spontaneous angina in patients with variant angina. *Circulation* 64:76-83, 1981
139. Chierchia S, Brunelli C, Simonetti I, et al: Sequence of events in angina at rest: primary reduction in coronary flow. *Circulation* 61:759-768, 1980
140. Santamore WP, Kent RL, Carey RA, et al: Synergistic effects of pressure, distal resistance, and vasoconstriction on stenosis. *Am J Physiol* 243:H236-H242, 1982
141. Brown BG, Bolson EL, Dodge HT: Dynamic mechanisms in human coronary stenosis. *Circulation* 70:917-922, 1984
142. Epstein SE, Cannon RO III, Talbot TL: Hemodynamic principles in the control of coronary blood flow. *Am J Cardiol* 56:4E-10E, 1985
143. Ganz P, Alexander RW: New insights into the cellular mechanisms of vasospasm. *Am J Cardiol* 56:11E-15E, 1985
144. Kaski JC, Crea F, Meran D, et al: Local coronary supersensitivity to diverse vasoconstrictive stimuli in patients with variant angina. *Circulation* 74:1255-1265, 1986
145. Brum JM, Sufan Q, Lane G, et al: Increased vasoconstrictor activity of proximal coronary arteries with endothelial damage in intact dogs. *Circulation* 70:1066-1073, 1984
146. Werns SW, Walton JA, Hsia HH, et al: Evidence of endothelial dysfunction in angiographically normal coronary arteries of patients with coronary artery disease. *Circulation* 79:287-291, 1989
147. Toyo-oka T, Aizawa T, Suzuki N, et al: Increased plasma levels of endothelin-1 and coronary spasm induction in patients with vasospastic angina pectoris. *Circulation* 83:476-483, 1991
148. Vrints CJM, Bult H, Hitter E, et al: Impaired endothelium-dependent cholinergic coronary vasodilation in patients with angina and normal coronary arteriograms. *J Am Coll Cardiol* 19:21-31, 1992
149. Levene DL, Freeman MR: α-Adrenoceptor-mediated coronary artery spasm. *JAMA* 236:1018-1022, 1976
150. Ricci DR, Orlick AE, Cipriano PR, et al: Altered adrenergic activity in coronary arterial spasm: insight into mechanism based on study of coronary arterial spasm: insight into mechanism based on study of coronary hemodynamics and the electrocardiogram. *Am J Cardiol* 43:1073-1079, 1979
151. Winniford MD, Filipchuk N, Hillis LD: Alpha-adrenergic blockade for variant angina: a long-term, double-blind, randomized trial. *Circulation* 67:1185-1188, 1983
152. Robertson RM, Bernard YD, Carr RK, et al: Alpha-adrenergic blockade in vasotonic angina: lack of efficacy of specific $alpha_1$-receptor blockade with prazosin. *J Am Coll Cardiol* 2:1146-1150, 1983
153. Yasue H, Horio Y, Nakamura N, et al: Induction of coronary artery spasm by acetylcholine in patients with variant angina: possible role of the parasympathetic nervous system in the pathogenesis of coronary artery spasm. *Circulation* 74:955-963, 1986
154. Okumura K, Yasue H, Horio Y, et al: Multivessel coronary spasm in patients with variant angina: a study with intracoronary injection of acetylcholine. *Circulation* 77:535-542, 1988
155. Ludmer PL, Selwyn AP, Shook TL, et al: Paradoxical vasoconstriction induced by acetylcholine in atherosclerotic coronary arteries. *N Engl J Med* 315:1046-1051, 1986
156. Okumura K, Yasue H, Matsuyama K, et al: A study on coronary hemodynamics during acetylcholine-induced coronary spasm in patients with variant angina: endothelium-dependent dilation in the resistance vessels. *J Am Coll Cardiol* 19:1426-1434, 1992
157. Brazenor RM, Angus JA: Ergometrine contracts isolated canine coronary arteries by a serotonergic mechanism: no role for alpha adrenoceptors. *J Pharmacol Exp Ther* 218:530-536, 1981
158. Müller-Schweinitzer E: The mechanism of ergometrine-induced coronary arterial spasm: in vitro studies on canine arteries. *J Cardiovasc Pharmacol* 2:645-655, 1980
159. Sakanashi M, Yonemura K-I: On the mode of action of ergometrine in the isolated dog coronary artery. *Eur J Pharmacol* 64:157-160, 1980
160. Cohen RA, Shepherd JT, Vanhoutte PM: 5-Hydroxytryptamine can mediate endothelium-dependent relaxation of coronary arteries. *Am J Physiol* 245:H1077-H1080, 1983
161. Freedman SB, Chierchia S, Rodriguez-Plaza L, et al: Ergonovine-induced myocardial ischemia: no role for serotonergic receptors? *Circulation* 70:178-183, 1984
162. McFadden EP, Clarke JG, Davies GJ, et al: Effect of intracoronary serotonin on coronary vessels in patients with stable angina and patients with variant angina. *N Engl J Med* 324:648-654, 1991
163. McFadden EP, Bauters C, Lablanche JM, et al: Effect of ketanserin on proximal and distal coronary constrictor responses to intracoronary infusion of serotonin in patients with stable angina, patients with variant angina, and control patients. *Circulation* 86:187-195, 1992
164. Sinzinger H, Feigl W, Silberbauer K: Prostacylin generation in atherosclerotic arteries (letter to the editor). *Lancet* 2:469, 1979
165. D'Angelo V, Villa S, Mysliwiec M, et al: Defective fibrinolytic and prostacyclin-like activity in human atheromatous plaques. *Thromb Haemost* 39:535-536, 1978
166. Maseri A: Role of coronary artery spasm in symptomatic and silent myocardial ischemia. *J Am Coll Cardiol* 9:249-262, 1987
167. Waters DD, Szlachcic J, Bourassa MG, et al: Exercise testing in patients with variant angina: results, correlation with clinical and angiographic features and prognostic significance. *Circulation* 65:265-274, 1982
168. De Servi S, Falcone C, Gavazzi A, et al: The exercise test in variant angina: results in 114 patients. *Circulation* 64:684-688, 1981
169. Severi S, Davies G, Maseri A, et al: Long-term prognosis of "variant" angina with medical treatment. *Am J Cardiol* 46:226-232, 1980
170. Conti CR: Coronary artery spasm: provocative testing (editorial). *Clin Cardiol* 17:353, 1994
171. Heupler FA Jr, Proudfit WL, Razavi M, et al: Ergonovine maleate provocative test for coronary arterial spasm. *Am J Cardiol* 41:631-640, 1978
172. Schroeder JS, Bolen JL, Quint RA, et al: Provocation of coronary

spasm with ergonovine maleate: new test with results in 57 patients undergoing coronary arteriography. *Am J Cardiol* 40:487-491, 1977

173. Chahine RA: The provocation of coronary artery spasm. *Cathet Cardiovasc Diagn* 6:1-5, 1980

174. Harding MB, Leithe ME, Mark DB, et al: Ergonovine maleate testing during cardiac catheterization: a 10-year perspective in 3,447 patients without significant coronary artery disease or Prinzmetal's variant angina. *J Am Coll Cardiol* 20:107-111, 1992

175. Bertrand ME, LaBlanche JM, Tilmant PY, et al: Frequency of provoked coronary arterial spasm in 1089 consecutive patients undergoing coronary arteriography. *Circulation* 65:1299-1306, 1982

176. Miwa K, Fujita M, Ejiri M, et al: Usefulness of intracoronary injection of acetylcholine as a provocative test for coronary artery spasm in patients with vasospastic angina. *Heart Vessels* 6:96-101, 1991

177. Heupler FA Jr: Provocative testing for coronary arterial spasm: risk, method and rationale. *Am J Cardiol* 46:335-340, 1980

178. Buxton A, Goldberg S, Hirshfeld JW, et al: Refractory ergonovine-induced coronary vasospasm: importance of intracoronary nitroglycerin. *Am J Cardiol* 46:329-334, 1980

179. Crevey BJ, Owen SF, Pitt B: Irreversible coronary occlusion related to administration of ergonovine. *Circulation* 64:853-856, 1981

180. Robertson RM, Wood AJJ, Vaughn WK, et al: Exacerbation of vasotonic angina pectoris by propranolol. *Circulation* 65:281-285, 1982

181. De Caterina R, Carpeggiani C, L'Abbate A: A double-blind, placebo-controlled study of ketanserin in patients with Prinzmetal's angina: evidence against a role for serotonin in the genesis of coronary vasospasm. *Circulation* 69:889-894, 1984

182. Kugiyama K, Yasue H, Okumura K, et al: Suppression of exercise-induced angina by magnesium sulfate in patients with variant angina. *J Am Coll Cardiol* 12:1177-1183, 1988

183. Waters DD, Théroux P, Crittin J, et al: Previously undiagnosed variant angina as a cause of chest pain after coronary artery bypass surgery. *Circulation* 61:1159-1164, 1980

184. David PR, Waters DD, Scholl J-M, et al: Percutaneous transluminal coronary angioplasty in patients with variant angina. *Circulation* 66:695-702, 1982

185. Corcos T, David PR, Bourassa MG, et al: Percutaneous transluminal coronary angioplasty for the treatment of variant angina. *J Am Coll Cardiol* 5:1046-1054, 1985

186. Yasue H, Takizawa A, Nagao M, et al: Long-term prognosis for patients with variant angina and influential factors. *Circulation* 78:1-9, 1988

187. Walling A, Waters DD, Miller DD, et al: Long-term prognosis of patients with variant angina. *Circulation* 76:990-997, 1987

188. Mark DB, Califf RM, Morris KG, et al: Clinical characteristics and long-term survival of patients with variant angina. *Circulation* 69:880-888, 1984

189. Nakamura M, Takeshita A, Nose Y: Clinical characteristics associated with myocardial infarction, arrhythmias, and sudden death in patients with vasospastic angina. *Circulation* 75:1110-1116, 1987

190. Waters DD, Bouchard A, Théroux P: Spontaneous remission is a frequent outcome of variant angina. *J Am Coll Cardiol* 2:195-199, 1983

191. Scholl J-M, Veau P, Benacerraf A, et al: Long-term prognosis of medically treated patients with vasospastic angina and no fixed significant coronary atherosclerosis. *Am Heart J* 115:559-564, 1988

192. Nobuyoshi M, Tanaka M, Nosaka H, et al: Progression of coronary atherosclerosis: Is coronary spasm related to progression? *J Am Coll Cardiol* 18:904-910, 1991

193. Kaski JC, Tousoulis D, McFadden E, et al: Variant angina pectoris: role of coronary spasm in the development of fixed coronary obstructions. *Circulation* 85:619-626, 1992

194. Raymond R, Lynch J, Underwood D, et al: Myocardial infarction and normal coronary arteriography: a 10 year clinical and risk analysis of 74 patients. *J Am Coll Cardiol* 11:471-477, 1988

195. Amromin GD, Gildenhorn HL, Solomon RD, et al: The synergism of X-irradiation and cholesterol-fat feeding on the development of coronary artery lesions. *J Atheroscler Res* 4:325-334, 1964

196. Lange RL, Reid MS, Tresch DD, et al: Nonatheromatous ischemic heart disease following withdrawal from chronic industrial nitroglycerin exposure. *Circulation* 46:666-678, 1972

197. Chaitman BR, Bourassa MG, Lespérance J, et al: Anomalous left coronary artery from pulmonary artery: an eight year angiographic follow-up after saphenous vein bypass graft. *Circulation* 51:552-555, 1975

198. Liberthson RR, Dinsmore RE, Fallon JT: Aberrant coronary artery origin from the aorta: report of 18 patients, review of literature and delineation of natural history and management. *Circulation* 59:748-754, 1979

199. Click RL, Holmes DR Jr, Vlietstra RE, et al: Anomalous coronary arteries: location, degree of atherosclerosis and effect on survival—a report from the Coronary Artery Surgery Study. *J Am Coll Cardiol* 13:531-537, 1989

200. Sim DN, Neill WA: Investigation of the physiological basis for increased exercise threshold for angina pectoris after physical conditioning. *J Clin Invest* 54:763-770, 1974

201. Kennedy CC, Spiekerman RE, Lindsay MI Jr, et al: One-year graduated exercise program for men with angina pectoris: evaluation by physiologic studies and coronary arteriography. *Mayo Clin Proc* 51:231-236, 1976

202. Kattus A: Medical vs surgical therapy for ischemic heart disease. *Chest* 58 Suppl 1:299-304, 1970

203. Kavanagh T, Shephard RJ, Chisholm AW, et al: Prognostic indexes for patients with ischemic heart disease enrolled in an exercise-centered rehabilitation program. *Am J Cardiol* 44:1230-1240, 1979

204. Schuler G, Schlierf G, Wirth A, et al: Low-fat diet and regular, supervised physical exercise in patients with symptomatic coronary artery disease: reduction of stress-induced myocardial ischemia. *Circulation* 77:172-181, 1988

205. Shephard RJ: Recurrence of myocardial infarction in an exercising population. *Br Heart J* 42:133-138, 1979

206. Eckstein RW: Effect of exercise and coronary artery narrowing on coronary collateral circulation. *Circ Res* 5:230-235, 1957

207. Bloor CM, White FC, Sanders TM: Effects of exercise on collateral development in myocardial ischemia in pigs. *J Appl Physiol* 56:656-665, 1984

208. Wenger NK: Does exercise training enhance collateral circulation? *Bibl Cardiol* No 36, 1976, pp 143-145

209. Shephard RJ: Some physiologic reasons for training the patient with angina. *Pract Cardiol* 8:59, 1982

210. Magder S, Linnarsson D, Gullstrand L: The effect of swimming on patients with ischemic heart disease. *Circulation* 63:979-986, 1981

211. Fox SM III, Naughton JP, Gorman PA: Physical activity and cardiovascular health. II. The exercise prescription: intensity and duration. *Mod Concepts Cardiovasc Dis* 41:21-24, 1972

212. Rothbaum DA: Coronary artery disease. *Cardiovasc Clin* 12 No 1:105-118, 1981

213. O'Rourke RA, Chatterjee K, Wei JY: Cardiovascular disease in the elderly. Coronary heart disease. *J Am Coll Cardiol* 10 Suppl A:52-56, 1987

214. Gersh BJ: Clinical manifestations of coronary heart disease in the elderly. In *Coronary Heart Disease in the Elderly.* Edited by NK Wenger, CD Furberg, E Pitt. New York, Elsevier Science Publishing Company, 1986, pp 276-302

215. Gersh BJ, Kronmal RA, Frye RL, et al: Coronary arteriography and coronary artery bypass surgery: morbidity and mortality in patients ages 65 years or older: a report from the Coronary Artery Surgery Study. *Circulation* 67:483-491, 1983

216. Mihalick MJ, Fisch C: Electrocardiographic findings in the aged. *Am Heart J* 87:117-128, 1974

217. Gersh BJ, Kronmal RA, Schaff HV, et al: Comparison of coronary artery bypass surgery and medical therapy in patients 65 years of age or older: a nonrandomized study from the Coronary Artery Surgery Study (CASS) registry. *N Engl J Med* 313:217-224, 1985

218. National Cooperative Study Group: Unstable angina pectoris. I. Report of protocol and patient population. *Am J Cardiol* 37:896-902, 1976

219. Munger TM, Oh JK: Unstable angina. *Mayo Clin Proc* 65:384-406, 1990

220. Théroux P: A pathophysiologic basis for the clinical classification and management of unstable angina. *Circulation* 75 Suppl 5:103-105, 1987

221. Braunwald E: Unstable angina: a classification. *Circulation* 80:410-414, 1989

222. Hultgren HN, Pfeifer JF, Angell WW, et al: Unstable angina: comparison of medical and surgical management. *Am J Cardiol* 39:734-740, 1977

223. Alison HW, Russell RO Jr, Mantle JA, et al: Coronary anatomy and arteriography in patients with unstable angina pectoris. *Am J Cardiol* 41:204-209, 1978

224. Davies MJ, Thomas AC: Plaque fissuring—the cause of acute myocardial infarction, sudden ischaemic death, and crescendo angina. *Br Heart J* 53:363-373, 1985

225. Sherman CT, Litvack F, Grundfest W, et al: Coronary angioscopy in patients with unstable angina pectoris. *N Engl J Med* 315:913-919, 1986

226. Davies MJ, Thomas A: Thrombosis and acute coronary-artery lesions in sudden cardiac ischemic death. *N Engl J Med* 310:1137-1140, 1984

227. Bresnahan DR, Davis JL, Holmes DR Jr, et al: Angiographic occurrence and clinical correlates of intraluminal coronary thrombus: role of unstable angina. *J Am Coll Cardiol* 6:285-289, 1985

228. Gorlin R, Fuster V, Ambrose JA: Anatomic-physiologic links between acute coronary syndromes (editorial). *Circulation* 74:6-9, 1986

229. Fuster V, Badimon L, Cohen M, et al: Insights into the pathogenesis of acute ischemic syndromes. *Circulation* 77:1213-1220, 1988

230. Curfman GD, Heinsimer JA, Lozner EC, et al: Intravenous nitroglycerin in the treatment of spontaneous angina pectoris: a prospective, randomized trial. *Circulation* 67:276-282, 1983

231. Figueras J, Lidon R, Cortadellas J: Rebound myocardial ischaemia following abrupt interruption of intravenous nitroglycerin infusion in patients with unstable angina at rest. *Eur Heart J* 12:405-411, 1991

232. Williams DO, Kirby MG, McPherson K, et al: Anticoagulant treatment of unstable angina. *Br J Clin Pract* 40:114-116, 1986

233. Théroux P, Ouimet H, McCans J, et al: Aspirin, heparin, or both to treat acute unstable angina. *N Engl J Med* 319:1105-1111, 1988

234. Lewis HD Jr, Davis JW, Archibald DG, et al: Protective effects of aspirin against acute myocardial infarction and death in men with unstable angina: results of a Veterans Administration Cooperative Study. *N Engl J Med* 309:396-403, 1983

235. Berglund U, Wallentin L: Influence on platelet function by heparin in men with unstable coronary artery disease. *Thromb Haemost* 66:648-651, 1991

236. Théroux P, Waters D, Lam J, et al: Reactivation of unstable angina after the discontinuation of heparin. *N Engl J Med* 327:141-145, 1992

237. Lubsen J, Tijssen JGP: Efficacy of nifedipine and metoprolol in the early treatment of unstable angina in the coronary care unit: findings from the Holland Interuniversity Nifedipine/Metoprolol Trial (HINT). *Am J Cardiol* 60 Suppl:18A-25A, 1987

238. Parodi O, Simonetti I, Michelassi C, et al: Comparison of verapamil and propranolol therapy for angina pectoris at rest: a randomized, multiple-crossover, controlled trial in the coronary care unit. *Am J Cardiol* 57:899-906, 1986

239. Yusuf S, Wittes J, Friedman L: Overview of results of randomized clinical trials in heart disease. II. Unstable angina, heart failure, primary prevention with aspirin, and risk factor modification. *JAMA* 260:2259-2263, 1988

240. Gottlieb SO, Weisfeldt ML, Ouyang P, et al: Effect of the addition of propranolol to therapy with nifedipine for unstable angina pectoris: a randomized, double-blind, placebo-controlled trial. *Circulation* 73:331-337, 1986

241. Held PH, Yusuf S, Furberg CD: Calcium channel blockers in acute myocardial infarction and unstable angina: an overview. *BMJ* 299:1187-1192, 1989

242. Parodi O, Maseri A, Simonetti I: Management of unstable angina at rest by verapamil: a double-blind cross-over study in coronary care unit. *Br Heart J* 41:167-174, 1979

243. Parodi O, Simonetti I, L'Abbate A, et al: Verapamil versus propranolol for angina at rest. *Am J Cardiol* 50:923-928, 1982

244. Théroux P, Taeymans Y, Morissette D, et al: A randomized study comparing propranolol and diltiazem in the treatment of unstable angina. *J Am Coll Cardiol* 5:717-722, 1985

245. Gerstenblith G, Ouyang P, Achuff SC, et al: Nifedipine in unstable angina: a double-blind, randomized trial. *N Engl J Med* 306:885-889, 1982

246. Hill JA, Feldman RL, Pepine CJ, et al: Randomized double-blind comparison of nifedipine and isosorbide dinitrate in patients with coronary arterial spasm. *Am J Cardiol* 49:431-438, 1982

247. Holland Interuniversity Nifedipine/Metoprolol Trial (HINT) Research Group: Early treatment of unstable angina in the coronary care unit: a randomised, double blind, placebo controlled comparison of recurrent ischaemia in patients treated with nifedipine or metoprolol or both. *Br Heart J* 56:400-413, 1986

248. Pepine CJ, Feldman RL, Hill JA, et al: Clinical outcome after treatment of rest angina with calcium blockers: comparative experience during the initial year of therapy with diltiazem, nifedipine, and verapamil. *Am Heart J* 106:1341-1347, 1983

249. Lubsen J: Medical management of unstable angina. What have we learned from the randomized trials? *Circulation* 82 Suppl 2:82-87, 1990

250. Grambow DW, Topol EJ: Effect of maximal medical therapy on refractoriness of unstable angina pectoris. *Am J Cardiol* 70:577-581, 1992

251. Lawrence JR, Shepherd JT, Bone I, et al: Fibrinolytic therapy in unstable angina pectoris: a controlled clinical trial. *Thromb Res* 17:767-777, 1980

252. Vetrovec GW, Leinbach RC, Gold HK, et al: Intracoronary thrombolysis in syndromes of unstable ischemia: angiographic and clinical results. *Am Heart J* 104:946-952, 1982

253. Ambrose JA, Hjemdahl-Monsen C, Borrico S, et al: Quantitative and qualitative effects of intracoronary streptokinase in unstable angina and non-Q-wave- infarction. *J Am Coll Cardiol* 9:1156-1165, 1987

254. Gotoh K, Minamino T, Katoh O, et al: The role of intracoronary thrombus in unstable angina: angiographic assessment and thrombolytic therapy during ongoing anginal attacks. *Circulation* 77:526-532, 1988

255. Freeman MR, Langer A, Wilson RF, et al: Thrombolysis in unstable angina. Randomized double-blind trial of t-PA and placebo. *Circulation* 85:150-157, 1992

256. Vejar M, Hackett D, Brunelli C, et al: Comparison of low-dose aspirin and coronary vasodilators in acute unstable angina. *Circulation* 81 Suppl 1:4-11, 1990

257. Pozzati A, Bugiardini R, Borhi A, et al: Transient ischaemia refractory to conventional medical treatment in unstable angina: angiographic correlates and prognostic implications. *Eur Heart J* 13:360-365, 1992

258. De Servi S, Berzuini C, Poma E, et al: Long-term survival and risk stratification in patients with angina at rest undergoing medical treatment. *Int J Cardiol* 22:43-50, 1989

259. Betriu A, Heras M, Cohen M, et al: Unstable angina. Outcome according to clinical presentation. *J Am Coll Cardiol* 19:1659-1663, 1992

CHAPTER

29

Myocardial ischemia clinical syndromes

C. Antianginal agents

Michael D. McGoon, M.D., and Clarence Shub, M.D.

ANGINA is a symptom complex reflecting inadequate oxygen supply for myocardial metabolic demands. Therapy must be directed toward reducing ischemia by promoting coronary blood flow or limiting myocardial oxygen consumption. Coronary blood flow is largely dependent upon (1) coronary arterial resistance, (2) the availability of coronary collateral vessels, (3) duration of diastole, and (4) aortic diastolic pressure. Improvement in coronary flow can be promoted by agents that (1) decrease coronary resistance either by direct vasodilatation or by reduction of intramyocardial tension, (2) promote development of and flow through collateral vessels, or (3) augment the duration of diastole (Table 29C-1).

The main determinants of myocardial oxygen consumption are (1) intramyocardial tension (which by the Laplace relation is a function of cavity volume and pressure), (2) myocardial contractility, and (3) heart rate. Reduction of myocardial metabolic demand can be promoted by agents that (1) limit intramyocardial tension by reducing intracavitary pressure development (especially by decreasing afterload) or by reducing ventricular volume (especially by increasing venous capacitance), (2) reduce the myocardial contractile state by decreasing the rate and extent of systolic tension development, or (3) slow the heart rate (see Table 29C-1).

NITRATES

Mode of action

Physicochemical features. The compounds of this class contain one or more nitrate groups covalently bound to the carbon atoms of an organic residue.

The ability of organic nitrates to produce vascular smooth muscle relaxation appears to be mediated by activation of guanylate cyclase and an increase in the rate of cyclic guanosine monophosphate synthesis.[1] Intermediate steps in this process involve the intracellular (and in some cases extracellular[2]) formation of nitric oxide from organic nitrates, a reaction that is facilitated by compounds containing sulfhydryl groups (thiols). Nitric oxide (which can also be released endogenously by endothelial cells[3] and therefore may be an endothelium-derived relaxing factor[4]) in turn reacts with thiols to form S-nitrosothiols, which activate guanylate cyclase.[5-9] Tolerance to the effects of nitrates that may occur after sustained exposure corresponds with inability to generate cyclic guanosine monophosphate,[10] possibly due to oxidation of sulfhydryl groups.

Cardiovascular effects (Fig 29C-1)

PERIPHERAL VASCULAR EFFECTS. Although the predominant site of action varies among the various agents, all of the organic nitrates and nitrites have the ability to produce vasodilatation. Nitroglycerin increases venous capacitance peripherally and in the splanchnic and pulmonary venous beds. The concomitant increase in venous pooling results in reduced preload on the heart similar to the effect of acutely reducing blood volume by phlebotomy and thereby decreases end-diastolic left ventricular volume and diastolic wall tension.[11] Dimin-

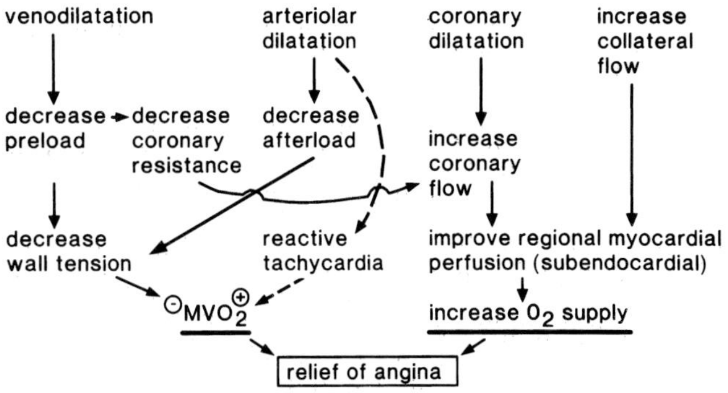

Fig 29C-1 Cardiovascular effects of nitrates and the mechanisms by which they reduce symptoms of angina. *Dashed arrows* indicate less clinically apparent effects than those indicated by *solid arrows*. MVO_2, myocardial oxygen uptake; O_2, oxygen; +, increase; −, decrease.

Table 29C-1 Potential means of improving myocardial oxygen demand/supply ratio

Parameter	Determinants	Effect of therapeutic agent	Mechanism of therapeutic effect
Coronary blood flow	Coronary resistance		
	Vascular tone	Decrease	Produce vasodilatation
	Intramyocardial tension	Decrease	Reduce diastolic volume or pressure (Laplace relation)
	Coronary collateral vessels	Increase	Promote development of collaterals or flow
	Duration of diastole	Increase	Slow heart rate
Myocardial oxygen consumption	Intramyocardial tension		
	Preload	Decrease	Reduce diastolic volume or pressure (Laplace relation)
	Afterload	Decrease	Limit systolic tension development, decrease end-systolic volume
	Contractile state	Decrease	Decrease rate and extent of systolic tension development
	Heart rate	Decrease	Decrease systolic work per minute

ished myocardial wall tension results in lessened myocardial oxygen demand.

Arteriolar resistance is also decreased by nitroglycerin[12] and especially by amyl nitrite. This reduction in afterload decreases systolic wall tension and increases ventricular emptying (decreased volume), which also limits myocardial oxygen consumption, but these effects are seldom obtained at clinical doses.[13]

CORONARY ARTERIAL EFFECTS. Nitrates enhance blood flow in normal canine coronary arteries[14] and produce vasodilatation in normal and stenotic human coronary arteries.[15-17] Nitroglycerin also decreases resistance in coronary collateral vessels.[18] Nitroglycerin appears to redistribute myocardial blood flow to ischemic subendocardial layers[19] and increase subendocardial Po_2.[20] Nitrates are potent vasodilators of epicardial coronary arteries, and they promote resolution of spontaneous or ergonovine-induced spasm.

Despite these direct coronary vascular effects, all of which promote myocardial oxygen supply, the administration of nitroglycerin to patients with coronary artery disease produces little or no effect on total coronary blood flow. Intracoronary nitroglycerin is ineffective in preventing atrial pacing-induced angina,[21] although coronary flow increases somewhat, especially to the least ischemic regions.[22] Conversely, systemic administration of nitroglycerin relieves pacing-induced angina in many patients yet also *reduces* coronary blood flow to both ischemic and nonischemic regions.[23] These observations suggest that coronary vasodilatation may be maximal in these patients to begin with or that the ability of nitroglycerin to reduce wall stress and oxygen consumption (which are indirect stimuli for maintaining increased coronary blood flow) predominates over direct coronary effects.

Rarely, nitroglycerin appears to aggravate myocardial ischemia,[24,25] a phenomenon termed "paradoxic angina." The proposed mechanism for this is that coronary arteriolar vasodilatation may lower coronary pressure distal to the stenosis and thus promote further collapse of the vessel lumen in the stenotic zone.[26,27] An alternative explanation may be that even moderate nitroglycerin-induced hypotension may decrease the transstenotic gradient enough to produce adverse effects on coronary flow.[28]

MYOCARDIAL EFFECTS. No direct myocardial effects have been attributed with certainty to these compounds. However, the net result of peripheral or coronary vascular vasodilatation is often to improve left ventricular function.[29,30]

Pharmacokinetics (Table 29C-2) and pharmacodynamics (Table 29C-3)

Organic nitrate esters are lipid-soluble compounds whose biotransformation into water-soluble denitrated metabolites reduces their biologic potency. The degradation of organic nitrates appears to be partly due to catalyzation by hepatic glutathione-organic nitrate reductase. Evidence from portosystemic shunted animals, however, suggests that the liver is not the only metabolizer of nitroglycerin; substantial clearance may occur in nonhepatic tissue, particularly the vasculature.[31]

Glyceryl trinitrate is predominantly converted to the dinitrate form. This is further converted to a mononitrate

Table 29C-2 Pharmacokinetic behavior of nitrates

Agent	Oral bioavailability, %	Plasma half-life	Route of elimination	Active metabolites
Nitroglycerin	Low	3 min	Hepatic, red blood cells, blood vessels	Yes, but weaker
Isosorbide dinitrate	60: sublingual 20-25: oral	60 min: sublingual 4 hr: oral	Hepatic*	Yes; 60% metabolized to isosorbide-5-mononitrate
Isosorbide-5-mononitrate	100	4-5.6 hr	Nonhepatic excretion	No

*Large first-pass hepatic clearance for oral doses, but total clearance exceeds hepatic blood flow, implying additional extrahepatic clearance.

quite slowly, and there is very little conversion of mononitrate to glycerol. Most of the urinary metabolites that are excreted are in a dinitrate form. These are 1,2-glycerol dinitrate and 1,3-glycerol dinitrate. They have about 1⁄10 the activity of nitroglycerin.

Many forms of nitroglycerin are used clinically:

1. Sublingual tablet
2. Buccal application
3. Oral tablet
4. Ointment
5. Dermal patch
6. Injection for intravenous use
7. Injection for intracoronary use
8. Aerosol

Nitroglycerin has the same pharmacokinetic characteristics regardless of formulation: short half-life, 60% protein absorption, and hepatic and vascular routes of elimination. The various formulations simply permit alternative routes of delivery, which result in different drug concentration profiles over time. Thus, the formulation used can be tailored to the desired clinical effect. Sublingual or transmucosal preparations produce a rapid onset of action; intravenous nitroglycerin achieves rapid effects and is quickly titratable; sustained-release oral preparations are of slower onset but achieve longer effective drug levels (not because of a longer half-life but because of persistent release into the bloodstream); transdermal preparations and retained transmucosal tablets similarly achieve prolonged steady-state drug levels in the blood.

Isosorbide dinitrate has an initial (α) half-life of just a few minutes and a further elimination (β) half-life lasting 2 to 4 hours. Isosorbide-5-mononitrate is the major metabolite and has a half-life of approximately 4 hours. About 60% of the administered isosorbide dinitrate is eliminated as isosorbide-5-mononitrate in the urine; the remainder is eliminated in the bound form as glucuronide. Isosorbide-5-mononitrate is available as an orally administered agent that has high oral bioavailability and is not hepatically metabolized (see Table 29C-2).

Nitrate tolerance

The development of vehicles to achieve prolonged absorption of nitroglycerin, which was intended to provide sustained clinical effect with ease of administration and enhanced compliance, has led to increased recognition of tolerance, a phenomenon once thought to have little clinical significance. Substantial evidence has accumulated that exposure to continuous levels of nitroglycerin leads to measurable decreases in, and even elimination of, therapeutic effect in terms of frequency of spontaneous electrocardiographic (ECG) ischemia,[32] coronary vasodilatation,[33] exercise ischemia,[34] exercise duration,[35,36] and pulmonary capillary wedge pressure.[37] This diminution of nitroglycerin's action can be observed in as little as 24 hours of constant exposure, which most often occurs with transdermal and intravenous routes of administration.

The predominant opinion currently is that tolerance develops as intracellular sulfhydryl groups, necessary for mediating the effect of nitroglycerin on vascular smooth muscle cells, are depleted. Consequently, attempts at counteracting this effect have involved either exogenous supplying of sulfhydryl groups in the form of *N*-acetylcysteine[38-40] or the amino acid methionine[41] or permitting the endogenous replenishment of sulfhydryl groups by intermittently interrupting nitroglycerin administration.[39,42-45] Intermittent nitrate administration carries the potential for development of withdrawal symptoms, such as decreased angina threshold, or protracted occurrence of side effects that do not attenuate over time.[34] With some exceptions,[46] these approaches have been successful in avoiding or attenuating tolerance. Concomitant administration of an angiotensin converting enzyme inhibitor, regardless of whether it contains a sulfhydryl group, may attenuate the development of tolerance.[47] Cross-tolerance between nitroglycerin and isosorbide dinitrate has been observed.[48]

Alternative explanations for tolerance include the possibilities that guanylate cyclase activity diminishes after prolonged treatment, that counteractive increases in neurohormones (such as catecholamines, arginine vasopressin, renin aldosterone, and angiotensin II) are provoked, and that intravascular blood volume increases.[49-51]

β-ADRENERGIC BLOCKING AGENTS

The response of the cardiovascular system to catecholamines is mediated by specific cell-membrane receptors. The action of a sympathomimetic amine is determined by

Table 29C-3 Indications for, dosages of, and pharmacodynamic features of nitrates

Agent	Rationale and indications	Dosage*	Onset of action, min	Peak effect, min	Duration of effect
Nitroglycerin					
Sublingual	Short-term prophylaxis, acutely abort angina	0.3-0.8 mg p.r.n.	2-5	4-8	10-30 min
Oral	Sustained prophylaxis	6.5-19.5 mg b.i.d.	15-40	40-120	3-6 hr†
Lingual aerosol	Short-term prophylaxis, acutely abort angina	0.4-0.8 mg p.r.n.	2-5	4-8	10-30 min
Buccal	Sustained prophylaxis	1.0-3 mg q5h during day	2-5	4-8	Sustained during 3- to 5-hr application†
2% ointment	Sustained prophylaxis	0.5-2.0 in. (about 15 mg/in.) h.s.	30-60	30-60	Sustained during 7-hr application†
Transdermal patch	Sustained prophylaxis	10-30 mg/24 hr; remove for 8-12 hr daily to prevent tolerance	30-60	30-60	Sustained during 24-hr application†
Intravenous	Acute unstable ischemia or infarct management, pulmonary edema, severe hypertension	5 μg/min; then titrate, usually to 30-80 μg/min	1	1-2	Sustained during infusion†
Isosorbide dinitrate					
Oral	Sustained prophylaxis	5-40 mg b.i.d.-t.i.d.	15-20	20-30	3-8 hr
Sublingual	Short-term prophylaxis, acutely abort angina	2.5-10 mg p.r.n.	2	5-10	½-2 hr
Isosorbide-5-mononitrate	Sustained prophylaxis, may be useful when hepatic or renal function is unpredictable	20 mg p.o. on arising and 7 hr later ("asymmetrical dosing")	45-60	90-180	4-8 hr
Erythrityl tetranitrate					
Oral	Sustained prophylaxis	10-30 mg t.i.d.	15-20	30-60	3-6 hr
Sublingual	Sustained prophylaxis	5-10 mg p.r.n.	5	5-10	1-3 hr
Pentaerythritol tetranitrate					
Oral	Sustained prophylaxis	10-40 mg q.i.d.	15-20	30-45	3-6 hr
Oral, sustained action	Sustained prophylaxis	80 mg b.i.d.	30	60	8-10 hr

*p.r.n., prophylactically or to abort angina.
†Tolerance would develop during long-term administration and thus alter profile of effects.

Table 29C-4 Adrenergic receptors

Tissue	Receptor type	Response to stimulation
Cardiac	$Beta_1$	Increase discharge rate of sinus node Increase AV node conduction velocity Decrease AV node refractoriness Increase contractility
Kidney	$Beta_1$	Renin release
Arterioles		
Coronary	Alpha	Constriction
	Beta	Dilatation
Skin	Alpha	Constriction
Skeletal muscle	Alpha	Constriction
	$Beta_2$	Dilatation
Pulmonary	Alpha	Constriction
	$Beta_2$	Dilatation
Splanchnic	Alpha	Constriction
	$Beta_2$	Dilatation
Veins	Alpha	Constriction
	$Beta_2$	Dilatation
Bronchi	$Beta_2$	Dilatation

AV, atrioventricular.

the type and site of receptor with which it interacts (Table 29C-4). Stimulation of β_1-receptors, which are located primarily in the myocardium, increases cardiac contractility, sinus discharge rate, and atrioventricular (AV) node conduction velocity, and decreases AV node refractoriness. The β_2-receptor, the predominant β-adrenergic receptor subtype in vascular and bronchial tissue, mediates arteriolar dilatation and bronchial smooth muscle relaxation.

The rationale for the use of β-adrenergic blockers in the management of angina is based on the ability of these drugs to inhibit the chronotropic and inotropic responses to catecholamines.

Mode of action

Physicochemical features. β-Adrenergic receptors are proteins or lipoproteins located in the plasma cell membrane in close association with, but distinct from, adenylate cyclase. The potency of a β-agonist in evoking a β-adrenergic response is directly related to its ability to occupy a receptor site. β-Adrenergic antagonists inhibit the effects of catecholamines by competitively blocking β-adrenergic receptor sites.

β-Adrenergic blockers are structurally similar to the specific β-adrenergic agonist isoproterenol (Fig 29C-2). The basic functional unit is an aromatic ring, a two-carbon side chain, and an alkyl-substituted secondary or tertiary amine. The larger the alkyl group, the greater is the affinity for the β-receptor.[52] The aromatic ring substituents apparently determine the degree of agonist or antagonist activity.[52,53] Although β-antagonists are available only as racemic mixtures of optical isomers, it is the (−) levorotatory isomers that possess β-blocking activity; the (+) dextrorotatory stereoisomers contribute only to the nonspecific effects of the agents.

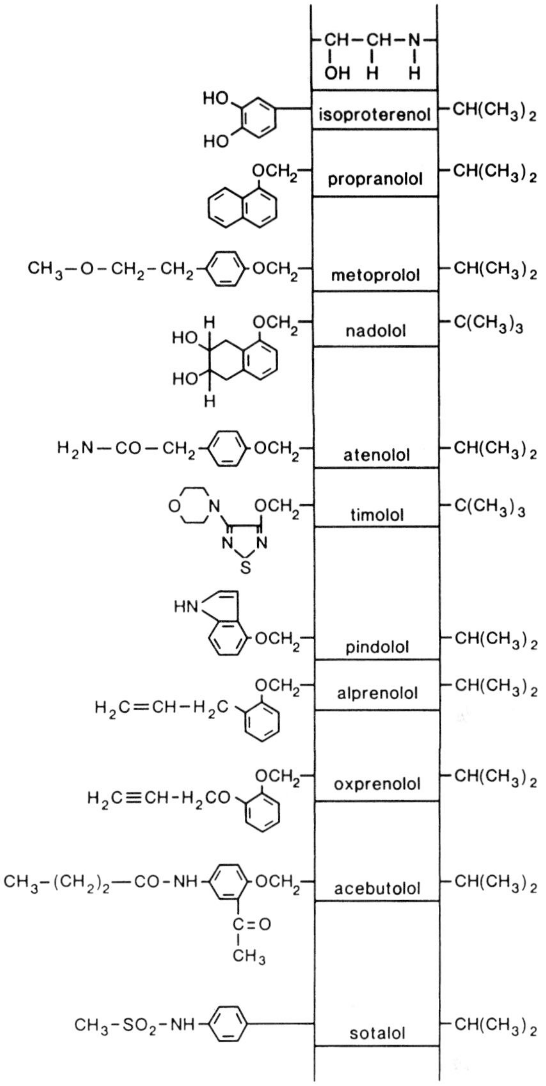

Fig 29C-2 All β-adrenergic blockers share the central structure of isoproterenol *(top),* and variation of the aromatic ring and amine imparts their individual characteristics.

Ancillary properties

CARDIOSELECTIVITY. The extent to which a β-adrenergic blocker is capable of blocking β_1- and not β_2-receptors determines its cardioselectivity.[54] Certain agents are more cardioselective than others: metoprolol, atenolol, and acebutolol are all relatively cardioselective (Table 29C-5). These drugs are up to 100 times more potent inhibitors of isoproterenol-induced increases in heart rate and contractility than they are of bronchial or

Table 29C-5 Dosages and ancillary properties of β-adrenergic blocking agents

Agent	Usual daily oral dose (doses/day)*	Need to adjust in renal failure	Cardioselective	ISA
Propranolol	160-480 mg (2-4)	Yes	0	0
Nadolol	40-320 mg (1)	Yes	0	0
Timolol	20-40 mg (2)	Yes	0	+/−
Sotalol	240-480 mg (1)	Yes	0	0
Pindolol	7.5-22.5 mg (3)	Yes	0	+ + +
Alprenolol	120-400 mg (2)	?	0	+ +
Oxprenolol	120-400 mg (2-3)	?	0	+ +
Atenolol	50-200 mg (1)	Yes	+	0
Metoprolol	100-200 mg (2-3)	?	+	0
Acebutolol	600-1,200 mg (1-2)	Yes	+	+
Esmolol	Up to 300 μg/kg/min	No (titrate)	+	0
Labetalol	200-800 mg (2)	No	0	0

ISA, intrinsic sympathomimetic activity.
*Sustained-action formulations are available for some drugs.

peripheral vascular dilatation.[53] Cardioselectivity is dose-dependent, since at higher doses (often in the usual clinical dose range) these agents also display β_2 antagonism and cardioselectivity is lost.[55,56] Noncardioselective β-blockers, on the other hand, inhibit both β_1- and β_2-receptors at all doses.

Cardioselectivity offers theoretic advantages in the clinical management of cardiac disease since there is less tendency to produce unwanted bronchoconstriction or peripheral arterial vasoconstriction.[56] Although there are fewer side effects and less decrease in rate of forced expiration in asthmatic patients and healthy volunteers, cardioselective agents may exacerbate bronchospasm in some patients,[52,56] and the likelihood of doing so increases at doses that are high enough to be clinically useful.

INTRINSIC SYMPATHOMIMETIC ACTIVITY. All β-antagonists block β-adrenergic receptors. Some agents, however, also possess partial agonist activity and, therefore, are capable of producing sympathetic stimulation.[57] Agents with this property, referred to as "intrinsic sympathomimetic activity," include pindolol, alprenolol, oxprenolol, and acebutolol (see Table 29C-5). The degree to which intrinsic sympathomimetic activity is clinically apparent depends in part on the underlying sympathetic activity of the person receiving the drug. In patients with minimal sympathetic activity, the β-blocking properties of the drug make little contribution and the stimulatory effects may predominate. Intrinsic sympathomimetic activity is not dose-dependent; the degree of intrinsic sympathomimetic activity remains the same at all doses, but the maximum response of the tissue is less than that for pure β-agonists. Drugs with intrinsic sympathomimetic activity may exert a small but probably clinically irrelevant bronchoprotective effect.[58-61]

MEMBRANE-STABILIZING ACTIVITY. Some β-adrenergic blockers, especially at higher doses, reduce the rate of rapid depolarization and maximal amplitude of the action potential in a "quinidine-like" fashion. This is considered a nonspecific effect that is unrelated to β-antagonism and is probably not involved in any clinical effect of these drugs at therapeutic doses.

Cardiovascular effects (Fig 29C-3). The therapeutic role of β-adrenergic blockers derives from their ability to limit myocardial oxygen consumption, especially during exercise, by attenuating heart rate response, myocardial contractility, and left ventricular wall tension in systole. The extent to which a β-adrenergic blocker produces these effects is a function of its potency, concentration, predominant site of action (selectivity), and degree of intrinsic sympathomimetic activity. In addition, the effect of the drug depends on the status of the sympathetic nervous system at the time the drug is administered and also apparently on genetic characteristics of the patient.[62]

HEART RATE. Heart rate generally declines in response

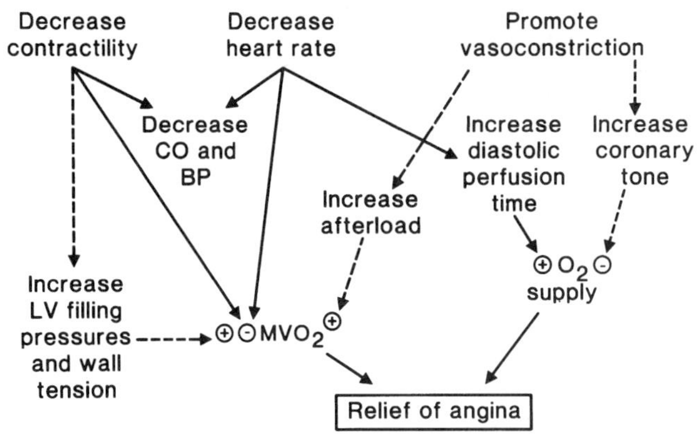

Fig 29C-3 Cardiovascular effects of β-adrenergic blockers and the mechanisms by which they reduce symptoms of angina. *Dashed arrows* indicate less clinically apparent effects than those indicated by *solid arrows*. *BP*, blood pressure; *CO*, carbon monoxide; *LV*, left ventricular; *MVO_2*, myocardial oxygen uptake; *O_2*, oxygen; +, increase; −, decrease.

to administration of a β-adrenergic blocking agent. The higher the baseline heart rate (reflecting more sympathetic activity), the greater is the reduction.[52,63] Agents with intrinsic sympathomimetic activity may cause less attenuation of resting heart rate.[59,64] When sympathetic activity is more intense, as occurs on assumption of an upright position, during exercise, with isoproterenol administration, or in patients with heart failure or hypotension, the negative chronotropic effects of β-adrenergic blockers with or without partial agonist properties are similar.[59,65] Nonselective antagonists may be more effective than cardioselective agents in reducing isoproterenol-induced tachycardia since, by limiting β-adrenergic peripheral vasodilatation, reflex stimulation of the heart rate is reduced.[52]

Reduction in heart rate is the main reason for the decline in cardiac output observed after the administration of β-adrenergic blockers. However, when heart rate is maintained by artificial cardiac pacing, cardiac output generally still decreases after β-blockade in both normal persons and patients with cardiac disease.[66-71] The reason for this decline is multifactorial—it is in part dependent upon negative inotropic effects and in part on augmentation of peripheral vascular resistance.

MYOCARDIAL EFFECTS. β-Adrenergic blockade generally depresses left ventricular function. In normal persons, β-adrenergic blockers may decrease left ventricular ejection fraction at rest and during exercise (in comparison with controls),[72] and elevate left ventricular end-diastolic pressure at rest and during exercise.

In patients with heart disease treated with β-adrenergic blockers, resting ejection fraction also tends to decrease[67,73] or remain unchanged,[74,75] but it may increase in patients with an ischemic functional response to exercise.[72,75,76] Left ventricular end-diastolic pressure may increase or remain unchanged at either activity level,[77-79] although a disproportionate increase in diastolic volume (and thus compliance) may occur.

Effects of β-adrenergic blockers on myocardial function can be summarized as follows:

- Minimal myocardial depression occurs in resting patients with or without coronary artery disease.
- Left ventricular performance (contractility) is decreased during exercise, independent of heart rate response, although decrease is less in patients with ischemic heart disease.
- Greatest reduction in left ventricular performance is in those with poor baseline performance (with high sympathetic activity).
- β-Adrenergic blockers with intrinsic sympathomimetic activity depress left ventricular function less at doses that reduce heart rate response to activity to the same degree that nonselective β-adrenergic blockers reduce it.
- Cardioselectivity does not influence negative inotropism.

PERIPHERAL VASCULAR EFFECTS. Peripheral vascular resistance contributes to left ventricular afterload and, thus, may affect cardiac output, myocardial wall tension, and oxygen demand. Preservation of adrenergic-mediated peripheral vasodilatation would theoretically improve these parameters at a given level of myocardial contractility and heart rate, whereas blockade of peripheral β-receptors would increase peripheral resistance by leaving α-adrenergic-mediated vasoconstriction unopposed. A number of studies support the notion that cardioselective β-adrenergic blockers, by not antagonizing β_2-dependent vasodilatation, cause less decline in cardiac output than nonselective agents, although little clinical advantage at usual doses is apparent.[63,80] β-Adrenergic blockers with intrinsic sympathomimetic activity may produce less increase in systemic vascular resistance.

CORONARY ARTERIAL EFFECTS. The effect of β-adrenergic blockade on the coronary arteries is to reduce coronary blood flow and increase coronary vascular resistance, both at rest and during exercise, in part because of relatively diminished myocardial oxygen demands but also because of inhibition of adrenergic vasodilation. Studies in animals and humans suggest that coronary flow is redistributed to favor ischemic and subendocardial zones.[81-84] This redistribution may help counteract the potential for coronary steal phenomena caused by nitrates. The potential coronary vasoconstrictive influence of β-adrenergic blockers is outweighed by concurrent reduction of myocardial oxygen demand and therefore is of little clinical significance except in occasional instances of coronary vasospasm contributing predominantly to ischemia (vasotonic angina).[85]

Pharmacokinetics (Table 29C-6)

All β-adrenergic blockers except atenolol and nadolol are well absorbed after oral administration. Bioavailability after oral administration varies, however, since some β-adrenergic blockers (especially propranolol, metoprolol, acebutolol, and alprenolol) undergo extensive hepatic metabolism and are subject to extensive first-pass

Table 29C-6 Pharmacokinetic behavior of β-adrenergic blocking agents

Agent	Absorption, % of oral dose	Bioavailability, %	Protein binding, %	Peak level, hr
Propranolol	>90	≃30	90-96	1-1½
Nadolol	≃30	≃30	≃30	3
Timolol	>90	≃75	≃10	...
Sotalol	...	...	...	...
Pindolol	>90	≃90	50-60	1-2
Alprenolol	>90	≃10	85	1-2
Oxprenolol	>90	≃40	...	≃1
Atenolol	≃50	≃40	<5	2-4
Metoprolol	95	50	10	1-2
Acebutolol	>90	≃40	≃25	2-3
Esmolol	...	...	...	1 min
Labetalol	>90	25	50	1-2

extraction, which reduces the amount of drug entering the systemic circulation. If the metabolite is active, as is the case for acebutolol, the β-antagonistic effect is not attenuated by first-pass extraction.

The more lipid-soluble the β-adrenergic blocking agent, the greater is the role of hepatic excretion. The drugs that undergo hepatic metabolism display the greatest intersubject variability in plasma concentration after equal oral doses, because of individual differences in genetically determined detoxification capabilities and variation in hepatic blood flow. In addition, hepatic metabolism of some β-adrenergic blockers is a saturable process at therapeutic doses. Plasma protein binding decreases the half-life of propranolol by promoting transport of the drug to the site of elimination.

The less lipid-soluble agents (especially nadolol, acebutolol, atenolol, and sotalol) are excreted proportionately more by the kidneys, and plasma levels between patients after equivalent doses are more uniform. These drugs are also less capable of crossing the blood-brain barrier and may be associated less with side effects involving the central nervous system.

Nearly all β-adrenergic blockers reach peak concentration in the blood about 1 to 3 hours after an oral dose; this corresponds to the time of maximum β-blocking activity. Elimination half-life varies widely; those with long half-lives (nadolol, atenolol, and sotalol) require less frequent administration. Although the half-life of acebutolol is short, that of its potent metabolite, diacetolol, is 8 to 13 hours, thus requiring less frequent dosing (see Table 29C-6). In general, the half-life of lipid-soluble agents is short compared to that of water-soluble β-adrenergic blockers.

Labetalol

Labetalol is an α- and β-adrenergic blocking agent that was first developed in 1971.[86] Although labetalol is less potent than phentolamine or propranolol at the α- and β-adrenergic receptors, respectively, the effect of simultaneous inhibition at these sites may have unique salutary effects in the treatment of angina.[87-89] The β-blocking potency of labetalol is four to six times greater than its α-blocking potency.[90] Labetalol reduces myocardial contractility, both by β-blockade and by a noradrenergic action probably attributable to membrane-stabilizing activity.[90] Resting[87] and exercise[90] heart rate are significantly decreased by labetalol. When compared with propranolol at equipotent β-adrenergic blocking doses, labetalol decreases, rather than increases, peripheral vascular resistance and causes a greater reduction in blood pressure,[90] most likely because of its blockade of α-receptor-mediated vasoconstriction. Cardiac output and pulmonary capillary wedge pressure at rest are unaffected by therapeutic doses of labetalol. Coronary vascular resistance is decreased, probably as a result of α-adrenergic blockade, with a resulting increase in coronary sinus blood flow at rest.[87]

CALCIUM-ENTRY BLOCKING AGENTS

In the myocardial cell, calcium provides the link between electrical excitation of the cell membrane and activation of intracellular contractile elements. Either the influx of calcium ions during the cardiac action potential or the membrane depolarization per se elicits the release of intracellular calcium stores. Calcium from these sources binds to the regulatory protein troponin and causes

Plasma half-life, hr	Lipid solubility	Route of elimination	Active metabolites
3.2-6	High	Hepatic	Yes (after oral doses only and rapidly excreted by kidney)
12-24	Low	Renal and biliary (90% unchanged)	No
3-5	Low	Hepatic and renal (≈20% unchanged)	No
8.5-17	Low	Renal (≈60% unchanged)	. . .
3-4	Mod	Renal (≈40% unchanged) and hepatic	No
2-3	High	Hepatic	Yes
1.5-2	High	Hepatic	. . .
6-9	Low	Renal (>40% unchanged) and hepatic	No
3-4	Mod	Hepatic	Yes (weak)
3-4	Low	Hepatic and renal	Yes (equipotent)
9 min	Low	Blood and tissue esterases	Yes (very weak)
6-8	Low	Hepatic	No

tropomyosin to be displaced. This permits interaction of the contractile proteins, actin and myosin, and splitting of ATP by myofibrillar ATPase.

The actin-myosin apparatus is also responsible for contraction of vascular smooth muscle and thus for vasoconstriction. The interaction of actin and myosin is regulated by calmodulin, a heat-stable protein that is structurally similar to the calcium-binding subunit of troponin. In vascular smooth muscle, when intracellular calcium concentration exceeds about 10^{-6} M, it binds to calmodulin (up to 4 moles of calcium per mole of calmodulin)[91] and produces a complex that in turn binds to and activates myosin light-chain kinase. Activated myosin kinase then phosphorylates the myosin light chain, and this leads to actin-myosin interaction and contraction.[92] Thus, in vascular smooth muscle, calcium acts as an activator, whereas in myocardium it functions as a derepressor. When cytoplasmic calcium concentration decreases to about 10^{-8} M, calmodulin dissociates from myosin kinase, myosin phosphorylation ends, and dephosphorylation (by myosin light-chain phosphatase) occurs. Smooth muscle relaxation ensues.

By limiting the transmembrane inward flux of calcium, these agents decrease the calcium-dependent processes of myocardial and vascular smooth muscle contraction. This results in a negative inotropic effect and vasodilation and in slowing of impulse formation and conduction in the sinoatrial and AV nodes.

In vivo, actions of calcium-entry blockers depend on a number of factors in addition to their direct action on isolated tissue. These factors include (1) the underlying coronary or peripheral vascular tone and reactivity, (2) baseline ventricular function, and (3) reflex responsiveness. Also, the interaction of various effects of a calcium-entry blocker may produce a response in the patient that is somewhat different from the response seen in experimental preparations. Thus, the negative inotropic effect of dihydropyridines is generally clinically inconsequential because of the pronounced reduction in afterload which is due to vasodilatation. The other agents may have more significant myocardial depressant effects clinically.

Dihydropyridines

Nifedipine was the first dihydropyridine approved for treatment of angina, but others also are now available: nicardipine, nisoldipine, nimodipine, felodipine, amlodipine and isradipine. Not all these agents are approved for use in angina, although studies have demonstrated efficacy.

Mode of action

PHYSICOCHEMICAL FEATURES. All dihydropyridines exert their effect by inhibiting influx of calcium ions through calcium channels of cardiac and vascular smooth muscle cells. By limiting calcium entry, they reduce calcium-mediated disinhibition of the myocardial contractile apparatus and prevent the intracellular concentration of calcium in vascular smooth muscle cells from reaching levels required for optimal binding to calmodulin.

CARDIOVASCULAR EFFECTS (FIG 29C-4). The dihydropyridines have similar actions from which they derive their antianginal qualities; they differ mainly in their pharmacokinetic profiles (Table 29C-7). For the purposes of describing the physiologic actions of this family, the well-documented effects of nifedipine are representative.

Coronary arterial effects. Nifedipine has a pronounced

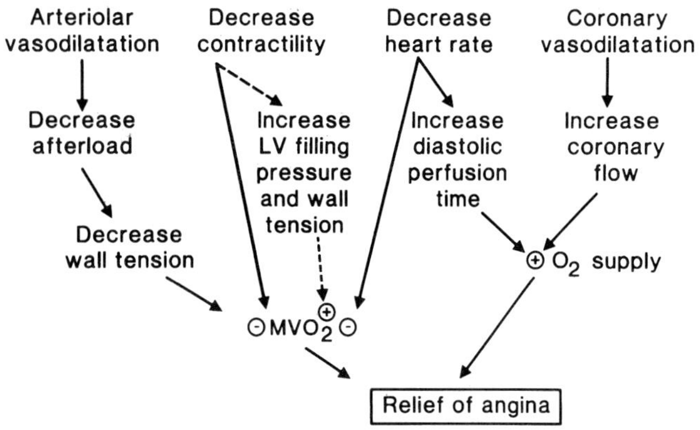

Fig 29C-4 Cardiovascular effects of calcium-entry blockers and the mechanisms by which they reduce symptoms of angina. The extent to which each type of calcium-entry blocker produces these effects varies. For example, verapamil exhibits a greater clinical effect on contractility than do the dihydropyridines (see text). *Dashed arrows* indicate less clinically apparent effects than those indicated by *solid arrows*. *LV*, left ventricular; *MVO_2*, myocardial oxygen uptake; *O_2*, oxygen; +, increase; −, decrease.

coronary vasodilatory effect; in experimental animals, mean coronary resistance decreases by about 40%[93] and coronary flow increases. The coronary vasodilator effect of nifedipine in animals has been confirmed by studies both in normal humans and in patients with coronary artery disease.[94,95] In patients with coronary artery disease, there is increased myocardial perfusion at rest in normally perfused as well as poststenotic regions after intracoronary or sublingual administration of nifedipine. Further augmentation of flow to normal and underperfused areas occurs during pacing-induced stress and exercise.

In addition to decreasing resistance and increasing flow through existing coronary arteries and collaterals,[96] nifedipine may promote the development of coronary collaterals.[97] Improved blood flow to previously underperfused areas may enhance local contractile performance,[96] although peripheral hemodynamic effects of nifedipine may contribute more significantly in improving regional wall motion abnormalities.

Nicardipine may diminish the progression of minor atherosclerotic lesions into potentially hemodynamically significant stenoses, an effect that correlates with its tendency to reduce blood pressure.[98] The mechanism relating these effects causally is unknown, and no effect on more advanced lesions has been observed. Similar observations have been made for nifedipine.[99]

Peripheral vascular effects. Nifedipine is a peripheral vasodilator that produces a decrease in mean systemic pressure[100] and peripheral arterial resistance[100,101] in experimental animals, normal persons, and coronary patients with or without mild to moderate left ventricular

Table 29C-7 Pharmacokinetic behavior of calcium-entry blockers

Agent	Absorption, % of oral dose	Bioavailability, % of oral dose	Protein binding, %	Peak level, hr	Plasma half-life, hr	Main route of elimination	Active metabolites
Dihydropyridines							
Nifedipine	90	65	95	0.5	4-5	Hepatic	No
Nifedipine XL	80	65	95	6	. . .	Hepatic	No
Nicardipine	90	15-40	98	½-2	2-8	Hepatic	No
Amlodipine	. . .	64-90	93	6-12	30-50	Hepatic	No
Isradipine	90-95	15-24	95	1-2	8	Hepatic	. . .
Felodipine	>90	20	>99	2.5-5	11-16	Hepatic	No
Papaverine derivative							
Verapamil	90	10-35	90	1-2	3-7	Hepatic	Yes
Verapamil SR	90	10-35	90	7-8	12	Hepatic	Yes
Benzothiazepine derivative							
Diltiazem	90	25-40	80	2-3	3-4½	Hepatic	Yes
Diltiazem SR	90	25-40	80	6-11	5-7	Hepatic	Yes
Diltiazem CD	~90	40	70-80	10-14	5-8	Hepatic	Yes
Bepridil	>90	. . .	>99	2-3	42	Hepatic	. . .

CD, "extended (one dose per day) release"; SR, "sustained release"; XL, "extended release."

failure. Since nifedipine has only a minor direct effect on the sinus node discharge rate at therapeutic doses, the resulting decrease in afterload may produce up to a 60% increase in heart rate[93,100] which may promote ischemia.[102] Indeed, nifedipine appears to inhibit the arterial baroreceptor reflex to vasoconstrictive stimuli by an apparent vagolytic action,[103] yet it produces a baroreceptor-mediated reflex increase in β-adrenergic tone in response to systemic vasodilatation.[104] The drug appears to be a more powerful arterial dilator than venodilator; hence, afterload reduction predominates over preload reduction. Lower afterload and accelerated heart rate increase cardiac output[93,100] and, unlike the effect of nitroglycerin, increase venous return.[93] During exercise, nifedipine-induced arteriolar vasodilatation occurs predominantly in nonexercising muscle.[105]

Myocardial effects. In vitro, nifedipine exhibits a powerful negative inotropic action. Clinically, hemodynamic indices of contractility generally are unaffected. Indeed, because of concurrent peripheral hemodynamic changes, the left ventricular systolic and end-diastolic pressures and volumes, ejection fraction, pulmonary wedge pressure, dp/dt, and velocity of circumferential fiber shortening are usually unchanged or improved,[106,107] and echocardiographically measured left ventricular end-systolic and end-diastolic diameters are decreased after nifedipine administration in patients with coronary artery disease.[108] Patients with poor baseline ventricular function derive the best response in terms of ventricular performance, predominantly because of reduction of afterload.[109] Nicardipine may have less direct myocardial or conduction depressant effect than nifedipine.[110] In addition, it appears to normalize ischemic diastolic dysfunction.[111,112]

VERAPAMIL

Verapamil inhibits transsarcolemmal inward calcium flux, with consequent coronary and peripheral arterial vasodilatory, negative inotropic, and electrophysiologic properties. The vascular and myocardial contractile effects account for the antianginal activity of verapamil.

Mode of action

Physicochemical features. Verapamil exists as optical isomers. The (+) isomer is the weaker calcium-entry blocker antagonist and may inhibit fast channels.[101,113] The (−) isomer alters the kinetics of the inward calcium channels by slowing activation, inactivation, and rate of recovery.[114] These actions have important effects on the electrophysiologic qualities of the myocardial cell. By the inhibition of inward calcium movement across the membranes of myocardial and vascular smooth muscle cells, activation of the contractile apparatus is diminished, and this results in decreased myocardial contractility and reduced smooth muscle tone. Verapamil binds to the inner surface of the plasmalemma,[115] and part of its action may be due to stereospecific inhibition of calcium-activated ATPase.[115]

CARDIOVASCULAR EFFECTS (SEE FIG 29C-4)

Coronary arterial effects. Verapamil has been shown to decrease coronary vascular resistance and increase myocardial blood flow in animals with[116] or without[117] experimental coronary arterial occlusion. In patients with coronary artery disease, coronary resistance may decrease and coronary flow increase acutely after intravenous or intracoronary administration of verapamil.[118,119] However, substantial concomitant decreases in aortic pressure and myocardial oxygen consumption may result in a lower coronary blood flow after verapamil therapy in coronary patients, both at rest and during atrial pacing.[120]

Peripheral vascular effects. Verapamil, when administered intravenously, has been found to cause an acute decrease in systemic arterial pressure and resistance in experimental animals, healthy humans, and patients with coronary artery disease.[120-124] Mean arterial pressure generally decreases by 10% to 20% and resistance by 20% to 35% after intravenous injection of a bolus at rest.

Myocardial effects. Verapamil is believed to decrease the metabolic demands of the myocardium in several ways. By electromechanical uncoupling, it decreases contractility.[121,122] Since verapamil has a potent afterload-reducing action, the clinical hemodynamic effects of its negative inotropism are generally trivial,[124] and cardiac output and ejection fraction are not compromised[123] and may increase.[123,124] Patients with poor baseline left ventricular function (ejection fraction ≤ 0.35 and pulmonary capillary wedge pressure ≥ 20 mm Hg), however, may be prone to further deterioration after verapamil.[123]

Because verapamil has a significant negative chronotropic effect, peripheral vasodilatation does not produce substantial increases in heart rate, and this therefore further minimizes myocardial metabolic demands. However, even when the heart is artificially paced in patients with coronary artery disease, myocardial lactate extraction is maintained at near resting levels after verapamil; this finding indicates that myocardial metabolic demands are decreased independently of the heart rate.

In the experimental acutely ischemic myocardium, the ability of verapamil to limit myocardial damage has been demonstrated by the use of ECG criteria,[116,125] coronary flow studies,[125] histologic techniques,[126] metabolic studies,[127] and autoradiography.[128] In vitro studies indicate that verapamil reduces hypoxic ultrastructural damage;[129] helps preserve mitochondrial respiration, ATP-generating capacity, and endogenous ATP and creatine kinase stores; and prevents overaccumulation of mitochondrial calcium.[130]

Verapamil also affects diastolic function of the myocardium. Studies in animals and patients indicate that verapamil increases left ventricular diastolic compliance[131] and peak filling rate.[132]

Diltiazem

Diltiazem, a benzothiazepine derivative, is structurally distinct from the papaverine-like compounds and dihydropyridines.

Mode of action

PHYSICOCHEMICAL FEATURES. Like other calcium-entry blockers, diltiazem acts by inhibiting the transmembrane inward flow of calcium through the slow channels of myocardial and vascular smooth muscle cells. In vitro studies suggest that its slow-channel effects predominate at low concentrations, whereas fast-channel inhibitory effects occur at relatively higher concentrations.[101,133-135] In common with other drugs of this class, its effects are due to the inhibitory action it exerts on the slow inward calcium current, which results in excitation-contraction uncoupling.[136,137]

CARDIOVASCULAR EFFECTS (SEE FIG 29C-4)

Coronary arterial effects. Diltiazem was originally developed as a coronary vasodilator, and early studies suggested that its preferential effect at clinically employed doses was coronary smooth muscle relaxation. Subsequent investigation has confirmed that diltiazem is an effective dilator of large coronary arteries and collateral vessels[138] and that it improves blood flow distal to experimental coronary arterial occlusions.[139] Diltiazem may also enhance the development of collateral channels,[140] although this may be in response to, and not a cause of, improved cardiac function and increased physical activity.[141] Radionuclide studies in animals indicate that diltiazem increases blood flow to both normal and ischemic myocardium,[142] and it may redistribute perfusion somewhat to the endocardium of ischemic zones[143] or to the border zones of transmurally ischemic myocardium.[142]

Peripheral vascular effects. The primary hemodynamic effects of diltiazem are related to its systemic vasodilating properties, which appear to be most prominent in the coronary and cerebral circulations.[144,145] Diltiazem produces a decrease in peripheral arterial blood pressure and systemic resistance.[138,144,146] Decreases in pulmonary arterial and capillary wedge pressure are less pronounced but may be significant in patients with higher baseline pressures.

Myocardial effects. Diltiazem exerts negative inotropic actions in vitro.[137] Clinically, however, depressed myocardial contractility is negligible even after β-adrenergic blockade, and cardiac output either decreases only slightly or increases. In acutely ischemic myocardium, diltiazem diminishes the decrease in ATP, reduces the production of lactic acid, and promotes recovery of myocardial function after reperfusion.[147-149]

Bepridil

Bepridil is a calcium-entry blocker structurally unrelated to the other calcium-entry blocker families. It has characteristics that may both enhance and detract from its capabilities as an antianginal agent. Notably, its half-life is longer than that of most other calcium-entry blockers (see Table 29C-7). However, because of its electrophysiologic effects induced by sodium-channel inhibition, it also possesses a potential for arrhythmogenesis that the other calcium-entry blockers lack. In general, this agent appears to be comparable to other calcium-entry blockers and may be superior when maximum doses of other agents are not optimally effective.[150]

Mode of action

PHYSICOCHEMICAL FEATURES. Bepridil inhibits the influx of calcium through voltage-dependent membrane channels and consequently reduces the calcium-dependent processes, similar to other calcium-entry blockers. It also inhibits sodium channels (like type I antiarrhythmic agents), sodium-calcium exchange, outward repolarizing potassium currents (like class III antiarrhythmic agents), and receptor-operated calcium channels in vascular smooth muscle cells.[151] In addition, bepridil appears to enter vascular smooth muscle cells and functions as a calmodulin antagonist.[151,152]

CARDIOVASCULAR EFFECTS

Coronary arterial effects. Bepridil appears to improve myocardial perfusion, as measured by thallium 201 scintigraphy, over that with placebo at any given workload.[153] The specific mechanisms have not been directly elucidated but presumably are similar to those of other calcium-entry blockers; coronary vasodilatation probably is contributory.

Peripheral vascular effects. Despite its effect on vascular smooth muscle, bepridil decreases blood pressure only when administered at relatively high doses in persons with normal ventricular function, and it has essentially no hypotensive effect or ability to lower either systemic or pulmonary resistance in patients with suboptimal left ventricular function.[153]

Myocardial effects. When compared with other antianginal agents (propranolol and diltiazem) in patients with coronary artery disease, bepridil exhibits relative improvements in both systolic and diastolic performance at rest and during exercise.[154] Whether these effects derive from a primary effect on ventricular relaxation and performance, are a consequence of decreased myocardial ischemia, or are a combination of each has not been established.

Pharmacokinetics

The pharmacokinetic characteristics of the calcium-entry blockers vary among the different structural groups of these medications. The pharmacokinetic profiles are summarized in Table 29C-7.

CLINICAL USE OF ANTIANGINAL AGENTS

Medical therapy, which includes altering risk factors and treating associated diseases, such as anemia, as well as judiciously using antianginal drugs, improves angina in most (80% to 90%) patients with chronic stable angina. If the patient does not have a response to this approach, coronary revascularization should be considered.

The goal of drug therapy is to minimize the frequency and severity of the anginal attacks and to improve the patient's functional capacity. The type of angina may help determine the choice of treatment. As a general approach, for angina caused by an excessive increase in myocardial oxygen demand, for example, classic effort-induced angina, a rational approach is to use drugs that decrease myocardial oxygen demand. For angina caused by increased coronary vasomotor tone (vasospastic or variant angina), coronary vasodilators should be used. Patients with both pathophysiologic mechanisms ("mixed" angina) may require combination therapy. In each of these circumstances, the patient's clinical response to treatment is the most important clinical gauge of therapeutic efficacy. In selected patients, additional testing is necessary, for example, exercise testing for those with effort-induced angina or ambulatory ECG ST-segment monitoring for those with vasospastic angina or silent ischemia.

Various drugs alter myocardial oxygen demand, improve myocardial perfusion, or do both, leading to decreased ischemia and improved systolic and diastolic function of the ischemic zone.

Measures designed to decrease myocardial oxygen demand exert their effects by reducing heart rate, systolic blood pressure, cardiac contractility, or left ventricular cavity dimension (in the dilated heart) and, thereby, decreasing ventricular wall tension (according to the Laplace relationship). Some therapeutic measures may exert beneficial influences by more than one mechanism; for example, a β-adrenergic blocking drug, by decreasing heart rate, prolongs diastole and, thus, improves coronary perfusion time and in addition decreases myocardial oxygen demand through its negative inotropic effects (see Fig 29C-3). In addition to causing coronary artery dilatation, nitrates reduce left ventricular size (preload effect) and decrease left ventricular end-diastolic pressure and myocardial systolic wall tension (see Fig 29C-1). Even though nitrates are effective coronary artery dilators, not all coronary lesions respond favorably to administration of nitrates. The reason may be related to preservation of healthy smooth vascular muscle in some coronary lesions and its ability to respond to vasodilator stimuli. Concentric coronary lesions with no areas of functioning smooth muscle cells would not be expected to respond to nitrate-induced vasodilatation.

Nitrates (see Table 29C-3)

Nitroglycerin in sublingual, buccal, or lingual aerosol form should be used prophylactically before physical activity and stressful situations that might be expected to precipitate anginal attacks. To be effective, sublingual nitroglycerin must be used properly. Potency is affected by the age of the tablet and the method of storage. In open air, 50% of the potency may be lost in 1 month. Cotton and gauze rapidly absorb nitroglycerin and may accelerate loss of potency, so that most forms of wrapping are counterproductive. Nitroglycerin tablets should be stored at room temperature in tightly stoppered dark-glass containers with no more than 100 tablets per container.

If the sublingual tablet is potent, a slight stinging sensation is usually noticed under the tongue. If this sensation is absent or if the tablet crumbles easily, the supply should be discarded and new tablets obtained. A new supply is advisable every 3 to 4 months in any event.

The patient should be advised to take the first dose while sitting or supine to determine whether there is a susceptibility to the hypotensive effects of the medication. If symptoms have not abated, two more doses can be taken 5 minutes apart. Failure to obtain relief after three doses should prompt urgent medical consultation.

The use and dosage of all formulations of longer acting nitrates should be tailored to the symptomatic response. The regimen should be guided also by the likelihood of tolerance developing if blood levels are sustained. Dosing schedules of two to three times daily during waking hours for oral preparations are usually sufficient. Topical or transdermal delivery should be interrupted daily, usually at night, for the necessary "drug holiday" (see "Nitrate Tolerance," above).

Adverse effects are not uncommon in patients treated with nitrates:

1. Hypotension, occasionally associated with bradycardia, may occur and, indeed, may lead to syncope. This side effect is potentiated by alcohol or hypovolemia. The hypotension may be alleviated by increasing the venous return (for example, by lying down).
2. Headaches may also be a significant problem, but tolerance often occurs after 1 or 2 weeks. Nitrates may aggravate vascular headaches and even initiate spells of "cluster headaches."
3. Methemoglobinemia used to occur with sodium nitrite. It is extremely rare with nitroglycerin, although it is more frequent with higher doses or prolonged administration of the intravenous form of the drug.
4. Studies in factory workers[155] with chronic industrial nitroglycerin exposure have shown that abrupt withdrawal can produce nonatherosclerotic ischemic heart disease, presumably due to coronary artery spasm. This observation suggests that caution should be exercised when high-dose nitrate treatment is withdrawn from patients.

β-Adrenergic blockers (see Table 29C-5)

Indications. β-Adrenergic blockers are indicated for symptomatic management of patients with stable and unstable exertional angina, in addition to other established uses, including treatment of hypertension and arrhythmias (see Part V and chapter 60B).

Contraindications and precautions. Cardiac side effects are predominantly related to slowing of the heart rate and depression of left ventricular function. Bradycardia may occur because of sinus slowing or the development of AV block. Drugs with intrinsic sympathomimetic activity may minimize or even protect against the occurrence of AV block. In large doses, β-adrenergic blockers can induce sinus arrest or sinoatrial block; thus, these agents are best avoided in patients with evidence of significant AV node disease or sick sinus syndrome. Left ventricular decompensation, when it occurs, is mainly limited to patients with significant left ventricular dysfunction who depend on increased sympathetic activity at rest in order to maintain adequate cardiac output. Even though some patients with poor left ventricular function due to ischemic heart disease may tolerate β-adrenergic blockade, initiation of therapy with these agents in such patients should be instituted only during careful hospital observation, and consideration should be given to hemodynamic monitoring.

All β-adrenergic blocking agents may provoke bronchospasm in susceptible persons. Cardioselective agents and drugs with intrinsic sympathomimetic activity have less tendency to increase airway resistance, but the risk is probably not insignificant at usual therapeutic doses. Thus, β-adrenergic blockers should be avoided if possible in patients with asthma or other obstructive disease of the airways. The advantage of using cardioselective agents in patients with the risk of bronchoconstriction is not only to minimize that risk somewhat but also to allow the more effective use of β_2-specific agonist inhalants if respiratory difficulty occurs.

Use of nonselective β-adrenergic blocking agents should be avoided in patients who are also taking clonidine, since these agents can potentiate the hypertensive rebound effect if use of clonidine is suddenly discontinued. β-Adrenergic blockers should be used with caution in conjunction with agents that may promote orthostatic hypotension (reserpine, methyldopa, and others), further depress sinus node function and AV node conduction (digitalis, calcium-entry blockers), or exacerbate ventricular dysfunction (calcium-entry blockers, especially verapamil). Drugs commonly used to advantage with β-adrenergic blocking agents may also have pharmacokinetic interactions; concomitant use of verapamil, for example, may decrease atenolol clearance,[156] leading to potentially significant morbidity.[157]

The dosage of those drugs that are excreted by renal mechanisms (atenolol, nadolol, pindolol, timolol, acebutolol, and sotalol) should be decreased in patients with renal failure.

Administration and dosage (see Table 29C-5). The degree of effective β-adrenergic blockade is best determined by heart rate attenuation during exercise, since heart rate at rest is relatively less affected by β-blockade, depends in part on the presence or absence of intrinsic sympathomimetic activity, and correlates poorly with clinical benefit. Calculation of double-product attenuation, measurement of ST-segment depression, and determination of duration of exercise can provide additional insight, but these methods are usually not required to establish the optimal dose. Symptomatic improvement is the standard of successful management, and dosage can be titrated on the basis of the patient's report of the frequency of the angina or the requirement for sublingual nitrates. Since variability of plasma levels between patients is high, determination of plasma concentration, particularly in refractory patients, may be a useful guide to adjusting the dosage. In general, therapeutic effect increases at larger doses and is limited only by the development of deleterious side effects.

Dose frequency is guided by the elimination half-life, but it appears that dose intervals of propranolol longer than would be expected on the basis of half-life are efficacious. At the same daily dose, propranolol is equally effective in terms of frequency of angina, exercise tolerance, exertional ECG changes, and double-product whether it is given in two or four divided doses.[158] Slow-release preparations of some β-adrenergic blocking agents have been developed and appear to be effective.

The discontinuation of a β-adrenergic blocker after prolonged administration requires special attention, since abrupt withdrawal of propranolol has been associated with a "rebound" increase in ischemic events, including unstable angina, ventricular arrhythmias, myocardial infarction, and sudden death.[159] Accumulating evidence suggests that withdrawal phenomena may be a function primarily of the development of increased receptor density during chronic β-adrenergic blockade which causes "hypersensitivity" to endogenous catecholamine stimulation after discontinuation of the drug.[160] Other potential factors include increased catecholamine turnover, enhanced affinity of catecholamines to receptor sites, and increased rate of cyclic AMP activation without change in receptor binding. It is also possible that during use of propranolol the underlying coronary artery disease has progressed or the patient's activity level has increased, and therefore more symptoms are produced after therapy is stopped than were present before it was started. Observations suggest that β-adrenergic blockers with intrinsic sympathomimetic activity are less likely to produce a "hypersensitivity" response after withdrawal.[161]

Thus, when use of a β-adrenergic blocker is stopped, the drug should not be withdrawn abruptly. Although gradual decrease of the dosage over 2 weeks probably substantially reduces withdrawal phenomena, one report suggests that immediate decrease to a low dosage, which is then maintained for 2 weeks before it is stopped altogether, is even more beneficial.[162]

Discontinuation of β-adrenergic blockade before cardiac surgery was once advocated; however, continuing low or moderate levels of β-blockade in patients with ischemic heart disease who are undergoing operation is appropriate.

Esmolol, a short-acting, intravenously administered β-adrenergic blocking agent, although not practical for the management of chronic angina pectoris, may be beneficial in patients with unstable angina by permitting rapid titration to the maximum tolerated dose.[163] This agent may be particularly useful when the potential for adverse effects is high, since cessation results in rapid reversal of side effects.[164]

Adverse and toxic effects. As mentioned earlier, cardiovascular side effects are related to depression of left ventricular function, sinus node dysfunction, and AV node conduction delay and hypotension. Symptoms range from pulmonary edema and shock due to decreased myocardial function to fatigue related to reduced cardiac output. Life-threatening syncope may result from the development of high-grade heart block or pronounced hypotension. The occurrence of these untoward events can be minimized by avoiding β-adrenergic blockade in patients with enlarged hearts or a history of heart failure in whom high sympathetic activity is essential and in patients with evidence of sinus node dysfunction or more than first-degree heart block.

Bronchospasm in susceptible persons is a relatively common side effect. Although compounds with cardioselective properties or intrinsic sympathomimetic activity may predispose less to elevation of airway resistance, the risk at therapeutic doses warrants avoiding β-adrenergic blockade altogether in asthmatic patients.

Table 29C-8 Dosages and pharmacodynamic features of calcium-entry blockers

Agent	Unit dose sizes, mg	Clinical daily oral dose, mg (doses/day)	Onset of action, min	Peak effect, hr
Dihydropyridines				
Nifedipine	10, 20	30-120 (3-6)	3 (sublingual) 20 (oral)	< ½ 1-2
Nifedipine XL	30, 60, 90	30-120 (1)	...	...
Nicardipine	20, 30	60-120 (3)	...	...
Amlodipine	2.5, 5, 10	5-10 (1)	...	...
Isradipine*	2.5, 5	2.5-10 (2)	120-180	...
Felodipine*	5, 10	5-20 (1)	120-300	...
Papaverine derivative				
Verapamil	40, 80, 120	240-480 (3-4)	30-120 (oral)	5
Verapamil SR	120, 180, 240	120-240 (1)	...	...
Benzothiazepine derivative				
Diltiazem	30, 60, 90, 120	180-360 (4)	15-30 (oral)	½
Diltiazem SR	60, 90, 120	120-240 (2)	30-60	...
Diltiazem CD	180, 240, 300	180-300 (1)	...	...
Bepridil	200, 300, 400	200-400 (1)	...	...

CD, "extended (one dose per day) release"; SR, "sustained release"; XL, "extended release."
*Not approved for use in treatment of angina.

Adverse circulatory effects include cold extremities, loss of pulses, worsened claudication, Raynaud's phenomenon,[156] and cyanosis due to decreased cardiac output and blockade of β_2-mediated peripheral vasodilatation. These effects may be less with cardioselective or sympathomimetic agents.

Other reported systemic effects are severe hypoglycemia in insulin-dependent diabetics and fasting patients, depression, hallucinations, nightmares, muscle cramps, gastrointestinal complaints, impotence, and rare hematologic reactions.[165] Occasionally, switching to a cardioselective agent or one with intrinsic sympathomimetic activity will reduce the risk of hypoglycemia,[166] and a less lipophilic agent will eliminate central nervous system side effects. Although no β-adrenergic blocker has a direct sedative effect, fatigability is a common complaint of patients. Muscle tremor during treatment with pindolol has been reported; it is perhaps due to β_2-receptor stimulation.

Calcium-entry blockers

The calcium-entry blockers are indicated for use in variant and chronic exertional angina. Usual doses and dosage regimens are shown in Table 29C-8.

Because of the differences in the pharmacologic effects of the various calcium-entry blockers, the profile of potential adverse effects and consequent precautionary measures is different for each type of calcium-entry blocker (Table 29C-9).

Combination therapy

The use of nitrates in combination with β-blockers is one of several rational therapeutic approaches. The salutary preload-lowering effect of nitrates tends to offset the potentially deleterious tendency of β-adrenergic blockers to increase left ventricular diastolic volume and pressures. In addition, the beneficial bradycardiac effect of β-adrenergic blockers blunts the troublesome reflex

Table 29C-9 Clinical features of calcium-entry blockers

Agent	Contraindications and precautions	Adverse effects (%)*	Drug interactions
Nifedipine	Drug sensitivity Hypotension Aortic stenosis Hepatic failure Heart failure	Dizziness, lightheadedness (27) Flushing (25) Edema (7) About 5% quit because of side effects	May increase serum digoxin level Cimetidine increases serum nifedipine May potentiate hypotensive response to contrast agents
Nicardipine	Drug sensitivity Hypotension Aortic stenosis Hepatic failure	Headache, peripheral edema, flushing, palpitation, nausea, dizziness, postural hypotension (< 10)	Cimetidine increases serum nicardipine Increases plasma cyclosporine level
Amlodipine	Drug sensitivity Hypotension Aortic stenosis Hepatic failure Heart failure	Peripheral edema (10) Headache, dizziness, flushing, palpitations, fatigue, nausea (< 10)	None known
Isradipine†	Drug sensitivity Hypotension	Headache (13) Dizziness, edema, palpitations, fatigue, flushing (< 10)	None known
Felodipine†	Drug sensitivity Hypotension Aortic stenosis Hepatic failure Heart failure	Peripheral edema (20) Headache (18) Flushing, dizziness, upper respiratory symptoms, weakness, cough, constipation, diarrhea, rash (< 10)	Increases serum digoxin level Cimetidine increases serum felodipine Caution with β-blockers
Verapamil	Drug sensitivity Significant sinus node dysfunction 2nd- or 3rd-degree AV block Hypotension Aortic stenosis Hepatic failure Heart failure or MI and pulmonary congestion Accessory bypass tract with atrial flutter or fibrillation	Constipation, dizziness, nausea, hypotension, headache, edema, heart failure, fatigue, dyspnea, bradycardia, rash (< 10)	Additive effects with β-blockers, may increase propranolol and metoprolol levels Increases serum digoxin level because of decreased renal clearance Rifampin decreases verapamil bioavailability May increase cyclosporine level
Diltiazem	Drug sensitivity Significant sinus node dysfunction 2nd- or 3rd-degree AV block Hypotension Aortic stenosis Hepatic failure Heart failure or MI and pulmonary congestion	Headache, bradycardia, peripheral edema, 1st-degree AV block (< 10)	Additive effects with β-blockers, increases propranolol level Cimetidine increases serum diltiazem Increases serum digoxin level
Bepridil	Drug sensitivity Hepatic failure Significant ventricular arrhythmias, sinus node dysfunction, or 2nd- or 3rd-degree AV block LBBB Long QT or other drugs that prolong QT Hypotension Low potassium or potassium-wasting diuretics Low magnesium	Proarrhythmia (prolongation of QT and torsades de pointes VT) (1) Nausea (20) Dizziness (20) Nervousness, headache, weakness (10) Palpitations, dyspnea, diarrhea, fatigue, syncope (< 10)	No or small increases in serum digoxin level Theoretic concern about increased proarrhythmia with type I antiarrhythmic agents, digitalis, tricyclic antidepressants

AV, atrioventricular; LBBB, left bundle-branch block; MI, myocardial infarction; VT, ventricular tachycardia.
*Not all adverse effects listed were necessarily significantly more frequent with the agent than with placebo.
†Not approved for use in angina.

tachycardia that can be induced by nitrates alone. If nitrate tolerance is avoided, this combination is effective in many patients. The combination of nitrates and dihydropyridines, such as nifedipine, may cause bothersome reflex tachycardia, hypotension, and headaches. Therefore, verapamil or diltiazem often is better tolerated in combination with nitrates.

The combination of verapamil or diltiazem with a β-adrenergic blocker has significant antianginal efficacy but causes a high frequency of adverse and potentially dangerous side effects, such as AV block.[167] Although combined use of verapamil and a β-adrenergic blocker has been considered potentially hazardous, verapamil (320 to 480 mg daily) and propranolol (median dose, 240 mg/day; range, 160 to 320 mg/day) have been used safely in combination for patients with angina (not in patients with overt heart failure or a resting ejection fraction of less than 30%).[168]

Possible adverse effects from combination therapy with verapamil and β-adrenergic blockers (because of their additive effects) include severe bradycardia, AV block (which may be sudden and dramatic),[169] hypotension, dizziness, and overt left ventricular failure. Thus, extreme caution should be exercised when the patient has preexisting left ventricular dysfunction, AV node conduction delay, or hypotension, because these conditions might worsen dramatically. This admonition is especially important when intravenous administration is planned. Intravenous administration of calcium can reverse the adverse effects of verapamil and may be lifesaving in an emergency.

Combination therapy with a β-adrenergic blocker and diltiazem usually is well tolerated, but sinus bradycardia and prolongation of AV conduction may occur.[170] The combination of diltiazem and propranolol has been shown to lead to greater improvement in exercise performance when directly compared with high-dose diltiazem monotherapy. Bradyarrhythmias may occur during therapy with the combination of β-adrenergic blockers and diltiazem (either low or high doses), but the combination of nifedipine or other dihydropyridines and β-adrenergic blockers is usually well tolerated. Other negative inotropic agents, such as disopyramide, should not be used concurrently with verapamil.

A dihydropyridine drug, for example, nifedipine, in combination with a β-adrenergic blocker[171] provides an additive therapeutic effect with few serious adverse effects. The addition of a β-adrenergic blocker blunts the reflex tachycardia that may occur with nifedipine; however, the intrinsic negative chronotropic and dromotropic effects of nifedipine may become "unmasked" by concomitant β-adrenergic blocker therapy because of inhibition of the reflex sympathetic activation that usually occurs with nifedipine alone. Severe hypotension may occur when nifedipine is added to a preexisting β-adrenergic blocker treatment program, and ischemia[172] or even overt cardiac failure[174] may rarely occur.

Combination therapy is not necessarily superior to monotherapy, is more likely to produce side effects, and in certain circumstances may even lead to worsening of ischemia.[173] For example, in a double-blind, randomized, crossover trial, the combination of nifedipine, isosorbide mononitrate, and atenolol was studied in patients already taking atenolol for stable angina.[174] There was no significant difference in angina attacks, nitroglycerin use, exercise duration, or exercise ECG indices of ischemia. Total exercise duration was longer in patients taking atenolol and isosorbide mononitrate than in those taking atenolol alone, but the mean difference was only 46 seconds. In some patients, exercise time was actually shorter with triple therapy than with atenolol and isosorbide mononitrate alone.

TREATMENT OF CLINICAL CONDITIONS POSSIBLY ASSOCIATED WITH ANGINA

In some clinical circumstances, certain classes of drugs may be preferable to others and may even be considered the drugs of first choice in the treatment of angina (Table 29C-10). The selection of a particular agent or combination of medications depends largely on its recognized effects (as summarized in Table 29C-11) and what effect it will have on a specific patient's clinical situation.

Left ventricular systolic failure

The cardiac effects of digitalis in patients with coronary heart disease are complex, and this drug may be beneficial, have no effect, or even be deleterious. The net response depends on status of left ventricular function, cardiac size, and interaction with other cardioactive and vasoactive drugs.

Digitalis may be useful in the treatment of congestive heart failure due to coronary heart disease, especially if cardiac dilatation and severe systolic dysfunction are present. The symptoms of heart failure and angina may be secondary to diastolic dysfunction. The latter responds poorly to digitalis therapy because of unfavorable effects on left ventricular relaxation.[175] The proarrhythmic effect of digitalis also may be enhanced in active ischemia. Angiotensin converting enzyme inhibitors are effective in patients with heart failure with or without coronary disease. However, captopril has been shown to decrease exercise tolerance and increase the severity of angina in patients with both angina and heart failure. This effect appears to be related to the magnitude of the captopril-induced hypotensive effect, especially during combination therapy.[176]

Because nitrates reduce left ventricular filling pressure and volume, these agents, usually in combination with diuretics, are preferred in patients with severe left ventricular systolic function. When a calcium-entry blocker is used, diltiazem is generally well tolerated, even with considerably impaired left ventricular systolic performance.[177] Diltiazem, however, has been reported to exacerbate heart failure.[178] Although dihydropyridines such as amlodipine and nicardipine have been used in patients with severe left ventricular dysfunction, other dihydropyridines have caused appreciable clinical deterioration in such patients.[179,180] If left ventricular function is normal or only mildly impaired (ejection fraction of

Table 29C-10 Treatment for patients who have angina in conjunction with other medical conditions

Clinical condition	Recommended drug (alternative drug)
Cardiac arrhythmias and conduction abnormalities	
Sinus bradycardia	Dihydropyridine (β-blocker with ISA)
Sinus tachycardia (not due to cardiac failure)	β-Blocker
Supraventricular tachycardia	Verapamil or β-blocker
Atrioventricular block	Dihydropyridine
Rapid atrial fibrillation	Verapamil or β-blocker
Ventricular arrhythmias	β-Blocker
Left ventricular dysfunction	
Congestive heart failure	
Mild-moderate (LVEF 35%-50%)	Dihydropyridine or diltiazem (verapamil or β-blocker cautiously)
Severe (LVEF <35%)	Nitrate, diuretic
Left-sided valvular heart disease*	
Aortic stenosis (mild)†	β-Blocker, calcium-entry blocker, or nitrate
Aortic regurgitation	Dihydropyridine
Mitral regurgitation	Dihydropyridine
Mitral stenosis‡	β-Blocker or verapamil
Miscellaneous	
Systemic hypertension	β-Blocker or calcium-entry blocker
Headaches	β-Blocker (verapamil or diltiazem)
COPD with bronchospasm or asthma	Dihydropyridine, verapamil, or diltiazem (low-dose β_1-selective blocker or β-blocker with ISA)
Hyperthyroidism	β-Blocker
Raynaud's syndrome	Dihydropyridine
Claudication	Calcium-entry blocker or nitrate (β-blocker)
Depression	Calcium-entry blocker or nitrate
Neurasthenia or fatigue states	Calcium-entry blocker or nitrate
Insulin-dependent diabetes mellitus	Calcium-entry blocker or nitrate

COPD, chronic obstructive pulmonary disease; ISA, intrinsic sympathomimetic activity; LVEF, left ventricular ejection fraction.
*Consideration should be given to surgical therapy for patients with severe valvular heart disease.
†Vasodilators might increase aortic valve gradient, and β-blockers or verapamil could cause left ventricular failure. Any of these drugs can cause hypotension and should be used with caution in patients with severe aortic stenosis.
‡If congestive heart failure (associated with normal left ventricular function) occurs in a patient with angina, severe mitral stenosis, and rapid atrial fibrillation, a β-blocker or verapamil (in combination with digitalis) may be used to decrease the heart rate.

more than 40%), β-adrenergic blockers or calcium-entry blockers usually are well tolerated.[123,181] β-Adrenergic blockers, by their negative inotropic and bradycardiac effects, increase cardiac size and increase wall stress. These alterations, in turn, may counteract their anti-ischemic effects. The antiarrhythmic effects of β-adrenergic blockers may be of benefit in these patients.

Hypertension

For the patient with angina and coexistent hypertension, lowering of blood pressure alone may alleviate the angina. Ideal agents are effective as monotherapy for both disorders. Calcium-entry blockers or β-adrenergic blockers are effective in this circumstance. Both classes of drugs allow regression of left ventricular hypertrophy. Occasionally, both drugs need to be combined for effective control of angina and hypertension. Because increased peripheral resistance is common in adults with long-standing hypertension, the use of a calcium-entry blocker is rational from the pharmacologic standpoint, especially in elderly patients and others with low-renin types of hypertension[182] or who experience side effects from β-adrenergic blockers.

The calcium-entry blockers as a group appear to be approximately equivalent in terms of their efficacy in patients with chronic hypertension and angina pectoris. In addition, the antihypertensive efficacy of the calcium-entry blockers is roughly comparable to that of β-adrenergic blockers. Calcium-entry blockers provide an alternative treatment to β-adrenergic blockade for patients in whom the latter is contraindicated, for example, those with concomitant asthma.

In patients with classic effort-induced angina and those with high-renin types of hypertension, β-adrenergic blockers may be preferable. The choice of a specific β-adrenergic blocker or calcium-entry blocker needs to be individualized by taking into account the cost of therapy and minimal interference with the patient's quality of life.

In general, direct-acting vasodilators, such as hydralazine and minoxidil, should not be used in patients with angina unless β-adrenergic blockers are administered concomitantly to blunt reflex tachycardia. Hydralazine administered to a patient with a nonfailing, nondilated ischemic heart may cause reflex tachycardia, which can worsen the ischemia. Hydralazine also seems to have a separate, positive inotropic effect on the heart,[183] which can increase myocardial oxygen demand. Despite the increased coronary flow noted with hydralazine, this drug can provoke ischemic events, including myocardial infarction, in patients with coronary artery disease.

Arrhythmias, conduction disturbances, bradycardia, and tachycardia

Patients with resting bradycardia or inadequate heart rate response to exercise might respond better to dihydropyridines, whereas patients with resting tachycardia (and normal left ventricular function) or an inappropriately fast heart rate response to exercise can be expected to respond better to β-adrenergic blocking agents.

Dihydropyridines are the calcium-entry blockers of choice for sinus or AV node disease. In selected, carefully monitored patients with sinus bradycardia, a β-adrenergic blocker with partial agonist activity may be an alternative. If the patient has a history of supraventricular tachycardia (especially if the electrophysiologic mechanism is AV node reentry), verapamil is the agent of choice. Diltiazem or a β-adrenergic blocker can be considered for alternative therapy. Verapamil, diltiazem, or a β-blocker can be used as adjunctive therapy to control ventricular rate in patients with atrial fibrillation or flutter. In patients who have ischemia-related ventricular arrhythmias, β-adrenergic blockers are preferable.

Renal failure

Calcium-entry blockers are metabolized in the liver, but many of their metabolites undergo renal excretion. Metabolites of nifedipine are inert, but the metabolites of verapamil and diltiazem retain some degree of biologic activity. The clinical significance of these observations is not known. Because the plasma half-life of diltiazem is similar in patients with and without renal failure, diltiazem ultimately may prove to be the calcium-entry blocker of choice in chronic renal failure.[184] Nifedipine has been reported to cause acute but reversible deterioration in renal function when given to patients with preexisting renal insufficiency.[185]

In patients with severe renal failure, water-soluble β-adrenergic blockers (which are excreted by the kidney) are best avoided. If such an agent is to be used, the dosage should be lowered, the dose intervals widened, and the patient monitored carefully for untoward effects (such as bradycardia). Lipid-soluble β-adrenergic blockers are preferable. If angina cannot be controlled with medical therapy and it limits dialysis, coronary angiography and coronary revascularization should be considered. Medical management of patients undergoing long-term hemodialysis may be difficult, because such patients often are chronically anemic and frequently have severe hypertension and experience fluid shifts, transient arrhythmias, and hemodynamic changes during dialysis that may provoke angina. Nadolol has a unique renovascular effect and preserves renal blood flow despite lowering cardiac output.[186]

Insulin-dependent diabetes mellitus

Therapy with β-adrenergic blockers may mask the symptoms associated with hypoglycemia (except sweating) and also may prolong hypoglycemia by inhibiting glycolysis. Ordinarily, these effects do not pose a problem for patients who are not taking insulin. If β-adrenergic blockers are to be used at all, β_1-selective agents at low doses are preferable. In general, however, calcium-entry blockers or nitrates are preferred.

Peripheral vascular disease

Nonselective β-adrenergic blockers theoretically may cause relatively unopposed peripheral α-receptor-mediated vasoconstriction and worsening of limb ischemia in patients with severe atherosclerosis obliterans. The clinical significance of this phenomenon is unclear.[187] β-Adrenergic blockers can be used in most patients with claudication if need be. Calcium-entry blockers or nitrates are preferable.

Depression

Clinical reports have yielded conflicting information about the association between β-adrenergic blockers and depression, and a causal effect has been questioned.[188] β-Adrenergic blockers increase sedation and fatigue and decrease alertness and vigor.[189] These factors should be taken into account when these drugs are prescribed for patients with a history of depression. In general, it is best to avoid β-adrenergic blockers in clinically depressed patients if possible and use calcium-entry blockers or nitrates.

Chronic lung disease with bronchospasm

In general, calcium-entry blockers or nitrates are preferred in patients with bronchospasm; β-adrenergic blockers should be avoided. All β-adrenergic blockers potentially can aggravate bronchospasm or even provoke an attack of acute bronchospasm. Cardioselective β-adrenergic blockers (such as atenolol or metoprolol in low doses) can be used cautiously in certain circumstances under close observation. The clinician should be aware

Table 29C-11 Summary of effects of antianginal agents (at usual therapeutic levels) on parameters of myocardial oxygen demand/supply ratio*

Parameter	Nitrates	Beta-adrenergic blockers: No ISA	ISA	Noncardioselective
Supply				
Coronary resistance				
Vascular tone	↓↓	↑	0↑	↑
Intramyocardial diastolic tension	↓↓↓	↑	0↑	↑
Coronary collateral circulation	↑	0	0	0
Duration of diastole	0(↓)	↑↑↑	↑↑	↑↑↑(0↓)
Demand				
Intramyocardial systolic tension				
Preload	↓↓↓	0↑	0↑	0↑
Afterload	↓	↓	↓	↓(↑)
Contractility	0(↑)	↓↓↓	↓↓	↓↓↓
Heart rate	0(↑)	↓↓↓	↓	↓↓↓(0↑)

ISA, intrinsic sympathomimetic activity.
* ↑, increase; ↓, decrease; 0, little or no definite effect. Number of arrows represents relative intensity of effect. Arrows in parentheses indicate reflex-mediated effects. See also Table 29C-1.
†Reflects decrease in systemic pressure rather than resistance.
From Shub C, Vlietstra RE, McGoon MD: Selection of optimal drug therapy for the patient with angina pectoris. *Mayo Clin Proc* 60:539-548, 1985. By permission, Mayo Foundation.

that cardioselectivity is lost as the dosage is increased.[190] Patients whose bronchospasm worsens while they are taking a β_1-selective agent still will have a response to β_2 stimulants, such as albuterol, whereas patients taking nonselective agents generally will not. Drugs with partial agonist activity are also less likely to provoke bronchospasm.

Angina in the elderly

Nitrates may not be well tolerated by the elderly, and hypotension can occur, presumably because of attenuated vasomotor and baroreceptor reflexes. Lower starting and maintenance doses of nitrates should be used in these patients. When used properly, nitrates can be effective, however.[191] Similarly, use of β-adrenergic blocking drugs may worsen borderline sinus node or AV node dysfunction. β-Adrenergic blockers given to the elderly are associated with higher plasma levels than those in younger patients, and side effects are increased, especially those related to the central nervous system, for example, fatigue.[192]

Calcium-entry blockers are being used increasingly in this group of patients. Diltiazem in low doses (180 mg daily) is the recommended initial therapy in the elderly. High-dose diltiazem monotherapy (greater than 240 mg daily) is associated with an increased incidence of conduction abnormalities, peripheral vasodilator effects, and other side effects.

REFERENCES

1. Murad F: Cyclic guanosine monophosphate as a mediator of vasodilation. *J Clin Invest* 78:1-5, 1986
2. Fung H-L, Chong S, Kowaluk E, et al: Mechanisms for the pharmacologic interaction of organic nitrates with thiols. Existence of an extracellular pathway for the reversal of nitrate vascular tolerance by N-acetylcysteine. *J Pharmacol Exp Ther* 245:524-530, 1988
3. Palmer RMJ, Ferrige AG, Moncada S: Nitric oxide release accounts for the biological activity of endothelium-derived relaxing factor (letter to the editor). *Nature* 327:524-526, 1987
4. Vanhoutte PM: The end of the quest? *Nature* 327:459-460, 1987
5. Ignarro LJ, Lippton H, Edwards JC, et al: Mechanism of vascular smooth muscle relaxation by organic nitrates, nitrites, nitroprusside and nitric oxide: evidence for the involvement of S-nitrosothiols as active intermediates. *J Pharmacol Exp Ther* 218:739-749, 1981
6. Kukovetz WR, Holzmann S, Straka M, et al: On the molecular mode of action of nitroglycerin. In *Vascular Neuroeffector Mechanisms: 4th International Symposium.* Edited by JA Bevan, M Fujiwara, RA Maxwell, et al. New York, Raven Press, 1983, pp 145-150
7. Napoli SA, Gruetter CA, Ignarro LJ, et al: Relaxation of bovine coronary arterial smooth muscle by cyclic GMP, cyclic AMP and analogs. *J Pharmacol Exp Ther* 212:469-473, 1980
8. Gruetter CA, Gruetter DY, Lyon JE, et al: Relationship between cyclic guanosine 3′:5′-monophosphate formation and relaxation of coronary arterial smooth muscle by glyceryl trinitrate, nitroprusside, nitrite and nitric oxide: effects of methylene blue and methemoglobin. *J Pharmacol Exp Ther* 219:181-186, 1981
9. Galvas PE, DiSalvo J: Concentration and time-dependent relationships between isosorbide dinitrate-induced relaxation and formation of cyclic GMP in coronary arterial smooth muscle. *J Pharmacol Exp Ther* 224:373-378, 1983
10. Keith RA, Burkman AM, Sokoloski TD, et al: Vascular tolerance to nitroglycerin and cyclic GMP generation in rat aortic smooth muscle. *J Pharmacol Exp Ther* 221:525-531, 1982
11. Williams JF Jr, Glick G, Braunwald E: Studies on cardiac

	Calcium-entry blockers		
Cardioselective	**Nifedipine**	**Verapamil**	**Diltiazem**
0↑	↓↓↓	↓↓↓	↓↓↓
↑	↓↓	0↑	0
0	↑	0	↑
↑↑↑(↓)	0↑(↓↓)	↑↑↑(↓)	↑↑(↓)
0↑	↓	↓0↑	0↓
↓(0↑)	↓↓↓	↓↓	↓↓
↓↓↓	↓↓(↑↑)	↓↓(↑)	↓(↑)
↓↓↓(↑)	0↓(↑↑)	↓↓↓(↑)	↓↓(↑)

dimensions in intact unanesthetized man. V. Effects of nitroglycerin. *Circulation* 32:767-771, 1965

12. Chiong MA, West RO, Parker JO: Influence of nitroglycerin on myocardial metabolism and hemodynamics during angina induced by atrial pacing. *Circulation* 45:1044-1056, 1972

13. Abrams J: A reappraisal of nitrate therapy. *JAMA* 259:396-401, 1988

14. Macho P, Vatner SF: Effects of nitroglycerin and nitroprusside on large and small coronary vessels in conscious dogs. *Circulation* 64:1101-1107, 1981

15. Badger RS, Brown BG, Gallery CA, et al: Coronary artery dilation and hemodynamic responses after isosorbide dinitrate therapy in patients with coronary artery disease. *Am J Cardiol* 56:390-395, 1985

16. Feldman RL, Marx JD, Pepine CJ, et al: Analysis of coronary responses to various doses of intracoronary nitroglycerin. *Circulation* 66:321-327, 1982

17. Simonetti I, Michelassi C, De Caterina R, et al: Dose- and time-related vasodilator response of conduit coronary arteries to intracoronary isosorbide dinitrate in human beings. *Am Heart J* 117:323-331, 1989

18. Goldstein RE, Stinson EB, Scherer JL, et al: Intraoperative coronary collateral function in patients with coronary occlusive disease: nitroglycerin responsiveness and angiographic correlations. *Circulation* 49:298-308, 1974

19. Horwitz LD, Gorlin R, Taylor WJ, et al: Effects of nitroglycerin on regional myocardial blood flow in coronary artery disease. *J Clin Invest* 50:1578-1584, 1971

20. Winbury MM, Howe BB, Weiss HR: Effect of nitroglycerin and dipyridamole on epicardial and endocardial oxygen tension: further evidence for redistribution of myocardial blood flow. *J Pharmacol Exp Ther* 176:184-199, 1971

21. Ganz W, Marcus HS: Failure of intracoronary nitroglycerin to alleviate pacing-induced angina. *Circulation* 46:880-889, 1972

22. Liu P, Houle S, Burns RJ, et al: Effect of intracoronary nitroglycerin on myocardial blood flow and distribution in pacing-induced angina pectoris: quantitative assessment by single-photon emission tomography. *Am J Cardiol* 55:1270-1276, 1985

23. Fuchs RM, Brinker FA, Guzman PA, et al: Regional coronary blood flow during relief of pacing-induced angina by nitroglycerin: implications for mechanism of action. *Am J Cardiol* 51:19-23, 1983

24. Russek HI, Urbach KF, Zohman BL: Paradoxical action of glyceryl trinitrate (nitroglycerin) in coronary patients. *JAMA* 158:1017-1021, 1955

25. Bove AA, Vlietstra RE: Paradoxical angina after nitroglycerin—another variant (letter to the editor). *N Engl J Med* 306:484-485, 1982

26. Santamore WP, Walinsky P: Altered coronary flow responses to vasoactive drugs in the presence of coronary arterial stenosis in the dog. *Am J Cardiol* 45:276-285, 1980

27. Malindzak GS Jr, Green HD, Stagg PL: Effects of nitroglycerin on flow after partial constriction of the coronary artery. *J Appl Physiol* 29:17-22, 1970

28. Gascho JA, Mahanes MS, Flanagan TL, et al: Effects of nitroglycerin-induced hypotension on myocardial blood flow in a two vessel occlusion-stenosis anesthetized canine model. *J Am Coll Cardiol* 6:856-863, 1985

29. McEwan MP, Berman ND, Morch JE, et al: Effect of intravenous and intracoronary nitroglycerin on left ventricular wall motion and perfusion in patients with coronary artery disease. *Am J Cardiol* 47:102-108, 1981

30. Chesebro JH, Ritman EL, Frye RL, et al: Regional myocardial wall thickening response to nitroglycerin: a predictor of myocardial response to aortocoronary bypass surgery. *Circulation* 57:952-957, 1978

31. Fung H: Pharmacokinetic determinants of nitrate action. *Am J Med* 76 Special Issue 6A:22-26, 1984

32. Nabel EG, Barry J, Rocco MB, et al: Effects of dosing intervals on the development of tolerance to high dose transdermal nitroglycerin. *Am J Cardiol* 63:663-669, 1989

33. Moreyra AE, Kostis JB: Effect of cutaneous nitroglycerin patches on coronary artery diameter: issues concerning development of tolerance. *J Am Coll Cardiol* 13:428-433, 1989

34. Waters DD, Juneau M, Gossard D, et al: Limited usefulness of intermittent nitroglycerin patches in stable angina. *J Am Coll Cardiol* 13:421-425, 1989
35. Colditz GA, Halvorsen KT, Goldhaber SZ: Randomized clinical trials of transdermal nitroglycerin systems for the treatment of angina: a meta-analysis. *Am Heart J* 116:174-180, 1988
36. Zimrin D, Reichek N, Bogin KT, et al: Antianginal effects of intravenous nitroglycerin over 24 hours. *Circulation* 77:1376-1384, 1988
37. Elkayam U, Kulick D, McIntosh N, et al: Incidence of early tolerance to hemodynamic effects of continuous infusion of nitroglycerin in patients with coronary artery disease and heart failure. *Circulation* 76:577-584, 1987
38. May DC, Popma JJ, Black WH, et al: In vivo induction and reversal of nitroglycerin tolerance in human coronary arteries. *N Engl J Med* 317:805-809, 1987
39. Packer M, Lee WH, Kessler PD, et al: Prevention and reversal of nitrate tolerance in patients with congestive heart failure. *N Engl J Med* 317:799-804, 1987
40. Horowitz JD, Henry CA, Syrjanen ML, et al: Combined use of nitroglycerin and N-acetylcysteine in the management of unstable angina pectoris. *Circulation* 77:787-794, 1988
41. Levy WS, Katz RJ, Wasserman AG: Methionine restores the venodilative response to nitroglycerin after the development of tolerance. *J Am Coll Cardiol* 17:474-479, 1991
42. Schaer DH, Buff LA, Katz RJ: Sustained antianginal efficacy of transdermal nitroglycerin patches using an overnight 10-hour nitrate-free interval. *Am J Cardiol* 61:46-50, 1988
43. Luke R, Sharpe N, Coxon R: Transdermal nitroglycerin in angina pectoris: efficacy of intermittent application. *J Am Coll Cardiol* 10:642-646, 1987
44. Cowan JC, Bourke JP, Reid DS, et al: Prevention of tolerance to nitroglycerin patches by overnight removal. *Am J Cardiol* 60:271-275, 1987
45. DeMots H, Glasser SS: Intermittent transdermal nitroglycerin therapy in the treatment of chronic stable angina. *J Am Coll Cardiol* 13:786-793, 1989
46. Parker JO, Farrell B, Lahey KA, et al: Nitrate tolerance: the lack of effect of N-acetylcysteine. *Circulation* 76:572-576, 1987
47. Katz RJ, Levy WS, Buff L, et al: Prevention of nitrate tolerance with angiotensin converting enzyme inhibitors. *Circulation* 83:1271-1277, 1991
48. Manyari DE, Smith ER, Spragg J: Isosorbide dinitrate and glyceryl trinitrate: demonstration of cross tolerance in the capacitance vessels. *Am J Cardiol* 55:927-931, 1985
49. Abrams J: Use of nitrates in ischemic heart disease. *Curr Probl Cardiol* 17:481-542, 1992
50. Dupuis J, Lalonde G, Lemieux R, et al: Tolerance to intravenous nitroglycerin in patients with congestive heart failure: role of increased intravascular volume, neurohumoral activation and lack of prevention with N-acetylcysteine. *J Am Coll Cardiol* 16:923-931, 1990
51. Packer M: What causes tolerance to nitroglycerin? The 100 year old mystery continues. *J Am Coll Cardiol* 16:932-935, 1990
52. Conolly ME, Kersting F, Dollery CT: The clinical pharmacology of beta-adrenoceptor-blocking drugs. *Prog Cardiovasc Dis* 19:203-234, 1976
53. Frishman W: Clinical pharmacology of the new beta-adrenergic blocking drugs. I. Pharmacodynamic and pharmacokinetic properties. *Am Heart J* 97:663-670, 1979
54. Dunlop D, Shanks RG: Selective blockade of adrenoceptive beta receptors in the heart. *Br J Pharmacol Chemother* 32:201-218, 1968
55. Frishman WH: β-Adrenoceptor antagonists: new drugs and new indications. *N Engl J Med* 305:500-506, 1981
56. Koch-Weser J: Metoprolol. *N Engl J Med* 301:698-703, 1979
57. Cocco G, Burkart F, Chu D, et al: Intrinsic sympathomimetic activity of beta-adrenoceptor blocking agents. *Eur J Clin Pharmacol* 13:1-4, 1978
58. Oh VMS, Kaye CM, Warrington SJ, et al: Studies of cardioselectivity and partial agonist activity in β-adrenoceptor blockade comparing effects on heart rate and peak expiratory flow rate during exercise. *Br J Clin Pharmacol* 5:107-120, 1978
59. Frishman WH, Kostic J: The significance of intrinsic sympathomimetic activity in beta-adrenoceptor blocking drugs. *Cardiovasc Rev Rep* 3:503-512, 1982
60. Benson MK, Berrill WT, Cruickshank JM, et al: A comparison of four β-adrenoceptor antagonists in patients with asthma. *Br J Clin Pharmacol* 5:415-419, 1978
61. Frishman W, Davis R, Strom J, et al: Clinical pharmacology of the new beta-adrenergic blocking drugs. V. Pindolol (LB-46) therapy for supraventricular arrhythmia: a viable alternative to propranolol in patients with bronchospasm. *Am Heart J* 98:393-398, 1979
62. Zhou H-H, Koshakji RP, Silberstein DJ, et al: Altered sensitivity to and clearance of propranolol in men of Chinese descent as compared with American whites. *N Engl J Med* 320:565-570, 1989
63. Frishman W, Silverman R: Clinical pharmacology of the new beta-adrenergic blocking drugs. II. Physiologic and metabolic effects. *Am Heart J* 97:797-807, 1979
64. Taylor SH, Silke B, Lee PS: Intravenous beta-blockade in coronary heart disease: is cardioselectivity or intrinsic sympathomimetic activity hemodynamically useful? *N Engl J Med* 306:631-635, 1982
65. Frishman W, Kostis J, Strom J, et al: Clinical pharmacology of the new beta-adrenergic blocking drugs. VI. A comparison of pindolol and propranolol in treatment of patients with angina pectoris: the role of intrinsic sympathomimetic activity. *Am Heart J* 98:526-535, 1979
66. Bloomfield DA, Sowton E: Rate-independent effects of propranolol: The differentiation between chronotropic, inotropic, and peripheral vascular responses. *Circ Res* 21 Suppl 3:243-247, 1967
67. Coltart DJ, Alderman EL, Robison SC, et al: Effect of propranolol on left ventricular function, segmental wall motion, and diastolic pressure-volume relation in man. *Br Heart J* 37:357-364, 1975
68. Sonnenblick EH, Braunwald E, Williams JF Jr, et al: Effects of exercise on myocardial force-velocity relations in intact unanesthetized man: relative roles of changes in heart rate, sympathetic activity, and ventricular dimensions. *J Clin Invest* 44:2051-2062, 1965
69. Donoso E, Cohn LJ, Newman BJ, et al: Effects of propranolol on patients with complete heart block and implanted pacemakers. *Circulation* 36:534-538, 1967
70. Bourdillon PD, Canepa-Anson R, Rickards AF: Hemodynamic effects of intravenous metoprolol. *Am J Cardiol* 44:1195-1200, 1979
71. Robinson C, Jackson G, Fisk C, et al: Haemodynamic effects of atenolol in patients with coronary artery disease. *Br Heart J* 40:22-28, 1978
72. Marshall RC, Wisenberg G, Schelbert HR, et al: Effect of oral propranolol on rest, exercise and postexercise left ventricular performance in normal subjects and patients with coronary artery disease. *Circulation* 63:572-583, 1981
73. Frishman W, Smithen C, Befler B, et al: Noninvasive assessment of clinical response to oral propranolol therapy. *Am J Cardiol* 35:635-644, 1975
74. Marshall RC, Berger HJ, Reduto LA, et al: Assessment of cardiac performance with quantitative radionuclide angiocardiography: effects of oral propranolol on global and regional left ventricular function in coronary artery disease. *Circulation* 58:808-814, 1978
75. Battler A, Ross J Jr, Slutsky R, et al: Improvement of exercise-induced left ventricular dysfunction with oral propranolol in patients with coronary heart disease. *Am J Cardiol* 44:318-324, 1979
76. Higginbotham MB, Morris KG, Coleman RE, et al: Chronic stable angina monotherapy: nifedipine versus propranolol. *Am J Med* 86 Suppl 1A:1-5, 1989
77. Hendry WG, Silke B, Taylor SH: Haemodynamic dose-response effects of i.v. metoprolol in coronary heart disease. *Eur J Clin Pharmacol* 19:323-327, 1981
78. Svendsen TL, Hartling OJ, Trap-Jensen J, et al: Adrenergic beta receptor blockade: hemodynamic importance of intrinsic sympathomimetic activity at rest. *Clin Pharmacol Ther* 29:711-718, 1981
79. Shubrooks SJ Jr, Zir LM, Dinsmore RE, et al: Left ventricular wall motion response to intravenous propranolol. *Circulation* 52:124-129, 1975
80. Sklar J, Johnston GD, Overlie P, et al: The effects of a cardioselective (metoprolol) and a nonselective (propranolol) beta-adrenergic blocker on the response to dynamic exercise in normal man. *Circulation* 65:894-899, 1982
81. Becker LC, Fortuin NJ, Pitt B: Effects of ischemia and antianginal drugs on the distribution of radioactive microspheres in the canine left ventricle. *Circ Res* 28:263-269, 1971
82. Gross GJ, Winbury MM: *Beta* adrenergic blockade on intramyocardial distribution of coronary blood flow. *J Pharmacol Exp Ther* 187:451-464, 1973
83. Rainwater J, Steele P, Kirch D, et al: Effect of propranolol on

myocardial perfusion images and exercise ejection fraction in men with coronary artery disease. *Circulation* 65:77-81, 1982

84. Buck JD, Hardman HF, Warltier DC, et al: Changes in ischemic blood flow distribution and dynamic severity of a coronary stenosis induced by beta blockade in the canine heart. *Circulation* 64:708-715, 1981

85. Robertson RM, Wood AJJ, Vaughn WK, et al: Exacerbation of vasotonic angina pectoris by propranolol. *Circulation* 65:281-285, 1982

86. Boakes AJ, Knight EJ, Prichard BNC: Preliminary studies of the pharmacological effects of 5-{1-hydroxy-2-[(1-methyl-3-phenylpropyl) amino]-ethyl}salicylamide (AH 5158) in man (abstract). *Clin Sci* 40:18P-19P, 1971

87. Gagnon R-M, Morissette M, Présant S, et al: Hemodynamic and coronary effects of intravenous labetalol in coronary artery disease. *Am J Cardiol* 49:1267-1269, 1982

88. Frishman WH, Strom JA, Kirschner M, et al: Labetalol therapy in patients with systemic hypertension and angina pectoris: effects of combined alpha and beta adrenoceptor blockade. *Am J Cardiol* 48:917-928, 1981

89. Frishman W, Halprin S: Clinical pharmacology of the new beta-adrenergic blocking drugs. VII. New horizons in beta-adrenoceptor blockade therapy: labetalol. *Am Heart J* 98:660-665, 1979

90. Brittain RT, Levy GP: A review of the animal pharmacology of labetalol, a combined α- and β-adrenoceptor-blocking drug. *Br J Clin Pharmacol* 3 Suppl 3:681-694, 1976

91. Hartshorne DJ: Biochemical basis for contraction of vascular smooth muscle. *Chest* 78:140-149, 1980

92. Adelstein RS, Hathaway DR: Role of calcium and cyclic adenosine 3′:5′ monophosphate in regulating smooth muscle contraction: mechanisms of excitation-contraction coupling in smooth muscle. *Am J Cardiol* 44:783-787, 1979

93. Gross R, Kirchheim H, von Olshausen K: Effects of nifedipine on coronary and systemic hemodynamics in the conscious dog. *Arzneimittelforsch* 29:1361-1368, 1979

94. Kaltenbach M, Schulz W, Kober G: Effects of nifedipine after intravenous and intracoronary administration. *Am J Cardiol* 44:832-838, 1979

95. Malacoff RF, Lorell BH, Mudge GH Jr, et al: Beneficial effects of nifedipine on regional myocardial blood flow in patients with coronary artery disease. *Circulation* 65 Suppl 1:32-37, 1982

96. Henry PD, Schuchleib R, Clark RE, et al: Effect of nifedipine on myocardial ischemia: analysis of collateral flow, pulsatile heat and regional muscle shortening. *Am J Cardiol* 44:817-824, 1979

97. Schmier J, Brückner UB, Mittmann U, et al: Intercoronary collaterals and intramyocardial blood distribution in dogs following nifedipine administration compared with controls. *Excerpta Medica International Congress Series* No 388, 1975, pp 42-49

98. Waters D, Lespérance J, Francetich M, et al: A controlled clinical trial to assess the effect of a calcium channel blocker on the progression of coronary atherosclerosis. *Circulation* 82:1940-1953, 1990

99. Lichtlen P, Hugenholtz PG, Rafflenbeul W, et al: Retardation of angiographic progression of coronary artery disease by nifedipine: results of the International Nifedipine Trial on Antiatherosclerotic Therapy (INTACT). *Lancet* 335:1109-1113, 1990

100. Matsumoto S, Ito T, Sada T, et al: Hemodynamic effects of nifedipine in congestive heart failure. *Am J Cardiol* 46:476-480, 1980

101. Henry PD: Comparative pharmacology of calcium antagonists: nifedipine, verapamil and diltiazem. *Am J Cardiol* 46:1047-1058, 1980

102. Casolo GC, Balli E, Poggesi L, et al: Increase in number of myocardial ischemic episodes following nifedipine administration in two patients: detection of silent episodes by Holter monitoring and role of heart rate. *Chest* 95:541-543, 1989

103. Millard RW, Lathrop DA, Grupp G, et al: Differential cardiovascular effects of calcium channel blocking agents: potential mechanisms. *Am J Cardiol* 49:499-506, 1982

104. Low RI, Takeda P, Mason DT, et al: The effects of calcium channel blocking agents on cardiovascular function. *Am J Cardiol* 49:547-553, 1982

105. Thomson A, Fletcher PJ, Harris PJ, et al: Regional distribution of cardiac output at rest and during exercise in patients with exertional angina pectoris before and after nifedipine therapy. *J Am Coll Cardiol* 11:837-842, 1988

106. Serruys PW, Brower RW, ten Katen HJ, et al: Regional wall motion from radiopaque markers after intravenous and intracoronary injections of nifedipine. *Circulation* 63:584-591, 1981

107. Majid PA, De Jong J: Acute hemodynamic effects of nifedipine in patients with ischemic heart disease. *Circulation* 65:1114-1118, 1982

108. Just H, von Mengden HJ, Kersting F, et al: Influence of nifedipine on left ventricular dimensions and contractility in patients with coronary artery disease: comparison with nitrates. *Excerpta Medica International Congress Series* No 388, 1978, pp 47-56

109. Ludbrook PA, Tiefenbrunn AJ, Reed FR, et al: Acute hemodynamic responses to sublingual nifedipine: dependence on left ventricular function. *Circulation* 65:489-498, 1982

110. Sorkin EM, Clissold SP: Nicardipine: a review of its pharmacodynamic and pharmacokinetic properties, and therapeutic efficacy, in the treatment of angina pectoris, hypertension and related cardiovascular disorders. *Drugs* 33:296-345, 1987

111. Sasayama S, Nakamura Y, Kawai C: Effects of nifedipine on left ventricular distensibility, relaxation and filling dynamics during pacing-induced myocardial ischemia. *Am J Cardiol* 63:102E-107E, 1989

112. Nakamura Y, Sasayama S, Nonogi H, et al: Effects of pacing-induced ischemia on early left ventricular filling and regional myocardial dynamics and their modification by nifedipine. *Circulation* 76:1232-1244, 1987

113. Bayer R, Kalusche D, Kaufmann R, et al: Inotropic and electrophysiological actions of verapamil and D 600 in mammalian myocardium. III. Effects of the optical isomers on transmembrane action potentials. *Naunyn Schmiedebergs Arch Pharmacol* 290:81-97, 1975

114. Antman EM, Stone PH, Muller JE, et al: Calcium channel blocking agents in the treatment of cardiovascular disorders. I. Basic and clinical electrophysiologic effects. *Ann Intern Med* 93:875-885, 1980

115. Mas-Oliva J, Nayler WG: The effect of verapamil on the Ca^{2+}-transporting and Ca^{2+}-ATPase activity of isolated cardiac sarcolemmal preparations. *Br J Pharmacol* 70:617-624, 1980

116. Da Luz PL, de Barros LFM, Leite JJ, et al: Effect of verapamil on regional coronary and myocardial perfusion during acute coronary occlusion. *Am J Cardiol* 45:269-275, 1980

117. Rowe GG, Stenlund RR, Thomsen JH, et al: The systemic and coronary hemodynamic effects of iproveratril. *Arch Int Pharmacodyn Ther* 193:381-390, 1971

118. Chew CYC, Brown BG, Singh BN, et al: Effects of verapamil on coronary hemodynamic function and vasomobility relative to its mechanism of antianginal action. *Am J Cardiol* 51:699-705, 1983

119. Babbitt DG, Perry JM, Forman MB: Intracoronary verapamil for reversal of refractory coronary vasospasm during percutaneous transluminal coronary angioplasty. *J Am Coll Cardiol* 12:1377-1381, 1988

120. Ferlinz J, Turbow ME: Antianginal and myocardial metabolic properties of verapamil in coronary artery disease. *Am J Cardiol* 46:1019-1026, 1980

121. Singh BN, Roche AHG: Effects of intravenous verapamil on hemodynamics in patients with heart disease. *Am Heart J* 94:593-599, 1977

122. Newman RK, Bishop VS, Peterson DF, et al: Effect of verapamil on left ventricular performance in conscious dogs. *J Pharmacol Exp Ther* 201:723-730, 1977

123. Chew CYC, Hecht HS, Collett JT, et al: Influence of severity of ventricular dysfunction on hemodynamic responses to intravenously administered verapamil in ischemic heart disease. *Am J Cardiol* 47:917-922, 1981

124. Vincenzi M, Morlino T, Allegri P, et al: Changes in cardiovascular function induced by verapamil in healthy subjects and in patients with ischemic heart disease. *Clin Cardiol* 4:15-21, 1981

125. Smith HJ, Singh BN, Nisbet HD, et al: Effects of verapamil on infarct size following experimental coronary occlusion. *Cardiovasc Res* 9:569-578, 1975

126. Reimer KA, Lowe JE, Jennings RB: Effect of the calcium antagonist verapamil on necrosis following temporary coronary artery occlusion in dogs. *Circulation* 55:581-587, 1977

127. Clements IP, Vlietstra RE, Dewey JD, et al: Protective effect of verapamil infusion on mitochondrial respiratory function in ischemic myocardium. In *Coronary Heart Disease.* Edited by M Kaltenbach, P Lichtlen, R Balcon, et al. Stuttgart, Georg Thieme Publishers, 1978, pp 284-296

128. DeBoer LWV, Strauss HW, Kloner RA, et al: Autoradiography with ^{99}Tc labeled albumin microspheres, a new method for delineation of ischemic tissue at risk of infarction: demonstration of the protective effect of verapamil (abstract). *Am J Cardiol* 45:485, 1980

129. Nayler WG, Grau A, Slade A: A protective effect of verapamil on hypoxic heart muscle. *Cardiovasc Res* 10:650-662, 1976

130. Nayler WG, Ferrari R, Williams A: Protective effect of pretreatment with verapamil, nifedipine and propranolol on mitochondrial function in the ischemic and reperfused myocardium. *Am J Cardiol* 46:242-248, 1980

131. Van Trigt P, Olsen CO, Pellom GL, et al: The effect of verapamil on the diastolic mechanics of the left ventricle (abstract). *Am J Cardiol* 47:411, 1981

132. Bonow RO, Leon MB, Rosing DR, et al: Effect of propranolol and verapamil on left ventricular diastolic filling in patients with coronary artery disease (abstract). *Circulation* 62 Suppl 3:85, 1980

133. Saikawa T, Nagamoto Y, Arita M: Electrophysiologic effects of diltiazem, a new slow channel inhibitor, on canine cardiac fibers. *Jpn Heart J* 18:235-245, 1977

134. Nabata H: Effects of calcium-antagonistic coronary vasodilators on myocardial contractility and membrane potentials. *Jpn J Pharmacol* 27:239-249, 1977

135. Nakajima H, Hoshiyama M, Yamashita K, et al: Effect of diltiazem on electrical and mechanical activity of isolated cardiac ventricular muscle of guinea pig. *Jpn J Pharmacol* 25:383-392, 1975

136. Lathrop DA, Valle-Aguilera JR, Millard RW, et al: Comparative electrophysiologic and coronary hemodynamic effects of diltiazem, nisoldipine and verapamil on myocardial tissue. *Am J Cardiol* 49:613-620, 1982

137. Morad M, Tung L, Greenspan AM: Effect of diltiazem on calcium transport and development of tension in heart muscle. *Am J Cardiol* 49:595-601, 1982

138. Joyal M, Cremer KF, Pieper JA, et al: Systemic, left ventricular and coronary hemodynamic effects of intravenous diltiazem in coronary artery disease. *Am J Cardiol* 56:413-417, 1985

139. Nakamura M, Koiwaya Y, Yamada A, et al: Effects of diltiazem, a new antianginal drug, on myocardial blood flow following experimental coronary occlusion. *Perspect Cardiovasc Res* 3:129-142, 1979

140. Nagao T, Murata S, Sato M: Effects of diltiazem (CRD-401) on developed coronary collaterals in the dog. *Jpn J Pharmacol* 25:281-288, 1975

141. Vanhoutte PM: Calcium entry blockers and cardiovascular failure. *Fed Proc* 40:2882-2887, 1981

142. Millard RW: Changes in cardiac mechanics and coronary blood flow of regionally ischemic porcine myocardium induced by diltiazem. *Chest* 78:193-199, 1980

143. Bache RJ, Dymek DJ: Effect of diltiazem on myocardial blood flow. *Circulation* 65 Suppl 1:19-26, 1982

144. Flaim SF, Zelis R: Clinical use of calcium entry blockers. *Fed Proc* 40:2877-2881, 1981

145. Nagao T, Sato M, Nakajima H, et al: Studies on a new 1,5-benzothiazepine derivative (CRD-401). II. Vasodilator actions. *Jpn J Pharmacol* 22:1-10, 1972

146. Hossack KF, Pool PE, Steele P, et al: Effects of diltiazem in angina on effort: a multicenter trial. *Am J Cardiol* 49:567-572, 1982

147. Bing RJ, Weishaar R, Rackl A, et al: Mechanisms of antianginal drugs. *Perspect Cardiovasc Res* 3:89-102, 1979

148. Weishaar R, Ashikawa K, Bing BJ: Effect of diltiazem, a calcium antagonist, on myocardial ischemia. *Am J Cardiol* 43:1137-1143, 1979

149. Sasayama S, Takahashi M, Nakamura M, et al: Effects of diltiazem on pacing-induced ischemia in conscious dogs with coronary stenosis: improvement of postpacing deterioration of ischemic myocardial function. *Am J Cardiol* 48:460-467, 1981

150. Singh BN: Comparative efficacy and safety of bepridil and diltiazem in chronic stable angina pectoris refractory to diltiazem. *Am J Cardiol* 68:306-312, 1991

151. Gill A, Flaim SF, Damiano BP, et al: Pharmacology of bepridil. *Am J Cardiol* 69:11D-16D, 1992

152. Barron E, Marshall RJ, Martorana M, et al: Comparative antiarrhythmic and electrophysiological effects of drugs known to inhibit calmodulin (TFP, W7 and bepridil). *Br J Pharmacol* 89:603-612, 1986

153. Narahara KA: Hemodynamic effects of bepridil in patients with coronary artery disease. *Am J Cardiol* 69:17D-24D, 1992

154. Zusman RM, Christensen DM, Higgins J, et al: Effects of antianginal therapy on left ventricular systolic and diastolic performance: comparison of the response to bepridil, propranolol, and diltiazem. *Am J Cardiol* 69:25D-30D, 1992

155. Lange RL, Reid MS, Tresch DD, et al: Nonatheromatous ischemic heart disease following withdrawal from chronic industrial nitroglycerin exposure. *Circulation* 46:666-678, 1972

156. Keech AC, Harper RW, Harrison PM, et al: Extent and pharmacokinetic mechanisms of oral atenolol-verapamil interaction in man. *Eur J Clin Pharmacol* 35:363-366, 1988

157. Findlay IN, MacLeod K, Gillen G, et al: A double blind placebo controlled comparison of verapamil, atenolol, and their combination in patients with chronic stable angina pectoris. *Br Heart J* 57:336-343, 1987

158. Thadani U, Parker JO: Propranolol in angina pectoris: comparison of therapy given two and four times daily. *Am J Cardiol* 46:117-123, 1980

159. Miller RR, Olson HG, Amsterdam EA, et al: Propranolol-withdrawal rebound phenomenon: exacerbation of coronary events after abrupt cessation of antianginal therapy. *N Engl J Med* 293:416-418, 1975

160. Aarons RD, Nies AS, Gal J, et al: Elevation of β-adrenergic receptor density in human lymphocytes after propranolol administration. *J Clin Invest* 65:949-957, 1980

161. Bolli P, Bühler FR, Raeder EA, et al: Lack of beta-adrenoreceptor hypersensitivity after abrupt withdrawal of long-term therapy with oxprenolol. *Circulation* 64:1130-1134, 1981

162. Rangno RE, Nattel S, Lutterodt A: Prevention of propranolol withdrawal mechanism by prolonged small dose propranolol schedule. *Am J Cardiol* 49:828-833, 1982

163. Wallis DE, Pope C, Littman WJ, et al: Safety and efficacy of esmolol for unstable angina pectoris. *Am J Cardiol* 62:1033-1037, 1988

164. Kirshenbaum JM, Kloner RF, McGowan N, et al: Use of an ultrashort-acting beta-receptor blocker (esmolol) in patients with acute myocardial ischemia and relative contraindications to beta-blockade therapy. *J Am Coll Cardiol* 12:773-780, 1988

165. Nawabi IU, Ritz ND: Agranulocytosis due to propranolol. *JAMA* 223:1376-1377, 1973

166. Deacon SP, Barnett D: Comparison of atenolol and propranolol during insulin-induced hypoglycaemia. *Br Med J* 2:272-273, 1976

167. Leon MB, Rosing DR, Bonow RO, et al: Combination therapy with calcium-channel blockers and beta blockers for chronic stable angina pectoris. *Am J Cardiol* 55:69B-80B, 1985

168. Leon MB, Rosing DR, Bonow RO, et al: Clinical efficacy of verapamil alone and combined with propranolol in treating patients with chronic stable angina pectoris. *Am J Cardiol* 48:131-139, 1981

169. Carrasco HA, Fuenmayor A, Barboza JS, et al: Effect of verapamil on normal sinoatrial node function and on sick sinus syndrome. *Am Heart J* 96:760-771, 1978

170. Hung J, Lamb IH, Connolly SJ, et al: The effect of diltiazem and propranolol, alone and in combination, on exercise performance and left ventricular function in patients with stable effort angina: a double-blind, randomized, and placebo-controlled study. *Circulation* 68:560-567, 1983

171. Dargie HJ, Lynch PG, Krikler DM, et al: Nifedipine and propranolol: a beneficial drug interaction. *Am J Med* 71:676-682, 1981

172. Boden WE, Korr KS, Bough EW: Nifedipine-induced hypotension and myocardial ischemia in refractory angina pectoris. *JAMA* 253:1131-1135, 1985

173. Packer M: Combined beta-adrenergic and calcium-entry blockade in angina pectoris. *N Engl J Med* 320:709-718, 1989

174. Akhras F, Jackson G: Efficacy of nifedipine and isosorbide mononitrate in combination with atenolol in stable angina. *Lancet* 338:1036-1039, 1991

175. Lorell BH, Isoyama S, Grice WN, et al: Effects of ouabain and isoproterenol on left ventricular diastolic function during low-flow ischemia in isolated blood-perfused rabbit hearts. *Circ Res* 63:457-467, 1988

176. Cleland JGF, Henderson E, McLenachan J, et al: Effect of captopril, an angiotensin-converting enzyme inhibitor, in patients with angina pectoris and heart failure. *J Am Coll Cardiol* 17:733-739, 1991

177. Walsh RW, Porter CB, Starling MR, et al: Beneficial hemodynamic effects of intravenous and oral diltiazem in severe congestive heart failure. *J Am Coll Cardiol* 3:1044-1050, 1984

178. Packer M, Lee WH, Medina N, et al: Comparative negative inotropic effects of nifedipine and diltiazem in patients with severe left ventricular dysfunction (abstract). *Circulation* 72 Suppl 3:275, 1985

179. Elkayam U, Weber L, McKay C, et al: Spectrum of acute hemodynamic effects of nifedipine in severe congestive heart failure. *Am J Cardiol* 56:560-566, 1985

180. Brooks N, Cattell M, Pidgeon J, et al: Unpredictable response to nifedipine in severe cardiac failure. *Br Med J* 281:1324, 1980

181. Ferlinz J, Easthope JL, Aronow WS: Effects of verapamil on

myocardial performance in coronary disease. *Circulation* 59:313-319, 1979

182. O'Rourke RA: Rationale for calcium entry-blocking drugs in systemic hypertension complicated by coronary artery disease. *Am J Cardiol* 56:34H-40H, 1985

183. Khatri I, Uemura N, Notargiacomo A, et al: Direct and reflex cardiostimulating effects of hydralazine. *Am J Cardiol* 40:38-42, 1977

184. Pozet N, Brazier JL, Hadj Aïssa A, et al: Pharmacokinetics of diltiazem in severe renal failure. *Eur J Clin Pharmacol* 24:635-638, 1983

185. Diamond JR, Cheung JY, Fang LST: Nifedipine-induced renal dysfunction: alterations in renal hemodynamics. *Am J Med* 77:905-909, 1984

186. Frishman W, Silverman R: Clinical pharmacology of the new beta-adrenergic blocking drugs. Part 3. Comparative clinical experience and new therapeutic applications. *Am Heart J* 98:119-131, 1979

187. Hiatt WR, Stoll S, Nies AS: Effect of β-adrenergic blockers on the peripheral circulation in patients with peripheral vascular disease. *Circulation* 72:1226-1231, 1985

188. Bright RA, Everitt DE: β-blockers and depression: evidence against an association. *JAMA* 267:1783-1787, 1992

189. Dimsdale JE, Newton RP, Joist T: Neuropsychological side effects of β-blockers. *Arch Intern Med* 149:514-525, 1989

190. Cruickshank JM: The clinical importance of cardioselectivity and lipophilicity in beta blockers. *Am Heart J* 100:160-178, 1980

191. Gersh BJ: Clinical manifestations of coronary heart disease in the elderly. In *Coronary Heart Disease in the Elderly.* Edited by NK Wenger, CD Furberg, E Pitt. New York, Elsevier Science Publishing Company, 1986, pp 276-302

192. Crooks J, O'Malley K, Stevenson IH: Pharmacokinetics in the elderly. *Clin Pharmacokinet* 1:280-296, 1976

CHAPTER

30

Acute myocardial infarction

A. Diagnosis and prognosis

Bernard J. Gersh, M.B.,Ch.B., D.Phil., and Ian P. Clements, M.D.

THE United States is experiencing a decline in the mortality from cardiovascular disease.[1] The reasons are multifactorial, but the decline could be due to decreased incidence rates, reduced in-hospital coronary deaths, and improved survival trends after hospital dismissal.[2-5] Despite these encouraging trends, the prevalence of coronary artery disease in developed countries has reached immense proportions, and this disorder continues to exact a terrible toll in human suffering, death, and overall cost to society. Cardiovascular disease remains the single most frequent cause of death in the United States and the United Kingdom,[1,6] and currently more than 1 million myocardial infarctions occur annually in the United States. There are about 700,000 coronary heart disease deaths per year. In a clinicopathologic study in Rochester, Minnesota, coronary heart disease was the cause of death in 32% of all adult autopsies, and among these, acute myocardial infarction was the cause of death in 39%.[7] Coronary heart disease accounts for 23% of all deaths and 52% of all cardiovascular mortality in women. Differences in mortality rates between men and women become less after age 65, and after age 75, women have a higher incidence of coronary heart disease than men and a similar rate of myocardial infarction.[8] These figures underscore the magnitude of the problem, and they emphasize that the diagnosis and management of acute myocardial infarction continue to be of the utmost concern to the practicing physician. Nonetheless, recent trends in the management of myocardial infarction and, in particular, the introduction of thrombolytic therapy raise the encouraging possibility that the mortality, both early and late, of acute myocardial infarction may radically change in the coming years.

CLINICAL HISTORY

Prodromal symptoms

Prodromal symptoms of myocardial infarction are common – the incidence ranges from 39% to 70% – although they are often overshadowed by the acute event.[9-12] An awareness of the prodromal symptoms of myocardial infarction and their potential significance should be instilled into both patients and physicians, since only about one-third of patients with prodromal symptoms consulted a physician before the acute event.[9,10,13]

Chest pain or an unstable pattern of angina is by far the most common prodromal symptom, and in many patients is the sole symptom.[9-11,13,14] Other prodromal symptoms, although less dramatic, are sufficiently common to warrant attention. These include dyspnea, tiredness, fatigue, weakness, general malaise, palpitations, dizziness, syncope, and ankle edema.[9-11,14]

Precipitating factors

The pathogenic mechanisms underlying acute myocardial infarction and transient silent myocardial ischemia are discussed in chapter 28A. The present section refers primarily to clinical events that antedate and may precipitate or "trigger" acute myocardial infarction.

Kinlen,[11] who reported the presenting features of acute infarction in an English community, implied that in only very few patients did heavy exertion precede the acute infarction. Other studies, performed mainly among younger patients, documented a much stronger association between acute infarction and physical exertion.[15,16] In 18.7% of patients in the Thrombolysis in Myocardial Infarction (TIMI) II trial, infarction occurred during moderate or marked physical activity, and this was more frequent in men, nonsmokers, and patients who had had exertional pain in the preceding 3 weeks, among other factors.

Acute myocardial infarction, sudden cardiac death, thrombotic strokes, and transient myocardial ischemia do not occur randomly throughout the day but show marked circadian variations, with a peak during the period from 6 a.m. to 12 noon[15,17-22] (Fig 30A-1). In a study from Germany of the weekly distribution of myocardial infarcts, a peak on Mondays occurred primarily among the working population, whereas nonworking patients had a more even weekly distribution.[23] In the TIMI II study of patients receiving thrombolytic therapy, 34.4% of infarctions began in the morning (6 a.m. to noon) (Fig 30A-2). Characteristics independently predicting a higher frequency in the morning hours were no history of angina, occurrence of the infarction on a weekday, no history of current smoking, and no use of a β-adrenergic blocking agent in the 24 hours before infarction.[24] In the Second International Study of Infarct Survival (ISIS-2) trial, the circadian pattern of acute myocardial infarction was similar among patients of five different geographic regions on three continents and in various subcategories of patients defined by age, sex, previous myocardial infarction, and aspirin intake before myocardial infarction. For reasons unknown, however, the circadian pattern was absent in diabetic patients[25] (Fig 30A-3). These data point strongly to the likelihood that acute ischemic events are precipitated by the physical and mental stresses of ordinary daily activities, with their consequent effects on myocardial oxygen demands, coronary vascular tone, plasma catecholamines, platelet aggregation, and fibrinolytic activity.[21,26] A plausible theory linking the triggering effects of daily activities to plaque rupture and subsequent thrombosis has been proposed.[21] A direct implication of

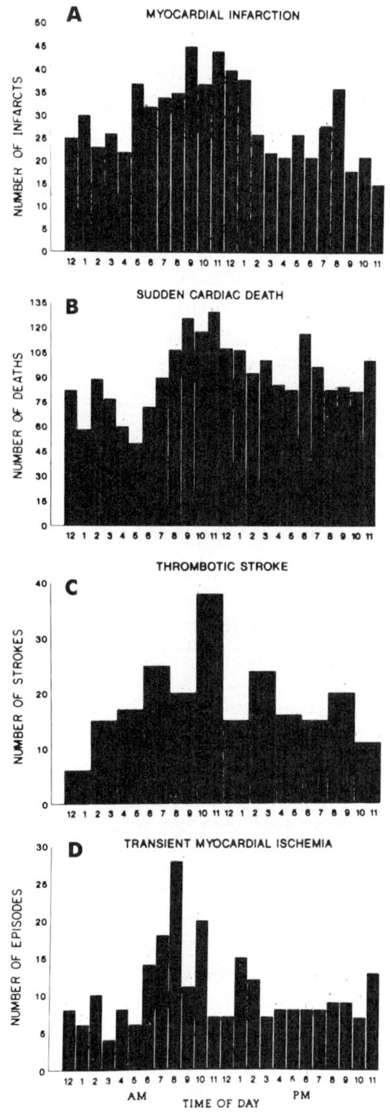

Fig 30A-1 Event rates according to the time of day in patients with acute myocardial infarction **(A),** sudden cardiac death **(B),** thrombotic stroke **(C),** and silent ischemia **(D).** (**A,** from Muller JE, Tofler GH, Stone PH: Circadian variation and triggers of onset of acute cardiovascular disease. *Circulation* 79:733-743, 1989. By permission of the American Heart Association. **B,** from Muller JE, Ludmer PL, Willich SN, et al: Circadian variation in the frequency of sudden cardiac death. *Circulation* 75:131-138, 1987. By permission of the American Heart Association. **C,** from Tsementzis SA, Gill JS, Hitchcock ER, et al: Diurnal variation of and inactivity during the onset of stroke. *Neurosurgery* 17:901-904, 1985. By permission of Congress of Neurological Surgeons. **D,** from Rocco MB, Barry J, Campbell S, et al: Circadian variation of transient myocardial ischemia in patients with coronary artery disease. *Circulation* 75:395-400, 1987. By permission of the American Heart Association.)

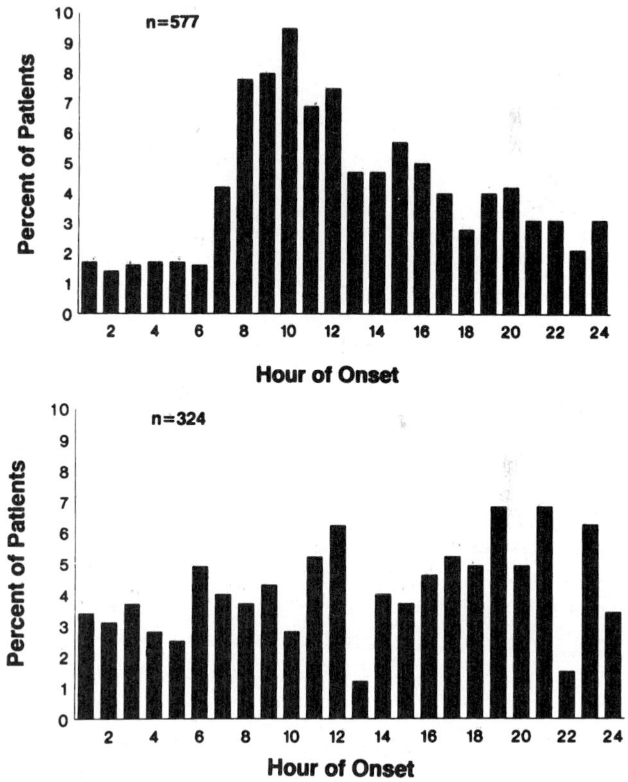

Fig 30A-2 Hourly frequency of the onset of myocardial infarction based on characteristics found to independently predict an increased frequency between 6 a.m. and noon: no β-blocker use in the 24 hours before infarction, no pain other than the index pain in the preceding 48 hours, occurrence of infarction on a weekday, and current nonsmoking status. **Top,** 577 patients with all four predictors. **Bottom,** 324 patients with no or one predictor. (From Tofler GH, Muller JE, Stone PH, et al: Modifiers of timing and possible triggers of acute myocardial infarction in the Thrombolysis in Myocardial Infarction Phase II [TIMI II] Study Group. *J Am Coll Cardiol* 20:1049-1055, 1992. By permission of American College of Cardiology.)

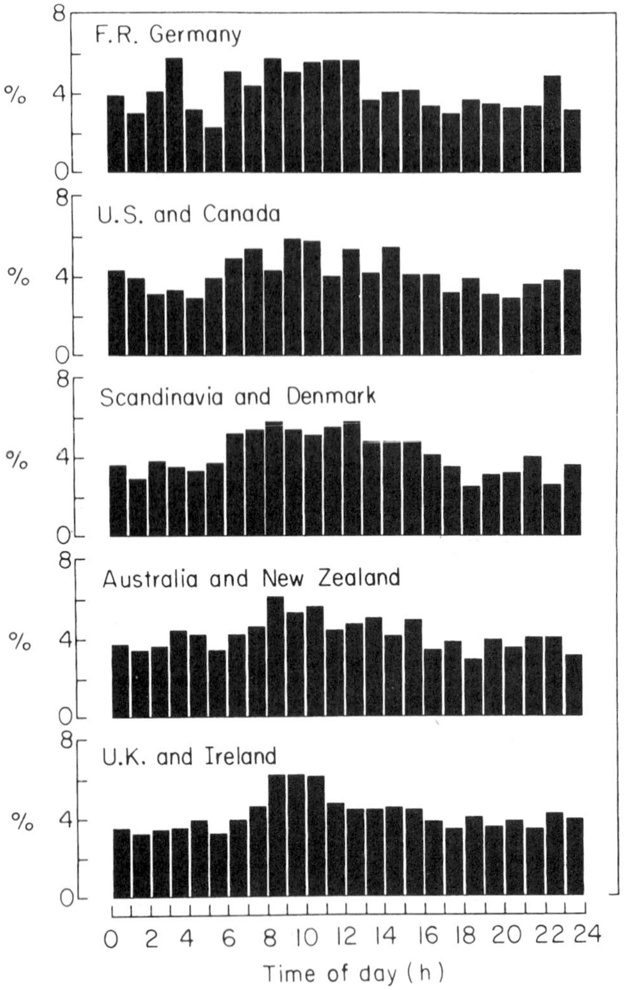

Fig 30A-3 Time of onset of symptoms of suspected acute myocardial infarction stratified by geographic subpopulations in the Second International Study of Infarct Survival. (From ISIS-2 [Second International Study of Infarct Survival] Collaborative Group: Morning peak in the incidence of myocardial infarction: experience in the ISIS-2 trial. *Eur Heart J* 13:594-598, 1992. By permission of European Society of Cardiology.)

these concepts is the need to provide pharmacologic protection during vulnerable periods.

Evidence also tends to incriminate emotional stress as a provocative factor in acute myocardial infarction in predisposed patients,[11,13,27,28] and investigations into the effects of mental stress on transient ischemia have documented both increased myocardial oxygen demand and decreased coronary blood flow.[21,25,29,30] Emotional stress also increases platelet aggregation, at least in part by sympathoadrenal stimulation.[31] An association between fatal myocardial infarction and the use of psychotropic drugs in young women has been suggested but remains unproven.[32]

Acute myocardial infarction undoubtedly occurs as a complication of general surgical procedures, particularly in patients with recent previous myocardial infarctions.[33,34] The mortality of postoperative myocardial infarction is high, especially in patients with known preoperative infarctions.[34-37] Perioperative acute myocardial infarction after coronary bypass grafting has declined, occurring in about 5% of patients.[38] As the number of hospital survivors of coronary bypass surgery grows, the incidence of late myocardial infarction is increasing. Such patients may have smaller myocardial infarcts and better residual left ventricular function because less jeopardized myocardium lies distal to the infarct-producing lesion in a native vessel.[39] One study suggested that acute myocardial infarction late after bypass surgery is usually caused by thrombotic occlusion of a saphenous vein graft.[24]

Other precursors of myocardial infarction, although uncommon, are cardiac trauma (both penetrating and blunt),[40-42] blast injury,[43] coronary artery dissection (spontaneous or associated with pregnancy),[44,45] nitroglycerin withdrawal in subjects with chronic industrial exposure,[46] ergot therapy,[47] serum sickness,[48] wasp stings,[49,50] and "allergic" coronary vasospasm.[51] A study of cardiovascular events during missile attacks on Israel in 1991 found that the peak incidence of acute myocardial infarction closely coincided with the onset of the Gulf War and that the rate of coronary care unit admissions reverted to normal after the first week of war despite continuing missile attacks. The effects of extreme emotional stress in patients with preexisting cardiac disease may be profound and potentially dangerous.[52] Emotional support, along with clinically relevant prognostic indicators of severity of myocardial infarction and comorbidity, may be an independent risk factor for mortality in patients who have experienced myocardial infarction.[53] Also, coronary arteriography together with percutaneous transluminal balloon angioplasty and percutaneous balloon valvuloplasty might be considered a cause of acute myocardial infarction.[54-57] The incidence of myocardial infarction after diagnostic arteriography was 2.5% in the Coronary Artery Surgery Study (CASS) registry[54] and 0.07% in the study from the Society for Cardiac Angiography; the complication rate is higher among patients undergoing percutaneous transluminal coronary angioplasty or percutaneous balloon valvuloplasty.[57,58]

Previously, the use of cocaine was considered not to be associated with serious cardiac events, but several reports now emphasize this drug's potential to precipitate acute myocardial infarction, malignant ventricular arrhythmias, myocarditis, sudden death, or a combination of these events, usually after intranasal use. The pathophysiology may include increased myocardial oxygen demands, small vessel vasoconstriction, and potentiation of sympathetic activity.[59-62] Myocardial infarction due to the self-administration of amphetamines[63] and glue sniffing[64] has been reported.

Symptoms

The cardinal symptom of myocardial infarction in patients who survive to reach the hospital is chest pain or discomfort. The pain is typically severe, but all gradations of intensity may be encountered, reflecting both different perceptions of pain and different degrees of stoicism.

Characteristically, the pain is described as crushing, dull, squeezing, constricting, viselike, bursting, or "a sensation of pressure without the chest." In one series, 81.6% of patients presented with chest pain, yet only 20% described it as crushing, constricting, or viselike pain.[11] Other relatively common adjectives used to describe the pain are "burning," "indigestion-like," and "aching." Occasionally, patients describe the pain as "sharp" or "stabbing," although this is certainly atypical and contrary to standard teaching.

The pain is usually retrosternal and in the left side of the chest but may radiate to the neck, jaw, shoulders, arms, and fingers. Epigastric pain is often encountered and may be a source of diagnostic confusion with other abdominal disorders. Pain sometimes occurs in unusual sites, including the back of the neck, occipital region, and interscapular region. Radiation to the back has been reported in 8% of patients.[11] In patients with preexisting angina pectoris, the pain of acute infarction is similar to the anginal episodes but is more severe, is present at rest, and is not fully relieved by nitroglycerin.

The pain of cardiac ischemia is gradual in onset, and peak intensity is not obtained until after several minutes. This contrasts with the situation in perforation of a peptic ulcer, for example, in which the maximal intensity of the pain is reached almost instantly. The duration of the chest discomfort in acute infarction varies but is usually longer than 30 minutes and is often hours. After relief of the acute episode, patients may describe a residual vague "heaviness," "bruising sensation," or "ache" in the chest that disappears in 24 to 48 hours.

Atypical presenting features

The clinical features of myocardial infarction may be atypical and sometimes so unobtrusive that the diagnosis is overlooked. Particularly in the elderly, the forms of clinical presentation of acute infarction are protean and are subject to the vagaries of memory. The diagnosis in this population is a pitfall for the unwary physician.[65,66] In one study, only 19% of elderly patients were said to have a classic onset with substernal or epigastric pain or discomfort.[65] Other modes of presentation were sudden dyspnea or an exacerbation of heart failure (20%), acute confusion (13%), stroke or pulmonary embolism (9%), sudden death (8%), syncope (7%), giddiness, vertigo, or faintness (6%), peripheral gangrene or increased claudication (5%), palpitations (4%), renal failure (3%), recurrent vomiting (3%), restlessness (1%), and diaphoresis (0.5%). Although others have suggested that the spectrum of presentation in the elderly may be similar to that in younger adults,[65,66] Bayer et al.[67] documented that the presenting symptoms varied significantly with increasing age (even among an elderly population). The frequency of "atypical" presentations, namely syncope, stroke, and acute confusion, is substantially higher among octogenarians, and in this age group, atypical symptoms are the rule.[67] In all age groups over 65 years, dyspnea and diaphoresis are prominent symptoms. A decline in the frequency of the latter with increasing age may be a manifestation of reduced autonomic tone. In only 2% of elderly patients are infarcts truly silent[68] (Table 30A-1).

Myocardial infarction presenting with pain confined to the ear has been reported recently and attributed to connections between visceral afferent vagal fibers and the trigeminal nerve nuclei.[69]

Painless, or silent, myocardial infarction has been recognized since Gallavardin's observation[70] in 1921 that patients may die of infarction without chest pain. The high prevalence of unrecognized myocardial infarction—23% of electrocardiographically documented infarctions—noted in the Framingham study[71] in 1973 does not appear to have changed, because it was 25% in the 1984 update of the Framingham data.[72,73] In a study of Japanese-American men in Hawaii aged 45 to 68 years, clinically unrecognized infarctions accounted for 22% of all nonfatal infarctions.[74] Unrecognized myocardial infarction occurs more commonly in elderly patients, insulin-dependent diabetics, and patients with a history of hypertension.[65,71-73,75-77] Among patients with known preexisting heart disease, the percentage of unrecognized infarcts increased from 18% among normotensive patients to 35% among men with definite hypertension; for women, this proportion increased from 27% to 49%.[73] A decreased sensitivity to pain has been suggested as the explanation for the relatively high incidence of painless myocardial infarction in diabetic persons[75] and in postoperative patients receiving analgesics.[78]

Unrecognized myocardial infarction was as likely as a recognized one to cause death, congestive heart failure, or stroke,[72] and in the Hawaiian study, the 10-year mortality among patients with unrecognized infarctions was worse than that among patients with recognized infarctions, even after adjusting for age and other possible determinants.[74] One clinical autopsy report, however, suggested that patients with clinically undetected infarcts had smaller infarcts, although the severity of coronary disease appeared to be similar in all groups.[79] Failure to seek medical attention and denial may be important factors in undetected myocardial infarction, and variations in sen-

Table 30A-1 Frequency of presenting symptoms of acute myocardial infarction among elderly patients grouped by age range

	Percentage of patients		
Symptom	Aged 65-74 yr	Aged 75-84 yr	Aged ≥85 yr
Chest pain	78	60	38
Dyspnea	41	44	43
Sweating	34	23	14
Syncope	3	18	18
Confusion	3	8	19
Stroke	2	7	7

Modified from Bayer AJ, Chadha JS, Farag RR, et al: Changing presentation of myocardial infarction with increasing old age. J Am Geriatr Soc 34:263-266, 1986 sitivity to bodily sensations and emotions may explain, in part, why patients delay in responding to symptoms of acute myocardial infarction, but why most patients fail to seek medical attention remains undetermined.[22,71,75] Delays in establishing a correct diagnosis and instituting monitoring, plus advanced age, may account for the high mortality reported in patients with atypical presentations of infarction.[80]

Associated symptoms

Gastrointestinal symptoms are believed to be more common in patients with inferoposterior myocardial infarction than in patients with anterior infarction.[81] Possibly, stimulation of cardiac sensory receptors, especially in the inferoposterior wall (analogous to the Bezold-Jarisch reflex), may cause reflex gastric dilatation in addition to bradycardia and hypotension.[82] Herlihy et al.,[83] in a study of 265 patients, showed that nausea or vomiting predicted not only myocardial infarction but also larger infarctions (whether inferior or anterior). Nausea and vomiting may accompany acute reperfusion, and the higher enzyme levels may not necessarily result from a large infarct but rather indicate successful reperfusion—whether spontaneous or otherwise.[84-87] A previous study suggested that vomiting soon after the onset of acute cardiac pain strongly indicates a transmural infarction.[88] Intractable hiccupping in patients with acute myocardial infarction has been reported.[89]

Profuse diaphoresis is a manifestation of the autonomic imbalance present during the early stages of acute myocardial infarction.[90] The phenomenon of angor animi, in which the patient experiences terror and a sense of impending doom, was first described by Latham[91] in 1845 to 1846, although Heberden[92] had previously referred to the sense of anxiety accompanying angina pectoris.

Occasionally the onset or early stages of acute myocardial infarction may be complicated by syncope, often as a result of an arrhythmia. True vasovagal syncope in response to pain occurs occasionally, and the relationship to posture provides a suggestive historical clue. Syncope may follow the administration of nitrates, and although the mechanism of bradycardia in nitrate-induced hypotension remains unclear, this reaction is documented and underscores the need for careful observation while nitrates are used in acute infarction.[93,94] Bradycardia may be elicited by decreased central blood volume.[95] The authors subjectively believe that nitroglycerin-induced hypotension and bradycardia in acute myocardial infarction are more frequent in volume-depleted patients.

PHYSICAL EXAMINATION

Any patient with acute myocardial infarction must have a detailed physical examination to guide immediate management and provide a baseline for comparison with subsequent events. Coexisting diseases in other systems can be identified, and this information may be crucial to subsequent management. Because the clinical course of many patients with acute myocardial infarction is labile, frequent reassessment of the physical findings is also needed.

General

The patient's general appearance may be markedly influenced by pain, anxiety, nausea, and the administration of analgesics. Pallor, restlessness, diaphoresis, cold extremities, and hypotension are common autonomic sequelae; these may respond to treatment, and the examination should be repeated after alleviation of such symptoms. No rectal examination is done in the early phase. Shock is accompanied by hypotension, clammy skin, and often agitation and confusion. Cheyne-Stokes respiration is an ominous feature. Tachypnea accompanies left ventricular failure and pulmonary edema. Patients who are in shock as a result of right ventricular infarction, however, can lie flat without breathlessness, in contrast to most patients with shock complicating extensive necrosis of the left ventricle, in whom pulmonary edema is common.

During the first few hours after an acute infarction, the patients are usually afebrile. A modest increase in temperature, rarely exceeding 39°C rectally, is common in the subsequent 24 to 48 hours; the temperature reaches a maximum on days 2 to 5, and 74% of patients are afebrile after 1 week.[96] Inasmuch as the fever is probably a nonspecific response to tissue necrosis, extensive infarcts may cause larger increases in temperature. Fever persisting beyond 5 to 7 days should stimulate a search for other causes.

Cardiovascular system

Pulse. The rate, regularity, and volume of the pulse vary with the underlying hemodynamic status, the autonomic milieu, and the presence or absence of arrhythmias. (This subject is discussed in detail in the section on arrhythmias.)

Peripheral pulses. A discrepant or absent pulse indicates atherosclerotic vascular disease, as does the presence of bruits. Systemic embolization can complicate myocardial infarction, and an initial detailed examination of the peripheral vasculature may prove indispensable in evaluating subsequent embolic or thrombotic events and must precede the use of invasive procedures, such as intra-aortic balloon counterpulsation, coronary angiography, and cardiac surgery. Peripheral vascular and cerebrovascular disease may increase the morbidity and mortality of these procedures.

Jugular venous pressure. In patients without previous myocardial infarction or chronic congestive cardiac failure, the jugular venous pressure is not usually elevated in acute myocardial infarction. Involvement of the right ventricle by infarction may reduce the compliance of this chamber, and the venous pressure is consequently elevated. If atrioventricular (AV) dissociation due to complete heart block or ventricular tachycardia is present, independent "a" wave activity may be visible.

Blood pressure. The blood pressure varies widely in acute myocardial infarction. Hypotension early in the clinical course results from pain, analgesic or nitrate administration, hypovolemia, left ventricular failure, or a reflex phenomenon. Bradycardia and hypotension are common in the early phase of myocardial infarction (the pathogenesis is discussed later in this chapter in the section on supraventricular arrhythmias).[90] In patients with cardiogenic shock, hypotension with a narrow pulse pressure is usual.

Mild hypotension (systolic blood pressure, 90 to 100 mm Hg) is common and may persist for 1 to 2 weeks, followed by a gradual increase in the blood pressure toward normal. In some patients, the pressure fails to return to previous levels.[97] One subgroup of these mildly hypotensive patients remain warm and well perfused, in contrast to those with hypotension and cardiac shock; although the precise mechanism is not yet determined, a disproportionate reduction in systemic vascular resistance has been implicated.[97] Clearly, systemic hypotension is not necessarily diagnostic of cardiogenic shock in patients with acute myocardial infarction.

A few persons with acute infarction have elevated blood pressure,[90,98] which may reflect underlying preexisting hypertension. In addition, an acute hypertensive reaction may occur in previously normotensive persons and in chronically hypertensive patients.[99] This acute, labile hypertensive response may result from sympathetic overactivity due to multiple mechanisms. (See the section below on arrhythmias and hypertension in acute infarction.)

Palpation. Palpation of the precordium may demonstrate cardiomegaly, which usually indicates chronic antecedent cardiac disease. A systolic outward impulse or "bulge," which is typically located superior to the cardiac apex and between the apex and the left sternal edge,[100] is a clinical manifestation of the regional wall motion abnormalities seen in experimental models of ischemia. This physical finding is common, particularly in patients with anterior myocardial infarction, and if it persists, it may herald the development of a left ventricular aneurysm. Usually these ischemic bulges are only present during the first 48 hours after the onset of symptoms. Other features on palpation include a presystolic impulse and, on occasion, a palpable third heart sound.

Auscultation. Heart sounds may be of normal intensity or soft, especially in the early phase of acute infarction or if the patient is hypotensive.[101] Impaired left ventricular function and left ventricular dp/dt reduce the intensity of S_1.[102] Left ventricular dysfunction due to acute ischemia uncommonly causes reversed splitting of S_2.[103] Conduction disturbances—namely, left and right bundle-branch block—characteristically affect the heart sounds, causing soft S_1 and paradoxic splitting of S_2 in left bundle-branch block and wide splitting of S_1 and S_2 in complete right bundle-branch block.

An atrial gallop (S_4) is almost invariable in acute infarction, probably indicating reduced left ventricular compliance. Its absence in a patient in whom acute infarction is suspected makes the diagnosis less likely unless atrial fibrillation is present, but the specificity of its presence is low.

A left ventricular S_3 gallop is less common than the atrial gallop but it is an ominous finding, implying significant ventricular dysfunction and increased left ventricular filling pressure[104] (Fig 30A-4). In contrast, the bedside estimation of ejection fraction (as opposed to filling pressure) based on physical findings, chest roentgenogram, electrocardiogram (ECG), patient history, and

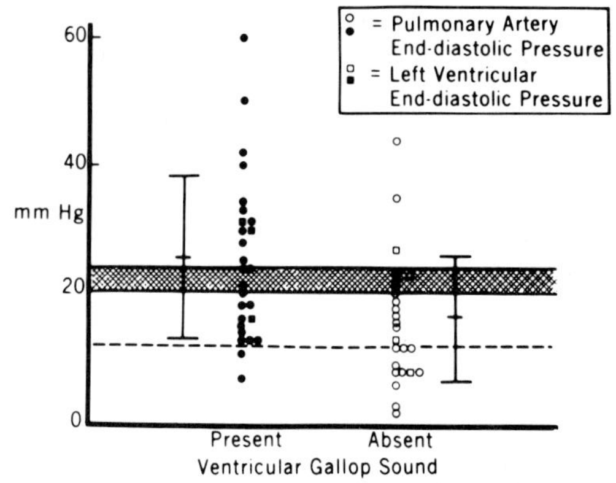

Fig 30A-4 Ventricular gallop sound *(VGS)* and left ventricular filling pressure in acute myocardial infarction *(dashed line,* 12 mm Hg; *shaded bar,* 20 to 24 mm Hg). Twenty-five of 27 patients with a VGS had abnormal elevations of pulmonary artery end-diastolic pressure *(PAEDP)* or left ventricular end-diastolic pressure *(LVEDP),* whereas 11 of 26 patients without a VGS had normal left ventricular filling pressure. Patients with a VGS and a PAEDP or LVEDP of less than 20 mm Hg could have received a volume expander for improvement of left ventricular function, and patients with a VGS and a PAEDP or LVEDP of more than 24 mm Hg would be candidates for reduction of blood volume for optimal ventricular performance. (From Riley CP, Russell RO Jr, Rackley CE: Left ventricular gallop sound and acute myocardial infarction. *Am Heart J* 86:598-602, 1973. By permission of CV Mosby Company.)

clinical course during admission was unreliable in a study of 98 patients with acute myocardial infarction.[14] Systolic and diastolic murmurs may be preexisting and require documentation. A new systolic murmur developing after acute infarction is a major complication. New diastolic murmurs in acute infarction are rare but could arise from movement of blood within a left ventricular aneurysm or as a result of blood flow through a stenosed coronary artery.[105] A pericardial friction rub is often audible (see chapter 30B). Characteristically, the rub appears 2 or 3 days after the onset of infarction, and although usually transient and intermittent, it may persist for days or weeks. Delayed onset of a rub or its persistence should raise the suspicion of postmyocardial infarction (Dressler's syndrome) (see chapter 30B).

Respiratory system

In left ventricular failure, auscultation may reveal moist rales over the lung bases. If acute pulmonary edema develops, coarse rales and wheezes become prominent over the entire lung fields. Interstitial pulmonary edema may, by increasing the work of breathing, result in tachypnea without any auscultatory findings.

Other systems

Examination of the abdomen may identify the features of right heart failure, which in patients with acute infarction usually suggest chronic preexisting heart failure. Acute right heart failure after myocardial infarction may occur with right ventricular infarction but is otherwise uncommon. Detection of an abdominal aortic aneurysm on abdominal palpation is valuable, particularly if procedures such as intra-aortic balloon counterpulsation are being considered.

Evaluation of the extremities for signs of deep vein thrombosis or superficial thrombophlebitis should be part of both the initial and subsequent daily examinations.

DIFFERENTIAL DIAGNOSIS

The differential diagnosis of myocardial infarction is outlined in Table 30A-2.

LABORATORY TECHNIQUES IN THE DIAGNOSIS AND EVALUATION OF ACUTE MYOCARDIAL INFARCTION

Electrocardiography

Serial ECGs are more helpful than an isolated recording, and records that antedate the onset of infarction are valuable. In our unit, the ECG is obtained daily for the first 3 days and during any recurrences of chest pain or arrhythmias. The ECG manifestations of myocardial infarction are described in detail in chapter 3A. This section correlates the ECG findings with clinically relevant and also controversial features of acute myocardial infarction.

Time course of the ECG changes in transmural infarction. In acute transmural myocardial infarction, ECG changes take place in the QRS complex, ST segments, and T waves. These are discussed in chapter 3A.

Persistent ST-segment elevation is of clinical interest in the light of the association between this ECG finding and left ventricular aneurysms.[125,126] ST-segment elevation resolves within 2 weeks after myocardial infarction in 95% of inferior infarctions but in only 40% of anterior infarctions; ST-segment elevation that persists more than 2 weeks after infarction does not subsequently resolve.[127] Persistent ST-segment elevation as found in anterior wall acute infarction suggests dyskinetic wall motion rather than an aneurysm; it is a feature of more extensive infarction and an adverse prognostic sign.[128] Persistent ST-segment elevation may also reflect an increase in the magnitude of the initial elevation rather than a decrease in the initial rate of resolution.

Diagnostic accuracy of the ECG in acute myocardial infarction. Pathologic and angiographic studies substantiate the value of the ECG in the diagnosis of acute myocardial infarction, but the technique has many limitations.[129,130] Data from the Multicenter Investigation of the Limitations of Infarct Size (MILIS) study of 3,697 patients with clinically suspected acute myocardial infarction showed a diagnostic sensitivity of the ECG alone of 81%, but the specificity was only 69%, with a predictive value of 72%.[131] The "canceling" of electrical events as a result of multiple infarctions in opposite myocardial planes may cause "pseudonormalization," with the disappearance of the pathologic Q wave, even among patients with infarctions large enough to have caused left ventricular dysfunction.[132] Among patients with any chest pain and no history of myocardial infarction, ST-segment elevation is highly predictive of evolving myocardial infarction.[133] In patients with less specific ECG features, other modalities under evaluation, for example, echocardiography and radionuclide imaging, may assume increasing importance in the determination of the "triage" process.[134] When a computer application of a complex scoring system was used, overall specificity was only 86%, and this was lower in men than in women and in older than in younger subjects.[135]

The ECG is reliable in localizing the left anterior descending coronary artery as the infarct-related artery in patients with anterior infarctions,[136] but for the right coronary artery, it is specific but not sensitive.[137,138] Occlusion of the left circumflex coronary artery is less likely to result in acute ECG changes because of its posterior location, but in patients with acute ST-segment elevation in the inferior leads, additional ST-segment elevation in the lateral leads with an isoelectric or elevated segment in standard lead I is helpful in differentiating circumflex-related from right coronary artery-related myocardial infarction. An abnormal R wave in lead V_1 is a specific but insensitive marker of circumflex-related coronary occlusion.[138] Anterolateral ST-segment depression during acute inferior infarction indicates either multivessel disease or an extensive area of myocardial jeopardy subserved by the infarct-related artery.[139] Conversely, the absence of ST-segment depression virtually precludes multivessel disease.

Transmural (Q-wave) vs. subendocardial (non-Q-wave) myocardial infarction. The ECG diagnosis of subendocardial infarction, in contrast to that of transmural infarction, is not definitive and is mainly inferential. Pathologically, subendocardial infarction involves less than half of the inner ventricular wall, an area that is electrically "inert" and that contributes little to the morphology of the QRS complex.[140,141] The most consis-

Table 30A-2 Differential diagnosis of acute myocardial infarction

Pericarditis and myopericarditis[106-110]
Dissecting aortic aneurysm
Pulmonary disorders
Pulmonary embolism
Spontaneous pneumothorax
Spontaneous interstitial emphysema of the lung[111]
Gastrointestinal disorders
Gallbladder disease[112]
Peptic ulcer perforation
Pancreatitis[113]
Rupture of the esophagus[114]
Spinal and chest wall diseases[115-117]
Acute cerebrovascular disease[118-124]
Anxiety state

tent, but not universal, findings are depression of the ST-segment and T-wave inversion, which persist usually for more than 24 hours in a regional or more widespread distribution. Changes may on occasion be transient. Fatal subendocardial infarctions can occur without significant changes in repolarization.[142] A definitive diagnosis of subendocardial myocardial infarction cannot be made on the basis of the ECG alone; symptoms or enzyme changes (or both) are required to support the conclusion.

In differentiating subendocardial infarction from transmural, the ECG lacks both sensitivity and specificity. Q-wave changes have been found in conventional ECG leads in patients with autopsy evidence of subendocardial infarction;[129,130,140,141,143] conversely, autopsy findings have revealed transmural infarction in subjects with the ECG changes of subendocardial infarction but no QRS alterations.[144]

Categorization of infarcts into transmural and subendocardial subtypes has been replaced by the designation of Q-wave and non-Q-wave myocardial infarction, respectively.[145,146] This takes into account the inability of the ECG to accurately reflect the histologic changes[142] but also implies that from a pathophysiologic, clinical, and prognostic standpoint, the two types of ECG infarct patterns have different implications (see chapter 30B).

ST-segment elevation, a reflection of transmural injury, is usually associated with complete occlusion of the infarct-related artery and thus is often considered an indication for thrombolytic therapy. Several studies, however, suggest that non-Q-wave infarctions ultimately develop in approximately 35% of such patients, and enzymatic, clinical, and angiographic evidence suggest early reperfusion as the result of spontaneous clot lysis or collateral blood flow.[147-149] In the prospective, multicenter Diltiazem Reinfarction Study, precordial ST-segment depression with upright T waves was an early ECG harbinger of posterior infarcts despite the initial masquerade as a non-Q-wave anterior infarction.[150]

Pseudoinfarction patterns. These patterns are discussed in chapter 3A.

Diagnosis of myocardial infarction in patients with left bundle-branch block or right ventricular pacing. Complete left bundle-branch block makes it difficult or impossible to diagnose acute or old myocardial infarction. Comparison with previous ECGs may be helpful, as are serial changes of the ST-T wave in leads showing negative QRS complexes. The effects of left and right bundle-branch block on the ECG in acute myocardial infarction are discussed in chapter 3A.

The MILIS study evaluated numerous previously proposed criteria for the diagnosis of acute myocardial infarction in patients with left bundle-branch block[151] (Fig 30A-5). Criteria that were highly specific (90% to 100%) and predictive (85% to 100%) for acute infarction were as follows: Q waves in at least two of leads I, aVL, V_5, and V_6; R-wave regression from leads V_1 through V_4; "late" notching of the upstroke of the S wave in at least two of leads V_3 through V_5; and primary (ST segment or T waves, or both, displaced toward the major QRS deflection) changes in two or more adjacent leads. No criterion was sensitive.

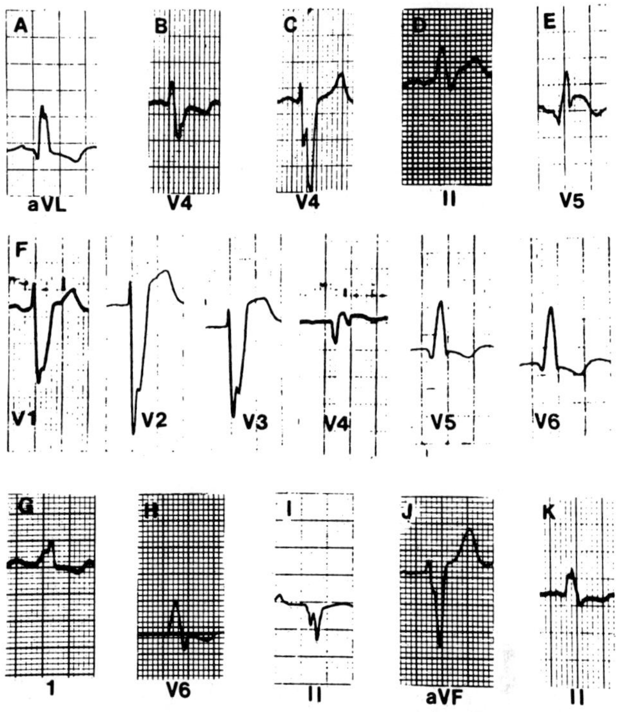

Fig 30A-5 Illustrations of the ECG criteria evaluated to diagnose myocardial infarction in patients with left bundle-branch block. **A,** pathologic Q wave in lead I, aVL, V_5, or V_6. **B,** notching of the upstroke (i.e., late notching) of the S wave in leads V_3 to V_5. **C,** notching of the downstroke or nadir (i.e., early notching) of the S wave in leads V_3 to V_5. **D,** primary ST-T wave changes (i.e., ST segment or T waves displaced toward the major QRS deflection). **E,** primary ST-segment changes only. **F,** R wave regression in leads V_1 to V_4 (in addition to Q waves in V_5 and V_6 and late notching of the S wave in V_3). **G,** notching of the upstroke of the R wave in lead I, aVL, V_5, or V_6 (i.e., Chapman's sign). **H,** terminal S wave (≥ 40 msec) in V_5 and V_6. **I,** pathologic Q wave in inferior leads (II, III, aVF). **J,** notching of S wave in lead aVF. **K,** notching of R wave in inferior leads.

Criteria that had a high specificity and positive predictive accuracy are shown in panels **A** through **F.** The morphologic observations documented in panels **G** through **K** were of little value. No criterion was sensitive. (From Hands ME, Cook EF, Stone PH, et al: Electrocardiographic diagnosis of myocardial infarction in the presence of complete left bundle-branch block. *Am Heart J* 116:23-30, 1988. By permission of CV Mosby Company.)

Ventricular pacing may mimic or obscure the Q waves of myocardial infarction. Nonetheless, during right ventricular pacing with a left bundle-branch morphology, the diagnosis of acute myocardial infarction can be made by careful attention to the changing morphology of the ST segments and T waves[152,153] (see Fig 30A-5). With right ventricular apical pacing that gives rise to a left bundle-branch morphology, the direction of the ST segment is opposite that of the mean QRS deflection. Thus, in leads with a dominantly downward QRS deflection, the ST segments show an upward concavity. During the early stage of acute myocardial infarction, primary ST-segment changes indicating acute injury accentuate those normally seen in leads with left bundle-branch block morphology and a negative QRS complex (see Fig 30A-5). Reports suggest that these primary ST changes are consistent only during the early stages of acute inferior and anteroseptal myocardial infarction and that they are detectable only when the electrode tip is in the apex of the right ventricle.[153]

Thus, changes in the ECG indicate myocardial infarction (acute or old) in left bundle-branch block or in right ventricular paced rhythm. However, ECGs must be recorded serially and studied along with clinical and laboratory findings.

Significance of "reciprocal" ST-segment depression. Depression of ST segments in leads facing the noninfarcted surface has been called "reciprocal" and has been explained as a purely electrical phenomenon or as a manifestation of ischemia "at a distance" due to multivessel disease.[154-156] In some instances, ST-segment depression may be a primary response due to changes in ionic gradients across the cell membrane.[157] This topic can be related to the prognostic importance of jeopardized areas of ischemic myocardium "at a distance" from the site of acute infarction[158] (Fig 30A-6). Using exercise testing and angiography in survivors of acute myocardial infarction, Jennings et al.[159] found that reciprocal ST-segment depression may reflect ischemia at a distance in some patients and is correlated with a high late morbidity and a high incidence of lethal arrhythmias. Conversely, a combined ECG and echocardiographic study from Camara et al.[160] suggested that reciprocal changes resulted not from remote ischemia but from factors determining the extent of ST-segment elevation, including infarct size, shape, and location.

Precordial ST-segment depression in patients with acute inferior myocardial infarction has been variously attributed to reciprocal projection of the elevated ST segments from the inferior leads, true posterior wall injury, or anterior ischemia. Data suggest that precordial ST-segment depression in infarction is a marker of extensive global and regional left ventricular dysfunction[156,161-165] and that it predicts a complicated hospital course,[162-164,166-168] particularly if the ST-segment depression is present for more than 24 to 48 hours.[162,163]

The "reciprocal" relationship between precordial ST-segment depression and inferior myocardial infarction is probably real but distorted by concomitant right ventricular and lateral wall involvement.[162,165,169] In addition, the height of the ST-segment elevation in the inferior leads, which may create reciprocal changes in the precordial leads, may in itself be a marker of the extent of ischemia. Anterior ST-segment depression is very common with inferior myocardial infarction, and although not a specific marker for posterior infarcts,[165] ST-segment depression has been found in several studies to be associated with more extensive inferior and inferoposterior wall infarction than with anteroseptal injury.[162,164-166]

Thus, in some patients with acute evolving inferior myocardial infarction, precordial anterior ST-segment depression reflects extensive left ventricular damage rather than a reciprocal change alone,[170] but this is unlikely to be due to anterior ischemia in the majority. In the individual patient, this ECG finding is of little

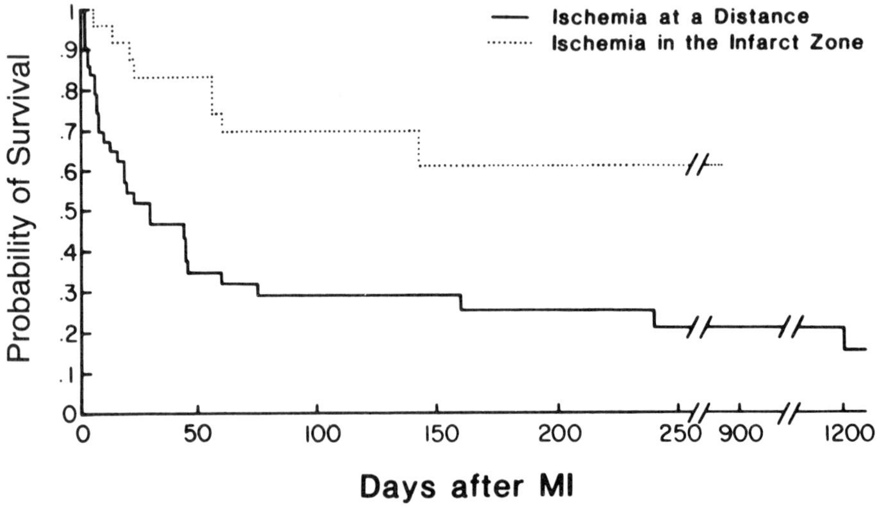

Fig 30A-6 Survival after infarction in patients with ischemia at a distance compared with survival in patients with ischemia in the infarct zone. The abscissa shows the days from acute myocardial infarction *(MI)* to death; the ordinate shows the probability of survival to a given time after infarction. The difference between the groups was significant ($P < 0.001$). (From Schuster EH, Bulkley BA: Early post-infarction angina: ischemia at a distance and ischemia in the infarct zone. *N Engl J Med* 305:1101-1105, 1981. By permission of Massachusetts Medical Society.)

predictive value because simple reciprocal changes cannot be excluded without further investigation. Nevertheless, accumulating evidence suggests that such patients, particularly if the ST-segment changes are persistent, form a high-risk group and may require further evaluation before dismissal. Conversely, among patients without initial precordial ST-segment depression, late survival after dismissal is excellent (92% at 5 years).[171] ST-segment changes as an indicator of right ventricular infarction are discussed in a later section of this chapter.

Inferior lead ST-segment depression during an acute anterior myocardial infarction appears to be primarily a reciprocal phenomenon.[170,171] Such depression is exaggerated when the site of the obstruction to the left anterior descending artery is more proximal, an indication of a more severe and larger infarction associated with a greater precordial degree of ST-segment elevation and, therefore, reciprocal ST-segment depression. In other patients with anterior infarcts, apparent inferior wall ischemia may be due to occlusion of a very long left anterior descending coronary artery that supplies part of the inferior wall after wrapping around the left ventricular apex. Alternatively, a previously occluded posterior descending coronary artery could be supplied by collaterals from the left anterior descending system, yielding ischemia at a distance.[172]

Inferior ST-segment elevation in anterior infarctions. In one study, when 25% or more of the inferior wall of the left ventricle was supplied by the left anterior descending coronary artery, there was significantly less acute inferior ST-segment depression. This implied that inferior wall transmural ischemia produced an injury current directed toward leads II, III, and aVF, thus attenuating the reciprocal ST-segment depression caused by the anterior wall injury.[172] A subsequent study showed that in addition to transmural ischemia of the inferior wall, ST-segment elevation in the inferior leads in patients with anterior infarction could result from a smaller mass of ischemic anterior wall myocardium, which in turn generated a weaker anterior lead-directed injury current and less reciprocal ST-segment depression in the inferior leads, allowing the inferior ST segments to move further upward.[173] A recent study by Sapin et al.[173] supported both hypotheses, showing that the extent of inferior ST-segment depression in patients with anterior infarcts was less in those with a left anterior descending artery that "wrapped around" the cardiac apex to the inferior wall and in those with distal occlusions, the latter occurrence suggesting a smaller mass of ischemic anterior myocardium (Fig 30A-7).

Precordial mapping. Attempts to reduce or limit the extent of myocardial necrosis during infarction have stimulated interest in the ECG as a tool to estimate infarct size. Earlier workers used multiple-lead precordial mapping of ST-segment shifts as an index of myocardial injury. Despite close correlations between epicardial and precordial ST-segment elevation in the animal model, serious practical and theoretic limitations exist to its use clinically, particularly in patients with pericarditis, electrolyte abnormalities, and conduction disturbances.[174] Because of these problems, QRS changes in multiple leads have been used to assess the extent of myocardial damage. The depth and number of Q waves and loss of the R wave might predict the extent and severity of ischemic damage.[174,175]

Wagner et al.[176] described a QRS scoring system for estimating infarct size and left ventricular function using the 12-lead ECG. The system is based on the duration of Q and R waves, the ratio of R-wave amplitude to

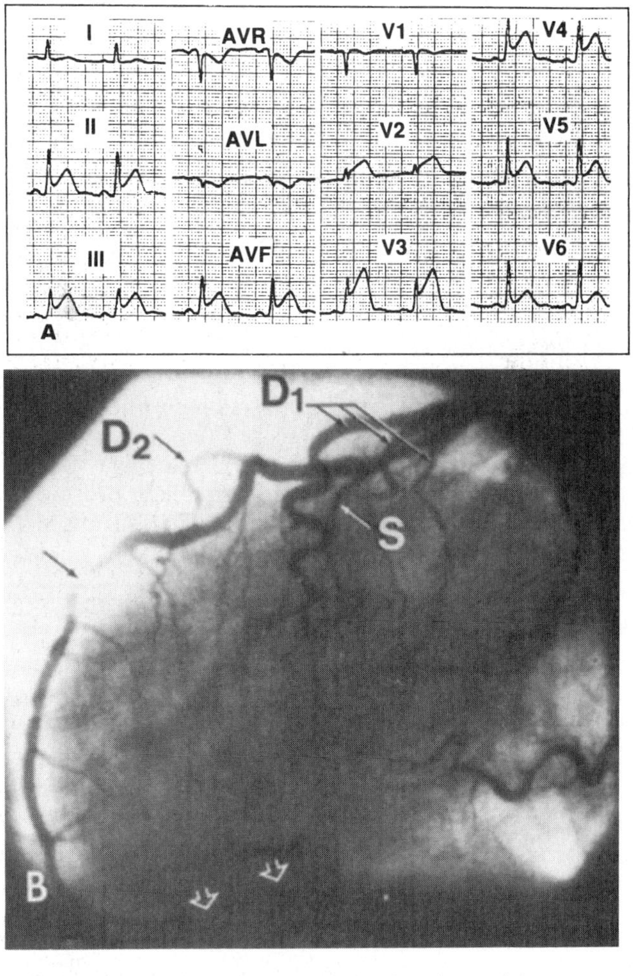

Fig 30A-7 **A,** electrocardiogram of patient with acute anterior myocardial infarction showing characteristic precordial lead ST-segment changes and inferior lead ST-segment elevation ("anterior-inferior" myocardial infarction). **B,** lateral projection of left anterior descending coronary artery in same patient 3 days after infarction. *Unlabeled solid arrow* indicates distal subtotal occlusion. *Double open arrows* indicate terminal portion of vessel on inferior wall of left ventricle. D_1, branching first diagonal vessel; D_2, second diagonal vessel; *S,* first septal perforating artery. (From Sapin PM, Musselman DR, Dehmer GJ, et al: Implications of inferior ST-segment elevation accompanying anterior wall acute myocardial infarction for the angiographic morphology of the left anterior descending coronary artery morphology and site of occlusion. *Am J Cardiol* 69:860-865, 1992. By permission of Excerpta Medica.)

Q-wave amplitude, and the R-to-S amplitude.[176,177] Others have suggested that the QRS scoring system is reliable as an estimate of infarct size in patients with anterior infarctions but may be misleading in patients with inferior infarctions.[178] Hindman et al.[179] compared the Sylvester QRS score, as a marker of both early and late prognosis, with the peak value of the MB fraction of creatine kinase (CK-MB) isoenzyme. For in-hospital morbidity and mortality, the QRS score was helpful, but only in patients with anterior infarcts. For late prognosis, the QRS score (as an indirect index of infarct size) was useful.[177,179]

A noninvasive, easily repeated determination of infarct size is needed, and although the ECG appears to have potential value, its limitations require further evaluation. Preceding thrombolytic or acute reperfusion therapy introduces major limitations of the ECG as an estimator of infarct size.[180]

Chest roentgenogram

The plain chest roentgenogram contributes little to the diagnosis of acute myocardial infarction but much to its management. It is also very helpful in excluding other conditions that may simulate infarction. A chest roentgenogram, preferably in the erect position, is part of the initial assessment and should be repeated daily for the first 3 days after admission. The radiographic appearances of the complications of myocardial infarction are discussed later in this chapter.

Erythrocyte sedimentation rate

The erythrocyte sedimentation rate is almost always increased after myocardial infarction. It is usually normal for the first few days (but may increase within a few hours of infarction) before increasing to a peak on the fourth or fifth day after infarction; it may remain elevated for several weeks and occasionally for several months. The elevated erythrocyte sedimentation rate is associated initially with an increase in plasma fibrinogen and α_2-globulin.[181] The increased rate does not correlate with the size of infarction or the prognosis.

Leukocyte count

Often there is an increase in the leukocyte count a few hours after the onset of chest pain in myocardial infarction; it peaks 2 to 4 days later and usually returns to normal within a week. The peak is usually 12,000 to 15,000 cells/mm^3 but may be as high as 20,000/mm^3. A very high leukocyte count or persistence of leukocytosis beyond a week should raise the question of a complication, such as infection, pericarditis, or embolism. The leukocytosis of infarction is present more often than fever and usually precedes it. In the differential count, the percentage of polymorphonuclear leukocytes usually increases, often with a slight shift to band forms. The elevated leukocyte count may be a response to stress with increased catecholamines and adrenal glucocorticoids, or to tissue necrosis, or to both.

Serum C-reactive protein

C-reactive protein (CRP), a very sensitive acute-phase reactant, was shown in one study to be increased in all patients with acute myocardial infarction, and there was a significant correlation between peak CRP and CK-MB values.[182] The CRP concentration may increase before the CK-MB[183] but appears to peak around 50 hours after the onset of pain, when the CK-MB value has already returned to normal.[182] Since CRP is a nonspecific response to tissue injury, increased levels in patients with chest pain who have a normal CK-MB value indicate a process other than acute infarction. Although not widely used, the CRP concentration, in conjunction with cardiac enzymes, appears to provide additional diagnostic information and to help detect complications after myocardial infarction.

Leukocytes

Rapid and accurate cell counters have demonstrated that a decrease in lymphocytes in relation to the total leukocyte count may be an early response to the stress of acute myocardial infarction. Thomason et al.[184] found that when lymphocytes decreased to less than 20.3% of all leukocytes in patients with acute chest pain, this marker was useful in detecting acute myocardial infarction in the absence of classical ECG changes. To use this marker, the authors of this study point out that other pathologic processes altering blood leukocyte proportions must be absent. The presence of ST elevation or a relative lymphocytopenia and elevated rapid myocardial CK-MB increased sensitivity for detection of acute myocardial infarction from 39% (ST elevation alone) to 65%.

Cardiac enzymes

In addition to the history and the ECG, the third criterion for the diagnosis of myocardial infarction is an increase in the serum levels of cardiac enzymes. Before the use of serum enzyme determinations, leukocytosis, increased erythrocyte sedimentation rate, and fever supported the diagnosis of myocardial infarction. In 1954, for the first time, a sensitive and much more specific laboratory test became available when it was shown that the serum level of glutamic-oxaloacetic transaminase, which catalyzes transfer of an amino group from aspartate to ketoglutaric acid and thus is now termed "aspartate transaminase," was increased after myocardial infarction.[185]

Myocardial injury but not simple ischemia causes a functional break in the sarcolemma and subsequent release of cytoplasmic constituents, including enzymes, into the extracellular fluid, where they are carried into the circulation via the venous blood flow or lymphatic drainage.[186-188] Small but significant venoarterial differences in enzyme activity can be measured after experimental myocardial infarction.[189] Depletion of enzymes from infarcted tissue can be correlated with increased blood levels.[190,191] The onset and duration of the abnormal increase in enzyme levels in the blood depend on characteristics of the enzyme, such as molecular weight, intracellular location (cytoplasm or mitochondria), degree of residual local myocardial perfusion, onset and degree of any reperfusion, local degradation, binding, degree of inactivation by plasma factors or lymph, volume of distribution, and rate of excretion by the kidney or removal by the reticuloendothelial system.

Aspartate transaminase. Myocardium has the highest concentration of aspartate transaminase (AST) of all organs, but it is also present in many other organs, including the liver, skeletal muscle, kidneys, and brain. Necrosis of 1 g or less of myocardium can produce a significant increase in serum activity of this enzyme. Thus the serum concentration of AST is a sensitive test for myocardial infarction; it has been found to be increased in at least 97% of patients who have autopsy evidence of myocardial infarction.[192] However, it is not very specific.

Lactic dehydrogenase and isoenzymes. Lactic dehydrogenase (LDH), which catalyzes the reversible transformation of pyruvate to lactate, is found in most tissues of the body, and therefore it, too, is not specific for myocardial infarction. Elevations can occur also in patients with myocarditis, liver disease or congestion, skeletal muscle disease or trauma (including intramuscular injections), pulmonary embolism, hemolysis, anemia (hemolytic, megaloblastic, or sickle cell), leukemia, acute or chronic renal disease, carcinomatosis (including many neoplasms), shock, and infarction of various viscera.[193]

The time course of increases in serum LDH is shown in Table 30A-3. In 282 patients with the clinical diagnosis of acute myocardial infarction, 86% had increased LDH activity, as did all 39 patients with myocardial infarction proved by autopsy.[192] The prolonged elevation—as long as 7 to 10 days—may be explained by release of enzymes from the inflammatory cells that surround and invade the area of myocardial necrosis. As noted above, congestive or embolic complications of myocardial infarction and renal infarction may also cause secondary (or primary) elevations of the serum concentration of LDH.

The lack of specificity of LDH and other myocardial enzymes led to the study of isoenzymes—different molecular forms of an enzyme that are often more organ-specific and that catalyze the same chemical reaction. LDH has five isoenzymes, which are tetramers of different combinations of H and M polypeptide subunits. Thus, the isoenzymes can be recognized electrophoretically; they are designated by numerals I through V, in relation to the speed of migration toward the anode. LDH-I and LDH-V are homotetramers of H and M chains, respectively. The remaining three isoenzymes are different hybrid combinations of H and M chains.

Myocardium, erythrocytes, and the kidneys contain large amounts of LDH-I and much lower amounts of LDH-II, whereas liver and skeletal muscle contain mainly LDH-IV and LDH-V. In normal subjects, more than half of the total LDH activity is composed of LDH-I and LDH-II, with more LDH-II than LDH-I. In myocardial infarction, this distribution is reversed. Elevation of LDH-I usually occurs within 12 to 24 hours of myocardial infarction and thus precedes the elevation of total LDH.[194,195] Some believe that a level of LDH-I more than 0.80 that of LDH-II is also consistent with myocardial necrosis.[195]

At least 95% to 100% of patients with acute myocardial infarction have had an elevation of serum LDH-I in at least one sample before 48 to 72 hours after infarction,[193,196] but in one study, 10 of 66 patients (15%) had less LDH-I than LDH-II by 48 to 72 hours after infarction. Thus, the absence of an abnormal ratio should not categorically exclude the diagnosis of infarction. With larger infarctions, LDH-I levels and the ratio of LDH-I to LDH-II increase sooner (sometimes as early as 8 hours), reach higher levels, and remain elevated for a longer time (up to 9 to 10 days). The increased ratio of LDH-I to LDH-II is not as sensitive as CK-MB.[195]

An appropriate increase and decrease in LDH-I and in the ratio of LDH-I to LDH-II should be sought to avoid false-positive results. Hemolysis (such as during venipuncture), hemolytic and megaloblastic anemias, renal injury or infarction, reduced renal function, and solid malignant tumors, especially of germ-cell origin (for example, advanced testicular carcinoma), all can cause an increase in LDH-I levels.

Because LDH-I reduces α-hydroxybutyric dehydrogenase (HBD) more rapidly than do the other isoenzymes of LDH, an increase in HBD activity coincides with the increase in LDH-I activity and is often measured in patients with acute myocardial infarction. Since HBD activity reflects LDH-I activity, it should not be considered a specific enzyme for myocardial infarction.

Creatine kinase and isoenzymes. CK catalyzes the transfer of high-energy phosphate from creatine phosphate to adenosine diphosphate. The time course of serum CK elevation is shown in Table 30A-3. In addition to myocardium, CK is found in high concentrations in skeletal muscle and in brain; there is little activity in the splanchnic viscera or the lung. Unlike the situation with other cardiac enzymes, there is a sex difference in the normal values: normal CK activity in women is two-thirds that in men.

Although an increase in serum CK is probably the most sensitive enzyme study for the laboratory diagnosis of acute myocardial infarction,[193,195-198] it is not entirely specific. False-positive elevations occur in about 15% of patients, mainly from minor skeletal muscle irritation or

Table 30A-3 Appearance, peak, and duration of activity of cardiac enzymes in the serum

Enzyme*	Time after onset of myocardial infarction: Appearance, hr	Peak, hr	Duration of activity, days
CK-MB	3-15	12-24	<1-3
CK	6-15	24	1-4
AST	8-12	24-48	3-5
LDH	24	48-72	7-14

*Abbreviations are as in the text.

injury (tremor associated with acute alcohol withdrawal; muscle contractions of convulsions or vigorous exercise; trauma associated with intramuscular injections, cardioversion, surgery, or snowmobiling; and muscle diseases), pericarditis, renal insufficiency or infarction, and sometimes diabetes mellitus and pulmonary embolism.[193] However, heart failure and liver disease do not cause increases in serum levels of CK.

As is seen in Table 30A-3, the appearance and peak are earlier and the duration is usually shorter than those of the other cardiac enzymes.

The three isoenzymes of CK are dimers (MM, MB, and BB), which are composed of the M and B monomers and can be detected by electrophoresis, column chromatography, or radioimmunoassay. The BB isoenzyme is found mainly in brain and kidney; MM and very small amounts of MB (1% or 2%) are found in skeletal muscle (including the tongue). The largest amount of MB (15% to 20%) is found in myocardium, the remainder being MM. Minor amounts of MB are present in the small intestine and diaphragm.[199-202] Methods for measuring CK-MB have been reviewed.[202] Normal serum contains CK-MB, but it cannot be detected by standard electrophoresis, and the normal value depends on the assay used to measure the isoenzyme.[201,202]

During an infarction, only about 15% of the CK-MB contained in the infarcted myocardium can be detected in the serum because of degradation locally (probably most important) or by lymph or blood.[203] The time course of increases in CK-MB levels is given in Table 30A-3. Note that the appearance of CK-MB and the peak of the increase are slightly earlier and the duration is usually shorter (because of more rapid clearance from the blood) than those for total CK. With small subendocardial infarctions, serum CK-MB usually peaks at 12 to 18 hours after the onset of symptoms and within 24 hours has returned to normal range (and below the sensitivity of conventional methods). Thus, the timing of blood sampling is critical in achieving maximal sensitivity of the CK-MB test. When the timing is proper, the sensitivity appears to approach 100%.[196,202] This requires drawing blood for CK-MB on admission, 12 to 18 hours after the onset of symptoms, and then every 12 hours for one or two more times.

For maximal specificity, one should be aware of the possible causes of false-positive increases in CK-MB levels. They can be divided into those of cardiac origin (injured myocardium) and those of noncardiac origin. Those of cardiac origin are other forms of myocardial damage and are not true false-positive findings for myocardial injury. In these instances, the degree and the timing of the increase in CK-MB should be noted as a possible means of differentiating the cause from acute infarction.

CARDIAC CAUSES OF CK-MB ELEVATION OTHER THAN MYOCARDIAL INFARCTION. Increased CK-MB levels can occur after cardioversion but only after substantial shocks (437 and 524 J); there is no increase with shocks of less than 400 J.[204] Mild elevation of CK-MB (the highest being three to four times the normal level detected by a very sensitive technique) may not be detected by standard electrophoresis. There may be an early peak level of CK-MB within 4 hours of cardioversion, which gradually decreases.[204] Thus, high-energy cardioversion may lead to a mild increase of CK-MB that differs substantially in its early time course in comparison with the finding with acute myocardial infarction. A similar early time course is found after myocardial contusion in patients with blunt chest trauma due to steering wheel injuries in auto accidents, in which increased CK-MB levels peak 4 to 8 hours after the accident and disappear by 24 hours.[205] The early CK-MB peaks appear to be due to uninhibited washout of the enzyme after myocardial injury in patients with good coronary blood flow. In myocardial contusion, however, the increase of CK-MB is often higher than that in cardioversion and thus reflects the severity of the trauma.

Cardiac surgery with manipulation of, dissection and incisions into, or possibly excision of myocardium causes increases in CK-MB levels. New myocardial preservation techniques using high-potassium solutions and hypothermia may cause release of myocardial enzymes and contribute to an increase of CK-MB with cardiopulmonary bypass surgery.[206,207] Analysis of the time course of the CK-MB increase (transient or persistent) has not been helpful in the diagnosis of perioperative infarction. Thus, the diagnosis of perioperative infarction with cardiac surgery cannot be made reliably on the basis of increased CK-MB alone.[208] In addition, inflammatory causes of injury, such as pericarditis and myocarditis, can cause increases in CK-MB for the duration of the inflammatory response.

Based on animal studies, transient or recurrent ischemia occurring without myocardial necrosis or injury does not increase CK-MB levels, whereas apparently similar ischemic insults that cause focal myocardial necrosis do increase CK-MB.[209,210] Similarly, in patients with exercise-induced ischemia lasting up to 15 minutes, increases of CK-MB levels do not occur as tested by radioimmunoassay.[187] Transient mild increases of CK-MB by radioimmunoassay and conventional electrophoresis occur within 6 to 8 hours of percutaneous transluminal coronary angioplasty in about 20% of patients. The increased CK-MB level returns to normal within 24 hours.[187,211] This may represent microinfarction with early washout of CK-MB. However, the prognosis in these asymptomatic patients with increased CK-MB levels is the same as that in patients without increased CK-MB levels.[187,211] Thus, we continue to dismiss asymptomatic patients 1 to 2 days after percutaneous transluminal coronary angioplasty regardless of the CK-MB elevation.

Although an increase in CK-MB was reported in five cases of atrial fibrillation (some chronic), there was no clear peak, and the cause remains unclear.[212,213] Similarly, it remains unclear why levels of CK were increased in coronary sinus blood after atrial pacing in patients with coronary artery disease who experienced angina but not in those who remained asymptomatic.[214]

INCREASES IN CK-MB LEVELS OF NONCARDIAC ORIGIN. The following situations can result in increased CK-MB levels:

Trauma

Skeletal muscle diseases (up to 3% to 5%)
Dermatomyositis, rhabdomyolysis, Duchenne's muscular dystrophy, and polymyositis, among others
Reye's syndrome[215,216]
Hypothyroidism
Labor and the peripartum period[146,217-220]

Current radioimmunoassays quantitate CK isoenzymes by the use of antibodies that are specific for the polypeptide subunits M or B. Assays specific for the B subunit are used to quantitate CK-MB in patients with myocardial infarction.[201,221,222] However, apparent increases may occur in patients with increased CK-BB, as in those with hypotension, renal disease, neurologic disease (including stroke), and carcinoma, including carcinomatosis and tumors of the prostate and the breast.[201,223-228]

Some conventional electrophoretic techniques may give nonspecific fluorescence in the region of CK-MB when high concentrations of certain drugs, such as aspirin and diazepam or other tranquilizers, are present. This finding may be interpreted as representing an increased level of CK-MB unless the electrophoresis is performed without creatine phosphate, the specific substrate for CK.[202]

RECOMMENDATIONS FOR ENZYME DETERMINATIONS INCLUDING CK-MB. Changes occur throughout the evolution of myocardial infarction, so that the diagnosis often requires serial measurements of enzymes. Sampling should be frequent enough to permit accurate diagnosis but within practical limits. To avoid interference from intramuscular injections, we administer morphine sulfate for analgesia intravenously.

Usually, testing of only one of the three cardiac enzymes is required. AST is not specific for myocardial infarction and is no longer measured for diagnosis. If the patient is seen within 24 hours of the onset of symptoms, only the CK and CK-MB levels are measured on admission, 12 hours after onset of symptoms, and every 12 hours over the next 12 to 36 hours, until the next sample beyond the peak is obtained. To keep costs to a minimum, an aliquot is frozen from each CK sample for measurement of the CK-MB at peak CK.[229] If findings reveal a definite evolution of a new Q wave or transmural myocardial infarction and symptoms along with a change in total CK, the diagnosis is certain without measuring CK-MB. CK-MB is useful in less definite cases.[196,202,229-232]

An increased level of CK-MB can occur when a normal peak of total CK has doubled or tripled from a patient's basal level of CK, and this increase usually represents definite myocardial injury.[202,233,234] Patients with this laboratory profile are usually 70 years of age or older, half of the time present with atypical symptoms (shortness of breath, syncope, weakness, or abdominal symptoms), and usually have ECG changes consistent with subendocardial infarction,[234] probably because of abundant collaterals associated with more severe disease. This laboratory profile can occur because serum CK-MB cannot increase without an associated increase in total CK by at least twofold and because the normal CK in some persons is on the low end of the scale; this suggests that each patient's basal level of CK should serve as the reference level.

Since conventional electrophoretic techniques are qualitative for CK-MB, usually cannot detect less than 12 units of CK-MB per liter,[235] and may detect atypical bands between CK-MM and CK-MB (which usually represent IgG-CK-BB complexes that are most often found in females and should not be missed if the usual MB isoenzyme control is run[236]), the diagnosis of infarction by conventional electrophoretic determinations of CK-MB when the peak total CK is normal is probably less sensitive and specific than that when CK-MB is measured quantitatively or when conventional electrophoretic determinations of CK-MB are made when total CK is increased.

Lack of an increase in CK-MB levels over 24 hours of observation in a patient without further chest pain rules out myocardial infarction and should expedite transfer of the patient from the coronary care unit for further diagnostic workup. However, the timing of the serum determination must be tailored to the circumstances. If interfering or primary events have occurred that can cause early increases in CK-MB levels, such as direct-current cardioversion, percutaneous transluminal coronary angioplasty, thrombolytic therapy for acute myocardial infarction, and blunt chest trauma, serum determinations are required at 2 to 4 hours, 12 hours, and 24 hours after the event to detect the early peak CK and CK-MB resulting from early washout in these circumstances. Early (less than 12 hours) and rapid release of CK-MB may occur spontaneously in nearly half of patients with acute myocardial infarction; it is associated with improvement in left ventricular function from admission to predismissal and suggests early spontaneous reperfusion.[237]

If patients are first seen at 24 hours or more after the onset of major symptoms of suspected myocardial infarction, the peak level of CK-MB may be missed or indeed none may be detected at all. In this situation, determination of CK-MB and LDH with isoenzymes is advisable on admission for the diagnosis of acute myocardial infarction. If these tests are not diagnostic, an infarct scan with technetium-99m pyrophosphate should be considered.

Echocardiography

Echocardiography is widely used in acute myocardial infarction. Specific applications are discussed in chapters 30B and 5. The attraction of portable echocardiography is its immediate accessibility in contrast to other sophisticated modalities, such as positron emission tomography, CT scanning, and magnetic resonance imaging.[238] Although the utility of echocardiography in the coronary care unit is undisputed, the incremental value of echocardiography over other techniques in specific situations and whether echocardiography should supplant some of the widely applied "standard" techniques remain to be determined.

The echocardiogram is useful in the assessment of left ventricular function, in the diagnosis or exclusion of acute infarction and its complications, as a determinant of early and late prognosis, and in monitoring the outcome of therapeutic interventions.[239] Potential applications under study include the assessment of the extent of myocardial jeopardy in the selection of patients for thrombolytic therapy, myocardial tissue characterization, and postinfarction exercise evaluation.

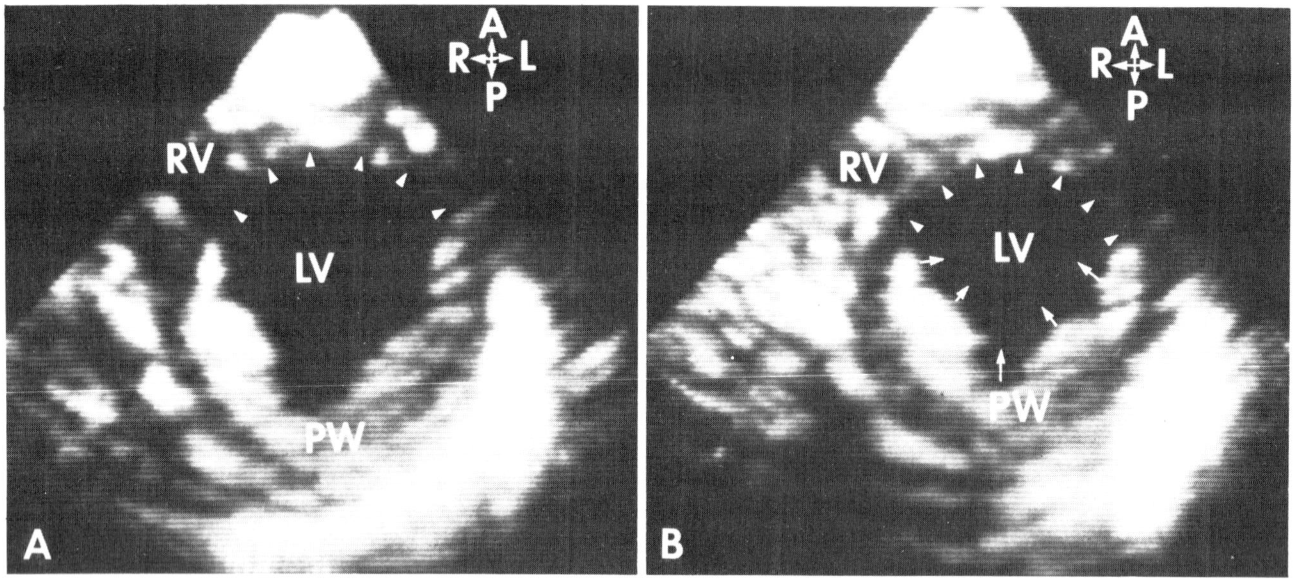

Fig 30A-8 Anteroseptal myocardial infarction. **A,** diastolic frame, parasternal short-axis view. Area of infarct *(arrowheads)* involves anterior ventricular septum and anterior left ventricular wall. Myocardium in this area is markedly thinned (compare with posterior wall). Left ventricle *(LV)* is mildly dilated. **B,** systolic frame, same patient and view. Infarcted area is akinetic, whereas remaining left ventricular segments are functioning normally (*arrows* represent inward motion of normally contracting walls). *A,* anterior; *L,* left; *P,* posterior; *PW,* posterior wall; *R,* right; *RV,* right ventricle. (From Reeder GS, Seward JB, Tajik AJ: The role of two-dimensional echocardiography in coronary artery disease: a critical appraisal. *Mayo Clin Proc* 57:247-258, 1982. By permission, Mayo Foundation.)

Assessment of left ventricular function. Two-dimensional echocardiography, with its spatial orientation and multiple views, allows one to visualize acutely infarcted myocardium and areas of regional hyperkinesia and remote asynergy[240,241] in both left and right ventricles[242-246] (Fig 30A-8) and is an excellent technique for assessing prognosis in acute myocardial infarction.[240] Good correlations with angiographic, radionuclide, and pathologic findings have been obtained.[247-250] Both the echocardiogram and the radionuclide angiogram are extremely reliable for anterior and apical wall motion abnormalities but are relatively less sensitive for wall motion abnormalities involving the inferior posterobasal and posterolateral left ventricular segments.[251] An inferior angulation view may improve the ability to detect posterior wall motion abnormalities.[252] Wall motion abnormalities alone may overestimate infarct size but, if extensive, can identify patients who need more aggressive intervention.[238] In serial studies in acute infarction, changes in ejection fraction between 0.05 and 0.1 were considered measurement errors or spontaneous variability, and complications such as extension were associated with greater fall in ejection fraction.[253,254]

Diagnosis. Two-dimensional echocardiography may be useful in the triage of patients with acute chest pain syndromes. Regional wall motion abnormalities correlate strongly with the subsequent diagnosis of acute myocardial infarction,[244,255] but the technique, although highly sensitive, is less reliable in patients with previous infarctions, previous coronary bypass surgery, or non-Q-wave infarcts, and the price of misclassification is potentially high. Two-dimensional echocardiography is useful in conjunction with other tests but should not be used as the sole diagnostic modality.[240] The exclusion of acute infarction may be facilitated by the echocardiographic detection of other abnormalities, for example, aortic dissection and pulmonary embolism.

Prognosis. Prognosis is highly correlated with left ventricular function, which can be quantified echocardiographically.[244,256,257] Nonetheless, ejection fraction may not necessarily correlate with the extent of infarction, since the former is modified by areas of compensatory hyperkinesis (in itself a favorable prognostic feature). A study by Nishimura et al.[257] at the Mayo Clinic (using an index of the extent and severity of regional wall motion abnormalities) defined a group at high risk for in-hospital complications by a left ventricular wall motion score index of 2 or greater. Over a 21-month period, 98% of patients with an index of less than 2.0 had no complications, whereas 62% with an index of 2.0 or greater had complications of recurrent infarction, congestive heart failure, angina, or death.[258] Whether these numbers are applicable to patients in the current infarct population, particularly those who undergo acute reperfusion therapy, is not established. Echocardiographically determined diastolic filling variables and, in particular, deceleration time have been shown to complement indices of systolic function in the identification of patients with postinfarction left ventricular failure.[73] Two-dimensional echocardiography has been useful in evaluating mechanisms of regional cardiac dilatation. In the first 3 days, the mechanism is dilatation of the infarcted segment or infarct expansion, a harbinger of left ventricular aneurysm formation and rupture.[259,260]

Complications. The role of echocardiography in the diagnosis of mechanical complications, for example, rupture, pericardial effusions, and left ventricular thrombi,[240,261-263] is discussed in chapter 30B. In critically ill patients in the coronary care unit (including those with mechanical complications), transesophageal echocardiography is superior to transthoracic echocardiography. The feasibility, safety, and clinical impact of transesophageal echocardiography were evaluated at the Mayo Clinic in 51 critically ill patients in intensive care units, most of whom were receiving mechanical ventilation.[264] In 59%, transesophageal echocardiography identified cardiovascular problems that were not clearly evident on transthoracic echocardiography.

Newer applications

1. In the selection of patients for thrombolytic therapy, two-dimensional echocardiography may be helpful in estimating the extent of infarcted or ischemic dysfunctioning myocardium. In an experimental preparation, Kaul et al.[265] used contrast echocardiography to determine the ischemic left ventricular area "at risk." Another interesting application of contrast echocardiography is its ability to assess collateral flow and myocardial viability.[266]
2. Chandraratna et al.,[267] using a technique of quantifying pixel intensity, suggested that echocardiography may help in myocardial tissue characterization. Normal, ischemic, and scarred myocardial tissue gave rise to specific amplitude distributions and frequency shifts when penetrated by an ultrasound signal.[268] Fitzgerald et al.[269] identified a number of features in the dog model that ultrasonically differentiate normal, ischemic, and infarcted myocardium. The future development of cardiac tissue characterization is tied to the availability of appropriate instrumentation, which cannot be obtained commercially at present.
3. The addition of Doppler echocardiography will stimulate investigations into the evaluation of diastolic function, cardiac output monitoring, and right-sided hemodynamics during acute myocardial infarction, but this technique is still under evaluation, particularly in acute myocardial infarction.[157]
4. Finally, exercise echocardiography appears to be very useful in the prognostic assessment of infarction survivors;[270] this is dealt with in chapter 5C.

Table 30A-4 Pathophysiologic classification of cardiac scintigraphic techniques

Myocardial perfusion ("cold-spot") scintigraphy
Radiolabeled particulate agents (macroaggregated albumin, microspheres)
Inert gases
Krypton-85
Xenon-133
Radionuclides of potassium, cesium, rubidium, thallium
^{99m}Tc-isonitriles
Metabolic substrates
Radiolabeled ammonia
Radiolabeled fatty acids
Infarct-avid ("hot-spot") scintigraphy
Nonimmunologic complexing with damaged cellular constituents
^{99m}Tc phosphates and diphosphonates
^{99m}Tc tetracycline
^{99m}Tc glucoheptonate
^{99m}Tc heparin
^{203}Hg mercurials
Immunologic complexing with damaged cellular constituents
^{131}I antibody to myosin
^{131}I antibody to myoglobin
^{99m}Tc antibody to myosin
Labeling of inflammatory infiltrate
Gallium-67 citrate
Indium-111 leukocytes
Ventricular function and wall motion scintigraphy
Positron imaging
Perfusion agents
^{13}N ammonia, ^{82}Rb rubidium, ^{15}O water
Metabolic agents
^{11}C palmitic acid
^{11}C glucose, ^{18}F fluorodeoxyglucose, ^{11}N glutamate, and other substances

Modified from Buja LM, Parkey RW, Bonte FJ, et al: Pathophysiology of "cold spot" and "hot spot" myocardial imaging agents used to detect ischemia or infarction. Cardiovasc Clin 10 No 2:105-123, 1979.

Radionuclide techniques

Several radionuclide techniques proposed for the diagnosis of myocardial infarction[271] are listed in Table 30A-4. Further uses of these procedures to obtain prognostic information are dealt with in a later section.

"Hot-spot" imaging. In infarct-avid "hot-spot" imaging (Fig 30A-9), various radionuclide-labeled compounds are concentrated in and around the area of infarction, and they give rise to a distinct area of isotope activity on the cardiac image—the "hot spot." Normal myocardium shows little or no isotope activity and thus is "cold" on imaging. Depending on the cellular and chemical characteristics of the infarct and peri-infarct zones, different radionuclides are taken up.

A transmural infarct consists of a central necrotic area with almost complete absence of blood flow and a peripheral area of tissue that is in jeopardy of infarction because of markedly reduced blood flow. The major necrotic central zone does not accumulate leukocytes in

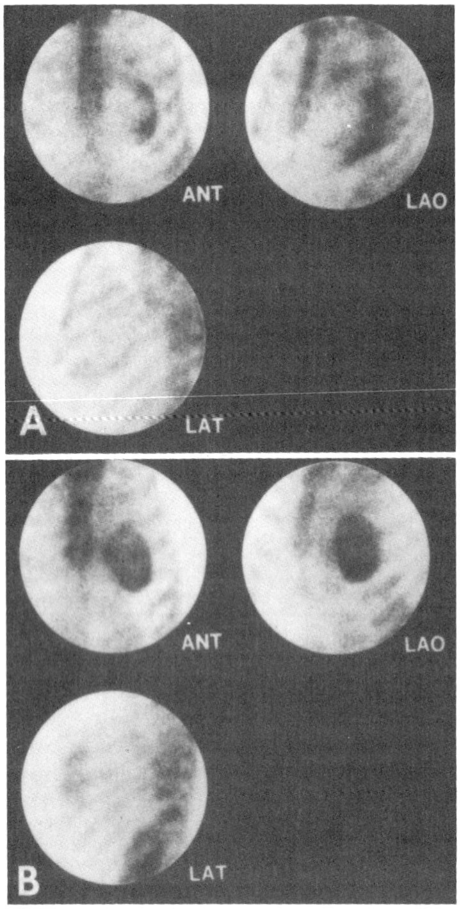

Fig 30A-9 "Hot-spot" imaging with ^{99m}Tc pyrophosphate. **A,** focal 4+ uptake in inferolateral myocardium. **B,** focal 4+ uptake in anterior myocardium. *ANT,* anterior; *LAO,* left anterior oblique; *LAT,* lateral. (From Wahner HW: Radioisotopes in medical diagnosis. In *Clinical Medicine.* Edited by JA Spittell Jr. Philadelphia, JB Lippincott Company, 1982, vol. 1, chapter 37, pp 1-92. By permission.)

the early hours and days after infarction; nor do the dead myocardial cells accumulate calcium.[272] Residual blood flow—20% to 40% of normal blood flow[273]—is required for the accumulation of calcium. This may occur in critically ischemic regions of jeopardized myocardium and is identified as spicules of calcium hydroxyapatite or calcium complexes with organic molecules.[274]

The biochemical and pathophysiologic changes of ischemia and infarction influence the uptake of various imaging agents. Technetium-99m (^{99m}Tc) pyrophosphate accumulates in ischemic myocardial cells in relation either to cellular calcium uptake[275] or to changes in cellular protein.[276] Myocardial release of myosin and myoglobulin in the infarcted zone is essential to labeling of these substances with radionuclide-tagged antibodies,[277,278] and similarly some blood flow is needed to allow the antibodies to reach these proteins. Leukocytosis is most pronounced initially in the peripheral zone, again probably in relation to residual blood flow, and this permits accumulation of leukocytes labeled with gallium-67 citrate[279] and indium-111.[280]

^{111}Indium-labeled antibody to myosin has a high ability to detect myocardial infarction[281,282] and is useful in patients with typical chest pain but no ECG evidence of infarction.[282] However, this technique cannot diagnose myocardial infarction early after onset, because a delay of 18 to 24 hours must occur between injection of the antibody and imaging to allow clearance from the blood pool before imaging.

"Cold-spot" imaging. Thallium-201 (^{201}Tl) and ^{99m}Tc sestamibi are the agents most commonly used clinically for perfusion imaging. The principle of perfusion imaging is that the radioactively labeled substance is distributed to the myocardium in proportion to blood flow.[283] Therefore, when the heart is imaged, the perfused myocardium shows accumulation of isotope on scintigrams, whereas areas of infarct are not seen and thus appear as "cold spots" on the scintigram.

Other perfusion agents include the inert gases krypton-85 and xenon-133 and potassium analogues, including isotopes of potassium, cesium, and rubidium.[284-288] Generally, these isotopes are unsuitable for clinical use because of their physical characteristics. However, rubidium-82 is now available from a generator[289] and may be available in the future.

Thallium-201 as ^{201}Tl chloride is cleared rapidly from the bloodstream by the myocardium. Eighty percent is extracted during the first myocardial passage of isotope.[283] At normal and low myocardial blood flows, the distribution of ^{201}Tl reflects myocardial blood flow accurately. At higher blood flows, however, ^{201}Tl uptake underestimates myocardial blood flow.[290] Uptake is facilitated by the Na,K-ATPase pump, and the integrity of this cellular enzyme is affected by myocardial ischemia or infarction. The myocardial clearance of these agents may be affected by digoxin, isoproterenol, and propranolol.[291]

Wackers et al.[292] studied the usefulness of ^{201}Tl imaging in myocardial infarction (Fig 30A-10). Its major advantage over ^{99m}Tc pyrophosphate is that failure of uptake of ^{201}Tl occurs as soon as blood flow is reduced to an area of myocardial infarction, and imaging can begin within 5 to 10 minutes of intravenous administration. Thus, this technique is highly sensitive for the detection of infarction, as Wackers et al.[292] found. However, this sensitivity is undermined by several factors. Old myocardial infarction appears as a "cold spot";[292] severe ischemia due to unstable angina pectoris also appears as a "cold spot."[293] An additional problem is related to delay in imaging after myocardial infarction. Wackers et al.[292] obtained 100% identification of myocardial infarction within 6 hours of the onset of symptoms in patients suffering a first infarct. In serial imaging, a partial or apparently complete filling in of these defects may occur. Thus, when patients were imaged for the first time 24 hours after the onset of symptoms, only about 80% of first acute infarcts were properly identified. This loss of sensitivity on later imaging was about 50% in patients with nontransmural myocardial infarction.[292]

^{201}Tl imaging is more sensitive than the ECG for

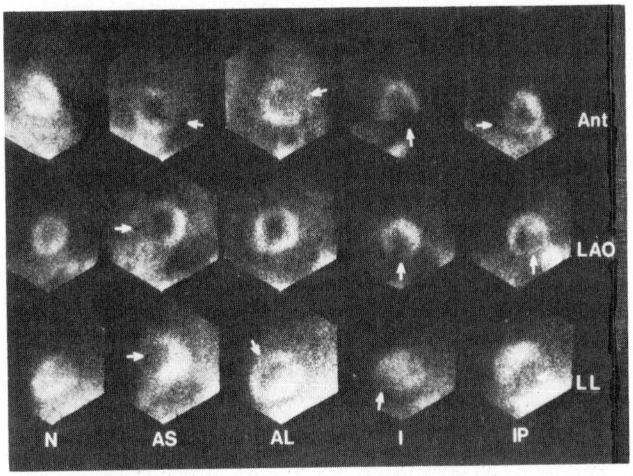

Fig 30A-10 Thallium-201 scintiscans of a normal subject *(N),* patient with anteroseptal infarction *(AS),* patient with anterolateral infarction *(AL),* patient with inferior infarction *(I),* and patient with inferoposterior infarction *(IP). Ant,* anterior; *LAO,* left anterior oblique; *LL,* left lateral; *arrows* indicate areas of decreased activity. (From Wackers FJT, Sokole EB, Samson G, et al: Value and limitations of thallium-201 scintigraphy in the acute phase of myocardial infarction. *N Engl J Med* 295:1-5, 1976. By permission of Massachusetts Medical Society.)

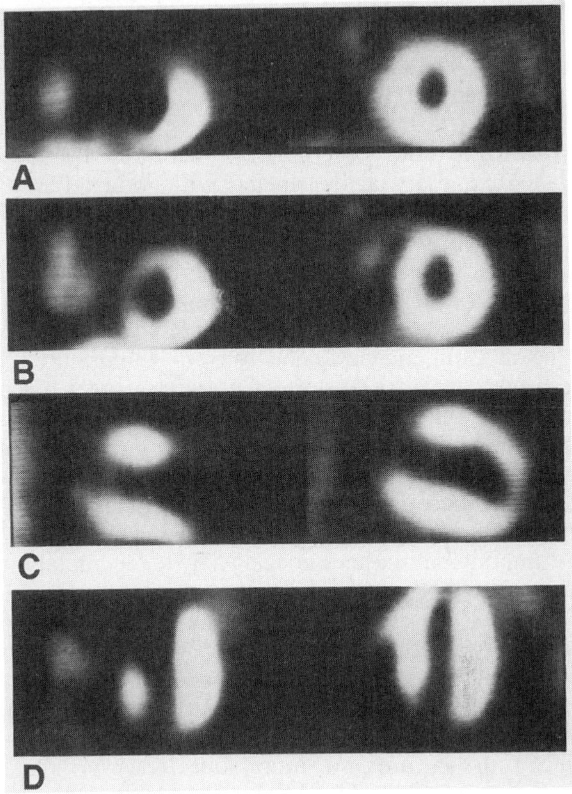

Fig 30A-11 Acute myocardial infarction involving the anterior, septal, and apical walls of the heart seen with technetium-99m isonitrile tomographic imaging *(left panels). Right panels* show myocardial salvage in the same patient after angioplasty. **A** and **B** are short-axis, **C** vertical long-axis, and **D** horizontal long-axis images. (From Behrenbeck T, Pellikka PA, Huber KC, et al: Primary angioplasty in myocardial infarction: assessment of improved myocardial perfusion with technetium-99m isonitrile. *J Am Coll Cardiol* 17:365-372, 1991. By permission of American College of Cardiology.)

identifying myocardial infarction but may not identify small infarcts (less than 7 g).[294] In patients with ECG abnormalities due to drugs such as quinidine or digoxin or in those with left bundle-branch block, paced rhythm, or other repolarization abnormalities, ^{201}Tl imaging may be extremely useful in identifying myocardial infarction.[295] ^{201}Tl imaging in patients undergoing thrombolysis is not useful in identifying myocardial recovery.[296]

Allowing for the various constraints of myocardial imaging, ^{201}Tl imaging early in the course of myocardial infarction may be useful diagnostically. Patients with acute myocardial ischemia (another group usually admitted to coronary care units), if imaged early after chest pain, may also benefit diagnostically and prognostically.[293]

^{99m}Tc sestamibi has evolved into a useful agent for perfusion imaging[297] and sometimes can replace ^{201}Tl for this purpose. Like ^{201}Tl, ^{99m}Tc sestamibi is distributed in relation to coronary blood flow except at high blood flow. This agent is bound to mitochondria[298] and, in contrast to ^{201}Tl, undergoes minimal redistribution. It has been used in the early hours after the onset of myocardial infarction for diagnosis of myocardial infarction[299] (Fig 30A-11). It has been particularly useful in patients with chest pain and equivocal ECG findings of myocardial ischemia or infarction.[300] Absence of a perfusion defect in these circumstances suggests that the chest pain is not due to myocardial ischemia, whereas a perfusion defect suggests that the chest pain is related to myocardial ischemia or infarction. The former circumstance indicates conservative management, and the latter suggests aggressive management of possible early myocardial infarction, with consideration of coronary angiography.

^{99m}Tc sestamibi imaging can be used to quantify the area at risk of infarction and the final infarct size in patients with acute myocardial infarction[301] if perfusion images are obtained in the early hours after onset and at hospital dismissal. The ability of intervention such as thrombolysis or coronary angioplasty to preserve myocardium can be assessed by this approach,[302] and it may be valuable in demonstrating the efficacy of other interventions in acute myocardial infarction.

Other radionuclide techniques in the diagnosis of myocardial infarction. Radionuclide angiography permits identification of left ventricular regional wall motion abnormalities in acute myocardial infarction.[303] However, this technique does not distinguish regional wall motion abnormalities due to acute infarction from those due to acute ischemia, old myocardial infarction, or other cardiac disease. When patients are known to have sustained an acute infarction and right ventricular infarction is suspected, radionuclide angiography, by revealing right ventricular infarction, may help confirm the diagnosis.[304]

Berger et al.[305] noted that combined imaging with ^{201}Tl and ^{99m}Tc pyrophosphate can be helpful: If a "cold spot" is seen on ^{201}Tl imaging early after infarction, a "hot spot" on subsequent ^{99m}Tc pyrophosphate imaging confirms an acute rather than an old infarction.

Myocardial infarction may be identified by labeled metabolites. Fatty acids labeled with iodine-123[306] or positron-emitting carbon-11[307] initially show a distribution reflecting mainly perfusion, and subsequently yield images depending on metabolism. Carbohydrate metabolites may be labeled with oxygen-15, carbon-11, or fluorine-18. Nitrogen-13-labeled ammonia behaves like a perfusion agent and yields positrons.[308] Rubidium-82[309] is also a myocardial perfusion agent, with a short half-life and a positron emitter, and it can be produced from a generator, unlike carbon-11, oxygen-15, fluorine-18, and nitrogen-13, which require a cyclotron for production. Interest in these isotopes is related to two features: (1) they may be incorporated into metabolites (^{123}I, ^{11}C, ^{15}O, ^{18}F), and thus subsequent imaging may reflect metabolism in the infarcted tissue; and (2) some are positron emitters (^{11}C, ^{13}N, ^{15}O, ^{18}F, ^{82}Rb), and thus positron-emission tomography is possible.[310] The use of positron-emission tomography has introduced the concept of metabolism-flow mismatch. Schelbert[311] showed that perfusion measured by ^{13}N-labeled ammonia may be considerably reduced in an area of infarction. However, glucose metabolism measured by ^{18}F-labeled deoxyglucose may be present in the infarct zone.

Viability. Myocardium after reperfusion subsequent to acute arterial occlusion does not return immediately to normal function, a phenomenon called "myocardial stunning."[312] Radionuclide perfusion agents can determine if myocardial stunning or myocardial necrosis is present in these circumstances. If, after reperfusion, the myocardium subtended by the reperfused infarct-related artery shows uptake of either ^{99m}Tc sestamibi or ^{201}Tl, that myocardium may be viable[313] and should return to mechanical function in the coming weeks or months. If ^{201}Tl imaging shows a defect that initially appears fixed but shows uptake 24 hours after injection, this region of myocardium is likely to be viable.[314] This information may guide the decision to perform angioplasty or coronary artery bypass grafting after thrombolysis. If myocardium supplied by a tightly stenosed infarct-related artery is viable, revascularization of this artery is supported.[315]

Viable myocardium in coronary artery disease may also be identified by the mismatch of perfusion and blood flow determined by positron emission tomography. If metabolism is present on a fluorine-13 2-deoxyglucose study in a region of absent blood flow determined by 13-ammonia images, a perfusion-metabolism mismatch, viable myocardium is suggested.[316]

Magnetic resonance imaging

Although magnetic resonance imaging (MRI) of the cardiovascular system is used in many centers, its role in the patient with an infarct remains primarily developmental. The present state of MRI of the cardiovascular system and its huge potential are comprehensively discussed elsewhere.[317]

Several studies suggest that MRI can delineate the area of acute infarction as a region of high signal density relative to the adjacent normal myocardium.[318,319] MRI may also differentiate healed infarcts from adjacent noninfarcted myocardium.[320] However, many of the MRI characteristics of infarction, although sensitive, are nonspecific, and Filipchuk et al.[321] noted increased myocardial signal intensity and a cavitary (chamber) signal in a significant percentage of asymptomatic volunteers. Although regions of scar and myocardial wall thinning have been well defined by MRI,[322] this definition has also been noted in segments not considered involved in the infarct.[321] The T2-weighted spin-echo technique is the most frequently used MRI method to visualize acute myocardial infarction, but image quality is often degraded by ghost artifacts from blood flow and respiratory and cardiac contractile motion. A recent study that used a velocity-compensated spin-echo pulse sequence demonstrated the potential for MRI to identify areas of transmural and nontransmural injury, myocardial hemorrhage, and possibly reversibly injured myocardium.[323] Experimental data on the animal model of ischemia in reperfusion suggest that MRI and intracellular sodium could conceivably be used to evaluate the response of specific regions of the myocardium to acute reperfusion and thrombolytic therapy.[324]

Ultrafast computed tomographic scanning

Ultrafast (or cine) CT scanning can provide highly quantitative images of the beating heart to define cardiac anatomy and function.[325-327] However, its role during the acute phase of myocardial infarction remains undefined. Although studies can be done quickly with little inconvenience to the patient, clinical justification is limited advocating this method as the means to define cardiac size and function during the first few days after infarction; such information can be obtained readily at the bedside by two-dimensional echocardiography or radionuclide angiography.

Ultrafast CT can be used in the early or late recovery phase to define the anatomic and physiologic effects of chronic ischemia or infarction. Precise definition of the size and extent of left ventricular aneurysm formation is possible, and ultrafast CT may be the most promising noninvasive method to quantitate the anatomic and mechanical consequences of postinfarction left ventricular remodeling.[328] Ultrafast CT has been shown to provide a highly sensitive and specific noninvasive method to define coronary bypass graft patency[329] and flow.[330] Finally, preliminary studies have suggested that ultrafast CT may provide quantitation of regional myocardial perfusion[331] to allow more precise definition of the physiologic significance of coronary artery stenoses.

FACTORS INFLUENCING PROGNOSIS AFTER MYOCARDIAL INFARCTION

Survival after myocardial infarction has been studied for over 50 years. Recently, survival has been modified by aggressive treatment regimens, including thrombolysis and other beneficial agents. However, limiting the analysis of survival factors to patients who survive to leave the hospital distorts the true prognosis after myocardial infarction. Death occurs commonly in the early minutes after myocardial infarction, and not all patients with myocardial infarction are either admitted to the hospital or seen by their physicians. In addition, myocardial infarction may be symptomatically silent in up to one-fourth of persons.[72] Thus, mortality after myocardial infarction may well be greater than the mortality of patients who survive to be dismissed from the hospital.

Mortality statistics after myocardial infarction

Approximately 1.5 million persons each year sustain a myocardial infarction in the United States.[332] In a study of patients experiencing myocardial infarction in the years 1940 to 1954, 36% of patients died in the hospital, and among those who survived, the cumulative mortality over the next 10 months was 14%.[333] The cumulative mortality of patients who survived for more than 8 weeks after the acute event was 39.3% at 5 years and 67.9% at 10 years. This study yields a horrifying mortality of 79% after 10 years. In the Framingham study,[334] the early mortality in patients in whom myocardial infarction developed was 22%; after 6 years, it was 46%. Including sudden death raised early mortality to 43%. A recent analysis[335] of 36 studies (36,561 patients) demonstrated declines between the 1960s and 1980s from 29% to 16% (in-hospital) and 31% to 18% (1-month) (Figure 30A-12). In this study, 5-year mortality between the 1960s and 1970s remained at 33%. No long-term studies are available for the 1980s.

Epidemiologic studies suggest that 40% to 70% of the true early mortality (within 30 days of the onset of infarction) occurs at the onset of infarction or before the patient seeks medical help.[336,337]

Over the past 5 to 10 years, several large studies have quantified the mortality in patients receiving conventional treatment with and without thrombolytic agents. Data indicate that hospital mortality in conventionally treated patients ranges from 4%[338] to 13%[339] and that these patients have a 1-year mortality of up to 19%.[340] Some studies have suggested declines in mortality for both in-hospital[341,342] and after-dismissal groups.[343,344]

Thrombolytic agents influence long-term mortality and reduce mortality at 1 year an average of 15% to 43%.[340,345] Patients treated with angioplasty of the infarct-related artery have very low mortality in the 6 months after acute infarction.[346] However, these recent studies do not include all patients with infarction, thus leaving the possibility that overall mortality from myocardial infarction is somewhat greater than suggested. Also, because of the wide ranges of mortality in studies of conventionally treated patients, it may be difficult to establish that an intervention is effective in reducing mortality without a concurrent controlled, randomized trial. Additionally, conventional treatment for patients with acute myocardial infarction is undergoing rapid change. In-hospital mortality ranges from 5% to 10%, with an additional 5% to 10% mortality at the end of 1 year. Subsequent yearly mortality averages 5% per year. Thus, over 50% of patients who suffer an acute myocardial infarction will be dead within 10 years of the event.

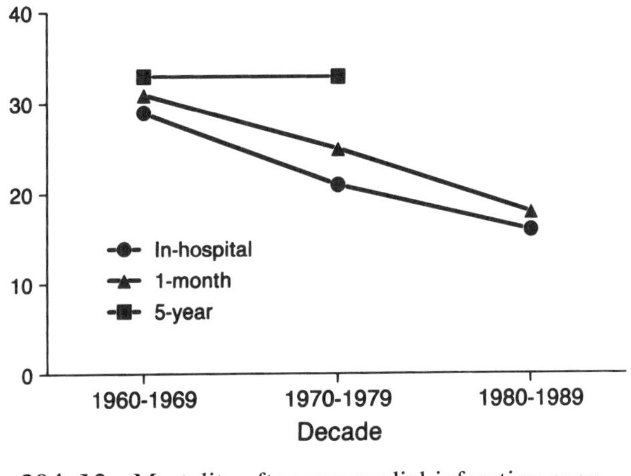

Fig 30A-12 Mortality after myocardial infarction over 30 years. (Data from de Vreede JJM, Gorgels APM, Verstraaten GMP, et al: Did prognosis after acute myocardial infarction change during the past 30 years? A meta-analysis. *J Am Coll Cardiol* 18:698-706, 1991.)

Pre-infarction patient characteristics and prognosis

Age, sex, and lifestyle. Hospital mortality increases with age,[347-349] being between 2% and 8% in patients less than 45 years of age and increasing linearly to 50% in patients more than 80 years old. Mortality is greater in women than in men at 1 month, 1 year, and 3 years.[350,351] Some studies suggest that the difference is related not to gender but to greater age and increased prevalence of other known risk factors in women than in men presenting with myocardial infarction. However, other studies suggest that women do have a greater mortality after infarction independent of other factors.[352] After adjustment for age and other factors, women had a greater in-hospital (relative odds, 1.72; 95% confidence interval, 1.45 to 2.04) and 1-year (1.32; 1.05 to 1.66) mortality than men. In the United States, mortality is greater in blacks than in whites, with the mortality in black women being the highest.[353-355] Risk factors such as hypertension, diabetes mellitus, and delay in arriving at the hospital are more common among blacks than among whites.[353] Deaths occurring 1 to 24 hours after the onset of symptoms are greater in younger patients.[356] In the prognostic index of Peel et al.[347] for grading severity of myocardial infarction, age over 65 was more heavily weighted than history of angina, mild hypotension, basal crepitations, or persistent ST-segment and T-wave changes. Norris et al.[348] also included age in their prognostic index, and increasing age was found to contribute significantly to mortality,[357-359] although not in all studies,[360,361] but the latter reports involved patients selected for study after they survived the acute episode. A high degree of life stress was associated with markedly increased mortality in one study[362] but not in another.[363] Elderly patients tend to receive thrombolysis less often than younger patients,[364] although the ISIS-2 but not the first Gruppo Italiano per lo Studio della Sopravvivenza nell'Infarto miocardico (GISSI) trial suggested a mortality benefit in older patients as well as in younger patients.

Prior angina and myocardial infarction. Angina pectoris before infarction is associated with an up to twofold increase in mortality after myocardial infarction.[357,365-367] In one study, prior angina pectoris influenced infarct mortality only in women.[368] Prognosis after infarction has not been correlated with type of angina, that is, whether chronic, stable, unstable, or resting. Mortality after myocardial infarction is influenced by the amount of left ventricle involved in the infarct. Thus, prior myocardial infarction would worsen prognosis, and, 2 to 3 years after myocardial infarction, patients with a history of prior infarction have been found to have twice the mortality of those without such a history.[333,365-367]

Hypertension. A history of hypertension before myocardial infarction adversely affected mortality at 1 month.[368] Longer-term mortality after infarction was also significantly increased in patients with a prior history of hypertension,[367-369] particularly in men[368] and in the older age groups.[369] Treatment of hypertension may ameliorate this detrimental effect.[370] Although these data support hypertension as adversely affecting mortality after myocardial infarction, some studies have not found this effect.[333,360] These latter studies have looked at relatively early mortality (6 months and 1 year). Interestingly, one study[367] found no influence of hypertension at 2 years but a significant effect after 5 years. Thus, hypertension may influence mortality several years after the occurrence of myocardial infarction.

Diabetes mellitus, hypercholesterolemia, and obesity. The presence of diabetes mellitus has increased early mortality after myocardial infarction in women but not in men.[368,371] Some studies found 6-month mortality and long-term mortality unaffected by diabetes[347,360] but a considerable increase in mortality was found in other studies in both men and women.[368,371] Diabetic patients with an increased glycosylated hemoglobin level had a worse prognosis than those with a normal level.[372] Hypercholesterolemia was not associated with increased mortality at 6 months,[360] but after 10 years, patients with hypercholesterolemia (≥ 275 mg/dL), particularly men, had double the mortality of patients with lesser cholesterol levels.[373] Obesity appeared not to influence mortality after infarction,[368,369,374] but in older patients (>65 years), obesity did increase 1-year mortality.[375]

Smoking. A history of cigarette smoking adversely influences long-term rather than short-term mortality after myocardial infarction. Cigarette smoking was not associated with a significantly greater 6-month mortality,[360] but more prolonged follow-up associated smoking with an increased risk of dying in patients who continued to smoke.[376,377] The Rochester, New York, group[378] showed a threefold greater mortality in smokers than in nonsmokers after myocardial infarction, an effect that persisted even in those who stopped smoking.

Prognostic indices

Prognostic indices have been developed to characterize mortality both in the hospital and during the convalescent period.[347,348,359,367,379] These indices attempt to predict long-term survival from a score based on historical, clinical, hemodynamic, and investigational data obtained in the early hours after myocardial infarction. Following thrombolysis, it is also possible to define mortality from

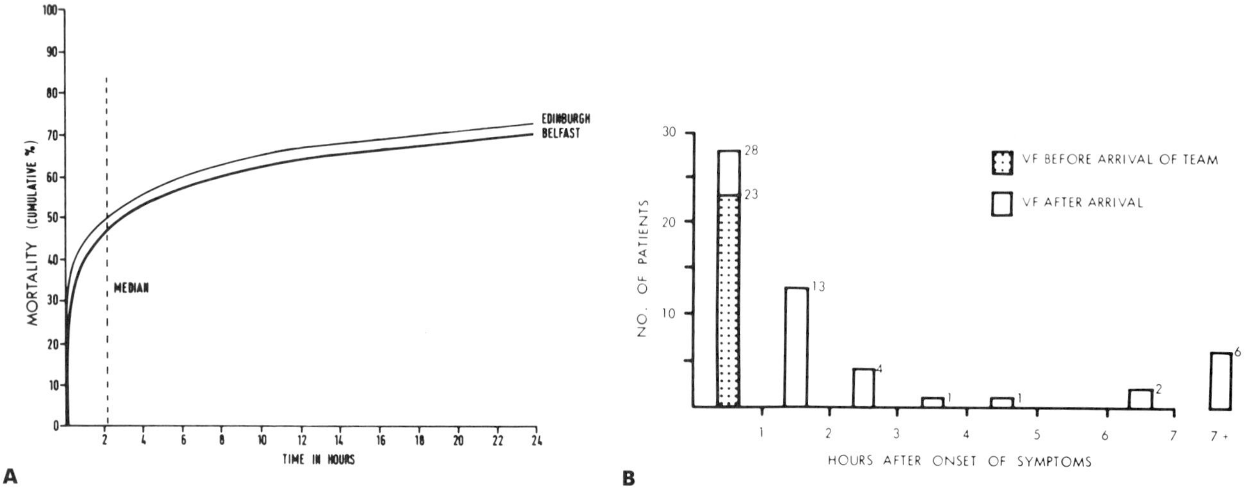

Fig 30A-13 **A,** cumulative mortality after myocardial infarction related to time after onset of symptoms. **B,** cumulative incidence of ventricular fibrillation *(VF)* after myocardial infarction related to time after onset of symptoms. (**A,** from Fulton M, Julian DG, Oliver MF: Sudden death and myocardial infarction. *Circulation* 40 Suppl 4:182-191, 1969. By permission of American Heart Association. **B,** from Pantridge JF, Webb SW, Adgey AAJ, et al: The first hour after the onset of acute myocardial infarction. *Prog Cardiol* 3:173-188, 1974. By permission of Lea & Febiger.)

readily available clinical indicators,[380] which resemble those identified with an adverse prognosis in patients not receiving thrombolysis. Factors identifying an adverse risk are age of 70 years or older, prior myocardial infarction, anterior infarction, atrial fibrillation, pulmonary rales, hypotension and sinus tachycardia, female gender, and diabetes mellitus. With none of these features, 6-week mortality was 1.5%, whereas the presence of four or more factors indicated a mortality of 17.2%.[380]

Time of initiation of treatment

Mortality from myocardial infarction is related to the time elapsed before treatment is started (Fig 30A-13,A). A mortality of 40% to 70% occurs within 1 hour of the onset of symptoms and infarction,[336,337] and sudden death may be the first manifestation of myocardial infarction. The incidence of life-threatening arrhythmias is high in the first hour after myocardial infarction.[90] Bradyarrhythmia with hypotension was found in 32% of patients within the first half hour of symptoms of infarction, and 62% of episodes of ventricular fibrillation occur in the first hour (see Fig 30A-13,B).

Fifteen percent of persons experience complete heart block in the first hour. Autonomic imbalance (sinus tachycardia without hypotension or hypertension, or sinus bradycardia with or without hypotension) occurred in 56% of all patients in the first hour after myocardial infarction.[90] The instability of the cardiovascular system immediately after a myocardial infarction supports the evidence that mortality is greatest in the early minutes after the event. This has prompted the advocacy of mobile intensive care ambulances, personnel to deal with rhythm and hemodynamic abnormalities,[90] and the training of large populations in cardiopulmonary resuscitation[381] (see Chapter 30B).

In the MILIS study, mortality was greater in patients who arrived at the emergency room 2 hours or more after the onset of symptoms than in patients treated earlier.[382] Early initiation of thrombolysis leads to a greater reduction in mortality and preservation of regional and global left ventricular function than does later initiation.[383,384] Thus, prompt, efficient treatment considerably improves prognosis after myocardial infarction.

Infarct characteristics and prognosis

A useful algorithm for weighting cardiac features contributing to prognosis is the Venn diagram propounded by O'Rourke[385] (Fig 30A-14). This shows the individual importance of residual cardiac function, the degree of potential myocardial ischemia, the role of cardiac arrhythmia in determining prognosis, and the additive feature of these factors. Many of the variables influencing prognosis reflect one or more of these prognostic determinants.

Infarct size and site. Both early and late (up to 4 years) mortality are adversely affected by increased infarct size,[386] which influences mortality more than infarct site. Congestive heart failure at admission to the hospital, which correlates well with infarct size, was considered the next best predictor of mortality.[386] Radionuclide "hot-spot" imaging to determine infarct size has confirmed the poor prognosis of patients with large myocardial infarcts.[387] Autopsy studies have shown that infarction of more than 40% of the left ventricle is associated with cardiogenic shock.[388] The amount of creatine kinase released by the myocardium is a means of quantifying the extent of myocardial infarction.[203,389]

Anterior infarcts tend to be large[386] and are more often associated with abnormalities of ventricular conduction[390] and persistent cardiac dysfunction.[391] Thus, they have a worse long-term prognosis than inferior infarcts.[392,393] Patients who have suffered a nontransmural myocardial infarction may also be designated as having a subendocardial or non-Q-wave myocardial infarction. These three terms, although not entirely synonymous, describe symptoms of acute infarction with ECG changes of ST depression or ST elevation in at least two contiguous ECG leads but without subsequent development of Q waves. Subendocardial rather than transmural infarction is believed to have occurred in these circumstances.

In-hospital mortality is lower in patients with non-Q-wave infarctions than in those with Q-wave infarctions.[394-396] Of note, the late mortality in patients with nontransmural infarction is the same as that in patients with transmural infarction.[149,395,397,398] Recurrent myocardial infarction, angina pectoris, and sudden death occur more commonly in the nontransmural group.[395,399-401] Patients with non-Q-wave infarctions with persistent ST-depression and in-hospital reinfarction seem at greatest risk from death within 3 months of infarction.[402]

Predismissal thallium stress studies are more likely to show ischemia in patients with non-Q-wave infarction than in those with Q-wave infarction.[403] The degree of infarct-related coronary artery occlusion is less in non-Q-wave than in Q-wave infarction.[147] However, the extent of coronary artery disease does not differ between nontransmural and transmural myocardial infarction.[395,404,405]

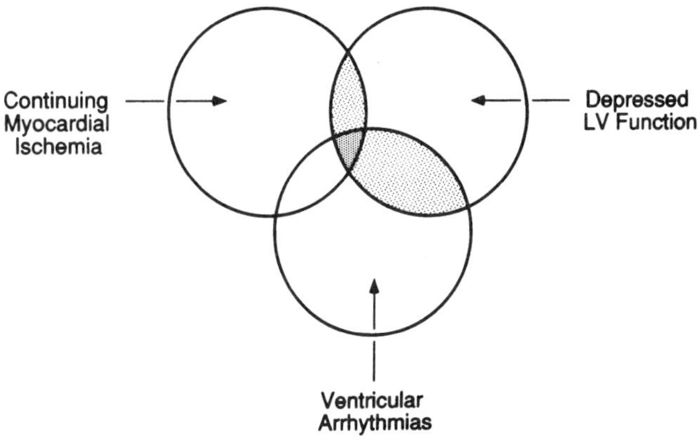

Fig 30A-14 Venn diagram indicating the interaction of the three major determinants of mortality after myocardial infarction. (From O'Rourke RA: Clinical decisions for postmyocardial infarction patients. *Mod Concepts Cardiovasc Dis* 55:55-60, 1986. By permission of American Heart Association.)

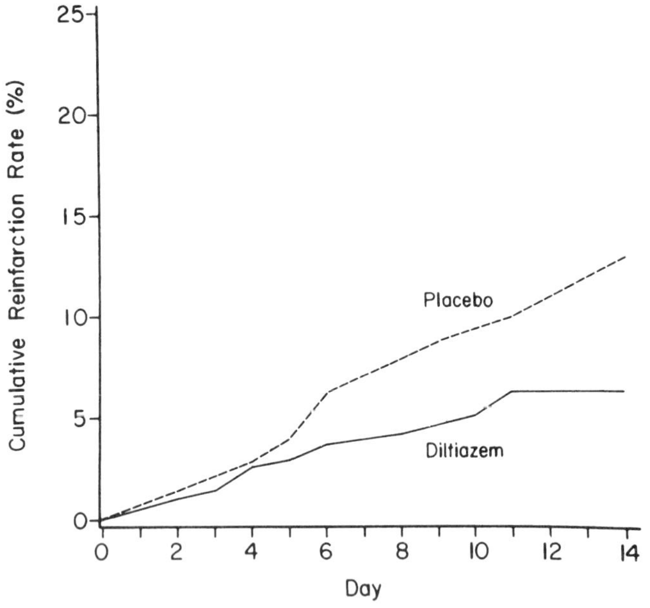

Fig 30A-15 Cumulative reinfarction rate in patients with non-Q-wave myocardial infarction. Diltiazem reduced the incidence of reinfarction from that with placebo. (From Gibson RS, Boden WE, Théroux P, et al: Diltiazem and reinfarction in patients with non-Q-wave myocardial infarction: results of a double-blind, randomized, multicenter trial. *N Engl J Med* 315:423-429, 1986. By permission of the journal.)

Some similarities in hospital course exist between patients with non-Q-wave infarction and patients receiving thrombolytic therapy. Non-Q-wave infarction may be associated with spontaneous thrombolysis in a few patients.[406]

Patients with non-Q-wave infarction represent a group in which intervention may lower the subsequent risk of ischemia and death[403,407-410] (Fig 30A-15). Thus, the patient with nontransmural infarction has a guarded prognosis despite an apparently benign course in the hospital.

Another group of patients identified as having a worsened prognosis are those with inferior infarction who have reciprocal ST-segment changes in the precordial ECG leads.[161]

Left ventricular dysfunction. Left ventricular dysfunction is of major prognostic significance in determining the hospital course of a patient[379] and influences prognosis in hospital survivors. Indicators of left ventricular dysfunction that have been examined for prognostic implications include clinical characteristics,[333,348,357,360,366] hemodynamic findings,[411] and noninvasive estimations, such as measurement of ejection fraction with radionuclides.[412] Patients who survived myocardial infarction without clinical or radiographic evidence of left ventricular dysfunction in the hospital had a 1-year posthospital mortality of 8%; those who had auscultatory signs of mild heart failure and those with frank pulmonary edema during hospitalization had mortality of 20% and 50%, respectively.[413] Peel et al.[347] and Norris et al.[348] included clinical and radiologic findings in their prognostic indices. The Killip classification of pulmonary edema can be used to grade left ventricular dysfunction after myocardial infarction, and increasing severity is associated with worsened prognosis in survivors.[414]

Disturbances in rhythm. Supraventricular arrhythmias, including sinus tachycardia, supraventricular tachycardia, atrial ectopy, atrial fibrillation, and flutter, may be associated with left heart failure and increased mortality after myocardial infarction.[333,361,415] Atrial fibrillation may have a more ominous significance than other atrial arrhythmias.[416] However, some studies have failed to confirm the prognostic significance of atrial rhythm problems.[366] Complete heart block in patients with inferior infarction was associated with a greater in-hospital mortality than the absence of complete block (20% vs. 4%) despite successful reperfusion in both groups.[417]

Ventricular fibrillation promptly controlled by cardioversion in the early hours of acute infarction has little prognostic impact.[418-421] However, if ventricular fibrillation occurs within 48 hours of the onset of symptoms, in-hospital mortality after myocardial infarction doubles.[422] Long-term mortality in patients with ventricular fibrillation or complex ventricular ectopy early in the course of infarction is less than 10% and appears to resemble that in patients without this complication.[418,423] However, ventricular fibrillation occurring later in the convalescent phase of infarction has a poorer prognosis, with a mortality of approximately 50% 1 or 2 years after infarction.[421,424] This is almost certainly a feature of its association with a large myocardial infarct and severe left ventricular dysfunction.

Patient characteristics after recovery from the acute event

Electrocardiogram and increased risk. See Table 30A-5.

Determination of prognosis at the end of hospital stay. Patients can be roughly divided into groups of high, medium, or low risk, depending on clinical characteristics and on noninvasive and invasive investigations. High-risk patients are fairly easy to identify, as noted throughout this section, and include those with severe left ventricular dysfunction, major abnormalities of the conduction system, significant ventricular arrhythmias, and unstable angina. The 1-year mortality in these patients is 30% or more. The medium-risk group may be identified among patients who have an uncomplicated hospital course. The 1-year mortality in this group is 10% to 20%. A low-risk group consists of those with a 5% mortality in the first year after infarction. In recent years, emphasis has been placed on identifying, among patients with an uncomplicated course, those who are at increased risk, with the goal of determining appropriate interventions to reduce risk.

Ventricular arrhythmias and ambulatory monitoring. The presence of ventricular arrhythmias on prolonged ECG monitoring may identify patients at medium risk (Fig 30A-16). Ventricular ectopy was found

Table 30A-5 Test features associated with an adverse prognosis after recovery from myocardial infarction

Test		Features associated with worsened prognosis
Electrocardiogram		Persistent infarct pattern[425]
		Left ventricular hypertrophy[426]
		Ventricular extrasystoles
		ST-segment depression
		Large, extensive Q waves
		Left ventricular conduction defects[427,428]
		Right bundle-branch block
		Atrial fibrillation
		Tall R wave in lead II
		T-wave inversion in lead V_5
		Abnormally negative P wave terminal force
		Q-T interval prolongation[429,430]
Prolonged ECG monitoring		Frequent ventricular extrasystoles
		Complex ventricular ectopy
Exercise ECG		Short duration of exercise
Signal-averaged ECG		Angina pectoris during procedure
		ST-segment depression ≥0.1 mV
Electrophysiology study		Heart rate variability
		Positive signal-averaged ECG
Radionuclide studies	Rest	Low left ventricular ejection fraction
		Low "first third" ejection fraction
		Increased left ventricular end-systolic volume
		Decreased ratio of systolic arterial pressure to left ventricular end-systolic volume
		Pronounced wall motion abnormalities
		Large thallium-201 perfusion defects
		Large ^{99m}Tc pyrophosphate myocardial uptake
		Persistently positive ^{99m}Tc pyrophosphate scintigram
	Exercise	Failure to increase left ventricular ejection fraction
		Increase in left ventricular end-systolic volume
		Decreased rise in ratio of systolic arterial pressure to left ventricular end-systolic volume index
		Extent of thallium-201 perfusion defects
Echocardiography		Extent of wall motion abnormalities
Cardiac catheterization		Left ventricular ejection fraction ≤40
		Proximal stenosis (≥70%) of left anterior descending coronary artery
		Left ventricular ejection fraction 0.21 to 0.49 and three-vessel coronary artery disease

in 72% to 85% of patients undergoing prolonged ECG monitoring (up to 8 hours) just before hospital dismissal.[431,432] About half these patients were considered to have disturbing ventricular ectopy, as defined by frequency, prematurity, aberrancy, bigeminy, paired ventricular ectopy, or ventricular tachycardia. The incidence of ventricular ectopy on a baseline ECG in patients surviving at least 3 months after myocardial infarction was 11.5%.[433] The presence of one or more ventricular premature complexes on the resting standard ECG in such patients over a 3-year period was associated with a twofold increase in mortality (21.7%), compared with patients in whom ventricular ectopy was absent (11.4%). The probability of death was increased when ventricular ectopy was more frequent or when it was present in pairs or runs. This relationship of ventricular ectopy to mortality appeared to be independent of other clinical characteristics, but it was aggravated by smoking, treatment with digitalis, or heart failure.

Sudden death often occurs in patients with significant ventricular ectopy at hospital dismissal.[433,434] The absence of ventricular ectopy was associated with a markedly

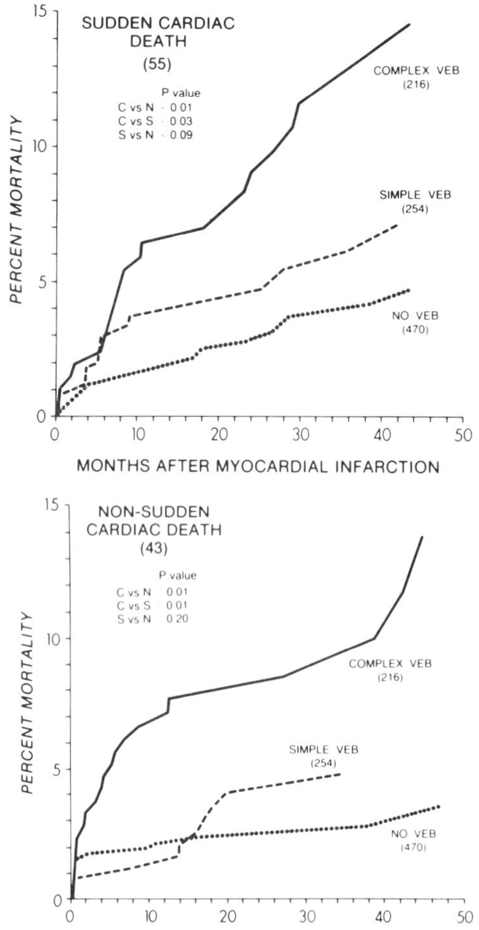

Fig 30A-16 Cumulative sudden **(upper)** and nonsudden **(lower)** cardiac mortality for patients with complex *(C)*, simple *(S)*, and no *(N)* ventricular ectopic beats *(VEB)*. (From Moss AJ, Davis HT, DeCamilla J, et al: Ventricular ectopic beats and their relation to sudden and nonsudden cardiac death after myocardial infarction. *Circulation* 60:998-1003, 1979. By permission of American Heart Association.)

diminished risk of sudden death.[434] However, another study found no correlation between ventricular ectopy and sudden death.[435] Interestingly, ST-segment abnormality was also more common in patients who died suddenly, suggesting that persistent ischemia may be a factor in causing ventricular ectopy in these patients.[434] One-hour ECG recordings demonstrated a threefold increase in the risk of sudden death with complex ventricular ectopy contrasted with the absence of such ectopy; again, ventricular ectopy made an independent contribution over other variables, including heart failure.[436] One-hour ECG recordings were found to be prognostically equivalent to 24-hour recordings.[437]

The predictive value of ventricular ectopy independent of other variables has also been found for nonsudden cardiac death.[438] Importantly, ventricular ectopy at hospital dismissal was of significant value in predicting mortality in the first 4 months after dismissal but not in the subsequent 8 months, and ventricular ectopy recorded 5 months after hospital dismissal had no prognostic significance in the next 7 months.[439] Ventricular ectopy at the time of hospital dismissal was also more common in patients who underwent a further infarction in the year after dismissal.[440] In a 5-year follow-up study, men who had complex ventricular ectopy died suddenly more commonly than those without ventricular ectopy (25% vs. 6%); this was also true to a lesser degree for nonsudden cardiac death (15% vs. 7%).[441] In this study, congestive heart failure had a greater influence on nonsudden cardiac death than did ventricular ectopy.

Although many of these studies support the independence of ventricular ectopy occurring early after hospital dismissal as a predictive factor, clearly left ventricular dysfunction plays an important role in the presence of ventricular ectopy. Patients with ventricular tachycardia had more severe cardiac impairment on clinical assessment,[442-444] as did those with lesser degrees of ectopy.[440,445] With the use of radionuclide angiography, an ejection fraction of 0.40 or less was more common in patients with significant ventricular ectopy.[446] This finding suggests that ventricular ectopy is not an independent predictor of cardiac mortality and that ventricular function is more important. A subsequent study by the same group[412] suggests that ventricular ectopy and poor cardiac function are excellent markers for patients prone to sudden death in the year after myocardial infarction. More recent studies[447-450] have demonstrated that ventricular ectopy has predictive prognostic value after myocardial infarction independent of ventricular function.

The Cardiac Arrhythmia Suppression Trial (CAST) found that among postinfarction patients in whom flecainide and encainide suppressed ventricular ectopy, late mortality was significantly higher in all subgroups than in patients receiving placebo or moricizine (Fig 30A-17). The current recommendation is that no class IC agent be used for asymptomatic or minimally symptomatic ventricular arrhythmias in survivors of myocardial infarction.

Of 48 survivors of myocardial infarction, 15 of 19 with repetitive ventricular responses on right ventricular stimulation had sudden death or symptomatic ventricular tachycardia in the subsequent 12 months, compared with 4 of 29 patients without such a response to pacing. A significant number of the patients who died suddenly in this study had relatively good ventricular function based on left ventricular ejection fraction.[451] Since there is a high (81%) frequency of complex ventricular ectopy after myocardial infarction, the validity of this factor in predicting subsequent cardiac events is compromised.

Measuring ST-segment depression on the 24-hour ECG has been suggested to identify patients at greater risk of dying or developing reinfarction,[452,453] particularly when patients cannot exercise.

Prolonged monitoring can also provide information on heart rate variability. Decreased variability in the hospital phase of acute myocardial infarction is associated with a worsened long-term prognosis,[454] especially when associated with an abnormal signal-averaged ECG.[455]

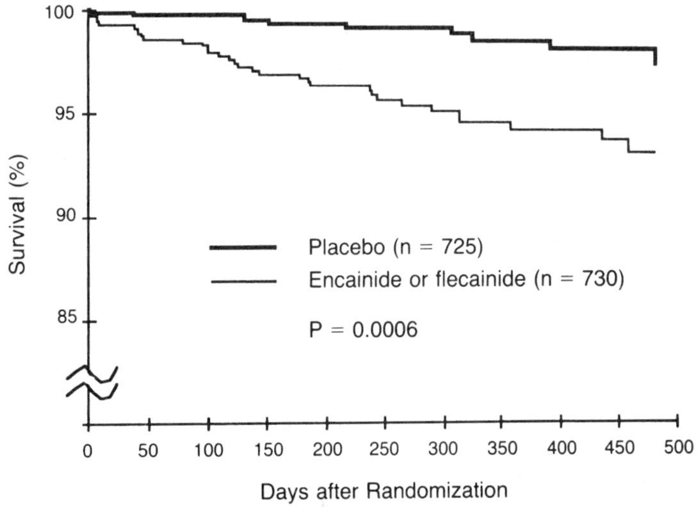

Fig 30A-17 Adverse effect of encainide or flecainide on mortality in the Cardiac Arrhythmia Suppression Trial (CAST). (From the Cardiac Arrhythmia Suppression Trial [CAST] Investigators: Preliminary report: effect of encainide and flecainide on mortality in a randomized trial of arrhythmia suppression after myocardial infarction. *N Engl J Med* 321:406-412, 1989. By permission of the journal.)

Electrophysiologic testing and use of signal-averaged electrocardiography. Electrophysiologic testing soon after myocardial infarction commonly induces ventricular arrhythmias,[456-459] including ventricular tachycardia and fibrillation, even in patients without a history of significant ventricular arrhythmias. In patients with a history of sustained ventricular tachycardia or fibrillation later in the course of infarction, electrophysiologic testing uniformly induced sustained ventricular arrhythmia[460,461] soon after infarction. However, induced ventricular arrhythmia was less common on later testing. The ability to induce and the type of ventricular arrhythmias depended on the electrophysiologic protocol.[462]

Several studies have demonstrated that inducibility does not indicate a particularly high risk,[456-458,463] although the opposite has been suggested.[464] Thus, inducible ventricular arrhythmias early in the postinfarction period are sensitive but not specific for late events.

The signal-averaged ECG is abnormal in about 35% of patients after myocardial infarction.[465] Such patients have a higher rate (17% to 29%) of sustained ventricular tachycardia or sudden death than patients with a normal signal-averaged ECG (1% to 4%).[464,465] The predictive value is greater in inferior than in anterior infarction. The signal-averaged ECG, 24-hour ECG, and radionuclide ejection fraction have independent predictive value.[466,467] Patients with abnormalities on all three tests have a 50% event rate, compared with the absence of events in patients without such abnormalities.[466] Thus, the signal-averaged ECG may be a valuable prognostic tool after myocardial infarction.

Exercise testing. It has been postulated that exercise testing in the late hospital course will identify patients who are at higher risk for death after surviving myocardial infarction (Fig 30A-18). Exercise testing was initially believed contraindicated in the convalescence phase of myocardial infarction, but in a review of 22 studies involving more than 3,300 patients, only 5 major arrhythmias and 2 deaths were reported.[468] Exercise was usually limited by symptoms or by a heart rate response of up to 120 to 130 beats/min, or 70% of maximal heart rate. However, some workers advocate symptom-limited stress testing before hospital dismissal. This approach yields more positive studies than lesser levels of exercise, but whether prognosis is better determined is unknown.[469]

Exercise testing can also screen for ventricular arrhythmias induced by exercise.[470-473] However, such arrhythmias are twice as likely to be found by prolonged ECG monitoring than by a stress ECG,[474-477] and ventricular ectopy with exercise usually occurs in patients in whom ectopy is found on prolonged ECG monitoring.[474] Exercise-induced ventricular ectopy may or may not provide additional prognostic information over ST-segment changes.[478,479]

Théroux et al.[480] noted an increased incidence of angina in the first year after infarction in patients who had angina during a submaximal exercise test 1 day before hospital dismissal after a myocardial infarction. A more striking finding in this study was a 27% 1-year mortality in patients who had ST-segment changes of 0.1 mV or more during the exercise test, compared with a 2% mortality in those without such ischemic exercise ST changes. Exercise-induced angina during such tests seems related to subsequent angina and the need for coronary artery bypass grafting[481,482] rather than to sudden death or reinfarction.[483] ST-segment depression may be more related to sudden death or reinfarction than to subsequent onset of angina.[471,475] Inability to complete a

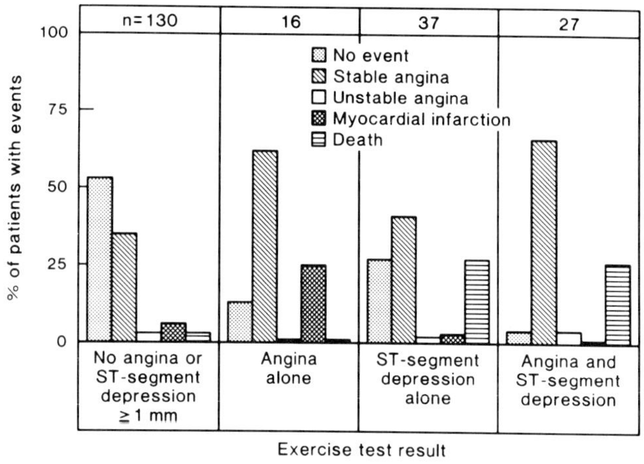

Fig 30A-18 Correlation between results of predismissal exercise testing and coronary events during the subsequent year after recovery from myocardial infarction. In this study, of the 20 persons who died in the first year, 17 (85%) had either ST-segment depression or a combination of ST-segment depression and angina at the time of the exercise test. (Data from Théroux P, Waters DD, Halphen C, et al: Prognostic value of exercise testing soon after myocardial infarction. *N Engl J Med* 301:341-345, 1979.)

limited exercise test after myocardial infarction is associated with poor prognosis,[481,484-487] and patients in whom stress testing is contraindicated have the highest subsequent mortality.[488] Overall, the stress test is most useful in identifying the lowest risk patient group. Such patients have the highest exercise duration, do not have ST-segment changes, and have increased blood pressure with exercise.[489-492] ST-segment changes seen on the exercise ECG after myocardial infarction are more likely to occur with angiographically determined multivessel coronary artery disease.[491-495] This is also evident in patients with non-Q-wave infarction.[496]

The prognostic importance of exercise-induced ST-segment changes remains undetermined.[497-499]

The combination of ST-depression on a 24-hour ECG and reduced left ventricular ejection fraction was associated with a fourfold increase in mortality compared with absence of these factors. This finding presumably indicates that ischemia is associated with reduced left ventricular function, both markers for an adverse prognosis.[500]

Radionuclide data and prognosis after myocardial infarction. The ability to measure ejection fraction accurately with radionuclide studies may allow improvement in prognostic ability. Since the extent of myocardial infarction may be a major determinant of prognosis, the ability to quantify infarct size with radionuclide methods may also be significant prognostically. Furthermore, assessment of prognosis can be enhanced by combining exercise testing with either perfusion imaging or radionuclide angiography.

Schulze et al.[412] demonstrated an 18% mortality in patients recovering from myocardial infarction who had an ejection fraction of less than 0.40, and a 31% mortality was seen in patients having an ejection fraction of 0.35 or less.[474] No deaths occurred in patients with ejection fractions of 0.40 or more. The mean follow-up period in this study was 7 months. Interestingly, the combination of complex ventricular ectopy on ambulatory monitoring and low ejection fraction identified all patients who died.

A resting left ventricular ejection fraction of less than 0.52 early in the course of infarction was associated with a twofold greater mortality at 1 year compared with an ejection fraction of more than 0.52.[501] Workers also analyzed the quantity of ventricular ejection in the first third of systole (first-third ejection fraction) early after the onset of infarction and found a high mortality in the first year when this quantity was 0.17 or less. Congestive heart failure developed more commonly in patients with an ejection fraction of less than 0.52. Left ventricular ejection fraction is less in patients with anterior than in those with inferior infarcts.[502,503] Exercise-induced changes in ejection fraction and cardiac volume measured by radionuclide angiography may be of predictive value (see Table 30A-5). Again, such studies are performed just before hospital dismissal.

Corbett et al.[504] performed radionuclide angiography with exercise before hospital dismissal in 61 patients who had had myocardial infarction. Exercise was performed in a stepwise manner until a heart rate of 130 beats/min was achieved, until symptoms of angina or dyspnea limited the exercise test, or until complex ventricular arrhythmias, ST-segment depression of 0.2 mV or more, or decreasing arterial pressure occurred. These subjects were then analyzed over a mean of 9.6 months for important cardiac events, including sudden death, cardiac death, recurrent infarction, unstable angina, angina requiring surgical management, persistent congestive heart failure, and limiting angina. Twenty-three patients had no cardiac event, and 38 had a cardiac event.

The best variables for identifying those who had cardiac events, with an accuracy of 84% to 90%, were changes, with exercise, in ejection fraction, end-systolic volume index, and ratio of systolic pressure to end-systolic volume index. Resting ejection fraction also had high predictive value. Patients who died were found to have had the lowest left ventricular ejection fraction and ratio of systolic arterial pressure to end-systolic volume index at rest and during exercise as well as the largest left ventricular end-systolic volume. Resting left ventricular ejection fraction is valuable for predicting mortality,[505] whereas evidence of ischemia, such as an ejection fraction decrease with exercise, predicts recurrent nonfatal ischemic events.[488]

Myocardial perfusion scintigraphy can measure the extent of infarction, and the larger the area of perfusion defects in patients with acute myocardial infarction, the graver the prognosis,[506-508] even when patients have no evidence of congestive heart failure. Small ^{201}Tl defects in acute myocardial infarction were associated with a much decreased 6-month mortality (7%) compared with larger defects (62%). When exercise stress testing was added to ^{201}Tl imaging in the convalescent phase of myocardial infarction,[509] myocardial ischemia seemed more often identified by perfusion defects than by ECG changes. The combination of ischemic ECG changes and ^{201}Tl perfusion defects with exercise was most accurate in identifying patients with multiple coronary arterial stenoses. Predismissal submaximal exercise ^{201}Tl scintigraphy was better able to identify both low-risk and high-risk groups of patients after myocardial infarction than were the stress ECG and the coronary arteriogram.[510] Positive results of thallium stress scintigraphy 3 days after reperfusion therapy in stable patients predicted a complicated hospital course. Most of the accumulated data on thallium stress testing and postinfarction prognosis were obtained before the thrombolytic or acute perfusion era. Whether the sensitivity and specificity of these studies will be similar in patients undergoing acute reperfusion therapy is unknown,[511] as is whether ^{201}Tl perfusion imaging with exercise is superior in prognostic ability to exercise radionuclide angiography. The role of pharmacologic stress-^{201}Tl perfusion imaging in determining prognosis after myocardial infarction remains to be explored.

A persistently positive ^{99m}Tc stannous pyrophosphate scintigram after acute myocardial infarction occurred in 9% to 54% of patients.[512-514] Forty-two percent of patients with a persistently positive scintigram had cardiac death, reinfarction, unstable angina pectoris, or decompensated heart failure 11.6 ± 6.9 months after scintigraphy, compared with 13% of patients with a negative scintigram. In the acute phase of myocardial infarction, a "doughnut" pattern with a large area of ^{99m}Tc pyrophosphate uptake indicates a poor prognosis.[387,515]

Some authors have proposed combining noninvasive testing to predict complications after myocardial infarction. The combination of a test to detect residual ischemia (exercise ECG or thallium perfusion study) with a test of ventricular function (echocardiogram or radionuclide angiogram) has high positive and negative predictive accuracies for complications.[516] In this study, knowledge of coronary artery anatomy did not enhance the predictive power of the noninvasive variables. Griffin et al.,[517] in a consecutive series of patients with Q-wave infarction, found that clinical variables (age, heart rate, mean blood pressure, and history of prior infarction) provided 78% of the discriminate accuracy in determining 1-year mortality; adding invasive hemodynamic data and radionuclide ejection fraction increased the predictive accuracy to 87% and 84%, respectively. This study indicates the power of clinical variables in predicting mortality.

Echocardiography. In-hospital mortality after myocardial infarction is strongly related to wall motion abnormality, as seen on the two-dimensional echocardiogram early after onset.[257,258,518-520] Patients with a marked wall motion abnormality had a high mortality (58%), whereas those with lesser abnormality had considerably lower immediate mortality (6%).[257] Long-term prognosis is worse in patients with markedly abnormal echo wall motion estimations.[248,521,522] Marked wall motion abnormality was usually associated with in-hospital (congestive heart failure, ventricular tachycardia, and ventricular fibrillation) and posthospital (congestive heart failure and severe angina) complications after myocardial infarction.[257,258]

Coronary arteriography. Performance of coronary arteriography in patients who have recovered from myocardial infarction[523] reveals that the increasing severity of coronary artery disease is related to a worsening prognosis in patients with chronic stable angina.[524,525]

More extensive coronary artery disease is present in patients with complex ventricular ectopy,[526] and no difference is seen in the spectrum of severity of coronary artery disease between patients with transmural and those with nontransmural myocardial infarction.[395,412] Early angiography in patients with nontransmural infarction and coronary artery bypass grafting has been performed in some centers, and long-term mortality has improved.[404] However, this may not be the proper course in patients with nontransmural infarction. A study correlating exercise testing with coronary angiography showed that patients with exercise-induced ischemia were more likely to have significant two- or three-vessel disease than those who had a satisfactory exercise test.[494,495]

Studies of patients with acute myocardial infarction who underwent coronary arteriography with left ventriculography before hospital dismissal showed that a left ventricular ejection fraction[526-528] of less than 0.40 and a history of prior myocardial infarction were the most important predictors of long-term mortality. Patients without symptoms after myocardial infarction have a good prognosis, so that angiography may be unneeded.[529,530]

High in-hospital mortality is associated with 70% or greater narrowing of the left anterior descending coronary artery proximal to the first septal branch.[531] This particular coronary artery lesion, if associated with significant disease elsewhere, also has an adverse effect on prognosis after recovery from myocardial infarction.[532,533] Since, for economic reasons, it is not feasible to offer coronary arteriography to all patients who recover from myocardial infarction, this test is best restricted to patients who have evidence of adverse clinical prognostic features, such as angina, ventricular ectopy, or exercise-induced ischemic changes.

Patients recovering from myocardial infarction who have left ventricular ejection fractions of 0.21 to 0.49 with severe three-vessel coronary artery disease have a worse prognosis than patients with a normal ejection fraction and similar coronary artery disease.[534] Lesser degrees of coronary artery disease did not influence prognosis in this study. Thus, noninvasive determinations of ejection fraction may help in selecting patients for coronary arteriography after myocardial infarction.

Influence of thrombolysis and a patent infarct-related artery. Some of the markers for adverse prognosis may be modified or negated in patients who have undergone thrombolysis. For example, patients undergoing thrombolysis were less likely to have inducible ventricular tachycardia on electrophysiologic testing[535] than those who did not. In addition, a positive signal-averaged ECG was less likely after thrombolysis,[536] although the positive signal-averaged ECG was still thought to be a marker for subsequent significant arrhythmias.

Other studies indicate that screening studies after thrombolysis for acute infarction retain their prognostic ability. Piccalo et al.[537] demonstrated that a negative stress test in these circumstances continued to identify a low-risk population after myocardial infarction.

A patent infarct-related artery is associated with a good in-hospital prognosis. However, 1-year mortality depends more on left ventricular function than on patency of the infarct-related artery.[538]

ST-depression on a 24-hour ECG was as frequent after thrombolysis and identified patients at high risk for events following infarction.[500] Low-level thallium tests have less ability to predict events in patients who receive thrombolysis than in those who do not.[539]

A patent infarct-related artery after myocardial infarction markedly enhances long-term survival. Cigarroa et al.[540] reported a 0% mortality in patients with antegrade flow compared with 18% in patients without antegrade infarct-related artery flow over a 46-month period. Patients who had angioplasty to open the infarct-related artery also showed a marked benefit in mortality compared with those whose infarct-related artery was closed.[541] Thus, a survival benefit may exist for an open infarct-related artery even if the opening of the artery is delayed to over 6 hours after the onset of symptoms.

After myocardial infarction, the left ventricle undergoes a remodeling process, particularly after anterior infarction, that leads to ventricular enlargement, ventricular aneurysm, and increased mortality.[542,543] Two approaches interfere with the remodeling process.

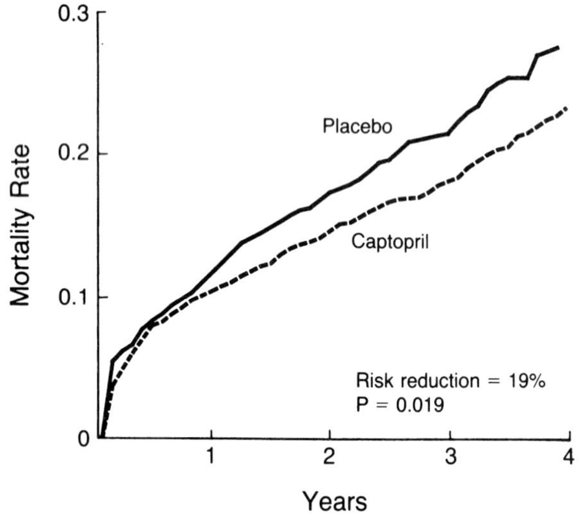

Placebo	1116	987	915	609	262
Captopril	1115	1000	938	614	288

Fig 30A-19 Cumulative mortality in patients receiving captopril or placebo after myocardial infarction. Mortality was reduced by 19% in the captopril-treated patients. The number of patients at risk at the beginning of each year is shown below the graph. (From Pfeffer MA, Braunwald E, Moyé LA, et al: Effect of captopril on mortality and morbidity in patients with left ventricular dysfunction after myocardial infarction: results of the Survival and Ventricular Enlargement Trial. *N Engl J Med* 327:669-677, 1992. By permission of the journal.)

Angiotensin-converting enzyme inhibitor limits ventricular enlargement after myocardial infarction and has been shown to decrease mortality (Fig 30A-19) in patients with left ventricular ejection fractions of 40% or less.[544] In this study, captopril administration was started 3 days after the onset of symptoms, and left ventricular ejection fraction was determined by radionuclide angiography. Earlier administration of angiotensin-converting enzyme inhibitors may be detrimental in acute infarction.[545]

A patent infarct-related artery also modifies the left ventricular remodeling process, leading to a limitation of ventricular enlargement.[546] This limitation probably contributes to the enhanced prognosis of patients with a patent rather than an occluded infarct-related artery after acute infarction.

Therapeutic implications of assessment of patients recovering from myocardial infarction

The goal of the noninvasive and invasive assessment of patients after recovery from myocardial infarction is to design therapy to prevent sudden death, reinfarction, congestive heart failure, and postinfarction angina. There is no doubt that having a myocardial infarction identifies patients with coronary artery disease. However, surgical intervention (bypass grafting) may be appropriate only in patients with three-vessel coronary artery disease and left main coronary artery disease—about one-third of all patients. The expense of using coronary arteriography in all patients recovering from myocardial infarction to identify this group seems excessive. A retrospective study[547] of patients recovering from myocardial infarction did suggest that bypass grafting may be more beneficial than medical therapy when a major part of the surviving ventricular muscle is supplied by critically narrowed (more than 70%) coronary arteries. These patients were more likely to have two- and three-vessel disease. Thus, consideration of an operative approach may be reasonable in this group. The CASS report[530] added a note of caution because after myocardial infarction, angina-free patients showed no difference in survival whether treated surgically or medically. However, most of these patients were considered for this study at least 3 weeks after their myocardial infarction.

To reduce the number of patients subjected to unnecessary arteriography, noninvasive tests should be used to identify patients at greater than average risk. Coronary angiography should be offered to all patients who have myocardial ischemia, based on clinical criteria such as the presence or absence of recurrent angina or angina equivalent. Provocative testing with limited exercise, with either ECG or radionuclide criteria, seems appropriate in all patients who have made a good recovery. Once the coronary artery anatomy and the severity of ischemia are known, a decision can be made whether to use anti-ischemic medication or coronary artery bypass grafting. As yet, no long-term study is available to clarify which of these courses is better, and the decision usually rests with the physician. The optimal time after myocardial infarction to offer bypass grafting is also unknown.

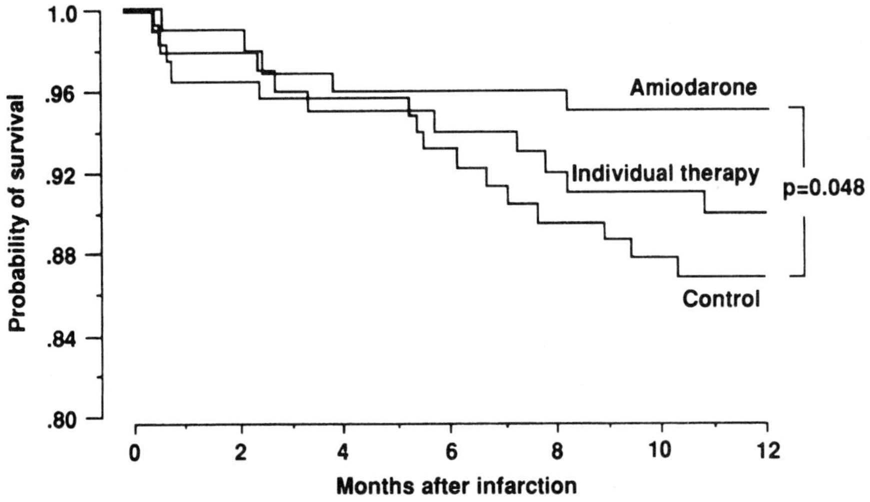

Fig 30A-20 Twelve-month mortality in three treatment groups of patients with asymptomatic ventricular arrhythmias: amiodarone, clinically guided antiarrhythmic therapy, and no treatment. Survival was best in patients treated with amiodarone. (From Burkart F, Pfisterer M, Kiowski W, et al: Effect of antiarrhythmic therapy on mortality in survivors of myocardial infarction with asymptomatic complex ventricular arrhythmias: Basel Antiarrhythmic Study of Infarct Survival [BASIS]. *J Am Coll Cardiol* 16:1711-1718, 1990. By permission of American College of Cardiology.)

Patients should be offered some form of prolonged ECG monitoring before hospital dismissal. Complex ventricular ectopy warrants consideration of the use of long-term antiarrhythmia drugs. A signal-averaged ECG obtained before dismissal from the hospital may be valuable in predicting the risk of life-threatening ventricular arrhythmias. Based on the CAST study, flecainide, encainide, and moricizine should not be given prophylactically to prevent sudden death after myocardial infarction, since these agents were associated with increased mortality compared with placebo.[548,549] More information is required to determine if long-term amiodarone treatment will improve mortality after myocardial infarction, as suggested by preliminary studies[550] (Figure 30A-20).

Since left ventricular dysfunction is such a strong predictor of long-term survival, the measurement of left ventricular ejection fraction with either a radionuclide angiogram or an echocardiogram may also be appropriate during the convalescent phase of myocardial infarction.

Since these noninvasive studies are not inexpensive, to be of value they should, if positive, be highly predictive of cardiac events after dismissal of the patient from the hospital. Noninvasive testing that yields such a result is not yet available.

An alternative therapeutic approach for patients who have recovered from myocardial infarction is a regimen that will prevent cardiac events. Such a regimen would, of course, include advice regarding appropriate diet, exercise, and discontinuance of smoking. The use of β-adrenergic blocking, calcium channel blocking, antiplatelet, anticoagulant, and antiarrhythmic agents and angiotensin-converting enzyme inhibitors has also been advocated.

REFERENCES

1. Levy RI: Declining mortality in coronary heart disease. *Arteriosclerosis* 1:312-325, 1981
2. Goldberg RJ, Gore JM, Alpert JS, et al: Incidence and case fatality rates of acute myocardial infarction (1975-1984): the Worcester Heart Attack Study. *Am Heart J* 115:761-767, 1988
3. Goldman L, Cook F, Hashimoto B, et al: Evidence that hospital care for acute myocardial infarction has not contributed to the decline in coronary mortality between 1973-1974 and 1978-1979. *Circulation* 65:936-942, 1982
4. Elveback LR, Connolly DC, Melton LJ III: Coronary heart disease in residents of Rochester, Minnesota. VII. Incidence, 1950 through 1982 *Mayo Clin Proc* 61:896-900, 1986
5. McCarthy E: Inpatient utilization of short-stay hospitals, by diagnosis. *Vital Health Stat,* series 13, Dec 1982, pp 1-82
6. Report of a Joint Working Party: The care of the patient with coronary heart disease. *J R Coll Physicians* 10:5-46, 1975
7. Spiekerman RE, Brandenburg JT, Achor RWP, et al: The spectrum of coronary heart disease in a community of 30,000: a clinicopathologic study. *Circulation* 25:57-65, 1962
8. Murdaugh CL, O'Rourke RA: Coronary heart disease in women: special considerations. *Curr Probl Cardiol* 13:73-156, 1988
9. Solomon HA, Edwards AL, Killip T: Prodromata in acute myocardial infarction. *Circulation* 40:463-471, 1969
10. Alonzo AA, Simon AB, Feinleib M: Prodromata of myocardial infarction and sudden death. *Circulation* 52:1056-1062, 1975
11. Kinlen LJ: Incidence and presentation of myocardial infarction in an English community. *Br Heart J* 35:616-622, 1973
12. Rosenblatt A, Selzer A: The nature and clinical features of myocardial infarction with normal coronary arteriogram. *Circulation* 55:578-580, 1977
13. Gelernt MD, Hochman JS: Acute myocardial infarction triggered by emotional stress. *Am J Cardiol* 69:1512-1513, 1992
14. Gadsboll N, Hoilund-Carlsen PF, Nielsen GG, et al: Interobserver agreement and accuracy of bedside estimation of right and left ventricular ejection fraction in acute myocardial infarction. *Am J Cardiol* 63:1301-1307, 1989
15. Tofler GH, Muller JE, Stone PH, et al: Modifiers of timing and possible triggers of acute myocardial infarction in the Thrombolysis in

Myocardial Infarction Phase II (TIMI II) Study Group. *J Am Coll Cardiol* 20:1049-1055, 1992

16. Green LH, Cohen SI, Kurland G: Fatal myocardial infarction in marathon racing. *Ann Intern Med* 84:704-706, 1976

17. Muller JE, Stone PH, Turi ZG, et al: Circadian variation in the frequency of onset of acute myocardial infarction. *N Engl J Med* 313:1315-1322, 1985

18. Muller JE, Ludmer PL, Willich SN, et al: Circadian variation in the frequency of sudden cardiac death. *Circulation* 75:131-138, 1987

19. Tsementzis SA, Gill JS, Hitchcock ER, et al: Diurnal variation of and inactivity during the onset of stroke. *Neurosurgery* 17:901-904, 1985

20. Rocco MB, Barry J, Campbell S, et al: Circadian variation of transient myocardial ischemia in patients with coronary artery disease. *Circulation* 75:395-400, 1987

21. Muller JE, Tofler GH, Stone PH: Circadian variation and triggers of onset of acute cardiovascular disease. *Circulation* 79:733-743, 1989

22. Kenyon LW, Ketterer MW, Gheorghiade M, et al: Psychological factors related to prehospital delay during acute myocardial infarction. *Circulation* 84:1969-1976, 1991

23. Willich SN, Löwel H, Lewis M, et al: Increased Monday risk of acute myocardial infarction in the working population (abstract). *Circulation* 86 Suppl 1:61, 1992

24. Grines CL, Booth DC, Nissen SE, et al: Mechanism of acute myocardial infarction in patients with prior coronary artery bypass grafting and therapeutic implications. *Am J Cardiol* 65:1292-1296, 1990

25. ISIS-2 (Second International Study of Infarct Survival) Collaborative Group: Morning peak in the incidence of myocardial infarction: experience in the ISIS-2 trial. *Eur Heart J* 13:594-598, 1992

26. Willich SN, Pohjola-Sintonen S, Bhatia SJS, et al: Suppression of silent ischemia by metoprolol without alteration of morning increase of platelet aggregability in patients with stable coronary artery disease. *Circulation* 79:557-565, 1989

27. Rahe RH, Romo M, Bennett L, et al: Recent life changes, myocardial infarction, and abrupt coronary death: studies in Helsinki. *Arch Intern Med* 133:221-228, 1974

28. Jenkins CD: Recent evidence supporting psychologic and social risk factors for coronary disease. *N Engl J Med* 294:987-994, 1976

29. Verrier RL, Hagestad EL, Lown B: Delayed myocardial ischemia induced by anger. *Circulation* 75:249-254, 1987

30. Rozanski A, Bairey CN, Krantz DS, et al: Mental stress in the induction of silent myocardial ischemia in patients with coronary artery disease. *N Engl J Med* 318:1005-1012, 1988

31. Grignani G, Soffiantino F, Zucchella M, et al: Platelet activation by emotional stress in patients with coronary artery disease. *Circulation* 83 Suppl 4:128-136, 1991

32. Thorogood M, Cowen P, Mann J, et al: Fatal myocardial infarction and use of psychotropic drugs in young women. *Lancet* 340:1067-1068, 1992

33. Goldman L, Caldera DL, Nussbaum SR, et al: Multifactorial index of cardiac risk in noncardiac surgical procedures. *N Engl J Med* 297:845-850, 1977

34. Tarhan S, Moffitt EA, Taylor WF, et al: Myocardial infarction after general anesthesia. *JAMA* 220:1451-1454, 1972

35. Mauney FM, Ebert PA, Sabiston DC Jr: Postoperative myocardial infarction: a study of predisposing factors, diagnosis, and mortality in a high-risk group of surgical patients. *Ann Surg* 172:497-502, 1970

36. Arkins R, Smessaert AA, Hicks RG: Mortality and morbidity in surgical patients with coronary artery disease. *JAMA* 190:485-488, 1964

37. Topkins MJ, Artusio JF Jr: Myocardial infarction and surgery: a five-year study. *Anesth Analg* 43:716-720, 1964

38. Schaff HV, Gersh BJ, Fisher LD, et al: Detrimental effect of perioperative myocardial infarction on late survival after coronary artery bypass. Report from the Coronary Artery Surgery Study (CASS). *J Thorac Cardiovasc Surg* 82:972-981, 1984

39. Crean PA, Waters DD, Bosch X, et al: Angiographic findings after myocardial infarction in patients with previous bypass surgery: explanations for smaller infarcts in this group compared with control patients. *Circulation* 71:693-698, 1985

40. Heitzman EJ, Heitzman GC: Myocardial infarction following penetrating wounds of the heart. *Am J Cardiol* 7:283-287, 1961

41. De Feyter PJ, Roos JP: Traumatic myocardial infarction with subsequent normal coronary arteriogram. *Eur J Cardiol* 6:25-31, 1977

42. Oliva PB, Hilgenberg A, McElroy D: Obstruction of the proximal right coronary artery with acute inferior infarction due to blunt chest trauma. *Ann Intern Med* 91:205-207, 1979

43. Keren A, Stessman J, Tzivoni D: Acute myocardial infarction caused by blast injury of the chest. *Br Heart J* 46:455-457, 1981

44. Ciraulo DA, Chesne RB: Coronary arterial dissection: an unrecognized cause of myocardial infarction, with subsequent coronary arterial patency. *Chest* 73:677-679, 1978

45. Shaver PJ, Carrig TF, Baker WP: Postpartum coronary artery dissection. *Br Heart J* 40:83-86, 1978

46. Lange RL, Reid MS, Tresch DD, et al: Nonatheromatous ischemic heart disease following withdrawal from chronic industrial nitroglycerin exposure. *Circulation* 46:666-678, 1972

47. Goldfischer JD: Acute myocardial infarction secondary to ergot therapy: report of a case and review of the literature. *N Engl J Med* 262:860-863, 1960

48. Roussak NJ: Myocardial infarction during serum sickness. *Br Heart J* 16:218-220, 1954

49. Levine HD: Acute myocardial infarction following wasp sting. report of two cases and critical survey of the literature. *Am Heart J* 91:365-374, 1976

50. Jones E, Joy M: Acute myocardial infarction after a wasp sting. *Br Heart J* 59:506-508, 1988

51. Gersh BJ, Bassendine MF, Forman R, et al: Coronary artery spasm and myocardial infarction in the absence of angiographically demonstrable obstructive coronary disease. *Mayo Clin Proc* 56:700-708, 1981

52. Meisel SR, Kutz I, Dayan KI, et al: Effect of Iraqi missile war on incidence of acute myocardial infarction and sudden death in Israeli civilians. *Lancet* 338:660-661, 1991

53. Berkman LF, Leo-Summers L, Horwitz RI: Emotional support and survival after myocardial infarction. A prospective, population-based study of the elderly. *Ann Intern Med* 117:1003-1009, 1992

54. Davis K, Kennedy JW, Kemp HG Jr, et al: Complications of coronary arteriography from the Collaborative Study of Coronary Artery Surgery (CASS). *Circulation* 59:1105-1112, 1979

55. Kennedy JW and the Registry Committee of the Society for Cardiac Angiography: Complications associated with cardiac catheterization and angiography. *Cathet Cardiovasc Diagn* 8:5-11, 1982

56. Gwost J, Stoebe T, Chesler E, et al: Analysis of the complications of cardiac catheterization over nine years. *Cathet Cardiovasc Diagn* 8:13-21, 1982

57. Bredlau CE, Roubin GS, Leimgruber PP, et al: In-hospital morbidity and mortality in patients undergoing electric coronary angioplasty. *Circulation* 72:1044-1052, 1985

58. Wyman RM, Safian RD, Portway V, et al: Current complications of diagnostic and therapeutic cardiac catheterization. *J Am Coll Cardiol* 12:1400-1406, 1988

59. Smith HWB III, Liberman HA, Brody SL, et al: Acute myocardial infarction temporally related to cocaine use: clinical, angiographic, and pathophysiologic observations. *Ann Intern Med* 107:13-18, 1987

60. Isner JM, Estes NAM III, Thompson PD, et al: Acute cardiac events temporally related to cocaine abuse. *N Engl J Med* 315:1438-1443, 1986

61. Mathias DW: Cocaine-associated myocardial ischemia: review of clinical and angiographic findings. *Am J Med* 81:675-678, 1986

62. Cregler LL, Mark H: Medical complications of cocaine abuse. *N Engl J Med* 315:1495-1499, 1986

63. Carson P, Oldroyd K, Phadke K: Myocardial infarction due to amphetamine. *Br Med J* 294:1525-1526, 1987

64. Cunningham SR, Dalzell GWN, McGirr P, et al: Myocardial infarction and primary ventricular fibrillation after glue sniffing. *Br Med J* 294:739-740, 1987

65. Pathy MS: Clinical presentation of myocardial infarction in the elderly. *Br Heart J* 29:190-199, 1967

66. Tinker GM: Clinical presentation of myocardial infarction in the elderly. *Age Ageing* 10:237-240, 1981

67. Bayer AJ, Chadha JS, Farag RR, et al: Changing presentation of myocardial infarction with increasing old age. *J Am Geriatr Soc* 34:263-266, 1986

68. Editorial: Presentation of myocardial infarction in the elderly. *Lancet* 2:1077-1078, 1986

69. Rothwell PM: Angina and myocardial infarction presenting with pain confined to the ear. *Postgrad Med J* 69:300-301, 1993

70. Gallavardin L: Symptômes et diagnostic de l'infarctus du myocarde. *J Med Lyon No 32,* 1921, pp 913-921

71. Margolis JR, Kannel WB, Feinleib M, et al: Clinical features of unrecognized myocardial infarction—silent and symptomatic: eighteen-year follow-up; the Framingham study. *Am J Cardiol* 32:1-7, 1973

72. Kannel WB, Abbott RD: Incidence and prognosis of unrecog-

nized myocardial infarction: an update on the Framingham Study. *N Engl J Med* 311:1144-1147, 1984
73. Oh JK, Ding ZP, Gersh BJ, et al: Restrictive left ventricular diastolic filling identifies patients with heart failure after acute myocardial infarction. *J Am Soc Echocardiogr* 5:497-503, 1992
74. Yano K, MacLean CJ: The incidence and prognosis of unrecognized myocardial infarction in the Honolulu, Hawaii, Heart Program. *Arch Intern Med* 149:1528-1532, 1989
75. Partamian JO, Bradley RF: Acute myocardial infarction in 258 cases of diabetes: immediate mortality and five-year survival. *N Engl J Med* 273:455-461, 1965
76. Bayliss RIS: The silent coronary. *Br Med J* 290:1093-1094, 1985
77. Aronow WS: Prevalence of presenting symptoms of recognized acute myocardial infarction and of unrecognized healed myocardial infarction in elderly patients. *Am J Cardiol* 60:1182, 1987
78. Master AM, Dack S, Jaffe HL: Postoperative coronary artery occlusion. *JAMA* 110:1415-1418, 1938
79. Cabin HS, Roberts WC: Quantitative comparison of extent of coronary narrowing and size of healed myocardial infarct in 33 necropsy patients with clinically recognized and in 28 with clinically unrecognized ("silent") previous acute myocardial infarction. *Am J Cardiol* 50:677-681, 1982
80. Uretsky BF, Farquhar DS, Berezin AF, et al: Symptomatic myocardial infarction without chest pain: prevalence and clinical course. *Am J Cardiol* 40:498-503, 1977
81. Ahmed SS, Gupta RC, Brancato RR: Significance of nausea and vomiting during acute myocardial infarction. *Am Heart J* 95:671-672, 1978
82. Johanssen UJ, Summers R, Mark AL: Gastric dilation during stimulation of cardiac sensory receptors. *Circulation* 63:960-964, 1981
83. Herlihy T, McIvor ME, Cummings CC, et al: Nausea and vomiting during acute myocardial infarction and its relation to infarct size and location. *Am J Cardiol* 60:20-22, 1987
84. Wei JY, Markis JE, Malagold M, et al: Cardiovascular reflexes stimulated by reperfusion of ischemic myocardium in acute myocardial infarction. *Circulation* 67:796-801, 1983
85. Esente P, Giambartolomei A, Gensini GG, et al: Coronary reperfusion and Bezold-Jarisch reflex (bradycardia and hypotension). *Am J Cardiol* 52:221-224, 1983
86. Wei JY: Nausea and vomiting during acute myocardial infarction (letter to the editor). *Am J Cardiol* 62:178, 1988
87. Vatner SF, Baig H, Manders WT, et al: Effects of coronary artery reperfusion on myocardial infarct size calculated from creatine kinase. *J Clin Invest* 61:1048-1056, 1978
88. Ingram DA, Fulton RA, Portal RW, et al: Vomiting as a diagnostic aid in acute ischaemic cardiac pain. *Br Med J* 281:636-637, 1980
89. Douthwaite AH: Intractable hiccuping in acute myocardial infarction (letter to the editor). *Br Med J* 2:709, 1971
90. Pantridge JF, Adgey AAJ, Geddes JS, et al: The Acute Coronary Attack. New York, Grune & Stratton, 1975, pp 26-42
91. Latham PM: Cited by Willius FA, Dry T: A History of the Heart and Circulation. Philadelphia, WB Saunders Company, 1948, p 134
92. Heberden W: Cited by Willius FA, Dry T: A History of the Heart and Circulation. Philadelphia, WB Saunders Company, 1948, p 134
93. Weissler AM, Warren JV, Estes EH Jr, et al: Vasodepressor syncope: factors influencing cardiac output. *Circulation* 15:875-882, 1957
94. Come PC, Pitt B: Nitroglycerin-induced severe hypotension and bradycardia in patients with acute myocardial infarction. *Circulation* 54:624-628, 1976
95. Sjöstrand T: Circulatory control via vagal afferents. VI. The bleeding bradycardia in the rat, its elicitation, and relation to the release of vasopressin. *Acta Physiol Scand* 89:39-50, 1973
96. Löfmark R, Nordlander R, Orinius E: The temperature course in acute myocardial infarction. *Am Heart J* 96:153-156, 1978
97. Thomas M, Malmcrona R, Shillingford J: Circulatory changes associated with systemic hypotension in patients with acute myocardial infarction. *Br Heart J* 28:108-117, 1966
98. Forrester JS, Chatterjee K, Swan HJC: Hemodynamic monitoring in patients with acute myocardial infarction. *JAMA* 226:60-61, 1973
99. Shell WE, Sobel BE: Protection of jeopardized ischemic myocardium by reduction of ventricular afterload. *N Engl J Med* 291:481-486, 1974
100. Hurst JW, Blackard E: Inspection and palpation of pulsations on the front of the chest (editorial). *Am Heart J* 56:159-164, 1958
101. Price WH, Brown AE: Alterations in intensity of heart sounds after myocardial infarction. *Br Heart J* 30:835-839, 1968
102. Shah PM: Hemodynamic determinants of the first heart sound. In Physiologic Principles of Heart Sounds and Murmurs. Edited by DF Leon, JA Shaver. New York, American Heart Association, 1975, pp 2-7
103. Yurchak PM, Gorlin R: Paradoxical splitting of the second heart sound in coronary heart disease. *N Engl J Med* 269:741-743, 1963
104. Riley CP, Russell RO Jr, Rackley CE: Left ventricular gallop sound and acute myocardial infarction. *Am Heart J* 86:598-602, 1973
105. Fearon RE, Cohen LS, O'Hara JM, et al: Diastolic murmurs due to two sequelae of atherosclerotic coronary artery disease: ventricular aneurysm and coronary artery stenosis. *Am Heart J* 76:252-258, 1968
106. Dec GW Jr, Waldman H, Southern J, et al: Viral myocarditis mimicking acute myocardial infarction. *J Am Coll Cardiol* 20:85-89, 1992
107. Barnes AR, Burchell HB: Acute pericarditis simulating acute coronary occlusion: a report of fourteen cases. *Am Heart J* 23:247-266, 1942
108. Spodick DH, Flessas AP, Johnson MM: Association of acute respiratory symptoms with onset of acute myocardial infarction: prospective investigation of 150 patients and matched control patients. *Am J Cardiol* 53:481-482, 1984
109. Miklozek CL, Crumpacker CS, Royal HD, et al: Myocarditis presenting as acute myocardial infarction. *Am Heart J* 115:768-776, 1988
110. Gardiner AJS, Short D: Four faces of acute myopericarditis. *Br Heart J* 35:433-442, 1973
111. Hamman L: Spontaneous mediastinal emphysema. *Bull Johns Hopkins Hosp* 64:1-21, 1939
112. Ryan ET, Pak PH, DeSanctis RW: Myocardial infarction mimicked by acute cholecystitis. *Ann Intern Med* 116:218-220, 1992
113. Spritzer HW, Peterson CR, Jones RC, et al: Electrocardiographic abnormalities in acute pancreatitis: two patients studied by selective coronary arteriography. *Milit Med* 134:687-693, 1969
114. Clain A, Heffernan SJ: Spontaneous rupture of the oesophagus: diagnosis and successful management. *Lancet* 2:1284-1286, 1956
115. Myers G, Freeman R, Scharf D, et al: Cervicoprecordial angina: diagnosis and management (abstract). *Am J Cardiol* 39:287, 1977
116. Kayser HL: Tietze's syndrome: a review of the literature. *Am J Med* 21:982-989, 1956
117. Epstein SE, Gerber LH, Borer JS: Chest wall syndrome: a common cause of unexplained cardiac pain. *JAMA* 241:2793-2797, 1979
118. Chou T-C, Susilavorn B: Electrocardiographic changes in intracranial hemorrhage. *J Electrocardiol* 2:193-196, 1969
119. Cropp GJ, Manning GW: Electrocardiographic changes simulating myocardial ischemia and infarction associated with spontaneous intracranial hemorrhage. *Circulation* 22:25-38, 1960
120. McLeod AA, Neil-Dwyer G, Meyer CHA, et al: Cardiac sequelae of acute head injury. *Br Heart J* 47:221-226, 1982
121. Badui E, Estañol B, Garcia-Rubi D: Coincidence of cerebrovascular accident and silent myocardial infarction. *Angiology* 33:702-709, 1982
122. Hussar AE, Pachter M: Myocardial infarction and fatal coronary insufficiency during electroconvulsive therapy. *JAMA* 204:1004-1007, 1968
123. Zhu WX, Olson DE, Karon BL, et al: Myocardial stunning after electroconvulsive therapy. *Ann Intern Med* 117:914-915, 1992
124. Dec GW Jr, Stern TA, Welch C: The effects of electroconvulsive therapy on serial electrocardiograms and serum cardiac enzyme values: a prospective study of depressed hospitalized inpatients. *JAMA* 253: 2525-2529, 1985
125. Gorlin R, Klein MD, Sullivan JM: Prospective correlative study of ventricular aneurysm: mechanistic concept and clinical recognition. *Am J Med* 42:512-531, 1967
126. Dubnow MH, Burchell HB, Titus JL: Postinfarction ventricular aneurysm: a clinicomorphologic and electrocardiographic study of 80 cases. *Am Heart J* 70:753-760, 1965
127. Mills RM Jr, Young E, Gorlin R, et al: Natural history of S-T segment elevation after acute myocardial infarction. *Am J Cardiol* 35:609-614, 1975
128. Arvan S, Varat MA: Persistent ST-segment elevation and left ventricular wall abnormalities: a 2-dimensional echocardiographic study. *Am J Cardiol* 53:1542-1546, 1984
129. Savage RM, Wagner GS, Ideker RE, et al: Correlation of postmortem anatomic findings with electrocardiographic changes in patients with myocardial infarction: retrospective study of patients with typical anterior and posterior infarcts. *Circulation* 55:279-285, 1977
130. Sullivan W, Vlodaver Z, Tuna N, et al: Correlation of electrocardiographic and pathologic findings in healed myocardial infarction. *Am J Cardiol* 42:724-732, 1978

131. Rude RE, Poole WK, Muller JE, et al: Electrocardiographic and clinical criteria for recognition of acute myocardial infarction based on analysis of 3,697 patients. *Am J Cardiol* 52:936-942, 1983

132. Abbott JA, Scheinman MM: Nondiagnostic electrocardiogram in patients with acute myocardial infarction: clinical and anatomic correlations. *Am J Med* 55:608-613, 1973

133. Miller DH, Kligfield P, Schreiber TL, et al: Relationship of prior myocardial infarction to false-positive electrocardiographic diagnosis of acute injury in patients with chest pain. *Arch Intern Med* 147:257-261, 1987

134. Hoffman JR, Igarashi E: Influence of electrocardiographic findings on admission decisions in patients with acute chest pain. *Am J Med* 79:699-707, 1985

135. Pahlm O, Haisty WK Jr, Wagner NB, et al: Specificity and sensitivity of QRS criteria for diagnosis of single and multiple myocardial infarcts. *Am J Cardiol* 68:1300-1304, 1991

136. Blanke H, Cohen M, Schlueter GU, et al: Electrocardiographic and coronary arteriographic correlations during acute myocardial infarction. *Am J Cardiol* 54:249-255, 1984

137. Bairey CN, Shah PK, Lew AS, et al: Electrocardiographic differentiation of occlusion of the left circumflex versus the right coronary artery as a cause of inferior acute myocardial infarction. *Am J Cardiol* 60:456-459, 1987

138. Huey BL, Beller GA, Kaiser DL, et al: A comprehensive analysis of myocardial infarction due to left circumflex artery occlusion: comparison with infarction due to right coronary artery and left anterior descending artery occlusion. *J Am Coll Cardiol* 12:1156-1166, 1988

139. Roubin GS, Shen WF, Nicholson M, et al: Anterolateral ST segment depression in acute inferior myocardial infarction: angiographic and clinical implications. *Am Heart J* 107:1177-1182, 1984

140. Prinzmetal M, Shaw CMcK Jr, Maxwell MH, et al: Studies on the mechanism of ventricular activity. VI. The depolarization complex in pure subendocardial infarction: role of the subendocardial region in the normal electrocardiogram. *Am J Med* 16:469-489, 1954

141. Sodi-Pallares D, Bisteni A, Medrano GA, et al: The activation of the free left ventricular wall in the dog's heart: in normal conditions and in left bundle branch block. *Am Heart J* 49:587-602, 1955

142. Levine HD: Subendocardial infarction in retrospect: pathologic, cardiographic, and ancillary features. *Circulation* 72:790-800, 1985

143. Cook RW, Edwards JE, Pruitt RD: Electrocardiographic changes in acute subendocardial infarction. I. Large subendocardial and large nontransmural infarcts. *Circulation* 18:603-612, 1958

144. Raunio H, Rissanen V, Romppanen T, et al: Changes in the QRS complex and ST segment in transmural and subendocardial myocardial infarctions: a clinicopathologic study. *Am Heart J* 98:176-184, 1979

145. Phibbs B: "Transmural" versus "subendocardial" myocardial infarction: an electrocardiographic myth. *J Am Coll Cardiol* 1:561-564, 1983

146. Spodick DH: Q-wave infarction versus S-T infarction. Nonspecificity of electrocardiographic criteria for differentiating transmural and nontransmural lesions. *Am J Cardiol* 51:913-915, 1983

147. Huey BL, Gheorghiade M, Crampton RS, et al: Acute non-Q wave myocardial infarction associated with early ST segment elevation: evidence for spontaneous reperfusion and implications for thrombolytic trials. *J Am Coll Cardiol* 9:18-25, 1987

148. Hackworthy RA, Vogel MB, Harris PJ: Relationship between changes in ST segment elevation and patency of the infarct-related coronary artery in acute myocardial infarction. *Am Heart J* 112:279-284, 1986

149. Gibson RS: Non-Q-wave myocardial infarction: diagnosis, prognosis, and management. *Curr Probl Cardiol* 13:1-72, 1988

150. Boden WE, Kleiger RE, Gibson RS, et al: Electrocardiographic evolution of posterior acute myocardial infarction: importance of early precordial ST-segment depression. *Am J Cardiol* 59:782-787, 1987

151. Hands ME, Cook EF, Stone PH, et al: Electrocardiographic diagnosis of myocardial infarction in the presence of complete left bundle branch block. *Am Heart J* 116:23-30, 1988

152. Barold SS, Wallace WA, Ong LS, et al: Primary ST and T wave abnormalities in the diagnosis of acute anterior myocardial infarction during permanent ventricular pacing. *J Electrocardiol* 9:387-390, 1976

153. Niremberg V, Amikam S, Roguin N, et al: Primary ST changes: diagnostic aid in paced patients with acute myocardial infarction. *Br Heart J* 39:502-505, 1977

154. Mirvis DM: Body surface distributions of repolarization forces during acute myocardial infarction. I. Isopotential and isoarea mapping. *Circulation* 62:878-887, 1980

155. Hellerstein HK, Katz LN: The electrical effects of injury at various myocardial locations. *Am Heart J* 36:184-220, 1948

156. Kyriakidis M, Antonopoulos A, Barbetseas J, et al: Correlation of reciprocal ST-segment depression after acute myocardial infarction with coronary angiographic findings. *Int J Cardiol* 36:163-168, 1992

157. Prinzmetal M, Toyoshima H, Ekmekci A, et al: Myocardial ischemia: nature of ischemic electrocardiographic patterns in the mammalian ventricles as determined by intracellular electrographic and metabolic changes. *Am J Cardiol* 8:493-503, 1961

158. Schuster EH, Bulkley BH: Early post-infarction angina: ischemia at a distance and ischemia in the infarct zone. *N Engl J Med* 305:1101-1105, 1981

159. Jennings K, Reid DS, Julian DG: "Reciprocal" depression of the ST segment in acute myocardial infarction. *Br Med J* 287:634-637, 1983

160. Camara EJN, Chandra N, Ouyang P, et al: Reciprocal ST change in acute myocardial infarction: assessment by electrocardiography and echocardiography. *J Am Coll Cardiol* 2:251-257, 1983

161. Shah PK, Pichler M, Berman DS, et al: Noninvasive identification of a high risk subset of patients with acute inferior myocardial infarction. *Am J Cardiol* 46:915-921, 1980

162. Gibelin P, Gilles B, Baudouy M, et al: Reciprocal ST segment changes in acute inferior myocardial infarction: clinical, haemodynamic and angiographic implications. *Eur Heart J* 7:133-139, 1986

163. Lembo NJ, Starling MR, Dell'Italia LJ, et al: Clinical and prognostic importance of persistent precordial (V_1-V_4) electrocardiographic ST segment depression in patients with inferior transmural myocardial infarction. *Circulation* 74:56-63, 1986

164. Ruddy TD, Yasuda T, Gold HK, et al: Anterior ST segment depression in acute inferior myocardial infarction as a marker of greater inferior, apical, and posterolateral damage. *Am Heart J* 112:1210-1216, 1986

165. Mukharji J, Murray S, Lewis SE, et al: Is anterior ST depression with acute transmural inferior infarction due to posterior infarction? A vectorcardiographic and scintigraphic study. *J Am Coll Cardiol* 4:28-34, 1984

166. Gibson RS, Crampton RS, Watson DD, et al: Precordial ST-segment depression during acute inferior myocardial infarction: clinical, scintigraphic, and angiographic correlations. *Circulation* 66:732-741, 1982

167. Salcedo JR, Baird MG, Chambers RJ, et al: Significance of reciprocal S-T segment depression in anterior precordial leads in acute inferior myocardial infarction: concomitant left anterior descending coronary artery disease? *Am J Cardiol* 48:1003-1008, 1981

168. Nasmith J, Marpole D, Rahal D, et al: Clinical outcomes after inferior myocardial infarction. *Ann Intern Med* 96:22-26, 1982

169. Lew AS, Maddahi J, Shah PK, et al: Factors that determine the direction and magnitude of precordial ST-segment deviations during inferior wall acute myocardial infarction. *Am J Cardiol* 55:883-888, 1985

170. Haraphongse M, Tanomsup S, Jugdutt BI: Inferior ST segment depression during acute anterior myocardial infarction: clinical and angiographic correlations. *J Am Coll Cardiol* 4:467-476, 1984

171. Quyyumi AA, Crake T, Rubens MB, et al: Importance of "reciprocal" electrocardiographic changes during occlusion of left anterior descending coronary artery. Studies during percutaneous transluminal coronary angioplasty. *Lancet* 1:347-350, 1986

172. Lew AS, Hod H, Cercek B, et al: Inferior ST segment changes during acute anterior myocardial infarction: a marker of the presence or absence of concomitant inferior wall ischemia. *J Am Coll Cardiol* 10:519-526, 1987

173. Sapin PM, Musselman DR, Dehmer GJ, et al: Implications of inferior ST-segment elevation accompanying anterior wall acute myocardial infarction for the angiographic morphology of the left anterior descending coronary artery morphology and site of occlusion. *Am J Cardiol* 69:860-865, 1992

174. Muller JE, Maroko PR, Braunwald E: Precordial electrocardiographic mapping, a technique to assess the efficacy of interventions designed to limit infarct size. *Circulation* 57:1-18, 1978

175. v. Essen R, Merx W, Doerr R, et al: QRS mapping in the evaluation of acute anterior myocardial infarction. *Circulation* 62:266-276, 1980

176. Wagner GS, Freye CJ, Palmeri ST, et al: Evaluation of a QRS scoring system for estimating myocardial infarct size. I. Specificity and observer agreement. *Circulation* 65:342-347, 1982

177. Palmeri ST, Harrison DG, Cobb FR, et al: A QRS scoring system for assessing left ventricular function after myocardial infarction. *N Engl J Med* 306:4-9, 1982

178. Eisen HJ, Barzilai B, Jaffe AS, et al: Relationship of QRS scoring system to enzymatic and pathologic infarct size: the role of infarct location. *Am Heart J* 115:993-1001, 1988
179. Hindman N, Grande P, Harrell FE Jr, et al: Relation between electrocardiographic and enzymatic methods of estimating acute myocardial infarct size. *Am J Cardiol* 58:31-35, 1986
180. Christian TF, Clements IP, Behrenbeck T, et al: Limitations of the electrocardiogram in estimating infarction size after acute reperfusion therapy for myocardial infarction. *Ann Intern Med* 114:264-270, 1991
181. Eastham RD, Morgan EH: Plasma-fibrinogen levels in coronary-artery disease. *Lancet* 2:1196-1197, 1963
182. de Beer FC, Hind CRK, Fox KM, et al: Measurement of serum C-reactive protein concentration in myocardial ischaemia and infarction. *Br Heart J* 47:239-243, 1982
183. Voulgari F, Cummins P, Gardecki TIM, et al: Serum levels of acute phase and cardiac proteins after myocardial infarction, surgery, and infection. *Br Heart J* 48:352-356, 1982
184. Thomson SP, Gibbons RJ, Smars PA, et al: Incremental value of the leukocyte differential and the rapid creatine kinase-MB isoenzyme for the early diagnosis of myocardial infarction. *Ann Intern Med* 122:335-341, 1995
185. LaDue JS, Wróblewski F, Karmen A: Serum glutamic oxaloacetic transaminase activity in human acute transmural myocardial infarction. *Science* 120:497-499, 1954
186. Sobel BE, Roberts R, Larson KB: Considerations in the use of biochemical markers of ischemic injury. *Circ Res* 38 Suppl 1:99-108, 1976
187. Beahrs MM, Chesebro JH, Markowitz H, et al: Does transient myocardial ischemia affect the serum levels of creatine kinase MB and myoglobulin measured by radioimmunoassay? (abstract) *Clin Res* 30:172A, 1982
188. Hearse DJ: Myocardial enzyme leakage. *J Mol Med* 2:185-200, 1977
189. Pasyk S, Bloor CM, Khouri EM, et al: Systemic and coronary effects of coronary artery occlusion in the unanesthetized dog. *Am J Physiol* 220:646-654, 1971
190. Jennings RB, Kaltenbach JP, Smetters GW: Enzymatic changes in acute myocardial ischemic injury. *Arch Pathol* 64:10-16, 1957
191. Shell WE, Kjekshus JK, Sobel BE: Quantitative assessment of the extent of myocardial infarction in the conscious dog by means of analysis of serial changes in serum creatine phosphokinase activity. *J Clin Invest* 50:2614-2625, 1971
192. Agress CM, Kin JHC: Evaluation of enzyme tests in the diagnosis of heart disease. *Am J Cardiol* 6:641-649, 1960
193. Sobel BE, Shell WE: Serum enzyme determinations in the diagnosis and assessment of myocardial infarction. *Circulation* 45:471-482, 1972
194. Karliner JS, Gander MP, Sobel BE: Elevated serum glyceraldehyde phosphate dehydrogenase activity following acute myocardial infarction. *Chest* 60:318-323, 1971
195. Vasudevan G, Mercer DW, Varat MA: Lactic hydrogenase isoenzyme determination in the diagnosis of acute myocardial infarction. *Circulation* 57:1055-1057, 1978
196. Irvin RG, Cobb FR, Roe CR: Acute myocardial infarction and MB creatine phosphokinase: relationship between onset of symptoms of infarction and appearance and disappearance of enzyme. *Arch Intern Med* 140:329-334, 1980
197. Smith AF: Diagnostic value of serum-creatine-kinase in a coronary-care unit. *Lancet* 2:178-182, 1967
198. Goldberg DM, Winfield DA: Diagnostic accuracy of serum enzyme assays for myocardial infarction in a general hospital population. *Br Heart J* 34:597-604, 1972
199. Roberts R, Sobel BE: Isoenzymes of creatine phosphokinase and diagnosis of myocardial infarction (editorial). *Ann Intern Med* 79:741-743, 1973
200. Smith AF: Separation of tissue and serum creatine kinase isoenzymes on polyacrylamide gel slabs. *Clin Chim Acta* 39:351-359, 1972
201. Homburger HA, Jacob GL: Creatine kinase radioimmunoassay and isoenzyme electrophoresis compared in the diagnosis of acute myocardial infarction. *Clin Chem* 26:861-866, 1980
202. Navin TR, Hager WD: Creatine kinase MB isoenzyme in the evaluation of myocardial infarction. *Curr Probl Cardiol* 3:1-32, 1979
203. Roberts R, Henry PD, Sobel BE: An improved basis for enzymatic estimation of infarct size. *Circulation* 52:743-754, 1975
204. Ehsani A, Ewy GA, Sobel BE: Effects of electrical countershock on serum creatine phosphokinase (CPK) isoenzyme activity. *Am J Cardiol* 37:12-18, 1976
205. Lindsey D, Navin TR, Finley PR: Transient elevation of serum activity of MB isoenzyme of creatine phosphokinase in drivers involved in automobile accidents. *Chest* 74:15-18, 1978
206. De Leiris J, Breton D, Feuvray D, et al: Lacticodehydrogenase release from perfused rat heart under the effect of abnormal media. *Arch Int Physiol Biochim* 77:749-762, 1969
207. Carlson CJ, Emilson B, Rapaport E: Serum MB-creatine phosphokinase isoenzyme in hypothermia (abstract). *Clin Res* 25:212A, 1977
208. Oldham HN Jr, Roe CR, Young WG Jr, et al: Intraoperative detection of myocardial damage during coronary artery surgery by plasma creatine phosphokinase isoenzyme analysis. *Surgery* 74:917-924, 1973
209. Ahmed SA, Williamson JE, Roberts R, et al: The association of increased plasma MB CPK activity and irreversible ischemic myocardial injury in the dog. *Circulation* 54:187-193, 1976
210. Geft IL, Fishbein MC, Ninomiya K, et al: Intermittent brief periods of ischemia have a cumulative effect and may cause myocardial necrosis. *Circulation* 66:1150-1153, 1982
211. Oh JK, Shub C, Ilstrup DM, et al: Creatine kinase release after successful percutaneous transluminal coronary angioplasty. *Am Heart J* 109:1225-1231, 1985
212. Varat MA, Mercer DW: Cardiac specific creatine phosphokinase isoenzyme in the diagnosis of acute myocardial infarction. *Circulation* 51:855-859, 1975
213. Smith AF, Radford D, Wong CP, et al: Creatine kinase MB isoenzyme studies in diagnosis of myocardial infarction. *Br Heart J* 38:225-232, 1976
214. Chiong MA, West R, Parker JO: Myocardial balance of inorganic phosphate and enzymes in man: effects of tachycardia and ischemia. *Circulation* 49:283-290, 1974
215. Alvira MM, Forman DT: Biochemical abnormalities in Reye's syndrome. *Ann Clin Lab Sci* 4:477-483, 1974
216. Roe CR, Schonberger LB, Gelbach SH, et al: Enzymatic alterations in Reye's syndrome: prognostic implications. *Pediatrics* 55:119-126, 1975
217. Goto I, Nagamine M, Katsuki S: Creatine phosphokinase isozymes in muscles: human fetus and patients. *Arch Neurol* 20:422-429, 1969
218. McNeely MDD, Berris B, Papsin FR, et al: Creatine kinase and its isoenzymes in the serum of women during pregnancy and the peripartum period. *Clin Chem* 23:1878-1880, 1977
219. Laboda HM, Britton VJ: Creatine kinase isoenzyme activity in human placenta and in serum of women in labor. *Clin Chem* 23:1329-1332, 1977
220. Bayer PM, Gabl F, Gergely T, et al: Isoenzyme der Creatinkinase in der Perinatalperiode. *J Clin Chem Clin Biochem* 15:349-352, 1977
221. Roberts R, Sobel BE, Parker CW: Radioimmunoassay of creatine kinase isoenzymes. *Science* 194:855-857, 1976
222. Rothkopf M, Boerner J, Stone MJ, et al: Detection of myocardial infarct extension by CK-B radioimmunoassay. *Circulation* 59:268-274, 1979
223. Mercer DW: Frequent appearance of creatine kinase isoenzyme BB in sera of critical-care patients (letter to the editor). *Clin Chem* 23:611-612, 1977
224. Chuga DJ, Bachner P: Creatine kinase isoenzyme BB in the serum of renal-disease patients, distinct from an albumin-like artifact (letter to the editor). *Clin Chem* 24:1286, 1978
225. Feld RD, Witte DL: Presence of creatine kinase BB isoenzyme in some patients with prostatic carcinoma. *Clin Chem* 23:1930-1932, 1977
226. Silverman LM, Dermer GB, Zweig MH, et al: Creatine kinase BB: a new tumor-associated marker. *Clin Chem* 25:1432-1435, 1979
227. Bell RD, Rosenberg RN, Ting R, et al: Creatine kinase BB isoenzyme levels by radioimmunoassay in patients with neurological disease. *Ann Neurol* 3:52-59, 1978
228. Thompson RJ, Rubery ED, Jones HM: Radioimmunoassay of serum creatine kinase-BB as a tumour marker in breast cancer. *Lancet* 2:673-675, 1980
229. Fisher ML, Carliner NH, Becker LC, et al: Serum creatine kinase in the diagnosis of acute myocardial infarction: optimal sampling frequency. *JAMA* 249:393-394, 1983
230. Roberts R, Gowda KS, Ludbrook PA, et al: Specificity of elevated serum MB creatine phosphokinase activity in the diagnosis of acute myocardial infarction. *Am J Cardiol* 36:433-437, 1975

231. Grande P, Christiansen C, Pedersen A, et al: Optimal diagnosis in acute myocardial infarction: a cost-effectiveness study. *Circulation* 61:723-728, 1980

232. Wagner GS: Optimal use of serum enzyme levels in the diagnosis of acute myocardial infarction: the perspective in 1980. *Arch Intern Med* 140:317-319, 1980

233. Dillon MC, Calbreath DF, Dixon AM, et al: Diagnostic problem in acute myocardial infarction: CK-MB in the absence of abnormally elevated total creatine kinase levels. *Arch Intern Med* 142:33-38, 1982

234. Heller GV, Blaustein AS, Wei JY: Implications of increased myocardial isoenzyme level in the presence of normal serum creatine kinase activity. *Am J Cardiol* 51:24-27, 1983

235. Yasmineh WG, Hanson NQ: Electrophoresis on cellulose acetate and chromatography on DEAE-Sephadex A-50 compared in the estimation of creatine kinase isoenzymes. *Clin Chem* 21:381-386, 1975

236. Homburger HA, Wold L, Jacob GL, et al: Metastable creatine kinase MM and complexes of creatine kinase BB and immunoglobulin G, "atypical" isoenzymes with similar electrophoretic mobility. *Clin Chem* 26:78-83, 1980

237. Ong L, Reiser P, Coromilas J, et al: Left ventricular function and rapid release of creatine kinase MB in acute myocardial infarction: evidence for spontaneous reperfusion. *N Engl J Med* 309:1-6, 1983

238. Kloner RA, Parisi AF: Acute myocardial infarction: diagnostic and prognostic applications of two-dimensional echocardiography. *Circulation* 75:521-524, 1987

239. Oh JK, Miller FA, Shub C, et al: Evaluation of acute chest pain syndromes by two-dimensional echocardiography: its potential application in the selection of patients for acute reperfusion therapy. *Mayo Clin Proc* 62:59-66, 1987

240. Nishimura RA: The role of echocardiography in acute myocardial infarction. In *Acute Myocardial Infarction.* Edited by BJ Gersh, SH Rahimtoola. New York, Elsevier Science Publishing Company, 1991, pp 144-164

241. Kan G, Visser CA, Lie KI, et al: Measurement of left ventricular ejection fraction after acute myocardial infarction: a serial cross sectional echocardiographic study. *Br Heart J* 51:631-636, 1984

242. Reeder GS, Seward JB, Tajik AJ: The role of two-dimensional echocardiography in coronary artery disease: a critical appraisal. *Mayo Clin Proc* 57:247-258, 1982

243. Meltzer RS, Woythaler JN, Buda AJ, et al: Two-dimensional echocardiographic quantification of infarct size alteration by pharmacologic agents. *Am J Cardiol* 44:257-262, 1979

244. Horowitz RS, Morganroth J, Parrotto C, et al: Immediate diagnosis of acute myocardial infarction by two-dimensional echocardiography. *Circulation* 65:323-329, 1982

245. Heger JJ, Weyman AE, Wann LS, et al: Cross-sectional echocardiography in acute myocardial infarction: detection and localization of regional left ventricular asynergy. *Circulation* 60:531-538, 1979

246. D'Arcy B, Nanda NC: Two-dimensional echocardiographic features of right ventricular infarction. *Circulation* 65:167-173, 1982

247. Kisslo JA, Robertson D, Gilbert BW, et al: A comparison of real-time, two-dimensional echocardiography and cineangiography in detecting left ventricular asynergy. *Circulation* 55:134-141, 1977

248. Shiina A, Tajik AJ, Smith HC, et al: Prognostic significance of regional wall motion abnormality in patients with prior myocardial infarction: a prospective correlative study of two-dimensional echocardiography and angiography. *Mayo Clin Proc* 61:254-262, 1986

249. Weiss JL, Bulkley BH, Hutchins GM, et al: Two-dimensional echocardiographic recognition of myocardial injury in man: comparison with postmortem studies. *Circulation* 63:401-408, 1981

250. Van Reet RE, Quinones MA, Poliner LR, et al: Comparison of two-dimensional echocardiography with gated radionuclide ventriculography in the evaluation of global and regional left ventricular function in acute myocardial infarction. *J Am Coll Cardiol* 2:243-252, 1984

251. Freeman AP, Giles RW, Walsh WF, et al: Regional left ventricular wall motion assessment: comparison of two-dimensional echocardiography and radionuclide angiography with contrast angiography in healed myocardial infarction. *Am J Cardiol* 56:8-12, 1985

252. Sharkey SW, Asinger RW, Elsperger KJ, et al: Two-dimensional echocardiographic detection of left ventricular posterior wall motion abnormalities using an inferior angulation view. *Am J Cardiol* 58:704-709, 1986

253. Kumar A, Minagoe S, Chandraratna PAN: Two-dimensional echocardiographic demonstration of restoration of normal wall motion after acute myocardial infarction. *Am J Cardiol* 57:1232-1235, 1986

254. Isaacsohn JL, Earle MG, Kemper AJ, et al: Postmyocardial infarction pain and infarct extension in the coronary care unit: role of two-dimensional echocardiography. *J Am Coll Cardiol* 11:246-251, 1988

255. Oh JK, Shub C, Miller FA Jr, et al: Role of two-dimensional echocardiography in the emergency room. *Echocardiography* 2:217-226, 1985

256. Gibson RS, Bishop HL, Stamm RB, et al: Value of early two-dimensional echocardiography in patients with acute myocardial infarction. *Am J Cardiol* 49:1110-1119, 1982

257. Nishimura RA, Tajik AJ, Miller FA Jr, et al: Role of two-dimensional echocardiography in the prediction of in-hospital complications after acute myocardial infarction. *J Am Coll Cardiol* 4:1080-1087, 1984

258. Nishimura RA, Reeder GS, Miller FA Jr, et al: Prognostic value of predischarge two-dimensional echocardiogram after acute myocardial infarction: preliminary observations. *Am J Cardiol* 53:429-432, 1984

259. Eaton LW, Weiss JL, Bulkley BH, et al: Regional cardiac dilatation after acute myocardial infarction: recognition by two-dimensional echocardiography. *N Engl J Med* 300:57-62, 1979

260. Erlebacher JA, Weiss JL, Weisfeldt ML: Early dilation of the infarcted segment in acute transmural myocardial infarction: role of infarct expansion in acute left ventricular enlargement. *J Am Coll Cardiol* 4:201-208, 1984

261. Asinger RW, Mikell FL, Elsperger J, et al: Incidence of left ventricular thrombosis after acute transmural myocardial infarction: serial evaluation by two-dimensional echocardiography. *N Engl J Med* 305:297-302, 1981

262. Ezekowitz MD, Wilson DA, Smith ED, et al: Comparison of indium-111 platelet scintigraphy and two-dimensional echocardiography in the diagnosis of left ventricular thrombi. *N Engl J Med* 306:1509-1512, 1982

263. Stratton JR, Lighty GW Jr, Pearlman AS, et al: Detection of left ventricular thrombus by two-dimensional echocardiography: sensitivity, specificity, and causes of uncertainty. *Circulation* 66:156-166, 1982

264. Oh JK, Seward JB, Khandheria BK, et al: Transesophageal echocardiography in critically ill patients. *Am J Cardiol* 66:1492-1495, 1990

265. Kaul S, Glasheen W, Ruddy TD, et al: The importance of defining left ventricular area at risk in vivo during acute myocardial infarction: an experimental evaluation with myocardial contrast two-dimensional echocardiography. *Circulation* 75:1249-1260, 1987

266. Sabia PJ, Powers ER, Ragosta M, et al: An association between collateral blood flow and myocardial viability in patients with recent myocardial infarction. *N Engl J Med* 327:1825-1831, 1992

267. Chandraratna PAN, Ulene R, Nimalasuriya A, et al: Differentiation between acute and healed myocardial infarction by signal averaging and color encoding two-dimensional echocardiography. *Am J Cardiol* 56:381-384, 1985

268. Tak T, Rahimtoola SH, Chandraratna PAN: Ultrasonic tissue characterization in ischemic heart disease and acute myocardial infarction. In *Acute Myocardial Infarction.* Edited by BJ Gersh, SH Rahimtoola. New York, Elsevier Scientific Publishing Company, 1991, pp 165-175

269. Fitzgerald PJ, McDaniel MD, Rolett EL, et al: Two-dimensional ultrasonic tissue characterization: backscatter power, endocardial wall motion, and their phase relationship for normal, ischemic, and infarcted myocardium. *Circulation* 76:850-859, 1987

270. Applegate RJ, Dell'Italia LJ, Crawford MH: Usefulness of two-dimensional echocardiography during low-level exercise testing early after uncomplicated acute myocardial infarction. *Am J Cardiol* 60:10-14, 1987

271. Buja LM, Parkey RW, Bonte FJ, et al: Pathophysiology of "cold spot" and "hot spot" myocardial imaging agents used to detect ischemia or infarction. *Cardiovasc Clin 10,* No 2:105-123, 1979

272. Buja LM, Parkey RW, Dees JH, et al: Morphologic correlates of technetium-99m stannous pyrophosphate imaging of acute myocardial infarcts in dogs. *Circulation* 52:596-607, 1975

273. Buja LM, Tofe AJ, Kulkarni PV, et al: Sites and mechanisms of localization of technetium-99m phosphorus radiopharmaceuticals in acute myocardial infarcts and other tissues. *J Clin Invest* 60:724-740, 1977

274. Buja LM, Dees JH, Harling DF, et al: Analytical electron microscopic study of mitochondrial inclusions in canine myocardial infarcts. *J Histochem Cytochem* 24:508-516, 1976

275. Buja LM, Parkey RW, Stokely EM, et al: Pathophysiology of technetium-99m stannous pyrophosphate and thallium-201 scintigraphy

of acute myocardial infarcts in dogs. *J Clin Invest* 57:1508-1522, 1976

276. Dewanjee MK, Kahn PC: Mechanism of localization of ^{99m}Tc-labeled pyrophosphate and tetracycline in infarcted myocardium. *J Nucl Med* 17:639-646, 1976

277. Beller GA, Khaw BA, Haber E, et al: Localization of radiolabeled cardiac myosin-specific antibody in myocardial infarcts: comparison with technetium-99m stannous pyrophosphate. *Circulation* 55:74-78, 1977

278. Parkey RW, Buja LM, Kulkarni P, et al: Localization of a specific I-131 antibody to myoglobin in myocardial tissue and factors which influence myoglobin release from cardiac cells (abstract). *J Nucl Med* 18:611, 1977

279. Kramer RJ, Goldstein RE, Hirshfeld JW Jr, et al: Accumulation of gallium-67 in regions of acute myocardial infarction. *Am J Cardiol* 33:861-867, 1974

280. Weiss ES, Ahmed AS, Thakur ML, et al: Imaging of the inflammatory response in ischemic canine myocardium with ^{111}indium-labeled leukocytes. *Am J Cardiol* 40:195-199, 1977

281. Johnson LL, Seldin DW, Becker LC, et al: Antimyosin imaging in acute transmural myocardial infarctions: results of a multicenter clinical trial. *J Am Coll Cardiol* 13:27-35, 1989

282. Jain D, Lahiri A, Raftery EB: Immunoscintigraphy for detecting acute myocardial infarction without electrocardiographic changes. *BMJ* 300:151-153, 1990

283. Weich HF, Strauss HW, Pitt B: The extraction of thallium-201 by the myocardium. *Circulation* 56:188-191, 1977

284. Cohen LS, Elliott WC, Gorlin R: Measurement of myocardial blood flow using krypton 85. *Am J Physiol* 206:997-999, 1964

285. Cannon PJ, Dell RB, Dwyer EM Jr: Measurement of regional myocardial perfusion in man with ^{133}xenon and a scintillation camera. *J Clin Invest* 51:964-977, 1972

286. Zaret BL, Strauss HW, Martin ND, et al: Noninvasive regional myocardial perfusion with radioactive potassium: study of patients at rest, with exercise, and during angina pectoris. *N Engl J Med* 288:809-812, 1973

287. Romhilt DW, Adolph RJ, Sodd VJ, et al: Cesium-129 myocardial scintigraphy to detect myocardial infarction. *Circulation* 48:1242-1251, 1973

288. Martin ND, Zaret BL, McGowan RL, et al: Rubidium-81: a new myocardial scanning agent. *Radiology* 111:651-656, 1974

289. Yano Y, Cahoon JL, Budinger TF: A precision flow-controlled Rb-82 generator for bolus or constant-infusion studies of the heart and brain. *J Nucl Med* 22:1006-1010, 1981

290. Strauss HW, Harrison K, Langan JK, et al: Thallium-201 for myocardial imaging: relation of thallium-201 to regional myocardial perfusion. *Circulation* 51:641-645, 1975

291. Hamilton GW, Narahara KA, Yee H, et al: Myocardial imaging with thallium-201: effect of cardiac drugs on myocardial images and absolute tissue distribution. *J Nucl Med* 19:10-16, 1978

292. Wackers FJT, Sokole EB, Samson G, et al: Value and limitations of thallium-201 scintigraphy in the acute phase of myocardial infarction. *N Engl J Med* 295:1-5, 1976

293. Wackers FJT, Lie KI, Liem KL, et al: Thallium-201 scintigraphy in unstable angina pectoris. *Circulation* 57:738-742, 1978

294. Mueller TM, Marcus ML, Ehrhardt JC, et al: Limitations of thallium-201 myocardial perfusion scintigrams. *Circulation* 54:640-646, 1976

295. Wackers FJ, Lie KI, Sokole E, et al: Thallium-201 for localization of acute myocardial infarction in the presence of left bundle branch block: correlation between site of infarction and ECG changes (abstract). *Circulation* 52 Suppl 2:54, 1975

296. Zaret BL, Wackers FJ: Radionuclide methods for evaluating the results of thrombolytic therapy. *Circulation* 76 Suppl 2:8-17, 1987

297. Holman BL, Jones AG, Lister-James J, et al: A new Tc-99m-labeled myocardial imaging agent, hexakis (t-butylisonitrile)-technetium(I) [Tc-99m TBI]: initial experience in the human. *J Nucl Med* 25:1350-1355, 1984

298. Piwnica-Worms D, Kronauge JF, Chiu ML: Uptake and retention of hexakis (2-methoxyisobutyl isonitrile) technetium(I) in cultured chick myocardial cells. Mitochondrial and plasma membrane potential dependence. *Circulation* 82:1826-1838, 1990

299. Gibbons RJ, Verani MS, Behrenbeck T, et al: Feasibility of tomographic 99mTc-hexakis-2-methoxy-2-methylpropyl-isonitrile imaging for the assessment of myocardial area at risk and the effect of treatment in acute myocardial infarction. *Circulation* 80:1277-1286, 1989

300. Christian TF, Clements IP, Gibbons RJ: Noninvasive identification of myocardium at risk in patients with acute myocardial infarction and nondiagnostic electrocardiograms with technetium-99m-sestamibi. *Circulation* 83:1615-1620, 1991

301. O'Connor MK, Hammell T, Gibbons RJ: In vitro validation of a simple tomographic technique for estimation of percentage myocardium at risk using methoxyisobutyl isonitrile technetium 99m (sestamibi). *Eur J Nucl Med* 17:69-76, 1990

302. Gibbons RJ, Holmes DR, Reeder GS, et al: Immediate angioplasty compared with the administration of a thrombolytic agent followed by conservative treatment for myocardial infarction. *N Engl J Med* 328:685-691, 1993

303. Rigo P, Murray M, Strauss HW, et al: Left ventricular function in acute myocardial infarction evaluated by gated scintiphotography. *Circulation* 50:678-684, 1974

304. Rigo P, Murray M, Taylor DR, et al: Right ventricular dysfunction detected by gated scintiphotography in patients with acute inferior myocardial infarction. *Circulation* 52:268-274, 1975

305. Berger HJ, Gottschalk A, Zaret BL: Dual radionuclide study of acute myocardial infarction: comparison of thallium-201 and technetium-99m stannous pyrophosphate imaging in man. *Ann Intern Med* 88:145-154, 1978

306. Machulla H-J, Stöcklin G, Kupfernagel C, et al: Comparative evaluation of fatty acids labeled with C-11, Cl-34m, Br-77, and I-123 for metabolic studies of the myocardium: concise communication. *J Nucl Med* 19:298-302, 1978

307. Sobel BE, Weiss ES, Welch MJ, et al: Detection of remote myocardial infarction in patients with positron emission transaxial tomography and intravenous ^{11}C-palmitate. *Circulation* 55:853-857, 1977

308. Harper PV, Schwartz J, Beck RN, et al: Clinical myocardial imaging with nitrogen-13 ammonia. *Radiology* 108:613-617, 1973

309. Budinger TK, Yano Y, Derenzo SE, et al: Infarction sizing and myocardial perfusion measurements using rubidium-82 and positron emission tomography (abstract). *Am J Cardiol* 45:399, 1980

310. Phelps ME, Hoffman EJ, Coleman RE, et al: Tomographic images of blood pool and perfusion in brain and heart. *J Nucl Med* 17:603-612, 1976

311. Schelbert HR: Current status and prospects of new radionuclides and radiopharmaceuticals for cardiovascular medicine. Semin Nucl Med 17:145-181, 1987

312. Braunwald E, Kloner RA: The stunned myocardium: prolonged, postischemic ventricular dysfunction. *Circulation* 66:1146-1149, 1982

313. Bonow RO, Dilsizian V: Thallium-201 and technetium-99m-sestamibi for assessing viable myocardium (editorial). *J Nucl Med* 33:815-818, 1992

314. Kiat H, Berman DS, Maddahi J, et al: Late reversibility of tomographic myocardial thallium-201 defects: an accurate marker of myocardial viability. *J Am Coll Cardiol* 12:1456-1463, 1988

315. Smucker ML, Beller GA, Watson DD, et al: Left ventricular dysfunction in excess of the size of infarction: a possible management strategy. *Am Heart J* 115:749-753, 1988

316. Brunken R, Tillisch J, Schwaiger M, et al: Regional perfusion, glucose metabolism, and wall motion in patients with chronic electrocardiographic Q wave infarction: evidence for persistence of viable tissue in some infarct regions by positron emission tomography. *Circulation* 73:951-963, 1986

317. Council on Scientific Affairs. Report of the Magnetic Resonance Imaging Panel: Magnetic resonance imaging of the cardiovascular system: present state of the art and future potential. *JAMA* 259:253-259, 1988

318. McNamara MT, Higgins CB, Schechtmann N, et al: Detection and characterization of acute myocardial infarction in man with use of gated magnetic resonance. *Circulation* 71:717-724, 1985

319. Johnston DL, Thompson RC, Liu P, et al: Magnetic resonance imaging during acute myocardial infarction. *Am J Cardiol* 57:1059-1065, 1986

320. Akins WE, Hill JA, Klaus W, et al: Assessment of left ventricular wall thickness in healed myocardial infarction by magnetic resonance imaging. *Am J Cardiol* 59:24-28, 1987

321. Filipchuk NG, Peshock RM, Malloy CR, et al: Detection and localization of recent myocardial infarction by magnetic resonance imaging. *Am J Cardiol* 58:214-219, 1986

322. Higgins CB, Lanzer P, Stark D, et al: Imaging by nuclear magnetic resonance in patients with chronic ischemic heart disease. *Circulation* 69:523-531, 1984

323. Johnston DL, Wendt RE III, Mulvagh SL, et al: Characterization of acute myocardial infarction by magnetic resonance imaging. *Am J Cardiol* 69:1291-1295, 1992
324. Cannon PJ, Maudsley AA, Sadek KH, et al: Sodium nuclear magnetic resonance imaging of myocardial tissue of dogs after coronary artery occlusion and reperfusion. *J Am Coll Cardiol* 7:573-579, 1986
325. Feiring AJ, Rumberger JA, Reiter SJ, et al: Determination of left ventricular mass in dogs with rapid-acquisition cardiac computed tomographic scanning. *Circulation* 72:1355-1364, 1985
326. Reiter SJ, Rumberger JA, Feiring AJ, et al: Precision of measurements of right and left ventricular volume by cine computed tomography. *Circulation* 74:890-900, 1986
327. Feiring AJ, Rumberger JA, Reiter SJ, et al: Sectional and segmental variability of left ventricular function: experimental and clinical studies using ultrafast computed tomography. *J Am Coll Cardiol* 12:415-425, 1988
328. Behrenbeck T, Gersh BJ, Bell MR, et al: Characterization of post-infarct remodeling of the left ventricle using ultrafast computed tomography (abstract). *Clin Res* 37:244A, 1989
329. Stanford W, Rooholamini M, Rumberger J, et al: Evaluation of coronary bypass graft patency by ultrafast computed tomography. *J Thorac Imaging 3,* No. 2:52-55, 1988
330. Rumberger JA, Feiring AJ, Hiratzka LF, et al: Quantification of coronary artery bypass flow reserve in dogs using cine-computed tomography. *Circ Res* 61 Suppl 2:117-123, 1987
331. Rumberger JA, Feiring AJ, Lipton MJ, et al: Use of ultrafast computed tomography to quantitate regional myocardial perfusion: a preliminary report. *J Am Coll Cardiol* 9:59-69, 1987
332. American Heart Association 1987 Heart Facts. Dallas, American Heart Association Center, 1987
333. Honey GE, Truelove SC: Prognostic factors in myocardial infarction. *Lancet* 1:1209-1212, 1957
334. Kannel WB, Sorlie P, McNamara PM: Prognosis after initial myocardial infarction: the Framingham study. *Am J Cardiol* 44:53-59, 1979
335. de Vreede JJ, Gorgels AP, Verstraaten GM, et al: Did prognosis after acute myocardial infarction change during the past 30 years? A meta-analysis. *J Am Coll Cardiol* 18:698-706, 1991
336. McNeilly RH, Pemberton J: Duration of last attack in 998 fatal cases of coronary artery disease and its relation to possible cardiac resuscitation. *Br Med J* 3:139-142, 1968
337. Fulton M, Julian DG, Oliver MF: Sudden death and myocardial infarction. *Circulation* 40 Suppl 4:182-191, 1969
338. National Heart Foundation of Australia Coronary Thrombolysis Group: Coronary thrombolysis and myocardial salvage by tissue plasminogen activator given up to 4 hours after onset of myocardial infarction. *Lancet* 1:203-208, 1988
339. Meinertz T, Kasper W, Schumacher M, et al: The German multicenter trial of anisoylated plasminogen streptokinase activator complex versus heparin for acute myocardial infarction. *Am J Cardiol* 62:347-351, 1988
340. Gruppo Italiano per lo studio della Streptochinasi nell'infarto miocardico (GISSI): Long-term effects of intravenous thrombolysis in acute myocardial infarction: final report of the GISSI study. *Lancet* 2:871-874, 1987
341. Pell S, Fayerweather WE: Trends in the incidence of myocardial infarction and in associated mortality and morbidity in a large employed population, 1957-1983. *N Engl J Med* 312:1005-1011, 1985
342. Goldberg RJ, Gore JM, Alpert JS, et al: Recent changes in attack and survival rates of acute myocardial infarction (1975 through 1981): the Worcester Heart Attack Study. *JAMA* 255:2774-2779, 1986
343. Gomez-Marin O, Folsom AR, Kottke TE, et al: Improvement in long-term survival among patients hospitalized with acute myocardial infarction, 1970 to 1980: The Minnesota Heart Survey. *N Engl J Med* 316:1353-1359, 1987
344. Stewart AW, Fraser J, Norris RM, et al: Changes in severity of myocardial infarction and three year survival rates after myocardial infarction in Auckland, 1966-7 and 1981-2. *Br Med J* 297:517-519, 1988
345. AIMS Trial Study Group: Long-term effects of intravenous anistreplase in acute myocardial infarction: final report of the AIMS study. *Lancet* 335:427-431, 1990
346. Grines CL, Browne KF, Marco J, et al: A comparison of immediate angioplasty with thrombolytic therapy for acute myocardial infarction. *N Engl J Med* 328:673-679, 1993
347. Peel AAF, Semple T, Wang I, et al: A coronary prognostic index for grading the severity of infarction. *Br Heart J* 24:745-760, 1962
348. Norris RM, Brandt PWT, Caughey DE, et al: A new coronary prognostic index. *Lancet* 1:274-278, 1969
349. Hoit BD, Gilpin EA, Henning H, et al: Myocardial infarction in young patients: an analysis of age subsets. *Circulation* 74:712-721, 1986
350. Wenger NK: Coronary disease in women. *Ann Rev Med* 36:285-294, 1985
351. Fiebach NH, Viscoli CM, Horwitz RI: Differences between women and men in survival after myocardial infarction. Biology or methodology? *JAMA* 263:1092-1096, 1990
352. Greenland P, Reicher-Reiss H, Goldbourt U, et al: In-hospital and 1-year mortality in 1,524 women after myocardial infarction. Comparison with 4,315 men. *Circulation* 83:484-491, 1991
353. Cooper RS, Simmons B, Castaner A, et al: Survival rates and prehospital delay during myocardial infarction among black persons. *Am J Cardiol* 57:208-211, 1986
354. Roig E, Castaner A, Simmons B, et al: In-hospital mortality rates from acute myocardial infarction by race in U.S. hospitals: findings from the National Hospital Discharge Survey. *Circulation* 76:280-288, 1987
355. Castaner A, Simmons BE, Mar M, et al: Myocardial infarction among black patients: poor prognosis after hospital discharge. *Ann Intern Med* 109:33-35, 1988
356. Hagstrom RM, Billings FT Jr, Ball COT, et al: The risk of sudden death following myocardial infarction. *Arch Environ Health* 15:450-454, 1967
357. Juergens JL, Edward JE, Achor RWP, et al: Prognosis of patients surviving first clinically diagnosed myocardial infarction. *Arch Intern Med* 105:444-450, 1960
358. Helmers C: Assessment of 3-year prognosis in survivors of acute myocardial infarction. *Br Heart J* 37:593-597, 1975
359. Moss AJ, DeCamilla J, Engstrom F, et al: The posthospital phase of myocardial infarction: identification of patients with increased mortality risk. *Circulation* 49:460-466, 1974
360. Bigger JT Jr, Heller CA, Wenger TL, et al: Risk stratification after acute myocardial infarction. *Am J Cardiol* 42:202-210, 1978
361. Vedin A, Wilhelmsen L, Wedel H, et al: Prediction of cardiovascular deaths and non-fatal reinfarctions after myocardial infarction. *Acta Med Scand* 201:309-316, 1977
362. Ruberman W, Weinblatt E, Goldberg JD, et al: Psychosocial influences on mortality after myocardial infarction. *N Engl J Med* 311:552-559, 1984
363. Shekelle RB, Gale M, Norusis M, et al: Type A score (Jenkins Activity Survey) and risk of recurrent coronary heart disease in the aspirin myocardial infarction study. *Am J Cardiol* 56:221-225, 1985
364. Smith SC Jr, Gilpin E, Ahnve S, et al: Outlook after acute myocardial infarction in the very elderly compared with that in patients aged 65 to 75 years. *J Am Coll Cardiol* 16:784-792, 1990
365. Norris RM, Caughey DE, Mercer CJ, et al: Prognosis after myocardial infarction: six-year follow-up. *Br Heart J* 36:786-790, 1974
366. Weinberg SL: Natural history six years after acute myocardial infarction: is there a low-risk group? *Chest* 69:23-28, 1976
367. Luria MH, Knoke JD, Wachs JS, et al: Survival after recovery from acute myocardial infarction: two and five year prognostic indices. *Am J Med* 67:7-14, 1979
368. Weinblatt E, Shapiro S, Frank CW: Prognosis of women with newly diagnosed coronary heart disease: a comparison with course of disease among men. *Am J Public Health* 63:577-593, 1973
369. Pell S, D'Alonzo CA: Immediate mortality of five-year survival of employed men with a first myocardial infarction. *N Engl J Med* 270:915-922, 1964
370. Connolly DC, Elveback LR, Oxman HA: Coronary heart disease in residents of Rochester, Minnesota, 1950-1975. III. Effect of hypertension and its treatment on survival of patients with coronary artery disease. *Mayo Clin Proc* 58:249-254, 1983
371. Stone PH, Muller JE, Hartwell T, et al: The effect of diabetes mellitus on prognosis and serial left ventricular function after acute myocardial infarction: contribution of both coronary disease and diastolic left ventricular dysfunction to the adverse prognosis. *J Am Coll Cardiol* 14:49-57, 1989
372. Oswald GA, Corcoran S, Yudkin JS: Prevalence and risks of hyperglycaemia and undiagnosed diabetes in patients with acute myocardial infarction. *Lancet* 1:1264-1267, 1984
373. Wong ND, Wilson PW, Kannel WB: Serum cholesterol as a prognostic factor after myocardial infarction: the Framingham Study. *Ann Intern Med* 115:687-693, 1991
374. Norris RM, Bensley KE, Caughey DE, et al: Hospital mortality in acute myocardial infarction. *Br Med J* 3:143-146, 1968

375. Hoit BD, Gilpin EA, Maisel AA, et al: Influence of obesity on morbidity and mortality after acute myocardial infarction. *Am Heart J* 114:1334-1341, 1987

376. Wilhelmsson C, Vedin JA, Elmfeldt D, et al: Smoking and myocardial infarction. *Lancet* 1:415-419, 1975

377. Sparrow D, Dawber TR, Colton T: The influence of cigarette smoking on prognosis after a first myocardial infarction: a report from the Framingham Study. *J Chronic Dis* 31:425-432, 1978

378. Moss AJ: Factors influencing prognosis after myocardial infarction. *Curr Probl Cardiol* 4:1-53, 1979

379. Henning H, Gilpin EA, Covell JW, et al: Prognosis after acute myocardial infarction: a multivariate analysis of mortality and survival. *Circulation* 59:1124-1134, 1979

380. Hillis LD, Forman S, Braunwald E, et al: Risk stratification before thrombolytic therapy in patients with acute myocardial infarction. *J Am Coll Cardiol* 16:313-315, 1990

381. Cobb LA, Werner JA, Trobaugh GB: Sudden cardiac death. I. A decade's experience with out-of-hospital resuscitation. *Mod Concepts Cardiovasc Dis* 49:31-36, 1980

382. Pantridge JF, Adgey AAJ: The prehospital phase of acute myocardial infarction. In *Textbook of Coronary Care.* Edited by LE Meltzer, AJ Dunning. Philadelphia, Charles Press, 1972, pp 95-106

383. Mathey DG, Sheehan FH, Schofer J, et al: Time from onset of symptoms to thrombolytic therapy: a major determinant of myocardial salvage in patients with acute transmural infarction. *J Am Coll Cardiol* 6:518-525, 1985

384. Fine DG, Weiss AT, Sapoznikov D, et al: Importance of early initiation of intravenous streptokinase therapy for acute myocardial infarction. *Am J Cardiol* 58:411-417, 1986

385. O'Rourke RA: Clinical decisions for postmyocardial infarction patients. *Mod Concepts Cardiovasc Dis* 55:55-60, 1986

386. Geltman EM, Ehsani AA, Campbell MK, et al: The influence of location and extent of myocardial infarction on long-term ventricular dysrhythmia and mortality. *Circulation* 60:805-814, 1979

387. Rude RE, Parkey RW, Bonte FJ, et al: Clinical implications of the technetium-99m stannous pyrophosphate myocardial scintigraphic "doughnut" pattern in patients with acute myocardial infarcts. *Circulation* 59:721-730, 1979

388. Page DL, Caulfield JB, Kastor JA, et al: Myocardial changes associated with cardiogenic shock. *N Engl J Med* 285:133-137, 1971

389. Norris RM, Whitlock RML, Barratt-Boyes C, et al: Clinical measurement of myocardial infarct size: modification of a method for the estimation of total creatine phosphokinase release after myocardial infarction. *Circulation* 51:614-620, 1975

390. Roos JC, Dunning AJ: Right bundle-branch block and left axis deviation in acute myocardial infarction. *Br Heart J* 32:847-851, 1970

391. Strauss HD, Ambos HD, Sobel BE, et al: Relationships between the site of infarction, infarct size, and mortality (abstract). *Am J Cardiol* 41:361, 1978

392. Kitchin AH, Pocock SJ: Prognosis of patients with acute myocardial infarction admitted to a coronary care unit. I. Survival in hospital. *Br Heart J* 39:1163-1166, 1977

393. Norris RM, Caughey DE, Deeming LW, et al: Prognosis following acute myocardial infarction. *NZ Med J* 77:12-18, 1973

394. Rigo P, Murray M, Taylor DR, et al: Hemodynamic and prognostic findings in patients with transmural and nontransmural infarction. *Circulation* 51:1064-1070, 1975

395. Schulze RA Jr, Pitt B, Griffith LSC, et al: Coronary angiography and left ventriculography in survivors of transmural and nontransmural myocardial infarction. *Am J Med* 64:108-113, 1978

396. Thanavaro S, Krone RJ, Kleiger RE, et al: In-hospital prognosis of patients with first nontransmural and transmural infarctions. *Circulation* 61:29-33, 1980

397. Hutter AM Jr, DeSanctis RW, Flynn T, et al: Nontransmural myocardial infarction: a comparison of hospital and late clinical course of patients with that of matched patients with transmural anterior and transmural inferior myocardial infarction. *Am J Cardiol* 48:595-602, 1981

398. Szklo M, Goldberg R, Kennedy HL, et al: Survival of patients with nontransmural myocardial infarction: a population-based study. *Am J Cardiol* 42:648-652, 1978

399. Scheinman MM, Abbott JA: Clinical significance of transmural versus nontransmural electrocardiographic changes in patients with acute myocardial infarction. *Am J Med* 55:602-607, 1973

400. Cannom DS, Levy W, Cohen LS: The short- and long-term prognosis of patients with transmural and nontransmural myocardial infarction. Am J Med 61:452-458, 1976

401. Marmor A, Sobel BE, Roberts R: Factors presaging early recurrent myocardial infarction ("extension"). *Am J Cardiol* 48:603-610, 1981

402. Schechtman KB, Capone RJ, Kleiger RE, et al: Differential risk patterns associated with 3 month as compared with 3 to 12 month mortality and reinfarction after non-Q wave myocardial infarction. *J Am Coll Cardiol* 15:940-947, 1990

403. Gibson RS, Beller GA, Gheorghiade M, et al: The prevalence and clinical significance of residual myocardial ischemia 2 weeks after uncomplicated non-Q wave infarction: a prospective natural history study. *Circulation* 73:1186-1198, 1986

404. Madigan NP, Rutherford BD, Frye RL: The clinical course, early prognosis, and coronary anatomy of subendocardial infarction. *Am J Med* 60:634-641, 1976

405. Théroux P, Kouz S, Bosch X, et al: Clinical and angiographic features of non-Q wave and Q wave myocardial infarction (MI) (abstract). *Circulation* 74 Suppl 2:203, 1986

406. DeWood MA, Stifter WF, Simpson CS, et al: Coronary arteriographic findings soon after non-Q-wave myocardial infarction. *N Engl J Med* 315:417-423, 1986

407. Gibson RS, Boden WE, Théroux P, et al: Diltiazem and reinfarction in patients with non-Q-wave myocardial infarction: results of a double-blind, randomized, multicenter trial. *N Engl J Med* 315:423-429, 1986

408. β-Blocker Heart Attack Trial Research Group: A randomized trial of propranolol in patients with acute myocardial infarction. I. Mortality results. JAMA 247:1707-1714, 1982

409. The MIAMI Trial Research Group: Mortality. *Am J Cardiol* 56:15G-22G, 1985

410. Klimt CR, Knatterud GL, Stamler J, et al: Persantin-aspirin reinfarction study. Part II. Secondary coronary prevention with Persantin and aspirin. *J Am Coll Cardiol* 7:251-268, 1986

411. Forrester JS, Diamond G, Chatterjee K, et al: Medical therapy of acute myocardial infarction by application of hemodynamic subsets (second of two parts). *N Engl J Med* 295:1404-1413, 1976

412. Schulze RA Jr, Strauss HW, Pitt B: Sudden death in the year following myocardial infarction: relation to ventricular premature contractions in the late hospital phase and left ventricular ejection fraction. *Am J Med* 62:192-199, 1977

413. Humphries JON, Taylor GJ, Mellits ED, et al: Predictors of clinical course after survival of myocardial infarction. *Trans Am Clin Climatol Assoc* 91:128-134, 1979

414. Killip T III, Kimball JT: Treatment of myocardial infarction in a coronary care unit: a two year experience with 250 patients. *Am J Cardiol* 20:457-464, 1967

415. Luria MH, Knoke JD, Margolis RM, et al: Acute myocardial infarction: prognosis and recovery. *Ann Intern Med* 85:561-565, 1976

416. Peel AAF, Semple T: Immediate prognosis in acute myocardial infarction. In *Textbook of Coronary Care.* Edited by LE Meltzer, AJ Dunning. Philadelphia, Charles Press, 1972, pp 152-172

417. Clemmensen P, Bates ER, Califf RM, et al: Complete atrioventricular block complicating inferior wall acute myocardial infarction treated with reperfusion therapy. *Am J Cardiol* 67:225-230, 1991

418. McNamee BT, Robinson TJ, Adgey AAJ, et al: Long-term prognosis following ventricular fibrillation in acute ischaemic heart disease. *Br Med J* 4:204-206, 1970

419. Stannard M, Sloman G: Ventricular fibrillation in acute myocardial infarction: prognosis following successful resuscitation. *Am Heart J* 77:573, 1969

420. Lawrie DM: Long-term survival after ventricular fibrillation complicating acute myocardial infarction. *Lancet* 2:1085-1087, 1969

421. Tofler GH, Stone PH, Muller JE, et al: Prognosis after cardiac arrest due to ventricular tachycardia or ventricular fibrillation associated with acute myocardial infarction (the MILIS Study). *Am J Cardiol* 60:755-760, 1987

422. Behar S, Goldbourt U, Reicher-Reiss H, et al: Prognosis of acute myocardial infarction complicated by primary ventricular fibrillation. *Am J Cardiol* 66:1208-1211, 1990

423. De Soyza N, Bennett FA, Murphy ML, et al: The relationship of paroxysmal ventricular tachycardia complicating the acute phase and ventricular arrhythmia during the late hospital phase of myocardial infarction to long-term survival. *Am J Med* 64:377-381, 1978

424. Lie KI, Liem KL, Durrer D: Management in hospital of ventricular fibrillation complicating acute myocardial infarction. *Br Heart J* 40 Suppl:78-82, 1978

425. Coronary Drug Project Research Group: The prognostic importance of the electrocardiogram after myocardial infarction: experience in the Coronary Drug Project. *Ann Intern Med* 77:677-689, 1972

426. Coronary Drug Project Research Group: Left ventricular hypertrophy patterns and prognosis: experience postinfarction in the Coronary Drug Project. *Circulation* 49:862-868, 1974

427. Waugh RA, Wagner GS, Haney TL, et al: Immediate and remote prognostic significance of fascicular block during acute myocardial infarction. *Circulation* 47:765-775, 1973

428. Ricou F, Nicod P, Gilpin E, et al: Influence of right bundle branch block on short- and long-term survival after acute anterior myocardial infarction. *J Am Coll Cardiol* 17:858-863, 1991

429. Schwartz PJ, Wolf S: QT interval prolongation as predictor of sudden death in patients with myocardial infarction. *Circulation* 57:1074-1077, 1978

430. Wheelan K, Mukharji J, Rude RE, et al: Sudden death and its relation to QT-interval prolongation after acute myocardial infarction: two-year follow-up. *Am J Cardiol* 57:745-750, 1986

431. Moss AJ, Schnitzler R, Green R, et al: Ventricular arrhythmias three weeks after acute myocardial infarction. *Ann Intern Med* 75:837-841, 1971

432. Vismara LA, DeMaria AN, Hughes JL, et al: Evaluation of arrhythmias in the late hospital phase of acute myocardial infarction compared to coronary care unit ectopy. *Br Heart J* 37:598-603, 1975

433. Coronary Drug Project Research Group: Prognostic importance of premature beats following myocardial infarction: experience in the Coronary Drug Project. *JAMA* 223:1116-1124, 1973

434. Vismara LA, Amsterdam EA, Mason DT: Relation of ventricular arrhythmias in the late hospital phase of acute myocardial infarction to sudden death after hospital discharge. *Am J Med* 59:6-12, 1975

435. Luria MH, Debanne SM, Osman MI: Long-term follow-up after recovery from acute myocardial infarction: observations on survival, ventricular arrhythmias, and sudden death. *Arch Intern Med* 145:1592-1595, 1985

436. Ruberman W, Weinblatt E, Goldberg JD, et al: Ventricular premature beats and mortality after myocardial infarction. *N Engl J Med* 297:750-757, 1977

437. Connolly SJ, Cairns JA, CAMIAT Pilot Study Group, et al: Comparison of one-, six-, and 24-hour ambulatory electrocardiographic monitoring for ventricular arrhythmia as a predictor of mortality in survivors of acute myocardial infarction. *Am J Cardiol* 69:308-313, 1992

438. Moss AJ, Davis HT, DeCamilla J, et al: Ventricular ectopic beats and their relation to sudden and nonsudden cardiac death after myocardial infarction. *Circulation* 60:998-1003, 1979

439. Moss AJ, DeCamilla JJ, Davis HP, et al: Clinical significance of ventricular ectopic beats in the early posthospital phase of myocardial infarction. *Am J Cardiol* 39:635-640, 1977

440. Rehnqvist N: Ventricular arrhythmias after an acute myocardial infarction: prognostic weight and natural history. *Eur J Cardiol* 7:169-187, 1978

441. Ruberman W, Weinblatt E, Goldberg JD, et al: Ventricular premature complexes and sudden death after myocardial infarction. *Circulation* 64:297-305, 1981

442. Anderson KP, DeCamilla J, Moss AJ: Clinical significance of ventricular tachycardia (three beats or longer) detected during ambulatory monitoring after myocardial infarction. *Circulation* 57:890-897, 1978

443. Kleiger RE, Miller JP, Thanavaro S, et al: Relationship between clinical features of acute myocardial infarction and ventricular runs two weeks to one year after infarction. *Circulation* 63:64-70, 1981

444. Bigger JT Jr, Weld FM, Rolnitzky LM: Prevalence, characteristics, and significance of ventricular tachycardia (three or more complexes) detected with ambulatory electrocardiographic recording in the late hospital phase of acute myocardial infarction. *Am J Cardiol* 48:815-823, 1981

445. Moss AJ, DeCamilla J, Mietlowski W, et al: Prognostic grading and significance of ventricular premature beats after recovery from myocardial infarction. *Circulation* 52 Suppl 3:204-210, 1975

446. Schulze RA Jr, Rouleau J, Rigo P, et al: Ventricular arrhythmias in the late hospital phase of acute myocardial infarction: relation to left ventricular function detected by gated cardiac blood pool scanning. *Circulation* 52:1006-1011, 1975

447. Bigger JT, Fleiss JL, Kleiger R, et al: The relationships among ventricular arrhythmias, left ventricular dysfunction, and mortality in the two years after myocardial infarction. *Circulation* 69:250-258, 1984

448. Kostis JB, Byington R, Friedman LM, et al: Prognostic significance of ventricular ectopic activity in survivors of acute myocardial infarction. *J Am Coll Cardiol* 10:231-242, 1987

449. Olson HG, Lyons KP, Troop P, et al: Prognostic implications of complicated ventricular arrhythmias early after hospital discharge in acute myocardial infarction: a serial ambulatory electrocardiography study. *Am Heart J* 108:1221-1228, 1984

450. The Multicenter Postinfarction Research Group: Risk stratification and survival after myocardial infarction. *N Engl J Med* 309:331-336, 1983

451. Greene HL, Reid PR, Schaeffer AH: The repetitive ventricular response in man: a predictor of sudden death. *N Engl J Med* 299:729-734, 1978

452. Petretta M, Bonaduce D, Bianchi V, et al: Characterization and prognostic significance of silent myocardial ischemia on predischarge electrocardiographic monitoring in unselected patients with myocardial infarction. *Am J Cardiol* 69:579-583, 1992

453. Currie P, Ashby D, Saltissi S: Prognostic significance of transient myocardial ischemia on ambulatory monitoring after acute myocardial infarction. *Am J Cardiol* 71:773-777, 1993

454. Kleiger RE, Miller JP, Bigger JT Jr, et al: Decreased heart rate variability and its association with increased mortality after acute myocardial infarction. *Am J Cardiol* 59:256-262, 1987

455. Farrell TG, Bashir Y, Cripps T, et al: Risk stratification for arrhythmic events in postinfarction patients based on heart rate variability, ambulatory electrocardiographic variables and the signal-averaged electrocardiogram. *J Am Coll Cardiol* 18:687-697, 1991

456. Roy D, Marchand E, Théroux P, et al: Programmed ventricular stimulation in survivors of an acute myocardial infarction. *Circulation* 72:487-494, 1985

457. Bhandari AK, Rose JS, Kotlewski A, et al: Frequency and significance of induced sustained ventricular tachycardia or fibrillation two weeks after acute myocardial infarction. *Am J Cardiol* 56:737-742, 1985

458. Santarelli P, Bellocci F, Loperfido F, et al: Ventricular arrhythmia induced by programmed ventricular stimulation after acute myocardial infarction. *Am J Cardiol* 55:391-394, 1985

459. Kuck K-H, Costard A, Schlüter M, et al: Significance of timing programmed electrical stimulation after acute myocardial infarction. *J Am Coll Cardiol* 8:1279-1288, 1986

460. Nestico PF, Hakki A-H, Felsher J, et al: Implications of abnormal right ventricular thallium uptake in acute myocardial infarction. *Am J Cardiol* 58:230-234, 1986

461. Roy D, Marchand E, Théroux P, et al: Long-term reproducibility and significance of provokable ventricular arrhythmias after myocardial infarction. *J Am Coll Cardiol* 8:32-39, 1986

462. Zehender M, Brugada P, Geibel A, et al: Programmed electrical stimulation in healed myocardial infarction using a standardized ventricular stimulation protocol. *Am J Cardiol* 59:578-585, 1987

463. Bhandari AK, Hong R, Kotlewski A, et al: Prognostic significance of programmed ventricular stimulation in survivors of acute myocardial infarction. *Br Heart J* 61:410-416, 1989

464. Denniss AR, Richards DA, Cody DV, et al: Prognostic significance of ventricular tachycardia and fibrillation induced at programmed stimulation and delayed potentials detected on the signal-averaged electrocardiograms of survivors of acute myocardial infarction. *Circulation* 74:731-745, 1986

465. Kuchar DL, Thorburn CW, Sammel NL: Late potentials detected after myocardial infarction: natural history and prognostic significance. *Circulation* 74:1280-1289, 1986

466. Gomes JA, Winters SL, Stewart D, et al: A new noninvasive index to predict sustained ventricular tachycardia and sudden death in the first year after myocardial infarction: based on the signal-averaged electrocardiogram, radionuclide ejection fraction and Holter monitoring. *J Am Coll Cardiol* 10:349-357, 1987

467. Kuchar DL, Thorburn CW, Sammel NL: Prediction of serious arrhythmic events after myocardial infarction: signal-averaged electrocardiogram, Holter monitoring and radionuclide ventriculography. *J Am Coll Cardiol* 9:531-538, 1987

468. Miller DH, Borer JS: Exercise testing early after myocardial infarction: risks and benefits. *Am J Med* 72:427-438, 1982

469. Juneau M, Colles P, Theroux P, et al: Symptom-limited versus low level exercise testing before hospital discharge after myocardial infarction. *J Am Coll Cardiol* 20:927-933, 1992

470. Ericsson M, Granath A, Ohlsén P, et al: Arrhythmias and symptoms during treadmill testing three weeks after myocardial infarction in 100 patients. *Br Heart J* 35:787-790, 1973

471. Smith JW, Dennis CA, Gassmann A, et al: Exercise testing three weeks after myocardial infarction. *Chest* 75:12-16, 1979

472. Jelinek MV, Lown B: Exercise stress testing for exposure of cardiac arrhythmia. *Prog Cardiovasc Dis* 16:497-522, 1974

473. Blackburn H, Taylor HL, Hamrell B, et al: Premature ventricular complexes induced by stress testing: their frequency and response to physical conditioning. *Am J Cardiol* 31:441-449, 1973

474. Borer JS, Rosing DR, Miller RH, et al: Natural history of left ventricular function during one year after acute myocardial infarction: comparison with clinical, electrocardiographic, and biochemical determinations. *Am J Cardiol* 46:1-12, 1980

475. DeBusk RF, Davidson DM, Houston N, et al: Serial ambulatory electrocardiography and treadmill exercise testing after uncomplicated myocardial infarction. *Am J Cardiol* 45:547-554, 1980

476. Ryan M, Lown B, Horn H: Comparison of ventricular ectopic activity during 24-hour monitoring and exercise testing in patients with coronary artery disease. *N Engl J Med* 292:224-229, 1975

477. Crawford M, O'Rourke RA, Ramakrishna N, et al: Comparative effectiveness of exercise testing and continuous monitoring for detecting arrhythmias in patients with previous myocardial infarction. *Circulation* 50:301-305, 1974

478. Markiewicz W, Houston N, DeBusk RF: Exercise testing soon after myocardial infarction. *Circulation* 56:26-31, 1977

479. Henry RL, Kennedy GT, Crawford MH: Prognostic value of exercise-induced ventricular ectopic activity for mortality after acute myocardial infarction. *Am J Cardiol* 59:1251-1255, 1987

480. Théroux P, Waters DD, Halphen C, et al: Prognostic value of exercise testing soon after myocardial infarction. *N Engl J Med* 301:341-345, 1979

481. Davidson DM, DeBusk RF: Prognostic value of a single exercise test three weeks after uncomplicated myocardial infarction. *Circulation* 61:236-242, 1980

482. Koppes GM, Kruyer W, Beckmann CH, et al: Response to exercise early after uncomplicated acute myocardial infarction in patients receiving no medication: long-term follow-up. *Am J Cardiol* 46:764-769, 1980

483. Granath A, Södermark T, Winge T, et al: Early work load tests for evaluation of long-term prognosis of acute myocardial infarction. *Br Heart J* 39:758-763, 1977

484. Bigger JT Jr, Dresdale RJ, Heissenbuttel RH, et al: Ventricular arrhythmias in ischemic heart disease: mechanism, prevalence, significance, and management. *Prog Cardiovasc Dis* 19:255-300, 1977

485. Krone RJ, Miller JP, Gillespie JA, et al: Usefulness of low-level exercise testing early after acute myocardial infarction in patients taking beta-blocking agents. *Am J Cardiol* 60:23-27, 1987

486. Fioretti P, Brower RW, Simoons ML, et al: Prediction of mortality during the first year after acute myocardial infarction from clinical variables and stress test at hospital discharge. *Am J Cardiol* 55:1313-1318, 1985

487. Krone RJ, Gillespie JA, Weld FM, et al: Low-level exercise testing after myocardial infarction: usefulness in enhancing clinical risk stratification. *Circulation* 71:80-89, 1985

488. Morris KG, Palmeri ST, Califf R, et al: Value of radionuclide angiography for predicting specific cardiac events after acute myocardial infarction. *Am J Cardiol* 55:318-324, 1985

489. Murray DP, Salih M, Tan LB, et al: Prognostic stratification of patients after myocardial infarction. *Br Heart J* 57:313-318, 1987

490. Handler CE: Submaximal predischarge exercise testing after myocardial infarction: prognostic value and limitations. *Eur Heart J* 6:510-517, 1985

491. Madsen EB, Gilpin E, Ahnve S, et al: Prediction of functional capacity and use of exercise testing for predicting risk after acute myocardial infarction. *Am J Cardiol* 56:839-845, 1985

492. Waters DD, Bosch X, Bouchard A, et al: Comparison of clinical variables and variables derived from a limited predischarge exercise test as predictors of early and late mortality after myocardial infarction. *J Am Coll Cardiol* 5:1-8, 1985

493. Dillahunt PH II, Miller AB: Early treadmill testing after myocardial infarction: angiographic and hemodynamic correlations. *Chest* 76:150-155, 1979

494. Fuller CM, Raizner AE, Verani MS, et al: Early post-myocardial infarction treadmill stress testing: an accurate predictor of multi-vessel coronary disease and subsequent cardiac events. *Ann Intern Med* 94:734-739, 1981

495. Schwartz KM, Turner JD, Sheffield LT, et al: Limited exercise testing soon after myocardial infarction: correlation with early coronary and left ventricular angiography. *Ann Intern Med* 94:727-734, 1981

496. Sia STB, MacDonald PS, Horowitz JD, et al: Usefulness of early exercise testing after non-Q-wave myocardial infarction in predicting prognosis. *Am J Cardiol* 57:738-744, 1986

497. Sami M, Kraemer H, DeBusk RF: The prognostic significance of serial exercise testing after myocardial infarction. *Circulation* 60:1238-1246, 1979

498. DeBusk RF, Haskell W: Symptom-limited vs heart-rate-limited exercise testing soon after myocardial infarction. *Circulation* 61:738-743, 1980

499. Saunamaki KI, Andersen JD: Clinical significance of the ST-segment response and other early exercise test variables in uncomplicated vs complicated myocardial infarction. *Eur Heart J* 8:603-610, 1987

500. Langer A, Minkowitz J, Dorian P, et al: Pathophysiology and prognostic significance of Holter-detected ST segment depression after myocardial infarction. *J Am Coll Cardiol* 20:1313-1317, 1992

501. Battler A, Slutsky R, Karliner J, et al: Left ventricular ejection fraction and first third ejection fraction early after acute myocardial infarction: value for predicting mortality and morbidity. *Am J Cardiol* 45:197-202, 1980

502. Shah PK, Pichler M, Berman DS, et al: Left ventricular ejection fraction determined by radionuclide ventriculography in early stages of first transmural myocardial infarction: relation to short-term prognosis. *Am J Cardiol* 45:542-546, 1980

503. Sanford CF, Corbett J, Nicod P, et al: Value of radionuclide ventriculography in the immediate characterization of patients with acute myocardial infarction. *Am J Cardiol* 49:637-644, 1982

504. Corbett JR, Dehmer GJ, Lewis SE, et al: The prognostic value of submaximal exercise testing with radionuclide ventriculography before hospital discharge in patients with recent myocardial infarction. *Circulation* 64:535-544, 1981

505. Ahnve S, Gilpin E, Henning H, et al: Limitations and advantages of the ejection fraction for defining high risk after acute myocardial infarction. *Am J Cardiol* 58:872-878, 1986

506. Gibson RS, Taylor GJ, Watson DD, et al: Prognostic significance of resting anterior thallium-201 defects in patients with inferior myocardial infarction. *J Nucl Med* 21:1015-1021, 1980

507. Silverman KJ, Becker LC, Bulkley BH, et al: Value of early thallium-201 scintigraphy for predicting mortality in patients with acute myocardial infarction. *Circulation* 61:996-1003, 1980

508. Hakki A-H, Nestico PF, Heo J, et al: Relative prognostic value of rest thallium-201 imaging, radionuclide ventriculography and 24 hour ambulatory electrocardiographic monitoring after acute myocardial infarction. *J Am Coll Cardiol* 10:25-32, 1987

509. Turner JD, Schwartz KM, Logic JR, et al: Detection of residual jeopardized myocardium 3 weeks after myocardial infarction by exercise testing with thallium-201 myocardial scintigraphy. *Circulation* 61:729-737, 1980

510. Gibson RS, Watson DD, Craddock GB, et al: Prediction of cardiac events after uncomplicated myocardial infarction: a prospective study comparing predischarge exercise thallium-201 scintigraphy and coronary angiography. *Circulation* 68:321-336, 1983

511. Topol EJ, Juni JE, O'Neill WW, et al: Exercise testing three days after onset of acute myocardial infarction. *Am J Cardiol* 60:958-962, 1987

512. Buja LM, Poliner LR, Parkey RW, et al: Clinicopathologic study of persistently positive technetium-99m stannous pyrophosphate myocardial scintigrams and myocytolytic degeneration after myocardial infarction. *Circulation* 56:1016-1023, 1977

513. Olson H, Lyons K, Aronow WS, et al: Prognostic implications of a persistently positive technetium-99m-pyrophosphate myocardial scintigram after acute myocardial infarction (abstract). *Clin Res* 26:96A, 1978

514. Olson HG, Lyons KP, Aronow WS, et al: Prognostic value of a persistently positive technetium-99m stannous pyrophosphate myocardial scintigram after myocardial infarction. *Am J Cardiol* 43:889-898, 1979

515. Holman BL, Chisholm RJ, Braunwald E: The prognostic implications of acute myocardial scintigraphy with ^{99m}Tc-pyrophosphate. *Circulation* 57:320-326, 1978

516. Candell-Riera J, Permanyer-Miralda G, Castell J, et al: Uncom-

plicated first myocardial infarction: strategy for comprehensive prognostic studies. *J Am Coll Cardiol* 18:1207-1219, 1991

517. Griffin BP, Shah PK, Diamond GA, et al: Incremental prognostic accuracy of clinical, radionuclide and hemodynamic data in acute myocardial infarction. *Am J Cardiol* 68:707-712, 1991

518. Heger JJ, Weyman AE, Wann S, et al: Cross-sectional echocardiographic analysis of the extent of left ventricular asynergy in acute myocardial infarction. *Circulation* 61:1113-1118, 1980

519. Gibson RS, Bishop HL, Stamm RB, et al: Value of early two-dimensional echocardiography in patients with acute myocardial infarction. *Am J Cardiol* 49:1110-1119, 1982

520. Horowitz RS, Morganroth J: Immediate detection of high-risk patients with acute myocardial infarction using two-dimensional echocardiographic evaluation of left ventricular regional wall motion abnormalities. *Am Heart J* 103:814-822, 1982

521. Kan G, Visser CA, Koolen JJ, et al: Short and long term predictive value of admission wall motion score in acute myocardial infarction: a cross sectional echocardiographic study of 345 patients. *Br Heart J* 56:422-427, 1986

522. Bhatnagar SK, Moussa MAA, Al-Yusuf AR: The role of prehospital discharge two-dimensional echocardiography in determining the prognosis of survivors of first myocardial infarction. *Am Heart J* 109:472-477, 1985

523. Russell RO Jr, Rogers WJ, Mantle JA, et al: Coronary arteriography within two months of acute myocardial infarction. *Cardiovasc Med* 2:679-682, 1977

524. Mock MB, Ringqvist I, Fisher LD, et al: Survival of medically treated patients in the Coronary Artery Surgery Study (CASS) registry. *Circulation* 66:562-568, 1982

525. Schulze RA Jr, Humphries JO'N, Griffith LSC, et al: Left ventricular and coronary angiographic anatomy: relationship to ventricular irritability in the late hospital phase of acute myocardial infarction. *Circulation* 55:839-943, 1977

526. Taylor GJ, Humphries JO'N, Mellits ED, et al: Predictors of clinical course, coronary anatomy, and left ventricular function after recovery from acute myocardial infarction. *Circulation* 62:960-970, 1980

527. Castaner A, Betriu A, Roig E, et al: Clinical course and risk stratification of myocardial infarct survivors with three-vessel disease. *Am Heart J* 112:1201-1209, 1986

528. Veenbrink TWG, vanderWerf T, Westerhof PW, et al: Is there an indication for coronary angiography in patients under 60 years of age with no or minimal angina pectoris after a first myocardial infarction? *Br Heart J* 53:30-35, 1985

529. Roubin GS, Harris PJ, Bernstein L, et al: Coronary anatomy and prognosis after myocardial infarction in patients 60 years of age and younger. *Circulation* 67:743-749, 1983

530. CASS Principal Investigators and Their Associates: Coronary Artery Surgery Study (CASS): a randomized trial of coronary artery bypass surgery; survival data. *Circulation* 68:939-950, 1983

531. Schuster EH, Griffith LS, Bulkley BH: Preponderance of acute proximal left anterior descending coronary arterial lesions in fatal myocardial infarction: a clinicopathologic study. *Am J Cardiol* 47:1189-1196, 1981

532. Platia EV, Grunwald L, Mellits ED, et al: Clinical and arteriographic variables predictive of survival in coronary artery disease. *Am J Cardiol* 46:543-552, 1980

533. Karimian HO, Joffe CD, Marcus DR, et al: The clinical importance of coronary arteriography after myocardial infarction. *Heart Lung* 8:87-91, 1979

534. Sanz G, Castañer A, Betriu A, et al: Determinants of prognosis in survivors of myocardial infarction: a prospective clinical angiographic study. *N Engl J Med* 306:1065-1070, 1982

535. Bourke JP, Young AA, Richards DA, et al: Reduction in incidence of inducible ventricular tachycardia after myocardial infarction by treatment with streptokinase during infarct evolution. *J Am Coll Cardiol* 16:1703-1710, 1990

536. Pedretti R, Laporta A, Etro MD, et al: Influence of thrombolysis on signal-averaged electrocardiogram and late arrhythmic events after acute myocardial infarction. *Am J Cardiol* 69:866-872, 1992

537. Piccalo G, Pirelli S, Massa D, et al: Value of negative predischarge exercise testing in identifying patients at low risk after acute myocardial infarction treated by systemic thrombolysis. *Am J Cardiol* 70:31-33, 1992

538. Brodie BR, Stuckey TD, Hansen CJ, et al: Importance of a patent infarct-related artery for hospital and late survival after direct coronary angioplasty for acute myocardial infarction. *Am J Cardiol* 69:1113-1119, 1992

539. Tilkemeier PL, Guiney TE, LaRaia PJ, et al: Prognostic value of predischarge low-level exercise thallium testing after thrombolytic treatment of acute myocardial infarction. *Am J Cardiol* 66:1203-1207, 1990

540. Cigarroa RG, Lange RA, Hillis LD: Prognosis after acute myocardial infarction in patients with and without residual anterograde coronary blood flow. *Am J Cardiol* 64:155-160, 1989

541. Ishihara M, Sato H, Tateishi H, et al: Benefits of late reperfusion on left ventricular function and survival (abstract). *J Am Coll Cardiol* 19 Suppl A:360, 1992

542. McKay RG, Pfeffer MA, Pasternak RC, et al: Left ventricular remodeling after myocardial infarction: a corollary to infarct expansion. *Circulation* 74:693-702, 1986

543. Meizlish JL, Berger HJ, Plankey M, et al: Functional left ventricular aneurysm formation after acute anterior transmural myocardial infarction. Incidence, natural history, and prognostic implications. *N Engl J Med* 311:1001-1006, 1984

544. Pfeffer MA, Braunwald E, Moye LA, et al: Effect of captopril on mortality and morbidity in patients with left ventricular dysfunction after myocardial infarction. Results of the Survival and Ventricular Enlargement trial. *N Engl J Med* 327:669-677, 1992

545. Swedberg K, Held P, Kjekshus J, et al: Effects of the early administration of enalapril on mortality in patients with acute myocardial infarction. Results of the Cooperative New Scandinavian Enalapril Survival Study II (CONSENSUS II). *N Engl J Med* 327:678-684, 1992

546. Lamas GA, Pfeffer MA, Braunwald E: Patency of the infarct-related coronary artery and ventricular geometry. *Am J Cardiol* 68:41D-51D, 1991

547. Rogers WJ, Smith LR, Oberman A, et al: Surgical vs nonsurgical management of patients after myocardial infarction. *Circulation* 62 Suppl 1:67-74, 1980

548. Echt DS, Liebson PR, Mitchell LB, et al: Mortality and morbidity in patients receiving encainide, flecainide, or placebo. The Cardiac Arrhythmia Suppression Trial. *N Engl J Med* 324:781-788, 1991

549. The Cardiac Arrhythmia Suppression Trial II Investigators: Effect of the antiarrhythmic agent moricizine on survival after myocardial infarction. *N Engl J Med* 327:227-233, 1992

550. Ceremuzynski L, Kleczar E, Krzeminska-Pakula M, et al: Effect of amiodarone on mortality after myocardial infarction: a double-blind, placebo-controlled, pilot study. *J Am Coll Cardiol* 20:1056-1062, 1992

CHAPTER

30

Acute myocardial infarction

B. Management and complications

Bernard J. Gersh, M.B.,Ch.B., D.Phil., James H. Chesebro, M.D., Ian P. Clements, M.D., and Peter B. Berger, M.D.

GENERAL MEASURES

Relief of pain and sedation

The relief of pain as quickly and safely as possible is an essential first step in managing acute myocardial infarction (MI). Patient well-being is the priority, but the secondary effects of persistent pain that increase myocardial oxygen demands by elevating blood pressure and heart rate provide an added stimulus for prompt, effective analgesia.[1] Intense chest pain is the most common presenting symptom, but ischemic pain may be replaced by symptoms resembling those of pericarditis. Recognition of this feature is important clinically because the prognostic import and the therapy of the two conditions differ. How pain is produced in acute MI has not been clearly elucidated. Ischemic injury may lead to the release of substances that stimulate pain-sensitive nerve endings, with prolonged pain reflecting hyperactivity of the nerve endings with hemodynamic and arrhythmic sequelae. Relief of pain may result when ischemia is reduced or as analgesic agents elevate pain thresholds. Whatever the mechanism, the physician must relieve pain as quickly and safely as possible.

The ideal drug for the treatment of pain in patients with acute infarction should produce rapid relief of pain and be free of adverse hemodynamic and systemic effects. No such drug is currently available. Table 30B-1 lists the pharmacologic agents used to relieve the pain of acute MI.

Anxiety and agitation often accompany pain, particularly early after the acute event.[32] Treatment with calm reassurance and, if necessary, minor tranquilizers such as diazepam or chlordiazepoxide is an important adjunct to the management of pain in these acutely ill patients. Nausea and vomiting are equally distressing symptoms, and specific therapy with antiemetics is often needed.

Diet

A liquid or soft diet is usually given in the first 24 hours after MI, followed by a 1,200-calorie, low-salt, low-cholesterol diet, unless otherwise indicated. Stimulants such as caffeine are to be avoided. Patients are weighed on admission, if the clinical condition is stable, and daily thereafter.

Bowel habits

A stool softener or laxative is given to prevent constipation and straining at stool, and a bedside commode is used on day one.

Oxygenation and ventilation

Most patients with acute MI, whether complicated or not, are hypoxemic.[6,33-35] The pathogenesis involved is influenced primarily by pulmonary congestion due to left ventricular failure, in addition to other factors such as pneumonia, preexisting chronic obstructive pulmonary disease (COPD), and atelectasis. Atelectasis is related to diminished respiratory excursions in patients who are heavily sedated or in pain. Pulmonary trauma in survivors of resuscitation after cardiac arrest may create major disturbances in pulmonary function.[33]

In patients who have arterial hypoxemia, the Pa_{O_2} should be restored to normal so that any increased oxygen delivery may benefit ischemic areas of the myocardium.[7,33,36] Increasing oxygen tension above normal is of no benefit and may be harmful, causing increased systemic vascular resistance and blood pressure.[37] Arterial punctures for oxygen saturation determinations are contraindicated if thrombolytic therapy is contemplated. If in doubt, oxygen should be administered, usually via a nasal cannula; 100% oxygen is delivered at 2 to 4 L/min for the first 3 to 4 days. The effect of this mild increase in inspired P_{O_2} on oxygen content and delivery of oxygen to the tissues is small, and therapy must be tailored to the patient's clinical, hemodynamic, and respiratory status. Regular chest physiotherapy is useful, particularly in the many coronary care unit patients who have COPD and a history of cigarette smoking.

A randomized trial suggested that continuous positive

Table 30B-1 Pharmacologic agents used to relieve pain in myocardial infarction

Agent	Route of administration	Mechanism of action	Contraindications and side effects	Comments
Nitroglycerin	Sublingual	Improves imbalance between overall myocardial oxygen supply and demand, especially in areas of regional ischemia; affects infarct size favorably[2,3]	Tachycardia and hypotension may develop in patients without left ventricular failure in whom relative hypovolemia develops[4]	Achieves pain relief comparable to that with IV morphine; ECG estimates of myocardial necrosis are significantly less than with morphine
Oxygen	Oral	Relieves breathlessness, anxiety, and pain when given in early hours;[5] corrects ventilation-perfusion inequalities producing hypoxemia[6] and reduces ischemia, dyspnea, infarct size, and pain[7]	With evidence of COPD, lower flow rates may be prudent[5]	Although a placebo effect may be involved, relief of anxiety and pain justifies routine use
Morphine	Intravenous; epidural and intrathecal administration effective but not widely used[1,8]	Combines potent analgesic effect with hemodynamic actions to reduce myocardial oxygen consumption and thus ventricular preload, heart rate, and ventricular afterload;[5,9,10] effectiveness lasts 7 to 9 hr;[1,11-13] hemodynamic actions probably are mediated through central depression of vasomotor centers, reducing sympathetic tone, and peripheral mechanisms, releasing histamine;[14,15] central narcotic action may alleviate distress and reduce work of breathing, which decreases tone[16-19]	Side effects include nausea and vomiting;[20] respiratory depression can occur,[10,11,17] and respiratory failure can develop;[20] should not be given intramuscularly	Recommended dosage is initial dose of 2-4 mg, additional doses of 3-6 mg every 5 to 10 min until pain is controlled (if respiratory or hemodynamic side effects are absent); if respiratory effects occur, can be reversed with naloxone in 0.4 mg increments IV to a total dose of 1.2 mg; facility for artificial ventilation must be available
Meperidine hydrochloride			Initially increases blood pressure, systemic vascular resistance, and pulse rate	When equipotent doses are used, has no clear advantage over morphine[17]
Pentazocine			Increases cardiac work by peripheral vasoconstriction[21] and may increase both pulmonary capillary wedge pressure and LVEDP[17,21]	Analgesic properties and potential for causing respiratory depression differ little from those of other narcotics

Table 30B-1 Pharmacologic agents used to relieve pain in myocardial infarction—cont'd

Agent	Route of administration	Mechanism of action	Contraindications and side effects	Comments
Nitrous oxide	Inhalation		Weak general anesthetic action can depress LOC, induce dreamlike states, and create difficulties in patient cooperation;[14] panic and dysphoric reactions may occur; rapid absorption from lung can cause atelectasis	Particularly effective in patients with mild to moderate pain and a useful adjunct to morphine when pain is severe;[22] effective in concentrations from 20% to 50% combined with oxygen[23]
Nalbuphine hydrochloride	Intravenous	Narcotic analgesic chemically and pharmacologically related to oxymorphone and naloxone	Can cause respiratory depression, which can be antagonized by 0.4 mg of naloxone, 10 mg of nalorphine, or 1 mg of levallorphan[24]	Ceiling for respiratory depression at higher doses may increase its safety for patients with severe pain unresponsive to usual dosages; has relatively few adverse hemodynamic effects; may produce less nausea and vomiting than other narcotics
β-adrenergic blocking agents	Intravenous	Reduce myocardial oxygen demand and, by reducing heart rate, prolong diastolic perfusion and improve oxygen supply-demand ratio; reduce pain due to ischemia[1,25-31]	Not used for patients with hypotension, bradycardia, conduction disturbances, heart failure, or asthma	Beneficial effect most pronounced in patients with a high rate-pressure product;[27,28] about 80% of CCU patients with presumed MI can tolerate β-blockade during acute phase[1]

CCU, coronary care unit; COPD, chronic obstructive pulmonary disease; ECG, electrocardiographic; IV, intravenous; LOC, level of consciousness; LVEDP, left ventricular end-diastolic pressure; MI, myocardial infarction.

airway pressure delivered by a face mask in patients with severe cardiogenic pulmonary edema produced early physiologic improvement and reduced the need for intubation and mechanical ventilation (35% in patients who received oxygen alone versus 0% in those who received oxygen plus continuous positive airway pressure).[15] This short-term study did not, however, establish whether or not long-term benefits occurred or whether a larger study would have shown an early mortality benefit.

Antithrombotic therapy

The American Heart Association endorsed anticoagulant therapy in the management of acute MI in 1948.[38-40] At that time, patients were treated by prolonged bed rest, and using anticoagulant therapy with heparin and dicumarol reduced mortality in the first 6 weeks after acute MI. The benefit resulted mainly from reducing the potentially fatal thromboembolic complications. The study in which these results were determined did not have appropriate randomization, however.

Benefits. The potential benefits and goals of anticoagulation in acute MI include the following: (1) prevention of venous thromboembolism, (2) reduction of arterial embolization (mainly to brain, extremities, or kidneys) from mural thrombi in the left ventricle, (3) reduction of clinical recurrence of myocardial infarction, reocclusion, and residual arterial thrombus burden (Fig 30B-1), and (4) reduction of total mortality from myocardial infarction. These goals will be discussed in relation to the potential benefits and risks of anticoagulant therapy.

VENOUS THROMBOEMBOLISM. Autopsy studies in patients who were treated with 3 weeks of bed rest, who had had no anticoagulants, and who died of MI showed that 16% of in-hospital deaths resulted from thromboemboli, usually involving the lungs.[41] Later studies, when the bed

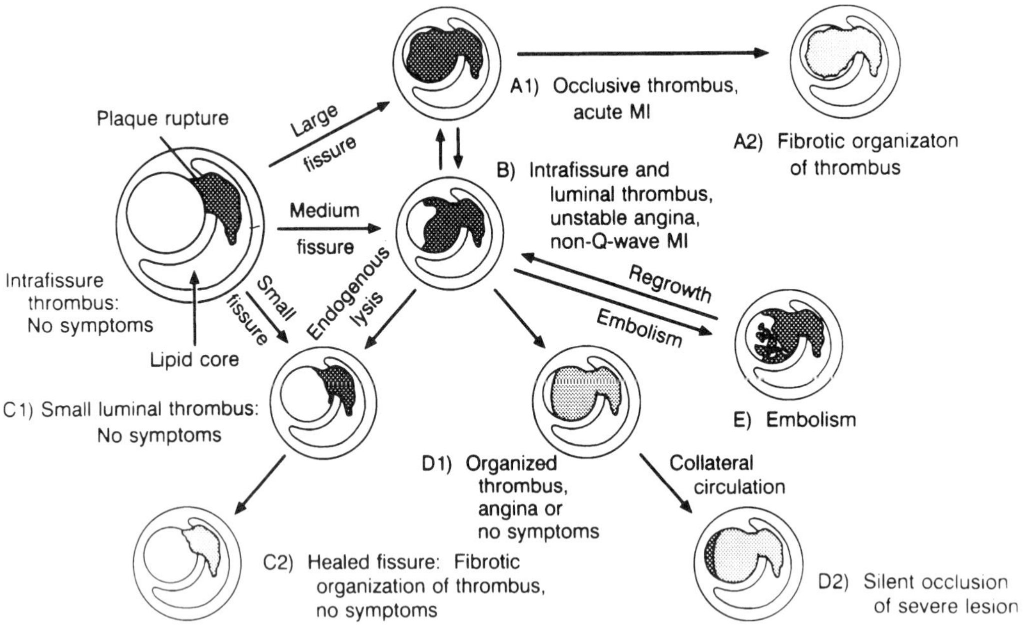

Fig 30B-1 Diagram showing major pathogenic modes of progression of coronary disease. Plaque disruption leads to formation of a fissure, with flowing blood contracting intra-arterial structures and forming an intrafissure thrombus. The fissure may be small, medium, or large and may progress immediately to various degrees of luminal obstruction (*A1, B,* and *C1*). Sudden progression with a large fissure may lead to occlusive thrombus and acute myocardial infarction *(A1).* Fibrotic organization of the thrombus *(A2)* or lysis of the thrombus with reopening of the lumen becoming partially obstructive *(B)* may occur. A medium-sized fissure may lead to immediate partial obstruction associated with unstable angina or non-Q-wave myocardial infarction *(B);* this may progress to total occlusion *(A1),* partial embolization *(E),* fibrotic organization *(D1),* endogenous lysis to a smaller thrombus *(C1),* no intraluminal thrombus *(E),* or fibrotic organization by fibromuscular proliferation (*A2, C2,* and *D1*). Severe residual stenosis *(D1)* may be associated with good collateral circulation and no symptoms. Because of very low antegrade flow and type II injury (endothelial denudation), this may silently occlude with fresh thrombus *(D2).* A small fissure may lead to a small thrombus without symptoms *(C1)* and undergo fibrotic organization with progression of disease without symptoms *(C2).*

rest was shorter, showed a much smaller contribution of embolic deaths to overall hospital mortality, with 0.6% of 499 untreated control patients having fatal pulmonary emboli (4.8% had clinically detectable pulmonary emboli) in the Veterans Administration Cooperative Clinical Trial[42]; no deaths resulted from pulmonary emboli in an untreated control group of 293 patients in a multicenter trial of streptokinase in acute myocardial infarction (4.4% had clinically detectable pulmonary emboli).[43] Since more than 90% of pulmonary emboli originate in veins of the legs or pelvis,[44] and since most are preventable with appropriate anticoagulant therapy, the incidence of deep vein thrombosis in patients with acute MI will be reviewed.

The diagnosis of deep vein thrombosis by physical examination alone is usually correct in only about 50% of cases.[45,46] Its true incidence can be overestimated by autopsy studies. Leg scanning with ^{125}I-labeled fibrinogen is the best noninvasive test for determining the incidence of early, asymptomatic, deep vein thrombosis in the calves and popliteal veins.[45-48] By this technique, the incidence ranged from 22% to 37%,[49-55] which is similar to the incidence in postoperative patients.[56] Deep vein thrombosis occurs much less often in patients who are admitted with chest pain but who do not experience MI (7% to 10%) compared with those in whom MI evolves (34% to 38%).[48-50] These observations and other in vivo tests of thromboembolic risk[57] suggest that a hypercoagulable state occurs after MI,[58] as after major surgery.[59]

Within 72 hours of acute infarction, more than 50% to 60% of leg vein thrombi have developed, and 75% within the first 5 to 7 days.[50,51,54] The conclusions are (1) the early formation of leg vein thrombi is in part but not solely or always related to prolonged immobilization, and (2) any therapeutic intervention to prevent venous thrombi should be started at the time of hospital admission, should be effective almost immediately, and should involve strategies for early mobilization.

Table 30B-2 Effect of anticoagulation on pulmonary emboli after acute myocardial infarction

Study*	No. of patients	Deaths due to PE, %		Clinical PE, %		Autopsy findings of PE or PI, %*	
		Control	AC	Control	AC	Control	AC
Hilden et al.[41]	800	4.0	1.4	. . .	. . .	28.0	5.0
BMR Council[65]	1,427	. . .	. . .	5.5‡	2.2‡	5.6†	1.2‡
VA Coop.[42]	999	0.6	0	4.8	2.0	PE 32.0	0
						PI 9.7	0

BMR Council, British Medical Research Council study; VA Coop., Veterans Administration Cooperative study; PE, pulmonary embolism; PI, pulmonary infarction; AC, anticoagulation.
*Percent of autopsies.
†Low-dose phenindione only (1 mg daily).
‡Therapeutic dose of phenindione (average, 72 mg daily) and heparin (for 36 hours).

Associated complications include heart failure and shock, which create stasis of blood; how quickly the patient is mobilized; and other patient characteristics. Thus, about one-third of all patients with acute MI experience deep venous thrombosis within a week, but the incidence increases to 40% to 50% in those with associated heart failure and to 50% to 60% in those with associated shock.[51,55] Similarly, leg vein thrombi were found in 9% of patients mobilized within the first 1 to 3 days after MI and in 63% of patients randomly selected to stay in bed for 5 days. When heart failure was present, only 22% of patients mobilized early had thrombi, compared with 80% of patients who were mobilized late after MI.[60] Other patient characteristics that increase the risk of leg vein thrombi include preexisting angina pectoris, history of MI or thromboembolism, obesity, varicose veins, arrhythmias, and especially age (there is a 12.5% incidence of leg vein thrombi in patients less than 50 years old compared with 71% in patients more than 70 years old, uncorrected for other risks noted).[55,59,61]

Regarding the *relation of deep leg vein thrombosis to the risk of pulmonary embolism,* studies by Kakkar and colleagues[45,62-64] reached the following conclusions: (1) calf vein thrombi remain confined to the calf 75% to 80% of the time and extend proximally to the popliteal, femoral, or iliac system 20% to 25% of the time; (2) if extension occurs, it is usually more than 3 days after the initial formation in the calf veins, and of the thrombi that extend proximally, 40% to 50% embolize to the lungs; and (3) iliofemoral thrombi form almost exclusively (90% to 95% of cases) from calf vein extension. Thus, approximately 10% of deep leg vein thrombi lead to clinical pulmonary embolism and this proves fatal in one-third of these patients.[62,64] Similarly, patients free of leg vein thrombi by ^{125}I-labeled fibrinogen leg scans had no pulmonary emboli (366 patients).[64] Thus, *patients who are mobilized within 3 days of infarction* not only *have a very low incidence of leg vein thrombi,* but, if thrombi were to occur, they would usually remain confined to the calf without extending proximally, in view of the minimum of 3 days required for extension. Patients who are mobilized early would therefore have a very minimal risk of pulmonary emboli. Anticoagulation significantly reduces the incidence of deep leg vein thrombi to 5% to 6% or less[50,52,54] and thus should reduce the risk of pulmonary emboli.

Clinically detectable pulmonary emboli continue to occur in about 4% to 5% of patients who are not anticoagulated or mobilized[42,43] and deaths primarily from pulmonary emboli in patients with acute MI are uncommon. The incidence of pulmonary emboli detected pathologically is usually considerably higher than the clinical estimate (Table 30B-2).

Hypoxemia can contribute substantially to arrhythmia and the risk of thromboembolic complications[66,67] and, thus, probably also to MI or infarct extension. *Anticoagulants are primarily preventive for pulmonary emboli* (Table 30B-2), but they do not necessarily affect the resolution of existing thromboemboli, as evidenced by persisting perfusion and diffusion abnormalities (at 2 weeks and 1 year after pulmonary emboli), which probably result from small peripheral pulmonary clots beyond the resolving capabilities of angiography or scanning.[68]

ARTERIAL THROMBOEMBOLISM. Left ventricular mural thrombi are the primary cause of arterial emboli in acute MI. The incidence of left ventricular mural thrombi in patients

Table 30B-3 Left ventricular mural thrombi at autopsy in acute myocardial infarction

Study	Patients with mural thrombus: No anticoagulation		Anticoagulation	
	No.	%	No.	%
Aber et al.[43]	10/24	42	. . .	. . .
VA Coop.[42]	15/31	48	5/23	22
Hilden et al.[41]	53/92	58	20/84	24

VA Coop., Veterans Administration Cooperative study.

Table 30B-4 Randomized studies on the effect of early anticoagulation on left ventricular thrombi in acute anterior myocardial infarction

Study	Study entry, hr	Treatment	No./total patients: Left ventricular thrombi* Treated	Control	Emboli Treated	Control
Nordrehaug et al.[89]	<12	Heparin/warfarin†	0/26	7/27	0/26	1/27
Arvan and Boscha[90]	<12	Heparin/warfarin†	4/13	6/17	1/13	1/17
Davis and Ireland[91]	<12	Heparin/warfarin†,‡	14/25	15/27	0/25	1/27
Gueret et al.[92]	<12	Heparin†	8/21	13/25	1/21	1/25
Turpie et al.[93]	<36	Heparin§,‖	10/95	28/88	1/95	4/88
SCATI[94]	<24	Heparin§	19/107	34/93	0/107	2/93
Totals			55/287(19%)	103/277(37%)	3/287(1%)	10/277(4%)
			$P < 0.001$		$P < 0.04$	

*Echocardiography 7 to 14 days and at dismissal.
†Adjusted for activated partial thromboplastin time, prothrombin time.
‡Control group received heparin, 5,000 U three times daily; 18 of 27 patients also received warfarin.
§12,500 U twice daily.
‖Control group received heparin, 5,000 U twice daily.

who die from acute MI has been 40% or more when anticoagulation is not used, compared with 20% to 25% with full anticoagulation (Table 30B-3). Thrombus formation appears to be initiated by platelet deposition to the damaged, akinetic, or dyskinetic endocardial surface, which is secondarily inflamed with a leukocyte response. This left ventricular thrombus formation may not differ appreciably from thrombus formation in arteries[69,70] except that (1) there is probably less endothelial damage since the first two to three layers of subendocardium usually survive because nutrients diffuse from the blood of the left ventricular cavity; (2) the inflammatory response to infarction may play a more important role and may contribute to the induction of tissue factor in the subendocardium; and (3) there is stasis in the infarcted (usually akinetic or dyskinetic) and often aneurysmal region, which contributes significantly to fibrin accumulation and explains why anticoagulants can significantly reduce the formation of mural thrombi.

The *incidence of mural thrombi is related to the size and location of the MI (almost always anterior)* and the presence of apical akinesis or dyskinesis.[71-75] Similarly, left ventricular aneurysms involve the anterior and apical segments and, in approximately 90% of patients, result from previous anteroseptal myocardial infarction.[73,76,77] The anatomic distribution of the left anterior descending coronary artery (which supplies the largest region of the myocardium, including the cardiac apex) and the configuration of the left ventricle, in which a much thinner wall of myocardium forms the cardiac apex, appear to account for the above observations. Thus, septal, posterior or inferior, and lateral locations of aneurysm are unusual. Approximately 50% to 60% of patients with left ventricular aneurysm have mural thrombus formation at the time of aneurysm resection.[76-82] Left ventricular *mural thrombus is most accurately detected by two-dimensional echocardiography;*[83-85] it is not reliably identified by left ventricular cineangiography.[76,77,82]

Two-dimensional echocardiography shows that *50% to 75% of left ventricular mural thrombi develop within the first 48 hours* after MI.[74] Most mural thrombi appear to develop within the 5 to 7 days of the acute event and resolve or become undetectable by two-dimensional echocardiography in most patients when they take oral anticoagulants for 1 to 3 months.[74,75] Approximately *20% of mural thrombi resolve spontaneously,* even without anticoagulant therapy. Other factors that favor resolution are resolution of apical dyskinesis and absence of cardiomyopathy due to ischemia.[74,75,86,87] *Patients with mural thrombus* detectable by two-dimensional echocardiography during hospitalization for acute MI *are at risk for future arterial embolization*[74,75,83,87,88] (Table 30B-4).

The *incidence of systemic emboli* after acute MI remains low—5% to 6% or less—and *is approximately 10% to 15% of the incidence of left ventricular mural thrombi.* (Table 30B-4).[41,42] The incidence of both mural thrombi at autopsy[41,42] (see Table 30B-3) and clinical cerebral emboli[38,42,65] (Table 30B-4 and 30B-5) was reduced in patients who were treated with anticoagulants.

The incidence of systemic embolization (includes acute events and patients with global left ventricular dysfunction) in patients with left ventricular aneurysm is also low (usually 5% to 6% or less) and is also about 10% to 15% of the incidence of mural thrombi confirmed at surgery, as seen from retrospective studies (Table 30B-6). Most systemic emboli in patients with left ventricular aneurysm occur in the early weeks to a few months after MI. In one study systemic embolism occurred only in patients who were not anticoagulated in the period immediately after acute myocardial infarction.[77] Recent small randomized

Table 30B-5 Cerebral emboli in acute myocardial infarction

Study	Patients, no.	Incidence, % Control	Anticoagulated
Wright et al.[38]	800	4.9	0.7
BMR Council[65]	1,427	2.5	1.1
VA Coop.[42]	999	3.8	0.8

BMR Council, British Medical Research Council study; VA Coop., Veterans Administration Cooperative study.

Table 30B-6 Mural thrombi confirmed at operation and embolization in left ventricular aneurysm

Study	Patients, no.	Mural thrombi, %	Emboli, %
Favaloro et al.[78]	130	99	6
Cooley and Hallman[79]	80	95	13
Kluge et al.[80]	36	69	0
Loop et al.[81]	400	53	5
Simpson et al.[82]	58	66	3
Reeder et al.[77]	100	46	5

studies in patients with acute anterior MI using two-dimensional echocardiography showed that anticoagulation decreases both the incidence of left ventricular mural thrombus and systemic embolization (see Table 30B-5). Delaying the start of subcutaneous heparin for 12 hours after administering thrombolytic therapy (streptokinase or recombinant tissue-type plasminogen activator [rt-PA]) in patients with anterior MI did not decrease the incidence of left ventricular mural thrombus (27%) compared with that in untreated control patients (30%).[95] Aspirin does not decrease the incidence of left ventricular thrombus.[96]

In patients with dilated cardiomyopathy (in which the whole ventricle contracts poorly) the incidence of systemic emboli in patients not treated with anticoagulants was 3.5 events per 100 patient-years but was zero in patients treated with anticoagulants.[97,98] Thus, the patient with dilated cardiomyopathy appears to need long-term anticoagulation.

RECURRENCE OF MI REOCCLUSION AND THROMBUS. Several early studies have shown no effect of anticoagulants on the short-term incidence of reinfarction.[42,65,99]Heparin markedly reduces the incidence of acute MI during the acute phase of unstable angina when most patients have subtotal occlusion.[100] Heparin appears to inactivate free thrombin near the thrombus but has a lesser effect on clot-bound thrombin.[101,102]

Clinical trials of heparin without thrombolytic therapy. Trials of heparin performed before thrombolytic trials suggested that heparin may be beneficial in acute MI.[39,103,104] Another meta-analysis showed a 22% reduction in reinfarction and a 17% reduction in death in patients treated with heparin compared with the control group.[105] The heparin dosage used in most studies was at least 20,000 U per day, and the average continuous intravenous dosage of heparin to maintain a therapeutic activated partial thromboplastin time (aPTT) between approximately 60 and 85 seconds was 30,500 U/24 hours in 11 studies.[101] These doses of heparin also reduced deep-vein thrombosis, pulmonary embolism, and stroke.[103]

Studies of heparin with thrombolytic therapy. Patients who have had interruption of their acute MI by thrombolysis have a residual high-grade coronary artery lesion that needs antithrombotic protection. These patients' risk of reocclusion of the infarct-related artery is less than 10% on combined heparin and aspirin therapy when the aPTT is maintained between 60 and 85 seconds.[106] When anticoagulation is discontinued or when the aPTT falls below twice the upper limit of normal in the hospital, reinfarction tends to occur.[107,108] Although reocclusion and recurrent ischemic events are unpredictable from quantitative or morphologic characteristics of the infarct-related artery,[109] they are inversely related to the adequacy of heparin therapy (measured by the aPTT).[110,111]

A single intravenous bolus (10,000 U) of heparin administered with rt-PA (1.5 mg/kg) over 4 hours (Thrombolysis and Angioplasty in Myocardial Infarction [TAMI]-III Trial) had no significant effect on coronary artery patency at 90 minutes (79% in both treatment groups).[112] Bolus dosing does not produce a sustained effect, and the dose used was below the effective dose used in animals. However, some randomized trials showed improvement of infarct-related artery patency days to weeks after acute MI (Table 30B-7). The benefit of heparin was greater in patients whose aPTT was more than 1.5 times control.[114,115] In this study, where patients receiving continued heparin therapy for 7 days had the same incidence of occlusion as patients receiving only aspirin plus dipyridamole, the mean aPTT was less than 60 seconds, and occlusion rates in both groups were high (about 20%).[116] Today's standard therapy to maximize patency and minimize reocclusion is the use of heparin plus aspirin.[106]

The frequency of recurrent ischemic events after thrombolytic therapy with streptokinase or urokinase is inversely related to the aPTT. The incidence of reocclusion and recurrent ischemia after thrombolysis with either streptokinase or rt-PA appears reduced by using aspirin with heparin[117] (Table 30B-8). Adequate heparin therapy (all aPTTs >1.5 times control) plus aspirin for 3 weeks improves patency and reduces residual stenosis of the infarct-related artery after streptokinase therapy for acute MI[118] (Table 30B-9). Heparin markedly attenuates the high procoagulant, thrombin activity (elevated plasma concentrations of fibrinopeptide A and thrombin-antithrombin III complexes) induced by streptokinase[119,120] and effectively inhibits the procoagulant activ-

Table 30B-7 Effect of intravenous heparin on infarct-related patency after thrombolytic therapy

Study	No. of patients	Treatment group	Control group	Time of angiography	Patency
TAMI-3[112]	134	rt-$PA_{(2)}$ + $H_{(3)}$	rt-$PA_{(2)}$ only	90 min	79% vs. 79% NS
Bleich et al.[113]	83	rt-PA + $H_{(5)}$	rt-PA only	Day 3	71% vs. 44% $P < 0.02$
HART[114]	205	rt-PA + $H_{(5)}$	rt-PA + $ASA_{(6)}$	18 hr	82% vs. 52% $P < 0.001$
ECSG-6[115]	652	rt-PA + $H_{(4)}$ + ASA	rt-PA + $ASA_{(7)}$	48-120 hr	83% vs. 75% $P < 0.01$
Australian NHF[116]	241	rt-PA + $H_{(4)}$	rt-PA + $H_{(4)}$ /24 hr and then $ASA/D_{(8)}$	7-10 days	81% vs. 80% NS

rt-PA: tissue-type plasminogen activator
(1) 100 mg/3-4 hr
(2) 1.5 mg/kg/4 hr

H: heparin
(3) bolus 10,000 U
(4) bolus 5,000 + 1,000 U/hr
(5) aPTT 1.5-2.0

ASA: aspirin
(6) 80 mg/day
(7) first day 250 mg IV (or 300 mg oral) and then 75-125 mg/day
(8) 300 mg/day + 300 mg dipyridamole (D)

Table 30B-8 Incidence of reocclusion and recurrent ischemia after thrombolysis in patients treated with or without aspirin (most also receiving heparin)[117]

	Reocclusion		
	Streptokinase	rt-PA	Ischemia
Aspirin	11% (197)	10% (222)	25% (2,977)
No aspirin	24% (334)	26% (179)	41% (721)

( ), total number of patients.
Modified from Roux S, Christeller S, Ludin E: Effects of aspirin on coronary reocclusion and recurrent ischemia after thrombolysis: a meta-analysis. *J Am Coll Cardiol* 19:671-677, 1992.

Table 30B-9 Adequate heparin therapy* improves infarct-related artery after streptokinase therapy[118]

	Adequate (n = 84)	Inadequate (n = 39)	P
Patency at 3 weeks, %	69	48	<0.02
Residual stenosis, %	57	74	<0.02

*All activated partial thromboplastin times more than 1.5 times control value.
Data from Cuccia C, Volterrani M, Volpini M, et al: Relationship between anticoagulation level ischemic events and angiographic characteristics of infarct-related artery following streptokinase in patients with acute myocardial infarction (abstract). *J Am Coll Cardiol* 19 Suppl A:92, 1992.

ity induced by plasmin, but higher concentrations than those usually achieved are required.[121]

Combined heparin and aspirin therapy should probably be continued throughout the hospitalization to keep rates of reocclusion at the lowest reported levels (under 7%).[106] According to the Antithrombotic Therapy in Acute Coronary Syndromes (ATACS) study, the heparin-aspirin combination should be converted to warfarin and low-dose aspirin to reduce recurrent infarction and ischemia in patients with non-Q-wave MI or unstable angina.[122]

Aspirin with and without thrombolytic therapy (Fig 30B-2). Aspirin in oral or intravenous loading doses of at least 2 mg/kg produces a rapid antithrombotic effect due to immediate and near-total inhibition of platelet cyclooxygenase and thus thromboxane A_2 production. With lower doses (0.5 to 1 mg/kg), full antiplatelet effect takes a few days. Doses less than 80 mg may not be reliably absorbed in all patients.[123,124]

In the second International Study of Infarct Survival (ISIS-II) of 17,000 patients with suspected acute myocardial infarction, the clinical efficacy of aspirin alone (160 mg/day) or combined with streptokinase was confirmed for inhospital reinfarction, vascular death, and total stroke[125] (Table 30B-10). Major bleeding episodes seen with aspirin alone were no different than with placebo. A meta-analysis of 32 angiographic studies showed that aspirin, usually combined with heparin, reduced coronary reocclusion and recurrent ischemia after thrombolysis[117] (see Table 30B-8). The lower incidence of reocclusion after thrombolysis in patients taking aspirin may account for the reduced mortality in patients on aspirin in ISIS-II. Aspirin may cover the added risk of thrombosis if the

Table 30B-10 Reinfarction, stroke, death, and bleeding complications in the Second International Study of Infarct Survival[125]

	Stroke, %	In-hospital reinfarction, %	Vascular death, %	Major bleeding, %
Streptokinase + aspirin	1.8	0.6	8.0	0.6
Aspirin alone	1.9	0.6	9.4	0.4
Streptokinase alone	3.8	0.7	9.2	0.5
Placebo	2.9	1.1	12.0/13.2	0.4/0.3

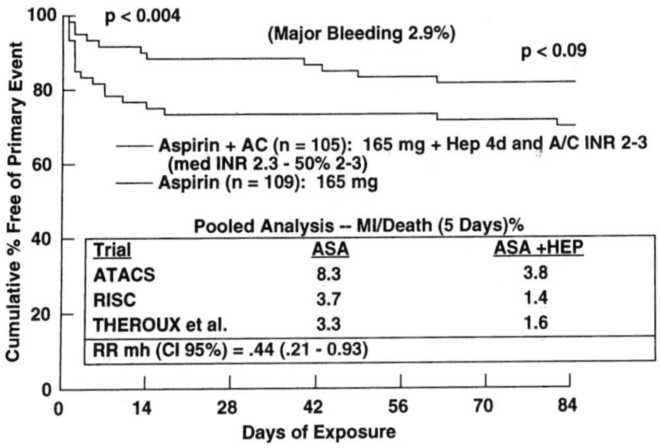

Fig 30B-2 The unstable angina in non-Q-wave infarction trial (ATACS) comparing anticoagulation (starting with heparin and switching to warfarin) plus aspirin versus aspirin alone, showing the incidence of ischemic events over the first 3 months for each group. *Boxed data,* antithrombotic therapy in unstable angina comparing heparin (HEP) plus aspirin (ASA) versus ASA alone in a pooled analysis for the end point of myocardial infarction or death from three randomized controlled trials after 5 days of therapy. (Modified from Cohen M, Adams PC, Parry G, et al: Combination antithrombotic therapy in unstable rest angina and non-Q-wave infarction in nonprior aspirin users. Primary end points analysis from the ATACS trial. *Circulation* 89:81-88, 1994.)

aPTT falls too low, as well as reducing the event rate from reactivation thrombosis when administered during cessation of heparin.[126]

Anticoagulation after hospital dismissal. After hospital dismissal there is continued reocclusion of the infarct-related artery. Coronary angiography performed 3 to 6 months after thrombolytic therapy in TAMI-6 and in the Antithrombotics and the Prevention of Reocclusion in Coronary Thrombolysis (APRICOT) trials showed an incidence of late reocclusion of 25% to 30% in previously patent infarct-related arteries.[127,128]

Thrombotic reocclusion is primarily mediated by highly thrombogenic thrombus covering the disrupted plaque (Fig 30B-3). In addition, the rheology of blood flow with residual stenosis and high shear forces contribute to increased thrombus formation. Hematologic factors that increase thrombogenicity include activated platelet aggregates; fibrin-bound and fibrin split product-bound thrombin, which activates factors VI and VIII, causing continued thrombin generation; plasmin activation of factor V to Va; lipids; and increased catecholamines.[58,102,129,130]

A double-blind randomized trial of the use of anticoagulants versus placebo in patients more than 60 years old who had their previous MI a median of 6 years before showed a significant reduction over 2 years in recurrent MI (15.9% in the placebo group vs. 5.7% in the anticoagulant-treated group, $P = 0.0001$) and in total mortality (13.4% in the placebo group vs. 7.6% in the treated group, $P = 0.017$).[131] Hemorrhagic events without death occurred in 0.7% in the placebo group and in 6.2% in the treated group over 2 years. The greater benefit in this trial compared with that in previous trials may have been due in part to the meticulous control of the anticoagulation; more than 70% to 80% of the thrombotests were within the therapeutic range or better. However, data concerning the two most important baseline risk factors related to mortality—the severity of underlying coronary artery disease and the status of left ventricular function—were unknown in these two groups of patients. In addition, all of the patients in the trial were maintained on anticoagulants for a median of 6 years before they entered the trial; this raised the question of whether this group was particularly anticoagulant responsive.

Clinical benefits from reperfusion by thrombolysis are lost with rethrombosis. The APRICOT trial attempted to prevent rethrombosis after hospital dismissal over the first 3 months, but a relatively low dose of intravenous heparin was administered and may have contributed to a suboptimal outcome in the heparin-coumadin group. In addition, the target INR of 2.8 to 4.0 was not achieved during hospitalization in at least 20% of patients.[128]

Two recent, well-designed randomized clinical trials of long-term anticoagulation after acute MI have shown that warfarin reduces reinfarction by approximately 25% over approximately 3 years in survivors of myocardial infarction (Tables 30B-11 and 30B-12).[132,133] The Coumadin-Aspirin Reinfarction Study (CARS) is testing a new approach, a combination of warfarin and low-dose aspirin

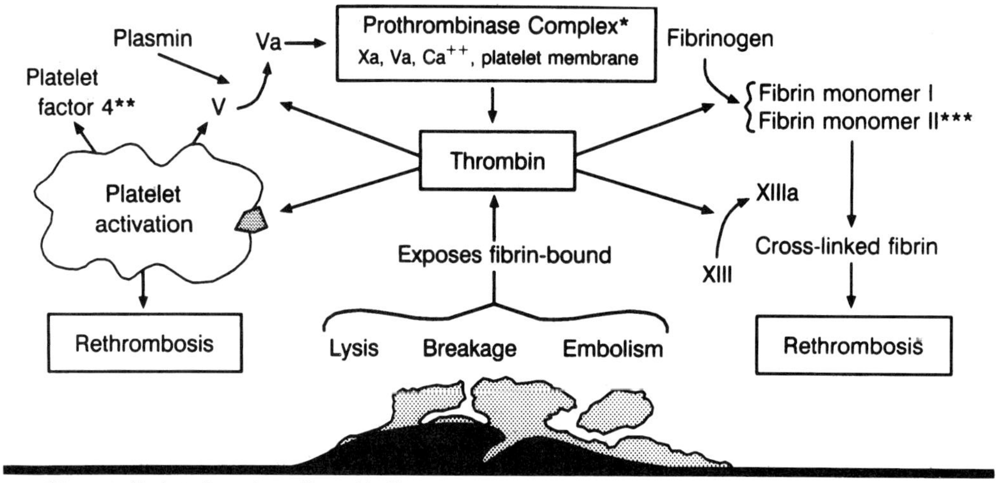

Fig 30B-3 Disturbance of thrombus by lysis (endogenous or exogenous), mechanical breakage (including coronary angioplasty), or spontaneous embolism exposes thrombin bound to fibrin. Thrombin activates platelets, activates factor V to Va (which leads to generation of more thrombin via the prothrombinase complex), converts fibrinogen to fibrin I and fibrin II, and activates factor XIII to XIIIa (which cross-links fibrin). These processes combine to produce rethrombosis. Heparin may only partially prevent rethrombosis because factor Xa within the prothrombinase complex is protected from heparin-antithrombin III, platelet factor 4 neutralizes heparin, and fibrin monomer II inhibits heparin-antithrombin III. (From Webster MWI, Chesebro JH, Fuster V: Antithrombotic therapy in acute myocardial infarction: enhancement of thrombolysis, reduction of reocclusion, and prevention of thromboembolism. In *Acute Myocardial Infarction*. Edited by BJ Gersh, SH Rahimtoola. New York, Elsevier Science Publishing Company, 1991, pp 333-348. By permission of Chapman & Hall.)

compared with aspirin alone in reducing the incidence of a combined end point of reinfarction, vascular death, and stroke in survivors of MI.

Mortality. Three retrospective studies[134-136] reported reduced mortality in hospitalized patients with acute MI who were treated with anticoagulants. Anticoagulation was also reported to be of value in improving long-term survival after MI in a collaborative analysis of nine controlled trials in men with a history of prolonged angina or previous MI[137] and in a 2-year study of patients over the age of 60.[131]

The value of heparin for reducing mortality remains suggestive compared with the reduced mortality during treatment with aspirin from meta-analyses and the prospective ISIS-II data. Uncertainty for heparin is in part due to delayed administration, delayed onset of action by the subcutaneous route, and low, inadequate, or unmonitored administration of a drug with variable dose-activity responses due to variable protein-binding and natural inhibitors within the circulation and thrombi. In addition, beneficial effects of short-term heparin are probably only measurable during its administration, since the long-term healing required after plaque disruption leaves a thrombotic surface for circulating blood and thrombosis is reactivated with early cessation of heparin therapy.[126]

The second Gruppo Italiano per lo Studio della Sopravvivenza nell' Infarto Miocardico (GISSI-2) trial and its international extension [138,139] compared the efficacy of streptokinase and rt-PA plus aspirin and whether added benefit resulted when subcutaneous heparin (12,500 U twice daily) was started 12 hours after the onset of thrombolytic therapy. GISSI-2 found no difference in overall mortality between the two thrombolytic agents, although streptokinase was associated with fewer strokes. The addition of delayed subcutaneous heparin had no effect on mortality at 35 days (9.3 vs. 9.4%, Table 30B-13). However, there was a significant reduction in in-hospital mortality when heparin was added to aspirin during the scheduled period of treatment (5.4 vs. 6.0%, $P < 0.05$; Table 30B-14). A significant difference in mortality favoring heparin was found when evaluating deaths that occurred in patients who did or did not receive the randomized therapy.

ISIS-3 compared streptokinase, rt-PA, and acylated plasminogen streptokinase activator complex (APSAC) plus aspirin with or without subcutaneous heparin (12,500 U twice daily, with a 4-hour delay from the start of thrombolytic therapy and no initial bolus) versus no heparin in 41,299 patients with acute MI.[140] No differences were found in mortality between thrombolytic agents and no reduction in reinfarction or 35-day mortality (10.3 vs. 10.6% with and without heparin; see Table

Table 30B-11 Warfarin after myocardial infarction (MI) in the Warfarin Re-Infarction Study (WARIS)*[132]

	Warfarin	Placebo	*P*
No. of patients	607	607	
Mortality, %	15	20	<0.03
Recurrent MI, %	14	20	<0.0007
Receiving β-blockers	14	22	
Not receiving β-blockers	13	19	
Cerebrovascular accident, %	3.3	7.2	<0.002
Serious bleeding, %	0.6	0	NS

*1,214 survivors of MI aged ≤75; randomized within 27 days of MI; average follow-up, 37 months.
Data from Smith P, Arnesen H, Holme I: The effect of warfarin on mortality and reinfarction after myocardial infarction. *N Engl J Med* 323:147-152, 1990.

Table 30B-12 Recurrent myocardial infarction (MI) and death with long-term anticoagulant therapy (ACRx) after MI in the Anticoagulants in the Secondary Prevention of Events in Coronary Thrombosis (ASPECT) trial

	Event rate/100 patient-years (intention to Rx)	
Event	ACRx (*n* = 1,700)	Placebo (*n* = 1,704)
Death, any cause	3.2	3.6
Vascular deaths	2.5	2.7
First recurrent MI	2.3	5.1
First cerebral event	0.7	1.2
Vascular event	4.8	7.9
Major bleeding	1.4	0.4

Double-blind, randomized, placebo-controlled trial (no aspirin); 3,404 survivors of MI within 6 weeks of dismissal; target prothrombin time, international normalized ratio of 2.8-4.8; mean follow-up of 37 months (range, 6 to 76). "Bad outcome," 24% lower than placebo.
Modified from Anticoagulants in the Secondary Prevention of Events in Coronary Thrombosis (ASPECT) Research Group: Effect of long-term oral anticoagulant treatment on mortality and cardiovascular morbidity after myocardial infarction. *Lancet* 343:499-503, 1994.

Table 30B-13 Randomized trials of adjunctive use of subcutaneous heparin with thrombolytic therapy: effect on mortality and bleeding complications

Study	Lytic agent	Adjunctive strategy	No. of patients	Mortality, %	Mortality or disabling stroke, %	Hemorrhagic stroke, %	Major bleeding, %
GISSI-2[138,139]	SK, t-PA	ASA	10,407	9.4	. . .	0.4	0.5*
		ASA+H-SC	10,361	9.3	. . .	0.3	1.0
ISIS-3[140]	SK, t-PA	ASA	20,643	10.6	. . .	0.4†	0.8†
	APSAC	ASA+H-SC	20,656	10.3	. . .	0.6	1.0
GUSTO[141]	SK	ASA+H-SC	9,841	7.2	7.7	0.5	0.3
	SK	ASA+H-IV	10,410	7.4	7.9	0.5	0.5
	Acc t-PA	ASA+H-IV	10,396	6.3‡	6.9	0.7§	0.4
	SK+t-PA	ASA+H-IV	10,374	7.0	7.6	0.9‡	0.6

Acc, accelerated; APSAC, acylated plasminogen-streptokinase activator complex; ASA, aspirin; GISSI, Gruppo Italiano per lo Studio della Sopravvivenza nell' Infarto Miocardico; GUSTO, Global Utilization of Streptokinase or Tissue-type Plasminogen Activator for Occluded Coronary Arteries; H-IV: intravenous heparin (aPTT, 60-85 sec); H-SC: subcutaneous heparin, 12,500 U twice daily, begun 4 hours (ISIS-3, GUSTO) or 12 hours (GISSI-2) after lytic therapy; ISIS, International Study of Infarct Survival; SK, streptokinase; t-PA, tissue-type plasminogen activator.
P * < 0.01, † < 0.05, ‡ < 0.001, and § = 0.03 compared with subcutaneous heparin; GUSTO trial did not compare heparin with no heparin.

Table 30B-14 Thrombolysis in acute myocardial infarction and adjunctive medical therapy: comparison of mortality in patients assigned to subcutaneous heparin plus aspirin or aspirin alone

Trial	Mortality, % ( ) total patients		
	ASA + heparin	ASA alone	*P*
ISIS-3[140]	7.4 (1,534)	7.9 (1,633)	0.06
GISSI-2[138,139]	5.4 (537)	6.0 (606)	0.05
Combined	6.8 (2,071)	7.3 (2,239)	0.01

Difference appeared only during treatment period (i.e., in hospital): ISIS-3, 0 to 7 days; GISSI-2, 0 to dismissal.

30B-13). During the scheduled 7 days of heparin, there was a trend toward lower mortality (see Table 30B-14) and a lower incidence of reinfarction (3.2 vs. 3.5%, P = 0.09) with heparin compared with no heparin. If both trials are pooled during the 7-day treatment period, heparin had lower mortality than no heparin (see Table 30B-14).

Since heparin administration was often "too little too late" in large clinical trials, the results of GISSI-2 and ISIS-3 trials have been criticized.[142] The delay of 4 to 12 hours for the start of subcutaneous heparin administered without a bolus most likely led to subtherapeutic aPTT levels during the first 24 to 48 hours,[143] when reocclusion, especially with tissue-type plasminogen activator (t-PA), is most likely to occur.[144]

The Studio sulla Calciparina Nell'Angina e nella Trombosi Ventricolare Nell'Infarto (SCATI) trial showed a significant reduction in mortality with heparin therapy in 711 patients with acute MI (433 admitted within 6 hours of symptoms) who received streptokinase (1,500,000 U/hr). Heparin was administered with an initial bolus of 2,000 U intravenously at the start of thrombolysis, followed 9 hours later by 12,500 U subcutaneously every 12 hours until hospital dismissal. No aspirin was given. Heparin treatment reduced in-hospital mortality from 8.8% to 4.5% (P = 0.05). Patients who received heparin without thrombolysis showed reduced in-hospital mortality (7.7% with heparin vs. 11.7% without heparin, P = 0.10). Recurrent ischemia was reduced from 19.6% to 14.2% (P = 0.08).

Although no anticoagulant therapy was mandated in the ISIS-2 trial,[139] more than 60% of patients received heparin intravenously or subcutaneously. Mortality was reduced in all treatment groups (streptokinase, aspirin, or both) as the intensity of planned heparin therapy increased. The lowest mortality occurred when streptokinase plus aspirin was combined with intravenous heparin (Table 30B-15).

The Global Utilization of Streptokinase and Tissue Plasminogen Activator for Occluded Coronary Arteries (GUSTO) trial (see Table 30B-13) was not designed to test the value of heparin, but the low absolute mortality rates and very low rates of reocclusion of 4.9% to 6.4% in all groups[106] suggest a beneficial effect of combined heparin and aspirin, since these are the lowest rates of reocclusion yet reported. No large-scale clinical trial has prospectively compared intravenous heparin plus aspirin with aspirin alone. However, heparin may be suboptimal as a thrombin inhibitor with mural thrombus, especially during thrombolysis. Newer, more potent direct thrombin inhibitors, such as hirudin, may improve the speed and extent of thrombolysis, improve the incidence of Thrombolysis in Myocardial Infarction (TIMI) grade 3 reperfusion with thrombolytic therapy, and reduce the residual stenosis and thrombus burden; this is being tested in TIMI-9b and GUSTO IIb.

Risks of anticoagulation. Proper selection of patients appears to be most important for reducing the risks of anticoagulation. The incidence of fatal bleeding due to therapy with heparin appears to be increased in patients more than 70 years old.[61] In one study of more than 8,000 patients, bleeding was associated with local disease in the bleeding organ in 64% of episodes and was more frequent in those over 65 years of age (in 3.8% followed for a mean of 7½ years) compared with those less than 65 years old (1.9%) but was significant for age in females only.[145] The increased risk of bleeding with age in patients receiving anticoagulants was not seen in another study.[131] Thus, most trials involving anticoagulants have excluded patients over age 70 as well as those with other known risks for bleeding (uncontrolled systemic hypertension, preexisting hemorrhagic diatheses, gastroduodenal ulceration,

Table 30B-15 Effect of heparin therapy "planned at entry" on 35-day vascular mortality in each of the treatment groups in the Second International Study of Infarct Survival[139]

Heparin	Mortality, % ( ) total patients			
	Streptokinase and aspirin	Streptokinase	Aspirin	Double placebo
Intravenous	6.4 (1,024)	8.3 (2,054)	8.7 (2,048)	13.1 (1,023)
Subcutaneous	7.6 (1,805)	9.0 (3,601)	9.4 (3,605)	13.5 (1,800)
None	9.6 (1,463)	10.1 (2,937)	9.8 (2,934)	12.9 (1,477)

malignancy, and hepatic disease). Bleeding in the SCATI trial[94] was 4.4% in those treated with heparin versus 0.6% in the control group. In general, bleeding is increased when heparin is combined with thrombolytic therapy (intracranial bleeding, 0.3% to 0.5%) but remains very low when heparin is used without lytic therapy (intracranial bleeding, 0.1% to 0.2% or less). Bleeding is also highly dependent on the intensity of therapy and remains minimal when the aPTT is controlled between 60 and 85 seconds compared with aPTTs in excess of 85 seconds (especially when combined with lytic therapy).[146,147] A meta-analysis of the ISIS trials showed that the incidence of intracranial bleeding increased with systolic blood pressure above 130 to 140 mm Hg on admission (personal communication, Peter Sleight, 1994).

Intracranial bleeding with warfarin therapy remains very low, with international normalized ratios (INRs) in the therapeutic range of 2.8 to 4.0 (see Tables 30B-11 and 30B-12). Long-term treatment with warfarin with the INR generally in the range of 2.0 to 3.0 results in an intracranial bleeding risk of approximately 0.3% per year in studies of warfarin therapy in nonvalvular atrial fibrillation.[148] The risk of bleeding probably increases with age above 75, especially if combined with an INR above 3.0 and higher systolic blood pressures.[148,149] High-dose aspirin therapy, especially over 325 mg, should be avoided with the use of warfarin, since this greatly increases the risk of bleeding, especially from the gastrointestinal tract.[150]

Use of low-dose heparin therapy in myocardial infarction. Heparin in low doses acts mainly by increasing the rate at which antithrombin III (antifactor Xa) combines with and inactivates activated factor X in the circulation.[151] A pronounced inhibition in clotting results from a modest interference in activity because factor X acts before thrombin does, at the beginning of the final stage of the coagulation cascade.[152]

With the subcutaneous route of administration, plasma concentrations of heparin increase only slightly but are maintained for hours.[153] Low-dose heparin allows effective antithrombotic therapy without significantly increasing the risk of bleeding, since there is no effect on the clotting time and only a mild to modest prolongation of the partial thromboplastin time.[153-155] Thus, laboratory monitoring is not required, and routine screening of the hemostatic mechanism before therapy is not necessary.[156]

Therapies such as low-dose heparin which reduce the incidence of venous thrombosis will also reduce the incidence of pulmonary emboli. Similar principles have been applied to the reduction of venous thrombosis with low-dose heparin in patients with acute MI (Table 30B-16), again without increasing the incidence of bleeding, even in patients who are at high risk for bleeding. Phlebography showed not only a reduction in calf vein thrombi but also a reduction in the incidence of propagation to the iliofemoral veins, which is of importance in preventing pulmonary emboli. It is important that therapy be started as soon as possible after admission for suspected or definite MI, since low-dose heparin is preventive but not therapeutic for venous thrombosis. The reduction of venous thrombosis and its propagation beyond the calf veins in patients with acute MI will also significantly reduce the risk of pulmonary emboli.

Therapeutic recommendations

ANTITHROMBOTIC THERAPY WITHOUT THROMBOLYTIC THERAPY. All patients with suspected acute MI should receive 160 to 325 mg of chewable aspirin as soon as possible. Daily doses of 80 to 160 mg should be continued indefinitely.

Meta-analysis of parenteral heparin therapy in acute MI showed a reduction in mortality by 17% to 22%, stroke by 50%, reinfarction by 22%, and pulmonary embolism by 54%.[105] Intravenous heparin and nitroglycerin therapy without lytic therapy resulted in patency of the infarct-related artery in 75% of patients after 10 to 14 days.[159] This suggests that all patients with ST elevation (involving Q-wave MI) should receive therapeutic heparin (aPTT, 60 to 85 sec) for the duration of the hospitalization. Results of the ATACS study in patients with non-Q-wave MI and unstable angina suggest that all patients should receive heparin plus aspirin (160 mg loading dose plus 80 mg daily thereafter) throughout the hospitalization.[122] This study also suggests that these patients should be switched from heparin to therapeutic warfarin (INR, 2.0 to 3.0) combined with aspirin, 80 mg per day, for at least 2 to 3 months after the infarction, but prospective studies of patients with MI are currently ongoing (CARS and CHAMPS studies).

Patients with anterior Q-wave MI are at increased risk for left ventricular mural thrombus and systemic embolization. They should receive therapeutic heparin treatment throughout hospitalization (aPTT, 60 to 85 sec) and switch to oral anticoagulation for approximately 3 months (INR 2.0 to 3.0), especially patients with persistent apical akinesis or dyskinesis.

Intravenous heparin should be administered with an intravenous bolus of 5,000 U (or approximately 70 U/kg) to saturate all heparin-binding proteins and endothelial-binding sites and followed by an intravenous infusion starting at 1,000 U/hr. A repeat aPTT should be done at

Table 30B-16 Effect of low-dose heparin therapy on venous thrombosis detected by ^{125}I-labeled fibrinogen leg scanning in patients with acute myocardial infarction: prospective randomized trials

Study	Dose interval	No. of patients with venous thrombosis/total no. (%) Control	Heparin
Handley et al.[52]	q12h	7/24 (29)	6/26 (23)
Warlow et al.[157]	q12h	11/64 (17)	2/63 (3)
Gallus et al.[154]	q8h	9/40 (23)	1/38 (3)
Emerson and Marks[158]	q12h	14/41 (34)	2/37 (5)

4 to 6 hours, at 12 hours, and at 24 hours, and the infusion adjusted to maintain the aPTT at 60 to 85 seconds. Intravenous heparin monitoring and dosage adjustment guidelines are outlined in chapter 28B, Table 28B-4.

ANTITHROMBOTIC THERAPY WITH THROMBOLYTIC THERAPY. Most large studies showing reduced mortality with thrombolytic therapy employing streptokinase or rt-PA also show a beneficial effect of adjunctive therapy with heparin, aspirin, or both. Angiographic data suggest that immediate heparin and aspirin are required to reduce simultaneous thrombosis and subsequent reocclusion. No studies have shown reocclusion rates less than 7% in patients who are not receiving heparin and aspirin.[106] The best therapy to maximize endogenous lysis of residual thrombus is not entirely known, but individual studies suggest that longer-term anticoagulant therapy, for at least 3 to 4 weeks, may be needed after thrombolysis.[118,160]

All patients without contraindications should receive 160 to 325 mg of chewable aspirin as soon as acute MI is suspected and continue daily and indefinitely with 80 to 160 mg per day.

Heparin should be administered as an intravenous bolus of 5,000 U (or approximately 70 U/kg) as soon as MI is suspected and followed immediately by an infusion of 1,000 U/hr to maintain the aPTT at 60 to 85 seconds, using the guidelines for intravenous heparin administration and monitoring outlined in chapter 28B, Table 28B-4. Because recent studies suggest that excessive heparin doses during thrombolysis contribute to intracranial hemorrhage,[146,147] maintenance of the aPTT between 60 and 85 seconds is advised for patients on thrombolytic therapy. The aPTT should be checked at 4 to 6 hours and again at 12 hours, and repeated 24 hours after the start of therapy. Intravenous therapy should be continued for 3 to 5 days and may be followed by subcutaneous heparin (minimum dosage, 12,500 U every 12 hours; average dose from five studies, 17,000 U every 12 hours[101]) to prolong the aPTT to 60 to 85 seconds for the remainder of the hospitalization. Patients receiving streptokinase may be treated with subcutaneous heparin from the beginning of thrombolytic therapy but should have a bolus of at least 5,000 U to achieve immediate therapeutic levels, especially in patients with acute anterior MI who may be at risk of developing left ventricular mural thrombus (two-thirds form within 48 hours). Less than 50% of patients achieve adequate anticoagulation with an aPTT >1.5 times control if 12,500 U is given every 12 hours as a fixed dose.

Switching heparin to warfarin and overlapping for 3 to 5 days (see guidelines in chapter 28B, Table 28B-6) until the prothrombin time is within therapeutic range (INR 2.0 to 3.0 when given with aspirin or 2.5 to 3.5 when administered alone) appear necessary to maximize potential endogenous lysis of residual thrombus and reduction of coronary events; this is currently being tested in prospective trials in acute MI. Therapeutic heparin is necessary in patients at risk of left ventricular mural thrombus (anterior Q-wave MI), since starting warfarin therapy without heparin therapy in patients with anterior MI increases the incidence of left ventricular mural thrombus to 62%, compared to 19% during therapeutic heparin use.[161]

Patients with moderate or worse residual stenosis or angiographically identified thrombus after thrombolysis are at particular risk for reocclusion and should be empirically anticoagulated with warfarin for 2 to 3 months to minimize residual stenosis, reocclusion, and reinfarction. While patients are on warfarin therapy, the aspirin dose should be reduced to 80 mg per day. Patients who develop recurrent angina, ischemia, or heart failure, have a positive rehabilitation exercise test, or show ST-segment changes with continuous monitoring are candidates for coronary angiography and possible revascularization.

All patients with acute MI are at risk for venous thromboembolism. The usual heparin therapy protects the infarct-related artery, prevents left ventricular mural thrombus, and prevents lower extremity deep venous thrombosis. Early mobilization of the patient, especially within the first 3 days of the acute event, greatly reduces the risk of deep venous thrombosis. Particular risk for deep venous thrombosis occurs in patients who remain bedridden and those with large infarcts or heart failure. Patients not fully anticoagulated or those with contraindications should receive low-dose heparin (5,000 U two or three times daily) before mobilization.

More potent direct thrombin inhibitors, such as hirudin, or inhibitors of platelets, such as glycoprotein IIa/IIIb receptor inhibitors (which also may need concomitant heparin or antithrombin therapy), may offer future alternatives and superiority compared with current therapies. However, until these newer therapies are fully evaluated, heparin and aspirin have an established and important role in the management of acute MI.

Physical activity and mobilization

This topic is discussed in chapter 14.

TECHNIQUES AND PRINCIPLES OF HEMODYNAMIC MONITORING

Clinical signs are often an inaccurate representation of the underlying hemodynamic profile, and this discrepancy is amplified by the pronounced variability in cardiac function during the early phase of acute MI.[162-167] In a patient population characterized by hemodynamic lability, constant hemodynamic monitoring provides a logical basis for the selection of therapy and its evaluation.[168]

Techniques

The introduction of the Swan-Ganz catheter and the development of portable image intensifiers greatly facilitated right heart catheterization during acute MI. Initially, introduction of the catheter required direct cutdown over the antecubital fossa, but more recently the Seldinger approach via the subclavian or the internal jugular vein has gained in popularity. Once the catheter is in the peripheral vein, it is advanced into the superior vena cava and right atrium. With inflation of the balloon and gradual advancement of the catheter, entry into the right ventricle and pulmonary artery is usually possible. The balloon allows the procedure to be performed without fluoroscopy, but fluoroscopic guidance is often useful in obtaining an ideal catheter position for prolonged monitoring. The

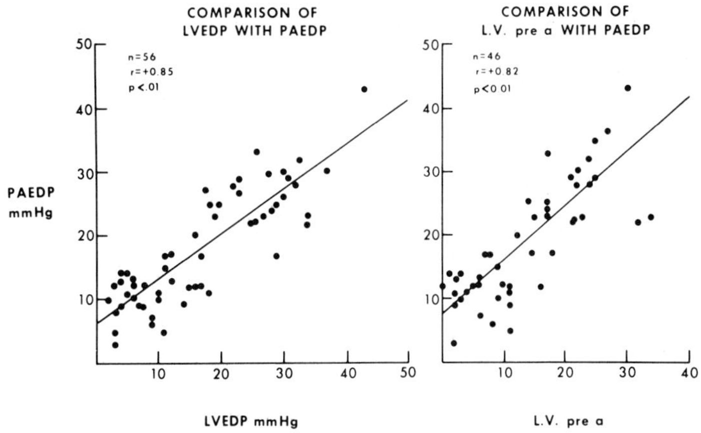

Fig 30B-4 Good correlation is seen between all comparisons of simultaneously recorded pulmonary end-diastolic pressure *(PAEDP)* and left ventricular end-diastolic pressure *(LVEDP) (left)* and between *PAEDP* and left ventricular *(L.V.)* pre-a pressure *(right)*. (From Scheinman M, Evans GT, Weiss A, et al: Relationship between pulmonary artery end-diastolic pressure and left ventricular filling pressure in patients in shock. *Circulation* 47:317-324, 1973. By permission of American Heart Association.)

use of fluoroscopy also reduces the amount of catheter manipulation in the right ventricle and can thereby reduce the incidence of mechanically provoked ventricular arrhythmias—an important consideration during the early phase of acute MI. With the catheter in the pulmonary artery, the pulmonary capillary wedge pressure is obtained by deflating the balloon, advancing it slightly, and then reinflating the balloon. Pulmonary capillary wedge pressure should be compared with pulmonary artery end-diastolic pressure while the balloon is deflated. If the two approximate each other, continuous monitoring of the pulmonary artery end-diastolic pressure is a practical method of monitoring left heart filling pressure[169,170] (Fig 30B-4).

Direct arterial measurement of systemic blood pressure not only is accurate but also provides an accessible site for arterial blood sampling. Percutaneous insertion is usually feasible, but in patients with severe peripheral vasoconstriction or impalpable pulses, a cutdown allowing direct visualization of the radial or brachial artery is needed. If the direct approach is employed, it is still advisable to puncture the artery with a needle and then insert the catheter, because an arteriotomy may cause leakage and bleeding around the site of catheter insertion.

Blood tends to clot in intracardiac catheters, so we use an anticoagulant in the flushing solution (2,500 units of heparin per 500 mL).[171] Regular flushing of venous catheters every 30 minutes is essential to the maintenance of satisfactory technical recordings during prolonged periods of monitoring.

Complications (Table 30B-17)

The uncertain value of the pulmonary artery catheter in some situations was recognized in a review by Matthay and Chatterjee,[172] which suggested guidelines aimed at minimizing the risk-benefit ratio. They emphasized the role of operator experience, early removal of the catheter once its uses are exhausted, awareness of potential pitfalls in pressure measurement, and the need to integrate the hemodynamic variables with other measures of tissue perfusion and clinical status. Serious complications are uncommon, occurring in 4.4% of cases in one series of 528 catheterizations.[173] Nonetheless, the potential for complications reinforces the need to carefully define the indications for hemodynamic monitoring.[173]

Misinterpretation of data. The consequences of therapeutic decisions based on erroneous hemodynamic measurements may be disastrous, and meticulous attention to accuracy is mandatory. A relatively common error is to misinterpret a "damped" pulmonary artery pressure as the mean pulmonary capillary wedge pressure. One can easily avoid this by remembering that the mean wedge pressure cannot be higher than the pulmonary artery end-diastolic pressure. Pressures should be recorded during held expiration or stable respiration, but in severely dyspneic patients this is not always possible. In this situation, pressures should be recorded at a similar time in the respiratory cycle. In patients on a respirator

Table 30B-17 Complications of intracardiac hemodynamic monitoring

Misinterpretation of data
Infection
Arrhythmias
Pulmonary infarction
Complications related to insertion
Pulmonary artery rupture
Ruptured valve chordae
Vena caval and atrial thrombosis

who require positive end-expiratory pressure, pulmonary capillary wedge pressure recorded from a catheter tip lodged within 1 cm or above the left atrium may inaccurately reflect left atrial pressure, according to a report by Shasby and associates.[174] This was particularly notable when the left atrial pressure was low. Catheters located below the level of the left atrium were accurate at all levels of positive end-expiratory pressure tested. The authors suggested that when positive end-expiratory pressure is used, the catheter position in relation to the left atrium should be confirmed on a lateral chest radiograph.

Changes in the patient's position in relation to the reference standard are a further cause of error, but this is easily avoidable. Accurate hemodynamic monitoring requires a thorough understanding of pressure waveforms, appreciation of the artifacts that may distort the waveforms, and attention to detail and recording techniques.

Infection. The incidence of infection can be kept low by strict adherence to sterile technique. Positive cultures from the tips of indwelling pulmonary artery catheters were obtained in 19% of 153 patients in a general intensive care unit at our institution.[175] A positive culture from the catheter tip was significantly associated with the known presence of a focus of infection before insertion and with retention of catheters for longer than 4 days.[175] Infection may result from contamination during placement or removal or from transient or persistent bacteremia. Infection is unlikely to result from pulmonary artery catheters, provided that they are used only in patients who have no evidence of sepsis, that repositioning is kept to a minimum, and that the catheter is removed within 72 hours.[176] Extrapolation from experience gained with temporary pacing suggests that infection is more common when the femoral vein is used as a portal of entry.[177]

Among patients undergoing flow-directed pulmonary artery catheterization, right-sided subendocardial lesions and sterile thrombi in addition to infective endocarditis with positive blood cultures were noted in approximately half.[178] Many of these lesions may be incidental autopsy findings, but the development from infected vegetations probably results directly from catheter-induced endocardial damage with concurrent or subsequent bacteremia.[178]

Pulmonary hemorrhage. This is a rare but catastrophic complication of hemodynamic monitoring; advanced age, pulmonary hypertension, and anticoagulant therapy are predisposing factors.[179] Treatment requires correction of coagulation disorders, transfusion, endobronchial intubation with aspiration, and the use of positive end-expiratory pressure. Pulmonary arteriography has been advocated, and successful therapeutic embolism of bleeding pulmonary artery pseudoaneurysms has been reported.[179]

Arrhythmias. Ventricular irritability is a feature of acute MI, particularly in the first few hours. Mechanical provocation with the catheter can cause ventricular tachycardia and fibrillation. Early reports of catheter use in intensive care units suggested that provocation of serious ventricular arrhythmias was infrequent.[168] However, Sprung and associates[180] reported ventricular arrhythmias in 29 of 60 critically ill patients undergoing right-sided Swan-Ganz catheterization; ventricular tachycardia developed in 20 patients and sustained ventricular tachycardia in 3. Factors possibly contributing to this high incidence of arrhythmias were the use of a triple-lumen catheter, a longer duration of manipulation because of technical problems in entering the pulmonary artery, and biochemical abnormalities such as ischemia, shock, acidosis, and electrolyte disturbances that can predispose the heart to arrhythmias. The best means of reducing the incidence of arrhythmic complications is to avoid vigorous catheter manipulation or coiling in the right ventricle, and fluoroscopy is helpful in this regard. A bolus of lidocaine, 50 to 75 mg, given before insertion of the catheter is recommended if no contraindications are seen. Complete heart block during balloon catheter insertion has also been reported, and is more likely in patients with preexisting left bundle-branch block.[181]

Pulmonary infarction. The catheter should never be left in the wedge position, nor should the balloon be inflated for a prolonged period, because vessel occlusion may lead to pulmonary infarction.[182] Such infarcts are usually minor, do not cause symptoms, and are diagnosed radiologically. This complication is avoidable by diligent monitoring of the pressure waveform and early recognition of spontaneous migration of the catheter into the wedge position.

Complications related to sites of insertion. Such complications usually reflect operator experience and attention to technique. The potential complications are described later in this chapter in relation to temporary pacemaker implantation.

Catheter knotting, pulmonary artery rupture, and ruptured tricuspid valve chordae tendineae. These complications are potentially serious but are fortunately rare[183-186] (Fig 30B-5). Careful attention to technique is essential. Care must be exercised in inflating the balloon, particularly when the location of the catheter tip in the pulmonary artery bed is unknown. Balloon inflation

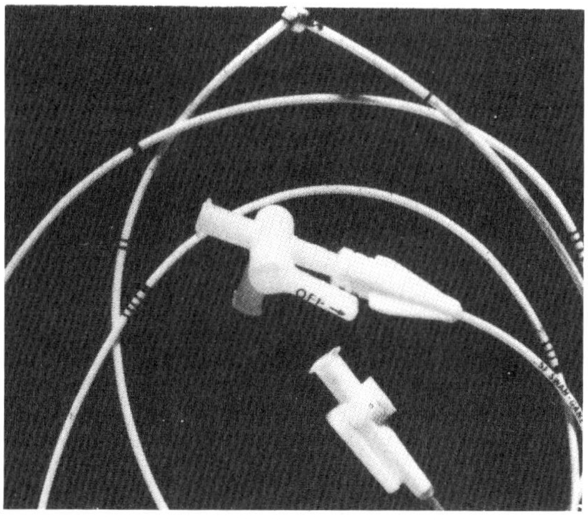

Fig 30B-5 Firm knot situated 14 cm from the tip of the flow-directed balloon-tipped catheter. (From Lipp H, O'Donoghue K, Resnekov L: Intracardiac knotting of a flow-directed balloon catheter [letter to the editor]. *N Engl J Med* 284:220, 1971. By permission.)

should be done with pressure monitoring and avoiding excessive catheter manipulation. The "wedge" time should be kept to a minimum, especially in patients with pulmonary hypertension. Guidelines for the safe use of these catheters have been published.[171,180,187]

Vena caval and atrial thrombosis. In the initial report of Swan-Ganz catheterization, thrombosis of the atrium and superior vena cava was described in one patient,[168] and subsequent reports substantiated this unusual complication and also noted perforation of the pulmonary valve.[175]

Hemodynamic data and calculations

Perhaps the most useful hemodynamic measurement is pulmonary capillary wedge pressure, which reflects left ventricular filling pressure.[171] Studies in patients with acute MI have emphasized that central venous pressure is often a poor guide to left ventricular filling pressure (Fig 30B-6). Discrepancies between the clinical and radiologic assessment of left ventricular filling pressure and measurement of the pulmonary capillary wedge pressure have also been stressed in previous studies.[163-166,169,170]

Direct measurement of the pulmonary capillary wedge pressure, systemic blood pressure, right atrial pressure, and cardiac index (the last often by thermodilution and use of the Fick principle)[188] permits the calculation of derived hemodynamic variables, specifically systemic and pulmonary vascular resistance, stroke volume, stroke index, and right and left ventricular work and stroke work index. Construction of a ventricular function curve by alteration of the preload with infusion of low-molecular-weight dextran or similar agents may help assess serial changes in cardiac performance and the response to therapeutic intervention.[171,189,190] Such curves have demonstrated that the "optimum" filling pressure in acute MI is higher than normal and lies between 16 and 20 mm Hg[189-191] (Fig 30B-7).

The use of pulmonary capillary wedge pressure or pulmonary artery end-diastolic pressure and right atrial pressure as indicators of left and right ventricular filling volume in the construction of ventricular function curves is based on several assumptions. Volume expansion is a clinical application of the Frank-Starling principle relating tension development to resting fiber length. In the intact left heart and in the absence of mitral valve disease, the pulmonary capillary wedge pressure is relatively far removed from end-diastolic fiber length and ventricular volume, particularly since the relation between pressure and volume depends partly on ventricular compliance. In the first few hours after infarction, quite pronounced changes occur in ventricular compliance; it initially increases and subsequently decreases.[192,193] These changes may radically alter estimates of ventricular filling volume based on pulmonary capillary wedge pressure, since that measurement is not a direct index of left

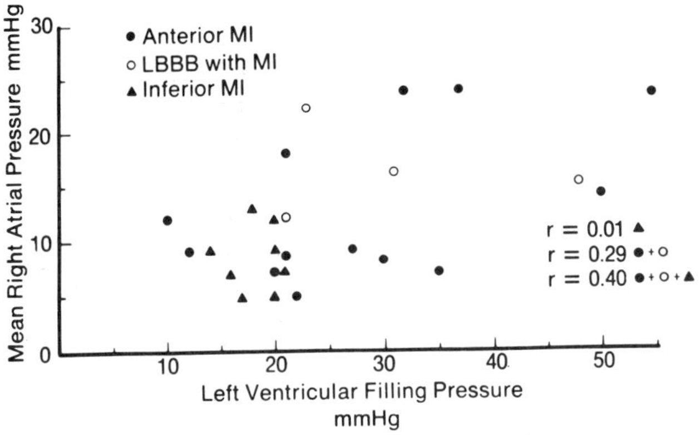

Fig 30B-6 Mean right atrial pressure is compared with left ventricular filling pressure measured as pulmonary artery end-diastolic pressure or left ventricular end-diastolic pressure in patients with acute myocardial infarction *(MI)*. There is no significant correlation between central venous and left ventricular filling pressures in anterior or inferior infarction or in left bundle-branch block *(LBBB),* and this prevents the electrocardiographic localization of the infarction. (From Rackley CE, Russell RO Jr: Coronary Care: Invasive Techniques for Hemodynamic Measurements. Dallas, American Heart Association, 1973, pp 1-36. By permission.)

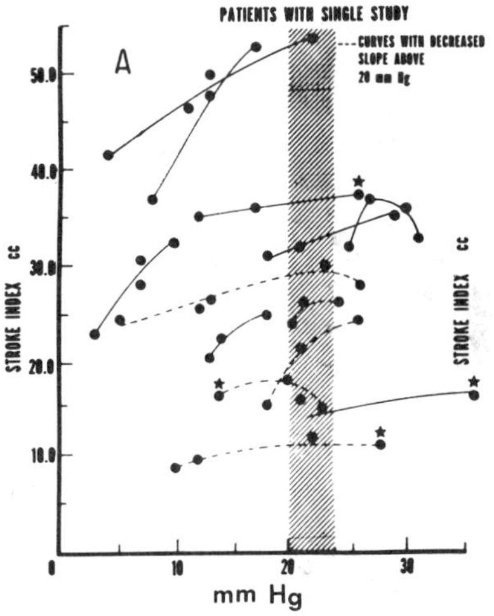

Fig 30B-7 Composite of ventricular function curves relating stroke index to left ventricular end-diastolic pressure or pulmonary artery end-diastolic pressure. In these patients with acute myocardial infarction, an increase in stroke index (and other descriptors of function) generally continued until the left ventricular filling pressure reached 20 to 24 mm Hg *(solid curves);* beyond this pressure, the curves tended to flatten or decrease *(dashed curves).* A *star* identifies each of the five curves whose ratio ΔSI/ΔFP (stroke index/filling pressure) was less than 0.30 mL/mm Hg. See text for further discussion. (From Russell RO Jr, Rackley CE, Pombo J, et al: Effects of increasing left ventricular filling pressure in patients with acute myocardial infarction. *J Clin Invest* 49:1539-1550, 1970. By permission of the American Society for Clinical Investigation.)

Table 30B-18 Clinical subsets of acute myocardial infarction

Subset	Pulmonary congestion	Peripheral hypoperfusion	Mortality %	Mortality No.	CI	PCP
I	No	No	1	1 of 75	2.7 ± 0.5	12 ± 7
II	Yes	No	11	4 of 36	2.3 ± 0.4	23 ± 5
III	No	Yes	18	4 of 22	1.9 ± 0.4	12 ± 5
IV	Yes	Yes	60	40 of 67	1.6 ± 0.6	27 ± 8

CI, cardiac index (liters/min per m^2); PCP, pulmonary capillary pressure (mm Hg).
From Forrester JS, Diamond GA, Swan HJC: Correlative classification of clinical and hemodynamic function after acute myocardial infarction. *Am J Cardiol* 39:137-145, 1977. By permission of Technical Publishing Company.

ventricular end-diastolic pressure. However, hemodynamic monitoring in acute MI is worthwhile and sometimes indispensable.

Other applications of specialized balloon catheters include continuous monitoring and sampling of mixed venous and pulmonary artery oxygen saturation.[194] A different multipurpose catheter incorporates electrodes in both the right ventricle and the right atrium for ventricular and atrial pacing.

Indications for hemodynamic monitoring

The indications for hemodynamic monitoring rely on clinical judgment. Monitoring has obvious value in the diagnosis and assessment of the complications and hemodynamic perturbations associated with acute MI, but is also valuable in assessing prognosis, response to therapy, and value of newer therapeutic interventions.[195] In general, hypotension and features suggesting peripheral hypoperfusion warrant hemodynamic monitoring. If compromised or even borderline hemodynamic status is suspected, monitoring should be done, particularly since the catheter can be withdrawn if the hemodynamic measurements are normal.

The major indications for hemodynamic monitoring are distinguishing between hypovolemia and pump failure and between ruptured ventricular septum and acute mitral regurgitation; management of severe left ventricular failure; differentiation of the adult respiratory distress syndrome from acute left ventricular failure; evaluation and management of low-cardiac-output syndromes; and diagnosis and therapy of pulmonary embolism, tamponade, and right ventricular infarction. Sometimes, as in differentiating ruptured ventricular septum from acute mitral regurgitation, echocardiography supplants the diagnostic role of hemodynamic monitoring.

In patients with left ventricular failure and acute MI, the clinical profile and hemodynamic spectrum vary but they dictate the therapy. Subdividing patients with acute MI into hemodynamic subsets that have therapeutic and prognostic implications arose from numerous investigations.[165,166,196,197] Swan-Ganz catheterization may be invaluable in categorizing and managing these patients[166,198] (Table 30B-18). Preload-reducing agents may be hazardous with low or normal wedge pressure (see

Table 30B-19 Recommendations for balloon flotation right heart catheterization in acute myocardial infarction

Class I

1. Severe or progressive congestive heart failure
2. Cardiogenic shock or progressive hypotension
3. Mechanical complications of acute infarction, such as a ventricular septal defect or papillary muscle rupture

Class IIA

1. Hypotension not responding rapidly to fluid administration in a patient without evidence of pulmonary congestion
2. Before giving a fluid challenge in a patient with circulatory insufficiency and suspected pulmonary congestion
3. As a diagnostic tool when there is suspicion of an intracardiac shunt, acute mitral insufficiency, or pericardial tamponade

Class IIB

1. Patients with acute myocardial infarction who are hemodynamically stable but have evidence of mild pulmonary congestion

Class III

1. Patients with acute myocardial infarction who are hemodynamically stable and do not have evidence of cardiac or pulmonary complications

Class I: usually indicated, always acceptable, and considered useful and effective; class II: acceptable, of uncertain efficacy, and may be controversial; A: weight of evidence in favor of usefulness and efficacy; B: not well established by evidence, can be helpful, and probably not harmful; class III: not indicated, may be harmful.
From Gunnar RM, Passamani ER, Bourdillon PD, et al: Guidelines for the early management of patients with acute myocardial infarction. A report of the American College of Cardiology/American Heart Association Task Force on Assessment of Diagnostic and Therapeutic Cardiovascular Procedures (Subcommittee to Develop Guidelines for the Early Management of Patients with Acute Myocardial Infarction). *J Am Coll Cardiol* 16:249-292, 1990. By permission of the American College of Cardiology.

subset III, Table 30B-18). Hypovolemic patients may have moderate hypotension, a pulmonary capillary wedge pressure of less than 10 mm Hg, and a cardiac index of less than 2.5 mg/min per m^2. Their clinical presentation may be misleading, and so they must be correctly identified and treated by volume repletion. Newer echocardiographic techniques have yet to be evaluated as determinants of therapy and prognosis.

"Inappropriate vasodilatation" with hypotension is rare and poorly understood. These patients are warm and well perfused yet hypotensive. Often no therapy is required, but recognition that the hypotension does not result from pump failure prevents unnecessary intervention. The possibility of gram-negative septicemia, which may cause similar hemodynamic changes, must be excluded (Tables 30B-19 and 30B-20).

LIMITATION OF SIZE OF MYOCARDIAL INFARCT

The degree of myocardial necrosis is directly related to the development of heart failure, cardiogenic shock, and death.[199-202] Loss of approximately 25% of the myocardial tissue frequently leads to heart failure, and loss in excess of 40% may result in cardiogenic shock and death as assessed by postmortem studies.[199-202] However, radionuclear studies using tomographic technetium-sestamibi imaging showed that the infarcted region may exceed 60% of the left ventricle in some patients who are dismissed from the hospital after acute MI.[203] The main factor influencing mortality after MI, or in any patient with coronary artery disease, is the degree of left ventricular dysfunction.[204-213] In addition, frequent and complex ventricular ectopy in the late hospital phase after acute MI also appears to influence mortality after a Q-wave infarction[206,207,210-213] (Table 30B-21).

Most of this ectopy appears to occur in patients with left ventricular dysfunction, especially those with ejection fractions less than 40%.[206,211-213] Rehabilitation exercise testing appears to allow identification of a high-risk subgroup in which most of the patients have ejection fractions less than 40% but some have ejection fractions greater than 40% and ischemic myocardium in jeopardy.[214,215]

Table 30B-20 Recommendations for intra-arterial pressure monitoring in acute myocardial infarction

Class I

1. Patients with severe hypotension (systolic pressure, <80 mm Hg) or cardiogenic shock
2. Patients receiving vasopressor agents

Class IIA

1. Patients receiving intravenous nitroprusside or other powerful arterial dilating agents
2. Hemodynamically stable patients receiving intravenous vasodilators for myocardial ischemia
3. Patients receiving intravenous inotropic agents
4. Patients with life-threatening arrhythmias

Class III

1. Patients with acute myocardial infarction who are hemodynamically stable

See Table 30B-19 for explanation of classification.
From Gunnar RM, Passamani ER, Bourdillon PD, et al: Guidelines for the early management of patients with acute myocardial infarction. A report of the American College of Cardiology/American Heart Association Task Force on Assessment of Diagnostic and Therapeutic Cardiovascular Procedures (Subcommittee to Develop Guidelines for the Early Management of Patients with Acute Myocardial Infarction). *J Am Coll Cardiol* 16:249-292, 1990. By permission of the American College of Cardiology.

Salvage of myocardium

Myocardial necrosis begins in the subendocardium and progresses outward toward the subepicardium at a rate that varies inversely with the amount of time that myocardial blood flow was below a critical level for cell survival.[216] With complete interruption of flow, cells die in 20 to 30 minutes; with residual flow through collateral vessels, cells may resist necrosis for hours.[217] Angiographic and pathoanatomic studies in patients suggest that myocardial necrosis may be limited by the presence of preexisting collaterals[218-221] and that angina preceding MI[218] or persistent chest pain up to the time of reperfusion[222] may be clinical clues to preexisting collateral circulation. After reperfusion in humans, full recovery of ischemic myocardium takes more than 3 days, but compensatory hyperkinesis may regress earlier. Thus, left ventricular function that varies or deteriorates early after acute MI may reflect regression of hyperkinesis in the noninfarcted region rather than extension of the infarct.[223]

Table 30B-21 Late sudden death after acute myocardial infarction

Ejection fraction after infarction, %	Repetitive VPB	Sudden death %	Sudden death No./total
>40	No	1.5	3/199
≤40	No	6.9	6/87
>40	Yes	7.2	4/55
≤40	Yes	25.5	12/47
		6.4	25/388

VPB, ventricular premature beats in couplets or runs.
Data from Mukharji J, Rude RE, Poole K, et al: Late sudden death following acute myocardial infarction: importance of combined presence of repetitive ventricular ectopy and left ventricular dysfunction (abstract). *Clin Res* 30:208A, 1982.

Factors influencing degree of ischemia or necrosis

Myocardial necrosis can be decreased by decreasing myocardial oxygen demand (heart rate, afterload, preload, and inotropic state), by increasing myocardial oxygen supply (via collateral circulation and especially with reperfusion), or by both.[224,225] Emergency intraaortic balloon pumping for acute anterior MI appeared to interrupt myocardial injury only if residual patency of the left anterior descending coronary artery (as demonstrated by early angiography) was present and balloon pumping was begun no more than 6 hours after onset of chest pain.[226] Pharmacologic and hemodynamic interventions that mainly decrease myocardial oxygen demands have not proved sufficiently efficacious to warrant their routine clinical use.[225] Some studies with β-adrenergic blockers and nitrates have given encouraging results.

β-Adrenergic blocking agents

β-Adrenergic blockers have little effect on blood flow to the ischemic zone[30] but mainly decrease myocardial oxygen demands (reflected by decreased arterial-coronary sinus oxygen difference and total coronary blood flow) by decreasing heart rate, blood pressure, cardiac and stroke indices, and inotropic effects.[227] The pulmonary artery wedge pressure response to propranolol in patients with acute MI shows only small and variable increases or decreases when the initial pressure is less than 25 mm Hg.[227,228] The decreased ischemia produced by these agents has been reflected in decreased myocardial lactate production and decreased ventricular arrhythmia, which may be related in part to blocking the lipolytic effects of catecholamines and thus decreasing the circulating levels of free fatty acids.[227-230]

Beneficial effects of β-blockers in patients with acute myocardial ischemia and infarction have been found by using precordial ST-segment mapping techniques.[29,231-236] Subtotal occlusion or collateral blood flow enhances both the clinical (less ischemic pain) and the electrocardiographic (ECG) responses,[234] probably because decreased myocardial demand has greater impact when there is greater residual blood supply. Although a β-blocker with intrinsic sympathomimetic activity, such as pindolol, has relieved ischemic chest pain, reduced ST-segment elevation, and improved regional wall abnormalities in patients with acute transmural MI,[235] this type of blocker did not significantly reduce infarct size in dogs[237] and failed to reduce mortality in patients after acute MI.[238] This may reflect the lack of reduced heart rate, a major determinant of myocardial oxygen consumption, in patients treated with β-blockers who have sympathomimetic activity.

Although acute administration of practolol (intravenously or orally) to patients with acute MI resulted in lower mortality compared with the placebo group, patients who had tachycardia at the time of entry had no major differences in the clinical course between those treated and the placebo group.[239]

Estimates of infarct size by enzyme release have correlated with subsequent death from pump failure,[240] the incidence of early and late ventricular arrhythmias,[241,242] and the extent of left ventricular dysfunction.[243,244] Only a few studies addressed the effect of acute β-blockade on indices of infarct size. In a small randomized trial of patients with uncomplicated MI, patients treated with propranolol (0.1 mg/kg of body weight intravenously, followed by 320 mg orally over the next 27 hours) within 4 hours after the onset of symptoms had less calculated creatine kinase (CK) release, less cumulative CK appearance into the plasma, and lower peak serum CK levels than control patients.[245]

In addition, patients with suspected MI treated with propranolol in the same dosage within 4 hours after the onset of symptoms had a significantly lower incidence of infarction by ECG criteria and lesser serum CK increases compared to patients in the control group.[246] Thus, threatened infarction might be prevented by acute β-blockade, as suggested by previous studies of acute propranolol therapy in patients with subtotal coronary artery occlusions[234] and by decreased incidence of proved MI in patients with suspected MI admitted to the hospital while on β-blocker therapy.[247]

Similarly, atenolol given intravenously within a median of 4 hours after the onset of symptoms decreased the frequency of acute MI, release of isoenzyme CK-MB, and ischemic pain.[26,248] In prospective, randomized, double-blind trials in patients, acute therapy with alprenolol administered within 12 hours,[249] metoprolol administered within 12 hours,[236] or timolol administered within 5 hours after the onset of symptoms of acute MI resulted in significant limitation of enzymatically estimated infarct size. Intravenous administration of metoprolol within 24 hours (median, 7 hours) after the onset of chest pain decreased 15-day mortality by 13% (4.9% to 4.3%, P = 0.29) and Q wave infarction from 54% to 51% of patients (P = 0.024; decreases were even greater when treatment was earlier, the heart rate times systolic pressure product was higher than the median), and estimated (enzymatic) infarct size was decreased (P = 0.07).[250-252] Intravenous atenolol therapy significantly decreased total mortality in patients with acute MI by 15% after 7 days, but most of this decrease in mortality occurred during the first 24 to 36 hours. No rebound effect occurred when treatment stopped after seven days. Mortality at 1 year showed a significant difference in favor of the atenolol group.[253] β-Blockers with partial agonist activity are not recommended, since they are either less effective in preventing CK release[254] or may even exacerbate CK release or necrosis.[255,256]

Early intravenous β-blockade followed by short-term oral therapy in acute MI has been studied in 30 randomized trials totaling nearly 28,000 patients. This therapy reduces the incidence of infarction by 10% to 15% in patients with threatened MI and reduces infarct size by 20% to 30%. This therapy also reduces the incidence of nonfatal reinfarction, nonfatal cardiac arrest, and mortality, each by about 15%. Treatment should start within 12 hours of the onset of symptoms to be effective. If patients are carefully selected, serious side effects are rare and reversible.[257]

Esmolol, a cardioselective β_1-adrenergic receptor blocker with a half-life of 9 minutes, may enable some patients with relative contraindication to β-blockers to receive and benefit from early β-blocker therapy. It can be useful for screening patients for subsequent therapy with β-blockers. Those who tolerate the esmolol infusion can be given a long-acting β-blocker. In patients with intolerance, the infusion can be stopped, and there is a rapid return to baseline hemodynamics.[258]

Immediate and deferred β-blockade after thrombolytic therapy in patients with acute MI were compared in phase II of the TIMI trial. Of the 1,434 patients enrolled in the β-blocker substudy, approximately half were randomized to each β-blocker group. Fifty-one percent of the patients in TIMI II were excluded from β-blocker therapy because of current β-blocker or calcium-channel blocker therapy on admission (45%), ventricular rate consistently less than 55 beats/min (27%), systolic blood pressure consistently less than 100 mm Hg (21%), rales involving one-third or more of the lung fields or pulmonary edema (16%), significant first-, second-, or third-degree heart block (12%), and asthma or COPD requiring long-term therapy with corticosteroids or β_2-stimulants (11%). Most of the patients (64%) were classified as not low risk, mainly because of anterior MI (56%), age 70 or older (9%), or prior MI (8%). TIMI II showed that immediate intravenous therapy with metoprolol is safe in patients who have evolving MI treated with thrombolysis with rt-PA. Immediate metoprolol therapy reduced the frequency of recurrent nonfatal MI from 4.6% in the deferred group to 2.4% in the immediate group ($P = 0.02$); this significant reduction was accounted for by a significant reduction of nonfatal reinfarction in the not-low-risk patients (from 5.6% in the deferred to 2.0% in the immediate group; $P = 0.005$). Immediate therapy also significantly reduced recurrent ischemia during hospitalization, from 21% in the deferred group to 15% in the immediate group ($P = 0.01$). Intracranial hemorrhage was less frequent in patients receiving immediate β-blocker therapy than in those receiving deferred therapy. No intracranial hemorrhage occurred within 6 days of entry in patients receiving 100 mg of rt-PA and assigned to immediate β-blocker therapy, whereas five patients in the deferred β-blocker group had hemorrhage ($P = 0.03$, not prospective end point). In patients who received 150 mg of rt-PA, intracranial hemorrhage within 6 days of entry occurred in two assigned to the immediate β-blocker group and in five assigned to the deferred β-blocker group (*P*, not significant). Immediate β-blocker therapy did not improve global left ventricular ejection fraction or infarct-zone function measured at hospital dismissal and did not alter total mortality from that in the deferred β-blocker group.[259,260]

Current recommendations. Acute β-blockade in patients not already on such therapy may be especially indicated for the hyperadrenergic state manifested by tachycardia, hypertension, or both without heart failure.[261] Patients already on β-blocker therapy when admitted for acute MI should continue therapeutic doses unless contraindicated. Patients not previously receiving β-blocker therapy who can be treated within the first 12 hours after the onset of symptoms of acute MI are candidates for short-term β-blocker therapy, especially those who continue to have ischemic pain.

β-Blocker therapy is rational,[262,263] safe, and more advantageous in patients who undergo thrombolytic therapy, because the slowing of MI appears to maximize myocardial salvage for reperfusion when therapy to decrease myocardial demand can be started within 1 to 2 hours of the onset of infarction[259,260,264] (Fig 30B-8). The clinical benefits of very early β-blockade are suggested by the TIMI IIB subgroup analysis; 696 patients treated with rt-PA within 2 hours of the onset of symptoms who received immediate β-blocker therapy had a significant reduction in mortality and reinfarction at 42 days compared with 694 patients in whom β-blocker therapy was delayed ($P < 0.01$). In patients treated after 2 hours, mortality and reinfarction were similar for immediate and deferred β-blocker therapy.[259] However, the reduced nonfatal reinfarction, recurrent ischemia, and intracranial hemorrhage in patients who received immediate β-blocker therapy and were treated with rt-PA provide compelling evidence for immediate β-blocker therapy, unless contraindicated, in all patients treated with thrombolytic therapy for acute MI.

From 20% to 50% of patients with acute MI may have contraindications to early therapy with a β-blocker.[236,249,259,260] These contraindications include (1) ventricular rate consistently below 50 beats/min; (2) systolic blood pressure consistently below 95 mm Hg; (3) significant first-degree atrioventricular (AV) delay

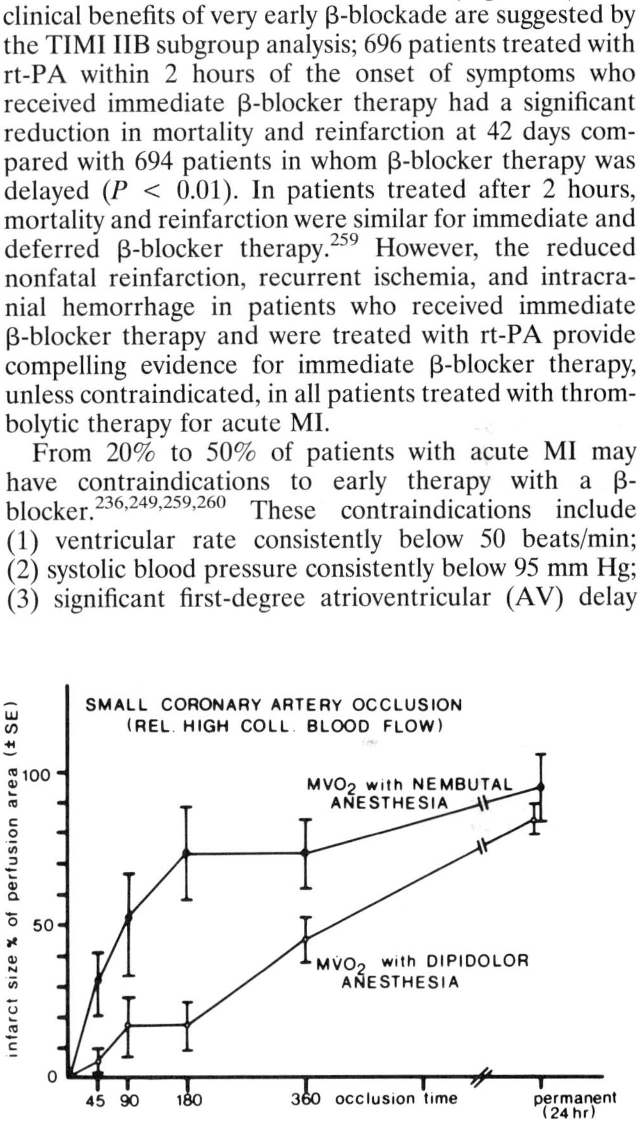

Fig 30B-8 Experimental coronary artery occlusion in control animals (pentobarbital [Nembutal] anesthesia) and animals with decreased myocardial oxygen consumption (*MVO_2*) due to slowing of heart rate by piritramide (Dipidolor) anesthesia showing the delay in myocardial necrosis early after coronary occlusion (especially the first 3 hours) in the latter group. However, with continued total coronary artery occlusion, reduction of MVO_2 does not lead to significant myocardial salvage by 24 hours. (From Schaper W, Schaper J: Der experimentelle Infarkt. Verh Dtsch Ges Herz Kreislaufforsch 45:1-6, 1979. By permission of Dr. Dietrich Steinkopff, Verlag GmbH & Co.)

(P-R interval, >0.24 sec) or second- or third-degree AV block; (4) asthma by history or significant wheezes on examination; and (5) rales extending more than one-third of the way up the lung fields or pulmonary congestion on chest radiograph. β-Blockade should be stopped if 3, 4, or 5 occurs; it should be maintained until recovery of the heart rate and blood pressure above the minimal outlined in 1 and 2 and then decreased to approximately half the dosage if the systolic arterial pressure falls below 90 mm Hg or the ventricular rate falls below 40 beats/min. β-Blockers with β-agonist properties, such as pindolol, have not proved effective, may be detrimental, and should not be used.

Acute β-blocker therapy includes the following alternatives in patients who have not been on maintenance therapy:

1. Propranolol, 0.1 mg/kg intravenously, in three equal doses at 5-minute intervals, followed 1 hour later by oral therapy averaging 40 mg (range, 20 to 80 mg) every 6 hours and adjusted to keep the heart rate below 60 beats/min and free of the contraindications noted above. Before each dose at acute administration, measure and record heart rate, arterial pressure (by cuff or intra-arterial measurement), and a standard ECG strip for AV block or delay. Invasive hemodynamic monitoring is not routinely required but could be used.
2. Metoprolol, 15 mg intravenously, in three equal doses at 2-minute intervals, followed by 50 mg orally every 6 hours (first tablet at 15 minutes after last injection) for 48 hours and then 100 mg twice daily. Use the same monitoring precautions as noted for propranolol.
3. Timolol, 1-mg bolus intravenously, repeated in 10 minutes; follow in another 10 minutes by a constant infusion (0.6 mg/hr) for 24 hours and then 10 mg orally twice daily.
4. Alprenolol, 5 mg intravenously and repeat in 10 minutes if heart rate or blood pressure does not decrease by 10% or more; 3 hours later, start 200 mg orally and continue twice daily.
5. Esmolol, a loading dose infusion of 500 μg/kg per minute for 1 minute, followed by a 4-minute maintenance infusion of 50 μg/kg per minute. If an adequate therapeutic effect is not observed within 5 minutes, repeat the loading dose and follow with a maintenance infusion of 100 μg/kg per minute (the average maintenance dosage). Continue the titration procedure, repeating the loading infusion and increasing the maintenance infusion by increments of 50 μg/kg per minute (for 4 minutes) using the same monitoring precautions as noted for propranolol. Maintenance dosages up to 200 μg/kg per minute may be used, but dosages as high as 300 μg/kg per minute provide little added effect, increase adverse effects, and are not recommended. After adequate heart rate control and stable clinical status are achieved, transition to an orally administered β-blocking agent can be accomplished as follows: Approximately 30 minutes after the first dose of the alternative oral β-blocker, reduce the esmolol infusion rate by 50%. After the second dose of the alternative agent, monitor the patient's response, and if satisfactory control is maintained for the first hour, discontinue the esmolol infusion.

Calcium channel blocking agents

Calcium channel blockers are approved for treatment of stable and unstable angina, systemic hypertension, and arrhythmias. Clinical trials show that verapamil is ineffective in reducing both mortality and the incidence of reinfarction.[265,266] Nifedipine administered alone, with β-blockade, or with thrombolytic therapy during infarction is ineffective in reducing mortality.[267-276] A significant potential problem with nifedipine is that it often causes reflex tachycardia and thus may increase myocardial oxygen consumption.[274,277]

Diltiazem either alone or with β-blockade does not reduce mortality during a Q-wave MI.[278,279] After a Q-wave MI in patients with good left ventricular function, a calcium channel blocker (diltiazem or verapamil) may be used in those who cannot tolerate a β-blocker. Calcium channel blockers should not be used in patients with acute MI who have (1) heart failure or pulmonary congestion on the chest radiograph, (2) a left ventricular ejection fraction of less than 40%, or (3) an anterior Q-wave infarction (in patients whose left ventricular function is not known), because these features have been associated with a greater risk of cardiac death or reinfarction in patients treated with diltiazem.[278]

Administration of diltiazem, 90 mg four times daily by mouth, started between 24 and 72 hours after the onset of a non-Q-wave MI significantly reduced reinfarction at 2 weeks and 1 year and also decreased the 1-year mortality.[280,281]

Current recommendations. Calcium channel blockers have no role in the acute phase of MI. For long-term survivors of Q-wave infarction, calcium channel blockade with diltiazem or verapamil may be useful in those who have good left ventricular function but cannot tolerate β-blockade or in those who need an adjunct to β-blockade. Diltiazem therapy helps reduce the incidence of transmural infarction and angina in patients after a non-Q-wave MI. Calcium channel blockers are contraindicated in patients who have had a MI and have heart failure, left ventricular dysfunction (ejection fraction of <40%), or a large anterior infarction.

Nitrates

Nitroglycerin can decrease myocardial oxygen demand by decreasing preload and afterload and thereby decreasing left ventricular wall tension.[282,283] It also can increase collateral blood flow to the ischemic zone.[284,285] Acute myocardial ischemia may respond differently, depending in part on the route of administration, dose of drug, and hemodynamic status of the patient.[286,287] Ischemia may be reduced in some patients regardless of the status of the left ventricular filling pressure.[288] Hypotension and tachycardia, which can be deleterious clinically, appear to be more likely with sublingual than with intravenous administration.[286,289] The hypotensive effect of nitroglycerin may be reversed by infusion of the α-adrenergic agonist phenylephrine, which decreases myocardial ischemia (determined by change in precordial ST-segment elevation) in some;[286] in other studies, it returned the arterial pressure to baseline levels and resulted in elevation of ST segments to baseline levels.[287] Thus, doses should be titrated and the response closely monitored.

Although decreases in mean arterial pressure of up to 25 mm Hg have been well tolerated,[287,288,290,291] studies[292-294] have aimed at a reduction in mean arterial pressure of 10% with nitroglycerin infusion. Intravenous infusion of nitroglycerin at up to approximately 50 μg/min usually does not increase heart rate.[287,288,290,291,295] At this level, it diminished ST elevation in one study; ST elevation was less diminished at infusion rates of 100 μg/min, and a slight increase in heart rate was noted, especially in patients without heart failure.[295] Severe hypotension and bradycardia may result (9% of patients, even in those without inferior infarction); they respond to leg elevation and atropine intravenously.[296] Clinical trials of intravenous nitroglycerin therapy generally show favorable results in indices of myocardial ischemia and infarct size as well as clinical results. Preliminary results[297] of a randomized trial of prolonged nitroglycerin therapy in 95 patients with acute MI showed reduced ST-segment elevation (by 30% in patients with anterior infarction, 30 minutes after the start of therapy), less R-wave decrease at initially ischemic sites, decreased frequency of serious ventricular arrhythmia, and, in patients with heart failure, a lower mortality (6% in treated vs. 20% in control) in the nitroglycerin-treated group.

In another randomized trial[291] of nitroglycerin infusion in 60 patients with acute MI, the treated group showed significantly reduced peak serum CK levels, rates of CK release, and calculated infarct sizes, especially when therapy was started within 8 hours after the onset of symptoms.

Effect on infarct-related artery. Nearly all considerations for nitroglycerin therapy in acute MI have been based on its effect on hemodynamics, the myocardium, and collateral circulation. No studies have focused specifically on the outcome of the infarct-related artery. Because the necessary adjunctive therapy is complex, the exact role of nitroglycerin is not easily evaluated. However, arterial injury is frequently accompanied by both thrombosis and vasoconstriction. The vasoconstriction has platelet-dependent, endothelium-dependent, and other cause-related components. Experimentally, intravenous administration of nitroglycerin titrated to reduce the mean arterial pressure by 10 mm Hg significantly reduced vasoconstriction and platelet deposition in deeply injured arteries.[298,299] Vasoconstriction can aggravate the problem of reocclusion and enhance platelet deposition and arterial thrombosis[300] (Fig 30B-9). Thus, intravenous administration of nitroglycerin during the first 24 hours in the treatment of MI by thrombolysis may have an empirical role.[300]

Current recommendations. Intravenous nitroglycerin therapy can be administered safely when titrated carefully to avoid hypotension (≥90 mm Hg systolic), tachycardia (heart rate increase ≤20%), or bradycardia (≥45-50 beats/min). Nitroglycerin appears most useful in patients with persistent or recurrent chest pain or with heart failure associated with MI. Other subgroups most likely to benefit might include patients with non-Q-wave or subendocardial infarction or patients who are admitted within 6 hours after the onset of symptoms, who are not candidates for reperfusion, and especially, who also have a history of chronic angina (>20 days before acute infarction); in patients with acute infarction and chronic angina, 77% had collateral circulation to the infarct-related artery[218] and theoretically might benefit most from nitroglycerin therapy.

A safe regimen of nitroglycerin starts with infusion at 10 μg/min and increases by 10 μg/min at 10-minute intervals to achieve a 10% reduction in systolic blood pressure, attain systolic blood pressure of 95 mm Hg, or achieve a maximal dose of 200 μg/min, whichever comes first. Although nitroglycerin administered sublingually in doses of 0.3 to 0.6 mg may be beneficial, this route of administration appears more hazardous because of variable absorption and possible induction of precipitous hypotension. The same dosage of nitroglycerin is rational, empirical therapy for approximately 24 hours during and after thrombolysis for acute MI to decrease the risk of reocclusion, as discussed earlier in this chapter.

Nitroprusside

Sodium nitroprusside is usually more balanced in decreasing preload and afterload than is nitroglycerin (usually stronger in decreasing preload). Several studies suggest that nitroglycerin is superior to nitroprusside for MI or ischemia. A comparative study[301] showed that, although the two drugs had directionally similar hemodynamic actions, nitroglycerin decreased and nitroprusside increased the sum of precordial ST-segment elevations in patients with acute anterior infarction.

In another clinical study,[302] nitroglycerin increased and nitroprusside decreased coronary blood flow to the ischemic zone in patients with collaterals demonstrated angiographically. Thus, it should be used in preference to nitroprusside in patients with acute myocardial ischemia and infarction.

The Veterans Administration Cooperative Study[303] included 812 patients with acute transmural infarction and left ventricular filling pressure of at least 12 mm Hg who were treated a mean of 17 hours after onset of symptoms. When the 48-hour infusion of nitroprusside was begun within 9 hours after symptom onset, early mortality rose compared with the placebo group (24% vs. 13%, respectively). However, late nitroprusside therapy (begun 9 or more hours after symptom onset) resulted in decreased mortality in the treated compared with the placebo group (14% vs. 22%). The use of nitrates was forbidden.

In another randomized trial[304] in 328 patients with acute transmural infarction within 12 hours (mean, 5 hours) after symptom onset, the group receiving nitroprusside infusion for 24 hours followed by isosorbide dinitrate (5 mg every 4 hours) for the next 6 days had a significantly lower early mortality: at 23 days, 3% compared with 11% in the placebo group. At 4 weeks, the mortality was still lower in the treated group: 5.5% compared with 12.1% in the control group. The mortality was also lower in the treated group at 24 hours (0 vs. 7 deaths, respectively) before isosorbide dinitrate was

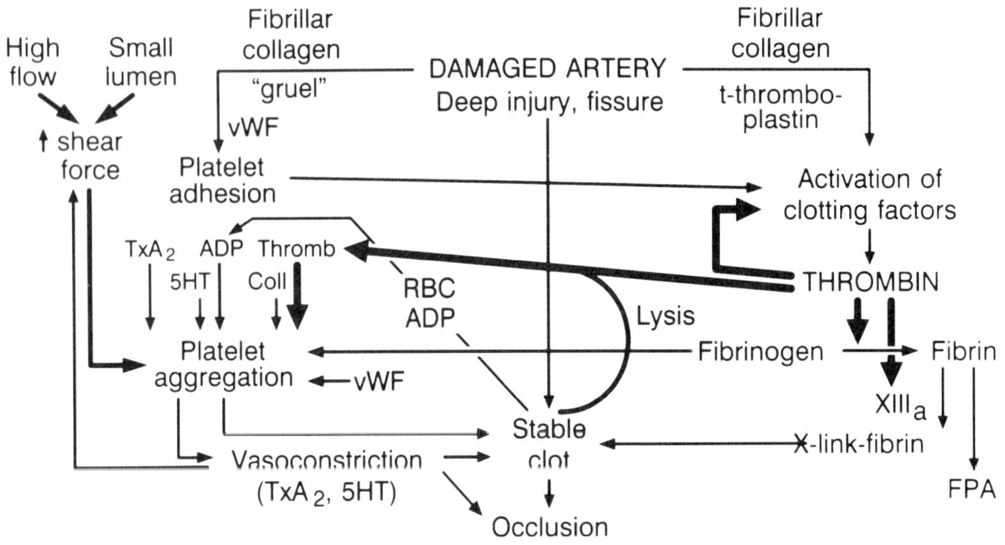

Fig 30B-9 Proposed mechanisms of thrombosis before and rethrombosis after thrombolysis. In rethrombosis, the arterial substrate for thrombosis is residual thrombus with fibrin-bound thrombin rather than injured artery. *Left,* platelet aggregation by collagen (from plaque or arterial media) and lipid "gruel" can occur by activation of five different membrane receptors: thromboxane A_2 *(TxA_2),* serotonin *(5HT),* adenosine diphosphate (*ADP;* some evidence of coupling to 5HT), collagen *(Coll),* and thrombin (*Thromb;* some evidence for coupling with collagen). Thrombin is probably the most potent primary activator of platelets. The first three activators of platelet-membrane receptors are platelet-containing substances that enhance activation and aggregation after the initial activation. The initial activation is probably and primarily via collagen and thrombin. The degree of vasoconstriction depends on the severity of platelet deposition (see text) and is probably mediated by platelet substances *(TxA_2, 5HT),* which contribute to increased shear forces, more platelet aggregation, and further occlusion and clot formation. Increased shear forces *(far left)* due to a small arterial lumen and high flow rates are also, in part, directly related to platelet deposition (see text). Factor VIII-von Willebrand's factor *(vWF)* is necessary for initial platelet adhesion and is also responsible for considerable platelet-to-platelet binding during aggregation. Fibrinogen also contributes to platelet-to-platelet binding at specific platelet-membrane glycoprotein IIb/IIIa receptors. *Right,* collagen and tissue thromboplastin *(t-thromboplastin)* initiate activation of the intrinsic and extrinsic clotting systems. The action between platelets and the coagulation system is also depicted by platelet activation of the clotting system and the activation of platelets by thrombin. Thrombin generation is increased by 280,000 times by formation of the prothrombinase complex, which requires four components (three clotting factors [factor Xa, factor Va, Ca^{++}] and the platelet phospholipid of the platelet membrane). *FPA,* fibrinopeptide A; *RBC,* red blood cells. (Modified from Chesebro JH, Fuster V: Antithrombotic therapy for acute myocardial infarction: mechanisms and prevention of deep venous, left ventricular, and coronary artery thromboembolism. *Circulation* 74 Suppl 3:1-10, 1986.)

begun. The incidence of cardiogenic shock, clinical signs of left-heart failure, and mean peak levels of CK-MB (only in the group with anterior infarction) all decreased significantly in the treated group. The study population was not restricted to patients with high left ventricular filling pressures, and there may have been more hypertensive patients in this study population with a higher-than-expected incidence of free wall, septal, or papillary muscle rupture in the placebo group.

Because of the deleterious results of early nitroprusside therapy in the study by Cohn et al.[303] (possibly a result of a "coronary steal"), nitroglycerin infusion is preferred to nitroprusside therapy for vasodilation whenever possible early after acute infarction. Hypertension without heart failure preferably is treated with β-adrenergic blockers (unless contraindicated). Hypertension not controlled by other means (especially if there is no further evidence of myocardial ischemia and symptom onset is more than 9 to 12 hours previously) may be treated with nitroprusside infusion, but routine use of nitroprusside therapy in acute

MI is not advised. Other vasodilators, such as trimethaphan, have been used to treat hypertension in patients with acute MI; in 14 patients, it resulted in a smaller-than-expected infarct size (enzymatically estimated).

Other possible adjuncts for salvage of ischemic myocardium

Intra-aortic balloon counterpulsation. This technique is discussed later in this chapter.

Magnesium therapy. Accumulating evidence from several small randomized trials suggests a beneficial role for the use of intravenously administered magnesium sulfate in the early phase of acute MI.[305] The mechanisms of benefit are unclear but include several potentially beneficial actions, such as coronary and systemic vasodilatation, platelet inhibition, antiarrhythmic effects, and the direct antagonism of intracellular calcium, which is increased in infarction. A recent randomized trial of 2,316 patients documented a 24% reduction in mortality in patients treated with the intravenous administration of magnesium sulfate compared to placebo.[306] What was surprising and particularly interesting in this trial was the reduction in the occurrence of left ventricular failure, which appeared to be the major mechanism whereby magnesium reduced mortality. This suggested a primary protective effect on the myocardium independent of other drugs, and at present it is reasonable to consider the routine administration of magnesium in patients with acute MI, although several larger randomized trials might clarify the role of magnesium further (ISIS-4, GISSI-III).

Reperfusion by thrombolysis

Reperfusion offers excellent potential for the salvage of ischemic myocardium early after acute transmural MI. Ischemia and necrosis progress from endocardium to epicardium at a rate dependent on time elapsed after interruption of blood flow, myocardial oxygen demand, and degree of hypoperfusion.[216-221,262] Necrosis can occur in 20 to 30 minutes with total deprivation of blood flow or may be delayed for several hours because of residual blood flow via subtotal occlusion or collateral circulation. Thus, goals for therapy should be based on influencing the three factors that determine the progression of necrosis—i.e., improve collateral blood flow to decrease hypoperfusion, decrease myocardial oxygen demand, and, most important, reestablish blood flow as quickly as possible (preferably within 2 to 4 hours after the onset of symptoms of acute infarction).

Agents. Possible thrombolytic agents[307-311] for use in acute MI include streptokinase, urokinase, and more fibrin-specific agents such as t-PA,[309] pro-urokinase,[310] and acylated streptokinase.[311]

Streptokinase, a nonenzyme protein with a molecular weight of 47,000 produced by Lancefield group C strains of β-hemolytic streptococci, is the most widely used thrombolytic agent. Streptokinase activates the fibrinolytic system indirectly by forming a complex with plasminogen or plasmin. The complex is strong, is formed extremely rapidly, and converts the inactive proenzyme and the enzyme into an effective plasminogen activator.[308] Streptokinase is much less expensive than urokinase, but it is antigenic and may produce fever, urticaria or rash (in less than 5% of patients), anaphylaxis (1 of 1,000 to 2,000 patients),[312] or, rarely, serum sickness.[313]

Although human plasma contains antibodies directed against streptokinase, the number of allergic reactions experienced by patients in the United States appears to be sufficiently low to obviate prophylactic corticosteroid therapy. The antibodies that bind to streptokinase inactivate it and are probably the main mechanism of its elimination. Because the antibody titer varies from person to person, the dose of streptokinase required to override the immunologic inhibition before fibrinolytic activation can be obtained also varies. However, 350,000 units of streptokinase will overcome the circulatory antibodies in 95% of a healthy population; individual requirements varied between 25,000 and 3,000,000 units.[314-316] A few days after streptokinase administration the antibody titer increases rapidly to 50 to 100 times the pretreatment value and remains high for 4 to 6 months, during which a repeat administration is usually impractical.[308]

Urokinase is a trypsin-like protease isolated from human urine or, more recently, from cultured human embryonic kidney cells, which accounts for its great expense. It may occur in large or small molecular forms (molecular weights 54,000 and 31,600). The latter probably is a degradation product of the former. Urokinase causes fibrinolysis by directly converting plasminogen to plasmin. Urokinase is inactivated by α_2-antiplasmin and α_2-macroglobulin, which also neutralize free plasmin in the blood.

Because streptokinase and urokinase are not specific for fibrin in converting of plasminogen to plasmin (Fig 30B-10), large amounts of plasmin are produced in the blood, causing α_2-antiplasmin, which rapidly inactivates free plasmin, to be quickly depleted and leaving increasing amounts of free plasmin in the blood. Plasmin is a nonspecific protease that hydrolyzes fibrin and other plasma proteins such as clotting factors (fibrinogen, prothrombin, and factors V and VIII), the first component of complement, and kallikreininogen. The result of plasmin excess with depletion of clotting factors and appearance of fibrin and fibrinogen split products, which have an anticoagulant effect, is a lytic state with potential for bleeding.[308]

Fortunately, the incidence of fatal hemorrhage associated with thrombolysis with intracoronary streptokinase is only 0.14% and occurs during the 24 to 72 hours after streptokinase administration while the patient is on full-dose heparin (suggesting that the relatively short-lived lytic state from intracoronary streptokinase was not involved). With intravenous streptokinase therapy with aspirin, heparin, or both, severe or major bleeding may occur in 0.3% to 0.5% of patients.[140,141] Because thrombolytic agents lyse thrombus but simultaneously enhance thrombosis, simultaneous antithrombotic therapy is needed to enhance thrombolysis and reduce reocclusion.[312] Streptokinase induces platelet aggregation by binding anti-streptokinase antibodies to the

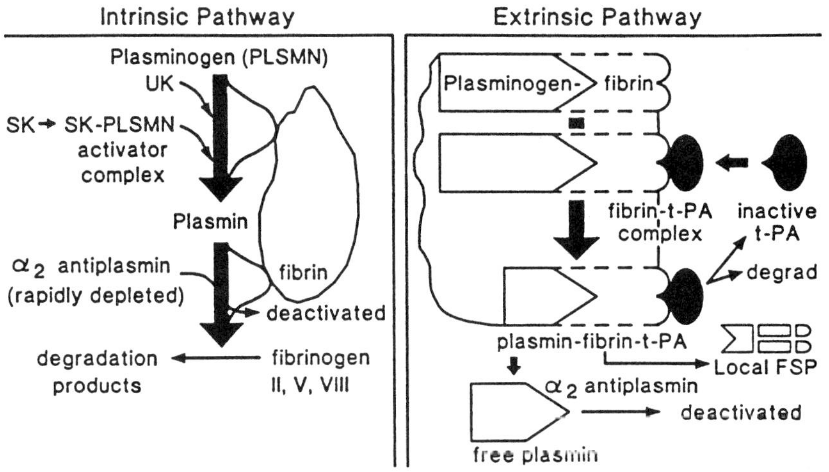

Fig 30B-10 Diagram of thrombolysis. The two most frequently used activators of the intrinsic pathway are streptokinase *(SK)* and urokinase *(UK)*. Urokinase directly converts plasminogen *(PLSMN)* to plasmin, whereas streptokinase forms the *SK-PLSMN* activator complex. Both lead to a large conversion of circulating PLSMN to plasmin *(broad arrow);* some fibrin-bound PLSMN is also converted to plasmin. α_2-Antiplasmin deactivates the circulating plasmin but becomes rapidly depleted, leaving an excess of plasmin, which acts as a nonspecific protease in the lysis of other circulating clotting factors (fibrinogen, factors II, V, and VIII) as well as the fibrin in the thrombus and produces a systemic lytic state. The extrinsic pathway of thrombolysis is activated by tissue plasminogen activator *(t-PA),* which by itself is inactive but is specifically activated by fibrin, thereby specifically activating the fibrin-bound plasminogen and localizing the formation of plasmin to the environment of the thrombus. The small amount of free plasmin generated is rapidly deactivated by α_2-antiplasmin. This essentially prevents lysis of circulating fibrinogen and other clotting factors or plasma proteins. Fibrin split products *(FSP)* are formed locally only from lysis of fibrin within the thrombus and appear to be readily dispersed, because they have not been detected in circulating blood thus far.

streptokinase-plasminogen complex on the platelet surface; this aggregation is partially inhibited by aspirin.[317] Thrombolytic agents generate plasmin, which activates factor V, which enhances thrombin generation and activity and results in the paradoxical elevation of fibrinopeptide A, a marker of thrombin activity on fibrinogen.[119] Since active thrombin binds to fibrin, fibrinolysis promotes the release of procoagulant thrombin from fibrin, which further promotes thrombosis via platelet activation and fibrin formation.[318] These mechanisms contribute to thrombosis during thrombolysis and, in part, explain why combined heparin and aspirin therapy has resulted in the lowest incidence of reocclusion thus far reported.[106]

Tissue-type plasminogen activator is a naturally occurring serum glycoprotein with a molecular weight of approximately 70,000. It was isolated from the culture fluid of human melanoma cells (mt-PA), is normally made by the vascular endothelium, and is indistinguishable in all properties and actions from the t-PA isolated from the human uterus and vessel wall and from the genetically produced recombinant t-PA (rt-PA). t-PA itself is essentially inactive; it requires fibrin as a cofactor for plasminogen activation and thus is only activated on the surface of a thrombus. The fibrin-t-PA complex converts plasminogen to plasmin, and lyses fibrin, only on the surface of the clot (see Fig 30B-10). Any free plasmin that may leave the clot surface is rapidly inactivated by α_2-antiplasmin.[308] In animal and human studies, t-PA appears to be nonantigenic, only minimally affects plasma proteins or hemostatic indices, and achieves thrombolysis after intravenous administration with only minimal (if any) systemic fibrinogenolytic activity or production of a lytic state. t-PA appears safer, faster acting, specific for clot lysis, and more effective (especially for older thrombus) than streptokinase or urokinase and is approximately twice as effective as streptokinase in opening the occluded infarct-related artery in patients with acute transmural MI.[309,319]

Acute MI is precipitated by disruption of vulnerable atherosclerotic plaques, which contain a lipid core covered by a fibrous cap infiltrated by macrophages that has become very thin and disrupts (usually at the margin).[320,321] The atheromatous fatty core is the most thrombogenic substrate of the human atherosclerotic plaque,[322] contains large amounts of tissue factor, and leads to marked thrombin generation and immediate deposition of platelets and fibrin(ogen). This thrombus that covers the disrupted atherosclerotic plaque is extremely thrombogenic and grows rapidly. Thrombus growth is partially inhibited by heparin but completely inhibited by hirudin.[323] Since hirudin inhibits thrombin only, its pivotal role in thrombus growth and formation may be seen. Thrombin activity is also necessary to maintain cohesion of in vivo platelet aggregates. Blocking thrombin activity with hirudin causes "dethrombosis" or dissolution of in vivo thrombi (90% dissolution within 1 hour) formed over deep arterial injury.[324] Only minute amounts of thrombin are necessary to activate platelet deposition. Thrombolysis increases thrombin generation by activating factor V to Va and also increases thrombosis during the lytic process by exposing underlying fibrin-bound thrombin, by releasing fibrin degradation products (which bind active thrombin and circulate), and by sensitizing platelets to increased activation.[312]

In patients with acute transmural MI indicated by chest pain for more than 20 to 30 minutes and ST-segment elevation, 80% to 87% have total thrombotic occlusion of the infarct-related artery within 6 hours after the onset of symptoms.[319,325] The proportion of patients with total occlusion decreases to approximately 65% between 6 and 24 hours after the onset of symptoms,[325] probably because of spontaneous thrombolysis. The effectiveness of a thrombolytic agent in opening arteries in patients is most accurately tested after baseline coronary angiography, because subtotal occlusion may vary from 5% to 33% in smaller studies.[326] However, today it is not considered practical or ethical to withhold thrombolytic therapy for baseline angiography, and thus a 20% patency at baseline is assumed, and angiographic measurements of reperfusion are now based on 60- or 90-minute patency of the infarct-related artery.[106,319]

Candidates and goals for thrombolysis. Candidates for thrombolysis are patients presenting with acute MI less than 12 hours after the onset of symptoms, with characteristic chest or myocardial ischemic pain lasting at least 20 minutes and accompanied by ECG changes of ≥ 0.1 mV of ST-segment elevation in two or more limb leads or ≥ 0.2 mV in two or more contiguous precordial leads.

Exclusion criteria are previous stroke, active bleeding, recent major trauma or major surgery (especially within 7 to 10 days), and noncompressible vascular punctures (such as aorta or subclavian arteries). As shown by the GUSTO trial, in which the oldest patient entered was 110 years old, age is no longer a contraindication.[141] Severe, uncontrolled hypertension (systolic blood pressure ≥ 180 mm Hg, unresponsive to initial therapy) is a relative contraindication to thrombolysis, but treatment may begin after better control (systolic pressure < 150 to 160 mm Hg) is gained with intravenous metoprolol or esmolol alone or combined with intravenous nitroprusside.

Patients over age 75 are six times less likely to receive thrombolytic therapy than younger patients.[327] However, the older the age, the larger the absolute benefit.[328] Analysis of patients 80 years of age or older in the ISIS-2 trial who received streptokinase and aspirin showed that 1-month mortality was reduced from 37% in the treated to 22% in the placebo group.[125] Additional analysis shows a clear-cut favorable benefit-to-risk ratio for thrombolytic treatment in elderly patients.[329] The bleeding risk associated with thrombolytic therapy is greater in the elderly.[330,331] The risk of stroke increases with age but also increases with the use of rt-PA compared with streptokinase.[332] In the ISIS-3 trial, the combined rate of stroke was 1.35% for t-PA and 1.0% for streptokinase.[140] In the GISSI-2 trial, there was also a small increase in the risk of stroke for use of rt-PA, most pronounced in patients over age 70; the stroke rate was 2.6% for rt-PA compared with 1.6% for streptokinase.[138] A weight-adjusted dose of duteplase rt-PA appears to markedly reduce the excess clustering of hemorrhagic events.[140] In the GUSTO trial, 12% of patients were age 75 or older, and overall mortality was slightly lower for rt-PA (19.3%) than for streptokinase (20.6%).[146]

IMPORTANT GOALS FOR THROMBOLYSIS. Critical goals for successful thrombolysis are accomplishing early reperfusion, reperfusion to normal flow of the infarct-related artery, reduction of mortality, preservation of left ventricular function, and continued patency of the infarct-related coronary artery. These goals are related and interdependent in that early reperfusion to normal flow and maintaining patency are necessary to reduce mortality and preserve left ventricular function, and maintaining patency and improving flow reserve of the coronary artery also depend on reducing the residual thrombus within the lumen of the coronary artery.

ACCOMPLISHING EARLY REPERFUSION. Factors contributing time delays in achieving reperfusion are outlined in Figure 30B-11. Average patient delays total 3.7 hours. Patient delays in seeking medical assistance vary but average about 50 minutes. Patient delays may be related to denial of a major problem, mistaking symptoms for a minor condition, being alone, being more advanced in age, or trying to contact a personal physician. Prior symptoms and history of angina or MI are not associated with reduced patient delays.[333]

Transportation delays in part depend on distance from a health care facility and the availability and training of local paramedical and ambulance systems. However, fewer than half of patients with probable acute MI use paramedic and ambulance systems for transport.[334] Paramedic transport time may be divided into 15-minute intervals for emergency call-to-site arrival, patient care on-site, and site-to-hospital intervals.[333]

The largest single component of delay, and thus the most modifiable, is in-hospital delay ("door-to-needle time").[335,336] If an ECG is done during transport or immediately upon arrival and staff are prepared, thrombolytic therapy may be started as early as 20 to 30 minutes after arrival. After starting drug therapy, time to reperfusion averages about 45 minutes.[337] Thus, future therapies should concentrate more on a high incidence of reperfusion to normal flow and less on the actual speed of reperfusion, and successful thrombolysis will mean treating the patient earlier. Other factors contributing to shortening time to drug administration are urban hospital location, admission to a teaching hospital, a high case volume of MI, storing drugs in the emergency room where the ER physician can make the decision to treat, and use of a simplified bolus regimen.[338,339]

Strategies for thrombolysis. Four possible intravenous

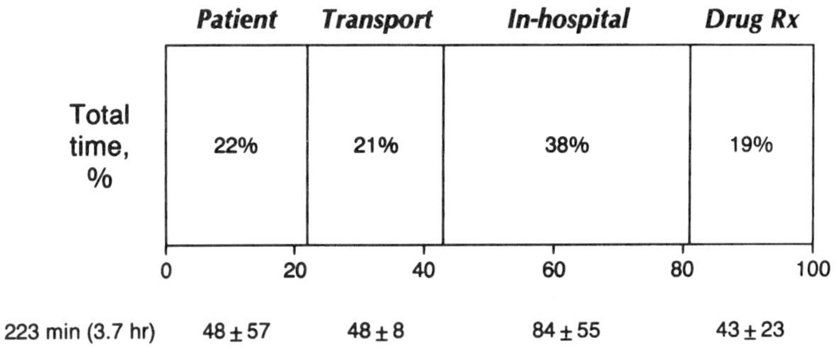

Fig 30B-11 Time delays in achieving reperfusion could be markedly diminished if therapy for reperfusion could be started just before transport or within 20 minutes of entry to the hospital. (Modified from Gersh BJ, Anderson JL: Thrombolysis and myocardial salvage: results of clinical trials and the animal paradigm—parodoxic or predictable? *Circulation* 88:296-306, 1993.)

thrombolytic strategies are given in Table 30B-22. In the GUSTO trial, the subcutaneous heparin treatment was continued for 7 days or until the patient was dismissed from the hospital. Intravenous heparin should be given for at least 48 hours and preferably for the duration of the hospitalization, especially in patients receiving rt-PA or having had an anterior transmural (Q-wave) MI.

Chewable aspirin should be administered as soon as possible after presentation in a dose of 160 to 325 mg followed by a daily dose of 80 to 160 mg indefinitely. In patients with prior allergic reaction to heparin, streptokinase may be administered with the chewable aspirin and without heparin, as initially done in GISSI and ISIS.[138,140]

Primary balloon angioplasty of the infarct-related artery may be done in hospitals with coronary angiography facilities during daylight and weekday hours when the catheterization laboratory is available for immediate intervention to open the infarct-related artery.[341,342] In the Mayo Clinic trial of Gibbons and colleagues, 108 patients were randomized to direct angioplasty versus rt-PA, with the first balloon inflation starting 277 minutes after the onset of chest pain and the rt-PA infusion starting a mean of 232 minutes after the onset of chest pain. Myocardial salvage was assessed by imaging with ^{99m}Tc-sestamibi, which showed 27% of the left ventricle salvaged by thrombolysis and 31% salvaged by direct angioplasty in patients with anterior MI. For patients with inferior MI, 7% was salvaged by thrombolysis and 5% of the left ventricle by angioplasty. Thus, in the treatment of acute MI, significant myocardium could be salvaged by either immediate angioplasty or the administration of thrombolytic agents in patients receiving concomitant aspirin and an immediate heparin bolus of 5,000 U followed by a 10,000 U bolus just before angioplasty and a continuous infusion of heparin for 5 days.[341]

In the Netherlands Study, 142 patients with acute MI were randomized to receive immediate angioplasty versus streptokinase; the results are in Table 30B-23. Immediate angioplasty after acute MI was associated with a higher rate of patency of the infarct-related artery, a less severe residual stenotic lesion, better left ventricular function, and less recurrent myocardial ischemia in infarction than in patients treated with intravenous streptokinase (1.5 million U intravenously over 1 hour). Intravenous heparin was administered to an aPTT of two or three times the normal value for at least 2 days.[343] This may have been too short, since reocclusion may occur throughout hospitalization.[319]

In the Primary Angioplasty in Myocardial Infarction (PAMI) study, 395 patients who presented within 12 hours of the onset of MI were treated with heparin and aspirin and randomly assigned to immediate percutaneous transluminal coronary angioplasty (PTCA) or to intravenous rt-PA followed by conservative care and radionuclide ventriculography within 24 hours and at 6 weeks. The in-hospital mortality rates in the rt-PA and PTCA groups were 6.5% and 2.6%, respectively (P = 0.06). In both treatment groups, intravenous heparin was administered for 3 to 5 days to a target aPTT of 1.5 to 2 times control.[342] Immediate PTCA reduced the combined occurrence of nonfatal MI or death, was associated with a lower rate of intracranial hemorrhage (none in the direct PTCA group and 2.0% in the rt-PA group), and resulted in similar left ventricular systolic function outcome.

Although patients appear to have a low incidence of posthospital chest pain and reinfarction after direct angioplasty, the angiographic incidence of restenosis may be as high as 55%.

REPERFUSION: IMPORTANCE OF NORMAL FLOW. Early patency of the infarct-related artery at 90 minutes after thrombolytic therapy is important for reduction of mortality and preservation of left ventricular function. Table 30B-24 shows the influence of TIMI flow at 90 minutes for predicting mortality at 30 days after thrombolysis for acute MI. Mortality was lowest for TIMI grade 3 flow regardless of the thrombolytic agent.[106]

Reperfusion to normal or TIMI 3 flow is also associated with improved left ventricular performance by global ejection fraction and by preserved regional wall motion (see Table 30B-24).[106] The effect of early patency on left ventricular function was evident as early as 90 minutes and persisted at 5 to 7 days.[106]

REDUCTION IN MORTALITY. Half of the mortality reduction occurs within 24 hours of thrombolysis. Diver-

Table 30B-22 Strategies for thrombolysis

1. Accelerated rt-PA in a bolus dose of 15 mg, 0.75 mg/kg body weight over a 30-minute period, not to exceed 50 mg, and 0.5 mg/kg up to 35 mg over the next 60 minutes with intravenous heparin in a bolus dose of 5,000 U and 1,000 U/hr (a dose of 1,200 U/hr is recommended for patients weighing more than 90 kg), with the dose adjusted to raise the activated partial thromboplastin time (aPTT) to between 60 and 85 seconds
2. Streptokinase, 1.5 million U over a 60-minute period with intravenous heparin as above
3. Streptokinase, 1.5 million U over a 60-minute period with subcutaneous heparin in a dose of 12,500 U twice daily, beginning 4 hours after the start of thrombolytic therapy*
   For acute anterior MI when heparin protection against left ventricular mural thrombus formation is desired immediately on admission, the subcutaneous dose of heparin at 12,500 U twice daily should be started immediately on admission, a bolus dose of heparin of 70 U/kg started simultaneously, and the aPTT adjusted to 60 to 85 seconds (average dose from five studies is 17,000 U every 12 hours)[101,146]
4. APSAC bolus dose of 30 mg injected over 5 minutes should be preceded by an intravenous bolus injection of 5,000 U of heparin[340]
   For patients with acute anterior MI, the bolus should be followed by a heparin infusion of 1,000 U/hr or subcutaneous heparin of 12,500 U every 12 hours to maintain the aPTT at 60 to 85 seconds for the duration of the hospitalization

*This is the treatment regimen tested in ISIS-3.[140]

gent survival rates were produced by stratification of patients according to their left ventricular function at 90 minutes; mortality was 3.9% among patients with ejection fractions above 45% and 14.7% among patients with ejection fractions ≤45% ($P < 0.001$).[106] The rate of patency and normality of flow of the infarct-related artery at 90 minutes best predicted mortality. Thus, the incidence of TIMI 3 flow for each of the treatment strategies in the GUSTO trial appears to be the mechanistic link for the mortality outcomes[106] (Table 30B-25). Other complications of acute MI and the allergic and anaphylactic reactions from thrombolytic therapy are significantly lower for the accelerated rt-PA and intravenous heparin group than for streptokinase and subcutaneous or intravenous heparin[146] (Table 30B-26).

In the first GISSI trial, patients were randomized within 12 hours after the onset of symptoms of MI. The treatments of streptokinase (1.5×10^6 U intravenously over 1 hour) or conventional care in the coronary care unit without thrombolysis were prospectively allocated by randomization. Patients were entered from January 1984 to June 1985 in 178 coronary care units (80% in Italy). The mortality differences for the entire group and by time after treatment[344] are summarized in Table 30B-27.

Table 30B-23 Results of the Netherlands study in 142 patients with acute myocardial infarction

	Immediate angioplasty	Streptokinase
Recurrent infarction, no. of pt	0	9
Unstable angina, no. of pt	4	14
Mean LVEF (%) before hospital dismissal	51	45
Infarct-related artery patent, % of pt	91	68
Residual stenosis (%) in infarct-related artery	36	76

LVEF, left ventricular ejection fraction.

Table 30B-24 TIMI flow grade at 90 minutes predicts mortality and ventricular function regardless of lytic agent[106]

		At 5 to 7 days	
TIMI flow grade	30-day mortality, %	Ejection fraction, %	Preserved RWM, % of group
3	4.4	61	39
2	7.4	56	27
1	8.9	54	22
0	8.9	56	18

RWM, regional wall motion; TIMI, Thrombolysis in Myocardial Infarction.

Table 30B-25 Lytic strategy, early and complete reperfusion, and mortality

	% of patients with	
Therapeutic strategy	TIMI 3 flow	Death
Accelerated rt-PA	54	6.3
rt-PA, SK	38	7.0
SK-IV	32	7.4
SK-SC	29	7.2

IV, intravenous; rt-PA, recombinant tissue plasminogen activator; SC, subcutaneous; SK, streptokinase; TIMI, Thrombolysis in Myocardial Infarction.

Table 30B-26 Other complications of myocardial infarction after thrombosis

Complication	SK and SC heparin (n = 8,669)	SK and IV heparin (n = 9,260)	Accelerated t-PA and IV heparin (n = 9,235)	Both thrombolytic agents and IV heparin (n = 9,193)	P value, accelerated t-PA vs. both SK groups
	Percent of patients				
Allergic reaction	5.7	5.8	1.6	5.4	<0.001
Anaphylaxis	0.7	0.6	0.2	0.6	<0.001
Congestive heart failure	17.5	16.8	15.2	16.8	<0.001
Cardiogenic shock	6.9	6.3	5.1	6.1	<0.001
Sustained hypotension	13.3	12.5	10.1	12.4	<0.001
Atrioventricular block*	9.5	8.7	7.3	8.4	<0.001
Sustained ventricular tachycardia	6.8	6.5	5.6	6.1	0.001
Ventricular fibrillation	7.1	6.9	6.3	6.9	0.02
Asystole	6.0	6.4	5.3	6.4	0.003
Atrial fibrillation or flutter	9.9	9.9	8.6	9.1	0.001
Reinfarction	3.4	4.0	4.0	4.0	0.26
Recurrent ischemia	19.9	19.6	19.0	18.8	0.14
Acute mitral regurgitation	1.6	2.6	1.3	1.4	0.11
Acute ventricular septal defect	0.5	0.4	0.4	0.6	0.59

IV, intravenous; SC, subcutaneous; SK, streptokinase; t-PA, tissue-type plasminogen activator.
From the GUSTO Investigators: An international randomized trial comparing four thrombolytic strategies for acute myocardial infarction. *N Engl J Med* 329:673-682, 1993. By permission of the journal.

Table 30B-27 Mortality in Gruppo Italiano per lo Studio della Sopravvivenza nell'Infarto Miocardico trial at 19 days: unblinded study of 11,815 patients*

Group	Streptokinase	Conventional care	P
	% Mortality		
Entire	10.6	13.0	<0.05
Rx ≤ 1 hr	8.1	15.3	0.0002
Rx ≤ 3 hr	8.6	11.8	<0.001
Rx 3-6 hr	11.3	13.4	<0.05
No prior MI	9.7	12.0	0.007

*Heparin was used at admission in 3% of patients and sometime during hospitalization in 17% of patients.

In ISIS-II, 17,187 patients entering 417 hospitals within 24 hours (median, 5 hours) after onset of suspected acute MI underwent randomization to placebo control versus treatments, as follows: (1) a 1-hour intravenous infusion of streptokinase, 1.5×10^6 U, (2) enteric coated aspirin, 160 mg/day for 1 month, (3) both active treatments, and (4) neither treatment. The results of vascular deaths are summarized in Figure 30B-12. Aspirin significantly reduced nonfatal reinfarction (1.0% vs. 2.0%) and nonfatal stroke (0.3% vs. 0.6%) and was not associated with any significant increase in cerebral hemorrhage or bleeding requiring transfusion. An excess of nonfatal reinfarction occurred when streptokinase was used alone, but this was avoided by the addition of aspirin. Those allocated to combined streptokinase and aspirin had significantly fewer reinfarctions (1.8% vs. 2.9%), strokes (0.6% vs. 1.1%), and deaths (8.0% vs. 13.2%) than those allocated to neither. Differences in vascular and all-cause mortality after treatment with streptokinase alone and by aspirin alone remained highly significant ($P < 0.001$ for each) after a median of 15 months' follow-up.[125]

Collaborative overview of early mortality from all randomized trials of more than 1,000 patients with suspected acute MI (GISSI-1,[344] ISAM,[345] AIMS,[346] ISIS-2,[125] ASSET,[347] USIM,[348] ISIS-3,[140] AMERAS,[349] and LATE[350]) showed benefit from fibrinolytic therapy in patients presenting with ST-elevation or bundle-branch block, irrespective of age, sex, blood pressure, heart rate, or previous history of MI or diabetes; it was greater when treatment was begun early. Among 45,000 patients, the relationship between benefit and delay from symptom onset to treatment showed highly significant absolute mortality reductions of about 30 patients per thousand for those presenting within 6 hours, of about 20 patients per thousand for those presenting 7 to 12 hours after onset of

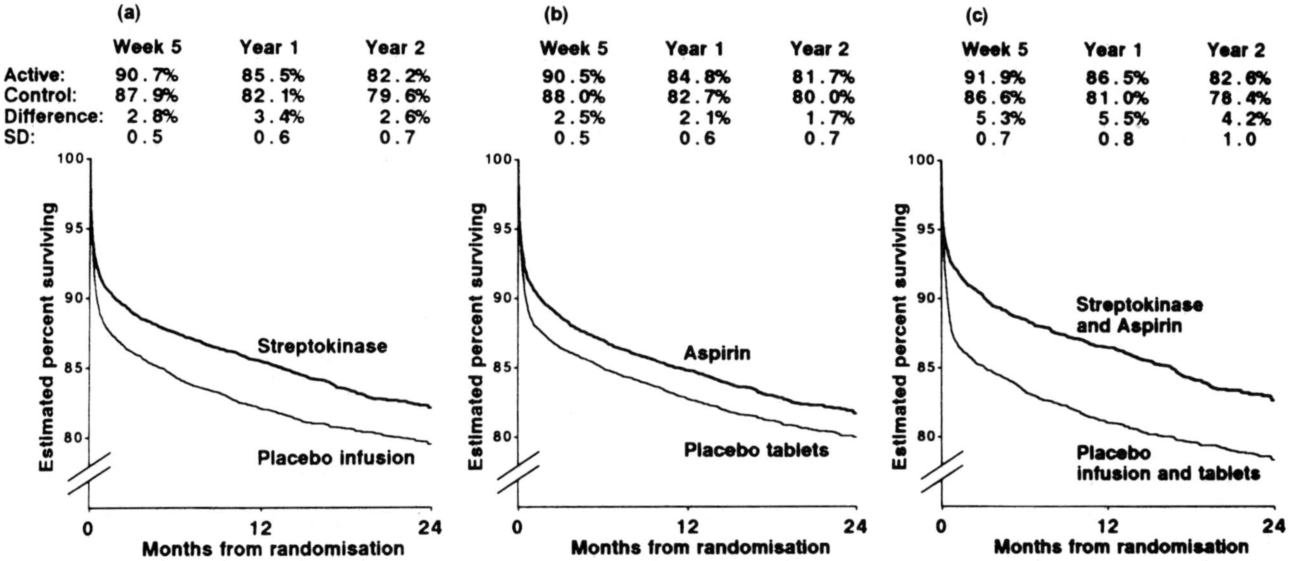

Fig 30B-12 Life-table estimates of 12-month and 24-month survival from the second International Study of Infarct Survival.[125] Median follow-up was 15 months and maximum was 34 months. (From ISIS-2 [Second International Study of Infarct Survival] Collaborative Group: Randomised trial of intravenous streptokinase, oral aspirin, both or neither among 17,187 cases of suspected acute myocardial infarction: ISIS-2. *Lancet* 2:349-360, 1988. By permission of the journal.)

symptoms, and a statistically uncertain benefit of about 10 per thousand for those presenting at 13 to 18 hours[351] (Table 30B-28).

MYOCARDIAL SALVAGE AND PRESERVATION OF LEFT VENTRICULAR FUNCTION. A major determinant of myocardial salvage in patients with acute transmural infarction is the time from onset of symptoms to thrombolytic therapy.[352] Similar amounts of myocardium may be salvaged by reperfusion with thrombolysis or primary angioplasty in patients treated within 2½ to 5 hours.[341] This salvage is often sufficient to maintain the mean ejection fraction within normal limits.[341] Both streptokinase and rt-PA, when administered within 4 to 6 hours, can preserve global left ventricular function, but early patency to normal flow (TIMI 3) is associated with more improvement of global and regional left ventricular function[106] (see Table 30B-24). Regional improvement may be noted as early as 90 minutes after thrombolytic therapy. There is also moderate improvement in measures of regional function over the course of a week in patients treated within 4 to 6 hours.[106,352-356]

ACUTE NORMAL PATENCY AND MAINTAINING PATENCY OF THE INFARCT-RELATED ARTERY. The GUSTO trial demonstrated the superiority of rt-PA to streptokinase in the improvement to normal patency and flow, survival, and overall clinical benefit.[357] Strategies for maintaining patency of the infarct-related artery in the hospital and thereafter have already been discussed.

ASSESSMENT OF THE PATIENT AFTER MI. Patients in whom recurrent angina or ischemia develops at rest or during mild effort, heart failure, or a positive stress test at a low level of exercise (especially stage 1 of the Bruce protocol) are candidates for coronary angiography and possible revascularization. Patients who cannot exercise may be at higher risk but may also be assessed with thallium or ^{99m}Tc-sestamibi myocardial perfusion with the "stress" of increased flow reserve with dipyridamole or adenosine. A recent study suggests that continuous ST-segment monitoring may be the major and only test that contributes significant prognostic information to judge the risk of cardiac death, recurrent MI, and unstable angina requiring admission to the hospital over the next year after MI when simple clinical variables are taken into account. Continuous ST-segment monitoring may someday be used as the screening test of choice after MI and exercise testing be reserved to answer specific questions in selected patients.[358]

Approximately 80% of recurrent ischemic events occur within the first 48 hours after thrombolysis,[144] depending on the type of antithrombotic therapy employed and its duration and adequacy after thrombolysis. Selective rather than routine predismissal coronary angiography appears indicated after thrombolytic therapy for acute MI. By the end of 1 year, coronary angiography had been performed one or more times in 99% of a routine catheterization group and in 59% of a selective catheterization group (for ischemia that occurred spontaneously or on predismissal exercise testing; $P < 0.001$); death (10.2% and 7.0%, respectively; $P = 0.10$) and nonfatal MI (8.6% and 9.0%, respectively; $P = 0.87$) were not significantly different between groups. Thus, selective coronary angiography exposes 40% fewer patients to the small but finite risk, inconvenience, and cost of the procedure without compromising 1-year survival or reinfarction

Table 30B-28 Combined (nine studies) absolute differences in mortality during days 0 to 35 by presentation features[351]

Summary for three periods

	Patients				
	Fibrinolytic (n = 29,315)		Control (n = 29,285)		
Deaths during days	No.	%	No.	%	Benefit per 1,000 (SD)
0-1	1,170	4.0	1,103	3.8	−2 (2)
2-35	1,650	5.9	2,254	8.0	21 (2)
0-35	2,820	9.6	3,357	11.5	18 (3)

Results for "uncertain" indication arm of ISIS-3 were included in all subdivisions: in summary, for patients with ST elevation or bundle-branch block in ISIS-3, the results were 84/782 fibrinolytic vs. 97/760 control for delay of 0-6 hr, 69/586 vs. 86/597 for 7-12 hr, and 68/445 vs. 59/431 for 13-24 hr; and for patients with other ECG changes, they were 104/1,713 vs. 65/1,682 for 0-6 hr, 47/694 vs. 42/674 for 7-12 hr, and 28/381 vs. 26/413 for 13-24 hr. Certain of the presentation features were not recorded in GISSI-1 (heart rate and diabetes), AIMS (diabetes), USIM (heart rate, prior MI, diabetes), and ASSET and LATE (these particular ECG categories), so that data from these trials could not be included in subdivisions by these features. If the value of some presentation feature was missing for a particular patient, that patient was excluded from subdivision of that feature. BBB, bundle-branch block; bpm, beats per minute; ECG, electrocardiogram; elev, elevation; MI, myocardial infarction; SBP, systolic blood pressure; SD, standard deviation.

Modified from Fibrinolytic Therapy Trialists' (FTT) Collaborative Group: Indications for fibrinolytic therapy in suspected acute myocardial infarction: collaborative overview of early mortality and major morbidity results from all randomised trials of more than 1000 patients. *Lancet* 343:311-322, 1994.

rates.[359] The incidences of death and nonfatal MI (16%), postdismissal revascularization (17%), and rehospitalization (28% to 38%) remain disturbingly high in both groups but may be reduced by improved antithrombotic therapy, such as combining warfarin with aspirin, and evaluation is continuing in prospective, randomized trials (CARS, CHAMPS, ASPECT II, and OASIS studies).

Current recommendations. Ischemic chest pain of 20 to 30 minutes duration with ST-segment elevation has a 99% chance of evolving into acute MI, with approximately 80% of the infarct-related arteries being occluded.[319] Thus, rapid reperfusion is required.

Patients with ischemic chest pain consistent with acute infarction or unstable angina may immediately be given heparin, a 5,000-U (approximately 70 U/kg) intravenous bolus followed by an intravenous infusion at 1,000 U/hr while simultaneously starting to take 160 to 325 mg of chewable aspirin. A 12-lead ECG may be obtained as soon as possible, and those with ST-segment elevation without contraindications may then be given thrombolytic therapy, which should be accelerated rt-PA for anterior and large infarctions (bolus of 15 mg, 0.75 mg/kg of body weight over a 30-minute period, not to exceed 50 mg, and 0.5 mg/kg, up to 35 mg, over the next 60 minutes while continuing with intravenous heparin). Patients with inferior infarction also benefit from accelerated rt-PA, but this has a smaller advantage over streptokinase. They may be treated with intravenous streptokinase, 1.5 million U over 60 minutes along with heparin. Patients at a hospital during weekdays and daylight hours with an accessible cardiac catheterization laboratory, an open procedure room, and a prepared team may undergo primary angioplasty of the infarct-related artery and appear to gain similar overall benefit.[341-343]

Patients who have relative contraindications to thrombolysis are probably better treated with primary angioplasty, which may be followed with a heparin infusion for 3 to 5 days along with daily aspirin.

The assessment of chest pain before and after thrombolytic therapy is a readily available and useful indicator for the efficacy of thrombolysis. In patients with moderate or severe chest pain and complete resolution of symptoms during thrombolysis, there was salvage of 79% to 89% of the area at risk.[360] Other independent predictors of arterial patency after thrombolytic therapy were early peak of CK activity at ≤ 12 hours after the start of thrombolysis and ≥ 50% reduction in ST-segment elevation. The occurrence of reperfusion arrhythmias was not an independent predictor of arterial patency. The combination of all three markers using a logistic regression procedure showed a sensitivity of 100%, a specificity of 90%, a positive predictive value of 97%, and a negative predictive value of 100% for coronary artery patency in 82 patients.[361] Another study showed that a rapid and progressive decrease in ischemic pain and ST-segment elevation are reliable markers of reperfusion with TIMI grade 3 flow. Because ST elevation and pain often fluctuate before resolving with reperfusion, very frequent or continuous monitoring of ST elevation is essential for reliable recognition of the time and presence of reperfusion. Accelerated idioventricular rhythm and sudden bradycardia are not specific to reperfusion and do not occur in all patients with reperfusion.[362] Continuous, quantitative ST-segment analysis is a sensitive and specific

Table 30B-28 Combined (nine studies) absolute differences in mortality during days 0 to 35 by presentation features[351] – cont'd

Details for total duration

Presentation features	Patients		Deaths during days 0-35				Benefit per 1,000 (SD)
			Fibrinolytic		Control		
	Fibrinolytic	Control	No.	%	No.	%	
Entry ECG							
BBB	1,007	1,025	188	18.7	242	23.6	49 (18)
ST elev, anterior	6,587	6,642	868	13.2	1,120	16.9	37 (6)
ST elev, inferior	6,556	6,484	493	7.5	542	8.4	8 (5)
ST elev, other	3,053	3,024	324	10.6	404	13.4	27 (8)
ST depression	1,779	1,784	271	15.2	247	13.8	−14 (11)
Other abnormality	3,988	3,963	209	5.2	230	5.8	6 (6)
Normal	995	990	30	3.0	23	2.3	−7 (7)
Hours from onset							
0-1	1,678	1,670	159	9.5	217	13.0	35 (11)
2-3	8,297	8,315	683	8.2	889	10.7	25 (5)
4-6	8,294	8,195	802	9.7	945	11.5	19 (5)
7-12	6,478	6,404	719	11.1	813	12.7	16 (6)
13-24	4,568	4,701	457	10.0	493	10.5	5 (6)
Age (yr)							
<55	8,082	8,158	278	3.4	373	4.6	11 (3)
55-64	9,911	9,678	709	7.2	864	8.9	18 (4)
65-74	8,487	8,496	1,144	13.5	1,372	16.1	27 (5)
75+	2,835	2,953	689	24.3	748	25.3	10 (13)
Sex							
Male	22,353	22,412	1,835	8.2	2,258	10.1	19 (3)
Female	6,962	6,873	985	14.1	1,099	16.0	18 (6)
SBP, mm Hg							
<100	1,263	1,182	365	28.9	415	35.1	62 (18)
100-149	17,979	18,063	1,731	9.6	2,081	11.5	19 (3)
150-174	7,907	8,005	569	7.2	694	8.7	15 (4)
175+	2,166	2,035	155	7.2	167	8.2	11 (8)
Heart rate, bpm							
<80	12,922	12,965	926	7.2	1,097	8.5	13 (3)
80-99	6,268	6,221	579	9.2	706	11.3	21 (5)
100+	3,095	3,126	537	17.4	646	20.7	33 (10)
Prior MI							
Yes	5,719	5,577	717	12.5	784	14.1	15 (6)
No	22,468	22,635	1,993	8.9	2,467	10.9	20 (3)
Diabetes							
Yes	2,236	2,260	303	13.6	391	17.3	37 (11)
No	19,423	19,424	1,697	8.7	1,981	10.2	15 (3)
All patients	29,315	29,285	2,820	9.6	3,357	11.5	18 (3)

noninvasive technique for following coronary artery patency during acute MI. Achievement of a steady state of the ST-segment within 100 minutes of streptokinase reperfusion indicates successful reperfusion, with 89% sensitivity and 82% specificity. All patients with subtotal occlusion achieved an ST-segment steady state before streptokinase infusion, whereas no patient with total occlusion did so. Thus, achievement of ST-segment steady state before streptokinase infusion was 100% sensitive and 100% specific for subtotal occlusion at the first angiogram.[363] Failure to achieve indicators of successful reperfusion by resolution of chest pain or ST-segment elevation in patients with large anterior MIs may be considered an indicator for urgent coronary angiography to open and salvage the infarct-related artery.

Recurrent ischemia may be treated adjunctively as

needed with nitrates, β-blocker therapy, and, if necessary, calcium blockers. Long-term β-blocker therapy may be used in patients with concomitant hypertension or angina.

Angiotensin-converting enzyme (ACE) inhibitor therapy after MI can attenuate left ventricular remodeling, improve survival, prevent development of heart failure, and probably reduce recurrent or new MI. Patients most likely to benefit are those with left ventricular ejection fractions of 40% or less. Oral therapy would optimally be started after 3 days and within 2 weeks of the postinfarction time period. Benefit for longer than 4 years has been observed. Hemodynamically active doses equivalent to 50 mg of captopril three times daily should be used, with a gradual increase in dosage often started at 6.25 mg three times daily to avoid hypotensive episodes. Three studies have shown the benefit of ACE inhibitors in patients with left ventricular dysfunction.[364-367] In the SAVE trial, 35% of patients treated with captopril were taking β-blocker therapy at baseline,[364] and 66% of patients in the enalapril-treated group of the CONSENSUS II trial were taking β-blocker therapy.[365] No adverse interactions occurred, and there may be benefit from both therapies.

Antithrombotic therapy should be administered as outlined earlier.

Future therapies. Future therapies for acute myocardial infarction may include bolus rt-PA to achieve an even higher incidence of reperfusion with normal flow, direct thrombin inhibition with hirudin (a specific and potent direct thrombin inhibitor that appears most promising and is currently being tested in the GUSTO II and TIMI-9 trials), or possibly glycoprotein IIb/IIIa inhibitor therapy in conjunction with thrombolysis. However, glycoprotein IIb/IIIa inhibitors have caused marked prolongations of the bleeding time and excessive bleeding from puncture sites when combined with heparin, inhibit only platelets without inhibiting fibrin (and thus will probably also require heparin or another antithrombin therapy), and have not been adequately tested with thrombolytic therapy to ascertain the potential danger for intracerebral bleeding. Combining a IIb/IIIa inhibitor with thrombolytic therapy may prove dangerous, but this is not based on actual trial results.

Percutaneous transluminal coronary angioplasty

Since the early 1980s, PTCA has been used as a primary or adjunctive therapy for acute MI with increasing frequency. PTCA may be performed without prior thrombolytic therapy or at several different stages following thrombolytic therapy (Table 30B-29). Each application has been studied in a prospective, randomized and controlled fashion.

Direct PTCA. Direct or primary PTCA refers to the use of PTCA without antecedent thrombolytic therapy during the early stages of acute myocardial infarction, when it might be expected to result in myocardial salvage. The recognition that direct PTCA is safe and effective may have been delayed by the emergence of thrombolytic therapy for the treatment of acute MI. Pooled data from five prospective randomized controlled trials of throm-

Table 30B-29 Applications of percutaneous transluminal coronary angioplasty (PTCA) in acute myocardial infarction

Direct (primary, lone, immediate) PTCA
- PTCA without antecedent thrombolytic therapy early enough to result in myocardial salvage (≤24 hours)

Immediate PTCA
- PTCA as soon as possible after administration of thrombolytic therapy in all patients with a significant residual stenosis

Rescue (salvage) PTCA
- PTCA within hours after thrombolytic therapy in patients in whom thrombolytic therapy has failed to restore patency to the infarct-related artery

Delayed (deferred) PTCA
- PTCA in the days after thrombolytic therapy in an attempt to reduce recurrent ischemia or infarction

Table 30B-30 Disadvantages of thrombolytic therapy and potential advantages of PTCA for the treatment of acute myocardial infarction

Disadvantages of thrombolytic therapy	Potential advantages of PTCA
Frequent contraindications[344,347]	Few contraindications
Unable to identify an occluded or patent artery before treatment[319,377-379]	Able to confirm the diagnosis of acute myocardial infarction
	Able to identify the severity and extent of coronary disease
Unable to diagnose treatment failures[319,377-379]	Can identify treatment failures and appropriate candidates for surgery
Early reperfusion rates of only 50% to 80%	Able to achieve reperfusion more rapidly and to achieve a higher reperfusion rate than thrombolytic therapy[380]
Despite treatment, most patients have a significant residual stenosis, which is associated with a greater frequency of recurrent ischemia[381]	Treats the occlusion and the residual stenosis at the same time; less recurrent ischemia
	Less expensive[341]

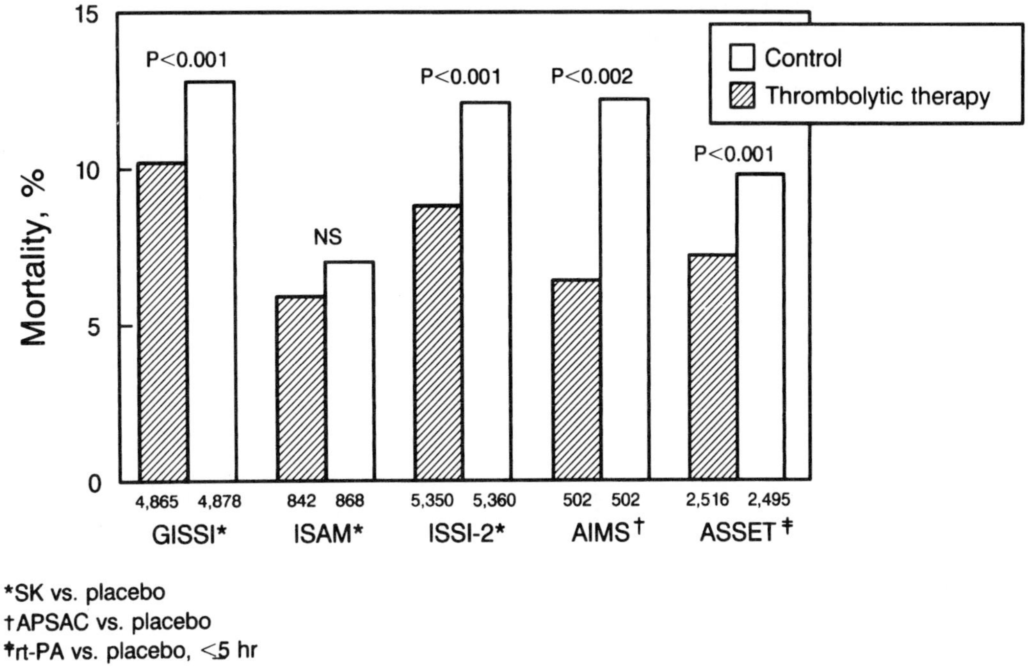

Fig 30B-13 Results from the five prospective controlled trials of thrombolytic therapy large enough to detect a reduction in mortality. Pooled data from these trials, involving more than 28,000 patients treated within 6 hours of symptom onset, reveal a 27% reduction in mortality with thrombolytic therapy in comparison with placebo. *AIMS,* APSAC Intervention Mortality Study; *APSAC,* acylated plasminogen streptokinase activator complex; *ASSET,* Anglo-Scandinavian Study of Early Thrombolysis; *GISSI,* Gruppo Italiano per lo Studio della Sopravvivenza nell'Infarto Miocardico; *ISAM,* Intravenous Streptokinase in Acute Myocardial Infarction; *ISSI,* International Study of Infarct Survival; *rt-PA,* recombinant tissue-type plasminogen activator; *SK,* streptokinase.

bolytic therapy reveal a 27% reduction in mortality with thrombolytic therapy when administered within 6 hours of the onset of symptoms[125,344-347] (Fig 30B-13). In addition, several smaller trials have shown that thrombolytic therapy improves left ventricular function through limitation of infarct size.[368-376]

PTCA is advocated as the initial treatment of acute MI in part because of disadvantages of thrombolytic therapy and in part because of potential advantages of PTCA (Table 30B-30). However, direct PTCA need not be superior to thrombolytic therapy to be the treatment chosen for many patients with acute MI. Most such patients either have contraindications to thrombolytic therapy or present with ECG abnormalities that have been shown not to benefit from thrombolytic therapy.[382,383]

The first report of patients undergoing PTCA without antecedent thrombolytic therapy was from the Mid-America Heart Institute in 1983;[384] shortly thereafter, these investigators reported the results of a larger number of patients who had undergone direct PTCA.[385] PTCA was able to open the infarct artery in greater than 90% of patients in these early reports, and the in-hospital mortality was less than 10%. Since then, patient series have documented successful opening of the infarct artery in 83% to 95% of patients, with in-hospital mortality rates of 6% to 9%[386-391] (Table 30B-31). Reocclusion occurred in 5% to 16% of patients. In view of these high survival rates, even though many patients included in these series would not have qualified for thrombolytic therapy due to co-morbidity and relative contraindications,[391] these results suggest that direct PTCA is a safe and effective form of reperfusion therapy.

The first prospective randomized trial of direct PTCA and thrombolytic therapy was reported in 1986 by O'Neill et al.[392] The study involved only 56 patients, and patients assigned to thrombolytic therapy received *intracoronary* streptokinase. However, the results suggested that PTCA and intracoronary thrombolytic therapy had similar efficacy; the group assigned to direct PTCA actually had greater improvement in left ventricular ejection fraction during the hospitalization, although this may have been due to differences in the baseline characteristics between the two treatment groups.[393]

In the Mayo Clinic Randomized Trial Comparing Immediate Angioplasty to Thrombolysis Followed by Conservative Treatment for Myocardial Infarction, the primary end point was myocardial salvage, as determined

Table 30B-31 Results of direct coronary angioplasty

Series	Year	No. of patients	Technical success, %	No. of patients: In-hospital mortality	Emergency CABG	Reocclusion
Pepine et al.[388]	1984	58	88	NR	NR	16
Rothbaum et al.[390]	1987	151	87	7	0	8
Marco et al.[389]	1987	43	95	9	0	5
Topol[386]	1988	47	96	6	0	16
Miller et al[387]	1987	81	92	8	2	8
O'Keefe et al.[391]	1989	500	94	7	2	15

CABG, coronary artery bypass surgery; NR, not reported.
Modified from Topol EJ: Mechanical interventions for acute myocardial infarction. In *Textbook of Interventional Cardiology*. Edited by EJ Topol. Philadelphia, WB Saunders Company, 1990, pp 269-299.

by tomographic imaging with technetium-99m-sestamibi.[341] The study randomized 103 patients within 12 hours of the onset of symptoms (mean duration of symptoms, 146 minutes) to either intravenous rt-PA or PTCA. The amount of myocardial salvage in the two treatment groups, expressed as an absolute percentage of the left ventricle, was similar (15% ± 19% vs. 13% ± 19%, P = NS), as was the mean predismissal left ventricular ejection fraction (0.50 ± 0.10 vs. 0.53 ± 0.11, P = NS), a secondary end point in the trial. An analysis of the cost of the two treatments indicated that angioplasty tended to be *less* expensive than thrombolysis ($21,400 ± $14,806 vs. $16,811 ± $8,827, $P = 0.09$), principally because of a lower frequency of recurrent ischemia and subsequent angioplasty in the group initially assigned to PTCA.

A second prospective trial from the Netherlands randomized 48 patients to intravenous streptokinase and 48 patients to direct PTCA.[343] Left ventricular ejection fraction before dismissal, the primary end point of the trial, was higher in the PTCA group (51% ± 11% vs. 45% ± 12%, $P = 0.004$), as was the proportion of patients with a patent infarct-related artery before hospital dismissal (91% vs. 68%, $P = 0.001$). Recurrent ischemia during the initial hospitalization occurred in 9% of PTCA patients, compared with 38% of streptokinase patients ($P = 0.001$). A trend toward lower mortality among patients in the PTCA group was observed (0% vs. 4% for thrombolytic therapy, $P = 0.13$). These investigators ultimately enrolled an additional 205 patients,[394] so that a total of 149 patients were randomized to streptokinase and 152 patients to PTCA. Inclusion of the additional patients not only supported the interim results, revealing a higher ejection fraction (50% ± 11% vs. 44% ± 11%) and a lower reinfarction rate (1% vs. 10%) in the PTCA group, but also revealed significantly lower mortality in the PTCA patients (2% vs. 7%, $P = 0.024$).

The PTCA in Acute Myocardial Infarction (PAMI) trial was a prospective study in which 395 patients were randomized to either intravenous rt-PA or direct PTCA.[342] The primary end point in the trial was combined mortality and reinfarction, which was lower in the PTCA group (5.1% vs. 12.0%, $P = 0.015$). A trend toward lower mortality was observed in the group assigned to PTCA (2.6% vs. 6.5% for rt-PA, $P = 0.06$); the mortality was significantly lower among high-risk patients (those older than 70, with a heart rate 100 beats/min on admission, or with anterior infarction) assigned to PTCA (2.0 vs. 10.4, $P = 0.01$). Recurrent ischemia was more frequent in the group assigned to thrombolytic therapy (28% vs. 10%, $P = 0.001$). A meta-analysis of these first three prospective randomized trials of direct coronary angioplasty and thrombolytic therapy suggests that although left ventricular ejection fraction is similar with these two treatments, mortality may be lower with direct PTCA (2.5%, 10 of 394, vs. 6.4%, 26 of 405, with thrombolytic therapy; $P = 0.013$). A meta-analysis of reinfarction in these trials also indicates that reinfarction rate among patients treated with direct PTCA is less common (2.5%, 10 of 394, vs. 7.7%, 31 of 405; $P = 0.0004$).[395] However, the high mortality rate in the PAMI and Netherlands trials resulted largely from a higher than expected hemorrhagic stroke rate, which was significantly greater than the stroke rate observed in the GISSI II and International trials; most of these were fatal.[138] In addition, the reinfarction rate in the two trials was significantly higher than expected, based on the observed reinfarction rate among patients in the TIMI II trial.

The speed with which reperfusion is achieved appears to be a critical determinant of the amount of benefit achieved. Until recently, it has been difficult to compare this speed between thrombolytic therapy and direct PTCA. Such comparison must include the time required to initiate each therapy and the *mean* time to reperfusion. Trials of thrombolytic therapy have not reported these times[377-379,396] whereas analyses of direct coronary angioplasty *have*.[384,397,398] The Mayo Clinic and the Netherlands trials provide the first detailed analyses of the time required to achieve reperfusion with direct PTCA.[341,343,380] Although patients assigned to thrombolytic therapy in these trials did not undergo early angiography, reperfusion rates from the TIMI I trial, in which early angiography was performed after thrombolytic therapy, may be used for comparison.[319,377] When

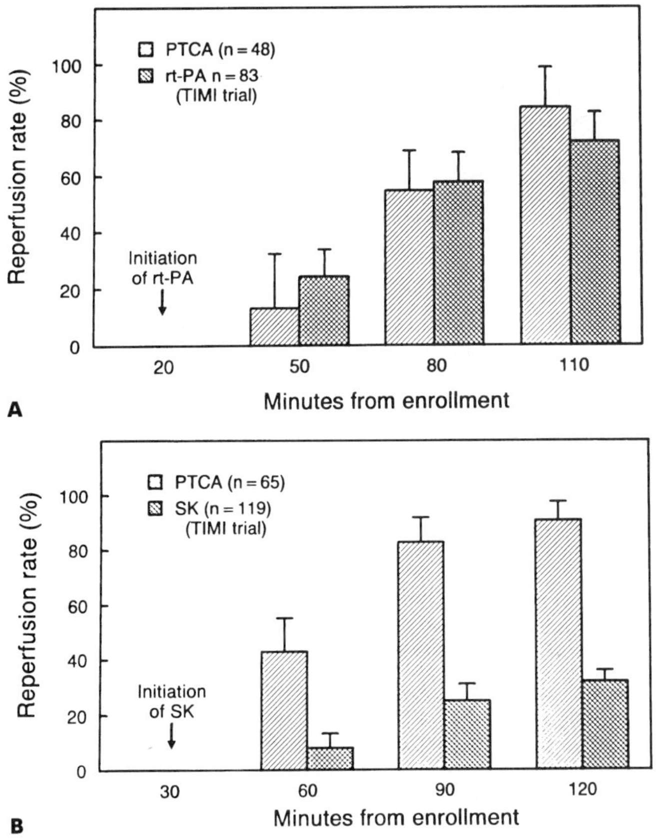

Fig 30B-14 The reperfusion rate for direct coronary angioplasty *(PTCA)* in the Mayo Clinic trial is compared with the previously published reperfusion rate for recombinant tissue-type plasminogen activator (t-PA) **(A),** and the reperfusion rate for direct PTCA in the Netherlands trial is compared with the previously published reperfusion rate for streptokinase *(SK)* **(B).** In these analyses, Thrombolysis in Myocardial Infarction (TIMI) grade 2 or 3 perfusion after thrombolytic therapy is considered to represent reperfusion. If only TIMI grade 3 perfusion is considered to represent reperfusion after thrombolytic therapy, direct PTCA compares favorably with the reperfusion rates of both rt-PA and SK. (Modified from Berger PB, Bell MR, Holmes DR Jr, et al: Time to reperfusion with direct coronary angioplasty and thrombolytic therapy in acute myocardial infarction. *Am J Cardiol* 73:231-236, 1994.)

the time required to initiate thrombolytic therapy is included and reperfusion rates rather than mean time to reperfusion are reported, comparison between the time required to achieve reperfusion with the two therapies can be performed. If TIMI grade 2 or 3 flow is considered to represent reperfusion after thrombolytic therapy, the reperfusion rate with direct coronary angioplasty in the Mayo Clinic trial is similar to the previously reported reperfusion rate for rt-PA, and the reperfusion rate for direct PTCA in the Netherlands trial compares favorably to the previously reported reperfusion rate for streptokinase (Fig 30B-14). However, recent evidence suggests that only TIMI grade 3 perfusion should be considered to represent reperfusion; the mortality with TIMI grade 2 perfusion more closely resembles that with grade 0 or 1 flow than that with normal TIMI 3 perfusion (Fig 30B-15).[399,400] If, as has been advocated, only TIMI grade 3 perfusion is considered to represent successful reperfusion,[399-403] direct PTCA compares favorably to previously reported reperfusion rates with both rt-PA and streptokinase. Accelerated administration of rt-PA has been reported to achieve TIMI 3 flow in 62% of patients;[396] streptokinase has been reported to achieve TIMI 3 flow in 18% of patients.[319]

Table 30B-32 Comparison of end points of thrombolytic therapy and direct percutaneous transluminal coronary angioplasty (PTCA)

Criterion	Thrombolysis	PTCA
Availability	Advantage	
Speed of reperfusion		Advantage
Patients reperfused		Advantage
Infarct size	Equivalent	Equivalent
Recurrent ischemia		Advantage
Reinfarction		Probable advantage
Mortality		Probable advantage
Total cost		Possible advantage

Thus, whether one therapy is superior may depend on which end point is considered for analysis (Table 30B-32). However, reports indicate that mortality from acute MI is considerably lower among patients treated with direct PTCA than among patients in the placebo groups of the large controlled trials of thrombolytic therapy and among historical controls who did not receive reperfusion therapy with thrombolytic therapy or direct PTCA.

On the basis of the proven benefit of thrombolytic therapy in acute MI and the results of these randomized studies of thrombolytic therapy and direct PTCA, direct PTCA should without question be considered the treatment of choice among patients with ST-segment elevation and true *contraindications* to thrombolytic therapy; these do not include age greater than 75 years,[125] presentation more than 6 hours after the onset of chest pain,[125] and recent cardiopulmonary resuscitation.[404] Patients with characteristics for which there are conflicting reports about the safety of thrombolytic therapy, including prior ischemic stroke,[330] and with characteristics that substantially increase the risk of thrombolytic therapy, including severe hypertension,[330] current coumadin therapy,[331] recent surgery, and gastrointestinal bleeding, should be treated with direct PTCA, if available.

Direct PTCA is also the treatment of choice in patients in whom thrombolytic therapy appears to be ineffective. Approximately 25% of patients with suspected MI present

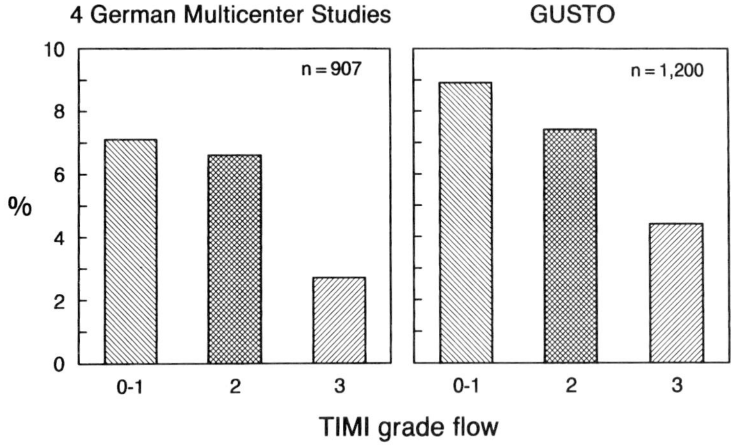

Fig 30B-15 Data from four German multicenter trials and the Global Utilization of Streptokinase or Tissue-type Plasminogen Activator for Occluded Coronary Arteries *(GUSTO)* trial reveal that the mortality of patients with Thrombolysis in Myocardial Infarction *(TIMI)* grade 2 perfusion 90 minutes after thrombolytic therapy more closely resembles that of patients with grade 0 or 1 perfusion than it does the mortality of patients with normal, TIMI 3, perfusion. (Modified from Vogt A, von Essen R, Tebbe U, et al: Impact of early perfusion status of the infarct-related artery on short-term mortality after thrombolysis for acute myocardial infarction: retrospective analysis of four German multicenter studies. *J Am Coll Cardiol* 21:1391-1395, 1993, and data from The GUSTO Angiographic Investigators: The effects of tissue plasminogen activator, streptokinase, or both on coronary-artery patency, ventricular function, and survival after acute myocardial infarction. *N Engl J Med* 329:1615-1622, 1993.)

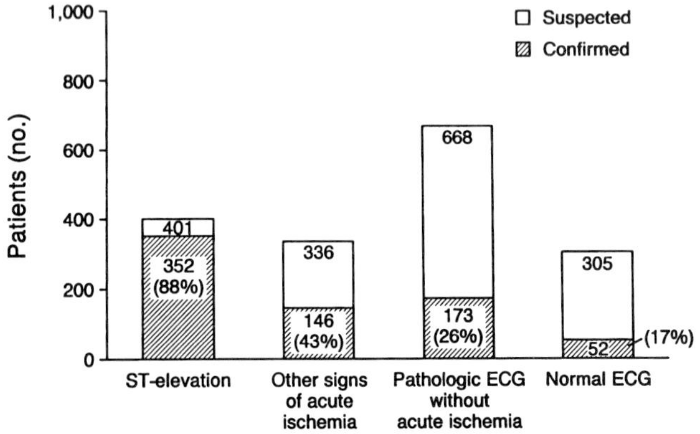

Fig 30B-16 Electrocardiographic findings among patients with suspected acute myocardial infarction, and the percentage of patients in whom myocardial infarction is subsequently confirmed. Most patients with suspected myocardial infarction do not have ST-segment elevation, and the diagnosis of myocardial infarction is less certain among patients without ST-segment elevation. (From Karlson BW, Herlitz J, Edvardsson N, et al: Eligibility for intravenous thrombolysis in suspected acute myocardial infarction. *Circulation* 82:1140-1146, 1990. By permission of American Heart Association.)

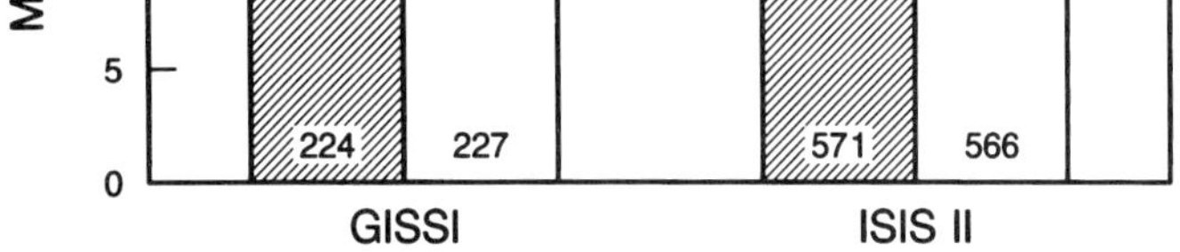

Fig 30B-17 Mortality in the Gruppo Italiano per lo Studio della Sopravvivenza nell'Infarto Miocardico (GISSI) and Second International Study of Infarct Survival (ISIS-II) trials among patients with ST-segment depression on the initial electrocardiogram. Mortality was similar among patients randomized to thrombolytic and nonthrombolytic therapy.

with ECG findings other than ST-segment elevation. The diagnosis of MI is less certain in such patients (Fig 30B-16),[382] and existing data indicate that most such patients do not benefit from thrombolytic therapy. In patients with ST-segment depression, the GISSI and ISIS-2 trials found mortality of nearly 20%; it was similar among patients randomized to thrombolytic and non-thrombolytic therapy[125,344] (Fig 30B-17). Why there is such high mortality among patients with initial ST-segment depression and why they do not benefit from thrombolytic therapy may be related to greater age[405] and increased prevalence of multivessel disease with collaterals to the infarct artery[406] in such patients. The only controlled thrombolysis trial to enroll patients with ST-segment depression in which early angiography was performed was the Mount Sinai–New York University Reperfusion Trial.[406] The results of this trial indicated that patients with ST-segment depression had a 24% 1-year mortality compared to a 12% mortality among patients with ST-segment elevation ($P=0.05$), and that they were more likely to have angiographically visible collateral blood vessels to the infarct artery than patients with ST-segment elevation (50% vs. 23%, $P=0.02$).

Direct PTCA might also be preferable among patients with bundle-branch block, especially left bundle-branch block. Right bundle-branch block does not preclude identification of ST-segment elevation; the diagnosis of MI is less certain among patients with left bundle-branch block, in whom ST-segment elevation cannot be identified. While there is conflicting evidence regarding whether patients with bundle-branch block benefit from thrombolytic therapy,[125,344] a strategy of coronary angiography followed by direct PTCA among patients with clinically suspected MI without supporting ischemic ECG changes provides the ability to confirm the diagnosis and to achieve reperfusion rapidly in patients with an occluded infarct-related artery.

The third group of patients in whom direct PTCA appears to be preferable to thrombolytic therapy includes those with congestive heart failure or cardiogenic shock. Although such patients represent only approximately 6% of patients with acute MI,[125,344] the mortality in these patients remains high, approximately 70%, despite thrombolytic therapy,[140,344] no better than the mortality of such patients initially described by Killip et al. in 1967.[407] The evidence suggesting that such patients may have improved survival comes from nonrandomized studies reporting the outcome of patients with cardiogenic shock undergoing direct PTCA[408-421] (Table 30B-33). Although the reperfusion rate achieved with PTCA, 73% from pooled data, is lower with cardiogenic shock than in most other situations, the mortality of patients in whom PTCA was successful, 30%, is considerably lower than the 70% mortality among patients with failed PTCA.[408-421] Thus, either PTCA failure contributes to the high mortality in patients with cardiogenic shock or, more likely, PTCA, when successful, reduces mortality among patients with cardiogenic shock.

Immediate PTCA. Because thrombolytic therapy achieves reperfusion in only 50% to 80% of patients at 90

Table 30B-33 Results of direct coronary angioplasty (PTCA) in the treatment of patients with cardiogenic shock

						Mortality if PTCA			
		Reperfusion achieved		Total mortality		Successful*		Unsuccessful	
Study	No. of patients	No.	%	No.	%	No.	%	No.	%
O'Neill et al.[408]	27	24/27	89	8/27	30	6/24	25	2/3	67
Shani et al.[409]	9	6/9	67	4/9	44	NA	...	NA	...
Heuser et al.[410]	10	6/10	60	4/10	40	1/6	17	3/4	75
Brown et al.[411]	28	17/28	61	16/28	57	7/17	41	9/11	82
Laramee et al.[412]	39	33/39	85	16/39	41	NA	...	NA	...
Lee et al.[413]	24	13/24	54	12/24	50	3/13	23	9/11	82
Lee et al.[414]	69	49/69	71	31/69	45	15/49	31	16/20	80
Gacioch et al.[415]	25	18/25	72	11/25	44	4/18	22	7/7	100
Disler et al.[416]	7	5/7	71	4/7	57	2/5	40	2/2	100
Verna et al.[417]	7	7/7	100	2/7	29	1/7	14	...	...
Meyer et al.[418]	25	22/25	88	12/25	48	9/22	41	3/3	100
Hibbard et al.[419]	45	28/45	62	20/45	44	8/28	29	12/17	71
Moosvi et al.[420]	38	25/33	76	18/38	47	11/29	38	7/9	78
Eltchanioff et al.[421]	33	25/33	76	12/33	36	6/25	24	6/8	75
Total	386	278/381	73	170/386	44	74/243	30	76/95	80

*The lower mortality among patients in whom coronary angioplasty was successful suggests either that angioplasty failure increases mortality or, more likely, that successful angioplasty reduces mortality among patients with cardiogenic shock.

From Bates ER, Topol EJ: Limitations of thrombolytic therapy for acute myocardial infarction complicated by congestive heart failure and cardiogenic shock. *J Am Coll Cardiol* 18:1077-1084, 1991. By permission of the American College of Cardiology.

minutes and most patients are left with a significant residual stenosis, predisposing them to recurrent ischemia and reocclusion, a strategy of PTCA immediately after the administration of thrombolytic therapy has been proposed. Termed "immediate PTCA," this strategy has now been studied in several prospective randomized trials[381,422,423] (see Fig 30B-17). Despite differences in the designs of these trials, the results indicate that immediate catheterization and PTCA after thrombolytic therapy does not reduce mortality or improve left ventricular function (Fig 30B-18), but may increase the number of hemorrhagic events and the need for coronary artery bypass surgery.

An additional trial has compared immediate coronary angioplasty after thrombolytic therapy to direct coronary angioplasty. O'Neill et al.[424] randomized 122 patients with acute MI either to streptokinase followed by immediate coronary angioplasty or to coronary angioplasty alone. There was no difference in the initial success rate of coronary angioplasty between the two groups or in the patency rate or ejection fraction at 6 months. However, hospitalization was longer and more costly in the patients assigned to initial streptokinase therapy, and there was also a greater need for emergency coronary artery bypass surgery.

On the basis of these data, immediate angioplasty appears to be the least desirable application of coronary angioplasty for acute MI and should not be done routinely.

Rescue coronary angioplasty. PTCA immediately after thrombolytic therapy does not appear to be beneficial, but what about PTCA in patients in whom the infarct-related artery remains occluded despite thrombolytic therapy? Such patients have a greater morbidity and mortality than patients in whom early reperfusion has been achieved.[425,426] If PTCA could successfully open the arteries in such patients, their morbidity and mortality would be lowered and approach those of patients in whom thrombolytic therapy *had* been successful in restoring blood flow. PTCA early after thrombolytic therapy in patients whose infarct-related artery remains occluded despite thrombolytic therapy has been termed "rescue PTCA." Early retrospective analyses of patients in whom rescue PTCA had been performed suggest that patients may have benefited from this approach[426-428] (Fig 30B-19). However, these studies included small numbers of patients and were subject to the limitations of all retrospective studies.

Until recently, the TAMI 5 study was the only prospective, randomized study of rescue coronary angioplasty reported to date.[429] In this study, 595 patients were randomly assigned to one of three thrombolytic regimens

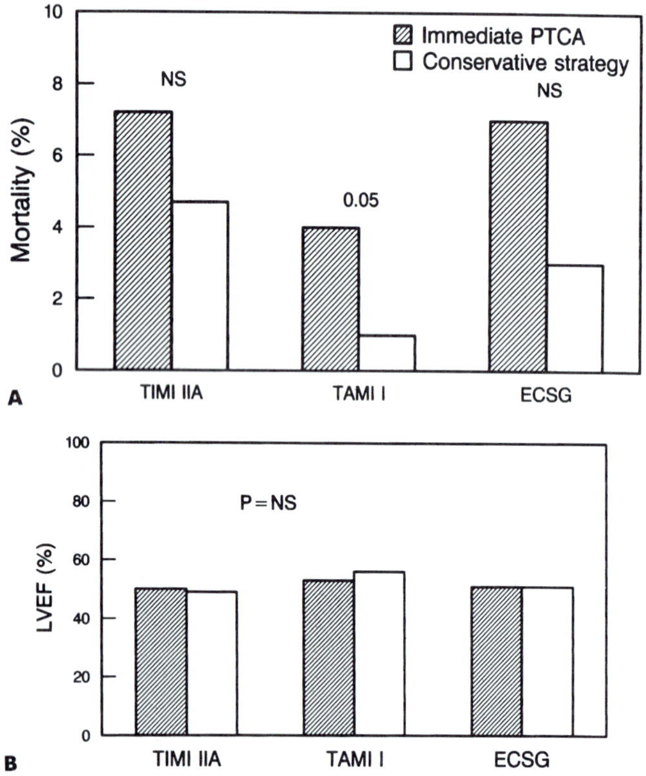

Fig 30B-18 Mortality **(A)** and left ventricular function **(B)** in three prospective, randomized trials comparing immediate coronary angioplasty with a conservative strategy. No benefit from a strategy of immediate percutaneous transluminal coronary angioplasty (PTCA) can be seen in these end points. *ECSG,* European Collaborative Study Group; *LVEF,* left ventricular ejection fraction; *TAMI,* Thrombolysis and Angioplasty in Myocardial Infarction; *TIMI,* Thrombolysis in Myocardial Infarction.

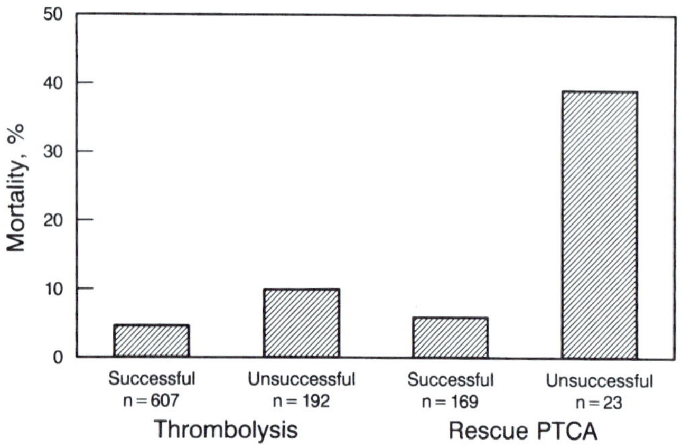

Fig 30B-19 Mortality among patients receiving thrombolytic therapy stratified according to whether early reperfusion of the infarct-related artery was achieved. Among patients with persistent occlusion who underwent rescue percutaneous transluminal coronary angioplasty *(PTCA),* mortality was nearly as low as that in patients in whom thrombolytic therapy had been successful. Mortality among patients in whom thrombolytic therapy and rescue PTCA were unsuccessful was high. (Modified from Abbottsmith CW, Topol EJ, George BS, et al: Fate of patients with acute myocardial infarction with patency of the infarct-related vessel achieved with successful thrombolysis versus rescue angioplasty. *J Am Coll Cardiol* 16:770-778, 1990.)

and subsequently underwent a second randomization either to immediate cardiac catheterization and PTCA if the infarct-related artery remained occluded or to delayed catheterization and PTCA 7 days after enrollment in the trial. Rescue PTCA was performed in 52 of the patients who underwent immediate catheterization and was successful in 43%. However, since catheterization was not performed immediately in the control group of patients receiving conservative therapy, the outcome of patients in whom rescue PTCA was performed could not be compared to that in patients whose infarct-related artery remained occluded following thrombolytic therapy who did not undergo PTCA. Rather, the entire group of 287 patients assigned to immediate catheterization was compared with the entire group of 288 patients undergoing delayed cardiac catheterization, reducing the power of the study to detect a benefit in the strategy of rescue PTCA. The results suggested that regional wall motion in the infarct zone was greater in the group assigned to immediate catheterization, although overall left ventricular function in the two groups was similar. No difference was noted in mortality, reinfarction, or recurrent ischemia between the two groups.

The success of rescue coronary angioplasty may depend on the thrombolytic agent used before PTCA. In the TAMI 5 study, rescue PTCA was more likely to be successful after the use of a non-fibrin-specific agent (urokinase or urokinase in combination with rt-PA) than following rt-PA alone.[429] A meta-analysis of the first five TAMI trials and data from the European Cooperative Study Group also support this observation.[422,426]

The first true study of rescue PTCA was recently reported. In the Randomized Evaluation of Salvage Angioplasty with Combined Utilization of Endpoints (RESCUE) trial, 151 patients with anterior infarction who underwent coronary angiography 90 minutes to 8 hours after thrombolytic therapy and who had occlusion of the infarct-related artery were randomized to PTCA or to a conservative strategy of medical therapy without immediate PTCA.[430] Although it may seem a forgone conclusion that patients with an anterior infarction and occlusion of the infarct-related artery despite thrombolytic therapy should undergo immediate PTCA, it must be remembered that between 50% and 70% of the patients in whom the infarct artery is occluded 90 minutes after thrombolytic therapy have "spontaneous" reperfusion within the next several hours as a result of late thrombolysis. Such patients may still have myocardial salvage and yet avoid the high reocclusion rates observed in previous studies of rescue angioplasty relative to patients in whom reperfusion was achieved by thrombolytic therapy alone. In the RESCUE trial, angioplasty was successful in 72 of the 78 patients randomized to PTCA. The mean resting ejection fraction assessed by equilibrium radionuclide ventriculography at 30 days was similar in the PTCA and conservative groups (40% ± 11% vs. 39% ± 12%, $P = 0.49$), although the mean ejection fraction with exercise was higher in the PTCA group (43% ± 15% vs. 38% ± 13%, $P = 0.04$). Mortality was similar in the PTCA and conservative groups (5% and 10%, respectively; $P = 0.18$), as was the frequency of severe heart failure (1% and 7%, respectively; $P = 0.11$), although the combined end point of death or severe heart failure occurred in fewer PTCA patients (6% vs. 17%, $P = 0.05$).[430,431]

Currently the strategy of rescue angioplasty is limited by the fact that catheterization must be performed in all patients to identify the few who have persistent occlusion of the infarct-related artery. If patients with persistent occlusion of the infarct-related artery after thrombolytic therapy could be identified noninvasively, catheterization and PTCA could be performed only in those patients without exposing all patients to the risks of coronary angiography during a lytic state. Early results suggest that analysis of creatine kinase isoenzymes or continuous monitoring of ST segments during thrombolytic therapy may allow for the rapid, noninvasive detection of reperfusion.[432,433] If a rapid, noninvasive marker of reperfusion can be discovered, rescue coronary angioplasty will be far easier and safer to apply because angiography will be performed only in the 30% to 50% of patients who remain occluded 90 minutes after thrombolytic therapy.

On the basis of current evidence, rescue angioplasty appears promising but as yet unproven and might best be reserved for patients with large infarctions in whom ischemic chest pain and certainly hemodynamic instability are present more than 60 minutes after thrombolytic therapy.

Deferred coronary angioplasty. Although approximately 85% of patients will have patent infarct-related arteries in the 24 to 48 hours of thrombolytic therapy, regardless of whether APSAC, rt-PA, or streptokinase is initially used, most such patients will have a significant residual stenosis. Since this is associated with an increased risk of abrupt closure, and many such patients will have spontaneous or exercise-induced ischemia, a strategy of deferred coronary angioplasty after thrombolytic therapy has been proposed. This refers to "prophylactic" coronary angioplasty to prevent postinfarction ischemia beyond the time in which myocardial salvage can be achieved.

Delayed coronary angioplasty has been the subject of two large trials[381,434] (Fig 30B-20). In the TIMI II trial, 3,339 patients received intravenous rt-PA within 4 hours of the onset of myocardial infarction and were randomized either to catheterization 18 to 48 hours following rt-PA and, if the coronary anatomy was suitable, coronary angioplasty or to a conservative strategy in which catheterization and angioplasty were performed only if spontaneous or exercise-induced ischemia occurred.[381,435] Although fully 41% of patients assigned to the conservative strategy underwent cardiac catheterization for recurrent ischemia within 14 days of infarction, no benefit was associated with an invasive strategy over a strategy of "watchful waiting" in terms of mortality and recurrent MI (the primary end points of the trial). However, an increased risk of emergency bypass surgery and bleeding complications was associated with the invasive strategy. Similar results were reported in the SWIFT (Should We Intervene Following Thrombolysis?) trial.[434] Few patients with congestive heart failure or hypotension were included in these trials; conclusions from these trials should be applied only to patients similar to those in the study

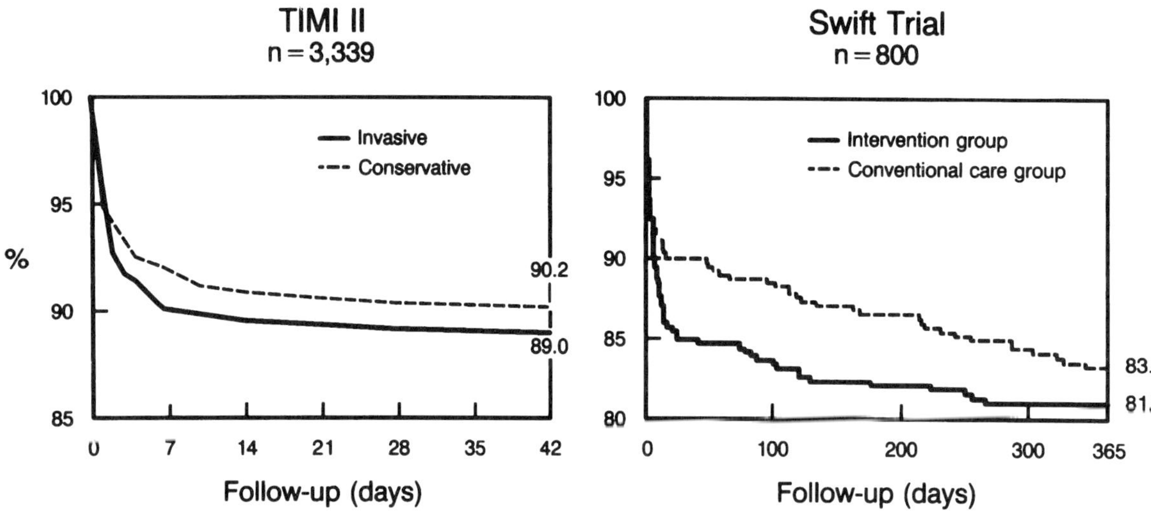

Fig 30B-20 Mortality and recurrent nonfatal myocardial infarction in the second Thrombolysis in Myocardial Infarction (TIMI II) and Should We Intervene Following Thrombolysis? (SWIFT) trials. An invasive strategy did not have a beneficial effect on mortality or recurrent infarction in either trial. (Modified from the TIMI Study Group: Comparison of invasive and conservative strategies after treatment with intravenous tissue plasminogen activator in acute myocardial infarction: results of the Thrombolysis in Myocardial Infarction (TIMI) Phase II Trial. *N Engl J Med* 320:618-627, 1989, and from SWIFT (Should We Intervene Following Thrombolysis?) Trial Study Group: SWIFT trial of delayed elective intervention vs conservative treatment after thrombolysis with anistreplase in acute myocardial infarction. *BMJ* 302:555-560, 1991. By permission.)

populations.[435] A third trial of elective coronary angioplasty after thrombolytic therapy compared with conservative therapy, in which coronary angioplasty was performed a mean of 9 days after admission, also revealed no benefit in patients without spontaneous or exercise-induced ischemia.[436]

Reperfusion by surgery

Some have advocated or discussed myocardial reperfusion by acute surgical revascularization.[437-442] This should be done within 4 to 5 hours after the onset of symptoms, which usually is logistically difficult when the patient is not already in a hospital (because of delays in admission and need for time for clinical evaluation, for mobilizing the catheterization team and performing the coronary arteriogram, and for mobilizing the surgical team and preparing for the operation). It is reasonable and logistically easier to perform the coronary bypass operation promptly in patients in whom acute infarction develops during coronary arteriography or PTCA or while awaiting coronary surgery in the hospital.[443,444] There is no evidence that surgical revascularization is superior to thrombolysis of the infarct-related artery, with or without PTCA, for salvage of ischemic myocardium in patients who have an evolving acute MI. Certainly, initial reperfusion by thrombolysis, with or without PTCA, is easier logistically, quicker, and less costly than bypass surgery.

Although thrombolysis for acute MI has been demonstrated to maintain or improve left ventricular function, presumably by the salvage of ischemic myocardium,[445] no randomized trials have been done using coronary bypass surgery at the time of acute infarction to demonstrate salvage of ischemic myocardium. However, 10% to 15% of patients who undergo thrombolysis for acute MI require aortocoronary bypass graft operation during hospitalization for recurrent ischemia, recurrent infarction, or cardiogenic shock not amenable to PTCA because of failure of the procedure to maintain patency of the infarct-related artery, left main coronary artery disease, or multivessel coronary artery disease causing recurrent ischemia or complicated by mural thrombus within the coronary artery.[260,319] Although it is advisable to clinically stabilize the patient with optimal medical treatment for the acute MI before proceeding to bypass operation, the urgency with which one proceeds depends on the severity and extent of ischemic and salvageable myocardium, the patient's clinical condition with maximal medical therapy, and the risk of delay versus the potential gain to be achieved with surgical revascularization.

DIAGNOSIS AND MANAGEMENT OF THE HEMODYNAMIC COMPLICATIONS OF ACUTE MI

Approach to the patient with persistent hypotension after acute MI

The diagnosis of cardiogenic shock carries a very poor prognosis despite newer forms of treatment, so it is incumbent upon the physician to search for treatable and reversible causes of persistent hypotension after acute infarction. Cardiogenic shock may be viewed as the result of a vicious cycle in which ischemia impairs ventricular performance, which leads to a reduction in arterial pressure and coronary perfusion, which may cause further ischemia and loss of cardiac contractility.[446-448] Thus, hypotension may be a cause or a consequence of cardiogenic shock. The search for a reversible cause of hypotension after MI must be prompt.

Pain, nausea, and vomiting. The most frequent accompaniments of acute MI are pain, nausea, and vomiting. These may cause profound but easily reversible hypotension and should never be overlooked. Problems related to oxygenation and acid-base balance produce hypoxia and acidosis, which can exacerbate hypotension. Correction of these disorders can occasionally lead to dramatic improvements in systemic hemodynamics, particularly in diabetic patients, in whom a MI may precipitate ketoacidosis. If the acidosis results from cardiogenic shock, however, it is usually irreversible. In the absence of these factors, the diagnostic possibilities are numerous (Table 30B-34).

Factitious hypotension. This entity may occasionally lead to confusion. Excess sympathetic activity producing spasm of smaller arteries can artificially lower the arm cuff blood pressure reading at the radial artery. Direct intravascular pressure measurement resolves the issue, but if this is measured through the radial artery and the waveform is poor, a more central arterial pressure may be required.[5]

Drugs. The hypotensive action of narcotics and tranquilizers discussed earlier in this chapter may be compounded by concomitant or preexisting therapy with other cardiac drugs, such as nitrates, diuretics, β-adrenergic blocking drugs, calcium entry blocking agents, antihypertensive drugs, and antiarrhythmia agents. Drug-induced hypotension complicating MI is common but reversible and warrants a high degree of clinical alertness.

The effects of nitrates and diuretics in increasing venous capacitance and reducing left ventricular filling pressure will be enhanced in hypovolemic patients.[449] Profound and even alarming hypotensive reactions may occur with the administration of nitrates in acute MI, and preexisting hypovolemia may be a contributory factor.[296]

A retrospective report by Bloch et al.[450] in 1976 raised the possibility that patients on long-term propranolol therapy (more than 80 mg/day) at the time of MI may be at greater risk of cardiac failure. This is unlikely to be a common problem because, despite the subsequent widespread use of β-blockers, no further reports imply an increased incidence of heart failure for patients in whom acute infarctions develop during long-term treatment with β-blockers. Furthermore, an Australian community-based study showed that among patients who were taking a β-blocker before the acute infarction, there was a clear benefit on early survival.[451] Nonetheless, the physician should be aware of the possibility, particularly among patients with hypotension and congestive heart failure, when there is no evidence of extensive acute necrosis or enzyme release. A disproportionate bradycardia or the lack of a compensatory tachycardia despite hypotension suggests a contribution from β-blockers to the syndrome.

Table 30B-34 Causes of hypotension during acute myocardial infarction

Pain, nausea, and vomiting
Factitious hypotension
Drugs
Analgesics
Tranquilizers
Nitrates
Diuretics
β-Blocking agents
Calcium entry blocking agents
Antihypertensive agents
Antiarrhythmia agents
Hypovolemia
Arrhythmias
Tachyarrhythmias
Bradyarrhythmias
Cardiac structural damage
Pump failure
Ruptured ventricular septum
Acute papillary muscle damage and mitral regurgitation
Left ventricular aneurysm (true and false)
Free wall rupture
Right ventricular infarction
Tamponade
Inappropriate vasodilatation
Miscellaneous
Pulmonary and systemic embolism
Pheumothorax
Bleeding
Septicemia

Pretreatment with antihypertensive and vasodilating agents may cause inappropriate hypotension during acute MI. Although the value of the judicious use of these drugs in acute infarction has been well established, it is advisable to avoid agents with long half-lives during the acute phase.

Most antiarrhythmia drugs have some negative inotropic action, and this may become manifest only when ventricular function is already compromised. Agents such as disopyramide, flecainide, and propranolol are more likely to cause hemodynamic depression than others such as lidocaine and procainamide. Nonetheless, the physician needs to tread a fine line between treating arrhythmias and avoiding the negative inotropic effects of certain antiarrhythmia agents.

Hypovolemia. Hypovolemia (relative or absolute) in acute infarction is readily explicable. Patients may be fluid-depleted as a result of vomiting, diaphoresis, anorexia, and fever, and the administration of narcotics or other cardioactive drugs may further reduce the ventricular filling pressure and exacerbate hypotension.

Hypotension and bradycardia as manifestations of the Bezold-Jarisch reflex should alert one to underlying hypovolemia. The clinical picture is commonly seen with clinical vasovagal episodes, namely, bradycardia and evidence of sympathetic withdrawal.[296] This is readily reversible with fluid repletion by means of isotonic saline or low-molecular-weight dextran.

Structural cardiac damage. Structural cardiac damage may occur within days, weeks, or months after the acute event, and its consequences can be catastrophic. Many of these conditions are potentially reversible and require prompt diagnosis and therapy.

Inappropriate vasodilatation. This unusual hemodynamic response to acute infarction was discussed earlier in this section.

Miscellaneous. Miscellaneous causes of hypotension (see Table 30B-34) are relatively infrequent. Attention to systems other than the cardiovascular is mandatory in coronary care management and essential to the diagnosis of most of these unusual but often serious complications.

Pulmonary and systemic emboli are well documented in MI, and pulmonary emboli may produce profound hypotension and shock. Pneumothorax may complicate cardiac arrest resuscitative procedures. Patients who are on artificial ventilators should be screened for the possibility of a tension pneumothorax.

The widespread use of anticoagulant and thrombolytic therapy in patients with acute infarction increases the risk of bleeding. "Silent" intra-abdominal or retroperitoneal bleeding may cause severe but reversible hypotension, and the diagnosis may be difficult.

The physician should always be alert to the possibility of septicemia, particularly gram-negative septicemia, as a cause of hypotension after MI. The diverse invasive procedures employed in the acute management of such patients provide a rich environment for infections. Hypotension caused by gram-negative septicemia is characterized, at least in the early treatable phase, by increased cardiac output and decreased systemic vascular resistance. The clinical presentation—warm, vasodilated extremities with hypotension—is striking. The importance of urgent diagnosis and therapy in this situation cannot be overemphasized, since the condition is eminently correctable if therapy is prompt.

Arrhythmias, both tachyarrhythmias and bradyarrhythmias, are a frequent and reversible cause of hypotension early and late after acute infarction, as discussed later in this chapter.

Cardiogenic shock

Insufficient tissue blood flow is the primary feature of circulatory shock, regardless of cause. Cardiogenic shock refers to profound circulatory failure primarily of cardiac origin. Low blood pressure itself does not necessarily indicate shock because, with decreased vascular resistance, perfusion can be normal at lower blood pressures. Similarly, tissue blood flow can be inadequate without marked hypotension when there is reflex vasoconstriction because blood flow depends on both perfusion pressure and vascular resistance. When cardiac output is limited, perfusion is preserved to the most vital organs—heart and brain—at the expense of less vital organs, such as skin, muscle, kidneys, liver, and splanchnic organs. Thus, cardiogenic shock resulting from acute MI is generally associated with most or all of these clinical signs: (1) peak systolic blood pressure <90 mm Hg (cuff pressure) or <80 mm Hg by intra-arterial measurement (or a reduction of >30 mm Hg below previous blood pressure); (2) peripheral vasoconstriction associated with cool, clammy, and often cyanotic skin, reflecting reflex sympathetic stimulation of vasoconstriction and diaphoresis; (3) urine output <20 mL/hr; (4) altered mental status (delirium, confusion, agitation, lethargy, obtundation, coma); and (5) persistence of shock after correction of contributing or secondary factors such as hypovolemia, drug toxicity, arrhythmia (including bradycardia), acidosis, and hypoxemia. When used without further description, the term "cardiogenic shock" generally implies a severe reduction in cardiac output caused by infarction of a large part of the left ventricle. The extent of myocardial loss required for the development of heart failure is believed to be $>25\%$ and for the development of cardiogenic shock to be 40% or more, based on autopsy studies.[199,202] However, nuclear studies with tomographic imaging reveal that myocardial loss of more than 40% of the left ventricle often occurs (especially in anterior infarction) without causing cardiogenic shock.[203]

Acute MI may result in the development of shock through four different mechanisms: (1) extensive left ventricular dysfunction due to the acute MI, with or without prior myocardial disease (prior infarction or cardiomyopathy, for example); (2) mechanical dysfunction in the right or left heart chambers due either to the infarction (papillary muscle dysfunction or rupture, ventricular septal defect, or tamponade) or preexisting mechanical dysfunction exacerbated by the acute infarction (severe valvular stenosis or regurgitation); (3) severe right ventricular dysfunction, with or without severe left ventricular dysfunction; and (4) changes in loading conditions due to the infarction or treatment of the infarction, including hypovolemia (due to vomiting, overdiuresis, etc.) or drug effects (such as excessive vasodilator therapy) superimposed on intrinsic myocardial disease. Only the first mechanism is generally considered to represent true *left ventricular* cardiogenic shock, since the other mechanisms generally respond to correction of the anatomic or contributing secondary factors, such as mechanical repair of the anatomic defect or correction of hypovolemia, drug toxicity, etc., and are not principally the result of left ventricular dysfunction. Cardiogenic shock in acute MI is most commonly caused by left ventricular dysfunction due to infarction and continuing ischemia, with the potential for salvage of considerable myocardium if reperfusion or revascularization is accomplished early. With the advent of coronary care units and the early recognition and treatment of arrhythmia, mortality from acute MI has decreased from 25% to 30% to approximately 10%;[452] cardiogenic shock is now the most common cause of death in patients with acute MI treated in coronary care units. With new methods of acute nonsurgical reperfusion of coronary arteries, the incidence of cardiogenic shock appears to have decreased to as low as 5% in published series of thrombolytic therapy intervention,[319,453] but the exclusion of patients with cardiogenic shock from these trials gives a falsely low impression of the incidence of cardiogenic shock.[454] Thus, the true incidence of cardiogenic shock in acute MI still may be as high as 10% to 15%.

History and physical examination. Rapid recognition of the patient with, or at risk of developing, cardiogenic shock and early therapeutic intervention are important. Initial rapid stabilization of the patient followed by aggressive and rapid therapy to limit infarct size and salvage ischemic myocardium is the cornerstone of therapy. Thus, patients with, or at high risk of developing, cardiogenic shock must be recognized and treated early and aggressively. They usually have a large anterior or anterolateral infarction. There may be a history of previous infarction.[202,455] Extension of recent infarction[456] or a stuttering progressive infarction[457,458] is also frequently present.

On physical examination, peripheral pulses may be thready or absent and rapid, and a narrow pulse pressure is often present. Body temperature may be low and cyanosis visible. Shallow, rapid respirations are common, although Cheyne-Stokes respirations may occur. Heart sounds are often distant because of the low output state; the third heart sound may be difficult to appreciate. A murmur of papillary muscle dysfunction may be present, although even severe mitral regurgitation may be present without a murmur.[459,460] Arrhythmias are common, including supraventricular and ventricular tachyarrhythmias, bradycardia, and AV block. Evidence of heart failure, such as pulmonary congestion and an elevated jugular venous pressure, is often present. If evidence of right heart failure, such as jugular venous distention and hepatic congestion is present *without* evidence of left heart failure, such as pulmonary congestion, a diagnosis of right ventricular infarction shoud be considered (see below). To identify causes of cardiogenic shock other than left ventricular dysfunction that require special treatment, including severe papillary dysfunction, cardiac tamponade, and predominantly right ventricular dysfunction, echocardiography with Doppler examination can supplement the physical examination.

Differential diagnosis. Right ventricular infarction occurs in approximately one-third of patients with inferior wall MI and is hemodynamically significant in approximately one-half of these patients; hemodynamically significant right ventricular infarction is rare in patients with anterior MI.[461] Prompt recognition of cardiogenic shock due to right ventricular infarction is clinically important, since it is generally reversible if certain therapy is initiated and other therapies are avoided. Administration of volume generally increases the cardiac output by reversing the relatively underfilled left ventricle; diuretics and nitroglycerine, which reduce filling of the left heart, should be avoided.[461] Occasionally, dopamine[462] or dobutamine[463] may be needed to increase the cardiac output in patients refractory to volume replacement.

Massive pulmonary embolism may cause circulatory shock and simulate a right ventricular MI or result from MI and prolonged bed rest. Generally, pulmonary artery pressures increase with a normal or low pulmonary capillary wedge pressure. Occasionally, only a mild increase in pulmonary artery pressure may be present if a previously normal right ventricle fails acutely. Pulmonary embolism can usually be distinguished from right ventricular infarction by the increased arterial-alveolar gradient and the nearly constant association of right ventricular infarction with inferior MI.

Tamponade may occur as a result of MI and rupture or, very rarely, hemorrhagic pericarditis and a bloody effusion occurring as a complication of thrombolytic and anticoagulant therapy; the presence of pulsus paradoxus and distention of the jugular veins should suggest the diagnosis. Echocardiography can both confirm the presence of a significant effusion and provide evidence that the effusion is hemodynamically significant. A nearly equal increase in diastolic pressure in all the right- and left-sided chambers is present in tamponade.

Laboratory findings. Findings in cardiogenic shock caused by left ventricular dysfunction are as follows: possible cardiomegaly on roentgenogram; pulmonary edema commonly; possible pleural effusions; ECG findings same as acute infarction, usually anterior; and possible evidence of prior MI. However, even extensive MI, both recent and remote, may be present without ECG evidence. Because a large anterior infarction usually involves the interventricular septum, conduction disturbances are common, especially right bundle-branch block and left anterior fascicular block.

Laboratory evidence of congestive heart failure, including congestive hepatitis; metabolic acidosis due to lacticacidemia, with secondary electrolyte abnormalities; respiratory failure, with hypocapnia and hypoxemia; and rhabdomyolysis due to skeletal muscle hypoperfusion may be seen. A leukocytosis is usually present. Renal hypoperfusion results in prerenal azotemia and leads to acute tubular necrosis, further contributing to metabolic acidosis.

Echocardiography. Echocardiography with Doppler examination can noninvasively assess several possible mechanisms of cardiogenic shock, including (1) the presence and extent of left ventricular dysfunction; (2) the extent of right ventricular dysfunction; (3) the presence of tamponade; and (4) mechanical problems in the right or left side of the heart, including severe valvular regurgitation, that may be silent.[459,460]

Hemodynamics. Hemodynamic measurements indicating cardiogenic shock due to left ventricular dysfunction include low cardiac output (cardiac index, <1.8 liters/min per m^2), arterial hypotension (systolic pressure, <80 mm Hg; mean, <60 mm Hg; diastolic, usually <50 mm Hg), and elevated left ventricular filling pressure (mean pulmonary artery wedge pressure >18 mm Hg). Usually there is tachycardia and an elevated total peripheral resistance (>33 Wood units). The low output is usually associated with a low stroke volume index (<20 mL/m^2), low stroke work index, and depressed isovolumic and ejection phase indices of contractility. If hemodynamically significant right ventricular infarction is present, the jugular venous pressure is usually 10 mm Hg or greater, with a right atrial to pulmonary capillary wedge pressure of 0.80 or greater.[461] Because right ventricular failure may be present or absent with left heart failure or profound cardiogenic shock, central venous pressure monitoring does not reflect the status of the left heart filling pressure and is ineffective for monitoring therapy.

Prevention. The most effective way to reduce mortality from cardiogenic shock in acute MI is to prevent its development. Measures that reduce MI size reduce the percentage of patients in whom cardiogenic shock develops, as demonstrated with thrombolytic therapy. Data from two large, prospective, randomized, placebo-controlled trials of thrombolytic therapy reveal 25% and 43% reductions in the percentage of patients with development of cardiogenic shock after thrombolytic therapy compared with the placebo arms in these trials[346,347] (Fig 30B-21). Given the equivalent[341,342] or greater[343] reduction in MI size achieved with coronary angioplasty compared with thrombolytic therapy and the ability to identify patients with coronary angiography who might benefit from immediate coronary artery bypass strategy, direct coronary angioplasty, like thrombolytic therapy, undoubtedly also reduces the percentage of patients in whom cardiogenic shock develops.

Therapy and management. Once cardiogenic shock has developed in patients with acute MI, a careful analysis of the history, physical examination, and laboratory data should be performed to determine the cause. Evidence for right ventricular infarction (which is almost exclusively associated with inferior MI), mechanical problems (including valve disease, myocardial rupture, and tamponade), and hypovolemia should be carefully sought; these disorders require specific treatment and have a very different prognosis from cardiogenic shock due to left ventricular dysfunction.

The mortality from cardiogenic shock due to left ventricular dysfunction, before the reperfusion era, among patients treated with medical therapy and intra-aortic balloon counterpulsation was approximately 80%.[413,464] Now in patients with acute MI complicated by severe congestive heart failure, hypotension, or cardiogenic shock, *early reperfusion is mandatory.* Although thrombolytic therapy reduces mortality in acute MI, the results of thrombolytic therapy in patients with cardiogenic shock have been disappointing[138,465,466] (Fig 30B-22), possibly because of lower reperfusion rates with a low cardiac output.[138,466] Thus, *angiography without antecedent thrombolytic therapy, followed by mechanical revascularization with either PTCA or bypass surgery, depending on the angiographic findings, is the preferred approach* (see Table 30B-33). If angioplasty or coronary artery bypass surgery is not immediately available, patients with acute MI and hemodynamic instability should probably be given thrombolytic therapy and should certainly be immediately transferred to the nearest center that has expertise in percutaneous or surgical revascularization. Although coronary angiography and angioplasty routinely performed immediately after thrombolytic therapy have not improved prognosis compared to a conservative strategy after thrombolytic therapy,[381,422,423] the trials evaluating this strategy included few patients with cardiogenic shock. If angiography after thrombolytic therapy reveals the infarct vessel to be occluded or subtotally occluded, "rescue" coronary angioplasty should be performed.[429,467] Although TIMI 2 or 3 flow was previously considered to represent "patency," coronary blood flow should be maximally increased in cardiogenic shock, and an infarct-related artery with TIMI 2 flow should be considered for immediate angioplasty (see Fig 30B-15). In addition, other arteries that are subtotally or totally occluded should probably be considered for immediate angioplasty, even though in general only the infarct-related artery is treated by angioplasty. Combining fibrin-specific and fibrin-nonspecific agents, such as rt-PA and streptokinase, with heparin and aspirin has been reported to reduce the reocclusion rate from "rescue"

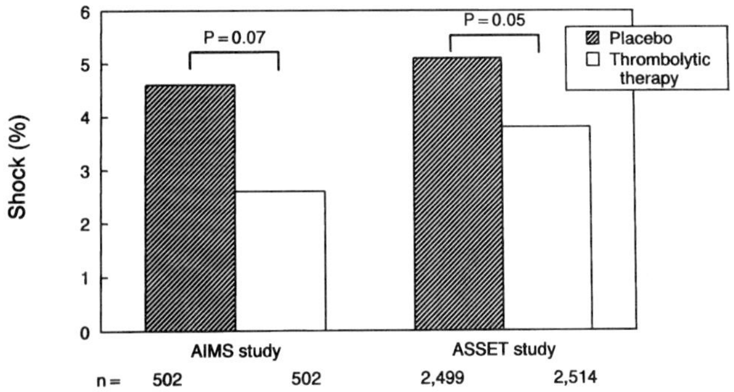

Fig 30B-21 Data from two prospective, randomized, placebo-controlled trials of thrombolytic therapy, the APSAC (acylated plasminogen-streptokinase activator complex) Intervention Mortality Study (AIMS) and Anglo-Scandinavian Study of Early Thrombolysis (ASSET) trials, revealing the effect of thrombolytic therapy on the percentage of patients in whom cardiogenic shock developed in these trials.

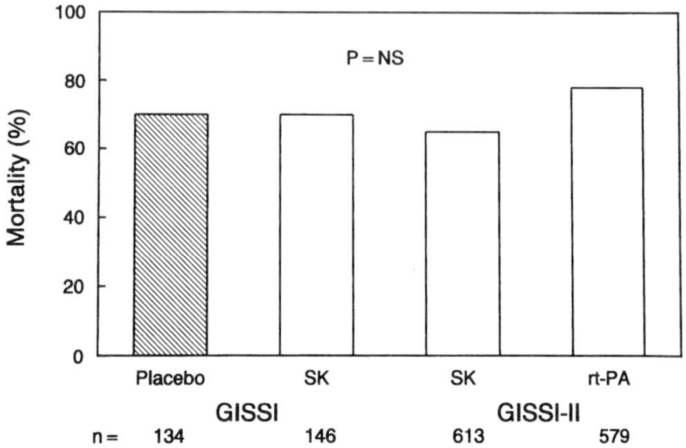

Fig 30B-22 Data from the Gruppo Italiano per lo Studio della Sopravvivenza nell'Infarto Miocardico (GISSI) and GISSI II international trials reveal a high mortality among patients in whom cardiogenic shock developed in these trials, regardless of whether they received thrombolytic therapy and of which thrombolytic agent they received. *rt-PA,* recombinant tissue-type plasminogen activator; *SK,* streptokinase.

angioplasty to 4% to 9% compared with 25% to 30% if rt-PA alone is used.[468-471] Survival is highly influenced by successful reperfusion;[467] in an analysis of pooled data from several patient series of direct coronary angioplasty, 70% of patients survived with successful angioplasty but only 30% survived if angioplasty was unsuccessful[466] (see Table 30B-33). Whether the use of an intra-aortic balloon pump helps maintain patency of the infarct artery and whether the benefits of aortic counterpulsation outweigh the risks is under investigation.[472] Patients in whom cardiogenic shock resolves with thrombolytic therapy should undergo "semielective" coronary angiography soon after thrombolysis, even without recurrent ischemia, to determine the need for revascularization with angioplasty or coronary bypass surgery.

The results of angioplasty appear to be better in patients with single-vessel disease than in those with multivessel disease.[413] Given the high mortality in patients with cardiogenic shock and multivessel disease, early coronary artery bypass graft surgery should be considered in patients with cardiogenic shock and multivessel disease, even if coronary angioplasty is successful. Early emergency coronary bypass grafting, combined with intra-aortic balloon pumping, has reduced mortality from cardiogenic shock to between 25% and 58%.[466,473-475]

Direct coronary angioplasty performed rapidly is preferable to thrombolytic therapy followed by coronary angiography and consideration of rescue angioplasty. Prospective randomized trials of coronary angioplasty compared with thrombolytic therapy have revealed that myocardial salvage is equivalent[341,342] or perhaps greater[343] with direct coronary angioplasty. In one trial, a mortality advantage among high-risk patients (defined as anterior infarction, age greater than 70 years, or a heart rate greater than 100 beats/min at admission) was seen on a post hoc analysis;[342] a meta-analysis of the three trials also suggests a lower mortality with coronary angioplasty.[395] Given the safety and efficacy of immediate angiography followed by direct coronary angioplasty, its ability to diagnose treatment failures and the extent and severity of coronary disease, its usefulness in selecting patients who might best be referred for immediate coronary artery bypass surgery, and the fact that thrombolytic therapy does not appear to be effective in cardiogenic shock and decreases the success rate of subsequent coronary angioplasty, immediate angiography without antecedent thrombolytic therapy, followed by angioplasty or surgical revascularization, appears to be the best reperfusion strategy for cardiogenic shock.[466]

Other therapies may also be important in the treatment of cardiogenic shock. Early recognition and aggressive management of pulmonary congestion and hypotension may greatly slow the rate of further myocardial necrosis[476] (see Fig 30B-8). The work of breathing may be far greater than at rest, significantly increasing myocardial work and oxygen demands and diverting much of the limited cardiac output to the respiratory muscles; thus, early intubation and respiratory assistance may be important. Furthermore, arterial hypoxemia can cause further deterioration of myocardial function. In part because of pulmonary venous hypertension and pulmonary congestion, pulmonary complications of cardiogenic shock are common. Secondary pneumonia may occur and must be looked for in patients with cardiogenic pulmonary edema, so that appropriate antibiotic therapy is initiated.

Although left ventricular filling pressure is usually increased, some patients with a high normal pulmonary artery wedge pressure (mean, 12 to 16 mm Hg) require increased left ventricular filling pressure to above normal (18 to 22 mm Hg) to maximize cardiac output by the Frank-Starling mechanism. Close observation must accompany volume expansion because the resultant increased left ventricular wall stress and filling pressure may lead to increased myocardial ischemia, pulmonary congestion, hypoxemia, and acidosis. If right heart failure due to right ventricular infarction is present and the left heart underfills, *further* volume should be administered to normalize left ventricular filling.[461] When right ventricular function normalizes in the days to weeks after MI, as is usual in patients who survive the acute phase of right ventricular infarction,[461] the extra volume can then be safely removed with diuretic therapy. In patients whose condition is refractory to volume replacement, inotropic support has been useful in normalizing cardiac output.[462,463]

INTRA-AORTIC BALLOON COUNTERPULSATION. Counterpulsation is the mainstay of support for the patient in cardiogenic shock while diagnostic and definitive therapeutic efforts are under way. Intra-aortic balloon pumping by gas inflation was first introduced in 1962 by Moulopoulos et al.[477] and was refined for clinical use by Krakauer et al.[478] Intra-aortic balloon counterpulsation became clinically practical with both selective coronary angiography and coronary bypass graft surgery. The development of percutaneous insertion of the intra-aortic balloon has allowed safe, rapid, and efficient insertion by experts in percutaneous arterial techniques. Intra-aortic balloon pumping is a particularly attractive therapeutic option because it decreases myocardial oxygen demand while simultaneously increasing myocardial oxygen supply and maintaining mean aortic pressure. The systolic unloading leads to a reduction in afterload and thus in left ventricular end-diastolic pressure, which helps reduce myocardial oxygen demand in ischemic segments. These hemodynamic changes may be particularly helpful in treating acute severe mitral regurgitation or a ventricular septal defect until definite surgical repair can be performed. This is also the only method that will augment diastolic aortic pressure without increasing myocardial oxygen demand, such as that occurring with catecholamine-mediated vasoconstriction. It can improve perfusion through subtotal stenoses and is indicated in all patients with cardiogenic shock for whom the decision to proceed with maximal diagnostic and therapeutic efforts has been made (except in patients who have absolute contraindications). The two absolute contraindications to intra-aortic balloon counterpulsation are aortic insufficiency that will worsen with diastolic augmentation and aortic dissection in which balloon insertion may increase the size of the false channel and further damage the aorta. Rapid, irregular rhythms make synchronized inflation of the balloon during diastole difficult and reduce the efficacy of intra-aortic balloon support. Severe peripheral vascular disease is a relative contraindication, as is a small body habitus; these may make proper placement of the intra-aortic balloon difficult and increase the vascular complication rate. Major vascular complications in patients with cardiogenic shock are common and may occur in up to one-third of patients.[479]

Indications for the initiation of intra-aortic balloon counterpulsation include cardiogenic shock or hemodynamic deterioration due to apparent primary pump failure or to mechanical lesions. Hemodynamic data that indicate the need for intra-aortic balloon counterpulsation are hypotension (<90 mm Hg systolic pressure, 60 mm Hg mean pressure, or >30 mm Hg below previous basal levels), increased pulmonary artery wedge pressure (>16 to 18 mm Hg), and a low cardiac index (≤ 2.0 liters/min per m^2).

The short-term survival of patients with cardiogenic shock treated medically with intra-aortic balloon pumping but without reperfusion therapy is very low, averaging about 20% at the time of hospital dismissal.[475,480-485] Although survival may be improved somewhat by intra-aortic balloon counterpulsation,[486] it is when used as an adjunct to mechanical reperfusion that intra-aortic balloon pumping achieves the greatest improvement in survival. Results of intra-aortic balloon pumping and surgery are from uncontrolled observational studies in which fewer than 50% of patients who were surgical candidates made it to the operating room. Those who underwent operation had a 50% survival at hospital dismissal.[475,487,488] Survival was considerably better if the operation took place within 16 hours of the onset of infarction.[475] Coronary angiography does not appear to increase mortality in cardiogenic shock when patients are supported by the intra-aortic balloon.[474,475,481,489]

Weaning from the intra-aortic balloon should begin within 24 or 38 hours of reperfusion or medical stabilization, if coronary bypass surgery is not planned. This is accomplished by gradually reducing the proportion of cardiac cycles during which the balloon inflates. When the patient's own circulation can be maintained at a pumping frequency of every fourth or greater cardiac cycle, the balloon can usually be removed successfully. It should not be completely stopped in situ because of the danger of thrombus formation.

Complications appear to be minimized by weaning the patient as soon as clinically feasible, using antithrombotic therapy with heparin, and having the balloon inserted into the aorta by a person skilled in intra-arterial techniques.[481,483,487,489-492] The major complications are related to ischemia of the leg associated with the balloon insertion. Leg ischemia appears enhanced by low cardiac output, generally is temporary, and usually disappears after removal of the balloon. Thromboembolism, such as peripheral emboli or arterial thrombosis at the site of balloon insertion, may occur even when the precautions are taken. Although hematologic complications are unusual, decreased platelet count (below 100,000/μL) have occurred related to the duration of balloon pumping.[491]

MECHANICAL PROBLEMS. Mechanical problems, such as ventricular septal rupture, mitral regurgitation due to papillary muscle dysfunction or rupture, and left ventricular aneurysms causing failure, are best treated surgically at a time dictated by the patient's hemodynamic status. If methods to achieve hemodynamic stabilization fail, early operation may be necessary.[459,493]

HEMODYNAMIC MONITORING. Immediate hemodynamic monitoring is unnecessary in many patients with MI and in some with hemodynamic instability. However, in patients whose clinical history, physical examination, and laboratory data provide unclear or conflicting data about ventricular filling pressures, pulmonary pressures, and cardiac output, invasive hemodynamic monitoring is essential to direct pharmacologic and other therapy; for example, whether volume replacement or diuretic therapy should be administered or whether inotropic therapy with or without vasodilator therapy is indicated. A pulmonary artery catheter provides information about right and left ventricular filling pressures and cardiac output, can detect right ventricular dysfunction and a ventricular septal defect (through analysis of waveforms, and oximetry), and can suggest the presence of severe mitral regurgitation (if large V waves are present on the pulmonary capillary wedge tracing). These three diagnoses require therapy quite different from that for cardiogenic shock due to left ventricular dysfunction. Intra-arterial monitoring of blood pressure can be helpful both for frequent blood drawing and for more accurate and continuous monitoring of blood pressure; cuff blood pressures may be falsely low by as much as 160 mm Hg below the intravascular pressure.[487,494] Measurement of ventricular filling pressures and cardiac output provides information about the severity of the problem and the prognosis.

ARRHYTHMIAS. Arrhythmias should be aggressively treated in patients with cardiogenic shock. The heart with significantly compromised left ventricular function is more vulnerable to decompensation by arrhythmia. Tachycardia reduces the time available for ventricular filling and coronary blood flow during diastole and increases myocardial oxygen demand, which could severely decrease left ventricular function when myocardial oxygen supply is limited by severe coronary disease. Bradycardia may precipitate decompensation when the stroke volume cannot increase normally to compensate for the bradycardia. Frequent premature beats, such as nonconducted atrial premature contractions or very early ventricular premature contractions that barely (if at all) open the aortic valve, can cause an effective bradycardia. Loss of synchronous AV contraction due to any form of AV dissociation (including accelerated junctional or ventricular rhythms) or AV block may also precipitate decompensation when ventricular function is already markedly decreased (and particularly in patients with right ventricular infarction).

Prompt treatment of arrhythmias helps decrease myocardial oxygen demand (especially reversal of tachyarrhythmias) and maintain circulatory support (by maintaining ventricular filling through an adequate heart rate and physiologic sequence of atrial and ventricular contraction). Among patients with predominant right ventricular dysfunction contributing to shock, complete heart block may develop in up to 40% of them; if this occurs, AV sequential pacing may be of much greater value than ventricular pacing alone in optimizing hemodynamics.

OTHER THERAPY. All other therapy should be aimed at decreasing myocardial oxygen demands, protecting and salvaging ischemic myocardium, and maintaining circulatory support long enough to improve myocardial blood flow by reperfusion. Basic measures for therapy of acute MI, such as relief of pain, sedation, and treatment of arrhythmia, should be carried out simultaneously. Relief of pain and sedation with morphine may help decrease autonomic contributions to circulatory impairment, such as excessive adrenergic stimulation producing tachyarrhythmias.

INOTROPIC SUPPORT. If hypotension and hypoperfusion persist after optimal adjustment of the left ventricular filling pressure, or if they develop rapidly before these adjustments can be made, patients may benefit from inotropic support with dopamine, dobutamine, or amrinone.

Dopamine is an endogenous catecholamine (the immediate precursor of norepinephrine) and at dosages as low as 1 to 5 μg/kg per minute causes stimulation of dopaminergic receptors and vasodilation of the renal, mesenteric, coronary, and cerebral vascular beds. This increases renal perfusion, sodium excretion, myocardial contractility, and cardiac output and decreases total peripheral resistance.[495-497] It may also increase cardiac output by improving contractility. Because vasodilation can be blocked by phenothiazines, such as chlorpromazine, and butyrophenones, such as haloperidol,[498] these drugs should be avoided in patients who require dopamine. At 5 to 8 μg/kg per minute, stimulation of β_1-adrenergic receptors of the myocardium predominates, increasing contractility, heart rate, and cardiac output. Above 8 μg/kg per minute, α-adrenergic receptors are stimulated directly and, at least in part, indirectly by the release of norepinephrine from sympathetic nerve terminals and by stimulation of serotonin- or tryptamine-sensitive receptors, leading to vasoconstriction and decreased renal blood flow.[495-499] Dosages of 10 to 15 μg/kg per minute may increase the pulmonary artery wedge pressure and lead to pulmonary congestion and arterial desaturation, at least in part due to vasoconstriction in both arteries and veins.[495-497,500] Above 20 μg/kg per minute, peripheral vasoconstriction becomes severe and coronary vasoconstriction may result.[495-497]

The balance between myocardial oxygen supply and demand must be considered when using dopamine in patients with acute MI or ischemic heart disease. Increased myocardial contractility, heart rate, arterial pressure, and left ventricular filling pressure, usually occurring at higher doses, increase myocardial oxygen demands; stimulation of dopamine receptors at lower doses causes vasodilation, increased sodium excretion, and decreased cardiac filling pressures and heart size, decreasing myocardial oxygen demand. Stimulation of dopamine receptors at lower doses dilates coronary arteries and increases blood flow,[501] whereas stimulation of α-adrenergic receptors at higher doses constricts coronary arteries and decreases coronary blood flow. However, life-threatening cardiogenic shock can often be quickly reversed by dopamine. If hypotension develops rapidly and is life-threatening, an intravenous infusion of dopamine can be started immediately at a dosage of 10 μg/kg per minute to increase the systolic blood pressure to 80 mm Hg. Because dopamine may exert deleterious effects through vasoconstriction, the dose should be carefully titrated whenever possible, and the minimum infusion necessary should be used.

Dobutamine is a synthetic catecholamine that acts directly and predominantly on β_1-adrenergic receptors and weakly on β_2- and α-adrenergic receptors. It has a favorable contractility-to-automaticity ratio and minimal chronotropic activity.[502,503] A potent inotrope that increases cardiac output, dobutamine decreases pulmonary artery wedge pressure and total peripheral resistance, redistributes cardiac output to the coronary and skeletal muscle circulation, and does not alter renal blood flow, mean arterial pressure, or heart rate when infused at 2.5 μg/kg per minute.[502-505] Significant hemodynamic tolerance to dobutamine has been observed, with more than 30% attenuation at 72 hours and more than 40% attenuation at 96 hours of continuous infusion.[506] If necessary, this attenuation may be overcome by increasing the infusion rate. As with any catecholamine, increased AV conduction may increase the ventricular response rate in patients with atrial fibrillation. The sinus rate may increase in some patients, especially at infusions of 7.5 μg/kg or more per minute and in most patients when infusion rates reach 15 μg/kg per minute.

Amrinone has both positive inotropic and vasodilatory effects.[507-509] The mechanism of action appears to be inhibition of phosphodiesterase III, an enzyme responsible for the degradation of cyclic adenosine monophosphate, resulting in increased intracellular calcium. Amrinone may also produce peripheral vasodilation by a direct effect on vascular smooth muscle.[508] It is useful in congestive heart failure complicating acute MI[510] and in patients whose condition is refractory to treatment with dopamine or dobutamine.[511]

For patients with cardiogenic shock who may require inotropic support and maintenance of coronary perfusion pressure, combined therapy with modest doses of dobutamine and dopamine, or dopamine and amrinone, may take advantage of the favorable effects of both drugs and minimize the deleterious side effects. Dobutamine and amrinone improve cardiac output, decrease pulmonary artery wedge pressure, have little effect on heart rate or blood pressure, and cause no release of norepinephrine from nerve endings. Dopamine has fewer sustained inotropic effects, may increase pulmonary artery wedge pressure, and is more likely to increase heart rate[512] but has vasopressor effects to maintain coronary perfusion pressure and increase renal blood flow and sodium excretion. Combined dobutamine and dopamine may be of greater benefit than either drug alone in patients in cardiogenic shock.[513] Combined therapy with dopamine and amrinone also appears promising.

Improved perfusion, not just increased arterial pressure, is the goal of therapy. Maintaining arterial pressure with a predominantly α-adrenergic agonist (such as norepinephrine or metaraminol) does not reduce mortality and may be detrimental to the heart by increasing myocardial oxygen demand and decreasing myocardial blood flow due to vasoconstriction in both the systemic and coronary arterial beds.[514] Although digitalis glycosides have a modest inotropic effect, their main role in cardiogenic shock is principally in the treatment of frequent or sustained supraventricular tachyarrhythmia. In cardiogenic shock, in which the primary problem is poor coronary perfusion, the ability of digitalis to improve cardiac performance (as it can in heart failure) and improve overall the ratio of myocardial oxygen supply to demand (as it can in the patient with cardiomegaly and ischemic heart disease) is markedly diminished. When a digitalis glycoside is used in cardiogenic shock to treat supraventricular tachyarrhythmias, the dosage should be decreased to approximately half that normally used, because of the increased myocardial sensitivity to digitalis in ischemia and the frequent presence of concomitant renal insufficiency.

Rupture of the ventricular free wall

Cardiac rupture, a dreaded complication of acute MI, is often sudden and unexpected.[515] In the coronary care unit era, cardiac rupture may have increased in frequency as a fatal event.[516] In a recent large series, cardiac rupture accounted for approximately one-third of in-hospital deaths after acute MI, the second most common mechanism after shock and cardiac failure.[517] The increase may be related in part to a reduction in the proportion of patients dying of acute arrhythmia. The relative infrequency of cardiac ruptures belies their importance, because if correctly and promptly diagnosed, ruptures are amenable to treatment. In a large autopsy series, patients dying of cardiac rupture had smaller infarcts than those dying of cardiogenic shock or arrhythmias (Fig 30B-23), an important finding that emphasizes the potential for a favorable long-term prognosis if the mechanical complication can be corrected.[518] Unfortunately, most ruptures involve the free wall rather than the septum and papillary muscles.[516] Although the time from rupture to death in free-wall rupture is short and the logistical constraints for surgical correction are formidable, septum and papillary muscle ruptures are far more amenable to therapy.

Incidence. An incidence of 8% to 17% of all infarct deaths, involving 1% to 3% of all infarct patients, is generally accepted,[515,516,518,519] but it may actually be higher, as suggested by larger epidemiologic studies.[520,521] Particularly high incidence rates reported from mental institutions[522] have raised the issue of continued activity of the patient after undetected MI as a cause of rupture, but this has not been confirmed in other series.[523,524]

Time of onset. Most ruptures occur within the first week of infarction; 32% occurred within the first 24 hours and 84% within the first week in one series.[525] In three large series, the median time to rupture was approxi-

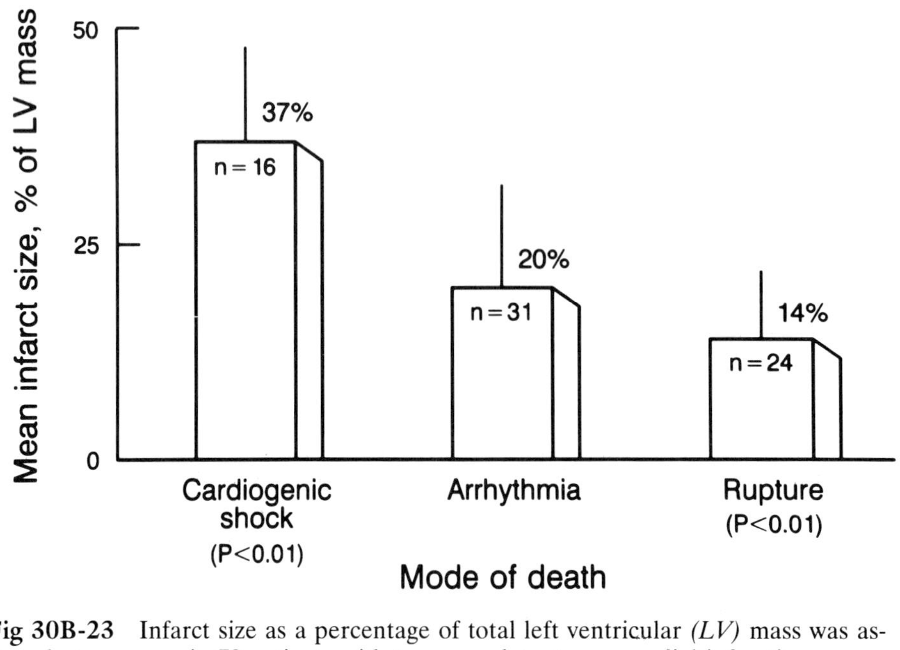

Fig 30B-23 Infarct size as a percentage of total left ventricular *(LV)* mass was assessed at necropsy in 78 patients with transmural acute myocardial infarction. Patients who died in cardiogenic shock had the largest infarcts (37% ± 11%) relative to left ventricular mass. Infarct size was 20% ± 12% in those patients who died of arrhythmias but was only 14% ± 8% (*P* <0.01 compared with other groups) in patients dying of cardiac rupture. (Data from Saffitz JE, Fredrickson RC, Roberts WC: Relation of size of transmural acute myocardial infarct to mode of death, interval between infarction and death and frequency of coronary arterial thrombus. *Am J Cardiol* 57:1249-1254, 1986.)

mately 4 days.[515,526,527] Occasionally, a patient with symptoms of acute MI actually has the onset of rupture, the antecedent MI having been silent.[528] In a Mayo Clinic study of 100 consecutive autopsy cases of rupture of the left ventricular free wall during acute MI, 49% of the deaths were actually out-of-hospital.[529] From pathologic studies, rupture may occur over a period of time, with a lag between the onset of the tear and epicardial breakthrough.[530] "Subacute" rupture with gradual leakage of blood contained by pericardial adhesions that appears as progressive but not catastrophic tamponade is an important clinical entity because of the possibility for surgical intervention and cure.[531-536] In a recent autopsy series, 95% of patients with free-wall rupture had associated hemopericardium with probable or definite tamponade.[536]

Pathology. Rupture probably results from intramural dissection or hematoma, with a circuitous pathway through the myocardium (Fig 30B-24). Approximately half the ruptures are serpiginous as opposed to simple "through and through" tears.[529] The most common site of rupture is the lateral aspect of the left ventricular free wall, but rupture of the right ventricle and of the atrium have been reported[515,529,537] (Fig 30B-25).

"Double" ruptures involving the free wall and ventricular septum are uncommon, and most are "junctional," involving the myocardium located directly anterior and posterior to the ventricular septum but without contact with either ventricular cavity. True double free-wall ruptures are rare.[538] Cardiac rupture is more common in women,[526,527,529] older patients, and patients experiencing a transmural infarction who lack collaterals; evidence of a previous infarct is present in only 15% to 25% of patients.[516,527,529,539,540] Mann and Roberts[538] noted that among patients dying of rupture, the amount of coronary artery narrowing was considerably less than that in patients dying of a first infarct without rupture.

Associated factors include previous history of hypertension,[519,522,529,541,542] and sustained hypertension.[515,526,527,543] The phenomenon of infarct expansion with recurrent chest pain, wall thinning, and disproportionate cardiac dilatation may cause rupture.[544] In a study of 110 autopsy patients by Schuster and Bulkley,[544] the incidence of rupture was 43% in the zone of expansion but only 1% in patients without expansion. The potential detrimental impact of steroids and nonsteroidal anti-inflammatory agents on infarct healing and rupture has been pointed out.[545] Anticoagulants may cause rupture.[524,542,546,547] Preliminary reports suggest that thrombolytic therapy, particularly if given late, may increase the risk of cardiac rupture within the first 24 hours,[548-550] although the overall incidence of rupture in one series was the same whether or not patients received thrombolytic therapy.[517] Late reperfusion increases the risk of rupture, but this does not outweigh the overall benefits of therapy, at least within the first 12 hours or in patients with recurrent pain.

Clinical features. The most common presentation is sudden hemodynamic collapse followed by rapid demise, with or without the clinical signs of tamponade. Electromechanical dissociation is frequent[551,552] but not necessarily pathognomonic of rupture, since it occurs in patients with cardiogenic shock without rupture. Other nonspecific ECG changes include tall, peaked T waves in the precordial leads,[553] ST-segment elevation or depression,[552] and bradyarrhythmias, including sinus bradycardia with junctional and idioventricular escape rhythms.[552,553] Rarely, the ECG may remain normal.[553]

Rupture may be preceded or heralded by episodes of recurrent pericardial pain with or without the features of a pericardial effusion or tamponade and hypotension.[551,554] Stabilization can result from pericardial blood clotting, extrinsic intrapericardial pressure, and adhesions

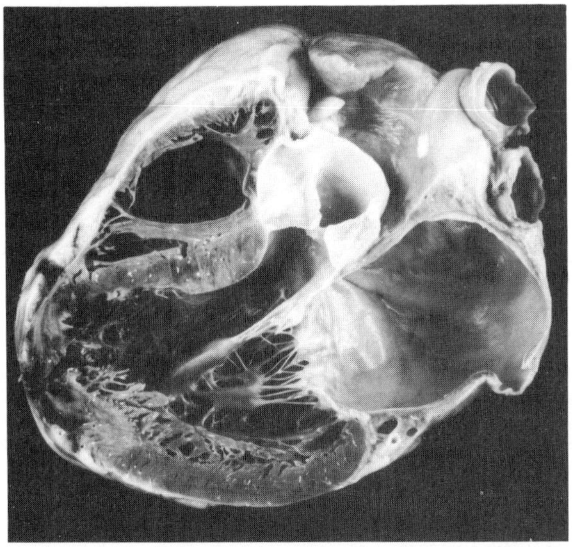

Fig 30B-24 Acute transmural apical myocardial infarction with rupture and fatal hemopericardium. (Courtesy of William D. Edwards, M.D.)

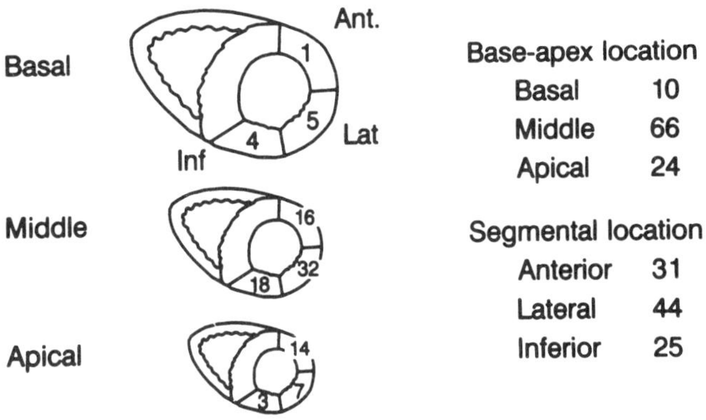

Fig 30B-25 Location of postinfarction ruptures of the left ventricular free wall in 100 autopsied subjects. (From Batts KP, Ackermann DM, Edwards WD: Postinfarction rupture of the left ventricular free wall: clinicopathologic correlates in 100 consecutive autopsy cases. *Hum Pathol* 21:530-535, 1990. By permission of WB Saunders Company.)

that partially seal the rupture and lead to a false aneurysm.[528,555-557] Echocardiographic features of effusion, tamponade, and right atrial or right ventricular wall compression are extremely helpful. The sensitivity and specificity of a combination of clinical, hemodynamic, and echocardiographic variables in subacute rupture were approximately 70% and 90%, respectively.[555,558]

Management. Successful treatment relies on prompt diagnosis and aggressive management. Cardiac rupture causing shock results in death within minutes, and intervention is logistically extremely difficult. However, in patients with a "subacute" course, there is time during which the diagnosis can be made and therapy initiated.[531-535,551,554,555]

The only definitive treatment is surgical, and as soon as the diagnosis has been made, all efforts should be directed toward attaining hemodynamic stability in preparation for immediate surgical intervention. Survival after acute rupture may be considered a function of early diagnosis, immediate preoperative therapy, and the interval before surgery. The inability to obtain a pulse during cardiopulmonary resuscitation may in itself suggest the diagnosis of cardiac rupture. Immediate pericardiocentesis, although not without risk, is of proven value in this situation and may buy time until a surgical team can be mobilized.[551,554,559,560] Pericardiocentesis may also establish the diagnosis, although distinction between pericardial aspirate and intraventricular blood is difficult.

Adjunctive measures include volume loading, use of inotropic agents, correction of acidosis, and, if necessary, administration of atropine in patients with bradyarrhythmias.[559] Urgent intra-aortic balloon counterpulsation helps stabilize hemodynamics.[561,562]

Successful surgical repair of free-wall rupture after MI is uncommon but has been documented with increasing frequency.[532,535,554,559-561,563-567] Operative mortality is high, which is not surprising, since many patients are transferred to the operating room while undergoing cardiopulmonary resuscitation.[567] A further stimulus, however, to the aggressive diagnosis and management of this complication is the excellent long-term prognosis reported in many survivors of the perioperative period.[535,551,559,563,566] Surgery done under cardiopulmonary bypass with infarctectomy and closure of the viable ventricular wall is preferred if sufficient time is available,[554,560-562,564,567] but alternative techniques include covering the rupture and surrounding the infarct muscle with a Teflon patch.[535] Closed heart repairs[551,554] using partial cardiopulmonary bypass and hypothermia[562] or partial bypass alone[563] have been successful.

Left ventricular false aneurysms

False aneurysms after acute MI should be considered with cardiac rupture; they are an uncommon sequela of free-wall rupture.[528,568-571]

Pathology. Figure 30B-26 illustrates the pathogenesis of false aneurysms after acute MI. Under ordinary circumstances, rupture leads to massive hemopericardium. Chesler et al.[568] suggested that no hemopericardium and a false aneurysm result from a prior pericardial reaction with adhesions overlying the infarcted site. These adhesions confine the escape of blood to a limited space and produce a false aneurysm consisting of a hematoma lined by pericardium and communicating with the left ventricular cavity.

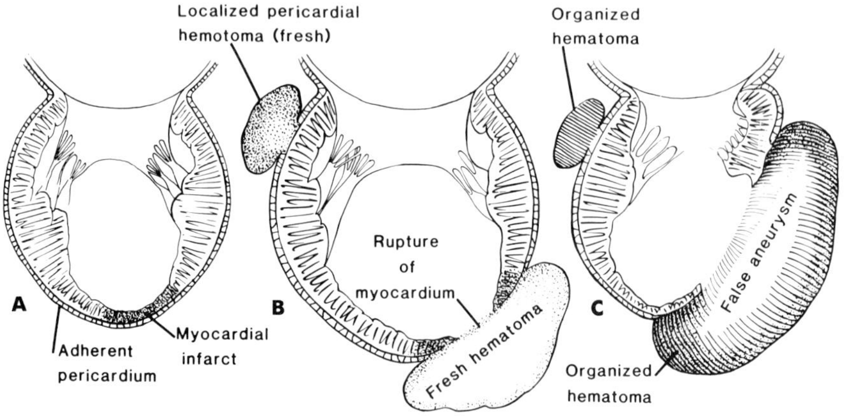

Fig 30B-26 Diagrammatic representation of the pathogenesis of false aneurysm. **A,** the primary stage is that of myocardial infarction associated with adhesions of the pericardium over the left ventricle. **B,** rupture of the left ventricular wall, resulting in a hematoma that communicates with the left ventricular cavity and also in a localized pericardial hematoma over the base of the heart. **C,** stage observed at autopsy, in which the fresh hematoma has become organized to form a false aneurysm and the edges of the perforation in the left ventricle have retracted from each other. Also, the localized pericardial hematoma has become organized. (From Chesler E, Korns ME, Semba T, et al: False aneurysms of the left ventricle following myocardial infarction. *Am J Cardiol* 23:76-82, 1969. By permission of Technical Publishing Company.)

The pathologic features of false aneurysm were summarized in nine autopsy patients with Van Tassel and Edwards.[528] The mouth of the aneurysm is small compared with the diameter of the fundus. The wall is composed of fibrous tissue, and is devoid of myocardial elements, thus constituting a pseudoaneurysm. The junction of the aneurysm in the left ventricle shows sudden interruption in continuity, and the parietal pericardium adheres to the outer surface of the false aneurysm[528] (Fig 30B-27). The distribution among the anatomic sites of the left ventricle in this series was even. In one series,[572] pseudoaneurysms were posterior or diaphragmatic in most patients in contrast to true left ventricular aneurysms, which are usually located anteriorly or laterally.[573,574]

Clinical features. Pseudoaneurysms tend to rupture;[528,572,573,575] in only 5 of the 23 cases reviewed by Gueron et al.[572] was the diagnosis made before death. The lethal consequences of this entity make a heightened awareness of the clinical features important. Rupture of a true left ventricular aneurysm may occur in its developing stage or 2 to 3 weeks after MI, but pseudoaneurysms can rupture at any time. Two cases of sudden death resulting from rupture of small chronic false aneurysms of the left ventricle have been reported;[573] in both the aneurysms were small, old (months or years), and clinically silent, as was the original MI. False aneurysms may cause progressive cardiac failure.[572,576,577]

The physical findings are nonspecific and are difficult to distinguish from true ventricular aneurysms. The precordial impulse may be abnormal and dyskinetic, and third and fourth heart sounds may be audible on auscultation. Flow through the narrow neck of the pseudoaneurysm causes apical systolic murmurs (often pansystolic) with radiation to the axilla.[572] Associated mitral regurgitation may be severe.[574] A to-and-fro murmur has been described.[569] A readily explicable but nonspecific feature is the presence of persistent pericardial friction rub.

The ECG may show persistent ST-segment elevation, as with true ventricular aneurysms, but in one series this sign was present in only five of nine patients.[528] Radiographically, there is an abnormal bulge on the lateral wall of the left ventricle (posteroanterior view), cardiomegaly, and a pericardial mass.[577,578] Progressive expansion of a paracardiac mass overlying the posterior left ventricle early after acute infarction is a valuable clue, occurring in approximately 20% of patients.[572,578]

Echocardiography. False aneurysms have a narrow neck in relation to fundal diameter, forming the basis of the real-time two-dimensional echocardiographic distinction between true and false aneurysms[579-583] (Fig 30B-28). M-mode echocardiography can demonstrate an echo-free extracardiac space behind the left ventricular posterior wall, but pseudoaneurysm cannot readily be differentiated from an extensive loculated pericardial effusion or a pericardial cyst by this technique alone.[576,579] The ratio of the maximum internal diameter of the neck to the maximum parallel internal dimension of the aneurysmal sac does not exceed 0.5 in false aneurysms, whereas it ranges from 0.9 to 1.0 in true aneurysms.[581,582]

Two patients had "pseudo-false" aneurysms that communicated with the left ventricle through a small orifice but had a wall containing myocardial tissue.[584] Preopera-

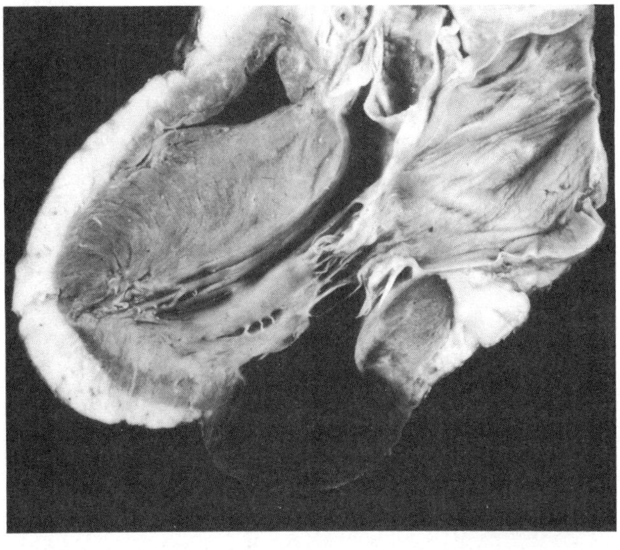

Fig 30B-27 Acute transmural inferior myocardial infarction with contained rupture (pseudoaneurysm) filled with thrombus. (Courtesy of William D. Edwards, M.D.)

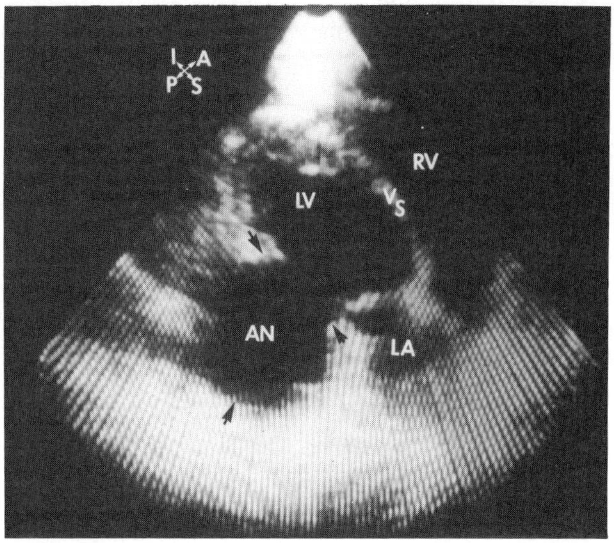

Fig 30B-28 Left ventricular false aneurysm, "off axis" echocardiographic parasternal view. False aneurysm *(AN)* arises from the posterobasal left ventricular wall. *Arrows* delineate the extent of the aneurysm and its narrow "neck," composed of remaining left ventricular wall. No thrombus is visible in this view. *A,* anterior; *I,* inferior; *LA,* left atrium; *LV,* left ventricle; *P,* posterior; *RV,* right ventricle; *S,* superior; *VS,* ventricular septum. (From Reeder GS, Seward JB, Tajik AJ: The role of two-dimensional echocardiography in coronary artery disease: a critical appraisal. *Mayo Clin Proc* 57:247-258, 1982. By permission, Mayo Foundation.)

tive diagnosis of these lesions by any technique appears unlikely.

Radionuclide angiography. Scintigraphic techniques have value in diagnosing false aneurysms,[578,585,586] but occasionally the site of the small communicating orifice exceeds the limits of resolution.[587]

Cineangiography. As with other diagnostic techniques, the size of the orifice in relation to the diameter of the fundus is an important radiographic feature, and the jetlike expulsion of contrast material during systole through a narrow orifice into the cavity may be visualized.[572,581] Limitations to angiography occur in separating true from false aneurysm, related to the anatomy of the lesion and the orientation of the x-ray beam.[582] Coronary arteriography is essential if concomitant coronary artery bypass surgery is being considered.

Management. The natural history of false aneurysms with their propensity to rupture mandates surgical therapy once the diagnosis has been made. Surgical management is not affected by symptoms, size, or chronicity, and removal and repair of the wall have been combined successfully with other procedures, such as mitral valve replacement and coronary bypass grafting.[574,588] Successful surgical repair may be performed both early and late after acute MI,[572,588,589] but the encouraging results obtained within weeks after infarction justify an aggressive early surgical approach.

In some cases of pseudoaneurysm the operation may be simpler than for true aneurysm because it might be possible to close the small communication into the left ventricle without resecting the entire aneurysmal wall.[584] Excellent long-term survival with considerable functional improvement can be achieved.[572,574,588,589]

True left ventricular aneurysm

This topic is discussed in chapter 31.

Rupture of the interventricular septum

Rupture of the interventricular septum is a calamitous but potentially reversible complication of acute MI. The typical presentation is a new systolic murmur associated with dramatic hemodynamic deterioration within the first few days after MI.

Incidence and natural history. Rupture of the interventricular septum occurs in 1% to 3% of all infarcts and accounts for 1% to 14% of peri-infarction deaths[590-592] and 12% of all cardiac ruptures. It is an early complication, occurring an average of 2 to 6 days after the onset of symptoms[593,594] in the Multicenter Investigation on the Limitation of Infarct Size (MILIS) study.[591] Progressive hemodynamic deterioration leading to death or surgical intervention is usual, and mortality is high. In 41 patients (1971 to 1975), 60% either died or required urgent surgery within 1 week, 20% had less rapid but relentless deterioration, 15% required surgery within weeks, and only 5% stabilized sufficiently to undergo elective surgery 2 to 9 months later.[595] Long-term survival without surgery is rare,[593] with the longest documented survival without surgery being 13 years.[596] In some patients with acquired septal defects at autopsy, old healed MI is present.[528]

Pathology and pathophysiology. As in free-wall rupture, hypertension preexisting or occurring during infarction has been incriminated as a causative factor in ventricular septal rupture,[541,597,598] but this is not a universal finding.[595,599] Septal rupture is more common in women[599] and in patients without previous MI[595] or angina.[594] In the MILIS study, rupture was 9.2 times more likely to occur in patients with all the following characteristics than in the remaining patients: (1) no history of previous angina or MI, (2) ST-segment elevation or signs of Q-wave development on the initial ECG, and (3) a peak CK-MB value (≥ 150 IU/L).[591]

In many patients with septal rupture, coronary artery disease may be limited, as seen by the incidence of single-vessel disease, which ranges from 24% to 69% in five large series, and by angiographic demonstration of poor septal collateral blood flow.[594,595,600-602]

In a speculative report on small numbers of patients, Boden and Sadaniantz[603] noted that the incidence of acute septal rupture after MI had increased fourfold since early 1983, when ibuprofen was widely prescribed for pericarditis.

Septal rupture has been reported in a patient with acute MI and normal coronary arteries with "muscular bridging."[604]

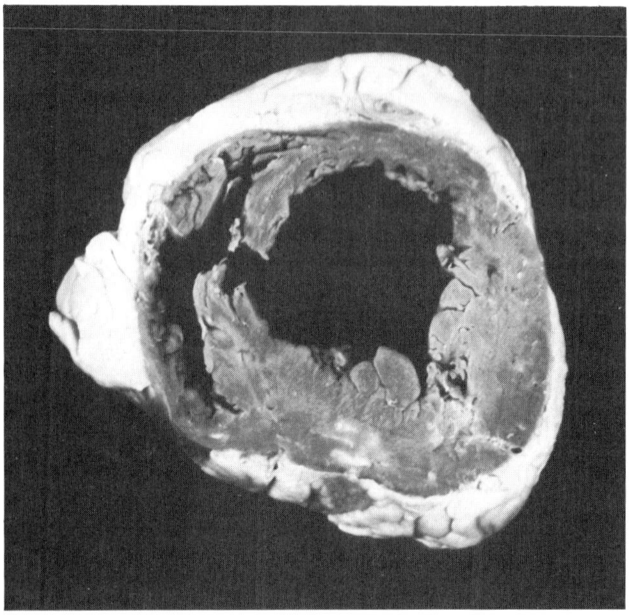

Fig 30B-29 Cross section viewed from the apex of the ventricular portion of the heart. A simple rupture of the ventricular septum is apparent as scars of an old inferior myocardial infarction. (From Edwards BS, Edwards WD, Edwards JE: Ventricular septal rupture complicating acute myocardial infarction: identification of simple and complex types in 53 autopsied hearts. *Am J Cardiol* 54:1201-1205, 1984. By permission of Cahners Publishing Company, a Division of Reed Publishing USA.)

Rupture usually results from dissection of the necrotic area, a funnel-shaped depression appearing at the site of rupture; in 20% of one series, ruptures were multiple. The distribution between anterior and inferior infarcts in patients with septal rupture is approximately equal.[594,600,605,606] A septal rupture nearly always involves the muscular septum, but the rupture site varies widely. Two types of ruptures occur: simple (direct through-and-through defects) and complex[607] (Figs 30B-29 and 30B-30). The latter were associated with extensive septal damage and a serpiginous dissection tract remote from the primary tear of the septum[607] and were far more frequently associated with inferior infarctions, particularly those involving the inferobasal rather than the anteroapical septum. Furthermore, complex ruptures were more likely to be associated with rupture of other structures, such as the free wall and papillary muscles.[607-609]

The worse prognosis of septal rupture in association with inferior than with anterior MI can be explained by some of the pathophysiologic features of complex rupture and associated right ventricular involvement.[599] An autopsy study identified a high incidence of right ventricular infarction in patients dying of septal rupture, and the greatest extent of right ventricular involvement was in patients with inferior infarcts.[599]

In a study of 25 patients by Moore et al.[592] (Fig 30B-31), the higher mortality in patients with inferior infarctions was attributed to more extensive right ventricular and septal dysfunction. Radford et al.[595] concluded that survival was related strongly to the presence of shock, but shock was not entirely attributable to left ventricular dysfunction with low left ventricular ejection fractions

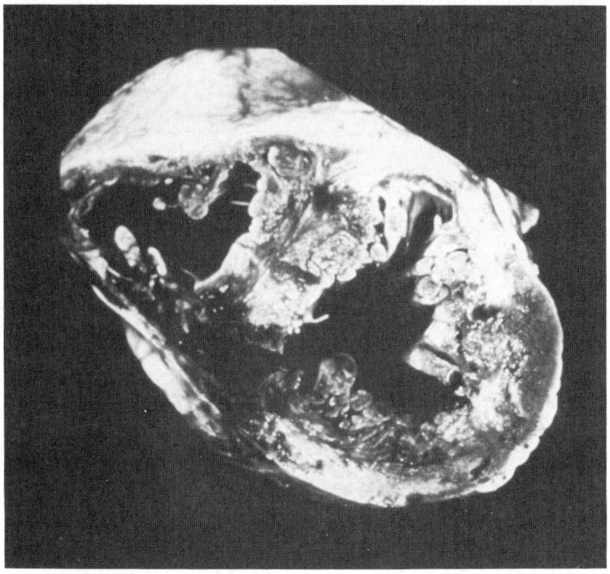

Fig 30B-30 Complex septal rupture with laceration and hemorrhage in the region of the inferobasal septum and involvement of the right ventricular free wall with additional rupture. (Courtesy of William D. Edwards, M.D.)

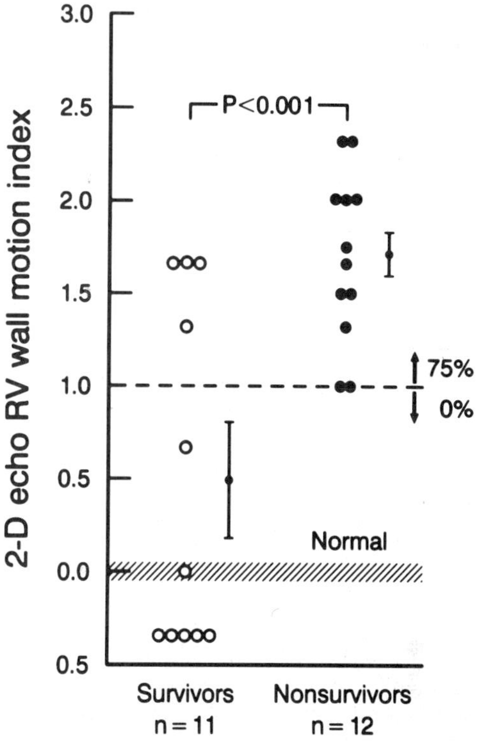

Fig 30B-31 Abnormal right ventricular *(RV)* function (increased right ventricular wall motion index) was present in all patients dying of acute septal rupture. Among survivors, right ventricular function was normal or mildly abnormal in most. *2-D echo,* two-dimensional echocardiography. (From Moore CA, Nygaard TW, Kaiser DL, et al: Postinfarction ventricular septal rupture: the importance of location of infarction and right ventricular function in determining survival. *Circulation* 74:45-55, 1986. By permission of American Heart Association.)

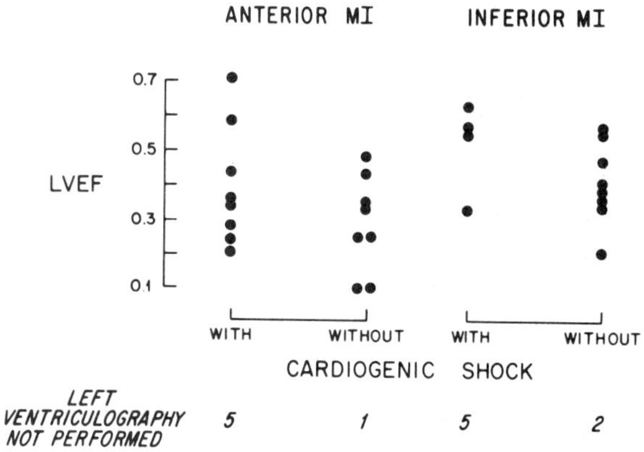

Fig 30B-32 Left ventricular ejection fraction *(LVEF)* in patients with and without cardiogenic shock. Ventricular septal rupture followed both anterior and inferior myocardial infarction *(MI).* (From Radford MJ, Johnson RA, Daggett WM Jr, et al: Ventricular septal rupture: a review of clinical and physiologic features and an analysis of survival. *Circulation* 64:545-553, 1981. By permission of American Heart Association.)

(Fig 30B-32). They emphasized the role of right ventricular dysfunction in the development of cardiogenic shock, particularly in patients with septal rupture and inferior MI.

Clinical features. The onset is usually dramatic, with a new pansystolic murmur developing in the first few days after acute MI. Sudden hemodynamic deterioration with hypotension and left ventricular failure is typical and is accompanied by florid evidence of right heart failure with a pronounced elevation in jugular venous pressure. The features of right heart failure may overshadow those of left ventricular failure. Exceptionally, rupture of the septum may produce serious hemodynamic derangements without a murmur.[610] The development of a systolic murmur during or after an acute MI can result from several causes, and the prognosis and therapy vary accordingly.

Differential diagnosis of new systolic murmurs. The differential diagnosis of conditions that are responsible for a new systolic murmur after MI is summarized in Table 30B-35.[610]

Diagnosis. On the ECG, conduction disturbances, including heart block, occur with septal rupture, but neither these nor other arrhythmias that have been described are specific for this condition.[593,611,612] The ECG changes noted at rupture include pronounced elevation in ST segments and supraventricular tachyarrhythmias.[613]

The chest radiograph reveals no features specific for the diagnosis. Pulmonary plethora is valuable, but early after rupture the most common feature is pulmonary venous hypertension, which is not as striking as in patients with ruptured papillary muscle and mitral regurgitation.[593,610,614]

Bedside right heart balloon-tipped catheterization used to confirm the diagnosis[593,615,616] is well documented, but advances in Doppler color-flow echocardiography have made the latter the diagnostic modality of choice, although pulmonary artery catheterization is still invaluable for medical management. A definitive diagnosis of a left-to-right shunt at ventricular level requires documentation of a "step-up" in oxygen saturation in the right ventricle or main pulmonary artery. The normal variability between superior vena caval and pulmonary artery saturations is 9%; anything greater may result from a left or right shunt.[617] In patients with severe acute mitral regurgitation, the transmission of large v waves to the pulmonary artery may produce a step-up in oxygen saturation in the right pulmonary artery, left pulmonary artery, or branches of these vessels[618] as opposed to the right ventricle and the main pulmonary artery in septal rupture. A further source of potential error may occur when extremely high pulmonary artery pressures (as in acute mitral regurgitation) produce a left-to-right shunt through a patent foramen ovale with a step-up at atrial level. Attention to technique, specifically to the site of sampling, eliminates these potential errors. Giant left atrial v waves may occur with interventricular septal rupture, simulating acute mitral regurgitation. These waves probably result from severe volume overload with reduced atrial and ventricular compliance.[619]

Echocardiography, particularly two-dimensional and Doppler echocardiographic techniques, is the best means for the differential diagnosis of septal rupture and acute mitral regurgitation[608,614,620-623] (Fig 30B-33). Two-dimensional echocardiography correctly localizes the site of septal rupture in most patients and assesses left and right ventricular function, but Doppler color-flow imaging is highly sensitive and specific and superior to two-dimensional echocardiography alone.[614,620,623] Carefully performed, echocardiography can rapidly exclude or confirm the diagnosis of ventricular septal rupture, and its ability to localize the site and evaluate the size of the shunt guides therapy and techniques for repair. Nonetheless, the timing of surgery and, in particular, very early surgery remains undetermined.[624]

Bedside radionuclide imaging can identify the site of rupture, confirm the presence of septal defect,[625] and quantitate shunt size.[625,626]

Left ventricular and coronary angiographic studies are undoubtedly useful in defining and locating the lesion and in excluding other defects, and they are essential if concomitant coronary artery bypass grafting is being considered.[600,627,628] One patient's septal defect was identified at angiography but bedside catheterization failed to show a step-up in oxygen saturation.[629] Cardiac catheterization and angiography carry a substantial risk, delay surgery, and have been associated with a higher operative mortality.[625,630]

Management. Immediate management includes vigorous medical treatment under monitoring conditions to achieve hemodynamic stability, even transiently.[631] Digitalization and use of other inotropes, attention to oxygenation, and judicious use of diuretics with monitoring are fairly standard measures. Vasodilating agents such as sodium nitroprusside may be valuable, but their effect on the size of the shunt is unpredictable.[632-634] They should be used with caution, since the net effect of the vasodilator on shunt size depends on its differential actions on the pulmonary and systemic vascular resistances.[632] The long-term use of sodium nitroprusside is limited by its potential for causing metabolic acidosis and neurotoxicity.

If medical therapy alone fails to provide stabilization, intra-aortic balloon counterpulsation may be effective

Table 30B-35 Differential diagnosis of new systolic murmurs after acute myocardial infarction

Rupture of the interventricular septum
Papillary muscle dysfunction
Papillary muscle rupture
Right ventricular infarction with tricuspid insufficiency
Mitral regurgitation due to left ventricular dilatation or true aneurysm
False aneurysm and rupture of the external wall
Massive pulmonary embolism with right heart failure and tricuspid insufficiency
Evolving pericardial friction rub

against progressive hemodynamic deterioration.[635,636] This intervention may reduce the size of the left-to-right shunt, enhance cardiac output and coronary blood flow, and decrease pulmonary wedge pressure.[636] Nonetheless, stability after balloon counterpulsation may be temporary.[636,637] Rapid, unexpected deterioration after apparent stabilization is common.[631,638]

Innovative experimental approaches to the medical therapy of septal rupture include inflation of a balloon in the pulmonary artery to increase the pulmonary vascular resistance and reduce left-to-right shunt. However, dysfunction of the right ventricle may be an important determinant of the hemodynamic response to acute rupture,[595] so this maneuver will probably not be widely applied clinically.[639]

Except occasionally, medical therapy alone is unlikely to provide sustained hemodynamic stability, and most patients die within 3 to 6 weeks.[595,640,641] In 139 cases

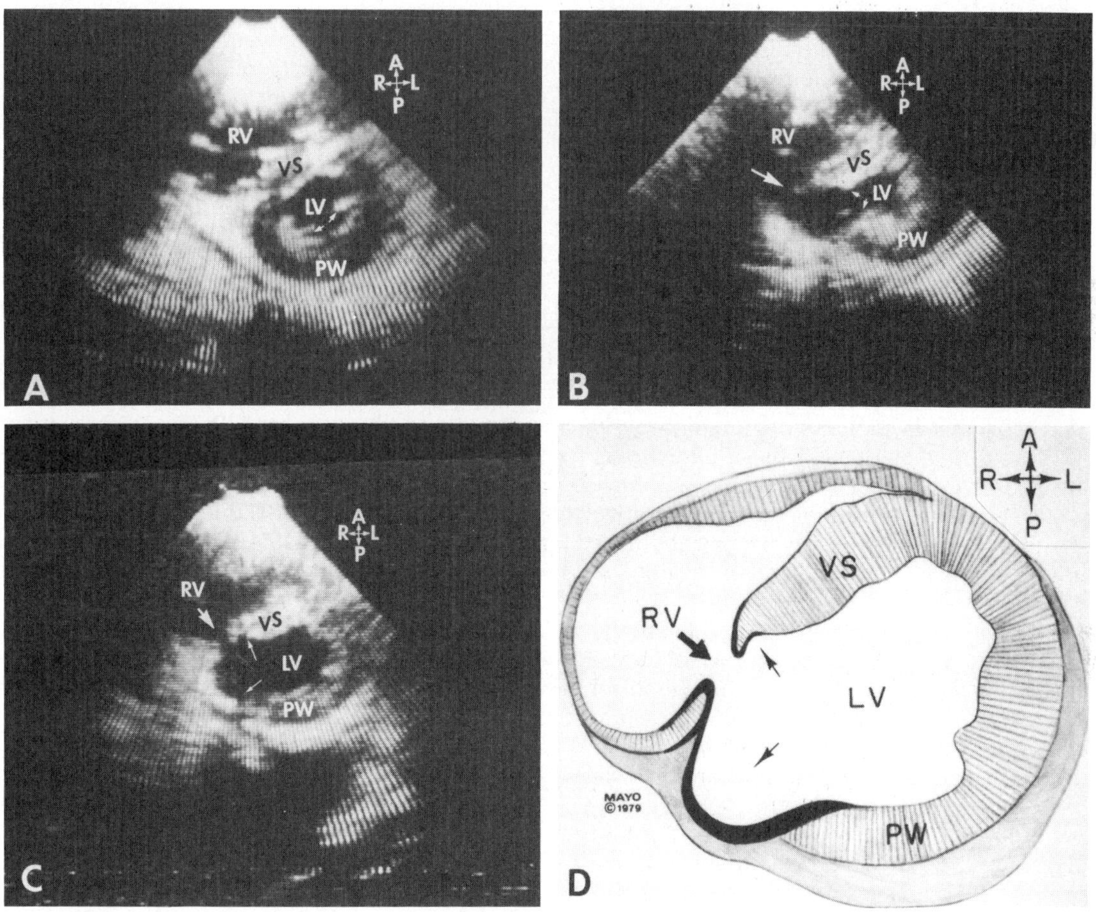

Fig 30B-33 Three echocardiographic parasternal short-axis views (tomographic sections 5 and 6). **A,** short-axis view of papillary muscle level *(arrows)* (section 6). Right ventricular *(RV)* dimension appeared increased. Left ventricular *(LV)* dimension was normal, and the circumference of the left ventricular myocardium from the ventricular septum *(VS)* to the posterior wall *(PW)* was intact and contracted normally. **B,** at the left ventricular apex (section 5), a large communication was visualized *(large arrow)* between the right ventricle and the left ventricle; it measured about 2 cm in diameter. At this level, the right ventricular dimension was inordinately large compared with the left ventricular dimension. **C,** section just inferior to the papillary muscles (sections 5 and 6) shows distinct, well-delineated *(small arrows)* thinning of the left ventricular myocardium. This involves approximately 25% of the circumferential area of the left ventricle. There is also a large defect *(large arrow)* in this portion of the ventricular septum. This thinned myocardium showed dyskinetic motion. **D,** graphic depiction of region shown in **C.** *A,* anterior; *L,* left; *P,* posterior; *R,* right. (From Scanlan JG, Seward JB, Tajik AJ: Visualization of ventricular septal rupture utilizing wide-angle two-dimensional echocardiography. *Mayo Clin Proc* 54: 381-384, 1979. By permission, Mayo Foundation.)

reported before 1977, fewer than 30% of patients without surgery survived for 2 weeks and only 20% for more than 30 days.[642] After the first report of a successful repair of acquired interventricular septal rupture in 1970,[643] the literature contains more than 200 reports of surgical therapy for this condition.[644] Although nearly all patients with septal rupture after MI require surgery, its timing and impact remain undetermined. Early observations by Mallory et al.[645] on the healing process after acute MI have had considerable influence on attitudes toward the timing of surgical intervention. They suggested that 3 weeks are required for adequate healing around the margins of the infarct and the site of rupture and for scar tissue formation sufficiently firm to hold sutures. Austen et al.[646] found low mortality in patients operated on 8 weeks after septal rupture as opposed to 3 weeks, probably in part because of tissue healing with less opportunity for breakdown of sutures.[647] However, this presumably also represents a natural selection of patients with less extensive infarcts, smaller defects, and lesser shunts, resulting in a lower operative mortality. The higher operative mortality in patients undergoing early surgery has led others to recommend that intervention be delayed as long as possible.[615]

Analyses of more recent surgical series differ in interpretation.[595,601,602,624,631,637,648-651] In general, these series show that mortality in patients operated on early after septal rupture is higher than in those undergoing later operation. However, patients who underwent early surgery were "sicker," having shock and severe congestive cardiac failure that necessitated early intervention, as opposed to those in whom hemodynamic stability could be maintained and surgery performed electively.

Radford et al.[595] stated that survival is not related to the timing of surgery but to the presence or absence of shock. Since no patient with shock survived with only medical therapy, they recommended early surgery in this group and in those without shock but with severe left ventricular failure.[595] Patients with posterior MIs appear to be at higher risk, and urgent surgery has also been recommended in this group.[649,650] In a multivariate analysis of data in 43 patients by Gaudiani et al.,[649] neither the timing of surgery nor technical problems related to early operation were considered to affect either mortality or long-term results.

In a retrospective analysis of 77 patients from the Mayo Clinic (1944 to 1985), no patients with cardiogenic shock survived without surgery.[594] The only survivors with cardiogenic shock underwent emergency operation within 48 hours. In a subsequent prospective study, nine consecutive patients (two with acute septal rupture and seven with acute mitral regurgitation) after MI who underwent emergency operation (several within hours of rupture) survived.[459] Currently, we recommend performing emergency operation immediately after diagnosis in all patients with acute septal rupture and cardiogenic shock or severe heart failure. In patients who are completely stable from a hemodynamic standpoint, delayed operation is reasonable,[652] but as emphasized earlier, constant vigilance and regular surveillance are necessary, since deterioration is frequent and unpredictable. Any deterioration on medical treatment prompts immediate operation.

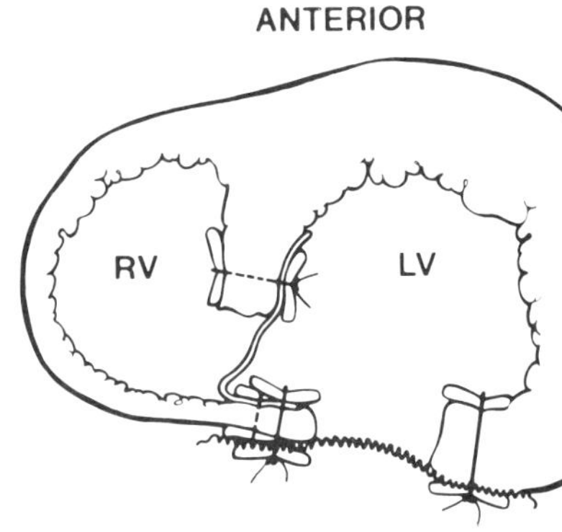

Fig 30B-34 Cross-sectional view of the completed repair of posterior septal rupture. *RV,* right ventricle; *LV,* left ventricle.

The initial surgical approach to septal rupture was a right ventriculotomy,[653] but a left-sided approach through the area of infarction is currently favored.[647,651,654] Its advantages are (1) exposure is not hampered by right ventricular trabeculations, (2) less viable muscle is destroyed, and (3) necrotic tissue can be excised.[608] The chances of recurrent left-to-right shunting through friable septal tissue have been reduced by various patch techniques and by buttressing the margins of the resection, creating a multilayered "sandwich" appearance[655] (Fig 30B-34). During the same surgical procedure, other complications coexisting with septal rupture may be successfully treated—for example, by aneurysmectomy or mitral valve replacement.[609,635,637,647] Concomitant coronary artery bypass surgery at the time of septal repair is advocated by most surgeons[600] but is not uniformly accepted.

Initial case reports of surgical repair of acute septal rupture[643] were followed in 1963 by the first report from the Mayo Clinic of a long-term survivor.[656] Subsequent series reported a high perioperative mortality of 25% to 53%,[616,624,630,647-651] but with time, early mortality has decreased,[637,652,657-660] remaining around 25%,[600] although one recent study reported 11%.[637] Mortality is increased in patients with inferior infarcts and right ventricular dysfunction.[659,660] In perioperative survivors, the late outcome is very encouraging, with a low subsequent mortality and well-preserved functional status.[459,589,594,637,648,649,651,659,661] Concomitant coronary bypass grafting may improve long-term survival but increases perioperative mortality[648] (Fig 30B-35).

Comment. A gathering consensus suggests that initial medical therapy be aimed at achieving hemodynamic stability with a view to prompt diagnosis and surgical intervention. In the few patients who have milder failure that is controllable medically, surgery can be undertaken electively, preferably after waiting a few weeks, and the results have been excellent. The timing of surgical

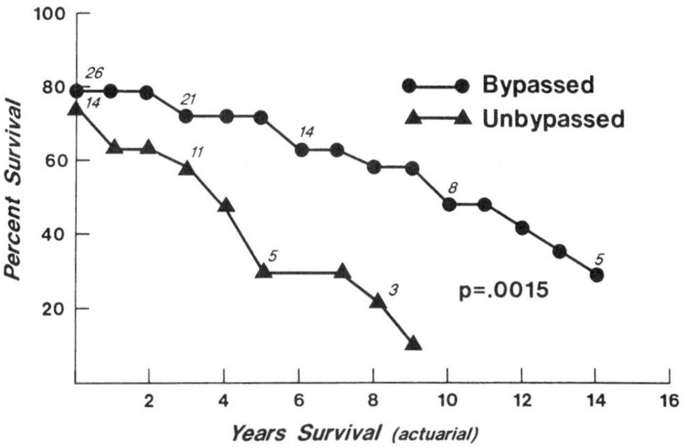

Fig 30B-35 Long-term survival of patients who did ("Bypassed") and did not ("Unbypassed") have coronary artery bypass grafting. Operative deaths are included in the determination. (From Muehrcke DD, Daggett WM Jr, Buckley MJ, et al: Postinfarct ventricular septal defect repair: effect of coronary artery bypass grafting. *Ann Thorac Surg* 54:876-883, 1992. By permission of the Society of Thoracic Surgeons.)

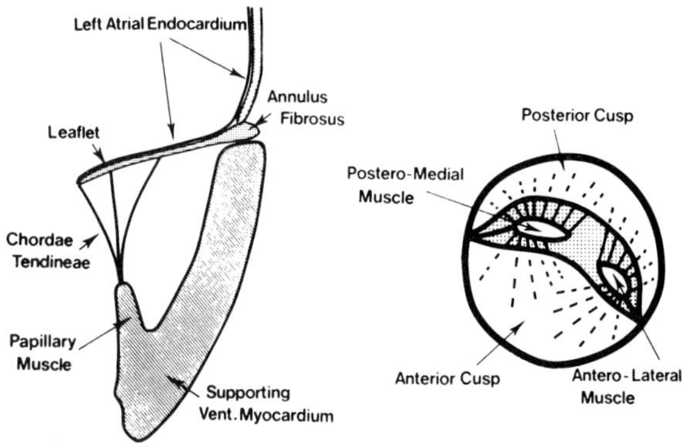

Fig 30B-36 Diagrams illustrating the morphologic composition of the mitral valve apparatus. *Left,* vertical section of the valve. The six valvular components are (1) the leaflet, which inserts into (2) the annulus fibrosus; (3) the left atrial endocardium, which continues to the free edge of the leaflet; (4) the fibrous chordae tendineae, which anchor the leaflet and are attached inferiorly to (5) the papillary muscles, which in turn arise from (6) the ventricular myocardium. *Right,* valve orifice viewed from above. The left side of the orifice is to the reader's right. The papillary muscle groups are arranged in anterolateral and posteromedial positions. Each papillary muscle supplies the adjacent halves of both valve cusps. (From Becker AE, Anderson RH: Mitral insufficiency complicating acute myocardial infarction. *Eur J Cardiol* 2:351-359, 1975. By permission of Excerpta Medica Foundation.)

intervention for patients with severe cardiac failure that is controllable medically remains uncertain.

Mitral regurgitation

Murmurs of mitral regurgitation are common (55% to 80%) in the early phase of acute MI. These are usually transient and highly variable, related to the dynamic nature of the ischemic process.[662] With contrast left ventriculography for diagnosis, 13% of patients entering phase I of the TIMI trial had mitral regurgitation, which was clinically silent in nearly all.[663] Persistence of the murmur beyond the acute phase and hemodynamically significant regurgitation are confined to a minority of patients. Because the mitral valve apparatus is intricate and its correct function depends on multiple components acting in concert, the cause of mitral regurgitation after myocardial infarction is multifactorial.

Pathophysiology. The mitral valve apparatus is composed of fibrous elements (the anuli fibrosi, the valve leaflets, and the chordae tendineae), the left atrial endocardium, and muscular elements (the papillary muscles together with the contiguous portion of the left ventricular free wall)[664] (Fig 30B-36). In chronic coronary artery disease, mitral regurgitation may result from left ventricular dilatation (which alters the spatial orientation of the papillary muscles), papillary muscle fibrosis, or dilatation of the annulus alone, although the last-named explanation is disputed.[665] In acute MI, mitral regurgitation has, for practical purposes, three main causes: papillary muscle ischemia or rupture, left ventricular dilatation or wall motion abnormalities, and chordal rupture resulting from infarction of the tip of the papillary muscle.

Papillary muscle rupture was first recognized in 1803 and first diagnosed ante mortem in 1948.[666] Sanders et al.[667] summarized 56 cases in the literature in 1957. Since then, several series totaling more than 160 patients have been reported.[459,460,612,635,646,668-671] The incidence at autopsy, irrespective of the cause of death, ranges from 0.04% to 0.11%.[672] In patients dying of acute MI, the reported incidence is 0.9%[672] to 5%.[669] Severe mitral regurgitation after acute MI is uncommon, but if the disorder is untreated, prognosis is very poor. Nonetheless, it is potentially reversible and amenable to surgical therapy; therefore, its infrequency belies its importance.

Acute MI involves primarily the muscular elements of the mitral apparatus and their mode of attachment to the fibrous elements. The papillary muscles prevent retroversion of the mitral valve leaflets into the left atrium during systole, primarily by maintaining chordal tension when the ventricular long-axis dimension shortens. Burch et al.[673,674] first described papillary muscle dysfunction, which has since been reviewed comprehensively.[664,665] The mechanisms of papillary muscle dysfunction include improper spatial orientation of the muscles and improper contraction of the muscles. Burch et al.[673,674] emphasized that a coordinate temporal sequence in the activation and contraction of the left ventricle and papillary muscle is necessary for complete competence of the mitral valve.

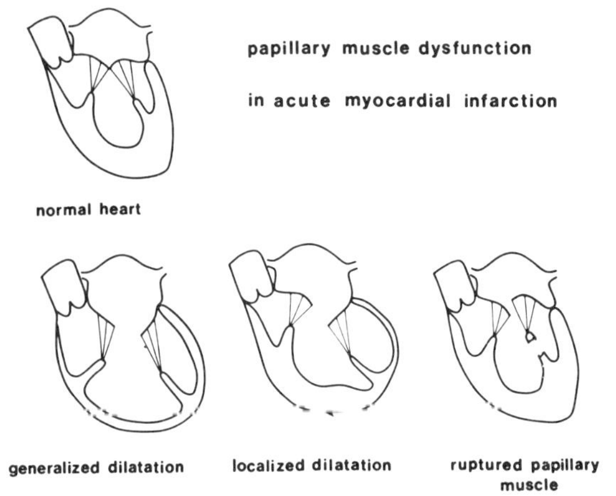

Fig 30B-37 Diagram illustrating the concept of papillary muscle dysfunction and its underlying pathologic processes. The processes illustrated demonstrate improper orientation of the muscles (localized and generalized dilatation) and improper contraction of the muscles (ruptured muscle). The third process underlying papillary muscle dysfunction is improper timing of papillary muscle contraction. (From Becker AE, Anderson RH: Mitral insufficiency complicating acute myocardial infarction. *Eur J Cardiol* 2:351-359, 1975. By permission of Excerpta Medica Foundation.)

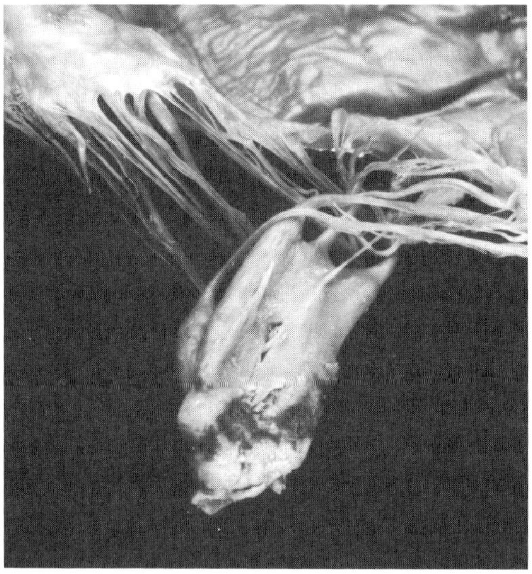

Fig 30B-38 Rupture of acutely infarcted posteromedial mitral papillary muscle, with acute mitral regurgitation. (Courtesy of William D. Edwards, M.D.)

The pathologic processes underlying papillary muscle dysfunction are illustrated in Figure 30B-37. Ventricular dilatation (local or regional) may result in mitral regurgitation by causing lateral and downward displacement of the papillary muscles. This causes a mechanical disadvantage, since the developed forces are applied tangentially to the valve leaflets, which are pulled down into the left ventricle and thus permit regurgitation.[664] Papillary muscle dysfunction may therefore arise without actual ischemia or necrosis of the muscle itself. Improper contraction of the papillary muscle due to either ischemia or necrosis may cause mitral regurgitation. However, isolated papillary muscle dysfunction does not necessarily cause mitral insufficiency, and some impairment of left ventricular contraction must be present for significant regurgitation to occur.[664,671,675-677] Rupture of the belly of a papillary muscle is the most severe and lethal manifestation of papillary muscle dysfunction after MI, and it causes acute, massive mitral regurgitation (Fig 30B-38). Rupture may be partial, occurring at one of the muscle heads supporting two or three chordae tendineae, or total, involving the entire muscle trunk. Total rupture is considered incompatible with life unless corrected urgently.

The arterial supply to the papillary muscles is tenuous, consisting of small vessels derived from the epicardial arteries, which in turn traverse the entire thickness of the left ventricular wall and the papillary muscles to reach their apices, the site of chordal attachment. The length of the arteries, their subendocardial location, and the thickness of the papillary muscles may account for their susceptibility to ischemia.[667,678] The posteromedial papillary muscle has a predominantly single blood supply from the posterior descending coronary artery and its terminal branches. Rupture of this muscle is 6 to 12 times more frequent than that of the anterolateral papillary muscle, which has a dual blood supply from the left anterior descending and circumflex vessels.[460,612,667,669,678,679]

Total rupture is reportedly more common than partial rupture.[612,669] Of 10 patients autopsied out of a series of 18 patients with papillary muscle rupture studied at our institution, only 2 had complete dehiscence of the muscle trunk, and the 8 others had partial rupture involving some of the chordal attachments; in 1 case, incomplete rupture of a single trunk was present.[460] Fatal rupture of both mitral and tricuspid papillary muscles has been described.[680]

In an autopsy series from the Mayo Clinic,[460] 5 of 10 infarcts were small (the area involved was less than 6 cm^2); infarction was inferoposterior in 9 cases, and this was limited to the subendocardium in 5. Only one patient had an infarct extending to involve the annulus, and two patients with complete dehiscence of the papillary muscle had extensive transmural infarcts. Wei et al.[669] reported a similar limited extent of infarction that involved, on average, 19% of the area of the left ventricle. Less than 25% of the left ventricle was involved in 10 of 13 patients. No patient in that series had infarction of the annulus, and in all patients the posterior wall was involved. The mechanism of rupture may be related to interstitial hemorrhages occurring with contraction band necrosis, and these may act as dissecting masses of blood.[681] The relatively small extent of left ventricular necrosis in most of these patients suggests that those with smaller infarcts may be prone to rupture because their relatively good ventricular function may result in a greater "shearing" force at the site of potential rupture.

Since these data were culled from autopsy findings in patients who died predominantly of cardiogenic shock, the limited extent of left ventricular damage suggests that death was due to the hemodynamic sequelae of acute mitral regurgitation. In patients with acute mitral regurgitation, severe left ventricular dysfunction is not a prerequisite for cardiogenic shock, as shown by Radford et al.[682] This has obvious implications for early surgical repair, particularly since sparing of the annulus suggests that mitral valve replacement would not require sutures into necrotic tissue.

All of the patients reported by Wei et al.[669] had coronary artery occlusion, and the right coronary artery was the site in the majority. In a recent Mayo Clinic series of 22 patients, single-vessel disease was present in 43% of patients.[679] The relatively limited extent of coronary artery disease in many of these patients also has obvious implications for surgical repair, although others have found more extensive coronary disease in those with mitral regurgitation.[683]

Clinical features. Several large studies have shown that the systolic murmur of papillary muscle dysfunction, although transient in most cases, is an adverse prognostic factor. It is associated with a higher incidence of prior MI, infarct extension, persistent chest pain, heart failure, and older age.[663,684,685] Early and late mortality is increased in patients with mitral regurgitation, even without an association with increased infarct size.[663,684]

In the early stages of acute MI, mild mitral regurgitation due to papillary muscle dysfunction cannot be differentiated reliably from regurgitation due to left ventricular dysfunction, and the two conditions may coexist.[673,674] Massive mitral regurgitation due to papillary muscle dysfunction or rupture is characterized by the dramatic onset of pulmonary edema, a new systolic murmur, or hypotension, usually 2 to 7 days after MI.[460,669] These patients are often very ill with massive pulmonary edema and occasionally no murmur.[683] The ECG may show typical changes of ST-T waves that correlate with papillary muscle dysfunction,[674] but others have considered these changes to be variable and nonspecific.[670] ECG evidence of left atrial enlargement points to significant mitral insufficiency.[683] The chest radiograph is also nonspecific, demonstrating severe pulmonary edema and often left ventricular enlargement, but, in contrast to patients with chronic mitral regurgitation, left atrial enlargement is absent.

Diagnosis. On bedside cardiac catheterization, the hemodynamics reflect the acute nature of the volume overload and the regurgitation of blood into a relatively normal-sized and noncompliant left atrium. The pulmonary artery pressure tracings demonstrate giant v waves (up to 70 to 100 mm Hg) and high mean wedge and pulmonary artery pressures.[615,686] There may also be a step-up in oxygen saturation in the peripheral pulmonary arteries as opposed to a step-up in the main pulmonary artery in patients with acute rupture of the interventricular septum.[618] Although these hemodynamic features are generally accepted as indicative of acute mitral regurgitation, caution should be exercised, in that similar findings have been described with acute interventricular septal rupture.[619] The usefulness of large v waves in the pulmonary capillary wedge tracings in establishing the diagnosis of mitral regurgitation has been assessed.[687,688] Fuchs et al.[687] found mitral regurgitation to be the commonest cause of large v waves, but this finding was neither sensitive nor specific for severe mitral regurgitation (Fig 30B-39). Both groups[687,688] concluded that large v waves in the wedge pressure waveform can be seen without mitral regurgitation and that the size of the v wave is related to factors that determine left atrial compliance. These studies, however, did not include patients with mitral regurgitation in acute MI and therefore do not establish sensitivity in this setting.

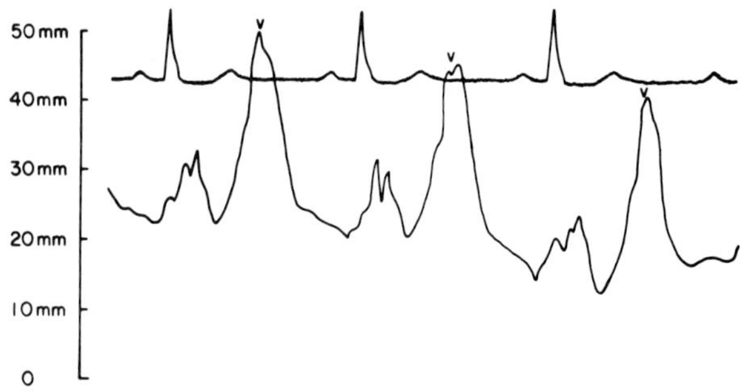

Fig 30B-39 Pulmonary capillary wedge tracing of a patient with large v waves. This patient had coronary artery disease and congestive heart failure but no clinical or angiographic evidence of significant mitral regurgitation. (From Fuchs RM, Heuser RR, Yin FCP, et al: Limitations of pulmonary wedge V waves in diagnosing mitral regurgitation. *Am J Cardiol* 49:849-854, 1982. By permission of Cahners Publishing Company, a Division of Reed Publishing USA.)

Use of bedside catheterization with observation of the pulmonary capillary wedge pressure waveform in the diagnosis of acute mitral regurgitation has limitations, particularly with low cardiac output and pulmonary hypertension.[679,687] Left ventriculography allows direct observation of the extent of regurgitation and the size of the left atrium in addition to the assessment of left ventricular function. In patients who are under consideration for surgery, coronary angiography should be performed during the same procedure.

Echocardiography has been a major advance in the noninvasive diagnosis of papillary muscle rupture.[624,668,689-695] Partial rupture of the papillary muscle has been directly visualized by two-dimensional echocardiography,[689] and complete rupture of the severed papillary muscle head and a flail segment of the mitral valve can be visualized. In the absence of the latter, the diagnosis is suggested by the appearance of a flail mitral leaflet. Color-flow imaging provides a semiquantitative technique for assessing the degree of mitral regurgitation,[696] but its utility is hampered by inadequate resolution. Transesophageal echocardiography is a further advance, but the most striking finding in patients with papillary muscle rupture is that left ventricular function is well preserved and hyperdynamic as a result of severe regurgitation into a low-impedance left atrium. This finding alone in the presence of hemodynamic deterioration should suggest a mechanical complication.

Medical management. The prognosis depends on the degree of rupture, the severity of mitral regurgitation, and ventricular function, but in patients with significant mitral regurgitation, it is usually poor.[682] Among patients seen in the presurgical era, an 83% mortality was found in the first 24 hours, and only 6% survived longer than 2 months.[667] Medical treatment alone is usually unsuccessful, although recent advances with vasodilator drugs and intra-aortic balloon counterpulsation have markedly improved the ability to stabilize hemodynamic status temporarily.

Aggressive medical management under monitoring conditions includes the use of vasodilators, which are particularly efficacious in acute mitral regurgitation because they reduce systemic vascular resistance and the amount of regurgitation and increase forward flow. Intravenous nitroprusside produces a dramatic hemodynamic improvement, with increases in forward stroke volume accompanied by reduced regurgitant fraction, height of the v wave, pulmonary capillary wedge pressure, and pulmonary artery pressure.[697] Hydralazine, parenterally and orally, may decrease the severity of regurgitation with resulting hemodynamic and clinical improvement.[698,699] Reduction of preload with high doses of oral nitrates or intravenous nitroglycerin is a useful adjunct to the use of vasodilators, which act primarily on the arterial system. Adjunctive therapy also includes use of diuretics, maintenance of acid-base status, and adequate oxygenation. Many patients have good left ventricular function, and inotropes or vasoconstrictor agents are usually not beneficial and may be harmful. The role of digitalis in this situation has not been determined.

If hemodynamic stability is not achieved promptly, intra-aortic balloon counterpulsation may be used to achieve the desired physiologic response; clinical and hemodynamic improvement results within 24 hours.[636] Nonetheless, improvement is usually temporary, and Gold et al.[636] found that complete correction of impaired circulatory dynamics is not usually obtained. Intra-aortic balloon counterpulsation should probably be confined to patients who are surgical candidates, for whom it allows further investigative procedures to be performed with low risk.

Surgical management. Figure 30B-40[460] illustrates the clinical course of 18 patients with papillary muscle rupture due to acute MI diagnosed at the Mayo Clinic between 1939 and 1981. It highlights the potential for sudden deterioration at varying times after the diagnosis despite apparent stabilization in some of the patients with heart failure alone.[460] Mitral regurgitation with heart failure and cardiogenic shock appears to pursue a relentless course to death.[460]

Replacement of the mitral valve in a patient with papillary muscle rupture is associated with a high perioperative mortality, ranging from 35% to 50% in patients in whom surgery is performed within 30 days of the acute event.[635,700]

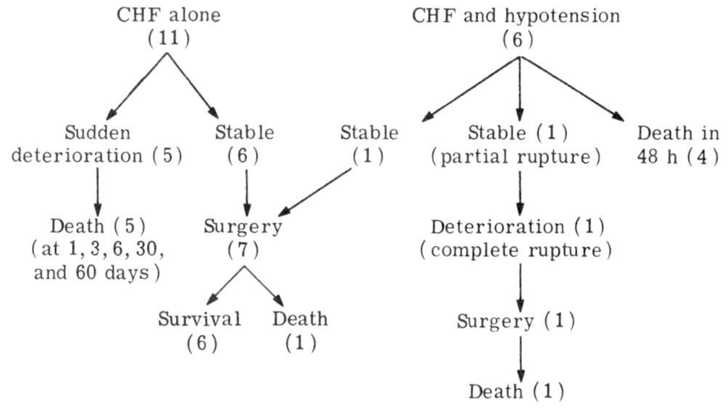

Fig 30B-40 Clinical course of patients with rupture of the papillary muscle. *CHF,* congestive heart failure. (From Nishimura RA, Schaff HV, Shub C, et al: Papillary muscle rupture complicating acute myocardial infarction: analysis of 17 patients. *Am J Cardiol* 51:373-377, 1983. By permission of Technical Publishing Company.)

Patients with papillary muscle rupture must be treated surgically. Earlier studies documenting a lower operative mortality (12% to 27%) when surgery was performed more than 3 months after the acute infarction led to the recommendation that surgery be delayed for at least 3 months.[700-703] However, this approach biases the selection process in favor of patients who can survive long enough to become surgical candidates, improving surgical survival but not necessarily overall patient survival.

Radford et al.[682] found that neither the angiographic extent of coronary artery disease nor the timing of mitral valve replacement was distinctly correlated with survival when the left ventricular ejection fraction was taken into account. These data strongly suggest that left ventricular function is the principal determinant of operative mortality and long-term survival.[567,682]

For patients with papillary muscle rupture, our approach has been modified by the potential for rapid and unpredictable deterioration despite initial hemodynamic stabilization.[459] Early, prompt surgical intervention is considered in all patients with suspected papillary muscle rupture, irrespective of their clinical presentation. Our initial prospective experience with this approach has been very encouraging, with only one death among the first nine patients reported (seven of whom had acute mitral regurgitation and two acute septal rupture).[459] Among 22 patients undergoing surgery for papillary muscle rupture at the Mayo Clinic during 1981 through 1990, perioperative mortality was 27%, but the 7-year actuarial survival rate was an encouraging 64% for perioperative survivors[679] (Fig 30B-41).

It has been strongly suggested that a policy of mitral valve repair, when feasible, is the preferred approach to patients with ischemic mitral regurgitation.[704,705] Whether this will apply to patients with rupture rather than papillary muscle dysfunction needs further evaluation.

In acute ischemic mitral regurgitation, emergency thrombolysis or angioplasty, or both, has successfully restored valve competence and hemodynamic stability.[685]

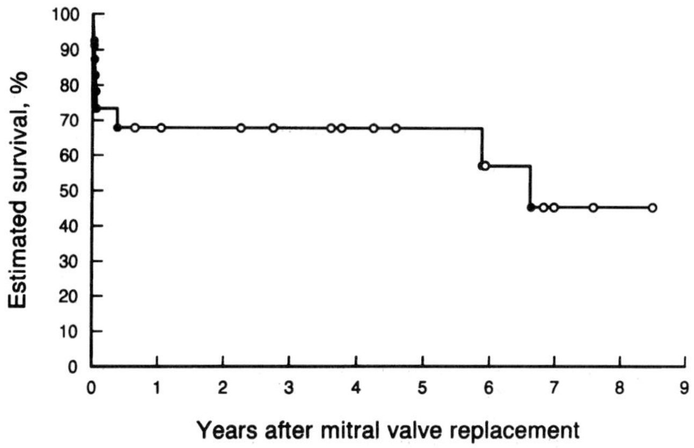

Fig 30B-41 Estimated survival after mitral valve replacement (21 patients) and mitral valve repair (1 patient) in patients with postinfarction rupture of a papillary muscle. Data include perioperative mortality, and points are plotted at times that correspond to the occurrence of deaths *(closed circles)* or to a change in the number of patients at risk of death (censored, alive) *(open circles)*. (From Kishon Y, Oh JK, Schaff HV, et al: Mitral valve operation in postinfarction rupture of a papillary muscle: immediate results and long-term follow-up of 22 patients. *Mayo Clin Proc* 67:1023-1030, 1992. By permission, Mayo Foundation for Medical Education and Research.)

Right ventricular infarction

Incidence. Although isolated right ventricular infarction without underlying cor pulmonale, right ventricular hypertrophy, or pulmonary embolism is rare,[706,707] such infarction is often combined with damage to the right ventricle.[708-719] The prevalence of right ventricular infarction in autopsy studies ranges from 14% to 34%.[709,711,719,720] In living patients with acute MI, clinical radionuclide evidence of right ventricular involvement was noted in 5% to 17%.[715,721] In patients with inferior (posterior) infarctions, concomitant right ventricular infarction was observed in 29% to 36%.[715,722]

Pathology. Autopsy findings have confirmed the association between right ventricular infarction and infarction of the posterior free wall of the left ventricle or the interventricular septum (or both).[711,719] Right ventricular MI uncommonly occurs in association with anteroseptal infarction, but in such cases, the right ventricular involvement is limited to the anterior right ventricular free wall in contiguity with the anterior left ventricular infarction.[718] Isner and Roberts[711] found the incidence of right ventricular infarction in autopsy cases with posterior infarction to be 25%, but in patients with infarction of the ventricular septum in addition to the posterior free wall, right ventricular damage was present in 50%.

The right ventricle is involved in different ways, depending on the pattern of extension from the left ventricle[711,714,723] (Fig 30B-42). Occasionally, right ventricular infarction may be confined to the papillary muscles of the right ventricle (usually the inferior papillary muscle).[711,714,723]

The distribution and severity of coronary atherosclerosis are similar in patients with and in those without right ventricular infarction.[711,719] Autopsy findings in patients with right ventricular infarction indicate a high incidence of severe stenosis of both the right and left anterior descending coronary arteries, with variable involvement of the circumflex and left main coronary arteries.[719] The site of right coronary artery occlusion is a major determinant of right ventricular infarction. Occlusion proximal to all or most of the right ventricular free-wall branches results in right ventricular infarction.[717] In patients in the TIMI-II trial with acute inferior myocardial infarctions who had thrombolytic therapy, complete occlusion of the infarct-related artery (as determined 18 to 48 hours following admission) was present in 48% of patients with right ventricular infarction compared with only 14% in those without right ventricular infarction.[721]

Explanations for the relative immunity of the right ventricle from infarction include the lower metabolic demands of the right ventricle,[724] the lower intracavitary pressures promoting collateral blood flow perfusion during both systole and diastole, and the excellent blood supply to the right ventricle. Right ventricular hypertrophy and pulmonary hypertension may predispose the heart to right ventricular infarction[706,707,724-726] but are by no means prerequisites or even common features of right ventricular infarction.[711,717-719,723] Severe disease in both right and left coronary arteries and the twofold greater incidence of recent coronary arterial occlusions (particularly of the right coronary artery) in patients with right ventricular infarction suggest that acute coronary artery lesions in patients with severe diffuse atherosclerotic disease might lead to right ventricular infarction by causing an abrupt decrease in collateral blood flow.[719] These conclusions are based on autopsy data and do not necessarily apply to the majority of patients with clinical features of right ventricular infarction, in whom the incidence of major complications and the mortality are low.[715]

Rupture of the heart is frequently associated with right ventricular infarction. It may involve more than one site, including the right ventricular free wall, ventricular septum, and left ventricular posterior wall.[538,717,727] Tricuspid insufficiency, both acute and chronic, may occur as a result of right ventricular papillary muscle dysfunction.[728-730] Although dilatation of the right ventricle is a common autopsy finding in right ventricular infarction, the incidence of right ventricular thrombus does not appear to be increased.[711]

Pathophysiology. The sequelae of right ventricular infarction range widely from minimal hemodynamic impairment to cardiogenic shock.[716] Structural damage to the right ventricle is far more common than major hemodynamic complications after infarction of this chamber. Furthermore, experimentally, isolated right ventricular damage is well tolerated,[731-736] as is surgical bypass of the right ventricle in the management of certain forms of congenital heart disease.[737,738]

Right ventricular infarction causes disproportionately

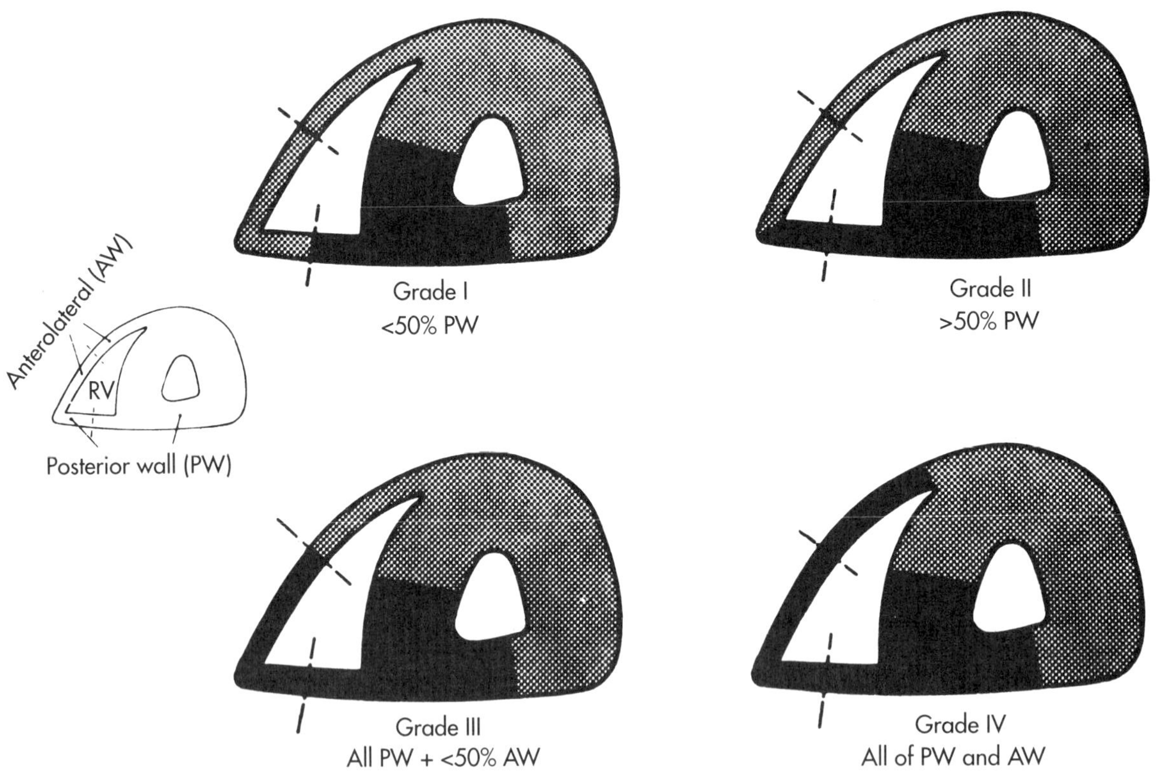

Fig 30B-42 Diagram of transverse slices of the right *(RV)* and left ventricles illustrating the scheme for grading the extent of right ventricular infarction. *AW,* anterolateral wall; *PW,* posterior wall. (From Isner JM, Roberts WC: Right ventricular infarction complicating left ventricular infarction secondary to coronary heart disease: frequency, location, associated findings and significance from analysis of 236 necropsy patients with acute or healed myocardial infarction. *Am J Cardiol* 42:885-894, 1978. By permission of Excerpta Medica.)

high right ventricular filling pressures,[710,714,739,740] probably because of impairment in contractility, compliance, or both. Pulmonary capillary wedge pressures are usually low in comparison with those normally found in acute infarction;[741] this reflects inadequate left ventricular preload caused, in part, by reduced right heart output.[710,716,742,743]

To identify the factors associated with systemic hypotension and right ventricular infarction, Lloyd et al.[716] compared hemodynamic findings in 19 patients with and without compromised systemic hemodynamic function. Hypotensive patients had higher right ventricular filling pressures and significantly higher wedge pressures. The increase in right heart filling pressure in hypotensive patients likely resulted from more extensive right ventricular damage. The significantly higher wedge pressure in hypotensive patients suggested that in patients with right ventricular infarction (whose right ventricular end-diastolic pressure was equal to or greater than the wedge pressure), an additional impairment of the left ventricular function was an important determinant of hypotension. The deleterious effect of elevated left ventricular end-diastolic pressure and wedge pressure on right ventricular performance was attributed to the direct relation between wedge pressure and pulmonary artery diastolic pressure, which in turn influences right ventricular afterload,[744] as illustrated in Figure 30B-43. Because the right ventricle has a large surface area in contrast to volume and the free wall is thin,[745] it is ill-adapted to compensate for increases in afterload. Probably in patients with right ventricular infarction, the extent of additional left ventricular dysfunction determines the hemodynamic outcome.[746]

The precise role of septal damage, so often associated with right ventricular infarction, in the pathogenesis of hypotension is as yet unclear, but paradoxic motion of the septum into the right ventricle may aid right ventricular ejection.[747] Clinical right ventricular infarction should not be considered an isolated disease of the right ventricle but rather a result of critical interaction between both ventricles.[716]

There is hemodynamic similarity between constrictive pericarditis and right ventricular infarction[713,716,739] (Fig 30B-44). The restraining effect of the pericardium, which is limited in its ability to dilate acutely,[748] coupled with pronounced right ventricular dilatation as seen in autopsy series,[711] might lead to pericardial restriction as a causal or contributory mechanism in the low-output syndrome seen in some patients with right ventricular infarction.[749] But some patients with shock due to right ventricular

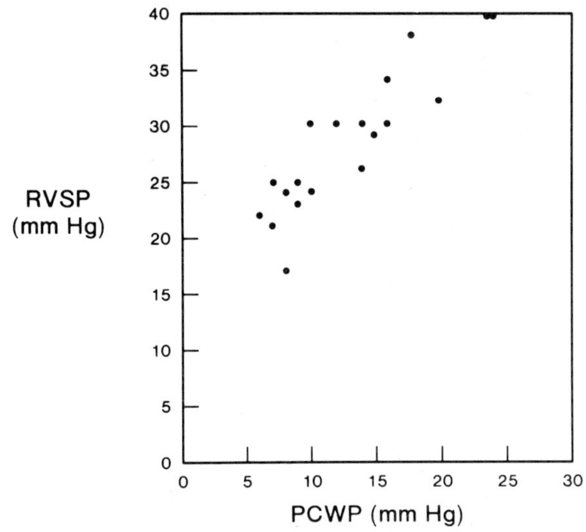

Fig 30B-43 Scatter diagram of right ventricular peak systolic pressure *(RVSP)* and pulmonary capillary wedge pressure *(PCWP)* in 19 patients. The correlation coefficient is 0.895 (*P* <0.001). (From Lloyd EA, Gersh BJ, Kennelly BM: Hemodynamic spectrum of "dominant" right ventricular infarction in 19 patients. *Am J Cardiol* 48:1016-1022, 1981. By permission of Cahners Publishing Company, a Division of Reed Publishing USA.)

infarction do not have the diastolic pressure equilibration characteristic of pericardial restriction (see Fig 30B-44), and alternative explanations must be sought. The "dip and plateau" configuration of the right ventricular diastolic pressure waveform in right ventricular infarction may result from reduced right ventricular compliance, as in restrictive cardiomyopathy.[716,750,751] Irrespective of the mechanism, hemodynamic compromise in patients with right ventricular infarction is exacerbated by decreased preload reserve depending on atrial systole, and the amplitude of the right atrial A wave is an important determinant of compromised right ventricular dysfunction and the compensatory role played by the atrium.[742]

Clinical features. The importance of right ventricular infarction is related to the fact that it is one of the relatively few potentially reversible causes of cardiogenic shock after acute MI.[710] The typical syndrome involves transmural inferior or direct posterior MI, jugular venous distention, and clear lung fields both clinically and radiologically.[710,715,716,740] A positive Kussmaul sign (which is both sensitive and specific[715,752]) and right ventricular third or fourth heart sounds provide additional evidence of right ventricular dysfunction (Table 30B-36). In addition to clear lung fields, a right pleural effusion may be present.[713,717]

In a few patients with hypotension or cardiogenic shock, the clinical presentation is striking. These patients lie still and flat in bed in dramatic contrast to the demeanor of most patients in cardiogenic shock, who usually have pulmonary edema. Conduction disturbances within the first 24 hours are frequent and tend to be more severe in

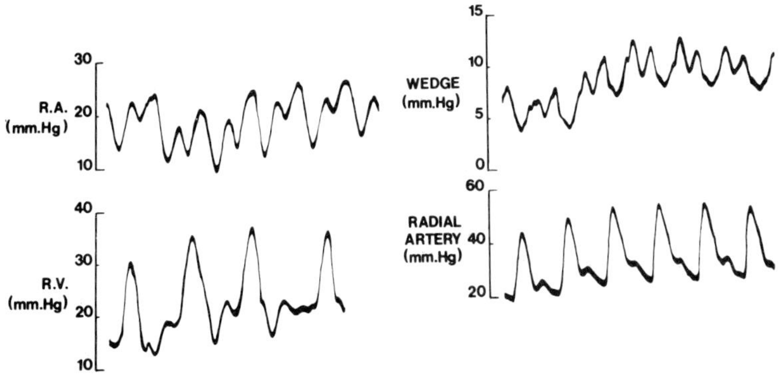

Fig 30B-44 Representative pressure recordings from a patient with right ventricular infarction. Right atrial *(R.A.),* right ventricular *(R.V.),* and pulmonary capillary wedge pressures were recorded sequentially. Right atrial pressure was elevated, with a prominent y descent. (The accompanying electrocardiographic tracing is not shown, but the timing of the y descent was established at the time of analysis.) Right ventricular end-diastolic pressure was elevated and exceeded pulmonary capillary wedge pressure. A "dip and plateau" pattern in the right ventricular diastolic pressure waveform is noted. In this patient, equalization of diastolic pressures of the left and the right sides of the heart is not present. The patient was very hypotensive, with a radial arterial systolic pressure of approximately 50 mm Hg. (From Lloyd EA, Gersh BJ, Kennelly BM: Hemodynamic spectrum of "dominant" right ventricular infarction in 19 patients. *Am J Cardiol* 48:1016-1022, 1981. By permission of Cahners Publishing Company, a Division of Reed Publishing USA.)

Table 30B-36 Clinical findings associated with right ventricular infarction

Hypotension
Elevated jugular venous pressure
Kussmaul's sign
Abnormal jugular venous pressure pattern (y ≥ x descent)
Tricuspid regurgitation
Right-sided S_3 and S_4
Pulsus paradoxus
High-grade atrioventricular block

From Dell'Italia LJ, O'Rourke RA: Pathophysiology and treatment of right ventricular myocardial infarction. In *Acute Myocardial Infarction.* Edited by BJ Gersh, SH Rahimtoola. New York, Elsevier Science Publishing Company, 1991, pp 271-283. By permission of Chapman & Hall.

patients with hypotension[710,716] (Table 30B-37). A low incidence of complete heart block was found by Cintron et al.[715] in patients without systemic hypotension. The murmurs of tricuspid insufficiency[728] and associated septal rupture[727,753] have been reported occasionally, and the former was documented on two-dimensional echocardiography in most patients with right ventricular infarction in one small study.[754]

Right ventricular infarction contributes to overall release of CK in patients with transmural inferior MI.[755] The presence of disproportionately high enzyme values in association with minimal depression of left ventricular function in inferior infarction should indicate possible right ventricular infarction.[755]

Diagnosis. Further diagnostic studies need not be undertaken in patients with clinical evidence of right ventricular infarction and no compromised systemic hemodynamics. In those with hypotension and clinical suspicion of right ventricular infarction, further evaluation is warranted. A definitive diagnosis leads to specific therapy and may ensure that inappropriate measures—for example, use of diuretics, which could further reduce right ventricular filling pressure and cardiac output—are avoided.

The ECG demonstrates the features of acute inferior MI (usually transmural), but direct posterior or lateral infarction may also be present. ST-segment elevation in the right precordial ECG leads points to the diagnosis of right ventricular MI.[756-760] As Isner[717] noted, the right-sided ECG changes are often subtle and typically evanescent. Croft et al.[758] concluded that ST-segment elevation of 0.1 mV or more in at least one right precordial lead (V_4R to V_6R) was highly sensitive (90%) and specific (91%) in detecting right ventricular infarction as defined on ^{99m}Tc stannous pyrophosphate scintigraphy (Fig 30B-45). A combination of leads V_4R to V_6R was a better indicator than any individual lead; leads V_1R to V_3R were less helpful. The pathogenesis of the ST-segment elevation in the right precordial leads may result either from transmural right ventricular damage or from associated infarction of the posterior interventricular septum, reflected through the "electrical window" constituted by the necrotic right ventricle.[758]

The sensitivity and specificity of precordial ST-segment elevation in the left-sided chest leads are less well established.[761] In patients with ST-segment elevation in the precordial leads unassociated with diagnostic changes in the inferior leads, ST-segment elevation was highest in lead V_1 or V_2 and decreased toward lead V_5 in patients with right ventricular infarction. In contrast, among patients with anterior left ventricular infarctions, the degree of ST-segment elevation was lowest in V_1 and increased toward lead V_5.[762]

Radionuclide techniques that demonstrate a disproportionate reduction in right ventricular ejection fraction or detect regional wall motion abnormalities in the right ventricle[742,763-765] help define the severity of right ventricular dysfunction. However, these abnormalities are not in themselves pathognomonic of right ventricular infarction. Both regional wall motion abnormalities and reduced right ventricular ejection fraction have been noted in patients without hemodynamic evidence of right ventricular infarction. Furthermore, these measurements do not distinguish between ischemia and necrosis.

Echocardiography helps distinguish between right ventricular infarction and cardiac tamponade.[713,717,754,766-768] Two-dimensional echocardiography assesses global right ventricular size and performance and segmental wall motion abnormalities.[717,754,766-768] It can also assess asso-

Table 30B-37 Incidence of electrocardiographic conduction disturbances (19 patients)

	Implantation of temporary pacemaker		Sinus bradycardia or sinus arrest		Second-degree heart block		Complete heart block	
Group*	No.	%	No.	%	No.	%	No.	%
I (6 cases)†	0	0	2	33	2	33	0	0
II (13 cases)	9	69	6	46	5	38	4	31

*Groups were determined according to systolic blood pressure on admission: group I, more than 100 mm Hg; group II, less than 100 mm Hg.
†One patient had atrial fibrillation with an irregular but slow ventricular response.
From Lloyd EA, Gersh BJ, Kennelly BM: Hemodynamic spectrum of "dominant" right ventricular infarction in 19 patients. *Am J Cardiol* 48:1016-1022, 1981. By permission of Cahners Publishing Company, a Division of Reed Publishing USA.

ciated valvular dysfunction, right-to-left shunts, and rupture. Although two-dimensional echocardiography is highly sensitive in detecting segmental wall motion abnormalities,[767] it is not specific for the presence of *hemodynamically important* right ventricular infarction. Therefore, right ventricular dilatation must be considered in addition to regional wall motion abnormalities in the diagnosis.

Although right ventricular infarction may be suspected clinically and structural damage to the chamber can be identified noninvasively, hemodynamic measurement and monitoring in patients with right ventricular infarction and systemic hypotension are crucial. The hemodynamic assessment is diagnostic, guides therapy, and monitors the results of treatment; bedside catheterization is probably indispensible to the management of patients with right ventricular infarction and hemodynamic complications. The possibility that right ventricular failure might follow occlusion of the right coronary artery, suggested by Herrick[769] in 1912, was supported by hemodynamic observations made more than 50 years later.[770,771]

The hemodynamic profile of "dominant" right ventricular infarction was first described by Cohn et al.[710] and has been repeatedly confirmed by others.[713,714,716,740,755,772] Characteristically, right ventricular filling pressure is equal to or greater than the left ventricular filling pressure, which in turn is either "normal" or minimally elevated. The pulmonary artery pressure is also normal or minimally elevated.[716] Hypovolemia may mask the "typical" hemodynamic characteristics of right ventricular infarction, but repeated measurements after volume loading may be extremely helpful.[740,767] A noncompliant pattern of the right atrial pressure waveform with a y descent streeper than the x descent is common (see Fig 30B-44), and differentiation from tamponade and constrictive pericarditis may be difficult.[713,716,739-741] A close relationship between right atrial pressure and pulmonary capillary wedge pressure or a severe noncompliant pattern in the right atrial pressure waveform was found to be 81.8% sensitive and 97.4% specific for the diagnosis of right ventricular infarction.[740] Depressed right ventricular function curves demonstrated by volume loading in

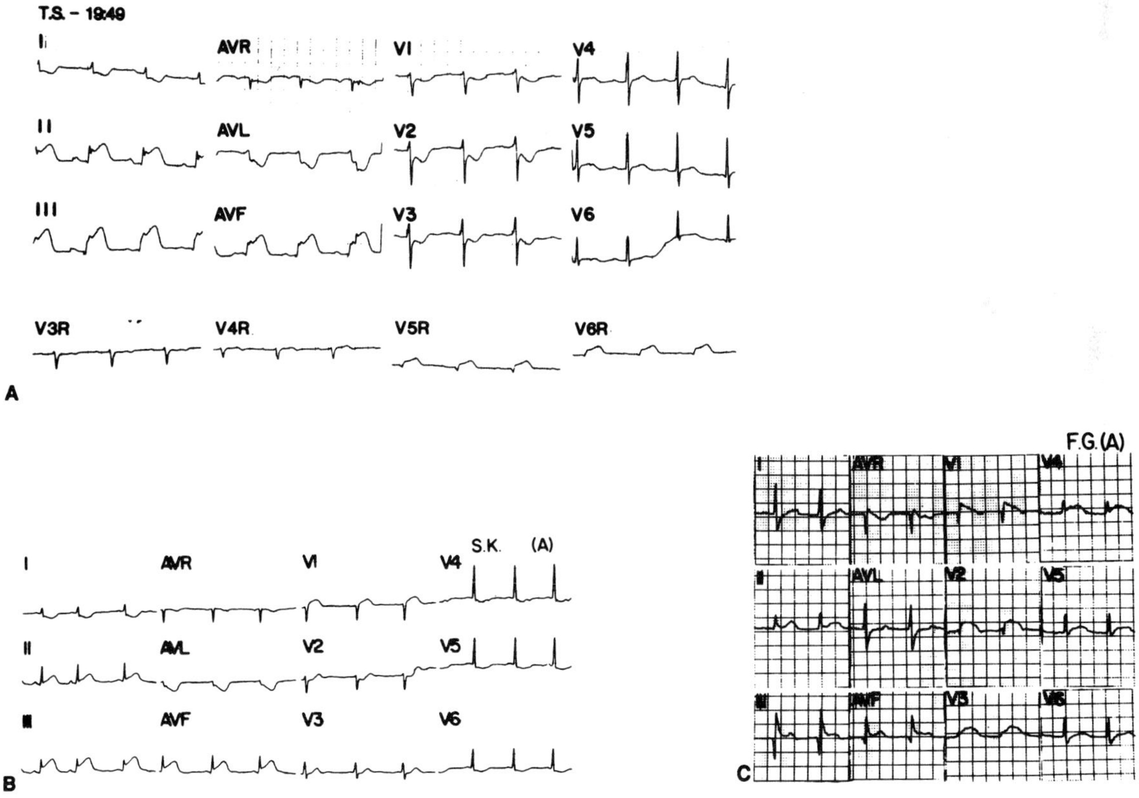

Fig 30B-45 Examples of ECG findings in three different patients with acute inferior myocardial infarction and associated right ventricular infarction. The signs of right ventricular infarction are ST-segment elevation in right-sided precordial leads V_5R and V_6R **(A)**, ST-segment elevation in lead V_1 **(B)**, and ST-segment elevation in V_1, V_2, V_3, V_4, and V_5 **(C)**. The patient represented in **C** had extensive right ventricular infarction with very little involvement of the left ventricle. (From Shah PK: New insights into the electrocardiogram of acute myocardial infarction. In *Acute Myocardial Infarction.* Edited by BJ Gersh, SH Rahimtoola. New York, Elsevier Science Publishing Company, 1991, pp 128-143. By permission of Chapman & Hall.)

patients with right ventricular infarction and infarction of the interventricular septum have been noted.[721]

In patients with interventricular septal rupture or severe tricuspid insufficiency complicating right ventricular infarction, bedside catheterization may demonstrate a step-up in oxygen saturation in the right ventricle or main pulmonary artery in septal rupture and prominent cv waves in the right atrium in tricuspid insufficiency.[728]

Differential diagnosis. Right ventricular infarction should be considered in any patient with hypotension and acute inferior MI. The most difficult condition to exclude is pericardial tamponade or constrictive pericarditis, although newer noninvasive techniques made this distinction easier. Rackley et al.[755] noted that an elevated systemic venous pressure in a patient with a normal pulmonary capillary wedge pressure may simulate acute pulmonary embolism. However, in right ventricular infarction, systolic pressures in the right ventricle and pulmonary artery are normal, in contrast to the mild elevation seen with acute pulmonary embolism and the larger elevation in patients with acute or chronic pulmonary embolism. Furthermore, dyspnea is absent in patients with right ventricular infarction in contrast to those with acute pulmonary embolism.

Prognosis and management. Right ventricular involvement during acute inferior MI (diagnosed by ST elevation in V_4R) is a strong independent predictor of major in-hospital complications (64% vs. 28%) and mortality (31% vs. 6%).[773] In patients without hypotension or shock, the early prognosis is excellent.[715,716,774] In those with hemodynamic complications, the outlook is less favorable.[713,742,743] The hospital mortality in patients with inferior and right ventricular infarction and complete AV block was 41% compared with an 11% mortality in patients with right ventricular infarction but no AV block, which was similar to that found in patients with inferior infarction without AV block and without right ventricular involvement.[775] Nonetheless, hypotension or shock in acute right ventricular infarction is potentially reversible, so the syndrome must be recognized and appropriate therapy instituted.[710,713,716,776,777] A further stimulus to the aggressive diagnosis and management of this condition is evidence that right (as opposed to left) ventricular function may improve rapidly after the initial ischemic insult[721,763,778,779] and further during the recovery phase.[763,780] Among patients receiving thrombolytic therapy, the 1-year mortality after dismissal in those with right ventricular infarction was encouragingly low at 3.5%, which was not significantly different from that among patients without right ventricular involvement.[721]

Major disturbances in conduction are frequent in these patients[710,716,775] (see Table 30B-37). In one series,[716] 69% of patients underwent temporary pacemaker implantation, although maintenance of an adequate heart rate alone produced minimal hemodynamic improvement. In patients with right ventricular infarction and significant left ventricular dysfunction, the 1-year prognosis is poor, but in those with hemodynamically significant right ventricular infarction, the long-term prognosis is excellent.[780]

The mainstay of therapy is fluid administration to increase right heart output and ventricular preload.[710,716] Validation of this approach in experimental right ventricular infarction has been obtained.[781] Inappropriate treatment, specifically the use of diuretic agents and other drugs that might further reduce ventricular preload and thus exacerbate systemic hypoperfusion,[782] must be rejected. The initial step is to administer fluids (either dextran or 0.9% saline), provided that the wedge pressure can be maintained at approximately 18 mm Hg or less, with the objective of maintaining adequate urinary output and systolic blood pressure of at least 100 mm Hg. Hemodynamic monitoring is essential. Patients may require as much as 100 or 200 mL of isotonic saline per hour.

For patients in whom the hemodynamics of right ventricular infarction are brought out by a volume challenge but in whom systemic perfusion is well maintained, no specific therapy is needed other than the avoidance of excessive preload reduction.

If fluid administration alone fails to produce a significant increase in right ventricular stroke work, cardiac output, and systemic blood pressure, the next step is to administer inotropic agents; dobutamine has been shown to be effective.[463] Theoretically, vasodilator agents would increase left ventricular ejection and thus augment right ventricular output by reducing right ventricular afterload, either through a direct action on the pulmonary vascular resistance or by reduction of left heart filling pressure[463,716,777,783] (see Fig 30B-43). In one series, however, nitroprusside did not produce any significant improvement in cardiac index or right ventricular ejection fraction.[463] It is likely that patients with severe right ventricular dysfunction in whom fluid replacement alone does not substantially increase stroke work are in the "flat" part of the right ventricular function curve. We recommend maintenance of adequate right and left ventricular filling pressures with volume loading and administration of agents that directly or indirectly reduce right and left ventricular afterload.[716,777] Dell'Italia et al.[780] found that an initial volume infusion had very little effect on systemic hemodynamics, which subsequently responded to inotropes. Differences between this series and earlier reports may be related to relative "hypovolemia" among the earlier cohorts of patients, in whom the diagnosis of right ventricular infarction may have been missed or treated initially and inappropriately with preload-reducing agents.

Preserving AV synchrony in right ventricular infarction is critical.[783-785] Dual-chamber temporary pacing systems are at times extremely helpful in managing patients with right ventricular infarction and conduction disturbances. In hypotensive patients with right ventricular infarction, atrial fibrillation should be considered an indication for emergency cardioversion.[783] A potential danger during temporary pacing in acute right ventricular infarction was suggested in a report by Sclarovsky et al.[786] of ventricular fibrillation complicating temporary pacing in five patients with clinical features of acute right ventricular infarction. Pacemaker perforation of the necrotic right ventricle is a theoretic possibility that requires consideration of softer pacing wires.

Hypertension

Hypertension detrimentally affects both the short-term and the long-term prognosis of acute MI.[787-791] Among patients receiving t-PA, the risk of intracranial hemorrhage was increased in those with "transient" hypertension immediately before infusion of t-PA.[792] Both the degree and the duration of systolic hypertension correlate with enzymatic estimates of infarct size,[791] presumably because of increased afterload and myocardial oxygen demands and ischemia. A universal objective in the patient with acute MI is to minimize afterload with its effects on myocardial oxygen demand. Reduction of ventricular afterload in hypertensive patients with acute infarction reduces infarct size and short-term mortality.[793]

Pathogenesis. Early after the onset of symptoms, an acute hypertensive reaction is commonly observed in patients who were previously normotensive, but this may also exaggerate blood pressure in chronically hypertensive patients.[793-795] Of 89 patients seen within 30 minutes of the onset of symptoms, 43% had evidence of sympathetic overactivity.[794] This acute response probably results from sympathetic arousal, and psychologic stimuli evoked by pain and distress probably play an important role in triggering sympathetic overactivity.[796] The response probably results from neurogenic reflexes arising from infarcted and contiguous areas of the ventricle or the proximal left coronary circulation.[795,797-799] Varying degrees of activation of and interaction between vagal and sympathetic afferent inputs from cardiac receptors to the central nervous system and input from the baroreceptors may account for the greater frequency of sympathetic overactivity in anterior MI.[794]

The clinical syndrome of the "hyperdynamic state" or "hyperfunction" after acute MI is well recognized. It is characterized by sinus tachycardia, increased blood pressures and cardiac output, and normal pulmonary capillary wedge pressure. Forrester et al.[800] found that 10% of their patients with acute infarction had left ventricular hyperfunction causing acute elevation of blood pressure. In some persons, acute MI evokes a generalized metabolic reaction characterized by sympathetic overactivity, presumably constituting a response to injury or stress.

Management. Hypertension in patients with the "hyperdynamic state" may respond to relief of pain and anxiety, and the diagnosis of resistant hypertension should not be made until both the pain and the anxiety have been treated. If hypertension persists, the most useful drugs are the β-adrenergic blocking agents. Our approach is to treat initially with intravenous administration of β-blocking agents. The very short half-life of esmolol makes it an attractive drug for patients in whom the potential for complications from β-blockers is considered to be increased. β-Blockers can usually be administered without the need for hemodynamic monitoring, but monitoring may be helpful and can increase the safety of β-blocker administration in "borderline" patients. Objectives are to reduce the systolic blood pressure to between 120 and 140 mm Hg, to maintain diastolic blood pressure above 60 mm Hg and mean blood pressure of above 80 mm Hg, and to reduce the pulse rate to 80 beats/min or less, provided that the wedge pressure does not exceed 18 mm Hg and the cardiac index does not fall below 2.2 to 2.5 liters/min per m^2. Sinus bradycardia of less than 50 beats/min contraindicates further doses of the drug.

Despite the low pulmonary capillary wedge pressure often noted in patients with the "hyperdynamic state," in our experience fluid replacement alone is of little value and surprisingly is usually accompanied by increased urine output. In some patients with acute infarction, renal function is increased with elevated glomerular filtration rates.[801] Salutary effects of β-blockade with sympathetic overactivity and acute infarction include reduced myocardial oxygen demand,[802] decreased lactate production,[803] reduced ventricular arrhythmias,[794,804] and diminished cumulative serum CK as an indicator of myocardial infarct size.[805,806] If the size of the infarct is to be limited by controlling blood pressure, this should probably be done within 4 to 6 hours after the onset of infarction.

In patients with hypertension after acute infarction in whom ischemic pain is persistent or recurrent, prompt control of blood pressure is mandatory. The choice of drug will depend in part on the presence or absence of left ventricular failure. With left ventricular failure as manifested by radiologic changes, a third heart sound, or an elevated pulmonary capillary wedge pressure, monitored blood pressure control is advisable. Although treatment may be initiated by sublingual and oral nitrates, intravenous nitroglycerin is particularly useful. The initial dose is 10 μg/min, and it is thereafter doubled every 10 minutes until blood pressure is controlled and the wedge pressure reduced to normal.[807] Intravenous sodium nitroprusside has been widely and successfully used in the control of postmyocardial infarction angina in hypertensive patients.[807] The initial dose should be small (10 μg/min); the dosage is gradually increased until blood pressure and wedge pressures have been satisfactorily reduced. Theoretically, intravenous nitroglycerin might be preferable to nitroprusside for reducing preload and afterload in early acute infarction because nitroprusside has been shown to increase infarct size in dogs.[198] The choice of drug, however, is determined somewhat by the severity of the hypertension because nitroprusside is a more effective afterload-reducing agent and is more suitable for patients with severe hypertension.

In the absence of heart failure, bronchospastic disease, or major disturbances in conduction, β-receptor blocking agents are effective in the control of postinfarction angina and hypertension. Tachycardia may result from the use of nitrates or nitroprusside, and the concomitant use of β-receptor-blocking agent may be extremely effective, provided that the pulmonary wedge pressure can be monitored.[807]

Regarding calcium antagonists, nifedipine and diltiazem have the most prominent dilating effect on small vessels and reduce blood pressure.[807] Logically, they appear useful in patients with continuing chest pain and hypertension after infarction, but further data are needed. The routine use of calcium channel blockers in acute MI is contraindicated.

In patients with chronic hypertension and acute MI, lowering blood pressure excessively compromises coronary artery blood flow. Currently, we maintain blood pressure approximately 20 to 40 mm Hg below control levels.[196,793,808] Control of angina and documentation of stable renal function and urine output measure adequate perfusion. Jugdutt et al.[3] found that blood pressure was reduced by 30% in hypertensive patients, but the greatest benefit was achieved by maintaining a mean blood pressure of at least 80 mm Hg. Other categories of patients with acute MI in whom control of elevated blood pressure is vital are those with acute interventricular septal rupture or mitral regurgitation.

In summary, hypertension after acute MI should be treated promptly and aggressively but carefully. Reasonable baseline levels are systolic blood pressures of 120 to 140 mm Hg and diastolic pressures above 60 mm Hg in patients who were previously normotensive and a level of 30 to 35 mm Hg below control[805] or a systolic blood pressure of approximately 150 mm Hg in patients with chronic hypertension and a mean blood pressure no lower than 80 mm Hg.[793] These guidelines apply in the absence of specific markers of the ideal coronary perfusion pressure in individual patients. Hemodynamic monitoring is useful, but recent data have emphatically shown that intravenous β-blocking agents can safely be given to most patients with acute MI, provided that attention is paid to clinical guidelines.[806,809]

PERICARDITIS

Traditionally, two forms of pericarditis after acute MI are recognized: "early" pericarditis, which occurs 24 to 72 hours after the onset of symptoms of infarction, and a "delayed" form, known as the "postmyocardial infarction syndrome," or "Dressler's syndrome,"[810-812] characterized by fever, persistent or recurrent pericarditis, and pericardial and pleural effusions occurring days or weeks after the infarction.[810,812-814] Current thinking suggests that these two entities are less distinct than originally thought and that no infallible line of demarcation can be drawn between early and delayed pericarditis.[813-819] Early pericarditis may blend imperceptibly into the postmyocardial infarction syndrome—which suggests a continuum between the two conditions.

Kossowsky et al.,[819] in reappraising Dressler's syndrome, concluded that separation of pericarditis after MI into two varieties is arbitrary and artificial. The change in impressions of the relationship between the two conditions was reinforced by Lichstein et al.[813] in a survey of 280 patients with acute MI during 1980. Early pericarditis was present in 6.4% of patients, none of whom developed Dressler's syndrome; this led to the conclusion that this syndrome has decreased in incidence and perhaps disappeared.[813] They believed that this decrease was most likely related to the diminished use of oral anticoagulants and to more aggressive treatment of pericarditis early after MI. Dressler's syndrome was diagnosed in 4 of 80 consecutive patients receiving anticoagulants unless specifically contraindicated; all four patients had "early" postinfarction pericarditis.[820]

Early pericarditis

Pericarditis is a short-lived although painful and disturbing complication of acute MI, but it is possibly the most common cause of recurring chest pain after admission to the hospital. Specific therapy usually alleviates the distressing symptoms. Symptoms must be differentiated from those of postinfarction angina.

Incidence and pathologic features. Probably the clinical diagnosis of pericarditis underestimates its true incidence, particularly since the pain and ECG changes may be attributed to recurrent ischemia.[811] Furthermore, the hallmark of pericarditis—the pericardial friction rub—is usually fleeting and may be missed unless frequent auscultation is performed.[814] The incidence of clinically diagnosed pericarditis determined by an audible friction rub or characteristic pain ranges from 6.7% to 20%.[813,815,821,822] The autopsy incidence of pericarditis ranges from 13% to 45%.[720,823,824] Typical ECG changes in pericarditis are present in only a small minority of patients with friction rubs.[822] In the MILIS study, pericarditis occurred in 25% of patients with Q-wave infarction and only 9% with non-Q-wave infarction.[821,825] The latter incidence reflects the imprecise correlation between the autopsy findings and the ECG diagnosis of Q-wave myocardial infarction[825,826] (see below). For pericarditis to be present during infarction, the infarct should extend to the epicardial surface. Nonetheless, pericarditis is not an invariable accompaniment of transmural MI, because the infarct may be separated from the pericardium either by a layer of muscle that obtains its blood supply from the epicardial vascular network[824] or by subepicardial adipose tissue.[827]

Clinical features. The pain of pericarditis is usually substernal, with radiation to the back, neck, or shoulders, but it may remain localized. In one series, 92% of patients with a friction rub complained of pain.[816] Enhancement of the pain by movement, particularly deep breathing, is characteristic, and the pain is best relieved by havingthe patient sit up and lean forward. The patient should be asked directly whether the pain differs from that experienced during the initial phase of acute infarction.

Again, the cardinal physical sign is the pericardial friction rub, which is typically evanescent. It is usually heard down the lower left sternal edge or medial to the apex, but the site may vary, and repeated auscultations may be needed. The onset of the pain of pericarditis preceded detection of the rub by 4 to 48 hours in 70% of patients in one analysis.[816]

The rub is most often heard on the second or third day after admission.[815,823,824,826] In a prospective study by Liem et al.,[826] pericarditis developed within 48 hours after acute MI in 80% and within 24 hours in 34%. Figure 30B-46 illustrates the time of appearance of friction rubs in relation to the onset of ischemic symptoms.[823] Detection of a rub on admission is less common but is well documented, particularly in patients resuscitated from

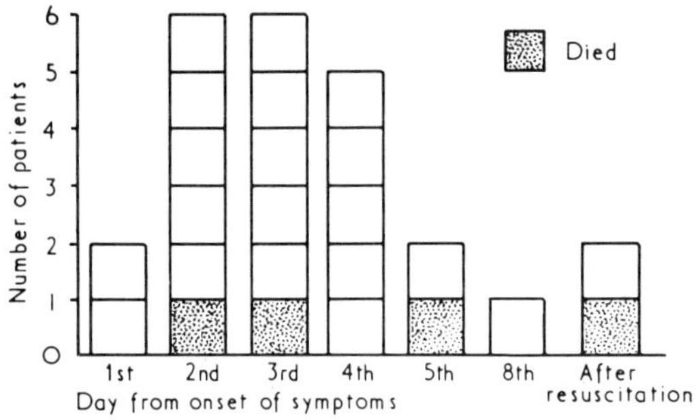

Fig 30B-46 Time of appearance of the friction rub of pericarditis after the onset of symptoms of infarction. (From Niarchos AP, McKendrick CS: Prognosis of pericarditis after acute myocardial infarction. *Br Heart J* 35:49-54, 1973. By permission.)

cardiac arrest.[815,823,824,826] More than 90% of friction rubs are diagnosed in the first 4 days, but late detection (5 to 11 days after infarction) has been reported.[815,823] Persistence of the rub for 3 days or less is usual.[823,824] In the 52 patients reported by Thadani et al.,[815] the rub remained audible for 1 to 6 days in 89% and for 8 to 16 days in 12%. Persistence of a friction rub for more than 3 days indicates a poor prognosis.[823,828]

An oral temperature exceeding 99°F was found in 94% of patients with pericarditis and in 72% of controls.[815] The duration of pyrexia is significantly longer in patients with pericarditis.[815,826] This may indicate more extensive myocardial necrosis or inflammation localized to the area overlying the MI.

Pericardial effusions are common in the early postinfarction period; with M-mode and two-dimensional echocardiography, they were noted in 26% to 37% of patients.[829-831] Pericardial effusions are usually small and not closely associated with a friction rub or typical chest pain; tamponade is very uncommon. As with pericardial friction rubs, effusions are more frequently associated with Q-wave and anterior infarctions.[829-831] After the administration of rt-PA, pericardial effusions were noted in 24% of patients by day 6, but they were generally small and tamponade did not develop.[832]

Electrocardiogram. The ECG changes accompanying pericarditis reflect subepicardial inflammation. In pericarditis complicating MI, the changes due to pericarditis may be masked by the ECG features of the underlying infarction. Pronounced concave ST-segment elevation in at least two of the limb leads and in most of the precordial leads is usual in pericarditis.[833] In patients with acute MI, the ST-segment elevation due to pericarditis may be mistaken as representing recurrent ischemia. A useful clue to pericarditis is that the changes in the ST-segment are not restricted to leads that show the features of infarction; that is, the repolarization changes are not confined to regional boundaries. Depression of the P-R segment further indicates pericarditis, although this finding is often difficult to evaluate.[834] Krainin et al.[822] studied 423 consecutive patients with acute MI; pericarditis was diagnosed clinically in 31, but only 1 had diagnostic ECG changes.

Clinical course and complications. Most clinical studies support the conclusion that pericarditis in acute infarction marks extensive myocardial damage and that this is reflected in a more complicated hospital course. The extent of myocardial necrosis in patients with pericarditis in comparison with controls is borne out by higher enzyme levels[815,823,826,828,835] and the degree of ST-segment elevation on admission.[824]

In the MILIS study,[821] pericarditis was associated with more extensive infarct size, a lower ejection fraction on admission, a greater incidence of heart failure, and atrial arrhythmias. Early mortality was 10% and 6% in patients with and without pericarditis, respectively, and mortality at 1 year was 18% and 12%. Much of the difference in late mortality could be explained by the lower ejection fraction in patients with pericarditis.[821] Most earlier series did not show any increase in early hospital mortality despite the more complicated course in patients with pericarditis.[815,816,823,826,836]

A similar trend was noted in patients with asymptomatic pericardial effusions during the early postinfarction period, because the incidences of congestive heart failure, ventricular arrhythmias, and markedly increased cardiac enzyme values were higher.[829-831] Among patients hospitalized with pericardial effusions, MI remains the most common clinical condition, and the most powerful predictor of subsequent cardiac tamponade is the size of the effusion echocardiographically.[832] Late mortality is also increased in patients with pericardial effusions, perhaps reflecting larger infarct size.[831]

An increased incidence of atrial arrhythmias (particularly atrial fibrillation) and ventricular arrhythmias is usual in postinfarction pericarditis.[815,823,826,835,837] The atrial arrhythmias may be related to involvement of the atrium or sinus node in the inflammatory process, but they could also result from an association with large infarcts and chamber dilatation. In a study of patients with a first Q-wave anterior MI, transient episodes of atrial fibrillation were more common in patients with hydropericardium than in those with or without pericarditis.[598] However, the most important factors discriminating the three groups were the height of the pulmonary artery wedge pressure and the extent of ventricular asynergy, and atrial fibrillation after Q-wave infarction was related not so much to the inflammatory infiltration involving the atria but to an increased atrial pressure resulting from the hemodynamics of left ventricular dysfunction. The greater frequency of AV block in patients with pericarditis is less readily explicable unless this further reflects extensive myocardial damage.[823,826] The reported incidence of congestive heart failure in patients with pericarditis varies.[815,823,824,828] The relative frequency of pleural and pulmonary parenchymal abnormalities in conjunction with pain-related tachycardia and tachypnea could lead to an overdiagnosis of congestive heart failure.[816]

Management. The treatment of early pericarditis is symptomatic, and reassurance to the patient that the pain is not due to recurrent ischemia is important. For pain, analgesics (aspirin and acetaminophen) usually suffice. Sawaya et al.[828] reported prompt and sustained relief of pain in 31 patients treated with salicylates at an average

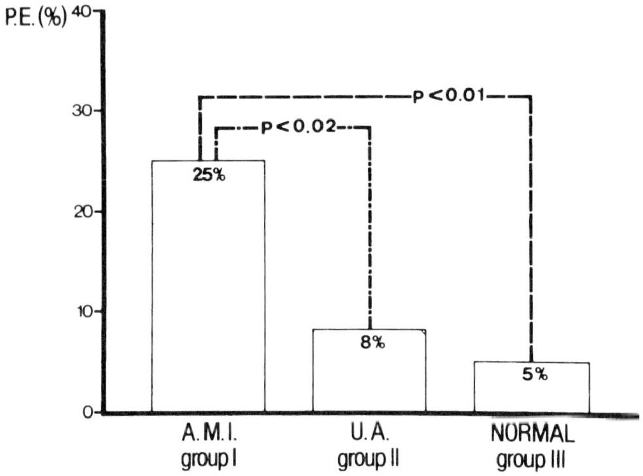

Fig 30B-47 Prevalence of pericardial effusion *(PE)* on the third day after admission in patients with acute myocardial infarction *(AMI)*, those with unstable angina *(UA)*, and subjects free from heart disease. (From Galve E, Garcia-Del-Castillo H, Evangelista A, et al: Pericardial effusion in the course of myocardial infarction: incidence, natural history, and clinical relevance. *Circulation* 73:294-299, 1986. By permission of American Heart Association.)

dose of 2 to 3 g per day for 14 days. In a prospective and a retrospective study, aspirin and indomethacin were found equally effective and safe in relieving the pain of pericarditis after acute infarction.[836] We use indomethacin as sparingly as possible and only until symptoms are relieved, because indomethacin may interfere with scar healing and may be loosely associated with cardiac rupture.[838,839] Yan et al.[840] prospectively evaluated an intravenous glucocorticoid preparation (40 mg of methylprednisolone sodium succinate) in 18 patients with postmyocardial infarction pericarditic pain unrelieved by opiates and found that the steroid preparation was effective within 3 to 4 hours. When aspirin (650 mg every 4 hours) was ineffective, intravenous dexamethasone (4 to 8 mg, repeated 6 hours later if needed) proved beneficial. In patients refractory to more conventional therapy, stellate ganglion blockade has been used.[841]

Despite the relative frequency of pericarditis and pericardial effusions early after acute MI,[823,829-831] the potentially disastrous complication of hemopericardium and tamponade is uncommon (Fig 30B-47).[832,842-845] Nonetheless, the risk of hemopericardium in patients receiving anticoagulants, although small, is definite.[816] A pericardial rub "early" after acute myocardial infarction may not in itself be a contraindication to anticoagulant therapy,[815,826] but Niarchos and McKendrick[823] reported 2 cases of hemopericardium out of 13 patients with pericarditis treated with anticoagulants, as opposed to none in 35 controls similarly treated. We withhold anticoagulant therapy in patients with the early development of pericarditis after acute MI. In those in whom the risk of thromboembolic complications is substantial or in patients undergoing acute coronary thrombolysis in whom prevention of reocclusion is a primary objective, anticoagulants may be administered, provided that one is able to deal promptly with any sign of cardiac tamponade.

Postmyocardial infarction (Dressler's syndrome)

Incidence. The postmyocardial infarction syndrome, or Dressler's syndrome, is an uncommon complication of acute MI; the incidence ranges from 0% to 4%.[815-817,823,824,828,846] Most reports suggest an incidence of 1% or less; as discussed previously, the entity may be disappearing.[813] Patients at highest risk for the postmyocardial infarction syndrome are those with "early" pericarditis.[815,816,823,824,828,847]

Clinical features. An average temperature of 101°F to 102°F is seen, although peaks to 103°F have been described. Persistence of fever beyond the tenth day after infarction, in the absence of any source of infection, may herald the onset of postmyocardial infarction syndrome.

Pain is usual and, in addition to the features described earlier, tends to recur. Among the 32 patients in Dressler's series, a pericardial friction rub appeared in the second week in 7 patients, in the third week in 11, later in the third week in 12, and at 10 weeks or later in 2.[812] Earlier documentation of a rub (within the first week) has been well described.[814,816-818]

Pericardial effusion is common, occurring in approximately 50% of patients.[810,817,848] The effusion may be serous, serosanguineous, or hemorrhagic,[849] even without anticoagulant therapy.[850] Aspiration of an effusion months after an acute MI in one patient yielded fluid described as suppurative and composed almost entirely of polymorphonuclear leukocytes; cultures of the effusion for bacteria and viral studies were negative.[851]

Pleurisy and pleural effusion were noted in 68% of Dressler's original patients. The effusions were usually small and were unilateral in about half the cases. Blood-stained pleural effusions are uncommon. A unilateral blood-stained effusion as a manifestation of Dressler's syndrome 2½ years after MI has been reported.[852] Patchy or linear pulmonary infiltrates on the chest radiograph are a prominent feature, noted in 28% to 61% of patients.[812] Whether they are immunologically mediated or atypical manifestations of heart failure or have some other cause is not known.[810,814,851]

Laboratory studies. Leukocytosis (involving predominantly polymorphonuclear cells), an increased erythrocyte sedimentation rate, and moderate anemia are found. The ECG may demonstrate the ST-segment changes characteristic of pericarditis, and the chest radiograph is helpful but not diagnostic. The progressive increase in the heart shadow on the chest radiograph or demonstration of an effusion echocardiographically favors a diagnosis of postmyocardial infarction syndrome.

Differential diagnosis. The conditions that could be confused with postmyocardial infarction syndrome are recurrent ischemia or infarction, congestive cardiac failure, pneumonia, atelectasis, bacterial endocarditis, and occult sepsis. Particular attention should be directed to the nature of the pain and to the constellation of signs and symptoms that make up this syndrome. The most difficult condition to exclude is pulmonary infarction. The onset after MI in both conditions may be similar, as may the radiologic features. A lung scan is often abnormal in either situation, and pulmonary angiography may occasionally be required to make the diagnosis. Nonetheless, the two conditions must be differentiated because anticoagulants are strongly indicated in pulmonary infarction but may be hazardous in postmyocardial infarction syndrome.

Etiology. Dressler originally thought that the syndrome represented an immune response to autoantigens released from necrotic myocardial tissue. Subsequent evidence has not been conclusive but tends to support his original premise. Humoral antiheart autoantibodies have been detected in patients with postmyocardial infarction syndrome and the related postcardiotomy syndrome,[853-856] but these are not specific for either condition.[857,858] Versey and Gabriel[859] measured the inactivation products of serum complement in 45 patients with acute MI. Activation of the complement cascade was found in only four patients, three of whom subsequently had postmyocardial infarction syndrome. This finding gave further weight to the possibility that this is an immune-complex disease incorporating antibodies that unite with myocardial antigen to form soluble complexes, which then activate the complement pathway.

Kennedy and Das[853] noted that both cellular and humoral immunity were abnormal during an exacerbation of postmyocardial infarction syndrome and were restored to normal on remission. They concluded that the clinical presentation of this syndrome, together with its other features, most closely resembles diseases designated as "rheumatoid" or "autoimmune" disorders. The possibility that postmyocardial infarction syndrome is due to reactivation of latent or dormant viral infections[860] has not been supported by the consistently negative viral studies in patients with Dressler's syndrome.[851,852] Dressler[810] postulated that anticoagulant therapy may play a role by causing leakage of blood into serous cavities; this supports the contention that the decreased use of oral anticoagulants in early pericarditis is partly responsible for the decline in the postmyocardial infarction syndrome.[813]

Complications. Major complications, although rare, have been well documented, but in general the postmyocardial infarction syndrome causes recurrent morbidity rather than mortality. The most serious and life-threatening complication is cardiac tamponade. The risk of pericardial hemorrhage in patients with Dressler's syndrome is increased by the use of anticoagulants.[810,816,849]

Hemorrhagic tamponade unrelated to anticoagulant therapy in patients with postmyocardial infarction pericarditis has been well described,[850,861] as has tamponade with nonhemorrhagic pericardial fluid.[862]

Among 31 patients with chronic or relapsing acute pericarditis, MI was the underlying cause in two patients. Pericardiectomy would appear to be an attractive option compared with the morbidity of long-term steroid administration in patients with multiple recurrences.[863]

Constrictive pericarditis after MI is rare. In a survey of 403 cases of pericarditis from the Mayo Clinic, none was considered a sequela of postmyocardial infarction pericarditis.[864] More recently, however, constrictive pericarditis after the postmyocardial infarction syndrome has been reported; at least two of the three patients were treated successfully by pericardiectomy.[865-867]

A link between the postmyocardial infarction syndrome and ventricular aneurysm has been noted, although the nature of the relationship is unclear.[847,868-870]

Therapy. The condition is usually self-limiting and may require no therapy other than reassurance. Pain often responds to simple analgesics,[849] and there are well-recorded cases of spontaneous resolution of symptoms.[817,846]

Treatment with corticosteroids usually brings dramatic relief of symptoms along with objective improvement in the pulmonary and pericardial lesions. Dressler[849] suggested an initial dosage of 40 to 60 mg daily to be slowly discontinued over a 4-week period. If symptoms recur with each attempt to reduce the dosage of steroids, a low-maintenance dosage of 5 to 10 mg daily may be required. A lower initial dosage, 30 to 40 mg daily for 10 to 14 days, has been found by others to be effective.[847] Although steroids are effective, they should be used with caution because of the tendency for relapse upon withdrawal.

Other successful anti-inflammatory agents are indomethacin,[814,817] butazolidin, and, exceptionally, mercaptopurine.[871] Colchicine was effective in nine patients with recurrent pericarditis, one of whom was classified as having a postmyocardial infarction syndrome.[872] A patient with recurrent angina pectoris and chronic (steroid-dependent) Dressler's syndrome who remained asymptomatic for at least 5 years after coronary artery surgery and pericardiectomy has been reported.[873]

Anticoagulants should be avoided in the postmyocardial infarction syndrome; their use is potentially hazardous and contraindicated. Other measures include aspiration of pleural effusions if respiration is hampered and constant awareness of the potential for tamponade, which would necessitate urgent pericardiocentesis.

EXTENSION OR RECURRENCE OF MI VERSUS EXPANSION

Early extension or recurrence of MI has a deleterious effect on prognosis because it increases the extent of total myocardial necrosis.[874,875] In addition, most patients with cardiogenic shock have had extension of their MI.[456]

Extension or early recurrence of infarction should be distinguished from expansion of acute infarction. In a necropsy study of 76 patients,[876] infarct expansion—acute dilation and thinning of the region of infarction due to intramural rupture of necrotic muscle fibers (without additional necrosis)—was common (observed in 59% of infarcts), was associated with large transmural infarcts (probably involving at least 17% of the ventricle), usually developed 5 to 7 days after infarction, and could produce acute dilation of the left ventricle with hemodynamic consequences. Expansion probably results from mechanical stretching by adjacent, normally contracting myocardium. It begins between 6 and 24 hours after infarction, progresses over days,[877] and may be important in the evolution of cardiac rupture and late aneurysm formation.[878-880]

A clinical study showed that patients with infarct expansion manifested by regional expansion with subsequent overall left ventricular dilation had a significantly greater mortality at 2 months, suggesting that infarct expansion with regional dilation may be an early lethal consequence of transmural infarction and an important mechanism of postinfarction cardiac dilation.[881] Both expansion and extension may be associated with ST-segment elevation. They may occur separately or together. However, extension was diagnosed in only 17% of infarcts at necropsy.[876]

Left ventricular end-systolic volume is the major determinant of survival after MI.[882-884] Left ventricular dilatation after MI appears to begin within the first 7 to 10 days, increases significantly over the following 6 weeks, and appears related to patency of the infarct-related artery.[885] Experimental reperfusion limits the expansion of the left ventricle by reducing the extent of transmural infarction, apparently by preserving a rim of epicardium.[216,886] If transmural infarction is limited to focal regions, expansion may not occur.[880] In addition, late reperfusion is associated with less expansion of the infarct, and this effect is independent of the extent of myocardial salvage or transmural infarction.[887] Reasons for this effect on "remodeling" or the processes of expansion and thinning of the infarct segment may be related to the rate of healing, the tensile strength, or the scar thickness of the infarcted segment that is reperfused.[888-890]

Several clinical studies suggest that reperfusion may limit infarct expansion independent of myocardial salvage and may reduce the development of left ventricular aneurysms even when thrombolytic therapy begins from 4 to 10 hours after the onset of symptoms.[891-893] In addition, preservation of the epicardial rim, even without significant myocardial salvage, may prevent myocardial rupture. The risk of cardiac rupture beyond the first 24 hours after thrombolysis was markedly reduced by streptokinase therapy in the GISSI trial.[548] In addition, a small study suggests that captopril may decrease progressive ventricular dilatation.[894]

The diagnosis of extension is overestimated if judged from ST-T changes or total serum CK levels;[895] these gave apparent incidences as high as 86% and 56%, respectively.[896] When CK-MB was used for the diagnosis of infarct extension, which increases the sensitivity and specificity for the diagnosis of initial or recurrent myocardial necrosis, the incidence ranged from approximately 10% to 40%, depending on the type of infarction, but overall was 14% to 30%,[895-904] which is comparable to the incidence observed at necropsy.[876] Among patients with subendocardial or nontransmural infarction, approximately 40% have recurrence, whereas in those with transmural infarction, 10% have recurrence.[898] Peak plasma CK and CK-MB levels were significantly lower at the initial infarction in patients who had a subsequent early recurrence than in those who did not,[895] which is compatible with the smaller or subendocardial infarct having the greater risk of extension. Over half of the recurrences occur within 10 days, with the remainder occurring within 14 to 18 days after the initial infarction.[898] This risk of early recurrence is understandable in view of the high incidence of subtotal occlusion with mural thrombus, which is very thrombogenic.[905-907]

Chest pain and ECG ST-T changes were sensitive indicators of early recurrence of infarction (90% and 80% sensitivity, respectively) but were not specific for recurrence (46% and 36% specificity, respectively). Among patients with early recurrence, 70% had new ST-T elevations, but Q waves developed in only 20% of patients with subendocardial infarction who had recurrence.[895] In other studies, a third to more than half of patients with extension were not detected clinically.[300,325,899-901,903-910] The site of early recurrent infarction indicated by ECG was the same as the initial site in 86% of patients. Thus, early recurrence and extension of infarct are nearly synonymous.

The clinical impact of early recurrence or infarct extent is great because early recurrence results in a significant decrease in global and regional left ventricular function (compared with improved or stable left ventricular function in the absence of recurrence)[895] and, most importantly, in a significant decrease in early survival.[895,898-901,903,904] In the largest study reported, early reinfarction was associated with increased early mortality mainly in patients with nontransmural infarction (Table 30B-38); most deaths occurred within 30 days of the initial infarction. Early reinfarction converts the mortality pattern of the patient with nontransmural infarction to that of a patient with transmural infarction without early recurrent infarction.[898] Risk factors associated with reinfarction in patients with nontransmural infarction include female sex, obesity (body weight >25% above optimal weight for height), and preceding recurrent chest pain (at least three episodes of anginal pain during hospitalization before extension).[895,898]

Table 30B-38 Short- and long-term mortality after myocardial infarction (MI): effect of early reinfarction

	Mortality, %			
	Nontransmural MI			
Time after initial MI	Without reinfarction	With reinfarction	Total	All transmural MI
3 weeks	8*	23*	10†	23†
9 months	23	34	27	30

*For mortality difference with and without early reinfarction, $P < 0.05$.
†For early mortality difference in nontransmural and transmural myocardial infarction, $P < 0.01$.
Data from Marmor A, Geltman EM, Schechtman K, et al. Recurrent myocardial infarction: clinical predictors and prognostic implications. *Circulation* 66:415-421, 1982.

Table 30B-39 Relationship of reocclusion rate to residual coronary artery stenosis after successful thrombolysis

Study	Reocclusion rate low			Reocclusion rate high		
	Reocclusion			Reocclusion		
	No./total	%	Lesion	No./total	%	Lesion
Harrison et al.[911]	0/12	0	>0.4 mm*	7/13†	54	≤0.4 mm
Badger et al.[912]	0/11	0	>0.6 mm*	5/12	57	≤0.6 mm*
Cowley‡[913]	3/22	14	<90%	10/14	71	≥90%
Serruys et al.[914]	2/33	6	<58%*	17/27	29	≥58%
Gash et al.[130]	1/7	14	<75%	5/17	29	≥75%
TIMI I§	1/30	3	>0.6 mm*	16/58	28	≤0.6 mm*

TIMI I, Thrombolysis in Myocardial Infarction, phase I.
*Quantitative angiography.
†Of 7 with reocclusions, 3 died, 3 had reinfarction, and 1 was asymptomatic.
‡Of 13 with reocclusions, 5 had reinfarction, 5 had unstable angina, and 3 were asymptomatic.
§Unpublished data.

Thus, nontransmural infarction is associated with modest initial necrosis (with additional myocardium in jeopardy) and modest mortality compared to transmural infarction but a high incidence (40%) of early recurrent infarction that should discourage early dismissal for an uncomplicated and benign situation. Instability of the patient with nontransmural infarction is probably related to the high incidence of subtotal occlusion of the infarct-related artery, the hemorrheologic factors of a high-grade residual lesion (Table 30B-39), the residual mural thrombus, the significant thrombogenicity of residual thrombus, and the apparent hyperthrombotic state in the early weeks after infarction, when a shortened platelet survival half-life is evident and the risk of reinfarction is greatest.[905-907,915]

When recurrent chest pain or a positive rehabilitation stress test is noted early after infarction, an aggressive approach should be considered. Coronary angiography and the possibility of PTCA or coronary bypass surgery should be considered. After nontransmural infarction, aggressive antithrombotic therapy should be considered: full-dose heparin infusion, 80 to 160 mg of aspirin a day, and 90 mg of diltiazem four times daily (in patients without left ventricular dysfunction). The Paris II trial of antiplatelet therapy showed a striking reduction in reinfarction in patients with non-Q-wave infarction.[916]

NON-Q-WAVE MI

Non-Q-wave MI occurs in up to 30% or 40% of patients with acute MI[917-919] and has distinct clinical, pathologic, and prognostic attributes. The term "non-Q-wave" implies that the ECG is diagnostic of this type of MI and that patients in whom this condition develops have symptoms of prolonged myocardial ischemia with acute ECG changes but without the subsequent development of Q waves. The acute ECG changes may include ST-segment elevation or depression.[920,921] Serum cardiac CK completes the clinical diagnostic triad and indicates that myocardial necrosis occurs in this condition. This infarction syndrome includes and shares a number of the features of subendocardial infarction. The latter term perhaps excludes patients presenting with ST elevation. "Nontransmural MI" is another term that may be used for non-Q-wave MI. However, from the ECG, it is often unclear whether a MI is transmural. Thus, the term "non-Q-wave infarction" has supplanted the terms "subendocardial" and "nontransmural MI."

The pathophysiology of this condition lies somewhere between chronic angina pectoris and Q-wave MI and resembles that of unstable angina pectoris. In unstable angina pectoris, the duration of ischemia is briefer and no myocardial necrosis occurs, whereas in non-Q-wave MI, ischemic symptoms are longer and myocardial necrosis occurs.

Angiographic studies in non-Q-wave MI often show a pattern of coronary atherosclerosis similar to that in chronic stable angina and Q-wave MI.[922,923] However, the angiographic hallmark of non-Q-wave infarction is a nonocclusive thrombus associated with an irregular disrupted atheromatous plaque.[924] In contrast, although plaque disruption is often present in Q-wave infarction, the thrombus occludes the infarct-related coronary artery.[925] The intravascular clotting sequence in non-Q-wave infarction has not progressed to the same extent as that in Q-wave MI. Interestingly, coronary anatomy and its relationship to thrombus in unstable angina and non-Q-wave infarction are similar.[926] DeWood et al.[924,925] noted that the incidence of an occluded coronary artery is low (20%) in the first 24 hours after symptoms of non-Q-wave infarction compared with that (80%) in patients with Q-wave infarction. Of note, the incidence of occluded coronary arteries increased with time after onset of non-Q-wave infarction in contrast to the decreasing incidence in Q-wave infarctions.

Elevation of CK-MB is less in patients with non-Q-wave

infarction than in those with Q-wave infarction,[927] and often an early peak of CK-MB is found.[921,928] Thus, autothrombolysis may occur in patients with non-Q-wave infarction early after the onset of symptoms,[929] producing a pattern of enzyme release similar to that in patients undergoing successful thrombolysis after Q-wave MI.

Apart from the ECG and cardiac enzyme analysis,[930] noninvasive tests are of little value in identifying non-Q-wave MI. ^{99m}Tc pyrophosphate ("hot-spot") imaging is often negative, as is "cold-spot" imaging with ^{201}Tl.[931,932] Wall motion abnormalities after non-Q-wave infarction may or may not be defined by echocardiography or radionuclide ventriculography.

Natural history studies in patients with non-Q-wave MI demonstrate a hospital and posthospital course distinct from that of patients with Q-wave MI. On balance, studies show a lower in-hospital mortality after non-Q-wave MI than after Q-wave infarction (10% and 20%, respectively), whereas subsequent mortality in patients with non-Q-wave infarction equals or exceeds that in Q-wave MI (31% compared with 26%).[917] The incidence of reinfarction is considerably higher in patients with non-Q-wave than in those with Q-wave infarction (16% compared with 6%).[917] Persistent ST-segment depression is a powerful predictor of a poor prognosis.[918,919]

The worsening prognosis after hospital dismissal and higher reinfarction rate have prompted the early identification of this condition and the rapid initiation of management designed to limit these complications.

One approach is early angiography, particularly in patients with recurrent pain or persistent ST-segment depression.[918,919] Since non-Q-wave infarction identifies a subgroup of patients with a tripling of mortality after hospital dismissal, revascularization before hospital dismissal may be justified, particularly if postinfarction ischemia occurs.[933] Surgical revascularization is done for multivessel disease and balloon angioplasty for single-vessel disease and selected multivessel disease. Patients who undergo such an aggressive approach have lower death and reinfarction rates than do medically managed patients.[933,934]

Medical management in these patients before revascularization should include heparinization. Intravenous administration of heparin reduces the incidence of infarction and reinfarction in patients with unstable angina pectoris and non-Q-wave infarction.[935,936] Antiplatelet agents, such as aspirin or the combination of aspirin and persantine, have been shown to reduce mortality and the rate of reinfarction in these patients.[937] Thus, the use of 80 to 325 mg of aspirin daily is recommended in patients with non-Q-wave MI. Diltiazem, 90 mg four times a day in the hospital, has also been shown to reduce the reinfarction rate in patients with non-Q-wave infarction.[938] Therefore, diltiazem can be recommended for the initial medical management of these patients, provided that ventricular function is reasonably well preserved (ejection fraction >0.40).[939] Other calcium channel blockers and β-blockers have not been shown to reduce reinfarction rates in these patients.[940-942] However, β-blockers, particularly the short-acting agent esmolol, may be valuable in controlling tachycardia or hypertension associated with an evolving non-Q-wave infarction.

The role of thrombolytic agents in non-Q-wave MI is unclear. Since intracoronary thrombosis is part of the pathophysiology of non-Q-wave infarction, thrombolytic agents (streptokinase or rt-PA) might prevent reinfarction and recurrent angina. In limited studies, this has not yet been proven.[943,944] Thrombus in non-Q-wave infarction may differ from that in Q-wave infarction. A consequence of this difference is that it may be resistant to conventional thrombolytic agents. This speculation remains to be explored.

The usefulness of noninvasive stress testing after non-Q-wave infarction must be defined further.[945] Clearly, for patients in whom unstable symptoms (reinfarction or recurrent ischemia) develop, no exercise testing is indicated; the patients proceed to revascularization. However, in patients who remain asymptomatic throughout their hospital course, noninvasive stress testing may help to differentiate those at low risk from those at high risk.[917,946] It may be reasonable to observe closely asymptomatic patients after non-Q-wave infarction who have a negative stress thallium study. These patients may be treated with aspirin and diltiazem rather than revascularization. However, if one is to be confident that this approach is appropriate, all patients with non-Q-wave infarction should have their coronary artery anatomy defined by coronary arteriography.

Several authors have pointed out the similarities between non-Q-wave MI and successful thrombolysis in Q-wave MI.[929,947] Both conditions may represent the consequences of thrombolysis; in the former, it is spontaneous, and in the latter, medically induced. Thus, both circumstances yield partially occluded vessels with an early peak in serum CK-MB concentration, and the subsequent hospital course in both conditions is complicated by reinfarction and recurrent angina pectoris.

Patients with non-Q-wave MI form an important subgroup of those with MI. Although the in-hospital mortality of this condition is less than that of Q-wave infarction, there is a subsequent tripling in mortality. Thus, the cardiologist must identify this condition and proceed with aggressive management, including coronary angiography and revascularization. In-hospital management should include aspirin, diltiazem, and heparin.

REFERENCES

1. Herlitz J, Hjalmarson Å, Waagstein F: Treatment of pain in acute myocardial infarction. *Br Heart J* 61:9-13, 1989
2. Kim YI, Williams JF Jr: Large-dose sublingual nitroglycerin in acute myocardial infarction: relief of chest pain and reduction of Q wave evolution. *Am J Cardiol* 49:842-848, 1982
3. Jugdutt BI, Warnica JW: Intravenous nitroglycerin therapy to limit myocardial infarct size, expansion, and complications: effect of timing, dosage, and infarct location. *Circulation* 78:906-919, 1988
4. Williams DO, Amsterdam EA, Mason DT: Hemodynamic effects of nitroglycerin in acute myocardial infarction: decrease in ventricular preload at the expense of cardiac output. *Circulation* 51:421-427, 1975
5. Gunnar RM, Passamani ER, Bourdillon PD, et al: Guidelines for the early management of patients with acute myocardial infarction. A report of the American College of Cardiology/American Heart Association Task Force on Assessment of Diagnostic and Therapeutic

Cardiovascular Procedures (Subcommittee to Develop Guidelines for the Early Management of Patients with Acute Myocardial Infarction). *J Am Coll Cardiol* 16:249-292, 1990

6. Fillmore SJ, Shapiro M, Killip T: Arterial oxygen tension in acute myocardial infarction. Serial analysis of clinical state and blood gas changes. *Am Heart J* 79:620-629, 1970
7. Maroko PR, Radvany P, Braunwald E, et al: Reduction of infarct size by oxygen inhalation following acute coronary occlusion. *Circulation* 52:360-368, 1975
8. Pasqualucci V: Advances in the management of cardiac pain. In *Advances in Pain Research and Therapy: Recent Advances in the Management of Pain.* Vol. 7. Edited by C Benedetti, CR Chapman, G Moricca. New York, Raven Press, 1984, pp 501-504
9. Ward JM, McGrath RL, Weil JV: Effects of morphine on the peripheral vascular response to sympathetic stimulation. *Am J Cardiol* 29:659-666, 1972
10. Thomas M, Malmcrona R, Fillmore S, et al: Haemodynamic effects of morphine in patients with acute myocardial infarction. *Br Heart J* 27:863-875, 1965
11. Scott ME, Orr R: Effects of diamorphine, methadone, morphine, and pentazocine in patients with suspected acute myocardial infarction. *Lancet* 1:1065-1067, 1969
12. Alderman EL: Analgesics in the acute phase of myocardial infarction. *JAMA* 229:1646-1648, 1974
13. Lasagna L, Beecher HK: The optimal dose of morphine. *JAMA* 156:230-234, 1954
14. Remetz MS, Cabin HS: Analgesic therapy in acute myocardial infarction. *Cardiol Clin* 6:29-36, February 1988
15. Bersten AD, Holt AW, Vedig AE, et al: Treatment of severe cardiogenic pulmonary edema with continuous positive airway pressure delivered by face mask. *N Engl J Med* 325:1825-1830, 1991
16. Timmis AD, Rothman MT, Henderson MA, et al: Haemodynamic effects of intravenous morphine in patients with acute myocardial infarction complicated by severe left ventricular failure. *Br Med J* 280:980-982, 1980
17. Lester R: Achieving pain relief with physiologic management and analgesic agents during acute myocardial infarction. In *Acute Coronary Care: Principles and Practice.* Edited by RM Califf, GS Wagner. Boston, Martinus Nijhoff, 1985, pp 299-309
18. Vismara LA, Leaman DM, Zelis R: The effects of morphine on venous tone in patients with acute pulmonary edema. *Circulation* 54:335-337, 1976
19. Vasko JS, Henney RP, Oldham HN, et al: Mechanisms of action of morphine in the treatment of experimental pulmonary edema. *Am J Cardiol* 18:876-883, 1966
20. Nielsen JR, Pedersen KE, Dahlstrøm CG, et al: Analgetic treatment in acute myocardial infarction: a controlled clinical comparison of morphine, nicomorphine and pethidine. *Acta Med Scand* 215:349-354, 1984
21. Alderman EL, Barry WH, Graham AF, et al: Hemodynamic effects of morphine and pentazocine differ in cardiac patients. *N Engl J Med* 287:623-627, 1972
22. Kerr F, Hoskins MR, Brown MG, et al: A double-blind trial of patient-controlled nitrous-oxide/oxygen analgesia in myocardial infarction. *Lancet* 1:1397-1400, 1975
23. Thompson PL, Lown B: Nitrous oxide as an analgesic in acute myocardial infarction. *JAMA* 235:924-927, 1976
24. Romagnoli A, Keats AS: Comparative hemodynamic effects of nalbuphine and morphine in patients with coronary artery disease. *Cardiovasc Dis Bull Texas Heart Inst* 5:19-24, 1978
25. Waagstein F, Hjalmarson AC: Double-blind study of the effect of cardioselective beta-blockade on chest pain in acute myocardial infarction. *Acta Med Scand* Suppl 587:201-207, 1975
26. Ramsdale DR, Faragher EB, Bennett DH, et al: Ischemic pain relief in patients with acute myocardial infarction by intravenous atenolol. *Am Heart J* 103:459-467, 1982
27. Herlitz J, Hjalmarson Å, Holmberg S, et al: Effect of metoprolol on chest pain in acute myocardial infarction. *Br Heart J* 51:438-444, 1984
28. The MIAMI Trial Research Group: Narcotic analgesics and other antianginal drugs. *Am J Cardiol* 56:30G-34G, 1985
29. The International Collaborative Study Group: Reduction of infarct size with the early use of timolol in acute myocardial infarction. *N Engl J Med* 310:9-15, 1984
30. Vatner SF, Baig H, Manders WT, et al: Effects of propranolol on regional myocardial function, electrograms, and blood flow in conscious dogs with myocardial ischemia. *J Clin Invest* 60:353-360, 1977
31. Buck JD, Hardman HF, Warltier DC, et al: Changes in ischemic blood flow distribution and dynamic severity of a coronary stenosis induced by beta blockade in the canine heart. *Circulation* 64:708-715, 1981
32. Hackett TP, Cassem NH, Wishnie HA: The coronary-care unit: an appraisal of its psychologic hazards. *N Engl J Med* 279:1365-1370, 1968
33. Rebuck AS, Cade JF, Campbell EJM: Pulmonary aspects of myocardial infarction. *Mod Concepts Cardiovasc Dis* 42:17-21, 1973
34. Fillmore SJ, Guimarães AC, Scheidt SS, et al: Blood-gas changes and pulmonary hemodynamics following acute myocardial infarction. *Circulation* 45:583-591, 1972
35. Pain MCF, Stannard M, Sloman G: Disturbances of pulmonary function after acute myocardial infarction. *Br Med J* 2:591-594, 1967
36. Thomas M, Malmcrona R, Shillingford J: Haemodynamic effects of oxygen in patients with acute myocardial infarction. *Br Heart J* 27:401-407, 1965
37. McNicol MW, Kirby BJ: Oxygen therapy in myocardial infarction. In *Textbook of Coronary Care.* Edited by LE Meltzer, AJ Dunning. Philadelphia, Charles Press, 1972, pp 521-530
38. Wright IS, Marple CD, Beck DF: Report of the committee for the evaluation of anticoagulants in the treatment of coronary thrombosis with myocardial infarction. *Am Heart J* 36:801-815, 1948
39. Chalmers TC, Matta RJ, Smith H Jr, et al: Evidence favoring the use of anticoagulants in the hospital phase of acute myocardial infarction. *N Engl J Med* 297:1091-1096, 1977
40. Selzer A: Use of anticoagulant agents in acute myocardial infarction: statistics or clinical judgment? *Am J Cardiol* 41:1315-1317, 1978
41. Hilden T, Iversen K, Raaschou F, et al: Anticoagulants in acute myocardial infarction. *Lancet* 2:327-331, 1961
42. Veterans Administration Cooperative Investigators: Anticoagulants in acute myocardial infarction: results of a cooperative clinical trial. *JAMA* 225:724-729, 1973
43. Aber CP, Bass NM, Berry CL, et al: Streptokinase in acute myocardial infarction: a controlled multicentre study in the United Kingdom. *Br Med J* 2:1100-1104, 1976
44. Wessler S, Kleiger RE, Cornfield J, et al: Coumarin therapy in acute myocardial infarction. *Arch Intern Med* 134:774-779, 1974
45. Flanc C, Kakkar VV, Clarke MB: The detection of venous thrombosis of the legs using ^{125}I-labeled fibrinogen. *Br J Surg* 55:742-747, 1968
46. Lambie JM, Mahaffy RG, Barber DC, et al: Diagnostic accuracy in venous thrombosis. *Br Med J* 2:142-143, 1970
47. Negus D, Pinto DJ, Le Quesne LP, et al: ^{125}I-labelled fibrinogen in the diagnosis of deep-vein thrombosis and its correlation with phlebography. *Br J Surg* 55:835-839, 1968
48. Kakkar V: The diagnosis of deep vein thrombosis using the ^{125}I fibrinogen test. *Arch Surg* 104:152-159, 1972
49. Murray TS, Lorimer AR, Cox FC, et al: Leg-vein thrombosis following myocardial infarction. *Lancet* 2:792-793, 1970
50. Nicolaides AN, Kakkar VV, Renney JTG, et al: Myocardial infarction and deep-vein thrombosis. *Br Med J* 1:432-434, 1971
51. Maurer BJ, Wray R, Shillingford JP: Frequency of venous thrombosis after myocardial infarction. *Lancet* 2:1385-1387, 1971
52. Handley AJ, Emerson PA, Fleming PR: Heparin in the prevention of deep vein thrombosis after myocardial infarction. *Br Med J* 2:436-438, 1972
53. Handley AJ: Low-dose heparin after myocardial infarction. *Lancet* 2:623-624, 1972
54. Wray R, Maurer B, Shillingford J: Prophylactic anticoagulant therapy in the prevention of calf-vein thrombosis after myocardial infarction. *N Engl J Med* 288:815-817, 1973
55. Simmons AV, Sheppard MA, Cox AF: Deep venous thrombosis after myocardial infarction: predisposing factors. *Br Heart J* 35:623-625, 1973
56. International Multicentre Trial: Prevention of fatal postoperative pulmonary embolism by low doses of heparin. *Lancet* 2:45-51, 1975
57. Chesebro JH, Fuster V, Pumphrey CW, et al: Improvement of shortened platelet survival half-life from the early to the late phase of myocardial infarction (abstract). Circulation 64 Suppl 4:197, 1981
58. Merlini PA, Bauer KA, Oltrona L, et al: Persistent activation of coagulation mechanism in unstable angina and myocardial infarction. *Circulation* 90:61-68, 1994

59. Ygge J: Changes in blood coagulation and fibrinolysis during the postoperative period. *Am J Surg* 119:225-232, 1970

60. Miller RR, Lies JE, Carretta RF, et al: Prevention of lower extremity venous thrombosis by early mobilization: confirmation in patients with acute myocardial infarction by ^{125}I-fibrinogen uptake and venography. *Ann Intern Med* 84:700-703, 1976

61. Emerson PA, Teather D, Handley AJ: The application of decision theory to the prevention of deep vein thrombosis following myocardial infarction. *Q J Med* 43:389-398, 1974

62. Kakkar VV, Howe CT, Flanc C, et al: Natural history of postoperative deep-vein thrombosis. *Lancet* 2:230-233, 1969

63. Kakkar VV: Venous thrombosis after myocardial infarction (letter to the editor). *Lancet* 1:258-259, 1972

64. Kakkar VV: Peripheral venous scanning with ^{125}I-tagged fibrinogen (reply to letter to the editor). *Lancet* 1:910, 1972

65. Report of the Working Party on Anticoagulant Therapy in Coronary Thrombosis to the Medical Research Council: Assessment of short-term anticoagulant administration after cardiac infarction. *Br Med J* 1:335-342, 1969

66. Steele P, Ellis JH Jr, Weily HS, et al: Platelet survival time in patients with hypoxemia and pulmonary hypertension. *Circulation* 55:660-662, 1977

67. Taussig HB: *Congenital Malformations of the Heart.* Vol 2. Second edition. Cambridge, Harvard University Press, 1960, pp 47-48

68. Sharma GVRK, Burleson VA, Sasahara AA: Effect of thrombolytic therapy on pulmonary-capillary blood volume in patients with pulmonary embolism. *N Engl J Med* 303:842-845, 1980

69. Deykin D: Thrombogenesis. *N Engl J Med* 276:622-628, 1967

70. Fuster V, Chesebro JH: Current concepts of thrombogenesis: role of platelets. *Mayo Clin Proc* 56:102-112, 1981

71. Jordan RA, Miller RD, Edwards JE, et al: Thrombo-embolism in acute and in healed myocardial infarction. I. Intracardiac mural thrombosis. *Circulation* 6:1-6, 1952

72. Phares WS, Edwards JE, Burchell HB: Cardiac aneurysms: clinicopathologic studies. *Proc Staff Meet Mayo Clin* 28:264-271, 1953

73. Schlichter J, Hellerstein HK, Katz LN: Aneurysm of the heart: a correlative study of one hundred and two proved cases. *Medicine (Baltimore)* 33:43-86, 1954

74. Asinger RW, Mikell FL, Elsperger J, et al: Incidence of left ventricular thrombosis after acute transmural myocardial infarction: serial evaluation by two-dimensional echocardiography. *N Engl J Med* 305:297-302, 1981

75. Keating EC, Gross SA, Schlamowitz RA, et al: Mural thrombi in myocardial infarctions: prospective evaluation by two-dimensional echocardiography. *Am J Med* 74:989-995, 1983

76. Swan HJC, Magnusson PT, Buchbinder NA, et al: Aneurysm of the cardiac ventricle: its management by medical and surgical intervention. *West J Med* 129:26-40, 1978

77. Reeder GS, Lengyel M, Tajik AJ, et al: Mural thrombus in left ventricular aneurysm: incidence, role of angiography, and relation between anticoagulation and embolization. *Mayo Clin Proc* 56:77-81, 1981

78. Favaloro RG, Effler DB, Groves LK, et al: Ventricular aneurysm: clinical experience. *Ann Thorac Surg* 6:227-243, 1968

79. Cooley DA, Hallman GL: Surgical treatment of left ventricular aneurysm: experience with excision of postinfarction lesions in 80 patients. *Prog Cardiovasc Dis* 11:222-228, 1968

80. Kluge TH, Ullal SR, Hill JD, et al: Dyskinesia and aneurysm of the left ventricle: surgical experience in 36 patients. *J Cardiovasc Surg* 12:273-280, 1971

81. Loop FD, Effler DB, Navia JA, et al: Aneurysms of the left ventricle: survival and results of a ten-year surgical experience. *Ann Surg* 178:399-404, 1973

82. Simpson MT, Oberman A, Kouchoukos NT, et al: Effect of anticoagulation on the incidence of mural thrombi and systemic embolization in patients with left venticular aneurysms (abstract). *Am J Cardiol* 41:398, 1978

83. DeMaria AN, Bommer W, Neumann A, et al: Left ventricular thrombi identified by cross-sectional echocardiography. *Ann Intern Med* 90:14-18, 1979

84. Reeder GS, Tajik AJ, Seward JB: Left ventricular mural thrombus: two-dimensional echocardiographic diagnosis. *Mayo Clin Proc* 56:82-86, 1981

85. Asinger RW, Mikell FL, Sharma B, et al: Observations on detecting left ventricular thrombus with two-dimensional echocardiography: emphasis on avoidance of false-positive diagnoses. *Am J Cardiol* 47:145-156, 1981

86. Asinger R, Mikell F, Elsperger J, et al: Long-term prospective evaluation of left ventricular thrombus (LVT) with transmural infarction (MI): when should anticoagulation be discontinued? (Abstract) *Circulation* 64 Suppl 4:197, 1981

87. Spirito P, Bellotti P, Chiarella F, et al: Prognostic significance and natural history of left ventricular thrombi in patients with acute anterior myocardial infarction: a two-dimensional echocardiographic study. *Circulation* 72:774-780, 1985

88. Funke Küpper AJ, Freek WA, Verheugt WJ, et al: Long-term treatment with oral anticoagulants in patients with left ventricular thrombosis after myocardial infarction (abstract). *Circulation* 72 Suppl 3:III-458, 1985

89. Nordrehaug JE, Johannessen KA, von der Lippe G: Usefulness of high-dose anticoagulants in preventing left ventricular thrombus in acute myocardial infarction. *Am J Cardiol* 55:1491-1493, 1985

90. Arvan S, Boscha K: Prophylactic anticoagulation for left ventricular thrombi after acute myocardial infarction: a prospective randomized trial. *Am Heart J* 113:688-693, 1987

91. Davis MJ, Ireland MA: Effect of early anticoagulation on the frequency of left ventricular thrombi after anterior wall acute myocardial infarction. *Am J Cardiol* 57:1244-1247, 1986

92. Gueret P, Dubourg O, Ferrier A, et al: Effects of full-dose heparin anticoagulation on the development of left ventricular thrombosis in acute transmural myocardial infarction. *J Am Coll Cardiol* 8:419-426, 1986

93. Turpie AGG, Robinson JG, Doyle DJ, et al: Comparison of high-dose with low-dose subcutaneous heparin to prevent left ventricular mural thrombosis in patients with acute transmural anterior myocardial infarction. *N Engl J Med* 320:352-357, 1989

94. SCATI (Studio sulla Calciparina Nell'Angina e nella Trombosi Ventricolare Nell'Infarto) Group: Randomised controlled trial of subcutaneous calcium-heparin in acute myocardial infarction. *Lancet* 2:182-186, 1989

95. Vecchio C, Chiarella F, Lupi G, et al: Left ventricular thrombus in anterior acute myocardial infarction after thrombolysis. A GISSI-2 connected study. *Circulation* 84:512-519, 1991

96. Kupper AJ, Verheugt FW, Peels CH, et al: Effect of low dose acetylsalicylic acid on the frequency and hematologic activity of left ventricular thrombus in anterior wall acute myocardial infarction. *Am J Cardiol* 63:917-920, 1989

97. Lapeyre AC III, Steele PM, Kazmier FJ, et al: Systemic embolism in chronic left ventricular aneurysm: incidence and the role of anticoagulation. *J Am Coll Cardiol* 6:534-538, 1985

98. Fuster V, Gersh BJ, Giuliani ER, et al: The natural history of idiopathic dilated cardiomyopathy. *Am J Cardiol* 47:525-531, 1981

99. Drapkin A, Merskey C: Anticoagulant therapy after acute myocardial infarction: relation of therapeutic benefit to patient's age, sex, and severity of infarction. *JAMA* 222:541-548, 1972

100. Theroux P, Waters D, Qiu S, et al: Aspirin versus heparin to prevent myocardial infarction during the acute phase of unstable angina. *Circulation* 88:2045-2048, 1993

101. Hirsh J: Heparin. *N Engl J Med* 324:1565-1574, 1991

102. Weitz JI, Hudoba M, Massel D, et al: Clot-bound thrombin is protected from inhibition by heparin-antithrombin III but is susceptible to inactivation by antithrombin III-independent inhibitors. *J Clin Invest* 86:385-391, 1990

103. Yusuf S, Sleight P, Held P, et al: Routine medical management of acute myocardial infarction. Lessons from overviews of recent randomized controlled trials. *Circulation* 82 Suppl 2:117-134, 1990

104. Lau J, Antman EM, Jimenez-Silva J, et al: Cumulative meta-analysis of therapeutic trials for myocardial infarction. *N Engl J Med* 327:248-254, 1992

105. MacMahon S, Collins R, Knight C, et al: Reduction in major morbidity and mortality by heparin in acute myocardial infarction. *Circulation* 78 Suppl 2:98, 1988

106. The GUSTO Angiographic Investigators: The effects of tissue plasminogen activator, streptokinase, or both on coronary-artery patency, ventricular function, and survival after acute myocardial infarction. *N Engl J Med* 329:1615-1622, 1993

107. Merx W, Dörr R, Rentrop P, et al: Evaluation of the effectiveness of intracoronary streptokinase infusion in acute myocardial infarction:

postprocedure management and hospital course in 204 patients. *Am Heart J* 102:1181-1187, 1981

108. Ganz W: Intracoronary thrombolysis in evolving myocardial infarction (editorial). *Ann Intern Med* 95:500-502, 1981

109. Ellis SG, Topol EJ, George BS, et al: Recurrent ischemia without warning: analysis of risk factors for in-hospital ischemic events following successful thrombolysis with intravenous tissue plasminogen activator. *Circulation* 80:1159-1165, 1989

110. Kaplan K, Davison R, Parker M, et al: Role of heparin after intravenous thrombolytic therapy for acute myocardial infarction. *Am J Cardiol* 59:241-244, 1987

111. Arnout J, Simoons M, de Bono D, et al: Correlation between level of heparinization and patency of the infarct-related coronary artery after treatment of acute myocardial infarction with alteplase (rt-PA). *J Am Coll Cardiol* 20:513-519, 1992

112. Topol EJ, George BS, Kereiakes DJ, et al: A randomized controlled trial of intravenous tissue plasminogen activator and early intravenous heparin in acute myocardial infarction. *Circulation* 79:281-286, 1989

113. Bleich SD, Nichols T, Schumacher R, et al: The role of heparin following coronary thrombolysis with tissue plasminogen activator (t-PA) (abstract). *Circulation* 80 Suppl II:113, 1989

114. Hsia J, Hamilton WP, Kleiman N, et al: A comparison between heparin and low-dose aspirin as adjunctive therapy with tissue plasminogen activator for acute myocardial infarction. *N Engl J Med* 323:1433-1437, 1990

115. de Bono DP, Simoons ML, Tijssen J, et al: Effect of early intravenous heparin on coronary patency, infarct size, and bleeding complications after alteplase thrombolysis: results of a randomized double blind European Cooperative Study Group trial. *Br Heart J* 67:122-128, 1992

116. Thompson PL, Aylward PE, Federman J, et al: A randomized comparison of intravenous heparin with oral aspirin and dipyridamole 24 hours after recombinant tissue-type plasminogen activator for acute myocardial infarction. *Circulation* 83:1534-1542, 1991

117. Roux S, Christeller S, Ludin E: Effects of aspirin on coronary reocclusion and recurrent ischemia after thrombolysis: a meta-analysis. *J Am Coll Cardiol* 19:671-677, 1992

118. Cuccia C, Volterrani M, Volpini M, et al: Relationship between anticoagulation level ischemic events and angiographic characteristics of infarct-related artery following streptokinase in patients with acute myocardial infarction (abstract). *J Am Coll Cardiol* 19 Suppl A:92, 1992

119. Eisenberg PR, Sherman LA, Jaffe AS: Paradoxic elevation of fibrinopeptide A after streptokinase: evidence for continued thrombosis despite intense fibrinolysis. *J Am Coll Cardiol* 10:527-529, 1987

120. Rapold HJ, de Bono D, Arnold AE, et al: Plasma fibrinopeptide A levels in patients with acute myocardial infarction treated with alteplase. Correlation with concomitant heparin, coronary artery patency, and recurrent ischemia. *Circulation* 85:928-934, 1992

121. Eisenberg PR, Miletich JP: Induction of marked thrombin activity by pharmacologic concentrations of plasminogen activators in nonanticoagulated whole blood. *Thromb Res* 55:635-643, 1989

122. Cohen M, Adams PC, Parry G, et al: Combination antithrombotic therapy in unstable rest angina and non-Q-wave infarction in nonprior aspirin users. Primary end points analysis from the ATACS trial. *Circulation* 89:81-88, 1994

123. Patrignani P, Filabozzi P, Patrono C: Selective cumulative inhibition of platelet thromboxane production by low-dose aspirin in healthy subjects. *J Clin Invest* 69:1366-1372, 1982

124. Clarke RJ, Mayo G, Price P, et al: Suppression of thromboxane A2 but not of systemic prostacyclin by controlled-release aspirin. *N Engl J Med* 325:1137-1141, 1991

125. ISIS-2 (Second International Study of Infarct Survival) Collaborative Group: Randomised trial of intravenous streptokinase, oral aspirin, both, or neither among 17,187 cases of suspected acute myocardial infarction: ISIS-2. *Lancet* 2:349-360, 1988

126. Theroux P, Waters D, Lam J, et al: Reactivation of unstable angina after the discontinuation of heparin. *N Engl J Med* 327:141-145, 1992

127. Topol EJ, Califf RM, Vandormael M, et al: A randomized trial of late reperfusion therapy for acute myocardial infarction. *Circulation* 85:2090-2099, 1992

128. Meijer A, Verheugt FW, Werter CJ, et al: Aspirin versus coumadin in the prevention of reocclusion and recurrent ischemia after successful thrombolysis: a prospective placebo-controlled angiographic study. Results of the APRICOT Study. *Circulation* 87:1524-1530, 1993

129. Fitzgerald DJ, Catella F, Roy L, et al: Marked platelet activation in vivo after intravenous streptokinase in patients with acute myocardial infarction. *Circulation* 77:142-150, 1988

130. Gash AK, Spann JF, Sherry S, et al: Factors influencing reocclusion after coronary thrombolysis for acute myocardial infarction. *Am J Cardiol* 57:175-177, 1986

131. Report of the Sixty Plus Reinfarction Study Research Group: A double-blind trial to assess long-term oral anticoagulant therapy in elderly patients after myocardial infarction. *Lancet* 2:989-994, 1980

132. Smith P, Arnesen H, Holme I: The effect of warfarin on mortality and reinfarction after myocardial infarction. *N Engl J Med* 323:147-152, 1990

133. Anticoagulants in the Secondary Prevention of Events in Coronary Thrombosis (ASPECT) Research Group: Effect of long-term oral anticoagulant treatment on mortality and cardiovascular morbidity after myocardial infarction. *Lancet* 343:499-503, 1994

134. Modan B, Shani M, Schor S, et al: Reduction of hospital mortality from acute myocardial infarction by anticoagulant therapy. *N Engl J Med* 292:1359-1362, 1975

135. Tonascia J, Gordis L, Schmerler H: Retrospective evidence favoring use of anticoagulants for myocardial infarctions. *N Engl J Med* 292:1362-1366, 1975

136. Szklo M, Tonascia JA, Goldberg R, et al: Additional data favoring use of anticoagulant therapy in myocardial infarction: a population-based study. *JAMA* 242:1261-1264, 1979

137. International Anticoagulant Review Group: Collaborative analysis of long-term anticoagulant administration after acute myocardial infarction. *Lancet* 1:203-209, 1970

138. Gruppo Italiano per lo Studio della Sopravvivenza nell'Infarto Miocardico: GISSI-2: a factorial randomised trial of alteplase versus streptokinase and heparin versus no heparin among 12,490 patients with acute myocardial infarction. *Lancet* 336:65-71, 1990

139. The International Study Group: In-hospital mortality and clinical course of 20,891 patients with suspected acute myocardial infarction randomised between alteplase and streptokinase with or without heparin. *Lancet* 336:71-75, 1990

140. ISIS-3 (Third International Study of Infarct Survival) Collaborative Group: ISIS-3: a randomised comparison of streptokinase vs tissue plasminogen activator vs anistreplase and of aspirin plus heparin vs aspirin alone among 41,299 cases of suspected acute myocardial infarction. *Lancet* 339:753-770, 1992

141. Topol E, Califf R, Van de Werf F, et al: An international randomized trial comparing four thrombolytic strategies for acute myocardial infarction. *N Engl J Med* 329:673-682, 1993

142. Delanty N, Fitzgerald DJ: Subcutaneous heparin during coronary thrombolysis. Too little, too late (editorial). *Circulation* 86:1636-1638, 1992

143. Kroon C, Ten Hove WR, De Boer A, et al: Highly variable anticoagulant response after subcutaneous administration of high-dose (12,500 IU) heparin in patients with myocardial infarction and healthy volunteers. *Circulation* 86:1370-1375, 1992

144. Ohman EM, Califf RM, Topol EJ, et al: Consequences of reocclusion after successful reperfusion therapy in acute myocardial infarction. *Circulation* 82:781-791, 1990

145. Roos V, van Joost HE: The cause of bleeding during anticoagulant treatment. *Acta Med Scand* 178:129-131, 1965

146. The Global Use of Strategies to Open Occluded Coronary Arteries (GUSTO) IIa Investigators: Randomized trial of intravenous heparin versus recombinant hirudin for acute coronary syndromes. *Circulation* 90:1631-1637, 1994

147. Antman EM: Hirudin in acute myocardial infarction. Safety report from the Thrombolysis and Thrombin Inhibition in Myocardial Infarction (TIMI) 9A Trial. *Circulation* 90:1624-1630, 1994

148. Atrial Fibrillation Investigators: Risk factors for stroke and efficacy of antithrombotic therapy in atrial fibrillation. Analysis of pooled data from five randomized controlled trials. *Arch Intern Med* 154:1449-1457, 1994

149. Stroke Prevention in Atrial Fibrillation Investigators: Warfarin versus aspirin for prevention of thromboembolism in atrial fibrillation: Stroke Prevention in Atrial Fibrillation II Study. *Lancet* 343:687-691, 1994

150. Chesebro JH, Fuster V, Elveback LR, et al: Trial of combined

warfarin plus dipyridamole or aspirin therapy in prosthetic heart valve replacement: danger of aspirin compared with dipyridamole. *Am J Cardiol* 51:1537-1541, 1983

151. Biggs R, Denson KWE, Akman N, et al: Antithrombin III, antifactor Xa and heparin. *Br J Haematol* 19:283-305, 1970

152. Wessler S: Prevention of venous thromboembolism by low-dose heparin. *Mod Concepts Cardiovasc Dis* 45:105-109, 1976

153. Bonnar J, Denson KWE, Biggs R: Subcutaneous heparin and prevention of thrombosis (letter to the editor). *Lancet* 2:539-540, 1972

154. Gallus AS, Hirsh J, Tuttle RJ, et al: Small subcutaneous doses of heparin in prevention of venous thrombosis. *N Engl J Med* 288:545-551, 1973

155. Kakkar VV, Field ES, Nicolaides AN, et al: Low doses of heparin in prevention of deep-vein thrombosis. *Lancet* 2:669-671, 1971

156. Sherry S: Low-dose heparin for the prophylaxis of pulmonary embolism (editorial). *Am Rev Respir Dis* 114:661-666, 1976

157. Warlow C, Beattie AG, Terry G, et al: A double-blind trial of low doses of subcutaneous heparin in the prevention of deep-vein thrombosis after myocardial infarction. *Lancet* 2:934-936, 1973

158. Emerson PA, Marks P: Preventing thromboembolism after myocardial infarction: effect of low-dose heparin or smoking. *Br Med J* 1:18-20, 1977

159. Rentrop KP, Feit F, Blanke H, et al: Effects of intracoronary streptokinase and intracoronary nitroglycerin infusion on coronary angiography patterns and mortality in patients with acute myocardial infarction. *N Engl J Med* 311:1457-1463, 1984

160. Nakagawa S, Hanada Y, Koiwaya Y, et al: Angiographic features in the infarct-related artery after intracoronary urokinase followed by prolonged anticoagulation: role of ruptured atheromatous plaque and adherent thrombus in acute myocardial infarction in vivo. *Circulation* 78:1335-1344, 1988

161. Kontny F, Dale J, Abildgaard U, et al: Adverse effect of warfarin in acute myocardial infarction: increased left ventricular thrombus formation in patients not treated with high-dose heparin. *Eur Heart J* 14:1040-1043, 1993

162. Riley CP, Russell RO Jr, Rackley CE: Left ventricular gallop sound and acute myocardial infarction. *Am Heart J* 86:598-602, 1973

163. Kostuk W, Barr JW, Simon AL, et al: Correlations between the chest film and hemodynamics in acute myocardial infarction. *Circulation* 48:624-632, 1973

164. Rotman M, Chen JTT, Seningen RP, et al: Pulmonary arterial diastolic pressure in acute myocardial infarction. *Am J Cardiol* 33:357-362, 1974

165. Forrester JS, Diamond G, Chatterjee K, et al: Medical therapy of acute myocardial infarction by application of hemodynamic subsets (first of two parts). *N Engl J Med* 295:1356-1362, 1976

166. Forrester JS, Diamond GA, Swan HJC: Correlative classification of clinical and hemodynamic function after acute myocardial infarction. *Am J Cardiol* 39:137-145, 1977

167. Shell WE, DeWood MA, Peter T, et al: Comparison of clinical signs and hemodynamic state in the early hours of transmural myocardial infarction. *Am Heart J* 104:521-528, 1982

168. Swan HJC, Ganz W, Forrester J, et al: Catheterization of the heart in man with use of a flow-directed balloon-tipped catheter. *N Engl J Med* 283:447-451, 1970

169. Rutherford BD, McCann WD, O'Donovan TPB: The value of monitoring pulmonary artery pressure for early detection of left ventricular failure following myocardial infarction. *Circulation* 43:655-666, 1971

170. Scheinman M, Evans GT, Weiss A, et al: Relationship between pulmonary artery end-diastolic pressure and left ventricular filling pressure in patients in shock. *Circulation* 47:317-324, 1973

171. Rackley CE, Russell RO Jr: *Coronary Care: Invasive Techniques for Hemodynamic Measurements.* Dallas, American Heart Association, 1973, pp 1-36

172. Matthay MA, Chatterjee K: Bedside catheterization of the pulmonary artery: risks compared with benefits. *Ann Intern Med* 109:826-834, 1988

173. Boyd KD, Thomas SJ, Gold J, et al: A prospective study of complications of pulmonary artery catheterizations in 500 consecutive patients. *Chest* 84:245-249, 1983

174. Shasby DM, Dauber IM, Pfister S, et al: Swan-Ganz catheter location and left atrial pressure determine the accuracy of the wedge pressure when positive end-expiratory pressure is used. *Chest* 80:666-670, 1981

175. Michel L, Marsh HM, McMichan JC, et al: Infection of pulmonary artery catheters in critically ill patients. *JAMA* 245:1032-1036, 1981

176. Applefeld JJ, Caruthers TE, Reno DJ, et al: Assessment of the sterility of long-term cardiac catheterization using the thermodilution Swan-Ganz catheter. *Chest* 74:377-380, 1978

177. Austin JL, Preis LK, Crampton RS, et al: Analysis of pacemaker malfunction and complications of temporary pacing in the coronary care unit. *Am J Cardiol* 49:301-306, 1982

178. Rowley KM, Clubb KS, Smith GJW, et al: Right-sided infective endocarditis as a consequence of flow-directed pulmonary-artery catheterization. *N Engl J Med* 311:1152-1156, 1984

179. Carlson TA, Goldenberg IF, Murray PD, et al: Catheter-induced delayed recurrent pulmonary artery hemorrhage. Intervention with therapeutic embolism of the pulmonary artery. *JAMA* 261:1943-1945, 1989

180. Sprung CL, Jacobs LJ, Caralis PV, et al: Ventricular arrhythmias during Swan-Ganz catheterization in the critically ill. *Chest* 79:413-415, 1981

181. Abernathy WS: Complete heart block caused by the Swan-Ganz catheter. *Chest* 65:349, 1974

182. Foote GA, Schabel SI, Hodges M: Pulmonary complications of the flow-directed balloon-tipped catheter. *N Engl J Med* 290:927-931, 1974

183. Lipp H, O'Donoghue K, Resnekov L: Intracardiac knotting of a flow-directed balloon catheter (letter to the editor). *N Engl J Med* 284:220, 1971

184. Cuasay RS, Lemole GM: Rupture of pulmonary artery by Swan-Ganz catheter: a cause of postoperative bleeding after open-heart operation. *Ann Thorac Surg* 32:415-419, 1981

185. Smith WR, Glauser FL, Jemison P: Ruptured chordae of the tricuspid valve: the consequence of flow-directed Swan-Ganz catheterization. *Chest* 70:790-792, 1976

186. Meister SG, Furr CM, Engel TR, et al: Knotting of a flow-directed catheter about a cardiac structure. *Cathet Cardiovasc Diagn* 3:171-175, 1977

187. Swan HJC, Ganz W: Guidelines for use of balloon-tipped catheter (letter to the editor). *Am J Cardiol* 34:119-120, 1974

188. Ganz W, Swan HJC: Measurement of blood flow by thermodilution. *Am J Cardiol* 29:241-246, 1972

189. Russell RO Jr, Rackley CE, Pombo J, et al: Effects of increasing left ventricular filling pressure in patients with acute myocardial infarction. *J Clin Invest* 49:1539-1550, 1970

190. Crexells C, Chatterjee K, Forrester JS, et al: Optimal level of filling pressure in the left side of the heart in acute myocardial infarction. *N Engl J Med* 289:1263-1266, 1973

191. Gorlin R: Practical cardiac hemodynamics. *N Engl J Med* 296:203-205, 1977

192. Swan HJC, Forrester JS, Diamond G, et al: Hemodynamic spectrum of myocardial infarction and cardiogenic shock: a conceptual model. *Circulation* 45:1097-1110, 1972

193. Forrester JS, Diamond G, Parmley WW, et al: Early increase in left ventricular compliance after myocardial infarction. *J Clin Invest* 51:598-603, 1972

194. Krauss XH, Verdouw PD, Hugenholtz PG, et al: On-line monitoring of mixed venous oxygen saturation after cardiothoracic surgery. *Thorax* 30:636-643, 1975

195. Rackley CE, Russell RO Jr, Mantle JA, et al: Modern approach to the patient with acute myocardial infarction. *Curr Probl Cardiol* 1:1-47, 1977

196. Forrester JS, Diamond G, Chatterjee K, et al: Medical therapy of acute myocardial infarction by application of hemodynamic subsets (second of two parts). *N Engl J Med* 295:1404-1413, 1976

197. Ratshin R, Rackley CE, Russell RO Jr: Hemodynamic evaluation of left ventricular function in shock complicating myocardial infarction. *Circulation* 45:127-139, 1972

198. Thirteenth Bethesda Conference: Emergency cardiac care. *Am J Cardiol* 50:365-420, 1982

199. Herman MV, Heinle RA, Klein MD, et al: Localized disorders in myocardial contraction: asynergy and its role in congestive heart failure. *N Engl J Med* 277:222-232, 1967

200. Braunwald E: The pathogenesis and treatment of shock in myocardial infarction. *Johns Hopkins Med J* 121:421-429, 1967

201. Harnarayan C, Bennett MA, Pentecost BL, et al: Quantitative study of infarcted myocardium in cardiogenic shock. *Br Heart J* 32:728-732, 1970

202. Page DL, Caulfield JB, Kastor JA, et al: Myocardial changes associated with cardiogenic shock. *N Engl J Med* 285:133-137, 1971

203. Gibbons RJ, Verani MS, Behrenbeck T, et al: Feasibility of tomographic ^{99m}Tc-hexakis-2-methoxy-2-methylpropyl-isonitrile imaging for the assessment of myocardial area at risk and the effect of treatment in acute myocardial infarction. *Circulation* 80:1277-1286, 1989

204. Vlietstra RE, Assad-Morell JL, Frye RL, et al: Survival predictors in coronary artery disease: medical and surgical comparisons. *Mayo Clin Proc* 52:85-90, 1977

205. Vlietstra RE, Frye RL, Elveback LR: Predicting survival in CAD (letter to the editor). *Circulation* 60:464, 1979

206. Schulze RA Jr, Strauss HW, Pitt B: Sudden death in the year following myocardial infarction: relation to ventricular premature contractions in the late hospital phase and left ventricular ejection fraction. *Am J Med* 62:192-199, 1977

207. Ruberman W, Weinblatt E, Goldberg JD, et al: Ventricular premature beats and mortality after myocardial infarction. *N Engl J Med* 297:750-757, 1977

208. Burggraf GW, Parker JO: Prognosis in coronary artery disease: angiographic, hemodynamic, and clinical factors. *Circulation* 51:146-156, 1975

209. Bruschke AVG, Proudfit WL, Sones FM Jr: Progress study of 590 consecutive nonsurgical cases of coronary disease followed 5-9 years. II. Ventriculographic and other correlations. *Circulation* 47:1154-1163, 1973

210. Moss AJ, Davis HT, DeCamilla J, et al: Ventricular ectopic beats and their relation to sudden and nonsudden cardiac death after myocardial infarction. *Circulation* 60:998-1003, 1979

211. The Multicenter Postinfarction Research Group: Risk stratification and survival after myocardial infarction. *N Engl J Med* 309:331-336, 1983

212. Mukharji J, Rude RE, Poole K, et al: Late sudden death following acute myocardial infarction: importance of combined presence of repetitive ventricular ectopy and left ventricular dysfunction (abstract). *Clin Res* 30:208A, 1982

213. Bigger JT Jr, Fleiss JL, Kleiger R, et al: The relationships among ventricular arrhythmias, left ventricular dysfunction, and mortality in the 2 years after myocardial infarction. *Circulation* 69:250-258, 1984

214. Corbett JR, Dehmer GJ, Lewis SE, et al: The prognostic value of submaximal exercise testing with radionuclide ventriculography before hospital discharge in patients with recent myocardial infarction. *Circulation* 64:535-544, 1981

215. Dewhurst NG, Muir AL: Comparative prognostic value of radionuclide ventriculography at rest and during exercise in 100 patients after first myocardial infarction. *Br Heart J* 49:111-121, 1983

216. Reimer KA, Lowe JE, Rasmussen MM, et al: The wavefront phenomenon of ischemic cell death. 1. Myocardial infarct size vs duration of coronary occlusion in dogs. *Circulation* 56:786-794, 1977

217. Fishbein MC, Hare CA, Gissen SA, et al: Identification and quantification of histochemical border zones during the evolution of myocardial infarction in the rat. *Cardiovasc Res* 14:41-49, 1980

218. Cortina A, Prieto-Granda J, Torre F, et al: Angiographic and functional correlation in patients with acute myocardial infarction (abstract). *Am J Cardiol* 49:947, 1982

219. Blumgart HL, Schlesinger MJ, Davis D: Studies on the relation of the clinical manifestations of angina pectoris, coronary thrombosis, and myocardial infarction to the pathologic findings: with particular reference to the significance of the collateral circulation. *Am Heart J* 19:1-91, 1940

220. Levin DC: Pathways and functional significance of the coronary collateral circulation. *Circulation* 50:831-837, 1974

221. Hamby RJ, Aintablian A, Schwartz A: Reappraisal of the functional significance of the coronary collateral circulation. *Am J Cardiol* 38:305-309, 1976

222. Rentrop P, Blanke H, Karsch KR, et al: Changes in left ventricular function after intracoronary streptokinase infusion in clinically evolving myocardial infarction. *Am Heart J* 102:1188-1193, 1981

223. Schmidt WG, Sheehan FH, von Essen R, et al: Evolution of left ventricular function after intracoronary thrombolysis for acute myocardial infarction. *Am J Cardiol* 63:497-502, 1989

224. Maroko PR, Kjekshus JK, Sobel BE, et al: Factors influencing infarct size following experimental coronary artery occlusions. *Circulation* 43:67-82, 1971

225. Rude RE, Muller JE, Braunwald E: Efforts to limit the size of myocardial infarcts. *Ann Intern Med* 95:736-761, 1981

226. Leinbach RC, Gold HK, Harper RW, et al: Early intraaortic balloon pumping for anterior myocardial infarction without shock. *Circulation* 58:204-210, 1978

227. Mueller HS, Ayres SM, Religa A, et al: Propranolol in the treatment of acute myocardial infarction: effect on myocardial oxygenation and hemodynamics. *Circulation* 49:1078-1087, 1974

228. Mueller HS, Ayres SM: The role of propranolol in the treatment of acute myocardial infarction. *Prog Cardiovasc Dis* 19:405-412, 1977

229. Ahumada GG, Karlsberg RP, Jaffe AS, et al: Reduction of early ventricular arrhythmia by acebutolol in patients with acute myocardial infarction. *Br Heart J* 41:654-659, 1979

230. Opie LH: Metabolism of free fatty acids, glucose, and catecholamines in acute myocardial infarction: relation to myocardial ischemia and infarct size. *Am J Cardiol* 36:938-953, 1975

231. Maroko PR, Libby P, Covell JW, et al: Precordial S-T segment elevation mapping: an atraumatic method for assessing alterations in the extent of myocardial ischemic injury; the effects of pharmacologic and hemodynamic interventions. *Am J Cardiol* 29:223-230, 1972

232. Pelides LJ, Reid DS, Thomas M, et al: Inhibition by β-blockade of the ST segment elevation after acute myocardial infarction in man. *Cardiovasc Res* 6:295-301, 1972

233. Waagstein F, Hjalmarson ÅC: Double-blind study of the effect of cardioselective beta-blockade on chest pain in acute myocardial infarction. *Acta Med Scand [Suppl]* 587:201-207, 1976

234. Gold HK, Leinbach RC, Maroko PR: Propranolol-induced reduction of signs of ischemic injury during acute myocardial infarction. *Am J Cardiol* 38:689-695, 1976

235. Heikkilä J, Nieminen MS: Failure of methylprednisolone to protect acutely ischemic myocardium: a contrast with subsequent beta-adrenergic blockade in man. *Chest* 73:577-582, 1978

236. Herlitz J, Elmfeldt D, Hjalmarson Å, et al: Effect of metoprolol on indirect signs of the size and severity of acute myocardial infarction. *Am J Cardiol* 51:1282-1288, 1983

237. Genth K, Hofmann M, Hofmann M, et al: The effect of β-adrenergic blockade on infarct size following experimental coronary occlusion. *Basic Res Cardiol* 76:144-151, 1981

238. The European Infarction Study Group: European Infarction Study (E.I.S.): a secondary beta-blocker prevention trial after myocardial infarction (abstract). *Circulation* 68 Suppl 3:294, 1983

239. Barber JM, Boyle DM, Chaturvedi NC, et al: Practolol in acute myocardial infarction. *Acta Med Scand [Suppl]* 587:213-216, 1976

240. Sobel BE, Bresnahan GF, Shell WE, et al: Estimation of infarct size in man and its relation to prognosis. *Circulation* 46:640-648, 1972

241. Cox JR Jr, Roberts R, Ambos HD, et al: Relations between enzymatically estimated myocardial infarct size and early ventricular dysrhythmia. *Circulation* 53 Suppl 1:150-155, 1976

242. Geltman EM, Ehsani AA, Campbell MK, et al: The influence of location and extent of myocardial infarction on long-term ventricular dysrhythmia and mortality. *Circulation* 60:805-814, 1979

243. Rogers WJ, McDaniel HG, Smith LR, et al: Correlation of angiographic estimates of myocardial infarct size and accumulated release of creatine kinase MB isoenzyme in man. *Circulation* 56:199-205, 1977

244. Morrison J, Coromilas J, Munsey D, et al: Correlation of radionuclide estimates of myocardial infarction size and release of creatine kinase-MB in man. *Circulation* 62:277-287, 1980

245. Peter T, Norris RM, Clarke ED, et al: Reduction of enzyme levels by propranolol after acute myocardial infarction. *Circulation* 57:1091-1095, 1978

246. Norris RM, Clarke ED, Sammel NL, et al: Protective effect of propranolol in threatened myocardial infarction. *Lancet* 2:907-909, 1978

247. Fox KM, Chopra MP, Portal RW, et al: Long-term beta blockade: possible protection from myocardial infarction. *Br Med J* 1:117-119, 1975

248. Yusuf S, Ramsdale D, Rossi P, et al: Reduction in infarct size, morbidity, and short-term mortality by early intravenous beta-blockade (abstract). *J Am Coll Cardiol* 1:676, 1983

249. Jürgensen HJ, Frederiksen J, Hansen DA, et al: Limitation of myocardial infarct size in patients less than 66 years treated with alprenolol. *Br Heart J* 45:583-588, 1981

250. The Miami Trial Research Group: Mortality. *Am J Cardiol* 56:15G-22G, 1985

251. The Miami Trial Research Group: Development of myocardial infarction. *Am J Cardiol* 56:23G-26G, 1985

252. The Miami Trial Research Group: Enzymatic estimation of infarct size. *Am J Cardiol* 56:27G-29G, 1985

253. Sleight P, For the ISIS-1 Trial Group: Beta-blockade early in acute myocardial infarction. *Am J Cardiol* 60:6A-10A, 1987

254. Manning AS, Keogh JM, Hearse DJ, et al: Beta-blockade and ischaemic injury: effects of partial agonist activity. *Cardiovasc Res* 14:619-623, 1980

255. Nayler WG: Protecting the ischaemic myocardium. In *Proceedings of a Symposium: Comparative Beta-Blockade and the Ischaemic Myocardium.* Edited by DG Julian. New York, Biomedical Information, 1981, pp 1-14

256. Heber ME, Rosenthal E, Thomas N, et al: Effect of labetalol on indices of myocardial necrosis in patients with suspected acute infarction. *Eur Heart J* 8:11-18, 1987

257. Held P, Yusuf S: Early intravenous beta-blockade in acute myocardial infarction. *Cardiology* 76:132-143, 1989

258. Kirshenbaum JM: Nonthrombolytic intervention in acute myocardial infarction. *Am J Cardiol* 64:25B-28B, 1989

259. Roberts R, Rogers WJ, Mueller HS, et al: Immediate versus deferred beta-blockade following thrombolytic therapy in patients with acute myocardial infarction: results of the Thrombolysis in Myocardial Infarction (TIMI) II-B study. *Circulation* 83:422-437, 1991

260. The TIMI Study Group: Comparison of invasive and conservative strategies after treatment with intravenous tissue plasminogen activator in acute myocardial infarction: results of the Thrombolysis in Myocardial Infarction (TIMI) Phase II Trial. *N Engl J Med* 320:618-627, 1989

261. Braunwald E, Muller JE, Kloner RA, et al: Role of beta-adrenergic blockade in the therapy of patients with myocardial infarction. *Am J Med* 74:113-123, 1983

262. Schaper W, Schaper J: Der experimentelle Infarkt. *Verh Dtsch Ges Herz Kreislaufforsch* 45:1-6, 1979

263. Lange R, Kloner RA, Braunwald E: First ultra-short-acting beta-adrenergic blocking agent: its effect on size and segmental wall dynamics of reperfused myocardial infarct in dogs. *Am J Cardiol* 51:1759-1767, 1983

264. Hammerman H, Kloner RA, Briggs LL, et al: Enhancement of reperfusion salvage by early beta-adrenergic blockade (abstract). *Circulation* 68 Suppl 3:187, 1983

265. Danish Multicenter Study Group on Verapamil in Myocardial Infarction: Verapamil in acute myocardial infarction. *Am J Cardiol* 54:24E-28E, 1984

266. Crea F, Deanfield J, Crean P, et al: Effects of verapamil in preventing early postinfarction angina and reinfarction. *Am J Cardiol* 55:900-904, 1985

267. Muller JE, Morrison J, Stone PH, et al: Nifedipine therapy for patients with threatened and acute myocardial infarction: a randomized, double-blind, placebo-controlled comparison. *Circulation* 69:740-747, 1984

268. Gottlieb SO, Weiss JL, Flaherty JT, et al: Effect of nifedipine on clinical course and left ventricular function in low risk acute myocardial infarction: a double-blind randomized trial (abstract). *Circulation* 70 Suppl 2:257, 1984

269. Branagan JP, Walsh K, Kelly P, et al: Effect of early treatment with nifedipine in suspected acute myocardial infarction. *Eur Heart J* 7:859-865, 1986

270. Walker L, MacKenzie G, Adgey J: Effect of nifedipine in the early phase of acute myocardial infarction on enzymatically estimated infarct size and arrhythmias (abstract). *Br Heart J* 57:83-84, 1987

271. Neufeld HN: Calcium antagonists in secondary prevention after acute myocardial infarction: the Secondary Prevention Reinfarction Nifedipine Trial (SPRINT). *Eur Heart J* 7 Suppl B:51-52, 1986

272. Moss AJ: Secondary prevention with calcium channel-blocking drugs in patients after myocardial infarction: a critical review. *Circulation* 75 Suppl 5:148-153, 1987

273. Sirnes PA, Overskeid K, Pedersen TR, et al: Evolution of infarct size during the early use of nifedipine in patients with acute myocardial infarction: the Norwegian Nifedipine Multicenter Trial. *Circulation* 70:638-644, 1984

274. Wilcox RG, Hampton JR, Banks DC, et al: Trial of early nifedipine in acute myocardial infarction: the Trent study. *BMJ* 293:1204-1208, 1986

275. Report of the Holland Interuniversity Nifedipine/Metoprolol Trial (HINT) Research Group: Early treatment of unstable angina in the coronary care unit: a randomised, double-blind, placebo controlled comparison of recurrent ischaemia in patients treated with nifedipine or metoprolol or both. *Br Heart J* 56:400-413, 1986

276. Erbel R, Pop T, Meinertz T, et al: Combination of calcium channel blocker and thrombolytic therapy in acute myocardial infarction. *Am Heart J* 115:529-538, 1988

277. Skolnick AE, Frishman WH: Calcium channel blockers in myocardial infarction. *Arch Intern Med* 149:1669-1677, 1989

278. The Multicenter Diltiazem Postinfarction Trial Research Group: The effect of diltiazem on mortality and reinfarction after myocardial infarction. *N Engl J Med* 319:385-392, 1988

279. Zannad F, Amor M, Karcher G, et al: Effect of diltiazem on myocardial infarct size estimated by enzyme release, serial thallium-201 single-photon emission computed tomography and radionuclide angiography. *Am J Cardiol* 61:1172-1177, 1988

280. Gibson RS, Boden WE, Theroux P, et al: Diltiazem and reinfarction in patients with non-Q-wave myocardial infarction: results of a double-blind, randomized, multicenter trial. *N Engl J Med* 315:423-429, 1986

281. Boden WE, Krone RJ, Kleiger RE, et al: Diltiazem reduces long-term cardiac event rate after non-Q wave infarction: Multicenter Diltiazem Post-Infarction Trial (MDPIT) (abstract). *Circulation* 78 Suppl 2:96, 1988

282. Smith ER, Redwood DR, McCarron WE, et al: Coronary artery occlusion in the conscious dog: effects of alterations in arterial pressure produced by nitroglycerin, hemorrhage, and alpha-adrenergic agonists on the degree of myocardial ischemia. *Circulation* 47:51-57, 1973

283. Gerry JL Jr, Schaff HV, Kallman CH, et al: Effects of nitroglycerin on regional myocardial ischemia induced by atrial pacing in dogs. *Circ Res* 48:569-576, 1981

284. Jugdutt BI, Becker LC, Hutchins GM, et al: Effect of intravenous nitroglycerin on collateral blood flow and infarct size in the conscious dog. *Circulation* 63:17-28, 1981

285. Fukuyama T, Schechtman KB, Roberts R: The effects of intravenous nitroglycerin on hemodynamics, coronary blood flow, and morphologically and enzymatically estimated infarct size in conscious dogs. *Circulation* 62:1227-1238, 1980

286. Boerer JS, Redwood DR, Levitt B, et al: Reduction in myocardial ischemia with nitroglycerin or nitroglycerin plus phenylephrine administered during acute myocardial infarction. *N Engl J Med* 293:1008-1012, 1975

287. Come PC, Flaherty JT, Baird MG, et al: Reversal by phenylephrine of the beneficial effects of intravenous nitroglycerin in patients with acute myocardial infarction. *N Engl J Med* 293:1003-1007, 1975

288. Flaherty JT, Come PC, Baird MG, et al: Effects of intravenous nitroglycerin on left ventricular function and ST segment changes in acute myocardial infarction. *Br Heart J* 38:612-621, 1976

289. Awan NA, Amsterdam EA, Vera Z, et al: Reduction of ischemic injury by sublingual nitroglycerin in patients with acute myocardial infarction. *Circulation* 54:761-765, 1976

290. Flaherty JT, Reid PR, Kelly DT, et al: Intravenous nitroglycerin in acute myocardial infarction. *Circulation* 51:132-139, 1975

291. Bussmann W-D, Passek D, Seidel W, et al: Reduction of CK and CK-MB indexes of infarct size by intravenous nitroglycerin. *Circulation* 63:615-622, 1981

292. Jaffe AS, Geltman EM, Tiefenbrunn AJ, et al: Reduction of infarct size in patients with inferior infarction with intravenous glyceryl trinitrate: a randomized study. *Br Heart J* 49:452-460, 1983

293. Flaherty JT, Becker LC, Bulkley BH, et al: A randomized prospective trial of intravenous nitroglycerin in patients with acute myocardial infarction. *Circulation* 68:576-588, 1983

294. Jugdutt BI, Sussex BA, Warnica JW, et al: Persistent reduction in left ventricular asynergy in patients with acute myocardial infarction by intravenous infusion of nitroglycerin. *Circulation* 68:1264-1273, 1983

295. Bussmann WD, Schöfer H, Kurita A, et al: Nitroglycerin in acute myocardial infarction. X. Effect of small and large doses of nitroglycerin on ST segment deviation: experimental and clinical results. *Clin Cardiol* 2:106-112, 1979

296. Come PC, Pitt B: Nitroglycerin-induced severe hypotension and bradycardia in patients with acute myocardial infarction. *Circulation* 54:624-628, 1976

297. Chiche P, Baligadoo SJ, Derrida JP: A randomized trial of prolonged nitroglycerin infusion in acute myocardial infarction (abstract). *Circulation* 60 Suppl 2:165, 1979

298. Lam JYT, Chesebro JH, Fuster V: Platelets, vasoconstriction, and nitroglycerin during arterial wall injury: a new antithrombotic role for an old drug. *Circulation* 78:712-716, 1988
299. Fischell TA, Derby G, Tse TM, et al: Coronary artery vasoconstriction routinely occurs after percutaneous transluminal coronary angioplasty: a quantitative arteriographic analysis. *Circulation* 78:1323-1334, 1988
300. Chesebro JH, Badimon L, Fuster V: New approaches to treatment of myocardial infarction. *Am J Cardiol* 65:12C-19C, 1990
301. Chiariello M, Gold HK, Leinbach RC, et al: Comparison between the effects of nitroprusside and nitroglycerin on ischemic injury during acute myocardial infarction. *Circulation* 54:766-773, 1976
302. Mann T, Cohn PF, Holman BL, et al: Effect of nitroprusside on regional myocardial blood flow in coronary disease: results in 25 patients and comparison with nitroglycerin. *Circulation* 57:732-738, 1978
303. Cohn JN, Franciosa JA, Francis GS, et al: Effect of short-term infusion of sodium nitroprusside on mortality rate in acute myocardial infarction complicated by left ventricular failure: results of a Veterans Administration Cooperative Study. *N Engl J Med* 306:1129-1135, 1982
304. Durrer JD, Lie KI, van Capelle FJL, et al: Effect of sodium nitroprusside on mortality in acute myocardial infarction. *N Engl J Med* 306:1121-1128, 1982
305. Teo KK, Yusuf S, Collins R, et al: Effects of intravenous magnesium in suspected acute myocardial infarction: overview of randomised trials. *BMJ* 303:1499-1503, 1991
306. Woods KL, Fletcher S, Roffe C, et al: Intravenous magnesium sulphate in suspected acute myocardial infarction: results of the second Leicester Intravenous Magnesium Intervention Trial (LIMIT-2). *Lancet* 339:1553-1558, 1992
307. Marder VJ: The use of thrombolytic agents: choice of patient, drug administration, laboratory monitoring. *Ann Intern Med* 90:802-808, 1979
308. Collen D: On the regulation and control of fibrinolysis: Edward Kowalski Memorial Lecture. *Thromb Haemost* 43:77-89, 1980
309. Collen D: Human tissue-type plasminogen activator: from the laboratory to the bedside. *Circulation* 72:18-20, 1985
310. Collen D, Stump D, Van de Werf F, et al: Coronary thrombolysis in dogs with intravenously administered human pro-urokinase. *Circulation* 72:384-388, 1985
311. Been M, de Bono DP, Muir AL, et al: Coronary thrombolysis with intravenous anisoylated plasminogen-streptokinase complex BRL 26921. *Br Heart J* 53:253-259, 1985
312. Zoldhelyi P, Fuster V, Chesebro JH: Antithrombins as conjunctive therapy in arterial thrombolysis. *Coron Artery Dis* 3:1003-1009, 1992
313. Alexopoulos D, Raine AEG, Cobbe SM: Serum sickness complicating intravenous streptokinase therapy in acute myocardial infarction. *Eur Heart J* 5:1010-1012, 1984
314. Johnson AJ, McCarty WR: The lysis of artificially induced intravascular clots in man by intravenous infusions of streptokinase. *J Clin Invest* 38:1627-1643, 1959
315. Verstraete M, Vermylen J, Amery A, et al: Thrombolytic therapy with streptokinase using a standard dosage scheme. *Br Med J* 1:454-456, 1966
316. Hirsh J, O'Sullivan EF, Martin M: Evaluation of a standard dosage schedule with streptokinase. *Blood* 35:341-349, 1970
317. Vaughn DE, Van Houtte E, Declerck PJ, et al: Streptokinase-induced platelet aggregation: prevalence and mechanism. *Circulation* 84:84-91, 1991
318. Bloom AL: The release of thrombin from fibrin by fibrinolysin. *Br J Haematol* 8:129-133, 1962
319. Chesebro JH, Knatterud G, Roberts R, et al: Thrombolysis in Acute Myocardial Infarction (TIMI) Trial, Phase I: a comparison between intravenous tissue plasminogen activator and intravenous streptokinase: clinical findings through hospital discharge. *Circulation* 76:142-154, 1987
320. Fuster V, Badimon L, Badimon JJ, et al: The pathogenesis of coronary artery disease and the acute coronary syndromes. *N Engl J Med* 326:242-250, 1992
321. Fuster V: Lewis A. Conner Memorial Lecture. Mechanisms leading to myocardial infarction: insights from studies of vascular biology. *Circulation* 90:2126-2146, 1994
322. Fernandez-Ortiz A, Badimon JJ, Falk E, et al: Characterization of the relative thrombogenicity of atherosclerotic plaque components: implications for consequences of plaque rupture. *J Am Coll Cardiol* 23:1562-1569, 1994
323. Meyer BJ, Badimon JJ, Mailhac A, et al: Inhibition of growth of thrombus on fresh mural thrombus. Targeting optimal therapy. *Circulation* 90:2432-2438, 1994
324. Wysokinski WE, McBane RD, Hassinger NL, et al: "Dethrombosis": effect of thrombin inhibition on thrombus propagation and maintenance (abstract). *Thromb Haemost* 69:692, 1993
325. DeWood MA, Spores J, Notske R, et al: Prevalence of total coronary occlusion during the early hours of transmural myocardial infarction. *N Engl J Med* 303:897-902, 1980
326. Rentrop KP: Thrombolytic therapy in patients with acute myocardial infarction. *Circulation* 71:627-631, 1985
327. Weaver WD, Litwin PE, Martin JS, et al: Effect of age on use of thrombolytic therapy and mortality in acute myocardial infarction. *J Am Coll Cardiol* 18:657-662, 1991
328. Muller DW, Topol EJ: Selection of patients with acute myocardial infarction for thrombolytic therapy. *Ann Intern Med* 113:949-960, 1990
329. Krumholz HM, Pasternak RC, Weinstein MC, et al: Cost effectiveness of thrombolytic therapy with streptokinase in elderly patients with suspected acute myocardial infarction. *N Engl J Med* 327:7-13, 1992
330. Gore JM, Sloan M, Price TR, et al: Intracerebral hemorrhage, cerebral infarction, and subdural hematoma after acute myocardial infarction and thrombolytic therapy in the Thrombolysis in Myocardial Infarction Study. *Circulation* 83:448-459, 1991
331. De Jaegere PP, Arnold AA, Balk AH, et al: Intracranial hemorrhage in association with thrombolytic therapy: incidence and clinical predictive factors. *J Am Coll Cardiol* 19:289-294, 1992
332. Maggioni AP, Franzosi MG, Santoro E, et al: The risk of stroke in patients with acute myocardial infarction after thrombolytic and antithrombotic treatment. *N Engl J Med* 327:1-6, 1992
333. Gersh BJ, Anderson JL: Thrombolysis and myocardial salvage. Results of clinical trials and the animal paradigm—paradoxic or predictable? *Circulation* 88:296-306, 1993
334. Weaver WD, Eisenberg MS, Martin JS, et al: Myocardial Infarction Triage and Intervention Project—phase I: patient characteristics and feasibility of prehospital initiation of thrombolytic therapy. *J Am Coll Cardiol* 15:925-931, 1990
335. Karagounis L, Ipsen SK, Jessop MR, et al: Impact of field-transmitted electrocardiography on time to in-hospital thrombolytic therapy in acute myocardial infarction. *Am J Cardiol* 66:786-791, 1990
336. Kereiakes DJ, Weaver WD, Anderson JL, et al: Time delays in the diagnosis and treatment of acute myocardial infarction: a tale of eight cities. *Am Heart J* 120:773-780, 1990
337. Anderson JL, Rothbard RL, Hackworthy RA, et al: Multicenter reperfusion trial of intravenous Anisoylated Plasminogen Streptokinase Activator Complex (APSAC) in acute myocardial infarction: controlled comparison with intracoronary streptokinase. *J Am Coll Cardiol* 11:1153-1163, 1988
338. Sharkey SW, Bruneete DD, Ruiz E, et al: An analysis of time delays preceding thrombolysis for acute myocardial infarction. *JAMA* 262:3171-3174, 1989
339. Gonzalez ER, Ornato JP, Jones LA, et al: Prospective multicenter assessment of critical factors delaying hospital thrombolytic therapy (abstract). *J Am Coll Cardiol* 17 Suppl A:247, 1991
340. Neuhaus KL, von Essen R, Tebbe U, et al: Improved thrombolysis in acute myocardial infarction with front-loaded administration of alteplase: results of the rt-PA-APSAC patency study (TAPS). *J Am Coll Cardiol* 19:885-891, 1992
341. Gibbons RJ, Holmes DR, Reeder GS, et al: Immediate angioplasty compared with the administration of a thrombolytic agent followed by conservative treatment for myocardial infarction. *N Engl J Med* 328:685-691, 1993
342. Grines CL, Browne KF, Marco J, et al: A comparison of immediate angioplasty with thrombolytic therapy for acute myocardial infarction. *N Engl J Med* 328:673-679, 1993
343. Zijlstra F, de Boer MJ, Hoorntje JC, et al: A comparison of immediate coronary angioplasty with intravenous streptokinase in acute myocardial infarction. *N Engl J Med* 328:680-684, 1993
344. Gruppo Italiano per lo Studio della Streptochinasi nell'Infarto Miocardico (GISSI): Effectiveness of intravenous thrombolytic treatment in acute myocardial infarction. *Lancet* 1:397-402, 1986
345. The I.S.A.M. Study Group: A prospective trial of intravenous streptokinase in acute myocardial infarction (I.S.A.M.). Mortality, morbidity, and infarct size at 21 days. *N Engl J Med* 314:1465-1471, 1986

346. AIMS Trial Study Group: Effect of intravenous APSAC on mortality after acute myocardial infarction: preliminary report of a placebo-controlled clinical trial. *Lancet* 1:545-549, 1988

347. Wilcox RG, von der Lippe G, Olsson CG, et al: Trial of tissue plasminogen activator for mortality reduction in acute myocardial infarction: Anglo-Scandinavian Study of Early Thrombolysis (ASSET). *Lancet* 2:525-530, 1988

348. Rossi P, Bolognese L: Comparison of intravenous urokinase plus heparin versus heparin alone in acute myocardial infarction. *Am J Cardiol* 68:585-592, 1991

349. EMERAS (Estudio Multicentrico Estreptoquinasa Republicas de America del Sur) Collaborative Group: Randomised trial of late thrombolysis in patients with suspected acute myocardial infarction. *Lancet* 342:767-772, 1993

350. LATE Study Group: Late Assessment of Thrombolytic Efficacy (LATE) study with alteplase 6-24 hours after onset of acute myocardial infarction. *Lancet* 342:759-766, 1993

351. Fibrinolytic Therapy Trialists' (FTT) Collaborative Group: Indications for fibrinolytic therapy in suspected acute myocardial infarction: collaborative overview of early mortality and major morbidity results from all randomised trials of more than 1000 patients. *Lancet* 343:311-322, 1994

352. Mathey DG, Sheehan FH, Schofer J, et al: Time from onset of symptoms to thrombolytic therapy: a major determinant of myocardial salvage in patients with acute transmural infarction. *J Am Coll Cardiol* 6:518-525, 1985

353. Stack RS, Phillips HR III, Grierson DS, et al: Functional improvement of jeopardized myocardium following intracoronary streptokinase infusion in acute myocardial infarction. *J Clin Invest* 72:84-95, 1983

354. Sheehan FH, Braunwald E, Canner P, et al: The effect of intravenous thrombolytic therapy on left ventricular function: a report on tissue-type plasminogen activator and streptokinase from the Thrombolysis in Myocardial Infarction (TIMI Phase I) Trial. *Circulation* 75:817-829, 1987

355. Morgan CD, Roberts RS, Haq A, et al: Coronary patency, infarct size and left ventricular function after thrombolytic therapy for acute myocardial infarction: results from the Tissue Plasminogen Activator: Toronto (TPAT) placebo-controlled trial. *J Am Coll Cardiol* 17:1451-1457, 1991

356. Bates ER, Califf RM, Stack RS, et al: Thrombolysis and Angioplasty in Myocardial Infarction (TAMI-1) trial: influence of infarct location on arterial patency, left ventricular function and mortality. *J Am Coll Cardiol* 13:12-18, 1989

357. Braunwald E: The open-artery theory is alive and well—again (editorial). *N Engl J Med* 329:1650-1652, 1993

358. Gill JB, Cairns JA, Roberts R, et al: Comparative incremental prognostic values of silent ischemia, exercise testing, and LV function over clinical variables in survivors of acute MI (abstract). *Circulation* 90 Suppl 1:501, 1994

359. Rogers WJ, Babb JD, Baim DS, et al: Selective versus routine predischarge coronary arteriography after therapy with recombinant tissue-type plasminogen activator, heparin and aspirin for acute myocardial infarction. *J Am Coll Cardiol* 17:1007-1016, 1991

360. Christian TF, Gibbons RJ, Hopfenspirger MR, et al: Severity and response of chest pain during thrombolytic therapy for acute myocardial infarction: a useful indicator of myocardial salvage and infarct size. *J Am Coll Cardiol* 22:1311-1316, 1993

361. Hohnloser SH, Zabel M, Kasper W, et al: Assessment of coronary artery patency after thrombolytic therapy: accurate prediction utilizing the combined analysis of three noninvasive markers. *J Am Coll Cardiol* 18:44-49, 1991

362. Shah PK, Cercek B, Lew AS, et al: Angiographic validation of bedside markers of reperfusion. *J Am Coll Cardiol* 21:55-61, 1993

363. Krucoff MW, Green CE, Satler LF, et al: Noninvasive detection of coronary artery patency using continuous ST-segment monitoring. *Am J Cardiol* 57:916-922, 1986

364. Pfeffer MA, Braunwald E, Moye LA, et al: Effect of captopril on mortality and morbidity in patients with left ventricular dysfunction after myocardial infarction. Results of the Survival and Ventricular Enlargement trial. *N Engl J Med* 327:669-677, 1992

365. Swedberg K, Held P, Kjekshus J, et al: Effects of the early administration of enalapril on mortality in patients with acute myocardial infarction. Results of the Cooperative New Scandinavian Enalapril Survival Study II (CONSENSUS II). *N Engl J Med* 327:678-684, 1992

366. The SOLVD Investigators: Effect of enalapril on mortality and the development of heart failure in asymptomatic patients with reduced left ventricular ejection fractions. *N Engl J Med* 327:685-691, 1992

367. Cohn JN: The prevention of heart failure—a new agenda (editorial). *N Engl J Med* 327:725-727, 1992

368. Kennedy JW, Martin GV, Davis KB, et al: The Western Washington Intravenous Streptokinase in Acute Myocardial Infarction Randomized Trial. *Circulation* 77:345-352, 1988

369. White HD, Norris RM, Brown MA, et al: Effect of intravenous streptokinase on left ventricular function and early survival after acute myocardial infarction. *N Engl J Med* 317:850-855, 1987

370. Guerci AD, Gerstenblith G, Brinker JA, et al: A randomized trial of intravenous tissue plasminogen activator for acute myocardial infarction with subsequent randomization to elective coronary angioplasty. *N Engl J Med* 317:1613-1618, 1987

371. National Heart Foundation of Australia Coronary Thrombolysis Group: Coronary thrombolysis and myocardial salvage by tissue plasminogen activator given up to 4 hours after onset of myocardial infarction. *Lancet* 1:203-208, 1988

372. O'Rourke M, Baron D, Keogh A, et al: Limitation of myocardial infarction by early infusion of recombinant tissue-type plasminogen activator. *Circulation* 77:1311-1315, 1988

373. Van de Werf F, Arnold AE, the European Cooperative Study Group for Recombinant Tissue-Type Plasminogen Activator: Intravenous tissue plasminogen activator and size of infarct, left ventricular function, and survival in acute myocardial infarction. *BMJ* 297:1374-1379, 1988

374. Armstrong PW, Baigrie RS, Daly PA, et al: Tissue plasminogen activator: Toronto (TPAT) placebo-controlled randomized trial in acute myocardial infarction. *J Am Coll Cardiol* 13:1469-1476, 1989

375. Bassand JP, Machecourt J, Cassagnes J, et al: Multicenter trial of intravenous anisoylated plasminogen streptokinase activator complex (APSAC) in acute myocardial infarction: effects on infarct size and left ventricular function. *J Am Coll Cardiol* 13:988-997, 1989

376. Meinertz T, Kasper W, Schumacher M, et al: The German Multicenter Trial of anisoylated plasminogen streptokinase activator complex versus heparin for acute myocardial infarction. *Am J Cardiol* 62:347-351, 1988

377. Mueller HS, Rao AK, Forman SA: Thrombolysis in Myocardial Infarction (TIMI): comparative studies of coronary reperfusion and systemic fibrinogenolysis with two forms of recombinant tissue-type plasminogen activator. *J Am Coll Cardiol* 10:479-490, 1987

378. Smalling RW, Schumacher R, Morris D, et al: Improved infarct-related arterial patency after high dose, weight-adjusted, rapid infusion of tissue-type plasminogen activator in myocardial infarction: results of a multicenter randomized trial of two dosage regimens. *J Am Coll Cardiol* 15:915-921, 1990

379. Topol EJ, Morris DC, Smalling RW, et al: A multicenter, randomized, placebo-controlled trial of a new form of intravenous recombinant tissue-type plasminogen activator (activase) in acute myocardial infarction. *J Am Coll Cardiol* 9:1205-1213, 1987

380. Berger PB, Bell MR, Holmes DR Jr, et al: Time to reperfusion with direct coronary angioplasty and thrombolytic therapy in acute myocardial infarction. *Am J Cardiol* 73:231-236, 1994

381. The TIMI Research Group: Immediate vs delayed catheterization and angioplasty following thrombolytic therapy for acute myocardial infarction: TIMI II A results. *JAMA* 260:2849-2858, 1988

382. Karlson BW, Herlitz J, Edvardsson N, et al: Eligibility for intravenous thrombolysis in suspected acute myocardial infarction. *Circulation* 82:1140-1146, 1990

383. Cragg DR, Friedman HZ, Bonema JD, et al: Outcome of patients with acute myocardial infarction who are ineligible for thrombolytic therapy. *Ann Intern Med* 115:173-177, 1991

384. Hartzler GO, Rutherford BD, McConahay DR, et al: Percutaneous transluminal coronary angioplasty with and without thrombolytic therapy for treatment of acute myocardial infarction. *Am Heart J* 106:965-973, 1983

385. Hartzler GO, Rutherford BD, McConahay DR: Percutaneous transluminal coronary angioplasty: application for acute myocardial infarction. *Am J Cardiol* 53:117C-121C, 1984

386. Topol EJ: Direct vs. sequential percutaneous transluminal coronary angioplasty. In *Acute Coronary Intervention.* Edited by EJ Topol. New York, Alan R Liss, 1988, pp 79-94

387. Miller PF, Brodie BR, Weintraub RA, et al: Emergency coronary

angioplasty for acute myocardial infarction. Results from a community hospital. *Arch Intern Med* 147:1565-1570, 1987

388. Pepine CJ, Prida X, Hill JA, et al: Percutaneous transluminal coronary angioplasty in acute myocardial infarction. *Am Heart J* 107:820-822, 1984

389. Marco J, Caster L, Szatmary LJ, et al: Emergency percutaneous transluminal coronary angioplasty without thrombolysis as initial therapy in acute myocardial infarction. *Int J Cardiol* 15:55-63, 1987

390. Rothbaum DA, Linnemeier TJ, Landin RJ, et al: Emergency percutaneous transluminal coronary angioplasty in acute myocardial infarction: a 3 year experience. *J Am Coll Cardiol* 10:264-272, 1987

391. O'Keefe JH Jr, Rutherford BD, McConahay DR, et al: Early and late results of coronary angioplasty without antecedent thrombolytic therapy for acute myocardial infarction. *Am J Cardiol* 64:1221-1230, 1989

392. O'Neill W, Timmis GC, Bourdillon PD, et al: A prospective randomized clinical trial of intracoronary streptokinase versus coronary angioplasty for acute myocardial infarction. *N Engl J Med* 314:812-818, 1986

393. Hlatky MA: Intracoronary streptokinase versus coronary angioplasty for acute myocardial infarction (letter to the editor). *N Engl J Med* 315:1093-1094, 1986

394. de Boer MJ, Hoorntje JC, Ottervanger JP, et al: Immediate coronary angioplasty versus intravenous streptokinase in acute myocardial infarction: left ventricular ejection fraction, hospital mortality and reinfarction. *J Am Coll Cardiol* 23:1004-1008, 1994

395. Simari RD, Berger PB, Bell MR, et al: Coronary angioplasty in acute myocardial infarction: primary, immediate adjunctive, rescue, or deferred adjunctive approach? *Mayo Clin Proc* 69:346-358, 1994

396. Carney RJ, Murphy GA, Brandt TR, et al: Randomized angiographic trial of recombinant tissue-type plasminogen activator (alteplase) in myocardial infarction. *J Am Coll Cardiol* 20:17-23, 1992

397. Kahn JK, Rutherford BD, McConahay DR, et al: Results of primary angioplasty for acute myocardial infarction in patients with multivessel coronary artery disease. *J Am Coll Cardiol* 16:1089-1096, 1990

398. Brodie BR, Weintraub RA, Stuckey TD, et al: Outcomes of direct coronary angioplasty for acute myocardial infarction in candidates and non-candidates for thrombolytic therapy. *Am J Cardiol* 67:7-12, 1991

399. GUSTO Investigators: Global utilization of streptokinase vs t-PA for occluded arteries. *N Engl J Med* (in press)

400. Vogt A, von Essen R, Tebbe U, et al: Impact of early perfusion status of the infarct-related artery on short-term mortality after thrombolysis for acute myocardial infarction: retrospective analysis of four German multicenter studies. *J Am Coll Cardiol* 21:1391-1395, 1993

401. Stadius ML: Angiographic monitoring of reperfusion therapy for acute myocardial infarction. TIMI grade 3 perfusion is the goal (editorial). *Circulation* 87:2055-2057, 1993

402. Anderson JL, Karagounis LA, Becker LC, et al: TIMI perfusion grade 3 but not grade 2 results in improved outcome after thrombolysis for myocardial infarction. Ventriculographic, enzymatic, and electrocardiographic evidence from the TEAM-3 Study. *Circulation* 87:1829-1839, 1993

403. Karagounis L, Sorensen SG, Menlove RL, et al: Does Thrombolysis in Myocardial Infarction (TIMI) perfusion grade 2 represent a mostly patent artery or a mostly occluded artery? Enzymatic and electrocardiographic evidence from the TEAM-2 study. *J Am Coll Cardiol* 19:1-10, 1992

404. Scholz KH, Tebbe U, Herrmann C, et al: Frequency of complications of cardiopulmonary resuscitation after thrombolysis during acute myocardial infarction. *Am J Cardiol* 69:724-728, 1992

405. Boden WE, Gibson RS, Schechtman KB, et al: ST segment shifts are poor predictors of subsequent Q wave evolution in acute myocardial infarction. A natural history study of early non-Q wave infarction. *Circulation* 79:537-548, 1989

406. Feit F, Rey M, Sherman W, et al: The Second Mt. Sinai-NYU Reperfusion Trial: incidence and significance of isolated ST-depression (i-ST ↓) at screening (abstract). *Circulation* 78 Suppl 2:212, 1988

407. Killip T III, Kimball JT: Treatment of myocardial infarction in a coronary care unit. A two year experience with 250 patients. *Am J Cardiol* 20:457-464, 1967

408. O'Neill W, Erbel R, Laufer N, et al: Coronary angioplasty therapy of cardiogenic shock complicating acute myocardial infarction (abstract). *Circulation* 72 Suppl 3:309, 1989

409. Shani J, Rivera M, Greengart A, et al: Percutaneous transluminal coronary angioplasty in cardiogenic shock (abstract). *J Am Coll Cardiol* 7 Suppl A:149, 1986

410. Heuser RR, Maddoux GL, Goss JE, et al: Coronary angioplasty in the treatment of cardiogenic shock: the therapy of choice (abstract). *J Am Coll Cardiol* 7 Suppl A:219, 1986

411. Brown TM Jr, Iannone LA, Gordon DR, et al: Percutaneous myocardial reperfusion (PMR) reduces mortality in acute myocardial infarction (MI) complicated by cardiogenic shock (abstract). *Circulation* 72 Suppl 3:309, 1985

412. Laramee LA, Rutherford BD, Ligon RW, et al: Coronary angioplasty for cardiogenic shock following myocardial infarction (abstract). *Circulation* 78 Suppl 2:634, 1988

413. Lee L, Bates ER, Pitt B, et al: Percutaneous transluminal coronary angioplasty improves survival in acute myocardial infarction complicated by cardiogenic shock. *Circulation* 78:1345-1351, 1988

414. Lee L, Erbel R, Brown TM, et al: Multicenter registry of angioplasty therapy of cardiogenic shock: initial and long-term survival. *J Am Coll Cardiol* 17:599-603, 1991

415. Gacioch GM, Topol EJ: Frontiers in cardiogenic shock management: integration of angioplasty and new support devices (abstract). *Circulation* 80 Suppl 2:624, 1989

416. Disler L, Haitas B, Benjamin J, et al: Cardiogenic shock in evolving myocardial infarction: treatment by angioplasty and streptokinase. *Heart Lung* 16:649-652, 1987

417. Verna E, Repetto S, Boscarini M, et al: Emergency coronary angioplasty in patients with severe left ventricular dysfunction or cardiogenic shock after acute myocardial infarction. *Eur Heart J* 10:958-966, 1989

418. Meyer P, Blanc P, Baudouy M, et al: Traitement du choc cardiogenique primaire par angioplastie transluminale coronarienne à la phase aigue de l'infarctus. *Arch Mal Coeur Vaiss* 83:329-334, 1990

419. Hibbard MD, Holmes DR Jr, Bailey KR, et al: Percutaneous transluminal coronary angioplasty in patients with cardiogenic shock. *J Am Coll Cardiol* 19:639-646, 1992

420. Moosvi AR, Villanueva L, Gheorghiade M, et al: Early revascularization improves survival in cardiogenic shock (abstract). *Circulation* 82 Suppl 3:308, 1990

421. Eltchaninoff H, Simpfendorfer C, Whitlow PL: Coronary angioplasty improves both early and 1 year survival in acute myocardial infarction complicated by cardiogenic shock (abstract). *J Am Coll Cardiol* 17 Suppl A:167, 1991

422. Simoons ML, Arnold AER, Betriu A, et al: Thrombolysis with tissue plasminogen activator in acute myocardial infarction: no additional benefit from immediate percutaneous coronary angioplasty. *Lancet* 1:197-203, 1988

423. Topol EJ, Califf RM, George BS, et al: A randomized trial of immediate versus delayed elective angioplasty after intravenous tissue plasminogen activator in acute myocardial infarction. *N Engl J Med* 317:581-588, 1989

424. O'Neill WW, Weintraub R, Grines CL, et al: A prospective, placebo-controlled, randomized trial of intravenous streptokinase and angioplasty versus lone angioplasty therapy of acute myocardial infarction. *Circulation* 86:1710-1717, 1992

425. Kennedy JW, Ritchie JL, Davis KB, et al: The Western Washington randomized trial of intracoronary streptokinase in acute myocardial infarction: a 12-month follow-up report. *N Engl J Med* 312:1073-1078, 1985

426. Abbottsmith CW, Topol EJ, George BS, et al: Fate of patients with acute myocardial infarction with patency of the infarct-related vessel achieved with successful thrombolysis versus rescue angioplasty. *J Am Coll Cardiol* 16:770-778, 1990

427. Fung AY, Lai P, Topol EJ, et al: Value of percutaneous transluminal coronary angioplasty after unsuccessful intravenous streptokinase therapy in acute myocardial infarction. *Am J Cardiol* 58:686-691, 1986

428. Holmes DR Jr, Gersh BJ, Bailey KR, et al: Emergency "rescue" percutaneous transluminal coronary angioplasty after failed thrombolysis with streptokinase: early and late results. *Circulation* 81 Suppl 4:51-56, 1990

429. Califf RM, Topol EJ, Stack RS, et al: Evaluation of combination thrombolytic therapy and timing of cardiac catheterization in acute myocardial infarction. Results of Thrombolysis and Angioplasty in Myocardial Infarction – phase 5 randomized trial. *Circulation* 83:1543-1556, 1991

430. Ellis SG, da Silva ER, Heyndrickx G, et al: Randomized comparison of rescue angioplasty with conservative management of patients with early failure of thrombolysis for acute anterior myocardial infarction. *Circulation* 90:2280-2284, 1994

431. Ellis SG, Van de Werf F, Ribeiro-daSilva E, et al: Present status of rescue coronary angioplasty: current polarization of opinion and randomized trials (editorial). *J Am Coll Cardiol* 19:681-686, 1992
432. Seacord LM, Abendschein DR, Nohara R, et al: Detection of reperfusion within 1 hour after coronary recanalisation by analysis of isoforms of the MM creatine kinase isoenzyme in plasma. *Fibrinolysis* 2:151-156, 1988
433. Dellborg M, Swedberg K: Dynamic QRS-complex and ST-segment vectorcardiographic monitoring in acute myocardial infarction (abstract). *Circulation* 80 Suppl 2:355, 1989
434. SWIFT (Should We Intervene Following Thrombolysis?) Trial Study Group: SWIFT trial of delayed elective intervention v conservative treatment after thrombolysis with anistreplase in acute myocardial infarction. *BMJ* 302:555-560, 1991
435. Mueller HS, Cohen LS, Braunwald E, et al: Predictors of early morbidity and mortality after thrombolytic therapy of acute myocardial infarction. Analyses of patient subgroups in the Thrombolysis in Myocardial Infarction (TIMI) trial, phase II. *Circulation* 85:1254-1264, 1992
436. Ellis SG, Mooney MR, George BS, et al: Randomized trial of late elective angioplasty versus conservative management for patients with residual stenoses after thrombolytic treatment of myocardial infarction. *Circulation* 86:1400-1406, 1992
437. Phillips SJ, Kongtahworn C, Zeff RH, et al: Emergency coronary artery revascularization: a possible therapy for acute myocardial infarction. *Circulation* 60:241-246, 1979
438. McIntosh HD, Buccino RA: Emergency coronary artery revascularization of patients with acute myocardial infarction: you can . . . but should you? (Editorial.) *Circulation* 60:247-250, 1979
439. DeWood MA, Spores J, Notske RN, et al: Medical and surgical management of myocardial infarction. *Am J Cardiol* 44:1356-1364, 1979
440. Berg R Jr, Selinger SL, Leonard JJ, et al: Immediate coronary artery bypass for acute evolving myocardial infarction. *J Thorac Cardiovasc Surg* 81:493-497, 1981
441. DeWood MA, Heit J, Spores J, et al: Anterior transmural myocardial infarction: effects of surgical coronary reperfusion on global and regional left ventricular function. *J Am Coll Cardiol* 1:1223-1234, 1983
442. Hammermeister KE: The effect of coronary bypass surgery on survival. *Prog Cardiovasc Dis* 25:297-334, 1983
443. Vlietstra RE, Holmes DR Jr, Reeder GS, et al: Balloon angioplasty in multivessel coronary artery disease. *Mayo Clin Proc* 58:563-567, 1983
444. Loop FD, Cheanvechai C, Sheldon WC, et al: Early myocardial revascularization during acute myocardial infarction. *Chest* 66:478-482, 1974
445. Markis JE, Malagold M, Parker JA, et al: Myocardial salvage after intracoronary thrombolysis with streptokinase in acute myocardial infarction: assessment by intracoronary thallium-201. *N Engl J Med* 305:777-782, 1981
446. Pasternak RC, Braunwald E, Alpert JS: Acute myocardial infarction. In *Harrison's Principles of Internal Medicine.* Edited by E Braunwald, KJ Isselbacher, RG Petersdorf, et al. New York, McGraw-Hill, 1986, pp 982-993
447. Braunwald E (ed): Protection of the ischemic myocardium. *Circulation* 53 Suppl 1:1-228, 1976
448. Braunwald E, Maroko PR: Limitation of infarct size. *Curr Probl Cardiol* 3:1-51, April 1978
449. Mantle JA, Russell RO Jr, Moraski RE, et al: Isosorbide dinitrate for the relief of severe heart failure after myocardial infarction. *Am J Cardiol* 37:263-268, 1976
450. Bloch A, Beller GA, DeSanctis RW: Chronic propranolol administration and acute myocardial infarction. *Am Heart J* 92:121-123, 1976
451. Nidorf SM, Parsons R, Thompson PL, et al: Prior beta blocker therapy improves 28 day post infarction survival (abstract). *J Am Coll Cardiol* 13 Suppl A:12, 1989
452. Resnekov L: Circulatory assistance for the failing heart. *Br Heart J* 35:1265-1270, 1973
453. Kennedy JW, Ritchie JL, Davis KB, et al: Western Washington randomized trial of intracoronary streptokinase in acute myocardial infarction. *N Engl J Med* 309:1477-1482, 1983
454. Pfeffer MA, Braunwald E, Cuddy TE, et al: Selection bias in the use of thrombolytic therapy in acute myocardial infarction (abstract). *Circulation* 80 Suppl 2:522, 1989
455. Wackers FJ, Lie KI, Becker AE, et al: Coronary artery disease in patients dying from cardiogenic shock or congestive heart failure in the setting of acute myocardial infarction. *Br Heart J* 1976;38:906-910
456. Alonso DR, Scheidt S, Post M, et al: Pathophysiology of cardiogenic shock: quantification of myocardial necrosis, clinical, pathologic, and electrocardiographic correlations. *Circulation* 48:588-596, 1973
457. Gutovitz AL, Sobel BE, Roberts R: Progressive nature of myocardial injury in selected patients with cardiogenic shock. *Am J Cardiol* 41:469-475, 1978
458. Geddes JS, Adgey AAJ, Pantridge JF: Prevention of cardiogenic shock. *Am Heart J* 99:243-254, 1980
459. Nishimura RA, Schaff HV, Gersh BJ, et al: Early repair of mechanical complications after acute myocardial infarction. *JAMA* 256:47-50, 1986
460. Nishimura RA, Schaff HV, Shub C, et al: Papillary muscle rupture complicating acute myocardial infarction: analysis of 17 patients. *Am J Cardiol* 51:373-377, 1983
461. Berger PB, Ryan TJ: Inferior myocardial infarction. High-risk subgroups. *Circulation* 81:401-411, 1990
462. Shah PK, Maddahi J, Berman DS, et al: Scintigraphically detected predominant right ventricular dysfunction in acute myocardial infarction: clinical and hemodynamic correlates and implications for therapy and prognosis. *J Am Coll Cardiol* 6:1264-1272, 1985
463. Dell'Italia LJ, Starling MR, Blumhardt R, et al: Comparative effects of volume loading, dobutamine, and nitroprusside in patients with predominant right ventricular infarction. *Circulation* 72:1327-1335, 1985
464. Ellis SG, O'Neill WW, Bates ER, et al: Implications for patient triage from survival and left ventricular functional recovery analyses in 500 patients treated with coronary angioplasty for acute myocardial infarction. *J Am Coll Cardiol* 13:1251-1259, 1989
465. Gruppo Italiano per lo Studio della Streptochinasi nell'Infarto Miocardico (GISSI): Long-term effects of intravenous thrombolysis in acute myocardial infarction: final report of the GISSI study. *Lancet* 2:871-874, 1987
466. Bates ER, Topol EJ: Limitations of thrombolytic therapy for acute myocardial infarction complicated by congestive heart failure and cardiogenic shock. *J Am Coll Cardiol* 18:1077-1084, 1991
467. Bengtson JR, Kaplan AJ, Pieper KS, et al: Prognosis in cardiogenic shock after acute myocardial infarction in the interventional era. *J Am Coll Cardiol* 20:1482-1489, 1992
468. Grines CL, Nissen SE, Booth DC, et al: A new thrombolytic regimen for acute myocardial infarction using combination half dose tissue-type plasminogen activator with full dose streptokinase: a pilot study. *J Am Coll Cardiol* 14:573-580, 1989
469. Topol EJ, Califf RM, George BS, et al: Coronary arterial thrombolysis with combined infusion of recombinant tissue-type plasminogen activator and urokinase in patients with acute myocardial infarction. *Circulation* 77:1100-1107, 1988
470. Califf RM, Topol EJ, George BS, et al: Characteristics and outcome of patients in whom reperfusion with intravenous tissue-type plasminogen activator fails: results of the Thrombolysis and Angioplasty in Myocardial Infarction (TAMI) I trial. *Circulation* 77:1090-1099, 1988
471. Baim DS, Diver DJ, Knatterude GL, et al: PTCA "salvage" for thrombolytic failures—implications from TIMI II-A (abstract). *Circulation* 78 Suppl 2:112, 1988
472. Ohman EM, George BS, White CJ, et al: The use of aortic counterpulsation to improve sustained coronary artery patency during acute myocardial infarction: results of a randomized trial (abstract). *J Am Coll Cardiol* 21 Suppl A:397, 1993
473. Mundth ED, Yurchak PM, Buckley MJ, et al: Circulatory assistance and emergency direct coronary-artery surgery for shock complicating acute myocardial infarction. *N Engl J Med* 283:1382-1384, 1970
474. Leinbach RC, Dinsmore RE, Mundth ED, et al: Selective coronary and left ventricular cineangiography during intraaortic balloon pumping for cardiogenic shock. *Circulation* 45:845-852, 1972
475. DeWood MA, Notske RN, Hensley GR, et al: Intraaortic balloon counterpulsation with and without reperfusion for myocardial infarction shock. *Circulation* 61:1105-1112, 1980
476. Chatterjee K, Parmley WW, Ganz W, et al: Hemodynamic and metabolic responses to vasodilator therapy in acute myocardial infarction. *Circulation* 48:1183-1193, 1973
477. Moulopoulos SD, Topaz S, Kolff WJ: Diastolic balloon pumping

(with carbon dioxide) in the aorta: a mechanical assistance to the failing circulation. *Am Heart J* 63:669-675, 1962

478. Krakauer JS, Rosenbaum A, Freed PS, et al: Clinical management ancillary to phase-shift balloon pumping in cardiogenic shock: preliminary comments. *Am J Cardiol* 27:123-128, 1971

479. Gunnar RM: Cardiogenic shock complicating acute myocardial infarction. *Circulation* 78:1508-1510, 1988

480. Leinbach RC, Gold HK, Dinsmore RE, et al: The role of angiography in cardiogenic shock. *Circulation* 48 Suppl 3:95-98, 1973

481. Scheidt S, Wilner G, Mueller H, et al: Intra-aortic balloon counterpulsation in cardiogenic shock: report of a co-operative clinical trial. *N Engl J Med* 288:979-984, 1973

482. Wajszczuk WJ, Krakauer J, Rubenfire M, et al: Current indications for mechanical cardiac assistance on the basis of experience with 104 patients (abstract). *Am J Cardiol* 33:176, 1974

483. Willerson JT, Curry GC, Watson JT, et al: Intraaortic balloon counterpulsation in patients in cardiogenic shock, medically refractory left ventricular failure and/or recurrent ventricular tachycardia. *Am J Med* 58:183-191, 1975

484. Hagemeijer F, Laird JD, Haalebos MMP, et al: Effectiveness of intraaortic balloon pumping without cardiac surgery for patients with severe heart failure secondary to a recent myocardial infarction. *Am J Cardiol* 40:951-956, 1977

485. Baron DW, O'Rourke MF: Long-term results of arterial counterpulsation in acute severe cardiac failure complicating myocardial infarction. *Br Heart J* 38:285-288, 1976

486. Lorente P, Gourgon R, Beaufils P, et al: Multivariate statistical evaluation of intraaortic counterpulsation in pump failure complicating acute myocardial infarction. *Am J Cardiol* 46:124-134, 1980

487. Scheidt S, Collins M, Goldstein J, et al: Mechanical circulatory assistance with the intraaortic balloon pump and other counterpulsation devices. *Prog Cardiovasc Dis* 25:55-76, 1982

488. Pierri MK, Zema M, Kligfield P, et al: Exercise tolerance in late survivors of balloon pumping and surgery for cardiogenic shock. *Circulation* 62 Suppl 1:138-141, 1980

489. McEnany MT, Kay HR, Buckley MJ, et al: Clinical experience with intraaortic balloon pump support in 728 patients. *Circulation* 58 Suppl 1:124-132, 1978

490. Beckman CB, Geha AS, Hammond GL, et al: Results and complications of intraaortic balloon counterpulsation. *Ann Thorac Surg* 24:550-557, 1977

491. McCabe JC, Abel RM, Subramanian VA, et al: Complications of intra-aortic balloon insertion and counterpulsation. *Circulation* 57:769-773, 1978

492. Gold HK, Leinbach RC, Buckley MJ, et al: Refractory angina pectoris: follow-up after intraaortic balloon pumping and surgery. *Circulation* 54 Suppl 3:41-46, 1976

493. Bardet J, Masquet C, Kahn J-C, et al: Clinical and hemodynamic results of intra-aortic balloon counterpulsation and surgery for cardiogenic shock. *Am Heart J* 93:280-288, 1977

494. Gunnar RM, Loeb HS, Pietras RJ, et al: Hemodynamic measurements in a coronary care unit. *Prog Cardiovasc Dis* 11:29-44, 1968

495. Goldberg LI: Cardiovascular and renal actions of dopamine: potential clinical applications. *Pharmacol Rev* 24:1-29, 1972

496. Goldberg LI, McDonald RH Jr, Zimmerman AM: Sodium diuresis produced by dopamine in patients with congestive heart failure. *N Engl J Med* 269:1060-1064, 1963

497. Rosenblum R, Tai AR, Lawson D: Dopamine in man: cardiorenal hemodynamics in normotensive patients with heart disease. *J Pharmacol Exp Ther* 183:256-263, 1972

498. Yeh BK, McNay JL, Goldberg LI: Attenuation of dopamine renal and mesenteric vasodilation by haloperidol: evidence for a specific dopamine receptor. *J Pharmacol Exp Ther* 168:303-309, 1969

499. Gilbert J-C, Goldberg LI: Characterization by cyproheptadine of the dopamine-induced contraction in canine isolated arteries. *J Pharmacol Exp Ther* 193:435-442, 1975

500. Loeb HS, Bredakis J, Gunnar RM: Superiority of dobutamine over dopamine for augmentation of cardiac output in patients with chronic low output cardiac failure. *Circulation* 55:375-381, 1977

501. Toda N, Goldberg LI: Effects of dopamine on isolated canine coronary arteries. *Cardiovasc Res* 9:384-389, 1975

502. Plachetka JR: Clinical pharmacology of dobutamine. *J Cardiovasc Med* 6:75-85, 1981

503. Tuttle RR, Mills J: Dobutamine: development of a new catecholamine to selectively increase cardiac contractility. *Circ Res* 36:185-196, 1975

504. Magorien RD, Unverferth DV, Brown GP, et al: Dobutamine and hydralazine: comparative influences of positive inotropy and vasodilation on coronary blood flow and myocardial energetics in nonischemic congestive heart failure. *J Am Coll Cardiol* 1:499-505, 1983

505. Robie NW, Goldberg LI: Comparative systemic and regional hemodynamic effects of dopamine and dobutamine. *Am Heart J* 90:340-345, 1975

506. Unverferth DV, Blanford M, Kates RE, et al: Tolerance to dobutamine after a 72-hour continuous infusion. *Am J Med* 69:262-266, 1980

507. Alousi AA, Farah AE, Lesher GY, et al: Cardiotonic activity of amrinone—Win 40680 [5-amino-3,4′-bipyridine-6(1H)-one]. *Circ Res* 45:666-677, 1979

508. Millard RW, Dube G, Grupp G, et al: Direct vasodilator and positive inotropic actions of amrinone. *J Mol Cell Cardiol* 12:647-652, 1980

509. Benotti JR, Grossman W, Braunwald E, et al: Hemodynamic assessment of amrinone. A new inotropic agent. *N Engl J Med* 299:1373-1377, 1978

510. Gunnicker M, Hess W: Preliminary results with amrinone in perioperative low cardiac output syndrome. *Thorac Cardiovasc Surg* 35:219-225, 1987

511. Heuer H, Frenking B, Gülker H: Effect of amrinone in acute severe cardiac failure. *Arzneim-Forsch/Drug Res* 38:567-570, 1988

512. Leier CV, Heban PT, Huss P, et al: Comparative systemic and regional hemodynamic effects of dopamine and dobutamine in patients with cardiomyopathic heart failure. *Circulation* 58:466-475, 1978

513. Richard C, Ricome JL, Rimailho A, et al: Combined hemodynamic effects of dopamine and dobutamine in cardiogenic shock. *Circulation* 67:620-626, 1983

514. Amsterdam EA, DeMaria AN, Hughes JL, et al: Myocardial infarction shock: mechanisms and management. In *Congestive Heart Failure: Mechanisms, Evaluation and Treatment.* Edited by DT Mason. New York, Dun-Donnelley Publishing Corporation, 1976, pp 365-396

515. Bates RJ, Beutler S, Resnekov L, et al: Cardiac rupture—challenge in diagnosis and management. *Am J Cardiol* 40:429-437, 1977

516. Reddy SG, Roberts WC: Frequency of rupture of the left ventricular free wall or ventricular septum among necropsy cases of fatal acute myocardial infarction since introduction of coronary care units. *Am J Cardiol* 63:906-911, 1989

517. Roldán I, López-Sendón J, Perdigão C, et al: Causes of death after thrombolytic therapy in acute myocardial infarction (abstract). *J Am Coll Cardiol* 19 Suppl A:154, 1992

518. Saffitz JE, Fredrickson RC, Roberts WC: Relation of size of transmural acute myocardial infarct to mode of death, interval between infarction and death and frequency of coronary arterial thrombus. *Am J Cardiol* 57:1249-1254, 1986

519. Lewis AJ, Burchell HB, Titus JL: Clinical and pathologic features of postinfarction cardiac rupture. *Am J Cardiol* 23:43-53, 1969

520. Spiekerman RE, Brandenburg JT, Achor RWP, et al: The spectrum of coronary heart disease in a community of 30,000: a clinicopathologic study. *Circulation* 25:57-65, 1962

521. Crawford MD, Morris JN: Ruptured ventricle: incidence in population of London, 1957-8. *Br Med J* 2:1624-1626, 1960

522. Jetter WW, White PD: Rupture of the heart in patients in mental institutions. *Ann Intern Med* 21:783-802, 1944

523. Kavelman DA: Myocardial rupture: a study in non-psychotic and psychotic patients. *Can Med Assoc J* 82:1105-1107, 1960

524. Maher JF, Mallory GK, Laurenz GA: Rupture of the heart after myocardial infarction. *N Engl J Med* 255:1-10, 1956

525. Rasmussen S, Leth A, Kjoller E, et al: Cardiac rupture in acute myocardial infarction: a review of 72 consecutive cases. *Acta Med Scand* 205:11-16, 1979

526. Delborg M, Held P, Swedberg K, et al: Rupture of the myocardium: occurrence and risk factors. *Br Heart J* 54:11-16, 1985

527. Mann JM, Roberts WC: Rupture of the left ventricular free wall during acute myocardial infarction: analysis of 138 necropsy patients and comparison with 50 necropsy patients with acute myocardial infarction without rupture. *Am J Cardiol* 62:847-859, 1988

528. Van Tassel RA, Edwards JE: Rupture of heart complicating myocardial infarction: analysis of 40 cases including nine examples of left ventricular false aneurysm. *Chest* 61:104-116, 1972

529. Batts KP, Ackermann DM, Edwards WD: Postinfarction rupture of the left ventricular free wall: clinicopathologic correlates in 100 consecutive autopsy cases. *Hum Pathol* 21:530-535, 1990

530. Becker AE, van Mantgem J-P: Cardiac tamponade: a study of 50 hearts. *Eur J Cardiol* 3:349-358, 1975

531. Greenberg MA, Gitler B: Left ventricular rupture in a patient with coexisting right ventricular infarction. *N Engl J Med* 309:539-542, 1983

532. Windsor HM, Chang VP, Shanahan MX: Postinfarction cardiac rupture. *J Thorac Cardiovasc Surg* 84:755-761, 1982

533. Feneley MP, Chang VP, O'Rourke MF: Myocardial rupture after acute myocardial infarction: ten year review. *Br Heart J* 49:550-556, 1983

534. Chandraratna PAN, Pitha JV, Nanna M, et al: Prolonged survival after cardiac rupture following myocardial infarction. *Chest* 81:643-644, 1982

535. Núñez L, de la Llana R, López Sendón J, et al: Diagnosis and treatment of subacute free wall ventricular rupture after infarction. *Ann Thorac Surg* 35:525-529, 1983

536. Roberts WC: Rupture of the left ventricular free wall during acute myocardial infarction without hemopericardium. *Am J Cardiol* 65:1033-1034, 1990

537. Lowe TE, Wartman WB: Myocardial infarction. *Br Heart J* 6:115-128, 1944

538. Mann JM, Roberts WC: Fatal rupture of both left ventricular free wall and ventricular septum (double rupture) during acute myocardial infarction: analysis of seven patients studied at necropsy. *Am J Cardiol* 60:722-724, 1987

539. Atkinson JB, Robinowitz M, McAllister HA, et al: Association of eosinophils with cardiac rupture. *Hum Pathol* 16:562-568, 1985

540. Shapira I, Isakov A, Burke M, et al: Cardiac rupture in patients with acute myocardial infarction. *Chest* 92:219-223, 1987

541. Roberts WC, Ronan JA Jr, Harvey WP: Rupture of the left ventricular free wall (LVFW) or ventricular septum (VS) secondary to acute myocardial infarction (AMI): an occurrence virtually limited to the first transmural AMI in a hypertensive individual (abstract). *Am J Cardiol* 35:166, 1975

542. Griffith GC, Hegde B, Oblath RW: Factors in myocardial rupture: an analysis of two hundred and four cases at Los Angeles County Hospital between 1924 and 1959. *Am J Cardiol* 8:792-798, 1961

543. Christensen DJ, Ford M, Reading J, et al: Effect of hypertension on myocardial rupture after acute myocardial infarction. *Chest* 72:618-622, 1977

544. Schuster EH, Bulkley BH: Expansion of transmural myocardial infarction: a pathophysiologic factor in cardiac rupture. *Circulation* 60:1532-1538, 1979

545. Silverman HS, Pfeifer MP: Relation between use of anti-inflammatory agents and left ventricular free wall rupture during acute myocardial infarction. *Am J Cardiol* 59:363-364, 1987

546. Capeci NE, Levy RL: The influence of anticoagulant therapy on the incidence of thromboembolism, hemorrhage, and cardiac rupture in acute myocardial infarction: correlation of clinical and autopsy data in 100 cases. *Am J Med* 26:76-80, 1959

547. Gans RH: Acute myocardial infarction with rupture of the ventricle. *Am Heart J* 41:332-339, 1951

548. Mauri F, De Biase AM, Franzosi MG, et al: Analisi delle cause di morte intraospedaliera [in-hospital causes of death in patients admitted to the GISSI study]. *G Ital Cardiol* 17(1):37-44, 1987

549. Honan MB, Harrell FE Jr, Reimer KA, et al: Cardiac rupture, mortality and the timing of thrombolytic therapy: a meta-analysis. *J Am Coll Cardiol* 16:359-367, 1990

550. Loukinen KL, O'Neill W, Laufer N, et al: Myocardial rupture complicating tissue plasminogen activator therapy of acute myocardial infarction (abstract). *J Am Coll Cardiol* 13 Suppl A:94, 1989

551. Cobbs BW Jr, Hatcher CR Jr, Robinson PH: Cardiac rupture: three operations with two long-term survivals. *JAMA* 223:532-535, 1973

552. Friedman HS, Kuhn LA, Katz AM: Clinical and electrocardiographic features of cardiac rupture following acute myocardial infarction. *Am J Med* 50:709-720, 1971

553. London RE, London SB: Rupture of the heart: a critical analysis of 47 consecutive autopsy cases. *Circulation* 31:202-208, 1965

554. O'Rourke MF: Subacute heart rupture following myocardial infarction: clinical features of a correctable condition. *Lancet* 2:124-126, 1973

555. Lopez-Sendon J, Gonzalez A, Lopez de Sa E, et al: Diagnosis of subacute ventricular wall rupture after acute myocardial infarction: sensitivity and specificity of clinical, hemodynamic and echocardiographic criteria. *J Am Coll Cardiol* 19:1145-1153, 1992

556. Edwards JE: The value and limitations of necropsy studies in coronary arterial disease. *Prog Cardiovasc Dis* 13:309-323, 1971

557. Datta BN, Bowes VF, Silver MD: Incomplete rupture of the heart with diverticulum formation. *Pathology* 7:179-185, 1975

558. Desoutter P, Halphen C, Haïat R: Two-dimensional echographic visualization of free ventricular wall rupture in acute anterior myocardial infarction. *Am Heart J* 108:1360-1361, 1984

559. Coma-Canella I, López-Sendón J, García AG, et al: Hemodynamic effect of dextran, dobutamine, and pericardiocentesis in cardiac tamponade secondary to subacute heart rupture. *Am Heart J* 114:78-84, 1987

560. Kendall RW, DeWood MA: Postinfarction cardiac rupture: surgical success and review of the literature. *Ann Thorac Surg* 25:311-315, 1978

561. Hochreiter C, Goldstein J, Borer JS, et al: Myocardial freewall rupture after acute infarction: survival aided by percutaneous intraaortic balloon counterpulsation. *Circulation* 65:1279-1282, 1982

562. Parr GVS, Pae WE Jr, Pierce WS, et al: Cardiogenic shock due to ventricular rupture: a surgical approach. *J Thorac Cardiovasc Surg* 82:889-891, 1981

563. FitzGibbon GM, Hooper GD, Heggtveit HA: Successful surgical treatment of postinfarction external cardiac rupture. *J Thorac Cardiovasc Surg* 63:622-630, 1972

564. Anagnostopoulos E, Beutler S, Levett JM, et al: Myocardial rupture: major left ventricular infarct rupture treated by infarctectomy. *JAMA* 238:2715-2716, 1977

565. Lillehei CW, Lande AJ, Rassman WR, et al: Surgical management of myocardial infarction: some promising concepts utilizing revascularization, mechanical circulatory assistance, operative treatment of severe complications, and cardiac replacement. *Circulation* 40 Suppl 4:315-333, 1969

566. West PN, Shaw RC, Weldon CS: Posterior ventricular aneurysm, severe mitral regurgitation, and rupture of the left ventricle after acute myocardial infarction: six-year survival after surgical correction. *Ann Thorac Surg* 25:236-239, 1978

567. Cohn LH: Surgical management of acute and chronic cardiac mechanical complications due to myocardial infarction. *Am Heart J* 102:1049-1060, 1981

568. Chesler E, Korns ME, Semba T, et al: False aneurysms of the left ventricle following myocardial infarction. *Am J Cardiol* 23:76-82, 1969

569. Cone RB, Hawley RL: Pseudoaneurysm of the heart following infarction. *Arch Pathol* 77:166-171, 1964

570. Roberts WC, Morrow AG: Pseudoaneurysm of the left ventricle: an unusual sequel of myocardial infarction and rupture of the heart. *Am J Med* 43:639-644, 1967

571. Bjornsson L: Pseudoaneurysm of the left ventricle of the heart: a rare complication of myocardial rupture following infarction – report of a case. *Am J Clin Pathol* 41:302-306, 1964

572. Gueron M, Wanderman KL, Hirsch M, et al: Pseudoaneurysm of the left ventricle after myocardial infarction: a curable form of myocardial rupture. *J Thorac Cardiovasc Surg* 69:736-742, 1975

573. Vlodaver Z, Coe JI, Edwards JE: True and false left ventricular aneurysms: propensity for the latter to rupture. *Circulation* 51:567-572, 1975

574. Buehler DL, Stinson EB, Oyer PE, et al: Surgical treatment of aneurysms of the inferior left ventricular wall. *J Thorac Cardiovasc Surg* 78:74-78, 1979

575. Ersek RA, Chesler E, Korns ME, et al: Spontaneous rupture of a false left ventricular aneurysm following myocardial infarction. *Am Heart J* 77:677-680, 1969

576. Van Mechelen R, van Hemel NM, van Rijk PP: Non-invasive diagnosis of pseudoaneurysm of the left ventricle. *Br Heart J* 40:812-816, 1978

577. Winzelberg GG, Miller SW, Okada RD, et al: Scintigraphic assessment of false left ventricular aneurysms. *AJR* 135:569-574, 1980

578. Onik G, Recht L, Edwards JE, et al: False left ventricular aneurysm: diagnosis by noninvasive means. *J Nucl Med* 21:177-182, 1980

579. Roelandt J, van den Brand M, Vletter WB, et al: Echocardiographic diagnosis of pseudoaneurysm of the left ventricle. *Circulation* 52:466-472, 1975

580. Reeder GS, Seward JB, Tajik AJ: The role of two-dimensional

echocardiography in coronary artery disease: a critical appraisal. *Mayo Clin Proc* 57:247-258, 1982

581. Catherwood E, Mintz GS, Kotler MN, et al: Two-dimensional echocardiographic recognition of left ventricular pseudoaneurysm. *Circulation* 62:294-303, 1980

582. Gatewood RP Jr, Nanda NC: Differentiation of left ventricular pseudoaneurysm from true aneurysm with two-dimensional echocardiography. *Am J Cardiol* 46:869-878, 1980

583. Weyman AE, Peskoe SM, Williams ES, et al: Detection of left ventricular aneurysms by cross-sectional echocardiography. *Circulation* 54:936-944, 1976

584. Stewart S, Huddle R, Stuard I, et al: False aneurysm and pseudo-false aneurysm of the left ventricle: etiology, pathology, diagnosis, and operative management. *Ann Thorac Surg* 31:259-265, 1981

585. Botvinick EH, Shames D, Hutchinson JC, et al: Noninvasive diagnosis of a false left ventricular aneurysm with radioisotope gated cardiac blood pool imaging: differentiation from true aneurysm. *Am J Cardiol* 37:1089-1093, 1976

586. Gould L, Yang DC-S, Martinucci L: Radionuclide diagnosis of left ventricular pseudoaneurysm. *Am Heart J* 104:1377-1378, 1982

587. Sweet SE, Sterling R, McCormick JR, et al: Left ventricular aneurysm after coronary bypass surgery: radionuclide diagnosis and surgical resection. *Am J Cardiol* 43:154-157, 1979

588. Scanlon PJ, Moran JM, Nemickas V, et al: Post-infarction left ventricular pseudoaneurysm properly diagnosed clinically and angiographically and successfully treated surgically. *Cathet Cardiovasc Diagn* 1:397-403, 1975

589. Rittenhouse EA, Sauvage LR, Mansfield PB, et al: False aneurysm of the left ventricle: report of four cases and review of surgical management. *Ann Surg* 189:409-415, 1979

590. Logue B, Bone D, Kaplan J: The diagnosis and management of mechanical defects due to myocardial infarction. *Cardiovasc Rev Rep* 1:446-459, 1980

591. Pohjola-Sintonen S, Muller JE, Stone PH, et al: Ventricular septal and free wall rupture complicating acute myocardial infarction: experience in the Multicenter Investigation of Limitation of Infarct Size. *Am Heart J* 117:809-818, 1989

592. Moore CA, Nygaard TW, Kaiser DL, et al: Postinfarction ventricular septal rupture: the importance of location of infarction and right ventricular function in determining survival. *Circulation* 74:45-55, 1986

593. Selzer A, Gerbode F, Kerth WJ: Clinical, hemodynamic, and surgical considerations of rupture of the ventricular septum after myocardial infarction. *Am Heart J* 78:598-607, 1969

594. Lemery R, Smith HC, Giuliani ER, et al: Prognosis in rupture of the ventricular septum after acute myocardial infarction and role of early surgical intervention. *Am J Cardiol* 70:147-151, 1992

595. Radford MJ, Johnson RA, Daggett WM Jr, et al: Ventricular septal rupture: a review of clinical and physiologic features and an analysis of survival. *Circulation* 64:545-553, 1981.

596. Landale DG, Schlappi JC: Thirteen-year survival with acquired interventricular septal defect after myocardial infarction. *Am Heart J* 64:33-37, 1962.

597. Edmondson HA, Hoxie HJ: Hypertension and cardiac rupture: a clinical and pathologic study of seventy-two cases, in thirteen of which rupture of the interventricular septum occurred. *Am Heart J* 24:719-733, 1942

598. Sugiura T, Iwasaka T, Takahashi N, et al: Factors associated with atrial fibrillation in Q wave anterior myocardial infarction. *Am Heart J* 121:1409-1412, 1991

599. Cummings RG, Reimer KA, Califf R, et al: Quantitative analysis of right and left ventricular infarction in the presence of postinfarction ventricular septal defect. *Circulation* 77:33-42, 1988

600. Muehrcke DD, Daggett WM Jr, Buckley MJ, et al: Postinfarct ventricular septal defect repair: effect of coronary artery bypass grafting. *Ann Thorac Surg* 54:876-882, 1992

601. Killen DA, Reed WA, Wathanacharoen S, et al: Postinfarction rupture of the interventricular septum. *J Cardiovasc Surg* 22:113-126, 1981

602. Hill JD, Lary D, Kerth WJ, et al: Acquired ventricular septal defects: evolution of an operation, surgical technique, and results. *J Thorac Cardiovasc Surg* 70:440-449, 1975

603. Boden WE, Sadaniantz A: Ventricular septal rupture during ibuprofen therapy for pericarditis after acute myocardial infarction. *Am J Cardiol* 55:1631-1632, 1985

604. Binetti G, Maresta A, Piovaccari G, et al: Aneurisma ventricolare e rottura del setto interventricolare postinfartuale in un caso con coronarie "normali." *G Ital Cardiol* 11:144-150, 1981

605. Longo EA, Cohen LS: Rupture of interventricular septum in acute myocardial infarction. *Am Heart J* 92:81-85, 1976

606. Mann JM, Roberts WC: Cardiac morphologic observations after operative closure of acquired ventricular septal defect during acute myocardial infarction: analysis of 16 necropsy patients. *Am J Cardiol* 60:981-987, 1987

607. Edwards BS, Edwards WD, Edwards JE: Ventricular septal rupture complicating acute myocardial infarction: identification of simple and complex types in 53 autopsied hearts. *Am J Cardiol* 54:1201-1205, 1984

608. Scanlan JG, Seward JB, Tajik AJ: Visualization of ventricular septal rupture utilizing wide-angle two-dimensional echocardiography. *Mayo Clin Proc* 54:381-384, 1979

609. Gowda KS, Loh CW, Roberts R: The simultaneous occurrence of a ventricular septal defect and mitral insufficiency after myocardial infarction. *Am Heart J* 92:234-236, 1976

610. Hutchins GM: Rupture of the intraventricular septum complicating myocardial infarction: pathological analysis of ten patients with clinically diagnosed perforations. *Am Heart J* 97:165-173, 1979

611. James TN: De subitaneis mortibus. XXIV. Ruptured interventricular septum and heart block. *Circulation* 55:934-946, 1977

612. Vlodaver Z, Edwards JE: Rupture of ventricular septum or papillary muscle complicating myocardial infarction. *Circulation* 55:815-822, 1977

613. Khan MM, Asgill ML, Mackinnon J: Electrocardiographic changes produced by septal rupture after acute myocardial infarction. *Ir J Med Sci* 150:144-151, 1981

614. Fortin DF, Sheikh KH, Kisslo J: The utility of echocardiography in the diagnostic strategy of postinfarction ventricular septal rupture: a comparison of two-dimensional echocardiography versus Doppler color flow imaging. *Am Heart J* 121:25-32, 1991

615. Meister SG, Helfant RH: Rapid bedside differentiation of ruptured interventricular septum from acute mitral insufficiency. *N Engl J Med* 287:1024-1025, 1972

616. Giuliani ER, Danielson GK, Pluth JR, et al: Postinfarction ventricular septal rupture: surgical considerations and results. *Circulation* 49:455-459, 1974

617. Hillis LD, Firth BG, Winniford MD: Variability of right-sided cardiac oxygen saturations in adults with and without left-to-right intracardiac shunting. *Am J Cardiol* 58:129-132, 1986

618. Tatooles CJ, Gault JH, Mason DT, et al: Reflux of oxygenated blood into the pulmonary artery in severe mitral regurgitation. *Am Heart J* 75:102-106, 1968

619. Drobac M, Schwartz L, Scully HE, et al: Giant left atrial V-waves in post-myocardial infarction ventricular septal defect. *Ann Thorac Surg* 27:347-349, 1979

620. Bansal RC, Eng AK, Shakudo M: Role of two-dimensional echocardiography, pulsed, continuous wave color flow Doppler techniques in the assessment of ventricular septal rupture after myocardial infarction. *Am J Cardiol* 65:852-860, 1990

621. Recusani F, Raisaro A, Sgalambro A, et al: Ventricular septal rupture after myocardial infarction: diagnosis by two-dimensional and pulsed Doppler echocardiography. *Am J Cardiol* 54:277-281, 1984

622. Miyatake K, Okamoto M, Kinoshita N, et al: Doppler echocardiographic features of ventricular septal rupture in myocardial infarction. *J Am Coll Cardiol* 5:182-187, 1985

623. Helmcke F, Mahan EF III, Nanda NC, et al: Two-dimensional echocardiography and Doppler color flow mapping in the diagnosis and prognosis of ventricular septal rupture. *Circulation* 81:1775-1783, 1990

624. Parry G, Goudevenos J, Adams PC, et al: Septal rupture after myocardial infarction: Is very early surgery really worthwhile? *Eur Heart J* 13:373-382, 1992

625. Wynne J, Fishbein MC, Holman BL, et al: Radionuclide scintigraphy in the evaluation of ventricular septal defect complicating acute myocardial infarction. *Cathet Cardiovasc Diagn* 4:189-197, 1978

626. Bedynek JL, Fenoglio JJ Jr, McAllister HA Jr: Rupture of the ventricular septum as a complication of myocardial infarction. *Am Heart J* 97:773-781, 1979

627. Crosby IK, Craver JM, Crampton RS, et al: Resection of acute posterior ventricular aneurysm with repair of ventricular septal defect after acute myocardial infarction. *J Thorac Cardiovasc Surg* 70:57-62, 1975

628. Lufschanowski R, Angelini P, Del Rio C, et al: Ventricular septal rupture secondary to myocardial infarction. *Chest* 65:59-63, 1974
629. Daggett WM: Surgical management of ventricular septal defects complicating myocardial infarction. *World J Surg* 2:753-764, 1978
630. Kaplan MA, Harris CN, Kay JH, et al: Postinfarctional ventricular septal rupture: clinical approach and surgical results. *Chest* 69:734-738, 1976
631. Montoya A, McKeever L, Scanlon P, et al: Early repair of ventricular septal rupture after infarction. *Am J Cardiol* 45:345-348, 1980
632. Tecklenberg PL, Fitzgerald J, Allaire BI, et al: Afterload reduction in the management of postinfarction ventricular septal defect. *Am J Cardiol* 38:956-958, 1976
633. DiSegni E, Kaplinsky E, Klein HO, et al: Treatment of ruptured interventricular septum with afterload reduction. *Arch Intern Med* 138:1427-1429, 1978
634. Khan MM, Patterson GC, O'Kane HO, et al: Management of ventricular septal rupture in acute myocardial infarction. *Br Heart J* 44:570-576, 1980
635. Buckley MJ, Mundth ED, Daggett WM, et al: Surgical management of ventricular septal defects and mitral regurgitation complicating acute myocardial infarction. *Ann Thorac Surg* 16:598-607, 1973
636. Gold HK, Leinbach RC, Sanders CA, et al: Intraaortic balloon pumping for ventricular septal defect or mitral regurgitation complicating acute myocardial infarction. *Circulation* 47:1191-1196, 1973
637. Skillington PD, Davies RH, Luff AJ, et al: Surgical treatment for infarct-related ventricular septal defects. Improved early results combined with analysis of late functional status. *J Thorac Cardiovasc Surg* 99:798-808, 1990
638. Gunnar RM, Loeb HS, Scanlon PJ, et al: Management of acute myocardial infarction and accelerating angina. *Prog Cardiovasc Dis* 22:1-30, 1979
639. Babb JD, Waldhausen JA, Zelis R: Balloon-induced right ventricular outflow obstruction: a new approach to control of acute interventricular shunting after myocardial infarction in canines and swine. *Circ Res* 40:372-379, 1977
640. Godley RW, Weyman AE, Feigenbaum H, et al: Patterns of mitral leaflet motion in patients with probable papillary muscle dysfunction (abstract). *Am J Cardiol* 43:411, 1979
641. Phaneuf DC, Waters DD, Théroux P, et al: Chronic oral vasodilator therapy to control heart failure in postinfarction ventricular septal defect. *Cathet Cardiovasc Diagn* 5:277-282, 1979
642. Kirklin JW, Barratt-Boyes BG: *Cardiac Surgery. Morphology, Diagnostic Criteria, Natural History, Techniques, Results, and Indications.* New York, John Wiley & Sons, 1986
643. Cooley DA, Belmonte BA, Zeis LB, et al: Surgical repair of ruptured interventricular septum following acute myocardial infarction. *Surgery* 41:930-937, 1957
644. Brandt B III, Wright CB, Ehrenhaft JL: Ventricular septal defect following myocardial infarction. *Ann Thorac Surg* 27:580-589, 1979
645. Mallory GK, White PD, Salcedo-Salgar J: The speed of healing of myocardial infarction: a study of the pathologic anatomy in seventy-two cases. *Am Heart J* 18:647-671, 1939
646. Austen WG, Sokol DM, DeSanctis RW, et al: Surgical treatment of papillary-muscle rupture complicating myocardial infarction. *N Engl J Med* 278:1137-1141, 1968
647. Kitamura S, Mendez A, Kay JH: Ventricular septal defect following myocardial infarction: experience with surgical repair through a left ventriculotomy and review of literature. *J Thorac Cardiovasc Surg* 61:186-199, 1971
648. Matsui K, Kay JH, Mendez M, et al: Ventricular septal rupture secondary to myocardial infarction: clinical approach and surgical results. *JAMA* 245:1537-1539, 1981
649. Gaudiani VA, Miller DC, Stinson EB, et al: Postinfarction ventricular septal defect: an argument for early operation. *Surgery* 89:48-54, 1981
650. Loisance DY, Cachera JP, Poulain H, et al: Ventricular septal defect after acute myocardial infarction: early repair. *J Thorac Cardiovasc Surg* 80:61-67, 1980
651. Forfar JC, Irving JB, Miller HC, et al: The management of ventricular septal rupture following myocardial infarction. *Q J Med* 49:205-217, 1980
652. Heitmiller R, Jacobs ML, Daggett WM: Surgical management of postinfarction ventricular septal rupture. *Ann Thorac Surg* 41:683-691, 1986
653. Daggett WM, Buckley MJ: The surgical treatment of postinfarction ventricular septal defect: indications, techniques, and results. In *Surgery for the Complications of Myocardial Infarction.* Edited by JM Moran, LL Michaelis. New York, Grune & Stratton, 1980, pp 211-230
654. Kopf GS, Meshkov A, Laks H, et al: Changing patterns in the surgical management of ventricular septal rupture after myocardial infarction. *Am J Surg* 143:465-472, 1982
655. Daggett WM: Surgical technique for early repair of posterior ventricular septal rupture. *J Thorac Cardiovasc Surg* 84:306-312, 1982
656. Payne WS, Hunt JC, Kirklin JW: Surgical repair of ventricular septal defect due to myocardial infarction. *JAMA* 183:603-605, 1963
657. Daggett WM, Buckley MJ, Akins CW, et al: Improved results of surgical management of postinfarction ventricular septal rupture. *Ann Surg* 196:269-277, 1982
658. Miyamoto AT, Lee ME, Kass RM, et al: Post-myocardial infarction ventricular septal defect: improved outlook. *J Thorac Cardiovasc Surg* 86:41-46, 1983
659. Jones MT, Schofield PM, Dark JF, et al: Surgical repair of acquired ventricular septal defect: determinants of early and late outcome. *J Thorac Cardiovasc Surg* 93:680-686, 1987
660. Keenan DJ, Monro JL, Ross JK, et al: Acquired ventricular septal defect. *J Thorac Cardiovasc Surg* 85:116-119, 1983
661. Weintraub RM, Thurer RL, Wei J, et al: Repair of postinfarction ventricular septal defect in the elderly. Early and long-term results. *J Thorac Cardiovasc Surg* 85:191-196, 1983
662. Heikkilä J: Mitral incompetence as a complication of acute myocardial infarction. *Acta Med Scand [Suppl]* 475:1-139, 1967
663. Lehmann KG, Francis CK, Dodge HT, et al: Mitral regurgitation in early myocardial infarction. Incidence, clinical detection, and prognostic implications. *Ann Intern Med* 117:10-17, 1992
664. Becker AE, Anderson RH: Mitral insufficiency complicating acute myocardial infarction. *Eur J Cardiol* 2:351-359, 1975
665. Roberts WC, Perloff JK: Mitral valvular disease: a clinicopathologic survey of the conditions causing the mitral valve to function abnormally. *Ann Intern Med* 77:939-975, 1972
666. Davison S: Spontaneous rupture of a papillary muscle of the heart: a report of three cases and a review of the literature. *J Mount Sinai Hosp NY* 14:941-953, 1948
667. Sanders RJ, Neubuerger KT, Ravin A: Rupture of papillary muscles: occurrence of rupture of the posterior muscle in posterior myocardial infarction. *Dis Chest* 31:316-323, 1957
668. Mintz GS, Victor MF, Kotler MN, et al: Two-dimensional echocardiographic identification of surgically correctable complications of acute myocardial infarction. *Circulation* 64:91-96, 1981
669. Wei JY, Hutchins GM, Bulkley BH: Papillary muscle rupture in fatal acute myocardial infarction: a potentially treatable form of cardiogenic shock. *Ann Intern Med* 90:149-152, 1979
670. DeBusk RF, Harrison DC: The clinical spectrum of papillary-muscle disease. *N Engl J Med* 281:1458-1467, 1969
671. Shelburne JC, Rubinstein D, Gorlin R: A reappraisal of papillary muscle dysfunction: correlative clinical and angiographic study. *Am J Med* 46:862-871, 1969
672. Cederqvist L, Söderström J: Papillary muscle rupture in myocardial infarction: a study based upon an autopsy material. *Acta Med Scand* 176:287-292, 1964
673. Burch GE, DePasquale NP, Phillips JH: Clinical manifestations of papillary muscle dysfunction. *Arch Intern Med* 112:112-117, 1963
674. Burch GE, DePasquale NP, Phillips JH: The syndrome of papillary muscle dysfunction. *Am Heart J* 75:399-415, 1968
675. Tsakiris AG, Rastelli GC, Amorim DdeS, et al: Effect of experimental papillary muscle damage on mitral valve closure in intact anesthetized dogs. *Mayo Clin Proc* 45:275-285, 1970
676. Mittal AK, Langston M Jr, Cohn KE, et al: Combined papillary muscle and left ventricular wall dysfunction as a cause of mitral regurgitation: an experimental study. *Circulation* 44:174-180, 1971
677. Merin G, Giuliani ER, Pluth JR, et al: Surgery for mitral valve incompetence after myocardial infarction. *Am J Cardiol* 32:322-324, 1973
678. Fox AC, Glassman E, Isom OW: Surgically remediable complications of myocardial infarction. *Prog Cardiovasc Dis* 21:461-484, 1979
679. Kishon Y, Oh JK, Schaff HV, et al: Mitral valve operation in postinfarction rupture of a papillary muscle: immediate results and long-term follow-up of 22 patients. *Mayo Clin Proc* 67:1023-1030, 1992
680. Perrault MA, Leclercq JF, Masquet C, et al: Infarctus massif biventriculaire avec rupture d'un pilier mitral et d'un pilier tricuspidien: étude anatomique. *Arch Mal Coeur* 70:1091-1095, 1977

681. Wei JY, Hutchins GM: The pathogenesis of papillary muscle rupture complicating myocardial infarction: hemorrhage accompanying contraction band necrosis. *Lab Invest* 39:204-209, 1978

682. Radford MJ, Johnson RA, Buckley MJ, et al: Survival following mitral valve replacement for mitral regurgitation due to coronary artery disease. *Circulation* 60 Suppl 1:39-47, 1979

683. Gahl K, Sutton R, Pearson M, et al: Mitral regurgitation in coronary heart disease. *Br Heart J* 39:13-18, 1977

684. Maisel AS, Gilpin EA, Klein L, et al: A murmur of papillary muscle dysfunction in acute myocardial infarction: clinical features and prognostic implications. *Am Heart J* 112:705-711, 1986

685. Barzilai B, Davis VG, Stone PH, et al: Prognostic significance of mitral regurgitation in acute myocardial infarction. *Am J Cardiol* 65:1169-1175, 1990

686. Walsh RA, O'Rourke RA: The diagnosis and management of acute left-sided valvular regurgitation. *Curr Probl Cardiol* 4:1-34, December 1979

687. Fuchs RM, Heuser RR, Yin FCP, et al: Limitations of pulmonary wedge V waves in diagnosing mitral regurgitation. *Am J Cardiol* 49:849-854, 1982

688. Pichard AD, Kay R, Smith H, et al: Large V waves in the pulmonary wedge pressure tracing in the absence of mitral regurgitation. *Am J Cardiol* 50:1044-1050, 1982

689. Nishimura RA, Shub C, Tajik AJ: Two dimensional echocardiographic diagnosis of partial papillary muscle rupture. *Br Heart J* 48:598-600, 1982

690. Bishop HL, Gibson RS, Stamm RB, et al: Role of two-dimensional echocardiography in the evaluation of patients with ventricular septal rupture postmyocardial infarction. *Am Heart J* 102:965-971, 1981

691. Farcot JC, Boisante L, Rigaud M, et al: Two dimensional echocardiographic visualization of ventricular septal rupture after acute anterior myocardial infarction. *Am J Cardiol* 45:370-377, 1980

692. Ahmad S, Kleiger RE, Conners J, et al: The echocardiographic diagnosis of rupture of a papillary muscle. *Chest* 73:232-234, 1978

693. Parisi AF, Moynihan PF, Folland ED, et al: Echocardiography in acute and remote myocardial infarction. *Am J Cardiol* 46:1205-1214, 1980

694. Erbel R, Schweizer P, Bardos P, et al: Two-dimensional echocardiographic diagnosis of papillary muscle rupture. *Chest* 79:595-598, 1981

695. Zone DD, Botti RE: Right ventricular infarction with tricuspid insufficiency and chronic right heart failure. *Am J Cardiol* 37:445-448, 1976

696. Helmcke F, Nanda NC, Hsiung MC, et al: Color Doppler assessment of mitral regurgitation with orthogonal planes. *Circulation* 75:175-183, 1987

697. Chatterjee K, Parmley WW, Swan HJC, et al: Beneficial effects of vasodilator agents in severe mitral regurgitation due to dysfunction of subvalvar apparatus. *Circulation* 48:684-690, 1973

698. Massie BM, Chatterjee K: Vasodilator therapy of pump failure complicating acute myocardial infarction. *Med Clin North Am* 63:25-51, January 1979

699. Greenberg BH, Massie BM, Brundage BH, et al: Beneficial effects of hydralazine in severe mitral regurgitation. *Circulation* 58:273-279, 1978

700. Kouchoukos NT: Surgical treatment of acute complications of myocardial infarction. In *Critical Care Cardiology.* Edited by CE Rackley. Philadelphia, FA Davis Company, 1981, pp 141-149

701. Gerbode FLA, Hetzer R, Krebber HJ: Surgical management of papillary muscle rupture due to myocardial infarction. *World J Surg* 2:791-796, 1978

702. Gann D, Colin C, Hildner FJ, et al: Mitral valve replacement in medically unresponsive congestive heart failure due to papillary muscle dysfunction. *Circulation* 56 Suppl 2:101-104, 1977

703. Glancy DL, Stinson EB, Shepherd RL, et al: Results of valve replacement for severe mitral regurgitation due to papillary muscle rupture or fibrosis. *Am J Cardiol* 32:313-321, 1973

704. Rankin JS, Feneley MP, Hickey MS, et al: A clinical comparison of mitral valve repair versus valve replacement in ischemic mitral regurgitation. *J Thorac Cardiovasc Surg* 95:165-177, 1988

705. Hickey MStJ, Smith LR, Muhlbaier LH, et al: Current prognosis of ischemic mitral regurgitation: implications for future management. *Circulation* 78 Suppl I:51-59, 1988

706. Kopelman HA, Forman MB, Wilson BH, et al: Right ventricular myocardial infarction in patients with chronic lung disease: possible role of right ventricular hypertrophy. *J Am Coll Cardiol* 5:1302-1307, 1985

707. Coma-Canella I, Gamallo C, Onsurbe PM, et al: Acute right ventricular infarction secondary to massive pulmonary embolism. *Eur Heart J* 9:534-540, 1988

708. Rigo P, Murray M, Strauss HW, et al: Left ventricular function in acute myocardial infarction evaluated by gated scintiphotography. *Circulation* 50:678-684, 1974

709. Wartman WB, Hellerstein HK: The incidence of heart disease in 2,000 consecutive autopsies. *Ann Intern Med* 28:41-65, 1948

710. Cohn JN, Guiha NH, Broder MI, et al: Right ventricular infarction: clinical and hemodynamic features. *Am J Cardiol* 33:209-214, 1974

711. Isner JM, Roberts WC: Right ventricular infarction complicating left ventricular infarction secondary to coronary heart disease: frequency, location, associated findings, and significance from analysis of 236 necropsy patients with acute or healed myocardial infarction. *Am J Cardiol* 42:885-894, 1978

712. Wackers FJT, Lie KI, Sokole EB, et al: Prevalence of right ventricular involvement in inferior wall infarction assessed with myocardial imaging with thallium-201 and technetium-99m pyrophosphate. *Am J Cardiol* 42:358-362, 1978

713. Lorell B, Leinbach RC, Pohost GM, et al: Right ventricular infarction: clinical diagnosis and differentiation from cardiac tamponade and pericardial constriction. *Am J Cardiol* 43:465-471, 1979

714. Erhardt LR: Right ventricular involvement in acute myocardial infarction. *Eur J Cardiol* 4:411-418, 1976

715. Cintron GB, Hernandez E, Linares E, et al: Bedside recognition, incidence, and clinical course of right ventricular infarction. *Am J Cardiol* 47:224-227, 1981

716. Lloyd EA, Gersh BJ, Kennelly BM: Hemodynamic spectrum of "dominant" right ventricular infarction in 19 patients. *Am J Cardiol* 48:1016-1022, 1981

717. Isner JM: Right ventricular myocardial infarction. *JAMA* 259: 712-718, 1988

718. Cabin HS, Clubb S, Wackers FJT, et al: Right ventricular myocardial infarction with anterior wall left ventricular infarction: an autopsy study. *Am Heart J* 113:16-23, 1987

719. Ratliff NB, Hackel DB: Combined right and left ventricular infarction: pathogenesis and clinicopathologic correlations. *Am J Cardiol* 45:217-221, 1980

720. Roeske WR, Savage RM, O'Rourke RA, et al: Clinicopathologic correlations in patients after myocardial infarction. *Circulation* 63:36-45, 1981

721. Berger PB, Ruocco NA Jr, Ryan TJ, et al: Frequency and significance of right ventricular dysfunction during inferior wall left ventricular myocardial infarction treated with thrombolytic therapy (results from the Thrombolysis in Myocardial Infarction [TIMI] II trial). *Am J Cardiol* 71:1148-1152, 1993

722. Kikis D, Esser H, Stiens R, et al: Mitbeteiligung des rechten Ventrikels beim akuten Myokardinfarkt. *Med Klin* 72:1372-1378, 1977

723. Erhardt LR: Clinical and pathological observations in different types of acute myocardial infarction: a study of 84 patients deceased after treatment in a coronary care unit. *Acta Med Scand* [Suppl] 560:1-78, 1974

724. Wade WG: The pathogenesis of infarction of the right ventricle. *Br Heart J* 21:545-554, 1959

725. Peter RH, Ramo BW, Ratliff N, et al: Collateral vessel development after right ventricular infarction in the pig. *Am J Cardiol* 29:56-60, 1972

726. James TN: The coronary circulation and conduction system in acute myocardial infarction. *Prog Cardiovasc Dis* 10:410-449, 1968

727. Grose R, Spindola-Franco H: Right ventricular dysfunction in acute ventricular septal defect. *Am Heart J* 101:67-74, 1981

728. McAllister RG, Friesinger GC, Sinclair-Smith BC: Tricuspid regurgitation following inferior myocardial infarction. *Arch Intern Med* 136:95-99, 1976

729. Vatterott PJ, Nishimura RA, Gersh BJ, et al: Severe isolated tricuspid insufficiency in coronary artery disease. *Int J Cardiol* 14:295-301, 1987

730. Korr KS, Levinson H, Bough EW, et al: Tricuspid valve replacement for cardiogenic shock after acute right ventricular infarction. *JAMA* 244:1958-1960, 1980

731. Kagan A: Dynamic responses of the right ventricle following extensive damage by cauterization. *Circulation* 5:816-823, 1952

732. Guiha NH, Limas CJ, Cohn JN: Predominant right ventricular dysfunction after right ventricular destruction in the dog. *Am J Cardiol* 33:254-258, 1974
733. Bakos ACP: The question of the function of the right ventricular myocardium: an experimental study. *Circulation* 1:724-732, 1950
734. Donald DE, Essex HE: Pressure studies after inactivation of the major portion of the canine right ventricle. *Am J Physiol* 176:155-161, 1954
735. Santamore WP, Lynch PR, Heckman JL, et al: Left ventricular effects on right ventricular developed pressure. *J Appl Physiol* 41:925-930, 1976
736. Starr I, Jeffers WA, Meade RH Jr: The absence of conspicuous increments of venous pressure after severe damage to the right ventricle of the dog with a discussion of the relation between clinical congestive failure and heart disease. *Am Heart J* 26:291-301, 1943
737. Glenn WWL: Circulatory bypass of the right side of the heart. IV. Shunt between superior vena cava and distal right pulmonary artery: report of clinical application. *N Engl J Med* 259:117-120, 1958
738. Fontan F, Baudet E: Surgical repair of tricuspid atresia. *Thorax* 26:240-248, 1971
739. Jensen DP, Goolsby JP Jr, Oliva PB: Hemodynamic pattern resembling pericardial constriction after acute inferior myocardial infarction with right ventricular infarction. *Am J Cardiol* 42:858-861, 1978
740. Lopez-Sendon J, Coma-Canella I, Gamallo C: Sensitivity and specificity of hemodynamic criteria in the diagnosis of acute right ventricular infarction. *Circulation* 64:515-525, 1981
741. Goldstein JA, Barzilai B, Rosamond TL, et al: Determinants of hemodynamic compromise with severe right ventricular infarction. *Circulation* 82:359-368, 1990
742. Zaus EA, Kearns WM Jr: Massive infarction of the right ventricle and atrium: report of a case. *Circulation* 6:593-598, 1952
743. Gewirtz H, Gold HK, Fallon JT, et al: Role of right ventricular infarction in cardiogenic shock associated with inferior myocardial infarction. *Br Heart J* 42:719-725, 1979
744. Reuben SR, Swadling JP, Gersh BJ, et al: Impedance and transmission properties of the pulmonary arterial system. *Cardiovasc Res* 5:1-9, 1971
745. Stool EW, Mullins CB, Leshin SJ, et al: Dimensional changes of the left ventricle during acute pulmonary arterial hypertension in dogs. *Am J Cardiol* 33:868-875, 1974
746. Berger HJ, Matthay RA, Davies RA, et al: Comparison of exercise right ventricular performance in chronic obstructive pulmonary disease and coronary artery disease: noninvasive assessment by quantitative radionuclide angiocardiography. *Invest Radiol* 14:342-353, 1979
747. Sharkey SW, Shelley W, Carlyle PF, et al: M-mode and two-dimensional echocardiographic analysis of the septum in experimental right ventricular infarction: correlation with hemodynamic alterations. *Am Heart J* 110:1210-1218, 1985
748. Silber EN, Katz LN: *Heart Disease.* New York, Macmillan Publishing Co, 1975, pp 11-12
749. Goldstein JA, Vlahakes GJ, Verrier ED, et al: The role of right ventricular systolic dysfunction and elevated intrapericardial pressure in the genesis of low output in experimental right ventricular infarction. *Circulation* 65:513-522, 1982
750. Shaper AG, Hutt MSR, Coles RM: Necropsy study of endomyocardial fibrosis and rheumatic heart disease in Uganda 1950-1965. *Br Heart J* 30:391-401, 1968
751. Coma-Canella I, Lopez-Sendon J: Ventricular compliance in ischemic right ventricular dysfunction. *Am J Cardiol* 45:555-561, 1980
752. Dell'Italia LJ, Starling MR, O'Rourke RA: Physical examination for exclusion of hemodynamically important right ventricular infarction. *Ann Intern Med* 99:608-611, 1983
753. Vijay NK, Grow JB Sr, Schoonmaker FW: Right ventricular and septal rupture from myocardial infarction: a case report. *Rocky Mountain Med J* 73:205-207, 1976
754. D'Arcy B, Nanda NC: Two-dimensional echocardiographic features of right ventricular infarction. *Circulation* 65:167-173, 1982
755. Rackley CE, Russell RO Jr, Mantle JA, et al: Right ventricular infarction and function. *Am Heart J* 101:215-218, 1981
756. Erhardt LR, Sjögren A, Wahlberg I: Single right-sided precordial lead in the diagnosis of right ventricular involvement in inferior myocardial infarction. *Am Heart J* 91:571-576, 1976
757. Candell-Riera J, Figueras J, Valle V, et al: Right ventricular infarction: relationships between ST segment elevation in V_4R and hemodynamic, scintigraphic, and echocardiographic findings in patients with acute inferior myocardial infarction. *Am Heart J* 101:281-287, 1981
758. Croft CH, Nicod P, Corbett JR, et al: Detection of acute right ventricular infarction by right precordial electrocardiography. *Am J Cardiol* 50:421-427, 1982
759. Klein HO, Tordjman T, Ninio R, et al: The early recognition of right ventricular infarction: diagnostic accuracy of the electrocardiographic V_4R lead. *Circulation* 67:558-565, 1983
760. Lopez-Sendon J, Coma-Canella I, Alcasena S, et al: Electrocardiographic findings in acute right ventricular infarction: sensitivity and specificity of electrocardiographic alterations in right precordial leads V_4R, V_3R, V_1, V_2 and V_3. *J Am Coll Cardiol* 6:1273-1279, 1985
761. Coma-Canella I, López-Sendón J, Alcasena S, et al: Electrocardiographic alterations in leads V_1 to V_3 in the diagnosis of right and left ventricular infarction. *Am Heart J* 112:940-946, 1986
762. Geft IL, Shah PK, Rodriguez L, et al: ST elevations in leads V_1 to V_5 may be caused by right coronary artery occlusion and acute right ventricular infarction. *Am J Cardiol* 53:991-996, 1984
763. Yasuda T, Okada RD, Leinbach RC, et al: Serial evaluation of right ventricular dysfunction associated with acute inferior myocardial infarction. *Am Heart J* 119:816-822, 1990
764. Baigrie RS, Haq A, Morgan CD, et al: The spectrum of right ventricular involvement in inferior wall myocardial infarction: a clinical, hemodynamic and noninvasive study. *J Am Coll Cardiol* 1:1396-1404, 1983
765. Starling MR, Dell'Italia LJ, Chaudhuri TK, et al: First transit and equilibrium radionuclide angiography in patients with inferior transmural myocardial infarction: criteria for the diagnosis of associated hemodynamically significant right ventricular infarction. *J Am Coll Cardiol* 4:923-930, 1984
766. Lopez-Sendon J, Garcia-Fernandez MA, Coma-Canella I, et al: Segmental right ventricular function after acute myocardial infarction: two-dimensional echocardiographic study in 63 patients. *Am J Cardiol* 51:390-396, 1983
767. Dell'Italia LJ, Starling MR, Crawford MH, et al: Right ventricular infarction: identification by hemodynamic measurements before and after volume loading and correlation with noninvasive techniques. *J Am Coll Cardiol* 4:931-939, 1984
768. Cecchi F, Zuppiroli A, Favilli S, et al: Echocardiographic features of right ventricular infarction. *Clin Cardiol* 7:405-412, 1984
769. Herrick JB: Clinical features of sudden obstruction of the coronary arteries. *JAMA* 59:2015-2020, 1912
770. Lassers BW, George M, Anderton JL, et al: Left ventricular failure in acute myocardial infarction. *Am J Cardiol* 25:511-522, 1970
771. Fluck DC, Valentine PA, Treister B, et al: Right heart pressures in acute myocardial infarction. *Br Heart J* 29:748-757, 1967
772. Ahnve S, Erhardt LR, Lindvall K, et al: Cardiac filling pressures in acute inferior myocardial infarction with and without right ventricular involvement. *Eur J Cardiol* 7:125-130, 1978
773. Zehender M, Kasper W, Kauder E, et al: Right ventricular infarction as an independent predictor of prognosis after acute inferior myocardial infarction. *N Engl J Med* 328:981-988, 1993
774. Daubert JC, Mattheyses M, Fourdilis M, et al: L'infarctus du ventricule droit. 2. Incidences pronostiques et thérapeutiques. *Arch Mal Coeur* 70:257-264, 1977
775. Mavric Z, Zaputovic L, Matana A, et al: Prognostic significance of complete atrioventricular block in patients with acute inferior myocardial infarction with and without right ventricular involvement. *Am Heart J* 119:823-828, 1990
776. Sharpe DN, Botvinick EH, Shames DM, et al: The noninvasive diagnosis of right ventricular infarction. *Circulation* 57:483-490, 1978
777. Raabe DS Jr, Chester AC: Right ventricular infarction. *Chest* 73:96-99, 1978
778. Steele P, Kirch D, Ellis J, et al: Prompt return to normal of depressed right ventricular ejection fraction in acute inferior infarction. *Br Heart J* 39:1319-1323, 1977
779. Hellman C, Zafrir N, Arditi A, et al: Improvement of ventricular function after acute right ventricular myocardial infarction (abstract). *Circulation* 62 Suppl 3:313, 1980
780. Dell'Italia LJ, Lembo NJ, Starling MR, et al: Hemodynamically important right ventricular infarction: follow-up evaluation of right ventricular systolic function at rest and during exercise with radionuclide ventriculography and respiratory gas exchange. *Circulation* 75:996-1003, 1987

781. Goldstein JA, Vlahakes GJ, Verrier ED, et al: Volume loading improves low cardiac output in experimental right ventricular infarction. *J Am Coll Cardiol* 2:270-278, 1983
782. Cohn JN: Right ventricular infarction revisited. *Am J Cardiol* 43:666-668, 1979
783. Isner JM, Fisher GP, Del Negro AA, et al: Right ventricular infarction with hemodynamic decompensation due to transient loss of active atrial augmentation: successful treatment with atrial pacing. *Am Heart J* 102:792-794, 1981
784. Topol EJ, Goldschlager N, Ports TA, et al: Hemodynamic benefit of atrial pacing in right ventricular myocardial infarction. *Ann Intern Med* 96:594-597, 1982
785. Love JC, Haffajee CI, Gore JM, et al: Reversibility of hypotension and shock by atrial or atrioventricular sequential pacing in patients with right ventricular infarction. *Am Heart J* 108:5-13, 1984
786. Sclarovsky S, Zafrir N, Strasberg B, et al: Ventricular fibrillation complicating temporary ventricular pacing in acute myocardial infarction: significance of right ventricular infarction. *Am J Cardiol* 48:1160-1166, 1981
787. Pell S, D'Alonzo CA: Immediate mortality of five-year survival of employed men with a first myocardial infarction. *N Engl J Med* 270:915-922, 1964
788. Peel AAF, Semple T, Wang I, et al: A coronary prognostic index for grading the severity of infarction. *Br Heart J* 24:745-760, 1962
789. Connolly DC, Elveback LR, Oxman HA: Coronary heart disease in residents of Rochester, Minnesota, 1950-1975. III. Effect of hypertension and its treatment on survival of patients with coronary artery disease. *Mayo Clin Proc* 58:249-254, 1983
790. Beard OW, Hipp HR, Robins M, et al: Initial myocardial infarction among 503 veterans: five-year survival. *Am J Med* 28:871-883, 1960
791. Fox KM, Tomlinson IW, Portal RW, et al: Prognostic significance of acute systolic hypertension after myocardial infarction. *Br Med J* 3:128-130, 1975
792. Althouse R, Maynard C, Olsufka M, et al: Risk factors for hemorrhagic and ischemic stroke in myocardial infarct patients treated with tissue plasminogen activator (abstract). *J Am Coll Cardiol* 13 Suppl A:153, 1989
793. Shell WE, Sobel BE: Protection of jeopardized ischemic myocardium by reduction of ventricular afterload. *N Engl J Med* 291:481-486, 1974
794. Pantridge JF, Adgey AAJ, Geddes JS, et al: The Acute Coronary Attack. New York, Grune & Stratton, 1975, pp 26-42
795. Dye LE, Urthaler F, MacLean WAH, et al: New arterial hypertension during myocardial infarction. *South Med J* 71:289-292, 1978
796. Ceremużyński L: Hormonal and metabolic reactions evoked by acute myocardial infarction. *Circ Res* 48:767-776, 1981
797. James TN, Isobe JH, Urthaler F: Analysis of components in a cardiogenic hypertensive chemoreflex. *Circulation* 52:179-192, 1975
798. Brown AM: Excitation of afferent cardiac sympathetic nerve fibres during myocardial ischaemia. *J Physiol* (Lond) 190:35-53, 1967
799. Malliani A, Schwartz PJ, Zanchetti A: A sympathetic reflex elicited by experimental coronary occlusion. *Am J Physiol* 217:703-709, 1969
800. Forrester JS, Chatterjee K, Swan HJC: Hemodynamic monitoring in patients with acute myocardial infarction. *JAMA* 226:60-61, 1973
801. Bennett ED, Brooks NH, Keddie J, et al: Increased renal function in patients with acute left ventricular failure: a possible homeostatic mechanism. *Clin Sci Molec Med* 52:43-50, 1977
802. Mueller HS, Ayres SM, Religa A, et al: Propranolol in the treatment of acute myocardial infarction: effect on myocardial oxygenation and hemodynamics. *Circulation* 49:1078-1087, 1974
803. Opie LH: Metabolism of free fatty acids, glucose, and catecholamines in acute myocardial infarction: relation to myocardial ischemia and infarct size. *Am J Cardiol* 36:938-953, 1975
804. Ahumada GG, Karlsberg RP, Jaffe AS, et al: Reduction of early ventricular arrhythmia by acebutolol in patients with acute myocardial infarction. *Br Heart J* 41:654-659, 1979
805. Sobel BE, Braunwald E: The management of acute myocardial infarction. In *Heart Disease: A Textbook of Cardiovascular Medicine.* Vol 2. Edited by E Braunwald. Philadelphia, WB Saunders Company, 1980, pp 1355-1386
806. Peter T, Norris RM, Clarke ED, et al: Reduction of enzyme levels by propranolol after acute myocardial infarction. *Circulation* 57:1091-1095, 1978
807. Chiariello M, Gold HK, Leinbach RC, et al: Comparison between the effects of nitroprusside and nitroglycerin on ischemic injury during acute myocardial infarction. *Circulation* 54:766-773, 1976
808. Kuo PT: Management of hypertensive complications in acute myocardial infarction. *Pract Cardiol* 5:197-200, 1979
809. Mueller HS, Rao PS, Fletcher J, et al: Propranolol during the evolution and subsequent ten days of myocardial infarction in man: hemodynamic, initial cardiac energetic, and neurohumoral responses. *Clin Cardiol* 2:393-403, 1979
810. Dressler W: The post-myocardial-infarction syndrome: a report on forty-four cases. *Arch Intern Med* 103:28-42, 1959
811. Likoff W: Pericarditis complicating myocardial infarction. *Am J Cardiol* 7:69-72, 1961
812. Dressler W: A post-myocardial-infarction syndrome: preliminary report of a complication resembling idiopathic, recurrent, benign pericarditis. *JAMA* 160:1379-1383, 1956
813. Lichstein E, Arsura E, Hollander G, et al: Current incidence of postmyocardial infarction (Dressler's) syndrome. *Am J Cardiol* 50:1269-1271, 1982
814. Khan AH: Pericarditis of myocardial infarction: review of the literature with case presentation. *Am Heart J* 90:788-794, 1975
815. Thadani U, Chopra MP, Aber CP, et al: Pericarditis after acute myocardial infarction. *Br Med J* 2:135-137, 1971
816. Toole JC, Silverman ME: Pericarditis of acute myocardial infarction. *Chest* 67:647-653, 1975
817. Kossowsky WA, Epstein PJ, Levine RS: Post myocardial infarction syndrome: an early complication of acute myocardial infarction. *Chest* 63:35-40, 1973
818. Stein I, Prussin G: The early appearance of the postmyocardial infarction syndrome. *Angiology* 20:262-268, 1969
819. Kossowsky WA, Lyon AF, Spain DM: Reappraisal of the postmyocardial infarction Dressler's syndrome. *Am Heart J* 102:954-956, 1981
820. Northcote RJ, Hutchison SJ, McGuinness JB: Evidence for the continued existence of the postmyocardial infarction (Dressler's) syndrome. *Am J Cardiol* 53:1201-1202, 1984
821. Tofler GH, Muller JE, Stone PH, et al: Pericarditis in acute myocardial infarction: characterization and clinical significance. *Am Heart J* 117:86-92, 1989
822. Krainin FM, Flessas AP, Spodick DH: Infarction-associated pericarditis: rarity of diagnostic electrocardiogram. *N Engl J Med* 311:1211-1214, 1984
823. Niarchos AP, McKendrick CS: Prognosis of pericarditis after acute myocardial infarction. *Br Heart J* 35:49-54, 1973
824. Lichstein E, Liu H-M, Gupta P: Pericarditis complicating acute myocardial infarction: incidence of complications and significance of electrocardiogram on admission. *Am Heart J* 87:246-252, 1974
825. Hutter AM Jr, DeSanctis RW, Flynn T, et al: Nontransmural myocardial infarction: a comparison of hospital and late clinical course of patients with that of matched patients with transmural anterior and transmural inferior myocardial infarction. *Am J Cardiol* 48:595-602, 1981
826. Liem KL, Lie KI, Durrer D, et al: Pericarditis in acute myocardial infarction. *Lancet* 2:1004-1006, 1975
827. Parkinson J, Bedford DE: Cardiac infarction and coronary thrombosis. *Lancet* 1:4-11, 1928
828. Sawaya JI, Mujais SK, Armenian HK: Early diagnosis of pericarditis in acute myocardial infarction. *Am Heart J* 100:144-151, 1980
829. Kaplan K, Davison R, Parker M, et al: Frequency of pericardial effusion as determined by M-mode echocardiography in acute myocardial infarction. *Am J Cardiol* 55:335-337, 1985
830. Galve E, Garcia-del-Castillo H, Evangelista A, et al: Pericardial effusion in the course of myocardial infarction: incidence, natural history, and clinical relevance. *Circulation* 73:294-299, 1986
831. Pierard LA, Albert A, Henrard L, et al: Incidence and significance of pericardial effusion in acute myocardial infarction as determined by two-dimensional echocardiography. *J Am Coll Cardiol* 8:517-520, 1986
832. Eisenberg MJ, Oken K, Guerrero S, et al: Prognostic value of echocardiography in hospitalized patients with pericardial effusion. *Am J Cardiol* 70:934-939, 1992
833. Fowler NO: The electrocardiogram in pericarditis. *Cardiovasc Clin* 5 No 3:255-267, 1973
834. Spodick DH: Diagnostic electrocardiographic sequences in acute pericarditis: significance of PR segment and PR vector changes. *Circulation* 48:575-580, 1973

835. McLean KH, Bett JHN, Saltups A: Pericarditis in acute myocardial infarction. *Aust NZ J Med* 5:1-2, 1975
836. Berman J, Haffajee CI, Alpert JS: Therapy of symptomatic pericarditis after myocardial infarction: retrospective and prospective studies of aspirin, indomethacin, prednisone, and spontaneous resolution. *Am Heart J* 101:750-753, 1981
837. Barman PC, Krishnaswami V, Geraci AR: Pericarditis in acute myocardial infarction. *NY State J Med* 73:645-648, 1973
838. Hammerman H, Kloner RA, Schoen FJ, et al: Indomethacin-induced scar thinning after experimental myocardial infarction. *Circulation* 67:1290-1295, 1983
839. Hammerman H, Schoen FJ, Braunwald E, et al: Drug-induced expansion of infarct: morphologic and functional correlations. *Circulation* 69:611-617, 1984
840. Yan V, Hunt D, Sloman G: Pericardial pain in acute myocardial infarction: double blind trial of steroid therapy. *Eur J Cardiol* 1:79-82, 1973
841. Weissbein AS, Heller FN: A method of treatment for pericardial pain. *Circulation* 24:607-612, 1961
842. Anderson MW, Christensen NA, Edwards JE: Hemopericardium complicating myocardial infarction in the absence of cardiac rupture: report of three cases. *Arch Intern Med* 90:634-645, 1952
843. Lange HF, Aarseth S: The influence of anticoagulant therapy on the occurrence of cardiac rupture and hemopericardium following heart infarction. II. A controlled study of a selected treated group based on 1,044 autopsies. *Am Heart J* 56:257-263, 1958
844. Goldstein R, Wolff L: Hemorrhagic pericarditis in acute myocardial infarction treated with bishydroxycoumarin. *JAMA* 146:616-621, 1951
845. Miller RL: Hemopericardium with use of oral anticoagulant therapy. *JAMA* 209:1362-1364, 1969
846. Davidson C, Oliver MF, Robertson RF: Post-myocardial-infarction syndrome. *Br Med J* 2:535-539, 1961
847. Bernstein A: The postmyocardial infarction syndrome of Dressler. *Br J Hosp Med* 17:560-571, 1977
848. Levin EJ, Bryk D: Dressler syndrome (postmyocardial infarction syndrome). *Radiology* 87:731-736, 1966
849. Dressler W: Management of pericarditis secondary to myocardial infarction. *Prog Cardiovasc Dis* 3:134-140, 1960
850. Dressler W, Yurkofsky J, Starr MC: Hemorrhagic pericarditis, pleurisy, and pneumonia complicating recent myocardial infarction. *Am Heart J* 54:42-49, 1957
851. Soloff LA: Pericardial cellular response during the postmyocardial infarction syndrome. *Am Heart J* 82:812-816, 1971
852. Domby WR, Whitcomb ME: Pleural effusion as a manifestation of Dressler's syndrome in the distant post-infarction period. *Am Heart J* 96:243-245, 1978
853. Kennedy HL, Das SK: Postmyocardial infarction (Dressler's) syndrome: report of a case with immunological and viral studies. *Am Heart J* 91:233-239, 1976
854. Gery I, Davies AM, Ehrenfeld EN: Heart-specific autoantibodies. *Lancet* 1:471-472, 1960
855. Van Der Geld H: Anti-heart antibodies in the postpericardiotomy and the postmyocardial infarction syndromes. *Lancet* 2:617-621, 1964
856. Engle MA, Ito T: The postpericardiotomy syndrome. *Am J Cardiol* 7:73-82, 1961
857. Heine WI, Friedman H, Mandell MS, et al: Antibodies to cardiac tissue in acute ischemic heart disease. *Am J Cardiol* 17:798-803, 1966
858. Ehrenfeld EN, Gery I, Davies AM: Specific antibodies in heart disease. *Lancet* 1:1138-1141, 1961
859. Versey JMB, Gabriel R: Soluble-complex formation after myocardial infarction. *Lancet* 2:493-494, 1974
860. Burch GE, Colcolough HL: Postcardiotomy and postinfarction syndromes—a theory. *Am Heart J* 80:290-291, 1970
861. Sawaya MP Jr, Favrot LK, Smith SC Jr: Hemorrhagic cardiac tamponade complicating the postmyocardial infarction syndrome in the absence of anticoagulation. *Heart Lung* 4:770-774, 1975
862. Tew FT, Mantle JA, Russell RO Jr, et al: Cardiac tamponade with nonhemorrhagic pericardial fluid complicating Dressler's syndrome. *Chest* 72:93-95, 1977
863. Fowler NO, Harbin AD III: Recurrent acute pericarditis: follow-up study of 31 patients. *J Am Coll Cardiol* 7:300-305, 1986
864. Connolly DC, Burchell HB: Pericarditis: a ten-year survey. *Am J Cardiol* 7:7-14, 1961
865. Beaufils P, Bardet J, Temkine J, et al: Syndrome de Dressler: Péricardite constrictive post-infarctus opérée avec succès. *Arch Mal Coeur* 68:651-656, 1975
866. Haïat R: Post-myocardial infarction constrictive pericarditis (letter to the editor). *Am Heart J* 101:358, 1981
867. Goldhaber SZ, Lorell BH, Green LH: Constrictive pericarditis: a case requiring pericardiectomy following Dressler's postmyocardial infarction syndrome. *J Thorac Cardiovasc Surg* 81:793-796, 1981
868. Blau N, Shen BA, Pittman DE, et al: Massive hemopericardium in a patient with postmyocardial infarction syndrome. *Chest* 71:549-552, 1977
869. Henrard L, Lisin N: Infarctus du myocarde et péricardite tardive. *Arch Mal Coeur* 72:862-867, 1979
870. Curry CL: The relationship between the post-myocardial infarction syndrome and post-infarction ventricular aneurysm. *J Natl Med Assoc* 64:480-482, 1972
871. Kossowsky WA, Kim K-S, Tobin MS: Antimetabolite therapy in the post-myocardial-infarction syndrome. *Am Heart J* 83:527-531, 1972
872. Guindo J, Rodríguez de la Serna A, Ramio J, et al: Recurrent pericarditis. Relief with colchicine. *Circulation* 82:1117-1120, 1990
873. Gibbons JA, Vieweg WVR: Dressler's syndrome and angina pectoris relieved by surgery. *Chest* 77:431-432, 1980
874. Geltman EM, Schechtman K, Ehsani AA, et al: The influence of infarct size on prognosis among patients with repeat infarction (abstract). *Circulation* 60 Suppl 2:163, 1979
875. Bloor CM, Roeske WR, O'Rourke RA: Clinical pathologic correlates in acute myocardial infarction. *Adv Cardiol* 23:14-24, 1978
876. Hutchins GM, Bulkley BH: Infarct expansion versus extension: two different complications of acute myocardial infarction. *Am J Cardiol* 41:1127-1132, 1978
877. Eaton LW, Bulkley BH: Expansion of acute myocardial infarction: its relationship to infarct morphology in a canine model. *Circ Res* 49:80-88, 1981
878. Schuster EH, Bulkley BH: Expansion of transmural myocardial infarction: a pathophysiologic factor in cardiac rupture. *Circulation* 60:1532-1538, 1979
879. Hochman JS, Bulkley BH: Pathogenesis of left ventricular aneurysms: an experimental study in the rat model. *Am J Cardiol* 50:83-88, 1982
880. Hochman JS, Bulkley BH: Expansion of acute myocardial infarction: an experimental study. *Circulation* 65:1446-1450, 1982
881. Eaton LW, Weiss JL, Bulkley BH, et al: Regional cardiac dilatation after acute myocardial infarction: recognition by two-dimensional echocardiography. *N Engl J Med* 300:57-62, 1979
882. White HD, Norris RM, Brown MA, et al: Left ventricular end-systolic volume as the major determinant of survival after recovery from myocardial infarction. *Circulation* 76:44-51, 1987
883. Hammermeister KE, DeRouen TA, Dodge HT: Variables predictive of survival in patients with coronary disease: selection by univariate and multivariate analyses from the clinical, electrocardiographic, exercise, arteriographic, and quantitative angiographic evaluations. *Circulation* 59:421-430, 1979
884. Norris RM, Barnaby PF, Brandt PWT, et al: Prognosis after recovery from first acute myocardial infarction: determinants of reinfarction and sudden death. *Am J Cardiol* 53:408-413, 1984
885. O'Keefe JH, Chesebro JH, Bove AA, et al: Prevention of left ventricular dilatation after myocardial infarction by successful thrombolysis (abstract). *J Am Coll Cardiol* 9:61A, 1987
886. Weisman HF, Bush DE, Mannisi JA, et al: Early reperfusion reduces the severity of infarct expansion (abstract). *Circulation* 70 Suppl 2:261, 1984
887. Hochman JS, Choo H: Limitation of myocardial infarct expansion by reperfusion independent of myocardial salvage. *Circulation* 75:299-306, 1987
888. Connelly CM, Vogel WM, Wiegner AW, et al: Effects of reperfusion after coronary artery occlusion on post-infarction scar tissue. *Circ Res* 57:562-577, 1985
889. Hale SL, Kloner RA: Left ventricular topographic alterations in the completely healed rat infarct caused by early and late coronary artery reperfusion. *Am Heart J* 116:1508-1513, 1988
890. Gaasch WH, Bing OHL, Pine MB, et al: Myocardial contracture during prolonged ischemic arrest and reperfusion. *Am J Physiol* 235:H619-H627, 1978
891. Nolan SE, Weiss JL, Shapiro EP, et al: Early tPA during acute

anterior myocardial infarction reduces infarct expansion: a randomized placebo controlled trial (abstract). *Circulation* 78 Suppl 2:438, 1988

892. Marino P, Zanolla L, Golia G, et al: Effects of intravenous streptokinase on left ventricular modeling after myocardial infarction: the GISSI trial (abstract). *Circulation* 78 Suppl II:275, 1988

893. Hamano Y, Minamino T, Katoh O, et al: Intracoronary thrombolysis limits the complication with left ventricular aneurysm in acute myocardial infarction (abstract). *Circulation* 78 Suppl 2:502, 1988

894. Pfeffer MA, Lamas GA, Vaughan DE, et al: Effect of captopril on progressive ventricular dilatation after anterior myocardial infarction. *N Engl J Med* 319:80-86, 1988

895. Marmor A, Sobel BE, Roberts R: Factors presaging early recurrent myocardial infarction ("extension"). *Am J Cardiol* 48:603-610, 1981

896. Reid PR, Taylor DR, Kelly DT, et al: Myocardial-infarct extension detected by precordial ST-segment mapping. *N Engl J Med* 290:123-128, 1974

897. Fraker TD Jr, Wagner GS, Rosati RA: Extension of myocardial infarction: incidence and prognosis. *Circulation* 60:1126-1129, 1979

898. Marmor A, Geltman EM, Schechtman K, et al: Recurrent myocardial infarction: clinical predictors and prognostic implications. *Circulation* 66:415-421, 1982

899. Baker JT, Bramlet DA, Lester RM, et al: Myocardial infarct extension: incidence and relationship to survival. *Circulation* 65:918-923, 1982

900. Strauss HD: Myocardial infarction extension: clinical significance. *Primary Cardiol* 8:1, 1982

901. Buda AJ, Macdonald IL, Dubbin JD, et al: Myocardial infarct extension: prevalence, clinical significance, and problems in diagnosis. *Am Heart J* 105:744-749, 1983

902. Gillespie TA, Ambos HD, Sobel BE, et al: Effects of dobutamine in patients with acute myocardial infarction. *Am J Cardiol* 39:588-594, 1977

903. Rothkopf M, Boerner J, Stone MJ, et al: Detection of myocardial infarct extension by CK-B radioimmunoassay. *Circulation* 59:268-274, 1979

904. Nasser FN, Chesebro JH, Homburger HA, et al: Myocardial infarct extension: diagnosis by CK-MB radioimmunoassay and clinical significance (abstract). *Clin Res* 29:226A, 1981

905. DeWood MA, Stifter WF, Simpson CS, et al: Coronary arteriographic findings soon after non-Q-wave myocardial infarction. *N Engl J Med* 315:417-423, 1986

906. Fuster V, Badimon L, Cohen M, et al: Insights into the pathogenesis of acute ischemic syndromes. *Circulation* 77:1213-1220, 1988

907. Badimon L, Lassila R, Badimon J, et al: Residual thrombus is more thrombogenic than severely damaged vessel wall. *Circulation* 78 Suppl II:119, 1988

908. Heras M, Chesebro JH, Thompson PL, et al: Prevention of early and late rethrombosis and further strategies after coronary reperfusion. In *Thrombolysis in Cardiovascular Disease.* Edited by DG Julian, W Kubler, RM Norris, et al. New York, M. Dekker, 1989

909. Penny WJ, Chesebro JH, Heras M, et al: Antithrombotic therapy for patients with cardiac disease. *Curr Probl Cardiol* 13:425-513, 1988

910. Heras M, Chesebro JH, Webster MWI, et al: Hirudin, heparin, and placebo during deep arterial injury in the pig. The in vivo role of thrombin in platelet-mediated thrombosis. *Circulation* 82:1476-1484, 1990

911. Harrison DG, Ferguson DW, Collins SM, et al: Rethrombosis after reperfusion with streptokinase: importance of geometry of residual lesions. *Circulation* 69:991-999, 1984

912. Badger RS, Brown BG, Kennedy JW, et al: Usefulness of recanalization to luminal diameter of 0.6 millimeter or more with intracoronary streptokinase during acute myocardial infarction in predicting "normal" perfusion status, continued arterial patency and survival at one year. *Am J Cardiol* 59:519-522, 1987

913. Cowley MJ: Personal communication

914. Serruys PW, Wijns W, Van den Brand M, et al: Is transluminal coronary angioplasty mandatory after successful thrombolysis? Quantitative coronary angiographic study. *Br Heart J* 50:257-265, 1983

915. Chesebro JH, Fuster V, Pumphrey CW, et al: Improvement of shortened platelet survival half-life from the early to the late phase of myocardial infarction (abstract). *Circulation* 64 Suppl 4:197, 1981

916. Paris II Research Group: Persantine-aspirin reinfarction study. Part II. Secondary coronary prevention with persantine and aspirin. *J Am Coll Cardiol* 7:251-268, 1986

917. Gibson RS: Non-Q-wave myocardial infarction: diagnosis, prognosis, and management. *Curr Probl Cardiol* 13:9-71, 1988

918. Schechtman KB, Capone RJ, Kleiger RE, et al: Risk stratification of patients with non-Q wave myocardial infarction. The critical role of ST segment depression. *Circulation* 80:1148-1158, 1989

919. Willich SN, Stone PH, Muller JE, et al: High-risk subgroups of patients with non-Q wave myocardial infarction based on direction and severity of ST segment deviation. *Am Heart J* 114:1110-1118, 1987

920. Ogawa H, Hiramori K, Haze K, et al: Classification of non-Q-wave myocardial infarction according to electrocardiographic changes. *Br Heart J* 54:473-478, 1985

921. Huey BL, Gheorghiade M, Crampton RS, et al: Acute non-Q-wave myocardial infarction associated with early ST segment elevation: evidence for spontaneous coronary reperfusion and implications for thrombolytic trials. *J Am Coll Cardiol* 9:18-25, 1987

922. Schulze RA Jr, Pitt B, Griffith LSC, et al: Coronary angiography and left ventriculography in survivors of transmural and nontransmural myocardial infarction. *Am J Med* 64:108-113, 1978

923. Fuster V, Frye RL, Connolly DC, et al: Arteriographic patterns early in the onset of the coronary syndromes. *Br Heart J* 37:1250-1255, 1975

924. DeWood MA, Stifter WF, Simpson CS, et al: Coronary arteriographic findings soon after non-Q-wave myocardial infarction. *N Engl J Med* 315:417-423, 1986

925. DeWood MA, Spores J, Notske R, et al: Prevalence of total coronary occlusion during the early hours of transmural myocardial infarction. *N Engl J Med* 303:897-902, 1980

926. Holmes DR Jr, Hartzler GO, Smith HC, et al: Coronary artery thrombosis in patients with unstable angina. *Br Heart J* 45:411-416, 1981

927. Sobel BE, Bresnahan GF, Shell WE, et al: Estimation of infarct size in man and its relation to prognosis. *Circulation* 46:640-648, 1972

928. Shell WE, DeWood MA, Kligerman M, et al: Early appearance of MB-creatine kinase activity in nontransmural myocardial infarction detected by a sensitive assay for the isoenzyme. *Am J Med* 71:254-262, 1981

929. Ong L, Reiser P, Coromilas J, et al: Left ventricular function and rapid release of creatine kinase MB in acute myocardial infarction: evidence for spontaneous reperfusion. *N Engl J Med* 309:1-6, 1983

930. Théroux P, Kouz S, Bosch X, et al: Clinical and angiographic features of non-Q wave and Q wave myocardial infarction (MI) (abstract). *Circulation* 74 Suppl 2:303, 1986

931. Corbett JR, Lewis M, Willerson JT, et al: ^{99m}Tc-pyrophosphate imaging in patients with acute myocardial infarction: comparison of planar imaging with single-photon tomography with and without blood pool overlay. *Circulation* 69:1120-1128, 1984

932. Wackers FJT, Sokole EB, Samson G, et al: Value and limitations of thallium-201 scintigraphy in the acute phase of myocardial infarction. *N Engl J Med* 295:1-5, 1976

933. Singh AK, Rivera R, Cooper GN Jr, et al: Early myocardial revascularization for postinfarction angina: results and long-term follow-up. *J Am Coll Cardiol* 6:1121-1125, 1985

934. Breyer RH, Engelman RM, Rousou JA, et al: Postinfarction angina: an expanding subset of patients undergoing coronary artery bypass. *J Thorac Cardiovasc Surg* 90:532-540, 1985

935. Telford AM, Wilson C: Trial of heparin versus atenolol in prevention of myocardial infarction in intermediate coronary syndrome. *Lancet* 1:1225-1228, 1981

936. Théroux P, Ouimet H, McCans J, et al: Aspirin, heparin, or both to treat acute unstable angina. *N Engl J Med* 319:1105-1111, 1988

937. Klimt CR, Knatterud GL, Stamler J, et al: Persantine-aspirin reinfarction study: Part II. Secondary coronary prevention with persantine and aspirin. *J Am Coll Cardiol* 7:251-269, 1986

938. Gibson RS, Boden WE, Theroux P, et al: Diltiazem and reinfarction in patients with non-Q-wave myocardial infarction: results of a double-blind, randomized, multicenter trial. *N Engl J Med* 315: 423-429, 1986

939. The Multicenter Diltiazem Postinfarction Trial Research Group: The effect of diltiazem on mortality and reinfarction after myocardial infarction. *N Engl J Med* 319:385-392, 1988

940. β-Blocker Heart Attack Trial Research Group: A randomized trial of propranolol in patients with acute myocardial infarction: I. Mortality results. *JAMA* 247:1707-1714, 1982

941. Neufeld NH: Calcium antagonists in secondary prevention after acute myocardial infarction: the Secondary Prevention Reinfarction Nifedipine Trial (SPRINT). *Eur Heart J* 7 Suppl B:51-52, 1986

942. The Danish Study Group on Verapamil in Myocardial Infarction: Verapamil in acute myocardial infarction. *Eur Heart J* 5:516-528, 1984

943. Mandelkorn JB, Wolf NM, Singh S, et al: Intracoronary thrombus in nontransmural myocardial infarction and in unstable angina. *Am J Cardiol* 52:1-6, 1983

944. Ambrose JA, Hjemdahl-Monsen C, Borrico S, et al: Quantitative and qualitative effects of intracoronary streptokinase in unstable angina and non-Q wave infarction. *J Am Coll Cardiol* 9:1156-1165, 1987

945. Krone RJ, Dwyer EM Jr, Greenberg H, et al: Risk stratification in patients with first non-Q wave infarction: limited value of the early low level exercise test after uncomplicated infarcts. *J Am Coll Cardiol* 14:31-37, 1989

946. Gibson RS, Beller GA, Gheorghiade M, et al: The prevalence and clinical significance of residual myocardial ischemia 2 weeks after uncomplicated non-Q wave infarction: a prospective natural history study. *Circulation* 73:1186-1198, 1986

947. Roberts R: Recognition, pathogenesis, and management of non-Q-wave infarction. *Mod Concepts Cardiovasc Dis* 56:17-21, 1987

CHAPTER

30

Acute myocardial infarction

C. Arrhythmias

Bernard J. Gersh, M.B.,Ch.B., D.Phil.

THE introduction of the coronary care unit[1] and modern techniques of cardiopulmonary resuscitation in the 1960s, including external cardiac massage,[2] synchronized cardioversion,[3] and direct-current defibrillation,[4] verified that death need not inexorably follow ventricular fibrillation in cases of acute myocardial infarction. The demonstration that ventricular fibrillation early after myocardial infarction could be reversed and, once reversed, was unlikely to recur[5] revolutionized approaches to the management of myocardial infarction.

The advent of the coronary care unit has reduced the in-hospital mortality of acute infarction by approximately 30%[6] and virtually abolished all hospital deaths due to primary arrhythmias. Of course, inasmuch as two-thirds of deaths after acute infarction occur before the patient reaches a hospital, it is obvious that the coronary care unit alone cannot substantially decrease the total community mortality from coronary artery disease.[6-8a] Evidence that arrhythmias are almost invariable in the early phases of acute infarction[8a-10] and that many deaths are associated with small infarcts[11] is a powerful incentive to initiate treatment as early as possible after the onset of symptoms, as is the potential for early reperfusion to salvage myocardium, with its beneficial effect on in-hospital and late prognosis. The era of acute reperfusion does not negate the value of an aggressive approach to arrhythmias that occur after infarction. By causing hemodynamic instability and increasing infarct size, arrhythmias may contribute significantly to hospital mortality. In addition, experimental evidence suggests that closely coupled ventricular premature beats may actually increase infarct size in comparison to the effect in controls or in animals with widely coupled premature beats.[12] Effective management of arrhythmias may help salvage ischemic myocardium and thus have a beneficial effect on both early and late prognosis in acute infarction.

BLOOD SUPPLY OF THE CONDUCTION SYSTEM

The normal anatomy of the conduction system is discussed in chapter 12. In this section, the blood supply of the conduction system is discussed, specifically in relation to arrhythmias and conduction disturbances complicating acute myocardial infarction.

The vascular supply to the sinus node is via a small artery that arises about 2 cm from the ostium of the right coronary artery in approximately 55% of persons and from the proximal part of the left circumflex coronary artery in 45%.[13,14] The artery encircles the superior vena cava before supplying the sinus node. The disputed existence of specialized atrial conduction pathways is discussed in chapter 22A. Nonetheless, the atria, including those regions thought by some to be the site of specialized tracts, receive their blood supply from the sinus node artery and the atrial branches of the circumflex coronary artery.

Figure 30C-1 is a diagram of the blood supply to the atrioventricular (AV) node and bundle branches. In approximately 80% of patients, the blood supply of the AV node is via the AV node branch of the dominant right coronary artery.[14] This vessel arises from the right coronary artery as it crosses the crux. In the remaining 20% of human hearts, the blood supply is via a branch of a dominant circumflex coronary artery or from both vessels.[14,15] Collateral flow to the AV node may be provided by Kugel's artery, which courses posteriorly into the lower portion of the interatrial septum from either the proximal right or the left coronary system.[15] The relative lack of AV node necrosis in patients with inferior infarcts and heart block[16] supports the existence of an extensive collateral network to the AV node via the septal branches of the left anterior descending coronary artery.[15,17,18]

The bundle of His and the interventricular septum have a dual blood supply that arises from branches of the AV node artery and the septal perforating branches of the left anterior descending coronary artery.[15]

The proximal right bundle branch is related to the membranous septum and the summit of the muscular septum[19] and is supplied by branches of the left anterior descending coronary artery or the AV node artery, or both. In its more distal portion, the long, thin structure runs within the ventricular septum and subsequently subendocardially toward the papillary muscle and parietal surface of the right ventricle. The distal right bundle

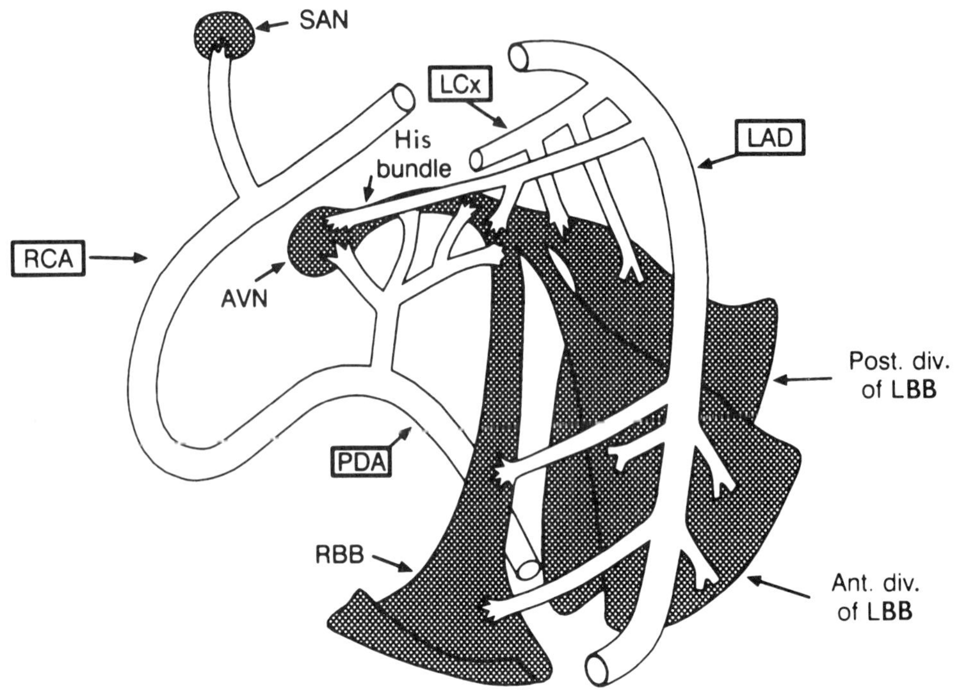

Fig 30C-1 Diagram of the conduction system and its blood supply. *SAN,* sinoatrial node; *AVN,* atrioventricular node; *LCx,* left circumflex coronary artery; *LAD,* left anterior descending coronary artery; *RCA,* right coronary artery; *PDA,* posterior descending branch of right coronary artery; *RBB,* right bundle branch; *LBB,* left bundle branch. (From DeGuzman M, Rahimtoola SH: What is the role of pacemakers in patients with coronary artery disease and conduction abnormalities? *Cardiovasc Clin* 13 No 1:191-207, 1983. By permission of FA Davis Company.)

branch is supplied by branches of the left anterior descending coronary artery and shares a blood supply with the anterior fascicle of the left bundle branch.

Figure 30C-1 illustrates the more extensive dual vascular supply to the main left bundle branch and the posteroinferior fascicle of the left bundle branch, which is supplied from the posterior descending and left anterior descending coronary arteries.[19,20]

Correlations among the site of infarction, the vascular anatomy, and the clinical disturbances in conduction are imprecise. This is not surprising in light of the multivessel distribution of coronary artery disease and the wide permutations of the collateral network.

VENTRICULAR ARRHYTHMIAS

Experimental and theoretical mechanisms

The pioneering efforts of Wiggers and Wégria[21] and Harris and Guevara Rojas[22] in the 1940s focused on the mechanisms of arrhythmias in acute myocardial infarction and expanded the concept of a vulnerable period for the induction of ventricular fibrillation by a stimulus occurring late in systole, first observed by DeBoer[23] in 1921. Harris and Guevara Rojas[22] described an early phase and a late phase of arrhythmias after experimental coronary artery occlusion in the dog and concluded that these changes were due to enhanced automaticity of fibers at the borders of the ischemic or infarcted zone. This conclusion was based in part on an inability to record, because of technical limitations, "continuous low-amplitude electrograms" in areas of slowed conduction.[24]

Subsequent animal studies identified three phases of arrhythmias after experimental coronary artery occlusion: an early phase, beginning minutes after occlusion and lasting at the most for 1 to 2 hours;[24-27] delayed arrhythmias, occurring 6 to 48 hours after occlusion;[28-31] and late arrhythmias, noted after 3 to 10 days.[30,32-35] The effects of coronary artery occlusion on the metabolism and ultrastructure of ventricular muscle cells are immediate, but the effects on the subendocardial Purkinje system may be delayed.[36] The variable time course of the biochemical consequences of ischemia in different tissues may account for the first two phases of ventricular arrhythmias.[36]

Modern methods of electrode design and signal amplification[25] altered the previous view that all arrhythmias after infarction were a result of enhanced automaticity; recent research underscores the potential importance of reentry mechanisms. The evolution of these ideas and the current electrophysiologic concepts of ischemic arrhythmias are the subject of comprehensive reviews.[14,24,36-38]

Early-onset arrhythmias. Arrhythmias occurring at varying times after the onset of experimental infarction most likely result from different mechanisms. Early-onset arrhythmias are probably a result of reentry.[38] The heterogeneity of the electrophysiologic properties between adjacent regions of perfused and nonperfused tissue is particularly important for the development of reentrant arrhythmias during acute ischemia. Important factors contributing to altered membrane depolarization and other electrophysiologic abnormalities in acute ischemia include the rapid loss of intracellular potassium ions and increased intracellular free calcium ions.[38,39] Han and Moe[40] in 1964 showed that ectopic activity after coronary artery occlusion in the dog may result from focal reexcitation in microreentry circuits because of pronounced asynchrony of recovery among adjacent fibers in the ischemic area. Current may flow from fibers undergoing early repolarization to those that are incompletely repolarized, and this may result in reexcitation of the repolarized cells and premature ventricular extrasystoles. Several studies subsequently verified that conduction was delayed in acutely ischemic tissue, with fractionated potentials prolonged well into the ST segment; an electrophysiologic substrate for reentry was thus identified[26,41] (Fig 30C-2). That an increase in heart rate causes fractionation of local electrograms is further support for reentry as a mechanism of these early-phase arrhythmias.[42] Waldo and Kaiser[25] in 1973 demonstrated continuous electrical activity that "bridged" sinus beats, and this finding strongly suggested that conduction in ischemic zones could be sufficiently slow to facilitate reentry. In 1974, Scherlag et al.,[29] using the dog model, substantiated a relation between delayed activation of the local electrogram and ventricular tachycardia or fibrillation due to reentry (Fig 30C-3). These and other experimental studies have modified our concepts of ventricular vulnerability. They imply that in the early-phase arrhythmias of experimental myocardial infarction, the coupling interval of an ectopic beat and its relation to the T wave are less important than the underlying electrophysiologic derangements in the ischemic myocardium. Stated differently, late-coupled premature beats in association with pronounced delays in conduction might have the same significance as early-cycle ventricular premature beats with normal repolarization.

Electrophysiologic phenomena such as slow conduction

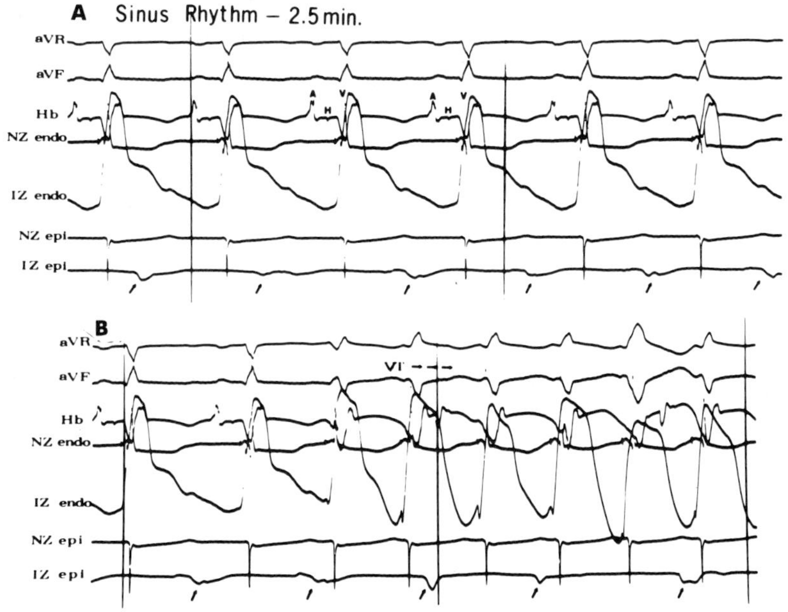

Fig 30C-2 Initiation of ventricular tachycardia *(VT)* associated with pronounced delay of localized epicardial activation. **A** and **B** are continuous records. There was a pronounced delay in and diminution of the epicardial potential in the ischemic zone *(arrows)* 2½ minutes after coronary artery ligation **(A).** Delayed activation was very localized, since it occurred in the ST segment without any change on the surface ECG. The occurrence of epicardial activation at the end of the refractory period of the ventricles *(second arrow* in **B)** corresponded to the onset of ventricular tachycardia, which went on to ventricular fibrillation. Intervals between time lines are 1 second. *NZ endo, IZ endo,* endocardium in control or normal zone (NZ) or ischemic zone (IZ); *NZ epi, IZ epi,* epicardium in control or normal zone or ischemic zone; *Hb,* His bundle electrogram. (From Scherlag BJ, Lazzara R: Ischemic arrhythmias: basic mechanisms. In *Cardiac Arrhythmias: Their Mechanisms, Diagnosis, and Management.* Edited by WJ Mandel. Philadelphia, JB Lippincott Company, 1980, pp 366-395. By permission.)

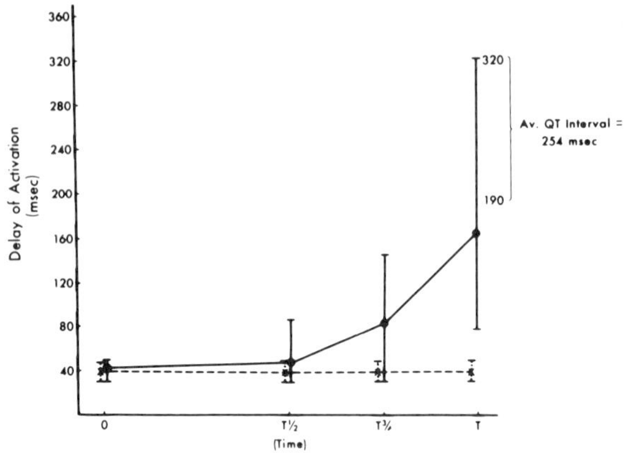

Fig 30C-3 Relationship between delay in epicardial activation in recorded electrograms (ordinate) and the time of onset (abscissa) of ventricular tachycardia normalized in each of 20 dogs. The average time of onset of ventricular tachycardia was 4 minutes in absolute terms. The potentials from the ischemic epicardium *(solid line)* showed variable but significantly greater average delay than did the potentials from the nonischemic epicardium *(broken line)*. This finding was particularly evident just before the onset of ventricular tachycardia, at which time some recorded potentials showed delayed activation well beyond the end of the average Q-T interval (254 msec; range, 190 to 320 msec). (From Scherlag BJ, El-Sherif N, Hope R, et al: Characterization and localization of ventricular arrhythmias resulting from myocardial ischemia and infarction. *Circ Res* 35:372-383, 1974. By permission of American Heart Association.)

and the ability of late-coupled ectopic beats to precipitate malignant arrhythmias may be understood at a cellular level. In ischemic cells (both muscle cells and His-Purkinje cells), recovery of the action potential is markedly prolonged, manifesting as postrepolarization refractoriness—that is, a prolongation of refractoriness that outlasts the action potential, Q-T interval, or repolarization.[24,43] Alterations in the "membrane responsiveness" curve in ischemic cells generate action potentials with a slowed rate of upstroke, leading to decreased conduction velocity. Postrepolarization refractoriness lays the foundation for nonuniform ventricular depolarization and repolarization, which prevent an orderly spread of excitation and create the milieu for reentry. Consequently, the extrasystolic impulse may result in a grossly irregular wave front and increase the potential for ventricular fibrillation. Ventricular fibrillation originates from the same conditions that predispose to reentry in the first place—namely, slowed conduction with temporal and asynchronous dispersion of recovery at numerous sites in the ventricle.[24,37]

Ischemia causes complex changes in both myocardial and systemic metabolism; its effect on the electrophysiology of the ischemic heart is the subject of detailed reviews.[14,36] In general, the "sicker" the patient and the larger the infarct, the more frequent are arrhythmias and the greater are the metabolic disturbances.[44] The consequences of myocardial ischemia—namely, hypoxia, accumulation of anaerobic metabolites, changes in pH, and alterations in intracellular and extracellular ionic concentrations—probably exert a multifactorial influence on the genesis of postinfarction arrhythmias, whether these are due to reentry or increased automaticity.[38,39] In addition to the influence of an altered extracellular environment, structural or irreversible metabolic changes in the cells themselves may markedly alter their electrophysiologic properties. In addition to the electrophysiologic properties of diseased tissue, which form the anatomic substrate of arrhythmias, the propensity for an arrhythmia to develop can be greatly influenced by changes in autonomic tone and, in particular, sympathetic overactivity.[14,36,38,39,45,46] Moreover, arrhythmias due to reentry or triggered activity cannot occur de novo without appropriate triggering factors, such as premature ventricular complexes.[38]

Delayed arrhythmias. Accumulating evidence implicates enhanced automaticity of ischemic subendocardial Purkinje fibers in the genesis of delayed arrhythmias 6 to 8 hours after experimental coronary occlusion. At this time, the bulk of the ischemic zone is inexcitable, but surviving subendocardial Purkinje fibers, which underlie the infarcted myocardium and are partly nourished by intracavitary blood, develop abnormal automaticity.[30,32,38,47] Surviving subendocardial Purkinje fibers in the infarcted zone display an increase in the slope of phase 4 spontaneous diastolic depolarization,[30,31,48] and this change is enhanced by catecholamines, hypoxia, and myocardial fiber stretch (all of which are present locally in the ventricle after acute myocardial infarction).[14] Using the canine model of infarction and programmed ventricular stimulation, Davis et al.[28] showed that delayed arrhythmias have characteristics of enhanced automaticity. These arrhythmias could not be induced by premature or rapid stimulation of the ventricles, and overdrive pacing caused either transient suppression or acceleration. These arrhythmias may correspond to the accelerated idioventricular parasystolic rhythms seen several hours or days after the onset of clinical acute myocardial infarction.[49]

Although the explanation that these arrhythmias are due to enhanced automaticity is plausible, the delay in repolarization of affected Purkinje fibers may lead to reentrant rhythms at this time.[24] Indeed, reentrant ventricular tachycardia may be indistinguishable electrocardiographically from accelerated ventricular rhythms due to enhanced automaticity.

Late arrhythmias. Late arrhythmias during the chronic completed phase of myocardial infarction are due to reentry, and the arrhythmogenic substrate at this stage is generally stable, unlike the situation during acute ischemia.[50] Reentry originates in areas of slow conduction in the border zone between normal and infarcted tissue.[32,34,50] The border zone is markedly heterogeneous from an electrophysiology standpoint and is characterized histologically by areas of viable myocardium interspersed with bands of collagen and connective tissue.[32,34,50,51] In summary, in the border zone of an infarct, the disruption of the normal architecture by scar tissue enhances nonuniform conduction, which leads to extremely slow conduction in some areas, regions of unidirectional block, and the development of reentry.[36,45] Additional evidence suggesting that enhanced automaticity is not present in animals at this time substantiates the conclusion that reentry is the likely mechanism of late arrhythmias after experimental coronary occlusion.[32-35]

Davis et al.[28] and Wit et al.[52] showed that ventricular tachycardia 3 to 5 days after coronary occlusion and reperfusion could be terminated and induced by programmed stimulation or overdrive pacing, a characteristic of both triggered automaticity and reentry. The failure of the tachycardia to be significantly influenced at 3 to 5 days by agents that blocked the slow calcium channel argued against triggered automaticity as a cause.[28]

The reentrant circuit is anatomically small but is likely to include the periphery of the infarcted zone.[35] A correlation between reentry arrhythmias in the dog occurring 3 to 5 days after myocardial infarction and chronic ventricular tachycardia is likely, because a similar model of reentrant ventricular tachycardia 3 weeks after experimental myocardial infarction has been developed.[35] The inducible, stable reentrant rhythms are possibly analogous to those seen clinically in chronic ischemic heart disease and in survivors from acute myocardial infarction.[35,53]

Arrhythmias occurring after experimental myocardial infarction have varied mechanisms, and they may respond differently to drugs. This characteristic has important clinical implications, but one should be aware of the caveats expressed by Scherlag and Lazzara[24]—that current information is insufficient to allow one to assume that experimental and clinical situations are necessarily the same.

Reperfusion arrhythmias. The potential role of coronary vasospasm and intracoronary thrombolysis early after acute myocardial infarction has led to a resurgence of interest in reperfusion arrhythmias. That ventricular tachycardia and ventricular fibrillation may follow opening of an occluded coronary artery has long been recognized.[54] Reperfusion arrhythmias differ from early postligation arrhythmias in their time course, degree of malignancy, and responsiveness to antiarrhythmic agents.[55,56] In dogs undergoing ligation followed by reperfusion, arrhythmias are more frequent than in those with permanent occlusion.[57]

The mechanisms underlying reperfusion in arrhythmias are incompletely understood.[56,58] They usually occur within a brief period after the restoration of coronary flow and are critically related to the degree of occlusion, rarely occurring if this is less than 10 minutes or longer than 30 minutes.[59] They do not respond to antiarrhythmic agents that usually suppress arrhythmias related to ischemia, which again implies a different mechanism.[60] The role of calcium overload, free oxygen radicals, and other ionic and electrical inhomogeneities needs further evaluation.[58]

Clinically, reperfusion arrhythmias do occur, but they are probably more benign than would be expected from experimental data. In the Intravenous Streptokinase in Acute Myocardial Infarction study, nonsustained ventricular tachycardia, bradycardia, and accelerated idioventricular rhythms were more frequent after streptokinase than after placebo, but the incidence of ventricular fibrillation was no different.[61] The mechanism of the bradycardia and hypotension after reperfusion of inferior infarcts may result from activation of the Bezold-Jarisch reflex due to stimulation of receptors in the posterior regions of the left ventricle.[62,63] The severity and frequency of reperfusion arrhythmias may possibly be a function of the method and rapidity of reperfusion as well as the degree of residual stenosis. For example, compared with intracoronary streptokinase, primary angioplasty was associated with a greater incidence of ventricular tachycardia and ventricular fibrillation after reperfusion.[64] As markers of successful reperfusion, however, arrhythmias are unreliable and relatively insensitive, although, some would claim, reasonably specific[65-68] (Fig 30C-4). As opposed to the experience with more benign ventricular arrhythmias, there is evidence to support an overall reduction in the incidence of ventricular fibrillation in patients receiving thrombolytic therapy. In a meta-analysis of six randomized trials involving more than 36,000 patients, the incidence of ventricular fibrillation of 5.2% in patients treated with thrombolytic therapy was 16% less than the 6.1% incidence in control patients, and this difference was statistically significant.[69]

Clinical ventricular arrhythmias

Incidence. The incidence of arrhythmias occurring immediately after the onset of chest pain exceeds that reported from coronary care units.[70] In a prospective study of 294 patients seen within 1 hour after the onset of symptoms, Pantridge et al.[8a] found incidences of 58% for ventricular ectopic beats, 9.5% for ventricular fibrillation, and 2% for ventricular tachycardia. Within 4 hours after onset of symptoms, the cumulative incidences were 93% for ventricular ectopy, 15.5% for ventricular fibrillation, and 4% for ventricular tachycardia. The strikingly high early incidence of ventricular fibrillation underscores the potential value of mobile coronary care units and community education and emphasizes that treatment must be sought promptly on recognition of symptoms. Delay in seeking admission to a hospital correlates with the incidence of sudden death.[71] In patients with myocardial infarction who survive to reach the coronary care unit, the subsequent incidence of ventricular fibrillation is significantly less (5.7%) than that in the prehospital phase.[72]

Ventricular arrhythmias after acute myocardial infarction can be classified as shown in Table 30C-1.

Warning arrhythmias. The concept of "warning arrhythmias," particularly the R-on-T phenomenon, has its origins in early experimental work on the vulnerable period for ventricular fibrillation. In the early experience of coronary care units, certain forms of ventricular premature complexes were recognized as harbingers of more serious ventricular arrhythmias that prompt aggressive therapy might avoid.[1] Lown[73] observed that "death, while sudden, is not unannounced." This concept has been challenged; experimental data have shown that repolarization may be prolonged and extend beyond the

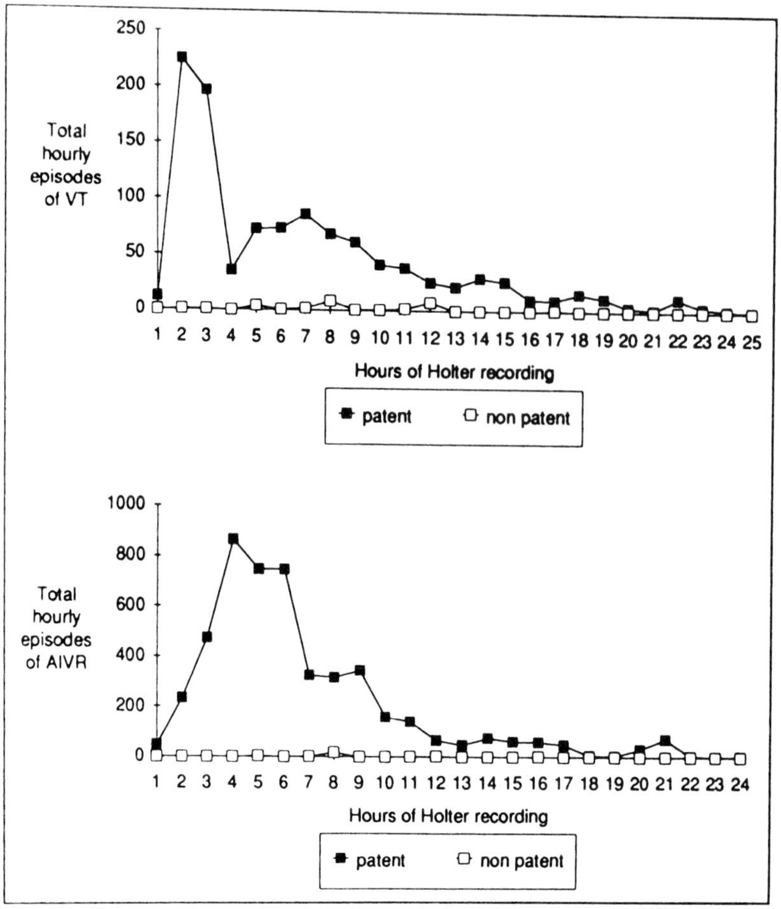

Fig 30C-4 Hourly total frequency of ventricular tachycardias (*VT*) and accelerated idioventricular rhythms (*AIVR*) according to coronary artery patency. (From Gressin V, Louvard Y, Pezzano M, et al: Holter recording of ventricular arrhythmias during intravenous thrombolysis for acute myocardial infarction. *Am J Cardiol* 69:152-159, 1992. By permission of Excerpta Medica.)

Table 30C-1 Clinical classification of ventricular arrhythmias after acute myocardial infarction

Ventricular ectopy—"warning arrhythmias"
Frequent ventricular ectopy—five or more per minute
Paired or multiform ectopy
Early (R-on-T) ectopy
Paroxysmal ventricular tachycardia ("malignant" ventricular tachycardia)
Accelerated idioventricular rhythm (idioventricular tachycardia)
Ventricular fibrillation
Primary
Secondary or complicating
Agonal
Precipitated by drugs or invasive procedures
Predismissal (late recovery phase) ventricular arrhythmias

T wave,[29,41,43,74] and these data indicate that the underlying electrophysiologic milieu may be more important than the coupling interval of the ventricular premature extrasystole. This possibility does not negate the concept that ventricular ectopy is an antecedent of malignant arrhythmias, but it does emphasize that late-coupled extrasystoles should not necessarily be considered benign. Several clinical studies have questioned the role of "warning arrhythmias" as precedents of ventricular tachycardia or fibrillation.[75-79] These studies showed that warning arrhythmias are common in acute myocardial infarction, the incidence of warning arrhythmias is similar in those with and without ventricular fibrillation, many patients have warning arrhythmias without ventricular fibrillation and vice versa, and ventricular premature extrasystoles initiating ventricular fibrillation are often late-coupled.

Paroxysmal ventricular tachycardia (malignant ventricular tachycardia). This arrhythmia is associated with a rapid rate, usually exceeding 140 beats/min. It is often self-limited, consisting of short runs of at least three consecutive ventricular premature beats, but sustained ventricular tachycardia causing hemodynamic impairment or degeneration into ventricular fibrillation is common. Ventricular tachycardia occurs in 3% to 15% of patients.[14] A relation between sympathetic overactivity may predispose the heart to early ventricular arrhythmias.[70]

Polymorphous ventricular tachycardia was noted in 1.2% of 771 consecutive patients admitted with acute myocardial infarction. The arrhythmia was resistant to multiple drugs and to overdrive pacing. Repeated cardioversion was effective in only three patients.[80] Verapamil was effective in three of four patients in whom it was tried, but it was concluded that in comparison with regular ventricular tachycardia, polymorphous ventricular tachycardia in acute infarction had a poor prognosis, six of nine patients dying during hospitalization and the remaining three within 6 months of dismissal. Another study concurred with the poor prognosis of polymorphous ventricular tachycardia within the first 2 weeks after myocardial infarction and noted that it is often associated with signs or symptoms of recurrent myocardial ischemia refractory to conventional drug therapy, although it may be suppressed by intravenously administered amiodarone, and coronary bypass surgery appears to be effective in preventing the recurrence.[81]

Sustained monomorphic ventricular tachycardia usually implies the development of a fixed arrhythmic substrate, which is most frequently seen in patients with extensive infarctions.[58] Sustained monomorphic ventricular tachycardia is relatively uncommon before day 2 or 3 of infarction, probably because of the time necessary for the substrate to evolve.[58] Nonetheless, its presence during the early phase of infarction is a harbinger of ventricular tachycardia in the late recovery phase and warrants investigation and therapy (see below).

Idioventricular rhythm (idioventricular tachycardia). Idioventricular rhythm has a slow rate – 60 to 120 beats/min – and is characterized by a wide QRS complex, usually unassociated with any hemodynamic disturbance. It occurs in 24% to 40% of patients after myocardial infarction[14,49] and is most common in inferior myocardial infarctions in the first 48 hours. In studies combining serial coronary angiography and continuous electrocardiographic (ECG) monitoring, accelerated idioventricular rhythms have been observed to be a reasonably sensitive and specific marker of successful reperfusion,[65,66,82] although this finding is disputed by others.[67] Perhaps its occurrence in the absence of thrombolytic therapy implies spontaneous reperfusion and a good prognosis.[58] Accelerated idioventricular rhythm usually occurs in brief, self-limited episodes and is more likely to become manifest when there is an underlying sinus bradycardia.[58] The postulated mechanism is enhanced automaticity of the subendocardial Purkinje fibers resembling the "delayed" phase of ventricular arrhythmias in the animal model. Clinical features that support the concept of enhanced automaticity are an association with escape beats and fusion beats, suppression by acceleration of the dominant rhythm, unifocal origin, and occasional association with parasystole. In some patients, accelerated idioventricular rhythms may be a manifestation of rapid automatic ventricular tachycardia with 2:1 or 3:1 exit block, and in this situation both forms of tachycardia are seen, the rate of the rapid ventricular tachycardia being a multiple of the rate of the idioventricular rhythm.[83] Sclarovsky et al.[84] described a multiform accelerated idioventricular rhythm with features suggesting multifocality. None of the patients were compromised hemodynamically, but the arrhythmia was abolished in most by verapamil.

The prognosis is generally good, and therapy is not indicated except for careful observation. Occasionally, the rhythm may compromise systemic hemodynamics or lead to ventricular fibrillation.[83,85] Talbot and Greaves[86] classified idioventricular rhythms after acute myocardial infarction into those with rates of less than 75 beats/min and those with rates of 75 to 120 beats/min. Rhythms with rates of less than 75 beats/min that occurred during periods of sinus slowing had an entirely benign course. There was, however, a significant association between "rapid," or true, ventricular tachycardia and idioventricular rhythms at rates faster than 75 beats/min.

Ventricular fibrillation. The clinical approach to and classification of ventricular fibrillation by Oliver et al.[87] is useful (Table 30C-2). Primary ventricular fibrillation occurs early after the onset of symptoms (Fig 30C-5) in patients without preceding cardiac failure, hypotension, or major arrhythmias, in contrast to the secondary form, which develops in patients with any of these three clinical conditions. In a series of 500 patients with acute myocardial infarction who were monitored either in an ambulance or in the hospital within 1 hour after the onset of symptoms, primary ventricular fibrillation occurred in 55 patients, in 54 of them within 10 hours after the onset of symptoms.[88]

Earlier studies suggested that if primary ventricular fibrillation were successfully treated, subsequent 2-year mortality was favorable.[89,90] In a community-wide

Table 30C-2 Types of ventricular fibrillation

	Patients no.	Immediate successful resuscitation, no.	Survivors, no.
All cases	44	33	23
Types			
Primary	15	15	13
Complicating shock or failure	17	12	5
Agonal	4	0	0
Pacemaker-induced	5	4	3
Drug-induced	3	2	2

Data from Oliver MJ, Julian DG, Donald KW: Problems in evaluating coronary care units: their responsibilities and their relation to the community. *Am J Cardiol* 20:465-474, 1967.

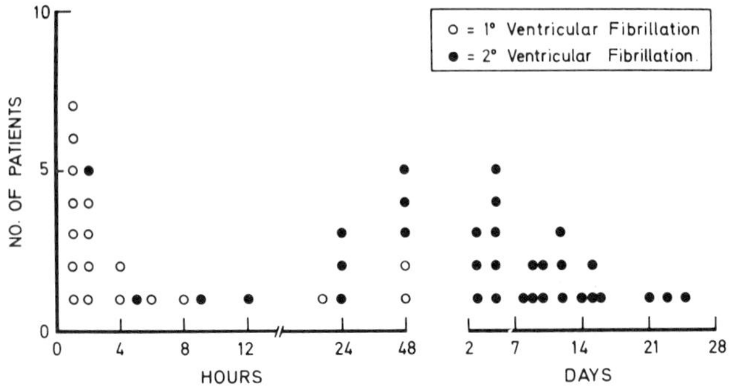

Fig 30C-5 Time of onset of the first episode of ventricular fibrillation in 51 patients with acute myocardial infarction. (From Jewitt D: The genesis of cardiac arrhythmias in acute myocardial infarction. *Prog Cardiol* 1:61-94, 1972. By permission of Lea & Febiger.)

study from Worcester, Mass., the long-term prognosis in patients dismissed from the hospital after resuscitation from early (1 to 2 days of admission) cardiac arrest was better than that among patients dismissed after "late" cardiac arrest.[91] Of relevance to the controversy surrounding the role of routine prophylactic lidocaine therapy (see below) are three studies that emphasized the higher in-hospital mortality in patients with sustained primary ventricular tachycardia, even though late survival after dismissal was no different for patients without such arrhythmias.[92-94] Another study, however, showed a difference in 2-year survival between those with and those without early ventricular fibrillation—57% and 77%, respectively.[95] In a case-control study, Schwartz et al.[96] found that the occurrence of primary ventricular fibrillation did not adversely affect long-term prognosis in patients with inferior infarcts but that patients with anterior infarcts had a marked increase in late mortality. Although there are attractions to the concept of preventing ventricular arrhythmias by prophylactic antiarrhythmic therapy, significant side effects militate against the benefit of such an approach. This controversial issue is discussed later in this chapter.

In secondary ventricular fibrillation, underlying ventricular dysfunction augurs a poor outcome, even if initial treatment is successful. Agonal ventricular fibrillation occurs in a patient dying of shock or advanced pump failure who has already lost one or more vital functions, such as respiration or blood pressure. Figure 30C-5 illustrates that primary ventricular fibrillation occurs early after myocardial infarction, and the prevention of this arrhythmia has been the focus of the controversy surrounding prophylactic lidocaine therapy. Patients receiving thrombolytic therapy in a large randomized trial had a reduction of about 20% in the frequency of secondary ventricular fibrillation (streptokinase, 1.4%; control, 2.9%), and the major effect was in patients treated within 3 hours after the onset of symptoms.[97] The prognosis of "late" ventricular fibrillation—between 48 hours and 18 days after acute myocardial infarction—was recently evaluated by Jensen et al.[98] in Copenhagen, Denmark. Late ventricular fibrillation showed a nonsignificant trend toward a poorer long-term prognosis than early ventricular fibrillation, but this result was almost entirely due to the higher incidence of heart failure in these patients.[98]

Arrhythmias in the late recovery phase. The prognostic implications of arrhythmias detected in the late recovery phase or in the first few weeks after myocardial infarction are dealt with in detail in chapter 30A. A large body of evidence strongly correlates frequent and complex ventricular ectopy with the occurrence of sudden and other forms of cardiac death in the year after myocardial infarction.[99-107] In the Multicenter Investigation of the Limitation of Infarct Size, patients with more than 10 premature ventricular complexes per hour had 3.4 times the risk of sudden cardiac death, independent of other clinical factors.

In the large Multicenter Study of Postinfarction Survivors (820 patients), Bigger et al.[108] identified 90 patients with nonsustained ventricular tachycardia and 2 patients with sustained ventricular tachycardia during ECG monitoring on an average of 11 ± 3 days after infarction. Ventricular tachycardia was associated with several other factors predictive of an adverse outcome, including older age, malignant ventricular arrhythmias during the early hospital phase, reduced left ventricular ejection fraction, and congestive heart failure. Even when adjusted for other risk factors, however, ventricular tachycardia nearly doubled the risk of dying in the next approximately 2 1/2 years.[107]

Moss et al.,[99] in a prospective study of 940 patients, identified complex ventricular premature extrasystoles as an independent predictor of cardiac mortality over an average follow-up of 3 years. In a study of 1,739 male survivors of acute myocardial infarction enrolled in the Health Insurance Plan of Greater New York, complex ventricular ectopy (that is, R-on-T, runs of two or more ventricular premature beats, or multiform or bigeminal complexes) was the strongest independent predictor of death, particularly sudden death, over a 5-year period.[101] The association between ventricular ectopy and a reduced ejection fraction in survivors of myocardial infarction has been emphasized,[102] and it was found that sudden death occurred mainly in patients with ejection fractions of less than 0.40 but that in this group of patients, sudden cardiac death occurred primarily in those with complex ventricular ectopia (Fig 30C-6). Bigger and Weld[103] underscored the importance of ventricular premature complexes, particularly repetitive ones, in the long-term prognosis of acute infarction. Persistent ST-segment abnormalities were more common in patients who had sudden death, a suggestion that persistent ischemia may be a factor causing ectopy.

The bulk of accumulated evidence points in a single direction. Late ventricular arrhythmias are an accompaniment of more extensive myocardial infarcts and are found in association with other factors predictive of an adverse outcome. Nonetheless, symptomatic, frequent, and complex ventricular ectopy with nonsustained ventricular tachycardia is also a powerful independent predictor of late mortality. Whether patients at particularly high risk can be identified by invasive electrophysi-

	EF≥0.40	EF<0.40
VPC Class 0-II	33	19
VPC Class III-V	3	26

Fig 30C-6 Division of 81 patients into subgroups by class of ventricular premature contraction *(VPC)* and ejection fraction *(EF)* is demonstrated. All sudden deaths occurred in patients in the subgroups with complicated VPCs (classes III to V) and ejection fractions of less than 0.40. Note the lack of patients with complicated VPCs and ejection fraction of 0.40 or more. (From Schulze RA Jr, Strauss HW, Pitt B: Sudden death in the year following myocardial infarction: relation to ventricular premature contractions in the late hospital phase and left ventricular ejection fraction. *Am J Med* 62:192-199, 1977. By permission of Technical Publishing Company.)

ologic testing in the early postinfarction period or by the use of the signal-averaged ECG is discussed in chapter 30A. In brief, invasive electrophysiologic testing in this situation appears to be of limited value. However, several studies have shown that late potentials on the signal-averaged ECG are a powerful predictor of late mortality and malignant ventricular arrhythmias (see chapter 30A). It should be emphasized that the evidence associating complex ventricular ectopy with arrhythmic and other cardiac mortality in survivors of acute myocardial infarction emanates from the prethrombolytic era. Accumulating evidence suggests that the predictive value of complex ectopy and ambulatory monitoring in the signal-averaged ECG might be substantially less in lower risk patients who have had thrombolytic therapy.[109] Newer modalities for risk stratification, such as heart rate variability, are promising.

What is of critical but as yet undetermined importance is whether suppression of ventricular ectopy by antiarrhythmic agents after infarction reduces sudden cardiac death.[104-107] This issue is the topic of a large multicenter investigation, the Cardiac Arrhythmia Suppression Trial (CAST), in which postinfarction patients with ventricular ectopy are randomized either to no therapy or to several drug regimens. One arm of the study was terminated prematurely because mortality was much higher in patients treated with encainide and flecainide than in those given a placebo.[110] The second CAST study (CAST-II) compared moricizine and placebo.[111] This trial was stopped early because the first 14-day period of treatment with moricizine after a myocardial infarction was associated with an excess of mortality in the treatment group, and it was thought highly unlikely that a long-term survival benefit from moricizine would have been observed had the trial been completed. The CAST trials have had a profound impact on clinical practice, and at this stage, pending further data on the long-term benefits or otherwise of amiodarone,[55] asymptomatic ventricular arrhythmias in survivors of infarction should not be treated.

Therefore, firm recommendations for the management of patients with asymptomatic ventricular arrhythmias appearing late after acute myocardial infarction cannot be made until the results of further large controlled trials are available. What is certain, however, is that if a drug regimen is prescribed for a patient, careful surveillance is essential not only to ensure drug efficacy but also, more importantly, to exclude a proarrhythmic effect. Guidelines based on a single day of monitoring were provided by Pratt et al.[112] in the Cardiac Arrhythmia Pilot Study. Whether documentation of an absence of a proarrhythmic effect on acute testing will be sustained long-term is as yet unknown.

Other approaches to the management of sustained ventricular arrhythmias after infarction, including arrhythmia surgery, implantation of artificial cardioverter-defibrillators, long-term antitachycardia pacing, and catheter ablation, are discussed in other chapters. The following section on management and treatment deals with arrhythmias during the acute phase of myocardial infarction.

Management of ventricular arrhythmias in acute myocardial infarction

In this section, only therapeutic modalities for *acute*-phase arrhythmias are discussed. Techniques for the control of late-phase malignant arrhythmias or arrhythmias after dismissal, including drug therapy, arrhythmia surgery, the implantable cardioverter-defibrillator, antitachycardia pacing, and catheter ablation, are described in other chapters.

Indications for treatment. The indications for treatment are as follows: (1) Ventricular extrasystoles. Despite the controversy over the issue of "warning arrhythmias" and their relation to ventricular tachycardia and fibrillation, there are appropriate indications for therapy: namely, ventricular premature complexes of six or more per minute or with multifocal or paired premature complexes, prolonged periods of bigeminal rhythm, and early coupled premature complexes (R-on-T phenomenon) or those occurring in short bursts of three or more in succession. (2) Accelerated idioventricular rhythm. In general, accelerated idioventricular rhythm does not require therapy other than close monitoring. In occasional patients, AV dissociation with loss of atrial transport may be important, and in such cases the ectopic rhythm can be overdriven by acceleration of the sinus node discharge rate with atropine. (3) Paroxysmal ventricular tachycardia and ventricular fibrillation. Control of these arrhythmias is mandatory and is a major function of the coronary care unit.

Prophylactic lidocaine therapy. The role of prophylactic lidocaine therapy in acute myocardial infarction is controversial. Support for prophylaxis arose in part from the observation that "warning arrhythmias" do not always precede malignant arrhythmias. If ventricular fibrillation is to be prevented, all patients should be treated, irrespective of whether complex ventricular ectopy is present. A further stimulus to prophylactic therapy is the relative inability to detect serious arrhythmias during routine monitoring.[113] In this regard, Harrison's comments[114] are fitting: "It is questionable whether warning arrhythmias really warn, and even if they do they are frequently not detected."

Reservations about prophylactic therapy with lidocaine hinge on doubts related to the efficacy of this drug in the first few hours after myocardial infarction[8a] (which might, in part, be related to subtherapeutic blood levels[115,116]). Concern about the toxicity of lidocaine was raised by a large trial of lidocaine and placebo in which a low incidence of ventricular fibrillation was found in both groups but a trend toward an increase in the incidence of asystole and hypotension was noted in the treated group.[117] In an excellent study of intravenously administered lidocaine by Lie et al.,[78] a striking reduction in the incidence of ventricular fibrillation was noted in treated patients: In the largest trial to date (6,024 patients), in which intramuscularly administered lidocaine was compared with placebo in the prehospital phase, there was a significant reduction in the incidence of ventricular fibrillation during the period when lidocaine levels were therapeutic.[118] Asystolic episodes were more frequent and more prolonged in lidocaine-treated patients, although there was no apparent increase in asystolic deaths.[118]

Although a 1981 study in which the results of several trials of lidocaine prophylaxis were pooled concluded that such therapy was beneficial, particularly in specific subgroups,[119] this conclusion was not borne out by a later overview of 14 randomized trials by MacMahon et al.[120] The 14 randomized trials included 9,155 patients receiving either placebo or lidocaine administered intramuscularly or intravenously. Overall, allocation of lidocaine was associated with a reduction in the odds of ventricular fibrillation of about one-third with a 95% confidence interval (range, 3% to 56% reduction), but there was no evidence of any beneficial effect on early mortality. In fact, the odds of early death were about one-third greater among patients allocated to lidocaine, although this difference was not statistically significant. MacMahon et al.[120] concluded that their overview of all the trial results did not provide definitive evidence on the efficacy or nonefficacy of prophylactic lidocaine therapy. They recommended that "future trials involve large numbers of patients in prolonged follow-up." Two other meta-analyses have similarly emphasized a lack of benefit from prophylactic administration of lidocaine in addition to the potential for harm by increasing the frequency of asystole.[121,122]

A recent meta-analysis by Antman and Berlin[123] documented the declining incidence of ventricular fibrillation between 1970 and 1990. This very important study estimated that the primary ventricular fibrillation rate was 4.51% in control patients in 1970 and decreased to 0.35% in 1990; the corresponding figures for the lidocaine-treated groups were 4.32% in 1970 and 0.11% in 1990. It would appear that in the 1990s, estimates of the risk-benefit ratio of lidocaine prophylaxis argue strongly against the routine prophylactic use of lidocaine in patients with acute myocardial infarction. In an accompanying editorial, Singh[124] drew the inescapable conclusion that "routine prophylactic lidocaine therapy in acute myocardial infarction is an idea whose time is all but gone" (Fig 30C-7). The mechanisms of the striking reduction in the incidence of ventricular fibrillation are probably multifactorial and most likely include the use of β-blockers, the advent of thrombolytic therapy, changes in admission criteria, a declining risk of hypokalemia, and the overall decline in mortality related to ischemic heart disease.[123]

The American College of Cardiology (ACC) and American Heart Association (AHA) Task Force report

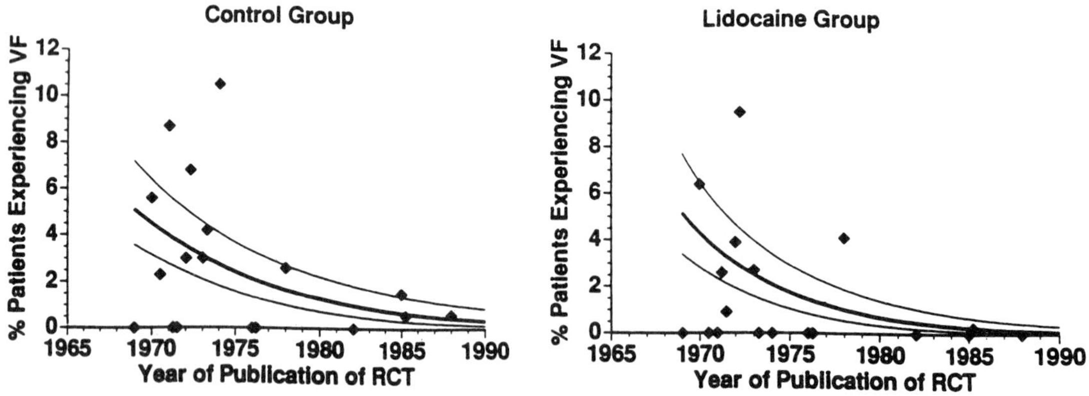

Fig 30C-7 Graphs show percentage of patients in the control (*left*) and lidocaine (*right*) groups of the randomized control trials (*RCT*) who experienced ventricular fibrillation (*VF*). Isolated points (♦) are the observed percentages for each RCT; dark curves are predicted values from the univariate logistic regression model using year of publication of the RCT as the predictor variable; the lighter curves are 95% confidence intervals. (From Antman EM, Berlin JA: Declining incidence of ventricular fibrillation in myocardial infarction: implications for the prophylactic use of lidocaine. *Circulation* 86:764-773, 1992. By permission of American Heart Association.)

classified the indication for prophylactic use of lidocaine as class IIB (not well established by evidence, can be helpful, and probably not harmful). Our feeling is that prophylactic use of lidocaine should not be routine unless myocardial infarction is strongly suspected and reliable defibrillation in an intensive care unit is unavailable. In some situations, the decision should be individualized, but the bulk of the available data now argues strongly against prophylactic antiarrhythmic therapy.

It has been suggested that β-blockade might offer an alternative to lidocaine, but, disappointingly, neither the Metoprolol in Acute Myocardial Infarction study group nor the First International Study of Infarct Survival found any difference in the incidence of ventricular fibrillation between patients receiving β-blockers and those receiving a placebo.[125,126]

In a double-blind, placebo-controlled trial of 434 patients, the effect of nifedipine on ventricular arrhythmias during the acute phase of myocardial infarction was studied. Nifedipine appeared to have no effect on the frequency of ventricular ectopy or on the incidence of major ventricular arrhythmias. However, there was a significant reduction in the number of patients with short runs of nonsustained ventricular tachycardia among those monitored during the 5 to 24 hours from the onset of pain. The significance of this finding is uncertain.[127] If lidocaine is to be administered, recommended dosages are as follows: (1) multiple injection technique, 50 mg intravenously at intervals of 5 minutes for a total dose of 200 to 300 mg;[128,129] (2) constant-infusion technique, 20 mg/min for a total dose of 3 to 5 mg/kg; and (3) bolus technique, 100 mg over 1 minute, and if this is not effective, a 50-mg bolus 5 or 10 minutes after the initial bolus. In patients in the prehospitalization phase of acute infarction, 400 mg of intramuscularly (deltoid) delivered lidocaine appeared protective. Maintenance dosages should range from 2 to 5 mg/min and should be started simultaneously with the loading dose. The maintenance dosage should be reduced by 50% in patients who have congestive heart failure, shock, and liver disease and in patients over the age of 70 years.[114,128] In patients receiving β-blockers, which reduce hepatic blood flow, and those receiving concomitant therapy with cimetidine or halothane, the maintenance dosage should also be halved.[123] Administration for 24 to 36 hours after infarction or until the diagnosis of infarction has been excluded is recommended. The drug should be infused with the aid of a calibration pump, and determination of lidocaine blood levels may be helpful in refractory cases or when toxicity is suspected.

General measures. Careful attention to factors that may contribute to the frequency and severity of arrhythmias is essential. Paramount among these is the correction of hypoxia.[130] Other circumstances that provoke arrhythmias include acid-base and electrolyte imbalance,[131] continued pain, and excessive anxiety.

The importance of the serum potassium concentration on admission and previous diuretic therapy in relation to the subsequent development of ventricular fibrillation was emphasized by Nordrehaug and von der Lippe.[132] The frequency of ventricular fibrillation was 17% in patients with hypokalemia, compared with 7% in patients with a serum potassium concentration of 3.6 mmol/L or greater, and in hypokalemic patients, ventricular fibrillation was noted significantly earlier (median, 0.3 hour compared with 7 hours).

Data from Abraham et al.[133] suggested that patients with acute myocardial infarction have altered lymphocyte potassium and magnesium concentrations. A subsequent study implied that a 2.4-g dose of magnesium sulfate compared with placebo in 94 patients with acute myocardial infarction significantly reduced the incidence of potentially lethal arrhythmias,[134] although this was not the case in a recent randomized trial in which the major effect of magnesium therapy was on cardiac failure (see above). Although the correct dosage and the long-term effects of this treatment need to be determined, it would seem prudent to correct both hypokalemia and hypomagnesemia in patients with acute myocardial infarction in the expectation that potentially fatal cardiac arrhythmias may be prevented. This plan of action may apply to other subsets of patients with coronary disease.

Because hypotension and heart failure predispose the heart to arrhythmias, correction of the underlying hemodynamic disturbance is necessary to complement specific antiarrhythmic measures. Bussmann et al.[135] showed that intravenous administration of nitroglycerin, which could improve myocardial ischemia and therefore ventricular function, reduced the frequency of non-life-threatening ventricular ectopic beats during the acute phase of myocardial infarction.

Cardioversion and defibrillation. Ventricular fibrillation or ventricular tachycardia with significant hemodynamic decompensation necessitates prompt cardioversion or defibrillation. A precordial "thump" may terminate ventricular tachycardia, presumably by mechanical stimulation, which can generate about 1 J of energy and thus preexcite the reentry circuit or perhaps abort triggered automaticity.[136] There is evidence that a precordial thump may convert ventricular tachycardia to fibrillation by stimulation during the vulnerable period.[128] This is more likely in patients with ventricular tachycardia who are receiving digitalis.[137] If the patient has collapsed, the chance, though small, that it might succeed and the minimal time lost in the attempt warrant use of the procedure, pending electrical defibrillation.[128]

Countershock should not be delayed, because the duration of hypotension or ventricular fibrillation is inversely related to the success of the procedure. An organized treatment protocol for the resuscitation of patients with ventricular tachycardia and ventricular fibrillation has been established.[138] Blind defibrillation may be attempted in a pulseless patient, but in a monitored setting with a defibrillator present, the recognition of ventricular fibrillation or pulseless ventricular tachycardia should lead to immediate nonsynchronized defibrillation of 200 J without intervening basic life support. If a pulse is not rapidly restored, subsequent shocks of 200 to 300 J, and again at 360 J, should follow.[128,138,139] Arguments for low-energy defibrillation have been proposed, and the efficacy of this approach, particularly in patients with primary ventricular fibrillation during the early phase of acute myocardial infarction, has been well demonstrated.[8b] For ventricular tachycardia, an initial shock of 50 J is usually effective. Appropriate support measures, including cardiopulmonary resuscitation and correction of metabolic disturbances, are crucial. When defibrillation is successful and ventricular fibrillation recurs repeatedly, antiarrhythmic agents administered intravenously may stabilize the myocardium until the period of electrical vulnerability resolves.[58] The treatment of first choice is lidocaine, 100 mg or 1.5 mg/kg as a bolus, and if this is unsuccessful, bretylium tosylate may be effective. Intravenously administered amiodarone may be useful as a last resort, but this is still investigational.

Antiarrhythmia drug therapy. The use of antiarrhythmia agents in acute myocardial infarction was addressed by the Thirteenth Bethesda Conference, and their dosage recommendations are adhered to in the following text.[128]

Lidocaine is the initial drug of choice and the mainstay of therapy. Although it appears to be less effective in patients with sympathetic overactivity manifesting as sinus tachycardia, particularly in the first hour after acute myocardial infarction, the effectiveness of lidocaine in the coronary care unit is not in dispute (Fig 30C-8). Loading and maintenance dosages were discussed earlier. Careful attention to signs of toxicity, both early and late, is necessary since the drug, although relatively safe, is not innocuous. These side effects are dose- and blood level-related and may be kept to a minimum by careful attention to the dosage schedule.

The efficacy of procainamide in acute myocardial infarction has been well established, and it has been used prophylactically.[140] Koch-Weser et al.[140] found that in patients with acute infarction, procainamide given orally at 3-hour intervals significantly reduced the incidence of ventricular fibrillation. Recommended intravenous dosages are 50 mg/min to a total dose of 1 g or until the arrhythmia disappears followed by maintenance dosages of 2 to 6 mg/min, which should be reduced after 12 hours on the basis of blood levels. When the loading dose is given, blood pressure and the ECG should be monitored, although the drug is usually well tolerated hemodynamically, even in patients with heart failure.[141] The incidence of high-grade AV block is small;[142] in patients with conduction disturbances and acute infarction, a temporary pacemaker may be needed before the drug is given.

Use of bretylium tosylate has been largely confined to patients with ventricular arrhythmias that are refractory to lidocaine or procainamide. Clinical studies have shown that parenteral bretylium is effective primarily in suppressing recurrent, resistant ventricular tachycardia or ventricular fibrillation,[143] and it raises the threshold for ventricular fibrillation in both normal and ischemic hearts. Its efficacy in ventricular tachycardia and in the prophylactic treatment of patients suffering from uncomplicated myocardial infarction is less certain.[128] In patients with recurrent, refractory ventricular fibrillation, bretylium may enhance the likelihood of successful defibrillation.[128,144]

The recommended rapid intravenous dosage is 5 to 10 mg/kg, which can be repeated in 1 to 2 hours if the arrhythmia persists. Maintenance therapy is administered at a constant infusion of 1 to 2 mg/min for no longer than 3 to 5 days.

A major limitation to the use of bretylium is hypotension. This is primarily orthostatic and occurs approximately 2 hours after the drug has been given; even in the supine position, significant reductions in blood pressure

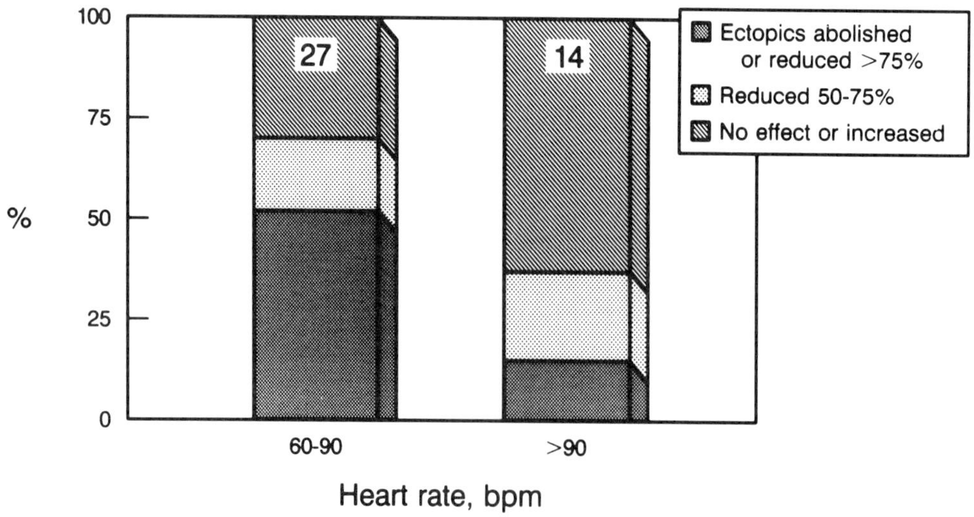

Fig 30C-8 Effect of lidocaine, 100 mg intravenously followed by 2 mg/min, on ventricular ectopic activity in 41 patients treated within 4 hours of the onset of symptoms. The heart rate was between 60 and 90/min in 27 patients and more than 90/min in 14. (From Pantridge JF, Webb SW, Adgey AAJ, et al: The first hour after the onset of acute myocardial infarction. *Prog Cardiol* 3:173-188, 1974. By permission of Lea & Febiger.)

may occur. Hypotension necessitated the withdrawal of bretylium in one-third of patients in one study.[81] The severity of hypotension may be reduced by slower infusion rates, with the drug given over 30 to 45 minutes, by maintenance of a supine position, and by the concomitant administration of fluids. In patients with acute myocardial infarction, use of bretylium may be hazardous. Not only does it interfere with adrenergic tone to cause hypotension but also its positive inotropic and chronotropic actions, related to the initial release of neuronal stores of catecholamines, may aggravate ischemia by increasing myocardial oxygen consumption.

Quinidine sulfate is effective in reducing the incidence of arrhythmias after acute myocardial infarction.[145] It may be administered orally or by intramuscular injection, but experience with the intravenous route in acute myocardial infarction is limited. The drug's ability to cause profound hypotension and conduction disturbances, particularly when the intravenous route is used, has prevented its wider application in acute myocardial infarction.

Phenytoin appears to be of little value in the acute management of ventricular arrhythmias after myocardial infarction. It has been reported to be of use in the prophylaxis of arrhythmias after recovery from myocardial infarction[146,147] and for the arrhythmias of digitalis toxicity. Nonetheless, it should be considered in the patient who is refractory to other forms of therapy, and there appears to be an additive effect when it is given simultaneously with lidocaine.[148] Emergency doses are 100 mg intravenously at 5-minute intervals until the arrhythmia has been abolished, side effects occur, or a total dose of 1,000 mg has been given.[128] After the loading dose, 500 mg is administered on each of the next 2 days in divided doses, modified according to body size. Adverse hemodynamic effects are uncommon but warrant caution, particularly in patients with ventricular dysfunction.

Mexiletine has been shown to be useful for the control of ventricular arrhythmias complicating acute myocardial infarction.[149] The drug was given to 59 patients with lidocaine-resistant arrhythmias and found to be effective in 69%. Side effects were common, however, and they were severe in 29% of patients. In another prospective study, mexiletine given as 250 mg every 8 hours was compared with procainamide given as 500 mg every 4 hours in 60 patients with arrhythmias requiring control with lidocaine within 48 hours of myocardial infarction. Both drugs were effective in comparison with placebo.[149] Clearly, mexiletine is not a drug of first choice but may be useful in patients with arrhythmias that are resistant to conventional agents.

Clinical studies using disopyramide either orally or intravenously have shown a significant reduction in complex ventricular ectopy in both clinical and experimental myocardial infarction.[150,151] In a study of patients with acute myocardial infarction, the clinical efficacy of intravenously administered disopyramide paralleled that of lidocaine; furthermore, disopyramide was found to be an effective alternative agent for patients with arrhythmia uncontrolled by lidocaine.[152]

The intravenous preparation is unavailable in the United States other than on an investigational basis, and the side effects of disopyramide, particularly the negative inotropic action, have limited its use in acute myocardial infarction.

Not surprisingly, tocainide, which is a lidocaine congener, has been shown to be effective in the prophylaxis and treatment of ventricular arrhythmias in both short-term and long-term periods after myocardial infarction.[153] For aprindine, the toxic-therapeutic ratio is narrow, particularly during the initial loading period, and the idiosyncratic reactions to the drug (agranulocytosis and jaundice) limit its use as a first-line drug in acute myocardial infarction.[154] Aprindine is not available for use in the United States.

Despite the wide spectrum of antiarrhythmic effects of amiodarone, an exceedingly long elimination half-life limits the drug's value during the acute phase of myocardial infarction. However, in urgent situations, high doses of amiodarone administered orally may be effective, and in this circumstance, the recommended dosage is 800 to 2,000 mg two to three times daily for 24 to 48 hours to achieve a blood level of 2 to 3 μg/mL.[153,155] Intravenous administration of amiodarone is not routinely available in the United States but is an alternative for intractable arrhythmias in the postinfarction period.

Sotalol, which has recently been made available in the United States, is attractive as an alternative in patients with arrhythmias refractory to other antiarrhythmia agents.[156]

The class 1C agents encainide, flecainide, and propafenone are effective suppressants of ventricular ectopic activity, but their long half-lives, the lack of an intravenous preparation, and their potentially negative inotropic effects have for practical purposes eliminated them in the management of the acute arrhythmias of myocardial infarction.

The role of β-adrenergic blocking agents specifically for the control of ventricular arrhythmias in acute myocardial infarction is not clear. There is evidence that sympathetic overactivity may initiate ventricular arrhythmias, particularly in the early hours after acute myocardial infarction.[14] Although ventricular arrhythmias after acute myocardial infarction may respond to β-adrenergic blockade,[157] results are variable, and the exact situation in which these agents may be effective has not been defined. A double-blind trial of metoprolol, 15 mg given intravenously soon after admission to 1,395 patients with suspected or proved acute myocardial infarction, demonstrated a prophylactic effect against ventricular fibrillation but a lack of effect on less serious ventricular arrhythmias.[158] Pooled results from all the randomized trials of early intravenous β-blockade in acute infarction showed only a very small, albeit statistically significant, difference in the incidence of ventricular fibrillation in treated and untreated patients, 2.2% compared with 2.6%.[58,126] It is rational to use β-blocking drugs for the treatment of arrhythmias related to persistent or recurrent ischemia, provided that ventricular function is adequate and there is no evidence of AV block, but not for specific ventricular arrhythmia prophylaxis.

In patients with persistent or recurrent ischemia and ventricular arrhythmias, a logical approach includes nitrates and, if circumstances allow, β-blocking or calcium-channel-blocking agents. Ventricular arrhythmias are related to the extent of myocardial injury and theoretically may respond to measures aimed at reducing infarct size.[159] Intra-aortic balloon counterpulsation has been effective in the control of ventricular irritability in this situation.[160]

Drug-induced arrhythmias. The relation between delayed repolarization (Q-T interval prolongation) and life-threatening arrhythmias has been well established and is discussed in chapters 24A and 22C. With respect to acute myocardial infarction, the occurrence of malignant arrhythmias is more likely in patients with prolonged Q-T intervals.[161,162] Antiarrhythmia agents such as quinidine and, to a lesser extent, disopyramide, amiodarone, and procainamide may precipitate or exacerbate ventricular arrhythmias. All drugs, including the investigational agents, have the potential to exacerbate arrhythmias. Although torsade de pointes is the most dramatic and characteristic manifestation of this syndrome, the physician should bear in mind the possibility of drug-induced exacerbation of arrhythmia (including diuretics that cause electrolyte depletion) in any patient who is refractory to conventional antiarrhythmia therapy. In this situation, the initial step is to discontinue use of the offending drug and correct any underlying electrolyte disturbances. Other measures that may be required are intravenous use of propranolol, temporary atrial or ventricular pacing, left stellate ganglionic blockade, and, rarely, the use of isoproterenol or glucagon to shorten the Q-T interval.

Each antiarrhythmic drug has the potential for proarrhythmia, and this is most often seen in patients with more extensive myocardial damage, poor left ventricular function, and a history of sustained ventricular tachycardia, but another important factor is ischemia[161] (Fig 30C-9). The last-named factor is particularly relevant in patients with acute myocardial infarction, but an interaction between ischemic myocardium and antiarrhythmic drugs such as encainide and flecainide has been noted and might explain the markedly increased risk of death in treated patients with non-Q-wave myocardial infarctions in CAST.[163]

Invasive electrophysiologic techniques. In acute myocardial infarction, the response of ventricular tachyarrhythmias to pacing is unpredictable. Bradycardia may favor reentry by increasing the temporal dispersion of refractoriness. Pacing or increasing the heart rate may reduce arrhythmogenesis by suppressing the automaticity of Purkinje fibers or by suppressing reentrant mechanisms.[14] Irrespective of the mechanism, atrial and ventricular overdrive pacing has been successfully used to terminate and prevent recurrent ventricular tachycardia.[164-166] The procedure can be dangerous if it accelerates the ventricular rate or introduces a stimulus during the vulnerable period and thereby produces a ventricular fibrillation.[24] It is advisable that the pacemaker rate be

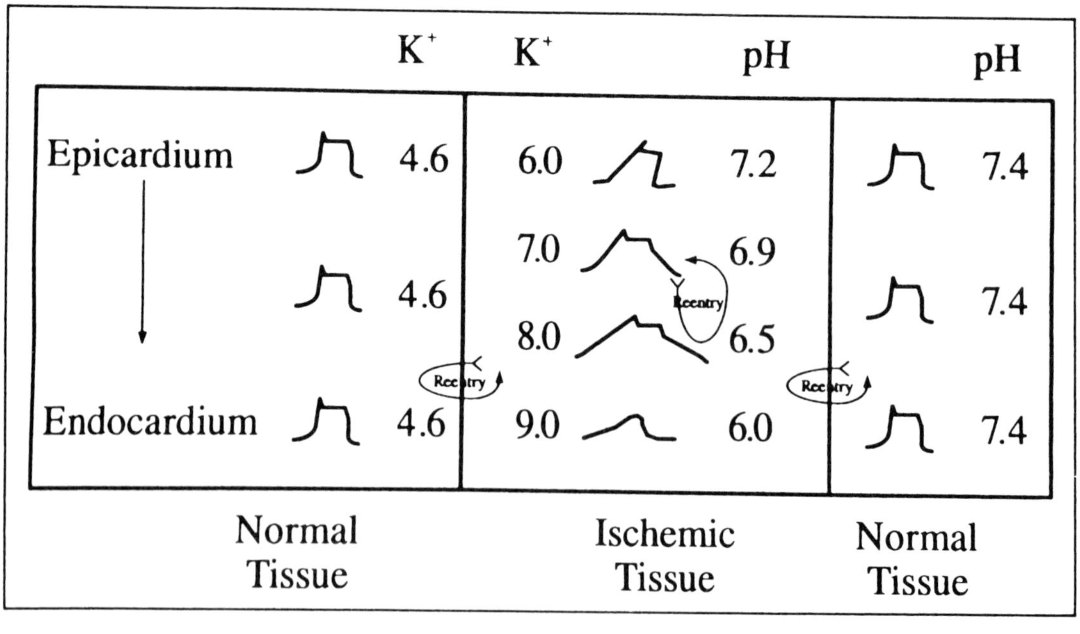

Fig 30C-9 Theoretical mechanism for enhanced potential of reentrant arrhythmias in ischemic tissue. Changes in potassium (K^+) and pH alter action potential and electrophysiologic properties, creating differences between normal and ischemic tissue as well as between epicardium and endocardium within ischemic regions. These differences in electrophysiologic parameters may be enhanced by antiarrhythmic drugs. (From Podrid PJ, Fogel RI: Aggravation of arrhythmia by antiarrhythmic drugs and the important role of underlying ischemia. *Am J Cardiol* 70:100-102, 1992. By permission of Excerpta Medica.)

maintained at the lowest rate consistent with the maintenance of sinus rhythm, keeping in mind the consequences of tachycardia on myocardial oxygen consumption.

Programmed ventricular stimulation to terminate recurrent ventricular arrhythmias in the acute coronary care unit is feasible.[167] Its role, both therapeutically and prognostically, in patients with late-onset arrhythmias[168] is discussed in chapter 30A.

The feasibility and effectiveness of applying low-energy countershock by means of an intravascular catheter in an acute cardiac care unit was reported by Yee et al.[169] in eight patients with recurrent ventricular tachyarrhythmias, two of whom had acute myocardial infarction. This provocative but preliminary report highlights the potential for a more expedient approach to the treatment of acute arrhythmias in myocardial infarction.

Surgery. The surgical approach to postinfarction arrhythmias is discussed in chapter 26.

SUPRAVENTRICULAR ARRHYTHMIAS

Sinus and junctional bradycardia

The incidence of sinus bradycardia in acute myocardial infarction ranges from 14% to 36%.[8c,14,86] Sinus bradycardia may occur in conjunction with sinus arrest or sinoatrial exit block and junctional escape rhythms. Table 30C-3 emphasizes the high incidence of sinus bradyarrhythmias within the first hour after the onset of symptoms;[8c] 70% of 82 patients with sinus or nodal bradycardia had posterior (inferior) infarction.

Mechanisms. Ischemic damage to the sinus node may account for sinus bradycardia in some patients, but two observations suggest that this mechanism is involved only in a minority of cases.[170,171] First, the association between sinus bradycardia and inferior (posterior) myocardial infarction exceeds the frequency that would be expected on the basis of the arterial supply to the sinus node[14] (see Table 30C-3 and Fig 30C-1). Second, the distribution of sinus bradycardia with time after the onset of symptoms, together with the response of the bradycardia to atropine, argues strongly against ischemic damage and points to autonomic imbalance with parasympathetic overactivity as the major cause of sinus bradycardia after acute myocardial infarction.[8c]

Abundant experimental evidence suggests that a cholinergic reflex is important in the genesis of sinus bradycardia after myocardial infarction. Stimulation, in the dog, of the lower interatrial septum in the area between the ostium of the coronary sinus and the posterior AV node (a region richly innervated with cholinergic ganglia and nerve endings) results in bradycardia and hypotension consistent with the Bezold-Jarisch reflex.[172] This area is vulnerable to ischemia in inferior infarction, and stimulation of stretch receptors in acutely ischemic regions could precipitate a vagally mediated reflex and result in bradycardia and vasodilation.[173] Regardless of the actual site of the neural components involved in these reflexes, it is highly likely that in patients with inferior or posterior infarction, a human counterpart of the Bezold-Jarisch reflex is responsible for sinus or nodal bradycardia and hypotension.[174]

Fear, pain, and despair may elicit an oxygen-conserving or "diving" reflex in animals[174] and vasovagal syncope in man.[175] These emotional disturbances are a prominent feature of early acute infarction. Peripheral venous pooling with a reduction in ventricular filling pressure is a feature of the vasovagal syndrome, and in acute infarction, reflex bradycardia is probably accentuated by medications such as morphine and nitrates.

These data do not exclude the possibility that sinus node ischemia or infarction causes both acute and chronic bradyarrhythmias with evidence of the sick sinus node syndrome in some patients.[171] In another study of patients with acute inferior myocardial infarction treated with thrombolytic therapy, sinus bradyarrhythmias and atrial tachyarrhythmias were postulated to be due to ischemia of the sinus node from coronary occlusion proximal to the origin of the sinus node artery.[170]

Clinical features. The significance of sinus bradycardia is related to the hemodynamic and electrophysiologic sequelae of a slow heart rate and the effect of increased vagal tone on mortality and infarct size. If sinus bradycardia is well tolerated without hypotension, an adverse effect on mortality is unlikely and bradycardia may even

Table 30C-3 Incidence of bradyarrhythmias in 331 patients with acute myocardial infarction in a coronary care unit

Arrhythmia	Total incidence, %	Incidence by site of infarction, % — Anterior (n = 158)	Inferior (n = 128)	Combined (n = 45)
Sinus bradycardia	100-30	35-22	53-41	12-27
Nodal bradycardia	20-6	5-3	11-8.5	4-9
First-degree AV block	38-11	11-7	17-13	8-18
Second-degree AV block	30-9	3-2	20-15.5	5-13
Third-degree AV block	29-9	7-4.5	15-12	7-16

From Jewitt D: The genesis of cardiac arrhythmias in acute myocardial infarction. *Prog Cardiol* 1:61-94, 1972. By permission of Lea & Febiger.

be salutary.[176,177] However, the acutely ischemic heart may be unable to compensate for a decrease in heart rate, the result being a reduction in blood pressure, cardiac output, and coronary flow. In sinus tachycardia with junctional escape rhythms, the loss of atrial transport and the possible negative inotropic effect of vagal stimulation could be additive.[178] Pronounced hypotension due to a reduction in coronary perfusion may increase infarct size,[179] although some have concluded the opposite.[180] A clinical study confined to small numbers of patients implicated bradycardia and hypotension as contributors to mortality in acute myocardial infarction.[177]

That bradycardia may predispose to ventricular arrhythmias has a sound experimental basis. In the dog, bradycardia has been shown to increase the temporal dispersion of refractoriness to favor reentry,[163] to facilitate the discharge of ectopic spontaneously depolarizing pacemaker foci,[174] and to reduce the ventricular fibrillation threshold.[174] Evidence to the contrary was provided by Epstein et al.,[180] who, in a different dog model of acute ischemia, could not substantiate any tendency for bradycardia or vagal stimulation to provoke ventricular arrhythmias. Although the experimental data on the relation between bradycardia and ventricular arrhythmias are conflicting, clinical evidence suggests that bradycardia after acute myocardial infarction increases the frequency of premature ventricular complexes and ventricular tachycardia.[1,8c,181] Bradycardia preceding ventricular fibrillation in the early phase of acute myocardial infarction has been noted.[70] Perhaps the arrhythmic sequelae of bradycardia are related to the time after the onset of myocardial infarction, since in hospitalized patients with sinus bradycardia the prognosis is good.[182]

Management. Sinus or nodal bradycardia associated with hypotension or frequent ventricular ectopy should be treated; if it is uncomplicated, no therapy is necessary. Intravenous administration of atropine in 0.3- to 0.5-mg doses up to a maximum of 2.0 mg is recommended, and the benefits may be striking. The lower doses (<0.5 mg) have been associated with a paradoxical bradycardia.[183] The importance of using small incremental doses and of monitoring carefully warrants emphasis, because elimination of vagal overactivity may unmask latent sympathetic overactivity and produce sinus tachycardia and, rarely, ventricular tachycardia or ventricular fibrillation.[8c,181] Inappropriate sinus tachycardia and the initiation of ventricular arrhythmias correlate with the use of larger doses of atropine.[181,184]

Complementary therapy includes the control of pain and anxiety and the avoidance of hypovolemia. The problem of hypovolemia should always be considered if sinus bradycardia is refractory to therapy. We do not advocate the use of isoproterenol except in an extreme emergency, pending temporary pacemaker implantation. A pacemaker is, however, rarely necessary.

Sinus tachycardia

Mechanisms and clinical features. Sinus tachycardia—as a marker of the sympathetic overactivity and autonomic instability that are characteristic of the early phase of acute myocardial infarction—was observed in 24% of patients within 30 minutes after the onset of symptoms and in 15% seen within 1 hour.[8c] When transient hypertension alone was accepted as a marker of sympathetic overactivity, the incidence increased to 35% of patients seen within 30 minutes, and a further 8% were unmasked by treatment of increased vagal tone.[8c] Sinus tachycardia occurs most often in patients with anterior myocardial infarction. The increase in sympathetic activity and circulating catecholamines is probably a result of neurogenic reflexes arising from infarcted and contiguous areas of the left ventricle.[185,186] Pain, fear, anxiety, fever, and hypovolemia are contributory processes. Sinus tachycardia is a compensatory mechanism in cardiac failure, cardiogenic shock, or pulmonary embolism but may follow administration of drugs such as atropine and isoproterenol. Another postulated mechanism for sympathetic overactivity and sinus tachycardia is augmented responsiveness of ischemic myocardium to circulating catecholamines.[45]

Sinus tachycardia is an adverse prognostic sign in acute myocardial infarction.[9,187] The problem is in part related to the link between sinus tachycardia and cardiac failure, since the cardiac failure reflects extensive muscle necrosis. Inasmuch as an increased heart rate increases myocardial oxygen demand and reduces the diastolic filling time, sinus bradycardia may be a cause and not simply a consequence of pump failure.[179] Indeed, both in-hospital and postdismissal mortality have been shown to be increased with increasing heart rate on admission, and on multivariate analysis, heart rate was an *independent* predictor of mortality[179] (Fig 30C-10). Sympathetic overactivity can unfavorably influence arrhythmogenesis by reducing the ventricular fibrillation threshold and facilitating both reentrant and automatic ventricular arrhythmias.[24,40]

Management. The foregoing discussion establishes a strong case for the prompt treatment of sinus tachycardia

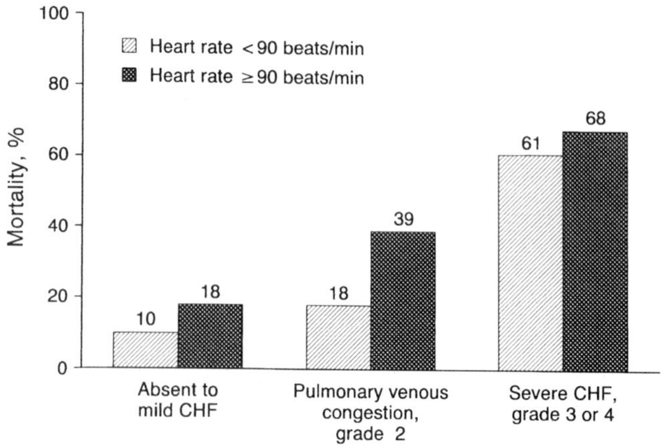

Fig 30C-10 Mortality from hospital dismissal to 1 year stratified by maximum heart rate in the coronary care unit. *CHF*, congestive heart failure. (Data from Hjalmarson Å, Gilpin EA, Kjekshus J, et al: Influence of heart rate on mortality after acute myocardial infarction. *Am J Cardiol* 65:547-553, 1990.)

in acute myocardial infarction. The first step is to correct any underlying causes, including pain, anxiety, and hypovolemia. In the absence of signs of cardiac failure or any other contraindications, intravenous β-blockade is usually safe and effective without the need for invasive monitoring. Our approach is to administer propranolol, metoprolol, or esmolol intravenously in an attempt to maintain the pulse rate below 80 beats/min and to follow this with a maintenance oral dose.[188]

If underlying cardiac failure is suspected, therapy should be guided by invasive hemodynamic monitoring. In our experience, there is a subgroup of patients with sinus tachycardia and baseline hemodynamics who have either normal or a mildly increased pulmonary capillary wedge pressure but in whom the administration of β-blocking agents results in a significant increase in wedge pressure or decrease in cardiac output. In these patients, sinus tachycardia may be masking latent cardiac failure with a sympathetic response to left ventricular dysfunction. Such patients may have a response to a judicious combination of β-blocking agents and either diuretics or vasodilators, but hemodynamic monitoring is essential.

Clearly, autonomic imbalance is a frequent and generally unfavorable accompaniment of the acute phase of myocardial infarction. A convincing incentive to the aggressive treatment of both sympathetic and parasympathetic overactivity is provided by evidence from Pantridge et al.[8c] Early therapeutic intervention in patients in their prospective study yielded a 10% mortality with a 3.3% incidence of cardiogenic shock, which compared favorably with results in a different series of patients seen within an hour of infarction but treated less aggressively.[189]

Atrial tachyarrhythmias

Incidence. Atrial tachyarrhythmias, consisting of atrial premature extrasystoles, atrial fibrillation, atrial flutter, and paroxysmal supraventricular tachycardia, are common; the reported incidence is as high as 44%.[190] These arrhythmias are often transient and recurrent. In approximately one-third of patients, several types of atrial tachyarrhythmias may occur in the same patient.[191] The incidence of atrial fibrillation is approximately 8% to 10%, with a range of 7.5% to 20%.[85,188,191-193] Atrial flutter is encountered less often, 3% to 4%,[191,194] and the incidence of supraventricular tachycardia varies widely, from 2% to 16%, depending on the definition.[85,191,194] Sustained paroxysmal supraventricular tachycardia is rare.[194]

Mechanisms. Experimental electrophysiologic studies have shown that both reentry and focal ectopic activity due to increased automaticity can cause atrial extrasystoles, atrial fibrillation, and supraventricular tachycardia.[14] The experimental induction of atrial fibrillation by atrial premature complexes occurring during the period of atrial vulnerability[195] has been substantiated clinically.[196] The electrophysiologic substrate for these arrhythmias is enhanced by the influence of hypoxia and ischemia on the refractory periods and conduction properties of the atrium. Furthermore, it is likely that autonomic instability plays a critical role in the genesis of these arrhythmias. Parasympathetic overactivity may augment the heterogeneity of refractoriness and conduction and as such can precipitate intra-atrial reentry arrhythmias and atrial fibrillation.[14,197] Supraventricular tachycardia in acute myocardial infarction may be a consequence of AV node reentry; although this mechanism has been well established in patients with ischemic heart disease, its role in acute infarction requires further clarification.[198] Nonparoxysmal junctional tachycardia, in which there is an automatic focus in the lower AV node or common His bundle, has been recognized in acute myocardial infarction and carries a poor prognosis.[199] The electrophysiologic mechanisms of supraventricular tachyarrhythmias have been well explored, but this does not apply to their occurrence in acute myocardial infarction in which the relative frequency of the various mechanisms is unknown.

At a macroscopic level, the pathogenesis of atrial arrhythmias in acute myocardial infarction is attributable to several mechanisms: (1) ischemia of the sinus node and atria, (2) pericarditis, and (3) hemodynamic mechanisms—that is, the consequences of left heart failure with hypoxia, atrial distention, and atrial hypertension. Sympathetic overactivity in this situation may also be contributory.

In some patients, ischemia of the sinus node and atrium as a result of occlusion of the sinus node artery is probably the cause of atrial arrhythmias.[170] This is, however, unlikely to be the responsible mechanism in most patients, because the transient nature of the arrhythmias and their equal frequency of occurrence in anterior and inferior myocardial infarction[191,192] are at variance with the blood supply to the sinoatrial node and with the natural history of ischemic necrosis. In most patients with atrial fibrillation complicating acute myocardial infarction, the arrhythmia develops more than 24 hours after the onset of infarction. One study suggested that "early" atrial fibrillation (within 3 hours of infarction) occurred with coexistent occlusion of the left circumflex artery proximal to the origin of the left atrial circumflex branch and impaired perfusion of the AV nodal artery.[200] Since both arteries contribute to perfusion of the left atrium, the implication is that acute left atrial ischemia is a pathophysiologic mechanism of early atrial fibrillation.[201]

Cristal et al.[190] observed that the prognosis was ominous in patients with atrial arrhythmias and anterior myocardial infarction but unaffected by similar arrhythmias in inferior infarction; thus, two different mechanisms were suggested. In inferior myocardial infarction, the arrhythmias may result from a small area of necrosis affecting the sinus node and the atrium. In contrast, in patients with anterior infarcts, atrial arrhythmias are largely an expression of pump failure, leading to atrial distention, hypoxia, and sympathetic overactivity.[190] A recent population-based study from Worcester, Mass.,[188] documented higher in-hospital and late mortality in patients with atrial fibrillation but suggested that this is mediated through other factors associated with a poor prognosis, although this arrhythmia remains a marker of underlying ventricular dysfunction and a compromised myocardium. Similarly, a large study from Italy documented the association of supraventricular tachyarrhythmias during the late hospital phase of acute myocardial infarction with subsequent death, but this was due to the relationship of supraventricular arrhythmias to cardiac enlargement and left ventricular dysfunction and was not an independent effect.[201] Stretching of the left atrial musculature may in itself be arrhythmogenic, and other studies correlate supraventricular arrhythmias, including atrial fibrillation, with increased left atrial dimension or pressures, left ventricular dysfunction, and advanced age.[192,202]

The subepicardial location of the sinoatrial node and its proximity to the pericardium explain the frequent association of pericarditis and atrial fibrillation after acute myocardial infarction and in pericarditis due to other causes.[170,191,192] In a series of 700 patients with acute myocardial infarction, pericarditis was present in 28% of patients with atrial fibrillation who did not have congestive heart failure, 8% of patients with atrial fibrillation and mild heart failure, and 9% of patients in sinus rhythm.[193] Thus, in patients without congestive heart failure, atrial fibrillation in acute myocardial infarction may be a consequence of pericarditis, whereas in those with heart failure, atrial tachyarrhythmias most likely are a result of left ventricular failure.[193] In an attempt to elucidate the role of inflammatory and hemodynamic factors in the genesis of atrial fibrillation in patients with a first Q-wave anterior infarction, Sugiura et al.[192] documented transient atrial fibrillation in 20% of patients with pericarditis, 14% without pericarditis (not significant), and 42% with hydropericardium. However, the important factors that discriminated the three groups on multivariate analysis were the height of the pulmonary artery wedge pressure and the extent of advanced ventricular asynergy, and it was concluded that atrial fibrillation after Q-wave anterior infarction was related not to the inflammatory infiltration involving the atria but to the increase in atrial pressure resulting from a hemodynamic change caused by more extensive myocardial damage. The possibility that supraventricular arrhythmias may be iatrogenic—for example, due to digitalis toxicity—should always be considered.

Clinical features. The association between atrial tachyarrhythmias and an adverse prognosis in many series is not surprising. Not only do these arrhythmias occur in conjunction with other adverse prognostic features of myocardial infarction but also the tachycardia and the loss of effective atrial contraction may increase the extent of ischemia by causing a decrease in cardiac output and blood pressure and an increase in myocardial energy requirements. In an examination of the effect of atrial fibrillation on subsequent clinical course, Liem et al.[193] showed that in patients with mild congestive heart failure, the development of atrial fibrillation caused clinical deterioration and an increase in mortality. In patients without heart failure and in those with previous severe congestive heart failure, the clinical course was not influenced by the arrhythmias.[193] In another series, only 20% of the patients tolerated the arrhythmia without difficulty.[191] A recent large population-based study suggested that atrial fibrillation is a common complication of myocardial infarction, occurring in 13% to 20% of patients, and that it is associated with higher in-hospital and long-term mortality.[188] Although this is probably mediated through other factors, it remains a marker of underlying ventricular dysfunction and a compromised myocardium.

The onset in most patients is within the first 3 days, and it is uncommon in the prehospital phase. This arrhythmia is typically transient, having had a duration of less than 4 hours in 71% of patients reported in one study. Several investigators have noted that the greater the duration of the arrhythmia and the later its onset, the higher the mortality.[177,192,193]

Management. The principles of management are to treat the underlying causes, to control the ventricular rate, and to prevent further clinical deterioration.

Frequent *atrial premature complexes*, particularly if early-coupled, are a harbinger of atrial tachyarrhythmias in approximately half the patients.[191] A case can be made for treating these patients with digoxin to improve hemodynamic status and control the ventricular rate in the event that they subsequently experience atrial flutter or fibrillation. In our institution, however, atrial premature complexes are not considered an indication for therapy other than careful observation and attention to underlying precipitating factors. The possibility that digoxin in acute myocardial infarction may adversely affect outcome by increasing myocardial oxygen demand underlies our current approach.[203]

Atrial fibrillation may be transient and recurrent. This characteristic limits the value of cardioversion unless the patient is severely symptomatic with hypotension or chest pain. Therapy is aimed at controlling the ventricular rate with digoxin, 0.5 mg intravenously (provided that the patient is not already receiving the drug), followed by 0.125 to 0.25 mg intravenously every 2 hours until a total dose of 1.5 mg over 24 hours has been given. After reversion to sinus rhythm, the likelihood of recurrence warrants maintenance therapy for 3 to 5 days. In acute myocardial infarction, chemical cardioversion with quinidine is of little value.

The use of verapamil or intravenous β-blockers to control the ventricular rate is acceptable, but the pharmacologic properties of these compounds mandate that heart failure and underlying conduction disease be excluded before their use. Safe administration of these drugs in acute infarction complicated by sustained atrial arrhythmias requires careful observation. If overt or occult cardiac failure is suspected, hemodynamic monitoring is useful. The use of β-adrenergic blocking agents in the management of atrial arrhythmias after myocardial infarction has been well established,[204] but the short half-life of esmolol makes it a particularly attractive drug when the hemodynamic situation is borderline.

Control of the ventricular rate with intravenously administered verapamil in eight patients with atrial fibrillation occurring within 72 hours after acute myocardial infarction was reported by Hagemeijer.[205] The drug was administered intravenously in 1-mg doses at 1-minute intervals to a total dose of 20 mg, or less if the arrhythmia was controlled, hypotension occurred, or pulmonary capillary wedge pressure was more than 15 mm Hg.

Attitudes concerning the management of atrial fibrillation in acute myocardial infarction are changing. In patients without overt heart failure or conduction disturbances, verapamil is increasingly being used as the drug of choice. Its beneficial effects on ischemia are an added reason for its use in this situation.

The approach to therapy for *atrial flutter* is similar to that for atrial fibrillation, except that medical management and control of the ventricular rate with drugs (particularly digitalis compounds) are less easily accomplished. Atrial flutter usually responds to low-energy synchronous-mode cardioversion (10 to 25 J), but the self-limited nature of the arrhythmia limits its use. β-Blocking agents and particularly verapamil are useful in controlling the ventricular rate in atrial flutter; reversion to sinus rhythm was noted in seven of eight patients in Hagemeijer's series.[205] The same caveats given for the use of these drugs in atrial fibrillation apply to their use in atrial flutter. Atrial flutter that is refractory to conventional drug therapy may respond to atrial overdrive pacing techniques.[194,206]

For *supraventricular tachycardia*, initial treatment should be carotid sinus massage or other vagal maneuvers. Edrophonium chloride should be used with great caution, since the excessive parasympathetic activity may cause hypotension or bradycardia. In acute myocardial infarction, sympathomimetic agents (for example, phenylephrine or metaraminol), which cause transient hypertension, should be avoided. Intravenous adenosine has been a major advance. If these maneuvers fail, our approach is to use digoxin intravenously (provided that the patient is not already receiving digoxin and that digitalis toxicity has been excluded) unless the hemodynamic status warrants urgent countershock. β-Blocking or calcium channel blocking agents may be of value, but data on their use in sustained supraventricular tachycardia in acute myocardial infarction are sparse.[204,207] On theoretical grounds, one can propose verapamil or diltiazem as the drug of choice if adenosine fails. It has the added advantage of not increasing the risk from subsequent electrical cardioversion if this becomes necessary.

If one can apply the therapeutic principles based on studies in patients without acute myocardial infarction, it is likely that supraventricular tachycardia due to AV node, intra-atrial, or sinus node reentry will respond to overdrive pacing or programmed stimulation techniques, and the overdrive atrial pacing may also suppress "automatic" atrial tachycardia.[208,209] Unfortunately, the minimal overdrive rate required to suppress the arrhythmia may be such as to exacerbate ischemia. Pacing is unlikely to be effective in the therapy of nonparoxysmal junctional tachycardia.[199] Experience with these techniques in acute myocardial infarction is limited.[194,206,209]

Permanent pacemaker implantation for sinus node dysfunction in acute myocardial infarction. Two systematic studies suggest that sinus node dysfunction in acute myocardial infarction is usually temporary but that careful follow-up is required.[210,211] Parameswaran et al.[211] noted the return of normal sinus rhythm in virtually all patients with sinus bradycardia during the acute phase of infarction, but in patients with sinus bradycardia and atrial tachyarrhythmias (tachycardia-bradycardia syndrome), the late prognosis was less benign. Five of the six survivors required prophylactic antiarrhythmia therapy or permanent pacemaker implantation, or both. Simonsen et al.[212] gave a more guarded long-term prognosis for patients with sinus node dysfunction in acute myocardial infarction. Over a mean follow-up of nearly 3 years, symptomatic arrhythmias were noted in 26%, and approximately 10% required permanent pacemaker implantation.

Atrioventricular conduction disturbances

The pathogenesis, prognosis, and management of conduction disturbances in acute myocardial infarction are related to the blood supply of the conduction system, the location of the infarction, the extent of damage to the myocardium and conduction system, and the presence of preexisting conduction disease (see Fig 30C-1). The conduction system may be involved at three levels: the AV node or junction, the bundle of His, and the bundle branches. The anatomy of blood supply of the conduction system has been discussed previously. It is unusual for conduction disease in acute myocardial infarction to be confined to the common His bundle, and for the purposes of this discussion the conduction defects are divided into those proximal and those distal to the common bundle of His and the bundle branches. Classifying the conduction disturbances according to the site of infarction, whether anterior or inferior, has pragmatic value but is an oversimplification, particularly when the vagaries of the blood supply, the collateral circulation, and the preexisting conduction disease are taken into account.

Incidence. The incidence of AV block (excluding bundle-branch block) in 331 patients with acute infarction admitted to the Hammersmith Hospital Coronary Care Unit is shown in Table 30C-3.[168] In the Worcester Heart Attack Study, the overall incidence of complete heart block in 4,762 patients with validated acute infarction hospitalized at 16 hospitals in the Worcester metropolitan area was 5.8%, but the incidence was 3.9% in patients with anterior infarcts and 7.7% in those with inferoposterior infarcts[213] (Table 30C-4). The ECG diagnosis and features of AV block are discussed in chapter 3A. Others report an overall incidence of AV block in acute myocardial infarction of 12% to 25%. In two recent large studies of patients with inferior myocardial infarctions entered into trials of thrombolytic therapy, the incidence of second- and third-degree heart block was 12% in one[208] and the incidence of complete AV block was 13% in the other.[214] First-degree AV block occurs in 2% to 13%, second-degree AV block in 3% to 10% (if due to proximal disease, this almost invariably occurs in type I or Wenckebach pattern), and third-degree, or complete, heart block in 3% to 15%.[10,19,20,215-217]

Proximal conduction disturbances in acute infarction. Proximal conduction disturbances are nearly always a result of inferoposterior infarction. An AV block usually appears within 2 to 72 hours after the onset of symptoms and tends to be transient[208,214] (Fig 30C-11). The average duration is 2 to 4 days, but the block may last as long as

Table 30C-4 Incidence rates and adjusted relative risks of complete heart block complicating acute myocardial infarction (AMI): Worcester Heart Attack Study

Year	All patients		Anterior AMI		Inferior/posterior AMI	
	Incidence rates (%)	Adjusted relative risk	Incidence rates (%)	Adjusted relative risk	Incidence rates (%)	Adjusted relative risk
1975	5.1	1.0*	3.6	1.0*	6.6	1.0*
1978	6.8	1.14† (0.70, 1.85)‡	4.9	1.11 (0.48, 2.55)	8.5	1.17 (0.64, 2.14)
1981	5.2	1.01 (0.61, 1.65)	3.5	0.62 (0.26, 1.49)	6.9	1.16 (0.63, 2.11)
1984	5.0	1.09 (0.63, 1.86)	3.5	0.96 (0.38, 2.40)	6.7	1.14 (0.59, 2.23)
1986	5.9	1.51 (0.86, 2.66)	3.7	0.72 (0.29, 1.74)	8.3	1.89 (0.94, 3.79)
1988	7.3	1.92 (1.09, 3.41)	4.6	0.94 (0.37, 2.34)	9.2	2.42 (1.20, 4.88)
Total	5.8		3.9		7.7	

*Referrent category.
†Risk for developing complete heart block relative to those patients hospitalized in 1975 after controlling for differences in baseline predictive characteristics.
‡95% confidence intervals.
From Goldberg RJ, Zevallos JC, Yarzebski J, et al: Prognosis of acute myocardial infarction complicated by complete heart block (the Worcester Heart Attack Study). *Am J Cardiol* 69:1135-1141, 1992. By permission of Excerpta Medica.

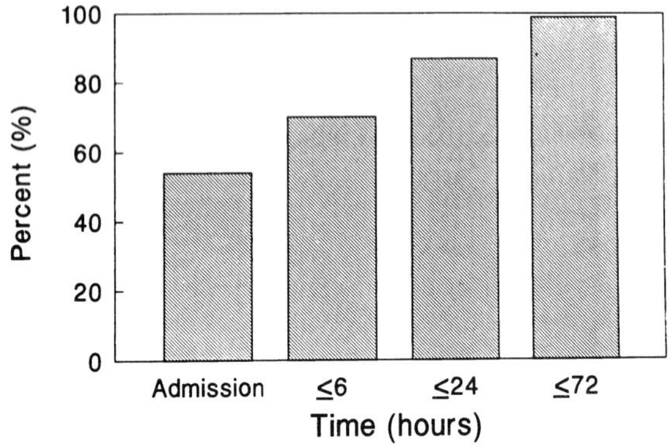

Fig 30C-11 Cumulative percentage of patients in whom complete atrioventricular block developed ≤6, ≤24, and ≤72 hours after onset of myocardial infarction. (From Clemmensen P, Bates ER, Califf RM, et al: Complete atrioventricular block complicating inferior wall acute myocardial infarction treated with reperfusion therapy. *Am J Cardiol* 67:225-230, 1991. By permission of Excerpta Medica.)

16 days;[208,214,216,218] permanent AV block is rare. Progression to complete heart block, if it occurs, is gradual; a preceding period of first- or second-degree AV block occurs in most patients.[216] Resolution of complete heart block is also gradual. In the event of complete heart block, the escape rate of 40 to 50 beats/min and the absence of asystolic pauses are compatible with the properties of a junctional escape pacemaker,[19,215] but slower ventricular rates, less than 40 beats/min, were noted in 44% of patients in one series.[216]

In 1980, Scheinman and Gonzalez[219] stated that classic type II second-degree AV block had not been documented in patients with acute inferior myocardial infarction. Evidence to the contrary was provided by data from the Multicenter Investigation of the Limitation of Infarct Size study,[220] but this was refuted in an editorial by Barold.[221] He stated that "the existence and significance of true type II second-degree AV block with a narrow QRS complex remains to be documented in acute myocardial infarction, particularly inferior wall infarction."

The high incidence of proximal AV block in inferoposterior myocardial infarction is related to the blood supply of the AV node from the branch of the dominant coronary artery, specifically the right coronary artery in 90% of patients. Pathologic studies demonstrate patency of the AV node artery in many patients, and examination of the conduction system has often failed to show necrosis of the AV node, His bundle, or bundle branches.[16] Rotman et al.[19] reviewed the data on 25 patients with posterior myocardial infarction and complete heart block and noted that even in patients with definite necrosis of the AV node and His bundle, necrosis was often not extensive and in many was confined to localized areas within or adjacent to the conducting system. In an autopsy study of 44 hearts with posteroinferior myocardial infarction, 97% of patients with AV block had acute necrosis of the prenodal atrial myocardium; this should be considered a suprahis-

Table 30C-5 Anatomic data from patients who underwent protocol coronary angiography 18 to 48 hours after admission to the hospital in whom heart block did and did not develop by 24 hours after hospital admission

	Heart block by 24 hr (n = 39)		No heart block by 24 hr (n = 723)		
	No.	%	No.	%	P*
Infarct-related artery					0.04
RCA	36	92.3	543	75.1	
LCx	2	5.1	153	21.2	
LAD	1	2.6	27	3.7	
Multivessel disease	13	34.2	246	35.0	NS
Collateral channels present	7	18.4	92	13.1	NS
Stenosis ≥60% in both the LAD and RCA	10	26.3	139	19.8	NS
Stenosis ≥60% in both the LCx and RCA	4	10.5	133	19.0	NS
Occluded infarct-related artery	11	28.2	112	15.5	0.04

LAD, left anterior descending coronary artery; LCx, left circumflex coronary artery; RCA, right coronary artery.
*Statistical significance is indicated by $P < 0.01$; NS = $P \geq 0.10$. All data are expressed as number of patients and percent of patient group.
From Berger PB, Ruocco NA Jr, Ryan TJ, et al: Incidence and prognostic implications of heart block complicating inferior myocardial infarction treated with thrombolytic therapy: results from TIMI II. *J Am Coll Cardiol* 20:533-540, 1992. By permission of American College of Cardiology.

ian structure and could provide an anatomic basis for the block in posteroinferior infarcts.[222] The transient nature of the AV block, the response to atropine, and the histopathologic findings indicate that disorders other than AV node infarction are major causes of conduction disturbances. Speculative but plausible explanations include hypersensitivity of the AV node to hypoxia[14,223] and edema with hydropic cell swelling and inflammation.[224] The heightened susceptibility of the AV node to increased vagal tone and the response to atropine suggest a prominent contribution from vasovagal mechanisms in this situation.

A provocative case report described a patient with AV block who did not have a response to atropine but had a response to aminophylline, a competitive antagonist of adenosine.[225] The primary role of aminophylline may be related to its antagonistic effect on adenosine, which is known to be an endogenous product of ischemia and hypoxia. Whether aminophylline is routinely effective in the management of AV block associated with inferior infarctions remains to be determined.

Complete heart block after acute inferoposterior infarction may infrequently be associated with escape rhythms with wide QRS complexes. This may be due to bundle-branch block (either preexisting or acute) or to a distally located escape focus.[218,226] In bundle-branch block, ECGs that antedate the onset of block are necessary in making the diagnosis. Lie et al.[217] showed that an escape rhythm with a left bundle-branch block morphology in acute inferior infarction was a result of bradycardia-dependent, or phase IV, bundle-branch block, whereas a right bundle-branch block morphology implied a distal escape focus. The mortality in their patients was not increased, and this finding, together with spontaneous regression, led to the conclusion that widened QRS complexes during complete heart block in acute inferior infarction are of no prognostic significance. Others have found the appearance of wide-complex escape beats to be more ominous.[218,226]

Prognosis and management. Proximal complete heart block in inferior infarction is associated with increased mortality, complication rate, and enzyme elevations. In two series, mortality rates in patients with and those without block were 28% and 13%[218] and 22% and 9%,[217] respectively. The excess mortality is primarily due to ventricular dysfunction. One study found that patients with advanced AV block had lower left and right ventricular ejection fractions and more extensive wall motion abnormalities than patients without block.[227] Of importance regarding the blood source of the AV node, which is supplied by the right coronary artery and by collateral flow from the left anterior descending coronary artery, a report from Bassan et al.[17] emphasized the association between AV block complicating posteroinferior infarcts and multivessel disease, specifically, greater prevalence of left anterior descending coronary artery obstruction. This was not the case in the study of patients in the Thrombolysis in Myocardial Infarction trial[208] (Table 30C-5).

Similar findings were reported in the two large studies of thrombolytic therapy. In the Thrombolysis and Angioplasty in Myocardial Infarction study group, complete AV block was a strong independent predictor of in-hospital mortality and in addition was associated with a higher reocclusion rate, ventricular tachyarrhythmias, congestive heart failure, hypotension, and a poor ejection fraction.[214] In this study, acute patency rates of the infarct artery after thrombolytic therapy were similar in patients with and without heart block, whereas in the study by Berger et al.,[208] coronary catheterization 18 to 48 hours after admission revealed occlusion of the infarct-related artery in 28.2% of patients with heart block compared with

Table 30C-6 Influence of high-degree atrioventricular block, infarct location, and heart failure on hospital mortality

Location of infarct and extent of heart failure	Bundle-branch block: With high-degree AVB: Patients, no.	With high-degree AVB: Hospital mortality, %	Without high-degree AVB: Patients, no.	Without high-degree AVB: Hospital mortality, %
Anterior-indeterminate				
Killip I + II	25	36	157	2
Killip III + IV	53	64	114	54
Inferior-posterior				
Killip I + II	17	20	41	2
Killip III + IV	7	80	25	28

AVB, atrioventricular block.
From Hindman MC, Wagner GS, JaRo M, et al: The clinical significance of bundle branch block complicating acute myocardial infarction. 1. Clinical characteristics, hospital mortality, and one-year follow-up. *Circulation* 58:679-688, 1978. By permission of American Heart Association.

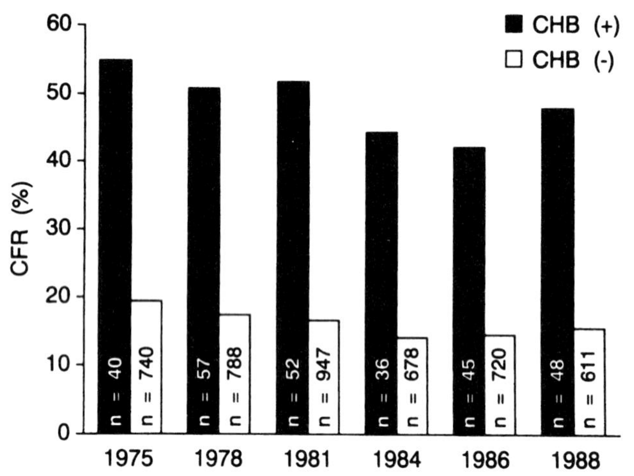

Fig 30C-12 In-hospital fatality rates (CFR) of acute myocardial infarction according to occurrence of complete heart block (CHB) and time period: Worcester Heart Attack Study. (From Goldberg RJ, Zevallos JC, Yarzebski J, et al: Prognosis of acute myocardial infarction complicated by complete heart block (the Worcester Heart Attack Study). *Am J Cardiol* 69:1135-1141, 1992. By permission of Excerpta Medica.)

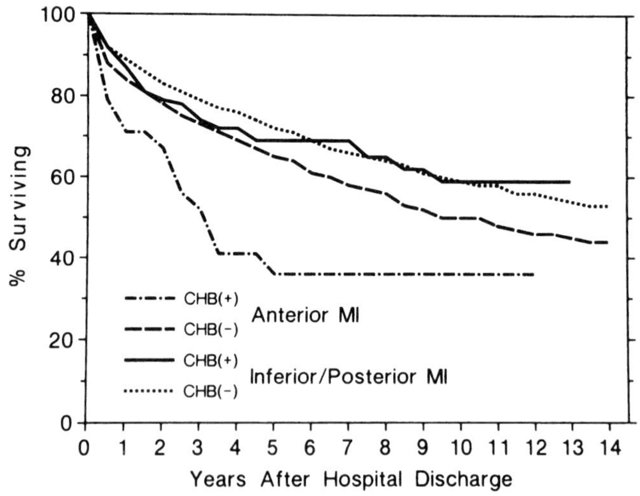

Fig 30C-13 Long-term survival after acute myocardial infarction (*MI*) according to occurrence of complete heart block (*CHB*) and to location of infarction: Worcester Heart Attack Study. (From Goldberg RJ, Zevallos JC, Yarzebski J, et al: Prognosis of acute myocardial infarction complicated by complete heart block (the Worcester Heart Attack Study). *Am J Cardiol* 69:1135-1141, 1992. By permission of Excerpta Medica.)

15.5% of those without. In this study, 21-day mortality was 9.9% in patients with heart block and 2.2% in those without, but a multivariate analysis suggested that mortality was due to severe cardiac dysfunction, and no patient was thought to have died as a result of the heart block or its treatment.

Rotman et al.[228] found that the development of high-degree AV block in inferior infarction did not alter the mortality in two categories—in patients without heart failure or shock and in those with severe heart failure preceding the onset of block. In most patients, mortality is the result of larger infarcts and pump failure, but in a subgroup of patients reported by Tans et al.[216]—namely, those with pump failure and an escape rhythm of less than 50 beats/min—temporary pacing was of striking benefit. This indicates that in some patients with complete heart block and inferoposterior infarction, the conduction disturbance may contribute to heart failure and extension of the infarct.[216] On the basis of these data, temporary pacemaker implantation is not routinely recommended for all patients with inferior infarction and high-grade AV block. In a subgroup of patients with inferior infarction and distal conduction disturbances (namely, bundle-branch block), the natural history appears different because the development of high-grade AV block is of adverse prognostic significance (Table 30C-6).

In the Worcester Heart Attack Study (Fig 30C-12), in-hospital mortality in patients with anterior infarcts and complete heart block was 63% compared with 18.8% in those without heart block. However, a similar trend was seen in patients with inferior-posterior infarcts; in-hospital mortality was 41.9% in those with third-degree heart block and 14% in those without ($P < 0.01$).[213] The impact of complete heart block on long-term outcome after hospital dismissal is illustrated in Figure 30C-13, in which no significant differences in long-term survival are apparent for patients with and without complete heart block in association with inferior-posterior wall infarction.

The occurrence and clinical implications of complete AV block among a large group of patients undergoing thrombolytic therapy in a randomized trial were analyzed.[229] The results were similar to those evidenced before the advent of reperfusion therapy, with an incidence of complete AV block of 10.4% in patients with inferior infarction and 2% in those with anterior infarction. Fifteen-day mortality was 20.1% in patients with AV block as opposed to 8.1% in those without.

The management of proximal conduction disturbances applies mainly to patients with acute inferoposterior infarction. The development of first-degree AV block warrants careful observation without the need for other therapy. Indications for the treatment of second- or third-degree AV block are as follows: (1) symptoms (dizziness, syncope, hypotension, shock, congestive heart failure, or recurrent chest pain), (2) development of bradycardia-related ventricular irritability, (3) asystolic pauses, and (4) a rate persistently below 40 beats/min without symptoms, particularly if the rhythm is that of complete heart block, with escape beats having a wide QRS configuration or resistance to atropine.

The drug of choice is atropine given intravenously. The response varies, and in some patients the chronotropic effects of atropine on the sinus node may exceed its dromotropic effects on the AV node and result in higher grades of AV block.[230] Isoproterenol is not used except in an emergency, pending temporary pacemaker implantation. The use of aminophylline in this situation requires further evaluation.

Distal conduction disturbances (bundle-branch block and AV block) in acute infarction

Pathogenesis. Distal conduction disturbances in acute infarction are associated predominantly with acute anterior infarcts.[20,231] Manifestations of distal conduction disease are bundle-branch block, which can be isolated, bifascicular, trifascicular, bilateral, or alternating; and type II Mobitz (second-degree or third-degree AV block). High-degree AV block is defined as type II second-degree AV block or third-degree AV block that develops after type II second-degree AV block or, often, suddenly without preceding second-degree AV block. The resulting escape rhythm arising from the distal conduction system is slow, has a wide QRS morphology, and is unstable, with a predisposition to asystole and Stokes-Adams attacks. The ECG features of these conduction abnormalities are discussed in chapter 3A.

Fundamental to the combination of distal conduction disturbances and anterior infarction is the proximity of the common His bundle, the proximal right and left bundle branches, and the anterior fascicle of the left bundle branch to the septum (see Fig 30C-1). Dependence of these structures on the septal arteries of the left anterior descending coronary artery and on the extensive dual network from the left and right coronary arteries, which supply much of the distal conduction system, accounts for the severe myocardial damage in patients with distal conduction disturbances that arise in anterior infarction. This reflects either extensive coronary artery disease or widespread necrosis involving the divergent components of the distal conduction system.

Conduction disturbances in anterior infarction should be considered markers of severe disease. Their natural history depends primarily on the extent of ischemic damage and secondarily on the instability of the escape rhythm in the advent of complete heart block. Clearly, treatment of the conduction disturbances, specifically complete heart block, influences only one component of the clinical course and is unlikely to have a major impact on either early or late mortality, except in certain subgroups of patients.

Clinical features. The occurrence of bundle-branch block in acute infarction is the subject of a detailed review by Roos and Dunning[232] of 21 clinical series (including their own) reported between 1969 and 1975. Three more recent studies,[231,233,234] including two large collaborative multicenter studies,[231,233] add substantially to our knowledge of this serious complication of acute infarction. These data include patients with infarcts located anteriorly, inferiorly, or indeterminately, but those with transmural anterior infarction predominate.

The overall incidence of distal conduction disturbances in acute myocardial infarction ranges from 9% to 35%,[20,231,232,234-240] with an average incidence of 20% to 25%. There is a growing impression, however, that during the era of "acute reperfusion," the frequency of distal conduction disturbances has declined. They occur predominantly in older patients. The most frequent types of bundle-branch block (BBB) are isolated left (L) BBB and isolated left anterior fascicular block (LAFB) followed by right (R) BBB plus LAFB and isolated RBBB. Isolated left posterior fascicular block (LPFB) and RBBB plus LPFB occur much less often.[20,231,232] Hospital mortality is high; it was 41.8% in the pooled data of Roos and Dunning,[232] 20% in the UCLA-USCMC series,[234] and 35% in the multicenter study of Hindman et al.,[231] as opposed to 12% in those without BBB (Table 30C-7). In the large database from San Diego, Calif., and Vancouver, Canada, among patients with anterior myocardial infarctions, BBB was associated with a 72% incidence of congestive heart failure and a 32% in-hospital mortality

Table 30C-7 Hospital mortality and risk of progression of high-degree AV block with distal conduction disturbances complicating acute myocardial infarction

Study	Nature of the conduction disturbance*						
	LBBB	RBBB	RBBB + LAFB	RBBB + LPFB	ABBB	CHB	High-degree AVB
				Mortality, %			
Roos and Dunning[232] (pooled data)	44.7	51.3	48	71.3	7	85	...
Hindman et al.[231] (multicenter study)	22	24	29	38	44	...	47
			Risk of progression to high-degree AVB, %				
Roos and Dunning[232] (pooled data)	15	27	31	42	...	...	...
Hindman et al.[233] (multicenter study)	13	14	27	29	44	...	...

*LBBB, isolated left bundle-branch block; RBBB, isolated right bundle-branch block; LAFB, left anterior fascicular block; LPFB, left posterior fascicular block; ABBB, alternating bundle-branch block; CHB, complete heart block; AVB, atrioventricular block.

compared with 52% and 8%, respectively, in patients without RBBB. Mortality 1 year after hospital dismissal was 17% in patients with RBBB as opposed to 7% in those without, and RBBB was an independent predictor of increased in-hospital and 1-year mortality when entered into a multivariate analysis. Nonetheless, the absence of left ventricular failure identifies a subgroup of patients with RBBB who have low in-hospital (4%) and 1-year postdismissal (5%) cardiac mortality. The wide range in figures reflects different patient populations, including criteria, and periods of study. Nonetheless, it is evident that BBB complicating acute infarction is a serious complication, one that is associated with a high mortality and a risk of sudden complete heart block, which further increases mortality.

In a minority of patients with BBB and inferoposterior infarction, hospital mortality was 17%, in comparison with a 9% mortality in 370 control patients without BBB.[231] Twenty percent of such patients had progression to high-degree AV block, although mortality was lower in those in whom progression to complete heart block was preceded by type I second-degree AV block. Even in patients with severe heart failure, the development of high-degree AV block influenced mortality independently[231] (see Table 30C-6).

Prognosis appears to be more favorable in patients with transient BBB.[232,241-243] Lie et al.[242] reported a mortality of 12.5% in patients with BBB of less than 6 hours' duration, 50% in those with BBB of 6 to 24 hours' duration, and no survivors in the few patients in whom BBB persisted. The potential reversibility of conduction disease due to ischemia was highlighted in a report demonstrating transient complete heart block during chest pain in a patient with a reversible septal perfusion defect on a thallium scan.[244] The prognosis in patients with preexisting BBB may be better than that in those in whom BBB appears during the acute infarction;[237] this presumably reflects primary conduction disease in the former and myocardial necrosis in the latter. Neither the aggregated data examined by Roos and Dunning[232] nor the two large studies[231,233,234] confirmed this; nonetheless, in some patients with preexisting conduction disease, high-degree AV block that is amenable to pacing may be a result of new but small areas of necrosis.[237] In an earlier study, Godman et al.[245] found that complete heart block was not frequent in patients with unilateral BBB, and because of the high subsequent mortality due to pump failure in addition to the morbidity of temporary pacing at that time, they advised against prophylactic pacing in patients without bifascicular or bilateral BBB.

Factors determining the risk of the progression of BBB to high-degree AV block were examined by Hindman et al.[233] (Table 30C-7 and Fig 30C-14). At risk were patients with "new" bilateral BBB, defined as RBBB plus LAFB, RBBB plus LPFB, and RBBB plus LBBB; at medium risk were patients with "new" RBBB or LBBB plus first-degree AV block or patients with "old" BBB plus first-degree AV block. In the absence of any of these three combinations of variables, the risk of progression to high-degree AV block was lower (9%). The UCLA-USCMC investigators reported similar findings, although they were unable to show an influence related to the "age" of the BBB.[20]

Lamas et al.,[220] using the database from the Multicenter Investigation for the Limitation of Infarct Size, developed a scoring system designed to predict the incidence of complete heart block and the need for prophylactic temporary pacing. Patients were assigned one point toward the total score for each of the following abnormalities of conduction: first-degree AV block, Mobitz I or Mobitz II second-degree block, left anterior hemiblock, left posterior hemiblock, RBBB, and LBBB. Figure 30C-15 illustrates the usefulness of this index: the risk of heart block developing in patients with a score of 0 was only 1.2%, increasing to 36.4% in patients with a score of 3 or more.

Immediate management. The role of prophylactic pacing in acute myocardial infarction (particularly ante-

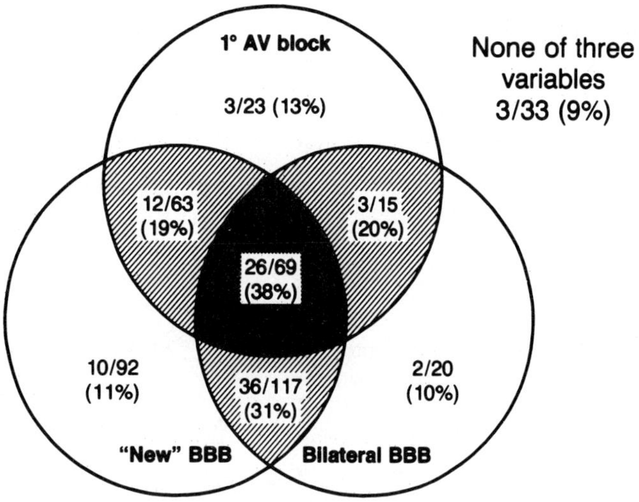

Fig 30C-14 Circles represent population subgroups with one of the three labeled variables. The areas of overlap represent patients with two or three variables. The denominator of each fraction indicates the total number of patients in that subgroup, and the numerator indicates the total number of patients in whom high-degree AV block developed. The percentage of patients with high-degree AV block in each subgroup is noted in parentheses. *BBB,* bundle-branch block. (From Hindman MC, Wagner GS, JaRo M, et al: The clinical significance of bundle branch block complicating acute myocardial infarction. 2. Indications for temporary and permanent pacemaker insertion. *Circulation* 58:689-699, 1978. By permission of American Heart Association.)

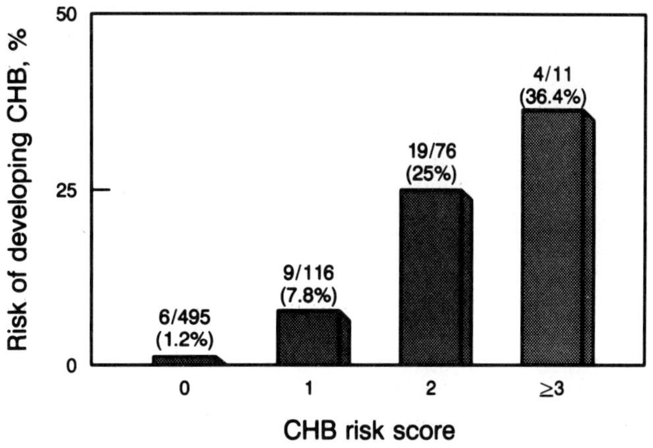

Fig 30C-15 Risk of complete heart block *(CHB)* developing on the basis of ECG conduction abnormalities. (From Lamas GA, Muller JE, Turi ZG, et al: A simplified method to predict occurrence of complete heart block during acute myocardial infarction. *Am J Cardiol* 57:1213-1219, 1986. By permission of Cahners Publishing Company, a Division of Reed Publishing USA.)

rior) complicated by distal conduction disturbances was the subject of extensive debate in the 1970s. The demonstration that death due to pump failure ranged from 25% to 91% (mean, 67%)[232] implied that pacing may have a negligible effect on mortality. Individual studies were unable to show any statistical benefit of pacing on survival, probably because of the small sample size in any single series. A valuable outcome of the two large multi-institutional studies[20,231] is the demonstration that cardiac failure is not an invariable accompaniment of BBB in acute myocardial infarction and that in more than half the patients, cardiac failure was either mild or absent[231] (see Table 30C-6). This strikingly emphasizes the adverse influence on mortality of high-degree AV block that is independent of pump failure or the site of infarction.

Although neither this study[231] nor its predecessors could document the statistical benefit of prophylactic temporary pacing, the issue has been largely resolved without resort to statistical proof. Most series describe patients whose lives were probably saved by pacing and in whom the onset of complete heart block was clinically undetectable and hemodynamically smooth.[246] Furthermore, in patients with BBB and acute infarction, ventricular arrhythmias are common and are a cause of death. The safety of antiarrhythmia drug therapy in patients with serious conduction disturbances is enhanced by prior placement of a temporary pacemaker.

Prophylactic temporary pacing is recommended in patients with BBB and acute infarction, who are considered to be at significant risk for high-degree AV block. This is performed in the hope that it will save the lives of some patients. Furthermore, since the risk of progression to complete heart block is high, prophylactic insertion of a pacemaker spares patients "the experience of resuscitation, with all the splendor and misery of cardiac technology."[232]

Table 30C-8 summarizes our current indications for prophylactic pacing in patients with acute myocardial infarction and distal conduction disturbances. The indications for temporary pacing as listed should not be considered definitive or be adhered to rigidly. Our recent approach has been modified by the development of external noninvasive temporary cardiac pacing.[247] In individual patients, particularly those with more borderline indications for temporary cardiac pacing, insertion of a temporary pacemaker may be avoided, provided that documentation of the ability of an external device to capture is obtained first. Indications for temporary pacing in Table 30C-8 are based to a large extent on the nature of the conduction disturbance and the site of infarction, whether anterior, inferior, or indeterminate. The indications for prophylactic pacing need also take into account the increased risk imposed by thrombolytic therapy and the availability of practical external pacemakers that can be used for standby indications or in an emergency.

The decision to pace a patient with certain ECG patterns of conduction disease is based in part on the natural history and on the assumption that these patterns indicate widespread or trifascicular disease. For example, definitive proof that prolongation of the P-R interval in association with bifascicular block is due to delay in the remaining fascicle would require an invasive electrophysiologic study; such a procedure is as invasive as temporary pacing and is probably not justified in the light of evidence that acute measurement of H-V intervals would add little to patient management.[248,249]

Table 30C-8 Indications for temporary pacing in acute myocardial infarction and distal conduction disturbances

High-grade AVB (type II second-degree AVB or CHB)
RBBB + LAFB (new or indeterminate onset)
RBBB + LPFB (new or indeterminate onset)
RBBB or LBBB plus first- or second-degree block (type I AVB)
Alternating RBBB or LBBB (irrespective of time of onset)
RBBB with alternating LAFB or LPFB (irrespective of time of onset)
"Masquerading" BBB
"Old" or preexisting RBBB + LAFB or LPFB + first-degree AVB
Patients with LBBB in whom flow-directed pulmonary artery catheterization is performed
Exceptions
Patients seen after termination of a transient bifascicular block (duration, <6 hr)

Abbreviations are as in Table 30C-7.

As can be seen from Table 30C-8 and from the ACC-AHA Task Force recommendations for temporary pacemakers in acute myocardial infarction, BBB that has been known to exist before myocardial infarction is considered a contraindication to temporary pacing. A reasonable exception, however, is LBBB in a patient in whom flow-directed pulmonary artery catheterization is considered. The potential exists for "traumatic" RBBB to cause complete heart block and asystole in the patient with underlying LBBB. This is a potential use of temporary pacing wires, which can be inserted via a balloon catheter, but in an emergency, an external, transcutaneous pacing unit is effective, provided that documentation of capture has been obtained.[247,250] In general, we monitor patients with isolated RBBB or LBBB by frequent 12-lead ECGs and resort to pacing if the conduction disorder progresses. Our experience conforms with that of others in that isolated RBBB or LBBB does not progress to complete heart block without passing through a phase of hemiblock, first-degree AV block, or second-degree AV block.[251] The association of anterior myocardial infarction and type I or Mobitz I second-degree AV block is unusual, but because it reflects widespread disease and is associated with a high mortality, it warrants temporary pacing.

Late management. Patients who survive the acute phase of myocardial infarction complicated by BBB (without high-degree AV block) remain at high risk for sudden death after hospital dismissal.[252] Most such deaths are due to underlying severe left ventricular dysfunction, and ventricular fibrillation is the most common cause of sudden death,[10,253] although complete heart block may occur in some patients.[233] Hauer et al.[254] showed that in survivors of BBB and acute myocardial infarction, 7 of 18 patients had potentially lethal complications, consisting of pulmonary edema, AV block, and recurrent ventricular tachycardia/ventricular fibrillation, within the first 6 weeks. They recommended a prolonged period of monitoring in these patients and showed that the 1-year prognosis in patients surviving the first 6 weeks was good and was not likely to be affected by prophylactic pacing.[254] Waters and Mizgala[255] did not advise permanent pacing in survivors of acute myocardial infarction with "incomplete bilateral bundle branch block" and drew attention to the frequency of fatal ventricular arrhythmias. A study from England (the Birmingham Permanent Pacemaker Trial) found no survival benefit with permanent pacing in survivors of acute myocardial infarction complicated by new left posterior hemiblock or RBBB with or without left anterior hemiblock. In this study, the H-V interval measured 2 or more weeks after infarction was not helpful.[256]

The potential role of invasive electrophysiologic testing to evaluate the conduction system before dismissal, including incremental pacing and programmed stimulation to assess the severity of infra-His conduction disease, is of great interest. Stressing the conduction system with the use of drugs such as procainamide should be part of such a study, particularly if it is contemplated that the patient will in the future need antiarrhythmic therapy for spontaneous or inducible arrhythmias.[257-259]

In a minority of patients whose hospital course is complicated by BBB followed by persistent high-degree AV block, permanent pacing is necessary.

More controversial is the issue of permanent pacing in patients with BBB in acute infarction in whom transient complete heart block or type II second-degree AV block has occurred. The poor prognosis after dismissal in patients with anterior myocardial infarction complicated by complete heart block is illustrated in Figure 30C-13. Several studies suggest that the long-term outcome in such patients is not improved by permanent pacing.[246,252,260] A different conclusion was drawn in the multicenter report by Hindman et al.[233] During the first year of follow-up, the incidence of sudden death and recurrent high-degree AV block was 10% in patients with permanent pacing in contrast to 65% in those without pacing. These data support those from previous reports,[261,262] and the recommendation to implant permanent pacemakers in survivors of acute myocardial infarction (particularly anterior infarction) complicated by BBB and transient high-degree AV block is currently followed at our institution. It is recognized that the benefits of pacing are decreased in survivors with severe cardiac dysfunction. The role of permanent pacing in survivors of acute myocardial infarction with BBB without the development of transient high-degree AV block is uncertain.

Temporary transvenous pacing in acute infarction

Techniques and complications of right-heart catheterization in the coronary care unit have been reviewed earlier in this chapter, and many apply to insertion of a temporary pacemaker. Specific aspects of this procedure are discussed here.

Sites of insertion. Hynes et al.[263] reviewed the Mayo Clinic experience with temporary pacemaker insertion in the coronary care unit in 1,022 consecutive patients between 1976 and 1981; 32% of the patient population had acute myocardial infarction.

In this 5-year span, use of the basilic vein declined (95.6% in 1976 but only 22.8% in 1980) in favor of the subclavian and internal jugular venous approaches; this trend continues. The internal jugular vein is currently the preferred route of access, and in our experience it is associated with fewer complications. Potential complications include pneumothorax, carotid artery puncture, and air embolism, but these should be minimal when close attention is paid to technique and experience is greater. Pacemaker insertion via the femoral vein has the attendant hazards of deep venous thrombosis, pulmonary embolism,[264] and infection,[265] and it is used only in an emergency, pending insertion at a more suitable site. When visible, the external jugular vein, usually the right, is an acceptable and safe route of access.

Devices. Bipolar electrodes, which eliminate the inconvenience and discomfort of a remote anode and the problem of extraneous electrical interference, are routinely used in our unit. There are, however, advantages to a unipolar system, particularly in acute myocardial infarction, because undersensing is less frequent and cathodal stimulation is theoretically less likely to cause ventricular fibrillation should a paced stimulus fall on the T wave in the vulnerable period.[208]

The most frequently used temporary pacing device is a single-chamber unit with the ability to pace on demand or asynchronously from the ventricle (VVI mode). Atrial leads (particularly those incorporating preformed J-shaped or looped electrodes) that can be used for temporary atrial pacing or for AV synchronous pacing are helpful and preferred in situations that require either the atrial transport contribution to hemodynamic stability or overdrive pacing.[266-268] Units that function in either the VVI mode (AV sequential pacing without atrial sensing)[266,267] or the DDD mode (both atrial and ventricular sensing in pacing) are now available.[268]

Balloon-pacing catheters are useful,[269] particularly because they do not, at least theoretically, require fluoroscopy for insertion and therefore may be helpful during emergencies. The increased rigidity of the more frequently used rigid catheters requires their placement under fluoroscopic control. However, the flexibility of balloon flotation catheters is a disadvantage in patients who are or are likely to become pacemaker-dependent, since they are less stable in maintaining a pacing position. An important advance has been the development of new balloon-tipped pulmonary artery pressure catheters that incorporate a separate right ventricular pacing port through which a flexible wire is passed into the apex of the right ventricle. Reliability of pacing compares favorably with that reported in the literature with standard transvenous pacing catheters.

Complications. Table 30C-9, as modified from Hynes et al.,[263] lists the complications related to temporary pacemaker implantation in 1,022 patients, including

Table 30C-9 Complications of temporary pacing in 1,022 consecutive patients

Complication	Patients, no.	%
Pericardial friction rub	54	5
Ventricular arrhythmias requiring electrical cardioversion	24	2
Perforation of the right ventricle	21	2
Inadvertent arterial puncture	11	1
Local infection	12	1
Phlebitis	6	1
Diaphragmatic stimulation	10	...
Pneumothorax	1	...
Cardiac tamponade	1	...

Modified from Hynes JK, Holmes DR Jr, Harrison CE: Five-year experience with temporary pacemaker therapy in the coronary care unit. *Mayo Clin Proc* 58:122-126, 1983.

subjects without acute infarcts. No mortality resulted from the procedure. The overall incidence of complications was 13.7% compared with 16.9% reported by Lumia and Rios.[270] The number of complications increased with the duration of pacemaker therapy; 68% of complications occurred in patients in whom the pacemaker had been in place for more than 72 hours.

Pacing system malfunction is common with temporary pacing (the incidence is 18% to 43%)[263,265,270] and manifests as a failure to sense or to pace, or both. Patients with acute myocardial infarction are possibly more liable to pacemaker malfunction because the electrode may be in contact with necrosed tissue.[271] This can lead to high thresholds or low intracardiac potentials and cause malfunction of sensing. Theoretically, these problems will be more frequent in patients with right ventricular infarction, and there are reports suggesting that such patients are at risk for pacemaker-induced ventricular fibrillation and ventricular tachycardia.[272,273] Right ventricular damage may promote failure of pacemaker capture.[274] It is well to remember that a demand pacemaker requires a finite time for the sensing mechanism to become operative. Since the likelihood of pacemaker-induced fibrillation due to a stimulus falling in the vulnerable period is greater at higher current strengths, the output of the generator should be set at a minimum when the pacemaker is initially activated. Thereafter, the output can be increased to threshold levels. The risk of pacemaker-induced ventricular fibrillation is minimized by careful attention to equipment, including the ECG recording machine, telemetry transmitter, and pacemaker generator. Leakage currents may be dangerous, and such accidents are inexcusable.

Infection (both local and systemic) is a potentially hazardous complication that can be minimized by the adoption of sterile conditions during insertion and while the temporary lead is in place. The shorter the time the lead is in place, the less likely the risk of infection, but if bacteremia does occur, the lead should be removed as soon as possible, cultures obtained, and appropriate antibiotic therapy begun. If a new lead has to be implanted, a different route of access must be obtained. Acute venous thrombosis of the upper extremity after insertion of permanent pacemaker leads is a potentially serious complication. The frequency of this complication in patients with acute myocardial infarction is unknown, but an awareness of the venous complications of transvenous pacing is important because prompt diagnosis and therapy may decrease the potential morbidity and mortality.

Thus, complications with temporary cardiac pacing are frequent and perhaps more so in acute myocardial infarction. Nonetheless, with experience and attention to detail, major morbidity can be kept low and mortality minimal.

REFERENCES

1. Lown B, Fakhro AM, Hood WB Jr, et al: The coronary care unit: new perspectives and directions. *JAMA* 199:188-198, 1967
2. Kouwenhoven WB, Jude JR, Knickerbocker GG: Closed-chest cardiac massage. *JAMA* 173:1064-1067, 1960
3. Lown B, Newman J, Amarasingham R, et al: Comparison of alternating current with direct current electroshock across the closed chest. *Am J Cardiol* 10:223-233, 1962
4. Lown B, Amarasingham R, Newman J: New method for terminating cardiac arrhythmias: use of synchronized capacitor discharge. *JAMA* 182:548-555, 1962
5. Cobb LA, Baum RS, Alvarez H III, et al: Resuscitation from out-of-hospital ventricular fibrillation: 4 years follow-up. *Circulation* 52 Suppl 3:223-228, 1975
6. Lown B, Wolf M: Approaches to sudden death from coronary heart disease. *Circulation* 44:130-142, 1971
7. Kuller L, Lilienfeld A: Epidemiological study of sudden and unexpected deaths due to arteriosclerotic heart disease. *Circulation* 34:1056-1068, 1966
8. Pantridge JF, Adgey AAJ, Geddes JS, et al: *The Acute Coronary Attack*. New York, Grune & Stratton, 1975, pp a, 26-42; b, 68-71; c, 43-78
9. Julian DG, Valentine PA, Miller GG: Disturbances of rate, rhythm and conduction in acute myocardial infarction: a prospective study of 100 consecutive unselected patients with the aid of electrocardiographic monitoring. *Am J Med* 37:915-927, 1964
10. Meltzer LE, Kitchell JB: The incidence of arrhythmias associated with acute myocardial infarction. *Prog Cardiovasc Dis* 9:50-63, 1966
11. Mower MM, Miller DI, Nachlas MM: Clinical features relevant to possible resuscitation in death after acute myocardial infarction. *Am Heart J* 67:437-444, 1964
12. Nattel S, Beau S, McCarragher G: Effect of frequent ventricular ectopy on myocardial infarct size in dogs. *Cardiovasc Res* 21:286-292, 1987
13. James TN: The coronary circulation and conduction system in acute myocardial infarction. *Prog Cardiovasc Dis* 10:410-449, 1968
14. Vieweg WVR, Alpert JS, Hagan AD: Origin of the sinoatrial and atrioventricular node arteries in right, mixed, and left inferior emphasis systems. *Cathet Cardiovasc Diagn* 1:361-373, 1975
15. Frink RJ, James TN: Normal blood supply to the human His bundle and proximal bundle branches. *Circulation* 47:8-18, 1973
16. Sutton R, Davies M: The conduction system in acute myocardial infarction complicated by heart block. *Circulation* 38:987-992, 1968
17. Bassan R, Maia IG, Bozza A, et al: Atrioventricular block in acute inferior wall myocardial infarction: harbinger of associated obstruction of the left anterior descending coronary artery. *J Am Coll Cardiol* 8:773-778, 1986
18. Kennel AJ, Titus JL: The vasculature of the human atrioventricular conduction system. *Mayo Clin Proc* 47:562-566, 1972

19. Rotman M, Wagner GS, Wallace AG: Bradyarrhythmias in acute myocardial infarction. *Circulation* 45:703-722, 1972

20. DeGuzman M, Rahimtoola SH: What is the role of pacemakers in patients with coronary artery disease and conduction abnormalities? *Cardiovasc Clin* 13 No. 1:191-207, 1983

21. Wiggers CJ, Wégria R: Ventricular fibrillation due to single, localized induction and condenser shocks applied during the vulnerable phase of ventricular systole. *Am J Physiol* 128:500-505, 1940

22. Harris AS, Guevara Rojas A: The initiation of ventricular fibrillation due to coronary occlusion. *Exp Med Surg* 1:105-122, 1943

23. DeBoer S: On the fibrillation of the heart. *J Physiol (Lond)* 54:400-409, 1921

24. Scherlag BJ, Lazzara R: Ischemic arrhythmias: basic mechanisms. In *Cardiac Arrhythmias: Their Mechanisms, Diagnosis, and Management*. Edited by WJ Mandel. Philadelphia, JB Lippincott Company, 1980, pp 366-395

25. Waldo AL, Kaiser GA: A study of ventricular arrhythmias associated with acute myocardial infarction in the canine heart. *Circulation* 47:1222-1228, 1973

26. Boineau JP, Cox JL: Slow ventricular activation in acute myocardial infarction: a source of re-entrant premature ventricular contractions. *Circulation* 48:702-713, 1973

27. Janse MJ, van Capelle FJL, Morsink H, et al: Flow of "injury" current and patterns of excitation during early ventricular arrhythmias in acute regional myocardial ischemia in isolated porcine and canine hearts: evidence for two different arrhythmogenic mechanisms. *Circ Res* 47:151-165, 1980

28. Davis J, Glassman R, Wit AL: Method for evaluating the effects of antiarrhythmic drugs on ventricular tachycardias with different electrophysiologic characteristics and different mechanisms in the infarcted canine heart. *Am J Cardiol* 49:1176-1183, 1982

29. Scherlag BJ, El-Sherif N, Hope R, et al: Characterization and localization of ventricular arrhythmias resulting from myocardial ischemia and infarction. *Circ Res* 35:372-383, 1974

30. Lazzara R, El-Sherif N, Scherlag BJ: Electrophysiological properties of canine Purkinje cells in one-day-old myocardial infarction. *Circ Res* 33:722-734, 1973

31. Friedman PL, Stewart JR, Wit AL: Spontaneous and induced cardiac arrhythmias in subendocardial Purkinje fibers surviving extensive myocardial infarction in dogs. *Circ Res* 33:612-626, 1973

32. El-Sherif N, Scherlag BJ, Lazzara R, et al: Re-entrant ventricular arrhythmias in the late myocardial infarction period. 1. Conduction characteristics in the infarction zone. *Circulation* 55:686-702, 1977

33. Karagueuzian HS, Fenoglio JJ Jr, Weiss MB, et al: Protracted ventricular tachycardia induced by premature stimulation of the canine heart after coronary artery occlusion and reperfusion. *Circ Res* 44:833-846, 1979

34. Michelson EL, Spear JF, Moore EN: Electrophysiologic and anatomic correlates of sustained ventricular tachyarrhythmias in a model of chronic myocardial infarction. *Am J Cardiol* 45:583-590, 1980

35. Garan H, Fallon JT, Ruskin JN: Sustained ventricular tachycardia in recent canine myocardial infarction. *Circulation* 62:980-987, 1980

36. Dillon SM, Allessie MA, Ursell PC, et al: Influences of anisotropic tissue structure on reentrant circuits in the epicardial border zone of subacute canine infarcts. *Circ Res* 63:182-206, 1988

37. Zipes DP: Electrophysiological mechanisms involved in ventricular fibrillation. *Circulation* 52 Suppl 3:120-130, 1975

38. Weiss JN, Nademanee K, Stevenson WG, et al: Ventricular arrhythmias in ischemic heart disease. *Ann Intern Med* 114:784-797, 1991

39. Opie LH, Nathan D, Lubbe WF: Biochemical aspects of arrhythmogenesis and ventricular fibrillation. *Am J Cardiol* 43:131-148, 1979

40. Han J, Moe GK: Nonuniform recovery of excitability in ventricular muscle. *Circ Res* 14:44-60, 1964

41. Williams DO, Scherlag BJ, Hope RR, et al: The pathophysiology of malignant ventricular arrhythmias during acute myocardial ischemia. *Circulation* 50:1163-1172, 1974

42. Hope RR, Williams DO, El-Sherif N, et al: The efficacy of antiarrhythmic agents during acute myocardial ischemia and the role of heart rate. *Circulation* 50:507-514, 1974

43. Lazzara R, El-Sherif N, Scherlag BJ: Disorders of cellular electrophysiology produced by ischemia of the canine His bundle. *Circ Res* 36:444-454, 1975

44. Gang ES, Bigger JT Jr, Livelli FD Jr: A model of chronic ischemic arrhythmias: the relation between electrically inducible ventricular tachycardia, ventricular fibrillation threshold and myocardial infarct size. *Am J Cardiol* 50:469-477, 1982

45. Denniss AR, Richards DA, Waywood JA, et al: Electrophysiological and anatomic differences between canine hearts with inducible ventricular tachycardia and fibrillation associated with chronic myocardial infarction. *Circ Res* 64:155-166, 1989

46. Schaal SF, Wallace AG, Sealy WC: Protective influence of cardiac denervation against arrhythmias of myocardial infarction. *Cardiovasc Res* 3:241-244, 1969

47. Spear JF, Michelson EL, Spielman SR, et al: The origin of ventricular arrhythmias 24 hours following experimental anterior septal coronary artery occlusion. *Circulation* 55:844-852, 1977

48. Karagueuzian HS, Fenoglio JJ Jr, Weiss MB, et al: Coronary occlusion and reperfusion: effects on subendocardial cardiac fibers. *Am J Physiol* 238:H581-H593, 1980

49. Rothfeld EL, Zucker IR, Parsonnet V, et al: Idioventricular rhythm in acute myocardial infarction. *Circulation* 37:203-209, 1968

50. Hope RR, Scherlag BJ, El-Sherif N, et al: Continuous concealed ventricular arrhythmias. *Am J Cardiol* 40:733-738, 1977

51. Gardner PI, Ursell PC, Fenoglio JJ Jr, et al: Electrophysiologic and anatomic basis for fractionated electrograms recorded from healed myocardial infarcts. *Circulation* 72:596-611, 1985

52. Wit AL, Wiggins JR, Cranefield PF: Some effects of electrical stimulation on impulse initiation in cardiac fibers: its relevance for the determination of the mechanisms of clinical cardiac arrhythmias. In *The Conduction System of the Heart: Structure, Function, and Clinical Implications*. Edited by HJJ Wellens, KI Lie, MJ Janse. Philadelphia, Lea & Febiger, 1976, pp 163-181

53. Josephson ME, Horowitz LN, Farshidi A, et al: Recurrent sustained ventricular tachycardia. 1. Mechanisms. *Circulation* 57:431-440, 1978

54. Porter WT: Further researches on the closure of the coronary arteries. *J Exp Med* 1:46-70, 1896

55. Cairns JA, Connolly SJ, Gent M, et al: Post-myocardial infarction mortality in patients with ventricular premature depolarizations: Canadian Amiodarone Myocardial Infarction Arrhythmia Trial Pilot Study. *Circulation* 84:550-557, 1991

56. Manning AS, Hearse DJ: Reperfusion-induced arrhythmias: mechanisms and prevention. *J Mol Cell Cardiol* 16:497-518, 1984

57. Baughman KL, Maroko PR, Vatner SF: Effects of coronary artery reperfusion on myocardial infarct size and survival in conscious dogs. *Circulation* 63:317-323, 1981

58. Woelfel A, Gettes LS: Tachyarrhythmias during acute myocardial infarction. In *Acute Myocardial Infarction*. Edited by BJ Gersh, SH Rahimtoola. New York, Elsevier Science Publishing Company, 1991, pp 236-248

59. Balke CW, Kaplinsky E, Michelson EL, et al: Reperfusion ventricular tachyarrhythmias: correlation with antecedent coronary occlusion tachyarrhythmias and duration of myocardial ischemia. *Am Heart J* 101:449-456, 1981

60. Naito M, Michelson EL, Kmetzo JJ, et al: Failure of antiarrhythmic drugs to prevent experimental reperfusion ventricular fibrillation. *Circulation* 63:70-79, 1981

61. I.S.A.M. Study Group: A prospective trial of intravenous streptokinase in acute myocardial infarction (I.S.A.M.): mortality, morbidity, and infarct size at 21 days. *N Engl J Med* 314:1465-1471, 1986

62. Koren G, Weiss AT, Ben-David Y, et al: Bradycardia and hypotension following reperfusion with streptokinase (Bezold-Jarisch reflex): a sign of coronary thrombolysis and myocardial salvage. *Am Heart J* 112:468-471, 1986

63. Wei JY, Markis JE, Malagold M, et al: Cardiovascular reflexes stimulated by reperfusion of ischemic myocardium in acute myocardial infarction. *Circulation* 67:796-801, 1983

64. Timmis GC, Ramos RG, Gangadharan V, et al: Determinants of reperfusion arrhythmias in a randomized trial of streptokinase vs angioplasty for acute myocardial infarction (abstract). *Circulation* 72 Suppl 3:219, 1985

65. Goldberg S, Greenspon AJ, Urban PL, et al: Reperfusion arrhythmia: a marker of restoration of antegrade flow during intracoronary thrombolysis for acute myocardial infarction. *Am Heart J* 105:26-32, 1983

66. Miller FC, Krucoff MW, Satler LF, et al: Ventricular arrhythmias during reperfusion. *Am Heart J* 112:928-932, 1986

67. Califf RM, O'Neil W, Stack RS, et al: Failure of simple clinical

measurements to predict perfusion status after intravenous thrombolysis. *Ann Intern Med* 108:658-662, 1988

68. Gressin V, Louvard Y, Pezzano M, et al: Holter recording of ventricular arrhythmias during intravenous thrombolysis for acute myocardial infarction. *Am J Cardiol* 69:152-159, 1992

69. Volpi A, Cavalli A: Secondary ventricular fibrillation complicating acute myocardial infarction. *Prim Cardiol* 18:28-34, October 1992

70. Adgey AAJ, Geddes JS, Mulholland HC, et al: Incidence, significance, and management of early bradyarrhythmia complicating acute myocardial infarction. *Lancet* 2:1097-1101, 1968

71. Goldstein S, Moss AJ, Greene W: Sudden death in acute myocardial infarction: relationship to factors affecting delay in hospitalization. *Arch Intern Med* 129:720-724, 1972

72. Carruth JE, Silverman ME: Ventricular fibrillation complicating acute myocardial infarction: reasons against the routine use of lidocaine. *Am Heart J* 104:545-550, 1982

73. Lown B: Electrical reversion of cardiac arrhythmias. *Br Heart J* 29:469-489, 1967

74. Naito M, Michelson EL, Kaplinsky E, et al: Role of early cycle ventricular extrasystoles in initiation of ventricular tachycardia and fibrillation: evaluation of the R on T phenomenon during acute ischemia in a canine model. *Am J Cardiol* 49:317-322, 1982

75. El-Sherif N, Myerburg RJ, Scherlag BJ, et al: Electrocardiographic antecedents of primary ventricular fibrillation: value of the R-on-T phenomenon in myocardial infarction. *Br Heart J* 38:415-422, 1976

76. Dhurandhar RW, MacMillan RL, Brown KWG: Primary ventricular fibrillation complicating acute myocardial infarction. *Am J Cardiol* 27:347-351, 1971

77. Lie KI, Wellens HJJ, Downar E, et al: Observations on patients with primary ventricular fibrillation complicating acute myocardial infarction. *Circulation* 52:755-759, 1975

78. Lie KI, Wellens HJ, van Capelle FJ, et al: Lidocaine in the prevention of primary ventricular fibrillation: a double-blind, randomized study of 212 consecutive patients. *N Engl J Med* 291:1324-1326, 1974

79. Roberts R, Ambos HD, Loh CW, et al: Initiation of repetitive ventricular depolarizations by relatively late premature complexes in patients with acute myocardial infarction. *Am J Cardiol* 41:678-683, 1978

80. Grenadier E, Alpan G, Maor N, et al: Polymorphous ventricular tachycardia in acute myocardial infarction. *Am J Cardiol* 53:1280-1283, 1984

81. Wolfe CL, Nibley C, Bhandari A, et al: Polymorphous ventricular tachycardia associated with acute myocardial infarction. *Circulation* 84:1543-1551, 1991

82. Ganz W, Geft I, Shah PK, et al: Intravenous streptokinase in evolving myocardial infarction. *Am J Cardiol* 53:1209-1216, 1984

83. Lichstein E, Ribas-Meneclier C, Gupta PK, et al: Incidence and description of accelerated ventricular rhythm complicating acute myocardial infarction. *Am J Med* 58:192-198, 1975

84. Sclarovsky S, Strasberg B, Fuchs J, et al: Multiform accelerated idioventricular rhythm in acute myocardial infarction: electrocardiographic characteristics and response to verapamil. *Am J Cardiol* 52:43-47, 1983

85. Kimball JT, Killip T: Aggressive treatment of arrhythmias in acute myocardial infarction: procedures and results. *Prog Cardiovasc Dis* 10:483-504, 1968

86. Talbot S, Greaves M: Association of ventricular extrasystoles and ventricular tachycardia with idioventricular rhythm. *Br Heart J* 38:457-464, 1976

87. Oliver MJ, Julian DG, Donald KW: Problems in evaluating coronary care units: their responsibilities and their relation to the community. *Am J Cardiol* 20:465-474, 1967

88. O'Doherty M, Tayler DI, Quinn E, et al: Five hundred patients with myocardial infarction monitored within one hour of symptoms. *Br Med J* 286:1405-1408, 1983

89. Stannard M, Sloman G: Ventricular fibrillation in acute myocardial infarction: prognosis following successful resuscitation. *Am Heart J* 77:573, 1969

90. Lawrie DM: Long-term survival after ventricular fibrillation complicating acute myocardial infarction. *Lancet* 2:1085-1087, 1969

91. Goldberg RJ, Gore JM, Haffajee CI, et al: Outcome after cardiac arrest during acute myocardial infarction. *Am J Cardiol* 59:251-255, 1987

92. Behar S, Goldbourt U, Reicher-Reiss H, et al: Prognosis of acute myocardial infarction complicated by primary ventricular fibrillation. *Am J Cardiol* 66:1208-1211, 1990

93. Tofler GH, Stone PH, Muller JE, et al: Prognosis after cardiac arrest due to ventricular tachycardia or ventricular fibrillation associated with acute myocardial infarction (the MILIS study). *Am J Cardiol* 60:755-761, 1987

94. Volpi A, Maggioni A, Franzosi MG, et al: In-hospital prognosis of patients with acute myocardial infarction complicated by primary ventricular fibrillation. *N Engl J Med* 317:257-261, 1987

95. Conley MJ, McNeer JF, Lee KL, et al: Cardiac arrest complicating acute myocardial infarction: predictability and prognosis. *Am J Cardiol* 39:7-12, 1977

96. Schwartz PJ, Zaza A, Grazi S, et al: Effect of ventricular fibrillation complicating acute myocardial infarction on long-term prognosis: importance of the site of infarction. *Am J Cardiol* 56:384-389, 1985

97. Volpi A, Cavalli A, Santoro E, et al: Incidence and prognosis of secondary ventricular fibrillation in acute myocardial infarction: evidence for a protective effect of thrombolytic therapy. *Circulation* 82:1279-1288, 1990

98. Jensen GVH, Torp-Pedersen C, Køber L, et al: Prognosis of late versus early ventricular fibrillation in acute myocardial infarction. *Am J Cardiol* 66:10-15, 1990

99. Moss AJ, Davis HT, DeCamilla J, et al: Ventricular ectopic beats and their relation to sudden and nonsudden cardiac death after myocardial infarction. *Circulation* 60:998-1003, 1979

100. Kotler MN, Tabatznik B, Mower MM, et al: Prognostic significance of ventricular ectopic beats with respect to sudden death in the late postinfarction period. *Circulation* 47:959-966, 1973

101. Ruberman W, Weinblatt E, Goldberg JD, et al: Ventricular premature complexes and sudden death after myocardial infarction. *Circulation* 64:297-305, 1981

102. Schulze RA Jr, Strauss HW, Pitt B: Sudden death in the year following myocardial infarction: relation to ventricular premature contractions in the late hospital phase and left ventricular ejection fraction. *Am J Med* 62:192-199, 1977

103. Bigger JT Jr, Weld FM: Analysis of prognostic significance of ventricular arrhythmias after myocardial infarction: shortcomings of Lown grading system. *Br Heart J* 45:717-724, 1981

104. Bastian BC, Macfarlane PW, McLauchlan JH, et al: A prospective randomized trial of tocainide in patients following myocardial infarction. *Am Heart J* 100:1017-1022, 1980

105. Chamberlain DA, Jewitt DE, Julian DG, et al: Oral mexiletine in high-risk patients after myocardial infarction. *Lancet* 2:1324-1327, 1980

106. Gottlieb SH, Achuff SC, Mellits ED, et al: Prophylactic antiarrhythmic therapy of high-risk survivors of myocardial infarction: lower mortality at 1 month but not at 1 year. *Circulation* 75:792-799, 1987

107. Rydén L, Arnman K, Conradson T-B, et al: Prophylaxis of ventricular tachyarrhythmias with intravenous and oral tocainide in patients with and recovering from acute myocardial infarction. *Am Heart J* 100:1006-1012, 1980

108. Bigger JT Jr, Fleiss JL, Rolnitzky LM, et al: Prevalence, characteristics and significance of ventricular tachycardia detected by 24-hour continuous electrocardiographic recordings in the late hospital phase of acute myocardial infarction. *Am J Cardiol* 58:1151-1160, 1986

109. Farrell TG, Bashir Y, Cripps T, et al: Risk stratification for arrhythmic events in postinfarction patients based on heart rate variability, ambulatory electrocardiographic variables and the signal-averaged electrocardiogram. *J Am Coll Cardiol* 18:687-697, 1991

110. The Cardiac Arrhythmia Suppression Trial (CAST) investigators: Preliminary report: effect of encainide and flecainide on mortality in a randomized trial of arrhythmia suppression after myocardial infarction. *N Engl J Med* 321:406-412, 1989

111. The Cardiac Arrhythmia Suppression Trial II investigators: Effect of the antiarrhythmic agent moricizine on survival after myocardial infarction. *N Engl J Med* 327:227-233, 1992

112. Pratt CM, Théroux P, Slymen D, et al: Spontaneous variability of ventricular arrhythmias in patients at increased risk for sudden death after acute myocardial infarction: consecutive ambulatory electrocardiographic recordings of 88 patients. *Am J Cardiol* 59:278-283, 1987

113. Vetter NJ, Julian DG: Comparison of arrhythmia computer and conventional monitoring in coronary-care unit. *Lancet* 1:1151-1154, 1975

114. Harrison DC: Should lidocaine be administered routinely to all patients after acute myocardial infarction? (Editorial.) *Circulation* 58:581-584, 1978

115. Lie KI, Liem KL, Louridtz WJ, et al: Efficacy of lidocaine in preventing primary ventricular fibrillation within 1 hour after a 300 mg intramuscular injection: a double-blind, randomized study of 300 hospitalized patients with acute myocardial infarction. *Am J Cardiol* 42:486-488, 1978

116. Darby S, Bennett MA, Cruickshank JC, et al: Trial of combined intramuscular and intravenous lignocaine in prophylaxis of ventricular tachyarrhythmias. *Lancet* 1:817-819, 1972

117. Dunn HM, McComb JM, Kinney CD, et al: Prophylactic lidocaine in the early phase of suspected myocardial infarction. *Am Heart J* 110:353-362, 1985

118. Koster RW, Dunning AJ: Intramuscular lidocaine for prevention of lethal arrhythmias in the prehospitalization phase of acute myocardial infarction. *N Engl J Med* 313:1105-1110, 1985

119. DeSilva RA, Hennekens CH, Lown B, et al: Lignocaine prophylaxis in acute myocardial infarction: an evaluation of randomised trials. *Lancet* 2:855-858, 1981

120. MacMahon S, Collins R, Peto R, et al: Effects of prophylactic lidocaine in suspected acute myocardial infarction: an overview of results from the randomized, controlled trials. *JAMA* 260:1910-1916, 1988

121. Hine LK, Laird N, Hewitt P, et al: Meta-analytic evidence against prophylactic use of lidocaine in acute myocardial infarction. *Arch Intern Med* 149:2694-2698, 1989

122. Yusuf S, Wittes J, Friedman L: Overview of results of randomized clinical trials in heart disease. I. Treatment following myocardial infarction. *JAMA* 260:2088-2093, 1988

123. Antman EM, Berlin JA: Declining incidence of ventricular fibrillation in myocardial infarction: implications for the prophylactic use of lidocaine. *Circulation* 86:764-773, 1992

124. Singh BN: Routine prophylactic lidocaine administration in acute myocardial infarction. An idea whose time is all but gone? (Editorial.) *Circulation* 86:1033-1035, 1992

125. The MIAMI Trial Research Group: Arrhythmias. *Am J Cardiol* 56:35G-38G, 1985

126. ISIS-I (First International Study of Infarct Survival) Collaborative Group: Randomized trial of intravenous atenolol among 16,027 cases of suspected myocardial infarction. ISIS-I. *Lancet* 2:57-66, 1986

127. Walker LJE, MacKenzie G, Adgey AAJ: Effect of nifedipine on arrhythmias in the acute phase of myocardial infarction. *Eur Heart J* 9:471-478, 1988

128. American College of Cardiology: Thirteenth Bethesda Conference: emergency cardiac care. *Am J Cardiol* 50:365-420, 1982

129. Wyman MG, Lalka D, Hammersmith L, et al: Multiple bolus technique for lidocaine administration during the first hours of an acute myocardial infarction. *Am J Cardiol* 41:313-317, 1978

130. Ayres SM, Grace WJ: Inappropriate ventilation and hypoxemia as causes of cardiac arrhythmias: the control of arrhythmias without antiarrhythmic drugs. *Am J Med* 46:495-505, 1969

131. Anderson R, Gardner FV, Honey H, et al: Relation between metabolic acidosis and cardiac dysrhythmias in acute myocardial infarction. *Br Heart J* 30:493-496, 1968

132. Nordrehaug JE, von der Lippe G: Hypokalaemia and ventricular fibrillation in acute myocardial infarction. *Br Heart J* 50:525-529, 1983

133. Abraham AS, Rosenman D, Meshulam Z, et al: Serum, lymphocyte, and erythrocyte potassium, magnesium, and calcium concentrations and their relation to tachyarrhythmias in patients with acute myocardial infarction. *Am J Med* 81:983-988, 1986

134. Abraham AS, Rosenmann D, Kramer M, et al: Magnesium in the prevention of lethal arrhythmias in acute myocardial infarction. *Arch Intern Med* 147:753-755, 1987

135. Bussmann W-D, Neumann K, Kaltenbach M: Effects of intravenous nitroglycerin on ventricular ectopic beats in acute myocardial infarction. *Am Heart J* 107:940-944, 1984

136. Cranefield PF: Action potentials, afterpotentials, and arrhythmias. *Circ Res* 41:415-423, 1977

137. Sclarovsky S, Kracoff OH, Agmon J: Acceleration of ventricular tachycardia induced by a chest thump. *Chest* 80:596-599, 1981

138. American Heart Association: *Textbook of Advanced Cardiac Life Support*. Dallas, American Heart Association, 1987, pp 235-248

139. Weaver WD, Thuman C, Compass MK, et al: Cited by Gunnar RM, Lambrew CT, Abrams W, et al: Task Force IV: Pharmacologic interventions. Emergency cardiac care. *Am J Cardiol* 50:393-408, 1982

140. Koch-Weser J, Klein SW, Foo-Canto LL, et al: Antiarrhythmic prophylaxis with procainamide in acute myocardial infarction. *N Engl J Med* 281:1253-1260, 1969

141. Greenspan AM, Horowitz LN, Spielman SR, et al: Large dose procainamide therapy for ventricular tachyarrhythmia. *Am J Cardiol* 46:453-462, 1980

142. Scheinman MM, Weiss AN, Shafton E, et al: Electrophysiologic effects of procaine amide in patients with intraventricular conduction delay. *Circulation* 49:522-529, 1974

143. Heissenbuttel RH, Bigger JT Jr: Bretylium tosylate: a newly available antiarrhythmic drug for ventricular arrhythmias. *Ann Intern Med* 91:229-238, 1979

144. Holder DA, Sniderman AD, Fraser G, et al: Experience with bretylium tosylate by a hospital cardiac arrest team. *Circulation* 55:541-544, 1977

145. Jones DT, Kostuk WJ, Gunton RW: Prophylactic quinidine for the prevention of arrhythmias after acute myocardial infarction. *Am J Cardiol* 33:655-660, 1974

146. Stone N, Klein MD, Lown B: Diphenylhydantoin in the prevention of recurring ventricular tachycardia. *Circulation* 43:420-427, 1971

147. Lovell RRH, Mitchell ME, Prineas RJ, et al: Phenytoin after recovery from myocardial infarction: controlled trial in 568 patients. *Lancet* 2:1055-1057, 1971

148. Yatteau RF, Wallace AG: Clinical pharmacology of antiarrhythmic agents in acute myocardial infarction. *Prog Cardiol* 1:95-119, 1972

149. Campbell RWF, Talbot RG, Dolder MA, et al: Comparison of procainamide and mexiletine in prevention of ventricular arrhythmias after acute myocardial infarction. *Lancet* 1:1257-1260, 1975

150. Jennings G, Model DG, Jones MBS, et al: Oral disopyramide in prophylaxis of arrhythmias following myocardial infarction. *Lancet* 1:51-54, 1976

151. Kus T, Sasyniuk BI: Effects of disopyramide phosphate on ventricular arrhythmias in experimental myocardial infarction. *J Pharmacol Exp Ther* 196:665-675, 1976

152. Sbarbaro JA, Rawling DA, Fozzard HA: Suppression of ventricular arrhythmias with intravenous disopyramide and lidocaine: efficacy comparison in a randomized trial. *Am J Cardiol* 44:513-520, 1979

153. Kreeger RW, Hammill SC: New antiarrhythmic drugs: tocainide, mexiletine, flecainide, encainide, and amiodarone. *Mayo Clin Proc* 62:1033-1050, 1987

154. Zipes DP, Troup PJ: New antiarrhythmic agents: amiodarone, aprindine, disopyramide, ethmozin, mexiletine, tocainide, verapamil. *Am J Cardiol* 41:1005-1024, 1978

155. Mostow ND, Vrobel TR, Noon D, et al: Rapid suppression of complex ventricular arrhythmias with high-dose oral amiodarone. *Circulation* 73:1231-1238, 1986

156. Hohnloser SH, Zabel M, van de Loo A, et al: Efficacy and safety of sotalol in patients with complex ventricular arrhythmias. *Int J Cardiol* 37:283-291, 1992

157. Gibson D, Sowton E: The use of beta-adrenergic receptor blocking drugs in dysrhythmias. *Prog Cardiovasc Dis* 12:16-39, 1969

158. Rydén L, Ariniego R, Arnman K, et al: A double-blind trial of metoprolol in acute myocardial infarction: effects on ventricular tachyarrhythmias. *N Engl J Med* 308:614-618, 1983

159. Roberts R, Husain A, Ambos HD, et al: Relation between infarct size and ventricular arrhythmia. *Br Heart J* 37:1169-1175, 1975

160. Hanson EC, Levine FH, Kay HR, et al: Control of postinfarction ventricular irritability with the intraaortic balloon pump. *Circulation* 62 Suppl 1:130-137, 1980

161. Podrid PJ, Fogel RI: Aggravation of arrhythmia by antiarrhythmic drugs and the important role of underlying ischemia. *Am J Cardiol* 70:100-102, 1992

162. Moss AJ, Schwartz PJ: Delayed repolarization (QT and QTU prolongation) and malignant ventricular arrhythmias. *Mod Concepts Cardiovasc Dis* 51:85-90, 1982

163. Akiyama T, Pawitan Y, Greenberg H, et al: Increased risk of death and cardiac arrest from encainide and flecainide in patients after non-Q-wave acute myocardial infarction in the Cardiac Arrhythmia Suppression Trial. *Am J Cardiol* 68:1551-1555, 1991

164. Kastor JA, DeSanctis RW, Harthorne JW, et al: Transvenous

atrial pacing in the treatment of refractory ventricular irritability. *Ann Intern Med* 66:939-945, 1967

165. Batchelder JE, Zipes DP: Treatment of tachyarrhythmias by pacing. *Arch Intern Med* 135:1115-1124, 1975

166. Moss AJ, Rivers RJ Jr, Griffith LSC, et al: Transvenous left atrial pacing for the control of recurrent ventricular fibrillation. *N Engl J Med* 278:928-931, 1968

167. Hartzler GO, Maloney JD: Programmed ventricular stimulation in management of recurrent ventricular tachycardia. *Mayo Clin Proc* 52:731-741, 1977

168. Jewitt D: The genesis of cardiac arrhythmias in acute myocardial infarction. *Prog Cardiol* 1:61-94, 1972

169. Yee R, Zipes DP, Gulamhusein S, et al: Low energy countershock using an intravascular catheter in an acute cardiac care setting. *Am J Cardiol* 50:1124-1129, 1982

170. Kyriakidis M, Barbetseas J, Antonopoulos A, et al: Early atrial arrhythmias in acute myocardial infarction: role of the sinus node artery. *Chest* 101:944-947, 1991

171. Alboni P, Baggioni GF, Scarfò S, et al: Role of sinus node artery disease in sick sinus syndrome in inferior wall acute myocardial infarction. *Am J Cardiol* 67:1180-1184, 1991

172. Jarisch A, Zotterman Y: Depressor reflexes from the heart. *Acta Physiol Scand* 16:31-51, 1949

173. Costantin L: Extracardiac factors contributing to hypotension during coronary occlusion. *Am J Cardiol* 11:205-217, 1963

174. Zipes DP: The clinical significance of bradycardic rhythms in acute myocardial infarction. *Am J Cardiol* 24:814-825, 1969

175. Engel GL: Psychologic stress, vasodepressor (vasovagal) syncope, and sudden death. *Ann Intern Med* 89:403-412, 1978

176. Norris RM, Mercer CJ, Yeates SE: Sinus rate in acute myocardial infarction. *Br Heart J* 34:901-904, 1972

177. Warren JV, Lewis RP: Beneficial effects of atropine in the pre-hospital phase of coronary care. *Am J Cardiol* 37:68-72, 1976

178. DeGeest H, Levy MN, Zieske H, et al: Depression of ventricular contractility by stimulation of the vagus nerves. *Circ Res* 17:222-235, 1965

179. Hjalmarson Å, Gilpin EA, Kjekshus J, et al: Influence of heart rate on mortality after acute myocardial infarction. *Am J Cardiol* 65:547-553, 1990

180. Epstein SE, Goldstein RE, Redwood DR, et al: The early phase of acute myocardial infarction: pharmacologic aspects of therapy. *Ann Intern Med* 78:918-936, 1973

181. Scheinman MM, Thorburn D, Abbott JA: Use of atropine in patients with acute myocardial infarction and sinus bradycardia. *Circulation* 52:627-633, 1975

182. Norris RM: Bradyarrhythmia after myocardial infarction (letter to the editor). *Lancet* 1:313-314, 1969

183. Chadda KD, Lichstein E, Gupta PK, et al: Effects of atropine in patients with bradyarrhythmia complicating myocardial infarction: usefulness of an optimum dose for overdrive. *Am J Med* 63:503-510, 1977

184. Massumi RA, Mason DT, Amsterdam EA, et al: Ventricular fibrillation and tachycardia after intravenous atropine for treatment of bradycardias. *N Engl J Med* 287:336-338, 1972

185. James TN, Isobe JH, Urthaler F: Analysis of components in a cardiogenic hypertensive chemoreflex. *Circulation* 52:179-192, 1975

186. Brown AM: Excitation of afferent cardiac sympathetic nerve fibres during myocardial ischaemia. *J Physiol (Lond)* 190:35-53, 1967

187. Jewitt DE, Balcon R, Raftery EB, et al: Incidence and management of supraventricular arrhythmias after acute myocardial infarction. *Lancet* 2:734-738, 1967

188. Goldberg RJ, Seeley D, Becker RC, et al: Impact of atrial fibrillation on the in-hospital and long-term survival of patients with acute myocardial infarction: a community-wide perspective. *Am Heart J* 119:996-1001, 1990

189. Mather HG, Pearson NG, Read KLQ, et al: Acute myocardial infarction: home and hospital treatment. *Br Med J* 3:334-338, 1971

190. Cristal N, Szwarcberg (Shahar) J, Gueron M: Supraventricular arrhythmias in acute myocardial infarction: prognostic importance of clinical setting; mechanism of production. *Ann Intern Med* 82:35-39, 1975

191. Liberthson RR, Salisbury KW, Hutter AM Jr, et al: Atrial tachyarrhythmias in acute myocardial infarction. *Am J Med* 60:956-960, 1976

192. Sugiura T, Iwasaka T, Takahashi N, et al: Factors associated with atrial fibrillation in Q wave anterior myocardial infarction. *Am Heart J* 121:1409-1412, 1991

193. Liem KL, Lie KI, Durrer D, et al: Clinical setting and prognostic significance of atrial fibrillation complicating acute myocardial infarction. *Eur J Cardiol* 4:59-62, 1976

194. DeSanctis RW, Block P, Hutter AM Jr: Tachyarrhythmias in myocardial infarction. *Circulation* 45:681-702, 1972

195. Brooks CMcC, Orias O, Gilbert JL, et al: Auricular fibrillation: relationship of 'vulnerable period' to 'dip' phenomenon of auricular excitability curve. *Am J Physiol* 164:301-306, 1951

196. Bennett MA, Pentecost BL: The pattern of onset and spontaneous cessation of atrial fibrillation in man. *Circulation* 41:981-988, 1970

197. Alessi R, Nusynowitz M, Abildskov JA, et al: Nonuniform distribution of vagal effects on the atrial refractory period. *Am J Physiol* 194:406-410, 1958

198. Bigger JT Jr, Goldreyer BN: The mechanism of supraventricular tachycardia. *Circulation* 42:673-688, 1970

199. Konecke LL, Knoebel SB: Nonparoxysmal junctional tachycardia complicating acute myocardial infarction. *Circulation* 45:367-374, 1972

200. Hod H, Lew AS, Keltai M, et al: Early atrial fibrillation during evolving myocardial infarction: a consequence of impaired left atrial perfusion. *Circulation* 75:146-150, 1987

201. Berisso MZ, Carratino L, Ferroni A, et al: Frequency, characteristics and significance of supraventricular tachyarrhythmias detected by 24-hour electrocardiographic recording in the late hospital phase of acute myocardial infarction. *Am J Cardiol* 65:1064-1070, 1990

202. Berisso MZ, Ferroni A, De Caro E, et al: Clinical significance of supraventricular tachyarrhythmias after acute myocardial infarction. *Eur Heart J* 7:743-748, 1986

203. Marcus FI: Use of digitalis in acute myocardial infarction (editorial). *Circulation* 62:17-19, 1980

204. Jewitt DE, Singh BN: The role of β-adrenergic blockade in myocardial infarction. *Prog Cardiovasc Dis* 16:421-438, 1974

205. Hagemeijer F: Verapamil in the management of supraventricular tachyarrhythmias occurring after a recent myocardial infarction. *Circulation* 57:751-755, 1978

206. Zeft HJ, Cobb FR, Waxman MB, et al: Right atrial stimulation in the treatment of atrial flutter. *Ann Intern Med* 70:447-456, 1969

207. Heng MK, Singh BN, Roche AHG, et al: Effects of intravenous verapamil on cardiac arrhythmias and on the electrocardiogram. *Am Heart J* 90:487-498, 1975

208. Berger PB, Ruocco NA Jr, Ryan TJ, et al: Incidence and prognostic implications of heart block complicating inferior myocardial infarction treated with thrombolytic therapy: results from TIMI II. *J Am Coll Cardiol* 20:533-540, 1992

209. Foster PR, Zipes DP: Pacing and cardiac arrhythmias. In *Cardiac Arrhythmias: Their Mechanisms, Diagnosis, and Management*. Edited by WJ Mandel. Philadelphia, JB Lippincott Company, 1980, pp 605-624

210. Hatle L, Bathen J, Rokseth R: Sinoatrial disease in acute myocardial infarction: long-term prognosis. *Br Heart J* 38:410-414, 1976

211. Parameswaran R, Ohe T, Goldberg H: Sinus node dysfunction in acute myocardial infarction. *Br Heart J* 38:93-96, 1976

212. Simonsen E, Nielson BL, Nielsen JS: Sinus node dysfunction in acute myocardial infarction. *Acta Med Scand* 208:463-469, 1980

213. Goldberg RJ, Zevallos JC, Yarzebski J, et al: Prognosis of acute myocardial infarction complicated by complete heart block (the Worcester Heart Attack Study). *Am J Cardiol* 69:1135-1141, 1992

214. Clemmensen P, Bates ER, Califf RM, et al: Complete atrioventricular block complicating inferior wall acute myocardial infarction treated with reperfusion therapy. *Am J Cardiol* 67:225-230, 1991

215. Norris RM: Heart block in posterior and anterior myocardial infarction. *Br Heart J* 31:352-356, 1969

216. Tans AC, Lie KI, Durrer D: Clinical setting and prognostic significance of high degree atrioventricular block in acute inferior myocardial infarction: a study of 144 patients. *Am Heart J* 99:4-8, 1980

217. Lie KI, Wellens JH, Schuilenburg RM, et al: Mechanism and significance of widened QRS complexes during complete atrioventricular block in acute inferior myocardial infarction. *Am J Cardiol* 33:833-839, 1974

218. Gupta PK, Lichstein E, Chadda KD: Heart block complicating acute inferior wall myocardial infarction. *Chest* 69:599-604, 1976

219. Scheinman MM, Gonzalez RP: Fascicular block and acute myocardial infarction. *JAMA* 244:2646-2649, 1980

220. Lamas GA, Muller JE, Turi ZG, et al: A simplified method to predict occurrence of complete heart block during acute myocardial infarction. *Am J Cardiol* 57:1213-1219, 1986

221. Barold SS: Narrow QRS Mobitz type II second-degree atrioventricular block in acute myocardial infarction: true or false? (Editorial.) *Am J Cardiol* 67:1291-1294, 1991

222. Bilbao FJ, Zabalza IE, Vilanova JR, et al: Atrioventricular block in posterior acute myocardial infarction: a clinicopathologic correlation. *Circulation* 75:733-736, 1987

223. Watanabe Y, Dreifus LS: Second degree atrioventricular block. *Cardiovasc Res* 1:150-158, 1967

224. Becker AE, Lie KI, Anderson RH: Bundle-branch block in the setting of acute anteroseptal myocardial infarction: clinicopathological correlation. *Br Heart J* 40:773-782, 1978

225. Wesley RC Jr, Lerman BB, DiMarco JP, et al: Mechanism of atropine-resistant atrioventricular block during inferior myocardial infarction: possible role of adenosine. *J Am Coll Cardiol* 8:1232-1234, 1986

226. Schamroth L, Ziady F, de Kock J: Acute inferior wall myocardial infarction associated with complete atrioventricular block and left posterior hemiblock. *Br Heart J* 37:471-474, 1975

227. Strasberg B, Pinchas A, Arditti A, et al: Left and right ventricular function in inferior acute myocardial infarction and significance of advanced atrioventricular block. *Am J Cardiol* 54:985-987, 1984

228. Rotman M, Wagner GS, Waugh RA: Significance of high degree atrioventricular block in acute posterior myocardial infarction: the importance of clinical setting and mechanism of block. *Circulation* 47:257-262, 1973

229. Maggioni AP, Franzosi MG, Santoro E, et al: Incidence and prognostic significance of complete atrio-ventricular block in 11,483 patients treated with reperfusion therapy after acute myocardial infarction in the GISSI-2 trial (abstract). *J Am Coll Cardiol* 21:87A, 1993

230. Castellanos A, Garcia HG, Rozanski JJ, et al: Atropine-induced multilevel block in acute inferior myocardial infarction: a possible indication for prophylactic pacing. *PACE* 4:528-537, 1981

231. Hindman MC, Wagner GS, JaRo M, et al: The clinical significance of bundle branch block complicating acute myocardial infarction. 1. Clinical characteristics, hospital mortality, and one-year follow-up. *Circulation* 58:679-688, 1978

232. Roos JC, Dunning AJ: Bundle branch block in acute myocardial infarction. *Eur J Cardiol* 6:403-424, 1978

233. Hindman MC, Wagner GS, JaRo M, et al: The clinical significance of bundle branch block complicating acute myocardial infarction. 2. Indications for temporary and permanent pacemaker insertion. *Circulation* 58:689-699, 1978

234. DeGuzman M, Ahmadpour H, Haywood LJ: Incidence, development, progress and outcome of atrioventricular block in acute myocardial infarction with bundle branch block: a ten year analysis (abstract). *Circulation* 64 Suppl 4:197, 1981

235. Col JJ, Weinberg SL: The incidence and mortality of intraventricular conduction defects in acute myocardial infarction. *Am J Cardiol* 29:344-350, 1972

236. Atkins JM, Leshin SJ, Blomqvist G, et al: Ventricular conduction blocks and sudden death in acute myocardial infarction: potential indications for pacing. *N Engl J Med* 288:281-284, 1973

237. Gann D, Balachandran PK, Sherif NE, et al: Prognostic significance of chronic versus acute bundle branch block in acute myocardial infarction. *Chest* 67:298-303, 1975

238. Rizzon P, Di Biase M, Baissus C: Intraventricular conduction defects in acute myocardial infarction. *Br Heart J* 36:660-668, 1974

239. Basualdo CAE, Haraphongse M, Rossall RE: Intraventricular blocks in acute myocardial infarction. *Chest* 67:75-78, 1975

240. Scheinman M, Brenman B: Clinical and anatomic implications of intraventricular conduction blocks in acute myocardial infarction. *Circulation* 46:753-760, 1972

241. Norris RM, Croxson MS: Bundle branch block in acute myocardial infarction. *Am Heart J* 79:728-733, 1970

242. Lie KI, Wellens HJ, Schuilenburg RM, et al: Factors influencing prognosis of bundle branch block complicating acute antero-septal infarction: the value of His bundle recordings. *Circulation* 50:935-941, 1974

243. Lichstein E, Gupta PK, Chadda KD: Long-term survival of patients with incomplete bundle-branch block complicating acute myocardial infarction. *Br Heart J* 37:924-930, 1975

244. Weiss AT, Hasin Y, Gotsman MS: Septal ischemia as a mechanism of complete atrioventricular block: demonstration by thallium scintigraphy. *Am J Cardiol* 51:1559-1560, 1983

245. Godman MJ, Lassers BW, Julian DG, et al: Complete bundle-branch block complicating acute myocardial infarction. *N Engl J Med* 282:237-240, 1970

246. Nimetz AA, Shubrooks SJ Jr, Hutter AM Jr, et al: The significance of bundle branch block during acute myocardial infarction. *Am Heart J* 90:439-444, 1975

247. Zoll PM, Zoll RH, Falk RH, et al: External noninvasive temporary cardiac pacing: clinical trials. *Circulation* 71:937-944, 1985

248. Harper R, Hunt D, Vohra J, et al: His bundle electrogram in patients with acute myocardial infarction complicated by atrioventricular or intraventricular conduction disturbances. *Br Heart J* 37:705-710, 1975

249. Gould L, Reddy CVR, Kim SG, et al: His bundle electrogram in patients with acute myocardial infarction. *PACE* 2:428-434, 1979

250. Falk RH, Zoll PM, Zoll RH: Safety and efficacy of noninvasive cardiac pacing: a preliminary report. *N Engl J Med* 309:1166-1168, 1983

251. Kennelly BM: To pace or not to pace. In *Advances in the Management of Arrhythmias*. Edited by DT Kelly. Australia, Telectronics, 1978, pp 388-393

252. Ginks WR, Sutton R, Oh W, et al: Long-term prognosis after acute anterior infarction with atrioventricular block. *Br Heart J* 39:186-189, 1977

253. Lie KI, Liem KL, Schuilenburg RM, et al: Early identification of patients developing late in-hospital ventricular fibrillation after discharge from the coronary care unit: a 5 1/2 year retrospective and prospective study of 1,897 patients. *Am J Cardiol* 41:674-677, 1978

254. Hauer RNW, Lie KI, Liem KL, et al: Long-term prognosis in patients with bundle branch block complicating acute anteroseptal infarction. *Am J Cardiol* 49:1581-1585, 1982

255. Waters DD, Mizgala HF: Long-term prognosis of patients with incomplete bilateral bundle branch block complicating acute myocardial infarction: role of cardiac pacing. *Am J Cardiol* 34:1-6, 1974

256. Watson RDS, Glover DR, Page AJF, et al: The Birmingham Trial of permanent pacing in patients with intraventricular conduction disorders after acute myocardial infarction. *Am Heart J* 108:496-501, 1984

257. Bhandari AK, Hong R, Kotlewski A, et al: Prognostic significance of programmed ventricular stimulation in survivors of acute myocardial infarction. *Br Heart J* 61:410-416, 1989

258. Hamer A, Vohra J, Hunt D, et al: Predictions of sudden death by electrophysiologic studies in high risk patients surviving acute myocardial infarction. *Am J Cardiol* 50:223-229, 1982

259. Richards DA, Cody DV, Denniss AR, et al: Ventricular electrical instability: a predictor of death after myocardial infarction. *Am J Cardiol* 51:75-80, 1983

260. Murphy E, DeMots H, McAnulty J, et al: Prophylactic permanent pacemakers for transient heart block during myocardial infarction? Results of a prospective study (abstract). *Am J Cardiol* 49:952, 1982

261. Ritter WS, Atkins JM, Blomqvist CG, et al: Permanent pacing in patients with transient trifascicular block during acute myocardial infarction. *Am J Cardiol* 38:205-208, 1976

262. Waugh RA, Wagner GS, Haney TL, et al: Immediate and remote prognostic significance of fascicular block during acute myocardial infarction. *Circulation* 47:765-775, 1973

263. Hynes JK, Holmes DR Jr, Harrison CE: Five-year experience with temporary pacemaker therapy in the coronary care unit. *Mayo Clin Proc* 58:122-126, 1983

264. Nolewajka AJ, Goddard MD, Brown TC: Temporary transvenous pacing and femoral vein thrombosis. *Circulation* 62:646-650, 1980

265. Austin JL, Preis LK, Crampton RS, et al: Analysis of pacemaker malfunction and complications of temporary pacing in the coronary care unit. *Am J Cardiol* 49:301-306, 1982

266. Hartzler GO, Maloney JD, Curtis JJ, et al: Hemodynamic benefits of atrioventricular sequential pacing after cardiac surgery. *Am J Cardiol* 40:232-236, 1977

267. Fields J, Berkovits BV, Ing EE, et al: Surgical experience with

temporary and permanent A-V sequential demand pacing. *J Thorac Cardiovasc Surg* 66:865-877, 1973

268. Littleford PO: Physiologic temporary pacing: techniques and indications. *Clin Prog Electrophysiol Pacing* 2:236, 1984

269. Lang R, David D, Klein HO, et al: The use of the balloon-tipped floating catheter in temporary transvenous cardiac pacing. *PACE* 4:491-496, 1981

270. Lumia FJ, Rios JC: Temporary transvenous pacemaker therapy: an analysis of complications. *Chest* 64:604-608, 1973

271. Sutton R, Chatterjee K, Leatham A: Heart-block following acute myocardial infarction: treatment with demand and fixed-rate pacemakers. *Lancet* 2:645-648, 1968

272. Sclarovsky S, Zafrir N, Strasberg B, et al: Ventricular fibrillation complicating temporary ventricular pacing in acute myocardial infarction: significance of right ventricular infarction. *Am J Cardiol* 48:1160-1166, 1981

273. Cueni TA, White RA, Burkart F: Pacemaker-induced ventricular tachycardia in patients with acute inferior myocardial infarction. *Int J Cardiol* 1:93-97, 1981

274. Belhassen B, Pelleg A, Lavotzkin J, et al: Conduction disturbances between a pacemaker electrode and the myocardium in right ventricular infarction. *J Electrocardiol* 14:101-103, 1981

CHAPTER

31

Coronary revascularization: indications and outcomes

Michael D. McGoon, M.D., Valentin Fuster, M.D., Bernard J. Gersh, M.B.,Ch.B., D.Phil., and Charles J. Mullany, M.B., B.S.

THE first coronary artery bypass graft operation was performed in 1964, and the first percutaneous transluminal coronary angioplasty (PTCA) was done in 1977. In the early 1990s, bypass graft operations were performed at a rate of approximately 380,000 per year in the United States and PTCA procedures at 340,000 per year.[1,2] This chapter focuses predominantly on issues pertaining to whether or not to recommend revascularization by coronary artery bypass grafting. Data on efficacy and outcome are distilled from various methods of study, which provide different perspectives from which to draw overall conclusions (Tables 31-1 and 31-2). Similar considerations apply to decisions about angioplasty and other recanalization procedures, but these are modified by factors such as differences in risk, discomfort, expense, recurrence of coronary artery stenosis, and need for repeat or subsequent alternative procedures.[35]

BENEFITS OF CORONARY REVASCULARIZATION

Relief of angina

Benefits. From 80% to 90% of patients with stable or unstable angina experience symptomatic improvement or become symptom-free after coronary artery bypass grafting operations.[13,14,22,29,36-38] Immediate symptomatic success rates for PTCA of 85% to 90% have been estimated.[1] Improvement occurs in similar proportions of patients with one-, two-, or three-vessel involvement or left main coronary artery stenosis who undergo coronary artery bypass grafting. Mitigation of symptoms appears to be related to adequacy of revascularization (Table 31-3) and to graft patency.[16] In addition to relieving symptoms, revascularization appears to impart a reduced risk of subsequent myocardial infarction in patients with three-vessel coronary artery disease[39,40] (Fig 31-1).

Table 31-1 Methodologic types of clinical trials comparing coronary bypass with medical treatment

Type	Controls	Strengths	Weaknesses	Representative studies
Retrospective, matched	Historical or life table	Simplicity Large study population	Comparability not ensured Selection bias	Buffalo General Hospital[3] Texas Heart Institute[4]
Registry	Concurrent, nonrandomized	Size Selection bias can be reduced by statistical adjustment[5]	Unrecorded baseline variables may prevent valid comparison	Seattle Heart Watch[6-11] Duke[12]
Prospective, randomized	Random assignment, with or without stratification	Removes investigator bias Balances groups for all variables (known or unknown)	Crossover Low participation rates Changes in therapy over time	VA[13-20] European[21-23] CASS[24-30] NCSG[31-34]

CASS, Coronary Artery Surgery Study; NCSG, National Cooperative Study Group for unstable angina; VA, Veterans Administration.

Table 31-2 Difficulties in comparing or pooling studies

Problems	Example	Study
Different study populations	Stable angina	
Symptomatic status	Mild	CASS
	42% class III or IV	ECSS
	60% class III	VA
Left ventricular function	Ejection fraction >50%	ECSS
	Any ejection fraction	VA
	Ejection fraction ≥35%	CASS
Degree of stenosis	≥75% narrowing	Duke
	≥50% narrowing	ECSS, VA
Distribution of disease	Left main stenosis excluded	NCSG
	Proximal LAD stenosis	CASS < ECSS
Different study periods (involving changing cardiovascular mortality, learning curve phenomenon, and changing techniques, drugs, and ancillary care)	1969-74	Seattle
	1969-80	Duke
	1972-74	VA
	1972-76	NCSG
	1973-76	ECSS
	1974-79	CASS
Different results in "comparable" groups		
Five-year survival in medical patients	85%	ECSS
	93%	Duke
Operative mortality	3.3%	ECSS
	5.8%	Duke

CASS, Coronary Artery Surgery Study; ECSS, European Coronary Surgery Study; LAD, left anterior descending coronary artery; NCSG, National Cooperative Study Group for unstable angina; VA, Veterans Administration.

Duration of benefit. Recurrence of angina in patients with initial lessening of symptoms after bypass grafting occurs at a rate of 3% to 20% per year.[41] Recurrence of symptoms is highly correlated with changes in the grafts of coronary arteries, including graft occlusion or severe stenosis, progression of a preexisting stenosis to occlusion, and development of new stenoses distal to the graft or in ungrafted arteries.[42]

Studies comparing the incidence of patency for the internal thoracic artery with that for the saphenous vein have shown superiority for the former. In patients with recurrent symptoms studied 3 to 10 years after revascularization, patency was only 26% for saphenous veins but 94% for internal thoracic arteries.[43] The patency rate of the internal thoracic artery at 7.5 years has been reported to be 94%, compared with 50% for the saphenous vein.[44] Other studies have also confirmed better patency of the internal thoracic artery than of saphenous vein grafts at 1 year (88.5% compared with 76.4%) and at 10 years (84.1% compared with 52.8%).[45] Despite the greater patency of the internal thoracic artery than of the saphenous vein, the use of the internal thoracic artery has not been definitely shown to extend the duration of relief from angina. Although Loop et al.[46] demonstrated improvement in survival and greater freedom from late myocardial infarction, reoperation, and late cardiac events in patients receiving an internal thoracic graft, the return of angina was not greatly different from that in patients with saphenous grafts only. This finding suggests that preservation of flow to the left anterior descending artery and septum is important in influencing survival of major cardiac events and that return of angina is more influenced by progression of disease in the right and circumflex systems.[47] Nevertheless, because of the increased patency of the internal thoracic artery and subsequent better survival, attempts are being made to provide nearly complete revascularization with both internal thoracic arteries or other arterial conduits, such as the gastroepiploic and inferior epigastric arteries.[48,49]

Among patients undergoing successful PTCA, restenosis occurs in approximately 40%, frequently with recurrence of symptoms. The incidence of restenosis has not been demonstrably affected by refinements in dilatation techniques or modification of adjunctive drug therapy strategies.

Implications for quality of life. Most studies have found few, if any, gains in work rehabilitation of surgically treated patients in comparison with those managed medically.[6,30,50-56] Our experience has been that employment declines progressively in both treatment groups.[55] Among postoperative patients, the strongest predictors of nonemployment are, in decreasing order, (1) postoperative angina, (2) preoperative unemployment, (3) employment as a laborer, and (4) age greater than 55 years.[55]

Revascularization appears to result in a significant reduction in subsequent cardiovascular hospitalizations, predominantly because of fewer admissions due to myocardial infarction.[57]

Prolongation of life

Survival of medically treated patients with angina is inversely related to the extent of coronary artery involvement[58,59] (Fig 31-2). Factors found at catheterization to be additionally associated with mortality are abnormal left ventricular function (Fig 31-3), left main coronary artery stenosis (see Fig 31-2), and increased left ventricular end-diastolic pressure. Important noninvasive predictors of mortality are a history of peripheral vascular disease, severe congestive heart failure, conduction defects, ventricular premature complexes at rest, and progressive or nocturnal chest pain.[58]

Randomized trials and registry studies have provided reliable indicators of the effect of coronary artery bypass grafting on survival. In the group of all patients with angina, there is generally a small but usually not statistically significant improvement in survival[29] (Fig 31-4). A

Table 31-3 Results with coronary revascularization correlated with degree of revascularization

	Revascularization		
Clinical result	**Complete***	**Partial†**	**None**
Free of angina, %	85	40	5
Negative treadmill exercise test, %	91	24	0

*All stenoses were more than 50%, with nonoccluded graft.
†One or more but not all grafts were occluded or one or more stenoses were not revascularized.

more important observation, however, is that certain subgroups can be defined in which survival is significantly enhanced by surgical intervention, as discussed below.

Left main coronary artery stenosis. The survival of patients with more than 50% narrowing of the diameter of the left main coronary artery is enhanced by coronary artery bypass grafting. The Veterans Administration (VA) Cooperative Study of stable angina,[20] the European Coronary Surgery Study (ECSS) group,[23] and the Collaborative Study in Coronary Artery Surgery (CASS)[26] all support this conclusion (Fig 31-5). The improvement in comparison with medical therapy is particularly pronounced when the stenosis is severe,[20,26] when left ventricular function is impaired, or when there is concomitant right coronary occlusion.[63]

Revascularization also improves survival in most patients with left main equivalent coronary disease (proximal disease in the left anterior descending and circumflex arteries).[64]

Three-vessel disease. Coronary artery bypass grafting tends to prolong survival in most patients who have stenotic lesions in all three coronary arteries[11,12,20,23] (Fig 31-6), although this improvement is not always statistically significant[60] or sustained.[61] This benefit resides predominantly among the population of patients with three-vessel disease and reduced left ventricular function[14,60] (Fig 31-7). Among these patients, the survival outcomes for both therapeutic modalities are at least somewhat worse than those for patients with normal left ventricular function; however, the disparity between medical and surgical outcomes is more pronounced, significantly favoring revascularization. The VA study and CASS suggest that there is little or no survival benefit from surgery in patients with three-vessel disease and no left ventricular dysfunction (unless, in the VA study, only the 10 institutions with low operative mortality are considered).[20] In contrast, the ECSS showed improved survival in patients with normal left ventricular function undergoing surgery for three-vessel disease.[65] This result may, in part, be due to differences in baseline patient characteristics (see Table 31-2). Analysis of CASS registry data[66] supports the conclusion that advanced anginal symptoms in patients with three-vessel disease and normal left ventricular function have a negative prognostic significance for medically treated, but not for surgically treated, patients (see Fig 31-1).

In general, *all available information suggests that among patients with stable angina and three-vessel coronary artery disease, those with worse prognostic indicators (significant ischemic symptoms or left ventricular dysfunction) have the most improved outcomes from revascularization.*

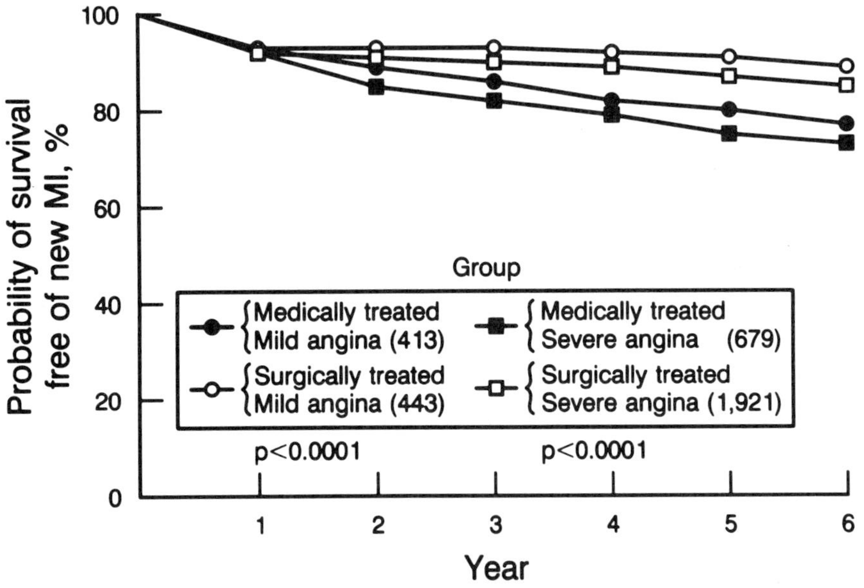

Fig 31-1 Nonrandomized patients with three-vessel disease in the Coronary Artery Surgery Study (CASS) registry evaluated in terms of survival free of myocardial infarction *(MI)*. Patients with either mild or severe angina had improved infarct-free survival if revascularization was performed.[39,40]

Two-vessel disease. For all patients with two-vessel coronary artery disease, the benefit from revascularization in terms of survival is less pronounced. Nevertheless, with the exception of the randomized CASS patients (Fig 31-8,A), a trend of improved survival has been noted as a result of surgical intervention in randomized trials (Fig 31-8,B and C) and registries.[8,12,67] Patients with significant angina do not seem to have any added benefit from surgery in terms of longevity if their left ventricular function is normal (Fig 31-9,A); however, as left ventricular function deteriorates, enhanced survival due to surgery becomes more definite[68] (Fig 31-9,B and C). Revascularization also appears to specifically benefit patients in

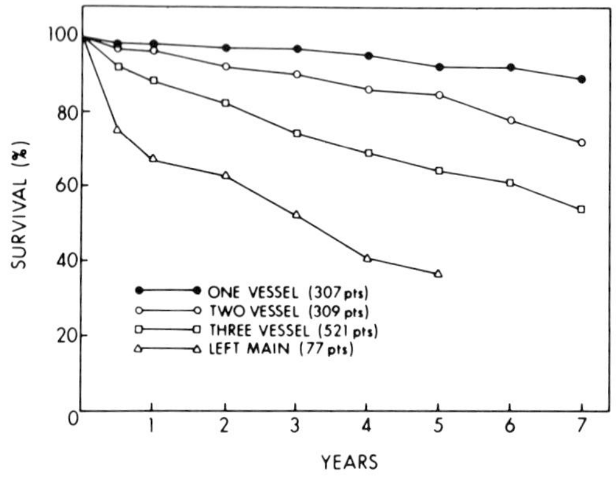

Fig 31-2 Cumulative survival with one-, two-, and three-vessel disease and left main coronary artery disease. (From Harris PJ, Harrell FE Jr, Lee KL, et al: Survival in medically treated coronary artery disease. *Circulation* 60:1259-1269, 1979. By permission of American Heart Association.)

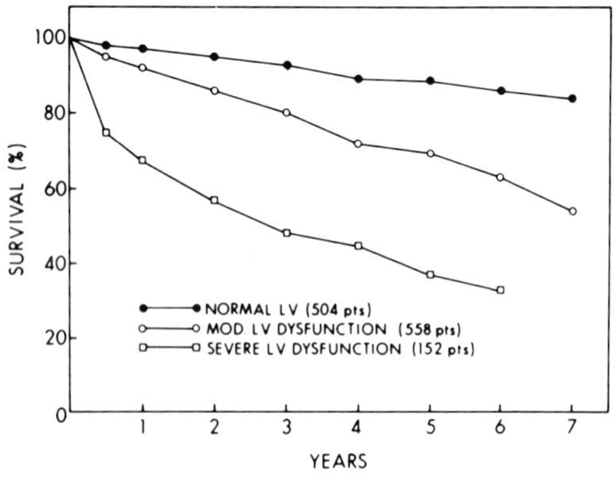

Fig 31-3 Cumulative survival related to the overall left ventricular *(LV)* contraction pattern. Moderate LV dysfunction represents an abnormal but not a diffusely abnormal LV contraction pattern. (From Harris PJ, Harrell FE Jr, Lee KL, et al: Survival in medically treated coronary artery disease. *Circulation* 60:1259-1269, 1979. By permission of American Heart Association.)

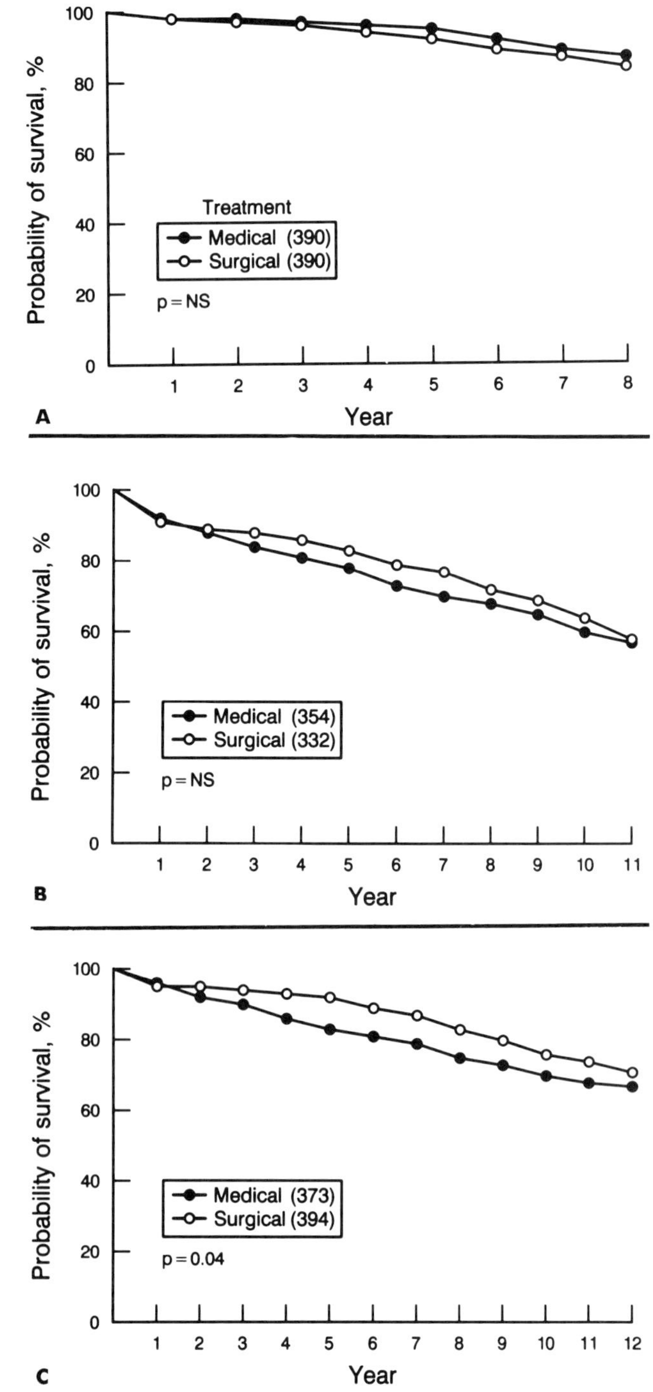

Fig 31-4 Actuarial survival of all randomized patients with coronary artery disease undergoing either medical or surgical treatment in the **(A)** CASS,[60] **(B)** Veterans Administration (VA) Coronary Artery Bypass Surgery Cooperative Study,[61] and **(C)** European Coronary Surgery Study (ECSS).[62]

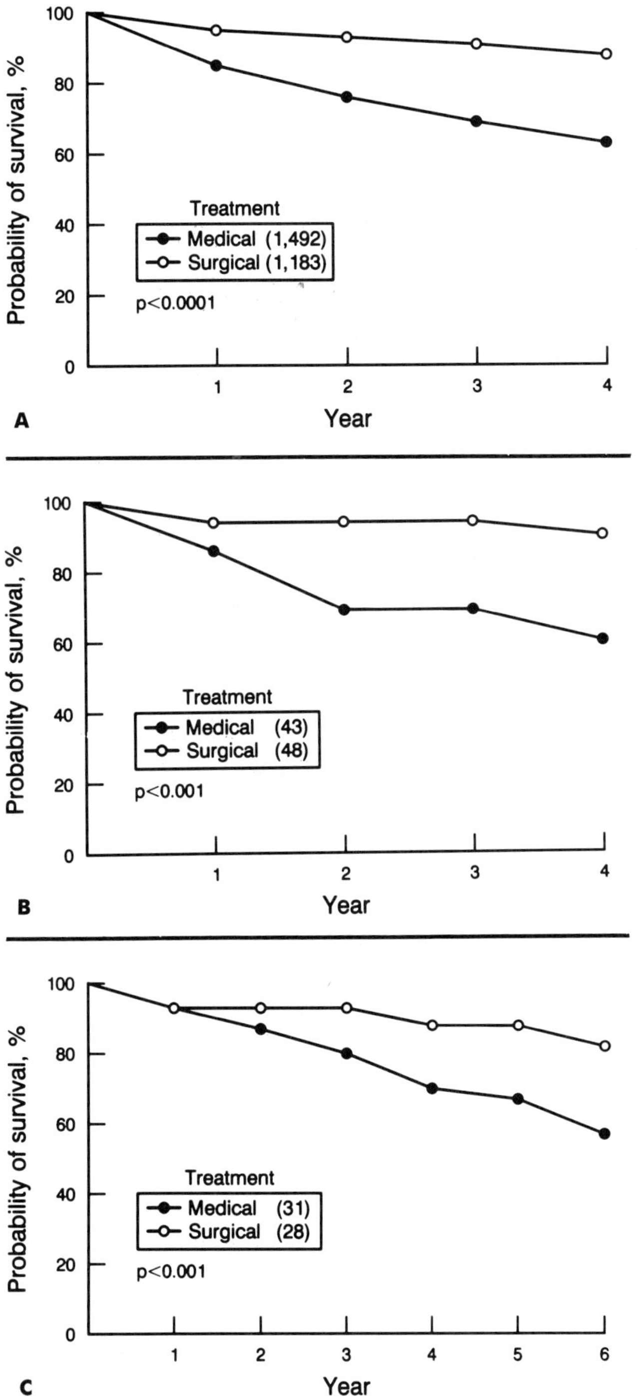

Fig 31-5 Actuarial survival of patients with left main coronary artery disease in the **(A)** CASS registry,[26] **(B)** VA study,[20] and **(C)** ECSS.[23]

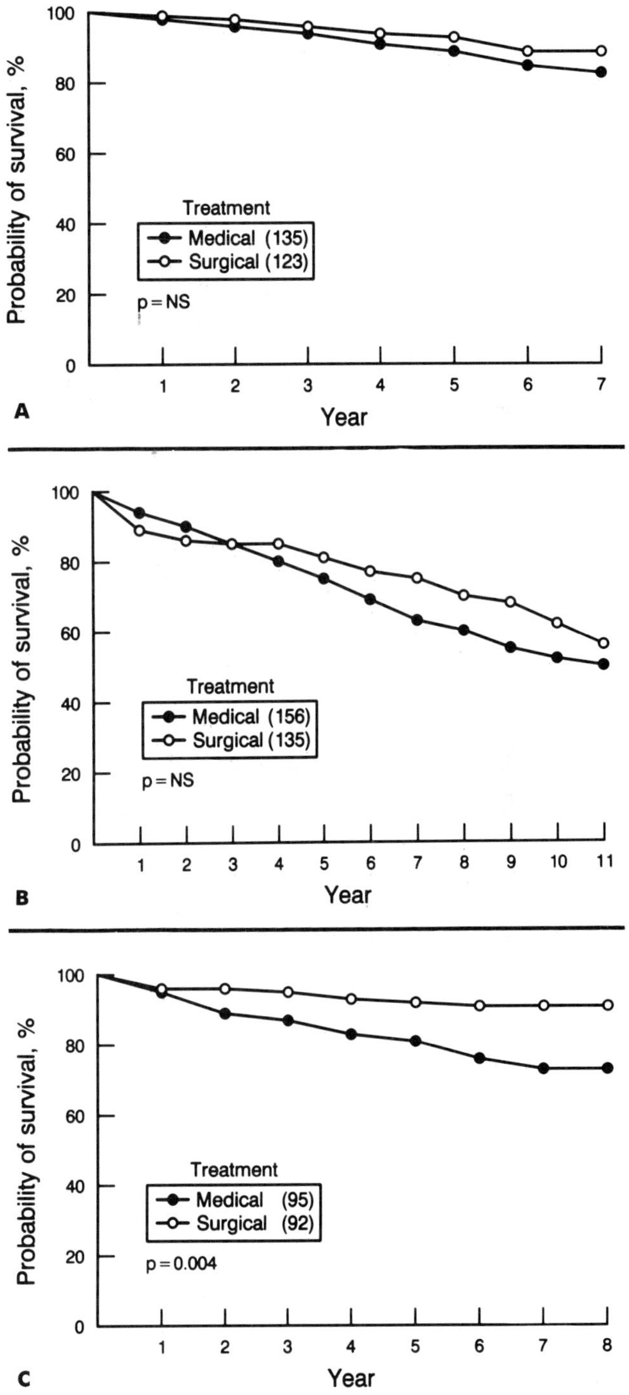

Fig 31-6 Actuarial survival for randomized patients with three-vessel coronary artery disease in the **(A)** CASS,[60] **(B)** VA study,[61] and **(C)** ECSS.[65]

whom one of the two stenosed vessels is the proximal left anterior descending artery.[65]

One-vessel disease. Coronary artery bypass grafting in patients with single-vessel involvement offers no documented improvement in longevity (Fig 31-10). The main rationale for single-vessel coronary artery bypass grafting is for relief of medically refractory angina[69] when catheter-based intervention is not feasible or has been unsuccessful.

Symptomatic status. Since improving survival would be the only indication for surgery in an asymptomatic or minimally symptomatic patient, it is useful to know whether these patients respond to surgery in the same way as the entire group of patients with coronary artery disease. Indeed, the Seattle Heart Watch registry study, which examined this point,[11] found that the results in minimally symptomatic patients essentially paralleled those in their entire cohort: surgery improved survival (borderline significance), the effect being greatest in those with three-vessel disease and moderately impaired left ventricular function. These results were further confirmed by CASS:[70] among patients with exercise-induced silent ischemia, the survival of those with single- or two-vessel disease was not improved by coronary bypass, whereas those with three-vessel disease had a 7-year survival of 85% after surgery, compared with 58% for patients not

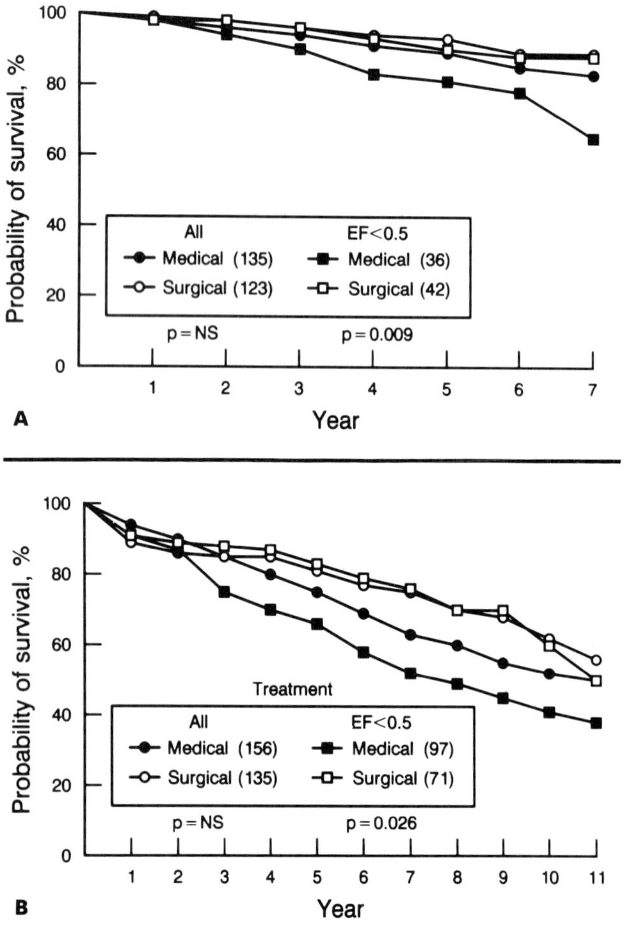

Fig 31-7 Actuarial survival for randomized patients with three-vessel coronary artery disease; all patients are compared with those in the subgroup having a left ventricular ejection fraction *(EF)* less than 50%. **A,** CASS.[60] **B,** VA study.[61]

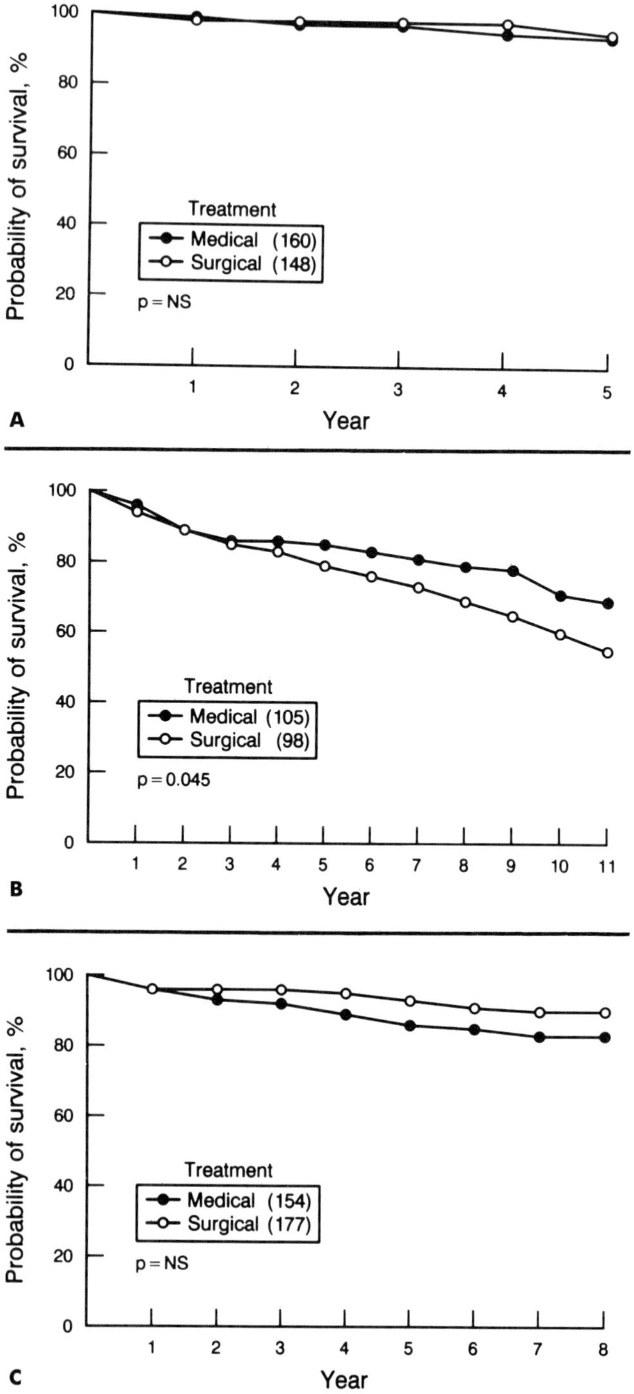

Fig 31-8 Actuarial survival for randomized patients with two-vessel coronary artery disease in the **(A)** CASS,[29] **(B)** VA study,[61] and **(C)** ECSS.[65]

operated on. The difference was even more pronounced for patients with concomitantly abnormal left ventricular function. Since asymptomatic patients with three-vessel disease and poor exercise capacity on exercise electrocardiography have a particularly poor prognosis, revascularization has been recommended for this group.[71] Generally, however, asymptomatic patients have a significantly better prognosis, even when not revascularized, than those with angina.

Gender. A higher operative mortality has been ob-

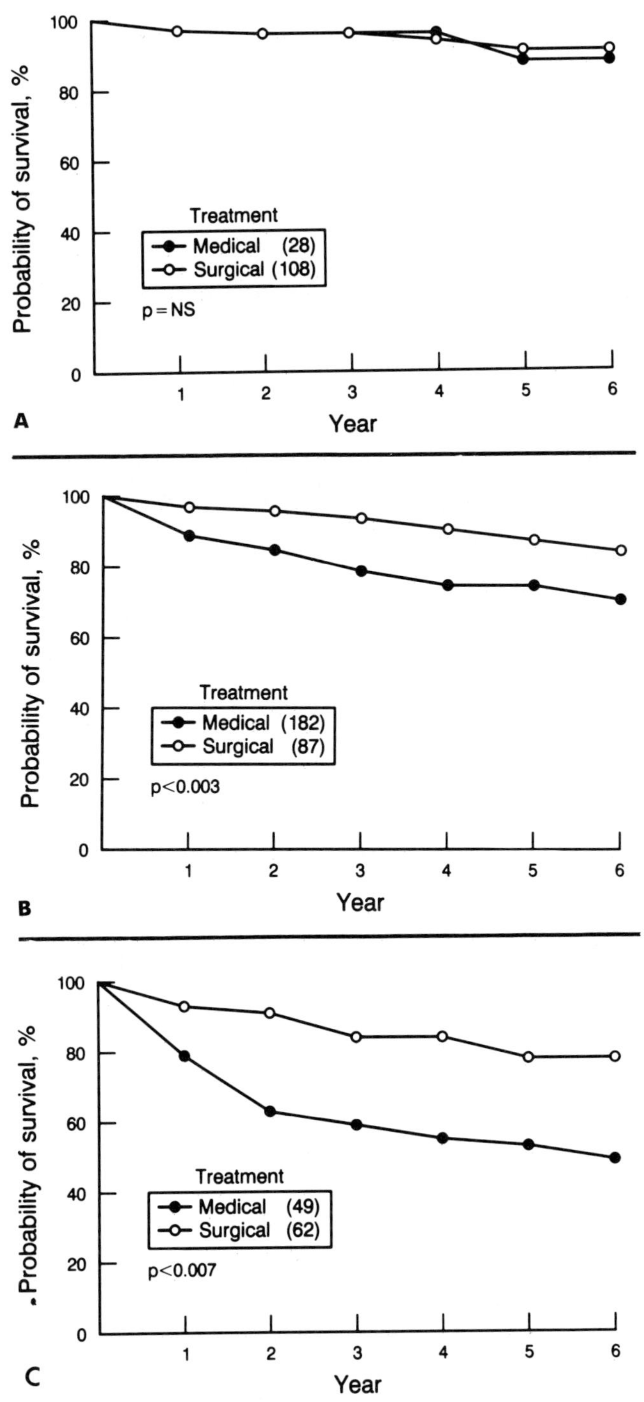

Fig 31-9 Actuarial survival for nonrandomized CASS registry patients with proximal two-vessel coronary artery disease, severe angina, and normal **(A)**, moderately abnormal **(B)**, and severely abnormal **(C)** left ventricular function.[68]

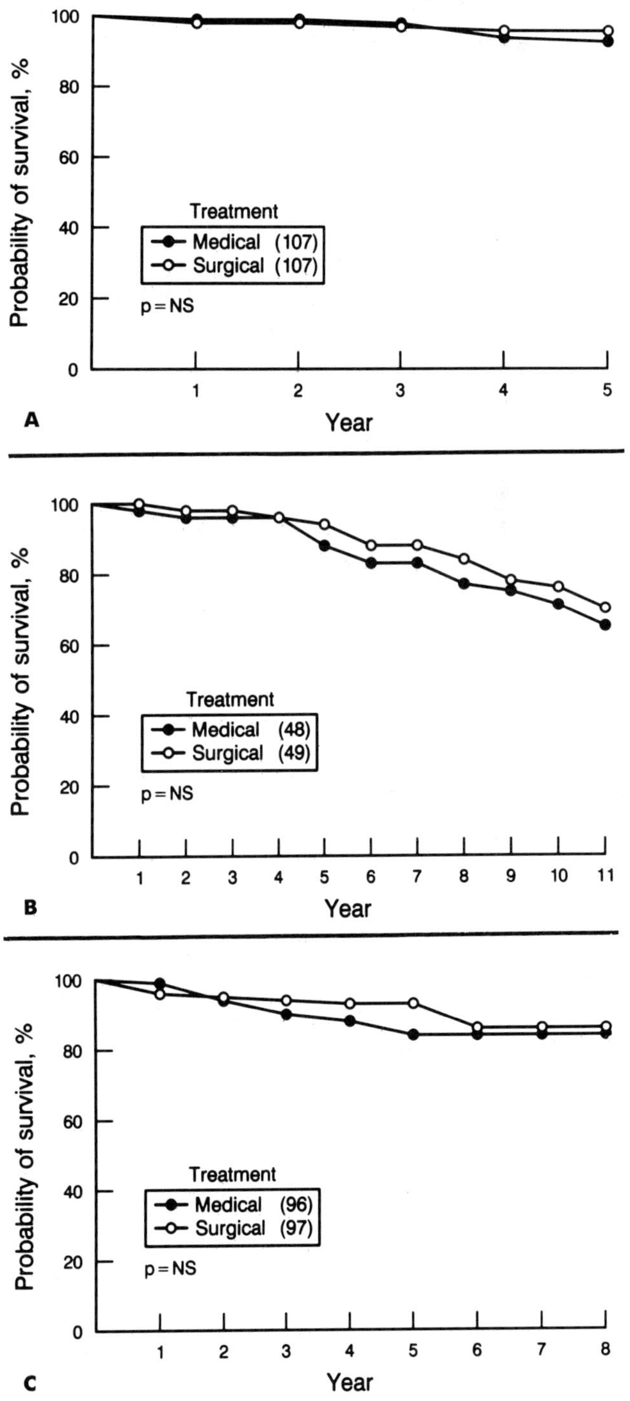

Fig 31-10 Actuarial survival for randomized patients with single-vessel coronary artery disease in the **(A)** CASS,[29] **(B)** VA study,[61] and **(C)** ECSS.[65]

served in women undergoing coronary artery surgery than in men, a result likely related to smaller body surface area.[72] Despite a lower long-term graft patency in women, survival is not different from that in men,[72] but long-term symptomatic relief is less.

Age. Coronary artery bypass surgery has been increasingly used in patients of advanced age, including octogenarians.[73,74] In a series of 159 elderly patients from the Mayo Clinic, the perioperative mortality of isolated coronary bypass surgery was 10.4%, but this was increased almost fourfold in patients with peripheral vascular disease and in those undergoing emergency procedures. The long-term outcome among elderly patients is favorable, particularly in those with normal or relatively mild left ventricular dysfunction and those without associated comorbid conditions. Successful bypass surgery among the elderly requires careful patient selection with meticulous attention to associated medical conditions that may influence early and late outcome, including peripheral vascular disease, cerebrovascular disease, and renal dysfunction (Fig 31-11).

Left ventricular function. Ejection fraction as an index of systolic left ventricular function is an important determinant of survival in both medically and surgically treated patients.[7,60,75] In patients with ejection fractions of less than 50%, survival appears to be enhanced by operation, at least if two or more vessels are involved. Regardless of the extent of coronary artery disease, patients with moderately depressed ejection fraction (25% to 49%) have improved survival after coronary artery bypass grafting. A significant improvement in

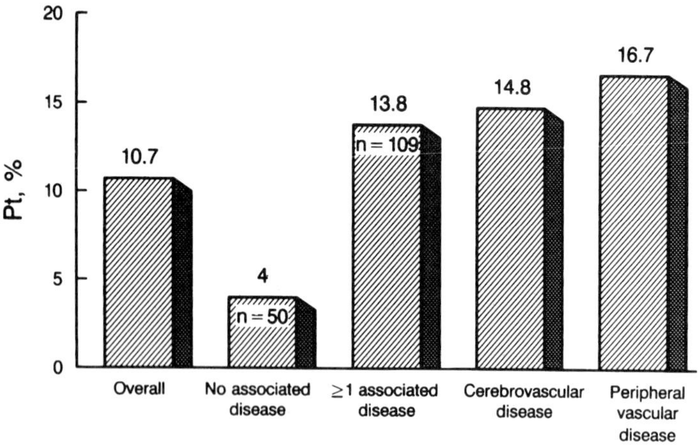

Fig 31-11 Percentage of patients aged 80 years or older who died perioperatively after coronary artery bypass graft surgery. Those with peripheral vascular disease had the highest perioperative risk of death. Patients without other associated disease (including vascular disease, diabetes, chronic obstructive pulmonary disease, creatinine ≥1.5 mg/dL, or mitral valve disease) had the best early survival. (Data from Mullany CJ, Darling GE, Pluth JR, et al: Early and late results after isolated coronary artery bypass surgery in 159 patients aged 80 years and older. *Circulation* 82 Suppl 4:229-236, 1990.)

surgical treatment of patients with ejection fractions of less than 25% to 36% has been reported.[76,77] It is fair to state that left ventricular dysfunction has become an indication for operation rather than a contraindication.

Use of the internal thoracic artery. Internal thoracic artery grafting has resulted in improved survival in patients undergoing coronary artery bypass surgery compared with that in matched patients receiving vein grafts alone.[46,78] This benefit applies even to patients who have poor left ventricular function[79] or who are older than 70 years.[80] Superior long-term patency of internal thoracic grafts is particularly important in young patients or those with diffuse disease, small vessels, or unsuitable saphenous veins, in whom the risk of subsequent reoperation is high. This has led to a greater use of arterial conduits, such as bilateral internal thoracic arteries, a gastroepiploic artery, and the inferior epigastric artery as free grafts.[48,49] Although the long-term benefits of these alternative conduits are not yet known, subsequent freedom from reoperation should be greater than that currently existing.

Improved myocardial function

Global left ventricular performance. Volumetric or hemodynamic indices of left ventricular function at rest generally do not change after coronary artery bypass grafting, regardless of graft patency. Angiographic and radionuclide evaluations of left ventricular performance during exercise before and after operation, however, have shown significant postoperative improvement of the exercise ejection fraction, stroke volume, and end-diastolic volume in most patients with patent grafts.[81,82]

Regional left ventricular performance. Regional left ventricular performance improves after coronary artery bypass grafting in patients with abnormal preoperative performance and patent grafts after surgery.[83,84] Conversely, graft occlusion or inadequate revascularization is associated with a decrease in regional performance.[83] Response to coronary artery bypass grafting can be predicted by preoperative interventional studies of regional left ventricular performance; thus, noninfarcted areas of hypokinesis which improve after the administration of nitroglycerin or inotropic stimulation can be expected to improve after successful revascularization.[85,86]

RISKS OF CORONARY ARTERY SURGERY

Operative mortality

The most immediate concern in evaluating the potential role of surgery for an individual patient is the possibility that the procedure itself will result in premature death. Fortunately, because of increased experience and improved techniques, the operative mortality has improved—from 3% to 10% (and up to 25% in some centers) in the late 1960s to 1% to 2.5%[36] in the late 1970s, where it has remained for *elective* coronary bypass surgery. *Total* operative mortality for bypass surgery, however, has increased (to approximately 8%) since the 1970s because an increased portion of patients have emergency operations or have complex or unstable disease.[87,88] Predictors of operative mortality include evidence of left ventricular dysfunction as manifested by congestive heart failure, cardiomegaly, left ventricular wall motion abnormalities, and elevated left ventricular end-diastolic pressure. Increasing age, female sex, and urgent operation[25,27,72,89] also increase operative mortality.

Myocardial infarction

The reported incidence of perioperative myocardial infarction ranges from 1.3% to 40%. Multiple factors influence perioperative infarction, including coronary anatomy and collateralization, adequacy of myocardial protection, duration of aortic cross-clamping, extent of coronary artery disease and need for endarterectomy, and urgency of surgery. Perioperative infarction is an important predictor of late survival.[90]

Incomplete revascularization and graft occlusion

Since survival, symptomatic results, and left ventricular function postoperatively depend in part on graft patency and completeness of revascularization,[91-93] the occurrence of graft disease is of major clinical importance. Early postoperative graft occlusion is usually due to inadequate vessel size, extensive disease, or poor distal runoff. At 1 to 5 years, the predominant cause of graft closure is fibrous intimal hyperplasia like that in early atherosclerotic disease. Subsequently, progressive atherosclerosis within the graft leads to a continual attrition of vein grafts. By 10 years, no more than 50% of saphenous grafts are still patent.

Aggressive management of risk factors is important after coronary artery bypass grafting. Adequate aerobic exercise, control of hypertension, cessation of smoking, and reduction in serum lipids are essential in the overall management of the patient. Increased serum lipid values are an important risk factor in graft atherosclerosis and thrombosis,[94,95] and reduction of serum cholesterol postoperatively has been shown to reduce the progression of graft disease.[96]

The rate of occlusion of grafts in the first postoperative year appears to be declining. This may be due to improved surgical technique and to the extensive use of platelet-inhibiting drugs. The use of aspirin, with or without dipyridamole, beginning in the immediate perioperative period has been shown to enhance graft patency.[97] Most of the surgical patients in the randomized trials of the 1970s received neither platelet-inhibiting drugs nor arterial conduits. Consequently, the long-term results of current surgery are expected to be better than the results in patients operated on in earlier years.[98]

Progression of disease in native coronary arteries

During the first postoperative year, progression of stenosis occurs primarily in arteries that have been grafted. In subsequent years, narrowing in nongrafted arteries occurs progressively, so that by 5 to 7 years after surgery, there is no difference in the severity of the disease in proximal segments of grafted and nongrafted arteries. Thus, by 5 to 7 years, approximately 50% of all vessels have had demonstrable progression of narrowing or the occurrence of new significant narrowing.

Reoperation

Because of the progressive recurrence of angina pectoris, particularly between 5 and 10 years after initial surgery, reoperation has become more frequent.[99] Predictors of reoperation include young age at initial operation,[99,100] absence of an internal thoracic artery graft, incomplete revascularization, New York Heart Association class III or IV functional status, and single- or double-vessel disease.[99] In general, operative mortality for reoperations has been higher than that for initial revascularization, although with greater experience, mortality for reoperative surgery will likely decline. Reported mortality ranges from 2.8% to 5.3%.[101-103] Reoperation can also be successfully done for the third or fourth time with acceptable mortality and morbidity.[104]

REFERENCES

1. Garratt KN, Holmes DR: PTCA: the benchmark for assessing new interventional devices. *J Myocardial Ischemia* 4:15-22, 1992
2. Graboys TB, Biegelson B, Lampert S, et al: Results of a second-opinion trial among patients recommended for coronary angiography. *JAMA* 268:2537-2540, 1992
3. Greene DG, Bunnell IL, Arani DT, et al: Long-term survival after coronary bypass surgery: comparison of various subsets of patients with general population. *Br Heart J* 45:417-426, 1981
4. Reul GJ Jr, Cooley DA: Long-term survival following aortocoronary artery bypass: analysis of 4,522 consecutive patients. *Eur Surg Res* 8:349-357, 1976
5. Hlatky MA, Califf RM, Harrell FE Jr, et al: Comparison of predictions based on observational data with the results of randomized controlled clinical trials of coronary artery bypass surgery. *J Am Coll Cardiol* 11:237-245, 1988
6. Hammermeister KE, DeRouen TA, English MT, et al: Effect of surgical versus medical therapy on return to work in patients with coronary artery disease. *Am J Cardiol* 44:105-111, 1979
7. Hammermeister KE, DeRouen TA, Dodge HT: Variables predictive of survival in patients with coronary disease: selection by univariate and multivariate analyses from the clinical, electrocardiographic, exercise, arteriographic, and quantitative angiographic evaluations. *Circulation* 59:421-430, 1979
8. Hammermeister KE, DeRouen TA, Dodge HT: Evidence from a nonrandomized study that coronary surgery prolongs survival in patients with two-vessel coronary disease. *Circulation* 59:430-435, 1979
9. Hammermeister KE, DeRouen TA, Dodge HT: Effect of coronary surgery on survival in asymptomatic and minimally symptomatic patients. *Circulation* 62 Suppl 1:98-102, 1980
10. DeRouen TA, Hammermeister KE, Dodge HT: Comparisons of the effects on survival after coronary artery surgery in subgroups of patients from Seattle Heart Watch. *Circulation* 63:537-545, 1981
11. Hammermeister KE, DeRouen TA, Dodge HT: Comparison of survival of medically and surgically treated coronary disease patients in Seattle Heart Watch: a nonrandomized study. *Circulation* 65 Suppl 2:53-59, 1982
12. Whalen RE, Harrell FE Jr, Lee KL, et al: Survival of coronary artery disease patients with stable pain and normal left ventricular function treated medically or surgically at Duke University. *Circulation* 65 Suppl 2:49-52, 1982
13. Veterans Administration Cooperative Group: Veterans Administration Cooperative Study of surgery for coronary arterial occlusive

disease. III. Methods and baseline characteristics, including experience with medical treatment. *Am J Cardiol* 40:212-225, 1977

14. Murphy ML, Hultgren HN, Detre K, et al: Treatment of chronic stable angina: a preliminary report of survival data of the randomized Veterans Administration Cooperative Study. *N Engl J Med* 297:621-627, 1977

15. Read RC, Murphy ML, Hultgren HN, et al: Survival of men treated for chronic stable angina pectoris: a cooperative randomized study. *J Thorac Cardiovasc Surg* 75:1-13, 1978

16. Peduzzi P, Hultgren HN: Effect of medical vs surgical treatment on symptoms in stable angina pectoris: the Veterans Administration Cooperative Study of surgery for coronary arterial occlusive disease. *Circulation* 60:888-900, 1979

17. Veterans Administration Coronary Bypass Surgery Cooperative Study Group: Long-term results of internal mammary artery implantation for coronary artery disease: a controlled trial. *Ann Thorac Surg* 29:234-242, 1980

18. Detre K, Peduzzi P, Murphy M, et al: Effect of bypass surgery on survival in patients in low- and high-risk subgroups delineated by the use of simple clinical variables. *Circulation* 63:1329-1338, 1981

19. Takaro T, Peduzzi P, Detre KM, et al: Survival in subgroups of patients with left main coronary artery disease: Veterans Administration Cooperative Study of surgery for coronary arterial occlusive disease. *Circulation* 66:14-22, 1982

20. Takaro T, Hultgren HN, Detre KM, et al: The Veterans Administration Cooperative Study of stable angina: current status. *Circulation* 65 Suppl 2:60-67, 1982

21. European Coronary Surgery Study Group: Coronary-artery bypass surgery in stable angina pectoris: survival at two years. *Lancet* 1:889-893, 1979

22. Second Interim Report by the European Coronary Surgery Study Group: Prospective randomised study of coronary artery bypass surgery in stable angina pectoris. *Lancet* 2:491-495, 1980

23. European Coronary Surgery Study Group: Prospective randomized study of coronary artery bypass surgery in stable angina pectoris: a progress report on survival. *Circulation* 65 Suppl 2:67-71, 1982

24. Davis K, Kennedy JW, Kemp HG Jr, et al: Complications of coronary arteriography from the Collaborative Study of Coronary Artery Surgery (CASS). *Circulation* 59:1105-1112, 1979

25. Kennedy JW, Kaiser GC, Fisher LD, et al: Multivariate discriminant analysis of the clinical and angiographic predictors of operative mortality from the Collaborative Study in Coronary Artery Surgery (CASS). *J Thorac Cardiovasc Surg* 80:876-885, 1980

26. Chaitman BR, Fisher LD, Bourassa MG, et al: Effect of coronary bypass surgery on survival patterns in subsets of patients with left main coronary artery disease: report of the Collaborative Study in Coronary Artery Surgery (CASS). *Am J Cardiol* 48:765-777, 1981

27. Kennedy JW, Kaiser GC, Fisher LD, et al: Clinical and angiographic predictors of operative mortality from the Collaborative Study in Coronary Artery Surgery (CASS). *Circulation* 63:793-802, 1981

28. Zimmern SH, Rogers WJ, Bream PR, et al: Total occlusion of the left main coronary artery: the Coronary Artery Surgery Study (CASS) experience. *Am J Cardiol* 49:2003-2010, 1982

29. CASS Principal Investigators and Their Associates: Coronary Artery Surgery Study (CASS): a randomized trial of coronary artery bypass surgery; survival data. *Circulation* 68:939-950, 1983

30. CASS Principal Investigators and Their Associates: Coronary Artery Surgery Study (CASS): a randomized trial of coronary artery bypass surgery; quality of life in patients randomly assigned to treatment groups. *Circulation* 68:951-960, 1983

31. National Cooperative Study Group to Compare Medical and Surgical Therapy: Unstable angina pectoris. I. Report of protocol and patient population. *Am J Cardiol* 37:896-902, 1976

32. National Cooperative Study Group to Compare Medical and Surgical Therapy: Unstable angina pectoris. II. In-hospital experience and initial follow-up results in patients with one, two and three vessel disease. *Am J Cardiol* 42:839-848, 1978

33. National Cooperative Study Group to Compare Medical and Surgical Therapy: Unstable angina pectoris. III. Results in patients with S-T segment elevation during pain. *Am J Cardiol* 45:819-824, 1980

34. National Cooperative Study Group to Compare Medical and Surgical Therapy: Unstable angina pectoris. IV. Results in patients with left anterior descending coronary artery disease. *Am J Cardiol* 48:517-524, 1981

35. Reeder GS: Angioplasty and the cost of myocardial revascularization: has its promise been fulfilled? (Editorial.) *Int J Cardiol* 15:287-292, 1987

36. Rahimtoola SH: Coronary bypass surgery for chronic angina—1981: a perspective. *Circulation* 65:225-241, 1982

37. Cosgrove DM, Loop FD, Sheldon WC: Results of myocardial revascularization: a 12-year experience. *Circulation* 65 Suppl 2:37-43, 1982

38. Lawrie GM, Morris GC Jr: Survival after coronary artery bypass surgery in specific patient groups. *Circulation* 65 Suppl 2:43-48, 1982

39. Myers WO, Schaff HV, Fisher LD, et al: Time to first new myocardial infarction in patients with severe angina and three-vessel disease comparing medical and early surgical therapy: a CASS registry study of survival. *J Thorac Cardiovasc Surg* 95:382-388, 1988

40. Myers WO, Gersh BJ, Fisher LD, et al: Time to first new myocardial infarction in patients with mild angina and three-vessel disease comparing medicine and early surgery: a CASS registry study of survival. *Ann Thorac Surg* 43:599-612, 1987

41. Gersh BJ, Califf RM, Loop FD, et al: Coronary bypass surgery in chronic stable angina. *Circulation* 79 Suppl 1:46-59, 1989

42. Campeau L, Lespérance J, Hermann J, et al: Loss of the improvement of angina between 1 and 7 years after aortocoronary bypass surgery: correlations with changes in vein grafts and in coronary arteries. *Circulation* 60 Suppl 1:1-5, 1979

43. Singh RN, Sosa JA, Green GE: Internal mammary artery versus saphenous vein graft: comparative performance in patients with combined revascularization. *Br Heart J* 50:48-58, 1983

44. Lytle BW, Loop FD, Cosgrove DM, et al: Long-term (5-12 years) sequential studies of internal mammary artery and saphenous vein coronary bypass grafts (abstract). *Circulation* 68 Suppl 3:114, 1983

45. Grondin CM, Campeau L, Lespérance J, et al: Comparison of late changes in internal mammary artery and saphenous vein grafts in two consecutive series of patients 10 years after operation. *Circulation* 70 Suppl 1:208-212, 1984

46. Loop FD, Lytle BW, Cosgrove DM, et al: Influence of the internal-mammary-artery graft on 10-year survival and other cardiac events. *N Engl J Med* 314:1-6, 1986

47. Kirklin JW, Akins CW, Blackstone EH, et al: Guidelines and indications for coronary artery bypass graft surgery: a report of the American College of Cardiology/American Heart Association Task Force on Assessment of Diagnostic and Therapeutic Cardiovascular Procedures (Subcommittee on Coronary Artery Bypass Graft Surgery). *J Am Coll Cardiol* 17:543-589, 1991

48. Pym J, Brown PM, Charrette EJP, et al: Gastroepiploic-coronary anastomosis: a viable alternative bypass graft. *J Thorac Cardiovasc Surg* 94:256-259, 1987

49. Buche M, Schoevaerdts JC, Chalant CH, et al: Multiple-vessel coronary revascularization using both in situ mammary arteries and a free inferior epigastric artery (letter to the editor). *J Thorac Cardiovasc Surg* 99:754-755, 1990

50. Russell RO Jr, Wayne JB, Kronenfeld J, et al: Surgical versus medical therapy for treatment of unstable angina: changes in work status and family income. *Am J Cardiol* 45:134-140, 1980

51. Barnes GK, Ray MJ, Oberman A, et al: Changes in working status of patients following coronary bypass surgery. *JAMA* 238:1259-1262, 1977

52. Anderson AJ, Barboriak JJ, Hoffmann RG, et al: Retention or resumption of employment after aortocoronary bypass operations. *JAMA* 243:543-545, 1980

53. Love JW: Employment status after coronary bypass operations and some cost considerations. *J Thorac Cardiovasc Surg* 80:68-72, 1980

54. Oberman A, Wayne JB, Kouchoukos NT, et al: Employment status after coronary artery bypass surgery. *Circulation* 65 Suppl 2:115-119, 1982

55. Smith HC, Hammes LN, Gupta S, et al: Employment status after coronary artery bypass surgery. *Circulation* 65 Suppl 2:120-125, 1982

56. Johnson WD, Kayser KL, Pedraza PM, et al: Employment patterns in males before and after myocardial revascularization surgery: a study of 2229 consecutive male patients followed for as long as 10 years. *Circulation* 65:1086-1093, 1982

57. Hamilton WM, Hammermeister KE, DeRouen TA, et al: Effect of coronary artery bypass grafting on subsequent hospitalization. *Am J Cardiol* 51:353-360, 1983

58. Harris PJ, Harrell FE Jr, Lee KL, et al: Survival in medically treated coronary artery disease. *Circulation* 60:1259-1269, 1979

59. Harris PJ, Lee KL, Harrell FE Jr, et al: Outcome in medically treated coronary artery disease: ischemic events; nonfatal infarction and death. *Circulation* 62:718-726, 1980

60. Passamani E, Davis KB, Gillespie MJ, et al: A randomized trial of coronary artery bypass surgery: survival of patients with a low ejection fraction. *N Engl J Med* 312:1665-1671, 1985

61. The Veterans Administration Coronary Artery Bypass Surgery Cooperative Study Group: Eleven-year survival in the Veterans Administration randomized trial of coronary bypass surgery for stable angina. *N Engl J Med* 311:1333-1339, 1984

62. Varnauskas E and the European Coronary Surgery Study Group: Twelve-year follow-up of survival in the randomized European Coronary Surgery Study. *N Engl J Med* 319:332-337, 1988

63. Rittenhouse EA, Sauvage LR, Mansfield PB, et al: Severe left main coronary arterial stenosis with right coronary arterial occlusion: results of bypass graft surgery. *Am J Cardiol* 49:645-650, 1982

64. Chaitman BR, Davis KB, Kaiser GC, et al: The role of coronary bypass surgery for 'left main equivalent' coronary disease: the Coronary Artery Surgery Study Registry. *Circulation* 74 Suppl 3:17-25, 1986

65. Varnauskas E and the European Coronary Surgery Study Group: Survival, myocardial infarction, and employment status in a prospective randomized study of coronary bypass surgery. *Circulation* 72 Suppl 5:90-101, 1985

66. Kaiser GC, Davis KB, Fisher LD, et al: Survival following coronary artery bypass grafting in patients with severe angina pectoris (CASS): an observational study. *J Thorac Cardiovasc Surg* 89:513-522, 1985

67. Pryor DB, Harrell FE Jr, Rankin JS, et al: The changing survival benefits of coronary revascularization over time. *Circulation* 76 Suppl 5:13-21, 1987

68. Mock MB, Fisher LD, Holmes DR Jr, et al: Comparison of effects of medical and surgical therapy on survival in severe angina pectoris and two-vessel coronary artery disease with and without left ventricular dysfunction: a Coronary Artery Surgery Study registry study. *Am J Cardiol* 61:1198-1203, 1988

69. Tyras DH, Kaiser GC, Barner HB, et al: The rationale for operative therapy of symptomatic single-vessel coronary artery disease. *J Thorac Cardiovasc Surg* 80:73-78, 1980

70. Weiner DA, Ryan TJ, McCabe CH, et al: Comparison of coronary artery bypass surgery and medical therapy in patients with exercise-induced silent myocardial ischemia: a report from the Coronary Artery Surgery Study (CASS) registry. *J Am Coll Cardiol* 12:595-599, 1988

71. Kent KM, Rosing DR, Ewels CJ, et al: Prognosis of asymptomatic or mildly symptomatic patients with coronary artery disease. *Am J Cardiol* 49:1823-1831, 1982

72. Loop FD, Golding LR, MacMillan JP, et al: Coronary artery surgery in women compared with men: analyses of risks and long-term results. *J Am Coll Cardiol* 1:383-390, 1983

73. Mullany CJ, Darling GE, Pluth JR, et al: Early and late results after isolated coronary artery bypass surgery in 159 patients aged 80 years and older. *Circulation* 82 Suppl 4:229-236, 1990

74. Ko W, Krieger KH, Lazenby WD, et al: Isolated coronary artery bypass grafting in one hundred consecutive octogenarian patients: a multivariate analysis. *J Thorac Cardiovasc Surg* 102:532-538, 1991

75. Mock MB, Ringqvist I, Fisher LD, et al: Survival of medically treated patients in the Coronary Artery Surgery Study (CASS) Registry. *Circulation* 66:562-568, 1982

76. Pigott JD, Kouchoukos NT, Oberman A, et al: Late results of surgical and medical therapy for patients with coronary artery disease and depressed left ventricular function. *J Am Coll Cardiol* 5:1036-1045, 1985

77. Alderman EL, Fisher LD, Litwin P, et al: Results of coronary artery surgery in patients with poor left ventricular function (CASS). *Circulation* 68:785-795, 1983

78. Cameron A, Kemp HG Jr, Green GE: Bypass surgery with the internal mammary artery graft: 15 year follow-up. *Circulation* 74 Suppl 3:30-36, 1986

79. Cameron A, Davis KB, Green GE, et al: Clinical implications of internal mammary artery bypass grafts: the Coronary Artery Surgery Study experience. *Circulation* 77:815-819, 1988

80. Gardner TJ, Greene PS, Rykiel MF, et al: Routine use of the left internal mammary artery graft in the elderly. *Ann Thorac Surg* 49:188-194, 1990

81. Kent KM, Borer JS, Green MV, et al: Effects of coronary-artery bypass on global and regional left ventricular function during exercise. *N Engl J Med* 298:1434-1439, 1978

82. Lim YL, Kalff V, Kelly MJ, et al: Radionuclide angiographic assessment of global and segmental left ventricular function at rest and during exercise after coronary artery bypass graft surgery. *Circulation* 66:972-979, 1982

83. Chesebro JH, Ritman EL, Frye RL, et al: Videometric analysis of regional left ventricular function before and after aortocoronary artery bypass surgery: correlation of peak rate of myocardial wall thickening with last postoperative graft flows. *J Clin Invest* 58:1339-1347, 1976

84. Brundage BH, Massie BM, Botvinick EH: Improved regional ventricular function after successful surgical revascularization. *J Am Coll Cardiol* 3:902-908, 1984

85. Chesebro JH, Ritman EL, Frye RL, et al: Left ventricular performance before and after aortocoronary artery bypass surgery. *Circulation* 65 Suppl 2:98-105, 1982

86. Chesebro JH, Ritman EL, Frye RL, et al: Regional myocardial wall thickening response to nitroglycerin: a predictor of myocardial response to aortocoronary bypass surgery. *Circulation* 57:952-957, 1978

87. Naunheim KS, Fiore AC, Wadley JJ, et al: The changing profile of the patient undergoing coronary artery bypass surgery. *J Am Coll Cardiol* 11:494-498, 1988

88. Gersh BJ, Schaff HV: The changing patient population and results of coronary bypass surgery. *Curr Opinion Cardiol* 3:894-900, 1988

89. Gersh BJ, Kronmal RA, Frye RL, et al: Coronary arteriography and coronary artery bypass surgery: morbidity and mortality in patients ages 65 years or older; a report from the Coronary Artery Surgery Study. *Circulation* 67:483-491, 1983

90. Schaff HV, Gersh BJ, Fisher LD, et al: Detrimental effect of perioperative myocardial infarction on late survival after coronary artery bypass: report from the Coronary Artery Surgery Study (CASS). *J Thorac Cardiovasc Surg* 88:972-980, 1984

91. Lawrie GM, Morris GC Jr, Silvers A, et al: The influence of residual disease after coronary bypass on the 5-year survival rate of 1274 men with coronary artery disease. *Circulation* 66:717-723, 1982

92. Frick MH, Harjola P-T, Valle M: Persistent improvement after coronary bypass surgery: ergometric and angiographic correlations at 5 years. *Circulation* 67:491-496, 1983

93. Gould BL, Clayton PD, Jensen RL, et al: Association between early graft patency and late outcome for patients undergoing artery bypass graft surgery. *Circulation* 69:569-576, 1984

94. Solymoss BC, Nadeau P, Millette D, et al: Late thrombosis of saphenous vein coronary bypass grafts related to risk factors. *Circulation* 78 Suppl 1:140-143, 1988

95. Stewart WJ, Goormastic M, Healy BP, et al: Clinical outcome ten years after coronary bypass: effects of cholesterol and triglycerides in 4913 pts (abstract). *J Am Coll Cardiol* 11 Suppl A:7, 1988

96. Blankenhorn DH, Nessim SA, Johnson RL, et al: Beneficial effects of combined colestipol-niacin therapy on coronary atherosclerosis and coronary venous bypass grafts. *JAMA* 257:3233-3240, 1987

97. Brown BG, Cukingnan RA, DeRouen T, et al: Improved graft patency in patients treated with platelet-inhibiting therapy after coronary bypass surgery. *Circulation* 72:138-146, 1985

98. Muhlbaier LH, Pryor DB, Rankin JS, et al: Observational comparison of event-free survival with medical and surgical therapy in patients with coronary artery disease: 20 years of follow-up. *Circulation* 86 Suppl 2:198-204, 1992

99. Cosgrove DM, Loop FD, Lytle BW, et al: Predictors of reoperation after myocardial revascularization. *J Thorac Cardiovasc Surg* 92:811-821, 1986

100. Rowe MH, Mullany CJ, White AL, et al: Early and late survival after coronary-artery surgery. *Med J Aust* 150:682-693, 1989

101. Foster ED, Fisher LD, Kaiser GC, et al: Comparison of operative mortality and morbidity for initial and repeat coronary bypass grafting: the Coronary Artery Surgery Study (CASS) registry experience. *Ann Thorac Surg* 38:563-569, 1984

102. Loop FD, Lytle BW, Gill CC, et al: Trends in selection and results of coronary artery reoperations. *Ann Thorac Surg* 36:380-388, 1983

103. Schaff HV, Orszulak TA, Gersh BJ, et al: The morbidity and mortality of reoperation for coronary artery disease and analysis of late results with use of actuarial estimate of event-free interval. *J Thorac Cardiovasc Surg* 85:508-514, 1983

104. Accola KD, Craver JM, Weintraub WS, et al: Multiple reoperative coronary artery bypass grafting. *Ann Thorac Surg* 52:738-744, 1991

CHAPTER

32

Aortic valvular stenosis

Emilio R. Giuliani, M.D., Lyle J. Olson, M.D., and Clarence Shub, M.D.

Aortic stenosis is the most common valvular lesion causing morbidity in man. In this chapter, the etiology, pathophysiology, evaluation, and management of valvular aortic stenosis in adults are reviewed.

The site of obstruction and cause of different types of left ventricular outflow obstruction, including valvular aortic stenosis and associated lesions, are summarized in Table 32-1. In most patients, obstruction is at the valvular level. Less frequently, obstruction is at the subvalvular level, as observed in hypertrophic obstructive cardiomyopathy (see chapter 20) or congenital discrete subaortic stenosis (see chapter 46). Rarely, the cause of obstruction is congenital supravalvular stenosis (see chapter 46).

PATHOANATOMY AND ETIOLOGY

Aortic valve stenosis is classified into four etiologic types on the basis of characteristic pathoanatomy: degenerative, bicuspid, rheumatic, and congenital[1-6] (see Table 32-1).

Degenerative aortic valvular stenosis

Degenerative aortic valve stenosis typically occurs in patients over age 65 years. Morphologically, it is characterized by a trileaflet aortic valve free of commissural fusion, with calcified nodular excrescences within the valve pockets that restrict leaflet motion. The orifice of the valve appears triradiate, a change attributed to hemodynamic trauma to the valve leaflets over many years. The process is common in patients older than 65 years, and stenosis generally is mild. However, progression of stenosis requiring surgical therapy is not uncommon, and it is now the most frequent indication for aortic valve replacement for aortic valve stenosis at our institution.[7]

Bicuspid aortic valvular stenosis

The congenitally bicuspid aortic valve (Fig 32-1) is differentiated from degenerative aortic valve disease by cusps of unequal size, the larger of which is conjoined and often contains a raphe at the site of fusion of two cusps. In most cases, the right and left cusps are fused, so that both coronary ostia arise above the conjoined cusp. Calcification of the raphe, annulus, and valve pockets produces a narrowed orifice shaped like an ellipse or a narrow slit. Prevalence of the bicuspid aortic valve is 1% to 2% in the general population, with men three to four times more likely to be affected than women.[3-5] The bicuspid valve may progress to calcific stenosis, be affected by aortic valve insufficiency or infective endocarditis, or be associated with aortic dissection.[8] Patients with coarctation of the aorta frequently have concurrent aortic valve regurgitation due to a bicuspid aortic valve and systemic arterial hypertension.

Because the pathologic changes of the bicuspid valve develop gradually during the early years of life, the murmur of stenosis may not appear until adolescence or adulthood, and symptoms may be delayed until a later age. In contrast, stenosis of the rheumatic type may be severe enough to be clinically manifest before the development of significant calcification.

Rheumatic aortic valvular stenosis

Rheumatic aortic valve stenosis is characterized by commissural fusion as well as cusp fibrosis and calcification; stenosis becomes more severe as more commissures are fused, and secondary calcification further hinders valve motion. Depending on the number of fused commissures and the nature of the fibrocalcific process, the stenotic orifice may assume a variety of irregular forms. Rheumatic postinflammatory disease accounts for 14% to 35% of cases of aortic stenosis and implies a previous chronic, apparently noninfectious, fibrosing process that produces morphologic changes indistinguishable from those of confirmed cases of chronic rheumatic valvular disease.[4] However, such valves should not necessarily be designated "rheumatic" on morphologic criteria alone, because these patients frequently do not have a history of acute rheumatic fever and because other nonrheumatic

Table 32-1 Left ventricular outflow obstruction: anatomic location, etiology, and clinical characteristics

Type (incidence)	Murmur first heard*	Symptoms first noted*	Associated aortic regurgitation, %	Other associated lesions
Valvular (90%)				
Congenital	Infancy	Infancy, adolescence	25	Miscellaneous, rare
Rheumatic	Adulthood†	Adulthood†	75	Mitral disease, 75%; tricuspid disease, 5%
Calcific bicuspid	Adolescence Adulthood	Adulthood Old age	40	Coarctation of aorta, rare
Calcific senile sclerotic	Old age	Old age	>25	...
Subvalvular (9%)				
Hypertrophic	Infancy Adulthood	Adolescence Old age	Rare	Mitral incompetence, 90%; miscellaneous, 10%
Discrete	Infancy	Infancy, adulthood	50-75	Miscellaneous, 50%
Supravalvular (<1%)	Infancy	Infancy, adulthood	Rare	Peripheral pulmonary stenosis, 25%-50%; miscellaneous, 10%

*Infancy, <1 yr; childhood, 1-14 yr; adolescence, 14-18 yr; adulthood, 18-65 yr; old age, >65 yr.
†Often in adolescence or even childhood in developing countries.

inflammatory processes may result in identical valvular pathoanatomy.

Rheumatic aortic valvular stenosis rarely manifests as an isolated valvular lesion; in most patients, there is associated mitral valve disease. Mild-to-moderate aortic valvular regurgitation frequently coexists. It is an acquired disease, and in contrast to congenital stenosis, signs and symptoms in most patients develop during adulthood.

Rare causes of aortic stenosis

Among the rare causes of valvular aortic stenosis are inborn errors of metabolism in which endogenous substances accumulate in the cusps and produce mechanical obstruction. Examples include homozygous type II hyperlipidemic states,[9] Fabry's disease,[10] and ochronosis.[11] Vegetations large enough to produce valvular obstruction may be seen in infective endocarditis (especially fungal)[12] and in systemic lupus erythematosus.[13,14]

PATHOGENESIS AND PATHOPHYSIOLOGY

The most common pathologic substrates causing obstruction of the aortic valve orifice are commissural fusion (either congenital or acquired) and cusp fibrosis with calcification. Each of these processes hinders cusp excursion and imparts valvular rigidity, thereby producing obstruction. Regardless of the underlying cause, most forms of aortic valvular stenosis with or without aortic insufficiency are associated with calcification.

Classically, the pathophysiologic characteristics of aortic valvular stenosis have been described in hydraulic terms. Accordingly, the pathophysiologic hallmark of aortic stenosis is a transvalvular pressure gradient. By long-standing convention, a peak-to-peak pressure gradient measured by cardiac catheterization exceeding 50 mm Hg in a patient with normal cardiac output has represented severe obstruction to left ventricular outflow; similarly, a gradient of 25 to 50 mm Hg is regarded as moderate stenosis, and less than 25 mm Hg is mild.[15]

An alternative measure of the severity of aortic valve stenosis is obtained by estimation of the aortic valve orifice area by the Gorlin formula.[16] This formula and its application in the patient with valvular aortic stenosis are described later in this chapter. The normal aortic valve has an orifice area of 3 to 5 cm^2 in average-sized adults. Reduction of the valve orifice by as much as 50% does not produce a significant pressure gradient, but as the stenosis becomes more severe, obstruction to the left ventricular outflow becomes clinically significant. Important valvular stenosis occurs when the orifice area is decreased to less than 30% of normal, so that an orifice dimension of 1 cm^2 or less is regarded as hemodynamically significant. By convention, an aortic valve orifice area less than 0.75 cm^2 (or 0.5 cm^2/m^2 of body surface area) is regarded as severe aortic valve stenosis.

Pathophysiologic sequelae of aortic valve obstruction include the development of left ventricular hypertrophy and associated increased left ventricular diastolic pressure (Fig 32-2). Initially, these compensatory changes may not be associated with symptoms or deleterious hemody-

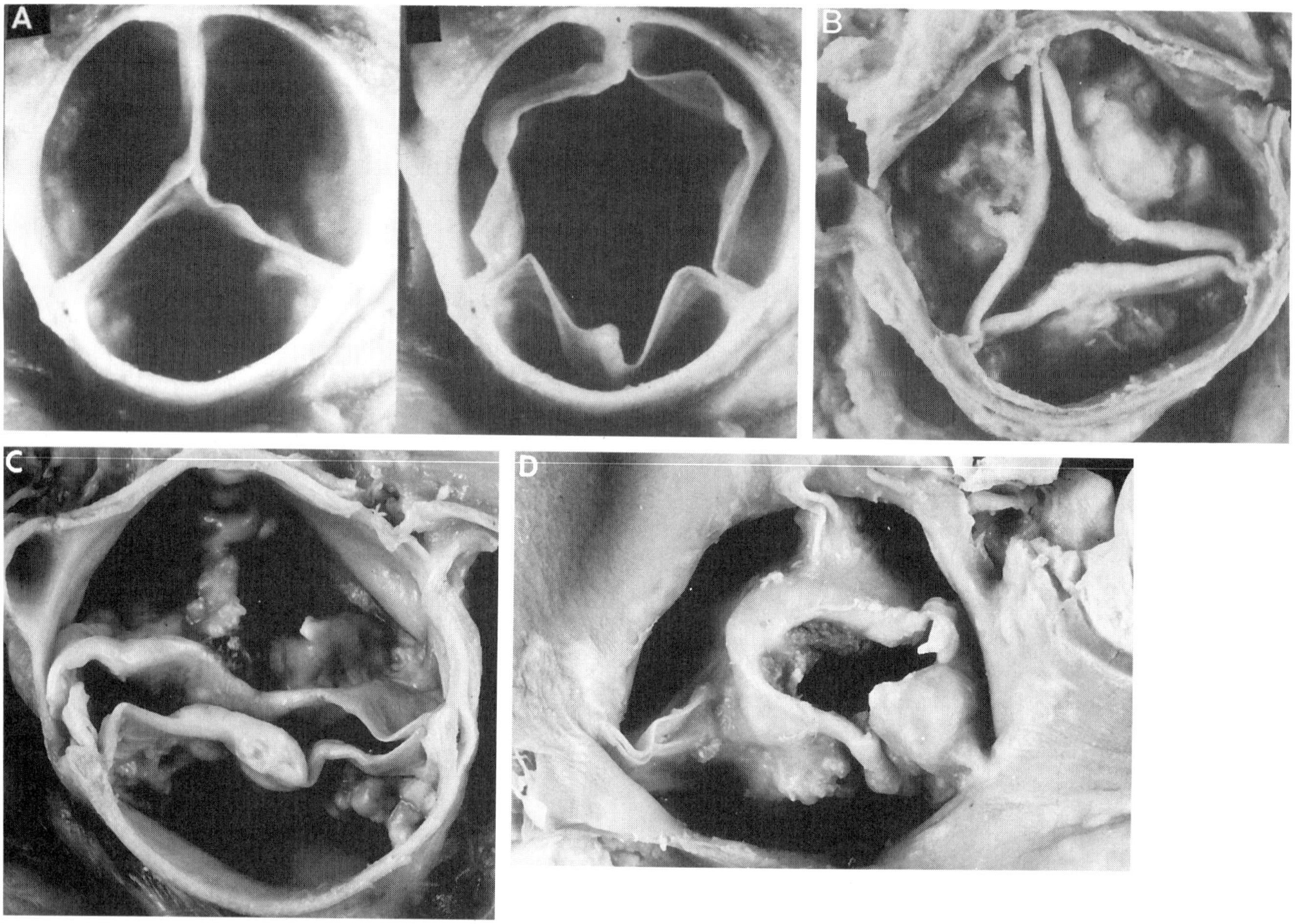

Fig 32-1 Etiologic types of aortic valvular stenosis. **A,** normal aortic valve closed *(left)* and opened *(right)*. **B,** degenerative aortic valvular stenosis. **C,** bicuspid aortic valvular stenosis. **D,** rheumatic aortic valvular stenosis. (**A,** from Olson LJ, Edwards WD, Tajik AJ: Aortic valve stenosis: etiology, pathophysiology, evaluation, and management. *Curr Probl Cardiol* 12:453-508, 1987. By permission, Mayo Foundation.)

namic effects, and patients may tolerate moderate-to-severe obstruction for many years without symptoms. However, progressive left ventricular hypertrophy to compensate for progressive valvular obstruction leads to a progressive increase in left ventricular diastolic pressure. This pressure increase does not necessarily signify left ventricular failure; instead, it reflects the diminished compliance of the hypertrophied left ventricular wall. The decrease in compliance of the left ventricle produces an increase in the afterload for the left atrium, which also responds with hypertrophy. Eventually, if aortic stenosis is untreated, mean left atrial pressure increases enough to produce pulmonary venous hypertension, which is then associated with pulmonary edema and right heart failure.

Increased left ventricular diastolic pressure and myocardial hypertrophy are characteristic of long-standing aortic valve stenosis, but left ventricular diastolic volume usually remains normal until late in the course of the disease. Increased left ventricular mass is generally not as great as that seen in aortic regurgitation or combined aortic stenosis and regurgitation.[17] Left ventricular hypertrophy associated with aortic valve stenosis is concentric and is an appropriate initial compensatory response to left ventricular outflow obstruction because hypertrophy enables maintenance of cardiac output and reduces wall stress.

Measurement of left ventricular wall thickness provides an assessment of the myocardial response to the pressure overload of left ventricular outflow tract obstruction. Although transvalvular pressure gradient and left ventricular pressure and volume are useful in the assessment of ventricular pump function in patients with aortic stenosis, direct assessment of myocardial contractile function may add useful information for patient management—information not apparent on the basis of pressure-volume data alone. Myocardial function can be assessed by relating changes in wall thickness and ventricular chamber dimension through application of

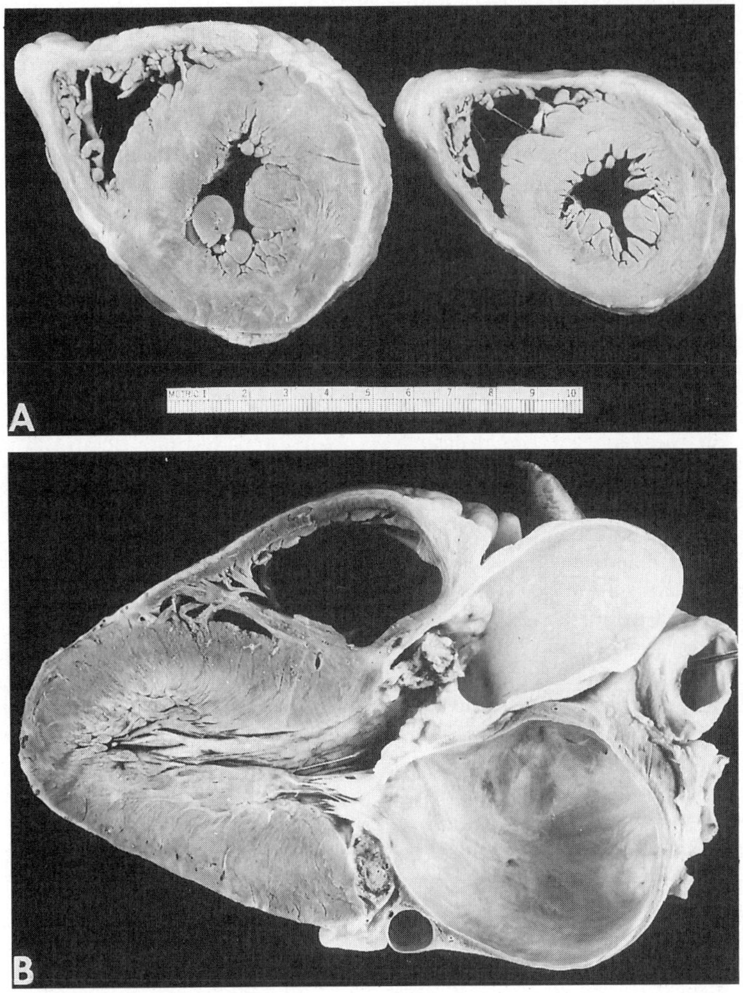

Fig 32-2 Left ventricular hypertrophy associated with aortic valvular stenosis. **A,** concentric hypertrophy with normal heart at right for comparison. **B,** left ventricle in long-axis orientation showing degenerative form of calcific aortic valvular stenosis with extension of calcium onto anterior mitral leaflet and ventricular septum. Left ventricle is hypertrophied and left atrium is dilated. Mitral annular calcification is also present. (**A,** from Olson LJ, Edwards WD, Tajik AJ: Aortic valve stenosis: etiology, pathophysiology, evaluation, and management. *Curr Probl Cardiol* 12:453-508, 1987. By permission, Mayo Foundation. **B,** from Edwards WD, Tajik AJ, Seward JB: Standardized nomenclature and anatomic basis for regional tomographic analysis of the heart. *Mayo Clin Proc* 56:479-497, 1981. By permission, Mayo Foundation.)

wall stress. Wall stress may be regarded as an expression of the extent to which intraventricular pressure is borne by individual myocardial fibers and is based on the Laplace relationship:

$$X = \frac{P \cdot r}{2 \cdot h}$$

in which X is wall stress, P is pressure, r is radius, and h is wall thickness. Several formulae based on the Laplace relationship have been developed for application to the heart.[18,19]

On the basis of estimated wall stress, patients with aortic valve stenosis may be categorized into those in whom normal wall stress is maintained and those in whom wall stress is increased. The Laplace relationship demonstrates that if the increase in ventricular pressure or dimension is not associated with simultaneous increase in wall thickness, wall stress is increased. Conversely, if wall thickness increases compensatorily with increase in pressure or dimension, wall stress may be maintained.

It has been observed that in patients who clinically appear to tolerate pressure overload, wall stress is not increased, because there is associated hypertrophy.[20-22] In other patients, however, little hypertrophy develops despite severe stenosis. In these patients, pressure overload is less well tolerated and left ventricular dilatation and failure may ensue. Presumably, the potential for hypertrophy at the myocardial fiber level is different in each patient. Thus, certain patients may be less able to tolerate a given hemodynamic pressure overload. In these patients, left ventricular failure may occur earlier in aortic valve obstruction with a lesser degree of aortic stenosis.

In most patients with severe aortic stenosis, cardiac output fails to increase normally during exercise. However, resting cardiac output decreases only late in the course of the disease. If cardiac output decreases at rest in a patient with aortic stenosis or if other associated heart disease produces a decrease in cardiac output, the transvalvular aortic pressure gradient also decreases. When a decrease in pressure gradient is associated with a decrease in cardiac output, estimation of the severity of aortic stenosis is difficult on the basis of the pressure gradient alone. In this situation, estimation of the aortic valve orifice area is generally regarded as a more accurate method for assessing the severity of stenosis. However, the Gorlin formula may not be reliable when cardiac output is low and valve area is less than 1.5 cm^2 (the range in which surgical decisions are most important).[23]

In the patient with aortic stenosis, coronary blood flow is increased at rest but is normal when corrected for left ventricular mass.[24] With severe aortic stenosis, however, myocardial oxygen supply at rest may be inadequate, even if the coronary arteries are normal, because the subendocardium is vulnerable to ischemia from the increased myocardial oxygen demand associated with increased left ventricular mass, increased intracavitary pressures, and prolonged ejection time. Furthermore, coronary blood flow may be impaired by increased intracavitary pressure, which compresses the subendocardial segments of the coronary arteries, and by decreased coronary perfusion gradient due to decreased diastolic aortic-left ventricular pressure gradient. These factors, which produce myocardial ischemia in the patient with aortic stenosis, are exacerbated during exercise.

Hence, the symptoms of the patient with aortic stenosis can be understood by considering the associated cardiac hemodynamic abnormalities. The most common symptoms are exertional dyspnea, angina, syncope, and presyncope. Exertional dyspnea is attributed to increased left ventricular diastolic pressure with consequent increased pulmonary vascular pressure producing dyspnea. Angina may or may not be associated with underlying coronary artery disease.[25,26] If coronary artery disease is absent, angina may be attributed to inadequate myocardial oxygen supply associated with the increased demands caused by left ventricular hypertrophy, increased intracavitary pressures, prolonged ejection time, and compression of the subendocardial segments of the coronary arteries during diastole as a consequence of increased intracavitary pressure. The tendency toward myocardial ischemia is increased during exercise because heart rate and diastolic pressure are increased. Coexistent coronary artery disease further compromises myocardial oxygen supply and exacerbates ischemia.

Syncope or presyncope may be exertional or, rarely, occur at rest. Exertional syncope may occur during or immediately after exertion when venous return decreases. With exertion, syncope is caused by decreased cerebral perfusion due to peripheral vasodilatation and the inability of the heart to increase cardiac output across a fixed stenotic valve orifice. There also may be a reflex decrease in peripheral resistance due to marked increases in left ventricular systolic pressure.[27] Syncope at rest occurs much less often than exertional syncope and is frequently associated with heart block or ventricular arrhythmias.

CLINICAL FEATURES

History and clinical course

The symptoms of aortic valvular stenosis include one or several of the following:[15,28-30] angina pectoris, sometimes atypical, occurs in about 60% of symptomatic patients; exertional dyspnea occurs in about 90% of symptomatic patients; exertional dizziness, syncope, or fatigability occurs in about 35% of symptomatic patients; infective endocarditis, systemic embolism, and dissecting aneurysm are infrequent complications.

Only about 35% of patients with symptomatic aortic stenosis are alive at the end of 5 years, and 90% have died by the end of 10 years[31] (Fig 32-3). This poor course applies only after the onset of symptoms; thus, there is a long latent period during which patients have asymptomatic mild or moderate obstruction.

Although aortic stenosis is a progressive disease, characterized by increasing valvular obstruction, the rate of progression varies greatly.[32-34] Increasing fibrosis and calcification of the aortic valve, with or without commissural fusion, cause progressive valve immobility and reduction of valve orifice area.[35] Serial catheterization studies have shown that progression of aortic stenosis occurs in 40% to 75% of patients, but generally this is not predictable. Left ventricular systolic function may undergo insidious deterioration that may not be recognized clinically. In serial studies, the change in aortic valve

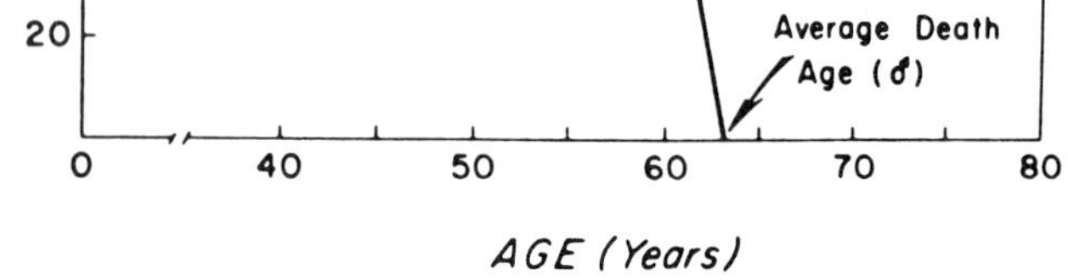

Fig 32-3 Natural history of aortic stenosis without operative treatment. (From Ross J Jr, Braunwald E: Aortic stenosis. *Circulation* 38 Suppl 5:61-67, 1968. By permission of American Heart Association.)

gradient can vary from 0 to as much as 44 mm Hg per year and is not influenced by the study interval.

The pattern of patients presenting with symptomatic severe aortic stenosis has changed. Today, most patients we see are elderly with senile aortic stenosis. The physical findings in elderly patients with severe aortic stenosis are different from those in younger patients.[36,37] The most important differences are the lower intensity of the systolic murmur and the wider pulse pressure.

Physical findings

A systolic murmur often is the sign that alerts the physician to the possibility of left ventricular outflow obstruction (Table 32-2). However, definitive diagnosis, identification of site, and quantitation of the obstruction are obtained by specific observations during auscultation of the heart and palpation of the carotid arteries and the apical impulse.

Inspection. In patients with severe stenosis, inspection of the thorax may reveal a localized systolic pulsation in the second right intercostal space due to poststenotic dilatation of the aorta.

Carotid pulse. Palpation of the carotid arteries in significant aortic valvular stenosis reveals highly characteristic findings and usually is the clue that distinguishes this lesion from other cardiac lesions associated with a systolic murmur. As an index of obstruction, the more severe the lesion, the more slowly the pulse rises to a late systolic peak (tardus) and the more decreased is the pulse volume (parvus). The exceptions to these characteristics of the carotid pulse occur in the younger[38] and older[39] age groups and in some patients with hypertension[40]—because of the dynamic nature of the carotid pulse in the young and the rigidity of the arteries in the aged.

Jugular venous pulse and pressure. These are normal except in the unusual patient in whom there is significant pulmonary arterial hypertension causing an increased jugular venous pressure or a prominent jugular "a" wave or both. Our experience and that of others[41] in aortic stenosis do not support Bernheim's concept that hypertrophy and bowing of the ventricular septum into the right ventricular outflow tract cause obstruction there and thus a prominent "a" wave.

Palpation. The apical impulse gives considerable information about the severity of the obstruction. With

Table 32-2 Left ventricular outflow obstruction: noninvasive differential diagnostic evaluation

Feature	Valvular	Subvalvular: HOC	Subvalvular: Discrete	Supravalvular
Incidence, %	90	9	<1	<1
Sex ratio, M:F	3:1	3:1	1:1	1:1
Carotid pulse	Parvus-tardus	Hyperkinetic (bisferious)	Parvus-tardus	±Parvus-tardus; R carotid pulse may be larger
Apical impulse	Forceful, sustained	Forceful, "double" or "triple"	Forceful, sustained	Forceful, sustained
Sounds	S_2 single in calcific; ejection click in congenital and rheumatic; S_4	S_2 may be paradoxic; S_4 loud	S_4	S_4
Systolic murmurs	+	+	+	+
Carotid transmission	+	−	+	R>L
Amyl nitrate	↑	↑	↑	↑
Valsalva	↓	↑	↓	↓
Squat	↑	↓	↑	↑
Diastolic murmur (aortic incompetence)	±	−	±	−
Electrocardiogram	LVH "strain pattern"	LVH "strain pattern"; deep septal Q; WPW rarely	LVH "strain pattern"	±LVH "strain pattern"
Chest roentgenogram				
Cardiothoracic ratio	N - ↑	N - ↑	N - ↑	N - ↑
Poststenotic aortic dilatation	↑ ↑	N	N - ↑	↓
Calcified valve	In calcific type	...	...	...

HOC, hypertrophic obstructive cardiomyopathy; L, left; LVH, left ventricular hypertrophy; N, normal; R, right; WPW, Wolff-Parkinson-White syndrome.

severe stenosis, the impulse is forceful and relatively well localized due to left ventricular hypertrophy, and it is sustained as a reflection of the prolonged effort of the left ventricle in ejecting the blood through the obstruction. The apical impulse may not be displaced to the left because the left ventricular hypertrophy may not be associated with dilatation. Presystolic distention of the hypertrophied left ventricle during left atrial systole is usually palpable and coincides with the auscultatory fourth heart sound. A palpable systolic thrill is commonly found when sought by careful palpation of the heart while the patient is leaning forward with expiration held. The thrill usually is maximal at the second right intercostal space but also can be felt in the carotid arteries and suprasternal notch, at the left sternal edge and at the apex. In some cases of calcific stenosis the thrill may be present at the apex only. The presence or absence of a thrill is related more to body type and aortic configuration than to the degree of stenosis.

Auscultation. An aortic systolic ejection click just following S_1, most evident at the apex and to the right of the sternum and uninfluenced by respiration, is present only when the stenotic aortic valve is very mobile[15,42-45] (Fig 32-4). Hence, the click may be present in congenital valvular stenosis, being an important sign that identifies the valvular level of obstruction. It may be the first indication of bicuspid aortic valve preceding the development of the murmur and stenosis. It is less common in rheumatic stenosis, and it is rare after the third decade because of increasing valvular calcification.

The S_2 in severe noncalcific valvular stenosis may be paradoxically split as a result of prolongation of left ventricular systole with delayed aortic valve closure. Characteristically, in severe calcific valvular stenosis the aortic closure is inaudible (except that in the senile type the calcification involves only the base of the three leaflets, which, therefore, may still be pliable); thus, S_2 is single with only the pulmonary component being detected. Moreover, in severe calcific valvular stenosis, S_2 may be completely inaudible as a result of the long systolic murmur enveloping P_2.

A fourth heart sound is present in severe aortic stenosis as a result of a forceful left atrial contraction in the presence of left ventricular hypertrophy with decreased compliance; in patients more than 45 years old this is an unreliable sign of severity because it can be present in the absence of aortic valvular stenosis.

A third heart sound appears only with the onset of left ventricular failure, except that it can be a normal finding in patients less than 35 years old.

The classic systolic murmur is maximally located at the second right intercostal space and is well transmitted to the carotid arteries and apex of the heart. In the presence of calcific valvular stenosis the murmur can be equally loud at the left sternal border or louder and very musical at the apex. The murmur is harsh and crescendo-decrescendo in character, starting after the S_1 and ending before or with the S_2. The severity of stenosis affects the time of peaking of the murmur and its duration. Murmurs associated with significant stenosis peak later in systole and extend to the S_2. The severity of stenosis correlates poorly with the loudness of the murmur. Soft murmurs in the presence of severe stenosis, sometimes heard with difficulty, may be present when there is left ventricular failure or in the presence of chronic obstructive lung disease or obesity. Conversely, loud murmurs may be present with mild stenosis; these murmurs, however, will be characterized by early peaking and short duration. The murmur of aortic valvular stenosis becomes softer during

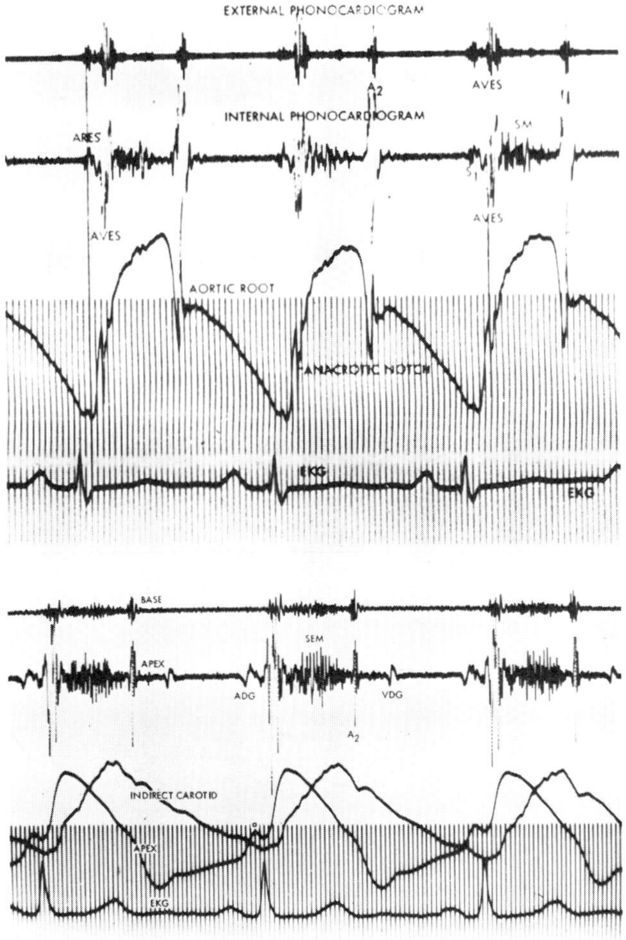

Fig 32-4 Phonocardiogram of aortic valvular stenosis. **Upper,** mild aortic stenosis, with prominent ejection sound introducing a short ejection murmur and ending well before a well-preserved aortic closure sound; the aortic ejection sound is coincident with the anacrotic notch recorded from the high-fidelity catheter in the central aorta. **Lower,** severe calcific aortic stenosis, with a long crescendo-decrescendo murmur and single S_2 and also a loud S_4; note the slow rise on the carotid tracing and the large presystolic heave on the apexcardiogram coincident with the atrial gallop. *ADG,* atrial diastolic gallop; *ARES,* aortic root ejection sound; *AVES,* aortic valve ejection sound; *SM,* systolic murmur; *VDG,* ventricular diastolic gallop. (Courtesy of James A. Shaver, M.D., University of Pittsburgh School of Medicine.)

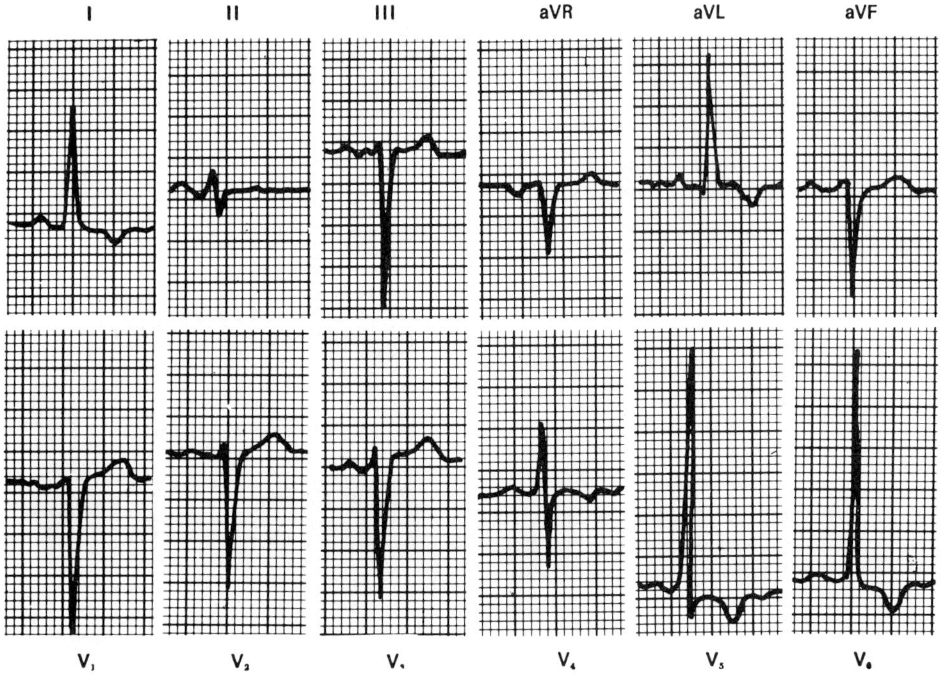

Fig 32-5 Electrocardiogram of patient with severe aortic valvular stenosis. Note increased QRS voltage consistent with left ventricular hypertrophy and ST-T changes consistent with strain pattern.

the straining phase of the Valsalva maneuver because the reduction in venous return results in a decreased forward flow. As in other types of left ventricular outflow obstruction, the murmur becomes louder with inhalation of amyl nitrite, because the decrease in peripheral resistance results in an increase in forward flow.

The association of a diastolic murmur of aortic incompetence is not infrequent and is an important sign because its presence suggests that the stenosis most likely is valvular (it also occurs in the rarer discrete subvalvular stenosis).

Electrocardiography

Except in hypertrophic obstructive cardiomyopathy, in most instances of left ventricular outflow obstruction there is a relationship between the degree of obstruction and the left ventricular hypertrophy assessed by QRS voltage criteria plus associated ST-T changes of the so-called strain pattern[28,29] (Fig 32-5). Hence, the electrocardiogram (ECG) is valuable for assessing progression by a comparison of serial tracings at appropriate intervals.[32]

In three-fourths of the patients with significant aortic valvular stenosis, the ECG is accurate in assessing the severity of the stenosis, but in the remainder it is not.[40] In some instances there may be a normal QRS voltage despite significant stenosis; this is more common in the elderly,[39] in whom voltage may decline, perhaps due to myocardial fibrosis, and in adolescents, in whom ST-T wave changes may precede QRS voltage criteria for hypertrophy and, rarely, the ECG is normal. In other instances there may be increased QRS voltage or ST-T wave changes despite mild stenosis; this is more common in thin-chested adolescents, who may have a high QRS voltage in the precordial leads but a normal QRS in leads III and aVF, or in adults in whom increased QRS voltage may be due to associated systemic hypertension, and ST-T wave changes may be due to digoxin effects or to coronary artery disease or may be nonspecific. Conduction defects (e.g., left axis deviation, bundle-branch block, and atrioventricular block) are found in approximately one-third of patients with aortic stenosis.[46] Left bundle-branch block may signal underlying left ventricular dysfunction. The presence of left atrial enlargement or atrial fibrillation should arouse suspicion of associated left ventricular dysfunction or mitral valve disease, or both. Ventricular ectopic activity[47] and complete atrioventricular block are rare.

Use of exercise testing to predict the severity of aortic stenosis has been reported in both children and adults.[48,49] The value of this technique in separating mild and severe cases has not been documented. A review of the literature shows that complications from exercise testing are rare when it is performed with appropriate caution and monitoring.[50-53] In tests of more than 500 patients with aortic stenosis, Linderholm et al.[54] did not have any complications. Despite the relative safety of exercise testing, American Heart Association and American College of Cardiology guidelines for its use list moderate to severe aortic stenosis as a contraindication.[55] Prospective studies of exercise testing in patients with aortic stenosis are needed to further evaluate its role in therapeutic decision-making.

Chest roentgenography

Chest roentgenography may be helpful diagnostically.[56] Despite severe aortic valvular stenosis, the heart size may be normal or minimally enlarged, but its shape is usually abnormal. The concentric left ventricular hypertrophy is manifested by rounding of the left lower cardiac border in the posteroanterior view (Fig 32-6). Left ventricular failure can be associated with an increase in size of the left ventricle, but a marked enlargement raises the suspicion that an associated lesion may be present. The same applies when the left atrium is markedly enlarged.

Poststenotic dilatation produces a prominence of the proximal ascending aorta to the right in the posteroanterior view and anteriorly in the lateral view; the aortic knob is normal. The degree of dilatation does not reflect the severity of the stenosis. Calcification of the aortic valve, demonstrated by fluoroscopy with an image-intensifier unit, or by two-dimensional echocardiography, is common in patients who are more than 40 years old and have isolated valvular stenosis.

Echocardiography

Two-dimensional echocardiography. Echocardiography has become the primary diagnostic laboratory modality for the evaluation of patients with aortic valvular stenosis. Two-dimensional (2D) echocardiography reliably demonstrates increased valve thickness and calcification as well as reduced leaflet excursion with systole, thereby qualitatively differentiating valvular stenosis from left ventricular outflow obstruction due to subvalvular or supravalvular disease.[57-62] Although calcification of the aortic valve leaflets is invariably associated with valvular

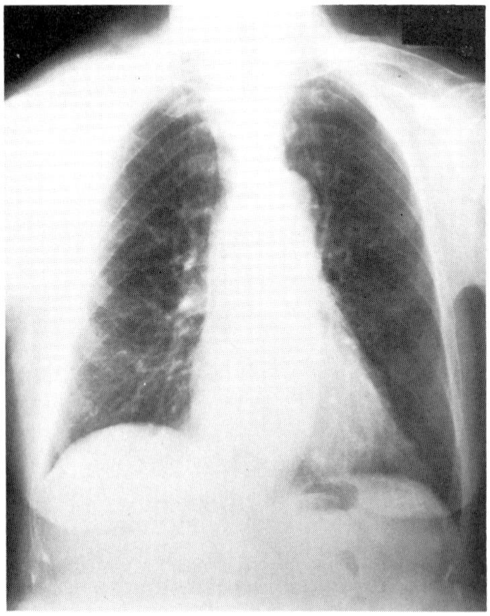

Fig 32-6 Chest roentgenogram of a patient with severe aortic valvular stenosis (gradient > 100 mm Hg). The heart size is normal or minimally enlarged. Note the round shape of the left lower cardiac border, indicating concentric left ventricular hypertrophy. (Courtesy of T. Schattenberg, M.D.)

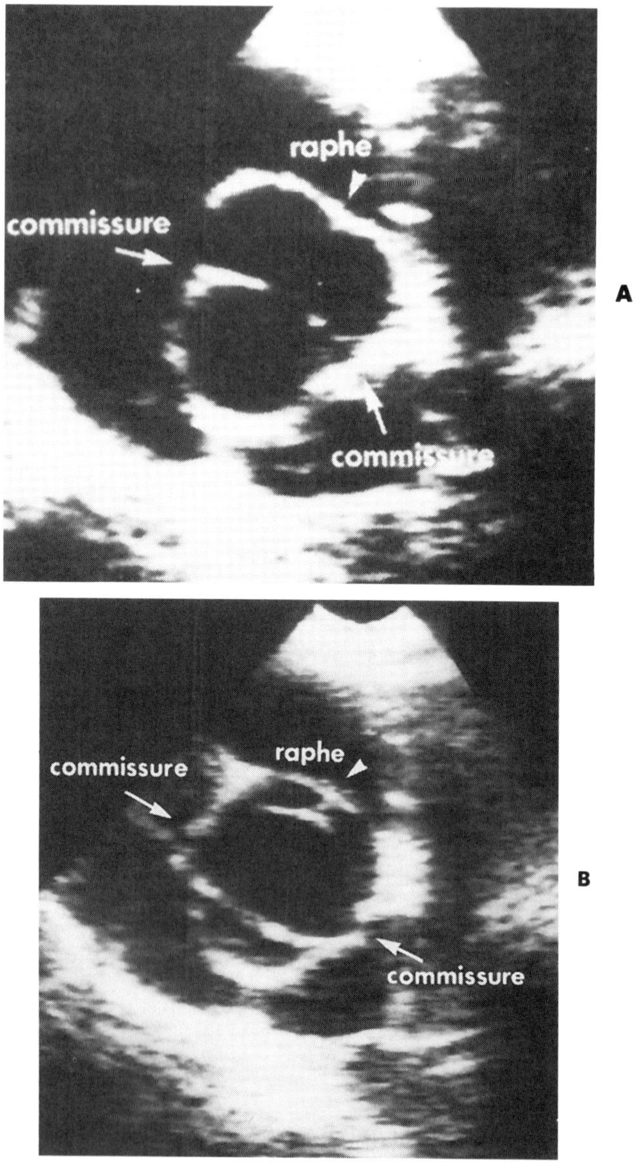

Fig 32-7 Parasternal short-axis view of a bicuspid aortic valve in diastole (**A**) and systole (**B**). Commissures are abnormally located at 4 o'clock and nearly 10 o'clock, with a raphe at 1 o'clock *(arrowhead)*. The oval appearance of the valve orifice during systole is characteristic. Inspection of valve opening and closure on real-time two-dimensional echocardiographic examination enables differentiation of a bicuspid valve from a tricuspid valve. (From Brandenburg RO Jr, Tajik AJ, Edwards WD, et al: Accuracy of 2-dimensional echocardiographic diagnosis of congenitally bicuspid aortic valve: echocardiographic-anatomic correlation in 115 patients. *Am J Cardiol* 51:1469-1473, 1983. By permission of Excerpta Medica.)

stenosis, the severity of calcification is not a reliable predictor of hemodynamic severity. This is especially true in young patients, in whom obstruction due to congenital rheumatic disease may not be associated with calcification. Systolic doming of the valve leaflets is frequently observed in association with significant stenosis when calcification is not prominent.[58,61] Echocardiography enables characterization of valve leaflet morphology with high sensitivity, including identification of a congenitally bicuspid aortic valve and commissural fusion associated with rheumatic disease[63,64] (Fig 32-7). However, dense calcification may make identification of cusp number, and hence morphology, difficult.

Other anatomic abnormalities frequently associated with aortic valvular stenosis demonstrated by 2D echocardiography are left ventricular hypertrophy, poststenotic dilatation of the aorta, other associated valvular lesions, and subaortic muscular hypertrophy, which may contribute to left ventricular outflow obstruction.

The hemodynamic severity of valvular stenosis may be estimated with confidence by combined 2D and M-mode echocardiography in some patients.[58-60] In patients with densely calcific aortic stenosis, severely decreased leaflet motion, and left ventricular hypertrophy, 2D echocardiography reliably predicts severe obstruction. Similarly, in patients with minimal aortic valve calcification, normal valve motion, and no left ventricular hypertrophy, 2D echocardiography reliably predicts that aortic stenosis is absent or trivial. However, many patients are not in either of these categories. In these patients, tomographic imaging is unreliable for prediction of the transvalvular gradient or semiquantitative assessment of the severity of stenosis.[58-60,65] Definitive assessment of the hemodynamic severity of aortic stenosis requires estimation of the transvalvular pressure gradient and aortic valve area by Doppler echocardiography.

Doppler echocardiography. The aim of the Doppler echocardiographic evaluation of the patient with aortic valve stenosis is measurement of the transvalvular pressure gradient and aortic valve orifice area. This can be accomplished in more than 97% of patients.[66]

Pressure gradient estimation in aortic stenosis by Doppler echocardiography requires measurement of the velocity of blood flow distal to the stenotic orifice. Transvalvular aortic velocity is increased in patients with aortic stenosis. The measurement of transvalvular aortic velocity by continuous-wave Doppler echocardiography enables estimation of maximal instantaneous and mean transvalvular pressure gradients by application of the modified Bernoulli equation.[66-71] The modified Bernoulli equation is expressed as $\Delta P = 4V^2$, in which ΔP represents the pressure gradient and V is the velocity of transvalvular blood flow measured by continuous-wave echocardiography. The pressure gradient is obtained by substituting the measured velocity for V in the modified Bernoulli equation.

Interpretation of data obtained by the Doppler echocardiographic method requires appreciation that the maximal instantaneous gradient represents an instantaneous pressure difference between the left ventricle and the aorta, whereas the commonly used peak-to-gradient measurement obtained by pullback of a single catheter at catheterization reflects the difference between peak left ventricular systolic and ascending aortic pressures, which are nonsynchronous events[67] (Fig 32-8). The Doppler-derived maximal instantaneous gradient always exceeds the peak-to-peak gradient obtained at cardiac catheterization. The peak-to-peak gradient is an arbitrary convention, is not physiologic, and is not directly comparable to the Doppler-derived maximal instantaneous gradient. The clinical utility of catheterization-measured peak-to-peak gradient may be attributed to the fortuitous correlation between peak-to-peak and mean gradients.

The validation of the Doppler method for gradient measurement has been proved in simultaneous Doppler echocardiographic and dual cardiac catheterization studies of aortic valve gradients. Extremely high correlation between maximal instantaneous gradient measured by Doppler imaging and that measured by dual catheters in the left ventricle and aorta has been demonstrated.[66,72,73] Similarly, the correlation of mean gradient measurements by catheterization and Doppler echocardiography in simultaneous studies has also been extremely high.[67] The hemodynamic severity of aortic valve stenosis by measurement of catheter pressure gradient is typically expressed as a peak-to-peak or mean gradient. Hence, the most clinically useful expression for the severity of aortic stenosis by Doppler echocardiography is provided by the mean gradient, which is directly comparable to the mean gradient obtained by catheterization.

Pressure gradient data alone correctly classify the hemodynamic severity of aortic stenosis in fewer than 50% of patients.[66] Hence, it is prudent to determine valve area as well as pressure gradient in all patients with aortic stenosis. The method for echocardiographic determination of aortic valve area is based on the physiologic principle that laminar flow through a conduit is equal to the mean velocity multiplied by the cross-sectional orifice dimension. At constant flow, the ratio of cross-sectional areas at two different sites is inversely proportional to the ratio of the respective mean velocities at those sites. This relationship is expressed by the equation

$$A_1 \times V_1 = A_2 \times V_2$$

in which A_1 is the cross-sectional area of the left ventricular outflow tract, A_2 is the cross-sectional area of the stenotic valve, V_2 is the mean velocity of blood flow distal to the obstruction, and V_1 is the mean velocity proximal to the obstruction. If the mean velocity of the stenotic valve is known, the stenotic area can be derived as flow divided by the mean velocity of the stenotic jet. Rearrangement of the continuity equation yields the aortic valve area:

$$A_2 = A_1 \times (V_1/V_2)$$

Because the systolic ejection time is the same and the time velocity curve follows a similar course for the left ventricular outflow tract and aortic valve flow, the peak velocity and peak left ventricular outflow tract velocity may be substituted for the mean velocities of the continuity equation.[67] In practice, A_1 is determined by 2D echocardiography and peak V_1 and V_2 are measured by

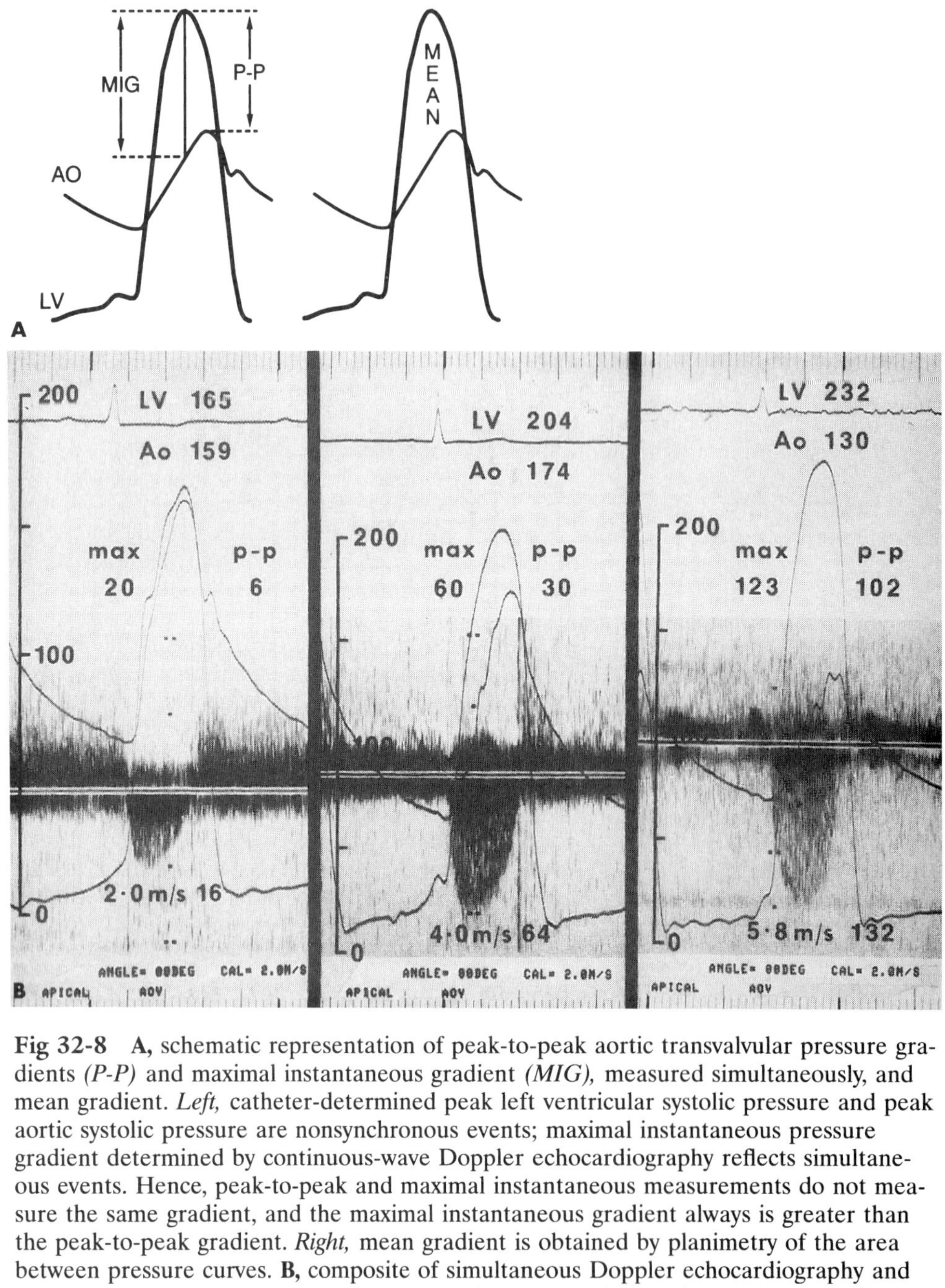

Fig 32-8 **A,** schematic representation of peak-to-peak aortic transvalvular pressure gradients *(P-P)* and maximal instantaneous gradient *(MIG),* measured simultaneously, and mean gradient. *Left,* catheter-determined peak left ventricular systolic pressure and peak aortic systolic pressure are nonsynchronous events; maximal instantaneous pressure gradient determined by continuous-wave Doppler echocardiography reflects simultaneous events. Hence, peak-to-peak and maximal instantaneous measurements do not measure the same gradient, and the maximal instantaneous gradient always is greater than the peak-to-peak gradient. *Right,* mean gradient is obtained by planimetry of the area between pressure curves. **B,** composite of simultaneous Doppler echocardiography and catheter pressure measurements in three patients with mild, moderate, and severe elevations of transvalvular aortic gradients due to aortic stenosis. Pressure gradients were measured by dual catheters in the left ventricle and ascending aorta. The maximal *(max)* catheter gradient is greater than the peak-to-peak *(p-p)* catheter gradient for each degree of severity of stenosis. The maximal Doppler-derived gradients accurately measure the simultaneously recorded maximal catheter gradient but overestimate the peak-to-peak catheter gradient. The Doppler calibrations are in 2 m/sec increments. *AO* or *Ao,* ascending aorta; *LV,* left ventricle. (**A,** from Olson LJ, Tajik AJ: Echocardiographic evaluation of valvular heart disease. In *Cardiac Imaging: A Companion to Braunwald's Heart Disease.* Edited by ML Marcus, HL Schelbert, DJ Skorton, et al. Philadelphia, WB Saunders Company, 1991, pp 419-448. By permission. **B,** from Currie PJ, Seward JB, Reeder GS, et al: Continuous-wave Doppler echocardiographic assessment of severity of calcific aortic stenosis: a simultaneous Doppler-catheter correlative study in 100 adult patients. *Circulation* 71:1162-1169, 1985. By permission of American Heart Association.)

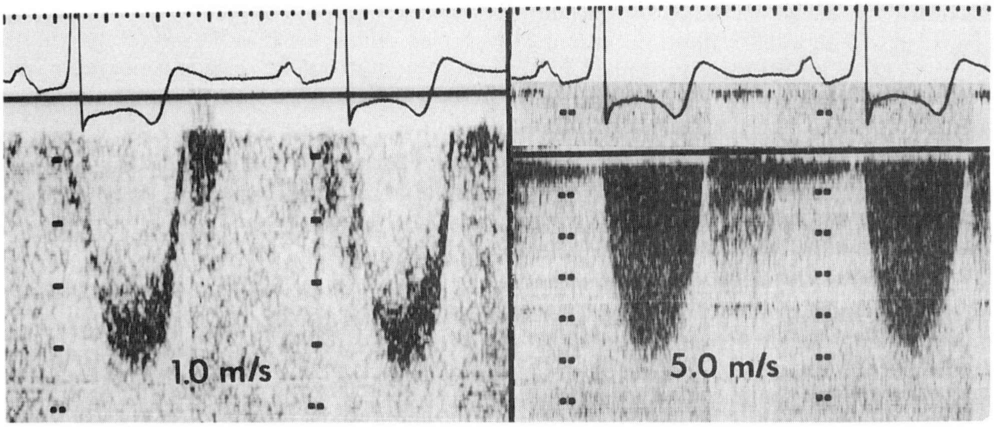

Fig 32-9 Determination of aortic valve area by use of the continuity equation. Velocity profiles of left ventricular outflow **(left)** and aorta **(right)** are measured by Doppler echocardiography in a patient with aortic stenosis. (From Olson LJ, Edwards WD, Tajik AJ: Aortic valve stenosis: etiology, pathophysiology, evaluation, and management. *Curr Probl Cardiol* 12:453-508, 1987. By permission, Mayo Foundation.)

pulsed- and continuous-wave Doppler echocardiography, respectively (Fig 32-9).

Investigators have consistently demonstrated the accuracy of Doppler echocardiography for the estimation of aortic valve area in adults with aortic stenosis in comparison with measurements obtained by cardiac catheterization using the Gorlin formula.[34,66,74-76] For patients in whom it is not possible to estimate the left ventricular outflow tract diameter by 2D echocardiography (and, hence, impossible to estimate aortic valve area), a highly sensitive index for the detection of severe aortic stenosis is provided by the ratio of V_1 to V_2. Severe aortic stenosis has been shown to be present in 92% of patients in whom V_1/V_2 is less than 0.25.[66] This index is independent of cardiac output and therefore may be used for serial evaluation.

DIAGNOSTIC PROBLEMS

Noninvasive studies

The wide range of clinical entities associated with a systolic murmur can create difficulties in making the diagnosis of left ventricular outflow obstruction. However, accurate examination of the contour of the carotid pulse permits differentiation of significant aortic valvular stenosis from most other cardiac lesions associated with a systolic murmur. Exceptions to this may occur in adolescents or in some patients with associated hypertension (both have a rather "dynamic" carotid pulse) or in some elderly patients with rigid or diseased carotid arteries in whom one or both carotid pulses can be diminished in volume or parvus. It is important to note that by "inching" the stethoscope back and forth from the aortic area to the carotid artery area, it usually is possible to distinguish a carotid bruit from a transmitted aortic valve murmur (if there is a continuous bruit, this distinction is more obvious). Then, comparing the pulse contours of both carotid arteries often will enable the clinician to differentiate significant carotid disease from significant aortic valvular stenosis.

When the acquired aortic valvular stenosis is not severe, the contour of the carotid pulse may be less definitive, and the diagnosis of aortic stenosis may be masked by other conditions. However, the murmur of aortic valvular stenosis should be distinguished at the bedside from similar murmurs of other conditions (see chapter 2).

The distinguishing features in patients with left ventricular outflow obstruction at different levels are presented in Table 32-2.

In chronic rheumatic mitral valvular regurgitation, the murmur is not crescendo-decrescendo. After the inhalation of amyl nitrite, the murmur decreases in intensity as a result of decreased peripheral resistance, which increases forward flow and reduces regurgitant flow. The intensity of the murmur does not increase after an ectopic beat, and, finally, clinical features other than the murmur are usually of diagnostic help. Doppler and 2D echocardiography frequently resolve questions.

Mitral regurgitation secondary to a flail posterior leaflet, due to either ruptured chordae tendineae or significant prolapse, causes the apical murmur to be transmitted to the base and to the carotid arteries, and it can become louder after inhalation of amyl nitrite because the increase in forward flow results in reduction of left ventricular volume, more "slack" in the supporting apparatus, and, thus, augmentation of regurgitation. In this differential diagnosis, particular attention should be paid to the hyperdynamic carotid pulse and apical impulse, both characteristic of the mitral but not of the aortic lesion. Doppler and two-dimensional echocardiography are very helpful in making the correct diagnosis.

Hypertrophic obstructive cardiomyopathy (HOC) may have an apical holosystolic component of mitral regurgitation as well as an upper left sternal border midsystolic component of left ventricular outflow obstruction. Hence, the diagnosis of HOC has to be kept in mind in patients with auscultatory features of both mitral incompetence and aortic stenosis. Characteristically, the murmur of HOC does not radiate to the neck, and it usually becomes louder during the straining phase of the Valsalva maneuver because the decrease in venous return results in reduction of left ventricular volume with augmentation of the dynamic obstruction. Other diagnostic features of HOC, such as the carotid pulse and the ECG, are helpful. In rare instances of advanced aortic valvular stenosis with severe left ventricular hypertrophy, the murmur also can be louder during the Valsalva maneuver; it is possible that some of these cases represent an association of aortic valvular disease and HOC. Echocardiography is the noninvasive procedure of choice for the diagnosis of HOC. Continuous wave Doppler echocardiography can help confirm the severity of left ventricular outflow tract obstruction.

When the murmur of aortic valvular stenosis is loud at the left sternal border, it may be mistaken for a murmur originating in the right heart, either from pulmonary stenosis or, more rarely, from an atrial septal defect. Such right-sided murmurs characteristically disappear within one or two beats into the straining phase of the Valsalva maneuver and return within one to two beats following release of Valsalva, whereas murmurs to the left heart lesions return later, that is, four or five beats after release of Valsalva. With release, the wide splitting of S_2 is a precise characteristic of isolated pulmonary stenosis or atrial septal defect. Echocardiography can confirm the diagnosis.

Finally, as in aortic valvular stenosis, aortic supravalvular and discrete subvalvular stenosis may be manifested by a murmur louder in the right upper sternal border and also by a carotid pulse that is tardus and parvus. However, in supravalvular aortic stenosis, the murmur is maximal below the right clavicle and distinctly radiates to the right carotid artery; about half of the patients characteristically have a greater pulse and systolic pressure in the right carotid and brachial arteries than in the left (usually, the systolic pressure in the right arm is no more than 15 mm Hg higher than in the left). Discrete subvalvular aortic stenosis is difficult to distinguish from aortic valvular stenosis, except that associated mild aortic regurgitation is common, an ejection click is rare, S_2 is not single, and 2D echocardiography usually is diagnostic.

Invasive studies

Indications. Invasive studies should be performed not on a routine basis[77] but in selected situations.[78,79] These situations should include the following.

1. Patients with clinical evidence of aortic stenosis and angina or patients in whom the probability of coronary artery disease is high. In these situations,

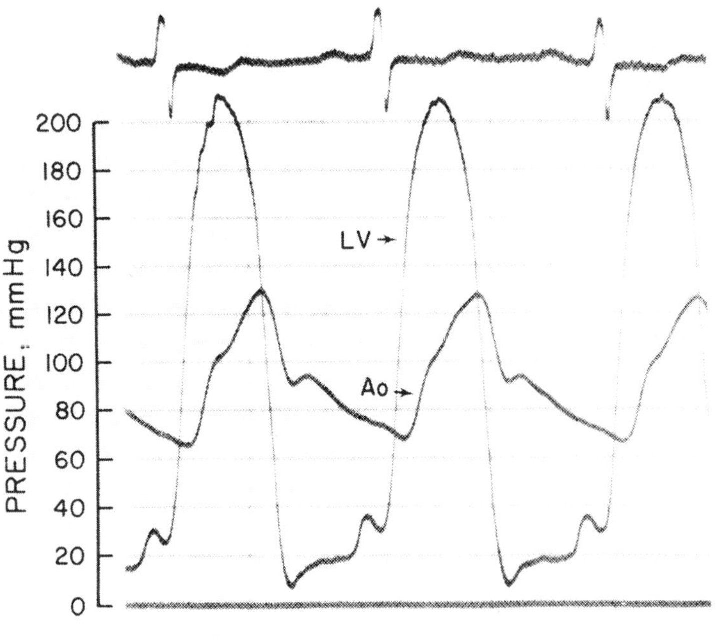

Fig 32-10 Left ventricular *(LV)* and aortic *(Ao)* pressure tracings in an elderly man with severe calcific aortic stenosis. The large "a" wave in the LV tracing is consistent with decreased compliance of the massively hypertrophied ventricle. The LV pressure was measured with a micromanometer catheter; aortic pressure was measured with a fluid-filled catheter system attached via tubing to a P23Db transducer. This accounts in part for the delay in onset of Ao upstroke relative to LV pressure rise. (From Grossman W: Profiles in valvular heart disease. In *Cardiac Catheterization and Angiography.* Edited by W Grossman. Philadelphia, Lea & Febiger, 1986, pp 359-381. By permission.)

coronary arteriography may be of help in identifying the group of patients with associated coronary disease – about one-third of the patients with angina.

2. Patients with clinical evidence of left ventricular outflow obstruction in whom the level of obstruction is not clearly defined by clinical examination or echocardiography. In these rare cases, catheterization should be done.
3. Major discordance between the clinical findings and results of Doppler echocardiography, especially in a patient with symptoms in whom aortic valve surgery is contemplated. Since Doppler echocardiography, when properly performed and interpreted, provides accurate hemodynamic data, in most patients it obviates cardiac catheterization.

Findings. The profiles have been described by Grossman[80] (Fig 32-10). At catheterization of a stenotic aortic valve, the valve usually is easier to cross when the catheter is inserted via the right brachial artery rather than via the femoral artery. When the aortic valve is difficult to cross, aortic root angiography may be helpful in indicating the position of the valve orifice; otherwise, the angiographic findings cannot be used as an indication of the severity of the stenosis.

Under conditions of rest and a normal cardiac output, a peak systolic gradient across the aortic valve of more than 50 mm Hg is considered severe.[15] A gradient of less than 25 mm Hg implies mild stenosis, and a gradient of 25 to 50 mm Hg implies moderate stenosis. With decreased cardiac output, there is a proportional decrease in the gradient; this is important to consider to avoid undergrading the severity of the stenosis (Fig 32-11). In this circumstance, the valve area *(A)* calculated by the Gorlin formula[81,82] may be more accurate than the pressure gradient as an estimate of the severity of the stenosis:

$$A = \frac{\text{CO}}{\text{SEP} \times 44.3 \times \sqrt{\text{gradient}}}$$

in which CO is cardiac output, SEP is systolic ejection period per minute (systolic ejection period per beat, as measured from the pressure tracings, multiplied by beats/min), and gradient is the gradient across the aortic valve.

COEXISTING CONDITIONS

Coronary artery disease

Controversy over whether the absence of chest pain rules out serious coronary disease appears to have been settled. Of patients without angina, some have been shown to have significant coronary artery disease.[83] The important question remains unanswered: Is it necessary to identify coexistent coronary artery obstructive disease in the patient with aortic stenosis?

Severe aortic stenosis[84] implies significant left ventricular hypertrophy producing an imbalance of supply and demand even in patients with angiographically normal coronary arteries. The reverse, if recognized, has not been acknowledged; that is, with regression of left ventricular hypertrophy, the lesions that were once functionally significant become functionally insignificant. Most animal

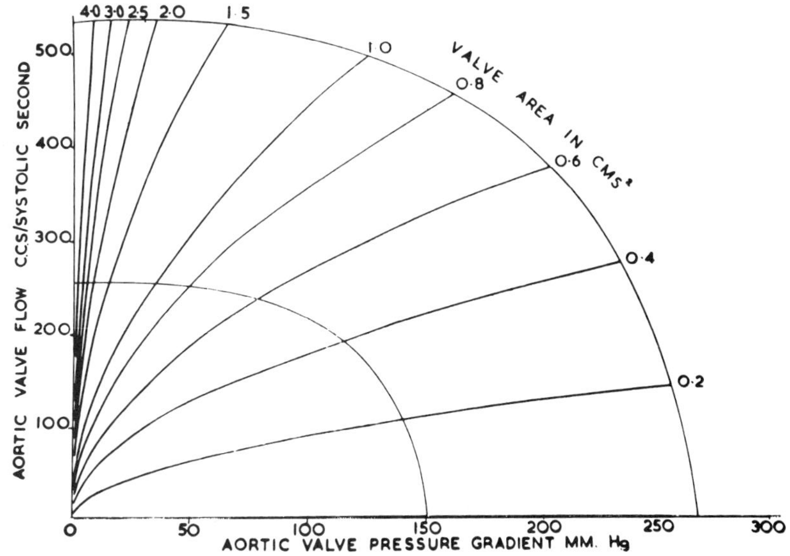

Fig 32-11 Interrelationship of aortic valve pressure gradient, aortic valve flow, and aortic valve area. As example, at valve area of 0.6 cm^2 and normal flow (250 mL/sec), the aortic valve pressure gradient is about 75 mm Hg; if the flow is 200 mL/sec, the pressure gradient is about 50 mm Hg. (From Herman MV, Cohn PF, Gorlin R: Resistance to blood flow by stenotic valves: calculation of orifice area. In *Cardiac Catheterization and Angiography.* Edited by W Grossman. Philadelphia, Lea & Febiger, 1980, pp 124-130. By permission.)

studies show that regression of left ventricular hypertrophy can occur rapidly, with return to near-normal left ventricular mass in 2 to 3 weeks.[85,86] Kennedy et al.,[87] Cody et al.,[88] and Drost[89] demonstrated a decrease in left ventricular mass in patients after aortic surgery for aortic stenosis.

Since the report of Flemma et al.,[90] many reports have appeared citing the results of combined aortic valve surgery and aortocoronary bypass surgery. From these reports, certain general conclusions can be made. First, it is technically possible to do both procedures at the same time. The hospital mortality is higher when both procedures are performed[91-93] than when aortic or coronary surgery is done alone. Cardiovascular causes continue to be a most important determinant of morbidity and late postoperative death.[93] Not all patients with coexistent coronary obstructive disease require bypass surgery. However, subsets of patients with left main coronary artery disease or its equivalent may benefit from the addition of bypass coronary surgery.[94]

Mitral annular calcification

Mitral annular calcification is associated with calcific aortic stenosis in 25% to 50% of patients. Patients with aortic stenosis and mitral annular calcification are older, have more severe aortic stenosis, and are more often female. Although these patients die more frequently from cardiac causes, no differences are apparent in 5- and 10-year actuarial survival rates.[95,96]

Pulmonary hypertension

Contrary to popular belief, pulmonary hypertension frequently (approximately 50%) accompanies isolated calcific aortic stenosis. Pulmonary hypertension is related to increased left ventricular end-diastolic pressure. Reactive and reversible vasoconstriction seems the likely cause of pulmonary hypertension, since the surgical results are excellent.[97,98]

Gastrointestinal bleeding

The association of chronic gastrointestinal bleeding and aortic stenosis remains problematical.[99] This association is called "Heyde syndrome."[100] Gastrointestinal operations are successful in preventing recurrent bleeding in a small percentage of patients, but valve replacement is frequently effective. It appears that for unexplained gastrointestinal bleeding associated with significant aortic stenosis, aortic valve replacement should be considered because of the likelihood of cure.[101]

MANAGEMENT

Principles of treatment

In aortic valvular stenosis, the appearance of symptoms is a strong indication for surgical intervention.[30] Symptoms are usually the manifestation of significant valvular obstruction. It is at this stage of the disease that the prognosis with nonoperative management is poorer than the prognosis with surgical intervention.[102]

Once symptoms appear, surgical intervention is indicated.[30,103,104] Management of asymptomatic patients with severe aortic stenosis remains problematic. Proponents for surgery in the asymptomatic patient argue that sudden death can occur as a first symptom; furthermore, left ventricular dysfunction develops in some patients, who, therefore, benefit less than patients with normal ventricular function preoperatively.[103]

Table 32-3 summarizes the pertinent reports in the literature addressing sudden death in the asymptomatic patient. On the basis of the latest data, we must conclude that sudden death is uncommon in an asymptomatic patient with aortic stenosis. Certainly, this risk is less than the mortality associated with aortic valve surgery, particularly in the older age group.

Chronic pressure overload due to aortic valve stenosis leads to progressive left ventricular hypertrophy, often of a marked degree. In addition to the increased muscle mass, interstitial connective tissue invariably is increased. Correction of this abnormal hemodynamic state by aortic valve replacement results in regression of left ventricular muscle mass.[108-110] Although the interstitial space changes little in the first 2 years postoperatively, the relative interstitial space (percentage of fibrosis) is significantly reduced at approximately 5 years after the operation in patients with aortic stenosis. These changes lead to a return toward normal function postoperatively in more than 50% of patients.

Unfortunately, aortic valve replacement does not always result in improvement of left ventricular performance. From 25% to 50% of patients with low preoperative ejection fractions do not have significant improvement postoperatively. This lack of left ventricular response may be secondary to factors unrelated to aortic valve stenosis. Factors such as progressive coronary atherosclerosis and imperfect myocardial preservation during surgery contribute to the poor results in some patients. Before recommending a palliative procedure to a person without symptoms, we must identify the subset of patients who do poorly postoperatively and determine if earlier intervention will help this group.

If surgical intervention is not yet indicated, the most important aspect in the medical management is close follow-up, at least on a yearly basis, to assess any deterioration that might prompt surgical intervention. This includes a detailed clinical evaluation and assessment of both systolic and diastolic function by echocardiography. In patients with rheumatic aortic stenosis, prophylaxis against recurrent rheumatic fever[111] is important (discussed in chapter 54). Specifically, such prophylaxis should be undertaken for at least 5 years after the last rheumatic attack (a time when the patient is still at high risk for recurrence) or until the patient has reached age 40 to 45 years, whichever is longer. Even the latter recommendation is not absolute, because rheumatic valvular and myocardial inflammation often appear to persist beyond this age.[112,113] Thus, judgment must be exercised[114] – e.g., the grandmother with rheumatic heart disease who is continually exposed to streptococcal

Table 32-3 Sudden death in asymptomatic patients with severe aortic stenosis

Study	Date	No. of patients	Follow-up, mo	Sudden deaths, no.	Comments
Dry and Willius[105]	1939	23	Autopsy	?	2 pt "apparently in good health"
Frank et al.[30]	1973	3	?	1	
Chizner et al.[104]	1980	10	29-84	0	
Kelly et al.[106]	1988	51	17 ± 9	0	2 deaths; more symptoms appeared
Pellikka et al.[107]	1990	143	6-48; mean, 20	0	30 pt had surgery within 3 mo of diagnosis; 2 deaths

infection in her grandchildren may need antibiotic protection for an indefinite period of time. Certain adults are at "high risk" for recurrence of rheumatic fever. These include those who had a recent attack or have had multiple attacks, those from a lower socioeconomic status, and those in certain professions (schoolteachers, physicians, nurses, allied medical personnel, military personnel). The need for daily prophylaxis in adults who have not had rheumatic fever for 10 years or more is less well established.

If atrial fibrillation occurs, these patients should be converted to sinus rhythm rapidly. If they have severe aortic stenosis, reversion to sinus rhythm becomes a matter of some urgency; if they are symptomatic at this time, conversion to sinus rhythm and treatment of symptoms is a medical emergency.[114] Aortic valve replacement must be seriously considered at this time.

Patients who present with heart failure should be hospitalized, treated, and stabilized. If no contraindications are present, aortic valve replacement is indicated.

The report by Cribier et al.[115] generated great interest for aortic balloon valvotomy in elderly patients with aortic valve stenosis. Initial reports on balloon valvotomy have described significant short-term hemodynamic and symptomatic improvement with a low incidence of complications. Subsequent follow-up studies, however, have shown that this technique is not the treatment of choice for most patients with calcific aortic stenosis, primarily because of the incompleteness of the procedure in relieving obstruction and because of a very high restenosis rate.[116-118]

The majority of patients that we now see with aortic stenosis are elderly—past 70 years of age—and have multiple coexisting medical problems and a significantly increased risk of cardiac surgery.[119] Mortality for patients 65 years or older undergoing aortic valve replacement has been reported as 10% to 16%.[120,121] In patients older than 80, the early mortality rate has been 31%.[122] Further, the natural history of this subgroup of elderly patients with severe symptomatic aortic stenosis who are not candidates for surgery because either they refuse operation or medical problems coexist is 57% alive at 1 year, 42% at 2 years, and 25% at 3 years.[123] For these reasons and because studies demonstrate the feasibility of percutaneous aortic balloon valvuloplasty in the elderly,[124] the balloon procedure may be useful in selected clinical situations.

The mechanisms of successful dilatation include fracture of calcific nodules, grossly inapparent microfractures of the leaflets, and stretching and splitting of fused commissures. The variation in mechanism of dilatation and cause of the aortic stenosis may be important factors in the time course of valvular restenosis in a given patient[125] (Fig 32-12).

Balloon valvuloplasty may be the procedure of choice in patients who are at high risk, including those with advanced age, previous myocardial infarction, or depressed left ventricular function, and in patients who oppose surgical intervention. Should restenosis occur, a second dilatation could be performed, with the recognition that the duration of symptomatic improvement will be limited. Patients in the second group are those who have severe symptomatic aortic stenosis and are in need of an urgent noncardiac operation.[126] However, although severe aortic stenosis has been reported to increase the risk of a noncardiac operation, recent advances in anesthetic management may alter this risk.[127] Finally, balloon aortic balloon aortic valvuloplasty is a valid therapeutic alternative as a bridge to subsequent aortic valve replacement.

Surgical technique

Operations for acquired aortic valvular stenosis are performed utilizing the standard techniques of extracorporeal circulation. Exposure of the valve typically requires ascending aortic cross-clamping and aortotomy as well as left atrial or ventricular venting. Particular care must be taken to preserve myocardial integrity during operations of this type, since left ventricular myocardial failure, already prevalent preoperatively, reduces tolerance to further ischemic stress.

Valve replacement consists of two basic steps: resection of the diseased valve and insertion of a substitute valve. In the absence of significant calcification of the aortic valve, its excision is simply accomplished by incising each cusp 2 or 3 mm away from and parallel to its base, thus leaving a scallop-shaped rim of the original valve to which the substitute valve can be attached. However, when calcification is severe, excision may be technically demanding. Calcific masses that are penetrating the annulus must be tediously curetted and teased from their beds, leaving the fibrous base of the cusps intact.

The issues relating to selection of the prosthetic valve

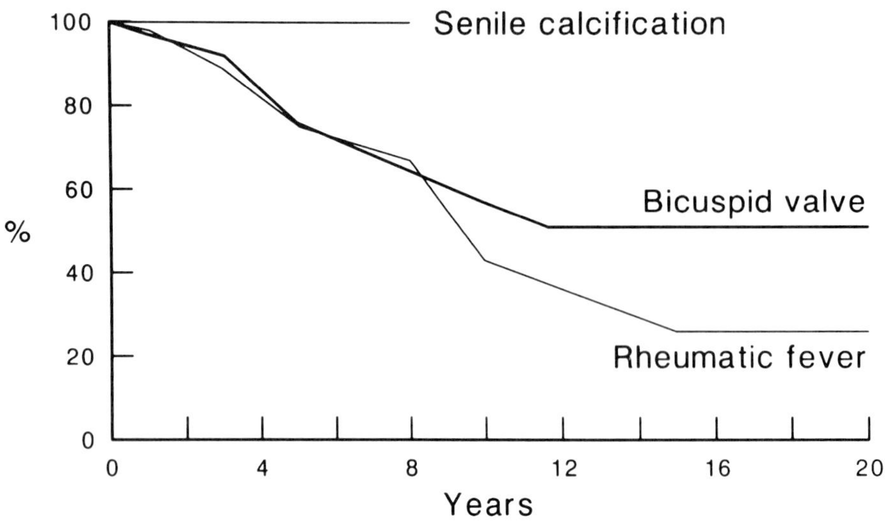

Fig 32-12 Freedom from reoperation in patients with rheumatic fever, bicuspid aortic valves, and senile calcification who have undergone aortic valve decalcification. (From King RM, Pluth JR, Giuliani ER, et al: Mechanical decalcification of the aortic valve. *Ann Thorac Surg* 42:269-272, 1986. By permission of the Society of Thoracic Surgeons.)

are discussed in chapter 37. The details of valve insertion are not described here, but obviously it is essential that the valve be securely, completely, and permanently attached to the aortic root at operation in order to prevent regurgitation around the prosthesis but attached in such a way as to ensure free movement of the valvular apparatus.

There is renewed interest in preserving, if possible, the native aortic valve. Ultrasonic decalcification of the annulus may prove to be a useful adjunct in aortic valve replacement. Initial results[128] are encouraging, but further experience is essential before a definite recommendation can be made.

Postoperative course

Details of the postoperative course and follow-up after valve replacement are discussed in chapter 37. The hospital mortality rate for replacement of the aortic valve is 7% or less, and most early deaths are related to arrhythmias resulting from advanced left ventricular hypertrophy and failure.[114,129,130] Because the work of the heart is immediately greatly decreased by elimination of the aortic gradient, cardiac performance tends to be excellent postoperatively, and the convalescence is rapid and smooth. Left ventricular hypertrophy regresses but usually not completely.

The literature dealing with late results of valve replacement is extensive.[131-137] Briefly, the 10-year survival after aortic valve replacement is 60% or better, and the 15-year survival is 50% or better.[114] Function is improved in the surviving patients. The late results of operation also depend on the status of the myocardium preoperatively.

ASYMPTOMATIC AORTIC STENOSIS IN NONCARDIAC SURGERY

Aortic stenosis has been shown to be a significant risk factor for noncardiac surgery.[138] Confronted with the clinical problem of an asymptomatic patient with documented severe aortic stenosis who must undergo elective noncardiac surgery, the physician has three management options: (1) prophylactic aortic valve surgery before the noncardiac operation, (2) prophylactic aortic balloon valvuloplasty,[139,140] and (3) acceptance of the increased risk of noncardiac surgery without preoperative mechanical intervention for the aortic valve but with careful intraoperative and postoperative monitoring.[127]

Several factors need to be taken into account when choosing among these three options.

1. Many of the patients are likely to be elderly and may be frail or have serious coexisting medical conditions.
2. The operative mortality risk for aortic valve replacement, ordinarily in the 5% to 7% range, increases considerably for aortic valve replacement in the elderly (approaching 15% to 30%), so that this approach is untenable in many circumstances.
3. Balloon aortic valvuloplasty, even in centers with considerable experience, has inherent risks, including serious vascular trauma at the femoral puncture site (requiring transfusions and surgical repair) and ventricular perforation with cardiac tamponade.[116] Although the procedure-related mortality is very low, deaths have occurred.[116,140] In addition, the rate of complications may be even higher in centers that have limited experience with the balloon valvuloplasty technique.

4. Some patients may be so physically limited or sedentary that clinical assessment of symptomatic status is not possible.

O'Keefe et al.[127] reported on a series of 48 consecutive elderly patients with significant aortic stenosis, 75% of whom had symptoms, who, because of serious coexisting medical illness or refusal to have aortic valve surgery, underwent noncardiac surgery at an acceptably low risk. In this series, there were no perioperative deaths and only minor perioperative hemodynamic abnormalities, which were promptly recognized and easily managed. Although this was a consecutive series, the patients were highly selected and had careful perioperative monitoring and anesthetic care. Intraoperative hypotension was promptly recognized and treated. It must be emphasized that these observations do not imply that patients with severe aortic stenosis can undergo noncardiac surgery with impunity, because such patients are known to be at increased risk. Patients with associated coronary artery disease or coexistent left ventricular dysfunction may not do as well.

REFERENCES

1. Edwards JE: Calcific aortic stenosis: pathologic features. *Proc Staff Meet Mayo Clin* 36:444-451, 1961
2. Roberts WC: The congenitally bicuspid aortic valve: a study of 85 autopsy cases. *Am J Cardiol* 26:72-83, 1970
3. Roberts WC: The structure of the aortic valve in clinically isolated aortic stenosis: an autopsy study of 162 patients over 15 years of age. *Circulation* 42:91-97, 1970
4. Pomerance A: Isolated aortic stenosis. In *The Pathology of the Heart.* Edited by A Pomerance, MJ Davies. Oxford, Blackwell Scientific Publications, 1975, pp 327-341
5. Subramanian R, Olson LJ, Edwards WD: Surgical pathology of pure aortic stenosis: a study of 374 cases. *Mayo Clin Proc* 59:683-690, 1984
6. Pomerance A: Pathogenesis of aortic stenosis and its relation to age. *Br Heart J* 34:569-574, 1972
7. Passik CS, Ackermann DM, Pluth JR, et al: Temporal changes in the causes of aortic stenosis: a surgical pathologic study of 646 cases. *Mayo Clin Proc* 62:119-123, 1987
8. Larson EW, Edwards WD: Risk factors for aortic dissection: a necropsy study of 161 cases. *Am J Cardiol* 53:849-855, 1984
9. Roberts WC, Ferrans VJ, Levy RI, et al: Cardiovascular pathology in hyperlipoproteinemia: anatomic observations in 42 necropsy patients with normal or abnormal serum lipoprotein patterns. *Am J Cardiol* 31:557-570, 1973
10. Silver MD: Obstruction to blood flow, related to the aortic valve. In *Cardiovascular Pathology.* Vol. 1. Edited by MD Silver. New York, Churchill Livingstone, 1983, pp 599-617
11. Gould L, Reddy CVR, DePalma D, et al: Cardiac manifestations of ochronosis. *J Thorac Cardiovasc Surg* 72:788-791, 1976
12. Roberts WC, Ewy GA, Glancy DL, et al: Valvular stenosis produced by active infective endocarditis. *Circulation* 36:449-451, 1967
13. Lerman BB, Thomas LC, Abrams GD, et al: Aortic stenosis associated with systemic lupus erythematosus. *Am J Med* 72:707-710, 1982
14. Pritzker MR, Ernst JD, Caudill C, et al: Acquired aortic stenosis in systemic lupus erythematosus. *Ann Intern Med* 93:434-436, 1980
15. Wood P: Aortic stenosis. *Am J Cardiol* 1:553-571, 1958
16. Gorlin R, Gorlin SG: Hydraulic formula for calculation of the area of the stenotic mitral valve, other cardiac valves, and central circulatory shunts. I. *Am Heart J* 41:1-45, 1951
17. Kennedy JW, Twiss RD, Blackmon JR, et al: Quantitative angiocardiography. III. Relationships of left ventricular pressure, volume, and mass in aortic valve disease. *Circulation* 38:838-845, 1968
18. Yin FCP: Ventricular wall stress. *Circ Res* 49:829-842, 1981
19. Mirsky I: Left ventricular stresses in the intact human heart. *Biophys J* 9:189-208, 1969
20. Hood WP Jr, Rackley CE, Rolett EL: Wall stress in the normal and hypertrophied human left ventricle. *Am J Cardiol* 22:550-558, 1968
21. Grossman W, Jones D, McLaurin LP: Wall stress and patterns of hypertrophy in the human left ventricle. *J Clin Invest* 56:56-64, 1975
22. Gunther S, Grossman W: Determinants of ventricular function in pressure-overload hypertrophy in man. *Circulation* 59:679-688, 1979
23. Cannon SR, Richards KL, Crawford M: Hydraulic estimation of stenotic orifice area: a correction of the Gorlin formula. *Circulation* 71:1170-1178, 1985
24. Bertrand ME, LaBlanche JM, Tilmant PY, et al: Coronary sinus blood flow at rest and during isometric exercise in patients with aortic valve disease: mechanism of angina pectoris in presence of normal coronary arteries. *Am J Cardiol* 47:199-205, 1981
25. Hancock EW: Aortic stenosis, angina pectoris, and coronary artery disease. *Am Heart J* 93:382-393, 1977
26. Green SJ, Pizzarello RA, Padmanabhan VT, et al: Relation of angina pectoris to coronary artery disease in aortic valve stenosis. *Am J Cardiol* 55:1063-1065, 1985
27. Mark AL, Kioschos JM, Abboud FM, et al: Abnormal vascular responses to exercise in patients with aortic valve stenosis. *J Clin Invest* 52:1138-1146, 1973
28. Anderson MW: The clinical course of patients with calcific aortic stenosis. *Proc Staff Meet Mayo Clin* 36:439-444, 1961
29. Schattenberg TT, Titus JL, Parkin TW: Clinical findings in acquired aortic valvular stenosis: effect of disease of other valves. *Am Heart J* 73:322-325, 1967
30. Frank S, Johnson A, Ross J Jr: Natural history of valvular aortic stenosis. *Br Heart J* 35:41-46, 1973
31. Ross J Jr, Braunwald E: Aortic stenosis. *Circulation* 38 Suppl 5:61-67, 1968
32. Larsen VH, Jensen BS: Spontaneous progression of valvular aortic stenosis. *Dan Med Bull* 32:69-72, 1985
33. Ng ASH, Holmes DR Jr, Smith HC, et al: Hemodynamic progression of adult valvular aortic stenosis. *Cathet Cardiovasc Diagn* 12:145-150, 1986
34. Otto CM, Pearlman AS, Gardner CL: Hemodynamic progression of aortic stenosis in adults assessed by Doppler echocardiography. *J Am Coll Cardiol* 13:545-550, 1989
35. Cheitlin MD, Gertz EW, Brundage BH, et al: Rate of progression of severity of valvular aortic stenosis in the adult. *Am Heart J* 98:689-700, 1979
36. Agarwal AK: Aortic stenosis: Ddx and Tx of the elderly patient. *Geriatrics* 40:105-107; 110-112, February 1985
37. Selzer A, Lombard JT: Clinical findings in adult aortic stenosis—then and now. *Eur Heart J* 9 Suppl E:53-55, 1988
38. Braunwald E, Goldblatt A, Aygen MM, et al: Congenital aortic stenosis. I. Clinical and hemodynamic findings in 100 patients. *Circulation* 27:426-462, 1963
39. Roberts WC, Perloff JK, Costantino T: Severe valvular aortic stenosis in patients over 65 years of age. *Am J Cardiol* 27:497-506, 1971
40. Forker AD, McCallister BD, Giuliani ER, et al: Atypical presentations of patients with calcific aortic stenosis: patients with normal ECG and patients with associated systemic hypertension. *JAMA* 212:774-779, 1970
41. Andersen JA, Hansen BF, Lyngborg K: Isolated valvular aortic stenosis: clinico-pathological findings in an autopsy material of elderly patients. *Acta Med Scand* 197:61-64, 1975
42. Perloff JK: Clinical recognition of aortic stenosis: the physical signs and differential diagnosis of the various forms of obstruction to left ventricular outflow. *Prog Cardiovasc Dis* 10:323-352, 1968
43. Giuliani ER, Brandenburg RO, Fuster V: Evaluation of cardiac murmurs. *Cardiovasc Clin* 10 No 3:1-18, 1980
44. Tavel ME: *Clinical Phonocardiography and External Pulse Reading.* Second edition. Chicago, Year Book Medical Publishers, 1973
45. De Leon AC Jr, Harvey WP: Pharmacological agents and auscultation. *Mod Concepts Cardiovasc Dis* 44:23-28, 1975
46. Thompson R, Mitchell A, Ahmed M, et al: Conduction defects in aortic valve disease. *Am Heart J* 98:3-10, 1979
47. Lombard JT, Selzer A: Valvular aortic stenosis: a clinical and hemodynamic profile of patients. *Ann Intern Med* 106:292-298, 1987
48. Forssell G, Jonasson R, Nordlander R, et al: Electrocardiographic prediction of the severity of aortic valvular stenosis. *Acta Med Scand* 215:43-46, 1984
49. Almendral JM, García-Andoain JM, Sánchez-Cascos A, et al:

Treadmill stress testing in the evaluation of patients with valvular heart disease: possible role in the assessment of functional capacity and severity of the lesion. *Cardiology* 69:42-51, 1982

50. Chandramouli B, Ehmke DA, Lauer RM: Exercise-induced electrocardiographic changes in children with congenital aortic stenosis. *J Pediatr* 87:725-730, 1975

51. James FW, Schwartz DC, Kaplan S, et al: Exercise electrocardiogram, blood pressure, and working capacity in young patients with valvular or discrete subvalvular aortic stenosis. *Am J Cardiol* 50:769-775, 1982

52. Nylander E, Ekman I, Marklund T, et al: Severe aortic stenosis in elderly patients. *Br Heart J* 55:480-487, 1986

53. Yano K, Kuriya T, Hashiba K: Simultaneous monitoring of electrocardiogram and arterial blood pressure during exercise-induced syncope in a patient with severe aortic stenosis – a case report. *Angiology* 40:143-148, February 1989

54. Linderholm H, Osterman G, Teien D: Detection of coronary artery disease by means of exercise ECG in patients with aortic stenosis. *Acta Med Scand* 218:181-188, 1985

55. Exercise Testing Task Force members: Guidelines for exercise testing: A report of the American College of Cardiology/American Heart Association Task Force on Assessment of Cardiovascular Procedures (Subcommittee on Exercise Testing). *J Am Coll Cardiol* 8:725-738, 1986

56. Klatte EC, Tampas JP, Campbell JA, et al: The roentgenographic manifestations of aortic stenosis and aortic valvular insufficiency. *AJR* 88:57-69, 1962

57. Chang S, Clements S, Chang J: Aortic stenosis: echocardiographic cusp separation and surgical description of aortic valve in 22 patients. *Am J Cardiol* 39:499-504, 1977

58. DeMaria AN, Bommer W, Joye J, et al: Value and limitations of cross-sectional echocardiography of the aortic valve in the diagnosis and quantification of valvular aortic stenosis. *Circulation* 62:304-312, 1980

59. Godley RW, Green D, Dillon JC, et al: Reliability of two-dimensional echocardiography in assessing the severity of valvular aortic stenosis. *Chest* 79:657-662, 1981

60. Weyman AE, Feigenbaum H, Dillon JC, et al: Cross-sectional echocardiography in assessing the severity of valvular aortic stenosis. *Circulation* 52:828-834, 1975

61. Weyman AE, Feigenbaum H, Hurwitz RA, et al: Localization of left ventricular outflow obstruction by cross-sectional echocardiography. *Am J Med* 60:33-38, 1976

62. Wong M, Tei C, Sadler N, et al: Echocardiographic observations of calcium in operatively excised stenotic aortic valves. *Am J Cardiol* 59:324-329, 1987

63. Brandenburg RO Jr, Tajik AJ, Edwards WD, et al: Accuracy of 2-dimensional echocardiographic diagnosis of congenitally bicuspid aortic valve: echocardiographic-anatomic correlation in 115 patients. *Am J Cardiol* 51:1469-1473, 1983

64. Nanda NL, Gramiak R: Evaluation of bicuspid valves by two-dimensional echocardiography (abstract). *Am J Cardiol* 41:372, 1978

65. Schwartz A, Vignola PA, Walker HJ, et al: Echocardiographic estimation of aortic-valve gradient in aortic stenosis. *Ann Intern Med* 89:329-335, 1978

66. Oh JK, Taliercio CP, Holmes DR Jr, et al: Prediction of the severity of aortic stenosis by Doppler aortic valve area determination: prospective Doppler-catheterization correlation in 100 patients. *J Am Coll Cardiol* 11:1227-1234, 1988

67. Currie PJ, Seward JB, Reeder GS, et al: Continuous-wave Doppler echocardiographic assessment of severity of calcific aortic stenosis: a simultaneous Doppler-catheter correlative study in 100 adult patients. *Circulation* 71:1162-1169, 1985

68. Currie PJ, Hagler DJ, Seward JB, et al: Instantaneous pressure gradient: a simultaneous Doppler and dual catheter correlative study. *J Am Coll Cardiol* 7:800-806, 1986

69. Hegranaes L, Hatle L: Aortic stenosis in adults: non-invasive estimation of pressure differences by continuous wave Doppler echocardiography. *Br Heart J* 54:396-404, 1985

70. Hatle L, Angelsen BA, Tromsdal A: Non-invasive assessment of aortic stenosis by Doppler ultrasound. *Br Heart J* 43:284-292, 1980

71. Stamm RB, Martin RP: Quantification of pressure gradients across stenotic valves by Doppler ultrasound. *J Am Coll Cardiol* 2:707-718, 1983

72. Callahan MJ, Tajik AJ, Su-Fan Q, et al: Validation of instantaneous pressure gradients measured by continuous-wave Doppler in experimentally induced aortic stenosis. *Am J Cardiol* 56:989-993, 1985

73. Smith MD, Dawson PL, Elion JL, et al: Correlation of continuous wave Doppler velocities with cardiac catheterization gradients: an experimental model of aortic stenosis. *J Am Coll Cardiol* 6:1306-1314, 1985

74. Otto CM, Pearlman AS, Comess KA, et al: Determination of the stenotic aortic valve area in adults using Doppler echocardiography. *J Am Coll Cardiol* 7:509-517, 1986

75. Skjaerpe T, Hegrenaes L, Hatle L: Noninvasive estimation of valve area in patients with aortic stenosis by Doppler ultrasound and two-dimensional echocardiography. *Circulation* 72:810-818, 1985

76. Zoghbi WA, Farmer KL, Soto JG, et al: Accurate noninvasive quantification of stenotic aortic valve area by Doppler echocardiography. *Circulation* 73:452-459, 1986

77. O'Rourke RA: Preoperative cardiac catheterization: its need in most patients with valvular heart disease. *JAMA* 248:745-750, 1982

78. Fuster V, Brandenburg RO, Giuliani ER, et al: Clinical approach and management of acquired valvular heart disease. *Cardiovasc Clin* 10 No 3:125-159, 1980

79. St John Sutton MG, St John Sutton M, Oldershaw P, et al: Valve replacement without preoperative cardiac catheterization. *N Engl J Med* 305:1233-1238, 1981

80. Grossman W: Profiles in valvular heart disease. In *Cardiac Catheterization and Angiography.* Edited by W Grossman. Philadelphia, Lea & Febiger, 1986, pp 359-381

81. Herman MV, Cohn PF, Gorlin R: Resistance to blood flow by stenotic valves: calculation of orifice area. In *Cardiac Catheterization and Angiography.* Edited by W Grossman. Philadelphia, Lea & Febiger, 1980, pp 124-130

82. Carabello BA, Grossman W: Calculation of stenotic valve orifice area. In *Cardiac Catheterization and Angiography.* Edited by W Grossman. Philadelphia, Lea & Febiger, 1986, pp 143-154

83. Vandeplas A, Willems JL, Piessens J, et al: Frequency of angina pectoris and coronary artery disease in severe isolated valvular aortic stenosis. *Am J Cardiol* 62:117-120, 1988

84. Lewis RC, Creus AB: Angina pectoris and aortic valve disease. *Cardiovasc Clin* 7:169-172, 1975

85. Cooper G IV, Satava RM, Harrison CE, et al: Normal myocardial function and energetics after reversing pressure-overload hypertrophy. *Am J Physiol* 226:1158-1165, 1974

86. Cutilletta AF: Regression of myocardial hypertrophy: III. Alterations in left ventricular performance. *J Mol Cell Cardiol* 14:695-701, 1982

87. Kennedy JW, Doces J, Steward DK: Left ventricular function before and following aortic valve replacement. *Circulation* 56:944-950, 1977

88. Cody RJ Jr, Stephens DD, Walker HJ, et al: Early post-operative changes in left ventricular dimensions and mass following valve replacement in adults with aortic stenosis. *J Cardiovasc Surg* 22:19-27, 1981

89. Drost H: Aortic valve replacement in aortic stenosis and regression of left ventricular hypertrophy. In *Cardiac Left Ventricular Hypertrophy.* Edited by HEDJ ter Keurs, JJ Schipperheyn. Boston, Martinus Nijhoff Publishers, 1983, p. 267

90. Flemma RJ, Johnson WD, Lepley D Jr, et al: Simultaneous valve replacement and aorta-to-coronary saphenous vein bypass. *Ann Thorac Surg* 12:163-170, 1971

91. Geha AS, Francis CK, Hammond GL, et al: Combined valve replacement and myocardial revascularization. *J Vasc Surg* 1:27-35, 1984

92. Galvin I, Mosieri J, Paneth M, et al: An analysis of isolated aortic valve surgery and combined procedures in patients over 70 years of age. *J Cardiovasc Surg* 29:577-581, 1988

93. Lytle BW, Cosgrove DM, Goormastic M, et al: Aortic valve replacement and coronary bypass grafting for patients with aortic stenosis and coronary artery disease: early and late results. *Eur Heart J* 9 Suppl E:143-147, 1988

94. Iung B, Drissi MF, Michel P-L, et al: Prognosis of valve replacement for aortic stenosis with or without coexisting coronary heart disease: a comparitive study. *J Heart Valve Dis* 2:430-439, 1993

95. Nair CK, Sketch MH, Ahmed I, et al: Calcific valvular aortic stenosis with and without mitral anular calcium. *Am J Cardiol* 60:865-870, 1987

96. Michel PL, Vitoux B, Dermine P, et al: Mitral calcification in aortic stenosis. *Eur Heart J* 9 Suppl E:77-82, 1988

97. Johnson LW, Hapanowicz MB, Buonanno C, et al: Pulmonary hypertension in isolated aortic stenosis: hemodynamic correlations and follow-up. *J Thorac Cardiovasc Surg* 95:603-607, 1988

98. Buonanno C, Johnson LW, Bowser MA, et al: Pulmonary hypertension in severe aortic stenosis: incidence, mechanisms, clinical and surgical implications. *G Ital Cardiol* 17:636-641, 1987

99. Mehta PM, Heinsimer JA, Bryg RJ, et al: Reassessment of the association between gastrointestinal arteriovenous malformations and aortic stenosis. *Am J Med* 86:275-277, 1989

100. Apostolakis E, Doering C, Kantartzis M, et al: Calcific aortic-valve stenosis and angiodysplasia of the colon: Heyde's syndrome—report of two cases. *Thorac Cardiovasc Surg* 38:374-376, 1990

101. King RM, Pluth JR, Giuliani ER: The association of unexplained gastrointestinal bleeding with calcific aortic stenosis. *Ann Thorac Surg* 44:514-516, 1987

102. Barnhorst DA, Oxman HA, Connolly DC, et al: Isolated replacement of the aortic valve with the Starr-Edwards prosthesis: a 9 year review. *J Thorac Cardiovasc Surg* 70:113-118, 1975

103. Turina J, Hess O, Sepulcri F, et al: Spontaneous course of aortic disease. *Eur Heart J* 8:471-483, 1987

104. Chizner MA, Pearle DL, deLeon AC Jr: The natural history of aortic stenosis in adults. *Am Heart J* 99:419-424, 1980

105. Dry TJ, Willius FA: Calcareous disease of the aortic valve: study of 228 cases. *Am Heart J* 17:138-157, 1939

106. Kelly TA, Rothbart RM, Cooper CM, et al: Comparison of outcome of asymptomatic to symptomatic patients older than 20 years of age with valvular aortic stenosis. *Am J Cardiol* 61:123-130, 1988

107. Pellikka PA, Nishimura RA, Bailey KR, et al: The natural history of adults with asymptomatic, hemodynamically significant aortic stenosis. *J Am Coll Cardiol* 15:1012-1017, 1990

108. Krayenbuehl HP, Hess OM, Monrad ES, et al: Left ventricular myocardial structure in aortic valve disease before, intermediate, and late after aortic valve replacement. *Circulation* 79:744-755, 1989

109. Harpole DH, Jones RH: Serial assessment of ventricular performance after valve replacement for aortic stenosis. *J Thorac Cardiovasc Surg* 99:645-650, 1990

110. Nakano S, Taniguchi K, Kawamoto T, et al: Postoperative reversibility of left ventricular hypertrophy and myocardial function in aortic valvular disease. *Jpn Circ J* 54:563-567, 1990

111. Committee on Prevention of Rheumatic Fever and Bacterial Endocarditis of the American Heart Association: Prevention of rheumatic fever. *Circulation* 55:1-4, 1977

112. Roberts WC, Virmani R: Aschoff bodies *at necropsy* in valvular heart disease: evidence from an analysis of 543 patients over 14 years of age that rheumatic heart disease, at least anatomically, is a disease of the mitral valve. *Circulation* 57:803-807, 1978

113. Edwards WD, Peterson K, Edwards JE: Active valvulitis associated with chronic rheumatic valvular disease and active myocarditis. *Circulation* 57:181-185, 1978

114. Rahimtoola SH, Chandraratna PAN: Valvular heart disease. In *Clinical Medicine.* Vol 6, Chap 15. Edited by JA Spittell Jr. Philadelphia, Harper & Row, Publishers, 1983, pp 1-51

115. Cribier A, Saoudi N, Berland J, et al: Percutaneous transluminal valvuloplasty of acquired aortic stenosis in elderly patients: an alternative to valve replacement? *Lancet* 1:63-67, 1986

116. Safian RD, Berman AD, Diver DJ, et al: Balloon aortic valvuloplasty in 170 consecutive patients. *N Engl J Med* 319:125-130, 1988

117. Litvack F, Jakubowski AT, Buchbinder NA, et al: Lack of sustained clinical improvement in an elderly population after percutaneous aortic valvuloplasty. *Am J Cardiol* 62:270-275, 1988

118. Nishimura RA, Holmes DR Jr, Reeder GS, et al: Doppler evaluation of results of percutaneous aortic balloon valvuloplasty in calcific aortic stenosis. *Circulation* 78:791-799, 1988

119. Craver JM, Goldstein J, Jones EL, et al: Clinical, hemodynamic, and operative descriptors affecting outcome of aortic valve replacement in elderly versus young patients. *Ann Surg* 199:733-740, 1984

120. Barnhorst DA, Giuliani ER, Pluth JR, et al: Open-heart surgery in patients more than 65 years old. *Ann Thorac Surg* 18:81-88, 1974

121. Magovern JA, Pennock JL, Campbell DB, et al: Aortic valve replacement and combined aortic valve replacement and coronary artery bypass grafting: predicting high risk groups. *J Am Coll Cardiol* 9:38-43, 1987

122. Edmunds LH Jr, Stephenson LW, Edie RN, et al: Open-heart surgery in octogenarians. *N Engl J Med* 319:131-136, 1988

123. O'Keefe JH Jr, Vlietstra RE, Bailey KR, et al: Natural history of candidates for balloon aortic valvuloplasty. *Mayo Clin Proc* 62:986-991, 1987

124. Brady ST, Davis CA, Kussmaul WC, et al: Percutaneous aortic balloon valvuloplasty in octogenarians: morbidity and mortality. *Ann Intern Med* 110:761-766, 1989

125. King RM, Pluth JR, Giuliani ER, et al: Mechanical decalcification of the aortic valve. *Ann Thorac Surg* 42:269-272, 1986

126. Roth RB, Palacios IF, Block PC: Percutaneous aortic balloon valvuloplasty: its role in the management of patients with aortic stenosis requiring major noncardiac surgery. *J Am Coll Cardiol* 13:1039-1041, 1989

127. O'Keefe JH Jr, Shub C, Rettke SR: Risk of noncardiac surgical procedures in patients with aortic stenosis. *Mayo Clin Proc* 64:400-405, 1989

128. Sheppard BB, Milliken JC, Nelson RJ, et al: Ultrasonic decalcification of the aortic annulus during aortic valve replacement. *Ann Thorac Surg* 52:59-65, 1991

129. Scott WC, Miller DC, Haverich A, et al: Determinants of operative mortality for patients undergoing aortic valve replacement. Discriminant analysis of 1,479 operations. *J Thorac Cardiovasc Surg* 89:400-413, 1985

130. Cohn LH, Allred EN, DiSesa VJ, et al: Early and late risk of aortic valve replacement: a 12 year concomitant comparison of the porcine bioprosthetic and tilting disc prosthetic aortic valves. *J Thorac Cardiovasc Surg* 88:695-705, 1984

131. McGoon DC: Valve replacement: a comparative analysis of long-term results. In *Cardiovascular Medicine.* Vol 1. Edited by JHK Vogel. New York, Raven Press, 1982, pp 277-284

132. Murphy DA, Levine FH, Buckley MJ, et al: Mechanical valves: a comparative analysis of the Starr-Edwards and Björk-Shiley prostheses. *J Thorac Cardiovasc Surg* 86:746-752, 1983

133. Zussa C, Ottino G, di Summa M, et al: Porcine cardiac bioprostheses: evaluation of long-term results in 990 patients. *Ann Thorac Surg* 39:243-250, 1985

134. Chaux A, Czer LSC, Matloff JM, et al: The St. Jude Medical bileaflet valve prosthesis: a 5 year experience. *J Thorac Cardiovasc Surg* 88:706-717, 1984

135. Baudet EM, Oca CC, Roques XF, et al: A 5½ year experience of the St. Jude Medical cardiac valve prosthesis. *J Thorac Cardiovasc Surg* 90:137-144, 1985

136. Brais MP, Bédard JP, Goldstein W, et al: Ionescu-Shiley pericardial xenografts: follow-up of up to 6 years. *Ann Thorac Surg* 39:105-111, 1985

137. Smith N, McAnulty JH, Rahimtoola SH: Severe aortic stenosis with impaired left ventricular function and clinical heart failure: results of a valve replacement. *Circulation* 58:255-264, 1978

138. Goldman L, Caldera DL, Nussbaum SR, et al: Multifactorial index of cardiac risk in noncardiac surgical procedures. *N Engl J Med* 297:845-850, 1977

139. Rahimtoola SH: Catheter balloon valvuloplasty of aortic and mitral stenosis in adults: 1987. *Circulation* 75:895-901, 1987

140. Hayes SN, Holmes DR Jr, Nishimura RA, et al: Palliative percutaneous aortic balloon valvuloplasty before noncardiac operations and invasive diagnostic procedures. *Mayo Clin Proc* 64:753-757, 1989

CHAPTER

33

Aortic regurgitation

Michael D. McGoon, M.D., Valentin Fuster, M.D., Clarence Shub, M.D., and Hartzell V. Schaff, M.D.

ANATOMIC CONSIDERATIONS

Diastolic regurgitation of blood from the aorta to the left ventricle through an incompetent aortic valve has various causes, which may be grouped into two general anatomic categories: those associated with intrinsic abnormalities of the aortic valvular apparatus, and those related to disease of the aortic root. Both anatomic abnormalities can present as a chronic variety, frequently progressive, or as an acute or a subacute variety (Table 33-1 and Fig 33-1).

Intrinsic valvular disease

Rheumatic. Rheumatic fever may cause mild aortic incompetence during the first episode, which may become hemodynamically and symptomatically significant years later. In operatively excised aortic valves having pure regurgitation, rheumatic disease is the most frequent cause. Rheumatic endocarditis leads to fibrosis, shortening, and contracture of the valve cusps, which results in malalignment (Fig 33-2). Inability of the cusps to coapt adequately, as a consequence of retraction, permits a regurgitant stream to flow during left ventricular relaxation. Impingement of the regurgitant jet upon the endocardium may produce a characteristic jet lesion on the left ventricular outflow tract. Documented rheumatic endocarditis only rarely causes pure isolated aortic regurgitation; usually, there is associated aortic stenosis due to cusp fusion or associated mitral valve disease or both.

Congenital. A common congenital cause of chronic aortic regurgitation in adults is bicuspid aortic valve (Fig 33-3). In most cases, the anterior cusp is larger and redundant, resulting in diastolic prolapse of the cusp into the left ventricle and chronic, progressive aortic regurgitation. Hypertension can favor this process. Thus, in cases of coarctation of the aorta, for example, the high incidence of an aortic bicuspid valve and hypertension explains the commonly associated aortic regurgitation in this condition. Uncommonly, rupture of a raphe strand in the bicuspid valve may produce an incompetent valve.

Degenerative myxomatous changes of the aortic valve may also be considered a congenital predisposition to development of chronic aortic regurgitation. Although occasionally associated with cystic medial necrosis of the aortic root, regurgitation may occur as a result of cusp prolapse alone.

Cusp fenestration is not a rare congenital anatomic anomaly but seldom produces clinically significant aortic regurgitation.

As discussed in chapter 41, ventricular septal defects, particularly those in a supracristal location, may be associated with chronic and progressively severe aortic regurgitation. This is likely due to weakening of the neighboring supporting aortic annulus, leading to malalignment of the valve cusps. A similar mechanism may account for the high incidence (about 65%) of aortic regurgitation, usually of trivial to moderate degree, occurring in patients with hypertrophic cardiomyopathy after ventricular myotomy and myectomy.[1]

Another condition that may cause aortic regurgitation is an aortico-left ventricular tunnel bypassing the aortic

Table 33-1 Aortic valvular regurgitation: clinical presentation in various anatomic and clinical types

Primary anatomic abnormality	Clinical presentation: Chronic	Clinical presentation: Acute or subacute
Intrinsic valvular disease	Rheumatic Bicuspid valve Myxomatous valve (prolapse) Associated congenital heart disease	Infective endocarditis Traumatic rupture Spontaneous prolapse
Disease of the ascending aorta	Marfan's syndrome Idiopathic Senile Chronic aortitis Syphilitic Connective tissue	Aortic dissection Acute aortitis (infective endocarditis) Chest trauma

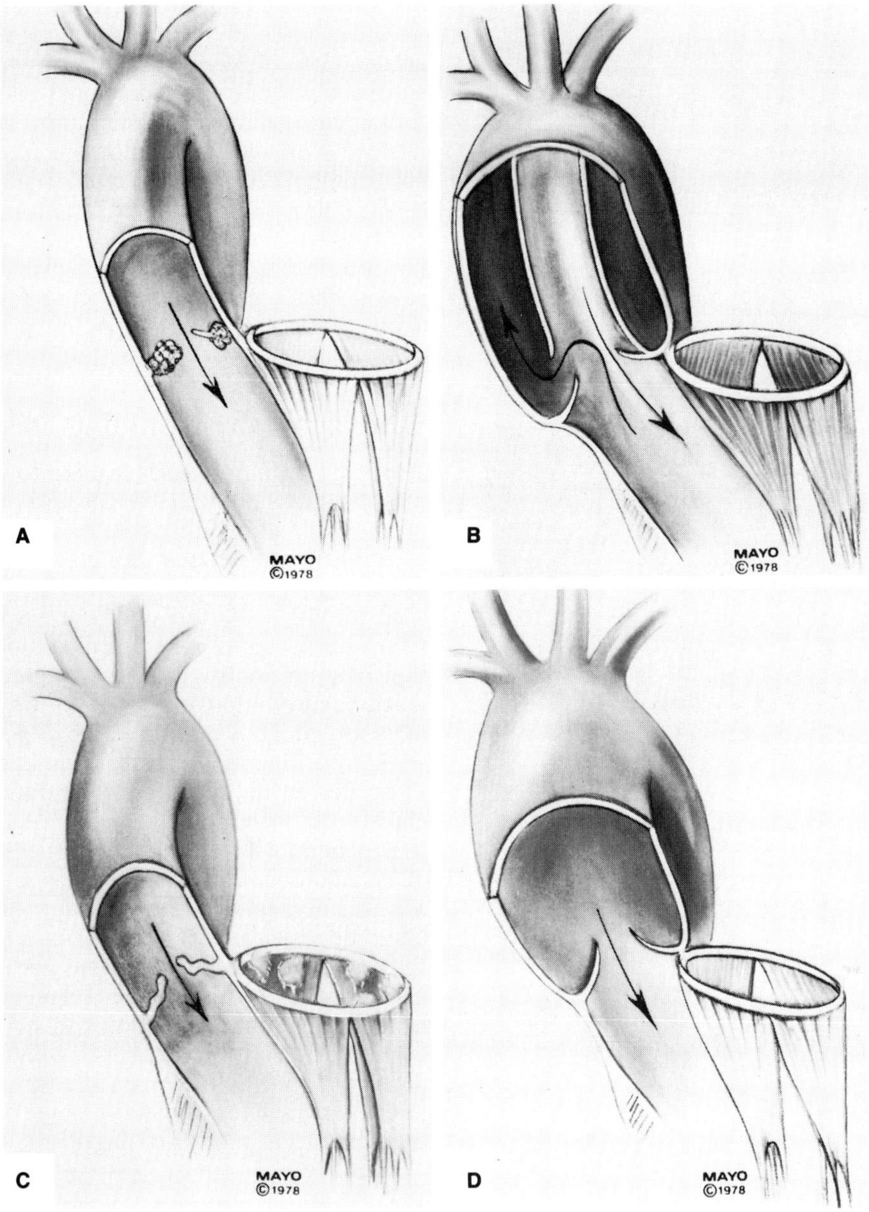

Fig 33-1 Types of aortic regurgitation. **A,** acute bacterial endocarditis. **B,** acute aortic dissection. **C,** chronic rheumatic valve disease with aortic regurgitation and mitral valve disease. **D,** chronic dilatation of the aortic root. (From Fuster V, Brandenburg RO, Giuliani ER, et al: Clinical approach and management of acquired valvular heart disease. *Cardiovasc Clin* 10 No 3:125-159, 1980. By permission, Mayo Foundation.)

valve just outside the annulus; this disorder can be either congenital or acquired secondary to infective endocarditis.

Infective endocarditis. Acute or subacute infection of the aortic valve usually involves a previously abnormal valvular apparatus, most commonly a congenitally bicuspid valve or a tricuspid aortic valve affected by rheumatic disease. Usually, acute or subacute valvular regurgitation is due to tissue destruction (Fig 33-4) – either of the cusps, leading to perforation, or of the cusp attachments, leading to prolapse. Infrequently, regurgitation results from the interposition of a vegetation between cusps that prevents complete closure. Rarely, bacterial invasion of perivalvular tissue may lead to an aortico-left ventricular tunnel that bypasses the aortic valve outside the annulus. The progression of hemodynamic deterioration and symptoms in infective endocarditis of the aortic valve depends largely on the rapidity and extent of valve destruction. Because of contracture of the healing cusps, regurgitation may progress even after the infection is cured (Fig 33-5).

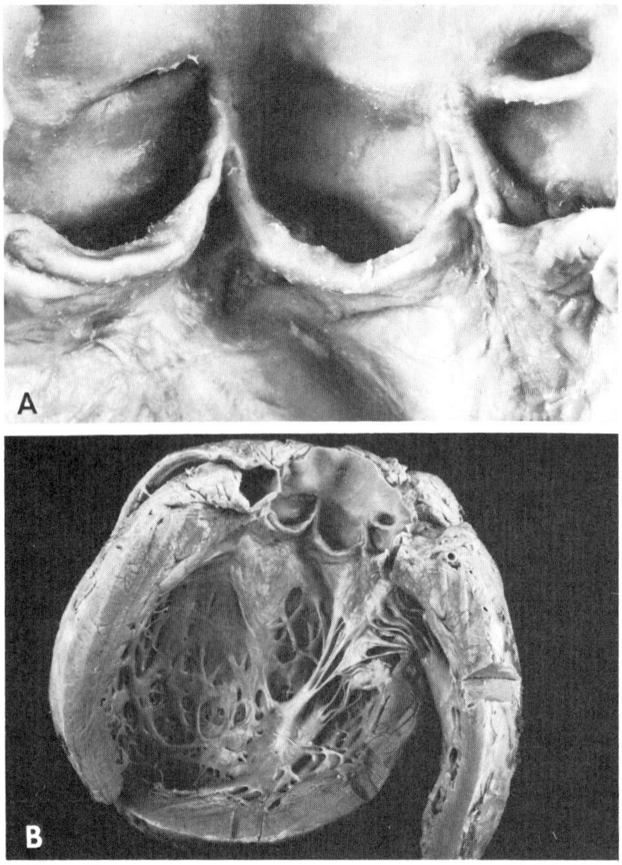

Fig 33-2 **A,** rheumatic aortic regurgitation due to scar retraction of cusps. (Courtesy of William D. Edwards, M.D.) **B,** rheumatic aortic regurgitation due to scar retraction of cusps without commissural fusion. Note the marked left ventricular dilatation and the subaortic regurgitant jet lesions. (Courtesy of William D. Edwards, M.D.)

Collagen disease. Aortic regurgitation associated with systemic lupus erythematosus may occur as a result of attenuation of valve tissue with secondary acute or subacute perforation. Occasional patients with rheumatoid arthritis have granulomas, fibrosis, and calcification usually involving the aortic root (see "Diseases of the Ascending Aorta," below) and valvular supporting structures or, less often, the cusps themselves.

Trauma. Penetrating or blunt chest trauma may produce laceration of the aortic valve structures. Rarely, severe straining may lead to cusp rupture and result in acute aortic regurgitation. Acute prolapse of an aortic cusp is rare.

Diseases of the ascending aorta

Aortic root abnormalities leading to valve incompetence may be grouped into two general categories: chronic primary dilatation and acute or subacute disruption.

Primary dilatation. Dilatation of the aortic root causes regurgitation by stretching and bowing of the valve cusps, relative shortening of the cusps, and widening of the commissures (Fig 33-6). Idiopathic aortic root dilatation may be one of the most common single causes of aortic regurgitation, especially in the elderly, accounting for approximately 30% of cases in one series.[2]

Various disease processes have been implicated in or associated with aortic root dilatation. These include (1) Marfan's syndrome, which in about 80% of patients is associated with progressive aortic dilatation as a result of cystic medial necrosis (the elastic fibers of the media are fragmented and the resulting clefts are filled with cystic deposits of metachromatic-staining mucoid material); (2) progressive idiopathic aortic dilatation, which also appears to result from changes of cystic medial necrosis; (3) senile dilatation and annuloaortic ectasia or aortitis of unknown cause; (4) syphilitic aortitis,[3] which develops about 15 to 25 years after the initial infection and is now rare; and (5) connective tissue disorders in the form of rheumatoid arthritis or ankylosing spondylitis, Reiter's

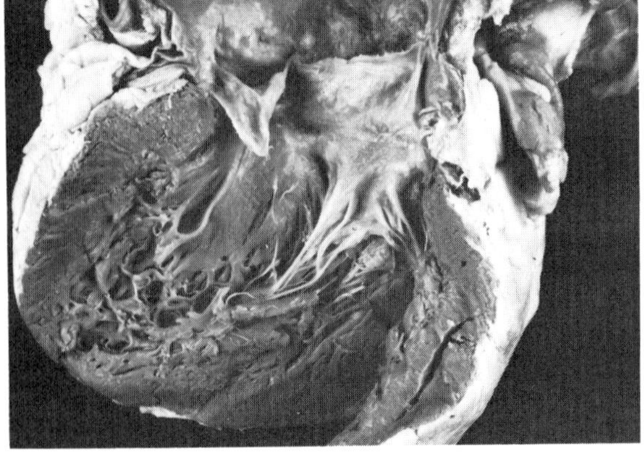

Fig 33-3 Aortic regurgitation due to prolapse of congenitally bicuspid aortic valve. (Courtesy of William D. Edwards, M.D.)

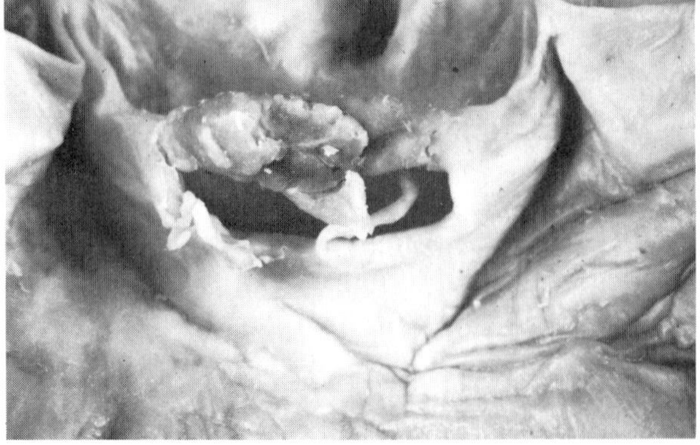

Fig 33-4 Aortic regurgitation due to active infective endocarditis with cuspid perforation. (Courtesy of William D. Edwards, M.D.)

syndrome, relapsing polychondritis, giant cell arteritis, osteogenesis imperfecta, and Whipple's disease.

In addition to affecting the aortic root and aortic valve annulus, the first two disease processes, as well as some of the connective tissue disorders, often involve the aortic and mitral leaflets.

Disruption. Acute or subacute destruction of the integrity of the aortic root may lead to disruption of the supporting structures of the valve, resulting in aortic regurgitation (see Fig 33-1). This occurs as laceration or dissection and consists of a longitudinal cleavage of the aortic media by a dissecting column of blood that usually does not completely encircle the lumen but tends to progress toward the aortic arch and descending aorta.

Usually the dissection occurs in patients with idiopathic dilatation of the ascending aorta, hypertension, or Marfan's syndrome, and it is less often associated with pregnancy; rarely it can result from blunt chest trauma or from acute aortitis complicating aortic valve infective endocarditis. It is thought by some that in Marfan's syndrome or in idiopathic dilatation of the ascending aorta, cystic medial necrosis weakens the aortic wall, resulting in hemorrhage from the vasa vasorum and perhaps secondary tearing of the intima. Others think that the intimal tear, perhaps favored by the hypertension commonly found in these patients, allows the intraluminal blood to dissect into the weakened aortic media, leading to the dissecting hematomas (see also chapter 58A).

Aortic regurgitation occurs in about 30% of cases of dissection of the aortic root; it develops as a result of one or a combination of secondary retraction of the cusp leading to poor alignment for closure, prolapse of a cusp, or extension of the medial tear into the cusp itself, leading to rupture.[4,5]

PATHOPHYSIOLOGY

Chronic aortic regurgitation (Fig 33-7)

The diastolic return of blood retrogradely into the left ventricle results in a large total systolic stroke volume in order to maintain effective forward cardiac output. At rest, effective stroke volume is maintained according to Starling's law: there is ejection of the increased left ventricular end-diastolic volume (which results from the diastolic regurgitation), with concomitant increase in total stroke volume and ejection fraction. Eccentric left ventricular hypertrophy also contributes to the increase in left ventricular performance. Left ventricular dilatation leads to myocardial fiber stretching and elongation. Chamber enlargement alone would lead to an increased wall stress at any given intraventricular pressure. However, sarcomere replication and hypertrophic thickening tend to normalize wall stress as described by the law of Laplace ($\sigma = \frac{Pa}{2h}$, in which σ is circumferential wall stress, P is intraventricular pressure, a is intraventricular radius, and h is wall thickness). Ventricular hypertrophy increases proportionately with radius, so that the ratio of wall thickness to cavity radius remains essentially normal.[6] In extremely dilated hearts (cor bovinum), total left ventricular mass may be markedly increased to more than a kilogram.

Because significant cardiac compensation is related to an increased ejection fraction, a "normal" ejection fraction suggests inadequate compensation in response to the regurgitant lesion.[7] In patients with advanced ventricular enlargement (greater than 150 mL/m^2), preload reserve is exhausted and no further compensation can occur.[8] Decreased ejection fraction leads to increased end-systolic volume, which, in turn, appears to be one of the most sensitive indices of myocardial dysfunction.[9] Ultimately, markedly increased left ventricular diastolic volume leads to high diastolic pressures;[10] increased left ventricular end-diastolic pressure thus is also a sign of decompensation.

The exertion-induced decrease in systemic vascular resistance and acceleration of heart rate that decreases the duration of diastole both decrease regurgitation.[11-13] Concomitant elevation of left ventricular diastolic pres-

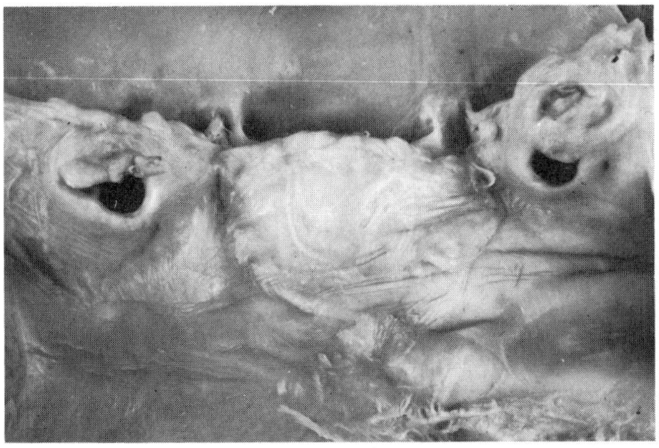

Fig 33-5 Aortic regurgitation due to healed infective endocarditis with cuspid perforations. (Courtesy of William D. Edwards, M.D.)

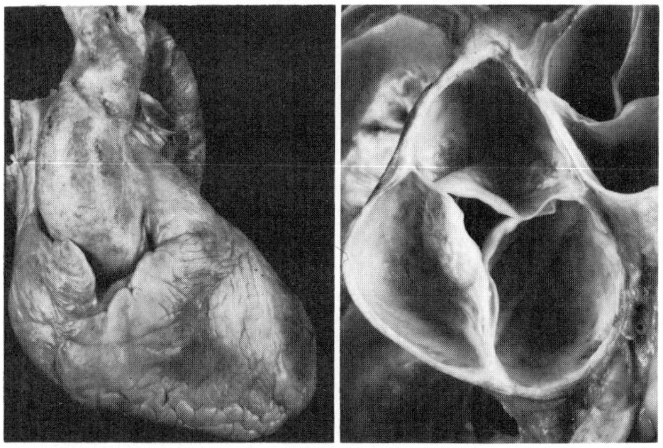

Fig 33-6 Aortic regurgitation due to idiopathic aortic root dilatation in an elderly man. Any disease process (such as aortitis or Marfan's syndrome) associated with dilatation of the ascending aorta potentially may produce aortic regurgitation. (Courtesy of William D. Edwards, M.D.)

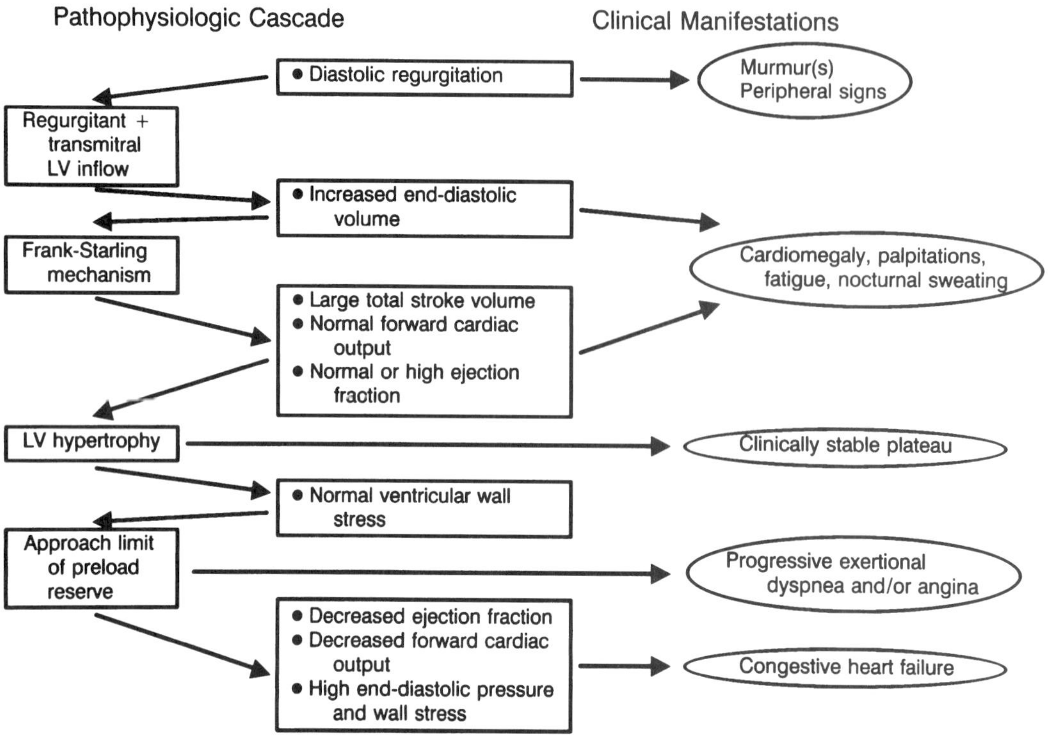

Fig 33-7 Pathophysiology of aortic regurgitation. *LV,* left ventricular.

sure may also contribute to this effect.[14] Regurgitant flow per beat is diminished at higher heart rates, while antegrade flow of blood across the mitral valve is maintained (at heart rates up to 150 beats/min). Despite a relative decrease in regurgitant flow during exercise, the increased venous return and left ventricular volume may lead to decompensation, with a decrease in exertional ejection fraction, stroke volume, and relative cardiac output.[9,15-18] This decrease in cardiac output may lead to exertional fatigability; the increases in left ventricular end-diastolic volume and pressure lead to pulmonary venous congestion with exertional dyspnea. Evidence suggests that an elevated pulmonary artery wedge pressure during exercise is correlated with lower rest and exercise ejection fractions.[19] Deterioration of ejection fraction with exercise cannot be predicted accurately in these patients by clinical parameters, including symptomatic status, heart size, and left ventricular hypertrophy, or by the ejection fraction measured at rest,[20,21] which may still be increased or normal in early decompensation. An abnormal response of the ejection fraction to exercise may antedate the development of symptoms; thus, evaluation of left ventricular exercise reserve by radionuclide ventriculography may uncover an abnormal contractile state in an asymptomatic patient.[22,23] Conversely, depressed ventricular function at rest does not preclude a normal ejection fraction with exercise.[24] The prognostic and therapeutic implications of such an observation, however, have not been established.[25] The left ventricular response to other stimuli (such as isometric exercise or vasopressor administration) may reveal indices of early left ventricular dysfunction.[26-28]

In addition to resting and exertional abnormalities of global ventricular function, patients with symptomatic left ventricular failure exhibit regional dysfunction, predominantly of the anterior, inferior, and septal segments.[29]

Diastolic function of the left ventricle also appears to be altered in patients with chronic volume overload and hypertrophy due to aortic regurgitation.[8,30,31] Abnormal early diastolic filling has been noted, and although the myocardium appears to relax normally in these hypertrophic hearts, the speed of diastolic relaxation of the entire ventricle is impaired.

Patients with chronic aortic regurgitation and normal coronary arteries occasionally experience anginal symptoms. The ratio of coronary blood flow to myocardial oxygen demand is adversely affected by aortic regurgitation in several ways. Increased left ventricular myocardial mass and, in advanced cases, increased wall tension augment total myocardial oxygen consumption. In addition, increased wall tension decreases the subendocardial perfusion gradient by exerting extravascular compression on intramyocardial coronary arterioles. Coronary blood flow, which occurs predominantly during diastole, is also decreased by the lower diastolic aortic pressure caused by the regurgitant valvular lesion. Finally, coronary arteriolar vasodilatory reserve is diminished in patients with chronic aortic regurgitation.[32]

Acute or subacute aortic regurgitation

When acutely developing aortic regurgitation is severe, dyspnea occurs due to the increases in left ventricular end-diastolic and pulmonary venous pressures which result from the abrupt regurgitation of a large volume of blood into a noncompliant left ventricle. With advanced left ventricular failure, the high left ventricular end-diastolic pressure tends to minimize the peripheral signs of aortic regurgitation and makes the diastolic murmur short, soft, and occasionally inaudible, thus obscuring the diagnosis; the increased heart rate and short diastole also may minimize the murmur. Because left ventricular dilatation and hypertrophy do not occur acutely, cardiac size on chest radiographs may be normal, except for a wide mediastinum if there is aortic dissection. For similar reasons the electrocardiogram (ECG) may remain unchanged.

CLINICAL SYNDROME

Salient aspects of clinical diagnoses and estimation of severity are summarized in Table 33-2.

History and clinical course

The course of aortic regurgitation (Fig 33-8) ranges from a trivial and slowly progressing regurgitation secondary to rheumatic fever to the severe, acute aortic regurgitation associated with infective endocarditis.

Chronic aortic regurgitation. A diastolic murmur may occur with the onset of rheumatic fever. The degree of regurgitation may be minimal, and longevity may not be affected, barring complicating events such as infective endocarditis. More often, after a period of about 10 years during which the only sign is a diastolic murmur, the aortic regurgitation becomes hemodynamically significant. Except for awareness of overactivity of the heart and neck vessels, this condition usually is well tolerated for periods ranging from 10 to 30 years. Ultimately, significant symptoms of left ventricular failure appear, consisting of exertional and episodic nocturnal dyspnea followed by progressive deterioration over 1 to 10 years. Angina pectoris is an infrequent and late event, occurring in about 20% of patients.[33] Finally, a late symptom is excessive perspiration, perhaps related to modifications of the autonomic nervous system. Whereas postural lightheadedness is often described in these patients, frank syncope is uncommon. In patients with Marfan's syndrome, dilatation of the aortic root is usually progressive, particularly during adolescence and early adulthood; in these instances, acute aortic dissection is a greater threat than the development of severe aortic regurgitation.

In patients with chronic aortic regurgitation, longevity is correlated roughly with degree of regurgitation and development of symptoms. If regurgitation is minimal, symptoms may never develop and longevity may not be shortened. Patients with mild to moderate degrees of regurgitation have a 10-year mortality rate of 5% to 15%, whereas those with "free" aortic regurgitation have a 10-year mortality rate of 30% and a 20-year mortality rate of greater than 50%.[34-36] The development of symptoms correlates with a poorer mortality rate: 50% of patients with free aortic regurgitation and angina are dead in 5 years, and nearly 50% of those with severe left ventricular failure are dead in 2 years.[35,37] Experience at the Mayo Clinic with patients in New York Heart Association functional class III or IV also suggests a poor prognosis: after 10 years, 96% of patients in class III or IV had died.[38] Spagnuolo et al.[39] found that 87% of high-risk patients (those with systolic blood pressure more than 140 mm Hg and diastolic blood pressure less than 40 mm Hg, left ventricular strain on the ECG, and moderate or marked cardiomegaly) experienced severe heart failure, angina, or death within 6 years, whereas only 8% of those without any risk factor had similar outcomes.

Table 33-2 Aortic regurgitation—clinical diagnosis and estimation of severity

	Mild*	Significant
Peripheral signs		
Diastolic blood pressure, mm Hg	>60	≤60
Capillary pulsation	−	+
Dynamic pulse and apex	−	+
Auscultation		
Diastolic murmur		
Duration	Short	Long
Intensity	Grade I	≥Grade II
Austin Flint murmur	−	+
Apical S_3	−	+
Cardiac size	Normal	Abnormal
Left ventricular hypertrophy	−	±

*Signs may be misinterpreted as mild when left ventricular end-diastolic pressure is high (e.g., acute and subacute forms).

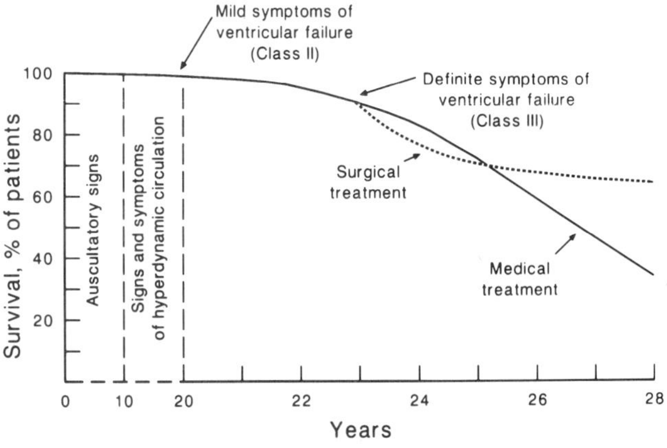

Fig 33-8 Scheme of clinical presentation and natural history of chronic aortic regurgitation.

Acute or subacute aortic regurgitation. Abrupt onset of aortic regurgitation is usually secondary to infective endocarditis or aortic dissection. Under these circumstances, the manifestations of the underlying disease generally predominate. When the acute aortic regurgitation is severe, compensatory mechanisms such as ventricular dilatation and hypertrophy are unable to develop, and symptoms occur due to the abrupt onset of regurgitant flow into a noncompliant chamber. Consequently, the high left ventricular end-diastolic pressure and pulmonary venous pressure produce significant dyspnea. The clinical course depends on the underlying disease, and this is discussed with aortic dissection (chapter 58A).

Physical findings

Careful evaluation in the office or at the bedside is essential for establishing the diagnosis of aortic regurgitation. This evaluation usually provides an estimation of the hemodynamic status of the patient and the etiologic basis of the lesion (Table 33-3).

Electrocardiogram

The ECG may be entirely normal in patients with chronic mild aortic regurgitation or with acute or subacute aortic regurgitation. Features of left ventricular hypertrophy are usually present in chronic moderate aortic regurgitation (Fig 33-9) but may be absent. The presence of a "strain"

Table 33-3 Physical findings in aortic regurgitation

Parameter	Sign	Description
General inspection of patient	de Musset's sign	Head nodding
	Müller's sign	Bobbing uvula
	Quincke's sign	Pulsatile blanching and flushing of nail bed with gentle pressure
Arterial pulse	Widened pulse pressure	Hemodynamically severe if >100 mm Hg. Not accurate in young patients with compliant vessels or in patients with acute aortic regurgitation
	Corrigan's "water-hammer" pulse	Sharp systolic upstroke and diastolic collapse of pulse
	Traube's sign	"Pistol shot" sound when femoral artery is auscultated
	Duroziez's sign	Biphasic femoral bruit during auscultation with gentle pressure
	Hill's sign	Systolic pressure in legs exceeding that in arms
Jugular venous pulse	Usually normal	Elevated if dilated aorta compresses superior vena cava
	"a" wave	Elevated if pulmonary hypertension develops
Precordial palpation	Apical impulse	Diffuse, hyperdynamic, displaced inferiorly and leftward. Double diastolic impulse in severe aortic regurgitation
	Base	Systolic thrill due to high flow. Diastolic thrill rarely present—suggests severe aortic regurgitation
Auscultation	First heart sound	Normal or decreased
	Systolic click	Early systolic click may be present before left ventricular decompensation occurs
	Second heart sound	Usually normal; occasionally decreased, absent, or paradoxically split. P_2 increased if pulmonary hypertension has developed
	Third heart sound	May be present even without left ventricular dysfunction, because of rapid early diastolic filling
	Diastolic murmur	High-pitched, blowing decrescendo murmur best heard at mid-low left sternal border. Loudest on right if aortic root is dilated. Duration rather than intensity correlates with severity. Intensity and duration are reduced by amyl nitrite. "Cooing" suggests cusp fenestration, perforation, eversion, or laceration
	Austin Flint murmur	Mid-diastolic or presystolic diastolic murmur best heard at apex is due to transmitral turbulence as mitral valve begins closing early
	Systolic murmur	Aortic ejection murmur due to high flow or concomitant stenotic disease. Holosystolic murmur may indicate mitral regurgitation due to left ventricular dysfunction

pattern of repolarization abnormality implies severe chronic aortic regurgitation: left ventricular enlargement, hypertrophy, elevated wall stress, and reduced fractional shortening.[40]

Among symptomatic patients with isolated aortic regurgitation at the Mayo Clinic, 22% had atrial fibrillation. In the absence of mitral valve disease, the presence of this rhythm may predict a relatively poor prognosis. Atrioventricular conduction delay is frequently noted late in the course of the disease.

Chest radiograph

As the severity of aortic regurgitation increases, dilation and enlargement of the left ventricle are more apparent (Fig 33-10). The apex is displaced laterally, inferiorly (seen below the diaphragmatic level), and somewhat posteriorly.

In aortic regurgitation the ascending aorta may be slightly dilated, but it may be very prominent in patients with coexisting aortic stenosis, in patients with primary dilatation of the aortic root, and in patients with acute dissection.

Left atrial enlargement indicates associated mitral valve disease or substantial left ventricular failure. Calcification of the aortic valve in pure aortic regurgitation is unusual; when present, coexisting aortic stenosis must be considered.

Echocardiography

Structural abnormalities of the aortic valve and distortions of the aortic annulus and root that lead to the aortic regurgitation often can be recognized. In cases of combined aortic valve stenosis and regurgitation echocardiographically, the aortic valve abnormality is readily apparent (see section on aortic stenosis). In infective endocarditis, aortic valve vegetations may be detected. Aneurysm or dissection of the ascending aorta may be evident (Fig 33-11).

Transesophageal echocardiography permits imaging of the ascending and descending thoracic aorta in almost all

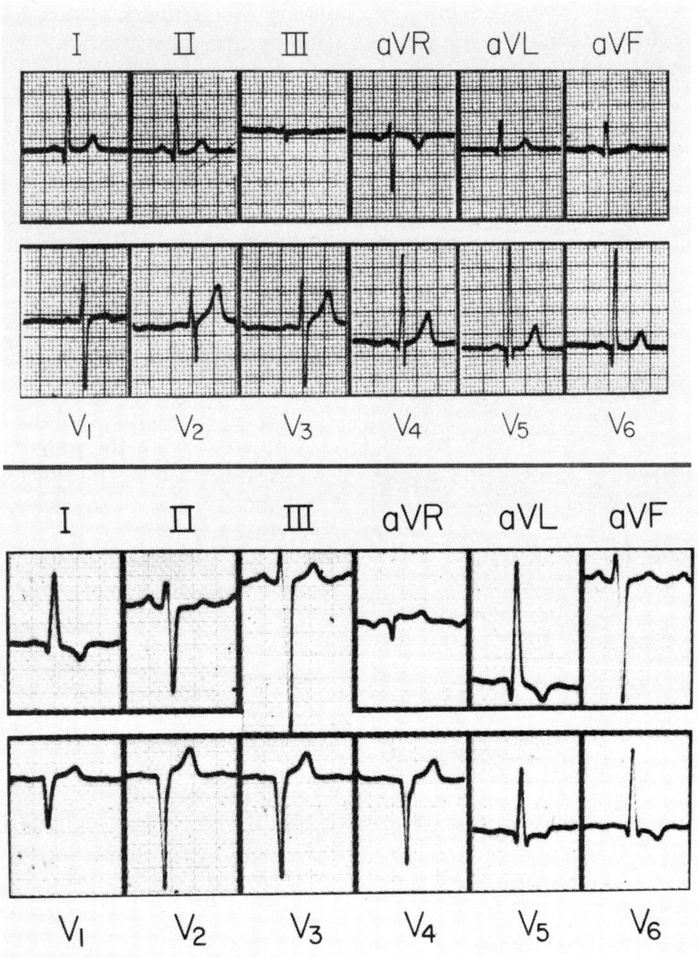

Fig 33-9 Electrocardiogram in chronic aortic regurgitation. **Upper,** pattern of left ventricular volume overload with prominent R, Q, and T waves in the left precordial leads. **Lower,** pattern of left ventricular hypertrophy with prominent R wave and ST-T changes in the left precordial leads and deep S wave in the right precordial leads.

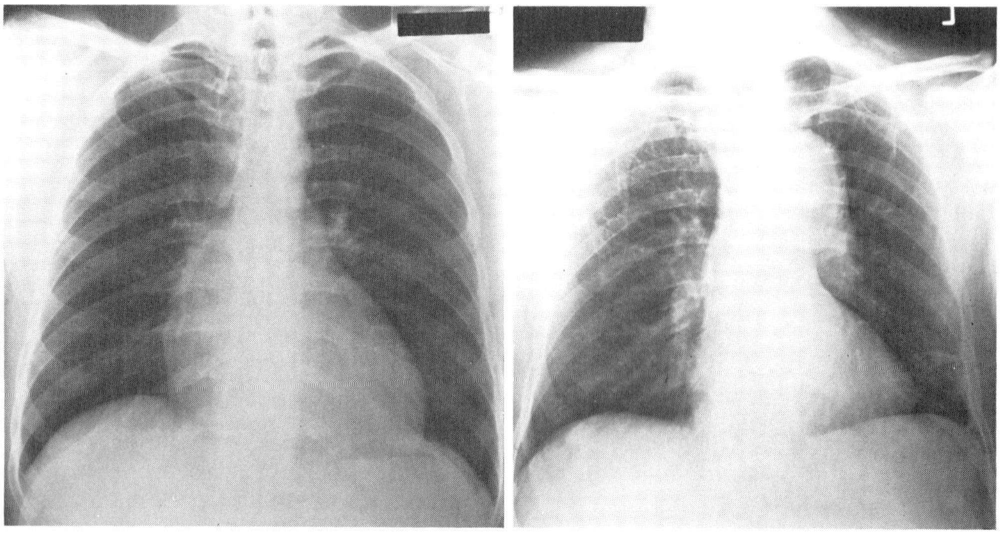

Fig 33-10 Chest roentgenograms. **Left,** rheumatic chronic aortic regurgitation, showing left ventricular enlargement with the characteristic elongation of the apex toward the left and inferiorly (seen below the diaphragmatic level). **Right,** acute aortic regurgitation secondary to acute aortic dissection, showing prominent mediastinum related to the aortic dissection and venous congestion secondary to left ventricular failure; the left ventricle is not dilated because it has not had enough time for distention.

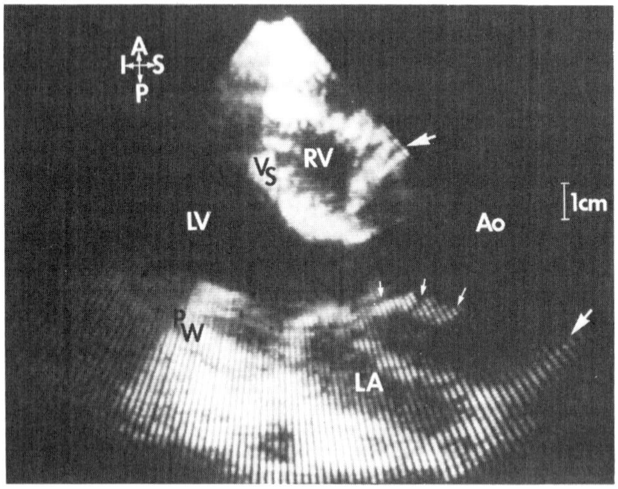

Fig 33-11 Two-dimensional echocardiogram (parasternal long-axis view) of aortic dissection, showing markedly dilated (6.5 cm) aortic root *(large arrows)* and an extraneous, linear, intra-aortic echo *(small arrows)* representing an intimal flap. (If an intimal flap is not seen, the combination of a dilated aortic root and an otherwise unexplained pericardial effusion is also suggestive of aortic dissection.) *A,* anterior; *Ao,* aorta; *I,* inferior; *LA,* left atrium; *LV,* left ventricle; *P,* posterior; *RV,* right ventricle; *S,* superior; *VS,* ventricular septum.

patients with suspected aortic dissection and compares favorably with both aortography and computed tomography scanning.[41] It offers many advantages, especially in emergency situations.[42] It is relatively easy to perform at the bedside, faster to obtain than aortography or computed tomography scanning, and avoids the potential risks of parenteral administration of contrast material. In some medical centers, the decision to proceed directly to surgery is made on the basis of this test without confirmatory aortography.

At times, the aortic valve itself may appear to be entirely normal on the echocardiogram despite the presence of aortic regurgitation.

Echocardiographic assessment of severity of aortic regurgitation and of myocardial dysfunction. If the left ventricle is not dilated in a patient with chronic aortic regurgitation, the aortic regurgitation usually is not hemodynamically significant. On the other hand, in cases of acute severe aortic regurgitation – e.g., ruptured aortic cusp secondary to infective endocarditis – the left ventricle may not be dilated but is hyperdynamic and may show premature closure of the mitral valve or decreased mitral valve deceleration time, or both, as assessed by Doppler scan. These findings suggest a marked increase in left ventricular diastolic pressure and should prompt the clinician to consider early surgical intervention.

Left ventricular diastolic and systolic dimensions (as indices of diastolic and systolic volumes) and derived ejection fraction or percentage fractional shortening (as indices of left ventricular systolic function) can be assessed and followed serially in patients with aortic regurgitation.

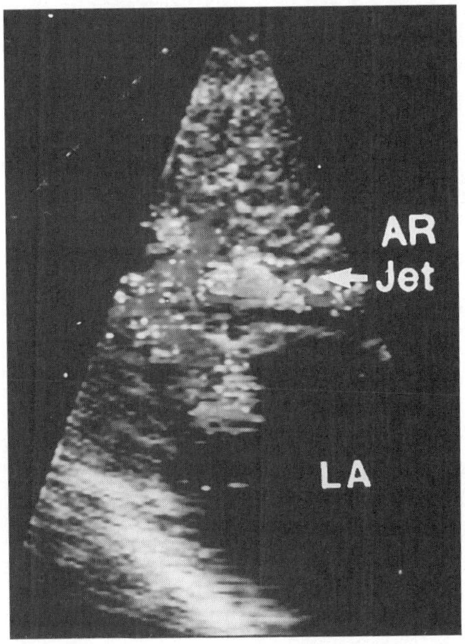

Fig 33-12 (see color plate after page 200) Doppler color-flow image of aortic regurgitation *(AR)* in the parasternal long-axis recording position. The diastolic regurgitant jet is shown *(arrow)*. *LA,* left atrium.

Other echocardiographic assessments of global left ventricular systolic function are based on estimates of left ventricular systolic wall stress—e.g., end-systolic wall stress or radius-to-thickness ratio. In this way the "appropriateness" of the degree of left ventricular hypertrophy (which theoretically allows normalization of systolic wall stress) can be studied. Indeed, preoperative echocardiographic estimates of systolic wall stress and end-systolic dimension have been shown to be 80% to 90% accurate in predicting postoperative normalization or persistence of left ventricular dilatation. However, assessment of wall stress by echocardiography still remains primarily a research tool and is not used widely in clinical practice.

Role of Doppler echocardiography. Doppler echocardiography is extremely sensitive in diagnosing the presence of aortic regurgitation and adds functional (flow) information to the echocardiographic examination[43] (Fig 33-12). Mild aortic regurgitation detected by Doppler echocardiography may not be audible by auscultation, but moderate or severe aortic regurgitation by Doppler criteria usually can also be detected clinically. The prevalence of Doppler-diagnosed aortic regurgitation in otherwise normal hearts increases with age and is presumably due to aortic sclerosis or aortic root dilatation (or both).[44] In most cases, the degree of regurgitation is trivial to mild and often inaudible by auscultation. In a prospective study of 211 normal volunteers who were under age 50, none of the subjects was found to have aortic regurgitation by color-flow imaging.[45]

Pulmonic regurgitation or mitral stenosis can be differentiated from aortic regurgitation by the Doppler technique. One of the most important roles of Doppler echocardiography is the assessment of severity of aortic regurgitation. Doppler measurements used for this purpose include

1. The width or area of the regurgitant jet by color-flow imaging relative to the width or area of the left ventricular outflow tract just beneath the aortic valve.[46-49]
2. The slope, deceleration time, or derived pressure half-time of the aortic regurgitant diastolic signal obtained by continuous-wave Doppler examination. The spectral pattern of the regurgitant jet velocity profile is determined by the instantaneous pressure difference between the ascending aorta and the left ventricle; the steeper the slope, the faster the rise in left ventricular diastolic pressures.[50-53] Indices of left ventricular diastolic filling also have been used to detect severe aortic regurgitation.[54] The rapid rise in left ventricular diastolic pressure with severe aortic regurgitation is reflected by an increased early inflow velocity and short deceleration time. Diastolic mitral regurgitation may also be observed.
3. The relative degree of flow reversal recorded from the descending thoracic aorta with use of pulsed-wave Doppler imaging.[52]
4. Assessment of regurgitant fraction by Doppler echocardiography using the continuity equation.[55]

A composite of the data from these techniques provides the best final assessment of the severity of aortic regurgitation.

In some medical centers, intraoperative echocardiography has been used to assess the severity of valvular regurgitation,[56] and in selected cases, the information obtained may influence the surgical approach during the operation. Intraoperative transesophageal echocardiography can also be used for this purpose.

Other imaging techniques

Other imaging modalities have demonstrated high levels of accuracy in assessing regurgitant flow, ventricular dimensions, and myocardial function. Cine magnetic resonance images correlate well with echocardiographic volumetric data and Doppler evaluation of regurgitant flow.[57,58] Radionuclide ventriculography can semiquantify regurgitant flow[59-61] as well as provide early evidence of ventricular decompensation provoked by exertion. As with all studies, radionuclide ventriculography is subject to variability of interpretation, so that one must interpret the results with caution, taking into account the entire clinical context.[62]

Invasive studies

Indications. In more than 90% of cases, invasive studies do not alter clinical decisions on management that are based on data obtained from Doppler echocardiographic techniques.[63] Although each patient must be assessed individually, the general guidelines for invasive studies are as follows:

1. Patients with angina pectoris or other possible

evidence of coronary disease who are being considered for aortic valve replacement. Preoperative coronary arteriography might be considered in patients over age 50 without clinical evidence of coronary artery disease.

2. When there is suspicion of a complex lesion associated with a diastolic murmur but the specific cause cannot be clearly determined by other means. These would include association of aortic regurgitation with ventricular septal defect, aortopulmonary window, or rupture of a sinus of Valsalva aneurysm into a cardiac chamber. At the present time, Doppler echocardiography may confirm these diagnoses; however, hemodynamic and angiographic studies are usually necessary prior to surgical correction.
3. Left ventricular dysfunction out of proportion to the apparent mild degree of aortic regurgitation assessed clinically.
4. Acute or subacute aortic regurgitation or progressive aortic root dilatation with or without significant physical findings. Angiography may be useful to assess the anatomy of the aorta and coronary ostia.

Aortic cineangiography is helpful for semiquantitative assessment of the severity and dynamics of the regurgitation. A scale of 1+ to 4+ is widely used. In 1+ (mild) regurgitation, a small amount of contrast medium enters the left ventricle in diastole; it is cleared with each beat and never fills the ventricular chamber. In 2+ (moderate) regurgitation, more contrast medium enters with each diastole and faint opacification of the entire chamber occurs. With 3+ (moderately severe) regurgitation, the left ventricular chamber is well-opacified and equal to the ascending aorta in density. In 4+ (severe) aortic regurgitation, dense opacification of the left ventricular chamber occurs on the first beat, and the left ventricle appears to be more densely opacified than the ascending aorta.

Another angiographic quantitative assessment of aortic regurgitation involves calculation of the regurgitant fraction (RF). This entails measurement of both total left ventricular stroke volume (TSV) from the left ventriculogram and the amount that goes forward by way of the aorta to the systemic circulation (the forward stroke volume, FSV) by a Fick or indicator-dilution technique: FSV = cardiac output/heart rate. TSV is calculated as the difference between end-diastolic and end-systolic left ventricular volumes: TSV = EDV − ESV. Regurgitant stroke volume (RSV, regurgitant volume/beat) is then given by RSV = TSV − FSV. RF is then calculated as RF = RSV/TSV. The accuracy of these angiographic calculations depends upon many factors; therefore, there is a trend at present to use radionuclide volumetric data, but this approach also is not free of error. In general the following definitions can be used: RF $<20\%$, mild aortic regurgitation; 20% to 40%, moderate; 40% to 60%, moderately severe; and $>60\%$, severe.

An important objective of cardiac catheterization is evaluation, by ventriculography, of left ventricular function by measuring ejection fraction. The other important measurements of ventricular function—end-systolic volume and left ventricular end-diastolic pressure—have already been mentioned as part of the evaluation at catheterization.

Finally, part of the angiographic evaluation of aortic regurgitation involves assessment of the aortic valve leaflets (mobility, calcification, number of cusps), the ascending aorta (extent and type of dilatation), and possible associated abnormalities (e.g., coronary lesions, sinus of Valsalva aneurysm, dissecting aneurysm of the aorta, and ventricular septal defect).

MANAGEMENT

Principles: medical versus surgical treatment

Patients with rheumatic aortic regurgitation should receive prophylaxis against rheumatic fever (by the same approach discussed in detail in the section on aortic stenosis and in chapter 54). In any patient with aortic regurgitation, antibiotic prophylaxis against bacterial endocarditis is advised prior to any surgical or dental manipulative procedure, the choice of antibiotic being determined by the location and type of procedure performed.

Patients with hemodynamically significant aortic regurgitation are candidates for surgery, particularly if significant symptoms have developed (see below). However, those patients in whom operation must be delayed or cannot be carried out for any reason may benefit from medical therapy alone. Various vasodilators, including nitroprusside, amyl nitrite, nitroglycerin, hydralazine, prazosin, and nifedipine, are capable of decreasing regurgitant flow by decreasing peripheral systemic resistance, which in turn may produce a reduction in left ventricular size and an increase in ejection fraction.[64-66] Reduction of left ventricular afterload may also decrease the regurgitant orifice area of the aortic valve by decreasing the diastolic transvalvular pressure gradient.[67] However, a substantial number of patients may not tolerate long-term use of vasodilators.[64,65] The use of digoxin is advisable in patients with severe aortic regurgitation and left ventricular dilatation or other evidence of depressed systolic function, regardless of symptomatic status. Angina may respond to administration of nitrates, but the benefit is generally less than that observed in patients with angina due primarily to coronary artery obstruction.

It is accepted that patients with moderate to severe symptoms deserve aortic valve replacement, both for symptomatic relief and for prolongation of life.[38,68] It is widely thought, however, that results would be enhanced if the operation were performed before significant symptoms developed and that timing of the operation should be based on the severity of aortic regurgitation and the degree of left ventricular dysfunction.[69] Previous attempts to define specific indicators for recommending operation were based on studies in which it was found that certain patient subgroups have increased operative mortality, poor late survival, or unimproved postoperative left ventricular function. It has been reasoned, therefore, that operative intervention should be undertaken *prior* to the development of characteristics that predict poor postoperative results. Suggested criteria included a cardiothoracic ratio greater than 0.64,[70,71] fractional shortening less than 25% to 29%,[68,72,73] end-systolic diameter greater than 55 mm,[72,73] end-diastolic radius-to-myocardial wall thickness ratio greater than 4.0,[74] ejection fraction less

Table 33-4 Timing of operation in patients with chronic aortic regurgitation

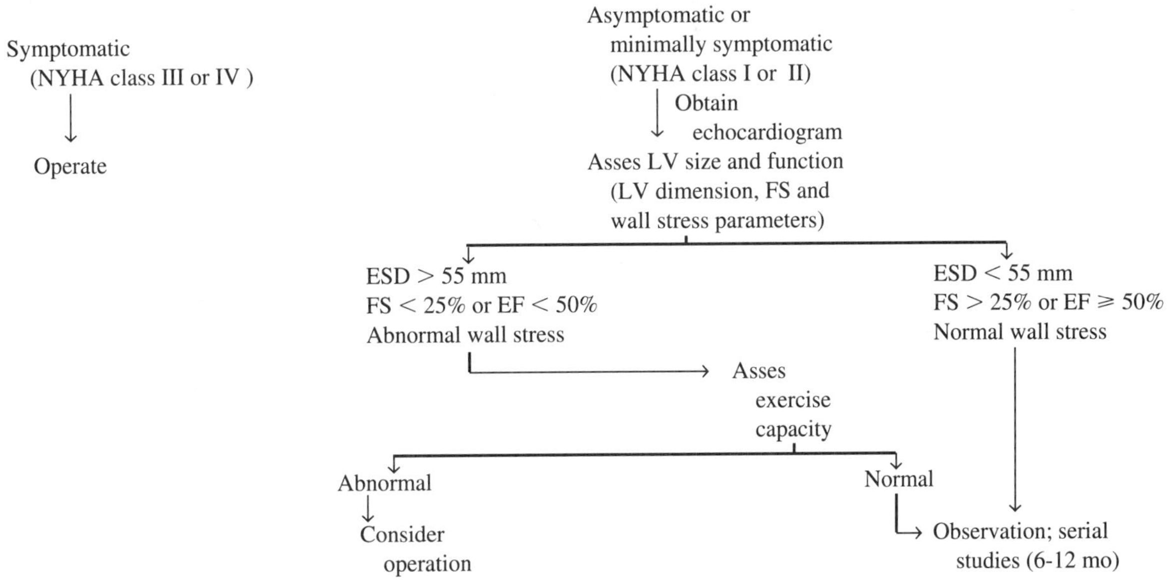

EF, ejection fraction; ESD, end-systolic dimension; FS, fractional shortening; LV, left ventricle; NYHA, New York Heart Association.

than 0.45 m^2, cardiac index less than 2.2 to 2.5 L/min per m^2,[70,75,76] and long duration of left ventricular dysfunction.[77]

Asymptomatic patients with evidence of left ventricular dysfunction (i.e., end-systolic diameter greater than 55 mm or fractional shortening less than 25% to 29%) have a high likelihood (67%) of having symptoms within 3 years,[73] suggesting that operation should be considered in these patients (Table 33-4). Our approach is to consider operation in asymptomatic or minimally symptomatic patients with such a degree of left ventricular dysfunction, particularly if their exercise capacity is impaired. Nevertheless, the degree of left ventricular dysfunction that places a patient in a higher risk category is still unclear. Radionuclide studies indicate that left ventricular exercise dysfunction may be present in up to two-thirds of asymptomatic patients with a normal resting ejection fraction.[15] This indicator may be too sensitive to warrant operation because long-term prognosis may still be excellent;[68] nevertheless, this may be a first warning to the physician that closer follow-up of the patient is needed.[68]

However, optimal management of patients with severe aortic valve insufficiency who have no cardiac symptoms is still controversial. Some clinicians favor medical management with afterload-reducing drugs, believing that risks of operation and late valve-related complications outweigh the potential benefit in limiting left ventricular hypertrophy and enlargement. Data from Bonow et al.[68] suggest that when aortic valve replacement is delayed until the onset of symptoms or left ventricular dysfunction, or both, survival with medical treatment is excellent, and aortic valve replacement can be performed with low risk and expectation of improvement in left ventricular size and function. In their experience, 58% of patients with normal systolic function and severe aortic valve insufficiency remained stable for 11 years after diagnosis. Thus, it seems safe to observe such patients and monitor left ventricular size and performance with serial echocardiographic studies. Additional prognostic information can be gained from measurement of left ventricular dimension (Table 33-5). For example, risk (per year) of death, symptoms, or left ventricular dysfunction was 2% for patients with left ventricular end-diastolic dimension less than 70 mm compared with 10% for those in whom this dimension was 70 mm or greater. For the asymptomatic patient with left ventricular enlargement and systolic dysfunction, valve replacement should be considered, especially if the patient is young and free of complicating medical illnesses that might be expected to increase operative mortality.

In deciding for or against operation in patients with aortic insufficiency, the clinician should also consider the influence of timing of the operation on prosthesis-related complications and late sudden cardiac events. Magnussen et al.[78] examined 121 patients who were alive 30 days after valve replacement for aortic regurgitation and found that only factors related to preoperative cardiac status and cardioplegic method predicted late valve-related complications, including thromboembolism; predicted 10-year event-free survival rates for low- and high-risk subgroups were, respectively, 98% and 46% for thromboembolism, 87% and 68% for all prosthesis-related complications, 100% and 0% for sudden cardiac-related events (myocardial infarction and arrhythmia), and 72% and 38% for combined prosthesis- and sudden cardiac-related morbidity and mortality. Of particular importance was the finding that in a multivariate model, these variables, which are related to the extent of cardiac disability, had far more

Table 33-5 Risk of late events in asymptomatic patients with severe chronic aortic regurgitation and normal left ventricular (LV) systolic function

Variable	Likelihood of death, symptoms, or LV dysfunction (per year), %
LV end-systolic dimension, mm	
>50	19
40-49	6
<40	0
LV end-diastolic dimension, mm	
≥70	10
<70	2
LV ejection fraction response to exercise, %	
Decrease >5	12
Decrease 0-5	4
Increase >0	1

From Bonow RO, Lakatos E, Maron BJ, et al: Serial long-term assessment of the natural history of asymptomatic patients with chronic aortic regurgitation and normal left ventricular systolic function. *Circulation* 84:1625-1635, 1991. By permission of American Heart Association.

impact on late valve-related complications than did the type of prosthesis. Thus, deciding to operate early in the course of aortic regurgitation may reduce the rate of these complications, increase longevity, and enhance the quality of life.

Asymptomatic patients with severe aortic regurgitation and normal resting left ventricular function do not generally require valve replacement prophylactically, since operative response is usually excellent if valve replacement is deferred until symptoms or ventricular dysfunction develops.

Surgical techniques

The precise pathogenesis of aortic regurgitation is largely irrelevant to its surgical management, because the indications for operation and the nature of the operation itself—namely, valve replacement—are basically similar regardless of cause of the condition. Before the availability of adequate replacement valves, attempts were made to reconstruct the aortic valve; however, experience demonstrated the inadequacy of reconstruction in most instances. The two most promising techniques were bicuspidization—in which the noncoronary cusp and sinus were excised and the aorta and aortic root were reconstructed and thereby made smaller—and patching of cusps that had been perforated by previous endocarditis. Neither technique gave early or late improvement dependably, and they have been largely abandoned.

Many young patients and their families want to avoid chronic anticoagulation with warfarin, which is necessary with mechanical prosthetic aortic valves, and attention has turned again to aortic valve repair. In recent years, valvuloplasty for aortic insufficiency has been attempted in children and young adults with rheumatic valvulitis[79,80] and in selected patients with bicuspid aortic valves.[81] Aortic valve insufficiency in young patients with rheumatic heart disease can sometimes be repaired with cusp extension, and this technique is particularly advantageous if the patient has associated mitral valve disease that can be repaired; there are, however, no data on late durability of such procedures.

In a few circumstances, repair of aortic regurgitation is clearly preferable to valve replacement. For example, in acute dissection of the ascending aorta, reconstruction of the ascending aorta (see below) may be combined with resuspension of the aortic layers at the level of the aortic commissures, thus frequently restoring valvular competence.[82,83] Of course, the cusps must be normal and the aortic root not dilated to warrant an attempt at reconstruction rather than replacement of the valve.

Replacement of the aortic valve is technically similar whether accomplished for aortic stenosis or for aortic regurgitation, except that the incompetent valve generally is neither heavily calcified nor small in diameter. Thus, valvular replacement usually is somewhat simpler technically for regurgitation.

Two types of conditions may offer special technical challenges. The first is bacterial endocarditis involving, and causing focal destruction of, the annulus of the aortic valve. When the process is limited, excision of the valve and evacuation and curettement of the annular abscess may prepare a tissue surface adequate for holding sutures for anchoring the replacement valve. However, there is increased risk of periprosthetic leak, recurrent endocarditis, or valvular dehiscence postoperatively.

In some situations, the process is so advanced that there is essentially no hope of anchoring a replacement valve securely at the annular level; one method for attempting salvage in this situation is to occlude the coronary ostia, place the replacement valve in the mid ascending aorta downstream from the annular abscesses and coronary arterial ostia, and then place saphenous vein bypass grafts between the distal ascending aorta and the epicardial coronary arteries. Another method is reconstruction of the aortic valve annulus (and sinotubular area, if necessary) with an aortic valve homograft or a pulmonary autograft. Fresh or cryopreserved, antibiotic-sterilized homografts appear to be more resistant to infection than stent-mounted bioprostheses or mechanical heart valves. Also, annular abscesses can be repaired by freehand suture techniques during implantation of homograft valves.[84]

The second condition that may complicate aortic valve replacement for regurgitation is a pathologic lesion in the ascending aorta. The types include acute or chronic dissection, dilatation, and frank aneurysm formation. The indications for operation and principles of operative technique for these different conditions of the ascending aorta are discussed in chapter 58A. This section focuses specifically on the techniques as they apply to the associated aortic regurgitation.

Longitudinal strip excision. In diffuse dilatation of an ascending aorta covered by normally vascularized adventitia and having a well-preserved wall, longitudinal strip excision combined with replacement of the incompetent aortic valve may restore a normal diameter to the ascending aorta. This can be accomplished, after the prosthetic valve is inserted, by excision of a strip 2 cm wide from each lip of the aortotomy before it is closed in the usual manner. A long aortotomy extending to the aortic cross-clamp is indicated. Arterial cannulation is performed in the arch of the aorta or peripherally to allow the cross-clamp to be placed just proximal to the origin of the innominate artery.

Layer approximation and obliteration of intimal tear. In acute aortic dissection involving the ascending aorta, a transversely oriented tear in the inside layer of the dissection is usually present about 1 to 4 cm downstream from the aortic valve. This allows communication between the lumen of the ascending aorta and the space between the layers of the dissection. After the aortic valvular involvement is dealt with, either by replacement or by resuspension as discussed above, the aortotomy is extended circumferentially at the level of the intimal tear as far around the aorta as it is involved by the dissection. The inner and outer layers of the dissection are then approximated by sandwiching them together between strips of felt material. This is accomplished along both the distal and the proximal edges of the circumferential aortotomy. Closing the aortotomy then obliterates the original tear.

Graft insertion. For aneurysms of the ascending aorta not amenable to any of the reparative procedures above, correction must involve insertion of an arterial graft that will function as the aortic wall for the involved segment. Several methods have been successful. We currently prefer to excise the diseased aortic segment and replace it with a prosthetic graft made of low-porosity woven synthetic polyester fiber (Dacron) or with a homograft; alternatively, the graft may be inserted within the lumen of the aorta. The graft is sutured proximally to the inner surface of the aorta at a level as close as possible to the downstream margins of the aortic annulus and coronary arterial ostia, and a zone of intact aortic root is left between the proximal end of the graft and the sewing ring of the prosthetic aortic valve. The distal attachment of the graft is to the inner surface of the aorta just proximal to the aortic cross-clamp.

Aortic graft as integral part of aortic valve prosthesis. When the graft technique noted above is used, progressive postoperative stretching and dilation of the sinus portion of the aorta between valvular prosthesis and aortic graft may occur, especially if this zone is lengthened by downstream displacement of the coronary arterial ostia, as may occur in Marfan's syndrome or the forme fruste of that condition. When annuloaortic ectasia is present, it is preferable to construct the aortic graft as an integral unit with the aortic valve prosthesis[85] (Fig 33-13). Coronary blood flow is provided by anastomosing coronary ostial buttons to fenestrations in the graft or by anastomosing segments of saphenous vein or Dacron grafts of smaller diameter to the coronary ostia and to the ascending aortic graft.[86]

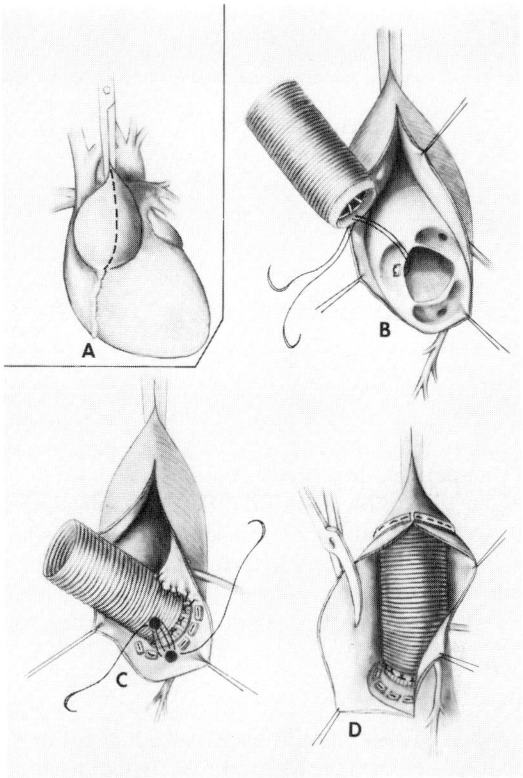

Fig 33-13 Aneurysm of the ascending aorta with associated aortic regurgitation. **A,** after extracorporeal circulation is instituted, ascending aorta is cross-clamped just proximal to origin of innominate artery. A longitudinal incision is made along the length of the aneurysm. **B,** aortic valve has been excised and first suture is placed to attach prosthetic valve to aortic annulus. The valve is incorporated in a composite ascending aortic graft. **C,** prosthesis has been attached to the aortic annulus, and the left coronary artery stoma has been sutured to a circular hole in the aortic graft. Sutures are being placed to attach, in a similar manner, the right coronary artery stoma to the graft. **D,** distal anastomosis has been completed. (Modified from Kouchoukos NT, Karp RB, Blackstone EH, et al: Replacement of the ascending aorta and aortic valve with a composite graft: results in 86 patients. *Ann Surg* 192:403-412, 1980.)

Postoperative course

Perioperative mortality ranges from 6% to 8% for patients with symptomatic predominant aortic regurgitation and 2% for minimally disabled patients.[87] Long-term postoperative survival varies widely among reports: mortality rates for the first 1 to 2 years range from 15% to 40%.[38,68,88,89] Mortality tends to be less in series of patients who were operated on more recently,[68,90] who were less compromised hemodynamically and had less severe symptoms,[75] or who were younger.[90,91] The long-

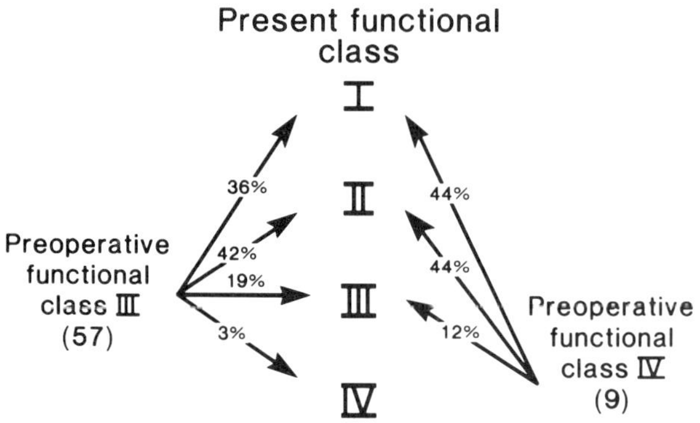

Fig 33-14 Follow-up functional class of patients who underwent isolated Starr-Edwards aortic valve replacement. Numbers in parentheses indicate number of patients in each preoperative functional class who were living at follow-up. (From McGoon MD, Fuster V, McGoon DC, et al: Aortic and mitral valve incompetence: long-term follow-up [10 to 19 years] of patients treated with the Starr-Edwards prosthesis. *J Am Coll Cardiol* 3:930-938, 1984. By permission of American College of Cardiology.)

term status of very symptomatic patients who underwent aortic valve replacement with the Starr-Edwards prosthesis during the years 1963 to 1971 at the Mayo Clinic has been examined.[91] Ten percent died within 30 days postoperatively. Among the survivors, probability of surviving to 1 year was 84%; to 3 years, 69%; to 10 years, 52%; and to 15 years, 40%. In this group of very symptomatic patients with aortic regurgitation, the surgical survival was significantly better than survival in similar patients treated medically.[38]

In the Mayo Clinic study, 80% of patients who had aortic valve replacement for aortic regurgitation and who were alive at the time of follow-up had improved symptomatically by at least one functional class (Fig 33-14). In addition, 39% of patients had become asymptomatic, which is remarkable, taking into account that preoperatively all these patients were in class III or IV.

About 60% of the patients with chronic aortic regurgitation have normal left ventricular diastolic diameter within 1 to 3 years after operation; this outcome appears to be related to favorable preoperative left ventricular systolic diameter or volume, diastolic radius-to-wall thickness ratio, end-systolic ventricular wall stress, ratio of regurgitant stroke volume to end-diastolic volume, and coronary blood flow.[74,92-95] Thus, in general, preoperative contractile state predicts postoperative left ventricular performance.[96-99] Patients who exhibit the greatest improvement in diastolic dimension and ejection fraction shortly after operation are also most likely to have even further improvement over the longer term.[100] Regression of left ventricular hypertrophy may also proceed over a period of years.[101] Despite the prognostic relevance of preoperative ventricular function, the substantial success rate of operation when the ventricle is compromised should warrant intervention in most patients without prohibitive contraindications.[102]

REFERENCES

1. Sasson Z, Prieur T, Skrobik Y, et al: Aortic regurgitation: a common complication after surgery for hypertrophic obstructive cardiomyopathy. *J Am Coll Cardiol* 13:63-67, 1989
2. Roman MJ, Devereux RB, Niles NW, et al: Aortic root dilatation as a cause of isolated, severe aortic regurgitation: prevalence, clinical and echocardiographic patterns, and relation to left ventricular hypertrophy and function. *Ann Intern Med* 106:800-807, 1987
3. Heggtveit HA: Syphilitic aortitis: a clinicopathologic autopsy study of 100 cases, 1950 to 1960. *Circulation* 29:346-355, 1964
4. Edwards JE: Lesions causing or simulating aortic insufficiency. *Cardiovasc Clin* 5 No 1:127-148, 1973
5. Murray CA, Edwards JE: Spontaneous laceration of ascending aorta. *Circulation* 47:848-858, 1973
6. Starling MR, Kirsh MM, Montgomery DG, et al: Mechanisms for left ventricular systolic dysfunction in aortic regurgitation: importance for predicting the functional response to aortic valve replacement. *J Am Coll Cardiol* 17:887-897, 1991
7. Mehmel HC, v. Olshausen K, Schuler G, et al: Estimation of left ventricular myocardial function by the ejection fraction in isolated, chronic, pure aortic regurgitation. *Am J Cardiol* 54:610-616, 1984
8. Ricci DR: Afterload mismatch and preload reserve in chronic aortic regurgitation. *Circulation* 66:826-834, 1982
9. Dehmer GJ, Firth BG, Hillis LD, et al: Alterations in left ventricular volumes and ejection fraction at rest and during exercise in patients with aortic regurgitation. *Am J Cardiol* 48:17-27, 1981
10. Osbakken M, Bove AA, Spann JF: Left ventricular function in chronic aortic regurgitation with reference to end-systolic pressure, volume and stress relations. *Am J Cardiol* 47:193-198, 1981
11. Laniado S, Yellin EL, Yoran C, et al: Physiologic mechanisms in aortic insufficiency. I. The effect of changing heart rate on flow dynamics. II. Determinants of Austin Flint murmur. *Circulation* 66:226-235, 1982
12. Firth BG, Dehmer GJ, Nicod P, et al: Effect of increasing heart rate in patients with aortic regurgitation: effect of incremental atrial pacing on scintigraphic, hemodynamic and thermodilution measurements. *Am J Cardiol* 49:1860-1867, 1982
13. Steingart RM, Yee C, Weinstein L, et al: Radionuclide ventriculographic study of adaptations to exercise in aortic regurgitation. *Am J Cardiol* 51:483-488, 1983
14. Gerson MC, Engel PJ, Mantil JC, et al: Effects of dynamic and isometric exercise on the radionuclide-determined regurgitant fraction in aortic insufficiency. *J Am Coll Cardiol* 3:98-106, 1984
15. Borer JS, Bacharach SL, Green MV, et al: Exercise-induced left ventricular dysfunction in symptomatic and asymptomatic patients with aortic regurgitation: assessment with radionuclide cineangiography. *Am J Cardiol* 42:351-357, 1978
16. Massie BM, Kramer BL, Loge D, et al: Ejection fraction response to supine exercise in asymptomatic aortic regurgitation: relation to simultaneous hemodynamic measurements. *J Am Coll Cardiol* 5:847-855, 1985
17. Boucher CA, Kanarek DJ, Okada RD, et al: Exercise testing in aortic regurgitation: comparison of radionuclide left ventricular ejection fraction with exercise performance at the anaerobic threshold and peak exercise. *Am J Cardiol* 52:801-808, 1983
18. Huxley RL, Gaffney FA, Corbett JR, et al: Early detection of left ventricular dysfunction in chronic aortic regurgitation as assessed by contrast angiography, echocardiography, and rest and exercise scintigraphy. *Am J Cardiol* 51:1542-1550, 1983
19. Kawanishi DT, McKay CR, Chandraratna PAN, et al: Cardiovascular response to dynamic exercise in patients with chronic symptomatic mild-to-moderate and severe aortic regurgitation. *Circulation* 73:62-72, 1986
20. Thompson R, Ross I, McHaffie D, et al: Left ventricular function in asymptomatic patients with severe aortic regurgitation: relation to clinical parameters and exercise performance. *Clin Cardiol* 5:523-530, 1982
21. Greenberg B, Massie B, Thomas D, et al: Association between the exercise ejection fraction response and systolic wall stress in patients with chronic aortic insufficiency. *Circulation* 71:458-465, 1985
22. Schuler G, von Olshausen K, Schwarz F, et al: Noninvasive assessment of myocardial contractility in asymptomatic patients with severe aortic regurgitation and normal left ventricular ejection fraction at rest. *Am J Cardiol* 50:45-52, 1982
23. Johnson LL, Powers ER, Tzall WR, et al: Ventricular volume and

ejection fraction response to exercise in aortic regurgitation. *Am J Cardiol* 51:1379-1385, 1983

24. Iskandrian AS, Hakki A-H, Manno B, et al: Left ventricular function in chronic aortic regurgitation. *J Am Coll Cardiol* 1:1374-1380, 1983
25. Gee DS, Juni JE, Santinga JT, et al: Prognostic significance of exercise-induced left ventricular dysfunction in chronic aortic regurgitation. *Am J Cardiol* 56:605-609, 1985
26. Shen WF, Roubin GS, Choong CY-P, et al: Evaluation of relationship between myocardial contractile state and left ventricular function in patients with aortic regurgitation. *Circulation* 71:31-38, 1985
27. Branzi A, Lolli C, Piovaccari G, et al: Echocardiographic evaluation of the response to afterload stress test in young asymptomatic patients with chronic severe aortic regurgitation: sensitivity of the left ventricular end-systolic pressure-volume relationship. *Circulation* 70: 561-569, 1984
28. Bolen JL, Holloway EL, Zener JC, et al: Evaluation of left ventricular function in patients with aortic regurgitation using afterload stress. *Circulation* 53:132-138, 1976
29. Osbakken MD, Bove AA, Spann JF: Left ventricular regional wall motion and velocity of shortening in chronic mitral and aortic regurgitation. *Am J Cardiol* 47:1005-1009, 1981
30. Eichhorn P, Grimm J, Koch R, et al: Left ventricular relaxation in patients with left ventricular hypertrophy secondary to aortic valve disease. *Circulation* 65:1395-1404, 1982
31. Rousseau MF, Pouleur H, Charlier AA, et al: Assessment of left ventricular relaxation in patients with valvular regurgitation. *Am J Cardiol* 50:1028-1036, 1982
32. Nitenberg A, Foult J-M, Antony I, et al: Coronary flow and resistance reserve in patients with chronic aortic regurgitation, angina pectoris and normal coronary arteries. *J Am Coll Cardiol* 11:478-486, 1988
33. Timmermans P, Willems JL, Piessens J, et al: Angina pectoris and coronary artery disease in severe aortic regurgitation. *Am J Cardiol* 61:826-829, 1988
34. Rapaport E: Natural history of aortic and mitral valve disease. *Am J Cardiol* 35:221-227, 1975
35. Hegglin R, Scheu H, Rothlin M: Aortic insufficiency. *Circulation* 38 Suppl 5:77-92, 1968
36. Bland EF, Wheeler EO: Severe aortic regurgitation in young people: a long-term perspective with reference to prognosis and prosthesis. *N Engl J Med* 256:667-672, 1957
37. Segal J, Harvey WP, Hufnagel C: A clinical study of one hundred cases of severe aortic insufficiency. *Am J Med* 21:200-210, 1956
38. McGoon MD, Fuster V, Pluth JR, et al: Medical and surgical long term follow-up (10-21 years) of chronic aortic incompetence (abstract). *Circulation* 64 Suppl 4:76, 1981
39. Spagnuolo M, Kloth H, Taranta A, et al: Natural history of rheumatic aortic regurgitation: criteria predictive of death, congestive heart failure, and angina in young patients. *Circulation* 44:368-380, 1971
40. Roman MJ, Kligfield P, Devereaux RB, et al: Geometric and functional correlates of electrocardiographic repolarization and voltage abnormalities in aortic regurgitation. *J Am Coll Cardiol* 9:500-508, 1987
41. Erbel R, Engberding R, Daniel W, et al: Echocardiography in diagnosis of aortic dissection. *Lancet* 1:457-461, 1989
42. Seward JB, Khandheria BK, Oh JK, et al: Transesophageal echocardiography: technique, anatomic correlations, implementation, and clinical applications. *Mayo Clin Proc* 63:649-680, 1988
43. Goldberg SJ, Allen HD: Quantitative assessment by Doppler echocardiography of pulmonary or aortic regurgitation. *Am J Cardiol* 56:131-135, 1985
44. Choong CY, Abascal VM, Weyman J, et al: Prevalence of valvular regurgitation by Doppler echocardiography in patients with structurally normal hearts by two-dimensional echocardiography. *Am Heart J* 117:636-642, 1989
45. Yoshida K, Yoshikawa J, Shakudo M, et al: Color Doppler evaluation of valvular regurgitation in normal subjects. *Circulation* 78:840-847, 1988
46. Cujec B, David T, Wilansky S, et al: Colour flow imaging in severe mitral and aortic regurgitation. *Can J Cardiol* 4:341-346, 1988
47. Baumgartner H, Kratzer H, Helmreich G, et al: Quantitation of aortic regurgitation by colour coded cross-sectional Doppler echocardiography. *Eur Heart J* 9:380-387, 1988
48. Perry GJ, Helmcke F, Nanda NC, et al: Evaluation of aortic insufficiency by Doppler color flow imaging. *J Am Coll Cardiol* 9:952-959, 1987
49. Smith MD, Grayburn PA, Spain MG, et al: Observer variability in the quantitation of Doppler color flow jet areas for mitral and aortic regurgitation. *J Am Coll Cardiol* 11:579-584, 1988
50. Nishimura RA, Tajik AJ: Determination of left-sided pressure gradients by utilizing Doppler aortic and mitral regurgitant signals: validation by simultaneous dual catheter and Doppler studies. *J Am Coll Cardiol* 11:317-321, 1988
51. Grayburn PA, Handshoe R, Smith MD, et al: Quantitative assessment of the hemodynamic consequences of aortic regurgitation by means of continuous wave Doppler recordings. *J Am Coll Cardiol* 10:135-141, 1987
52. Shaw PM: Doppler assessment of aortic regurgitation: correlation with hemodynamics and angiography. *Herz* 11:318-322, 1986
53. Beyer RW, Ramirez M, Josephson MA, et al: Correlation of continuous-wave Doppler assessment of chronic aortic regurgitation with hemodynamics and angiography. *Am J Cardiol* 60:852-856, 1987
54. Oh JK, Hatle LK, Sinak LJ, et al: Characteristic Doppler echocardiographic pattern of mitral inflow velocity in severe aortic regurgitation. *J Am Coll Cardiol* 14:1712-1717, 1989
55. Rokey R, Sterling LL, Zoghbi WA, et al: Determination of regurgitant fraction in isolated mitral or aortic regurgitation by pulsed Doppler two-dimensional echocardiography. *J Am Coll Cardiol* 7:1273-1278, 1986
56. Goldman ME, Fuster V, Guarino T, et al: Intraoperative echocardiography for the evaluation of valvular regurgitation: experience in 263 patients. *Circulation* 74 Suppl 1:143-149, 1986
57. Pflugfelder PW, Landzberg JS, Cassidy MM, et al: Comparison of cine MR imaging with Doppler echocardiography for the evaluation of aortic regurgitation. *AJR* 152:729-735, 1989
58. Utz JA, Herfkens RJ, Heinsimer JA, et al: Valvular regurgitation: dynamic MR imaging. *Radiology* 168:91-94, 1988
59. Voth E, Sciagrà R, Schicha H, et al: Significance of gated equilibrium radionuclide ventriculography in quantification and follow up of valvular regurgitation. *Eur J Nucl Med* 14:467-471, 1988
60. Kelbaek H, Aldershvile J, Svendsen JH, et al: Combined first pass and equilibrium radionuclide cardiographic determination of stroke volume for quantitation of valvular regurgitation. *J Am Coll Cardiol* 11:769-773, 1988
61. Philippe L, Mena I, Darcourt J, et al: Evaluation of valvular regurgitation by factor analysis of first-pass angiography. *J Nucl Med* 29:159-167, 1988
62. Cornyn JW, Massie BM, Greenberg B, et al: Reproducibility of rest and exercise left ventricular ejection fraction and volumes in chronic aortic regurgitation. *Am J Cardiol* 59:1361-1365, 1987
63. Slater J, Gindea AJ, Freedberg RS, et al: Comparison of cardiac catheterization and Doppler echocardiography in the decision to operate in aortic and mitral valve disease. *J Am Coll Cardiol* 17:1026-1036, 1991
64. Greenberg B, Massie B, Bristow JD, et al: Long-term vasodilator therapy of chronic aortic insufficiency: a randomized double-blinded, placebo-controlled clinical trial. *Circulation* 78:92-103, 1988
65. Dumesnil JG, Tran K, Dagenais GR: Beneficial long-term effects of hydralazine in aortic regurgitation. *Arch Intern Med* 150:757-760, 1990
66. Scognamiglio R, Fasoli G, Ponchia A, et al: Long-term nifedipine unloading therapy in asymptomatic patients with chronic severe aortic regurgitation. *J Am Coll Cardiol* 16:424-429, 1990
67. Reimold SC, Byrne JG, Caguioa ES, et al: Load dependence of the effective regurgitant orifice area in a sheep model of aortic regurgitation. *J Am Coll Cardiol* 18:1085-1090, 1991
68. Bonow RO, Lakatos E, Maron BJ, et al: Serial long-term assessment of the natural history of asymptomatic patients with chronic aortic regurgitation and normal left ventricular systolic function. *Circulation* 84:1625-1635, 1991
69. Turina J, Turina M, Rothlin M, et al: Improved late survival in patients with chronic aortic regurgitation by earlier operation. *Circulation* 70 Suppl 1:147-152, 1984
70. Samuels DA, Curfman GD, Friedlich AL, et al: Valve replacement for aortic regurgitation: long-term follow-up with factors influencing the results. *Circulation* 60:647-654, 1979
71. Louagie Y, Brohet C, Robert A, et al: Factors influencing postoperative survival in aortic regurgitation: analysis by Cox regression model. *J Thorac Cardiovasc Surg* 88:225-233, 1984

72. Cunha CLP, Giuliani ER, Fuster V, et al: Preoperative M-mode echocardiography as a predictor of surgical results in chronic aortic insufficiency. *J Thorac Cardiovasc Surg* 79:256-265, 1980

73. Henry WL, Bonow RO, Rosing DR, et al: Observations on the optimum time for operative intervention for aortic regurgitation. II. Serial echocardiographic evaluation of asymptomatic patients. *Circulation* 61:484-492, 1980

74. Gaasch WH, Carroll JD, Levine HJ, et al: Chronic aortic regurgitation: prognostic value of left ventricular end-systolic dimension and end-diastolic radius/thickness ratio. *J Am Coll Cardiol* 1:775-782, 1983

75. Greves J, Rahimtoola SH, McAnulty JH, et al: Preoperative criteria predictive of late survival following valve replacement for severe aortic regurgitation. *Am Heart J* 101:300-308, 1981

76. Forman R, Firth BG, Barnard MS: Prognostic significance of preoperative left ventricular ejection fraction and valve lesion in patients with aortic valve replacement. *Am J Cardiol* 45:1120-1125, 1980

77. Bonow RO, Rosing DR, Maron BJ, et al: Reversal of left ventricular dysfunction after aortic valve replacement for chronic aortic regurgitation: influence of duration of preoperative left ventricular dysfunction. *Circulation* 70:570-579, 1984

78. Magnussen K, Lund O, Knudsen MA, et al: Valve replacement for aortic regurgitation: earlier operation may reduce the rate of late complications related to the prostheses. *Thorac Cardiovasc Surg* 38:295-301, 1990

79. Duran C, Kumar N, Gometza B, et al: Indications and limitations of aortic valve reconstruction. *Ann Thorac Surg* 52:447-453, 1991

80. Kumar N, Gometza B, al Halees Z, et al: Surgery for aortic regurgitation in the young: repair versus replacement. *J Cardiovasc Surg (Torino)* 33:7-13, 1992

81. Cosgrove DM, Rosenkranz ER, Hendren WG, et al: Valvuloplasty for aortic insufficiency. *J Thorac Cardiovasc Surg* 102:571-577, 1991

82. Fann JI, Glower DD, Miller DC, et al: Preservation of aortic valve in type A aortic dissection complicated by aortic regurgitation. *J Thorac Cardiovasc Surg* 102:62-73, 1991

83. Jex RK, Schaff HV, Piehler JM, et al: Repair of ascending aortic dissection: influence of associated aortic valve insufficiency on early and late results. *J Thorac Cardiovasc Surg* 93:375-384, 1987

84. Tuna IC, Orszulak TA, Schaff HV, et al: Results of homograft aortic valve replacement for active endocarditis. *Ann Thorac Surg* 49:619-624, 1990

85. Gott VL, Pyeritz RE, Cameron DE, et al: Composite graft repair of Marfan aneurysm of the ascending aorta: results in 100 patients. *Ann Thorac Surg* 52:38-45, 1991

86. Svensson LG, Crawford ES, Hess KR, et al: Composite valve graft replacement of the proximal aorta: comparison of techniques in 348 patients. *Ann Thorac Surg* 54:427-437, 1992

87. McGoon DC: Editor's comment: an alternative viewpoint. *J Thorac Cardiovasc Surg* 79:169-172, 1980

88. Schwarz F, Baumann P, Manthey J, et al: The effect of aortic valve replacement on survival. *Circulation* 66:1105-1110, 1982

89. Clark DG, McAnulty JH, Rahimtoola SH: Valve replacement in aortic insufficiency with left ventricular dysfunction. *Circulation* 61:411-421, 1980

90. Scott WC, Miller DC, Haverich A, et al: Determinants of operative mortality for patients undergoing aortic valve replacement: discriminant analysis of 1,479 operations. *J Thorac Cardiovasc Surg* 89:400-413, 1985

91. McGoon MD, Fuster V, McGoon DC, et al: Aortic and mitral valve incompetence: long-term follow-up (10 to 19 years) of patients treated with the Starr-Edwards prosthesis. *J Am Coll Cardiol* 3:930-938, 1984

92. Kumpuris AG, Quinones MA, Waggoner AD, et al: Importance of preoperative hypertrophy, wall stress and end-systolic dimension as echocardiographic predictors of normalization of left ventricular dilatation after valve replacement in chronic aortic insufficiency. *Am J Cardiol* 49:1091-1100, 1982

93. Fioretti P, Roelandt J, Tirtaman C, et al: Value of the regurgitant volume to end diastolic volume ratio to predict the regression of left ventricular dimensions after valve replacement in aortic insufficiency. *Eur Heart J* 8 Suppl C:15-20, 1987

94. Kawachi K, Kitamura S, Oyama C, et al: Relations of preoperative hemodynamics and coronary blood flow to improved left ventricular function after valve replacement for aortic regurgitation. *J Am Coll Cardiol* 11:925-929, 1988

95. Taniguchi K, Nakano S, Hirose H, et al: Preoperative left ventricular function: minimal requirement for successful late results of valve replacement for aortic regurgitation. *J Am Coll Cardiol* 10:510-518, 1987

96. Mirsky I, Henschke C, Hess OM, et al: Prediction of postoperative performance in aortic valve disease. *Am J Cardiol* 48:295-303, 1981

97. Toussaint C, Cribier A, Cazor JL, et al: Hemodynamic and angiographic evaluation of aortic regurgitation 8 and 27 months after aortic valve replacement. *Circulation* 64:456-463, 1981

98. Boucher CA, Bingham JB, Osbakken MD, et al: Early changes in left ventricular size and function after correction of left ventricular volume overload. *Am J Cardiol* 47:991-1004, 1981

99. Stone PH, Clark RD, Goldschlager N, et al: Determinants of prognosis of patients with aortic regurgitation who undergo aortic valve replacement. *J Am Coll Cardiol* 3:1118-1126, 1984

100. Bonow RO, Dodd JT, Maron BJ, et al: Long-term serial changes in left ventricular function and reversal of ventricular dilatation after valve replacement for chronic aortic regurgitation. *Circulation* 78:1108-1120, 1988

101. Monrad ES, Hess OM, Murakami T, et al: Time course of regression of left ventricular hypertrophy after aortic valve replacement. *Circulation* 77:1345-1355, 1988

102. Carabello BA, Usher BW, Hendrix GH, et al: Predictors of outcome for aortic valve replacement in patients with aortic regurgitation and left ventricular dysfunction: a change in the measuring stick. *J Am Coll Cardiol* 10:991-997, 1987

CHAPTER

34

Mitral stenosis

Rick A. Nishimura, M.D., Robert O. Brandenburg, M.D., Emilio R. Giuliani, M.D., and Dwight C. McGoon, M.D.

ETIOLOGY

In the adult, mitral stenosis is almost invariably secondary to rheumatic heart disease. The absence of a history of acute rheumatic fever in many patients with mitral stenosis has led to speculation regarding a viral cause, but no definite proof of this has been found.[1] Many patients without a classic history of acute rheumatic fever do have a history of recurrent streptococcal tonsillitis or pharyngitis, suggesting that a smoldering type of rheumatic fever may have occurred. Mitral stenosis can occur in a pure state or can be associated with varying degrees of mitral incompetence, aortic valvular disease, or, less often, organic tricuspid valvular disease.

In the mitral valve, the rheumatic pathologic process causes leaflet thickening and calcification, commissural fusion, or chordal fusion—one or all of these processes may occur.[2] The result is a funnel-shaped apparatus in which the area of the mitral orifice is decreased, and eventually mitral valve flow is decreased.[3] The decrease in flow is the result of interchordal fusion, which obliterates the secondary orifices, and of commissural fusion, which narrows the principal orifice.[4]

NATURAL HISTORY AND SYMPTOMS

Whatever the pathologic process involved, the area of the orifice must decrease by half or more before clinical symptoms will develop (normal, 4 to 6 cm^2). At this point, the resistance to flow causes an increase in left atrial pressure to maintain normal left ventricular filling.[5] In addition, left atrial decompression is slowed in proportion to the degree of obstruction. The increased left atrial pressure may persist if tachycardia shortens the diastolic period. Left atrial dilatation and hypertrophy will be sequelae of this process, and the augmented left atrial systole will maintain reasonably normal diastolic flow for a time.[6] Eventually, however, the dilated, scarred left atrium becomes the site of abnormal electrical activity in the form of atrial fibrillation. Initially this will be paroxysmal but eventually will become chronic. The loss of atrial systole causes significant impairment in ventricular filling and makes forward flow increasingly dependent on the diastolic filling period. Consequently, only mild increases in heart rate may cause severe left atrial hypertension. Left atrial hypertension eventually causes pulmonary venous congestion and interstitial and intra-alveolar edema. Lung compliance is reduced and mild airway obstruction occurs.[7]

These factors explain the various evolving types of dyspnea—that is, effort-induced dyspnea, paroxysmal nocturnal dyspnea, orthopnea, and dyspnea associated with pulmonary edema. It also explains the recumbent cough and hemoptysis that may be associated with rupture of bronchial veins during bronchitis or later be the frothy, bloody sputum of pulmonary edema.[8]

The symptoms tend to progress gradually, but there will be brief periods of increased severity of symptoms due to respiratory infections, unusual physical or emotional stress, paroxysmal atrial fibrillation, pregnancy, or pulmonary embolism. In the more advanced stages of mitral stenosis, pulmonary venous hypertension leads to progressive pulmonary arteriolar constriction associated with intimal and medial hyperplasia. This development protects the pulmonary capillaries from excessive pressure which would result in transudation of fluid into the interstitial tissues and alveoli of the lung. However, it leads to pulmonary arterial hypertension with resultant right ventricular hypertrophy and eventually to right ventricular failure with tricuspid incompetence, hepatic congestion, visceral congestion, ascites, and edema.

Effort fatigue predominates early, followed by symptoms related to the hepatic and visceral congestion. A frequent complication of this congestion is pulmonary embolism with pulmonary infarction. Additional complications are atrial fibrillation, which eventually becomes chronic in more than 50% of patients after recurrent paroxysms over a period of years, especially in those patients who have a large left atrium and are more than 40 years old,[9] and systemic embolism, which occurs in 10% to 20% of patients,[10,11] especially if atrial fibrillation and a large left atrium are present.[12,13] Chest discomfort of anginal type occurs in a small number of patients with mitral stenosis (10% to 15%). This symptom may be due to associated coronary atherosclerosis, coronary emboli, or right ventricular hypertension, but after investigation, no cause may be found.[8] An unusual symptom is hoarseness caused by left vocal cord paralysis due to left recurrent laryngeal nerve paralysis. This is not secondary to the enlarged left atrium but is caused by compression of the left recurrent laryngeal nerve between the enlarged hypertensive pulmonary artery, the aorta, and the ligamentum arteriosum.[14]

The classic natural history of mitral stenosis has changed over the past few decades in North America. A 10-10-10 sequence was described in the past: it took 10 years from the time of acute rheumatic fever for the stenosis to be recognized by auscultation, another 10 years for it to produce symptoms, and another 10 years for the patient to reach a stage of serious or total disability.[8,15] In current times, there are different subsets of patient presentations due to a milder, more delayed course of the disease process. In one subset, the patients present in their third to fourth decade of life with moderate New York Heart Association functional class II-III symptoms; severe pulmonary hypertension and right heart failure have not yet occurred. These patients are predominantly women and usually have very pliable, noncalcified valves. The initial presentation of symptoms may also occur in older patients, usually in the seventh to eighth decade of life. These patients have heavily calcified, fibrotic valves and may well have right heart decompensation from severe pulmonary hypertension. A slowly progressive disease process in conjunction with gradual limitation of activity is probably responsible for this type of presentation in the elderly patient. With the immigration to the United States of patients from Southeast Asia and other Third World countries, where the disease process is much more progressive, severe mitral stenosis may be seen in the very young.[16]

PHYSICAL FINDINGS

The general appearance of patients with mitral stenosis is usually normal. Only infrequently, in patients with severe pulmonary vascular disease and a low cardiac output, is the malar erythrocyanosis noted. The arterial pulse is usually normal, except that in patients with a low cardiac output and atrial fibrillation it will be reduced. The jugular venous pulse may be normal, it may suggest pulmonary hypertension with a large "a" wave or right ventricular failure with elevated "a" and v waves, or it may reveal evidence of organic tricuspid valve disease.

The left ventricular impulse is "tapping" in quality and somewhat difficult to detect except in the left lateral decubitus position. The obstruction to flow through the mitral valve prevents detection of a presystolic impulse or an early diastolic filling wave. In the presence of a pliable anterior mitral valve leaflet, a delayed first heart sound is palpable. The delay in the first sound contrasted with the left ventricular impulse is a measure of the severity of the mitral stenosis.[17] In the presence of significant pulmonary hypertension, a hypertrophied right ventricle will produce an outward impulse that can be seen and palpated along the left sternal edge. Occasionally, the right ventricular impulse will extend all the way to the cardiac apex. Also, in the presence of significant pulmonary hypertension, the pulmonic closure sound can be palpated over the second left intercostal space.

The cardinal auscultatory features of mitral stenosis are discussed in chapter 2. They consist of accentuation of the first heart sound, an early diastolic opening snap, and an early, mid-diastolic rumble with presystolic accentuation. Mitral stenosis in its early or milder form is often unrecognized unless the physician listens carefully at the apex, with the patient in the left lateral decubitus position, and uses the bell of the stethoscope to detect the low-frequency diastolic murmurs. Mild exercise or amyl nitrite can be used to accentuate the diastolic murmur. A shorter interval between A_2 and the opening snap is associated with increasing severity of stenosis. Auscultatory variations will be dependent on valve mobility, flow, and cardiac rhythm. When the valve is calcified and immobile, the opening snap will be absent and the first heart sound will be soft. With atrial fibrillation, the presystolic murmur is usually absent. In a patient with severe pulmonary hypertension and a low cardiac output, the large, hypertensive right ventricle will occupy the apex, and these two factors combined may result in so-called silent mitral stenosis.[18] A holodiastolic murmur during long diastolic periods indicates a persisting gradient and hence severe stenosis.[19] In the presence of pulmonary arterial hypertension, the pulmonic component of the second heart sound is accentuated and may be followed by the diastolic murmur of pulmonic valve incompetence.[20] Finally, because of the frequent association of mitral valve incompetence with aortic or tricuspid valvular disease, these corresponding murmurs also may be present.

NONINVASIVE STUDIES

The chest roentgenogram is helpful in both confirming the diagnosis and assessing the severity of the stenosis. A large

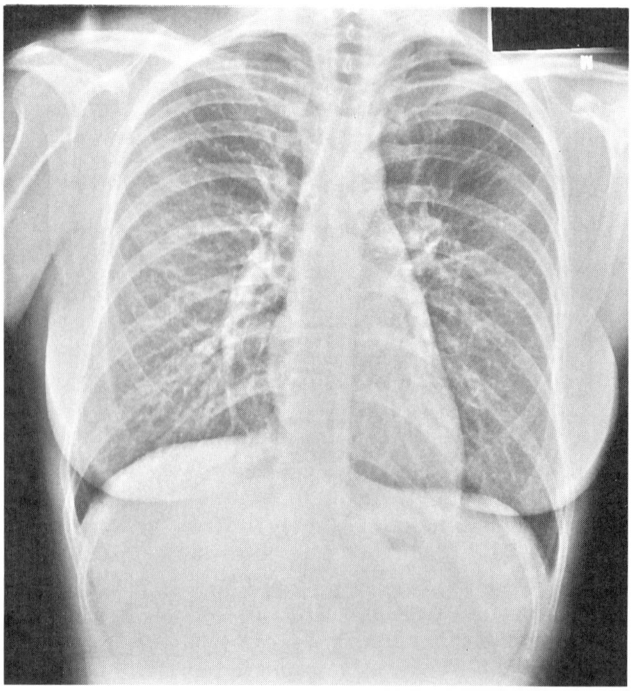

Fig 34-1 Left atrial enlargement and normal left ventricular contour in a patient with mitral stenosis.

left atrial shadow, dilated upper lobe veins, and evidence of alveolar or interstitial edema with 1- to 3-cm horizontal lines in the costophrenic angles (Kerley's B lines) all are consistent with significant mitral stenosis. In the presence of pulmonary arterial hypertension, the central pulmonary arteries are prominent, and there will be a sudden decrease in the vascular markings in the peripheral lung fields associated with right ventricular enlargement that will be seen best in the lateral film (Fig 34-1).

The electrocardiogram (ECG) is often normal except for a prolonged, bifid P wave in lead 2 and a prominent late negative deflection in V_1 related to left atrial enlargement. Atrial fibrillation is the most common abnormal rhythm. Despite severe degrees of right ventricular hypertrophy, the ECG commonly will disclose only right axis deviation with S waves in leads 1 and V_6 and an rSr′ in lead V_1 (Fig 34-2).

ECHOCARDIOGRAPHY IN MITRAL STENOSIS

Echocardiography has become the diagnostic tool of choice in the evaluation of mitral stenosis. The refinement of two-dimensional echocardiographic imaging and the introduction of Doppler echocardiography have produced an accurate, noninvasive method for determination of the severity of mitral stenosis. Other pertinent information obtainable from an echocardiographic examination of a patient with mitral stenosis includes extent of calcification and fibrosis of the mitral valve, presence of atrial thrombi, chamber size and function, and presence of other valvular abnormalities.

Prior to the late 1950s, no accurate noninvasive diagnostic method was available for confirmation of the clinical suspicion of mitral stenosis. In 1957, Edler and Gustafson[21] observed a decreased rate of diastolic closure of the mitral valve, typical of mitral stenosis, on M-mode echocardiography. M-mode echocardiography was at one time a highly accurate method for qualitative assessment of mitral stenosis. However, with the advent of two-dimensional echocardiography, most of these M-mode findings are of historical interest only (Fig 34-3).

Two-dimensional echocardiography

The two-dimensional echocardiographic examination has become an essential tool in the evaluation of mitral stenosis because it permits visualization of mitral valve motion in different tomographic planes in real time. It has become the standard for the diagnosis of mitral stenosis. In addition, the feasibility of mitral valve commissurotomy or percutaneous balloon valvuloplasty can be evaluated, and information can be obtained about chamber size and function and about other valvular abnormalities.

Findings on the parasternal long-axis view can be diagnostic for mitral stenosis (Fig 34-4). In mitral stenosis, there is thickening and calcification of the valve leaflets, which results in heavy, dense echoes from the valve. Mitral valve opening is restricted, seen as decreased excursion of the leaflets during diastole. The diagnostic feature of mitral stenosis is "doming" of the anterior leaflet in diastole – i.e., the body of the leaflet separates more widely than the edges (see Fig 34-4). The posterior leaflet is frequently immobile or severely restricted in diastolic movement. The maximum diastolic separation of the edges of both leaflets in the long-axis view indicates the approximate severity of mitral stenosis and should be used in conjunction with a short-axis view for quantitation.

Quantitation of the severity of mitral stenosis can be achieved by directly measuring the mitral valve orifice on the short-axis view[22-29] (Fig 34-5). This method is reliable

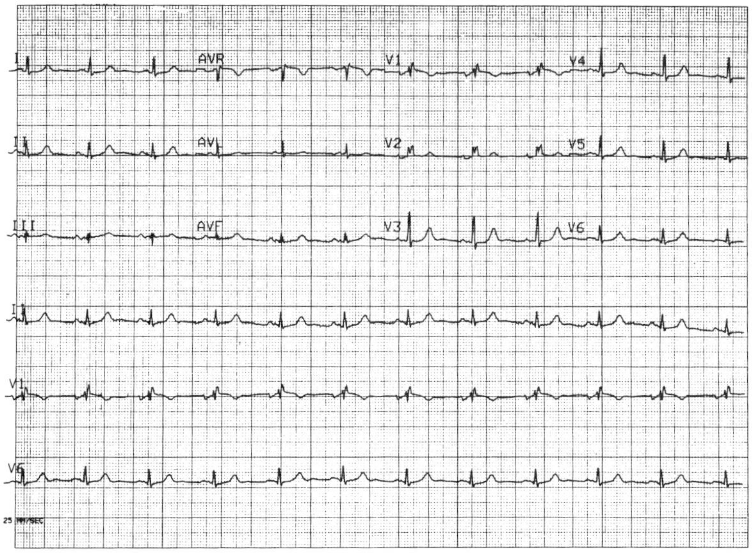

Fig 34-2 Mild right axis deviation and left atrial enlargement in a typical electrocardiogram from a patient with mitral stenosis.

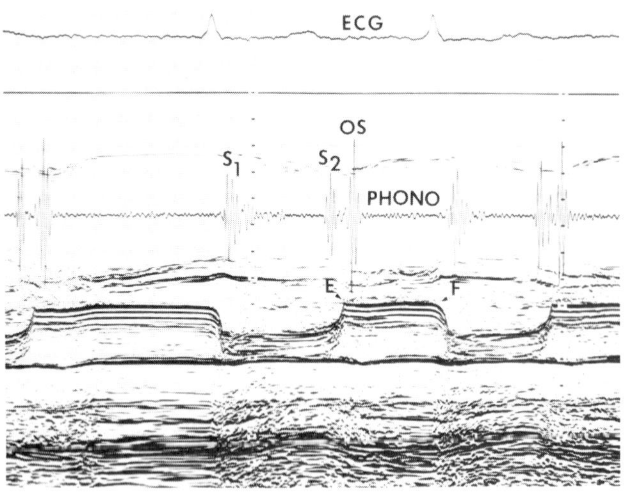

Fig 34-3 M-mode echocardiogram showing mitral stenosis. Heavy, dense echoes emanate from the anterior mitral valve leaflet, representing fibrosis and calcification. The E-to-F slope is flat, and there is no A point because the patient is in atrial fibrillation. The posterior leaflet is immobile. *ECG,* electocardiogram; *PHONO,* phonocardiogram; S_1, first heart sound; S_2, second heart sound; *OS,* opening snap.

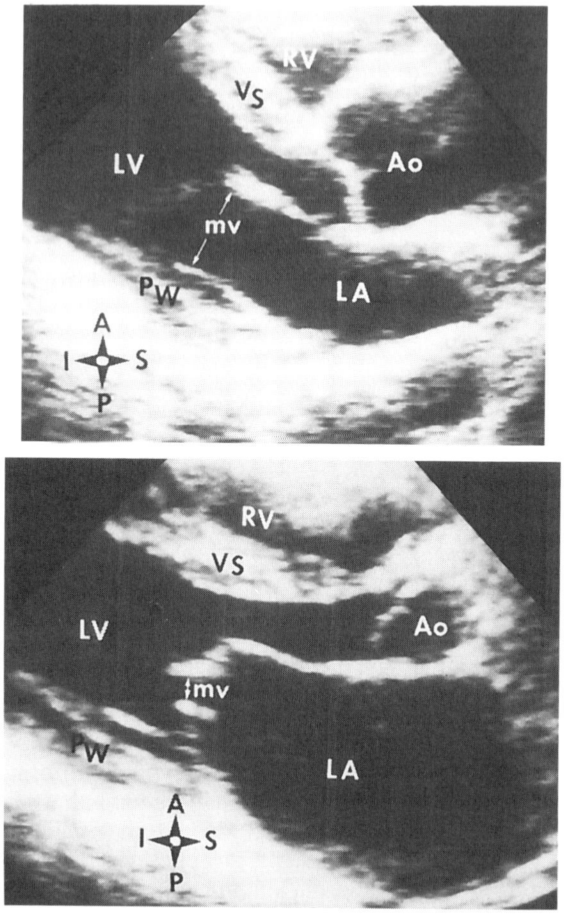

Fig 34-4 Two-dimensional echocardiograms in long-axis view. **Top,** normal heart during diastole. The mitral valve leaflets *(mv)* open widely *(arrows)* and are parallel to the ventricular septum *(VS)* and posterior wall *(PW).* **Bottom,** mitral stenosis during diastole. The anterior mitral valve leaflet demonstrates "doming," and the posterior leaflet is immobile, resulting in a restricted mitral valve orifice *(arrows).* The left atrium *(LA)* is enlarged. *A,* anterior; *Ao,* aorta; *I,* inferior; *LV,* left ventricle; *P,* posterior; *RV,* right ventricle; *S,* superior.

and reproducible.[25] There is excellent correlation between mitral valve area measured from a two-dimensional echocardiogram and the area measured directly on surgical or pathologic specimens.

The mitral valve orifice in the short-axis view must be scanned superiorly and inferiorly to find the smallest orifice. Because of doming of the anterior leaflet, a short-axis tomographic plane may overestimate the mitral valve orifice if not directly cut through the edges of the leaflets. Measuring the smallest separation at the tips of the leaflets on the long-axis view and comparing it to the anterior-posterior diameter at the mitral valve orifice on the short-axis view is important to document that the proper tomographic plane is taken. By use of a freeze frame in diastole, the opening can then be subjected to planimetry to give an accurate mitral valve area.

Although considered to be the standard for quantitation of mitral stenosis, two-dimensional echocardiographic measurement of mitral valve area has inherent drawbacks. There frequently are areas of dropout for which an assumption must be made as to the outline of the mitral valve orifice. Gain setting was a problem in the past, because using too high a gain could cause high divergent echoes. However, with the newer imaging techniques now available, this is rarely a problem. Lastly, the dense echoes reflected from a heavily calcified mitral valve or mitral valve annulus make it very difficult for the valve orifice to be measured (Fig 34-6). It is in these situations that Doppler echocardiography has become a valuable adjunct to the two-dimensional examination.

The two-dimensional echocardiogram has become the diagnostic modality of choice in determining suitability for commissurotomy or percutaneous mitral balloon valvuloplasty. Four major factors are well visualized by two-dimensional echocardiography: (1) valve mobility, (2) leaflet thickening, (3) degree of calcification, and (4) subvalvular fusion. A mitral valve score has been developed for semiquantitation.[30,31] A value of 1 to 4 is given for each of these characteristics, with 1 representing least involvement and 4 severe involvement. The mitral valve score is the sum of the four values. It has been shown that percutaneous mitral balloon valvuloplasty can be safely accomplished with excellent results if the score is less than 8. A score greater than 10, however, is associated with a higher risk of complications, less optimal results, and a high restenosis rate.[30-32] Calcification in the commissures may be another predictor of poor outcome.

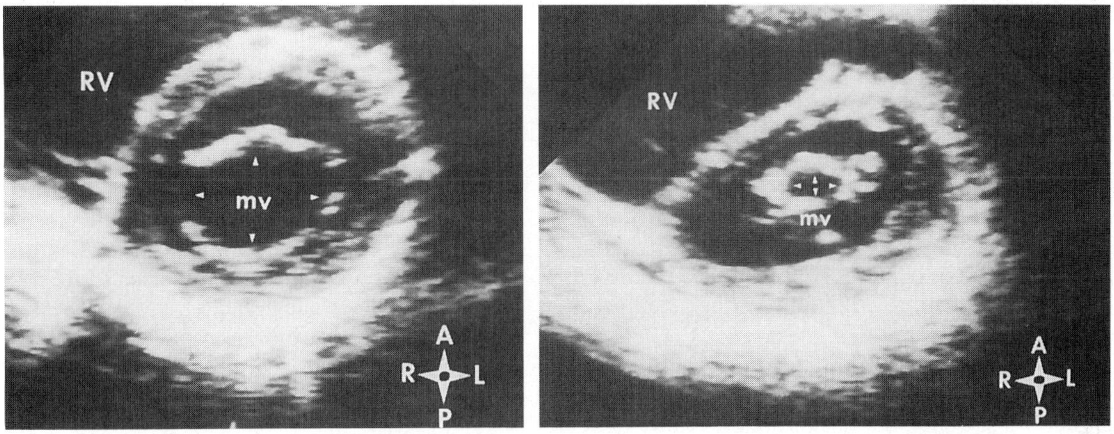

Fig 34-5 Two-dimensional echocardiograms in short-axis view. **Left,** normal mitral valve during diastole. The mitral valve leaflets *(mv)* are thin and mobile, resulting in an unrestricted mitral valve orifice *(arrows).* **Right,** mitral stenosis during diastole. There is severe restriction of opening of both anterior and posterior mitral valve leaflets, resulting in a significant left ventricular inflow obstruction *(arrows).* There is minimal calcification of the mitral valve leaflets. Note the enlarged right ventricle *(RV)* with flattening of the septum from pulmonary hypertension. *A,* anterior; *L,* left; *P,* posterior; *R,* right.

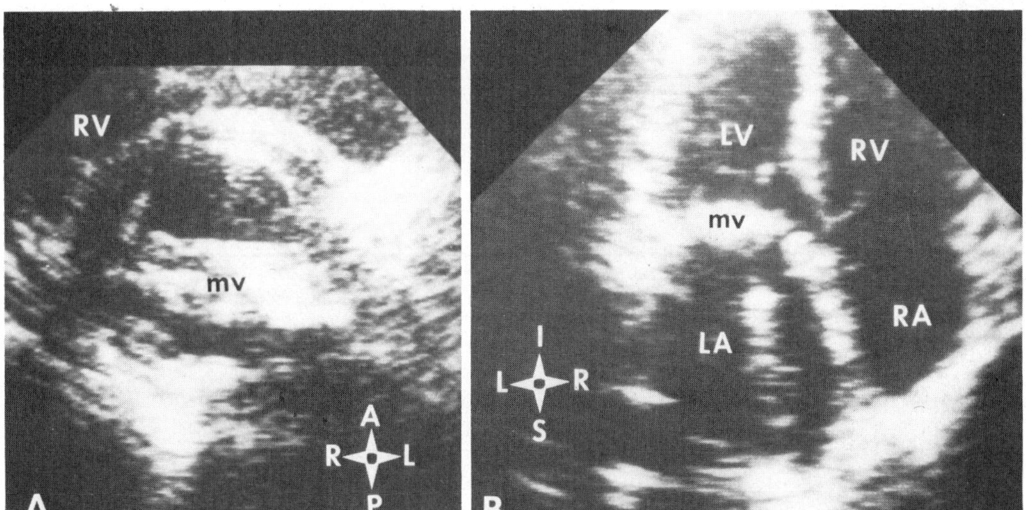

Fig 34-6 Two-dimensional echocardiogram in short-axis view (**A**) and four-chamber view (**B**) showing mitral stenosis. The mitral valve leaflets *(mv)* are heavily calcified, resulting in dense echoes from the valve. The degree of opening cannot be assessed because of the heavy calcification. The left atrium *(LA),* right ventricle *(RV),* and right atrium *(RA)* are enlarged in the four-chamber view. *A,* anterior; *I,* inferior; *L,* left; *LV,* left ventricle; *P,* posterior; *R,* right; *S,* superior.

In evaluating a patient for percutaneous mitral balloon valvuloplasty, it is essential to know if there is a thrombus present in the left atrium or left atrial appendage, since the multiple large catheters used during the procedure may cause dislodgment. Precordial two-dimensional echocardiography has a low sensitivity for detection of atrial thrombi because of the distance of this structure from the transducer. Transesophageal echocardiography provides reliable high-resolution images of the left atrium and left atrial appendage[33] and is very useful in ruling out thrombi before valvuloplasty.[34]

The two-dimensional echocardiographic examination is useful for diagnosis of other causes of left ventricular inflow obstruction. The other causes of left ventricular inflow obstruction include cor triatriatum, left atrial myxoma, supravalvular mitral ring, and parachute mitral valve.[35]

Information about the secondary effects of mitral stenosis can be gained from the two-dimensional echocardiographic examination. This technique permits measurement of the extent of dilatation of the left atrium and right-sided chambers. If the left ventricle is enlarged, coexistent regurgitant lesions must be considered. In addition, a decrease in left ventricular function or regional wall abnormalities would suggest the presence of coronary artery disease or a primary myopathic process. Because rheumatic heart disease may involve other valves, both the tricuspid and aortic valves can be visualized and assessed.

Doppler echocardiography

Two-dimensional echocardiography can portray mitral valve morphology and movement. Doppler echocardiography provides information concerning the flow of blood across the mitral valve and is highly accurate in the diagnosis as well as the quantitation of mitral stenosis.

Table 34-1 Severity of mitral stenosis

	Mean gradient	Mitral valve area, cm^2	Diastolic half-time, msec
Mild	0-4	>1.5	<150
Moderate	5-10	1.0-1.5	150-220
Severe	>10	<1.0	>220

In patients with mitral stenosis, there is a diastolic gradient between the left atrium and the left ventricle. The transmitral continuous-wave Doppler velocity curve thus consists of a high initial diastolic velocity (greater than 1.5 m/sec) and a slow rate of decline of the initial velocity (Fig 34-7).

There are several methods by which information may be gained from the Doppler signal to estimate the severity of mitral stenosis (Table 34-1). Instantaneous pressure drop (ΔP) between two chambers can be calculated from the Doppler velocity (V) by using a modified Bernoulli equation ($\Delta P = 4 \times V^2$). The mitral valve Doppler velocity tracing can be used to determine the mean pressure gradient across the mitral valve. The correlation between simultaneous cardiac catheterization measurements and pressure gradients calculated from Doppler echocardiography is excellent[36-40] (Fig 34-8). Because of catheter "whip" artifacts and inherent problems with pulmonary capillary wedge pressures, conventional right and left heart catheterization may provide inaccurate measure-

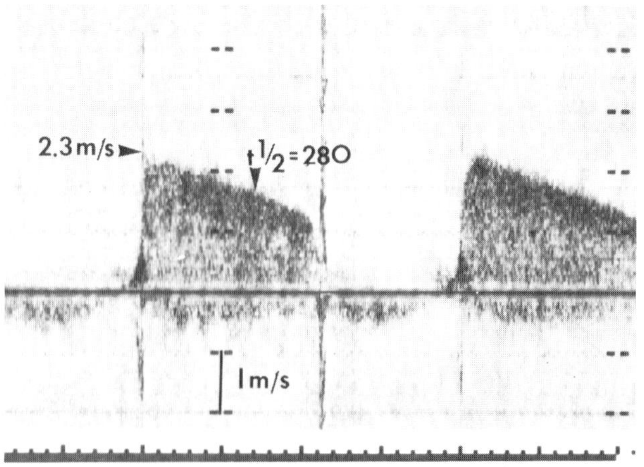

Fig 34-7 Continuous-wave Doppler echocardiogram of the mitral valve from a patient with mitral stenosis. The initial peak diastolic velocity is markedly increased to 2.3 m/sec, corresponding to a left ventricle-left atrium pressure gradient of 21 mm Hg. The diastolic slope is delayed, resulting in a diastolic half-time ($t_{½}$) of 280 msec, equivalent to a mitral valve area of 0.8 cm^2.

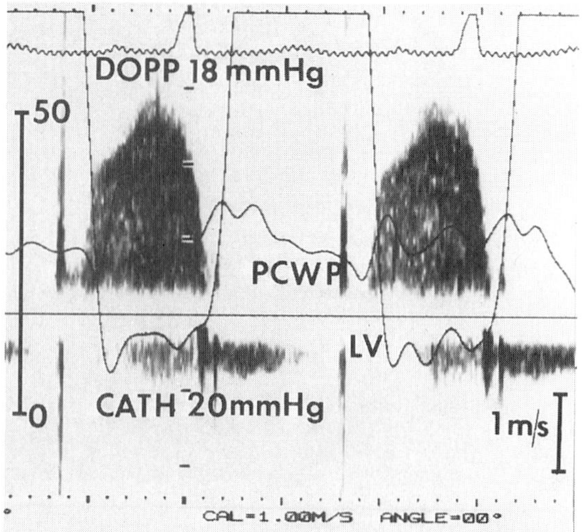

Fig 34-8 Simultaneous left ventricular *(LV)* and pulmonary capillary wedge pressure *(PCWP)* tracing and the continuous-wave Doppler mitral flow velocity curve *(DOPP)* in a patient with mitral stenosis. The mean gradient by cardiac catheterization *(CATH)* is similar to the mean gradient by Doppler echocardiography.

ments of transmitral gradients.[41,42] Since the transmitral Doppler velocity is technically easy to obtain from the apical position, Doppler echocardiography should be considered the optimal method to measure mean gradient in a patient with mitral stenosis.

The second method for quantitation of the severity of mitral stenosis uses diastolic half-time ($t_{1/2}$) (see Fig 34-7). As the stenosis becomes more severe, the decline in diastolic pressure gradient between the left atrium and the left ventricle is slower. The rate of decline can be measured by the $t_{1/2}$, which is the time it takes for the gradient to decrease to 50%. This is an accurate measurement of the severity of mitral stenosis because it is inversely proportional to the mitral valve area and is independent of heart rate, coexistent mitral regurgitation, or variation in R-R interval (seen with atrial fibrillation). The $t_{1/2}$ is calculated from the Doppler tracing by converting the initial peak velocity in early diastole to a pressure drop. The initial pressure drop is divided by 2 and transformed back to velocity. The time it takes the Doppler signal to reach this velocity from the initial peak velocity is the $t_{1/2}$. Another way to measure $t_{1/2}$ is to obtain a deceleration time, which is the time from the initial peak velocity to the point at which an extrapolation of the deceleration of flow reaches the baseline. Multiplication of the deceleration time by 0.29 provides a measurement of $t_{1/2}$ (see chapter 5B). Normally the $t_{1/2}$ is 20 to 60 msec; in mitral stenosis, it reaches 90 to >300 msec. Hatle et al.[43] found that by dividing 220 by the $t_{1/2}$, a value for the mitral valve area can be obtained directly. Measurement of the diastolic $t_{1/2}$ by Doppler echocardiography is accurate and reproducible in the evaluation of the severity of mitral stenosis[39,40,43] (Table 34-1 and Fig 34-9).

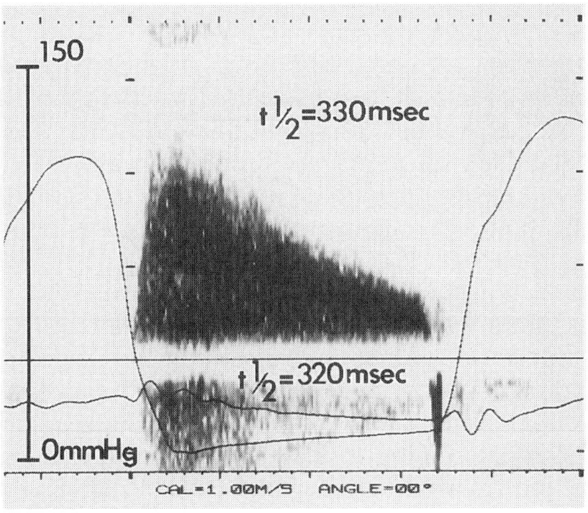

Fig 34-9 Simultaneous pulmonary capillary wedge and left ventricular pressures along with the continuous-wave Doppler velocity curve in a patient with mitral stenosis. The diastolic half-time ($t_{1/2}$) by cardiac catheterization correlates well with the diastolic half-time by Doppler echocardiography. (From Nishimura RA, Tajik AJ: Quantitative hemodynamics by Doppler echocardiography: a noninvasive alternative to cardiac catheterization. *Prog Cardiovasc Dis* 36:309-342, 1994. By permission of WB Saunders Company.)

The diastolic $t_{1/2}$ is dependent on factors other than the severity of the obstruction. These factors include compliance of the left atrium and left ventricle. Since there is a significant change in the compliance of both cardiac chambers immediately after an acute intervention, such as commissurotomy or balloon valvuloplasty, the diastolic $t_{1/2}$ becomes inaccurate.[44-46] Therefore, the diastolic $t_{1/2}$ should not be used in assessing the acute results of these interventions, although it again becomes accurate several days after the procedure.[46] Other factors that influence left ventricular compliance, such as severe aortic regurgitation and myocardial dysfunction, may cause inaccuracies in the diastolic $t_{1/2}$. Therefore, in the evaluation of a patient with mitral stenosis by Doppler echocardiography, the results of the mitral valve area calculated by the diastolic $t_{1/2}$ should be correlated with other factors, such as clinical history, two-dimensional echocardiographic appearance of the mitral valve, and measured mean gradient. If there is a discrepancy among these variables, other methods of calculating mitral valve area should be pursued.

One other method is the use of the continuity equation, in which flow through the mitral valve is equated with flow through another valve orifice,[47,48] preferably the left ventricular outflow tract.

$$\text{Flow}_{MV} = \text{Area}_{LVO}$$
$$\text{Area}_{MV} \times \text{TVI}_{MV} = \text{Area}_{LVO} \times \text{TVI}_{LVO}$$
$$\text{Area}_{MV} = (\text{Area}_{LVO} \times \text{TVI}_{LVO}) \div \text{TVI}_{MV}$$

in which MV is the mitral valve, LVO is the left ventricular outflow tract, TVI is the time velocity integral of the Doppler velocity curves, Area_{LVO} is the area of the left ventricular outflow tract as measured on two-dimensional echocardiography, and Area_{MV} is the calculated mitral valve area. If concomitant aortic or mitral regurgitation is absent, this is an accurate method for calculating mitral valve area.[47,48] Proximal flow acceleration may also be used to calculate mitral valve area.

Doppler echocardiography is useful in the evaluation of other valvular abnormalities coexistent with mitral stenosis. It can detect and semiquantitate coexistent aortic or mitral regurgitation. Evaluation of the tricuspid valve for stenosis or regurgitation is done in the same manner as for the mitral valve. In addition, if tricuspid regurgitation is present, right ventricular and, in many cases, pulmonary artery systolic pressure can be estimated by determining the peak systolic velocity.[49]

DIAGNOSTIC PROBLEMS AND INDICATIONS FOR INVASIVE STUDIES

The diagnosis and severity of mitral stenosis can usually be determined clinically with ease on the basis of the history and clinical examination. In some situations, the clinical diagnosis of mitral stenosis becomes more difficult, such as when severe pulmonary hypertension or severe chronic obstructive pulmonary disease is present. Other disease states, such as severe aortic regurgitation, atrial septal defect, and dilated cardiomyopathy, may have findings on examination that mimic mitral stenosis. However, with the widespread use of two-dimensional and Doppler echocardiography, these rarely present a significant problem.

The results of the history, clinical examination, and two-dimensional and Doppler echocardiography can be used to determine the diagnosis and severity of mitral stenosis in most instances. Cardiac catheterization should not be required for evaluation of mitral valve hemodynamics at rest, although it may be useful in determining the degree of coexistent regurgitant lesions. In patients with symptoms of angina pectoris or risk factors for coronary artery disease, coronary angiography should be performed if intervention is contemplated.

Since the decision to intervene depends on the patient's symptoms, it is important to determine the relationship of mitral valve hemodynamics to the production of symptoms. In a patient with severe mitral stenosis and New York Heart Association functional class III-IV symptoms, it is clear that improving mitral valve hemodynamics will be beneficial. Conversely, in a patient with mild mitral stenosis and minimal or no symptoms, continued observation is warranted. However, diagnostic problems arise when there is a discrepancy between measured mitral valve hemodynamics and symptoms. In this circumstance, exercise hemodynamics are very useful. These can be done either by right and left heart catheterization with exercise or by exercise Doppler echocardiography, examining the response of the mitral valve gradients and pulmonary pressures to exercise.

MANAGEMENT

After an attack or attacks of acute rheumatic fever, the only treatment indicated for the next 15 to 25 years is prophylaxis with antibiotics. The duration of therapy is arbitrary and judgmental, but treatment is usually appropriate until age 30 years. Higher doses of antibiotics are used temporarily for surgical or dental procedures even though infective endocarditis is rare in isolated mitral stenosis.

With the onset of mild symptoms of effort dyspnea and fatigue, only counseling on general measures is usually necessary. The patient is urged to avoid unusual physical stresses—the advisability of a prudent lifestyle with adequate rest and a physical activity program consistent with the clinical state is emphasized. Since the gradient in mitral stenosis depends highly on diastolic filling, the use of β-blockers to decrease the heart rate response to exercise may result in significant improvements in exercise tolerance in patients with mild-to-moderate symptoms.

Intervention in the patient with mitral stenosis is clearly indicated if symptoms are debilitating, that is, New York Heart Association functional class III or IV. Because the left ventricle is protected by the stenotic mitral valve, there is no need to intervene in the patient with minimal symptoms to prevent left ventricular dysfunction, such as that occurring in patients with regurgitant lesions. Thus, the symptomatic response to the stenotic mitral valve determines the timing of intervention. In patients whose symptoms are out of proportion to measured mitral valve hemodynamics, exercise testing is recommended to gain an objective measurement of exercise tolerance. Because the rheumatic process is slowly progressive, many patients gradually decrease their daily activity without becoming aware of significant limitations imposed by the mitral stenosis. Concomitant Doppler echocardiography can add hemodynamic information to that of the exercise test.

In a subgroup of patients who claim not to have symptoms, increasing pulmonary hypertension develops from severe mitral stenosis. Intervention has been recommended in these patients to prevent irreversible pulmonary vascular disease and subsequent right heart failure. These patients are usually significantly limited on objective exercise testing but, because of their sedentary daily activity, have not experienced symptoms; they should undergo an interventional procedure.

The decision to proceed with an interventional procedure is usually made on the basis of history or objective exercise testing, or both. The patient with minimal or no symptoms can be followed conservatively with a yearly careful history and examination. In patients with more severe symptoms, the decision to intervene should be tempered by the knowledge that many patients with mitral stenosis can undergo operative intervention without the insertion of a valvular prosthesis, that is, percutaneous mitral balloon valvuloplasty or surgical commissurotomy. Thus, the decision to operate is made earlier in the patient with a mobile, noncalcified mitral valve in whom valvuloplasty or commissurotomy is an option than in the patient with a heavily calcified mitral valve in whom mitral valve replacement is necessary. If a patient has moderate symptoms, New York Heart Association functional class II+, especially if they are progressing, intervention is reasonable if valvuloplasty or commissurotomy can be performed. Alternatively, the patient with a heavily calcified valve in whom commissurotomy is not possible should be operated on only if symptoms are of class III-IV severity.

If the initial significant presenting symptom is acute pulmonary edema, it is most often precipitated by the onset of paroxysmal atrial fibrillation with a rapid ventricular rate. Formerly, the therapeutic approach was intravenous treatment with digoxin to slow the ventricular rate, morphine, oxygen, and intravenous heparin. This has been modified in that verapamil or diltiazem (given intravenously) may be substituted for digoxin. Oral digitalis therapy would then be started to maintain a slow ventricular rate, and, if conversion to a normal sinus rhythm does not occur, a group IA or group IC agent could be added in an attempt to obtain pharmacologic conversion under ECG monitoring. If this is not successful, elective electrical direct current cardioversion can be carried out.

In chronic, sustained, or recurrent atrial fibrillation, digoxin, verapamil, diltiazem, or a β-blocker can be used to control the ventricular response. If the patient's symptoms resolve or are minimal after treatment of atrial fibrillation, medical therapy will delay surgical intervention for a number of years.

Thromboembolic problems continue to be one of the most troublesome complications of mitral stenosis. Systemic thromboembolism is particularly likely to occur with the onset of atrial fibrillation, and consequently intravenous heparin therapy should be started promptly when this event occurs. It has also seemed appropriate for patients to be receiving long-term anticoagulant therapy when conversion from atrial fibrillation to normal sinus rhythm is planned. All clinicians encounter difficult judgmental problems in selecting patients for long-term anticoagulant therapy in the presence of mitral stenosis.

Patients particularly at risk seem to be those who have chronic atrial fibrillation and a large left atrium. Systemic arterial emboli have been noted, however, in patients with normal sinus rhythm and with only a slightly enlarged left atrium. The authors have generally followed the premise that long-term anticoagulant therapy is indicated for patients with mitral stenosis who are in chronic atrial fibrillation or have a history of recurrent paroxysmal atrial fibrillation and who have significant enlargement of the left atrium or a history of a thromboembolic event. In elderly patients, the risk of bleeding with anticoagulant therapy is clearly increased and must be weighed against the risks of the thromboembolic tendency.

INTERVENTIONS FOR TREATMENT OF MITRAL STENOSIS

The treatment of the patient with severe, symptomatic mitral stenosis has undergone significant changes in the past decade. Mitral commissurotomy, the first intracardiac surgical intervention performed in large numbers for acquired heart disease, is still a highly effective procedure. The closed approach has gradually given way to an open approach using cardiopulmonary bypass, for reasons outlined below. In percutaneous mitral balloon valvuloplasty, one or more large balloons are inserted percutaneously and inflated across the stenotic mitral valve.[50-57] It can alleviate symptoms to an extent comparable to closed commissurotomy and is becoming the procedure of choice in some institutions for treatment of mitral stenosis in properly selected patients.

These three procedures (closed commissurotomy, open commissurotomy, and percutaneous mitral balloon valvuloplasty) are most effective in patients with pliable, noncalcified valves. In patients with heavily calcified, fibrotic valves and subvalvular fusion, mitral valve replacement is the procedure of choice. The morphologic state of the mitral valve can be determined preoperatively by the physical examination (a loud first heart sound and a crisp opening snap, indicating a pliable valve) and confirmed by two-dimensional echocardiography.

Percutaneous mitral balloon valvuloplasty

Percutaneous mitral balloon valvuloplasty was first introduced in the mid-1980s as a nonsurgical approach for the treatment of severe mitral stenosis.[51,58] Inflating one or more large balloons across the mitral valve relieves stenosis in selected patients. The overall results of the procedure depend greatly on such factors as leaflet morphology and operator experience. Thus, the decision to proceed with percutaneous mitral balloon valvuloplasty is based not only on the patient's symptoms but also on the degree and type of involvement of the mitral valve apparatus and the facilities available to the patient.

The technique of percutaneous mitral balloon valvuloplasty is technically challenging.[50] It requires a transseptal puncture so that balloons can be placed by a femoral venous route into the right atrium, into the left atrium, and then through the mitral valve (Fig 34-10). Various

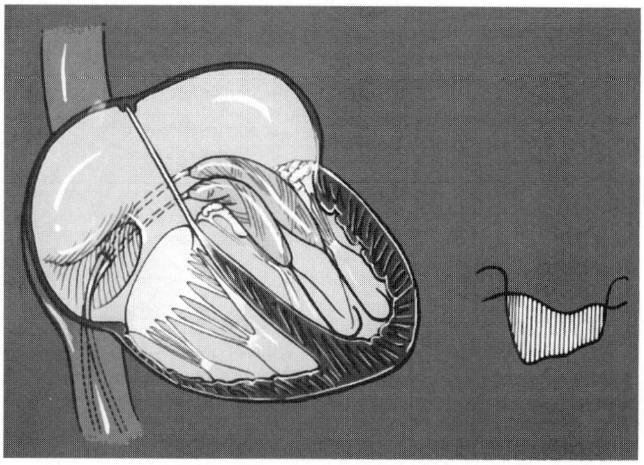

Fig 34-10 Drawing of a dual-balloon technique for mitral balloon valvuloplasty. One or more large balloons are placed across the fossa ovalis from the right atrium to the left atrium. The balloons are then passed across the mitral valve partially into the left ventricle. During inflation, both balloons straddle the mitral valve and produce a splitting of fused commissures. (From Nishimura RA, Holmes DR Jr, Reeder GS: Percutaneous balloon valvuloplasty. *Mayo Clin Proc* 65:198-220, 1990. By permission of Mayo Foundation for Medical Education and Research.)

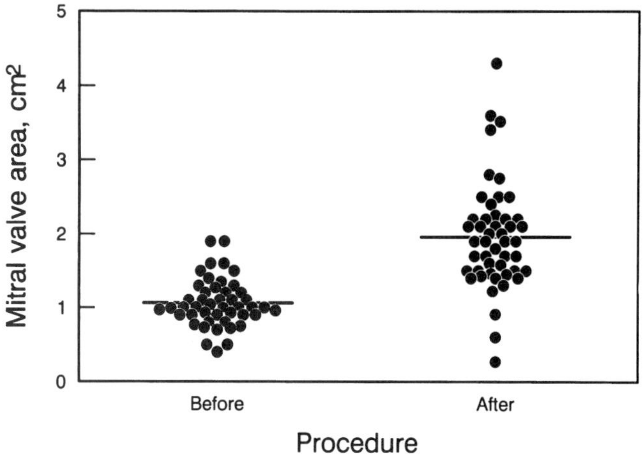

Fig 34-11 Initial Mayo Clinic experience with the first 50 patients undergoing percutaneous mitral balloon valvuloplasty. Mean mitral valve area increased from 1 cm^2 before the procedure to 2 cm^2 after the procedure. (Modified from Nishimura RA, Holmes DR Jr, Reeder GS: Percutaneous balloon valvuloplasty. *Mayo Clin Proc* 65:198-220, 1990.)

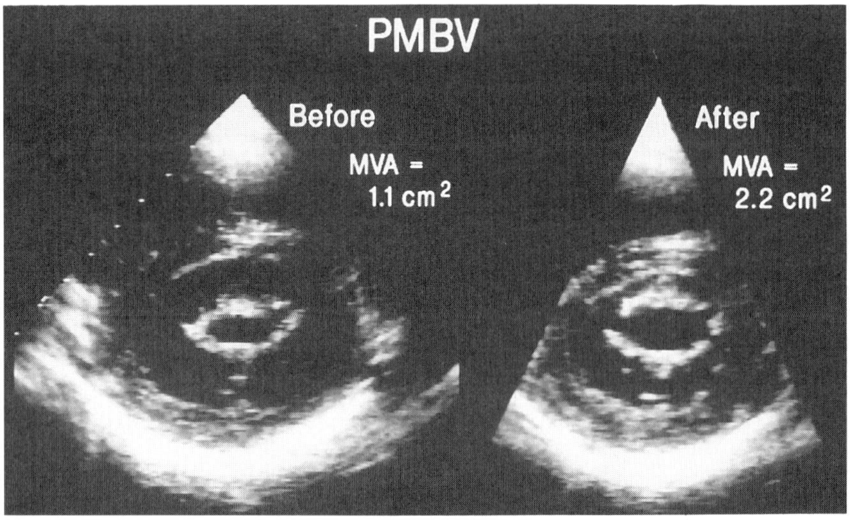

Fig 34-12 Two-dimensional short-axis echocardiographic views of the mitral valve before **(left)** and after **(right)** percutaneous mitral balloon valvuloplasty *(PMBV)* show that splitting of fused commissures significantly increased mitral valve area *(MVA)*.

methods are currently used, including those accomplished with a large single balloon, dual balloons,[59] and a specially designed pillow-shaped balloon (the Inoue balloon).[58] There are no proven benefits to any one technique, although final valve area tends to be larger with the dual-balloon technique and the chance of major complications is perhaps less with the self-stabilizing Inoue balloon.[60]

When successful, percutaneous mitral balloon valvuloplasty significantly improves hemodynamics and greatly reduces symptoms on short-term follow-up.[31,53,55-57,61-66] Usually, the mean gradient is reduced by 50% and the initial mitral valve area is doubled (Fig 34-11). Percutaneous mitral balloon valvuloplasty, like surgical commissurotomy, splits fused commissures[67,68] (Fig 34-12). Thus, the final hemodynamic results in selected patients after percutaneous mitral balloon valvuloplasty are similar to those achieved by surgical commissurotomy in selected patients.[64]

Major complications can occur during the procedure. These include cardiac tamponade (2% to 7%), systemic embolization (2% to 3%), emergency surgery (2% to 6%), and death (1% to 4%).[50,61,63-65,69] The degree of mitral regurgitation usually increases by one grade in 30% to 40% of patients and by two grades in 10% of patients; severe mitral regurgitation develops in 2% to 3% of patients.[31] Residual atrial septal defects are common, occurring in 18% to 20% of patients, with a Qp:Qs of more than 1.3 in 7% to 8% of patients.[57,61] Most of these septal defects appear to close during short-term follow-up.[57] A steep operator curve is associated with this procedure for both the occurrence of complications and the rate of success.[70] Thus, it has been recommended that this procedure be limited to use by experienced operators in hospitals with facilities for cardiac surgery.[50,61]

The morphology of the mitral valve apparatus is closely related to success in patients undergoing percutaneous mitral balloon valvuloplasty.[31,50,62] In patients with pliable, noncalcified valves, the initial success rate is higher, the complication rate lower, and the event-free rate on follow-up higher. Conversely, in patients with calcified, fibrotic valves and subvalvular fusion, the rate of complications increases, the initial success rate is lower, and long-term outcome is better. The type of valve morphology can be estimated by physical examination, because patients with loud intensity of the first heart sound and a crisp opening snap have more pliable valves. Direct visualization of valve morphology is possible on two-dimensional echocardiographic examination (Fig 34-13), and an echocardiographic score has been devised for semiquantitation of mitral valve morphology.[31] In this scoring system, a grade from 1 to 4 is assigned for leaflet mobility, leaflet thickening, subvalvular thickening, and calcification, with 1 being the least and 4 the most involvement. The sum of the individual grades equals the mitral valve score. In patients with a score of less than 8, the chance of a good outcome (final mitral valve area of more than 1.5 cm^2 or an increase in mitral valve area of at least 25%) is 84%, whereas in patients with a score of greater than 8, 58% have suboptimal results.[62] In the initial Mayo Clinic experience (Fig 34-14), the final mitral valve area was inversely related to the echocardiographic score and only patients with a score exceeding 8 had complications.[50] For follow-up, the event-free (free of mitral valve replacement, repeat percutaneous mitral balloon valvuloplasty, and cardiac death) survival rates at 1 and 2 years, respectively, were 91% and 94% in those with a score of 8 or lower and 72% and 58% in those with a score higher than 8.[64] Even in patients with higher scores, mitral valvuloplasty may be successful if the commissures are not heavily calcified.

In patients with noncalcified, mobile mitral valve

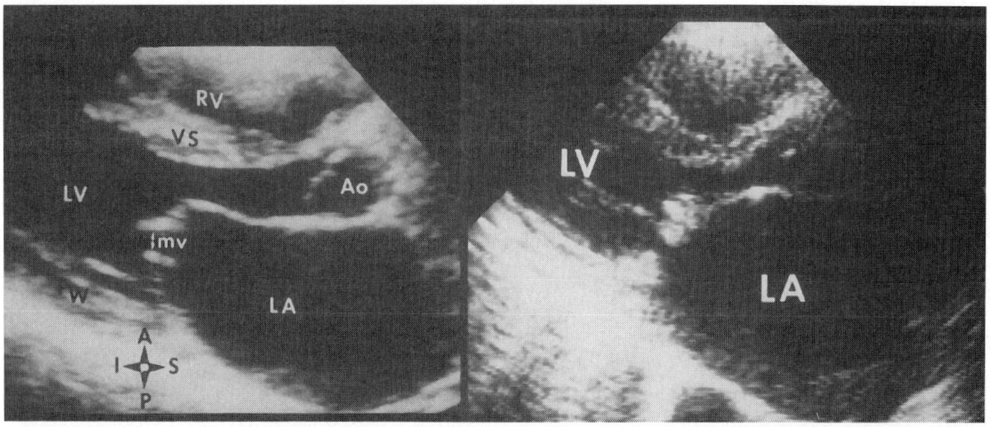

Fig 34-13 Parasternal long-axis views in two patients with mitral stenosis. **Left,** pliable, noncalcified valve with a score of 6. **Right,** heavily calcified, fibrotic valve with subvalvular fusion and a score of 12 (see text). *A,* anterior; *Ao,* aorta; *I,* inferior; *LA,* left atrium; *LV,* left ventricle; *mv,* mitral valve; *P,* posterior; *PW,* posterior wall; *RV,* right ventricle; *S,* superior; *VS,* ventricular septum.

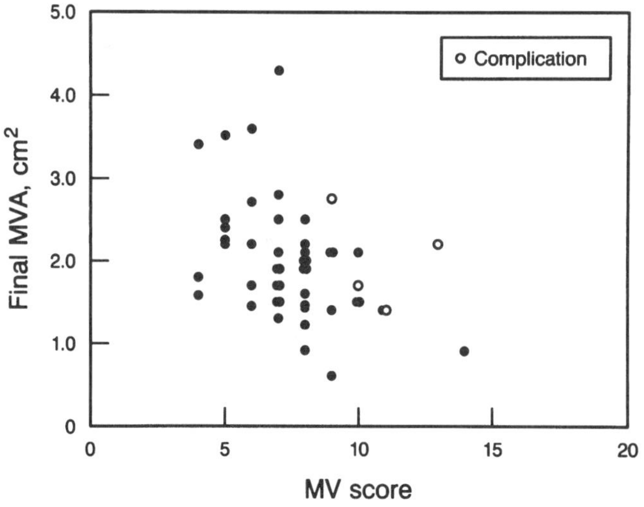

Fig 34-14 Scatterplot of the initial mitral valve *(MV)* score and the final mitral valve area *(MVA)* in the first 50 patients undergoing percutaneous mitral balloon valvuloplasty at the Mayo Clinic shows an inverse relationship between the two measurements. All complications *(open circles)* occurred in patients with scores of 9 or greater. (Modified from Nishimura RA, Holmes DR Jr, Reeder GS: Percutaneous balloon valvuloplasty. *Mayo Clin Proc* 65:198-220, 1990.)

leaflets who need intervention, percutaneous mitral balloon valvuloplasty is considered the initial treatment of choice in many institutions. In this select subgroup of patients, the procedure can be performed with low risk and a high success rate. Although follow-up is limited, in patients with a score of less than 8, the 5-year event-free survival rate was 84%, similar to that expected after surgical commissurotomy.[64] The cost of percutaneous mitral balloon valvuloplasty is about 10% of that of an open heart procedure. The length of hospital stay is less than 2 days, and the patient can return to daily activities shortly thereafter. However, the patients who truly benefit from this procedure form a select subgroup, and balloon valvuloplasty should be performed only in institutions having experience with the technique. Continuing follow-up is required to determine whether the long-term results will be comparable to those obtained by surgical commissurotomy.

In the workup of patients with severe, symptom-producing mitral stenosis who might be considered candidates for balloon valvuloplasty, echocardiography should be performed to determine mitral valve morphology. If the score is less than 8 or the commissures are not heavily calcified, transesophageal echocardiography should be done to rule out an atrial clot[34] or significant mitral regurgitation, which would preclude valvuloplasty. If an experienced operator is available, percutaneous mitral balloon valvuloplasty is a reasonable option in these patients. In patients with more calcified mitral valve leaflets or thickened subvalvular fusion, surgery should then be performed. At operation, the valve can be inspected and the decision made on whether open commissurotomy or mitral valve replacement should be done.

Mitral commissurotomy

In those socioeconomic situations in which cost is not an overwhelming consideration, the "closed" mitral commissurotomy has appropriately gradually given way to use of the open approach with use of the heart-lung machine. The closed approach is still preferred in some areas.

Closed approach. Closed commissurotomy is performed without the use of cardiopulmonary bypass—the heart is functioning and maintaining the circulation. A finger is passed into the left atrium via its appendage, and usually a dilating instrument is passed through a stab

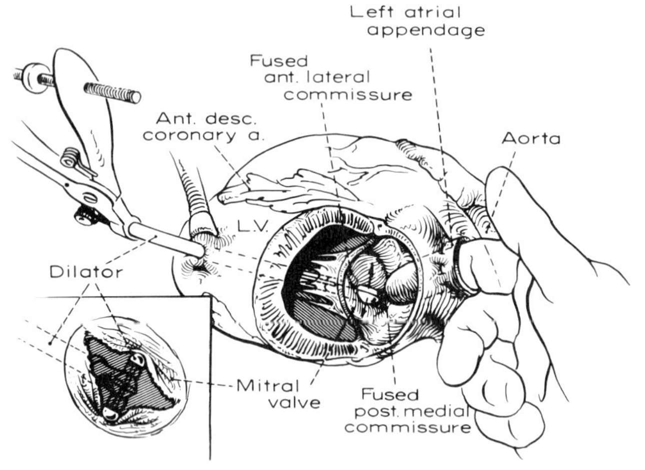

Fig 34-15 Technique of closed mitral commissurotomy using a mitral dilating instrument. (From Ellis FH Jr, Boolukos GPN, Connolly DC: Reoperation for mitral stenosis. *Arch Surg* 85:675-681, 1962. By permission of the American Medical Association.)

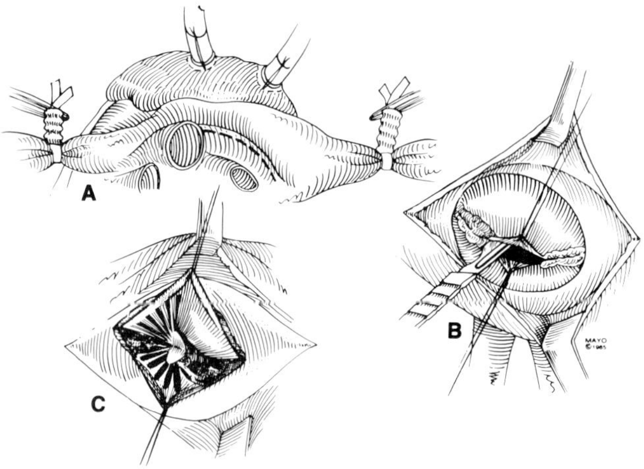

Fig 34-16 Technique of open mitral commissurotomy. **A,** the approach is through an incision into the left atrium just behind the right atrium and the interatrial groove. **B,** note the curved configuration of the mitral orifice and the fused commissures. Sharp dissection is used to open the commissures. **C,** the commissural incision can be extended through the corresponding commissural pillar of fused chordae and even into the papillary muscle to achieve maximal mobility of the leaflets. (By permission, Mayo Foundation.)

wound at the apex of the left ventricle and then into the orifice of the mitral valve, where the instrument is opened so that the valve commissures are split (Fig 34-15). Occasionally, particularly in young patients with relatively recent onset of severe mitral stenosis, finger pressure alone is sufficient to fracture the adhesions binding the two mitral leaflets at their commissures. Fortunately, the pathology of a stenotic mitral valve is such that the dilation procedure can be successful in the vast majority of patients—that is, the fusion of the commissures is more susceptible to fracture than are the leaflets themselves. Because of this fortunate situation, the results of closed mitral commissurotomy have been excellent.

COMMENT. The closed approach has given way to use of the open approach for several reasons. The closed operation provides the surgeon with less absolute control over the operative conditions. Some valves are "leathery," so that the commissures are difficult to split without fear of tearing the leaflets. Furthermore, if intraoperative complications develop, such as ventricular fibrillation, hemorrhage, or acute mitral insufficiency due to significant tearing of the valve, recovery is more hectic or less probable than if cardiopulmonary bypass were used. Additionally, closed mitral commissurotomy is often difficult to teach and to learn, because only the operating surgeon can feel what is being done within the heart. Therefore, much more so than for other operations, the surgical resident must go through a learning experience of trial and error while gaining familiarity with the precise amount of tension to be exerted on the dilator, etc. Also, entry into the heart with the finger and instruments incurs a risk of thromboembolism from unsuspected or unencountered thrombus in the atrium or left ventricle. Furthermore, experience has demonstrated a very low risk associated with open-heart repair of mitral stenosis, the expected mortality being no more than 2% for open mitral commissurotomy.

Open approach. In performing open mitral commissurotomy, extracorporeal circulation and cardioplegic myocardial protection are instituted in the usual manner. Typically, the left atrium is incised longitudinally just lateral to the interatrial groove on the right aspect of the atria. When it is established that tricuspid exposure also will be needed, and especially when the atria are significantly dilated, exposure of the mitral valve via a right atriotomy and an atrial septotomy is preferred. After careful study of the valve, the surgeon must decide whether commissurotomy is feasible.

Sometimes the commissurotomy is begun by using a valve dilator. In any case, the commissures are identified by placing traction on the leaflets. Some surgeons prefer incising the commissures from the annulus toward the orifice, and others do it in the opposite direction. It is important to appreciate that the mitral orifice, and hence its commissures, is so oriented that in the closed position the valve forms a distinct curvilinear configuration, with the concavity oriented anteriorly (Fig 34-16).

As the commissure is progressively being opened, usually by sharp dissection, it is important that the surgeon be oriented appropriately with respect to the underlying fan of chordae so that the incision is always in the middle of the commissure rather than deviating into either the anterior or posterior leaflet. Typically, dense fusion of the chordae deep to the valve is encountered. This fused mass should be incised and separated, thus restoring as much mobility as possible to the leaflets. At times it is appropriate to carry the incision of fused chordae down into the papillary muscle and, at times, even to fenestrate the mass of fused chordae in an effort to simulate the presence of individual chordae.

After obtaining as complete a restoration of the mitral orifice as possible, it is essential not to allow the existence of any mitral insufficiency to go unrecognized or unrelieved. Various techniques to test the valve's competence during operation should be used, such as distending the left ventricle gently with fluid or blood. Further confirmation of the valve's competence after reinstitution of normal circulation can be provided by recording double dye-dilution curves or by intraoperative contrast echocardiography. If insufficiency of more than a mild degree has been induced, it must be repaired by annuloplasty or plastic repair of leaflets; if this is not feasible, the valve may need to be replaced. Open operation on the mitral valve should include closure of the orifice into the left atrial appendage in order to minimize the chance of thromboembolism later.

The management of mitral valvular insufficiency is discussed in chapter 35.

Postoperative care

Pulmonary hypertension with consequent stiffening of the lungs is nearly universally present preoperatively and does not subside immediately after mitral commissurotomy. For this reason, the work of ventilation is usually found to be increased postoperatively, thus requiring careful evaluation as to the appropriate time to discontinue ventilatory assistance. Usually, such assistance is required at least throughout the first postoperative night and at times for an additional period.

In patients who had maintained a sinus rhythm preoperatively, atrial fibrillation not uncommonly develops postoperatively, sometimes in a paroxysmal fashion. Therefore, patients who came to operation in sinus rhythm should have sinus rhythm restored before dismissal from the hospital. For patients with long-standing preoperative atrial fibrillation, cardioversion probably should be postponed until several months postoperatively; the likelihood of persisting sinus rhythm after early postoperative cardioversion is small in this situation.

Thromboembolism is a distinct risk both before and after operation for mitral stenosis, ranging from 1% to 27% per patient-year, depending on administration of anticoagulant treatment, rhythm, and whether a commissurotomy had been done.[71] Long-term (indefinitely) anticoagulation with warfarin is indicated in postcommissurotomy patients who are in atrial fibrillation or whose valve could not be enlarged adequately at operation, especially if embolism had occurred previously, the left atrium is markedly enlarged, and the rheumatic involvement had been prolonged.

Results of operation

The hospital mortality associated with mitral commissurotomy is low, no more than 1% or 2%, and a little lower than the risk associated with mitral valve replacement. The few deaths that do occur are predominantly related to an inadequate performance of the myocardium with resultant acute or subacute cardiac failure.

The late result of operation depends mainly on the degree to which normal mitral valve function was restored by operation. Thus, the symptomatic result and long-term survival will be most improved in the young patient who has a pliable, noncalcified valve with a relatively recent, relatively fibrinous type of adherence of the anterior and posterior leaflets at their commissures. Such valves can be restored to essentially normal function. These patients should enjoy complete relief of the symptoms and signs of their mitral stenosis. At the other extreme, a patient who has a valve that is so immobilized as to be nearly in need of replacement might obtain only limited benefit from commissurotomy, and probably would become a candidate for reoperation and valve replacement within just a few years.

The pathologic state of the mitral valve does not remain static after mitral commissurotomy but continues to progress. The likelihood that reoperation will be required 10, 20, or even 30 years postoperatively should be carefully explained to the patient preoperatively.

The overall late results of open mitral commissurotomy are relatively good. In a study by Smith et al.[71] the risk of death by 8 years postoperatively, determined actuarially, was 14%, the risk of reoperation among survivors was 16%, and the risk of thromboembolism among survivors not reoperated on was 11%. Similarly, in the early experience at the Mayo Clinic, survival after closed transventricular commissurotomy was 79%, 67%, and 55% at 10, 15, and 20 years postoperatively. Probability of surviving without mitral valve reoperation was 57% at 10 years and 24% at 20 years.[72] The issue of whether open or closed commissurotomy provides better long-term relief of mitral stenosis has not been settled. In the experience of Hickey et al.,[73] technique (open versus closed) was not a risk factor for a second mitral commissurotomy, subsequent mitral valve replacement, thromboembolism, or poor functional result.

REFERENCES

1. Burch GE, Colcolough HL: Viral valvulitis. *Am Heart J* 78:119-123, 1969
2. Rusted IE, Scheifley CH, Edwards JE: Studies of the mitral valve. II. Certain anatomic features of the mitral valve and associated structures in mitral stenosis. *Circulation* 14:398-406, 1956
3. Roberts WC, Perloff JK: Mitral valvular disease: a clinicopathologic survey of the conditions causing the mitral valve to function abnormally. *Ann Intern Med* 77:939-975, 1972
4. Eliot RS, Edwards JE: Pathology of rheumatic fever and chronic valvular disease. In *The Heart, Arteries and Veins.* Fourth edition. Edited by JW Hurst, RB Logue, RC Schlant, et al. New York, McGraw-Hill Book Company, 1978, pp 952-965
5. Reichek N, Shelburne JC, Perloff JK: Clinical aspects of rheumatic valvular disease. *Prog Cardiovasc Dis* 15:491-537, 1973
6. Stott DK, Marpole DGF, Bristow JD, et al: The role of left atrial transport in aortic and mitral stenosis. *Circulation* 41:1031-1041, 1970
7. Wilhelmsen L: Lung mechanics in rheumatic valvular disease. *Acta Med Scand [Suppl]* 489:1-114, 1968
8. Wood P: An appreciation of mitral stenosis. Part I. Clinical features. *Br Med J* 1:1051-1063, 1954
9. Probst P, Goldschlager N, Selzer A: Left atrial size and atrial fibrillation in mitral stenosis: factors influencing their relationship. *Circulation* 48:1282-1287, 1973
10. Coulshed N, Epstein EJ, McKendrick CS, et al: Systemic embolism in mitral valve disease. *Br Heart J* 32:26-34, 1970
11. Deverall PB, Olley PM, Smith DR, et al: Incidence of systemic embolism before and after mitral valvotomy. *Thorax* 23:530-536, 1968
12. Abernathy WS, Willis PW III: Thromboembolic complications of rheumatic heart disease. *Cardiovasc Clin* 5 No 2:131-175, 1973

13. Daley R, Mattingly TW, Holt CL, et al: Systemic arterial embolism in rheumatic heart disease. *Am Heart J* 42:566-581, 1951

14. Case records of the Massachusetts General Hospital (Case 19-1989). *N Engl J Med* 320:1260-1268, 1989

15. Rowe JC, Bland EF, Sprague HB, et al: The course of mitral stenosis without surgery: ten- and twenty-year perspectives. *Ann Intern Med* 52:741-749, 1960

16. Tandon R, Potti S, Mathur VS, et al: Critical rheumatic mitral stenosis in children. *Indian Pediatr* 9:171-173, 1972

17. Floyd J, Willis PW IV, Craige E: The apex impulse in mitral stenosis: graphic explanation of the palpable movements at the cardiac apex. *Am J Cardiol* 51:311-314, 1983

18. Harvey WP: Silent valvular heart disease. *Cardiovasc Clin* 5 No 2:77-95, 1973

19. Craige E: Phonocardiographic studies in mitral stenosis. *N Engl J Med* 257:650-654, 1957

20. McArthur JD, Sukumar IP, Munsi SC, et al: Reassessment of Graham Steell murmur using platinum electrode technique. *Br Heart J* 36:1023-1027, 1974

21. Edler I, Gustafson A: Ultrasonic cardiogram in mitral stenosis: preliminary communication. *Acta Med Scand* 159:85-90, 1957

22. Wann LS, Weyman AE, Feigenbaum H, et al: Determination of mitral valve area by cross-sectional echocardiography. *Ann Intern Med* 88:337-341, 1978

23. Nichol PM, Gilbert BW, Kisslo JA: Two-dimensional echocardiographic assessment of mitral stenosis. *Circulation* 55:120-128, 1977

24. Henry WL, Griffith JM, Michaelis LL, et al: Measurement of mitral orifice area in patients with mitral valve disease by real-time, two-dimensional echocardiography. *Circulation* 51:827-831, 1975

25. Martin RP, Rakowski H, Kleiman JH, et al: Reliability and reproducibility of two dimensional echocardiographic measurement of the stenotic mitral valve orifice area. *Am J Cardiol* 43:560-568, 1979

26. Glover MU, Warren SE, Vieweg WVR, et al: M-mode and two-dimensional echocardiographic correlation with findings at catheterization and surgery in patients with mitral stenosis. *Am Heart J* 105:98-102, 1983

27. Motro M, Schneeweiss A, Lehrer E, et al: Correlation between cardiac catheterization and echocardiography in assessing the severity of mitral stenosis. *Int J Cardiol* 1:25-34, 1981

28. Naito M, Morganroth J, Mardelli TJ, et al: Rheumatic mitral stenosis: cross-sectional echocardiographic analysis. *Am Heart J* 100:34-40, 1980

29. Nicolosi GL, Atkins F, Dunn M: Echocardiographic evaluation of mitral stenosis in predicting mitral valve replacement vs commissurotomy: relation to hemodynamic measurements. *Chest* 77:147-154, 1980

30. Rediker DE, Block PC, Abascal VM, et al: Mitral balloon valvuloplasty for mitral restenosis after surgical commissurotomy. *J Am Coll Cardiol* 11:252-256, 1988

31. Abascal VM, Wilkins GT, Choong CY, et al: Mitral regurgitation after percutaneous balloon mitral valvuloplasty in adults: evaluation by pulsed Doppler echocardiography. *J Am Coll Cardiol* 11:257-263, 1988

32. Block PC: Who is suitable for percutaneous balloon mitral valvotomy? (Editorial.) *Int J Cardiol* 20:9-14, 1988

33. Seward JB, Khandheria BK, Oh JK, et al: Transesophageal echocardiography: technique, anatomic correlations, implementation, and clinical applications. *Mayo Clin Proc* 63:649-680, 1988

34. Kronzon I, Tunick PA, Glassman E, et al: Transesophageal echocardiography to detect atrial clots in candidates for percutaneous transseptal mitral balloon valvuloplasty. *J Am Coll Cardiol* 16:1320-1322, 1990

35. Snider AR, Roge CL, Schiller NB, et al: Congenital left ventricular inflow obstruction evaluated by two-dimensional echocardiography. *Circulation* 61:848-855, 1980

36. Holen J, Aaslid R, Landmark K, et al: Determination of pressure gradient in mitral stenosis with a non-invasive ultrasound Doppler technique. *Acta Med Scand* 199:455-460, 1976

37. Hatle L, Brubakk A, Tromsdal A, et al: Noninvasive assessment of pressure drop in mitral stenosis by Doppler ultrasound. *Br Heart J* 40:131-140, 1978

38. Holen J, Simonsen S: Determination of pressure gradient in mitral stenosis with Doppler echocardiography. *Br Heart J* 41:529-535, 1979

39. Knutsen KM, Bae EA, Sivertssen E, et al: Doppler ultrasound in mitral stenosis: assessment of pressure gradient and atrioventricular pressure half-time. *Acta Med Scand* 211:433-436, 1982

40. Stamm RB, Martin RP: Quantification of pressure gradients across stenotic valves by Doppler ultrasound. *J Am Coll Cardiol* 2:707-718, 1983

41. Hosenpud JD, McAnulty JH, Morton MJ: Overestimation of mitral valve gradients obtained by phasic pulmonary capillary wedge pressure. *Cathet Cardiovasc Diagn* 9:283-290, 1983

42. Schoenfeld MH, Palacios IF, Hutter AM Jr, et al: Underestimation of prosthetic mitral valve areas: role of transseptal catheterization in avoiding unnecessary repeat mitral valve surgery. *J Am Coll Cardiol* 5:1387-1392, 1985

43. Hatle L, Angelsen B, Tromsdal A: Noninvasive assessment of atrioventricular pressure half-time by Doppler ultrasound. *Circulation* 60:1096-1104, 1979

44. Reid CL, McKay CR, Chandraratna PA, et al: Mechanisms of increase in mitral valve area and influence of anatomic features in double-balloon, catheter balloon valvuloplasty in adults with rheumatic mitral stenosis: a Doppler and two-dimensional echocardiographic study. *Circulation* 76:628-636, 1987

45. Come PC, Riley MF, Diver DJ, et al: Noninvasive assessment of mitral stenosis before and after percutaneous balloon mitral valvuloplasty. *Am J Cardiol* 61:817-825, 1988

46. Chen CG, Wang YP, Guo BL, et al: Reliability of the Doppler pressure half-time method for assessing effects of percutaneous mitral balloon valvuloplasty. *J Am Cardiol* 13:1309-1313, 1989

47. Nakatani S, Masuyama T, Kodama K, et al: Value and limitations of Doppler echocardiography in the quantification of stenotic mitral valve area: comparison of the pressure half-time and the continuity equation methods. *Circulation* 77:78-85, 1988

48. Nakatani S, Nagata S, Beppu S, et al: Acute reduction of mitral valve area after percutaneous balloon mitral valvuloplasty: assessment with Doppler continuity equation method. *Am Heart J* 121:770-775, 1991

49. Currie PJ, Seward JB, Chan K-L, et al: Continuous wave Doppler determination of right ventricular pressure: a simultaneous Doppler-catheterization study in 127 patients. *J Am Coll Cardiol* 6:750-756, 1985

50. Nishimura RA, Holmes DR Jr, Reeder GS: Percutaneous balloon valvuloplasty. *Mayo Clin Proc* 65:198-220, 1990

51. Lock JE, Khalilullah M, Shrivastava S, et al: Percutaneous catheter commissurotomy in rheumatic mitral stenosis. *N Engl J Med* 313:1515-1518, 1985

52. Kveselis DA, Rocchini AP, Beekman R, et al: Balloon angioplasty for congenital and rheumatic mitral stenosis. *Am J Cardiol* 57:348-350, 1986

53. McKay CR, Kawanishi DT, Rahimtoola SH: Catheter balloon valvuloplasty of the mitral valve in adults using a double-balloon technique: early hemodynamic results. *JAMA* 257:1753-1761, 1987

54. Palacios I, Block PC, Brandi S, et al: Percutaneous balloon valvotomy for patients with severe mitral stenosis. *Circulation* 75:778-784, 1987

55. McKay CR, Kawanishi DT, Kotlewski A, et al: Improvement in exercise capacity and exercise hemodynamics 3 months after double-balloon, catheter balloon valvuloplasty treatment of patients with symptomatic mitral stenosis. *Circulation* 77:1013-1021, 1988

56. Zaibag MA, Ribeiro PA, Kasab SA, et al: One-year follow-up after percutaneous double balloon mitral valvotomy. *Am J Cardiol* 63:126-127, 1989

57. Palacios IF, Block PC, Wilkins GT, et al: Follow-up of patients undergoing percutaneous mitral balloon valvotomy: analysis of factors determining restenosis. *Circulation* 79:573-579, 1989

58. Inoue K, Owaki T, Nakamura T, et al: Clinical application of transvenous mitral commissurotomy by a new balloon catheter. *J Thorac Cardiovasc Surg* 87:394-402, 1984

59. Al Zaibag M, Ribeiro PA, Al Kasab S, et al: Percutaneous double-balloon mitral valvotomy for rheumatic mitral-valve stenosis. *Lancet* 1:757-761, 1986

60. Rihal CS, Nishimura RA, Reeder GS, et al: Percutaneous balloon mitral valvuloplasty: comparison of double and single (Inoue) balloon techniques. *Cathet Cardiovasc Diagn* 29:183-190, 1993

61. Herrmann HC, Kleaveland JP, Hill JA, et al: The M-Heart Percutaneous Balloon Mitral Valvuloplasty Registry: initial results and early follow-up. *J Am Coll Cardiol* 15:1221-1226, 1990

62. Abascal VM, Wilkins GT, O'Shea JP, et al: Prediction of successful outcome in 130 patients undergoing percutaneous balloon mitral valvotomy. *Circulation* 82:448-456, 1990

63. Lefèvre T, Bonan R, Serra A, et al: Percutaneous mitral

valvuloplasty in surgical high risk patients. *J Am Coll Cardiol* 17:348-354, 1991

64. Cohen DJ, Kuntz RE, Gordon SPF, et al: Predictors of long-term outcome after percutaneous balloon mitral valvuloplasty. *N Engl J Med* 327:1329-1335, 1993

65. Babic UU, Pejcic P, Djurisic Z, et al: Percutaneous transarterial balloon mitral valvuloplasty: 30 months experience. *Herz* 13:91-99, 1988

66. Nobuyoshi M, Hamasaki N, Kimura T, et al: Indications, complications, and short-term clinical outcome of percutaneous transvenous mitral commissurotomy. *Circulation* 80:782-792, 1989

67. Kaplan JD, Isner JM, Karas RH, et al: In vitro analysis of mechanisms of balloon valvuloplasty of stenotic mitral valves. *Am J Cardiol* 59:318-323, 1987

68. Block PC, Palacios IF, Jacobs ML, et al: Mechanism of percutaneous mitral valvotomy. *Am J Cardiol* 59:178-179, 1987

69. Block PC: Early results of mitral balloon valvuloplasty (MBV) for mitral stenosis: report from the NHLBI Registry (abstract). *Circulation* 78 Suppl 2:489, 1988

70. Rihal CS, Nishimura RA, Holmes DR Jr: Percutaneous balloon mitral valvuloplasty. The learning curve. *Am Heart J* 122:1750-1756, 1991

71. Smith WM, Neutze JM, Barratt-Boyes BG, et al: Open mitral valvotomy: effect of preoperative factors on result. *J Thorac Cardiovasc Surg* 82:738-751, 1981

72. Rihal CS, Schaff HV, Frye RL, et al: Long-term follow-up of patients undergoing closed transventricular mitral commissurotomy: a useful surrogate for percutaneous balloon mitral valvuloplasty? *J Am Coll Cardiol* 20:781-786, 1992

73. Hickey MS, Blackstone EH, Kirklin JW, et al: Outcome probabilities and life history after surgical mitral commissurotomy: implications for balloon commissurotomy. *J Am Coll Cardiol* 17:29-42, 1991

CHAPTER

35

Mitral regurgitation

Michael D. McGoon, M.D., Hartzell V. Schaff, M.D., Maurice Enriquez-Sarano, M.D., Valentin Fuster, M.D., and Mark J. Callahan, M.D.

ANATOMIC CONSIDERATIONS

Mitral regurgitation may occur as a result of one of three general anatomic abnormalities: (1) primary alteration of the mitral valve leaflets or commissures; (2) anatomic or functional defects of the tensor apparatus; or (3) alteration of left ventricular and left atrial function (Fig 35-1 and Table 35-1). Any of the three anatomic varieties can present as a chronic, acute, or subacute problem.

Alteration of mitral leaflets or commissures

Rheumatic. Pure rheumatic mitral regurgitation is seen in about 10% of patients with rheumatic mitral valve disease.[1] Usually, mitral regurgitation is associated with mitral stenosis and fusion of the commissures (Fig 35-2). Severe rheumatic mitral regurgitation requiring surgical correction is still frequent in developing countries[2] but is now rare in developed countries.[3] Retractile fibrosis of the leaflets and chordae causes loss of coaptation due to fixation of the posterior leaflet and retraction of anterior leaflet tissue (Fig 35-3). Secondary dilatation of the mitral annulus tends to further decrease the contact between leaflets.

Mitral valve prolapse. Systolic prolapse of one of the mitral leaflets into the left atrium is a frequent cause of mild or, much less commonly, significant mitral regurgitation. Although prolapse of a mitral valve leaflet is present in 6% to 10% of otherwise healthy young people, predominantly females,[4] most of these valves are not incompetent. Mitral valve prolapse accounts for about 12% of all mitral regurgitation[1] but is the most common cause (38% to 62%) of isolated pure mitral regurgitation.[3] It may be associated with various conditions, including Marfan's syndrome, Ehlers-Danlos syndrome, thoracic skeletal abnormalities, other congenital cardiac abnormalities such as atrial septal defect or supravalvular aortic stenosis, and hypertrophic cardiomyopathy. Usually, however, no demonstrable abnormality other than mitral valve prolapse is present.[1]

Mitral regurgitation usually results from a combination of leaflet and annular enlargement producing systolic leaflet billowing.[5] Macroscopically, the valve leaflet area and length are increased,[6] and interchordal hooding of the leaflets is noted[7] (Fig 35-4). Microscopically, the valves are myxomatous, with deposition of mucopolysaccharides in a thickened spongiosa layer encroaching on the fibrosa layer. The elastic content of the valves is markedly increased.[8] Myxomatous changes in the annulus may result in annular dilatation and calcification.[9] Myxomatous infiltration also may involve other valves and cause regurgitation.[10] Mitral regurgitation may progress because of dilatation of the annulus or chordal rupture. The latter complication occurs more frequently in men than in women.[11] Other complications, such as infective endocarditis, thrombus formation, thromboembolism, and sudden death, are infrequent[12,13] and are observed most often in patients with significant mitral regurgitation.[14]

A second form of mitral valve prolapse—in which one or more of the chordae-papillary muscle "units" appear to be relatively long with respect to the left ventricular volume—permits mitral leaflet prolapse at the end of systole.[15] A third form of mitral prolapse is associated with abnormalities in regional left ventricular function.[16]

Calcification of mitral annulus. Spontaneous calcification of the mitral ring may prohibit effective closure of the mitral valve and cause mitral regurgitation, particularly in middle-aged and elderly women.

Calcification of the mitral annulus decreases systolic annular constriction and prevents normal leaflet coaptation in systole, both of which may lead to mitral regurgitation. Mitral annular calcification may be accelerated by other cardiovascular conditions such as systemic hypertension, hypertrophic obstructive cardiomyopathy, and aortic stenosis (Fig 35-5). Occasionally, the calcium may invade the conduction system, leading to conduction defects.

Infective endocarditis. Infective endocarditis accounts for about 5% of cases of mitral regurgitation. Vegetations may cause a mild degree of regurgitation by interposition between the leaflets. Severe endocarditic regurgitation is more often related to chordal rupture (Fig 35-6) than to either destruction of mitral tissue at the edges of the leaflets or perforation of the leaflets (Fig 35-7).

Congenital abnormalities (see Part VIII). Congenital cleft of the anterior mitral valve leaflet (Fig 35-8) rarely

The assistance of William D. Edwards, M.D., who reviewed this chapter, is gratefully acknowledged.

Table 35-1 Anatomic and clinical types of mitral valve regurgitation

	Clinical presentation	
Anatomic type	**Chronic**	**Acute or subacute**
Leaflets	Rheumatic Prolapse (myxomatous) Annular calcification Connective tissue Congenital cleft	Infective endocarditis
Tensor apparatus (chordae-papillary muscle)	Prolapse (elongated chordae-papillary muscle)	Idiopathic rupture Myocardial infarction with rupture Infective endocarditis with rupture Chronic leaflet abnormality with rupture
Myocardium	Regional (coronary disease, prolapse) Diffuse (dilated cardiomyopathy) Hypertrophic obstructive cardiomyopathy	

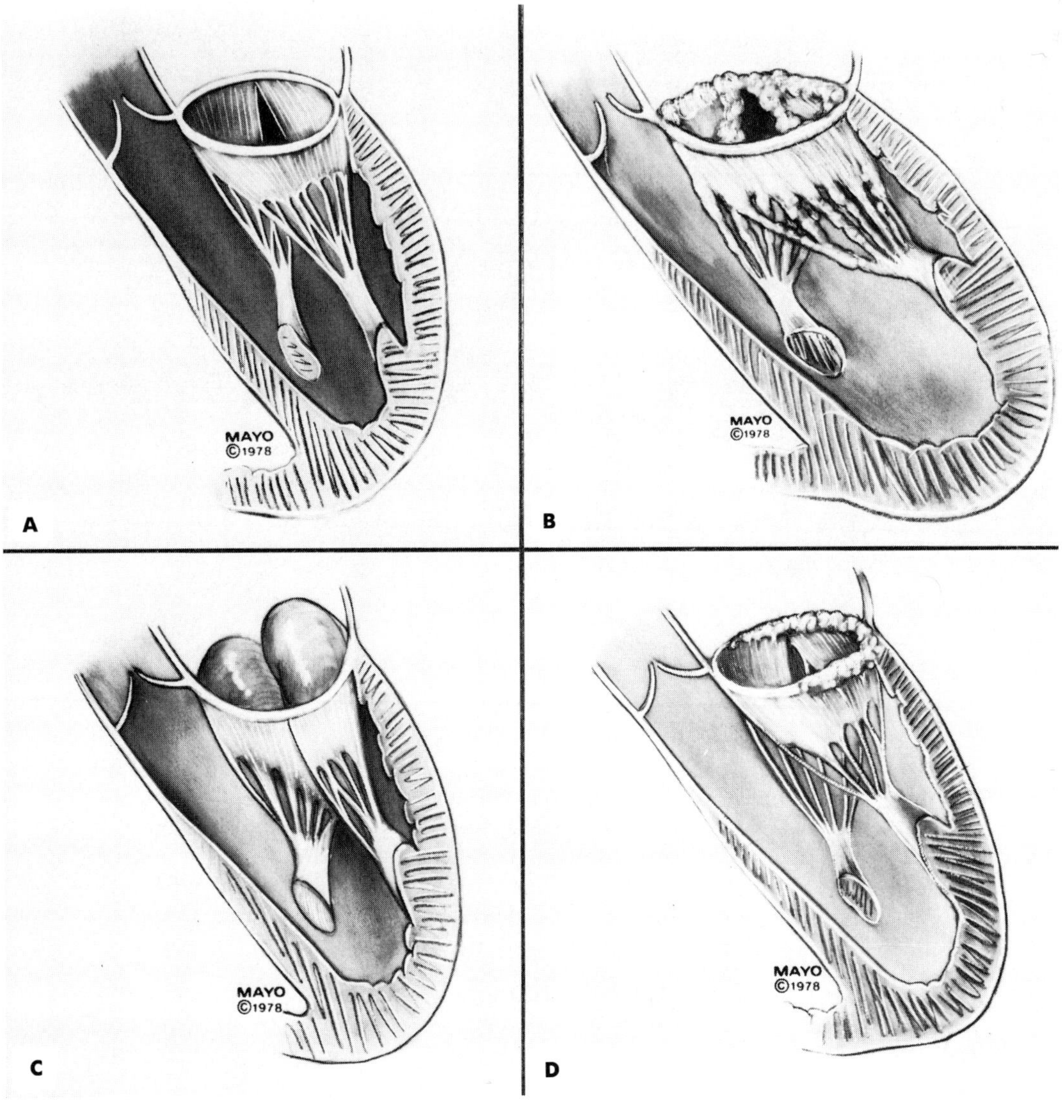

Fig 35-1 Types of mitral regurgitation. **A,** normal mitral valve; **B,** chronic rheumatic valve disease; **C,** chronic myxomatous valve prolapse; **D,** chronic annular calcification

Continued.

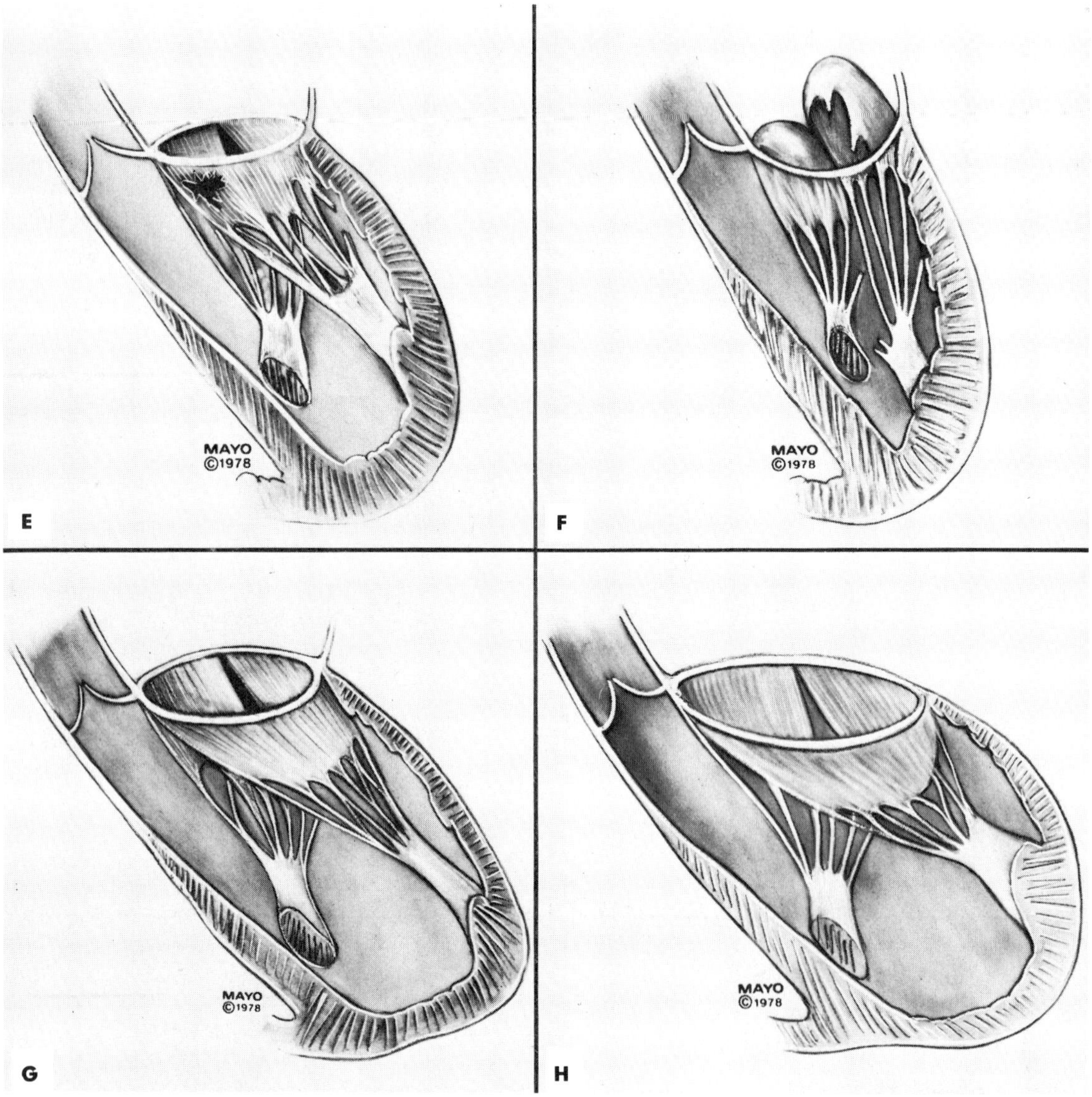

Fig 35-1, cont'd. **E,** acute infectious endocarditis (note perforation of a mitral valve leaflet and rupture of a chorda tendinea); **F,** flail mitral leaflet as result of acute idiopathic rupture of several chordae tendineae; **G,** chronic regional myocardial dysfunction leading to mitral regurgitation; **H,** chronic diffuse myocardial dysfunction leading to mitral regurgitation. (From Fuster V, Brandenburg RO, Giuliani ER, et al: Clinical approach and management of acquired valvular heart disease. *Cardiovasc Clin* 10 No 3:125-159, 1980. By permission, Mayo Foundation.)

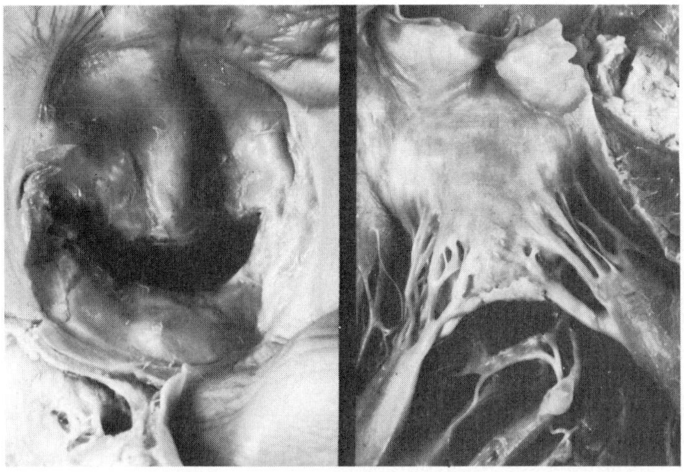

Fig 35-2 Rheumatic mitral stenosis and regurgitation due to leaflet and chordal fibrocalcific thickening. (Courtesy of William D. Edwards, M.D.)

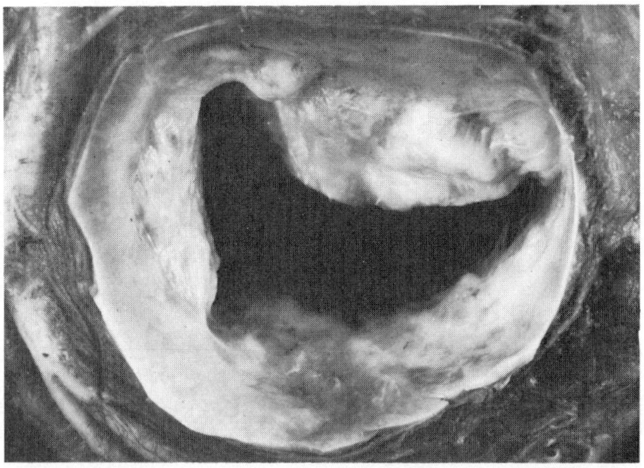

Fig 35-3 Rheumatic mitral regurgitation due to scar retraction of leaflets without appreciable commmissural fusion (Courtesy of William D. Edwards, M.D.)

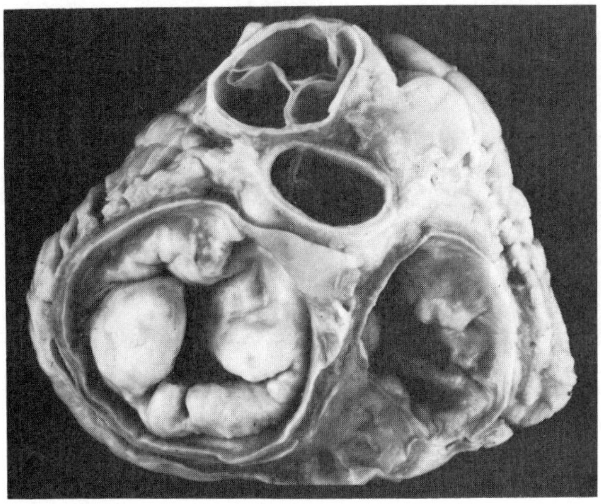

Fig 35-4 Mitral regurgitation due to floppy mitral valve (mitral valve prolapse) with annular dilatation and leaflet redundancy. (Courtesy of William D. Edwards, M.D.)

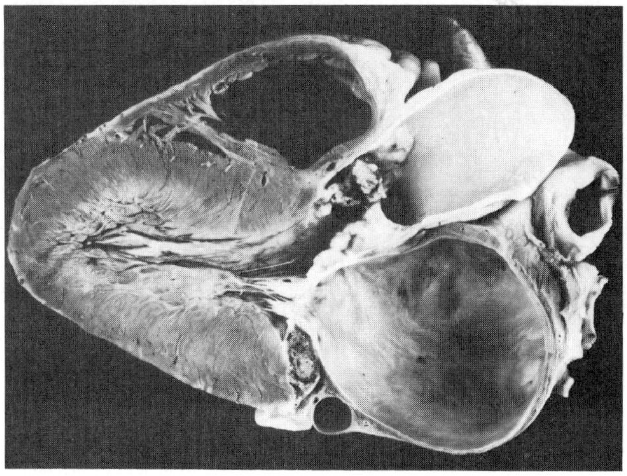

Fig 35-5 Mild degenerative mitral regurgitation due to subannular calcification of posterior leaflet and extension of calcific excrescences from stenotic aortic valve onto anterior mitral leaflet. (Courtesy of William D. Edwards, M.D.)

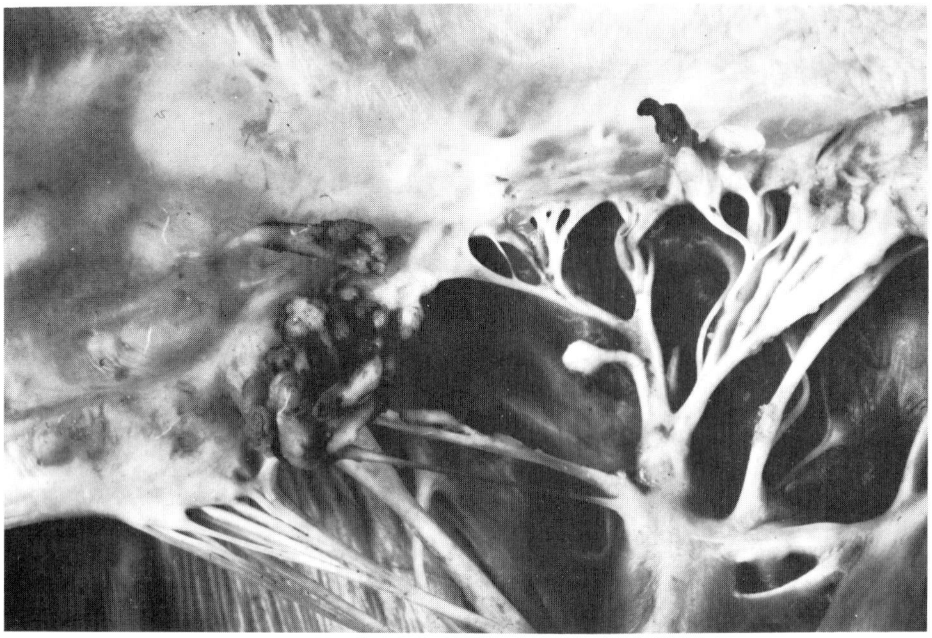

Fig 35-6 Mitral regurgitation due to infective endocarditis with rupture of chordae tendineae. (Courtesy of William D. Edwards, M.D.)

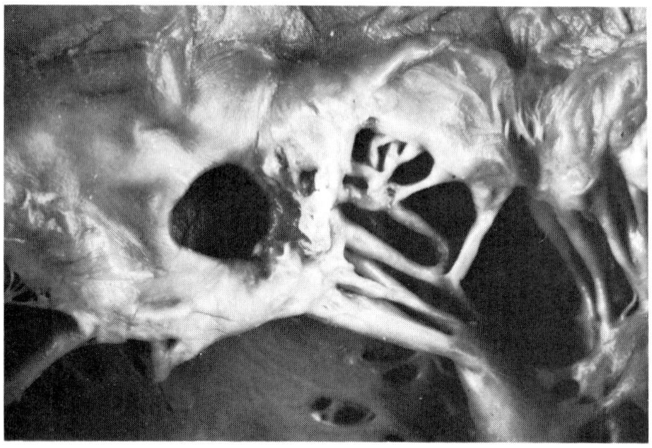

Fig 35-7 Mitral regurgitation due to infective endocarditis with perforation of anterior leaflet. (Courtesy of William D. Edwards, M.D.)

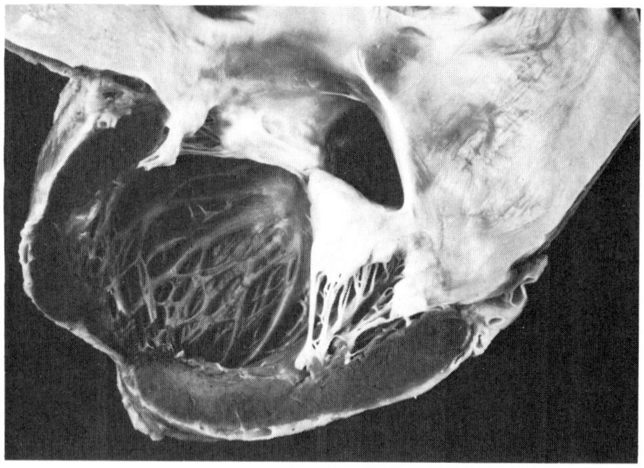

Fig 35-8 Mitral regurgitation due to congenitally cleft anterior mitral leaflet and primum atrial septal defect in partial atrioventricular canal. (Courtesy of William D. Edwards, M.D.)

is encountered without other features of persistent atrioventricular (AV) canal. When present, however, it can produce significant mitral regurgitation,[15] the degree of which generally corresponds to the width of the cleft. Corrected transposition with Ebstein's anomaly of the left AV valve[15] and anomalous mitral arcade are rare congenital causes of mitral incompetence.

Connective tissue disorders. Marfan's syndrome and Ehlers-Danlos syndrome may cause mitral regurgitation secondary to mitral prolapse. In addition, hypereosinophilic syndrome,[15] carcinoid tumors,[17] ergot-related lesions,[18] systemic lupus erythematosus, and Hurler's syndrome may cause mitral regurgitation by immobilization of mitral leaflets.

Defective tensor apparatus

Ruptured chordae tendineae. Approximately 20% of cases of mitral regurgitation are attributable to rupture of the chordae tendineae.[15] A floppy valve is observed in

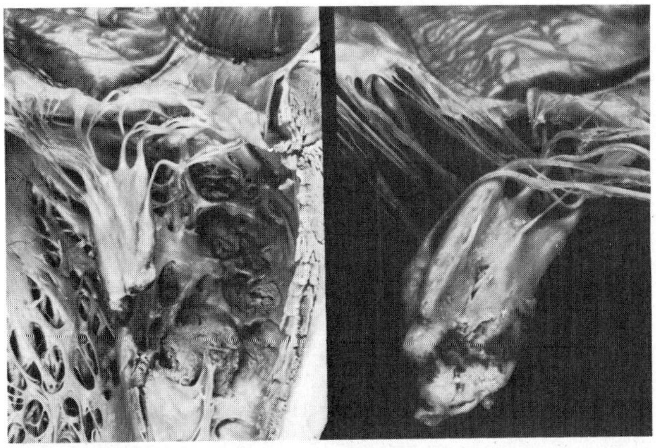

Fig 35-9 Acute mitral regurgitation due to rupture of infarcted posteromedial mitral papillary muscle. (Courtesy of William D. Edwards, M.D.)

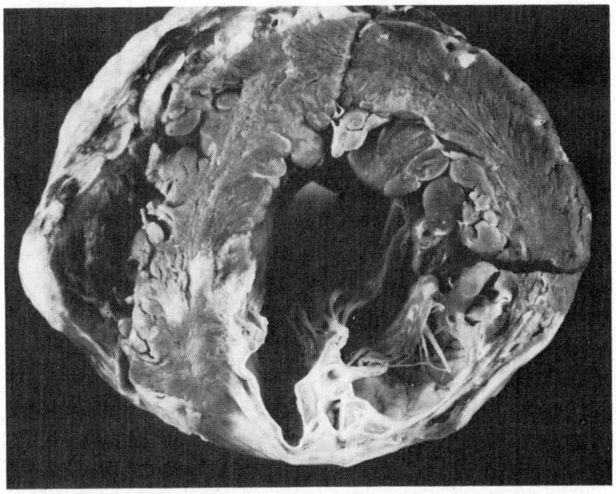

Fig 35-10 Postinfarction mitral regurgitation due to scarring of inferior left ventricular free wall and posteromedial mitral papillary muscle and to dilatation of left ventricular chamber. (Courtesy of William D. Edwards, M.D.)

most patients (73%) requiring operation for chordal rupture.[3] Frequently, no clinically demonstrable cause of rupture can be discerned. Endocarditis of anterior leaflet chordae resulting in rupture not uncommonly is due to the development of a jet lesion and infection secondary to aortic valve endocarditis. Blunt thoracic trauma or direct perforating injury also may cause chordae tendineae rupture.

Ruptured papillary muscle. Total transection of a left ventricular papillary muscle may be produced by chest trauma or myocardial infarction (Fig 35-9). In the former, rupture of the ventricular septum or free wall is frequently associated, as well as severe noncardiac injury. In the latter, infarction may be either transmural or subendocardial and usually involves the adjacent ventricular wall. Rupture usually occurs in the first week after infarction and involves the posteromedial papillary muscle four times more frequently than the anterolateral one.[15] Complete rupture is a hemodynamically catastrophic event and usually is fatal because the equivalent of nearly 60 chordae tendineae are disrupted. Partial rupture of a papillary muscle (i.e., transection of one or two pillars of the papillary muscle) is more frequent, and survival is possible if left ventricular function is adequate. However, risk of progression to complete rupture warrants immediate surgical attention.[19]

Papillary muscle dysfunction. Fibrosis of an infarcted papillary muscle may lead to dysfunction and distortion such that closure of the valve apparatus is imperfect during systole (Fig 35-10). Mitral annular enlargement is also frequently a component of infarct-related mitral regurgitation.[20] Approximately 10% of cases of mitral regurgitation are attributable to intact but dysfunctional papillary muscles.[1] The posteromedial papillary muscle is supplied by the posterior descending right coronary artery and becomes ischemic or infarcted more frequently than does the anterolateral papillary muscle, which is supplied by both diagonal and marginal branches of the left coronary system and by the right coronary artery. Apart from coronary artery disease, other conditions may cause foci of necrosis or fibrosis with dysfunction of the papillary muscle, such as hypertension, focal myocarditis, dilated cardiomyopathy, left ventricular outflow obstruction, acute aortic or mitral regurgitation, systemic endocardial fibroelastosis, cardioneuropathies, and infiltrative disease.

Alteration of left ventricular and left atrial function

Diffuse left ventricular enlargement, as in dilated cardiomyopathy, or a regional left ventricular abnormality, as in myocardial infarction, can result in an alteration of the position and directional axis of tension of the papillary muscles as well as in dilatation of the mitral ring, all of which may produce mitral regurgitation (Fig 35-11). Such conditions may contribute to mitral regurgitation by their effects on papillary muscle dysfunction and on the contractility of the mitral annulus. Left atrial and left ventricular enlargement associated with any type of chronic mitral regurgitation "begets more mitral regurgitation" and therefore perpetuates a vicious cycle. Abnormal position, anchoring, or tensing of the papillary muscles may contribute to the occurrence of mitral regurgitation in hypertrophic cardiomyopathy (see chapter 20) or in congenital anomalies (parachute mitral valve, accessory papillary muscle).

PATHOPHYSIOLOGY
Chronic mitral regurgitation

The abnormal anatomy of the defective mitral valve creates a regurgitant orifice. The systolic pressure gradient between the left ventricle and the left atrium produces flow through the orifice that over the duration of the cardiac cycle results in a regurgitant volume constituting a portion (regurgitant fraction) of the total stroke volume.

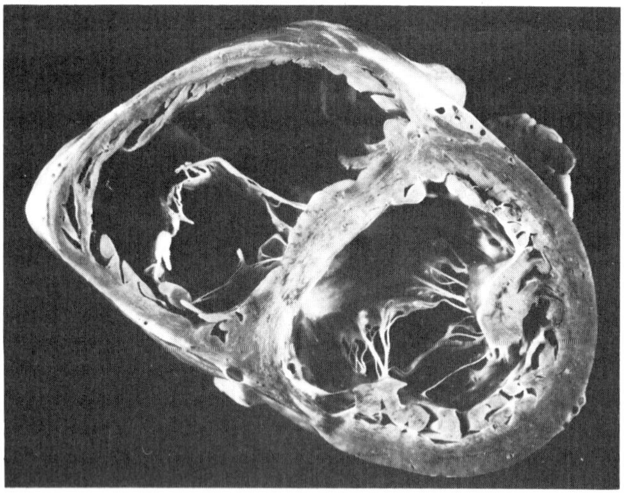

Fig 35-11 Mitral and tricuspid regurgitation due to biventricular dilatation in idiopathic dilated cardiomyopathy. (Courtesy of William D. Edwards, M.D.)

The regurgitant volume interferes with left atrial function and reenters the left ventricle in diastole, modifying left ventricular loading and function.

The regurgitant orifice is dynamic, with characteristics that depend on the type and severity of the lesion. In severe mitral regurgitation, the orifice is open throughout systole and permits holosystolic regurgitant flow. A small regurgitant orifice decreases in size as left ventricular size decreases throughout systole; regurgitation thus predominantly occurs early in systole. Mitral valve prolapse, conversely, is augmented as ventricular contraction progresses, so that regurgitation tends to be greatest in late systole. The reduction of regurgitant volume by vasodilators appears to be mediated by changes in left ventricular volume and, consequently, in the size of the regurgitant orifice.[21-23]

In mitral regurgitation, a portion of the left ventricular stroke volume is ejected retrogradely into a chamber of relatively low impedance, the left atrium, which results in left atrial systolic expansion.[24] The decrease in resistance to outflow is proportional to the regurgitant volume and the compliance of the left atrium. The resulting favorable loading conditions may mask significant left ventricular contractile dysfunction, especially when compared with comparable regurgitation in aortic regurgitation.[25,26] During diastole, the left ventricle accepts not only the usual pulmonary venous return of blood but also the blood previously ejected into the left atrium through the incompetent valve. The systolic escape of blood into the left atrium and its subsequent return during diastole produces a large total left ventricular stroke volume.

Despite relatively normal left ventricular end-diastolic pressure, in significant chronic mitral regurgitation the volume load produces left ventricular hypertrophy concomitantly with dilatation of the chamber, so that the wall mass-to-chamber volume ratio remains normal and, according to the Laplace relationship, the wall tension is minimized. A compensated state thus may be preserved for an extended period, during which indices of myocardial function, such as ejection fraction, remain normal or supranormal and ventricular emptying is augmented. With time, left ventricular function deteriorates slowly and symptoms develop. However, because of the persistent low-resistance pathway for ejection, the actual extent of left ventricular myocardial depression may not be apparent until the regurgitant pathway is eliminated by operation.[24] In addition, impaired left ventricular relaxation may contribute to deterioration of overall ventricular function.[27] Myocardial tissue from patients with chronic mitral regurgitation and severe left ventricular failure has an increased proportion of interstitial fibrotic tissue.

Acute or subacute mitral regurgitation

Some of the pathophysiologic and clinical features of acute or subacute mitral regurgitation are different from those of chronic mitral regurgitation. During the acute or subacute phase, there is insufficient time for left atrial or left ventricular enlargement to occur, and, therefore, the left cardiac diastolic and pulmonary venous pressures tend to be high; this explains the characteristic presentation of acute or subacute dyspnea at rest or on exercise despite normal cardiac size on the chest radiograph and a normal electrocardiogram. The noncompliance of the left atrial and left ventricular chambers also accounts for the palpatory evidence of distention of the left atrium during systole and of the left ventricle during early diastole and for the auscultatory evidence of loud third and fourth heart sounds. Noncompliance of the left atrial chamber may be associated with a very high left atrial pressure and resistance to the systolic regurgitant flow; therefore, the systolic murmur of mitral regurgitation in this condition can be short, soft, and occasionally inaudible, which obscures the diagnosis.

CLINICAL SYNDROME

History and clinical course

Chronic mitral regurgitation. Patients with gradual progression of mitral regurgitation have a prolonged asymptomatic interval of up to 20 years or more after the initiating event, and symptoms first appear in middle age or beyond (Fig 35-12). In most cases, left atrial compliance and size increase to accommodate the regurgitant volume and effectively protect against marked increase in pulmonary vascular pressures. Consequently, symptoms of pulmonary congestion are less prominent and occur late in the course of the disease.

Lassitude, fatigue, and generalized weakness, reflecting low cardiac output as a result of the large regurgitant volume of blood ejected into an enlarged left atrium, tend to predominate as early symptoms rather than frank dyspnea or pulmonary edema, which are more likely to occur with mitral stenosis. Similarly, the development of atrial fibrillation in about three-fourths of the patients[1] and the occurrence of systemic emboli tend to be associated with an enlarged left atrium ($\geqslant$5 cm) noted at

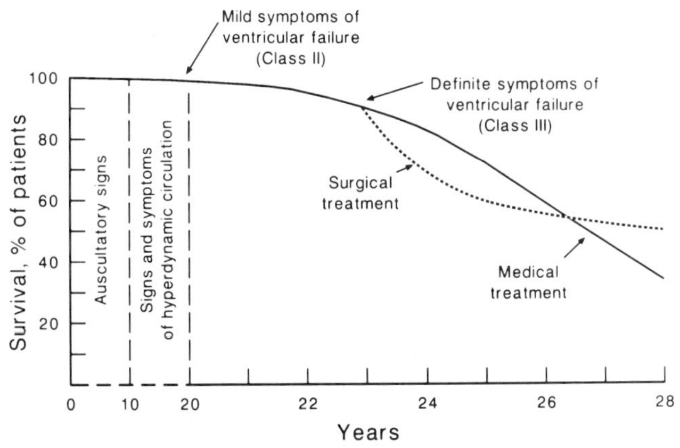

Fig 35-12 Scheme of the clinical presentation and natural history of chronic mitral regurgitation.

echocardiography. As left ventricular function deteriorates, exertional dyspnea, orthopnea, and paroxysmal nocturnal dyspnea become more prominent. The superimposition of acutely exacerbated regurgitation on chronic mitral regurgitation, which may occur with chordal rupture, infective endocarditis, or increased left ventricular afterload, produces a more catastrophic picture in which pulmonary symptoms predominate.

A significant number of patients with mitral valve prolapse suffer from anxiety, atypical chest pains, palpitations, and a wide spectrum of symptoms. In some patients the anxiety syndrome seems to be precipitated by the knowledge that they have cardiac disease. In a small group of patients, particularly those with redundant mitral leaflets or associated prolapse of other valves, the symptoms may have an organic basis—hemodynamically significant mitral incompetence, focal myocardial ischemia resulting from tension on the papillary muscles (atypical angina), or significant arrhythmias (palpitations). Finally, in a small proportion of these patients, the occurrence of systemic embolization that causes transient ischemic attacks, amaurosis fugax, or even acute hemiplegia has been observed.

The observed longevity of patients with chronic mitral regurgitation depends, in part, on the point in the disease process at which follow-up is begun. In unselected patients treated medically, 80% lived for 5 years and 60% for 10 years after diagnosis.[28] More homogeneous and selected groups of medically managed patients in New York Heart Association functional class II or III had a 5-year survival of about 55% and a 10-year survival of about 20%;[29] patients in functional class III or IV had a 5-year survival of about 40% and 10-year survival of about 15%. Ejection fraction is a powerful predictor of survival and appears to exceed more load-independent indices in predicting survival of patients not operated on.[30] Depression of right ventricular ejection fraction also appears to predict diminished longevity.[31]

The longevity of patients with mitral valve prolapse tends to be equal to that of the normal population with two exceptions. First, in about 15% of patients the mitral regurgitation progresses to a significant degree, and therefore their longevity may be decreased. This is rare in patients with isolated clicks. Second, longevity can be affected by the risk of infective endocarditis, although the incidence appears to be low and is almost negligible in patients with isolated clicks or minor echocardiographic alterations.

Acute or subacute mitral regurgitation. It usually is easy to distinguish the four common types of acute mitral regurgitation clinically. In *infective endocarditis,* there usually are other manifestations of the disease, although this may not be apparent in the elderly patient; most often there is only mild to moderate mitral regurgitation, but occasionally preexisting mild mitral regurgitation from another cause is transformed into severe regurgitation when complicated by infective endocarditis. *Idiopathic rupture of chordae tendineae,* the commonest cause of acute mitral regurgitation in an otherwise healthy person, usually causes symptoms suddenly. *Rupture of chordae tendineae as a complication of any of the other etiologic processes* affecting the valvular leaflets should be suspected in the absence of other obvious causes (e.g., onset of atrial fibrillation, pneumonitis, or increase in salt intake) when there is unexplained hemodynamic deterioration in a patient known previously to have had mild mitral regurgitation. *Acute myocardial infarction* often results in transient or permanent mild mitral regurgitation; however, sometimes the mitral regurgitation is severe, particularly in instances of significant papillary muscle dysfunction or rupture. The latter usually leads to death in hours or a few days unless surgical treatment is undertaken.

Physical findings

Blood pressure and arterial pulse. The peripheral arterial pulses are often normal but may be of small amplitude relative to the hyperdynamic apical impulse. The upstroke of the arterial pulsation is frequently brisk, but of low amplitude.

Precordial palpation. In patients with significant mitral regurgitation, the apical impulse is brief, laterally displaced, and somewhat diffuse. Despite its brevity, it is hyperactive—i.e., the amplitude is increased. A ventricular filling impulse related to the increased return of diastolic volume may be palpable at the apex in early diastole. Not infrequently, an abnormal left parasternal systolic impulse may be observed or palpated. An apical thrill may be present and usually indicates severe mitral regurgitation.

Auscultation. In rheumatic chronic mitral regurgitation, the first heart sound usually is normal or decreased in intensity; however, if mitral stenosis is also present, it may be increased.

In patients with mitral valve prolapse, systolic nonejection clicks are frequently heard and may be single or multiple. The clicks usually are heard best at the apex or left sternal border, tend to occur in mid or late systole, and are believed to be produced by the prolapsing leaflet and by the sudden tensing of the elongated chordae tendineae. Any maneuver that decreases left ventricular volume (see below) will result in an earlier occurrence of the prolapse and a click or clicks during systole. Patients with mitral valve prolapse may exhibit various other abnormal systolic sounds, including honks, whoops, or squeaks, which occasionally can be heard without a stethoscope (even by the patients themselves).

The second heart sound usually is normal. An accentuated pulmonic component indicates pulmonary hypertension. The aortic component may be early, because of shortened ventricular systole that causes persistent wide splitting of the second heart sound.

A third heart sound heard at the apex with the bell of the stethoscope is common. It tends to occur especially in moderate or severe mitral regurgitation, because of the high diastolic flow into the ventricle, and therefore does not necessarily imply significant left ventricular dysfunction or high left ventricular filling pressures.

Fourth heart sounds are unusual in chronic mitral regurgitation, even with normal sinus rhythm, because of the flaccidity of the left atrium. In acute mitral regurgitation, a fourth sound is common because the left atrial and left ventricular chambers are noncompliant.

The auscultatory hallmark of mitral regurgitation is a *systolic murmur* that typically is holosystolic, beginning with the first heart sound and often lasting to or past aortic closure. Usually the murmur is medium to high pitched, blowing in quality, and of relatively stable intensity throughout systole. The intensity of the murmur does not correlate well with the severity of regurgitant flow. The murmur is best heard with the diaphragm of the stethoscope placed firmly over the apex. Usually the apical murmur radiates to the axilla, unless prolapse or flail leaflet is present as a result of ruptured chordae. If the posterior leaflet is flail, the regurgitant stream is baffled anteriorly, and the radiation may be most audible over the sternum, where it may be confused with the murmur of aortic stenosis (Fig 35-13); conversely, a flail anterior leaflet directs the stream posteriorly, so that the murmur radiates to the back and spine and, in rare cases, to the occipital portion of the skull. The murmur may be notably short, soft, or absent in acute severe mitral regurgitation or in a severe prosthetic perivalvular leak.

Characteristically, the mitral regurgitation murmur is constant at different cycle lengths; this helps to differentiate this murmur from that of aortic stenosis or idiopathic obstructive cardiomyopathy. In addition, the murmur of mitral regurgitation typically increases when loading conditions of the left ventricle are increased, as occurs with squatting, leg elevation, isometric exercise, or phenylephrine administration. It decreases when loading is decreased, as with standing or amyl nitrite inhalation (for more details of dynamic auscultation, see chapter 2).

In contrast to rheumatic mitral regurgitation, the murmur of mitral valve prolapse is only holosystolic when the prolapse and mitral incompetence are severe; more often, it is present in a click-crescendo or crescendo-click-decrescendo pattern in mid to late systole. The onset and intensity of the murmur are variable. As a rule, a decrease in left ventricular volume (standing, amyl nitrite) allows the leaflets to prolapse earlier in systole, so that the murmur begins sooner, whereas increase in ventricular volume (squatting, leg raising) delays the onset.

A diastolic rumble is not uncommon, even without superimposed mitral stenosis, although it usually is short, begins after the third heart sound, and tapers rapidly. It is caused by high diastolic transmitral flow and thus reflects severe mitral regurgitation.

Electrocardiogram

About 75% of patients with significant mitral regurgitation have atrial fibrillation, consistent with a significantly enlarged left atrium.[1] Patients with normal sinus rhythm nearly always have evidence of left atrial enlargement—i.e., P mitrale configuration (broad notched P waves in lead II and biphasic P waves in lead V_1). The QRS

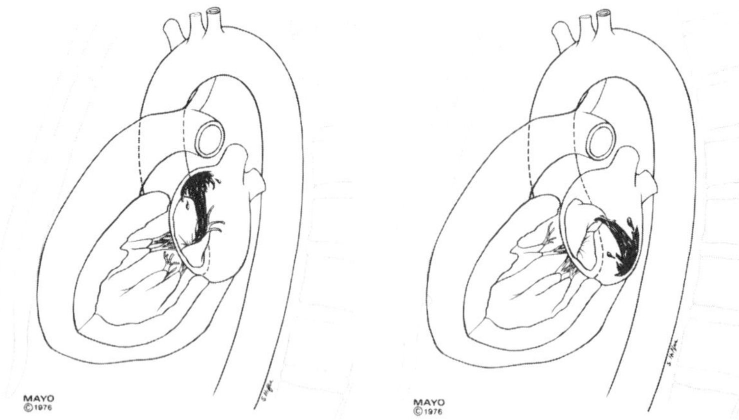

Fig 35-13 Characteristic directions of regurgitant blood flow in mitral regurgitation due to flail mitral leaflets. **Left,** flail posterior leaflet; **right,** flail anterior leaflet. (See text regarding transmission of murmurs.) (From Giuliani ER, Brandenburg RO, Fuster V: Evaluation of cardiac murmurs. *Cardiovasc Clin* 10 No 3:1-18, 1980. By permission, Mayo Foundation.)

complex and axis usually are normal and associated with nonspecific ST-segment and T-wave alterations.

Chest roentgenogram

The thoracic cage is normal except that some patients with mitral valve prolapse or the Marfan syndrome have a high prevalence of pectus excavatum, scoliosis, straight spine, or thin chest, which can cause lateral displacement of the normal heart and mimic cardiomegaly. True cardiomegaly with left ventricular and left atrial enlargement is a common finding in significant chronic mitral regurgitation and is uncommon in acute mitral regurgitation (Fig 35-14). Left atrial enlargement may be recognized by straightening of the left heart border, by a characteristic right-sided double density (right and left atrial borders superimposed), and, occasionally, by elevation of the left mainstem bronchus. The radiographic size of the left atrium provides a rough guide to the severity and duration of the mitral regurgitation.

In patients with mitral regurgitation, the pulmonary vasculature is usually normal until late in the disease when significant venous pulmonary hypertension develops. The resulting redistribution of flow to the upper lobes and interstitial edema cause Kerley B lines. Frank pulmonary edema may be evident in acute onset or exacerbation of mitral regurgitation.

Mitral annular calcification, one of the frequent causes of mitral regurgitation, often appears as a dense, coarse, "C"-shaped opacity, particularly in lateral or oblique films or fluoroscopic projections.

Echocardiography

Echocardiography has a central role in the evaluation of mitral regurgitation. Two-dimensional echocardiography with directed M-mode measurements, pulsed- and continuous-wave Doppler assessment, color-flow imaging, and transesophageal methods all contribute to characterization of mitral regurgitation in terms of (1) mitral valve morphology, (2) severity of regurgitation, and (3) ventricular and atrial function.

Morphologic characterization

ALTERATIONS OF MITRAL LEAFLET OR COMMISSURES. Rheumatic mitral valve disease often produces some decrease in orifice size (stenosis) and may also produce regurgitation. In the presence of stenosis, recognition of regurgitation by M-mode or two-dimensional echocardiography alone can be difficult unless the regurgitant volume is large enough to cause volume overload of the left ventricle and dilatation with systolic expansion of the left atrium (Fig 35-15). Doppler techniques complement this evaluation. Color-flow estimation of regurgitant jet severity in rheumatic mitral valve disease has been shown to correlate well with angiographic grading.[32]

Mitral valve prolapse is defined by both M-mode and two-dimensional characteristics. In M-mode images, the leaflet echo dips posteriorly to a line drawn between the C and D points of the mitral valve echogram. Typical M-mode echocardiographic patterns of mitral valve prolapse include pansystolic posterior bowing ("hammocking") and mid to late systolic posterior "buckling" of the mitral valve.

For the two-dimensional echocardiographic analysis of

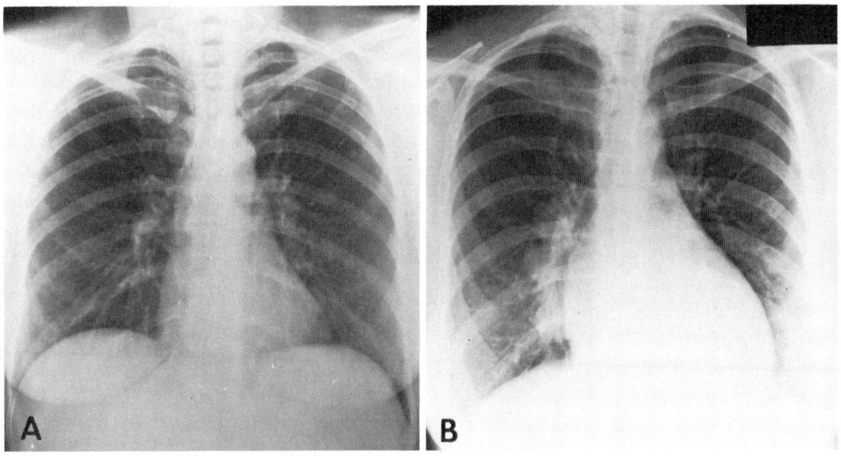

Fig 35-14 Chest roentgenograms. **A,** acute mitral regurgitation secondary to infective endocarditis. Despite near-normal roentgenographic appearance, the patient was in New York Heart Association class III and at cardiac catheterization had a left ventricular end-diastolic pressure of 35 mm Hg. **B,** chronic mitral regurgitation showing left ventricular enlargement with the characteristic elongation of the apex toward the left and inferiorly and left atrial enlargement with straightening or prominence of the mid left heart border and right-sided double density. (**A,** from Fuster V, Brandenburg RO, Giuliani ER, et al: Clinical approach and management of acquired valvular heart disease. *Cardiovasc Clin* 10 No 3:125-159, 1980. By permission of FA Davis Company.)

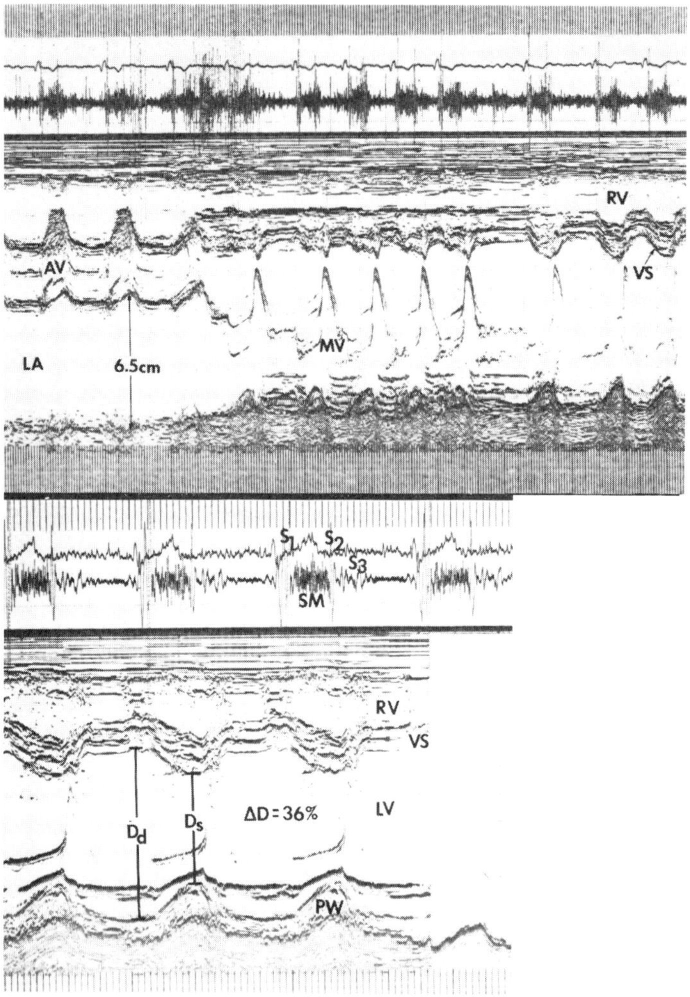

Fig 35-15 M-mode echocardiograms, showing indirect patterns of mitral regurgitation. **Upper,** dilated, hyperdynamic left ventricle (pattern of "left ventricular volume overload") along with enlarged left atrium and increased excursion of the mitral valve. This combination is strongly suggestive of mitral regurgitation. **Lower,** use of echocardiogram in mitral regurgitation to assess function of left ventricle *(LV)*. Measurements of left ventricular dimensions are shown. Note the normal fractional shortening (ΔD) of 36%. On top, a simultaneous phonocardiogram displays pansystolic murmur *(SM)* and third heart sound (S_3). S_1, first heart sound; S_2, second heart sound; D_d, left ventricular internal dimension in diastole; D_s, left ventricular internal dimension in systole; *PW,* posterior wall; *VS,* ventricular septum; and *RV,* right ventricle. (**Lower,** from Shub C: The role of echocardiography in clinical practice. In *Clinical Medicine.* Vol 6, Chap 34. Edited by JA Spittell Jr. Philadelphia, Harper & Row, Publishers, 1982, pp 1-44. By permission.)

mitral valve prolapse (Fig 35-16), the heart may be examined in multiple planes. An imaginary line is constructed from the base of the anterior leaflet attachment at the aortic root to the base of the posterior leaflet attachment at the mitral annulus. If the leaflet tissue bows into the left atrium beyond that line, prolapse is diagnosed. Prolapse of either or both leaflets can be identified in this manner. Approximately 10% of patients with the click-murmur syndrome do not have echocardiographic evidence of mitral prolapse. Conversely, echocardiographic evidence of mitral prolapse may be present without either a systolic click or a murmur. If the classic auscultatory features of a systolic nonejection click and a mid to late apical systolic murmur are present, mitral valve prolapse cannot be excluded, even if the echocardiographic findings are normal. About 10% of patients with mitral valve prolapse also have tricuspid valve prolapse.[10,33]

Occasionally, a "pseudoprolapse" pattern can be produced by improper recording techniques. Varying the

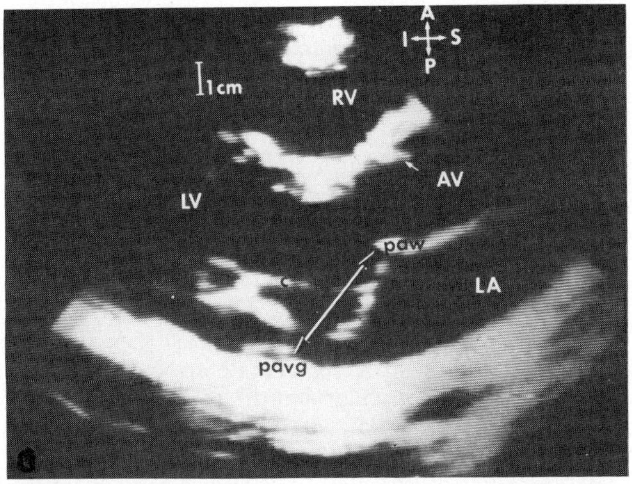

Fig 35-16 Mitral valve prolapse. Two-dimensional echocardiogram shows long-axis parasternal view of prolapse. Note imaginary line *(large arrow)* drawn from posterior AV groove *(pavg)* to posterior aortic wall *(paw)*. Prolapse is said to occur when the mitral valve appears superior to (to the right of) this line. S_1, *first heart sound; RV,* right ventricle; *LV,* left ventricle; *AV,* aortic valve; *c,* chorda; *A,* anterior; *P,* posterior; *I,* inferior; and *S,* superior. (From Shub C: The role of echocardiography in clinical practice. In *Clinical Medicine.* Vol 6, Chap 34. Edited by JA Spittell Jr. Philadelphia, Harper & Row, Publishers, 1982, pp 1-44. By permission.)

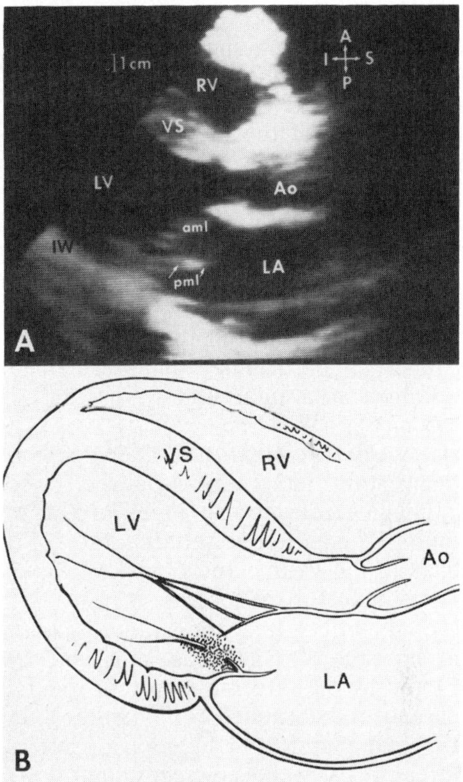

Fig 35-17 **A,** long-axis view of left ventricle *(LV)* in systole, demonstrating flail posterior mitral leaflet *(pml)* due to ruptured chordae. *RV,* right ventricle; *VS,* ventricular septum; *Ao,* aorta; *aml,* anterior mitral leaflet; *LA,* left atrium; *IW,* inferior wall. **B,** drawing corresponding to ultrasonographic plane shown in **A.** (From Nasser FN, Giuliani ER: *Clinical Two-Dimensional Echocardiography.* Chicago, Year Book Medical Publishers, 1983, p 85. By permission.)

transducer position may affect the appearance of the mitral valve pattern, and improper angulation of the transducer may cause a mitral valve contour that simulates prolapse. A pattern suggesting prolapse may occur in the presence of pericardial effusion.

Mitral annular calcification produces dense, linear echoes behind the mitral valve, which often obscure the details of the posterior leaflet. The echocardiogram reveals an irregular calcific density in the left AV groove. The calcium may extend into the ventricular side of the annulus and onto the posterior mitral leaflet.

Although echocardiography is the procedure of choice for detecting, localizing, and characterizing mitral valvular vegetations,[34] not all patients with infective endocarditis have echocardiographically demonstrable vegetations. Nevertheless, when definite vegetations (>2 mm) are present, the echocardiogram has been shown, by correlative surgical and autopsy studies, to be both sensitive and specific in detecting them. Transesophageal echocardiography images the mitral apparatus at a closer range and with higher resolution than permissible with conventional echocardiography.[35,36] It is indicated for the evaluation of patients in whom infective endocarditis is suspected but vegetations cannot be identified. Relatively fresh vegetations may appear shaggy and often do not seem to interfere with valve motion. Established or healed vegetations may have a denser appearance due to fibrosis or calcification. Mitral valve vegetations often evolve into flail structures that flutter from atrium to ventricle and back during the cardiac cycle. These may consist of valve tissue, chordal tissue, and healed vegetation. These long-standing vegetations typically persist for years without change. On the other hand, they may embolize platelet material or fragments of vegetation, even in the absence of active infection.

Defective tensor apparatus. Redundance of chordae or rupture of several chordae may produce minor valve prolapse or dysfunction. More extensive rupture of chordae tendineae may produce a flail mitral leaflet. The term "flail leaflet" describes free movement of part or all of a leaflet into the atrium during systole and into the ventricle in a chaotic way during diastole. Most cases involve only part of the leaflet. The two-dimensional echocardiographic examination permits a full examination of the flail structure (Fig 35-17). Flail movement, coarse fluttering of chordal or leaflet tissue, ruptured chordal tissue appearing as coiled masses, and loose, string-like structures all may be seen in the complete scan of the abnormal structure. Long- and short-axis views in the parasternal position and the apical four-chamber view probably afford the best images.

Two-dimensional echocardiography can detect abnormalities of the papillary muscle such as calcification, thinning, and scar formation. There may be an anomaly of the number of papillary muscles, of the distribution of the papillary heads, or of the muscle tissue. Rupture of a portion of a papillary muscle may be seen. Apart from direct visualization of primary papillary muscle abnormalities, the visualization of an underlying left ventricle abnormality—e.g., thinning and hypokinesis of the inferior wall in coronary disease—may be an important part of the evaluation. Mitral regurgitation of various degrees of severity is a frequent accompaniment of left ventricular dysfunction, particularly that occurring after inferior wall myocardial infarction.[37]

Severity of regurgitation

SEMIQUANTITATIVE METHODS. The appearance of the mitral regurgitant jet when visualized by color-flow Doppler imaging provides an index of the severity of regurgitation. The jet length, jet area, ratio of jet area to left atrial area, and width of the jet at the orifice have been suggested as indicators of severity.[38-41]

However, the utility of jet appearance is constrained by technical limitations[42] (such as gain and frame rate setting[43]) and by the intrinsic nature of regurgitant jets. Jet appearance is determined by momentum[44] (a function of velocity and therefore a function of left ventricular systolic pressure) as well as by regurgitant flow. Furthermore, jets are limited by the left atrium,[44] so that a jet can appear larger in a large atrium.[45,46] A severe but eccentric regurgitant stream may appear small because it impinges on a nearby atrial wall. Transesophageal color-flow imaging has higher resolution and superior visualization but is subject to the same potential inaccuracies as transthoracic imaging.

The pulmonary venous velocity profile measured by transesophageal Doppler echocardiography may reflect the degree of mitral regurgitation.[47,48] Systolic reversal of flow in the pulmonary veins suggests severe regurgitation but is affected also by left atrial pressure and the direction of the jet.[49]

QUANTITATIVE METHODS. The goal of quantitative methodology is to measure variables that accurately indicate the amount of regurgitation on the basis of regurgitant volume per beat or regurgitant fraction. The effective regurgitant orifice (ERO) can be calculated as a quantitative expression of the mitral regurgitant lesion. This calculation is based on the following logic:[50,51]

$$\text{Flow through an orifice} = \text{area of the orifice} \times \text{velocity}$$

Thus,

$$\text{Regurgitant flow} = \text{regurgitant orifice area} \times \text{regurgitant velocity}$$

Consequently, the effective regurgitant orifice can be calculated:

$$\text{ERO} = \text{regurgitant flow/regurgitant velocity}$$

When integrated over the cardiac cycle, this is

$$\text{ERO} = \text{regurgitant volume/regurgitant TVI}$$

in which TVI is the time velocity integral of the regurgitant jet, and regurgitant volume is determined by obtaining the difference between diastolic mitral volume and systolic transaortic stroke volume.

Practical quantitation of mitral regurgitation can be performed by any of four methods:

1. *Quantitative Doppler imaging.* Regurgitant volume is calculated as the difference between mitral and aortic stroke volumes measured by pulsed-wave Doppler echocardiography.[52,53]
2. *Quantitative two-dimensional echocardiography.* Regurgitant volume is measured as the difference between total stroke volume determined by planimetry of left ventricular end-diastolic and end-systolic volumes and aortic stroke volume determined by the quantitative Doppler method.[54,55]
3. *Amplitude-weighted mean velocity.* The proportionality of stroke volumes through the mitral and aortic valves is determined by measuring the amplitude-weighted velocities by continuous-wave Doppler echocardiography.[56] This permits calculation of regurgitant fraction.[57]
4. *Proximal isovelocity surface area.* Color-flow mapping is used to determine precisely the velocity of blood converging on the regurgitant orifice.[58,59] The value determined permits calculation of regurgitant flow[60] and effective regurgitant orifice.[50]

Use of echocardiography and radionuclide techniques in evaluation of secondary myocardial dysfunction and timing of operation for chronic mitral regurgitation. In a patient with chronic mitral regurgitation, if the left ventricle is not dilated and hyperdynamic, the mitral regurgitation usually is not hemodynamically significant. On the other hand, in acute severe mitral regurgitation—e.g., rupture of valvular structures secondary to infective endocarditis—the left ventricle may not be dilated but is hyperdynamic. In chronic mitral regurgitation, myocardial function can be assessed and followed serially on the basis of left ventricular diastolic and systolic dimensions (as a reflection of diastolic and systolic volumes) and derived ejection fraction and percentage fractional shortening (as a reflection of left ventricular systolic function).

Attempts to more accurately assess global left ventricular function have been made. Descriptors of left ventricular function that have been reported to correlate with postoperative results include end-systolic wall stress/end-systolic volume index (ESWS/ESVI) ratio[61] and the tension-volume ejection fraction (ESWS/ESVIX ejection fraction).[62] Although these measurements may be useful in judging relatively load-independent left ventricular function and have retrospective predictive capability, it is not clear that measurement in the individual patient is clinically useful, in part because of the difficulty in defining end-systole.[63]

Imaging data can help the clinician make a decision regarding the timing of mitral valve operation. Echocardiographic evaluation, as discussed previously, can provide anatomic and functional data about the ventricle and valve. Radionuclide ventriculography can provide important information on degree of regurgitation and myocar-

Table 35-2 Timing of operation in chronic mitral regurgitation

Symptomatic (class III-IV)
↓
Operate

Asymptomatic or minimally symptomatic (class I-II)
↓ Radionuclide studies; Echocardiography
Assess EF (and other parameters of systolic function)

→ EF normal or low
↓
Consider operation

→ EF increased
↓
Observation; serial studies (6-12 mo)

EF, ejection fraction.
*See text.

dial reserve during stress.[64-66] Above-normal left ventricular systolic function is generally thought to imply a better long-term prognosis in symptomatic patients; in such cases, operation may be advised only to ameliorate symptoms. The long-term postoperative results are worse in symptomatic patients with preoperative left ventricular systolic dysfunction. Some patients have normal or decreased left ventricular function before the onset of symptoms and are also at increased postoperative risk because this already implies some ventricular decompensation. For the asymptomatic or minimally symptomatic patient the approach remains controversial. Our present scheme of evaluation is as shown in Table 35-2.

Invasive studies

Cardiac catheterization is useful to assess hemodynamic status, severity of mitral regurgitation, left ventricular function, and coronary anatomy.

Characteristic hemodynamic findings include reduced forward cardiac output and increased pulmonary capillary wedge pressure. Marked pulmonary hypertension is rarely present.[67] A prominent v wave is more frequently observed in acute mitral regurgitation than in chronic lesions (Fig 35-18). Other conditions also may produce v waves, including ventricular septal defect or significantly reduced atrial compliance in the absence of mitral regurgitation.[68]

Severity of regurgitation can be described qualitatively by left ventricular angiography. Observed degree and duration of left atrial opacification can be used to grade the degree of regurgitation (Table 35-3).

Another angiographic quantitative assessment of mitral regurgitation involves calculation of the regurgitant frac-

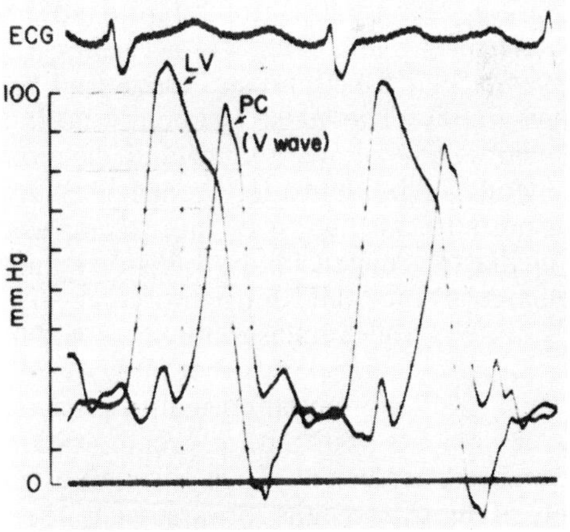

Fig 35-18 Left ventricular *(LV)* and pulmonary capillary wedge *(PC)* pressure tracings in a patient with ruptured chordae tendineae and acute mitral regurgitation. The giant v wave results from regurgitation of blood into a relatively small and noncompliant left atrium. Electrocardiogram *(ECG)* illustrates the time of the PCV wave, whose peak follows ventricular repolarization, as manifested by the T wave of the ECG. (From Grossman W: Profiles in valvular heart disease. In *Cardiac Catheterization and Angiography.* Third edition. Edited by W Grossman. Philadelphia, Lea & Febiger, 1986, pp 359-381. By permission.)

Table 35-3 Grading of mitral regurgitation

Severity grade	Description
1+	A small amount of contrast material enters the left atrium in systole, does not fill the atrium, and is progressively cleared with each beat
2+	More contrast material enters the left atrium during the first several beats, and the entire atrium is faintly opacified
3+	The left atrium becomes well opacified, equal in density to the left ventricle
4+	Complete, dense opacification of the left atrium occurs on the first beat

tion (RF). Total left ventricular stroke volume (TSV) is determined from the left ventriculogram, and the amount that is ejected forward into the aorta (the forward stroke volume, FSV) is calculated by Fick or indicator-dilution technique. The TSV is the difference between end-diastolic and end-systolic left ventricular volumes (EDV − ESV = TSV); regurgitant stroke volume (RSV) per beat is TSV minus FSV, and regurgitant fraction (RF) is RSV/TSV. The accuracy of these angiographic calculations depends on many factors; therefore, at present there is a trend toward use of radionuclide volumetric data; however, these are not free of error. Given the inaccuracies, in general RF $<20\%$ corresponds to mild mitral regurgitation, 20% to 40% to moderate, 40% to 60% to moderately severe, and $>60\%$ to severe.

Left ventricular function can be assessed by quantitative angiography. The most frequently used indices of function are end-systolic volume and ejection fraction. Simultaneous high-fidelity left ventricular pressure recording permits calculation of more complex variables, including diastolic distensibility, wall stress, maximum left ventricular elastance, and left ventricular stiffness. The clinical utility of these measurements is not fully established.

Regional wall motion abnormalities have been observed in patients with mitral regurgitation and no significant coronary lesions. Thus, coronary angiography is the only definitive means of assessing the need for coronary revascularization at the time of mitral valve surgery.

MANAGEMENT

Principles

Patients with rheumatic mitral regurgitation should receive antirheumatic fever prophylaxis (chapter 54). In any patient with mitral regurgitation, antibiotic therapy for prophylaxis against bacterial endocarditis is advised for any surgical or dental manipulative procedure, the choice of antibiotic being determined by the location and type of procedure performed. Maintenance of sinus rhythm is not as important with mitral regurgitation as it is with mitral stenosis. Unless there is a clear decrease in function after onset of atrial fibrillation, most patients with severe mitral regurgitation probably should be left in atrial fibrillation, with the rate controlled pharmacologically; these patients should be considered for surgical therapy, after which they can be converted to sinus rhythm. Oral anticoagulant therapy is indicated in three groups of patients:[69] patients with intermittent or chronic atrial fibrillation, patients with sinus rhythm but a large left atrium (>55 mm by M-mode echocardiography), and patients with a history of previous systemic embolism.

Patients with mild mitral prolapse need reassurance. Endocarditis prophylaxis cannot be strongly recommended in patients whose only abnormal feature is a nonejection systolic click. Patients with mitral valve prolapse in whom the risk of endocarditis developing is higher (presence of regurgitation or thickened leaflets) should receive prophylaxis.[70] Patients with mild prolapse and a history of palpitations, light-headedness, dizziness, or syncope should undergo ambulatory ECG monitoring or treadmill exercise testing. The results of these tests are usually unrewarding or overinterpreted; nevertheless, in patients with significant and complex arrhythmias, propranolol has been the drug of choice thus far. In addition, β-adrenergic blockers may be of some benefit in patients with ischemic pain related to coronary disease and perhaps in some patients with regional ischemia resulting from tension on the papillary muscles produced by the prolapsing valve.[71] Because the decrease in left ventricular size induced by nitrates may intensify the prolapse and the possible resultant ischemia, these agents should be used with caution. Finally, although its value has not been established, antithrombotic therapy may be considered as prophylactic in rare patients with mild mitral prolapse who have experienced unexplained central neurologic events.

Patients with hemodynamically significant mitral regurgitation should be considered for mitral valve repair or replacement, particularly if symptoms are present. Appropriate timing of the operation is critical: delay in correction may lead to worsening of hemodynamic status and irreversible myocardial deterioration. Premature operation subjects patients to unnecessary perioperative risk as well as potential late complications of prostheses if valve replacement is necessary.

Several markers of left ventricular dysfunction have been identified that correlate with outcome of operation. Risk of early death after mitral valve replacement for mitral regurgitation is increased in patients with significant cardiomegaly (cardiothoracic ratio >0.78), very large left atrium, and severely compromised hemodynamic status (cardiac index <1.5 L/min/m^2, systolic pulmonary artery pressure >100 mm Hg, and left ventricular end-diastolic pressure >20 mm Hg).[72] Preoperative ESWS/ESVI has reportedly correlated with patient outcome after valve repair. Such an index is attractive because it can be estimated noninvasively and used for follow-up in patients with mitral regurgitation.[73] In our experience, however, ESWS/ESVI and other measures of end-systolic volume and pressure do not predict early postoperative left ventricular dysfunction or subsequent mortality or lack of clinical improvement.[63]

The degree of left ventricular dysfunction generally is underestimated by conventional assessment of systolic function in patients with chronic mitral regurgitation. This conclusion is emphasized by the observation that there is a marked decrease in ejection fraction and a high incidence of left ventricular dysfunction after successful surgical correction.[74,75] These observations, along with evidence that ejection fraction predicts postoperative probability of survival,[76] imply that operation should be undertaken before the disease has produced even relatively mild evidence of left ventricular dysfunction.

Nevertheless, precise hemodynamic and volumetric criteria to determine truly optimal timing have not been established. The decision for or against operation is also influenced by the suitability of the valve for repair. As discussed below, mitral valve reconstruction appears to have a lower operative risk than mitral valve replacement, and the incidence of late valve complications is much lower in patients who have had valve repair than in those with mitral valve prostheses.[77,78]

Operation is recommended for patients with severe mitral regurgitation who are clearly symptomatically limited, particularly those in functional class III or IV. Exception to this policy may be taken for patients with advanced left ventricular dysfunction who are considered to have a high perioperative risk and poor late functional outcome, although no precise lower limit of acceptable left ventricular function has been established. Such patients, as well as those whose operation must be delayed or cannot be carried out for any reason, should be treated medically.

Vasodilators decrease regurgitant flow by decreasing peripheral systemic resistance; the enhanced forward stroke volume permits increased cardiac output, which minimizes the symptoms of fatigability, and the decrease in regurgitant flow, together with the associated decrease in left ventricular end-diastolic pressure, decreases dyspnea. The use of digoxin and diuretics is also advisable in patients with severe mitral regurgitation. Nevertheless, mitral valve operation may be the only alternative despite increased early postoperative risk. Pulmonary hypertension also should not be a contraindication to mitral valve operation, since gratifying symptomatic results and improvement of pulmonary hemodynamics have been obtained.[79]

Asymptomatic patients or those with mild symptoms (class II) who have significant mitral regurgitation may be considered candidates for operation, especially if serial examination reveals progressive cardiac enlargement or development of atrial fibrillation and especially if valve repair is anticipated. Asymptomatic patients or patients with mild symptoms who have normal or low ejection fraction may have ventricular decompensation and should be considered for operation; patients with increased ejection fraction should be reexamined every 6 to 12 months.

Surgical technique

Mitral valve reconstruction. There is increasing enthusiasm among surgeons for valve repair rather than replacement. The frequency with which valvuloplasty can be used in patients with mitral regurgitation varies with the experience of the operating team and the spectrum of underlying valve disease; repair is more often feasible in patients with degenerative valve disease than in patients with regurgitation caused by rheumatic valvulitis or endocarditis. In our current practice, valve repair is performed in over 90% of patients referred for primary correction of acquired mitral valve insufficiency. If the patient is in sinus rhythm, long-term postoperative anticoagulation is not required after reconstruction of the valve. Evidence also suggests that preservation of chordae tendineae and papillary muscles has a beneficial effect on postoperative left ventricular function.[80-82]

If the valve is free of significant calcification or fibrotic immobility, regurgitation is caused by leaflet prolapse or annular dilatation, or both. There are many causes of prolapse, including chordal rupture and elongation. For annular dilatation, reduction in the circumference of the mitral orifice, i.e., annuloplasty, has become the standard method of repair. Commissural annuloplasty has been used successfully by Reed et al.[83] and by Kay et al.[84] Because localized "bunching" as a result of this approach tended to distort tensions on the valve, the concept of concentrically shortening the posterior mitral valve annulus by suturing it to a rigid, cloth-covered ring was developed by Carpentier et al.;[85] a similar, but flexible, ring was developed by Durán et al.[86] We and others have modified the concept of valve annuloplasty further by using a partial ring that subtends only the posterior portion of the mitral valve annulus and, thus, avoids any sutures near the anterior mitral leaflet.[87-89] This method has several advantages, including lessening of operative time and prevention of damage or distortion to the anterior leaflet of the mitral valve.

If a chorda or set of chordae is ruptured, a section of the corresponding leaflet will flail upward into the left atrium. Immobilization of this flail section by plicating it upon itself[90] (Fig 35-19) (or by excising the flail section and then repairing the leaflet) will overcome the problem of localized prolapse. However, the resulting reduction in surface area of the leaflet could itself enhance residual regurgitation; therefore, annuloplasty has become a routine part of the repair.

A perforation in a leaflet as a result of infective endocarditis, especially if located at the base of the anterior leaflet, may be closed by using a patch of synthetic material.

It is important to assess adequacy of mitral valve reconstruction before completion of the operation. The first method is careful inspection of the valve immediately after repair; the surgeon can fill the left ventricle with saline and observe, through the left atrium, any mitral valve leakage. The second important method of intraoperative assessment of the mitral valve is transesophageal echocardiography with Doppler color-flow mapping.[91] This technique is used routinely to assess the results of valve repair. Transesophageal echocardiography can gauge the presence and severity of residual mitral valve leakage, permit visualization of the anatomical features of the repair, and provide an estimate of ventricular function.

Echocardiography is essential for identification of

systolic anterior motion of the mitral valve, which may occur early after mitral valve repair in 5% to 10% of patients; systolic anterior motion of the mitral valve may cause residual regurgitation. This condition, however, almost always improves with intravascular volume replacement and amelioration of the hyperdynamic circulation immediately after bypass.

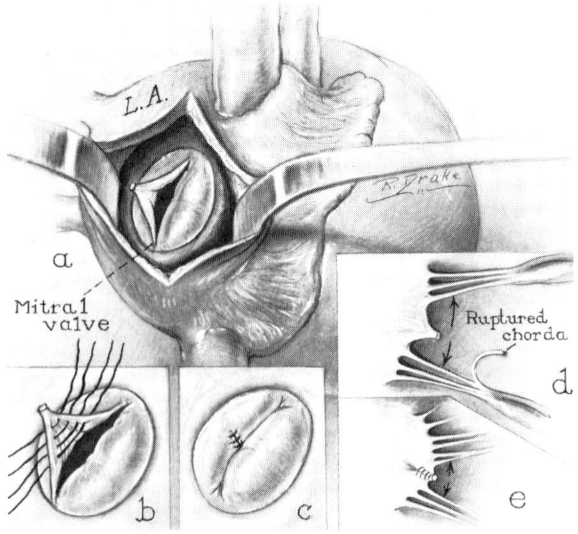

Fig 35-19 Plication repair of flail portion of posterior mitral leaflet, due to rupture of chordae. After plication, the adjacent intact chordae support the entire free margin of the leaflet. (From McGoon DC: Repair of mitral insufficiency due to ruptured chordae tendineae. *J Thorac Cardiovasc Surg* 39:357-362, 1960. By permission of CV Mosby Company.)

The third method to assess residual mitral regurgitation at the end of operation is double-sampling dye curves. Indocyanine green dye is injected into the left ventricular cavity while blood is aspirated from the aorta and left atrium. The blood is drawn through a densitometer connected to a recording instrument that inscribes curves of the concentration of dye in the aorta and left atrium. If no dye appears in left atrial blood until recirculation time has elapsed (no regurgitation) or if it appears in small amounts (< 15% in the left atrium compared with the aorta), the result can be considered satisfactory.

Valve replacement. When reconstruction of the incompetent mitral valve is believed to be impossible, or, if attempted, is unsuccessful, then replacement must be performed. The choice of prosthetic valves and the criteria for selecting among them are described elsewhere (chapter 37). In brief, the dilemma with respect to the mitral valve, as with the aortic valve, is the choice between a prosthetic valve of excellent durability but with the hazard of thromboembolism and a biologic valve with undefined long-term durability but less tendency to cause thromboembolism.[69] Because of the frequent association of atrial fibrillation,[69] chronic anticoagulant therapy is probably wise for most patients even after replacement of the mitral valve with a bioprosthesis, so that the hope of avoiding the risks of anticoagulation is not necessarily a factor in choosing a substitute valve for the mitral position.[92]

Late results

Information on valve replacement is discussed in detail in chapter 37. For patients with symptoms preoperatively, exertional dyspnea and fluid retention are greatly improved after correction of mitral regurgitation, and the

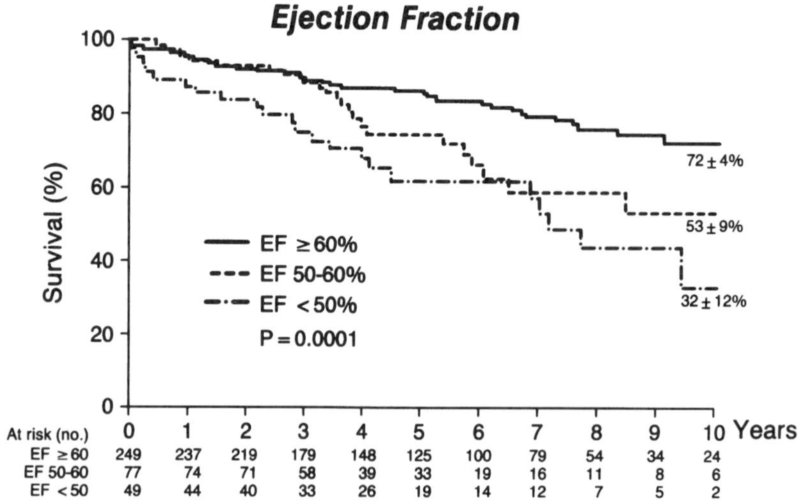

Fig 35-20 Late survival after correction of mitral regurgitation. Patients are stratified by preoperative echocardiographic ejection fraction. (From Enriquez-Sarano M, Tajik AJ, Schaff HV, et al: Echocardiographic prediction of survival after surgical correction of organic mitral regurgitation. *Circulation* 90:830-837, 1994. By permission of American Heart Association.)

Table 35-4 Operative mortality after mitral valve replacement or repair

Patients	Mortality, % Replacement	Repair	P
All	10.3	2.6	0.002
Age ≥75 yr	30.8	6.8	0.0005
Age <75 yr	5.7	1.3	0.036

From Enriquez-Sarano M, Schaff HV, Orszulak TA, et al: Valve repair improves the outcome of surgery for mitral regurgitation. A multivariate analysis. *Circulation* 91:1022-1028, 1995. By permission of American Heart Association.

subsequent course depends on several factors, including adequacy of ventricular function and surgical methods (Fig 35-20). For patients with degenerative mitral valve disease, mitral valve repair rather than prosthetic replacement significantly improves survival. Our studies show that the 5- and 10-year survival rates are 83% and 68%, respectively, after mitral valve repair and 69% and 52% after mitral valve replacement.[93]

It also appears that operative mortality is lower after valve repair than after valve replacement for mitral regurgitation. Overall mortality after repair of mitral valve regurgitation is approximately 3% (Table 35-4).

The postoperative hemodynamic response to correction of mitral regurgitation depends on the degree to which ventricular function is depressed preoperatively. In echocardiographic studies of patients who survive mitral valve repair or replacement for mitral regurgitation, ejection fraction decreased from an average of 58% preoperatively to 50% postoperatively.[94] Postoperative left ventricular dysfunction (ejection fraction of <50%) occurs in approximately 40% of patients and carries an especially poor prognosis; 8 years postoperatively, survival of patients with left ventricular dysfunction was only 38% compared with 69% for patients with postoperative ejection fractions of >50%. Thus, it appears prudent to advise operation for patients with severe mitral regurgitation when the ejection fraction is ≤60%, even for those who do not have symptoms or have little limitation in activity. This advice is especially pertinent if valve repair can be performed.

REFERENCES

1. Selzer A, Katayama F: Mitral regurgitation: clinical patterns, pathophysiology and natural history. *Medicine (Baltimore)* 51:337-366, 1972
2. Turner E, Wisenbaugh T, Sinovich V, et al: Morphologic patterns in patients undergoing reoperation after repair of rheumatic mitral regurgitation. *Am J Cardiol* 71:455-457, 1993
3. Olson LJ, Subramanian R, Ackermann DM, et al: Surgical pathology of the mitral valve: a study of 712 cases spanning 21 years. *Mayo Clin Proc* 62:22-34, 1987
4. Procacci PM, Savran SV, Schreiter SL, et al: Prevalence of clinical mitral-valve prolapse in 1169 young women. *N Engl J Med* 294:1086-1088, 1976
5. Pini R, Devereux RB, Greppi B, et al: Comparison of mitral valve dimensions and motion in mitral valve prolapse with severe mitral regurgitation to uncomplicated mitral valve prolapse and to mitral regurgitation without mitral valve prolapse. *Am J Cardiol* 62:257-263, 1988
6. Waller BF, Morrow AG, Maron BJ, et al: Etiology of clinically isolated, severe, chronic, pure mitral regurgitation: analysis of 97 patients over 30 years of age having mitral valve replacement. *Am Heart J* 104:276-288, 1982
7. Lucas RV Jr, Edwards JE: The floppy mitral valve. *Curr Probl Cardiol* 7:1-48, 1982
8. Lis Y, Burleigh MC, Parker DJ, et al: Biochemical characterization of individual normal, floppy and rheumatic human mitral valves. *Biochem J* 244:597-603, 1987
9. Ormiston JA, Shah PM, Tei C, et al: Size and motion of the mitral valve annulus in man. II. Abnormalities in mitral valve prolapse. *Circulation* 65:713-719, 1982
10. Rippe JM, Angoff G, Sloss LJ, et al: Multiple floppy valves: an echocardiographic syndrome. *Am J Med* 66:817-824, 1979
11. Wilcken DE, Hickey AJ: Lifetime risk for patients with mitral valve prolapse of developing severe valve regurgitation requiring surgery. *Circulation* 78:10-14, 1988
12. Düren DR, Becker AE, Dunning AJ: Long-term follow-up of idiopathic mitral valve prolapse in 300 patients: a prospective study. *J Am Coll Cardiol* 11:42-47, 1988
13. Nishimura RA, McGoon MD, Shub C, et al: Echocardiographically documented mitral-valve prolapse: long-term follow-up of 237 patients. *N Engl J Med* 313:1305-1309, 1985
14. MacMahon SW, Hickey AJ, Wilcken DEL, et al: Risk of infective endocarditis in mitral valve prolapse with and without precordial systolic murmurs. *Am J Cardiol* 59:105-108, 1987
15. Edwards JE: Pathology of mitral incompetence. In *Cardiovascular Pathology*. Vol 1. Edited by MD Silver. New York, Churchill Livingstone, 1983, pp 575-598
16. Malcolm AD, Canković-Darracott S, Chayen J, et al: Biopsy evidence of left ventricular myocardial abnormality in patients with mitral-leaflet prolapse and chest pain. *Lancet* 1:1052-1055, 1979
17. Pellikka PA, Tajik AJ, Khandheria BK, et al: Carcinoid heart disease. Clinical and echocardiographic spectrum in 74 patients. *Circulation* 87:1188-1196, 1993
18. Redfield MM, Nicholson WJ, Edwards WD, et al: Valve disease associated with ergot alkaloid use: echocardiographic and pathologic correlations. *Ann Intern Med* 117:50-52, 1992
19. Kishon Y, Oh JK, Schaff HV, et al: Mitral valve operation in postinfarction rupture of a papillary muscle: immediate results and long-term follow-up of 22 patients. *Mayo Clin Proc* 67:1023-1030, 1992
20. Izumi S, Miyatake K, Beppu S, et al: Mechanism of mitral regurgitation in patients with myocardial infarction: a study using real-time two-dimensional Doppler flow imaging and echocardiography. *Circulation* 76:777-785, 1987
21. Keren G, Bier A, Strom JA, et al: Dynamics of mitral regurgitation during nitroglycerin therapy: a Doppler echocardiographic study. *Am Heart J* 112:517-525, 1986
22. Keren G, Laniado S, Sonnenblick EH, et al: Dynamics of functional mitral regurgitation during dobutamine therapy in patients with severe congestive heart failure: a Doppler echocardiographic study. *Am Heart J* 118:748-754, 1989
23. Yoran C, Yellin EL, Becker RM, et al: Dynamic aspects of acute mitral regurgitation: effects of ventricular volume, pressure and contractility on the effective regurgitant orifice area. *Circulation* 60:170-176, 1979
24. Gehl LG, Mintz GS, Kotler MN, et al: Left atrial volume overload in mitral regurgitation: a two dimensional echocardiographic study. *Am J Cardiol* 49:33-38, 1982
25. Wisenbaugh T, Spann JF, Carabello BA: Differences in myocardial performance and load between patients with similar amounts of chronic aortic versus chronic mitral regurgitation. *J Am Coll Cardiol* 3:916-923, 1984
26. Nwasokwa O, Camesas A, Weg I, et al: Differences in left ventricular adaptation to chronic mitral and aortic regurgitation. *Chest* 95:106-110, 1989
27. Rousseau MF, Pouleur H, Charlier AA, et al: Assessment of left ventricular relaxation in patients with valvular regurgitation. *Am J Cardiol* 50:1028-1036, 1982
28. Rapaport E: Natural history of aortic and mitral valve disease. *Am J Cardiol* 35:221-227, 1975

29. Hammermeister KE, Fisher L, Kennedy JW, et al: Prediction of late survival in patients with mitral valve disease from clinical, hemodynamic, and quantitative angiographic variables. *Circulation* 57:341-349, 1978

30. Ramanathan KB, Knowles J, Connor MJ, et al: Natural history of chronic mitral insufficiency: relation of peak systolic pressure/end-systolic volume ratio to morbidity and mortality. *J Am Coll Cardiol* 3:1412-1416, 1984

31. Hochreiter C, Niles N, Devereux RB, et al: Mitral regurgitation: relationship of noninvasive descriptors of right and left ventricular performance to clinical and hemodynamic findings and to prognosis in medically and surgically treated patients. *Circulation* 73:900-912, 1986

32. Yoshikawa J, Yoshida K, Akasaka T, et al: Value and limitations of color Doppler flow mapping in the detection and semiquantification of valvular regurgitation. *Int J Card Imaging* 2:85-91, 1987

33. Werner JA, Schiller NB, Prasquier R: Occurrence and significance of echocardiographically demonstrated tricuspid valve prolapse. *Am Heart J* 96:180-186, 1978

34. Martin RP, Meltzer RS, Chia BL, et al: Clinical utility of two dimensional echocardiography in infective endocarditis. *Am J Cardiol* 46:379-385, 1980

35. Shively BK, Gurule FT, Roldan CA, et al: Diagnostic value of transesophageal compared with transthoracic echocardiography in infective endocarditis. *J Am Coll Cardiol* 18:391-397, 1991

36. Birmingham GD, Rahko PS, Ballantyne F III: Improved detection of infective endocarditis with transesophageal echocardiography. *Am Heart J* 123:774-781, 1992

37. Loperfido F, Biasucci LM, Pennestrí F, et al: Pulsed Doppler echocardiographic analysis of mitral regurgitation after myocardial infarction. *Am J Cardiol* 58:692-697, 1986

38. Spain MG, Smith MD, Grayburn PA, et al: Quantitative assessment of mitral regurgitation by Doppler color flow imaging: angiographic and hemodynamic correlations. *J Am Coll Cardiol* 13:585-590, 1989

39. Tribouilloy C, Shen WF, Quere JP, et al: Assessment of severity of mitral regurgitation by measuring regurgitant jet width at its origin with transesophageal Doppler color flow imaging. *Circulation* 85:1248-1253, 1992

40. Miyatake K, Izumi S, Okamoto M, et al: Semiquantitative grading of severity of mitral regurgitation by real-time two-dimensional Doppler flow imaging technique. *J Am Coll Cardiol* 7:82-88, 1986

41. Helmcke F, Nanda NC, Hsiung MC, et al: Color Doppler assessment of mitral regurgitation with orthogonal planes. *Circulation* 75:175-183, 1987

42. Losordo DW, Pastore JO, Coletta D, et al: Limitations of color flow Doppler imaging in the quantification of valvular regurgitation: velocity of regurgitant jet, rather than volume, determines size of color Doppler image. *Am Heart J* 126:168-176, 1993

43. Stevenson JG: Two-dimensional color Doppler estimation of the severity of atrioventricular valve regurgitation: important effects of instrument gain setting, pulse, repetition frequency, and carrier frequency. *J Am Soc Echo* 2:1-10, 1989

44. Thomas JD, Liu CM, Flachskampf FA, et al: Quantification of jet flow by momentum analysis. An in vitro color Doppler flow study. *Circulation* 81:247-259, 1990

45. Enriquez-Sarano M, Tajik AJ, Bailey KR, et al: Color flow imaging compared with quantitative Doppler assessment of severity of mitral regurgitation: influence of eccentricity of jet and mechanism of regurgitation. *J Am Coll Cardiol* 21:1211-1219, 1993

46. Cape EG, Yoganathan AP, Weyman AE, et al: Adjacent solid boundaries alter the size of regurgitant jets on Doppler color flow maps. *J Am Coll Cardiol* 17:1094-1102, 1991

47. Castello R, Pearson AC, Lenzen P, et al: Effect of mitral regurgitation on pulmonary venous velocities derived from transesophageal echocardiography color-guided pulsed Doppler imaging. *J Am Coll Cardiol* 17:1499-1506, 1991

48. Klein AL, Obarski TP, Stewart WJ, et al: Transesophageal Doppler echocardiography of pulmonary venous flow: a new marker of mitral regurgitation severity. *J Am Coll Cardiol* 18:518-526, 1991

49. Klein AL, Stewart WJ, Bartlett J, et al: Effects of mitral regurgitation on pulmonary venous flow and left atrial pressure: an intraoperative transesophageal echocardiographic study. *J Am Coll Cardiol* 20:1345-1352, 1992

50. Vandervoort PM, Rivera JM, Mele D, et al: Application of color Doppler flow mapping to calculate effective regurgitant orifice area. An in vitro study and initial clinical observations. *Circulation* 88:1150-1156, 1993

51. Enriquez-Sarano M, Seward JB, Bailey KR, et al: Effective regurgitant orifice area: a noninvasive Doppler development of an old hemodynamic concept. *J Am Coll Cardiol* 23:443-451, 1994

52. Lewis JF, Kuo LC, Nelson JG, et al: Pulsed Doppler echocardiographic determination of stroke volume and cardiac output: clinical validation of two new methods using the apical window. *Circulation* 70:425-431, 1984

53. Enriquez-Sarano M, Bailey KR, Seward JB, et al: Quantitative Doppler assessment of valvular regurgitation. *Circulation* 87:841-848, 1993

54. Blumlein S, Bouchard A, Schiller NB, et al: Quantitation of mitral regurgitation by Doppler echocardiography. *Circulation* 74:306-314, 1986

55. Gorge G, Erbel R, Brennecke R, et al: High-resolution two-dimensional echocardiography improves the quantification of left ventricular function. *J Am Soc Echocardiogr* 5:125-134, 1992

56. Jenni R, Ritter M, Eberli F, et al: Quantification of mitral regurgitation with amplitude-weighted mean velocity from continuous wave Doppler spectra. *Circulation* 79:1294-1299, 1989

57. Enriquez-Sarano M, Kaneshige AM, Tajik AJ, et al: Amplitude-weighted mean velocity: clinical utilization for quantitation of mitral regurgitation. *J Am Coll Cardiol* 22:1684-1690, 1993

58. Recusani F, Bargiggia GS, Yoganathan AP, et al: A new method for quantification of regurgitant flow rate using color Doppler flow imaging of the flow convergence region proximal to a discrete orifice. An in vitro study. *Circulation* 83:594-604, 1991

59. Bargiggia GS, Tronconi L, Sahn DJ, et al: A new method for quantitation of mitral regurgitation based on color flow Doppler imaging of flow convergence proximal to regurgitant orifice. *Circulation* 84:1481-1489, 1991

60. Chen C, Koschyk D, Brockhoff C, et al: Noninvasive estimation of regurgitant flow rate and volume in patients with mitral regurgitation by Doppler color mapping of accelerating flow field. *J Am Coll Cardiol* 21:374-383, 1993

61. Ejini M, Sasayama S, Fujita M, et al: Importance of regurgitant fraction for left ventricular end-systolic wall stress to end-systolic volume ratio in patients with chronic mitral regurgitation. *Jpn Circ J* 52:426-430, 1988

62. Breisblatt W, Goodyer AVN, Zaret BL, et al: An improved index of left ventricular function in chronic mitral regurgitation. *Am J Cardiol* 57:1105-1108, 1986

63. Kontos GJ Jr, Schaff HV, Gersh BJ, et al: Left ventricular function in subacute and chronic mitral regurgitation: effect on function early postoperatively. *J Thorac Cardiovasc Surg* 98:163-169, 1989

64. Kelbæk H, Aldershvile J, Svendsen JH, et al: Combined first pass and equilibrium radionuclide cardiographic determination of stroke volume for quantitation of valvular regurgitation. *J Am Coll Cardiol* 11:769-773, 1988

65. Philippe L, Mena I, Darcourt J, et al: Evaluation of valvular regurgitation by factor analysis of first-pass angiography. *J Nucl Med* 29:159-167, 1988

66. Sciagrà R, Voth E, Tebbe U, et al: Evaluation of three methods for quantifying valvular regurgitation using gated equilibrium radionuclide ventriculography. *Eur Heart J* 8:1109-1118, 1987

67. Alexopoulos D, Lazzam C, Borrico S, et al: Isolated chronic mitral regurgitation with preserved systolic left ventricular function and severe pulmonary hypertension. *J Am Coll Cardiol* 14:319-322, 1989

68. Fuchs RM, Heuser RR, Yin FC, et al: Limitations of pulmonary wedge V waves in diagnosing mitral regurgitation. *Am J Cardiol* 49:849-854, 1982

69. Pumphrey CW, Fuster V, Chesebro JH: Systemic thromboembolism in valvular heart disease and prosthetic heart valves. *Mod Concepts Cardiovasc Dis* 51:131-136, 1982

70. Devereux RB, Kramer-Fox R, Kligfield P: Mitral valve prolapse: causes, clinical manifestations, and management. *Ann Intern Med* 111:305-317, 1989

71. Winkle RA, Lopes MG, Goodman DJ, et al: Propranolol for patients with mitral valve prolapse. *Am Heart J* 93:422-427, 1977

72. Dalby AJ, Firth BG, Forman R: Preoperative factors affecting the outcome of isolated mitral valve replacement: a 10 year review. *Am J Cardiol* 47:826-834, 1981

73. Carabello BA, Spann JF: The uses and limitations of end-systolic indexes of left ventricular function. *Circulation* 69:1058-1064, 1984

74. Crawford MH, Souchek J, Oprian CA, et al: Determinants of survival and left ventricular performance after mitral valve replacement. Department of Veterans Affairs Cooperative Study on Valvular Heart Disease. *Circulation* 81:1173-1181, 1990
75. Enriquez-Sarano M, Tajik AJ, Schaff HV, et al: Echocardiographic prediction of left ventricular function after correction of mitral regurgitation: results and clinical implications. *J Am Coll Cardiol* 24:1536-1543, 1994
76. Enriquez-Sarano M, Tajik AJ, Schaff HV, et al: Echocardiographic prediction of survival after surgical correction of organic mitral regurgitation. *Circulation* 90:830-837, 1994
77. Orszulak TA, Schaff HV, Danielson GK, et al: Mitral regurgitation due to ruptured chordae tendineae: early and late results of valve repair. *J Thorac Cardiovasc Surg* 89:491-498, 1985
78. Oliveira DBG, Dawkins KD, Kay PH, et al: Chordal rupture. II: Comparison between repair and replacement. *Br Heart J* 50:318-324, 1983
79. Cámara ML, Aris A, Padró JM, et al: Long-term results of mitral valve surgery in patients with severe pulmonary hypertension. *Ann Thorac Surg* 45:133-136, 1988
80. David TE, Uden DE, Strauss HD: The importance of the mitral apparatus in left ventricular function after correction of mitral regurgitation. *Circulation* 68 Suppl 2:76-82, 1983
81. David TE, Burns RJ, Baccus CM, et al: Mitral valve replacement for mitral regurgitation with and without preservation of chordae tendineae. *J Thorac Cardiovasc Surg* 88:718-725, 1984
82. Goldman ME, Mora F, Fuster V, et al: Is mitral valvuloplasty superior to mitral valve replacement for preservation of left ventricular function? An intraoperative two-dimensional echocardiographic study (abstract). *J Am Coll Cardiol* 7:160A, 1986
83. Reed GE, Pooley RW, Moggio RA: Durability of measured mitral annuloplasty: seventeen-year study. *J Thorac Cardiovasc Surg* 79:321-325, 1980
84. Kay GL, Kay JH, Zubiate P, et al: Mitral valve repair for mitral regurgitation secondary to coronary artery disease. *Circulation* 74 Suppl 1:88-98, 1986
85. Carpentier A, Chauvaud S, Fabiani JN, et al: Reconstructive surgery of mitral valve incompetence: ten-year appraisal. *J Thorac Cardiovasc Surg* 79:338-348, 1980
86. Durán CG, Revuelta JM, Gaite L, et al: Stability of mitral reconstructive surgery at 10-12 years for predominantly rheumatic valvular disease. *Circulation* 78 Suppl 1:91-96, 1988
87. Cooley DA, Frazier OH, Norman JC: Mitral leaflet prolapse: surgical treatment using a posterior annulus collar prosthesis. *Bull Texas Heart Inst* 3:438, 1976
88. Chang CH, Lin PJ, Chang JP, et al: Long-term results of polytetrafluoroethylene mitral annuloplasty. *Ann Thorac Surg* 57:644-647, 1994
89. Fundaro P, Salati M, Cialfi A, et al: Polytetrafluoroethylene posterior annuloplasty for mitral regurgitation (letter to the editor). *Ann Thorac Surg* 50:165-166, 1990
90. McGoon DC: Repair of mitral insufficiency due to ruptured chordae tendineae. *J Thorac Cardiovasc Surg* 39:357-362, 1960
91. Freeman WK, Schaff HV, Khandheria BK, et al: Intraoperative evaluation of mitral valve regurgitation and repair by transesophageal echocardiography: incidence and significance of systolic anterior motion. *J Am Coll Cardiol* 20:599-609, 1992
92. Edmunds LH Jr: Thromboembolic complications of current cardiac valvular prostheses. *Ann Thorac Surg* 34:96-106, 1982
93. Enriquez-Sarano M, Schaff HV, Orszulak TA, et al: Valve repair improves the outcome of surgery for mitral regurgitation. A multivariate analysis. *Circulation* 91:1022-1028, 1995
94. Enriquez-Sarano M, Tajik AJ, Schaff HV, et al: Echocardiographic prediction of left ventricular function after correction of mitral regurgitation: results and clinical implications. *J Am Coll Cardiol* 24:1536-1543, 1994

CHAPTER

36

Tricuspid valve disease

Emilio R. Giuliani, M.D., John J. Lynch, M.D., and Robert O. Brandenburg, M.D.

Tricuspid valve disease of clinical importance is relatively uncommon. The observations by King[1] in the 19th century on the function of the right atrioventricular (AV) valve remain the foundation on which additional observations have been added to form our present knowledge of the tricuspid valve in both health and disease. Silver et al.[2] in 1971 and Wooley[3] in 1981 published excellent reviews on the subject.

ANATOMIC CONSIDERATIONS

In order to appreciate fully the pathophysiologic consequences of tricuspid valve disease, it is important to understand the tricuspid valve as a functioning unit. This valve is made up of six anatomic structures whose integrated function is essential if the valve is to perform normally (Table 36-1). The tricuspid valve is divided into three leaflets – anterior, posterior, and septal. The majority of the chordae tendineae insert on the free edges of the leaflets. The free edges of the anterior and septal leaflets contain notches; the free edge of the posterior leaflet contains scallops similar to those on the leaflets of the mitral valve. The belly of the leaflets lies between the free edge and the basal zone, which is the area of attachment to the annulus.[4]

Generally there are two major papillary muscles: one gives rise to chordae that attach to both the anterior and the posterior leaflets; the other gives rise to chordae extending to the posterior and septal leaflets. One or more smaller papillary muscles also give rise to chordae attached to these leaflets. In addition, chordae arise from the ventricular wall and attach to the ventricular surface of the septal leaflet. These chordae arise more often from the ventricular septum and attach to the underlying surface of the septal leaflet.

The tricuspid annulus represents a portion of the "skeleton" of the heart and, because of attachments of the ventricular and atrial muscle fibers, plays an important role in normal valve function. Tsakiris et al.[5] demonstrated that, with atrial systole, there is approximately 25% decrease in the maximum valve circumference as a result of atrial contraction. They also showed that the tricuspid annular motion associated with atrial systole was distinctly different from that seen with ventricular systole. From these observations, it was concluded that atrial systole contributes to normal tricuspid valve closure. Okamoto et al.[6] demonstrated that this contribution may initiate the closure of the tricuspid valve but is not capable of closing it tightly. The chordae tendineae, papillary muscles, and ventricular myocardium all are important as supporting structures for the tricuspid leaflets. An abnormality of any of these structures may produce dysfunction of the tricuspid valve. An important area of anatomy is the triangle of Koch, because the conducting tissue passing from the atrium to the ventricle lies within it.[7] These electrical pathways must be intact to ensure a normal sequence of activation and normal valve function.

TRICUSPID STENOSIS

The most common cause of tricuspid stenosis is rheumatic involvement of the tricuspid valve. This is usually associated with mitral and aortic involvement and only rarely with aortic involvement alone[8] (Table 36-2). Isolated tricuspid stenosis of rheumatic cause has been reported but is extremely rare; the majority of patients with tricuspid stenosis also have tricuspid regurgitation.[8-12] The incidence of organic tricuspid valve involvement in rheumatic heart disease, as reported in the literature, varies depending on the definition of involvement, the method used for diagnosis, and the patient's country of origin. Friedberg[13] stated that microscopic evidence of rheumatic inflammation was almost as common in the tricuspid valve as in the mitral valve. Others have reported

We appreciate the review of this chapter by W.D. Edwards, M.D.

Table 36-1 Anatomy of tricuspid valve unit

Tricuspid valve leaflets
Chordae tendineae
Papillary muscles
Tricuspid valve annulus
Right atrium
Right ventricle
Electrical conducting pathways

Table 36-2 Ages and associated valvular lesions in 29 patients with rheumatic tricuspid disease*

	Valvular lesions	
Age, yr	Mitral	Combined (aortic & mitral)
10-19	0	1
20-29	0	1
30-39	2	5
40-49	2	11
50-59	2	5
60-69	0	0
Total	6	23

*Based on 48 consecutive patients requiring tricuspid valve surgery.

Table 36-3 Clinical symptoms in 29 patients with rheumatic tricuspid disease

Symptom	No.	Percent
Fatigue	29	100
Dyspnea	29	100
Edema	28	97
Ascites	16	55
Orthopnea/PND*	1	4

*Paroxysmal nocturnal dyspnea.

an incidence of 5% to 10% among patients with rheumatic heart disease.[9,10,13-18] Reports from India indicate an incidence of 35% to 45%.[19-21] Some observers have reported an incidence of tricuspid stenosis of 2% to 3% in patients with rheumatic heart disease when detailed cardiac catheterization studies were done.[22-24]

The pathologic features of tricuspid rheumatic involvement are similar to those of mitral valve disease but are of a much milder degree.[19-25]

Other causes of tricuspid stenosis are rare. Nonrheumatic tricuspid stenosis usually is not associated with other cardiac defects. The causes include congenital tricuspid stenosis,[26-29] fibroelastosis,[30] endomyocardial fibrosis,[31] carcinoid heart disease,[32] systemic lupus erythematosus,[23] right atrial myxoma,[33] tumors,[34-40] endocarditis,[41] catheter entanglements,[42,43] diseases of the pericardium,[44-46] unruptured aneurysm of the sinus of Valsalva,[39] cardiac hydatid disease,[40] and pacemaker lead.[47] All produce similar hemodynamic abnormalities.

Pathophysiology of tricuspid stenosis

In the adult, the tricuspid valve orifice area is approximately 7 cm^2. Although little has been published on this subject, it appears that significant tricuspid stenosis occurs only at an orifice area of less than 2 cm^2. The initial hemodynamic changes are an increase in right atrial pressure and a decrease in right ventricular stroke volume. The degree of right atrial pressure increase is related to the severity of the stenosis and the compliance of the right atrium. The classic findings in patients with sinus rhythm are a large right atrial "a" wave and often a large v wave because of the association of tricuspid regurgitation. A shallow y trough is seen in all cases of significant tricuspid stenosis and is the result of slow atrial emptying. Because pure tricuspid stenosis is rare, the usual hemodynamic findings are the result of combined tricuspid stenosis and regurgitation. Right ventricular volumes usually are normal or low if stenosis predominates but are increased when there is a significant degree of tricuspid regurgitation. The cardiac index may be low, depending on the severity of the tricuspid valve disease as well as the severity of any associated mitral or aortic valve disease.

Transtricuspid gradients generally are small during rest. Killip and Lukas[48] have indicated that any gradient more than 1.9 mm Hg indicates tricuspid stenosis. These small gradients may be missed on routine withdrawal tracings, and it has been stressed that the end-diastolic tricuspid gradient is insensitive and does not indicate the severity of tricuspid stenosis.[24,48,49] Therefore, a planned, detailed technique of evaluation must be used. This small tricuspid gradient increases with inspiration and decreases during expiration. This is mainly due to a decrease in right ventricular end-diastolic pressure with inspiration. Although changes occur in the volume in the right atrium (augmented right atrial filling with inspiration), there is little respiratory change in right atrial pressure. The most reliable method appears to be the use of two matched catheters across the tricuspid valve so that pressures may be recorded simultaneously, and measurements should be made throughout the respiratory cycle. Recently, provocation with intravenous solution of saline to amplify the transvalvular pressure gradient in rheumatic tricuspid stenosis has been reported.[50] Doppler echocardiography can now accurately assess instantaneous and mean valve gradients.

Natural history and clinical course

The natural history of rheumatic tricuspid stenosis is dictated by the associated valvular lesions.[51] The majority of patients with rheumatic tricuspid disease are women between the ages of 30 and 60. In most cases, the symptoms are related to the associated mitral or aortic valve disease. The most common manifestation of tricuspid involvement is fatigue and is undoubtedly secondary to decreased cardiac output.[52] Dyspnea and abnormal fluid accumulation occur in that order of frequency (Table 36-3). Pulmonary edema, hemoptysis, orthopnea, and paroxysmal nocturnal dyspnea are infrequent in patients with tricuspid valve disease in spite of associated severe mitral stenosis.

Table 36-4 Clinical profile in rheumatic tricuspid valve disease

Female, age 30-60
Associated mitral or aortic valve disease
Absence of symptoms of pulmonary venous hypertension
Major symptoms
Fatigue
Dyspnea
Edema
Ascites

Physical examination

Physical appearance. Rheumatic tricuspid stenosis should be suspected in a woman between 30 and 60 years old who presents with symptoms of fatigue and fluid retention and auscultatory findings of rheumatic mitral or aortic valve disease (Table 36-4).

Arterial and venous pulse. In patients with sinus rhythm, there is a large "a" wave.[53] The height of this wave varies from patient to patient. Patients with atrial fibrillation show a distinct irregular systolic v wave followed by a slow y descent.[51] Although difficult to appreciate, a slow y descent is diagnostic of obstruction at the valvular level (Fig 36-1). The arterial pulse reflects changes in rhythm and left ventricular stroke volume.

Auscultation. The finding of a "tricuspid" diastolic murmur is the hallmark of tricuspid valve obstruction. The murmur of tricuspid stenosis is best heard along the left parasternal region at the fourth and fifth ribs.[54] Rarely, it is best heard over the lower sternum or to the right of the sternum. In patients with sinus rhythm, the presystolic murmur begins before the murmur of mitral stenosis, has a higher mixed frequency component than the murmur of mitral stenosis, is crescendo-decrescendo in its configuration, and terminates before the first heart sound. This is in sharp contrast to the presystolic murmur of mitral stenosis, which is crescendo and ends with the first heart sound[55] (Fig 36-2). The murmur increases in intensity during inspiration (Carvallo's sign)[54] (Fig 36-3). While making this observation, one should not expose the patient to prolonged inspiratory and expiratory apnea. The best way to appreciate the change in intensity of the murmur is to listen as the patient is breathing slowly, deeply, and continuously. Occasionally, having the patient stop breathing for 2 to 3 seconds at the end of inspiration increases the chance of hearing the subtle diastolic murmur.

During atrial fibrillation, the diastolic murmur of tricuspid stenosis is heard in early diastole or middiastole (Fig 36-4). The murmur begins after the tricuspid opening snap when this is present. The murmur is high frequency and decrescendo and is heard best along the lower left sternal border or over the xiphoid. As in sinus rhythm, the murmur increases in intensity with inspiration, an observation first documented by Rivero-Carvallo[56] and often referred to as "Carvallo's sign." The murmurs of aortic and pulmonary insufficiency are similar to the murmur of tricuspid stenosis, both in location and in quality. The murmur of aortic insufficiency begins immediately with the aortic component of the second heart sound, and the murmur of pulmonary insufficiency begins immediately after the pulmonary component.

The opening snap of the tricuspid valve only rarely can be distinguished from the mitral opening snap and therefore is of limited value in the diagnosis of tricuspid

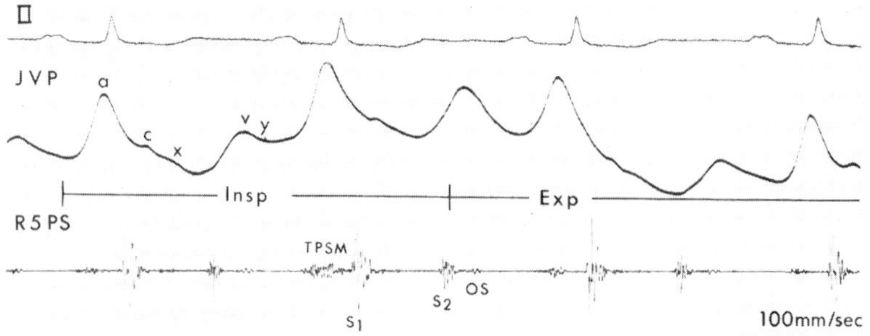

Fig 36-1 Rheumatic tricuspid stenosis in 43-year-old woman. Electrocardiogram shows sinus rhythm with the large P-wave configuration of left atrial enlargement (due to associated mitral disease). Note large "a" wave and gentle x and y descents. *Exp,* expiration; *Insp,* inspiration; *JVP,* jugular venous pulse; *OS,* opening snap; *R5PS,* right fifth parasternal; *TPSM,* tricuspid presystolic murmur. (From Giuliani ER, Brandenburg RO, Fuster V: Evaluation of cardiac murmurs. *Cardiovasc Clin* 10 No 3:1-18, 1980. By permission of FA Davis Company.)

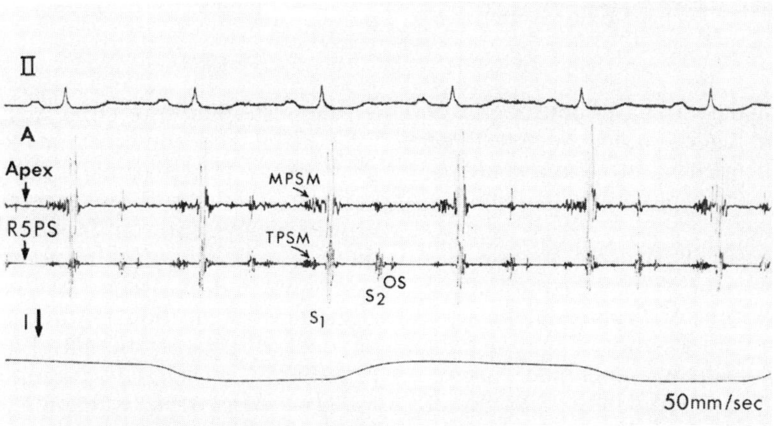

Fig 36-2 Mitral, aortic, and tricuspid rheumatic valvular stenosis confirmed at autopsy. *R5PS,* right fifth parasternal; *TPSM,* tricuspid presystolic murmur (note early onset, higher frequency, and increased intensity during inspiration compared to mitral presystolic murmur *[MPSM]*); *I,* inspiration. (From Giuliani ER, Brandenburg RO, Fuster V: Evaluation of cardiac murmurs. *Cardiovasc Clin* 10 No 3:1-18, 1980. By permission of FA Davis Company.)

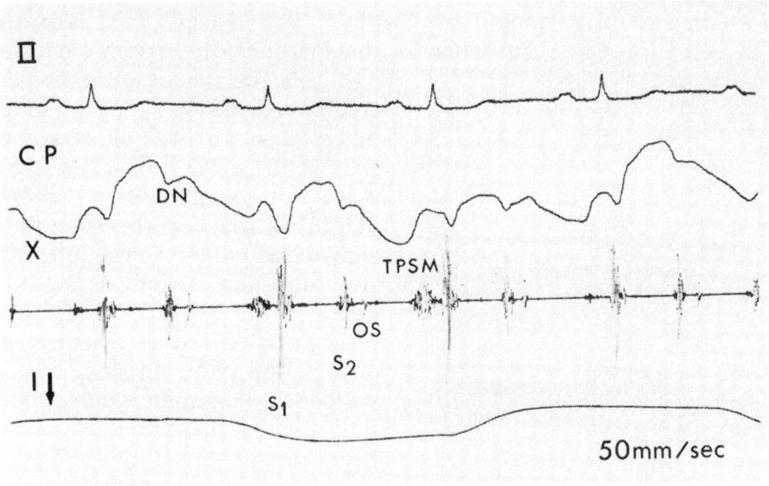

Fig 36-3 Tricuspid stenosis in 50-year-old patient. Note characteristic diamond-shaped tricuspid presystolic murmur ending before the first heart sound and increasing in intensity during inspiration *(I)*. *II,* lead II of the ECG; *CP,* carotid pulse; *DN,* dicrotic notch; *X,* xiphoid; *TPSM,* tricuspid presystolic murmur. (From Giuliani ER, Brandenburg RO, Fuster V: Evaluation of cardiac murmurs. *Cardiovasc Clin* 10 No 3:1-18, 1980. By permission of FA Davis Company.)

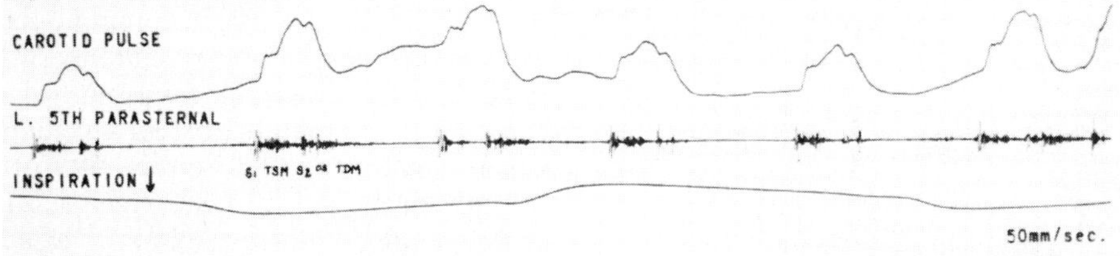

Fig 36-4 Tricuspid stenosis and atrial fibrillation. Note characteristics of diastolic murmur similar to those of aortic regurgitation. *OS,* opening snap; *TDM,* tricuspid diastolic murmur; *TSM,* tricuspid systolic murmur.

stenosis. Because it is unusual not to have some degree of tricuspid incompetence or regurgitation, an associated systolic murmur is normally present. Atrial and ventricular filling sounds are not present in patients with dominant tricuspid stenosis.

Thus, the clinical diagnosis of tricuspid stenosis depends on the presence of a giant "a" wave (if in normal sinus rhythm), a slow y descent of the jugular pulse, a tricuspid diastolic murmur, and absence of both a right ventricular impulse and a palpable pulmonic closure. These findings are usually encountered in the presence of associated mitral and aortic valvular disease.

Noninvasive evaluation

Electrocardiogram and chest roentgenogram. The electrocardiogram may give a clue to the diagnosis of tricuspid stenosis. When the height of the P wave in lead II is more than 2.5 mm, right atrial enlargement is suggested (Fig 36-5). Often the P wave will show a double-peaked configuration in the presence of mitral stenosis. Other findings may be present as a reflection of mitral valve disease, including a QRS frontal axis shifted to the right and evidence of right ventricular hypertrophy.[52]

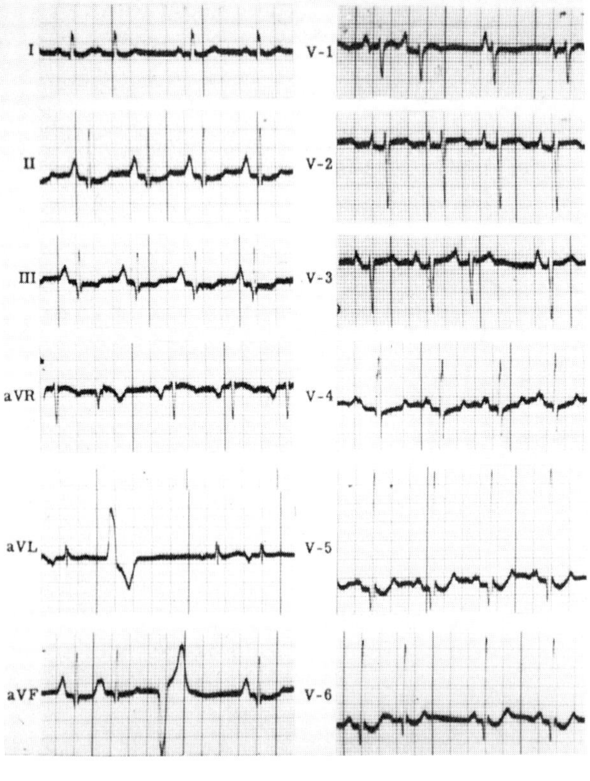

Fig 36-5 Electrocardiogram from 37-year-old patient with rheumatic mitral and tricuspid disease. Patient is in sinus rhythm. Note the tall, peaked P waves in leads II, III, and aVF, and in right precordial leads, indicative of right atrial dilatation.

The posteroanterior chest roentgenogram often shows right atrial and superior vena caval shadows that are prominent. The maximal distance of the right atrial border of the heart from the midline often exceeds 5 cm. Cardiomegaly is present in virtually all cases. Additional findings reflecting the hemodynamic changes of the associated mitral or aortic lesions often are present. Although calcification is often seen fluoroscopically in patients with rheumatic mitral and aortic disease, calcification of the rheumatic tricuspid valve is rarely seen.[52]

Echocardiogram. Evaluation of the tricuspid valve has historically been difficult because no true standard has been established to assess the valve. Although reliable information can be obtained by cardiac catheterization, a catheter across the tricuspid valve can potentially induce error in pressure measurements.[7] With the development of two-dimensional and color-flow Doppler echocardiography, this structure can be assessed in a way previously unknown. Although physical examination is helpful in determining whether tricuspid stenosis or regurgitation is present, it is not as sensitive as Doppler ultrasonography.[57] The tricuspid valve is an anterior cardiac structure that lies beneath the sternum in an anteromedial position. Typically, the valve is examined echocardiographically by combining the parasternal long-axis right ventricular inflow view with the short-axis parasternal view of the right ventricular outflow and tricuspid valve and with the apical four-chamber view. Intermediate views are also helpful in defining the tricuspid valve structure.[58] The views obtained by the examiner should focus on the valve structural unit, encompassing not only the valve leaflets but also the chordae tendineae, papillary muscle and muscular supporting structures, tricuspid annulus, right atrium, and right ventricle.

Echocardiographic examination detects many similarities in leaflet and annular motion in systole and diastole between right-sided and left-sided AV valves. However, there are also important differences. The tricuspid valve comprises three unequally sized leaflets, the anterior leaflet being larger than both the posterior and the septal leaflets. The septal leaflet of the tricuspid valve typically inserts more apically in the ventricular septum than the septal leaflet of the mitral valve. Three papillary muscles usually support the valve leaflets, with insertion of the chordae tendineae into these muscular groups.[58,59] However, not all chordae of the tricuspid valve have this relationship, and the chordal support may be directly into the infundibulum wall surface or the muscular trabeculae of the right ventricular free wall.

Examination of the tricuspid valve is best divided into structural and physiologic components of valve function. Leaflet thickness, mobility, and insertion positions are all important in assessing tricuspid valve disease. In the congenital anomaly—Ebstein's anomaly—the tricuspid valve is malformed and either part or all of the valve is apically displaced into the right ventricular cavity. The septal leaflet, most commonly affected, is displaced apically at its insertion into the ventricular septum. The anterior leaflet is least often displaced.[58]

The structural abnormalities of the tricuspid valve can lead to functional abnormality characterized by either restrictive inflow disease (i.e., tricuspid stenosis) or valvular regurgitant disease (i.e., tricuspid regurgitation).

The echocardiographic appearance of tricuspid stenosis is similar to that of mitral stenosis. Specifically, the leaflets tend to be thickened, with diastolic doming and restricted orifice size.[7] The supporting chordae tendineae also tend to be thickened, and the commissures may be fused. The added continuous-wave and pulsed-wave Doppler analyses of the tricuspid stenosis jet help to quantitate the severity of stenosis.[57,60,61] The Doppler waveform is typically affected by respirations, and care must be taken to evaluate pressure gradients in that light. Although the pressure half-time formula to quantitate stenosis has not been as well validated in tricuspid stenosis as in mitral stenosis, data suggest that there is good correlation with cardiac catheterization and the use of a Doppler-derived tricuspid valve (TV) area by a modified pressure half-time (PT½) method: TV area = 190/PT½.[60,61] Doppler analysis can also provide rapid, noninvasive assessment of the maximum and mean pressure gradients across the tricuspid valve.

Diagnostic problems

Associated valvular lesions. The importance of identifying tricuspid disease in the presence of mitral or aortic stenosis is clear from the many reports in the literature about lack of clinical improvement because of unrelieved tricuspid stenosis in patients who have undergone a surgical procedure on a mitral or aortic valve.[62-64] The diagnosis of rheumatic tricuspid stenosis may be made clinically and confirmed echocardiographically. Invasive studies are rarely necessary to support the diagnosis. It is important that the clinician maintain a high level of acuity and examine carefully for evidence of tricuspid stenosis, particularly in a woman between 30 and 60 years old who has evidence of rheumatic mitral involvement (see Table 36-4).

Cardiac tumors. Diagnostic problems arise when the clinical presentation of a cardiac tumor suggests obstruction of the tricuspid valve. This diagnosis should be considered in any patient whose findings suggest tricuspid stenosis in the absence of clinical findings of mitral and aortic disease.

MYXOMA. Right atrial myxomas (Fig 36-6) account for approximately 25% of cardiac intracavitary myxomas.[65] The systemic symptoms of fever, anorexia, and weight loss suggest the diagnosis of an atrial myxoma, infective endocarditis, or vasculitis. Clues to the correct diagnosis are changing auscultatory findings, absence of clinical findings of mitral or aortic valve disease, and negative blood cultures. Rarely, a tumor may be calcified, and the diagnosis can then be made from the chest roentgenogram or at chest fluoroscopy. The diagnosis of right atrial myxoma now can be made with a high degree of reliability by using two-dimensional echocardiography.[66-68] Therefore, angiography is not necessary and may be hazardous. If precordial echocardiographic images are unsatisfactory, transesophageal echocardiography can provide rapid, confident delineation of this entity.

METASTATIC TUMORS. Metastatic tumors involving the heart are 20 times more common than primary tumors. Cardiac metastases are found in approximately 20% of autopsies performed after a patient has died of cancer. Clinical diagnosis of cardiac involvement due to secondary spread to the pericardium and into intracardiac structures continues to be uncommon, and the diagnosis is based largely on echocardiographic findings. Cardiac valve involvement is uncommon and rarely is recognized clinically. However, certain tumors, particularly hypernephromas and melanomas, may mimic or produce tricuspid stenosis both clinically and hemodynami-

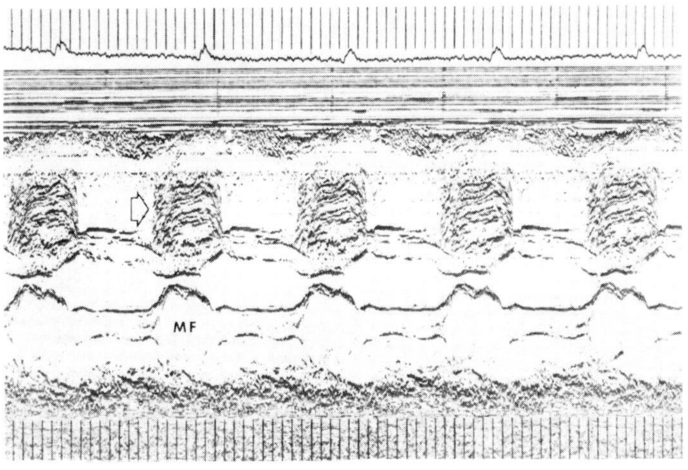

Fig 36-6 M-mode echocardiogram obtained through the ventricular chambers, demonstrating a mass of echoes *(large arrow)* filling the tricuspid funnel. At operation, large right atrial myxoma was found. *MF,* mitral valve funnel. (From Giuliani ER, Nasser FN: Two-dimensional echocardiography in acquired heart diseases—Part II. *Curr Probl Cardiol* 5:1-54, March 1981. By permission of Year Book Medical Publishers.)

cally.[36,37] The use of echocardiography and magnetic resonance imaging should prevent errors in diagnosis and eliminate the need for invasive studies.

Iatrogenic problems. The increasing use of catheters, cardiac pacing, and monitoring has introduced a new cause of obstruction at the level of the tricuspid valve. Between 1% and 2% of patients with endocardial pacing have clinical evidence of thrombosis. The risk of venous thrombosis should be kept in mind, particularly in patients with AV sequential pacing systems requiring multiple leads. When thrombosis interferes with tricuspid valve function, appropriate surgical intervention is indicated.

Constrictive pericarditis. Constrictive pericarditis with systemic venous congestion may simulate tricuspid disease. However, in constrictive pericarditis, the jugular venous pulse shows a prominent y descent in contrast to the gentle or absent y trough seen in tricuspid stenosis. In addition, there seldom is a murmur of tricuspid regurgitation. If the constriction is significant, a paradoxic arterial pulse can be demonstrated. Those with calcification of the pericardium are readily identified by posteroanterior and lateral chest roentgenograms. In difficult cases, echocardiography, computed tomography, magnetic resonance imaging, or cardiac catheterization may be necessary.

TRICUSPID VALVE REGURGITATION
Anatomic considerations

Congenital anomalies or acquired disease of any portion of the tricuspid valve unit may produce regurgitation of this valve[69] (Table 36-5). Less common causes are transvenous pacemakers and catheters,[70,71] coronary heart disease,[72,73] chest trauma,[74,75] thyrotoxicosis,[76] and orthotopic cardiac transplantation.[77] The most common congenital abnormality is tricuspid valve prolapse.[78] A less common congenital cause of tricuspid regurgitation is displacement of the attachment of the tricuspid leaflets (Ebstein's anomaly). The most common acquired abnormality that produces clinically significant tricuspid regurgitation is dilatation of the tricuspid annulus[79,80] (Figs 36-7 and 36-8). The next most common is abnormalities of the leaflets of the tricuspid valve.

A more recent problem is tricuspid incompetence after orthotopic heart transplantation.[81] Data suggest that one-third of patients have tricuspid regurgitation at the end of 1 year. Frequency and severity increase with time.[81] Its appearance postoperatively is independent of preoperative mean pulmonary artery pressure, pulmonary vasculature resistance, and the cumulative number of rejection episodes. The appearance of tricuspid valve regurgitation in recipients of orthotopic heart transplants may be due to mismatched size of the donor heart and

Table 36-5 Anatomic considerations in tricuspid valve regurgitation

Congenital
- Tricuspid valve prolapse
- Ebstein's anomaly
- AV canal defect
- Congenital tricuspid dysplasia

Acquired
- Obstructive
  - Tricuspid stenosis
  - Right atrial tumor
  - Pacemaker leads
  - Pericardial disease
- Regurgitant
  - Dilated annulus
  - Infective endocarditis
  - Right ventricular hypertension
  - Traumatic
  - Prolapse
  - Right ventricular infarction
  - Cardiomyopathy
  - Chronic heart failure

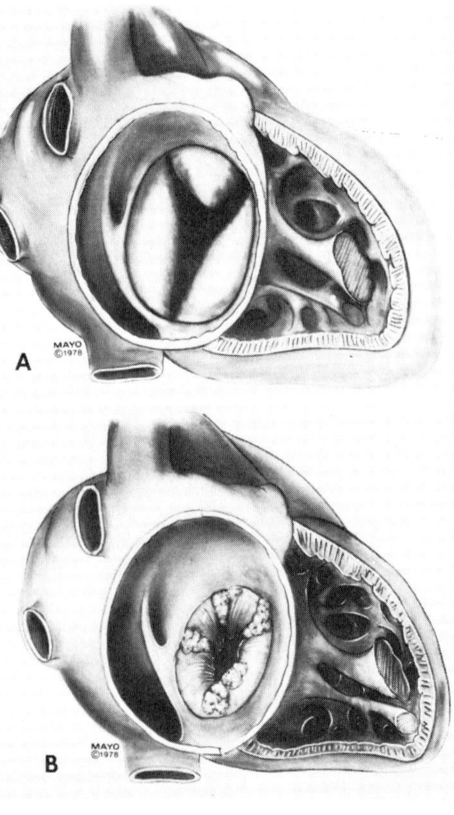

Fig 36-7 Types of tricuspid valve regurgitation. **A,** functional tricuspid incompetence secondary to dilatation and abnormal right ventricular function. **B,** organic rheumatic tricuspid disease with regurgitation. (From Fuster V, Brandenburg RO, Giuliani ER, et al: Clinical approach and management of acquired valvular heart disease. *Cardiovasc Clin* 10 No 3:125-159, 1980. By permission, Mayo Foundation.)

recipient pericardial activity. Although rarely of any hemodynamic significance, this complication can be detected by intraoperative echocardiography and managed, if necessary, by pericardial reduction-plasty.[82]

In more that 20% of 95 apparently healthy, nonathletic women aged 24 to 65, Doppler echocardiography detected tricuspid regurgitation. The significance of this finding is unknown. It did not seem to impair their physical exercise performance.[83]

Dilated tricuspid annulus. The tricuspid valve orifice area is decreased during atrial systole and ventricular systole, supporting the concept that "contraction" of the tricuspid valve annulus contributes to normal closure of this valve. Because fibrous structures cannot contract, we assume that this change in tricuspid valve orifice is related to the function of the atrial and ventricular musculature attached to the tricuspid annulus. It follows then that any abnormality of these two chambers, such as idiopathic dilatation of the right atrium, atrial fibrillation, or change in structure, volume, or pressure of the right ventricle, will impair function of the tricuspid annulus and be the cause of tricuspid regurgitation. Tricuspid regurgitation is due most commonly to dilatation of the tricuspid annulus secondary to chronic heart failure, left-sided rheumatic valvular heart disease, or, less often, chronic cor pulmonale.

Tricuspid valve prolapse. Prolapse of one or more leaflets of the tricuspid valve, producing tricuspid regurgitation, is a definite entity that might be secondary to other cardiac anomalies or disease processes or might be a primary structural defect. In the following discussion, we will be referring only to those patients whose tricuspid valve prolapse is due to a primary abnormality of the tricuspid valve leaflets, chordae, and papillary muscles.

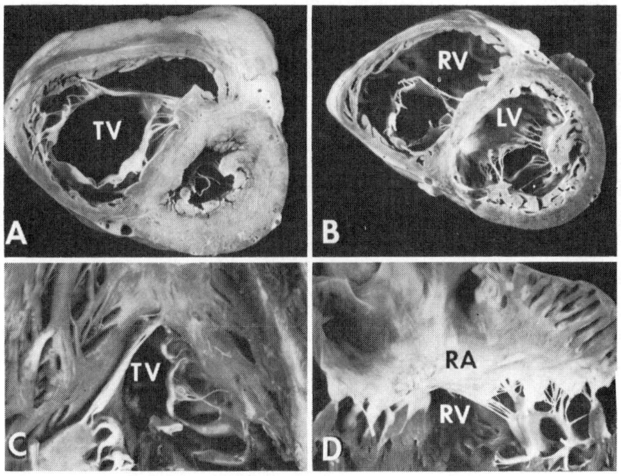

Fig 36-8 Pathology of tricuspid valve disease. **A,** tricuspid regurgitation due to annular dilatation in 58-year-old man with thromboembolic pulmonary hypertension. **B,** tricuspid and mitral regurgitation in 50-year-old man with idiopathic dilated cardiomyopathy. **C,** rheumatic tricuspid regurgitation in 54-year-old woman. **D,** tricuspid stenosis and regurgitation in 55-year-old woman with carcinoid heart disease. (Courtesy of W.D. Edwards, M.D.) (**D,** from Callahan JA, Wroblewski EM, Reeder GS, et al: Echocardiographic features of carcinoid heart disease. *Am J Cardiol* 50:762-768, 1982. By permission of Technical Publishing Company.)

Until clear definitions of the normal echocardiographic, angiocardiographic, and anatomic findings for the tricuspid valve are available, the true incidence of tricuspid valve prolapse will not be known. Tricuspid valve prolapse represents a wide spectrum of findings from very mild abnormalities of the tricuspid leaflets or supporting structures to severe changes to the tricuspid valve unit.[84-88] The majority are of intermediate degree.

The few studies available suggest that the incidence of tricuspid valve prolapse is 2% to 3% in the general population.[89] The frequency of tricuspid valve prolapse is significantly higher in patients who have mitral valve prolapse, the reported prevalence rate being 40% to 50%.[90-93] Approximately 10% of patients with atrial septal defect have echocardiographic evidence of tricuspid valve prolapse.[94] Prolapse has been reported secondary to pulmonary hypertension;[95,96] chronic obstructive pulmonary disease; right heart failure of any form or Ehlers-Danlos syndrome;[97] and interference by pacemaker leads.[98]

Abnormalities of leaflet tissue. Congenital cleft of the tricuspid valve leaflets is uncommon. Destruction of leaflet tissue has been reported in association with calcified right atrial myxoma,[65] and it certainly occurs in infective endocarditis, particularly in persons who are intravenous drug abusers. Although relatively rare, infective endocarditis involving the tricuspid valve may cause significant tricuspid insufficiency by destroying leaflets or chordae[99] or by producing contraction and thickening of leaflets or chordae during healing of the infection. Occasionally, large vegetations will interfere with normal valve function.

Approximately one-third of all patients with rheumatic valvular heart disease have documented rheumatic tricuspid valvulitis.[19-21] The resulting structural abnormalities cause incompetence of the valve, usually of a mild degree and often subclinical in nature. These structural changes frequently include thickening, shortening, and fibrous fusion of the supporting chordae, thus contributing to regurgitation and usually some degree of tricuspid valve stenosis.[25]

Leaflet mobility may be impaired by a number of disease entities other than rheumatic valvulitis. These conditions include carcinoid syndrome, hypereosinophilic syndrome, and systemic lupus erythematosus.

Abnormalities of supporting structures. Although acute disruption of the supporting structures of the tricuspid valve may be the result of nonpenetrating cardiac trauma[75,100] or infective endocarditis, the most frequent cause is acute myocardial infarction. Infarction of the right ventricle alone is rare.[101] It accompanies infarction of the left ventricle in approximately 15% of cases.[102] This occurs primarily in patients who have infarction of the posterior ventricular wall with or without septal involvement.

Pathophysiology of tricuspid regurgitation

It is important to understand the normal volume, pressure, and flow relationships among the chambers of the vena cava, right atrium, and right ventricle. Changes in right atrial/right ventricular compliance alter the normal flow pattern, as does the presence of tricuspid disease. Normally, forward flow continues from the cava to the right atrium during ventricular systole and terminates at the end of systole. Flow into the right atrium starts again in early diastole and continues until atrial systole, when there is a small reversal flow ("a" wave in the jugular venous pulse).[3] In patients with tricuspid regurgitation, this flow pattern is altered by a decreased flow into the right atrium during ventricular systole or, in more severe cases, reversal of flow from right ventricle to right atrium to the caval systems. With mild tricuspid regurgitation and a normal right atrial pressure-volume relationship, this reversal of flow is mild. In severe regurgitation there is alteration in right atrial compliance and large volume and pressure changes in the right atrium, and the reversed flow may occur throughout ventricular systole with forward flow from the vena cava to the right atrium occurring only during diastole. Regurgitant fraction at times may equal the forward flow. The net effect of this abnormality is to limit cardiac output, causing fatigue and shortness of breath.[3]

Increased pressure within the right atrium is reflected in a retrograde fashion to the caval system and, in turn, to the venous system of all organs. Chronic venous hypertension results in dysfunction of the liver, kidneys, gastrointestinal tract, brain, and other less vital organs. The net effect of these hemodynamic changes—i.e., a decrease in cardiac output and chronic venous hypertension—is sodium and fluid accumulation, causing edema, effusions, and ascites.

Natural history and clinical course

The natural history and clinical course of isolated tricuspid regurgitation are unknown because it is a rare clinical entity. When it is due to a connective tissue disorder, it is the natural history of that systemic disease. When it results from rheumatic left valvular heart disease, the clinical course and natural history are dictated by the left heart lesions.

Physical examination

Physical appearance. The physical appearance of a patient with significant tricuspid regurgitation is impressive. The large, abnormal venous neck pulsations are obvious during the history-taking. Indeed, patients may present with this complaint alone. On examination, the precordium is hyperactive, suggesting intracardiac shunt, and there is a dynamic, sustained precordial lift due to right ventricular dilatation and hypertrophy. When the regurgitation is severe, the patients may demonstrate a rocking or to-and-fro motion of the lower thorax.[103] A large, pulsating liver and pulsations of varicose veins of the lower extremities also may be present;[55,104,105] the latter may be demonstrated only by elevating the leg to the proper height.

Arterial and venous pulse. The arterial pulse reflects the underlying abnormality of both the electrical and mechanical functions of the heart. If the patient is in sinus rhythm with a low cardiac output (low stroke volume), the arterial pulse will be regular, small in volume but normal in its upstroke and runoff. In a patient who has atrial fibrillation, the carotid pulse will be irregular. The prominent jugular venous pulsations, especially the systolic wave and the rapid y descent, may be the most important findings on examination. The venous pulsations of the deep jugular system are most prominent when the patient is in the recumbent position. However, if the venous pressure is significantly increased, then the head of the bed and the upper torso of the patient must be elevated to obtain the ideal level to evaluate these pulses. The systolic or v wave is often very prominent and indeed may be palpable and confused with the arterial pulse. At times, the pulsations are of such great magnitude that the lower ear lobe will move, as seen in aortic regurgitation. A venous systolic thrill and murmur in the neck may be felt and heard in some cases of severe tricuspid insufficiency.[106]

Auscultation. The auscultatory hallmark of tricuspid valve regurgitation is the systolic murmur heard over the lower sternum and xiphoid that increases in intensity with inspiration, first described by Rivero-Carvallo.[105] The mechanism of this change in intensity of murmur is the same as that in tricuspid stenosis; that is, it is due to an increase in systemic venous return and tricuspid flow secondary to the inspiratory decrease in intrapleural pressure. The murmur may not increase with inspiration, particularly in a patient with markedly increased venous pressure. The systolic murmur may be early, limited to midsystole or late systole, or it may be pansystolic. A tricuspid opening snap rarely may occur. Right ventricular third heart sounds may be identified in patients with tricuspid regurgitation. Their location along the left lower sternal border and their augmentation during inspiration identify them as right-sided in origin. In occasional patients, severe tricuspid regurgitation is not associated with a murmur. This is especially apt to occur in long-standing post-traumatic tricuspid regurgitation. Reversed splitting of the second sound has been reported.[107]

Noninvasive evaluation. The electrocardiogram and chest roentgenogram are rarely diagnostic, except in Ebstein's anomaly. They do reflect the underlying changes in chamber size and ventricular hypertrophy.

Echocardiography. Two-dimensional echocardiography helps to define structural causes and specific valve deformities related to tricuspid regurgitation. Combined with continuous-wave, pulsed-wave, and color-flow Doppler imaging, it has been used to attempt to quantitate the severity of tricuspid regurgitation.[57,59] Pulsed-wave Doppler tracing of the regurgitant jet into the right atrium and flow-reversal patterns noted in the inferior vena cava and hepatic veins are semiquantitative methods for assessing the severity of tricuspid regurgitation. Relation of the color-flow jet area to the right atrial area also offers a semiquantitative assessment of tricuspid regurgitation. Tricuspid regurgitation is frequently seen in patients with increased right heart pressures and, to a lesser degree, in normal persons.[57,59,108-110] Subclinical tricuspid regurgitation can be detected in the normal population because of the high sensitivity of this method in detecting minor degrees of incompetence.[110]

The tricuspid regurgitant jet velocity profile can also be used to give an accurate noninvasive measurement of the difference in the upper right ventricular pulmonary artery systolic pressures between the right atrium and the right ventricle.[57,108,109,111] Currie et al.[108] found excellent correlation between pressures recorded at cardiac catheterization and those derived from the continuous-wave velocity of tricuspid regurgitation during Doppler echocardiography. In a study of 127 patients in whom pressures were measured simultaneously by Doppler echocardiography and catheterization, there was a high correlation of the pressure gradient between the right ventricle and the right atrium ($r = 0.96$). The modified Bernoulli equation ($P_1 - P_2 = 4V^2$) was used to determine the pressure gradient across the tricuspid valve.[111] Again, tricuspid regurgitation was a common finding in this patient population. Saline contrast enhancement of the tricuspid regurgitant jet detected by color-flow imaging has improved the detection of the peak velocities determined by the Doppler spectral analysis.[112]

Transesophageal echocardiography has enabled visualization of the near-field images of the right atrium and atrial septum as well as the tricuspid valve leaflets. Use of both the longitudinal and transverse planes obtained by the biplane transducer and the intermediate planes now obtained with the multiplane transducer increases detail in the analysis of the tricuspid valve and its associated structures.

Management

Medical. The medical management of patients with tricuspid valve disease may be divided into two parts. One part is treatment of the underlying cause of the tricuspid disease – e.g., in the case of infective endocarditis, use of the proper antimicrobial drugs. The other part is the medical treatment of congestive heart failure and includes the use of inotropic agents, low sodium intake, diuretics, and vasodilating agents (see chapter 17).

One of the most common and serious complications after tricuspid valve replacement, even in patients with adequate anticoagulation, is prosthetic valve thrombosis.[113] Tricuspid Bjork-Shiley prostheses, in particular, appear to be at high risk.[114] Before the advent of thrombolytic therapy, surgery was necessary in these cases. Now it is possible to successfully treat these valves with either streptokinase or recombinant human tissue-type plasminogen activator.[115,116]

Balloon valvotomy. The first successful percutaneous double-balloon valvotomy for tricuspid stenosis was reported by Al Zaibag et al.[117] in January 1987, and the validity of this technique has been confirmed by others.[118] Subsequent reports demonstrated the feasibility of concurrent balloon dilatation of tricuspid stenosis and calcific mitral stenosis,[119] tricuspid stenosis and pulmonary stenosis,[120] and mitral, aortic, and tricuspid stenosis.[121]

Successful balloon valvuloplasty for stenosis of a porcine bioprosthesis in a tricuspid valve position has also been reported.[122] Bourdillon et al.[123] reported on a complication of tricuspid percutaneous balloon valvuloplasty, namely, the development of severe tricuspid regurgitation requiring replacement of the tricuspid valve. The pathologic findings in this case indicate that fracture of the fused commissure of the stenotic tricuspid valve can be achieved by balloon dilatation. It appears that patients with pure tricuspid stenosis or minimal tricuspid regurgitation are potential candidates for this procedure. Further experience and long-term follow-up will be necessary before the role of percutaneous balloon valvuloplasty for tricuspid stenosis is known.

Surgical. Historically, surgical tricuspid valve disease was primarily caused by rheumatic valvulitis. Infrequently, congenital anomaly,[124] trauma,[125] or a right atrial tumor[126] was the cause. In recent years, however, infective endocarditis and congenital disorders have become more prominent as reasons for surgical intervention (Table 36-6). Although tricuspid endocarditis is seen in persons not addicted to drugs,[127,128] it is encountered with increasing frequency in the addict, and the addicted patient presents a unique set of problems.[129]

During the past quarter of a century, the surgical approach to the tricuspid valve has evolved gradually. Generally, if the valve was stenotic secondary to a rheumatic process, the patient received a prosthetic valve. Today, valvotomy is often attempted, and success has been considerable.[118,119,121,130] If surgery becomes necessary, every attempt at reconstruction is made before the valve is replaced.

The approach to the problem of tricuspid regurgitation remains unsettled and continues to evolve. If tricuspid regurgitation is mild, particularly as evaluated echocardiographically, nothing is done to the valve, although some surgeons still may do an annuloplasty. Tricuspid annuloplasty is performed if tricuspid regurgitation is moderate to severe. Repairing or restructuring the tricuspid valve[131] is often a part of the procedure. Basically, this technique is an adaptation of that developed for the mitral valve; however, because of the differences in both anatomy and physiology, certain modifications must be made. Three methods are widely used for tricuspid annuloplasty. In the De Vega method, sutures are used to tighten the annulus from the anterior leaflet to the posterior leaflet and thus induce deformation of the valve opening. Because a single thread is used for tightening, the leaflets show seams or folds. The Kay-Boyd method involves suture of the annulus of the posterior leaflet alone. Generally, this technique is not sufficient to prevent massive tricuspid regurgitation induced by enlargement of the anteroposterior annulus with elongated anterior and posterior leaflets. In the Carpentier-Edwards method, the tricuspid annulus is evenly sutured onto a hard ring with a specific form to correct the valve opening to a normal form and thus provide stable control of regurgitation. It has been noted, however, that this method may cause right ventricular dysfunction because it stabilizes the tricuspid opening. The Carpentier-Edwards method may be the most reliable in treating severe massive tricuspid regurgitation.[132]

REPLACING THE VALVE. Generally, operative mortality is substantially greater when tricuspid replacement is involved,[133] and late performance of most prosthetic

Table 36-6 Etiologic distribution of 363 surgically excised tricuspid valves

Classification	Year of study					Total	
	1963-1967	1968-1972	1973-1977	1978-1982	1983-1987	No.	%
Postinflammatory disease	65	72	30	11	16	194	53
Congenital disorder	6	15	17	20	35	93	26
Pulmonary venous hypertension	9	28	8	3	8	56	15
Infective endocarditis	2	2	1	3	3	11	3
Carcinoid syndrome	0	0	0	1	4	5	1
Trauma	0	1	0	0	0	1	<1
Iatrogenic	0	0	0	1	0	1	<1
Indeterminate	0	1	1	0	0	2	<1
Total	82	119	57	39	66	363	100

From Hauck AJ, Freeman DP, Ackermann DM, et al: Surgical pathology of the tricuspid valve: a study of 363 cases spanning 25 years. *Mayo Clin Proc* 63:851-863, 1988. By permission, Mayo Foundation for Medical Education and Research.

valves in a tricuspid position is distinctly less satisfactory than that of the same valve placed in either the aortic or the mitral position. The main problem with the prosthetic tricuspid prosthesis is the increased incidence of obstruction, the basis of which is the geometric configuration of the right ventricle, which allows the prosthesis to become compressed between the right ventricular free wall and the septum. Compression can result in narrowing of the flow pathway and ultimate entrapment of the poppet or interference with disk movement. Additional problems are structural valve failure, thrombosis, prosthetic valve endocarditis, and anticoagulant-related hemorrhage. Bioprosthetic valves have shown acceptable long-term durability, even in the younger age group.[134] For this reason, when replacement is absolutely necessary because reconstruction is impossible, a stent-mounted tissue valve is preferred. A frame-mounted tissue valve of the largest possible size should be used.

TRICUSPID VALVE ENDOCARDITIS. The traditional approach to the surgical treatment of tricuspid valve endocarditis is tricuspidectomy with or without prosthetic valve replacement.[135-137] Tricuspid valve excision, unfortunately, results in severe tricuspid regurgitation, which may not be tolerated in one-third of the patients, even without coexisting pulmonary disease.[135] Frequently, subsequent insertion of a prosthetic valve is necessary in these patients. If valve replacement is performed and the choice is a mechanical device, obstruction, anticoagulation in patients who are not dependable, and risk of reinfection (since most drug users continue to use intravenous drugs) present major long-term management problems. If a bioprosthetic valve is used, the problems are reinfection because of continued use of narcotics and need for reoperation because most patients are young. Because of these problems, a more aggressive attempt to preserve the native tricuspid valve has been advocated. "Vegetectomy"[138] only may be adequate to cure the infections. Generally, reconstruction of the tricuspid valve is necessary and frequently successful.[132,138] This approach carries with it a lower risk for reinfection and low short- and long-term mortality.[138]

REFERENCES

1. King TW: An essay on the safety-valve function in the right ventricle of the human heart and on the gradations of this function in the circulation of warm-blooded animals. *Guys Hosp Rep* 2:104-178, 1837
2. Silver MD, Lam JHC, Ranganathan N, et al: Morphology of the human tricuspid valve. *Circulation* 43:333-348, 1971
3. Wooley CF: Rediscovery of the tricuspid valve. *Curr Probl Cardiol* 6:1-41, April 1981
4. Virmani R: The tricuspid valve (editorial). *Mayo Clin Proc* 63:943-946, 1988
5. Tsakiris AG, Mair DD, Seki S, et al: Motion of the tricuspid valve annulus in anesthetized intact dogs. *Circ Res* 36:43-48, 1975
6. Okamoto M, Tsubokura T, Kajiyama G, et al: Diastolic atrioventricular valve closure and regurgitation following atrial contraction: their relation to timing of atrial contraction. *Clin Cardiol* 12:149-153, 1989
7. Kratz J: Evaluation and management of tricuspid valve disease. *Cardiol Clin* 9:397-407, 1991
8. Mittal SR, Upadhyay S, Saxena R: Rheumatic tricuspid stenosis without involvement of the mitral valve. *Int J Cardiol* 24:112-115, 1989
9. Loya YS, Mashru MR, Patil RB, et al: Isolated tricuspid stenosis: a case report with review of literature. *Indian Heart J* 41:270-273, 1989
10. Finnegan P, Abrams LD: Isolated tricuspid stenosis. *Br Heart J* 35:1207-1210, 1973
11. Fujii S, Funaki K, Denzumi N: Isolated rheumatic tricuspid regurgitation and stenosis. *Clin Cardiol* 9:353-355, 1986
12. Hauck AJ, Freeman DP, Ackermann DM, et al: Surgical pathology of the tricuspid valve: a study of 363 cases spanning 25 years. *Mayo Clin Proc* 63:851-863, 1988
13. Friedberg CK: *Diseases of the Heart.* Vol 2. Third edition. Philadelphia, WB Saunders Company, 1966, p 1162
14. Clawson BJ: Rheumatic heart disease: an analysis of 796 cases. *Am Heart J* 20:454-474, 1940
15. Lannigan R: *Cardiac Pathology.* London, Butterworth, 1966, p 115
16. Daniels SJ, Mintz GS, Kotler MN: Rheumatic tricuspid valve disease: two-dimensional echocardiographic, hemodynamic, and angiographic correlations. *Am J Cardiol* 51:492-496, 1983
17. Cooke WT, White PD: Tricuspid stenosis: with particular reference to diagnosis and prognosis. *Br Heart J* 3:147-165, 1941
18. Smith JA, Levine SA: The clinical features of tricuspid stenosis: a study of trivalvular stenosis. *Am Heart J* 23:739-760, 1942

19. Chopra P, Tandon HD: Pathology of chronic rheumatic heart disease with particular reference to tricuspid valve involvement. *Acta Cardiol* 32:423-434, 1977

20. Edwards WD, Peterson K, Edwards JE: Active valvulitis associated with chronic rheumatic valvular disease and active myocarditis. *Circulation* 57:181-185, 1978

21. Roy S, Tandon HD: Pathology of acute rheumatic fever. *Ann Ind Acad Med Sci* 8:47-53, 1972

22. Yu PN, Harken DE, Lovejoy FW Jr, et al: Clinical and hemodynamic studies of tricuspid stenosis. *Circulation* 13:680-691, 1956

23. Gibson R, Wood P: The diagnosis of tricuspid stenosis. *Br Heart J* 17:552-562, 1955

24. Sanders CA, Harthorne JW, DeSanctis RW, et al: Tricuspid stenosis: a difficult diagnosis in the presence of atrial fibrillation. *Circulation* 33:26-33, 1966

25. Rusted IE, Scheifley CH, Edwards JE: Studies of the mitral valve. II. Certain anatomic features of the mitral valve and associated structures in mitral stenosis. *Circulation* 14:398-406, 1956

26. Mehl SJ, Kaltman AJ, Kronzon I, et al: Combined tricuspid and pulmonic stenosis: clinical, echocardiographic, hemodynamic, surgical, and pathological features. *J Thorac Cardiovasc Surg* 74:55-60, 1977

27. Cox JN, de Seigneux R, Bolens M, et al: Tricuspid atresia, hypoplastic right ventricle, intact ventricular septum and congenital absence of the pulmonary valve. *Helv Paediatr Acta* 30:389-398, 1975

28. Greenwood RD: Ossification of the right auriculo ventricular opening of the heart. *J Indiana State Med Assoc* 69:88-89, 1976

29. Oeconomos NS, Camilaris DH, Petritis J, et al: Congenital tricuspid valvular stenosis. *J Cardiovasc Surg* 16:100-103, 1975

30. Dennis JL, Hansen AE, Corpening TN: Endocardial fibroelastosis. *Pediatrics* 12:130-139, 1953

31. Davies JNP, Ball JD: The pathology of endomyocardial fibrosis in Uganda. *Br Heart J* 17:337-359, 1955

32. Ridker PM, Chertow GM, Karlson EW, et al: Bioprosthetic tricuspid valve stenosis associated with extensive plaque deposition in carcinoid heart disease. *Am Heart J* 121:1835-1838, 1991

33. Lyons HA, Kelly JJ Jr, Nusbaum N, et al: Right atrial myxoma: a clinical study of a patient in whom diagnosis was made by angiocardiography during life (surgically removed). *Am J Med* 25:321-326, 1958

34. Thomas JH, Panoussopoulos DG, Jewell WR, et al: Tricuspid stenosis secondary to metastatic melanoma. *Cancer* 39:1732-1737, 1977

35. De Cock KM, Gikonyo DK, Lucas SB, et al: Metastatic tumour of right atrium mimicking constrictive pericarditis and tricuspid stenosis. *Br Med J* 285:1314, 1982

36. Borow KM, Henschke C, Sloss LJ, et al: Tricuspid stenosis masquerading as right ventricular failure in a patient with a prosthetic mitral valve. *Cathet Cardiovasc Diagn* 7:409-415, 1981

37. Nishida H, Grooters RK, Coster D, et al: Metastatic right atrial tumor in colon cancer with superior vena cava syndrome and tricuspid obstruction. *Heart Vessels* 6:125-127, 1991

38. Cunha CLP, Giuliani ER, Callahan JA, et al: Echophonocardiographic findings in patients with prosthetic heart valve malfunction. *Mayo Clin Proc* 55:231-242, 1980

39. Gibbs KL, Reardon MJ, Strickman NE, et al: Hemodynamic compromise (tricuspid stenosis and insufficiency) caused by an unruptured aneurysm of the sinus of Valsalva. *J Am Coll Cardiol* 7:1177-1181, 1986

40. Mancuso L, Bondí F, Marchí S, et al: Cardiac hydatid disease with clinical features resembling tricuspid stenosis. *Am Heart J* 113:1234-1236, 1987

41. Silverman NA, Levitsky S, Spigos DG, et al: Massive hemoptysis and recurrent tricuspid infective endocarditis in a heroin addict. *Chest* 82:195-196, 1982

42. Greco MA, Senesh JD, Aleksic S, et al: Tricuspid stenosis secondary to entanglement of ventriculoatrial catheter in the valve leaflets. *Surg Neurol* 18:34-36, 1982

43. Lee ME, Chaux A: Unusual complications of endocardial pacing. *J Thorac Cardiovasc Surg* 80:934-940, 1980

44. Beaver WL, Dillon JC, Jolly W: Pseudo-tricuspid stenosis: a rare entity. *Chest* 71:772-774, 1977

45. Cintron GB, Snow JA, Fletcher RD, et al: Pericarditis mimicking tricuspid valvular disease. *Chest* 71:770-772, 1977

46. Wray TM, Prochaska J, Fisher RD, et al: Traumatic pericardial hematoma simulating tricuspid valve obstruction. *Johns Hopkins Med J* 137:147-150, 1975

47. Enia F, Lo Mauro R, Meschisi F, et al: Right-sided infective endocarditis with acquired tricuspid valve stenosis associated with transvenous pacemaker: a case report. *PACE* 14:1093-1097, 1991

48. Killip T III, Lukas DS: Tricuspid stenosis: physiologic criteria for diagnosis and hemodynamic abnormalities. *Circulation* 16:3-13, 1957

49. Kitchin A, Turner R: Diagnosis and treatment of tricuspid stenosis. *Br Heart J* 26:354-379, 1964

50. Ribeiro PA, Al Zaibag M, Al Kasab S, et al: Provocation and amplification of the transvalvular pressure gradient in rheumatic tricuspid stenosis. *Am J Cardiol* 61:1307-1311, 1988

51. Gutner RN: Trivalvular rheumatic stenosis: documentation of disease progression by serial cardiac catheterization. *Am J Med Sci* 280:185-191, 1980

52. Abraham KA, Cherian G, Durairaj M, et al: Clinical and haemodynamic appraisal of rheumatic tricuspid stenosis. *J Assoc Physicians India* 25:341-346, 1977

53. Messer AL, Hurst JW, Rappaport MB, et al: A study of the venous pulse in tricuspid valve disease. *Circulation* 1:388-393, 1950

54. Schilder DP, Harvey WP: Confusion of tricuspid incompetence with mitral insufficiency: a pitfall in the selection of patients for mitral surgery. *Am Heart J* 54:352-367, 1957

55. Giuliani ER, Brandenburg RO, Fuster V: Evaluation of cardiac murmurs. *Cardiovasc Clin* 10 No 3:1-18, 1980

56. Rivero-Carvallo JM: El diagnóstico de la estenosis tricuspídea. *Arch Inst Cardiol Mex* 20:1-11, 1950

57. Hatle L, Angelsen B: *Doppler Ultrasound in Cardiology: Physical Principles and Clinical Applications.* Second revised edition. Philadelphia, Lea & Febiger, 1985, pp 170-176

58. Weyman AE: *Cross-Sectional Echocardiography.* Philadelphia, Lea & Febiger, 1982, pp 338-341

59. Feigenbaum H: *Echocardiography.* Fourth edition. Philadelphia, Lea & Febiger, 1986, pp 301-310

60. Fawzy ME, Mercer EN, Dunn B, et al: Doppler echocardiography in the evaluation of tricuspid stenosis. *Eur Heart J* 10:985-990, 1989

61. Pérez JE, Ludbrook PA, Ahumada GG: Usefulness of Doppler echocardiography in detecting tricuspid valve stenosis. *Am J Cardiol* 55:601-602, 1985

62. Hollman A: Tricuspid valvotomy. *Lancet* 1:535-537, 1956

63. Trace HD, Bailey CP, Wendkos MH: Tricuspid valve commissurotomy with a one-year follow-up. *Am Heart J* 47:613-618, 1954

64. Pantridge JF, Marshall RJ: Tricuspid stenosis. *Lancet* 1:1319-1322, 1957

65. Zitnik RS, Giuliani ER: Clinical recognition of atrial myxoma. *Am Heart J* 80:689-700, 1970

66. Giuliani ER, Nasser FN: Two-dimensional echocardiography in acquired heart diseases – Part I. *Curr Probl Cardiol* 5:1-47, February 1981

67. Fyke FE III, Seward JB, Edwards WD, et al: Primary cardiac tumors: experience with 30 consecutive patients since the introduction of two-dimensional echocardiography. *J Am Coll Cardiol* 5:1465-1473, 1985

68. Goli VD, Thadani U, Thomas SR, et al: Doppler echocardiographic profiles in obstructive right and left atrial myxomas. *J Am Coll Cardiol* 9:701-703, 1987

69. Waller BF: Etiology of pure tricuspid regurgitation. *Cardiovasc Clin* 17 No 2:53-95, 1987

70. Rubio PA, Al-Bassam MS: Pacemaker-lead puncture of the tricuspid valve: successful diagnosis and treatment. *Chest* 99:1519-1520, 1991

71. Stewart D, Leman RB, Kaiser J, et al: Catheter-induced tricuspid regurgitation: incidence and clinical significance. *Chest* 99:651-655, 1991

72. Vatterott PJ, Nishimura RA, Gersh BJ, et al: Severe isolated tricuspid insufficiency in coronary artery disease. *Int J Cardiol* 14:295-301, 1987

73. Feng WC, Singh AK, Moran JM: Tricuspid regurgitation with postinfarction ventricular septal defect. *Ann Thorac Surg* 49:659-660, 1990

74. Noera G, Sanguinetti M, Pensa P, et al: Tricuspid valve incompetence caused by nonpenetrating thoracic trauma. *Ann Thorac Surg* 51:320-322, 1991

75. Moront M, Lefrak EA, Akl BF: Traumatic rupture of the interventricular septum and tricuspid valve: case report. *J Trauma* 31:134-136, 1991

76. Talwar KK, Bajaj R, Kothari SS, et al: Tricuspid regurgitation in thyrotoxicosis – case report. *Indian Heart J* 39:353-355, 1987

77. Lewen MK, Bryg RJ, Miller LW, et al: Tricuspid regurgitation by Doppler echocardiography after orthotopic cardiac transplantation. *Am J Cardiol* 59:1371-1374, 1987

78. Froom P, Krivisky M, Ribak J, et al: Systolic tricuspid leaflet prolapse in asymptomatic young men. *Clin Cardiol* 12:697-700, 1989

79. Glancy DL, Marcus FI, Cuadra M, et al: Isolated organic tricuspid valvular regurgitation: causes and consequences. *Am J Med* 46:989-996, 1969

80. Sbar S, Daicoff G, Nightingale D, et al: Chronic tricuspid insufficiency. *South Med J* 66:917-920, 1973

81. Herrmann G, Simon R, Haverich A, et al: Left ventricular function, tricuspid incompetence, and incidence of coronary artery disease late after orthotopic heart transplantation. *Eur J Cardiothorac Surg* 3:111-118, 1989

82. Haverich A, Albes JM, Fahrenkamp G, et al: Intraoperative echocardiography to detect and prevent tricuspid valve regurgitation after heart transplantation. *Eur J Cardiothorac Surg* 5:41-45, 1991

83. Michelsen S, Hurlen M, Otterstad JE: Prevalence of tricuspid and pulmonary regurgitation diagnosed by Doppler in apparently healthy women. Possible influence on their physical performance? *Eur Heart J* 9:61-67, 1988

84. Iteld BJ, Kelly WM, Phillips JH: Precordial honk in association with tricuspid valve prolapse. *South Med J* 75:72-74, 1982

85. Bashour T, Lindsay J Jr: Midsystolic clicks originating from tricuspid valve structures: a sequela of heroin-induced endocarditis. *Chest* 67:620-621, 1975

86. Sassé L, Froelich CR: Echocardiographic tricuspid prolapse and nonejection systolic click. *Chest* 73:869-870, 1978

87. Doi YL, Sugiura T, Bishop RL, et al: High-speed echophonocardiographic detection of tricuspid valve prolapse in mitral valve prolapse with discrepancy in onset of systolic murmur. *Am Heart J* 103:301-303, 1982

88. Tei C, Shah PM, Tanaka H: Phonographic-echographic documentation of systolic honk in tricuspid prolapse. *Am Heart J* 103:294-295, 1982

89. Rippe JM, Angoff G, Sloss LJ, et al: Multiple floppy valves: an echocardiographic syndrome. *Am J Med* 66:817-824, 1979

90. Mardelli TJ, Morganroth J, Chen CC, et al: Tricuspid valve prolapse diagnosed by cross-sectional echocardiography. *Chest* 79:201-205, 1979

91. Ogawa S, Hayashi J, Sasaki H, et al: Evaluation of combined valvular prolapse syndrome by two-dimensional echocardiography. *Circulation* 65:174-180, 1982

92. Morganroth J, Jones RH, Chen CC, et al: Two dimensional echocardiography in mitral, aortic and tricuspid valve prolapse: the clinical problem, cardiac nuclear imaging considerations and a proposed standard for diagnosis. *Am J Cardiol* 46:1164-1177, 1980

93. Maranhão V, Gooch AS, Yang SS, et al: Prolapse of the tricuspid leaflets in the systolic murmur-click syndrome. *Cathet Cardiovasc Diagn* 1:81-90, 1975

94. Chandraratna PAN, Littman BB, Wilson D: The association between atrial septal defect and prolapse of the tricuspid valve: an echocardiographic study. *Chest* 73:839-842, 1978

95. Lense LD, Kronzon I, Danilowicz D, et al: Echocardiographic findings in a patient with primary pulmonary hypertension. *Cathet Cardiovasc Diagn* 2:87-91, 1976

96. Karayannis E, Stefadouros MA, Abdulla AM, et al: Use of echocardiography in the diagnosis of prolapsed tricuspid valve. *J Med Assoc Georgia* 67:205-208, 1978

97. Leier CV, Call TD, Fulkerson PK, et al: The spectrum of cardiac defects in the Ehlers-Danlos syndrome, types I and III. *Ann Intern Med* 92:171-178, 1980

98. Gibson TC, Davidson RC, DeSilvey DL: Presumptive tricuspid valve malfunction induced by a pacemaker lead: a case report and review of the literature. *PACE* 3:88-95, 1980

99. Kisslo J, von Ramm OT, Haney R, et al: Echocardiographic evaluation of tricuspid valve endocarditis: an M mode and two dimensional study. *Am J Cardiol* 38:502-507, 1976

100. Todd RB: A case of rupture of the chordae tendineae of the tricuspid valve of the heart, with remarks. *Dublin Q J Med Sci* 5:1-11, 1848

101. Wade WG: The pathogenesis of infarction of the right ventricle. *Br Heart J* 21:545-554, 1959

102. Isner JM, Roberts WC: Right ventricular infarction complicating left ventricular infarction secondary to coronary heart disease: frequency, location, associated findings and significance from analysis of 236 necropsy patients with acute or healed myocardial infarction. *Am J Cardiol* 42:885-894, 1978

103. Friedberg CK: *Physical Diagnosis in Cardiovascular Disease.* New York, Grune & Stratton, 1969

104. Hallock P, Clarke WO: Significance of generalized systolic pulsation of veins, with report of a case in which there was marked pulsation of varicose veins. *Am Heart J* 22:410-416, 1941

105. Rivero-Carvallo JM: Signo para el diagnóstico de las insuficiencias tricuspídeas. *Arch Inst Cardiol Mex* 16:531-540, 1946

106. Amidi M, Irwin JM, Salerni R, et al: Venous systolic thrill and murmur in the neck: a consequence of severe tricuspid insufficiency. *J Am Coll Cardiol* 7:942-945, 1986

107. Strickland NH, Gibson DG: Reversed splitting of the second heart sound due to tricuspid regurgitation. *Int J Cardiol* 20:412-415, 1988

108. Currie PJ, Seward JB, Chan KL, et al: Continuous wave Doppler determination of right ventricular pressure: a simultaneous Doppler-catheterization study in 127 patients. *J Am Coll Cardiol* 6:750-756, 1985

109. Popp RL, Yock PG: Noninvasive intracardiac pressure measurement using Doppler ultrasound. *J Am Coll Cardiol* 6:757-758, 1985

110. Yock PG, Schnittger I, Popp RL: Is continuous wave Doppler too sensitive in diagnosing pathologic valvular regurgitation? (Abstract.) *Circulation* 70 Suppl 2:381, 1984

111. Skjaerpe T, Hatle L: Noninvasive estimation of pulmonary artery pressure by Doppler ultrasound in tricuspid regurgitation. In *Cardiac Doppler Diagnosis.* Vol. 1. Edited by MP Spencer. The Hague, Martinus Nijhoff Publishers, 1984, pp 247-254

112. Waggoner AD, Barzilai B, Pérez JE: Saline contrast enhancement of tricuspid regurgitant jets detected by Doppler color flow imaging. *Am J Cardiol* 65:1368-1371, 1990

113. Beeuwsaert R, Denef B, De Geest H: Diagnosis and treatment of obstruction of a tricuspid Björk-Shiley prosthesis. *Acta Cardiol (Brux)* 38:13-25, 1983

114. Björk VO, Henze A: Ten years' experience with the Björk-Shiley tilting disc valve. *J Thorac Cardiovasc Surg* 78:331-341, 1979

115. Mosseri M, Rosenheck S, Galoon E, et al: Successful treatment of an immobile and thrombosed prosthetic tricuspid valve by fibrinolysis with a single dose of streptokinase (letter to the editor). *Isr J Med Sci* 24:114-116, 1988

116. Matsuda M, Matsuda Y, Okuda F, et al: Thrombolysis of tricuspid Björk-Shiley prosthesis with tissue-type plasminogen activator. *Jpn Circ J* 52:583-587, 1988

117. Al Zaibag M, Ribeiro P, Al Kasab S: Percutaneous balloon valvotomy in tricuspid stenosis. *Br Heart J* 57:51-53, 1987

118. Robalino BB, Whitlow PL, Marwick T, et al: Percutaneous balloon valvotomy for the treatment of isolated tricuspid stenosis. *Chest* 100:867-869, 1991

119. Sharma S, Loya YS, Daxini BV, et al: Concurrent double balloon valvotomy for combined rheumatic mitral and tricuspid stenosis. *Cathet Cardiovasc Diagn* 23:42-46, 1991

120. Chen CR, Lo ZX, Huang ZD, et al: Concurrent percutaneous balloon valvuloplasty for combined tricuspid and pulmonic stenoses. *Cathet Cardiovasc Diagn* 15:55-60, 1988

121. Konugres GS, Lau FYK, Ruiz CE: Successive percutaneous double-balloon mitral, aortic, and tricuspid valvotomy in rheumatic trivalvular stenoses. *Am Heart J* 119:663-666, 1990

122. Benedick BA, Davis SF, Alderman E: Balloon valvuloplasty for fungal endocarditis induced stenosis of a bioprosthetic tricuspid valve. *Cathet Cardiovasc Diagn* 21:248-251, 1990

123. Bourdillon PDV, Hookman LK, Morris SN, et al: Percutaneous balloon valvuloplasty for tricuspid stenosis: hemodynamic and pathological findings. *Am Heart J* 117:492-495, 1989

124. McFaul RC, Davis Z, Giuliani ER, et al: Ebstein's malformation: surgical experience at the Mayo Clinic. *J Thorac Cardiovasc Surg* 72:910-915, 1976

125. Tachovsky TJ, Giuliani ER, Ellis FH Jr: Prosthetic valve replacement for traumatic tricuspid insufficiency: report of a case originally diagnosed as Ebstein's malformation. *Am J Cardiol* 26:196-199, 1970

126. Smith ST, Hautamaki K, Lewis JW Jr, et al: Transthoracic and transesophageal echocardiography in the diagnosis and surgical management of right atrial myxoma. *Chest* 100:575-576, 1991

127. Grover A, Anand IA, Varma J, et al: Profile of right-sided endocarditis: an Indian experience. *Int J Cardiol* 33:83-88, 1991

128. Anderson JR, Scott P, Nair RU: Conservative surgery in multiple cusp involvement in tricuspid valve endocarditis. *Br Heart J* 66:244-245, 1991

129. Cannon NS, Cabbs CS: Infective endocarditis in drug addicts. In *Infective Endocarditis.* Edited by D Kaye. Baltimore, University Park Press, 1976, pp 111-127

130. Ribeiro PA, Al Zaibag M, Idris MT: Percutaneous double balloon tricuspid valvotomy for severe tricuspid stenosis: 3-year follow-up study. *Eur Heart J* 11:1109-1112, 1990

131. Yada I, Tani K, Shimono T, et al: Preoperative evaluation and surgical treatment for tricuspid regurgitation associated with acquired valvular heart disease. *J Cardiovasc Surg* 31:771-777, 1990

132. Sutlic Z, Schmid C, Borst HG: Repair of flail anterior leaflets of tricuspid and mitral valves by cusp remodeling. *Ann Thorac Surg* 50:927-930, 1990

133. Mullany CJ, Gersh BJ, Orszulak TA, et al: Repair of tricuspid valve insufficiency in patients undergoing double (aortic and mitral) valve replacement: perioperative mortality and long-term (1 to 20 years) follow-up in 109 patients. *J Thorac Cardiovasc Surg* 94:740-748, 1987

134. Kawachi Y, Masuda M, Tominaga R, et al: Comparative study between St. Jude medical and bioprosthetic valves in the right side of the heart. *Jpn Circ J* 55:553-562, 1991

135. Straumann E, Stulz P, Jenzer HR: Tricuspid valve endocarditis in the drug addict: a reconstructive approach ("vegetectomy"). *Thorac Cardiovasc Surg* 38:291-294, 1990

136. Barbour DJ, Roberts WC: Valve excision only versus valve excision plus replacement for active infective endocarditis involving the tricuspid valve. *Am J Cardiol* 57:475-478, 1986

137. Jagger JD, McCaughan BC, Pawsey CGK: Tricuspid valve endocarditis cured by excision of a single vegetation. *Am Heart J* 112:626-627, 1986

138. Allen MD, Slachman F, Eddy AC, et al: Tricuspid valve repair for tricuspid valve endocarditis: tricuspid valve "recycling." *Ann Thorac Surg* 51:593-598, 1991

CHAPTER

37

Prosthetic valves

Hartzell V. Schaff, M.D.

A prosthesis is defined as an artificial device designed to replace a part of the body. In this instance, "artificial" means "not genuine or original." Thus, it is appropriate to refer to all currently used replacement cardiac valves as "prosthetic valves," with the probable exception of the transplanted autologous pulmonary valve.[1,2] Such prosthetic valves may be classified according to at least two characteristics—the origins of their material components and their mode of function.

In regard to the origins of their material components, valves are designated as either "tissue valves" or "nontissue valves" (Fig 37-1). Tissue valves are made up (usually only in part) of materials obtained from animals or humans and therefore are sometimes referred to by the synonymous term "bioprostheses." A tissue valve could be unmounted (or freestanding), but now it almost always is mounted inside a frame that is suitable for suturing the valve to the annulus of the resected host valve. Tissue valves are usually semilunar in design—that is, they mimic (or actually are) the aortic valve. Efforts to achieve dependable function of a valve mimicking the chordae-supported mitral type of design have been unrewarding. Examples of tissue valves are the homograft aortic valve, the heterograft (porcine) aortic valve (e.g., Hancock, Carpentier-Edwards), a bovine pericardial semilunar valve (e.g., Ionescu-Shiley, Carpentier-Edwards pericardial), a homograft dura mater valve, and a human autograft fascia lata valve. Nontissue valves, also called mechanical valves, include all other types of prosthetic valves that do not incorporate tissues generated by living bodies.

According to their mode of function, valves are designated as "central flow valves," "lateral flow valves," or "semicentral flow valves." Tissue valves are of the central flow variety, and it is appropriate to include the newer bileaflet nontissue valve known as the St. Jude valve in this category. The lateral flow variety of prosthetic valve is represented by the ball valve, the disk valve, and any other valve having a centrally situated occluder, regardless of geometric design. The semicentral flow type of valve is exemplified by the tilting disk prosthesis.

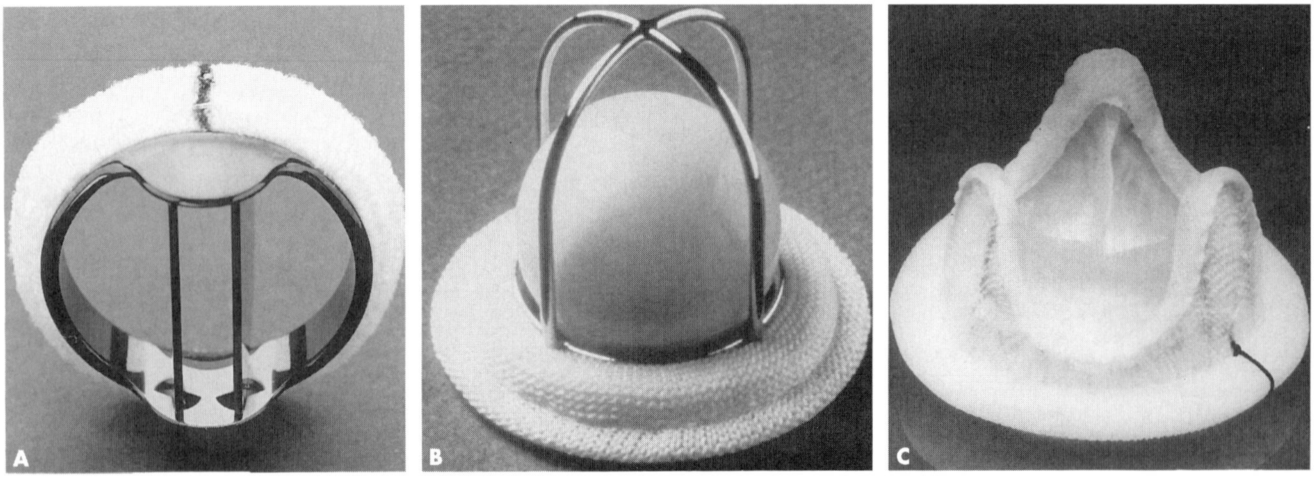

Fig 37-1 Popular types of valve prostheses. **A,** bileaflet St. Jude prosthesis in fully open position (there are two lateral major flow orifices and a minor central orifice). **B,** Starr-Edwards prosthesis (model 6120). **C,** porcine heterograft (frame-mounted, glutaraldehyde-preserved).

NONTISSUE VALVES

Ball valve

Description. The ball valve is a lateral flow nontissue prosthesis consisting of a ring to which is attached a cage, and in the cage a spherical poppet moves passively from a closed position seated in the ring to an open position out in the cage. The Starr-Edwards ball valve prosthesis is the classic and currently popular example of this class of valve. The ring and cage, made of an alloy known as Stellite 21, are cast and polished as a unit; the poppet is of solid Silastic. Except on its inner surface where the ball seats, the ring is covered with a cloth suitable for suturing and anchoring the valve in the annulus. The mitral valve prosthesis (Model 6120) has four struts in its cage, and the aortic valve prosthesis (Model 1260) has only three struts. Other types of ball valves have been available in the past but, for various reasons, either are not available or are less used at present.

Durability. The durability of the Starr-Edwards bare-strut Silastic ball valve prosthesis has been excellent for the past 2 decades. In fact, almost the only concern about its long-term performance is related to the possibility of alteration in the ball poppet itself, a change known as "ball variance." This change can occur as a result of abrasion injury or lipid infiltration, or both.[3-5] Whatever the true mechanisms for the occurrence of ball variance may have been, design changes were made in the Starr-Edwards aortic prosthesis in 1965 to decrease trauma to the ball during function of the valve (a minor design change in 1968 gave rise to the 1260 model, which has been manufactured unaltered since then). Since these changes were made, ball variance in Starr-Edwards valves has virtually vanished. The process of ball variance may still be taking place but at a much reduced rate, so that it may appear as a complication only 2 or more decades after implantation, but no evidence for this has become apparent as yet. Thus, the durability of the Starr-Edwards 1260 (aortic) and 6120 (mitral) ball valves is a very persuasive comparative advantage for this valve.

Hemodynamics. The hemodynamic performance of a valve varies with the size of the valve, other conditions being constant. The system used by Edwards Laboratories for identifying the size of the valves is arbitrary and must be translated into logical information about the diameter of the annulus into which it would fit snugly. The translation table for the aortic and mitral prostheses and a summary of hemodynamic performance for various valve sizes are presented in Table 37-1. The 2M (mitral) size is almost always smaller than desirable for the adult heart;[6] the mean transvalvular pressure gradient for the commonly used 3M or 4M sizes is 3 to 10 mm Hg, and calculated "effective" orifice area has been reported to be 1.4 to 2.9 cm^2.[7] For the aortic valve, postoperative studies of valve sizes customarily used in adults (10A or larger) have indicated an average mean systolic aortic gradient of 15 mm Hg and a calculated "effective" orifice area of 1.5 cm^2.[8] Similar gradients and orifice areas have been calculated by Doppler techniques.[9] Thus, the hemodynamic function of this valve is satisfactory in comparison with that of the diseased valve it replaces, but it is not perfect, especially because of its lateral flow characteristic, which results from the poppet remaining in the pathway of blood flow while in the open position.

Thromboembolism. The ball valve prosthesis carries a significant risk of thromboembolism that has continued throughout 2 decades of follow-up. Experience has shown clearly that anticoagulation achieved by use of warfarin is

Table 37-1 Tissue annulus diameters of Starr-Edwards valves and summary of hemodynamic data

Prosthesis size	Annulus diameter, mm	Peak systolic (aortic) or mean diastolic (mitral) gradient, mm Hg	Calculated orifice area, cm^2
		Aortic Valve	
6A	16	NA	NA
7A	18	NA	NA
8A	21	29	0.9
9A	23	18-28	1.1-1.2
10A	24	13-23	1.3-1.4
11A	26	11-21	1.3-1.5
12A	27	13-22	1.7-1.8
		Mitral Valve	
00M	NA	NA	NA
0M	NA	NA	NA
1M	26	10	1.4
2M	28	4-8	1.4-2.4
3M	30	3-10	1.4-2.2
4M	32	3-5	1.9-2.9
5M	34	5	2.6

NA, not available.

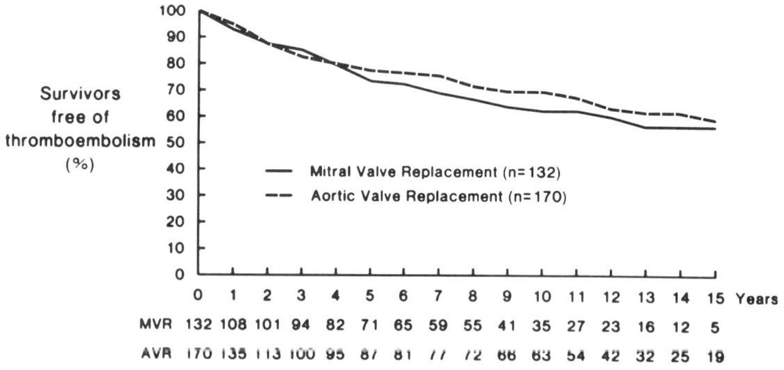

Fig 37-2 Percentage of survivors free of thromboembolism plotted against time (years) in patients with isolated Starr-Edwards mitral or aortic prostheses. The number of patients seen at each follow-up interval is given below the horizontal axis. *MVR,* mitral valve replacement; *AVR,* aortic valve replacement. (From Fuster V, Pumphrey CW, McGoon MD, et al: Systemic thromboembolism in mitral and aortic Starr-Edwards prostheses: a 10-19-year follow-up. *Circulation* 66 Suppl I:1-157–1-161, 1982. By permission of American Heart Association.)

highly effective in reducing but not in eliminating this risk. Determination of the true incidence of thromboembolism is not possible, because many such events undoubtedly occur without being noticed at all; others give only transient evidence, and a minority cause residual damage. Thus, the interpretation of whether an embolism did or did not occur is highly subjective, and criteria fluctuate considerably among investigators. Furthermore, the patient's preoperative status affects the postoperative incidence of thromboembolism.[10] Late follow-up studies by Starr's group indicate that for the bare-strut ball valves inserted during the 1960s, the risk of thromboembolism was about 6% per year with mitral replacement and about 4% per year with aortic replacement; for the same valves inserted more recently, the incidence fell to 1% or 2% for each.[11-14] These early high incidences of thromboembolism agree well with the Mayo overall findings for the same valves, although in our study the incidences were similar for aortic and mitral valves[15] (Fig 37-2). Further, our data also support the concept of reduced thromboembolic risk in the more current era.[7] For example, linearized risk of thromboembolism in patients having Starr-Edwards valve replacement at the Mayo Clinic between 1979 and 1981 was less than two events per 100 patient-years, whereas it was more than four events per 100 patient-years for patients undergoing operation from 1962 through 1971 (Tables 37-2 and 37-3). There is evidence that risk is higher in the initial 2 to 5 years and decreases thereafter.[16]

Survival. In clinical practice, late patient survival rates are related more closely to preoperative patient characteristics than to the type of prosthesis chosen for insertion.[10] These patient-related factors include advanced functional class preoperatively, atrial or ventricular enlargement, a history of prior heart surgery, advanced age, and untreated associated disease.[17] Nevertheless, it is helpful to note that most studies of late death after placement of the bare-strut Starr-Edwards valve in either the aortic or the mitral position show a mean incidence very close to 4% per year; the value is somewhat higher in the first postoperative year and lower thereafter.[11-18] Contrary to the incidence of thromboembolism, this incidence of death is independent of the valve type (Fig 37-3).

Tilting-disk valves

The concept of a tilting-disk valve came to Gott et al.,[19] who in 1964 reported use of a hinged bileaflet valve; to Cruz et al.,[20] who developed a pivoting-disk prosthesis for experimental study beginning in 1963; and to Pierce et al.,[21] who studied a hinged tilting-disk valve in 1968. Wada et al.[22] in Japan developed a hingeless tilting-disk valve, which was made available to surgeons around the world, including Björk, who, with Donald Shiley, developed the hingeless mechanism of the Björk-Shiley valve.[23] Other tilting-disk designs are those developed by Kaster and Lillehei,[24] the basic design of which is used in the Omni-Science valve, and the Medtronic-Hall prosthesis developed by Karl V. Hall and Robert Kaster.[25]

St. Jude medical valve. Currently, the most popular tilting-disk valve is the St. Jude Medical heart valve. Its basic design is descended from the central hinging Gott-Daggett valve and the central flow, hingeless, double-leaflet Lillehei-Kalke valve.[26,27] The bileaflet configuration of the St. Jude Medical valve was designed by Possis and Nicoloff to provide central, evenly distributed flow to wash all exposed surfaces and maximize the effective orifice area. The valve is constructed of pyrolitic carbon, and its two leaflets open to an 85° position, or almost parallel to the bloodstream, so that a nearly full orifice is achieved (e.g., the 21-mm valve has an orifice area of 2.06 cm^2). The leaflets rotate on a fulcrum by means of an ear protruding from each end of each leaflet and fitting into a precisely machined depression on the inner surface of the orifice ring.

DURABILITY. Clinical experience with the St. Jude Medical heart valve began in October 1977, and mechanical failure of the prosthesis has been reported infre-

Table 37-2 Linearized risk of thromboembolism from different prosthetic heart valves

Type of prosthetic valve	Year of implantation	Events per 100 patient-years: Aortic	Events per 100 patient-years: Mitral
Starr-Edwards			
Mayo Clinic	1979-1981	1.9	1.6
	1962-1971	4.6	4.5
University of Oregon	1973-1979	3.4	0.8
	1965-1972	5.0	6.6
Stanford University	1965-1976	. . .	3.4
Björk-Shiley		1.0-3.0	1.0-4.0
Medtronic-Hall	1977-1987	1.4	1.4
St. Jude Medical		1.1	1.8
Bioprosthetic		0.5-2.0	3.0-4.0

Table 37-3 Actuarial risk of thromboembolism from different prosthetic heart valves

Type of prosthetic valve	Year of implantation	% of patients free of thromboembolism at 5 yr: Aortic	% of patients free of thromboembolism at 5 yr: Mitral
Starr-Edwards			
Mayo Clinic	1979-1981	91	93
	1962-1971	75	78
University of Oregon	1973-1979	87	96
	1965-1972	77	68
Massachusetts General Hospital	1973-1977	90	83
Stanford University	1965-1976	86	62
National Heart Hospital	1975-1980	80	. . .
	1966-1971	93	. . .
University of Louvain	1965-1980	. . .	81
Björk-Shiley		94-97	81-89
Bioprosthetic*		94-98	86-98

*Patients with bioprosthetic valves do not require long-term warfarin therapy unless they are in atrial fibrillation or have an enlarged left atrium (50 mm or more by echocardiography).

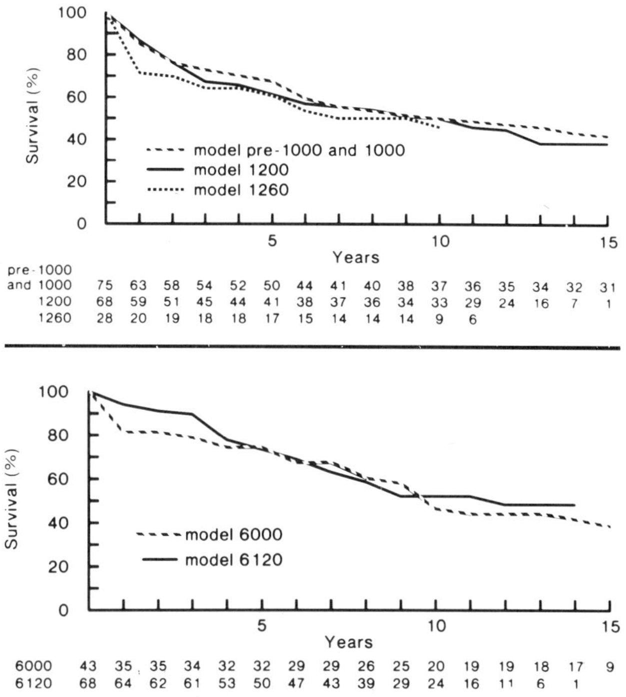

Fig 37-3 Actuarial survival of patients, shown by valve model implanted. Hospital deaths are excluded. Number of survivors at each time interval is shown below the horizontal axis. The expected survival, on the basis of age and sex distribution, is from the 1970 life table for the West North Central states. **Upper,** with isolated Starr-Edwards aortic valve replacement for symptomatic aortic incompetence. **Lower,** with isolated Starr-Edwards mitral valve replacement for symptomatic mitral incompetence. Model 6310 is not depicted because of small sample size. (From McGoon MD, Fuster V, McGoon DC, et al: Aortic and mitral valvular incompetence: long-term follow-up [10-19 years] of patients treated with the Starr-Edwards prosthesis. *J Am Coll Cardiol* 3:930-938, 1984. By permission of American College of Cardiology.)

quently.[28,29] According to the manufacturer, there have been only six episodes of leaflet escape reported from over 60,000 valves implanted.[30] The longest and most complete follow-up has been reported by Arom et al.,[31] who found no structural failure or evidence of valve wear among 1,298 patients followed for a total of 4,360 patient-years (longest, 10 years).

HEMODYNAMICS. A number of reports confirm the hemodynamic advantage of the central flow design of the St. Jude Medical valve. Transvalvular gradients and calculated orifice areas of the St. Jude valve are equal to or better than those of the Björk-Shiley valve and the Medtronic-Hall prosthesis,[32-35] and the valve is suitable for patients with small aortic annulus diameter (e.g., 19 or 21 mm), especially for those with small body surface areas (Fig 37-4).

THROMBOEMBOLISM. If anticoagulation is adequate, thromboembolic risk after valve replacement with the St.

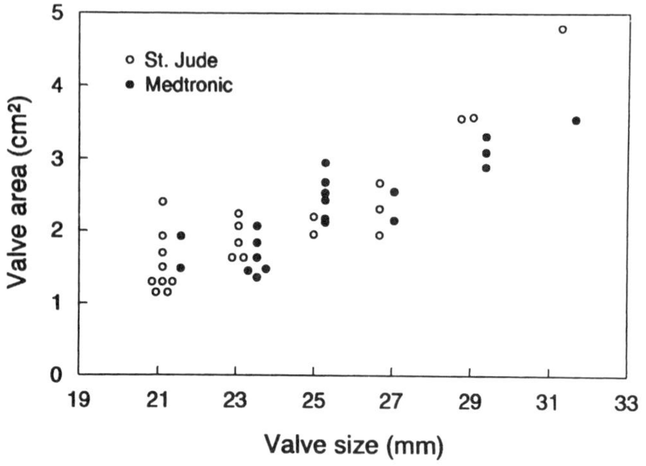

Fig 37-4 Valve area (cm²) is plotted as a function of valve size (mm) for the St. Jude Medical and Medtronic aortic valve prostheses. (From Tatineni S, Barner HB, Pearson AC, et al: Rest and exercise evaluation of St. Jude Medical and Medtronic Hall prostheses: influence of primary lesion, valvular type, valvular size, and left ventricular function. *Circulation* 80 Suppl 1:16-23, 1989. By permission of American Heart Association.)

Jude prosthesis is low (see Table 37-2), approximately 1.5% per year overall (1.1% per year after aortic valve replacement and 1.8% per year after mitral valve replacement).[31] Kopf et al.[36] suggested that the extent of anticoagulation with warfarin can be reduced safely in patients with St. Jude valves so that the prothrombin time is 1.3 to 1.5 times control rather than 1.5 to 2.0 times control. With this regimen of less intense anticoagulation, risk of thromboembolism was only 0.7% per patient-year and risk of hemorrhage was 1.3% per patient-year.

Thrombotic obstruction of St. Jude valves has been reported,[37-39] and the risk appears to be greater in valves in the atrioventricular position than in those in the aortic position, especially in patients with inadequate anticoagulation with warfarin.

Björk-Shiley valve. Although the Björk-Shiley valve is no longer marketed in the United States, knowledge of its clinical performance and limitations is imperative, because the valve was widely used in the 1970s and early 1980s; the Shiley Company has claimed that over 270,000 valves were distributed.[30] As seen in Table 37-4, the original Björk-Shiley prosthesis has undergone evolutionary changes.[40-42] The tilting disk of the earliest model was made of Delrin, and this was changed to pyrolitic carbon in 1971. In 1975, a ring-shaped radiopaque marker was inserted into the disk. The disk was redesigned in 1978 to have a convexoconcave shape, and the retaining struts were altered so that the pivot point of the disk moved 2.5 mm away from the orifice ring. These changes were intended to decrease stagnation of flow in the pivot area and along the smaller prosthetic orifice in an effort to minimize risk of valve thrombosis and reduce flow gradients.[41] The convexoconcave (CC) disk opened to an angle of 60° (60° CC), and in later models not sold in the United States, the angle of the disk opening was increased to 70° (70° CC).

Table 37-4 Development of the Björk-Shiley tilting disk valve

Model	Distribution period
Delrin disk	1969 to 1979
Pyrolytic carbon conical disk	1971 to 1977
Pyrolytic carbon spherical disk	1975 to present
60° convexoconcave disk	1976 to 1986
70° convexoconcave disk	1980 to 1983 (never sold in USA)
Monostrut valve	1982 to present (not yet sold in USA)

The most attractive feature of Björk-Shiley valves is the good hemodynamic function, especially in small (19 mm and 21 mm) valve sizes.[43-45] The valve also has two distinct disadvantages, however. First, obstruction can develop because of interference with disk opening; disk immobilization has occurred from entrapment of suture material or valvular chordae.[46] Perhaps the most common cause of disk malfunction is thrombotic obstruction, a serious and potentially fatal complication that is minimized but not eliminated by adequate anticoagulation.[47-50] The incidence of this serious complication varies according to the adequacy of anticoagulation management, but apparently it can occur even in well-controlled patients; if anticoagulation is interrupted, this risk is a definite disadvantage of the prosthesis. In Honolulu, 4.4% of patients (5.9% of mitral and 2.7% of aortic prostheses) experienced this event within a few years of follow-up.[47] In South Africa, the incidence of thrombotic occlusion was 8% after insertion of the mitral prosthesis,[48] but patients in this study were poorly anticoagulated and received the earlier model.

The most serious complication with the Björk-Shiley valve is catastrophic failure due to strut fracture, which was first reported in the 60° CC valve in September 1978; by June 14, 1987, there were reports of 213 outlet strut fractures among approximately 83,000 prostheses implanted.[42] Most (76%) fractures occurred in large valve sizes (29 mm, 31 mm, and 33 mm), but outlet strut fracture has been reported in 21-mm, 23-mm, 25-mm, and 27-mm Björk-Shiley CC valves. Risk of strut fracture ranges from 0.21 event per 100 patient-years for small valves (21 to 27 mm) to 0.318 event per 100 patient-years for large valves (29 to 33 mm) manufactured between Feb. 1, 1981, and June 30, 1982. In vitro analysis suggests that excessive stress on the outlet strut could occur during closure of the prostheses.

In October 1985, 29-mm, 31-mm, and 33-mm CC Björk-Shiley valves manufactured from March 1982 through June 1982 were recalled, and in November 1986, all unimplanted CC valves were voluntarily recalled because of risk of outlet strut fracture. At present, it does not appear that elective reoperation for explantation of intact CC Björk-Shiley valves with 60° opening angle is indicated, because cumulative risk of catastrophic failure is lower than the risk of reoperation. This conclusion will have to be reexamined as more data accumulate.

Additional information on risk of outlet strut fracture will be crucial for management of patients who have Björk-Shiley valves. Risk of strut fracture appears to cluster into four groups based on valve size and date of manufacture.[42] (1) Small valves (21 to 27 mm) appear to have a very low risk of strut fracture, approximately 0.02% per year. (2) Large valves (29 to 33 mm) processed before Feb. 1, 1981, also have a low risk (0.05% per year) of strut fracture. (3) Large valves processed between Feb. 1, 1981, and June 30, 1982, have the highest risk of fracture (average, 0.32% per year), but this risk seems to decrease with time. (4) Large valves processed after June 30, 1982, have a relatively low risk of fracture (0.08% per year).

More recent data suggest that risk of strut fracture may be higher than previously estimated. Among 2,303 patients in the Netherlands with 60° CC or 70° CC Björk-Shiley heart valves and mean postoperative follow-up of 6.6 years,[51] 42 failures due to outlet strut fracture occurred, and multivariate analysis identified wide opening angle (70° CC), large valve size (29 mm diameter or larger), and young age (less than 50 years) as risk factors for outlet strut fracture. For large 70° CC mitral valves, cumulative risk of strut fracture after 8 years was 17.4%, and unlike the analysis above, this excessive risk applied to late as well as to early batches of valves. In patients with large 60° CC mitral valves, the cumulative risk after 8 years was 4.2%, and incidence rates were constant over time. Overall survival since implantation was better for patients with 60° CC prostheses than for those with 70° CC prostheses, and the adjusted hazard ratio for mortality for patients receiving a 70° CC prosthesis was 1.5. In this study, the necropsy rate was only 24%, suggesting that the reported incidence of strut fracture for the 70° CC is underestimated. If these rates of strut fracture are confirmed by other series, elective replacement of the valve might be indicated for patients who are at high risk and are otherwise in good health.[52]

Diagnosis of outlet strut fracture should be considered in any patient with a CC Björk-Shiley valve who has evidence of acute cardiac failure and symptoms of progressive dyspnea, chest pain, or a decreased level of consciousness. Absence of prosthetic valve sounds and evidence of cardiogenic shock may be present. Diagnosis of outlet strut fracture can be made with an overpenetrated chest radiograph, preferably taken in two views; typical radiographic findings are absence of the strut or occluded disk (or both) and localization of the strut occluder in an extra-anatomic location. Immediate operation and valve rereplacement are mandatory for patient survival.

At present, there are no reliable methods for identification of valves at high risk aside from follow-up and careful analysis of subgroups stratified according to date of manufacture and valve size. For example, analyses such as those reported above indicate that the early production series of the 29- to 31-mm 70° CC Björk-Shiley heart valves, which were not sold in the United States, have an uncommonly high risk of outlet strut fracture. The hazard function for mechanical failure among these valves has remained essentially constant over a 7-year follow-up period, and the cumulative 7-year actuarial incidence of mechanical failure is 12.5%. Lindblom et al.[53] and Ericsson et al.[54] advised prophylactic replacement of these valves in selected patients.

TISSUE VALVES

To avoid the limitation of prosthetic valves, particularly their thrombogenic tendency, attention was turned early to the use of tissue valves, initially the homograft aortic valve. Unfortunately, the availability of such valves in the fresh state is limited—a problem that has not been easily overcome, at least in the United States. Cryopreservation has expanded the duration of viability of homograft valves and is currently the preferred method of preservation.[55] Late function of cryopreserved valves is uncertain, and earlier sterilization and preservation methods caused accelerated degeneration of such homograft valves. Improved methods for the preservation of porcine valves, developed to overcome these problems, led to the wide use of such valves in clinical practice.

Porcine valve prostheses

Description. In 1965 in Paris, Carpentier and associates began the era of xenograft valve replacement using formaldehyde-preserved porcine valves, but the ultimate universal degeneration of such valves led to glutaraldehyde preservation, which causes cross-linkage and hence more permanent strengthening of the valve's collagen fibers. Such a valve was implanted in 1968.[56] Subsequently, Hancock Laboratories, and later Edwards Laboratories, prepared and distributed such valves. The Hancock valve is treated with 0.2% glutaraldehyde; the Carpentier-Edwards valve is treated with 0.625%. The Hancock valve is mounted on a rigid Stellite ring having flexible polypropylene support pillars, whereas the Carpentier-Edwards valve is mounted on a totally flexible Elgiloy frame.

Hemodynamics. Because the porcine valve is of natural design with central flow characteristics, it was somewhat unanticipated that one of its limitations would be its hemodynamic characteristics.[57] This limitation results from two factors—the necessity for a stent or frame interposed between the valve and the host annulus and, in the aortic position, the anatomic characteristics of the right coronary cusp of the porcine valve. This cusp is broadly mounted on the crest of the ventricular septum, which limits its excursion in the processed product; this results in significant gradients across the valve, particularly when small valves are required. In an effort to minimize this limitation, Hancock Laboratories developed a composite valve in which the right coronary cusp is excised and replaced by the noncoronary cusp from another animal. One study of the modified orifice valve, however, showed very little improvement in performance.[58] Thus, the hemodynamic performance of the porcine valve is little different from that of the nontissue prosthetic valves,[9] except that in small sizes the transvalvular gradient may be worse.

Thromboembolism. Extensive comparisons have been made of the risks of thromboembolism with tissue and nontissue prostheses.[59] As seen in Tables 37-2 and 37-3, the risks are similar (incidence of failure: aortic, 2% per year; mitral, 4%), with the very important difference, however, that most of the patients with a tissue valve in the aortic position and about half the patients with a tissue valve in the mitral position are not anticoagulated, whereas all patients with prosthetic valves are routinely anticoagulated. In fact, the greatest risk of systemic embolism with tissue prostheses is in patients who have a mitral prosthesis and atrial fibrillation.[60] There is no apparent difference in thromboembolic potential between the Hancock and the Carpentier-Edwards mitral prostheses.[61] A review study by Edmunds[61] found that the risk of anticoagulation was 0.17% per year for mortality and 2.2% per year for morbidity. Thus, the reduced requirement for anticoagulation constitutes a significant advantage for the tissue valve except for the first 3 postoperative months. During this time, the incidence of thromboembolism is high and most patients require anticoagulation.

Durability. For the earlier recipients of "first-generation" porcine valves, the duration of follow-up extends to 15 years. Clearly, the risk per year that a given valve will deteriorate is a function of its length of service. Thus, the risk of valvular malfunction cannot be linearized but should be stated as an actuarial incidence. The incidence seems to accelerate beginning at about 6 years[62] and to vary, particularly in patients who were younger than 35 years at operation.[63] In the experience of Magilligan et al.,[62] freedom from structural valve degeneration was 71% at 10 years and 31% at 15 years (Fig 37-5). Burdon et al.[64] found that freedom from structural valve deterioration of porcine valves after 10 and 15 years was significantly higher for aortic valve (85% and 63%) than for mitral valve (78% and 45%) prostheses ($P = 0.001$). Risk of reoperation was also higher for mitral valves (57%) than for aortic valves (43%) at 15 years. Among the first-generation bioprostheses, there is no apparent advantage of one type of porcine valve over another[65,66] (Fig 37-6). Thus, late degeneration is a serious drawback for the porcine valve, and patients and their families should understand this problem preoperatively. Fortunately, tissue valve failure tends to be noncatastrophic, so that reoperation usually can be accomplished electively and at little more risk than for the initial procedure.[67]

Some progress has been made in the processing of porcine bioprostheses. Glutaraldehyde fixation under low pressure appears to preserve the microarchitecture of the cusps, and this change may improve valve durability and retard calcification.[68]

Bovine pericardial prosthesis

In an effort to overcome the hemodynamic limitation of the porcine bioprosthetic valve, Ionescu et al.[69] preserved bovine pericardium by treatment with glutaraldehyde and mounted it on a frame. This minimized the loss of diameter caused by the stent itself.

Unfortunately, medium-term follow-up of the Ionescu-Shiley valve has been disappointing.[70-72] It appears that cusp tear at the attachment of pericardium to the commissures and mineralization lead to premature valve failure, and this is true for both mitral and aortic valves.[70,73] Multiple factors are involved in premature

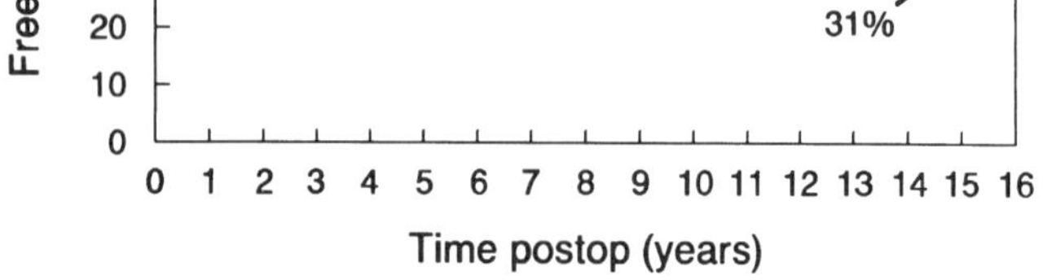

Fig 37-5 Freedom from valve degeneration (all porcine valves). Ten years postoperatively, 71% of patients were free of valve degeneration, and by 15 years postoperatively, only 31% of patients were free of structural failure. (Modified from Magilligan DJ Jr, Lewis JW Jr, Stein P, et al: The porcine bioprosthetic heart valve: experience at 15 years. *Ann Thorac Surg* 48:324-330, 1989.)

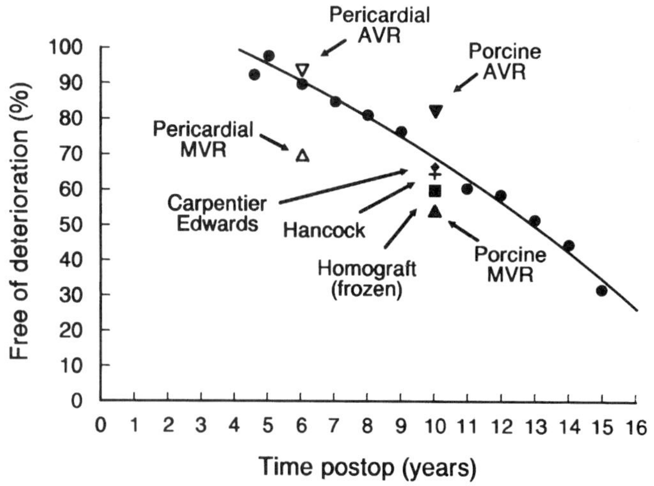

Fig 37-6 Data from Magilligan et al.[62] have been replotted, and the percentages of patients free of valve failure are shown in the closed circles. Additional data from current series of tissue valves suggest that the failure rate for bioprosthetic valves is roughly similar for the first-generation Hancock and Carpentier-Edwards valves and for frozen homografts. Pericardial heterografts seem to deteriorate earlier, although truly long-term data are not yet available. *AVR*, aortic valve replacement; *MVR*, mitral valve replacement.

degeneration of pericardial valves, and design features of the Ionescu-Shiley valve may predispose to leaflet tears at the commissures. However, tissue degeneration with disrupted collagen and absent or disrupted elastin fibers has been observed in Ionescu-Shiley, Mitroflow, and Hancock pericardial valves.[74] The early experience with a bovine pericardial valve of a different design by the Edwards company shows promise of better durability than was found in these first-generation pericardial bioprostheses.[75]

PROSTHESIS-RELATED PROBLEMS

Patients with prosthetic heart valves are not cured. Rather, they still have myocardial or ventricular dysfunction, which may lead to late mortality, including sudden unexplained death (see previous sections for the different types of valvular heart disease). In addition, patients with prosthetic heart valves have serious complications related to the prosthesis itself (Table 37-5). Some of these complications have been discussed in the descriptions of the different prosthetic valves (e.g., thromboembolism); for completeness, a brief summary of the other, less common, complications is presented here.

Prosthetic valve noise

Although minor compared with other potential complications of artificial heart valves, noise from prostheses is often a great concern to patients before operation. Bioprostheses are essentially free of noise aside from midsystolic ejection murmurs, which are inaudible to patients. Mechanical valves have opening and closing clicks that may be heard by patients, and the intensity of the sound is related to the design of the valve and the morphology of the patient. Older model ball and cage valves with metal poppets were excessively noisy in some patients, but currently available caged-ball prostheses with Silastic poppets and tilting-disk valves rarely disturb patients.

Table 37-5 Prosthesis-related problems

1. Prosthesis endocarditis
2. Prosthesis dehiscence
3. Prosthesis dysfunction
   - Obstructon—usually thrombotic, occasionally resulting from 1 or 2
   - Regurgitation
   - Hemolysis
   - Structural failure
4. Thromboembolism
5. Hemorrhage with anticoagulant therapy
6. Valve prosthesis-patient mismatch
7. Prosthesis replacement—often because of 1, 2, or 3; occasionally because of 4, 5, or 6

Modified from Rahimtoola SH, Chadraratna PAN: Valvular heart disease. In *Clinical Medicine.* Vol 6, Chap 15. Edited by JA Spittell Jr. Philadelphia, Harper & Row, Publishers, 1982, pp. 1-51.

Laurens et al.[76] measured the sound produced by the CarboMedics, Björk-Shiley monostrut, and St. Jude Medical prostheses and surveyed patients for symptoms that might be related to valve noise. The Björk-Shiley monostrut valve was slightly louder than the other two prostheses. More importantly, 14% of all patients had complaints related to the valve sound, including sleep disturbance, irritation, nervousness, and fear, and more patients with a Björk-Shiley monostrut prosthesis could hear their valve or had complaints than those with the other two prostheses. Younger patients and patients with a mitral valve prosthesis could hear their valve more often than older patients or patients after aortic valve replacement. Similarly, Moritz et al.[77] found that Duromedics, Edwards, and Björk-Shiley monostrut valves were significantly louder than St. Jude Medical and CarboMedics valves, and louder valves were more often heard by the patients and caused more complaints during both sleep and daytime.

Prosthetic valve endocarditis

The risk of prosthetic endocarditis is about 1% per patient-year.[78] Despite therapy, infections in the early postoperative period are difficult to cure and have a high mortality (about 85%); early reoperation is usually recommended. Mortality from late postoperative infection (2 months or more after valve replacement) is approximately 40%, the same as that from native valve endocarditis. About half the patients can be treated successfully with medication alone. For patients who have no response to medical treatment or have evidence of heart failure, annular invasion, repeated embolism, prosthesis dysfunction, or gram-negative, staphylococcal, fungal, or *Serratia* infection, the infected valve should be replaced. The importance of adequate antibiotic prophylaxis for prevention of endocarditis cannot be overemphasized.

Clinical detection of prosthesis dehiscence and prosthesis failure

Prosthesis dehiscence usually is the result of a suture or sutures pulling out of the tissues. It may result from infection, inadequate surgical technique, or poor quality of the patient's tissue. The most common cause for dysfunction of well-established devices is thrombotic obstruction.[50] This complication is not common, but the results can be hemodynamically catastrophic and require immediate diagnosis and reoperation; it is a particular problem with the Björk-Shiley valve and the St. Jude valve. The incidence of sudden prosthesis thrombosis after placement of a Björk-Shiley valve is three to four times higher in the mitral than in the aortic position. Failure is more common with tissue valves than with mechanical prostheses because of leaflet deterioration or calcification; progressive prosthetic incompetence is the rule. Obstruction is being reported with increasing frequency in patients with heterografts in place for 6 to 7 years or more. The tissue valves currently in use are unlikely to provide the long-term performance of the ball-and-cage valve mechanical prosthesis.

Table 37-6 Ascultatory findings in patients with normally functioning prosthetic heart valves

Prosthesis	Aortic	Mitral
Starr-Edwards ball valve	Sharp opening sound after S_1*	Sharp opening sound 70-150 msec after S_2
	Sharp closing sound at S_2	Sharp closing sound at S_1
	Ball "rattles" during systole	Ball "rattles" during diastole
	SEM	SEM
Björk-Shiley	Soft opening sound after S_1	Soft opening sound 70-150 msec after S_2
	Sharp closing sound at S_2	Sharp closing sound at S_1
	SEM	
Heterograft	SEM	Diastolic rumble† SEM

SEM, systolic ejection murmur.
*Absence of opening or closing sounds with mechanical prosthesis usually signifies severe prosthesis dysfunction.
†Indicates bioprosthetic obstruction or prosthesis-patient mismatch.
Modified from Rahimtoola SH, Chandraratna PAN: Valvular heart disease. In *Clinical Medicine.* Vol. 6, Chap 15. Edited by JA Spittell Jr. Philadephia, Harper & Row, Publishers, 1982, pp 1-51.

The diagnosis of prosthesis dehiscence or failure should be made on the basis of complete clinical evaluation; of particular importance are the auscultatory features and the use of noninvasive techniques, especially Doppler echocardiography.[79] The auscultatory findings to expect with some normally functioning prostheses are listed in Table 37-6. Minor aortic regurgitation murmurs, heard with variable frequency in patients with aortic prostheses, may represent periprosthetic or transvalvular leaks. Occasionally, such leaks become hemodynamically significant or cause refractory hemolysis. Mitral regurgitation murmurs with mitral prostheses are less common. In fact, severe perivalvular mitral regurgitation and occasionally aortic regurgitation may be inaudible on physical examination, a factor to remember when considering possible causes of deterioration of function in a patient.

Echocardiography is the primary diagnostic method for identifying prosthetic valve malfunction. Transesophageal echocardiography can demonstrate thrombus or vegetations; impairment of leaflet, disk, or poppet motion; and, in some cases of partial dehiscence, rocking of the prosthetic sewing ring. Also, pulsed-wave, color-flow mapping can assess regurgitation, and continuous-wave interrogation in experienced hands can accurately predict and evaluate transvalvular gradients[79] (Fig 37-7).

Hemolysis

Some degree of hemolysis is present with all mechanical prostheses but not with bioprostheses.[80] The St. Jude valve appears to have an especially low incidence of clinically important hemolysis.[81] However, important hemolysis may occur with perivalvular leak or severe prosthesis obstruction, regardless of prosthesis type. The serum lactate dehydrogenase concentration is usually the simplest and most reliable index of hemolysis in patients with prosthetic valves. A sudden increase in this value may indicate prosthesis dysfunction or perivalvular leak or, with a cloth-covered prosthesis, cloth tear. Therapy with iron and folate usually corrects anemia. Valve replacement occasionally may be required for severe, refractory hemolytic anemia.

Anticoagulant therapy and hemorrhage

Long-term anticoagulation therapy is associated with bleeding episodes. The incidence of minor hemorrhages is 2% to 4% per year; for major hemorrhages it is 1% to 2% per year, and for death it is 0.2% to 0.5% per year.[80] The incidence of these complications is much higher when aspirin is included in the regimen with warfarin.[82] Risk of bleeding is related not only to the care with which therapy with warfarin is monitored and adjusted but also to the desired level of anticoagulation. The international normalized ratio (INR) method of standardizing the reporting of prothrombin time adjusts for differences due to variations in thromboplastin reagents.[83]

Previously, most centers in the United States followed a recommendation for maintaining the prothrombin time ratio at 1.5 to 2.0 for patients with prosthetic heart valves, and many experts continue to advise an INR value of 4.0 for such patients.[84] Recent evidence suggests that a protocol of moderate anticoagulation (prothrombin time ratio, 1.5; INR, 2.65) is as effective as a high-intensity regimen (prothrombin time ratio, 2.5; INR, 9) in preventing thromboembolism after cardiac valve replacement; importantly, the risks of major and minor bleeding episodes are reduced by 50% in patients receiving a moderate level of anticoagulation.[85,86]

We interpret these data as follows. For patients who have bileaflet tilting disk prostheses in the aortic position, we recommend a target INR of 2 to 2.5, and patients are advised to take aspirin in a low dose (81 mg/day).[87] More intense anticoagulation is used for patients with mechanical valves in the mitral position, especially if the cardiac rhythm is atrial fibrillation; for these patients, we suggest an INR target value of 3.5 to 4 in conjunction with low-dose aspirin.

Valve prosthesis-patient mismatch

No prosthesis in current use has an effective orifice as large as that of the native valve.[80] Therefore, all patients with prosthetic heart valves have mild to moderate stenosis; in other words, patients with aortic valve prostheses have obstruction to left ventricular outflow ("aortic stenosis"), and patients with mitral valve prostheses have obstruction to left atrial emptying ("mitral stenosis").[88,89] This is most important when, for technical reasons, a small prosthesis must be placed in a large patient. The resulting patient-prosthesis mismatch contributes to incomplete relief of symptoms.

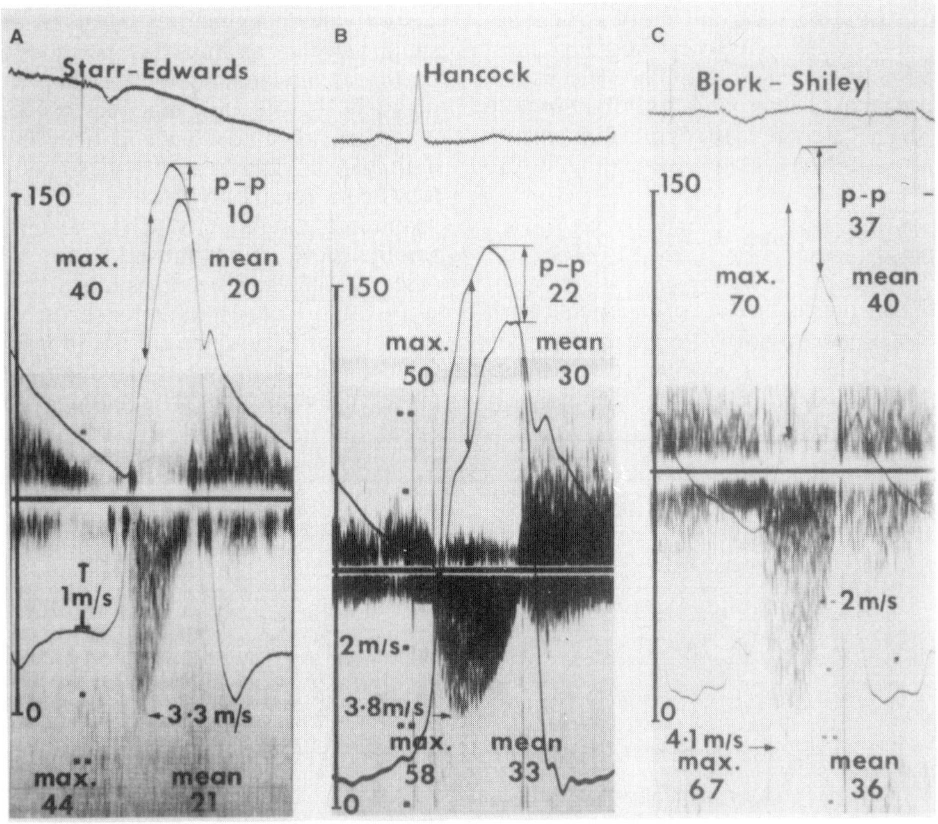

Fig 37-7 Simultaneous Doppler-catheter pressure recordings from three patients with three different aortic valve types (**A,** Starr-Edwards; **B,** Hanock; and **C,** Björk-Shiley) in whom left ventricular and ascending aortic pressure measurements were obtained by dual-catheter technique. Note the close correlation between Doppler- and catheter-derived maximal *(max.)* and mean gradients throughout a broad range of measured gradients. The peak-to-peak *(p-p)* gradients are lower than both the maximal and the mean gradients. (From Burstow DJ, Nishimura RA, Bailey KR, et al: Continuous wave Doppler echocardiographic measurement of prosthetic valve gradients: a simultaneous Doppler-catheter correlative study. Circulation 80:504-514, 1989. By permission of American Heart Association.)

FOLLOW-UP

All patients need appropriate antibiotics for prophylaxis against infective endocarditis. Patients with rheumatic heart disease continue to need antibiotics as prophylaxis against recurrence of rheumatic carditis. Adequate anticoagulation is needed for some patients; at present, this means anticoagulation with sodium warfarin unless this therapy is specifically contraindicated. Anticoagulation is needed in all patients with any type of mechanical prosthesis, in patients with bioprostheses who are in atrial fibrillation, and in all patients with bioprostheses during the first 3 months postoperatively.

During the first 6 weeks after operation, most attention is usually directed toward relieving postoperative discomfort and readjusting cardiac medications.[90] A plan of graduated activity is started that, in most cases, enables the patient to return to full activity in 6 weeks, but hard physical labor with the upper extremities should be prohibited for 3 to 6 months to allow proper healing of the sternum. If atrial fibrillation appears for the first time in the perioperative period, cardioversion is attempted before dismissal. If the arrhythmia persists, another attempt is made at the 6-week examination. Most patients continue to take digoxin, and other medications are administered as needed.

The postpericardiotomy syndrome occurs in 10% to 25% of patients and is characterized by fever and pleuropericarditis. It usually develops in postoperative week 2 or 3 but can appear as late as 1 year after operation and sometimes recurs.[91] Although this syndrome usually is self-limiting, most patients benefit from taking anti-inflammatory drugs, such as aspirin and indomethacin. Recognizing this syndrome is important to avoid a needless quest for pulmonary emboli or endocarditis, which might otherwise be suspected.

The workup on subsequent visits should include a complete history and physical examination. The main focus of the examination is on physical signs related to functioning of the prosthesis. At certain intervals, depending on the patient's needs, electrocardiogram, chest radiograph, complete blood cell count, blood electrolyte and lactate dehydrogenase values, and prothrombin time should be obtained. An early echocardiogram is important because it serves as a baseline for evaluating future recordings.

SUMMARY

Even after more than a quarter century of experience with valve replacement, no one type of valve has emerged as exclusively superior (Table 37-7). Patient variables are also important in the selection of a valve (Table 37-8). Tissue valves degenerate much faster in the young. A small valvular annulus favors choosing a valve having better hemodynamic performance. If pregnancy is planned, if a bleeding tendency exists or anticoagulation is contraindicated, or if patient compliance for the anticoagulation program is questionable, the tissue valve may be preferable. Anticoagulation is often considered a requirement in patients with atrial fibrillation or left atrial thrombus even if a tissue valve were to be used, so in this case a tissue valve becomes less appealing.

The record of survival after replacement with a specific type of prosthetic valve has not proved to be a good basis for comparison between valves or for selecting one in preference to another. The reason is that patient variables

Table 37-7 Comparison of prosthetic valves*

Criterion	Ball valve	Tilting-disk valve	Porcine valve	Pericardial valve
Decreased incidence of thromboembolism	...	...	+	+
Hemodynamics	...	+	...	+
Durability	+	?†	...	...

*+, Valve possesses this quality.
†Because model innovations are recent, length of follow-up experience is limited.

Table 37-8 Factors affecting choice of valve for individual patient*

Factor	Ball valve	Tilting-disk valve	Porcine valve	Pericardial valve
Young age	+	+	...	...
Small annulus	...	+	...	+
Pregnancy desired	...	...	+	+
Bleeding history	...	...	+	+
Atrial fibrillation	+	+	...	...
Anticoagulation compliance doubtful	...	...	+	+

*+, Valve possesses this quality.

Table 37-9 Valves used at the Mayo Clinic from January 1992 through December 1992*

	Mechanical prostheses			Bioprostheses			
	SJM	SE	MH	Intact	CE	HG†	All valves
Aortic	101	11	16	41	136	17	322
Mitral	56	36		8	22		122
Tricuspid	5	3			13		21
Pulmonary						56	56
Composite‡	9		7			2	18
Total	171	50	23	49	171	75	539

SJM, St. Jude Medical; SE, Starr-Edwards; MH, Medtronic-Hall; CE, Carpentier-Edwards; HG, cryopreserved homograft.
*The total of 539 valve prostheses does not include 128 annuloplasty rings used for mitral or tricuspid valve repair.
†Includes two pulmonary autografts with homograft replacement of pulmonary valve.
‡Ascending aortic graft with integral aortic valve replacement.

apparently have a much stronger influence on survival than do the variables related to the prosthesis, and the many studies of comparative survivals for the various valves consistently show no advantage of one over the others. Consistent guidelines with clear definitions for reporting performance of prosthetic heart valves should help in future comparisons of various prostheses.[92]

Practices in choosing a valve for use at a given institution or by a given surgeon vary greatly. The incidence of use of various valves at the Mayo Clinic during a recent year is shown in Table 37-9.

REFERENCES

1. Ross D, Jackson M, Davies J: Pulmonary autograft aortic valve replacement: long-term results. *J Card Surg* 6 Suppl:529-533, 1991
2. Elkins RC, Santangelo K, Stelzer P, et al: Pulmonary autograft replacement of the aortic valve: an evolution of technique. *J Card Surg* 7:108-116, 1992
3. Krosnick A: Death due to migration of the ball from an aortic-valve prosthesis. *JAMA* 191:1083-1084, 1965
4. Ablaza SGG, Blanco G, Maranhão V, et al: Fatal extrusion of the ball from a Starr-Edwards aortic valve prosthesis: report of a case. *J Thorac Cardiovasc Surg* 50:401-409, 1965
5. Pierie W, Raible D, Siposs G, et al: Valve replacement: durability of silicone rubber (abstract). *Circulation* 32 Suppl 2:171-172, 1965
6. Glancy DL, O'Brien KP, Reis RL, et al: Hemodynamic studies in patients with 2M and 3M Starr-Edwards prostheses: evidence of obstruction to left atrial emptying. *Circulation* 39 Suppl 1:113-118, 1969
7. Schaff HV, Chesebro JH: Experience with the Starr-Edwards Silastic ball valve. *Cardiol Clin* 3 (No 3):405-416, 1985
8. Bristow JD, Kremkau EL: Hemodynamic changes after valve replacement with Starr-Edwards prostheses. *Am J Cardiol* 35:716-724, 1975
9. Williams GA, Labovitz AJ: Doppler hemodynamic evaluation of prosthetic (Starr-Edwards and Björk-Shiley) and bioprosthetic (Hancock and Carpentier-Edwards) cardiac valves. *Am J Cardiol* 56:325-332, 1985
10. Mitchell RS, Miller DC, Stinson EB, et al: Significant patient-related determinants of prosthetic valve performance. *J Thorac Cardiovasc Surg* 91:807-816, 1986
11. Teply JF, Grunkemeier GL, Sutherland HD, et al: The ultimate prognosis after valve replacement: an assessment at twenty years. *Ann Thorac Surg* 32:111-118, 1981
12. Miller DC, Oyer PE, Stinson EB, et al: Ten to fifteen year reassessment of the performance characteristics of the Starr-Edwards Model 6120 mitral valve prosthesis. *J Thorac Cardiovasc Surg* 85:1-18, 1983
13. Miller DC, Oyer PE, Mitchell RS, et al: Performance characteristics of the Starr-Edwards Model 1260 aortic valve prosthesis beyond ten years. *J Thorac Cardiovasc Surg* 88:193-203, 1984
14. Perier P, Deloche A, Chauvaud S, et al: Comparative evaluation of mitral valve repair and replacement with Starr, Björk, and porcine valve prostheses. *Circulation* 70 Suppl I:I-187-I-192, 1984
15. Fuster V, Pumphrey CW, McGoon MD, et al: Systemic thromboembolism in mitral and aortic Starr-Edwards prostheses: a 10-19-year follow-up. *Circulation* 66 Suppl I:I-157-I-161, 1982
16. Mikaeloff P, Van Haecke P, Frieh JP, et al: Facteurs pronostiques après remplacement valvulaire mitral par la prothèse de Starr-Edwards modèle 6120. *Arch Mal Coeur* 74:799-807, 1981
17. Barnhorst DA, Oxman HA, Connolly DC, et al: Long-term follow-up of isolated replacement of the aortic or mitral valve with the Starr-Edwards prosthesis. *Am J Cardiol* 35:228-233, 1975
18. McGoon MD, Fuster V, McGoon DC, et al: Aortic and mitral valve incompetence: long-term follow-up (10 to 19 years) of patients treated with the Starr-Edwards prosthesis. *J Am Coll Cardiol* 3:930-938, 1984
19. Gott VL, Daggett RL, Whiffen JD, et al: A hinged-leaflet valve for total replacement of the human aortic valve. *J Thorac Cardiovasc Surg* 48:713-723, 1964
20. Cruz AB Jr, Kaster RL, Simmons RL, et al: Flow characteristics of the meniscus prosthetic heart valve. *J Thorac Cardiovasc Surg* 49:813-817, 1965
21. Pierce WS, Behrendt DM, Morrow AG: A hinged prosthetic cardiac valve fabricated of rigid components: experimental evaluations in vitro and in vivo. *J Thorac Cardiovasc Surg* 56:229-235, 1968
22. Wada J, Komatsu S, Ikeda K, et al: A new hingeless valve. In *Prosthetic Heart Valves.* Edited by LA Brewer III. Springfield, Illinois, Charles C Thomas, Publisher, 1969, pp 304-314
23. Björk VO: A new tilting disc valve prosthesis. *Scand J Thorac Cardiovasc Surg* 3:1-10, 1969
24. Kaster RL, Lillehei CW, Starek PJK: The Lillehei-Kaster pivoting disc aortic prosthesis and a comparative study of its pulsatile flow characteristics with four other prostheses. *Trans Am Soc Artif Intern Organs* 16:233-243, 1970
25. Hall KV: The Medtronic Hall heart valve: background, latest results, and future work. *Ann Thorac Surg* 48:S47-S48, 1989
26. Wang JH: The design simplicity and clinical elegance of the St. Jude Medical heart valve. *Ann Thorac Surg* 48 Suppl 3:S55-S56, 1989
27. Gott VL, Daggett RL, Young WP: Development of a carbon-coated, central-hinging, bileaflet valve. *Ann Thorac Surg* 48 Suppl 3:S28-S30, 1989
28. Antunes MJ: Mechanical failure of a St. Jude Medical prosthesis (letter to the editor). *Am J Cardiol* 68:841-842, 1991
29. Orsinelli DA, Becker RC, Cuénoud HF, et al: Mechanical failure of a St. Jude Medical prosthesis. *Am J Cardiol* 67:906-908, 1991
30. Carlson D, Stephenson LW: Mechanical cardiac valves: current status. *Cardiol Clin* 3 (No 3):439-443, 1985
31. Arom KV, Nicoloff DM, Kersten TE, et al: Ten years' experience with the St. Jude Medical valve prosthesis. *Ann Thorac Surg* 47:831-837, 1989
32. Tatineni S, Barner HB, Pearson AC, et al: Rest and exercise evaluation of St. Jude Medical and Medtronic Hall prostheses: influence of primary lesion, valvular type, valvular size, and left ventricular function. *Circulation* 80 Suppl I:I16-I23, 1989
33. Horstkotte D, Haerten K, Seipel L, et al: Central hemodynamics at rest and during exercise after mitral valve replacement with different prostheses. *Circulation* 68 Suppl II:161-168, 1983
34. Wortham DC, Tri TB, Bowen TE: Hemodynamic evaluation of the St. Jude Medical valve prosthesis in the small aortic anulus. *J Thorac Cardiovasc Surg* 81:615-620, 1981
35. Thormann J, Gottwik M, Schlepper M, et al: Hemodynamic alterations induced by isoproterenol and pacing after aortic valve replacement with the Björk-Shiley or St. Jude Medical prosthesis. *Circulation* 63:895-904, 1981
36. Kopf GS, Hammond GL, Geha AS, et al: Long-term performance of the St. Jude Medical valve: low incidence of thromboembolism and hemorrhagic complications with modest doses of warfarin. *Circulation* 76 Suppl III:III-132-III-136, 1987
37. Bowen TE, Tri TB, Wortham DC: Thrombosis of a St. Jude Medical tricuspid prosthesis: case report. *J Thorac Cardiovasc Surg* 82:257-262, 1981
38. Nuñez L, Iglesias A, Sotillo J: Entrapment of leaflet of St. Jude Medical cardiac valve prosthesis by miniscule thrombus: report of two cases. *Ann Thorac Surg* 29:567-569, 1980
39. Cassidy JM, Smith MD, Gurley JC, et al: Detection of thrombosis of St. Jude Medical prostheses by transesophageal echocardiography. *Am Heart J* 122:1466-1469, 1991
40. Åberg B, Henze A: Comparison between the *in vitro* flow dynamics of the standard and the convexo-concave Björk-Shiley tilting disc valve prostheses. *Scand J Thorac Cardiovasc Surg* 13:177-189, 1979
41. Björk VO: The improved Björk-Shiley tilting disk valve prosthesis. *Scand J Thorac Cardiovasc Surg* 12:81-84, 1978.
42. Hiratzka LF, Kouchoukos NT, Grunkemeier GL, et al: Outlet strut fracture of the Björk-Shiley 60° convexo-concave valve: current information and recommendations for patient care. *J Am Coll Cardiol* 11:1130-1137, 1988
43. Björk VO, Olin C: The hydrodynamic performance of the paediatric size Björk-Shiley disc valve prosthesis. *Scand J Thorac Cardiovasc Surg* 6:1-5, 1972
44. Björk VO, Henze A, Holmgren A, et al: Evaluation of the 21 mm Björk-Shiley tilting disc valve in patients with narrow aortic roots: a clinical, haemodynamic and angiographic study. *Scand J Thorac Cardiovasc Surg* 7:203-213, 1973
45. Schaff HV, Borkon AM, Hughes C, et al: Clinical and hemodynamic evaluation of the 19 mm Björk-Shiley aortic valve prosthesis. *Ann Thorac Surg* 32:50-57, 1981
46. Williams DB, Pluth JR, Orszulak TA: Extrinsic obstruction of the Björk-Shiley valve in the mitral position. *Ann Thorac Surg* 32:58-62, 1981

47. Moreno-Cabral RJ, McNamara JJ, Mamiya RT, et al: Acute thrombotic obstruction with Björk-Shiley valves: diagnosis and surgical considerations. *J Thorac Cardiovasc Surg* 75:321-329, 1978

48. Copans H, Lakier JB, Kinsley RH, et al: Thrombosed Björk-Shiley mitral prostheses. *Circulation* 61:169-174, 1980

49. Björk VO, Henze A: Management of thrombo-embolism after aortic valve replacement with the Björk-Shiley tilting disc valve: medicamental prevention with dicumarol in comparison with dipyridamole-acetylsalicylic acid. Surgical treatment of prosthetic thrombosis. *Scand J Thorac Cardiovasc Surg* 9:183-191, 1975

50. Kontos GJ Jr, Schaff HV, Orszulak TA, et al: Thrombotic obstruction of disc valves: clinical recognition and surgical management. *Ann Thorac Surg* 48:60-65, 1989

51. van der Graaf Y, de Waard F, van Herwerden LA, et al: Risk of strut fracture of Björk-Shiley valves. *Lancet* 339:257-261, 1992

52. Birkmeyer JD, Marrin CAS, O'Connor GT: Should patients with Björk-Shiley valves undergo prophylactic replacement? *Lancet* 340:520-523, 1992

53. Lindblom D, Rodriguez L, Björk VO: Mechanical failure of the Björk-Shiley valve: updated follow-up and considerations on prophylactic rereplacement. *J Thorac Cardiovasc Surg* 97:95-97, 1989

54. Ericsson A, Lindblom D, Semb G, et al: Strut fracture with Björk-Shiley 70° convexo-concave valve: an international multi-institutional follow-up study. *Eur J Cardiothorac Surg* 6:339-346, 1992

55. O'Brien MF, Stafford EG, Gardner MA, et al: A comparison of aortic valve replacement with viable cryopreserved and fresh allograft valves, with a note on chromosomal studies. *J Thorac Cardiovasc Surg* 94:812-821, 1987

56. Carpentier A, Lemaigre G, Robert L, et al: Biological factors affecting long-term results of valvular heterografts. *J Thorac Cardiovasc Surg* 58:467-482, 1969

57. Cosgrove DM, Lytle BW, Gill CC, et al: In vivo hemodynamic comparison of porcine and pericardial valves. *J Thorac Cardiovasc Surg* 89:358-368, 1985

58. Rossiter SJ, Miller DC, Stinson EB, et al: Hemodynamic and clinical comparison of the Hancock modified orifice and standard orifice bioprostheses in the aortic position. *J Thorac Cardiovasc Surg* 80:54-60, 1980

59. Cohn LH, Allred EN, Cohn LA, et al: Early and late risk of mitral valve replacement: a 12 year concomitant comparison of the porcine bioprosthetic and prosthetic disc mitral valves. *J Thorac Cardiovasc Surg* 90:872-880, 1985

60. Zussa G, Ottino G, di Summa M, et al: Porcine cardiac bioprostheses: evaluation of long-term results in 990 patients. *Ann Thorac Surg* 39:243-250, 1985

61. Edmunds LH Jr: Thromboembolic complications of current cardiac valvular prostheses. *Ann Thorac Surg* 34:96-106, 1982

62. Magilligan DJ Jr, Lewis JW Jr, Stein P, et al: The porcine bioprosthetic heart valve: experience at 15 years. *Ann Thorac Surg* 48:324-329, 1989

63. Magilligan DJ Jr, Lewis JW Jr, Jara FM, et al: Spontaneous degeneration of porcine bioprosthetic valves. *Ann Thorac Surg* 30:259-265, 1980

64. Burdon TA, Miller DC, Oyer PE, et al: Durability of porcine valves at fifteen years in a representative North American patient population. *J Thorac Cardiovasc Surg* 103:238-251, 1992

65. Perier P, Deloche A, Chauvaud S, et al: A 10-year comparison of mitral valve replacement with Carpentier-Edwards and Hancock porcine bioprostheses. *Ann Thorac Surg* 48:54-59, 1989

66. Starr A, Grunkemeier GL: The expected lifetime of porcine valves [editorial]. *Ann Thorac Surg* 48:317-318, 1989

67. Husebye DG, Pluth JR, Piehler JM, et al: Reoperation on prosthetic heart valves: an analysis of risk factors in 552 patients. *J Thorac Cardiovasc Surg* 86:543-551, 1983

68. Barratt-Boyes BG, Ko PH, Jaffe WM: The zero pressure fixed Medtronic Intact porcine valve: clinical results over a 6-year period, including serial echocardiographic assessment. *J Card Surg* 6 Suppl:606-612, 1991

69. Ionescu MI, Pakrashi BC, Mary DAS, et al: Replacement of heart valves with frame-mounted tissue grafts. *Thorax* 29:56-67, 1974

70. Pelletier LC, Carrier M, Leclerc Y, et al: Porcine versus pericardial bioprostheses: a comparison of late results in 1,593 patients. *Ann Thorac Surg* 47:352-360, 1989

71. Teoh KH, Ivanov J, Weisel RD, et al: Survival and bioprosthetic valve failure: ten-year follow-up. *Circulation* 80 Suppl:I8-I15, 1989

72. Nistal F, Garcia-Martinez V, Fernández D, et al: Degenerative pathologic findings after long-term implantation of bovine pericardial bioprosthetic heart valves. *J Thorac Cardiovasc Surg* 96:642-651, 1988

73. Walley VM, Keon CA, Khalili M, et al: Ionescu-Shiley valve failure I: Experience with 125 standard-profile explants. *Ann Thorac Surg* 54:111-116, 1992

74. Trowbridge EA, Lawford PV, Crofts CE, et al: Pericardial heterografts: why do these valves fail? *J Thorac Cardiovasc Surg* 95:577-585, 1988

75. Perier P, Mihaileanu S, Fabiani J-N, et al: Long-term evaluation of the Carpentier-Edwards pericardial valve in the aortic position. *J Card Surg* 6 Suppl:589-594, 1991

76. Laurens RRP, Wit HP, Ebels T: Mechanical heart valve prostheses: sound level and related complaints. *Eur J Cardiothorac Surg* 6:57-61, 1992

77. Moritz A, Steinseifer U, Kobinia G, et al: Closing sounds and related complaints after heart valve replacement with St Jude Medical, Duromedics Edwards, Björk-Shiley Monostrut, and Carbomedics prostheses. *Br Heart J* 67:460-465, 1992

78. Heimberger TS, Duma RJ: Infections of prosthetic heart valves and cardiac pacemakers. *Infect Dis Clin North Am* 3(2):221-245, 1989

79. Burstow DJ, Nishimura RA, Bailey KR, et al: Continuous wave Doppler echocardiographic measurement of prosthetic valve gradients: a simultaneous Doppler-catheter correlative study. *Circulation* 80:504-514, 1989

80. Rahimtoola SH, Chandraratna PAN: Valvular heart disease. In *Clinical Medicine.* Vol 6, Chap 15. Edited by JA Spittell Jr. Philadelphia, Harper & Row, Publishers, 1982, pp 1-51

81. DiSesa VJ, Collins JJ Jr, Cohn LH: Hematological complications with the St. Jude valve and reduced-dose Coumadin. *Ann Thorac Surg* 48:280-283, 1989

82. Chesebro JH, Fuster V, Elveback LR, et al: Trial of combined warfarin plus dipyridamole or aspirin therapy in prosthetic heart valve replacement: danger of aspirin compared with dipyridamole. *Am J Cardiol* 51:1537-1541, 1983

83. Butchart EG, Lewis PA, Kulatilake ENP, et al: Anticoagulation variability between centres: implications for comparative prosthetic valve assessment. *Eur J Cardiothorac Surg* 2:72-81, 1988

84. Loeliger EA: Therapeutic target values in oral anticoagulation—justification of Dutch policy and a warning against theso-called moderate-intensity regimens. *Ann Hematol* 64:60-65, 1992

85. Saour JN, Sieck JO, Mamo LAR, et al: Trial of different intensities of anticoagulation in patients with prosthetic heart valves. *N Engl J Med* 322:428-432, 1990

86. Wilson DB, Dunn MI, Hassanein K: Low-intensity anticoagulation in mechanical cardiac prosthetic valves. *Chest* 100:1553-1557, 1991

87. Turpie AG, Gent M, Laupacis A, et al: A comparison of aspirin with placebo in patients treated with warfarin after heart-valve replacement. *N Engl J Med* 329:524-529, 1993

88. Rahimtoola SH: The problem of valve prosthesis-patient mismatch. *Circulation* 58:20-24, 1978

89. Rahimtoola SH, Murphy E: Valve prosthesis—patient mismatch: a *long-term sequela. Br Heart J* 45:331-335, 1981

90. Morton MJ, Rahimtoola SH: How to follow patients with prosthetic heart valves. *J Cardiovasc Med* 5:475-495, 1980

91. Nishimura RA, Fuster V, Burgert SL, et al: Clinical features and long-term natural history of the postpericardiotomy syndrome. *Int J Cardiol* 4:443-450, 1983

92. Edmunds LH Jr, Clark RE, Cohn LH, et al: Guidelines for reporting morbidity and mortality after cardiac valvular operations. *Ann Thorac Surg* 46:257-259, 1989

CHAPTER

38

The scope of the problem

Carole A. Warnes, M.D.

CONGENITAL heart disease may be defined as a significant structural malformation of the heart or great vessels that is present at birth. The incidence of congenital heart disease is approximately 8 per 1,000 live births.[1] As discussed in chapter 12, congenital heart disease is caused by imperfect embryogenesis. Therefore, the ideal remedy for this problem would be to elucidate and then eradicate abnormal embryogenesis. Indeed, genetic advances in pediatric cardiology[2,3] offer hope for future prevention. Furthermore, noninvasive diagnostic techniques applied in fetal life or at birth,[4,5] as well as innovative nonsurgical interventional approaches,[6,7] offer a much more optimistic view in the care of these patients.

In the past several decades, dramatic changes have occurred in the management of the infant born with congenital heart disease. Significant advances have been made in surgical repair, anesthesia, intensive care, and noninvasive diagnosis, so that increasing numbers of infants born with congenital cardiac anomalies are surviving to adulthood. This has led to a "new community" of adult survivors with congenital cardiac anomalies.[8,9] This new population is made up of two groups of patients. One group consists of persons who have survived naturally without previous surgery; they usually have mild anomalies, such as a bicuspid aortic valve or atrial septal defect, but some have more complex anomalies, such as tetralogy of Fallot, pulmonary atresia, and univentricular atrioventricular connection. There is a larger group, however, who have had previous surgery, either a palliative procedure, such as an aortopulmonary shunt, or complete repair. The types of lesions encountered in patients seen in the first 3 years of the Adult Congenital Heart Disease Clinic at the Mayo Clinic are shown in Table 38-1. The patients who have had previous cardiac surgery cannot be considered completely "cured," and many encounter other cardiac problems later in life. The only congenital cardiac anomaly completely cured by surgery is the successfully ligated patent ductus arteriosus; thereafter, patients can lead a normal life and do not need antibiotic prophylaxis for endocarditis. Although excellent and uncomplicated survival is possible when several simple lesions are repaired early in life, some of these lesions may pose problems; for example, in a patient with a successfully repaired secundum atrial septal defect, atrial arrhythmias may still develop in adulthood.

Patients who have had more complex lesions repaired may encounter several problems.[10] Biologic valves and conduits used in many surgical repairs eventually calcify and need replacement, and they are always susceptible to endocarditis. Arrhythmias are frequent sequelae and may on occasion be life threatening. Ventricular dysfunction is common for many reasons: left ventricular dysfunction due to volume overload from a surgically created shunt, for example, or right ventricular dysfunction after tetralogy repair when there is residual pulmonary regurgitation or a ventricular septal defect. Since the introduction of more effective myocardial protection in the 1970s, serious ventricular dysfunction without residual lesions has become less common. When repair is performed at an early age, myocardial failure may be avoided, but the incidence of myocardial failure has been equaled, if not exceeded, by the increased number of survivors with complex lesions in whom ventricular failure before 40 years of age is probable if not inevitable.[11]

These patients also need informed advice about routine matters, such as exercise, employment, insurance, and driving capability.[12]

Because of these problems, the cardiologist caring for these patients must be familiar not only with the anatomic and physiologic characteristics of each anomaly but also with the anticipated residua and sequelae specific for each lesion. The cardiologist must also be familiar with the best management strategies and the preferred means of further surgical intervention when necessary. This is a heavy responsibility for adult cardiologists, who are usually more familiar with acquired than with congenital heart disease. Many of the patients have been seen for years by a pediatric cardiologist and often encounter difficulties finding an adult cardiologist who has expertise with congenital heart disease. They may feel "aban-

Table 38-1 Frequency of cardiac anomalies during the first 6 years of the Adult Congenital Heart Disease Clinic

	Number of anomalies	
	Natural history	Postoperative
Aortic stenosis, coarctation of aorta	26	36
Pulmonary stenosis	16	13
Primary and secondary atrial septal defects, anomalous pulmonary veins	77	36
Ventricular septal defect	29	20
Ebstein's anomaly	49	18
Eisenmenger's syndrome	22	2
Tetralogy of Fallot, pulmonary atresia, truncus arteriosus	10	114
Single ventricle, tricuspid atresia	12	62
Corrected transposition of the great arteries	11	15
Transposition of the great arteries	0	29
Miscellaneous	67	31
Total	319	376

doned" by their pediatrician, who cared for them successfully for many years, and these problems, in addition to the major obstacle of obtaining medical insurance, frequently prevent these patients from securing adequate cardiac follow-up.

Conversely, adult patients seen by pediatric cardiologists may feel uncomfortable in a pediatric outpatient setting and be discouraged from continuing follow-up. Female patients may need counseling about contraception and pregnancy management, and since all patients may be subject to acquired cardiac disease, their management may be suboptimal in this setting.

SUMMARY

Congenital heart disease in adults is still a largely unrecognized subspecialty but is emerging as a discipline that requires special expertise. Tertiary facilities are now established to take care of these patients and their special problems.[13] The skills and dedication of the pediatric cardiologist must be matched by those of the adult cardiologist, and education, training, and research need to be further developed. In the United States alone, well over one-half million patients with congenital heart disease have reached adulthood. Much time, money, and effort have been spent to secure their survival. Most patients are eager to work, "contribute" to society, and lead as normal a life as possible. Their lot can surely be enhanced by expert medical care.

REFERENCES

1. Mitchell SC, Korones SB, Berendes HW: Congenital heart disease in 56,109 births: incidence and natural history. *Circulation* 43:323-332, 1971
2. Burn J: Genetic advances in paediatric cardiology. *Curr Opin Cardiol* 3:43-49, 1988
3. Boughman JA, Ferencz C, Neill CA: Genetic advances in pediatric cardiology. *Curr Opin Cardiol* 4:53-59, 1989
4. Williams RG: Fetal cardiology. *Curr Opin Cardiol* 4:60-63, 1989
5. DiSessa TG: Recent developments in qualitative and quantitative assessment of congenital heart disease. *Curr Opin Cardiol* 4:76-83, 1989
6. Deanfield JE: Interventional catheterization in congenital heart disease. *Curr Opin Cardiol* 3:87-91, 1988
7. Rocchini AP: Interventional catheterization. *Curr Opin Cardiol* 4:93-96, 1989
8. Somerville J: Congenital heart disease in adults and adolescents. *Br Heart J* 56:395-397, 1986
9. Perloff JK (Chairman): 22nd Bethesda Conference: congenital heart disease after childhood: an expanding patient population. *J Am Coll Cardiol* 18:311-342, 1991
10. Perloff JK: Adults with surgically treated congenital heart disease: sequelae and residua. *JAMA* 250:2033-2036, 1983
11. Laks H, Pearl JM: The surgeon's responsibility. Operation and reoperation: the UCLA experience. *J Am Coll Cardiol* 18:327-329, 1991
12. Cetta F, Warnes CA: Adults with congenital heart disease: patient knowledge of endocarditis prophylaxis. *Mayo Clin Proc* 70:50-54, 1995
13. Somerville J, Webb GD, Skorton DJ, et al: Medical center experiences. *J Am Coll Cardiol* 18:315-318, 1991

CHAPTER

39

Congenital echocardiography

Donald J. Hagler, M.D.

ECHOCARDIOGRAPHY has played an ever-increasing role in the clinical management of patients with congenital heart disease. Several previous chapters have been devoted to the general application of ultrasound in cardiology; this chapter deals with specifics of its application to congenital heart disease. The current generally accepted broad applications of echocardiography to congenital heart disease can include (1) anatomic assessment; (2) hemodynamic and functional assessment, including Doppler, color-flow, and contrast modalities; (3) stress echocardiography; (4) fetal echocardiography; (5) transesophageal echocardiography; and (6) intraoperative echocardiography. Recent innovations have also included intravascular and three-dimensional reconstruction techniques for congenital cardiac disease.

PHYSICIAN TRAINING

Clear guidelines for adequate pediatric echocardiographic training, including both general and specific directions for fetal and transesophageal echocardiography, have been issued by the Society of Pediatric Echocardiography in conjunction with the American Society of Echocardiography.[1-4]

THE ECHOCARDIOGRAPHIC EXAMINATION

As discussed in earlier chapters, echocardiographic examinations are generally goal-oriented. For all practical purposes, however, a complete and thorough examination is necessary in the initial review of any patient with congenital heart disease to adequately exclude the multiple and varied features of complex forms of the disease.

For most pediatric examinations, a comfortable, quiet atmosphere helps soothe and relax the anxious patient. The presence and assistance of the parents are almost always helpful in allaying the child's fears. For patients older than 2 years, special facilities to allow audiovisual entertainment through videotaped children's stories and cartoons have been particularly useful in preoccupying and quieting the pediatric patients in our echocardiographic laboratory.

For the most terrified and uncontrolled patient younger than 3 years, sedation may be the only effective method to obtain an adequate echocardiographic examination. The echocardiographic examination for complex congenital heart disease may require 45 to 60 minutes to complete. With the additional 30 to 45 minutes that may be necessary for adequate sedation, it is imperative that 1 to 2 hours be allocated in the patient's schedule to adequately accomplish the echocardiographic examination.

Many pediatric echocardiographic laboratories use chloral hydrate for effective prolonged sedation for echocardiography at an oral dose of 75 to 100 mg/kg. Unfortunately, this agent has several side effects that make its use generally unsatisfactory. The taste is terrible. Children immediately dislike it and frequently begin gagging and may vomit with the first taste. Sometimes the drug may be repeated at one-third to one-half the first dose if much of it has been regurgitated. The onset of effect may not occur for more than 30 minutes. Some children become only very agitated after drug administration.

Because of these effects, other agents have been tried. Midazolam given intranasally at a dose of 0.1 to 0.3 mg/kg has the advantage of very rapid onset. However, effective sedation lasts only about 30 minutes and may be only a calming effect rather than a truly hypnotic one. The drug may be given again at the lower dosage after 15 minutes.

Some have recommended rectal thiopental at a dose of 5 to 10 mg/kg, repeated if necessary in 30 minutes at one-half the dose. However, greater precautions for respiratory arrest must be made, including observation by a nurse and pulse oximetry. For in-patient sedation, the American Academy of Pediatrics has recommended routine sedation for radiologic procedures with pentobarbital administered intravenously at a dose of 2 to 3 mg/kg, with subsequent increments of 0.5 to 1 mg/kg until a hypnotic effect is achieved. Continuous observation by a nurse and pulse oximetry are also recommended.

In general, echocardiographic examination in the pediatric patient includes all the parasternal, apical, subcostal, and suprasternal notch views previously described. In addition, because of the varied location of cardiac structures in association with congenital abnormalities of cardiac situs, complete echocardiographic examinations may also require scans from and examination techniques for a variety of unusual locations, including bilateral parasternal and high parasternal sites. For the pediatric examination, patient growth and the variable size of cardiac structures observed in congenital cardiac defects require particular attention to provide a detailed examination, including multiple measurements of cardiac chamber, great artery, and valvular dimensions as well as specific measurements of the congenital defects encountered during the examination. In addition, it is imperative that adequate ranges of normal values be available for all the M-mode, two-dimensional, and Doppler echocardiographic measurements obtained.

A SEGMENTAL APPROACH TO ECHOCARDIOGRAPHIC EXAMINATION

A segmental approach to the echocardiographic study has been particularly important in the echocardiographic assessment of the anatomic details of most forms of congenital heart disease. For practical purposes, this approach has been extracted from the methods published and used by pathologists to categorize and classify forms of congenital cardiac disease.[5,6] The segmental approach to an echocardiographic examination has been mandatory for complete evaluation of complex congenital cardiac defects, including abnormalities of visceral, atrial, and cardiac vessel situs.

Early M-mode echocardiographic reports advocated a segmental approach to echocardiographic study.[7] However, not until the advent of two-dimensional imaging could the precise mechanism for segmental analysis of situs connections, ventricular anatomy, and chamber position be accurately detailed echocardiographically for a complete diagnostic assessment.[8,9] Table 39-1 outlines the stepwise segmental approach for prospective two-dimensional echocardiographic study of complex congenital heart disease. It effectively details the anatomic features of the cardiac and extracardiac morphology that should be echocardiographically defined for a complete segmental echocardiographic diagnosis. Although the practical echocardiographic examination may not proceed in a segmental fashion, the anatomic details obtained during the examination should be sufficient to allow a segmental stepwise approach to the echocardiographic diagnosis. A complete echocardiographic study should include appropriate views and analyses for adequate determination of (1) atrial and visceral situs, (2) atrioventricular (AV) connections and AV valve morphology, (3) ventricular situs and morphology, and (4) great artery relationships and extracardiac course.

Table 39-1 Segmental approach for prospective two-dimensional echocardiographic study of complex congenital heart disease

1. **Atrial and visceral situs**
   - Caval position and connection
   - Hepatic veins
   - Coronary sinus
   - Pulmonary venous connection
2. **AV connections and AV valve morphology**
   - Commitment (AV malalignment-overriding, crisscross)
   - Insertion (chordal attachment-straddling)
   - Leaflet numbers
   - Papillary muscles (position, number, abnormality-parachute)
   - Leaflet abnormalities (cleft, thickening-stenosis)
3. **Ventricular situs and morphology**
   - Cardiac position (levocardia, dextrocardia, mesocardia)
   - Ventricular relations (anterior, posterior, superior, inferior, right, left)
   - AV valve attachment
   - Shape (ellipsoid, crescentic, triangular)
   - Trabecular pattern
   - Papillary muscles (two discrete or multiple irregular)
4. **Great artery relations and extracardiac course**
   - Position (normal, side-by-side, D-malposed, L-malposed)
   - Ventriculoarterial connection
   - Override
   - AV valve continuity (subvalvular conus)
   - Identification
     - Posterior course and bifurcation of pulmonary artery
     - Anterior and superior course of aorta
   - Aortic arch location (right, left arch) and brachiocephalic branching pattern
   - Arch anomalies (hypoplasia, coarctation, patent ductus arteriosus)

Atrial and visceral situs

Figure 39-1 sequentially illustrates the typical echocardiographic observations of the abdominal viscera to be made in an assessment of visceral situs. Since visceral and atrial situs are usually concordant, an echocardiographic assessment of visceral situs may allow a determination of atrial situs by correctly correlating visceral and atrial situs with systemic and pulmonary venous connections. Each case, however, must be individually reviewed to anticipate possible exceptions when the atrial and visceral situs are ambiguous and possibly discordant. Figure 39-1,A depicts situs solitus with a normal left-sided stomach and spleen and right-sided liver. The echocardiographic short- and long-axis scans of the liver easily demonstrate the hepatic and inferior vena caval connections superiorly to the right atrium. The spleen can be visualized with a long-axis scan over the left lateral aspect of the lower chest and abdomen, and in some cases, composite short-axis scans (Fig 39-2) can demonstrate all the anatomic features associated with visceral situs solitus. Similarly, situs inversus totalis and situs ambiguus can be accurately demonstrated by these abdominal short- and long-axis visceral scans. Figure 39-3 illustrates an example of situs ambiguus. The patient has a large midline liver with an interrupted inferior vena cava and hemiazygous continuation. The long-axis scans in this figure demonstrate the aorta and the posterior hemiazygos vein. In addition, the

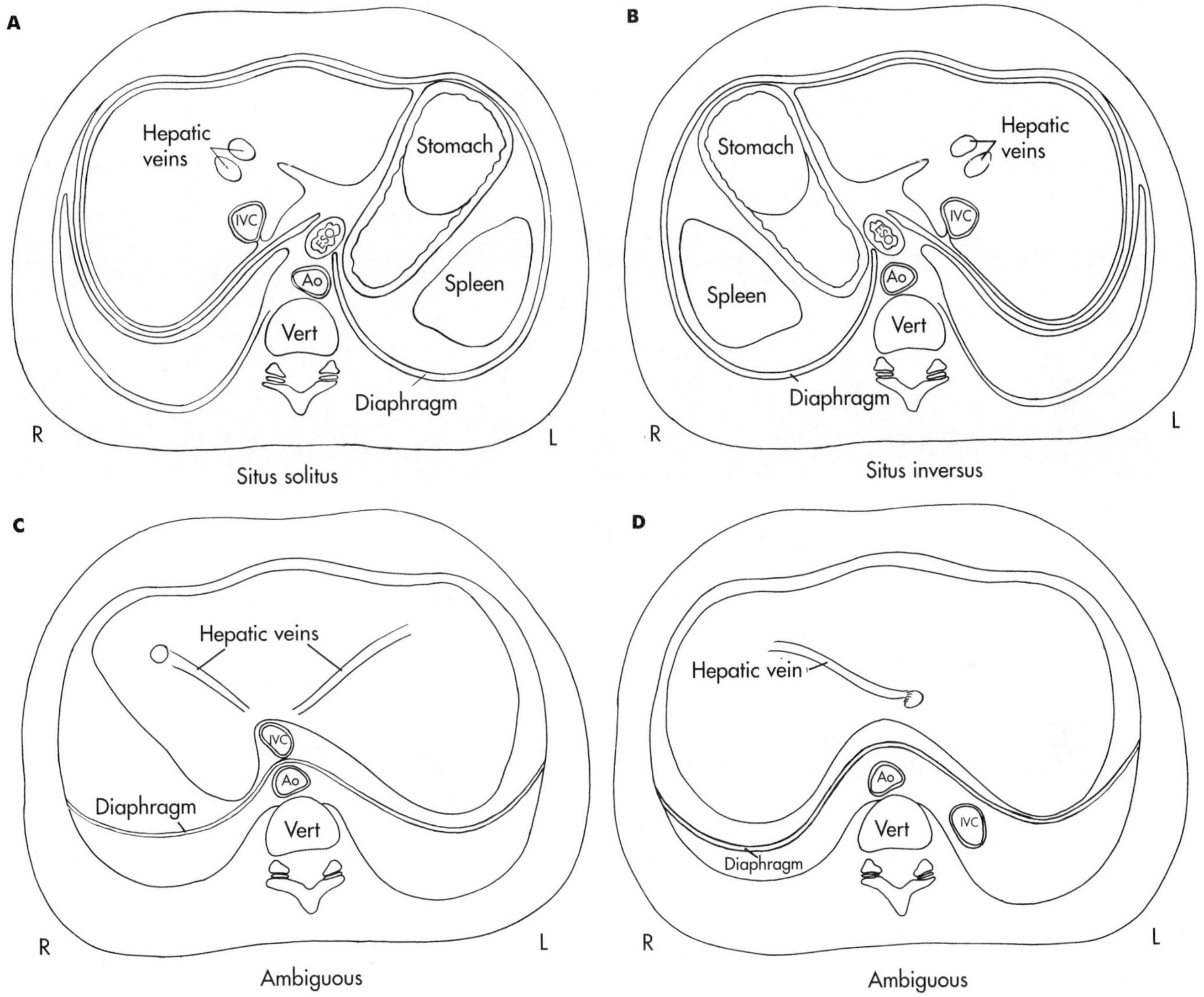

Fig 39-1 Anatomic-echocardiographic findings on subcostal short-axis scans of the abdomen. **A**, situs solitus, with the liver mass on the patient's right (*R*). Note that the inferior vena cava (*IVC*) is the intrahepatic portion and the descending abdominal aorta (*Ao*) is retroperitoneal and posterior to the diaphragm. **B**, situs inversus, with visceral structure completely inverted left to right from situs solitus. **C**, ambiguous visceral situs with a large midline liver mass and no spleen (asplenia). The intrahepatic portion of the IVC is present but maintains an unusual relation with the abdominal aorta, which is directly posterior, slightly off midline, and directly anterior to the vertebral body (*Vert*). **D**, situs ambiguus with associated interruption of the hepatic portion of the IVC and a hemiazygous continuation of the IVC as it courses superiorly and retroperitoneally (posterior to the diaphragm) along the left side of the vertebral body. *ESO*, esophagus; *L*, left. (By permission, Mayo Foundation.)

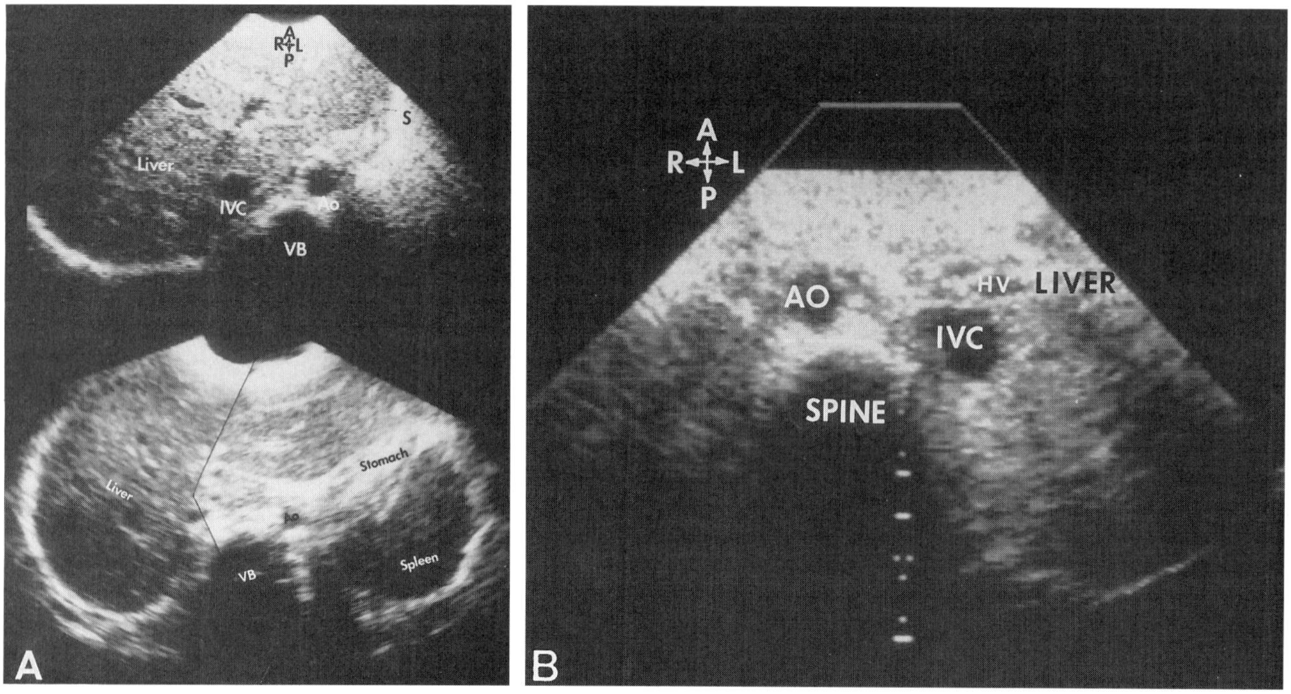

Fig 39-2 **A**, composite subcostal short-axis scans in situs solitus. All anatomic structures depicted in Figure 39-1,A are shown. **B**, subcostal short-axis scan in situs inversus totalis illustrating the anatomy depicted in Figure 39-1,B. *A*, anterior; *Ao* or *AO*, descending abdominal aorta; *HV*, hepatic vein; *IVC*, inferior vena cava; *L*, left; *P*, posterior; *R*, right; *S*, stomach; *VB*, vertebral body.

separate hepatic venous connection to the common atrium may be bilateral with situs ambiguus. Since situs ambiguus may be associated with asplenia (usually observed in so-called right isomerism) and polysplenia (usually observed in left isomerism), the echocardiographic demonstration of multiple spleens, as shown in Figure 39-4, is helpful in this pathologic distinction. The constellation of cardiac defects associated with left isomerism (bilateral left-sidedness) is then expected rather than the cardiac defects more often associated with right isomerism (bilateral right-sidedness). The inability to find any evidence of a spleen on ultrasound examination of the abdomen points to a diagnosis of asplenia and right isomerism.

After an assessment of visceral situs has established some basis for determination of atrial situs, the atrial situs itself may be more precisely determined by other characteristics in Table 39-1, such as caval position and atrial connections, location and drainage of the coronary sinus (usually identifying the right atrium), and pulmonary venous connections (usually associated with the left atrium). Determination of extracardiac anatomy, required in an assessment of venous connections, has been particularly improved in recent years with the development of high-frequency, high-resolution ultrasonic imaging. This has been especially helpful in the neonatal period, because soft tissue density and high-frequency transducers allow excellent resolution of these anatomic features. Utilization of 5- and 7.5-MHz transducer imaging provides an excellent opportunity to accurately define the extracardiac anatomy to determine systemic and pulmonary venous connections.

The addition of color-flow imaging has substantially improved our ability to recognize venous return via these extracardiac connections and to correlate them with other associated anatomy in a cross-sectional format. Apical two-dimensional images in Figure 39-5 show a dilated coronary sinus draining to the right atrium, and high left parasternal scans in Figure 39-6 use color-flow imaging to reveal left superior vena caval flow via the coronary sinus into the right atrium. Similarly, a high right parasternal short-axis scan in Figure 39-7 utilizes color-flow imaging to accurately portray normal pulmonary venous connections to the left atrium in a newborn infant. Use of the combined techniques of high-resolution two-dimensional imaging and the color-flow imaging has substantially improved our ability to accurately define atrial and visceral situs.

AV connections and AV valve morphology

The next logical step in the segmental approach is an assessment of AV connections and AV valve morphology. Included in this very important aspect of the two-dimensional echocardiographic assessment is a determination of the ventricular commitment of each AV valve

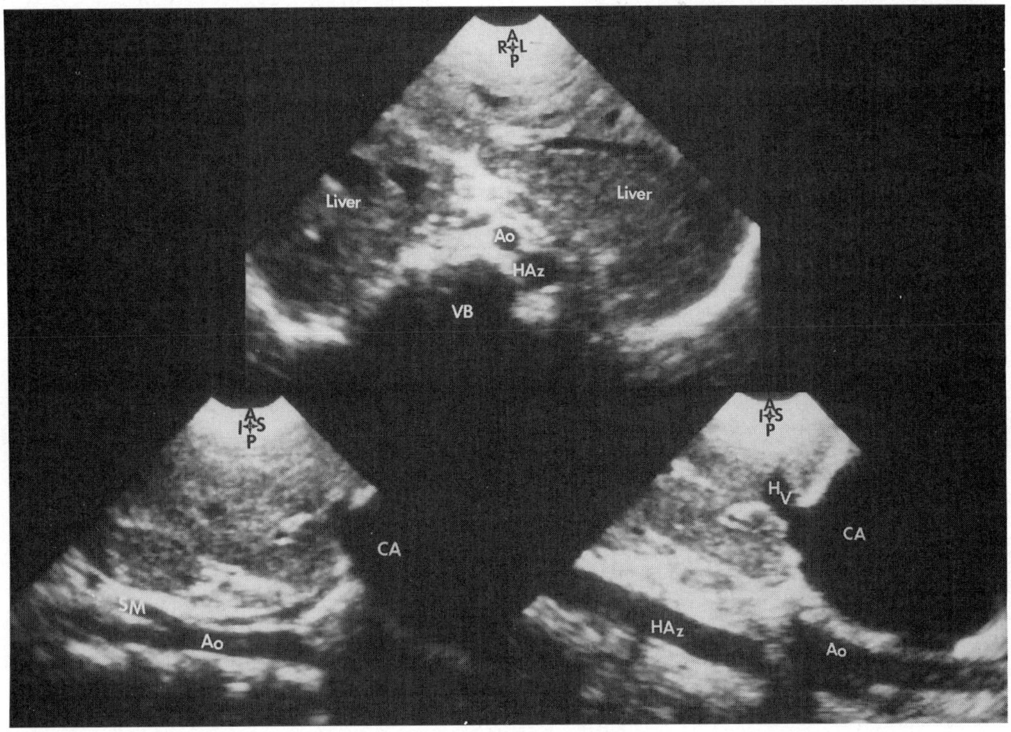

Fig 39-3 Subcostal scans in a patient with situs ambiguus. **Top**, short-axis scan. A hemiazygous (*HAz*) continuation of the inferior vena cava is observed in a retroperitoneal location posterior to the aorta (*Ao*) and to the left of the vertebral body (*VB*). The liver is large and spans across the midline. **Bottom left and right**, longitudinal scans of the abdomen show the hemiazygos vein coursing superiorly and located posterior to the aorta. Note that the left hepatic vein (*HV*) separately enters the common atrium (*CA*). *A*, anterior; *I*, inferior; *L*, left; *P*, posterior; *R*, right; *S*, superior; *SM*, superior mesenteric artery. (From Seward JB, Tajik AJ, Edwards WD, et al: *Two-Dimensional Echocardiographic Atlas*. Vol. 1: *Congenital Heart Disease*. New York, Springer-Verlag, 1987. By permission, Mayo Foundation.)

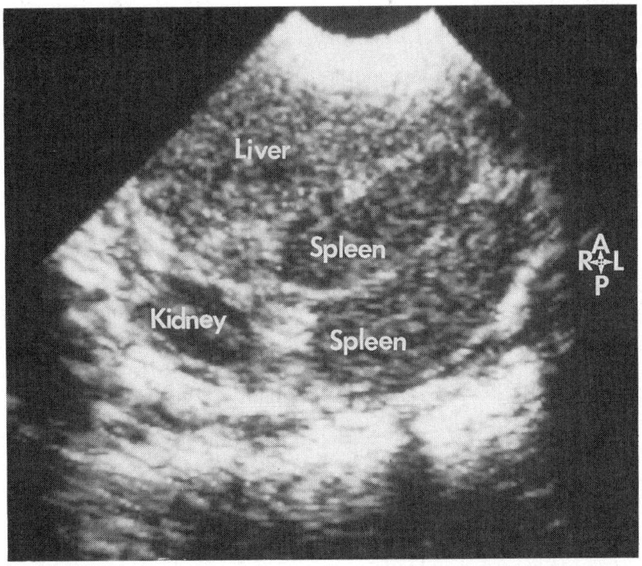

Fig 39-4 Subcostal short-axis scan demonstrating multiple spleens in a patient with polysplenia and bilateral left-sidedness. *A*, anterior; *L*, left; *P*, posterior; *R*, right.

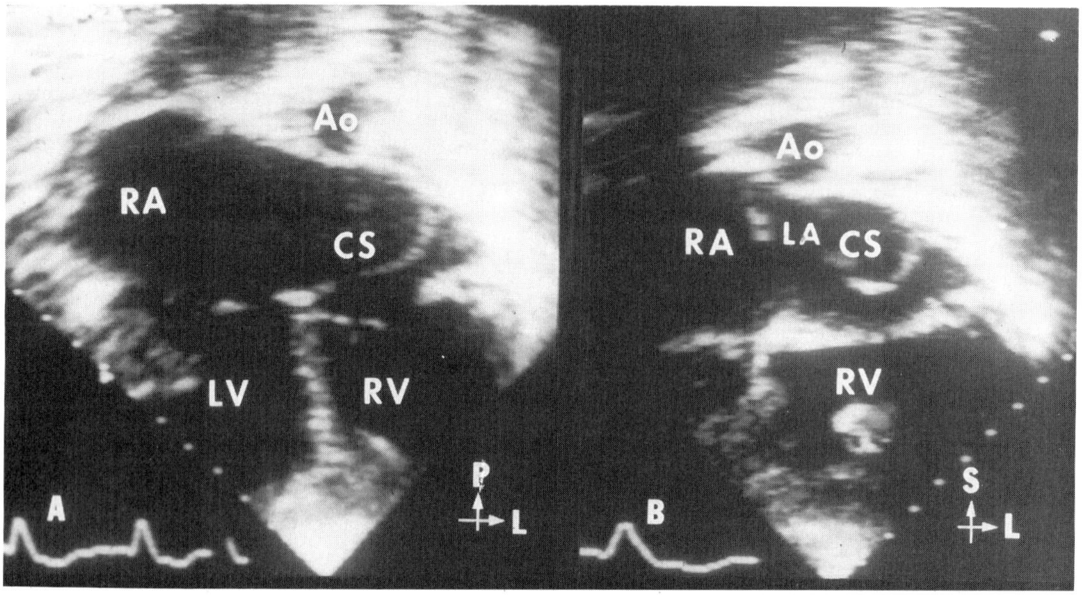

Fig 39-5 Apical two-dimensional images show (**A**) the orifice of the coronary sinus (*CS*) entering the right atrium (*RA*) and (**B**) a dilated coronary sinus coursing superiorly along the lateral wall of the left atrium (*LA*). These findings are consistent with a persistent left superior vena cava to the right atrium via the coronary sinus. Note also that the left atrium drains into the morphologic right ventricle (*RV*), consistent with atrioventricular discordance. *Ao*, aorta; *L*, left; *LV*, left ventricle; *P*, posterior; *S*, superior.

and with that an assessment of whether AV valve override or straddling is present.[10] The anatomic features distinguishing AV overriding from AV valve straddling are illustrated in Figure 39-8. As shown, AV valve override results from a malalignment of the atrial and ventricular septa, allowing the AV valve to override the ventricular septum. AV valve straddling, an abnormality of the AV valve tensor apparatus, consists of abnormal chordal attachments into the contralateral ventricle through a ventricular septal defect. Overriding and straddling may occur independently or may coexist in the same valve. From a surgical perspective, AV valve straddling is the more serious defect, since it may adversely affect the ability to adequately repair the ventricular septal defect.

Figure 39-8 also illustrates three types of AV valve straddling. Type A straddling consists of chordal attachments into the contralateral ventricle near the crest of the ventricular septum (within 1 cm of the crest of the septum). Type B straddling results when a chordal attachment inserts in the contralateral ventricle but along the ventricular septal surface, usually from a distinct papillary muscle attachment. Type C straddling occurs with chordal attachments inserting onto the free wall, usually well separated from the surface of the ventricular septum. The types of AV valve straddling also are related in severity and the ability to assess surgical repair without valve deformity or replacement. Thus, types A and B often may be successfully surgically repaired without valve replacement, whereas type C usually cannot. AV valve straddling may affect either valve or both simultaneously. Figure 39-9 shows echocardiographic examples of tricuspid and mitral valve straddling.

The degree of AV valve override or malalignment of the AV septum best defines the degree of commitment of the respective atrium to the ventricle. If the degree of AV valve override exceeds a 50% commitment to the contralateral ventricle because both AV valves are predominantly committed to one ventricle, this type of AV connection may be better defined as a univentricular AV connection. In univentricular AV connection, a large ventricular chamber functions as the single ventricular chamber providing flow to systemic and pulmonary circuits. The other ventricular chamber, with a diminutive or no AV connection, is then rudimentary in structure and function. Univentricular AV connections may be best categorized in a functional and anatomic format into double-inlet, single-inlet, and common-inlet forms (Figure 39-10). Such abnormalities of AV valve commitment are fully characterized by apical four-chamber and short-axis projections, which show the commitment of the AV valves to a main ventricular chamber in double-inlet ventricle, the absence of one AV connection in single-inlet univentricular connection, and a common AV valve receiving the inlet from both atria in common-inlet ventricle. All three forms of univentricular AV connection can be associated with hypoplasia of the contralateral ventricle. The hypoplastic ventricle or chamber may function as a rudimentary accessory chamber or as a

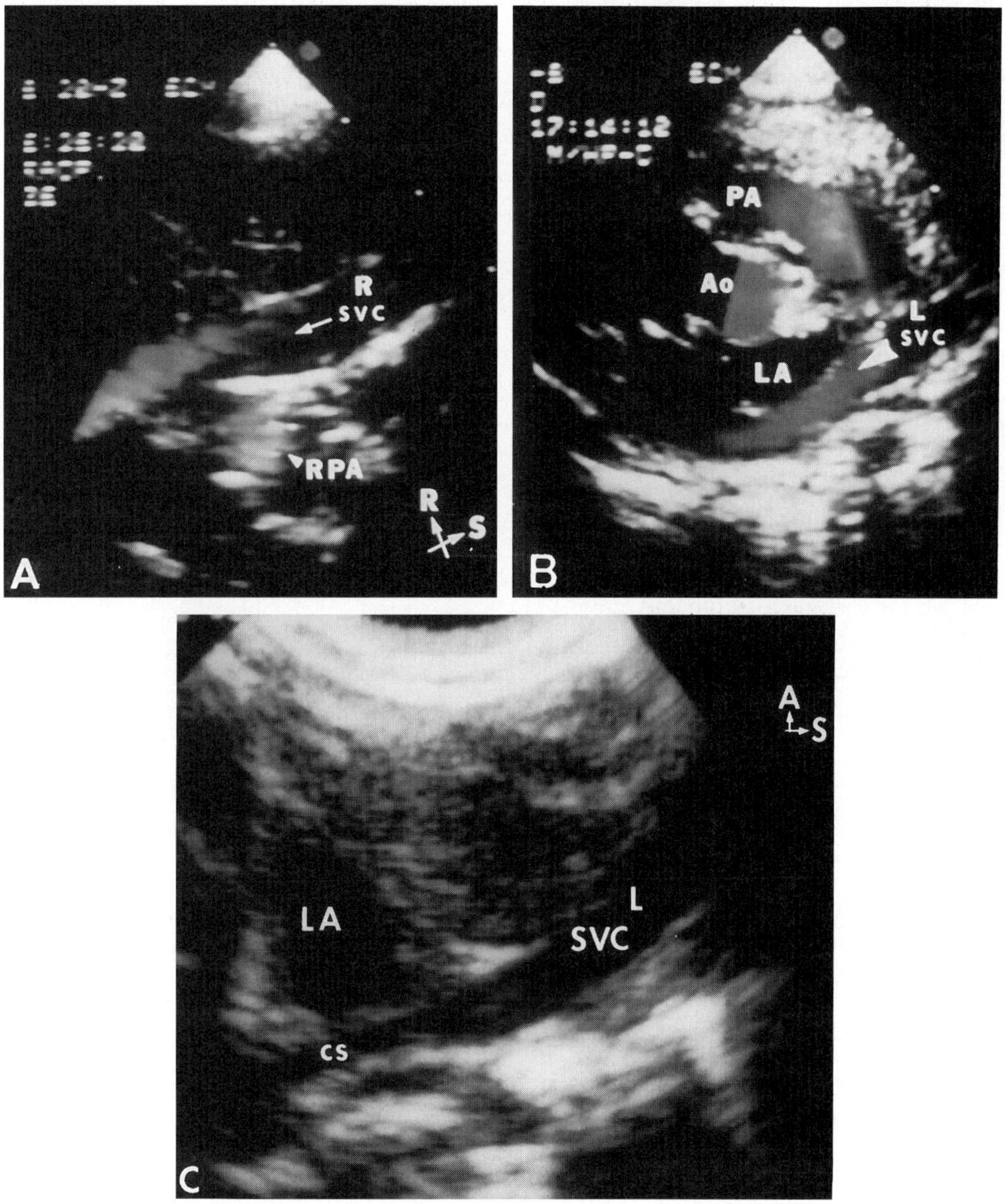

Fig 39-6 (see color plate after page 1512) High left and right parasternal scans demonstrating with color-flow imaging a right superior vena cava (*RSVC*) in **A** and a left superior vena cava (*LSVC*) in **B** and **C** draining via the coronary sinus (*cs*) to the right atrium. In **A**, the right pulmonary artery (*RPA*) is observed in short axis as it courses posterior to the RSVC. In **C**, the most superior portion of the LSVC is observed. In **B**, color flow shows the LSVC flow and its position anterior to the left pulmonary artery (*PA*). *A*, anterior; *Ao*, aorta; *L*, left; *LA*, left atrium; *R*, right; *S*, superior.

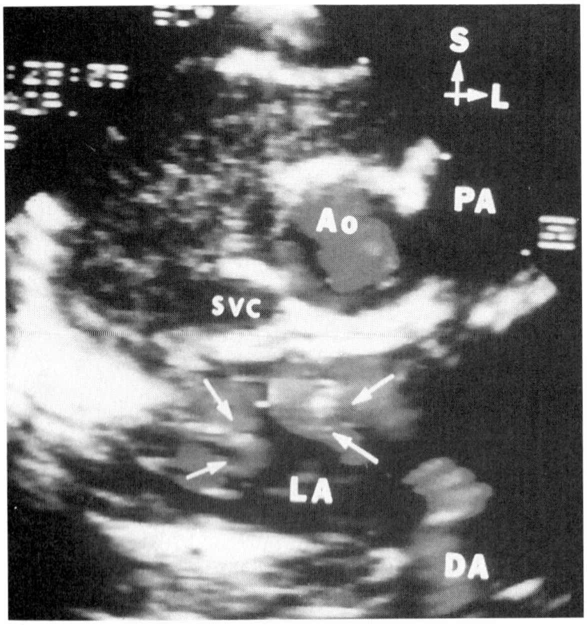

Fig 39-7 (see color plate after page 1512) High right parasternal short-axis scan in a neonate demonstrates with color-flow imaging normal pulmonary venous drainage to the left atrium (*LA*). All four pulmonary veins produce separate color-flow jets (*arrows*) entering the four quadrants of the left atrium. In addition, the superior vena cava (*SVC*) is noted in cross section to the right of the ascending aorta (*Ao*). *DA*, descending aorta; *L*, left; *PA*, pulmonary artery; *S*, superior.

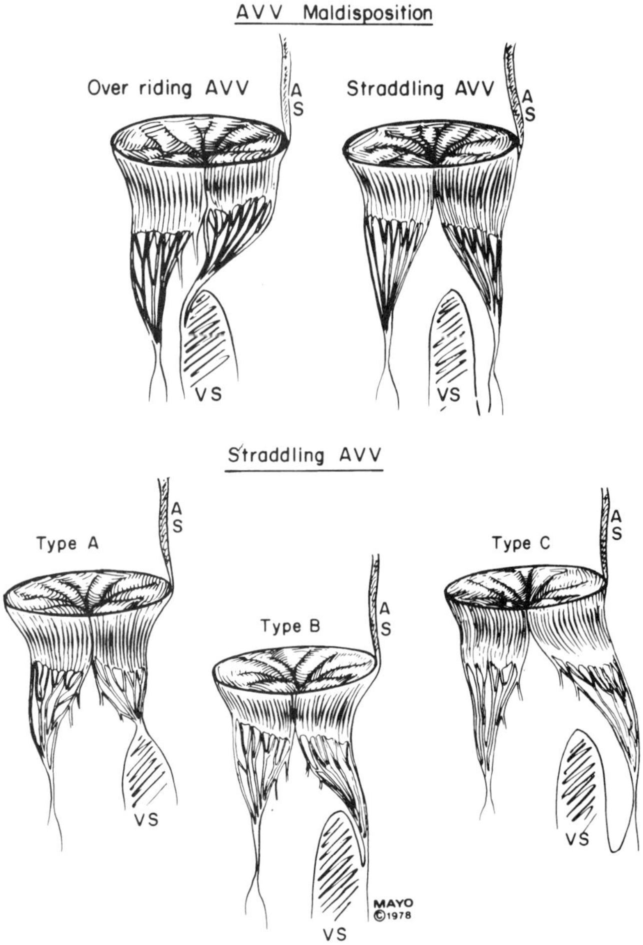

Fig 39-8 **Top**, anatomic features differentiating overriding from straddling atrioventricular valve (*AVV*). **Bottom**, three types of atrioventricular valve straddling. See text for detailed discussion. *AS*, atrial septum, *VS*, ventricular septum. (From Seward JB, Tajik AJ, Edwards WD, et al: *Two-Dimensional Echocardiographic Atlas*. Vol. 1: *Congenital Heart Disease*. New York, Springer-Verlag, 1987, p 206. By permission, Mayo Foundation.)

hypoplastic outlet chamber communicating to one or both great arteries. Figure 39-11 shows the typical echocardiographic examples of univentricular AV connections: double-inlet ventricle, in which a large main ventricular chamber receives the inflow of two separate and distinctly functioning AV valves; single-inlet ventricle, in which a single AV valve provides the only ventricular access into a large main ventricular chamber and the other AV valve is atretic; and common-inlet ventricle, in which both atria drain via a common AV valve into a large main ventricular chamber.

Ventricular situs and morphology

In the segmental approach for two-dimensional echocardiographic study of complex congenital heart disease, a determination of ventricular situs and morphology should be considered now. Included is an assessment of cardiac base-apex axis, basically determining the location of the apex of the heart and its projection to the left, as in levocardia, to the right, as in dextrocardia, or to the midline, as in mesocardia. In Figure 39-12, a subcostal four-chamber view, findings are consistent with atrial situs solitus with dextrocardia (isolated dextrocardia). The cardiac apex clearly points to the right, an indication of dextrocardia. In addition to gross cardiac position, this view reveals the relationship of the morphologic right ventricle to the left ventricle. Thus, some echocardiographic assessment of the anatomic features allowing a determination of ventricular morphology is required.

The most important and reliable method to determine ventricular morphology has been an assessment of the level of AV valve attachment to the ventricular septum. Thus, with an apical four-chamber view (see Fig 39-12), the point of attachment of the tricuspid valve (identifying a morphologic right ventricle) at the inlet ventricular septum is more inferior than the point of attachment of the mitral valve (identifying the morphologic left ventricle). The portion of the inlet septum separating the points of attachment of the tricuspid and mitral valves in this way can be clearly defined as the AV septum. In addition, other characteristics of AV valve and ventricular

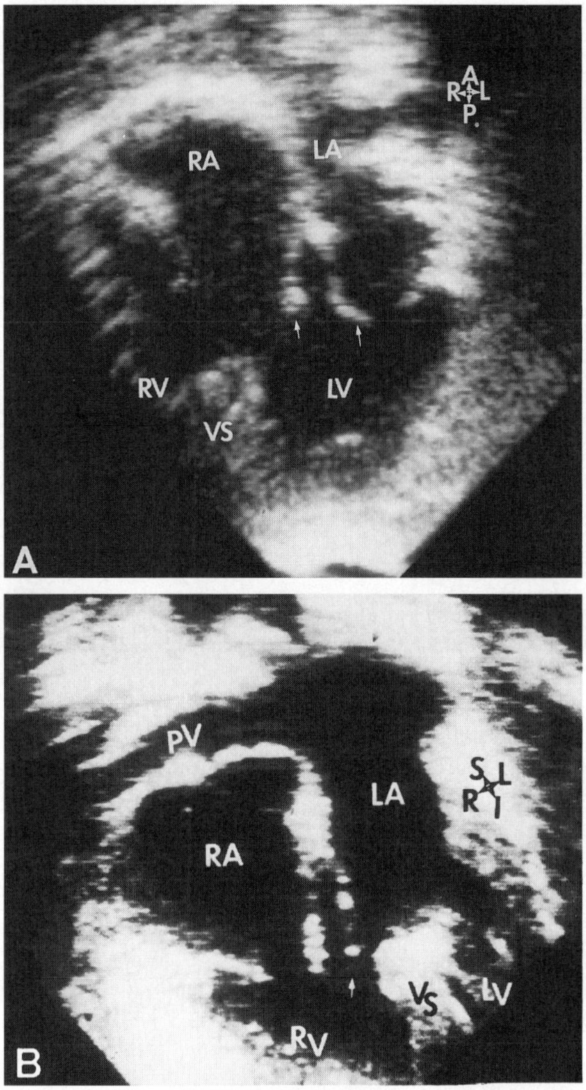

Fig 39-9 Apical four-chamber views of atrioventricular valve override and straddling. **A**, severe tricuspid valve override and type C tricuspid valve straddling. The exact point of tricuspid valve attachment in the left ventricle (*LV*) is not evident but attachment is to the left ventricular posterior wall. *Arrows* indicate mitral and tricuspid leaflets in the left ventricle. **B**, mitral valve override and type A straddling are demonstrated with a chordal attachment (*arrow*) to the right upper ventricular septum (*VS*). In both examples, the ventricular septal defect is large and involves the inlet septum. *A*, anterior; *I*, inferior; *L*, left; *LA*, left atrium; *P*, posterior; *PV*, pulmonary vein; *R*, right; *RA*, right atrium; *RV*, right ventricle; *S*, superior.

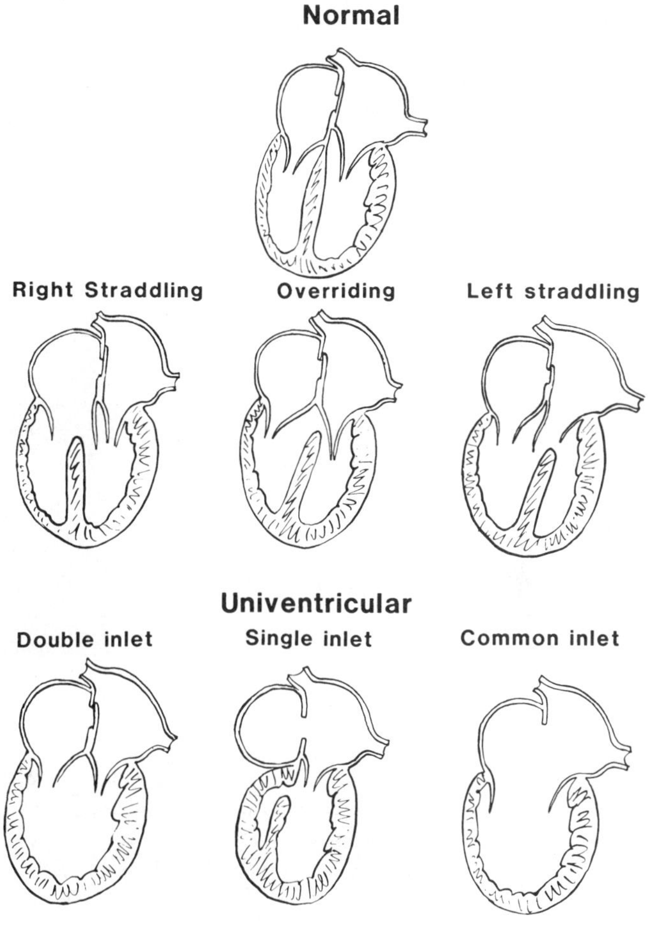

Fig 39-10 Normal, straddling, overriding, and univentricular atrioventricular connections. See text for detailed discussion. (From Seward JB, Tajik AJ, Edwards WD, et al: *Two-Dimensional Echocardiographic Atlas*. Vol. 1: *Congenital Heart Disease*. New York, Springer-Verlag, 1987, p 205. By permission, Mayo Foundation.)

morphology may be used, as listed in Table 39-1, including morphology and number of papillary muscles, and the presence or absence of conus separating the AV valves from the semilunar valves can provide an accurate echocardiographic assessment of ventricular morphology. Figure 39-13 also illustrates this section of the inlet ventricular septum and the relative points of attachment of the tricuspid and mitral valves. The right panel, depicting the basal portion of an apical long-axis view, shows the normal relationships of the tricuspid and aortic valves and their attachments at the membranous ventricular septum. The membranous septum is divided by the attachment of the tricuspid valve into an AV component separating the left ventricle from the right atrium and an interventricular component separating the left and right ventricles. This important anatomic landmark near the crux of the heart should be routinely inspected during the echocardiographic examination.

Great artery relations and extracardiac course

The final step in a prospective two-dimensional study of complex congenital heart disease is an assessment of the relation of the great arteries and their respective extracardiac courses. This requires determining not only the

Fig 39-11 Apical echocardiographic scans demonstrating three types of univentricular atrioventricular connection (double-inlet, single-inlet, and common-inlet). **Top**, double-inlet ventricle. Both right (*r*) and left (*l*) atrioventricular valves are predominantly committed to a large (main) ventricular chamber (*MVC*). **Bottom left**, single-inlet ventricle. A single left (*L*) atrioventricular valve is the only ventricular access emptying into a large MVC. The right atrioventricular valve (*arrowhead*) is atretic but does not seem committed to the same ventricular chamber. **Bottom right**, common-inlet ventricle. Both atria empty via a large common atrioventricular valve (*arrows*) into a common ventricular chamber. Complete morphologic details of the ventricles are not determined in these single scan planes. *AS*, atrial septum; *I*, inferior; *L*, left; *LA*, left atrium; *R*, right; *RA*, right atrium; *S*, superior. (From Seward JB, Tajik AJ, Edwards WD, et al: *Two-Dimensional Echocardiographic Atlas*. Vol. 1: *Congenital Heart Disease*. New York, Springer-Verlag, 1987, p 222. By permission, Mayo Foundation.)

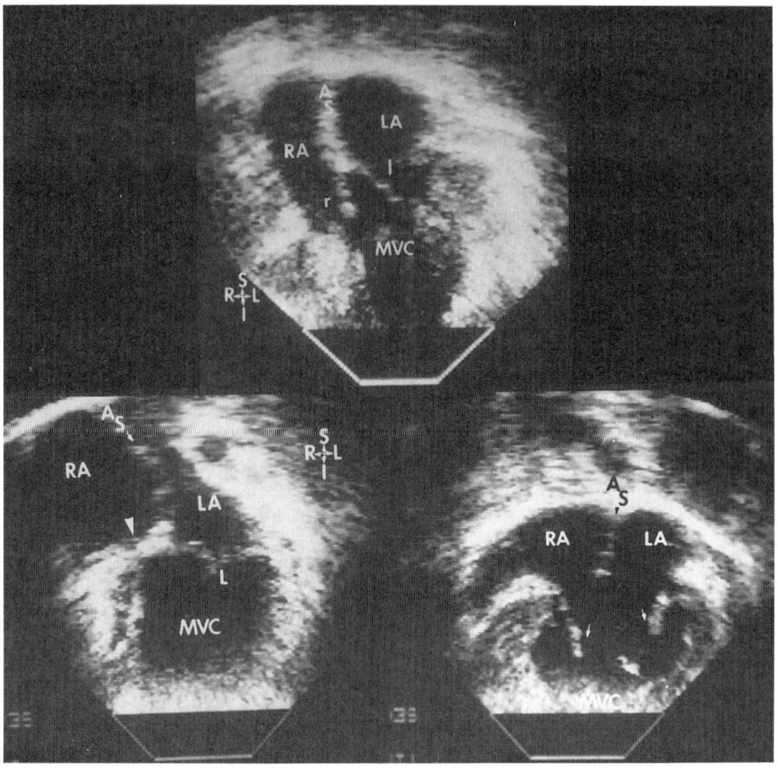

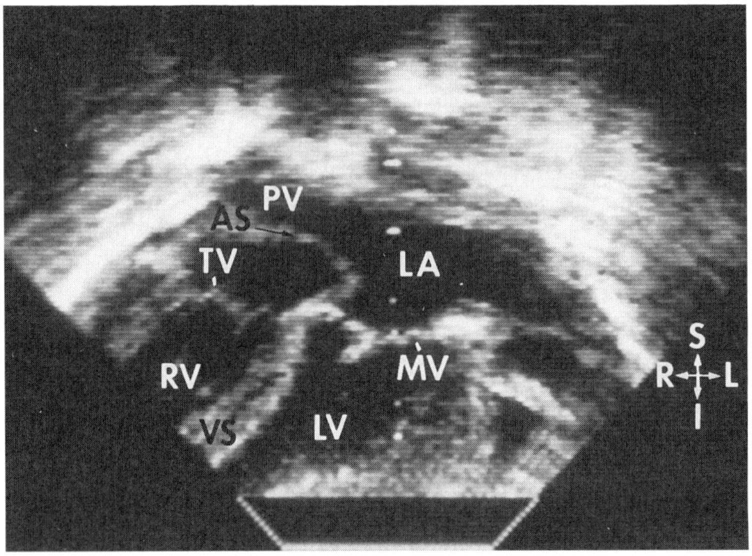

Fig 39-12 Subcostal four-chamber view in a 4-month-old patient with situs solitus and isolated dextrocardia. Pulmonary venous drainage enters the morphologic left atrium (*LA*) on the left. Ventricular morphology is identified by relative points of insertion of the atrioventricular valves. The morphologic tricuspid valve (*TV*) inserts at a lower position along the ventricular septum (*VS*) than the morphologic mitral valve (*MV*). Morphologic left ventricle (*LV*) also has an ellipsoid configuration and a smoother-walled appearance. The left atrium connects with the morphologic left ventricle, with atrioventricular concordance. The unusual curved appearance of the atrial septum (*AS*) is related partly to associated left juxtaposed atrial appendages and partly to isolated dextrocardia with the ventricular mass pulled to the right and the atria positioned normally. *I*, inferior; *L*, left; *PV*, pulmonary vein; *R*, right; *RV*, right ventricle; *S*, superior. (From Huhta JC, Hagler DJ, Seward JB, et al: Two-dimensional echocardiographic assessment of dextrocardia: a segmental approach. *Am J Cardiol* 50:1351-1360, 1982. By permission of Excerpta Medica.)

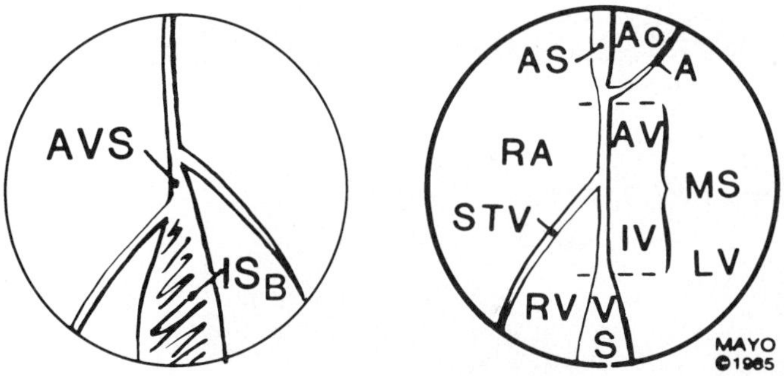

Fig 39-13 Anatomic details of the "crux" of the heart. **Left panel**, apical four-chamber view of basal inlet septum (IS_B) and atrioventricular septum (*AVS*). Note that the AVS is created with attachment of the right-sided tricuspid valve lower than that of the mitral valve on the left. This allows a potential communication between the left ventricle and the right atrium through the AVS. **Right panel**, membranous septum (*MS*) also has interventricular (*IV*) and atrioventricular (*AV*) components produced by attachment of the septal tricuspid valve (*STV*) leaflet on the septum inferior to the attachment of the aortic (*Ao*) valve leaflet (*A*) on the left side. This allows a potential communication from left ventricle (*LV*) to right atrium (*RA*) through the atrioventricular septum. *AS*, atrial septum; *RV*, right ventricle; *VS*, ventricular septum. (By permission, Mayo Foundation.)

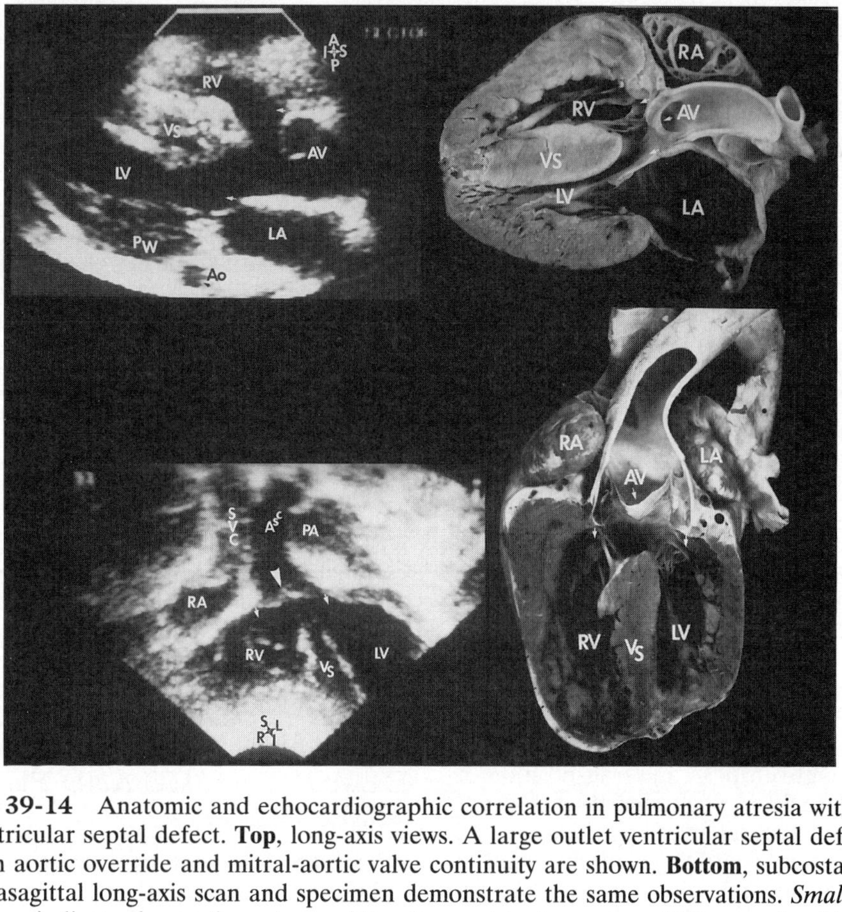

Fig 39-14 Anatomic and echocardiographic correlation in pulmonary atresia with ventricular septal defect. **Top**, long-axis views. A large outlet ventricular septal defect with aortic override and mitral-aortic valve continuity are shown. **Bottom**, subcostal parasagittal long-axis scan and specimen demonstrate the same observations. *Small arrows* indicate the aortic root overriding the ventricular septum (*VS*); *arrowhead* indicates the aortic valve (*AV*). *A*, anterior; *Ao*, aorta; *ASC*, ascending aorta; *I*, inferior; *L*, left; *LA*, left atrium; *LV*, left ventricle; *P*, posterior; *PA*, pulmonary artery; *PW*, posterior wall; *R*, right; *RA*, right atrium; *RV*, right ventricle; *S*, superior; *SVC*, superior vena cava.

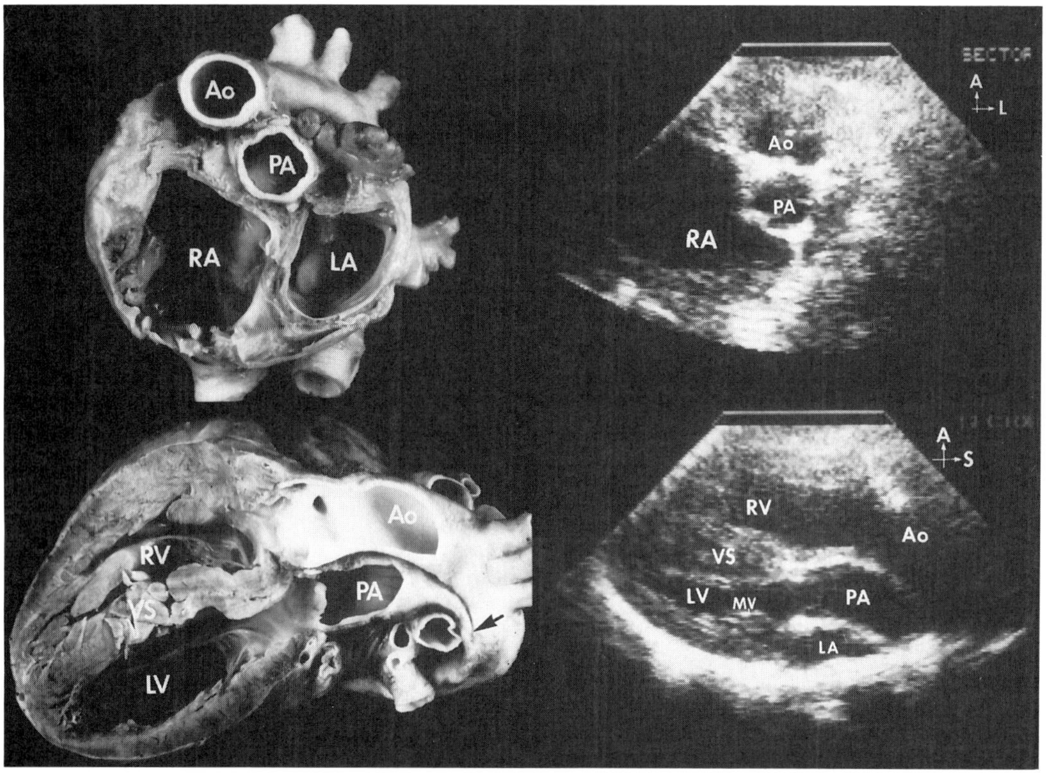

Fig 39-15 Echocardiographic-pathologic correlation of the anatomic features of ventriculoarterial discordance with AV concordance (complete transposition) of the great arteries. The long-axis sections (*bottom panels*) show the ventriculoarterial discordance with the posterior pulmonary artery (*PA*) coursing posteriorly to the lungs. In the *top panels*, the great artery relationships are shown, with the aorta (*Ao*) in a right anterior position relative to the pulmonary artery. *A*, anterior; *L*, left; *LA*, left atrium; *LV*, left ventricle; *MV*, mitral valve; *RA*, right atrium; *RV*, right ventricle; *S*, superior; *VS*, ventricular septum. (From Daskalopoulos DA, Edwards WD, Driscoll DJ, et al: Correlation of two-dimensional echocardiographic and autopsy findings in complete transposition of the great arteries. *J Am Coll Cardiol* 2:1151-1157, 1983. By permission of American College of Cardiology.)

position of one great artery relative to the other but also the respective relationships of the great arteries to the ventricles. The ventriculoarterial connections and the presence and degree of arterial override should be assessed. An accurate determination of these characteristics is particularly important for a precise depiction of a variety of conotruncal abnormalities, ranging from simple malalignment ventricular septal defect to tetralogy of Fallot, double-outlet right ventricle, and transposition of the great arteries. Figure 39-14 illustrates several of the features described for an assessment of ventriculoarterial connections and great artery-ventricle relation. As noted in Table 39-1, great artery identification is also part of this assessment, allowing recognition of the conotruncal abnormalities. Figure 39-15 illustrates anatomic and echocardiographic findings in complete transposition of the great arteries. The posterior course and bifurcation of the pulmonary artery provide reliable echocardiographic features for its identification. The final portion of the examination includes a careful assessment of the extracardiac course and branching patterns of the great arteries, identifying the situs of the aortic arch and the brachiocephalic branching. This type of examination also allows recognition of associated anomalies, such as patent ductus arteriosus and coarctation of the aorta.

HEMODYNAMIC AND FUNCTIONAL ASSESSMENT

As echocardiography has slowly replaced cardiac catheterization in the assessment of congenital heart disease, it has been imperative that echocardiography provide a reliable determination of the hemodynamic and functional cardiac abnormalities observed in congenital heart disease. Obviously, M-mode and two-dimensional echocardiography provide important information about myo-

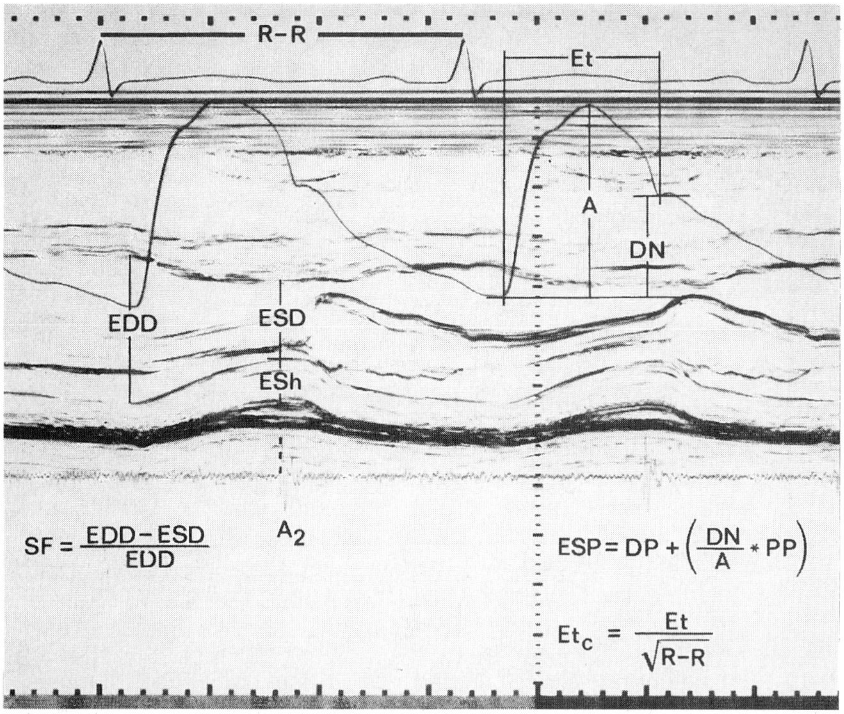

Fig 39-16 An M-mode echocardiogram of the left ventricle with simultaneously recorded electrocardiogram, carotid pulse tracing, and phonocardiogram used for calculating end-systolic wall stress and velocity of fiber shortening. The end-diastolic dimension (*EDD*) and end-systolic dimension (*ESD*) of the left ventricle and the end-systolic posterior wall thickness (*ESh*) are derived from the echocardiogram, with the largest cavity dimensions and the aortic component of the second heart sound (A_2) used to mark end-diastole and end-systole, respectively. The end-systolic pressure (*ESP*) is determined from the carotid pulse tracing by linear interpolation. The pulse tracing is calibrated from cuff blood pressure measurements. The ejection time (*Et*) is measured from the carotid pulse tracing. *A*, distance from nadir to apex of pulse tracing; *DN*, distance from nadir of pulse tracing to dicrotic arch; *DP*, diastolic pressure; Et_c, ejection time adjusted for heart rate; *PP*, pulse pressure; *R-R*, R-R interval; *SF*, shortening fraction. (From Sanders SP: Echocardiography. In *Fetal and Neonatal Cardiology*. Edited by WA Long. Philadelphia, WB Saunders Company, 1990, p 304. By permission.)

cardial systolic function along with reliable determinations of chamber, great artery, and myocardial wall dimensions.

In addition to the standard M-mode measurements of chamber dimensions and assessment of left ventricular systolic function predicted by shortening fraction (EDD − ESD/EDD) and ejection fraction ($EDD^2 - ESD^2/EDD^2$),[11] a variety of systolic measurements are available from echocardiographic examination. The rate-corrected velocity of circumferential fiber shortening (Vcf_c) or the average rate of change of the left ventricular circumference in diameters per second can be determined by standard M-mode measurements $Vcf_c = EDD - ESD/EDD \cdot Et_c$, in which EDD is end-diastolic diameter, ESD is end-systolic diameter, and Et_c is the ejection time divided by the square root of the R-R interval. As illustrated in Figure 39-16, the ET can be determined from simultaneously recorded carotid pulse tracings or directly from the aortic valve M-mode tracing. Use of the heart-rate-adjusted ejection time (Et_c) removes any effect of heart rate on the velocity of fiber shortening. The heart-rate-adjusted mean velocity of fiber shortening depends on afterload but is independent of preload.[12] Colan et al.[13] described the practical application of systolic measurements of velocity of fiber shortening and wall stress to congenital heart disease and normal pediatric values. Figure 39-17 compares rate-corrected velocity of fiber shortening with left ventricular end-systolic wall stress to provide a reliable predictor of the myocardial contractility that is not influenced by preload and reflects appropriate changes in afterload.

Two-dimensional echocardiography provides a reproducible mechanism for estimating ventricular volume. Estimates of left ventricular volume have proven the most

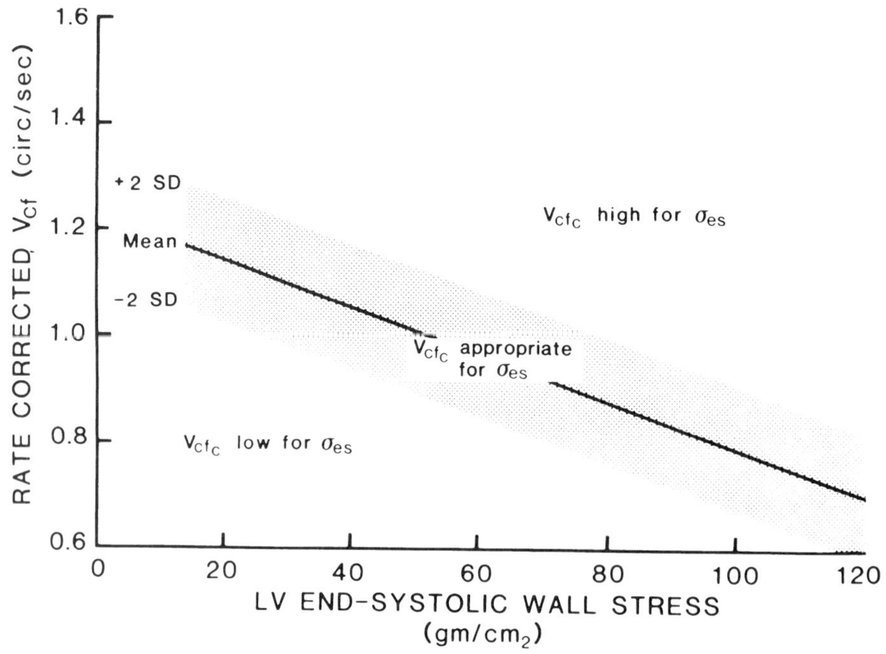

Fig 39-17 Relation of rate-corrected velocity of circumferential fiber shortening (V_{cfc}) to end-systolic wall stress (σ_{es}). Shaded area is the normal range with two standard deviations from the mean. Changes in contractility move the relation above or below the normal range. (From Colan SD, Borow KM, Neumann A: Left ventricular end-systolic wall stress-velocity of fiber shortening relation: a load-independent index of myocardial contractility. *J Am Coll Cardiol* 4:715-724, 1984. By permission of American College of Cardiology.)

reliable and easily obtained in patients with congenital cardiac defects.[14] Estimation of left ventricular volume is often used in evaluating volume overload conditions, determining left ventricular mass, assessing severity of ventricular hypoplasia, and approximating ejection fraction and left ventricular stroke volume. Volume estimates in which the biplane Simpson's rule algorithm is used with apical two- and four-chamber views, as described by Silverman et al.,[14] appear to provide the most reproducible estimates in patients with congenital heart disease. Although some underestimation of ventricular volumes may be encountered in direct angiographic comparisons, the reproducibility of this method allows a reliable mechanism for long-term patient follow-up. Because right ventricular abnormalities are a frequent concomitant of congenital heart disease, estimates of right ventricular volume are also of significant importance for the pediatric cardiologist. However, because of the irregular shape and heavy trabeculation in the right ventricle, volume estimates are more problematic than those for the left ventricle. Nevertheless, methods utilizing apical or subcostal four-chamber and long-axis views provide some mechanism for volume estimation.[15]

Doppler echocardiography and color-flow imaging

As described in chapter 5B, the application of Doppler techniques to echocardiography has provided a critical mechanism for noninvasive assessment of significant hemodynamic abnormalities.[16,17] The application of Doppler techniques in congenital heart disease has been essential in noninvasively predicting the severity of obstructive cardiac lesions. Pulsed- and continuous-wave Doppler techniques have provided the additional "physiologic" and "hemodynamic" data that, combined with careful and complete two-dimensional echocardiographic examination, enhance the prospect of managing critically ill neonates noninvasively and without confirmatory cardiac catheterization.[18] Figure 39-18 demonstrates typical continuous-wave Doppler echocardiographic findings in a 20-year-old patient with severe coarctation of the aorta. The hemodynamic data are consistent with a severe degree of obstruction and prolonged diastolic flow through the coarctation site. The systolic flow velocities suggest a coarctation peak systolic gradient of approximately 30 mm Hg.

Similarly, the noninvasive ability to accurately predict right ventricular and pulmonary artery systolic pressures is of great importance for congenital heart defects often affecting right ventricular hemodynamics. With Doppler interrogation of tricuspid valve insufficiency, one can predict the right ventricular-to-right atrial systolic pressure gradient,[19] and with the addition of an estimate of the right atrial mean pressure (usually assumed to be 10 mm Hg in infants and children unless there is evidence of right heart failure), one can predict the right ventricular systolic pressure. If Doppler interrogation of the pulmonary

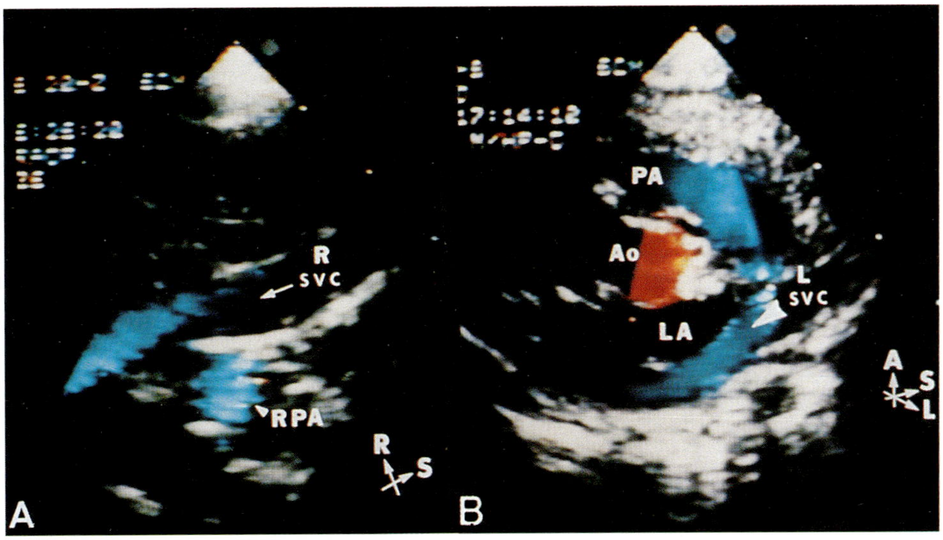

Fig 39-6 See page 1505

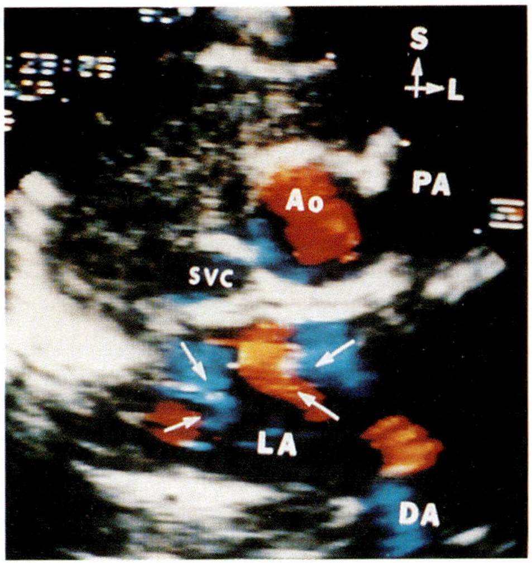

Fig 39-7 See page 1506

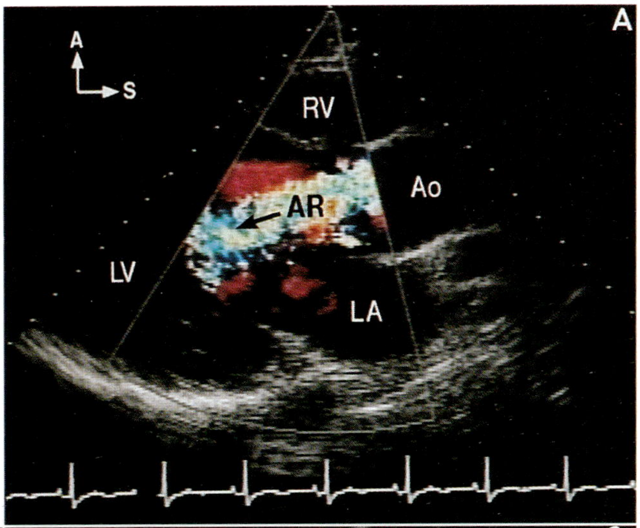

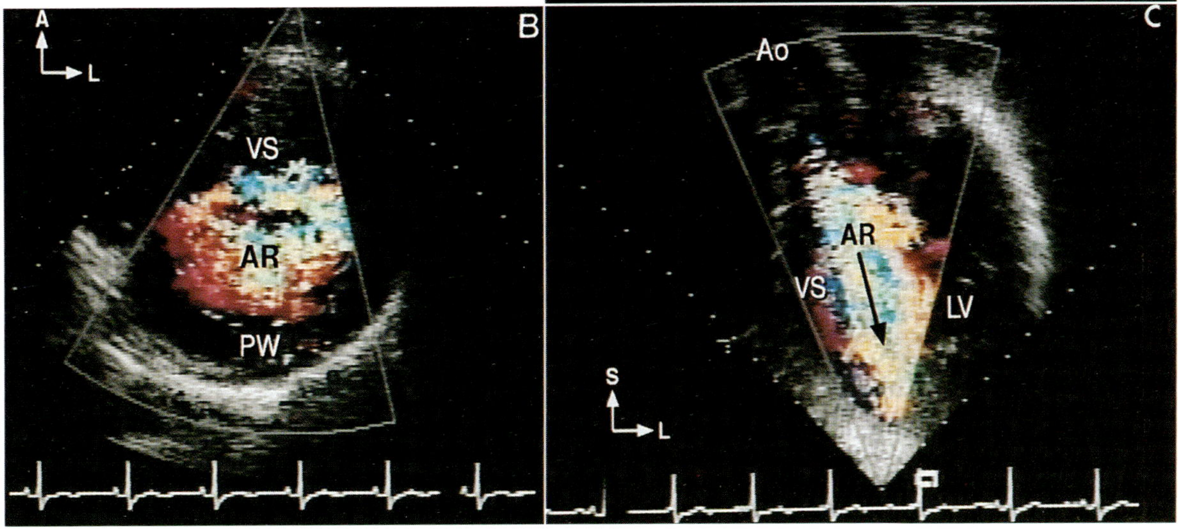

Fig 39-20 See page 1515

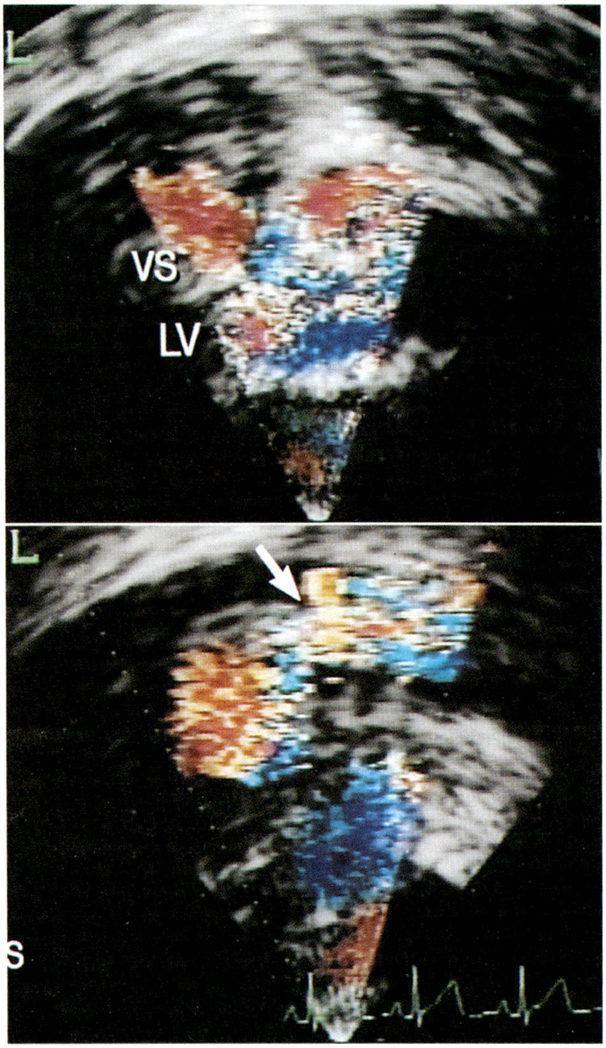

Fig 39-23 See page 1518

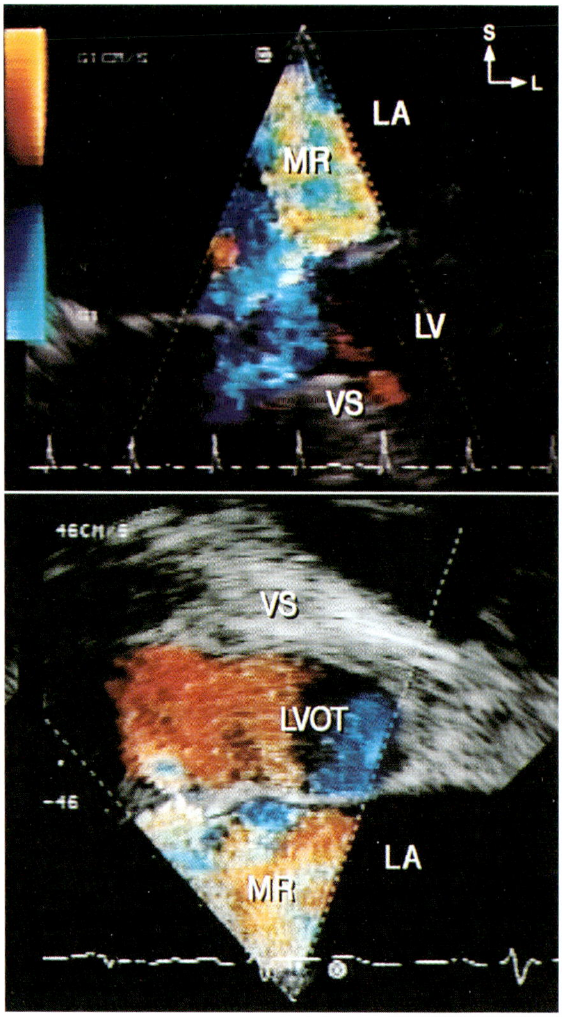

Fig 39-26 See page 1520

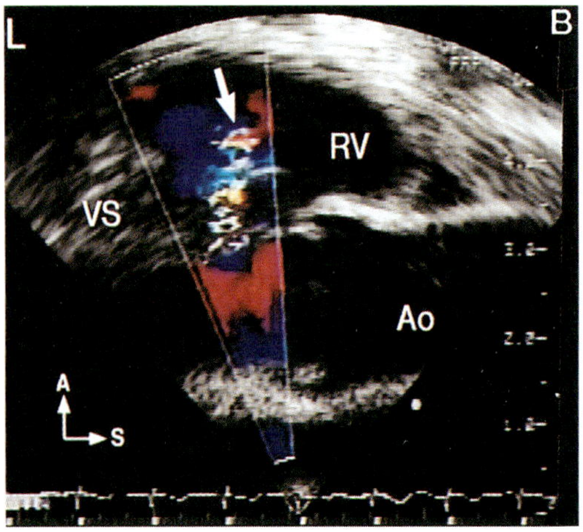

Fig 39-25 See page 1519

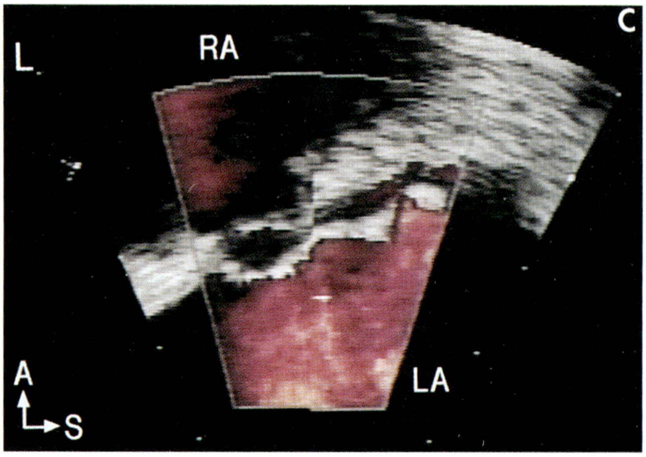

Fig 39-27 See page 1521

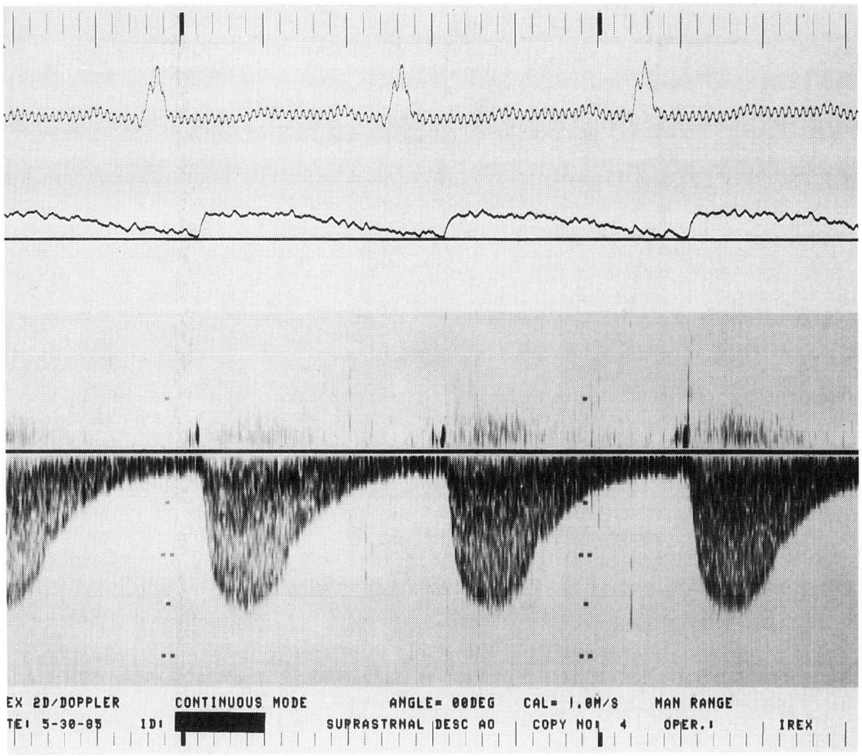

Fig 39-18 Continuous-wave Doppler interrogation of the descending aorta in a 20-year-old patient with coarctation of the aorta. Note double density in the recorded velocity tracing, indicating two separate velocities recorded. The lower velocity, of approximately 1.6 m/sec (V_1), originates from the proximal portion of the descending aorta, and the higher velocity, of 3.2 m/sec (V_2), is recorded through the coarctation site. Since the pressure gradient is predicted by $4(V_2^2 - V_1^2)$, one would estimate the coarctation gradient to be approximately 30 mm Hg.

outflow tract indicates no outflow tract gradient, one can assume that the right ventricular and the pulmonary artery pressures are nearly equal and therefore provide an estimate of the pulmonary artery systolic pressure. When a ventricular septal defect is present, continuous-wave Doppler echocardiography can also be used to predict the right ventricular systolic pressure with interrogation of the ventricular septal defect shunt jet. A low-velocity shunt jet of less than 2 m/sec predicts nearly equal right and left ventricular pressures. Higher velocity jets must be carefully assessed, with the recognition that earlier activation of the left ventricle may create a transient interventricular pressure gradient that is not reflected in the actual measured peak-to-peak ventricular pressures. High-velocity pansystolic flow greater than 4 m/sec usually indicates a significant left-to-right ventricular pressure gradient.

Figure 39-19 shows Doppler and catheter pressure tracings obtained simultaneously during cardiac catheterization. As observed in similar studies of aortic stenosis and tricuspid regurgitation, the peak Doppler velocities accurately predict the maximal instantaneous gradient between the right ventricle and the left ventricle, and the mean Doppler velocity accurately predicts the mean catheter-measured gradients. The catheter-measured peak-to-peak gradients are therefore in between these two but not accurately reflected by either. As observed in this example, with very high pansystolic velocities recorded, the measured peak-to-peak gradient is actually relatively close to the maximal gradient and could be approximated by the maximal Doppler velocity.

The application of color-flow imaging to congenital heart disease has had a profound effect on noninvasive evaluation and clinical management. One of the earlier recognized benefits of Doppler color-flow imaging is the remarkable rapidity with which correct diagnosis, recognition of anatomy, and detection of associated anomalies can be attained. Color-flow imaging has frequently predicted unsuspected septal defects and valvular regurgitation precisely and rapidly. In Figure 39-20, a composite of longitudinal, short-axis, and apical long-axis scans, severe aortic regurgitation is observed with color-flow imaging. Recent efforts have attempted to determine regurgitant and shunt volumes by use of prevolume isovelocity spectral analysis.[20] Additionally, color-flow imaging has greatly improved our ability to characterize complex anatomic details of extracardiac structures and connections. Recent technology providing high-resolution two-dimensional imaging (7.0 MHz) with added digital expansion (ZOOM) in combination with dual-frequency

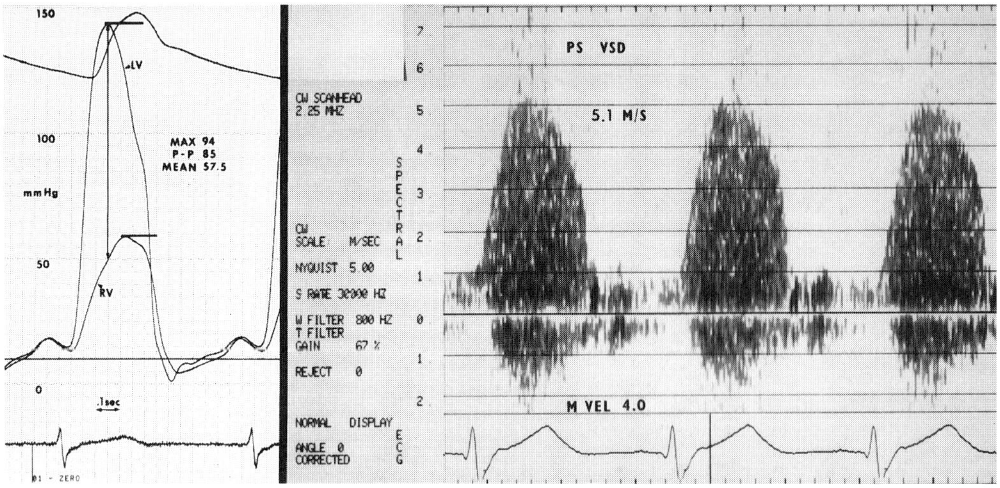

Fig 39-19 Simultaneously recorded right and left ventricular pressures and continuous-wave Doppler interrogation in a patient with a restrictive ventricular septal defect (*VSD*). Note that VSD Doppler velocity is pansystolic and exceeds 5.0 m/sec. The Doppler predicted maximum VSD gradient is approximately 100 mm Hg, whereas the catheter-measured maximum VSD gradient is 94 mm Hg. The difference between the simultaneous catheter-measured peak systolic right and left ventricular pressures is slightly less at 85 mm Hg.

(5.0 MHz) Doppler color-flow imaging has substantially improved noninvasive management of infants with a variety of complex congenital heart disease. Figures 39-6 and 39-7 demonstrate the application of high-resolution imaging and color-flow Doppler imaging to provide detailed information of cross-sectional intracardiac and extracardiac structural relationships and flow phenomena occurring within those structures.[21,22] Without the availability of color-flow imaging, clear recognition and precise demonstration of anatomic relations and connections would not be possible.

Stress echocardiography

Current applications of stress echocardiography, including bicycle and treadmill exercise echocardiography and dobutamine stress echocardiography, are described in chapter 5C. Its application to patients with congenital heart disease has in recent years gained greatest attention primarily for assessment and follow-up in patients undergoing corrective surgical procedures, such as the arterial switch procedure, modified Fontan procedure, and coronary reimplantation for aortic root disease or anomalous coronary origin.[23]

Combined application of continuous-wave Doppler imaging with stress echocardiography also has become particularly important in echocardiographic assessment of congenital obstructive cardiac lesions. With these techniques, additional hemodynamic data can be provided to improve noninvasive assessment of the severity of obstructive lesions. As noted in chapter 5B, the Doppler-derived mean gradient has been the most representative measure of the degree of obstruction across a stenotic valve and has correlated best with simultaneously recorded catheter gradients. However, resting valve gradients may not adequately reflect the hemodynamic changes that occur in children and young adults during strenuous exercise. Thus, application of continuous-wave Doppler echocardiography during stress testing can provide this additional information, predicting changes in maximal and mean gradients during exercise.[24] In our laboratory, supine bicycle exercise combined with continuous-wave Doppler examination has provided the best mechanism for stress-Doppler testing. In patients too young to adequately exercise on the bicycle, simple running in place or jumping exercise may provide another mechanism for stress-Doppler testing.

FETAL ECHOCARDIOGRAPHY

Routine use of echocardiography in fetal diagnosis of congenital heart disease has an ever-increasing role in current pediatric cardiology practice. As a screening procedure, it provides an ideal mechanism for early detection and management of patients with congenital heart disease. Numerous previous studies documented the utility of fetal echocardiography for accurate diagnosis and patient management.[25-30] Unlike postnatal echocardiography, the fetal echocardiogram often "stands alone" as the sole diagnostic tool available for fetal heart disease.

Although a number of clinical applications of fetal echocardiography are evident from previous reports, including management of fetal cardiac arrhythmias, screening of diabetic or high-risk pregnancies, screening

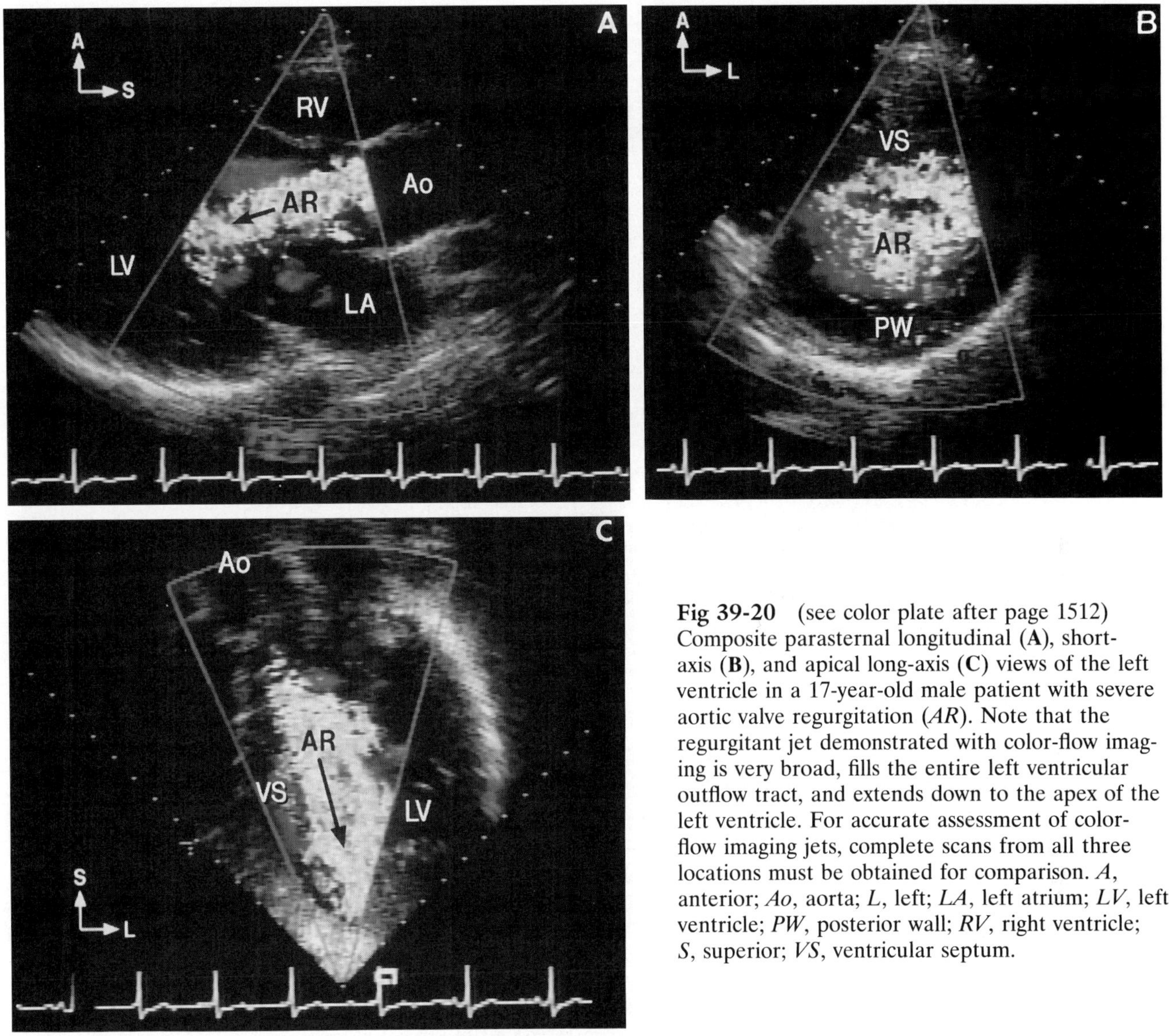

Fig 39-20 (see color plate after page 1512) Composite parasternal longitudinal (**A**), short-axis (**B**), and apical long-axis (**C**) views of the left ventricle in a 17-year-old male patient with severe aortic valve regurgitation (*AR*). Note that the regurgitant jet demonstrated with color-flow imaging is very broad, fills the entire left ventricular outflow tract, and extends down to the apex of the left ventricle. For accurate assessment of color-flow imaging jets, complete scans from all three locations must be obtained for comparison. *A*, anterior; *Ao*, aorta; *L*, left; *LA*, left atrium; *LV*, left ventricle; *PW*, posterior wall; *RV*, right ventricle; *S*, superior; *VS*, ventricular septum.

for known toxic drug use (phenytoin, lithium), and screening of siblings or children of patients with congenital heart disease, the most significant role and clinical benefit of fetal echocardiography have been in evaluation of fetuses recognized by routine fetal ultrasound screening to have significant extracardiac defects or an abnormal cardiac "four-chamber view." Earlier fears that fetal recognition of congenital heart disease would simply result in early termination of such fetuses[31,32] have not been realized, since obstetricians, pediatric cardiologists, and cardiac surgeons have learned through fetal echocardiography to recognize those fetuses with cardiac lesions that can be effectively managed and treated postnatally. To date, therapeutic interventions guided by fetal echocardiography (e.g., balloon valvotomy) have experienced rather disappointing results. However, the future development of this application of fetal echocardiography will warrant careful observation.

The fetal echocardiographic examination itself requires substantial expertise for recognition of congenital heart disease as well as considerable skill at rapid mental reconstruction of three-dimensional images. Little has been published to date on a reliable approach for reproducible demonstration of fetal visceral, atrial, and cardiac situs. However, application of the physical principles of ultrasound and a review of the current standards for electronic manipulation of ultrasound images may provide important clues for reliable fetal examination. Figure 39-21 schematically illustrates such a review. The initial instrument setup requires that the "imaging electronics" be set in the standard mode, so that the image obtained from the "notched" half of the ultrasound probe is electronically placed on the right half of the video screen. It is important at this point that no electronic left-to-right image switching or reversal be made. A long-axis view of the entire fetus is first obtained. With the

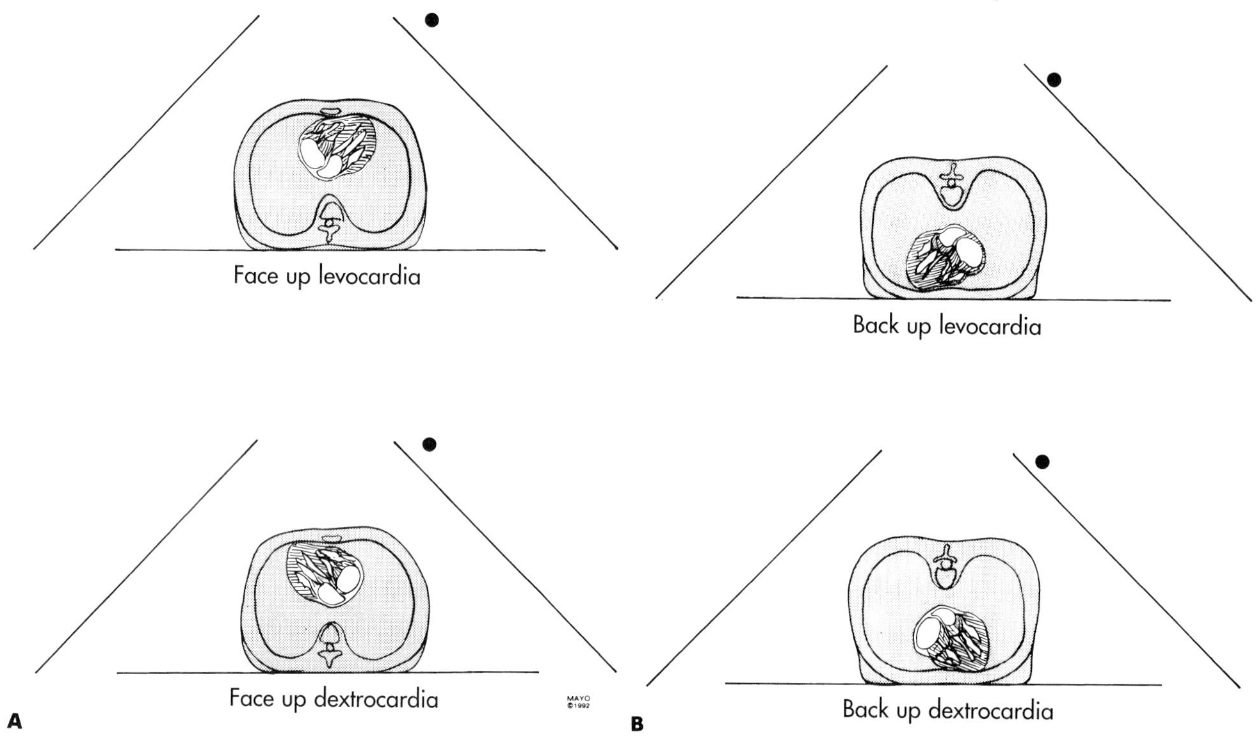

Fig 39-21 Schematic video image orientation for echocardiographic study of fetuses assuming supine (**A**) or prone (**B**) fetal positions as described. Illustrated are the expected cardiac axes for levocardia and dextrocardia. (From Cordes TM, O'Leary PW, Seward JB, et al: Distinguishing right from left: a standardized technique for fetal echocardiography. *J Am Soc Echocardiogr* 7:47-53, 1994. **A**, by permission, Mayo Foundation. **B**, by permission of American Society of Echocardiography.)

ultrasound probe notch pointing to the fetal head, the image of the fetal head is oriented to the examiner's right side of the video screen. Since the initial transducer orientation is guided by the fetal head rather than the maternal position, the superior-inferior axis orientation of the fetus does not affect the orientation of the video images obtained. When the ultrasound probe is rotated 90°, a standard short-axis (cross-sectional) view of the fetus is obtained. In this orientation, short-axis scans through the fetal chest and abdomen can allow clear recognition of the right and left sides of the fetus. The right-to-left orientation of the fetal image then depends only on the anterior-posterior fetal orientation to the ultrasound probe. For example, if the fetal face is up and is located in the anterior, or near, field of the imaging transducer, the fetal video image is oriented so that the left side of the fetus is seen on the viewer's right side of the video screen. If the fetal back is up and is located in the anterior, or near, field of the imaging transducer, the fetal video image is oriented so that the right side of the fetus is placed on the right side of the video screen. Once the anatomic right and left sides of the fetus are recognized, appropriateness of visceral and cardiac situs can be echocardiographically determined. Figure 39-21 illustrates the two examples of fetal orientation and also shows the expected observations in levocardia and dextrocardia, and in Figure 39-22, the actual fetal ultrasound examination demonstrates examples of levocardia and dextrocardia.

TRANSESOPHAGEAL ECHOCARDIOGRAPHY

The application of transesophageal echocardiography (TEE) to congenital heart disease has been relatively slow and in many instances limited to intraoperative evaluation.[32-34] The primary limitations have been the general unavailability of suitable equipment for pediatric use and the more frequent need for anesthesia support for use in children. The technical development of small, high-resolution probes suitable for use in neonates and children has been disappointingly slow. The application of biplane and multiplane technology for TEE in adult heart disease has clearly indicated the superiority of these imaging methods and systems and demonstrates that a multiplanar approach is best for satisfactory TEE evaluation of congenital heart disease. When similar high-quality miniaturized probes become available for neonates weighing 3.0 kg, TEE will assume the important role in clinical diagnosis of congenital heart disease that it has

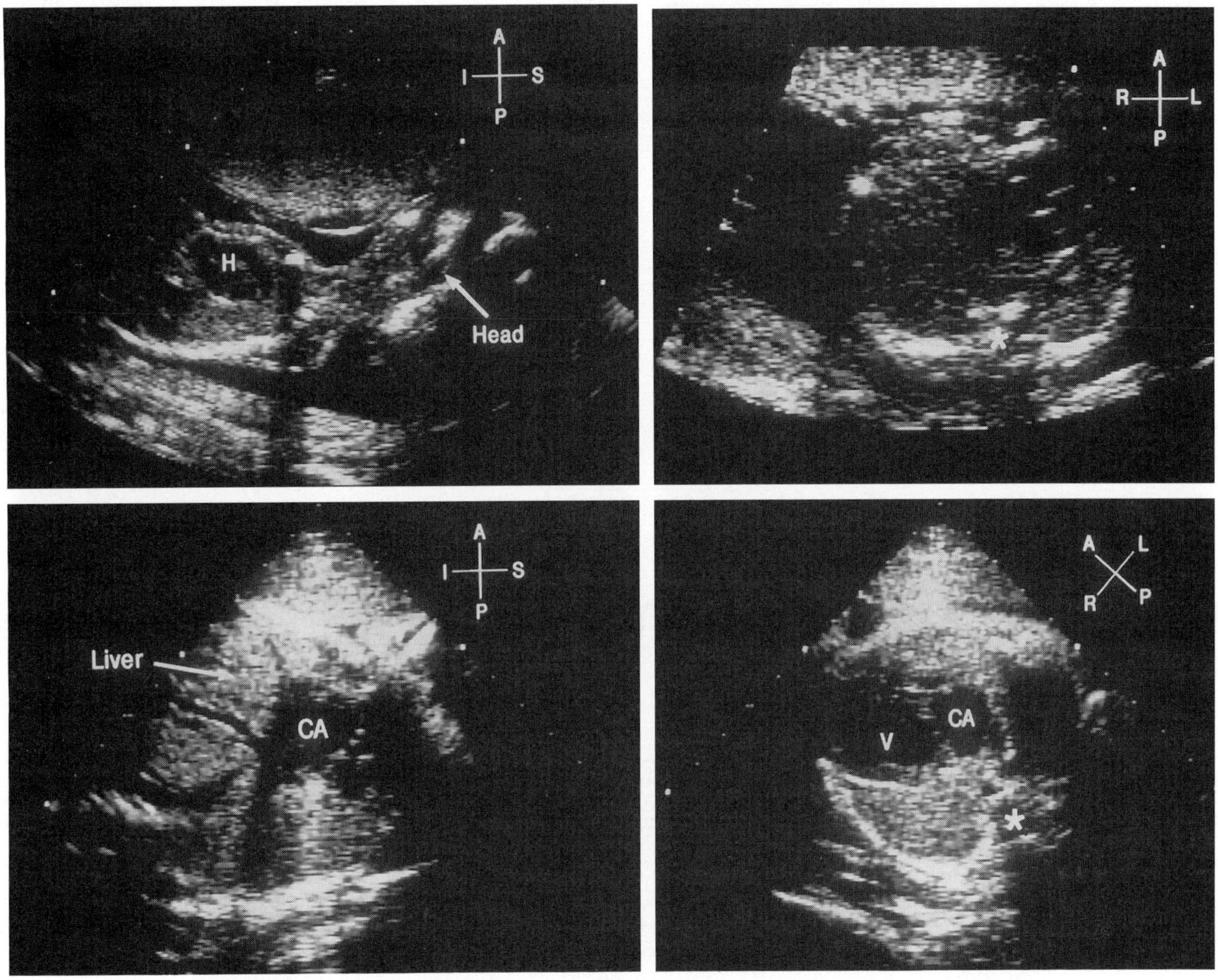

Fig 39-22 Fetal echocardiographic study with long- and short-axis scans demonstrates normal visceral and cardiac situs (**top left and right**) and situs ambiguus with dextrocardia (**bottom left and right**). *A*, anterior; *CA*, common atrium; *H*, heart; *I*, inferior; *L*, left; *P*, posterior; *R*, right; *S*, superior; *V*, ventricle. (**Bottom right**, from Cordes TM, O'Leary PW, Seward JB, et al: Distinguishing right from left: a standardized technique for fetal echocardiography. *J Am Soc Echocardiogr* 7:47-53, 1994. By permission of American Society of Echocardiography.)

achieved for acquired cardiac disease. It is hoped that this will be relatively soon. Current technology provides a 5-MHz biplane probe with 24 elements per plane on an endoscopic shaft 7 mm in diameter that allows two-dimensional and color-flow imaging. Although this has substantially improved image quality and diagnostic accuracy, image resolution, Doppler and color-flow capability, and probe maneuverability are inadequate. A 7.5-MHz multiplanar, high-resolution (48 to 64 elements) probe capable of pulsed-wave, continuous-wave, and color-flow Doppler study and incorporated on the 7-mm shaft would have the imaging capability required for neonates and infants.

In general, neonatal echocardiography provides excellent transthoracic images. However, the usefulness of TEE in providing further important details of cardiac and extracardiac anatomy, in improving cardiac resolution in older children, and in being easily accessible for cardiac diagnosis under difficult conditions, such as in the operating room or postoperatively in the intensive care unit, clearly indicates the importance of this imaging modality for congenital heart disease. In older children with congenital heart disease and in many patients after repair of congenital heart disease, transthoracic images may be of poor quality, so that adequate echocardiographic evaluation is impossible. Preoperative TEE examination may sufficiently improve anatomic resolution so that further invasive studies are unnecessary. Patients with complex cardiac and extracardiac connections after such procedures as the Mustard and modified Fontan seem particularly to benefit from TEE study.

Resolution of the detailed anatomy of cardiac structures and demonstration of flow phenomena with color-flow imaging are particularly important features of TEE, providing improved hemodynamic and clinical evaluation.[35,36] In Figure 39-23, longitudinal scan plane images in a 2-year-old patient with tetralogy of Fallot reveal a somewhat unusual feature of partial obstruction of the ventricular septal defect by the septal leaflet of the tricuspid valve. Color-flow imaging shows that turbulent flow of the right-to-left shunt accelerates at the site of the ventricular septal defect. The longitudinal scan also clearly demonstrates the infundibular obstruction in this patient. For comparison, the longitudinal scan plane in Figure 39-24 produces a more typical long-axis view in an older patient with tetralogy of Fallot. In Figure 39-25, longitudinal plane images in a 5-year-old patient with a supracristal ventricular septal defect and a prolapsed aortic valve leaflet, color-flow imaging clearly demonstrates the left-to-right shunt and its disturbing effect on the aortic valve leaflet. As evident in these views, longitudinal scan plane images are extremely useful.

The information available from multiple image planes is particularly important for rapid and comprehensive collation of complex congenital cardiac defects. Figure 39-26 demonstrates horizontal and longitudinal scan plane images in patients with AV septal defects. Because of the relative proximity of the ultrasound probe to the posterior aspect of the heart, resolution of the crux of the heart, which is primarily affected by this cardiac defect, is striking. This allows improved resolution of details of small ventricular septal defects, as observed in interme-

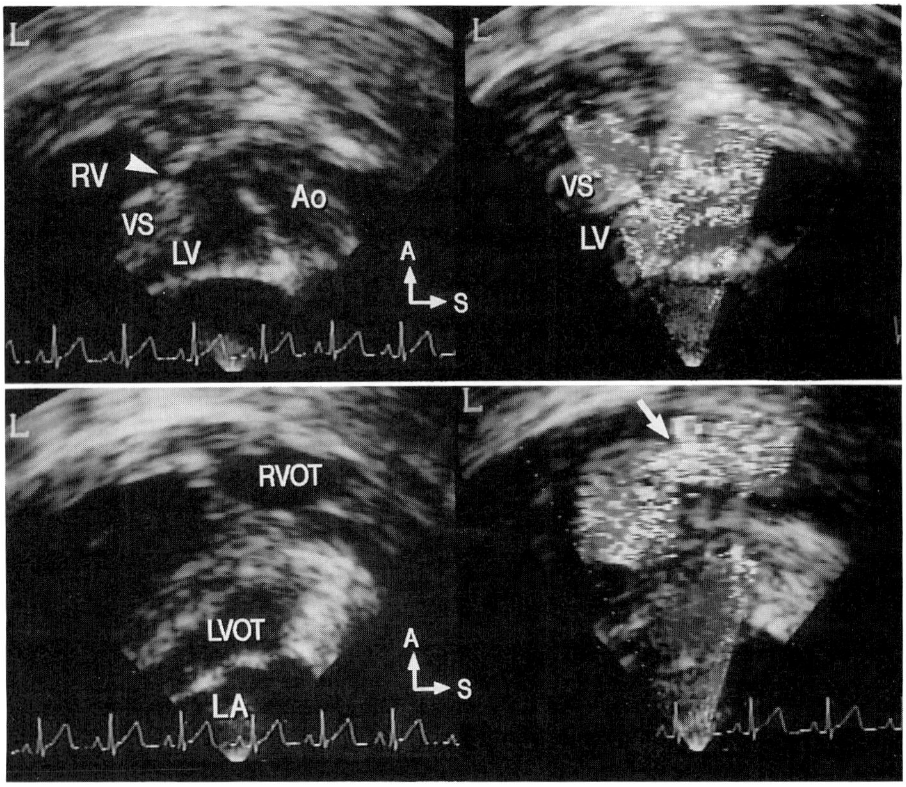

Fig 39-23 Longitudinal (*L*) scan transesophageal echocardiographic images in a 2-year-old patient with tetralogy of Fallot. **Top**, although the ventricular septal defect was moderately large, allowing aortic override typical of tetralogy, the longitudinal plane images demonstrated that the defect was partially obstructed by the tricuspid septal leaflet, resulting in a functionally restrictive defect (*arrowhead*). The color-flow image (see color plate after page 1512). illustrates the turbulence of the right-to-left shunt at the site of the defect, with aliased flow. **Bottom**, longitudinal plane images in the same patient show obstruction of the infundibular right ventricular outflow tract (*RVOT*) typical of that in tetralogy of Fallot. Color flow (see color plate after page 1512) demonstrates systolic turbulence and aliasing at the outflow narrowing (*arrow*). *A*, anterior; *Ao*, aorta; *LA*, left atrium; *LV*, left ventricle; *LVOT*, left ventricular outflow tract; *RV*, right ventricle; *S*, superior; *VS*, ventricular septum.

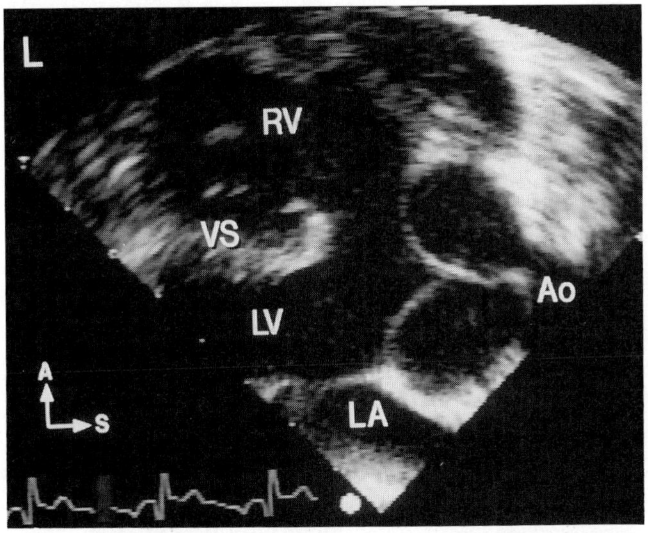

Fig 39-24 Typical longitudinal (*L*) scan transesophageal echocardiographic image, long-axis view, in a 56-year-old patient with tetralogy of Fallot. The high-resolution image is nearly identically oriented to a typical parasternal long-axis view. Note the large outlet ventricular septal defect with aortic override. *A*, anterior; *Ao*, aorta; *LA*, left atrium; *LV*, left ventricle; *RV*, right ventricle; *S*, superior; *VS*, ventricular septum.

diate forms of AV septal defects, and improved recognition of AV valve abnormalities and regurgitant jets with color-flow imaging.

TEE also has a significant role in the successful deployment of new interventional catheterization devices, such as the atrial septal and ductal devices.[37] Figure 39-27 shows images from longitudinal scan planes recorded during successful placement of an atrial septal closure device for patent foramen ovale and right-to-left shunting. After the device was placed, no further evidence of right-to-left intracardiac shunt appeared with color-flow imaging and contrast echocardiography. As better and smaller TEE probes become available for pediatric use, practical application of TEE in the catheterization laboratory may also include routine use to monitor other therapeutic procedures, such as balloon atrial septostomy and balloon valvotomy.

INTRAOPERATIVE ECHOCARDIOGRAPHY

Early experience with intraoperative echocardiography demonstrated that epicardial imaging provided important information on the results of surgical repair of congenital cardiac defects.[34,38-41] Although our initial study of epicardial imaging demonstrated that significant residual defect could be recognized postoperatively, we also noted several technical difficulties with this intraoperative ap-

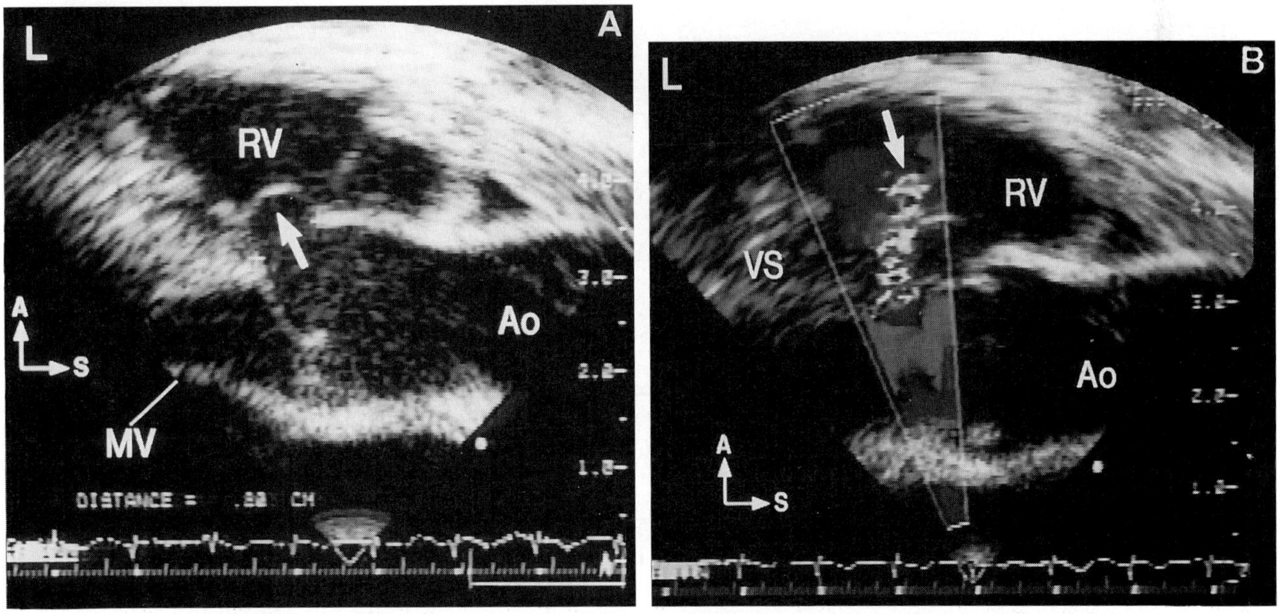

Fig 39-25 Longitudinal (*L*) plane transesophageal echocardiographic images in 5-year-old patient with a supracristal ventricular septal defect. **A**, the *crosshairs* indicate the size of the defect, and the *arrow* points to the right coronary cusp prolapsing through the defect. **B,** with color-flow imaging (see color plate after page 1512), the systolic left-to-right shunt through the defect is observed (*arrow*). The jet appears to distort the prolapsing aortic leaflet. *A*, anterior; *Ao*, aorta; *MV*, mitral valve; *RV*, right ventricle; *S*, superior; *VS*, ventricular septum.

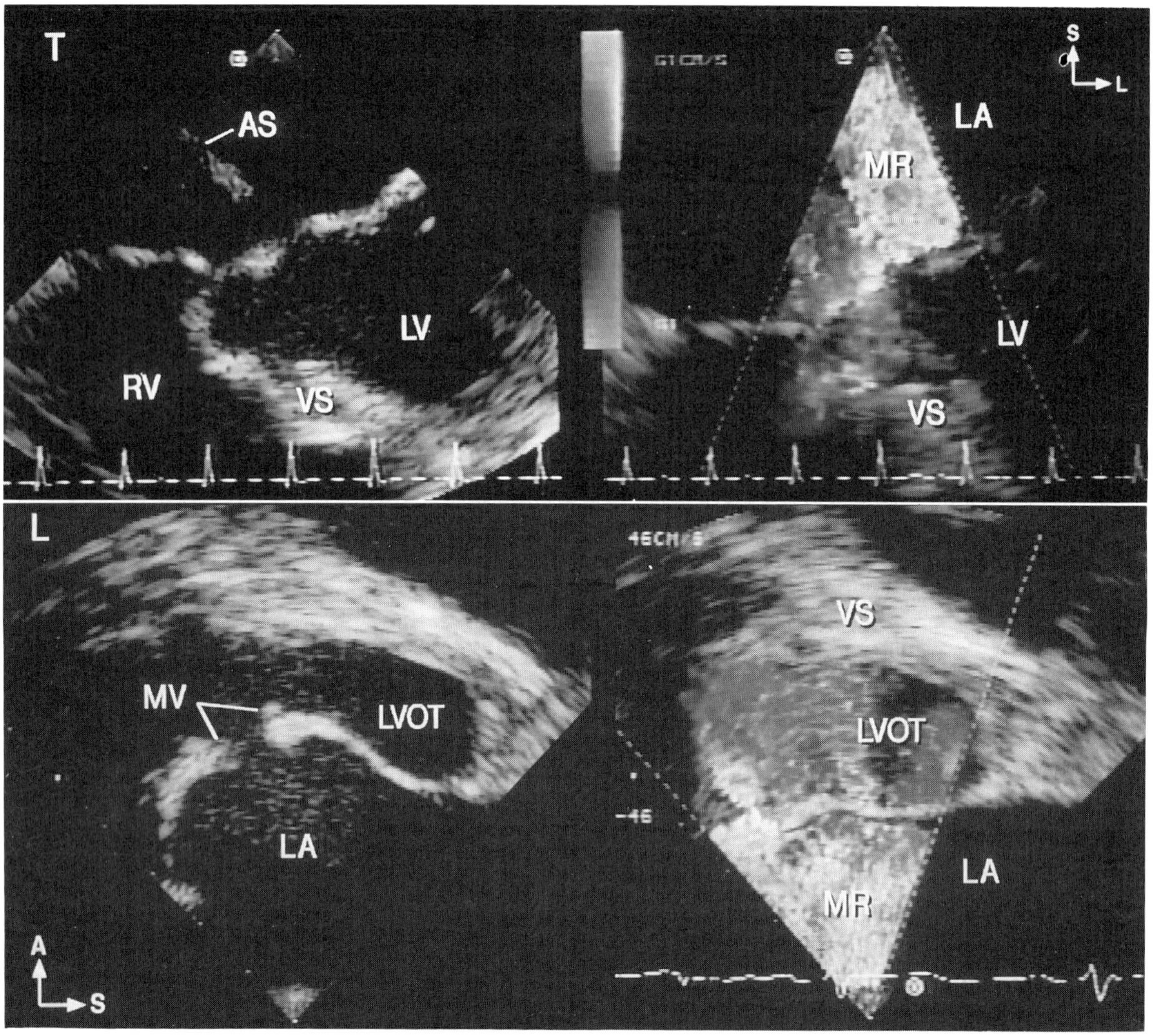

Fig 39-26 Transesophageal echocardiography in atrioventricular canal defect. **Top**, horizontal (*T*) plane images in a 3-year-old patient with an intermediate form of atrioventricular canal defect. There is a large ostium primum atrial septal defect. The membranous portion of the ventricular septum (*VS*) also bulges into the right ventricle. With color-flow imaging (see color plate after page 1512), a small left-to-right shunt is observed coursing through a membranous defect. In addition, color-flow imaging demonstrates a large, broad jet of mitral regurgitation (*MR*) originating from the mitral valve cleft and entering the left atrium (*LA*). **Bottom**, longitudinal (*L*) plane images in a 48-year-old patient who had previous repair of a partial form of atrioventricular canal defect. A residual cleft in the anterior mitral valve (*MV*) leaflet is observed, and with color-flow imaging (see color plate after page 1512) it is evident that this is the source of a severe degree of mitral regurgitation. The scans also demonstrate that the left ventricular outflow tract (*LVOT*) is widely patent. *A*, anterior; *AS*, atrial septum; *L*, left; *LV*, left ventricle; *RV*, right ventricle; *S*, superior.

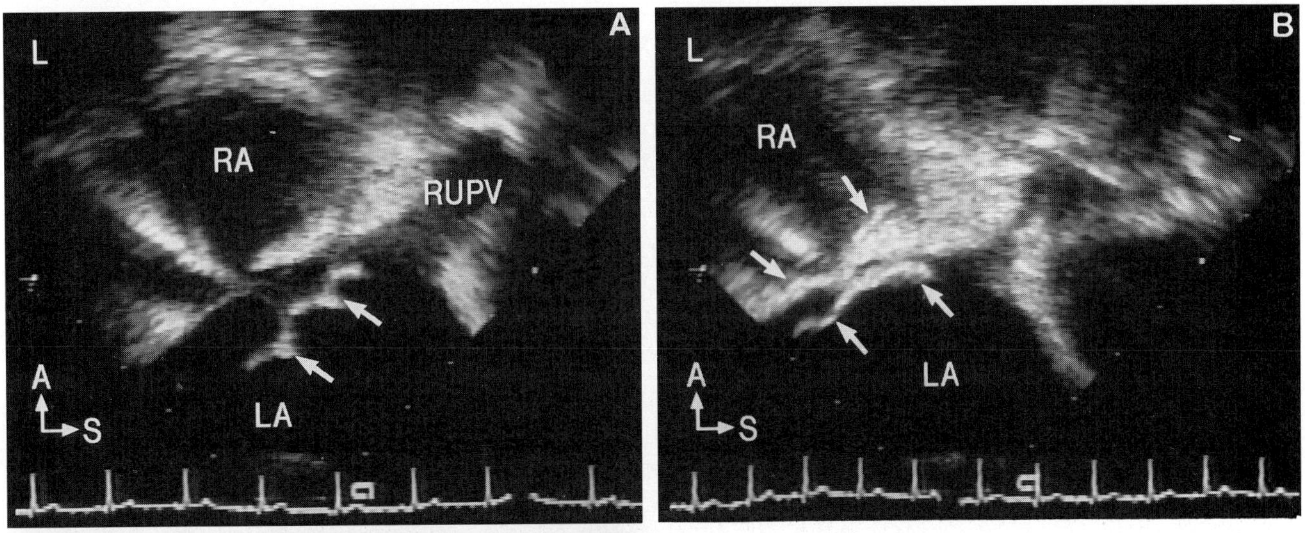

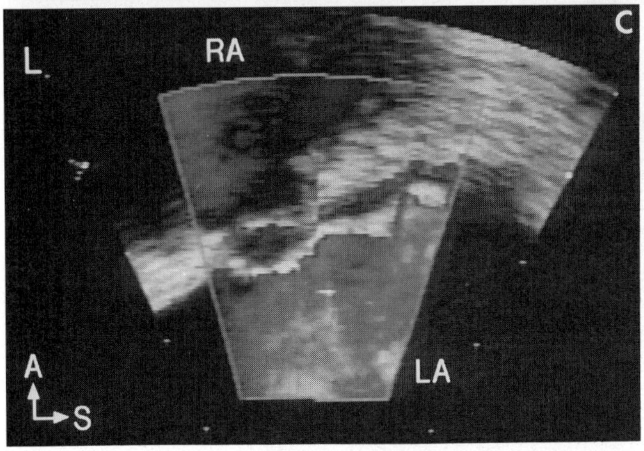

Fig 39-27 Sequential transesophageal echocardiographic images in the longitudinal (*L*) plane during placement of an atrial septal closure device in a patient with patent foramen ovale and multiple previous strokes. **A**, initial deployment of the device (*arrows*) in the left atrium (*LA*). **B**, further deployment placing portion of the device (*arrows*) in the right atrium (*RA*). **C** (see color plate after page 1512), after release, the device is properly positioned and there is no further evidence of right-to-left shunt with color-flow imaging. *A*, anterior; *RUPV*, right upper pulmonary vein; *S*, superior.

proach.[38] With the advent of smaller and biplane probes for transesophageal use, much of the initial enthusiasm for intraoperative study switched to the transesophageal approach. Although the direct epicardial approach initially had several distinct advantages, including easier recognition of residual ventricular septal defects and easier demonstration of right heart structures, recent improvements in resolution resulting from higher-element transducers and biplane imaging have favored the transesophageal approach.

Transesophageal imaging offers the clear advantages of a longer and repeated time period for accurate and more precise delineation of complex anatomic details and changing hemodynamics; a complete lack of any interference or disruption of the surgical field, cardiac function, or surgical routines; a greater number of imaging planes and views; and improved imaging of posterior left heart structures.[41] In a review of approximately 105 patients who underwent cardiac surgery for congenital heart disease at the Mayo Clinic from 1990 to 1992 and had biplane intraoperative TEE, we found that approximately 7% of the patients had significant postoperative echocardiographic findings that warranted immediate return to cardiopulmonary bypass and repair of residual cardiac lesions.[42] An additional 16% had significant postoperative findings on TEE examination that were not severe enough to warrant reoperation. The lesions requiring reoperation were significant residual ventricular septal defect, residual AV valve abnormalities, residual outflow tract obstructive lesions, and stenosis of the connection between the right atrium and the pulmonary artery after the modified Fontan procedure. Significant residual lesions demonstrated with TEE after repair of congenital cardiac defects are shown in Figure 39-28. In addition, the preoperative demonstration of significant details of intracardiac anatomy and sites of valvular insufficiency in a patient with AV septal defect provided important guidelines for subsequent surgical repair. Although some postoperative TEE observations may not be significant in the long term, it is clear from this experience that intraoperative TEE has had a substantial and important effect on the operative management of congenital heart disease. The efficacy and safety of intraoperative TEE observed thus far[43] suggest that its routine intraoperative use will be preferred over the intraoperative epicardial approach.

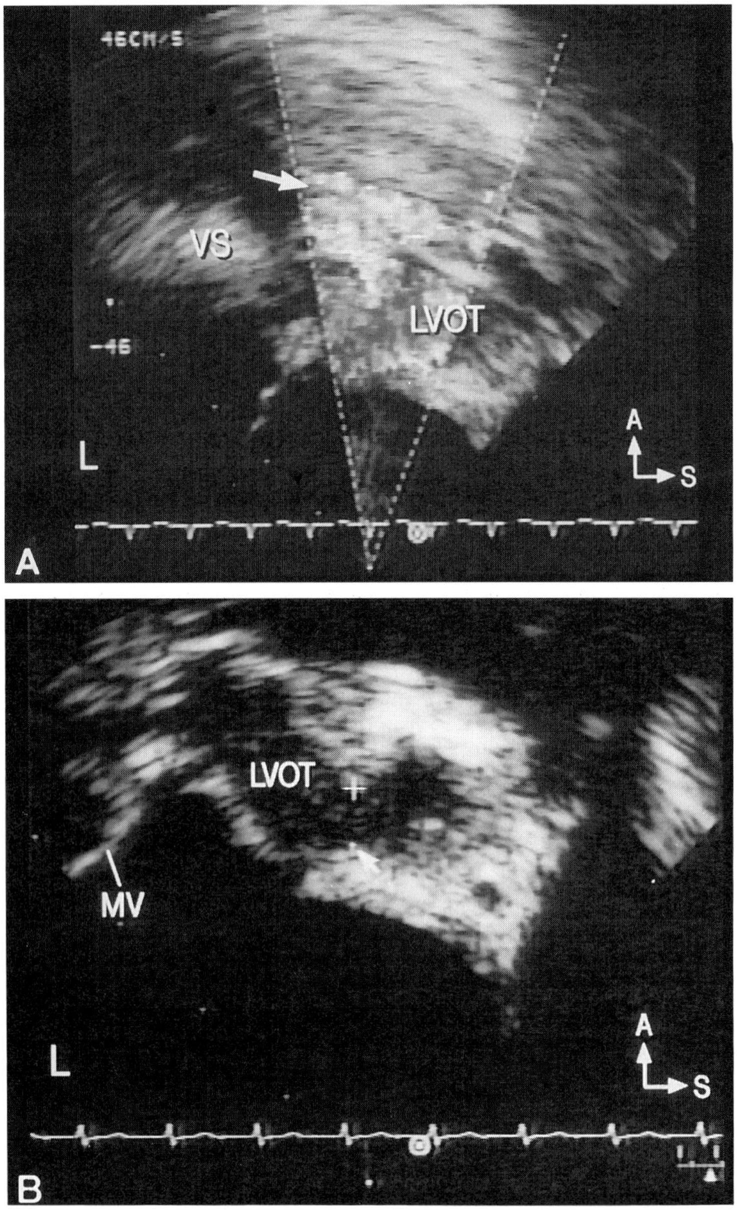

Fig 39-28 Longitudinal (*L*) plane left ventricular outflow tract (*LVOT*) scans in patients with residual lesions. **A** (see color plate after page 200), patient who had subaortic resection for fibromuscular obstruction. Although the outflow tract is widely patent, a moderate left-to-right (*arrow*) shunt through a ventricular septal defect created during the subaortic resection is readily apparent. Cardiopulmonary bypass was immediately resumed and the defect closed. **B**, patient who had subaortic stenosis after previous repair of a complete AV canal defect. After patch enlargement of the LVOT, a persistent muscular narrowing was evident (*markers*). Cardiopulmonary bypass was resumed and the muscular obstruction successfully removed. *A*, anterior; *MV*, mitral valve; *S*, superior; *VS*, ventricular septum.

CONCLUSION

As outlined in this chapter, the application of cardiac ultrasonography to congenital heart disease has several unique features. The heavy reliance on cardiac ultrasonography for clinical decision-making in congenital heart disease has become increasingly evident with the proliferation of echocardiographic modalities for clinical assessment. High-resolution two-dimensional imaging, Doppler echocardiography, color-flow imaging, TEE, and fetal studies have dramatically increased the noninvasive diagnostic capabilities of the pediatric cardiologist. Even though the noninvasive diagnostic capabilities have resulted in a reduction in the number of cardiac catheterization procedures performed at most institutions, the goal for improved echocardiographic imaging is not replacement of invasive catheterization. Instead, echocardiographic techniques should be directed to work in a collaborative and complementary fashion to provide the best diagnostic information for clinical and surgical management.

REFERENCES

1. Meyer RA, Hagler D, Huhta J, et al: Guidelines for Physician Training in Pediatric Echocardiography. Recommendations of the Society of Pediatric Echocardiography Committee on Physician Training. *Am J Cardiol* 60:164-165, 1987
2. Meyer RA, Hagler D, Huhta J, et al: Guidelines for Physician Training in Fetal Echocardiography. Recommendations of the Society of Pediatric Echocardiography Committee on Physician Training. *J Am Soc Echocardiogr* 3:1-3, 1990
3. Pearlman AS, Gardin JM, Martin RP, et al: Guidelines for Optimal Physician Training in Echocardiography. Recommendations of the American Society of Echocardiography Committee for Physician Training in Echocardiography. *J Am Soc Echocardiogr* 1:278-286, 1988
4. Pearlman AS, Gardin JM, Martin RP, et al: Guidelines for Physician Training in Transesophageal Echocardiography. Recommendations of the American Society of Echocardiography Committee for Physician Training in Echocardiography. *J Am Soc Echocardiogr* 5:187-194, 1992
5. Van Praagh RS, Van Praagh S, Vlad P, et al: Anatomic types of congenital dextrocardia: diagnostic and embryologic implications. *Am J Cardiol* 13:510-531, 1964
6. Calcaterra G, Anderson RH, Lau KC, et al: Dextrocardia--value of segmental analysis in its categorisation. *Br Heart J* 42:497-507, 1979
7. Solinger R, Elbl F, Minhas K: Deductive echocardiographic analysis in infants with congenital heart disease. *Circulation* 50:1072-1096, 1987
8. Hagler DJ, Tajik AJ, Seward JB, et al: Atrioventricular and ventriculoarterial discordance (corrected transposition of the great arteries): wide-angle two-dimensional echocardiographic assessment of ventricular morphology. *Mayo Clin Proc* 56:591-600, 1981
9. Huhta JC, Hagler DJ, Seward JB, et al: Two-dimensional echocardiographic assessment of dextrocardia: a segmental approach. *Am J Cardiol* 50:1351-1360, 1982
10. Rice MJ, Seward JB, Edwards WD, et al: Straddling atrioventricular valve: two-dimensional echocardiographic diagnosis, classification and surgical implications. *Am J Cardiol* 55:505-513, 1985
11. Quinones MA, Waggoner AD, Reduto LA, et al: A new, simplified and accurate method for determining ejection fraction with two-dimensional echocardiography. *Circulation* 64:744-750, 1981
12. Quinones MA, Gaasch WH, Cole JS, et al: Echocardiographic determination of left ventricular stress-velocity relations in man. With reference to the effects of loading and contractility. *Circulation* 51:689-700, 1975
13. Colan SD, Borow KM, Neumann A: Left ventricular end-systolic wall stress-velocity of fiber shortening relation: a load-independent index of myocardial contractility. *J Am Coll Cardiol* 4:715-724, 1984
14. Silverman NH, Ports TA, Snider AT, et al: Determination of left ventricular volume in children: echocardiographic and angiographic comparisons. *Circulation* 62:548-557, 1980
15. Silverman NH, Hudson S: Evaluation of right ventricular volume and ejection fraction in children by two-dimensional echocardiography. *Pediatr Cardiol* 4:197-204, 1983
16. Hagler DJ, Seward JB, Tajik AJ, et al: Functional assessment of the Fontan operation: combined M-mode, two dimensional and Doppler echocardiographic studies. *J Am Coll Cardiol* 4:756-764, 1984
17. Riggs TW, Rodriguez R, Snider AR, et al: Doppler echocardiographic evaluation of right and left ventricular diastolic function in normal neonates. *J Am Coll Cardiol* 13:700-705, 1989
18. Hagler DJ, Tajik AJ, Seward JB, et al: Noninvasive assessment of pulmonary valve stenosis, aortic valve stenosis and coarctation of the aorta in critically ill neonates. *Am J Cardiol* 57:369-372, 1986
19. Currie PJ, Seward JB, Chan K-L, et al: Continuous wave Doppler determination of right ventricular pressure: a simultaneous Doppler-catheterization study in 127 patients. *J Am Coll Cardiol* 6:750-756, 1985
20. Enriquez-Sarano M, Bailey KR, Seward JB, et al: Quantitative Doppler assessment of valvular regurgitation. *Circulation* 87:841-848, 1993
21. Smyllie JH, Sutherland GR, Keeton BR: The value of Doppler color flow mapping in determining pulmonary blood supply in infants with pulmonary atresia with ventricular septal defect. *J Am Coll Cardiol* 14:1759-1765, 1989
22. Hagler DJ: Doppler color flow imaging and determination of pulmonary blood supply in infants with pulmonary atresia with ventricular septal defect (editorial). *J Am Coll Cardiol* 14:1766-1767, 1989
23. Vogel M, Smallhorn JF, Trusler GA, et al: Echocardiographic analysis of regional left ventricular wall motion in children after the arterial switch operation for complete transposition of the great arteries. *J Am Coll Cardiol* 15:1417-1423, 1990
24. Teien D, Wendel H, Holm S, et al: Estimation of Doppler gradients at rest and during exercise in patients with recoarctation of the aorta. *Br Heart J* 65:155-157, 1991
25. Rustico MA, Benettoni A, D'Ottavio G, et al: Fetal echocardiography: the role of the screening procedure. *Eur J Obstet Gynecol Reprod Biol* 36:19-25, 1990
26. Allan LD, Chita SK, Sharland GK, et al: The accuracy of fetal echocardiography in the diagnosis of congenital heart disease. *Int J Cardiol* 25:279-288, 1989
27. Allan LD, Cook A, Sullivan I, et al: Hypoplastic left heart syndrome: effects of fetal echocardiography on birth prevalence. *Lancet* 337:959-961, 1991
28. Kleinman CS, Donnerstein RL: Ultrasonic assessment of cardiac function in the intact human fetus. *J Am Coll Cardiol* 5 Suppl:84-94, 1985
29. Kleinman CS, Hobbins JC, Jaffe CC, et al: Echocardiographic studies of the human fetus: prenatal diagnosis of congenital heart disease and cardiac dysrhythmias. *Pediatrics* 65:1059-1067, 1980
30. Copel JA, Morotti R, Hobbins JC, et al: The antenatal diagnosis of congenital heart disease using fetal echocardiography: Is color flow mapping necessary? *Obstet Gynecol* 78:1-8, 1991
31. Veille JC, Mahowald MB, Sivakoff M: Ethical dilemmas in fetal echocardiography. *Obstet Gynecol* 73:710-714, 1989
32. Martin GR, Ruckman RN: Fetal echocardiography: a large clinical experience and follow-up. *J Am Soc Echocardiogr* 3:4-8, 1990
33. Stümper OFW, Elzenga NJ, Hess J, et al: Transesophageal echocardiography in children with congenital heart disease: an initial experience. *J Am Coll Cardiol* 16:433-441, 1990
34. Ritter SB: Transesophageal real-time echocardiography in infants and children with congenital heart disease. *J Am Coll Cardiol* 18:569-580, 1991
35. Kronzon I, Tunick PA, Freedberg RS, et al: Transesophageal echocardiography is superior to transthoracic echocardiography in the diagnosis of sinus venosus atrial septal defect. *J Am Coll Cardiol* 17:537-542, 1991
36. Stümper OFW, Sreeram N, Elzenga NJ, et al: Diagnosis of atrial situs by transesophageal echocardiography. *J Am Coll Cardiol* 16:442-446, 1990
37. Hellenbrand WE, Fahey JT, McGowan FX, et al: Transesophageal echocardiographic guidance of transcatheter closure of atrial septal defect. *Am J Cardiol* 66:207-213, 1990

38. Hagler DJ, Tajik AJ, Seward JB, et al: Intraoperative two-dimensional Doppler echocardiography: a preliminary study for congenital heart disease. *J Thorac Cardiovasc Surg* 95:516-522, 1988

39. Hsu Y-H, Santulli T Jr, Wong A-L, et al: Impact of intraoperative echocardiography on surgical management of congenital heart disease. *Am J Cardiol* 67:1279-1283, 1991

40. Sreeram N, Kaulitz R, Stümper OFW, et al: Comparative roles of intraoperative epicardial and early postoperative transthoracic echocardiography in the assessment of surgical repair of congenital heart defects. *J Am Coll Cardiol* 16:913-920, 1990

41. Stümper O, Sutherland GR, Sreeram N, et al: The role of intraoperative ultrasound examination in patients undergoing a Fontan-type procedure. *Br Heart J* 65:204-210, 1991

42. O'Leary PW, Hagler DJ, Seward JB, et al: Biplane intraoperative transesophageal echocardiography in congenital heart disease (abstract). *J Am Soc Echocardiogr* 5:323, 1992

43. Lunn RJ, Oliver WC Jr, Hagler DJ, et al: Aortic compression by transesophageal echocardiographic probe in infants and children undergoing cardiac surgery. *Anesthesiology* 77:587-590, 1992

CHAPTER

40

Atrial septal defect

Carole A. Warnes, M.D., Valentin Fuster, M.D., David J. Driscoll, M.D., and Dwight C. McGoon, M.D.

ANATOMIC CONSIDERATIONS

Atrial septal defect was described by Rokitansky in 1875, but it was not until 1941 that Bedford et al. drew attention to its clinical features.[1] If one excludes congenital bicuspid aortic valve and mitral valve prolapse, atrial septal defect is the most common form of congenital heart disease found among adolescents and adults (see chapter 38). About 75% of the atrial septal defects are of the ostium secundum type, 20% are of the ostium primum type, and 5% are of the sinus venosus type[2-4] (Fig 40-1). More rare types of atrial septal defects include a defect posterior and inferior to the fossa ovalis (i.e., between the fossa and the inferior vena cava) and a defect in the position normally occupied by the coronary sinus (when the left superior vena cava drains into the left atrium).[5]

The ostium secundum defect is located in the region of the fossa ovalis and occasionally is associated with prolapse of the mitral valve and mitral regurgitation. The reason for this association is unknown,[6,7] although abnormal left ventricular geometry is responsible, in part, for the prevalence of mitral valve prolapse in the absence of any connective tissue abnormality of leaflets or chordae tendineae.[8] The association of ostium secundum defect and mitral stenosis (Lutembacher's syndrome), presumably rheumatic, is now uncommon, but the clinical characteristics have been well described.[1] It is important to recognize that a patent foramen ovale, which persists in more than 5% of normal adolescents or adults, is not a true atrial septal defect in which septal tissue is deficient; the foramen ovale normally permits right-to-left flow in utero but no flow after birth. In pathologic conditions with high right atrial pressures, right-to-left shunting occurs through the patent foramen ovale, and it may also be found in normal adults when the normal interatrial pressure gradient is transiently reversed by a provocative maneuver such as coughing or the Valsalva maneuver.[9] It has been suggested that a patent foramen ovale is more common in young patients with ischemic stroke, the implication being that paradoxical embolism is responsible.[10] With chronically increased left atrial pressure and stretching of the septum, left-to-right flow through the defect may occur.

The ostium primum defect, or partial form of AV canal defect, is characterized by absence of the septum superior to the AV valves. Because of the deficiency of the AV septum, the AV valves insert at the same level, and there is usually an associated cleft in the anterior mitral leaflet, with varying degrees of mitral regurgitation. Less commonly, the mitral valve has a double orifice.[11] Rarely does mild tricuspid incompetence occur, even though hypoplasia of the septal tricuspid leaflet is usual.

The sinus venosus defect is located high in the septum and usually is associated with "partial anomalous pulmonary venous connection" in which the right upper and middle lobe veins connect to the superior vena cava or right atrium.[12] An atrial septal defect is uncommon when the anomalous pulmonary veins arise from the left lung or when the inferior vena cava receives anomalous pulmonary veins from the right lung, which often is hypoplastic.[5,13,14]

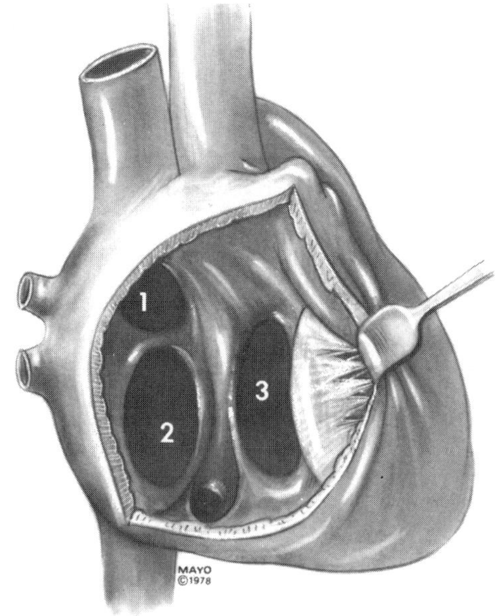

Fig 40-1 Types of atrial septal detect: **1,** sinus venosus; **2,** ostium secundum; and **3,** ostium primum. (From Fuster V, Brandenburg RO, McGoon DC, et al: Clinical approach and management of congenital heart disease in the adolescent and adult. *Cardiovasc Clin* 10 No 3:161-197, 1980. By permission, Mayo Foundation.)

PATHOPHYSIOLOGY

Most atrial septal defects are sufficiently large to allow equalization of the pressures in the two atria. In the uncomplicated state the flow is in a left-to-right direction across the defect. Although the pulmonary blood flow may exceed normal considerably (four times normal is not uncommon), the pulmonary vascular resistance is normal or lower than normal and the pulmonary arterial pressure is nearly normal. The pulmonary arterial "wedge" or left atrial pressure also is normal.

The left-to-right shunt through the atrial septal defect results because compliance of the right ventricle is greater than that of the left ventricle. A large left-to-right shunt is unusual in infancy because the right ventricular wall is relatively thick and stiff, but this condition diminishes after the first few weeks of life, permitting left-to-right shunting if an atrial septal defect is present. In adult patients, the right ventricle may become stiffer because of pulmonary stenosis, pulmonary hypertension, or cardiomyopathy, and this may diminish or even reverse the shunt, leading to the development of cyanosis. Conversely, problems affecting left ventricular compliance (aortic stenosis, coronary artery disease, systemic hypertension) increase flow across the defect and even lead to right-sided heart failure. Left-to-right flow through an uncomplicated atrial septal defect begins in ventricular systole and usually lasts throughout diastole, peaking in early diastole and becoming augmented in late diastole during atrial contraction. The magnitude and direction of shunt flow reflect the phasic variation of the interatrial pressure difference during the cardiac cycle.[15,16]

It is important to note that the right pulmonary veins typically are more closely related to the secundum atrial septal defect than are the left pulmonary veins. Consequently, the greater portion of the blood shunted through an ostium secundum atrial septal defect comes from the right lung rather than from the left; thus, partial anomalous pulmonary venous "drainage" occurs commonly, even in the absence of an anomalous pulmonary venous connection. Also, the ostium of the inferior vena cava is closely allied to the atrial septum near the fossa ovalis, which explains the common occurrence of a small (<5%) right-to-left shunt from the inferior cava through the secundum atrial septal defect. A few patients with atrial septal defect have a large right-to-left shunt and cyanosis despite absence of pulmonary hypertension; such patients have a large eustachian valve of the inferior vena cava that deflects the caval blood toward the septal defect and left atrium.[17] Another rare cause of cyanosis in atrial septal defect is direct connection of an associated left superior vena cava into the left atrium.[17]

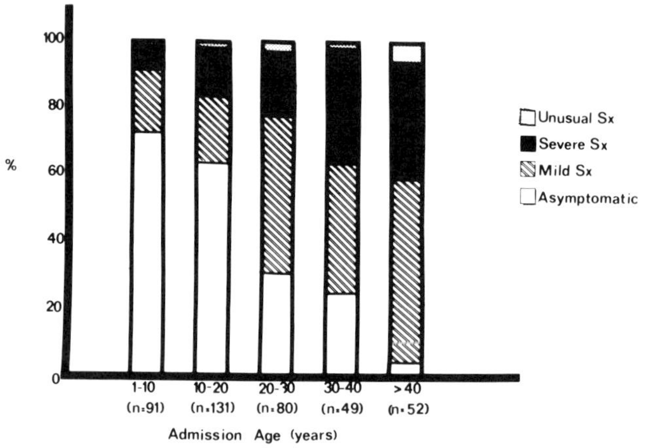

Fig 40-2 Symptoms *(Sx)* increase with advancing age in untreated patients with atrial septal defect. (From Hamilton WT, Haffajee CI, Dalen JE, et al: Atrial septal defect secundum: clinical profile with physiologic correlates in children and adults. *Cardiovasc Clin* 10 No 1:267-277, 1979. By permission of FA Davis Company.)

CLINICAL SYNDROME

History and clinical course[1,2,18-23]

Of the different types of atrial septal defect, the ostium secundum type occurs more often in females—the female-to-male ratio varies from 1.5:1 to 3.5:1. In some instances, particularly associated with the Holt-Oram syndrome[18,19] (see "Physical Findings," below) and with significantly prolonged P-R interval,[20,21] the defect occurs in families.[22] In childhood, isolated atrial septal defects are usually well tolerated. The most significant feature in the clinical history is the discovery of a murmur, often not until the patient is more than 5 years old. During childhood and adolescence, most patients remain asymptomatic; after that, symptoms increase with advancing age (Fig 40-2). Exertional dyspnea, as a result of the rigidity or noncompliance of the lungs (large pulmonary blood flow), and mild fatigability with exercise, presumably as a result of decreased left ventricular stroke volume, commonly develop only in the third and fourth decades of life. Then, the patient's condition may deteriorate chiefly for three reasons: (1) advent of atrial arrhythmias, especially fibrillation or flutter; (2) development of pulmonary vascular obstructive disease and pulmonary hypertension, leading to a decrease in the left-to-right shunt and possible development of a right-to-left shunt with cyanosis and atypical chest pain (a significant degree of pulmonary hypertension, with a pulmonary vascular resistance above 7 units · m^2, occurs in about 15% of patients); and (3) development of right heart failure related to the above two conditions or, more often, related to the chronic volume overload of the right ventricle, which can be further increased in older patients by the usual decrease in left ventricular distensibility or the development of left heart failure.

With unrepaired atrial septal defect, survival into adulthood is the rule, and many patients live to advanced ages. Death related to this malformation is most often the result of heart failure. Less commonly it is related to a pulmonary infection (susceptibility to pulmonary infections is present at all ages), pulmonary arterial thrombosis or embolism, or paradoxic brain embolism or abscess. Infective endocarditis is very rare in isolated atrial septal defect but can occur if there is associated mitral valve prolapse with mitral incompetence. There are three main

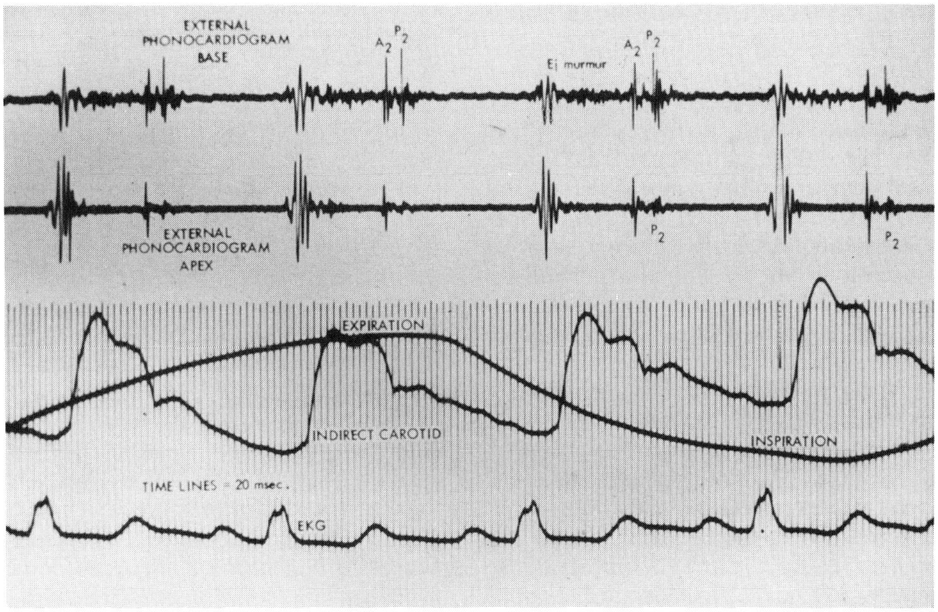

Fig 40-3 Wide, fixed splitting in patient with large atrial septal defect. Note also the shunt ejection *(EJ)* systolic murmur. A_2, aortic component; P_2, pulmonic component.

exceptions to the above clinical course of isolated atrial septal defect.

1. Occasionally in infancy, there is a large left-to-right shunt leading to heart failure. If the patient survives, heart failure tends to subside by age 1 or 2, and the course usually becomes that of a typical atrial septal defect.[23]

2. With the ostium primum type of defect, although the clinical course is similar to that with the ostium secundum and sinus venosus types of defects, patients with severe mitral incompetence have symptoms that are more severe and are apt to occur earlier in life.

3. In some instances, when the left-to-right shunt is relatively small, patients can remain asymptomatic for more than 5 decades.

Physical findings

The diagnosis of atrial septal defect usually is made in the office or at the bedside on the basis of the physical examination. Chest radiographs, electrocardiograms (ECGs), and echocardiograms document the clinician's clinical impression.

Physical appearance. Adults with atrial septal defects have a normal physical appearance, but children with a large left-to-right shunt may be thin and small and exhibit a left precordial bulge.[1] Cyanosis and digital clubbing occur when pulmonary hypertension reverses the interatrial shunt. An ostium secundum atrial septal defect is suspected in the presence of the Holt-Oram syndrome.[24] In this syndrome, one or both thumbs are hypoplastic or absent; an extreme of the syndrome is the absence or malformation of the radii or of arms, with or without underdeveloped hands[18-20] (see chapter 68).

Arterial and venous pulses. The arterial pulse is usually normal. The jugular venous pulse is usually normal in height, although the crests of the "a" and v waves tend to be equal, reflecting the left atrial pressure contour.[25,26] In patients with pulmonary hypertension, there is a dominant "a" wave. Elevated jugular venous pressure is encountered only in patients with associated left ventricular failure or mitral stenosis because the atrial intercommunication prevents right atrial pressure from significantly exceeding left atrial pressure.

Precordial palpation. The left ventricular impulse is absent or is overshadowed by a dominant right ventricle, eliciting an impulse in the low left sternal border.[27] Although not always distinguishable, the right ventricular impulse of the volume overload phase (large left-to-right shunt) tends to be hyperdynamic and brief, whereas the impulse of the pressure overload complication (pulmonary hypertension) tends to be less dynamic and more sustained. The dilated pulmonary trunk often is palpable in the second left intercostal space.

Auscultation. Three features are important.[1]

1. A typical wide and fixed splitting of the second heart sound, which is the most important diagnostic clue[28,29] (Fig 40-3). The term "fixed" refers to the essentially constant time lag throughout the respiratory cycle between the sounds of aortic and pulmonary valve closures. The width of the split is due to a delay in the pulmonic component (P_2), in part because the duration of right ventricular mechanical systole increases with the larger volume of blood ejected and in part because the considerable vasodilatation of the pulmonary vasculature delays the intra-arterial pulmonary tension necessary to close the pulmonary valve.[30] The splitting is fixed because normal phasic differences in stroke volume between the two ventricles associated with respiratory fluctuations of systemic venous return are prevented by the atrial septal defect. In partial anomalous pulmonary venous connec-

tion with *intact* atrial septum, the second heart sound is widely or persistently split, but the duration of the split is not fixed.

2. A soft systolic murmur (maximum, grade 3), crescendo-decrescendo in shape and "superficial" in quality (proximity of the dilated pulmonary trunk to the chest wall), which is heard maximally in the second left intercostal space. The ejection of a large right ventricular stroke volume into a dilated pulmonary trunk accounts for this murmur; on occasion, and by similar mechanisms, systolic turbulence can be generated in the dilated peripheral pulmonary arteries, with transmission to other areas of the thorax.

3. An early to mid-diastolic murmur,[29,31] "superficial" and low-pitched in character, which is confined to the low left sternal border but sometimes is heard at the apex because the apex is occupied by the right ventricle. This murmur is due to greatly increased diastolic flow across the tricuspid orifice (relative tricuspid stenosis) and is a useful sign of a large left-to-right shunt.[32] Contrary to the murmur of true tricuspid stenosis, this flow murmur does not increase with inspiration, because the atrial septal defect prevents respiratory fluctuations in right ventricular stroke volume, as discussed above. Indeed, the lack of respiratory variation in the murmur sometimes may lead to its being confused with the murmur of aortic incompetence; in addition, the frequently superficial character of the tricuspid diastolic and pulmonary systolic murmurs may simulate pericardial rubs.

In atrial septal defect with pulmonary hypertension, the above three auscultatory features differ significantly.[33,34]

1. The wide fixed splitting of the second heart sound persists as long as a significant left-to-right shunt is present. However, P_2 is loud, which may overshadow the perception of the aortic component (A_2); in addition, with abolition or reversal of the shunt, the wide split disappears.

2. The pulmonic systolic murmur is replaced by a shorter murmur due to the ejection of a normal or decreased stroke volume into a dilated pulmonary trunk. Such a murmur is preceded by a typical pulmonic ejection systolic click. Occasionally, when the pulmonary hypertension and right ventricular enlargement lead to dilatation of the tricuspid ring, a holosystolic murmur of tricuspid incompetence can be elicited in the low left sternal border or, sometimes, at the apex.

3. The diastolic tricuspid flow murmur may vanish. Occasionally, when the pulmonary hypertension leads to pulmonary valvular incompetence, a high-frequency, early diastolic murmur of Graham Steell may develop.

Electrocardiogram

Unless coronary artery disease or systemic hypertension modifies the tracings, the ECG in atrial septal defect can reveal four important features:

1. Most patients are in normal sinus rhythm, but after the third decade the incidence of supraventricular arrhythmias increases, especially atrial fibrillation or flutter, which occurs in about 10% of patients by age 30 and about 20% by age 50.[35]

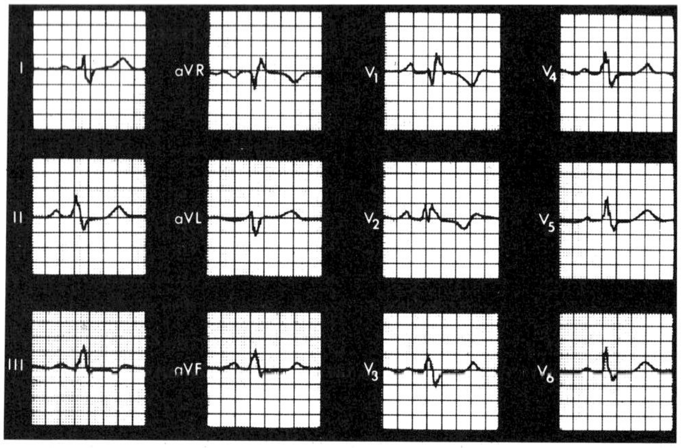

Fig 40-4 ECG of 32-year-old man with ostium secundum atrial septal defect. Note right ventricular conduction delay (rsR′ pattern over the right precordial leads) (frontal QRS axis about +100°). (From Fuster V, Danielson GK: Congenital heart disease in the adult. In *Office Management of Medical and Surgical Heart Disease: A Concise Guide for Physicians.* Edited by LI Bonchek, HL Brooks. Boston, Little, Brown & Company, 1981, pp 183-217. By permission.)

2. The P-R interval often is prolonged,[1,36,37] especially in older patients, and this is related to intra-atrial conduction delay rather than to slowing of conduction across the atrioventricular (AV) node.[38] However, a markedly prolonged P-R interval (220 msec) due to impaired AV conduction tends to occur in the familial type of atrial septal defect[20,21,39,40] and in rare cases may lead to complete heart block. Interestingly, some members of these families may have P-R prolongation even in the absence of an associated atrial septal defect.[33]

3. The ECG hallmark, present in 90% of patients with atrial septal defect, is an rSr′ complex or rSR′ complex with a slight increase in QRS duration recorded from right precordial leads[1,35,37,41] (Fig 40-4). In the rSr′ complex, the r′ and slight increase in QRS duration are related to prolongation of the rightward, superior, and anterior terminal forces caused by hypertrophy of the right ventricular crista.[42-44] A similar rSr′ complex is seen in about 5% of normal subjects, but the r′ is usually less wide and less slurred than in atrial septal defect. A progressive increase in the height (mV) of r′ leading to an rsR′ complex indicates progressive hypertrophy of the free right ventricular wall, related to a chronic large left-to-right shunt, and usually suggests the presence of progressive pulmonary vascular obstructive disease and pulmonary hypertension;[35] reciprocal changes occur in the left precordial leads with the R waves diminishing and the S waves becoming deeper.

4. In ostium secundum and sinus venosus types of defects, the mean QRS axis in the frontal plane usually is downward or slightly to the left or right (right-axis deviation occurs in those patients with pulmonary hypertension); in addition, depolarization is typically clockwise with Q waves in leads II and III.[23,37,42] On the other hand,

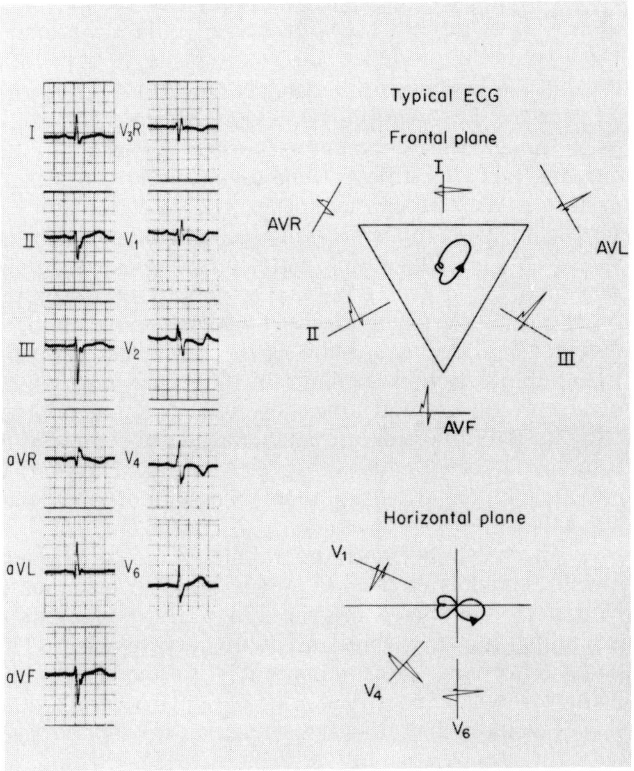

Fig 40-5 Typical ECG of partial AV canal defect. Note left axis deviation (QRS axis about −70°) and right ventricular conduction delay. The schematically reconstructed frontal loop shows a counterclockwise superiorly directed QRS loop. (From Ongley PA, Pongpanich B, Spangler JG, et al: The electrocardiogram in atrioventricular canal. In *Atrioventricular Canal Defects.* Edited by RH Feldt. Philadelphia, WB Saunders Company, 1976, pp 51-75. By permission.)

as an important clue in ostium primum defects, the mean QRS axis is almost always upward and to the left (marked left-axis deviation) (Fig 40-5) and sometimes reaches the right; depolarization is typically counterclockwise with Q waves in leads I and aVL.[3,37,41,45-47] The characteristic frontal plane QRS pattern in ostium primum defect is related to an unusual congenital disposition of the AV conduction system.[46-48] Only rarely, the QRS pattern in an ostium secundum defect can mimic that in ostium primum;[21,22,49] the reverse is even rarer.[50]

Chest radiograph

The following three features are of interest[1] (Fig 40-6).

1. Only about 15% of patients with atrial septal defect have a normal-sized heart on the chest radiograph; this is more frequent in the younger patients.[35] The remainder have some degree of cardiomegaly, occasionally severe (Fig 40-7), which is mainly related to right atrial enlargement producing a rightward convexity in the frontal view. A less important cause is enlargement of the right ventricle and outflow tract, which results in some promi-

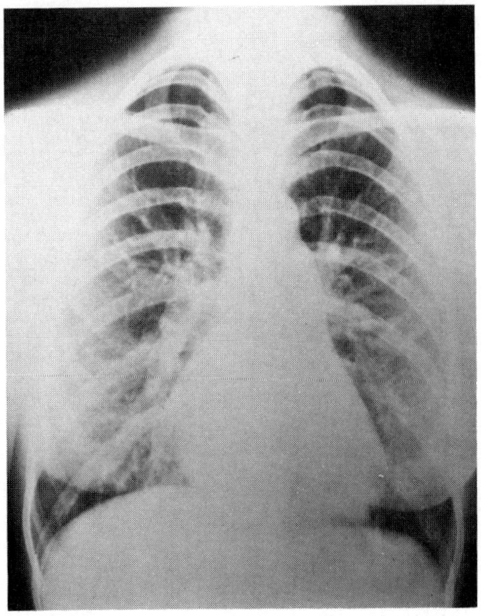

Fig 40-6 Chest radiograph of 34-year-old woman with ostium secundum atrial septal defect and large left-to-right shunt. Note mild cardiomegaly, prominent pulmonary trunk and pulmonary arteries, and increased pulmonary blood flow. (From Fuster V, Danielson GK: Congenital heart disease in the adult. In *Office Management of Medical and Surgical Heart Disease: A Concise Guide for Physicians.* Edited by LI Bonchek, HL Brooks. Boston, Little, Brown & Company, 1981, pp 183-217. By permission.)

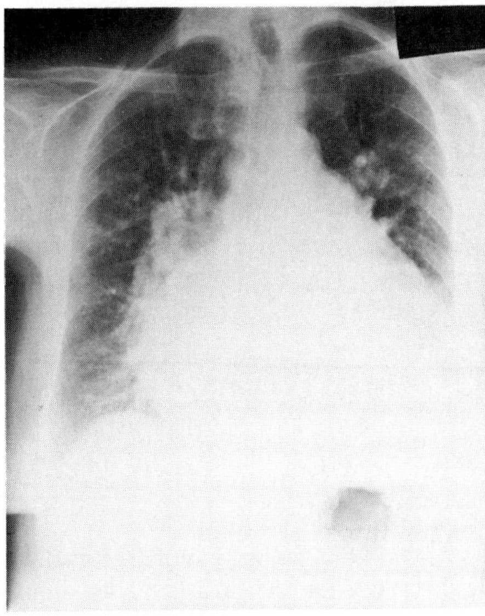

Fig 40-7 Chest radiograph showing cardiomegaly and congestive heart failure in an elderly woman with atrial septal defect. (From Fuster V, Brandenburg RO, McGoon DC, et al: Clinical approach and management of congenital heart disease in the adolescent and adult. *Cardiovasc Clin* 10 No 3:161-197, 1980. By permission of FA Davis Company.)

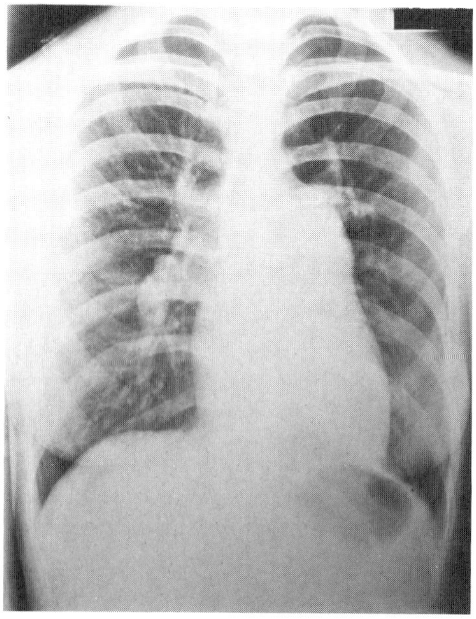

Fig 40-8 Chest radiograph of 35-year-old woman with atrial septal defect. There is severe pulmonary vascular obstructive disease with prominence of the main pulmonary artery and decreased peripheral pulmonary vascularity. (From Fuster V, Brandenburg RO, McGoon DC, et al: Clinical approach and management of congenital heart disease in the adolescent and adult. *Cardiovasc Clin* 10 No 3:161-197, 1980. By permission of FA Davis Company.)

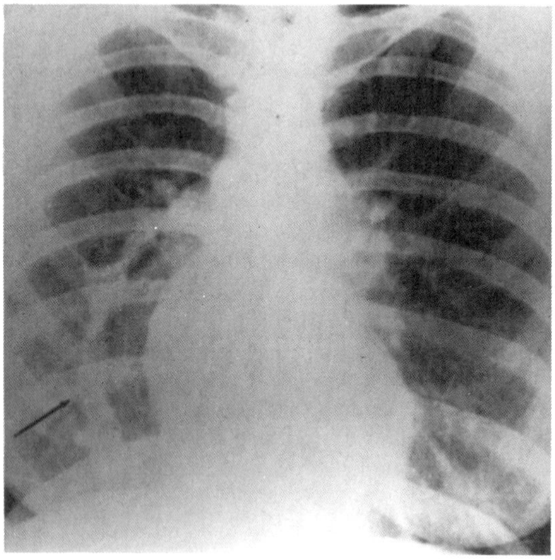

Fig 40-9 Partial anomalous pulmonary venous connection to the inferior vena cava. A large anomalous vessel *(arrow)* is seen in the right lower pulmonary field; the vessel becomes broader as it proceeds inferiorly before entering the inferior vena cava. The pulmonary arterial vasculature is slightly increased. (From Edwards JE, Carey LS, Neufeld HN, et al: *Congenital Heart Disease: Correlation of Pathologic Anatomy and Angiocardiography.* Vol. 1. Philadelphia, WB Saunders Company, 1965, pp 191-234. By permission.)

nence of the left midcardiac border and lifting of the apex.[51] In the lateral view, the large, volume-overloaded right ventricle produces anterior bowing of the upper third of the sternum[51] and displaces the heart posteriorly, so that the left ventricular shadow overlaps the spine, even though that chamber is normal in size.[52] In this circumstance, the inferior vena cava shadow can be seen as usual in the retrocardiac space; otherwise, when the left ventricle is truly dilated, it tends to be within the cardiac shadow.[52] The left atrium is not enlarged because a major portion of the increased pulmonary venous return streams directly into the right atrium through the atrial septal defect. Close approximation of the septal defect to the right pulmonary veins explains the difference in streaming between right and left lungs. The left atrium is enlarged only in the following three circumstances: an ostium primum defect with mitral regurgitation, atrial fibrillation, and a secundum atrial septal defect in patients older than 40 years.

2. The most specific radiographic feature of the left-to-right shunt is in the lung fields—that is, evidence of increased pulmonary arterial blood flow or plethora extending to the peripheral pulmonary vessels.[32] This feature becomes more apparent with increasing age, being evident in nearly 80% of patients over age 40.[35]

3. The pulmonary trunk is almost always dilated, as is its right branch; the left branch is hidden behind the dilated pulmonary trunk.[51] With the development of pulmonary vascular obstructive disease and pulmonary hypertension, the right pulmonary artery can appear as a very large inverted comma with an abrupt cutoff; the peripheral pulmonary arterial vasculature is replaced by clear or ischemic lung fields[53] (Fig 40-8).

The different types of partial anomalous pulmonary venous connection and atrial septal defect are not distinctive radiographically. The anomalous connection of the right pulmonary vein to the inferior vena cava is of particular interest. The large venous trunk can be recognized in the frontal chest film as a density that takes a downward course along the lower right border of the heart, widening as it approaches the angle formed by the heart and diaphragm; this density resembles a curved Turkish sword (scimitar sign) (Fig 40-9). In this condition, the scimitar sign often coexists with hypoplasia of the right lung, the heart being shifted into the right chest.[5,13,14,54]

Echocardiogram

Use of two-dimensional echocardiography improves the accuracy in diagnosing atrial septal defect by providing direct visualization of the atrial septum. Multiple echocardiographic windows can be used to visualize an atrial septal defect, but the subcostal four-chamber view is usually the best, because the ultrasound beam is nearly perpendicular to the plane of the atrial septum (Fig 40-10). The limbus of the normal fossa ovalis may, however, have a thicker refractile rim producing artifactual "echo fallout" in the mid-atrial septum. Because of this, a diagnosis of secundum atrial septal defect should not be made on the basis of this finding alone.[55]

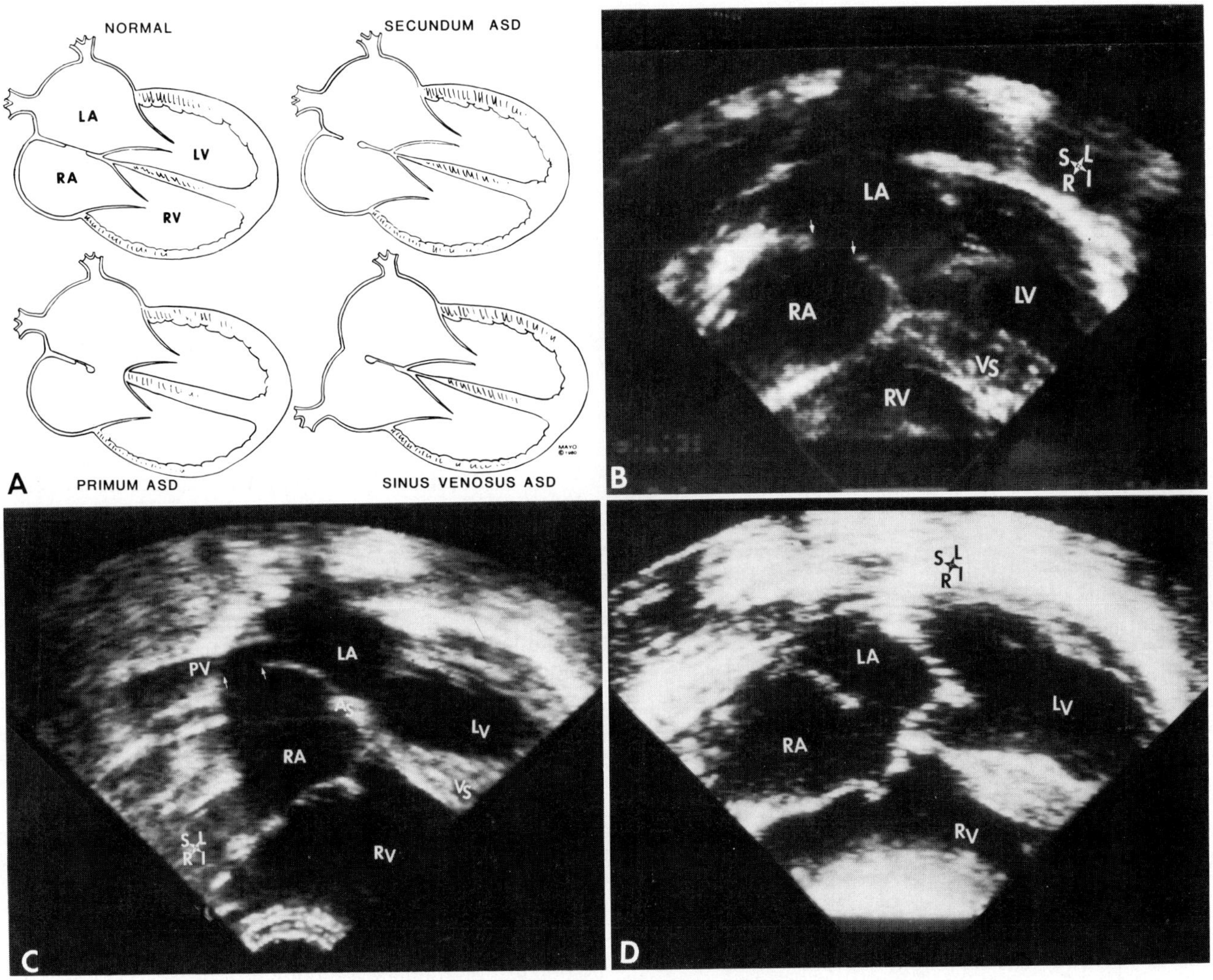

Fig 40-10 Diagrams (**A**) of two-dimensional echocardiographic appearance of atrial septum in subcostal views and two-dimensional echocardiograms (**B, C, D**) from the subcostal four-chamber view, showing the types of atrial septal defect *(ASD)*. **A,** normal septum and various types of ASD. In a normal heart, note thinning of area of the fossa ovalis, a potential cause for echo "dropout" and a false-positive reading of ASD in the standard precordial views; compare with the ostium secundum type of ASD. Note characteristic locations for primum and sinus venosus ASDs. **B,** secundum ASD *(arrows)* located in the central portion of the atrial septum in the region of the fossa ovalis. **C,** sinus venosus defect *(arrows)* posterior to the fossa ovalis and just beneath the orifice of the superior vena cava. In this example, a pulmonary vein *(PV)* anomalously enters the right atrium *(RA)*. **D,** primum ASD *(arrows)* in the inferior portion of the atrial septum. The AV valves insert at the same level onto the crest of the ventricular septum. *I,* inferior; *L,* left; *LA,* left atrium; *LV,* left ventricle; *R,* right; *RV,* right ventricle; *S,* superior; *VS,* ventricular septum. (**A,** from Shub C: The role of echocardiography in clinical practice. In *Clinical Medicine.* Vol. 6, Chap 34. Edited by JA Spittell Jr. Philadelphia, Harper & Row, Publishers, 1984, pp 1-44. By permission, Mayo Foundation. **B, C, D,** from Seward JB, Tajik AJ, Edwards WD, et al: *Two-Dimensional Echocardiographic Atlas.* Vol. 1. *Congenital Heart Disease.* New York, Springer-Verlag, 1987. By permission, Mayo Foundation.)

Diagnostic accuracy is improved by the use of pulsed-wave Doppler mapping along the atrial septum, color Doppler echocardiography,[56] and echodetectable contrast material (indocyanine green and saline). Rapid intravenous injection of such a material during imaging of the atrial septum confirms a left-to-right shunt at the atrial level if there is negative washout of bubbles in the right atrium. Echoes moving from right atrium to left atrium confirm a right-to-left shunt.[57,58] Sinus venosus defects are the most difficult to visualize, but transesophageal echocardiography has improved the diagnostic yield[59,60] Right ventricular and pulmonary artery pressures can be reliably estimated by continuous-wave Doppler echocardiography when there is associated tricuspid regurgitation.

In ostium primum defect, the apical four-chamber view is superior for demonstrating the defect in the basal part of the atrial septum and the insertion of both septal portions of the AV valves at the same level to the crest of the ventricular septum (usually, the tricuspid valve inserts lower than the mitral valve). The parasternal short-axis view is best for identification and quantification of the cleft in the anterior mitral leaflet; in this view there is diastolic separation of the anterior mitral leaflet echoes (Fig 40-11).

Associated mitral regurgitation may be visualized by color Doppler echocardiography. Occasionally, the mitral valve leaflets may have attachments to a single papillary muscle—"parachute" mitral valve. Other associated lesions that may be visualized are subaortic stenosis, aneurysm of the membranous ventricular septum, and persistent left superior vena cava.

Transesophageal echocardiography has significantly improved the diagnostic yield of atrial septal defect. If right atrial or right ventricular size and right-sided volume overload are increased and the atrial septum is not well delineated on transthoracic echocardiography, transesophageal echocardiography will permit detailed visualization of the atrial septum. In addition, when a sinus venosus defect is present, the common association of anomalous right pulmonary vein can be delineated along with its entry site (usually into the superior vena cava or the superior vena cava-right atrial junction).

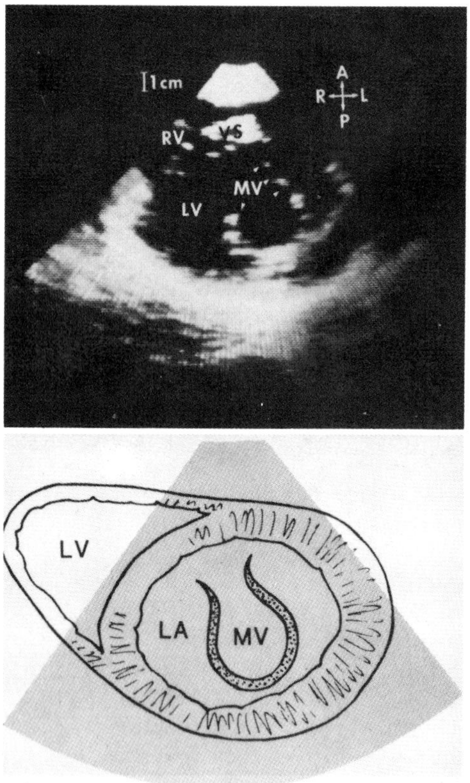

Fig 40-11 **Upper,** short-axis view obtained parasternally at level of mitral valve in patient with primum AV canal defect and cleft anterior mitral valve. Note abnormal motion of cleft mitral valve *(arrowheads).* **Lower,** drawing corresponding to ultrasonographic plane above. *A,* anterior; *L,* left; *LV,* left ventricle; *MV,* mitral valve; *P,* posterior; *R,* right; *RV,* right ventricle; *VS,* ventricular septum. (From Nasser FN, Giuliani ER: *Clinical Two-Dimensional Echocardiography.* Chicago, Year Book Medical Publishers, 1983, pp 229-254. By permission.)

DIAGNOSTIC PROBLEMS AND INDICATIONS FOR INVASIVE STUDIES

The diagnosis of atrial septal defect is sometimes overlooked in three clinical situations: (1) in older patients[61] in whom the most apparent presenting features are cardiomegaly (see Fig 40-7) and supraventricular arrhythmia, both easily misinterpreted as resulting from coronary or hypertensive heart disease or cardiomyopathy; (2) in patients with chronic obstructive pulmonary disease or obesity in whom the auscultatory and roentgenographic features of atrial septal defect are obscured by the pulmonary problem or thick chest wall; and (3) in patients in whom the diastolic flow murmur and right ventricular hypertrophy may suggest mitral stenosis, particularly if the delayed pulmonary component of the second heart sound is confused with an opening snap.

Conversely, an atrial septal defect is easily overdiagnosed in two clinical situations: (1) in young patients, mostly females with a thin chest, pectus excavatum, or straight back, in whom the second heart sound is widely split (this occurs only in the supine position), a pulmonary flow systolic murmur is easily heard, and the lung fields may show increased vascular pattern; and (2) in two groups of patients with left-to-right shunts who have clinical features of atrial septal defect, except that the widely split second heart sound is not fixed but varies with respiration—those who have systemic arteriovenous fistula whose peripheral continuous murmur has been overlooked and those with partial anomalous pulmonary venous connection and intact atrial septum.

With adequate two-dimensional echocardiographic imaging in conjunction with color Doppler study or injection of contrast material, the interatrial shunt and its physiologic consequences can be adequately documented. Cardiac catheterization appears indicated only in the following circumstances: (1) when inadequate noninvasive studies fail to demonstrate an atrial septal defect but show right ventricular volume overload without any other obvious cause (with transesophageal echocardiography, this situation is rare); (2) when there is associated mitral regurgitation but the degree of regurgitation is uncertain (this occurs in patients with ostium primum defects); (3) when features suggest pulmonary hypertension (see Fig 40-8) that could preclude surgery or compromise the surgical result; and (4) when associated coronary artery disease is suspected on clinical grounds and, therefore, coronary arteriography is justified.

At cardiac catheterization, the diagnosis may be readily confirmed by passage of the catheter across the atrial defect. The site at which the catheter crosses suggests the nature of the defect:[62] if high in the cardiac silhouette, a sinus venosus defect; if midseptal, a patent foramen ovale or ostium secundum defect; if low, an ostium primum defect. Prior to crossing the defect or in those instances in which the atrial septal defect cannot be crossed, the defect can be suspected when there is increased oxygen saturation of right atrial blood compared with blood from the superior and inferior venae cavae. An increase of 10% in oxygen saturation in one series of blood samples through the catheter or an increase of 5% in two series usually indicates an interatrial communication. A ventricular septal defect with insufficiency of the tricuspid valve, a left ventricular right atrial shunt, or a complete AV canal can produce similar findings. Anomalous connection of some or all of the pulmonary veins to the right atrium can result in arterialization of blood in the right atrium; accurate differentiation usually can be made by selective angiocardiography or from indicator dilution curves combined with the clinical assessment.[3]

Generally, right ventricular pressure is not increased, although as a result of the increased pulmonary flow, peak systolic gradients as high as 40 mm Hg across a normal pulmonic valve have been encountered. Pulmonary artery pressure usually is normal, as is the calculated pulmonary arterial resistance (less than 4 units · m^2). Studies of adult patients have documented a greater frequency of pulmonary hypertension and increased pulmonary artery resistance. The degree of increase in pulmonary artery resistance reflects the degree of pulmonary vascular obstruction and usually is mild to moderate; severe pulmonary vascular obstructive disease (pulmonary artery resistance greater than 7 units · m^2) is infrequent.[63]

Angiocardiography is rarely used for the diagnosis of atrial septal defect because echocardiography and cardiac catheterization are satisfactory diagnostic procedures. However, in ostium primum defects, the left ventricular angiogram during diastole demonstrates a narrowed outflow tract of the left ventricle, which is related to the deformed and abnormally attached opened anterior mitral leaflet (the gooseneck) (Fig 40-12), which is of diagnostic importance.[64,65] In atrial septal defect, angiocardiographic volume studies in young children have shown significant increases in right ventricular end-diastolic volume and right ventricular stroke index, with normal values for right ventricular ejection fraction.[66] However, studies in older children and adults have suggested decreases in right ventricular function.[67] In

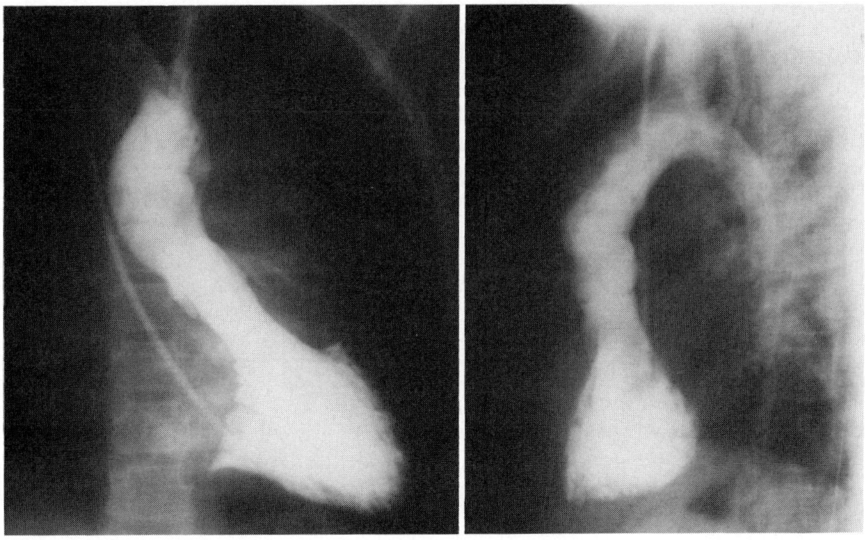

Fig 40-12 Frontal **(left)** and lateral **(right)** left ventriculograms of patient with partial AV canal. Frontal view shows elongation and narrowing of left ventricular outflow tract. Right side of ventricular silhouette is scalloped and indented, and this correlates with abnormal attachment of mitral valve. Lateral view shows intact ventricular septum on edge and confirms absence of interventricular shunting, as expected in this form of defect. (From Feldt RH, Edwards WD, Puga FJ, et al: Atrial septal defects and atrioventricular canal. In *Moss' Heart Disease in Infants, Children, and Adolescents.* Edited by FH Adams, GC Emmanouilides. Baltimore, Williams & Wilkins, 1983, pp 118-134. By permission.)

addition, a decrease in left ventricular stroke work has also been reported,[68] but this is considered to be rare.[69]

MANAGEMENT

Medical versus surgical treatment

Infective endocarditis is rare in patients with atrial septal defect, and therefore antibiotic coverage at the time of dental or surgical procedures is unnecessary unless there is associated mitral valve disease. Restriction of activity also is not necessary.

Operation is recommended for all patients with uncomplicated atrial septal defect of a size that produces clinical evidence of hemodynamic derangement (this occurs when the left-to-right shunt is 30% or greater), even if the patient has few or no symptoms. This approach is based on evidence that the hemodynamic derangement tends to progress,[35,70-74] whereas the operative risks are very low and the long-term results of operation are excellent.[35,75-77] Operative closure is recommended electively after diagnosis in children because the risk of operation would not be lessened by deferring operation, certain irreversible changes in the right atrium and ventricle and left ventricle could be avoided, and cardiovascular performance could be restored and enjoyed early rather than imposing suboptimal conditions for an extended period.

There are three clinical situations in which surgical closure of an atrial septal defect may be debatable: (1) the older patient in whom, as a result of age, surgical mortality may be increased; (2) the patient with associated mitral incompetence in whom mitral valve replacement may be required; (3) the patient with atrial septal defect and pulmonary hypertension in whom the surgical result may be poor. Regarding patients in the older age groups, from 1955 through 1978, 66 patients between the ages of 60 and 78 years underwent surgical repair of their atrial septal defect at our institution.[61] Eighteen patients had additional surgical procedures. There were four deaths—an operative mortality of 6%. If one excludes the operative deaths, survival curves for these patients are identical to those of persons matched for age and sex in the general population (Fig 40-13). By contrast, without operation, adults with atrial septal defect appear to die at an earlier age than do normal adults of the same age and sex.[35,61,70-72] Most importantly, despite some increase in the incidence of postoperative complications, most of the patients in this elderly population have very significant symptomatic and hemodynamic improvement postoperatively.[78] Thus, we advise closure of atrial septal defects, even in the older patient, unless there is some serious medical contraindication.

Regarding atrial septal defect and significant mitral incompetence when there is reason to believe that mitral valve replacement may be required, operative intervention may be postponed in the asymptomatic patient with good ventricular function. This conservative attitude is justified because of the higher surgical risk and the need for long-term anticoagulation if a prosthetic valve is used (in general, mitral valve repair can be accomplished without long-term need for anticoagulants).

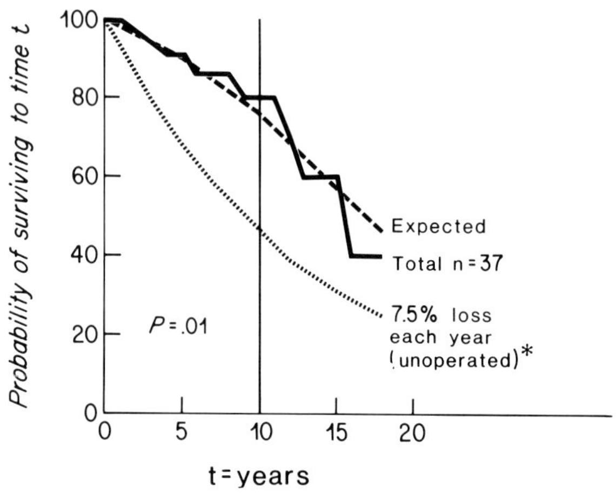

Fig 40-13 Long-term survival after closure of atrial septal defect in the elderly. Data from Campbell[70] and from St John Sutton et al.[61]

Finally, regarding pulmonary hypertension, from 1953 through 1978, 40 patients had isolated secundum atrial septal defect with total pulmonary resistance higher than 7 units · m^2.[63] In all patients, the pulmonary hypertension developed in adulthood between the third and fifth decades. Fourteen of these patients had medical treatment, 26 had surgical treatment, and all were followed for a mean of 12 years. The results supported the following conclusions: in patients with total pulmonary resistance between 7 and 14 units · m^2, surgical treatment is preferable; in patients with total pulmonary resistance greater than 14 units · m^2, medical treatment is preferable. In borderline situations (e.g., total pulmonary resistance of 12 to 15 units · m^2 and a systemic oxygen saturation value of 92% or greater), surgical treatment is favored. In patients in whom there is associated significant mitral regurgitation and venous hypertension, a high total pulmonary resistance—even higher than 14 units · m^2—is not a clear contraindication for surgical treatment. We may assume that part of the increased pulmonary resistance results from the venous hypertension and therefore is reversible. We have had success in some of these patients with this approach.

Surgical technique

Operation for secundum atrial septal defect is accomplished by using the standard approach and techniques of extracorporeal circulation, with one exception. For cosmetic reasons, in girls and young women it is acceptable to utilize a right anterolateral thoracotomy instead of a median sternotomy. The right atriotomy should avoid the region of the sinus node.

Closure of a secundm type of defect of the fossa ovalis may be by direct suture, especially in children or young adults in whom stretching and thinning of the atrial septum has not become marked and the muscular atrial septum at the perimeter of the fossa ovalis is well developed and sturdy. Almost always, the closure is by a continuous suture running parallel to the longitudinal axis of the body (Fig 40-14). If the septal defect is unusually large, leaving a rather narrow rim of intact septum, and if the remaining septum is stretched, thin, and wispy, it is best to close the defect with some type of synthetic or biologic patch. Elastic knitted polyester fiber (Dacron) is suitable (Fig 40-15). In closing the defect—whether by suture or with a patch—suturing, probing, retracting, or other trauma to the region of the sinus or AV node must be avoided.

When the right pulmonary veins connect to the right atrium in association with a secundum atrial septal defect, a patch is virtually always required, and the repair is almost as simple as that for isolated atrial septal defect. When the right pulmonary veins connect to the superior vena cava, they are usually veins draining the upper lobe,

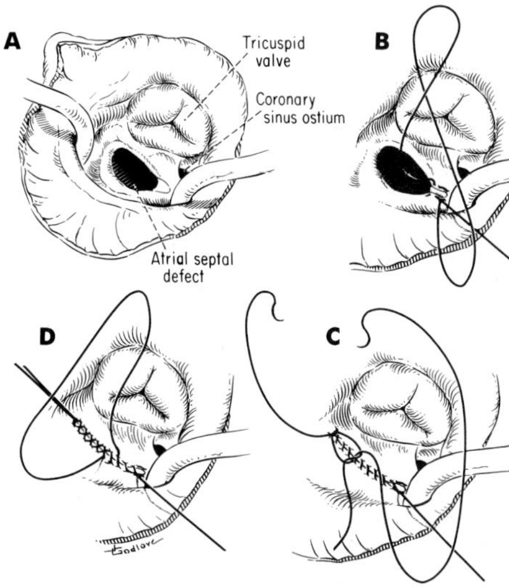

Fig 40-14 Direct closure of secundum atrial septal defect. A longitudinally oriented double-layer continuous suture approximates the margins of the secundum atrial septal defect. Inferiorly, the sutures grasp not only the flimsy remnants of the septum primum but also the muscular margins representing the septum secundum. (From Danielson GK: Surgical considerations in congenital heart disease. In *Cardiac and Vascular Diseases.* Vol 1. Edited by HL Conn Jr, O Horwitz. Philadelphia, Lea & Febiger, 1971, pp 686-746. By permission.)

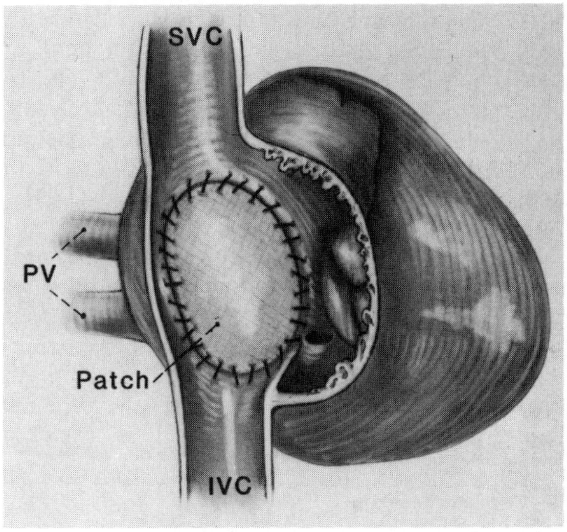

Fig 40-15 Patch closure of secundum atrial septal defect. *SVC*, superior vena cava; *IVC*, inferior vena cava: *PV*, pulmonary veins.

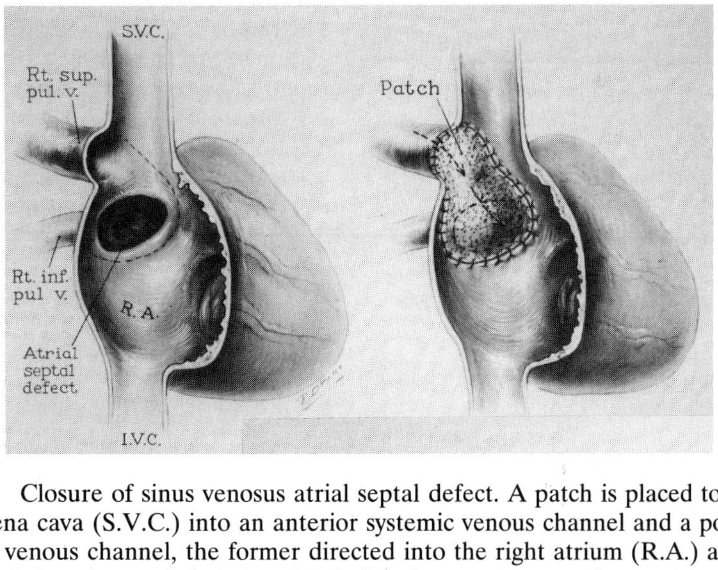

Fig 40-16 Closure of sinus venosus atrial septal defect. A patch is placed to divide the superior vena cava (S.V.C.) into an anterior systemic venous channel and a posterior pulmonary venous channel, the former directed into the right atrium (R.A.) and the latter into the left atrium. *inf.*, inferior; *I.V.C.*, inferior vena cava; *pul. v.*, pulmonary vein; *Rt.*, right; *sup.*, superior. (From Kirklin JW, Ellis FH Jr, Wood EH, et al: Treatment of anomalous pulmonary venous connections in association with interatrial communications. *Surgery* 39:389-398, 1956. By permission of CV Mosby Company.)

or upper and middle lobes, of the lung; usually, an atrial septal defect is present, and it typically lies superior to the fossa ovalis, between it and the orifice of the superior vena cava. This septal defect is the sinus venosus type. The vena cava is larger than normal because it carries both pulmonary and caval venous blood and can be partitioned, by a patch, into pulmonary and systemic venous flow pathways (Fig 40-16).

The rare coronary sinus type of atrial septal defect can be difficult to identify. Because it consists of a fenestration of the wall between the coronary sinus and the left atrium, the actual defect is not readily seen. Its presence can be verified by passing a probe or the end of a clamp through the ostium of the coronary sinus and through the fenestration into the left atrium. It can be closed either by incising the atrial septum and closing the fenestration from the left atrial side or by letting the fenestration remain open and simply closing the ostium of the coronary sinus. In the latter approach, myocardial venous effluent would be diverted to the left atrium, resulting in a small right-to-left intracardiac shunt; also, care must be taken to protect the AV node from harm.

Repair of the partial type of AV canal has two principal objectives: careful approximation and alignment of the edges of the cleft in the mitral valve, and closure of the ostium primum atrial septal defect with a patch (Fig 40-17). The aim is to close the cleft in such a way as to optimize the competence of the mitral valve. Fortunately, thickened ridges typically are present along the edges of the cleft, and these are of identical length, probably as a result of closure of these edges against each other during systole throughout life. It has been learned not only that accurate approximation of these ridges provides optimal alignment of the valve but also that the ridges themselves provide strength for the suture line. In instances in which incompetence of the valve has been minimal preoperatively and accurate orientation of the edges of the cleft does not seem possible, it may be best not to suture this cleft but to leave the mitral valve alone. In some hearts, mitral annuloplasty may be effective in decreasing the degree of persistent mitral regurgitation even after cleft repair. Almost never is mitral repair so unsuccessful that replacement of the mitral valve should be performed at the time of the primary repair. The interatrial communication is closed by a patch of pericardium or prosthetic material. This patch is attached to the junction of the mitral and tricuspid valves along the crest of the ventricular septum, with special care taken to avoid injury to the bundle of His near the junction of the ventricular septum and the posterior annulus of the AV valve.

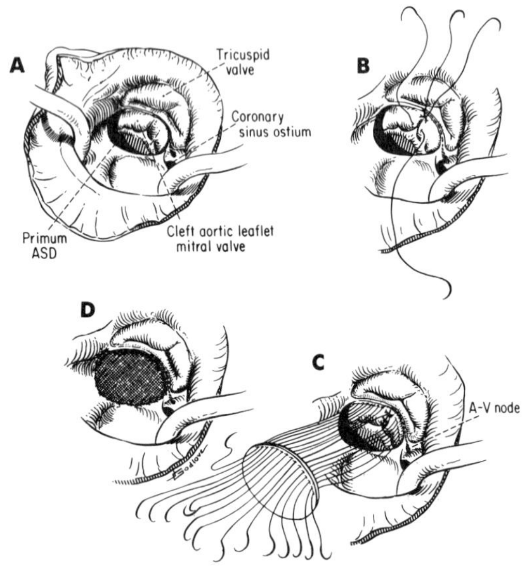

Fig 40-17 Repair of partial AV canal. **A,** surgical exposure through long atriotomy with wide mobilization of venous cannulae. **B,** beginning closure of cleft in anterior mitral leaflet. **C,** sutures placed between patch and junction of atrial and tricuspid valves for closure of ostium primum atrial septal defect *(ASD)*. **D,** repair completed. (From Danielson GK: Endocardial cushion defects. In *Pediatric Surgery.* Third edition, Vol. 1. Edited by MM Ravitch, KJ Welch, CD Benson, et al: Chicago, Year Book Medical Publishers, 1979, pp 720-726. By permission.)

During repair of any atrial septal defect, the possibility that air can find its way into the left heart to produce systemic air embolism is the most significant technical hazard. This can be avoided by discontinuing pulmonary ventilation as cardiopulmonary bypass is first begun, by cross-clamping the ascending aorta while the heart is open, and by providing continuous suction through a slotted needle tack vent in the most anterior surface of the ascending aorta.

Transcatheter closure of atrial septal defects has been investigated for several years, but thus far no definitive device or technique has been successful enough to be advocated.[79,80]

Postoperative course

The risk of death from elective repair of an uncomplicated ostium secundum atrial septal defect is less than 1%; it is slightly higher with ostium primum defects.[81] In a series of 79 consecutive operations for secundum atrial septal defect in patients 40 to 60 years old, no hospital deaths occurred.[75] Even among the 66 patients more than age 60, there were no hospital deaths except in 4 patients who required other procedures in addition to closure of the atrial septal defect, giving an overall risk of 6% in this elderly group.[61] Finally, 22 patients with atrial septal defect and moderate pulmonary hypertension (total pulmonary resistance between 7 and 14 units $\cdot$ m^2) underwent operation, with only two deaths.[63]

Late follow-up of patients who have survived closure of an atrial septal defect indicates that their life expectancy has been restored to approximately that of their age group, even in the elderly patients[61] (see Fig 40-13) and in the group with moderate pulmonary hypertension[63] (Fig 40-18). But most important, in all of these groups of patients there is an excellent symptomatic improvement postoperatively. The largest proportion is completely asymptomatic[35,61,63,75-77,81] (Fig 40-19). A residual left-to-right shunt is reported to occur in ap-

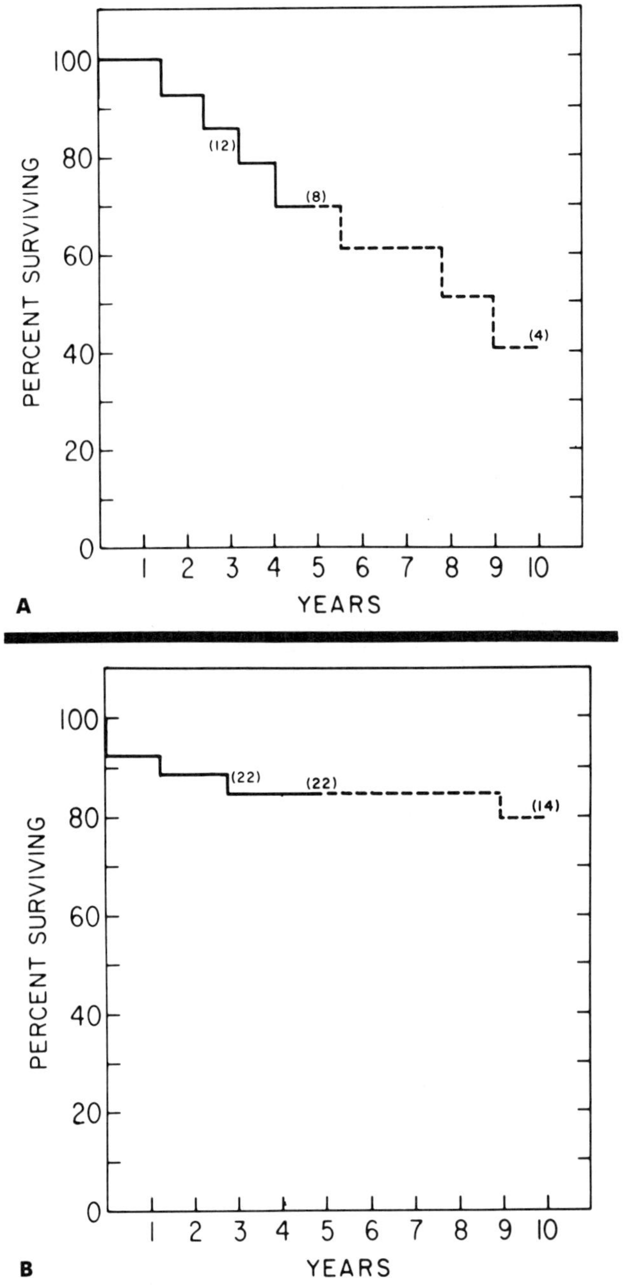

Fig 40-18 Observed survival to 10 years in 14 medically treated patients (**A**) and 26 surgically treated patients (**B**) with atrial septal defect and pulmonary vascular obstructive disease. Parentheses enclose number of living patients under observation at 3, 5 and 10 years. (From Steele PM, Fuster V, Cohen M, et al: Isolated atrial septal defect with pulmonary vascular obstructive disease—long-term follow-up and prediction of outcome after surgical correction. *Circulation* 76:1037-1042, 1987. By permission of American Heart Association.)

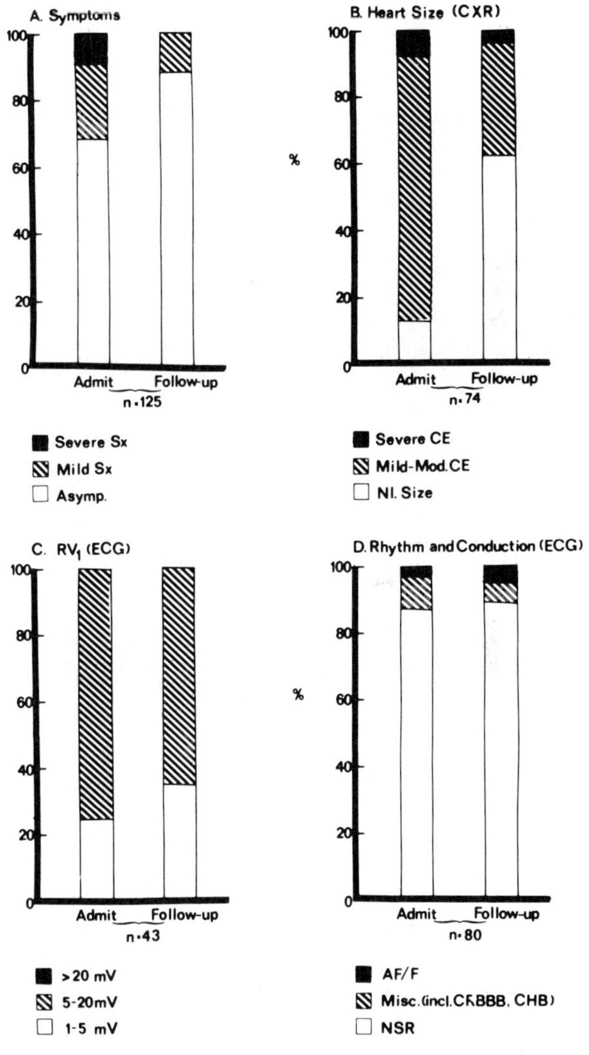

Fig 40-19 In patients seen at admission and again at follow-up at least 1 year after repair of the atrial septal defect, improvement is noted in symptoms and in heart size (**A** and **B**) but there is little change in the ECG (**C** and **D**). *Sx,* symptoms; *CXR,* chest radiograph; *CE,* cardiac enlargement; *Nl,* normal; *RV_1,* R wave in lead V_1; *ECG,* electrocardiogram; *AF/F,* atrial fibrillation or flutter; *CRBBB,* complete right bundle-branch block; *CHB,* complete heart block; *NSR,* normal sinus rhythm. (From Hamilton WT, Haffajee CI, Dalen JE, et al: Atrial septal defect secundum: clinical profile with physiologic correlates in children and adults. *Cardiovasc Clin* 10 No 1:267-277, 1979. By permission of FA Davis Company.)

proximately 5% to 10% of patients, although the degree of shunt tends to be small.[82] A long-term follow-up study (27 to 32 years) of 123 patients who underwent repair of an isolated secundum or sinus venosus defect suggested that patients operated on before age 25 have an excellent prognosis; older patients require careful, regular supervision.[83] Cardiorespiratory exercise capacity after surgical closure of atrial septal defect has been reported to be influenced by age at the time of operation, the best results occurring when surgery is performed in childhood.[84]

On auscultation a faint midsystolic ejection murmur, probably related to residual dilatation of the pulmonary artery, may be present in many patients after successful repair of the atrial septal defect.[82] A widely split, but not fixed, second heart sound, also probably related to residual dilatation of the pulmonary artery, can be detected in a few patients. Finally a murmur of mitral incompetence may be present in patients with associated mitral valve prolapse and frequently after repair of the cleft mitral valve; in a few of these patients, subsequent mitral valve replacement has been required.[85]

Regarding postoperative electrical abnormalities, right intraventricular conduction disturbance, with or without right ventricular hypertrophy, persists postoperatively (see Fig 40-19), although the decrease in the height of the R wave in lead V_1 suggests small involution of right ventricular hypertrophy;[35] in addition, in ostium primum defects the left-axis deviation persists. Although most patients are in normal sinus rhythm postoperatively, there is no evidence that preexisting arrhythmias are significantly ameliorated by operation, nor can it be stated that the operation prevents the late appearance of supraventricular arrhythmias.[35] In fact, significant supraventricular arrhythmias—in the form of sick sinus syndrome after repair of sinus venosus defects, paroxysmal atrial tachycardia, and atrial fibrillation-flutter—occur postoperatively in approximately 5% of the patients.[86] These arrhythmias may develop weeks, months, or even years after the operation.[77]

Radiographic evidence of cardiomegaly long after successful repair of an atrial septal defect has been noted in 20% to 30% of patients[35,87,88] (see Fig 40-19). In a large number of these patients the persistent enlargement appears to be due to failure of regression of the previously enlarged right ventricle and right atrium and thus is considered as myocardial dysfunction secondary to the preoperative right-sided volume overload[67,76] (see below). Persistent enlargement of the main pulmonary artery is usually seen even if the postoperative hemodynamic status is normal.[87]

Regarding ventricular function, residual right ventricular dilatation and dysfunction occur postoperatively in some of the patients, particularly in those older at the time of operation.[89,90] This can be attributed to the preoperative long-standing volume overload or, rarely, to some residual pulmonary hypertension.[63] There have been a few reports of occasional abnormal left heart function after operation;[91-93] this has been attributed to increasing filling of a previously "underloaded" left ventricle, to acquired disease (i.e., systemic hypertension or coronary disease), or to altered compliance of the left ventricle as a result of mechanical transmission of the enlarged right ventricle occasionally seen in patients operated on later in life.[67]

Thromboembolism causing cerebrovascular accidents or pulmonary embolism is a recognized but rare complication after closure of atrial septal defect; it is unrelated to the type of closure but may be related to the presence of atrial fibrillation.[94] It is our practice to anticoagulate all adult patients who have sustained atrial fibrillation after atrial septal defect closure.

The incidence of infective endocarditis does not appear to be increased after repair of atrial septal defects; therefore, antibiotic prophylaxis is considered unnecessary except in patients who have associated mitral valve prolapse or in those with ostium primum defects and residual mitral incompetence.[76]

The result of repair of partial AV canal (ostium primum defects) has been satisfactory throughout the experience with this operation. Repair of partial AV canal (ostium primum defects) in 47 of 52 adult patients ranging up to 57 years in age resulted in three operative deaths (6% operative mortality) and two late deaths.[81] Two patients required mitral valve replacement. All surviving patients were in New York Heart Association class I or II, and no patient required subsequent implantation of a permanent pacemaker. All four patients over 60 years of age survived operation and achieved continuing benefit from operation.[95] In an earlier study[96] of patients of all ages, the incidence of late deaths was found to be small, a fraction of 1% per year, and usually these deaths were related to arrhythmias or to the necessity for late mitral valve replacement.

REFERENCES

1. Perloff JK: *The Clinical Recognition of Congenital Heart Disease.* Second edition. Philadelphia, WB Saunders Company, 1978, pp 277-379
2. Fuster V, Brandenburg RO, McGoon DC, et al: Clinical approach and management of congenital heart disease in the adolescent and adult. *Cardiovasc Clin* 10 No 3:161-197, 1980
3. DuShane JW, Weidman WH, Brandenburg RO, et al: Differentiation of interatrial communications by clinical methods: ostium secundum, ostium primum, common atrium, and total anomalous pulmonary venous connection. *Circulation* 21:363-371, 1960
4. Swan HJC, Kirklin JW, Becu LM, et al: Anomalous connection of right pulmonary veins to superior vena cava with interatrial communications: hemodynamic data in eight cases. *Circulation* 16:54-66, 1957
5. Edwards JE, Carey LS, Neufeld HN, et al: *Congenital Heart Disease: Correlation of Pathologic Anatomy and Angiocardiography.* Vol 1. Philadelphia, WB Saunders Company, 1965, pp 191-234
6. Betriu A, Wigle ED, Felderhof CH, et al: Prolapse of the posterior leaflet of the mitral valve associated with secundum atrial septal defect. *Am J Cardiol* 35:363-369, 1975
7. Devereux RB, Perloff JK, Reichek N, et al: Mitral valve prolapse. *Circulation* 54:3-14, 1976
8. Schreiber TL, Feigenbaum H, Weyman AE: Effect of atrial septal defect repair on left ventricular geometry and degree of mitral valve prolapse. *Circulation* 61:888-896, 1980
9. Dubourg O, Bourdarias J-P, Farcot J-C, et al: Contrast echocardiographic visualization of cough-induced right to left shunt through a patent foramen ovale. *J Am Coll Cardiol* 4:587-594, 1984
10. Lechat P, Mas JL, Lascault G, et al: Prevalence of patent foramen ovale in patients with stroke. *N Engl J Med* 318:1148-1152, 1988
11. Warnes CA, Somerville J: Double mitral valve orifice in atrioventricular defects. *Br Heart J* 49:59-64, 1983

12. Davia JE, Cheitlin MD, Bedynek JL: Sinus venosus atrial septal defect: analysis of fifty cases. *Am Heart J* 85:177-185, 1973

13. Kittle CF, Crockett JE: Vena cava bronchovascular syndrome – a triad of anomalies involving the right lung: anomalous pulmonary vein, abnormal bronchi and systemic pulmonary arteries. *Ann Surg* 156:222-233, 1962

14. Mascarenhas E, Javier RP, Samet P: Partial anomalous pulmonary venous connection and drainage. *Am J Cardiol* 31:512-518, 1973

15. Joffe HS: Effect of age on pressure-flow dynamics in secundum atrial septal defect. *Br Heart J* 51:469-472, 1984

16. Pollick C, Sullivan H, Cujec B, et al: Doppler color-flow imaging assessment of shunt size in atrial septal defect. *Circulation* 78:522-528, 1988

17. Maillis MS, Cheng TO, Meyer JF, et al: Cyanosis in patients with atrial septal defect due to systemic venous drainage into the left atrium. *Am J Cardiol* 33:674-678, 1974

18. Massumi RA, Nutter DO: The syndrome of familial defects of heart and upper extremities (Holt-Oram syndrome). *Circulation* 34:65-76, 1966

19. Silverman ME, Copeland AJ Jr, Hurst JW: The Holt-Oram syndrome: the long and the short of it. *Am J Cardiol* 25:11-17, 1970

20. Bizarro RO, Callahan JA, Feldt RH, et al: Familial atrial septal defect with prolonged atrioventricular conduction: a syndrome showing the autosomal dominant pattern of inheritance. *Circulation* 41:677-683, 1970

21. Emanuel R, O'Brien K, Somerville J, et al: Association of secundum atrial septal defect with abnormalities of atrioventricular conduction or left axis deviation: genetic study of 10 families. *Br Heart J* 37:1085-1092, 1975

22. Nora JJ, McNamara DG, Fraser FC: Hereditary factors in atrial septal defect. *Circulation* 35:448-456, 1967

23. Hunt CE, Lucas RV Jr: Symptomatic atrial septal defect in infancy. *Circulation* 47:1042-1048, 1973

24. Holt M, Oram S: Familial heart disease with skeletal malformations. *Br Heart J* 22:236-242, 1960

25. Thiron J-M, Cribier A, Cazor J-L, et al: Variations in height of jugular "a" wave in relation to heart rate in normal subjects and in patients with atrial septal defect. *Br Heart J* 44:37-43, 1980

26. Parikh DN, Fisher J, Moses JW, et al: Determinants and importance of atrial pressure morphology in atrial septal defect. *Br Heart J* 51:473-479, 1984

27. Eddleman EE Jr, Holt JH, Bancroft WH Jr: Computer analysis of the kinetocardiogram from patients with atrial septal defects. *Am Heart J* 71:435-445, 1966

28. Leatham A: The second heart sound key to auscultation of the heart. *Acta Cardiol (Brux)* 19:395-416, 1964

29. Leatham A, Gray I: Auscultatory and phonocardiographic signs of atrial septal defect. *Br Heart J* 18:193-208, 1956

30. Shaver JA, O'Toole JD: The second heart sound: newer concepts. I. Normal and wide physiological splitting. *Mod Concepts Cardiovasc Dis* 46:7-12, 1977

31. Nadas AS, Ellison RC: Phonocardiographic analysis of diastolic flow murmurs in secundum atrial septal defect and ventricular septal defect. *Br Heart J* 29:684-688, 1967

32. Rees A, Farru O, Rodriguez R: Phonocardiographic, radiological, and haemodynamic correlation in atrial septal defect. *Br Heart J* 34:781-786, 1972

33. Brammell HL, Vogel JHK, Pryor R, et al: The Eisenmenger syndrome: a clinical and physiologic reappraisal. *Am J Cardiol* 28:679-692, 1971

34. Perloff JK: Auscultatory and phonocardiographic manifestations of pulmonary hypertension. *Prog Cardiovasc Dis* 9:303-340, 1967

35. Hamilton WT, Haffajee CI, Dalen JE, et al: Atrial septal defect secundum: clinical profile with physiologic correlates in children and adults. *Cardiovasc Clin* 10 No 1:267-277, 1979

36. Anderson PAW, Rogers MC, Canent RV Jr, et al: Atrioventricular conduction in secundum atrial septal defects. *Circulation* 48:27-31, 1973

37. Pryor R, Woodwark GM, Blount SG Jr: Electrocardiographic changes in atrial septal defects: ostium secundum defect versus ostium primum (endocardial cushion) defect. *Am Heart J* 58:689-700, 1959

38. Levin AR, Haft JI, Engle MA, et al: Intracardiac conduction intervals in children with congenital heart disease: comparison of His bundle studies in 41 normal children and 307 patients with congenital cardiac defects. *Circulation* 55:286-294, 1977

39. Björnstad PG: Secundum type atrial septal defect with prolonged PR interval and autosomal dominant mode of inheritance. *Br Heart J* 36:1149-1154, 1974

40. Pease WE, Nordenberg A, Ladda RL: Familial atrial septal defect with prolonged atrioventricular conduction. *Circulation* 53:759-762, 1976

41. Lee Y-C, Scherlis L: Atrial septal defect: electrocardiographic, vectorcardiographic, and catheterization data. *Circulation* 25:1024-1041, 1962

42. Burch GE, DePasquale, NP: *Electrocardiography in the Diagnosis of Congenital Heart Disease.* Philadelphia, Lea & Febiger, 1967

43. Boineau JP, Spach MS, Ayers CR: Genesis of the electrocardiogram in atrial septal defect. *Am Heart J* 68:637-651, 1964

44. Moore EN, Boineau JP, Patterson DF: Incomplete right bundle-branch block: an electrocardiographic enigma and possible misnomer. *Circulation* 44:678-687, 1971

45. Toscano-Barbosa E, Brandenburg RO, Burchell HB: Electrocardiographic studies of cases with intracardiac malformations of the atrioventricular canal. *Proc Staff Meet Mayo Clin* 31:513-523, 1956

46. Boineau JP, Moore EN, Patterson DF: Relationship between the ECG, ventricular activation, and the ventricular conduction system in ostium primum ASD. *Circulation* 48:556-564, 1973

47. Feldt RH, DuShane JW, Titus JL: The atrioventricular conduction system in persistent common atrioventricular canal defect: correlations with electrocardiogram. *Circulation* 42:437-444, 1970

48. Goodman DJ, Harrison DC, Cannom DS: Atrioventricular conduction in patients with incomplete endocardial cushion defect. *Circulation* 49:631-637, 1974

49. Tan K-T, Takao A, Hashimoto A, et al: Electrocardiogram of secundum type atrial septal defect simulating endocardial cushion defect. *Br Heart J* 37:209-215, 1975

50. Morgan BC, Ricketts HJ, Winterscheid LC: Inferior clockwise frontal plane forces in a child with endocardial cushion defect. *Am Heart J* 82:275-276, 1971

51. Elliott LP, Schiebler GL: *X-Ray Diagnosis of Congenital Cardiac Disease.* Springfield, Illinois, Charles C Thomas, Publisher, 1968

52. Keats TE, Rudhe U, Foo GW: Inferior vena caval position in the differential diagnosis of atrial and ventricular septal defects. *Radiology* 83:616-621, 1964

53. Wood P: The Eisenmenger syndrome or pulmonary hypertension with reversed central shunt. *Br Med J* 2:701-709; 755-762, 1958

54. Massumi RA, Alwan AO, Hernandez TJ, et al: The scimitar syndrome: a physiologic explanation for the associated dextroposition of the heart, maldevelopment of the right lung and its artery, and for the systemic collateral supply to the lung. *J Thorac Cardiovasc Surg* 53:623-633, 1967

55. Dillon JC, Weyman AE, Feigenbaum H, et al: Cross-sectional echocardiographic examination of the interatrial septum. *Circulation* 55:115-120, 1977

56. Khanderia BK, Shub C, Tajik AJ, et al: Utility of color flow imaging for visualizing shunt flow in atrial septal defect. *Int J Cardiol* 23:91-98, 1989

57. Seward JB, Tajik AJ, Hagler DJ, et al: Peripheral venous contrast echocardiography. *Am J Cardiol* 39:202-212, 1977

58. Weyman AE, Wann LS, Caldwell RL, et al: Negative contrast echocardiography: a new method for detecting left-to-right shunts. *Circulation* 59:498-505, 1979

59. Morimoto K, Matsuzaki M, Tohma Y, et al: Diagnosis and quantitative evaluation of atrial septal defect by transesophageal 2-D color Doppler echocardiography (abstract). *Circulation* 76 Suppl 4:39, 1987

60. Kronzon I, Tunick PA, Freedberg RS, et al: Transesophageal echocardiography is superior to transthoracic echocardiography in the diagnosis of sinus venosus atrial septal defect. *J Am Coll Cardiol* 17:537-542, 1991

61. St John Sutton MG, Tajik AJ, McGoon DC: Atrial septal defect in patients ages 60 years or older: operative results and long-term postoperative follow-up. *Circulation* 64:402-409, 1981

62. Taketa RM, Sahn DJ, Simon AL, et al: Catheter positions in congenital cardiac malformations. *Circulation* 51:749-757, 1975

63. Steele PM, Fuster V, Cohen M, et al: Isolated atrial septal defect with pulmonary vascular obstructive disease – long-term follow-up and prediction of outcome after surgical correction. *Circulation* 76:1037-1042, 1987

64. Baron MG, Wolf BS, Steinfeld L, et al: Endocardial cushion defects: specific diagnosis by angiocardiography. *Am J Cardiol* 13:162-175, 1964

65. Rastelli GC, Kirklin JW, Titus JL: Anatomic observations on complete form of persistent common atrioventricular canal with special reference to atrioventricular valves. *Mayo Clin Proc* 41:296-308, 1966

66. Graham TP Jr, Jarmakani JM, Atwood GF, et al: Right ventricular volume determinations in children: normal values and observations with volume or pressure overload. *Circulation* 47:144-153, 1973

67. Graham TP Jr: Ventricular performance in adults after operation for congenital heart disease. *Am J Cardiol* 50:612-620, 1982

68. Levin AR, Liebson PR, Ehlers KH, et al: Assessment of left ventricular function in secundum atrial septal defect: evaluation by determination of volume, pressure and external systolic time indices. *Pediatr Res* 9:894-899, 1975

69. St John Sutton MG, Tajik AJ, Mercier L-A, et al: Assessment of left ventricular function in secundum atrial septal defect by computer analysis of the M-mode echocardiogram. *Circulation* 60:1082-1090, 1979

70. Campbell M: Natural history of atrial septal defect. *Br Heart J* 32:820-826, 1970

71. Adams CW: A reappraisal of life expectancy with atrial shunts of the secundum type. *Dis Chest* 48:357-375, 1965

72. Craig RJ, Selzer A: Natural history and prognosis of atrial septal defect. *Circulation* 37:805-815, 1968

73. Dave KS, Pakrashi BC, Wooler GH, et al: Atrial septal defect in adults: clinical and hemodynamic results of surgery. *Am J Cardiol* 31:7-13, 1973

74. Markman P, Howitt G, Wade EG: Atrial septal defect in the middle-aged and elderly. *Q J Med* 34:409-426, 1965

75. Danielson GK, McGoon DC: Surgical considerations in treating adults with congenital heart disease. *Cardiovasc Clin* 10 No 1:543-561, 1979

76. Rahimtoola SH, Kirklin JW, Burchell HB: Atrial septal defect. *Circulation* 38 Suppl 5:2-12, 1968

77. McNamara DG, Latson LA: Long-term follow-up of patients with malformations for which definitive surgical repair has been available for 25 years or more. *Am J Cardiol* 50:560-568, 1982

78. Harjula A, Kupari M, Kyösola K, et al: Early and late results of surgery for atrial septal defect in patients aged over 60 years. *J Cardiovasc Surg* 29:134-139, 1988

79. Lock JE, Cockerham JT, Keane JF, et al: Transcatheter umbrella closure of congenital heart defects. *Circulation* 75:593-599, 1987

80. Sideris EB, Sideris SE, Fowlkes JP, et al: Transvenous atrial septal defect occlusion in piglets with a "buttoned" double-disk device. *Circulation* 81:312-318, 1990

81. Hynes JK, Tajik AJ, Seward JB, et al: Partial atrioventricular canal defect in adults. *Circulation* 66:284-287, 1982

82. Gersony WM, Krongrad E: Evaluation and management of patients after surgical repair of congenital heart diseases. *Prog Cardiovasc Dis* 18:39-56, 1975

83. Murphy JG, Gersh BJ, McGoon MD, et al: Long-term outcome after surgical repair of isolated atrial septal defect: follow-up at 27 to 32 years. *N Engl J Med* 323:1645-1650, 1990

84. Reybrouck T, Bisschop A, Dumoulin M, et al: Cardiorespiratory exercise capacity after surgical closure of atrial septal defect is influenced by the age at surgery. *Am Heart J* 122:1073-1078, 1991

85. Feldt RH, Edwards WD, Puga FJ, et al: Atrial septal defects and atrioventricular canal. In *Moss' Heart Disease in Infants, Children, and Adolescents*. Third edition. Edited by FH Adams, GC Emmanouilides. Baltimore, Williams & Wilkins, 1983, pp 118-134

86. Clark DS, Hirsch HD, James DM, et al: Electrocardiographic changes following surgical treatment of congenital cardiac malformations. *Prog Cardiovasc Dis* 17:451-465, 1975

87. Young D: Later results of closure of secundum atrial septal defect in children. *Am J Cardiol* 31:14-22, 1973

88. Amplatz K, Formanek A, Knight L, et al: Radiographic changes in the postoperative patient. *Prog Cardiovasc Dis* 17:403-438, 1975

89. Pearlman AS, Borer JS, Clark CE, et al: Abnormal right ventricular size and ventricular septal motion after atrial septal defect closure: etiology and functional significance. *Am J Cardiol* 41:295-301, 1978

90. Liberthson RR, Boucher CA, Strauss HW, et al: Right ventricular function in adult atrial septal defect: preoperative and postoperative assessment and clinical implications. *Am J Cardiol* 47:56-60, 1981

91. Flamm MD, Cohn KE, Hancock EW: Ventricular function in atrial septal defect. *Am J Med* 48:286-294, 1970

92. Davies H, Oliver GC, Rappaport WJ, et al: Abnormal left heart function after operation for atrial septal defect. *Br Heart J* 32:747-753, 1970

93. Popio KA, Gorlin R, Teichholz LE, et al: Abnormalities of left ventricular function and geometry in adults with atrial septal defect: ventriculographic, hemodynamic and echocardiographic studies. *Am J Cardiol* 36:302-308, 1975

94. Hawe A, Rastelli GC, Brandenburg RO, et al: Embolic complications following repair of atrial septal defects. *Circulation* 39 Suppl 1:185-191, 1969

95. Hynes JK, Tajik AJ, Seward JB, et al: Partial atrioventricular canal defect in elderly patients (aged 60 years or older). *Am J Cardiol* 50:59-62, 1982

96. McMullan MH, McGoon DC, Wallace RB, et al: Surgical treatment of partial atrioventricular canal. *Arch Surg* 107:705-710, 1973

CHAPTER

41

Ventricular septal defect

Carole A. Warnes, M.D., Valentin Fuster, M.D., David J. Driscoll, M.D., and Dwight C. McGoon, M.D.

ANATOMIC CONSIDERATIONS

Isolated ventricular septal defect is one of the most common forms of congenital heart disease encountered in infants and children, with an incidence of 1.5 to 2.5 per 1,000 live births.[1,2] A ventricular septal defect may be found as an integral part of another anomaly, such as tetralogy of Fallot or pulmonary atresia; but in this chapter, only isolated ventricular septal defect is discussed.

Isolated ventricular septal defects can occur in different anatomic locations, and there is still some debate about the ideal nomenclature. About 75% of defects are located in the membranous septum, closely related to the aortic valve, and may be called "perimembranous," with the prefix "peri" underscoring the variable extension into the adjacent portions of the muscular septum.[3] This descriptive term, however, includes different types of ventricular septal defects with difficult natural histories, making inclusion under one heading unattractive to clinicians. Similarly, a proposed classification based entirely on echocardiographic findings does not appear to be of practical advantage.[4] A simple classification relating the defect to the contiguous valve—subvalvular—or its site in the muscular septum may be used[5] (Fig 41-1). Subvalvular ventricular septal defects lie beneath atrioventricular (AV) valves or semilunar valves, or both, without any interposed muscle tissue between the hole and the valve cusps, which form a border or limiting boundary. Defects are thus described as subaortic, subpulmonary, doubly committed subarterial (subpulmonary and subaortic), subtricuspid, and inlet (lying beneath the septal leaflets of both AV valves and extending posteriorly close to the crux). Muscular defects are those bordered by muscle and not immediately related to AV or semilunar valves. They may be classified according to their position in the muscular septum and may be apical, central, or outlet (in the outflow tract of the right ventricle). Muscular defects are occasionally multiple, producing a septum resembling Swiss cheese.

An important point is the frequent spontaneous closure of ventricular septal defects of both types, subvalvular and muscular.[6-11] It has been estimated that 40% of ventricular septal defects close in infancy, and about 60% do so by age 5; occasionally, spontaneous closure occurs in older children or even adults. However, the larger the initial defect, the less likely is spontaneous closure—that is, although initially large defects can close spontaneously, when the pulmonary arterial pressure is near the systemic pressure the rate of spontaneous closure is probably less than 5%.[12,13] Spontaneous closure of a ventricular septal defect occasionally can be associated with the develop-

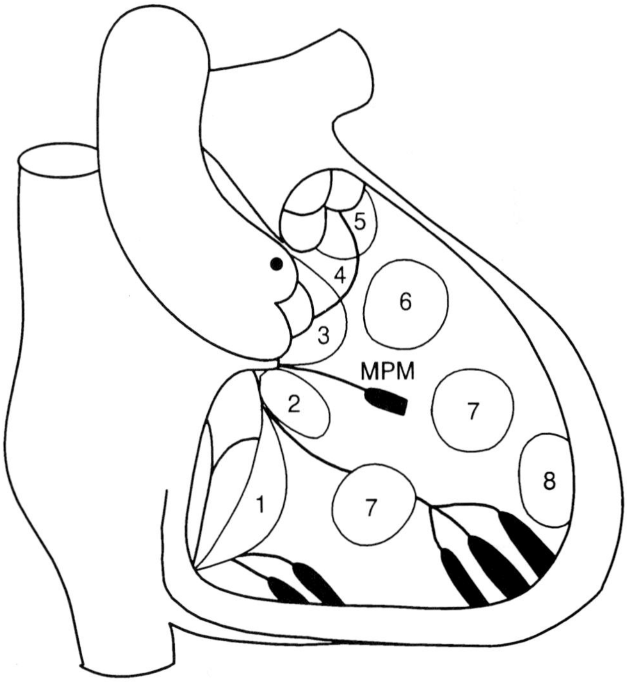

Fig 41-1 Anatomic diagram illustrating the position of ventricular septal defects. *1* to *5,* subvalvular; *6* to *8,* muscular. *1,* inlet; *2,* subtricuspid; *3,* subaortic; *4,* subarterial doubly committed; *5,* subpulmonary; *6,* outlet; *7,* central; *8,* apical. *MPM,* medial papillary muscle. (From Capelli H, Andrade JL, Somerville J: Classification of the site of ventricular septal defect by 2-dimensional echocardiography. *Am J Cardiol* 51:1474-1480, 1983. By permission of Cahners Publishing Company, a Division of Reed Publishing USA.)

ment of a blind septal aneurysm, usually without ill effect.[14,15]

PATHOPHYSIOLOGY

The primary variable that determines the physiologic state of the patients is the size of the defect. With a small or medium-sized defect, the size limits the magnitude of the left-to-right shunt. However, with a large defect—that is, approximately the size of the aortic orifice—there is essentially no resistance to flow across the opening, and the relative resistance offered by the systemic and pulmonary circulations regulates the magnitude of flow across the defect.[16]

Age is another important variable. With the child's early growth, the size of the defect can decrease relative to the body surface, and the defect even may close. After birth, the small muscular pulmonary arteries of the normal infant change from a small lumen and a thick medial muscle layer to thin-walled structures with increased lumen size. The rate of decrease in pulmonary vascular resistance that accompanies these changes is such that the right ventricular pressure is approximately at adult levels within 7 to 10 days after birth.[17,18] During the first few months of life, pulmonary vascular resistance usually decreases gradually, so that in patients with ventricular septal defect there is augmentation of the left-to-right shunt. After the first year of life, the fate of the pulmonary vascular resistance depends mainly on the size of the ventricular septal defect; it tends to increase in patients in whom the defect remains large.

In adolescents and adults, ventricular septal defect usually presents in one of three different forms: as a small septal defect without significant left-to-right shunt or hemodynamic derangement; as a large defect with secondary severe pulmonary vascular obstructive disease and with cyanosis as a result of a right-to-left shunt; or as a large defect with a large left-to-right shunt that has induced secondary infundibular pulmonary stenosis, leading to an anatomic-clinical syndrome difficult to differentiate from acyanotic or cyanotic tetralogy of Fallot.

Small ventricular septal defects. These are defined as defects whose size imposes a high resistance to flow with a resultant large pressure difference between the two ventricles during ventricular systole, a small left-to-right shunt ($Qp/Qs < 1.5$), normal right heart pressures (normal ratio of pulmonary artery pressure [PAP] to systemic arterial pressure [SP]), and essentially normal work characteristics of the ventricles.[16] There is little or no tendency for an increase in pulmonary vascular resistance. The pressure is greater in the left ventricle throughout the cardiac cycle and can result in a continuous left-to-right shunt across the defect. However, usually only a holosystolic murmur throughout ventricular systole can be heard associated with the large pressure gradient across the defect (Fig 41-2); the absence of a murmur during diastole, although flow continues across the defect, is most likely related to the lack of turbulence due to the small quantity of blood being shunted at this time.[16] The majority of these small defects close in the first 3 years of life.

Medium-sized ventricular septal defects. Although large enough to permit a moderate-to-large shunt ($Qp/Qs = 1.5\text{-}2$), these defects are small enough to offer some resistance to flow and therefore result in a lower peak systolic pressure in the right ventricle than in the left ventricle ($PAP/SP \leq 0.5$). There is considerable variation in the size of the defect in this group; however, in these patients the area of the defect generally is less than 1 cm^2/m^2 of body surface area.[16,19] It is unusual for this group to have a marked increase in pulmonary vascular resistance; most have moderate to large left-to-right shunts, with volume overload of the left atrium and left ventricle and left ventricular hypertrophy. Right ventricu-

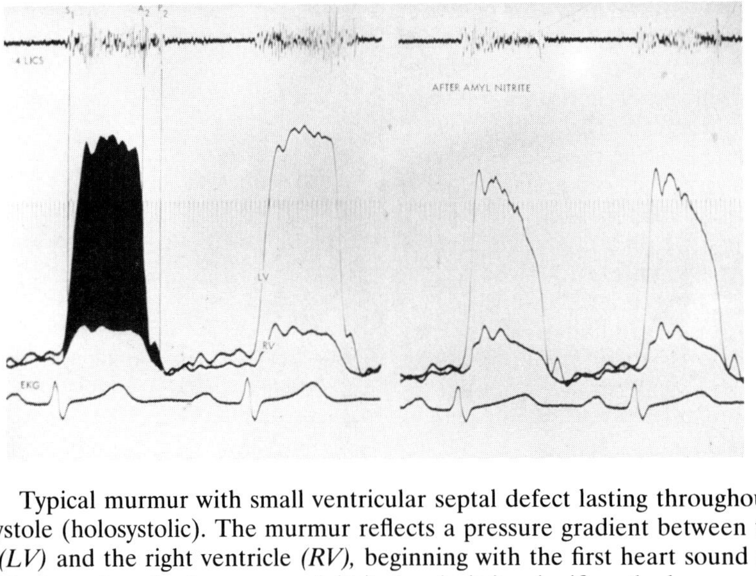

Fig 41-2 Typical murmur with small ventricular septal defect lasting throughout ventricular systole (holosystolic). The murmur reflects a pressure gradient between the left ventricle *(LV)* and the right ventricle *(RV)*, beginning with the first heart sound (S_1) and ending with the pulmonic closure sound (P_2). Amyl nitrite significantly decreases the intensity of the murmur (see text). A_2, aortic component of second heart sound.

lar systolic work and muscle mass vary according to the increase in right ventricular pressure. Because of the significant left-to-right shunt, and therefore the increased return to the left heart, the holosystolic murmur of ventricular septal defect is associated with a mitral flow middiastolic murmur and a left ventricular filling sound (third heart sound). In addition, the left-to-right shunt and left-sided volume overload can produce radiographic evidence of left ventricular enlargement and a pattern of increased pulmonary flow as well as electrocardiographic (ECG) evidence of left ventricular hypertrophy. In infants these medium-sized ventricular septal defects are associated with a moderate-to-large shunt. As the child becomes larger, the relative size and degree of shunt become smaller. This is why these moderate-sized defects are not seen frequently in adults—either they become small or they close in the first few years of life.[20]

Large ventricular septal defects. Ventricular septal defects are considered large when their area is greater than 1 cm^2/m^2 of body surface area; these approximate the size of the aortic orifice. Because of the nonrestrictive or nearly nonrestrictive character of the defect, blood is ejected into the systemic and pulmonary circuits at nearly the same pressure, so that pulmonary hypertension at nearly systemic pressure is obligatory[21] (PAP/SP > 0.5). Because of the normal tendency for gradual decrease in pulmonary vascular resistance within the first 3 months of life, a large left-to-right shunt (Qp/Qs > 2) ensures a large volume overload of the left ventricle, which may result in its failure. In addition, these large defects produce not only the clinical findings described for the moderate-sized types but also evidence of pulmonary hypertension.

With the exception of a few patients in whom the defect spontaneously closes, patients with unrepaired large defects die or, as adolescents or adults, present with severe pulmonary vascular obstructive disease or with secondary protective infundibular pulmonary stenosis. In the group with severe pulmonary vascular obstructive disease, the left-to-right shunt tends to decrease and to become a right-to-left shunt; this conversion is apt to result in cyanosis, disappearance of the murmurs related to the left-to-right shunt, and, most importantly, appearance of clinical evidence of severe pulmonary hypertension, the so-called Eisenmenger's complex.[22] Secondary significant infundibular pulmonary stenosis can also result in a decrease of the left-to-right shunt or even in shunt reversal and cyanosis; both the acyanotic and cyanotic stages are clinically indistinguishable from tetralogy of Fallot.[23]

CLINICAL SYNDROME

History and clinical course

The clinical state of the patient depends primarily on the size of the defect, the state of pulmonary vascular resistance, and the changes in these two variables with age.[8,16,20,23,24] Another important variable is the site of the ventricular septal defect, which may also determine whether the defect will close spontaneously. Defects in the muscular septum frequently close or get smaller, as do subtricuspid defects, which are often closed by the septal cusp of the tricuspid valve. It has been reported that in patients with follow-up from birth, as many as 45% of ventricular septal defects close spontaneously.[11] In contrast, subaortic defects do not usually close spontaneously, because the superior border is the aortic valve. Small subpulmonary defects (also known as "supracristal defects") may be manifested by aortic regurgitation, because the right coronary cusp prolapses into the defect.

Small ventricular septal defects. The clinical course is benign throughout infancy and childhood. In those patients in whom spontaneous closure of the defect does not occur, the only danger is endocarditis, and this is rarc before the age of 2 years.

Medium-sized ventricular septal defects. Although common in infancy, such defects are rarely seen in adolescents and adults. Less rare, however, is the adolescent or adult who presents with a moderate left-to-right shunt. This is related either to a large ventricular septal defect partially occluded by the septal leaflet of the tricuspid valve[25] or to a large ventricular septal defect that has led to an "acquired" protective moderate infundibular pulmonary stenosis.[26] Because of the moderate left-to-right shunt with increased congestion of the lungs, these patients may present with some exertional dyspnea in contrast with those who have small defects.

Large ventricular septal defects. In patients with large defects, from age 1 to 12 months severe symptoms are due primarily to left ventricular failure secondary to the large left-to-right shunt. The initial symptoms consist of tachypnea, excessive sweating due to increased sympathetic tone, and fatigue when feeding. The history usually describes an infant who has these symptoms beginning usually during the first month and progressing in severity as the pulmonary vascular resistance decreases. However, some infants with large defects do not normally have a decrease in pulmonary vascular resistance in the first few months of life and so develop only mild to moderate left-to-right shunting and no evidence of left ventricular failure. Most infants in whom left ventricular failure develops improve with medical therapy; hypertrophy of the left ventricle, enabling this chamber to handle large flows, probably accounts for some of this improvement.

In addition, between 6 and 24 months of age, relief of symptoms is associated with a gradual decrease in the magnitude of the left-to-right shunt, as a result of various factors: (1) There may be a decrease in size or spontaneous closure of the defect; however, this occurs only rarely in these large defects. (2) Progressive increase in the pulmonary vascular resistance may lead to pulmonary vascular obstructive disease; this is by far the most frequent natural course of the large defects. (3) Occasionally, a protective hypertrophy of the outflow tract of the right ventricle develops and produces obstruction in this area. Such obstruction may be mild or moderate, in which case the patient may present in adolescence or adulthood with a moderate left-to-right shunt (as with medium-sized ventricular septal defect). Most commonly, the obstruction is severe and a tetralogy of Fallot type of clinical syndrome develops.[23]

The natural course of the large defects makes it clear

that these patients must be studied hemodynamically within the first year of life. It is at this age that they commonly begin to develop significant pulmonary vascular obstructive disease, and, unless surgical correction is then offered, they usually soon become inoperable.[20] In fact, because the progression of the pulmonary vascular obstructive disease leads to a decrease in the left-to-right shunt, after age 12 to 24 months, the majority of these patients may be asymptomatic except for frequent respiratory infections. It is in adolescence or early adulthood that the pulmonary vascular obstructive disease becomes so severe that a right-to-left shunt ensues and cyanosis becomes apparent – the Eisenmenger complex. Incidentally, the term "Eisenmenger's syndrome" is used to indicate any defect that allows free communication between the pulmonary and systemic circuits with a predominant right-to-left shunt secondary to a marked increase in pulmonary vascular resistance.[16] Chest pain resembling angina, exertional syncope, hemoptysis, cerebral thrombosis related to high hematocrit value, and cerebral abscess related to paradoxic septic emboli all have been described.[14,27,28] Death commonly occurs in the third decade, although exceptional patients may reach the fifth or, rarely, the seventh decade.[29,30] Death can be sudden, and its risk is particularly high in pregnant women with this disease.[31]

Physical findings

Isolated ventricular septal defect in adolescents and adults usually presents in one of three forms: a small defect without significant hemodynamic derangement; a large defect with secondary severe pulmonary vascular obstructive disease and with cyanosis as a result of right-to-left shunt; and a large defect with secondary infundibular pulmonary stenosis, which is difficult to differentiate from acyanotic or cyanotic tetralogy of Fallot. The physical findings are quite different in the three different forms.[14,16]

Small ventricular septal defects. Because the hemodynamic derangement is mild, adolescents and adults with small defects have a healthy physical appearance. Arterial and venous pulses are normal. On palpation the apical impulse is normal; a systolic thrill is usually palpable along the left sternal border, unless the defect is very small. Apart from this thrill, auscultation provides the pathognomonic and sole physical finding of this mild condition – a loud holosystolic murmur that can be plateau, crescendo, or crescendo-decrescendo and is localized in the low left sternal border. Unlike that in most cases of mitral regurgitation, the murmur of ventricular septal defect has high-frequency components well heard with the diaphragm of the stethoscope and some components of lower frequency that give it a characteristic harsh quality. The aortic component of the second heart sound (A_2) may be masked by the loud vibrations that end with the pulmonic closure sound (P_2) (see Fig 41-2).

In patients with muscular defects or very small defects, there may be short murmurs that cut off in midsystole, presumably because of closure of the defect by systolic contraction of septal musculature. On the other hand, the unusual patient who presents in adolescence or adulthood with a medium-sized defect or moderate left-to-right shunt may have, in addition to the holosystolic murmur, a third heart sound and a short early middiastolic rumble, both resulting from the increased left-sided volume overload. Also, for the same reason, such patients have a hyperdynamic precordium detectable on palpation. Finally, in the unusual supracristal type of ventricular septal defect, the murmur is maximal in the second or first left intercostal space.

Large ventricular septal defect with pulmonary vascular obstructive disease. Within the first 2 years of life, patients with large ventricular septal defects present with the clinical features resulting from the large volume overload of the left ventricle. After age 2, patients with these large defects usually develop progressive pulmonary vascular obstructive disease; therefore, they usually present in adolescence or adulthood with these features – the physical findings of pulmonary hypertension associated with some left-to-right and right-to-left shunts.

PHYSICAL APPEARANCE. Patients usually have poor growth and development, and the left anterior thorax may bulge outward because of the years of left ventricular hyperdynamic enlargement early in life. Fewer than 5% of the patients have the features of Down's syndrome. When the shunt is reversed, symmetric cyanosis and clubbing appear; the degree of cyanosis varies from trivial to marked and generally worsens with effort and the passage of time.

ARTERIAL AND VENOUS PULSES. The arterial pulse is usually normal. The jugular venous pulse pressure may be elevated due to right ventricular failure; the jugular "a" wave may be prominent because of decreased compliance due to right ventricular hypertrophy. In some patients, large jugular systolic v waves may be apparent because of tricuspid regurgitation resulting from the high right ventricular pressure. Nevertheless, in many patients the jugular venous pressure and pulse may be relatively normal – that is, the right ventricle may be able to cope with the pulmonary hypertension by reason of its hypertrophy and the decompressing effect of the septal defect.

PRECORDIAL PALPATION. In early childhood, large ventricular septal defects with large left-to-right shunts result in volume overload and a palpable dilated and dynamic left ventricle. In contrast, in adolescence or adulthood the pulmonary vascular obstructive disease results in significant decrease of the left-to-right shunt, and therefore the left ventricular impulse is trivial or absent. Instead, as a result of right ventricular hypertrophy, the right ventricular impulse becomes palpable in the xiphoid region, although it is relatively quiet because of the decompressing effect of the septal defect. A dilated hypertensive pulmonary trunk is often palpated, together with a long pulmonic component of the second heart sound.

AUSCULTATION. When the pulmonary vascular obstructive disease tends to abolish the significant left-to-right shunt, the holosystolic murmur of ventricular septal defect vanishes and auscultatory signs of pulmonary hypertension prevail. Flow into the dilated pulmonary trunk causes a pulmonic ejection sound. This is followed by a short, soft, midsystolic murmur in the second left interspace. The second heart sound is quite loud because of the pulmonic component. Very commonly, it is single because the right and left ventricles, which are in communication, may reach an equilibrium in overload and performance that leads to simultaneous closure of both semilunar valves.[32] Quite often, the loud second heart sound is closely followed by a high-frequency diastolic murmur of pulmonary incompetence (Graham Steell's murmur), which is due to dilatation of the pulmonic valve ring as a result of the pulmonary hypertension.

Large ventricular septal defect with acquired infundibular pulmonary stenosis. In a few patients with large ventricular septal defects, progressive "acquired" infundibular stenosis may develop from the time of infancy and may range from a mild type to, most commonly, a severe type.[23,26,33-37] Accordingly, the physical findings in adolescence or adulthood may range from those of a large ventricular septal defect with pulmonary vascular obstructive disease when the stenosis is mild and nonprotective to those of a tetralogy of Fallot when the stenosis is severe.

Electrocardiogram

With a small ventricular septal defect, the ECG usually is normal; however, a few patients with small defects demonstrate an rsr′ in lead V_1. In the unusual patients who present in adolescence or adulthood with a medium-sized defect or moderate left-to-right shunt, the ECG may show evidence of left ventricular hypertrophy and volume overload reflected in leads V_5 and V_6 by tall R waves, deep narrow Q waves, and tall, peaked T waves;[38-40] in addition, mild right ventricular hypertrophy may be evident in lead V_1, as reflected by an rsR′ pattern.[14]

In adolescent or adult patients with large ventricular defects and pulmonary vascular obstructive disease, evidence of left ventricular hypertrophy is usually absent because the volume work by the left ventricle is essentially normal. In such patients, the most important ECG feature is the presence of an rsR′ pattern or, more commonly, a tall monophasic R wave in the right precordial leads, reflecting significant right ventricular hypertrophy[14,16] (Fig 41-3). Reciprocal changes tend to occur in the left precordial leads, with the R waves diminishing and the S waves becoming deeper. Marked right-axis deviation with deep S waves in lead I, II, or III is common. Finally, peaked or tall P waves are uncommon, analogous to the normal jugular venous "a" wave in these patients.[14]

In patients with a large ventricular septal defect and acquired significant infundibular pulmonary stenosis, the ECG shows the pattern of right ventricular hypertrophy. That is, it is similar to the ECG of patients with tetralogy of Fallot (see chapter 49) and to the ECG described in patients with large ventricular septal defect and pulmonary vascular obstructive disease (see Fig 41-3).

Chest radiograph

The chest radiograph also is a useful mirror of the hemodynamic disturbance in isolated ventricular septal defect. With a small ventricular septal defect, it usually shows normal heart size and normal pulmonary vascularity; occasionally, patients who had a large communication in infancy that subsequently became small may have slight residual cardiomegaly.[14] In the unusual patients who present in adolescence or adulthood with a medium-sized defect or moderate left-to-right shunt, the chest radiograph may show slight cardiomegaly and increased pulmonary vascular markings in both the central and the peripheral portions of the lung fields.

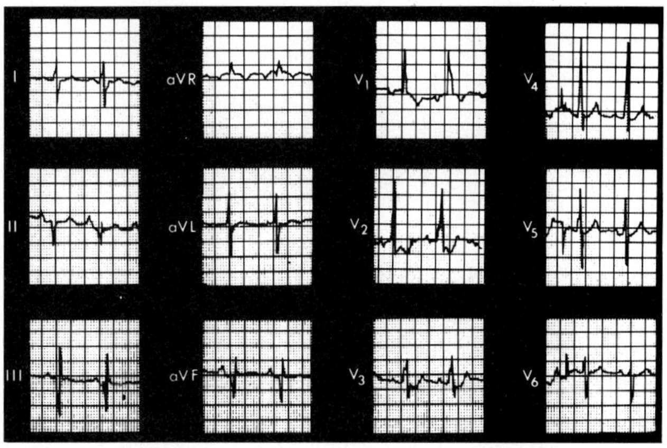

Fig 41-3 Electrocardiogram of 25-year-old woman with ventricular septal defect complicated by pulmonary vascular obstructive disease. Note prominent and monophasic R wave in the right precordial leads, deep S wave in the left precordial leads, and marked right-axis deviation with deep S waves in the standard leads, suggesting severe right ventricular hypertrophy. (From Fuster V, Danielson GK: Congenital heart disease in the adult. In *Office Management of Medical and Surgical Heart Disease: A Concise Guide for Physicians.* Edited by LI Bonchek, HL Brooks. Boston, Little, Brown & Company, 1981, pp 183-217. By permission.)

In adolescent and adult patients with large ventricular septal defects and pulmonary vascular obstructive disease, the cardiac size is normal or nearly normal, because the left ventricular overload and hypertrophy of early life have partially or totally regressed. Characteristically, the apex is tilted upward, reflecting right ventricular hypertrophy, particularly of the outflow tract (Fig 41-4). Most importantly, in the lung fields, centrally the pulmonary trunk and its main branches are markedly dilated whereas in the outer third there is an abrupt decrease in vascularity—the "pruning effect."[41] This disparity between the central and the peripheral pulmonary vascularity is typical of all types of pulmonary hypertension secondary to pulmonary vascular obstructive disease.

In patients with a large ventricular septal defect and acquired significant infundibular pulmonary stenosis, the chest radiograph may be indistinguishable from that in tetralogy of Fallot (see chapter 49)—that is, cardiac size and shape as in patients with right ventricular hypertrophy secondary to pulmonary vascular obstructive disease but with lung fields revealing decreased vascularity both centrally and peripherally.

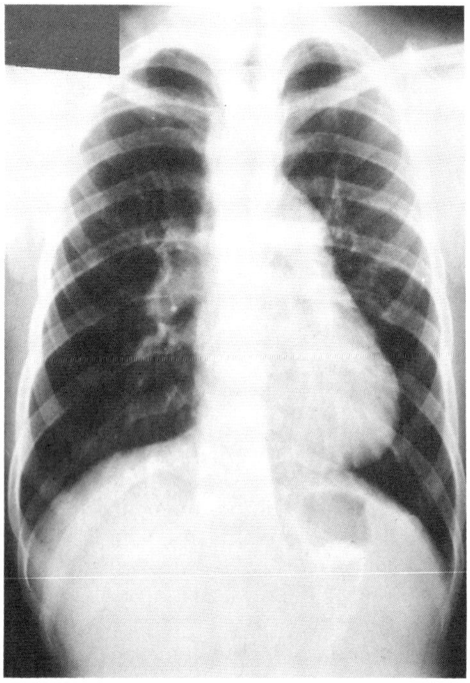

Fig 41-4 Chest radiograph of 22-year-old man with ventricular septal defect complicated by pulmonary vascular obstructive disease. Note nearly normal cardiac size with apex tilted upward, marked dilatation of central pulmonary arteries, and decreased peripheral pulmonary vascularity. (From Fuster V, Danielson GK: Congenital heart disease in the adult. In *Office Management of Medical and Surgical Heart Disease: A Concise Guide for Physicians.* Edited by LI Bonchek, HL Brooks. Boston, Little, Brown & Company, 1981, pp 183-217. By permission.)

Echocardiogram

Two-dimensional echocardiography is extremely useful for visualization of defects (Fig 41-5), and with pulsed-wave and color Doppler examination, the sensitivity with experienced echocardiographers may be 90%.[42,43] The continuous-wave Doppler velocity across the defect can also be measured to provide an estimate of interventricular pressure gradient and, thus, to provide a noninvasive determination of right ventricular and pulmonary artery pressure in patients with an isolated ventricular septal defect.[44,45] The sensitivity of color Doppler echocardiography is less accurate in patients with multiple ventricular septal defects when pressures in the two ventricles are similar, because small amounts of interventricular shunting through small muscular defects may be missed. This is particularly true in small infants.[46]

The size of the ventricular septal defect may be estimated on the basis of findings from echocardiography. The width of the jet on color-flow imaging roughly correlates with defect size. Computer analysis of the color-flow jet, examining the proximal isovelocity surface area, may become a method to directly calculate shunt volume. Volumetric flow analysis by pulsed-wave Doppler study can be used to estimate Qp/Qs. Other indirect findings, such as right ventricular size, pulmonary artery size, and tricuspid regurgitation velocity (for calculation of right ventricular systolic pressure), provide further information about shunt size.

DIAGNOSTIC PROBLEMS AND INDICATIONS FOR INVASIVE STUDIES

The wide range of clinical manifestations and complex lesions associated with ventricular septal defects can cause confusion in some cases. Here we will discuss first the diagnostic problems of the three most common types of presentation in adolescents and adults.

Small ventricular septal defects. This presentation can be confused with three clinical conditions.

1. Mild pulmonary valvular stenosis. However, this condition always has distinguishing auscultatory features. The murmur of pulmonary stenosis is heard best at the upper left sternal border and radiates toward the left clavicle; inhalation of amyl nitrite results in an early increase in venous return and makes the murmur of pulmonary stenosis louder, whereas in ventricular septal defect the murmur becomes softer because the peripheral dilating effects of this drug decrease the left-to-right shunt (see Fig 41-2). In pulmonary stenosis, the second heart sound is widely split, and there is an ejection systolic click. In some patients with small ventricular septal defect, a septal aneurysm develops, which results in an early to midsystolic click that can lead to further confusion with pulmonary valvular stenosis.
2. Occasional patients with mild mitral incompetence have only a murmur best heard close to the sternum, and this may be difficult to distinguish from the murmur of a small ventricular septal defect.
3. Hypertrophic obstructive cardiomyopathy may be confused with small ventricular septal defect, although the increased loudness of the murmur after the Valsalva maneuver or inhalation of amyl nitrite, the ECG pattern of hypertrophy, and the specific echocardiographic features all distinguish the two conditions.

Therefore, despite the differential signs described above, on some occasions we are not able to clearly distinguish among small ventricular septal defect, mild pulmonary valvular stenosis, and mild mitral incompetence. Echocardiography permits differentiation of these lesions, so that cardiac catheterization usually is unnecessary.

Large ventricular septal defects with severe pulmonary vascular obstructive disease. The clinical features can be similar to those exhibited by patients with pulmonary hypertension secondary to the other types of systemic-pulmonary communication or by patients with primary pulmonary hypertension. Because the long-term prognosis depends on the underlying cause of the pulmonary hypertension, we think that cardiac catheterization is indicated to verify the diagnosis and to quantitate the pulmonary vascular disease. In addition, the

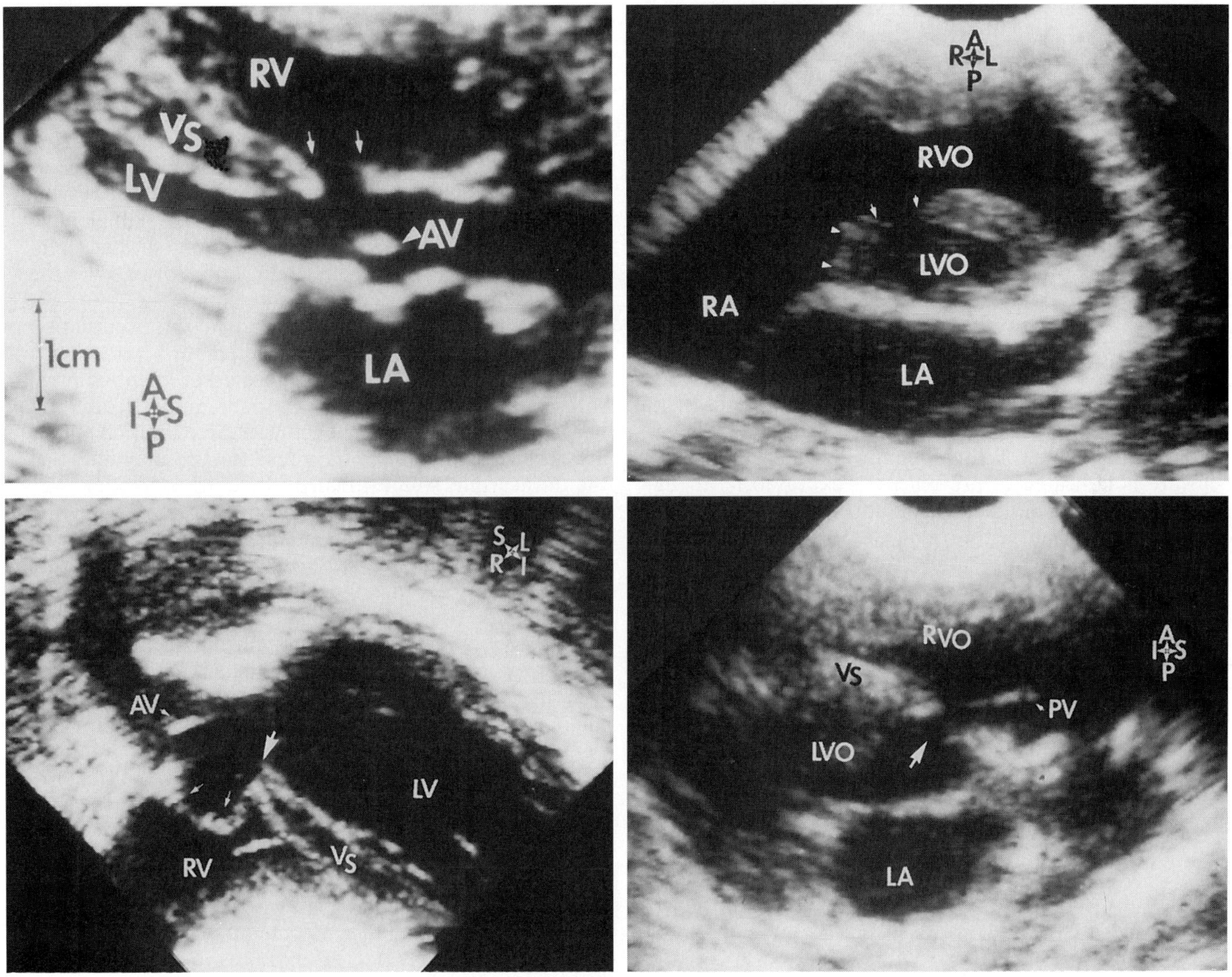

Fig 41-5 Two-dimensional echocardiographic views of ventricular septal defects. **A,** parasternal long-axis scan with slight medial tilt of the transducer. A large membranous ventricular septal defect *(arrows)* is visualized just beneath the aortic valve *(AV)*. **B,** parasternal short-axis scan at the level of the left ventricular outflow tract *(LVO)* shows a ventricular septal defect that is subtricuspid *(arrows)* and partially closed by the septal leaflet of the tricuspid valve *(arrowheads)*. **C,** subcostal four-chamber scan at aortic valve level demonstrating an aneurysm of the membranous septum *(small arrows)*. A large membranous ventricular septal defect is visualized *(large arrow)*. This patient had a very small left-to-right shunt. **D,** parasternal short-axis scan showing a ventricular septal defect *(large arrow)* that is subpulmonary. These defects are also called "outflow" or "supracristal" defects. *A,* anterior; *I,* inferior; *L,* left; *LA,* left atrium; *LV,* left ventricle; *P,* posterior; *PV,* pulmonary valve; *R,* right; *RA,* right atrium; *RV,* right ventricle; *RVO,* right ventricular outflow tract; *S,* superior; *VS,* ventricular septum. (From Seward JB, Tajik AJ, Edwards WD, et al: *Two-Dimensional Echocardiographic Atlas.* Vol. 1. *Congenital Heart Disease.* New York, Springer-Verlag, 1987, p. 377. By permission, Mayo Foundation.)

cyanotic patient occasionally has another type of congenital defect that is amenable to surgical repair but has been missed clinically and echocardiographically. This emphasizes the need for cardiac catheterization in most patients who have clinical evidence of severe pulmonary hypertension, unless the underlying cause is obvious.

Large ventricular septal defects with infundibular pulmonary stenosis. These cases are indistinguishable from tetralogy of Fallot and, therefore, the clinical and diagnostic approaches are similar to those discussed for that condition.

Left ventricular to right atrial shunt. The rare entity of a congenital shunt from left ventricle to right atrium[47] may be confused with a ventricular septal defect, although it may be distinguished by a systolic v wave in the venous pulse and a murmur that is transmitted to the right and upward.

Ventricular septal defect and aortic regurgitation. Ventricular septal defects beneath the aortic valve produce prolapse of the aortic cusp, which may cause significant aortic regurgitation in childhood.[23,48-50] Although the defects are frequently small, prophylactic closure is indicated to prevent progressive aortic regurgitation.[51] For patients in whom aortic regurgitation has already developed, closure of the defect with aortic valvuloplasty can be accomplished with low mortality and significant reduction in aortic regurgitation.[50]

Summary. For the appropriate management of adolescents and adults with isolated ventricular septal defects, we consider cardiac catheterization to be justified in all cases except those that meet the clinical criteria for small defects. It is important to emphasize that all patients who presumably have large defects detected after birth should be studied within the first year of life; this may lead to appropriate surgical management at that early age, prior to the onset of complicating pulmonary vascular obstructive disease. Cardiac catheterization at infancy will document the presence of the defect or defects, the magnitude of shunting across the defect (Qp/Qs), the pulmonary and systemic pressures (PAP/SP), the pulmonary vascular resistance (Rp), and the workload of the two ventricles as assessed by the intracardiac shunting and pressures. At this early age, with Rp not yet increased, evaluation of Qp/Qs and PAP/SP usually is sufficient to assess the size of the defect. In addition, cardiac catheterization at this early age will document or rule out the presence of associated defects.

The exact approach for obtaining all of this information is discussed in chapter 10A. In brief, first right heart catheterization is performed with measurement of pressures and oxygen saturation in the pulmonary circuit, right heart, and femoral artery. Then, indicator-dilution curves are recorded to confirm the presence and magnitude of the intracardiac shunt. Finally, left ventricular cineangiocardiography is performed to localize more precisely the site (Fig 41-6) and number of ventricular septal defects (important information for the surgeon if operation is required). Bargeron et al.[52,53] at the University of Alabama developed a long-axis oblique view that has proved to be very useful in visualizing the ventricular septum, in accurately delineating the size and number of defects, and in evaluating the left ventricular outflow

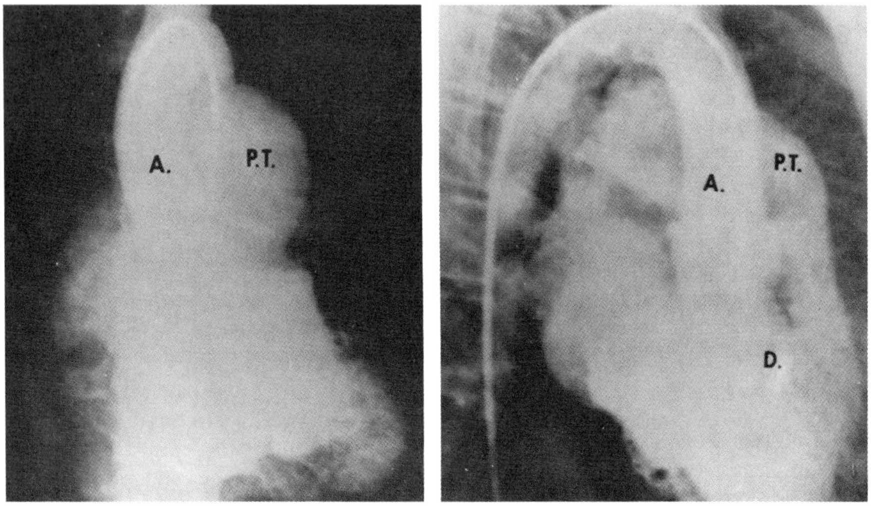

Fig 41-6 Selective left ventriculogram, frontal **(left)** and lateral **(right)** views. The tip of the catheter is positioned in the left ventricle. The contrast agent passes through the ventricular septal defect *(D.)* into the outflow tract of the right ventricle and thence into the pulmonary trunk *(P.)*. Contrast agent also opacifies the aorta *(A.)*. In the lateral view the crista supraventricularis is represented by the irregular island of radiolucency lying immediately above the defect. Therefore, the defect lies immediately inferior to the crista supraventricularis (membranous type of defect). (From Edwards JE, Carey LS, Neufeld HN, et al: *Congenital Heart Disease: Correlation of Pathologic Anatomy and Angiocardiography.* Vol. 1. Philadelphia, WB Saunders Company, 1965, pp 81-122. By permission.)

tract. In patients with a diastolic murmur suggesting aortic incompetence, an aortogram is required for detection and estimation of the degree of aortic incompetence.

Cardiac catheterization later in childhood, in adolescence, and in adulthood will document the presence of the defect, and, if the defect is large, the presence of secondary infundibular pulmonary stenosis or pulmonary vascular obstructive disease. The degree of pulmonary vascular obstructive disease must be known for the appropriate management of the patient. It can be assessed by estimating the total pulmonary vascular resistance (PAP/Qp) or, even more accurately, the pulmonary arteriolar resistance ([PAP − left atrial pressure]/Qp).

MANAGEMENT

Medical versus surgical treatment

Management of an isolated ventricular septal defect requires accurate diagnosis of the defect and evaluation of the physiologic variables. It also depends on the age of the patient. Particularly in the case of an infant or child, detailed communication with the parents is important because they should be informed of the implications of repeated evaluations and the clinical courses that can ensue. Management is simplest for the child with a small defect—follow-up with emphasis on the continuing benign nature of the defect and reassurance to the family that the child should be raised in a normal manner except for the use of antibiotic prophylaxis at the time of dental or surgical procedures.

To understand the few indications for surgical closure of a ventricular septal defect in adolescence or adulthood, it is essential to understand the pros and cons of the operation. In general terms, although patients who have an isolated ventricular septal defect usually are candidates for operative closure of the defect, judgment is required in determining the advisability and timing of operation in individual cases.[54,55] The reasons for this include the fact that small ventricular septal defects often will close spontaneously over the course of months or years. Even if spontaneous closure does not occur, the ill effects of a small ventricular septal defect may not warrant the risk and other disadvantages of surgical intervention. Another factor of importance has been the record of greater risk of operative closure of the defect in early infancy than at 1 or 2 years of age.[54,56,57] Finally, the proper timing of operation is significantly influenced by the observation that the progression and irreversibility of pulmonary vascular obstructive changes are closely related to the age of the patient.[58]

From the interplay of these considerations, a general plan of management for the infant with a ventricular septal defect can be formulated. The diagnosis now is usually recognized within the first months of life and confirmed by cardiac catheterization. Thus, if the ventricular septal defect is sufficiently large to allow near equalization of ventricular pressures (PAP/SP $\geq$ 0.75), operation is urgently indicated whenever cardiac failure occurs and is not responsive to medical management. The reason is that the risk of hospital death from closing the ventricular septal defect in infancy, which is between 10% and 20%, is lower than the risk of continued uncontrollable cardiac failure. Some surgical teams may still favor banding of the pulmonary artery in this setting for the infant,[59] but the trend is clearly toward closure of the defect.[60] If cardiac failure can be controlled medically or has not developed, careful observation is indicated, with repeat cardiac catheterization by 12 to 15 months of age; if PAP/SP remains $\geq$ 0.75, surgical closure of the ventricular septal defect is advised. This is because delay in closure of the defect may result in progressive pulmonary vascular obstructive disease, and then closure of the defect at an older age might not prevent progressive increase in pulmonary vascular resistance postoperatively. Furthermore, additional delay would not be expected to decrease the risk of operation further (about 2% by age 18 to 24 months), and also the likelihood of spontaneous closure of such a large defect after this age would be remote.

If repeat catheterization at 12 to 15 months of age suggests that the defect is becoming smaller (PAP/SP has become $<$ 0.75), further postponement of operation is advisable. The reasons are that the likelihood of progressive development of pulmonary vascular obstructive disease is more remote in the presence of decreasing pulmonary hypertension and that because the defect has become relatively smaller, it is likely to continue to diminish in size.

Similarly, if at the original diagnostic catheterization the PAP/SP was found to be $<$ 0.75 and cardiac failure did not appear or was well controlled, operation would be postponed.

These two groups of patients having PAP/SP $<$ 0.75 from the beginning or after 15 months should be followed clinically. If there are no signs of changing hemodynamic status, repeat catheterization can be deferred until about age 4 years. At that time, even with PAP/SP $\leq$ 0.5, operative closure of the ventricular septal defect is considered to be advisable if a large pulmonary blood flow is present (Qp/Qs = 1.5-2). This is because the hemodynamic burden is significant and may handicap the growing child or cause irreversible left ventricular changes and because the defect is of moderate size and is not showing evidence of progressive closure. If Qp/Qs is 1.3 to 1.5, further observation is warranted because of the remaining hope that progressive closure could yet occur. If Qp/Qs $<$ 1.3, operation probably can be avoided altogether, and spontaneous closure would be considered likely.

With the passage of time, fewer adult or nearly adult patients with a large or moderately large ventricular septal defect will be appearing for care, because they will have been operated on at an earlier age. However, those older patients who do appear can be placed in one of the following categories:

1. Small ventricular septal defect with PAP/SP about normal and Qp/Qs $<$ 1.3. Operation is believed unnecessary in these cases, because the hemodynamic burden is slight and the risk of infective endocarditis is less than the small risk of operation.[61] If Qp/Qs is between about 1.3 and 1.5, the situation is borderline, and judgments must be individualized.
2. Medium-sized ventricular septal defect or moderate

left-to-right shunt (PAP/SP $\leq$ 0.5 and Qp/Qs 1.5 to 2). This is rarely seen in adolescents and adults. Operation is advisable for the same reasons as those for the medium-sized defects detected in childhood.

3. Large ventricular septal defect with PAP/SP > 0.75 but with small Qp/Qs due to significant pulmonary vascular obstructive disease judged by Rp > 7 units · m^2. Classically, cases have been defined as inoperable when Rp exceeds 10 units · m^2. However, we observed that in patients more than 3 years old, Rp of 7 to 10 units · m^2 does not necessarily predict a good surgical result.[29] Operation is not recommended for this group of patients with high Rp because of high operative and late mortality rates and persistence of severe pulmonary hypertension postoperatively.[62] Furthermore, lung biopsy does not appear to add much to the prognostic value of the pulmonary vascular resistance obtained at catheterization.[63] Cardiopulmonary transplantation is the only therapeutic option in these patients with advanced pulmonary vascular obstructive disease.
4. Large ventricular septal defect with acquired significant infundibular pulmonary stenosis. In this situation with hemodynamics resembling those in tetralogy of Fallot, the principles of surgical management are similar to those in tetralogy of Fallot (see chapter 49).

See chapter 61 for a discussion of inoperable cases with severe pulmonary vascular obstructive disease and right-to-left shunt (cyanosis in the Eisenmenger syndrome).

Transcatheter closure of ventricular septal defects

As the list of successful transcatheter closures of various congenital cardiac defects expands, attempts are being made to close ventricular septal defects with these devices. Although closure has been successfully accomplished,[64] most ventricular septal defects cannot be managed with this technique or a modification of it, particularly those close to the membranous septum, where the umbrella device probably would interfere with the aortic or tricuspid valve (or both). Whether these devices will in the future have a place in the closure of muscular defects, however, remains to be evaluated.

Surgical technique

Standard techniques of open heart surgery are used except that, in infants, profound systemic hyperthermia and intermittent circulatory arrest may be useful. The cardiac approach may be via a right ventriculotomy, a right atriotomy, or even a left ventriculotomy in the case of one or more apically situated muscular septal defects. The choice among these approaches must be individualized, depending upon the location of the defect and the preference of the surgeon. Defects located in the vicinity of the membranous ventricular septal defect often can be satisfactorily closed via a right atriotomy[65,66] by retracting the septal and anterior leaflets of the tricuspid valve. This is even true of many posterior septal defects, which are tucked under the septal leaflet.

For a ventricular septal defect of the conal septum (supracristal type), the transatrial approach is not appropriate, and a high right ventriculotomy is required. When a right ventriculotomy is required, it should be kept as short as possible and should avoid as many epicardial coronary branches as possible. It should be placed over the outflow tract rather than over the trabeculated portion of the ventricle as much as possible. With recognition of these preferences, it becomes inconsequential whether

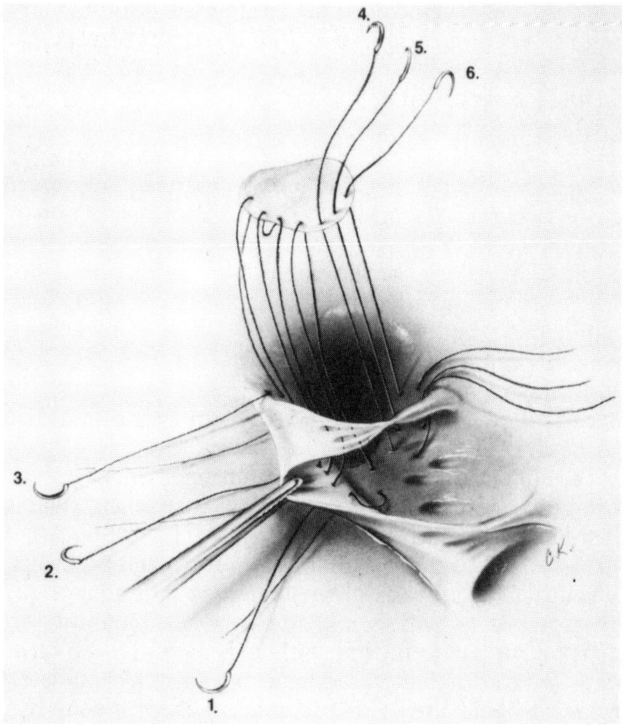

Fig 41-7 The authors' technique for closure of a typical ventricular septal defect by using a patch. The patient's head is to the left; upward in the illustration corresponds to an anterior location. The forceps are retracting the septal leaflet of the tricuspid valve so as to expose the critical posteroinferior angle of the ventricular septal defect. Note that the base of the septal leaflet is being attached to the posterior rim of the patch. Suture 1 is perhaps the most critical in avoiding the bundle of His; it sandwiches the patch between the right surface of the ventricular septum at the posteroinferior angle of the ventricular septal defect and the base of the septal leaflet. Suture 2 anchors the posterior rim of the patch to the base of the septal leaflet, and suture 3 represents the transition from the attachment of the patch to the base of the septal leaflet to attachment to the muscle of the superior rim of the defect. Sutures 4, 5, and 6 attach the inferior rim of the patch to the right surface of the ventricular septum, the sutures being placed somewhat shallowly in the ventricular septum to avoid encirclement of the bundle of His. The subsequent sutures that will attach the patch to the anterior half of the rim of the defect can be placed deeply and securely because they will be remote from the conduction bundle.

the ventriculotomy is oriented transversely or longitudinally.

The great majority of ventricular septal defects require use of a patch for secure closure, about the only exception being small muscular defects. Thus, the likelihood of complete or permanent closure and of avoidance of heart block is best ensured by the tension-free repair allowed by patch closure. In most hearts with the most common type of ventricular septal defect, the membranous type, there is no posterior rim to the defect, its posterior limit being the tricuspid annulus itself. The bundle of His traverses this area. It is preferred to anchor the patch, along this posterior limit of the defect, to the base of the adjacent septal tricuspid leaflet, just 2 mm or so from its attachment (hinge) to the annulus, thus avoiding heart block but achieving secure attachment (Fig 41-7).

When aortic insufficiency is associated with a subaortic ventricular septal defect, visualization of the aortic valve via a separate aortotomy is advisable because prolapse of an aortic cusp (usually the right coronary cusp) is usually the cause for the insufficiency. An attempt to reconstruct the aortic valve is warranted, and the technique of Trusler et al.[67] has been especially successful. More recently, Chauvaud et al.[68] reported that triangular resection of the prolapsed cusp, annuloplasty, and reinforcement of the aortic wall offer a better result than plication of the prolapsed cusp or cusps. If, at the time of operation, reconstruction of the aortic valve is not feasible or is unsuccessful, replacement of the valve should be performed, but only in instances in which insufficiency is large.

Leung et al.[50] reported their experience with 25 patients with ventricular septal defect and aortic regurgitation who had septal defect closure and aortic valvuloplasty and an average follow-up of 10 years. The aortic regurgitation was first noted at age 1.3 to 12 years (mean, 5.2 years) and progressed in 11 during observation. At the time of operation, 60% had a small shunt (<1.7:1) and all but two had moderate to severe regurgitation. There were no operative deaths, and after surgery 18 patients had a significant reduction in aortic regurgitation and 7 had stabilization but no improvement in the degree of regurgitation; 3 of the latter group required subsequent valve replacement. Rhodes et al.[69] reported that aortic valvuloplasty was more effective in patients operated on before age 10 than in those older than 15 years at the time of operation (46% and 14%, respectively). The durability of the valvuloplasty was 76% at 12 years and 51% at 18 years. Thus, successful valvuloplasty can be accomplished and can avoid or delay valve replacement.[51,70]

Postoperative course

The risk of death from elective repair of an uncomplicated ventricular septal defect is less than 2%. It is increased by the presence of associated anomalies, multiple ventricular septal defects, or, especially, associated severe pulmonary vascular obstructive disease.[23,71]

Thus far, late follow-up of patients who have survived closure of a ventricular septal defect indicates that their life expectancy has been restored to that of their same age group (except in those over age 3 at operation and having pulmonary vascular obstructive disease).[72] However, because most patients were operated on in childhood, and in the last 3 decades, longer follow-up is needed to confirm this good survival compared with a control adult and elderly population. In addition to the favorable survival, most patients are improved symptomatically after closure of a ventricular septal defect, whether or not the hemodynamic result is perfect. Although a residual ventricular septal defect is surprisingly common, occurring in 14% to 25% of cases in reported series,[73] usually it is not hemodynamically significant.[74]

On auscultation, a faint pulmonary midsystolic murmur is commonly present after closure of the ventricular septal defect.[23] In those patients with a systolic murmur louder than grade 2/6, a residual ventricular septal defect should be considered.[71] It is estimated that 5% to 8% of patients with isolated ventricular septal defect develop the aortic diastolic murmur of aortic regurgitation; often, this is not obvious preoperatively in infants but develops and progresses later in life.[75]

Regarding postoperative electrical abnormalities, 50% to 90% of patients who undergo repair through a right ventriculotomy and up to 40% of those whose defect is repaired by using the transatrial approach manifest right bundle-branch block.[76,77] In most cases, this conduction abnormality is peripheral—that is, secondary to disruption of distal Purkinje's fibers incident to ventriculotomy—but in a few cases it appears to be proximal—secondary to direct damage of the proximal right bundle branch by the ventricular septal defect patch.[71,76,77] Complete AV block was a common complication in the 1950s, but improved knowledge of the course of the conduction system and consequent changes in surgical approach have reduced the incidence rate of this complication to less than 2%.[24,74] Other postoperative atrial and ventricular arrhythmias have been described and probably explain the occasional sudden death at a long time after operation.[24,78] It has been suggested that residual cardiomegaly or development of myocardial dysfunction secondary to progressive pulmonary vascular obstructive disease may trigger such occasionally fatal arrhythmias.[71]

Radiographic evidence of some degree of cardiomegaly after closure of the ventricular septal defect has been observed in about 25% of patients. Of these patients, about one-third have a residual ventricular septal defect or pulmonary vascular obstructive disease that has progressed rather than regressed after operation.[71] Otherwise, in the large majority of patients with a large defect and high pulmonary blood flow, there is an immediate postoperative decrease in the size of the heart and pulmonary arteries.[79]

In those patients who have no residual ventricular defect and undergo operation before age 3, significant residual pulmonary hypertension or ventricular dysfunction is only rarely observed.[71,80,81] On the other hand, in patients over age 3 at operation, significant and progressive pulmonary vascular obstructive disease or ventricular dysfunction at rest or on exercise frequently is seen.[29,71,80,82]

The incidence of infective endocarditis decreases dramatically after successful repair of a ventricular septal defect. If the defect is completely closed, the risk of endocarditis is similar to that in the general population. However, because small residual defects are frequent, antibiotic prophylaxis is still recommended for all patients after ventricular septal defect repair.[79]

REFERENCES

1. Hoffman JIE, Rudolph AM: The natural history of ventricular septal defects in infancy. *Am J Cardiol* 16:634-653, 1965
2. Nora JJ, Fraser FL: *Medical Genetics: Principles and Practice.* Philadelphia, Lea & Febiger, 1974
3. Perloff JK: *The Clinical Recognition of Congenital Heart Disease.* Philadelphia, WB Saunders Company, 1987
4. Baker EJ, Leung MP, Anderson RH, et al: The cross sectional anatomy of ventricular septal defects: a reappraisal. *Br Heart J* 59:339-351, 1988
5. Capelli H, Andrade JL, Somerville J: Classification of the site of ventricular septal defect by 2-dimensional echocardiography. *Am J Cardiol* 51:1474-1480, 1983
6. Alpert BS, Mellits ED, Rowe RD: Spontaneous closure of small ventricular septal defects: probability rates in the first five years of life. *Am J Dis Child* 125:194-196, 1973
7. Bloomfield DK: The natural history of ventricular septal defect in patients surviving infancy. *Circulation* 29:914-955, 1964.
8. Campbell M: Natural history of ventricular septal defect. *Br Heart J* 33:246-257, 1971
9. Hoffman JIE: Natural history of congenital heart disease; problems in its assessment with special reference to ventricular septal defects. *Circulation* 37:97-125, 1968
10. Li MD, Keith JD: Spontaneous closure of ventricular septal defect. *Am Heart J* 80:432-433, 1970
11. Moe DG, Guntheroth WG: Spontaneous closure of uncomplicated ventricular septal defect. *Am J Cardiol* 60:674-678, 1987
12. Mesko ZG, Jones JE, Nadas AS: Diminution and closure of large ventricular septal defects after pulmonary artery banding. *Circulation* 48:847-855, 1973
13. Yasui H, Yoshitoshi M, Myamoto AT, et al: Ventricular septal defect: selection of patients and timing for surgery. *Am Heart J* 93:40-50, 1977
14. Perloff JK: *The Clinical Recognition of Congenital Heart Disease.* Second edition. Philadelphia, WB Saunders Company, 1978, pp 396-441
15. Hoeffel JC, Henry M, Flizot M, et al: Radiologic patterns of aneurysms of the membranous septum. *Am Heart J* 91:450-456, 1976
16. Graham TP Jr, Bender HW, Spach MS: Ventricular septal defect. In *Moss' Heart Disease in Infants, Children, and Adolescents.* Third edition. Edited by FH Adams, GC Emmanouilides. Baltimore, Williams & Wilkins, 1983, pp 134-154
17. Dammann JF Jr, Ferencz C: The significance of the pulmonary vascular bed in congenital heart disease. III. Defects between the ventricles or great vessels in which both increased pressure and blood flow may act upon the lungs and in which there is a common ejectile force. *Am Heart J* 52:210-231, 1956
18. Rudolph AM: The effects of postnatal circulatory adjustments in congenital heart disease: E. Mead Johnson Award Address, October, 1964. *Pediatrics* 36:763-772, 1965
19. Savard M, Swan HJC, Kirklin JW, et al: Hemodynamic alterations associated with ventricular septal defects. In *Symposium on Congenital Heart Disease.* Edited by AD Bass, GK Moe. Washington DC, American Association for the Advancement of Science, 1960, pp 141-164
20. Fuster V, Brandenburg RO, McGoon DC, et al: Clinical approach and management of congenital heart disease in the adolscent and adult. *Cardiovasc Clin* 10 No 3:161-197, 1980
21. Tikoff G, Kuida H: Pathophysiology of heart failure in congenital heart disease. *Mod Concepts Cardiovasc Dis* 41:1-6, 1972
22. Abbot ME: Congenital heart disease. In *Nelson Loose-Leaf Medicine: A Perpetual System of Living Medicine.* Vol. 4. New York, T Nelson & Sons, 1931, pp 207-321
23. Engle MA, Kline SA: Ventricular septal defect in the adult. *Cardiovasc Clin* 10 No 1:279-309, 1979
24. Weidman WH, Blount SG Jr, DuShane JW, et al: Clinical course in ventricular septal defect. *Circulation* 56 Suppl 1:56-69, 1977
25. Hoffman JIE, Rudolph AM, Nadas AS, et al: Pulmonic stenosis, ventricular septal defect, and right ventricular pressure above systemic level. *Circulation* 22:405-411, 1960
26. Shepherd RL, Glancy DL, Jaffe RB, et al: Acquired subvalvular right ventricular outflow obstruction in patients with ventricular septal defect. *Am J Med* 53:446-455, 1972
27. Clarkson PM, Frye RL, DuShane JW, et al: Prognosis for patients with ventricular septal defect and severe pulmonary vascular obstructive disease. *Circulation* 38:129-135, 1968
28. Brammell HL, Vogel JHK, Pryor R, et al: The Eisenmenger syndrome: a clinical and physiologic reappraisal. *Am J Cardiol* 28:679-692, 1971
29. Fuster V, Ritter DG, McGoon DC: Medical and surgical long-term followup of ventricular septal defect with pulmonary vascular obstructive disease (abstract). *Am J Cardiol* 43:346, 1979
30. Warnes CA, Boger JE, Roberts WC: Eisenmenger ventricular septal defect with prolonged survival. *Am J Cardiol* 54:460-462, 1984
31. Pitts JA, Crosby WM, Basta LL: Eisenmenger's syndrome in pregnancy: does heparin prophylaxis improve the maternal mortality rate? *Am Heart J* 93:321-326, 1977
32. Sutton G, Harris A, Leatham A: Second heart sound in pulmonary hypertension. *Br Heart J* 30:743-756, 1968
33. Gasul BM, Dillon RF, Vrla V, et al: Ventricular septal defects: their natural transformation into those with infundibular stenosis or into the cyanotic or noncyanotic type of tetralogy of Fallot. *JAMA* 164:847-853, 1957
34. Gotsman MS: Increasing obstruction to the outflow tract in Fallot's tetralogy. *Br Heart J* 28:615-621, 1966
35. Maron BJ, Ferrans VJ, White RI Jr: Unusual evolution of acquired infundibular stenosis in patients with ventricular septal defect: clinical and morphologic observations. *Circulation* 48:1092-1103, 1973
36. Watson H, Lowe KG: Functional adaptations of the right ventricular outflow tract in congenital heart disease. *Br Heart J* 27:408-412, 1965
37. Walker WJ, Garcia-Gonzalez E, Hall RJ, et al: Interventricular septal defect: analysis of 415 catheterized cases, ninety with serial hemodynamic studies. *Circulation* 31:54-65, 1965
38. DuShane JW, Weidman WH, Brandenburg RO, et al: The electrocardiogram in children with ventricular septal defect and severe pulmonary hypertension: correlation with response to pulmonary arterial pressure to surgical repair. *Circulation* 22:49-54, 1960
39. Papadopoulous C, Lee Y-C, Scherlis L: Isolated ventricular septal defect: electrocardiographic, vectorcardiographic and catheterization data. *Am J Cardiol* 16:359-368, 1965
40. Witham AC, McDaniel JS: Electrocardiogram, vectorcardiogram and hemodynamics in ventricular septal defect. *Am Heart J* 79:335-346, 1970
41. Vickers CW, Kincaid OW, DuShane JW, et al: Ventricular septal defect and severe pulmonary hypertension: radiologic considerations in selection of patients for surgery. *Radiology* 75:69-79, 1960
42. Stevenson JG, Kawabori I, Dooley T, et al: Diagnosis of ventricular septal defect by pulsed Doppler echocardiography: sensitivity, specificity and limitations. *Circulation* 58:322-326, 1978
43. Ortiz E, Robinson PJ, Deanfield JE, et al: Localisation of ventricular septal defects by simultaneous display of superimposed colour Doppler and cross sectional echocardiographic images. *Br Heart J* 54:53-60, 1985
44. Murphy DJ Jr, Ludomirsky A, Huhta JC: Continuous-wave Doppler in children with ventricular septal defect: noninvasive estimation of interventricular pressure gradient. *Am J Cardiol* 57:428-432, 1986
45. Silbert DR, Brunson SC, Schiff R, et al: Determination of right ventricular pressure in the presence of a ventricular septal defect using continuous wave Doppler ultrasound. *J Am Coll Cardiol* 8:379-384, 1986
46. Ludomirsky A, Huhta JC, Vick W III, et al: Color Doppler detection of multiple ventricular septal defects. *Circulation* 74:1317-1322, 1986
47. Edwards JE, Carey LS, Neufeld HN, et al: *Congenital Heart Disease: Correlation of Pathologic Anatomy and Angiocardiography.* Vol. 1. Philadelphia, WB Saunders Company, 1965, pp 81-122
48. Nadas AS, Thilenius OG, LeFarge CG, et al: Ventricular septal defect with aortic regurgitation: medical and pathologic aspects. *Circulation* 29:862-873, 1964

49. Tatsuno K, Konno S, Sakakibara S: Ventricular septal defect with aortic insufficiency: angiocardiographic aspects and a new classification. *Am Heart J* 85:13-21, 1973

50. Leung MP, Beerman LB, Siewers RD, et al: Long-term followup after aortic valvuloplasty and defect closure in ventricular septal defect with aortic regurgitation. *Am J Cardiol* 60:890-894, 1987

51. Colan SD: Long-term results after repair of congenital heart disease. *Curr Opin Cardiol* 4:111-117, 1989

52. Bargeron LM Jr, Elliott LP, Soto B, et al: Axial cineangiography in congenital heart disease. Section I. Concept, technical and anatomic considerations. *Circulation* 56:1075-1083, 1977

53. Elliott LP, Bargeron LM Jr, Bream PR, et al: Axial cineangiography in congenital heart disease. Section II. Specific lesions. *Circulation* 56:1084-1093, 1977

54. Blackstone EH, Kirklin JW, Bradley EL, et al: Optimal age and results in repair of large ventricular septal defects. *J Thorac Cardiovasc Surg* 72:661-679, 1976

55. Fisher RD, Faulkner SL, Sell CG, et al: Operative closure of isolated defects of the ventricular septum: planned delay. *Ann Thorac Surg* 26:351-356, 1978

56. Ching E, DuShane JW, McGoon DC, et al: Total correction of ventricular septal defect in infancy using extracorporeal circulation: surgical considerations and results of operation. *Ann Thorac Surg* 12:1-9, 1971

57. Sigmann JM, Perry BL, Behrendt DM, et al: Ventricular septal defect: results after repair in infancy. *Am J Cardiol* 39:66-71, 1977

58. DuShane JW, Krongrad E, Ritter DG, et al: The fate of raised pulmonary vascular resistance after surgery in ventricular septal defect. In *The Child With Congenital Heart Disease After Surgery.* Edited by BSL Kidd and RD Rowe. Mount Kisco, NY, Futura Publishing Company, 1976, pp 299-312

59. Girod DA, Hurwitz RA, King H, et al: Recent results of two-stage surgical treatment of large ventricular septal defect. *Circulation* 50 Suppl 2:9-13, 1974

60. McNicholas KW, Bowman FO Jr, Hayes CJ, et al: Surgical management of ventricular septal defects in infants. *J Thorac Cardiovasc Surg* 75:346-352, 1978

61. Corone P, Doyon F, Gaudeau S, et al: Natural history of ventricular septal defect: a study involving 790 cases. *Circulation* 55:908-915, 1977

62. Cartmill TB, DuShane JW, McGoon DC, et al: Results of repair of ventricular septal defect. *J Thorac Cardiovasc Surg* 52:486-499, 1966

63. Bush A, Busst CM, Haworth SG, et al: Correlations of lung morphology, pulmonary vascular resistance, and outcome in children with congenital heart disease. *Br Heart J* 59:480-485, 1988

64. Lock JE, Block PC, McKay RG, et al: Transcatheter closure of ventricular septal defects. *Circulation* 78:361-368, 1988

65. Hudspeth AS, Cordell AR, Meredith JH, et al: An improved transatrial approach to the closure of ventricular septal defects. *J Thorac Cardiovasc Surg* 43:157-163, 1962

66. Lincoln C, Jamieson S, Joseph M, et al: Transatrial repair of ventricular septal defects with reference to their anatomic classification. *J Thorac Cardiovasc Surg* 74:183-190, 1977

67. Trusler GA, Moes CAF, Kidd BSL: Repair of ventricular septal defect with aortic insufficiency. *J Thorac Cardiovasc Surg* 66:394-402, 1973

68. Chauvaud S, Serraf A, Mihaileanu S, et al: Ventricular septal defect associated with aortic valve incompetence: results of two surgical managements. *Ann Thorac Surg* 49:875-880, 1990

69. Rhodes LA, Keane JF, Keane JP, et al: Long follow-up (to 43 years) of ventricular septal defect with audible aortic regurgitation. *Am J Cardiol* 66:340-345, 1990

70. Hitchcock JF, Suijker WJL, Ksiezycka E, et al: Management of ventricular septal defect with associated aortic incompetence. *Ann Thorac Surg* 52:70-73, 1991

71. McNamara DG, Latson LA: Long-term follow-up of patients with malformations for which definitive surgical repair has been available for 25 years or more. *Am J Cardiol* 50:560-568, 1982

72. Moller JH, Patton C, Varco RL, et al: Late results (30 to 35 years) after operative closure of isolated ventricular septal defect from 1954 to 1960. *Am J Cardiol* 68:1491-1497, 1991

73. Keith JD: Ventricular septal defect. In *Heart Disease in Infancy and Childhood.* Third edition. Edited by JD Keith, RD Rowe, P Vlad. New York, Macmillan Publishing Co, 1978, pp 320-379

74. Kirklin JW, DuShane JW: Indications for repair of ventricular septal defects. *Am J Cardiol* 12:75-79, 1963

75. Keane JR, Plauth WH Jr, Nadas AS: Ventricular septal defect with aortic regurgitation. *Circulation* 56 Suppl 1:72-77, 1977

76. Vetter VL, Horowitz LN: Electrophysiologic residua and sequelae of surgery for congenital heart defects. *Am J Cardiol* 50:588-604, 1982

77. Okoroma EO, Guller B, Maloney JD, et al: Etiology of right bundle-branch block pattern after surgical closure of ventricular-septal defects. *Am Heart J* 90:14-18, 1975

78. Friedli B, Kidd BSL, Mustard WT, et al: Ventricular septal defect with increased pulmonary vascular resistance: late results of surgical closure. *Am J Cardiol* 33:403-409, 1974

79. Amplatz K, Formanek A, Knight L et al: Radiographic changes in the postoperative patient. *Prog Cardiovasc Dis* 17:403-438, 1975

80. Graham TP Jr, Jarmakani JM, Atwood GF, et al: Right ventricular volume determinations in children: normal values and observations with volume or pressure overload. *Circulation* 47:144-153, 1973

81. Cordell D, Graham TP Jr, Atwood GF, et al: Left heart volume characteristics following ventricular septal defect closure in infancy. *Circulation* 54:294-298, 1976

82. Maron BJ, Redwood DR, Hirschfeld JW Jr, et al: Postoperative assessment of patients with ventricular septal defect and pulmonary hypertension: response to intense upright exercise *Circulation* 48:864-874, 1973

CHAPTER

42

Patent ductus arteriosus and other aorticopulmonary and coronary abnormal communications

David J. Driscoll, M.D., Valentin Fuster, M.D., and Hartzell V. Schaff, M.D.

ANATOMIC CONSIDERATIONS

Patent ductus arteriosus is encountered commonly in infants, but this malformation constitutes only about 2% of all the congenital heart defects found in adults, the reason probably being that most of the cases are easily identified early in life because of the continuous murmur, and appropriate operation is undertaken. The ductus arteriosus is an isolated defect in more than 75% of the cases encountered in infants and in almost all the cases in adults.

During fetal life the ductus arteriosus is an important vascular channel that connects the left pulmonary artery at its origin from the pulmonary trunk to the descending aorta just distal to the left subclavian artery. If there is a right aortic arch, the ductus arteriosus may be on the right, joining the right pulmonary artery and the right aortic arch just distal to the right subclavian artery. Rarely, the ductus may be bilateral. During fetal life the ductus serves as a normal conduit for the major portion of right ventricular output—the blood flowing into the descending aorta[1] (Fig 42-1). Normally, the ductus arteriosus closes functionally within the first 24 hours after birth and anatomically within the first 4 weeks.[2-5] Premature infants, particularly those with the lowest body weights, have a high incidence of patent ductus arteriosus; 75% of patent ductus arteriosus in premature infants close within the first 3 months after birth, whereas only 40% in nonpremature infants close within 3 months. If there has been no closure after 3 months, the chances of closure at a later age are small.

Other aorticopulmonary communications are briefly discussed later in this chapter.

PATHOPHYSIOLOGY

The hemodynamic consequences of persistent patency of the ductus arteriosus depend chiefly upon two factors: the size of the communication and the pulmonary vascular resistance.[6] Patent ductus arteriosus in adults usually presents in one of three different forms: a small ductus without significant hemodynamic derangement; a medium ductus with or without mild left ventricular failure; and a large ductus with secondary severe pulmonary vascular obstructive disease and cyanosis.

Small patent ductus arteriosus. This is manifested by a small left-to-right shunt (Qp/Qs < 1.5) and normal ratio of pulmonary artery pressure (PAP) to systemic arterial

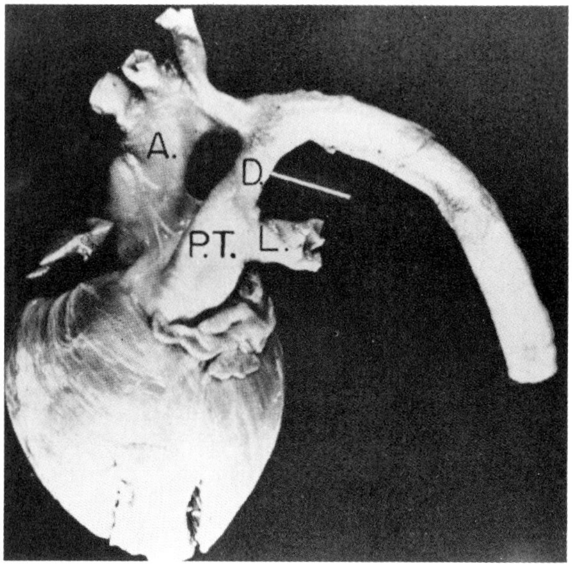

Fig 42-1 Heart and great vessels from newborn infant, showing position of ductus arteriosus *(D.)*. Although the ductus arteriosus is a branch of the left pulmonary artery *(L.)*, the general contour of its course conforms with that of the pulmonary trunk *(P.T.)*. *A.*, aortic arch with branches arising from it. (From Edwards JE, Carey LS, Neufeld HN, et al: *Congenital Heart Disease: Correlation of Pathologic Anatomy and Angiocardiography.* Vol. 1. Philadelphia, WB Saunders Company, 1965, pp 5-80. By permission.)

pressure (SP). The pressure gradient across the defect and normal pulmonary vascular resistance favor the left-to-right shunt throughout the cardiac cycle, which is easily identified clinically by the detection of a continuous murmur about the left infraclavicular area.

Medium-sized patent ductus arteriosus. The shunt is moderate to large (Qp/Qs = 1.5 to 2), yet small enough to offer some resistance to flow, and therefore results in a lower peak systolic pressure in the pulmonary artery than in the aorta (PAP/SP ≤ 0.5). It is unusual for this group to have markedly increased pulmonary vascular resistance. Because of the significant left-to-right shunt and, therefore, increased return to the left heart, there is volume overload of the left atrium and left ventricle, leading to the clinical manifestations described below.

Large patent ductus arteriosus. Because of the nonrestrictive or nearly nonrestrictive character of the defect, blood is ejected into the systemic and pulmonary circuits at nearly the same pressure, so that pulmonary hypertension at near systemic pressure is obligatory. Because of the physiologic gradual decrease in the pulmonary vascular resistance within the first 3 months of life, a large left-to-right shunt ensues and the large volume overload of the left ventricle tends to result in left ventricular failure. In addition, these large defects exhibit not only the clinical findings of the medium-sized defects but also clinical evidence of pulmonary hypertension. If the defect is not closed surgically and these patients survive into childhood and adulthood, one of two different anatomicoclinical courses occurs. The first is a relative decrease in the size of the ductus compared with the growth of the other cardiovascular structures; this results in a medium defect with its clinical characteristics. The second is the development of severe pulmonary vascular obstructive disease, which, with the large type of patent ductus arteriosus, can occur at any time from age 3 until early adulthood; in this group of patients the left-to-right shunt tends to decrease and revert to a right-to-left shunt, with cyanosis, disappearance of the continuous murmur, and other clinical, radiographic, and electrocardiographic (ECG) features of severe pulmonary hypertension.

CLINICAL SYNDROME

History and clinical course

Patent ductus arteriosus predominates in females (sex ratio, 2:1 to 3:1).[7] The prenatal history can be of interest because patent ductus arteriosus occasionally may result from maternal rubella during gestation.[8] Another interesting point is the much higher incidence of patent ductus arteriosus in people born at high altitudes compared with those born at sea level.[9]

Small patent ductus arteriosus. The clinical course usually is benign.[7,10] In some cases, late spontaneous closure of the small ductus has been described, but this probably is rare.[9] Any patient with a patent ductus arteriosus has a small risk of infective endarteritis;[7,11,12] the risk increases slightly with advancing age, and the infection occurs at the site of impact of the ductus stream against the pulmonary artery wall.[13] Aneurysm formation of the ductus is also a rare complication; a large dilatation, even of the closed or nonpatent ductus,[14,15] leading to a mediastinal mass, rupture, or dissection has been described.[13,16]

Medium-sized patent ductus arteriosus. In general, these patients remain asymptomatic, except after the third decade of life, when shortness of breath can begin to develop as a result of the increased pulmonary flow or mild left ventricular failure secondary to the left ventricular volume overload. The long-term survival of these patients is significantly decreased compared with a control population.[7,10]

Large patent ductus arteriosus. From age 1 week to 12 months, in patients with isolated large ductus arteriosus severe symptoms are due primarily to increased pulmonary venous pressure.[6,11,15] The initial symptoms consist of tachypnea, excessive sweating due to increased sympathetic tone, and fatigue when feeding. These symptoms usually are described as beginning within the first week of life in the premature infant or in the second or third month of age in the full-term infant. The symptoms become more severe as the pulmonary vascular resistance decreases. Unless medical or surgical treatment is initiated, the majority of patients die. In the medically treated patients, symptoms tend to improve between 6 and 24 months of age; this is mainly because of compensating left ventricular hypertrophy, progressive increase in the pulmonary vascular resistance which decreases the magnitude of the left-to-right shunt, and, in some patients, decrease in size of the ductus.

Unless there is a relative reduction in the size of the ductus, children with a large patent ductus arteriosus tend to develop pulmonary vascular obstructive disease. Indeed, in adolescence or early adulthood, the pulmonary vascular obstructive disease is so severe that a right-to-left shunt ensues and cyanosis becomes apparent. Chest pain resembling angina, exertional shortness of breath and syncope, hemoptysis, and cerebral abscess related to paradoxic septic emboli all can occur.[11] However, because of the anatomy and preferential flow of the unoxygenated blood toward the lower extremities in these patients with a ductus and reversed shunt, it is not unusual that leg fatigue and selective cyanosis of only the lower extremities dominate the clinical picture.[11,17,18] Fortunately, because of earlier surgical intervention, such patients will be rarely seen in the future.

Physical findings

Small patent ductus arteriosus. In accordance with the very mild hemodynamic derangement, adolescents and adults with a small ductus have a healthy physical appearance; however, in rare instances, patients who were affected by maternal rubella may grow poorly and have cataract, deafness, or mental retardation.[11] Arterial and venous pulses are normal. On palpation, the apical impulse is normal; rarely, there is a continuous thrill in the first or second left intercostal space.

Auscultation provides the pathognomonic and sole physical finding of this condition – the "continuous" murmur. This murmur typically is loudest in the first or second intercostal space beneath the left clavicle and can radiate along the upper left sternal border; the classic murmur of a small ductus is soft and high frequency in quality, rises to a peak in later systole, continues without interruption through the second sound, which it envelops, and then declines in intensity during the course of diastole. At the beginning of systole the flow into the pulmonary trunk is chiefly from the right ventricle rather than through the duct; during the course of the systole, the contribution from the ductus progressively increases; then, during diastole, the flow into the pulmonary artery is from the ductus alone and vanishes progressively as the gradient between the aorta and pulmonary artery decreases. Because in the neonatal period the pulmonary vascular resistance is high, the continuous left-to-right shunt through the small ductus and, therefore, the continuous murmur are not clinical features of that period.

Medium-sized patent ductus arteriosus. As a result of the runoff from the aorta, the peripheral pulses are bounding, and the pulse pressure widens. The jugular venous pulse is normal. On palpation, the left ventricular impulse may by dynamic, related to the moderate left ventricular volume overload. In addition, a continuous thrill may be present in the first or second left intercostal space. On auscultation, there is the continuous murmur described above for small patent ductus, but with this larger ductus the murmur is more noisy and "machine-like" in character. In addition, because of the significant left-to-right shunt and, therefore, increased return to the left heart, there is an associated mitral flow middiastolic murmur and a left ventricular filling sound (third heart sound).

Large patent ductus arteriosus with pulmonary vascular obstructive disease. If there is no reduction in the size of the ductus after age 2 years, progressive pulmonary vascular obstructive disease usually develops in patients with a large ductus. These patients usually present in adolescence or adulthood with the physical findings of pulmonary hypertension associated with some right-to-left shunt. Their physical appearance frequently shows the preferential cyanosis as well as clubbing of the lower extremities (Table 42-1). However, because a small amount of unsaturated blood may enter the left subclavian artery, the fingers of the left hand also may be mildly cyanosed and clubbed; only infrequently are the fingers of the right hand affected.[11] The arterial pulse is usually normal. As a result of right ventricular hypertrophy, the right ventricular impulse becomes palpable in the xyphoid region; in addition, a dilated hypertensive pulmonary trunk is often palpated together with a loud pulmonic component of the second heart sound.[19]

On auscultation[20] as pulmonary vascular obstructive disease and pulmonary hypertension progress, the systolic portion of the ductus murmur shortens and ultimately vanishes altogether, leaving a silent duct (right-to-left flow through a patent ductus does not generate a murmur). Flow into the dilated pulmonary trunk causes a pulmonic ejection sound, which is followed by a short, soft, pulmonic systolic murmur. The second heart sound is quite loud because of the pulmonic component and is closely split (or sometimes single). Often, the loud second heart sound is closely followed by a high-frequency diastolic murmur of pulmonary incompetence (Graham Steell's murmur).

Table 42-1 Differential diagnostic features among the most common shunt defects associated with pulmonary vascular obstructive disease

Feature	Atrial septal defect	Ventricular septal defect	Patent ductus arteriosus
Age at presentation, yr	>30	3-15	3-15
Cyanosis of extremities	Generalized	Generalized	Lower
R wave in lead V_1	rsR′	Monophasic	Monophasic

Electrocardiogram

When the patent ductus arteriosus is small, the ECG is normal. In adults with medium-sized ductus and a moderate left-to-right shunt, the ECG shows evidence of left ventricular hypertrophy.

In adolescent or adult patients with large patent ductus arteriosus and pulmonary vascular obstructive disease, the ECG is quite similar to that in ventricular septal defect complicated by pulmonary vascular obstructive disease[21] (see chapter 41, Fig 41-3).

Chest radiograph

When the ductus is small, the radiograph usually shows normal heart size and normal pulmonary vascularity.

In adults with a medium-sized ductus and a moderate left-to-right shunt (Fig 42-2), the chest radiograph may show some cardiomegaly related to the left ventricular and left atrial volume overloads. There is an increase in the peripheral pulmonary vascular markings and also in the size of the central pulmonary arteries related to the increased pulmonary flow. Finally, because of the increased flow reaching the aorta (a specific characteristic of this shunt defect), the ascending aorta or the aortic knob, or both, may appear prominent.

In adolescent or adult patients with large patent ductus arteriosus and pulmonary vascular obstructive disease, the chest radiograph is similar to that in ventricular septal defect complicated by pulmonary vascular obstructive disease (see chapter 41, Fig 41-4). Because the left cardiac volume overload and hypertrophy of early life have partially or totally regressed, the cardiac size is normal or nearly normal. Characteristically, the apex is tilted upward, reflecting right ventricular hypertrophy, particularly of the outflow tract. Most importantly, in the lung fields, the pulmonary trunk and its main branches are markedly

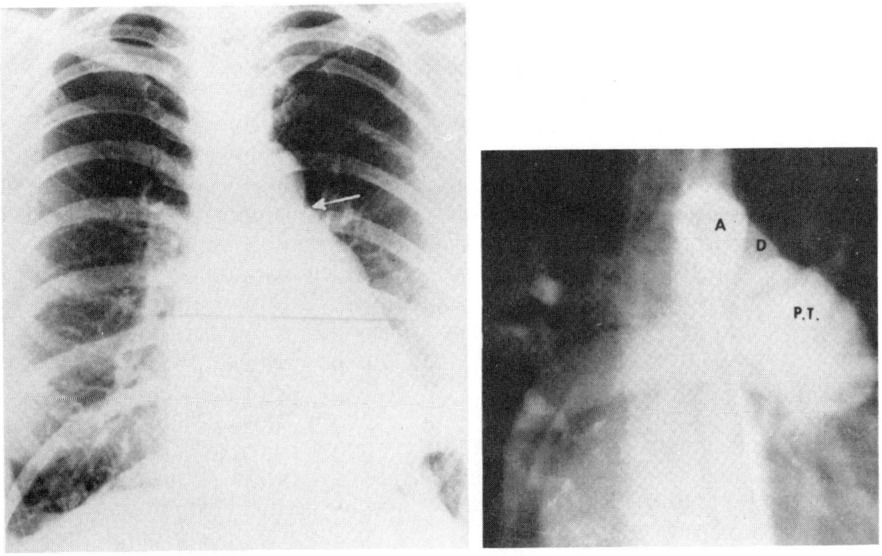

Fig 42-2 Left, anteroposterior radiograph of 38-year-old woman with medium-sized patent ductus arteriosus. Note cardiomegaly related to left ventricular and left atrial enlargement as shown by the left cardiac border. There is an increase in the peripheral pulmonary vascular markings and in the size of the central pulmonary arteries. The aortic knob is prominent. *Arrow* points to a faint convex density at the junction of the outlines of the aorta and pulmonary trunk. This density represents the ductus. It is more likely to be seen in older children and in adults than in infants. **Right,** selective aortography, frontal view, in 8-year-old boy. The tip of the catheter is in the ascending aorta *(A)*. Contrast material injected into the aorta results in opacification of the pulmonary trunk *(P.T.)* through the ductus *(D)*, which is also faintly opacified. This illustration points out the significance of the convex density filling the aorticopulmonary angle in the left panel of this figure. (From Edwards JE, Carey LS, Neufeld HN, et al: *Congenital Heart Disease: Correlation of Pathologic Anatomy and Angiocardiography.* Vol. 1. Philadelphia, WB Saunders Company, 1965, pp 5-80. By permission.)

dilated and may show calcification centrally,[22] but in the outer third there is an abrupt decrease in vascularity.

Echocardiogram

Direct visualization of patent ductus arteriosus with two-dimensional echocardiography usually can be achieved.[23,24] Simultaneous use of Doppler echocardiography for detection of the presence of a continuous disturbance of flow into the left pulmonary artery also is useful in determining the presence of a ductus arteriosus.[25] The combination of M-mode, two-dimensional, and Doppler techniques is useful in providing an index of the left-sided volume overload and function and in estimating pulmonary artery pressures.

DIAGNOSTIC PROBLEMS AND INDICATIONS FOR INVASIVE STUDIES

We will discuss only the diagnostic problems of the most common presentations in adults.

Small and medium-sized patent ductus arteriosus. These have to be distinguished from other conditions also associated with a continuous murmur or with systolic and diastolic murmurs simulating a continuous murmur. Such conditions, some of them rare, are briefly and specifically described here, because the majority are also congenital lesions that may be manifested in the adult and because they can be mistaken for a patent ductus.

VENOUS HUM. The venous hum[11,26,27] is frequently heard, in children and young adults, over the base of the neck, usually best on the right side. It disappears in the supine position or with gentle compression of the neck veins and varies with rotation of the head and with respiration.

MAMMARY SOUFFLE. This is an innocent, continuous murmur that is sometimes heard during late pregnancy and the early postpartum period in lactating women.[28] Its maximal intensity is anywhere over either side of the heart, but there is a tendency for it to be somewhat louder in the second or third right or left intercostal space, on either side or perhaps bilaterally. Contrary to the typical ductus murmurs, the mammary souffle is louder and peaks in systole, tends to vanish in the upright position, and, typically, is abolished by local compression exerted by the stethoscope or a finger.

AORTICOPULMONARY WINDOW. This is a rare congenital opening between the aorta and the pulmonary trunk just above the aortic valve.[11,29-32] In an analysis[33] of the patients reported in the literature, the lesion occurred in association with other anomalies in approximately half of all cases. If the defect is small or medium-sized, the clinical picture is similar to that of a patent ductus arteriosus, except that the continuous murmur is lower and more medial in location. However, most commonly, this defect presents in infants as a large left-to-right shunt; in adults, it presents without a murmur and with the clinical features of severe pulmonary vascular obstructive disease. Anatomically, identification of two semilunar valves at echocardiography distinguishes the aorticopulmonary window from truncus arteriosus.

RUPTURE OF ANEURYSM OF SINUSES OF VALSALVA. The aortic sinuses are almost entirely intracardiac. Occasionally, small congenital aneurysms can develop, undetectable on chest radiographs, and can rupture acutely into a cardiac chamber, producing continuous or systolic and diastolic murmurs that can mimic a patent ductus arteriosus. Congenital aneurysms almost always originate in the right or in the noncoronary sinus, and if they rupture it is into the right ventricle or right atrium, respectively.[29,34] Occasionally, the ruptured aneurysm is acquired as a result of infective endocarditis.[35,36] Finally, congenital aortic sinus aneurysm may be associated with ventricular septal defect.[29,37,38]

FISTULAS OF CORONARY CIRCULATION. With both coronary arteries arising normally from the aorta, a fistula of the coronary circulation is defined as a fistulous branch of a coronary artery communicating directly with a cardiac chamber, generally a right cardiac chamber.[11,29,39-42] Occasionally, the fistula drains into a great vessel, mainly into the pulmonary trunk.[40,43,44] The coronary artery that forms the fistula characteristically is dilated, elongated, and tortuous;[29,45,46] however, the fistula itself tends to be unrecognized radiographically. The left-to-right shunt usually is small or, at most, moderate in degree.[11,29,41,47]

Patients with small shunts characteristically are asymptomatic, and, as with a small patent ductus arteriosus, the only clinical feature is a continuous murmur. If the continuous murmur is distinctly louder in either systole or diastole, this helps to distinguish the fistula of the coronary circulation from a patent ductus arteriosus. If the continuous murmur peaks in the vicinity of the second heart sound, the configuration serves no useful purpose in this differential diagnosis, but the atypical location of the murmur may be helpful in pointing out the possibility of fistula.[11,48] A number of coronary artery fistulas are first discovered at thoracotomy performed for the mistaken diagnosis of patent ductus arteriosus.[40,48,49] Progressive enlargement of the shunt[29,45,46] and secondary infective endocarditis[50,51] have been documented.

In the moderate-sized to large left-to-right shunts, the continuous murmur is associated with the clinical features of volume overload (as described above for the other shunts, as in patent ductus arteriosus).[11] Cardiac failure may develop, but usually not until the fourth, fifth, or sixth decade. In addition, in some of these patients with large fistulas, as a result of diversion of blood from the normal coronary artery into the fistulous branch, features of myocardial ischemia have been documented.[43,44,52,53] These fistulas with a significant shunt should be treated by suture-ligation of the fistula; the results tend to be good.[54-56]

ANOMALOUS ORIGIN OF CORONARY ARTERY FROM PULMONARY TRUNK. Most commonly, this refers to an anomalous origin of the left coronary artery from the pulmonary trunk.[11,42,54,57,58] The lack of antegrade perfusion of the anomalous left coronary artery and the diversion of blood from the normal right coronary system to the left both lead to left ventricular ischemia, fibrosis, and enlargement plus associated mitral incompetence. The overall left-to-right shunt is small and may generate a continuous murmur as in patent ductus arteriosus. Differentiating features are similar to those described above for the fistulas of the coronary circulation, but echocardiography is approaching the status of definitive diagnostic tool.[59-61]

Interestingly, although anomalous origin of the right coronary artery from the pulmonary trunk is much more rare than origin of the left coronary artery, its identification in the adult population may be more common. This is because that condition is less prone to cause ischemia early in life and is associated with good survival into adulthood. New surgical vascular procedures for use early and later in life are now being proposed.[54,62]

PULMONARY ARTERIOVENOUS FISTULAS. These may cause continuous murmurs which, in distinction to ductus arteriosus, usually are localized at sites over the lungs and removed from the precordial area.[63] This disorder may be associated with mild cyanosis and a normal heart size; it is suspected in the presence of a mass on the chest radiograph, especially with hereditary hemorrhagic telangiectasia (Rendu-Osler-Weber disease), which very commonly is the basis of the fistula. A solitary fistula or multiple fistulas confined to one lobe can be treated by lobectomy, particularly to avoid complications such as significant cyanosis, hemoptysis, infective arteritis, paradoxic embolus, or cerebral abscess.

PERIPHERAL PULMONARY ARTERY STENOSIS OR COARCTATION OF THE AORTA. These entities are discussed in later sections and only rarely can be confused with ductus arteriosus. The widespread location of a long systolic murmur extending into diastole or, less commonly, continuous murmur plus other clinical, radiographic, and ECG features point to the correct diagnosis.

BRONCHIAL COLLATERAL VESSELS. These vessels produce widespread continuous murmurs. The correct diagnosis can be suspected in this situation because such collaterals typically occur in those congenital cardiac conditions that are associated with cyanosis and a decrease in pulmonary blood flow.

Large patent ductus arteriosus with severe pulmonary vascular obstructive disease. These patients can present with clinical features similar to those exhibited by patients with pulmonary hypertension from other causes. The features that differentiate it from other types of pulmonary hypertension have been discussed above (see Table 42-1) as well as in the preceding chapters on shunt defects.

Invasive studies. In children or adults, diagnostic cardiac catheterization is needed only infrequently, unless there is a suspicion of one of the above conditions, of pulmonary vascular obstructive disease, or of abnormalities associated with the patent ductus (e.g., congenital coronary disease).

In the majority of patients the catheter can be manipulated from the pulmonary artery across the ductus arteriosus into the descending aorta by probing near the takeoff of the left pulmonary artery. With a small ductus, typically there is an increase in oxygen saturation of 3% to 5% between the right ventricle and pulmonary artery, but there may be no detectable shunt by oximetry. All pressures are usually normal. With a moderate-sized ductus, there is usually an increase in oxygen saturation of about 10% to 20% between the right ventricle and pulmonary artery. The pulmonary and right ventricular systolic pressures can approach half of the systemic pressures (due to the wide aortic pulmonary communication), mean pressure in the left atrium and end-diastolic pressure in the left ventricle may be increased (due to the volume overload), and the aortic or systemic pulse pressure may widen (due to runoff into the pulmonary artery).

At angiography, a left anterior oblique view, which "opens up" the aortic arch after injection of contrast medium into the ascending aorta or aortic arch, permits visualization of the ductus and pulmonary artery.

In the adult patient with a large ductus and pulmonary vascular obstructive disease, there may be a slight increase in the pulmonary artery oxygen saturation (due to some remaining left-to-right shunt) and a low systemic oxygen saturation, which typically is lower in the descending aorta than in the ascending aorta (due to right-to-left shunting through the ductus). Pulmonary and right ventricular systolic pressures are near systemic levels (due to the increased pulmonary vascular resistance), left atrial and left ventricular end-diastolic pressures return to normal (due to the decreased volume overload), and the aortic or systemic pulse pressure narrows (due to less runoff into the pulmonary artery).

For angiographic visualization of the ductus in these patients with predominant right-to-left shunt, the contrast medium is injected into the pulmonary artery.

MANAGEMENT

Medical versus surgical treatment

In a report from the Cleveland Clinic on long-term follow-up (mean of 18 years) in 117 adults with persistent ductus arteriosus, about two-thirds of the patients had surgical closure and about one-third were treated medically.[64] The outcome was mixed, since the study population included, among other differences, patients of different ages and with different sizes of ductus.

As with ventricular septal defect, the great challenge is to identify, within the first 2 years of life, those patients with a large ductus, because the majority of these patients will develop severe pulmonary vascular obstructive disease. The different types of patent ductus arteriosus that present in adults are managed as follows.

Small and medium-sized patent ductus arteriosus. Three major risks exist: (1) development of infective endocarditis; (2) deposition of calcium in the walls of the ductus (this occurs very commonly, is progressive with age, and can compromise the surgical results); and (3) left ventricular failure and decreased life expectancy in patients with medium-sized defects. Because of these risks and the almost negligible operative mortality in children, the mere presence of a ductus arteriosus is an indication for operation. The operative management of patent ductus arteriosus in the adult involves certain complicating features (see below).

Large patent ductus arteriosus with severe pulmonary vascular obstructive disease. As judged from the data obtained in patients with large left ventricular septal defect, we think that pulmonary vascular resistance greater than 10 units · m^2 indicates severe pulmonary vascular obstructive disease and contraindicates closure of the shunt in adolescents or adults. Our medical approach to these patients with pulmonary hypertension is similar to that described for ventricular septal defect complicated by pulmonary vascular obstructive disease (see chapter 41).

Surgical technique in the adult

The surgical management of patent ductus arteriosus in the adult involves certain complicating features that are much less common in the infant or child. In addition to the more precise evaluation of pulmonary vascular resistance and its implications with respect to indications for operation, there are several potential structural alterations in the region of the ductus that require special consideration with respect to operative technique. These problems include the common presence of pulmonary hypertension, the reported incidences ranging from 21%[65] to 81%;[66] a tendency for the ductus to be giant in size in adults, as occurred in nearly 50% in the series of John et al.;[66] the common occurrence of calcification in the adult ductus, which raises the risk of catastrophic hemorrhage on application of a clamp in this area; and finally, the prior or concurrent presence of infective endocarditis in the ductus, which occurs in approximately 4%[66] of patients (operation is better accomplished at least 6 weeks after eradication of the infection).

As a result of these technically complicating features often present in the adult patient with a patent ductus, the operative procedure often requires modification from the standard operation for division or multiple ligation of the ductus used in infants and children.

Our own preference for the giant, short, calcified ductus associated with severe pulmonary hypertension has been a modification of the technique for closing a ductus encountered incidentally at the time of open heart surgery[67] (Fig 42-3). A median sternotomy is used, extracorporeal circulation is implemented in the usual manner, and, as systemic hypothermia is induced, clamps are placed across the right, left, and main pulmonary arteries. Cooling is continued to the level of 15°C to 18°C. The rate of perfusion is then decreased to 0.5 L/min/m^2 or less, the clamps on the pulmonary arteries are released, and the pulmonary artery is entered and emptied of blood by aspiration. Depending upon the characteristics of the vessel wall at the pulmonary orifice of the ductus, either the ductus can be transected entirely from the pulmonary artery along with or without a surrounding margin of pulmonary artery or the orifice of the ductus can be closed with a prosthetic patch. Care must be taken to avoid entry of air into the aorta. By utilizing these special techniques,

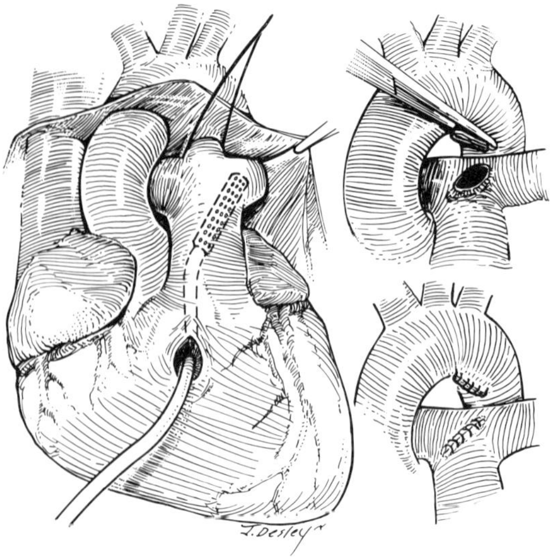

Fig 42-3 Closure of patent ductus during open heart operation. During extracorporeal circulation, with the pressures in the great arteries greatly decreased, it may be possible to isolate the ductus sufficiently for placement of a single cross-clamp. In that case, the ductus is cut out of the pulmonary artery and both the resulting orifice in the pulmonary artery and the stump of the ductus are closed by direct suture. If the ductus is heavily calcified and aneurysmal, profound hypothermia is instituted (see text for technique) and the ductus is transected from the pulmonary artery during circulatory arrest, thus avoiding the necessity of cross-clamping it. (From McGoon DC: Closure of patent ductus during open-heart surgery. *J Thorac Cardiovasc Surg* 48:456-464, 1964. By permission of CV Mosby Company.)

the risk of closure of a patent ductus in an adult has been substantially decreased, to about 3%.

Postoperative course

The overall risk of death from repair of this lesion at all ages is less than 2%; it is less than 1% when small infants and patients with pulmonary hypertension are excluded.[68,69] Reports of long-term results of operation for patent ductus arteriosus are surprisingly sparse.[7,70] When the ductus is divided in children under 3 years of age who have no other major cardiovascular defects, late sequelae are rare and long-term results are excellent. In patients over age 3, preoperative significantly increased pulmonary vascular resistance and pulmonary hypertension can persist or even progress postoperatively.[71] On the other hand, patients who have a hemodynamically significant patent ductus arteriosus and are 50 to 70 years old with cardiomegaly and left cardiac failure but without high pulmonary vascular resistance may have excellent long-term results after operation.

Auscultation postoperatively reveals a soft systolic ejection murmur in some patients, probably related to persistent dilatation of the main pulmonary artery.[69] A continuous murmur related to recanalization of the interrupted ductus has been observed but should not occur with the current surgical methods of closure.[72]

Regarding postoperative electrical abnormalities, left ventricular hypertrophy regresses promptly after repair of the patent ductus arteriosus.[73] In patients with high pulmonary vascular resistance and pulmonary hypertension preoperatively, right ventricular hypertrophy may not regress, indicating persistence of the hypertension.

Radiographically, in most patients with preoperative cardiomegaly there is a decrease in heart size beginning within days and continuing as long as a full year.[74] The pulmonary artery and ascending aorta may remain prominent despite surgical repair, but the caliber of peripheral pulmonary vascular markings should decrease promptly within 2 to 4 weeks. Ductal aneurysm after operative closure of a patent ductus arteriosus is rare; if it occurs, it may be seen as a left mediastinal mass.[74] Inadvertent injury to the phrenic nerve at thoracotomy may cause diaphragmatic paralysis with elevation of a hemidiaphragm apparent on the chest radiograph; this is well tolerated and tends to persist for several months or occasionally years, but is rarely permanent.[75]

The increased risk of infective endocarditis disappears after successful repair of patent ductus arteriosus; therefore, antibiotic prophylaxis is considered unnecessary except in patients who have other associated cardiac abnormalities.[76]

Nonsurgical closure

The first successful application of a transcatheter closure technique for patent ductus arteriosus suitable for use in infants and children was reported by Rashkind and Cuaso[77] in 1979. Later, a multi-institutional report of 156 patients revealed a successful result in about two-thirds, but postrelease embolization of the occluder occurred in 15% (with subsequent removal of the device).[78] Using a modified technique, Wessel et al.[79] reported successful transcatheter closure in 22 of 23 children. In the experience of Hosking et al.,[80] embolization of the Rashkind device occurred in 4 of 190 patients and other complications occurred in 3.6% of patients. The prevalence of residual shunting was 38% at 1 year, 18% at 2 years, and 8% at 40 months. Importantly, reocclusion was successful in all nine patients in whom it was attempted. Other devices promise to improve the success rate of closure of larger patent ductus.[81,82] Clearly, skilled physicians properly trained may soon perform transcatheter closure of an uncomplicated patent ductus arteriosus routinely as the best alternative to surgical closure.

REFERENCES

1. Rudolph AM: The changes in the circulation after birth: their importance in congenital heart disease. *Circulation* 41:343-359,1970
2. Hiraishi S, Misawa H, Oguchi K, et al: Two-dimensional Doppler echocardiographic assessment of closure of the ductus arteriosus in normal newborn infants. *J Pediatr* 11:755-760,1987
3. Reller MD, Ziegler ML, Rice MJ, et al: Duration of ductal shunting in healthy preterm infants: an echocardiographic color flow Doppler study. *J Pediatr* 112:441-446,1988
4. Drayton MR, Skidmore R: Ductus arteriosus blood flow during first 48 hours of life. *Arch Dis Child* 62:1030-1034, 1987

5. Ramsay JM, Murphy DJ Jr, Vick GW III, et al: Response of the patent ductus arteriosus to indomethacin treatment. *Am J Dis Child* 141:294-297,1987

6. Fuster V. Brandenburg RO, McGoon DC, et al: Clinical approach and management of congenital heart disease in the adolescent and adult. *Cardiovasc Clin* 10 No 3:161-197,1980

7. Campbell M: Natural history of persistent ductus arteriosus. *Br Heart J* 30:4-13,1968

8. Campbell M: Place of maternal rubella in the aetiology of congenital heart disease. *Br Med J* 1:691-696, 1961

9. Alzamora-Castro V, Battilana G, Abugattas R, et al: Patent ductus arteriosus and high altitude. *Am J Cardiol* 5:761-763, 1960

10. Coggin CJ, Parker KR, Keith JD: Natural history of isolated patent ductus arteriosus and the effect of surgical correction: twenty years' experience at The Hospital for Sick Children, Toronto. *Can Med Assoc J* 102:718-720, 1970

11. Perloff JK: *The Clinical Recognition of Congenital Heart Disease.* Second edition. Philadelphia, WB Saunders Company, 1978, pp 524-560

12. Espino-Vela J, Zamora C: Patent ductus arteriosus: the natural history after the first year of life. In *The Natural History and Progress in Treatment of Congenital Heart Defects.* Springfield, Illinois, Charles C Thomas, Publisher, 1971, pp 39-50

13. Espino-Vela J, Cardenas N, Cruz R: Patent ductus arteriosus: with special reference to patients with pulmonary hypertension. *Circulation* 38 Suppl 5:45-60, 1968

14. Falcone NW, Perloff JK, Roberts WC: Aneurysm of the nonpatent ductus arteriosus. *Am J Cardiol* 29:422-426, 1972

15. Heymann MA: Patent ductus arteriosus. In *Moss' Heart Disease in Infants, Children and Adolescents.* Third edition. Edited by FH Adams, GC Emmanouilides. Baltimore, Williams & Wilkins, 1983, pp 158-171

16. Das JB, Chesterman JT: Aneurysms of the patent ductus arteriosus. *Thorax* 11:295-302,1956

17. Williams B, Ling J-T, Leight L, et al: Patent ductus arteriosus and osteoarthropathy. *Arch Intern Med* 111:346-350, 1963

18. Davies DH, Gazetopoulos N: Dyspnoea and differential hypercapnia in the "Eisenmenger ductus." *Guys Hosp Rep* 115:175-181, 1966

19. Brammell HL, Vogel JHK, Pryor R, et al: The Eisenmenger syndrome: a clinical and physiologic reappraisal. *Am J Cardiol* 28:679-692,1971

20. Perloff JK: Auscultatory and phonocardiographic manifestations of pulmonary hypertension. *Prog Cardiovasc Dis* 9:303-340, 1967

21. Burch GE, DePasquale NP: *Electrocardiography in the Diagnosis of Congenital Heart Disease.* Philadelphia, Lea & Febiger, 1967

22. Timpanelli AE, Steinberg I: Calcification of the pulmonary artery in patent ductus arteriosus with reversal of blood flow: report of four cases. *Am J Med* 30:405-417, 1961

23. Smallhorn JF: Patent ductus arteriosus—evaluation by echocardiography. *Echocardiography* 4:101-118,1987

24. Sahn DJ, Allen HD: Real-time cross-sectional echocardiographic imaging and measurement of the patent ductus arteriosus in infants and children. *Circulation* 58:343-354, 1978

25. Ritter SB: Recent advances in color-Doppler assessment of congenital heart disease. *Echocardiography* 5:457-475, 1988

26. Jones FL Jr: Frequency, characteristics and importance of the cervical venous hum in adults. *N Engl J Med* 267:658-660, 1962

27. Cutforth R, Wiseman J, Sutherland RD: The genesis of the cervical venous hum. *Am Heart J* 80:488-492,1970

28. Tabatznik B, Randall TW, Hersch C: The mammary souffle of pregnancy and lactation. *Circulation* 22:1069-1073,1960

29. Edwards JE, Carey LS, Neufeld HN, et al: *Congenital Heart Disease: Correlation of Pathologic Anatomy and Angiocardiography.* Vol 1. Philadelphia, WB Saunders Company, 1965, pp 5-80

30. Morrow AG, Greenfield LJ, Braunwald E: Congenital aortopulmonary septal defect: clinical and hemodynamic findings, surgical technic, and results of operative correction. *Circulation* 25:463-476, 1962

31. Neufeld HN, Lester RG, Adams P Jr, et al: Aorticopulmonary septal defect. *Am J Cardiol* 9:12-25, 1962

32. Blieden LC, Moller JH: Aorticopulmonary septal defect: an experience with 17 patients. *Br Heart J* 36:630-635, 1974

33. Kutsche LM, Van Mierop LHS: Anatomy and pathogenesis of aorticopulmonary septal defect. *Am J Cardiol* 59:443-447,1987

34. Sakakibara S, Konno S: Congenital aneurysm of the sinus of Valsalva: anatomy and classification. *Am Heart J* 63:405-424, 1962

35. Conde CA, Meller J, Donoso E, et al: Bacterial endocarditis with ruptured sinus of Valsalva and aorticocardiac fistula. *Am J Cardiol* 35:912-917, 1975

36. Weyman AE, Dillon JC, Feigenbaum H, et al: Premature pulmonic valve opening following sinus of Valsalva aneurysm rupture into the right atrium. *Circulation* 51:556-560,1975

37. Burchell HB, Edwards JE: Aortic sinus aneurysm with communications into the right ventricle and associated ventricular septal defect. *Proc Staff Meet Mayo Clin* 26:336-340, 1951

38. Yacoub MH, Lise M, Muir J: Aneurysms of two sinuses of Valsalva with a ventricular septal defect and aortic regurgitation. *Br Heart J* 31:661-663, 1969

39. Upshaw CB Jr: Congenital coronary arteriovenous fistula: report of a case with an analysis of seventy-three reported cases. *Am Heart J* 63:399-404, 1962

40. Edis AJ, Schattenberg TT, Feldt RH, et al: Congenital coronary artery fistula: surgical considerations and results of operation. *Mayo Clin Proc* 47:567-571, 1972

41. Neufeld HN, Lester RG, Adams P Jr, et al: Congenital communication of a coronary artery with a cardiac chamber or the pulmonary trunk ("coronary artery fistula"). *Circulation* 24:171-179, 1961

42. Takahashi M: Congenital and acquired coronary artery abnormalities in children. *Curr Opin Cardiol* 4:71-75, 1989

43. Eie H, Hillestad L: Arterio-venous fistulae of the coronary arteries: a report of six cases. *Scand J Thorac Cardiovasc Surg* 5:34-38, 1971

44. Gobel FL, Anderson CF, Baltaxe HA, et al: Shunts between the coronary and pulmonary arteries with normal origin of the coronary arteries. *Am J Cardiol* 25:655-661, 1970

45. Davison PH, McCracken BH, McIlveen DJS: Congenital coronary arterio-venous aneurysm. *Br Heart J* 17:569-572, 1955

46. Harris A, Jefferson K, Chatterjee K: Coronary arteriovenous fistula with aneurysm of coronary sinus. *Br Heart J* 31:400-403, 1969

47. Jaffe RB, Glancy DL, Epstein SE, et al: Coronary arterial-right heart fistulae: long-term observations in seven patients. *Circulation* 47:133-143, 1973

48. Sakakibara S, Yokoyama M, Takao A, et al: Coronary arteriovenous fistula: nine operated cases. *Am Heart J* 72:307-314, 1966

49. Querimit AS, Rowe GG: Localization of coronary arteriovenous fistula by indicator-dilution curves. *Am J Cardiol* 27:114-119, 1971

50. Stansel HC Jr, Fenn JE: Coronary arteriovenous fistula between the left coronary artery and persistent left superior vena cava complicated by bacterial endocarditis. *Ann Surg* 160:292-296, 1964

51. Tsagaris TJ, Hecht HH: Coronary artery aneurysm and subacute bacterial endarteritis. *Ann Intern Med* 57:116-121, 1962

52. De Nef JJE, Varghese PJ, Losekoot G: Congenital coronary artery fistula: analysis of 17 cases. *Br Heart J* 33:857-862, 1971

53. Morgan JR, Forker AD, O'Sullivan MJ Jr, et al: Coronary arterial fistulas: seven cases with unusual features. *Am J Cardiol* 30:432-436, 1972

54. Lurie PR, Takahashi M: Abnormalities and diseases of the coronary vessels. In *Moss' Heart Disease in Infants, Children, and Adolescents.* Third edition. Edited by FH Adams, GC Emmanouilides. Baltimore, Williams & Wilkins, 1983, pp 501-516

55. Cooley DA, Ellis PR Jr: Surgical considerations of coronary arterial fistula. *Am J Cardiol* 10:467-474, 1962

56. Oldham NH Jr, Ebert PA, Young WG, et al: Surgical management of congenital coronary artery fistula. *Ann Thorac Surg* 12:503-511,1971

57. Askenazi J, Nadas AS: Anomalous left coronary artery originating from the pulmonary artery: report of 15 cases. *Circulation* 51:976-987, 1975

58. Talner NS, Halloran KH, Mahdavy M, et al: Anomalous origin of the left coronary artery from the pulmonary artery: a clinical spectrum. *Am J Cardiol* 15:689-695, 1965

59. King TC, Saffitz JE: Acute right ventricular infarction resulting from intracardiac infusion of hyperosmotic hyperalimentation solutions. *Am J Cardiol* 55:1659-1660, 1985

60. Jureidini SB, Nouri S, Pennington DG: Anomalous origin of the left coronary artery from the pulmonary trunk: repair after diagnostic cross sectional echocardiography. *Br Heart J* 58:173-175, 1987

61. Diamant S, Luber JM Jr, Brunson SC, et al: Two-dimensional and pulsed Doppler echocardiography in anomalous origin of the left coronary artery from the pulmonary artery: pre and postoperative studies. *Am Heart J* 113:195-198, 1987

62. Grace RR, Angelini P, Cooley DA: Aortic implantation of anomalous left coronary artery arising from pulmonary artery. *Am J Cardiol* 39:608-613, 1977

63. Moyer JH, Glantz G, Brest AN: Pulmonary arteriovenous fistulas: physiologic and clinical considerations. *Am J Med* 32:417-435, 1962

64. Fisher RG, Moodie DS, Sterba R, et al: Patent ductus arteriosus in adults – long-term follow-up: nonsurgical versus surgical treatment. *J Am Coll Cardiol* 8:280-284, 1986

65. Black LL, Goldman BS: Surgical treatment of the patent ductus arteriosus in the adult. *Ann Surg* 175:290-293, 1972

66. John S, Muralidharan S, Jairaj PS, et al: The adult ductus: review of surgical experience with 131 patients. *J Thorac Cardiovasc Surg* 82:314-319, 1981

67. McGoon DC: Closure of patent ductus during open-heart surgery. *J Thorac Cardiovasc Surg* 48:456-464, 1964

68. McNamara DG, Latson LA: Long-term follow-up of patients with malformations for which definitive surgical repair has been avaliable for 25 years or more. *Am J Cardiol* 50:560-568, 1982

69. Rowe RD: Patent ductus arteriosus. In *Heart Disease in Infancy and Childhood.* Third edition. Edited by JD Keith, RD Rowe, P Vlad. New York, Macmillan Publishing Company, 1978, pp 418-451

70. Lucht U, Søndergaard T: Late results of operation for patent ductus arteriosus. *Scand J Thorac Cardiovasc Surg* 5:223-226, 1971

71. Neutze JM: Follow up of high resistance patients after shunt surgery. *NZ Med J* 64 Cardiac Suppl:37-38, 1965

72. Jones JC: Twenty-five years' experience with the surgery of patent ductus arteriosus. *J Thorac Cardiovasc Surg* 50:149-165, 1965

73. Clark DS, Hirsch HD, Tamer DM, et al: Electrocardiographic changes following surgical treatment of congenital cardiac malformations. *Prog Cardiovasc Dis* 17:451-465, 1975

74. Amplatz K, Formanek A, Knight L, et al: Radiographic changes in the postoperative patient. *Prog Cardiovasc Dis* 17:403-438, 1975

75. Morriss JH, McNamara DG: Residuae, sequelae, and complications of surgery for congenital heart disease. *Prog Cardiovasc Dis* 18:1-25, 1975

76. Manning JA: Endocarditis prophylaxis in the child with congenital heart disease after survery. In *The Child With Congenital Heart Disease After Surgery.* Edited by BSL Kidd, RD Rowe. Mount Kisco, New York, Futura Publishing Company, 1976, pp 447-450

77. Rashkind WJ, Cuaso CC: Transcatheter closure of patent ductus arteriosus: successful use in a 3.5 kilogram infant. *Pediatr Cardiol* 1:3-8,1979

78. Rashkind WJ, Mullins CE, Hellenbrand WE, et al: Nonsurgical closure of patent ductus arteriosus: clinical applications of the Rashkind PDA occluder system. *Circulation* 75:583-592, 1987

79. Wessel DL, Keane JF, Parness I, et al: Outpatient closure of the patent ductus arteriosus. *Circulation* 77:1068-1071, 1988

80. Hosking MCK, Benson LN, Musewe N, et al: Transcatheter occlusion of the persistently patent ductus arteriosus: forty-month follow-up and prevalence of residual shunting. *Circulation* 84:2313-2317, 1991

81. Saveliev VS, Prokubovski VI, Kolody SM, et al: Patent ductus arteriosus: transcatheter closure with a transvenous technique. *Radiology* 184:341-344, 1992

82. Bridges ND, Perry SB, Parness I, et al: Transcatheter closure of a large patent ductus arteriosus with the Clamshell septal umbrella. *J Am Coll Cardiol* 18:1297-1302, 1991

CHAPTER

43

Medical management of cyanosis, including Eisenmenger's syndrome

Carole A. Warnes, M.D.

Cyanotic patients, especially those with pulmonary hypertension are more dependent for continued life and health on medical decisions that are comparatively routine for patients without cyanosis. Patients with pulmonary hypertension are especially vulnerable to any intervention that causes vasodilatation and a decrease in peripheral resistance. The results are an increased right-to-left shunt, cerebral hypoxia, and the induction of a potentially lethal arrhythmia. Causes of vasodilatation include drugs (e.g., nitrates, angiotensin converting enzyme inhibitors), radioiodine contrast material, and spinal or general anesthesia. Avoidance of common producers of vasodilatation such as hot tubs, prolonged hot showers, alcohol, and dehydration is very important.

HEMATOLOGIC DISORDERS

One of the major consequences of cyanosis is disturbance of the hematopoietic system resulting in erythrocytosis. This is not analogous to polycythemia vera, since only the red cells are increased in number, the white blood cell count is usually normal, and the platelets are either normal in number or, more commonly, decreased.

The increase in red blood cell mass causes the most concern in adults with cyanosis, and the more severe the cyanosis, the higher the hematocrit. Concern arises because the increased viscosity that results from the erythrocytosis increases the risk of red blood cell "sludging," with the potential for thrombus formation and subsequent cerebrovascular accident.[1] The risk of cerebrovascular accident, however, although higher than normal, appears not to be substantially increased, partly, perhaps, because the shear rate in the cerebral microcirculation is high and helps maintain cerebral blood flow in erythrocytosis. Thus, therapy aimed at reducing the hematocrit is frequently not necessary.[2] Furthermore, most cyanotic patients have a stable, well-compensated erythropoietic system, and phlebotomy potentially destabilizes this well-balanced equilibrium. Most patients tolerate a hemoglobin concentration up to 20 mg/dL with a corresponding hematocrit of approximately 65%. If values are above those levels, patients often complain of headache and poor concentration. Therapeutic phlebotomy of one unit of red cells alleviates these symptoms. Concomitant fluid replacement with dextrose or saline must *always* be done to avoid dehydration, increased viscosity, and hypotension. Replacement is especially important in patients with pulmonary hypertension. Phlebotomy should be performed only when necessary and never more than four times a year. More frequent phlebotomies result in microcytosis and iron-deficient red cells, often with a relative anemia. This problem is the most common one associated with cyanotic heart disease. It should always be remembered that patients with cyanosis need higher hematocrits than normal persons, and the aim is not to reduce the hemoglobin level to the normal range. Iron deficiency anemia causes a reduction in exercise capacity, and since microcytes are less deformable than normal red cells, there is more risk of red cell "sludging,"[3,4] and, paradoxically, the risk of stroke is increased.[5] Thus, overzealous ordering of phlebotomies should be avoided.

Once iron deficiency anemia has developed, its treatment is also complex. Therapy with regular doses of iron supplements may result in a rapid rebound erythrocytosis. A reasonable approach is to give one tablet of ferrous sulfate a day and check the response in 1 week.[2] If the hemoglobin value is rising rapidly, administration of iron is discontinued; if not, the patient continues to take iron and the full blood count is determined in approximately 2 weeks.

CLOTTING DIATHESIS

Patients with cyanosis also have abnormalities of the coagulation system. The platelets are usually low in number and do not exhibit normal function.[6] The levels of vitamin K-dependent clotting factors (prothrombin, factors VII and IX) and factor V are usually below normal, and commonly the prothrombin time and activated partial thromboplastin times are prolonged.[7,8] Thus, patients are at increased risk for spontaneous bleeding (e.g., in the gut). The risk can be exaggerated when cyanotic patients are given anticoagulants, aspirin, or other antiplatelet agents. In general, therefore, these agents should be avoided, and any use should be for specific reasons with careful and frequent monitoring.

CEREBRAL ABSCESS

The potential for paradoxical embolus and cerebral abscess exists in all cyanotic patients. Whenever such a patient presents with new neurologic symptoms, however transient, or even a personality change, blood should be obtained for culture, endocarditis ruled out, and cerebral abscess excluded.

RENAL DYSFUNCTION

Adults with cyanotic heart disease invariably have impairment of the glomerular filtration rate, which may be reflected by an increased serum creatinine value.[9] The histopathologic substrate in the kidney appears to be thickening of the basement membrane with hypercellular and congested glomeruli.[10] The abnormal renal function is, in large part, responsible for impaired urate clearance from the body and increased uric acid levels associated with cyanosis.[9,11] Particular care must be given around the time of cardiac catheterization, for example, when the combination of dehydration and a contrast medium load may seriously jeopardize renal function. For the patient with significant cyanosis, the author's policy is to admit the patient the night before cardiac catheterization for intravenous hydration. Cardiac catheterization should always be performed by experienced investigators giving the minimum amount of contrast load necessary with concomitant fluid replacement. After the procedure, urine output and fluid replacement should be carefully watched.

URIC ACID AND GOUT

The reported incidence of gout is approximately 0.3% in the general population[12] and 2% in cyanotic congenital heart disease.[13] In patients with Eisenmenger's syndrome, it is approximately 5%.[14] The high uric acid levels occur mainly because of impaired urate excretion by the kidney but also in part because of increased uric acid production secondary to high red cell turnover.[9] Frank gout, however, is uncommon, so that treatment with allopurinol is unnecessary unless clinical gout is manifested.

ACNE

Many cyanotic adults have a significant problem with facial and truncal acne. This not only causes cosmetic concerns but also is a potential source of infection. Treatment is the same as that for noncyanotic patients, but long-term use of antibiotics may mask symptoms of endocarditis and induce antibiotic resistance.

SCOLIOSIS

Scoliosis is common in patients with congenital heart disease, especially those who are cyanotic. It is particularly frequent in those who have had a lateral thoracotomy. It may be severe enough to warrant orthopedic procedures such as insertion of a Harrington rod and may also compromise pulmonary function.

ARTHROPATHY

Some adult cyanotic patients complain of pain in the ankles and knees, which is associated with hypertrophic osteoarthropathy. This periostitis is manifested on radiographs as a thin radiopaque line of new bone at the distal end of the diaphyses.[15] The joints are usually not involved, but effusion and pain in the joints may occur, and the overlying soft tissue may be warm and tender.[16] Correction of cyanosis alleviates the problem. Relief of the pain can be achieved by conventional anti-inflammatory agents, although care must be taken with nonsteroidal agents, which may exacerbate the bleeding diathesis.

ALTITUDE AND AIR TRAVEL

At an altitude of 8,000 feet, the atmospheric Po_2 is considerably less than at sea level, and profoundly cyanotic patients may notice acute symptomatic deterioration. Living at high altitude is best avoided by persons with significant cyanosis, since both symptoms and the degree of erythrocytosis tend to be exaggerated. Travel at 40,000 feet in commercial aircraft has a similar effect, because the ambient Po_2 also decreases. Patients with mild cyanosis usually experience no discomfort, but those with severe cyanosis should ensure that a container of oxygen is available and that they maintain adequate hydration throughout the trip.

PREGNANCY AND CONTRACEPTION

Women with significant cyanosis are unlikely to carry a pregnancy to term. Many spontaneously abort in the first trimester, and in others with less severe hypoxia, poor fetal growth and dysmaturity may occur. These risks correlate approximately with the degree of hypoxia; the higher the maternal hemoglobin and hematocrit values, the less likely the fetus is to reach term. Whittemore[17] reported that among cyanotic mothers whose hematocrit was 65% or more, 80% of all pregnancies ended in spontaneous abortion; the incidence was 60% in mildly cyanotic mothers. Few fetuses survive if the maternal hemoglobin exceeds 18 g/dL.[18] Maternal cyanosis handicaps fetal growth, and surviving offspring usually have a lower birth weight than normal. Pregnancy also poses a danger for the mother because of a right-to-left shunt and the risks of thrombus and paradoxical embolus. Thrombophlebitis, therefore, must be treated promptly to reduce the risk for cerebral embolus. Meticulous attention must be paid to leg care throughout pregnancy and the puerperium for all cyanotic women. Similarly, care must be taken with intravenous injections to avoid air bubbles.

Women with Eisenmenger's syndrome should be counseled strongly against pregnancy. The maternal mortality is approximately 50%,[19] and even those who deliver successfully often die in the ensuing 48 hours, frequently because of massive pulmonary infarct. Women with Eisenmenger's syndrome who become pregnant should be advised to have a termination, but this should be performed under optimal conditions with careful cardiac monitoring, adequate hydration, and absolute avoidance of systemic hypotension, which is potentially fatal.

Contraceptive advice should be carefully considered in all women with cyanotic heart disease. In general (especially for those with pulmonary hypertension), estrogen-containing contraceptive pills should be avoided because of the increased risk of thrombus. Progesterone-only medication may be a reasonable option. Barrier methods of contraception provide a safe alternative, provided that they are strictly adhered to. Intrauterine devices are not appropriate because of the risks of infection and sepsis. For women with Eisenmenger's syndrome, tubal ligation offers a safe alternative, with the same provisos if general anesthesia is chosen. Laparoscopic tubal sterilization under local anesthesia appears to be a relatively safe option.[20]

NONCARDIAC SURGERY

Even minor surgical procedures (e.g., appendectomy) pose significant risks for cyanotic patients, especially those with Eisenmenger's syndrome, and emergency procedures pose a greater hazard than elective ones. For patients with severe cyanosis and hematocrits of more than 65%, elective surgical procedures may be preceded by phlebotomy and fluid replacement, which help to correct the hemostatic defects and minimize the significant risks of bleeding in the perioperative period.[21,22] With this approach, platelet function may be restored to normal for at least 3 weeks. Special attention should be paid to hydration, renal function, and the development of sepsis. Antibiotic prophylaxis should be used when appropriate.

General anesthesia poses special risks for patients with Eisenmenger's syndrome, and when possible, cardiac anesthesiologists should be involved with the patient's case. Although not without risk, insertion of a Swan-Ganz catheter facilitates rapid recognition of alterations in pulmonary wedge pressure so that preload can be maintained. An oximetric Swan-Ganz catheter may help alert the physician to minor decreases in oxygen saturation, which may signify increased right-to-left shunting. Intra-arterial monitoring permits awareness of small changes in blood pressure so that hypotension can be avoided.

REFERENCES

1. Friedland RP, Grant S: Hematocrit, viscosity and cerebral blood flow. *Am Heart J* 97:404-405,1979
2. Perloff JK, Rosove MH, Child JS, et al: Adults with cyanotic congenital heart disease: hematologic management. *Ann Intern Med* 109:406-413,1988
3. Linderkamp O, Klose HJ, Betke K, et al: Increased blood viscosity in patients with cyanotic congenital heart disease and iron deficiency. *J Pediatr* 95:567-569, 1979
4. Hutton RD: The effect of iron deficiency on whole blood viscosity in polycythaemic patients. *Br J Haematol* 43:191-199,1979
5. Rosove MH, Perloff JK, Hocking WG, et al: Chronic hypoxaemia and decompensated erythrocytosis in cyanotic congenital heart disease. *Lancet* 2:313-315, 1986
6. Ware JA, Reaves WH, Horak JK, et al: Defective platelet aggregation in patients undergoing surgical repair of cyanotic congenital heart disease. *Ann Thorac Surg* 36:289-294, 1983
7. Henricksson P, Värendh G, Lundström N-R: Haemostatic defects in cyanotic congenital heart disease. *Br Heart J* 41:23-27, 1979
8. Rosove MH, Hocking WG, Harwig SSL, et al: Studies of β-thromboglobulin, platelet factor 4, and fibrinopeptide A in erythrocytosis due to cyanotic congenital heart disease. *Thromb Res* 29:225-235, 1983
9. Ross EA, Perloff JK, Danovitch GM, et al: Renal function and urate metabolism in late survivors with cyanotic congenital heart disease. *Circulation* 73:396-400, 1986
10. Spear GS: The glomerular lesion of cyanotic congenital heart disease. *Johns Hopkins Med J* 140:185-188, 1977
11. Young D: Hyperuricemia in cyanotic congenital heart disease (letter to the editor). *Am J Dis Child* 134:902-903, 1980
12. Wyngaarden JB: Gout. In *The Metabolic Basis of Inherited Disease.* Second edition. Edited by JB Stanbury, JB Wyngaarden, DS Fredrickson. New York, McGraw-Hill Book Company, 1966, p 668
13. Somerville J: Gout in cyanotic congenital heart disease. *Br Heart J* 23:31-34, 1961
14. Young D, Mark H: Fate of the patient with Eisenmenger syndrome. *Am J Cardiol* 28:658-669, 1971
15. Singh H, Parkash A, Saini M, et al: Bone changes in congenital cyanotic heart disease. *Br Heart J* 34:412-417, 1972
16. Frand M, Koren G, Rubinstein Z: Reversible hypertrophic osteoarthropathy associated with cyanotic congenital heart disease. *Am J Dis Child* 136:687-689, 1982
17. Whittemore R: Congenital heart disease: its impact on pregnancy. *Hosp Pract* 18:65-74, December 1983
18. Neill CA, Swanson S: Outcome of pregnancy in congenital heart disease (abstract). *Circulation* 24:1003, 1961
19. Gleicher N, Midwall J, Hochberger D, et al: Eisenmenger's syndrome and pregnancy. *Obstet Gynecol Surv* 34:721-741, 1979
20. Snabes MC, Poindexter AN III: Laparoscopic tubal sterilization under local anesthesia in women with cyanotic heart disease. *Obstet Gynecol* 78:437-440, 1991
21. Maurer HM, McCue CM, Robertson LW, et al: Correction of platelet dysfunction and bleeding in cyanotic congenital heart disease by simple red cell volume reduction. *Am J Cardiol* 35:831-835, 1975
22. Colón-Otero G, Gilchrist GS, Holcomb GR, et al: Preoperative evaluation of hemostasis in patients with congenital heart disease. *Mayo Clin Proc* 62:379-385, 1987

CHAPTER

44

Atrioventricular canal defect

Robert H. Feldt, M.D., David J. Driscoll, M.D., Valentin Fuster, M.D., and Hartzell V. Schaff, M.D.

ANATOMIC CONSIDERATIONS

The term "atrioventricular canal defect" includes a spectrum of congenital cardiac malformations that have similar embryologic origins. Defective development of the endocardial cushions results in this spectrum. The primitive endocardial cushions normally fuse centrally to produce two distinct and separate atrioventricular (AV) valve orifices. In addition, they participate in formation of the ventricular septum and, by "bowing upward," contact the downward-growing atrial septum primum to obliterate the ostium primum. Thus, aberrations in endocardial cushion formation, migration, and fusion with other primitive intracardiac structures result in significant congenital cardiac malformations. Although several classifications exist for this defect, we prefer that outlined in Table 44-1 as modified from Rastelli et al.,[1] McGoon et al.,[2] and Titus and Rastelli.[3]

Only the complete forms of AV canal are discussed in this chapter. Discussions of ostium primum atrial septal defect and ventricular septal defect of the AV canal type are in chapters 40 and 41, respectively.

In the New England Regional Infant Cardiac Program, 119 (5%) of 2,381 newborn infants with congenital heart disease had an AV canal defect.[4] Seventy-one of these 119 (60%) had complete AV canal, and 21 (18%) had an ostium primum type of atrial septal defect without interventricular communication. Assuming an incidence of congenital heart disease of 0.8% in the general population, the incidence of AV canal defect is 1 in 250,000 live births. In this study there was a predominance of females (70 females to 49 males). Congenital cardiac defects, especially AV canal defects, are relatively common in patients with Down's syndrome: approximately 40% of these patients have congenital heart disease, and 40% of those with congenital heart disease have an AV canal defect. The complete form of AV canal defect is more common than other forms in patients with Down's syndrome (43 of the 54 patients with Down's syndrome in the New England Regional Infant Cardiac Program had complete AV canal).

The central AV portion of the cardiac septum and the contiguous mitral and tricuspid valves are abnormal in complete AV canal. Specifically, the inferior aspect of the atrial septum is absent (persistent ostium primum), and the basilar portion of the ventricular septum is deficient.[3] From the left ventricular aspect, the ventricular septal defect is located in the left ventricular outflow tract. Deficiency of the ventricular septum together with abnormally cephalad displacement of the aortic valve produces an elongated left ventricular outflow tract.

The medial portions of the mitral and tricuspid valve annuli are absent in complete AV canal. Thus, a common

Table 44-1 Classification of AV canal defects

Incomplete or partial AV canal
Without interventricular communication
Ostium primum atrial septal defect with cleft mitral valve
Common atrium with AV valve malformation
Isolated cleft of anterior leaflet of mitral valve
Cleft or partial absence of septal leaflet of tricuspid valve
Small defects of the AV septum (Gerbode defect)
Ventricular septal defect of AV canal type
Intermediate type AV canal
Ostium primum type atrial septal defect of AV canal type, with interventricular communication (usually hemodynamically restrictive) but two complete AV valve rings (usually with cleft mitral or tricuspid valve leaflets)
Complete AV canal
Ostium primum type atrial septal defect continuous with interventricular communication (usually hemodynamically unrestrictive) and a common AV valve
Common anterior AV valve leaflet is divided and is attached by chordae to crest of ventricular septum
Common anterior AV valve leaflet is partially divided and is attached to right ventricular medial papillary muscles
Common anterior AV valve leaflet is undivided and not attached to septum by chordae

Modified from Rastelli et al.,[1] McGoon et al.,[2] and Titus and Rastelli.[3]

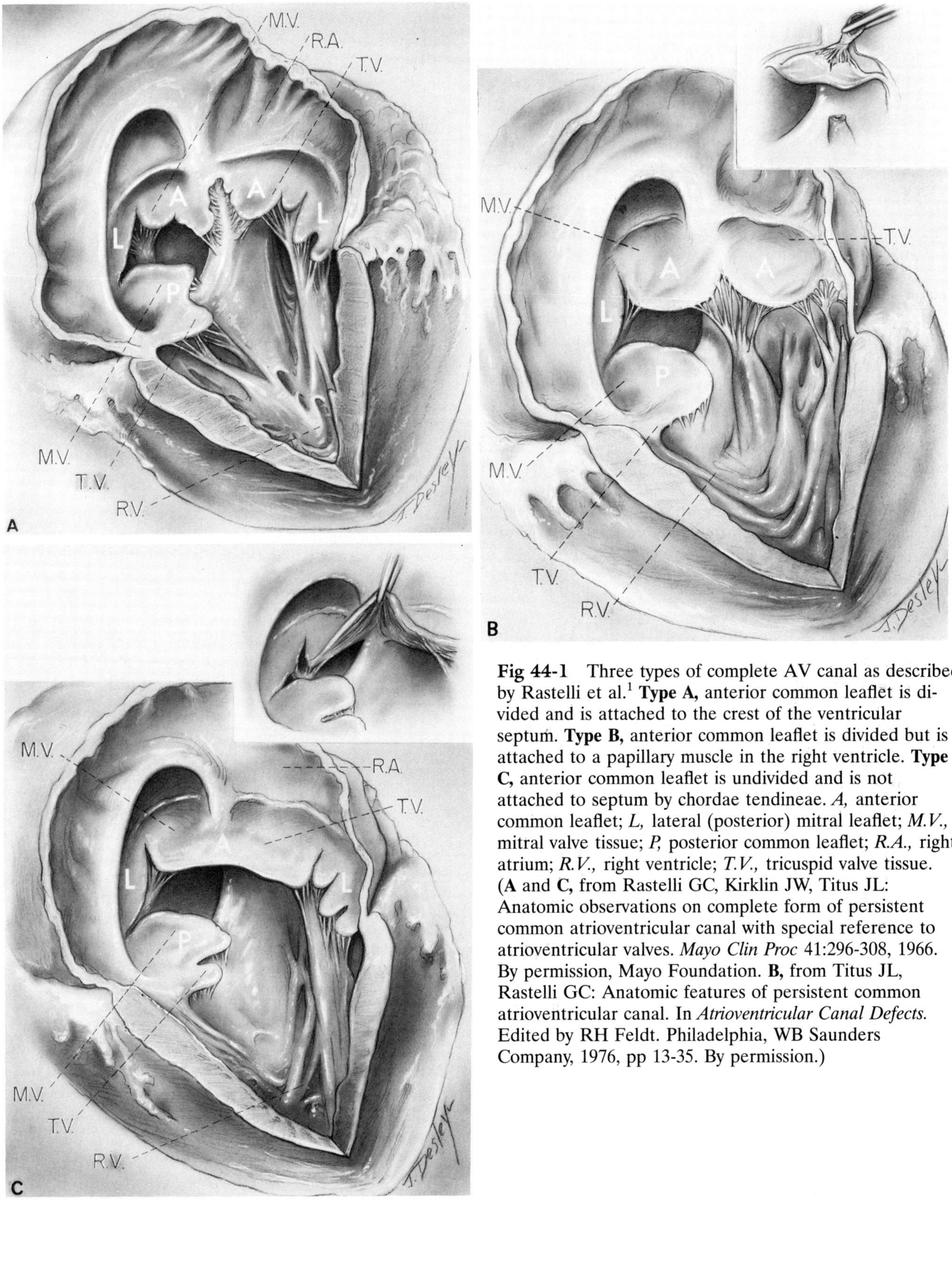

Fig 44-1 Three types of complete AV canal as described by Rastelli et al.[1] **Type A,** anterior common leaflet is divided and is attached to the crest of the ventricular septum. **Type B,** anterior common leaflet is divided but is attached to a papillary muscle in the right ventricle. **Type C,** anterior common leaflet is undivided and is not attached to septum by chordae tendineae. *A,* anterior common leaflet; *L,* lateral (posterior) mitral leaflet; *M.V.,* mitral valve tissue; *P,* posterior common leaflet; *R.A.,* right atrium; *R.V.,* right ventricle; *T.V.,* tricuspid valve tissue. (**A** and **C,** from Rastelli GC, Kirklin JW, Titus JL: Anatomic observations on complete form of persistent common atrioventricular canal with special reference to atrioventricular valves. *Mayo Clin Proc* 41:296-308, 1966. By permission, Mayo Foundation. **B,** from Titus JL, Rastelli GC: Anatomic features of persistent common atrioventricular canal. In *Atrioventricular Canal Defects.* Edited by RH Feldt. Philadelphia, WB Saunders Company, 1976, pp 13-35. By permission.)

AV valve exists. The posterior mitral valve leaflet usually is normal but may be deficient or contain an accessory orifice. When an accessory orifice is present, the chordae from the accessory orifice usually attach to a single papillary muscle. Rastelli et al.[1] classified complete AV canal on the basis of the anatomy of the common anterior AV valve leaflet (Fig 44-1). In their type A complete AV canal, the common anterior AV valve leaflet is divided and attached to the crest of the ventricular septum by chordae. In type B, it is divided and chordae tendineae from the midportions of the divided anterior leaflet are attached to the right ventricular medial papillary muscle. In type C, the leaflet is undivided and not attached to the ventricular septum (so-called free-floating anterior leaflet). Type A is the most common form, constituting 80% of cases of complete AV canal. Type B is the rarest form. Type C most commonly occurs with associated cardiac malformations such as pulmonary valve stenosis or transposition of the great arteries. Type C is especially common in patients with Down's syndrome.

PATHOPHYSIOLOGY

Patients with complete AV canal develop congestive heart failure as a result of and proportional to the degree of left-to-right shunt through the septal defect and the degree of AV valve insufficiency. Although the net intracardiac shunt is left-to-right, some right-to-left shunt also occurs.[5] Growth failure occurs in many infants with complete AV canal. Because of the increased pulmonary blood flow, congestive failure, and associated mitral regurgitation, pulmonary vascular obstructive disease eventually develops in patients with complete AV canal if it is not corrected surgically. Pulmonary vascular obstructive disease may develop particularly rapidly in infants with Down's syndrome associated with complete AV canal; the reasons for this are incompletely defined.[6]

CLINICAL SYNDROME

History and clinical course

Patients with complete AV canal attract medical attention early in life because of signs and symptoms of congestive heart failure, including tachypnea, tachycardia, poor feeding, sweating, and growth failure. Without surgical correction, only 54% of babies with complete AV canal survive to 6 months of age, 35% to 12 months of age, 15% to 24 months of age, and 4% to 5 years of age.[7] Rarely does such a patient reach adulthood in an operable condition. Patients who do survive without operation invariably develop pulmonary vascular obstructive disease. As pulmonary vascular obstructive disease worsens, the signs and symptoms of congestive heart failure and pulmonary congestion may abate; eventually, increasing cyanosis and polycythemia occur.

Physical findings

Physical appearance. In the first 2 to 3 years of life, the majority of patients with complete AV canal are acyanotic, but about 30% will have mild cyanosis. Infants with severe heart failure appear undernourished with poorly developed subcutaneous fat stores. Those patients who survive childhood without surgical correction tend to become cyanotic.

Precordial palpation. Within the first 2 to 3 years of life, the cardiac precordial impulses are overactive, and the impulse at the lower left sternal border (right ventricular impulse) is prominent, reflecting right ventricular hypertension. Because of the pulmonary hypertension, closure of the pulmonary valve may be palpable at the upper left sternal border.

Auscultation. In infancy, the first cardiac sound usually is normal. The pulmonary component of the second heart sound is increased. A grade 2/6 to 3/6 precordial systolic murmur, resulting from flow of blood through the ventricular septal defect or through the pulmonary valve, usually is present. Mitral insufficiency is usually present and is manifested by a high-frequency, blowing systolic murmur heard at the cardiac apex and radiating into the left axilla. A low-frequency apical diastolic murmur, reflecting antegrade flow through the AV valve, usually is audible.

Electrocardiogram

In complete AV canal the electrocardiogram is characterized by a superior QRS axis, first-degree AV block, and right and left ventricular hypertrophy. Particularly if there is left ventricle-to-right atrium shunting of blood, tall, peaked P waves reflecting right atrial enlargement may be present. The frontal plain vectorcardiographic loop is directed superiorly and rotates counterclockwise or in a "figure of 8" pattern. The abnormal QRS axis and prolonged AV conduction have been attributed to morphological aberration of the cardiac conduction tissue.[8]

Chest radiograph

Cardiomegaly and increased pulmonary vascular markings are characteristic. As pulmonary vascular obstructive disease develops in patients who have not had operative correction, the cardiac size and pulmonary vascular markings may regress while the central pulmonary artery size increases.

Echocardiography

Two-dimensional echocardiographic techniques have supplanted cardiac catheterization and angiography in the diagnosis of AV canal and in the delineation of specific features of the AV valve morphology and valvular attachments.[9] A key feature of the echocardiographic diagnosis of complete AV canal is the absence of attachment of the medial aspects of the AV valves to the septum (Fig 44-2). Also, chordae attaching the anterior leaflet to the septum or papillary muscles can be appreciated; thus, it occasionally is possible to define the exact type of AV valve malformation (Rastelli type A, B, or C).

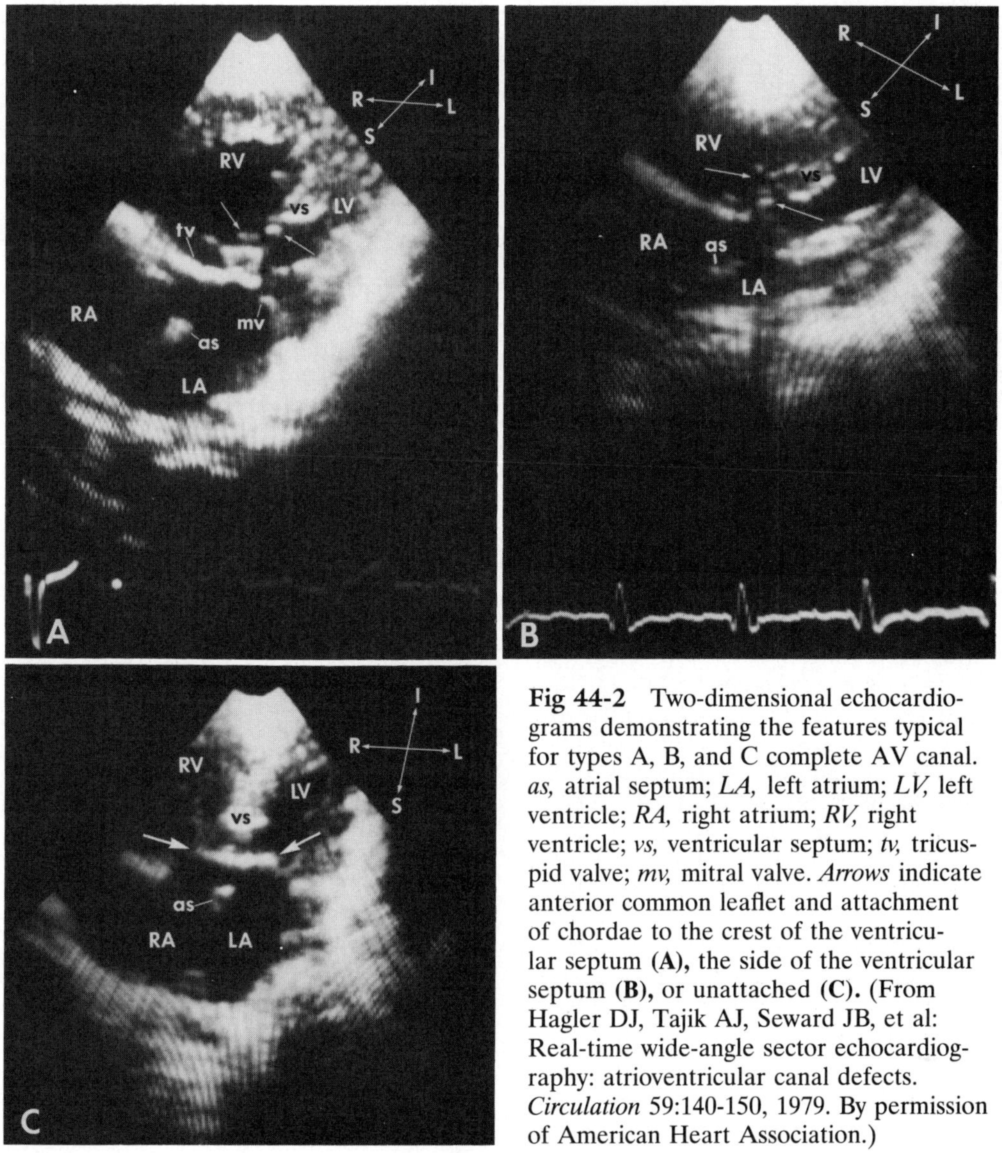

Fig 44-2 Two-dimensional echocardiograms demonstrating the features typical for types A, B, and C complete AV canal. *as,* atrial septum; *LA,* left atrium; *LV,* left ventricle; *RA,* right atrium; *RV,* right ventricle; *vs,* ventricular septum; *tv,* tricuspid valve; *mv,* mitral valve. *Arrows* indicate anterior common leaflet and attachment of chordae to the crest of the ventricular septum **(A),** the side of the ventricular septum **(B),** or unattached **(C).** (From Hagler DJ, Tajik AJ, Seward JB, et al: Real-time wide-angle sector echocardiography: atrioventricular canal defects. *Circulation* 59:140-150, 1979. By permission of American Heart Association.)

DIAGNOSTIC PROBLEMS AND INVASIVE STUDIES

Catheterization is indicated to assess hemodynamically the degree of pulmonary vascular obstructive disease in order to determine operability. There is evidence for left-to-right and right-to-left atrial and ventricular shunting by oximetry but, in the absence of significant pulmonary vascular obstructive disease, the net shunt is left to right. In 39 patients with a complete AV canal, the right ventricle-to-left ventricle pressure ratio was less than 0.3 in none, between 0.3 and 0.6 in 1, between 0.7 and 0.8 in none, and above 0.8 in 38.[5] Obviously, the lower pressure ratio is associated with a smaller ventricular septal defect. It is important to measure pulmonary artery pressure and calculate pulmonary arteriolar resistance to determine suitability for operative correction. The left ventricular angiographic appearance of complete AV canal is quite characteristic and has been described as a "gooseneck" (Fig 44-3). This appearance is created by the abnormal caudad displacement of the AV valves and cephalad position of the aortic valve. Because of the deficient ventricular septum, the right border of the left ventricle is concave on the anteroposterior projection of the left ventricular angiogram during diastole.

MANAGEMENT

Medical versus surgical treatment

Infants who have complete AV canal with congestive heart failure should be treated with digitalis and diuretic drugs. If growth failure continues despite optimal doses of these drugs, formulas with increased caloric content can

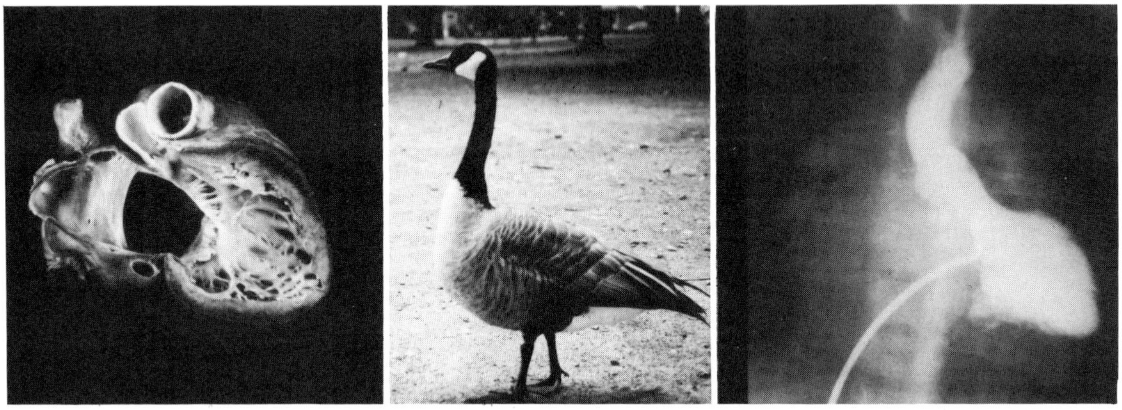

Fig 44-3 **Right,** left ventricular angiogram demonstrating typical appearance in complete AV canal. **Left,** pathologic specimen. "Gooseneck" appearance of pathologic specimen and angiogram is apparent. (We are grateful to Dr. William Edwards for the photograph of the necropsy specimen and the goose.)

be used in an attempt to augment caloric intake. If congestive heart failure is refractory to medical therapy or if growth failure continues, surgical intervention will be necessary. In any case, because pulmonary vascular obstructive disease may become severe and may even progress in older patients after intracardiac repair, repair for complete AV canal should be performed before age 1. For patients presenting for care who are more than 1 year old, operation is indicated if pulmonary resistance does not exceed 8 to 10 units · m^2.

Operative correction includes closure of the interatrial and interventricular septal defects with prosthetic material, either as a single patch or separate ventricular (subvalvular) and atrial septal patches. Also required is suspension of the medial aspects of the left and at least part of the right AV valve leaflets from the patch material. Rarely, a competent mitral valve cannot be fashioned from native valve tissue and replacement of the left AV valve with a prosthesis is necessary. Significant associated cardiac malformations should be repaired also.

Operative mortality for complete AV canal varies among institutions, but for patients more than 6 months old without significant pulmonary vascular obstructive disease, operative mortality is approximately 10%.[10-16] Operative mortality in infants less than 6 months old is higher than in those more than 6 months old at the time of operation. The role of pulmonary artery banding in infants with complete AV canal and refractory pulmonary edema and congestive heart failure still is being debated.[16,17] Most investigators agree that pulmonary artery banding is not useful in the presence of severe AV valve regurgitation. Many surgeons and pediatric cardiologists believe that intracardiac repair is preferable to pulmonary artery banding in infants of all ages.

Chin et al.[18] identified the following anatomic features that may adversely affect outcome of operation: (1) marked deficiency of AV valve tissue, (2) ventricular hypoplasia, (3) malalignment of the common AV valve and ventricles, (4) double-orifice mitral valve, (5) solitary left ventricular papillary muscle group, and (6) additional ventricular septal defects.

Successful management and long-term good results in patients with AV canal depend on early recognition of the defect, an understanding of the important associated defects, realization that pulmonary vascular disease may develop in the first 12 to 18 months of life, and accurate surgical repair. Perioperative management of children with this defect and Down's syndrome is especially challenging, and these patients require careful and cautious follow-up.

REFERENCES

1. Rastelli GC, Kirklin JW, Titus JL: Anatomic observations on complete form of persistent common atrioventricular canal with special reference to atrioventricular valves. *Mayo Clin Proc* 41:296-308, 1966
2. McGoon DC, Puga FJ, Danielson GK: Atrioventricular canal. In *Gibbon's Surgery of the Chest.* Vol. 2. Fourth edition. Edited by DC Sabiston Jr, FC Spencer. Philadelphia, WB Saunders Company, 1983, pp 1051-1066
3. Titus JL, Rastelli GC: Anatomic features of persistent common atrioventricular canal. In *Atrioventricular Canal Defects.* Edited by RH Feldt. Philadelphia, WB Saunders Company, 1976, pp 13-35
4. Report of the New England Regional Infant Cardiac Program. *Pediatrics* 65 Suppl:441-444, 1980
5. Park JM, Ritter DG, Mair DD: Cardiac catheterization findings in persistent common atrioventricular canal. In *Atrioventricular Canal Defects.* Edited by RH Feldt. Philadelphia, WB Saunders Company, 1976, pp 76-86
6. Cooney TP, Thurlbeck WM: Pulmonary hypoplasia in Down's syndrome. *N Engl J Med* 307:1170-1173, 1982
7. Berger TJ, Blackstone EH, Kirklin JW, et al: Survival and probability of cure without and with operation in complete atrioventricular canal. *Ann Thorac Surg* 27:104-111, 1979
8. Feldt RH, Titus JL: The conduction system in persistent common atrioventricular canal. In *Atrioventricular Canal Defects.* Edited by RH Feldt. Philadelphia, WB Saunders Company, 1976, pp 36-43
9. Hagler DJ, Tajik AJ, Seward JB, et al: Real-time wide-angle sector echocardiography: atrioventricular canal defects. *Circulation* 59:140-150, 1979
10. Rastelli GC, Ongley PA, Kirklin JW, et al: Surgical repair of the complete form of persistent common atrioventricular canal. *J Thorac Cardiovasc Surg* 55:299-308, 1968

11. Kahn DR, Levy J, France NE, et al: Recent results after repair of atrioventricular canal. *J Thorac Cardiovasc Surg* 73:413-415, 1977

12. McGoon DC, McMullan MH, Mair DD, et al: Correction of complete atrioventricular canal in infants. *Mayo Clin Proc* 48:769-772, 1973

13. Studer M, Blackstone EH, Kirklin JW, et al: Determinants of early and late results of repair of atrioventricular septal (canal) defects. *J Thorac Cardiovasc Surg* 84:523-542, 1982

14. Bender HW Jr, Hammon JW Jr, Hubbard SG, et al: Repair of atrioventricular canal malformation in the first year of life. *J Thorac Cardiovasc Surg* 84:515-520, 1982

15. Minale C, von Bernuth G, Bardos P, et al: Repair of complete atrioventricular canal in early childhood. *Thorac Cardiovasc Surg* 30:88-90, 1982

16. Silverman N, Levitsky S, Fisher E, et al: Efficacy of pulmonary artery banding in infants with complete atrioventricular canal. *Circulation* 68 Suppl 2:148-152, 1983

17. Williams WH, Guyton RA, Michalik RE, et al: Individualized surgical management of complete atrioventricular canal. *J Thorac Cardiovasc Surg* 86:838-844, 1983

18. Chin A, Keane JF, Norwood WI, et al: Repair of complete common atrioventricular canal in infancy. *J Thorac Cardiovasc Surg* 84:437-445, 1982

CHAPTER

45

Coarctation of the aorta

Carole A. Warnes, M.D., Valentin Fuster, M.D., and Dwight C. McGoon, M.D.

ANATOMIC CONSIDERATIONS

Coarctation of the aorta was described over 200 years ago by the Prussian anatomist Johann Friedrich Meckel,[1] and the clinical findings were outlined about 100 years ago.[2] Corrective surgery for this condition was introduced more than 50 years ago.[3,4]

Coarctation of the aorta is usually discovered in infants or children; only about 20% of the cases are diagnosed for the first time in adolescents or adults. The majority (95%) of coarctations are below the left subclavian artery and above the ductus arteriosus ("preductal coarctation") or just at or below the ductus ("postductal coarctation"). The coarctation usually consists of a discrete infolding of the left posterolateral aspect of the aortic wall, causing the lumen to narrow eccentrically; secondary dilatation commonly develops in the proximal aorta and left subclavian artery and also distal to the coarctation. The preductal type of coarctation most commonly is discovered in early infancy because it is usually severe and is associated with other significant congenital anomalies[5,6] such as ventricular septal defect, proximal tubular hypoplasia of the aortic arch, transposition of the great arteries, or mitral valve disease. The postductal type can be discovered in adulthood because it tends to be less severe and usually is not associated with other significant congenital anomalies. Indeed, in patients who survive infancy the degree of aortic coarctation tends to progress, but this may not become clinically apparent until adulthood.[7,8]

As a result of the condition, there is progressive development of systemic collaterals from the subclavian and axillary arteries through the internal mammary, scapular, and intercostal arteries (Fig 45-1). Other associated anomalies or complications may become apparent initially in adulthood. A bicuspid aortic valve, which has been reported to occur in between 40% and 80% of the cases,[9,10] can lead to calcific aortic stenosis, infective endocarditis, or, less commonly, significant aortic valvular incompetence. Other complications include rupture of an aneurysm of the circle of Willis and rupture or dissection in the neighborhood of the coarctation. Coarctation of the aorta is the most common cardiovascular abnormality in Turner's syndrome.[11]

Only 5% of the coarctations are localized either proximal to the left subclavian artery or, rarely, in the abdominal aorta.[12,13] Interruption of the aortic arch is a separate entity, but usually it has the same location, clinical features, and associated congenital anomalies as the coarctation manifested in early infancy;[6,14] nevertheless, it is out of the scope of a chapter mainly related to adolescence and adulthood.

PATHOPHYSIOLOGY

The most important pathophysiologic consequence of coarctation of the aorta is systemic proximal hypertension with abnormal differences between upper and lower extremity pulses and systolic blood pressures. During exercise, the pressure gradient across the zone of coarc-

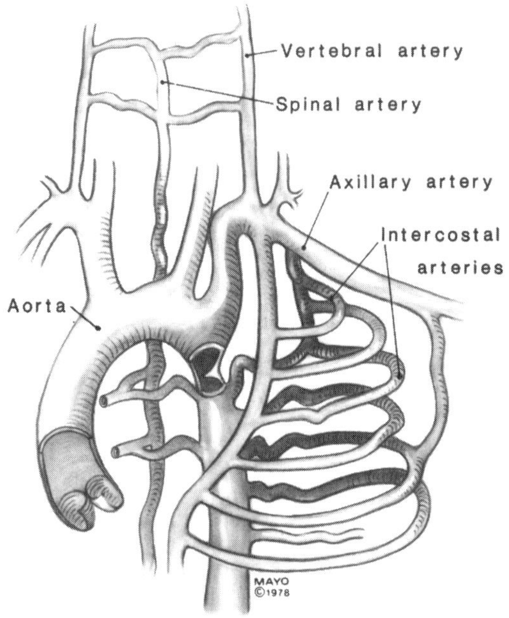

Fig 45-1 Postductal coarctation of the aorta with well-developed collateral circulation. (From Fuster V, Brandenburg RO, McGoon DC, et al: Clinical approach and management of congenital heart disease in the adolescent and adult. *Cardiovasc Clin* 10 No 3:161-197, 1980. By permission, Mayo Foundation.)

tation increases, and a large increase occurs in upper body systolic blood pressure.[15] The mechanical component of the coarctation does not always fully explain the systemic hypertension. That is, after surgical repair, systemic hypertension may persist[16-19] and the arteriolar resistance has been found to be high in the proximal vascular beds.[20] For this reason, a role of the renin/angiotensin system has been considered.

Collateral circulation to bypass the constriction of coarctation of the aorta may begin to develop in utero, particularly in patients with severe postductal coarctation. In severe preductal coarctation, the opened ductus arteriosus tends in part to provide collateral circulation by shunting blood right to left toward the lower part of the body. In those patients who survive infancy, the development of collateral vessels tends to be clinically apparent by auscultation and chest radiographs by 5 to 10 years of age.[6] The majority of the collateral vessels come from the subclavian arteries, from which branches, in turn, lead to dilated intercostal, internal mammary, and epigastric arteries; the anterior spinal artery is also involved as a collateral channel (see Fig 45-1).

From a pathophysiologic point of view it is important to comment on the five major complications of coarctation of the aorta:[6] cardiac failure, aortic valve disease, rupture or dissection in the neighborhood of the coarctation, endarteritis, and rupture of an aneurysm of the circle of Willis.

Cardiac failure is not uncommon in infants with severe preductal coarctation. Left ventricular failure tends to occur because of associated anomalies (such as ventricular septal defect or mitral valve disease) or because of pressure overload. Right heart failure also may occur in patients with severe postductal coarctation because of pulmonary hypertension. In an adult with coarctation of the aorta, left ventricular failure may occur as a result of hypertension associated with coronary artery disease or aortic valve disease.

Calcified aortic stenosis may occur in long-term survivors of surgical treatment[15] because of the high incidence of bicuspid aortic valve that, with time, tends to become calcified.[9,10,16,21] In addition, as a result of the association of systemic hypertension with the abnormal aortic valve, aortic valve regurgitation may occur.

Rupture or dissection of the aorta may originate either in the proximal dilated ascending aorta,[22] being in part related to the hypertension and local stress, or just beyond the coarctation[22,23] as a result of the jet of blood across the coarctation, which erodes the intimal area.[5] This is also the most common site of infective endarteritis.[5,24] Nevertheless, in patients with coarctation of the aorta, infective endarteritis at the site of coarctation occurs less frequently than endocarditis on the bicuspid valve.[5,24,25]

Intracerebral hemorrhage[24,26,27] is another complication of coarctation of the aorta and appears to be related to the combination of an increased incidence of aneurysms of the circle of Willis in this condition (in about 10% of cases)[24] plus the presence of hypertension, which in part may precipitate the rupture. However, cerebrovascular accidents late postoperatively have been described in nonhypertensive patients.[28]

CLINICAL SYNDROME

History and clinical course

Among symptomatic infants with coarctation of the aorta, the frequency of associated anomalies is high.[5] Generally, they have a severe preductal type of coarctation with associated ventricular septal defect, mitral incompetence, or other anomalies; the ductus arteriosus tends to remain open to provide circulation to the lower part of the body. The cardiac failure may be left- or right-sided, and the mortality rate is highest in the first two months of life. Among the small proportion of symptomatic infants in whom the coarctation is the only anomaly, many improve on medical management and become asymptomatic by early childhood.[5,6]

Coarctation of the aorta first recognized in adolescents or young adults is not usually associated with symptoms. In patients over age 30, symptoms and major complications leading to death are common.[8] The initial clue to coarctation of the aorta in the adolescent or young adult is the discovery of systemic hypertension or an abnormality on a routine chest radiograph, particularly notching of the ribs. In this clinical context, a search for absent or weak and delayed femoral pulses is important for confirmation of the diagnosis. The early symptoms may be headaches related to hypertension, the feeling of prominent arterial pulsations in the neck, and leg fatigue.[6] About half of these patients die within the first 3 decades of life, and more than three-fourths are dead by age 50 years.[5,8,24,29] Longer survival is uncommon[6,8,30,31] (Fig 45-2).

The main complications leading to death within the first 3 decades are rupture of the aorta, infective endocarditis or endarteritis, and cerebral hemorrhage. Patients surviving into the fourth decade have an increasing incidence of cardiac failure. Thus, in adolescents and adults, coarctation of the aorta tends to produce minor symptoms at

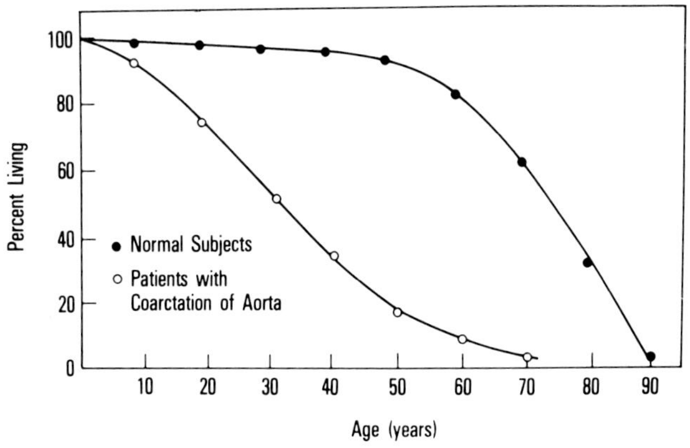

Fig 45-2 Survival plotted as a function of age for 465 patients with coarctation of the aorta who did not undergo surgical correction and survived the first year of life and for 1,000 normal subjects who survived the first year. (From Maron BJ: Coarctation of the aorta in the adult. *Cardiovasc Clin* 10 No 1:311-319, 1979. By permission of FA Davis Company.)

most, but the complications usually are dramatic and lead to death. Rupture of the aorta or dissecting aneurysm occurs most frequently in the third or fourth decade of life;[22,29,32,33] it originates either in the proximal dilated ascending aorta or in a postcoarctation aneurysm, which may result in bleeding into the esophagus.[22-24,33,34] Therefore, episodes of hematemesis or melena predict the disaster in these patients. Infective endarteritis or endocarditis may occur at any time, but most commonly it is within the second to fourth decades of life.[8,24,33] The complication of intracerebral hemorrhage due to rupture of an aneurysm of the circle of Willis tends to occur in the second or third decade of life.[24,33] The increasing incidence of left ventricular failure in older patients is the result of hypertension associated with coronary artery disease or of aortic valve disease related to bicuspid aortic valve.

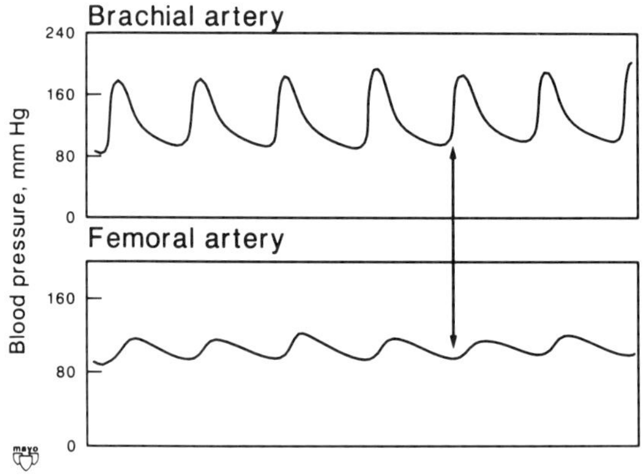

Fig 45-3 Simultaneous brachial and femoral arterial pressure pulses in patient with severe coarctation of the aorta. Femoral pulses were palpable but smaller and delayed with respect to brachial pulses. The important difference between upper and lower extremity pressures is in systolic, not diastolic, levels.

Physical findings

Physical appearance. In general, appearance, growth and development are normal with the following exceptions:[6] occasional association of Turner's syndrome[11,35,36] (see chapter 68); infants and children with cardiac failure appear very ill or may have cyanosis of the lower extremities only (see preductal coarctation under "Pathophysiology"); and occasional adults who appear with an athletic chest but with narrow hips and thin legs or with an undeveloped left arm when the coarctation compromises the origin of the subclavian artery.

Blood pressure, arterial pulse, and venous pulse. In infants with coarctation of the aorta, the brachial and radial pulses usually are easily palpable but the femoral pulses are weak or absent. Measurement by the flush[37] or Doppler ultrasound[38] technique in both arms and one leg reveals hypertension in the upper limbs and hypotension in the lower limbs. Among patients who survive infancy and reach adolescence or adulthood, practically all have a pressure gradient (systolic rather than diastolic) and most have a pulse difference between the upper and lower extremities (Fig 45-3). One study[39] revealed that 89% of these patients had systolic hypertension in the upper extremities; femoral pulses were absent in 40% of patients, were weakly palpable with a pulse lag (when compared simultaneously with the brachial pulses) in 44% of patients, and were normal in only 16% of patients. Exercise may exaggerate the systolic blood pressure gradient between arms and legs.[15,40] Other arterial pulse features in patients with coarctation of the aorta are forceful carotid and suprasternal pulsations[33] and palpable collateral vessels in the muscles of the back.

In the clinical context of hypertension, particularly in the young, weak and delayed femoral pulses or absence of them is the clinical diagnostic hallmark of coarctation of the aorta.

Precordial palpation. The left ventricular impulse is forceful and sustained in those patients with significant hypertension and left ventricular hypertrophy. A visible and palpable impulse in the right parasternal region may be apparent in dilatation of the ascending aorta; in addition, a systolic thrill in the suprasternal region is common.

Auscultation. An ejection systolic click is present when there is an associated bicuspid aortic valve.[41] The second heart sound (aortic component) is loud as a result of hypertension. A fourth heart sound may be generated by the association of hypertension with left ventricular hypertrophy. Murmurs may originate from three sources: arterial collaterals, the coarctation itself, and the bicuspid aortic valve[6] (Fig 45-4). Collateral systolic murmurs tend to be delayed in systole and are spread widely over the thorax, especially anteriorly. The coarctation itself can be responsible for a systolic murmur, especially heard over the spine in the midthoracic region; such a murmur may extend into diastole in the form of a continuous murmur. Finally, an associated bicuspid aortic valve may generate an aortic systolic murmur that may be difficult to distinguish from murmurs of collateral circulation, and, occasionally, may generate a diastolic murmur of aortic regurgitation.

Electrocardiogram

Among adolescents and adult patients with isolated coarctation of the aorta, the electrocardiogram can be entirely normal, particularly if the coarctation is mild and there is no significant hypertension. On the other hand, in more severe coarctation with chronic significant hypertension, the electrocardiogram usually reveals the high-voltage pattern of left ventricular hypertrophy with or without repolarization changes of strain.

Chest radiograph

The chest radiograph may show subtle but characteristic features[6] (Fig 45-5). Irregularities or notching of the inferior margins of the posterior ribs results from collateral flow through dilated and pulsatile intercostal arteries;

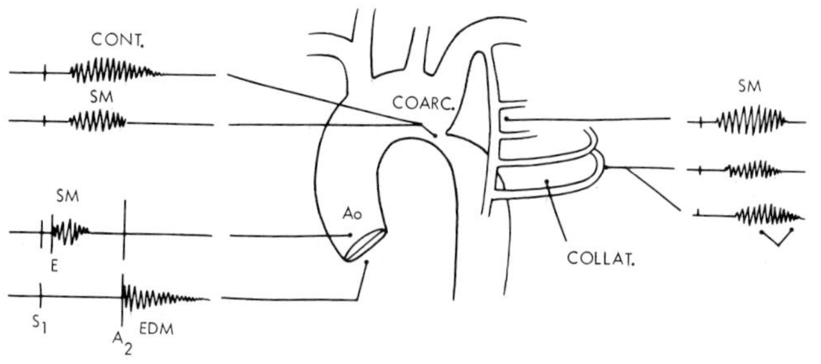

Fig 45-4 Schematic illustration of principal murmurs heard in patients with coarctation of the aorta. Lower left side shows auscultatory events associated with bicuspid aortic valve—namely, an aortic ejection sound *(E),* a short midsystolic murmur *(SM),* and an early diastolic murmur *(EDM)* of aortic regurgitation. At upper left are shown the continuous *(CONT.)* and delayed systolic *(SM)* murmurs that originate in the coarctation itself and are best heard posteriorly over the thoracic spine. At right are shown collateral arterial murmurs that are crescendo-decrescendo in shape and delayed in onset and termination because of origin in vessels that are some distance from the heart. These collateral murmurs are best designated "delayed systolic murmurs." (From Perloff JK: *The Clinical Recognition of Congenital Heart Disease.* Second edition. Philadelphia, WB Saunders Company, 1978, pp 126-154. By permission.)

these are evident usually after 6 years of age and only if the coarctation is significant. A "3" configuration of the aortic knob represents the coarctation site with proximal and distal dilatations; a mirror image of this, an "E" configuration, is seen on the barium-filled esophagus. Finally, there may be a slight prominence of the left ventricle representing hypertrophy and dilatation.

Echocardiogram

The echocardiogram is useful in determining the associated abnormalities such as the status of the aortic and mitral valves and the presence or absence of left ventricular hypertrophy. Discrete coarctation of the aorta also may be demonstrated by two-dimensional echocardiography.[42] Weyman et al.[43] were among the first to study the feasibility of diagnosing coarctation of the aorta. They were able to visualize this area in 16 of 18 patients. In each case there was a localized area of restricted aortic diameter in the region of the left subclavian artery and corresponding to the angiographic appearance of the coarctation (Fig 45-6).

Doppler studies are useful in identifying coarctation of the aorta,[5] and continuous-wave sampling from the suprasternal notch down the descending aorta demonstrates increased velocities from turbulent flow. Calculation of the pressure drop across the coarctation by the modified Bernoulli equation may correspond well with the gradient measured at cardiac catheterization,[44] particularly when the precoarctation velocity is included in the equation.[45] In some patients, however, agreement is poor

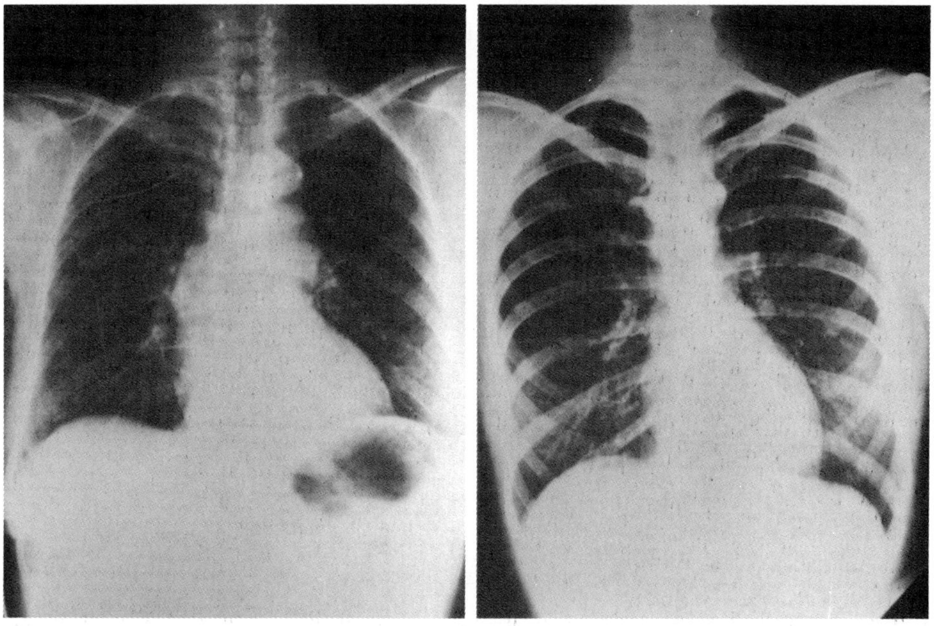

Fig 45-5 **Left,** coarctation of aorta with "3" sign seen along upper aspect of left cardiac silhouette; indentation just below aortic arch represents coarcted segment with poststenotic dilatation below this. **Right,** no other characteristics of aortic coarctation are present except notching beneath the undersurface of the ribs, evident on the left side.

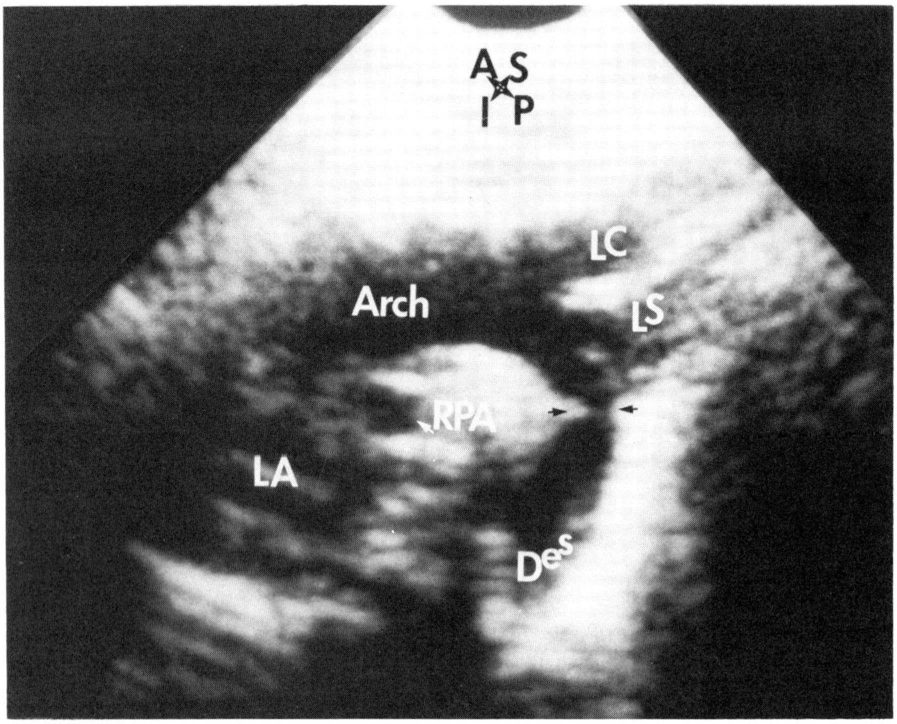

Fig 45-6 An echocardiogram from a suprasternal long-axis view shows marked narrowing of the descending thoracic aorta *(Des)* in a patient with coarctation *(black arrows)*. The coarctation appears as a ledge-like indentation just distal to the left subclavian artery *(LS)*. *A,* anterior; *Arch,* aortic arch; *I,* inferior; *LA,* left atrium; *LC,* left common carotid artery; *P,* posterior; *RPA,* right pulmonary artery; *S,* superior. (From Seward JB, Tajik AJ, Edwards WD, et al: *Two-Dimensional Echocardiographic Atlas.* Vol 1. *Congenital Heart Disease.* New York, Springer-Verlag, 1987, p 482. By permission, Mayo Foundation.)

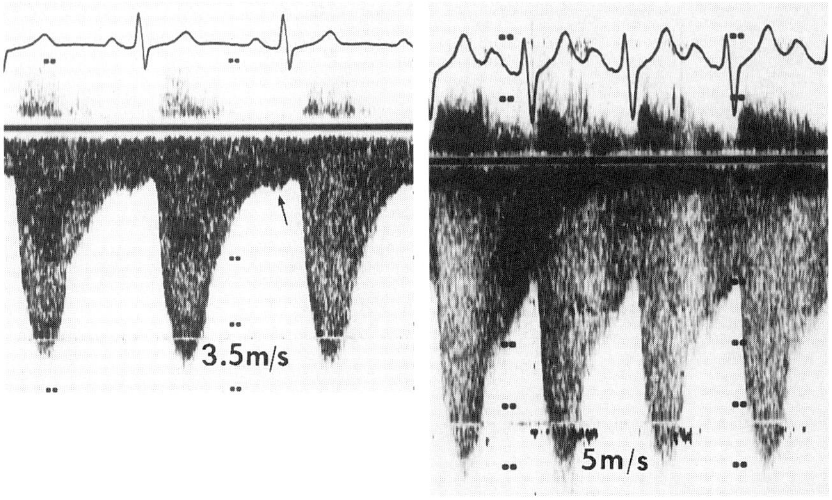

Fig 45-7 Continuous-wave Doppler recordings down the descending aorta in a patient with coarctation of the aorta. **Left,** resting recording with a peak systolic velocity of 3.5 m/sec indicates a maximum instantaneous gradient of approximately 49 mm Hg. Note the persistence of high-velocity flow (approximately 1 m/sec) in diastole *(arrow)*. **Right,** with exercise, the peak velocity increases to 5 m/sec (100 mm Hg maximum instantaneous gradient) and the diastolic flow also is increased, to 2 m/sec. These measurements are consistent with severe coarctation.

between the coarctation gradients measured invasively and those measured by Doppler echocardiography.[46] The discrepancy occurs because it may be difficult to align the Doppler beam with flow and is more frequent when there is a long tubular stenosis rather than a discrete one, since this invalidates the Bernoulli equation.[47,48] A high peak systolic gradient (>40 mm Hg) may be more specific in detecting a significant coarctation in addition to the persistence of high-velocity flow during diastole.[49] Exercise may exaggerate these abnormalities[50] (Fig 45-7).

In addition to echocardiography and Doppler studies, digital subtraction angiography[51] and magnetic resonance imaging[52] are evolving as less invasive diagnostic techniques than cardiac catheterization and conventional angiography in patients with coarctation of the aorta.

DIAGNOSTIC PROBLEMS AND INDICATIONS FOR INVASIVE STUDIES

It is easy to diagnose coarctation of the aorta, but unfortunately this diagnosis frequently is overlooked. Two points are important in this regard: (1) the possibility of coarctation of the aorta should be suspected in any patient under age 50 who has hypertension, and (2) simultaneous palpation of the radial and femoral pulses should be performed as part of any routine cardiovascular examination.

In patients with a coarctation involving the orifice of the left subclavian artery, the left radial and femoral pulses are equally weak; in these patients the diagnosis of coarctation will be clarified if the right radial and carotid pulses are routinely used for comparison with the femoral pulses.

In patients with coarctation but without significant hypertension (because of excellent collateral circulation), this collateral circulation also can provide good femoral pulses, and the only diagnostic clue is significant rib notching on the radiograph.

In patients with congenital coarctation of the abdominal aorta, rib notching may be absent, at least in the upper ribs, but a continuous abdominal bruit occasionally is present.

In patients with pseudocoarctation or kinking of the aorta with incidental hypertension, the diagnosis of coarctation may be excluded in general because the abnormal aortic arch on chest radiographs is not associated with rib notching, and the radial and femoral pulses are synchronous. Nevertheless, because these patients can have associated peripheral vascular disease and because pseudocoarctation creates a murmur well heard in the back, the differential diagnosis of true coarctation may be difficult.

In children or adults with the typical clinical findings of isolated coarctation, confirmation of the diagnosis by cardiac catheterization and angiography is unnecessary. However, these invasive studies are justified when the clinical diagnosis is uncertain, as in those rare clinical presentations outlined above, and when echocardiography and other noninvasive modalities (e.g., magnetic resonance imaging) are not diagnostic. Because the pressure gradient across the coarctation may not be severe (it depends on the degree of coarctation and of collateral vessels) when the diagnosis is confirmed at catheterization and angiography,[53] in order to assess severity the physician must evaluate the clinical, hemodynamic, and angiographic data together.[5] Finally, catheterization is mandatory in those infants with symptomatic coarctation because the surgeon needs to know about possible associated anomalies and the anatomy of the aortic arch prior to operation.

MANAGEMENT

Medical versus surgical treatment

Medical treatment of coarctation is justified only as a prelude to definitive repair. Management consists of periodic examinations to detect deterioration in the hemodynamic state, control of hypertension, advice to avoid strenuous exercise, and protection against bacterial endarteritis at the level of the lesion or bacterial endocarditis if a bicuspid aortic valve is also present.

Balloon dilation angioplasty of coarctation of the aorta was first reported in 1983,[54] and the procedure has gained increasing popularity.[55,56] In most patients, short-term success in gradient reduction and increase in coarctation diameter has been reported,[57,58] but since balloon dilatation relieves the coarctation by tearing the intima and media,[59,60] aortic aneurysm is an important complication. The incidence of aneurysm varies widely.

The Valvuloplasty and Angioplasty of Congenital Anomalies (VACA) Registry has confirmed that native coarctations can be effectively dilated in both infants and older children.[61] After 141 procedures on patients aged 3 days to 29 years, there were 24 complications (17%), most related to the arterial puncture. There were, however, one death and two early and six late "aneurysms." Since most aneurysms appeared late after angioplasty, there remains concern that the true incidence of this complication has not yet emerged. Because the natural history of these aneurysms remains uncertain, the role of angioplasty is still in question.[61] Recoarctation may also occur.

Although some reports have suggested that improved "long-term" results occur when the initial balloon dilatation is performed after infancy,[62] others have suggested that because of the high mortality rates after surgical repair, balloon angioplasty is the procedure of choice in the neonate and infants under 1 year of age.[63]

Successful angioplasty of coarctation has also been performed in adolescents and adults up to 55 years of age.[64,65]

Some authors have suggested that balloon angioplasty is more successful for coarctation resulting from postoperative restenosis than for native coarctation,[52,66] and the assumption has been that circumferential scar tissue prevents aortic rupture and makes aneurysm formation unlikely. The VACA Registry reported results in 200 patients (mean age, 7 years) with recoarctation.[67] Pressure differences of 20 mm Hg or less were found in 79.4% of the patients, but five died of complications related to the procedure (2.5%), one of aortic rupture.

Surgical treatment for coarctation of the aorta has been an acceptable form of management for this anomaly since the first reported repair in 1945.[3] Although there is general agreement about the necessity for urgent operation in patients with coarctation and heart failure or severe upper limb hypertension, controversy still exists about the optimal age for repair in the relatively symptom-free patient. A Mayo Clinic study[16] suggests that surgery should be offered about or after age 1 year in most patients with secondary hypertension or symptoms, or both, the outcome being more favorable in patients operated on within the first decade of life than in those operated on later. Evidence that residual hypertension and late complications are directly related to age at surgical correction[16,19,68] and an improving technical ability to relieve the coarctation permanently and adequately in infants[69,70] have led to a trend to recommend elective repair of coarctation at younger ages, even less than 2 years of age.[71-73] Some patients who may not have had surgical correction during childhood and thus appear with uncorrected coarctation of the aorta in adulthood should be considered as candidates for elective repair of the coarctation because their late result appears to be significantly better than the natural history of unrepaired coarctation of the aorta.[8,16,17,74]

Surgical technique

Some controversy remains as to the preferred technique for correction of coarctation in infants: by end-to-end anastomosis, by patch grafting, or by the subclavian flap method.[69-71,73,75] Surgical correction of coarctation in the adult usually can be accomplished by resection of the coarcted segment and end-to-end anastomosis. Technical problems relating to associated aneurysmal changes of the intercostal arteries or aorta or to atherosclerotic changes of the aorta (primarily distal to the coarctation) may require interposition of an arterial graft and may pose a particular challenge. Thus, the operative risk in the adolescent and adult may be somewhat greater than the negligible risk of coarctation repair during childhood beyond infancy. A catastrophic complication of coarctation repair is paraplegia, which results from spinal cord ischemia and has a reported incidence of 0.3% to 1.5%.[76-78] Some studies have suggested that perioperative monitoring of cortical somatosensory evoked potentials may help to identify patients at risk.[78,79]

Postoperative course

The long-term operative results have been evaluated in a large retrospective study at the Mayo Clinic[16] involving 646 patients who had undergone operative repair of isolated coarctation of the aorta between 1946 and 1981. The median age at operation was 16 years (range, 1 week to 72 years). Thirty-two patients (5%) were less than 1 year old at operation, and only 72 patients (11%) were more than 35 years old.

By estimated survival analysis, survival for the whole group appeared to be quite good—91% of patients alive at 10 years, 84% at 20 years, and 72% at 30 years. The mean age at death was 38 years, confirming the report by others[17] that these surgically treated patients often die at a young age. Of the late deaths, 37% were due to coronary artery disease. This high incidence of death from premature coronary artery disease was more pronounced as patients were followed for longer periods of time. In addition, 13% of the late deaths occurred suddenly without an apparent cause but with the likelihood that some were related to coronary disease. Nine percent of the late deaths were due to heart failure (caused by severe aortic regurgitation in 5% and by hypertensive heart disease in 4%). Seven percent of the deaths were from stroke, which was hemorrhagic in 4%; thus, the incidence of death due to intracranial hemorrhage in the whole group was less than 1%. Seven percent of the deaths were due to a ruptured aortic aneurysm; the importance of this as a cause of sudden death in patients operated on for coarctation has been reported.[80] Seven percent of the deaths occurred after subsequent cardiovascular surgery, and 20% of the deaths were related to other causes.

With respect to survival, the age at operation was found to be highly prognostic: the older the patient, the higher the probability of death; specifically, for patients younger than 14 years at the time of initial coarctectomy, survival at 20 years was 91%, and for patients 14 years old or older at the time of the operation, survival was 79%[16] (Fig 45-8). Systolic blood pressure preoperatively and postoperatively also were found to be significant predictors of death: the higher the pressure, the higher the probability of death. It appears that the duration of preoperative hypertension is critically important in determining the degree of arterial disease and hence the likelihood of subsequent cardiovascular events. Postoperatively, this

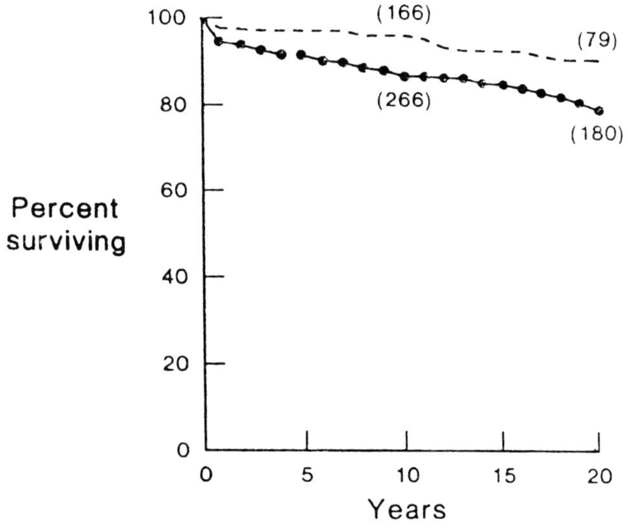

Fig 45-8 Observed survival curves to 20 years in patients younger than 14 years *(broken line)* and 14 years or older *(solid line)* at the time of initial coarctectomy. Numbers within parentheses represent patients under observation at 10 and 20 years. (From Cohen M, Fuster V, Steele PM, et al: Coarctation of the aorta: long-term follow-up and prediction of outcome after surgical correction. *Circulation* 80:840-845, 1989. By permission of American Heart Association.)

arterial pathologic process is accelerated if the patient is male or if hypertension is present.

In terms of clinical course, in the Mayo Clinic study the vast majority of survivors functioned normally—83% of the patients were asymptomatic. The frequency of future cardiovascular events in these patients is illustrated by the high incidence of subsequent cardiovascular operations: 14% of the patients underwent further operation at some stage during the follow-up period. Aortic valve replacement was performed in 7%, when a bicuspid valve had become incompetent or stenosed. Reoperation because of coarctation was required in 3% of the patients; half of these were less than 1 year old at the initial operation, giving an incidence of reoperation for coarctation in infants of 24%. This high incidence in infants has been previously reported[72,73,75,81] and suggests that patients should not undergo operation until at least 1 year old, unless repair in individual infants is clearly indicated and the most recent techniques are used. Two percent of patients had a mitral valve operation, 1% underwent coronary artery bypass grafting, and 1% had surgical repair of an aortic aneurysm.

Several authors have reported a significant incidence of aortic aneurysm formation at the site of previous patch aortoplasty.[82-85] The incidence varies from 5% to 25%, and formation may occur 3 to 18 years after the surgical procedure. Most patients in whom the diameter of the aneurysm exceeds that of the diaphragmatic aorta by 1:5 or greater have progressive dilatation within 3 to 5 years.[86]

Despite a satisfactory decrease in blood pressure in most patients soon after operation,[81,87,88] there is a significant incidence of hypertension that increases with longer follow-up.[17,89] Thirty years after coarctation repair, only 32% of patients are expected to be normotensive[68] and 25% are very significantly hypertensive.[16]

REFERENCES

1. Jarcho S: Coarctation of the aorta (Meckel, 1750; Paris, 1791). *Am J Cardiol* 7:844-852,1961
2. Flexner J: Coarctation of the aorta (adult type): clinical and experimental studies. *Am Heart J* 11:572-580, 1936
3. Crafoord C, Nylin G: Congenital coarctation of the aorta and its surgical treatment. *J Thorac Surg* 14:347-361, 1945
4. Gross RE, Hufnagel CA: Coarctation of the aorta: experimental studies regarding its surgical correction. *N Engl J Med* 233:287-293, 1945
5. Gersony WM: Coarctation of the aorta. In *Moss' Heart Disease in Infants, Children, and Adolescents.* Third edition. Edited by FH Adams, GC Emmanouilides. Baltimore, Williams & Wilkins, 1983, pp 188-199
6. Perloff JK: *The Clinical Recognition of Congenital Heart Disease.* Second edition. Philadelphia, WB Saunders Company, 1978, pp 126-154; 735-753
7. Ostermiller WE Jr, Somerndike JM, Hunter JA, et al: Coarctation of the aorta in adult patients. *J Thorac Cardiovasc Surg* 61:125-130, 1971
8. Campbell M: Natural history of coarctation of the aorta. *Br Heart J* 32:633-640, 1970
9. Edwards JE: Congenital malformations. H. Malformations of aorta arch system. In *Pathology of the Heart.* Second edition. Edited by SE Gould, Springfield, Illinois, Charles C Thomas, Publisher, 1960, pp 449-462
10. Tawes RL Jr, Berry CL, Aberdeen E: Congenital bicuspid aortic valves associated with coarctation of the aorta in children. *Br Heart J* 31:127-128, 1969
11. Nora JJ, Torres FG, Sinha AK, et al: Characteristic cardiovascular anomalies of XO Turner syndrome, XX and XY phenotype and XO/XX Turner mosaic. *Am J Cardiol* 25:639-641, 1970
12. Bahabozorgui S, Nemir P Jr: Coarctation of the abdominal aorta. *Am J Surg* 111:224-229, 1966
13. Taylor DG, Grainger RG, Matthews HL, et al: Suprarenal abdominal aortic obstruction. *Br J Surg* 53:195-198, 1966
14. Sissman NJ: Anomalies of the aortic arch complex. In *Moss' Heart Disease in Infants, Children, and Adolescents.* Third edition. Edited by FH Adams, GC Emmanouilides. Baltimore, Williams & Wilkins, 1983, pp 199-215
15. Cumming GR, Mir GH: Exercise haemodynamics of coarctation of the aorta: acute effects of propranolol. *Br Heart J* 32:365-369, 1970
16. Cohen M, Fuster V, Steele PM, et al: Coarctation of the aorta: long-term follow-up and prediction of outcome after surgical correction. *Circulation* 80:840-845, 1989
17. Maron BJ, Humphries JO'N, Rowe RD, et al: Prognosis of surgically corrected coarctation of the aorta: a 20-year postoperative appraisal. *Circulation* 47:119-126, 1973
18. James FW, Kaplan S: Systolic hypertension during submaximal exercise after correction of coarctation of aorta. *Circulation* 50 Suppl 2:27-33, 1974
19. Nanton MA, Olley PM: Residual hypertension after coarctectomy in children. *Am J Cardiol* 37:769-772, 1976
20. Šamánek M, Goetzová J, Fišerová J, et al: Differences in muscle blood flow in upper and lower extremities of patients after correction of coarctation of the aorta. *Circulation* 54:377-381, 1976
21. Smith DE, Matthews MB: Aortic valvular stenosis with coarctation of the aorta: with special reference to the development of aortic stenosis upon congenital bicuspid valves. *Br Heart J* 17:198-206, 1955
22. Edwards JE: Aneurysms of the thoracic aorta complicating coarctation. *Circulation* 48:195-201, 1973
23. Whyte D, Lu AT: Coarctation of the aorta with aneurysm and rupture into the esophagus: report of a case and review of the literature. *J Pediatr* 49:461-464, 1956
24. Edwards JE, Carey LS, Neufeld HN, et al: *Congenital Heart Disease: Correlation of Pathologic Anatomy and Angiocardiography.* Vol 1. Philadelphia, WB Saunders Company, 1965, pp 677-704
25. Kieffer SA, Linde LM, Kegel SM, et al: Mycotic aneurysm distal to coarctation of the aorta: report of an unusual case and review of the literature. *J Thorac Cardiovasc Surg* 42:507-513, 1961
26. Woltman HW, Shelden WD: Neurologic complications associated with congenital stenosis of the isthmus of the aorta: a case of cerebral aneurysm with rupture and a case of intermittent lameness presumably related to stenosis of the isthmus. *Arch Neurol Psychiatry* 17:303-316, 1927
27. Shearer WT, Rutman JY, Weinberg WA, et al: Coarctation of the aorta and cerebrovascular accident: a proposal for early corrective surgery. *J Pediatr* 77:1004-1009, 1970
28. Simon AB, Zloto AE: Coarctation of the aorta: longitudinal assessment of operated patients. *Circulation* 50:456-464, 1974
29. Reifenstein GH, Levine SA, Gross RE: Coarctation of the aorta: a review of 104 autopsied cases of the "adult type," 2 years of age or older. *Am Heart J* 33:146-168, 1947
30. Karnell J: Coarctation of the aorta. *Circulation* 38 Suppl 5:35-44, 1968
31. Jarcho S: Coarctation of the aorta (Reynaud, 1828). *Am J Cardiol* 9:591-597, 1962
32. Anagnostopoulos CE, Prabhakar MJS, Kittle CF: Aortic dissections and dissecting aneurysms. *Am J Cardiol* 30:263-273, 1972
33. Campbell M, Baylis JH: The course and prognosis of coarctation of the aorta. *Br Heart J* 18:475-495, 1956
34. Robicsek F, Taylor FH, Sanger PW: Studies on the poststenotic dilation. IV. Spontaneous perforation of the aorta distal to the coarctation. *Angiology* 12:68-72, 1961
35. Youker JE, Roe BB: Aneurysm of the aortic sinuses and ascending aorta in Turner's syndrome. *Am J Cardiol* 23:89-93, 1969
36. Goldberg MB, Scully AL, Solomon IL, et al: Gonadal dysgenesis in phenotypic female subjects: a review of eighty-seven cases, with cytogenetic studies in fifty-three. *Am J Med* 45:529-543, 1968
37. Goldring D, Wohltmann H: Flush method for blood pressure determinations in newborn infants. *J Pediatr* 40:285-289, 1952
38. Hernandez A, Goldring D, Hartmann AF Jr: Measurement of blood pressure in infants and children by the Doppler ultrasonic technique. *Pediatrics* 48:788-794, 1971

39. Strafford MA, Griffiths SP, Gersony WM: Coarctation of the aorta: a study in delayed detection. *Pediatrics* 69:159-163, 1982

40. Dahlbäck O, Dahn I, Westling H: Hemodynamic observations in coarctation of the aorta: with special reference to the blood pressure above and below the stenosis at rest and during exercise. *Scand J Clin Lab Invest* 16:339-346, 1964

41. Hancock EW: The ejection sound in aortic stenosis. *Am J Med* 40:569-577, 1966

42. Sahn DJ, Allen HD, McDonald G, et al: Real-time cross-sectional echocardiographic diagnosis of coarctation of the aorta: a prospective study of echocardiographic-angiographic correlations. *Circulation* 56: 762-769, 1977

43. Weyman AE, Caldwell RL, Hurwitz RA, et al: Cross-sectional echocardiographic detection of aortic obstruction. 2. Coarctation of the aorta. *Circulation* 57:498-502, 1978

44. Robinson PJ, Wyse RKH, Deanfield JE, et al: Continuous wave Doppler velocimetry as an adjunct to cross sectional echocardiography in the diagnosis of critical left heart obstruction in neonates. *Br Heart J* 52:552-556, 1984

45. Aldousany AW, DiSessa TG, Alpert BS, et al: Significance of the Doppler-derived gradient across a residual aortic coarctation. *Pediatr Cardiol* 11:8-14, 1990

46. Houston AB, Simpson IA, Pollock JCS, et al: Doppler ultrasound in the assessment of severity of coarctation of the aorta and interruption of the aortic arch. *Br Heart J* 57:38-43, 1987

47. Gibbs JL: Ultrasound and coarctation of the aorta (editorial). *Br Heart J* 64:109-110, 1990

48. Teirstein PS, Yock PG, Popp RL: The accuracy of Doppler ultrasound measurement of pressure gradients across irregular, dual, and tunnellike obstructions to blood flow. *Circulation* 72:577-584, 1985

49. Carvalho JS, Redington AN, Shinebourne EA, et al: Continuous wave Doppler echocardiography and coarctation of the aorta: gradients and flow patterns in the assessment of severity. *Br Heart J* 64:133-137, 1990

50. Teien D, Wendel H, Holm S, et al: Estimation of Doppler gradients at rest and during exercise in patients with recoarctation of the aorta. *Br Heart J* 65:155-157, 1991

51. Chernin MM, Pond GD, Bjelland JC, et al: Evaluation of double aortic arch and aortic coarctation by intravenous digital subtraction angiography (IV DSA). *J Cardiovasc Surg* 28:581-584, 1987

52. Soulen RL, Kan J, Mitchell S, et al: Evaluation of balloon angioplasty of coarctation restenosis by magnetic resonance imaging. *Am J Cardiol* 60:343-345, 1987

53. Freed MD, Keane JF: Profiles in congenital heart disease. In *Cardiac Catheterization and Angiography.* Second edition. Edited by W Grossman. Philadelphia, Lea & Febiger, 1980, pp 377-400

54. Sperling DR, Dorsey TJ, Rowen M, et al: Percutaneous transluminal angioplasty of congenital coarctation of the aorta. *Am J Cardiol* 51:562-564, 1983

55. Rocchini AP: Interventional catheterizaton. *Curr Opinion Cardiol* 4:93-96, 1989

56. Cooper SG, Sullivan ID, Wren C: Treatment of recoarctation: balloon dilation angioplasty. *J Am Coll Cardiol* 14:413-419, 1989

57. Morrow WR, Vick GW III, Nihill MR, et al: Balloon dilation of unoperated coarctation of the aorta: short- and intermediate-term results. *J Am Coll Cardiol* 11:133-138, 1988

58. Wren C, Peart I, Bain H, et al: Balloon dilatation of unoperated aortic coarctation: immediate results and one year follow up. *Br Heart J* 58:369-373, 1987

59. Lock JE, Niemi T, Burke BA, et al: Transcutaneous angioplasty of experimental aortic coarctation. *Circulation* 66:1280-1286, 1982

60. Lock JE, Castaneda-Zuniga WR, Bass JL, et al: Balloon dilatation of excised aortic coarctations. *Radiology* 143:689-691, 1982

61. Tynan M, Finley JP, Fontes V, et al: Balloon angioplasty for the treatment of native coarctation: results of Valvuloplasty and Angioplasty of Congenital Anomalies Registry. *Am J Cardiol* 65:790-792, 1990

62. Beekman RH, Rocchini AP, Dick M II, et al: Percutaneous balloon angioplasty for native coarctation of the aorta. *J Am Coll Cardiol* 10:1078-1084, 1987

63. Rao PS, Thapar MK, Galal O: Follow-up results of balloon angioplasty of native coarctation in neonates and infants. *Am Heart J* 120:1310-1314, 1990

64. Tyagi S, Arora R, Kaul UA, et al: Balloon angioplasty of native coarctation of the aorta in adolescents and young adults. *Am Heart J* 123:674-680, 1992

65. Fawzy ME, Dunn B, Galal O, et al: Balloon coarctation angioplasty in adolescents and adults: early and intermediate results. *Am Heart J* 124:167-171, 1992

66. Hess J, Mooyaart EL, Busch HJ, et al: Percutaneous transluminal balloon angioplasty in restenosis of coarctation of the aorta. *Br Heart J* 55:459-461, 1986

67. Hellenbrand WE, Allen HD, Golinko RJ, et al: Balloon angioplasty for aortic recoarctation: results of Valvuloplasty and Angioplasty of Congenital Anomalies Registry. *Am J Cardiol* 65:793-797, 1990

68. Presbitero P, Demarie D, Villani M, et al: Long term results (15-30 years) of surgical repair of aortic coarctation. *Br Heart J* 57:462-467, 1987

69. Waldhausen JA, Nahrwold DL: Repair of coarctation of the aorta with a subclavian flap. *J Thorac Cardiovasc Surg* 51:532-533, 1966

70. Bergdahl LAL, Blackstone EH, Kirklin JW, et al: Determinants of early success in repair of aortic coarctation in infants. *J Thorac Cardiovasc Surg* 83:736-742, 1982

71. Waldhausen JA, Whitman V, Werner JC, et al: Surgical intervention in infants with coarctation of the aorta. *J Thorac Cardiovasc Surg* 81:323-325, 1981

72. Campbell DB, Waldhausen JA, Pierce WS, et al: Should elective repair of coarctation of the aorta be done in infancy? *J Thorac Cardiovasc Surg* 88:929-936, 1984

73. Harlan JL, Doty DB, Brandt B III, et al: Coarctation of the aorta in infants. *J Thorac Cardiovasc Surg* 88:1012-1019, 1984

74. Maron BJ: Coarctation of the aorta in the adult. *Cadiovasc Clin* 10 No 1:311-319, 1979

75. Cobanoglu A, Teply JF, Grunkemeier GL, et al: Coarctation of the aorta in patients younger than three months: a critique of the subclavian flap operation. *J Thorac Cardiovasc Surg* 89:128-135, 1985

76. Brewer LA III, Fosburg RG, Mulder GA, et al: Spinal cord complications following surgery for coarctation of the aorta: a study of 66 cases. *J Thorac Cardiovasc Surg* 64:368-379, 1972

77. Lerberg DB, Hardesty RL, Siewers RD, et al: Coarctation of the aorta in infants and children: 25 years of experience. *Ann Thorac Surg* 33:159-169, 1982

78. Keen G: Spinal cord damage and operations for coarctation of the aorta: aetiology, practice and prospects. *Thorax* 42:11-18, 1987

79. Pollock JC, Jamieson MP, McWilliam R: Somatosensory evoked potentials in the detection of spinal cord ischemia in aortic coarctation repair. *Ann Thorac Surg* 41:251-254, 1986

80. Forfang K, Rostad H, Sörland S, et al: Late sudden death after surgical correction of coarctation of the aorta: importance of aneurysm of the ascending aorta. *Acta Med Scand* 206:375-379, 1979

81. Jacobsen JR, Wennevold A, Boesen I: Coarctation of the aorta operated upon in infancy: long-term follow-up. *Eur J Cardiol* 10:123-129, 1979

82. Rheuban KS, Gutgesell HP, Carpenter MA, et al: Aortic aneurysm after patch angioplasty for aortic isthmic coarctation in childhood. *Am J Cardiol* 58:178-180, 1986

83. Bromberg BI, Beekman RH, Rocchini AP, et al: Aortic aneurysm after patch aortoplasty repair of coarctation: prospective analysis of prevalence, screening tests and risks. *J Am Coll Cardiol* 14:734-741, 1989

84. McGoldrick JP, Brown IW, Ross DN: Coarctation of aorta: late aneurysm formation with Dacron onlay patch grafting. *Ann Thorac Surg* 45:89-90, 1988

85. Clarkson PM, Brandt PWT, Barratt-Boyes BG, et al: Prosthetic repair of coarctation of the aorta with particular reference to Dacron onlay patch grafts and aneurysm formation. *Am J Cardiol* 56:342-346, 1985

86. Mendelsohn AM, Crowley DC, Lindauer A, et al: Rapid progression of aortic aneurysms after patch aortoplasty repair of coarctation of the aorta. *J Am Coll Cardiol* 20:381-385, 1992

87. Nanton MA, Olley PM: Residual hypertension after coarctectomy in children. *Am J Cardiol* 37:769-772, 1976

88. Wright JL, Burchell HB, Wood EH, et al: Hemodynamic and clinical appraisal of coarctation four to seven years after resection and end-to-end anastomosis of the aorta. *Circulation* 14:806-814, 1956

89. Björk VO, Bergdahl L, Jonasson R: Coarctation of the aorta: the world's longest follow-up. *Adv Cardiol* 22:205-215, 1978

CHAPTER

46

Left-sided outflow obstruction

Valentin Fuster, M.D., Carole A. Warnes, M.D., David J. Driscoll, M.D., and Hartzell V. Schaff, M.D.

ANATOMIC CONSIDERATIONS

Congenital left-sided outflow obstruction, particularly at the aortic valvular level, is often encountered in adults. Less frequently, the obstruction is at the subvalvular level; very rarely, it is at the supravalvular level[1,2] (Fig 46-1).

Valvular aortic stenosis

About 30% of the cases are diagnosed in adolescents or young adults. This anomaly may be due to a unicuspid valve, to hypoplasia of the annulus, or, most commonly, to a valve that is congenitally bicuspid due to cuspal fusion or incomplete cuspal division. There are two extremes in the spectrum of congenital aortic valvular stenosis. One is aortic atresia,[3] which may be associated with mitral atresia and is the most common type of congenital heart disease that causes death in the first week of life; this entity is beyond the scope of this chapter. The other is the nonstenotic bicuspid aortic valve, which is the most common congenital heart defect, estimated to be present in 1% of the population; as a result of progressive calcification, this defect is a frequent cause of acquired calcific aortic valvular stenosis, which is commonly observed in the middle-aged and elderly, as described in detail in chapter 32.

Subvalvular aortic stenosis

There may be a fixed, localized membrane situated 0.5 to 2 cm below the level of the aortic valve and attached to the septum and base of the anterior mitral leaflet. More commonly, there is a fibromuscular membrane or a tunnel with a significant muscular component, which on occasion is difficult to differentiate from hypertrophic obstructive cardiomyopathy.

Associated aortic valvular regurgitation frequently is present and may be progressive; the incidence and severity of aortic valve regurgitation are greater in adults than in children.[4-6] The mechanism responsible for the aortic valve leakage is believed to be repetitive trauma caused by the jet of blood through the subvalvular stenosis impinging on the aortic valve cusps at the beginning of systole. Moreover, both clinical and experimental evidence suggest that the aortic valve in subaortic stenosis closes early, and early closure may lead to enhanced damage to the valve leaflets.[7] Histologic studies indicate

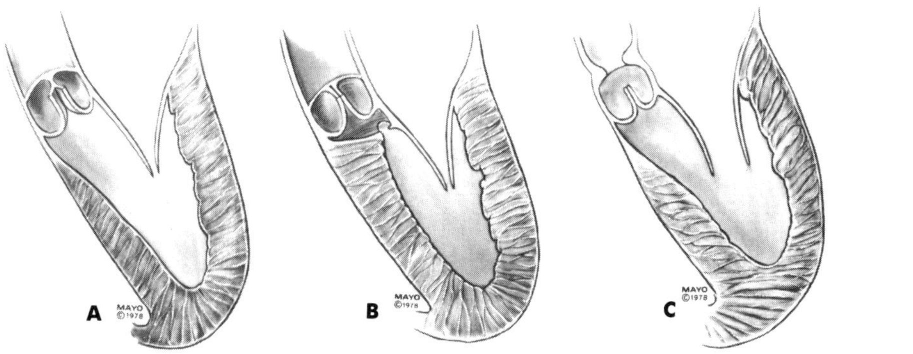

Fig 46-1 Types of congenital left-sided outflow obstruction. **A,** aortic valvular stenosis; **B,** discrete subaortic stenosis; **C,** aortic supravalvular stenosis. (From Fuster V, Brandenburg RO, McGoon DC, et al: Clinical approach and management of congenital heart disease in the adolescent and adult. *Cardiovasc Clin* 10 No 3:161-197, 1980. By permission, Mayo Foundation.)

Table 46-1 Characteristics of left-sided outflow obstructions

Type	Murmur first heard*	Symptoms first noted*	Associated aortic incompetence, % of patients	Other associated lesions
Valvular (90%)				
Congenital	Infancy	Infancy; adolescence	25	Miscellaneous, rare
Rheumatic	Adulthood†	Adulthood†	75	Mitral disease, 75%; tricuspid disease, 5%
Calcific bicuspid	Adolescence; adulthood	Adulthood; old age	40	Coarctation of aorta, rare
Calcific senile sclerotic	Old age	Old age	Rare	. . .
Subvalvular (9%)				
Hypertrophic	Infancy; adulthood	Adolescence; old age	Rare	Mitral incompetence, 90%; miscellaneous, 10%
Discrete	Infancy	Infancy; adulthood	50-75	Miscellaneous, 50%
Supravalvular (<1%)	Infancy	Infancy; adulthood	Rare	Peripheral pulmonary stenosis, 25%-50%; miscellaneous, 10%

*Infancy, <1 year old; childhood, ages 1 to 14 years; adolescence, ages 14 to 18 years; adulthood, ages 18 to 65 years; old age, >65 years old.
†Often in adolescence or even in childhood in developing areas.

that fibroelastic tissue may extend from the subaortic lesion into the aortic cusps.[8]

Aortic subvalvular stenosis in the form of hypertrophic obstructive cardiomyopathy is not discussed in this chapter because it is only rarely present at birth and hence is not ordinarily considered a congenital lesion; the entity is discussed in detail in chapter 20.

Supravalvular aortic stenosis

The obstruction occurs just above the coronary ostium. There are two main anatomic types: the hourglass type, which is the most common, and the hypoplastic type, characterized by uniform narrowing of the ascending aorta. Frequently associated lesions include peripheral pulmonary arterial stenosis; very rarely, there is stenosis of the branches of the aortic arch. The coronary arteries are subjected to high perfusion pressure, which may cause premature coronary atherosclerosis; moreover, the coronary ostium may be obstructed by the adjacent stenotic ring or the frequently encountered adherence of an aortic valve cusp to the obstructing shelf.

PATHOPHYSIOLOGY

When congenital aortic stenosis is not severe in infancy, it tends to become severe with age.[9,10] Unlike in acquired aortic valvular stenosis, the symptoms in congenital aortic stenosis tend to appear only with the more severe degrees of stenosis.[11] The pathophysiology of the different symptoms is similar to that in acquired valvular stenosis,[10] described in chapter 32.

CLINICAL FEATURES

With each of the three different types of obstructive lesions, there is a systolic murmur at birth, but the clinical symptoms may not develop until early adulthood (Table 46-1). The symptoms include exertional dyspnea, exertional dizziness or syncope, and exertional angina.

Aortic valvular stenosis

Apart from age at presentation, other clinical features distinguish congenital from rheumatic or senescent forms of aortic valvular stenosis[10-13] (Table 46-2). In congenital aortic valvular stenosis, symptoms tend to appear only with the more severe degrees of left ventricular outflow obstruction. The contour of the carotid pulse is not a good index for judging severity of stenosis because it is more dynamic and variable in infants than in adults. Because the aortic valve of these young patients is rarely calcified, an early systolic click is heard, the aortic component of the second heart sound is preserved, and fluoroscopy is not diagnostic. The electrocardiogram (ECG) may disclose ST-T wave changes preceding the voltage criteria for left ventricular hypertrophy, although a normal tracing does not exclude a significant stenosis.[14]

Echocardiography has an important role in the detection of bicuspid aortic valve. Valve morphology and the status of the left ventricle can be assessed by M-mode and two-dimensional echocardiography.[10] Doppler echocardiography is an accurate, noninvasive method for determining the degree of valvular stenosis and provides a semiquantitative method for evaluating the degree of

Table 46-2 Aortic valvular stenosis

Clinical feature	Young (congenital)	Middle-aged or elderly (calcified)
Progressive	Yes	Yes
Symptoms	Aortic gradient 75-100 mm Hg	Aortic gradient 50-75 mm Hg
Abnormal carotid pulse	Unreliable sign	Reliable sign
Click	Present	Absent
Aortic closure sound (A_2)	Present	Absent
Electrocardiogram	Unreliable	More reliable (left ventricular hypertrophy pattern)

valvular regurgitation. Recognition of bicuspid aortic valve is clinically important because of the increased risk of infective endocarditis, calcification, progressive valvular stenosis, or valvular regurgitation (see chapter 32). Because echocardiography is noninvasive and well tolerated, it is ideal for charting the progression of left ventricular outflow obstruction, the response of the left ventricle, and the adequacy of treatment with surgery or balloon dilatation.

Although congenital aortic stenosis may occur in patients with a single cusp or three leaflets, a bicuspid aortic valve is a common finding.[15,16] The number of cusps present often can be counted in the short-axis cross-sectional view of the aortic valve (Fig 46-2). Systolic doming in the long-axis parasternal view of the echocardiogram (Fig 46-3) often is diagnostic. Also, continuous-wave Doppler echocardiographic examination of the aortic valve provides noninvasive quantitative assessment of the aortic valve gradient and aortic valve area.[17,18]

Discrete subaortic stenosis

Most of the clinical features are so similar to those of congenital aortic valvular stenosis that differentiation is difficult[12,13,19,20] (Tables 46-2 and 46-3). However, the absence of an early systolic click and the presence of auscultatory features of aortic valvular regurgitation are more common findings in discrete subaortic stenosis than in congenital aortic valvular stenosis.

Several investigators[21-25] have demonstrated the utility of two-dimensional echocardiography in discrete subaortic stenosis. Furthermore, it has been suggested that two-dimensional echocardiography with Doppler evaluation is superior to angiography in detecting and characterizing these lesions.[26] Patterns of obstruction of cross-sectional anatomy revealed by two-dimensional echocardiography are as follows:[27] The discrete membrane appears as a distinct mini-echo within the outflow tract (Fig 46-4), and the fibromuscular lesion appears as a diffuse or shelf-like obstruction of the left ventricular outflow tract. Echocardiography with Doppler examination also is valuable in the postoperative reevaluation of patients for residual obstruction or development of new fibromuscular obstructions.[4,25]

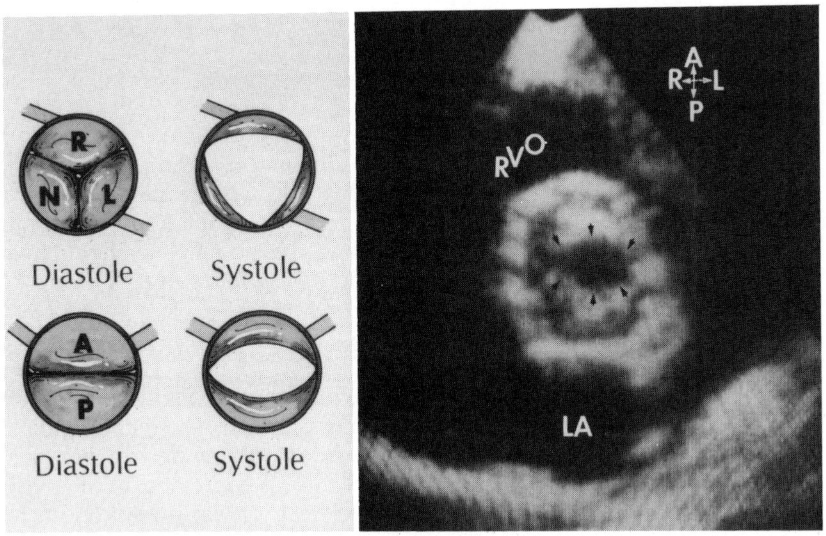

Fig 46-2 **Left,** diagram of normal tricuspid (top) and bicuspid (bottom) aortic valves in diastole and systole. *R,* right cusp; *L,* left cusp; *N,* noncoronary cusp; *A,* anterior; *P,* posterior. **Right,** two-dimensional echocardiographic appearance of bicuspid aortic valve in systole. *Arrowheads,* aortic orifice; *A,* anterior; *P,* posterior; *R,* right; *L,* left; *LA,* left atrium; *RVO,* right ventricular outflow tract. (From Shub C: The role of echocardiography in clinical practice. In *Clinical Medicine.* Vol. 6, Chap 34. Edited by JA Spittell Jr. Philadelphia, Harper & Row, Publishers, 1982, pp 1-44. By permission.)

Table 46-3 Noninvasive differential diagnostic evaluation of left-sided outflow obstruction

Feature	Valvular	Subvalvular: Hypertrophic	Subvalvular: Discrete	Supravalvular
Incidence, %	90	9	<1	<1
Sex ratio, M/F	3/1	3/1	1/1	1/1
Carotid pulse	Parvus tardus	Hyperkinetic (bisferious)	Parvus tardus	Parvus tardus present or absent; R carotid pulse may be larger
Apical impulse	Forceful, sustained	Forceful, "double" or "triple"	Forceful, sustained	
Sounds	S_2 single in calcific; ejection click in congenital and rheumatic; S_4	S_2 may be paradoxic; S_4 loud	S_4	S_4
Systolic murmurs	+	+	+	+
Carotid transmission	+	−	+	R > L
Amyl nitrite	↑	↑	↑	↑
Valsalva	↓	↑	↓	↓
Squat	↑	↓	↑	↑
Diastolic murmur (aortic regurgitation)	±	−	±	−
Electrocardiogram	LVH; "strain pattern"	LVH; "strain pattern"; deep septal Q; WPW rarely	LVH; "strain pattern"	LVH and "strain pattern" present or absent
Chest roentgenogram				
Cardiothoracic ratio	N-↑	N-↑	N-↑	N-↑
Poststenotic aortic dilatation	↑↑	N	N-↑	↓
Calcified valve	Only in calcific type	...	...	...

LVH, left ventricular hypertrophy; N, normal; WPW, Wolff-Parkinson-White syndrome; ↑, increased; ↓, decreased.

Supravalvular aortic stenosis

One-third of the cases represent transmission as a familial dominant trait; one-third are nonfamilial and are associated with idiopathic infantile hypercalcemia with characteristic elfin facies and mental retardation, although not exclusive to this type (Fig 46-5); and one-third represent sporadic disease.[12,28,29] To make the diagnosis, one must look for the following characteristic features (see Tables 46-1 and 46-3): 50% of the patients with supravalvular stenosis have a characteristically greater pulse and systolic pressure in the right carotid and brachial arteries than in the left (in normal subjects, the systolic pressure in the right arm is no more than 15 mm Hg higher than in the left); the systolic murmur is maximal below the right clavicle and radiates primarily to the right carotid artery; a diastolic murmur or an ejection click is absent almost invariably; and when associated peripheral stenosis of the pulmonary arteries is present, a separate systolic or continuous murmur is heard over the corresponding area of the thorax. The chest radiographs and ECGs are similar to those in the other types of left-sided outflow obstruction.

Two-dimensional echocardiography has proved helpful in identifying and characterizing the type and extent of supravalvular aortic stenosis, and correlation with angiocardiographic data is good.[22,30] If multiple views are used, it should be possible to identify and quantify the type, extent, and severity of this lesion.

DIAGNOSTIC PROBLEMS

The wide range of clinical entities associated with systolic murmurs can create difficulties in making the diagnosis of a left-sided outflow obstructive lesion. In our experience, the diagnosis, particularly of aortic valvular stenosis in adolescence or early adulthood, may be overlooked in three clinical situations.

1. When the murmur is louder at the apex, it may be mistaken for mitral regurgitation. Hence, it is important to remember the following differential features: the murmur of chronic mitral regurgitation is not crescendo-decrescendo; with inhalation of amyl nitrite, it decreases in intensity as a result of decreased peripheral resistance, which increases forward flow and reduces regurgitant

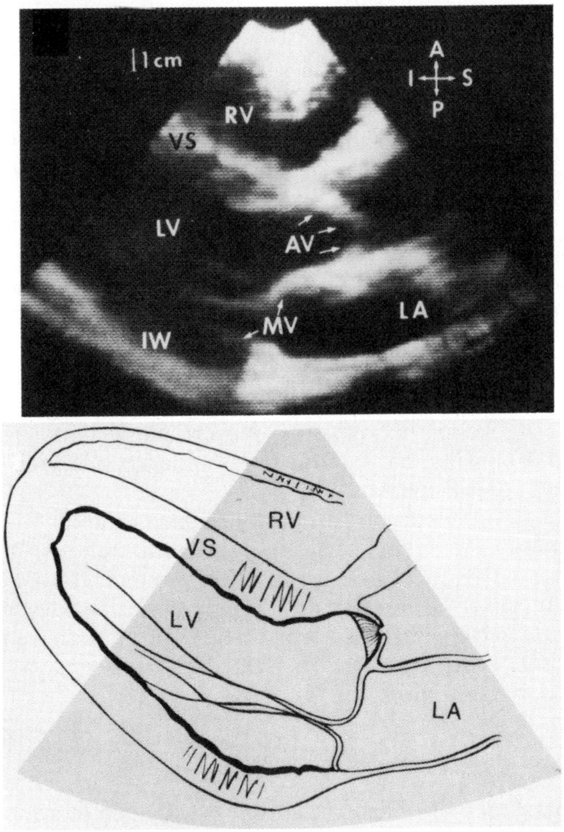

Fig 46-3 **Top**, long-axis view of left ventricle (*LV*), demonstrating doming produced by bicuspid aortic valve (*AV*) (*arrows*). **Bottom**, drawing corresponding to ultrasonographic plane. *A*, anterior; *I*, inferior; *IW*, inferior wall; *LA*, left atrium; *MV*, mitral valve; *P*, posterior; *RV*, right ventricle; *S*, superior; *VS*, ventricular septum. (From Nasser FN, Giuliani ER: *Clinical Two-Dimensional Echocardiography*. Chicago, Year Book Medical Publishers, 1983, pp 88-105. By permission.)

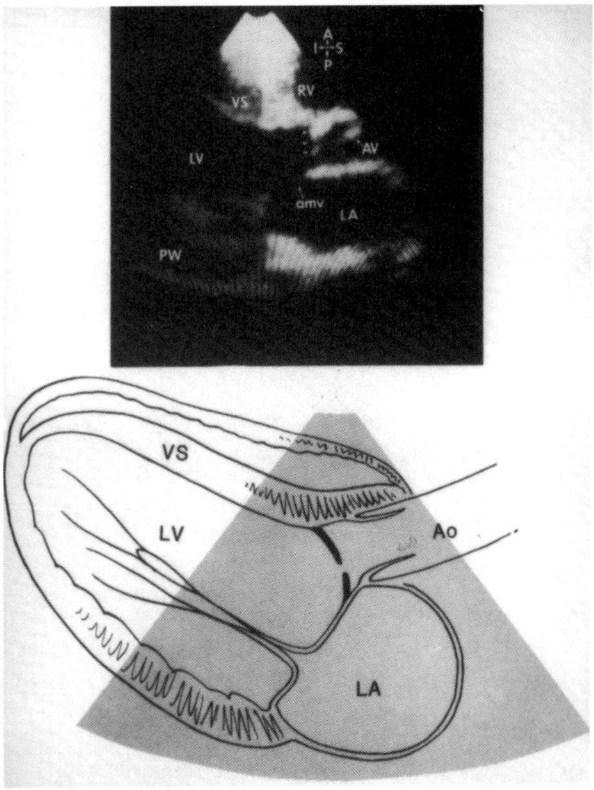

Fig 46-4 **Top**, long-axis view of left ventricle (*LV*), demonstrating subvalvular fibrous diaphragm (*arrowheads*) preoperatively. **Bottom**, drawing corresponding to ultrasonographic plane. *A*, anterior; *amv*, anterior mitral valve; *Ao*, aorta; *AV*, aortic valve; *I*, inferior; *LA*, left atrium; *P*, posterior; *PW*, posterior wall; *RV*, right ventricle; *S*, superior; *VS*, ventricular septum. (From Nasser FN, Giuliani ER: *Clinical Two-Dimensional Echocardiography*. Chicago, Year Book Medical Publishers, 1983, pp 88-105. By permission.)

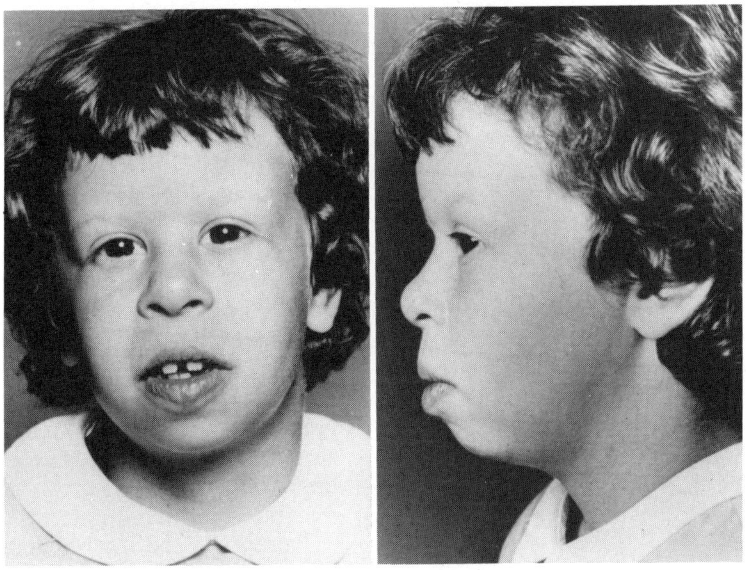

Fig 46-5 Facial appearance of girl with supravalvular aortic stenosis, bilateral stenosis of pulmonary arteries, mental retardation, and infantile hypercalcemia. Chin is small, mouth is large, lips are patulous, nose is blunt and upturned, eyes are wide-set, forehead is broad, cheeks are baggy, and teeth are malformed.

flow; it does not increase after an ectopic beat; and clinical features other than the murmur are usually of diagnostic help. Echocardiography differentiates the lesions.

2. When the murmur is loud at the left sternal border, it may be mistaken for a murmur originating in the right side of the heart, either from pulmonary stenosis or, more rarely, from an atrial septal defect. Such murmurs characteristically disappear within one or two beats during the Valsalva maneuver and return promptly in one or two beats after release. The wide persistent splitting of the second heart sound is characteristic of isolated pulmonary stenosis or atrial septal defect. Again, noninvasive techniques such as echocardiography usually confirm the diagnosis.

3. The murmur of hypertrophic obstructive cardiomyopathy may have an apical holosystolic component and an upper left sternal border midsystolic component. Hence, this diagnosis must be kept in mind in patients with auscultatory features of both mitral regurgitation and aortic stenosis. Characteristically, the murmur of hypertrophic obstructive cardiomyopathy does not radiate to the neck, and it usually becomes louder during the straining phase of the Valsalva maneuver because the decrease in venous return results in reduction of left ventricular volume with augmentation of the dynamic obstruction. Other clinical and noninvasive diagnostic features, particularly those disclosed by echocardiography, are confirmatory.

Once the clinician identifies the murmur of left-sided outflow obstruction and has excluded hypertrophic obstructive cardiomyopathy, diagnostic consideration must be given not only to the likelihood of aortic valvular stenosis but also to the other, less frequent types of obstruction already discussed.

In young patients with aortic valvular stenosis, the usual clinical symptoms and signs as well as the ECG findings are less reliable for the assessment of severity than in older patients with calcific aortic valvular stenosis. Noninvasive assessment of the exact site and severity of left-sided outflow obstruction can reliably be made by two-dimensional and Doppler echocardiographic techniques, which permit accurate noninvasive follow-up.[31] In patients with poor echocardiographic images, conventional transthoracic echocardiography may fail to image discrete subvalvular aortic stenosis, but transesophageal echocardiography improves the diagnostic imaging.[32] Other techniques, such as magnetic resonance imaging and ultrafast computed tomography (Imetron) scanning, also provide excellent views of the left ventricular outflow area. Rarely, cardiac catheterization may be indicated for patients with supravalvular aortic stenosis to determine the exact aortic anatomy and distribution of hypoplasia before surgical intervention.

MANAGEMENT

Balloon valvuloplasty

Since the first description of balloon aortic valvuloplasty in 1984,[33] several studies have suggested that congenital aortic stenosis can be relieved with this technique.[34-36] The procedure can be accomplished with low mortality and morbidity and appears more likely to be successful when the valve is thin and pliable and is bicuspid rather than unicuspid.[37] The mechanism by which stenosis is relieved appears to be separation of fused commissures. Aortic regurgitation is the complication that causes most concern, but the degree of valve leakage after dilatation is variable and difficult to predict.[37] Other complications of balloon valvuloplasty are loss of the femoral pulse, transient arrhythmias, and trauma to the mitral valve.[37] Because results of long-term evaluation of these patients are not yet available, reliable comparison with the surgical alternatives is not possible. Nevertheless, initial results are promising, but patients who undergo this procedure need careful follow-up.

Balloon dilatation has also been used in small numbers of patients for relief of discrete subaortic stenosis,[38,39] but since a discrete obstruction with only a small gradient may still cause turbulence and progressive damage to the aortic valve and subsequent aortic regurgitation, removal of the obstruction by surgical excision seems a more reasonable option.

Surgical treatment

It has been established that the occurrence of symptoms secondary to aortic valvular stenosis implies a poor prognosis unless surgical intervention is accomplished promptly. One of the problems in the management of aortic valvular stenosis in the younger age groups is that many of the patients with a severe stenotic lesion are asymptomatic. The possibility of sudden death in such patients becomes an important consideration, as does the concern that persistence of such high levels of obstruction, even in the asymptomatic patient, might result in irreversible impairment of left ventricular function. Because of these factors, there is general agreement that patients with congenital aortic valvular stenosis who have peak systolic gradients greater than 70 to 75 mm Hg should undergo valvotomy.

In older patients with congenitally bicuspid aortic valve and acquired valvular stenosis, the incidence of sudden death in those without symptoms is low, and symptoms tend to develop with less severe gradients. For these reasons, we advise surgical correction in the adult patient when the first clinical symptoms develop. Consideration for earlier intervention may be given if rapidly increasing hemodynamic severity of left ventricular outflow obstruction or progressive, severe left ventricular hypertrophy develops.

There also is general agreement that patients with congenital valvular aortic stenosis who have peak systolic gradients of less than 50 mm Hg can be followed without surgical treatment. However, as shown in Figure 46-6, approximately 40% of such patients require surgical treatment during long-term follow-up.

Patients in the intermediate group—those with gradients between 50 and 75 mm Hg—require individualized management. Comparisons between medically and surgically treated patients in this category indicated the preference for surgical management of patients having gradients greater than 50 mm Hg. Indeed, in the Natural

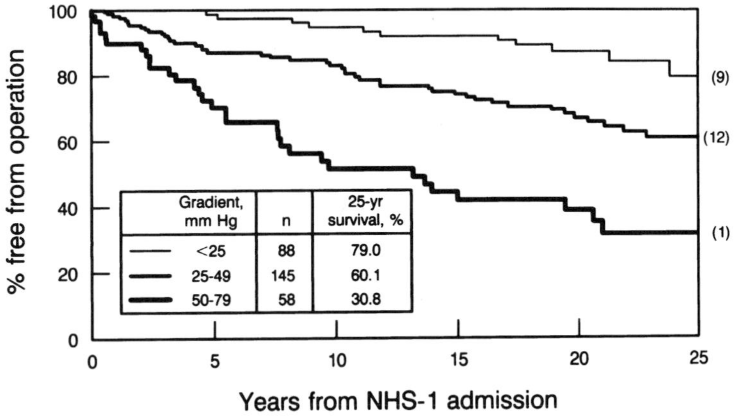

Fig 46-6 Survival free of reoperation for patients with congenital valvular aortic stenosis who were at least 2 years of age at the time of admission to the First Natural History Study (NHS-1). Patients were managed medically by protocol and are stratified by gradient at admission (<25, 25-49, and 50-79 mm Hg). (From Keane JF, Driscoll DJ, Gersony WM, et al: Second Natural History Study of Congenital Heart Defects. Results of treatment of patients with aortic valvar stenosis. *Circulation* 87 Suppl 1:16-27, 1993. By permission of American Heart Association.)

History Study of Congenital Heart Defects, almost 70% of patients who had initial gradients of 50 to 80 mm Hg had undergone surgical treatment of congenital aortic stenosis by 25 years of follow-up[40] (see Fig 46-6). Because a more nearly complete and permanent repair seems achievable for subaortic stenosis, there is even greater security in recommending operation for subaortic stenosis when the peak systolic gradient reaches 50 mm Hg or greater.[4] The same is true for supravalvular aortic stenosis, for which relief is also highly effective.[12,41]

Before surgical intervention becomes indicated, the most important aspect in the medical management of all these patients is close follow-up, at least on a yearly basis, to assess any deterioration that might prompt surgical intervention. We also advise the patient to avoid strenuous competitive exercise and to use antimicrobial prophylaxis against infective endocarditis.

Surgical technique

Most adults who require operation for congenital aortic valvular stenosis after age 20 have so much calcification superimposed on the valve that the only appropriate procedure is valve replacement (see chapter 32). However, in young adults who do not exhibit secondary calcification, aortic valvotomy is preferred whenever a reasonably adequate valvular opening can be achieved, in an effort to defer as long as possible the disadvantages of replacing the valve with a substitute valve.

From the technical standpoint, the only significant debatable point with respect to valvotomy is management of the fused cusp of the bicuspid valve. The question is whether to incise the region of the raphe; incision in this area carries with it the risk of producing significant aortic insufficiency, but it improves the probability of significantly relieving the degree of stenosis. Because the postoperative course of patients with residual stenosis seems better than that of those in whom significant aortic regurgitation has been produced, it seems better to err on the side of avoiding incisions in the region of the raphe if the risk of producing an insufficiency of the valve seems significant.[12,42,43]

Correction of discrete subaortic stenosis requires the excision of a deep wedge of fibromuscular tissue from the anterior septal aspect of the left ventricular outflow tract, which is done through an aortotomy. Usually, the membrane is excised sharply and myectomy follows. The surgeon must apply careful judgment in the compromise between the two opposing objectives of operation—namely, wide and deep excision of the obstructing portion of the septum and avoidance of heart block or injury to the surrounding structures (Fig 46-7). The myectomy consists of a deep excision of muscle that protrudes into the left ventricular outflow tract. The excision is created in a straight line beginning just below the nadir of the right aortic valve cusp and extending toward the parietal left ventricular wall. The width of the resected muscle is determined on the left side by the anterior leaflet of the mitral valve and on the right by a point beneath the nadir of the right aortic valve cusp.

More severe and complicated forms of subaortic obstruction sometimes require extensive operations. In the 1970s and early 1980s, patients with severe recurrent tunnel obstruction and aortic annulus hypoplasia were treated by insertion of a Hancock conduit between the left ventricular apex and the ascending aorta or the descending aorta.[14] More recently, patients with similar pathologic features have been treated by Konno-Rastan aortoventriculoplasty, in which the aortic valve is replaced by a mechanical valve prosthesis.[44-46] Some patients with additional mild aortic annular hypoplasia can be treated with myectomy and annular enlargement, according to

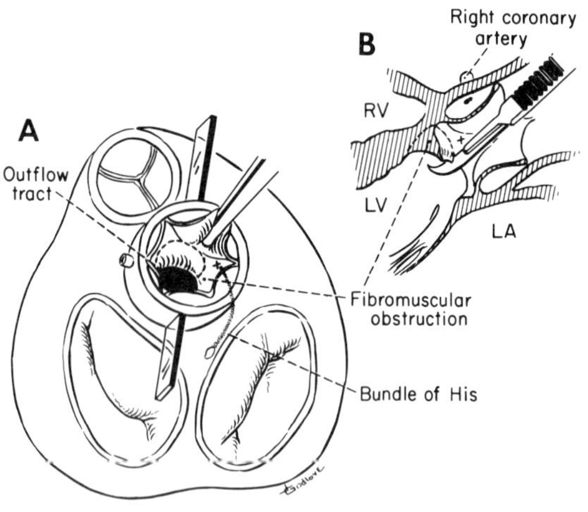

Fig 46-7 Relief of subvalvular aortic stenosis. Deep excision of the fibromuscular tissue of the anterior septum is usually indicated, as illustrated by the *broken line*. *X* indicates the danger zone for the bundle of His. **A**, right coronary cusp of the aortic valve is being retracted with forceps. *LA*, left atrium; *LV*, left ventricle; *RV*, right ventricle. (From McGoon DC: Technics of open-heart surgery for congenital heart disease. *Curr Probl Surg* April:1-42, 1968. By permission of Year Book Medical Publishers.)

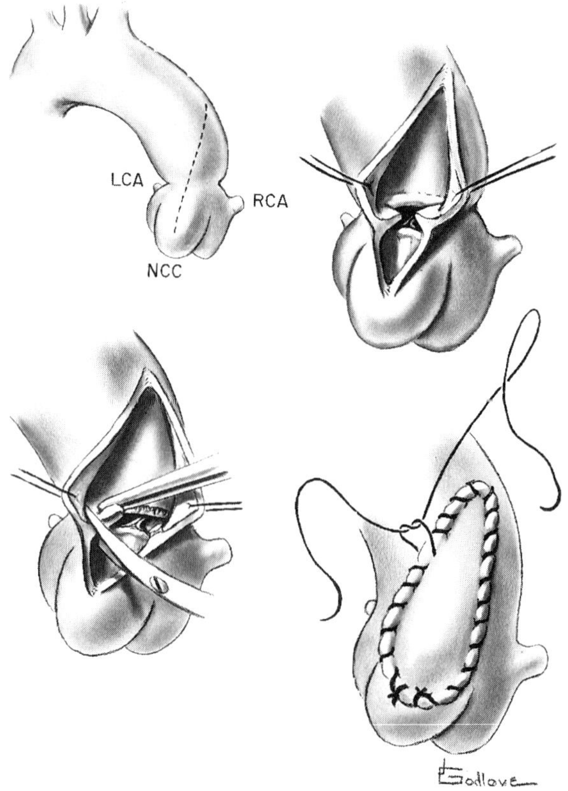

Fig 46-8 Teardrop-shaped patch repair of discrete form of supravalvular aortic stenosis. After the stenotic ridge is excised, a generous teardrop-shaped autologous pericardial patch is sutured into place. *LCA*, left coronary artery; *NCC*, noncoronary cusp; *RCA*, right coronary artery. (From van Son JAM, Danielson GK, Puga FJ, et al: Supravalvular aortic stenosis: long-term results of surgical treatment. *J Thorac Cardiovasc Surg* 107:103-114, 1994. By permission of Mosby-Year Book.)

Nicks et al.[47] and Manouguian and Seybold-Epting.[48] In the latter techniques, the aortotomy is directed toward the commissure between the left and the noncoronary aortic valve cusps and extended through the fibrous trigone onto[47] or into[48] the anterior leaflet of the mitral valve. Subsequently, the subannular incision and the ascending aorta are closed with a patch in conjunction with insertion of a prosthetic heart valve.[48]

Although the subvalvular stenosis is commonly of the discrete, localized fibromuscular type and only about one-fourth of the patients with subaortic stenosis have a more diffuse muscular encroachment of the septum on the outflow tract, adequate relief of subaortic stenosis nevertheless requires resection of myocardium as well as fibrous tissue in virtually all patients.[4,12,19,20,42,43] In situations of severe tunnel subaortic stenosis in which the aortic valve annulus is nearly normal in size, a modification of the Konno-Rastan operation can be used.[49,50] For this procedure, an oblique aortotomy is made toward the commissure between the left and the right aortic cusps, and the obstructing membrane and muscle are excised from the area immediately below the valve. Then, a longitudinal or transverse incision is made in the right ventricular outflow tract, and the interventricular septum is incised longitudinally from the base toward the apex. Through this incision any remaining membrane can be excised, and a wide septal myectomy is easily accomplished. The ventricular septal incision and the right ventriculotomy are then closed with a patch.

The classic correction of the discrete form of supravalvular aortic stenosis involves an obliquely oriented aortotomy that extends through the stenotic hourglass deformity down into the expanded portion of the noncoronary sinus of Valsalva and down to the basal attachment of the noncoronary cusps.[29,41] The thickened ridge on the inner aspect of the hourglass is carefully trimmed away between commissural attachments, and then the diameter of the base of the aorta is markedly enlarged by placing a wide teardrop-shaped patch of synthetic material or pericardium to close the aortotomy (Fig 46-8). When the stenotic zone is particularly diminutive, a more radical type of repair, advocated by Doty et al.,[51] is accomplished by patch graft enlargement not only into the noncoronary sinus of Valsalva but also into the right coronary sinus (Fig 46-9). In the long tubular form of supra-aortic stenosis, palliation can be achieved by extensive patch graft enlargement of the entire ascending aorta and even of the aortic arch after induction of profound hypothermia and partial or complete circulatory arrest[41] (Fig 46-10).

Postoperative course

The risk of operation for relief of the various types of left ventricular outflow tract obstruction is not great, currently

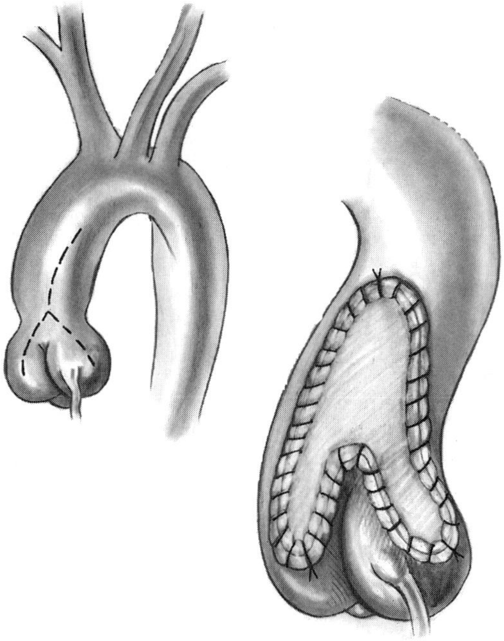

Fig 46-9 Pantaloon-shaped patch repair of discrete form of supravalvular aortic stenosis. After excision of the supravalvular ridge, a pantaloon-shaped pericardial patch is sutured into place. (From van Son JAM, Danielson GK, Puga FJ, et al: Supravalvular aortic stenosis: long-term results of surgical treatment. *J Thorac Cardiovasc Surg* 107:103-114, 1994. By permission of Mosby-Year Book.)

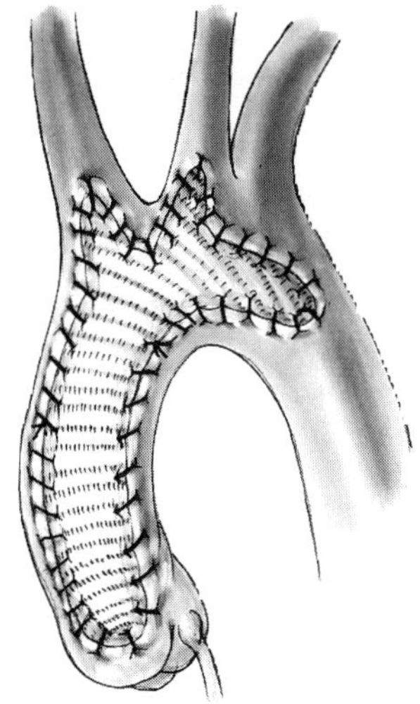

Fig 46-10 Repair of diffuse supravalvular aortic stenosis with involvement of the proximal arch vessels by means of a polyester fiber (Dacron) patch carried into the aortic arch and proximal innominate and left common carotid arteries. (From van Son JAM, Danielson GK, Puga FJ, et al: Supravalvular aortic stenosis: long-term results of surgical treatment. *J Thorac Cardiovasc Surg* 107:103-114, 1994. By permission of Mosby-Year Book.)

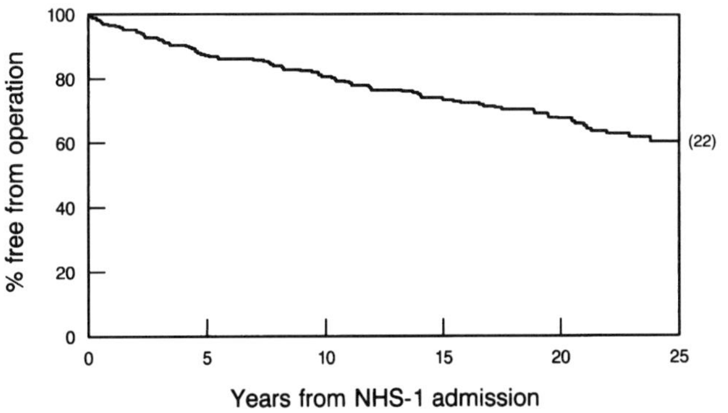

Fig 46-11 Survival free of reoperation for patients with congenital valvular aortic stenosis who were treated surgically at the time of admission to the First Natural History Study (NHS-1). (From Keane JF, Driscoll DJ, Gersony WM, et al: Second Natural History Study of Congenital Heart Defects. Results of treatment of patients with aortic valvar stenosis. *Circulation* 87 Suppl 1:16-27, 1993. By permission of American Heart Association.)

ranging from 1% to 5% in patients beyond infancy. The chief drawback to the operation, however, is the nearly consistent presence of a residual gradient of varying degree postoperatively. This is particularly evident after aortic valvotomy, because the bicuspid or unicuspid aortic valve cannot be opened to the extent that a normal valve would without the virtual certainty of creating serious regurgitation of the valve.[10,12,42,43] Thus, aortic valvotomy generally is classified as a palliative procedure.[12] Patients undergoing aortic valvotomy must be informed of the probability that reoperation for aortic valve replacement will be required in the future, possibly within 2 to 3 decades, and also that periodic examinations will be required throughout life, probably annually. When comparative data are available,[10] the long-term prognosis for patients with congenital aortic stenosis, including the valvular variety, is significantly better after surgical treatment. Nevertheless, adverse events postoperatively are not uncommon;[10,42] there is a high incidence of residual stenosis and reoperation. One long-term study[52] reported the probability of reoperation to be 44% at 22 years. In the Natural History Study of Congenital Heart Defects, the incidence of reoperation approached 40% by 25 years after initial operation[40] (Fig 46-11). Infective endocarditis is still an important problem after valvotomy, and antibiotic prophylaxis must be continued postoperatively.

Overall late survival of patients having correction of subaortic stenosis is approximately 75% at 20 years postoperatively, and late outcome is better in patients with discrete subaortic stenosis (10-year survival, 91%) than in those with tunnel subaortic stenosis (10-year survival, 79%). Late reoperation may be necessary in as many as 10% to 15% of patients because of recurrent or residual stenosis or aortic valve regurgitation, or both.

Late survival after repair of supravalvular aortic stenosis is also good, and the chief determinant of poor late outcome is associated aortic valvular disease (Fig 46-12).

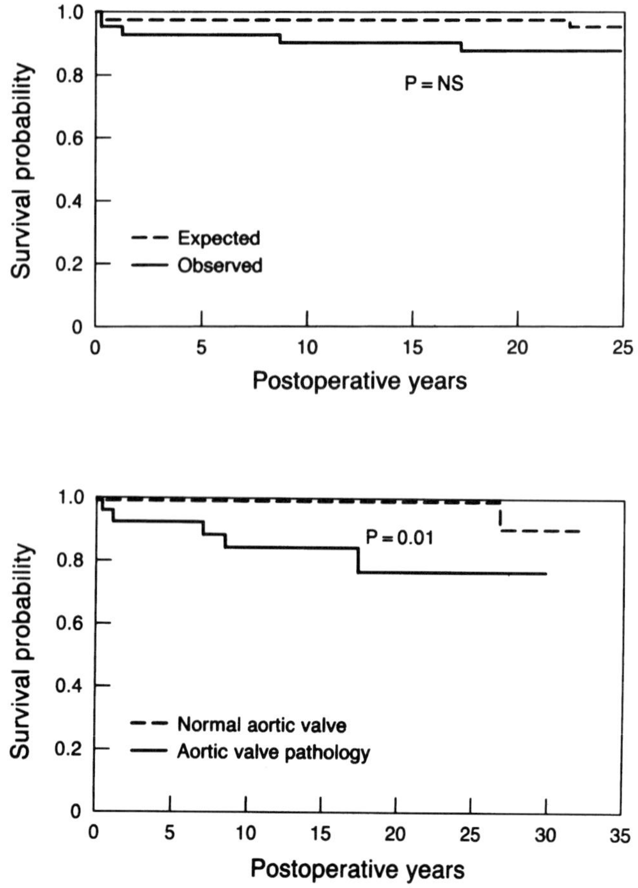

Fig 46-12 Survival of patients dismissed alive after repair of supravalvular aortic stenosis. The **upper panel** also shows expected survival of an age- and sex-matched population. The **lower panel** demonstrates survival of the same patients stratified according to whether they did or did not have associated aortic valve disease. (From van Son JAM, Danielson GK, Puga FJ, et al: Supravalvular aortic stenosis: long-term results of surgical treatment. *J Thorac Cardiovasc Surg* 107:103-114, 1994. By permission of Mosby-Year Book.)

Another concern in the late management of patients with supravalvular aortic stenosis is development of coronary artery disease. Presumably, aortic root hypertension causes intimal thickening and accelerated atherosclerosis.

REFERENCES

1. Edwards JE: Pathology of left ventricular outflow tract obstruction. *Circulation* 31:586-599, 1965
2. Fuster V, Brandenburg RO, McGoon DC, et al: Clinical approach and management of congenital heart disease in the adolescent and adult. *Cardiovasc Clin* 10:161-197, 1980
3. Roberts WC, Perry LW, Chandra RS, et al: Aortic valve atresia: a new classification based on necropsy study of 73 cases. *Am J Cardiol* 37:753-756, 1976
4. van Son JA, Schaff HV, Danielson GK, et al: Surgical treatment of discrete and tunnel subaortic stenosis. Late survival and risk of reoperation. *Circulation* 88 Suppl 2:159-169, 1993
5. Brown J, Stevens L, Lynch L, et al: Surgery for discrete subvalvular aortic stenosis: actuarial survival, hemodynamic results, and acquired aortic regurgitation. *Ann Thorac Surg* 40:151-155, 1985
6. Douville EC, Sade RM, Crawford FA Jr, et al: Subvalvar aortic stenosis: timing of operation. *Ann Thorac Surg* 50:29-33, 1990
7. Sabbah HN, Stein PD: Mechanism of early systolic closure of the aortic valve in discrete membranous subaortic stenosis. *Circulation* 65:399-402, 1982
8. Feigl A, Feigl D, Lucas RV Jr, et al: Involvement of the aortic valve cusps in discrete subaortic stenosis. *Pediatr Cardiol* 5:185-189, 1984
9. Cohen LS, Friedman WF, Braunwald E: Natural history of mild congenital aortic stenosis elucidated by serial hemodynamic studies. *Am J Cardiol* 30:1-5, 1972
10. Friedman WF, Novak V, Johnson AD: Congenital aortic stenosis in adults. *Cardiovasc Clin* 10:235-251, 1979
11. Wagner HR, Weidman WH, Ellison RC, et al: Indirect assessment of severity in aortic stenosis. *Circulation* 56 Suppl 2:120-123, 1977
12. McGoon DC, Geha AS, Scofield EL, et al: Surgical treatment of congenital aortic stenosis. *Dis Chest* 55:388-394, 1969
13. Braunwald E, Goldblatt A, Aygen MM, et al: Congenital aortic stenosis. I. Clinical and hemodynamic findings in 100 patients. *Circulation* 27:426-450; 460-462, 1963
14. Ellison RC, Wagner HR, Weidman WH, et al: Congenital valvular aortic stenosis: clinical detection of small pressure gradient. *Am J Cardiol* 37:757-761, 1976
15. Fowles RE, Martin RP, Abrams JM, et al: Two-dimensional echocardiographic features of bicuspid aortic valve. *Chest* 75:434-440, 1979
16. Spencer FC, Neill CA, Sank L, et al: Anatomical variations in 46 patients with congenital aortic stenosis. *Am Surg* 26:204-216, 1960
17. Hatle L, Angelsen B: *Doppler Ultrasound in Cardiology: Physical Principles and Clinical Applications*. Philadelphia, Lea & Febiger, 1982, pp 22-24; 35-37; 89-97
18. Hatle L, Angelsen BA, Tromsdal A: Non-invasive assessment of aortic stenosis by Doppler ultrasound. *Br Heart J* 43:284-292, 1980
19. Sung C-S, Price EC, Cooley DA: Discrete subaortic stenosis in adults. *Am J Cardiol* 42:283-290, 1978
20. Newfeld EA, Muster AJ, Paul MH, et al: Discrete subvalvular aortic stenosis in childhood. Study of 51 patients. *Am J Cardiol* 38:53-61, 1976
21. Popp RL, Silverman JF, French JW, et al: Echocardiographic findings in discrete subvalvular aortic stenosis. *Circulation* 49:226-231, 1974
22. Weyman AE, Feigenbaum H, Hurwitz RA, et al: Localization of left ventricular outflow obstruction by cross-sectional echocardiography. *Am J Med* 60:33-38, 1976
23. Weyman AE, Feigenbaum H, Hurwitz RA, et al: Cross-sectional echocardiography in evaluating patients with discrete subaortic stenosis. *Am J Cardiol* 37:358-365, 1976
24. Sahn DJ, Henry WL: Clinical applications of real-time two-dimensional scanning in congenital heart disease. *Cardiovasc Clin* 9:295-316, 1978
25. Reeder GS, Danielson GK, Seward JB, et al: Fixed subaortic stenosis in atrioventricular canal defect: a Doppler echocardiographic study. *J Am Coll Cardiol* 20:386-394, 1992
26. Wilcox WD, Seward JB, Hagler DJ, et al: Discrete subaortic stenosis: two-dimensional echocardiographic features with angiographic and surgical correlation. *Mayo Clin Proc* 55:425-433, 1980
27. Nasser FN, Giuliani ER: *Clinical Two-Dimensional Echocardiography*. Chicago, Year Book Medical Publishers, 1983, pp 88-105
28. Lewis AJ, Ongley PA, Kincaid OW, et al: Supravalvular aortic stenosis. Report of a family with peculiar somatic features and normal intelligence. *Dis Chest* 55:372-379, 1969
29. Rastelli GC, McGoon DC, Ongley PA, et al: Surgical treatment of supravalvular aortic stenosis. Report of 16 cases and review of literature. *J Thorac Cardiovasc Surg* 51:873-882, 1966
30. Weyman AE, Caldwell RL, Hurwitz RA, et al: Cross-sectional echocardiographic characterization of aortic obstruction. 1. Supravalvular aortic stenosis and aortic hypoplasia. *Circulation* 57:491-497, 1978
31. Currie PJ, Hagler DJ, Seward JB, et al: Instantaneous pressure gradient: a simultaneous Doppler and dual catheter correlative study. *J Am Coll Cardiol* 7:800-806, 1986
32. Mugge A, Daniel WG, Wolpers HG, et al: Improved visualization of discrete subvalvular aortic stenosis by transesophageal color-coded Doppler echocardiography. *Am Heart J* 117:474-475, 1989

33. Lababidi Z, Wu JR, Walls JT: Percutaneous balloon aortic valvuloplasty: results in 23 patients. *Am J Cardiol* 53:194-197, 1984

34. Walls JT, Lababidi Z, Curtis JJ, et al: Assessment of percutaneous balloon pulmonary and aortic valvuloplasty. *J Thorac Cardiovasc Surg* 88:352-356, 1984

35. Choy M, Beekman RH, Rocchini AP, et al: Percutaneous balloon valvuloplasty for valvar aortic stenosis in infants and children. *Am J Cardiol* 59:1010-1013, 1987

36. Rocchini AP, Beekman RH, Ben Shachar G, et al: Balloon aortic valvuloplasty: results of the Valvuloplasty and Angioplasty of Congenital Anomalies Registry. *Am J Cardiol* 65:784-789, 1990

37. Sholler GF, Keane JF, Perry SB, et al: Balloon dilation of congenital aortic valve stenosis. Results and influence of technical and morphological features on outcome. *Circulation* 78:351-360, 1988

38. Suarez de Lezo J, Pan M, Sancho M, et al: Percutaneous transluminal balloon dilatation for discrete subaortic stenosis. *Am J Cardiol* 58:619-621, 1986

39. Lababidi Z, Weinhaus L, Stoeckle H Jr, et al: Transluminal balloon dilatation for discrete subaortic stenosis. *Am J Cardiol* 59:423-425, 1987

40. Keane JF, Driscoll DJ, Gersony WM, et al: Second Natural History Study of Congenital Heart Defects. Results of treatment of patients with aortic valvar stenosis. *Circulation* 87 Suppl 1:16-27, 1993

41. van Son JAM, Danielson GK, Puga FJ, et al: Supravalvular aortic stenosis: long-term results of surgical treatment. *J Thorac Cardiovasc Surg* 107:103-114, 1994

42. Jones M, Barnhart GR, Morrow AG: Late results after operations for left ventricular outflow tract obstruction. *Am J Cardiol* 50:569-579, 1982

43. Morrow AG, Goldblatt A, Braunwald E: Congenital aortic stenosis. II. Surgical treatment and the results of operation. *Circulation* 27:450-462, 1963

44. Konno S, Imai Y, Iida Y, et al: A new method for prosthetic valve replacement in congenital aortic stenosis associated with hypoplasia of the aortic valve ring. *J Thorac Cardiovasc Surg* 70:909-917, 1975

45. Rastan H, Koncz J: Plastic enlargement of the left ventricular outflow tract. A new operative method. *Thoraxchir Vask Chir* 23:169-175, 1975

46. Rastan H, Koncz J: Aortoventriculoplasty: a new technique for the treatment of left ventricular outflow tract obstruction. *J Thorac Cardiovasc Surg* 71:920-927, 1976

47. Nicks R, Cartmill T, Bernstein L: Hypoplasia of the aortic root. The problem of aortic valve replacement. *Thorax* 25:339-346, 1970

48. Manouguian S, Seybold-Epting W: Patch enlargement of the aortic valve ring by extending the aortic incision into the anterior mitral leaflet. New operative technique. *J Thorac Cardiovasc Surg* 78:402-412, 1979

49. Misbach GA, Turley K, Ullyot DJ, et al: Left ventricular outflow enlargement by the Konno procedure. *J Thorac Cardiovasc Surg* 84:696-703, 1982

50. Cooley DA, Garrett JR: Septoplasty for left ventricular outflow obstruction without aortic valve replacement: a new technique. *Ann Thorac Surg* 42:445-448, 1986

51. Doty DB, Polansky DB, Jenson CB: Supravalvular aortic stenosis. Repair by extended aortoplasty. *J Thorac Cardiovasc Surg* 74:362-371, 1977

52. Hsieh KS, Keane JF, Nadas AS, et al: Long-term follow-up of valvotomy before 1968 for congenital aortic stenosis. *Am J Cardiol* 58:338-341, 1986

CHAPTER

47

Pulmonary stenosis with intact ventricular septum

Carole A. Warnes, M.D., Valentin Fuster, M.D., and Dwight C. McGoon, M.D.

ANATOMIC CONSIDERATIONS

Isolated pulmonary valvular stenosis is a common form of congenital heart disease found among adults.[1] Less frequently, the obstruction is at the supravalvular level. Also infrequently among adults, pulmonary stenosis may be part of another anomaly such as tetralogy of Fallot, transposition of the great arteries, double-outlet right ventricle, or endocardial cushion defect. This chapter will deal only with isolated pulmonary stenosis—so-called pulmonary stenosis with intact ventricular septum.

Pulmonary valvular stenosis

Typically, this anomaly consists of a dome-shaped valve with a central opening and fused commissures (Fig 47-1). Less commonly, the valve is dysplastic with three leaflets and a narrow pulmonary orifice. If the foramen ovale is not anatomically sealed, the severe forms of pulmonary stenosis with high right-sided pressures may result in a right-to-left shunt at the atrial level. The extreme form of pulmonary stenosis is pulmonary atresia with intact ventricular septum; this entity will not be discussed further because, if untreated, most of these patients die in the first few weeks of life.

Pulmonary subvalvular stenosis

This lesion consists of hypertrophy of the infundibular muscle, causing obstruction. The isolated form is very rare; more commonly, it develops secondarily in response to an underlying ventricular septal defect or is secondary to significant pulmonary valvular stenosis (see Fig 47-1). We exclude from this chapter discussion of infundibular pulmonary stenosis that occurs as part of other complex anomalies such as tetralogy of Fallot or in association with hypertrophic obstructive cardiomyopathy.

Pulmonary supravalvular stenosis

This anomaly, which is also named "peripheral pulmonary artery stenosis," consists of single or multiple, discrete or diffuse stenotic lesions involving the main pulmonary

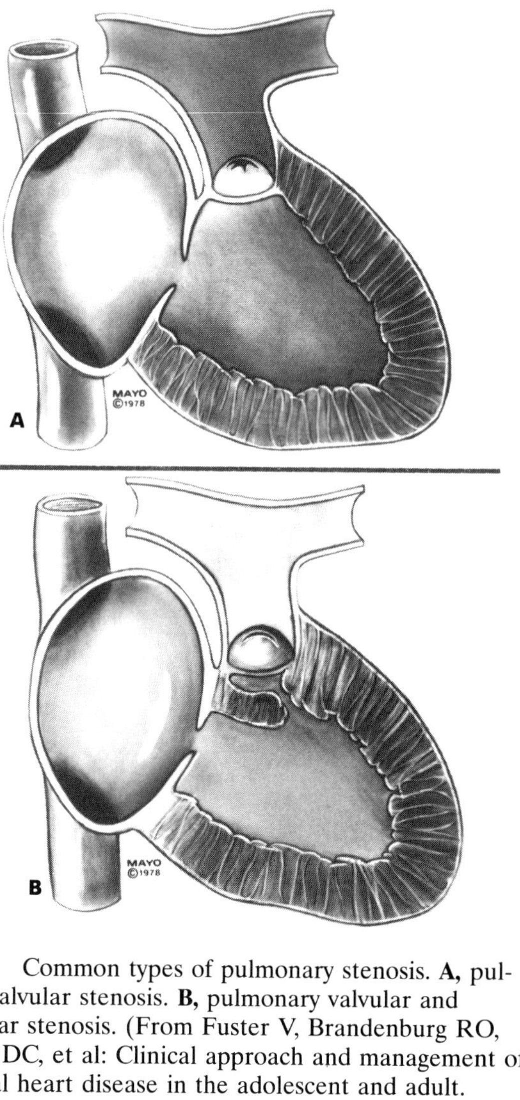

Fig 47-1 Common types of pulmonary stenosis. **A,** pulmonary valvular stenosis. **B,** pulmonary valvular and subvalvular stenosis. (From Fuster V, Brandenburg RO, McGoon DC, et al: Clinical approach and management of congenital heart disease in the adolescent and adult. *Cardiovasc Clin* 10 No 3:161-197, 1980. By permission, Mayo Foundation.)

artery or its main or small branches. Most commonly, this lesion occurs as part of tetralogy of Fallot. In this chapter we will deal with the infrequent isolated type and the form associated with supravalvular aortic stenosis.

CLINICAL FEATURES

The three different types of obstruction usually cause a systolic murmur that can be heard in neonates. However, clinical symptoms develop only in about 25% of the patients because progression of the disease is the exception rather than the rule, in contrast with aortic stenosis.[2,3] The symptoms may develop at any time from infancy to adulthood and most commonly reflect significant stenosis. With a transvalvular gradient greater than 75 mm Hg, symptoms include easy fatigability, exertional dyspnea, angina or syncope, and central cyanosis in those few cases with a right-to-left shunt through a patent foramen ovale.[2-5]

Pulmonary valvular stenosis

The small percentage of patients with the dysplastic type of valvular stenosis have noncardiac abnormalities described as Noonan's syndrome.[6-9] They include small stature, mild mental retardation, triangle-shaped face, webbed neck, ptosis, hypertelorism, low-set ears, and pectus excavatum. The syndrome may be familial,[10] and in some families the parents may show minor stigmas of Noonan's syndrome. Although pulmonic stenosis is the commonest associated cardiac abnormality, many other forms of congenital heart disease also may occur.

The following features suggest severe stenosis[2,4,11] (gradient greater than 75 mm Hg): a giant "a" wave in the jugular venous pulse, reflecting decreased compliance of the hypertrophic right ventricle;[2] an easily palpable right ventricular impulse in the lower left parasternal region;[12,13] auscultatory evidence of a fourth heart sound accentuated by inspiration, resulting from strong right atrial contraction and the noncompliant hypertrophied right ventricle; a loud, long systolic murmur, loudest in the second left intercostal space and peaking in late systole (as the severity of pulmonic stenosis increases, right ventricular ejection and the murmur are prolonged [Fig 47-2]); the pulmonic component of the second heart sound is widely separated from the aortic component and is soft or, with the most severe forms, absent (again, as the severity of pulmonic stenosis increases and the valve becomes more rigid, right ventricular ejection is prolonged and P_2 becomes delayed and softer); and the electrocardiogram (ECG) discloses significant right ventricular hypertrophy, with an R in V_1 of 10 mm and an inverted T wave, or an R in V_1 and an S in V_6 of 35 mm (Fig 47-3). In addition, an ejection systolic click, maximal at the base of the heart and louder in expiration,[14] results from the pliable pulmonic valve in mild to moderate pulmonic stenosis (Fig 47-4).

The chest radiograph in pulmonary valve stenosis typically demonstrates a normal heart size with poststenotic dilatation and a normal pulmonary vascular pattern. Two exceptions to this rule are as follows: (1) When right ventricular failure supervenes, pulmonary blood flow decreases and vascular markings diminish. (2) In cyanotic

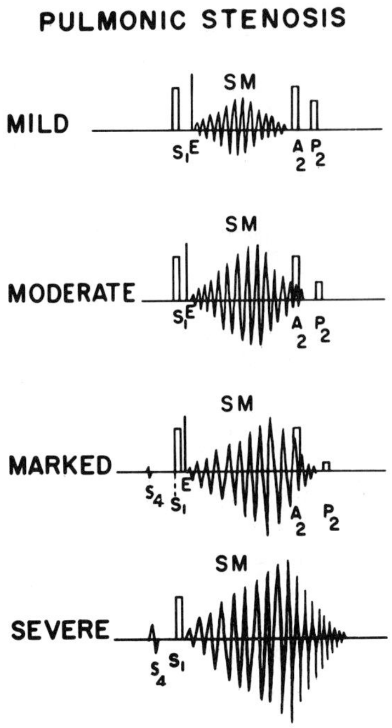

Fig 47-2 Schematic illustration of phonocardiograms in mild to severe valvular pulmonic stenosis. S_1, first heart sound; *E,* ejection sound; *SM,* systolic murmur; A_2, aortic component of second heart sound; P_2, pulmonic component of second heart sound; S_4, fourth heart sound. (From Perloff JK: *The Clinical Recognition of Congenital Heart Disease.* Second edition. Philadelphia, WB Saunders Company, 1978, pp 185-221. By permission.)

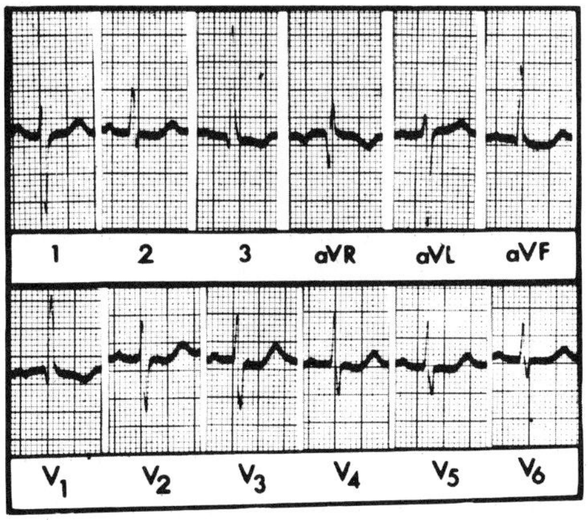

Fig 47-3 Electrocardiogram of patient with valvular pulmonic stenosis and gradient of 100 mm Hg. Right ventricular hypertrophy is manifested by significant right-axis deviation and an R complex in lead V_1. (From Perloff JK: *The Clinical Recognition of Congenital Heart Disease.* Second edition. Philadelphia, WB Saunders Company, 1978, pp 185-221. By permission.)

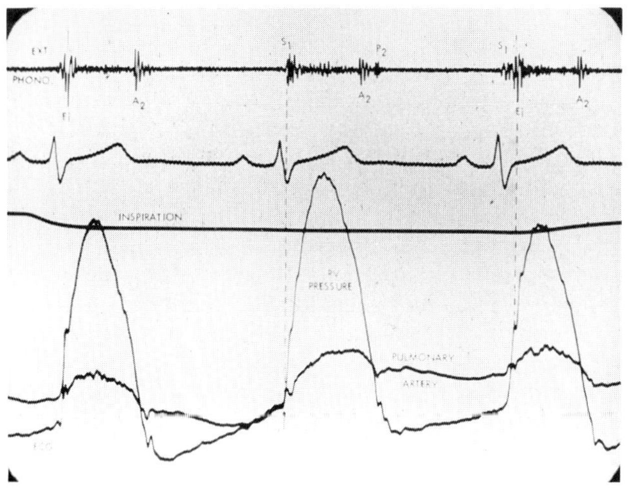

Fig 47-4 Mechanism responsible for variation in intensity of ejection sound *(Ej)* with respiration. With inspiration, venous return increases, causing equalization of diastolic pressure in pulmonary artery and right ventricle and resultant preopening of pulmonic valve in diastole. As a result, during isometric contraction there is no doming of the valve and no opening sound. In next cycle, there is a diastolic gradient at the time of isometric contraction, doming of the valve, and a loud pulmonic ejection sound *(P_2)*. *A_2*, aortic component of second heart sound; *RV*, right ventricular; *S_1*, first heart sound.

patients with an atrial right-to-left shunt, pulmonary flow and vascular markings are reduced.

With stenosis at valve level, disproportionate enlargement of the left branch often accompanies dilatation of the main pulmonary artery (Fig 47-5,A), which occasionally enlarges to aneurysmal proportions (Fig 47-5,B).

Two-dimensional echocardiography is a useful and reliable method for determining the presence of valvular pulmonary stenosis.[15,16] In almost all patients, the valve can be identified from standard and, particularly, high parasternal short-axis views. The leaflets may appear thickened and the valve domes in systole with restricted separation of the leaflet tips (Fig 47-6). Additional information may be obtained by measuring the pulmonary annulus to determine whether it is hypoplastic; similarly, poststenotic dilatation of the main pulmonary artery may be evaluated. Right ventricular hypertrophy and dilatation may also be examined. Doppler evaluation of the stenotic pulmonary valve has now virtually supplanted cardiac catheterization in most patients. With use of continuous-wave Doppler ultrasound across the stenotic valve, the peak gradient may reliably be calculated by applying the modified Bernoulli equation.[17,18] Usually, the transducer is placed in the left parasternal area and the ultrasound beam is directed through the main axis of the pulmonary artery, although the peak velocity may be obtained from other windows, such as subcostal and apical, and at the suprasternal notch.[19]

Pulmonary subvalvular stenosis

The clinical features are similar to those in patients with isolated pulmonary valvular stenosis. However, the ab-

A

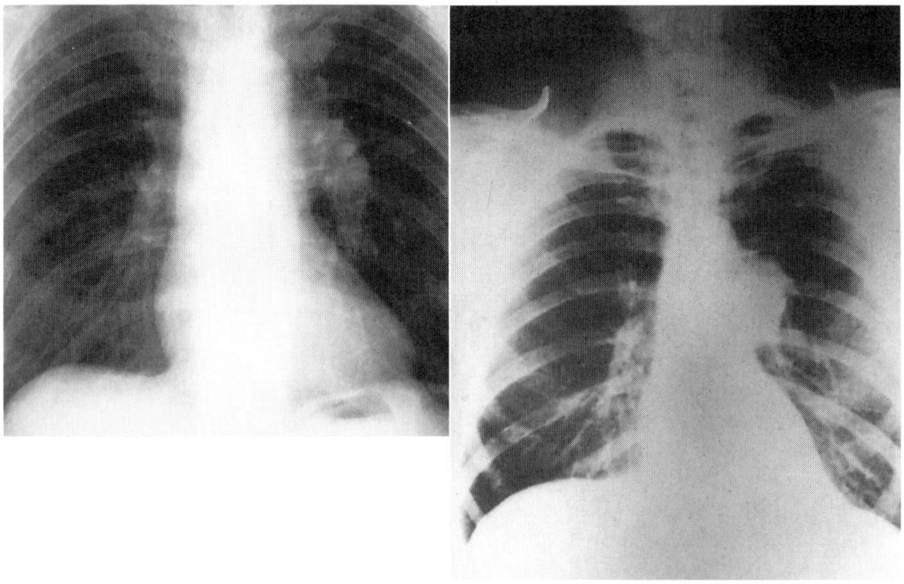

B

Fig 47-5 **A,** chest radiograph of severe valvular pulmonary stenosis. The main pulmonary artery is dilated (poststenotic dilatation), and dilatation extends into the left branch. **B,** posteroanterior view of pulmonary artery aneurysmal dilatation. Such aneurysms may be associated with relatively small pulmonary gradients (in this case, 25 mm Hg) and complete absence of symptoms.

sence of an early systolic click, the prominence of the systolic murmur at the mid left sternal border, and the absence of radiographic poststenotic dilatation of the main pulmonary artery favor the diagnosis of infundibular stenosis;[11] this holds whether the infundibular stenosis is associated with valvular stenosis or with a small ventricular septal defect. Two-dimensional echocardiography may document the infundibular stenosis.

Pulmonary supravalvular stenosis

This anomaly may be an isolated anatomic entity with or without stigmas of congenital rubella, or it may be associated with any of the anatomicoclinical varieties of supravalvular aortic stenosis. The clinical picture is similar to that of pulmonary valvular or subvalvular stenosis. However, the systolic murmur is most prominent at the upper left sternal border, axillae, and posterior lung fields, and it usually extends into early diastole.[11]

DIAGNOSTIC PROBLEMS AND INDICATIONS FOR INVASIVE STUDIES

In adolescents and adults, the diagnosis of isolated pulmonary stenosis can be made with reasonable confidence by clinical means. There are five conditions that can resemble pulmonary stenosis, but usually they all are easily distinguishable.

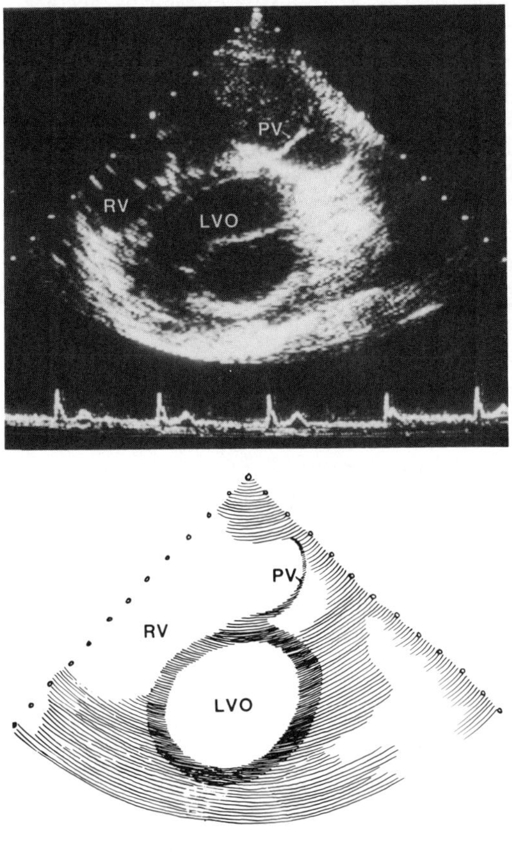

Fig 47-6 Moderate pulmonary stenosis by cardiac catheterization in 16-year-old boy. Tomographic view of right ventricular outflow tract and pulmonary valve *(PV)* demonstrates doming of the pulmonary valve. *LVO,* left ventricular outflow; *RV,* right ventricle. (Courtesy of T.T. Schattenburg, M.D.)

1. Atrial septal defect, in common with pulmonary stenosis, usually exhibits an ejection systolic murmur, wide splitting of the second heart sound, and ECG evidence of right ventricular hypertrophy. However, in atrial septal defect, splitting of the second heart sound is fixed, an early ejection click is not heard, there is roentgenographic evidence of cardiac enlargement or increased pulmonary flow, and, most important, the echocardiogram reveals right ventricular volume overload.

2. Small ventricular septal defect, particularly of the supracristal type, may produce a murmur similar to that of pulmonary valvular stenosis. However, after inhalation of amyl nitrite, the murmur of ventricular septal defect becomes softer because the left-to-right shunt decreases as a result of peripheral vasodilation, whereas the murmur of pulmonary stenosis becomes louder as a result of the increased venous return.

3. In mild left-sided outflow obstruction, the murmur may be difficult to distinguish from that of pulmonary stenosis. However, during the Valsalva maneuver, the murmur of aortic stenosis becomes softer after the fifth heartbeat, whereas in pulmonary stenosis this response occurs within the first three heartbeats. Also, after the release, the murmur of aortic stenosis returns to its normal intensity after the fifth heartbeat, whereas in pulmonary stenosis this occurs within the first three heartbeats. Finally, in patients with hypertrophic obstructive cardiomyopathy affecting the right or left side of the heart or both, the systolic murmurs become louder during the Valsalva maneuver because the decrease in venous return results in smaller ventricular volume with consequent increase in the dynamic obstruction.

4. In acyanotic or pink tetralogy of Fallot, the most important differential features from isolated pulmonary stenosis are absence of a large jugular venous presystolic "a" wave and a decrease in the systolic murmur after amyl nitrite inhalation because the right-to-left shunt increases as a result of peripheral vasodilation whereas in isolated pulmonary stenosis the murmur becomes louder because of increasing venous return and hence increasing pulmonary flow.

5. The cyanotic form of tetralogy of Fallot, as well as the other cyanotic cardiac conditions, usually can be differentiated from isolated pulmonary stenosis with cyanosis due to right-to-left shunt across the foramen ovale by the above features and by others discussed in chapter 49.

In adolescents and adults, the diagnosis and estimation of severity of pulmonary valvular stenosis usually are made easily on clinical grounds and the site and severity of obstruction determined by two-dimensional and Doppler echocardiography. Right ventricular pressure can be determined by measuring the tricuspid regurgitant velocity; therefore, diagnostic cardiac catheterization before intervention is usually not needed. We think that a hemodynamic study to measure the pressure gradient across the stenosis and an angiographic study to localize the narrowing are necessary in the following clinical conditions: (1) when significant infundibular or supravalvular stenosis is suspected, because the surgical approach is different; (2) when there is cyanosis, because the clinical differentiation from other complex cyanotic cardiac anomalies is inexact; and (3) when the clinical symptoms are out of proportion to the other clinical features, because the measurement of the exact gradient can be of help in the interventional decision. In addition, in some institutions, catheterization is routinely performed in all patients in whom the stenosis is suspected to be severe and confirmation is sought prior to intervention.

MANAGEMENT

Most studies of the natural history of pulmonary stenosis[3,5,20-22] show that gradients often increase in patients with moderate to severe stenosis and the stenosis becomes more severe, whereas most patients with mild pulmonary stenosis remain in that category at follow-up. Patients younger than 1 or 2 years, however, tend to have a higher chance than older patients of moving into the moderate or severe category.[20,21] The prognosis for patients with pulmonary stenosis who have reached adulthood without right ventricular failure or symptoms is reported to be good, with minimal risk of bacterial endocarditis, right ventricular failure, or death.[3,5] On the other hand, impaired cardiac output in response to exercise has been found in patients with severe stenosis,[23] and right ventricular myocardial changes are the rule in patients with long-standing right ventricular hypertension.[24]

It is appropriate, therefore, to perform pulmonary valvotomy (either percutaneously with a balloon or surgically) at any age in patients with significant pulmonary stenosis who have related symptoms, such as easy fatigability, dyspnea on exertion, cyanosis, and congestive heart failure. Even if such disability is absent, the benefits of relief of the stenosis outweigh the disadvantages for patients with gradients across the pulmonary outflow tract of greater than 75 mm Hg during peak systole and in most instances for those with gradients as low as 50 or 60 mm Hg. In patients with gradients of less than 50 mm Hg, the indications for valvuloplasty or valvotomy are less well defined, and because of the benign natural history of the disease process and the ease with which echo-Doppler studies can noninvasively determine pulmonary valve gradients, simple follow-up appears appropriate.[25]

Balloon pulmonary valvuloplasty

Percutaneous balloon pulmonary valvuloplasty as it is now used was first described by Kan et al. in 1982.[26] The technique has been used in neonates, infants, children, and adults and is now considered to be the procedure of choice for treatment of congenital pulmonary valve stenosis.[27-31] The circumferential pressure exerted by balloon inflation is likely to tear the weakest part of the valve. This may be the fused commissures, but if these cannot be torn, tears in the valve cusps or avulsion of the valve leaflets can occur.[32-34]

Because the technique is relatively new, long-term results are not yet available. Early and intermediate-term results, however, appear to be excellent, and even though there may be residual infundibular hypertrophy and subpulmonary obstruction immediately after dilatation, these appear to regress.[35,36] The outcome may be less successful if the pulmonary valve is dysplastic.[36,37] Restenosis after pulmonary valvuloplasty has been reported[27,28] and appears more likely to occur if the immediate postvalvuloplasty gradient is greater than 30 mm Hg.[38] Pulmonary regurgitation has been reported in 79% of patients at intermediate follow-up[37,38] and although this has not been a problem, clearly it must be watched on long-term follow-up studies.

Surgical technique

Surgical treatment for valvular pulmonic stenosis has been available for more than 40 years, since the first description by Brock.[39] Because balloon valvuloplasty is a recent development, it is difficult to compare balloon with surgical pulmonary valvuloplasty. Certainly in adults, or in the absence of congestive heart failure and cyanosis, surgical pulmonary valvotomy can be accomplished at a risk of less than 1%,[40] although the procedure has largely been replaced by balloon valvuloplasty. When the surgical approach is chosen, the use of cardiopulmonary bypass and mild systemic hypothermia is preferred. The pulmonary valve is approached through an incision in the pulmonary artery, and valvulotomy is accomplished by accurate incision of the rudimentary commissures. Inspection and sounding of the infundibular portion of the right ventricle is always accomplished in order to identify the rare associated instance of fixed organic obstruction of the outflow tract. The long-standing issue as to the management of outflow tract hypertrophy and functional stenosis is being clarified by accumulating evidence that such outflow tract hypertrophy and residual stenosis will regress in the absence of fixed infundibular obstruction, and therefore resection of secondary infundibular hypertrophy at the time of operation usually is not required.[41]

Postoperative course

The late result of operation, despite the common occurrence of trivial pulmonary valvular insufficiency,[42] is excellent in the patient who was uncompromised preoperatively. In the Joint Study on Congenital Heart Disease,[3] only 5% of patients who underwent operation for valvular pulmonary stenosis had a right ventricle-to-pulmonary artery residual peak systolic pressure gradient of 50 mm Hg or more. Such occasional residual gradients tend to persist from the time of the operation rather than develop late postoperatively. Although infundibular stenosis tends to resolve in most cases,[41] the occasional persistence of a ventricle-to-pulmonary artery gradient and a low cardiac output syndrome may be related to significant residual infundibular stenosis.[43] Although long-term survival is excellent for patients operated on for isolated pulmonary stenosis, it decreases among patients undergoing operation at relatively advanced age (over 21 years old), probably because of the sequelae of long-standing right ventricular hypertrophy.[44]

After a successful pulmonary valve operation, usually there is persistence of a short midsystolic murmur and a short, low-pitched diastolic murmur of pulmonary insufficiency (unlike the high-pitched Graham Steell diastolic murmur of pulmonary hypertension). In most cases, there is a gradual reduction in the ECG pattern of right ventricular hypertrophy, although the pattern does not return entirely to normal in a substantial number of patients.[42,45] Lack of improvement in the ECG by 3 years after the operation suggests significant pulmonary stenosis.[42] Late postoperative supraventricular and ventricular arrhythmias are rare. Although only about 25% of patients continue to have some degree of cardiomegaly late postoperatively, dilatation of the main pulmonary artery segment usually persists even after an ideal surgical result.[42]

REFERENCES

1. Fuster V, Brandenburg RO, McGoon DC, et al: Clinical approach and management of congenital heart disease in the adolescent and adult. *Cardiovasc Clin* 10 No 3:161-197, 1980
2. Kaplan S, Adolph RJ: Pulmonic valve stenosis in adults. *Cardiovasc Clin* 10 No 1:327-339, 1979
3. Nugent EW, Freedom RM, Nora JJ, et al: Clinical course in pulmonary stenosis. *Circulation* 56 Suppl 1:38-47, 1977
4. Ellison RC, Freedom RM, Keane JF, et al: Indirect assessment of severity in pulmonary stenosis. *Circulation* 56 Suppl 1:14-23, 1977
5. Johnson LW, Grossman W, Dalen JE, et al: Pulmonic stenosis in the adult: long-term follow-up results. *N Engl J Med* 287:1159-1163, 1972
6. Noonan JA, Ehmke DA: Associated noncardiac malformations in children with congenital heart disease (abstract). *J Pediatr* 63:468-469, 1963
7. Noonan JA: Hypertelorism with Turner phenotype: a new syndrome with associated congenital heart disease. *Am J Dis Child* 116:373-380, 1968
8. Duncan WJ, Fowler RS, Farkas LG, et al: A comprehensive scoring system for evaluating Noonan syndrome. *Am J Med Genet* 10:37-50, 1981
9. Nora JJ, Nora AH, Sinha AK, et al: The Ullrich-Noonan syndrome (Turner phenotype). *Am J Dis Child* 127:48-55, 1974
10. Bolton MR, Pugh DM, Mattioli LF, et al: The Noonan syndrome: a family study. *Ann Intern Med* 80:626-629, 1974
11. Perloff JK: *The Clinical Recognition of Congenital Heart Disease.* Second edition. Philadelphia, WB Saunders Company, 1978, pp 185-221
12. Schmidt RE, Craige E: Precordial movements over the right ventricle in children with pulmonary stenosis. *Circulation* 32:241-250, 1965
13. Holt JH Jr, Eddleman EE Jr: The precordial movements in adults with pulmonic stenosis. *Circulation* 35:492-500, 1967
14. Hultgren HN, Reeve R, Cohn K, et al: The ejection click of valvular pulmonic stenosis. *Circulation* 40:631-640, 1969
15. Weyman AE, Hurwitz RA, Girod DA, et al: Cross-sectional echocardiographic visualization of the stenotic pulmonary valve. *Circulation* 56:769-774, 1977
16. Nasser FN, Giuliani ER: *Clinical Two-Dimensional Echocardiography.* Chicago, Year Book Medical Publishers, 1983, pp 88-105
17. Lima CO, Sahn DJ, Valdes-Cruz LM, et al: Noninvasive prediction of transvalvular pressure gradient in patients with pulmonary stenosis by quantitative two-dimensional echocardiographic Doppler studies. *Circulation* 67:866-871, 1983
18. Kosturakis D, Allen HD, Goldberg SJ, et al: Noninvasive quantification of stenotic semilunar valve areas by Doppler echocardiography. *J Am Coll Cardiol* 3:1256-1262, 1984
19. Frantz EG, Silverman NH: Doppler ultrasound evaluation of valvar pulmonary stenosis from multiple transducer positions in children requiring pulmonary valvuloplasty. *Am J Cardiol* 61:844-849, 1988
20. Mody MR: The natural history of uncomplicated valvular pulmonic stenosis. *Am Heart J* 90:317-321, 1975
21. Wennevold A, Jacobsen JR: Natural history of valvular pulmonary stenosis in children below the age of two years: long-term follow-up with serial heart catheterizations. *Eur J Cardiol* 8:371-378, 1978
22. Hayes CJ, Gersony WM, Driscoll DJ, et al: Second Natural History Study of Congenital Heart Defects: Results of treatment of patients with pulmonary valvar stenosis. *Circulation* 87 Suppl 1:28-37, 1993
23. Howitt G: Haemodynamic effects of exercise in pulmonary stenosis. *Br Heart J* 28:152-160, 1966
24. Jones M, Ferrans VJ: Myocardial ultrastructure in children and adults with congenital heart disease. *Cardiovasc Clin* 10 No 1:501-530, 1979
25. Rao PS: Indications for balloon pulmonary valvuloplasty (editorial). *Am Heart J* 116:1661-1662, 1988
26. Kan JS, White RI Jr, Mitchell SE, et al: Percutaneous balloon valvuloplasty: a new method treating congenital pulmonary-valve stenosis. *N Engl J Med* 307:540-542, 1982
27. Tynan M, Baker EJ, Rohmer J, et al: Percutaneous balloon pulmonary valvuloplasty. *Br Heart J* 53:520-524, 1985
28. Kveselis DA, Rocchini AP, Snider AR, et al: Results of balloon valvuloplasty in the treatment of congenital valvar pulmonary stenosis in children. *Am J Cardiol* 56:527-532, 1985
29. Radtke W, Keane JF, Fellows KE, et al: Percutaneous balloon valvotomy of congenital pulmonary stenosis using oversized balloons. *J Am Coll Cardiol* 8:909-915, 1986
30. Rao PS, Fawzy ME, Solymar L, et al: Long-term results of balloon pulmonary valvuloplasty of valvar pulmonic stenosis. *Am Heart J* 115:1291-1296, 1988
31. Stanger P, Cassidy SC, Girod DA, et al: Balloon pulmonary valvuloplasty: results of the Valvuloplasty and Angioplasty of Congenital Anomalies Registry. *Am J Cardiol* 65:775-783, 1990
32. Walls JT, Lababidi Z, Curtis JJ: Assessment of percutaneous balloon pulmonary and aortic valvuloplasty. *J Thorac Cardiovasc Surg* 88:352-356, 1984
33. Benson LN, Smallhorn JS, Freedom RM, et al: Pulmonary valve morphology after balloon dilatation of pulmonary valve stenosis. *Cathet Cardiovasc Diagn* 11:161-166, 1985
34. Khan MAA, Yousef SA, Mullins CE: Percutaneous transluminal balloon pulmonary valvuloplasty for the relief of pulmonary valve stenosis with special reference to double-balloon technique. *Am Heart J* 112:158-166, 1986
35. Fontes VF, Sousa JEMR, Esteves CA, et al: Pulmonary valvuloplasty—experience of 100 cases. *Int J Cardiol* 21:335-342, 1988
36. Thapar MK, Rao PS: Significance of infundibular obstruction following balloon valvuloplasty for valvar pulmonic stenosis. *Am Heart J* 118:99-103, 1989
37. Musewe NN, Robertson MA, Benson LN, et al: The dysplastic pulmonary valve: echocardiographic features and results of balloon dilatation. *Br Heart J* 57:364-370, 1987
38. Rao PS: Balloon pulmonary valvuloplasty: a review. *Clin Cardiol* 12:55-74, 1989
39. Brock RC: Pulmonary valvulotomy for the relief of congenital pulmonary stenosis: report of three cases. *Br Med J [Clin Res]* 1:1121-1126, 1948
40. Danielson GK, Exarhos ND, Weidman WH, et al: Pulmonic stenosis with intact ventricular septum: surgical considerations and results of operation. *J Thorac Cardiovasc Surg* 61:228-234, 1971
41. Griffith BP, Hardesty RL, Siewers RD, et al: Pulmonary valvulotomy alone for pulmonary stenosis: results in children with and without muscular infundibular hypertrophy. *J Thorac Cardiovasc Surg* 83:577-583, 1982
42. McNamara DG, Latson LA: Long-term follow-up of patients with malformations for which definitive surgical repair has been available for 25 years or more. *Am J Cardiol* 50:560-568, 1982
43. Nadas AS: Pulmonic stenosis: indications for surgery in children and adults. *N Engl J Med* 287:1196-1197, 1972
44. Kopecky SL, Gersh BJ, McGoon MD, et al: Long-term outcome of patients undergoing surgical repair of isolated pulmonary valve stenosis: follow-up at 20-30 years. *Circulation* 78:1150-1156, 1988
45. Clark DS, Hirsch HD, Tamer DM, et al: Electrocardiographic changes following surgical treatment of congenital cardiac malformations. *Prog Cardiovasc Dis* 17:451-465, 1975

CHAPTER

48

Ebstein's anomaly of the tricuspid valve

David J. Driscoll, M.D., Valentin Fuster, M.D., and Gordon K. Danielson, M.D.

ANATOMIC CONSIDERATIONS

In 1866, Wilhelm Ebstein described the tricuspid valve malformation that today bears his name.[1] It is a relatively rare form of congenital heart disease, occurring in 1 per 1,000 autopsies of patients with congenital heart disease or 1 per 210,000 live births[2] and constituting less than 1% of all forms of congenital heart disease.[2] Equal numbers of males and females are affected.

Ebstein's anomaly consists of abnormally developed tricuspid valve leaflets that are attached abnormally to an enlarged tricuspid valve annulus, right ventricle, and valve-support apparatus. The attachments of the septal and posterior (inferior) leaflets may be displaced from the tricuspid annulus toward the right ventricular apex. The commissure between these two leaflets usually is the point of maximal displacement[3,4] (Fig 48-1). In one-third of the cases, the attachment of these leaflets is not truly displaced, but the leaflets are adherent to the ventricular wall. Often, these leaflets are dysplastic and small. The anterior tricuspid valve leaflet usually is attached to the tricuspid valve annulus but is enlarged, elongated ("sail-like"), abnormally adherent, or tethered to the right ventricle and may be fenestrated and contain fibrous strands (Fig 48-2). The leaflet may be attached to the ledge separating the inlet and trabecular portions of the right ventricle.[3] Extensive attachment of this leaflet along the ledge can obstruct blood flow from the right atrium and the atrialized portion of the right ventricle to the body of the right ventricle. In approximately 10% of cases, this abnormal attachment together with fusion of the leaflet commissures results in complete obstruction of inflow to the body of the right ventricle.[3] In the majority of cases, however, the abnormal tricuspid valve leaflets and attachments allow tricuspid regurgitation. The degree of tethering of the anterior tricuspid valve leaflet, particularly of the free edge, is an important consideration in the reconstruction of this valve.

The abnormal attachment of the tricuspid valve leaflets produces anatomic separation of the proximal part of the right ventricular inlet (the so-called atrialized portion of the right ventricle) from the trabecular portion or body of the right ventricle (see Fig 48-2). However, the atrialized portion of the right ventricle contracts in unison with the right ventricle. In Ebstein's anomaly the right ventricular cavity usually is dilated, the free wall is thin, and there is a decrease in the number of right ventricular muscle fibers.[4] The atrium itself usually is dilated and, with the atrialized portion of the right ventricle, the combined chamber dimension can be massive. The eustachian valve may be prominent.[3]

Ebstein's malformation may not be limited to abnormalities of the right side of the heart. It may be associated with left ventricular dysfunction and mitral valve prolapse.[5-7] An atrial septal defect or patent foramen ovale is present in 30% to 78% of patients with Ebstein's anomaly.[3,8] The presence of an interatrial communication creates a right-to-left interatrial shunt, which accounts for the cyanosis in many patients with Ebstein's anomaly.

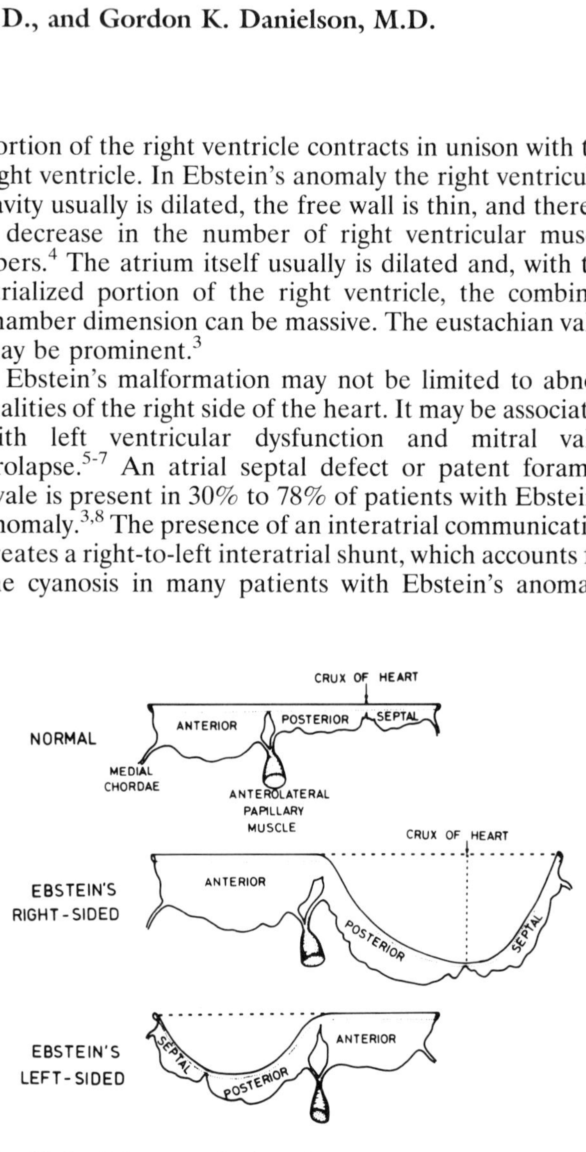

Fig 48-1 Diagram of tricuspid valve leaflet, showing point of maximal displacement of posterior and septal leaflets. The valve tissue has been laid flat. (From Anderson KR, Zuberbuhler JR, Anderson RH, et al: Morphologic spectrum of Ebstein's anomaly of the heart: a review. *Mayo Clin Proc* 54:174-180, 1979. By permission, Mayo Foundation.)

Ebstein's anomaly has been associated with pulmonary valve stenosis, ventricular septal defect, pulmonary hypertension, bicuspid aortic valve, and right aortic arch. Patients with ventricular inversion (corrected transposition of the great arteries) may have a malformation of the left-sided morphological tricuspid atrioventricular (AV) valve that is similar to Ebstein's anomaly in some respects but different in others.[9]

In the Mayo Clinic series of 189 patients operated on, the prevalence of an accessory AV pathway (Kent bundle) was 15%.[10] Nearly always, these are right-sided free-wall or posterior septal accessory pathways.[10] This accounts in part for the high incidence of palpitations and supraventricular tachycardia observed in patients with Ebstein's anomaly.

The AV valves normally form by a process of delamination of the valvular tissue from the ventricular surface. The embryologic basis of Ebstein's anomaly probably is an abnormal or incomplete delamination process; certainly, this could explain the broad spectrum of anatomic malformations observed. Ebstein's anomaly probably is inherited in a multifactorial fashion, with a risk of 1% if there is one affected sibling. There appears to be an association between maternal lithium ingestion during pregnancy and Ebstein's anomaly in offspring.

PATHOPHYSIOLOGY

The pathophysiology of Ebstein's anomaly mainly depends on the degree of incompetence of the tricuspid valve.[11] Other contributing factors are the presence of an atrial septal defect or patent foramen ovale, the degree of impairment of right ventricular and left ventricular function, the presence of an accessory AV conduction pathway, and, occasionally, the presence of tricuspid stenosis.

It has been postulated that antegrade blood flow from the right atrium to the right ventricle is impeded by systolic contraction of the atrialized portion of the right ventricle.[12] Also, during atrial contraction, the relaxation and dilation of the atrialized portion of the ventricle may affect antegrade blood flow.[12] Presumably, this may contribute to the decreased systemic blood flow and the symptoms of fatigue.

The presence of an atrial septal defect usually allows a net right-to-left interatrial shunt, producing cyanosis and polycythemia. The volume of the right-to-left shunt, and hence the degree of cyanosis, is related to the severity of tricuspid insufficiency (or stenosis) and the compliance of the right ventricle.

Shiina et al. [13] found that in patients with the anatomic features of Ebstein's anomaly the decreased functional capacity was related to (1) small functional right ventricle; (2) valve leaflet abnormalities in the form of extreme dysplasia of the tricuspid valve septal leaflet, absence of the septal leaflet, the degree of displacement of the anterior leaflet, and the degree of tethering of the anterior leaflet; and (3) aneurysmal dilation of the right ventricular outflow tract. More recently, left ventricular dysfunction was correlated at echocardiography with the degree of downward displacement of the tricuspid valve and paradoxical septal motion.[14] Indeed, such left ventricular dysfunction secondary to abnormality of contiguous structures can also contribute to the decreased functional capacity seen preoperatively or even postoperatively in some patients with Ebstein's anomaly.

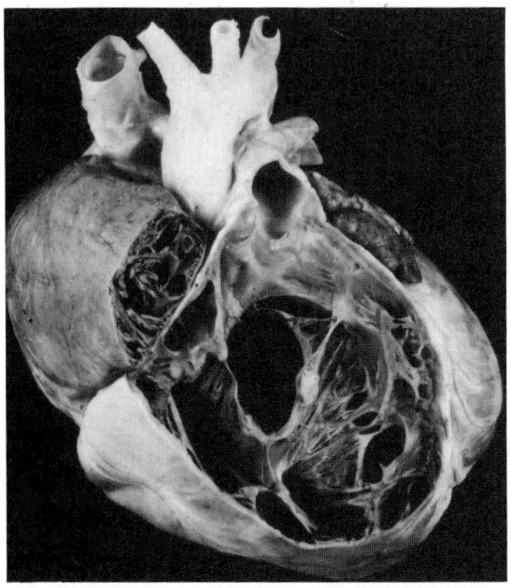

Fig 48-2 Pathologic specimen, showing large sail-like anterior leaflet of tricuspid valve and separation of right atrium, atrialized portion of right ventricle, and right ventricle.

CLINICAL SYNDROME

History and clinical course

Symptoms in childhood or later in life vary markedly, as would be expected from the variations in anatomic abnormalities. Although in a few patients with mild malformations of the tricuspid valve there are no symptoms, the majority of patients have cyanosis and dyspnea [15] (Table 48-1). Thus, the frequent right-to-left shunt at the atrial level results in cyanosis, and in addition the low arterial oxygen tension contributes to the dyspnea, perhaps by stimulating the carotid bodies and increasing ventilation. Furthermore, it is possible that in patients with right-sided cardiac failure the dyspnea results in part from inadequate perfusion of the exercising muscles, which has been thought to provoke reflex ventilatory stimulation. Palpitations in the form of paroxysmal atrial arrhythmias and peripheral edema are less frequent.

In infants, the clinical spectrum of Ebstein's anomaly ranges from acyanosis and no symptoms to distress and marked cyanosis. However, many infants with Ebstein's anomaly who are cyanotic gradually become less cyanotic as pulmonary blood flow increases. The infusion of PGE_1 may stabilize these babies sufficiently to allow time for the pulmonary arteriolar resistance to decrease and the pulmonary blood flow to increase. Therefore, it is important to avoid early aggressive surgical management of cyanotic newborns with Ebstein's anomaly who do not have anatomic obstruction to right ventricular inflow or outflow of blood.

Based on our study of 67 patients with Ebstein's

Table 48-1 Clinical findings at diagnosis of Ebstein's anomaly in 67 patients

Finding	No.	%
Dyspnea	40	60
Cyanosis	41	61
Palpitations	8	12
Edema	7	10
Functional class*		
I	13	19
II	24	36
III	23	34
IV	7	10
Electrocardiogram abnormal	67	100
Chest radiograph abnormal	67	100
Cardiomegaly absent	5	7
Cardiomegaly present	62	93

*New York Heart Association.

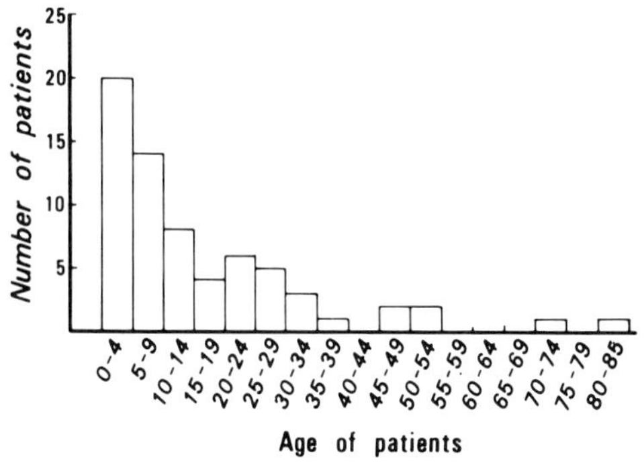

Fig 48-3 Distribution of ages at time of diagnosis in 67 patients with proved Ebstein's anomaly of tricuspid valve. (From Giuliani ER, Fuster V, Brandenburg RO, et al: Ebstein's anomaly: the clinical features and natural history of Ebstein's anomaly of the tricuspid valve. *Mayo Clin Proc* 54:163-173, 1979. By permission, Mayo Foundation.)

anomaly who had a mean follow-up of 12 years and a maximum of 26 years, predictors of mortality were significant functional incapacity (New York Heart Association class III or IV), degree of cardiomegaly (cardiothoracic ratio >0.65), systemic arterial blood oxygen desaturation (<90%), and diagnosis in infancy.[15] Otherwise, patients with Ebstein's anomaly have occasionally been noted to live into the seventh and eighth decades. Others have died in infancy and early childhood.

Physical findings

Physical appearance. In a study at the Mayo Clinic, the mean age at the time of diagnosis was 14 years[15] (Fig 48-3). Growth and development are generally normal. Cyanosis and digital clubbing are apparent in patients with associated intracardiac right-to-left shunts. Some patients have a distinctive violaceous hue, particularly of the malar area, the posterior aspects of the arms, and the lateral aspects of the torso. Usually, these patients have at least mild polycythemia, and systemic arterial blood oxygen desaturation can be demonstrated during exercise if it is not apparent at rest. This violaceous hue also can be apparent in patients without a demonstrable right-to-left shunt; presumably in these patients this results from severely reduced cardiac output. Because of cardiomegaly, patients with Ebstein's anomaly have a prominent precordium.

Arterial and venous pulsations. The arterial and venous pulsations usually are normal, even in the presence of tricuspid insufficiency. The jugular venous pulsations may not have the characteristic large systolic v wave noted with tricuspid insufficiency unassociated with Ebstein's anomaly; presumably, this is because of poor transmission of the venous pulse wave retrogradely in the presence of a dilated, compliant right atrial cavity.

Precordial palpation. Despite marked cardiomegaly, the apical precordial impulse may be normal, albeit displaced.

Auscultation. The auscultatory signs may be the first findings to alert the clinician to the possibility of Ebstein's anomaly. These can best be summarized as a multiplicity of sounds and murmurs, all originating from the right side of the heart. The first heart sound is widely split, and is due to delay in the second component, which originates in the malformed tricuspid apparatus, probably the large anterior leaflet. The second heart sound is widely and persistently split by the delay in pulmonary valve closure due to the right bundle-branch block. The intensity of the pulmonic component of the second heart sound may be normal, or it may be soft as a result of low pulmonary pressure when there is right-to-left shunt. Both atrial and ventricular filling sounds are relatively common and contribute to the multiple sounds and cadence quality so often noted in patients with Ebstein's anomaly. Because the sounds originate in the right side of the heart, they become louder during inspiration. A systolic murmur of tricuspid regurgitation that increases with inspiration is heard along the left sternal border and is almost always present in patients with Ebstein's anomaly. Frequently, there also are diastolic and presystolic murmurs of low intensity due to functional anatomic or tricuspid stenosis. These murmurs also become louder with inspiration.

Electrocardiogram

Classically, the electrocardiogram is characterized by first-degree AV block, tall, peaked P waves consistent with right atrial enlargement, and right bundle-branch block pattern (Fig 48-4). Patients with ventricular preexcitation will have a short P-R interval and a δ wave. The absence of ventricular preexcitation on the surface electrocardiogram does not exclude the presence of an accessory AV conduction pathway.

Chest radiographs

In Ebstein's anomaly, the cardiac silhouette may vary from nearly normal (Fig 48-5, left) to a configuration that is

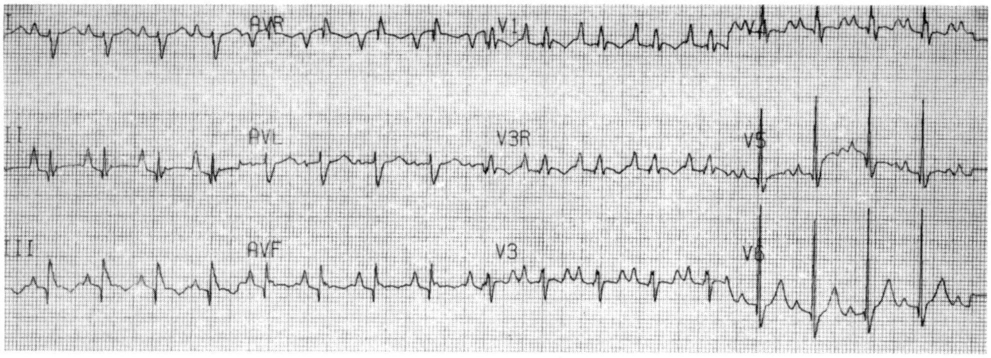

Fig 48-4 Electrocardiogram from 15-year-old boy with Ebstein's anomaly. Note prominent P wave, prolonged AV conduction, and delay in right ventricular conduction.

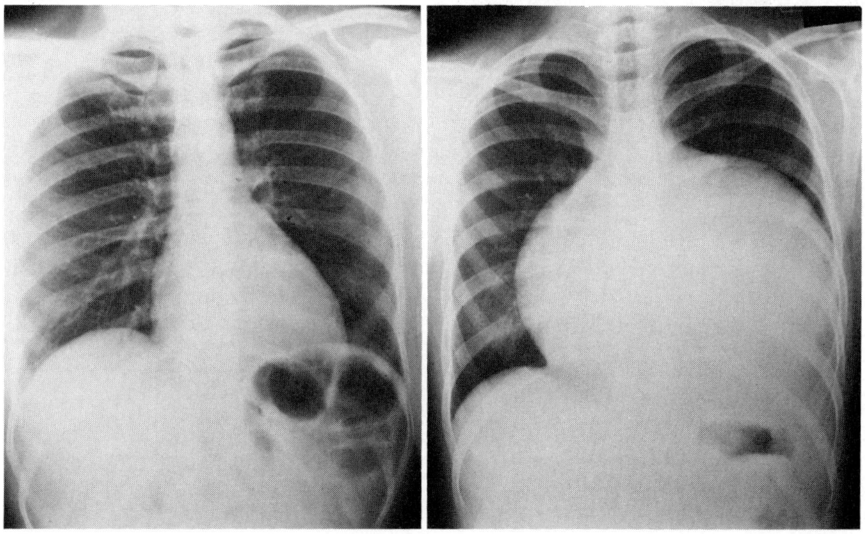

Fig 48-5 Chest radiographs in patients with Ebstein's anomaly. **Left,** in 17-year-old asymptomatic girl, heart is only slightly enlarged. **Right,** in 3-year-old symptomatic girl, there is marked cardiomegaly. (From Giuliani ER, Fuster V, Brandenburg RO, et al: Ebstein's anomaly: the clinical features and natural history of Ebstein's anomaly of the tricuspid valve. *Mayo Clin Proc* 54:163-173, 1979. By permission, Mayo Foundation.)

fairly typical for this disease (Fig 48-5, right). The typical contour is found in the great majority of cases and consists of a balloon-shaped heart, similar to that seen with pericardial effusion, with a narrow waist. The enlarged right atrium is responsible for the most impressive features and in some cases makes up almost the entire cardiac silhouette. In the posteroanterior view, the right atrium produces a rightward curvature. Dilation of the right ventricular outflow tract produces varying degrees of displacement of the upper left cardiac border. It is this combination of leftward displacement of the base of the heart together with rightward convexity caused by the enlarged right atrium that accounts for the globular cardiac silhouette. In cyanotic patients, the vascular pattern is decreased because of the right-to-left shunt.

Echocardiography

Echocardiography has revolutionized the diagnostic approach to evaluation of patients with Ebstein's anomaly.[15] An experienced echocardiographer can usually provide enough anatomic details so that cardiac catheterization is unnecessary.[16]

Two-dimensional echocardiography is now the diagnostic modality of choice for the assessment of Ebstein's anomaly (Fig 48-6). By using two-dimensional echocardiographic techniques, the degree of malformation of the tricuspid valve (leaflet displacement, degree of tethering, dysplasia, absence) can be appreciated and has been correlated with functional capacity and with whether or not surgical repair can be accomplished without the use of a prosthetic valve.[13,16] In the evaluation of tricuspid

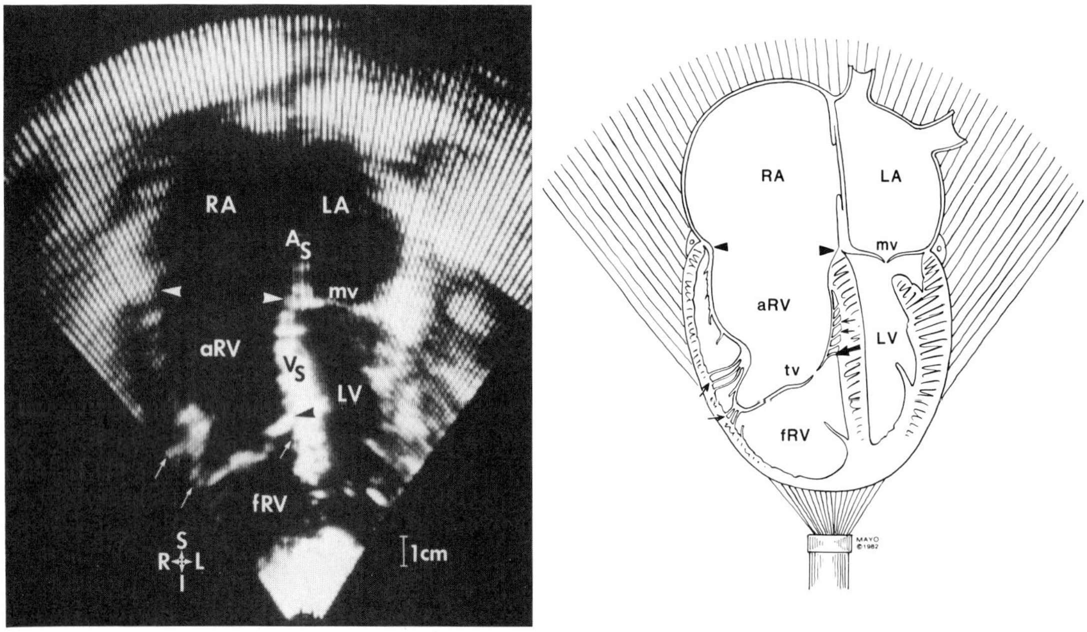

Fig 48-6 Two-dimensional echocardiogram (four-chamber view) and interpretive diagram, showing features typical of Ebstein's anomaly. *RA,* right atrium; *LA,* left atrium; *mv,* mitral valve; *LV,* left ventricle; *fRV,* functional right ventricle; *tv,* tricuspid valve; *aRV,* atrialized right ventricle; A_s, atrial septum; V_s, ventricular septum; *I,* inferior; *L,* left; *R,* right; *S,* superior; *arrows,* tethering of leaflets. (From Shiina A, Seward JB, Edwards WD, et al: Two-dimensional echocardiographic spectrum of Ebstein's anomaly: detailed anatomic assessment. *J Am Coll Cardiol* 3:356-370, 1984. **Left,** by permission of American College of Cardiology. **Right,** by permission, Mayo Foundation.)

valve function, semiquantitation of tricuspid regurgitation is accomplished by pulsed-wave Doppler interrogation of the hepatic vein as well as Doppler color-flow imaging of the extent of the tricuspid regurgitant jet into the right atrium.[17] Color-flow imaging also allows the diagnosis of left-to-right or right-to-left shunting across the atrial septum. Other associated abnormalities such as ventricular septal defects and pulmonic stenosis can be detected by two-dimensional and Doppler echocardiography.

Cardiac catheterization

In most adolescents and adults, cardiac catheterization and angiography are unnecessary for evaluation of Ebstein's anomaly. Pulmonary artery angiography is necessary to define areas of pulmonary artery distortion when operation is contemplated for patients who have had a systemic-to-pulmonary artery anastomosis. It may also be necessary for assessment in patients with suspected pulmonary artery hypoplasia. Coronary angiography to exclude concomitant coronary artery disease is indicated for patients older than 50 years and for patients younger than 50 who have signs or symptoms of coronary artery disease or compelling risk factors for coronary artery disease. Invasive electrophysiologic studies may be necessary to localize accessory electrical bypass tracks. In the majority of patients with Ebstein's anomaly, the right atrial pressure is found to be moderately increased, and the pulse contour most often shows a dominant v wave with a steep y descent. However, in patients with a markedly dilated right atrium, the atrial pressure pulse contour may be normal despite the presence of severe tricuspid regurgitation. Right ventricular systolic pressure most often is normal, although patients with severe tricuspid regurgitation may have an increased right ventricular end-diastolic pressure. Pulmonary artery pressure is normal or, occasionally, decreased in patients with severe tricuspid regurgitation and a large right-to-left shunt at atrial level. In patients with an associated atrial septal defect, oximetry will demonstrate a shunt. With a right-to-left shunt, intracardiac dye-dilution curves injected from the inferior or superior vena cava will also show this shunt by early appearance of dye at the systemic arterial sampling site.

The tricuspid regurgitation, enlarged right atrium, displaced tricuspid valve apparatus, ventricular size and function, and presence of associated defects can be demonstrated angiographically (Fig 48-7). Furthermore, cineangiography has established a correlation between the functional severity and the nature of the distal tricuspid valve attachments, which are classified in three different subgroups.[18]

In cyanotic newborns with Ebstein's anomaly, contrast medium injected into the right ventricle may regurgitate to the right atrium with little or no appearance of it in the

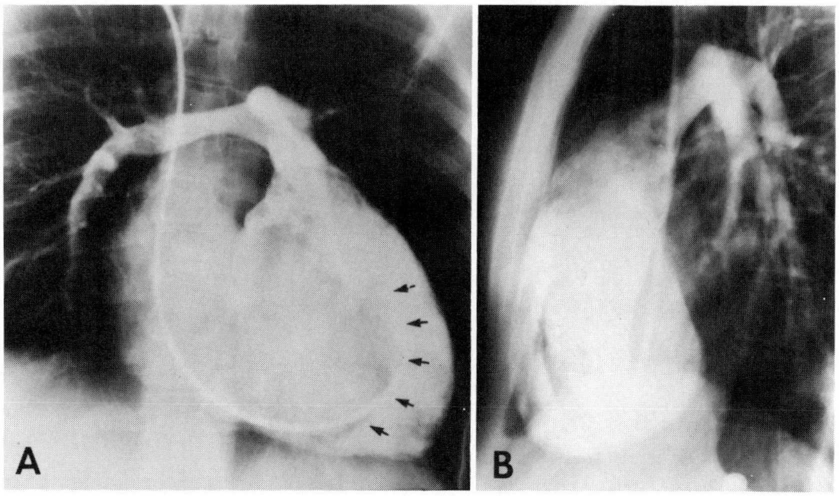

Fig 48-7 Anteroposterior (**A**) and lateral (**B**) right ventriculograms from 21-year-old woman. Anteroposterior view shows large sail-like anterior leaflet *(arrows)* displaced well to left of spine. Severe tricuspid regurgitation is evident. Lateral projection displays pronounced anterior displacement of abnormal anterior tricuspid leaflet. (From Giuliani ER, Fuster V, Brandenburg RO, et al: Ebstein's anomaly: the clinical features and natural history of Ebstein's anomaly of the tricuspid valve. *Mayo Clin Proc* 54:163-173, 1979. By permission, Mayo Foundation.)

pulmonary artery, suggesting anatomic obstruction to right ventricular outflow. However, this also occurs in the absence of anatomic obstruction to right ventricular outflow if pulmonary resistance is increased. Patency of the right ventricular outflow tract must be established by other techniques.[19] By using aortography performed near the ductus arteriosus, the pulmonary artery can be visualized, and the presence of pulmonary regurgitation allows visualization of a patent right ventricular outflow tract. Certainly, advancement of a catheter from the right atrium into the pulmonary artery establishes patency between these two structures. The presence of equal systolic pressures in the pulmonary artery and right ventricle would be consistent with a patent right ventricular outflow tract.

MANAGEMENT

Medical versus surgical treatment

The management of Ebstein's malformation requires a choice between nonoperative and operative interventions. The protracted natural history (which is typical of this anomaly), in contrast to the uncertain long-term results of surgical intervention, supports continuation of the policy of postponing surgical intervention until the onset of significant or progressive disability. In a study at the Mayo Clinic,[10,15] adverse prognostic factors included (1) functional class III or IV, (2) moderate to severe cardiomegaly (cardiothoracic ratio >0.65), (3) moderately severe or progressive cyanosis, (4) disability occurring during infancy, (5) paradoxical emboli, (6) right ventricular outflow tract obstruction, and (7) progressive increase in heart size. It seems appropriate, therefore, that the presence of any of these features should lead to careful consideration of operative intervention. In addition, intractable supraventricular tachycardia associated with an accessible accessory AV conduction pathway may require earlier surgical intervention. Because of improved surgical results, progression of symptoms and signs, especially cyanosis and cardiomegaly, is a relative indication for operation.

Surgical technique

The surgical approach to Ebstein's anomaly has evolved over the past 30 years. In the 1950s, systemic-to-pulmonary artery shunts were created to increase pulmonary blood flow. This was not very successful, especially in patients without anatomic obstruction to pulmonary blood flow. Better results were obtained by Glenn et al.[20] with a superior vena cava-to-pulmonary artery connection. In 1958, Hunter and Lillehei[21] tried repositioning the septal and posterior tricuspid valve leaflets, but this had no apparent success.[22] Barnard and Schrire[23] successfully replaced the tricuspid valve with a prosthesis in 1963. Reconstruction of the tricuspid valve was attempted in 1969 by Hardy and Roe.[24] At present, three approaches are available for the surgical repair of Ebstein's anomaly—namely, replacement of the valve[6,25-27] with either a mechanical or a "biological" prosthesis, plastic reconstruction of the valve,[8] or both valve replacement and cardiac reconstruction.[28]

It is important to emphasize that this anomaly includes a wide spectrum of malformations, the unifying characteristic feature being displacement of the tricuspid orifice down into the ventricle to reside at the junction of the inlet

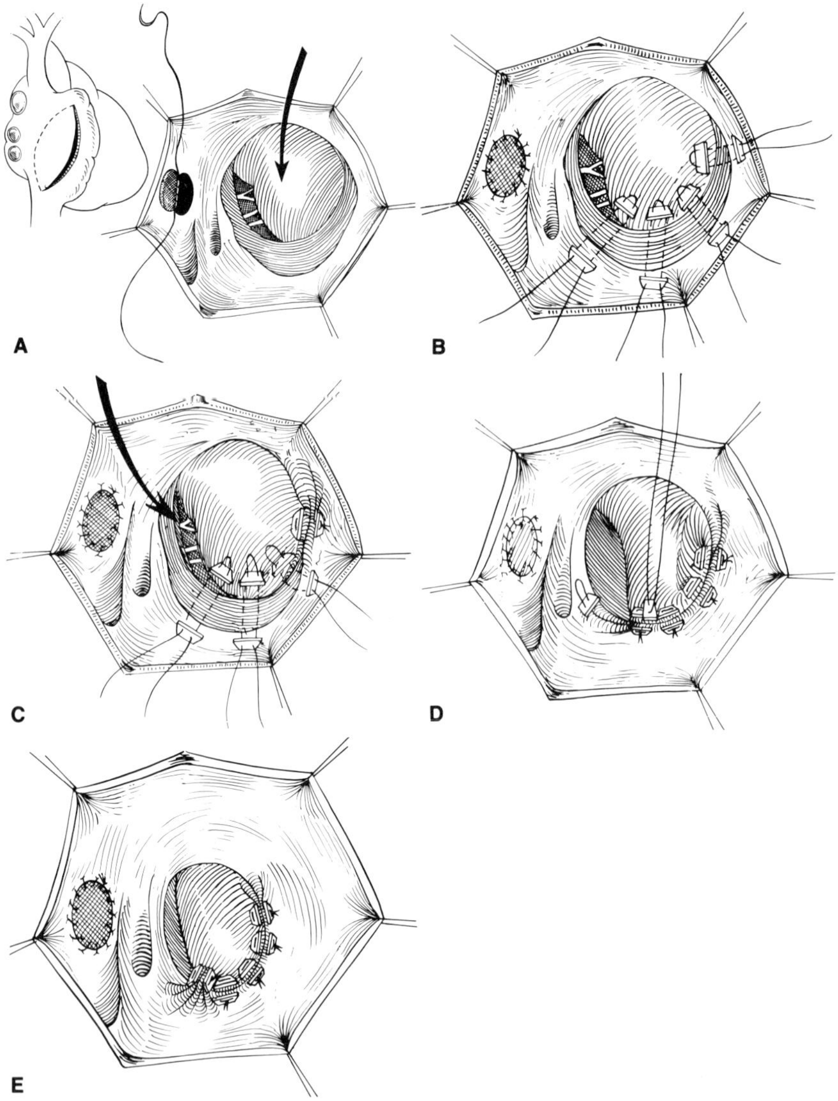

Fig 48-8 Diagram of reconstruction of tricuspid valve. **A,** an incision is made in right atrium, and redundant portion of right atrium is excised. **B,** atrial septal defect is closed. **C,** mattress sutures are placed in the atrialized portion of the right ventricle and the sutures are secured. *Arrow* indicates displaced septal leaflet. **D** and **E,** posterior tricuspid annuloplasty. (Modified from Danielson GK, Maloney JD, Devloo RAE: Surgical repair of Ebstein's anomaly. *Mayo Clin Proc* 54:185-192, 1979. By permission, Mayo Foundation.)

and trabecular ventricular zones of the ventricle.[29] It is the septal and inferior (lateral) leaflets of the tricuspid valve that show ventricular displacement of their annular attachments, whereas the anterior leaflet of the valve is typically enlarged and remains attached at the true annulus. When the enlarged anterior leaflet of the deformed valve remains pliable and mobile, repair of the valve rather than replacement is the technique of choice[8,10,30] (Fig 48-8). In such patients the operative management consists of: (1) electrophysiologic mapping for identification of the specialized conduction tissue, (2) closure of the atrial septal defect or patent foramen ovale, (3) plication of the atrialized portion of the right ventricle, (4) reduction of the size of the tricuspid annulus by a posterior annuloplasty, and (5) correction of associated anomalies, such as relief of pulmonary stenosis or division of accessory conduction pathways.

Early and late results

Danielson achieved excellent results after valve reconstruction.[8,10,30,31] Between 1972 and February 1991, 189 patients with Ebstein's anomaly underwent surgical repair at the Mayo Clinic. They ranged in age from 11 months to

64 years. In 58%, tricuspid valve reconstruction was possible. Hospital mortality was 6.3%. None had permanent complete heart block. All 28 patients who had one or more accessory conduction pathways (Wolff-Parkinson-White syndrome) underwent successful division of the pathway or pathways as part of operative treatment. At follow-up of more than 1 postoperative year, 92.9% of patients were in New York Heart Association class I or II. There were 10 late deaths, most sudden and presumably secondary to cardiac arrhythmia. Four patients (3.6%) required reoperation for valve replacement after valve reconstruction (1 to 14 years later).

REFERENCES

1. Ebstein W: Ueber einen sehr seltenen Fall von Insufficienz der Valvula tricuspidalis, bedingt durch eine angeborene hochgradige Missbildung derselben. *Arch Anat Physiol,* 1866, pp 238-254
2. Keith JD, Rowe RD, Vlad P: *Heart Disease in Infancy and Childhood.* New York, Macmillan Company, 1958, p 34
3. Anderson KR, Zuberbuhler JR, Anderson RH, et al: Morphologic spectrum of Ebstein's anomaly of the heart: a review. *Mayo Clin Proc* 54:174-180, 1979
4. Anderson KR, Lie JT: The right ventricular myocardium in Ebstein's anomaly: a morphometric histopathologic study. *Mayo Clin Proc* 54:181-184, 1979
5. Monibi AA, Neches WH, Lenox CC, et al: Left ventricular anomalies associated with Ebstein's malformations of the tricuspid valve. *Circulation* 57:303-306, 1978
6. Ng R, Somerville J, Ross D: Ebstein's anomaly: late results of surgical correction. *Eur J Cardiol* 9:39-52, 1979
7. Adams JCL, Hudson R: A case of Ebstein's anomaly surviving to the age of 79. *Br Heart J* 18:129-132, 1956
8. Danielson GK, Fuster V: Surgical repair of Ebstein's anomaly. *Ann Surg* 196:499-503, 1982
9. Anderson KR, Danielson GK, McGoon DC, et al: Ebstein's anomaly of the left-sided tricuspid valve: pathological anatomy of the valvular malformation. *Circulation* 58 Suppl 1:87-91, 1978
10. Danielson GK, Driscoll DJ, Mair DD, et al: Operative treatment of Ebstein's anomaly. *J Thorac Cardiovasc Surg* 104:1195-1202, 1992
11. Lev M, Liberthson RR, Joseph RH, et al: The pathologic anatomy of Ebstein's disease. *Arch Pathol* 90:334-343, 1970
12. Danielson GK: Ebstein's anomaly. In *Gibbon's Surgery of the Chest.* Vol. 2. Fourth edition. Edited by DC Sabiston Jr, FC Spencer. Philadelphia, WB Saunders Company, 1983, pp 1204-1210
13. Shiina A, Seward JB, Edwards WD, et al: Two-dimensional echocardiographic spectrum of Ebstein's anomaly: detailed anatomic assessment. *J Am Coll Cardiol* 3:356-370, 1984
14. Benson LN, Child JS, Schwaiger M, et al: Left ventricular geometry and function in adults with Ebstein's anomaly of the tricuspid valve. *Circulation* 75:353-359, 1987
15. Giuliani ER, Fuster V, Brandenburg RO, et al: Ebstein's anomaly: the clinical features and natural history of Ebstein's anomaly of the tricuspid valve. *Mayo Clin Proc* 54:163-173, 1979
16. Shiina A, Seward JB, Tajik AJ, et al: Two-dimensional echocardiographic-surgical correlation in Ebstein's anomaly: preoperative determination of patients requiring tricuspid valve plication vs replacement. *Circulation* 68:534-544, 1983
17. Reeder GS, Currie PJ, Hagler DJ, et al: Use of Doppler techniques (continuous-wave, pulsed-wave, and color flow imaging) in the noninvasive hemodynamic assessment of congenital heart disease. *Mayo Clin Proc* 61:725-744, 1986
18. Leung MP, Baker EJ, Anderson RH, et al: Cineangiographic spectrum of Ebstein's malfunction: its relevance to clinical presentation and outcome. *J Am Coll Cardiol* 11:154-161, 1988
19. Freedom RM, Culham G, Moes F, et al: Differentiation of functional and structural pulmonary atresia: role of aortography. *Am J Cardiol* 41:914-920, 1978
20. Glenn WWL, Browne M, Whittemore R: Circulatory bypass of the right side of the heart: cava-pulmonary artery shunt—indications and results (report of a collected series of 537 cases). In *The Heart and Circulation in the Newborn and Infant.* Edited by DE Cassels. New York, Grune & Stratton, 1966, pp 345-357
21. Hunter SW, Lillehei CW: Ebstein's malformation of the tricuspid valve: study of a case together with suggestion of a new form of surgical therapy. *Dis Chest* 33:297-304, 1958
22. Lillehei CW, Kalke BR, Carlson RG: Evolution of corrective surgery for Ebstein's anomaly. *Circulation* 35 Suppl 1:111-118, 1967
23. Barnard CN, Schrire V: Surgical correction of Ebstein's malformation with prosthetic tricuspid valve. *Surgery* 54:302-308, 1963
24. Hardy KL, Roe BB: Ebstein's anomaly: further experience with definitive repair. *J Thorac Cardiovasc Surg* 58:553-560, 1969
25. Barbero-Marcial M, Verginelli G, Awad M, et al: Surgical treatment of Ebstein's anomaly: early and late results in twenty patients subjected to valve replacement. *J Thorac Cardiovasc Surg* 78:416-422, 1979
26. Bove EL, Kirsh MM: Valve replacement for Ebstein's anomaly of the tricuspid valve. *J Thorac Cardiovasc Surg* 78:229-232, 1979
27. Melo J, Saylam A, Knight R, et al: Long-term results after surgical correction of Ebstein's anomaly: report of two cases. *J Thorac Cardiovasc Surg* 78:233-235, 1979
28. Timmis HH, Hardy JD, Watson DG: The surgical management of Ebstein's anomaly: the combined use of tricuspid valve replacement, atrioventricular plication, and atrioplasty. *J Thorac Cardiovasc Surg* 53:385-391, 1967
29. Zuberbuhler JR, Allwork SP, Anderson RH: The spectrum of Ebstein's anomaly of the tricuspid valve. *J Thorac Cardiovasc Surg* 77:202-211, 1979
30. Danielson GK, Maloney JD, Devloo RAE: Surgical repair of Ebstein's anomaly. *Mayo Clin Proc* 54:185-192, 1979
31. Mair DD, Seward JB, Driscoll DJ, et al: Surgical repair of Ebstein's anomaly: selection of patients and early and late operative results. *Circulation* 72 Suppl 2:70-76, 1985

CHAPTER

49

Tetralogy of Fallot

Carole A. Warnes, M.D., David J. Driscoll, M.D., Valentin Fuster, M.D., and Francisco J. Puga, M.D.

ANATOMIC CONSIDERATIONS

Tetralogy of Fallot consists of a ventricular septal defect, pulmonary stenosis, a rightward shift of the aortic root so that the aorta "overrides" the ventricular septal defect, and right ventricular hypertrophy. Although Etienne-Louis-Arthur Fallot is credited with the classic description of this lesion (1888), Nils Stensen was the first to describe it, in 1671.[1,2]

The ventricular septal defect is located in the posterior portion of the ventricular septum and involves the membranous septum. Typically, it is situated directly beneath the aortic valve.[3] Except in extremely rare cases, the ventricular septal defect is unrestrictive – that is, it allows equalization of right and left ventricular pressures. The bundle of His courses along the posteroinferior margin of the ventricular septal defect.[3] The papillary muscle of the conus is small, displaced, and attached to the inferior edge of the ventricular septal defect. An atrial septal defect is present in approximately 15% of the cases.

Essentially all patients with tetralogy of Fallot have some degree of infundibular narrowing. This is created by the superior displacement of parietal and septal bands and the anterior position of the infundibular septum. Many patients also have pulmonary valvular stenosis, which may be associated with a hypoplastic pulmonary valve annulus and a bicuspid pulmonary valve. In addition, the pulmonary artery may range from normal size to severely hypoplastic (Fig 49-1). One pulmonary artery (usually the left) originates from the aorta rather than from the main pulmonary artery in approximately 3% of cases.[3]

The aortic root and valve annulus typically are enlarged, which, along with the underlying septal defect (lack of supporting tissue inferior to the valve), may contribute to development of aortic insufficiency in some patients. A right aortic arch is present in 25% of patients with tetralogy of Fallot. Hurwitz et al.[4] found important coronary arterial anomalies in 10% of patients with tetralogy of Fallot. Anomalous origin of the left anterior descending coronary artery from the right coronary artery occurred in 3%, and a small left anterior descending coronary artery associated with a relatively large conal branch of the right coronary artery occurred in 7%.

Tetralogy of Fallot is one of the two most common forms of cyanotic congenital heart disease (transposition of the great arteries is the other) and constitutes 10% of all forms of congenital heart disease.[5] The inheritance pattern is multifactorial, with a recurrence risk for siblings of approximately 2.5%.[6] Zellers et al.[7] reported a 1% to 2% occurrence of congenital heart defect in live-born offspring of probands with tetralogy of Fallot.

The embryologic basis of tetralogy of Fallot is similar to that of pulmonary atresia with ventricular septal defect. Unequal division of the conal truncus results in the diminutive right ventricular outflow tract. The ventricular septal defect results from abnormal union of the conal and truncal septal swellings and the muscular ventricular septum.

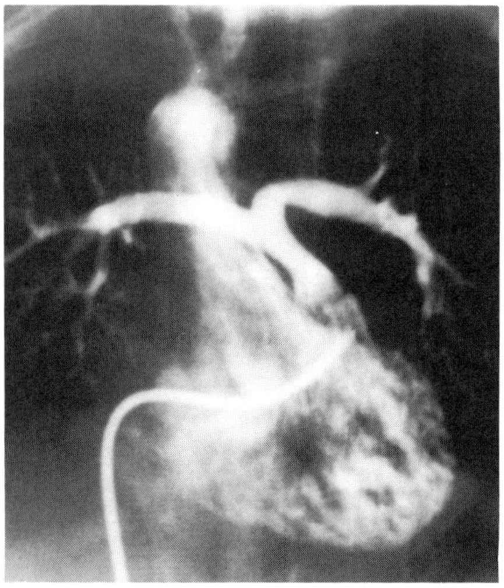

Fig 49-1 Right ventricular angiogram demonstrating anatomy of tetralogy of Fallot. The pulmonary arteries are hypoplastic. The right ventricle is enlarged. The aorta fills with contrast material via the interventricular communication.

PATHOPHYSIOLOGY

The pathophysiology of tetralogy of Fallot is variable, depending on the volume of pulmonary blood flow. This flow is determined by the degree of right ventricular outflow obstruction and the presence and size of the ductus arteriosus or systemic-to-pulmonary artery collateral vessels and surgically created shunts. The majority of patients have decreased pulmonary blood flow and a predominant right-to-left interventricular shunt. Thus, these patients will have cyanosis, erythrocytosis, dyspnea, and fatigue. The degree of cyanosis and polycythemia is proportional to the pulmonary blood flow.

Some patients with relatively mild right ventricular outflow obstruction or significant volume of pulmonary blood flow supplied by a patent ductus arteriosus, systemic-to-pulmonary artery collateral vessels, or surgically created shunt may not have cyanosis. Indeed, occasional patients with tetralogy of Fallot may have increased pulmonary blood flow and signs and symptoms of congestive heart failure. Generally, the degree of right ventricular outflow obstruction increases with age, producing progressively decreasing pulmonary blood flow and increasing cyanosis.

In newborn infants, some pulmonary blood flow is supplied by the patent ductus arteriosus. An abrupt decrease in pulmonary blood flow—and increase in cyanosis and perhaps progressive acidosis—can occur when the ductus arteriosus closes. Thus, it is critical to identify the sources and reliability of pulmonary blood flow in all cyanotic infants so that, if necessary, interventions to increase pulmonary blood flow can be performed before the ductus arteriosus closes.

Cyanotic patients with tetralogy of Fallot have increased risk of stroke from systemic arterial embolism or in situ thrombosis. Long-standing hypoxemia and increased right ventricular pressure may contribute to myocardial fibrosis and decreased ventricular function.

Infants and children can have hypercyanotic ("hypoxemic" or "tet") spells. These consist of agitation, hyperpnea, dyspnea, increased cyanosis, hypoxemia, and acidosis. The spells can progress to unconsciousness, seizures, and death. The mechanism of these spells is poorly understood but certainly involves an abrupt decrease of pulmonary blood flow and increased right-to-left intracardiac shunt. One proposed mechanism has been that spasm of the pulmonary infundibular muscle occurs. However, anything that results in a relative decrease in the ratio of pulmonary to systemic vascular resistance could precipitate such a spell.

HISTORY AND CLINICAL COURSE

Most infants with tetralogy of Fallot are cyanotic at birth. The cyanosis may increase in intensity as the ductus arteriosus closes. If hypoxemia is severe, acidosis and death can result. In a few instances, because of a reasonably normal pulmonary blood flow, cyanosis may not be clinically detectable, and the malformation is not recognized in the newborn. However, in these cases, a murmur is audible early in the first year of life and frequently is detected during a "well baby" examination. As the infant grows, the relative pulmonary blood flow decreases, and cyanosis and erythrocytosis appear or increase in severity. Patients with unrepaired tetralogy of Fallot are at risk for the complications resulting from right-to-left intracardiac shunt and erythrocytosis, which include stroke and brain abscess. The hypercyanotic spells are uncommon before 2 months of age and after childhood. They may be fatal.

Hunter[8] described the squatting that is characteristic of children with tetralogy of Fallot. The children squat to obtain relief from their dyspnea. Presumably, squatting produces kinking of the iliofemoral arteries, resulting in increased systemic vascular resistance which favors increased pulmonary blood flow. Squatting also could produce an increase in mixed venous oxygen concentration by decreasing the return of poorly oxygenated blood from the large muscle masses of the lower extremities.

Survival to adulthood is uncommon without surgery, but several reports have described survival to the fifth and sixth decades. Adults may present with endocarditis affecting the aortic valve or with a cerebrovascular accident. Right ventricular failure does not occur until at least the fifth decade and may be precipitated by aortic regurgitation or atrial arrhythmias.[9]

Physical findings

Most patients with tetralogy of Fallot are cyanotic and have terminal digital clubbing. Infants and children with marked hypoxemia may fail to grow.

Arterial and venous pulsations. The arterial pulses usually are normal. The pulse pressure may be increased if there is significant systemic-to-pulmonary artery collateral circulation or a large patent ductus arteriosus. Unless there is ventricular failure, the jugular venous pulsations are normal.

Precordial palpations. Because of increased right ventricular pressure, the cardiac impulse at the lower left sternal border (the right ventricular impulse) is prominent. The aorta is large and relatively anteriorly placed, so closure of the aortic valve may be palpable at the upper left sternal border. A thrill produced by the turbulent blood flow through the right ventricular outflow tract may be felt at the upper left sternal border.

Auscultation. The first heart sound is normal. Occasionally, an aortic ejection click is audible over the cardiac apex. The second heart sound is increased in intensity (due to the anterior position of the aorta) and usually single, although occasionally a pulmonary component is audible. Continuous murmurs may be present if the ductus arteriosus is patent or there are systemic-to-pulmonary artery communications or surgically created shunts. With marked erythrocytosis, the murmurs may be inaudible. In contrast to isolated pulmonary stenosis, in which the intensity of the murmur is related directly to the severity of the stenosis, in tetralogy of Fallot the murmur becomes less intense as the severity of the stenosis increases. Indeed, during a hypercyanotic spell, the murmur is diminished and may be inaudible. In older patients, aortic insufficiency can occur accompanied by the characteristic murmur.

Electrocardiogram

Right-axis deviation and right ventricular hypertrophy are apparent by electrocardiography. The presence of left-axis deviation should alert the examiner to the possible association of an AV canal malformation and tetralogy of Fallot.

Chest radiograph

Characteristically, the cardiac size is normal and the pulmonary vascular markings are decreased. The apex of the heart is "uptilted" because of right ventricular hypertrophy. Because the right ventricular outflow tract and main pulmonary artery are hypoplastic, the "main pulmonary artery segment" may be absent along the left upper cardiac border. This produces a so-called boot-shaped (coeur en sabot) appearance of the heart. A right aortic arch is apparent in 25% of cases. A discrepancy of pulmonary vascular markings between the right and left lungs should suggest origin of one pulmonary artery from the aorta or stenosis of a branch pulmonary artery.

DIAGNOSTIC PROBLEMS AND INDICATIONS FOR INVASIVE STUDIES

Cardiac catheterization

Right-to-left intracardiac shunting through the ventricular septal defect is apparent by oximetry. The degree of systemic arterial blood oxygen saturation is proportional to the pulmonary blood flow. Right ventricular pressure is equal to left ventricular pressure. Ventriculography will reveal a large ventricular septal defect and pulmonary, subpulmonary, or suprapulmonary valve stenosis (see Fig 49-1). The aortic root is enlarged and located cephalad to the ventricular septal defect. Systemic-to-pulmonary artery collateral vessels or a patent ductus arteriosus can be visualized during ventriculography or aortography. It is important to exclude the rare circumstance of multiple ventricular septal defects. This usually can be established from the lateral projection of the left or right ventriculogram because the ventricular septum is aligned in the sagittal plane in tetralogy of Fallot.

The size and distribution of the pulmonary arteries and sources of blood supply to the pulmonary arteries must be established for planning precise surgical intervention. Delineation of coronary artery anatomy, specifically identification of anomalous origin of the left anterior descending coronary artery from the right coronary artery, is critical to proper surgical management.

With severe right ventricular outflow tract obstruction, placement of the catheter into the pulmonary artery can produce critical obstruction to pulmonary blood flow and result in severe hypoxemia. Thus, systemic arterial blood oxygen saturation should be monitored closely during this maneuver. Particularly in infants and children, cardiac catheterization and angiography can precipitate hypercyanotic spells. The risk of this can be minimized by ensuring adequate hydration during and after cardiac catheterization.

Echocardiography

Two-dimensional echocardiography demonstrates the subaortic ventricular septal defect and an enlarged aorta "overriding" the ventricular septum. These features are also present in truncus arteriosus and pulmonary atresia with ventricular septal defect. The size of the proximal pulmonary arteries can be assessed, but distal features of pulmonary architecture cannot be outlined. Also, it is difficult to exclude multiple ventricular septal defects and coronary abnormalities by echocardiography.

MANAGEMENT

Before repair

During infancy, adequate pulmonary blood flow must be maintained. As the patent ductus arteriosus closes, pulmonary blood flow may become inadequate. When severe hypoxemia develops, the ductus arteriosus can be maintained patent by infusing prostaglandin E_1 while surgical intervention to establish a systemic-to-pulmonary artery anastomosis is being organized. Selection of the optimal anastomosis is controversial, but most surgeons and cardiologists prefer a Blalock-Taussig or a modified Blalock-Taussig anastomosis because it is associated with less distortion of the pulmonary artery than are direct aorticopulmonary anastomoses. However, in small infants the incidence of occlusion is higher with Blalock-Taussig shunts than with direct aorticopulmonary anastomoses.

Because of the presence of erythrocytosis in these growing children, iron deficiency may occur with tetralogy of Fallot, and this should be corrected. It is erroneous to withhold iron treatment for fear of accentuating erythrocytosis. Iron replacement results in increased mean cell hemoglobin concentration and oxygen-carrying capacity. Indeed, hypercyanotic spells may be precipitated by relative anemia and can be eliminated in some instances by iron replacement.

It is critical to recognize and to treat hypercyanotic spells. The treatment of these should be stepwise. Initially, the infant should be cuddled and held in a comfortable but knee-chest position. Oxygen can be administered if the procedure does not increase the child's agitation. If these simple maneuvers are inadequate, morphine (0.01 to 0.1 mg/kg) should be given subcutaneously. These measures usually will terminate the spell. However, if they do not, an intravenous infusion should be started, intravascular volume should be expanded, and sodium bicarbonate should be administered to correct acidosis secondary to hypoxemia. If the spell continues, an infusion of phenylephrine can be given to increase systemic vascular resistance. If this is unsuccessful, propranolol may be given intravenously but should be used with extreme caution and in very small amounts. Rarely, general anesthesia will be necessary to terminate a spell, and occasionally surgical creation of a systemic-to-pulmonary artery anastomosis will be needed.

Timing of operation

There is a tendency to perform primary complete intracardiac repair even in infants. Kirklin et al.[10] demonstrated that this is an acceptable approach if pulmonary artery size is adequate. However, if pulmonary transannular right ventricular outflow patch reconstruction is required to relieve right ventricular hypertension and if the patient's body surface area (BSA) is 0.48 m^2 or less, these authors found it to be safer to perform a two-stage repair; the first stage is designed to increase pulmonary blood flow.

The adult patient with uncorrected tetralogy of Fallot is becoming more and more rare. It is universally accepted that the prognosis for patients who have undergone complete repair is vastly improved over that of patients not operated on or undergoing only surgical palliation. Although there may still be disagreement as to the timing of complete repair – during infancy or at 2 to 4 years of age – there is no disagreement that corrective operation preferably should be accomplished by early childhood rather than being deferred until later. This policy has developed as a result of the poor prognosis of uncorrected or merely palliated tetralogy of Fallot rather than because there is documentation of an increased operative or late risk after correction during adulthood.[11] Recent improvements in surgical management and enhanced myocardial protection[12] as well as palliative balloon dilatation of the pulmonary valve[13,14] are moving the interventional time in tetralogy of Fallot toward infancy or the first year of life.

Surgical technique

The procedure has two basic steps – namely, closure of the ventricular septal defect and relief of the pulmonary stenosis.[10,15-18] The ventricular septal defect is repaired in a manner similar to that used for an isolated ventricular septal defect because attachment of the patch to the rim of the dextrorotated aortic annulus merely shifts the plane in which the patch lies within the heart. Relief of outflow tract obstruction is first attempted by careful pulmonary valvotomy and resection of hypertrophied bundles of muscle of the crista supraventricularis, particularly the parietal band. This can be accomplished by working through the ventriculotomy. The desired objective is to relieve the stenosis, at least to a degree that will give assurance that the right ventricular systolic pressure after repair will be no greater than about 0.65 times the systolic pressure in the left ventricle. This ratio can be estimated by measuring the diameter of the enlarged outflow tract with the help of calibrated sounds. From charts derived from studies of patients with tetralogy[19] it can be anticipated that the postrepair right ventricular-to-left ventricular systolic pressure ratio (RVP/LVP) will be 0.65 or less if the pulmonary arterial outflow tract diameter is at least 13 mm for a patient with a BSA of 1.0 m^2, 15 mm for a BSA of 1.5 m^2, and 18 mm for a BSA of 2.0 m^2. Usually, the residual confinement of the right ventricular outflow tract is located at the pulmonary annulus as well as at the infundibular zone. In such instances, if adequate relief of the outflow tract stenosis (RVP/LVP < 0.65) is not achieved by the above measures, the ventriculotomy must be extended across the pulmonary annulus and onto the pulmonary trunk with excision of the pulmonary valve leaflets (especially if they are rigid or calcified); this

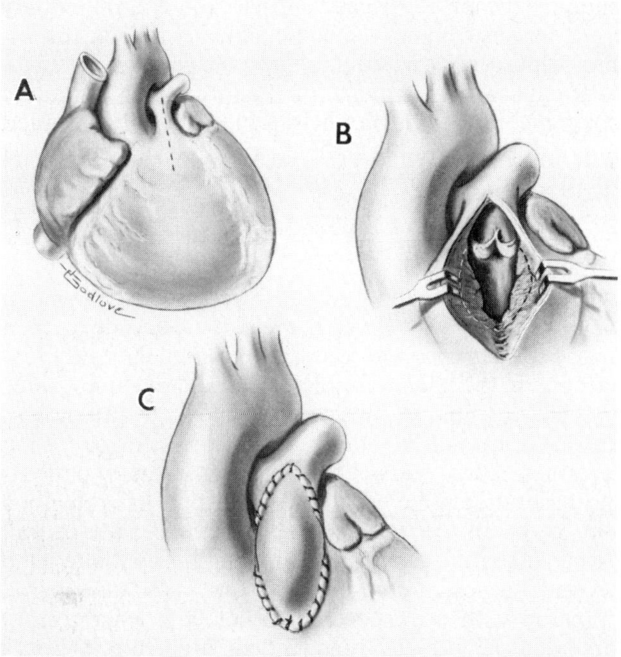

Fig 49-2 Patch graft reconstruction of hypoplastic right ventricular outflow tract and pulmonary trunk. **A,** a longitudinal incision is made along the entire length of the pulmonary trunk, across the pulmonary annulus, and along the hypoplastic portion of the outflow tract. **B,** commissural fusion is relieved and, in some instances, fibrotic or calcified cusps are entirely excised. The hypertrophic margins of the ventriculotomy are thinned by excising their inner portions. **C,** a teardrop-shaped patch of pericardium or synthetic material is sutured to the margins of the incision. The patch is of a size just sufficient to relieve stenosis and achieve a streamlined configuration to the outflow tract. (From Danielson GK: Surgical considerations in congenital heart disease. In *Cardiac and Vascular Diseases.* Vol. 1. Edited by HL Conn Jr, O Horwitz. Philadelphia, Lea & Febiger, 1971, pp 686-746. By permission.)

extended cardiotomy is closed with a teardrop-shaped patch of pericardium or synthetic material (Fig. 49-2). This is called a "transannular patch reconstruction."

Occasionally, the peripheral pulmonary arteries are too small to allow closure of the ventricular septal defect with an acceptably low right ventricular pressure. In these cases, a staged operation is necessary as has been described for pulmonary atresia with ventricular septal defect (see chapter 50) or by creating a systemic-to-pulmonary artery anastomosis.

Surgical repair in the adult is not significantly different from that accomplished in children.

Special surgical considerations are necessary for patients with anomalous origin of the left anterior descending artery from the right coronary artery.[20] It is critical that the anomalous artery be preserved. In such situations it frequently is necessary to interpose an extracardiac conduit between the right ventricle and the pulmonary artery because it may be impossible to relieve the infundibular stenosis without injuring the coronary arteries.

Patients with tetralogy of Fallot should continue bacterial endocarditis prophylaxis indefinitely. Continued long-term evaluation of patients after tetralogy of Fallot repair is warranted.

Results of operation

The results of complete operative repair of tetralogy of Fallot are good.[11,21-23] Even in the earliest decade of open cardiac surgery (prior to 1965), the hospital mortality rate for repair in the adult was only 10%,[10] and the innovations of surgical technique, myocardial protection, and patient care have substantially decreased the risks of operation since those early years. The long-term status of patients who have undergone corrective operation has remained quite good. In the Mayo Clinic experience, the overall 32-year actuarial survival rate among 163 patients who survived surgery between 1955 and 1960 was 86%, compared with an expected rate of 96% in a control population (Fig 49-3). Independent predictors of long-term survival were older age at operation and a higher ratio of right ventricular to left ventricular systolic pressure after surgery. Late sudden death from cardiac causes occurred in 10 of 163 patients during a 32-year period. The 30-year probability of survival without reoperation was 88%; the most common reason for late reoperation was recurrent or residual ventricular septal defect.

Arciniegas et al.[23] reported a combined early and late mortality of 7.7% for 209 patients operated on between 1964 and 1970. There was only one case of surgical complete AV block. Eighty-seven percent of the patients had a good result, 5.1% had a fair result, and 7.6% had a poor result.

Malignant ventricular arrhythmia is now considered the major cause of sudden death after tetralogy repair. Several factors have been associated with an increased incidence of ventricular arrhythmias, including right ventricular hypertension,[22,24] residual ventricular septal defect,[25-27] older age at surgery,[25,28] and duration of cardiopulmonary bypass.[29] Thus, the combination of prolonged right ventricular hypertrophy with fibrosis, together with right ventriculotomy or pulmonary regurgitation, or both, contributes to right ventricular dysfunction and supports the concept that early repair might help prevent the right ventricular "substrate" of the arrhythmia. Since the incidence of ventricular arrhythmias on Holter monitoring ($\geq$ grade 2 of the Lown classification) may be found in approximately 45% of patients at follow-up,[25,28,30,31] it remains difficult to determine which patients are at risk of sudden death. It seems rational, however, to perform periodic Holter monitoring and exercise testing to screen for sustained ventricular tachycardia.

Exercise performance improves after repair of tetralogy of Fallot. Wessel et al.[32] found that males averaged 82% of predicted work performance and females averaged 86%. Similarly, Hannon et al.[33] reported maximum oxygen

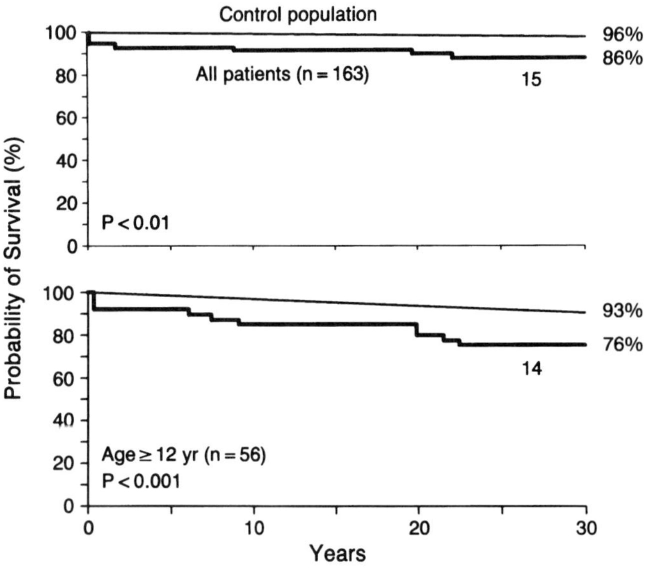

Fig 49-3 Long-term survival of patients who had complete repair of tetralogy of Fallot. **Top,** actuarial survival rate up to 32 years after surgery for 163 patients and the expected survival rate in an age- and sex-matched control population. **Bottom,** actuarial survival rate up to 30 years for patients 12 years old or older at the time of operation and comparison with a control population. Values below the curves are the numbers of patients who were alive and had completed the period of actuarial follow-up. (From Murphy JG, Gersh BJ, Mair DD, et al: Long-term outcome in patients undergoing surgical repair of tetralogy of Fallot. *N Engl J Med* 329:593-599, 1993. By permission of the journal.)

uptake to be 70% of normal for 24 patients 1 to 16 years after repair of tetralogy of Fallot. Some investigators[34-36] have documented an abnormal cardiac output response to exercise, which probably reflects abnormal right ventricular function. There may be an indirect relationship between exercise capacity and age at time of intracardiac repair.[37]

Right ventricular outflow tract reconstruction to relieve pulmonary stenosis frequently produces pulmonary insufficiency. Fortunately, this is well tolerated in most cases. Later, however, it may cause right ventricular dilatation and failure, with secondary tricuspid regurgitation and supraventricular and ventricular arrhythmias. Reoperation to insert a new pulmonary valve (often with tricuspid annuloplasty) can be accomplished with a low operative risk and good hemodynamic results.[38]

Pseudoaneurysm formation of the right ventricular outflow tract patch can occur (Fig 49-4). Rosenthal et al.[39] observed this in 8 of 135 patients who had right ventricular outflow patch reconstruction. Three of these eight patients had peripheral pulmonary stenosis. In general, reoperation is indicated for rapid progressive enlargement of the pseudoaneurysm.

Another late complication after repair of tetralogy of Fallot is aortic valve insufficiency, which may be due to

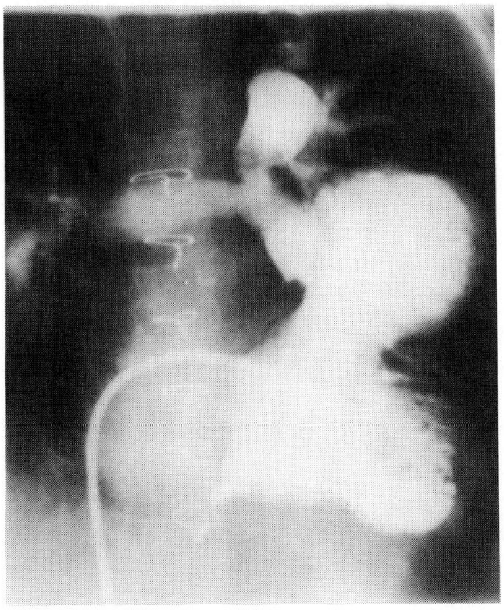

Fig 49-4 Right ventricular angiogram demonstrating aneurysm of right ventricular outflow tract. Also, stenoses are present in right and left proximal arteries.

bacterial endocarditis or direct traumatic injury during earlier repair.[9] However, a unique cause of late aortic insufficiency is central incompetence of the cusps due to annular dilatation. This seems to be a problem particularly in patients who undergo repair late in life; in such patients, the aorta accepts the output of the left and right ventricles for many years, and this volume overload may be worsened by aortopulmonary shunts and systemic collateral blood flow to the lungs. Even after repair, which eliminates right-to-left shunting of blood, the aorta remains large, and inadequate central coaptation of the cusps may lead to severe insufficiency and the need for valve replacement. All adults and adolescents undergoing repair of tetralogy of Fallot or pulmonary atresia with ventricular septal defect should have careful preoperative assessment of aortic valve competence by echocardiography or aortography.

The three principal primary causes for continuing or recurrent disability after correction of tetralogy of Fallot are myocardial structural and fibrotic changes secondary to longstanding preoperative or postoperative (or both) increase in myocardial work demands or to inadequate intraoperative protection of the myocardium; disturbances of cardiac rhythm; and residual hemodynamic defects. Complete diagnostic reevaluation usually is required to identify the cause or causes of disability. Medical supportive therapy is indicated if the myocardium is the primary fault. Antiarrhythmia drugs, electrophysiologic evaluation and testing, and even surgical intervention for ablation of arrhythmogenic loci[40,41] may be required for control of rhythm disturbances.

In patients with significant residual hemodynamic abnormality, reoperation must be strongly considered. In a study of 41 patients who had undergone reoperation after total correction of tetralogy of Fallot,[42] the reoperation involved closure of a residual ventricular septal defect in 28 patients, relief of residual ventricular outflow tract gradient in 11, tricuspid valve replacement, repair, or annuloplasty in 6, aneurysmorrhaphy or excision of an outflow tract aneurysm in 5, insertion of a right ventricle-to-pulmonary outflow tract valve in 3, closure of a patent foramen ovale or atrial septal defect in 3, repair of a residual surgical shunt in 3, mitral valve replacement in 1, and aortic valve repair in 1. The risk of reoperation declined to negligible levels in this study[42] during the last decade of experience. Only one late death occurred after a mean follow-up of 5.3 years. Studies such as this one indicate that even a small shunt through a residual ventricular septal defect may cause clinical deterioration and that this deterioration can be reversed by reoperation, especially when other associated defects, such as pulmonary insufficiency and tricuspid insufficiency, may be present. Thus, reoperation probably should be recommended when an outflow tract gradient greater than 50 mm Hg at rest is present or when an isolated ventricular septal defect allows a pulmonary flow greater than 1.5 times systemic flow.

REFERENCES

1. Bartholini T: *Acta medica & philosophica Hafniensia.* Vol 1. Hafniae, Petri Haubold, 1671 & 1672, pp 202-203
2. Goldstein HI: Discussion. *Bull Hist Med* 22:525-526, 1948
3. Rowe RD: Tetralogy of Fallot. In *Heart Disease in Infancy and Childhood.* Third edition. Edited by JD Keith, RD Rowe, P Vlad. New York, Macmillan Publishing Company, 1978, pp 470-505
4. Hurwitz RA, Smith W, King H, et al: Tetralogy of Fallot with abnormal coronary artery: 1967 to 1977. *J Thorac Cardiovasc Surg* 80:129-134, 1980
5. Report of the New England Regional Infant Cardiac Program. *Pediatrics* 65:388, 1980
6. Nora JJ: Etiologic aspects of heart diseases. In *Moss' Heart Disease in Infants, Children, and Adolescents.* Third edition. Edited by FH Adams, GC Emmanouilides. Baltimore, Williams & Wilkins, 1983, pp 2-10
7. Zellers TM, Driscoll DJ, Michels VV: Prevalence of significant congenital heart defects in children of parents with Fallot's tetralogy. *Am J Cardiol* 65:523-526, 1990
8. Hunter W: Three cases of mal-conformation in the heart. *Medical Observations Inquiries (Lond)* 6:291-309, 1784
9. Capelli H, Ross D, Somerville J: Aortic regurgitation in tetrad of Fallot and pulmonary atresia. *Am J Cardiol* 49:1979-1983, 1982
10. Kirklin JW, Blackstone EH, Pacifico AD, et al: Routine primary repair vs two-stage repair of tetralogy of Fallot. *Circulation* 60:373-386, 1979
11. Fuster V, McGoon DC, Kennedy MA, et al: Long-term evaluation (12 to 22 years) of open heart surgery for tetralogy of Fallot. *Am J Cardiol* 46:635-642, 1980
12. Touati GD, Vouché PR, Amodeo A, et al: Primary repair of tetralogy of Fallot in infancy. *J Thorac Cardiovasc Surg* 99:396-402, 1990
13. Qureshi SA, Kirk CR, Lamb RK, et al: Balloon dilatation of the pulmonary valve in the first year of life in patients with tetralogy of Fallot: a preliminary study. *Br Heart J* 60:232-235, 1988
14. Sreeram N, Saleem M, Jackson M, et al: Results of balloon pulmonary valvuloplasty as a palliative procedure in tetralogy of Fallot. *J Am Coll Cardiol* 18:159-165, 1991
15. Lillehei CW, Cohen M, Warden HE, et al: Direct vision intracardiac surgical correction of the tetralogy of Fallot, pentalogy of Fallot, and pulmonary atresia defects: report of first ten cases. *Ann Surg* 142:418-442, 1955
16. Tucker WY, Turley K, Ullyot DJ, et al: Management of symptomatic tetralogy of Fallot in the first year of life. *J Thorac Cardiovasc Surg* 78:494-499, 1979
17. Puga FJ, DuShane JW, McGoon DC: Treatment of tetralogy of Fallot in children less than 4 years of age. *J Thorac Cardiovasc Surg* 64:247-253, 1972

18. Stephenson LW, Friedman S, Edmunds LH Jr: Staged surgical management of tetralogy of Fallot in infants. *Circulation* 58:837-841, 1978
19. Kirklin JW, Blackstone EH: Editorial on papers by Naito, Wessel, and their colleagues. *J Thorac Cardiovasc Surg* 80:594-599, 1980
20. Humes RA, Driscoll DJ, Danielson GK, et al: Tetralogy of Fallot with anomalous origin of left anterior descending coronary artery: surgical options. *J Thorac Cardiovasc Surg* 94:784-787, 1987
21. Poirier RA, McGoon DC, Danielson GK, et al: Late results after repair of tetralogy of Fallot. *J Thorac Cardiovasc Surg* 73:901-908, 1977
22. Garson A Jr, Nihill MR, McNamara DG, et al: Status of the adult and adolescent after repair of tetralogy of Fallot. *Circulation* 59:1232-1240, 1979
23. Arciniegas E, Farooki ZQ, Hakimi M, et al: Early and late results of total correction of tetralogy of Fallot. *J Thorac Cardiovasc Surg* 80:770 778, 1980
24. Garson A Jr, Gillette PC, Gutgesell HP, et al: Stress-induced ventricular arrhythmia after repair of tetralogy of Fallot. *Am J Cardiol* 46:1006-1012, 1980
25. Kavey R-EW, Blackman MS, Sondheimer HM: Incidence and severity of chronic ventricular dysrhythmias after repair of tetralogy of Fallot. *Am Heart J* 103:342-350, 1982
26. Kavey R-EW, Thomas FD, Byrum CJ, et al: Ventricular arrhythmias and biventricular dysfunction after repair of tetralogy of Fallot. *J Am Coll Cardiol* 4:126-131, 1984
27. Burns RJ, Liu PP, Druck MN, et al: Analysis of adults with and without complex ventricular arrhythmias after repair of tetralogy of Fallot. *J Am Coll Cardiol* 4:226-233, 1984
28. Deanfield JE, McKenna WJ, Presbitero P, et al: Ventricular arrhythmia in unrepaired and repaired tetralogy of Fallot. Relation to age, timing of repair, and haemodynamic status. *Br Heart J* 52:77-81, 1984
29. Vaksmann G, Fournier A, Davignon A, et al: Frequency and prognosis of arrhythmias after operative "correction" of tetralogy of Fallot. *Am J Cardiol* 66:346-349, 1990
30. Chandar JS, Wolff GS, Garson A Jr, et al: Ventricular arrhythmias in postoperative tetralogy of Fallot. *Am J Cardiol* 65:655-661, 1990
31. Kobayashi J, Hirose H, Nakano S, et al: Ambulatory electrocardiographic study of the frequency and cause of ventricular arrhythmia after correction of tetralogy of Fallot. *Am J Cardiol* 54:1310-1313, 1984
32. Wessel HU, Cunningham WJ, Paul MH, et al: Exercise performance in tetralogy of Fallot after intracardiac repair. *J Thorac Cardiovasc Surg* 80:582-593, 1980
33. Hannon JD, Danielson GK, Puga FJ, et al: Cardiorespiratory response to exercise after repair of tetralogy of Fallot. *Tex Heart Institute J* 12:393-400, 1985
34. Rocchini AP: Hemodynamic abnormalities in response to supine exercise in patients after operative correction of tetrad of Fallot after early childhood. *Am J Cardiol* 48:325-330, 1981
35. Bjarke B: Oxygen uptake and cardiac output during submaximal and maximal exercise in adult subjects with totally corrected tetralogy of Fallot. *Acta Med Scand* 197:177-186, 1975
36. Epstein SE, Beiser GD, Goldstein RE, et al: Hemodynamic abnormalities in response to mild and intense upright exercise following operative correction of an atrial septal defect or tetralogy of Fallot. *Circulation* 47:1065-1075, 1973
37. James FW, Kaplan S, Schwartz DC, et al: Response to exercise in patients after total surgical correction of tetralogy of Fallot. *Circulation* 54:671-679, 1976
38. Finck SJ, Puga FJ, Danielson GK: Pulmonary valve insertion during reoperation for tetralogy of Fallot. *Ann Thorac Surg* 45:610-613, 1988
39. Rosenthal A, Gross RE, Pasternac A: Aneurysms of right ventricular outflow patches. *J Thorac Cardiovasc Surg* 63:735-740, 1972
40. Harken AH, Horowitz LN, Josephson ME: Surgical correction of recurrent sustained ventricular tachycardia following complete repair of tetralogy of Fallot. *J Thorac Cardiovasc Surg* 80:779-881, 1980
41. Garson A Jr, Randall DC, Gillette PC, et al: Prevention of sudden death after repair of tetralogy of Fallot: treatment of ventricular arrhythmias. *J Am Coll Cardiol* 6:221-227, 1985
42. Uretzky G, Puga FJ, Danielson GK, et al: Reoperation after correction of tetralogy of Fallot. *Circulation* 66 Suppl 1:202-208, 1982

CHAPTER

50

Pulmonary atresia and ventricular septal defect

Douglas D. Mair, M.D., William D. Edwards, M.D., Paul R. Julsrud, M.D., and Francisco J. Puga, M.D.

ANATOMIC CONSIDERATIONS

Pulmonary valve atresia and ventricular septal defect is considered pathologically to represent the most severe end of the spectrum of tetralogy of Fallot. Although this designation is justifiable and helps to explain the intracardiac pathologic anatomy, delineating the extracardiac pathologic anatomy and planning the most effective management are often much more difficult for this lesion than for tetralogy. The reason is that the anatomy of the pulmonary blood supply in this deformity is extremely variable. Although in the standard variety of tetralogy of Fallot the pulmonary arteries are occasionally hypoplastic and have anomalies of peripheral arborization, they are much more commonly normal in size and distribution. In addition, in tetralogy of Fallot, well-developed systemic-to-pulmonary collateral vessels are very unusual. In pulmonary atresia and ventricular septal defect, however, there are often severe abnormalities in the size and distribution of the pulmonary arteries and well-developed systemic collateral vessels supplying all or portions of the lung parenchyma.

Although a corrective operation was first performed more than 20 years ago for this condition in patients who had well-developed pulmonary arterial trees, severe abnormalities of the pulmonary arteries were then considered inoperable or eligible only for surgical palliation. However, in recent years new surgical techniques have evolved that make eventual surgical correction a possibility for a significant proportion of patients with this lesion, even though often two or more "staged" procedures are necessary to accomplish this ultimate goal.

This entity is characterized anatomically by the absence of any direct continuity between the right ventricle and the pulmonary arteries. The extent of pulmonary artery atresia is quite variable and involves the central pulmonary arteries (that is, those outside the lungs) either proximally or diffusely.[1] At surgery or autopsy, the atretic arterial segment may be recognized as a solid elastic cord in about three-fourths of the cases but remains unidentifiable in the other cases, even after careful and exhaustive dissection. Most commonly, the pulmonary valve and a proximal portion of the pulmonary trunk are involved. Rarely, only the pulmonary valve is imperforate. When the atretic segment involves only the pulmonary valve and the pulmonary trunk, so that the right and left pulmonary arteries maintain free communication with each other, the central pulmonary arteries are considered confluent. In contrast, when the atretic process extends beyond the bifurcation and, therefore, interrupts this continuity, nonconfluence exists. The identification of the presence or absence of pulmonary artery confluence is very important in surgical decision-making for this lesion.[2]

The blood supplied to the lungs is derived entirely from the systemic arterial circulation.[3-7] These sources are the ductus arteriosus, systemic-to-pulmonary collateral arteries, and plexuses of bronchial or pleural arteries. On rare occasions, a coronary artery-to-pulmonary artery fistula is the source of pulmonary blood supply (Fig 50-1). Ductal and collateral sources may coexist in the same patient but only very rarely coexist in the same lung.[1] A single systemic arterial source to a lung is termed a "unifocal blood supply," whereas multiple channels constitute a multifocal blood supply.

The caliber of the central pulmonary arteries varies considerably and appears to be related directly to the amount of blood flow and indirectly to the anatomic sources of blood supply.[1] When the ductus or collateral arteries anastomose proximally to the central pulmonary arteries or their lobar branches, the central vessels may be only mildly hypoplastic or even normal in size. In contrast, when multiple collateral arteries are anastomosed more distally, at segmental or subsegmental levels, the central pulmonary arteries tend to be quite hypoplastic. Furthermore, stenoses of the systemic arterial channels, either congenital or acquired, are frequently observed and are generally associated with appreciable hypoplasia of the central pulmonary arteries because of diminished blood flow.[1,7]

The various patterns of intrapulmonary arterial distribution may be quite complex; they appear to be determined primarily by the types of systemic blood supply.[1,7] When a ductus supplies confluent central pulmonary

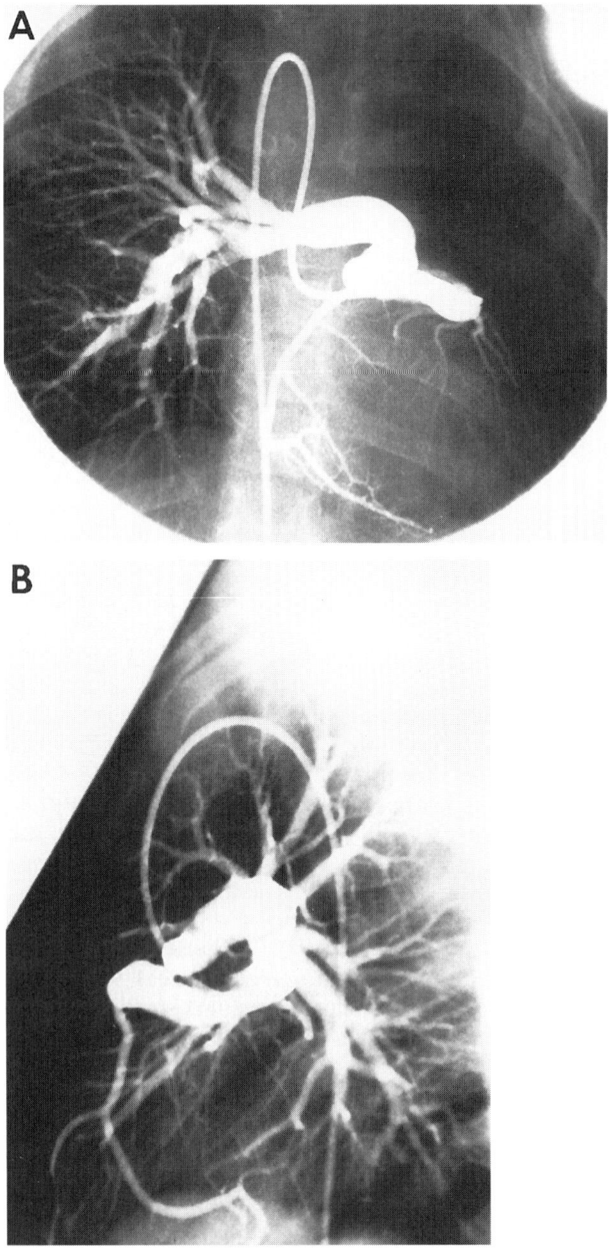

Fig 50-1 Fistula from left coronary artery to right pulmonary artery. **A**, systemic collateral arteries arising from the descending aorta supply the left pulmonary artery. **B**, in lateral view, note the aneurysmal dilatation of the proximal left coronary artery and the stenosis at its communication with the right pulmonary artery.

arteries, the intrapulmonary arteries of both lungs are normal. However, when nonconfluent central pulmonary arteries are present, the homolateral lung has a unifocal blood supply and a normal arterial distribution, but the contralateral lung usually has a multifocal blood supply from several collateral arteries and a fragmented intrapulmonary arterial distribution (arborization abnormality).[1] When both lungs are supplied by multiple collateral channels, intrapulmonary arborization abnormalities are the rule and the ductus is congenitally absent.

The ductus arteriosus, when present, is usually a unilateral structure and is associated with confluent pulmonary arteries in more than 80% of cases.[1] Rarely, bilateral ducti may occur with nonconfluent pulmonary arteries. Unlike collateral arteries, the ductus does not branch before joining the central pulmonary arteries and tends to be less tortuous than collaterals. Since the ductus, when present, is widely patent during fetal life, the pulmonary arteries are normal in size at the time of birth. However, normal postnatal ductal narrowing usually occurs and produces distal stenoses in 35% to 50% of the cases and a nonpatent ligamentum arteriosum in many of the remainder.[1] As a result, blood flow to the lungs is diminished, and relative hypoplasia of the pulmonary arteries becomes progressively more severe as the child grows.

Collateral arteries, when present, arise most commonly from the descending thoracic aorta, less commonly from the subclavian arteries, and rarely from the abdominal aorta or its branches. Their number and diameter may vary greatly. Stenoses are present in nearly 60% of collateral arteries and tend to occur near the aortic or intrapulmonary anastomoses; they may be discrete or segmental.[1] Anastomoses between the central pulmonary arteries (or their branches) and the collateral arteries are observed in about 40% of subjects and may occur at the hilum or within the lung. In the remaining 60%, the collateral arteries enter the pulmonary hilum, travel with the bronchi as pulmonary arteries, and supply a variable number of bronchopulmonary segments. Although the central pulmonary arteries are confluent in about two-thirds of the cases, they usually supply only a portion of each lung, owing to the coexistence of multiple collateral arteries and arborization abnormalities.[1]

Small arterial plexuses that follow the bronchi or spread over the pleural surfaces may be observed angiocardiographically in more than one-half of the patients. They may arise from the aorta and its thoracic branches or from the systemic collateral arteries. It is thought that these vessels enlarge and proliferate postnatally in response to regional reduction in pulmonary blood flow.

The ductus arteriosus is a precarious sole source of pulmonary blood supply,[5] and its tendency to close necessitates a surgical shunt in early infancy in many cases. Collateral arteries appear to be a more stable source of pulmonary blood flow, presumably because of their multiple numbers. However, stenosis of collaterals may develop progressively, so that these vessels become inadequate sources of pulmonary blood flow as the patient grows. Furthermore, because of hyperperfusion of some bronchopulmonary segments and hypoperfusion of others in the same patient, the pulmonary vascular bed has exhibited a variety of histopathologic lesions, ranging from hypertensive pulmonary vascular disease to stasis thrombosis.[1]

As in tetralogy of Fallot, the ventricular septal defect may be membranous or infundibular. Since it is also a malalignment defect that is roofed by the overriding aorta, it tends to be larger than isolated membranous or infundibular defects. Rarely, the ventricular septal defect may be obstructed by accessory tricuspid valvular tissue.[8]

In most cases, the origin and distribution of the coronary arteries are normal, although the conus artery tends to be quite prominent. Reported anomalies include higher than normal origin of the coronary ostia, the previously mentioned coronary artery-to-pulmonary artery fistula, and transposition patterns in which the right coronary artery arises from the left anterior aortic sinus and travels across the right ventricular infundibulum.[9]

The conduction system in patients with pulmonary atresia and ventricular septal defect tends to be normal. An important surgical consideration is the fact that the bundle of His is closely related to the rim of membranous ventricular septal defects but is relatively remote from the border of infundibular defects.[10]

Pulmonary atresia with ventricular septal defect may be associated with other anomalies, including persistent left superior vena cava to the coronary sinus, partial or total anomalous pulmonary venous connection, tricuspid stenosis or atresia, complete atrioventricular canal, complete or corrected transposition of the great arteries, dextrocardia, and the asplenia and polysplenia syndromes.[9]

PATHOPHYSIOLOGY

The natural history and pathophysiology of pulmonary atresia and ventricular septal defect are variable, depending primarily on the source and adequacy of the pulmonary blood supply. Infants in whom a patent ductus arteriosus is the primary source of pulmonary blood flow may become critically hypoxemic in the first days of life as the ductus begins to close and will succumb within a short time if ductal patency is not maintained with the use of prostaglandin E_2 or if a surgical shunt is not established to provide an alternative source of pulmonary blood supply. In patients whose pulmonary blood supply is primarily achieved through systemic-to-pulmonary artery collaterals, the natural history can vary greatly, because it depends on the adequacy of pulmonary blood supply via these channels. On rare occasions, such patients during infancy may have excessive pulmonary blood flow through these collateral vessels and exhibit the manifestations of congestive heart failure, even during the neonatal period. A rare patient may require banding of one or more of these collateral vessels to decrease the amount of pulmonary blood flow and control congestive heart failure. More commonly, however, the pulmonary blood supply is not excessive and the patients gradually become cyanotic and polycythemic as the pulmonary blood supply via these collateral vessels becomes inadequate as the patient grows. These patients often need palliative surgery during early childhood to increase pulmonary blood flow and to encourage growth of the pulmonary arteries, which are frequently hypoplastic. At this institution, however, we have seen patients who have reached adulthood without having had palliative surgery, including several who have lived beyond 40 years of age strictly by virtue of pulmonary blood supply achieved by the systemic-to-pulmonary artery collateral vessels.

HISTORY AND CLINICAL COURSE

The diagnosis of pulmonary atresia and ventricular septal defect usually is made during early infancy, although on occasion the patient with large pulmonary blood flow who is cyanotic may escape detection during the first few months of life and occasionally even live several years before an abnormality is suspected. Although early palliative surgery is not necessary in all infants with this condition, most patients beyond infancy referred to the Mayo Clinic have had a palliative surgical procedure performed in an attempt to maintain adequate pulmonary blood flow and, in some instances, to encourage growth of hypoplastic pulmonary arteries. Both palliated and nonpalliated patients with this condition tend to become more cyanotic and polycythemic as growth occurs and outstrips their pulmonary blood supply, which remains stable or decreases as their systemic-to-collateral or surgically created shunts become stenotic. Such patients exhibit increasing cyanosis, clubbing of the fingernails and toenails, and decreased exercise tolerance. Because they have a right-to-left shunt and are polycythemic, they are at risk of thromboembolic complications, including stroke and brain abscess. These patients usually have good myocardial function during childhood, but if the anomaly is not corrected, myocardial failure may develop in adolescence or early adulthood as a result of chronic arterial hypoxemia and, in some instances, volume overload on the left ventricle.

Physical findings

Cyanosis, which may be profound, is usually present in the early neonatal period in these patients, with the exception of the uncommon patient with a large patent ductus arteriosus or well-developed systemic-to-pulmonary collaterals. Cyanosis may be mild immediately after birth and increases in severity during the first several days of extrauterine life as the ductus begins to close. It is not uncommon for the degree of cyanosis and the arterial oxygen tension, as measured by periodic blood gas determinations, to fluctuate considerably over the first several days as the ductus arteriosus constricts and relaxes. Once the neonatal period is past, the degree of cyanosis in such patients usually increases gradually as the patient's growth outstrips the pulmonary blood flow available through the patent ductus arteriosus, systemic-to-pulmonary collaterals, surgically created systemic-to-pulmonary artery shunts, or established right ventricular-to-pulmonary artery continuity.

Growth and development in such patients are usually delayed, although if pulmonary blood flow is adequate and systemic hypoxemia only mild, this may not be the case. Because heart failure secondary to excessive pulmonary blood flow is uncommon in these patients, growth failure on this basis is infrequently seen.

Peripheral pulses and blood pressure usually are normal in the neonatal period, even in patients with a patent ductus arteriosus, because the runoff into the lungs is not excessive during the first few weeks. In clearly cyanotic patients, the pulses remain normal. However, in patients beyond the neonatal period in whom pulmonary blood flow through a patent ductus arteriosus, collateral vessels, and surgically created shunts is substantial, the pulses are accentuated, the pulse pressure is widened, and only minimal cyanosis may be present. Signs of heart failure, such as hepatomegaly and venous distention, are rare in these patients.

The cardiac impulse is usually most prominent at the lower left sternal border and is secondary to the "lift" caused by the enlarged right ventricle. A systolic thrill can sometimes be felt along the lower left sternal border.

Auscultation reveals a normal first heart sound and a single second sound. A systolic murmur is frequently audible along the lower left sternal border but is usually not more than grade 3/6 in intensity. Because the right ventricular outflow tract is atretic, there is no separate loud systolic ejection murmur at the upper left sternal border. If a patent ductus arteriosus is present or a surgical shunt has been created, a continuous murmur is usually heard over the upper left chest after the first 4 to 6 weeks of life. If systemic-to-pulmonary collateral vessels are present, continuous murmurs are also heard, often most prominently over the back, because these vessels usually originate from the descending aorta.

Electrocardiogram

The electrocardiographic findings in this condition are similar to those in tetralogy of Fallot. Right ventricular hypertrophy and right axis deviation of the frontal QRS axis are the rule. In patients with increased pulmonary blood flow, a small subgroup, combined ventricular hypertrophy and left atrial enlargement may be found. The electrocardiogram often helps differentiate this condition from pulmonary atresia with intact ventricular septum, in which right ventricular hypoplasia is the rule and in which diminutive anteriorly directed QRS forces are seen and left ventricular preponderance is in evidence.

Chest radiograph

In the posteroanterior chest radiograph of patients with pulmonary atresia and ventricular septal defect, the heart frequently has a characteristic appearance likened to the shape of a boot (that is, coeur en sabot). This x-ray finding is due to levorotation of the heart, which produces a prominent left upturned cardiac apex secondary to right ventricular hypertrophy. There is also a concavity in the region of the main pulmonary artery due to the underdevelopment of the subpulmonary infundibulum. The frequency of a right-sided aortic arch is greater in patients with pulmonary atresia and ventricular septal defect (about 50%) than in those with tetralogy of Fallot (only 20% to 25%).[4] The pulmonary vascular markings usually have a heterogeneous reticular appearance that does not conform to the usual arborization pattern of pulmonary vessels. This appearance is due to the collateral arteries from the systemic circulation, which are frequently quite large and supply blood flow to the pulmonary arteries. In patients with small or stenotic collateral vessels, the lung fields may exhibit greatly diminished vascular markings. In the uncommon patient with a large patent ductus arteriosus and normally developed central pulmonary artery, a chest radiograph may show enlarged central pulmonary arteries with increased peripheral vascularity.

Echocardiography

Parasternal long-axis scans demonstrate the classic intracardiac anatomy of pulmonary atresia with ventricular septal defect. In this view, a large subaortic ventricular septal defect is seen with various degrees of aortic override. The parasternal short-axis scan demonstrates that the right ventricular outflow tract ends blindly. However, a more posterior segment of the main pulmonary artery, not in continuity with the right ventricle, may be demonstrated. The short-axis scan may also help to delineate coronary artery anomalies sometimes seen in this condition or the occasional coronary artery-to-pulmonary artery fistula.

Suprasternal notch scans are particularly important for assessment of aortic arch anatomy, brachiocephalic branching, and the presence and size of the central pulmonary arteries (Fig 50-2). Long-axis scans from the suprasternal notch demonstrate the side of the aortic arch and upper descending aortic collaterals if they are present. The suprasternal notch short-axis scan demonstrates the proximal right and main pulmonary arteries (see Fig 50-2). Precise measurements of right pulmonary artery size from this scan are possible for assessing adequacy for surgical repair or palliative shunting. This view also demonstrates the proximal right pulmonary artery in the patient with a previous Waterston shunt and enables assessment of any distortion or hypoplasia of the proximal right pulmonary artery secondary to this operation. With transducer angulation to the left and counterclockwise, the main and proximal left pulmonary arteries may be demonstrated. Unfortunately, the more distal aspects of the right and left pulmonary artery trees are not demonstrable echocardiographically, and angiocardiography is necessary to visualize these vessels. Blalock-Taussig anastomoses often may not be visualized beyond their proximal course from the subclavian artery. However,

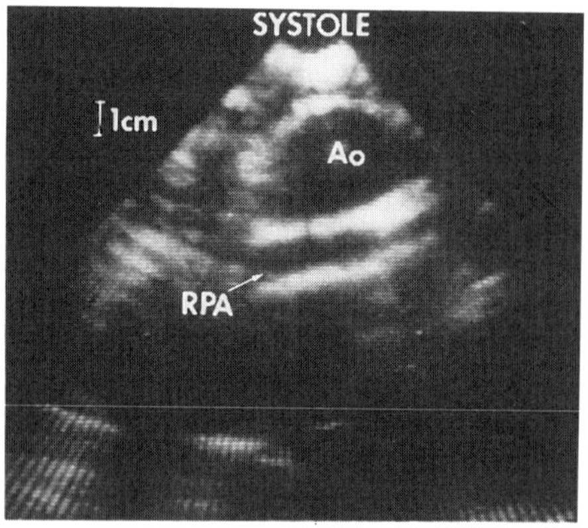

Fig 50-2 Suprasternal notch short-axis scan in patient with pulmonary atresia, ventricular septal defect, and a prior Waterston shunt. Note hypoplasia of right pulmonary artery (*RPA*). *Ao*, aorta.

continuous-wave Doppler interrogation may allow some assessment of the flow pattern (continuous or systolic only) and some prediction of the gradient through the shunt site. Continuous-flow velocities greater than 4 m/sec are usually associated with normal pulmonary artery pressure.

DIAGNOSTIC PROBLEMS AND INDICATIONS FOR INVASIVE STUDIES

Differential diagnosis

Differential diagnosis in these patients depends on the adequacy of their pulmonary blood supply and the resultant degree of cyanosis manifested. In the very cyanotic newborn with this condition, the differential diagnosis includes severe tetralogy of Fallot, transposition of the great arteries, tricuspid atresia, double-outlet right ventricle or single ventricle with severe pulmonary stenosis or pulmonary atresia, and total anomalous pulmonary venous connection with pulmonary venous obstruction. In the less common patient with pulmonary atresia and ventricular septal defect in whom the pulmonary blood supply is normal or increased, the differential diagnosis includes lesions in which cyanosis is minimal and evidence of heart failure may be present. Such lesions include ventricular septal defect, large isolated patent ductus arteriosus, double-outlet right ventricle or single ventricle without significant pulmonary stenosis, persistent truncus arteriosus, and total anomalous pulmonary venous connection without pulmonary venous obstruction. The physical examination often gives important clues to the correct diagnosis, and when it is complemented with an electrocardiogram and chest radiograph, an accurate clinical diagnosis can often be made. The advent of echocardiography has provided a noninvasive means by which an accurate primary diagnosis can be made, although, as noted above, angiocardiography is necessary to delineate all details of pulmonary blood supply.

Cardiac catheterization

Although the diagnosis in patients with pulmonary atresia and ventricular septal defect can be made echocardiographically and some palliative shunting procedures performed on this basis, cardiac catheterization and angiography are mandatory before patients can be considered for definitive operation. Angiography is necessary to delineate the presence, size, and distribution of the two pulmonary arteries and to ascertain the extent of collateral blood supply to the lungs, information that is critical in surgical decision-making. Venous catheterization reveals normal right atrial pressure unless tricuspid incompetence is present and no step-up of oxygenation at the atrial level unless an associated atrial septal defect is present. When the catheter enters the right ventricle, pressures at systemic levels are measured because of the presence of a large ventricular septal defect. With the right ventricular outflow tract atretic, the catheter will not enter the pulmonary arteries from the right ventricle, but it can easily be manipulated from the right ventricle through the ventricular septal defect into the ascending aorta. Aortic pressure is normal if the pulmonary blood flow is normal or reduced, but a widened pulse pressure may be present if there is a large runoff into the lungs through a patent ductus arteriosus, collateral vessels, or a previously constructed shunt. Systemic arterial desaturation is present, the degree depending on the adequacy of pulmonary blood flow.

In pulmonary atresia and ventricular septal defect, the two pulmonary arteries are under low pressure and the pulmonary resistance is normal in most patients. In a few instances, however, patients with a large patent ductus arteriosus, a large communication between a systemic collateral vessel and the pulmonary arteries, a large fistula connecting the coronary artery to the pulmonary arteries, or a shunt anastomosis that has become too large (particularly common in Waterston and Potts shunts) have increased pressure in the pulmonary arteries, and if this condition has been present for some time, they are at risk for development of hypertensive pulmonary vascular obstructive disease. In such instances, it is usually easy to enter the two pulmonary arteries through the large communication present, measure the pressure, and determine pulmonary flow by the Fick principle. With this information, pulmonary arteriolar resistance can be calculated for insight into the degree of hypertensive vascular disease present.

To begin the angiographic evaluation of the patient with this lesion, we have found it preferable to make an injection in the left ventricular cavity while the patient is positioned to achieve a 70° left anterior oblique view combined with 20° of cranial angulation. The resulting angiocardiographic projection displays the middle portion and most of the upper intraventricular septum tangentially. The left ventricular injection in this position demonstrates the superiorly located, malaligned ventricular septal defect characteristic of this lesion while excluding additional muscular septal defects. An injection into the aortic root with the patient in the same position demonstrates the coronary artery anatomy. Of surgical importance is the origin of the left anterior descending coronary artery from the right coronary artery, an anomaly that occurs in 5% to 10% of these patients.[11] If the surgeon is not aware that the left anterior descending coronary artery originates from the right coronary artery and crosses the right ventricular outflow tract, it may be transected at the time of the right ventriculotomy, with disastrous results. It is particularly important to define coronary anatomy preoperatively if a previous surgical procedure within the pericardial sac could have resulted in the formation of epicardial adhesions that would obscure the coronary anatomy from the surgeon's view.

Angiographic delineation of the anatomy of the pulmonary blood supply is of critical importance in the proper management of these patients. Although it may be done by cineangiography, a large-film radiographic format with use of biplane serial film angiocardiography is advantageous in this situation because it provides the large field of view required to visualize both lung fields simultaneously and also makes possible photographic subtraction techniques that have proved useful in demonstrating the anatomy.[12]

Determining whether there is a confluence of the proximal right and left pulmonary arteries is of paramount importance. In addition, the angiographer must accomplish a detailed analysis of the systemic arterial blood supply to the pulmonary arterial tree, including identification of the degree of communication among the various vascular pathways. If a pulmonary artery confluence is present, systemic-to-pulmonary collateral vessels may communicate directly with it or connect to it indirectly by another branch of the collateral artery. In addition, systemic collaterals may not communicate with central pulmonary arteries but instead terminate by connecting with peripheral pulmonary artery branches.[1]

Frequently, an upper descending aortogram is obtained first to demonstrate the number and location of the systemic-to-pulmonary artery collateral vessels (Fig 50-3,A). Selective injection in these collateral vessels is then performed to delineate the extent of pulmonary arterial tree supplied by each collateral vessel and determine what type of pulmonary artery connection is present (Fig 50-3,B). During the process of assessing the adequacy of the pulmonary arterial tree, both the central and the peripheral pulmonary arteries must be well demonstrated. This demonstration allows detection of discrete stenoses or tubular hypoplasia involving the pulmonary arteries as well as the degree to which the central and peripheral pulmonary arteries communicate. Both the size and the peripheral distribution of the pulmonary arteries are important in surgical decision-making for these patients.

If the initial aortogram does not identify a pulmonary artery confluence and selective injection of the significant systemic-to-pulmonary artery collaterals also fails to identify such a confluence, a pulmonary vein wedge injection is frequently helpful in identifying existing hypoplastic central pulmonary arteries (Fig 50-4). In pulmonary venous wedge angiography, an end-hole catheter is advanced into a pulmonary vein to a wedge position. A transseptal approach may be required if the atrial septum is intact and a patent foramen ovale is not present.

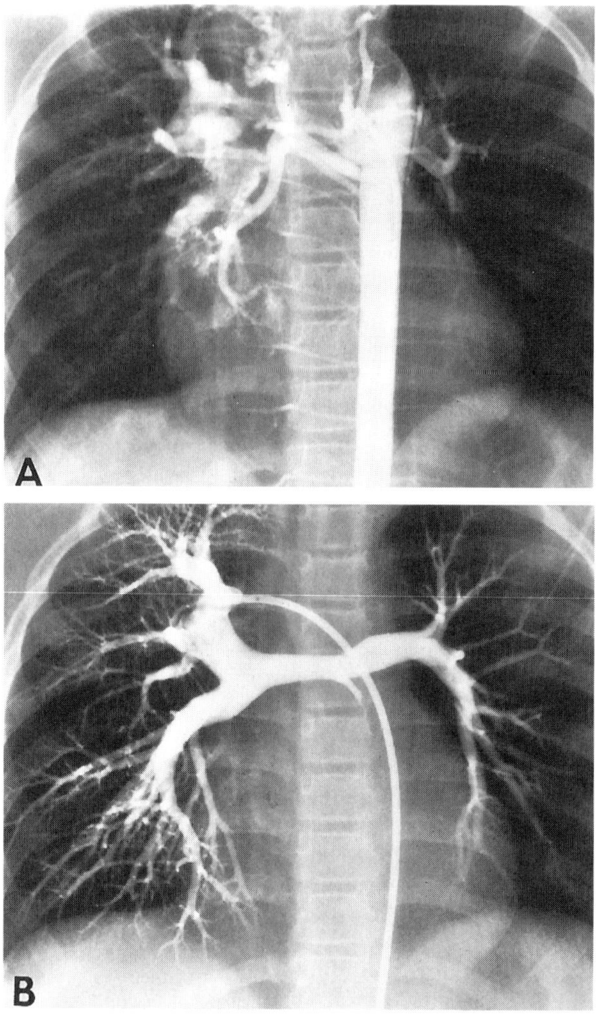

Fig 50-3 **A**, descending aortogram shows multiple systemic collateral vessels, but confluent pulmonary arteries are not seen. **B**, selective injection of a systemic collateral vessel in the same patient demonstrates a well-developed pulmonary artery confluence. (From Davis GD, Fulton RE, Ritter DG, et al: Congenital pulmonary atresia with ventricular septal defect: angiographic and surgical correlates. *Radiology* 128:133-144, 1978. By permission of Radiological Society of North America.)

MANAGEMENT

Although medical treatment with digitalis and diuretics may be indicated in the occasional patient with this lesion who is in heart failure and although phlebotomy may relieve the side effects of extreme polycythemia in patients with severe hypoxemia, the treatment of this condition is essentially surgical. In patients with this deformity, the anatomy of pulmonary blood flow is complex and different in every case; often, therefore, determining the best surgical course to follow is not easy. A number of patients have two pulmonary arteries that are confluent and of sufficient size and distribution to permit complete repair, even during early infancy, which consists of establishing continuity between the right ventricle and the pulmonary artery and closing the ventricular septal defect. Many patients, however, have hypoplasia or a limited distribution of the two pulmonary arteries, so that palliative surgery is required before correction can be attempted as a second- or third-stage procedure.[13] Palliation may involve establishing continuity between the right ventricle and the pulmonary artery while leaving the ventricular septal defect open in an attempt to increase pulmonary blood flow and pulmonary artery size.[14] In some cases, shunts between the aorta and the pulmonary artery are used to achieve the same goal, although in recent years the more widely used approach in this institution has been establishment of right ventricle-to-pulmonary artery continuity. Unifocalization of segments not in continuity with the two confluent pulmonary arteries in an attempt to establish sufficient parenchymal segmental distribution to permit later definitive repair has also been done at this institution.[2,15]

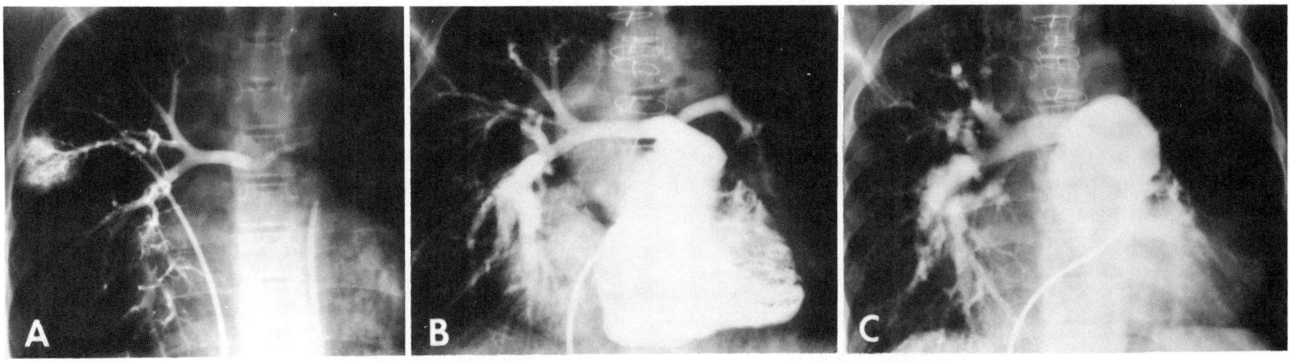

Fig 50-4 **A**, pulmonary vein wedge injection demonstrates a hypoplastic pulmonary artery confluence. **B**, same patient shortly after establishment of a right ventricular-to-pulmonary artery connection. **C**, 1 year later, after complete repair. Note pulmonary artery enlargement.

Experience here in more than 200 patients has established that 90% are candidates for surgical help and that approximately 75% of these eventually become candidates for definitive correction, although some may need several operations in a staged approach.[2]

In a number of patients, severe central hypoplasia of the pulmonary arteries precludes complete repair because an intolerably high right ventricular pressure would result at the end of repair. When the central pulmonary arterial areas, as measured radiographically, appear to be less than 50% of normal, single-stage complete reconstruction of the anomaly is contraindicated. Under these circumstances, a preliminary operation designed to promote enlargement of the pulmonary arteries is indicated.[13,14] Although establishment of extracardiac systemic-to-pulmonary artery shunts has been shown to promote enlargement of the pulmonary arteries, anastomosis to these diminutive arteries is often accompanied by severe distortion, scarring, and interruption of the pulmonary arterial confluence, with resulting inadequate growth of one or both branches.

We prefer to establish continuity between the right ventricle and the hypoplastic pulmonary arterial confluence by interposition of a tube graft. This procedure can be accomplished under extracorpeal circulation or by use of a "closed heart" technique that appears to minimize the magnitude of this preliminary step.[14] The procedure results in acceptable palliation of cyanotic infants and in reliable and rapid enlargement of the central pulmonary arteries, so that about 50% of patients thus treated and followed up for 2 years become candidates for complete repair of the anomaly (see Fig 50-4). In addition to achieving palliation, the procedure provides direct access to pulmonary arteriography, which allows precise delineation of the peripheral arborization of these vessels and the nature of the arterial perfusion of each pulmonary arterial segment.

Patients with pulmonary atresia, ventricular septal defect, and hypoplastic confluent pulmonary arteries usually have abnormalities of peripheral pulmonary artery arborization, with multiple systemic collateral arteries supplying those segments of lung parenchyma not reached by the central pulmonary arteries.[1,7] These abnormal sources of pulmonary arterial flow must be thoroughly mapped before surgery so that a proper sequence of treatment can be planned.[16] Conditions for complete repair that must be met in patients subjected previously to right ventricular outflow reconstruction are several. They include central pulmonary arterial area greater than 50% of normal, predominant left-to-right intracardiac shunt, the equivalent of one whole lung in the number of pulmonary arterial segments supplied by the central pulmonary artery confluence, and, when present, repairable flow-constricting stenotic lesions to the pulmonary arterial outflow. In a series of patients at this institution who met these criteria and submitted to complete repair of the anomaly, the mean ratio of right ventricular-to-left ventricular peak systolic pressure after repair was 0.66, indicating an adequate pulmonary arterial bed.[13]

Inadequate peripheral arborization of the central pulmonary arteries precludes complete repair in a significant proportion of these patients unless unifocalization procedures are carried out to bring more pulmonary segments into continuity with the central pulmonary artery confluence.[15] In these patients, a substantial number of pulmonary arterial segments are supplied not by the confluence but through systemic collateral arteries arising from the descending aorta or the brachiocephalic arteries. In the planning of unifocalization procedures, a careful angiographic and hemodynamic study of the systemic collateral arteries and their draining intrapulmonary arterial branches is mandatory.[16] Selection criteria for unifocalization include pulmonary arterial segments supplied by discrete systemic collateral arteries showing evidence of stenotic lesions that have protected their peripheral pulmonary arterioles from the consequences of persistent exposure to increased pressure. The unifocalization procedure must bypass the systemic collateral portion that is subjected to progressive intimal hyperplasia. These procedures are usually performed through lateral thoracotomies, and, when possible, anastomosis of the unifocalized pulmonary arterial segment to the central pulmonary arteries is achieved directly.[15] Unfortunately, anatomic constraints at times have forced use of prosthetic materials for reconstruction of lobar confluency. At present, a small number of patients treated in this fashion have reached an anatomic and hemodynamic condition permitting successful completion of the repair with acceptable postrepair ratios of right ventricular-to-left ventricular peak systolic pressure[15] (Fig 50-5).

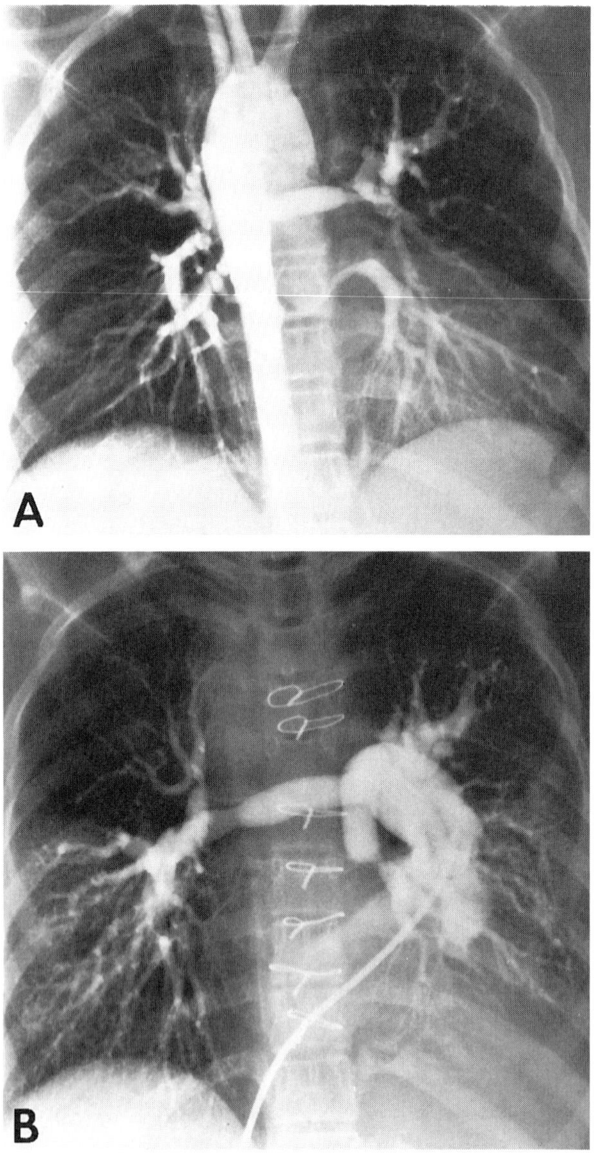

Fig 50-5 **A**, upper descending aortogram demonstrates nonconfluent pulmonary arteries supplied by multiple systemic collateral vessels. **B**, same patient after bilateral unifocalization procedures and complete repair. (From Puga FJ, Leoni FE, Julsrud PR, et al: Complete repair of pulmonary atresia, ventricular septal defect, and severe peripheral arborization abnormalities of the central pulmonary arteries: experience with preliminary unifocalization procedures in 38 patients. *J Thorac Cardiovasc Surg* 98:1018-1029, 1989. By permission of Mosby-Year Book.)

A lack of continuity between the right and the left pulmonary arteries may occur naturally, such as at the site of closure of a patent ductus arteriosus or when each pulmonary arterial branch has a separate blood supply from a ductus or from systemic collateral arteries. In many patients, unfortunately, nonconfluence of the pulmonary arterial branch is a result of previous surgical attempts at palliation that distort and scar the arteries at the site of the anastomosis, most frequently seen in patients with prior Waterston shunts. Purposeful interruption of the pulmonary arterial confluence by the surgeon is observed during construction of the Glenn anastomosis (connection of the superior vena cava to the right pulmonary artery) or with construction of the end-to-end Blalock-Taussig shunt. We have advocated not using the Waterston shunt for palliation in patients with this condition for this reason and support the concept that surgical interruption of the pulmonary arterial confluence in the patient with pulmonary atresia and ventricular septal defect is destructive and should be abandoned.

An infant with naturally occurring nonconfluence who is in need of surgical treatment cannot simply have a surgical shunt to the more available pulmonary artery, because this maneuver promotes the development of only that pulmonary artery. Rather, an effort should be made at the time of initial palliation to reconstruct the confluence so that systemic-to-pulmonary artery shunting results in increased blood supply to both lungs. This reconstruction is particularly possible when the site of luminal obstruction is the site of entry of the ductus arteriosus. For patients with short gaps in continuity of the pulmonary arteries reachable through a median sternotomy approach, such as those after the Waterston anastomosis, single-stage corrective repair is possible. Total dismantling of the shunt and patch angioplasty of the scarred pulmonary artery are mandatory to achieve a good surgical result. A different problem exists in patients with large segmental gaps in the pulmonary confluence. Reconstruction of the pulmonary confluence demands the insertion of a prosthetic tube graft from pulmonary artery to pulmonary artery, interruption of extracardiac sources of pulmonary blood flow, closure of the ventricular septal defect, and insertion of a valve prosthetic conduit between the right ventricle and the newly established pulmonary arterial confluence.[2] Single-stage repair in such patients is possible when the most proximal ends of the individual pulmonary arteries are accessible through a median sternotomy or through a bilateral transsternal thoracotomy, but the procedure is formidable and it may be wise in some patients to stage the reconstruction. Although the early results are good and such procedures can be accomplished with a low surgical mortality in selected patients, the long-term result depends on the durability of the implanted prosthetic conduits.

Hypoplastic nonconfluent pulmonary arteries are not amenable to single-stage reconstruction and have often been subjected to multiple attempts at surgical palliation. Surgical shunting into the small pulmonary arteries may be very rewarding because of the palliation achieved and the induced rapid enlargement of these vessels. Because of extensive mediastinal collateralization, exposure of these small arteries at the hilus may be difficult. If such a situation is encountered, we prefer to expose the pulmonary arteries within the major pulmonary fissure, a constant site where dissection is less risky and more predictable.[2,15] A simple, small Gore-Tex shunt from the subclavian arteries can be created in all these patients with various degrees of palliation achieved, depending on the size of the shunted vessel and its distribution. Nonetheless, when such a pulmonary artery is moderately hypoplastic and fully distributed, offering the potential for eventual complete repair, anastomosis of a large-sized conduit (14 to 16 mm) with proximal anastomosis to a small window in the ascending aorta accomplishes the same physiologic result but offers a more favorable anatomic arrangement for final reconstruction, since the proximal end of the graft is then available anteriorly.

In patients with less complex forms of this condition in whom the pulmonary arteries are well developed with good distribution and the atretic pulmonary artery segment is short, surgical repair can be accomplished in a manner similar to that for tetralogy of Fallot, and the late prognosis and potential areas of concern in these patients are identical to those for the patient with tetralogy. However, a significant number of patients with this condition require an extracardiac valved conduit to establish continuity between the right ventricle and the pulmonary artery, and in such patients problems related to the durability of these conduits can occur.[17] Experience has shown that most heterograft conduits, at least those placed during childhood, eventually need replacement because of obstruction developing either at the valve or, as a result of a fibrin peel, within the graft. However, this procedure can usually be accomplished with a low surgical risk, and evidence is accumulating that such conduits placed during adolescence or adulthood may last for many years. There is additional evidence that fresh, antibiotic-sterilized homograft conduits obtained from cadavers may be quite durable, even when placed during childhood, and the increasing availability of such conduits and their use may decrease the need for reoperation because of future conduit obstruction. Generally, therefore, it is thought that in patients with this lesion who, after repair, have a pulmonary artery pressure that is near normal, late prognosis should not be distinctly different from that in the patient with tetralogy of Fallot.

It is less certain what the long-term results will be in patients who, after repair, have some residual pulmonary artery and right ventricular hypertension secondary to pulmonary artery hypoplasia or maldistribution, because corrective surgery in such patients has been performed only during the past 20 years. Follow-up results to date have been very encouraging, but additional data are clearly necessary before definitive conclusions can be drawn. Similarly, long-term prognosis is uncertain for patients with this condition in whom pulmonary artery anatomy dictates that only palliation is possible, but again many of them, if well palliated, will continue to function quite well into early adulthood.

As with patients who have tetralogy of Fallot, patients with this condition who become parents run a higher risk than normal of their children being afflicted with a congenital heart lesion. Women who have had correction and who have pulmonary artery pressures that are normal or only slightly increased seem to tolerate pregnancy well. However, for women in whom significant pulmonary artery hypertension persists after correction, pregnancy is probably not advisable. Likewise, in palliated patients who remain hypoxemic, pregnancy clearly carries an increased risk to both the mother and the fetus.

REFERENCES

1. Liao P-K, Edwards WD, Julsrud PR, et al: Pulmonary blood supply in patients with pulmonary atresia and ventricular septal defect. *J Am Coll Cardiol* 6:1343-1350, 1985
2. Puga FJ: Surgical treatment of pulmonary atresia and ventricular septal defect. *Prog Pediatr Cardiol* 1 No 1:37-49, 1992
3. Jefferson K, Rees S, Somerville J: Systemic arterial supply to the lungs in pulmonary atresia and its relation to pulmonary artery development. *Br Heart J* 34:418-427, 1972
4. McGoon MD, Fulton RE, Davis GD, et al: Systemic collateral and pulmonary artery stenosis in patients with congenital pulmonary valve atresia and ventricular septal defect. *Circulation* 56:473-479, 1977
5. Haworth SG: Collateral arteries in pulmonary atresia with ventricular septal defect: a precarious blood supply. *Br Heart J* 44:5-13, 1980
6. Fäller K, Haworth G, Taylor JFN, et al: Duplicate sources of pulmonary blood supply in pulmonary atresia with ventricular septal defect. *Br Heart J* 46:263-268, 1981
7. Rabinovitch M: Pathology and anatomy of pulmonary atresia and ventricular septal defect. *Prog Pediatr Cardiol* 1 No 1:9-17, 1992
8. Fisher EA, Thanopoulos BD, Eckner FAO, et al: Pulmonary atresia with obstructed ventricular septal defect. *Pediatr Cardiol* 1:209-217, 1980
9. Bharati S, Paul MH, Idriss FS, et al: The surgical anatomy of pulmonary atresia with ventricular septal defect: pseudotruncus. *J Thorac Cardiovasc Surg* 69:713-721, 1975
10. Davies MJ, Anderson RH, Becker AE: *The Conduction System of the Heart*. London, Butterworths, 1983, pp 121-124
11. Berry BE, McGoon DC: Total correction for tetralogy of Fallot with anomalous coronary artery. *Surgery* 74:894-898, 1973
12. Fulton RE, Davis GD: Congenital pulmonary atresia: photographic subtraction as an aid in recognizing hypoplastic pulmonary arteries. *AJR* 131:1003-1007, 1978
13. Millikan JS, Puga FJ, Danielson GK, et al: Staged surgical repair of pulmonary atresia, ventricular septal defect, and hypoplastic, confluent pulmonary arteries. *J Thorac Cardiovasc Surg* 91:818-825, 1986
14. Puga FJ, Uretzky G: Establishment of right ventricle-hypoplastic pulmonary artery continuity without the use of extracorporeal circulation. *J Thorac Cardiovasc Surg* 83:74-80, 1982
15. Puga FJ, Leoni FE, Julsrud PR, et al: Complete repair of pulmonary atresia, ventricular septal defect, and severe peripheral arborization abnormalities of the central pulmonary arteries: experience with preliminary unifocalization procedures in 38 patients. *J Thorac Cardiovasc Surg* 98:1018-1029, 1989
16. Mair DD, Julsrud PR: Diagnostic evaluation of pulmonary atresia in ventricular septal defect: cardiac catheterization and angiography. *Prog Pediatr Cardiol* 1 No 1:23-36, 1992
17. Agarwal KC, Edwards WD, Feldt RH, et al: Pathogenesis of nonobstructive fibrous peels in right-sided porcine-valved extracardiac conduits. *J Thorac Cardiovasc Surg* 83:584-589, 1982

CHAPTER

51

Truncus arteriosus

David J. Driscoll, M.D., and Gordon K. Danielson, M.D.

ANATOMIC CONSIDERATIONS

Truncus arteriosus is a congenital cardiac malformation in which the pulmonary arteries, the aorta, and the coronary arteries originate from one great artery. It was described by Buchanan[1] in 1864 and was classified into four major types by Collett and Edwards[2] in 1949. Truncus arteriosus occurs in approximately 1 per 11,616 live births and constitutes 0.7% of all cases of congenital heart disease.[3] The classification of Collett and Edwards is based on the origin of the pulmonary arteries from the truncus: type I, a single pulmonary artery arises from the truncus; type II, the right and left pulmonary arteries originate from the truncus close together but independently; type III, the right and left pulmonary arteries arise independently from opposite sides of the truncus (Fig 51-1). What had been described as type IV truncus arteriosus (absence of the pulmonary arteries) no longer is considered to be a form of truncus arteriosus but rather is a type of pulmonary artery atresia with ventricular septal defect. Originally, Collett and Edwards included an aortic-pulmonary window as the fifth type of truncus arteriosus. At present, however, the term "truncus arteriosus" is reserved for Collett and Edwards types I to III. Even type III can be disputed because in these hearts the origin of the pulmonary arteries is from a posterolateral position on the aorta rather than directly laterally. Type I is the most common (48% to 68%), type II is the second most common (29% to 34%), and type III is the least common (6% to 10%).[2,4-6]

The origin of the pulmonary arteries from the truncus arteriosus usually is unobstructed. However, in a study of autopsy specimens, Calder et al.[5] found 14% with partial obstruction of the pulmonary arteries. Portions of the truncal valve leaflets produced the obstruction in 10 patients, and there was pulmonary arterial stenosis in 2 patients. Unilateral absence of one pulmonary artery occurs in 8% to 16% of patients.[5,7] The pulmonary artery that most commonly is absent is contralateral to the aortic arch.

The aortic arch is right-sided in 21% to 34% of cases[7] and interrupted in 11% to 19%. When interrupted, a patent ductus arteriosus provides continuity between the pulmonary artery and the descending thoracic aorta.

The truncal valve is tricuspid in 61% to 72% of cases, is quadricuspid in 15% to 31%, is bicuspid in 6% to 12%, and has five or six cusps in fewer than 2%.[5-8] The truncal valve is insufficient in approximately 15% of cases and may be stenotic in 11%.[5] Truncal valve stenosis or insufficiency is associated with thickened and dysplastic cusps, prolapse of unsupported cusps, and dilation of the truncal valve annulus.

The left coronary artery usually originates from the left posterior sinus of the truncal valve and the right coronary artery, from the right anterior aspect of the truncus.[5] There is a single coronary ostium, or two coronary ostia located close together, in 13% of cases.[5] Because the left anterior descending coronary artery usually is small and displaced leftward, portions of the myocardium of the right ventricular outflow tract may be supplied by a relatively large conal branch of the right coronary artery.[7] A left dominant coronary artery system occurs in 27% of cases, three times more commonly than in the normal population.[7] Rarely, a coronary artery arises from the pulmonary artery.[4,9]

A large ventricular septal defect located between the limbs of the septomarginal band and beneath the truncal valve cusps is associated with truncus arteriosus. Rarely, the ventricular septum is intact [10-12] or the defect in it is restrictive.[13] The truncus arteriosus is positioned above the ventricular septal defect in 68% to 83% of cases but originates to the right of the ventricular septal defect (above the right ventricle) in 11% to 29% and to the left of the ventricular septum (above the left ventricle) in 4% to 6%. Usually, a muscular margin separates the defect from the conduction tissue, but if not, the conduction tissue is located along the left aspect of the posterior-inferior rim of the defect. There is fibrous continuity of the mitral and truncal valve annuli in essentially all cases, and in addition, in some instances there also is continuity of the tricuspid and truncal valve annuli.

In addition to a right aortic arch, interrupted aortic arch, unilateral absence of the pulmonary artery, and coronary artery abnormalities, truncus arteriosus may be associated with patent ductus arteriosus (30% of cases),[8] aberrant origin of the right subclavian artery (4% to 10% of cases),[7] secundum atrial septal defect (9% to 20% of cases),[7] persistence of the left superior vena cava, tricuspid valve stenosis, tricuspid valve atresia, partial anomalous pulmonary venous connection, or, very rarely, mitral valve stenosis or atresia.

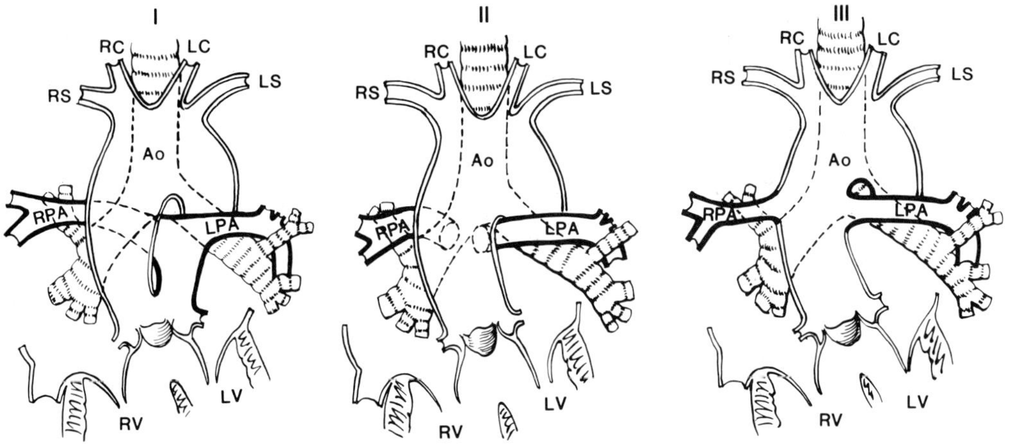

Fig 51-1. Diagram of truncus arteriosus types I, II, and III. *RC* and *LC*, right and left carotid arteries; *RS* and *LS*, right and left subclavian arteries; *Ao*, aorta; *RPA* and *LPA*, right and left pulmonary arteries; *RV* and *LV*, right and left ventricles. (From Edwards JE, McGoon DC: Absence of anatomic origin from heart of pulmonary arterial supply. *Circulation* 47:393-398, 1973. By permission of American Heart Association.)

Associated extracardiac anomalies have been reported in 21% to 30% of cases and include skeletal anomalies, hydroureter, and bowel malrotation. The DiGeorge syndrome or partial DiGeorge syndrome has been associated with conal and truncal abnormalities and is important to recognize because transfusion of lymphocytes into these patients can precipitate a fatal graft-vs.-host reaction.

The truncus and conus arteriosus are partitioned by the spiral formation of the dextrodorsal and sinistroventral truncal ridges and sinistroventral and dextrodorsal conal ridges. This spiral partitioning allows the aorta to originate from the left ventricle and the pulmonary artery from the right ventricle. The membranous portion of the ventricular septum is formed from merging of the lower portion of the conus ridges and the endocardial cushions and crest of the muscular ventricular septum.[2] Truncus arteriosus results from absence or abnormal development of the conal and truncal septa. Because of abnormal conal septal development, the anterior tricuspid valve leaflet and medial tricuspid papillary muscle may be malformed.[7]

PATHOPHYSIOLOGY

The pathophysiology of truncus arteriosus is related to the presence, and the degree, of obstruction to pulmonary blood flow and truncal valve incompetence or stenosis. In most instances there is little or no restriction to pulmonary blood flow, and pulmonary and systemic artery pressures are equal. Increased pulmonary blood flow may result in left ventricular failure, pulmonary venous hypertension, and congestive heart failure. Presumably, because of increased pulmonary artery blood flow and pulmonary venous hypertension, pulmonary vascular obstructive disease develops relatively rapidly in most patients with truncus arteriosus. For reasons that are unclear, pulmonary vascular obstructive disease develops more rapidly in patients with truncus arteriosus than in patients with only a large ventricular septal defect and similar pulmonary artery blood pressure and flow. Persistence of the shunt throughout the cardiac cycle may be implicated. If the patient survives infancy and early childhood, the pulmonary blood flow decreases as pulmonary vascular obstructive disease develops and pulmonary resistance increases. Eventually, a net right-to-left shunt develops, causing increasing cyanosis and progressive ventricular fibrosis and failure. The presence of truncal valve insufficiency or stenosis accentuates the degree of congestive heart failure and pulmonary venous hypertension.

CLINICAL SYNDROME

History and clinical course

Patients with truncus arteriosus usually are identified shortly after birth because of congestive heart failure, cyanosis, or failure to thrive. Without operative intervention their prognosis is very poor. Marcelletti et al.[14] examined the natural history of truncus arteriosus in 23 patients not treated surgically. The oldest patient was age 16 when first seen and was still alive 10 years later, but with very severe pulmonary obstructive vascular disease. Ten patients died in infancy, 1 died between 1 and 7 years of age, and 3 died after age 7—a mortality of 61%. Severe congestive heart failure is the usual cause of death. Without operation, few patients with truncus arteriosus reach adulthood.

Physical findings

Physical appearance. Patients with unrestricted pulmonary blood flow frequently show poor growth and poor subcutaneous fat development. Patients with restricted pulmonary blood flow tend to thrive and grow. However, as restriction of pulmonary blood flow increases, cyanosis increases.

Arterial and venous pulsations. Except for jugular venous distention with congestive heart failure, the venous pulsations usually are normal. The arterial pulse pressure is increased in patients with normal or only moderately increased pulmonary vascular resistance and in those with truncal valve regurgitation. The lower extremity pulses may be diminished or absent in patients with coarctation of the aorta or interrupted aortic arch and a restrictive patent ductus arteriosus.

Precordial palpation. The apical impulse is prominent, overactive, and displaced laterally to the left in patients with increased pulmonary blood flow or truncal valve insufficiency. The degree of overactivity is proportional to the pulmonary blood flow or truncal valve insufficiency. The right ventricular impulse at the left lower sternal border is overactive. Closure of the truncal valve frequently is palpable at the upper left sternal border.

Auscultation. The first heart sound usually is normal. The second heart sound is increased in intensity, and although frequently single, it can be split despite the presence of only one semilunar valve. An apical ejection click is common. A holosystolic or ejection murmur is audible in the majority of patients. A low-frequency apical diastolic murmur resulting from abnormally increased blood flow through the mitral valve orifice is present in patients with increased pulmonary blood flow. An early diastolic decrescendo murmur is associated with truncal valve insufficiency. Continuous murmurs are unusual unless pulmonary arterial stenosis is present.

Electrocardiogram

The electrocardiogram is characterized by sinus rhythm, right-axis deviation, and biventricular hypertrophy. As the pulmonary blood flow diminishes due to development of pulmonary vascular obstructive disease, the electrocardiographic manifestations of left ventricular hypertrophy may regress relative to right ventricular hypertrophy.

Chest radiograph

Except in cases with decreased pulmonary blood flow, the chest radiograph is characterized by moderate cardiomegaly and increased pulmonary vascular markings. With normal or decreased pulmonary blood flow the cardiac size may be normal. Asymmetry of the pulmonary vascular markings suggests associated unilateral absence of a pulmonary artery.[7] In 21% to 34% of patients, the aortic arch is right-sided, and this finding associated with increased pulmonary vascular markings suggests the diagnosis of truncus arteriosus.

DIAGNOSTIC PROBLEMS AND INDICATIONS FOR INVASIVE STUDIES

Prior to the introduction of two-dimensional echocardiography, cardiac catheterization and angiography were necessary to confirm the diagnosis of truncus arteriosus. Oximetry reveals characteristic combined right-to-left and left-to-right shunt at the ventricular and great artery locations. Although the blood oxygen saturations of the aorta and pulmonary artery frequently are similar, in some instances streaming of oxygenated and deoxygenated blood from the ventricles can result in differences. Blood pressures in the right ventricle and left ventricle typically are equal. Left atrial pressure will be increased relative to the pulmonary blood flow and the degree of congestive heart failure. Except in the presence of truncal valve stenosis, peak systolic ventricular, truncal, and aortic

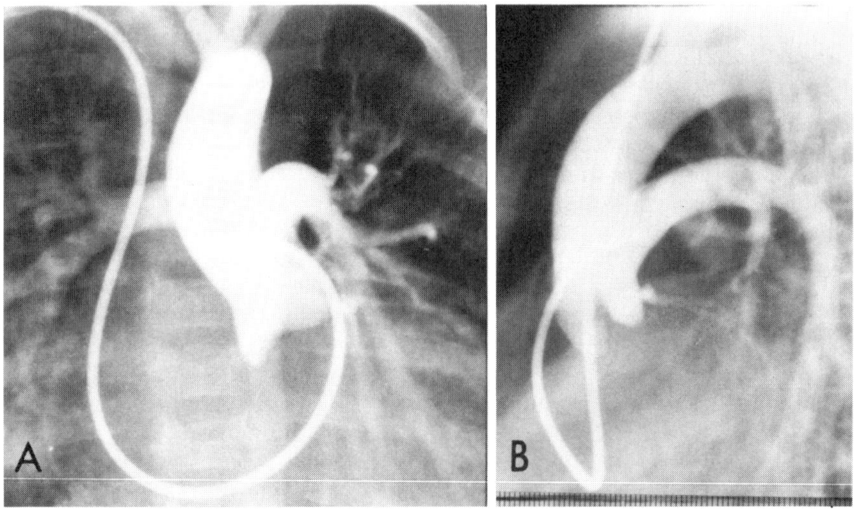

Fig 51-2. Anteroposterior (**A**) and lateral (**B**) angiographic projections after injection of contrast medium into the truncal root. Origin of pulmonary arteries from the truncus is apparent. (From Mair DD, Edwards WD, Fuster V, et al: Truncus arteriosus. In *Moss' Heart Disease in Infants, Children, and Adolescents.* Third edition. Edited by FH Adams, GC Emmanouilides. Baltimore, Williams & Wilkins, 1983, pp 400-410. By permission.)

blood pressures are equal. Also, in the absence of pulmonary artery obstruction, pulmonary artery and aortic pressures are equal. Calculated systemic vascular resistance usually is normal, and pulmonary vascular resistance can be normal or markedly increased, depending on the degree of pulmonary vascular obstructive disease.

Angiocardiography

Angiocardiography is utilized to visualize the origin of the pulmonary arteries from the truncus, the size and number of ventricular septal defects, the presence or absence of pulmonary artery obstruction, the presence or absence of truncal valve insufficiency, absence of a pulmonary artery, coronary arterial anomaly, and associated structural defects (Fig 51-2). In infants with severe congestive heart failure, injection of contrast medium for angiocardiography can cause hypotension and death.

Echocardiography

The diagnosis of truncus arteriosus and associated anomalies can be made by using two-dimensional echocardiography (Fig 51-3). The truncus arteriosus, the origin and division of the pulmonary arteries, and the ventricular septal defect can be visualized. In selected cases, interruption of the aortic arch can be appreciated. With Doppler techniques, truncal valve stenosis can be quantitated and regurgitation can be semiquantitated. Associated intracardiac shunts and intracardiac pressures can be identified and measured. In some cases, surgical intervention can be undertaken on the basis of clinical findings and echocardiography without invasive cardiac catheterization studies.

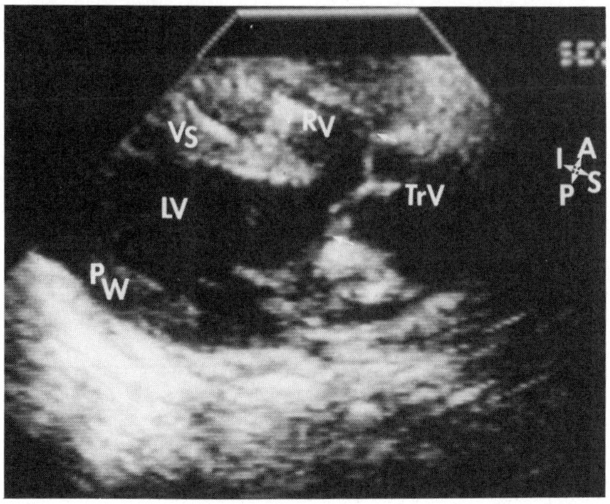

Fig 51-3. Two-dimensional echocardiogram (parasternal long-axis view) showing origin of pulmonary arteries from truncal root. *LV,* left ventricle; *PW,* posterior wall; *RV,* right ventricle; *TrV,* truncal valve; *VS,* ventricular septum. (From Mair DD, Edwards WD, Fuster V, et al: Truncus arteriosus. In Moss' *Heart Disease in Infants, Children, and Adolescents.* Third edition. Edited by FH Adams, GC Emmanouilides. Baltimore, Williams & Wilkins, 1983, pp 400-410. By permission.)

MANAGEMENT

Closure of the ventricular septal defect, establishment of continuity of the right ventricle and pulmonary arteries, and repair of associated malformations before the occurrence of significant pulmonary vascular obstructive disease are the basic treatment tenets.[15,16] (Fig 51-4). Medical management of congestive heart failure with digitalis and diuretic drugs is an adjunct to rather than a substitute for surgical therapy.

Complete repair should be performed within the first 6 months of life for patients with nonobstructed pulmonary blood flow. Of course, at this age a relatively small conduit will have to be used to establish continuity of the right ventricle with the pulmonary artery. Thus, reoperation will be necessary to implant a larger conduit later in life. If recently described techniques to establish continuity of the right ventricle and the pulmonary artery without the need for a prosthetic conduit prove successful and are applicable to infants,[17,18] reoperation for conduit replacement may be obviated. However, a major concern with nonvalved repair in infancy is whether the resultant pulmonary insufficiency will increase early mortality, because most patients have increased pulmonary artery pressure and resistance postoperatively.

Early complete repair offers the best chance to prevent development of fatal pulmonary vascular obstructive disease. Pearl et al.[19] described the results in 32 infants operated on before 1 year of age (average, 3.5 months) between 1982 and 1990. Overall early mortality was 15.6%, and late mortality was 7.4%. For patients operated on before 1 month of age, mortality was 7%. Much of the mortality was associated with complex forms of truncus arteriosus, especially associated interrupted aortic arch. In the most recent 4 years of Pearl and associates' experience, there were no early deaths among 22 patients without interrupted aortic arch.

Banding of the pulmonary artery is not preferred to complete repair except in circumstances in which complete repair is not feasible. Because the segment of main pulmonary artery in type I truncus arteriosus is very short, banding of that structure frequently results in kinking of one pulmonary artery (usually the right pulmonary artery) and inadequate protection of the other lung from pulmonary vascular obstructive disease. Individual banding of each pulmonary artery more effectively controls pulmonary blood flow, but there is a tendency for such bands to migrate peripherally and distort the pulmonary arteries or occlude the upper lobe branches. In addition, it is difficult to adjust the tightness of these bands to be effective but not to exceed the critical closing pressure of the tiny pulmonary artery.

Unfortunately, not all patients with truncus arteriosus have had repair as infants, and repair must be considered at an older age. If significant pulmonary vascular obstructive disease is present, closure of the ventricular septal defect may be fatal and is contraindicated. Pulmonary resistance <8 units $\cdot$ m^2 is associated with an acceptable

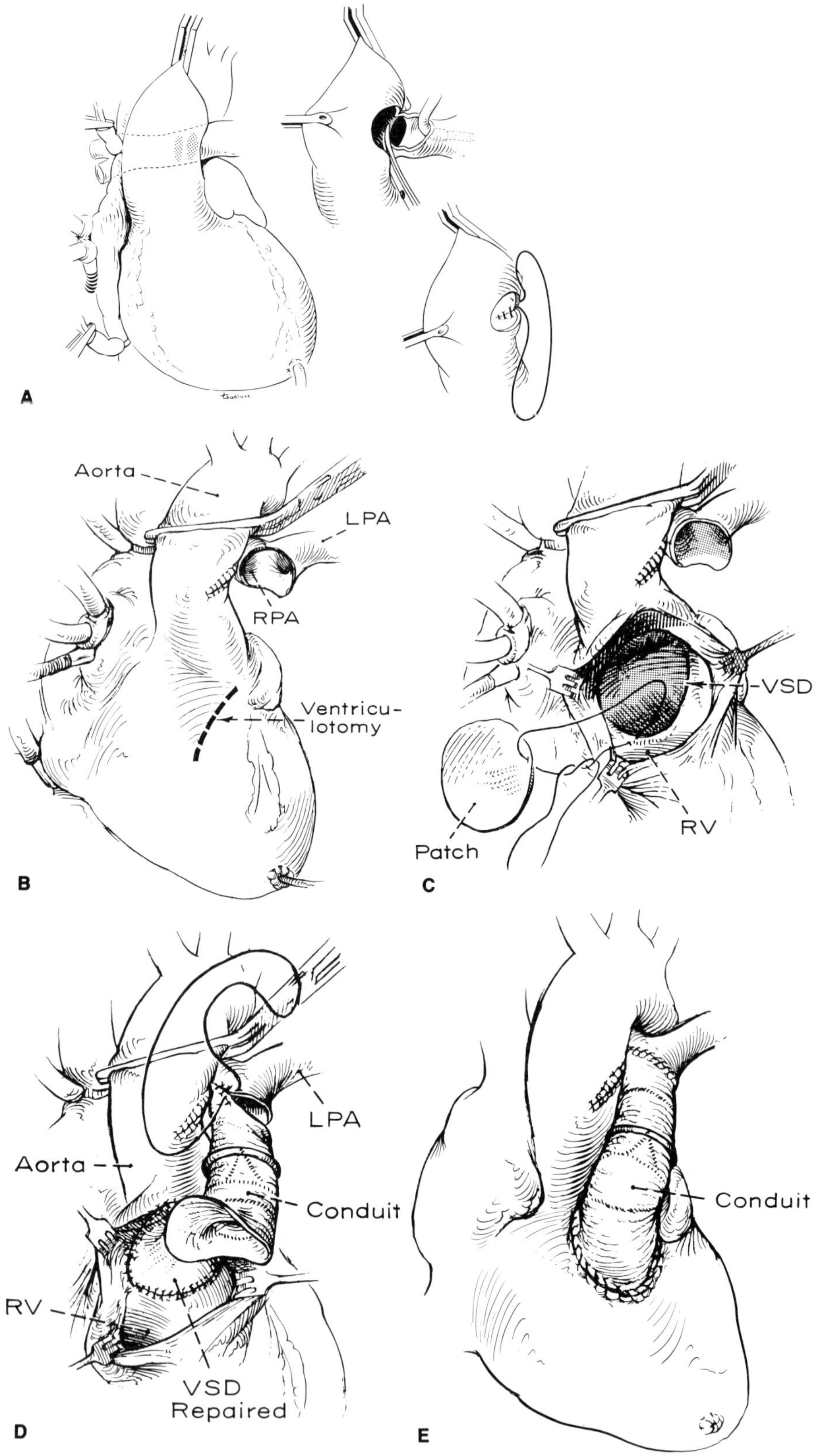

Fig 51-4. Surgical technique for complete repair of truncus arteriosus. **A,** origin of the pulmonary artery is separated from truncal root. **B,** right ventriculotomy is performed. **C,** ventricular septal defect *(VSD)* is closed with a prosthetic patch. **D** and **E,** valve-containing conduit (preferably a homograft) is anastomosed to the proximal pulmonary artery **(D)** and right ventricle *(RV)* **(E).** *LPA,* left pulmonary artery; *RPA,* right pulmonary artery. (**A,** from McGoon DC, Rastelli GC, Ongley PA: An operation for the correction of truncus arteriosus. *JAMA* 205:69-73, 1968. By permission of American Medical Association. **B-E,** from Lofland GK: Truncus arteriosus. In *Surgery of the Chest.* Vol. 1. Fifth edition. Edited by DC Sabiston Jr, FC Spencer. Philadelphia, WB Saunders Company, 1990, pp 1359-1366. By permission.)

operative outcome.[20] Marcelletti et al.[20] reported operative mortalities of 14% for 42 patients with a pulmonary resistance < 8 units · m^2 and 39% (with five late deaths) for 28 patients with pulmonary resistance > 8 units · m^2. Unfortunately, the progression of pulmonary vascular obstructive disease may not be halted by repair in some patients, regardless of the level of pulmonary resistance preoperatively. No method is available for identification of these unfortunate patients preoperatively.

Fyfe et al.[21] reviewed the outcome of 19 patients with truncus arteriosus and congenital or acquired unilateral absence of a pulmonary artery. The combined early and late mortality for this group was 68%; it was 33% for patients with pulmonary resistance < 8 units · m^2 and 82% for those with pulmonary resistance > 8 units · m^2.

Management of significant truncal valve stenosis or insufficiency is a technical challenge. In infants, repair of an insufficient truncal valve is occasionally possible. In older patients, replacement of the truncal valve is usually necessary.

All patients with truncus arteriosus require continued medical care even after definitive surgical repair. Acquired conduit stenosis and conduit valve malfunction remain problems and must be identified before excessive right ventricular hypertension develops. As with patients with tetralogy of Fallot, some late deaths after repair of truncus arteriosus probably are related to ventricular arrhythmias. Right ventricular hypertension or severe pulmonary insufficiency may increase the risk of serious ventricular arrhythmias. All patients should continue prophylaxis against bacterial endocarditis.

REFERENCES

1. Buchanan A: Malformation of heart: undivided truncus arteriosus; heart otherwise double. *Trans Pathol Soc Lond* 15:89-91, 1864
2. Collett RW, Edwards JE: Persistent truncus arteriosus: a classification according to anatomic types. *Surg Clin North Am,* August 1949, pp 1245-1270
3. Kidd BSL: Persistent truncus arteriosus. In *Heart Disease in Infancy and Childhood.* Third edition. Edited by JD Keith, RD Rowe, P Vlad. New York, Macmillan Publishing Co, 1978, pp 457-469
4. Bharati S, McAllister HA Jr, Rosenquist GC, et al: The surgical anatomy of truncus arteriosus communis. *J Thorac Cardiovasc Surg* 67:501-510, 1974
5. Calder L, Van Praagh R, Van Praagh S, et al: Truncus arteriosus communis: clinical, angiocardiographic, and pathologic findings in 100 patients. *Am Heart J* 92:23-38, 1976
6. Crupi G, Macartney FJ, Anderson RH: Persistent truncus arteriosus: a study of 66 autopsy cases with special reference to definition and morphogenesis. *Am J Cardiol* 40:569-578, 1977
7. Mair DD, Edwards WD, Fuster V, et al: Truncus arteriosus. In *Moss' Heart Disease in Infants, Children, and Adolescents.* Third edition. Edited by FH Adams, GC Emmanouilides. Baltimore, Williams & Wilkins, 1983, pp 400-410
8. Van Praagh R, Van Praagh S: The anatomy of common aorticopulmonary trunk (truncus arteriosus communis) and its embryologic implications: a study of 57 necropsy cases. *Am J Cardiol* 16:406-425, 1965
9. Daskalopoulos DA, Edwards WD, Driscoll DJ, et al: Fatal pulmonary artery banding in truncus arteriosus with anomalous origin of circumflex coronary artery from right pulmonary artery. *Am J Cardiol* 52:1363-1364, 1983
10. Bain CWC, Parkinson J: Common aorto-pulmonary trunk: a rare congenital defect. *Br Heart J* 5:97-100, 1943
11. Thiene G, Bortolotti U: Truncus arteriosus communis with intact ventricular septum (letter to the editor). *Br Heart J* 43:605-606, 1980
12. Carr I, Bharati S, Kusnoor VS, et al: Truncus arteriosus communis with intact ventricular septum. *Br Heart J* 42:97-102, 1979
13. Rosenquist GC, Bharati S, McAllister HA, et al: Truncus arteriosus communis: truncal valve anomalies associated with small conal or truncal septal defects. *Am J Cardiol* 37:410-412, 1976
14. Marcelletti C, McGoon DC, Mair DD: The natural history of truncus arteriosus. *Circulation* 54:108-111, 1976
15. McGoon DC, Rastelli GC, Ongley RA: An operation for the correction of truncus arteriosus. *JAMA* 205:69-73, 1968
16. Di Donato RM, Fyfe DA, Puga FJ, et al: Fifteen-year experience with surgical repair of truncus arteriosus. *J Thorac Cardiovasc Surg* 89:414-422, 1985
17. Sharma BK, Pilato M, Ott DA: Surgical repair of type II truncus arteriosus without a conduit. *Ann Thorac Surg* 50:479-481, 1990
18. Barbero-Marcial M, Riso A, Atik E, et al: A technique for correction of truncus arteriosus types I and II without extracardiac conduits. *J Thorac Cardiovasc Surg* 99:364-369, 1990
19. Pearl J, Laks H, Drinkwater DC Jr, et al: Repair of truncus arteriosus in infancy. *Ann Thorac Surg* 52:780-786, 1991
20. Marcelletti C, McGoon DC, Danielson GK, et al: Early and late results of surgical repair of truncus arteriosus. *Circulation* 55:636-641, 1977
21. Fyfe DA, Driscoll DJ, Di Donato RM, et al: Truncus arteriosus with single pulmonary artery: influence of pulmonary vascular obstructive disease on early and late operative results. *J Am Coll Cardiol* 5:1168-1172, 1985

CHAPTER

52

Tricuspid atresia and single ventricle

David J. Driscoll, M.D., Hartzell V. Schaff, M.D., and Gordon K. Danielson, M.D.

DEFINITION AND HISTORICAL AND ANATOMIC CONSIDERATIONS

Tricuspid atresia

In tricuspid atresia, there is complete agenesis of the tricuspid valve and no direct communication between the right atrium and right ventricle.[1] Tricuspid atresia was described in 1906 by Kühne[2] and is the third most common form of cyanotic congenital heart disease.[3] It occurs in 0.6 to 1.0 birth per 10,000 live births[2] and represents approximately 2.7% of cases of congenital heart disease.[1]

The location of the atretic valve frequently is represented by a dimple in the muscular floor of the right atrium. The right ventricle consists mainly of conus with an underdeveloped sinus portion. The size of the right ventricle in tricuspid atresia is quite variable. An interatrial communication is necessary for survival. A patent foramen ovale is most common (80%); there can be a secundum atrial septal defect or, rarely, an ostium primum type of atrial septal defect.[1]

Tricuspid atresia is classified according to the positions of the great arteries and the presence or absence of a ventricular septal defect, pulmonary atresia, or pulmonary stenosis[4,5] (Table 52-1). It is apparent from this classification that tricuspid atresia can be associated with increased or decreased pulmonary blood flow. With normally related great arteries, the majority of patients will have decreased pulmonary blood flow; with dextrotransposed great arteries, increased pulmonary blood flow is more common. In patients with normally related great arteries, pulmonary blood flow usually is limited by a restrictive ventricular septal defect rather than by pulmonary valve stenosis. However, with dextrotransposed great arteries, if pulmonary blood flow is limited, it is limited by pulmonary valve stenosis. With pulmonary atresia, pulmonary blood flow usually is limited and is dependent on persistent patency of a ductus arteriosus or systemic-to-pulmonary artery collateral vessels.

Additional cardiovascular malformations are present in 18% of patients with normally related great arteries and 63% of patients with transposed great arteries. These malformations include persistence of the left superior vena cava (16%), coarctation of the aorta (8%), a patent ductus arteriosus (3%), and right aortic arch (3% to 8%).[1,6] Left juxtaposed atrial appendages occur in 10% to 40% of patients with tricuspid atresia and transposed great arteries.[7,8] Additional extracardiac anomalies occur in 20%.[8]

The conduction system is abnormal in tricuspid atresia. There is early origin of the left bundle from the common bundle.[1] This accounts for the abnormally superior QRS axis and counterclockwise frontal plane vectorcardiographic loop. Approximately 7% of patients with tricuspid atresia manifest arrhythmias. Ventricular preexcitation

Table 52-1 Classification of tricuspid atresia

Type	Description	Relative frequency, % Clinical	Relative frequency, % Autopsy
I	Normally related great arteries	70	69
I-A	No VSD; pulmonary atresia		9
I-B	Restrictive VSD; pulmonary stenosis		51
I-C	Large VSD; no pulmonary stenosis		9
II	Dextrotransposition of great arteries	23	28
II-A	VSD; pulmonary atresia		2
II-B	VSD; pulmonary stenosis		8
II-C	VSD; no pulmonary stenosis		18
III	Levotransposition of great arteries	7	3

VSD, ventricular septal defect.
Adapted from Rosenthal and Dick.[1]

with the Wolff-Parkinson-White syndrome has been reported in association with tricuspid atresia.

Tricuspid atresia results from malalignment of the ventricular septum and the atrioventricular (AV) canal. The ventricular septum is shifted toward the right, and the malaligned ventricular septum blocks the right AV valve orifice.[1,6]

Single ventricle

The terms "single ventricle," "common ventricle," and "univentricular heart" include a spectrum of malformations unified by the presence of one completely formed ventricular chamber that receives both tricuspid and mitral valves or a common AV valve. Tricuspid and mitral atresia are excluded by this definition. Unfortunately, the terminology of this entity has become quite confusing. We will use the nomenclature of Van Praagh et al.[9] as later modified by Hallermann et al.[10] Van Praagh et al. categorized single, or common (synonymous), ventricle depending on the morphology of the ventricular mass: type A, morphological left ventricle with rudimentary outflow pouch consisting of right ventricular infundibulum; type B, morphological right ventricle without left ventricular sinus (a remnant of the left ventricular cavity may be present as a "slit-like" nonfunctional accessory chamber or pouch); type C, ventricle consisting of portions of both right ventricular and left ventricular mass (ventricular septum absent or rudimentary); and type D, ventricle that does not have characteristics of right ventricular or left ventricular mass (absence of right ventricular and left ventricular sinuses). These four types can be classified further depending on whether D or L looping occurred and on the spatial relationship of the great arteries (normal [I], D-transposed [II], or L-transposed [III]). In the series of Van Praagh et al., 78% of cases were type A, 5% were type B, 7% were type C, and 10% were type D. There were essentially equal numbers with D-transposed and L-transposed great arteries (42% and 43%, respectively). Fifteen percent had normally related great arteries.

Detailed postmortem examination of the heart frequently is necessary to classify hearts according to the Van Praagh nomenclature. Fortunately, Hallermann et al.[10] simplified the Van Praagh et al. classification on the basis of angiographic features of the heart that are obtained before the patient dies. Ritter et al.[11] pointed out that frequently it is difficult to distinguish among types B, C, and D with available clinical imaging techniques, so they[10,11] included B and D with type C (thus, the designation "C" represents the three groups in which there is no outlet chamber). The designation "A" is retained for those with an apparent outlet chamber. The numbers I, II, and III are retained to refer to the relationship of the great arteries as above. Table 52-2 shows the incidences of these types of single ventricle encountered in a large clinical experience.[11]

It bothers some people to use the term "single ventricle" or "univentricular heart" when, in fact, two chambers (a dominant ventricle and an outlet chamber or accessory pouch) are present in the ventricular mass. One can rationalize using this nomenclature if a ventricle is considered to be a ventricle only if it consists of a sinus portion that contains tensor apparatus of the AV valves and an outflow tract or infundibulum derived from the bulbus cordis.[12] Others have introduced the term "double-inlet left ventricle" (Table 52-3).

Single ventricle occurs in approximately 1 per 6,500 live births and constitutes 1.5% of cases of congenital heart disease. The reported male-to-female ratio ranges from 1.25:1 to 2:1.[9,11,15]

The embryologic basis of single ventricle is faulty alignment of the AV canal with the developing ventricle such that both AV valves are oriented toward one ventricle.[15] Subpulmonary obstruction may result from posterior deviation of the infundibular septum.[16]

Associated congenital cardiac lesions are common.[11]

Table 52-2 Distribution of anatomic types of single ventricle in 145 cases in clinical practice

Type	% of total	Pulmonic stenosis, % of type
A-I	6	44
A-II	10	50
A-III	47	45
C-I	4	68
C-II	20	76
C-III	13	94

Data from Ritter et al.[11]

Table 52-3 Various classifications of single ventricle

	Nomenclature	
Author(s)	With outlet chamber	Without outlet chamber
Van Praagh et al.[9]	Single or common ventricle, type A	Single or common ventricle, types B, C, and D
Hallermann et al.[10]	Single or common ventricle, type A	Single or common ventricle, type C
Lev et al.[12]	Single ventricle	Common ventricle
de la Cruz and Miller[13]	Double-inlet left ventricle	Single or common ventricle
Somerville et al.[14]	Common ventricle	Common ventricle

Modified from McGoon et al.[19]

Pulmonary stenosis is the most frequent, occurring in 51% of cases. Pulmonary stenosis is present in 81% of cases without an outlet chamber and in 43% of those with an outlet chamber. It occurs most frequently (94%) in cases without an outlet chamber and with L-transposition of the great arteries. It is least common (36%) in cases with an outlet chamber and D-transposition of the great arteries. Interatrial septal defects occur in 27% of cases. Fifteen percent of cases are associated with isolated levocardia, dextrocardia, or dextrocardia and situs inversus. Other associated defects include right AV valve insufficiency (12%), patent ductus arteriosus (8%), common AV valve (4%), coarctation of the aorta (3%), and pulmonary atresia (3%).

Keeton et al.[17] categorized the coronary artery anatomy in 26 patients with single ventricle; 21 had an outlet chamber and 5 did not. The majority of patients had a left dominant coronary artery pattern. In general, the left coronary artery originated from the left posterior aortic sinus, and the right coronary artery originated from the right posterior aortic sinus. In most patients with an outlet chamber, right and left delimiting arteries originating from the right and left coronary arteries, respectively, outlined the outlet chamber.

The conduction system is abnormal and variably located in single ventricle. In patients with an outlet chamber and those with AV and ventriculoarterial discordance (L-loop), there is an anomalously located anterior AV node. In patients without an outlet chamber, the location of the AV node is unpredictable – it can be located posteriorly, laterally, or anteriorly.[18] The common bundle encircles the subpulmonary outflow tract anteriorly and is closely related to the pulmonary valve attachments when the outlet chamber is leftward and anterior. When the outlet chamber is rightward and anterior, the common bundle is inferior and posterior to the pulmonary valve annulus. In patients without an outlet chamber, the common bundle is located posteriorly in the ventricular muscle mass.[19,20]

PATHOPHYSIOLOGY

The pathophysiology of tricuspid atresia or single ventricle depends on the presence and severity of pulmonary stenosis, AV valve insufficiency, ventricular function, and subaortic obstruction. Patients with significant pulmonary stenosis are cyanotic and, with time, develop polycythemia. Patients without pulmonary stenosis have increased pulmonary blood flow and may have signs and symptoms of pulmonary congestion and congestive heart failure. Patients with type I-A, I-B, II-A, or II-B tricuspid atresia (see Table 52-1) have restricted pulmonary blood flow, may have significant hypoxemia, and frequently require operative intervention to increase pulmonary blood flow. Patients with type I-C or II-C have increased pulmonary blood flow, minimal cyanosis, significant pulmonary hypertension, and congestive heart failure and frequently require operative intervention, especially during infancy, to decrease pulmonary blood flow.

Decreased ventricular function and AV valve insufficiency can develop in patients with tricuspid atresia or single ventricle and long-standing ventricular volume overload or inherent abnormalities of one or both AV valves. Increasing symptoms of congestive heart failure can occur as AV valve insufficiency and ventricular function worsen.

The development of subaortic obstruction is an important complication in patients with tricuspid atresia or single ventricle. The risk of death at the time of corrective operation is markedly increased for such patients.[21] In patients with tricuspid atresia, subaortic obstruction may occur in the presence of transposed great arteries and a ventricular septal defect that decreases in size. Subaortic obstruction may be accentuated after surgical placement of a pulmonary artery band because of marked ventricular hypertrophy. Because of the abnormally positioned AV node and common bundle, patients with A-III single ventricle have an unusually high incidence of spontaneous or surgically acquired AV block. McGoon et al.[19] reported a 17% incidence of preoperative AV block and an additional 30% incidence of AV block after cardiac septation.

HISTORY AND CLINICAL COURSE

Tricuspid atresia

Because of apparent cyanosis, congestive heart failure, or growth failure, essentially no patient with tricuspid atresia escapes medical detection by adolescence.[22,23] Indeed, all but one patient with tricuspid atresia evaluated at Boston Children's Hospital required hospitalization by 6 months of age.[1] Hypoxic spells occur in 16% to 45% of infants less than 6 months old with tricuspid atresia.[1] Without palliative treatment, 50% of patients with tricuspid atresia die by age 6 months, 60% by 1 year, and 90% by 10 years.[6] However, with the refined diagnostic and surgical techniques now available, many patients are surviving to adolescence or adulthood.

Brain abscess occurs in 1.3% to 5% of patients with tricuspid atresia – one episode of brain abscess per 273 patient-years.[24,25] Brain abscess must be suspected in any patient with cyanotic heart disease, headache, focal neurologic signs, or seizures. Of course, cerebrovascular accidents may occur in cyanotic patients with polycythemia.

Bacterial endocarditis occurs in 17% to 25% of patients with tricuspid atresia who have had a surgical systemic-to-pulmonary artery anastomosis – one episode of bacterial endocarditis per 72 patient-years.[7,26] Because patients with tricuspid atresia and normally related great arteries usually have restricted pulmonary blood flow, pulmonary vascular obstructive disease is unusual in types I-A and I-B. It does occur in patients with tricuspid atresia, normally related great arteries, and unrestricted pulmonary blood flow (type I-C).[6,27] Because patients with tricuspid atresia and transposed great arteries usually have unrestricted pulmonary blood flow, they are at risk for development of pulmonary vascular obstructive disease.

Single ventricle

The presence of congenital heart disease is apparent at an early age in most patients with single ventricle. The appearance of cyanosis, tachypnea, or poor weight gain attracts medical attention in the neonatal period or early infancy. Occasionally, patients with ample pulmonary blood flow escape detection for several months. Without treatment, long-term survival of patients with single ventricle is poor. Of 182 infants with single ventricle at the Sick Children's Hospital in Toronto, Ontario, 117 (64%) died. Fifty percent of the deaths were in the first month of life and 74% were in the first 6 months. Moodie et al.[28] assessed survival in 83 patients who were not operated on; most had survived infancy before inclusion in the study. Fifty percent of the patients with type A single ventricle were dead by 14 years after diagnosis (yearly death rate, 4.8%). Survival was even worse for patients with type C single ventricle; 50% were dead by 4 years after diagnosis. The presence of pulmonic stenosis did not appear to influence survival. The causes of death for patients with type A single ventricle included congestive heart failure in 20%, arrhythmia in 20%, and sudden, unexplained death in 10%.

Thoracolumbar scoliosis is more common in patients with cyanotic congenital heart disease than in children without heart disease. Scoliosis can be progressive and, if severe, significantly compromise respiratory function. Appropriate orthopedic consultation should be obtained for all patients with significant scoliosis.

Physical findings

Physical appearance. Patients with decreased pulmonary blood flow are cyanotic and have clubbing of the terminal digits. Patients with abnormally increased pulmonary blood flow and chronic congestive heart failure may grow poorly and have decreased subcutaneous fat development.

Arterial and venous pulses. The arterial pulses usually are normal. The jugular venous pulses usually are normal. However, they may be prominent if congestive heart failure is present, and a prominent "a" wave may be apparent in the presence of right AV valve stenosis and absence of an interatrial communication in patients with single ventricle or, if the interatrial communication becomes restrictive, in patients with tricuspid atresia. Patients with AV valve insufficiency can have a prominent v wave and a pulsatile liver.

Precordial palpation. The apical impulse is displaced laterally to the left and is overactive. The degree of overactivity is relative to the volume overload of the left ventricle, which is related to the pulmonary blood flow and presence and degree of mitral insufficiency. A palpable thrill at the mid to lower left sternal border may suggest the presence of a restrictive ventricular septal defect. Closure of the semilunar valves may be palpable in tricuspid atresia with transposed great arteries. The liver is pulsatile when the interatrial communication is restrictive. Because of a relatively anteriorly located aorta in many patients with single ventricle, aortic valve closure may be palpable at the upper left sternal border.

Auscultation

TRICUSPID ATRESIA. Cardiac murmurs are present in 80% of patients with tricuspid atresia.[6] A low-frequency holosystolic murmur or ejection murmur frequently is audible. This emanates from turbulent blood flow through the ventricular septal defect or stenotic pulmonary valve. Patients who have had a systemic or pulmonary artery communication have a continuous murmur. A superior vena cava-to-pulmonary artery (Glenn) anastomosis does not create a murmur. A murmur of mitral insufficiency may be heard, but frequently other murmurs obscure it.

SINGLE VENTRICLE. The first heart sound may be increased in intensity. The second heart sound usually is single and increased in intensity. Most patients have a relatively loud systolic murmur resulting from pulmonary stenosis or flow through a bulboventricular foramen (the opening from the ventricular chamber into the overflow chamber). Patients with increased pulmonary blood flow may have a middiastolic apical murmur from increased blood flow through the AV valves.

Electrocardiogram

For tricuspid atresia, the usual rhythm is sinus with tall peaked P waves indicative of right atrial enlargement (Fig 52-1). The frontal plane vectorcardiographic loop is oriented to the left and superiorly. In 7% of cases (usually associated with transposed great arteries), the frontal plane QRS axis is normal (0° to +90°); in 4% of cases, the axis may be to the right.[6] The right ventricular electrocardiographic forces are diminished, and usually there is evidence of left ventricular hypertrophy with discordant QRS and T waves. The P-R interval is prolonged in approximately 15% of cases,[1] presumably due to prolonged atrial conduction time because AV node function usually is normal. Rarely, ventricular preexcitation (Wolff-Parkinson-White syndrome) occurs in patients with tricuspid atresia.

The electrocardiogram most characteristic of single ventricle is the one associated with an A-III single ventricle (Fig 52-2). Because of embryologic L-looping, septal depolarization is reversed from normal (i.e., the forces are directed posteriorly and leftward). This produces a Q wave in lead V_1 and absence of a Q wave in lead V_6. In addition, most patients have evidence of anterior ventricular enlargement.

Chest radiograph

Most patients with tricuspid atresia or single ventricle have cardiomegaly.[10] The pulmonary vascular markings are increased in patients with increased pulmonary blood flow and decreased in those with significant pulmonic stenosis. The right atrium may be prominent in patients with tricuspid atresia.

Exercise testing

Exercise tolerance is decreased with increasing age. In our laboratory, the maximum oxygen uptake with exercise was 44% of predicted and decreased progressively with increasing age.[29] Systemic arterial blood oxygen saturation decreased from a mean of 86% at rest to 63% with exercise. Ventilation is abnormal. The upper limit of ventilatory capacity is reached at a relatively low oxygen uptake. The resting ventilatory equivalent for oxygen was abnormally increased (59%) and increased further with exercise, to 65% in our patients.

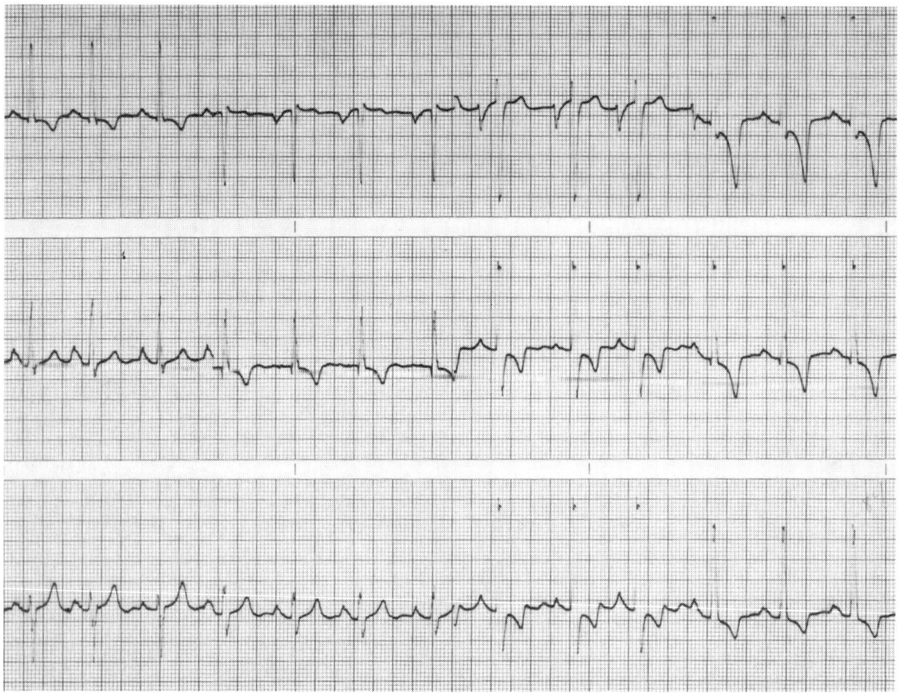

Fig 52-1 Typical electrocardiographic pattern for tricuspid atresia: left-axis deviation of the frontal plane QRS axis, and evidence of right atrial enlargement and left ventricular hypertrophy.

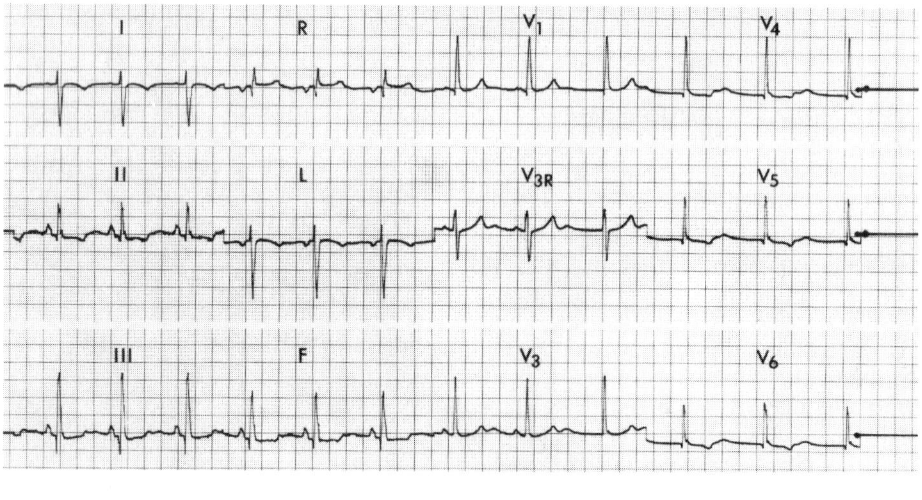

Fig 52-2 Electrocardiogram characteristic of A-III single ventricle.

DIAGNOSTIC PROBLEMS AND INDICATIONS FOR INVASIVE STUDIES

Cardiac catheterization and angiography

The goals of cardiac catheterization must include establishing (1) the type of tricuspid atresia or single ventricle, (2) for patients with single ventricle, the presence and location of an outlet chamber, (3) the spatial relationship of the aorta and pulmonary artery and the ventriculoarteriolar relationships, (4) the presence and location of obstruction to pulmonary or systemic blood flow, (5) the degree of AV valve insufficiency, (6) pulmonary artery pressure and arteriolar resistance, (7) pulmonary artery size, distribution, and distortion from previous operation, (8) ventricular end-diastolic pressure and ventricular ejection fraction, (9) the presence of associated lesions, and (10) the presence or absence of AV fistulae in a previously established Glenn anastomosis. This information is critical when patients are considered for the modified Fontan operation. Infants with tricuspid atresia, mitral atresia, or double-inlet ventricle with a stenotic AV valve may benefit from cardiac catheterization and balloon or blade atrial septectomy.

Echocardiography

Two-dimensional echocardiography has supplanted invasive cardiac catheterization studies for many aspects of the evaluation of a patient with tricuspid atresia or single ventricle. The basic intracardiac anatomy, great vessel relationships, associated cardiac defects, presence of pulmonary stenosis, and size of the bulboventricular foramen can be assessed with two-dimensional echocardiography. Doppler echocardiography techniques can quantitate pulmonary stenosis, bulboventricular foramen obstruction, and degree of AV valve insufficiency. Echocardiographic techniques clearly are superior to angiography for assessing AV valve morphology, overriding, and straddling.

MANAGEMENT

The principles of management are similar for patients with tricuspid atresia and single ventricle. Medical management for infants with restricted pulmonary blood flow and severe hypoxemia includes infusion of prostaglandin E_1 to maintain patency of the ductus arteriosus until a systemic-to-pulmonary artery anastomosis can be constructed. The use of balloon atrial septostomy in infants with tricuspid atresia is controversial. Some investigators have recommended balloon atrial septostomy for all infants with tricuspid atresia. Other investigators point out that the intra-atrial communication is unrestrictive in most of these patients and that balloon atrial septostomy is indicated only for those with a small interatrial communication. Blade atrial septostomy is useful in older children in whom an intra-atrial communication that once was adequate has become restricted. Balloon or blade septostomy may also be helpful in patients with mitral atresia and a restrictive atrial septal defect.

Patients with increased pulmonary blood flow or decreased ventricular function and congestive heart failure benefit from digitalis, diuretic drugs, and, perhaps, afterload-reducing agents. Patients with pulmonary vascular obstructive disease and polycythemia who are not candidates for corrective operation can have venoclysis for reduction of erythrocyte mass for symptomatic relief from headache and fatigue associated with extreme polycythemia. Medical management should also be directed toward prevention of bacterial endocarditis or treatment of bacterial endocarditis if it occurs. Patients with a right-to-left shunt are at increased risk for brain abscess, and brain abscess must be identified and appropriately treated.

There are three categories of surgical approach to patients with tricuspid atresia or single ventricle: (1) palliative operations to increase (systemic-to-pulmonary artery shunts) or decrease (pulmonary artery banding) pulmonary blood flow, (2) ventricular septation, and (3) ventricular exclusion (Fontan) procedures. Patients with decreased and increased pulmonary blood flow may obtain symptomatic improvement from systemic-to-pulmonary artery (or Glenn) anastomosis and pulmonary artery banding, respectively. Usually these procedures are necessary early in life. However, these palliative procedures have distinct disadvantages. Systemic-to-pulmonary artery shunts can kink and distort the pulmonary artery, so that subsequent definitive repair is more difficult or impossible. Increasing pulmonary blood flow too much increases the ventricular volume load and may contribute to ventricular failure. A Glenn anastomosis does not increase ventricular volume overload but occasionally has been associated with the late development of ipsilateral pulmonary arteriovenous fistulae. Distal migration of a pulmonary artery band can cause distortion of a pulmonary artery. In patients with an outlet chamber, pulmonary artery banding has been associated with accelerated diminution in diameter (stenosis) of the bulboventricular foramen.

The septation operation[19] involves placing a large synthetic patch within the single functioning ventricle of the anomaly to divide the AV valves and the ventricular chamber into two parts – one to function as the pulmonary ventricle and the other as the systemic ventricle. The procedure is extremely complex and subject to many technical and anatomic challenges. As a result, the relatively high early and late mortality rates have greatly dampened enthusiasm for the procedure at this time. On the basis of studies by Feldt et al.[30] and McKay et al.,[31] if septation procedures are to be used, they should be restricted to patients with an anterior and leftward subaortic outlet chamber (type A-III), normal AV valves, absence of bulboventricular foramen obstruction, no prior palliative procedures, and absence of congestive heart failure and profound polycythemia. Indeed, the modified Fontan operation probably is superior to ventricular septation procedures.

The concept of ventricular exclusion described by Fontan and Baudet[32] can be used for the management of patients with tricuspid atresia and for patients with single ventricle. Fontan and his associates constructed a Glenn anastomosis to direct superior vena caval systemic venous return to the right lung, directed inferior vena caval systemic venous return to the pulmonary artery with a valve-containing conduit connecting the right atrium and pulmonary artery, inserted a valve into the inferior vena cava, closed the interatrial communication, and obliterated the connection of the ventricle to the pulmonary artery. Although this procedure has been modified considerably, the concept of directing systemic venous return from the right atrium directly to the pulmonary arteries or via a hypoplastic right ventricle has retained the eponymous designation "the Fontan procedure."

There is considerable debate about the most efficacious modification of the Fontan operation. Nearly all investigators think that a prosthetic valve in the inferior vena cava or atrial-to-pulmonary artery connection is unnecessary. In addition, the most efficacious method of directing systemic venous return to the pulmonary arteries is yet to be defined.

Choussat et al.[33] outlined 10 criteria for low-risk operability: (1) age at operation between 4 and 15 years, (2) presence of sinus rhythm, (3) normal systemic venous return, (4) normal right atrial volume, (5) mean pulmonary artery pressure ≤ 15 mm Hg, (6) pulmonary arteriolar resistance <4 U · m^2, (7) ratio of pulmonary artery diameter to aortic diameter >0.75, (8) left ventricular ejection fraction $\geq 60\%$, (9) competent mitral valve, and (10) no adverse effects from prior pulmonary artery operation. Experience has shown that these should be considered guidelines, and the absence of one or more of them is not necessarily an absolute contraindication to the use of the modified Fontan procedure. For example, sequential AV pacemaker systems can be implanted to establish synchronous AV contraction for patients with complete AV block. Innovative baffle techniques can be used to redirect blood flow from unusual vena caval attachments to the pulmonary artery. A significant increase in pulmonary vascular resistance is an absolute contraindication to the Fontan operation. AV valve regurgitation can be managed with repair of the valve, but the need to repair the valve or replace the mitral valve in patients with single ventricle presents an important risk factor for good long-term survival.

Humes et al.[34] reported the results of the Fontan operation for 135 patients with tricuspid atresia operated on at the Mayo Clinic between 1973 and 1985. There were 14 (10%) hospital and 13 late deaths. For those who survived the operation (including the first 30 postoperative days), 1- and 5-year survival rates were 95% and 87%, respectively. Of the 80 patients who had complete long-term follow-up with information, 92% were in New York Heart Association Class I or II, 97% worked or attended school, 52% were taking no cardiac medications, and 13% (10 patients) had persistent ascites or edema.

Between 1973 and 1985, 120 patients with the double-inlet left ventricle form of single ventricle had a modified Fontan operation at the Mayo Clinic.[34] There were 18 hospital deaths and 10 late deaths. However, current hospital mortality is approximately 8% for this group of patients. Predicted survival after hospital dismissal in the study by Humes et al. was 96% at 1 year and 85% at 5 years. Only a minority of these patients fulfilled all 10 of the criteria for a low-risk operation outlined by Choussat et al.[33]

Recently, results of a long-term follow-up study of the initial 352 patients undergoing a Fontan operation at the Mayo Clinic were reported.[35] This study encompassed 125 patients with tricuspid atresia, 114 with univentricular heart, and 113 with complex forms of single ventricle. The 1-, 5-, and 10-year survival rates were 77%, 70%, and 60%, respectively. In a multivariate model, the following factors contributed to poorer survival: types of single ventricle other than tricuspid atresia, earlier calendar year of operation, heteroataxia syndromes, young age at operation, increased mean pulmonary artery pressure, AV valve dysfunction, and poorer preoperative New York Heart Association classification. Five years after operation, 40% of the survivors were taking no cardiac medications and 60% continued to require one or more cardiac medications. Late postoperative problems included arrhythmias in approximately 20% of patients and hypoproteinemia or protein-losing enteropathy in 7% to 10% of patients. Although excellent results can be achieved with the Fontan operation, it is important to select patients for this operation judiciously to ensure good long-term results.

REFERENCES

1. Rosenthal A, Dick M II: Tricuspid atresia. In *Moss' Heart Disease in Infants, Children, and Adolescents*. Third edition. Edited by FH Adams, GC Emmanouilides. Baltimore, Williams & Wilkins, 1983, pp 271-283
2. Kühne M: Über zwei Falle kongenitaler Atresie des Ostium venosum dextrum. *Jahrb Kinderheilkd* 63:235-249, 1906
3. Rao PS (ed): *Tricuspid Atresia*. Mount Kisco, New York, Futura Publishing Company, 1982, pp 13-24
4. Edwards JE, Burchell HB. Congenital tricuspid atresia: a classification. *Med Clin North Am* July 1949, pp 1177-1196
5. Tandon R, Edwards JE: Tricuspid atresia: a re-evaluation and classification. *J Thorac Cardiovasc Surg* 67:530-542, 1974
6. Vlad P: Tricuspid atresia. In *Heart Disease in Infancy and Childhood*. Third edition. Edited by JD Keith, RD Rowe, P Vlad. New York, Macmillan Publishing Company, 1978, pp 518-541
7. Dick M, Fyler DC, Nadas AS: Tricuspid atresia: clinical course in 101 patients. *Am J Cardiol* 36:327-337, 1975
8. Report of the New England Regional Infant Cardiac Program. *Pediatrics* 65 Suppl:388; 392-403, 1980
9. Van Praagh R, Ongley PA, Swan HJC: Anatomic types of single or common ventricle in man: morphologic and geometric aspects of 60 necropsied cases. *Am J Cardiol* 13:367-386, 1964
10. Hallermann FJ, Davis GD, Ritter DG, et al: Roentgenographic features of common ventricle. *Radiology* 87:409-423, 1966
11. Ritter DG, Seward JB, Moodie D, et al: Univentricular heart (common ventricle): preoperative diagnosis; hemodynamic, angiocardiographic and echocardiographic features. *Herz* 4:198-205, 1979
12. Lev M, Liberthson RR, Kirkpatrick JR, et al: Single (primitive) ventricle. *Circulation* 39:577-591, 1969
13. de la Cruz MV, Miller BL: Double-inlet left ventricle: two pathological specimens with comments on the embryology and on its relation to single ventricle. *Circulation* 37:249-260, 1968
14. Somerville J, Becu L, Ross D: Common ventricle with acquired subaortic obstruction. *Am J Cardiol* 34:206-214, 1974
15. Kidd BSL: Single ventricle. In *Heart Disease in Infancy and Childhood*. Third edition. Edited by JD Keith, RD Rowe, P Vlad. New York, Macmillan Publishing Company, 1978, pp 405-417
16. Elliott LP, Anderson RH, Bargeron LM Jr, et al: Single or univentricular heart. In *Moss' Heart Disease in Infants, Children, and Adolescents*. Third edition. Edited by FH Adams, GC Emmanouilides. Baltimore, Williams & Wilkins, 1983, pp 386-400
17. Keeton BR, Lie JT, McGoon DC, et al: Anatomy of coronary arteries in univentricular hearts and its surgical implications. *Am J Cardiol* 43:569-580, 1979
18. Anderson RH, Arnold R, Thapar MK, et al: Cardiac specialized tissue in hearts with an apparently single ventricular chamber (double inlet left ventricle). *Am J Cardiol* 33:95-106, 1974
19. McGoon DC, Danielson GK, Ritter DG, et al: Correction of the univentricular heart having two atrioventricular valves. *J Thorac Cardiovasc Surg* 74:218-226, 1977
20. Bharati S, Lev M: The course of the conduction system in single ventricle with inverted (L-) loop and inverted (L-) transposition. *Circulation* 51:723-730, 1975
21. Barber G, Hagler DJ, Edwards WD, et al: Surgical repair of univentricular heart (double inlet left ventricle) with obstructed anterior subaortic outlet chamber. *J Am Coll Cardiol* 4:771-778, 1984
22. Bohm R, Schmidt K-H, Günther KH, et al: Tricuspid atresia and ventricular septal defect in a 31-year-old woman. *Cardiologia (Basel)* 53:11-18, 1968
23. Jordan JC, Sanders CA: Tricuspid atresia with prolonged survival: a report of two cases with a review of the world literature. *Am J Cardiol* 18:112-119, 1966
24. Dick M II, Rosenthal A: The clinical profile of tricuspid atresia. In *Tricuspid Atresia*. Edited by PS Rao. Mount Kisco, New York, Futura Publishing Company, 1982, pp 83-111
25. Fischbein CA, Rosenthal A, Fischer EG, et al: Risk factors for

brain abscess in patients with congenital heart disease. *Am J Cardiol* 34:97-102, 1974

26. Taussig HB, Keinonen R, Momberger N, et al: Long-time observations on the Blalock-Taussig operation. IV. Tricuspid atresia. *Johns Hopkins Med J* 132:135-145, 1973

27. Tingelstad JB, Lower RR, Howell TR, et al: Pulmonary artery banding in tricuspid atresia without transposed great arteries. *Am J Dis Child* 121:434-437, 1971

28. Moodie DS, Ritter DG, Tajik AJ, et al: Long-term follow-up in the unoperated univentricular heart. *Am J Cardiol* 53:1124-1128, 1984

29. Driscoll DJ, Danielson GK, Puga FJ, et al: Exercise tolerance and cardiorespiratory response to exercise after the Fontan operation for tricuspid atresia on functional single ventricle. *J Am Coll Cardiol* 7:1087-1094, 1986

30. Feldt RH, Mair DD, Danielson GK, et al: Current status of the septation procedure for univentricular heart. *J Thorac Cardiovasc Surg* 82:93-97, 1981

31. McKay R, Pacifico AD, Blackstone EH, et al: Septation of the univentricular heart with left anterior subaortic outlet chamber. *J Thorac Cardiovasc Surg* 84:77-87, 1982

32. Fontan F, Baudet E: Surgical repair of tricuspid atresia. *Thorax* 26:240-248, 1971

33. Choussat A, Fontan F, Besse P, et al: Selection criteria for Fontan's procedure. *Pediatr Cardiol* 1978, pp 559-566

34. Humes RA, Porter CJ, Mair DD, et al: Intermediate follow-up and predicted survival after the modified Fontan procedure for tricuspid atresia and double-inlet ventricle. *Circulation* 76 Suppl 3:67-71, 1987

35. Driscoll DJ, Offord KP, Feldt RH, et al: Five- to fifteen-year follow-up after Fontan operation. *Circulation* 85:469-496, 1992

CHAPTER

53

Dextrotransposition of the great arteries

David J. Driscoll, M.D., and Francisco J. Puga, M.D.

ANATOMIC CONSIDERATIONS

D-transposition of the great arteries implies that the positions of the aorta and pulmonary artery are reversed relative to the ventricular septum. The pulmonary artery arises from the morphological left ventricle and the aorta, from the morphological right ventricle (Fig 53-1). The atrioventricular (AV) connections are normal. Thus, there is AV concordance and ventriculoarterial discordance. Forty percent of patients with D-transposition of the great arteries have an associated ventricular septal defect. Pulmonic stenosis occurs in 6% with intact ventricular septum and 31% with ventricular septal defect.[1] Most have a patent ductus arteriosus at birth that subsequently closes.

The left coronary artery arises from the left aortic sinus, and the right coronary artery arises from the posterior aortic sinus. In 31 of 149 cases,[2] the circumflex coronary artery and right coronary artery originated from the posterior aortic sinus.

D-transposition of the great arteries results from abnormal conotruncal formation. Two theories exist regarding the mechanism for this. Van Praagh et al.[3] suggested that the normal pulmonary conus fails to form but a subaortic conus forms. This prevents the normal twisting of the aorta and pulmonary trunks, and these vessels remain aligned with the inappropriate ventricle. The second theory is based on abnormal fusion and lack of spiralling of the conal and truncal swellings.[4]

PATHOPHYSIOLOGY

In D-transposition of the great arteries, the systemic and pulmonary circulatory systems are parallel rather than in series. In the absence of associated anomalies, systemic venous blood returns to the systemic arterial system and pulmonary venous blood returns to the pulmonary arterial system—a situation incompatible with life. For survival, a communication must exist between these two systems. In most cases, a patent foramen ovale allows interatrial mixing of oxygenated and deoxygenated blood. Additional possible sites of mixing include a patent ductus arteriosus and a ventricular septal defect. In general, the degree of systemic arterial hypoxemia is inversely related to the number of mixing sites and the presence of pulmonic stenosis.

The volume of oxygenated blood (from left atrium, left ventricle, or pulmonary artery) that traverses a communication to reach the systemic circulation (right atrium, right ventricle, aorta) represents effective systemic blood flow, and the volume of deoxygenated blood (from right atrium, right ventricle, aorta) that traverses a communication and reaches the pulmonary circulation (left atrium, left ventricle, pulmonary artery) represents effective pulmonary blood flow. Usually, a relatively larger volume of blood than the effective systemic blood flow or effective pulmonary blood flow recirculates through the systemic circulation (the physiologic right-to-left shunt) or the

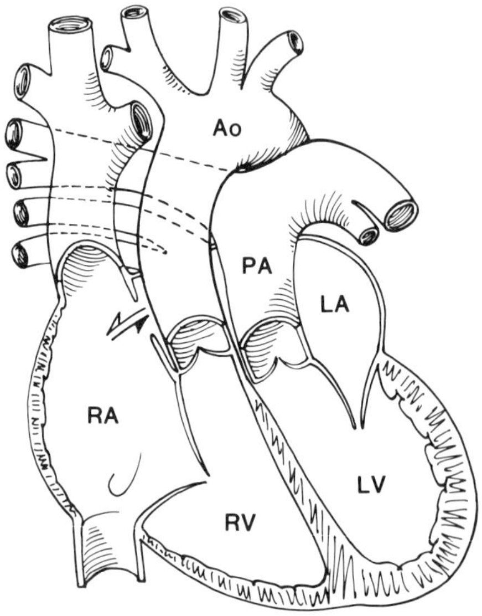

Fig 53-1 Diagram of D-transposition of the great arteries. The aorta *(Ao)* originates from the right ventricle *(RV)*, and the pulmonary artery *(PA)* originates from the left ventricle *(LV)*. *LA*, left atrium; *RA*, right atrium.

pulmonary circulation (the physiologic left-to-right shunt).[5] Because of this, pulmonary blood flow usually is increased in patients who have transposition of the great arteries and intact ventricular septum. Pulmonary blood flow may be decreased in patients who have transposition of the great arteries with ventricular septal defect and pulmonic stenosis.

CLINICAL SYNDROME
History and clinical course

Essentially all patients with D-transposition of the great arteries attract medical attention in infancy, usually early in infancy because of cyanosis or congestive heart failure or both. Without treatment, 30% of these patients die in the first week of life, 50% in the first month, 70% in the first 6 months, and 90% before the end of the first year.[5]

Transposition of the great arteries is more common in infants whose mothers are diabetic than in those whose mothers are not diabetic. Only 9% of patients with transposition of the great arteries have associated extracardiac anomalies.[5]

Because palliative and definitive operations for transposition of the great arteries may affect the cardiac conduction system, patients who have had these procedures (atrial septectomy, Mustard and Senning procedures) may have arrhythmias. For example, Hagler et al.[6] reported that 17 of 48 patients had junctional rhythm and 8 of 48 had a history of supraventricular tachycardia after the Mustard operation.

Pulmonary vascular obstructive disease develops more rapidly in patients with transposition of the great arteries and associated ventricular septal defect than in those with ventricular septal defect alone. Some adolescents and young adults who have not had definitive repair in infancy or childhood will have this complication. These patients will have continued cyanosis and polycythemia and are subject to the complications of right-to-left shunt and polycythemia, including stroke and brain abscess. Infants and young children with associated ventricular septal defect and pulmonic stenosis and those with intact ventricular septum and either dynamic or fixed left ventricular outflow obstruction can have hypercyanotic episodes resembling the spells observed in patients with tetralogy of Fallot.[5]

Physical findings

Physical appearance. Babies with transposition of the great arteries tend to be well developed but cyanotic. Cyanotic older infants and children exhibit terminal digital clubbing.

Arterial and venous pulses. The arterial and venous pulses usually are normal. The jugular venous pulses may be abnormal if superior vena cava or inferior vena cava obstruction develops after the Mustard or Senning operation.

Precordial palpation. The cardiac impulse at the lower left sternal border (right ventricular impulse) is prominent. Closure of the aortic component of the second heart sound may be palpable at the upper left sternal border.

Auscultation. The first cardiac sound usually is normal. Because of the relatively anterior location of the aorta, the second heart sound is accentuated and usually is single. However, in some cases the second heart sound can be split. Characteristically, infants with transposition of the great arteries and intact ventricular septum without pulmonary stenosis have only a soft or no cardiac murmur. Patients with a ventricular septal defect or pulmonary stenosis or both have a holosystolic murmur audible at the lower left sternal border. A middiastolic low-frequency murmur frequently is audible at the cardiac apex due to increased pulmonary blood flow across the mitral valve.

Electrocardiogram

In the newborn the electrocardiogram may be normal. However, in all other patients it is characterized by right-axis deviation and right ventricular hypertrophy.

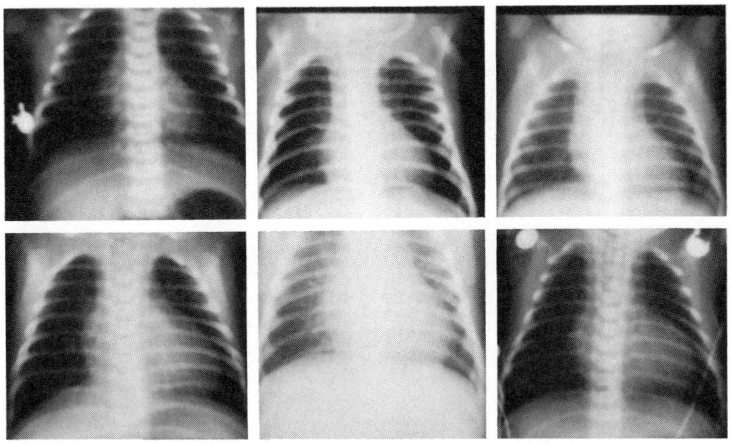

Fig 53-2 Chest radiographs from six infants with D-transposition of the great arteries. Cardiac size varies from normal to increased; pulmonary vascular markings vary from plethoric to oligemic.

After operation (particularly after the Mustard operation), the P-wave voltage may be diminished, and there is a relatively high incidence of sinus node dysfunction manifested by sinus bradycardia, junctional rhythm, and supraventricular tachycardia. The electrocardiogram may be normal for patients who have had the arterial switch procedure.

Chest radiograph

Cardiomegaly with increased pulmonary vascular markings is the most common radiographic appearance in infants with transposition of the great arteries. However, depending on the presence of associated intracardiac anomalies, the chest radiograph may be characterized by oligemic lung fields and a normal heart size (Fig 53-2). The superior mediastinal shadow may appear narrow in patients with transposition of the great arteries, but this is not a particularly helpful sign because it may occur normally or in patients with other complex forms of congenital heart disease. There is no chest radiographic appearance absolutely typical for transposition of the great arteries.

DIAGNOSTIC PROBLEMS AND INDICATIONS FOR INVASIVE STUDIES

Cardiac catheterization

Prior to the introduction of echocardiography, a basic tenet of pediatric cardiology was that cardiac catheterization should be performed as an emergency procedure for all cyanotic newborns. Initial survival of patients with transposition of the great arteries is related to the degree of mixing of systemic and pulmonary venous return. Hence, rapid and accurate diagnosis is essential so that venous mixing can be promptly optimized. Rashkind and Miller[7] described a technique used during catheterization to increase interatrial venous mixing by tearing the valve of the fossa ovalis with a balloon-tipped catheter. This technique allows survival of many infants with transposition of the great arteries who otherwise would die. By using a cutting catheter device described by Park et al.,[8] interatrial mixing can be increased in older infants and children in whom the valve of the fossa ovalis is too fibrous or too thick to be torn with a balloon-tipped catheter.

Right atrial blood pressure usually is normal. The finding of similar right atrial and left atrial blood pressures does not establish the presence of a large, unrestrictive interatrial communication. In the newborn, right ventricular blood pressure is typically equal to systemic arterial blood pressure. The left ventricular blood pressure will depend on the presence and size of a ventricular septal defect, the degree of pulmonic stenosis or dynamic left ventricular outflow obstruction, the degree of pulmonary vascular obstructive disease, and the age of the patient.

Angiocardiography delineates the abnormal ventriculoarterial relationships and presence of associated abnormalities (Fig 53-3).

The indications for cardiac catheterization have changed with the introduction of echocardiography, prostaglandin E_1 treatment, and the arterial switch procedure

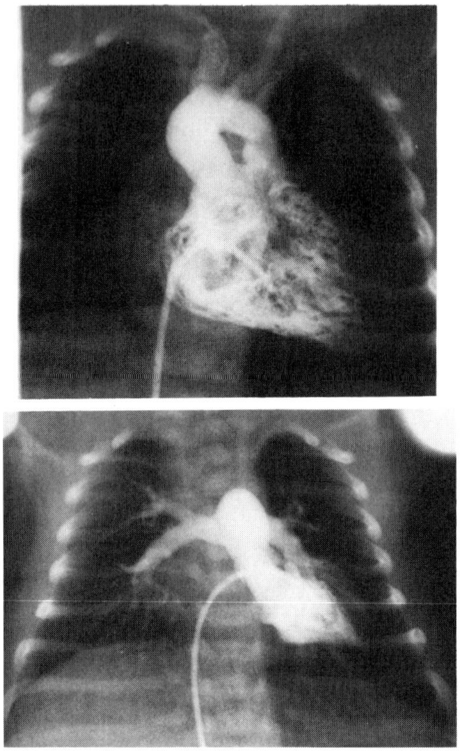

Fig 53-3 Angiograms demonstrating D-transposition of the great arteries.

for repair of transposition of the great arteries. Some surgeons are comfortable performing the arterial switch procedure in the newborn on the basis of echocardiographic delineation of the cardiac anatomy. Other surgeons think it is important to exclude certain congenital coronary artery anomalies by angiography before proceeding with operation. Since the presence of an atrial septal defect to allow adequate intracardiac mixing can be ascertained by echocardiography, not all babies with transposition of the great arteries require cardiac catheterization for balloon atrial septostomy.

Echocardiography

With two-dimensional echocardiography, the aorta and pulmonary artery can be identified by the posterior curvature of the aorta and the bifurcation of the pulmonary artery.[9] The presence of associated defects can be assessed and the size of the interatrial communication can be measured. Thus, emergency cardiac catheterization may be unnecessary if the diagnosis is apparent from echocardiography and adequate sites for intracardiac mixing are identified. Indeed, even balloon atrial septostomy has been performed with echocardiographic guidance.

MANAGEMENT

Critically ill newborns with transposition of the great arteries may benefit from infusion of prostaglandin E_1.[10] Enlargement of the interatrial communication (Rashkind balloon septostomy, Park blade septostomy, or Blalock-Hanlon septectomy) is important and is urgently required in patients with limited mixture of systemic and pulmonary venous returns. Digitalis and diuretic agents may be beneficial for patients with cardiomegaly and evidence of congestive heart failure.

Two general categories of definitive operative procedures are available for transposition of the great arteries: (1) rerouting of systemic and pulmonary venous returns in the atria to direct systemic venous return to the left ventricle and pulmonary venous return to the right ventricle (Senning and Mustard procedures[11,12]) and (2) establishing continuity between the left ventricle and aorta and between the right ventricle and pulmonary artery (Rastelli procedure, Kaye-Damus-Stansel procedure, and Jatene procedure).

The Senning and Mustard procedures have been used for more than 25 years. At present, the operative mortality for these procedures is less than 5% for patients who have transposition of great arteries with no significant associated abnormalities and 10% to 29% for patients with associated abnormalities.[13] Gutgesell and McNamara[14] assessed survival of a cohort of 62 infants who had transposition of the great arteries with intact ventricular septum; all had had balloon atrial septostomy shortly after birth and a Mustard operation at approximately 12 months of age. Eighty-seven percent were alive at 3 months, 77% at 1 year, and 66% at 2 years. Tynan[15] reported 65% survival at 1 year and 55% at 2 years after balloon atrial septostomy. At the Mayo Clinic, incidence of late death among 118 survivors of the Mustard operation performed between 1964 and 1973 was 21%.[16] Causes of death included progressive pulmonary vascular obstructive disease, arrhythmias, and residual or recurrent hemodynamic problems.

The Mustard or Senning procedure without closure of the ventricular septal defect ("palliative Mustard or Senning procedure")[17] has been used to improve the quality of life of patients with transposition of the great arteries, ventricular septal defect, and such severe pulmonary vascular obstructive disease that closure of the ventricular septal defect was contraindicated. With pulmonary resistance > 10 units · m^2, the ventricular septal defect cannot be closed safely. However, rerouting sys-

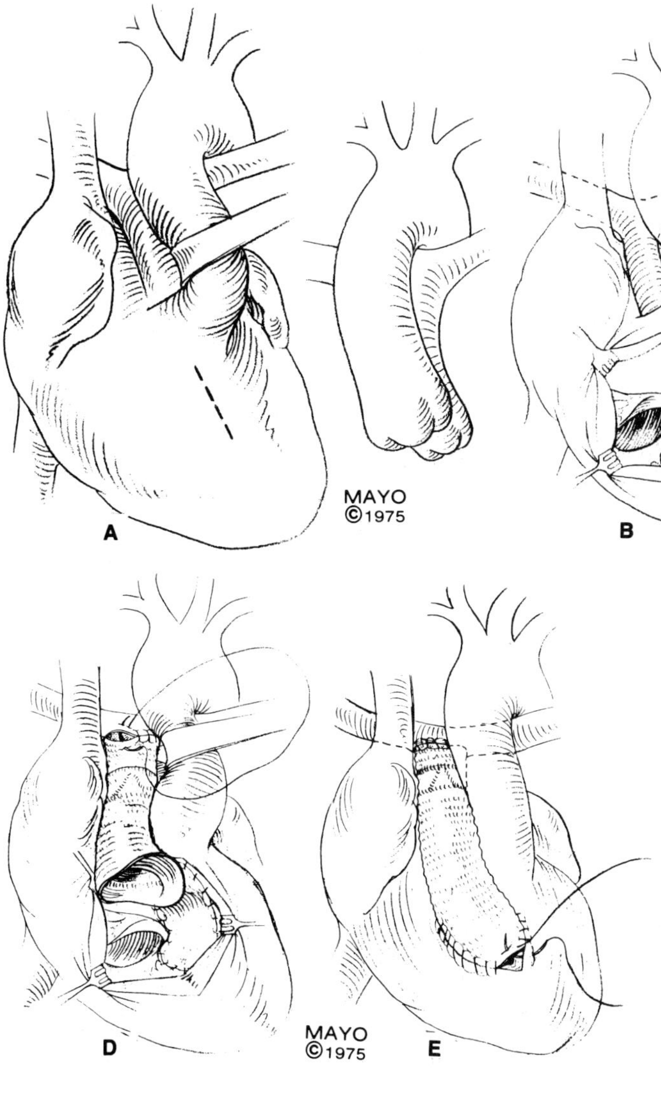

Fig 53-4 Rastelli operation. **A,** longitudinal ventriculotomy. **B,** tricuspid orifice and ventricular septal defect; *shaded area* represents tissue to be resected to enlarge the septal defect. **C,** septal defect is closed by patch to form a tunnel extending from left ventricle through septal defect and into the aorta; the pulmonary trunk has been divided and its proximal orifice has been oversewn. **D** and **E,** continuity between right ventricle and pulmonary artery is achieved by means of an extracardiac conduit. (From Marcelletti C, Mair DD, McGoon DC, et al: The Rastelli operation for transposition of the great arteries: early and late results. *J Thorac Cardiovasc Surg* 72:427-434, 1976. By permission, Mayo Foundation.)

temic and venous returns without closing the ventricular septal defect improves systemic arterial blood oxygen saturation in these patients. This improvement is typically much greater than simple reversal of the preoperative systemic and pulmonary arterial blood oxygen saturations.

In 1969, the Rastelli procedure was described;[18] it restores left ventricular and aortic continuity and right ventricular and pulmonary artery continuity in patients with transposition of the great arteries, ventricular septal defect, and pulmonary stenosis. The ventricular septal defect is closed so that blood ejected from the left ventricle is directed through the ventricular septal defect and exits through the aorta. The pulmonary artery is transected, and a conduit is interposed between the right ventricle and the distal main pulmonary artery (Fig 53-4). Marcelletti et al.[19] reported results of the Rastelli procedure in 59 patients operated on between 1968 and 1975. There were 11 (19%) postoperative deaths and 5 late deaths. In the last 25 patients in this series, however, the mortality was only 8%. Eleven patients required reoperation, mostly for conduit obstruction; undoubtedly, this number will increase with time. The survival after this operation compares very favorably to results after the Mustard procedure in patients with ventricular septal defect (26% mortality) or ventricular septal defect and pulmonic stenosis (28.5% mortality).[13] The major disadvantage of this procedure is progressive conduit obstruction or obstruction of the valve within the conduit. Several innovative operative techniques have been described recently to obviate a prosthetic conduit for establishment of continuity between the right ventricle and the pulmonary artery. The short- and middle-term results of these techniques are unknown.

In 1975, Kaye,[20] Damus,[21] and Stansel[22] independently reported a technique to establish left ventricular and aortic continuity and right ventricular and pulmonary artery continuity in patients with transposition of the great arteries and intact ventricular septum. The pulmonary artery is transected, and the distal opening of the proximal pulmonary artery stump is anastomosed end-to-side to the ascending aorta. Blood from the left ventricle is ejected through this stump into the aorta. The right ventricle is connected to the proximal main pulmonary artery by using a conduit.

Currently, the best surgical option for infants with transposition of the great arteries and a normal pulmonary valve is the arterial switch procedure described by Jatene et al.[23] and modified by others. In this procedure, the main pulmonary artery and proximal aorta are transected, the proximal main pulmonary artery is anastomosed to the distal aorta, and the proximal aorta is anastomosed to the distal pulmonary artery. The coronary ostia have to be transferred to the "new" aorta. This "arterial switch" can be performed only if the left ventricle has been subjected to systemic pressure and is capable of assuming the challenge of sustaining high-pressure blood propulsion. Thus, the procedure is reserved for infants with systemic pressure in the left ventricle, patients with associated ventricular septal defect and systemic pressure in the left ventricle, or patients in whom the left ventricle has been prepared by prior pulmonary artery banding. Several investigators[24-27] have reported the results of relatively large series of infants in whom the arterial switch procedure was used for correction. As experience with this operation has increased, the operative mortality has decreased. At present, the operative mortality with experienced surgeons is less than 10% and in some institutions is less than 5%. The short- to middle-term results of this procedure appear to be excellent.

The arterial switch procedure likely will provide better long-term results than atrial switch procedures (Senning or Mustard). However, the fate of the coronary arteries after the arterial switch procedure, the incidence and severity of supravalvar pulmonic or aortic stenosis at the sites of great artery anastomoses, and the fate of the pulmonary valve subjected to prolonged systemic arterial pressure remain to be determined.

REFERENCES

1. Kidd BSL: Complete transposition of the great arteries. In *Heart Disease in Infancy and Childhood.* Third edition. Edited by JD Keith, RD Rowe, P Vlad. New York, Macmillan Publishing Co, 1978, pp 590-611
2. Shaher RM, Puddu GC: Coronary arterial anatomy in complete transposition of the great vessels. *Am J Cardiol* 17:355-361, 1966
3. Van Praagh R, Layton WM, Van Praagh S: The morphogenesis of normal and abnormal relationships between the great arteries and the ventricles: pathologic and experimental data. In *Etiology and Morphogenesis of Congenital Heart Disease.* Edited by R Van Praagh, A Takao. Mount Kisco, New York, Futura Publishing Company, 1980, pp 271-316
4. Van Mierop LHS: Pathology and pathogenesis of the common cardiac malformations. *Cardiovasc Clin* 2 No 1:27-59, 1970
5. Paul MH: Transposition of the great arteries. In *Moss' Heart Disease in Infants, Children, and Adolescents.* Third edition. Edited by FH Adams, GC Emmanouilides. Baltimore, Williams & Wilkins, 1983, pp 296-333
6. Hagler DJ, Ritter DG, Mair DD, et al: Clinical, angiographic, and hemodynamic assessment of late results after Mustard operation. *Circulation* 57:1214-1220, 1978
7. Rashkind WJ, Miller WW: Creation of an atrial septal defect without thoracotomy: a palliative approach to complete transposition of the great arteries. *JAMA* 196:991-992, 1966
8. Park SC, Neches WH, Zuberbuhler JR, et al: Clinical use of blade atrial septostomy. *Circulation* 58:600-606, 1978
9. Daskalopoulos DA, Edwards WD, Driscoll DJ, et al: Correlation of two-dimensional echocardiographic and autopsy findings in complete transposition of the great arteries. *J Am Coll Cardiol* 2:1151-1157, 1983
10. Driscoll DJ, Kugler JD, Nihill MR, et al: The use of prostaglandin E_1 in a critically ill infant with transposition of the great arteries. *J Pediatr* 95:259-261, 1979
11. Senning Å: Surgical correction of transposition of the great vessels. *Surgery* 45:966-980, 1959
12. Mustard WT: Successful two-stage correction of transposition of the great vessels. *Surgery* 55:469-472, 1964
13. Arciniegas E, Farooki ZQ, Hakimi M, et al: Results of the Mustard operation for dextro-transposition of the great arteries. *J Thorac Cardiovasc Surg* 81:580-587, 1981
14. Gutgesell HP, McNamara DG: Transposition of the great arteries: results of treatment with early palliation and late intracardiac repair. *Circulation* 51:32-38, 1975
15. Tynan M: Survival of infants with transposition of great arteries after balloon atrial septostomy. *Lancet* 1:621-623, 1971
16. Mair DD, Hagler DJ: Late results of the Mustard operation for transposition of the great arteries. *Excerpta Medica International Congress Series No 470,* 1978, pp 784-789
17. Mair DD, Ritter DG, Danielson GK, et al: The palliative Mustard operation: rationale and results. *Am J Cardiol* 37:762-768, 1976
18. Rastelli GC, McGoon DC, Wallace RB: Anatomic correction of transposition of the great arteries with ventricular septal defect and subpulmonary stenosis. *J Thorac Cardiovasc Surg* 58:545-551, 1969

19. Marcelletti C, Mair DD, McGoon DC, et al: The Rastelli operation for transposition of the great arteries: early and late results. *J Thorac Cardiovasc Surg* 72:427-434, 1976

20. Kaye MP: Anatomic correction of transposition of great arteries. *Mayo Clin Proc* 50:638-640, 1975

21. Damus PS: Letter to the editor. *Ann Thorac Surg* 20:724-725, 1975

22. Stansel HC Jr: A new operation for *d*-loop transposition of the great vessels. *Ann Thorac Surg* 19:565-567, 1975

23. Jatene AD, Fontes VF, Paulista PP, et al: Successful anatomic correction of transposition of the great vessels: a preliminary report. *Arq Bras Cardiol* 28:461-464, 1975

24. Bical O, Hazan E, Lecompte Y, et al: Anatomic correction of transposition of the great arteries associated with ventricular septal defect: midterm results in 50 patients. *Circulation* 70:891-897, 1984

25. Losay J, Planche C, Gerardin B, et al: Midterm surgical results of arterial switch operation for transposition of the great arteries with intact septum. *Circulation* 82 Suppl 4:146-150, 1990

26. Wernovsky G, Jonas RA, Colan SD, et al: Results of the arterial switch operation in patients with transposition of the great arteries and abnormalities of the mitral valve or left ventricular outflow tract. *J Am Coll Cardiol* 16:1446-1454, 1990

27. Idriss FS, Ilbawi MN, DeLeon SY, et al: Arterial switch in simple and complex transposition of the great arteries. *J Thorac Cardiovasc Surg* 95:29-36, 1988

CHAPTER

54

Rheumatic fever and Kawasaki disease

David J. Driscoll, M.D.

RHEUMATIC FEVER

Acute rheumatic fever is a multisystem inflammatory disorder resulting from a preceding group A β-hemolytic streptococcal infection. Except for its cardiac effects, acute rheumatic fever is a self-limiting, relatively benign disorder. Unfortunately, the cardiac effects of acute rheumatic fever are serious and may be chronic and life-threatening.

Epidemiology

The incidence of acute rheumatic fever varies with geographic location and the population studied but ranges from 3 to 61 per 100,000 schoolchildren.[1-3] The highest incidence of acute rheumatic fever occurs in children 5 to 14 years of age.[2] Acute rheumatic fever is rare in children younger than 4 years of age but does occur.[2] Acute rheumatic fever is most common during the winter and spring, a seasonal variation similar to that of streptococcal pharyngitis.[2,4]

The incidence of initial attacks of acute rheumatic fever is increased in disadvantaged populations, presumably because of crowded living conditions that facilitate the spread of streptococcal infection.[5-8] Although initial occurrences of rheumatic fever may be increased, there is evidence that rheumatic fever recurrence is unrelated to overcrowding or socioeconomic status.[9]

Recently, there have been reports[10] of localized epidemics of acute rheumatic fever in the United States, and the reason for this resurgence is unclear. Some investigators[10] postulate a change in susceptibility to the disease based on genetic mechanisms or changes in the virulence of the streptococcal organism; possibly, there is an increased prevalence of mucoid strains of the streptococcus.

The streptococcus

The streptococcus is composed of a core of cytoplasm surrounded by a cytoplasmic membrane and a cell wall, which in turn is surrounded by a capsule that constitutes the external surface of the organism. The capsule is composed of hyaluronate, which is nonantigenic.[11] The cell wall is composed of three layers: the outermost protein layer, the middle carbohydrate layer, and the innermost mucopeptide protoplast layer.

The protein layer contains the proteins designated M, T, and R. The M protein is the most important because it determines the virulence of the organism, stimulates formation of opsonizing and precipitating antibodies, and may impede phagocytosis.[11,12] Lancefield[13] and Dochez et al.[14] classified group A streptococci into serologic types on the basis of the M protein. Acute rheumatic fever can result from infection by any of the serotypes of group A β-hemolytic streptococci, whereas glomerulonephritis is associated with only a limited number of the serotypes. Antibodies produced against the M protein antigen can impart long-lasting immunity against reinfection by that specific serotype. The middle layer of the cell wall, the carbohydrate layer, provides the group specification of the streptococcus. *N*-Acetylglucosamine is the group-specific carbohydrate for group A streptococci. The mucopeptide innermost layer of the cell wall forms the skeletal component of the cell and is responsible for the shape of the cell. The mucopeptide can cause a chronic relapsing arthritis and synovitis in rats.[15] The cytoplasmic membrane is an antigenic lipoprotein, which cross-reacts with several mammalian tissue antigens, including human glomerular basement membrane.[16] Rabbit antiserum to the streptococcal membrane structure binds to human sarcolemmal antigen.[17,18]

The streptococcus produces a number of extracellular

products, some of which are involved in the disease-causing effects of the microorganism.[19] Erythrogenic toxin is pyrogenic and is responsible for the rash of scarlet fever. Streptolysin-O is cardiotoxic and leukotoxic, and it is responsible for hemolysis of erythrocytes. Streptolysin-O will elicit an antibody response, antistreptolysin-O, in 70% to 85% of infected persons, and this forms the basis of a useful assay of invasive streptococcal infection.[1] Early and effective antibiotic treatment of streptococcal infections can suppress this antibody response. The antigenicity of streptolysin-O is inhibited by lipid extracts (probably cholesterol) of rabbit skin, and this property may be responsible for the lack of association between streptococcal skin infections and acute rheumatic fever. Free cholesterol neutralizes streptolysin-O, but serum cholesterol, not in a free state, is a poor inhibitor of streptolysin-O.[20] Streptolysin-S produces the hemolysis characteristic of β-hemolytic streptococci when cultured on sheep blood agar. Extracellular proteinase can cause myocardial necrosis. Streptokinase activates plasma proteins and converts plasminogen to plasmin. Diphosphopyridine nucleotidase elicits an antibody response (antidiphosphopyridine nucleotidase) in 87% of patients with acute rheumatic fever and is a useful adjunct to the antistreptolysin-O titer in identifying patients with invasive streptococcal disease.[11] There are four deoxyribonucleases (A, B, C, and D), all of which are antigenic.[21,22] Deoxyribonuclease B is produced in the largest quantities in response to group A streptococcal infection and is the most consistent of the deoxyribonucleases. Antideoxyribonuclease antibodies are useful indicators of invasive streptococcal disease.

Pathogenesis

Although it is clear that invasive group A streptococcal infection is causally related to acute rheumatic fever, the pathogenesis of this relationship is unclear. Most likely, acute rheumatic fever is an autoimmune disease in which invasive streptococcal infection evokes an antibody response by the host, and this antibody attacks antigenically similar host tissues.[23] Four streptococcal-host cross-reactive antigen-antibody systems have been identified:[23] (1) cardiac myofiber-smooth muscle antigen cross-reacting with streptococcal cell wall and cell membrane antigen; (2) heart valve fibroblast antigen cross-reacting with streptococcal cell membrane antigen; (3) subthalamic and caudate nuclei antigen cross-reacting with streptococcal cell membrane antigen; and (4) heart valve and connective tissue antigen cross-reacting with streptococcal group A carbohydrate antigen. Although heart-reactive antibody can be identified in patients with acute rheumatic fever, these antibodies can, at times, also be identified in patients with streptococcal infection but without acute rheumatic fever.

It is possible that streptococcal extracellular products play a role in the pathogenesis of acute rheumatic fever. Although some of these products are cardiotoxic, the effects of these toxins in vitro do not mimic the chronic granulomatous lesions seen in acute rheumatic fever.[12]

Clinical manifestations[11,24,25]

Fever and arthritis are the two most common initial presenting features of acute rheumatic fever. Three-fourths of patients with acute rheumatic fever have joint pain. Classically, the large joints, such as knees, ankles, elbows, and wrists, are involved and are tender, swollen, and erythematous. The pain migrates from one joint to another, each joint being involved for approximately 1 to 5 days. The arthritis persists for 2 to 4 weeks. In general, the severity of the joint symptoms is inversely proportional to the severity of cardiac involvement.[11]

Carditis occurs in 40% to 50% of patients with the first attack of acute rheumatic fever. It may be a presenting feature, but it more commonly occurs after the onset of arthritis. The endocardium, myocardium, and pericardium may be involved. Carditis may be recognized by the appearance of a new significant cardiac murmur, such as mitral regurgitation or aortic regurgitation, cardiomegaly, or signs and symptoms of congestive heart failure or pericarditis. Congestive heart failure may present initially as fatigue, anorexia, unexplained shortness of breath, or cough. Chest pain may be the first manifestation of pericarditis. Carditis may be insidious and be apparent only by the presence of tachycardia that is disproportionate to fever during sleep. Also, an arrhythmia may be the first manifestation of carditis.

Chorea is a late manifestation of acute rheumatic fever, but acute rheumatic fever must be considered in the differential diagnosis of patients with chorea, particularly those between the ages of 7 and 14 years. Rheumatic chorea is more common in girls than boys and is a rare manifestation of acute rheumatic fever after puberty.

Erythema marginatum is an unusual manifestation of acute rheumatic fever but, if present, is helpful in establishing the diagnosis, particularly in association with other manifestations of the disorder. Erythema marginatum is not pathognomonic for acute rheumatic fever because it can occur also as a manifestation of drug reactions. Erythema marginatum occurs predominantly on the trunk and medial aspect of the proximal parts of the extremities. The eruption begins as pink, slightly raised, nonpruritic macules. The borders of the lesions migrate peripherally as the central areas assume normal skin appearance. Heat applied to the skin can accentuate the appearance of erythema marginatum.[11]

Subcutaneous nodules occur in 7% to 20% of patients with acute rheumatic fever. They occur on extensor surfaces, over the spine, and on the scalp. They are nontender, nonpruritic, firm, painless masses. Usually the diagnosis of acute rheumatic fever already has been established by the time subcutaneous nodules appear. In general, subcutaneous nodules occur in patients with relatively severe carditis.

Acute rheumatic fever also may present with abdominal pain, epistaxis, or pneumonia. Patients with unsuspected acute rheumatic fever have undergone laparotomy because of an incorrect diagnosis of acute appendicitis.

Many conditions share clinical manifestations with acute rheumatic fever (Table 54-1). Many of these conditions are acute self-limiting processes that do not

Table 54-1 Differential diagnosis of rheumatic fever

Juvenile rheumatoid arthritis
Acute transient synovitis
Innocent murmur with a febrile illness
Viral myocarditis
Bacterial arthritis
Sickle cell anemia
Periarteritis nodosa
Kawasaki disease
Lupus erythematosus
Dermatomyositis
Henoch-Schönlein purpura
Legg-Calvé-Perthes disease
Slipped capital femoral epiphysis
Leukemia
Habit spasms, tics
Lyme disease

Table 54-2 Diagnosis of rheumatic fever

Jones criteria	Modified Jones criteria
Major	
Carditis	Carditis
Arthralgia	Polyarthritis
Chorea	Chorea
Subcutaneous nodules	Subcutaneous nodules
Recurrences of acute rheumatic fever	Erythema marginatum
Minor	
Rash	Prior acute rheumatic fever
Anemia	Arthralgia
Fever	Fever
Elevated erythrocyte sedimentation rate	Elevated erythrocyte sedimentation rate, serum C-reactive protein
Leukocytosis	Leukocytosis
Epistaxis	Prolonged P-R interval on ECG
Abdominal pain	
Precordial pain	
Rheumatic pulmonary disease	
Plus	
	Evidence of prior streptococcal infection (throat culture, scarlet fever, increased antistreptococcal antibodies)

require long-term prophylaxis and are unassociated with an increased risk of cardiac dysfunction. Although it is important to identify a person with acute rheumatic fever, it is equally important not to mislabel patients who do not have acute rheumatic fever. The diagnosis of acute rheumatic fever can be made if the patient exhibits two of the major manifestations or one major manifestation and two minor manifestations *and* has evidence of previous streptococcal infection (Table 54-2).

It must be stressed that evidence of a streptococcal infection should be present *in addition to* the major and minor manifestations. Some investigators think that the diagnosis of acute rheumatic fever should not be made unless evidence of a preceding streptococcal infection is present.[26] The one exception is the diagnosis of acute rheumatic fever on the basis of otherwise unexplained chorea. All patients with suspected acute rheumatic fever should have a throat culture and appropriate antistreptococcal enzyme assays to detect any evidence of streptococcal infection. The antistreptolysin-O antibody will be abnormally elevated or an increase or decrease of more than two tube dilutions can be documented in 70% to 85% of patients with acute rheumatic fever. A single value of 500 units is considered indicative of streptococcal infection, and a value of 333 units is of borderline significance.[11] If the antistreptolysin-O titer is 333 units or less, additional antistreptococcal antibody assays should be obtained. These include antideoxyribonuclease B, antinicotinamide adenine dinucleotidase, antihyaluronidase, and antistreptokinase. When three different streptococcal antibodies are measured, more than 95% of patients with acute rheumatic fever will have abnormal elevation of at least one.[27] The streptozyme test includes an assay for antibodies against five extracellular antigens of group A streptococci (streptolysin-O, hyaluronidase, streptokinase, deoxyribonuclease B, and nicotinamide adenine dinucleotidase).[28,29] Unfortunately, false-positive streptozyme tests are common, and the streptozyme test should not be used as a screening test. The streptozyme test is useful in conjunction with a negative or borderline antistreptolysin-O titer. A negative streptozyme test and a negative or borderline antistreptolysin-O titer indicate that streptococcal infection is unlikely.[30]

Treatment

The treatment of patients with acute rheumatic fever depends, to some degree, on the specific manifestations of the rheumatic fever.[11,24,26] All patients, regardless of their manifestations, should have a therapeutic course of antibiotics tailored to eradicate any streptococcal infection. This should be initiated after a throat culture has been obtained to assess whether streptococci are present, but the antibiotics should be administered even in the absence of a positive throat culture. One intramuscular injection of benzathine penicillin G (600,000 to 1,200,000 units) or a 10-day course of penicillin G (200,000 to 250,000 units four times a day) is recommended. Patients who are allergic to penicillin should receive erythromycin for 10 days (Table 54-3).

Aspirin was recommended for the treatment of acute rheumatic fever by Maclagan[31] in 1876. Although salicy-

Table 54-3 Treatment for streptococcal pharyngitis

Antibiotic	Duration (days)	Weight	Dose	Route
Benzathine penicillin G	1	>60 lb	1,200,000 units	Intramuscular
		<60 lb	600,000 units	Intramuscular
Penicillin V (phenoxy-methyl penicillin)	10	. . .	40 mg/kg per day, not to exceed 750 mg/day; for adults and most children, 250 mg b.i.d. or t.i.d. is recommended	Oral
Erythromycin	10	. . .		Oral
estolate			20-40 mg/kg per day in two to four divided doses; maximum dose of 1 g/day	
ethylsuccinate			40 mg/kg per day in two to four divided doses; maximum dose of 1 g/day	

lates reduce fever and arthritis, there is no evidence that salicylate therapy prevents carditis or permanent damage to the heart.[11] Hench et al.[32] were the first to use steroids in the treatment of patients with acute rheumatic fever. There have been several studies in which the incidence of cardiac disease seemed to be reduced with the use of steroids.[33-35] However, there were methodologic problems with these studies, and the results probably are inconclusive.[11] In 1955, the results of a combined United Kingdom and United States study indicated no significant differences among patients treated with aspirin, cortisone, or ACTH and the incidence of rheumatic heart disease.[36] The incidence of residual heart disease was related directly to the initial severity of the cardiac disease. Thus, although aspirin and steroids remain the mainstay of treatment for patients with acute rheumatic fever, "there has been no clear and consistent demonstration that cardiac damage is prevented or minimized by either salicylates or steroids even if used early in the course of the illness, in high or low dosages, or for long or short periods of time."[11]

Aspirin is the only anti-inflammatory agent that is recommended for the treatment of acute rheumatic fever characterized by arthritis alone or associated with minimal carditis. Minimal carditis includes the presence of minimal cardiomegaly or prolonged P-R interval on the electrocardiogram alone or a grade 1/6 to 2/6 apical systolic murmur. The dosage of aspirin is 90 to 120 mg/kg/day, or enough to maintain a serum salicylate level of 15 to 25 mg/dL.[26] One to 2 weeks of aspirin treatment is recommended when arthritis alone is present, and 2 to 4 weeks is recommended when minimal carditis is present in addition to arthritis.

If carditis is moderately severe or severe, the patient should be treated with prednisone (2 mg/kg/day, not to exceed 60 mg/day) for 1 to 4 weeks. Shortly after or concomitantly with stopping steroid therapy, aspirin (90 to 120 mg/kg/day) should be begun and continued for 1 ½ to 6 months.[1,37] Aspirin probably should be continued until active inflammation subsides (until the erythrocyte sedimentation rate is normal). Congestive heart failure may be treated with a digitalis preparation and diuretic drugs. If congestive heart failure is severe, oxygen inhalation may be helpful. Occasionally, operative repair or replacement of a severely compromised cardiac valve may be necessary during acute rheumatic fever if signs and symptoms of severe congestive heart failure are unresponsive to medical therapy.[38]

The importance of bed rest in the treatment of acute rheumatic fever is based on clinical observation and little scientific investigation.[11,39-41] In general, patients with chorea will prefer bed rest because of ataxia, and patients with arthritis will prefer bed rest because of joint pain. Bed rest for patients with carditis should be tempered by the severity of the carditis, congestive heart failure, and arrhythmias.

Rheumatic chorea is treated by maintaining the patient in a quiet environment. If choreiform movements are severe, the patient's bed rails may have to be cushioned to prevent inadvertent injury. The patient can be sedated with phenobarbital, chlorpromazine, or diazepam. Chorea should be treated for as long as it persists.

Sequelae

The only serious sequela of acute rheumatic fever is cardiac damage, particularly cardiac valvular damage. In general, the severity of chronic rheumatic cardiac disease is proportional to the severity of the initial carditis during the episode of acute rheumatic fever. The clinical features of chronic rheumatic valvular disease depend on the valve affected and the severity of the valvular dysfunction. Also, specific treatment for chronic rheumatic valvular disease is dependent upon the severity of the valve dysfunction.

Although valvular heart disease is the most common cardiac manifestation of acute rheumatic fever, certain forms of congestive cardiomyopathy may be a late sequela of acute rheumatic fever.

Prevention

There are three aspects to the prevention of acute rheumatic fever and its sequelae: (1) prevention of acute rheumatic fever by accurate and prompt recognition and treatment of streptococcal pharyngitis, (2) prevention of recurrent acute rheumatic fever through compulsive ongoing prophylaxis against streptococcal infection, and (3) prevention of bacterial endocarditis in persons with chronic rheumatic cardiac valve disease.

It is difficult to distinguish clinically between streptococcal pharyngitis and viral pharyngitis.[42,43] However, an abrupt onset of tender cervical lymphadenopathy, tonsillopharyngeal exudate, headache, anorexia, abdominal pain, and vomiting suggests the possibility of streptococcal pharyngitis. Streptococcal pharyngitis can be present, however, without these signs and symptoms. The presence of upper respiratory tract symptoms such as rhinitis and conjunctivitis suggests a viral cause for the pharyngitis, but streptococcal infection can cause nasopharyngitis or be associated with a concomitant viral respiratory tract infection. A throat culture is necessary for an accurate diagnosis of streptococcal pharyngitis. The culture should be obtained by vigorously swabbing both tonsillar pillars and posterior pharynx, and streaking on one-sixth of a 5% sheep blood agar plate. The plate is incubated for 24 hours and then observed for evidence of streptococcal growth. The presence of streptococci in the throat of a patient with pharyngitis does not, however, indicate that the organism and the pharyngitis are causally related. In as many as 50% of patients from whom streptococci are isolated from the pharynx, and who may be carriers of the organism, it is not responsible for the disease process. Whether a patient is a carrier or the pharyngitis is caused by a new streptococcal infection can be ascertained by an abnormal increase in antistreptococcal antibodies. However, by the time this assessment has been completed, it would be too late to provide adequate treatment with appropriate antibiotics to prevent acute rheumatic fever. Thus, from a practical standpoint, one must treat all patients with pharyngitis who have a positive throat culture, recognizing that chronic carriers of streptococci may be treated unnecessarily.

Antibiotic therapy for streptococcal pharyngitis will effectively prevent acute rheumatic fever if the treatment is begun within 7 to 8 days after the onset of the pharyngitis. The antibiotic therapy can be delayed until the result of a throat culture is available. However, antibiotic therapy should be started immediately for patients with symptoms of pharyngitis and prior acute rheumatic fever and for patients who are at increased risk of spreading streptococcal infection, such as medical personnel and teachers. Antibiotics can then be discontinued in these patients if the throat culture does not reveal streptococcal infection. The recommended antibiotic regimens are listed in Table 54-3. Patients should *not* be treated with tetracycline, because some strains of streptococci are resistant to this antibiotic. Also, sulfonamide drugs should not be used because these drugs may suppress but not eradicate the streptococcal infection.

Siblings and other household contacts of a patient with *acute rheumatic fever* should have a throat culture and, if the culture is positive, be treated with appropriate antibiotics even though asymptomatic. Household contacts of an index patient with *streptococcal pharyngitis* who have or recently had symptoms suggestive of streptococcal disease should have a throat culture and, if the result is positive, be treated with appropriate antibiotics. Except during specific outbreaks of streptococcal disease, culturing specimens from asymptomatic household contacts of patients with streptococcal pharyngitis is thought to be unnecessary.[44]

It is essential to prevent recurrent attacks of rheumatic fever. A high risk of recurrence is associated with (1) symptoms of pharyngitis, (2) young age, (3) a brief time since the last episode of acute rheumatic fever, (4) existing rheumatic heart disease, (5) the number of prior attacks of acute rheumatic fever, and (6) oral rather than parenteral prophylaxis.[9] Prophylaxis should be begun during the initial episode of rheumatic fever.[45] Parenteral administration of 1.2 million units of benzathine penicillin every 4 weeks is the most effective prophylactic regimen. Reliable patients who have a history of excellent compliance in the use of drugs can receive oral prophylaxis with sulfadiazine (1 g/day for patients weighing more than 60 lb and 0.5 g/day for those less than 60 lb), penicillin G (200,000 to 250,000 units by mouth twice a day), or erythromycin (250 mg by mouth twice a day). Because of possible poor compliance with drug regimens, most children and adolescents should receive intramuscular prophylaxis.

The duration of secondary rheumatic fever prophylaxis is controversial, but the following guidelines may be helpful. Patients who had rheumatic fever without carditis should receive prophylaxis for 5 years or to age 21, whichever is longer. Patients who had rheumatic fever with healed carditis but no valvular disease should receive prophylaxis for 10 years or well into adulthood, whichever is longer. Patients with residual carditis (persistent valvular disease) should receive prophylaxis until at least age 40 years, for at least 10 years after the last episode, or perhaps for life.[46]

Patients with rheumatic cardiac valve disease require prophylaxis against endocarditis for dental manipulation, bronchoscopy, tonsillectomy, adenoidectomy, genitourinary and gastrointestinal instrumentation, and unclean wounds. There is controversy as to whether or not endocarditis prophylaxis is necessary for uncomplicated endotracheal intubation. The penicillin regimen designed for prophylaxis against recurrent rheumatic fever is inadequate for prophylaxis against bacterial endocarditis because of the emergence of penicillin-resistant oral streptococci in patients receiving penicillin for rheumatic fever prophylaxis.[47] Thus, for patients receiving monthly or daily penicillin prophylaxis for acute rheumatic fever, erythromycin should be used for bacterial endocarditis prophylaxis. One gram of erythromycin in adults or 20 mg/kg in children (not to exceed 1 g) should be given as an initial dose 1½ to 2 hours before the procedure, and 500 mg in adults or 10 mg/kg in children (not to exceed 500 mg) 6 hours after the initial dose. For gastrointestinal and genitourinary tract surgery and instrumentation, antibiotics that are effective against gram-negative organisms (ampicillin, streptomycin, or gentamicin) should be used in addition to erythromycin.[48]

KAWASAKI DISEASE

Kawasaki disease is a generalized vasculitis of unknown cause.[49-51] The peak incidence occurs in children between 1 and 2 years of age, and 85% of cases occur in children younger than 5 years. Although the inflammatory component is self-limited, the disease can produce coronary artery and other systemic arterial aneurysms, thromboses, and obstructions. These are the important sequelae of Kawasaki disease, and they can result in significant morbidity and mortality.

There is no specific laboratory test for Kawasaki disease. The diagnosis is based on clinical features (Table 54-4). In general, fever that persists at least 5 days and at least four of the five clinical findings listed in Table 54-4 are necessary to establish the diagnosis. However, there are "atypical cases" of Kawasaki disease with classic coronary artery aneurysms but fewer than four of the clinical findings listed in Table 54-4.

Evidence of myocardial inflammation occurs in approximately 25% of patients with Kawasaki disease. Coronary aneurysms develop in 15% to 20% of cases of Kawasaki disease, but they resolve in at least 50% of the cases. The following are risk factors for development of coronary aneurysms: age less than 1 year at the time of disease, fever for more than 14 days, anemia, white blood cell count greater than 30,000, marked increase in the sedimentation rate, prolonged increase of C-reactive protein, and aneurysms of noncoronary systemic arteries. The most important risk factors for coronary artery obstruction are giant (greater than 8 mm in diameter) coronary aneurysms.

The goals of treatment are to prevent the development of coronary artery aneurysms and to reduce discomfort from the acute inflammatory illness. There has been debate over whether aspirin treatment reduces the incidence of coronary artery aneurysms, but despite this debate, aspirin is used because it relieves symptoms. There is good evidence that intravenously administered gamma globulin, particularly when given early in the course of the illness, reduces the incidence of coronary artery aneurysms, and this treatment is now standard.

Treatment after the acute phase of Kawasaki disease (more than 4 weeks after onset) is not well defined. Recently, the American Heart Association published guidelines for the long-term management of patients with Kawasaki disease.[52] In patients without coronary artery aneurysms, low doses of aspirin (3 to 5 mg/kg per day) are usually continued for 6 to 8 weeks. For patients with coronary artery aneurysms, low doses of aspirin are continued at least until all aneurysms have resolved. For patients with giant aneurysms, dipyridamole (3 to 6 mg/kg per day) or warfarin can be used in conjunction with low-dose aspirin.

The long-term fate of patients with persistent but nonobstructive coronary aneurysms and of those in whom the aneurysms have resolved is unclear. Presumably, these patients should have continued medical surveillance.

Table 54-4 Principal clinical features of Kawasaki disease

Peripheral extremity changes: erythema and edema of hands and feet, membranous desquamation of fingertips
Polymorphous exanthem
Bilateral nonexudative, painless bulbar conjunctival injection
Erythema and cracking of lips, strawberry tongue, diffuse injection of oral and pharyngeal mucosae
Acute, nonpurulent cervical lymphadenopathy

REFERENCES

1. Wannamaker LW: Rheumatic fever. In *Nelson Textbook of Pediatrics.* Eleventh edition. Edited by VC Vaughan III, RJ McKay Jr, RE Behrman, Philadelphia, WB Saunders Company, 1979, pp 682-695
2. Annegers JF, Pillman NL, Weidman WH, et al: Rheumatic fever in Rochester, Minnesota, 1935-1978. *Mayo Clin Proc* 57:753-757, 1982
3. Brownell KD, Bailen-Rose F: Acute rheumatic fever in children: incidence in a borough of New York City. *JAMA* 224:1593-1597, 1973
4. Stollerman GH: *Rheumatic Fever and Streptococcal Infection.* New York, Grune & Stratton, 1975
5. Collins SD: The incidence of rheumatic fever as recorded in general morbidity surveys of families. *Public Health Rep* Suppl 198:1-59, 1947
6. Gordis L, Lilienfeld A, Rodriguez R: Studies in the epidemiology and preventability of rheumatic fever—II: socio-economic factors and the incidence of acute attacks. *J Chronic Dis* 21:655-666, 1969
7. Quinn RW, Federspiel CF: The incidence of rheumatic fever in metropolitan Nashville, 1963-1969. *Am J Epidemiol* 99:273-280, 1974
8. Quinn RW: Rheumatic heart disease and crowding: a survey of rural and urban Connecticut school children. *Am J Public Health* 38:1071-1081, 1948
9. Spagnuolo M, Pasternack B, Taranta A: Risk of rheumatic-fever recurrences after streptococcal infections: prospective study of clinical and social factors. *N Engl J Med* 285:641-647, 1971
10. Bisno AL: Group A streptococcal infections and acute rheumatic fever. *N Engl J Med* 325:783-793, 1991
11. Markowitz M, Kuttner AG: Rheumatic fever: diagnosis, management and prevention. *Major Probl Clin Pediatr* 2:1-242, 1965
12. Zabriskie JB: Rheumatic fever: a streptococcal-induced autoimmune disease? *Pediatr Ann* 11:383-396, 1982
13. Lancefield RC: Specific relationship of cell composition to biological activity of hemolytic streptococci. *Harvey Lect* 36:251-290, 1941
14. Dochez AR, Avery OT, Lancefield RC: Studies on the biology of streptococcus. I. Antigenic relationships between strains of streptococcus haemolyticus. *J Exp Med* 30:179-213, 1919
15. Cromartie WJ, Craddock JG, Schwab JH, et al: Arthritis in rats after systemic injection of streptococcal cells or cell walls. *J Exp Med* 146:1585-1602, 1977
16. Rapaport FT, Markowitz AS, McCluskey RT, et al: Induction of renal disease with antisera to Group A streptococcal membranes. *Transplant Proc.* 1:981-984, 1969
17. Kaplan MH, Frengley JD: Autoimmunity to the heart in cardiac

disease: current concepts of the relation of autoimmunity to rheumatic fever, postcardiotomy and postinfarction syndromes and cardiomyopathies. *Am J Cardiol* 24:459-473, 1969

18. Zabriskie JB, Freimer EH: An immunological relationship between Group A streptococcus and mammalian muscle. *J Exp Med* 124:661-678, 1966
19. Halbert SP, Keatinge SL: The analysis of streptococcal infections. VI. Immunoelectrophoretic observations on extracellular antigens detectable with human antibodies. *J Exp Med* 113:1013-1028, 1961
20. Kaplan EL, Wannamaker LW: Suppression of the antistreptolysin O response by cholesterol and by lipid extracts of rabbit skin. *J Exp Med* 144:754-767, 1976
21. Wannamaker LW: The differentiation of three distinct desoxyribonucleases of group A streptococci. *J Exp Med* 107:797-812, 1958
22. Wannamaker LW: Characterization of a fourth desoxyribonuclease of group A streptococci (abstract). *Fed Proc* 21:231, 1962
23. Kaplan MH: Rheumatic fever, rheumatic heart disease, and the streptococcal connection: the role of streptococcal antigens cross-reactive with heart tissue. *Rev Infect Dis* 1:988-996, 1979
24. Wannamaker LW, Kaplan EL: Acute rheumatic fever. In *Moss' Heart Disease in Infants, Children, and Adolescents.* Edited by FH Adams, GC Emmanouilides. Baltimore, Williams & Wilkins, 1983, pp 534-552
25. Goldring D: Acute rheumatic fever. In *Textbook of Pediatric Infectious Diseases.* Vol 1. Edited by RD Feigin, JD Cherry. Philadelphia, WB Saunders Company, 1981, pp 280-287
26. Kaplan EL: Acute rheumatic fever. *Pediatr Clin North Am* 25:817-829, November 1978
27. Stollerman GH, Lewis AJ, Schultz I, et al: Relationship of immune response to group A streptococci to the course of acute, chronic and recurrent rheumatic fever. *Am J Med* 20:163-169, 1956
28. Janeff J, Janeff D, Taranta A, et al: A screening test for streptococcal antibodies. *Lab Med* 2:38-40, July 1971
29. Bisno AL, Ofek I: Serologic diagnosis of streptococcal infection: comparison of a rapid hemagglutination technique with conventional antibody tests. *Am J Dis Child* 127:676-681, 1974
30. Markowitz M: The changing picture of rheumatic fever. *Arthritis Rheum* 20:369-374, 1977
31. Maclagan T: The treatment of acute rheumatism by salicin. *Lancet* 1:342-343; 383-384, 1876
32. Hench PS, Slocumb CH, Barnes AR, et al: The effects of the adrenal cortical hormone 17-hydroxy-11-dehydrocorticosterone (compound E) on the acute phase of rheumatic fever: preliminary report. *Proc Staff Meet Mayo Clin* 24:277-297, 1949
33. Markowitz M, Kuttner AG: The effect of intensive and prolonged therapy with cortisone and hydrocortisone in first attacks of rheumatic carditis. *Pediatrics* 16:325-332, 1955
34. Roy SB, Massell BF: Comparison of large and small doses of hormones in the treatment of acute rheumatic carditis. *Circulation* 14:44-47, 1956
35. Dorfman A, Gross JI, Lorincz AE: The treatment of acute rheumatic fever. *Pediatrics* 27:692-706, 1961
36. United Kingdom and United States Joint Report: The treatment of acute rheumatic fever in children: a cooperative clinical trial of ACTH, cortisone and aspirin. *Circulation* 11:343-371, 1955
37. Bouillaud J: *New Researches on Acute Articular Rheumatism.* Translated by J Kitchen. Philadelphia, Haswell, Barrington, and Haswell, 1837
38. Kinsley RH, Girdwood RW, Milner S: Surgical treatment during the acute phase of rheumatic carditis. *Surg Annu* 13:299-323, 1981
39. Robertson HF, Schmidt RE, Feiring W: The therapeutic value of early physical activity in rheumatic fever: preliminary report. *Am J Med Sci* 211:67-73, 1946
40. Simon AJ, Mack I, Rosenblum P: Accelerated rehabilitation in rheumatic fever. *Am J Dis Child* 83:454-462, 1952
41. Lendrum BL, Simon AJ, Mack I: Relation of duration of bed rest in acute rheumatic fever to heart disease present 2 to 14 years later. *Pediatrics* 24:389-394, 1959
42. Kaplan EL, Top FH Jr, Dudding BA, et al: Diagnosis of streptococcal pharyngitis: differentiation of active infection from the carrier state in the symptomatic child. *J Infect Dis* 123:490-501, 1971
43. Wannamaker LW: Perplexity and precision in the diagnosis of streptococcal pharyngitis. *Am J Dis Child* 124:352-358, 1972
44. Report of the Committee on Infectious Diseases. *American Academy of Pediatrics.* Twenty-second edition. 1991
45. Committee Report of the American Heart Association: Prevention of rheumatic fever. *Circulation* 55:1-4, 1977
46. Dajani A, et al: Treatment of acute streptococcal pharyngitis and prevention of rheumatic fever: a statement for health professionals by the Committee on Rheumatic Fever, Endocarditis, and Kawasaki Disease of the Council on Cardiovascular Disease in the Young, The American Heart Association. *Circulation* (in press)
47. Sprunt K, Redman W, Leidy G: Penicillin resistant alpha streptococci in pharynx of patients given oral penicillin. *Pediatrics* 42:957-968, 1968
48. American Heart Association Committee Report: Prevention of bacterial endocarditis. *Circulation* 70:1123A-1127A, 1984
49. Gersony WM: Diagnosis and management of Kawasaki disease. *JAMA* 265:2699-2703, 1991
50. Newburger JW, Takahashi M, Beiser AS, et al: A single intravenous infusion of gamma globulin as compared with four infusions in the treatment of acute Kawasaki syndrome. *N Engl J Med* 324:1633-1639, 1991
51. Kawasaki T: Kawasaki disease. *Cardiology in the Young* 1:184-191, 1991
52. Dajani A (Chairman), Taubert KA, Takahashi M, et al: Guidelines for long-term management of patients with Kawasaki disease: report from the Committee on Rheumatic Fever, Endocarditis, and Kawasaki Disease in the Young, American Heart Association. *Circulation* 89:916-922, 1994

CHAPTER

55

The pericardium

Sharonne N. Hayes, M.D., and Gordon K. Danielson, M.D.

ANATOMY, FUNCTION, AND DYSFUNCTION OF THE PERICARDIUM

The pericardium is a bilayer fibroserous sac made up of an inner layer, the epicardium or visceral pericardium, that adheres to the heart surface and an outer layer, the parietal pericardium, that has fibrous attachments to the diaphragm, sternum, and costal cartilages and prevents excessive motion of the heart. The lining of the pericardium encloses the heart and the proximal portion of the great vessels. Serosal cells that line the pericardial space possess microvilli that participate in fluid and electrolyte balance with the heart and vascular system and also reduce friction associated with cardiac motion. Neuroreceptors and mechanoreceptors are present that may provide feedback regulation of the circulatory system. The pericardial space normally contains up to 50 mL of fluid.

The reaction of the pericardium to acute injury is limited to exudation of fluid, fibrin, and cells. The mode of clinical presentation of pericardial disease depends on both the cause and the stage or acuity of the pericardial inflammatory reaction. The major clinical manifestations are inflammatory pericarditis, effusion with or without tamponade, and constrictive pericarditis caused by fibrous scarring and calcification. This clinical spectrum may be, but is not necessarily, progressive. Pericardial disease can appear acutely, as pericarditis or cardiac tamponade; chronically, as relapsing pericarditis, chronic effusion, or chronic constriction; or subacutely, as effusive constrictive pericarditis.

The causes of pericardial disease are many (Table 55-1), but the range of possible causes can be narrowed by taking the history and presenting signs and symptoms into account. The general categories are as follows:

Idiopathic disease. This category includes many instances of presumed acute viral pericarditis for which serologic and cultural data are not available as well as pericardial diseases of uncertain cause. It is the most common diagnosis in patients with acute pericarditis.

Infections. Viruses are probably responsible for most cases of benign acute pericarditis. Tuberculosis may be manifested by subacute or chronic constrictive pericarditis. Bacterial and other infections are less common causes of pericardial disease.

Autoimmune and related diseases. Pericarditis is a common complication of many connective tissue disorders, including systemic lupus erythematosus (idiopathic or drug-induced), rheumatoid arthritis, and acute rheumatic fever, as well as a less common accompaniment of nearly all these disorders. Pericarditis may appear acutely or subacutely, either accompanying a flare of disease activity or alone as a primary disease process. Pericarditis associated with late post-myocardial infarction syndrome (Dressler's) and postpericardiotomy syndrome may also be in this category.

Neoplastic diseases. Malignant lesions may affect the pericardium as a primary process, by direct local extension of tumor, or by distant metastasis.

Acute myocardial infarction. Most cases of pericarditis associated with acute myocardial infarction actually represent myopericarditis. Infarcted myocardium produces a local inflammatory response that involves the pericardium. The recognition of this type of pericarditis is important, since the source of chest pain that develops after myocardial infarction may be either recurrent ischemia or pericardial inflammation.

Trauma. Penetrating and closed chest trauma, particularly due to motor vehicle accidents, remain important causes of pericardial injury and tamponade. Iatrogenic causes of pericardial disease have become more important with the advent of more aggressive invasive diagnostic and therapeutic methods that have an increased risk of cardiac perforation with resulting tamponade or inflammation. Cardiac surgery, by definition, damages the pericardium. Evidence of pericardial injury (friction rubs, electrocardiographic [ECG] changes) is common after cardiac surgical procedures.

Metabolic diseases. Uremic pericarditis may take the form of acute pericarditis or tamponade. Large pericardial effusions can accompany myxedema.

Radiation. Radiation may produce an acute pericarditis or constrictive pericarditis many years after radiation therapy. This cause of pericardial disease has become more common as more patients are cured of primary malignant disease.

Miscellaneous. This category includes a large number of

Table 55-1 Etiologic classification of pericardial disease

Idiopathic
Infection
- Viral
  - Coxsackie A and B, echovirus, influenza, cytomegalovirus, mumps, hepatitis B, varicella, infectious mononucleosis, adenovirus
- Bacterial
  - Pneumococcus, staphylococcus, streptococcus, meningococcus, gonococcus, salmonella, *Legionella pneumophila, Haemophilus influenzae,* tularemia
- Tuberculosis
- Fungal
  - Histoplasmosis, coccidioidomycosis, aspergillosis, blastomycosis
- Parasite
  - Toxoplasmosis, amebiasis, echinococcus
- Other
  - Mycoplasma, *Nocardia,* brucellosis, typhoid fever, Q fever, *Rickettsia,* Lyme disease

Autoimmune and related diseases
- Post-cardiac injury syndrome
  - Dressler's or late post-myocardial infarction syndrome, postpericardiotomy syndrome, post-trauma syndrome
- Connective tissue and inflammatory disorders
  - Systemic lupus erythematosus, rheumatoid arthritis, rheumatic fever, scleroderma, mixed connective tissue disease, adult Still's disease, polyarteritis nodosa, Wegener's granulomatosis, giant cell arteritis, Reiter's syndrome, ankylosing spondylitis, Whipple's disease, dermatomyositis, inflammatory bowel disease
- Drugs
  - Procainamide, hydralazine, isoniazid, penicillin, minoxidil, phenylbutazone, diphenylhydantoin
- Post-cardiac transplantation

Acute myocardial infarction
Neoplasm
- Primary, secondary (lung, breast, leukemia, lymphoma, melanoma)

Radiation
Metabolic
- Uremia, myxedema, cholesterol, gout

Trauma
- Closed chest injury, penetrating chest injury, thoracic surgery, intravascular diagnostic and therapeutic procedures, esophageal rupture, cardiac or great vessel rupture

Aortic dissection
Miscellaneous
- Amyloidosis, sarcoidosis, chylopericardium, thalassemia, pregnancy, acute pancreatitis

varied conditions that have been associated with pericardial disease.

A careful history should elicit any preexisting illness; exposure; current or previous drug, radiation, or surgical therapy; trauma; signs or symptoms of ischemic heart disease; and any other complaints that might suggest a condition associated with pericardial disease.

ACUTE INFLAMMATORY PERICARDITIS

Acute or subacute pericarditis is usually an inflammatory, fibrinous reaction with minimal accumulation of pericardial fluid. Echocardiography may demonstrate a small to moderate effusion without evidence of hemodynamic compromise (tamponade). Many agents and conditions can cause pericarditis, but they tend to be included in the general categories outlined in Table 55-1. Determining the cause of pericarditis is important, since specific therapy is often available for either the pericarditis itself or the underlying condition.

Clinical presentation

Although pericarditis can be silent, pain is usually the cardinal symptom and the presenting complaint. Unfortunately, the "typical" pain of pericarditis is neither pathognomonic nor diagnostic. The quality, intensity, and location can vary greatly. The onset of pain may be sudden or gradual. It is most often precordial but may be substernal or referred to the neck, arms, back, or trapezius ridge. The pain usually is described as sharp and pleuritic and is exacerbated by inspiration, cough, swallowing, or body movement. However, it may also be dull and exactly mimic myocardial ischemia. It is often relieved by sitting upright or leaning forward and exacerbated by recumbency. Low-grade fever, anorexia, malaise, or a recent upper respiratory infection is common. Tachypnea with shallow breathing to avoid respiration-induced pain may be present, but dyspnea per se is usually not present unless it is related to a coexisting illness.

A pericardial friction rub is pathognomonic for pericarditis. Its absence, however, does not exclude the diagnosis, especially since pericardial rubs can be evanescent, with varying intensity and character over a several-hour period. Pericardial rubs usually have a superficial scratchy, grating, or squeaky character. Most (52%) are made up of three components, with sounds corresponding to atrial systole, ventricular systole, and ventricular diastole.[1] Biphasic (33%) and monophasic (15%) rubs are somewhat less common but are important because they may obscure or be mistaken for the murmurs of mitral regurgitation, tricuspid regurgitation, or aortic stenosis. Pericardial friction rubs can be auscultated almost anywhere on the precordium but are usually heard best at the left lower sternal border and between the lower left sternal border and the apex. Rubs are heard best when firm pressure is applied to the diaphragm while the patient is sitting up and leaning forward during both inspiration and held expiration. Rubs are occasionally palpable (23%).[1] When the "classic" three-component friction rub

Table 55-2 Typical electrocardiographic changes in acute pericarditis

Stage	Description
I	ST-segment (J point) elevation (concave upward) in all ventricular leads with ST-segment depression in aVR, V_1, and V_2. PR-segment depression may be present.
II	ST segments return to baseline and T waves begin to flatten. PR-segment depression is common.
III	T-wave inversion, most prominent in leads most affected with ST-segment elevation.
IV	Gradual return to normal ECG pattern.

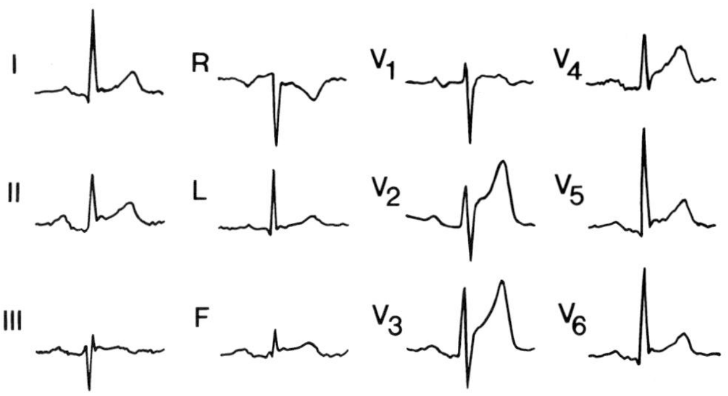

Fig 55-1 Electrocardiogram from a 65-year-old man who had severe pleuritic anterior chest pain for 6 hours. This is a fairly typical stage I pattern with concave upward ST-segment elevation in the precordial leads and I, II, and aVF; slight ST-segment depression in aVR; and PR-segment depression in I, II, aVF, and V_2 through V_6. This patient with recurrent inflammatory pericarditis had a good response to indomethacin, and an ECG 2 weeks later was completely normal.

is present, there is little doubt about the diagnosis. Two-component and, especially, one-component rubs must be differentiated from cardiac murmurs. Serial examinations in several positions may demonstrate the disappearance of a friction rub or changes in the number of components. Unusual location of a precordial sound, absence of expected radiation, or respiration changes may also help differentiate a pericardial friction rub from a murmur. Although friction rubs tend to become louder with inspiration, more than half are unchanged or become softer.[1]

Diagnostic tests

Electrocardiogram. The pericardium is electrically "silent." ECG abnormalities seen during pericarditis reflect subepicardial myocarditis. If the "typical" ECG changes of pericarditis described by Spodick[2] are seen in association with chest pain, the diagnosis can be made with great certainty. These changes usually occur in four stages (Table 55-2). The appearance of a typical stage I ECG is highly specific for pericarditis (Fig 55-1). Stage I changes usually occur soon after the development of chest pain and show concave upward ST segment elevation in all leads except aVR and V_1, upright T waves, and depressed or isoelectric PR segments.[2] PR-segment depression occurs in about 80% of patients with acute pericarditis.[2] The transition from stage I to stage III occurs relatively rapidly over hours to days. Progression to stage IV (normalization) may take months. Many patients with pericarditis have atypical ECGs at presentation. These include normal tracings, absence of one or more stages, isolated PR-segment depression,[2] localized abnormalities or nonspecific ST-segment and T-wave abnormalities that may simulate early repolarization,[3] myocardial ischemia, and injury. These atypical abnormalities may be suggestive but are not diagnostic of pericarditis. Serial ECGs often clarify the diagnosis or suggest another probable cause of chest pain. The appearance of the ST segments in patients with early repolarization variant should not change over time.

Most patients with pericarditis are tachycardic, but arrhythmias related to pericarditis are relatively infrequent. They are usually atrial in origin and are more likely to represent an underlying myocardial or metabolic abnormality than pericarditis itself.[4,5]

Chest radiography. The cardiac silhouette in acute pericarditis is usually normal. If a moderate or large pericardial effusion is present, there may be globular enlargement. Pleural effusions are common. The appearance of adenopathy, pulmonary mass, infiltrate, or other extracardiac abnormalities may aid in determining the cause of pericarditis.

Echocardiography. Two-dimensional echocardiography is sensitive and specific for the diagnosis of pericardial effusion[6] and may reveal additional information, such as loculation or tamponade. Most importantly, the finding of segmental wall motion abnormalities suggestive of ischemia or infarction in a patient with a consistent ECG alters therapy considerably. Although the finding of pericardial effusion can help confirm the diagnosis of pericarditis, its absence does not preclude the diagnosis. Pericardial effusion was found in only 54% of patients with acute idiopathic pericarditis.[7] Two-dimensional echocardiography can also localize many loculated effusions and can define intrapericardial hematoma[8] or mass.

Magnetic resonance imaging (MRI) and computed tomography (CT). In inflammatory pericarditis, very few indications exist for the use of CT or MRI. Echocardiography provides a low-cost and portable screening examination in suspected pericardial disease. However, if the echocardiogram is ambiguous or discordant with clinical findings, CT and MRI can provide additional important information.

MRI clearly delineates the pericardium without contrast or radiation exposure, has a wide viewing area unaffected by lung and bone interfaces, and can provide tissue characterization of effusions, masses, and cysts. It can detect very small or loculated effusions that may be missed by echocardiography,[9] can accurately assess pericardial thickness, and can easily differentiate pleural from pericardial effusion. The size and extent of pericardial masses also can be accurately delineated.

CT provides easy recognition and determination of the size and distribution of pericardial effusions, the degree of pericardial thickening and calcification, and the delineation of cysts and masses.[10,11] Ultrafast, or cine, CT may provide additional functional information.

Laboratory studies. In acute idiopathic pericarditis, patients may have mild leukocytosis and increased sedimentation rate. The frequent simultaneous occurrence of myocarditis may result in mildly increased creatine kinase and creatine kinase-MB values. In general, laboratory findings are consistent with the underlying disease process rather than pericarditis per se, and the goal of laboratory testing should be to determine the underlying cause and to differentiate suspected pericarditis from other pathologic conditions. A carefully elicited history should guide the selection of diagnostic studies, such as tuberculin skin test, blood culture, sensitive thyrotropin, urea and creatinine, and serologic tests for infection and autoimmune disease. "Routine" pericardiocentesis has a very low diagnostic yield;[7] therefore, pericardial aspiration or biopsy is indicated primarily in prolonged or complicated cases, when bacterial or neoplastic pericarditis is suspected, or in patients with tamponade. In this selected group of patients, the yield is significantly higher and the aspirated fluid should undergo thorough examination.

Differential diagnosis

The diagnosis of acute pericarditis is straightforward if the patient has characteristic pain, ECG changes, and a pericardial friction rub. When these features are not present or are atypical, echocardiography and chest radiography can be very helpful in excluding acute myocardial infarction, aortic dissection, pneumonia, pneumothorax, and rib fractures (Table 55-3). Serial physical examinations are critical.

Table 55-3 Differential diagnosis of pericarditis

Acute myocardial infarction or angina
Pleuritis (pneumonia, pulmonary embolus)
Aortic dissection
Spontaneous pneumothorax
Rib fracture with chest wall pain
Pulmonary infarction

Management of specific causes of acute pericarditis

Virtually any of the causes of pericardial disease in Table 55-1 can be manifested as acute inflammatory pericarditis. Many of these, such as tuberculosis, are more likely to be subacute or chronic and are discussed later.

Idiopathic and viral pericarditis. Acute inflammatory pericarditis is usually a self-limited illness, lasting 1 to 4 weeks. Treatment is aimed at relieving symptoms and modifying the inflammatory response. Aspirin (4 to 8 g daily), indomethacin (25 to 50 mg three or four times a day), or ibuprofen (200 to 400 mg three or four times a day) is often effective in relieving pain, fever, and malaise within 24 to 48 hours. Bed rest is recommended until pain and fever have resolved. Therapy should be continued for approximately 2 weeks. Steroids usually provide rapid and effective relief of symptoms but should be avoided, because use is associated with a high rate of recurrence of symptoms when discontinued.

Acute myocardial infarction. Pericarditis in acute myocardial infarction can occur when myocardial injury involves the epicardium. Symptoms and signs usually appear within the first 5 days of the clinical event. Symptoms and signs of pericarditis occurring after this period are usually classified as post-myocardial infarction (Dressler's) syndrome, but some investigators[12] believe that episodes of pericarditis occurring early and late after myocardial infarction are simply different manifestations of a single disease process. We have chosen to discuss these two entities separately. Pericarditis may be asymptomatic, the diagnosis being made solely by auscultation of a friction rub, or be manifested by new, severe pleuritic pain that usually has a different character from that of the infarction. Friction rubs occur in up to 20% of serially examined patients. Rubs are detected most often 2 or 3 days after infarction and are more common in Q-wave infarction and patients with lower ejection fraction than in non-Q-wave infarction.[13,14] The ECG rarely shows typical, diagnostic, stage I changes, even in patients with classic symptoms and friction rub.[15] Pericardial effusion is common after myocardial infarction but does not necessarily represent pericarditis. If a rub is absent, pericardial effusion associated with myocardial infarction is more likely due to congestive heart failure or other hemodynamic abnormalities than to pericarditis.[16] However, pericardial effusion in myocardial infarction, regardless of the cause, is associated with increased hospital mortality.[14,17] The use of thrombolytic therapy does not appear to increase the incidence of pericardial effusion or pericarditis[16,18,19] and may decrease pericardial involvement because of reduced infarct size.[14] Thrombolytic therapy may be a risk factor for early hemorrhagic pericarditis and tamponade.[20]

Specific treatment is usually unnecessary unless pain is present. Treatment is similar to that of acute idiopathic pericarditis. Progression to tamponade or constrictive pericarditis is rare.[21] There is no consensus on how anticoagulant agents affect this form of pericarditis, but unless there is a convincing indication for their use, they are best avoided.

Post-cardiac injury syndrome. Instances of pericarditis occurring or persisting more than 1 or 2 weeks after myocardial infarction (Dressler's syndrome)[22] or cardiac surgery (postpericardiotomy syndrome) or related to iatrogenic cardiac perforation[23-25] or blunt trauma[26] all probably have a similar pathophysiologic basis, but the mechanism remains obscure. One hypothesis is that blood in the pericardial space provokes an autoimmune response, possibly triggered in some instances by a newly acquired or reactivated viral infection.[27] Fever, malaise, chest pain, pleuropericarditis, increased sedimentation rate, leukocytosis, pleural effusion, and pulmonary infiltrates are usually present.[28] Pericardial effusions are common and may become large.

Dressler's syndrome was once a common complication of myocardial infarction but is now relatively rare. The reason may be decreased use of oral anticoagulants and more aggressive treatment of early post-myocardial infarction pericarditis.[29] Postpericardiotomy syndrome is more common, occurring in 10% to 30% of patients after cardiac operations. Patients who have a history of pericarditis or who have taken steroids in the past have an increased incidence, but this may be related more to the underlying indication for the use of steroids (suppression of inflammatory response) than to steroid use itself.[30]

Post-cardiac injury syndrome is usually a self-limited but often prolonged and disabling illness. Treatment is symptomatic, with bed rest and ibuprofen, indomethacin, or aspirin for 1 to 2 weeks. Rehospitalization may be required for pain control or to assess the development of cardiac tamponade. Treatment may reduce the incidence of recurrent symptoms.[31] Steroid use should be avoided if possible. Associated cardiac tamponade may occur and is treated with pericardiocentesis and anti-inflammatory drugs.

Recurrent (relapsing) pericarditis. Acute inflammatory pericarditis of idiopathic, viral, post-cardiac injury, or traumatic type is usually self-limited, but 15% to 30% of patients have one or more recurrences during the following months or years. Fowler and Harbin[32] defined recurrent pericarditis as pericarditis that occurs in the absence of underlying active systemic disease or a new inciting incident in a patient who has had definite pericarditis 3 or more months before the recurrent symptoms. These attacks are characterized by pain exacerbated by respiration, malaise, and fever and are usually less severe than the initial episode. Rarely, recurrent episodes are more severe. The development of constrictive pericarditis or tamponade is rare. The most common complication is severe, protracted, disabling pain.

Treatment of recurrent episodes is similar to treatment of initial episodes. Unfortunately, a few of these patients have refractory symptoms even after a course of nonsteroidal anti-inflammatory drugs. Steroids are best avoided because they may prolong attacks. Recurrences are often triggered when prednisone dosage is tapered to 15 to 20 mg/day or less. A combination of nonsteroidal anti-inflammatory drugs and prednisone, as well as prolongation of steroid tapering for several months, may allow withdrawal. Several reported case series suggest that colchicine (0.5 to 1.5 mg/day) is effective in relieving symptoms during withdrawal of steroids and might prevent recurrence of pericarditis.[33-35] The duration of therapy may need to be prolonged (more than 1 year), and colchicine has not been effective in all steroid-dependent patients. Radical pericardiectomy is justified if a prolonged trial of medical therapy is unsuccessful. If the removal of pericardium is as complete as anatomically possible, most patients remain free of recurrent attacks of pericarditis.[36]

Infection. Pericarditis due to bacterial infection other than tuberculosis is uncommon. It is usually associated with immunosuppressive therapy, burns, malignancy, bacteremia with staphylococcal or streptococcal organisms, pneumonia with empyema, or thoracic surgery. The diagnosis is often missed because the characteristic features of acute pericarditis are often absent and the other clinical features are often attributed to the underlying infectious process.[37] Therefore, purulent pericarditis commonly results in cardiac tamponade and the need for pericardial aspiration. The symptoms of circulatory deterioration often develop abruptly in a patient with cough, dyspnea, night sweats, and a spiking fever who has been treated for days or weeks for a thoracic infection (often postoperative) or for infective endocarditis that results in rupture of a myocardial abscess.[38]

Prompt pericardial aspiration, culture, and appropriate antibiotic therapy are indicated. Surgical therapy is frequently necessary, because these effusions are often loculated and cannot be drained completely percutaneously. Most patients require pericardiectomy, but subxiphoid pericardial drainage is sometimes adequate,[39] especially in debilitated patients.

Fungal and protozoal pericarditis are uncommon and usually occur in immunocompromised patients who have systemic infections. The exception is histoplasmosis pericarditis, which is usually self-limited.[40] Treatment is aimed at eradicating the underlying infection. Surgical therapy is occasionally required.

Autoimmune and connective tissue disorders

SYSTEMIC LUPUS ERYTHEMATOSUS. Pericarditis is the most common cardiac manifestation of systemic lupus erythematosus. Signs and symptoms of pericarditis occur in 30% to 50% of patients with systemic lupus erythematosus and in up to 75% when echocardiographic and pathologic findings are considered.[41,42] The presentation is usually that of acute pericarditis with or without tamponade,[43-47] although rare instances of constrictive pericarditis have been reported.[48,49]

Recurrences are common and are often associated with myocarditis and active systemic lupus erythematosus. Echocardiography is useful to confirm the diagnosis and to define coexistent myocardial dysfunction and valvular disease. It is critical to differentiate typical inflammatory pericarditis from infectious or uremic pericarditis in these frequently immunocompromised and nephritic patients. Diagnostic pericardiocentesis is indicated if infection is suspected, especially if symptoms have not remitted with steroid therapy. Treatment of symptomatic lupus pericarditis is with moderate to high doses of prednisone.

Pericarditis occurs in drug-induced lupus syndromes but is less common than in spontaneous systemic lupus erythematosus. Hydralazine, procainamide, and isoniazid are common offending agents. Treatment includes withdrawal of the suspected drug and symptomatic administration of nonsteroidal anti-inflammatory drugs.

RHEUMATOID ARTHRITIS. Pericarditis occurs clinically in fewer than 10% of patients with rheumatoid arthritis but in up to 50% by echocardiographic and pathologic criteria.[50-52] It is more common in patients with active serositis.[51] Tamponade and constrictive pericarditis are relatively uncommon complications, but constriction has been reported despite inactive systemic disease.[53-56] Acute symptomatic pericarditis is treated with moderate doses of corticosteroids or nonsteroidal anti-inflammatory drugs. Constriction is treated with pericardiectomy.[57,58]

RHEUMATIC FEVER. Clinical pericarditis occurs in 5% to 10% of patients with acute rheumatic fever[59] and is usually diagnosed by the finding of a friction rub. Chest pain is usually not a prominent feature. Pericardial effusion, if present, is usually small and rarely produces tamponade. Constrictive pericarditis does not appear to occur. Rarely, acute pericarditis is the only manifestation of acute rheumatic fever,[60,61] but more commonly, pericarditis signifies more severe myocardial and valvular involvement[59] and a poorer prognosis. Pericarditis does not alter the treatment of rheumatic fever.

OTHER. Pericardial involvement is also relatively common in juvenile rheumatoid arthritis, adult Still's disease, mixed connective tissue disease, and scleroderma. It has been reported rarely in many other autoimmune-related conditions, including polyarteritis nodosa, Wegener's granulomatosis, systemic sclerosis, sarcoidosis, giant cell arteritis, Reiter's syndrome, ankylosing spondylitis, Whipple's disease, dermatomyositis, and inflammatory bowel disease. Pericarditis in these conditions often signifies a more active disease process. Treatment is usually directed at the underlying disease and at relieving symptoms.

Uremia. The cause of uremic pericarditis is not entirely clear. Although a prompt response to dialysis in many uremic patients with pericarditis suggests a correctable toxic-metabolic reaction, pericarditis develops in many patients while they are receiving adequate dialysis.[62] Because this type of pericarditis may not resolve with intensification of dialysis, nonsteroidal anti-inflammatory drugs, or steroids, concern has been raised that a different cause is responsible for dialysis-associated pericarditis.[62-64] Most patients present with signs or symptoms similar to those of other forms of acute pericarditis. Friction rubs occur in nearly all patients.[64] Pericardial effusions are noted in almost 90% of patients[62] and may become large. Cardiac tamponade occurs relatively frequently (10% to 20%) and may cause significant hemodynamic instability during dialysis. In hemodynamically stable patients with uremia who may be inadequately dialysed, treatment of pericarditis is the institution or intensification of dialysis. Indomethacin and systemic steroids are rarely effective in altering the course of the disease.[65] If symptoms persist or if tamponade develops, pericardiocentesis should be done promptly. Intrapericardial instillation of steroids may reduce symptoms and recurrent effusion.[66] Pericardiectomy is indicated in refractory or recurrent cases or when constriction occurs.[62,64]

Radiation. Radiation-induced pericarditis has become increasingly common, occurring in up to 30% of patients after chest irradiation.[67] In a 5-year period at one center, almost 7% of all patients with pericarditis had radiation-induced pericarditis.[68] Radiation pericarditis appears to be dose-dependent,[69] and recognition of this relation has led to changes in dose and treatment fields to minimize cardiac exposure. The most common tumors associated with radiation pericarditis are lymphoma and breast and lung cancers.

Radiation pericarditis occurs in several forms. Acute pericarditis occurring during radiation treatment is usually associated with large tumors contiguous to the heart. The inflammatory response may be due to inflammation and necrosis of nearby tumor. Symptoms often resolve spontaneously even if radiation is continued. Delayed pericarditis appears months or even years after irradiation, either as acute pericarditis or as subacute effusion, chronic effusive-constrictive disease, or constrictive disease.[70]

Acute pericarditis without effusion or hemodynamic embarrassment is treated symptomatically as previously described. Patients with tamponade require pericardiocentesis. When operation is required for recurrent or persistent effusion or for constriction, extensive pericardiectomy should be performed. Late success of surgical therapy is related to the amount of pericardium removed.[71] Patients with radiation-induced constrictive pericarditis may have higher perioperative and late mortality than patients with other causes of constriction,[72,73] and pericardial disease may complicate myocardial revascularization and other cardiac operations in irradiated patients.[74] Since the most critical differential diagnosis is recurrent tumor, diagnostic pericardial aspiration or biopsy is sometimes required, even in asymptomatic patients. Pericardial fluid in radiation pericarditis is almost invariably an exudate with a high protein content.[70] Cytology should be performed routinely.

CARDIAC TAMPONADE AND LARGE PERICARDIAL EFFUSIONS

Large pericardial effusions and cardiac tamponade may occur as a result of almost any of the causes listed in Table 55-1, but the most common causes at our institution are malignancy, cardiac surgical procedures, iatrogenic disorders (predominantly catheter-related), trauma to the

Table 55-4 Causes of tamponade

	%
Malignancy	38
Surgical procedure	23
Idiopathy	12
Ischemic complication	5
Catheter complication	5
Infection	5
Miscellaneous	12

heart, inflammatory or autoimmune diseases, and uremia (Table 55-4). Hemopericardium causing tamponade can occur with dissection or rupture of an aortic aneurysm or cardiac rupture. Very large pericardial effusions can occur without symptoms if they accumulate slowly, allowing the parietal pericardium to stretch gradually. However, if as little as 100 mL of fluid enters the pericardial space rapidly, significant impairment of cardiac filling can occur and result in tamponade. Small localized pericardial effusions, especially when they compress the atria, can cause significant hemodynamic embarrassment. This may occur after cardiac surgery or trauma, and a high degree of awareness is necessary to make the diagnosis. Pneumopericardium, most often caused by chest trauma, local disease extension, or iatrogenic complications, has a high incidence of tamponade.[75]

Pathophysiology of cardiac tamponade

Normally, intrapericardial pressure is essentially equal to intrapleural pressure and is slightly negative in inspiration and positive in expiration. When intrapericardial fluid accumulates, the pressure rises slowly at first and then rapidly as the pericardium reaches its maximum volume. The effect of increased pericardial fluid on pericardial pressure depends on both the volume of fluid and the distensibility of pericardium. Central venous pressure is normally slightly higher than intrapericardial pressure, so that the normal venous-to-cardiac gradient is maintained. When intrapericardial pressure increases to equilibrate with central venous pressure, ventricular end-diastolic pressure and mean atrial pressure increase to support cardiac filling and systemic arterial pressure decreases. The resultant decrease in ventricular volume and filling causes a drop in stroke volume and cardiac output. Reflex increases in systemic vascular resistance and adrenergic tone provide some compensation at first, but as tamponade progresses, these mechanisms are no longer adequate to provide systemic perfusion.

Echocardiographic studies have supported the concept that tamponade is associated with decreased blood flow into the left side of the heart during inspiration and increased flow into the right side.[76] This occurrence is a result of the greater volume of blood that can be accommodated in the pulmonary vascular bed. Recent studies in experimental animals have supported this, showing that, with inspiration, flow to the right side of the heart is augmented and flow to the left side is decreased.[77,78] Hence, impairment of left-sided ouput with inspiration is caused primarily not by an inspiratory increase in intrapericardial pressure but rather by selective impairment of filling of the left side of the heart[79] (Fig 55-2).

All the factors that contribute to this selective decrease in left-sided filling during inspiration are not yet known, but the following observations are pertinent. Echocardiographic studies show evidence of increased right ventricular volume and a shift of the interventricular septum toward the left ventricle. The increased right ventricular volume further increases pressure in the pericardium and tends to compress the left ventricle further and reduce its volume. Experimental cardiac tamponade in dogs has shown a reversal of the normal gradient from pulmonary venous to left atrial pressure during inspiration, with resulting reversal of blood flow in the pulmonary veins.[80] When cardiac tamponade is severe enough to embarrass

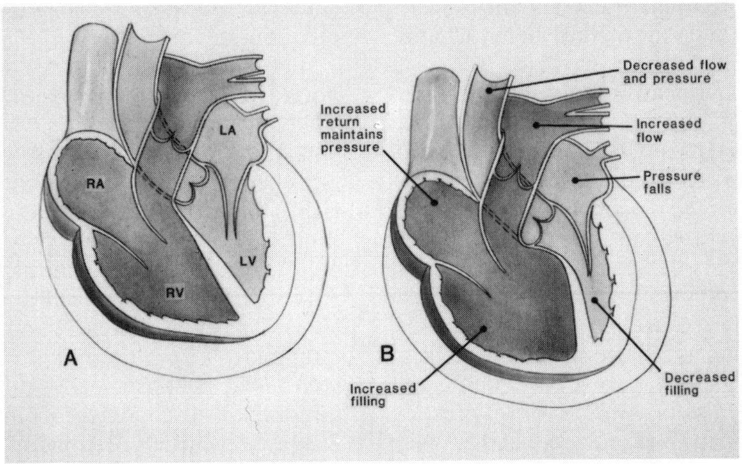

Fig 55-2 Diagram of expiration (**A**) and early inspiration (**B**) in the presence of cardiac tamponade. Increased intrapericardial pressure produces increased diastolic pressures and results in increased resistance to ventricular filling. With inspiration, however, there is increased flow to the right heart associated with a shift of the interventricular septum to the left. Filling of the left heart is reduced by a combination of factors (see text). There may be premature midsystolic closing of the aortic valve and delayed opening of the mitral valve. *RA,* right atrium; *LA,* left atrium; *RV,* right ventricle; *LV,* left ventricle.

both ventricles, the filling of the left and right chambers is determined by their filling pressures. Since pulmonary venous pressure is transiently below systemic pressure during inspiration, filling of the right ventricle is favored, and, as noted, this predilection tends to impede and lessen left ventricular filling. Expiration reverses this situation: pulmonary venous pressure increases to or above systemic venous pressure, and the result is increased left ventricular filling. Studies in patients show that these respiratory changes are transient and are limited to the initial phase of inspiration and expiration.[81]

The hemodynamic changes in cardiac tamponade represent a continuum ranging from subtle changes in left and right ventricular filling detectable only by sensitive Doppler or invasive techniques to gross hemodynamic derangement with hypotension, tachycardia, and multiorgan failure due to hypoperfusion.[78,82,83] Early recognition and treatment are critical, and currently employed sensitive diagnostic techniques allow both.

Clinical presentation

Beck's triad, consisting of hypotension, increased systemic venous pressure, and a small, quiet heart,[84] is typical of acute cardiac tamponade caused by a sudden increase in pericardial fluid and pressure due to trauma, aortic dissection, or cardiac rupture. More commonly, tamponade develops more gradually. Blood pressure may be nearly normal, and the cardiac silhouette may be enlarged. Large effusions without tamponade may cause no symptoms, but because subtle hemodynamic aberrations can be detected in most of these patients,[82,83] large amounts of pericardial fluid may affect ventricular volume and function even when no clinical signs or symptoms are present. Patients with early tamponade may have chest discomfort, cough, hoarseness, tachypnea, and dyspnea. If tamponade is severe, hypotension, dyspnea, pallor, cyanosis, anxiety, diaphoresis, and, ultimately, hemodynamic collapse can occur.

Initial clinical signs of tamponade are usually increased central venous pressure and a slight increase in heart rate. Central venous pressure is almost always increased except when hypovolemia is so severe that central venous pressure is reduced to normal. This condition has been termed "low-pressure tamponade."[85,86] As tamponade progresses, the heart sounds become distant, the heart rate increases, and the blood pressure and pulse pressure decrease. Pericardial rubs are present in 50% of cases.

Pulsus paradoxus, defined as an inspiratory decrease in systolic blood pressure of greater than 10 to 20 mm Hg or greater than 50% of the pulse pressure, is often present. When pulse pressure is already markedly reduced or when there is severe hypotension, pulsus paradoxus may not be detectable. Other conditions in which pulsus paradoxus may not be detected include advanced left ventricular hypertrophy or congestive heart failure in which left ventricular filling pressure is maintained, atrial septal defect in which pressures are equalized, and severe aortic regurgitation. Pulsus paradoxus may also be present in constrictive pericarditis, restrictive cardiomyopathy, obstructive lung disease, massive pulmonary embolus, and hypovolemic shock. The mechanism of pulsus paradoxus appears to be the inspiratory enhancement of right ventricular filling at the expense of left ventricular filling due to fixed cardiac volume.[77,87,88] Although the pattern of venous pulsation is rarely useful in tamponade, there may be a prominent x descent. Inspiratory distention of the neck veins (Kussmaul's sign) is uncommon unless there is underlying constriction.[89]

Diagnostic tests

Electrocardiogram. The ECG may be normal or show changes of acute pericarditis. Sinus tachycardia is common. Voltage may be low. Electrical alternans due to swinging motion of the heart within a pericardial effusion is not a common finding but when present is useful, since it is a relatively specific sign.[90,91]

Chest radiograph. The chest radiograph may be normal if the effusion is small, or the cardiac silhouette may be globular if a large effusion is present. Pleural effusions are common. Aortic size and contour should be examined to assess possible dissection.

Echocardiography. Patients with tamponade almost always have significant pericardial effusions. Echocardiography allows rapid detection and quantitation of pericardial fluid in nearly all patients. Patients with suspected tamponade who do not have obvious effusion can benefit from transesophageal echocardiography, which is useful when precordial images are poor or effusions are localized, especially postoperatively.[92-95] Echocardiography can also accurately distinguish many causes of hemodynamic compromise in patients who are not found to have an effusion or who may have a compressing mass or hematoma.[96] Transthoracic echocardiography in tension pneumopericardium may show complete or systolic phase loss of the cardiac image (the "air gap sign"), since air is a poor conductor of ultrasound.[97]

Two-dimensional and Doppler criteria for the diagnosis of cardiac tamponade have been developed. These echocardiographic signs reflect the altered pressure and filling hemodynamics. Two-dimensional echocardiographic features of tamponade include right atrial and right ventricular diastolic collapse,[98-101] reciprocal variation in ventricular chamber size through the respiratory cycle,[71] and lack of inspiratory vena caval collapse.[102] Although relatively specific, these signs are frequently absent, especially in early tamponade or when significant pulmonary hypertension is present. Left atrial or left ventricular collapse may occur in isolated left ventricular tamponade or in severe pulmonary hypertension.[103-105]

More recently, pulsed-wave Doppler echocardiographic features of tamponade have been described. Analyzing atrioventricular valve and venous flow profiles with pulsed Doppler technique along with nasal respirometry allows a noninvasive assessment of altered cardiac filling hemodynamics during various phases of the respiratory cycle.[88,106,107]

A normal Doppler profile across the mitral valve shows an initial peak (E wave) followed by a smaller peak (A wave) without respiratory variation. With cardiac tam-

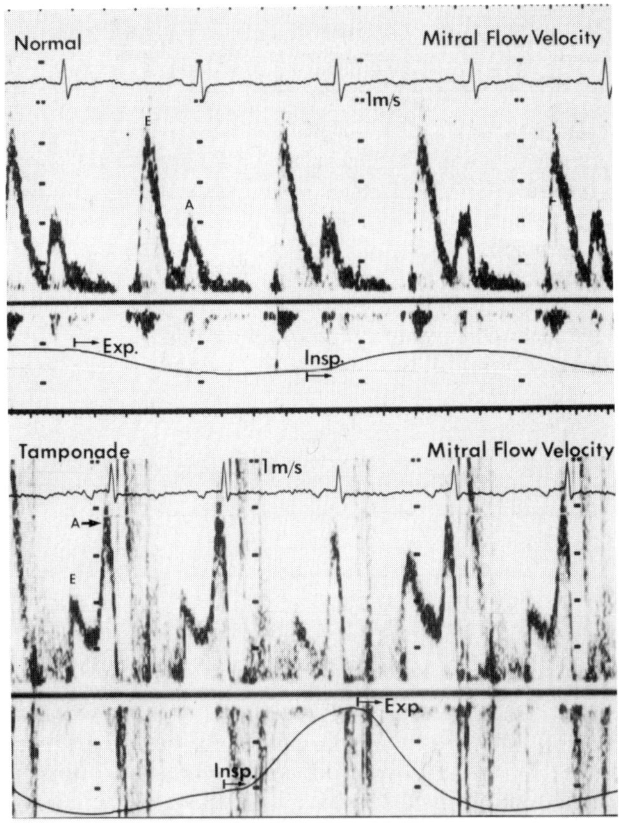

Fig 55-3 Mitral flow velocity profiles from normal control subject **(upper)** and from patient with cardiac tamponade **(lower).** In profile from patient, note decrease in peak early filling velocity *(E)* on first beat of inspiration *(Insp.)* in comparison with preceding beat during apnea and increase on first beat of expiration *(Exp.)*. In contrast, minimal variation is evident during respiration in normal subject. *A,* peak atrial filling velocity. (From Burstow DJ, Oh JK, Bailey KR, et al: Cardiac tamponade: characteristic Doppler observations. *Mayo Clin Proc* 64:312-324, 1989. By permission, Mayo Foundation for Medical Education and Research.)

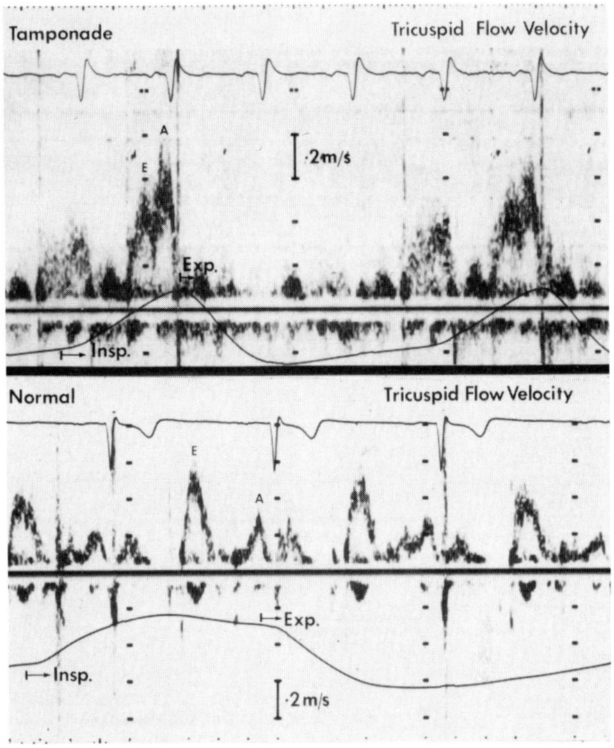

Fig 55-4 Tricuspid flow velocity profiles. **Upper,** from patient with cardiac tamponade. Note increase in flow velocity during inspiration *(Insp.)*. On first beat of expiration *(Exp.),* note total loss of tricuspid flow velocity. **Lower,** from normal control subject. Note increase in tricuspid peak early filling velocity *(E)* during inspiration, consistent with normal inspiratory increase in right ventricular filling. During expiration, no appreciable decrease in tricuspid E is evident. *A,* peak atrial filling velocity. (From Burstow DJ, Oh JK, Bailey KR, et al: Cardiac tamponade: characteristic Doppler observations. *Mayo Clin Proc* 64:312-324, 1989. By permission, Mayo Foundation for Medical Education and Research.)

ponade, there is an inspiratory decrease in mitral inflow velocity (Fig 55-3). The normal flow across the tricuspid valve is similar to mitral flow but with lower velocity and slightly increasing velocity with inspiration. With cardiac tamponade, there is an exaggerated increase in flow velocity with inspiration and a marked decrease at expiration (Fig 55-4). Normal Doppler flow in the superior vena cava and hepatic veins consists of forward flow into the right atrium during systole and diastole, with a higher velocity during systole and a slight increase in velocity with inspiration. With cardiac tamponade, systolic flow velocity increases during inspiration and decreases with expiration. Diastolic flow velocity decreases or disappears with expiration (Fig 55-5). There is an inspiratory increase in isovolumic relaxation time.

Similar reciprocal inspiratory changes in right and left ventricular stroke volumes have also been identified by analysis of aortic and pulmonary Doppler flow profiles.[77,78] In patients with tamponade, Doppler-assessed pulmonary venous flow, which reflects left atrial filling, shows a relative increase in the proportion of left atrial filling during ventricular systole over that during diastole and an inspiratory decrease in systolic left atrial filling.[108] Significant right or left ventricular dysfunction can make both the two-dimensional and the Doppler signs of tamponade less reliable.[108,109]

The respiratory variations in transvalvular velocities and variations in venous filling patterns in cardiac tamponade reflect the greater interdependence of the ventricles that develops when the heart becomes constrained by fluid. Filling of one ventricle influences filling of the other in a reciprocal manner. Likewise, changes in mitral inflow velocity reflect respiratory variation in preload. The pulmonary venous-to-left atrial gradient,

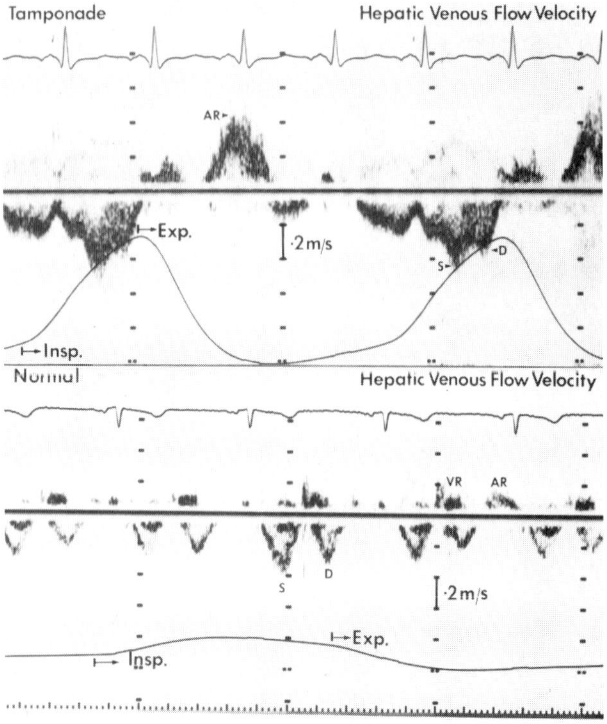

Fig 55-5 Hepatic venous flow velocity profiles. **Upper,** from same patient with cardiac tamponade illustrated in Figure 55-4 **Upper.** Note increase in flow velocity during inspiration *(Insp.)*. On first beat of expiration *(Exp.)*, note total loss of both systolic *(S)* and diastolic *(D)* forward flow and considerable increase in reverse flow with atrial contraction *(AR)*. These findings correspond to total loss of tricuspid flow velocity seen during expiration (Fig 55-4 **Upper**) in cardiac tamponade. **Lower,** from normal control subject. Note inspiratory increase in both systolic *(S)* and diastolic *(D)* forward flow velocities. During expiration, no substantial decrease in forward flow is evident; however, reverse flow is minimally increased at end-systole *(VR)* and with atrial contraction *(AR)*. (From Burstow DJ, Oh JK, Bailey KR, et al: Cardiac tamponade: characteristic Doppler observations. *Mayo Clin Proc* 64:312-324, 1989. By permission, Mayo Foundation for Medical Education and Research.)

normally unaffected by respiratory changes, varies with respiration in patients with tamponade. Doppler echocardiography provides a sensitive method to detect even very early hemodynamic changes related to pericardial effusion.

Catheterization. Although invasive methods are rarely required for the diagnosis of tamponade, characteristic hemodynamic changes are found. Stroke volume is decreased, and intrapericardial and intracardiac diastolic pressures are increased and equalized or nearly equalized.[81] The right atrial pressure waveform shows a predominant systolic x descent with a smaller or absent y descent. There is an inspiratory decrease in left ventricular and arterial systolic pressure (pulsus paradoxus) with a reciprocal increase in right ventricular systolic pressure.[77]

Table 55-5 Common causes of malignant pericardial disease

Metastatic
Lung
Breast
Lymphoma
Leukemia
Melanoma
Ovarian
Adenocarcinoma of unknown primary origin
Primary (rare)
Mesothelioma
Angiosarcoma
Fibrosarcoma
Pheochromocytoma
Lymphoma
Teratoma

Management of specific causes of effusion and cardiac tamponade

Patients who are in shock or who are hemodynamically unstable require urgent pericardiocentesis. Volume expansion and transfusion have little place in the management of tamponade when definitive therapy is available with pericardiocentesis, especially under echocardiographic guidance, as described below in the "Pericardial Aspiration" section. A pericardial drainage catheter should be inserted until the cause and rate of fluid accumulation have been ascertained. In most instances of tamponade, catheter drainage is the definitive therapy. However, many patients with iatrogenic ventricular puncture, trauma, or aortic dissection require further surgical intervention. Our experience with echocardiographically guided pericardiocentesis has been so favorable, however, that this procedure is performed whenever possible before the patient is sent to surgery to minimize the inherent risks of anesthesia induction.[71]

Patients with few symptoms and subtle changes on noninvasive testing can be managed by close follow-up or elective echocardiographically guided pericardiocentesis for therapy and diagnosis.

Neoplasm. Pericardial effusion with or without cardiac tamponade is the most common presentation of malignant pericardial disease, but effusive-constrictive and constrictive disease also occur when tumor has encased the heart. Occasionally, tamponade can develop quite rapidly, especially in hemorrhagic effusions. Primary tumors of the pericardium are rare and do not usually produce symptoms until they are advanced. Secondary tumors, such as pulmonary and breast malignant lesions, commonly involve the pericardium through local spread. Lymphoma, leukemia, and melanoma have a high rate of pericardial metastasis (Table 55-5). These may appear as an intrapericardial mass, diffuse pericardial thickening, or multiple discrete tumor deposits. While it is uncommon for metastatic pericardial disease to develop without other distant metastatic lesions,[110] tamponade is occasionally the presenting symptom of extracardiac malignant disease.[7,111-113]

Patients are often without symptoms in the early stages but may note dyspnea, cough, or nonspecific chest pain. Echocardiography should be performed to define pericardial thickness, to determine the size of any effusion or mass, and to assess left ventricular function and hemodynamics for tamponade or constriction. CT and MRI provide enhanced definition of contiguous structures and may define the location and extent of extracardiac malignant disease.[114,115]

If the patient does not have tamponade, no specific therapy is indicated. Diagnostic pericardiocentesis is useful in differentiating malignant pericardial disease from other causes of pericardial effusion. Although hemorrhagic effusion has no predictive value, the finding of malignant cells on cytologic examination is diagnostic. False-negative results do occur, however, especially in lymphoma and mesothelioma.[112] Closed pericardial biopsy can be considered if suspicion is high and cytologic findings are negative, but it may not be diagnostic because of the random distribution of tumor on the pericardium.[112,116] Although pericardial effusion in a patient with cancer can be an ominous sign, the incidence of idiopathic and radiation pericarditis is high and only one-half of patients with malignant disease and signs and symptoms of pericardial disease have malignant pericarditis.[112]

In patients with tamponade, our policy has been to perform echocardiographically guided pericardiocentesis with routine percutaneous catheter drainage for several days. Of patients treated in this manner, 30% to 40% require no further treatment.[117-119] There is no consensus on the treatment of patients whose effusions recur. Repeat pericardiocentesis with or without sclerotherapy, intrapericardial instillation of cancer chemotherapeutic agents, percutaneous balloon pericardiostomy, subxiphoid surgical drainage, and radiation therapy have all been suggested. Because of the limited survival of most patients with malignant pericardial effusions (usually weeks to months), complete pericardiectomy provides no clear survival advantage over more limited resections and causes a higher operative morbidity.[120] The condition and prognosis of the patient, as well as the availability of effective systemic therapy, may help determine the best course of treatment. The goal of treatment should be to make the patient as comfortable as possible with minimal risk and distress.

Trauma. Closed chest injury can result in pericarditis and effusion, especially if there has been epicardial injury. This occurrence is usually self-limited, but tamponade and postcardiac injury syndrome occasionally ensue.[121] Penetrating cardiac injury is much more likely to result in acute tamponade and hemodynamic collapse, which may be due to pericardial hemorrhage, myocardial rupture, or injury to the great vessels. Rupture of the esophagus into the pericardial space can lead to tamponade and an intense inflammatory and infectious pericarditis that requires early surgical intervention.

Pericardial effusion is common after cardiac surgery (50% to 85%), but most effusions are small and loculated and do not worsen. Although effusion is more commonly detected after coronary artery bypass surgery, cardiac tamponade, while rare, appears more commonly after valve replacement surgery, perhaps because of anticoagulant therapy.[95]

Postoperative intrapericardial hemorrhage with or without hematoma formation can cause localized cardiac tamponade, especially if the atria are compressed. This form of tamponade is particularly difficult to recognize, because clinical deterioration can be striking and there may be very little free pericardial fluid. Transesophageal echocardiography has proven very useful in diagnosing localized effusions and hematomas and in documenting their hemodynamic significance.[92-94,96]

Probably the most commonly encountered cause of trauma-induced effusion and tamponade is iatrogenic cardiac puncture during diagnostic and therapeutic procedures. Virtually every procedure that introduces a catheter or wire into the heart or coronary arteries has produced cardiac tamponade.[25] Patients often complain of sudden onset of chest pain, which may be pleuritic, and they may become tachycardic and hypotensive. Urgent echocardiography and echocardiographically guided pericardiocentesis with catheter drainage are usually sufficient, but if bleeding is brisk or continues for several days, surgical intervention may be required.

Myxedema. An enlarged cardiac silhouette on the chest radiograph and low-amplitude QRS and T waves on the ECG are the most frequent presenting clinical cardiac abnormalities in myxedema. The accompanying pericardial effusion accounts for these abnormalities, but the exact cause of the effusion is unclear. The cardiac abnormalities occasionally lead to the diagnosis of thyroid deficiency, but usually the other clinical features of myxedema predominate, and the cardiac findings are incidental. Some patients not only have pericardial effusion but also have pleural effusion, ascites, and fluid in the uvea of the eye. These abnormalities all occur without any evidence of cardiac failure and, therefore, suggest the probability of altered capillary permeability. Cardiac tamponade is extremely rare but has been reported. The incidence of pericardial effusion in hypothyroidism has become quite low, since the condition is now usually diagnosed before overt myxedema occurs.[122]

Treatment is thyroid hormone replacement. The pericardial effusion with its associated roentgenographic and ECG changes resolves in a few months.

CONSTRICTIVE PERICARDITIS

Constrictive pericarditis occurs when fibrous or calcific thickening and contraction of either the parietal or epicardial pericardium, or both, occur, preventing normal diastolic filling of the heart. The diagnosis of constrictive pericarditis is difficult and challenging to make, both because its clinical presentation is subtle and diverse and because current diagnostic tools are imperfect. Common causes of constrictive pericarditis are listed in Table 55-6. Although tuberculosis still causes most cases of constrictive pericarditis in many developing countries,[123] it has

Table 55-6 Causes of constrictive pericarditis

Common
- Idiopathic
- Irradiation
- Postsurgical

Uncommon
- Infectious: tuberculous, bacterial, fungal
- Neoplastic disease
- Connective tissue disorder
- Uremia
- Trauma
- Sarcoid
- Methysergide therapy
- Epicardial implantable defibrillator patches

Table 55-7 Frequency of appearance of signs and symptoms in constrictive pericarditis

	%
Edema	55-90
Dyspnea	50-80
Fatigue	30-50
Jugular venous distention	40-95
Hepatomegaly	30-90
Ascites	30 70
Pulsus paradoxus	8-40
Kussmaul's sign	15-75
Pericardial knock	5-40
Pericardial rub	5-25
Fever	5
Atrial fibrillation	10-35

been quite rare in the United States over the past 2 decades. A revival of tuberculous pericarditis is expected to occur because of the increased incidence of tuberculosis in patients with human immunodeficiency virus infection and other diseases associated with immunocompromised states as well as increased immigration from countries where tuberculosis is endemic.

No specific cause is found in most cases of constrictive pericarditis (more than 80% in our experience).[36] Radiation and cardiac surgical procedures are increasingly recognized causes of constrictive pericarditis, each representing almost 30% of reported series of patients.[124-126] Constrictive pericarditis after cardiac surgery is rare, occurring in 0.025% to 0.3% of patients,[36] but because of the large number of cardiac operations performed, it accounts for an important proportion of total cases of constrictive pericarditis. It can occur anywhere from 2 weeks to 17 years after any operation in which the pericardium is opened.[127-129] It may be more common in patients in whom the postpericardiotomy syndrome develops.[129]

Effusive constrictive pericarditis is a somewhat poorly defined clinical entity that usually appears subacutely with signs and symptoms of tamponade or constriction. The patients usually have moderate to large effusions along with increased central venous pressure, so that the diagnosis of cardiac tamponade is initially highly suspect. Despite adequate pericardiocentesis, however, the signs, symptoms, and physiologic factors remain abnormal and are usually consistent with constriction. Pericardial thickness is usually increased. Effusive constrictive disease may be more common after irradiation and in patients with rheumatoid arthritis. The diagnosis of residual constriction after removal of pericardial fluid requires a high degree of suspicion, but subsequent therapy with complete pericardiectomy is similar to that of "classic" constrictive pericarditis and appears to be successful.

Pathophysiology

Constrictive pericarditis appears to be an extension of the inflammatory process seen in acute pericarditis or trauma. Over time, either because of continuing systemic disease or continued inflammatory stimulus, the pericardium thickens, undergoes fibrosis, and ultimately calcifies. As in cardiac tamponade, the intrapericardial volume is fixed and intrapleural pressure is transmitted poorly to the heart through the thick pericardium. There is ventricular interdependence as well as dissociation between intracardiac and intrathoracic pressures. This leads to elevation and equilibration of diastolic pressures in all four chambers of the heart. There is a reciprocal relationship between left-sided and right-sided filling because of this interventricular coupling. In inspiration, left ventricular filling is compromised and right ventricular filling is favored. Early diastolic filling is rapid but stops abruptly as the stiff pericardium reaches its limit of distensibility. Ventricular diastolic pressure then rises rapidly and increases the atrial pressure, producing a pressure plateau from middle to end diastole. Venous filling of the right atrium is predominantly diastolic, which is in contrast to the normal pattern or that found in tamponade. Central venous pressure is always increased, often leading to hepatic congestion, ascites, and peripheral edema.

Clinical presentation

Dyspnea, edema, and fatigue, which often develop insidiously over months to years, are the most common symptoms of constrictive pericarditis. In late stages of the disease, ascites, anorexia, weakness, cachexia, and multiorgan failure occur. Nocturnal dyspnea, orthopnea, and chest discomfort are uncommon. Symptoms are often nonspecific, and the prominence of edema and ascites frequently leads to the mistaken diagnosis of cirrhosis. However, the neck veins are always distended, a characteristic finding not present in cirrhosis (Table 55-7).

Patients are frequently tachycardic, with normal or low blood pressure. Atrial fibrillation is common. Because of the marked elevation of venous pressure, jugular venous pulsations may become apparent only when the patient is sitting or standing and may persist after a good diuresis. A prominent diastolic y descent as well as an x descent may be appreciated but may be difficult to distinguish in tachycardic patients. The normal inspiratory drop in venous pressure does not occur, because changes in intrathoracic pressure are not transmitted through the thickened pericardium. Inspiratory distention of the neck veins (Kussmaul's sign) is frequently present but may also be present in congestive heart failure, right ventricular infarction, or restrictive cardiomyopathy; the mechanism may be the transmission of intra-abdominal pressure through the distended and compliant venous system to the superior vena cava.[130] Heart sounds are normal or soft, and murmurs are usually not heard. A pericardial knock may be heard or palpated in early diastole, and it may represent the rapid deceleration of blood entering the ventricles due to pericardial constraint. It occurs 90 to 120 msec after the aortic component of the second heart sound and may be difficult to differentiate from a classic third heart sound or the opening snap of mitral stenosis.[131] Signs of pleural effusion may be present. An enlarged and pulsatile liver is common, and ascites may be more prominent than peripheral edema, especially in young patients.

Diagnostic tests

Electrocardiogram. The ECG is usually unhelpful in assessing constrictive pericarditis, often showing nonspecific ST and T-wave abnormalities, low voltage, or atrial fibrillation.

Chest radiograph. The chest radiograph frequently shows cardiac enlargement, but there is rarely evidence of pulmonary congestion or hypertension. Pleural effusions are common. Intrapericardial calcification occurs in up to 50% of cases (Fig 55-6). There may be linear "eggshell calcification" or an irregular and scattered distribution of calcium anywhere over the heart.[132,133] When present with clinical signs of constriction, pericardial calcification is virtually diagnostic of constrictive pericarditis, but

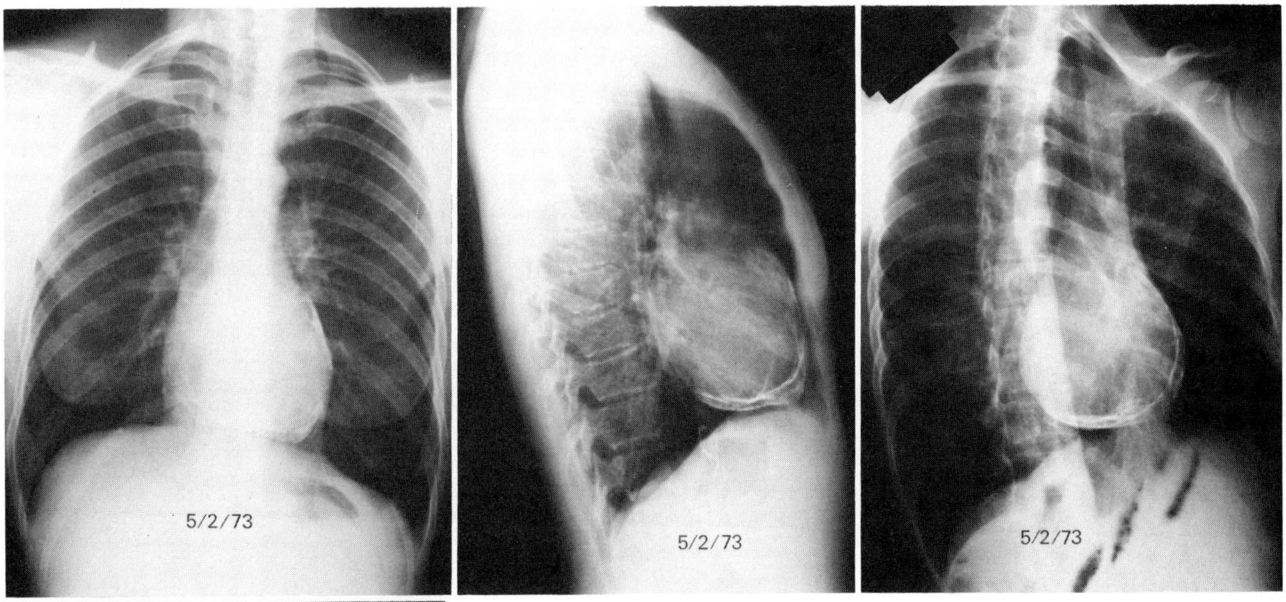

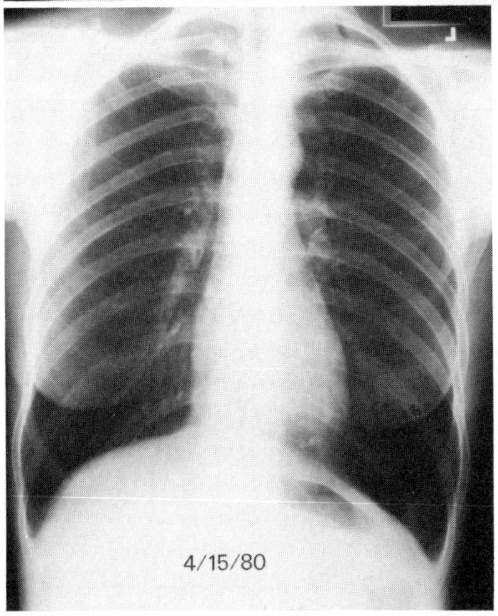

Fig 55-6 **Upper,** chest radiographs in a 48-year-old woman with constrictive pericarditis with calcification. Periodic edema and pericardial calcium had been noted 7 years earlier. Fatigue and dyspnea on effort were present for 1 year. The jugular venous pressure was 20 cm H_2O. A prominent y descent was present, along with a third heart sound. Pericardial resection was carried out in 1973. **Lower,** in 1980, the patient was asymptomatic, and the radiograph was normal.

calcium may be present without constriction, and constrictive pericarditis can be severe without evidence of calcification.

Echocardiography. The M-mode and two-dimensional echocardiographic features of constrictive pericarditis are nonspecific. Pericardial thickening, diastolic flattening of the left ventricular posterior wall,[134,135] abnormal septal motion,[136] inspiratory displacement of the atrial septum toward the left atrium,[137] and early opening of the pulmonic valve[134,135] have been described. Himelman et al.[138] showed that the finding of one or more of three disorders—early diastolic septal bounce, vena cava plethora with blunted respiratory motion, and pericardial adhesion with lack of pericardial sliding—improves sensitivity and specificity in differentiating constrictive pericarditis from restrictive cardiomyopathy or inconsequential pericardial thickening. These findings all suggest constrictive physiology but are not diagnostic. Two-dimensional echocardiography is useful primarily for distinguishing various other cardiac abnormalities (silent valvular disease and cardiomyopathy) that may simulate constrictive pericarditis. This aspect and other diagnostic procedures were reviewed by Nishimura et al.[139]

More recently, Hatle et al.[140] described the Doppler echocardiographic features of constrictive pericarditis, specifically in relation to the hemodynamic differences between constrictive and restrictive physiology. As described in patients with tamponade who have constrictive pericarditis, respiratory variation occurs in early diastolic filling velocities across the mitral and tricuspid valves. With inspiration, the early diastolic mitral velocity decreases and tricuspid velocity increases. The opposite occurs with expiration. These findings were not present in patients with restrictive cardiomyopathy. In addition, Appleton et al.[141] described the venous inflow features of patients with constrictive pericarditis. Patients with constrictive physiology had a marked decrease in diastolic forward flow and an increase in flow reversal during expiration. This finding coincides with an increase in filling of the left side of the heart seen in the mitral inflow signal (Fig 55-7). Transesophageal Doppler interrogation of the pulmonary veins has demonstrated a typical pattern

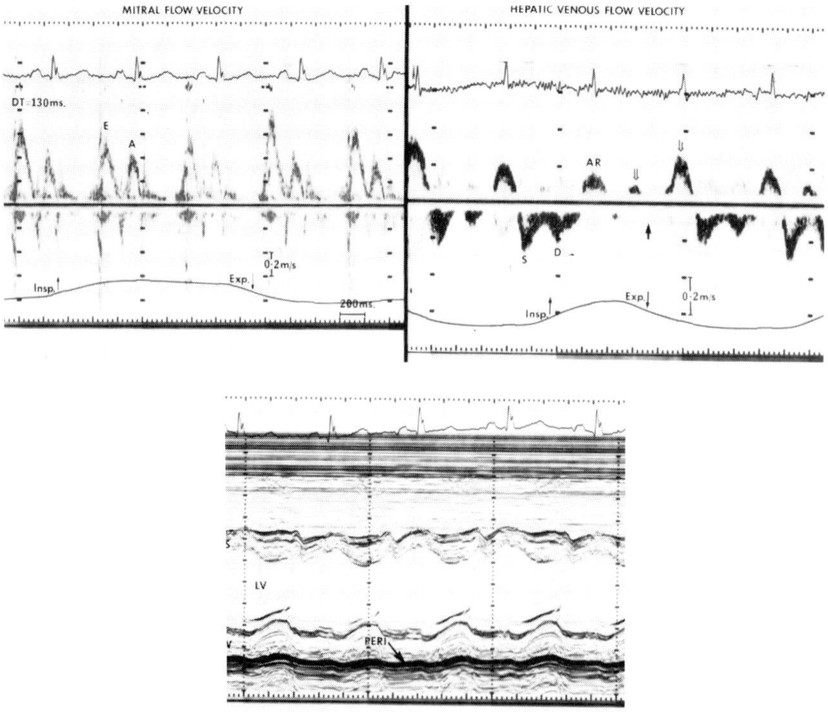

Fig 55-7 Composite picture showing mitral, hepatic Doppler flow patterns and M-mode echocardiogram in constrictive pericarditis. The mitral inflow velocity *(E,A)* markedly decreases on inspiration *(Insp.)* and increases on expiration *(Exp.)*. Hepatic venous flow velocity demonstrates marked decrease in diastolic forward flow *(solid arrow)* and increase in flow reversals *(open arrows)* on expiration. The pericardium is thickened on the M-mode strip. *A,* peak late mitral velocity; *AR,* atrial reversal; *D,* diastolic forward flow; *DT,* deceleration time; *E,* peak early filling velocity; *LV,* left ventricle; *PERI,* pericardium; *PW,* posterior wall; *S,* systolic forward flow velocity. (From Khandheria BK, Burstow DJ: Pericardial disease: echocardiographic developments. *Curr Opin Cardiol* 3:411-415, 1988. By permission of Gower Academic Journals.)

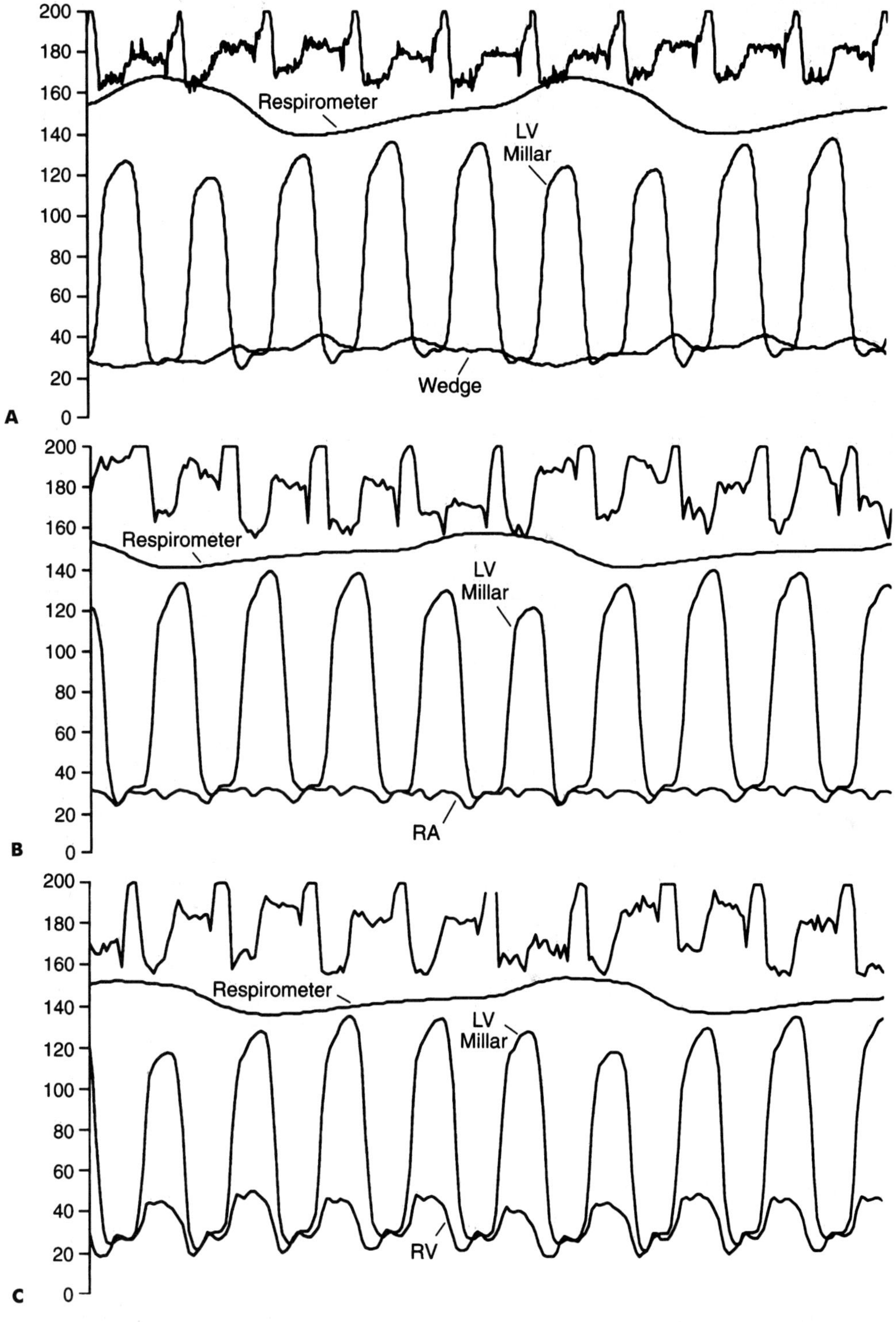

Fig 55-8 A-C, high-fidelity manometer tip catheter pressure tracings in a patient with constrictive pericarditis. There are elevation and equalization of left ventricular *(LV),* pulmonary capillary wedge *(Wedge),* right ventricular *(RV),* and right atrial *(RA)* end-diastolic pressures. The LV and RV tracings **(C)** reflect rapid early diastolic filling followed by a diastolic plateau (square root sign). Dynamic respiratory changes demonstrate an inspiratory decrease in the wedge-LV gradient, resulting in reduced LV filling **(A)** as well as dissociation between RV and LV filling pressure changes **(C).**

in constrictive pericarditis: biphasic antegrade flow with systolic flow greater than diastolic flow, expiratory enhancement of diastolic flow, and inspiratory diminution of both systolic and diastolic flows. Normal pulmonary venous flow is minimally affected by respiration.[142]

The Doppler finding of pure constrictive hemodynamics in patients with a clinical picture of constrictive pericarditis predicts improvement in symptoms and normalization of Doppler hemodynamics after pericardiectomy. These patients can usually be confidently operated on without invasive studies.[143]

Cardiac catheterization. Classically, the sine qua non of constriction is increased and equal or nearly equal diastolic pressures in all four chambers of the heart. The ventricular pressures reflect rapid early filling followed by a diastolic plateau (square root sign)[79] (Fig 55-8). Eighty-five percent of filling occurs in the first 30% to 40% of diastole, compared with 35% of filling in normals.[131] There are prominent and equal x and y descents in the right atrial tracing. The cardiac index is low normal or decreased.[144] Dynamic respiratory changes can be assessed by simultaneous right and left ventricular pressure curves. During inspiration, right ventricular pressure increases coincident with a decrease in left ventricular pressure, indicating dissociation of intrathoracic and intracardiac pressures as well as increased ventricular interaction.

Computed tomography and magnetic resonance imaging. Both CT and MRI provide accurate assessment of pericardial thickness.[10,11,145-148] MRI has a slight disadvantage, since it may not differentiate calcium from fibrosis.[149] Although not all patients with thickened pericardium (>2 to 4 mm) have constriction,[140] the finding of normal thickness strongly militates against constrictive pericarditis. This is helpful in differentiating restrictive cardiomyopathy from constrictive pericarditis.[145,150,151] (Fig 55-9). However, exceptions occur, and we have seen cases of constrictive pericarditis in which the pericardium had a normal thickness. The pericardium is usually thickened in patients who have undergone a cardiac surgical procedure in which the pericardial space is obliterated. Consequently, evidence of pericardial thickening in those patients is of little help in determining whether constriction is present.[11] Cine computed tomography provides measurements of both pericardial thickness and left and right ventricular filling fraction. The combination of anatomic and physiologic data shows promise in differentiating patients with and without constriction.[152]

Differential diagnosis

The clinical picture of constrictive pericarditis can mimic hepatic or renal disease as well as right ventricular failure or malignant disease. The history, noninvasive imaging, and routine laboratory testing combined with examination of the neck veins can usually promptly differentiate these entities. The most difficult and important differential diagnosis to make is that of restrictive cardiomyopathy. The treatment of constrictive pericarditis is surgical and can lead to dramatic improvement, whereas medical management is usually all that can be offered to patients with restrictive cardiomyopathy, whose long-term prognosis is often quite poor. Clinical presentation and cause provide few insights, but patients with a history of tuberculosis, radiation therapy, or surgery may be more likely to have constrictive pericarditis. Invasive hemodynamics alone cannot reliably differentiate the two dis-

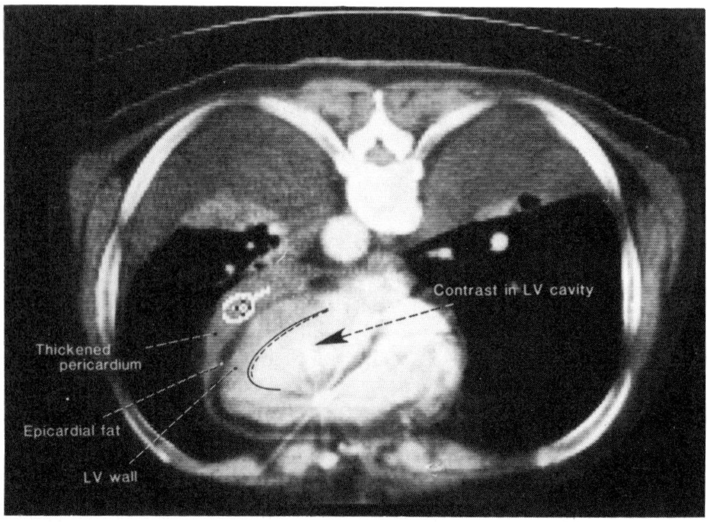

Fig 55-9 Computed tomographic scan of the chest in a 59-year-old patient who had undergone coronary artery bypass graft surgery and returned to the hospital 2 weeks after dismissal. He was complaining of dyspnea and fatigue and was noted to have a high jugular venous pressure. Suspicion of pericardial constriction was supported by the thickened pericardium noted on the scan. *LV,* left ventricle.

eases, since there is considerable overlap between almost any of the measured variables.

Doppler echocardiographic studies have greatly enhanced our understanding of the hemodynamic differences between restrictive myocardial disease and constrictive pericarditis. Patients with constrictive pericardial disease have respiratory variation in early diastolic filling velocities across the mitral and tricuspid valves. With inspiration, tricuspid velocity increases and mitral velocity decreases. With expiration, the reverse occurs.[140] In constrictive pericarditis, there is a higher Doppler pulmonary venous systolic-diastolic ratio and greater respiratory variation in pulmonary venous diastolic flow.[153] These findings are not present in patients with restrictive myocardial disease. If the classic Doppler findings are not present in patients thought to have constrictive pericarditis, cardiac catheterization may be required. Both restrictive cardiomyopathy and constrictive pericarditis may have elevation and equalization of end-diastolic pressures. However, in constrictive pericarditis, there is a discordance between right ventricular and left ventricular systolic pressures during inspiration.

Endomyocardial biopsy is occasionally useful, since the finding of myocardial abnormalities (such as amyloid infiltration, myocarditis, and fibrosis) may suggest a primary restrictive cause rather than a constricting pericardium. This finding may obviate additional exploratory thoracotomy.[154] Caution must be exercised, however, since restriction and constriction can coexist.[154-156] An abnormal endomyocardial biopsy specimen does not completely exclude constrictive pericarditis.

The classic clinical findings, characteristic Doppler tracings,[140,141,143,153] and thickened or calcified pericardium[145,146,150,152] all strongly point to constrictive pericarditis. These patients should undergo operation without further testing. If there is a discrepancy present, cardiac catheterization or endomyocardial biopsy, or both, may be helpful. In the end, despite the best efforts, a few patients require exploratory thoractomy, which remains the definitive means to make the diagnosis.

Management of constrictive pericarditis

Transient constriction has been reported in acute idiopathic pericarditis,[157] bacterial pericarditis, immune-mediated pericarditis,[158] and acute tuberculous pericarditis[159,160] and after cardiac surgery.[161] Early and aggressive management of pericardial inflammation, or antibiotics or treatment with combination chemotherapy for tuberculosis, during the acute phase may be indicated in many of these patients rather than immediate surgery. If such treatment produces a response, the patients presumably have constriction due to a thickened and inelastic pericardium from edema and inflammation rather than from irreversible fibrosis. The definitive therapy for constrictive pericarditis is pericardiectomy that is as complete as possible, especially the removal of all constricting pericardium and epicardium around the left and right ventricles. Rarely, there is constriction or compression of the venae cavae, right or left atrium, or right ventricular outflow tract; in any of these instances, pericardiectomy should be extended to the affected area as well. Our experience has shown that incomplete pericardiectomy leads to a higher incidence of inadequate relief of symptoms and need for reoperation.[36,162]

CONGENITAL DEFECTS AND ABNORMALITIES OF THE PERICARDIUM

Congenital defects

Congenital partial or complete absence of the pericardium is rare; we identified 15 patients from approximately 34,000 (0.044%) who underwent cardiovascular surgery.[163] Their ages ranged from 4 days to 68 years (median, 7 years; mean, 19.5 years). Partial and complete left-sided defects accounted for most of the cases in our experience and in reported series. Right-sided defects and total pericardial absence are much less common. All types may be associated with other congenital heart defects. Nearly all patients are asymptomatic, but a few have vague chest pain, dyspnea, or syncope.[164-166] Rarely, sudden death can occur if the heart becomes incarcerated in the defect.

In the past, congenital pericardial defects were difficult to diagnose; none of our 15 patients had this diagnosis made preoperatively. Physical findings are nonspecific but may include a systolic murmur or axillary displacement of the apical impulse.[165] Chest radiography in patients completely lacking the left pericardium often shows displacement of the heart to the left and prominence of pulmonary arteries and less often shows interposition of lung tissue between the aorta and the main pulmonary artery or between the base of the heart and the left hemidiaphragm. In partial left defects, the heart is in the normal position but there may be a bulge in the cardiac silhouette, often in the location of the left atrial appendage. ECG changes are nonspecific but may disclose right-axis deviation or right bundle-branch block.[164]

Echocardiography in patients with complete absence of the pericardium may show an enlarged right ventricle and abnormal interventricular septal motion, mimicking right ventricular volume overload.[167] Echocardiography of partial defects may show herniation of the left atrial appendage or other structures through the defect. CT and MRI are useful in defining tomographic anatomy.[168-170] Acquired defects of the pericardium, either traumatic or postoperative, have been reported to cause symptoms and cardiac strangulation.[171,172]

Complete absence of the left or right pericardium is nearly always asymptomatic and requires no treatment. Partial deficiency of the pericardium is also usually asymptomatic, and discovery occurs at the time of operation for some other condition. Occasional cases require surgical intervention for relief of symptoms. At one time, moderate-sized defects were considered a hazard because of their potential for herniation and cardiac strangulation, and the recommendation was made that these defects should be prophylactically repaired. Subsequent experience has shown that pericardial defects are rarely of clinical importance, and we and others[164] recommend surgery only for patients with symptoms.

Many procedures have been suggested for surgical management of symptomatic, moderate-sized pericardial defects, including primary closure, partial pericardiectomy, pericardioplasty, atrial appendectomy, and patch closure. In many cases, all that is needed is longitudinal pericariotomy performed by extension of the existing pericardial defect. This relieves tension on the pericardium and prevents herniation of the heart or its appendages through the partial pericardial defect. If the left atrial appendage herniates through a partial defect, the defect may be closed with a patch.

Cysts

Pericardial cysts usually are manifested as an asymptomatic rounded, well-demarcated mass at the right (60% to 90%) or left (10% to 40%) costophrenic angle on chest radiography.[173] Echocardiography demonstrates a thin-walled, sharply defined echolucent mass.[174] CT and MRI yield a similar diagnostic appearance.[175,176] Pericardial cysts do not usually cause symptoms or increase in size over time and should be treated conservatively. If there is any question about the diagnosis, pericardial cysts may be aspirated under echocardiographic or fluoroscopic guidance so that the fluid can be examined.

SURGICAL PROCEDURES FOR PERICARDIAL DISORDERS

Pericardial aspiration

When pericardiocentesis is necessary to obtain pericardial fluid for diagnosis or to relieve a large effusion or cardiac tamponade, we prefer to perform it under echocardiographic guidance.[177] Our experience with echocardiographically guided pericardiocentesis now exceeds 600 patients. The location and size of the pericardial effusion can be visualized in most patients, and the area of maximal fluid collection that is closest to the body wall, and therefore safest to enter, can be identified. With the widespread availability and portability of ultrasound equipment, we no longer perform ECG-guided pericardiocentesis, and in only rare instances have we found it necessary to perform a "blind" pericardiocentesis.

Callahan et al.[177,178] described the technique and subsequent results in detail. Two-dimensional echocardiography is used to locate the position on the chest or abdomen where pericardial fluid is closest to the transducer and free of intervening structures. The transducer angulation is noted along with the optimal entry point that avoids the heart, liver, and lungs (Fig 55-10). The point and the direction of entry are marked on the skin. A short

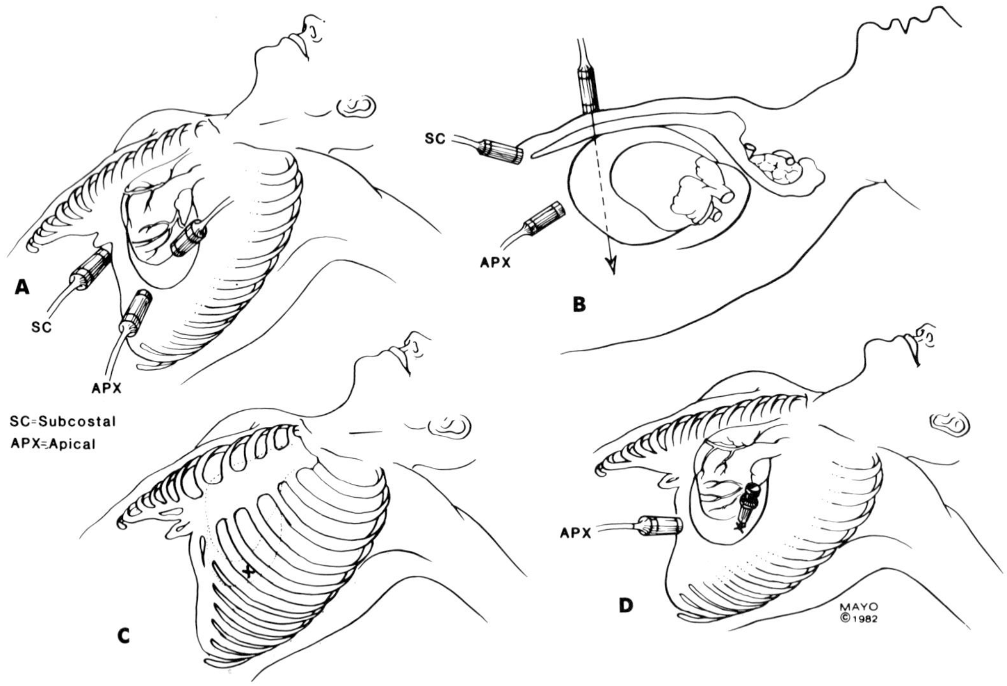

Fig 55-10 Diagram of echocardiographically directed pericardiocentesis. **A,** echo transducers in parasternal, apical, and subcostal positions. Pericardial fluid is represented as loculated effusion over apex. **B,** lateral view shows selected direction of ultrasound beam to avoid contact with heart. **C,** selected point of needle entry *(X)* marked on patient's skin. **D,** remote transducer monitors needle entry into pericardial sac through selected point *(X)* on skin. (From Callahan JA, Seward JB, Tajik AJ, et al: Pericardiocentesis assisted by two-dimensional echocardiography. *J Thorac Cardiovasc Surg* 85:877-879, 1983. By permission, Mayo Foundation.)

(5.7 cm), 14- to 16-gauge, Teflon-sheathed, radiopaque needle is usually used. In some cases, a longer (15.2 cm), 18-gauge, Teflon-sheathed needle may be needed to drain a large, loculated effusion that is confined entirely behind the heart. The needle is inserted into the pericardial space, the Teflon sheath is advanced, and the steel needle is removed. The position of the sheath can be visualized by two-dimensional echocardiography directly or by contrast techniques.[179] Removal of fluid is monitored by two-dimensional echocardiography from a transducer position outside the sterile field. Aspirated fluid should be cultured for bacteria, *Mycobacterium tuberculosis,* and fungus. Cell counts, cytologic examination for malignant cells, and protein and glucose determinations are useful in discovering the cause of the effusion.

For most patients with large effusions or cardiac tamponade and for those who may have infectious, malignant, or loculated[180] effusions, we insert a pericardial drainage catheter to encourage complete evacuation of fluid, to monitor the rate of fluid or blood drainage, and to prevent early recurrence of tamponade. Insertion is accomplished by advancing a short guide wire through the Teflon catheter and exchanging the catheter for a vascular dilator and introducer sheath system (6F to 8F) by means of standard percutaneous technique. A 60-cm pigtail catheter is passed into the pericardial space through the introducer.[118] The catheter is left in place for several days, and fluid is withdrawn manually every 1 to 12 hours as indicated by fluid volume. Complications of the procedure are rare;[118,178] they include pneumothorax, syncope, right ventricular wall puncture, and infection.

Tube drainage of the pericardium

In patients with recurrent, loculated, or viscous effusions or in patients with infectious pericarditis, better drainage than that provided by simple needle or catheter aspiration can be achieved by the insertion of a drainage tube into the pericardial space. This is done under direct exposure through a subxiphoid approach. If necessary, local anesthesia supplemented with monitored intravenous sedation can be substituted for general anesthesia. The xiphoid process is excised, and the dissection is carried superiorly beneath the costal margin to enter the pericardial sac. Loculated spaces are freed by finger exploration about the heart. A catheter or soft chest tube is then placed posteriorly for continued drainage. If needed, a second catheter can be placed anteriorly to allow through-and-through irrigation of the pericardial space. Pericardial biopsy for tissue examination and culture can also be performed.[181] A similar approach combined with limited pericardial resection can be used instead of formal pericardiectomy in debilitated patients with uremic pericarditis or malignant pericardial disease.[182-184]

Percutaneous balloon pericardiotomy

In some patients with recurrent moderate-to-large pericardial effusions, especially those with malignant pericardial disease, percutaneous balloon pericardiotomy has been performed. Several investigators[185,186] reported successful short-term results in such patients after producing a pericardial opening percutaneously by inflation of a balloon dilating catheter, 20 mm in diameter and 3 cm long, as it straddled the pericardium. Ziskind et al.[186] considered the procedure successful in 46 of 50 patients after a mean of 3.6 ± 3.3 months. Complications included bleeding and recurrent tamponade requiring operation in four patients. The authors suggested that percutaneous balloon pericardiotomy may be most useful in managing large pericardial effusions in patients with malignant conditions in whom life expectancy is limited and in whom it is desirable to avoid a more invasive procedure. However, information from the surgical literature showed that the long-term results of surgical creation of an opening in the pericardium for treatment of effusions were disappointing when the amount of pericardium resected was small.[36,71] In addition, prolonged catheter drainage usually treats the initial event with a low ($<20\%$) incidence of recurrence in most patients. Thus, we rarely find an indication for balloon pericardiotomy.

Thoroscopic pericardiectomy[187,188] and laparoscopic pericardial-peritoneal windows[189,190] have recently been reported as alternative methods for treating malignant effusions, but published experience is limited to single case reports.[187-190]

Pericardiectomy

Effusive disease. Pericardiectomy can vary in extent from a postage stamp fenestration to nearly total excision of the pericardium. Experience has indicated the advisability of more radical resection of the pericardium rather than lesser procedures for most patients. After limited pericardial resection (pericardial window), adhesions develop from the lung to the heart, and the margins of the resected pericardium have a tendency to seal down to the surface of the heart, thus closing the window. Also, the remaining pericardium continues to produce fluid. Late development of complications or need for reoperation is far more common after the window procedure than after more extensive pericardiectomy.[71] We prefer an anterior fifth intercostal space incision and believe that most patients are best served by complete pericardiectomy.

The subxiphoid approach for drainage of pericardial effusions has numerous advocates. Because of the poor general condition of some patients, the less traumatic procedure of subxiphoid drainage may be in their best immediate interest despite the higher probability of late complications. This concern is of less significance for patients with malignant effusion, because their survival interval is generally short. When the subxiphoid approach is used, resection of the largest accessible portion of the pericardium seems to be indicated, since early failures are more common with small windows than with larger windows.[191]

Constrictive pericarditis. The hemodynamic effects of chronic constriction are recognized to be due to impairment of ventricular filling, and postoperative catheterization studies have demonstrated persistent hemodynamic abnormalities when there has been incomplete decortication of the ventricles. We believe that maximal

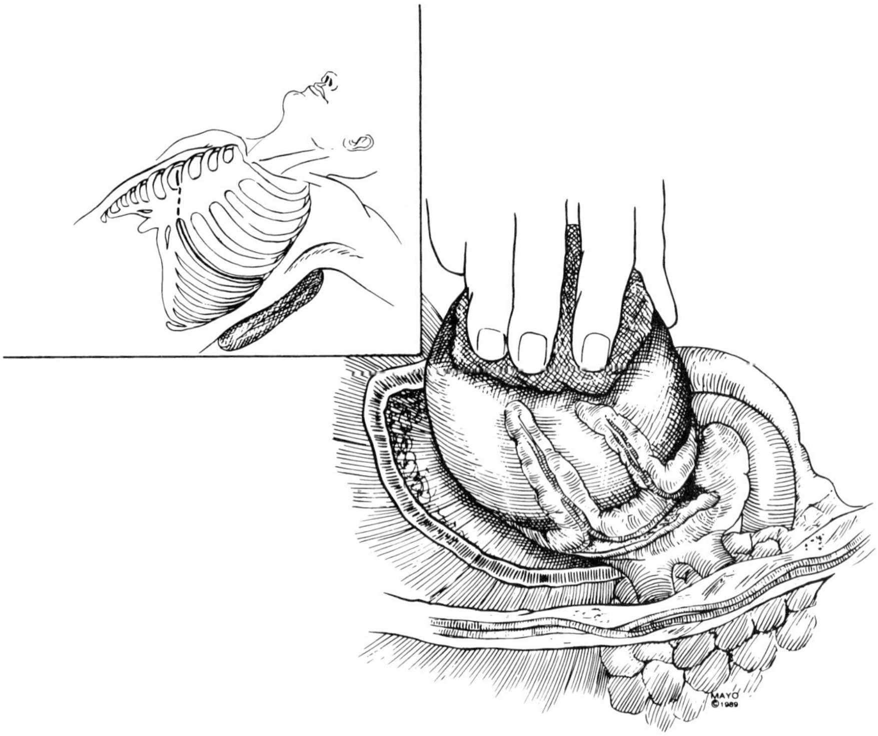

Fig 55-11 Diagram of our preferred approach for pericardiectomy through a fifth left intercostal space anterolateral thoracotomy, with extension of the incision across the sternum into the right fourth interspace as necessary *(inset)*. Constrictive tissues are removed from all ventricular surfaces from the right phrenic nerve to the left pulmonary veins. The phrenic nerves are preserved on pedicles, and the pericardium is removed from the diaphragm. Pericardiectomy through a median sternotomy, usually with cardiopulmonary bypass, has been used in selected cases of reoperation. (From Tuna IC, Danielson GK: Surgical management of pericardial diseases. *Cardiol Clin* 8:683-696, 1990. By permission, Mayo Foundation.)

exposure of the ventricular surfaces is most easily accomplished by a left anterolateral thoracotomy in the fifth intercostal space; it can be extended across the sternum into the right fourth intercostal space if more exposure of the right side of the heart is required (Fig 55-11). For us, this approach has provided optimal exposure of the critical ventricular surfaces of the heart with minimal manipulation and retraction of the heart, and it has the advantage of avoiding cardiopulmonary bypass and therefore systemic heparinization with its associated bleeding problems. Median sternotomy is used in some centers, but cardiopulmonary bypass often is required to gain access to the lateral and diaphragmatic surfaces of the posteriorly situated left ventricle. We have used median sternotomy, usually in conjunction with cardiopulmonary bypass, in selected patients who had a previous cardiac procedure, who had previous incomplete pericardiectomy, or who required repair of additional cardiac lesions.

We believe it is important to remove all diaphragmatic pericardium in contact with the right and left ventricles, including the pericardium posterior to the left phrenic nerve (except for a pedicle that contains the phrenic nerve), because we have seen patients who have had incomplete relief of symptoms or who have required reoperation for constriction when this had not been done. Constriction of the venae cavae, atria, or atrioventricular groove is uncommon in constrictive pericarditis, and resection of the pericardium overlying these structures is not pursued vigorously because of the hazard of hemorrhage, particularly if the pericardium is densely calcified, unless a definite and important gradient can be demonstrated.

As the heart is freed, it expands into the pericardial incision and contracts more vigorously. This is accompanied by a decrease in right atrial pressure as the dissection progresses and the pericardium is excised. After the parietal pericardium is removed, the visceral pericardium (epicardium) may be found to be minimally involved or merely edematous. In other patients, it may be thickened, opaque, and severely constrictive. When this is the case, the heart does not expand fully and atrial pressures remain elevated. We have encountered several patients who required urgent or late reoperation because constrictive epicardium had not been resected at the time of initial pericardiectomy. Resection of all thickened and constrictive epicardium is as important to a good result as complete resection of the parietal pericardium. The proper depth of decortication is achieved when the coronary arteries are exposed and the myocardium is visible between them.

Calcification of a fibrous epicardial peel may occur. When this is accompanied by areas of invasion of the underlying myocardium by calcium, it may be necessary to leave islands of partially resected calcium in those areas. Uncommonly, dense calcification in the atrioventricular groove may produce focal constriction of the right ventricular outflow tract or displacement of the atria, mimicking valvular stenosis. Resection of calcium in both of these situations may be expedited and made safer by the availability of ultrasound debridement.[36]

Total operative mortality in our institutional experience of 313 patients (1936-1990) was 14%. Mortality has decreased significantly in the recent experience (overall mortality less than 6%) even though the median age at operation has increased from 45 to 60 years. Early mortality arose primarily as a result of low cardiac output in a technically adequate pericardiectomy. In patients dying of low cardiac output, cardiac dilatation frequently was observed after decortication and autopsy findings showed cardiac dilatation and "disuse" myocardial atrophy.[36]

Univariate analysis defined that the most significant factor influencing operative mortality was the preoperative clinical condition of the patient. The operative risk was 1% for patients in New York Heart Association class I or II, 10% for class III, and 46% for class IV. The difference in operative mortality between groups was highly significant ($P < 0.001$). The major nonfatal complication after pericardiectomy was also low cardiac output, which appeared in one-third of the operative survivors. Sixty-four percent were treated with digitalis glycosides, volume expansion, and afterload reduction, and 36% required the addition of inotropic support. Fifteen percent of the latter also required intra-aortic balloon counterpulsation.

Long-term follow-up of operative survivors extended to 43 years (mean, 9 years). Five-year survival was improved among patients with preoperative New York Heart Association classes I and II symptoms compared with those in classes III and IV. Beyond 5 years, survival was similar among all groups and followed that of an age- and sex-matched control population. Most survivors were in class I or II. A few patients failed to improve because of underlying myocardial disease, such as amyloid infiltration, radiation injury, or myocarditis. Early and late surgical results will continue to improve if the diagnosis of constrictive pericarditis can be established early and if pericardiectomy is performed before marked constriction causes myocardial damage, multiorgan failure, and clinical deterioration to class III or IV.

Recurrent (relapsing) pericarditis. Recurrent pericarditis is a poorly understood condition, but the symptoms, including chest pain, fever, pleural effusions, and severe malaise, can be debilitating. For patients who do not have a response to anti-inflammatory agents and for those who have recurrent symptoms when steroid dosage is tapered (steroid dependency), complete pericardiectomy is usually effective. For recurrent pericarditis, we believe it is especially important to remove all accessible parietal pericardium from the right pulmonary veins anterolaterally over the heart to the left pulmonary veins, leaving the phrenic nerves on pedicles, and from the great vessels superiorly to and including the diaphragmatic pericardium inferiorly and behind the heart to the transverse sinus. Perhaps the complete extent of our resections accounts for the improved surgical results compared with those in early reports.[32] In a series of 20 patients, we noted 85% immediate freedom from further attacks of acute pericarditis and an additional 10% freedom from further attacks after 1 year. (A few patients have some symptoms for a number of months postoperatively.) Only one (5%) of these patients had recurrent symptoms more than 1 year after radical pericardiectomy; sometimes pleuritic symptoms were also present, so that identifying the exact origin of the pain was difficult. There were no operative or hospital deaths, and most patients were dismissed from the hospital 1 week after operation.

This favorable experience in patients with recurrent pericarditis leads us to recommend radical pericardiectomy for those who have had multiple attacks, for those who are steroid-dependent, and for those who do not tolerate medications required for relief of symptoms. Patients are grateful to be relieved of the burden of the physical and economic hardships caused by multiple disabling attacks of pericarditis. Radical pericardiectomy also provides tissue for diagnosis, and the late appearance of cardiac tamponade or constriction, although uncommon, can be avoided completely.

REFERENCES

1. Spodick DH: The pericardial rub: prospective, multiple observer investigation of pericardial friction in 100 patients. *Am J Cardiol* 35:357-362, 1975
2. Spodick DH: Diagnostic electrocardiographic sequences in acute pericarditis: significance of PR segment and PR vector changes. *Circulation* 48:575-580, 1973
3. Bruce ME, Spodick DH: Atypical electrocardiogram in acute pericarditis: characteristics and prevalence. *J Electrocardiol* 13:61-66, 1980
4. Spodick DH: Arrhythmias during acute pericarditis: a prospective study of 100 consecutive cases. *JAMA* 235:39-41, 1976
5. Spodick DH: Frequency of arrhythmias in acute pericarditis determined by Holter monitoring. *Am J Cardiol* 53:842-845, 1984
6. Horowitz MS, Schultz CS, Stinson EB, et al: Sensitivity and specificity of echocardiographic diagnosis of pericardial effusion. *Circulation* 50:239-247, 1974
7. Permanyer-Miralda G, Sagristá-Sauleda J, Soler-Soler J: Primary acute pericardial disease: a prospective series of 231 consecutive patients. *Am J Cardiol* 56:623-630, 1985
8. Fyke FE III, Tancredi RG, Shub C, et al: Detection of intrapericardial hematoma after open heart surgery: the roles of echocardiography and computed tomography. *J Am Coll Cardiol* 5:1496-1499, 1985
9. Mulvagh SL, Rokey R, Vick GW, et al: Usefulness of nuclear magnetic resonance imaging for evaluation of pericardial effusions, and comparison with two-dimensional echocardiography. *Am J Cardiol* 64:1002-1009, 1989
10. Isner JM, Carter BL, Bankoff MS, et al: Computed tomography in the diagnosis of pericardial heart disease. *Ann Intern Med* 97:473-479, 1982
11. Moncada R, Baker M, Salinas M, et al: Diagnostic role of computed tomography in pericardial heart disease: congenital defects, thickening, neoplasms, and effusions. *Am Heart J* 103:263-282, 1982
12. Kossowsky WA, Lyon AF, Spain DM: Reappraisal of the postmyocardial infarction Dressler's syndrome. *Am Heart J* 102:954-956, 1981
13. Tofler GH, Muller JE, Stone PH, et al: Pericarditis in acute

myocardial infarction: characterization and clinical significance. *Am Heart J* 117:86-92, 1989
14. Correale E, Maggioni AP, Romano S, et al: Comparison of frequency, diagnostic and prognostic significance of pericardial involvement in acute myocardial infarction treated with and without thrombolytics. Gruppo Italiano per lo Studio della Sopravvivenza nell'Infarto Miocardico (GISSI). *Am J Cardiol* 71:1377-1381, 1993
15. Krainin FM, Flessas AP, Spodick DH: Infarction-associated pericarditis: rarity of diagnostic electrocardiogram. *N Engl J Med* 311:1211-1214, 1984
16. Sugiura T, Iwasaka T, Takayama Y, et al: Factors associated with pericardial effusion in acute Q wave myocardial infarction. *Circulation* 81:477-481, 1990
17. Sugiura T, Iwasaka T, Tarumi N, et al: Clinical significance of pericardial effusion in Q-wave inferior wall acute myocardial infarction. *Am J Cardiol* 73:862-864, 1994
18. Sugiura T, Iwasaka T, Takahashi N, et al: Prognostic significance of hydropericardia and pericardial friction rub in Q-wave acute myocardial infarction. *Am J Cardiol* 67:533-534, 1991
19. Belkin RN, Mark DB, Aronsen L, et al: Pericardial effusion after intravenous recombinant tissue-type plasminogen activator for acute myocardial infarction. *Am J Cardiol* 67:496-500, 1991
20. Renken J, De Bruyne B, Benit E, et al: Cardiac tamponade early after thrombolysis for acute myocardial infarction: a rare but not reported hemorrhagic complication. *J Am Coll Cardiol 17:280-285, 1991*
21. Ramsdale DR, Epstein EJ, Coulshed N: Constrictive pericarditis after myocardial infarction. *Br Heart J* 56:476-478, 1986
22. Dressler W: The post-myocardial-infarction syndrome: a report of forty-four cases. *Arch Intern Med* 103:28-42, 1954
23. Peter RH, Whalen RE, Orgain ES, et al: Postpericardiotomy syndrome as a complication of percutaneous left ventricular puncture. *Am J Cardiol* 17:86-90, 1966
24. Kaye D, Frankl W, Arditi LU: Probable postcardiotomy syndrome following implantation of a transvenous pacemaker: report of the first case. *Am Heart J* 90:627-630, 1975
25. Peters RW, Scheinman MM, Raskin S, et al: Unusual complications of epicardial pacemakers: recurrent pericarditis, cardiac tamponade and pericardial constriction. *Am J Cardiol* 45:1088-1094, 1980
26. Tabatznik B, Isaacs JP: Postpericardiotomy syndrome following traumatic hemopericardium. *Am J Cardiol* 7:83-96, 1961
27. Engle MA, Gay WA Jr, McCabe J, et al: Postpericardiotomy syndrome in adults: incidence, autoimmunity and virology. *Circulation* 64 Suppl 2:58-60, 1981
28. Stelzner TJ, King TE Jr, Antony VB, et al: The pleuropulmonary manifestations of the postcardiac injury syndrome. *Chest* 84:383-387, 1983
29. Lichstein E, Arsura E, Hollander G, et al: Current incidence of postmyocardial infarction (Dressler's) syndrome. *Am J Cardiol* 50:1269-1271, 1982
30. Miller RH, Horneffer PJ, Gardner TJ, et al: The epidemiology of the postpericardiotomy syndrome: a common complication of cardiac surgery. *Am Heart J* 116:1323-1329, 1988
31. Horneffer PJ, Miller RH, Pearson TA, et al: The effective treatment of postpericardiotomy syndrome after cardiac operations: a randomized placebo-controlled trial. *J Thorac Cardiovasc Surg* 100:292-296, 1990
32. Fowler NO, Harbin AD III: Recurrent acute pericarditis: follow-up study of 31 patients. *J Am Coll Cardiol* 7:300-305, 1986
33. Guindo J, de la Serna AR, Ramió J, et al: Recurrent pericarditis: relief with colchicine. *Circulation* 82:1117-1120, 1990
34. Millaire A, de Groote P, Decoulx E, et al: Treatment of recurrent pericarditis with colchicine. *Eur Heart J* 15:120-124, 1994
35. Adler Y, Zandman-Goddard G, Ravid M, et al: Usefulness of colchicine in preventing recurrences of pericarditis. *Am J Cardiol* 73:916-917, 1994
36. Tuna IC, Danielson GK: Surgical management of pericardial diseases. *Cardiol Clin* 8:683-696, 1990
37. Sagrista-Sauleda J, Barrabes JA, Permanyer-Miralda G, et al: Purulent pericarditis: review of a 20-year experience in a general hospital. *J Am Coll Cardiol* 22:1661-1665, 1993
38. Rubin RH, Moellering RC Jr: Clinical, microbiologic and therapeutic aspects of purulent pericarditis. *Am J Med* 59:68-78, 1975
39. Bulkley BH, Klacsmann PG, Hutchins GM: A clinicopathological study of post-thoracotomy purulent pericarditis: a continuing problem of diagnosis and therapy. *J Thorac Cardiovasc Surg* 73:408-412, 1977
40. Wheat LJ, Stein L, Corya BC, et al: Pericarditis as a manifestation of histoplasmosis during two large urban outbreaks. *Medicine (Baltimore)* 62:110-119, 1983
41. Harvey AM, Shulman LE, Tumulty PA, et al: Systemic lupus erythematosus: review of the literature and clinical analysis of 138 cases. *Medicine (Baltimore)* 33:291-437, 1954
42. Copeland GD, von Capeller D, Stern TN: Systemic lupus erythematosus: a clinical report of 47 cases with pathologic findings in 18. *Am J Med Sci* 236:318-328, 1958
43. Kahl LE: The spectrum of pericardial tamponade in systemic lupus erythematosus. Report of ten patients. *Arthritis Rheum* 35:1343-1349, 1992
44. Reiner JS, Furie RA: Cardiac tamponade as an initial manifestation of systemic lupus erythematosus. *J Rheumatol* 16:1127-1129, 1989
45. Carroll N, Barrett JA: Systemic lupus erythematosus presenting with cardiac tamponade. *Br Heart J* 51:452-453, 1984
46. Averbuch M, Bojko A, Levo Y: Cardiac tamponade in the early postpartum period as the presenting and predominant manifestation of systemic lupus erythematosus. *J Rheumatol* 13:444-445, 1986
47. Ehrenfeld M, Asman A, Shpilberg O, et al: Cardiac tamponade as the presenting manifestation of systemic lupus erythematosus. *Am J Med* 86:626-627, 1989
48. Doherty NE, Siegel RJ: Cardiovascular manifestations of systemic lupus erythematosus. *Am Heart J* 110:1257-1265, 1985
49. Doherty NE, Feldman G, Maurer G, et al: Echocardiographic findings in systemic lupus erythematosus. *Am J Cardiol* 61:1144, 1988
50. Prakash R, Atassi A, Poske R, et al: Prevalence of pericardial effusion and mitral-valve involvement in patients with rheumatoid arthritis without cardiac symptoms: an echocardiographic evaluation. *N Engl J Med* 289:597-600,1973
51. Bonfiglio T, Atwater EC: Heart disease in patients with seropositive rheumatoid arthritis: a controlled autopsy study and review. *Arch Intern Med* 124:714-719, 1969
52. Bacon PA, Gibson DG: Cardiac involvement in rheumatoid arthritis: an echocardiographic study. *Ann Rheum Dis* 33:20-24, 1974
53. Hara KS, Ballard DJ, Ilstrup DM, et al: Rheumatoid pericarditis: clinical features and survival. *Medicine (Baltimore)* 69:81-91, 1990
54. Escalante A, Kaufman RL, Quismorio FP, et al: Cardiac compression in rheumatoid pericarditis. *Semin Arthritis Rheum* 20:148-163, 1990
55. Franco AE, Levine HD, Hall AP: Rheumatoid pericarditis: report of 17 cases diagnosed clinically. *Ann Intern Med* 77:837-844, 1972
56. Hakala M, Pettersson T, Tarkka M, et al: Rheumatoid arthritis as a cause of cardiac compression. Favourable long-term outcome of pericardiectomy. *Clin Rheumatol* 12:199-203, 1993
57. Liss JP, Bachmann WT: Rheumatoid constrictive pericarditis, treated by pericardiectomy: report of a case and review of the literature. *Arthritis Rheum* 13:869-876, 1970
58. Burney DP, Martin CE, Thomas CS, et al: Rheumatoid pericarditis: clinical significance and operative management. *J Thorac Cardiovasc Surg* 77:511-515, 1979
59. Massell BF, Fyler DC, Roy SB: The clinical picture of rheumatic fever: diagnosis, immediate prognosis, course, and therapeutic implications. *Am J Cardiol* 1:436-449, 1958
60. Pader E, Elster SK: Studies of acute rheumatic fever in the adult. I. Clinical and laboratory manifestations in thirty patients. *Am J Med* 26:424-441, 1959
61. Malpas JS, Landon J: Rheumatic fever in the young adult. *Ann Rheum Dis* 19:262-267, 1960
62. Rutsky EA, Rostand SG: Treatment of uremic pericarditis and pericardial effusion. *Am J Kidney Dis* 10:2-8, 1987
63. Marini PV, Hull AR: Uremic pericarditis: a review of incidence and management. *Kidney Int* 2 Suppl:163-166, 1975
64. Luft FC, Gillman JK, Weyman AE: Pericarditis in the patient with uremia. Clinical and echocardiographic evaluation. *Nephron* 25:160-166, 1980
65. Spector D, Alfred H, Siedlecki M, et al: A controlled study of the effect of indomethacin in uremic pericarditis. *Kidney Int* 24:663-669, 1983
66. Buselmeier TJ, Davin TD, Simmons RL, et al: Treatment of intractable uremic pericardial effusion: avoidance of pericardiectomy with local steroid instillation. *JAMA* 240:1358-1359, 1978
67. Martin RG, Ruckdeschel JC, Chang P, et al: Radiation-related pericarditis. *Am J Cardiol* 35:216-220, 1975
68. Gutierrez CA, Just-Viera JO: Clinical spectrum of radiation induced pericarditis. *Am Surg* 49:113-115, 1983

69. Stewart JR, Fajardo LF: Dose response in human and experimental radiation-induced heart disease. Application of nominal standard dose (NSD) concept. *Radiology* 99:403-408, 1971

70. Stewart JR, Fajardo LF: Radiation-induced heart disease: an update. *Prog Cardiovasc Dis* 27:173-194, 1984

71. Piehler JM, Pluth JR, Schaff HV, et al: Surgical management of effusive pericardial disease: influence of extent of pericardial resection on clinical course. *J Thorac Cardiovasc Surg* 90:506-516, 1985

72. Ni Y, von Segesser LK, Turina M: Futility of pericardiectomy for postirradiation constrictive pericarditis? *Ann Thorac Surg* 49:445-448, 1990

73. Karram T, Rinkevitch D, Markiewicz W: Poor outcome in radiation-induced constrictive pericarditis. *Int J Radiat Oncol Biol Phys* 25:329-331, 1993

74. Hicks GL Jr: Coronary artery operation in radiation-associated atherosclerosis: long-term follow-up. *Ann Thorac Surg* 53:670-674, 1992

75. Cummings RG, Wesly RLR, Adams DH, et al: Pneumopericardium resulting in cardiac tamponade. *Ann Thorac Surg* 37:511-518, 1984

76. D'Cruz IA, Cohen HC, Prabhu R, et al: Diagnosis of cardiac tamponade by echocardiography: changes in mitral valve motion and ventricular dimensions, with special reference to paradoxical pulse. *Circulation* 52:460-465, 1975

77. Gonzalez MS, Basnight MA, Appleton CP: Experimental cardiac tamponade: a hemodynamic and Doppler echocardiographic reexamination of the relation of right and left heart ejection dynamics to the phase of respiration. *J Am Coll Cardiol* 18:243-252, 1991

78. Picard MH, Sanfilippo AJ, Newell JV, et al: Quantitative relation between increased intrapericardial pressure and Doppler flow velocities during experimental cardiac tamponade. *J Am Coll Cardiol* 18:234-242, 1991

79. Shabetai R, Fowler NO, Guntheroth WG: The hemodynamics of cardiac tamponade and constrictive pericarditis. *Am J Cardiol* 26:480-489, 1970

80. Golinko RJ, Kaplan N, Rudolph AM: The mechanism of pulsus paradoxus during acute pericardial tamponade. *J Clin Invest* 42:249-257, 1963

81. Reddy PS, Curtiss EI, O'Toole JD, et al: Cardiac tamponade: hemodynamic observation in man. *Circulation* 58:265-272, 1978

82. Reddy PS, Curtiss EI, Uretsky BF: Spectrum of hemodynamic changes in cardiac tamponade. *Am J Cardiol* 66:1487-1491, 1990

83. Schutzman JJ, Obarski TP, Pearce GL, et al: Comparison of Doppler and two-dimensional echocardiography for assessment of pericardial effusion. *Am J Cardiol* 70:1353-1357, 1992

84. Beck CS: Two cardiac compression triads. *JAMA* 104:714-716, 1935

85. Antman EM, Cargill V, Grossman W: Low pressure-cardiac tamponade. *Ann Intern Med* 91:403-406, 1979

86. Hayes SN, Freeman WK, Gersh BJ: Low pressure cardiac tamponade: diagnosis facilitated by Doppler echocardiography. *Br Heart J* 63:136-140, 1990

87. Santoro IH, Neumann A, Carroll JD, et al: Pulsus paradoxus: a definition revisited. *J Am Soc Echocardiogr* 4:408-412, 1991

88. Leeman DE, Levine MJ, Come PC: Doppler echocardiography in cardiac tamponade: exaggerated respiratory variation in transvalvular blood flow velocity integrals. *J Am Coll Cardiol* 11:572-578, 1988

89. Spodick DH: Kussmaul's sign in pericardial disease (letter to the editor). *Am J Cardiol* 42:1060, 1978

90. Niarchos AP: Electrical alternans in cardiac tamponade. *Thorax* 30:228-233, 1975

91. Usher BW, Popp RL: Electrical alternans: mechanism in pericardial effusion. *Am Heart J* 83:459-463, 1972

92. Torelli J, Marwick TH, Salcedo EE: Left atrial tamponade: diagnosis by transesophageal echocardiography. *J Am Soc Echocardiogr* 4:413-414, 1991

93. Kochar GS, Jacobs LE, Kotler MN: Right atrial compression in postoperative cardiac patients: detection by transesophageal echocardiography. *J Am Coll Cardiol* 16:511-516, 1990

94. Simpson IS, Munsch C, Smith EEJ, et al: Pericardial haemorrhage causing right atrial compression after cardiac surgery: role of transoesophageal echocardiography. *Br Heart J* 65:355-356, 1991

95. Pepi M, Muratori M, Barbier P, et al: Pericardial effusion after cardiac surgery: incidence, site, size, and haemodynamic consequences. *Br Heart J* 72:327-331, 1994

96. Hutchison SJ, Smalling RG, Albornoz M, et al: Comparison of transthoracic and transesophageal echocardiography in clinically overt or suspected pericardial heart disease. *Am J Cardiol* 74:962-965, 1994

97. Reid CL, Chandraratna AN, Kawanishi D, et al: Echocardiographic detection of pneumomediastinum and pneumopericardium: the air gap sign. *J Am Coll Cardiol* 1:916-921, 1983

98. Gillam LD, Guyer DE, Gibson TC, et al: Hydrodynamic compression of the right atrium: a new echocardiographic sign of cardiac tamponade. *Circulation* 68:294-301, 1983

99. Schiller NB, Botvinick EH: Right ventricular compression as a sign of cardiac tamponade: an analysis of echocardiographic ventricular dimensions and their clinical implications. *Circulation* 56:774-779, 1977

100. Armstrong WF, Schilt BF, Helper DJ, et al: Diastolic collapse of the right ventricle with cardiac tamponade: an echocardiographic study. *Circulation* 65:1491-1496,1982

101. Singh S, Wann LS, Schuchard GH, et al: Right ventricular and right atrial collapse with cardiac tamponade—a combined echocardiographic and hemodynamic study. *Circulation* 70:966-971, 1984

102. Himelman RB, Kircher B, Rockey DC, et al: Inferior vena cava plethora with blunted respiratory response: a sensitive echocardiographic sign of cardiac tamponade. *J Am Coll Cardiol* 12:1470-1477, 1988

103. Fusman B, Schwinger ME, Charney R, et al: Isolated collapse of left-sided heart chambers in cardiac tamponade: demonstration by two-dimensional echocardiography. *Am Heart J* 121:613-616, 1991

104. D'Cruz IA, Kensey K, Campbell C, et al: Two-dimensional echocardiography in cardiac tamponade occurring after cardiac surgery. *J Am Coll Cardiol* 5:1250-1252, 1985

105. Frey MJ, Berko B, Palevsky H, et al: Recognition of cardiac tamponade in the presence of severe pulmonary hypertension. *Ann Intern Med* 111:615-617, 1989

106. Burstow DJ, Oh JK, Bailey KR, et al: Cardiac tamponade: characteristic Doppler observations. *Mayo Clin Proc* 64:312-324, 1989

107. Appleton CP, Hatle LK, Popp RL: Cardiac tamponade and pericardial effusion: respiratory variation in transvalvular flow velocities studied by Doppler echocardiography. *J Am Coll Cardiol* 11:1020-1030, 1988

108. Hoit BD, Ramrakhyani K: Pulmonary venous flow in cardiac tamponade: influence of left ventricular dysfunction and the relation to pulsus paradoxus. *J Am Soc Echocardiogr* 4:559-570, 1991

109. Hoit BD, Fowler NO: Influence of acute right ventricular dysfunction on cardiac tamponade. *J Am Coll Cardiol* 18:1787-1793, 1991

110. DeLoach JF, Haynes JW: Secondary tumors of heart and pericardium: review of the subject and report of one hundred thirty-seven cases. *Arch Intern Med* 91:224-249, 1953

111. Lopez JM, Delgado JL, Tovar E, et al: Massive pericardial effusion produced by extracardiac malignant neoplasms. *Arch Intern Med* 143:1815-1816, 1983

112. Posner MR, Cohen GI, Skarin AT: Pericardial disease in patients with cancer: the differentiation of malignant from idiopathic and radiation-induced pericarditis. *Am J Med* 71:407-413, 1981

113. Muir KW, Rodger JC: Cardiac tamponade as the initial presentation of malignancy: Is it as rare as previously supposed? *Postgrad Med J* 70:703-707, 1994

114. Glazer GM, Gross BH, Orringer MB, et al: Computed tomography of pericardial masses: further observations and comparison with echocardiography. *J Comput Assist Tomogr* 8:895-899, 1984

115. Lund JT, Ehman RL, Julsrud PR, et al: Cardiac masses: assessment by MR imaging. *AJR* 152:469-473, 1989

116. Edoute Y, Malberger E, Kuten A, et al: Cytologic analysis of pericardial effusion complicating extracardiac malignancy. *Am J Cardiol* 69:568-571, 1992

117. Rinkevich D, Borovik R, Bendett H, et al: Malignant pericardial tamponade. *Med Pediatr Oncol* 18:287-291, 1990

118. Kopecky SL, Callahan JA, Tajik AJ, et al: Percutaneous pericardial catheter drainage: report of 42 consecutive cases. *Am J Cardiol* 58:633-635, 1986

119. Weinberg BA, Conces DJ Jr, Waller BF: Cardiac manifestations of noncardiac tumors. Part I: Direct effects. *Clin Cardiol* 12:289-296, 1989

120. Park JS, Rentschler R, Wilbur D: Surgical management of pericardial effusion in patients with malignancies: comparison of subxiphoid window versus pericardiectomy. *Cancer* 67:76-80, 1991

121. Reid CL, Kawanishi DT, Rahimtoola SH, et al: Chest trauma: evaluation by two-dimensional echocardiography. *Am Heart J* 113:971-976, 1987

122. Kabadi UM, Kumar SP: Pericardial effusion in primary hypothyroidism. *Am Heart J* 120:1393-1395, 1990

123. Bashi VV, John S, Ravikumar E, et al: Early and late results of

pericardiectomy in 118 cases of constrictive pericarditis. *Thorax* 43:637-641, 1988

124. Cameron J, Oesterle SN, Baldwin JC, et al: The etiologic spectrum of constrictive pericarditis. *Am Heart J* 113:354-360, 1987

125. Seifert FC, Miller DC, Oesterle SN, et al: Surgical treatment of constrictive pericarditis: analysis of outcome and diagnostic error. *Circulation* 72 No 3:264-273, 1985

126. Lurie K, Shultz J, Remole S, et al: Constrictive pericardial disease caused by epicardial implantable cardiac defibrillator patches: treatment by pericardial stripping and nonthoracotomy lead system implantation. *Am Heart J* 128:623-625, 1994

127. Ng AS, Dorosti K, Sheldon WC: Constrictive pericarditis following cardiac surgery—Cleveland Clinic experience. Report of 12 cases and review. *Cleve Clin Q* 51:39-45, 1984

128. Kutcher MA, King SB III, Alimurung BN, et al: Constrictive pericarditis as a complication of cardiac surgery: recognition of an entity. *Am J Cardiol* 50:742-748, 1982

129. Killian DM, Furiasse JG, Scanlon PJ, et al: Constrictive pericarditis after cardiac surgery. *Am Heart J* 118:563-568, 1989

130. Meyer TE, Sareli P, Marcus RH, et al: Mechanism underlying Kussmaul's sign in chronic constrictive pericarditis. *Am J Cardiol* 64:1069-1072, 1989

131. Tyberg TI, Goodyer AVN, Langou RA: Genesis of pericardial knock in constrictive pericarditis. *Am J Cardiol* 46:570-575, 1980

132. Miller SW: *Cardiac Angiography.* Boston, Little, Brown & Company, 1984

133. Plum GE, Bruwer AJ, Clagett OT: Chronic constrictive pericarditis: roentgenologic findings in 35 surgically proved cases. *Proc Staff Meet Mayo Clin* 32:555-566, 1957

134. Engel PJ, Fowler NO, Tei CW, et al: M-mode echocardiography in constrictive pericarditis. *J Am Coll Cardiol* 6:471-474, 1985

135. Chandraratna PA, Aronow WS, Imaizumi T: Role of echocardiography in detecting the anatomic and physiologic abnormalities of constrictive pericarditis. *Am J Med Sci* 283:141-146, 1982

136. Gibson TC, Grossman W, McLaurin LP, et al: An echocardiographic study of the interventricular septum in constrictive pericarditis. *Br Heart J* 38:738-743, 1976

137. Vilacosta I, San Román Calvar JA, Iturralde Prieto E, et al: Transesophageal echocardiographic features of the atrial septum in constrictive pericarditis. *Am J Cardiol* 68:271-273, 1991

138. Himelman RB, Lee E, Schiller NB: Septal bounce, vena cava plethora, and pericardial adhesion: informative two-dimensional echocardiographic signs in the diagnosis of pericardial constriction. *J Am Soc Echocardiogr* 1:333-340, 1988

139. Nishimura RA, Connolly DC, Parkin TW, et al: Constrictive pericarditis: assessment of current diagnostic procedures. *Mayo Clin Proc* 60:397-401, 1985

140. Hatle LK, Appleton CP, Popp RL: Differentiation of constrictive pericarditis and restrictive cardiomyopathy by Doppler echocardiography. *Circulation* 79:357-370, 1989

141. Appleton CP, Hatle LK, Popp RL: Central venous flow velocity patterns can differentiate constrictive pericarditis from restrictive cardiomyopathy (abstract). *J Am Coll Cardiol* 9 Suppl A:119, 1987

142. Schiavone WA, Calafiore PA, Currie PJ, et al: Doppler echocardiographic demonstration of pulmonary venous flow velocity in three patients with constrictive pericarditis before and after pericardiectomy. *Am J Cardiol* 63:145-147, 1989

143. Oh JK, Hatle LK, Seward JB, et al: Diagnostic role of Doppler echocardiography in constrictive pericarditis. *J Am Coll Cardiol* 23:154-162, 1994

144. Gaasch WH, Peterson KL, Shabetai R: Left ventricular function in chronic constrictive pericarditis. *Am J Cardiol* 34:107-110, 1974

145. Masui T, Finck S, Higgins CB: Constrictive pericarditis and restrictive cardiomyopathy: evaluation with MR imaging. *Radiology* 182:369-373, 1992

146. Soulen RL, Stark DD, Higgins CB: Magnetic resonance imaging of constrictive pericardial disease. *Am J Cardiol* 55:480-484, 1985

147. Stark DD, Higgins CB, Lanzer P, et al: Magnetic resonance imaging of the pericardium: normal and pathologic findings. *Radiology* 150:469-474, 1984

148. Sechtem U, Tscholakoff D, Higgins CB: MRI of the normal pericardium. *Am J Radiol* 147:239-244, 1986

149. Sechtem U, Tscholakoff D, Higgins CB: MRI of the abnormal pericardium. *Am J Radiol* 147:245-252, 1986

150. Isner JM, Carter BL, Bankoff MS, et al: Differentiation of constrictive pericarditis from restrictive cardiomyopathy by computed tomographic imaging. *Am Heart J* 105:1019-1025, 1983

151. Reinmuller R, Gurgan M, Erdmann E, et al: CT and MR evaluation of pericardial constriction: a new diagnostic and therapeutic concept. *J Thorac Imaging* 8:108-121, 1993

152. Oren RM, Grover-McKay M, Stanford W, et al: Accurate preoperative diagnosis of pericardial constriction using cine computed tomography. *J Am Coll Cardiol* 22:832-838, 1993

153. Klein AL, Cohen GI, Pietrolungo JF, et al: Differentiation of constrictive pericarditis from restrictive cardiomyopathy by Doppler transesophageal echocardiographic measurements of respiratory variations in pulmonary venous flow. *J Am Coll Cardiol* 22:1935-1943, 1993

154. Schoenfeld MH, Supple EW, Dec GW Jr, et al: Restrictive cardiomyopathy versus constrictive pericarditis: role of endomyocardial biopsy in avoiding unnecessary thoracotomy. *Circulation* 75:1012-1017, 1987

155. Garrett J, O'Neill H, Blake S: Constrictive pericarditis associated with sarcoidosis (letter to the editor). *Am Heart J* 107:394, 1984

156. Lui CY, Makoui C: Severe constrictive pericarditis as an unsuspected cause of death in a patient with idiopathic hypereosinophilic syndrome and restrictive cardiomyopathy. *Clin Cardiol* 11:502-504, 1988

157. Sagristà-Sauleda J, Permanyer-Miralda G, Candell-Riera J, et al: Transient cardiac constriction: an unrecognized pattern of evolution in effusive acute idiopathic pericarditis. *Am J Cardiol* 59:961-966, 1987

158. Oh JK, Hatle LK, Mulvagh SL, et al: Transient constrictive pericarditis: diagnosis by two-dimensional Doppler echocardiography. *Mayo Clin Proc* 68:1158-1164, 1993

159. Agrawal S, Radhakrishnan S, Sinha N: Echocardiographic demonstration of resolving intrapericardial mass in tuberculous pericardial effusion. *Int J Cardiol* 26:240-241, 1990

160. Long R, Younes M, Patton N, et al: Tuberculous pericarditis: long-term outcome in patients who received medical therapy alone. *Am Heart J* 117:1133-1139, 1989

161. Ansinelli RA, Weeks KD, Key TS: Effect of steroids on postoperative constrictive pericarditis. *Am J Cardiol* 51:1238-1240, 1983

162. McCaughan BC, Schaff HV, Piehler JM, et al: Early and late results of pericardiectomy for constrictive pericarditis. *J Thorac Cardiovasc Surg* 89:340-350, 1985

163. van Son JAM, Danielson GK, Schaff HV, et al: Congenital partial and complete absence of the pericardium. *Mayo Clin Proc* 68:743-747, 1993

164. Nasser WK: Congenital absence of the left pericardium. *Am J Cardiol* 26:466-470, 1970

165. Morgan JR, Rogers AK, Forker AD: Congenital absence of the left pericardium: clinical findings. *Ann Intern Med* 74:370-376, 1971

166. Southworth H, Stevenson CS: Congenital defects of the pericardium. *Arch Intern Med* 61:223-240, 1938

167. Payvandi MN, Kerber RE: Echocardiography in congenital and acquired absence of the pericardium: an echocardiographic mimic of right ventricular volume overload. *Circulation* 53:86-92, 1976

168. Baim RS, McDonald IL, Wise DJ, et al: Computed tomography of absent pericardium. *Radiology* 135:127-128, 1980

169. Gutierrez FR, Shackelford GD, McKnight RC, et al: Diagnosis of congenital absence of the left pericardium by MR imaging. *J Comput Assist Tomogr* 9:551-553, 1985

170. Schiavone WA, O'Donnell JK: Congenital absence of the left portion of parietal pericardium demonstrated by nuclear magnetic resonance imaging. *Am J Cardiol* 55:1439-1440, 1985

171. Hwang JJ, Lien WP, Chen JJ, et al: Traumatic rupture of the pericardium with a peculiar chest radiographic finding. *Cardiology* 83:415-418, 1993

172. Ohshima H, Takeuchi H, Yamaguchi T, et al: Late cardiac strangulation due to an iatrogenic pericardial defect. *Chest* 104:977-978, 1993

173. Feigin DS, Fenoglio JJ, McAllister HA, et al: Pericardial cysts: a radiologic-pathologic correlation and review. *Radiology* 125:15-20, 1977

174. Hynes JK, Tajik AJ, Osborn MJ, et al: Two-dimensional echocardiographic diagnosis of pericardial cyst. *Mayo Clin Proc* 58:60-63, 1983

175. Rogers CI, Seymour EQ, Brock JG: Atypical pericardial cyst location: the value of computed tomography. *J Comput Assist Tomogr* 4:683-684, 1980

176. Amparo EG, Higgins CB, Farmer D, et al: Gated MRI of cardiac and paracardiac masses: initial experience. *AJR* 143:1151-1156, 1984

177. Callahan JA, Seward JB, Tajik AJ, et al: Pericardiocentesis assisted by two-dimensional echocardiography. *J Thorac Cardiovasc Surg* 85:877-879, 1983

178. Callahan JA, Seward JB, Nishimura RA, et al: Two-dimensional echocardiographically guided pericardiocentesis: experience in 117 consecutive patients. *Am J Cardiol* 55:476-479, 1985

179. O'Sullivan J, Heads A, Hunter S: Microbubble image enhancement and pericardiocentesis. *Int J Cardiol* 42:95-96, 1993

180. Pandian NG, Brockway B, Simonetti J, et al: Pericardiocentesis under two-dimensional echocardiographic guidance in loculated pericardial effusion. *Ann Thorac Surg* 45:99-100, 1988

181. Van Trigt P, Douglas J, Smith PK, et al: A prospective trial of subxiphoid pericardiotomy in the diagnosis and treatment of large pericardial effusion. A follow-up report. *Ann Surg* 218:777-782, 1993

182. Chan A, Rischin D, Clarke CP, et al: Subxiphoid partial pericardiectomy with or without sclerosant instillation in the treatment of symptomatic pericardial effusions in patients with malignancy. *Cancer* 68:1021-1025, 1991

183. Wall TC, Campbell PT, O'Connor CM, et al: Diagnosis and management (by subxiphoid pericardiotomy) of large pericardial effusions causing cardiac tamponade. *Am J Cardiol* 69:1075-1078, 1992

184. Campbell PT, Van Trigt P, Wall TC, et al: Subxiphoid pericardiotomy in the diagnosis and management of large pericardial effusions associated with malignancy. *Chest* 101:938-943, 1992

185. Palacios IF, Tuzcu EM, Ziskind AA, et al: Percutaneous balloon pericardial window for patients with malignant pericardial effusion and tamponade. *Cathet Cardiovasc Diagn* 22:244-249, 1991

186. Ziskind AA, Pearce AC, Lemmon CC, et al: Percutaneous balloon pericardiotomy for the treatment of cardiac tamponade and large pericardial effusions: description of technique and report of the first 50 cases. *J Am Coll Cardiol* 21:1-5, 1993

187. Mack MJ, Aronoff RJ, Acuff TE, et al: Present role of thoracoscopy in the diagnosis and treatment of diseases of the chest. *Ann Thorac Surg* 54:403-408, 1992

188. van der Schelling GP, Michielsen D, Hendrickx L, et al: Thoracoscopic pericardial fenestration, a first experience of a new approach. *Acta Chir Belg* 94:272-273, 1994

189. Ready A, Black J, Lewis R, et al: Laparoscopic pericardial fenestration for malignant pericardial effusion (letter to the editor). *Lancet* 339:1609, 1992

190. Sastic JW, Stalter KD, Goddard RL: Laparoscopic pericardial window. *J Laparoendosc Surg* 2:263-266, 1992

191. Santos GH, Frater RW: The subxiphoid approach in the treatment of pericardial effusion. *Ann Thorac Surg* 23:467-470, 1977

CHAPTER

56

Tumors of the heart

Hartzell V. Schaff, M.D., J. T. Lie, M.D., and Emilio R. Giuliani, M.D.

CURRENT management of cardiac neoplasms began after Goldberg et al.[1] first visualized an intracardiac tumor by means of contrast angiography in 1952 and Crafoord[2] successfully removed an atrial myxoma with use of extracorporeal circulation, reported in 1955. Thereafter, rapid advances were made in intracardiac operative techniques, which permitted the resection of most primary cardiac tumors with low mortality. Because many intracardiac tumors are benign, resection often leads to complete cure.[3]

Advances in noninvasive diagnostic techniques, particularly in ultrasound and magnetic resonance imaging (Fig 56-1), have made the diagnosis of cardiac tumors simple and accurate. At present, the greatest impediment to successful treatment of a patient with a cardiac tumor is no longer the pathologic condition itself but rather a lack of clinical alertness on the part of the primary physician, which results in a delay in proper diagnosis and treatment. Delay in diagnosis is caused by two factors. First, primary cardiac tumors are rare, and the incidence in unselected autopsy series is 0.0001% to 0.5%.[4-11] Thus, the average physician rarely encounters a patient with a primary cardiac tumor during his or her professional career. Second, patients have widely varying presentations; some tumors produce no clinical signs or symptoms, and others mimic valvular heart disease, subacute bacterial endocarditis, or other systemic disorders.

GENERAL CONSIDERATIONS

Tumors that originate in the heart itself, termed "primary" cardiac neoplasms, can be either malignant or benign and can often be classified as either intracavitary or intramyocardial, depending on their pattern of growth (Table 56-1). The heart can also be affected by secondary neoplasms; these are largely malignant tumors and have either metastasized to the myocardium via hematogenous or lymphocytic routes or have extended directly into the myocardium from surrounding intrathoracic structures. Secondary cardiac neoplasms are 6 to 40 times more common than primary tumors.[7,11-13]

Cardiac tumors are unlike many other neoplasms in that even if they are benign, they require surgical intervention. The heart has limited tolerance for space-occupying lesions; all but very small tumors pose a significant threat to the patient, either because of systemic complications or because of interference with normal cardiac function. Thus, rather than maintaining a complacent attitude because about 75% of primary cardiac neoplasms are benign, clinicians should adopt aggressive strategies for diagnosis and treatment because of the potentially favorable outcome for patients with these lesions.

PRINCIPAL BENIGN CARDIAC TUMORS (TABLE 56-2)

Cardiac myxomas: general clinical considerations

Cardiac myxoma is the most common primary tumor of the heart, accounting for about 50% of all such lesions.[5,6,14] Although these tumors occur in all age groups, most are diagnosed in the third to the sixth decade of life,[5,8,14-19] and most studies suggest a slight preponderance in women. Myxomas are rare in children,[20] and among the benign cardiac tumors of childhood, myxomas are less common than rhabdomyomas, fibromas, and teratomas.[5] Although most cardiac myxomas appear sporadically, there have been several reports of familial occurrence of the tumors.[21-26] In addition, the clinical and pathologic features of a syndrome of cardiac myxomas, spotty pigmentation (lentiginosis), and endocrine overactivity have been recognized by Carney et al.[27,28] and confirmed by others.[29-33] Patients with a familial pattern of myxomas are generally younger than patients with nonfamilial tumors and may have multicentric tumors in atypical locations.[34]

Pathology. Cardiac myxomas can arise from the endocardial surface of any of the four cardiac chambers, and they usually grow slowly in an intracavitary fashion. Approximately 75% of these tumors originate in the left atrium and 18% in the right atrium; the few remaining tumors are about equally distributed between the two ventricles.[5,8,11,18,35,36] Approximately 95% of atrial myxomas are single, but they can be multiple in one or more cardiac chambers.[8,34] Approximately 85% of atrial tumors, either right- or left-sided, originate from the atrial septum, usually in the vicinity of the fossa ovalis.[5] Of the atrial myxomas that do not originate from the septum, most arise from the posterior atrial wall.[5] Ventricular myxomas, on the other hand, usually originate from the free wall and not from the interventricular septum.[5] Biatrial myxomas originate either from the fossa ovalis and extend through the foramen ovale into each atrial chamber as a dumbbell tumor or from two separate atrial sites.[37-44]

The external appearance of cardiac myxomas is variable[5-8] (Fig 56-2). Most myxomas have a short stalk with a 1- or 2-cm attachment to the endocardium. They are gelatinous and papillary, and their friability explains their tendency to embolize. A much smaller percentage are smooth, spherical, and hard; these tend to be sessile rather than pedunculated. It has been speculated that sessile tumors represent the retained stalk after embolization of a pedunculated tumor.[4,11] Occasionally, areas of hemorrhage are grossly visible within the tumor, and rarely calcification of the tumor is noted.[8] Calcification appears to be more common in right than in left atrial myxomas.[26,45] Although myxomas as large as 15 cm in diameter have been noted, the average size at diagnosis is approximately 6 cm.[5]

Most myxomas have an abundant mucoid matrix (Fig 56-3), which stains weakly positive with the periodic acid-Schiff technique and more strongly with alcian blue. The staining characteristics of the matrix suggest that it is an acid mucopolysaccharide, probably related to chondroitin sulfate C. Throughout the matrix are small nests of polygonal cells with eosinophilic cytoplasm. The surface of the tumor is covered by a single layer of these endothelial cells, which also line multiple clefts that invaginate the superficial part of the tumor. The surface cells often appear to be contiguous with the underlying tumor cells. Ultrastructurally, the polygonal cells resemble multipurpose mesenchymal cells, suggesting the origin of the tumor.[5,46] Mitoses are only rarely visualized. Evidence of recurrent hemorrhage is often present in the form of hemosiderin-laden macrophages and degenerated collagen fibers with adherent iron and calcium.

Most investigators believe that myxomas are true neoplasms that are usually benign. Salyer et al.[47,48] have

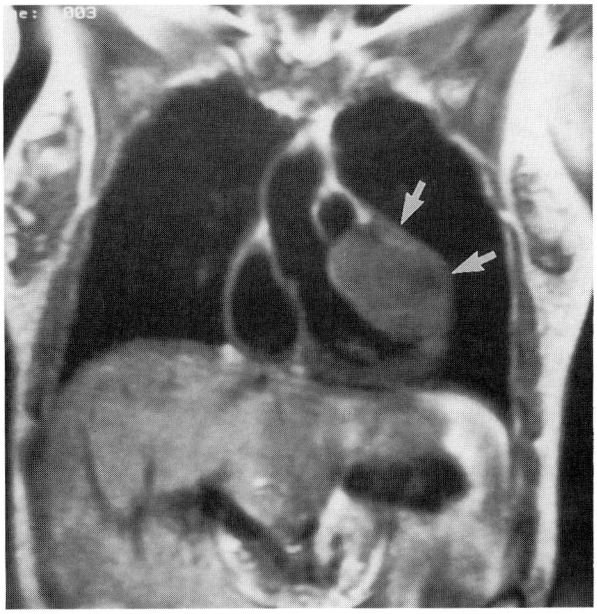

Fig 56-1 Coronal magnetic resonance image demonstrating cardiac fibroma (*arrows*) in left ventricular wall. (From Ehman RL, Julsrud PR: Magnetic resonance imaging of the heart: current status. *Mayo Clin Proc* 64:1134-1146, 1989. By permission, Mayo Foundation for Medical Education and Research.)

Table 56-1 Common types of primary tumors of the heart

Benign
- Myxoma
- Rhabdomyoma
- Fibroma
- Lipoma and lipomatous hypertrophy of the atrial septum
- Atrioventricular node tumor
- Papillary fibroelastoma
- Hemangioma

Malignant
- Angiosarcoma
- Rhabdomyosarcoma
- Fibrosarcoma

Table 56-2 Summary of surgically excised benign cardiac tumors (Mayo Clinic, 1957 through March 1991)

Type of tumor	No.	Sex, F:M	Mean age, yr	Site of tumor
Myxoma	80	51:25*	53	LA 64, RA 16
Fibroma	9	5:4	14.2	LV 5, RV 1, VS 2, LA 1
Lipomatous tumor	5	0:5	60.4	RA 4, RV 1
Fibroelastic papilloma	7	4:3	47.4	AV 3, MV 2, LV 1, TV 1
Hamartoma	1	1:0	1.2	LV 1

AV, aortic valve; LA, left atrium; LV, left ventricle; MV, mitral valve; RA, right atrium; RV, right ventricle; TV, tricuspid valve; VS, ventricular septum.
*Some patients had more than one tumor.
From Tazelaar HD, Locke TJ, McGregor CGA: Pathology of surgically excised primary cardiac tumors. *Mayo Clin Proc* 67:957-965, 1992. By permission, Mayo Foundation for Medical Education and Research.

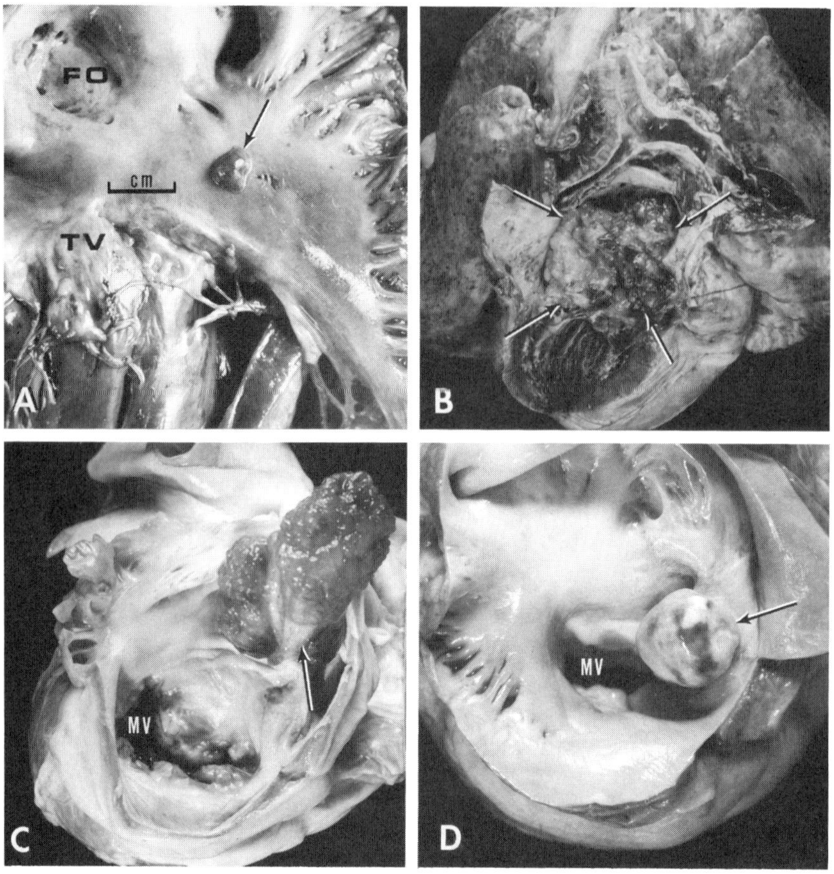

Fig 56-2 Variable gross features of cardiac myxomas. **A,** miniature right atrial myxoma (*arrow*) located anterior to the fossa ovalis (*FO*) and above the tricuspid valve (*TV*). **B,** giant left atrial myxoma (*arrows*) that fills the entire left atrial cavity. **C,** pedunculated, papillary left atrial myxoma with its pedicle attached to the fossa ovalis (*arrow*). It is mobile and can prolapse into the mitral valve orifice (*MV*). **D,** sessile, spherical left atrial myxoma (*arrow*) attached to the atrial septum without a pedicle and partially obstructing the mitral valve orifice (*MV*). (From Wold LE, Lie JT: Cardiac myxomas: a clinicopathologic profile. *Am J Pathol* 101:219-240, 1980. By permission of American Association of Pathologists.)

argued that myxomas are endocardial thrombi that have organized with fibrosis followed by an influx of fluid from surrounding granulation tissue to form the myxoma matrix. However, histologic, ultrastructural, and tissue culture studies provide persuasive evidence that myxomas are true neoplasms.[5-8,46,49-57]

Myxomas are known to recur after incomplete resection,[35] and tumor emboli may enlarge with or without local vascular invasion. These characteristics support a neoplastic origin of myxomas, with variable malignant potential.[58-62] Wold and Lie[8] suggested that metastasizing myxomas are probably myxosarcomas, which are difficult to differentiate from benign tumors histologically. Todo et al.[63] reported bona fide cerebral metastasis of malignant cardiac myxoma; their patient had rapid recurrence of the cardiac tumor, which contained sarcomatous components histologically identical to the tumors of the brain. In a retrospective study correlating DNA histograms with clinical outcome, 40% of patients with a DNA tetraploid pattern had recurrent tumor during a follow-up period that averaged 13 years.[64] None of the tumors with a normal DNA ploidy pattern recurred; thus, DNA flow cytometry may be a useful tool for predicting biologic behavior of cardiac myxomas.

Clinical features. Myxomas become symptomatic by three primary mechanisms: (1) obstruction of intracardiac blood flow by the tumor, (2) fragmentation with embolization of the tumor, and (3) production of systemic effects resulting from the presence of the tumor.[14,17,19,65] Unfortunately, none of the signs or symptoms produced by these mechanisms is specific for myxoma; they are consistent with a wide variety of cardiac and noncardiac disorders. If the symptoms are obstructive, the specific cardiac chamber in which a myxoma is located is closely related to the symptoms produced. Atrial myxomas are relatively slow growing, and some tumors cause no

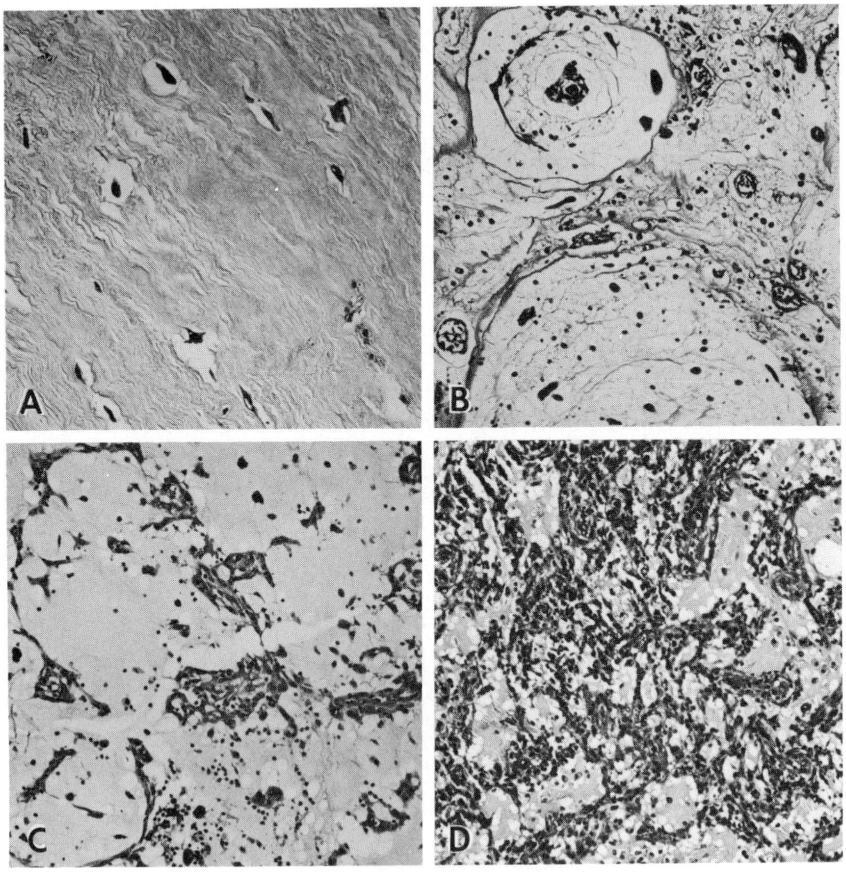

Fig 56-3 Variable histologic features of cardiac myxomas. **A,** individual stellate cells scattered in a dense collagenous stroma in a hypocellular left atrial myxoma. **B,** perivascular distribution of myxoma cells in mucinous lacunae. **C,** cords and clusters of syncytial myxoma cells in an amorphous mucoid matrix. **D,** hypercellular myxoma mimicking an epithelial cell tumor. (Hematoxylin and eosin; ×115.) (From Wold LE, Lie JT: Cardiac myxomas: a clinicopathologic profile. *Am J Pathol* 101:219-240, 1980. By permission of American Association of Pathologists.)

symptoms and are discovered incidentally at autopsy.[8,18]

Systemic effects. In earlier clinical reviews, systemic constitutional symptoms were reported in 90% of patients with cardiac myxoma,[65] but this incidence may decrease in current practice as more myxomas are diagnosed by echocardiography in asymptomatic patients. Systemic manifestations most often take the form of weight loss, fatigue, fever, and arthralgias.[7,14,15,19,26,35,36,65-67] Less common clinical findings are skin rash, clubbing, and Raynaud's phenomenon.[17] Laboratory abnormalities include anemia (often hemolytic), increased erythrocyte sedimentation rate, leukocytosis, thrombocytopenia, polycythemia, and hypergammaglobulinemia.[8,19,65,68-74] The exact cause of these constitutional symptoms and laboratory abnormalities is unclear. A generalized systemic or immunologic response to either necrotic tumor tissue or specific myxomatous protein has been proposed.[75] The increased immunoglobulins are usually of the IgG class.[17,56] Although actual circulating immune complexes have not been identified, the association of increased immunoglobulins and hypocomplementemia strongly suggests that a tumor-specific antigen-antibody complex is activating complement pathways.[76] Such complexes and the systemic reaction to them probably explain the symptoms that suggest collagen vascular disease, most often vasculitis, which patients with myxoma are known to have at presentation.[77-80] The systemic symptoms associated with cardiac myxomas may be caused by the constitutive production of interleukin-6 (IL-6), a potent hepatocyte-stimulating factor and B-cell differentiating factor. Jourdan et al.[81] found that IL-6 levels were 14 to 23 times higher from tumor cells of a patient with immunologic manifestations than from patients without these characteristics.

The constitutional responses to myxoma described above have been noted in the absence of any cardiac findings.[77,80] In general, all of these responses are reversible on removal of the tumor,[26,76,77,80] although persistence of symptoms has been noted after resection.[74] In some cases, the constitutional manifestations of myxoma so dominate the clinical picture that corticosteroid treatment is instituted for what is thought to be a systemic disease.[18,76,80] In these situations, the true diagnosis is usually made after embolic or cardiac manifestations of the tumor become apparent.[77] The constitutional symptoms of myxoma can be elicited by a tumor in any intracardiac location. The sequelae of embolic or obstructive symptoms of the tumor depend, of course, on the specific location of the tumor within the heart.

Clinical features specific to left atrial myxomas

Embolization. Systemic embolization of tumor fragments has been noted in 30% to 60% of patients with left-sided myxomas.[4,5,17,34,82,83] In most embolic events, actual tumor fragments appear to be involved, and it is not unusual for the diagnosis of a left-sided myxoma to be made by histologic examination of embolized material.[84-90] In most instances, the embolus is relatively small, although massive embolization has been reported,[86-90] including instances of embolization of the entire tumor.[89] Tumor emboli have been noted in virtually all systemic locations,[83] although they are most often detected in the brain, kidneys, lower extremities, or aortoiliac region.[87] Frequently, embolization to multiple sites is evident, and this can lead to a clinical diagnosis of bacterial endocarditis, especially when systemic manifestations are also present.[91,92] Presumed infection of the tumor with subsequent positive blood cultures has lent support to the diagnosis of endocarditis. This points up the necessity of considering a diagnosis of myxoma in all patients with these clinical findings.

Coronary artery embolization, a dramatic but rare manifestation of left-sided cardiac myxomas, should be considered in young patients with no prior history of coronary artery disease.[93-96]

Embolization to the central nervous system is noted in approximately one-fourth of patients with left atrial myxomas,[97] and an acute central nervous system event may be the first clinical manifestation of myxoma. Embolization to the cerebral hemispheres, brain stem, cerebellum, retina, and spinal cord has been reported.[83,95-109] Although emboli usually take the form of cerebral infarction with stroke, a pattern of transient ischemic attacks has been noted.[97,110]

In rare instances, tumor fragments continue to grow and thus create a symptom complex compatible with an expanding intracranial mass.[61,97,98] A more unusual delayed complication of embolized myxoma is arterial aneurysms at the site of embolization.[59,60,62,97,103,106,107] These aneurysms enlarge progressively and can cause neurologic symptoms years after removal of the primary tumor. Rupture of such an aneurysm has also been reported.[59,111] Aneurysmal changes in the cerebral vasculature in patients with atrial myxoma have been detected angiographically[62,111,112] and documented histologically.[103,111] The mechanism of aneurysm formation has not been firmly established. It has been postulated that a tumor embolus weakens the arterial wall and allows viable myxoma cells to penetrate the damaged endothelium; this leads to further weakening of the media and aneurysmal dilatation.[103,107] Rarely, these mechanisms can create neurologic symptoms many years after resection of a primary cardiac myxoma.[106]

Clinical symptoms caused by cerebrovascular embolization of myxoma, whether immediate or delayed, are not diagnostic. A cerebral arteriogram demonstrating multiple filling defects with aneurysm or pseudoaneurysm should arouse clinical suspicion of an embolizing myxoma.

Obstructive symptoms. Left atrial tumors may prolapse into the mitral funnel and produce mitral stenosis. If a tumor prevents coaptation of the mitral leaflet during systole, mitral insufficiency can result. The resulting signs and symptoms therefore closely mimic those of primary mitral valvular disease; these include dyspnea, orthopnea, paroxysmal nocturnal dyspnea, cough, acute pulmonary edema, and hemoptysis. Less specific findings are vague chest pains, fatigue, and weight loss.[66] These symptoms can occur suddenly or slowly over the course of several months, and they may be persistent or intermittent. Classically, symptoms can be elicited by a change in body position; however, this clinical feature is probably less often encountered than is implied from the literature. Complete obstruction to mitral valvular flow can lead to syncope and sudden death.[66]

If obstruction to left atrial blood flow is chronic, secondary pulmonary hypertension may develop and eventually lead to right ventricular hypertrophy and failure. Similar symptoms can be caused by tumor obstruction to pulmonary venous flow.[15,16] Finally, a mobile, calcified left atrial tumor can destroy the mitral valve—the so-called wrecking-ball effect—and lead to severe mitral regurgitation.[61]

Physical findings. Physical findings in left atrial myxoma vary with the pathophysiologic changes. Obstruction to left atrial flow leads to findings of pulmonary vascular congestion and, in long-standing cases of myxoma, right heart failure. The first heart sound is often loud and widely split. In patients with pulmonary hypertension, the pulmonary component of the second heart sound is prominent.[66] Frequently, an early diastolic sound, termed the tumor "plop," is noted (Fig 56-4). This sound presumably results from the sudden impact of the tumor against the endocardial wall with tensing of the tumor stalk.[113,114] The tumor "plop" follows the first heart sound at an interval intermediate between that of an opening snap and a third heart sound. The sound is of lower frequency than the usual opening snap; however, in many instances such a differentiation can be quite difficult. The usual heart murmur is an apical diastolic rumble, comparable to that in pure valvular mitral stenosis, and is caused by obstruction to atrial blood flow by the tumor. When the tumor interferes with closure of the valve, the typical apical holosystolic murmur of mitral insufficiency can be noted. On occasion, the quality of murmurs varies with the position of the body, presumably because of movement of the tumor.

Electrocardiogram and chest radiograph. The electrocardiographic (ECG) findings in patients with left atrial myxoma are nonspecific and reflect the changes in

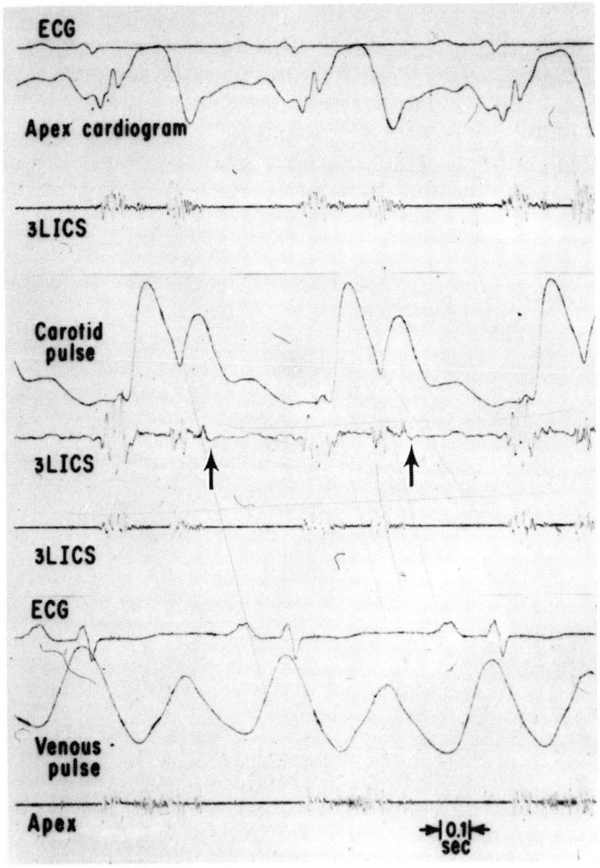

Fig 56-4 Phonocardiograms of a 36-year-old woman with a left atrial myxoma. Typical vibrations can be noted in the phonocardiogram during isovolumic contraction (S_1 to onset of ejection) and during isovolumic relaxation (P_2 to early diastolic sound – "tumor plop"). A characteristic notching is noted on the upstroke of the apexcardiogram. 3LICS, third left intercostal space. (From Zitnik RS, Giuliani ER, Burchill HB: Left atrial myxoma: phonocardiographic clues to diagnosis. Am J Cardiol 23:588-591, 1969. By permission of American College of Cardiology.)

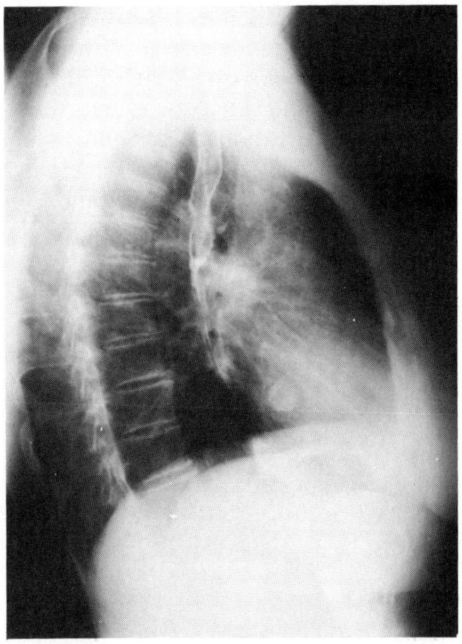

Fig 56-5 Lateral chest radiograph demonstrating calcified left atrial myxoma.

chamber size and rhythm resulting from obstruction to blood flow through the left atrium or from mitral valvular dysfunction. Most patients with myxoma have normal sinus rhythm, although atrial fibrillation or flutter is occasionally seen when left atrial enlargement is pronounced.[14,15,19,66] Left atrial enlargement and nonspecific T-wave and ST-segment abnormalities can be seen, as can right ventricular hypertrophy and left ventricular hypertrophy in patients with pulmonary hypertension and mitral insufficiency, respectively.[19]

Plain chest radiographs may be normal or they can reveal findings compatible with chronic mitral valvular dysfunction – that is, mild-to-moderate left atrial enlargement, pulmonary vascular congestion, and left ventricular enlargement. A giant left atrium is an unusual roentgenographic feature in patients with myxoma and is helpful in differentiating myxoma and chronic mitral valvular disease.[66] Occasionally, calcification of a myxoma can be visualized on the plain chest radiograph (Fig 56-5), although this feature is usually better defined on fluoroscopic examination, in which the movement of the tumor can be seen. Calcification within the left atrium is, of course, not pathognomonic of a left atrial myxoma; a wide variety of cardiac tumors are known to become calcified.[115-117] In addition, many other pericardial structures are known to undergo calcification – for example, cardiac valves, intraluminal thrombi, atrial walls, and coronary arteries.

Echocardiographic examination. Echocardiography is an excellent initial screening test for suspected atrial myxomas.[118-124] With transesophageal echocardiography, invasive studies are not required for either diagnosis or preoperative surgical guidance[120,125] (Fig 56-6). Two-dimensional echocardiography provides accurate assessment of tumor size, point of attachment to the cardiac wall, degree of tumor mobility, and effect of the tumor on overall cardiac function. The two-dimensional method is sensitive in the detection of small tumors,[123] permits visualization of tumors that do not encroach on the mitral funnel, and provides visualization of all four cardiac chambers for assessment of the possibility of multiple tumors. Nevertheless, an unfavorable acoustic density of some tumors can result in false-negative two-dimensional studies as well.[126] In addition, the improved visualization of the entire left atrium provided by the two-dimensional technique allows differentiation of tumor from the more prevalent intra-atrial thrombus, which can produce a similar mass effect. A thrombus often produces a layered echo appearance that allows one to distinguish between the two conditions.[124] The visualization of an intra-atrial mass with characteristic tumor echoes is sufficient diagnosis for surgical intervention. Transesophageal echocardiography may be the optimal approach for imaging atrial tumors, because it provides excellent resolution of right and left atrial masses and adjacent structures[127,128] (Fig 56-7). Transesophageal echocardiography is also useful for diagnosis of paracardiac masses, which may mimic cardiac tumors.[129] Ultrafast computed tomography scanning and magnetic resonance imaging are also excellent techniques for the diagnosis of atrial masses.[130]

Cardiac catheterization. Intracardiac pressure tracings are often abnormal in patients with myxoma,[131-133] but these are rarely of diagnostic value. Right-sided cardiac catheterization usually reveals increases in pulmonary arterial and pulmonary arterial capillary wedge

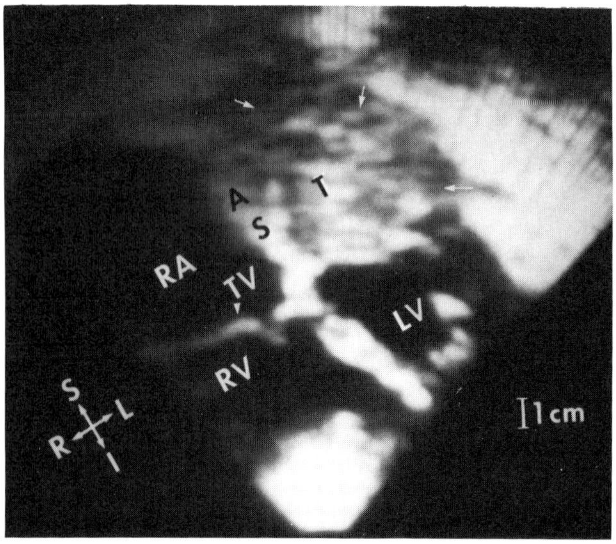

Fig 56-6 Two-dimensional echocardiogram in a patient with left atrial myxoma (*T;* also delineated by *arrows*). *AS,* atrial septum; *RA,* right atrium; *TV,* tricuspid valve; *RV,* right ventricle; *LV,* left ventricle; *S,* superior; *L,* left; *I,* inferior; *R,* right. (From Giuliani ER, Nasser FN: Two-dimensional echocardiography in acquired heart diseases—Part II. *Curr Probl Cardiol* 5:1-54, March 1981. By permission of Year Book Medical Publishers.)

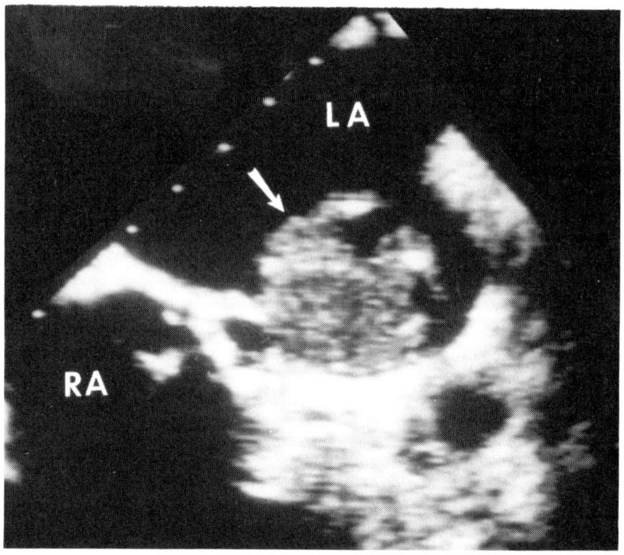

Fig 56-7 Transesophageal echocardiogram in a patient with left atrial myxoma (*arrow*). *LA,* left atrium; *RA,* right atrium.

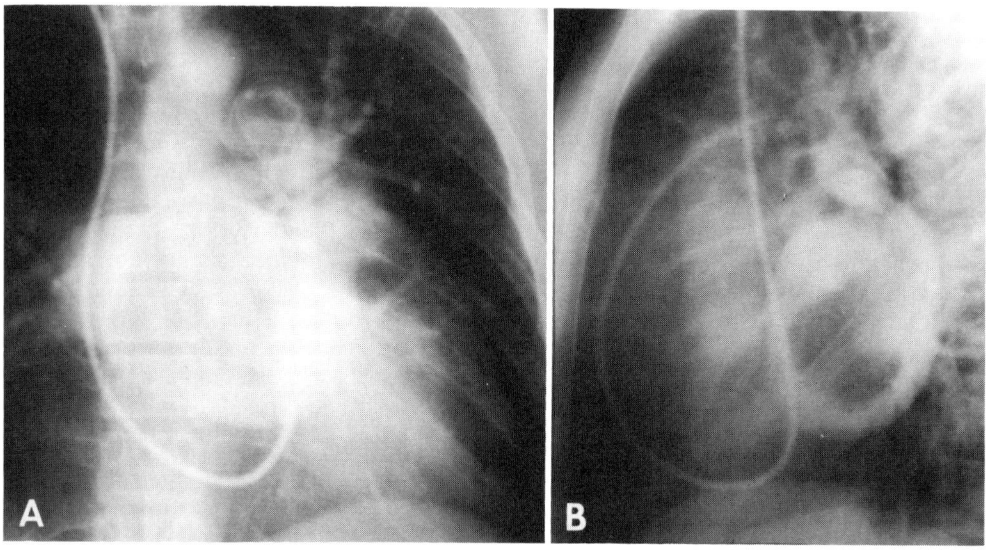

Fig 56-8 Anteroposterior (**A**) and lateral (**B**) angiographic studies in a patient with left atrial myxoma.

pressures compatible with obstruction to left-sided blood flow.

Angiography. Although angiography is no longer used as the initial diagnostic approach, physicians are well advised to be familiar with the angiographic appearance of cardiac tumors because occasionally the diagnosis does not become clear until cardiac catheterization is done.[119]

Tumors create a filling defect in the dye, and movement of the tumor can often be noted (Fig 56-8). The exact point of origination of the tumor is often not detectable angiographically. False-positive studies occur and are frequently a result of intracardiac thrombus, although valvular vegetations, septal aneurysms, and unusual streaming of nonopacified blood can also result in the appearance of a mass effect.[115]

Occasionally, mitral valvular insufficiency results in opacification of the left atrium via a left ventricular injection. More often, however, a pulmonary arterial injection with filming during the levo phase is more profitable in identifying left atrial tumors. Because of the threat of tumor embolization, a transseptal approach should generally be avoided.

Differential diagnosis in left atrial myxoma. Myxomas become symptomatic primarily through interference with intracardiac blood flow or valve function, embolization of tumor fragments or associated thrombus, or constitutional symptoms associated with the tumor. Most often, symptoms related to mechanical interference of mitral valve function predominate, and the tumor must be differentiated from mitral valvular disease. Factors in the patient's history, physical examination, and evaluation that help in distinguishing between these two entities are summarized in Table 56-3.

The diagnosis of left-sided myxoma should always be considered in a patient who has multiple systemic emboli, even if actual tumor fragments are not histologically identified as the embolic material. The association of multiple small embolic events and the constitutional symptoms commonly associated with myxoma often lead to the initial diagnosis of any of a wide variety of systemic diseases. Thus, the combination of fever, increased erythrocyte sedimentation rate, heart murmur, and multiple small emboli often raises a consideration of infective endocarditis[66,91,92] or acute rheumatic fever.[134] Vasculitis is frequently suspected when fever, increased erythrocyte sedimentation rate, skin rash, joint pains, and multiple systemic small arterial aneurysms related to tumor emboli dominate the clinical picture.[66,72,74,76-80] When pure embolic symptoms predominate, the clinical picture is often initially most compatible with stroke,[97,100,102-105,135] myocardial infarction,[94,95] or acute arterial insufficiency,[83-88] depending on the distribution of the embolized artery.

Clinical features specific to right atrial myxomas

Approximately one-fifth of cardiac myxomas arise in the right atrium. Tumors in this location produce symptoms by mechanisms similar to those of their left-sided counterparts.

Intracavitary growth of a right atrial myxoma leads to obstruction of right ventricular inflow, occasionally associated with interference with tricuspid valvular function. The result is increased systemic venous pressure, manifested by hepatomegaly, peripheral edema, and ascites.[136-138] Obstructed venous return leads to a low cardiac output and exertional dyspnea, syncope, and associated cyanosis.

Increased right atrial pressures resulting from obstructed blood flow can lead to opening of a presumably previously closed foramen ovale and subsequent right-to-left shunting.[139-141]

Chronic, recurrent embolization of tumor fragments can lead to pulmonary hypertension and, consequently, right heart failure.[136-138,142-144] Frequently, this heart failure is of relatively short duration, and it is often not responsive to the usual measures of digitalization and diuresis.

Right atrial myxomas are also associated with constitutional symptoms, which are similar to those encountered with tumors in the left atrium.[136-138] Constitutional symptoms can also dominate the clinical presentation.[145] Nonspecific laboratory abnormalities are seen with right atrial myxomas.

Table 56-3 Features differentiating left atrial myxoma from mitral valve disease

Parameter	Myxoma	Mitral valve disease
History	Short duration	Chronic
	Associated constitutional symptoms	No associated constitutional symptoms
	Syncope occasionally noted	Syncope rare
Symptoms	Occasionally episodic	Progressive
Physical examination	Tumor "plop"	Opening snap
	Murmurs varying with position	Murmurs constant
	Associated valve disease unusual	Associated valve disease common
Electrocardiogram	Sinus rhythm	Atrial fibrillation
Chest radiograph	Tumor calcification	Valve calcification
	Left atrium small	Left atrium enlarged
Echocardiogram	Characteristic findings	Characteristic findings

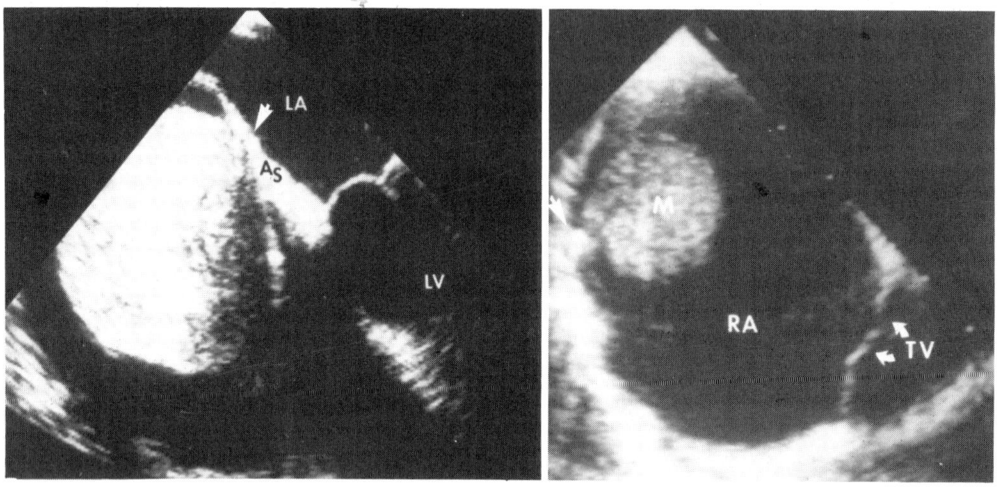

Fig 56-9 Transesophageal echocardiogram in a patient with right atrial myxoma (*arrows*). *AS,* atrial septum; *LA,* left atrium; *LV,* left ventricle; *M,* myxoma; *RA,* right atrium; *TV,* tricuspid valve. (Courtesy of J. Oh, M.D.)

Clinical findings. Right atrial obstruction is detected clinically by the observation of an increased jugular venous "a" wave. If tricuspid insufficiency has been created, a prominent v wave is also apparent. Auscultation reveals, in early systole, a wide splitting of the first heart sound, presumably due to delayed closure of the tricuspid valve as a result of the tumor's location. This delay in tricuspid closure may be associated with an early systolic sound related to brief tricuspid insufficiency.[66,146] A late diastolic rumbling murmur, varying with respiration or body position, reflects the obstructed flow through the tricuspid orifice. More severe interruption of normal tricuspid function leads to the classic systolic murmur of tricuspid insufficiency.[66] Rarely, an early diastolic sound corresponding to motion of the tumor is noted; however, this is not found as often as the tumor "plop" of the left atrial myxoma.

Noninvasive evaluation. The ECG in patients with right atrial myxoma is often normal.[137] When abnormalities are noted, they frequently reflect the pathophysiologic changes created by the tumor; right atrial hypertrophy, right axis deviation, low voltage, right bundle-branch block, and occasionally atrial fibrillation are noted.[137]

The chest radiograph is often normal, although signs of right-sided prominence can be noted. Calcification of right atrial myxomas is occasionally seen.[115-117]

As is the case with left-sided tumors, right atrial myxomas are best visualized with two-dimensional echocardiography and especially with the transesophageal technique[127,147-149] (Fig 56-9).

Invasive investigation. Pressure-wave tracings during cardiac catheterization reveal increased venous pressure above the tumor obstruction. This is often associated with a slow y descent reflecting the delayed right atrial emptying. If the tumor moves rapidly through the tricuspid valve during diastole, the y descent can become quite rapid as the atrial volume suddenly diminishes. As described with left atrial myxoma,[132] a notch in the upstroke of the right ventricular pressure curve can be noted with prolapsing tumors, reflecting displacement of the tumor into the right atrium from the right ventricle during systole.[150] Contrast angiography often demonstrates right atrial myxomas (Fig 56-10); however, catheter manipulation within the right atrium should be avoided; the injection should be made in the vena cava.

Differential diagnosis in right atrial myxoma. Right atrial myxomas are often confused with organic tricuspid valvular disease. Rheumatic tricuspid valvular disease, a frequent cause of tricuspid stenosis, is virtually always associated with clinically significant rheumatic mitral disease. Thus, the absence of associated mitral valvular disease in a patient with signs of tricuspid stenosis should raise the possibility of a right atrial myxoma. In addition, patients with myxoma often have a shorter symptomatic period than those with organic tricuspid valvular disease. Patients with right atrial myxoma frequently have normal sinus rhythm and may have increased erythrocyte sedimentation rates and serum levels of gamma globulins, features that are not present in patients with tricuspid valvular disease. Patients who present with increased systemic venous pressure, perhaps associated with other findings of right heart failure, must be differentiated from patients with constrictive pericarditis, chronic cor pulmonale, pulmonary thromboembolism, caval syndromes, Ebstein's anomaly, and carcinoid heart disease. All patients presenting with right heart obstruction should be evaluated with two-dimensional echocardiography.

Ventricular myxomas

Fewer than 10% of all myxomas arise in the ventricles; the distribution between these two chambers is approximately equal.[5,8] Constitutional symptoms appear to be less frequent with ventricular myxomas than with those arising in the atria.[151-154] Right ventricular myxomas become

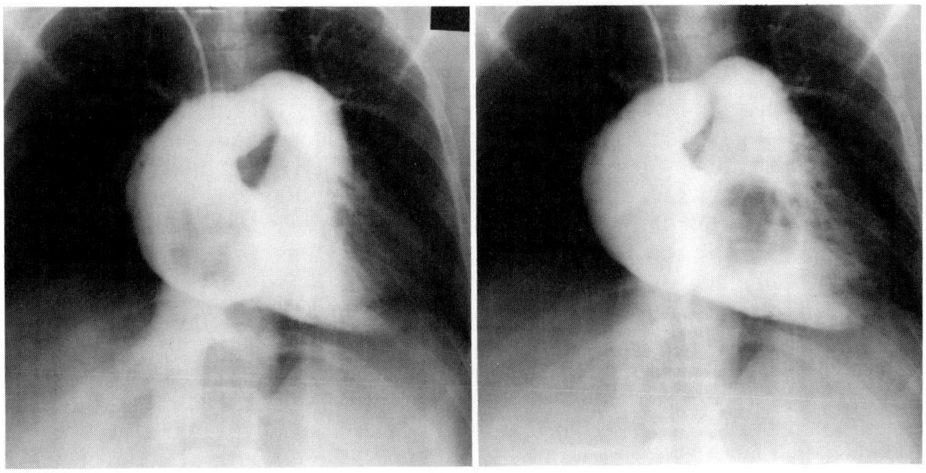

Fig 56-10 Angiocardiogram of a 26-year-old woman who presented with fever, anemia, and sedimentation rate of 112 mm in 1 hour (Westergren). **Left,** defect (mass) is in the right atrium during systole. **Right,** large mass is entering the right ventricular chamber during diastole. At surgery a large right atrial myxoma was successfully removed with reversal of all symptoms and findings. (From Giuliani ER, Brandenburg RO, Fuster V: Cardiac tumors. In *Clinical Medicine.* Edited by JA Spittell Jr. Hagerstown, Maryland, Harper & Row, Publishers, 1983, vol 6, chapter 24, pp 1-10. By permission.)

symptomatic primarily through obstruction to blood flow,[152,155-157] whereas left ventricular myxomas become symptomatic through both obstruction and systemic embolization.[153,154]

Right ventricular myxomas can present with syncope related to tricuspid or pulmonary valvular obstruction or, if obstruction is incomplete, with exertional dyspnea or chest pain. Physical examination often reveals a harsh ejection murmur in the pulmonary area, and thus pulmonary valvular or infundibular stenosis becomes the most frequent consideration in the differential diagnosis. Rarely, a tumor arising in the right atrium can prolapse completely through the tricuspid valve and interfere with both tricuspid and pulmonary valvular function.[158] Phonocardiographic studies of patients with right ventricular myxoma[151] have confirmed the presence of a prominent diastolic vibration, which corresponds to a sudden halting of tumor movement. Diagnosis is commonly made by echocardiographic examination.[159] Cardiac catheterization has revealed pulmonary outflow tract gradients of more than 50 mm Hg, a finding that has erroneously been diagnosed as reflecting pulmonic stenosis.[155]

Left ventricular myxomas often obstruct the left ventricular outflow tract and lead to symptoms of syncope or chest pain and physical findings similar to those seen in valvular aortic stenosis, from which the condition must be differentiated.[153,154] Echocardiographic examination is again definitive, although with a mass in the left ventricular outflow tract, a distinction must be made between tumor and thrombus. Left ventricular thrombi are usually located in the left ventricular apex and rarely in the outflow tract; they are often complications of acute myocardial infarction or dilated cardiomyopathy.

Surgical treatment of cardiac myxomas

Every myxoma is potentially amenable to surgical resection. In a patient without a history of cardiac disease in whom a typical myxoma is diagnosed by two-dimensional echocardiographic techniques, surgery should be undertaken promptly without cardiac catheterization or other invasive studies. This avoids the risk of tumor embolization related to catheter manipulation[125,160] and minimizes the delay between diagnosis and operation. Asymptomatic coronary artery disease is the only pathologic condition that would be inapparent to the operating surgeon under these conditions. Symbas et al.[161] emphasized that mortality is significant between the time of diagnosis and the operative intervention as a result of massive embolization or total obstruction to intracardiac blood flow. Because of this observation, operation should be undertaken promptly in any patient in whom the diagnosis of intracardiac myxoma has been made.

Operations for myxomas are performed by means of a median sternotomy and with standard cardiopulmonary bypass techniques. The general principles of surgical management of these lesions are, first, avoiding undue manipulation of the heart, which could lead to tumor embolization during the procedure; second, attempting to excise the endocardial origin of the tumor in an effort to prevent recurrence; third, carefully removing any loose tumor fragments from the cardiac chambers after the tumor has been removed; and fourth, carefully inspecting the cardiac valves that had contacted the tumor to assess for traumatic damage. The use of cardioplegic arrest provides a quiet operating field and enhances the probability of removing the friable tumors intact.

The approach to these tumors should be individualized

and should take into account the location of the tumor and its size. A small left atrial tumor arising from the area of the fossa ovalis can be approached through the right atrium with an en bloc excision of the tumor and its point of attachment to the atrial septum. The resulting atrial septal defect can be closed with either a pericardial or a prosthetic patch. Larger left atrial myxomas arising from the septum are often best evaluated through separate incisions into each atrium. In this way, the point of attachment can be clearly delineated from the left side and the septal resection can be carried out from the right side. Left atrial tumors arising from sites other than the atrial septum can be approached through the left atrium alone. For these tumors, it would seem prudent to remove the endocardium at the point of insertion of the tumor stalk and to consider coagulating this area as well in an effort to minimize the chance of tumor recurrence. Right ventricular tumors can be approached either through a right ventriculotomy or through the right atrium with exposure through the tricuspid valve, depending on the exact location of the tumor. In general, a full-thickness excision of the ventricular wall at the point of tumor origin does not appear to be warranted; however, excision of a portion of the endocardium in this region should be attempted. Left ventricular myxomas can be most safely approached through either the mitral or the aortic valve, depending on the location of the tumor. Associated valvular disease at the time of tumor removal may require valvular replacement or annuloplasty.

The results of surgical resection of cardiac myxomas are excellent.[18,19,35,36,67,138,162,163] Current operative mortality is well below 5%. Immediate hemodynamic improvement is noted. The vast majority of constitutional symptoms resolve completely, and the risk of embolism is eliminated. The potential for recurrence of atrial myxomas was initially reported by Read et al.,[58] and subsequent follow-up studies indicated that the risk of recurrence is approximately 5%.[35,163] Every effort should be made to remove the point of origin of the tumor, with preservation of surrounding valves and conduction tissue. It is likely, however, that tumor recurrence is, in many instances, metachronous and takes place in a previously unappreciated group of patients with a tendency for multicentric tumors. In our experience, there were no recurrences among 50 patients with sporadic myxomas treated by generally conservative resections in whom the average follow-up was 10.5 years.[34] In contrast, patients with myxomas and features of the complex of myxomas, spotty pigmentation, and endocrine overactivity and patients with synchronous myxomas or a family history of myxoma are at high risk for metachronous tumors. These patients should have a thorough search of all four cardiac chambers at the time of initial exploration and complete excision of the area of attachment to the atrial septum when tumors arise there. For patients at high risk, regular follow-up with two-dimensional echocardiography is required.

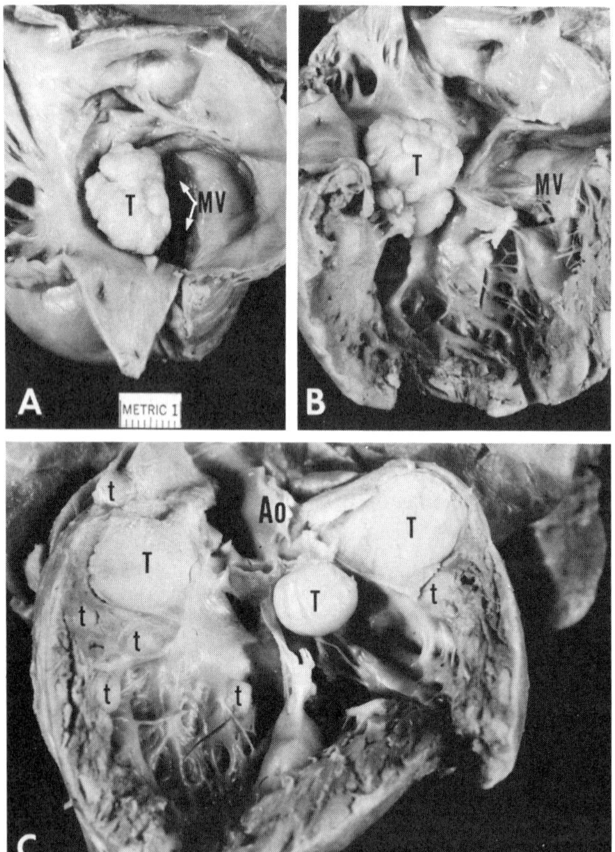

Fig 56-11 Multiple intracavitary and intramural rhabdomyomas in a male newborn infant. Large polypoid tumors (*T*) are shown obstructing the mitral valve (*MV*) orifice in **A** (left atrium viewed from above) and **B** (opened left ventricular inflow tract) and causing subaortic (A_o) left ventricular outflow obstruction in **C.** Note small satellite tumors (*t*) scattered throughout the left ventricular wall in **C.** (Case previously reported by Mair et al.[166])

OTHER BENIGN CARDIAC NEOPLASMS

Rhabdomyoma

Rhabdomyoma is the most common cardiac tumor in infants and children; it is rarely seen in patients more than 15 years of age.[5,7,164-166] Pathologically, the tumors are well-circumscribed, nonencapsulated, grayish nodules originating from the myocardium. They most often arise from the ventricular surfaces and affect the right and left sides equally.[164] The tumors are variable in size and cause symptoms either by obstructing intracardiac blood flow or by interfering with normal cardiac conduction (Fig 56-11). A diffuse form of the disease that affects the entire heart and leads to global heart failure appears to be very rare.[167] Histologically, rhabdomyomas are composed of large, vacuolated cells that contain abundant glycogen (Fig 56-12). Glycogen is readily identified by the periodic acid-Schiff reaction. Myofibrils extend from the centrally placed nucleus and create the classic "spider cell" appearance. Mitotic figures are distinctly absent.

The neoplastic nature of rhabdomyomas remains controversial.[164,165] On the basis of extensive light and electron microscopic examination, it is generally accepted

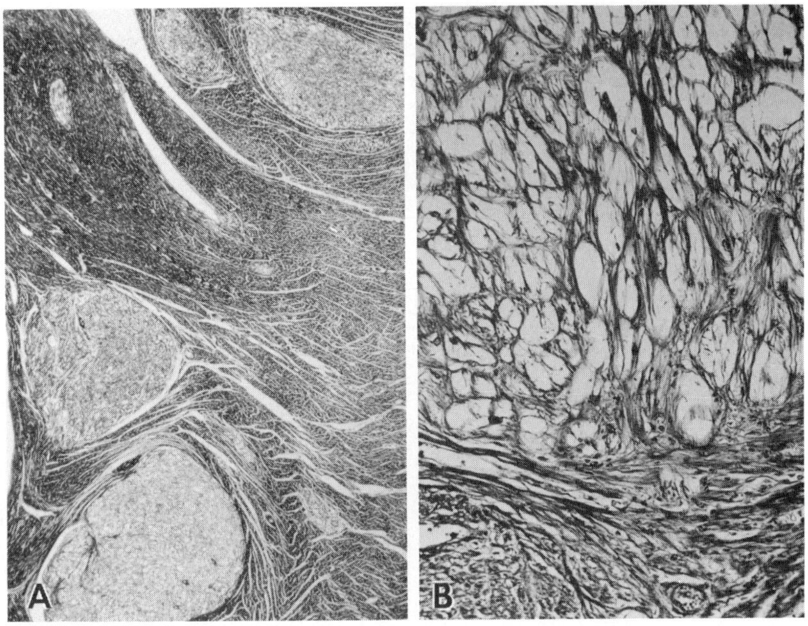

Fig 56-12 **A,** histologic appearance of intramural rhabdomyomas of various sizes, well demarcated from normal myocardium. **B,** ballooned-out, large vacuolated cells of rhabdomyoma. Vacuolated areas in alcohol-fixed tissue show abundant intracytoplasmic glycogen. (Hematoxylin and eosin; **A** ×12; **B** ×290.)

that rhabdomyomas originate from cardiac muscle cells and appear to represent hamartomas rather than true tumors. They have a congenital origin and have very limited potential for growth. Tuberous sclerosis appears to be associated with cardiac rhabdomyomas in approximately 30% of cases.

Infiltration of the myocardium in the vicinity of the conduction system can lead to a wide variety of cardiac arrhythmias, including fatal complete atrioventricular (AV) block.[165] The large tumors that project into the cardiac cavities can produce progressive heart failure, either chronically or acutely, depending on the location and mobility of the tumor mass. Such tumors can simulate congenital obstruction of any of the cardiac valves, and diagnoses of tetralogy of Fallot, mitral atresia, and congenital aortic stenosis have been reported.[165,166,168] Although the diagnosis is often suggested by echocardiography,[168,169] most of these very sick children come to cardiac catheterization and angiography, at which time the lesion usually can be readily visualized.

The mortality from rhabdomyoma that presents in infancy is high. The fact that approximately 90% of these tumors are multiple was initially used to justify nonoperative management. However, because the tumors have little propensity for further growth, there is currently a very definite role for surgical resection, even if subtotal, of a tumor or portion of a tumor causing significant symptoms. Successful resection of these tumors has been performed in children as young as 12 days of age by means of cardiopulmonary bypass with circulatory arrest.[165] Even if the tumor has been only partially resected, symptoms are usually relieved, and follow-up catheterization has not revealed significant regrowth of tumor, although follow-up has not been long in patients so treated.[165] Indeed, for many of these children, the presence or absence of tuberous sclerosis becomes the more important factor in determining ultimate prognosis.[170]

Fibroma

Fibromas are benign myocardial tumors that can be found in patients of any age, but the overwhelming majority are seen in patients younger than 10 years.[5,165,171] The tumors are virtually always solitary and are usually located in the left ventricular free wall or the interventricular septum. The tumor is usually firm and white and is quite well circumscribed but not encapsulated. Although these tumors do not invade or metastasize, they interdigitate with the adjacent myocardium.[5] Histologically, the fibroma consists of mature fibroblasts and associated hyalinized fibrous tissue (Fig 56-13). There are often multiple foci of calcification, which can be seen on routine chest roentgenography. Mitotic figures are quite rare.

Cardiac fibromas may mimic a broad spectrum of cardiac diseases, because they usually appear with congestive heart failure, heart murmurs, or sudden death.[171] Congestive failure is usually related to interference with myocardial contraction, although significant valvular dysfunction can also occur.[171] Significant arrhythmia is found in association with cardiac fibroma in approximately 30% of cases, and sudden death is a frequent mode of presentation and is presumably due to interference with cardiac conduction by the tumor.

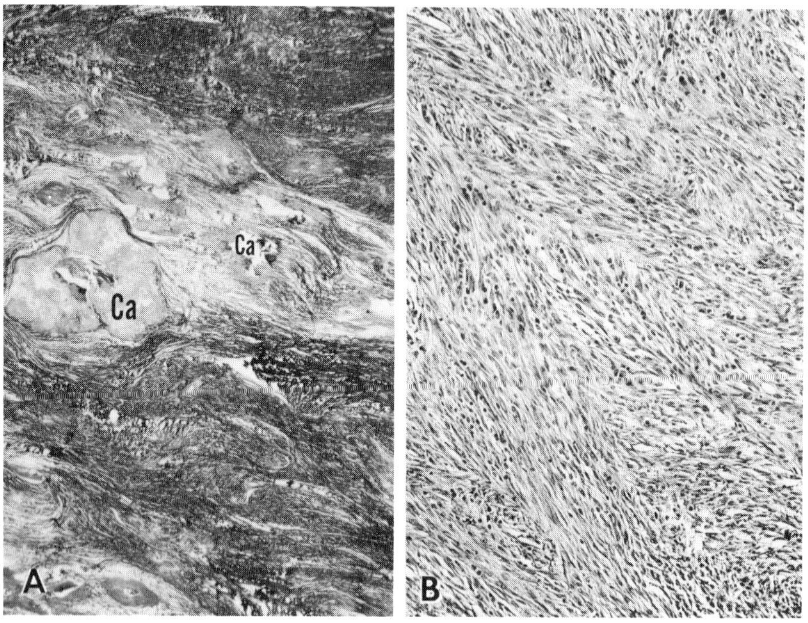

Fig 56-13 **A,** cardiac fibroma showing typical microscopic foci of dystrophic calcification (*Ca*) in hyalinized fibrous tissue. **B,** cellular area with interlacing fibroblasts. (Hematoxylin and eosin; **A** ×12; **B** ×115.)

Cardiac fibromas can occasionally be suggested by plain chest roentgenography when an irregular contour of the left heart border and calcification within the cardiac silhouette are noted. Although two-dimensional echocardiographic examination can detect many fibromas, magnetic resonance imaging provides excellent resolution of tumor and surrounding myocardium (see Fig 56-1). Angiography was used in the past to establish the diagnosis of fibromas, but often a tumor that does not project into the ventricle is not identified by standard contrast radiographic techniques.

Resection of even large intramural cardiac fibromas has become feasible by means of current techniques of cardiopulmonary bypass. A dissection plane between the tumor and the adjacent myocardium can usually be established. In many cases, the tumor can be enucleated, and myocardial integrity can be reestablished without the need for prosthetic materials.

Septal tumors are considerably more challenging than those involving the left ventricular free wall. Although complete resection of the fibroma is the therapeutic goal of the cardiac surgeon, excellent palliation has been obtained by removal of only that portion of the tumor that interferes with valvular function or compromises left ventricular chamber size.[171,172] It has been pointed out, however, that the potential for sudden death in these patients probably remains.[171] Two-dimensional echocardiography appears to be an excellent means of observing these patients for possible regrowth of tumor. The long-term outcome for patients in whom myocardial fibromas have been completely resected is good.[171] A huge unresectable left ventricular fibroma in a 17-year-old girl was successfully managed by cardiac transplantation.[173]

Lipoma and lipomatous hypertrophy of the atrial septum

Lipomas are benign tumors that can be found throughout the heart or pericardium. Most are small and asymptomatic; however, truly massive tumors are occasionally encountered.[165] Tumors that arise from the epicardial surface can protrude into the pericardial space and compromise cardiac function by compression or by an associated pericardial effusion. Myocardial or endocardial lipomas can become symptomatic through interference with cardiac conduction or through obstruction to intracardiac blood flow. Histologically, lipomas are encapsulated and consist of mature fat cells with varying amounts of associated fibrous tissue. Symptomatic lipomas can usually be readily resected by standard techniques.[174,175]

Lipomatous hypertrophy of the atrial septum (LHAS) was first recognized by Prior[176] in 1964 as an entity to be differentiated from true lipoma of the heart. It is characterized by excessive accumulation of nonencapsulated adipose tissue in the atrial septum cephalad and caudad to the fossa ovalis but always sparing the fossa (Fig 56-14). In most cases, LHAS measures more than 2 cm in maximum width, whereas the thickness of most of the atrial septum is less than 1.5 cm. Microscopically, LHAS is composed of mature adipose tissue with entrapped myocardial fibers scattered throughout but mainly in the periphery. Fetal fat, a hallmark of LHAS, is present in

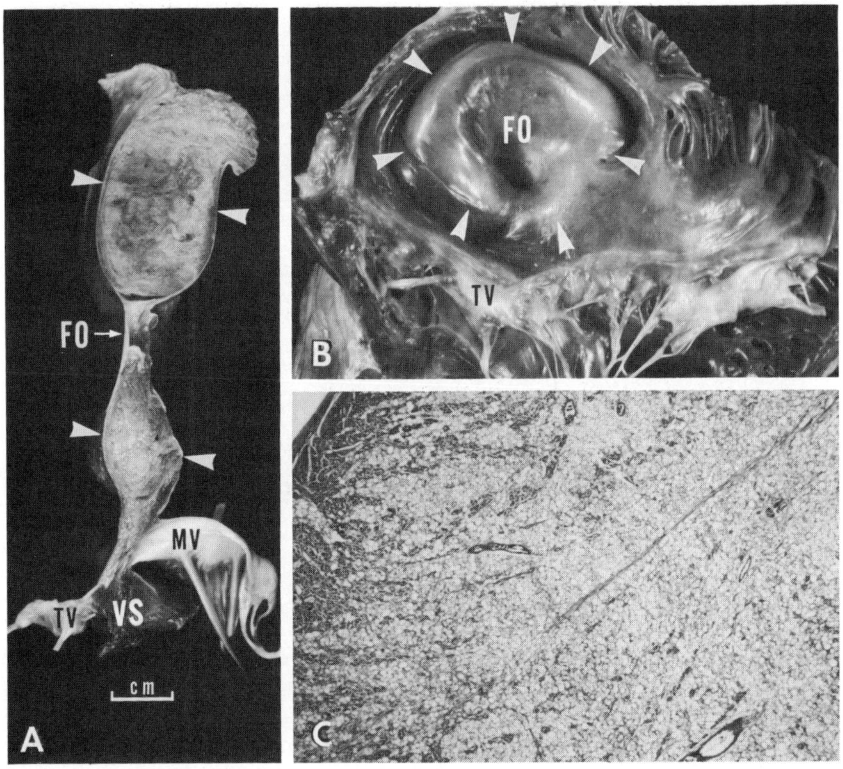

Fig 56-14 **A,** sagittal section of atrial septum showing lipomatous hypertrophy (*arrowheads*) above and below fossa ovalis (*FO*) and its relationship to the tricuspid valve (*TV*), mitral valve (*MV*), and crest of the ventricular septum (*VS*). **B,** a clue to this lesion is an easily palpable protuberant mass (*arrowheads*) around the fossa ovalis (*FO*) and above the tricuspid valve (*TV*) when the atrial septum is inspected in the opened right atrium. **C,** typical histologic appearance of nonencapsulated adipose tissue with variable amounts of fetal fat and trapped myocardial fibers in a greatly expanded atrial septum. (Hematoxylin and eosin; **C** ×15.)

variable amounts, and the entrapped cardiac myocytes may show hypertrophy or atrophic or vacuolated degenerative changes.

To date, close to 100 cases of LHAS have been reported.[4,176-183] It occurs commonly but not exclusively in elderly and obese or overweight persons. In many cases, LHAS has been an incidental finding at autopsy; some of these lesions are considered to be the anatomic basis of otherwise unexplained supraventricular arrhythmias and sudden death in both elderly and young persons.[177-181] Antemortem detection of LHAS is now possible by computed tomographic cardiac imaging,[182] two-dimensional echocardiography,[183] and magnetic resonance imaging.[130,184,185] The lesion should be included in the differential diagnosis of intracardiac thrombi and tumors. Since a cause-and-effect relationship between supraventricular arrhythmias and LHAS would be difficult to prove, the role of surgical ablation of LHAS remains uncertain.

Atrioventricular node tumor

Heterotopic epithelial replacement of the AV node (so-called mesothelioma of the AV node or AV node tumor[5,186,187]) is a rare cause of congenital heart block and sudden death. About 50 cases of this unusual lesion have been reported and have occurred predominantly in female patients from infancy to age 86 years.[187] The lesion, usually less than 1 cm in size and confined to the AV node, is virtually impossible to diagnose clinically and can be recognized at autopsy only by histologic examination of the AV conduction tissue (Fig 56-15).

The behavior of these tumors is not well understood. They are clearly associated with complete heart block and sudden death. On the other hand, symptoms of heart block are often noted in later life, suggesting a long asymptomatic period for the tumor. They are not necessarily associated with symptoms, having been found incidentally at postmortem examination.

It appears that this tumor becomes symptomatic only through interference with cardiac conduction. This being so, it is difficult to explain an apparent intolerance to electronic pacing that occurs in some of the patients.[186] In any event, the diagnosis of such a tumor should be considered in patients with intermittent heart block or cardiac arrest, particularly in younger patients. Because of the size and location of these tumors and the rarity with which they are diagnosed before death, there is no

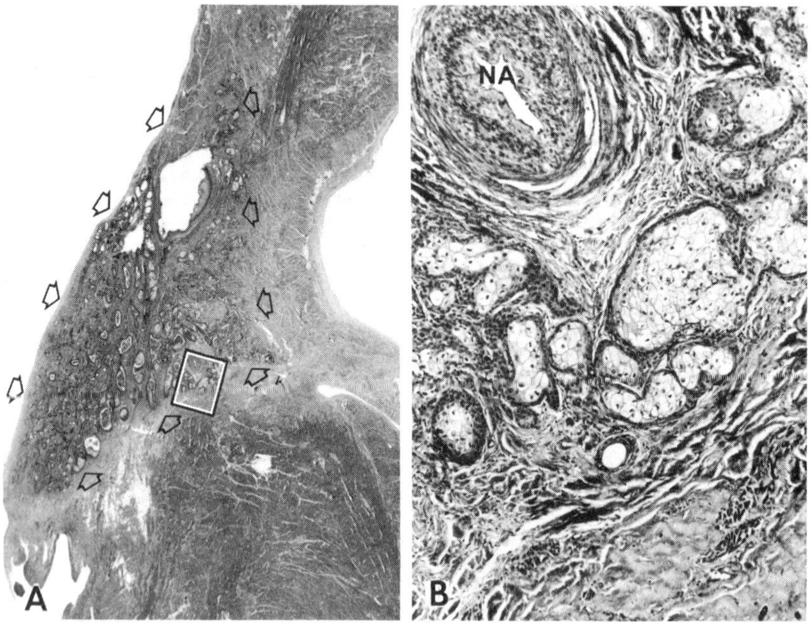

Fig 56-15 **A,** epithelial heterotopia replacing AV node (so-called AV node tumor or mesothelioma of the AV node) in the atrial septum (*arrows*) of a young woman who had congenital heart block and died suddenly at age 25. **B,** higher magnification of boxed area in **A,** showing clusters of typical squamous epithelium of dermoid cyst adjacent to the AV node artery (*NA*).(Hematoxylin and eosin; **A** ×6; **B** ×115.) (Case reported by Lie et al.[187])

currently accepted role for surgical intervention. Nevertheless, resection with subsequent electronic pacing seems theoretically feasible.

Papillary fibroelastoma

Papillary fibroelastomas are rare benign tumors that originate from the cardiac valves or adjacent endocardium.[5] The tumors are most often incidental findings at postmortem examination; however, they can occasionally interfere with valvular function or, if situated on the aortic valve, can cause symptomatic coronary ostial obstruction.[5] The tumors have a frondlike appearance not unlike the sea anemone. Histologically, the fronds consist of a central core of dense connective tissue surrounded by a layer of loose connective tissue covered by endothelial cells.[5] The tumors tend to originate from the atrial side of the AV valves and often, but not universally, occur on the ventricular surface of the semilunar valves (Fig 56-16). The aortic valve is most often involved in adults, in whom these tumors are usually encountered.

The relationship of these tumors to Lambl's excrescences is debatable. Boone et al. stated that Lambl's excrescences are similar in microscopic appearance to papillary fibroelastomas, but Lambl's excrescences are smaller and broader based. Some Lambl's excrescences and fibroelastomas are indistinguishable by microscopy. A clinical distinction is useful because of the potential for embolization of papillary fibroelastomas, which are thought to occur as a result of degenerative changes along the line of closure of valves.

Surgical resection of a symptomatic papillary fibroelastoma appears to be indicated, because stroke and fatal coronary artery embolization have been reported.[188] In most cases, the fibroelastoma can be excised from the valve and prosthetic replacement is not necessary.

Hemangioma

Hemangiomas are benign proliferations of endothelial cells that form vascular structures.[5] They are of various sizes and can be found throughout the myocardium (Fig 56-17). They are rare and are usually encountered as incidental findings at postmortem examination. Burke et al.[189] recently presented the clinical and histopathologic features of cardiac hemangiomas in 10 patients whose ages ranged from 2 weeks to 65 years (mean, 32 years). Eight patients had no other cardiovascular abnormalities, one patient had associated intra-atrial lipoma, and one had an anomalous origin of the left coronary artery. One patient had other hemangiomas of the oral cavity and small intestine. The tumors were manifested in a variety of ways, including pericardial effusion and sudden death. Of importance is the finding that all six tumors discovered in life were resected successfully.

MALIGNANT PRIMARY TUMORS OF THE HEART

Approximately one-fourth of all cardiac tumors are malignant.[5,7] Virtually all these are sarcomas affecting adults; a malignant tumor arising in the pediatric age

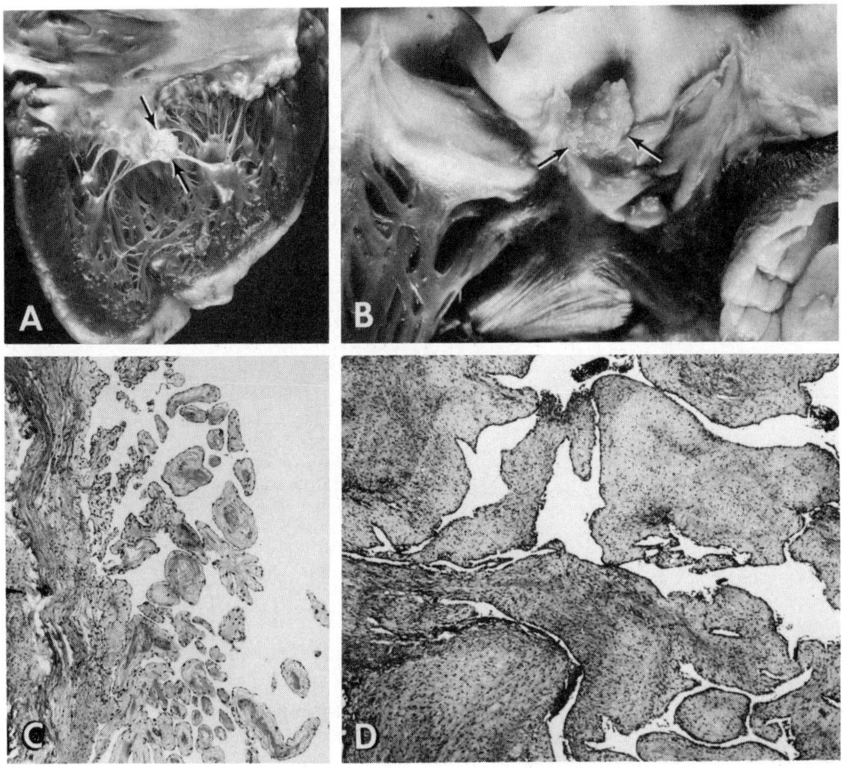

Fig 56-16 Papillary tumors (*arrows*) of the mitral valve (**A**) and the pulmonary valve (**B**) may look alike in gross appearance but are histologically dissimilar. **C**, typical fibroelastoma of the cardiac valve. Endothelium-covered papillary fronds have a collagen core surrounded by loose connective tissue that is rich in elastic fibers. **D**, typical myxoma of the cardiac valve. Its histology and ultrastructure are indistinguishable from those of intracavitary cardiac myxomas. (Hematoxylin and eosin; **C** and **D**, ×30.)

group is rare.[165] Histologically, these tumors assume a wide variety of morphological subtypes, most frequently angiosarcomas, rhabdomyosarcomas, and fibrosarcomas (Fig 56-18). From a clinical point of view, however, histologic characterization is largely an academic exercise. In general, these tumors are universally fatal, and the interval between diagnosis and death is very short.[190]

The potential for successful cure of these tumors is limited because of their aggressive biologic behavior. Sarcomas infiltrate the heart extensively, so that complete resection is not possible. In addition, the tumors tend to extend locally into the pericardium, lung, and other surrounding structures. Finally, approximately 80% of these tumors have distant metastasis at the time of discovery.[191] As mentioned for the pathologic description of cardiac myxomas, myxomas that are subsequently found to metastasize widely most likely represent myxosarcomas.[192,193]

Most of these tumors become manifest through cardiac symptoms; however, congestive heart failure can result from tumor infiltration of the cardiac valves, intracavity obstruction to blood flow, or diffuse infiltration of the myocardium with loss of effective pump function.[5,191] Extracardiac extension can result in symptomatic pericardial effusions, and acute tamponade can occur. Occasionally, the first manifestation of a malignant cardiac tumor is symptomatic metastasis. Finally, occasional patients present with the nonspecific symptoms of disseminated malignant disease, such as weight loss and anemia.

Angiosarcomas occur most often in adult males and most commonly involve the right atrium.[5,194-198] The predilection for the right heart often leads to a presentation with right-sided congestive heart failure or pericardial effusions. Although cure has not been achieved, palliation can be obtained in selected patients with surgical excision.

Rhabdomyosarcomas and fibrosarcomas appear to affect males and females equally and have no predilection for a particular cardiac chamber.[5] No patients with these malignant lesions have been cured, although adjuvant radiation therapy with chemotherapy in selected cases might offer some palliation of cardiac symptoms.[199,200] Although primary surgical resection of these tumors can rarely be accomplished,[199] its role in the total management of these disorders remains to be established.

SECONDARY TUMORS OF THE HEART

Secondary cardiac tumors—neoplasms that originate elsewhere and spread to the heart—are virtually all

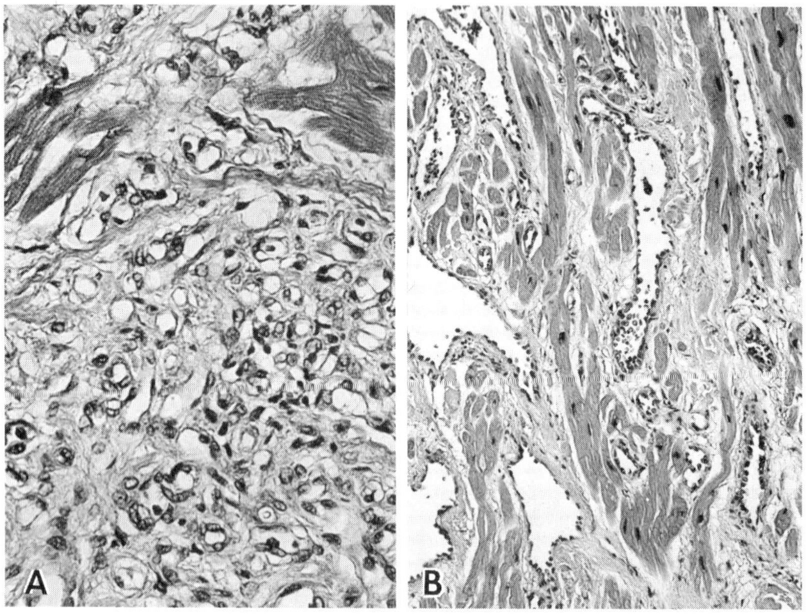

Fig 56-17 Variable histologic appearance in different areas of the same intracardiac hemangioma with biventricular involvement in a 17-year-old boy who died suddenly. **A,** capillary hemangioma. **B,** cavernous hemangioma. (Hematoxylin and eosin; ×115.)

A

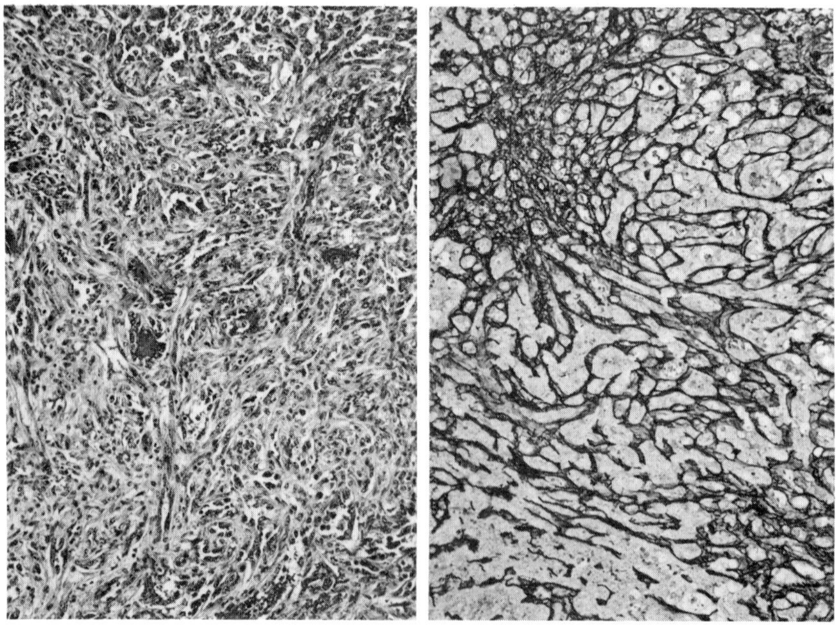

B

Fig 56-18 **A,** angiosarcoma with closely packed spindle cells masking the vascular pattern of the tumor. **B,** reticulum stain of the same microscopic field reveals an underlying network of vascular channels. (**A,** hematoxylin and eosin; ×115; **B,** reticulum stain; ×115.)

Table 56-4 Types of malignant tumors that metastasize to the heart and pericardium, in decreasing order of frequency

		Metastasis in heart or pericardium	
Primary malignant tumor	**Total no. of cases**	**No.**	**%**
Melanoma	59	22	37
Leukemia	215	54	25
Bronchogenic carcinoma	402	86	21
Carcinoma of breast	289	55	19
Lymphoma (Hodgkin's and non-Hodgkin's)	285	37	13
Carcinoma of esophagus	65	8	12
Carcinoma of ovary	115	11	10
Carcinoma of pancreas	168	14	8
Squamous carcinoma of lip, tongue, pharynx, and vocal cord	50	4	8
Carcinoma of bladder	86	5	6
Carcinoma of stomach	308	18	6
Renal cell carcinoma	95	5	5
Carcinoma of prostate	186	7	4
Carcinoma of colon	214	8	3
Carcinoma of cervix	92	2	2
Carcinoma of thyroid	50	1	2
Hepatoma	62	1	2

Data from Fine G: Neoplasms of the pericardium and heart. In *Pathology of the Heart and Blood Vessels.* Third edition. Edited by SE Gould. Springfield, Illinois, Charles C Thomas, Publisher, 1968, pp 851-883.

malignant. In incidence, secondary tumors outnumber those that originate in the heart by as much as 40 times in some series.[7,12,13] There is, however, considerable variation in the incidence of cardiac metastasis discovered at postmortem examination in patients dying of malignant disease – from 1.5% to 18.3%[7,12,201,202] (Table 56-4). The incidence of cancer metastatic to the heart appears to be increasing;[201,202] perhaps this increase is related to prolongation of survival in patients with malignant disease, which allows more time for metastasis to develop.

In absolute numbers, bronchogenic carcinoma, carcinoma of the breast, lymphoma, and leukemia account for the overwhelming majority of cardiac metastatic lesions (Fig 56-19). Of any one specific tumor type, however, malignant melanoma has the greatest propensity to such metastasis, 50% to 65% of melanoma patients being so affected.[203]

Tumors spread to the heart by direct extension from surrounding intrathoracic structures, by hematogenous spread, or by lymphatic spread.[203] Direct extension occurs most often in patients with bronchogenic carcinoma, which can extend through the pericardium into the left atrium. Other mediastinal tumors can behave similarly. Direct extension into the heart can also occur via the blood vessels; extension of hypernephroma into the heart via the inferior vena cava is the most common example. Finally, malignant pericardial effusions from noncardiac neoplasms can lead to the implantation of viable cells on the epicardial surface.

Blood-borne metastasis theoretically can occur from any malignant tumor. The embolized tumor cells lodge in the myocardium and grow; and because the myocardium has the greatest blood supply, this area is most often involved, whereas the valves and endocardium are least often affected.[11] When one excludes tumors that have propagated into the right atrium from the vena cava, metastasis appears to occur in equal incidence in the right and left sides of the heart.[203]

In whatever form they take, cardiac metastatic lesions usually occur in patients with extensive carcinomatosis.[7,12,201-204] Rarely is the metastasis the first manifestation of the malignant disease,[205] and most myocardial metastatic lesions are asymptomatic.

Cardiac metastasis can be suspected on the basis of the patient's tumor cell type and cardiac examination. The diagnosis can be substantiated by two-dimensional echocardiographic examination (Fig 56-20). Occasionally, angiography delineates obstructing intracavitary metastatic lesions. Tumors that are associated with a pericardial effusion can often be diagnosed by cytologic examination of the pericardial fluid.

Patients with metastatic cardiac disease can rarely be cured. In some instances, however, the symptoms from these metastatic lesions are so profound that they overshadow other manifestations of the patient's neoplastic burden. Consequently, efforts at early diagnosis and palliation are often justified in these patients. For tumors that are radiosensitive, external-beam irradiation has provided significant palliation of a variety of cardiac symptoms.[206] Recurrent malignant pericardial effusions can initially be treated with pericardiocentesis; however, reaccumulation usually occurs. In many of these patients,

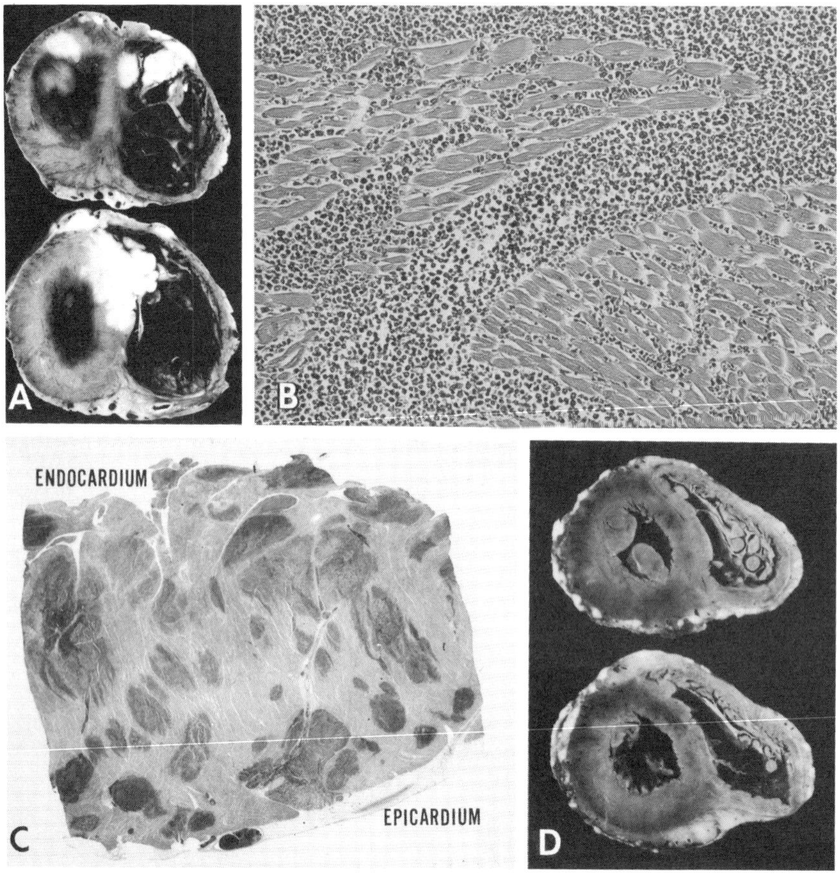

Fig 56-19 Metastatic tumors of the heart. **A,** gross appearance of extensive lymphoma involvement of the heart. **B,** diffuse and dense lymphoma infiltration of the myocardium. Note that individual myofibers are intact. **C,** extensive subendocardial, intramural, and subepicardial metastases of melanoma. **D,** epicardial metastases of carcinoma of the breast. Note the absence of intramural metastases. (Hematoxylin and eosin; **B** ×120; **C** ×3.)

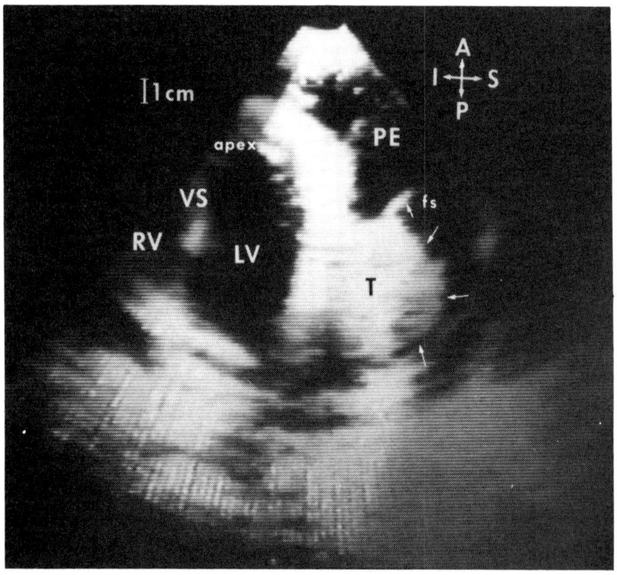

Fig 56-20 Frame from modified four-chamber two-dimensional echocardiographic section of a patient with large pericardial effusion (*PE*). The patient had had a mastectomy several years previously for adenocarcinoma. Note the large tumor mass within the pericardial space and attached to the epicardium (*T, arrows*) and also the fibrous strands (*fs*) extending from the tumor. Note scale. *A,* anterior; *I,* inferior; *LV,* left ventricle; *P,* posterior; *RV,* right ventricle; *S,* superior; *VS,* ventricular septum.

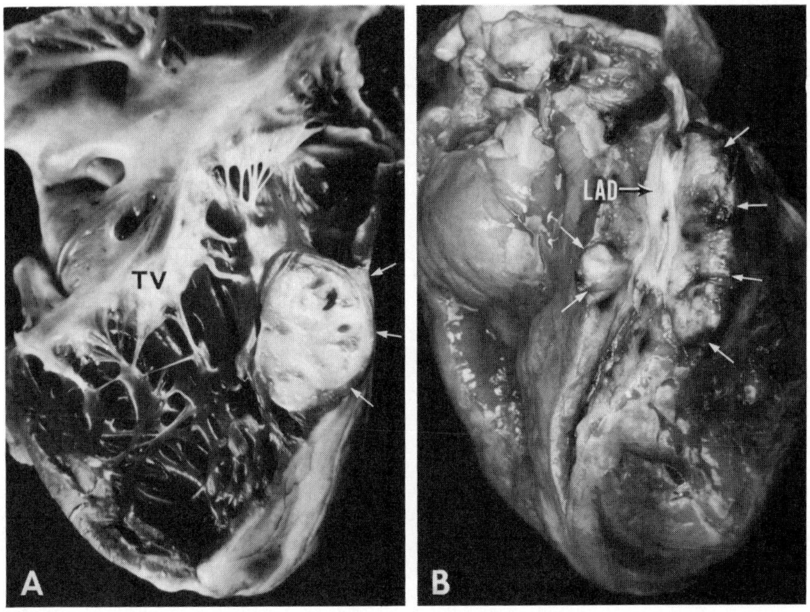

Fig 56-21 Clinically significant and potentially resectable metastatic tumors of the heart. **A,** solitary metastatic synovial sarcoma in the trabecula septomarginalis (*arrows*), causing right ventricular outflow tract obstruction. *TV,* tricuspid valve. **B,** discrete epicardial metastases of bronchogenic carcinoma (*arrows*), compressing the left anterior descending (*LAD*) coronary artery. Note that the artery is relatively free of atherosclerosis.

surgical resection of the accessible pericardium via a left anterior thoracotomy offers excellent control of the effusion.[207]

Surgical intervention has a small but definite role in patients with secondary cardiac tumors.[207,208] Metastatic tumors originating from a localized portion of the heart and leading to obstruction to intracardiac blood flow theoretically are the most amenable to resection[208,209] (Fig 56-21). The greatest benefit would be expected in patients in whom the primary tumor was controlled and in whom there had been a significant disease-free interval between control of the primary tumor and the detection of the cardiac metastatic lesions.

REFERENCES

1. Goldberg HP, Glenn F, Dotter CT, et al: Myxoma of the left atrium: diagnosis made during life with operative and postmortem findings. *Circulation* 6:762-767, 1952
2. Crafoord C: Discussion. In *International Symposium on Cardiovascular Surgery: Studies in Physiology, Diagnosis and Techniques.* Edited by CR Lam. Philadelphia, WB Saunders Company, 1955, pp 202-203
3. Murphy MC, Sweeney MS, Putnam JB Jr, et al: Surgical treatment of cardiac tumors: a 25-year experience. *Ann Thorac Surg* 49:612-617, 1990
4. McAllister HA, Fenoglio JJ: Tumors of the cardiovascular system. In *Atlas of Tumor Pathology, Fascicle 15, Second Series.* Washington, DC, Armed Forces Institute of Pathology, 1978
5. McAllister HA Jr: Primary tumors and cysts of the heart and pericardium. *Curr Probl Cardiol* 4:1-51, May 1979
6. Heath D: Pathology of cardiac tumors. *Am J Cardiol* 21:315-327, 1968
7. Prichard RW: Tumors of the heart: review of the subject and report of one hundred and fifty cases. *Arch Pathol* 51:98-128, 1951
8. Wold LE, Lie JT: Cardiac myxomas: a clinicopathologic profile. *Am J Pathol* 101:219-240, 1980
9. Leach WB: Primary neoplasms of the heart. *Arch Pathol* 44:198-204, 1947
10. Straus R, Merliss R: Primary tumor of the heart. *Arch Pathol* 39:74-78, 1945
11. Fabian JT, Rose AG: Tumours of the heart: a study of 89 cases. *S Afr Med J* 61:71-77, 1982
12. DeLoach JF, Haynes JW: Secondary tumors of heart and pericardium: review of the subject and report of the one hundred thirty-seven cases. *Arch Intern Med* 91:224-249, 1953
13. Griffiths GC: A review of primary tumors of the heart. *Prog Cardiovasc Dis* 7:465-479, 1965
14. Zitnik RS, Giuliani ER: Clinical recognition of atrial myxoma. *Am Heart J* 80:689-700, 1970
15. Goodwin JF, Stanfield CA, Steiner RE, et al: Clinical features of left atrial myxoma. *Thorax* 17:91-110, 1962
16. Greenwood WF: Profile of atrial myxoma. *Am J Cardiol* 21:367-375, 1968
17. Peters MN, Hall RJ, Cooley DA, et al: The clinical syndrome of atrial myxoma. *JAMA* 230:695-701, 1974
18. Bulkley BH, Hutchins GM: Atrial myxomas: a fifty year review. *Am Heart J* 97:639-643, 1979
19. St John Sutton MG, Mercier L-A, Giuliani ER, et al: Atrial myxomas: a review of clinical experience in 40 patients. *Mayo Clin Proc* 55:371-376, 1980
20. Pridie RB: Left atrial myxomas in childhood: presentation with emboli—diagnosis by ultrasonics. *Thorax* 27:759-763, 1972
21. Kleid JJ, Klugman J, Haas J, et al: Familial atrial myxoma. *Am J Cardiol* 32:361-364, 1973
22. Powers JC, Falkoff M, Heinle RA, et al: Familial cardiac myxomas: emphasis on unusual clinical manifestations. *J Thorac Cardiovasc Surg* 77:782-788, 1979
23. Liebler GA, Magovern GJ, Park SB, et al: Familial myxomas in four siblings. *J Thorac Cardiovasc Surg* 71:605-608, 1976
24. Siltanen P, Tuuteri L, Norio R, et al: Atrial myxoma in a family. *Am J Cardiol* 38:252-256, 1976

25. Farah MG: Familial atrial myxoma. *Ann Intern Med* 83:358-360, 1975
26. Crawford FA Jr, Selby JH Jr, Watson D, et al: Unusual aspects of atrial myxoma. *Ann Surg* 188:240-244, 1978
27. Carney JA, Gordon H, Carpenter PC, et al: The complex of myxomas, spotty pigmentation, and endocrine overactivity. *Medicine (Baltimore)* 64:270-283, 1985
28. Carney JA: Differences between nonfamilial and familial cardiac myxoma. *Am J Surg Pathol* 9:53-55, 1985
29. Handley J, Carson D, Sloan J, et al: Multiple lentigines, myxoid tumours and endocrine overactivity; four cases of Carney's complex. *Br J Dermatol* 126:367-371, 1992
30. Wallace TM, Levin HS, Ratliff NB, et al: Evaluation and management of Carney's complex: an illustrative case. *Cleve Clin J Med* 58:248-256, 1991
31. van Gelder HM, O'Brien DJ, Staples ED, et al: Familial cardiac myxoma. *Ann Thorac Surg* 53:419-424, 1992
32. Ichiba Y, Nishizaki Y, Tanizaki M: Cushing's syndrome due to primary pigmented nodular adrenocortical disease with cardiac myxomas and mucocutaneous lentigines. *Acta Paediatr* 81:91-92, 1992
33. Yen RS, Allen B, Ott R, et al: The syndrome of right atrial myxoma, spotty skin pigmentation, and acromegaly. *Am Heart J* 123:243-244, 1992
34. McCarthy PM, Piehler JM, Schaff HV, et al: The significance of multiple, recurrent, and "complex" cardiac myxomas. *J Thorac Cardiovasc Surg* 91:389-396, 1986
35. Richardson JV, Brandt B III, Doty DB, et al: Surgical treatment of atrial myxomas: early and late results of 11 operations and review of the literature. *Ann Thorac Surg* 28:354-358, 1979
36. Attar S, Lee Y-C, Singleton R, et al: Cardiac myxoma. *Ann Thorac Surg* 29:397-405, 1980
37. Dashkoff N, Boersma RB, Nanda NC, et al: Bilateral atrial myxomas: echocardiographic considerations. *Am J Med* 65:361-366, 1978
38. Fitterer JD, Spicer MJ, Nelson WP: Echocardiographic demonstration of bilateral atrial myxomas. *Chest* 70:282-284, 1976
39. Tway KP, Shah AA, Rahimtoola SH: Multiple biatrial myxomas demonstrated by two-dimensional echocardiography. *Am J Med* 71:896-899, 1981
40. Yipintsoi T, Donavanik L, Bhamarapravati N, et al: Bilateral atrial myxoma with successful removal: report of a case. *Dis Chest* 52:828-834, 1967
41. Gustafson AG, Edler IG, Dahlbäck OK: Bilateral atrial myxomas diagnosed by echocardiography. *Acta Med Scand* 201:391-394, 1977
42. Zajtchuk R, Fitterer JD, Strevey TE, et al: Bilateral atrial myxomas: preoperative diagnosis and successful removal. *J Thorac Cardiovasc Surg* 69:291-294, 1975
43. Cumming GR, Finkel K: Intracardiac myxoma involving the right and left atria in a young patient. *J Pediatr* 58:559-567, 1961
44. Imperio J, Summers D, Krasnow N, et al: The distribution patterns of biatrial myxomas. *Ann Thorac Surg* 29:469-473, 1980
45. Fauvre F, Johns VJ Jr, Jutzy RV: Cardiac myxomas: report of eight cases with successful excision. *West J Med* 127:284-291, 1977
46. Ferrans VJ, Roberts WC: Structural features of cardiac myxomas: histology, histochemistry, and electron microscopy. *Hum Pathol* 4:111-146, 1973
47. Salyer WR, Salyer DC: Myxoma-like features of organizing thrombi in arteries and veins. *Arch Pathol* 99:307-311, 1975
48. Salyer WR, Page DL, Hutchins GM: The development of cardiac myxomas and papillary endocardial lesions from mural thrombus. *Am Heart J* 89:4-17, 1975
49. Fine G, Morales A, Horn RC Jr: Cardiac myxoma: a morphologic and histogenetic appraisal. *Cancer* 22:1156-1162, 1968
50. Stovin PGI, Heath D, Khaliq SU: Ultrastructure of the cardiac myxoma and the papillary tumour of heart valves. *Thorax* 28:273-285, 1973
51. Feldman PS, Horvath E, Kovacs K: An ultrastructural study of seven cardiac myxomas. *Cancer* 40:2216-2232, 1977
52. Kelly M, Bhagwat AG: Ultrastructural features of a recurrent endothelial myxoma of the left atrium. *Arch Pathol* 93:219-226, 1972
53. Bashey RI, Nochumson S: Cardiac myxoma: biochemical analyses and evidence for its neoplastic nature. *NY State J Med* 79:29-32, 1979
54. Coltart DJ, Billingham ME, Popp RL, et al: Left atrial myxoma: diagnosis, treatment, and cytological observations. *JAMA* 234:950-953, 1975
55. Fisher ER, Hellstran HR: Evidence in support of the neoplastic nature of cardiac myxoma. *Am Heart J* 60:630-640, 1960
56. Glasser SP, Bedynek JL, Hall RJ, et al: Left atrial myxoma: report of a case involving hemodynamic, surgical, histologic and histochemical characteristics. *Am J Med* 50:113-122, 1971
57. Chopra P, Sharma VK: Left atrial myxoma: a morphologic and histogenetic study. *Jpn Heart J* 22:353-361, 1981
58. Read RC, White HJ, Murphy ML, et al: The malignant potentiality of left atrial myxoma. *J Thorac Cardiovasc Surg* 68:857-867, 1974
59. DeSousa AL, Muller J, Campbell RL, et al: Atrial myxoma: a review of the neurological complications, metastases, and recurrences. *J Neurol Neurosurg Psychiatry* 41:1119-1124, 1978
60. Steinmetz EF, Calanchini PR, Aguilar MJ: Left atrial myxoma as a neurological problem: a case report and review. *Stroke* 4:451-458, 1973
61. Frank RA, Shalen PR, Harvey DG, et al: Atrial myxoma with intellectual decline and cerebral growths on CT scan. *Ann Neurol* 5:396-400, 1979
62. New PFJ, Price DL, Carter B: Cerebral angiography in cardiac myxoma: correlation of angiographic and histopathological findings. *Radiology* 96:335-345, 1970
63. Todo T, Usui M, Nagashima K: Cerebral metastasis of malignant cardiac myxoma. *Surg Neurol* 37:374-379, 1992
64. McCarthy PM, Schaff HV, Winkler HZ, et al: Deoxyribonucleic acid ploidy pattern of cardiac myxomas: another predictor of biologically unusual myxomas. *J Thorac Cardiovasc Surg* 98:1083-1086, 1989
65. Goodwin JF: Diagnosis of left atrial myxoma. *Lancet* 1:464-468, 1963
66. Harvey WP: Clinical aspects of cardiac tumors. *Am J Cardiol* 21:328-343, 1968
67. Paulsen W, Nolewajka AJ, Boughner DR, et al: Left atrial myxoma: report of six cases and review of the literature. *Can Med Assoc J* 123:518-523, 1980
68. MacGregor GA, Cullen RA: The syndrome of fever, anaemia, and high sedimentation rate with an atrial myxoma. *Br Med J* 2:991-993, 1959
69. Levinson JP, Kincaid OW: Myxoma of the right atrium associated with polycythemia: report of successful excision. *N Engl J Med* 264:1187-1192, 1961
70. Vuopio P, Nikkilä EA: Hemolytic anemia and thrombocytopenia in a case of left atrial myxoma associated with mitral stenosis. *Am J Cardiol* 17:585-589, 1966
71. Gould L, Freiberg A, Lewnes GC, et al: Right atrial myxoma: associated with thrombocytopenia and bacterial endocarditis. *NY State J Med* 78:2081-2083, 1978
72. Huston KA, Combs JJ Jr, Lie JT, et al: Left atrial myxoma simulating peripheral vasculitis. *Mayo Clin Proc* 53:752-756, 1978
73. Willman VL, Symbas PN, Mamiya RT, et al: Unusual aspects of intracavitary tumors of the heart: report of two cases. *Dis Chest* 47:669-671, 1965
74. Selzer A, Sakai FJ, Popper RW: Protean clinical manifestations of primary tumors of the heart. *Am J Med* 52:9-18, 1972
75. Boss JH, Bechar M: Myxoma of the heart: report based on four cases. *Am J Cardiol* 3:823-828, 1959
76. Byrd WE, Matthews OP, Hunt RE: Left atrial myxoma presenting as a systemic vasculitis. *Arthritis Rheum* 23:240-243, 1980
77. Kaminsky ME, Ehlers KH, Engle MA, et al: Atrial myxoma mimicking a collagen disorder. *Chest* 75:93-95, 1979
78. Leonhardt ETG, Kullenberg KP-G: Biatrial atrial myxomas with multiple arterial aneurysms: a syndrome mimicking polyarteritis nodosa. *Am J Med* 62:792-794, 1977
79. Buchanan RRC, Cairns JA, Kraag G, et al: Left atrial myxoma mimicking vasculitis: echocardiographic diagnosis. *Can Med Assoc J* 120:1540-1542, 1979
80. Thomas MH: Myxoma masquerading as polyarteritis nodosa. *J Rheumatol* 8:133-137, 1981
81. Jourdan M, Bataille R, Seguin J, et al: Constitutive production of interleukin-6 and immunologic features in cardiac myxomas. *Arthritis Rheum* 33:398-402, 1990
82. O'Neil MB Jr, Grehl TM, Hurley EJ: Cardiac myxomas: a clinical diagnostic challenge. *Am J Surg* 138:68-74, 1979
83. Silverman J, Olwin JS, Graettinger JS: Cardiac myxomas with systemic embolization: review of the literature and report of a case. *Circulation* 26:99-103, 1962
84. Koikkalainen K, Kostiainen S, Luosto R: Left atrial myxoma revealed by femoral embolectomy: a case report and review of the literature. *Scand J Thorac Cardiovasc Surg* 11:33-35, 1977

85. Thompson JR, Simmons CR: Arterial embolus: manifestation of unsuspected myxoma. *JAMA* 228:864-865, 1974

86. Khan MAR, Mujahed MA: Atrial myxoma producing a saddle embolus in a child. *Thorax* 25:634-636, 1970

87. Bradham RR, Gregorie HB Jr, Howell JS Jr, et al: Aortic obstruction from embolizing cardiac myxoma. *J SC Med Assoc* 75:7-10, 1979

88. Tornvall G, Olin C: Massive embolization of cardiac myxoma: a case report. *Acta Med Scand* 206:123-126, 1979

89. Schweiger MJ, Hafer JG Jr, Brown R, et al: Spontaneous cure of infected left atrial myxoma following embolization. *Am Heart J* 99:630-634, 1980

90. Yeoh NTL, Clegg JF: Massive embolism from cardiac myxoma. *Angiology* 32:819-821, 1981

91. Corrigan E, Newhall D, Raymond RD: Left atrial myxoma—presenting as bacterial endocarditis. *RI Med J* 61:410-412, 1978

92. Rajpal RS, Leibsohn JA, Liekweg WG, et al: Infected left atrial myxoma with bacteremia simulating infective endocarditis. *Arch Intern Med* 139:1176-1178, 1979

93. Tanabe J, Williams RL, Diethrich EB: Left atrial myxoma: association with acute coronary embolization in an 11-year-old boy. *Pediatrics* 63:778-781, 1979

94. Balk AHM, Wagenaar SS, Bruschke AVG: Bilateral cardiac myxomas and peripheral myxomas in a patient with recent myocardial infarction. *Am J Cardiol* 44:767-770, 1979

95. Sybers HD, Boake WC: Coronary and retinal embolism from left atrial myxoma. *Arch Pathol* 91:179-182, 1971

96. Frenay JJJE, Bonte J, Franken P, et al: Left atrial myxoma with left retinal emboli, right hemiparesis and myocardial infarction: neurologic and echocardiographic diagnosis; surgical treatment. *Acta Neurol Belg* 81:215-222, 1981

97. Sandok BA, von Estorff I, Giuliani ER: CNS embolism due to atrial myxoma: clinical features and diagnosis. *Arch Neurol* 37:485-488, 1980

98. Rankin LI, DeSousa AL: Metastatic atrial myxoma presenting as intracranial mass. *Chest* 74:451-452, 1978

99. Hirose G, Kosoegawa H, Takado M, et al: Spinal cord ischemia and left atrial myxoma. *Arch Neurol* 36:439, 1979

100. Joynt RJ, Zimmerman G, Khalifeh R: Cerebral emboli from cardiac tumors. *Arch Neurol* 12:84-91, 1965

101. Cogan DG, Wray SH: Vascular occlusions in the eye from cardiac myxomas. *Am J Ophthalmol* 80:396-403, 1975

102. Tipton BK, Robertson JT, Robertson JH: Embolism to the central nervous system from cardiac myxoma: report of two cases. *J Neurosurg* 47:937-940, 1977

103. Burton C, Johnston J: Multiple cerebral aneurysms and cardiac myxoma. *N Engl J Med* 282:35-36, 1970

104. Yufe R, Karpati G, Carpenter S: Cardiac myxoma: a diagnostic challenge for the neurologist. *Neurology (Minneap)* 26:1060-1065, 1976

105. Barber F, Rosen P, Okin T: Atrial myxoma presenting as stroke. *Ann Emerg Med* 11:316-318, 1982

106. Sandok BA, von Estorff I, Giuliani ER: Subsequent neurological events in patients with atrial myxoma. *Ann Neurol* 8:305-307, 1980

107. Roeltgen DP, Weimer GR, Patterson LF: Delayed neurologic complications of left atrial myxoma. *Neurology (NY)* 31:8-13, 1981

108. Hutton JT: Atrial myxoma as a cause of progressive dementia. *Arch Neurol* 38:533, 1981

109. Maroon JC, Campbell RL: Atrial myxoma: a treatable cause of stroke. *J Neurol Neurosurg Psychiatry* 32:129-133, 1969

110. Yarnell PR, Spann JF Jr, Dougherty J, et al: Episodic central nervous system ischemia of undetermined cause: relation to occult left atrial myxoma. *Stroke* 2:35-40, 1971

111. Price DL, Harris JL, New PFJ, et al: Cardiac myxoma: a clinicopathologic and angiographic study. *Arch Neurol* 23:558-567, 1970

112. Stoane L, Allen JH Jr, Collins HA: Radiologic observations in cerebral embolization from left heart myxomas. *Radiology* 87:262-266, 1966

113. Bass NM, Sharratt GP: Left atrial myxoma diagnosed by echocardiography, with observations on tumour movement. *Br Heart J* 35:1332-1335, 1973

114. Martinez-Lopez JI: Sounds of the heart in diastole. *Am J Cardiol* 34:594-601, 1974

115. Abrams HL, Adams DF, Grant HA: The radiology of tumors of the heart. *Radiol Clin North Am* 9:299-326, August 1971

116. Davis GD, Kincaid OW, Hallerman FJ: Roentgen aspects of cardiac tumors. *Semin Roentgenol* 4:384-394, 1969

117. Steiner RE: Radiologic aspects of cardiac tumors. *Am J Cardiol* 21:344-356, 1968

118. Schattenberg TT: Echocardiographic diagnosis of left atrial myxoma. *Mayo Clin Proc* 43:620-627, 1968

119. Giuliani ER, Lemire F, Schattenberg TT: Unusual echocardiographic findings in a patient with left atrial myxoma. *Mayo Clin Proc* 53:469-473, 1978

120. Donahoo JS, Weiss JL, Gardner TJ, et al: Current management of atrial myxoma with emphasis on a new diagnostic technique. *Ann Surg* 189:763-767, 1979

121. DePace NL, Soulen RL, Kotler MN, et al: Two dimensional echocardiographic detection of intraatrial masses. *Am J Cardiol* 48:954-960, 1981

122. Bulkley BH, Weiss JL: Atrial myxomas: triumph of machine over man (editorial). *Chest* 75:537-539, 1979

123. Lappe DL, Bulkley BH, Weiss JL: Two-dimensional echocardiographic diagnosis of left atrial myxoma. *Chest* 74:55-58, 1978

124. Echt DS, Green SE, Popp RL: Advancing the diagnosis of left atrial myxoma (editorial). *Chest* 82:522-524, 1982

125. Dunnigan A, Oldham HN, Serwer GA, et al: Left atrial myxoma: is cardiac catheterization essential? *Am J Dis Child* 135:420-421, 1981

126. Come PC, Riley MF, Markis JE, et al: Limitations of echocardiographic techniques in evaluation of left atrial masses. *Am J Cardiol* 48:947-953, 1981

127. Obeid AI, Marvasti M, Parker F, et al: Comparison of transthoracic and transesophageal echocardiography in diagnosis of left atrial myxoma. *Am J Cardiol* 63:1006-1008, 1989

128. Reeder GS, Khandheria BK, Seward JB, et al: Transesophageal echocardiography and cardiac masses. *Mayo Clin Proc* 66:1101-1109, 1991

129. Lestuzzi C, Nicolosi GL, Mimo R, et al: Usefulness of transesophageal echocardiography in evaluation of paracardiac neoplastic masses. *Am J Cardiol* 70:247-251, 1992

130. Lund JT, Ehman RL, Julsrud PR, et al: Cardiac masses: assessment by MR imaging. *AJR* 152:469-473, 1989

131. Pitt A, Pitt B, Schaefer J, et al: Myxoma of the left atrium: hemodynamic and phonocardiographic consequences of sudden tumor movement. *Circulation* 36:408-416, 1967

132. Sung RJ, Ghahramani AR, Mallon SM, et al: Hemodynamic features of prolapsing and nonprolapsing left atrial myxoma. *Circulation* 51:342-349, 1975

133. Bower PJ, Ritter DG, Callahan JA, et al: Unusual hemodynamic findings of diagnostic value in a case of left atrial myxoma. *Am J Cardiol* 23:592-596, 1969

134. Lortscher RH, Toews WH, Nora JJ, et al: Left atrial myxoma presenting as rheumatic fever. *Chest* 66:302-303, 1974

135. Meyer JS, Charney JZ, Rivera VM, et al: Cerebral embolization: prospective clinical analysis of 42 cases. *Stroke* 2:541-554, 1971

136. Vidne B, Atsmon A, Aygen M, et al: Right atrial myxoma: case report and review of the literature. *Isr J Med Sci* 7:1196-1200, 1971

137. Hansen JF, Lyngborg K, Andersen M, et al: Right atrial myxoma. *Acta Med Scand* 186:165-171, 1969

138. Sannerstedt R, Varnauskas E, Paulin S, et al: Right atrial myxoma: report of a case and review of the literature. *Am Heart J* 64:243-254, 1962

139. Talley RC, Baldwin BJ, Symbas PN, et al: Right atrial myxoma: unusual presentation with cyanosis and clubbing. *Am J Med* 48:256-260, 1970

140. Goldschlager A, Popper R, Goldschlager N, et al: Right atrial myxoma with right to left shunt and polycythemia presenting as congenital heart disease *Am J Cardiol* 30:82-86, 1972

141. Meyers SN, Shapiro JE, Barresi V, et al: Right atrial myxoma with right to left shunting and mitral valve prolapse. *Am J Med* 62:308-314, 1977

142. Heath D, Mackinnon J: Pulmonary hypertension due to myxoma of the right atrium: with special reference to the behavior of emboli of myxoma in the lung. *Am Heart J* 68:227-235, 1964

143. Muroff LR, Johnson PM: Right atrial myxoma presenting as nonresolving pulmonary emboli: case report. *J Nucl Med* 17:890-892, 1976

144. Tai AR, Gross H, Siegelman SS: Right atrial myxoma and pulmonary hypertension. *NY State J Med* 70:2996-3000, 1970

145. Willey RF, Matthews MB, Walbaum PR: An unusual case of large right atrial myxoma. *Br Heart J* 44:108-110, 1980

146. Barlow J, Fuller D, Denny M: A case of right atrial myxoma: with special reference to an unusual phonocardiographic finding. *Br Heart J* 24:120-125, 1962

147. Come PC, Kurland GS, Vine HS: Two dimensional echocardiography in differentiating right atrial and tricuspid valve mass lesions. *Am J Cardiol* 44:1207-1212, 1979

148. Stern MJ, Cohen MV, Fish B, et al: Clinical presentation and non-invasive diagnosis of right heart masses. *Br Heart J* 46:552-558, 1981

149. Roudaut R, Pouget B, Videau P, et al: Right atrial myxoma in an asymptomatic child: echocardiographic diagnosis. *Eur Heart J* 1:453-459, 1980

150. Roguin N, Amikam S, Riss E: Prolapsing right atrial myxoma: clinical and haemodynamic considerations. *Br Heart J* 39:577-580, 1977

151. Hada Y, Wolfe C, Murray GF, et al: Right ventricular myxoma: case report and review of phonocardiographic and auscultatory manifestations. *Am Heart J* 100:871-877, 1980

152. Bortolotti U, Mazzucco A, Valfré C, et al: Right ventricular myxoma: review of the literature and report of two patients. *Ann Thorac Surg* 33:277-284, 1982

153. De Paiva EC, Macieira-Coelho E, Amram SS, et al: Intracavitary left ventricular myxoma. *Am J Cardiol* 20:260-262, 1967

154. Meller J, Teichholz LE, Pichard AD, et al: Left ventricular myxoma: echocardiographic diagnosis and review of the literature. *Am J Med* 63:816-823, 1977

155. Chandraratna PAN, San Pedro S, Elkins RC, et al: Echocardiographic, angiocardiographic, and surgical correlations in right ventricular myxoma simulating valvar pulmonic stenosis. *Circulation* 55:619-622, 1977

156. Zager J, Smith JO, Goldstein S, et al: Tricuspid and pulmonary valve obstruction relieved by removal of a myxoma of the right ventricle. *Am J Cardiol* 32:101-104, 1973

157. Snyder SN, Smith DC, Lau FYK, et al: Diagnostic features of right ventricular myxoma. *Am Heart J* 91:240-248, 1976

158. Frishman W, Factor S, Jordan A, et al: Right atrial myxoma: unusual clinical presentation and atypical glandular histology. *Circulation* 59:1070-1075, 1979

159. Ports TA, Schiller NB, Strunk BL: Echocardiography of right ventricular tumors. *Circulation* 56:439-447, 1977

160. Pindyck F, Peirce EC II, Baron MG, et al: Embolization of left atrial myxoma after transseptal cardiac catheterization. *Am J Cardiol* 30:569-571, 1972

161. Symbas PN, Hatcher CR Jr, Gravanis MB: Myxoma of the heart: clinical and experimental observations. *Ann Surg* 183:470-474, 1976

162. Miller JI, Mankin HT, Broadbent JC, et al: Primary cardiac tumors: surgical considerations and results of operation. *Circulation* 45 Suppl 1:134-138, 1972

163. Rosman HS, Goodwin JF, Cleland WP, et al: Two decades of atrial tumour. *Eur Heart J* 3:100-106, 1982

164. Fenoglio JJ Jr, McAllister HA Jr, Ferrans VJ: Cardiac rhabdomyoma: a clinicopathologic and electron microscopic study. *Am J Cardiol* 38:241-251, 1976

165. Arciniegas E, Hakimi M, Farooki ZQ, et al: Primary cardiac tumors in children. *J Thorac Cardiovasc Surg* 79:582-591, 1980

166. Mair DD, Titus JL, Davis GD, et al: Cardiac rhabdomyoma simulating mitral atresia. *Chest* 71:102-105, 1977

167. Shrivastava S, Jacks JJ, White RS, et al: Diffuse rhabdomyomatosis of the heart. *Arch Pathol Lab Med* 101:78-80, 1977

168. Mahoney L, Schieken RM, Doty D: Cardiac rhabdomyoma simulating pulmonic stenosis. *Cathet Cardiovasc Diagn* 5:385-388, 1979

169. Milner S, Abramowitz JA, Levin SE: Rhabdomyoma of the heart in a newborn infant: diagnosis by echocardiography. *Br Heart J* 44:224-227, 1980

170. Houser S, Forbes N, Stewart S: Rhabdomyoma of the heart: a diagnostic and therapeutic challenge. *Ann Thorac Surg* 29:373-377, 1980

171. Williams DB, Danielson GK, McGoon DC, et al: Cardiac fibroma: long-term survival after excision. *J Thorac Cardiovasc Surg* 84:230-236, 1982

172. Yamaguchi M, Hosokawa Y, Ohashi H, et al: Cardiac fibroma: long-term fate after excision. *J Thorac Cardiovasc Surg* 103:140-145, 1992

173. Jamieson SW, Gaudiani VA, Reitz BA, et al: Operative treatment of an unresectable tumor of the left ventricle. *J Thorac Cardiovasc Surg* 81:797-799, 1981

174. Moulton AL, Jaretzki A, Bowman FO Jr, et al: Massive lipoma of the heart. *NY State J Med* 76:1820-1825, 1976

175. Tuna IC, Julsrud PR, Click RL, et al: Tissue characterization of an unusual right atrial mass by magnetic resonance imaging. *Mayo Clin Proc* 66:498-501, 1991

176. Prior JT: Lipomatous hypertrophy of cardiac interatrial septum: a lesion resembling hibernoma, lipoblastomatosis and infiltrating lipoma. *Arch Pathol* 78:11-15, 1964

177. Page DL: Lipomatous hypertrophy of the cardiac interatrial septum: its development and probable clinical significance. *Hum Pathol* 1:151-163, 1970

178. Hutter AM Jr, Page DL: Atrial arrhythmias and lipomatous hypertrophy of the cardiac interatrial septum. *Am Heart J* 82:16-21, 1971

179. Crocker DW: Lipomatous infiltrates of the heart. *Arch Pathol Lab Med* 102:69-72, 1978

180. Reyes CV, Jablokow VR: Lipomatous hypertrophy of the cardiac interatrial septum: a report of 38 cases and review of the literature. *Am J Clin Pathol* 72:785-788, 1979

181. Voigt J, Agdal N: Lipomatous infiltration of the heart: an uncommon cause of sudden, unexpected death in a young man. *Arch Pathol Lab Med* 106:497-498, 1982

182. Isner JM, Swan CS II, Mikus JP, et al: Lipomatous hypertrophy of the interatrial septum: in vivo diagnosis. *Circulation* 66:470-473, 1982

183. Fyke FE III, Tajik AJ, Edwards WD, et al: Diagnosis of lipomatous hypertrophy of the atrial septum by two-dimensional echocardiography. *J Am Coll Cardiol* 1:1352-1357, 1983

184. Kriegshauser JS, Julsrud PR, Lund JT: MR imaging of fat in and around the heart. *AJR* 155:271-274, 1990

185. Ehman RL, Julsrud PR: Magnetic resonance imaging of the heart: current status. *Mayo Clin Proc* 64:1134-1146, 1989

186. James TN, Galakhov I: De subitaneis mortibus. XXVI. Fatal electrical instability of the heart associated with benign congenital polycystic tumor of the atrioventricular node. *Circulation* 56:667-678, 1977

187. Lie JT, Lufschanowski R, Erickson EE: Heterotopic epithelial replacement (so-called "mesothelioma") of the atrioventricular node, congenital heart block, and sudden death. *Am J Forensic Med Pathol* 1:131-137, 1980

188. Amr SS, Abu al Ragheb SY: Sudden unexpected death due to papillary fibroma of the aortic valve: report of a case and review of the literature. *Am J Forensic Med Pathol* 12:143-148, 1991

189. Burke A, Johns JP, Virmani R: Hemangiomas of the heart: a clinicopathologic study of ten cases. *Am J Cardiovasc Pathol* 3:283-290, 1990

190. Burke AP, Cowan D, Virmani R: Primary sarcomas of the heart. *Cancer* 69:387-395, 1992

191. Silverman NA: Primary cardiac tumors. *Ann Surg* 191:127-138, 1980

192. Larrieu AJ, Jamieson WRE, Tyers GFO, et al: Primary cardiac tumors: experience with 25 cases. *J Thorac Cardiovasc Surg* 83:339-346, 1982

193. Mahar LJ, Lie JT, Groover RV, et al: Primary cardiac myxosarcoma in a child. *Mayo Clin Proc* 54:261-266, 1979

194. Strohl KP: Angiosarcoma of the heart: a case study. *Arch Intern Med* 136:928-929, 1976

195. Glancy DL, Morales JB, Roberts WC: Angiosarcoma of the heart. *Am J Cardiol* 21:413-419, 1968

196. Rossi NP, Koischos JM, Aschenbrener CA, et al: Primary angiosarcoma of the heart. *Cancer* 37:891-894, 1976

197. Herrmann MA, Shankerman RA, Edwards WD, et al: Primary cardiac angiosarcoma: a clinicopathologic study of six cases. *J Thorac Cardiovasc Surg* 103:655-664, 1992

198. Putnam JB Jr, Sweeney MS, Colon R, et al: Primary cardiac sarcomas. *Ann Thorac Surg* 51:906-910, 1991

199. Schwartz JE, Schwartz GP, Judson PL, et al: Complete resection of a primary cardiac rhabdomyosarcoma: case report, review of the literature, and management recommendations. *Cardiovasc Dis Bull Tex Heart Inst* 6:413-424, 1979

200. Baldelli P, De Angeli D, Dolara A, et al: Primary fibrosarcoma of the heart. *Chest* 62:234-236, 1972

201. Hanfling SM: Metastatic cancer to the heart: review of the literature and report of 127 cases. *Circulation* 22:474-483, 1960

202. Malaret GE, Aliaga P: Metastatic disease to the heart. *Cancer* 22:457-466, 1968

203. Smith LH: Secondary tumors of the heart. *Rev Surg* 33:223-231, 1976

204. Berge T, Sievers J: Myocardial metastases: a pathological and electrocardiographic study. *Br Heart J* 30:383-390, 1968

205. Birmingham CL, Peretz DI: Metastatic carcinoma presenting as obstruction to the right ventricular outflow tract: report of a case and review of the literature. *Am Heart J* 97:229-232, 1979

206. Cham WC, Freiman AH, Carstens PHB, et al: Radiation therapy of cardiac and pericardial metastases. *Radiology* 114:701-704, 1975

207. Piehler JM, Pluth JR, Schaff HV, et al: Surgical management of effusive pericardial disease: influence of extent of pericardial resection on clinical course. *J Thorac Cardiovasc Surg* 90:506-514, 1985

208. Ravikumar TS, Topulos GP, Anderson RW, et al: Surgical resection for isolated cardiac metastases. *Arch Surg* 118:117-120, 1983

209. Magovern GJ, Yusuf MF, Liebler GA, et al: The surgical μ-section and chemotherapy of metastatic osteogenic sarcoma of the right ventricle. *Ann Thorac Surg* 29:76-80, 1980

CHAPTER

57

Cardiac trauma

Fletcher A. Miller, Jr., M.D.

In our age of high-speed travel, deceleration accidents are common, and lesions due to nonpenetrating cardiac trauma are recognized with increasing frequency.[1] An escalating rate of violent crime has led to a parallel increase in penetrating cardiac injuries. Lesions due to cardiac trauma may be clinically silent or masked by damage to other organs but nevertheless may result in serious or fatal complications.[1-13] Accurate, early diagnosis of such lesions is crucial. To this end, clinicians must be well versed in the applications and limitations of traditional diagnostic tools in detecting cardiac trauma as well as in the efficient use of modern imaging techniques.

There were 10 million motor vehicle accidents in the United States during 1992; these led to disability in 1,400,000 instances and to 35,800 deaths (data obtained from the National Safety Council, Chicago, IL). One therefore can assume that, at a minimum, 1,435,800 persons experienced enough deceleration to have sustained cardiac injury. Cardiac contusion occurs clinically in 9% to 21% of patients subjected to significant blunt chest trauma.[1,12,13] Using a conservative proportion, 10%, we arrive at an estimate of *at least* 143,580 cases of nonpenetrating cardiac trauma in 1992. The importance of recognizing cardiac trauma is underscored by its lethal potential. It is the most common unsuspected fatal visceral injury in trauma patients.[1]

ETIOLOGY

Direct blows to the chest injure the heart by compressing it between the sternum and the thoracic spine. Compression may contuse the heart directly or may lead to ischemic necrosis via coronary injury. Because the heart is suspended within the chest by the great vessels, deceleration can cause it to swing, like a pendulum, resulting in contrecoup injury. Cardiac contusion has been clearly documented after crush injuries involving only the legs and abdomen. Therefore, sudden increase in intrathoracic pressure is a third mechanism of nonpenetrating cardiac injury.[14]

Most cases of nonpenetrating cardiac trauma result from motor vehicle accidents. Such injuries also may be caused by falls from rooftops or other elevations or by blows from nonpenetrating objects such as baseballs, golf balls, hockey pucks, helmets, and fists.[15] Leg and abdominal crush injuries typically follow accidents related to operation of heavy equipment or to cave-ins that result in burial of the lower torso and legs. Fetal cardiac contusion after blunt trauma to the abdomen of a pregnant woman has been reported.[16] In the hospital, external chest compression during cardiopulmonary resuscitation may lead to cardiac injury. When attending a victim of one of these accidents, the physician must always consider the potential for cardiac damage.

PATHOLOGY

Table 57-1 presents a classification of traumatic lesions of the heart and great vessels. Rupture of the aorta is included because it also is a common sequela to blunt chest injury. Each of the three layers of the heart can be affected by trauma. It therefore would be appropriate to use the term "cardiac contusion" as a general descriptor of traumatic injuries to the heart; "pericardial contusion," "myocardial contusion," and "endocardial contusion" can be used to specify the layer involved. Table 57-2 lists the incidence of various traumatic cardiac lesions in three autopsy series.[3,17,18]

Pericardium

Evidence of pericarditis has been found in almost all autopsies performed in cases of severe blunt chest trauma.[4] As an isolated lesion, this is usually of no consequence--unless accompanied by significant bleeding. Parietal pericardial lesions may vary from small punctate areas of hemorrhage to large lesions with associated hematoma. Microscopically, the small lesions usually are composed of hemorrhage into the fibrous stroma of the parietal pericardium; the inner lining of mesothelial cells remains intact. A hemopericardium may accumulate slowly if due to rupture of a pericardiophrenic vessel or very rapidly if due to rupture of a ventricle, atrium, or coronary artery. In subacute cases, the parietal and visceral pericardial surfaces are usually coated with organizing hemorrhage.[3]

Pericardial laceration is usually accompanied by myocardial contusion or laceration.[4] In contrast, myocardial laceration or rupture has been reported to occur frequently without pericardial injury.[3] The pericardial lac-

Table 57-1 Traumatic cardiac lesions

I. Pericardial
  A. Hemorrhagic pericarditis
  B. Pericardial laceration
    1. Asymptomatic
    2. Herniation with cardiac strangulation
  C. Tamponade
    1. Rupture of pericardial vessel
    2. Rupture of coronary artery
    3. Rupture of cardiac chamber
  D. Purulent pericarditis, due to associated rupture of esophagus
  E. Pneumopericardium
  F. Recurrent pericarditis
  G. Constrictive pericarditis
  H. Intrapericardial diaphragmatic hernia
II. Myocardial
  A. Contusion
    1. Subepicardial
    2. Subendocardial
    3. Transmural
  B. Ischemic infarction, secondary to traumatic occlusion of coronary artery
  C. Myocardial hematoma
  D. Myocardial laceration
  E. Myocardial rupture
    1. Ventricular
    2. Ventricular septum
    3. Atrial
    4. Atrial septum
    5. Papillary muscles
  F. Aneurysm
  G. Pseudoaneurysm
  H. Diffuse calcification ("myocarditis ossificans")
III. Endocardial
  A. Thrombus
    1. Asymptomatic
    2. Systemic or pulmonary emboli
IV. Valvular
  A. AV valves
    1. Chordal rupture
    2. Papillary muscle rupture
    3. Torn leaflet
  B. Semilunar valves
    1. Avulsion of cusp
    2. Avulsion of commissure
    3. Torn cusp
    4. Intimal tear in adjacent aorta with cusp displacement
    5. Sinus of Valsalva aneurysm with cusp displacement
V. Coronary artery
  A. Intimal tear/thrombosis
  B. Laceration
  C. Arteriovenous fistula
  D. Arteriocameral fistula
VI. Aorta and pulmonary artery
  A. Rupture
    1. Pseudoaneurysm (with varying amounts of circumference involved)
    2. Exsanguination
  B. Aneurysm

eration itself is of no consequence unless accompanied by significant hemorrhage or by herniation of the heart through the pericardial defect. The former may lead to exsanguination (usually into the left pleural cavity). The latter varies from remaining asymptomatic to causing cardiac strangulation, which may be fatal.[3]

If the pericardial portion of the central tendon of the diaphragm is ruptured, abdominal contents may herniate into the pericardial space. The English literature contains fewer than 70 cases of intrapericardial diaphragmatic hernia in adults. The force of the trauma is transmitted through the abdominal viscera to the diaphragm. Rupture of the pericardial portion of the central tendon may be isolated, or it may be associated with tears of either hemidiaphragm or with massive disruption of the entire diaphragm. Once the central tendon ruptures, negative intrathoracic pressure is transmitted to the peritoneum.

Table 57-2 Autopsy series: nonpenetrating cardiac trauma

Finding	Parmley et al.[3] (546 cases)*	Bright and Beck[17] (168 cases)	Beasley[18] (44 cases)
Rupture	273 [80]	159	36
Right ventricle	56 [10]	31	4
Left ventricle	46 [13]	37	7
Right atrium	35 [6]	36	8
Left atrium	24 [2]	30	6
Ventricular septum	25 [5]	11	3
Atrial septum	18 [7]	1	8
Multichamber	69 [37]	13	
Myocardial contusion/laceration	105 [24]	11	33†
Pericardial laceration	18 [18]		11
Hemopericardium	13 [12]	76	21
Valve laceration/rupture	23 [4]	‡	4
Aortic	2 [2]		
Pulmonary	4		
Tricuspid	8		
Mitral	8 [1]		
Mitral and tricuspid	1 [1]		
Papillary muscle laceration/rupture	24		1
Coronary artery laceration/rupture	7 [3]		1

*[ ], additional cases with associated aortic rupture.
†Contusion; in 27 cases, myocardial laceration also occurred.
‡Valve ruptures were excluded because in 1935 "rupture of a valve seems to offer no possibility for operative repair."[17]

The gradient from the abdomen to the pericardial space increases with respiration. Therefore, with time, more and more of the abdominal viscera may be drawn into the pericardial space. Omentum is present in all cases, transverse colon and stomach are each present in about one-half of the cases, jejunum in about one-third, and the left lobe of the liver in about one-fifth. Symptoms result from strangulation of the abdominal viscera or from cardiac tamponade.[19-23]

Purulent pericarditis may result if chest trauma leads to rupture of the esophagus.[3] Pneumopericardium results from a traumatic communication between the pericardial cavity and the airway or the esophagus.[24]

Once traumatized, the pericardium may become inflamed recurrently, analogous to the Dressler and postcardiotomy syndromes. In such cases, the fluid usually is clear, there is associated fibrinous exudate on the epicardial surface, and focal infiltration of polymorphonuclear leukocytes and lymphocytes occurs. Rarely, this fluid accumulates to the point of tamponade.[2,3,25]

A dense, fibrous pericardial peel may develop as the consequence of traumatic hemopericardium. The resultant constrictive pericarditis usually does not appear until at least 1 year after the injury.[8,25,26]

Myocardium

Myocardial contusion occurs either as an isolated lesion or in conjunction with other complications, such as laceration and rupture. The area of contusion may be transmural or may be limited to the subepicardial or subendocardial region. The contused area may be recognized by patchy petechial lesions on the epicardial surface. These not infrequently are the outer surface of a pyramidal lesion that reaches deep into the myocardium. When the lesion involves the endocardial surface, there is a risk of mural thrombus formation and systemic or pulmonary embolism.[3]

In a radionuclide angiographic study of 77 victims of blunt chest trauma, Sutherland et al.[27] found that 42 (55%) of the patients had regional wall motion abnormalities. These most likely were due to myocardial contusion. Twenty-seven patients (64% of those with abnormalities) had right ventricular wall motion abnormalities, seven (17%) had left ventricular abnormalities, seven had biventricular abnormalities, and one patient had dyskinesis isolated to the ventricular septum. Similarly, in an echocardiographic study, Frazee et al.[28] found wall abnormalities in 22 of 58 patients studied (38%). The right ventricle was involved in 14 cases, the left ventricle in 7, and the ventricular septum in 2. It would appear, then, that the anteriorly located right ventricle is injured more often, the left ventricle being relatively protected by its posterior location.

Microscopically, the changes that occur after myocardial contusion are similar to those following ischemic infarction. With contusion, however, the transition from normal to abnormal tissue usually is more abrupt, and massive interstitial hemorrhage is more common. Also, cellular laceration and fragmentation are more likely with contusion. Polymorphonuclear cell infiltration begins within 24 hours after the injury and is followed by edema, necrosis, and loss of striations and nuclear integrity.[3,13,14,17,26]

The contused myocardium is nourished by a normal to increased blood supply. Extravasated blood in the area of the contusion produces deposits of hemosiderin, which are commonly seen during the first 3 months.[13,26] The injured area usually heals with a patchy scar interspersed with areas of normal myocardium. Transmural injury may lead to formation of a left or right ventricular aneurysm. Calcium may deposit in the area of contusion. Ossification of the traumatized myocardium is an unusual complication ("myocarditis ossificans").[29]

When chest trauma results in coronary artery occlusion, via an intimal tear or thrombus, ischemic infarction follows.[4] The pathologic features and possible complications are the same as those resulting when coronary occlusion complicates atherosclerosis.

Lacerations, typically with ragged edges, may involve the atria or ventricles and may be superficial or extend deep into the myocardium. Intramural hematoma is a potential complication.[3]

Cardiac rupture is a common lesion in autopsy series dealing with trauma (see Table 57-2). Bright and Beck[17] found that in 168 cases of nonpenetrating cardiac trauma, death was due to isolated free wall rupture in 134 instances. In the Parmley et al. series,[3] 546 deaths were due to cardiac injury. In 353 cases, death was due to rupture of the heart; multiple-chamber rupture occurred in 106 of these cases and aortic rupture in 80. Isolated rupture of the free wall occurred in 161 cases. The left and right ventricles ruptured with approximately equal frequency; the less common atrial ruptures involved the right atrium more often than the left. If the rupture is contained by pericardial adhesions, a pseudoaneurysm results. Otherwise, if the pericardium is intact, rupture of a cardiac chamber leads to rapid tamponade. If the pericardium has also been ruptured, the result is exsanguination, usually into the left pleural cavity.

Rupture of the atrial septum after blunt chest trauma is rare. There were 25 cases of atrial septal rupture in the Parmley et al. series,[3] 1 case in the series of Bright and Beck,[17] and 8 cases in a smaller series from our institution.[18] Such defects usually involve the area of the foramen ovale and frequently are associated with other traumatic lesions. Rupture of the atrioventricular (AV) septum can occur, leading to shunting from left ventricle to right atrium.

Ventricular septal defects are also relatively rare after blunt chest trauma. Thirty of the 546 trauma victims in the Parmley et al. series[3] and 11 of the 52 patients in the Bright and Beck series[17] had ventricular septal ruptures. Ruptures of the muscular septum are most common, followed in frequency by combined involvement of the muscular and membranous portions, with isolated membranous involvement being least common. There often are multiple defects. The conduction system may be involved simultaneously, producing intraventricular conduction delay or heart block. Traumatic ventricular septal defects are frequently associated with large areas of contused myocardium.

Rupture of the papillary muscles results in sudden, massive AV valvular regurgitation. Rupture occurs more commonly with the mitral than with the tricuspid valve.[26] Less severe regurgitation results if the muscles are only contused or partially lacerated.

Myocardial rupture localized to free wall, septum, or papillary muscle may occur immediately after a deceleration accident. Alternatively, rupture may be delayed[4,26,30,31] until necrosis has caused the myocardium to soften. This event typically occurs within 2 weeks after the initial injury but may occur even later. Berkery et al.[32] described a case in which delayed rupture of the ventricular septum was witnessed via two-dimensional echocardiography. A 26-year-old victim of a high-speed deceleration injury presented with physical findings of severe tricuspid regurgitation. The initial echocardiogram demonstrated the flail tricuspid valve leaflets and a ventricular septal hematoma. At 3 days, a small pericardial effusion had developed and the echocardiographic examination also demonstrated thinning and expansion of the septal segment previously occupied by hematoma. At 15 days, a loud murmur developed and the two-dimensional examination identified a large septal defect. This potential for delayed myocardial rupture must be borne in mind by physicians who care for victims of deceleration accidents.

Valvular injuries

Valvular insufficiency due to nonpenetrating trauma is rare. There was a 9% incidence of valvular injury in the Parmley et al. series[3] (23 cases of valve laceration or rupture and 24 cases of papillary muscle rupture). AV valve trauma was more common than aortic valve trauma. Valve rupture may occur immediately with trauma or may be delayed for several days to 2 weeks after the initial injury while necrosis is causing the damaged valve tissue to soften. In some cases, rupture occurs immediately, but the resultant murmur does not appear for several days because the cardiac output is initially reduced by tamponade, hemorrhage, or myocardial contusion. In some instances of aortic valve injury, the murmur is transient. In such cases, the initial regurgitation is thought to be due to valvular and perivalvular edema. Valvular insufficiency resolves as the edema subsides.[4] This same mechanism was identified for transient post-traumatic AV valvular regurgitation by Dodd et al.[33] Thirty-six hours after a 9-year-old was struck by a car, Doppler echocardiography revealed severe mitral and tricuspid regurgitation. Although no flail mitral or tricuspid valve segment was identified, prominence of the posteromedial papillary muscle suggested contusion and edema. The patient's condition stabilized with medical therapy, and at 1 week only mild residual mitral regurgitation was noted by Doppler echocardiography.

AV valvular insufficiency may be caused not only by papillary muscle rupture but also by traumatic rupture of chordae tendineae, direct rupture of the valve leaflets, or contusion (without rupture) of the papillary muscles. Aortic valve injury presumably arises from a sudden increase in intrathoracic (and hence intra-aortic) pressure during diastole.[34] This usually follows a direct blow to the chest. However, it has also been reported with crush injuries and with severe muscular straining (including one instance after labor and delivery). Involvement of the right coronary cusp is slightly more common than involvement of the left or noncoronary cusp.[35] Valvular insufficiency may result from perforation of a cusp, fenestration at the free margin, avulsion of the cusp at its base, avulsion of a commissural attachment, or an intimal tear in the aorta adjacent to the valve.[35-38] In the last situation, the cusp closest to the aortic intimal tear is usually displaced downward by thrombus in the aortic wall or by formation of a sinus of Valsalva aneurysm. Traumatic rupture of the aorta, particularly rupture of the posterior or right sinus of Valsalva, results in shunting from aorta to right atrium or right ventricle.[39-41]

Coronary artery trauma

Of the 546 cases in the Parmley et al. series,[3] 10 involved rupture of a coronary artery. This leads to hemopericardium, and tamponade usually develops rapidly. Ischemia or infarction may occur distal to the site of coronary artery rupture or laceration.

Although rare, occlusion of major coronary arteries has been reported after nonpenetrating cardiac trauma.[4,13,42-47] Traumatic intimal tears can lead to occlusion of the vessel. Alternatively, occlusion can result from compression of the lumen by hemorrhage and thrombus within the coronary artery wall. Transmural anterior infarction has been reported to occur after traumatic occlusion of the left anterior descending artery; transmural inferior infarcts have been reported after traumatic occlusion of either the circumflex or the right coronary artery. Once traumatic-ischemic infarction has occurred, the possible outcomes are identical to those for patients whose coronary occlusion is the result of atherosclerotic coronary disease. The patient may even be left with residual angina pectoris.

Blunt chest trauma can result in coronary artery fistulae.[4,46-48] An arteriovenous fistula results when a communication develops between a coronary artery and the coronary sinus or great cardiac vein; an arteriocameral fistula results from arterial communication with the right atrium or with the ventricles. In 7 of 10 reported cases, shunting was from the right coronary artery to the right atrium; 1 each of the other 3 cases involved a right coronary arteriovenous connection, a connection from the left anterior descending coronary artery to the right ventricle, and a fistula from the left anterior descending coronary artery to the left ventricle. Large shunts can lead to high-output left ventricular failure. Angina occurs when the fistula creates a coronary steal syndrome.

DIAGNOSIS: GENERAL ASPECTS

Overview

Cardiac trauma must be suspected whenever a patient has sustained significant blunt or penetrating chest or upper abdominal trauma or crush injuries of the legs or abdomen. The clinician's most valuable tool, in such instances, is a high degree of awareness. Patients who are conscious and oriented must be questioned carefully about chest pain and dyspnea. Physical examination should be directed to detection of signs of tamponade, valvular injury, or intracardiac shunting. A chest radiograph should be studied with particular attention to signs of pericardial or pleural effusion, pulmonary venous hypertension, and injury to the thoracic aorta. Serial electrocardiograms should be obtained in all cases, and the appearance of new abnormalities should be considered a clue to potential cardiac trauma. Although serial creatine kinase (CK) (and perhaps lactate dehydrogenase) isoenzyme concentrations are neither completely sensitive nor specific for myocardial contusion, they should be determined until the values begin to decrease from their peaks.

In some instances, these diagnostic modalities will raise a question of pericardial effusion, myocardial contusion, valvular injury, or intracardiac shunting. In such cases, surface echocardiography should be performed, including spectral Doppler and color-flow imaging. Usually, this examination accurately delineates these lesions. If no window is available for surface echocardiography, transesophageal echocardiography can be used to detect the full range of potential traumatic cardiac lesions. One of the various types of radioisotope scans is a reasonable alternative if the only clinical concern is the amount of myocardial injury.

If shunting or valvular injury is diagnosed, the severity of the lesions can usually be accurately assessed by a combination of spectral Doppler and color-flow imaging. If the windows for surface echocardiography do not permit adequate quantitation, transesophageal echocardiography should be performed. In such cases, catheterization and ventriculography are necessary only if a transesophageal study is contraindicated (because of, for example, an unstable cervical lesion). Coronary angiography is necessary if a traumatic coronary lesion is suspected.

History

Ventricular tachycardia and fibrillation or exsanguination may occur soon after chest trauma, [4,7,9] and therefore death may occur before medical assistance becomes available. If the victim lives long enough to be thoroughly evaluated, cardiac trauma must be suspected whenever the mechanism of injury has been sufficient. By far the most common circumstance leading to the cardiac injury is an automobile accident in which the driver's chest strikes the steering wheel. The speed of the automobile need not be greater than 20 miles per hour.[13]

Patients who are conscious and oriented should be questioned about chest pain. Both patient and physician must have discrimination to separate cardiac pain from pain due to chest wall injury or rib or sternal fractures. Some patients, however, describe substernal discomfort that is identical in quality to that of myocardial infarction.[5,12,13] This symptom may be delayed in onset for up to 6 to 8 hours after the initial injury,[5] and it may be associated with diaphoresis and nausea and vomiting. Alternatively, the physician may be able to obtain a history compatible with pericarditis: pleuritic pain aggravated by twisting or coughing and eased by sitting forward. Dyspnea in chest trauma may be due to primary pulmonary damage, such as contusion or pneumothorax. However, the emergency room physician must always remember that such dyspnea might also be the result of serious traumatic cardiac lesions.

Clinicians must also be mindful of potential traumatic cardiac complications at times remote from the initial injury. Constrictive pericarditis and recurrent pericarditis typically develop months to years after the initial injury. In addition, traumatic valvular or myocardial lesions may not be apparent on the initial examination and may be asymptomatic for various times afterward. Therefore, including questions about chest trauma is important whenever one is obtaining a cardiac history.

Physical examination

Chest bruises or lacerations and rib, clavicular, or sternal fractures are evidence that significant forces were applied to the chest during an accident. However, *serious cardiac injuries often occur without any external evidence of chest injury*.[2,4,13] Cardiac trauma is frequently found in patients whose injuries are remote from the chest—such as pelvic or long-bone fractures, cranial injuries, or rupture or laceration of abdominal viscera.

An unexplained rapid pulse rate may be the most obvious direct clue to cardiac damage. Similarly, unexplained hypotension may point to serious cardiac difficulty. In patients with trauma, one should always try to elicit pulsus paradoxus as a sign of cardiac tamponade. An increased jugular venous pressure has the same significance. Patients who present after rupture of a cardiac chamber almost invariably have severe hypotension and often have cyanosis of the upper torso, face, neck, and arms due to the marked increase in venous pressure.

Chest palpation should be performed quickly. A dyskinetic segment may be palpable if an entire thickness of myocardium has been contused. Systolic, diastolic, or continuous thrills may accompany ruptures of the valves, ventricular septum, or a sinus of Valsalva. With large pericardial fluid accumulations, the apex is impalpable.

On auscultation, a triphasic friction rub indicates pericardial trauma. This must be differentiated from the continuous murmurs that result from coronary arteriovenous fistula or from a ruptured sinus of Valsalva. Narrowing of the thoracic aorta by hematoma may result in an intrascapular systolic murmur.[4] With tamponade, the heart sounds are muffled.

Chest trauma can lead to aortic, mitral, or tricuspid regurgitation and to atrial or ventricular septal defects. These will be accompanied by specific physical signs, as detailed below. If constrictive pericarditis develops, it is often accompanied by typical signs, including a rapid y descent and a Kussmaul pattern to the jugular venous pulse and a pericardial knock on auscultation.

Chest radiograph

The chest radiograph is useful for demonstrating associated chest injuries, such as rib and sternal fractures and

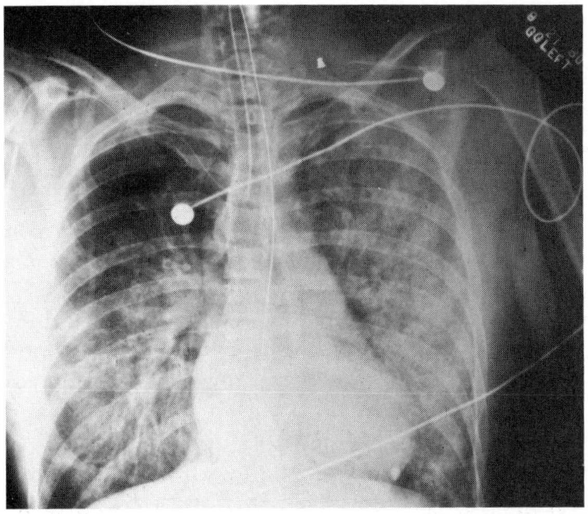

Fig 57-1 Chest radiograph from 22-year-old woman who sustained a steering-wheel injury during a single-car accident. Note the pulmonary infiltrates, most prominent on the left, due to pulmonary contusion. This patient required intubation; suctioning brought up copious amounts of bright-red blood. Echocardiography demonstrated thinning of the inferoapical left ventricular myocardium and an attached thrombus.

pulmonary contusion (Fig 57-1). It generally is of little help for the cardiac trauma itself. However, it may aid in detecting pericardial effusion, sometimes suggested by a separation between the parietal pericardial shadow and a lucent line of epicardial fat.[49] Large fluid accumulations may result if hemorrhage into the pericardium is slow. This event leads to the classic "water bottle" cardiac silhouette. In such cases, serial chest radiographs demonstrate progressive cardiomegaly as fluid accumulates (Fig 57-2). Other clues to significant pericardial effusion are enlargement of the azygous and superior vena caval shadows. Air within the pericardial space (pneumopericardium) indicates communication with the bronchial tree or esophagus.[50] A large pleural fluid accumulation (especially on the left) must always raise the question of thoracic aortic rupture, or of a myocardial or coronary artery laceration or rupture, accompanied by a torn pericardium.

Electrocardiogram

Before use of isoenzyme determinations and noninvasive cardiac imaging techniques, the diagnosis of cardiac contusion was made when a patient who had sustained significant chest trauma presented with new electrocardiographic (ECG) abnormalities. The ECG still serves as a useful, inexpensive screening tool.

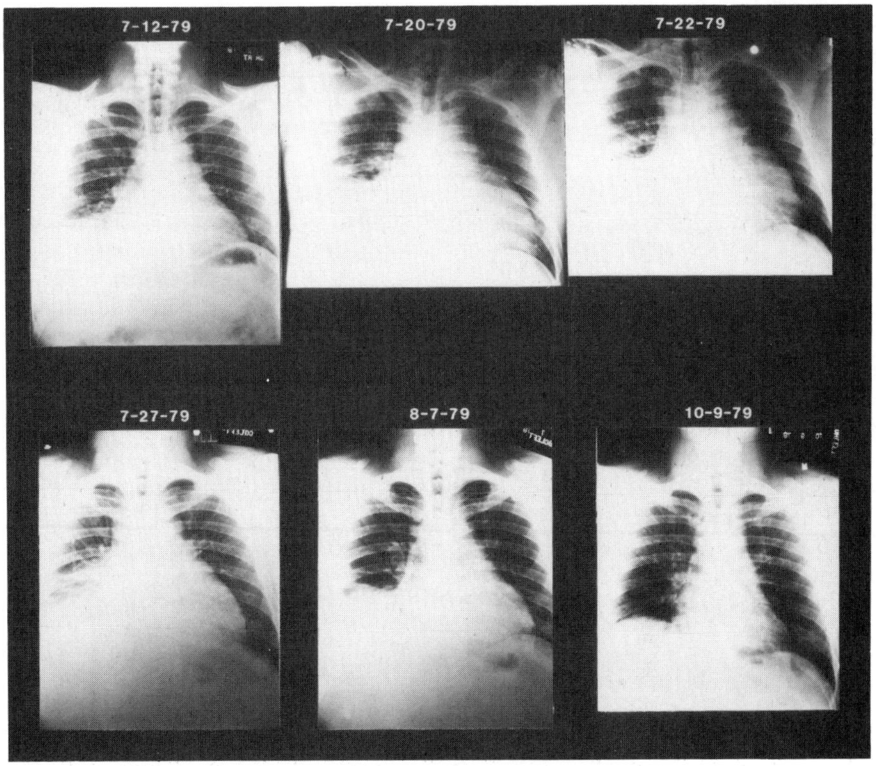

Fig 57-2 Serial chest radiographs from 27-year-old man whose chest struck the steering wheel during a single-car accident. The admission radiograph (7-12-79) demonstrated mild cardiomegaly and a left pleural effusion. A pericardial friction rub was heard on day 2. The heart size increased for several days and stabilized by 7-22-79. Thereafter, the heart size gradually decreased and was normal by 10-9-79. The time course of radiographic changes suggests pericardial effusion. This was confirmed by echocardiography. His ECGs are shown in Figure 57-4.

Abnormalities on the standard ECG occur in up to 50% of cases of significant chest trauma.[51] The most common change is T-wave flattening or inversion in one or more leads. The next most frequent change is slight ST-segment depression. Current of injury (localized ST-segment elevation) is a relatively rare ECG change after blunt chest trauma.[52-57] These changes are nonspecific. In some cases they reflect myocardial injury (subepicardial, subendocardial, or transmural); however, many other causes for ECG abnormalities are often present, including hypoxia, acidosis, pulmonary contusion, and central nervous system injury.

The development of pathologic Q waves is a more specific indicator of myocardial damage. This change is identical to that seen with ischemic transmural myocardial infarction (as discussed in chapter 3A) but may occur even when myocardial necrosis develops without changes in the coronary arteries. Although new Q waves should alert the clinician to probable myocardial contusion, their absence does not exclude significant cardiac injury. Cases have been reported in which the ECG remained entirely normal despite definite cardiac damage.[58]

The anterior location of the right ventricle makes it particularly vulnerable during chest trauma. Therefore, isolated contusion of the right ventricle is relatively common. The right ventricle may be silent electrocardiographically, because its depolarization frequently is overshadowed by that of the thicker ventricular septum and left ventricular free wall.[59] However, T-wave changes in the anterior precordial leads may be due to right ventricular injury. This situation is illustrated in Figures 57-3 and 57-4. The sensitivity for detecting right ventricular injury can be increased by use of right precordial chest leads.[60]

The average time course of ECG changes due to myocardial contusion is different from that due to ischemic infarction. ECG changes may occur within hours after chest trauma. However, these changes are frequently delayed for 48 hours and may not appear for up to 5 days after chest injury.[5] Although changes have been noted to persist for years after myocardial contusion, they usually resolve during the first month.[54,56-58]

Diffuse ST elevation after chest injury should immediately suggest traumatic pericarditis (see Fig 57-4). The ST segments are typically "concave-up," and this pattern is often accompanied by sinus tachycardia. PR-segment depression is an even more specific indicator of pericardial injury. If these changes are accompanied by gener-

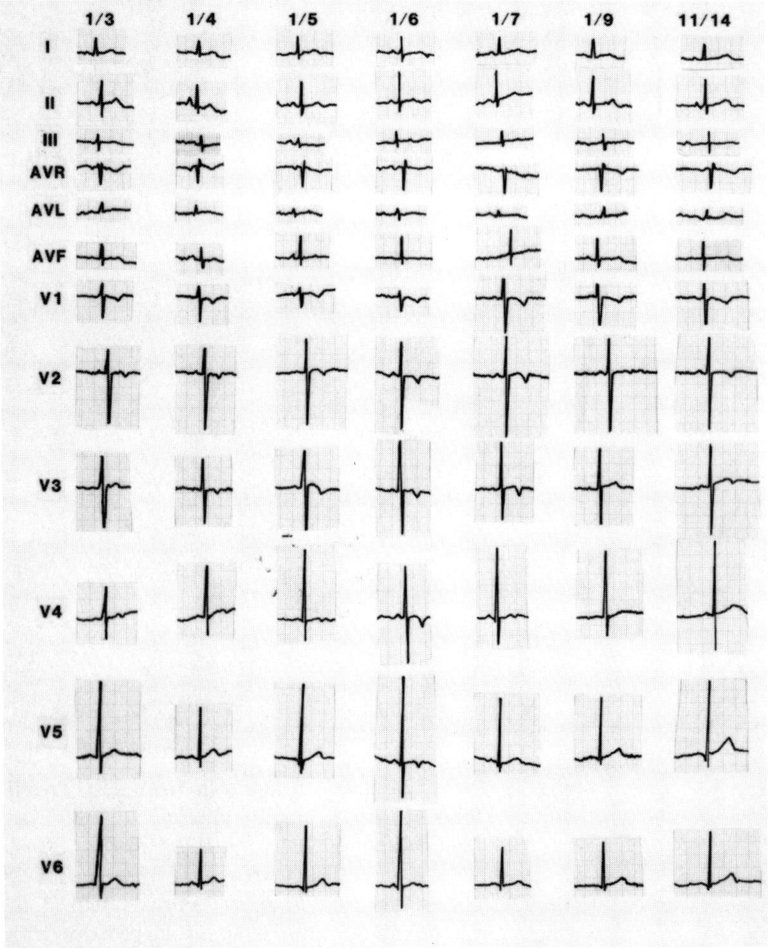

Fig 57-3 Serial ECGs from a 20-year-old man who sustained rib fractures and chest lacerations during a single-car accident. On 1/3 tracing, T waves are inverted in leads V_1 and V_2. T-wave inversion progressed such that by 1/6 it extended from V_1 to V_5. By 11/14 T-wave changes had largely resolved. Two-dimensional echocardiography showed that this patient had a right ventricular contusion with associated mural thrombus.

alized low voltage or electrical alternans, it is likely that the heart is freely swinging within a large collection of pericardial fluid.

Abnormalities of conduction. All types of conduction disturbances have been found after significant chest trauma, including first-, second-, and third-degree heart block, left anterior hemiblock, left bundle-branch block, and right bundle-branch block alone or with left anterior hemiblock or left posterior hemiblock. These abnormalities are usually transient. Patients rarely require a temporary pacemaker.[1,3,12,52-54,61,62]

Abnormalities of rate and impulse formation. Sinus tachycardia is almost always present in cardiac trauma. It may be due to the cardiac injury itself or to hypoxia, shock, pain, or emotional upset. Sinus bradycardia is rare after cardiac trauma, but at least one case of "sick sinus behavior" induced by chest injury has been reported.[63] In this patient, periods of sinus arrest preceded death; at autopsy, a large area of hemorrhage and necrosis was found within the sinoatrial node. Also, in a series of 27 patients with blunt chest trauma, Markiewicz et al.[64] described one patient who died suddenly on the sixth day with asystole.

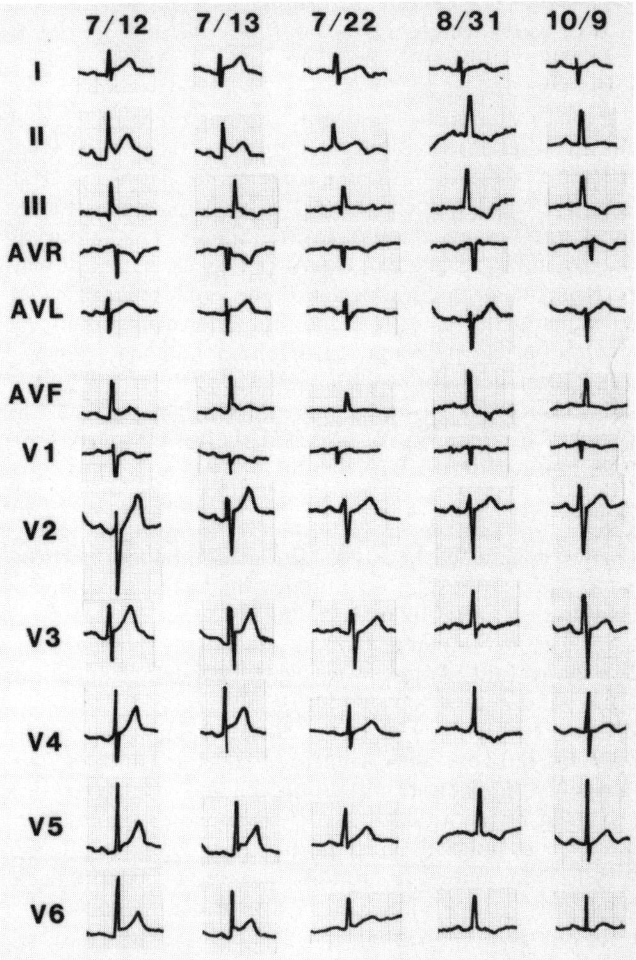

Fig 57-4 Serial ECGs from 27-year-old man whose chest radiographs are shown in Figure 57-2. The 7/12 tracing shows ST-segment elevation involving the inferior, anterior, and apical leads as well as lead I. This distribution supports the diagnosis of traumatic pericarditis (which was confirmed by echocardiography). The 7/12 and 7/13 tracings also show PR-segment depression in lead II. The ST elevations gave way to diffuse T-wave inversions (8/31). By 10/9 the ECG had largely returned to normal.

Atrial premature complexes often accompany cardiac trauma.[1,4,6,12,13,52,54,56,61,63,65] Instances of paroxysmal supraventricular tachycardia (with and without block) have been reported. Atrial fibrillation and flutter appear to be the most common arrhythmias associated with cardiac trauma, probably because of the high incidence of pericardial involvement.

Ventricular arrhythmias also are often seen after significant chest trauma.[1,4,6,12,13,52,54,56,61,63,65] Ventricular fibrillation occurs frequently after experimental cardiac trauma, and the frequency is increased if the experimental animal is given alcohol intravenously (enough to create mild intoxication) before the blow. This circumstance also leads to a high incidence of electromechanical dissociation.[62] Thus, cardiac trauma may lead to sudden death, particularly if the victim was intoxicated. In some such cases, autopsy reveals little or no pathologic evidence of cardiac damage despite the malignant arrhythmia.

Ventricular arrhythmias also occur in patients who initially survive and are hospitalized. In a study by Potkin et al.[66] of 100 patients, Holter monitoring was initiated within 12 hours after chest injury and was continued for 24 to 48 hours; 54% of patients had premature ventricular complexes, and 27% were in Lown class III or greater, including 3 patients with ventricular tachycardia. Hiatt et al.[67] described one instance of delayed-onset ventricular tachycardia in a series of 79 patients after blunt chest trauma, and Frazee et al.,[28] in a series of 58 patients with blunt chest trauma, noted that ventricular fibrillation occurred on day 3 in one patient. Ventricular tachycardia resulting from dyskinetic ventricular wall motion years after chest trauma has also been reported.[61]

Cardiac enzymes

In unselected series of patients with blunt chest trauma, CK-MB has been found, in trace or greater amounts, in 13% to 85% of patients.[24,30,31,39] This large range most likely is due to differences in sampling frequency among the series rather than to differences in isoenzyme determination. For accurate detection of CK-MB in patients after blunt chest trauma, measurement must be done immediately on presentation and must be repeated frequently during the first 24 hours. The MB fraction is much more labile than the MM fraction. After blunt chest trauma, the CK-MB fraction peaks in 6 to 24 hours;[68] persistence beyond 24 hours is most common in patients with shock or severe hypoxemia. Among 140 patients with blunt chest trauma, Fabian et al.[69] found that 119 had at least trace elevation of CK-MB. Of these, 53% had increases only on admission or at 6 hours, or both. By 24 hours, CK-MB had become undetectable in 74% of these patients. Given the differences in pathophysiology, it is certainly not surprising that CK-MB usually peaks earlier after blunt chest trauma than after ischemic myocardial infarction.

An increase in the CK-MB fraction is by no means a perfect screen for cardiac damage in patients with trauma. False-negative results certainly occur. In our initial series of seven patients in whom the diagnosis was made by echocardiography, two had normal CK-MB values (and normal ECGs).[70] This experience is shared by Reif et al.[71] A cardiac complication requiring treatment developed in 9 of 115 patients admitted with blunt chest trauma. Three of the nine had normal ECGs on admission, and CK-MB became elevated in only one. Furthermore, Potkin et al.[66] found the CK-MB value to be normal in four of five trauma cases in which microscopic proof of cardiac damage was determined at autopsy.

False-positive increases also occur, particularly if there has been an associated crush injury. However, significant elevation of CK-MB after blunt trauma most often indicates cardiac injury. Michelson[72] found that trauma victims with an increased CK-MB value had a much higher incidence of localized ECG changes than did those without this increase. In a small group of chest trauma patients studied by Reynolds and Jones,[68] cardiac complications were found only in the group that had both ECG abnormalities and increased CK-MB values. In a Mayo Clinic series of chest trauma victims,[73] 7 of 15 patients with increased CK-MB values had two-dimensional echocardiographic changes due to cardiac contusion. Fabian et al.[69] found that CK-MB elevation correlated with significant arrhythmias after chest injury in 92 patients. In a retrospective study of 342 patients with blunt trauma, Healey et al.[74] also found a strong correlation between CK-MB elevation and development of cardiac complications. In fact, cardiac complications developed in *all* their patients with severe CK-MB elevation (greater than 200 U/L).

Therefore, although CK-MB determination as an isolated test is not sufficient to make a diagnosis of cardiac contusion, it is a useful adjunct to the clinical examination and the ECG. Curiously, no studies are yet available to determine whether the addition of measurement of lactate dehydrogenase isoenzymes increases the sensitivity or specificity of enzyme analysis in the diagnosis of cardiac trauma.

Echocardiography

Echocardiography is ideal for detecting significant cardiac trauma.[70] High-resolution echocardiographic instruments can easily be transported to the patient's bedside—either in the emergency room or in the intensive care unit. Furthermore, diagnostic information is available as soon as the echocardiographic transducer is placed on the patient's chest or abdomen. This potential for immediate feedback is unique among the various cardiac imaging modalities and is obviously highly desirable in this clinical setting, since therapeutic decisions need to be made quickly if they are to be lifesaving. Patients with chest and abdominal trauma present a difficult challenge to the echocardiographer, because imaging windows may be limited by chest tubes, abdominal incisions and rigidity, or rib and sternal injuries. However, we have examined a large number of trauma victims and have been able to obtain diagnostic images in the vast majority of cases, particularly since we routinely supplement the transthoracic examination with subcostal imaging of the heart. Shah (see Symbas[75]) had a similar favorable experience applying echocardiography to the diagnosis of cardiac trauma. Furthermore, when surface echocardiographic images are inadequate, transesophageal echocardiography can provide diagnostic imaging in nearly 100% of cases. As with surface echocardiography, the transesophageal study can be performed quickly and at the patient's bedside, with clinically relevant information available as soon as the probe enters the esophagus. Contraindications to transesophageal echocardiography include injuries to the cervical spine and traumatic disruption of the esophagus.

Even in the most technically challenging cases, cardiac motion should be evident during the surface echocardiographic examination. If images are *completely absent* from apical, subcostal, and parasternal transducer positions, a chest radiograph should be obtained. This situation usually indicates pneumothorax, extensive subcutaneous emphysema, or pneumopericardium, because air prevents the transmission of ultrasound. Pneumomediastinum and pneumopericardium may also inhibit imaging from the transesophageal approach.

Two-dimensional echocardiography has become the standard for detection of pericardial effusion, so that this technique is particularly useful for patients who have sustained chest trauma (Fig 57-5). When there is clinical uncertainty, pulsed-wave Doppler echocardiography can be used to quickly check for cardiac tamponade. Furthermore, echocardiographic guidance makes pericardiocentesis easier and safer.[76] As illustrated in Figure 57-5, pleural effusions can also be rapidly detected by echocardiography (and thoracentesis can be performed under ultrasound guidance).

Echocardiography provides direct visualization of the right and left ventricles. Myocardial thinning and segmental wall motion abnormalities due to myocardial contusion can be easily identified.[71,72,77-79] As previously mentioned, if surface echocardiographic images are inadequate for specific regional wall motion analysis, transesophageal echocardiography almost always provides diagnostic information.[80,81] With echocardiography, it is easy to differentiate right from left ventricular injury or right ventricular contusion from cardiac tamponade. Figure 57-6 illustrates surface echocardiographic diagnosis of a large left ventricular contusion after a motor vehicle accident. Structural complications such as aneurysm, pseudoaneurysm, and mural thrombi can also be directly visualized by echocardiography.

Ruptures of the atrial and ventricular septa and traumatic abnormalities of the semilunar and AV valves can be directly visualized by two-dimensional echocardiography.[72,82-84] Figure 57-7 shows the echocardiographic appearance of a traumatically ruptured tri-

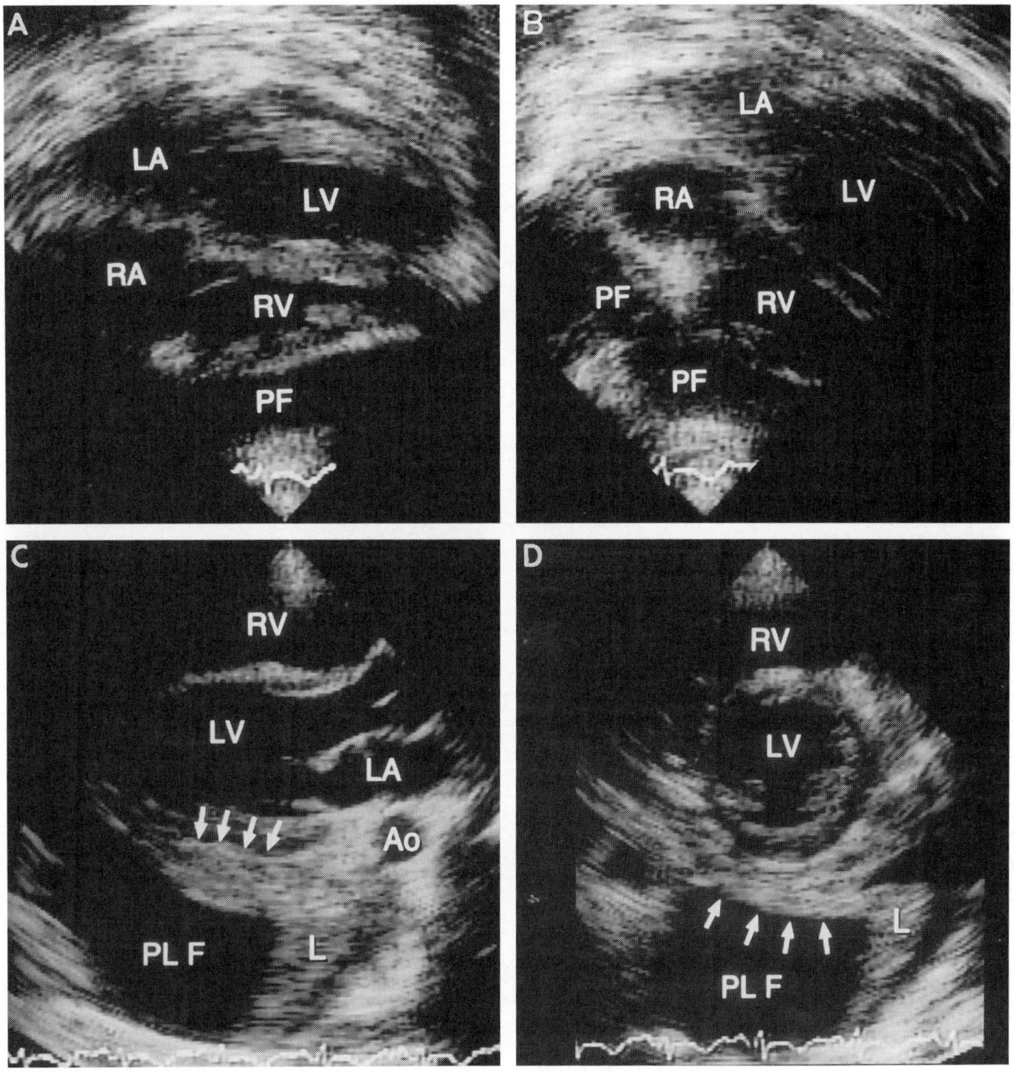

Fig 57-5 Two-dimensional echocardiogram from 22-year-old woman who suffered nonpenetrating cardiac trauma during a motor vehicle accident. **A,** subcostal four-chamber view (anatomic orientation) demonstrating pericardial fluid (*PF*) around the right ventricle (*RV*). This fluid was found to be hemorrhagic during echocardiographically guided pericardiocentesis. **B,** subcostal view with angulation to demonstrate that the fluid also surrounds the right atrium (*RA*). **C,** parasternal long-axis view of the right ventricle, left ventricle (*LV*), left atrium (*LA*), and descending thoracic aorta (*Ao*) demonstrates a large left pleural fluid collection (*PLF*) with atelectatic lung (*L*). *Arrows* point to thickened pericardium (which, at this point, most likely represents coagulum). **D,** parasternal short-axis view also demonstrates the thickened pericardium (*arrows*) and adjacent atelectatic lung within the large left pleural effusion.

cuspid valve. Spectral Doppler analysis and color-flow imaging are used to confirm severe tricuspid regurgitation resulting from the rupture. The combination of two-dimensional imaging, color-flow imaging, and spectral Doppler analysis can be used to quantitate the volume of traumatic shunts or regurgitant lesions.

Transesophageal echocardiography can be used not only as an adjunct for cardiac diagnosis but also as a means to diagnose or exclude traumatic lesions of the thoracic aorta, including transection and intramural hematoma.[80,85] Figure 57-8 shows a false aneurysm of the descending thoracic aorta resulting from a motor vehicle accident. This was diagnosed by transesophageal echocardiography with color-flow imaging, prompting immediate surgical repair. Transesophageal echocardiography also allows definition of traumatic lesions of the aortic sinuses. In addition, this technique has been used to accurately diagnose coronary artery fistula.[86]

The role of echocardiography in potential cardiac trauma has not been fully defined. It is certainly not indicated in every case, as discussed below. However, it would seem reasonable to apply this versatile diagnostic modality in all trauma cases in which aortic or valvular injury, intracardiac shunting, severe myocardial contusion, or pericardial effusion is suspected.

Radionuclide techniques

Technetium pyrophosphate has been used to image myocardial contusions in both clinical and experimental situations.[66,87-91] In the clinical setting, technetium pyrophosphate scans have been positive ("hot spot") 12 to 24 hours after cardiac trauma in some instances; in these cases, the scans usually revert to normal by 5 days.[87,89] Long-term persistence of activity may indicate aneurysm formation.[92,93] Abnormal cardiac uptake usually can be differentiated from abnormal uptake due to chest wall injury through the use of left anterior oblique and lateral views.[94] At institutions using technetium scanning in chest trauma victims, the scan has been most useful in patients with nonspecific ECG changes. However, there have been cases of clear-cut cardiac damage in which scanning results have been negative. Therefore, one cannot rule out myocardial contusion on the basis of a negative technetium pyrophosphate scan.[66,89]

Single photon emission computed tomography (SPECT) thallium scanning is useful for the diagnosis of ischemic myocardial infarction. Thallium is taken up wherever perfusion is intact, and there is no uptake ("cold spot") in areas to which blood flow has ceased. The major pathophysiologic difference between myocardial contusion and ischemic myocardial infarction is that with the former, perfusion to the damaged area is usually intact. Nevertheless, thallium imaging has been applied successfully in some cases of myocardial contusion.[94] Experience with this technique in potential cardiac trauma is small, and data on its prognostic accuracy are conflicting. In 40 patients sustaining blunt chest trauma, McCarthy et al.[95] found that the sensitivity of SPECT-thallium for prediction of cardiac complications was significantly less than

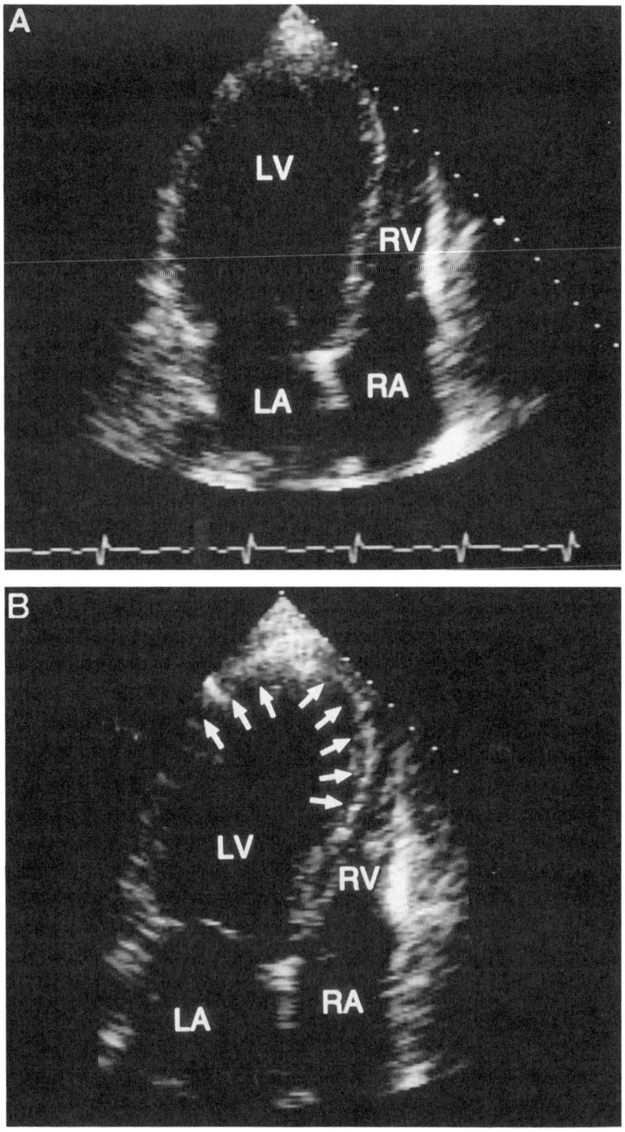

Fig 57-6 Two-dimensional echocardiogram from a 45-year-old woman who suffered a deceleration injury during a motor vehicle accident. **A**, apical four-chamber view, diastolic frame. The right ventricle (*RV*), right atrium (*RA*), and left atrium (*LA*) are normal. The left ventricle (*LV*) is moderately enlarged. **B**, this systolic frame demonstrates normal contraction of the basal left ventricle with akinesis of the apical-septal and lateral apical segments (*arrows*). Her left ventricular ejection fraction was 35%. The diagnosis of myocardial contusion was made after coronary angiography, which demonstrated normal coronary arteries. Follow-up echocardiography 2 months later demonstrated a left ventricular ejection fraction of 60% with only mild residual hypokinesis of the anterior left ventricle.

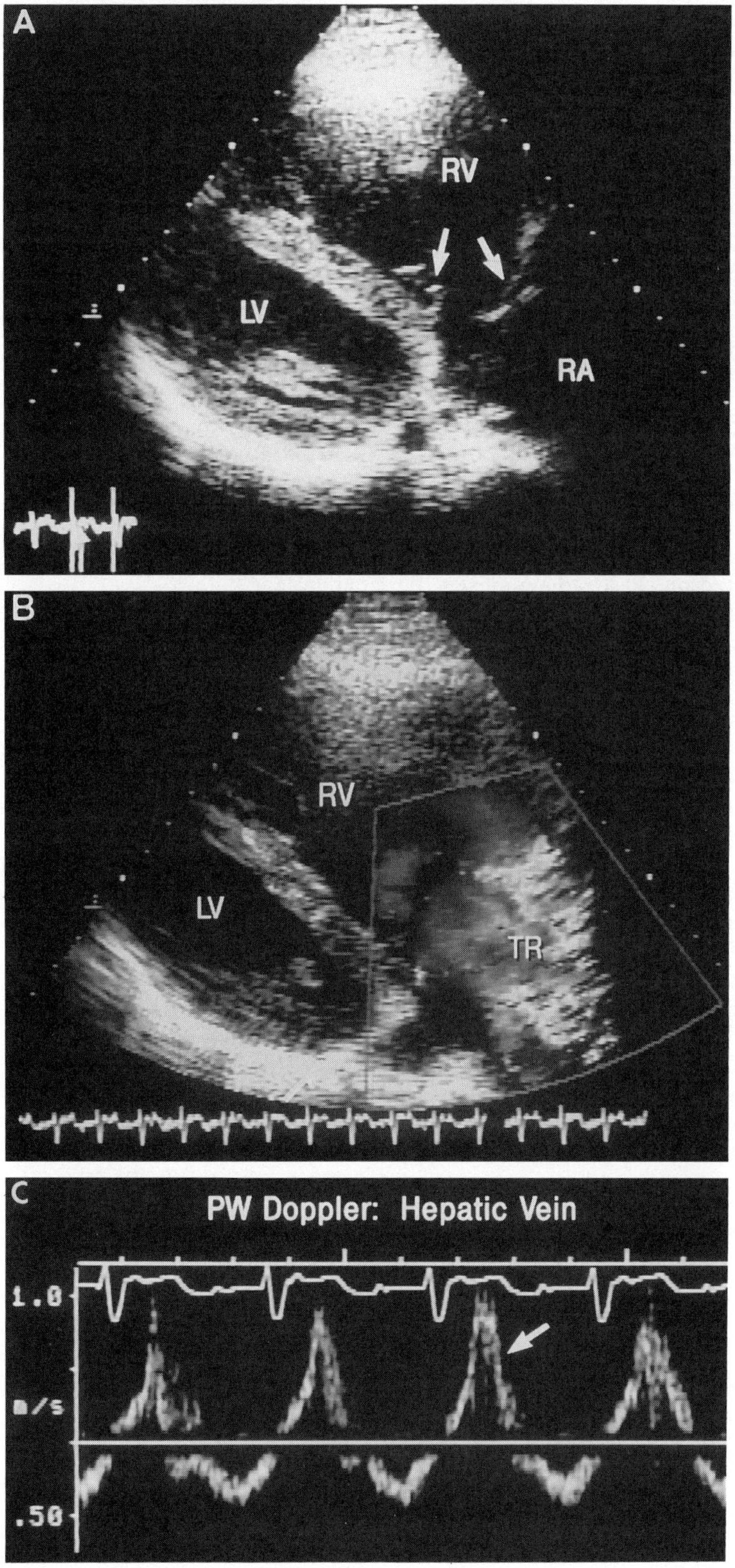

Fig 57-7 **A,** surface echocardiographic study, parasternal right ventricular inflow view. In this systolic frame, the anterior tricuspid valve leaflet (*right arrow*) is flail and has moved beyond the tricuspid annulus into the enlarged right atrium (*RA*). The septal tricuspid leaflet (*left arrow*) is properly supported. The right ventricle (*RV*) is markedly enlarged. The left ventricular chamber (*LV*) is normal. **B**, color-flow imaging (color not shown) reveals severe tricuspid regurgitation (*TR*). Color signals fill the enlarged right atrium in systole. There is color aliasing but no turbulence. This is characteristic of laminar flow, which is seen only when there is a huge regurgitant orifice. **C,** the severity of tricuspid regurgitation is underscored by pulsed-wave (*PW*) Doppler imaging from an enlarged hepatic vein. Systolic flow in the hepatic vein is completely reversed and hence recorded above the baseline (*arrow*). There is normal diastolic forward flow (below the baseline).

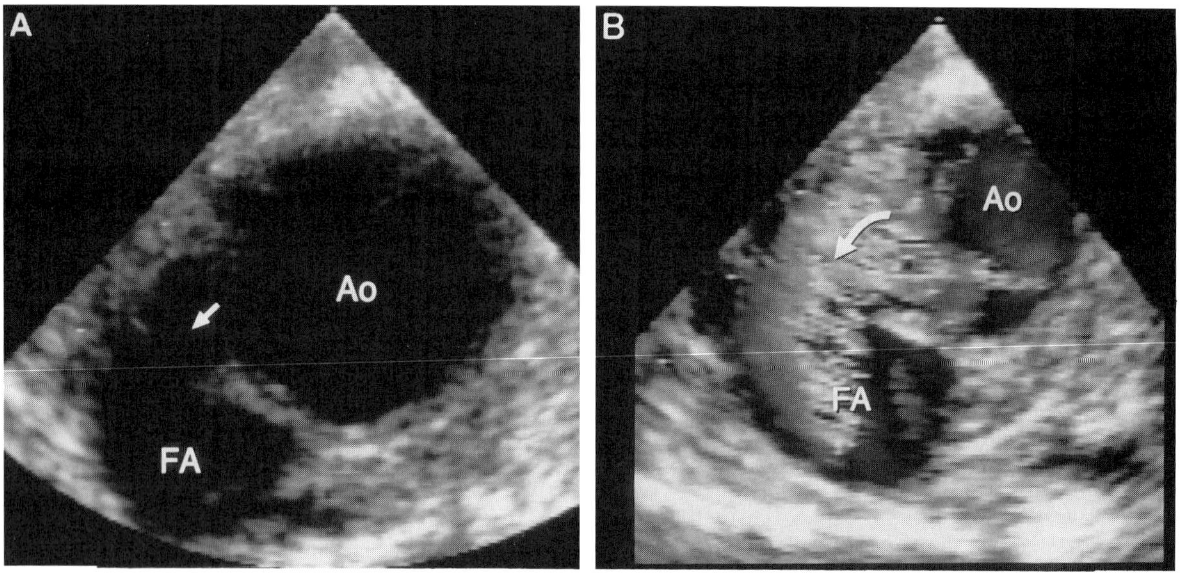

Fig 57-8 Transesophageal echocardiographic images from a study of the descending thoracic aorta in a 58-year-old man who complained of chest and hip pain after a motor vehicle accident. The transesophageal echocardiographic study was prompted by widening of the mediastinum noted on chest radiographs. **A**, horizontal-plane image demonstrating rupture of aortic wall (*arrow*) with formation of false aneurysm (*FA*). **B**, color-flow imaging (color not shown) confirms communication of descending thoracic aorta (*Ao*) and false aneurysm. The patient was taken immediately to surgery, and the aorta was found to be almost completely transected at the isthmus.

the predictive accuracy of the admission ECG. However, Holness and Waxman,[96] in 125 patients, and Godbe et al.,[97] in 175 patients, found that SPECT-thallium defects after blunt chest trauma predicted significant rhythm disturbances. Because of the small number of available studies, and particularly because patients must be transported to the nuclear laboratory for SPECT-thallium imaging, this modality has not become clearly established for the diagnosis of cardiac contusion. The place of newer scanning agents is even less well established. One clinical study of cardiac contusion demonstrated a positive correlation between scanning abnormalities on indium-111 antimyosin scintigraphy and regional wall motion abnormalities by echocardiography.[98] No studies are yet available on the applicability of sestamibi scanning for myocardial contusion.

Radionuclide angiography has also been applied to the diagnosis of myocardial contusion. This modality provides blood pool imaging and allows delineation of wall motion abnormalities, differentiation of right from left ventricular contusions, and determination of ejection fraction for both the right and the left ventricles.[27,99-101] Traumatic aneurysms have also been identified.[94] Therefore, radionuclide angiography is a reasonable diagnostic alternative when severe myocardial contusion is suspected and echocardiography is not readily available.

Catheterization and angiography

With the current diagnostic power of noninvasive imaging techniques, the role of invasive hemodynamics and contrast angiography for cardiac trauma has become far less important. Angiography occasionally is necessary to differentiate ruptured sinus of Valsalva aneurysms from coronary arteriovenous or arteriocameral fistulae, although transesophageal echocardiography is rapidly supplanting invasive angiography in this situation. The major current diagnostic indication for angiography with cardiac trauma is delineation of coronary artery anatomy in patients with transmural myocardial damage. In such cases, coronary angiography differentiates severe cardiac contusion from traumatic coronary artery occlusion with ischemic ventricular infarction[102,103] (see Fig 57-6). Of course, for hemodynamically unstable cases, Swan-Ganz catheterization is invaluable for continuous guidance of vasodilator, inotropic, and pressor therapy.

DIAGNOSIS: SPECIFIC TRAUMATIC CARDIAC LESIONS

Cardiac rupture

Patients who survive traumatic cardiac rupture to reach the emergency room with vital signs invariably are in shock, are restless, and have air hunger.[26] If the pericardium is intact, signs of tamponade may be present. Jugular venous pressure elevation, the most useful sign, is so severe in this situation that many patients have cyanosis of the upper torso, neck, and face.[104] The venous waveform may not be apparent with the patient supine. If it is detectable, a predominantly negative waveform (i.e., rapid x descent) typically is present. When the structure of the neck prohibits accurate inspection of the venous pattern, the severe increase in venous pressure is evident once a central venous pressure line is inserted. Pulsus paradoxus can be elicited in patients with an audible blood pressure. This pattern may also be apparent after a peripheral artery has been cannulated for monitoring purposes. It is very important to realize, however, that in many of these patients, hypotension is the only clinical clue to tamponade.[105-107]

Rapid bleeding into the pericardial space can result in tamponade with the accumulation of only 100 to 200 mL of fluid, because the rapidity of the collection does not allow the pericardium to stretch gradually and increase its compliance.[108] Therefore, one should not be surprised to see severe hemodynamic compromise without the massive fluid accumulation that precedes tamponade in more common situations (such as with malignant effusions). Electrical alternans is *not* present on the ECG, and heart size usually is *normal* on the chest radiograph.[105,106,109]

When myocardial rupture is associated with pericardial rupture, the patient has signs of pleural effusion and exsanguination.[26,104,110,111] The pleural effusion often is evident on physical examination and usually is obvious on a chest radiographic or ultrasound examination. The hemothorax is usually on the left. However, rupture of the right atrium at the junction with the superior or inferior vena cava (accompanied by pericardial rupture) results in bleeding into the right pleural space.[112]

In addition to demonstrating pleural effusion, the main utility of the chest radiograph in this situation is in initial assessment of the thoracic aorta. The pericardium covers a portion of the ascending aorta; hence, rupture of the proximal ascending aorta can lead to tamponade. In addition, three survivors of *combined* cardiac and aortic rupture have been reported.[113] If there are any abnormal mediastinal signs on the chest radiograph and if the patient's condition permits, emergency aortography[114] or computed tomography[115] of the chest can be used to document or exclude aortic rupture before surgical exploration.

If two-dimensional echocardiography is available on an emergency basis, we believe that the patient should remain in the emergency room for ultrasound scanning rather than be moved for aortography or computed tomography. By this means, pericardial or pleural effusion can be quickly confirmed while surgical personnel carry out initial resuscitative measures.[105,106] Alternatively, if the clinical situation demands immediate thoracotomy, transesophageal echocardiography can be performed without interrupting the surgical procedure. Since in most such instances the patients are not placed on cardiopulmonary bypass, intraoperative transesophageal echocardiography can be used to thoroughly inspect for traumatic defects of the heart and thoracic aorta.

Pericardial effusion

Bleeding from a traumatized coronary artery or pericardiophrenic vessel or from a contused, hemorrhagic area of epicardium is usually less vigorous than bleeding from cardiac rupture. If the rate of hemorrhage is sufficiently slow, the pericardium gradually stretches, and large amounts of blood can accumulate without severe hemodynamic compromise. The clinician may elicit a history of pericardial pain or detect a triphasic friction rub on auscultation. Serial chest radiographs show progressive cardiomegaly (see Fig 57-2). ECG changes of pericarditis may appear. Echocardiography demonstrates a large echo-free space, usually surrounding the left ventricle, apex, right ventricle, and right atrium. As the fluid collection grows, the heart begins to swing freely within it. At this point, electrical alternans appears on the ECG. Doppler echocardiographic demonstration of intracardiac pulsus paradoxus alerts the clinician to cardiac compression.

Recurrent pericarditis

Pericarditis may appear immediately after blunt chest trauma or, less commonly, at a time remote from the initial injury,[2,7] and it may recur for years thereafter. Just as with the postmyocardial infarction (Dressler) and postcardiotomy syndromes, the mechanism is assumed to be an autoimmune phenomenon.[48] The first episode often occurs a few weeks after trauma, but it may not occur until several months later.[12,48] Patients present with pericardial pain as well as systemic manifestations, including fever and sweats.[14] Physical examination primarily reveals an increased pulse rate and a pericardial friction rub. ECG manifestations of pericarditis often appear. The chest radiograph may demonstrate pneumonitis or pleural effusions, and the erythrocyte sedimentation rate is usually increased. In particularly severe episodes, an "anemia of chronic disease" can develop, in which serum iron levels are low and marrow stores are normal.

Intrapericardial diaphragmatic hernia

If the central pericardial portion of the diaphragm ruptures as a result of blunt trauma, abdominal viscera can herniate into the pericardial space. The stomach and transverse colon most commonly herniate.[116] The patient might have symptoms of chest or abdominal pain, nausea, and dyspnea. However, many patients have remained without symptoms for intervals of up to 10 years after the initial injury.[21,23] During the symptom-free interval, more and more abdominal viscera may be pulled into the pericardial space, eventually leading to distress. Epigastric pain was present in 55% of the 21 patients reported by Meng et al.[19] Intermittent vomiting, with or without distention, was present in 45%. Palpitations and dyspnea also were present in 45% of the cases. Thirty-six percent of the patients noted a "gurgling" sound in the chest, and 18% experienced weight loss. The symptoms often were aggravated by eating and relieved by belching or vomiting.

On physical examination, decreased breath sounds and bowel sounds in the chest are the most prominent findings. The point of maximum cardiac impulse is absent, and heart sounds are muffled. Distention occurs if the transverse colon becomes obstructed after herniation into the pericardial space. Signs of cardiac tamponade due to compression of the heart by abdominal viscera also may develop.

Gas bubbles within the cardiac silhouette on the chest radiograph are clues to intrapericardial diaphragmatic hernia. If a nasogastric tube is placed, its tip may be seen within the cardiac silhouette rather than in the abdomen. Once the diagnosis is suspected, a barium swallow study can be used to confirm the diagnosis by opacification of the intrapericardial organs. Echocardiography has also proven useful for this diagnosis.[117,118]

Constrictive pericarditis

Experimentally, superficial trauma to the myocardium is sufficient to result in constrictive pericarditis.[25] Clinically, this is a rare complication of cardiac trauma.[2,8,13,14] Although it may develop within weeks of the initial injury, it most frequently appears 6 months to 1 year later. The clinical diagnosis of cardiac constriction is described in chapter 55.

Myocardial contusion and ischemic myocardial infarction

Myocardial damage after blunt trauma may be due either to direct contusion of the myocardium or to traumatic coronary artery occlusion with ischemic infarction. The area of necrosis may be transmural or may be isolated to the subendocardial or subepicardial region.

It is likely that many instances of myocardial contusion go unnoticed amid an array of more obvious injuries. Small contusions probably heal completely or produce small areas of fibrosis that remain clinically silent. At the other end of the spectrum, transmural contusions are found by clinicians who seek the proper clues.

The conscious patient with myocardial contusion may give a history of pain identical in character and radiation to that experienced by patients with ischemic myocardial infarction[75] (chapter 29B). Possible manifestations of a large contusion are increased pulse rate, hypotension, and moist rales due to pulmonary edema. A dyskinetic segment may be apparent on inspection and palpation of the precordium. A fourth heart sound almost always is present, and a third heart sound is heard if there is sufficient left ventricular dysfunction.

Difficulty in establishing a diagnosis of myocardial contusion arises from lack of a single test that is perfectly sensitive and specific for the diagnosis. Currently, the combination of serial ECGs, serial CK-MB fraction determinations, and echocardiography appears to be the most efficient means of making an accurate diagnosis of myocardial contusion. Echocardiography allows real-time tomographic images of the ventricles. Areas of transmural contusion or ischemic infarction are detected as segmental areas of hypokinesis, akinesis, or dyskinesis. With time, the akinetic and dyskinetic regions may become thin and hyperrefractile, indicating scar formation.[70] As previously mentioned, radionuclide angiography can be used to detect regional ventricular wall motion abnormalities when echocardiography is not feasible. Perfusion techniques, such as SPECT with thallium and sestamibi, are also likely to be useful adjuncts to electrocardiography and cardiac enzyme determinations in diagnosing myocardial contusion.

Considerable controversy exists about the use of sophisticated imaging techniques for the diagnosis of cardiac contusion. The controversy centers not on the accuracy of these modalities for supporting a diagnosis of myocardial contusion but rather on the clinical importance of establishing this diagnosis. During the 1980s, there was considerable enthusiasm for use of echocardiography or nuclear cardiology imaging to screen for myocardial contusion, and monitoring in the intensive care unit was extended once such a diagnosis was established. From a series of studies of more than 3,100 patients, it has now become apparent that clinically important complications of myocardial contusions rarely occur in patients who are hemodynamically stable.[69,74,78,79,95,99,100,101,119-123] Important complications for patients sustaining blunt chest trauma can usually be predicted from serial ECGs (ST-segment shifts, new bundle-branch blocks or hemiblocks, or new Q waves), severe elevation of CK-MB fraction, and high Injury Severity Scale score. Furthermore, serious cardiac rhythm disturbances and congestive heart failure secondary to myocardial contusion almost always appear within 12 hours of chest injury. In reviewing 18 studies of the utility of CK-MB determination, electrocardiography, echocardiography, and radionuclide angiography for predicting clinically significant complications of myocardial contusion, Christensen and Sutton[124] noted that the results of CK-MB determinations and radionuclide angiography were nonspecific and that echocardiography was useful if decompensation occurred but not as a screening tool.

On the other hand, Reif et al.,[71] in a study of 115 patients, found that chest trauma patients with abnormal echocardiographic findings had a significantly higher level of cardiac complications requiring therapy. Although delayed clinically significant cardiac complications are rare after blunt chest trauma, a definite potential exists for severe rhythm disturbances or serious hemodynamic abnormalities with large myocardial contusions. These complications are more likely if the myocardium is infarcted secondary to coronary artery trauma. Although echocardiography as a primary screening tool for the diagnosis of myocardial contusion is not medically or economically sensible, it certainly is reasonable to use this bedside imaging technique as an adjunct in appropriate situations. A scheme for the diagnosis of clinically important myocardial contusion is illustrated in Figure 57-9.

Clinical investigation of imaging studies for patients with blunt chest trauma have lagged behind similar studies for patients with ischemic myocardial infarction. For patients with chest trauma, simple identification of wall motion abnormalities has been used to attempt to predict clinically significant cardiac complications. From the experience with myocardial infarction, it is obvious that not only wall motion abnormalities but also overall extent of ventricular dysfunction predicts major in-hospital cardiac events.[125-127] Rather than simply identifying whether patients with chest trauma have wall motion abnormalities, echocardiography should be used to determine the extent of ventricular contusion. This extent can

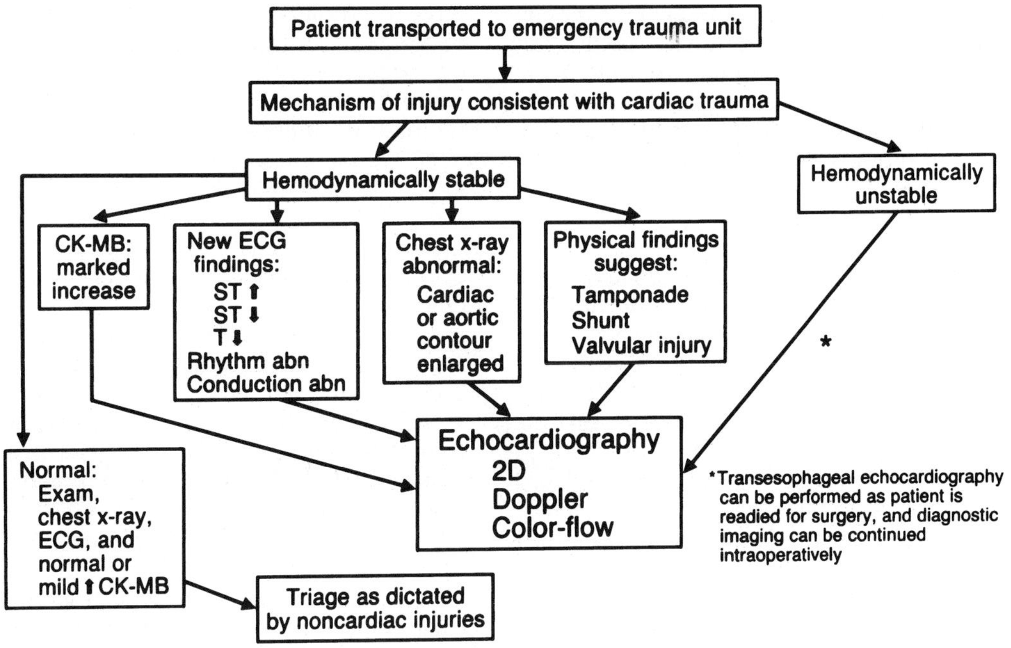

Fig 57-9 Flow diagram for use of echocardiography in patients with potential cardiac trauma.

be established by use of a wall motion score index standardized by the American Society of Echocardiography.[128]

If a large region of myocardial damage is detected, consideration should be given to coronary angiography, which allows differentiation of ischemic infarction due to coronary artery trauma from direct contusion of the myocardium. Alternatively, exercise echocardiography or exercise nuclear testing can be performed once the patient has recovered sufficiently. Exercise-induced ischemia would argue for a significant coronary artery lesion.

Aneurysms and pseudoaneurysms

Traumatic occlusion of the left anterior descending coronary artery may result in the formation of a left ventricular aneurysm.[129] Even without coronary occlusion, contusion of the myocardium can lead to an aneurysm of either the right or the left ventricle.[77,130] Whether or not coronary occlusion has occurred, true aneurysms can be complicated by mural thrombi with distal embolization, congestive heart failure, or life-threatening ventricular arrhythmias.[2]

Right ventricular aneurysms are difficult to detect clinically. Dyskinetic motion of the chest may be apparent at the left sternal border and may be accompanied by third or fourth heart sounds, which increase with inspiration. With left ventricular aneurysm, dyskinesis may be visible and palpable over the precordium, and apical third and fourth heart sounds usually are evident.

Left ventricular aneurysm is suggested by ST-segment elevation that persists for more than a few weeks after the initial chest trauma. Cardiomegaly is noted on the chest radiograph, and there may also be an unusual bulge or acute angulation of the left heart contour. Pseudoaneurysms have a similar appearance. In chronic cases, calcification of the aneurysm may be evident on either the posteroanterior or the lateral view.

Right and left ventricular aneurysms are clearly defined by two-dimensional echocardiography. This technique also allows detection of associated mural thrombus. True aneurysms typically have a wide neck; the width of the segment connecting uninvolved ventricle with the aneurysmal portion includes the entire short axis of the ventricle. False aneurysms are contained ruptures of the myocardium and therefore typically have a narrow-necked appearance by two-dimensional echocardiography. At times, the neck is not even apparent, and the false aneurysm appears as a cystic area adjacent to a contused or infarcted segment of myocardium. Color-flow imaging and pulsed-wave Doppler interrogation of the cystic area identify to-and-fro signals, thereby confirming communication with the ventricle.

Intracardiac shunts

The hemodynamics of traumatic ventricular septal defects depend on the size of the rupture as well as on the extent of associated left or right ventricular contusion. The patient often is acutely ill with dyspnea and shock. The ventricular septal defect is first apparent when a thrill is noted along the left sternal border, associated with a holosystolic murmur that radiates throughout the precordium and is loudest at the left sternal border. With large shunts, an apical mid-diastolic rumble signals the increased flow across the mitral valve. The auscultatory findings may not become apparent until low output due to hemorrhage or tamponade is corrected. Alternatively, these findings may not appear for several days after chest trauma because the rupture itself is delayed.[2,32]

Post-traumatic atrial septal defects per se do not lead to acute hemodynamic compromise. Characteristic signs that may be present on physical examination are fixed splitting of the second heart sound and a systolic ejection murmur in the pulmonary area. Large shunts lead to marked increase in flow across the tricuspid valve, resulting in a mid-diastolic rumble heard best at the left lower sternal border. A pattern of incomplete right bundle-branch block eventually may appear on the ECG.[48]

With traumatic atrial or ventricular septal defects, heart size usually is normal on the initial chest radiograph. Left-to-right shunting often results in pulmonary plethora. With large shunts, pulmonary artery enlargement eventually develops.

Ruptures of the atrial and ventricular septa can be directly visualized by two-dimensional echocardiography and color-flow imaging.[83,84,131-134] Defects of the AV septum also can be visualized. Transesophageal echocardiography is particularly useful for evaluating atrial septal defects. With rupture of either the ventricular or the atrial septum, the size of the defect can usually be directly measured by two-dimensional echocardiography, and the size of the shunt can be determined from the color-flow examination.

The left-to-right shunt can also be quantified by use of oximetry during passage of a flow-directed catheter at the bedside. Samples should be obtained from various sites within the right ventricle as well as in the vena cava, right atrium, and pulmonary artery. A sample must be obtained simultaneously from a systemic artery.

Traumatic sinus of Valsalva aneurysms may be asymptomatic. If the aneurysm ruptures, however, the patient usually experiences acute distress with symptoms of low cardiac output and either systemic or pulmonary venous hypertension. Aneurysms of the posterior sinus rupture into the right atrium; aneurysms of the right and left sinuses rupture into the right and left ventricles, respectively. Ruptures into the left ventricle are associated with physical findings similar to those of acute aortic regurgitation. Ruptures into the right side of the heart lead to jugular venous distention and are characterized by the appearance of a *continuous* murmur.

Sinus of Valsalva aneurysms can be identified by two-dimensional echocardiography. The ruptured portion of the sinus typically takes on the appearance of a "wind sock" protruding into the appropriate cardiac chamber. Color-flow imaging defines the shunt.

Mural thrombi

When myocardial contusion involves the endocardium, a mural thrombus may form. The incidence of mural thrombi in this situation is unknown. Thrombi may form in either ventricle. On two-dimensional echocardiography, large thrombi appear as rounded masses attached to abnormally contracting ventricular wall segments. Small or laminated thrombi are more difficult to detect, but newer high-frequency transducers usually allow differentiation of thrombus from adjacent myocardium.

Valvular lesions

Traumatic aortic valve injury. Aortic valve rupture is often accompanied by sudden pain in the chest or epigastrum.[14,75] This usually is severe and described as "tearing" in quality. It frequently radiates to the neck and arms and sometimes to the upper part of the back. In approximately half the cases, patients or relatives note an unusual sound in the chest. Faintness and syncope are frequently encountered soon after the rupture.[26,35,38] Because the left ventricle is unprepared to accept sudden regurgitation, traumatic aortic valve rupture is usually followed by acute pulmonary edema with restlessness, dyspnea, cough, and hemoptysis.[35]

In acute traumatic aortic regurgitation, the left ventricular diastolic pressure may increase to such an extent that it approaches the aortic pressure early in diastole. In such cases, an aortic diastolic murmur is brief or even nonexistent. If the patient survives, the aortic diastolic pressure eventually decreases as the left ventricle becomes more compliant. The typical peripheral signs of aortic regurgitation then appear (see chapter 2). The diastolic murmur also becomes more prominent. The torn, perforated, or avulsed aortic cusp vibrates with high frequency in diastole. Vibration gives rise to a characteristic pure-tone murmur that has been described in many ways, including "cooing dove," "angry bee," "seagull," and "croaking frog." A short, rough, early systolic murmur also usually is present as a result of high-volume flow across the injured valve.[26,35,37,38]

In acute injury, the ECG may show little more than a compensatory sinus tachycardia. In chronic cases, a pattern of left ventricular hypertrophy with strain develops. In the acute stage, the chest radiograph usually shows a normal heart size and may demonstrate lung-field patterns typical of pulmonary edema. Cardiomegaly due to left ventricular enlargement appears later in the course.

Two-dimensional echocardiography can be used to visualize the prolapsing cusp vibrating rapidly in the left ventricular outflow tract during diastole. With lesser degrees of cusp injury, one may see reverse-doming of the aortic valve in diastole or lack of diastolic coaptation of the cusps. Abnormalities of the aortic root immediately adjacent to the aortic valve can be visualized, particularly with transesophageal echocardiography. Sinus of Valsalva aneurysm and aortic mural hematoma can both displace adjacent aortic cusps, with resultant severe regurgitation.

With acute, severe aortic regurgitation, the marked increase in left ventricular diastolic pressure may diminish the color jet of aortic regurgitation. However, Doppler findings, including greatly reduced pressure half-time of aortic regurgitation, reduced mitral valve deceleration time, and diastolic mitral regurgitation, alert the echocardiographer to the severe hemodynamic consequences of the acute aortic valve lesion.

Traumatic mitral valve lesions. In the autopsy series of Parmley et al.,[3] rupture of AV valves was more common than rupture of the aortic valve. However, rupture of the AV valves usually was associated with other significant cardiac injuries—frequently with cardiac rupture. This explains why rupture of the aortic valve has been reported more frequently than rupture of the mitral valve in clinical series.[26] Nevertheless, isolated mitral valve rupture may result from blunt chest trauma. Complete rupture of a left-sided papillary muscle results in massive mitral regurgitation and severe hemodynamic compromise. Lesser degrees of traumatic mitral regurgitation result from rupture of a secondary papillary muscle, rupture of chordae tendineae, or, rarely, a tear in one of the leaflets.[135,136] Various degrees of regurgitation can also result from simple contusion of a papillary muscle.

As with traumatic aortic regurgitation, traumatic mitral rupture severely overloads an unprepared left ventricle. Increased diastolic pressure is transmitted to a normal-sized left atrium and then directly to the lungs, resulting in varying degrees of dyspnea. Findings on physical examination are characteristic of mitral regurgitation (see chapter 2). There are no cardiac findings that are specific for traumatic regurgitation. An apical systolic thrill is present in fewer than 50% of the cases.[137] The chest radiograph usually reveals a normal heart size and evidence of pulmonary venous hypertension. With the more severe lesions, a pattern of florid pulmonary edema is evident.

Papillary muscle rupture can be directly visualized by two-dimensional echocardiography, particularly from the esophageal window.[138] If regurgitation is due to ruptured chordae, the ruptured chord and flail segment of mitral leaflet are identified in the left atrium during systole. Contusion of a papillary muscle renders it hypokinetic and echo-dense on two-dimensional imaging, and the overlying left ventricular wall segments are often hypokinetic. Noncontused segments of the left ventricle are *hyperdynamic* because of left ventricular volume overload. The mitral regurgitant jet can be detected by color Doppler imaging, and the spatial extent of the jet within the left atrium is proportional to its severity. Severe mitral regurgitation frequently causes systolic reversed flow in one or more pulmonary veins. This anomaly can be documented with pulsed Doppler interrogation. Echocardiography with Doppler and color-flow imaging can also be used to calculate the regurgitant volume and regurgitant orifice area.

Swan-Ganz catheterization affords an indication of severe, acute regurgitation: large v waves in the pulmonary artery wedge tracing. In some cases, it is necessary to document the degree of mitral regurgitation with contrast left ventriculography.

Traumatic tricuspid valve lesions. Numerous cases of traumatic tricuspid regurgitation have been reported.[72,82,139-149] As in mitral valve trauma, regurgitation can result from rupture of a papillary muscle, ruptured chordae, torn leaflets, or simple papillary muscle contusion.

Symptoms typically develop rapidly in patients with ruptured papillary muscles, although the diagnosis is often obscured by associated injuries. In those with ruptured chordae or torn leaflets, the onset of symptoms often is insidious. Syncope has occurred shortly after tricuspid valve injury. Many patients have noted prominent neck vein pulsations. Exertional dyspnea and fatigue are the most common early symptoms. Symptoms and signs of right heart failure eventually develop in most patients. Cyanosis has developed in about one-fourth of cases because of stretching of the right atrium with resultant enlargement of a patent foramen ovale and right-to-left shunting. Aside from potential cyanosis, the physical signs of traumatic regurgitation are no different from those of other causes. It should be remembered that in severe regurgitation, the murmur may be soft or absent.

In all cases, the chest radiograph eventually shows cardiomegaly due to enlargement of the right atrium and right ventricle. Incomplete or complete right bundle-branch block has been present on the ECG in almost every instance. Left- or right-axis deviation is also common. Atrial fibrillation has been noted in several cases and may lead to a rapid increase in symptoms.

Two-dimensional echocardiography allows visualization of the enlarged right atrium and right ventricle as well as direct visualization of the tricuspid abnormality (see Fig 57-7). The involved leaflet moves with a flail motion beyond the usual point of coaptation in systole.[150-154] Color-flow imaging documents the degree of regurgitation. With severe lesions, systolic flow is reversed in the hepatic veins, as detected by color or pulsed-wave Doppler imaging. Right-to-left shunting across the foramen ovale can be visualized with color-flow imaging or after intravenous injection of agitated saline, particularly during transesophageal echocardiography.[155]

Werne et al.[156] and Pellegrini et al.[157] reported cases of simultaneous rupture of mitral and tricuspid valves. Both lesions can be identified by echocardiography, and valve repair or replacement can be guided by intraoperative transesophageal echocardiography.

Coronary artery lesions

Coronary artery rupture results in hemopericardium. Diagnostic techniques for this complication have been discussed above. Either coronary artery rupture or traumatic coronary artery occlusion can lead to ischemic myocardial infarction. Appropriate diagnostic techniques are identical to those for myocardial infarction occurring as a complication of atherosclerotic coronary artery disease (see chapter 30A).

Patients with traumatic coronary artery fistula may remain asymptomatic.[47] Large coronary artery fistulae initially precipitate myocardial infarction. With time, large shunts can lead to high-output failure. The patient complains of exertional dyspnea or exertional fatigue. Angina may also occur as the result of a coronary steal syndrome. On examination, the left ventricular apex is hyperdynamic, and a continuous murmur is audible at the left sternal border or apex. There is usually accentuation of the murmur in diastole.[48] Typically, there is an interval of several weeks to months between the initial injury and detection of the murmur. During this time, the fistula increases in size.[46] The ECG commonly reveals evidence of myocardial infarction. Coronary angiography is most commonly used for delineation of a coronary arteriovenous or arteriocameral fistula. The proximal portion of the involved coronary artery is usually dilated, and abnormal drainage through the fistula is evident. The size of the shunt can be determined by oximetry. More recently, coronary fistulae have been fully defined by transesophageal echocardiography.[86]

MANAGEMENT

Prevention

Nowhere in the field of cardiology is there such a tremendous potential for prevention of illness as in cardiac trauma. Most cardiac injuries result from motor vehicle accidents. Although we will never be able to eliminate such accidents, we already have the capability to lower the incidence and minimize the effects.

In 1992, there were 10,000,000 motor vehicle accidents in the United States, resulting in 1,400,000 disabilities and 35,800 deaths. About half of all fatal accidents involve intoxication. It is foolish for us, as a society, to continue to allow lives (particularly those of our children) to be wasted at the hands of irresponsible individuals who choose to drive while intoxicated. It is hoped that the current trend of stiffer penalties for intoxicated drivers is the beginning of the end for the tremendous injustice that results from allowing intoxicated drivers use of our public thoroughfares.

Strict enforcement of speed limits also decreases the number of traffic accidents and injuries. Of course, this must be coupled with a proper level of funding for highway maintenance, police monitoring, and driver education programs.

A disproportionate number of fatalities from motor vehicle accidents involve motorcycles, often as single vehicular crashes. Being in a large vehicle obviously increases the odds of surviving a motor vehicle accident. The other major measures that successfully limit morbidity when properly used are seat belts, child restraints, and air bags. Widespread education regarding these preventive measures is necessary. As physicians, we must assume some of the responsibility for such education, much as we assume responsibility for informing our patients about the dangers of cigarette smoking or excessive intake of salt or lipid.

Initial triage

A patient who has sustained a deceleration accident or crush injury and survives to reach the emergency room must be rapidly but thoroughly investigated for life-threatening cardiac trauma. Continuous ECG monitoring should be initiated immediately. Ventricular and supraventricular arrhythmias should be treated exactly as if the patient had acute myocardial infarction.

The airway and overall respiratory status should be assessed quickly. When necessary, intubation should be performed. If physical examination and chest radiographs demonstrate a pneumothorax or significant hemothorax, a chest tube should be placed.

Large-bore intravenous lines should be inserted for the administration of fluids and medication. One of these lines should be placed for measurement of central venous or right atrial pressure. If there is any evidence of left ventricular failure, a Swan-Ganz catheter is useful for monitoring both left and right heart pressures and for determining cardiac output. Hypotension is most easily monitored by placement of a small catheter in a peripheral artery. If the patient is hypotensive or unconscious, a urinary catheter should be placed. Strict recording of intake and output is mandatory.

If there is evidence of cardiac tamponade or severe left ventricular failure, immediate intervention is required. Tamponade should be relieved with pericardiocentesis while preparations are made for an immediate exploratory thoracotomy to detect and repair cardiac rupture. Left ventricular failure is treated with inotropic, diuretic, or vasodilator drugs as dictated by the hemodynamic measurements. Further diagnostic procedures can then be performed to determine the cause of the failure.

Simultaneously, the trauma team should be assessing the patient for other life-threatening lesions. Injuries to the central nervous system, vertebrae, lungs, great vessels, and abdominal viscera and major fractures should be managed as soon as any cardiac or respiratory failure has been controlled. Once the patient has been completely stabilized, further work-up can proceed to identify less acute cardiac lesions.

Management of specific problems

Arrhythmias and conduction disturbances. Supraventricular and ventricular arrhythmias should be approached exactly as they would be in patients with acute myocardial infarction. Vigorous attempts should be made to correct hypoxia, anemia, acidosis, and electrolyte imbalances. When necessary, specific antiarrhythmic medications should be administered. If subsequent testing identifies myocardial injury, monitoring should be continued for several days. Depending on the severity of the initial arrhythmia, 24-hour ambulatory monitoring can be used toward the end of the hospitalization.

Conduction disturbances also should be treated as in acute myocardial infarction. Symptomatic sinus bradycardia or Mobitz I block should be treated first with atropine. In rare instances of traumatic Mobitz II or complete heart block, a temporary transvenous pacemaker should be placed.

Rupture of free wall. The most lethal mechanical complication of cardiac trauma is rupture of one of the free walls of the heart. However, not all patients who sustain cardiac rupture die instantly. In the Parmley et al. series,[3] 23 of the 353 victims survived the rupture for periods varying from 30 minutes to 7 days. In the Bright and Beck series,[17] 30 of the 159 patients with free wall rupture survived for 1 hour or more. As first-response and transport teams have become more efficient, an increasing number of patients with cardiac rupture arrive in the emergency room with vital signs.

There has been a corresponding increase in reports of patients surviving traumatic cardiac rupture because of prompt surgical attention. Survivors have been reported with traumatic rupture of each of the four chambers.[31,104-106,110-113,158-161] In nearly all reported cases of survival after traumatic cardiac rupture, cardiorrhaphy was performed less than 5 hours after the initial injury.[104] It is only through rapid diagnosis and surgical intervention that such patients can be saved.

Pericardiocentesis becomes a temporizing measure in patients with cardiac rupture. The bleeding is often so rapid that clots form (in contrast to other causes of hemopericardium), and removal of fluid may be difficult.[26] Nevertheless, removal of as little as 75 mL of fluid may provide dramatic hemodynamic improvement, because of the steep pericardial compliance curve. A catheter should be left in the pericardial space for continuous irrigation. Meanwhile, the patient should be supported with fluids and pressor agents. A chest tube should be inserted if the patient has right or left hemothorax.

From the moment cardiac rupture is suspected, preparations for surgical repair must be initiated. Pevec et al.,[107] in a review of 61 survivors of cardiac rupture secondary to nonpenetrating trauma, noted that 41% of the surgical repairs were made in less than 1 hour. Fulda et al.[109] reported on 59 patients requiring emergency surgery for cardiac rupture secondary to blunt trauma. Each patient had signs of life at the scene of the accident or during transport, but only 29 (49%) had vital signs on admission to the emergency trauma unit. The diagnosis of cardiac rupture was made by emergency thoracotomy in the 30 patients who arrived in cardiac arrest. For the remaining 29 patients, urgent thoracotomy was carried out in 41% and a subxiphoid pericardial window was created in 34%. The overall mortality in this group of 59 patients was 76%, although the authors noted that mortality was 52% for patients with vital signs on admission to the emergency trauma unit.

Therefore, if blood pressure is unobtainable and the patient is comatose on presentation, the thorax must be opened in the emergency room without delay. Otherwise, the patient can be transferred to the operating room. Most operations can be performed without cardiopulmonary bypass. Induction of anesthesia, with intermittent positive-pressure breathing, causes both vasodilation and decreased venous return,[26,48] which can lead to cardiovascular collapse in a patient with cardiac rupture who is barely compensated. Therefore, the surgeon must be prepared to open the chest immediately on induction. Median sternotomy provides access to the ventricles and both atria. Once the defect has been located and repaired, the heart should be inspected and palpated for evidence of other lesions. If the patient has become hemodynamically stable, repair of coexisting cardiac lesions should be postponed to allow full diagnostic evaluation and consideration of all therapeutic options.[14]

In suspected cardiac rupture, diagnosis should proceed simultaneously with surgical exploration. This demand can be met by transesophageal echocardiography. The esophageal transducer can be inserted while the patient is being prepared for surgery, and imaging can proceed throughout the surgical procedure so long as the patient is not placed on cardiopulmonary bypass. With this strategy, the echocardiographer can search for associated cardiac and aortic lesions while the surgeon performs pericardial drainage and cardiorrhaphy.

Clinicians must be aware that rupture of a cardiac free wall may not occur until 2 weeks or longer after the initial trauma.[4,14,26] Such ruptures are catastrophic, just as they are with ischemic myocardial infarction. Chest pain and dyspnea are followed quickly by collapse with severe hypotension, usually accompanied by sinus bradycardia or junctional rhythm. Jugular venous distention may be readily apparent. Generating a blood pressure by external chest compressions is extremely difficult. In such a situation, one must proceed as outlined above. Pressor agents, fluids, and pericardiocentesis are temporizing measures; exploration and cardiorrhaphy should be carried out as rapidly as possible.

Pericardial effusion. A large pericardial fluid collection per se is not an indication for pericardiocentesis. To date, there is no evidence that prophylactic centesis prevents either recurrent or constrictive pericarditis. The fluid may resolve spontaneously and without sequelae (as in the case illustrated in Figure 57-2). The two indications for tapping a traumatic pericardial fluid collection are tamponade and suspicion that the effusion is purulent.

With a slowly collecting traumatic effusion, one certainly should not wait to intervene until the patient becomes hypotensive. Pericardiocentesis should be carried out as soon as there is evidence of restricted ventricular filling. The earliest signs are increased jugular venous or central venous pressure and pulsus paradoxus. If the patient is being monitored carefully, these signs are elicited well before the development of sinus tachycardia—which is ominous, usually heralding collapse. The safest method for pericardiocentesis relies on echocardiographic guidance[76] (see chapter 55). Pericardiocentesis can be carried out with a multiholed catheter (such as a pigtail). The catheter is left indwelling until intermittent suctioning yields no fluid for 24 to 48 hours and a repeat echocardiogram verifies that there has been no significant reaccumulation.

If a significant amount of fluid does reaccumulate after these measures, surgical exploration is necessary. The bleeding site should be identified and controlled. If the source proves to be diffuse oozing from the epicardial surface, a pericardiectomy should be performed.

After blunt trauma, the usual source of septic pericarditis is an associated esophageal rupture.[3] In addition to symptoms and signs of pericarditis, the patient has symptoms and signs of infection: malaise, fever, chills, and sweats. Tamponade may develop. A trauma victim who is febrile and has a significant pericardial effusion by echocardiography requires diagnostic pericardiocentesis. Positive cultures confirm the diagnosis and guide antibiotic therapy. The patient then requires a wide pericardiectomy and surgical drainage.

Pericardial laceration. This is rarely an isolated lesion. It most frequently accompanies myocardial laceration, contusion, or rupture.[4,14] Of the 546 trauma cases discussed by Parmley et al.,[3] 18 involved isolated pericardial laceration. Clark et al.[151] reviewed 142 cases of traumatic pericardial rupture. Most are left pleuropericardial tears, and chest radiographs may demonstrate displacement of the cardiac silhouette to the left. Less commonly, the tears involve the diaphragmatic right pleuropericardium or superior mediastinal pericardium. Most such tears are discovered incidentally during surgery for other lesions. Repair is indicated to prevent herniation of the heart, which can cause cardiac strangulation, and to prevent herniation of abdominal contents.

Recurrent pericarditis. Development of tamponade is rare with episodes of recurrent pericarditis. If the patient has recurrences, each episode is treated as if it were nonspecific pericarditis: salicylates or indomethacin is administered in anti-inflammatory dosages. If episodes are prolonged or recur in rapid succession, treatment is by pericardiectomy, which is both safe and curative.[162]

Intrapericardial diaphragmatic hernia. Once an intrapericardial diaphragmatic hernia has been diagnosed, surgical repair is indicated, because this lesion can cause tamponade or strangulated bowel.[19] A transabdominal approach provides the best exposure; the hernia contents can be reduced to their proper positions within the abdomen. The diaphragmatic defect is closed with nonabsorbable suture. The prognosis is generally excellent after surgical repair.[116]

Constrictive pericarditis. Constrictive pericarditis may develop rapidly when purulent pericarditis is present. The thick peel surrounding the heart must then be removed at the time the pericardial space is opened for drainage. In all other trauma cases in which constriction develops, the onset is typically delayed beyond 6 months and usually is insidious. It is important that the thickened pericardium be removed as completely as possible as soon as the diagnosis of constriction has been made. Once the pericardium calcifies, spicules extend into the myocardium, and surgical repair carries increased risk.

Myocardial contusion and ischemic myocardial infarction. Myocardial damage occurring after blunt trauma may be due to direct contusion of the myocardium or to traumatic coronary artery occlusion and ischemic infarction. In the instance of coronary artery trauma, the resultant myocardial damage is managed in the same way as myocardial infarction due to atherosclerosis. Chest pain is treated with nitroglycerin, β-blockers, or calcium channel blockers on the basis of individual circumstances. Continuous rhythm monitoring, initiated in the emergency room, is maintained for up to several days, depending on the amount of myocardial damage detected by echocardiography. The patient is initially kept at complete bed rest and then is supervised through a program of gradually increasing activities over 1 to 2 weeks (as allowed by other injuries). Heavy isometric activities should be completely avoided, because of both the potential for serious ventricular arrhythmias and the risk of delayed myocardial rupture. In most cases of right or left ventricular contusion, function rapidly improves. In the series by Sutherland et al.,[27] wall motion abnormalities decreased or resolved in 84% of the patients by 8 days; the abnormalities worsened in four patients and remained unchanged in one.

After chest trauma, if the myocardial contusion or ischemic infarction is large enough, signs of pump failure appear. In such cases, a flow-directed catheter should be inserted at the bedside and used for measurement of right atrial, right ventricular, pulmonary artery, and pulmonary artery wedge pressures as well as cardiac index. Continuous monitoring allows a rational approach to therapy with preload- and afterload-reducing agents and inotropes. Intravenous vasodilatation should be changed to oral administration of an angiotensin-converting enzyme inhibitor. If side effects do not appear, this therapy should be continued as long as significant ventricular dysfunction persists.

The trend at present is to intervene early in acute ischemic myocardial infarction. Patients with chest trauma seen shortly after the injury who have hyperacute ECG changes should be considered for coronary angiography. This will differentiate current of injury due to direct contusion from that due to coronary occlusion. Certainly, thrombolytic agents *cannot* be administered (by either systemic or intracoronary route) in these trauma cases. However, in some instances it is possible to open an occluded vessel with percutaneous transluminal coronary angioplasty or to bypass the occlusion surgically. The decision to proceed with either of these last two options must recognize that both require heparinization. Associated injuries, such as splenic rupture, certainly influence the decision.

Noncardiac surgical procedures are associated with increased risk during the first few months after ischemic myocardial infarction, including trauma involving coronary occlusion. It is not known if this same risk applies to direct myocardial contusion, but unless coronary angiography is done at once, myocardial infarction cannot be differentiated from myocardial contusion. Therefore, in patients with trauma who have definite myocardial damage, *elective* surgical procedures (e.g., repair of associated traumatic lesions) should be postponed for several weeks. Of course, if postponement would result in a threat to life or a threat of permanent disfigurement or disability, surgical repair should be performed without delay despite the additional risk. In such cases, the surgeon must inform the patient and the family of the increased risk of the procedure.

Aneurysms and pseudoaneurysms. Whether or not coronary occlusion has occurred, true aneurysms can be complicated by mural thrombi with distal embolization, congestive failure, or life-threatening ventricular arrhythmias. A surgical approach is indicated when such complications cannot be managed medically. For ventricular tachycardia, the extent of the resection should be guided by intraoperative electrophysiologic mapping.

Pseudoaneurysm formation is a rare complication of nonpenetrating cardiac trauma. Pseudoaneurysms are ruptures of the myocardium that have been contained only by an adherent segment of pericardium. There is significant risk of subsequent pericardial rupture with exsanguination. For this reason, whenever a pseudoaneurysm is recognized (by its *narrow-necked* appearance on two-dimensional echocardiography or contrast ventriculography), immediate surgical repair should be considered.

Intracardiac shunts. If trauma has resulted in a ventricular septal defect with a large shunt causing hemodynamic instability, emergency surgical closure may be unavoidable. However, every attempt should be made to stabilize the patient in order to delay surgical repair. Stabilization usually requires inotropic, vasodilator, and pressor agents administered intravenously. If these are insufficient and aortic trauma has been excluded, intra-aortic balloon pumping can be used. The goal of such hemodynamic support therapy is to allow development of scar tissue that will firmly hold suture lines at the time of septal repair.

If the left-to-right shunt is small, the patient should merely be observed for the development of symptoms and instructed in the use of infective endocarditis prophylaxis. Small post-traumatic ventricular septal defects usually remain small and thus never lead to pulmonary hypertension. In fact, some post-traumatic ventricular septal defects have closed spontaneously.[134,163]

Isolated traumatic atrial septal defects are managed exactly like their congenital counterparts, with large defects requiring elective suture or patch closure.[83,164] Even smaller atrial septal tears should be closed if the patient has a history of deep venous thrombosis, since the defect can serve as a portal for paradoxical embolism. This argument becomes more compelling if there is associated right ventricular contusion.

Rupture of the AV septum results in a left ventricle-to-right atrium shunt. Rupture of a traumatic sinus of Valsalva aneurysm usually results in shunting from the aorta to the right atrium or right ventricle. These defects expose the right heart to systemic pressure and usually produce symptoms and require surgical repair.

Mural thrombi. Frequently, choice of therapy for traumatic mural thrombi is dictated by a contraindication to anticoagulants because of hemorrhage from associated injuries. When there are no associated injuries, the therapeutic decision is more problematic. Some authors argue that anticoagulants should *never* be used in myocardial trauma because theoretically they enlarge the hemorrhagic contusion. However, because embolization can occur,[6] our policy has been to anticoagulate when a mural thrombus is clearly identified and there is no contraindication due to associated trauma.[70]

Valvular lesions. Therapy for traumatic valvular regurgitation depends on the volume of leakage and on the severity of resultant hemodynamic disturbance. Instruction in prophylaxis for infective endocarditis should be accomplished in all instances. Beyond that, each case must be handled individually—just as with nontraumatic valvular regurgitation. Long-term survival after medical therapy alone has been recorded for each valvular lesion. When surgery is indicated, preferential consideration should always be given to valvuloplasty[37] rather than to valve replacement. Management of traumatic aortic, mitral, and tricuspid regurgitation will now be considered in further detail.

TRAUMATIC AORTIC VALVE INJURY. Aortic valve injury due to nonpenetrating trauma was first reported by Plenderleath in 1830.[165] Severe, acute aortic regurgitation may lead to death immediately or in the ensuing hours or days. Howard[35] reported a large series of traumatic aortic valve ruptures in 1928. Patients who did not succumb immediately had a mean survival of 40 months. One patient survived 10 years and one 11 years. Such long-term survival may be enhanced today by use of vasodilators, particularly angiotensin-converting enzyme inhibitors.

Patients who have acute pulmonary edema should be taken to the operating room for emergency treatment. Intravenous administration of vasodilators and inotropes guided by a Swan-Ganz catheter should be used to support the patient while the operating room is readied. For patients who survive the initial trauma and remain asymptomatic, follow-up and consideration of operation should be the same as those for any other patient with chronic aortic regurgitation.

Blunt trauma causes aortic regurgitation by direct valvular injury or by distorting the root adjacent to the valve. Direct valvular lesions include cusp tears and avulsion of the commissures or cusps. The first surgical approach to traumatic aortic regurgitation was in 1954 by Leonard et al.,[166] who inserted a Hufnagel valve in the descending thoracic aorta. Since that time, multiple successful surgical approaches have been reported.[167-169] Reconstruction of the traumatized valve should always be considered at the time of operation. Successful valvuloplasty after aortic valve trauma was reported by Loop et al.,[37] Haskins et al.,[170] and Bex et al.[171] Valve repair can be guided by intraoperative transesophageal echocardiography, and results can be assessed by serial follow-up surface echocardiographic studies. The patient reported by Ovil et al.[172] had a normal-appearing valve by Doppler echocardiographic evaluation 2 years after aortic valvuloplasty.

TRAUMATIC MITRAL VALVE LESIONS. Therapy for mitral valve injury depends on the severity of the regurgitation, left ventricular size and function, and whether or not symptoms are present. In mild cases, counseling on infective endocarditis prophylaxis is all that is necessary. If regurgitation is severe, particularly with symptoms or progressive left ventricular enlargement, surgery must be considered. In this situation, vasodilator therapy should be viewed as temporizing. With massive traumatic mitral regurgitation, acute surgical intervention is necessary. The patient can be supported with intravenously administered inotropes, pressors, and vasodilators while the operating room is being readied. In such severe cases, intra-aortic balloon pumping may also be necessary to support the patient until surgical correction.

Valve replacement is the traditional approach to traumatic mitral regurgitation. However, successful mitral repair has been reported after blunt chest trauma.[137,138] Valvuloplasty, guided by intraoperative transesophageal echocardiography, should now be considered the surgical treatment of choice for traumatic mitral valve disease.

TRAUMATIC TRICUSPID VALVE LESIONS. The clinical course of patients with isolated traumatic tricuspid regurgitation is usually benign. Several patients with significant regurgitation and follow-up of more than 15 years have had only mild symptoms.[139,142,144,145] However, right heart failure eventually develops in most patients. This is the standard indication for valve surgery.[144] Valve replacement has consistently been successful. Recently, tricuspid valve repair has also been successful after blunt cardiac trauma. It has been possible to reimplant torn papillary muscles and chordae, to replace torn chordae with artificial chordae or chordae fashioned from pericardium, and to repair torn tricuspid leaflets. Tricuspid repairs are usually supported with annuloplasty.[150,152,153,173-178] In patients with cyanosis, closure of the foramen ovale is accomplished at the time of operation.

Symptoms of right heart failure may persist after tricuspid valve replacement[139] because of irreversible myocardial changes. We favor early surgery after echocardiographic identification of severe traumatic tricuspid regurgitation, since this strategy is most likely to preserve right ventricular function. Early surgery also increases the odds of successful repair by minimizing annular enlargement and preventing degeneration of the flail tricuspid structures.[179]

Coronary artery lesions. Coronary artery ruptures most often lead to acute tamponade. If the traumatized coronary artery is small, it is simply ligated at the time of surgical exploration. Otherwise, proximal ligation must be combined with bypass grafting to the distal coronary segment.

In rare instances, blunt trauma has led to coronary artery occlusion. Management is identical to that for any other ischemic myocardial infarction, except that standard anticoagulants may be contraindicated because of associated injuries. Such associated injuries also preclude interventional therapy with thrombolytic agents. However, it is conceivable that percutaneous transluminal coronary angioplasty or coronary artery bypass surgery could be carried out immediately in an attempt to limit the size of the traumatic ischemic infarction. This strategy should be considered only with large infarcts causing hemodynamic disturbances.

Indications for repair of traumatic coronary arteriovenous or arteriocameral fistulae include congestive heart failure and angina. Surgical treatment for traumatic fistula is usually more satisfactory than that for congenital arteriovenous fistula because there are typically fewer connections with the recipient chamber in traumatic cases. If medical therapy is chosen rather than surgical repair, the patient should be instructed in the use of prophylaxis for infective endocarditis.[46]

PENETRATING CARDIAC TRAUMA

Etiology

Penetrating cardiac trauma most commonly follows knife or gunshot wounds. Other objects, such as ice picks, occasionally are involved. Rarely, penetrating trauma to the heart is caused by fractured ribs or sternal fragments. Cardiac trauma is usually associated with a penetrating precordial wound, but the heart also may be injured when the external wound involves more remote portions of the chest, neck, or upper abdomen.[14,75]

Pathology

Penetrating trauma may be limited to the pericardium and a single cardiac chamber. The frequency with which each chamber is injured is in direct proportion to the area each projects on the anterior chest wall. Thus, the right ventricle is penetrated most often, followed in frequency by the left ventricle, the right atrium, and the left atrium.[4,14] Gunshot wounds typically involve more than one chamber. Penetrating wounds commonly involve the ventricular septum,[180-182] whereas laceration of the atrial septum is unusual.[183] Late sequelae of penetrating cardiac trauma include aneurysms[184] and pseudoaneurysms, the latter occurring more commonly by this mechanism than with nonpenetrating cardiac trauma.[185,186]

Injury to the cardiac valves has been reported after penetrating cardiac trauma.[180,183,187] The incidence of such injuries has not been determined. Valvular regurgitation may result from direct lacerations of the cusps or leaflets or from laceration of the chordae or papillary muscles.

Coronary artery injury occurs less commonly with penetrating cardiac trauma than with nonpenetrating.[4] A coronary artery laceration frequently leads to tamponade as well as to ischemic myocardial infarction. Coronary arteriovenous or arteriocameral fistula may form subsequently.[46,47]

Missiles most often penetrate the cardiac chambers directly. Less commonly, they are carried to the right heart after penetrating the venous system. Missiles may lodge within the myocardium or may become entrapped in the atrial appendages, trabeculae, or chordae tendineae. Missiles projecting into the atrial or ventricular cavities may become enmeshed in fibrin and later covered with endothelium, thereby causing no subsequent problems. Before endothelialization there is an obvious risk of embolization, and the missile also serves as a potential source for infective endocarditis.[14] Because of heavy trabeculation, missiles tend to lodge securely in the right ventricle; missile embolization is much more frequent from the left ventricle.

Pathophysiology

The hemodynamics of penetrating cardiac trauma depend on the status of the pericardial laceration. If it remains open, shock develops as a consequence of hemorrhage into the pleural space. If the pericardial wound seals off (e.g., with clot), shock develops as a consequence of tamponade.

Cardiac lesions created by knives or ice picks are usually discrete, with little or no damage to surrounding tissue. Ventricular wounds may seal off completely, whereas atrial wounds are less likely to do so. If a penetrating wound is small or partially seals off, bleeding is slow enough to allow for defibrination. Blood within the pericardial space therefore remains liquid.[26]

Gunshot wounds typically result in various degrees of cellular damage immediately adjacent to the area of penetration. Spontaneous closure is rare. Because the myocardial wound invariably is large, bleeding is so brisk that defibrination does not occur. In such instances, the blood within the pericardial or pleural space usually clots.[26]

Diagnosis

The clinician must suspect cardiac trauma anytime a patient presents with a penetrating wound of the chest, neck, or upper abdomen. If penetrating cardiac trauma has occurred, either tamponade or hemorrhagic shock and an associated hemothorax are present. In either case, symptoms and signs are identical to those described under nonpenetrating trauma with myocardial rupture.

Many patients with penetrating cardiac trauma die shortly after the injury. Stabbing victims will more likely survive to reach the emergency room than victims of gunshot.[4,188,189] Even when the patient survives to reach medical attention, the situation is usually desperate. The diagnosis is therefore frequently confirmed during exploratory thoracotomy or median sternotomy and cardiorrhaphy.[190-193] After such emergency measures, ancillary diagnostic procedures become necessary to detect associated intracardiac injuries. In some cases, the patient is hemodynamically stable long enough to permit such ancillary techniques before surgical repair. If emergency intraoperative transesophageal echocardiography is available, diagnosis of secondary cardiac lesions can proceed while the surgeon is attending the primary lesion.[75]

ECG evidence of pericarditis, bundle-branch block, or injury current frequently appears within the first few hours after penetrating trauma. ST-segment elevation (which is much more common in this condition than with nonpenetrating trauma) usually persists for several days. Thereafter, the T waves usually flatten or invert. In most instances, the ECG normalizes within the first few months, although changes may persist for years.[54]

The cardiac silhouette on the chest radiograph rarely yields clues to acute penetrating injury unless a missile has lodged within the heart. Fluoroscopy may be used in an attempt to differentiate missiles lodged in the myocardium from those lying within a cardiac chamber. Neither acute valvular insufficiency nor acute tamponade causes cardiomegaly to appear on the chest radiograph. However, severe, acute valvular regurgitation results in radiographic findings of pulmonary edema. After penetrating trauma, pleural fluid on the chest radiograph obligates the clinician to rule out a penetrating wound of the heart or a great vessel. Mediastinal widening on the chest radiograph is another important clue to injury of a great vessel.

In penetrating trauma, echocardiography has most often been applied for diagnosis of intracardiac lesions after the primary free-wall lesion has been repaired.[180-183,187,194] Two-dimensional echocardiography, with spectral Doppler and color-flow imaging, has proven particularly valuable for diagnosis of penetrating defects of the valves and septa. Surface, transesophageal, and epicardial echocardiographic procedures are also useful for accurate localization of intracardiac missiles.[195] After coronary artery injury, echocardiography defines overall left ventricular dysfunction as well as specific regional abnormalities, and it is particularly useful for detection of true and false aneurysms.

Echocardiography can also be used to accurately diagnose pericardial effusion and tamponade after penetrating cardiac injury.[196] It is critical that the echocardiographer and surgeons recognize the significance of small pericardial effusions in this clinical situation.[197] As previously mentioned, acute cardiac hemorrhage can lead to tamponade with only 100 to 200 mL of blood in the pericardial space. Echocardiography-guided pericardiocentesis may be used as a temporizing measure while the patient is being prepared for cardiorrhaphy. With large wounds, the pericardial blood will not be defibrinated and clots will form within the pericardial sac, rendering centesis relatively ineffective—even with use of a large-bore catheter.[75]

Plummer et al.[198] retrospectively reviewed 10 years of emergency unit experience with penetrating cardiac injuries. Forty-nine patients were identified, of whom 21 were triaged according to standard clinical evaluation and 28 were immediately evaluated with echocardiography. The average time to diagnosis and disposition for surgical therapy was 15 ± 11.4 minutes in the echocardiography group and 42.4 ± 21.7 minutes in the nonechocardiography group. This rapid triage contributed to 100% survival in the echocardiography group, whereas survival was only 57.1% for the nonechocardiography group. Neurologic outcome was also improved for the patients who were triaged by echocardiography. We believe that use of echocardiography for diagnosis of penetrating cardiac injuries will increase, particularly with increasing availability of emergency intraoperative transesophageal echocardiography.

Coronary artery lacerations often must be approached surgically without the benefit of coronary angiography. After primary repair, angiography may become necessary if a coronary arteriovenous or arteriocameral fistula is suspected. As noted previously, transesophageal echocardiography can often define the origin, course, and drainage site for coronary fistula, thereby obviating invasive angiography.

Treatment

When a patient is transported to the emergency room with suspected penetrating cardiac trauma, preparation should be made for immediate surgery. If the patient is in extremis, thoracotomy should be performed in the emergency room. Otherwise, supportive measures should be administered while the operating room is readied. Attar et al.,[188] in a review of 109 penetrating cardiac injuries treated at their institution, divided the patients into four groups of increasing hemodynamic stability at the time of presentation. The 38 patients in the first group were lifeless at the time of presentation, the 16 patients in the second group were agonal, the 33 patients in the third group were in shock, and the 22 patients in the fourth group were hemodynamically stable on admission to the emergency unit. Thoracotomy was performed immediately in the emergency room for 36 of the 38 patients in the first group and for all 16 patients in the second group; urgent thoracotomy was performed in the operating room for 24 of the 33 patients in the third group and for 20 of the 22 patients in the fourth group. Survival rates were 31% for group 1, 69% for group 2, 79% for group 3, and 82% for group 4, for an overall survival rate of 61%. As expected, the survival rate for gunshot wounds (40%) was significantly less than that for stab wounds (78%). Significant success rates with emergency room thoracotomy for penetrating cardiac injuries have also been published by Mitchell et al.[193] (15%), Mandal and Oparah[189] (30%), Kavolius et al.[191] (27%), and Knott-Craig et al.[190] (46%). The last-named authors quote an impressive overall hospital mortality rate of only 8.5% for 129 patients with cardiac stab wounds. As keys to their success, they emphasize aggressive transfusion to improve cardiac filling in the face of tamponade, empirical correction of acidosis with bicarbonate, minimal delays to emergency thoracotomy, and rapid drainage of pleural and pericardial spaces. Symbas[75] emphasizes use of light anesthesia or no anesthesia, depending on the patient's condition, and minimal positive pressure ventilation until after the pericardium has been opened, to avoid complete hemodynamic collapse.

Victims of penetrating cardiac trauma whose hemodynamic status is marginal or stable should be supported in the emergency room until arrangements are made for urgent thoracotomy or median sternotomy in the operating room. In preparation for surgery, the patient should be intubated and ventilated. A Swan-Ganz catheter should be inserted, not only to allow continuous measurement of left and right heart pressures but also to supply a central port for administration of blood and volume expanders. If tamponade is diagnosed, temporizing pericardiocentesis should be performed. A transesophageal echocardiographic probe should be inserted for intracardiac monitoring and diagnosis.

Once the patient reaches the operating room, the chest is opened and the pericardial sac exposed. If the sac is tense with bloody effusion, it is opened and the blood and clots are evacuated. Thereafter, the source of bleeding is identified and controlled. Myocardial wounds are usually sutured. Rarely, when the wound is too large to allow approximation of the edges, cardiopulmonary bypass is instituted and the defect is closed with a patch. Lacerations of large coronary arteries are either repaired primarily or bypassed. If the lacerated artery is small and not amenable to repair, it is simply ligated to control hemorrhage.[26,75]

During emergency surgical procedures for penetrating cardiac injuries, the surgeon seeks signs of associated internal cardiac injuries, such as a thrill indicative of ventricular septal defect or valvular laceration. Increasing use of intraoperative transesophageal echocardiography allows more precise identification of such defects. Occasionally the associated valvular or septal injury is so significant that the patient remains hemodynamically unstable after repair of the external cardiac injury. For such patients, cardiopulmonary bypass must be instituted and the valvular or septal laceration immediately repaired. Usually, however, the patient's hemodynamic condition stabilizes after repair of the external cardiac injury. In such instances, associated internal cardiac injuries are not approached during the primary surgical procedure. This delay allows methodical clinical and echocardiographic evaluation during the recovery period to determine whether the residual lesions are significant enough to warrant surgical repair.

When bullets, pellets, or shrapnel have caused penetrating cardiac wounds, every attempt should be made to identify their location intraoperatively so that they can be removed if accessible. Missiles completely embedded in the myocardium or lodging in the pericardial space are generally well tolerated. These can be left alone if they cannot be easily removed at the time of cardiorrhaphy. Every effort must be made to retrieve missiles that are only partially embedded or are freely mobile, because of the potential for embolism and for infective endocarditis. In addition, missiles that have lodged adjacent to coronary arteries should be removed, because of their potential to erode the vessel. Hartzler[199] reported bioptome catheter removal of a small missile from the right ventricle, obviating cardiotomy.

CONCLUSION

We live in an era of high-speed motor vehicles that have led, particularly in combination with alcohol use, to an increase in nonpenetrating cardiac trauma. An alarming increase in violent crimes has led to a parallel increase in penetrating cardiac trauma. Clinical expertise is required to diagnose cardiac injuries accurately in the milieu of multisystem trauma. First and foremost, the clinician must be highly aware of the possibility of cardiac trauma whenever the mechanism of injury is sufficient. Traditional cardiovascular diagnostic modalities should be judiciously supplemented with echocardiography for precise definition of traumatic cardiac lesions.

Both penetrating and nonpenetrating cardiac trauma can be lethal. Severe hemodynamic distress most often occurs coincident with the initial injury but may be delayed for several hours or days. Most patients have been in excellent health before the cardiac injury. The prognosis for full functional recovery is therefore excellent if the clinician heeds the warning provided by life-threatening rhythm and hemodynamic disturbances and responds quickly and aggressively.

REFERENCES

1. Jones JW, Hewitt RL, Drapanas T: Cardiac contusion: a capricious syndrome. *Ann Surg* 181:567-573, 1975
2. Jackson DH, Murphy GW: Nonpenetrating cardiac trauma. *Mod Concepts Cardiovasc Dis* 45:123-128, 1976
3. Parmley LF, Manion WC, Mattingly TW: Nonpenetrating traumatic injury of the heart. *Circulation* 18:371-396, 1958
4. Cohn PF, Braunwald E: Traumatic heart disease. In *Heart Disease: A Textbook of Cardiovascular Medicine.* Vol 2. Edited by E Braunwald. Philadelphia, WB Saunders Company, 1980, pp 1583-1596
5. Ferré GA, Steward WD: Cardiac contusion. *Clin Orthop* 53:123-130, 1967
6. Pomerantz M, Delgado F, Eiseman B: Unsuspected depressed cardiac output following blunt thoracic or abdominal trauma. *Surgery* 70:865-870, 1971
7. Liedtke AJ, DeMuth WE Jr: Nonpenetrating cardiac injuries: a collective review. *Am Heart J* 86:687-697, 1973
8. Rasaretnam R, Paul ATS: Constrictive pericarditis following mild non-penetrating trauma. *Aust NZ J Med* 5:57-62, 1975
9. Doty DB, Anderson AE, Rose EF, et al: Cardiac trauma: clinical

and experimental correlations of myocardial contusion. *Ann Surg* 180:452-459, 1974
10. DeMuth WE Jr, Zinsser HF Jr: Myocardial contusion. *Arch Intern Med* 115:434-442, 1965
11. Leading Article: Cardiac contusion. *Br Med J* 4:606, 1975
12. Symbas PN: Cardiac trauma. *Am Heart J* 92:387-396, 1976
13. Saunders CR, Doty DB: Myocardial contusion. *Surg Gynecol Obstet* 144:595-603, 1977
14. Symbas PN: Traumatic heart disease. *Curr Probl Cardiol* 7:1-35, June 1982
15. Abrunzo TJ: Commotio cordis: the single, most common cause of traumatic death in youth baseball. *Am J Dis Child* 145:1279-1282, 1991
16. Sherer DM, Abramowicz JS, Babkowski R, et al: Extensive fetal intrathoracic injuries sustained in a motor vehicle accident. *Am J Perinatol* 10:414-416, 1993
17. Bright EF, Beck CS: Nonpenetrating wounds of the heart: a clinical and experimental study. *Am Heart J* 10:293-321, 1935
18. Beasley HK: *Nonpenetrating Cardiac Injury.* Thesis, Mayo Graduate School of Medicine (University of Minnesota), Rochester, 1967
19. Meng RL, Straus A, Milloy F, et al: Intrapericardial diaphragmatic hernia in adults. *Ann Surg* 189:359-366, 1979
20. Aldhoheyan A, Jain SK, Hamdy M, et al: Traumatic intrapericardial diaphragmatic hernia. *Injury* 23:331-332, 1992
21. Mayor-Davies JA, Britz RS, Soares MJ: Intrapericardial herniation. A report of 2 cases. *S Afr J Surg* 29:55-56, 1991
22. Girzadas DV Jr, Fligner DJ: Delayed traumatic intrapericardial diaphragmatic hernia associated with cardiac tamponade. *Ann Emerg Med* 20:1246-1247, 1991
23. Beless DJ, Organ BC: Delayed presentation of intrapericardial diaphragmatic hernia, an unusual cause of colon obstruction. *Ann Emerg Med* 20:415-417, 1991
24. Van Gelderen WF: Stab wounds of the heart: two new signs of pneumopericardium. *Br J Radiol* 66:794-796, 1993
25. Sbokos CG, Karayannacos PE, Kontaxis A, et al: Traumatic hemopericardium and chronic constrictive pericarditis. *Ann Thorac Surg* 23:225-229, 1977
26. Symbas PN: *Trauma to the Heart and Great Vessels.* New York, Grune & Stratton, 1978
27. Sutherland GR, Driedger AA, Holliday RL, et al: Frequency of myocardial injury after blunt chest trauma as evaluated by radionuclide angiography. *Am J Cardiol* 52:1099-1103, 1983
28. Frazee RC, Mucha P Jr, Farnell MB, et al: Objective evaluation of blunt cardiac trauma. *J Trauma* 26:510-520, 1986
29. Grossman CM: Posttraumatic ossification of the myocardium. *J Trauma* 14:85-89, 1974
30. Hilton T, Mezei L, Pearson AC: Delayed rupture of tricuspid papillary muscle following blunt chest trauma. *Am Heart J* 119:1410-1412, 1990
31. Pollak S, Stellwag-Carion C: Delayed cardiac rupture due to blunt chest trauma. *Am J Forensic Med Pathol* 12:153-156, 1991
32. Berkery W, Hare C, Warner RA, et al: Nonpenetrating traumatic rupture of the tricuspid valve: formation of ventricular septal aneurysm and subsequent septal necrosis: recognition by two-dimensional Doppler echocardiography. *Chest* 91:778-780, 1987
33. Dodd DA, Johns JA, Graham TP Jr: Transient severe mitral and tricuspid regurgitation following blunt chest trauma. *Am Heart J* 114:652-654, 1987
34. Chi S, Blair TC, Gonzalez-Lavin L: Rupture of the normal aortic valve after blunt chest trauma. *Thorax* 32:619-622, 1977
35. Howard CP: Aortic insufficiency due to rupture by strain of a normal aortic valve. *Can Med Assoc J* 19:12-24, 1928
36. Rowland TW: Traumatic aortic insufficiency in children: case report and review of the literature. *Pediatrics* 60:893-895, 1977
37. Loop FD, Hofmeier G, Groves LK: Traumatic disruption of the aortic valve. *Cleve Clin Q* 38:187-194, 1971
38. Levine RJ, Roberts WC, Morrow AG: Traumatic aortic regurgitation. *Am J Cardiol* 10:752-763, 1962
39. Wei J, Chang C-Y, Chang Y-C: Traumatic sinus of Valsalva fistula. *Ann Thorac Surg* 52:852-854, 1991
40. Murray EG, Minami K, Körtke H, et al: Traumatic sinus of Valsalva fistula and aortic valve rupture. *Ann Thorac Surg* 55:760-761, 1993
41. Garcia-Ramirez JR, Holcombe DJ, Garcia-Gregory JA: Posttraumatic aortico-right ventricular fistula: a case study. *J Louisiana State Med Soc* 142:31-33, 1990
42. Stewart JSS: Primary traumatic coronary thrombosis. *Br Med J* 1:739-740, 1967
43. Stern T, Wolf RY, Reichart B, et al: Coronary artery occlusion resulting from blunt trauma. *JAMA* 230:1308-1309, 1974
44. Oren A, Bar-Shlomo B, Stern S: Acute coronary occlusion following blunt injury to the chest in the absence of coronary atherosclerosis. *Am Heart J* 92:501-505, 1976
45. Wainwright RJ, Edwards AC, Maisey MN, et al: Early occlusion and late stricture of normal coronary arteries following blunt chest trauma. *Chest* 78:796-798, 1980
46. Anderson GP, Adicoff A, Motsay GJ, et al: Traumatic right coronary arterial-right atrial fistula. *Am J Cardiol* 35:439-443, 1975
47. Austin SM, Applefeld MM, Turney SZ, et al: Traumatic left anterior descending coronary artery to right ventricle fistula: report of two cases. *South Med J* 70:581-584, 1977
48. Cheitlin MD, Abbott JA: The internist's role in the recognition and management of cardiovascular trauma. *Med Clin North Am* 63:201-221, January 1979
49. Soulen RL, Freeman E: Radiologic evaluation of traumatic heart disease. *Radiol Clin North Am* 9:285-297, August 1971
50. Hipona FA, Paredes S: The radiologic evaluation of patients with chest trauma: cardiovascular system. *Med Clin North Am* 59:65-93, January 1975
51. Gozo EG Jr, Cohen HC, Pick A: Traumatic bifascicular intraventricular block. *Chest* 61:294-296, 1972
52. Warburg E: *Subacute and Chronic Pericardial and Myocardial Lesions Due to Non-penetrating Traumatic Injuries: A Clinical Study.* London, Oxford University Press, 1938
53. Dolara A, Morando P, Pampaloni M: Electrocardiographic findings in 98 consecutive non-penetrating chest injuries. *Dis Chest* 52:50-56, 1967
54. Weisz GM, Blumenfeld Z, Barzilai A: Electrocardiographic changes in traumatized patients. *JACEP* 5:329-331, 1976
55. Kissane RW, Fidler RS, Koons RA: Electrocardiographic changes following extenal chest injury to dogs. *Ann Intern Med* 11:907-935, 1937
56. Chung EK, Renn J: Electrocardiographic changes in nonpenetrating trauma to the chest. *Acta Cardiol (Brux)* 25:418-423, 1970
57. Watson JH, Bartholomae WM: Cardiac injury due to nonpenetrating chest trauma. *Ann Intern Med* 52:871-880, 1960
58. Pearce W, Blair E: Significance of the electrocardiogram in heart contusion due to blunt trauma. *J Trauma* 16:136-140, 1976
59. Schamroth L: *The Electrocardiology of Coronary Artery Disease.* Oxford, Blackwell Scientific Publications, 1975, pp 13-18
60. Erhardt LR, Sjögren A, Wahlberg I: Single right-sided precordial lead in the diagnosis of right ventricular involvement in inferior myocardial infarction. *Am Heart J* 91:571-576, 1976
61. Fox KM, Rowland E, Krikler DM, et al: Electrophysiological manifestations of non-penetrating cardiac trauma. *Br Heart J* 43:458-462, 1980
62. Liedtke AJ, De Muth WE: Effects of alcohol on cardiovascular performance after experimental nonpenetrating chest trauma. *Am J Cardiol* 35:243-250, 1975
63. Bharati S, Chervony A, Gruhn J, et al: Atrial arrhythmias related to trauma to sinoatrial node. *Chest* 61:331-335, 1972
64. Markiewicz W, Best LA, Burstein S, et al: Echocardiographic evaluation after blunt trauma of the chest. *Int J Cardiol* 8:269-274, 1985
65. Taylor HB: Transient cardiac arrhythmia induced by nonpenetrating trauma to the chest. *Am Heart J* 46:557-564, 1953
66. Potkin RT, Werner JA, Trobaugh GB, et al: Evaluation of noninvasive tests of cardiac damage in suspected cardiac contusion. *Circulation* 66:627-631, 1982
67. Hiatt JR, Yeatman LA Jr, Child JS: The value of echocardiography in blunt chest trauma. *J Trauma* 28:914-922, 1988
68. Reynolds M, Jones JW: CPK-MB isoenzyme determinations in blunt chest trauma. *JACEP* 8:304-306, 1979
69. Fabian TC, Cicala RS, Croce MA, et al: A prospective evaluation of myocardial contusion: correlation of significant arrhythmias and cardiac output with CPK-MB measurements. *J Trauma* 31:653-659, 1991
70. Miller FA Jr, Seward JB, Gersh BJ, et al: Two-dimensional echocardiographic findings in cardiac trauma. *Am J Cardiol* 50:1022-1027, 1982

71. Reif J, Justice JL, Olsen WR, et al: Selective monitoring of patients with suspected blunt cardiac injury. *Ann Thorac Surg* 50:530-533, 1990
72. Michelson WB: CPK-MB isoenzyme determinations: diagnostic and prognostic value in evaluation of blunt chest trauma. *Ann Emerg Med* 9:562-567, 1980
73. King RM, Mucha P Jr, Seward JB, et al: Cardiac contusion: a new diagnostic approach utilizing two-dimensional echocardiography. *J Trauma* 23:610-614, 1983
74. Healey MA, Brown R, Fleiszer D: Blunt cardiac injury: Is this diagnosis necessary? *J Trauma* 30:137-146, 1990
75. Symbas PN: Traumatic heart disease. *Curr Probl Cardiol* 16:539-582, 1991
76. Callahan JA, Seward JB, Tajik AJ, et al: Pericardiocentesis assisted by two-dimensional echocardiography. *J Thorac Cardiovasc Surg* 85:877-879, 1983
77. Motro M, Barzilay Z, Schneeweiss A, et al: Isolated right ventricular infarction and aneurysm due to blunt chest trauma: valve of two-dimensional echocardiography and radionuclide angiography. *Am Heart J* 101:679-680, 1981
78. Norton MJ, Stanford GG, Weigelt JA: Early detection of myocardial contusion and its complications in patients with blunt trauma. *Am J Surg* 160:577-581, 1990
79. Helling TS, Duke P, Beggs CW, et al: A prospective evaluation of 68 patients suffering blunt chest trauma for evidence of cardiac injury. *J Trauma* 29:961-965, 1989
80. Brooks SW, Young JC, Cmolik B, et al: The use of transesophageal echocardiography in the evaluation of chest trauma. *J Trauma* 32:761-765, 1992
81. Orliaguet G, Jacquens Y, Riou B, et al: Combined severe myocardial and pulmonary contusion: early diagnosis with transesophageal echocardiography and management with high-frequency jet ventilation: case report. *J Trauma* 34:455-457, 1993
82. Bardy GH, Talano JV: Right ventricular failure in a young man after chest trauma. *Arch Intern Med* 142:615-616, 1982
83. Baumgartel ED: Cardiac rupture from blunt trauma with atrial septal defect. *Arch Surg* 127:347-348, 1992
84. Jebara VA, Acar C, Dervanian P, et al: Traumatic ventricular septal defects. Report of 3 cases with tricuspid valve rupture in 2 cases. *J Cardiovasc Surg* 33:253-255, 1992
85. Shapiro MJ, Yanofsky SD, Trapp J, et al: Cardiovascular evaluation in blunt thoracic trauma using transesophageal echocardiography (TEE). *J Trauma* 31:835-839, 1991
86. Rubin DA, Zaki AM, Zaghlol S, et al: Visualization of coronary artery fistula with transesophageal echocardiography. *J Am Soc Echocardiogr* 5:173-175, 1992
87. Go RT, Doty DB, Chiu CL, et al: A new method of diagnosing myocardial contusion in man by radionuclide imaging. *Radiology* 116:107-110, 1975
88. Chiu CL, Roelofs JD, Go RT, et al: Coronary angiographic and scintigraphic findings in experimental cardiac contusion. *Radiology* 116:679-683, 1975
89. Brantigan CO, Burdick D, Hopeman AR, et al: Evaluation of technetium scanning for myocardial contusion. *J Trauma* 18:460-463, 1978
90. Coleman J, Gonzalez A, Harlaftis N, et al: Myocardial contusion: diagnostic value of cardiac scanning and echocardiography. *Surg Forum* 27:293-294, 1976
91. Bayer MJ, Burdick D: Diagnosis of myocardial contusion in blunt chest trauma. *JACEP* 6:238-242, 1977
92. Datz FL, Lewis SE, Parkey RW, et al: Radionuclide evaluation of cardiac trauma. *Semin Nucl Med* 10:187-192, 1980
93. Rosenthall L: Intravenous radionuclide angiography in the diagnosis of trauma. *Semin Nucl Med* 4:395-409, 1974
94. McConnell BJ, McConnell RW, Guiberteau MJ: Radionuclide imaging in blunt trauma. *Radiol Clin North Am* 19:37-51, March 1981
95. McCarthy MC, Pavlina PM, Evans DK, et al: The value of SPECT-thallium scanning in screening for myocardial contusion. *Cardiovasc Intravent Radiol* 14:238-240, 1991
96. Holness R, Waxman K: Diagnosis of traumatic cardiac contusion utilizing single photon-emission computed tomography. *Crit Care Med* 18:1-3, 1990
97. Godbe D, Waxman K, Wang FW, et al: Diagnosis of myocardial contusion: quantitative analysis of single photon emission computed tomographic scans. *Arch Surg* 127:888-892, 1992
98. Hendel RC, Cohn S, Aurigemma G, et al: Focal myocardial injury following blunt chest trauma: a comparison of indium-111 antimyosin scintigraphy with other noninvasive methods. *Am Heart J* 123:1208-1215, 1992
99. Gunnar WP, Martin M, Smith RF, et al: The utility of cardiac evaluation in the hemodynamically stable patient with suspected myocardial contusion. *Am Surg* 57:373-377, 1991
100. Dubrow TJ, Mihalka J, Eisenhauer DM, et al: Myocardial contusion in the stable patient: What level of care is appropriate? *Surgery* 106:267-273, 1989
101. McLean RF, Devitt JH, Dubbin J, et al: Incidence of abnormal RNA studies and dysrhythmias in patients with blunt chest trauma. *J Trauma* 31:968-970, 1991
102. Fléjou Y, Roland E, Ecoiffier J. The place of angiography in the evaluation of traumatic injuries to the heart and coronary arteries. *Cardiovasc Radiol* 2:47-50, 1979
103. Katz S, Gimmon (Goldschmidt) Z, Lewis BS, et al: Coronary angiography after traumatic myocardial contusion. *J Trauma* 19:126-128, 1979
104. Trueblood HW, Wuerflein RD, Angell WW: Blunt trauma rupture of the heart. *Ann Surg* 177:66-69, 1973
105. Schiavone WA, Ghumrawi BK, Catalano DR, et al: The use of echocardiography in the emergency management of nonpenetrating traumatic cardiac rupture. *Ann Emerg Med* 20:1248-1250, 1991
106. Baxa MD: Cardiac rupture secondary to blunt trauma: a rapidly diagnosable entity with two-dimensional echocardiography. *Ann Emerg Med* 20:902-904, 1991
107. Pevec WC, Udekwu AO, Peitzman AB: Blunt rupture of the myocardium. *Ann Thorac Surg* 48:139-142, 1989
108. Hancock EW: Cardiac tamponade. *Med Clin North Am* 63:223-237, January 1979
109. Fulda G, Brathwaite CE, Rodriguez A, et al: Blunt traumatic rupture of the heart and pericardium: a ten-year experience (1979-1989). *J Trauma* 31:167-172, 1991
110. Noon GP, Boulafendis D, Beall AC Jr: Rupture of the heart secondary to blunt trauma. *J Trauma* 11:122-127, 1971
111. Layton TR, DiMarco RF, Pellegrini RV: Rupture of the left atrium from blunt trauma. *J Trauma* 19:117-118, 1979
112. O'Sullivan MJ Jr, Spagna PM, Bellinger SB, et al: Rupture of the right atrium due to blunt trauma. *J Trauma* 12:208-214, 1972
113. Howanitz EP, Buckley D, Galbraith TA, et al: Combined blunt traumatic rupture of the heart and aorta: two case reports and review of the literature. *J Trauma* 30:506-508, 1990
114. Siderys H, Strange PS: Rupture of the heart due to blunt trauma: successful treatment utilizing cardiopulmonary bypass. *J Thorac Cardiovasc Surg* 62:84-86, 1971
115. Fonner BT, Vogelzang RL: Right atrial rupture due to blunt trauma: CT evaluation. *Comput Med Imaging Graph* 16:27-29, 1992
116. Larrieu AJ, Wiener I, Alexander R, et al: Pericardiodiaphragmatic hernia. *Am J Surg* 139:436-440, 1980
117. van Loenhout RMM, Schiphorst TJMJ, Wittens CHA, et al: Traumatic intrapericardial diaphragmatic hernia. *J Trauma* 26:271-275, 1986
118. Vijayaraghavan SB: Diaphragmatic eventration into the pericardial sac: sonographic diagnosis. *J Clin Ultrasound* 16:510-512, 1988
119. Foil MB, Mackersie RC, Furst SR, et al: The asymptomatic patient with suspected myocardial contusion. *Am J Surg* 160:638-642, 1990
120. Wisner DH, Reed WH, Riddick RS: Suspected myocardial contusion: triage and indications for monitoring. *Ann Surg* 212:82-86, 1990
121. Baxter BT, Moore EE, Moore FA, et al: A plea for sensible management of myocardial contusion. *Am J Surg* 158:557-561, 1989
122. Miller FB, Shumate CR, Richardson JD: Myocardial contusion: When can the diagnosis be eliminated? *Arch Surg* 124:805-807, 1989
123. Cachecho R, Grindlinger GA, Lee VW: The clinical significance of myocardial contusion. *J Trauma* 33:68-71, 1992
124. Christensen MA, Sutton KR: Myocardial contusion: new concepts in diagnosis and management. *Am J Crit Care* 2:28-34, 1993
125. Nishimura RA, Tajik AJ, Shub C, et al: Role of two-dimensional echocardiography in the prediction of in-hospital complications after acute myocardial infarction. *J Am Coll Cardiol* 4:1080-1087, 1984

126. Kan G, Visser CA, Koolen JJ, et al: Short and long term predictive value of admission wall motion score in acute myocardial infarction: a cross sectional echocardiographic study of 345 patients. *Br Heart J* 56:422-427, 1986

127. Jaarsma W, Visser CA, van Eenige MJ, et al: Predictive value of two-dimensional echocardiographic and hemodynamic measurements on admission with acute myocardial infarction. *J Am Soc Echocardiogr* 1:187-193, 1988

128. Schiller NB, Shah PM, Crawford M, et al: Recommendations for quantitation of the left ventricle by two-dimensional echocardiography. *J Am Soc Echocardiogr* 2:358-367, 1989

129. Silver GM, Spampinato N, Favaloro RG, et al: Ventricular aneurysms and blunt chest trauma. *Chest* 63:628-631, 1973

130. Singh R, Nolan SP, Schrank JP: Traumatic left ventricular aneurysm: two cases with normal coronary angiograms. *JAMA* 234:412-414, 1975

131. Burns JMA, Houston AB, Dunn FG: Colour Doppler flow mapping in the diagnosis of traumatic ventricular septal defect. *Int J Cardiol* 29:245-246, 1990

132. Moront M, Lefrak EA, Akl BF: Traumatic rupture of the interventricular septum and tricuspid valve: case report. *J Trauma* 31:134-136, 1991

133. Rutherford EJ, White KS, Maxwell JG, et al: Immediate isolated intraventricular septal defect from nonpenetrating thoracic trauma. *Am Surg* 59:353-354, 1993

134. Ilia R, Goldfarb B, Wanderman KL, et al: Spontaneous closure of a traumatic ventricular septal defect after blunt trauma documented by serial echocardiography. *J Am Soc Echocardiogr* 5:203-205, 1992

135. Turabian M, Chan K-L: Rupture of mitral chordae tendineae resulting from blunt chest trauma: diagnosis by transesophageal echocardiography. *Can J Cardiol* 6:180-182, 1990

136. Shammas NW, Kaul S, Stuhlmuller JE, et al: Traumatic mitral insufficiency complicating blunt chest trauma treated medically: a case report and review. *Crit Care Med* 20:1064-1068, 1992

137. Bailey CP, Vera CA, Hirose T: Mitral regurgitation from rupture of chordae tendineae due to "steering wheel" compression. *Geriatrics* 24:90-105, September 1969

138. Spangenthal EJ, Sekovski B, Bhayana JN, et al: Traumatic left ventricular papillary muscle rupture: the role of transesophageal echocardiography in diagnosis and surgical management. *J Am Soc Echocardiogr* 6:536-538, 1993

139. Brandenburg RO, McGoon DC Campeau L, et al: Traumatic rupture of the chordae tendineae of the tricuspid valve: successful repair twenty-four years later. *Am J Cardiol* 18:911-915, 1966

140. Jahnke EJ Jr, Nelson WP, Aaby GV, et al: Tricuspid insufficiency: the result of nonpenetrating cardiac trauma. *Arch Surg* 95:880-886, 1967

141. Liu S-M. Sako Y, Alexander CS: Traumatic tricuspid insufficiency. *Am J Cardiol* 26:200-204, 1970

142. Tachovsky TJ, Giuliani ER, Ellis FH Jr: Prosthetic valve replacement for traumatic tricuspid insufficiency: report of a case originally diagnosed as Ebstein's malformation. *Am J Cardiol* 26:196-199, 1970

143. Morgan JR, Forker AD: Isolated tricuspid insufficiency. *Circulation* 43:559-564, 1971

144. Croxson MS, O'Brien KP, Lowe JB: Traumatic tricuspid regurgitation: long-term survival. *Br Heart J* 33:750-755, 1971

145. Cahill NS, Beller BM, Linhart JW, et al: Isolated traumatic tricuspid regurgitation: prolonged survival without operative intervention. *Chest* 61:689-691, 1972

146. Bryant LR, Mobin-Uddin K, Dillon ML, et al: Cardiac valve injury with major chest trauma. *Arch Surg* 107:279-283, 1973

147. Marvin RF, Schrank JP, Nolan SP: Traumatic tricuspid insufficiency. *Am J Cardiol* 32:723-726, 1973

148. Kessler KM, Foianini JE, Davia JE, et al: Tricuspid insufficiency due to nonpenetrating trauma. *Am J Cardiol* 37:442-444, 1976

149. Shahidnoorai S, Ameli M: Post traumatic tricuspid insufficiency: When to intervene? *J Cardiovasc Surg* 32:585-588, 1991

150. Linka A, Ritter M, Turina M, et al: Acute tricuspid papillary muscle rupture following blunt chest trauma. *Am Heart J* 124:799-802, 1992

151. Clark DE, Wiles CS III, Lim MK, et al: Traumatic rupture of the pericardium. *Surgery* 93:495-503, 1983

152. Hirata K, Kyushima M, Asato H, et al: Tricuspid regurgitation due to blunt chest trauma. Report of a case and review of the literature. *Jpn Heart J* 34:361-375, 1993

153. Naja I, Pomar JL, Barriuso C, et al: Traumatic tricuspid regurgitation. *J Cardiovasc Surg* 33:256-258, 1992

154. Longhini C, Brunazzi MC, Musacci GF, et al: Two-dimensional echocardiography in post traumatic tricuspid incompetence. *Acta Cardiol* 38:525-535, 1983

155. Kantor G, Devitt JH: Blunt cardiac injury and intraoperative hypoxaemia. *Can J Anaesth* 40:515-517, 1993

156. Werne C, Sagraves SG, Costa C: Mitral and tricuspid valve rupture from blunt trauma sustained during a motor vehicle collision. *J Trauma* 29:113-115, 1989

157. Pellegrini RV, Copeland CE, DiMarco RF, et al: Blunt rupture of both atrioventricular valves. *Ann Thorac Surg* 42:471-472, 1986

158. Brathwaite CE, Rodriguez A, Turney SZ, et al: Blunt traumatic cardiac rupture: a 5-year experience. *Ann Surg* 212:701-704, 1990

159. Mock CN, Campbell R, Burchard KW: Survival after blunt traumatic rupture of the left ventricle. *Am Surg* 56:561-565, 1990

160. McKeown PP, Rosemurgy A, Conant P: Blunt traumatic rupture of pulmonary vein, left atrium, and bronchus. *Ann Thorac Surg* 52:1171-1172, 1991

161. Savolainen HO, Jarvinen AA, Vihtonen KM: Left atrial rupture following blunt thoracic injury. Case report. *Scand J Thorac Cardiovasc Surg* 25:231-234, 1991

162. Wychulis AR, Connolly DC, McGoon DC: Surgical treatment of pericarditis. *J Thorac Cardiovasc Surg* 62:608-617, 1971

163. Pirzada FA, McDowell JW, Cohen EM, et al: Traumatic ventricular septal defect: sequential hemodynamic observations. *N Engl J Med* 291:892-895, 1974

164. Jenson BP, Hoffman I, Follis FM, et al: Surgical repair of atrial septal rupture due to blunt trauma. *Ann Thorac Surg* 56:1172-1174, 1993

165. Plenderleath D: Cited by Loop FD, Hofmeier G, Groves LK[37]

166. Leonard JJ, Harvey WP, Hufnagel CA: Cited by Chi S, Blair TC, Gonzalez-Lavin L[34]

167. German DS, Shapiro MJ, Willman VL: Acute aortic valvular incompetence following blunt thoracic deceleration injury: case report. *J Trauma* 30:1411-1412, 1990

168. Devineni R, McKenzie FN: Avulsion of a normal aortic valve cusp due to blunt chest injury. *J Trauma* 24:910-912, 1984

169. Reiland-Smith J, Weintraub RM, Sellke FW: Traumatic aortic valve injury sustained despite the deployment of an automobile air bag. *Chest* 103:1603, 1993

170. Haskins CD, Shapira N, Rahman E, et al: Repair of traumatic rupture of the aortic valve. *Arch Surg* 127:231-232, 1992

171. Bex JP, Grande A, Deveze JL: Traumatic aortic insufficiency (letter to the editor). *Ann Thorac Surg* 51:694-695, 1991

172. Ovil Y, Wahi R, Liu P, et al: Aortic valvoplasty for traumatic aortic insufficiency: a 2-year follow-up. *Ann Thorac Surg* 49:143-144, 1990

173. Kleikamp G, Schnepper U, Körtke H, et al: Tricuspid valve regurgitation following blunt thoracic trauma. *Chest* 102:1294-1296, 1992

174. Pasic M, von Segesser L, Carrel T, et al: Severe tricuspid regurgitation following blunt chest trauma: indication for emergency surgery. *Eur J Cardiothorac Surg* 6:455-457, 1992

175. Noera G, Sanguinetti M, Pensa P, et al: Tricuspid valve incompetence caused by nonpenetrating thoracic trauma. *Ann Thorac Surg* 51:320-322, 1991

176. Bayezid O, Mete A, Turkay C, et al: Traumatic tricuspid insufficiency following blunt chest trauma. *J Cardiovasc Surg* 34:69-71, 1993

177. Dontigny L, Baillot R, Panneton J, et al: Surgical repair of traumatic tricuspid insufficiency: report of three cases. *J Trauma* 33:266-269, 1992

178. Katz NM, Pallas RS: Traumatic rupture of the tricuspid valve: repair by chordal replacements and annuloplasty. *J Thorac Cardiovasc Surg* 91:310-314, 1986

179. van Son JA, Danielson GK, Schaff HV, et al: Traumatic tricuspid valve insufficiency. Experience in thirteen patients. *J Thorac Cardiovasc Surg* 108:893-898, 1994

180. Demetriades D, Charalambides C, Sareli P, et al: Late sequelae of penetrating cardiac injuries. *Br J Surg* 77:813-814, 1990

181. Sisto D, Hoffman D, Fernandes S, et al: Surgical correction of posttraumatic VSD via the right atrium. *Chest* 100:1316-1318, 1991

182. Nobre A, Sreeram N, McKay R: Traumatic ventricular septal defect: serial follow-up with Doppler ultrasound. *Int J Cardiol* 33:326-327, 1991
183. Cha EK, Mittal V, Allaben RD: Delayed sequelae of penetrating cardiac injury. *Arch Surg* 128:836-839, 1993
184. Bavaria JE, Miller JM, Josephson ME, et al: Endocardial resection in the treatment of ventricular tachycardia secondary to cardiac trauma. *J Cardiovasc Surg* 32:50-52, 1991
185. Kakos GS, Williams TE Jr, Kilman JW, et al: Traumatic left ventricular aneurysms after penetrating chest injury. *Ann Surg* 174:202-206, 1971
186. Aronstam EM, Strader LD, Geiger JP, et al: Traumatic left ventricular aneurysms. *J Thorac Cardiovasc Surg* 59:239-242, 1970
187. Xie SW, Picard MH: Two-dimensional and color Doppler echocardiographic diagnosis of penetrating missile wounds of the heart: chronic complications from intracardiac course of a bullet. *J Am Soc Echocardiogr* 5:81-84, 1992
188. Attar S, Suter CM, Hankins JR, et al: Penetrating cardiac injuries. *Ann Thorac Surg* 51:711-715, 1991
189. Mandal AK, Oparah SS: Unusually low mortality of penetrating wounds of the chest. Twelve years' experience. *J Thorac Cardiovasc Surg* 97:119-125, 1989
190. Knott-Craig CJ, Dalton RP, Rossouw GJ, et al: Penetrating cardiac trauma: management strategy based on 129 surgical emergencies over 2 years. *Ann Thorac Surg* 53:1006-1009, 1992
191. Kavolius J, Golocovsky M, Champion HR: Predictors of outcome in patients who have sustained trauma and who undergo emergency thoracotomy. *Arch Surg* 128:1158-1162, 1993
192. Böstman LA, Salo JA, Böstman OM: Stab wounds to the pericardium and heart: an analysis of 85 consecutive patients. *Eur J Surg* 158:271-275, 1992
193. Mitchell ME, Muakkassa FF, Poole GV, et al: Surgical approach of choice for penetrating cardiac wounds. *J Trauma* 34:17-20, 1993
194. Brathwaite CE, Weiss RL, Baldino WA, et al: Multichamber gunshot wounds of the heart: the utility of transesophageal echocardiography. *Chest* 101:287-288, 1992
195. Reeves WC, Movahed A, Chitwood WR, et al: Utility of precordial, epicardial and transesophageal two-dimensional echocardiography in the detection of intracardiac foreign bodies. *Am J Cardiol* 64:406-409, 1989
196. Freshman SP, Wisner DH, Weber CJ: 2-D echocardiography: emergent use in the evaluation of penetrating precordial trauma. *J Trauma* 31:902-905, 1991
197. Bolton JWR, Bynoe RP, Lazar HL, et al: Two-dimensional echocardiography in the evaluation of penetrating intrapericardial injuries. *Ann Thorac Surg* 56:506-509, 1993
198. Plummer D, Brunette D, Asinger R, et al: Emergency department echocardiography improves outcome in penetrating cardiac injury. *Ann Emerg Med* 21:709-712, 1992
199. Hartzler G: Percutaneous transvenous removal of a bullet embolus to the right ventricle. *J Thorac Cardiovasc Surg 80:153-155, 1980*

CHAPTER

58

Acquired diseases of the aorta

A. Thoracic aorta

Peter C. Spittell, M.D.

THE heart gives rise to the aorta and is continuous anatomically and functionally with it, yet the aorta itself is not a part of the heart. Although this book does not deal comprehensively with the vascular system as a separate entity, the intimacy between the heart and the aorta warrants inclusion of the following summary of acquired diseases affecting the thoracic aorta.

The location of the thoracic aorta within the chest accounts for several unique aspects of diseases affecting it:

1. They are commonly not diagnosed early.
2. They are often first recognized as a result of a finding on a chest radiograph.
3. They are confused at times with other, nonvascular, masses and neoplasms.[1,2]
4. Their protean manifestations are related to direct involvement of adjacent structures by the aortic disorder or the indirect involvement of various organ systems whose arterial blood supply arises from the thoracic aorta.

The organization of this chapter is based on the structural changes involving the aorta which give rise to the various clinical presentations. Within that framework, the various causes of acquired aortic disease are discussed. Preliminarily, however, a few general comments regarding the causes of aortic disease may be useful.

ETIOLOGIC FACTORS IN DISORDERS OF THE THORACIC AORTA

Acquired diseases of the thoracic aorta result from a broad spectrum of causes, which include aging, atherosclerosis, hypertension, inflammation, infection, degenerative changes, trauma, and neoplasia.

Aging

Like that of all arteries, the wall of the thoracic aorta consists of endothelium, a basement membrane, elastic and collagen fibers, and smooth muscle (Fig 58A-1). By virtue of the large amount of elastic tissue in the media, the thoracic aorta and its major branches are adapted to receiving (they distend with systole) and transmitting (they recoil during diastole) the pulsatile blood flow from left ventricular ejection. With aging, the intima and media thicken, the internal elastic lamella degenerates, and the circumference of the aorta increases;[3,4] there is gradual disruption of elastic lamellae and degeneration of smooth muscle in the media,[5] with resultant loss of elasticity. This aging process is best considered a "physiologic arteriosclerosis," representing more an adaptive type of response of the vessel wall to hemodynamic stress[6] than a forerunner of atherosclerosis.

Atherosclerosis

This widespread entity is characterized by the accumulation in the intima of lipid and carbohydrate, with resulting fibrosis and calcification[7] (see chapter 28A).

Hypertension

Hypertension accelerates both the aging process and atherosclerosis. Hypertension is also common in patients with penetrating aortic ulcer.[8] Furthermore, hypertension appears to be the dominant etiologic factor in most cases of aortic dissection,[9] although degenerative changes superimposed on congenital structural deficiency (the Marfan syndrome) and arteritis may account for some.

Inflammation

Certain of the systemic arteritides may involve the thoracic aorta or its major branches.

Infection

Infection in the thoracic aorta is of two main types: mycotic aneurysm and syphilitic aortitis. The aorta is the artery most often involved by mycotic aneurysms (Fig 58A-2), the favored site being the root and ascending aorta in the classic study by Stengel and Wolferth.[10] In syphilis, arterial involvement is a late manifestation, and the ascending and arch portions of the aorta are the most commonly involved sites.

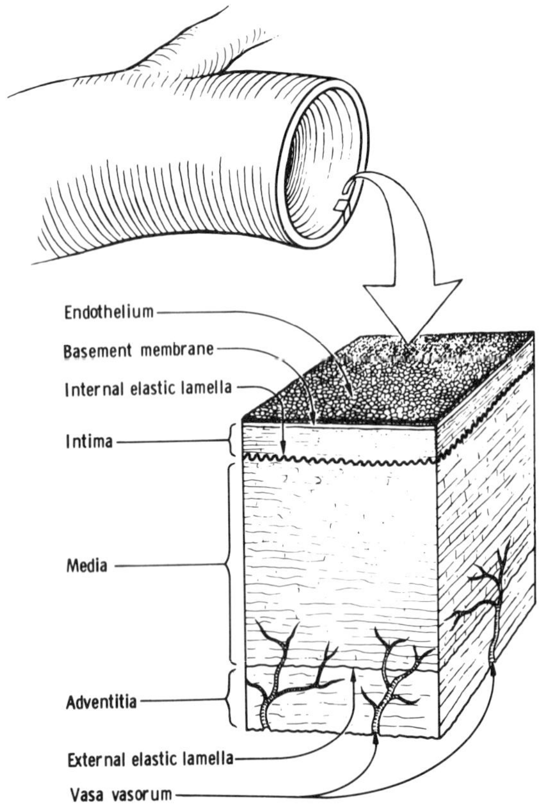

Fig 58A-1 Schematic drawing of the structural organization of the vascular wall. (From Lie JT: The structure of the normal vascular system and its reactive changes. In *Allen-Barker-Hines Peripheral Vascular Diseases.* Fifth edition. Edited by JL Juergens, JA Spittell Jr, JF Fairbairn II. Philadelphia, WB Saunders Company, 1980, pp 51-81. By permission, Mayo Foundation.)

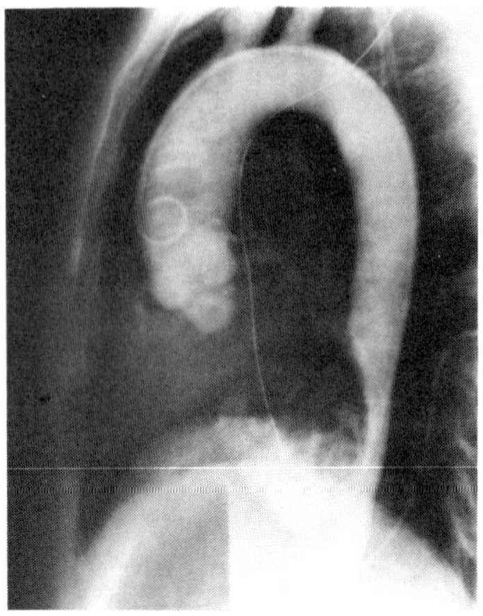

Fig 58A-2 Thoracic aortogram demonstrating mycotic aneurysm of the descending aorta.

Trauma

Although penetrating wounds and invasive angiographic procedures can traumatize the thoracic aorta, the most frequent trauma is that associated with sudden deceleration resulting in laceration at the isthmus.

Neoplasia

Primary neoplasms of the thoracic aorta are rare and are seldom diagnosed ante mortem. They are most frequently sarcomas and when symptomatic can give rise to occlusive disease of the thoracic aorta or be a source for arterial emboli.[11]

CLINICAL PRESENTATION OF AORTIC DISEASE

The structural changes and, hence, the clinical presentations of aortic disease include occlusive disease, aneurysmal disease, aortic dissection, penetrating aortic ulcer, traumatic rupture, and nonstenosing aortitis.

Occlusive disease

Atherosclerosis. Occlusive disease of the thoracic aorta is uncommon, because atherosclerosis, the principal cause of occlusive arterial disease, involves the thoracic aorta to a much lesser degree than it does the abdominal aorta and the arteries of the lower extremities. The principal changes due to atherosclerosis seen in the thoracic aorta are tortuosity and diffuse dilatation. Any occlusive disease involves the origin of some branches of the arch, principally the left subclavian and occasionally the innominate artery, and this involvement commonly is asymptomatic.

In some patients, atherosclerotic occlusion of the origin of the left or right subclavian artery may cause intermittent claudication of the arm of sufficient degree to warrant surgical treatment. Of greater import, however, is complete occlusion of the origin of either subclavian artery. Collateral blood flow to the arm may be derived principally from the cerebral circulation via reversed flow through the ipsilateral vertebral artery—so-called subclavian steal. This results in episodes of transient cerebral ischemia, especially when the ipsilateral arm is exercised. A similar situation may occur on the right side if the obstruction occurs at the origin of the innominate artery, in which case flow in the right carotid artery can "reverse" to enter the right subclavian artery. In addition to the symptoms of transient cerebral ischemia, physical signs of this condition include reduced arm and wrist pulses and reduced blood pressure on the affected side. The astute examiner, when palpating both radial arterial pulses simultaneously, may also detect a delay in pulsation on the affected side.[12]

Acquired coarctation of the thoracic aorta due to focally obstructive calcific atherosclerotic disease is rare but has been reported.[13] Patients who have symptoms present with upper extremity hypertension and reduced blood pressure in the lower extremities, with or without intermittent claudication.

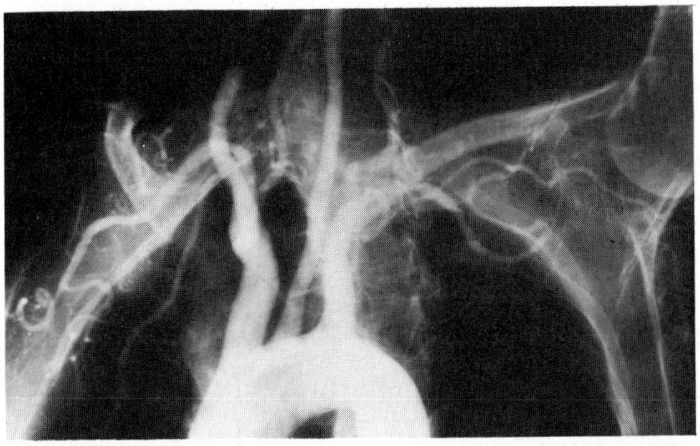

Fig 58A-3 Arch aortogram in 71-year-old woman with giant cell arteritis who presented with a complaint of bilateral arm claudication and had no detectable pulses in either arm. Angiographic findings are occlusion of both axillary arteries and stenotic segments in subclavian arteries. Takayasu's arteritis can look similar but occurs in a younger age group. Arteriosclerosis can be difficult to distinguish from giant cell arteritis. (From Fulton RE, Stanson AW, Forbes GS, et al: Vascular imaging: angiography, ultrasound, and computed tomography. In *Allen-Barker-Hines Peripheral Vascular Diseases.* Fifth edition. Edited by JL Juergens, JA Spittell Jr, JF Fairbairn II. Philadelphia, WB Saunders Company, 1980, pp 139-215. By permission, Mayo Foundation.)

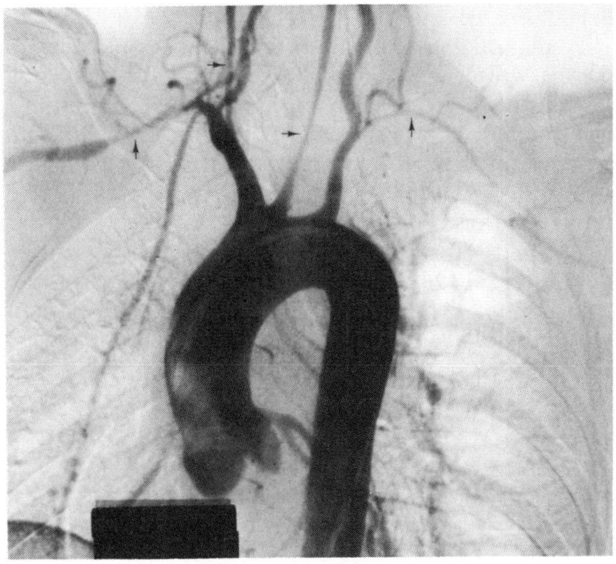

Fig 58A-4 Arch aortogram in 28-year-old woman with Takayasu's disease (idiopathic medial aortopathy and arteriopathy). Note severe narrowing of both common carotid arteries (*horizontal arrows*) and both subclavian arteries (*vertical arrows*). The left axillary artery is occluded in mid-course. (From Sheps SG, McDuffie FC: Vasculitis. In *Allen-Barker-Hines Peripheral Vascular Diseases.* Fifth edition. Edited by JL Juergens, JA Spittell Jr, JF Fairbairn II. Philadelphia, WB Saunders Company, 1980, pp 493-553. By permission, Mayo Foundation.)

Giant cell arteritis. The dominant clinical symptom of giant cell arteritis (formerly called "temporal arteritis" or "cranial arteritis") is usually headache; the most frequent and dreaded complication is blindness. The dominant physical finding is prominent, inflamed, or tender temporal arteries. Significant involvement of the aorta and large arteries has been recognized with increasing frequency.

Giant cell arteritis is a subacute or chronic inflammatory process with local and systemic manifestations. It is generally seen in persons older than 55 years, and it is about twice as common in women as in men. Involvement of the thoracic aorta and its branches may be minimal and asymptomatic, but when it is more extensive it can result in occlusion of one or more branches of the aortic arch,[14,15] dilatation or saccular aneurysm of the aorta,[16] or even aortic dissection.[17]

Diagnosis is typically made by biopsy of the superficial temporal artery. However, angiography is useful in confirming the diagnosis of aortic involvement and in differentiating this disorder from atherosclerotic occlusion. The ascending aorta may be dilated, and there may be thickening of its wall; involvement of branches of the arch, when present, is often bilateral, with segmental areas of smooth, tapered arterial occlusion in the absence of atherosclerotic changes (Fig 58A-3).

Management of the patient with aortic or large-artery involvement by giant cell arteritis is principally by administration of corticosteroids in adequate doses (beginning with 45 to 60 mg of prednisone daily) to suppress the arteritis. Arterial changes are reversible with adequate therapy, but when corticosteroid therapy has been insufficient to suppress the universally elevated erythrocyte sedimentation rate, there may be progressive involvement of the aorta and resultant dissection or rupture.[17]

Takayasu's disease. This disorder, also called "pulseless disease" and "idiopathic medial aortopathy and arteriopathy," is also a syndrome of arteritis of the aorta and its branches. In contrast to patients with giant cell arteritis, most of those with this type of arteritis are younger than 40; it also occurs more commonly in women—more than 80% of cases.

Many, but not all, patients have an early subacute phase with nonspecific systemic symptoms. The disease often goes unrecognized until the signs and symptoms of the occlusive arterial phase develop. The clinical manifestations of occlusion may include cerebrovascular insufficiency, arterial insufficiency of the upper or lower extremities, or mesenteric insufficiency, depending on the location of the aortitis and arteritis. Hypertension is very common; it occurs as a result of acquired aortic coarctation or involvement of the renal arteries by the arteritis.

Aortography is of great value in the diagnosis of Takayasu's disease. Segmental narrowing of a variable length of descending or abdominal aorta or narrowing of the origin of major branches of the aorta (Fig 58A-4) occurs as a result of thickening of the aorta or arterial wall. This usually allows distinction of Takayasu's disease from other causes of the aortic arch syndrome.[18] Although aneurysmal dilatation of the thoracic aorta can occur in Takayasu's disease,[19,20] it is not common or distinctive in this disorder.

Therapy with corticosteroids, sometimes combined with anticoagulant therapy, is effective for patients in the early phase of the disease in controlling systemic symptoms and return of pulses. For the patient in the later occlusive phase, surgical treatment to bypass the obstruction may be indicated to relieve hypertension caused by the acquired coarctation or renal artery stenosis.[21] Similarly, other occlusive arterial lesions may require surgical treatment for relief of ischemic manifestations.[16]

Aneurysmal disease

Etiology. Being mainly atherosclerotic, thoracic aortic aneurysms are more common in men than in women and occur most often in the sixth and seventh decades of life. Another important cause of thoracic aortic aneurysm which may be overlooked is trauma associated with incomplete aortic rupture in sudden deceleration (to be discussed later). Aneurysmal dilatation of the ascending aorta is a well-known clinical event in patients with the Marfan syndrome. In this condition, a number of abnormalities of the aortic media, including defective organization of collagen[22] and accumulation of mucopolysaccharide,[23] probably account for the loss of strength and resulting dilatation of the aorta. Perhaps less appreciated is the condition termed "annuloaortic ectasia" by Ellis et al.[24] It is characterized by dilatation of the aortic root in patients (the majority of them men) without other stigmas of the Marfan syndrome. These patients typically have aortic regurgitation and are prone to aortic dissection and sudden death.[25] Dilatation of the aortic root causing severe aortic regurgitation has been observed in some patients, apparently resulting only from associated systemic hypertension.[26] Aortitis associated with a number of conditions, including giant cell and Takayasu's arteritis, rheumatoid arthritis and ankylosing spondylitis, Behçet's disease, relapsing polychondritis, and Reiter's syndrome, can cause dilatation of the aorta, usually in the root and ascending portion, which results at times in associated aortic valve regurgitation.[18] The aorta is also the most common site of infectious arteritis and mycotic aneurysm.[7]

Pathogenesis. Whatever the underlying cause, the development of an aneurysm is related to weakening of the media of the artery. Once dilatation begins, the enlargement tends to be progressive, because the lateral pressure increases with widening of the lumen and slowing of flow (Bernoulli theorem). Furthermore, wall tension at constant arterial pressure increases with increasing diameter (Laplace's law).[27] Systemic hypertension enhances aneurysm formation.[28] Commonly, aneurysms contain laminated mural thrombus (Fig 58A-5), which, although it may retard enlargement, may also embolize to various regions of the distal arterial circulation.

At the cellular level, subtle defects in collagen and elastin, combined with an accelerated breakdown of these molecules by an increase in proteolytic enzyme activity or a decrease in the levels of protease inhibitors (or both), may play a significant role in the formation of aortic aneurysms.[29]

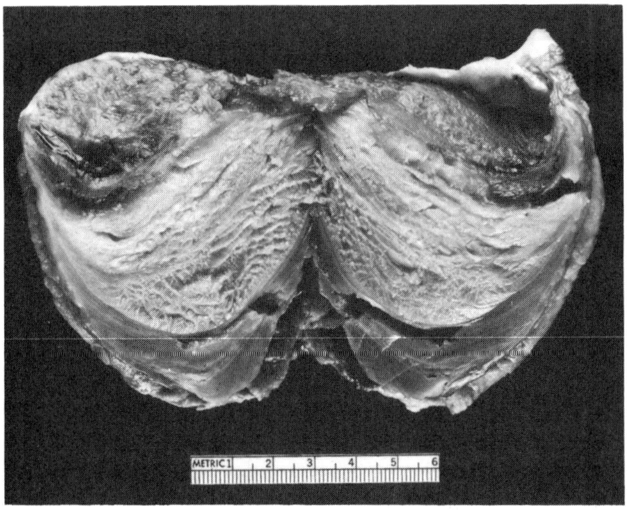

Fig 58A-5 Resected thoracic aortic aneurysm containing laminated thrombus. (From Spittell JA Jr: Some practical clinical aspects of aneurysms. *GP* 32 No. 1:78-85, 1965. By permission of the American Academy of Family Physicians.)

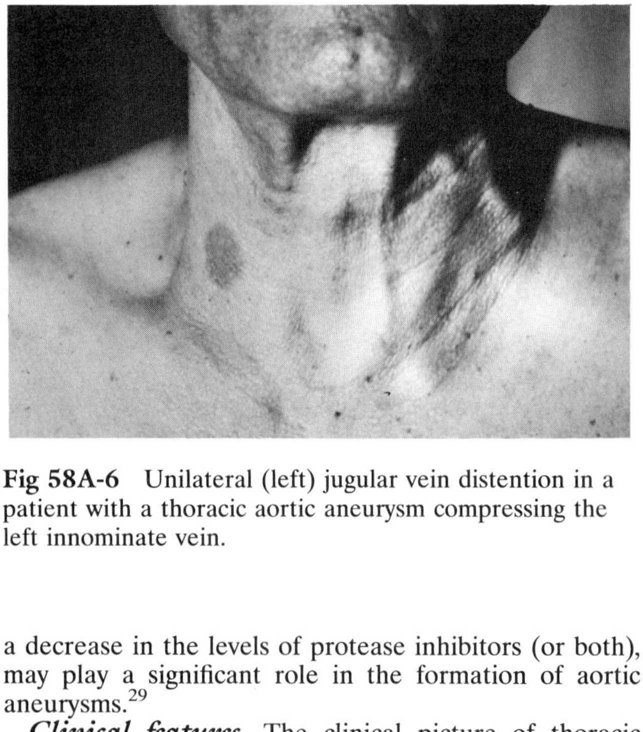

Fig 58A-6 Unilateral (left) jugular vein distention in a patient with a thoracic aortic aneurysm compressing the left innominate vein.

Clinical features. The clinical picture of thoracic aortic aneurysm is quite variable. Most aneurysms are asymptomatic, being discovered on the chest radiograph at the time of examination for another purpose.[30,31] When symptoms develop, the aneurysm is usually large enough to encroach on surrounding structures and cause back pain, dyspnea, dysphagia, cough, hoarseness, or stridor.

Commonly, aneurysms cause no physical signs, but when there is venous compression (Fig 58A-6), compression of other structures (e.g., fixation of a vocal cord), or

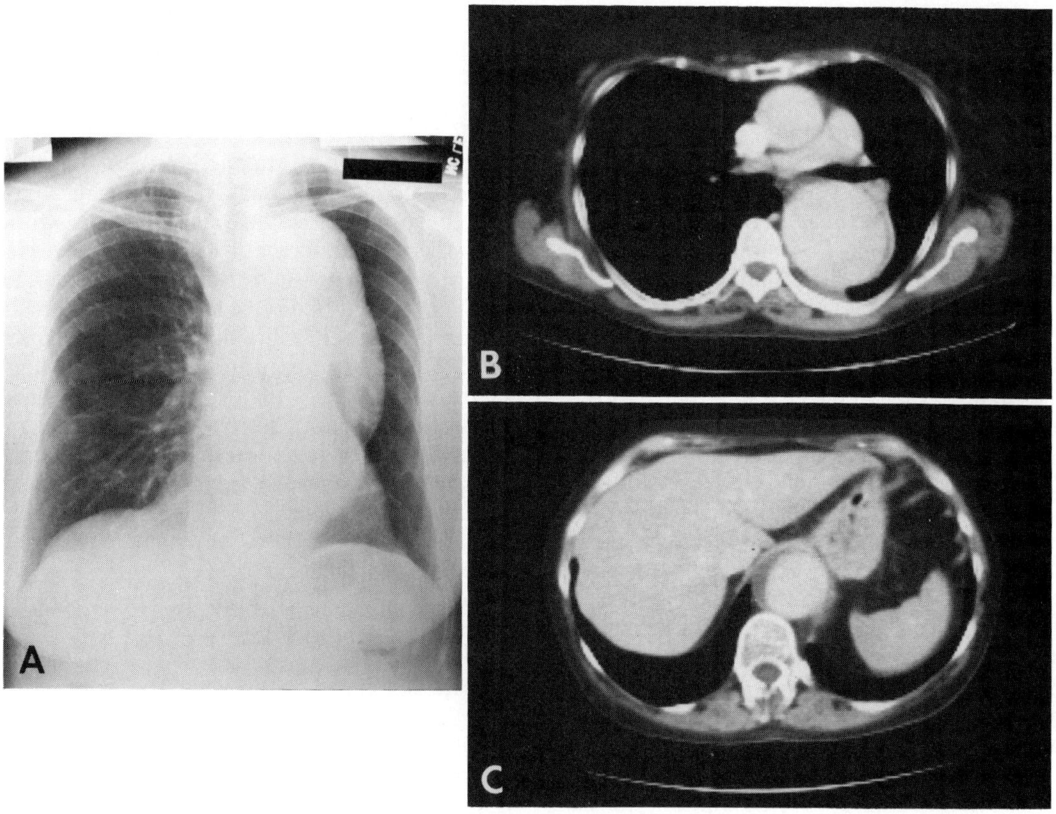

Fig 58A-7 **A,** chest radiograph demonstrating large thoracic aortic aneurysm which caused distention of the left external jugular vein and pulsation of the entire left anterior chest wall. **B,** computed tomography scan with contrast enhancement in same patient demonstrates a normal-caliber ascending aorta anteriorly and the aneurysm extending from about the level of the left subclavian artery to below the level of the diaphragm (**C**), where thrombus is evident in the right side of the aneurysm.

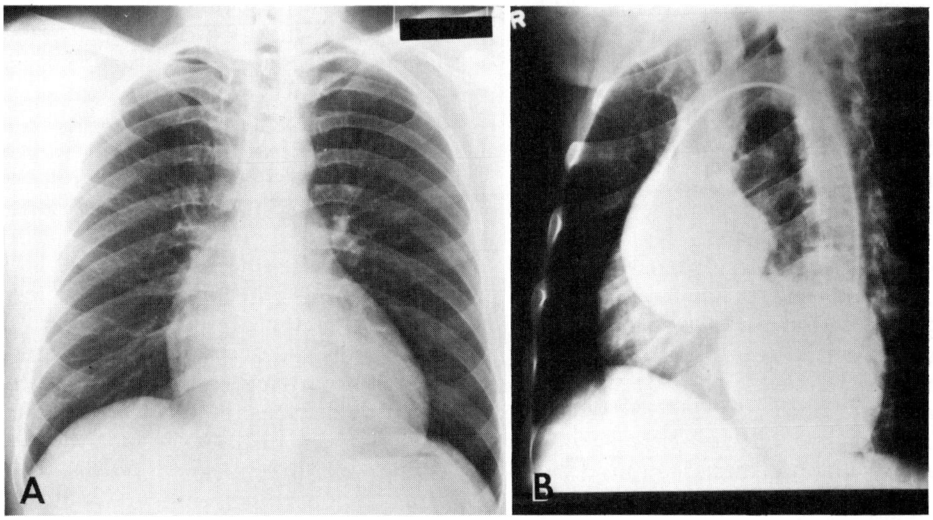

Fig 58A-8 Chest radiograph (**A**) and thoracic aortogram (**B**) of an ascending aortic aneurysm. (From Spittell JA Jr: Clinical aspects of aneurysmal disease. *Curr Probl Cardiol* 5 No 5:1-36, 1980. By permission of Year Book Medical Publishers.)

encroachment on the chest wall (Fig 58A-7), corresponding findings may be noted.

Radiologic features. On a plain radiograph, an aneurysm appears as a rounded or smooth density in the central portion of the chest, if it is not obscured by other structures (Fig 58A-8,A). Unless there is calcification in its wall, the aneurysm may be difficult to differentiate from intrathoracic tumor in the central chest or from simple elongation and torsion of the aorta.

Aortography has been the classic method to diagnose thoracic aortic aneurysms (Fig 58A-8,B), but computed tomography, particularly with intravenous contrast media enhancement, has become the standard imaging procedure (Fig 58A-7,B and C). Computed tomography is more sensitive than plain radiographs and angiography for detecting intimal calcification and intraluminal thrombus.[32,33] Magnetic resonance imaging and transthoracic and transesophageal two-dimensional echocardiography are also able to establish the diagnosis of thoracic aortic aneurysm.[34-37]

Prognosis. Factors that seem to worsen the prognosis are diastolic hypertension, large aneurysm (greater than 6 cm in diameter), and associated coronary and cerebrovascular disease.

Management. Because of the poor prognosis for the untreated patient with a thoracic aortic aneurysm, surgical treatment is justified, unless associated conditions contraindicate an operation. Based on the studies of natural history,[30,31] the following would seem to be reasonable indications for surgical treatment:

1. An aneurysm that is symptomatic.
2. An aneurysm with a diameter of 6 cm or greater.
3. An aneurysm enlarging under observation.
4. An aneurysm in a person with systemic hypertension.

The surgical approach to the repair of an aortic aneurysm depends on its location and extent. Special problems attend operations on the thoracic aorta compared with operations on the infrarenal aorta. Neither the ascending nor the arch portion of the aorta should be cross-clamped for repair of an aneurysm without the use of heart-lung bypass, adjunctive hypothermia, and myocardial protection. Even cross-clamping of the aorta at a point just distal to the left subclavian artery involves a substantial risk (4% to 18%)[38] of inducing severe ischemia of the spinal cord with resultant postoperative irreversible paraplegia. Attempts to reduce the incidence of spinal cord ischemia, including systemic hypothermia, rapid repair, temporary aortic shunt bypass, femorofemoral extracorporeal circulation, intrathecal papaverine, and left atrial-to-distal arterial aortic bypass, have been used with limited success. Risk factors for spinal cord ischemia or infarction include female sex and intraoperative hypotension (mean arterial pressure below 55 mm Hg).[39]

In general, fusiform aneurysms are opened and stripped clean of thrombus and atherosclerotic intima, after which an aortic vascular prosthesis is sutured to the luminal aspect of the proximal and distal nonaneurysmal aorta. The less common saccular aneurysm is usually transected at its neck, and aortic integrity is reconstituted by direct suturing or by a patch of vascular graft material. If aortic annular dilatation results from proximal extension of the aortic aneurysm, thus causing aortic valvular regurgitation, repair is effected by one of two methods. Either the valve and ascending aorta are replaced separately, the narrow rim of aortic root from which the coronary arteries arise being allowed to remain, or a composite graft is attached proximally at the annulus, after resection of the natural valve, and attached distally just beyond the aneurysm.[40,41] The composite graft consists of a replacement aortic valve that is inserted into the proximal end of a tubular aortic vascular crimped-fabric graft. In the use of such a composite graft, buttons of the aortic wall containing the coronary ostia must be implanted into appropriately placed windows in the proximal portion of the graft. For aneurysms that extend to involve the aortic arch, the graft being inserted for repair is incised for a few centimeters along its convexity, and the arch vessels are implanted into this window, usually as a single button of aorta containing the ostia of all three arch branches.[42] For operations of the type just described, protection of the brain must be provided, either by profound hypothermia or by separate perfusion of the cerebral circulation through special cannulation of carotid arteries.[42]

With technical improvements, including myocardial and cerebral protection, avoidance of air embolism, preclotting of fabric grafts, and use of improved suture materials, the risk of these seemingly formidable procedures has been reduced to rather satisfactory levels—namely, in the range of 3% to 10%, depending on the size and location of the aneurysm and the general condition of the patient.

Aortic dissection

Etiology. The exact cause of aortic dissection is not known, but multiple factors may be involved. It now appears that cystic medial necrosis—formerly considered the prerequisite for aortic dissection—is not the underlying cause;[43] furthermore, the histopathologic changes seen in these patients do not differ from those in the aortas of age-matched controls.[44] Investigations suggest that the changes commonly seen in the media of otherwise normal persons result from a process of injury and repair consequent to hemodynamic forces.[43,45]

The above views are consonant with those of Roberts,[9] who expressed the belief that systemic hypertension, which is present in as many as 70% of patients with aortic dissection, has a direct weakening effect on the arterial media and is a common denominator, although not the sole cause, of dissection. The high frequency of aortic dissection in the presence of coarctation of the aorta supports the causative role of hypertension. The adverse effect of hypertension on the vasa vasorum could have an added deleterious influence on the nutrition of the media.[46]

Other etiologic factors in aortic dissection are suggested by its occurrence in a number of different conditions that affect the aorta. It is commonly believed that structural aortic wall abnormalities seen in the Marfan syndrome result in the complication of aortic dissection. However, Roberts[9] questioned this, and he found normal histologic features of the aorta in all three of his patients with the Marfan syndrome who had suffered aortic dissection, and these patients had hypertension. In the Marfan syndrome, the histopathologic changes in the aorta have not been found to differ from those seen in controls.[44,45] In fact, Roberts believes it inappropriate to consider that the intimal and medial tears in the wall of an aortic root aneurysm accompanying the Marfan syndrome are indicative of true longitudinal aortic dissection. From these observations, it appears that the aortic aneurysms and root aneurysms seen in the Marfan syndrome and, perhaps, in other heritable connective tissue disorders affecting the aorta are due to a biochemical derangement that is not manifested by histologic alterations. Findings of chemical abnormalities of collagen in the Ehlers-Danlos syndrome[47,48] and the Marfan syndrome[22] which mimic those found in certain animals fed lathyrogens or copper-deficient diets[23] support the likelihood of an underlying metabolic aberration.

Stanson et al.[8] and Hussain et al.[49] described the precipitation of intramedial thoracic aortic dissection via ulceration of atheromatous plaques that extend through the intima and into the media (Fig 58A-9). They termed this lesion "penetrating aortic ulcer" to distinguish it from classic aortic dissection.

Although the event is uncommon, aortic dissection may complicate arteritis, notably giant cell arteritis.[17] The fact that the cellular infiltrate, muscle fiber necrosis, and fragmentation of elastic fibers of the media are seen mainly in the ascending aorta,[44] the usual location of the site of dissection, suggests that the location of the arteritis is a factor in the dissection.

An unusual association, perhaps related to abnormal hemodynamics and wall stresses in the ascending aorta, is the increased incidence of aortic dissection in patients having a congenitally bicuspid or unicommissural aortic valve.[50-52]

Whether an endocrine factor is involved in the cause of some cases of aortic dissection is not clear. A slightly increased incidence of aortic dissection in pregnancy has been reported. Etiologic factors such as hypertension,[9] coarctation, or connective tissue disorder[53] have not always been identified for each patient having dissection.

A rare cause of aortic dissection is trauma, either direct, such as that associated with intra-aortic balloon pumping[54] or arterial cannulation during cardiac operation,[55] or indirect, as a result of sudden deceleration. In the latter case, the tear is usually located in the region of the aortic isthmus.

Pathogenesis. The traditional and logical explanation for the development of aortic dissection is that a transverse tear develops in the intima and inner layer of the media of the aorta; this defect produces a flap, which traps the pulsatile flow of blood beneath it, and this is followed by longitudinal tearing of the aortic wall through its media. Thus, an inner intima-medial layer is separated

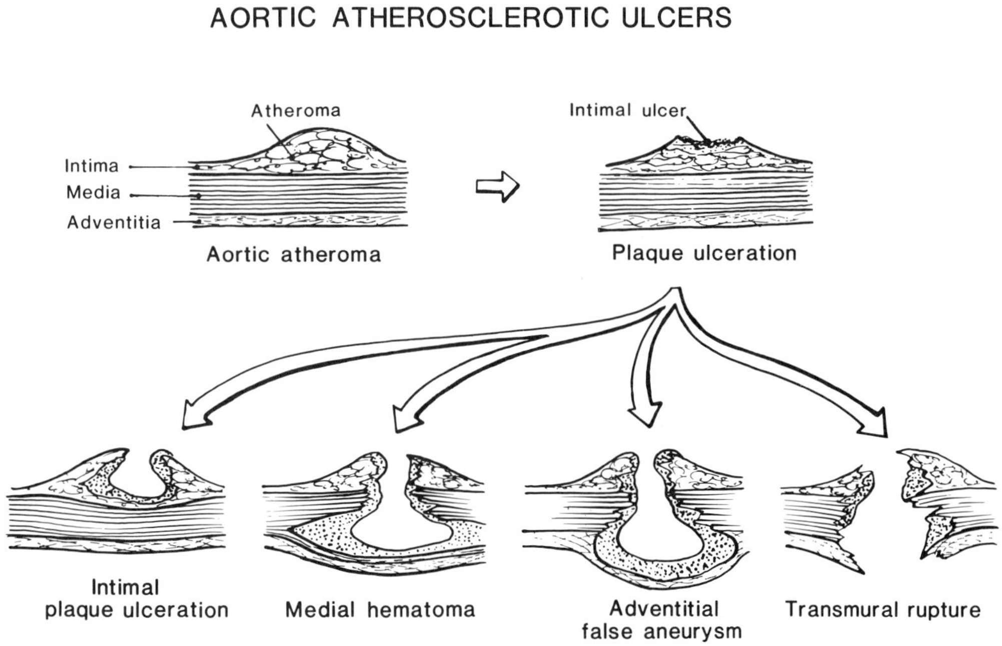

Fig 58A-9 Evolution of penetrating aortic ulcer. Ulcerated atheroma may extend into the media and expose it to pulsatile aortic flow. Extension of ulcer into the media may precipitate a medial hematoma (localized dissection), pseudoaneurysm, or transmural rupture. Ulcer crater may become filled with thrombus and result in considerable underestimation of the involved aortic segment. (From Stanson AW, Kazmier FJ, Hollier LH, et al: Penetrating atherosclerotic ulcers of the thoracic aorta: natural history and clinicopathologic correlations. *Ann Vasc Surg* 1:15-23, 1986. By permission.)

by liquid or clotted blood from an outer media-adventitial layer, but the dissection is not typically circumferential in the aorta; it usually spares a strip of ascending and arch portions of the aorta on its concave aspect and the posterior strip of descending thoracic aorta from which the intercostal arteries arise. It is not clear at present, however, whether the intimal tear is the primary event or is secondary to the development of an intramural hematoma in the media. The intimal tear is most often located in the ascending aorta, less often in the descending aorta, and infrequently in the transverse arch of the aorta. The increased frequency of the intimal tear in the ascending aorta may be related to the greater fixation of this portion of the aorta and to its greater hemodynamic stresses.

Once initiated, the dissection may extend proximally or distally in the aorta or in both directions. When the dissection encounters branches of the aorta, it may occlude them, extend into their walls, or pass around their origins. The dissection may rupture through the external layer at any point, or it may rupture back into the aortic lumen and create a second communication between the false and true lumens. Rupture of the external layer into a body cavity or space is the most common cause of death in aortic dissection; congestive heart failure, usually due to aortic regurgitation, is the second most common cause.

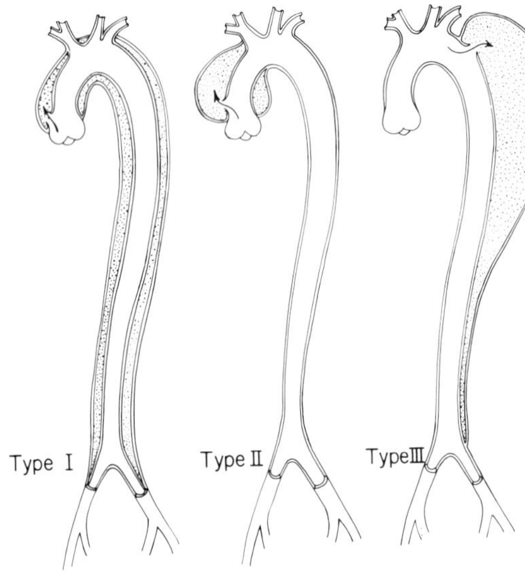

Fig 58A-10 Classification of aortic dissection: type I, primary tear in ascending aorta and dissection involving the aortic arch and distal aorta for a variable distance; type II, dissection involving only the ascending aorta; type III, primary tear in the subclavian artery and extending distally for a variable distance. Others classify aortic dissection into only two types, those involving the ascending aorta (types I and II above) and those originating in the descending aorta (type III above). (Modified from De Bakey ME, Henly WS, Cooley DA, et al: Surgical management of dissecting aneurysms of the aorta. *J Thorac Cardiovasc Surg* 49:130-148, 1965.)

The classification of aortic dissection originally proposed by De Bakey et al.[56] (Fig 58A-10) has been useful for those who deal with aortic dissection. The primary tear in more than 95% of cases is located in one of two locations: either in the ascending aorta a few centimeters above the aortic valve (type I or II) or just distal to the origin of the left subclavian artery in the descending thoracic aorta (type III). For practical purposes, since types I and II have a similar prognosis, there are really two types—those with the tear in the ascending aorta and those with the tear in the descending aorta, also called "proximal" and "distal," respectively, by some.[57] To cover the unusual situation in which a dissection beginning in the descending aorta dissects retrogradely to involve the ascending aorta, Dailey et al.[58] classified proximal dissections as type A and distal dissections without proximal extension as type B.

Clinical features. A cardinal maxim when a patient is encountered who has chest pain is to always consider the diagnosis of aortic dissection. Aortic dissection is usually a catastrophic illness, and it is associated with clinical findings of ischemia involving various organ systems, singly or in various combinations, and of cardiac disease. Often, the clinical findings will change as the dissection progresses.

Aortic dissection is two to three times more common in men than in women, and it usually occurs between the ages of 40 and 70 years.

The pain of aortic dissection is typically sudden in onset, severe, and described as "ripping" or "tearing." It usually begins in the chest, either anteriorly or posteriorly, and extends down the back to the hips and lower extremities if the dissection extends distally. At times the pain begins in the epigastrium or in an unusual location such as the neck, head, or shoulders.

On examination, the patient with acute aortic dissection often appears pale and sweaty, as if in shock, but has moderate or even severe hypertension. Hypertension, it should be emphasized, is the most common finding in aortic dissection. Other cardiovascular findings include tachycardia, murmurs, friction rubs, bruits, changes in arterial pulses, and, on occasion, venous distention.

Cardiac murmurs are usually heard at the base of the heart and may be systolic or diastolic or both. A diastolic murmur of aortic regurgitation indicates involvement of the ascending aorta. Pericardial friction rub is infrequent, but when present in the patient with aortic dissection, it is an ominous sign indicating involvement of the root of the aorta or leakage of blood into the pericardial sac. Systolic bruits may be heard over partially occluded arteries. Diminished or absent pulses in one or more extremities may be noted, and at times severe ischemia of an arm or leg is seen in the patient with acute aortic dissection.[59,60]

In 40% or more of patients with aortic dissection, there are neurologic findings varying from syncope to focal weakness due to involvement of the circulation to the brain or spinal cord.[61]

If the dissection has extended into the abdominal aorta, the aorta is usually tender and may be enlarged to palpation. On rare occasions, pressure on mediastinal structures by the enlarged thoracic aorta may cause hoarseness, dysphagia, or venous distention, even to the point of superior vena caval obstruction. The venous distention is uniquely pulseless because of the caval obstruction, or it may involve only the left arm and cervical regions if the left innominate vein alone is occluded.

There is no typical pattern of clinical laboratory findings in acute aortic dissection. The most common electrocardiographic finding is left ventricular hypertrophy as a result of systemic hypertension. Arrhythmias of any type may be seen but are not common. The picture of myocardial ischemia or infarction may occur when the dissection involves the coronary ostia, and if there has been leakage of blood into the pericardium, the electrocardiogram can show changes suggestive of pericarditis.

From the foregoing, it is not surprising that the diagnosis of aortic dissection can be elusive. In our experience it has been misdiagnosed most often as acute myocardial infarction, cerebrovascular accident, acute isolated peripheral arterial occlusion, and acute abdominal conditions.[62,63] In a recent review, a correct initial clinical impression of aortic dissection was made in 62% of patients overall, a finding emphasizing the need for continued improvement in the prompt recognition of this potentially lethal disease.[64]

The availability of effective therapy has made it more important not only that the diagnosis be made promptly but also that the location of the primary intimal tear be determined. Finding the site of the tear usually requires contrast angiography, but certain clinical findings strongly suggest involvement of the ascending aorta (Table 58A-1), which usually means that the primary intimal tear is also located there.

Roentgenography and other imaging. Developments in the diagnosis of aortic dissection have been exceedingly rapid in recent years. The most common findings on the chest radiograph are abnormalities in the region of the aortic knob,[65] including an increase in diameter (Fig 58A-11)—a double density due to superimposition of the enlarged aorta and deviation of the trachea toward the right. However, the chest radiograph may show no suggestive findings in 20% of cases, so a normal chest radiograph does not exclude aortic dissection. Chest radiographs are of the greatest help when previous films are available and comparison demonstrates an increase in the size of the aortic shadow (see Fig 58A-11).

The detection of aortic dissection by echocardiography has been reported by a number of investigators since 1972. With the evolution of two-dimensional echocardiography, the value of this noninvasive procedure as a screening method for the detection of dissection of the ascending aorta and aortic arch is established.[66,67] The introduction

Table 58A-1 Clinical features suggesting type I or type II dissecting aneurysm

Initial pain in anterior chest
Decreased or absent pulses and blood pressure in right arm
Decreased right carotid artery pulsation
Aortic diastolic murmur
Pericardial friction rub
Evidence of myocardial ischemia or infarction on electrocardiogram

From Spittell JA Jr: Clinical aspects of aneurysmal disease. *Curr Probl Cardiol* 5 No 5:1-36, 1980. By permission of Year Book Medical Publishers.

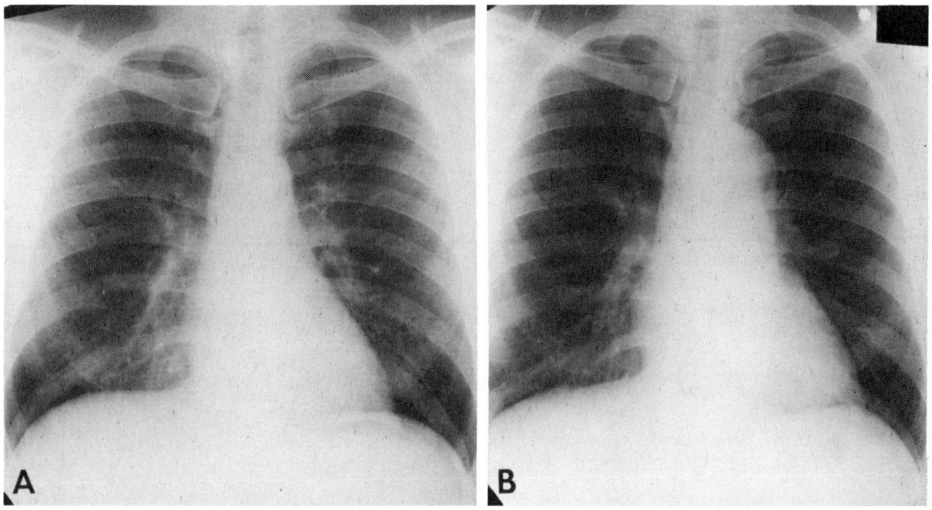

Fig 58A-11 Chest radiographs of a patient with an acute dissecting aneurysm. Film **A** was taken 20 months before the event. Film **B** was taken at the time of acute dissection and shows widening of the supracardiac aortic shadow. (From Spittell JA Jr, Wallace RB: Aortic dissection. *Am Fam Physician* 1 No 3:89-98, 1970. By permission of the American Academy of Family Physicians.)

of transesophageal echocardiography has enhanced the diagnostic value of echocardiography for the detection of aortic dissection in any part of the aorta.[68,69] With the addition of color-flow Doppler imaging, the true and false lumens are readily identified. Indeed, in a multicenter study,[68] the accuracy of transthoracic, suprasternal, and transesophageal echocardiography in the detection of aortic dissection was equal to that of computed tomography. The more recent introduction of biplane transesophageal echocardiography has further improved the specificity of this modality in the detection of aortic dissection, especially in the evaluation of ascending aortic involvement.[70] The availability of this procedure for rapid bedside examination without the risks associated with the use of contrast material and ionizing radiation makes it likely that it will become the standard for assessing aortic dissection.[71,72]

Computed tomography with intravenous injection of contrast medium has likewise been used with success in the diagnosis of aortic dissection.[73] Although quite reliable for demonstrating the dissection, computed tomography has the limitations of not demonstrating sites of reentry in the lower thoracic and abdominal aorta, aortic regurgitation, or involvement of branches of the aorta. In addition, computed tomography tends to miss involvement of the ascending aorta by dissection, a failing that could have serious clinical consequences in view of the success of surgery in this condition.[74]

With magnetic resonance imaging, the entire aorta can be visualized without the need for contrast media. Intimal flaps, differential flow in the true and false lumens, and thrombus formation in the false lumen are readily identified. In addition, magnetic resonance imaging demonstrates the site of entry to a dissection and associated aortic regurgitation.[75] Where available, this procedure may replace aortography in some patients.[37]

Aortography (Fig 58A-12) has been, and still is in some centers, the definitive diagnostic procedure in aortic dissection, although even it may occasionally fail to demonstrate a false lumen or an intimal flap. The diagnostic aortographic features are opacification of the false lumen, deformity of the true lumen by the false lumen, widening of the aorta, narrowing or occlusion of branches of the aorta, and presence of an intimal flap. For the present, aortography remains the procedure of choice to demonstrate involvement of branch vessels.

Prognosis. In most studies of untreated patients, 70% die in the first 2 weeks after onset of the dissection, and of those who survive the acute phase, one-half or more will die in the ensuing year.[76] The most common cause of death is rupture of the outer layer of the aorta, with exsanguination. Reentry of the false channel into the aortic lumen (formerly considered "healing") is no protection against fatal rupture of the dissection.[76] In general, younger patients, patients without hypertension or other cardiovascular disease, and patients with the primary tear in the descending aorta have a better prognosis than older and hypertensive patients and those with dissection of the ascending aorta.

Management. Ideally, in the patient suffering an acute aortic dissection, a definitive diagnosis should be established as soon as possible. This should be followed promptly by decisions regarding the preferred means of therapy and then expeditious implementation of that therapy. Location of the primary tear, definition of the extent of the dissection, and demonstration of any aortic regurgitation or any major arterial obstruction are essential for appropriate management.

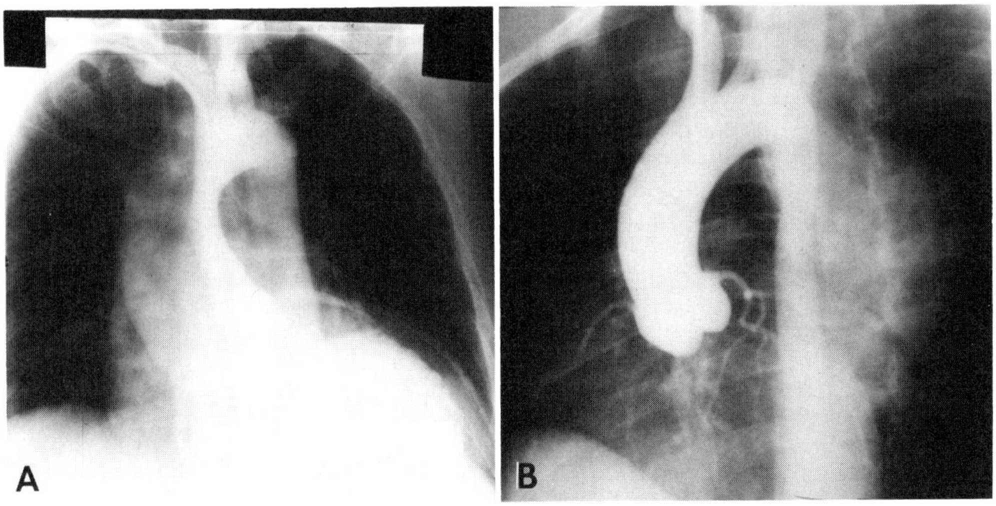

Fig 58A-12 Thoracic aortograms. **A,** dissection of the ascending aorta (type I). **B,** dissection of the descending thoracic aorta (type III). Both demonstrate deformity of the true lumen of a widened aorta. (**A** from Spittell JA Jr, Wallace RB: Aortic dissection. *Am Fam Physician* 1 No 3:89-98, 1970. By permission of the American Academy of Family Physicians.)

Initially, the patient suspected of having aortic dissection should be placed in an intensive care unit where appropriate monitoring and close observation are possible. The objectives are control of pain and pharmacologic treatment to stabilize the dissection and to control any hypertension that is present.

Effective therapy of aortic dissection has evolved as a result of the development of suitable cardiovascular surgical techniques[56] and the evolution of a pharmacologic approach to the control of forces that tend to continue or extend the dissection. The goals of therapy are to stabilize the dissection, prevent rupture, and repair damage that causes complications. Thus, most centers take an individualized approach, which involves pharmacologic therapy initially and then—depending on the location, extent, and complication of the dissection—surgical treatment or continued pharmacologic management or both.

After the type and extent of aortic dissection have been determined by imaging, definitive therapy can be planned. It is generally agreed that results with surgical therapy are better than those with pharmacologic therapy in types I and II (proximal, type A) dissection,[77-79] and thus immediate operation is recommended for these patients, just as soon as appropriate preparation can be made. In type III (distal, type B) dissection, opinions differ about the indications for and timing of any operation. Our practice has been to advise surgical treatment for type III dissections after 2 to 3 weeks of pharmacologic therapy if the dissection becomes stable and the patient's general condition does not contraindicate this approach. If pharmacologic therapy does not relieve pain and stabilize the dissection, prompt surgical therapy is indicated.

The objectives of surgical treatment are the elimination of the threat of external rupture, prevention of extension or recurrence of dissection, repair of aortic regurgitation (if present), and restoration of patency to any major arteries occluded by the dissection. In general, the objectives are achieved by resection of the portion of the aorta in which the initial tear is located, closure with sutures of any remaining false channel at the proximal and distal transection of the aorta, resuspension or replacement of an incompetent aortic valve, and relief of any occluded major branch of the aorta.[80]

The surgical approaches to the regions of the aorta involved in the intimal tear are similar to those described earlier in this chapter (the section on management of aneurysmal disease). Postoperatively, since hypertension and the force of left ventricular ejection apparently play a key role in the cause (and hence the risk of recurrence) of aortic dissection, careful long-term control should be pursued by means of a drug program that includes one or more agents, such as propranolol, that reduce the force of left ventricular ejection. If necessary to control blood pressure, drugs such as reserpine or guanethidine are added. Regular observation at least annually, including chest roentgenography, is advisable.

The pharmacologic approach to the management of dissection, originally proposed by Wheat et al.,[81] is designed to lessen the force of ventricular ejection and lower the blood pressure, which are the factors that have been demonstrated experimentally to initiate and extend arterial dissection.[82] For initial treatment, agents having a prompt action are favored, so that intravenous administration is necessary. The drugs available are propranolol, metoprolol, esmolol, labetalol, and sodium nitroprusside.[83] When sodium nitroprusside is chosen to lower the blood pressure, it should be used in combination with propranolol, because nitroprusside, being a vasodilator, may actually increase the force of ventricular ejection, an effect that is undesirable in aortic dissection.[84] Another option is intravenous administration of labetalol (20-mg bolus followed by continuous infusion to maintain systolic blood pressure around 110 mm Hg), which has both selective α- and nonselective β-adrenergic blocking actions. Later, orally administered labetalol, 200 mg twice daily, may be substituted.[83] Ideally, the systolic blood pressure should be reduced to between 110 and 120 mm Hg, if renal function permits.

Long-term pharmacologic therapy is advised by some for the management of stable type III aortic dissection and also for patients with proximal dissection but who do not undergo operation for some reason. Postoperatively, such a program should include one or more of the drugs that decrease the force of left ventricular contraction and should have as its goal maintenance of blood pressure at 130/90 mm Hg or lower, if tolerated by the patient and the patient's renal and cerebral circulation. Again, regular evaluation including a chest radiograph is desirable several times a year initially and later once or twice a year. These examinations are done to detect any aortic regurgitation or aneurysmal enlargement that might indicate the need for surgical intervention.

Traumatic rupture of the thoracic aorta

Pathogenesis. Trauma to the thoracic aorta may result from crushing injury and deceleration as well as from penetrating injuries, or it may be iatrogenic from intraaortic procedures. Aortic rupture from sudden deceleration is the most common traumatic condition of the thoracic aorta encountered clinically. Rupture of the thoracic aorta as a result of sudden deceleration may vary in degree from incomplete laceration to complete transection. The injury occurs most often as a result of automobile accidents but may also occur in falls from heights or compression by heavy objects.[85] With horizontal deceleration, as in automobile accidents, 80% of the aortic ruptures occur at the isthmus of the thoracic aorta just distal to the origin of the left subclavian artery and near the attachment of the ligamentum arteriosum, the point of aortic fixation where the shearing stress is maximal.[86]

Clinical features. Traumatic aortic rupture should be suspected whenever an injury involves sudden deceleration or chest trauma, either blunt or penetrating.

The presence of chest contusions or penetrating wounds, rib or sternal fractures,[87] hypertension in the arms,[88,89] decreased or absent pulses in the leg,[90] or evidence of fluid in the left side of the chest[91] are clues that should bring to mind the possibility of aortic rupture.

Radiologic features. The only finding on roentgenography of the chest may be widening of the mediastinum[92] (Fig 58A-13). The presence of left pleural fluid along with the mediastinal widening is an even stronger clue.[91]

Diagnosis. Given the proper setting and findings that are consistent with the diagnosis, thoracic aortography or magnetic resonance imaging should be carried out as soon as possible to confirm the diagnosis and localize the aortic rupture (see Fig 58A-13). Computed tomography[93] and transesophageal echocardiography[94] are also useful initial screening tests in patients with suspected traumatic rupture of the thoracic aorta.

Prognosis. Most patients with traumatic aortic rupture die before they reach a hospital, but Parmley et al.[85] estimated that as many as 20% may survive long enough to permit diagnosis and treatment. Some patients will survive the aortic laceration and later present with so-called chronic traumatic thoracic aortic aneurysm; about half of these lesions become unstable and enlarge at some time in their course, but there are no criteria to predict which will do so.[95]

Treatment. In the acute setting, extreme alertness, prompt diagnosis by aortography, and immediate surgical repair are necessary. Ordinarily, end-to-end anastomosis is not feasible, so a prosthetic graft is interposed after resection of the lacerated area.[96]

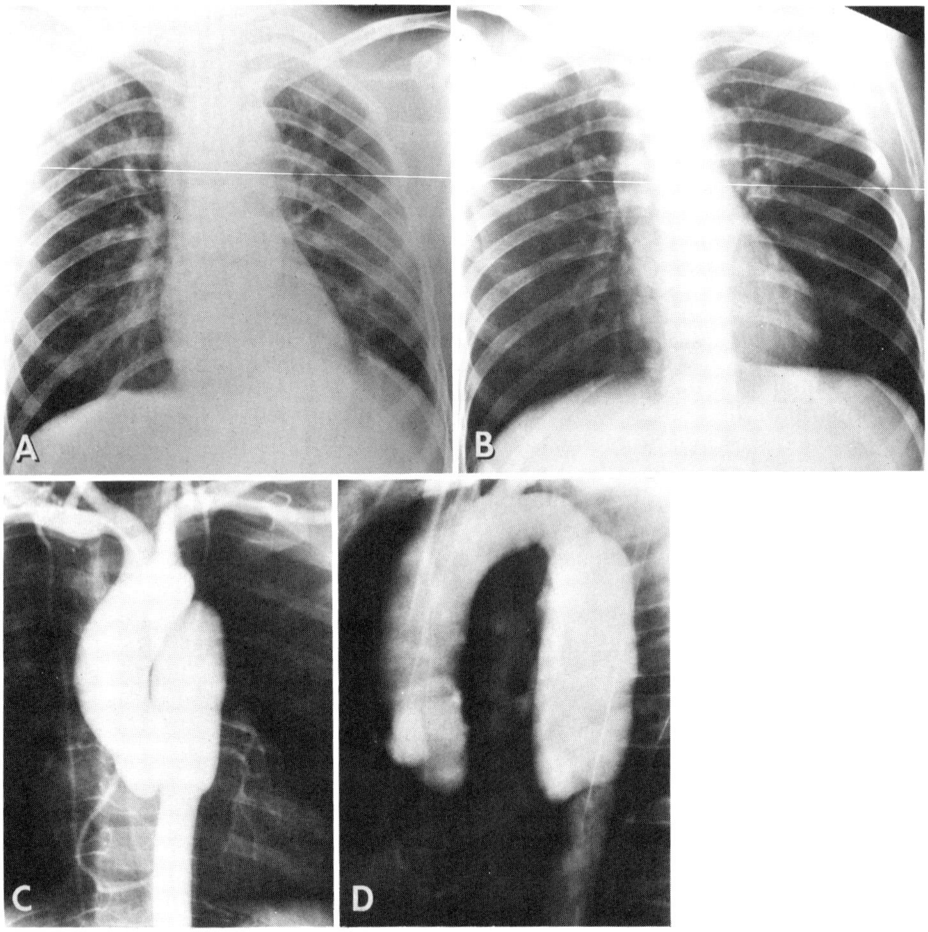

Fig 58A-13 **A,** chest radiograph of 12-year-old girl involved in an automobile accident in which she sustained severe chest injury. Note the questionably widened superior mediastinum. **B,** twelve days later, after surgery for pelvic fractures, the mediastinum was widened and the arch was prominent. Anteroposterior **(C)** and lateral **(D)** views of thoracic aortograms show false aneurysm at the site of laceration. At operation, there was circumferential intimal laceration of the aorta with only adventitial tissue containing the aneurysm, which was successfully repaired. (From Fulton RE, Stanson AW, Forbes GS, et al: Vascular imaging: angiography, ultrasound, and computed tomography. In *Allen-Barker-Hines Peripheral Vascular Diseases.* Fifth edition. Edited by JL Juergens, JA Spittell Jr, JF Fairbairn II. Philadelphia, WB Saunders Company, 1980, pp 139-215. By permission, Mayo Foundation.)

For chronic traumatic thoracic aortic aneurysm, we and others[95,97] favor surgical treatment – even though some of these patients may survive without it for long periods – because of the unpredictable course of this lesion and the low morbidity and mortality of surgical repair.

Aortitis

Although not a particularly common primary problem, aortitis, because of its diverse etiology and its occasional role in aortic regurgitation and in aortic dilatation and dissection, is an important disorder of the thoracic aorta.

Etiology. Inflammatory change can occur in the wall of the aorta in response to any type of injury. A way of classifying aortitis that permits a systematic consideration is shown in Table 58A-2. Both giant cell arteritis and Takayasu's disease have already received attention in this chapter in the discussion of the arteritides under the heading of "Occlusive Disease."

Pathogenesis. Syphilitic aortitis affects the ascending aorta most commonly, the arch next, and the descending thoracic aorta least frequently. With the initial infection, the spirochetes travel to the aorta, where they produce inflammation in the media, adventitia, and vasa vasorum. Fibrosis replaces the degenerative muscle fibers; this weakens the wall and produces the characteristic wrinkling of the intima as a late manifestation some 10 to 30 years after the initial infection.

Infections other than syphilis may cause an infectious aortitis and produce an aneurysm or involve an existing aneurysm. In the case of infectious aortitis, the primary lesion appears to be in the vasa vasorum, leading to an abscess in the arterial wall. The aorta is the artery most often involved with mycotic aneurysm.[2,98] It is interesting that staphylococcus has replaced streptococcus as the predominant organism in recent years.[99]

For the noninfectious types of aortitis, the pathogenesis and cause are obscure. Various investigators have conjectured about infectious agents and cell-mediated immune mechanisms in some types of aortitis, but such theories remain unproved. In most types, however, the aortic involvement appears to be an expression of the systemic nature of the underlying illness and vasculitis.[16] The basic lesions involve primarily the media, and to some extent the adventitia, and are often focal, except in rheumatic fever and rheumatoid arthritis, in which intimal involvement also occurs, producing a panaortitis.[100] Takayasu's aortitis differs from other types in that in some patients it can produce aortic narrowing ("acquired" coarctation); some authors have raised the question of whether cases of atypical descending thoracic aortic and abdominal aortic coarctation in reality represent end-stage Takayasu's aortitis.[18]

Aortic regurgitation may result from dilatation of the aortic ring in all forms of aortitis that affect the ascending aorta.

Clinical features. Syphilitic aortitis, unless complicated, is usually asymptomatic. With aneurysm formation, usually saccular in type, there may be signs of compression of other mediastinal structures; rarely, bony erosion occurs. When aortic regurgitation develops, of course the widened pulse pressure and diastolic blowing murmur are noted.

In the patient with a mycotic aneurysm, the findings are those of infective endocarditis, but no specific signs of mycotic aneurysm occur unless it encroaches on a surrounding structure or it ruptures. With other types of aortitis, the clinical signs are those of the underlying disease. With giant cell arteritis and Takayasu's aortitis, occlusion of one or more of the branches of the arch may occur. In the patient with the stenosing form of Takayasu's aortitis, the clinical findings are related to occlusive disease of the branches of the aorta.

Table 58A-2 Classification of aortitis

- I. Nonstenosing aortitis
  - A. Infectious
    1. Syphilitic aortitis
    2. Infectious arteritis (mycotic aneurysm)
  - B. Noninfectious
    1. Giant cell arteritis
    2. Takayasu's disease
    3. Rheumatoid arthritis and ankylosing spondylitis
    4. Relapsing polychondritis
    5. Rheumatic fever
    6. Miscellaneous types
- II. Stenosing aortitis
  - A. Takayasu's aortitis

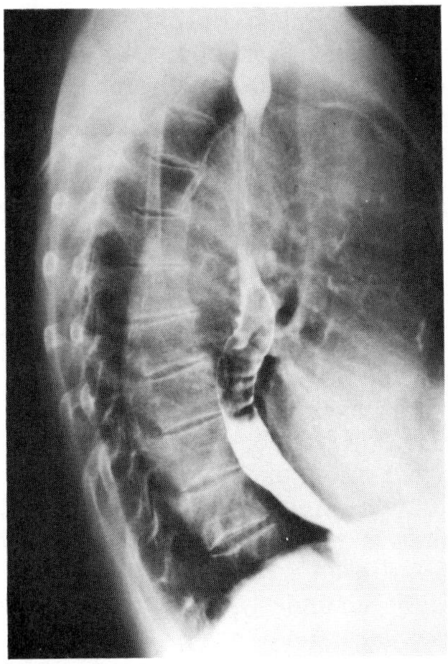

Fig 58A-14 Chest radiograph (lateral projection) demonstrating linear calcification of the wall of the ascending and transverse portions of the thoracic aorta due to syphilitic aortitis.

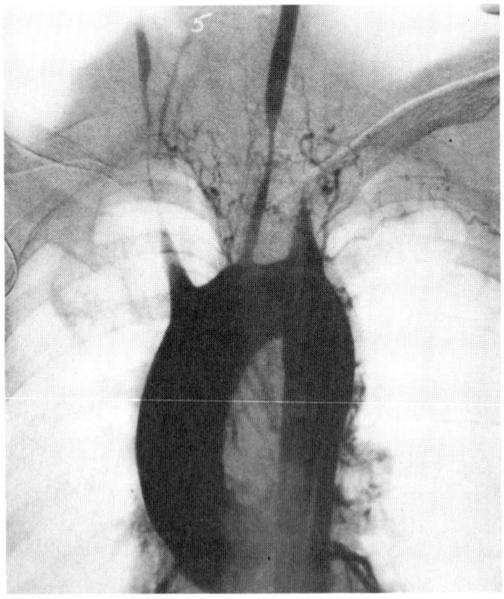

Fig 58A-15 Subtraction view of a thoracic arch aortogram in a man with Takayasu's aortitis. Note occlusion or stenosis of all branches of the aortic arch.

Radiologic features. The diagnosis of aortitis often arises from the findings on a chest radiograph suggesting dilatation of the ascending aorta or aneurysm. Linear calcification of the ascending aorta is most suggestive of syphilitic aortitis (Fig 58A-14); calcification can also be seen with other types of aortitis but does not usually involve the ascending aorta.

Aortography is valuable for demonstration of the extent of aortic dilatation, aneurysmal changes (see Fig 58A-2), and any occlusion that may be present (Fig 58A-15).

Diagnosis. The diagnosis of aortitis is usually inferred from any related clinical or chest roentgenographic findings. The various effects of aortitis are confirmed by aortography. Differentiation of the type of aortitis depends on associated findings of syphilis (serologic findings and characteristic calcification) or an associated systemic illness.

Prognosis. The prognosis for patients with syphilitic aortitis is about the same as that for the general population,[101,102] and death from its complications, other than aneurysm, is unusual. The prognosis for syphilitic aortic aneurysm, on the other hand, is poor, particularly when it is large enough to cause symptoms.[103]

Aortic rupture or dissection is a potential complication of giant cell arteritis. Otherwise, the prognosis of aortitis is generally that of the underlying systemic disorder.

Treatment. The preventive value of adequate therapy of early syphilis is the most important therapeutic aspect of syphilitic aortitis. Therapy of other types of aortitis is basically that of the underlying disorder. Management of any aneurysm, aortic regurgitation, or arterial occlusive disease is the same as that for such a lesion when it is due to other causes.

REFERENCES

1. Sos TA, Sniderman KW, Wixson D: Pitfalls in the plain film evaluation of the thoracic aorta: the mimicry of aneurysms and adjacent masses and the value of aortography. Part II. Descending thoracic aorta. *Cardiovasc Radiol* 2:77-83, 1979

2. Shahian DM, Javid H, Faber LP, et al: Lesions of the thoracic aorta and its arch branches simulating neoplasm. *J Thorac Cardiovasc Surg* 81:251-263, 1981

3. Movat HZ, More RH, Haust MD: The diffuse intimal thickening of the human aorta with aging. *Am J Pathol* 34:1023-1031, 1958

4. Wellman WE, Edwards JE: Thickness of the media of the thoracic aorta in relation to age. *Arch Pathol* 50:183-188, 1950

5. Adams CWM, Bayliss OB: The relationship between diffuse intimal thickening, medial enzyme failure and intimal lipid deposition in various human arteries. *J Atheroscler Res* 10:327-339, 1969

6. Lie JT: The structure of the normal vascular system and its reactive changes. In *Allen-Barker-Hines Peripheral Vascular Diseases.* Fifth edition. Edited by JL Juergens, JA Spittell Jr, JF Fairbairn II. Philadelphia, WB Saunders Company, 1980, pp 51-81

7. Fuster V, Kottke BA, Juergens JL: Atherosclerosis. In *Allen-Barker-Hines Peripheral Vascular Diseases.* Fifth edition. Edited by JL Juergens, JA Spittell Jr, JF Fairbairn II. Philadelphia, WB Saunders Company, 1980, pp 219-235

8. Stanson AW, Kazmier FJ, Hollier LH, et al: Penetrating atherosclerotic ulcers of the thoracic aorta: natural history and clinicopathologic correlations. *Ann Vasc Surg* 1:15-23, 1986

9. Roberts WC: Aortic dissection: anatomy, consequences, and causes. *Am Heart J* 101:195-214, 1981

10. Stengel A, Wolferth CC: Mycotic (bacterial) aneurysms of intravascular origin. *Arch Intern Med* 31:527-554, 1923

11. Tejada E, Becker GJ, Waller BF: Malignant myxoid emboli as the presenting feature of primary sarcoma of the aorta (myxoid malignant fibrous histiocytoma): a case report and review of the literature. *Clin Cardiol* 14:425-430, 1991

12. Patel A, Toole JF: Subclavian steal syndrome—reversal of cephalic blood flow. *Medicine (Baltimore)* 44:289-303, 1965

13. Sadony V, Kayambo GH, Walz M, et al: Acquired coarctation due to calcified thrombus in atherosclerosis of the descending thoracic aorta. Two cases and a review. *Eur J Cardiothorac Surg* 3:464-467, 1989

14. Hunder GG, Ward LE, Burbank MK: Giant-cell arteritis producing an aortic arch syndrome. *Ann Intern Med* 66:578-582, 1967

15. Pollock M, Blennerhassett JB, Clarke AM: Giant cell arteritis and the subclavian steal syndrome. *Neurology (Minneap)* 23:653-657, 1973

16. Sheps SG, McDuffie FC: Vasculitis. In *Allen-Barker-Hines Peripheral Vascular Diseases.* Fifth edition. Edited by JL Juergens, JA Spittell Jr, JF Fairbairn II. Philadelphia, WB Saunders Company, 1980, pp 493-553

17. Klein RG, Hunder GG, Stanson AW, et al: Large artery involvement in giant cell (temporal) arteritis. *Ann Intern Med* 83:806-812, 1975

18. Lande A, Berkmen YM: Aortitis: pathologic, clinical and arteriographic review. *Radiol Clin North Am* 14:219-240, August 1976

19. Cull DL, Parent FN III, Wheeler JR, et al: Thoracic aortic ectasia in a patient with Takayasu's disease. *Ann Vasc Surg* 5:470-472, 1991

20. Seo JW, Park IA, Yoon DH, et al: Thoracic aortic aneurysm associated with aortitis—case reports and histological review. *J Korean Med Sci* 6:75-82, 1991

21. Ishikawa K: Survival and morbidity after diagnosis of occlusive thromboaortopathy (Takayasu's disease). *Am J Cardiol* 47:1026-1032, 1981

22. Boucek RJ, Noble NL, Gunja-Smith Z, et al: The Marfan syndrome: a deficiency in chemically stable collagen cross-links. *N Engl J Med* 305:988-991, 1981

23. Pyeritz RE, McKusick VA: Basic defects in the Marfan syndrome (editorial). *N Engl J Med* 305:1011-1012, 1981

24. Ellis PR, Cooley DA, De Bakey ME: Clinical considerations and surgical treatment of annulo-aortic ectasia: report of successful operation. *J Thorac Cardiovasc Surg* 42:363-370, 1961

25. Lemon DK, White CW: Annuloaortic ectasia: angiographic, hemodynamic and clinical comparison with aortic valve insufficiency. *Am J Cardiol* 41:482-486, 1978

26. Waller BF, Zoltick JM, Rosen JH, et al: Severe aortic regurgitation from systemic hypertension (without aortic dissection) requiring

aortic valve replacement: analysis of four patients. *Am J Cardiol* 49:473-477, 1982

27. Johansen K: Aneurysms. *Sci Am* 247:110-125, 1982
28. Roberts WC: The hypertensive diseases: evidence that systemic hypertension is a greater risk factor to the development of other cardiovascular diseases than previously suspected. *Am J Med* 59:523-532, 1975
29. Griepp RB, Ergin MA, Lansman SL, et al: The natural history of thoracic aortic aneurysms. *Semin Thorac Cardiovasc Surg* 3:258-265, 1991
30. Joyce JW, Fairbairn JF II, Kincaid OW, et al: Aneurysms of the thoracic aorta: a clinical study with special reference to prognosis. *Circulation* 29:176-181, 1964
31. Pressler V, McNamara JJ: Thoracic aortic aneurysm: natural history and treatment. *J Thorac Cardiovasc Surg* 79:489-497, 1980
32. Posniak HV, Demos TC, Marsan RE: Computed tomography of the normal aorta and thoracic aneurysms. *Semin Roentgenol* 24:7-21, 1989
33. Sanders JH Jr, Malave S, Neiman HL, et al: Thoracic aortic imaging without angiography. *Arch Surg* 114:1326-1329, 1979
34. Kamp O, van Rossum AC, Torenbeek R: Transesophageal echocardiography and magnetic resonance imaging for the assessment of saccular aneurysm of the transverse thoracic aorta. *Int J Cardiol* 33:330-333, 1991
35. DeMaria AN, Bommer W, Neumann A, et al: Identification and localization of aneurysms of the ascending aorta by cross-sectional echocardiography. *Circulation* 59:755-761, 1979
36. Mintz GS, Kotler MN, Segal BL, et al: Two dimensional echocardiographic recognition of the descending thoracic aorta. *Am J Cardiol* 44:232-238, 1979
37. Lois JF, Gomes AS, Brown K, et al: Magnetic resonance imaging of the thoracic aorta. *Am J Cardiol* 60:358-362, 1987
38. Crawford ES, Rubio PA: Reappraisal of adjuncts to avoid ischemia in the treatment of aneurysms of descending thoracic aorta. *J Thorac Cardiovasc Surg* 66:693-703, 1973
39. Lynch DR, Dawson TM, Raps EC, et al: Risk factors for the neurologic complications associated with aortic aneurysms. *Arch Neurol* 49:284-288, 1992
40. Singh MP, Bentall HH: Complete replacement of the ascending aorta and the aortic valve for the treatment of aortic aneurysm. *J Thorac Cardiovasc Surg* 63:218-225, 1972
41. Selle JG, Robicsek F, Daugherty HK, et al: Technical options in repairing the diseased ascending aorta with aortic valve involvement. *Ann Thorac Surg* 32:578-583, 1981
42. Cooley DA, Ott DA, Frazier OH, et al: Surgical treatment of aneurysms of the transverse aortic arch: experience with 25 patients using hypothermic techniques. *Ann Thorac Surg* 32:260-270, 1981
43. Hirst AE, Gore I: Is cystic medionecrosis the cause of dissecting aortic aneurysm? (Editorial.) *Circulation* 53:915-916, 1976
44. Hasleton PS, Leonard JC: Dissecting aortic aneurysms: a clinicopathological study. II. Histopathology of the aorta. *Q J Med* 48:63-76, 1979
45. Schlatmann TJM, Becker AE: Pathogenesis of dissecting aneurysm of aorta: comparative histopathologic study of significance of medial changes. *Am J Cardiol* 39:21-26, 1977
46. Spittell JA Jr, Wallace RB: Dissecting aneurysm of the aorta (dissecting hematoma, aortic dissection). In *Allen-Barker-Hines Peripheral Vascular Diseases.* Fifth edition. Edited by JL Juergens, JA Spittell Jr, JF Fairbairn II. Philadelphia, WB Saunders Company, 1980, pp 403-413
47. Steinmann B, Tuderman L, Peltonen L, et al: Evidence for a structural mutation of procollagen type I in a patient with the Ehlers-Danlos syndrome type VII. *J Biol Chem* 255:8887-8893, 1980
48. Byers PH, Holbrook KA, Barsh GS, et al: Altered secretion of type III procollagen in a form of type IV Ehlers-Danlos syndrome: biochemical studies in cultured fibroblasts. *Lab Invest* 44:336-341, 1981
49. Hussain S, Glover JL, Bree R, et al: Penetrating atherosclerotic ulcers of the thoracic aorta. *J Vasc Surg* 9:710-717, 1989
50. Edwards WD, Leaf DS, Edwards JE: Dissecting aortic aneurysm associated with congenital bicuspid aortic valve. *Circulation* 57:1022-1025, 1978
51. Larson EW, Edwards WD: Risk factors for aortic dissection: a necropsy study of 161 cases. *Am J Cardiol* 53:849-855, 1984
52. Roberts CS, Roberts WC: Dissection of the aorta associated with congenital malformation of the aortic valve. *J Am Coll Cardiol* 17:712-716, 1991
53. Bixler D, Antley RM: Familial aortic dissection with iris anomalies – a new connective tissue disease syndrome? *Birth Defects* 12 No. 5:229-234, 1976
54. Lefemine AA, Kosowsky B, Madoff I, et al: Results and complications of intraaortic balloon pumping in surgical and medical patients. *Am J Cardiol* 40:416-420, 1977
55. Nicholson WJ, Crawley IS, Logue RB, et al: Aortic root dissection complicating coronary bypass surgery. *Am J Cardiol* 41:103-107, 1978
56. De Bakey ME, Henly WS, Cooley DA, et al: Surgical management of dissecting aneurysms of the aorta. *J Thorac Cardiovasc Surg* 49:130-148, 1965
57. Slater EE, DeSanctis RW: The clinical recognition of dissecting aortic aneurysm. *Am J Med* 60:625-633, 1976
58. Dailey PO, Trueblood HW, Stinson EB, et al: Management of acute aortic dissections. *Ann Thorac Surg* 10:237-246, 1970
59. O'Donovan TPB, Osmundson PJ, Payne WS: Painless dissecting aneurysm of the aorta: report of a case. *Circulation* 29:782-786, 1964
60. Cambria RP, Brewster DC, Gertler J, et al: Vascular complications associated with spontaneous aortic dissection. *J Vasc Surg* 7:199-209, 1988
61. Moersch FP, Sayre GP: Neurologic manifestations associated with dissecting aneurysm of the aorta. *JAMA* 144:1141-1148, 1950
62. Spittell JA Jr: Differential diagnosis of dissecting aneurysm. *Prog Cardiovasc Dis* 14:225-229, 1971
63. Eagle KA, Quertermous T, Kritzer GA, et al: Spectrum of conditions initially suggesting acute aortic dissection but with negative aortograms. *Am J Cardiol* 57:322-326, 1986
64. Spittell PC, Spittell JA Jr, Joyce JW, et al: Clinical features and differential diagnosis of aortic dissection: experience with 236 cases (1980 through 1990). *Mayo Clin Proc* 68:642-651, 1993
65. Earnest F IV, Muhm JR, Sheedy PF II: Roentgenographic findings in thoracic aortic dissection. *Mayo Clin Proc* 54:43-50, 1979
66. Victor MF, Mintz GS, Kotler MN, et al: Two dimensional echocardiographic diagnosis of aortic dissection. *Am J Cardiol* 48:1155-1159, 1981
67. Rubenson DS, Fowles RE, Miller DC, et al: Spontaneous dissection of the ascending aorta diagnosed by two-dimensional echocardiography. *Chest* 80:587-591, 1981
68. Erbel R, Daniel W, Visser C, et al: Echocardiography in diagnosis of aortic dissection. *Lancet* 1:457-460, 1989
69. Börner N, Erbel R, Braun B, et al: Diagnosis of aortic dissection by transesophageal echocardiography. *Am J Cardiol* 54:1157-1158, 1984
70. Omoto R, Kyo S, Matsumura M, et al: Evaluation of biplane color Doppler transesophageal echocardiography in 200 consecutive patients. *Circulation* 85:1237-1247, 1992
71. Lee E, Schiller NB: How useful is transesophageal echocardiography? *Choices Cardiol* 3:176-179, 1989
72. Adachi H, Omoto R, Kyo S, et al: Emergency surgical intervention of acute aortic dissection with the rapid diagnosis by transesophageal echocardiography. *Circulation* 84 Suppl 3:14-19, 1991
73. Moncada R, Salinas M, Churchill R, et al: Diagnosis of dissecting aortic aneurysm by computed tomography. *Lancet* 1:238-241, 1981
74. Morgan JM, Oldershaw PJ, Gray HH: Use of computed tomographic scanning and aortography in the diagnosis of acute dissection of the thoracic aorta. *Br Heart J* 64:261-265, 1990
75. Nienaber CA, Spielmann RP, von Kodolitsch Y, et al: Diagnosis of thoracic aortic dissection. Magnetic resonance imaging versus transesophageal echocardiography. *Circulation* 85:434-447, 1992
76. McCloy RM, Spittell JA Jr, McGoon DC: The prognosis in aortic dissection (dissecting aortic hematoma or aneurysm). *Circulation* 31: 665-669, 1965
77. Appelbaum A, Karp RB, Kirklin JW: Ascending vs descending aortic dissections. *Ann Surg* 183:296-300, 1976
78. Miller DC, Stinson EB, Oyer PE, et al: Operative treatment of aortic dissections: experience with 125 patients over a sixteen-year period. *J Thorac Cardiovasc Surg* 78:365-381, 1979
79. Glower DD, Speier RH, White WD, et al: Management and long-term outcome of aortic dissection. *Ann Surg* 214:31-41, 1991
80. Jex RK, Schaff HV, Piehler JM, et al: Repair of ascending aortic dissection: influence of associated aortic valve insufficiency on early and late results. *J Thorac Cardiovasc Surg* 93:375-384, 1987

81. Wheat MW Jr, Palmer RF, Bartley TD, et al: Treatment of dissecting aneurysms of the aorta without surgery. *J Thorac Cardiovasc Surg* 50:364-371, 1965
82. Prokop EK, Palmer RF, Wheat MW Jr: Hydrodynamic forces in dissecting aneurysms: in-vitro studies in a Tygon model and in dog aortas. *Circ Res* 27:121-127, 1970
83. Grubb BP, Sirio C, Zelis R: Intravenous labetalol in acute aortic dissection. *JAMA* 258:78-79, 1987
84. Palmer RF, Lasseter KC: Nitroprusside and aortic dissecting aneurysm (letter to the editor). *N Engl J Med* 294:1403-1404, 1976
85. Parmley LF, Mattingly TW, Manion WC: Penetrating wounds of the heart and aorta. *Circulation* 17:953-973, 1958
86. Cammack K, Rapport RL, Paul J, et al: Deceleration injuries of the thoracic aorta. *Arch Surg* 79:244-251, 1959
87. Greendyke RM: Traumatic rupture of aorta: special reference to automobile accidents. *JAMA* 195:527-530, 1966
88. Fox S, Pierce WS, Waldhausen JA: Acute hypertension: its significance in traumatic aortic rupture. *J Thorac Cardiovasc Surg* 77:622-625, 1979
89. Jahnke EJ Jr, Fisher GW, Jones RC: Acute traumatic rupture of the thoracic aorta: report of six consecutive cases of successful early repair. *J Thorac Cardiovasc Surg* 48:63-77, 1964
90. Eiseman B, Rainer WG: Clinical management of posttraumatic rupture of the thoracic aorta. *J Thorac Surg* 35:347-358, 1958
91. Stoney RJ, Roe BB, Redington JV: Rupture of thoracic aorta due to closed-chest trauma. *Arch Surg* 89:840-846, 1964
92. Pate JW, Butterick OD, Richardson RL: Traumatic rupture of the thoracic aorta. *JAMA* 203:1022-1024, 1968
93. Raptopoulos V, Sheiman RG, Phillips DA, et al: Traumatic aortic tear: screening with chest CT. *Radiology* 182:667-673, 1992
94. Snow CC, Appelbe AF, Martin TD, et al: Diagnosis of aortic transection by transesophageal echocardiography. *J Am Soc Echocardiogr* 5:100-102, 1992
95. Fleming AW, Green DC: Traumatic aneurysms of the thoracic aorta: report of 43 patients. *Ann Thorac Surg* 18:91-101, 1974
96. Duhaylongsod FG, Glower DD, Wolfe WG: Acute traumatic aortic aneurysm: the Duke experience from 1970 to 1990. *J Vasc Surg* 15:331-342, 1992
97. Quaini E, Colombo T, Donatelli F, et al: Chronic traumatic aneurysms of the descending thoracic aorta. *Tex Heart Inst J* 12:143-146, 1985
98. Mundth ED, Darling RC, Alvarado RH, et al: Surgical management of mycotic aneurysms and the complications of infection in vascular reconstructive surgery. *Am J Surg* 117:460-469, 1969
99. Anderson CB, Butcher HR Jr, Ballinger WF: Mycotic aneurysms. *Arch Surg* 109:712-717, 1974
100. Heggtveit HA, Hennigar GR, Morrione TG: Panaortitis. *Am J Pathol* 42:151-172, 1963
101. Rich C Jr, Webster B: The natural history of uncomplicated syphilitic aortitis. *Am Heart J* 43:321-332, 1952
102. Irvine RE: Outcome of uncomplicated syphilitic aortitis. *Br Med J* 1:832-834, 1956
103. Kampmeier RH: Saccular aneurysm of the thoracic aorta: a clinical study of 633 cases. *Ann Intern Med* 12:624-651, 1938

CHAPTER

58

Acquired diseases of the aorta

B. Abdominal aorta

Thom W. Rooke, M.D., and Anthony W. Stanson, M.D.

With the exception of atherosclerosis (and related complications), most of the diseases of the abdominal aorta are relatively uncommon. Recent advances in imaging technology, including computerized tomographic scanning, ultrasound and Doppler, magnetic resonance, and angiography, have not only improved our ability to diagnose problems with the aorta but also provided new tools for studying the causes, pathogenesis, prevalence, and natural history of aortic disease.

PATHOLOGIC CONDITIONS AFFECTING THE ABDOMINAL AORTA

Atherosclerosis

Atherosclerosis is the most common pathologic condition affecting the abdominal aorta (Figs 58B-1 and 58B-2). The details of atherogenesis and plaque formation are complex and have been discussed in detail elsewhere (see chapter 28). Risk factors for aortic atherosclerosis are similar to those for other arteries and include smoking, genetic factors, hypertension, diabetes, hyperlipidemia, male sex, advanced age, and a variety of others.[1] There may be a relationship between certain risk factors and the pattern of atherosclerosis distribution; for example, patients with disease limited exclusively to the aortoiliac region tend to be younger, have a higher incidence of smoking and hyperlipidemia, and have a lower incidence of diabetes and hypertension than those with more diffuse disease.[2] The mechanisms by which different risk factors affect the distribution of disease remain unknown.

Aortic disease is seen frequently in conjunction with atherosclerosis in other arteries, such as the coronary, carotid, renal, and iliofemoral arteries.[3] The significance of this association is twofold: 1. The possibility of diffuse vascular disease needs to be considered when patients are found to have abdominal aortic disease, especially when surgery to correct the aortic problem is being contemplated (see "Diagnosis and Evaluation of Abdominal Aortic Disease," below). 2. The possibility of significant occult aortic atherosclerosis should be considered in patients found to have peripheral vascular disease in other sites.

Degenerative disorders

A wide variety of nonatherosclerotic, so-called degenerative disorders can affect the abdominal aorta. In some instances, these disorders occur as the result of normal or pathologic processes originating within the aorta itself, whereas in others they reflect "reactive" or "adaptive" responses by the aorta to systemic events.

Normal aging. The abdominal aorta normally undergoes age-related changes in structure and composition.[4] The *intimal layer* becomes diffusely thickened (more so in the distal than in the proximal portion) and accumulates collagen and lipid. The *elastic lamella* thickens, accumulates calcium, and may eventually break down. The *medial layer* undergoes biochemical changes that affect the composition of mucopolysaccharides, hyaluronic acid, chondroitin sulfate, and heparan sulfate. Smooth muscle cells decrease in number. In conjunction with the continuing age-related histologic remodeling, the diameter of the aorta increases. The normal changes seen with aging can be accelerated and influenced by a variety of pathologic conditions, including atherosclerosis and hypertension.

Calcific medial sclerosis. Calcific sclerosis involves the widespread deposition of calcium into the media of the aorta and large arteries of the extremities. Although calcific sclerosis is typically a benign, isolated occurrence, it may also develop in association with atherosclerosis, hypertension, or diabetes and can be an intricate part of the pathologic picture caused by these conditions. The cause of calcific sclerosis is unknown, but the condition may reflect a healing response to occult medial injury.[5] In some individuals, a more malignant form of calcific medial sclerosis occurs at a relatively young age (as early as infancy) and may cause significant morbidity.[6]

Cystic medial necrosis (Erdheim's cystic medial necrosis). Although more common in the thoracic aorta, this relatively uncommon disorder occasionally affects the abdominal aorta. The hallmark of the disease is medial accumulation of mucoid material into microscopic collections that resemble cysts. Associated with this is generalized disruption or loss (or both) of elastic and collagen

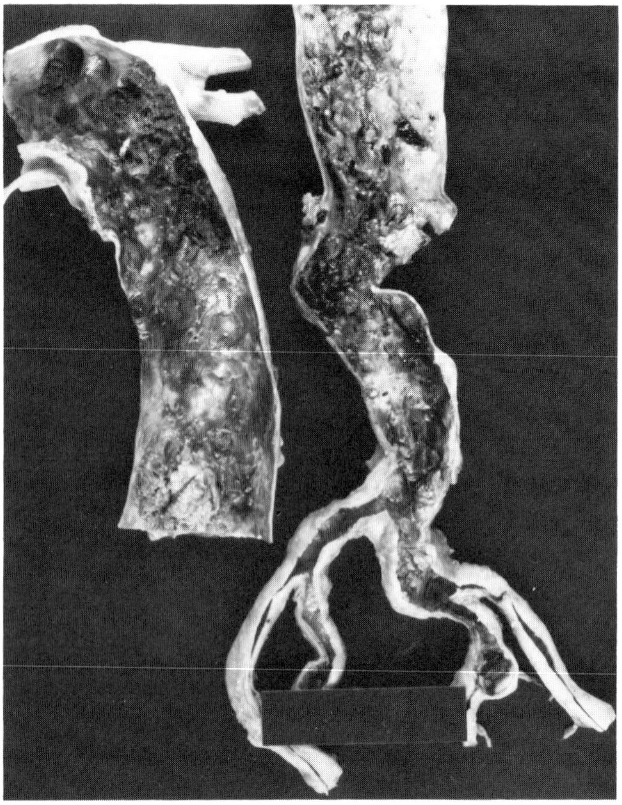

Fig 58B-1 Severe atheromatous disease of the aorta in autopsy specimen.

fibers, smooth muscle, and mucopolysaccharides; however, no true necrosis occurs. Although the terms "cystic" and "necrosis" are therefore inaccurate, the concept of cystic medial necrosis has become well established in the literature and is unlikely to be replaced. The histologic findings of cystic medial necrosis may be isolated or occur in association with other pathologic conditions, the best known of which is the genetically determined Marfan syndrome. Progressive aortic dilatation and sudden dissection (see chapter 58A) are the most serious potential consequences of this condition; these complications typically originate in the thoracic aorta but may progress distally to involve the abdominal aorta as well.

Other disorders. Numerous other "degenerative" conditions can affect the abdominal aorta. For the most part, these are rare and beyond the scope of this chapter. Some, like the *Ehlers-Danlos* syndrome (Fig 58B-3) (in which the collagen structure in the aortic wall is defective), are due to genetic errors; they are "acquired" only in the sense that problems with the aorta (or other vessels) such as dilatation and aneurysm formation may not develop until later in life. Arteriomegaly (Fig 58B-4) is a rare condition that often involves the abdominal aorta in conjunction with the iliofemoral and popliteal arteries. Histologically, there is noninflammatory degeneration of the internal elastic lamina and elastic tissues of the media that causes enlargement or aneurysm formation.[7] Pregnancy[8] and tuberous sclerosis[9] may also predispose to poorly understood changes that can weaken the aorta.

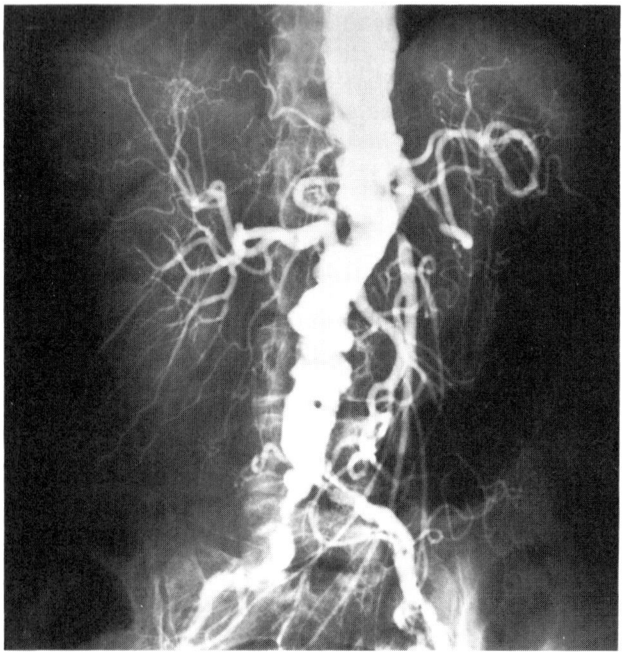

Fig 58B-2 Abdominal aortogram reveals severe atheromatous disease of the abdominal aorta and iliac arteries.

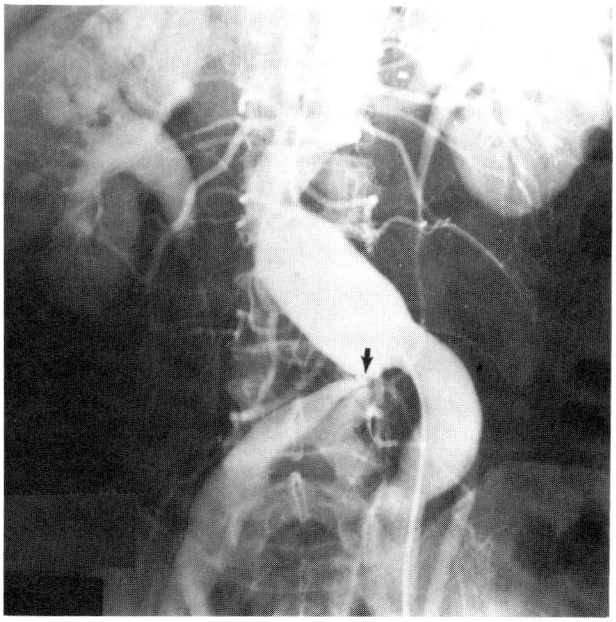

Fig 58B-3 Abdominal aortogram in a patient with Ehlers-Danlos syndrome shows an aneurysm of the aorta and iliac arteries and dissection *(arrow)* of the right common iliac artery.

Inflammatory disorders

The causes of most noninfectious inflammatory conditions of the abdominal aorta are unknown. These uncommon entities, which typically involve other large vessels as well, display a wide spectrum of pathologic and clinical manifestations. The names included here reflect those used most commonly at the Mayo Clinic.

Takayasu's disease. Takayasu's disease[10] is an inflammatory condition involving the aorta and its major branches (Fig 58B-5). It primarily affects women (in more than 80% of cases) and the young (less than 40 years of age), although exceptions to these rules occur. The disease has a worldwide distribution but appears to be more common in Asia than elsewhere. Histologically, the aorta shows focal or diffuse involvement of all layers. Typical features of the disease are intimal thickening, destruction of the muscular and elastic tissues, infiltration by lymphocytes and plasma cells, and inflammatory involvement of the vasa vasorum. In the acute stages of the disease, giant cells and granulomas are present. The inflammatory process usually causes scarring, shortening, and narrowing of the vessel, although dilatation and aneurysm formation can also occur.

Temporal arteritis. This disease involves a giant cell granulomatous destruction of the aorta and large vessels similar to that seen in Takayasu's arteritis. However, the population affected is markedly different; almost all patients with temporal arteritis are over 50 years of age, and the ratio of women to men (about 2:1) is less striking than that for Takayasu's. The extent to which the abdominal aorta is involved is variable; although pathologic involvement of the aorta and large branch vessels is common, the arteriographic findings in these vessels tend to be minimal. The abdominal aorta probably is involved less frequently than in Takayasu's disease.

Other inflammatory disorders. Very rarely, inflammatory conditions such as focal necrotizing arteritis, relapsing polychondritis, Behçet's syndrome, and Kawasaki's disease can involve the abdominal aorta. Little is known about the underlying causes for these conditions.

Inflammatory aneurysms. As many as 15%[11] of abdominal aortic aneurysms are of the so-called inflammatory variety.[12,13] In this condition, the aneurysm (presumably of atherosclerotic origin) becomes intensely inflamed (Fig 58B-6). The cause of the inflammatory response is unknown, although proposed mechanisms have included immunologic reactions to atheromatous debris or blood products that have leaked from the aorta; there is no conclusive evidence to support either of these theories.[14] A similarity between the histologic changes of inflammatory aneurysm and *retroperitoneal fibrosis* has also been noted,[14] raising uncertainty about whether inflammatory aneurysms are a variant form of retroperitoneal fibrosis or a separate and distinct pathologic entity.

Along with the usual intimal and medial destructive features of atherosclerosis, the inflammatory aneurysm shows infiltration by various inflammatory cell types (lymphocytes, plasma cells, and possibly neutrophils) into the adventitia, with subsequent formation of thick granulation tissue. Macroscopically, the inflammatory aneurysm has a smooth, fibrotic, gray-white surface. Reactive changes may involve surrounding structures, including the

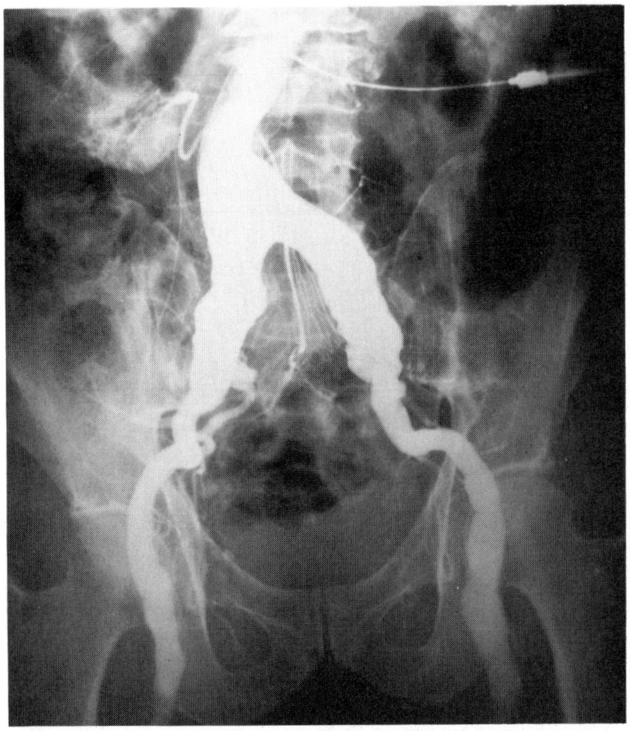

Fig 58B-4 Abdominal aortogram in a patient with arteriomegaly reveals multiple aneurysms: aorta and common iliac, hypogastric, and common femoral arteries.

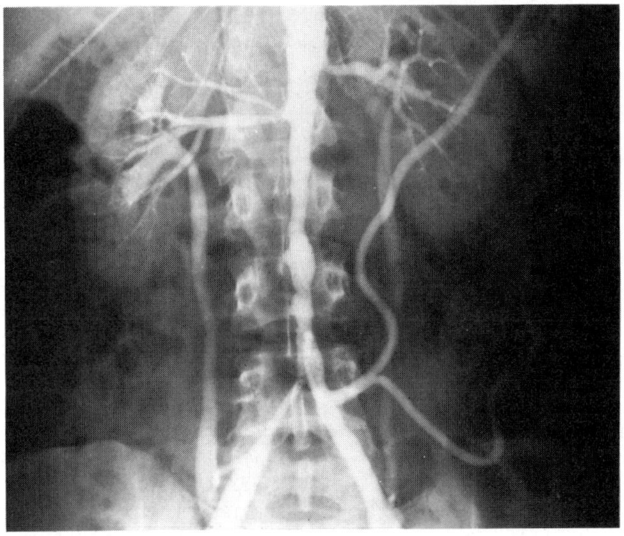

Fig 58B-5 Abdominal aortogram in a patient with Takayasu's disease shows a diffuse, irregular lumen with moderate narrowing of the aorta and stenosis of both renal and common iliac arteries. The inferior mesenteric artery is enlarged and supplies collateral flow to the occluded superior mesenteric artery.

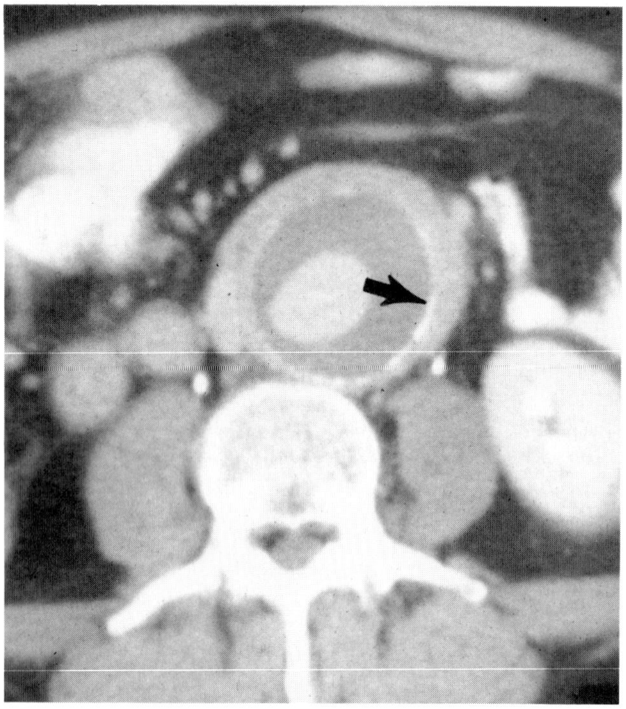

Fig 58B-6 Computed tomography scan of infrarenal abdominal aorta shows inflammatory aneurysm. The tissue thickness beyond the intimal calcification *(arrow)* is the inflamed adventitia.

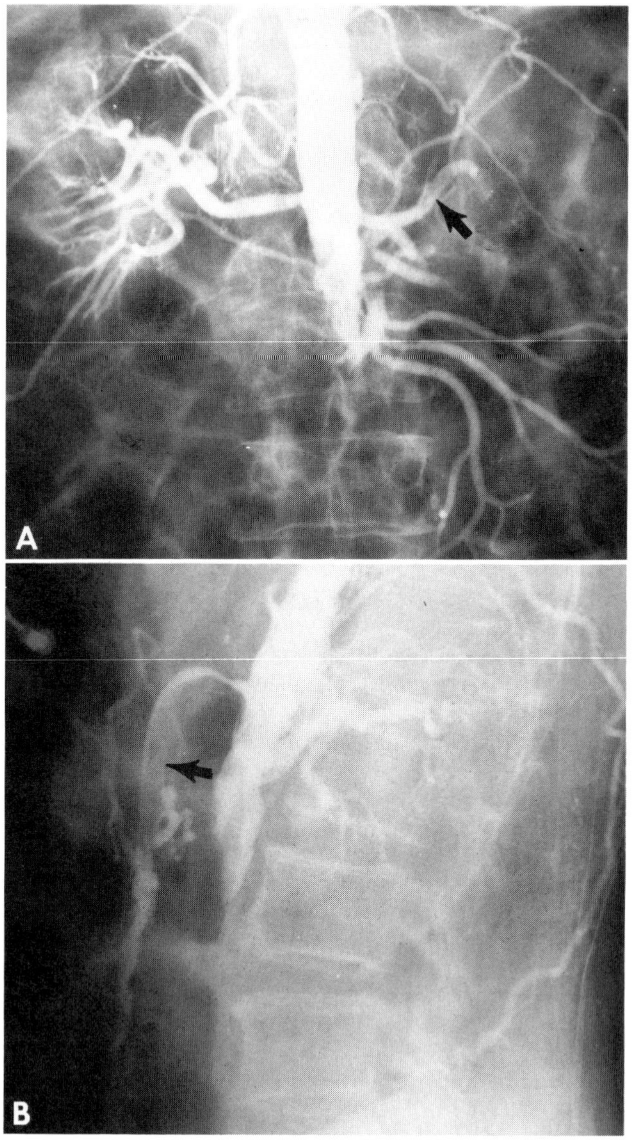

Fig 58B-7 Abdominal aortogram in a patient with embolic occlusion of the infrarenal aorta. Emboli *(arrows)* are also in the left renal artery **(A)** and superior mesenteric artery **(B)**.

ureters, intestines, nerves, and blood vessels, causing them to become densely adherent to the aorta. Surgical resection is therefore much more complicated for an inflammatory aneurysm than for noninflamed aneurysms. Inflammatory abdominal aneurysms are difficult to diagnose clinically; clues to the diagnosis include the triad of abdominal pain, weight loss, and elevated erythrocyte sedimentation rate.[15]

Trauma

Trauma in various forms may affect the abdominal aorta.[16-19] Gunshot (and other penetrating) wounds of the abdomen and back are relatively common and may cause catastrophic disruption of the aorta. Significant injury to the aorta can also result from nonpenetrating trauma, including falls, automobile accidents (especially when lap seat belts are used), and blows to the abdomen. Iatrogenic complications of invasive cardiovascular procedures (such as catheterization, translumbar aortography, and balloon counterpulsation pumping) and surgery (such as clamp injuries) represent a growing source of abdominal aortic trauma.[20-22] Intervertebral disk surgery (especially L4-5 laminectomy) is a well-documented cause of arteriovenous fistula.[23]

Miscellaneous conditions

Infection. Infection of the abdominal aorta (or other arteries) often occurs when there is a structural abnormality of the vessel; examples are atherosclerosis or preexisting abdominal aortic aneurysm,[24] trauma affecting the aorta, coarctation, and prosthetic grafts. The patient in whom abdominal aortic infection develops may be immunocompromised, have sepsis, or have bacterial endocarditis, although cases of infection occurring without any identified predisposing factor occur.[25] The most common infective organisms are gram-positive (pneumococci, other streptococci, and staphylococci), but gram-negative, anaerobic, and fungal causes are not rare.[26] Salmonella is an unusually aggressive arterial wall pathogen and may account for a significant number of aortic infections, some of which rupture or form aneurysms.[27] Syphilis, a common cause of a thoracic aneurysm in the

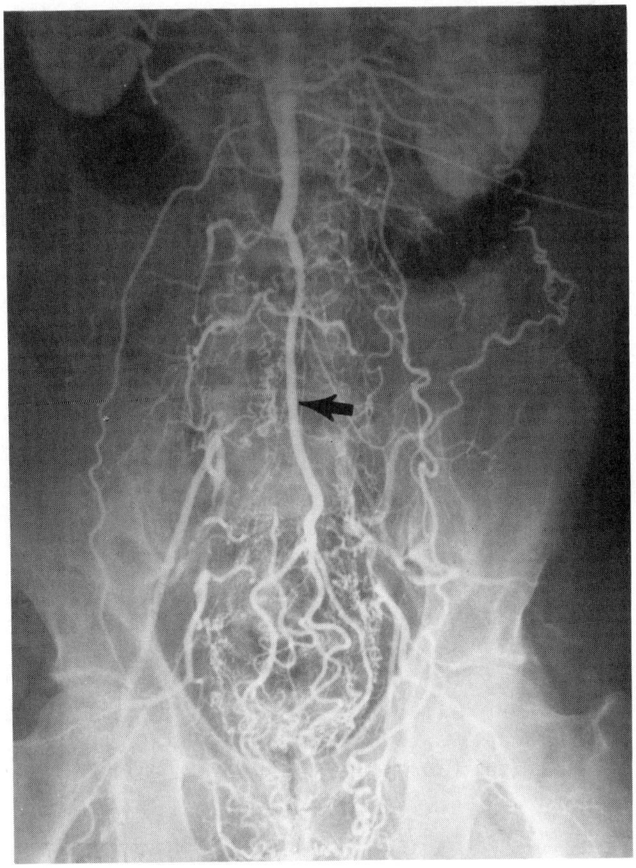

Fig 58B-8 Abdominal aortogram in a patient with occlusion of the infrarenal aorta secondary to atheromatous disease. The major midline collateral is the inferior mesenteric artery *(arrow)*. Lumbar arteries also supply collaterals to the right common iliac artery and both hypogastric arteries.

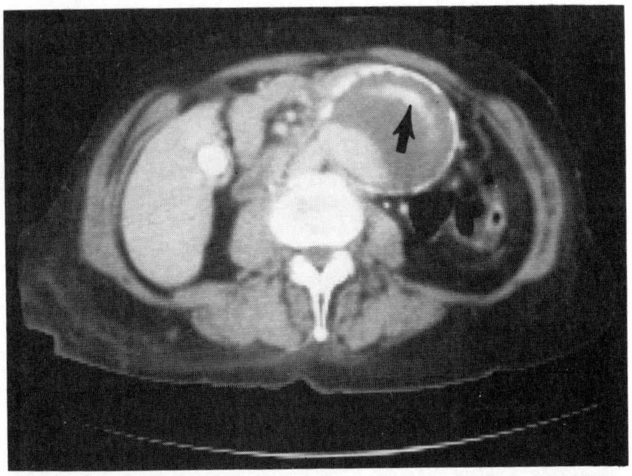

Fig 58B-9 Computed tomography scan of infrarenal aorta shows aneurysm with large amount of thrombus with calcification *(arrow)*. The peripheral, circumferential calcification is atheromatous disease of the intima.

past, is rarely associated with the abdominal aorta but may cause aneurysm formation.

Tumor. Primary tumors affecting the abdominal aorta are exceedingly rare.[28] Intraluminal tumors and sarcomas are remote possibilities. Much more commonly, the aorta can be affected by malignant lesions that metastasize or extend from nearby structures.

Embolism. The terminal aorta is subject to acute occlusion by large emboli (Fig 58B-7). These typically originate in the heart and may be due to mural thrombus (atrial or ventricular), valvular lesions, or cardiac myxoma. Large emboli confined to the aorta are usually limited to the terminal portion at the bifurcation ("saddle emboli").

SEQUELAE OF ABDOMINAL AORTIC DISEASE

Obstruction

Most of the previously outlined pathologic conditions that affect the abdominal aorta directly or indirectly cause obstruction of the vessel. Acute total aortic occlusion is potentially a catastrophic event and can produce severe bilateral lower extremity ischemia or renal occlusion (or both). In contrast, subtotal or gradual occlusion is often well tolerated, because of partially maintained intraluminal flow or development of collateral vessels (Fig 58B-8). Atherosclerosis is the most common cause of abdominal aortic obstruction, and therefore symptoms of aortic occlusion occur most frequently in patients who are older, are male, are smokers, and have other cardiovascular risk factors. When the triad of (1) impotence, (2) bilateral hip and buttock claudication, and (3) absent or decreased femoral pulses is seen in men, it is referred to as "Leriche's syndrome" and is virtually diagnostic of aortic occlusion. Although aortic occlusive disease most frequently impairs blood flow to the lower extremities (causing claudication or ischemia), it may also contribute to impaired renal and mesenteric perfusion. Thus, hypertension, renal failure, and intestinal ischemia are also potential sequelae of abdominal aortic obstruction.

Aneurysm

The abdominal aorta is considered aneurysmal when it enlarges to a diameter of 2.5 to 3.0 cm or greater (Fig 58B-9). The overall incidence of abdominal aortic aneurysm varies with the population investigated;[29] one study of high-risk individuals (60 to 75 years of age, male, with hypertension or coronary artery disease) suggested an incidence of 9%.[30] Aneurysms increase in size at a highly variable rate (typically, 0.2 to 0.8 cm per year), although the factors that affect the rate of growth are largely unknown.[29,31-33] Some aneurysms remain stable in size for years, whereas others grow rapidly.

Atherosclerosis is usually associated with abdominal aortic aneurysm, being present in an estimated 99% of all cases.[34] Not surprisingly, risk factors such as hypertension, age, smoking, and family history of abdominal aortic aneurysm are of etiologic importance. Various histologic and biochemical factors also appear to play a significant

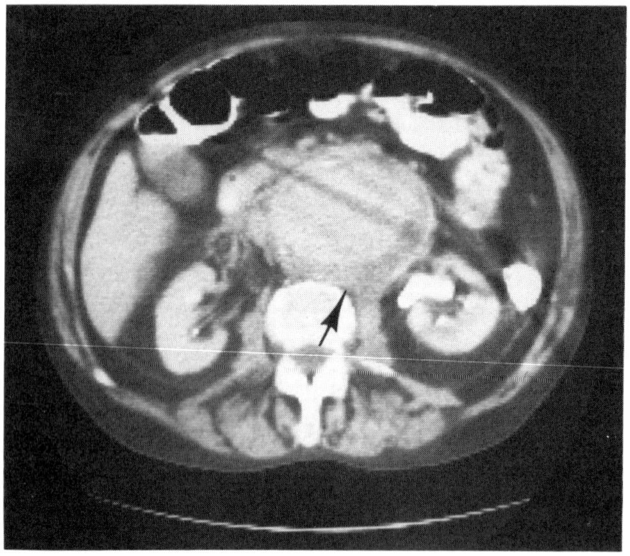

Fig 58B-10 Computed tomography scan of infrarenal aorta shows rupturing aneurysm. The *arrow* indicates tissue reaction where a recess of retroperitoneal fat should normally be found.

role in aneurysm formation; these include changes in smooth muscle function,[35] aortic wall elastin and collagen content,[35] and local or circulating elastase and collagenase activity.[36,37]

A major problem in diagnosing abdominal aortic aneurysm is that most are relatively asymptomatic and therefore unsuspected. Abdominal palpation during physical examination often misses those smaller than 4.5 cm;[38] unfortunately, aneurysms of this size already have the potential to rupture. The yearly incidence of rupture depends on aneurysm size; the rates for aneurysms with diameters of 5.0 cm, 5.7 cm, and 7.0 cm are 4.1%, 6.6%, and 19%, respectively.[29] Routine screening with duplex ultrasound scanning in high-risk individuals and those who are obese (which makes palpation of aneurysms difficult) has therefore been recommended by some authors.[30] Pain may signal the presence of an abdominal aortic aneurysm when the aneurysm is expanding rapidly or beginning to rupture. Inflammatory aneurysms also may be manifested by pain. New-onset pain associated with a known aneurysm is an indication for an immediate evaluation and treatment if necessary.

The most disastrous consequence of abdominal aortic aneurysm is rupture (Fig 58B-10), with an overall mortality of 78%.[29] The surgical mortality for those surviving long enough to undergo emergency surgery is 40% to 50%,[39] in contrast to an average elective repair mortality of 5% or less.[40] Other complications of abdominal aortic aneurysm are (1) mural thrombus formation with distal embolization, (2) dissection, (3) thrombosis with aortic occlusion, (4) rupture into the vena cava or other vein with subsequent arteriovenous fistula formation, and (5) erosion into the duodenum with formation of an aortoduodenal fistula. To prevent these adverse consequences, elective repair should be considered whenever possible by the time an asymptomatic abdominal aortic aneurysm reaches 6 cm.[34]

Dissection

Dissection of the abdominal aorta typically occurs by one of two mechanisms: (1) distal propagation of a dissection originating in the thoracic aorta and (2) dissection around an atherosclerotic ulcer (or other entry site) located in the abdominal aorta. Atherosclerosis is the usual predisposing factor for dissection, although various degenerative, inflammatory, and traumatic conditions can also be responsible. Dissection into the media creates an intimal "flap" that may give rise to a "false" lumen or channel running parallel to the "true" lumen (Fig 58B-11). When entry and exit sites across the intimal flap are present, blood can flow through the false lumen; subsequent enlargement of the false lumen may compromise flow in the true lumen. Occasionally, a combination of thrombosis, obstruction by the intimal flap, and compression by an expanding false channel causes obstruction of both the true and the false lumens. Other complications include involvement and obstruction of aortic branch vessels, external rupture through the vessel wall, and distal embolization of thrombi.

Perforation

Perforation of the abdominal aorta usually occurs in association with pathologic conditions that weaken the vessel wall or as the result of trauma. Depending on the site and circumstances of the perforation, bleeding may occur into the adjacent vein (arteriovenous fistula)[41,42] (Fig 58B-12), bowel (aortoenteric fistula), peritoneal cavity, or retroperitoneal space. Retroperitoneal bleeding can result from perforation occurring during the course of interventional cardiovascular procedures; although the flank or abdominal pain that typically occurs should alert the clinician to the possibility of retroperitoneal bleeding, it may remain undiagnosed until life-threatening amounts of blood have been lost.

The "penetrating ulcer" is an unusual entity that can result in aortic perforation.[43] Arising within an atherosclerotic plaque, it penetrates through the intima and into the media, where containment by the adventitia (or tissues superficial to the aorta) may give rise to a false aneurysm. Pain in the lumbar region or abdomen is a frequent presenting feature.

Distal embolization

Certain disease processes, especially atherosclerosis, may turn the abdominal aorta into a source of peripheral emboli. Laminated mural thrombus[44] and cholesterol fragments from plaques are the most common substrate for emboli. The so-called coral reef atherosclerotic lesion (Fig 58B-13) is a unique type of protruding, shaggy plaque that frequently produces recurrent atheroemboli.[45]

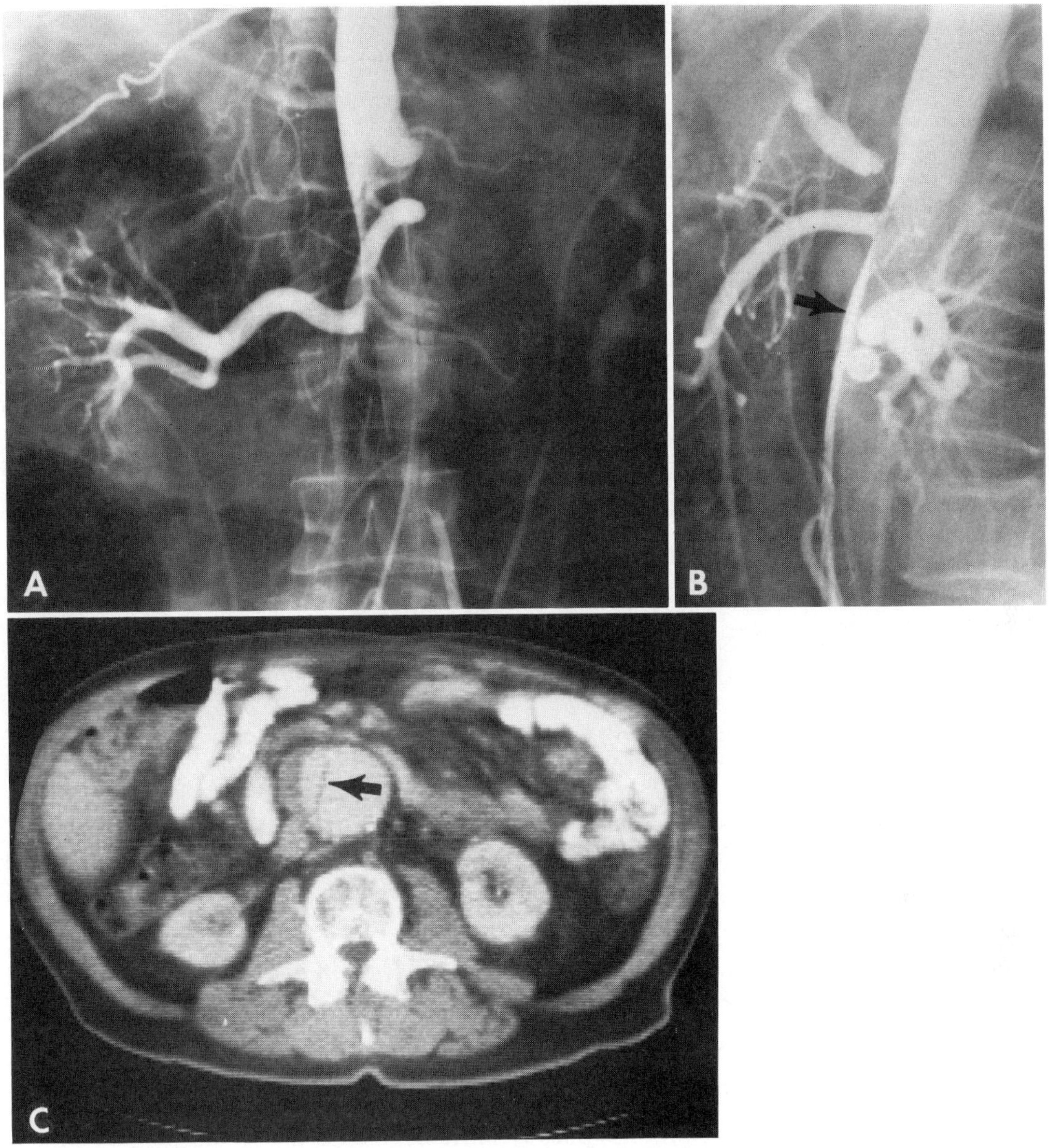

Fig 58B-11 **A** and **B,** abdominal aortogram shows dissection from the thoracic region extending to the aortic bifurcation. The true lumen is narrowed *(arrow).* The left renal artery does not fill from this lumen. **C,** computed tomography scan of infrarenal aorta reveals aortic dissection. *Arrow* indicates intimal flap.

Postgrafting complications

Significant complications are an occasional consequence of aortic replacement surgery. Perioperative infection is one of the most serious (Fig 58B-14), occurring in 0.77% of one large series.[46] Staphylococcus alone or in combination with other organisms appears to be the most common infective agent (seen in 34% of the above-mentioned series), but other gram-positive, gram-negative, and anaerobic[47] bacteria are important. Extra-anatomic bypass with subsequent removal of the infected graft is usually required to treat aortic graft infections. Late complications occur less frequently than perioperative ones; erosion by the graft into the bowel is the most common and serious.

DIAGNOSIS AND EVALUATION OF ABDOMINAL AORTIC DISEASE

Atherosclerosis with aortic obstruction or aneurysm formation (or both) is by far the most common abdominal aortic pathologic condition seen in general medical or cardiologic practice. Evaluation is complicated because

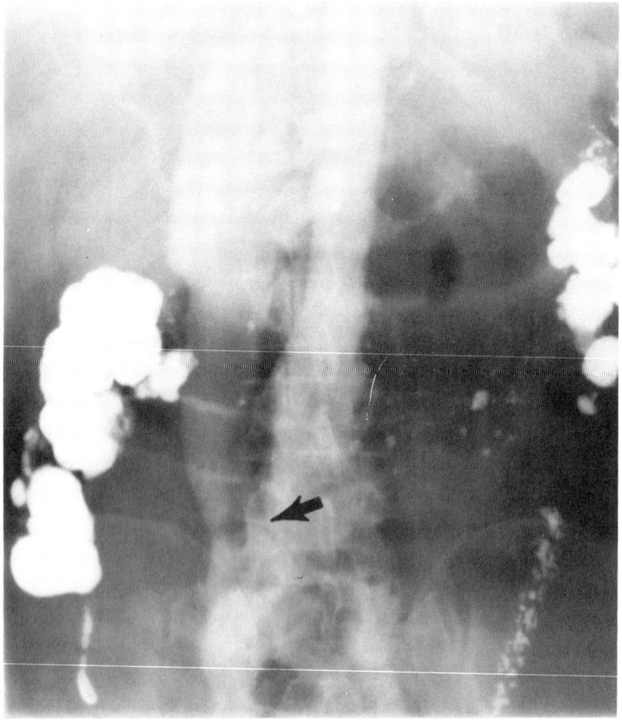

Fig 58B-12 Abdominal aortogram in a patient with a fistula *(arrow)* from an aortic aneurysm to the inferior vena cava.

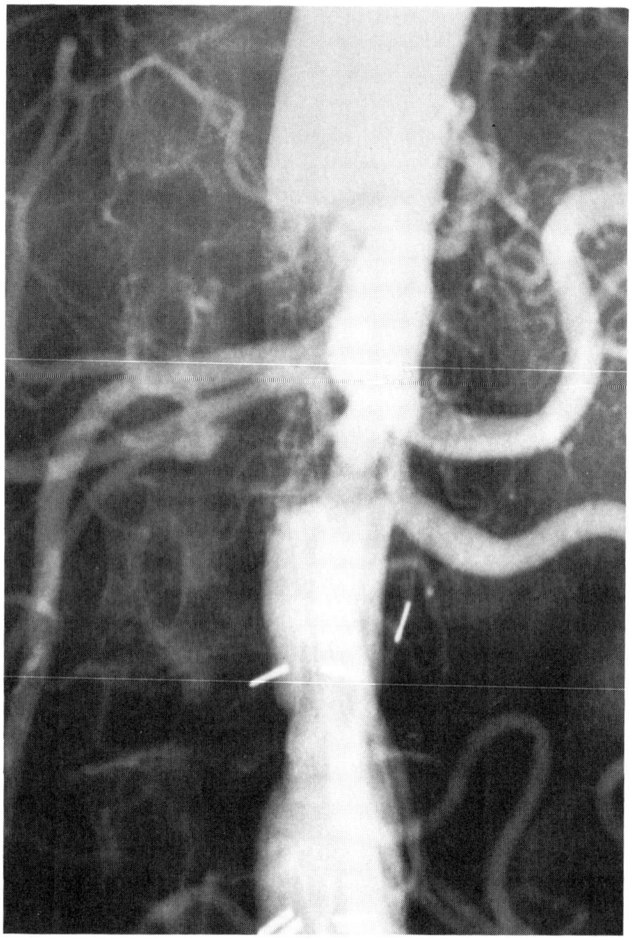

Fig 58B-13 Abdominal aortogram shows a large atheromatous plaque of the aorta at the level of the visceral arteries. The aortic lumen is narrow.

atherosclerosis is a global process and frequently affects arteries elsewhere in the body, often doing so asymptomatically. For most patients, the goal of the physician is therefore threefold: (1) Investigate the nature and severity of the aortic problem; (2) assess whether peripheral vessels (such as the carotids, renals, mesenterics, and iliofemorals) are also affected by disease and in need of treatment; and (3) determine whether (and to what extent) the heart and coronary arteries are diseased, especially if surgical correction of the aortic problem is being contemplated. The importance of evaluating diffuse atherosclerosis, especially coronary artery disease, in patients with aortic disease cannot be overemphasized, because most deaths in this group are due to cardiac causes.

History and physical examination

A detailed history that includes information about the patient's general health is essential. When the aortic problem has symptoms associated with it, specific questioning about the character, duration, localization, and so forth, of the symptoms is indicated. Cardiovascular risk factors should also be noted, along with any family history of cardiovascular or aortic disease. The clinician should determine if there is evidence of lower extremity disease (such as claudication or rest pain), carotid disease (previous stroke, endarterectomy, transient ischemic attack, or other unexplained neurologic symptoms), and coronary artery disease (angina, previous myocardial infarction, or coronary artery bypass grafting). A history of other conditions that could put the patient at risk for surgery, such as renal disease and chronic obstructive pulmonary disease, should be sought and assessed.

Although palpation of the abdomen for an aortic aneurysm should be a routine part of the physical examination in any patient over 50 years of age, particular care must be paid to the abdominal examination when abdominal aortic disease is known or suspected. During a complete physical examination, extra emphasis must be placed on (1) determination of the blood pressure in the arms and legs, (2) examination of the heart and lungs, (3) palpation of all pulses with auscultation for bruits (looking in particular for occult carotid disease), and (4) inspection of the lower extremity skin for evidence of ischemia (such as skin breakdown, discoloration, and hair loss) and distal embolization.

Laboratory studies

The appropriateness of different laboratory studies varies among patients. Patients thought to have active bleeding should have their hemoglobin checked, and the concen-

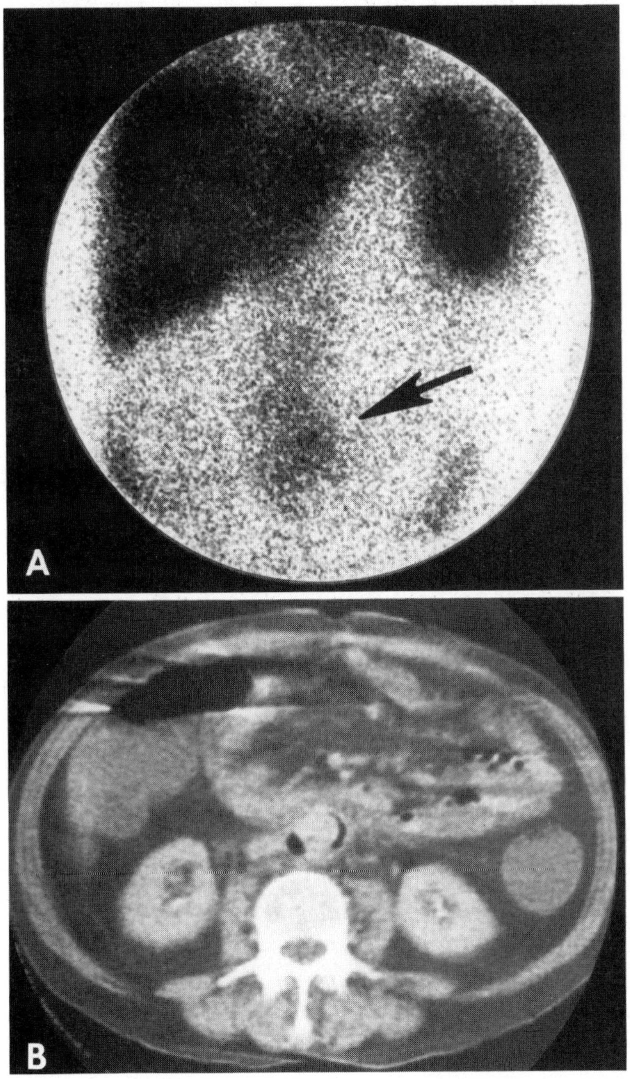

Fig 58B-14 **A,** isotope scan of the abdomen with use of neutrophils labeled with indium 111. *Arrow* indicates accumulation of tagged white blood cells at the infected aortic graft. **B,** computed tomography scan of infrarenal aorta. An aortic graft is infected, as demarcated by air around the graft.

tration of urea or creatinine (or both) should be determined in patients with possible renal impairment. The erythrocyte sedimentation rate is a valuable test for diagnosing many types of vasculitis and assessing their response to treatment. An increase in the erythrocyte sedimentation rate or white blood cell count along with fever and local signs may provide a clue to graft infection. Lipids should be checked in all patients with atherosclerosis in whom no recent determinations have been made (see chapter 13).

Functional testing

Functional testing is important not only for assessing the presence and severity of aortic occlusive disease but also for determining whether problems coexist in the coronary and carotid vessels. Noninvasive thigh pressure measurements (taken before and after lower extremity exercise, if necessary) are decreased by aortic occlusive disease and therefore provide a useful index of the severity of the disease in the aortoiliac system. The resting electrocardiogram gives information about previous infarction or other cardiac abnormalities; ischemic changes in the electrocardiogram occurring with exercise suggest the presence of underlying coronary artery disease, which may be significant (see chapter 3B). In some patients, the coronary status is better determined by radionuclide studies, such as multiple-gated acquisition scanning (which also gives information about cardiac function) and exercise thallium scanning (see chapter 6). In patients who cannot exercise, dipyridamole thallium scanning is an excellent alternative,[48,49] provided that there is no hemodynamically significant carotid disease (the hypotension induced by dipyridamole administration is potentially dangerous in patients with carotid occlusive disease). When carotid disease is present, adenosine can be used instead of dipyridamole.[50] Stress echocardiogram testing with intravenous dobutamine infusion also appears to be useful in this situation.[51] The carotid arteries can be noninvasively screened for significant disease, when indicated, by use of the oculoplethysmograph or Doppler echo scanning (transcranial or duplex).[52-54]

Since it is difficult to predict which patients with abdominal aortic aneurysm (or many other abdominal aortic problems) will have severe coronary artery disease, our policy is to use noninvasive functional cardiac testing liberally in these patients. However, decisions about whether to perform coronary arteriography and subsequent bypass grafting (or angioplasty) are then made on an individual basis, taking into account factors such as the estimated extent and severity of coronary artery disease (using symptoms and information obtained by noninvasive testing), exercise capacity of the patient, and urgency of the aortic surgery. Advances in anesthesia, surgical technique, and perioperative care have made it possible to operate on the abdominal aorta even when substantial coronary artery disease exists. Coronary disease can therefore often be managed medically, at least initially, with coronary revascularization reserved for a later date. However, the long-term cardiac follow-up of these patients remains critical, since cardiac disease is still the major late cause of death in patients successfully undergoing aortic surgery.[55]

Vascular imaging

Angiography has long been the standard in vascular imaging, and it remains so in many situations today. For example, it is still indicated in the workup of abdominal aortic aneurysms when significant distal disease or renal disease is suspected and to identify multiple renal arteries. However, a variety of newer technologies are now accepted as equal or superior to angiography in certain circumstances. For example, *ultrasound imaging* is an inexpensive and highly reliable method of studying abdominal aortic aneurysms, including screening and

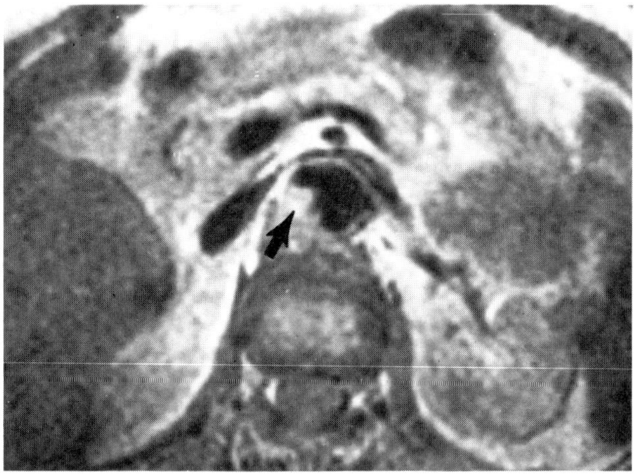

Fig 58B-15 Magnetic resonance scan of the abdominal aorta. The flowing blood (lumens of veins and arteries) is black. Large atheromatous plaque is in the aorta *(arrow)*.

following changes in size. Studies of aortic wall structure may also be performed with ultrasound scanning. Advances in *duplex scanning* (ultrasound imaging combined with Doppler) are making it possible to assess branch vessel flow to the kidneys and digestive tract as well. *Transthoracic and transesophageal cardiac echocardiography* can be used to evaluate resting cardiac function and to detect abnormalities originating in or extending from the thoracic aorta. *Computed tomographic scanning* is also an excellent way to study aneurysmal disease as well as dissection, graft infection,[56] perforation, and occlusion. *Magnetic resonance imaging* is rapidly developing into a modality for diagnosing aortic disease in a totally noninvasive way (Fig 58B-15). *Radionuclide studies,* such as indium-labeled white blood cell scanning, have proven to be useful for detecting infections in aortic grafts and aneurysms, especially when results of other studies are negative.[57,58]

TREATMENT OF ABDOMINAL AORTIC DISEASE

Medical

Risk factor reduction. Because atherosclerosis is the major disease process affecting the abdominal aorta,

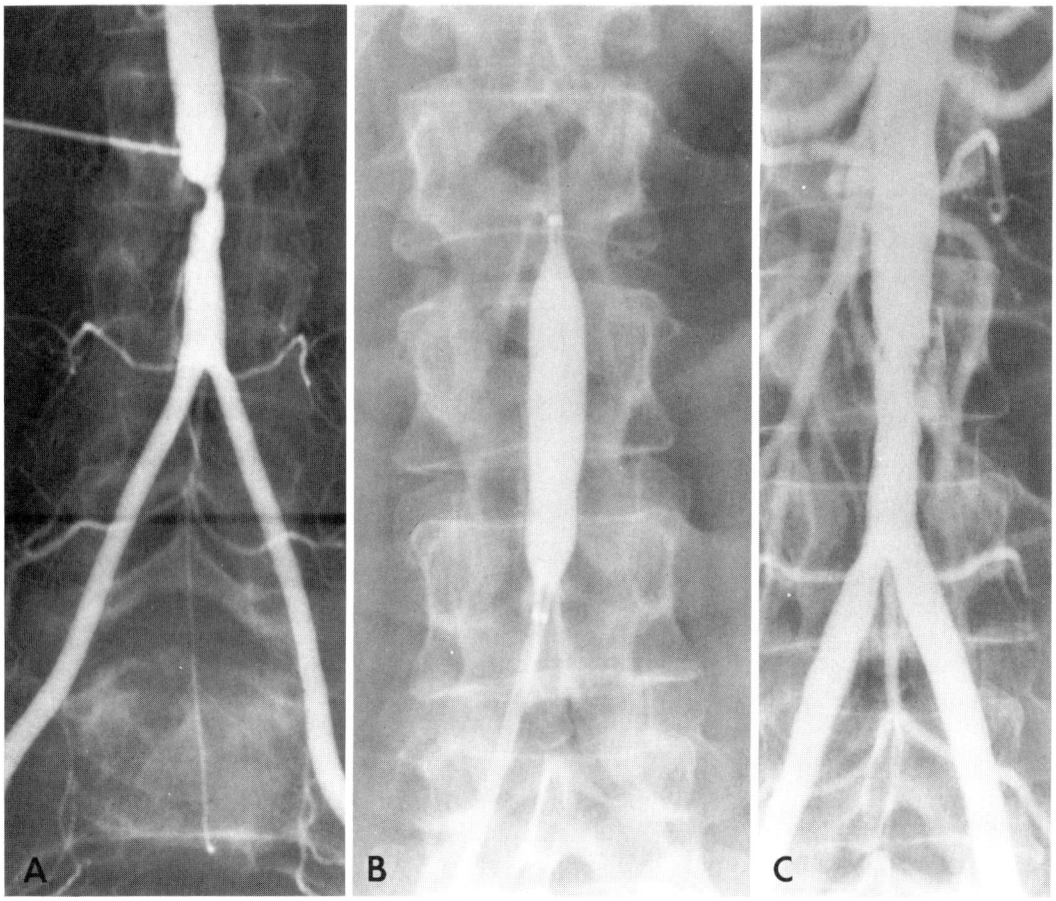

Fig 58B-16 Transluminal angioplasty of a stenotic atheromatous plaque. **A,** aortogram. **B,** dilatation balloon inflated. **C,** result after angioplasty.

medical efforts should be aimed at reducing risk factors and therefore preventing disease or slowing its progression. This is especially true considering how difficult it is to treat existing atherosclerosis medically. Getting patients to stop smoking is of prime importance; control of diabetes, hypertension, and lipids should also be attempted with dietary measures and, when indicated, drug therapy.

Drugs. Inflammatory conditions such as arteritis (and, in some situations, inflammatory aneurysm) can be treated with steroids, with the erythrocyte sedimentation rate used as a guide to the adequacy of therapy. Treatment may require months, and significant regression of vessel stenosis can occur during this time. Infections involving the abdominal aorta or grafts usually require prolonged administration of antibiotics and adjuvant surgery.

Acute abdominal aortic occlusion due to embolism or thrombosis may be treated in certain instances with any of the thrombolytic agents. Successful therapy may restore flow, although surgery is often required to correct residual underlying problems.

Surgery

Surgery remains the mainstay of treatment for many diseases of the abdominal aorta, especially aneurysms, dissections, perforations, and fixed obstructive disorders. *Grafting* using synthetic materials is performed with a straight aortic tube graft or, if necessary, a bifurcated aortoiliac or aortofemoral graft. The overall perioperative mortality with elective abdominal aortic aneurysm repair ranges from 0% to 16%, depending on the subgroups analyzed.[29,55] In high-risk subjects, extra-anatomic bypass with thrombosis of the aneurysm has been advocated, although this procedure remains controversial.[59-61] Surgical procedures must be specifically tailored to the disease process; the details on these surgical procedures are beyond the scope of this work.

Angioplasty

Balloon angioplasty and recanalization with mechanical methods (Fig 58B-16) are alternative ways to relieve obstructions in the abdominal aorta and elsewhere.[62,63] In certain situations, these techniques appear promising, although the long-term results are unknown at this time.

REFERENCES

1. Imura T, Yamamoto K, Satoh T, et al: Atherosclerotic change in the human abdominal aorta in vivo in relation to coronary heart disease and risk factors. *Atherosclerosis* 73:149-155, 1988

2. Hallett JW Jr, Brewster DC, Darling RC: *Patient Care in Vascular Surgery.* Second edition. Boston, Little, Brown and Company, 1987, pp 171-172

3. Allardice JT, Allwright GJ, Wafula JMC, et al: High prevalence of abdominal aortic aneurysm in men with peripheral vascular disease: screening by ultrasonography. *Br J Surg* 75:240-242, 1988

4. Lie JT: The structure of the normal vascular system and its reactive changes. In *Peripheral Vascular Diseases.* Edited by JL Juergens, JA Spittell Jr, JF Fairbairn II. Fifth edition. Philadelphia, WB Saunders Company, 1980, pp 51-81

5. Lie JT, Juergens JL: Degenerative arterial diseases other than atherosclerosis. In *Peripheral Vascular Diseases.* Fifth edition. Edited by JL Juergens, JA Spittell Jr, JF Fairbairn II. Philadelphia, WB Saunders Company, 1980, pp 237-251

6. Moran JJ: Idiopathic arterial calcification of infancy: a clinicopathologic study. *Pathol Annu* 10:393-417, 1975

7. Hollier LH, Stanson AW, Gloviczki P, et al: Arteriomegaly: classification and morbid implications of diffuse aneurysmal disease. *Surgery* 93:700-708, 1983

8. Schnitker MA, Bayer CA: Dissecting aneurysm of the aorta in young individuals, particularly in association with pregnancy: with report of a case. *Ann Intern Med* 20:486-511, 1944

9. Smith RB III, Sewell CW: Congenital aortic aneurysms. In *Aortic Surgery.* Edited by JJ Bergan, JST Yao. Philadelphia, WB Saunders Company, 1989, pp 469-482

10. Hall S, Barr W, Lie JT, et al: Takayasu arteritis: a study of 32 North American patients. *Medicine (Baltimore)* 64:89-99, 1985

11. Walker DI, Bloor K, Williams G, et al: Inflammatory aneurysms of the abdominal aorta. *Br J Surg* 59:609-614, 1972

12. Baskerville PA, Blakeney CG, Young AE, et al: The diagnosis and treatment of peri-aortic fibrosis ('inflammatory' aneurysms). *Br J Surg* 70:381-385, 1983

13. Crawford JL, Stowe CL, Safi HJ, et al: Inflammatory aneurysms of the aorta. *J Vasc Surg* 2:113-123, 1985

14. Gaylis H, Isaacson C: Abdominal aortic inflammatory aneurysms. In *Aortic Surgery.* Edited by JJ Bergan, JST Yao. Philadelphia, WB Saunders Company, 1989, 267-292

15. Pennell RC, Hollier LH, Lie JT, et al: Inflammatory abdominal aortic aneurysms: a thirty-year review. *J Vasc Surg* 2:859-869, 1985

16. Goldstone J: The infected infra-renal aortic graft. *Acta Chir Scand Suppl* 538:72-86, 1987

17. Mattox KL: Aortic trauma. *Curr Opinion Cardiol* 3:723-728, 1988

18. Sĕbesta P, Pirk J. Filipova H: Superior mesenteric artery syndrome following abdominal aortic aneurysm resection and replacement. *Thorac Cardiovasc Surg* 35:378-381, 1987

19. Lock JS, Huffman AD, Johnson RC: Blunt trauma to the abdominal aorta. *J Trauma* 27:674-677, 1987

20. Rooke TW: Vascular complications of interventional procedures. In *Interventional Cardiology.* Edited by DR Holmes Jr, RE Vlietstra. Philadelphia, FA Davis Company, 1989, pp 340-358

21. Bunt TJ, Manship L, Moore W: Iatrogenic vascular injury during peripheral revascularization. *J Vasc Surg* 2:491-498, 1985

22. Cullen PJ, Leahy AL, McBride KD, et al: Angiographically-induced infection of the aorta. *Ann Vasc Surg* 1:386-388, 1986

23. Boyd DP, Farha GJ: Arteriovenous fistula and isolated vascular injuries secondary to intervertebral disk surgery: report of four cases and review of the literature. *Ann Surg* 161:524-531, 1965

24. Perry MO: Infected aortic aneurysms. *J Vasc Surg* 2:597-599, 1985

25. Johansen K: Infected and other unusual aneurysms. In *Aortic Surgery.* Edited by JJ Bergan, JST Yao. Philadelphia, WB Saunders Company, 1989, pp 293-303

26. Ewart JM, Burke ML, Bunt TJ: Spontaneous abdominal aortic infections: essentials of diagnosis and management. *Am Surg* 49:37-50, 1983

27. MacLellan DG, Sandland AM, Spelman DW, et al: Ruptured abdominal aortic aneurysm: a complication of Salmonella bovismorbificans infection. *Aust N Z J Surg* 53:371-373, 1983

28. Josen AS, Khine M: Primary malignant tumor of the aorta. *J Vasc Surg* 9:493-498, 1989

29. Taylor LM Jr, Porter JM: Basic data related to clinical decision-making in abdominal aortic aneurysms. *Ann Vasc Surg* 1:502-504, 1986

30. Lederle FA, Walker JM, Reinke DB: Selective screening for abdominal aortic aneurysms with physical examination and ultrasound. *Arch Intern Med* 148:1753-1756, 1988

31. Guirguis EM, Barber GG: The natural history of abdominal aortic aneurysms. *Am J Surg* 162:481-483, 1991

32. Limet R, Sakalihassan N, Albert A: Determination of the expansion rate and incidence of rupture of abdominal aortic aneurysms. *J Vasc Surg* 14:540-548, 1991

33. Kaufman JA, Bettmann MA: Prognosis of abdominal aortic aneurysms: a population-based study. *Invest Radiol* 26:612-614, 1991

34. Olcott C IV, Mehigan JT: Aneurysms of the abdominal aorta and peripheral arteries. In *Diagnosis and Management of Peripheral Vascular Disease.* Edited by DC Miller, AJ Roon. Menlo Park, California, Addison-Wesley Publishing Company, 1982, pp 199-210

35. Powell J, Greenhalgh RM: Cellular, enzymatic, and genetic factors in the pathogenesis of abdominal aortic aneurysms. *J Vasc Surg* 9:297-304, 1989

36. Brown SL, Backstrom B, Busuttil RW: A new serum proteolytic enzyme in aneurysm pathogenesis. *J Vasc Surg* 2:393-399, 1985

37. Zarins CK, Runyon-Hass A, Zatina MA, et al: Increased collagenase activity in early aneurysmal dilatation. *J Vasc Surg* 3:238-248, 1986

38. Sommerville RL, Allen EV, Edwards JE: Bland and infected arteriosclerotic abdominal aortic aneurysms: a clinicopathologic study. *Medicine (Baltimore)* 38:207-221, 1959

39. Donaldson MC, Rosenberg JM, Bucknam CA: Factors affecting survival after ruptured abdominal aortic aneurysm. *J Vasc Surg* 2:564-570, 1985

40. Graham M, Chan A: Ultrasound screening for clinically occult abdominal aortic aneurysm. *Can Med Assoc J* 138:627-629, 1988

41. Petetin L, Pelouze GA, Mercier V, et al: Rupture of abdominal aortic aneurysm into the inferior vena cava: a study of seven cases. *Ann Vasc Surg* 1:572-577, 1987

42. Celoria GM, Friedmann P, Rhee SW, et al: Fistulas between the aorta and the left renal vein. *J Vasc Surg* 6:191-193, 1987

43. Cooke JP, Kazmier FJ, Orszulak TA: The penetrating aortic ulcer: pathologic manifestations, diagnosis, and management. *Mayo Clin Proc* 63:718-725, 1988

44. Gagliardi J-M, Batt M, Khodja R-H, et al: Mural thrombus of the aorta. *Ann Vasc Surg* 2:201-204, 1988

45. Qvarfordt PG, Reilly LM, Sedwitz MM: "Coral reef" atherosclerosis of the suprarenal aorta: a unique clinical entity. *J Vasc Surg* 1:903-908, 1984

46. O'Hara PJ, Hertzer NR, Beven EG, et al: Surgical management of infected abdominal aortic grafts: review of a 25-year experience. *J Vasc Surg* 3:725-731, 1986

47. Brook I: Role of anaerobic bacteria in aortofemoral graft infection. *Surgery* 104:843-845, 1988

48. Strawn DJ, Guernsey JM: Dipyridamole thallium scanning in the evaluation of coronary artery disease in elective abdominal aortic surgery. *Arch Surg* 126:880-884, 1991

49. Leppo J, Plaja J, Gionet M, et al: Noninvasive evaluation of cardiac risk before elective vascular surgery. *J Am Coll Cardiol* 9:269-276, 1987

50. Coyne EP, Belvedere DA, Vande Streek PR, et al: Thallium-201 scintigraphy after intravenous infusion of adenosine compared with exercise thallium testing in the diagnosis of coronary artery disease. *J Am Coll Cardiol* 17:1289-1294, 1991

51. Sawada SG, Segar DS, Ryan T, et al: Echocardiographic detection of coronary artery disease during dobutamine infusion. *Circulation* 83:1605-1614, 1991

52. Sutton KC, Wolfson SK Jr, Kuller LH: Carotid and lower extremity arterial disease in elderly adults with isolated systolic hypertension. *Stroke* 18:817-822, 1987

53. Biedert S, Winter R, Betz H, et al: The detection of intracranial carotid artery disease by continuous-wave Doppler sonography. *Neuroradiology* 28:296-303, 1986

54. Kenagy JW: Comparison of duplex scanning and contrast arteriography: a community hospital experience. *J Vasc Surg* 2:591-593, 1985

55. Hertzer NR: Basic data concerning associated coronary disease in peripheral vascular patients. *Ann Vasc Surg* 1:616-620, 1987

56. Mark AS, McCarthy SM, Moss AA, et al: Detection of abdominal aortic graft infection: comparison of CT and In-labeled white blood cell scans. *AJR* 144:315-318, 1985

57. Brunner MC, Mitchell RS, Baldwin JC, et al: Prosthetic graft infection: limitations of indium white blood cell scanning. *J Vasc Surg* 3:42-48, 1986

58. Lawrence PF, Dries DJ, Alazraki N, et al: Indium 111-labeled leukocyte scanning for detection of prosthetic vascular graft infection. *J Vasc Surg* 2:165-172, 1985

59. Schwartz RA, Nichols WK, Silver D: Is thrombosis of the infrarenal abdominal aortic aneurysm an acceptable alternative? *J Vasc Surg* 3:448-455, 1986

60. Schanzer H, Papa MC, Miller CM: Rupture of surgically thrombosed abdominal aortic aneurysm. *J Vasc Surg* 2:278-280, 1985

61. Inahara T, Geary GL, Mukherjee D, et al: The contrary position to the nonresective treatment for abdominal aortic aneurysm. *J Vasc Surg* 2:42-46, 1985

62. Morag B, Rubinstein Z, Kessler A, et al: Percutaneous transluminal angioplasty of the distal abdominal aorta and its bifurcation. *Cardiovasc Intervent Radiol* 10:129-133, 1987

63. el Ashmaoui A, Do DD, Triller J, et al: Angioplasty of the terminal aorta: follow-up of 20 patients treated by PTA or PTA with stents. *Eur J Radiol* 13:113-117, 1991

CHAPTER

59

Systemic disease with cardiac involvement

Lyle J. Olson, M.D., and Roger L. Click, M.D., Ph.D.

Many systemic diseases affect the heart, the manifestations of which depend on the anatomic site and extent of involvement. Clinical syndromes observed in the patient with systemic disease involving the heart include heart failure, arrhythmia with syncope or sudden death, and thromboembolism. Cardiac involvement may be the predominant clinical manifestation in the individual patient. In other patients, cardiac disease may be subclinical, discovered either incidentally or at postmortem examination.

Systemic diseases involving the heart may be categorized according to general etiologic origin (Table 59-1). Of these broad categories, infectious (chapter 19A), endocrine (chapter 63), neoplastic (chapter 56), and chemical, drug, and physical toxicities (chapter 19A) are covered elsewhere in this text; genetic diseases with systemic manifestations, including cardiac involvement, are reviewed in chapter 68.

This chapter reviews selected connective tissue, nutritional, metabolic, and neurologic diseases as well as sarcoidosis and miscellaneous disorders with cardiac involvement.

CONNECTIVE TISSUE DISEASE

The connective tissue diseases are systemic disorders of generalized inflammation of blood vessels. Symptoms are most prominent in the joints, muscles, and serosal surfaces of the pleura and pericardium. Because of a predilection for patients to present with arthritis, these disorders are often termed "rheumatic." However, the major morbidity and mortality are due to complications of heart, kidney, and central nervous system involvement.

Specific rheumatic disorders that may involve the heart are systemic lupus erythematosus, progressive systemic sclerosis, rheumatoid arthritis, ankylosing spondylitis, mixed connective tissue disease, and relapsing polychondritis (Table 59-2). Other disorders of diffuse vasculitis that also affect the heart are periarteritis nodosa, Wegener's granulomatosis, allergic granulomatosis, giant cell arteritis, and Behçet's syndrome (Table 59-3). Takayasu's arteritis, which affects primarily the great vessels, is discussed in chapter 58A.

Table 59-1 Systemic diseases with cardiac involvement

Connective tissue
Metabolic
Nutritional
Sarcoid
Hematologic
Neurologic
Infectious
Endocrine
Neoplastic
Chemical, drug, and physical toxicities
Miscellaneous

Table 59-2 Rheumatic disorders with cardiac involvement

Systemic lupus erythematosus
Progressive systemic sclerosis
Rheumatoid arthritis
Ankylosing spondylitis
Mixed connective tissue disease
Relapsing polychondritis

Table 59-3 Vasculitides with cardiac involvement

Periarteritis nodosa
Wegener's granulomatosis
Allergic granulomatosis
Giant cell arteritis
Behçet's syndrome

Systemic lupus erythematosus

Systemic lupus erythematosus (SLE) is an immunologic disorder of unknown cause affecting the skin, joints, lungs, kidneys, central nervous system, and heart. Although SLE may be acute, fulminating, and rapidly progressive, the clinical course is characterized by exacerbations and remissions. Most deaths are due to renal, central nervous system, or infectious complications; cardiac involvement is a less common cause of death or disability. The 10-year survival rate generally exceeds 80%.

Pathology. Antinuclear and anticytoplasmic antibodies circulate in the serum of patients, and immune complex deposition is characteristic of the disease. Serum complement is decreased in most patients, an observation that aids in the discrimination of this disorder from other connective tissue diseases.[1] Most patients have positive lupus erythematosus cell preparations. Pericarditis is the most frequent pathologic abnormality found at cardiac necropsy in patients with SLE, identified in 75%.[2]

The characteristic pathologic lesion of valvular disease is the Libman-Sacks vegetation, observed in a high proportion of autopsy cases.[3-5] Vegetations are typically 1 to 4 mm in diameter, sterile, and granular. They may be single or multiple and scattered over the endocardium of the valve, the valve rings, the chordae tendineae, and the endocardium of the atria or ventricles; all valve leaflets may be involved. Hematoxylin bodies (believed to be the histologic counterpart to lupus erythematosus cells) may be identified within the sterile vegetations. Vegetations are similar to those of nonthrombotic endocarditis or marantic endocarditis[3-5] (Fig 59-1).

The histologic lesions of myocarditis are focal collections of inflammatory cells, including polymorphonuclear leukocytes, lymphocytes, plasma cells, and macrophages,

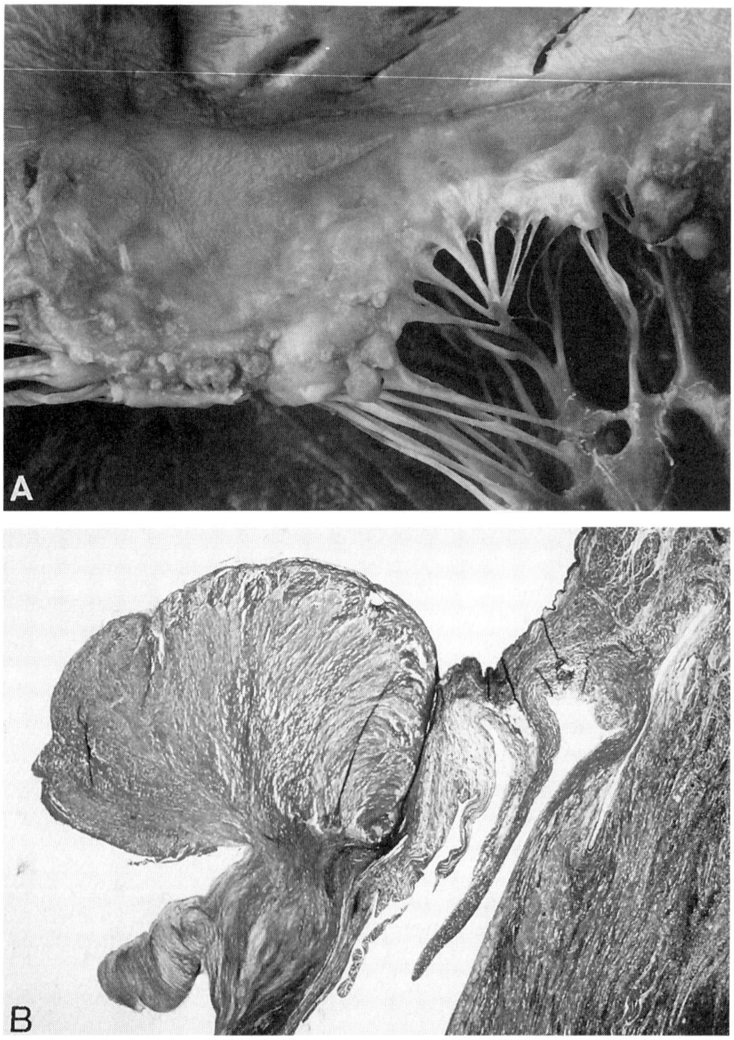

Fig 59-1 **A,** vegetations of Libman-Sacks endocarditis from a 25-year-old woman with systemic lupus erythematosus involving the mitral valve. Distribution of the vegetations at the leaflet margins is characteristic. **B,** histologic section of valvular vegetation in patient with Libman-Sacks endocarditis.

with associated interstitial edema. Hematoxylin bodies may also be seen within the lesions and fibrinoid changes observed in interstitial areas, especially in a perivascular distribution. When present, myocarditis is often associated with systemic myositis and antibodies to nuclear ribonucleoprotein.[6] The histologic inflammatory changes observed are similar in cardiac and skeletal muscle. Pathologic abnormalities of the coronary arteries include focal fibrinoid necrosis and thromboembolic obstruction, although these are rarely associated with myocardial necrosis.[2,4,7,8]

Clinical manifestations. Approximately one-third of patients with SLE have clinical evidence of cardiac involvement, including pericarditis, endocarditis, myocarditis, and coronary artery disease (arteritis or atherosclerosis).[2,4,7,8] Heart failure may be due to endocardial or myocardial disease. Arrhythmias are frequent and have been associated with myocarditis, hypertension, and uremia. Although a frequent finding at autopsy, pericarditis is less frequently diagnosed in life. Complications include tamponade, constrictive pericardial disease, and purulent pericarditis.[7,9,10]

Physical findings include pericardial friction rub, murmurs associated with aortic and mitral valve disease, and, less commonly, signs and symptoms of heart failure. Hypertension is frequent and is usually associated with renal involvement.

Like pericarditis, the endocarditis of SLE may be subclinical, identified only at autopsy. However, clinically significant valvular dysfunction occurs most often in the form of aortic or mitral valve regurgitation; valvular stenosis is less frequently observed. Though unusual, extensive scarring and deformation may affect the valves.[11-13] The development of valvulitis has been associated with antiphospholipid antibodies, thrombocytopenia, and recurrent thromboses.[12] Valvular disease increases the risk of infective endocarditis, which may be superimposed on the Libman-Sacks lesions.

Myocarditis is unusual but when observed may be associated with life-threatening complications, including heart failure, conduction block, and ventricular arrhythmias. The epicardial coronary arteries are not frequently involved in SLE. However, in patients who have undergone extensive therapy with corticosteroids, coronary artery disease may be more prevalent.[4] Patients treated with steroids are at increased risk for hypercholesterolemia and systemic hypertension, which may promote accelerated coronary atherosclerosis.

Extracardiac complications of SLE may produce secondary cardiovascular disease, which is more commonly observed than primary lupus heart disease. Systemic hypertension may lead to heart failure, and renal failure may promote uremic pericarditis. Infants born to women with SLE have an increased risk of SLE[14] and congenital heart block.[15-17]

Primary treatment utilizes anti-inflammatory agents, including corticosteroids, nonsteroidal anti-inflammatory drugs, and cytotoxic agents. Treatment of hypertension, heart failure, and arrhythmias is conventional. In occasional patients, pericardial effusion may require drainage, and valvular heart disease may require surgery.

Progressive systemic sclerosis

Progressive systemic sclerosis (PSS), also referred to as "scleroderma," is characterized by fibrous thickening of the skin and associated degenerative disease of the fingers, esophagus, bowel, kidneys, lung, and heart. Age at onset is the third to fifth decade, with women affected twice as often as men. Although the primary cause is unknown, evidence implicates a diffuse vascular lesion. Vascular disease is frequently manifested by Raynaud's phenomenon.[18,19]

Pathology. Vascular lesions are characterized by intimal proliferation and adventitial scarring of capillaries and arterioles.[19,20] Biventricular dilatation with fibrous scarring may be observed despite patent epicardial coronary arteries and normal valves. Pericarditis may be present, but constriction is rare.[21,22] Myocardial necrosis associated with patency of coronary arteries in association with contraction band necrosis suggests transient occlusion due to vasospasm and subsequent reperfusion as the mechanism of cardiac involvement (i.e., Raynaud's phenomenon of the heart).[21,23,24] In pulmonary vascular disease, pathologic findings are similar to those in idiopathic primary pulmonary hypertension and Eisenmenger's syndrome, including plexiform lesions and necrotizing arteritis.

Clinical manifestations. Skin involvement is predominant in most patients, although others may have minimal skin disease with severe visceral involvement. Approximately 90% of patients have Raynaud's phenomenon, esophageal dysfunction, and sclerotic skin.[19] The CREST (calcinosis cutis, Raynaud's phenomenon, esophageal abnormality, sclerodactyly, telangiectasia) syndrome is a PSS variant with mild skin disease but severe lung disease with pulmonary hypertension.[18,19] Clinical evidence of cardiovascular disease is detected less often than autopsy studies would suggest. Cardiac disease includes heart failure, arrhythmias, myocardial infarction, angina pectoris, and sudden death.

PSS may be associated with pulmonary fibrosis and secondary pulmonary hypertension with cor pulmonale. A primary pulmonary vascular lesion occurs and is also associated with progressive right heart failure. Pulmonary arterial pressure may become systemic and is frequently refractory to therapy. PSS also causes renal disease with systemic hypertension and renal failure; secondary cardiovascular disease is common, including biventricular failure and uremic pericarditis.

Thallium scintigraphy may demonstrate reversible perfusion defects in patients with angina pectoris but angiographically proven normal coronary arteries, suggesting myocardial microcirculatory dysfunction. Symptoms and perfusion defects may abate with administration of nifedipine.[25] Reversible cold-induced myocardial perfusion defects have also been demonstrated.[26]

Pericarditis is reported in a minority of patients with PSS. Most often, the probable cause is renal failure, although it may occur when no other cause is recognized. PSS is not known to cause primary valvular heart disease.

Nonspecific immunologic abnormalities observed in PSS include increased circulating levels of gamma globulin, cryoglobulin, antinuclear antibody, and rheumatoid factor. Electrocardiographic abnormalities are nonspecific and include atrial and ventricular arrhythmias and conduction block.[27] Chest radiography often demonstrates cardiomegaly associated with extensive fibrosis.

Cardiovascular disease secondary to systemic and pulmonary hypertension is common because of the predilection of PSS to affect the renal and pulmonary arterial circulations; included are biventricular failure, cor pulmonale, and uremic pericarditis. Because the primary cause of PSS is unknown, there is no specific therapeutic intervention; similarly, no known effective therapy is available for PSS with cardiac involvement. Treatment is supportive and includes standard care for the complications of cardiovascular involvement. Nifedipine may attenuate digital vasospasm (Raynaud's) and relieve myocardial ischemia.[28] Angiotensin-converting enzyme inhibition is of value for progressive renal disease.

Polymyositis

Polymyositis occurs as either a distinct entity characterized by diffuse inflammation of skeletal muscle or as part of a connective tissue overlap syndrome in association with PSS, SLE, or polyarteritis. Polymyositis primarily affects proximal striated muscles and may involve connective tissue, including skin and joints. When the skin is affected, the syndrome is referred to as "dermatomyositis."

Pathology. Autopsy studies have demonstrated histologic evidence of myocarditis in approximately 25% of cases.[29] In patients with evidence of myocarditis at autopsy, congestive heart failure was present before death. The disease may also affect the conduction system and coronary arteries.

Clinical manifestations. Pulmonary complications, especially pneumonitis, are prevalent because of respiratory muscle weakness and esophageal dysmotility promoting aspiration. Cardiac involvement may be subclinical or overt. In one series, 72% of patients with polymyositis had evidence of cardiac involvement by noninvasive investigation.[30] Electrocardiographic manifestations include atrial tachyarrhythmias, atrioventricular conduction abnormalities, bundle-branch block, and nonspecific repolarization abnormalities.[31] Congestive heart failure may also be observed.

Therapeutic intervention with immunosuppression, including corticosteroids, may ameliorate systemic muscle weakness but has not been shown to alter progression of cardiac disease. Conduction block may require pacemaker implantation.

Rheumatoid arthritis

Rheumatoid arthritis is the most common of the connective tissue diseases, may be familial, and affects women more often than men. It is characterized by fever, weight loss, anemia, lymphadenopathy, subcutaneous rheumatoid nodules, and arthritis with deforming erosion of the joints; pleuritis and vasculitis occur less commonly. Cardiovascular involvement is uncommon.

Pathology. Cardiac involvement may include pericarditis, valvulitis, coronary vasculitis, and myocarditis. Rheumatoid pericarditis is demonstrated in approximately 30% of autopsied cases.[32] Rheumatoid nodules may involve the myocardium, including the conduction system, and the endocardium, including the valves, and may lead to valvular perforation. Coronary artery disease appears to be more prevalent in patients with rheumatoid arthritis than in controls.[33-35]

Clinical manifestations. Pericarditis is the most frequent manifestation of cardiac involvement, usually identified by a friction rub or by pericardial effusion during echocardiography. However, the disease seldom progresses to tamponade or constriction.[36,37]

Significant valvular disease is uncommon, but occasionally surgical intervention is required for regurgitant aortic or mitral valve disease.[38]

Chest pain syndromes may be due to serositis or coronary artery disease. Electrocardiographic abnormalities are nonspecific but may include conduction block requiring permanent pacemaker implantation.[39] Sudden death, possibly due to coronary artery disease or heart block, has been reported.

Ankylosing spondylitis

Ankylosing spondylitis is a chronic inflammatory disorder of the articulations of the spine and adjacent soft tissues. It primarily affects young men, commencing in the third decade of life. The cause is unknown, but genetic, environmental, and infectious origins have been postulated. The major morbidity of the disorder is due to the development of chronic back pain, deforming dorsal kyphosis, and fusion of the costovertebral and sacroiliac joints, with immobilization of the spine. The HLA-B27 antigen appears to be a genetic marker for the disease. Cardiac disease is most often manifested as aortic regurgitation; less often, mitral regurgitation and heart block are observed.[40]

Pathology. Characteristic findings include aortic annulus and root enlargement associated with a sclerosing inflammatory lesion that may extend proximally and distally to the aortic valve. Occasionally, the lesion extends to the anterior mitral leaflet and the crest of the ventricular septum (Fig 59-2). Hence, mitral regurgitation and conduction disturbances are often observed.[41,42] Pericarditis has been described.[43]

Clinical manifestations. Cardiovascular disease associated with ankylosing spondylitis is due to aortic and mitral regurgitation and heart block. The prevalence of aortic valve regurgitation increases with the duration of the illness and may affect as many as 50% of patients who have had ankylosing spondylitis for 30 years.[41] Progression of valvular regurgitation may eventually require valve replacement.[44] Conduction defects may include heart block requiring pacemaker implantation.

Medical therapy for ankylosing spondylitis consists of administration of anti-inflammatory drugs. In more severe cases, corticosteroids may be used.

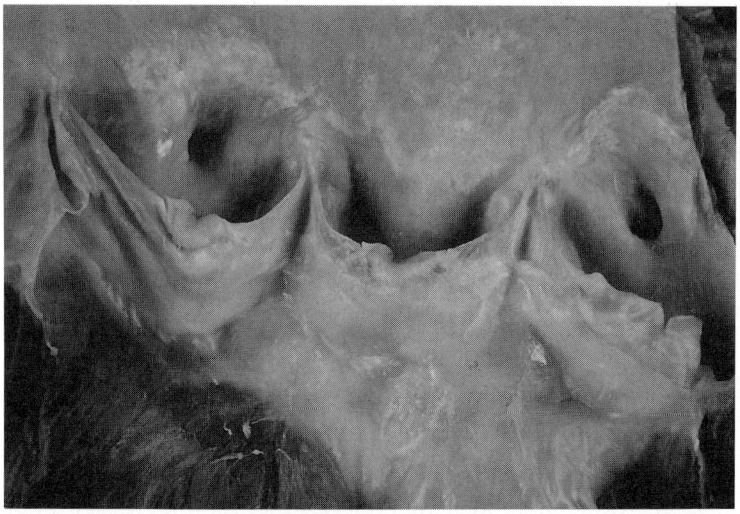

Fig 59-2 Characteristic fibrosis of ankylosing spondylitis at junction of mitral and aortic valves.

Mixed connective tissue disease

Mixed connective tissue disease is a syndrome with features of SLE, PSS, polymyositis, and rheumatoid arthritis. High titers of circulating antibodies to nuclear ribonucleoprotein are frequently identified in affected patients.

Cardiac manifestations include pericardial disease with effusion and pericarditis, including increased pericardial thickness, as well as myocarditis and valvular heart disease, especially mitral regurgitation. Arrhythmias and disorders of cardiac conduction, including sinus arrest and bundle-branch block, have also been described.[45-47]

Relapsing polychondritis

Relapsing polychondritis is an extremely rare disease of remissions and exacerbations of progressive inflammation of cartilaginous structures throughout the body, most commonly affecting auricular and nasal cartilage.

Cardiovascular disease may occur in as many as one-fourth of patients. Vasculitis of medium to large arteries frequently develops, causing aneurysm formation with fatal rupture. Aortic and mitral valve regurgitation may be observed due to involvement with dilatation of valvular annuli. Corticosteroids are the mainstay of therapy. In patients with progressive aortic and mitral valve regurgitation, surgery may be indicated.[48-50]

Periarteritis nodosa

Periarteritis nodosa, also referred to as "polyarteritis nodosa," is characterized by focal necrotizing inflammation primarily affecting small and medium-sized arteries and arterioles. Organ systems affected are the skin, kidneys, spleen and lymph nodes, gastrointestinal tract, musculoskeletal system, nervous system, and heart. This disorder is regarded as distinct from other forms of necrotizing angiitis (see below), including giant cell arteritis, Wegener's granulomatosis, hypersensitivity angiitis, and Behçet's disease, although overlapping features make classification difficult.[51]

Pathology. Vasculitis is characterized by inflammatory infiltration of media and adventitia, typically most prominent in the subepicardial coronary arteries and distal extramural coronary arteries. Advanced lesions involve the full thickness of the vessel wall, including the intima. Complications include focal aneurysmal enlargement due to vascular wall necrosis and thrombosis. As the lesions heal, intimal proliferation may be observed, which leads to coronary artery stenosis and predisposes to thrombosis with myocardial infarction.[52,53]

Clinical manifestations. Cardiac involvement, especially of the coronary arteries, is frequently observed and is complicated by myocardial infarction. Coronary arteriography demonstrates aneurysm formation, which produces a characteristic beaded appearance. Rarely, coronary arterial aneurysms rupture and produce hemopericardium. Other complications of primary cardiac involvement in periarteritis nodosa are pericarditis and conduction system disease.[54,55] Conduction system disease is due to a predilection for vasculitis to involve the sinoatrial and atrioventricular nodal arteries.[53]

Systemic hypertension, reported in up to 90% of patients with periarteritis nodosa, predisposes to secondary cardiovascular disease.[51] Hypertension occurs in association with chronic renal failure due to renal vasculitis. The development of systemic hypertension in association with renal failure and coronary artery disease also predisposes this group of patients to the development of heart failure, which may be seen in up to 60%.[51,56]

Prognosis is generally related to the stage of renal

disease. Corticosteroids are the mainstay of therapy, although they exacerbate coexisting hypertension. The efficacy of anticoagulant therapy to prevent thrombosis is unknown. Congestive heart failure, hypertension, and arrhythmias are treated in the conventional manner.

Giant cell arteritis

Giant cell arteritis is a disorder of major arteries, including the aorta and particularly the temporal arteries, that occurs in an older age group and tends to affect women more than men. There may be associated polymyalgia rheumatica.

Pathologically, this disorder is characterized by severe intimal proliferation, which may be associated with thrombosis. Histologically, periarteritis with focal areas of necrosis of the media and replacement with granulation tissue is associated with characteristic multinucleated giant cells. The carotid system is most often involved, but the aorta and other large arteries may also be affected.[57-59] Cardiac involvement by arteritis has been described, including manifestations of angina pectoris, myocardial infarction, and sudden death.[60-63] This disorder has been successfully managed with corticosteroids.[64]

Wegener's granulomatosis

Wegener's granulomatosis is a multisystem disease associated with necrotizing granulomas of the respiratory tract and with a focal necrotizing angiitis, which may affect the kidneys, causing glomerulitis, and the cardiovascular system. The respiratory tract and the kidneys are the main sites of involvement.[65,66] However, Wegener described cardiovascular involvement in one of three of his early cases, and coronary arteritis and myocarditis have also been reported.[67] Complications of cardiac involvement include myocardial infarction attributed to coronary arteritis as well as myocarditis, endocarditis, valvulitis, and conduction system disease. Myocarditis has been estimated to occur in 25% of affected individuals.[67]

Recognition of this syndrome is important, as it may be lethal without therapy. Current therapeutic agents include cyclophosphamide, azathioprine, corticosteroids, and antibiotics. Resolution of cardiovascular complications with therapy has been reported.[66]

Behçet's disease

Behçet's disease is a diffuse vasculitis typically manifested by recurrent oral and genital ulcers and eye disease with iritis and uveitis. Cardiovascular disease is observed in approximately 5% of patients, with manifestations that include thrombophlebitis, angiitis and aneurysms of large arteries, pericarditis, myocarditis, and valvular heart disease. Patients may present with signs and symptoms of heart failure, arrhythmias, and pericarditis.[68,69]

Allergic granulomatosis

Patients typically present with a respiratory illness manifested by pulmonary infiltrates with asthma and fever, frequently associated with a peripheral eosinophilia. The heart may also be a target organ, with myocarditis and complications of coronary arteritis similar to those reported for periarteritis nodosa.[70] Pathologically, the disease is recognized by abundant eosinophils within granulomatous collections of epithelial and giant cells.

NUTRITIONAL HEART DISEASE

Nutritional heart disease may be due to either obesity or various deficiency states of malnutrition (Table 59-4). Of these, obesity is by far the most common disorder affecting persons in the United States, whereas the malnutrition syndromes predominate in underdeveloped nations.

Obesity

Whether their obesity is lifelong or of adult onset, obese persons are predisposed to hypercholesterolemia, hypertriglyceridemia, insulin resistance with glucose intolerance, and hypertension. Hence, the obese patient is particularly predisposed to the development of coronary artery disease and heart failure. Hypoventilation syndromes and obstructive sleep apnea are more common in the obese and are associated with the development of pulmonary hypertension and cor pulmonale.

Pathology. There are no specific abnormalities of the heart characteristic of obesity. Gross inspection reveals increased pericardial fat and fatty infiltration of the myocardium. Increased left ventricular wall thickness is frequently observed, and it may affect the right ventricle. Histologically, findings are also nonspecific and include myocyte hypertrophy.[71,72]

Clinical manifestations. The prevalence of congestive heart failure is increased in markedly obese patients and has been estimated to be 10%.[73] On physical examination, gallop rhythms may be detected but murmurs are seldom present. Findings of congestive heart failure are frequent, including peripheral edema, hepatic congestion, and hypertension. Chest radiography typically demonstrates cardiomegaly, and the most frequent electrocardiographic abnormality is left-axis deviation.

In the massively obese individual, blood volume and cardiac output are increased in proportion to excess body weight.[74,75] Cardiac catheterization frequently reveals systemic and pulmonary hypertension. Left ventricular

Table 59-4 Classification of nutritional heart disease

Obesity
Malnutrition
Starvation, anorexia nervosa
Marasmus
Kwashiorkor
Thiamine deficiency
Selenium deficiency

end-diastolic pressures are increased at rest and with exercise. Left ventricular diastolic dysfunction is frequently observed and is associated with left ventricular hypertrophy and diminished diastolic compliance.[76] With weight loss, the characteristic hemodynamic aberrations are frequently reversible.[77,78]

The primary treatment of heart failure associated with obesity is achieved through weight reduction. Additional measures include dietary sodium restriction and administration of cardiac glycosides, vasodilators, and diuretics. This group of patients should also be carefully screened for coronary artery disease.

More than 50% of patients with the sleep apnea syndrome are obese.[79] They are typically middle-aged men with moderate to severe obesity. Nocturnal apneas are frequently associated with arterial oxygen tensions of 50 mm Hg or less with concurrent elevation of carbon dioxide tension. Cardiac arrhythmias are frequent, as is pulmonary hypertension.

A syndrome of chronic hypoventilation with cyanosis and somnolence, with hypoxemia, hypercapnia, respiratory acidosis, and polycythemia, is observed in approximately 5% of extremely obese patients.[80] Hypoventilation is reversible with weight reduction, and improvement in respiratory function and decrease in pulmonary artery pressures are associated with weight loss.

Malnutrition

Malnutrition associated with cardiovascular disease may be either primary (causative) or secondary (a complication of cardiac disease). Malnutrition may be secondary to starvation, protein-calorie deficiencies of childhood causing the syndromes of marasmus and kwashiorkor, or specific vitamin or trace element deficiencies. Marasmus and kwashiorkor typically occur in underdeveloped nations. However, starvation can be observed in developed countries also, particularly the syndrome of anorexia nervosa.

Pathology. Gross evaluation of the heart demonstrates loss of subepicardial fat, atrophy, and thinning of the ventricular myocardium. Histologic evaluation demonstrates myocyte atrophy, frequently associated with interstitial edema. Other nonspecific findings are fibrosis and degeneration of the conduction system and vacuolization (in kwashiorkor).[77,81]

Clinical manifestations. Heart failure, sudden death, and subclinical cardiac dysfunction may develop in patients with protein-calorie malnutrition or starvation. Symptoms are nonspecific and include weakness, depression, anorexia, diarrhea, and alopecia. Edema and ascites may be associated with decreased plasma oncotic pressure due to low circulating levels of plasma albumin. Physical examination does not demonstrate specific abnormalities of the cardiovascular system. Patients are frequently hypotensive and bradycardiac.

Nonspecific electrocardiographic abnormalities are bradycardia and ventricular arrhythmia, including sustained ventricular tachycardia, often associated with prolongation of the Q-T interval.[81,82] Serum electrolytes are frequently abnormal, with reduced concentrations of sodium, magnesium, phosphorus, calcium, and potassium. Deficiencies of magnesium and calcium may contribute to the development of heart failure and sudden death, and hypokalemia has also been implicated in sudden death. Cardiac catheterization studies of patients with protein-calorie malnutrition have demonstrated prolonged circulation time, bradycardia, hypotension, and reduced cardiac and stroke index and intravascular volumes. Ventricular filling pressures tend to be low, and vascular resistance is high in the most severely malnourished.[83]

Primary therapy is nutritional rehabilitation. However, refeeding must be undertaken cautiously, because overt heart failure is often observed in the refeeding phase. Heart failure has been attributed to an exacerbation of hypophosphatemia associated with dietary supplementation high in carbohydrates.[84]

Specific vitamin or trace element deficiencies

Deficiencies of vitamins and trace elements have been associated with cardiovascular disease. Like other disorders of malnutrition, they are infrequently observed in the Western world but may be common in underdeveloped nations.

Thiamine deficiency. Thiamine pyrophosphatase is a cofactor for the pyruvate oxidase system and the transketolase reaction; hence, it has a central role in carbohydrate metabolism. Diets high in carbohydrate increase the basal thiamine requirement.

Thiamine deficiency causes beriberi, which may appear with peripheral neuropathy, central nervous system disease, and high-output heart failure. It is rarely diagnosed in the Western world, but it has been suggested that it is systematically underdiagnosed, particularly in alcoholics.[85] Beriberi heart disease has reappeared in Asia, particularly among young people with a diet high in carbohydrate and polished rice.[86]

In the Western world, thiamine is found widely in foods, particularly flour and cereals, which are fortified with this nutrient; hence, nutritional deficiency is uncommon. However, inadequate absorption from the gastrointestinal tract may occur in malabsorption states, alcoholism, and folate deficiency. Thiamine may also be lost as a result of hemodialysis, diarrhea, and diuretic therapy.

PATHOLOGY. Cardiac necropsy demonstrates nonspecific abnormalities, including cardiac hypertrophy, vacuolization, interstitial edema, and lymphocytic infiltration.[87]

CLINICAL MANIFESTATIONS. The patient usually has a history of inadequate dietary intake of thiamine-containing food for several months. There may be associated high alcohol consumption as well as other evidence of malnutrition. Symptoms of weakness, fatigue, palpitations, dyspnea, and edema develop over a period of weeks, suggesting heart failure. There may be associated dysesthesias of the extremities and an associated peripheral neuropathy.

Abnormalities on cardiovascular physical diagnosis include low diastolic blood pressure with widened pulse pressure, a hyperactive precordium, and bounding peripheral pulses; tachycardia and gallop rhythms may be noted. Heart murmurs may be appreciated and are often functional.

The electrocardiogram may be normal. When abnormal, the findings are nonspecific and often include right-axis deviation and T-wave abnormalities.[88] Sinus tachycardia is common, and there may be low amplitude of the QRS and T waves as well as prolongation of the Q-T interval. Chest radiography demonstrates cardiomegaly, which may be associated with pulmonary congestion and pleural effusion. Hemodynamic characterization demonstrates increased cardiac output and low systemic vascular resistance, the hallmark of beriberi heart disease. Cardiac output may be extremely high. However, in alcoholics with beriberi heart disease, left ventricular systolic function may be reduced.[89-91]

Beriberi heart disease responds promptly to thiamine replacement. Patients should be hospitalized and thiamine administered parenterally at a dose of 100 mg; this is followed by 50 to 100 mg orally per day. The typical response is a decrement of heart rate, with diuresis producing resolution of systemic and pulmonary congestion. Cardiac size decreases, and electrocardiographic abnormalities resolve.[90-92]

Patients typically do not have a response to digitalis and diuretics alone without thiamine replacement. However, digitalis and diuretics are important to support the left ventricle, which may fail after correction of the peripheral vasodilatation associated with thiamine deficiency.

Selenium deficiency. Keshan disease, a cardiomyopathy due to selenium deficiency, occurs in China in agricultural areas poor in selenium.[93,94] This disorder is characterized by congestive heart failure, typically in infants and children. Dietary supplementation with selenium prevents the disorder. In industrialized nations, the disorder is extremely uncommon; however, it has been reported in patients receiving total parenteral nutrition with inadequate selenium replacement.[95,96]

Rapid weight loss

Rapid weight loss, such as that associated with stringent weight reduction diets, has been associated with sudden death. Q-T interval prolongation with ventricular arrhythmias has been reported in association with massive weight loss and may identify patients at increased risk.[97] Other electrolyte abnormalities, including hypokalemia and hypomagnesemia, may be important. Pathologic examination has demonstrated decreased myocardial fiber size and cardiac atrophy similar to those reported for malnutrition.

Malnutrition secondary to cardiac disease

Heart disease may cause malnutrition.[98] Typically, the presentation is cardiac cachexia, in which severe underlying heart disease is associated with anorexia and weight loss. There may be decreased intestinal absorption associated with gastrointestinal hypoxia. Decreased protein intake is then associated with cardiac atrophy, and a vicious cycle of heart failure and superimposed malnutrition follows. In advanced disease, patients have markedly increased morbidity and mortality in comparison to patients with similar degrees of heart disease without cachexia. This is particularly evident in patients undergoing open heart surgery.[98]

Table 59-5 Metabolic heart disease

Disorder	Enzyme deficiency	Cardiac manifestations	Inheritance
Mucopolysaccharidoses		Valvular; CHF	AR
Type I	L-iduronidase		
Type II	Iduronate-2-sulfatase		
Type III	Deficiency of enzymes for degradation of heparan sulfate		
Type IV	Deficiency of enzymes for degradation of keratan sulfate		
Type VI	*N*-acetylgalactosamine-4-sulfatase		
Glycogen storage disease		CHF	AR
Type II	Acid α-glucosidase		
Type III	Amylo-1,6-glucosidase		
Type IV	Branching enzyme		
Gaucher's disease	Glucosylceramidase	CHF, constrictive pericarditis, pulmonary hypertension	AR
Fabry's disease	α-Galactosidase	CHF, syncope, sudden death	X-linked recessive
Ochronosis	Homogentisic acid oxidase	Valvular heart disease	AR
Oxalosis	Glyoxylate aminotransferase	Conduction system, CHF	AR
Refsum's syndrome	Phytanic acid α-hydroxylase	Conduction system, syncope, sudden death	AR

AR, autosomal recessive; CHF, congestive heart failure.

METABOLIC HEART DISEASE

Various disorders of metabolism, most often of an identified enzymatic deficiency, may cause cardiovascular disease. These disorders are rare and are generally identified in the pediatric age group. However, some of those affected live into adulthood (Table 59-5).

Mucopolysaccharidoses

The mucopolysaccharidoses are a related group of disorders caused by heritable deficiencies of enzymes required to metabolize the mucopolysaccharides, including heparan sulfate, dermatan sulfate, and keratan sulfate.[99] Seven different mucopolysaccharidoses have been described. Cardiac involvement has been described in types I, II, III, IV, and VI.

Pathology. In type I disease, there is cardiac chamber enlargement with increased thickness of endocardium and chordae tendineae.[100] Fibrous nodules may be observed to affect the valves, which are thickened and may be characterized by aneurysmal dilatation of leaflet tissue. The epicardial coronary arteries often have severe stenoses. Histologically, characteristic clear cells (Hurler's cells) containing the mucopolysaccharides heparan sulfate and dermatan sulfate are found within the coronary arteries, valves, myocardium, and aorta.[100,101] Pathologic findings are less well described for the other mucopolysaccharidoses.

Clinical manifestations. Specific cardiovascular manifestations vary according to type. In type I disease, heart failure is frequent and may be due to coronary artery disease, a poorly compliant left ventricle, or valvular heart disease.[102] Death typically occurs in childhood and is due to heart failure or sudden death.

There is no specific therapy for this group of genetic disorders. Valvular heart disease and coronary artery disease have also been reported in the other mucopolysaccharidoses with recognized cardiac involvement.[103-109] Palliative valvular heart surgery has been performed.[107,109]

Glycogen storage disease (glycogenoses)

Like the mucopolysaccharidoses, a group of glycogenoses may involve the heart. The disorders result in accumulation of biochemically normal glycogen in excessive amounts within lysosomes. Types II, III, and IV are recognized to produce cardiac involvement.[110-113] Disease is inherited in an autosomal recessive fashion, affecting both sexes equally. The organ systems most affected are the heart, skeletal muscle, and liver.

Pathology. The cardiac chambers are grossly enlarged, primarily because of increased wall thickness. Histologically, glycogen is deposited throughout the myocardium, with associated diffuse vacuolization[110] (Fig 59-3).

Clinical manifestations. Patients may be recognized by a complex of signs, including hyperglossia, hypotonia, and other associated neurologic deficits.[110] Cardiovascular manifestations of the diseases are frequently predominant and recognized early in life. Sudden death in infancy is not uncommon. Other patients succumb to heart failure.

Characteristic electrocardiographic abnormalities include an appearance suggestive of left ventricular hypertrophy, with tall broad QRS complexes and a short P-R interval. Deep Q waves are also observed.[114] Chest radiography reveals cardiomegaly and pulmonary congestion. Echocardiography typically demonstrates increased ventricular wall thickness.

Diagnosis is by demonstration of the specific enzyme defect, which has been described by use of endomyocardial biopsy tissue.[113] No specific therapy is available; treatment is supportive and palliative.

Gaucher's disease

This disorder is an autosomal recessive glucosylceramide lipidosis due to a deficiency of glucosylceramidase causing a lysosomal storage disease. Infantile, juvenile, and adult forms of the disease have been described, primarily on the basis of degrees of neurologic involvement. Diagnosis is established by the demonstration of Gaucher's cells and the associated specific enzyme defect.

Infiltration of the myocardium with Gaucher's cells reduces ventricular compliance, producing heart failure. Systolic function may be impaired. Constrictive pericarditis and pulmonary hypertension have also been described.[115,116]

Fabry's disease

This disorder is an X-linked recessive disorder of glycosphingolipid metabolism due to a deficiency of the lysosomal enzyme α-galactosidase resulting in the deposition of ceramide trihexoside in all tissues. The disease is fully expressed in the male, whereas heterozygous females are less affected and have a near-normal life expectancy. Occasional women with severe cardiac involvement have been reported.[117]

Accumulation of the glycolipid occurs in myocardium, valvular tissue, cardiac conduction system, and vascular endothelium, yielding a heterogeneous group of cardiovascular disorders (Fig 59-4). Electrocardiographic abnormalities include various arrhythmias, conduction defects, and appearance of left ventricular hypertrophy. Clinically, the patient may present with heart failure, syncope, or sudden death. Antemortem diagnosis by endomyocardial biopsy has been described.[118]

Ochronosis (alkaptonuria)

Ochronosis is due to deficiency of the enzyme homogentisic oxidase. It is a rare autosomal recessive disorder that may cause myocardial, coronary artery, or valvular heart disease. Patients present in adulthood with signs and symptoms of degenerative joint disease. These patients may be recognized by characteristic blue sclera.

Cardiac disease is due to ochronotic pigment granules deposited within the collagenous and fibrous tissue of the heart. Calcific aortic and mitral valve diseases have been described, and pigmented coronary plaques have been observed in patients with myocardial infarction. Whether pigmented granules within the myocardium, valves, or coronary arteries represent the primary disorder or are incidental is not certain.[119]

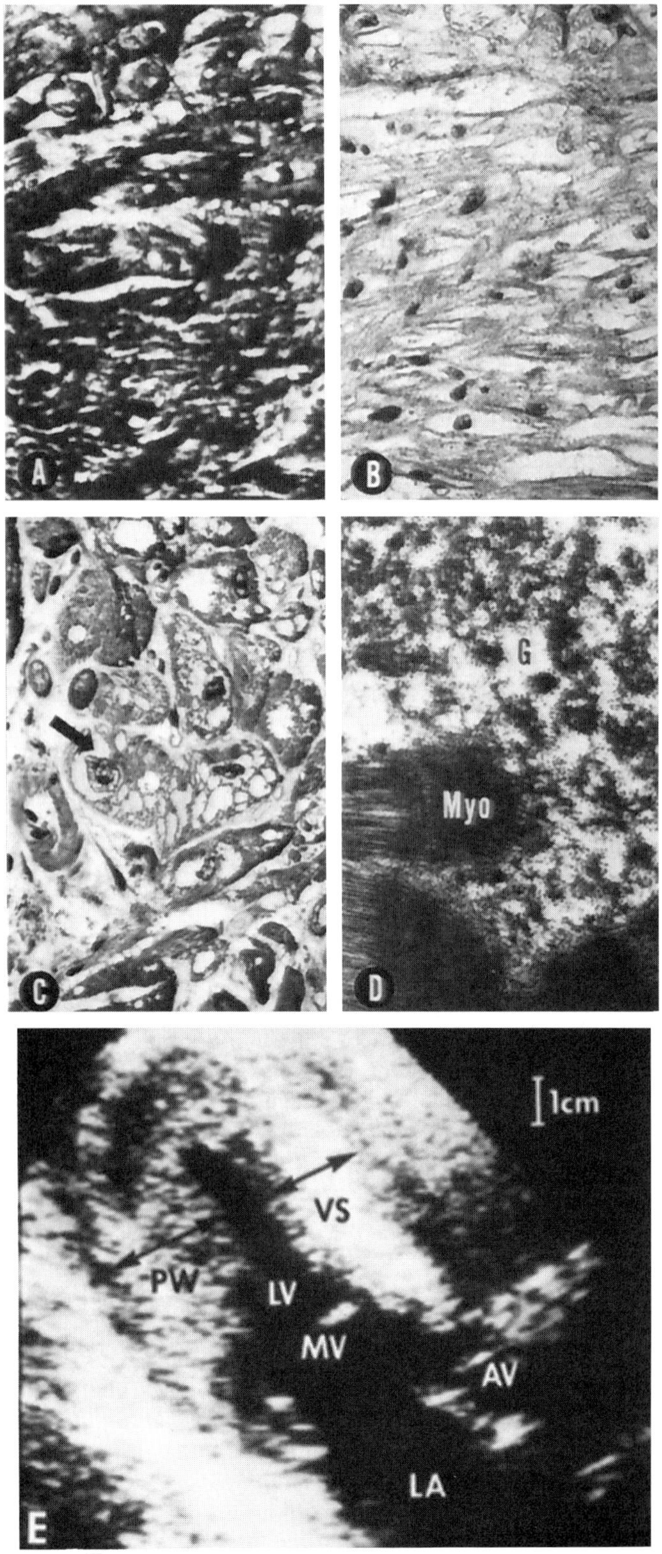

Fig 59-3 Photomicrographs of endomyocardial biopsy specimens from patient with glycogen storage disease, type III. **A-C,** light microscopy. Glycogen within myocardial cells reacts intensely with periodic acid-Schiff base **(A)** but is digested from the specimens by diastase **(B).** In plastic-embedded tissues stained with toluidine blue **(C),** sarcoplasmic glycogen appears as pale lakes *(arrow).* **D,** transmission electron microscopy. Glycogen granules *(G)* accumulate between bundles of myofilaments *(Myo).* Magnification: **A-C,** ×350; **D,** ×40,000. **E,** two-dimensional echocardiographic image, apical long-axis view, diastole. The ventricular septum *(VS)* and posterior wall *(PW)* are markedly thickened, measuring more than 2 cm *(arrows).* No systolic anterior motion of the mitral leaflets or compromise of the left ventricular outflow tract occurred during systole. *AV,* aortic valve; *LA,* left atrium; *LV,* left ventricle; *MV,* mitral valve leaflets. (From Olson LJ, Reeder GS, Noller KL, et al: Cardiac involvement in glycogen storage disease. III. Morphologic and biochemical characterization with endomyocardial biopsy. *Am J Cardiol* 53:980-981, 1984. By permission of Excerpta Medica.)

Oxalosis

Primary oxalosis is a rare heritable autosomal recessive disorder that leads to diffuse deposition of oxalate crystals. Calcium oxalate crystals may be deposited in the myocardium, coronary arteries, and cardiac conduction system. If overt heart disease develops, conduction system disease usually predominates, although heart failure may also be observed.[120] Hemodialysis may reduce the deposits of calcium oxalate.

Refsum's syndrome

Refsum's syndrome is a rare autosomal recessive disorder of lipid metabolism associated with phytanic acid accumulation. Neurologic features are most prominent, including mixed sensory and motor neuropathies, retinitis pigmentosa with night blindness, cerebellar ataxia, and nerve deafness due to phytanic acid accumulation within myelin sheaths. Cardiomyopathy has been observed. Phytanic acid accumulation has been observed within the sinus node and conduction system. Myocardial cells are atrophic, and there is associated fibrosis. Electrocardiographic abnormalities include conduction abnormalities, Q-T prolongation, and heart block. Patients may be affected by syncope or sudden death. Treatment requires a diet low in phytanic acid.[121]

MUSCULAR DYSTROPHIES

Cardiac involvement is characteristic of the progressive nonmyotonic muscular dystrophies, including the Duchenne, Becker, Erb, and Landouzy-Dejerine types. It is also characteristic of myotonic muscular dystrophy (Table 59-6). The muscular dystrophies with cardiac involvement are inherited. Cardiac involvement is frequently a prominent part of these disorders, particularly the myotonic and Duchenne types, although all may manifest cardiovascular involvement.[122-125]

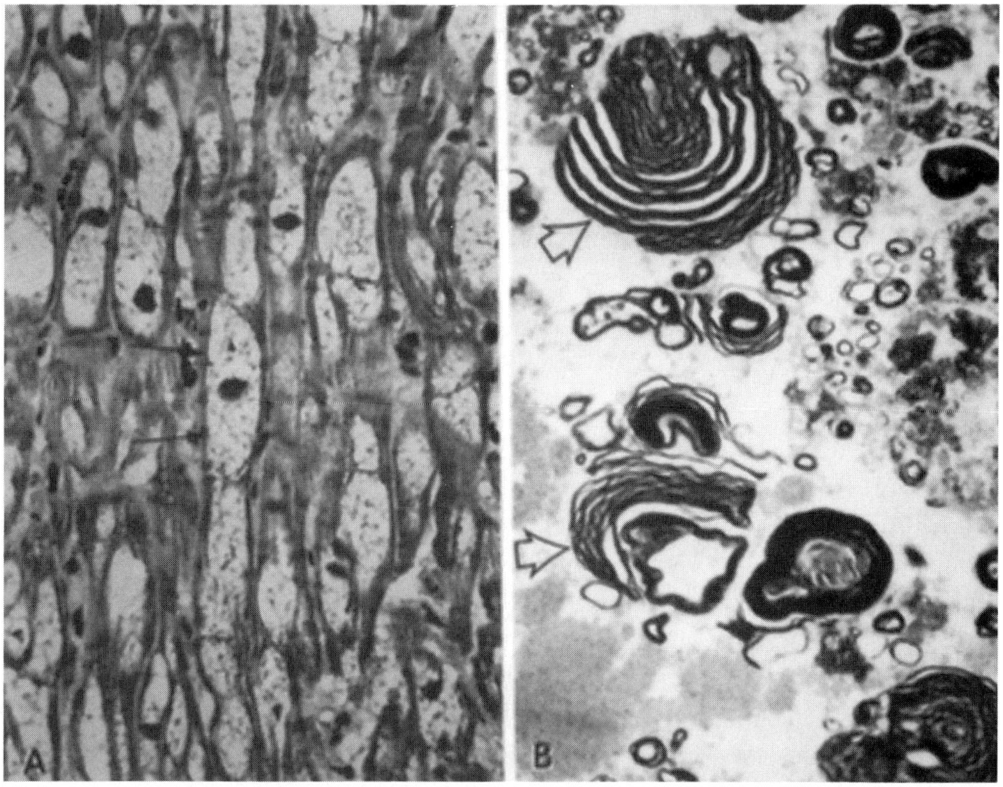

Fig 59-4 Fabry's disease: biopsy specimen from the right ventricle. **A,** light microscopy of longitudinal section shows extensive deposits of glycolipid in sarcoplasm, displacing contractile elements *(arrows)*. **B,** transmission electron microscopy shows lamellar whorls *(arrows)* and membranous sacs containing glycolipid; ×5,000. (From Broadbent JC, Edwards WD, Gordon H, et al: Fabry cardiomyopathy in the female confirmed by endomyocardial biopsy. *Mayo Clin Proc* 56:623-628, 1981. By permission, Mayo Foundation).

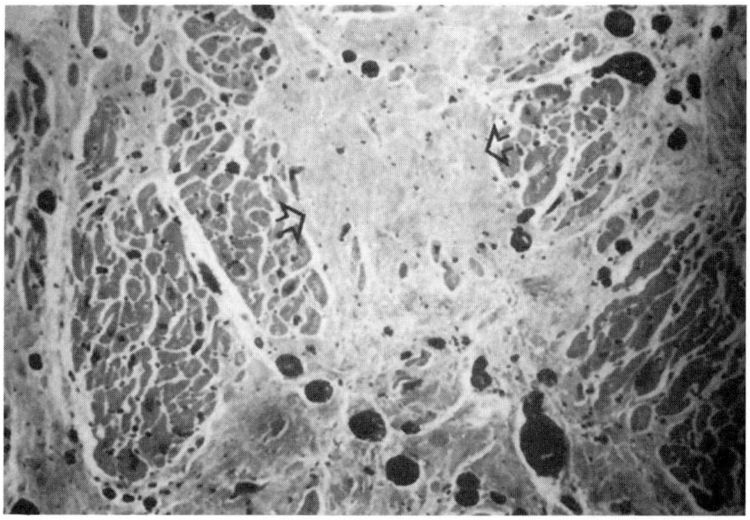

Fig 59-5 Myocardium in Duchenne's muscular dystrophy. Note extensive fibrosis *(arrows)*. (Courtesy of William D. Edwards, M.D.)

Table 59-6 Selected clinical features of muscular dystrophies

Type	Inheritance	Age at onset	Cardiac manifestations	Noncardiac manifestations	ECG abnormalities
Myotonic	AD	Early	Arrhythmias, CHF, heart block, sudden death	Cataracts, baldness, gonadal atrophy, mental retardation	Primary AVB, bundle-branch block, ventricular ectopy
Nonmyotonic Duchenne's	X-linked	1-6 yr	CHF, sudden death	Muscular pseudohypertrophy, scoliosis, respiratory failure	Sinus tachycardia, tall R waves right precordium, increased R:S ratio, deep Q waves from I, aVL, V_5, and V_6
Becker's	X-linked	Adult	CHF	Muscular pseudohypertrophy	Conduction block
Erb's	AR	1st-6th decade	Arrhythmia, CHF	Shoulder and pelvic pain, weakness	Primary AVB, conduction block
Landouzy-Dejerine	AD	12-20 yr	Arrhythmia, conduction block, CHF	Facial weakness, weakness of pectoralis and trapezius muscles	Primary AVB, conduction block
Emery-Dreifuss	X-linked	Adult	Sudden death	Weakness of peroneal and humeral muscles	Atrial arrhythmias, conduction block

AD, autosomal dominant; AR, autosomal recessive; AVB, atrioventricular block; CHF, congestive heart failure; ECG, electrocardiographic.

Pathology

The cardiac pathology of myotonic muscular dystrophy has been well characterized; it consists of multichamber enlargement with ventricular hypertrophy. Histologic abnormalities are nonspecific and include fatty infiltration with variation in size of myocardial fibers and interstitial fibrosis.[126] Electron microscopy demonstrates more characteristic abnormalities, including prominent I bands with myofibrillar degeneration and abnormal mitochondria. These findings may be observed before the onset of overt heart disease.[127] Careful examination of the sinus node and atrioventricular conduction systems has demonstrated loss of specialized conduction tissue, with replacement fibrosis and fat. The characteristic cardiac pathologic finding of Duchenne's muscular dystrophy is selective transmural scarring of the posterobasal region of the left ventricle, with or without extension to the lateral or inferior wall[122] (Fig 59-5). Duchenne's has been related to a deficiency of dystrophin, a muscle cell protein.[128]

Clinical manifestations

The clinical picture is most often dominated by the neurologic manifestations of the specific disease. Occasionally, cardiac disease is the presenting feature in the myotonic type. Cardiac manifestations include atrial or ventricular arrhythmias, conduction block, heart failure, and sudden death.

Electrocardiographic findings are frequently abnormal, manifesting first-degree atrioventricular block, particularly in the myotonic type, and ventricular conduction defects in the myotonic and nonmyotonic types[125-127,129-132] (Fig 59-6). Distinctive electrocardiographic findings are seen in Duchenne's and may be the earliest manifestation of heart disease; they consist of tall R waves over the right precordium and an increased ratio of the RS amplitude and deep Q waves in the limb leads.[122,124] Therapy for the cardiovascular involvement of the dystrophies is conventional for heart failure, arrhythmias, and conduction block.

MISCELLANEOUS

Amyloidosis (see also chapter 21)

Amyloidosis is a syndrome characterized by the extracellular deposition of amyloid protein within organ parenchyma. Amyloid deposition may be focal or diffuse, be confined to a single organ or involve multiple organ systems, and occur with or without overt organ dysfunction.[133,134] Many distinct diseases form the amyloid syndrome; each type is distinguished by a characteristic amyloid protein. Diseases known to cause functional

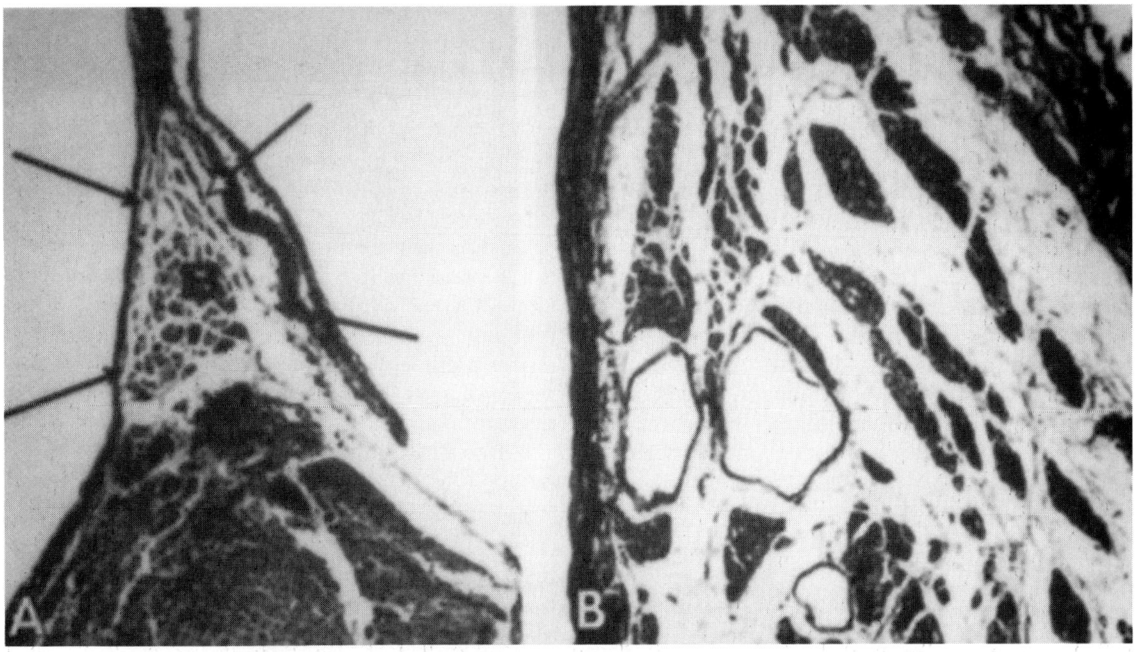

Fig 59-6 Cardiac conduction system in myotonic dystrophy. **A,** section of bundle of His *(arrows)* showing decreased number of fibers and replacement by fibrous and fatty tissues. **B,** higher magnification. (From Kennel AJ, Titus JL, Merideth J: Pathologic findings in the atrioventricular conduction system in myotonic dystrophy. *Mayo Clin Proc* 49:838-842, 1974. By permission, Mayo Foundation.)

cardiac impairment due to amyloid infiltration may be classified as primary, secondary, familial, or senile.[135]

In primary systemic amyloidosis, cardiac involvement, the leading cause of death, produces end-stage cardiac failure or death from arrhythmia in 40% of patients. Furthermore, once heart failure occurs, median survival is 5 months.[136] Median survival for patients with senile systemic amyloidosis or familial amyloidosis is less dismal, although mortality is also high.[132,137] Primary systemic amyloidosis is caused by the deposition of a monoclonal immunoglobulin. Multiple myeloma causes diffuse deposition of monoclonal immunoglobulin and creates a clinical picture very similar to that associated with primary systemic amyloidosis.[133] Secondary amyloidosis occurs in association with chronic infectious or inflammatory diseases and, occasionally, neoplastic disorders; it is extremely uncommon for overt cardiovascular disease to be associated with this disorder.[135]

Pathology. Pathologic examination of the heart demonstrates both focal and diffuse and microscopic and macroscopic evidence of amyloid. The amyloid fibers infiltrate the endocardium, myocardium, and pericardium as well as the valves, coronary arteries, and conduction system. On gross examination of advanced cases, the ventricular walls are extremely thickened and the ventricular chamber dimensions decreased. The atria are extremely dilated.

Clinical manifestations. The symptomatic presentation of cardiac amyloidosis is extremely variable. The most common initial manifestation is congestive heart failure.[132] Other frequent cardiovascular manifestations are syncope associated with either heart block or left ventricular outflow tract obstruction, ischemic syndromes due to occlusion of coronary arteries, and sudden death.[132,138] Physical examination of the patient with cardiac amyloidosis yields signs of congestive heart failure.

On diagnostic evaluation, the electrocardiogram often shows low voltage and disorders of conduction, and pseudoinfarction patterns may be present.[132] The primary diagnostic modality for the assessment of the patient with suspected or proven cardiac amyloidosis is echocardiography. Characteristic features in advanced disease are markedly increased ventricular wall thickness, increased myocardial echogenicity, and increased valve thickness. Left ventricular cavity dimension is reduced, and systolic function is normal or decreased. Pericardial effusions are also frequently observed. Ventricular wall thickness and diastolic function variables have been demonstrated to be of prognostic usefulness.[136,139-142]

Therapy is supportive and palliative; no therapy has been proven efficacious for the underlying disease. Diuretic therapy is the mainstay of congestive heart failure, because these patients may be predisposed to digoxin toxicity and intolerant of vasodilators as a result of hypotension or renal insufficiency. Occasionally, patients benefit from cardiac pacing.

Hemochromatosis (see also chapter 21)

Hemochromatosis is a storage disorder characterized by increased body stores of iron causing organ dysfunction. Hemochromatosis may be considered to be primary (genetic) or acquired; cardiac involvement is not uncommon. The genetic variant is characterized by autosomal recessive transmission and may lead to multiple organ failure in untreated patients. In older series, cardiac failure was the leading cause of death.[143] The incidence of this disorder, once believed to be approximately 1 in 10,000, has been revised upward to 2 to 3 per thousand, and as many as 6% to 10% of the population may be heterozygous for the disorder.[144]

Acquired hemochromatosis is a complication of chronic exogenous iron administration, usually in the form of repeated blood transfusions for chronic refractory anemia. Excessive dietary iron may also be a cause of the acquired form.

Pathology. Histologically, stainable iron is exclusively sarcoplasmic and is not observed in the interstitium (Fig 59-7). Iron may be found in the endocardial, myocardial, and epicardial layers of the heart, with slightly greater deposition in the epicardial layers. The intracellular location of iron characterizes the disorder as a storage disease rather than an infiltrative process.[145,146]

Clinical manifestations. Classically, the disorder is characterized by the tetrad of heart disease, liver disease, diabetes mellitus, and increased skin pigmentation. In current clinical practice, however, this is rarely seen. Patients may present with arthropathy and endocrine disorders as well as heart and liver disease.[147]

Cardiovascular manifestations of the disorder are

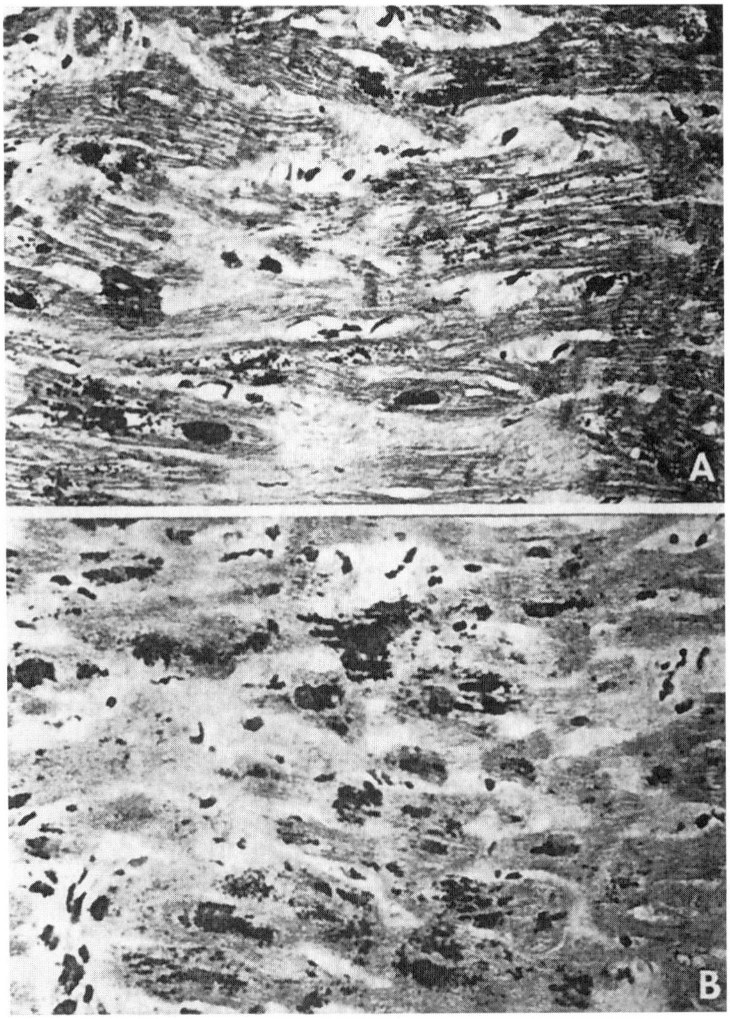

Fig 59-7 Endomyocardial biopsy specimens stained for iron in two patients with hemochromatosis. Iron deposition is limited to myocytes and tends to be perinuclear. **A,** mild (grade 2); **B,** severe (grade 4). (Gomori iron; original magnification, ×100.) (From Olson LJ, Edwards WD, Holmes DR Jr, et al: Endomyocardial biopsy in hemochromatosis: clinicopathologic correlates in six cases. *J Am Coll Cardiol* 13:116-120, 1989. By permission of American College of Cardiology.)

nonspecific. Patients may present with heart failure or arrhythmia. In advanced disease, physical examination demonstrates findings of heart failure, including increased venous pressure, gallop rhythms, edema, and hepatomegaly. Electrocardiographic features are also nonspecific and may include low-voltage QRS, atrial and ventricular arrhythmias, and repolarization abnormalities. In patients with heart failure, chest radiography reveals cardiomegaly and pulmonary congestion.[146]

The hemodynamic and morphologic abnormalities of cardiac hemochromatosis have been described as either dilated or restrictive.[146,148] In patients with the genetic form, wall thickness is typically normal by echocardiography. Echocardiographic features of hemochromatosis heart disease are generally those of dilated cardiomyopathy with increased left ventricular cavity dimension and depressed systolic function.[149] It appears that in secondary hemochromatosis associated with transfusion for chronic anemia, left ventricular mass is more likely to be increased.[150]

Cardiac dysfunction associated with iron overload may be reversed by iron removal via chelation or phlebotomy. Because cardiac hemochromatosis is potentially reversible and may mimic idiopathic dilated or restrictive cardiomyopathy, it is recommended that endomyocardial biopsy tissue from patients with unexplained heart failure be stained for iron.[146,151,152] In patients with established cardiac hemochromatosis, serial endomyocardial biopsy may be useful to monitor depletion of myocardial iron.

Cardiac involvement in hemochromatosis should be considered in any patient with unexplained heart failure. Screening for systemic iron overload includes determination of transferrin saturation and ferritin concentration in serum. The combined specificity and sensitivity of these two screening tests is approximately 95% for the detection of iron overload in patients with genetic hemochromatosis.[142] If screening tests suggest iron overload, histologic confirmation is necessary. Generally, this is accomplished by liver biopsy; however, endomyocardial biopsy is useful in patients whose primary clinical manifestations are cardiac.[146]

Carcinoid

The carcinoid syndrome is a rare cause of acquired valvular heart disease. Cardiac involvement is recognized in most patients with the syndrome and is a frequent cause of death.[153]

Carcinoid tumors arise most often from the gastrointestinal tract and rarely from bronchial tissue. The carcinoid syndrome is caused by metastatic disease and consists of cutaneous flushing, diarrhea, bronchoconstriction, and formation of cardiac endocardial plaque. Cardiac lesions are believed to be caused by high concentrations of circulating vasoactive substances, including serotonin and bradykinin secreted by metastatic lesions. These substances are inactived by the lungs; hence, left-sided cardiac lesions are unusual unless there is a coexistent right-to-left shunt.

Pathology. A fibrous plaque may form at the surface of the tricuspid and pulmonic valves and cause thickened, retracted, and rigid valves that are both stenotic and regurgitant (Fig 59-8). The endocardium and intima of the vena cava and pulmonary artery may also be involved.[154]

Clinical manifestations. Cardiac complications generally become manifest late in the course of disease. The combined effects of tricuspid and pulmonic valve disease lead to progressive right heart failure, a common cause of death. Hence, edema, ascites, fatigue, and shortness of breath dominate the clinical picture.[153]

Physical examination yields findings of right heart failure due to tricuspid and pulmonary valve disease. Accordingly, patients have edema, hepatomegaly, increased jugular venous pressure, and murmurs of combined tricuspid and pulmonic stenosis and regurgitation. Electrocardiographic abnormalities are nonspecific. Chest radiography demonstrates cardiomegaly.

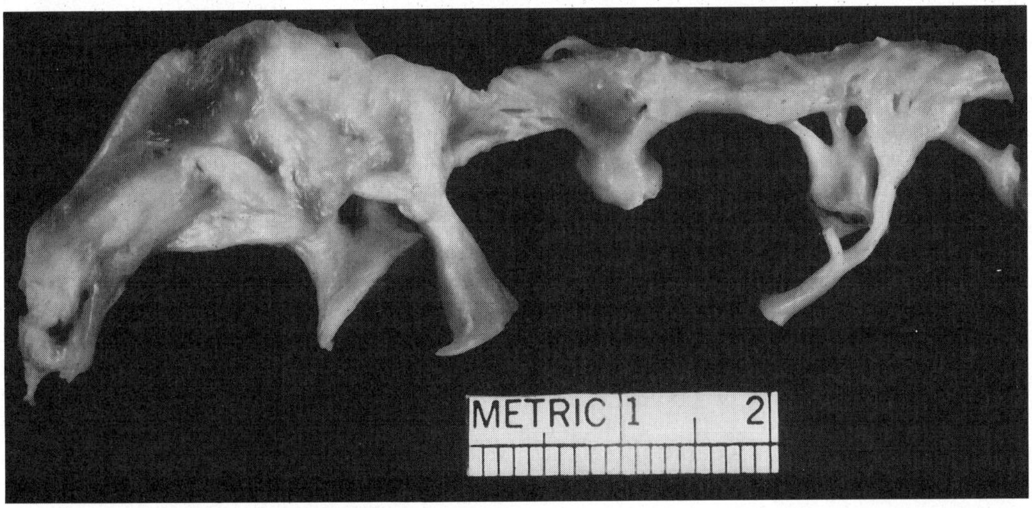

Fig 59-8 Surgically excised tricuspid valve from patient with carcinoid heart disease. Valvular involvement by carcinoid yields the characteristic appearance.

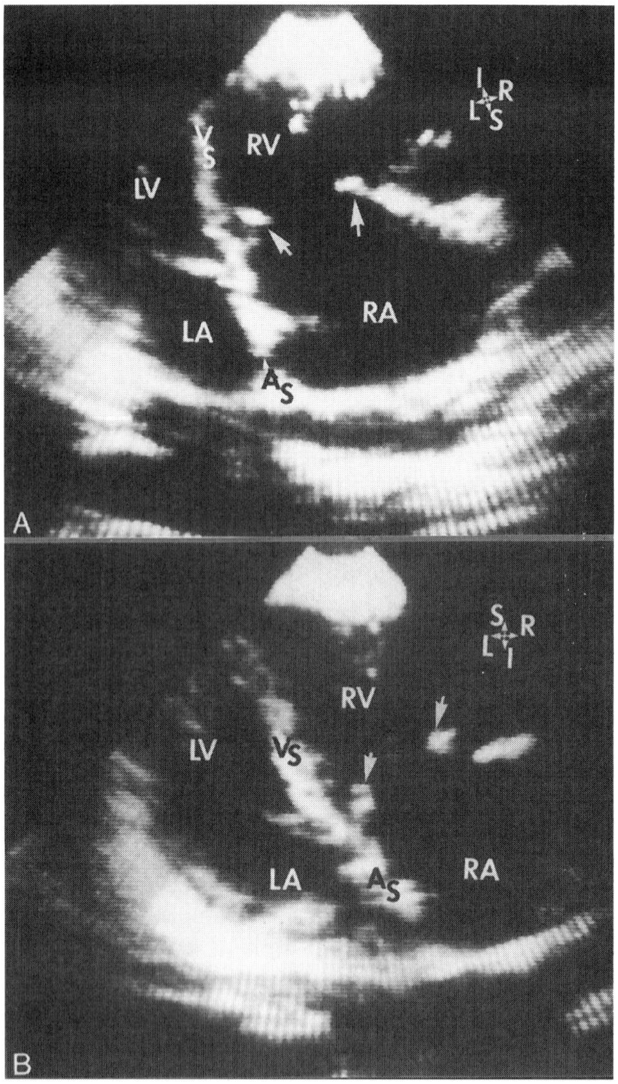

Fig 59-9 Carcinoid syndrome. Four-chamber view demonstrates enlarged right ventricle *(RV)* and right atrium *(RA)*. **A,** diastolic frame; **B,** systolic frame. Anterior and septal leaflets of the tricuspid valve are thickened and retracted as well as fixed in a semiopen position. *AS,* atrial septum; *I,* inferior; *L,* left; *LA,* left atrium; *LV,* left ventricle; *R,* right; *S,* superior; *VS,* ventricular septum. (From Callahan JA, Wroblewski EM, Reeder GS, et al: Echocardiographic features of carcinoid heart disease. *Am J Cardiol* 50:762-768, 1982. By permission of Excerpta Medica.)

Echocardiography is a useful and sensitive noninvasive method to recognize the characteristic morphologic abnormalities of carcinoid heart disease.[153,155] The appearance of the tricuspid valve is distinctive, characterized by thickened and retracted leaflets with diminished mobility and incomplete coaptation. The leaflets may remain in a fixed and semiopen position throughout the cardiac cycle, yielding a stenotic and incompetent valve (Fig 59-9). The pulmonic valve, usually more difficult to observe by transthoracic imaging, often demonstrates similar morphology, with increased valve thickness, retraction, fusion of commissures, and a semiopen, fixed position with combined stenosis and regurgitation.

Optimal treatment requires resection of the carcinoid tumor. When this is not feasible, palliation of heart failure typically requires digitalis and diuretic. Occasional patients benefit from surgical replacement of the tricuspid or pulmonic valves or resection of myocardial metastatic lesions.[156]

Sarcoidosis

Sarcoidosis, a granulomatous disorder of unknown cause, is manifested by lymphadenopathy, pulmonary infiltrates, and skin or eye lesions and most often affects young adults. Organ systems less commonly involved are the liver, spleen, mucous membranes, muscles, nervous system, and heart.[157]

Pathology. The characteristic feature is noncaseating granulomas dispersed among multiple organs.[157] Granulomas may be observed in any portion of the heart, although involvement of the intraventricular septum and left ventricular free wall is most common. The disease may be focal or diffuse and associated with lymphocytic myocarditis. Transmural myocardial involvement may occur, with replacement of the ventricular wall by sarcoid tissue, which may produce an aneurysm[158] (Fig 59-10).

Clinical manifestations. Overt clinical manifestations of sarcoid heart disease are observed in fewer than 5% of patients, although the disease may be found in 20% to 30% of cases at autopsy. The most common clinical problem is pulmonary disease in which diffuse infiltration causes severe pulmonary dysfunction, which leads to cor pulmonale in late stages of the disease.

Myocardial involvement is typically manifested by heart block, ventricular arrhythmias, sudden death, and congestive heart failure. Ventricular aneurysms may form.[159] Sudden death is the most common manifestation of primary cardiac sarcoidosis. In nonfatal cardiac arrest, the most frequent manifestation of myocardial sarcoid is conduction system disease. Congestive heart failure is usually of the dilated type. Myocardial involvement may produce restrictive heart disease, as the ventricular wall becomes stiff and hypocontractile.[157,158]

Antemortem diagnosis depends on demonstration of characteristic histologic changes, typically in noncardiac organ systems; biopsy tissue is often obtained from lymph nodes, liver, or lung. Endomyocardial biopsy may demonstrate cardiac involvement, but because heart disease is focal, a negative biopsy finding does not exclude the diagnosis.

The mainstay of therapy for systemic sarcoidosis is corticosteroid administration, which has been associated with improvement of ventricular function and amelioration of arrhythmias and conduction abnormalities. Permanent pacemaker implantation is indicated in patients with advanced heart block. Ventricular aneurysm resection has been reported for the treatment of ventricular tachycardia.[160]

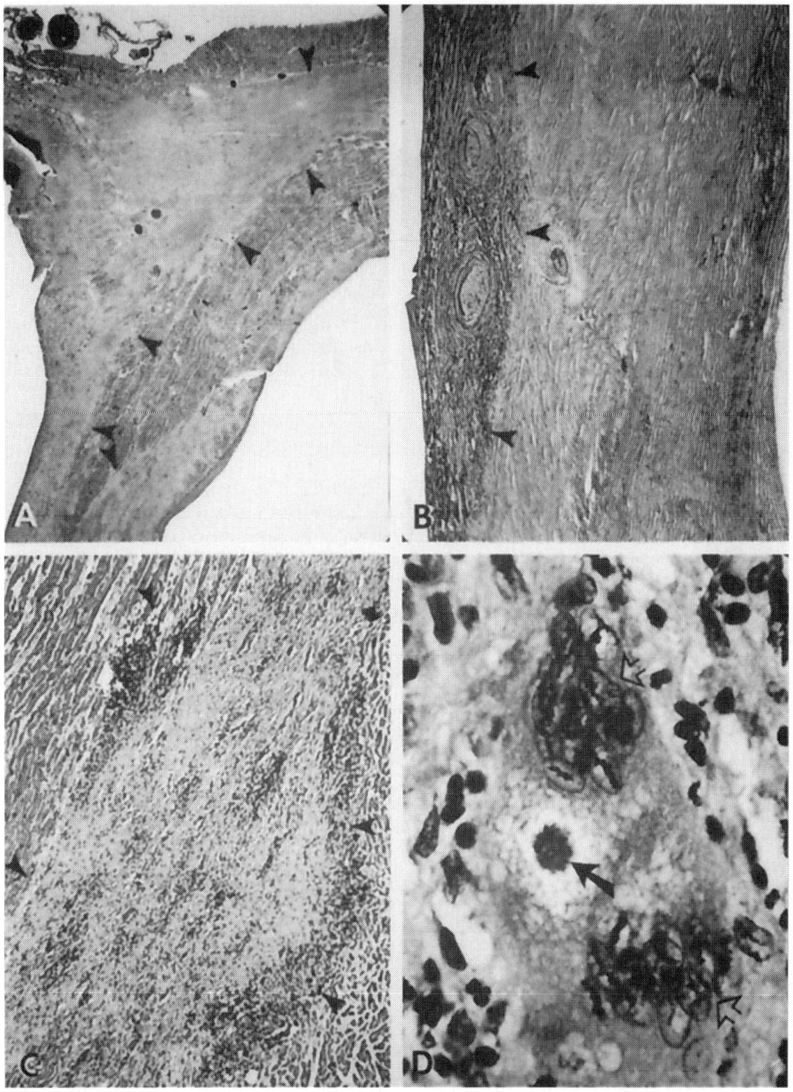

Fig 59-10 Myocardium in sarcoid heart disease. **A,** magnification of transverse section through base of right heart and left ventricles, including the ventricular septum, showing extensive areas of fibrosis replacing myocardium *(arrowheads)*. **B,** atrioventricular node *(arrowheads)* adjacent to central fibrous body and surrounding three small arteries, showing inflammatory reaction. **C,** inflammatory lesion in left ventricular wall *(arrowheads)*. **D,** noncaseating granuloma in left ventricular wall. Fibrinoid change with many Anichkov's ("caterpillar") interstitial cells *(open arrows)* and crystalloid *(solid arrow)*.

Kawasaki disease

Kawasaki disease (mucocutaneous lymph node syndrome) is an acute febrile illness of unknown cause that most often affects children. However, young adults may also contract the illness. The diagnosis is established when five of six criteria are satisfied: (1) fever that is unresponsive to antibiotics and that has lasted 2 weeks; (2) bilateral congestion of ocular conjunctiva; (3) erythema, dryness, and fissuring of the lips and papillae of the tongue and erythema of the oral and pharyngeal mucosa; (4) erythema and induration of the palms and soles and desquamation of the fingertips; (5) eczema of the thorax without vesicles or crusts, usually on days 5 to 7; and (6) cervical lymphadenopathy. There are no specific confirmatory diagnostic laboratory studies.[161]

Cardiac pathology is characterized by complications of coronary arteritis, including aneurysm formation, rupture, and thrombosis with myocardial infarction. Aneurysms may regress within 2 years of the onset of the acute illness. Myocarditis, pericarditis, and conduction system disease have also been observed.[162-164]

Sickle cell disease

Homozygous sickle cell disease is estimated to be present in 0.15% of black Americans. The cardiovascular system is frequently involved in sickle cell anemia. However, cardiovascular involvement tends to be noncardiac, with the primary manifestations consisting of renal and pulmonary infarction and pulmonary thrombosis.

The myocardium appears to be relatively protected against infarction in patients with sickle cell disease. However, acute myocardial infarction has been described. Despite the relative protection of the myocardium against complications of sickling cells, cardiac complications of the disease are observed, including cardiac enlargement due to hypertension, coronary artery disease, and complications of repeated blood transfusion, with myocardial iron deposition producing acquired hemochromatosis.[165]

Electrocardiographic findings are abnormal in as many as 70% of patients. Chest radiography demonstrates cardiomegaly in a similarly high proportion of patients. Electrocardiographic abnormalities are nonspecific and may include septal Q waves. Echocardiographic studies have demonstrated increased diameter of left ventricular mass with impairment of both systolic and diastolic function.[166]

REFERENCES

1. Woods VL Jr, Zvaifler NJ: Pathogenesis of systemic lupus erythematosus. In *Textbook of Rheumatology*. Vol. 2. Third edition. Edited by WN Kelley, ED Harris Jr, S Ruddy, et al. Philadelphia, WB Saunders Company, 1989, pp 1077-1100
2. Hejtmancik MR, Wright JC, Quint R, et al: The cardiovascular manifestations of systemic lupus erythematosus. *Am Heart J* 68:119-130, 1964
3. Gross L: Cardiac lesions in Libman-Sacks disease, with consideration of its relationship to acute diffuse lupus erythematosus. *Am J Pathol* 16:375-408, 1940
4. Bulkley BH, Roberts WC: The heart in systemic lupus erythematosus and the changes induced in it by corticosteroid therapy. A study of 36 necropsy patients. *Am J Med* 58:243-264, 1975
5. Baggenstoss AH: Visceral lesions in disseminated lupus erythematosus. *Proc Staff Meet Mayo Clin* 27:412-419, 1952
6. Borenstein DG, Fye WB, Arnett FC, et al: The myocarditis of systemic lupus erythematosus: association with myositis. *Ann Intern Med* 89:619-624, 1978
7. Harvey AM, Shulman LE, Tumulty PA, et al: Systemic lupus erythematosus: review of the literature and clinical analysis of 138 cases. *Medicine (Baltimore)* 33:291-437, 1954
8. Kong TQ, Kellum RE, Haserick JR: Clinical diagnosis of cardiac involvement in systemic lupus erythematosus: a correlation of clinical and autopsy findings in thirty patients. *Circulation* 26:7-11, 1962
9. Doherty NE, Siegel RJ: Cardiovascular manifestations of systemic lupus erythematosus. *Am Heart J* 110:1257-1265, 1985
10. Ansari A, Larson PH, Bates HD: Cardiovascular manifestations of systemic lupus erythematosus: current perspective. *Prog Cardiovasc Dis* 27:421-434, 1985
11. Galve E, Candell-Riera J, Pigrau C, et al: Prevalence, morphologic types, and evolution of cardiac valvular disease in systemic lupus erythematosus. *N Engl J Med* 319:817-823, 1988
12. Chartash EK, Lans DM, Paget SA, et al: Aortic insufficiency and mitral regurgitation in patients with systemic lupus erythematosus and the antiphospholipid syndrome. *Am J Med* 86:407-412, 1989
13. Straaton KV, Chatham WW, Reveille JD, et al: Clinically significant valvular heart disease in systemic lupus erythematosus. *Am J Med* 85:645-650, 1988
14. Lockshin MD, Bonfa E, Elkon K, et al: Neonatal lupus risk to newborns of mothers with systemic lupus erythematosus. *Arthritis Rheum* 31:697-701, 1988
15. McCue CM, Mantakas ME, Tingelstad JB, et al: Congenital heart block in newborns of mothers with connective tissue disease. *Circulation* 56:82-90, 1977
16. Winkler RB, Nora AH, Nora JJ: Familial congenital complete heart block and maternal systemic lupus erythematosus. *Circulation* 56:1103-1107, 1977
17. Reichlin M, Friday K, Harley JB: Complete congenital heart block followed by anti-Ro/SSA in adult life. Studies of an informative family. *Am J Med* 84:339-344, 1988
18. Botstein GR, LeRoy EC: Primary heart disease in systemic sclerosis (scleroderma): advances in clinical and pathologic features, pathogenesis, and new therapeutic approaches. *Am Heart J* 102:913-919, 1981
19. Campbell PM, LeRoy EC: Pathogenesis of systemic sclerosis: a vascular hypothesis. *Semin Arthritis Rheum* 4:351-368, 1975
20. Norton WL, Nardo JM: Vascular disease in progressive systemic sclerosis (scleroderma). *Ann Intern Med* 73:317-324, 1970
21. Sackner MA, Heinz ER, Steinberg AJ: The heart in scleroderma. *Am J Cardiol* 17:542-559, 1966
22. McWhorter JE IV, LeRoy EC: Pericardial disease in scleroderma (systemic sclerosis). *Am J Med* 57:566-575, 1974
23. Weiss S, Stead EA Jr, Warren JV, et al: Scleroderma heart disease: with consideration of certain other visceral manifestations of scleroderma. *Arch Intern Med* 71:749-776, 1943
24. Bulkley BH: Progressive systemic sclerosis: cardiac involvement. *Clin Rheum Dis* 5:131-149, 1979
25. Follansbee WP, Curtiss EI, Medsger TA Jr, et al: Physiologic abnormalities of cardiac function in progressive systemic sclerosis with diffuse scleroderma. *N Engl J Med* 310:142-148, 1984
26. Kahan A, Devaux JY, Amor B, et al: Nifedipine and thallium-201 myocardial perfusion in progressive systemic sclerosis. *N Engl J Med* 314:1397-1402, 1986
27. Follansbee WP, Curtiss EI, Rahko PS, et al: The electrocardiogram in systemic sclerosis (scleroderma). Study of 102 consecutive cases with functional correlations and review of the literature. *Am J Med* 79:183-192, 1985
28. Rodeheffer RJ, Rommer JA, Wigley F, et al: Controlled double-blind trial of nifedipine in the treatment of Raynaud's phenomenon. *N Engl J Med* 308:880-883, 1983
29. Haupt HM, Hutchins GM: The heart and cardiac conduction system in polymyositis-dermatomyositis: a clinicopathologic study of 16 autopsied patients. *Am J Cardiol* 50:998-1006, 1982
30. Gottdiener JS, Sherber HS, Hawley RJ, et al: Cardiac manifestations in polymyositis. *Am J Cardiol* 41:1141-1149, 1978
31. Denbow CE, Lie JT, Tancredi RG, et al: Cardiac involvement in polymyositis: a clinicopathologic study of 20 autopsied patients. *Arthritis Rheum* 22:1088-1092, 1979
32. Khan AH, Spodick DH: Rheumatoid heart disease. *Semin Arthritis Rheum* 1:327-337, 1972
33. Baggenstoss AH, Rosenberg EF: Unusual cardiac lesions associated with chronic multiple rheumatoid arthritis. *Arch Pathol* 37:54-60, 1944
34. Roberts WC, Kehoe JA, Carpenter DF, et al: Cardiac valvular lesions in rheumatoid arthritis. *Arch Intern Med* 122:141-146, 1968
35. Cathcart ES, Spodick DH: Rheumatoid heart disease: a study of the incidence and nature of cardiac lesions in rheumatoid arthritis. *N Engl J Med* 266:959-964, 1962
36. Liss JP, Bachmann WT: Rheumatoid constrictive pericarditis, treated by pericardiectomy. Report of a case and review of the literature. *Arthritis Rheum* 13:869-876, 1970
37. Franco AE, Levine HD, Hall AP: Rheumatoid pericarditis. Report of 17 cases diagnosed clinically. *Ann Intern Med* 77:837-844, 1972
38. Newman JH, Cooney LM Jr: Cardiac abnormalities associated with rheumatoid arthritis: aortic insufficiency requiring valve replacement. *J Rheumatol* 7:375-378, 1980
39. Ahern M, Lever JV, Cosh J: Complete heart block in rheumatoid arthritis. *Ann Rheum Dis* 42:389-397, 1983
40. Julkunen H: Rheumatoid spondylitis: clinical and laboratory study of 149 cases compared with 182 cases of rheumatoid arthritis. *Acta Rheum Scand Suppl* 4:24-28, 1962
41. Bulkley BH, Roberts WC: Ankylosing spondylitis and aortic regurgitation. Description of the characteristic cardiovascular lesion from study of eight necropsy patients. *Circulation* 48:1014-1027, 1973
42. Kawasuji M, Hetzer R, Oelert H, et al: Aortic valve replacement and ascending aorta replacement in ankylosing spondylitis: report of

three surgical cases and review of the literature. *Thorac Cardiovasc Surg* 30:310-314, 1982

43. Davidson P, Baggenstoss AH, Slocum CH, et al: Cardiac and aortic lesions in rheumatoid spondylitis. *Proc Staff Meet Mayo Clin* 38:427-435, 1963

44. Roberts WC, Hollingsworth JF, Bulkley BH, et al: Combined mitral and aortic regurgitation in ankylosing spondylitis. Angiographic and anatomic features. *Am J Med* 56:237-243, 1974

45. Singsen BH, Bernstein BH, Kornreich HK, et al: Mixed connective tissue disease in childhood. A clinical and serologic survey. *J Pediatr* 90:893-900, 1977

46. Rakovec P, Kenda MF, Rozman B, et al: Panconductional defect in mixed connective tissue disease: association with Sjögren's syndrome. *Chest* 81:257-259, 1982

47. Alpert MA, Goldberg SH, Singsen BH, et al: Cardiovascular manifestations of mixed connective tissue disease in adults. *Circulation* 68:1182-1193, 1983

48. McAdam LP, O'Hanlan MA, Bluestone R, et al: Relapsing polychondritis: prospective study of 23 patients and a review of the literature. *Medicine (Baltimore)* 55:193-215, 1976

49. Hemry DA, Moss AJ, Jacox RF: Relapsing polychondritis, a "floppy" mitral valve, and migratory polytendonitis. *Ann Intern Med* 77:576-580, 1972

50. Hughes RA, Curry N, Lessof MH: Relapsing polychondritis. *Proc R Soc Med* 64:664-666, 1971

51. Alarçon-Segovia D: The necrotizing vasculitides. A new pathogenetic classification. *Med Clin North Am* 61:241-260, 1977

52. Moskowitz RW, Baggenstoss AH, Slocum CH: Histopathologic classification of periarteritis nodosa: a study of 56 cases confirmed at necropsy. *Proc Staff Meet Mayo Clin* 38:345-357, 1963

53. Thiene G, Valente M, Rossi L: Involvement of the cardiac conducting system in panarteritis nodosa. *Am Heart J* 95:716-724, 1978

54. Frohnert PP, Sheps SG: Long-term follow-up study of periarteritis nodosa. *Am J Med* 43:8-14, 1967

55. Holsinger DR, Osmundson PJ, Edwards JE: The heart in periarteritis nodosa. *Circulation* 25:610-618, 1962

56. Zeek PM: Periarteritis nodosa and other forms of necrotizing angiitis. *N Engl J Med* 248:764-772, 1953

57. Huston KA, Hunder GG, Lie JT, et al: Temporal arteritis: a 25-year epidemiologic, clinical, and pathologic study. *Ann Intern Med* 88:162-167, 1978

58. Hamilton CR Jr, Shelley WM, Tumulty PA: Giant cell arteritis: including temporal arteritis and polymyalgia rheumatica. *Medicine (Baltimore)* 50:1-27, 1971

59. Klein RG, Campbell RJ, Hunder GG, et al: Skip lesions in temporal arteritis. *Mayo Clin Proc* 51:504-510, 1976

60. Lie JT: Disseminated visceral giant cell arteritis: histopathologic description and differentiation from other granulomatous vasculitides. *Am J Clin Pathol* 69:299-305, 1978

61. Martin JF, Kittas C, Triger DR: Giant cell arteritis of coronary arteries causing myocardial infarction. *Br Heart J* 43:487-489, 1980

62. Paulley JW: Coronary ischaemia and occlusion in giant cell (temporal) arteritis. *Acta Med Scand* 208:257-263, 1980

63. Säve-Söderbergh J, Malmvall B-E, Andersson R, et al: Giant cell arteritis as a cause of death. Report of nine cases. *JAMA* 255:493-496, 1986

64. Hunder GG, Sheps SG, Allen GL, et al: Daily and alternate-day corticosteroid regimens in treatment of giant cell arteritis: comparison in a prospective study. *Ann Intern Med* 82:613-618, 1975

65. Fauci AS, Wolff SM: Wegener's granulomatosis: studies in eighteen patients and a review of the literature. *Medicine (Baltimore)* 52:535-561, 1973

66. Fauci AS, Haynes BF, Katz P, et al: Wegener's granulomatosis: prospective clinical and therapeutic experience with 85 patients for 21 years. *Ann Intern Med* 98:76-85, 1983

67. Forstot JZ, Overlie PA, Neufeld GK, et al: Cardiac complications of Wegener granulomatosis: a case report of complete heart block and review of the literature. *Semin Arthritis Rheum* 10:148-154, 1980

68. Lie JT: Cardiac and pulmonary manifestations of Behçet syndrome *Pathol Res Pract* 183:347-355, 1988

69. Lewis PD: Behçet's disease and carditis. *Br Med J* 1:1026-1027, 1964

70. Lanham JG, Elkon KB, Pusey CD, et al: Systemic vasculitis with asthma and eosinophilia: a clinical approach to the Churg-Strauss syndrome. *Medicine (Baltimore)* 63:65-81, 1984

71. Amad KH, Brennan JC, Alexander JK: The cardiac pathology of chronic exogenous obesity. *Circulation* 32:740-745, 1965

72. Alexander JK, Pettigrove JR: Obesity and congestive heart failure. *Geriatrics* 22:101-108, 1967

73. Alexander JK, Amad KH, Cole VW: Observations on some clinical features of extreme obesity, with particular reference to cardiorespiratory effects. *Am J Med* 32:512-524, 1962

74. Kaltman AJ, Goldring RM: Role of circulatory congestion in the cardiorespiratory failure of obesity. *Am J Med* 60:645-653, 1976

75. Alexander JK, Dennis EW, Smith WG, et al: Blood volume, cardiac output, and distribution of systemic blood flow in extreme obesity. *Cardiovasc Res Center Bull* 1:39-44, 1962

76. Alexander JK, Woodard CB, Quinones MA, et al: Heart failure from obesity in medical complications of obesity. In *Proceedings of the Serono Symposia. Vol. 26.* Edited by M Manseni, B Lewis. London, Academic Press, 1979, p 175

77. Alexander JK, Peterson KL: Cardiovascular effects of weight reduction. *Circulation* 45:310-318, 1972

78. Backman L, Freyschuss U, Hallberg D, et al: Reversibility of cardiovascular changes in extreme obesity. Effects of weight reduction through jejunoileostomy. *Acta Med Scand* 205:367-373, 1979

79. Weitzman ED: The syndrome of hypersomnia and sleep-induced apnea (editorial). *Chest* 75:414-415, 1979

80. MacGregor MI, Block AJ, Ball WC Jr: Serious complications and sudden death in the Pickwickian syndrome. *Johns Hopkins Med J* 126:279-295, 1970

81. Wharton BA, Balmer SE, Somers K, et al: The myocardium in kwashiorkor. *Q J Med* 38:107-116, 1969

82. Keys A, Henschel A, Taylor HL: The size and function of the human heart at rest and in semi-starvation and in subsequent rehabilitation. *Am J Physiol* 150:153-169, 1947

83. Viart P: Hemodynamic findings in severe protein-calorie malnutrition. *Am J Clin Nutr* 30:334-348, 1977

84. Wharton BA, Howells GR, McCance RA: Cardiac failure in kwashiorkor. *Lancet* 2:384-387, 1967

85. Anonymous: Cardiovascular beriberi (editorial). *Lancet* 1:1287, 1982

86. Kawai C, Wakabayashi A, Matsumura T, et al: Reappearance of beriberi heart disease in Japan. A study of 23 cases. *Am J Med* 69:383-386, 1980

87. Rowlands DT Jr, Vilter CF: A study of the cardiac stigmata in prolonged human thiamine deficiency. *Circulation* 21:4-12, 1960

88. Schrire V, Gant J: The electrocardiographic changes associated with beri-beri heart disease: an analysis of 50 case studies at Groote Schuur Hospital, Cape Town, during a period of five years. *S Afr J Lab Clin Med* 5:195-235, 1959

89. Blacket RB, Palmer AJ: Haemodynamic studies in high output beri-beri. *Br Heart J* 22:483-501, 1960

90. Akbarian M, Yankopoulos NA, Abelmann WH: Hemodynamic studies in beriberi heart disease. *Am J Med* 41:197-212, 1966

91. Seftel HC, Metz J, Lakier JB: Cardiomyopathies in Johannesburg Bantu. I. Aetiology and characteristics of beriberi heart disease. *S Afr Med J* 46:1707-1713, 1972

92. Pereira VG, Masuda Z, Katz A, et al: Shoshin beriberi: report of two successfully treated patients with hemodynamic documentation. *Am J Cardiol* 53:1467, 1984

93. Keshan Disease Research Group, Chinese Academy of Medical Sciences: Observations on effect of sodium selenite in prevention of Keshan disease. *Chin Med J (Engl)* 92:471-476, 1979

94. Keshan Disease Research Group, Chinese Academy of Medical Sciences: Epidemiologic studies on the etiologic relationship of selenium and Keshan disease. *Chin Med J (Engl)* 92:477-482, 1979

95. Johnson RA, Baker SS, Fallon JT, et al: An occidental case of cardiomyopathy and selenium deficiency. *N Engl J Med* 304:1210-1212, 1981

96. Fleming CR, Lie JT, McCall JT, et al: Selenium deficiency and fatal cardiomyopathy in a patient on home parenteral nutrition. *Gastroenterology* 83:689-693, 1982

97. Bistrian BR, Blackburn GL, Vitale J, et al: Prevalence of malnutrition in general medical patients. *JAMA* 235:1567-1570, 1976

98. Abel RM, Fischer JE, Buckley MJ, et al: Malnutrition in cardiac surgical patients. Results of a prospective, randomized evaluation of early postoperative parenteral nutrition. *Arch Surg* 111:45-50, 1976

99. Neufelde EF, Muenzer J: The mucopolysaccharidoses. In *The Metabolic Basis of Inherited Disease.* Vol. 2. Sixth edition. Edited by CR

Scriver, AL Beaudet, WS Sly, et al. New York, McGraw-Hill Information Services Company, 1989, pp 1565-1587

100. Renteria VG, Ferrans VJ, Roberts WC: The heart in the Hurler syndrome: gross, histologic and ultrastructural observations in five necropsy cases. *Am J Cardiol* 38:487-501, 1976

101. Brosius FC III, Roberts WC: Coronary artery disease in the Hurler syndrome. Qualitative and quantitative analysis of the extent of coronary narrowing at necropsy in six children. *Am J Cardiol* 47:649-653, 1981

102. Krovetz LJ, Lorincz AE, Schiebler GL: Cardiovascular manifestations of the Hurler syndrome: hemodynamic and angiocardiographic observations in 15 patients. *Circulation* 31:132-141, 1965

103. Schieken RM, Kerber RE, Ionasescu VV, et al: Cardiac manifestations of the mucopolysaccharidoses. *Circulation* 52:700-705, 1975

104. Gross DM, Williams JC, Caprioli C, et al: Echocardiographic abnormalities in the mucopolysaccharide storage diseases. *Am J Cardiol* 61:170-176, 1988

105. Nagashima K, Endo H, Sakakibara K, et al: Morphological and biochemical studies of a case of mucopolysaccharidosis II (Hunter's syndrome). *Acta Pathol Jpn* 26:115-132, 1976

106. Cain H, Egner E, Kresse H: Mucopolysaccharidosis III A (Sanfilippo disease type A). Histochemical, electron microscopical and biochemical findings. *Beitr Pathol* 160:58-72, 1977

107. Herd JK, Subramanian S, Robinson H: Type 3 mucopolysaccharidosis: report of a case with severe mitral valve involvement. *J Pediatr* 82:101-104, 1973

108. Factor SM, Biempica L, Goldfischer S: Coronary intimal sclerosis in Morquio's syndrome. *Virchows Arch A Pathol Anat Histol* 379:1-10, 1978

109. Ireland MA, Rowlands DB: Mucopolysaccharidosis type IV as a cause of mitral stenosis in an adult. *Br Heart J* 46:113-115, 1981

110. Hers H-G, Van Hoof F, de Barsy T: Glycogen storage diseases. In *The Metabolic Basis of Inherited Disease.* Vol. 1. Sixth edition. Edited by CR Scriver, AL Beaudet, WS Sly, et al. New York, McGraw-Hill Information Services Company, 1989, pp 424-452

111. Blieden LC, Moller JH: Cardiac involvement in inherited disorders of metabolism. *Prog Cardiovasc Dis* 16:615-631, 1974

112. Miller CG, Alleyne GA, Brooks SE: Gross cardiac involvement in glycogen storage disease type 3. *Br Heart J* 34:862-864, 1972

113. Olson LJ, Reeder GS, Noller KL, et al: Cardiac involvement in glycogen storage disease. III. Morphologic and biochemical characterization with endomyocardial biopsy. *Am J Cardiol* 53:980-981, 1984

114. Ehlers KH, Hagstrom JWC, Lukas DS, et al: Glycogen-storage disease of the myocardium with obstruction to left ventricular outflow. *Circulation* 25:96-109, 1962

115. Edwards WD, Hurdey HP III, Partin JR: Cardiac involvement by Gaucher's disease documented by right ventricular endomyocardial biopsy. *Am J Cardiol* 52:654, 1983

116. Tamari I, Motro M, Neufeld HN: Unusual pericardial calcification in Gaucher's disease. *Arch Intern Med* 143:2010-2011, 1983

117. Desnick RJ, Bishop DF: Fabry disease: α-Galactosidase deficiency; Schindler's disease: α-*N*-acetyigalactosaminidase deficiency. In *The Metabolic Basis of Inherited Disease.* Vol. 2. Sixth edition. Edited by CR Scriver, AL Beaudet, WS Sly, et al. New York, McGraw-Hill Information Services Company, 1989, pp 1751-1796

118. Broadbent JC, Edwards WD, Gordon H, et al: Fabry cardiomyopathy in the female confirmed by endomyocardial biopsy. *Mayo Clin Proc* 56:623-628, 1981

119. Lichtenstein L, Kaplan L: Hereditary ochronosis: pathologic changes observed in two necropsied cases. *Am J Pathol* 30:99-125, 1954

120. Coltart DJ, Hudson RE: Primary oxalosis of the heart: a cause of heart block. *Br Heart J* 33:315-319, 1971

121. Gordon N, Hudson REB: Refsum's syndrome: heredopathia atactica polyneuritiformis: a report of three cases, including a study of the cardiac pathology. *Brain* 82:41-55, 1959

122. Perloff JK, de Leon AC Jr, O'Doherty D: The cardiomyopathy of progressive muscular dystrophy. *Circulation* 33:625-648, 1966

123. Moorman JR, Coleman RE, Packer DL, et al: Cardiac involvement in myotonic muscular dystrophy. *Medicine (Baltimore)* 64:371-387, 1985

124. D'Orsogna L, O'Shea JP, Miller G: Cardiomyopathy of Duchenne muscular dystrophy. *Pediatr Cardiol* 9:205-213, 1988

125. James TN: Observations on the cardiovascular involvement, including the cardiac conduction system, in progressive muscular dystrophy. *Am Heart J* 63:48-56, 1962

126. Kennel AJ, Titus JL, Merideth J: Pathologic findings in the atrioventricular conduction system in myotonic dystrophy. *Mayo Clin Proc* 49:838-842, 1974

127. Motta J, Guilleminault C, Billingham M, et al: Cardiac abnormalities in myotonic dystrophy. Electrophysiologic and histopathologic studies. *Am J Med* 67:467-473, 1979

128. Ervasti JM, Ohlendieck K, Kahl SD, et al: Deficiency of a glycoprotein component of the dystrophin complex in dystrophic muscle. *Nature* 345:315-319, 1990

129. Payne CA, Greenfield JC Jr: Electrocardiographic abnormalities associated with myotonic dystrophy. *Am Heart J* 65:436-440, 1963

130. Gottdiener JS, Hawley RJ, Gay JA, et al: Left ventricular relaxation, mitral valve prolapse, and intracardiac conduction in myotonia atrophica: assessment by digitized echocardiography and noninvasive His bundle recording. *Am Heart J* 104:77-85, 1982

131. Prystowsky EN, Pritchett EL, Roses AD, et al: The natural history of conduction system disease in myotonic muscular dystrophy as determined by serial electrophysiologic studies. *Circulation* 60:1360-1364, 1979

132. Kyle RA, Greipp PR: Amyloidosis (AL). Clinical and laboratory features in 229 cases. *Mayo Clin Proc* 58:665-683, 1983

133. Perloff JK, Roberts WC, de Leon AC Jr, et al: The distinctive electrocardiogram of Duchenne's progressive muscular dystrophy. An electrocardiographic-pathologic correlative study. *Am J Med* 42:179-188, 1967

134. Kyle RA, Bayrd ED: Amyloidosis: review of 236 cases. *Medicine (Baltimore)* 54:271-299, 1975

135. Kyle RA, Gertz MA: Cardiac amyloidosis (editorial). *Int J Cardiol* 28:139-141, 1990

136. Cueto-Garcia L, Reeder GS, Kyle RA, et al: Echocardiographic findings in systemic amyloidosis: spectrum of cardiac involvement and relation to survival. *J Am Coll Cardiol* 6:737-743, 1985

137. Olson LJ, Gertz MA, Edwards WD, et al: Senile cardiac amyloidosis with myocardial dysfunction. Diagnosis by endomyocardial biopsy and immunohistochemistry. *N Engl J Med* 317:738-742, 1987

138. Oh JK, Tajik AJ, Edwards WD, et al: Dynamic left ventricular outflow tract obstruction in cardiac amyloidosis detected by continuous-wave Doppler echocardiography. *Am J Cardiol* 59:1008-1010, 1987

139. Klein AL, Hatle LK, Burstow DJ, et al: Doppler characterization of left ventricular diastolic function in cardiac amyloidosis. *J Am Coll Cardiol* 13:1017-1026, 1989

140. Klein AL, Hatle LK, Burstow DJ, et al: Comprehensive Doppler assessment of right ventricular diastolic function in cardiac amyloidosis. *J Am Coll Cardiol* 15:99-108, 1990

141. Klein AL, Hatle LK, Taliercio CP, et al: Serial Doppler echocardiographic follow-up of left ventricular diastolic function in cardiac amyloidosis. *J Am Coll Cardiol* 16:1135-1141, 1990

142. Klein AL, Hatle LK, Taliercio CP, et al: Prognostic significance of Doppler measures of diastolic function in cardiac amyloidosis. A Doppler echocardiography study. *Circulation* 83:808-816, 1991

143. Milder MS, Cook JD, Stray S, et al: Idiopathic hemochromatosis, an interim report. *Medicine (Baltimore)* 59:34-49, 1980

144. Edwards CQ, Kushner JP: Screening for hemochromatosis. *N Engl J Med* 328:1616-1620, 1993

145. Olson LJ, Edwards WD, McCall JT, et al: Cardiac iron deposition in idiopathic hemochromatosis: histologic and analytic assessment of 14 hearts from autopsy. *J Am Coll Cardiol* 10:1239-1243, 1987

146. Olson LJ, Edwards WD, Holmes DR Jr, et al: Endomyocardial biopsy in hemochromatosis: clinicopathologic correlates in six cases. *J Am Coll Cardiol* 13:116-120, 1989

147. Finch SC, Finch CA: Idiopathic hemochromatosis, an iron storage disease. A. Iron metabolism in hemochromatosis. *Medicine (Baltimore)* 34:381-430, 1955

148. Cutler DJ, Isner JM, Bracey AW, et al: Hemochromatosis heart disease: an unemphasized cause of potentially reversible restrictive cardiomyopathy. *Am J Med* 69:923-928, 1980

149. Olson LJ, Baldus WP, Tajik AJ: Echocardiographic features of idiopathic hemochromatosis. *Am J Cardiol* 60:885-889, 1987

150. Henry WL, Nienhuis AW, Wiener M, et al: Echocardiographic abnormalities in patients with transfusion-dependent anemia and secondary myocardial iron deposition. *Am J Med* 64:547-555, 1978

151. Short EM, Winkle RA, Billingham ME: Myocardial involvement

in idiopathic hemochromatosis. Morphologic and clinical improvement following venesection. *Am J Med* 70:1275-1279, 1981

152. Skinner C, Kenmure AC: Haemochromatosis presenting as congestive cardiomyopathy and responding to venesection. *Br Heart J* 35:466-468, 1973

153. Pellikka PA, Tajik AJ, Khandheria BK, et al: Carcinoid heart disease. Clinical and echocardiographic spectrum in 74 patients. *Circulation* 87:1188-1196, 1993

154. Ross EM, Roberts WC: The carcinoid syndrome: comparison of 21 necropsy subjects with carcinoid heart disease to 15 necropsy subjects without carcinoid heart disease. *Am J Med* 79:339-354, 1985

155. Callahan JA, Wroblewski EM, Reeder GS, et al: Echocardiographic features of carcinoid heart disease. *Am J Cardiol* 50:762-768, 1982

156. Lundin L, Hansson HE, Landelius J, et al: Surgical treatment of carcinoid heart disease. *J Thorac Cardiovasc Surg* 100:552-561, 1990

157. Silverman KJ, Hutchins GM, Bulkley BH: Cardiac sarcoid: a clinicopathologic study of 84 unselected patients with systemic sarcoidosis. *Circulation* 58:1204-1211, 1978

158. Roberts WC, McAllister HA Jr, Ferrans VJ: Sarcoidosis of the heart. A clinicopathologic study of 35 necropsy patients (group 1) and review of 78 previously described necropsy patients (group 11). *Am J Med* 63:86-108, 1977

159. Jain A, Starek PJ, Delany DL: Ventricular tachycardia and ventricular aneurysm due to unrecognized sarcoidosis. *Clin Cardiol* 13:738-740, 1990

160. Lull RJ, Dunn BE, Gregoratos G, et al: Ventricular aneurysm due to cardiac sarcoidosis with surgical cure of refractory ventricular tachycardia. *Am J Cardiol* 30:282-287, 1972

161. Kawasaki T: Acute febrile mucocutaneous syndrome with lymphoid involvement with specific desquamation of the fingers and toes in children. *Arerugi* 16:178-222, 1967

162. Suzuki A, Kamiya T, Ono Y, et al: Follow-up study of coronary artery lesions due to Kawasaki disease by serial selective coronary arteriography in 200 patients. *Heart Vessels* 3:159-165, 1987

163. Fujiwara H, Kawai C, Hamashima Y: Clinicopathologic study of the conduction systems in 10 patients with Kawasaki's disease (mucocutaneous lymph node syndrome). *Am Heart J* 96:744-750, 1978

164. Takahashi M, Mason W, Lewis AB: Regression of coronary aneurysms in patients with Kawasaki syndrome. *Circulation* 75:387-394, 1987

165. Lippman SM, Niemann JT, Thigpen T, et al: Abnormal septal Q waves in sickle cell disease. Prevalence and causative factors. *Chest* 88:543-548, 1985

166. Balfour IC, Covitz W, Davis H, et al: Cardiac size and function in children with sickle cell anemia. *Am Heart J* 108:345-350, 1984

CHAPTER

60

Cardiovascular manifestations of hypertension

A. Diagnosis

Prince K. Zachariah, M.D., Ph.D., and Sheldon G. Sheps, M.D.

Systemic hypertension is a very common condition and a major contributor to cardiovascular morbidity and mortality. Untreated hypertension is associated with a shortening of the life expectancy by 10 to 20 years,[1] although the average untreated patient survives close to 20 years.[2] Both systolic and diastolic blood pressures form a continuum, and the frequency of hypertension in any population depends on the dividing line that is used for a designation of hypertension. If one uses as the definition one casual diastolic blood pressure of 95 mm Hg or more, 15% to 20% of the adult population in the United States were hypertensive in the early 1960s.[3] However, the frequency of hypertension in the United States appears to be changing. If one uses as the definition of hypertension in adults a systolic blood pressure of at least 140 mm Hg or a diastolic blood pressure of at least 90 mm Hg, or both, there were about 50 million people, or 26% of Americans older than 17 years, with hypertension reported between 1988 and 1991. This represents a decline of 8 million adults since the study conducted from 1976 to 1980. However, 21.5 million people, or 11.2% of adult Americans, were successfully controlling their blood pressure in 1988-1991. The prevalence rate of blood pressure elevation is higher in blacks than in whites, is intermediate in Hispanics, and increases with age. Regional differences in prevalence rate, severity, and cardiovascular complications of hypertension have also been reported.

An understanding of the frequency of the types of hypertension and the prevalence of potentially curable secondary hypertension is essential to the development of an appropriate diagnostic strategy in dealing with hypertensive patients. An analysis of a 3-year survey of adult hypertensive patients at the Mayo Clinic showed that of the total number, only 0.18% underwent surgery for renovascular hypertension, 0.04% for pheochromocytoma, and 0.01% for primary aldosteronism.[4] A similarly low incidence of secondary hypertension, less than 1%, was found in a study of 10,940 mildly hypertensive adults in a hypertension detection and follow-up program.[5] Other studies have shown a much higher incidence of secondary forms of hypertension, but those studies have been based largely on the intensive study of referred hypertensive patients. For example, at the Cleveland Clinic, the incidence of potentially curable hypertension was 6%. The hypertensive group studied included 4% with renovascular hypertension, 0.2% with pheochromocytoma, and 0.5% with primary aldosteronism. In the same study of 4,939 hypertensive patients, there were also 5% with chronic renal disease, 1% with coarctation of the aorta, and 0.2% with Cushing's syndrome.[6] In a study of 331 patients in a community-based referral clinic, 11 patients with oral contraceptive-induced hypertension were found (not analyzed in the Cleveland Clinic and Mayo Clinic studies); also, 7 had renovascular disease, 3 had polycystic kidney disease, 3 had chronic renal disease, and 2 had endocrine hypertension with no other types of secondary hypertension identified.[7]

An appropriate approach to the diagnosis of hypertension takes cognizance of the low frequency of curable secondary hypertension, the huge expense that would be involved in a comprehensive diagnostic survey of all hypertensive patients, and the knowledge that antihypertensive drug therapy is very effective in favorably altering the course of hypertensive disease in most patients.[5]

During the 1970s, task forces of the National High Blood Pressure Education Program and the National Heart, Lung, and Blood Institute were charged with providing practical recommendations for the management of high blood pressure. The task forces culminated in the formation of the Joint National Committee on Detection, Evaluation, and Treatment of High Blood Pressure, which has issued several reports and lists of recommendations, the most recent of which was published in 1993.[8] The recommendations of this committee dominate current thinking pertaining to the diagnosis and treatment of hypertension.

DETECTION

The diagnosis of hypertension begins with detection, but it should not end there. Considerable progress has been made in the initial detection of high blood pressure by encouraging all health care professionals to measure the blood pressure routinely at each patient visit. Additionally, many cases of hypertension are detected by blood pressure screening programs or when an individual determines his or her own blood pressure at automatic blood pressure stations at shopping centers, airports, banks, fire stations, and so on. Emphasis on this aspect of detection has resulted in 79% of the population having had a blood pressure check in the past year.

The standard method for indirect measurement of blood pressure is to employ an air-inflated, arm-occluding cuff, a calibrated mercury sphygmomanometer, and a stethoscope to detect Korotkoff sounds. The size of the bladder in the air-inflated, arm-occluding cuff is an important determinant of the indirectly measured blood pressure, and the size of the bladder should be correlated with the size of the patient's arm, the circumference being used as the guideline. The American Heart Association recently published new standards of cuff size (Table 60A-1). The length of the bladder is also of some importance; the American Heart Association Committee recommends a bladder length of approximately 2 to 2.5 times the bladder width.

The measurement of blood pressure in extremely obese persons is subject to error if the correct arm-occluding cuff is not used; a "thigh cuff" is often suitable in patients with very large arms. An alternative method is a standard arm cuff applied to the forearm. Korotkoff sounds can usually be detected by auscultating with the stethoscope over the radial artery to obtain both systolic and diastolic blood pressures. Occasionally these sounds are difficult to hear, and in such cases the systolic pressure can be checked by palpation of the radial artery or, more accurately, by the use of a Doppler ultrasound blood-flow-detecting instrument to indicate the systolic blood pressure.

The blood pressure should be measured with the subject seated and resting comfortably with the back and arm supported. The arms should be free of constricting garments. Both systolic and diastolic pressures should be recorded on the basis of the Korotkoff sounds. Auscultatory gap is related to phases II and III Korotkoff sounds and can be eliminated by raising the arm before inflating the cuff. The best determination of diastolic pressure for children is the phase IV Korotkoff sound.

Table 60A-1 Recommended bladder dimensions for blood pressure cuff

Name of cuff	Bladder size, cm	Arm circumference, cm
Newborn	3 × 6	≤6
Infant	5 × 10	6-10
Child	8 × 16	10-16
Small adult	10 × 20	16-25
Adult	13 × 26	26-32.5
Large adult	16 × 32	32-40
Adult thigh	20 × 40	≥40

Blood pressure should be recorded from both arms at the time of the initial examination. For the greatest accuracy, blood pressure in each arm should be taken simultaneously through use of a Y tube and two observers. A substantial difference in the blood pressures obtained in the two arms may be a sign of significant occlusive arterial disease involving the innominate or either subclavian artery. On subsequent examinations, the blood pressure from the arm with the higher reading should be used as the reference point relative to the diagnosis of hypertension.

The blood pressure should be determined with the patient standing as well as while sitting. In normal persons, a change in position from supine to standing results in a slight decrease in systolic blood pressure, a slight increase or no change in diastolic blood pressure, and a mild increase in heart rate. The standing blood pressure is of particular importance in certain clinical situations. These include patients whose history suggests symptomatic postural hypotension; a drop in blood pressure of 30/15 mm Hg with standing compared with the supine position corroborates the clinical importance of this maneuver.[9] It is particularly important to check orthostatic blood pressure in elderly patients who have problems after meals. Other patients in whom it is important to check the standing blood pressure are those who are receiving antihypertensive drug therapy and those suspected by reason of history or physical findings of having secondary hypertension. In particular, a pronounced postural drop in the blood pressure with standing may be a clue to severe sodium restriction in patients with renal parenchymal hypertension and chronic renal failure and also an indication of too vigorous antihypertensive therapy with agents capable of producing orthostatic hypotension.

The Joint National Committee on Detection, Evaluation, and Treatment of High Blood Pressure has recommended a series of arbitrary blood pressure classifications that are widely accepted (Table 60A-2). Other definitions of hypertension, equally arbitrary, have also gained acceptance. The World Health Organization definition since 1959 for epidemiologic studies of hypertension specifies three categories: (1) normal—below 140 mm Hg systolic, 90 mm Hg diastolic; (2) hypertensive—above 160 mm Hg systolic, 95 mm Hg diastolic; and (3) borderline—140 to 159 mm Hg systolic and 90 to 94 mm Hg diastolic.[10]

Statistical definitions for hypertension have also been advocated. For example, one such attempt was to define normal pressures as those occurring within 1 standard deviation of mean values, with departures of 2 standard deviations or more being considered abnormal and an indication of hypertension.[11] Such statistical definitions have not gained acceptance for adult patients, but the task force on blood pressure control in children has suggested that systolic and diastolic blood pressures more than the 95th percentile on at least two separate occasions, when measured several months apart, should prompt further

Table 60A-2 Classification of blood pressure for adults aged 18 years and older*

Category	Systolic, mm Hg	Diastolic, mm Hg
Normal†	< 130	< 85
High normal	130-139	85-89
Hypertension‡		
Stage 1 (mild)	140-159	90-99
Stage 2 (moderate)	160-179	100-109
Stage 3 (severe)	180-209	110-119
Stage 4 (very severe)	≥ 210	≥ 120

*Not taking antihypertensive drugs and not acutely ill. When systolic and diastolic pressures fall into different categories, the higher category should be selected to classify the individual's blood pressure status. For instance, 160/92 mm Hg should be classified as stage 2, and 180/120 mm Hg should be classified as stage 4. Isolated systolic hypertension is defined as a systolic blood pressure of 140 mm Hg or more and a diastolic blood pressure of less than 90 mm Hg and staged appropriately (e.g., 170/85 mm Hg is defined as stage 2 isolated systolic hypertension).

In addition to classifying stages of hypertension on the basis of average blood pressure levels, the clinician should specify presence or absence of target-organ disease and additional risk factors. For example, a patient with diabetes and a blood pressure of 142/94 mm Hg plus left ventricular hypertrophy should be classified as having "stage 1 hypertension with target-organ disease (left ventricular hypertrophy) and with another major risk factor (diabetes)." This specificity is important for risk classification and management.

†Optimal blood pressure with respect to cardiovascular risk is less than 120 mm Hg systolic and less than 80 mm Hg diastolic. However, unusually low readings should be evaluated for clinical significance.

‡Based on the average of two or more readings taken at each of two or more visits after an initial screening.

From the Joint National Committee on Detection, Evaluation, and Treatment of High Blood Pressure: The Fifth Report of the Joint National Committee on Detection, Evaluation, and Treatment of High Blood Pressure (JNC V). *Arch Intern Med* 153:154-183, 1993.

Table 60A-3 Recommendations for follow-up based on initial set of blood pressure measurements for adults age 18 and older

Initial screening blood pressure, mm Hg*		
Systolic	**Diastolic**	**Follow-up recommended†**
< 130	< 85	Recheck in 2 years
130-139	85-89	Recheck in 1 year‡
140-159	90-99	Confirm within 2 months
160-179	100-109	Evaluate or refer to source of care within 1 month
180-209	110-119	Evaluate or refer to source of care within 1 week
≥ 210	≥ 120	Evaluate or refer to source of care immediately

*If the systolic and diastolic categories are different, follow recommendation for the shorter time follow-up (e.g., 160/85 mm Hg should be evaluated or referred to source of care within 1 month).

†The scheduling of follow-up should be modified by reliable information about past blood pressure measurements, other cardiovascular risk factors, or target-organ disease.

‡Consider providing advice about lifestyle modifications

evaluation.[12] Systolic and diastolic blood pressures are a continuum, and actuarial studies have indicated a relationship between mortality and blood pressure levels from the lowest to the highest levels of both systolic and diastolic blood pressures for both men and women.[13] No studies have clearly demonstrated a dividing line for the threshold of risk.

After an initial high blood pressure value has been obtained, the blood pressure should be determined on subsequent examinations. The Joint National Committee on Detection, Evaluation, and Treatment of High Blood Pressure has made recommendations for follow-up based on the initial blood pressure measurements in adults (Table 60A-3). The Joint National Committee arrived at the opinion that elevated systolic blood pressure is as good a predictor of risk as diastolic blood pressure, but they chose only the diastolic blood pressure as a basis for establishing a diagnosis of hypertension and recommending disposition, because the goals for treating systolic blood pressure have not yet been established.

One attempt to clarify the problem inherent in a variable and labile blood pressure is to record the blood pressure repeatedly over time.[14] Studies comparing single casual readings, the average of three consecutive readings, the average of multiple readings in a 2-hour period, and the average of readings obtained over 24 hours show that the overall 24-hour average is lower than that with the three other methods. However, the average values for a 2 hour period between 8 a.m. and 10 a.m. correlate closely with the 24-hour averages despite differences in the absolute numbers, and the mean of three consecutive readings in a 15-minute period is of intermediate reliability between the 2-hour and the single-reading approach.

Ambulatory blood pressure monitors for diagnosis and treatment in hypertensive patients have become increasingly popular in recent years. Noninvasive ambulatory blood pressure monitoring provides multiple recordings during the patient's normal daily activities. The supplementary information obtained may be valuable in confirming the presence or absence of elevated blood pressures in "white-coat hypertension" and in determining the efficacy of antihypertensive medications in treated hypertensive patients. However, the clinical indications for ambulatory blood pressure recordings are not fully established. A proposed list of clinical indications is outlined in Table 60A-4. Noninvasive continuous blood pressure recordings are particularly useful in identifying short-lived events, such as episodic hypertension due to pheochromocytoma, hypotension induced by antihypertensive drugs, and hypotension secondary to autonomic failure.

Isolated systolic hypertension (systolic blood pressure ≥ 160 mm Hg) frequently occurs in the elderly population. Approximately 29 million people in the United States were over the age of 65 years in 1990, and 45% of the

Table 60A-4 Uses for automated ambulatory blood pressure monitoring

Office, or "white-coat," hypertension
Evaluation of drug resistance
Evaluation of nocturnal blood pressure changes
Episodic hypertension
Hypotensive symptoms associated with antihypertensive medications or autonomic dysfunction
Carotid sinus syncope and pacemaker syndromes

Table 60A-5 Adverse effects of systemic hypertension on the heart

Production of left ventricluar hypertrophy
Impaired coronary circulation leading to myocardial ischemia
Dysrhythmias from cardiac electrophysiologic abnormalities
Cardiac failure from systolic or diastolic dysfunction (or both)
Acceleration of occlusive coronary artery disease

Data from Frohlich ED, Apstein C, Chobanian AV, et al: The heart in hypertension. *N Engl J Med* 327:998-1008, 1992.

population have isolated systolic hypertension. Two-thirds of the people over age 65 years also have elevation of systolic and diastolic blood pressures greater than 140 and 90 mm Hg, respectively. With late onset of diastolic hypertension in the older population or hypertension in the elderly that no longer responds to previously effective regimens, a secondary cause of hypertension, such as renovascular stenosis, should be suspected.

New data describing the efficacy of antihypertensive treatment in decreasing the incidence of cardiovascular events caused by isolated systolic hypertension became available with the completion of the Systolic Hypertension in the Elderly Program in 1991. The active treatment group was found to have a relative risk of 0.64 ($P < 0.0003$) for stroke compared with the placebo group.[15] If nonpharmacologic therapy is not successful in reducing isolated systolic hypertension, administration of antihypertensive drugs is recommended, but the systolic blood pressure should be lowered cautiously to 140-160 mm Hg. This is particularly important in patients who have preexisting atherosclerotic disease of the coronary arteries and carotids.

Physical exercise regularly increases the systolic blood pressure along with the physiologic increases in heart rate and cardiac output. In normal persons, the systolic pressure increases from 7 to 10 mm Hg per MET (MET = basal oxygen requirements of the body at rest, sitting quietly; it is usually considered to be 3.5 mL O_2/kg · min). At peak physical effort, values of systolic blood pressure may range from as low as 190 to more than 240 mm Hg. Sedentary persons or cardiac patients may be unable to generate an adequate blood pressure increase during effort. Systolic blood pressure occasionally may increase inordinately. Although this is probably indicative of a hypertensive response, the pathologic implications of this response have not been established.[16]

EVALUATION

After hypertension as defined has been detected, evaluation of the patient should answer three questions: (1) Is target organ damage present? (2) Are cardiovascular risk factors other than hypertension present? (3) Does the patient have primary or a form of secondary (possibly curable) hypertension?[17] Most routine evaluations are limited to assessing target organ damage and identifying associated cardiovascular risk factors with no exhaustive search for secondary hypertension. Cardiovascular risk factors are discussed in chapter 13.

Assessment of target organ damage

The severity of hypertension as indicated by the level of blood pressure, both systolic and diastolic, correlates with the development of target organ damage and other morbid events. Antihypertensive treatment has been shown to reduce these events significantly.[18,19]

The heart. Systemic hypertension adversely affects the heart in a number of significant ways, contributing to the necessity of controlling hypertension (Table 60A-5). Hypertension and coronary heart disease often occur together, and the complications and course of the heart disease are determined by both factors.[20] However, hypertensive heart disease with pronounced left ventricular hypertrophy can occur in the absence of coronary artery disease.[21]

The adverse consequences of hypertension in the form of cardiac morbidity and mortality are now well known.[22] In the Framingham Study, for example, definite hypertension preceded congestive heart failure in 75% of the cases.[23] The risk of cardiac failure was three times higher in hypertensive patients with left ventricular hypertrophy as demonstrated on the electrocardiogram (ECG) than in those without this abnormality. Furthermore, 35% of men and 20% of women were dead within 5 years of the appearance of signs of left ventricular hypertrophy on the ECG. An even higher mortality was reported by Sokolow and Perloff[24] in a group of untreated hypertensive patients who had ECG evidence of left ventricular hypertrophy and repolarization abnormalities.

Concentric left ventricular hypertrophy is the usual major cardiac consequence of hypertension, although asymmetric hypertrophy, particularly involving the interventricular septum, may occur in borderline hypertension.[25]

Systemic hypertension is a classic example of left ventricular pressure overload (afterload). At the onset of left ventricular hypertrophy from pressure overload, the myocardial cells undergo major biochemical changes, including RNA-mediated protein synthesis and a diminution in ATPase.[26] The contractility of the myocardium is decreased per unit of myocardial mass in chronic pressure overload, but overall ventricular performance is maintained by an increase in cardiac mass.[27]

The progression from ventricular hypertrophy to cardiac failure occurs in stages. Meerson[28] hypothesized three such stages of progression. In the first stage, one of adaptation, the left ventricle responds to a chronic pressure overload with an increase in active muscle units, producing a period of stable hyperfunction. This response results in cardiac performance sufficient to escape clinical detection. In the early second stage of left ventricular hypertrophy, dysfunction of the left ventricle may be detected during cardiac catheterization by a decreased rate of left ventricular ejection, decreased stroke volume, and a shift of the Frank-Starling curve to the right.[29] The compensatory hypertrophy is initially unrecognized clinically, but subsequently the appearance of a fourth heart sound and ECG evidence of a left atrial abnormality indicate reduced compliance of the left ventricle.[30]

In the second stage, there is echocardiographic evidence of abnormally increased ventricular septal or posterobasal free-wall thickness. This was present in 61% of subjects with mild to moderate hypertension in one study, even though fewer than 10% of the subjects had abnormal 12-lead ECGs or chest radiographs.[31] Later in the second stage, ECG evidence of left ventricular hypertrophy becomes evident, along with enlargement of the left ventricle detected on the chest radiograph.[24]

The third stage occurs when the compensatory mechanisms are no longer sufficient to counterbalance the effects of chronic left ventricular pressure overload. It is the stage of overt heart failure, with left ventricular dilatation, pulmonary edema, and ultimately pulmonary hypertension, right ventricular hypertrophy, and failure.

Left ventricular hypertrophy represents a major independent risk factor for cardiac arrhythmias and sudden death.[32] Echocardiography provides the most sensitive and specific diagnosis of left ventricular enlargement, but its use is limited because of cost. However, left ventricular hypertrophy in patients at high risk of coronary artery atherosclerosis should be identified early with echocardiography, so that aggressive management can be instituted to reduce life-threatening cardiac arrhythmias and sudden death. Diastolic dysfunction leading to slow filling of the left ventricle has been recognized. Abnormal left ventricular compliance is in part responsible for the diastolic dysfunction, but the cause of this is not fully understood. This entity is commonly seen in hypertensive patients whose blood pressures were not fully controlled for several months to years. The presenting symptom is progressively worsening dyspnea on exertion, or there are symptoms of left ventricular failure. Two newer imaging methods, gated magnetic resonance imaging and ultrafast (cine) computed tomography, are being used to better evaluate cardiac function and wall thickness, but their cost currently prohibits routine use.[33] However, echocardiographic measurements in expert hands can also make a reliable diagnosis of diastolic dysfunction and estimate the ejection fraction.

The arteries. Target organ damage in hypertension other than for the cardiac manifestations described above relates to the pathologic changes in the arterial system and their consequences. The brain and kidneys bear the major brunt of target organ damage. However, the aorta itself may suffer.

The systemic arterial system from the aorta to the capillaries consists of three different segments, classified according to wall structures: (1) large elastic arteries—the aorta and its proximal branches, (2) the muscular arteries, and (3) small arteries that lead to prearterioles, arterioles, and finally capillaries. Hypertension affects each of the basic three segments in somewhat different patterns.

Evidence has been mounting that reduced vascular compliance is a surrogate for hypertensive cardiovascular disease. As an adaptive mechanism to increased cardiac output, pressure is shifted to high peripheral resistance by hypertrophy of the vascular wall. It may be important to reduce peripheral vascular resistance to allow regression of vascular hypertrophy in antihypertensive therapy.[34]

DISSECTING ANEURYSMS OF THE AORTA. Aortic dissection occurs predominantly in patients with hypertension. Approximately 80% of patients with aortic dissection have elevations of blood pressure to more than 140/90 mm Hg, and about 95% of such patients have been found to have cardiomegaly at autopsy, defined as a heart weight of more than 350 g in women and 400 g in men.[35] Generalized aortic dilatation also occurs more commonly in hypertensive than in normotensive persons. Elastic tissue in the aorta decreases with age, and this permits the higher intra-aortic pressure to enlarge the aorta.[36] This may lead to dilatation of the aortic root and aortic valve insufficiency (see chapter 58A).

Degeneration of the aortic media is believed to be the pathologic prerequisite for the development of aortic dissection. Usually this consists of deterioration of collagen and elastic tissue, often with cystic changes.[37] The precise relationships of medial degeneration and hypertension in the causation of aortic dissection remain speculative, although abnormal hemodynamic forces applied to the aorta are thought to be of major importance.

HIGH INTRAVASCULAR PRESSURE AS A CAUSE OF ATHEROSCLEROSIS. Hypertension is generally acknowledged to be a major risk factor in the development of atherosclerosis in large elastic and muscular arteries. Three naturally occurring conditions demonstrate this relationship conclusively: (1) In coarctation of the aorta, atherosclerosis develops to a far greater degree in the high-pressure segment proximal to the stenosis than in the low-pressure distal segment. (2) In anomalous origin of the left coronary artery from the low-pressure pulmonary artery, when such patients have survived to middle life there is a paucity of atherosclerosis in the left coronary system compared with the right coronary system, which in such patients arises from the high-pressure aortic root.[38] (3) Atherosclerosis of the pulmonary artery occurs in long-standing pulmonary hypertension. This is in contrast to its absence in the normal low-pressure pulmonary artery.[39]

The brain. It has become clear from epidemiologic studies that hypertension is the major risk factor for the

Table 60A-6 Stroke events in the Systolic Hypertension in the Elderly Program

Treatment group	No. of subjects	No. of events		
		Nonfatal	Fatal	Total*
Active	2,365	96	10	103
Placebo	2,371	149	14	159

Relative risk reduction at 95% confidence: 36%.
*Three participants in the active treatment group and four in the placebo group had both fatal and nonfatal strokes. Only the nonfatal strokes were counted in the total number of events.
From Phillips SJ, Whisnant JP: Hypertension and the brain. *Arch Intern Med* 152:938-945, 1992. By permission of American Medical Association.

development of cerebrovascular disease.[40] Systolic as well as diastolic hypertension is a risk factor. For each increase of 10 mm Hg in systolic blood pressure above the normal range, there is a corresponding 10% increase in the incidence of stroke.[41] Treatment of diastolic hypertension reduces the incidence of stroke by about 40%, and treatment of isolated systolic hypertension in persons aged 60 or older has been shown to reduce the incidence of stroke by more than 33%[42] (Table 60A-6).

The cerebrovascular complications of hypertension are mediated by arterial disorders of several types. Atherosclerosis in the extracranial arteries and in the circle of Willis is responsible for most strokes with large parenchymal cerebral infarctions. Hypertension predisposes the patient to atherosclerosis in these vessels, although large parenchymal cerebral infarcts occur commonly in normotensive patients also. Cerebral embolism from carotid atherosclerosis is a common cause of occlusion of the trunks of the anterior middle and posterior cerebral arteries and their cortical branches. Carotid atherosclerosis can also produce stroke because of local impairment of flow, although it is possible for complete occlusion of a carotid artery to occur with no consequent stroke.

The second type of brain involvement of major importance in hypertension is more specifically related to a high arterial pressure. Lacunes have been defined as the small trabeculated cavities often found in the deeper parts of the brain in hypertensive subjects. They are the remnants of small infarcts and range in diameter from 0.5 to 15 mm. The responsible arterial lesion in lacunes occurs at the bifurcation of small penetrating intracerebral arteries and consists of miliary saccular aneurysms. These lesions, which were first described by Charcot and Bouchard in 1869, occur almost entirely in hypertensive patients and consist of fibrinoid necrosis in the arterial wall, which produces asymmetric aneurysms. The lesions are located predominantly in the region of the central nervous system where the lacunar infarcts occur—namely, in the putamen, thalamus, pons, cerebellum, and subcortex. Fibrinoid necrosis may lead to occlusion of the arteries and will result in lacunar infarcts, or focal intracerebral hemorrhage may occur with rupture of the wall of the small saccular aneurysms.[43] Lacunar infarcts typically produce pure motor or sensory deficits without speech or visual impairment and with rapid improvement in several weeks. Intracerebral microaneurysms occur commonly in hypertensive patients—in 46% at autopsy compared with 7% in normotensive age- and sex-matched subjects in one study.[44]

Primary intracerebral hemorrhage almost always occurs in hypertensive persons.[45] These account for approximately 10% of all strokes in the United States. In other parts of the world, hemorrhagic stroke in hypertensive patients poses a larger problem. In certain parts of Japan, for example, hemorrhagic stroke is the most frequent cause of death in hypertensive subjects.[46] The majority of primary intracerebral hemorrhages are located in the cerebral hemispheres; a small proportion are found in the brain stem or cerebellum. Symptoms and the clinical picture depend on the site of the hemorrhage. When the hemorrhage occurs into the ventricles or subarachnoid space, a stiff neck is typical, but this sign may be absent when the intracranial bleeding is confined to the cerebral parenchyma. Computed tomography has greatly aided in the diagnosis of primary intracerebral hemorrhage.

The syndrome of malignant hypertension may result in another central nervous system complication of acute hypertension. Typically, such patients have retinopathy with papilledema, the diagnostic hallmark of acute hypertensive encephalopathy. Focal neurologic findings in these patients occur infrequently, although seizures and cortical blindness are occasionally present. The arterial lesions in hypertensive encephalopathy are predominantly severe arteriolar spasm. It is theorized that high cerebral perfusion pressure occurs with a failure of the normal autoregulatory mechanisms, and this leads to exudation of plasma through the capillaries and the development of cerebral edema.[47]

The skin. A rare complication of hypertension in recent years is leg ulcers due to hypertensive arteriolar disease (hypertensive ischemic ulcers of the leg). Typical histopathologic changes in the ulcer and adjacent skin consist of an increase in the thickness of the arteriolar wall and a decrease in the diameter of the lumen. Additionally, there may be hyaline degeneration in the media, intimal proliferation, and mild periarteritis.[48] Similar arteriolar changes have been found in the hypertensive patients who did not have ulceration of the skin. Hypertensive ischemic ulcers predominate in women in and beyond the sixth decade who have had chronic poorly controlled hypertension.

The kidneys. Hypertension is associated with end-stage renal disease, which is becoming a major health problem that should continue to worsen through the year 2000. Four subgroups of hypertensive patients are at high risk for end-stage renal disease (Table 60A-7). These groups should receive special attention in efforts to control high blood pressure.[49]

In the hypertensive kidney, many glomeruli appear normal by light microscopy in the early stages of the disease. However, electron microscopic examination of

Table 60A-7 Hypertensive patients with high risk for end-stage renal disease

Blacks
Patients with chronic renal failure
Diabetics
Elderly patients

the apparently normal glomeruli has revealed thickening of the capillary basement membranes.[50] Patients with severe essential hypertension have moderately thickened glomerular basement membranes, wrinkled glomerular scars, and completely hyalinized glomeruli.

Abnormalities in renal function which appear early in hypertensive subjects are a reduction in renal plasma flow and an increase in filtration fraction.[51] Despite these changes, the glomerular filtration rate (GFR) remains normal. The GFR decreases only after nephrosclerosis is well developed. Elevation of serum levels of creatinine, reflecting the reduced GFR, is thus a relatively late development in the course of benign essential hypertension.

Rapidly progressive renal failure rarely occurs in essential hypertension unless the hypertension is extremely severe and is in the "malignant" phase. In such a case, the renal failure may progress in a matter of weeks, with an increasing creatinine concentration reflecting a reduction of the GFR and of the renal plasma flow as measured by *p*-aminohippurate clearance.

An early sign of vascular and renal complications is microalbuminuria. Radioimmunoassay is the most accurate quantitative test for microalbuminuria, but other methods of screening can be used. It has been suggested that this test be used routinely for early detection of nephropathy to arrest the progress of renal insufficiency.[52]

Between 2% (Keith, Wagener, Barker group 2) and 59% (Keith, Wagener, Barker group 4) of untreated hypertensive subjects progress to end-stage renal failure and death.[53] Since hypertension is a potentially reversible cause of chronic renal failure, this complication should be markedly reduced by effective control of blood pressure.[18,19]

Investigation for secondary hypertension

In posing the question of whether the patient has primary or secondary hypertension, an overriding concern is the potential for cure of hypertension. Many factors determine whether it is worthwhile to seek a cure as opposed to control with antihypertensive drugs. The age of the patient and the severity of the hypertension are the most important considerations, and the presence or absence of other atherosclerotic risk factors is also important.

High blood pressure may occur as an important finding in a large number of diseases and clinical syndromes and as a result of the action of a great many different exogenous agents[54] (Table 60A-8). However, the vast majority of patients who present with mild to moderate hypertension as the major abnormality have primary (essential) hypertension. Probably fewer than 5% of all hypertensive persons have secondary hypertension, and only a portion of these cases are truly curable. The major secondary forms of hypertension that should be differentiated from primary hypertension in persons presenting with high blood pressure as the dominant abnormality are renovascular hypertension, certain renal parenchymal diseases, pheochromocytoma, primary aldosteronism, coarctation of the aorta, and hypertension due to oral contraceptives.

Primary hypertension is a diagnosis of exclusion; thus, the diagnosis depends partly on the vigor and thoroughness with which the possibility of secondary hypertension is pursued. As noted earlier, the aggressive investigation for secondary hypertension is particularly indicated in the young or the severely hypertensive patient and also in those whose hypertension does not respond to standard antihypertensive drug therapy, those who have specific clues in the history or on physical examination suggesting secondary hypertension, and those who have other major cardiovascular risk factors.

The basic elements of the evaluation of the hypertensive patient are reviewed below.

Clinical history

After the initial detection of hypertension, one should obtain a pertinent history, focusing on major factors that help to determine the type and extent of investigation of the hypertensive patient needed and to establish a basis for proper management. Historical information of prior blood pressure determinations should be obtained, including blood pressures on routine examinations, insurance examinations, pre-employment examinations, or hypertension-detection programs. In women who have been pregnant, the blood pressures during pregnancy provide important historical information about possible toxemia of pregnancy.[55] The rapidity of onset of hypertension may be important in providing a clue to secondary hypertension of various types in which the hypertension may be sudden and severe, in contrast to the usual course in primary hypertension, which is typically mild at onset with gradual progression. Sudden worsening of chronic hypertension should also be sought in the history, because this also may be a clue to secondary hypertension—for example, renal artery atherosclerosis and renovascular hypertension complicating primary hypertension.

The history should include detailed information about prior antihypertensive therapy, including specific agents, response to therapy, side effects from the drugs, and patient compliance. Drugs that may have potential adverse interactions with antihypertensive agents should be recorded. As an example, the hypotensive effect of guanethidine may be nullified by tricyclic antidepressant drugs.

The family history is important because primary hypertension is an inheritable disorder to a degree. In particular, the progeny of two hypertensive patients are very prone to acquire primary hypertension.[56] Although a strong family history of hypertension does not exclude

Table 60A-8 Secondary hypertension: diseases in which high blood pressure may occur

I. Systolic and diastolic hypertension

- Renovascular diseases
  - Atherosclerosis
  - Fibromuscular disease
  - Thrombosis
  - Embolism
  - Dissecting renal artery aneurysms
  - Atherosclerotic renal artery aneurysms
  - Extrinsic renal artery compression (from tumors or cysts)
  - Congenital hypoplasia of the renal artery
  - Neurofibromatosis
  - Transplant rejection fibrosis
  - Arteriovenous fistulas
  - Vasculitis (associated with periarteritis nodosa, systemic lupus erythematosus, scleroderma)
  - Intercapillary glomerular sclerosis (Kimmelstiel-Wilson disease)
- Renal parenchymal diseases
  - Polycystic kidneys
  - Glomerulonephritis
    - Membranoproliferative
    - Acute poststreptococcal
    - Chronic membranous
    - Focal sclerosing
    - Septic embolic
  - Chronic pyelonephritis
  - Renal cortical atrophy due to vesical-ureteral reflux
  - Ureteral obstruction
  - Prostatic obstruction
  - Perirenal hematoma
  - Renal vein thrombosis
  - Tumors (renin-producing juxtaglomerular cell tumor, Wilms' tumor)
  - Unclassified end-stage renal disease
  - Urate nephropathy
  - Analgesic nephropathy
  - Postirradiation nephropathy
  - Congenital hypoplastic kidney
  - Renal trauma
  - Liddle's syndrome
  - Gordon's syndrome
- Endocrine diseases
  - Cushing's syndrome
  - Congenital adrenal hyperplasia (11-hydroxylase deficiency)
  - Hypogonadism and mineralocorticoid excess (17-hydroxylase deficiency)
  - Primary aldosteronism
  - Acromegaly
  - Myxedema
  - Pheochromocytoma
  - Extra-adrenal chromaffin tumors
- Central nervous system diseases (neurogenic hypertension)
  - Psychogenic
  - Increased intracranial pressure
    - Encephalitis
    - Brain tumors
    - Respiratory acidosis
  - Acute poliomyelitis
  - Polyneuritis
  - Spinal cord section
  - Familial dysautonomia
  - Acute porphyria
- Exogenous agents*
  - Estrogen-containing oral contraceptives
  - Sodium
    - Sodium chloride
    - Sodium bicarbonate
    - Sodium-containing medications
  - Lithium
  - Mineralocorticoids
  - Anabolic or adrenogenic steroids
  - Nonsteroidal anti-inflammatory drugs
  - Direct or indirect sympathomimetics (e.g., ephedrine, phenylephrine)
  - Tricyclic antidepressants
  - Monoamine oxidase inhibitors in conjunction with high tyramine ingestion
  - Ergot alkaloids
  - Heavy-metal poisons (e.g., lead, arsenic)
  - Cyclosporine
  - Erythropoietin
  - Street drugs
- Miscellaneous
  - Coarctation of the aorta
  - Toxemia of pregnancy
  - Hypercalcemia
  - Increased intravascular volume (e.g., polycythemia, postoperative state)
  - Burns
  - Carcinoid syndrome
  - Insect stings (e.g., spider, scorpion)
  - Rebound hypertension
    - Sudden withdrawal of clonidine
    - Withdrawal of methyldopa, β-adrenergic receptor blockers, postganglionic sympathetic-blocking drugs

II. Systolic hypertension with wide pulse pressure

- Increased cardiac output or increased stroke volume
  - Arteriovenous fistula
  - Thyrotoxicosis
  - Hyperkinetic heart disease
  - Aortic valve insufficiency
  - Patent ductus arteriosus
  - Paget's disease of bone
  - Severe anemia
  - Beriberi
- Decreased compliance of aorta
  - Arteriosclerosis

*Data from Messerli FH, Frohlich ED: High blood pressure: a side effect of drugs, poisons, and food. *Arch Intern Med* 139:682-687, 1979.

secondary hypertension, it often appropriately lessens the extent to which the clinician chooses to investigate for possible secondary hypertension. Some secondary forms of hypertension have major hereditary manifestations, and the family history may be important in providing a clue to such conditions as pheochromocytoma, neurofibromatosis, hereditary renal parenchymal diseases, or multiple endocrine neoplasia type IIA.[57]

The history should include information about other major cardiovascular risk factors, especially cigarette smoking.[58] Hypertension and smoking are a particularly lethal combination. The family history of early cardiovascular death or of diabetes and hyperlipidemia is important in assessing the role of hypertension and possible cardiovascular morbidity in an individual patient.

The history is also important in relation to major target-organ complications from hypertension, particularly hypertensive and atherosclerotic heart disease, hypertensive and atherosclerotic central nervous system disease, and the renal complications of hypertension.

Exogenous agents may be of major importance in the cause of hypertension or in the worsening of primary hypertension[54] (see Table 60A-8). A dietary history of sodium chloride intake in its obvious and hidden forms is pertinent in every hypertensive patient. Other, more subtle forms of large sodium ingestion in the form of sodium bicarbonate or nonabsorbable antacids containing sodium should be elicited by history. Oral contraceptives containing estrogen are perhaps the commonest cause of curable hypertension seen in the United States, and the history of the type used and the duration of use should be obtained. Medications such as mineralocorticoids, lithium, sympathomimetics, ergot alkaloids, cyclosporine, and erythropoietin may cause or worsen hypertension and should be mentioned in the history. Licorice, available in chewing tobacco only in the United States, may produce hypertension as a result of the action of glycyrrhizic acid, and the history is of major importance in making this diagnosis in a patient who presents with clinical features suggesting primary aldosteronism.

Certain features in the history are highly suggestive of specific types of secondary hypertension. Flank pain, hematuria, or a history of renal trauma may be an important clue to renovascular hypertension. A history of proteinuria, pyelitis of pregnancy, renal stones, dysuria, fever, or chills may be a clue to parenchymal renal disease as a cause of hypertension. The initial clue to pheochromocytoma may come from the patient's history of headaches, sweating, palpitations, tachycardia, thoracic and epigastric distress, and weight loss. Hyperthyroidism associated with hypertension may be suspected from heat intolerance and loss of weight, and myxedema associated with hypertension may be suspected from a specific history of cold intolerance. Weakness, paralysis, tetany, paresthesias, and polyuria are historical clues to the presence of primary aldosteronism.

Physical examination

The general appearance of the patient may provide an important clue to certain endocrine conditions in which hypertension occurs; for example, in patients with acromegaly, myxedema, Graves' disease, or Cushing's syndrome, the diagnosis often is suspected at first glance. Closer inspection of a hypertensive patient may reveal neurofibromatosis, and the hypertension in such patients may be of a secondary type due either to pheochromocytoma or to renal artery stenosis caused by arterial dysplasia. Other neuroectodermal dysplasias that have been associated with pheochromocytoma and that also may be detected by inspection are tuberous sclerosis, Sturge-Weber syndrome, and ataxia-telangiectasia. A variant of multiple endocrine neoplasia type IIB has a high association with pheochromocytoma and is manifested by an abnormal phenotype, including orofacial neuromas. Inspection may also detect urochrome pigmentation as a possible sign of renal failure.

Careful examination of the optic fundus may reveal manifestations of retinopathy from increased cranial pressure caused by hypertension. Swelling of the optic disk in papilledema results in elevation and blurring of the disk, retinal hard exudates, venous congestion, and splinter hemorrhages and infarcts. Patients presenting with headache, nausea, vomiting, diplopia, ataxia, or altered consciousness may have increased intracranial pressure due to hypertension.[59]

Cardiac examination of the hypertensive patient is directed most specifically at the detection of hypertensive heart disease. In hypertensive patients, the cardiac rhythm is usually a regular sinus rhythm, although atrial fibrillation may occur in hypertensive heart disease, particularly when there is enlargement of the left atrium. Palpation of the precordium, which is optimally performed with the patient in the left lateral decubitus position, may reveal a sustained and perhaps (though not necessarily) broadened apical impulse as a result of left ventricular hypertrophy. Displacement of the point of maximum impulse to the left, in the absence of other cardiac disease, implies cardiac dilatation and is a relatively late finding in hypertensive heart disease. Auscultatory abnormalities of the heart sounds in hypertensive heart disease include paradoxic splitting of S_2, which is uncommon, however. The aortic component of S_2 is often accentuated and has a tambour quality. A fourth heart sound (S_4) occurs very commonly in hypertensive patients. The presence of S_3 usually indicates a failing left ventricle, a sign of an advanced stage of hypertensive heart disease. A grade 1/6 or 2/6 ejection murmur audible at the apex and base and heard in early or mid systole occurs frequently in the hypertensive patient. A well-documented, although uncommon, decrescendo diastolic murmur of aortic regurgitation has also been observed. This murmur is often transmitted to the right and left sternal borders and is due to dilatation of the aortic root and not to intrinsic aortic valve disease. The aortic regurgitation is usually very mild, and the murmur may vary in intensity from one examination to the next. The aortic regurgitation is rarely severe enough to alter the characteristics of the carotid artery pulses. When cardiac decompensation complicates hypertensive heart disease, the jugular venous pressure will be elevated, usually with the appearance of characteristic "a" and v waves.

The peripheral arterial pulses should be carefully palpated in all hypertensive patients. Reduction of pulses in one or both arms or legs can be a clue to aortic dissection complicating hypertension. Additionally, reduction of the pulse in one arm accompanied by a significantly lower blood pressure may be due to subclavian artery stenosis, and in such a patient blood pressure determinations from the involved arm would provide inaccurate information about the true state of the hypertension. Coarctation of the aorta will produce absent or markedly diminished femoral pulses when the coarctation is severe, but when it is mild it may result in only mild reduction of the femoral pulses. In such instances, the examiner should carefully time the appearance of the femoral pulse with the radial or brachial pulse to determine whether they are simultaneous, as in the normal person, or there is a substantial delay in the femoral pulse, as is seen in coarctation of the aorta.

The presence of arterial bruits should be sought by careful auscultation over the carotid and subclavian arteries, from the posterior thorax, throughout the abdomen, and over the femoral arteries. Coarctation of the aorta may result in pronounced collateral circulation with bruits heard widely, including in many areas in the posterior thorax. Systolic bruits in the upper quadrants of the abdomen may be important clues to renal artery stenosis. If the bruit extends into diastole (by definition a continuous bruit), the stenosis of the artery giving rise to the bruit is of severe degree. Another condition that can produce a continuous bruit is a renal arteriovenous malformation, with which there may be associated renovascular hypertension. Bruits over the carotid, subclavian, and femoral arteries may be an indication of a dissecting aortic hematoma complicating hypertension or may be clues to atherosclerosis of the involved arteries, in the cause of which hypertension may be a major factor.

Examination of the abdomen, in addition to the search for bruits, should include palpation for renal masses, as can occur in patients with polycystic kidneys. The examination should also carefully assess the width and intrinsic pulsation of the abdominal aorta in a search for an abdominal aortic aneurysm.

Examination of the skin of the legs of hypertensive patients may reveal current or previous hypertensive ischemic ulcers.

Laboratory tests

The Joint National Committee on Detection, Evaluation, and Treatment of High Blood Pressure made the following recommendations in 1993: A few laboratory tests should be performed routinely before therapy is begun. These include urinalysis; complete blood cell count; blood glucose (fasting, if possible), potassium, calcium, creatinine, uric acid, cholesterol (total and high-density lipoprotein), and triglyceride levels (an automated blood chemistry system is usually less expensive); and electrocardiography. Some of these tests are needed for determining the severity of cardiovascular disease and possible causes of hypertension. Others are related to cardiovascular risk factors or provide baseline values for judging biochemical effects of therapy. Other tests—such as urinary microalbumin determination, assessment of cardiac anatomy and function by echocardiography, and determination of plasma renin and urinary sodium—are additional measures occasionally useful in assessing cardiovascular status in selected cases.[8]

Some of the recommended laboratory tests provide clues to secondary hypertension (urinalysis, chest radiograph, potassium, creatinine, hematocrit, calcium, thyroid function, plasma renin activity, catecholamines, excretory urogram); some assess target-organ manifestations of hypertension (ECG, chest radiograph, creatinine); some look for other atherosclerotic risk factors or correlates of the course of hypertensive disease (cholesterol, blood glucose, plasma renin activity); and some are necessary for pretreatment baseline information in cases in which antihypertensive medications, notably diuretics, are likely to alter the test values (potassium, sugar, uric acid, creatinine, calcium).

Urinalysis. The urinalysis is of value as a possible clue to renal and renovascular hypertension. Renal parenchymal disease as a cause for hypertension can usually be ruled out by a normal urinalysis. The absence of significant proteinuria ordinarily excludes renal parenchymal hypertension. However, proteinuria is present in nearly half of all untreated hypertensive patients, and so it is of no special diagnostic significance unless protein is present in amounts exceeding grade 1.

In addition to the examination for protein, the specimen should be analyzed for specific gravity or osmolality to assess the concentrating ability of the kidney. Impairment of the concentrating ability occurs in chronic renal failure and, less commonly, in patients with hypokalemia or hypercalcemia.

The urine should also be examined for cells, bacteria, and formed elements. Blood casts or red blood cell casts are indicators of active glomerular disease. Microscopic hematuria may be a clue to glomerulonephritis and to renovascular disease or polycystic kidney disease.

Other urine examinations. Urine cultures should be obtained in patients who have a history suggestive of urinary tract infection. Asymptomatic bacilluria occurs with increased frequency in patients with hypertension of any cause and is important as a possible complication of polycystic disease or pyelonephritis. Urine cultures should be obtained by clean-catch midstream techniques. Occasionally, this will not yield satisfactory specimens or will be impossible; in such circumstances, urine may have to be obtained for culture by suprapubic aspiration. Catheterization of the patient to obtain urine for cultures should be avoided.

Twenty-four-hour urine collections may be analyzed for products of catecholamine metabolism (see under "Pheochromocytoma" later in this chapter). Additionally, quantitation of the potassium in a 24-hour specimen may be helpful in differentiating renal from nonrenal loss of potassium in the evaluation of hypokalemia, because patients with primary aldosteronism usually excrete more than 30 mEq of potassium per day. The 24-hour creatinine level may be obtained as needed for calculation of creatinine clearance. Quantitation of urinary sodium excretion is useful in two circumstances: (1) as a baseline estimate of dietary intake in preparing a management program for the patient or in looking for excess sodium as an etiologic agent in hypertension, and (2) as necessary information to correlate with plasma renin activity if such a test is to be done, since accurate interpretation of plasma renin activity requires correlation with the state of sodium balance.

Blood chemistry studies

POTASSIUM CONCENTRATION. The serum potassium determination is a valuable baseline for subsequent diuretic antihypertensive therapy. Additionally, the serum potassium concentration is important because hypokalemia may be the first clue to the presence of primary aldosteronism as a cause of hypertension.[60] The serum potassium level is usually, but not always, reduced to less than 3.5 mEq/L in primary aldosteronism. Hypokalemia in patients taking diuretics is difficult to interpret. If the hypertension is not severe, withdrawal of the diuretic for 1 month should return the serum potassium level to normal in most forms of hypertension, but the potassium level will usually remain significantly reduced with primary aldosteronism. Hypokalemia may also be a clue to licorice gluttony and should prompt questions concerning licorice intake when hypokalemia is observed in a patient with hypertension.

CREATININE CONCENTRATION. The serum creatinine level is a good index of the level of renal function. It is assumed that serum creatinine is released from muscle stores in a constant rate in steady-state conditions and is cleared by the kidney at a rate approximately that of inulin clearance; thus, the serum creatinine level provides a practical estimate of the GFR for a patient who is in a steady state.[61] The creatinine level may provide a clue to acute or chronic renal insufficiency in the hypertensive patient and serve as a baseline before the initiation of antihypertensive drug therapy. When more precise information about the GFR is required, a 24-hour creatinine clearance can be done.

CHOLESTEROL LEVEL. A combination of hypertension and hyperlipidemia increases the risk of atherosclerosis.[58] For this reason, the hypertensive patient should be screened for lipid disorders. In addition to the cholesterol determinations recommended by the Joint National Committee on Detection, Evaluation, and Treatment of High Blood Pressure, many physicians would also elect to determine the serum triglycerides and high-density lipoprotein cholesterol, particularly in persons younger than age 60 years. Therapy should be directed toward all atherosclerotic risk factors simultaneously in the hypertensive patient.

Electrocardiogram. The main reason for including the ECG among the minimal laboratory tests in the hypertensive workup is that it provides easily obtainable information about the presence of left ventricular hypertrophy, which is an excellent indicator of hypertensive heart disease. Left ventricular hypertrophy may serve as an independent predictor of the course of patients with untreated hypertension.[24] Of course, additional information pertinent to possible coexisting coronary heart disease, other cardiac disorders, and coexisting cardiac arrhythmias will be provided by the ECG.

Echocardiogram. Advances in echocardiography have enabled physicians to better evaluate whether and to what extent left ventricular hypertrophy and diastolic dysfunction are present in patients with hypertension. In addition, limited echocardiography, a procedure designed to evaluate only left ventricular wall thickness and mass, is being investigated as a method to perform routine cost-effective evaluation of left ventricular hypertrophy.[62]

Chest radiograph. Cardiac enlargement as a manifestation of hypertensive heart disease is an independent predictor of the course of untreated hypertension.[24] However, this change occurs relatively late in the course of primary hypertension. In addition to providing pertinent information about hypertensive heart disease, the chest radiograph may also reveal atherosclerotic aneurysmal disease of the thoracic aorta or provide a clue to dissecting aneurysms, which commonly involve the thoracic aorta. Hypertension is the major predisposing condition in the cause of dissecting aneurysms of the aorta. Notching of the ribs or abnormalities of the thoracic aorta in the region of the arch and descending thoracic aorta may be the initial clue to coarctation of the aorta as a cause of hypertension and should be searched for routinely when the chest radiograph from a hypertensive patient is examined.

Other laboratory tests. In young hypertensive patients or severely hypertensive patients of any age, a more thorough investigation than that so far described is warranted, particularly in a search for potentially curable forms of hypertension.

Plasma renin activity was once thought to be related to complications in hypertensive patients. Specifically, low levels of plasma renin activity were reported to be associated with a benign course.[63] Subsequent studies, including a 5-year prospective study, failed to show a correlation between low plasma renin activity and absence of myocardial infarction and stroke.[64,65] Renin levels have also been used to predict the response to various antihypertensive drugs but are not generally considered necessary before the initiation of drug therapy. The state of sodium balance must be taken into consideration in interpreting renin levels. Plasma renin activity decreases as patients become older, probably as a result of generalized nephrosclerotic changes and destruction of the juxtaglomerular tissue.

MAJOR DISEASE ENTITIES ASSOCIATED WITH SECONDARY HYPERTENSION

Renovascular disease

Renovascular disease is of major importance as the most frequently encountered form of secondary hypertension that is reversible by surgery[66] or, more recently, by percutaneous transluminal angioplasty.[67] Stenosis of the renal artery is most commonly produced by atherosclerosis. This process usually involves the orifice or the proximal 1 to 2 cm of the main renal artery. A functional abnormality as well as an anatomic abnormality should be demonstrated to document a diagnosis of renovascular hypertension in patients with renal artery stenosis.[68] Atherosclerosis of the renal artery has been observed many times in persons who are normotensive and in patients with preexisting primary hypertension.[68,69] Nevertheless, the incidence of hypertension is much greater in persons with atherosclerosis of the renal arteries than in those with normal renal arteries. Atherosclerosis of the renal artery often coexists with atherosclerosis in other major arterial systems, notably the aorta, the peripheral arteries to the lower extremities, and the coronary and cerebral circulations.

Fibromuscular dysplasia is the second most common cause of renal artery stenosis. Although other arterial systems, notably the carotid and iliac arteries, are involved with fibromuscular dysplasia, the disorder rarely produces clinically significant disease except for renovascular hypertension. Thus, fibromuscular dysplasia as a cause of renovascular hypertension should be sought, particularly in young hypertensive females.

Less frequent causes of renal artery obstruction are thrombosis, embolism, dissecting hematoma extending from the aorta, localized dissecting renal artery aneurysms, congenital hypoplasia of the renal artery, neurofibromatosis, transplant rejection fibrosis, arteritis, atherosclerotic aneurysms, and extrinsic pressure from renal cysts or perihilar tumors.[70-73] Renal ischemia in hypertension may also result from congenital or acquired arteriovenous fistulas or congenital malformation.[74] Rarely, renal artery stenosis with demonstrable abnormalities of renal function may be a transient phenomenon.[75]

A reduction of the renal arterial lumen by 60% of its diameter or 84% of its cross-sectional area has been demonstrated as necessary before a significant decrease in pressure occurs distal to renal artery stenosis.[76]

It is theorized that the lower blood pressure distal to a renal artery stenosis stimulates the production of renin. This proteolytic enzyme is secreted almost exclusively by the kidneys. Synthesis of renin occurs at the vascular pole of the glomerulus, in the macula densa, or in the granules of the juxtaglomerular apparatus or the afferent arteriole. Renin acts on a substrate protein in plasma to release angiotensin I, which is converted to angiotensin II, a potent pressor agent that is also the major stimulus to biosynthesis and secretion of aldosterone by the zona glomerulosa of the adrenal cortex. Aldosterone enhances the reabsorption of sodium by the renal tubule and thus serves to increase the effective blood volume. Thus, there are two basic mechanisms of importance in the initiation and maintenance of hypertension due to renal artery stenosis: the renin-angiotensin pressor effect and the increase in effective blood volume as a result of aldosterone.[77] Release of renin and the generation of angiotensin II are inversely related to the state of sodium balance. During sodium depletion, plasma renin and angiotensin II levels are high; conversely, during sodium loading, renin secretion is suppressed.

Most patients with renovascular hypertension have few characteristics in their history or abnormalities on physical examination which point specifically to renovascular hypertension. Nevertheless, clues that may be present that should intensify the search for a renovascular cause of hypertension include the development of hypertension before the age of 30 years, sudden onset of severe hypertension, abrupt worsening of an established hypertension, and hematuria or flank pain suggesting renal infarction. Bruits heard in the upper quadrants of the abdomen, to the right or left of the abdominal aorta, are the most frequently encountered signs suggesting renal artery stenosis, but they are observed in only about 50% of such patients. The bruits are usually systolic and of medium pitch. High-pitched continuous bruits or those that extend throughout systole and into diastole are less often present in patients with renovascular hypertension but are more suggestive of severe renal artery stenosis, particularly from fibromuscular dysplasia. Other stenotic arteries in the abdomen may, of course, produce bruits, the abdominal aorta also being a frequent source. Aortic bruits tend to be lower in pitch and to be localized over the abdominal aorta with transmission toward the iliac arteries.

Excretory urography. Excretory urography is a widely available radiographic procedure that aids in the diagnosis of renovascular hypertension. In addition, the excretory urogram is helpful in the diagnosis of chronic renal disease, pyelonephritis, polycystic kidneys, renal tumors, renal stones, urinary tract obstruction, and adrenal masses, all of which may be related to hypertension. Multiple films made during the first 5 minutes after the injection of contrast medium improve the diagnostic value of the test for renovascular disease. The rapid-sequence excretory urogram reveals abnormalities in more than 80% of patients with renovascular hypertension due to unilateral main renal artery stenosis.[78] Abnormal findings on excretory urograms are evident much less commonly when there is bilateral renal artery disease[79] or when stenosis involves only secondary branches of the renal arteries. The kidneys should be compared with regard to their overall size and contour. A difference in length of 1.5 cm or more is suggestive of renovascular disease, as is the impression of an overall reduction of renal mass of one kidney. However, anatomic variations and rotation of the kidney must be considered in evaluating the comparative renal masses. Decreasing size of one kidney demonstrated on serial examinations suggests renovascular disease. The contour of the kidney may be grossly abnormal in renovascular disease when there has been infarction or severe ischemia of one segment of the kidney. A contracted renal pelvis and caliceal system demonstrated on the excretory urogram suggests a reduced rate of urine formation. If this finding occurs in only one kidney, it is highly suggestive of renal artery stenosis.

Another infrequently encountered abnormality detectable on excretory urography is notching of the ureter as a result of indentation by greatly enlarged ureteral collateral arteries; this usually occurs in young patients with fibromuscular renal artery stenosis. With major renal artery occlusion, the appearance of contrast medium may be delayed in the affected kidney. This is most likely to be observed in the films taken 2 or 3 minutes after injection of the contrast agent. In a cooperative study of roentgenographic aspects of renovascular hypertension, delayed appearance time was the single most frequently noted abnormality in unilateral renovascular disease, having been present in 59% of patients with significant stenosis.[78] Similarly, in a study of bilateral disease, delayed appearance time was the single most commonly noted abnormality, observed in 43.3% of cases.[79] In films taken 20 minutes or more after injection, there may be a greater density of contrast medium on the ischemic side owing to more rapid excretion of the opaque medium by the nonischemic kidney.

The hypertensive urogram (a rapid-sequence excretory urogram in which films are taken on multiple occasions within the first 5 minutes after intravenous administration of contrast material and also at intervals for up to 20 minutes) as a screening test for renovascular hypertension has come under criticism because of its low sensitivity and specificity. In one study of hypertensive patients being screened, the incidence of positive rapid-sequence excretory urograms was 0.8%, and the true positive rate for prediction of cure or improvement of hypertension from surgical treatment of renal artery stenosis was 60.2%.[80]

Radioisotope renography and renal imaging. Because of recent advances in percutaneous transluminal renal angioplasty and surgical revascularization, radioisotope renography has received increasing interest as a means to detect renovascular hypertension. Typically, *o*-[^{131}I] iodohippurate (OIH) is used as the radionuclide to make qualitative measurements of kidney function. However, technetium kidney scans are gradually replacing OIH because of their higher sensitivity and specificity. Normal results from renography show three phases: (1) a rapid increase in activity corresponding to the arrival of the nuclide in the tissue, (2) a slower increase lasting 2 to 5 minutes until peak radioactivity, indicating relative renal blood flow, and (3) rapid excretion of the radionuclide from the kidney.[81]

The radioisotope renogram is characteristically abnormal for the affected kidney in patients with significant unilateral renal artery stenosis.[82] The slope of the second segment of the renogram may be less steep than normal, with a delay in time of peak radioactivity and a delay in the excretory segment. The abnormalities vary with the severity of the stenosis and with renal function. Alterations of excretion from the kidneys, such as those produced by ureteral obstruction, also alter the excretory segment of the renogram. Significant bilateral renal artery stenosis and segmental renal artery stenosis produce changes in the radioisotope renogram which are less characteristic than those just described, and the tests are more difficult to interpret than those obtained from patients with unilateral renal artery stenosis.

The renal images show the size, shape, and location of the kidneys, and they will identify renal neoplasms, cysts, and abscesses. Information is also obtained about the relative quality of renal perfusion and renal secretory function. Congenital abnormalities such as horseshoe kidneys, pelvic kidney, and fetal lobulation are readily identified. In patients with renovascular disease, areas of hypoperfusion and infarction can be identified.[83] Radioisotope renography is particularly useful in certain situations. These include testing patients who are sensitive to radiographic contrast media and also obtaining objective data by which to follow the course of patients with renal and renovascular disease.

The value of radioisotope renography after administration of the angiotensin-converting enzyme inhibitor captopril is increasingly recognized, and the results are promising for identifying patients with renovascular stenosis. The report of the Consensus Conference on Captopril Renography, published in 1991,[84] includes standardized grading criteria for response to captopril renography, recommendations for which radionuclide preparation should be used, and information on who should undergo captopril renography. Most studies have reported sensitivities from 80% to 95% and specificities from 50% to 94%. Captopril renography has the advantage over the captopril test, discussed below, of not necessitating discontinuation of antihypertensive medications, except for angiotensin-converting enzyme inhibitors, to attain higher sensitivity.

The rationale for the captopril-stimulation radionuclide studies is that captopril removes the angiotensin-II-dependent, efferent arteriolar resistance that results in a reduction of the transcapillary forces during glomerular filtration and, thereby, reduces renal function of the kidney distal to the stenosis.[85] Studies published so far of a selected group of patients with unilateral renal artery stenosis showed that the sensitivity and specificity of radionuclide renography was greater after captopril administration than before. Additional randomized prospective studies are needed before this diagnostic study can be widely recommended.

Plasma renin activity. Measurement of plasma renin activity is another test used in the diagnosis of renovascular hypertension. In this procedure, renal vein renin activity is used to assess the contribution of each kidney to renovascular hypertension. The renin activity from the involved kidney in unilateral renovascular hypertension is almost always more than 1.5 times greater than that from the uninvolved kidney. In bilateral renal artery stenosis, a ratio of more than 1.5:1 (more affected kidney to less affected kidney) is usually found, particularly under circumstances of sodium depletion and diuretic administration. Plasma renin activity has a low specificity, however, and its primary use is in the exclusion of renovascular disease based on low plasma renin values and normal plasma creatinine.[81]

Preparation of patients with suspected renal artery stenosis for the stimulation of renal vein renins can be achieved either by extreme salt restriction or volume depletion by the use of furosemide. The captopril test, which measures plasma renin activity after administration of the angiotensin-converting enzyme inhibitor captopril, has been shown to have high specificity and sensitivity, especially in patients whose serum creatinine level is less than 1.5 mg/dL or who have been withdrawn from medication. The captopril test is even more effective because of its relatively low cost and safety.[81] Administration of captopril 30 minutes before renal vein renin sampling can also enhance lateralization of renal vein renins. Peripheral plasma renin stimulation by captopril, a promising technique with increased sensitivity and specificity for detecting renovascular hypertension, has been extensively reviewed.[85,86] This test provides a simple, less costly, and useful approach for identifying patients with renovascular disease in a general population of patients with uncomplicated hypertension.

Duplex ultrasound. Duplex ultrasound of the renal arteries has been applied to the diagnosis of renal artery stenosis with some success. Various criteria developed for diagnosis have given sensitivities ranging from 31% to 91% and specificities from 88% to 100%.[87] Problems that remain unsolved with this technique are the frequency with which multiple renal arteries are not identified and the number of patients, currently about 15%, in whom studies are technically unsatisfactory, particularly in the lack of diagnostic information from the left renal artery.[88] When satisfactory data have been successfully obtained, the technique has been useful in natural history studies of renal artery stenosis and in assessing the results of angioplasty and renal artery bypass surgery.[89]

Renal arteriography. Renal arteriography can be used to determine the presence of atherosclerotic lesions along the renal artery, but it has the inherent risks of an invasive procedure, such as arteriotomy, dye injection, and catheter manipulation. Although advances have been made in digital subtraction technology that reduce the amount of dye necessary for the procedure, the possibility of mistakenly treating hemodynamically irrelevant stenoses on the basis of anatomic appearance recommends the use of noninvasive tests, such as those mentioned above. In addition, advances have been made in magnetic resonance imaging of the renal arteries. This technique has many of the same failings as invasive arteriography, such as inability to discern the physiologic significance of the stenoses. Finally, the high cost of magnetic resonance imaging procedures virtually precludes routine use, especially since less expensive noninvasive tests with comparable accuracy are available.[81]

Renal parenchymal disease

Chronic renal failure is a common cause of secondary hypertension. It complicates the course of disease in many diverse renal parenchymal diseases (see Table 60A-8). Hypertension appears more frequently, is more severe, and appears earlier in the course of the disease in some renal parenchymal disorders, with less overall impairment of renal function. Notable in this category are several types of the acute nephritic syndrome, especially membranoglomerulonephritis, which has an incidence of associated hypertension of 25%,[90] and acute postinfectious glomerulonephritis, with an incidence of hypertension of 81%.[91] Polycystic kidney disease also is complicated by hypertension in more than 70% of patients, usually appears in the fourth or fifth decade, and occurs with relatively good renal function and occasionally even with normal renal function.[92]

Membranoproliferative glomerulonephritis occurs in two forms and is a distinct histopathologic entity characterized by mesangial cell proliferation with interposition of mesangial cell cytoplasm between the endothelium and the basement membrane.[93] Type 1 is distinguished by the presence of deposits in the subendothelial area of the capillary wall. Type 2 has an electron-dense transformation of the glomerular and tubular basement membranes and is often termed "dense deposit disease."[94] Serum complement abnormalities occur in both types.[95] Hematuria, acute nephritis with edema and hypertension, severe proteinuria with nephrotic syndrome, and rapidly progressive glomerulonephritis have all been documented. Acute postinfectious glomerulonephritis usually occurs 10 to 14 days after an infection with β-hemolytic streptococci in the pharynx or occasionally in the skin. The presentation is often with hypertension, edema, and smoky-appearing urine. Renal biopsy, although rarely indicated clinically during the acute phase, reveals the diffuse glomerulonephritis in which all glomeruli are similarly affected.[96] Proliferation of endothelial and mesangial cells characterizes the inflammatory lesion.

Polycystic kidneys occur in an infantile and an adult form.[97] In this disorder, normal renal tissue is gradually encroached upon by multiple cysts of the renal parenchyma. Although the condition is bilateral, one kidney may be involved to a greater extent than the other. The adult familial type of disease is inherited as an autosomal dominant trait with virtually complete penetrance. Both kidneys are usually palpable; however, occasionally only one can be felt. Excretory urography displays diagnostic abnormalities consisting of enlarged kidneys, elongation of the renal pelvis, flattening of the calyces, and indentations due to the cysts. Additionally, ultrasonography and computed tomography will accurately identify the cystic abnormalities within the renal parenchyma. The patients will often experience abdominal distress, which may be severe and colicky, particularly if associated with hematuria and the passage of clots. Occasionally, the hematuria may be severe. Superimposed pyelonephritis and renal calculi may complicate the course of polycystic kidney disease.

In most of the other renal parenchymal diseases, hypertension develops when renal insufficiency is moderately severe.[98] Usually, the serum creatinine level is in the range of 4 to 5 mg/dL or the blood urea value exceeds 100 mg/dL, but there are wide variations among patients.

Renin-producing tumors have been identified as very rare causes of hypertension. These tumors are usually juxtaglomerular cell tumors[99] or Wilms' tumors.[100] Additionally, undifferentiated lung carcinoma has been identified as a renin-producing tumor.[101] In patients with renin-producing juxtaglomerular cell tumors, the typical presentation is for a young severely hypertensive patient to have secondary aldosteronism and elevated renin levels. Renal vein renin studies lateralize the high renin activity to one kidney. Arteriography may not accurately identify the tumor because it may be very small.

Hypertension complicating ureteral or prostatic obstruction may be ameliorated by relief of the obstruction and thus is an important, although infrequent, type of secondary renal hypertension. Excretory urography is diagnostic.

Endocrine diseases

Primary aldosteronism. Hypersecretion of aldosterone in the absence of a stimulus defines primary aldosteronism. A unilateral adrenal adenoma is the usual cause (80% to 85%).[60] Primary aldosteronism occurs more commonly in women than in men, in a ratio of approximately 2:1. It usually develops in persons between the ages of 30 and 50 years. Second in frequency to unilateral adrenal adenomas as a cause of primary aldosteronism is adenomatous hyperplasia with multiple small bilateral adrenal adenomas. The distinction between hyperplasia and adenoma is important, because the hypertension associated with hyperplasia is less frequently cured by surgery. A third cause of primary aldosteronism is adrenocortical carcinoma, which accounts for fewer than 5% of all cases of primary aldosteronism.[102]

Unprovoked hypokalemia in a hypertensive patient is the usual first clue to the presence of primary aldosteronism. Only when the process is well established do symptoms occur that are attributable to potassium depletion, which may include polyuria, weakness, fatigue, and muscle cramps. In addition to the hypokalemia, other laboratory findings include possible hypernatremia, metabolic alkalosis, impaired urine-concentrating ability, and ECG abnormalities, including prominent U waves. The algorithm for screening and diagnostic confirmation of primary aldosteronism is presented in Figure 60A-1. Some medications may interfere with the diagnostic tests for primary aldosteronism, and administration should be discontinued before diagnostic procedures. The course of treatment depends on whether the cause is unilateral adrenal adenoma or bilateral hyperplasia. This information is usually obtained through computed tomography scanning or magnetic resonance imaging. An algorithm for this diagnostic differentiation is in Figure 60A-2.[103]

The definitive test for primary aldosteronism is the documentation of inadequate suppression of aldosterone secretion by volume expansion.[60] Volume expansion can be induced by a 2- to 3-day diet containing 200 to 300 mEq/day of sodium. Normally, the aldosterone excretion rate should be less than 20 μg in 24 hours after 3 days of such a diet. Alternative methods of volume expansion include intravenous administration of saline or a high-salt intake supplemented by 0.2 mg of fludrocortisone daily for 3 days.

Inappropriate suppression of plasma renin activity occurs in primary aldosteronism. Plasma renin activity is sampled after the patient has been upright for 4 hours and either has received furosemide, 80 mg twice a day on the day preceding the test and 40 mg on the morning of the

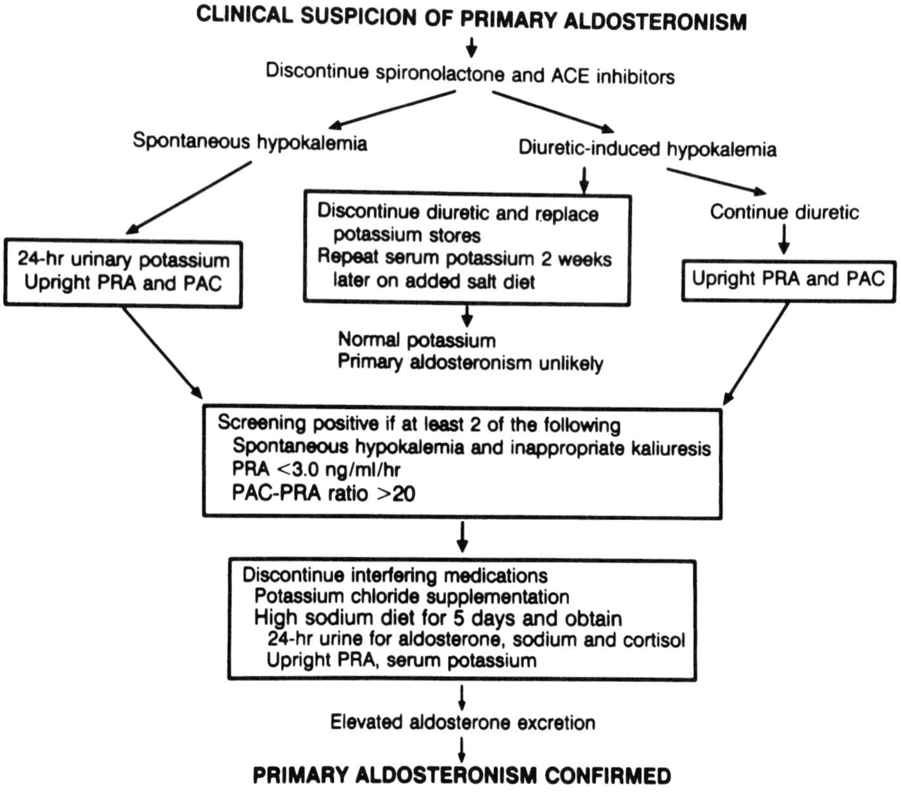

Fig 60A-1 Algorithm for screening and diagnostic confirmation of primary aldosteronism. *ACE,* angiotensin-converting enzyme; *PAC,* plasma aldosterone concentration; *PRA,* plasma renin activity. (From Young WF Jr, Hogan MJ, Klee GG, et al: Primary aldosteronism: diagnosis and treatment. *Mayo Clin Proc* 65:96-110, 1990. By permission, Mayo Foundation for Medical Education and Research.)

test, or has been receiving a low-sodium diet containing 20 mEq of sodium and 90 mEq of potassium for 3 days before the test, supplemented by 50 mg of hydrochlorothiazide daily for 3 days.

Cushing's syndrome. Hypertension is a prominent feature in Cushing's syndrome and is due to the mineralocorticoid effects of the hyperfunctioning adrenal tissue. An additional mechanism of hypertension may be related to an increase in renin substrate production, resulting in increased angiotensin II levels. Other manifestations of Cushing's syndrome are prominent and are due to glucocorticoid excess. These include hyperglycemia, diabetes mellitus, central fat distribution, decreased muscle mass, myopathy, easy bruisability of the skin with thin skin and striae, osteopenia with decreased bone matrix formation, and impaired calcium absorption. Adrenal androgen excess may also occur in Cushing's syndrome and produce hirsutism, oligomenorrhea, deepening of the voice, and balding.

Cushing's syndrome is most often iatrogenic. When excess exogenous steroid administration is excluded, Cushing's syndrome is usually due to bilateral adrenal hyperplasia resulting from increased adrenocorticotropic hormone (ACTH). The increased ACTH may be from the pituitary or, less commonly, from nonendocrine tumors, notably those in the lung. Less often, Cushing's syndrome is caused by primary adrenal tumors, either adenoma or carcinoma.[104]

Screening tests for Cushing's syndrome include the measurement of 24-hour urinary excretion of cortisol and the dexamethasone suppression test.[105] In the latter, 1 mg of dexamethasone is administered at bedtime, and serum cortisol is measured the next day between 7 a.m. and 10 a.m. In normal subjects, plasma cortisol levels under these circumstances should be less than 5 ng/dL. In addition, the 2-mg, low-dose dexamethasone suppression test is used in screening for Cushing's syndrome. To determine the cause of Cushing's syndrome, the overnight 8-mg, high-dose dexamethasone suppression test is now used. This may be replaced in the future by an outpatient version of the dexamethasone test or by a corticotropin-releasing hormone stimulation test that can be performed on an outpatient basis. The overnight test is combined with repeated measurements of ACTH by radioimmunoassay. Imaging procedures to localize the cause of Cushing's syndrome should be performed on the basis of the results of these tests[106] (Fig 60A-3).

Rare adrenal causes of hypertension include the congenital steroid biosynthetic defects. These usually produce hypertension in childhood. The 11β-hydroxylase defect is associated with androgen excess; in the 17α-hydroxylase defect, the sex steroids are deficient.

Pheochromocytoma. A pheochromocytoma is a catecholamine-producing tumor derived from chromaffin tissue; approximately 90% of these tumors arise in the adrenal medulla. Of the extra-adrenal pheochromocyto-

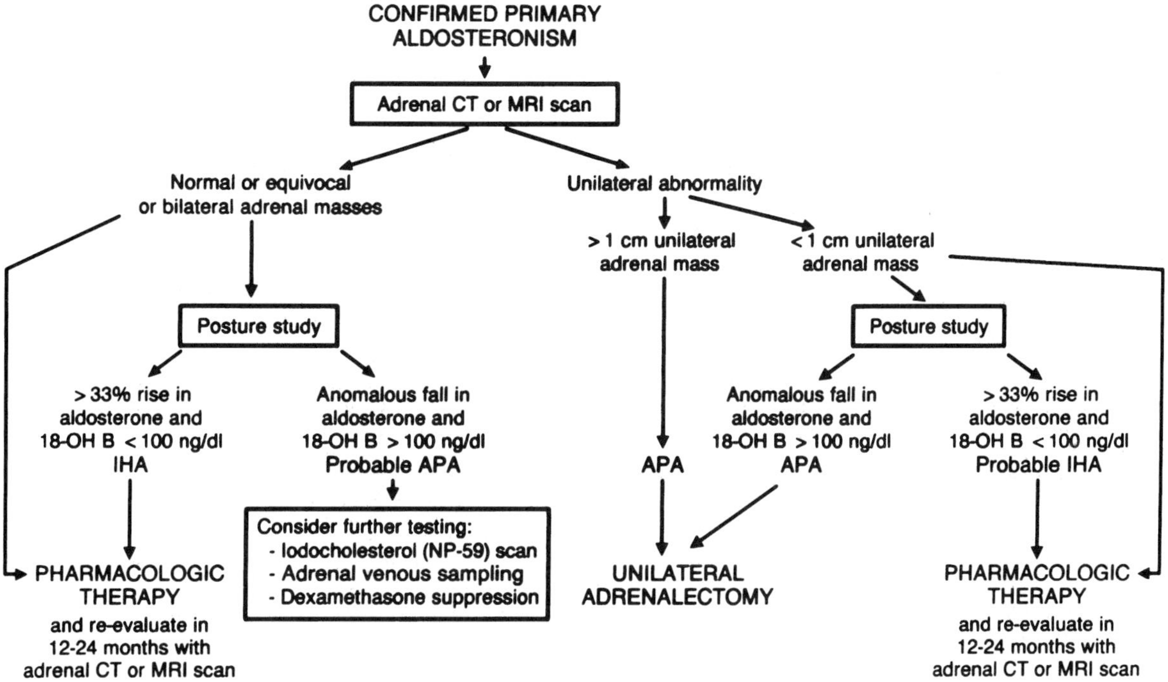

Fig 60A-2 Algorithm for diagnostic differentiation between aldosterone-producing adenoma *(APA)* and bilateral idiopathic hyperaldosteronism *(IHA)*. *CT,* computed tomography; *MRI,* magnetic resonance imaging; 18-OH B, 18-hydroxycorticosterone. (From Young WF Jr, Hogan MJ, Klee GG, et al: Primary aldosteronism: diagnosis and treatment. *Mayo Clin Proc* 65:96-110, 1990. By permission, Mayo Foundation for Medical Education and Research.)

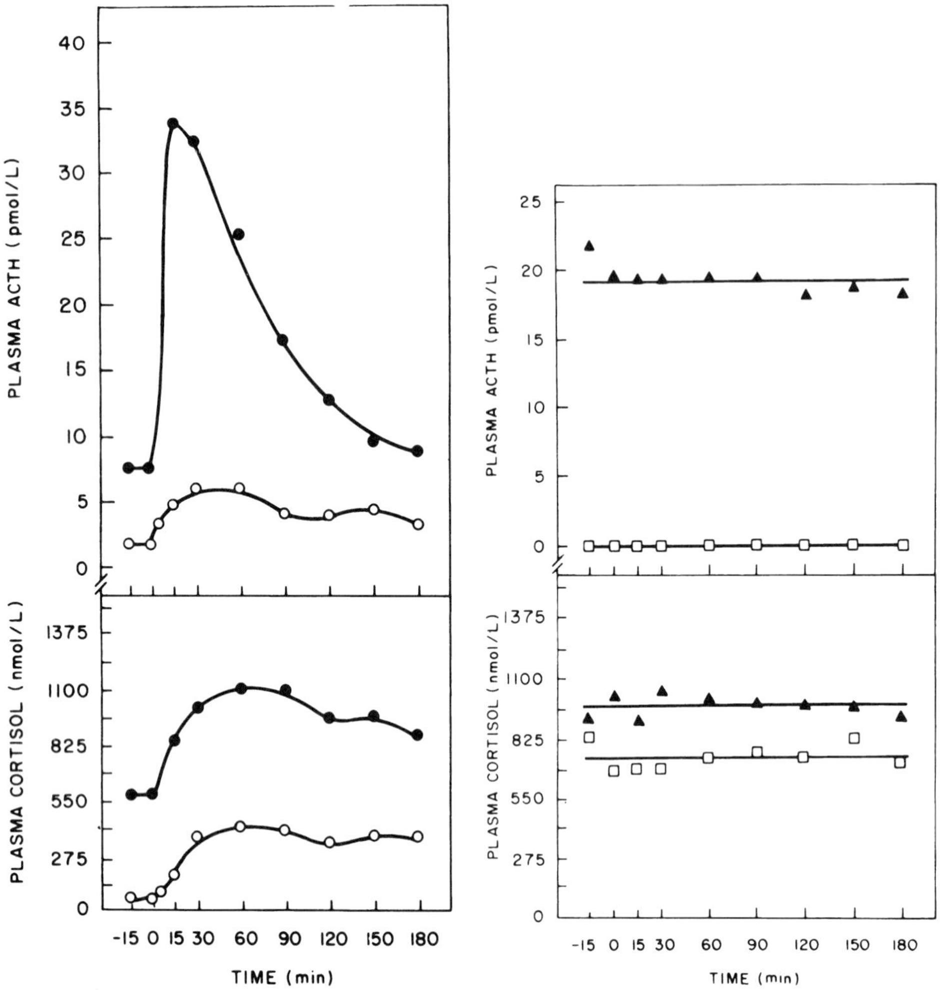

Fig 60A-3 Responses of plasma adrenocorticotropin *(ACTH)* and cortisol to ovine corticotropin-releasing hormone in, **left,** controls *(open circles)* and patients with the pituitary Cushing syndrome *(closed circles)* and, **right,** patients with the ectopic ACTH syndrome *(closed triangles)* and adrenal tumor *(open squares).* (From Chrousos GP, Schulte HM, Oldfield EH, et al: The corticotropin-releasing factor stimulation test: an aid in the evaluation of patients with Cushing's syndrome. *N Engl J Med* 310:622-626, 1984. By permission of the journal and modified from Chrousos GP [Moderator]: NIH conference. Clinical applications of corticotropin-releasing factor. *Ann Intern Med* 102:344-358, 1985.)

mas, most occur within the abdomen, but a small proportion are found in the chest or, even more rarely, in the neck. The tumors are characteristically very vascular, and 10% or fewer are malignant. The malignancy of these tumors cannot be established by histologic study or electron microscopy. The diagnosis of malignancy depends on finding tumor cells characteristic of pheochromocytoma in areas where chromaffin cells do not normally occur. Approximately 10% of pheochromocytomas are multicentric and 5% are bilateral. Bilateral tumors occur particularly in the pluriglandular neoplastic syndrome, which also includes medullary carcinoma of the thyroid and has an autosomal dominant pattern of inheritance. In a flow cytometry study of nuclear DNA ploidy of 75 pheochromocytomas with 10-year follow-up, the tumor remained benign in patients with a normal DNA histogram, whereas 30% to 40% of tetraploid, polyploid, or aneuploid histograms showed evidence of or subsequent development of malignant tumor.[107]

The adrenal medulla shares with the sympathetic nervous system the characteristic of synthesizing catecholamines, the major ones of which are dopamine, norepinephrine, and epinephrine. Important metabolic products of catecholamine metabolism are vanillylmandelic acid, normetanephrines, and metanephrines. Dopamine has a direct inotropic effect on the heart as well as decreasing peripheral resistance and causing mesenteric and renal vasodilatation. Norepinephrine is primarily an α-agonist, causing both arterial and venous vasoconstriction, and the major component of the hypertension occurring in cases of pheochromocytoma is due to the action of this catecholamine. Epinephrine has both α- and β-adrenergic effects; the β-adrenergic effects increase myocardial contractility, increase the heart rate, and produce peripheral vasodilatation.

The spells produced in a patient with pheochromocytoma during paroxysmal release of catecholamines may be spectacular in their clinical presentation. In addition to hypertensive crisis, common major manifestations are headache, sweating, palpitations, and pronounced pallor. Other symptoms that occur with pheochromocytoma spells in 10% to 40% of such patients include nausea, trembling, weakness, nervousness, epigastric pain, chest pain, dyspnea, flushing sensation, numbness or paresthesia, and blurring of vision.[108] Although hypertension may be intermittent in patients with pheochromocytoma, it is more often sustained, occurring in approximately 65% of patients with this condition.

The diagnosis of pheochromocytoma is made by the demonstration of abnormal catecholamine production and metabolism. Twenty-four-hour urinary excretion of metanephrines is a commonly performed screening test for pheochromocytoma; it has a high degree of accuracy and gives very few false-negative results. The test should not be performed within 72 hours after excretory urography, because methylglucamine, which is often present in many iodinated contrast media, may cause metanephrine values to be falsely normal in patients with pheochromocytoma. Another widely employed screening test for pheochromocytoma is the 24-hour urinary excretion of vanillylmandelic acid.[109]

In a patient who is strongly suspected of having pheochromocytoma, either because of the clinical history or because of abnormalities in the 24-hour urinary levels of metanephrine or vanillylmandelic acid, additional tests of urinary catecholamines should be performed. Norepinephrine, epinephrine, and dopamine can be quantitated by high-pressure liquid chromatography. Methyldopa, methenamine mandelate, and labetalol can produce false-negative results for these tests and should not be administered for 48 hours before the test.[110]

Pheochromocytoma and sustained hypertension will usually be detected by the 24-hour urine catecholamine studies described. It is customary to document the abnormalities with several urine samples. A single voided urine metanephrine determination has also been reported to be diagnostic.[111]

When a patient is suspected of having a pheochromocytoma but does not have sustained hypertension, the diagnosis may be established by collecting a urine specimen at the time of the symptomatic episode or by provocative pharmacologic tests with glucagon or histamine. Evaluation of fractionated plasma-free catecholamines by the technique of high-pressure liquid chromatography accurately measures separately unconjugated norepinephrine, epinephrine, and dopamine. When combined with a pharmacologic provocative test with glucagon or histamine, these measurements may be diagnostic in a patient with a paroxysmally secreting pheochromocytoma.

Diagnostic studies to localize a pheochromocytoma preoperatively have progressed rapidly in recent years. Computed tomography and magnetic resonance imaging are the two main procedures used to localize tumors, because of the advantages of noninvasive techniques and high accuracy. Magnetic resonance imaging is particularly useful and surpasses computed tomography scanning in localization of tumors outside the adrenal gland.[110] Computed tomography has largely replaced nephrotomography, angiography, and ultrasonography.[112,113] Computed tomography scanning is less hazardous than angiography and more accurate than the other methods.

If computed tomography scanning fails to identify the location of a pheochromocytoma, a [^{131}I]metaiodobenzylguanidine (MIBG) scan is recommended. The uptake of [^{131}I]MIBG into the adrenergic vesicles helps to localize the catecholamine-producing tissue. The suspected metastatic pheochromocytoma can also be identified with the [^{131}I] MIBG scan; approximately 10% of the results are false-negative and 1% to 2% are false-positive.[114]

Coarctation of the aorta

Coarctation of the aorta is a common congenital cardiovascular defect and is a frequent cause of secondary hypertension in children and infants. Most patients with coarctation of the aorta have the condition diagnosed before they reach adult life, and this condition is infrequently found today as a cause of hypertension in adult hypertensive patients.[6]

The coarctation usually occurs in the area of the ductus arteriosus and represents a localized obstruction, which may vary in severity from very mild to very severe. Less common locations for coarctation of the aorta are in the proximal aortic arch, lower descending aorta, and abdominal aorta. A bicuspid aortic valve is often present in patients with coarctation of the aorta, having occurred in 45% of such patients in one series.[115] In the same series of 100 specimens, there were one or more associated anomalies in 87% exclusive of the bicuspid aortic valve. The associated anomalies were tubular hypoplasia of the aortic arch, ventricular septal defect, patent ductus arteriosus, subaortic stenosis, and transposition of the great vessels. In older children and adults, collateral vessels develop to bypass the coarctation if it is more than a minor narrowing. In the usual type of coarctation, the major collateral vessels are branches of the subclavian arteries—transverse cervical, transverse scapular, and internal mammary arteries. These arteries communicate primarily with intercostal and superficial epigastric arteries.

Coarctation of the aorta results in systolic and diastolic hypertension in the upper body above the level of the coarctation. Although the evidence is conflicting, it appears that the hypertension is partly due to the mechanical obstruction from the coarctation itself and that an additional component is related to abnormalities in the renin-angiotensin system.[116] Rarer cases include coarctation of the thoracic and abdominal aorta and are often associated with renovascular disease.

Physical examination should provide the clue to the diagnosis of coarctation of the aorta in most patients. The femoral pulses may be absent or markedly reduced or, in the case of mild coarctation, be abnormal only in that there is a delay in the pulse compared with the brachial or radial pulse. Thus, it is advisable to palpate the pulses in the upper extremity and the femoral pulse simultaneously. When collateral circulation has developed sufficiently, bruits and prominent pulsations can be detected by auscultation and palpation in the posterior intercostal and periscapular areas. Other auscultatory abnormalities may be present, depending on associated congenital cardiac defects. Ophthalmoscopic examination may provide a clue to coarctation of the aorta in the hypertensive patient by demonstrating markedly tortuous arterioles, an observation made primarily in adult patients with coarctation. The diagnosis of coarctation of the aorta is strongly supported when the blood pressure is found to be elevated in the upper extremities and reduced in the lower extremities. This difference can often be magnified by having the patient exercise and measuring the blood pressure in the upper and lower extremities in the immediate postexercise period. In the normal person, the lower extremity-to-arm systolic blood pressure ratio will remain more than 1.0 after exercise. When there is substantial narrowing of the aorta as in coarctation, the blood pressure in the lower extremity will drop after exercise in contrast to an increase in the arm pressure; this reduces the lower extremity-to-arm ratio to less than 1.0.

Abnormalities on the chest radiograph that may suggest coarctation of the aorta in the usual position include a notch in the left border of the aorta near the arch, producing an appearance suggesting the number "3." Dilated intercostal arteries produce the abnormality of notching of the inferior borders, most often seen in the fourth through the eighth ribs. Additional abnormalities may be related to left ventricular hypertrophy if the hypertension has been severe and long-standing. Computed tomography with contrast medium will accurately delineate coarctation of the aorta, and magnetic resonance imaging and transesophageal echocardiography provide an alternative to arteriography in the diagnosis of aortic coarctation, but arteriography remains the definitive diagnostic study for most patients.

Central nervous system disease

An acute increase in intracranial pressure will produce an increase in systemic blood pressure accompanied by bradycardia. Brain tumors producing increased intracranial pressure, and particularly cerebellar and other posterior fossa tumors, have been etiologically associated with hypertension.[117] The hypertension may be paroxysmal and be associated with increased catecholamines and thus simulate the picture of pheochromocytoma.

Hypertension has been observed in patients with spinal cord section or severe spinal cord injury.[118] This occurs particularly if the level of injury is above T-6. The mechanism is thought to be sympathetic nervous system overactivity, with uncontrolled release of pressor amines due to stimuli from below the level of spinal cord injury.

Hypertension has also been observed in patients with acute idiopathic polyneuritis of the Guillain-Barré type,[119] and it was a frequent finding in acute poliomyelitis when this condition was epidemic.

Toxemia of pregnancy

Preeclampsia, the toxemia of late pregnancy characterized by hypertension, proteinuria, and edema, must be differentiated from primary or essential hypertension occurring coincidentally with pregnancy. Preeclampsia tends to occur suddenly in a young primigravida woman after the 20th week of pregnancy. Primiparous eclamptic women are no more prone than women in the general population to the development of sustained hypertension later in life, but there is a considerable increase in the prevalence of hypertension among multiparous women who have had eclampsia.[120] Attempts to temporize in severe midterm preeclampsia have resulted in often disastrous consequences for the mother and fetus and should be avoided. Usually, the safest course for the mother is interruption of gestation. Various laboratory tests (Table 60A-9) may be useful in diagnosing preeclampsia and differentiating it from essential or secondary hypertension.[121]

Oral contraceptives

Although oral contraceptive use is associated with only a small increase in mean blood pressure, the average increase being 5 to 6 mm Hg systolic and 1 to 2 mm Hg diastolic, the use of these estrogen-containing pills is currently the commonest form of curable hypertension in

Table 60A-9 Laboratory evaluation of women with hypertension that developed after midpregnancy

Test	Rationale
Hemoglobin and hematocrit	Hemoconcentration supports diagnosis of preeclampsia and is an indicator of severity. Values may be decreased, however, if hemolysis accompanies the disease
Blood smear	Signs of microangiopathic hemolytic anemia (e.g., schistocytes) favor diagnosis of preeclampsia and may be present when blood pressure is only mildly elevated
Platelet count	Decreased levels suggest severe preeclampsia
Urinalysis	If qualitative dipstick result is 1+ or greater, a quantitative measurement of protein excretion should be done. Hypertensive gravid women with proteinuria should be considered to have preeclampsia (pure or superimposed) until proved otherwise
Serum creatinine level	Abnormal or rising levels, especially when associated with oliguria, suggest severe preeclampsia
Serum uric acid level	Increased levels aid in the differential diagnosis of preeclampsia and are an indicator of disease severity
Serum oxaloacetic transaminase	Abnormal values suggest severe preeclampsia with hepatic involvement
Lactic acid dehydrogenase	Elevated levels are associated with both hemolysis and hepatic involvement and suggest severe preeclampsia
Serum albumin	Values may be decreased even in the absence of heavy proteinuria and may be related to "capillary leak" or hepatic involvement in preeclampsia

From Lefant C (Chairman): National High Blood Pressure Education Program Working Group Report on High Blood Pressure in Pregnancy. *Am J Obstet Gynecol* 163:1691-1712, 1990. By permission of Mosby–Year Book.

the United States. About 5% of women will acquire hypertension, defined as blood pressure of 140/90 mm Hg or more, within 5 years of starting to take the contraceptive pill. The incidence of hypertension is about three to six times higher in contraceptive pill users compared with nonusers.[122,123] Hypertension associated with estrogen-containing contraceptive pills is more likely to occur in women over 35 years of age and in those with a strong family history of hypertension, and it is slightly more likely to occur in women who are hypertensive during pregnancy.[124] The hypertension induced by contraceptive pills is usually mild, and in about half of the women it subsides in 3 to 6 months after use of the pill has been discontinued. In the other half, the hypertension persists, and in a small number it may be severe. Renal damage has been reported in women taking contraceptives.[125]

Estrogen use in postmenopausal women has been associated with the occurrence of hypertension,[126] but the magnitude of the problem has not been fully documented.

Cyclosporine, erythropoietin, and lithotripsy

Other associated types of hypertension include cyclosporine-associated hypertension (CAH),[127] erythropoietin-associated hypertension (EAH),[128] and hypertension after external shock wave lithotripsy.[129] CAH usually appears as mild to moderate hypertension, but severe hypertension may develop rapidly in some patients. The mechanism of CAH is still largely unknown, but it is a volume-dependent form of hypertension. Possibly the most promising treatment of CAH is with calcium channel blockers. Unlike diuretics, these agents do not deplete blood volume. Depletion can compound cyclosporine's nephrotoxic effects, particularly in renal transplant patients. Calcium antagonists also interact with cyclosporine to increase blood volumes, possibly allowing reduction of the cyclosporine dose.

Erythropoietin, used to increase blood levels in renal failure, is also associated with hypertension. EAH is directly related to the rising blood mass as the target hematocrit is approached and occurs in approximately 25% of patients. EAH can often be controlled by adjusting fluid removal during dialysis, but in some cases antihypertensive therapy is required.

Studies indicate that hypertension may develop after external shockwave lithotripsy, although in some studies the incidence decreased with time after the procedure, suggesting that in some patients blood pressure elevation may be transient. Hypertension may be due to acute vascular injury that is sometimes associated with the procedure. Other trials are investigating this phenomenon.

REFERENCES

1. Bechgaard P: A 40 years' follow-up study of 1000 untreated hypertensive patients. *Clin Sci Molec Med* Suppl 3:673s-675s, 1976

2. Perera GA: Hypertensive vascular disease: description and natural history. *J Chronic Dis* 1:33-42, 1955

3. National Health Survey: Blood pressure of adults by race and area, United States, 1960-1962. Washington, DC, National Center for Health Statistics, United States Department of Health, Education and Welfare, series 11, no 5, 1964

4. Tucker RM, Labarthe DR: Frequency of surgical treatment for hypertension in adults at the Mayo Clinic from 1973 through 1975. *Mayo Clin Proc* 52:549-555, 1977

5. Hypertension Detection and Follow-Up Program Cooperative Group: Five-year findings of the Hypertension Detection and Follow-Up program. I. Reduction in mortality of persons with high blood pressure, including mild hypertension: II. Mortality by race-sex and age. *JAMA* 242:2562-2571; 2572-2577, 1979

6. Gifford RW Jr: Evaluation of the hypertensive patient with emphasis on detecting curable causes. *Millbank Mem Fund Q* 47 pt 2, no 3:170-186, 1969

7. Ferguson RK: Cost and yield of the hypertensive evaluation: experience of a community-based referral clinic. *Ann Intern Med* 82:761-765, 1975

8. Joint National Committee on Detection, Evaluation, and Treatment of High Blood Pressure: The Fifth Report of the Joint National Committee on Detection, Evaluation, and Treatment of High Blood Pressure. *Arch Intern Med* 153:154-183, 1993

9. Thomas JE, Schirger A: Idiopathic orthostatic hypotension: a study of its natural history in 57 neurologically affected patients. *Arch Neurol* 22: 289-293, 1970

10. World Health Organization, First Report of the Expert Committee on Cardiovascular Diseases in Hypertension: Hypertension and coronary heart disease: classification and criteria for epidemiological studies. *WHO Tech Rep Ser* 168:1-28, 1959

11. Master AM, Dublin LI, Marks HH: The normal blood pressure range and its clinical implications. *JAMA* 143:1464-1470, 1950

12. National Heart, Lung, and Blood Institute's Task Force on Blood Pressure Control in Children: Report of the Task Force on Blood Pressure Control in Children. *Pediatrics* 59 Suppl:797-820, 1977

13. Society of Actuaries: *Build and Blood Pressure Study.* Vol. 1 and 2. Chicago, Society of Actuaries, 1959

14. Weber MA, Drayer JIM, Wyle FA, et al: A representative value for whole-day BP monitoring. *JAMA* 248:1626-1628, 1982

15. SHEP Cooperative Research Group: Prevention of stroke by antihypertensive drug treatment in older persons with isolated systolic hypertension. Final results of the Systolic Hypertension in the Elderly Program (SHEP). *JAMA* 265:3255-3264, 1991

16. American Heart Association Committee on Exercise: *Exercise Testing and Training of Individuals with Heart Disease or at High Risk for Its Development: A Handbook for Physicians.* Dallas, Texas, American Heart Association, 1975

17. 1988 Joint National Committee: The 1988 Report of the Joint National Committee on Detection, Evaluation, and Treatment of High Blood Pressure. *Arch Intern Med* 148:1023-1038, 1988

18. Veterans Administration Cooperative Study Group on Antihypertensive Agents: Effect of treatment on morbidity and hypertension: results in patients with diastolic blood pressure averaging 115 through 129 mm Hg. *JAMA* 202:1028-1034, 1967

19. Veterans Administration Cooperative Study Group on Antihypertensive Agents: Effects of treatment on morbidity in hypertension. II. Results in patients with diastolic blood pressure averaging 90 through 114 mm Hg. *JAMA* 213:1143-1152, 1970

20. Cohn JN, Limas CJ, Guiha NH: Hypertension and the heart. *Arch Intern Med* 133:969-979, 1974

21. Frohlich ED, Tarazi RC, Dustan HP: Clinical-physiological correlations in the development of hypertensive heart disease. *Circulation* 44:446-455, 1971

22. Truett J, Cornfield J, Kannel W: A multivariate analysis of the risk of coronary heart disease in Framingham. *J Chronic Dis* 20:511-524, 1967

23. McKee PA, Castelli WP, McNamara PM, et al: The natural history of congestive heart failure: the Framingham Study. *N Engl J Med* 285:1441-1446, 1971

24. Sokolow M, Perloff D: The prognosis of essential hypertension treated conservatively. *Circulation* 23:697-713, 1961

25. Safar ME, Lehner JP, Vincent MI, et al: Echocardiographic dimensions in borderline and sustained hypertension. *Am J Cardiol* 44:930-935, 1979

26. Zak R, Rabinowitz M: Molecular aspects of cardiac hypertrophy. *Annu Rev Physiol* 41:539-552, 1979

27. Pfeffer J, Pfeffer M, Fletcher P, et al: Alterations of cardiac performance in rats with established spontaneous hypertension. *Am J Cardiol* 44:994-998, 1979

28. Meerson FZ: The myocardium in hyperfunction, hypertrophy and heart failure. *Circ Res* 25 Suppl 2:1-163, 1969

29. Frohlich ED: Clinical significance of hemodynamic findings in hypertension. *Chest* 64:94-99, 1973

30. Tarazi RC, Frohlich ED, Dustan HP: Left atrial abnormality and ventricular preejection period in hypertension. *Dis Chest* 55:214-218, 1969

31. Savage DD, Drayer JIM, Henry WL, et al: Echocardiographic assessment of cardiac anatomy and function in hypertensive subjects. *Circulation* 59:623-632, 1979

32. Frohlich ED: Cardiac hypertrophy in hypertension. *N Engl J Med* 317:831-833, 1987

33. Frohlich ED, Apstein C, Chobanian AV, et al: The heart in hypertension. *N Engl J Med* 327:998-1008, 1992

34. Julius S: Transition from high cardiac output to elevated vascular resistance in hypertension. *Am Heart J* 116:600-606, 1988

35. Roberts WC: The hypertensive diseases: evidence that systemic hypertension is a greater risk factor to the development of other cardiovascular diseases than previously suspected. *Am J Med* 59:523-532, 1975

36. Schlatmann TJM, Becker AE: Histologic changes in the normal aging aorta: implications for dissecting aortic aneurysm. *Am J Cardiol* 39:13-20, 1977

37. Schlatmann TJM, Becker AE: Pathogenesis of dissecting aneurysm of aorta: comparative histopathologic study of significance of medical changes. *Am J Cardiol* 39:21-26, 1977

38. Burch GE, DePasquale NP: The anomalous left coronary artery: an experiment of nature (editorial). *Am J Med* 37:159-161, 1964

39. Heath D, Wood EH, DuShane JW, et al: The relation of age and blood pressure to atheroma in the pulmonary arteries and thoracic aorta in congenital heart disease. *Lab Invest* 9:259-272, 1960

40. Kannel WB, Dawber TR, Sorlie P, et al: Components of blood pressure and risk of atherothrombotic brain infarction: the Framingham Study. *Stroke* 7:327-331, 1976

41. Kannel WB, Wolf P, Dawber TR: Hypertension and cardiac impairments increase stroke risk. *Geriatrics* 33:71-83, September 1978

42. Phillips SJ, Whisnant JP: Hypertension and the brain. The National High Blood Pressure Education Program. *Arch Intern Med* 152:938-945, 1992

43. Fisher CM: The arterial lesions underlying lacunes. *Acta Neuropathol (Berl)* 12:1-15, 1969

44. Cole FM, Yates PO: The occurrence and significance of intracerebral micro-aneurysms. *J Pathol Bacteriol* 93:393-411, 1967

45. Kannel WB, Wolf PA, Verter J, et al: Epidemiologic assessment of the role of blood pressure in stroke: the Framingham Study. *JAMA* 214:301-310, 1970

46. Hatano S: Hypertension in Japan: a review. In *Epidemiology and Control of Hypertension.* Edited by O Paul. New York, Stratton Intercontinental Medical Book Corporation, 1975, pp 63-95

47. Strandgaard S, Olesen J, Skinhøj E, et al: Autoregulation of brain circulation in severe arterial hypertension. *Br Med J* 1:507-510, 1973

48. Schnier BR, Sheps SG, Juergens JL: Hypertensive ischemic ulcer: a review of 40 cases. *Am J Cardiol* 17:560-565, 1966

49. NHBPEP Working Group Report on Hypertension and Chronic Renal Failure, U.S. Department of Health and Human Services, August 1990

50. Jones DB: Arterial and glomerular lesions associated with severe hypertension: light and electron microscopic studies. *Lab Invest* 31:303-313, 1974

51. Reubi FC: *Clearance Tests in Clinical Medicine.* Springfield, Illinois, Charles C Thomas, Publisher, 1963

52. Kaplan NM: Microalbuminuria: a risk factor for vascular and renal complications of hypertension. *Am J Med* 92:8S-12S, 1992

53. Smith DE, Odel HM, Kernohan JW: Causes of death in hypertension. *Am J Med* 9:516-527, 1950

54. Messerli FH, Frohlich ED: High blood pressure: a side effect of drugs, poisons, and food. *Arch Intern Med* 139:682-687, 1979

55. Walters WAW: Review: the significance and management of raised blood pressure in pregnancy. *Aust NZ J Obstet Gynecol* 19:17-22, 1979

56. Pickering GW: *High Blood Pressure.* New York, Grune & Stratton, 1955

57. Carney JA, Sizemore GW, Sheps SG: Adrenal medullary disease in multiple endocrine neoplasia, type 2: pheochromocytoma and its precursors. *Am J Clin Pathol* 66:279-290, 1976

58. Kannel WB: Hypertension, blood lipids, and cigarette smoking as co-risk factors for coronary heart disease. *Ann NY Acad Sci* 304:128-139, 1978

59. Whiting AS, Johnson LN: Papilledema: clinical clues and differential diagnosis. *Am Fam Physician* 45:1125-1134, 1992

60. Weinberger MH, Grim CE, Hollifield JW, et al: Primary aldos-

teronism: diagnosis, localization, and treatment. *Ann Intern Med* 90:386-395, 1979

61. Kassirer JP: Clinical evaluation of kidney function: glomerular function. *N Engl J Med* 285:385-389, 1971

62. National High Blood Pressure Education Program, Working Group Report on the Heart in Hypertension, September 1991

63. Brunner HR, Laragh JH, Baer L, et al: Essential hypertension: renin and aldosterone, heart attack and stroke. *N Engl J Med* 286:441-449, 1972

64. Birkenhager WH, Kho TL, Schalekamp MADH, et al: Renin levels and cardiovascular morbidity in essential hypertension: a prospective study. *Acta Clin Belg* 32:168-172, 1977

65. Kaplan NM: The prognostic implications of plasma renin in essential hypertension. *JAMA* 231:167-170, 1975

66. Foster JH, Maxwell MH, Franklin SS, et al: Renovascular occlusive disease: results of operative treatment. *JAMA* 231:1043-1048, 1975

67. Schwarten DE: Transluminal angioplasty of renal artery stenosis: 70 experiences. *AJR* 135:969-974, 1980

68. Foster JH, Dean RH, Pinkerton JA, et al: Ten years' experience with the surgical management of renovascular hypertension. *Ann Surg* 177:755-764, 1973

69. Holley KE, Hunt JC, Brown AL Jr, et al: Renal artery stenosis: a clinical-pathologic study in normotensive and hypertensive patients. *Am J Med* 37:14-22, 1964

70. Rosenfeld JB, Cohen L, Garty I, et al: Unilateral renal hypoplasia with hypertension (Ask-Upmark kidney). *Br Med J* 2:217-218, 1973

71. Aquino MA, Lubash GD: Hypertension due to vascular lesions in neurofibromatosis. *South Med J* 64:756-757, 1971

72. Kihara I, Fujimaki S: A case of renovascular hypertension caused by aortitis of Takayasu's type. *Acta Pathol Jpn* 18:37-48, 1968

73. Weidmann P, Siegenthaler W, Ziegler WH, et al: Hypertension associated with tumors adjacent to renal arteries. *Am J Med* 47:528-533, 1969

74. Maldonado JE, Sheps SG: Renal arteriovenous fistula. *Postgrad Med* 40:263-269, 1966

75. Thind GS, Baum S, Kuroda K: Transient renal-artery stenosis: disappearance of the arteriographic and renal venous renin abnormalities. *N Engl J Med* 278:1201-1203, 1968

76. Haimovici H, Zinicola N: Experimental renal-artery stenosis: diagnostic significance of arterial hemodynamics. *J Cardiovasc Surg (Torino)* 3:259-262, 1962

77. Laragh JH: Vasoconstriction-volume analysis for understanding and treating hypertension: the use of renin and aldosterone profiles. *Am J Med* 55:261-274, 1973

78. Bookstein JJ, Abrams HL, Buenger RE, et al: Radiologic aspects of renovascular hypertension. Part 2. The role of urography in unilateral renovascular disease. *JAMA* 220:1225-1230, 1972

79. Bookstein JJ, Maxwell MH, Abrams HL, et al: Cooperative study of radiologic aspects of renovascular hypertension: bilateral renovascular disease. *JAMA* 237:1706-1709, 1977

80. Thornbury JR, Stanley JC, Fryback DG: Hypertensive urogram: a nondiscriminatory test for renovascular hypertension. *AJR* 138:43-49, 1982

81. Mann SJ, Pickering TG: Detection of renovascular hypertension. State of the art: 1992. *Ann Intern Med* 117:845-853, 1992

82. Burbank MK, Hunt JC, Tauxe WN, et al: Radioisotopic renography: diagnosis of renal arterial disease in hypertensive patients. *Circulation* 27:328-338, 1963

83. Robertson JS: Nuclear medicine procedures in nephrology. In *Renal Function Tests: Clinical Laboratory Procedures and Diagnosis.* Edited by CG Duarte. Boston, Little, Brown & Company, 1980, pp 269-289

84. Nally JV Jr, Chen C, Fine E, et al: Diagnostic criteria of renovascular hypertension with captopril renography. A consensus statement. *Am J Hypertens* 4:749S-752S, 1991

85. Nally JV: The captopril tests: a new concept in detecting renovascular hypertension? *Cleve Clin J Med* 56:395-401, 1989

86. Gosse P, Dupas JY, Reynaud P, et al: Captopril test in the detection of renovascular hypertension in a population with low prevalence of the disease: a prospective study. *Am J Hypertens* 2:191-193, 1989

87. Greene ER, Avasthi PS, Hodges JW: Noninvasive Doppler assessment of renal artery stenosis and hemodynamics. *JCU* 15:653-659, 1987

88. Robertson R, Murphy A, Dubbins PA: Renal artery stenosis: the use of duplex ultrasound as a screening technique. *Br J Radiol* 61:196-201, 1988

89. Taylor DC, Kettler MD, Moneta GL, et al: Duplex ultrasound scanning in the diagnosis of renal artery stenosis: a prospective evaluation. *J Vasc Surg* 7:363-369, 1988

90. Habib R, Kleinknecht C, Gubler MC, et al: Idiopathic membranoproliferative glomerulonephritis in children: report of 105 cases. *Clin Nephrol* 1:194-214, 1973

91. Burke FG, Ross S: Acute glomerulonephritis: a review of ninety cases. *J Pediatr* 30:157-170, 1947

92. Nash DA Jr: Hypertension in polycystic kidney disease without renal failure. *Arch Intern Med* 137:1571-1575, 1977

93. West CD: Pathogenesis and approaches to therapy of membranoproliferative glomerulonephritis (editorial). *Kidney Int* 9:1-7, 1976

94. Churg J, Sobin LH: *Renal Disease: Classification and Atlas of Glomerular Diseases.* Tokyo-New York, Igaku Shoin, 1982, pp 54, 83

95. Schreiber RD, Müller-Eberhard HJ: Complement and renal disease. *Contemp Issues Nephrol* 3:67-105, 1979

96. Lewy JE, Salinas-Madrigal L, Herdson PB, et al: Clinicopathologic correlations in acute poststreptococcal glomerulonephritis: a correlation between renal functions, morphologic damage and clinical course of 46 children with acute poststreptococcal glomerulonephritis. *Medicine (Baltimore)* 50:453-501, 1971

97. Danovitch GM: Clinical features and pathophysiology of polycystic kidney disease in man. In *Cystic Diseases of the Kidney.* Edited by KD Gardner Jr. New York, John Wiley & Sons, 1976, pp 125-150

98. Franklin WA, Jennings RB, Earle DP: Membranous glomerulonephritis: long-term serial observations on clinical course and morphology. *Kidney Int* 4:36-56, 1973

99. Conn JW, Cohen EL, Lucas CP, et al: Primary reninism: hypertension hyperreninemia and secondary aldosteronism due to renin-producing juxtaglomerular cell tumors. *Arch Intern Med* 130:682-696, 1972

100. Ganguly A, Gribble J, Tune B, et al: Renin-secreting Wilms' tumor with severe hypertension: report of a case and brief review of renin-secreting tumors. *Ann Intern Med* 79:835-837, 1973

101. Genest J, Rojo-Ortega JM, Kuchel O, et al: Malignant hypertension with hypokalemia in a patient with renin-producing pulmonary carcinoma. *Trans Assoc Am Physicians* 88:192-200, 1975

102. Salassa RM, Weeks RE, Northcutt RC, et al: Primary aldosteronism and malignant adrenocortical neoplasia. *Trans Am Clin Climatol Assoc* 86:163-172, 1975

103. Young WF Jr, Hogan MJ, Klee GG, et al: Primary aldosteronism: diagnosis and treatment. *Mayo Clin Proc* 65:96-110, 1990

104. Gold EM: The Cushing syndromes: changing views of diagnosis and treatment. *Ann Intern Med* 90:829-844, 1979

105. Crapo L: Cushing's syndrome: a review of diagnostic tests. *Metabolism* 28:955-977, 1979

106. Kaye TB, Crapo L: The Cushing syndrome: an update on diagnostic tests. *Ann Intern Med* 112:434-444, 1990

107. Hosaka Y, Rainwater LM, Grant CS, et al: Pheochromocytoma: nuclear deoxyribonucleic acid patterns studied by flow cytometry. *Surgery* 100:1003-1010, 1986

108. Thomas JE, Rooke ED, Kvale WF: The neurologist's experience with pheochromocytoma: a review of 100 cases. *JAMA* 197:754-758, 1966

109. Kuchel O, Buu NT, Fontaine A, et al: Free and conjugated plasma catecholamines in hypertensive patients with and without pheochromocytoma. *Hypertension* 2:177-186, 1980

110. Sheps SG, Jiang NS, Klee GG, et al: Recent developments in the diagnosis and treatment of pheochromocytoma. *Mayo Clin Proc* 65:88-95, 1990

111. Kaplan NM, Kramer NJ, Holland OB, et al: Single-voided urine metanephrine assays in screening for pheochromocytoma. *Arch Intern Med* 137:190-193, 1977

112. Korobkin M, White EA, Kressel HY, et al: Computed tomography in the diagnosis of adrenal disease. *AJR* 132:231-238, 1979

113. Stewart BH, Bravo EL, Haaga J, et al: Localization of pheochromocytoma by computed tomography. *N Engl J Med* 299:460-461, 1978

114. Sheps SG, Jiang N-S, Klee GG: Diagnostic evaluation of pheochromocytoma. *Endocrinol Metab Clin North Am* 17:397-414, 1988

115. Becker AE, Becker MJ, Edwards JE: Anomalies associated with coarctation of aorta: particular reference to infancy. *Circulation* 41:1067-1075, 1970

116. Alpert BS, Bain HH, Balfe JW, et al: Role of the renin-angiotensin-aldosterone system in hypertensive children with coarctation of the aorta. *Am J Cardiol* 43:828-834, 1979

117. Evans CH, Westfall V, Atuk NO: Astrocytoma mimicking the features of pheochromocytoma. *N Engl J Med* 286:1397-1399, 1972

118. Bors E: The challenge of quadriplegia: some personal observations in a series of two hundred thirty-three cases. *Bull Los Angeles Neurol Soc* 21:105-123, 1956

119. Davidson DLW, Jellinek EH: Hypertension and papilledema in the Guillain-Barré syndrome. *J Neurol Neurosurg Psychiatry* 40:144-148, 1977

120. Chesley LC, Annitto JE, Cosgrove RA: The remote prognosis of eclamptic women: sixth periodic report. *Am J Obstet Gynecol* 124:446-459, 1976

121. Lenfant C (Chairman): National High Blood Pressure Education Program Working Group Report on High Blood Pressure in Pregnancy. *Am J Obstet Gynecol* 163:1691-1712, 1990

122. Fisch IR, Frank J: Oral contraceptives and blood pressure. *JAMA* 237:2499-2503, 1977

123. Ramcharan S, Pellegrin FA, Hoag E: The occurrence and course of hypertensive disease in users and nonusers of oral contraceptive drugs. In *Oral Contraceptives and High Blood Pressure.* Edited by MJ Fregly, MS Fregly. Gainesville, Florida, The Dolphin Press, 1974, pp 1-15

124. Pritchard JA, Pritchard SA: Blood pressure response to estrogen-progestin oral contraceptive after pregnancy-induced hypertension. *Am J Obstet Gynecol* 129:733-739, 1977

125. Schoolwerth AC, Sandler RS, Klahr S, et al: Nephrosclerosis postpartum and in women taking oral contraceptives. *Arch Intern Med* 136:178-185, 1976

126. Pfeffer RI: Estrogen use, hypertension and stroke in postmenopausal women. *J Chronic Dis* 31:389-398, 1978

127. Porter GA, Bennett WM, Sheps SG: Cyclosporine-associated hypertension. National High Blood Pressure Education Program. *Arch Intern Med* 150:280-283, 1990.

128. Nissenson AR, Nimer SD, Wolcott DL: Recombinant human erythropoietin and renal anemia: molecular biology, clinical efficacy, and nervous system effects. *Ann Intern Med* 114:402-416, 1991

129. Smith LH, Drach G, Hall P, et al: National High Blood Pressure Program (NHBPEP) review paper on complications of shock wave lithotripsy for urinary calculi. *Am J Med* 91:635-641, 1991

CHAPTER

60

Cardiovascular manifestations of hypertension

B. Therapy

Mahlon K. Burbank, M.D., and Prince K. Zachariah, M.D., Ph.D.

More than 50 million Americans have elevated blood pressure (systolic blood pressure of 140 mm Hg or greater or diastolic blood pressure of 90 mm Hg or greater, or both) or are taking antihypertensive medication.[1] Black and older persons have a high prevalence of hypertension. Hypertension is just one of the causes of increased mortality from coronary heart disease and stroke, but in the past 2 decades, since the development of adequate therapy for increased blood pressure, the mortality from coronary heart disease has decreased nearly 50% and that from stroke, 57%.[2] This decline in mortality is believed to be due primarily to changes in lifestyle and to medical intervention directed at minimizing three major cardiovascular risk factors: cigarette smoking, hypertension, and hypercholesterolemia.

WHOM TO TREAT

"Normal" systemic blood pressure in the past has been considered to be 140 mm Hg or less systolic and 90 mm Hg or less diastolic. The World Health Organization had defined blood pressures greater than 160 mm Hg systolic and greater than 95 mm Hg diastolic to be abnormal and indicative of hypertension. In October 1992, however, the Fifth Report of the Joint National Committee on Detection, Evaluation, and Treatment of High Blood Pressure[1] reclassified normal blood pressures and hypertension as illustrated in Table 60B-1.

It should be noted that evidence for target-organ damage (Table 60B-2) should lead to more aggressive therapy and that detection and modification of cardiovascular risk factors—dyslipoproteinemia, cigarette smoking, diabetes mellitus, obesity, and physical inactivity—are considered essential parts of therapy.

DETECTION

Various strategies have been used to detect and to determine successful treatment of hypertension. Use of repeated office visits over several weeks is common unless the pressure is particularly high. Ambulatory recording with a fully automatic pressure measurement device has become the standard at the Mayo Clinic. While using this system, patients can carry out their usual activities.

The monitor weighs less than a pound. It measures and records blood pressure and heart rate by the oscillometric method every 10 minutes over a short term (6 hours). A report is generated by a computer. Whether for most patients such a device is more reliable than multiple pressure readings obtained in a physician's office is under study.[3]

The Joint National Committee[1] recommends the following for office readings:

1. Patients should be seated with arm bared, supported, and at heart level. They should not have smoked or ingested caffeine within 30 minutes before measurement.
2. Measurement should begin after 5 minutes of rest.
3. The proper cuff size must be used to ensure an accurate measurement. The bladder should nearly (at least 80%) or completely encircle the arm.
4. Measurements should be taken with a mercury sphygmomanometer, a recently calibrated aneroid manometer, or a calibrated electronic device.
5. Both systolic and diastolic pressures should be recorded. The disappearance of sound (phase V) should be used for the diastolic reading.
6. Two or more readings separated by 2 minutes should be averaged. If the first two readings differ by more

Table 60B-1 Classification of blood pressure for adults 18 years old and older*

Category	Systolic, mm Hg	Diastolic, mm Hg
Normal†	<130	<85
High normal	130-139	85-89
Hypertension‡		
Stage 1 (mild)	140-159	90-99
Stage 2 (moderate)	160-179	100-109
Stage 3 (severe)	180-209	110-119
Stage 4 (very severe)	≥210	≥120

*Not taking antihypertensive drugs and not acutely ill. When systolic and diastolic pressures are in different categories, the higher category should be selected to classify the individual's blood pressure status. For instance, 160/92 should be classified as stage 2 and 180/120 as stage 4. Isolated systolic hypertension is defined as systolic pressure ≥140 mm Hg and diastolic pressure <90 mm Hg and staged accordingly (e.g., 170/85 mm Hg is defined as stage 2 isolated systolic hypertension).
†Optimal blood pressure with respect to cardiovascular risk is systolic pressure <120 mm Hg and diastolic pressure <80 mm Hg. However, unusually low readings should be evaluated for clinical significance.
‡On the basis of the average of two or more readings taken at each of two or more visits after an initial screening.
Note: In addition to classifying stages of hypertension on the basis of average blood pressure levels, the clinician should specify presence or absence of target-organ disease and additional risk factors. For example, for a patient with diabetes, a blood pressure of 142/94 mm Hg, and left ventricular hypertrophy, the description should be "stage 1 hypertension with target-organ disease (left ventricular hypertrophy) and with another major risk factor (diabetes)." This specificity is important for risk classification and management.

Table 60B-2 Manifestations of target-organ disease

Organ system	Manifestations
Cardiac	Clinical, electrocardiographic, or radiologic evidence of coronary artery disease Left ventricular hypertrophy or "strain" by electrocardiography or left ventricular hypertrophy by echocardiography Left ventricular dysfunction or cardiac failure
Cerebrovascular	Transient ischemic attack or stroke
Peripheral vascular	Absence of one or more major pulses in the extremities (except for dorsalis pedis), with or without intermittent claudication; aneurysm
Renal	Serum creatinine ≥130 μmol/L (1.5 mg/dL) Proteinuria (1+ or greater) Microalbuminuria
Retinopathy	Hemorrhages or exudates, with or without papilledema

than 5 mm Hg, additional readings should be obtained.

Sometimes it is more effective to obtain blood pressure measurements for both diagnosis and monitoring at home or at work. Use of inexpensive manual or automatic devices by the patient or family can avoid the so-called white-coat hypertension of an office visit.

WHAT WE NEED TO KNOW

Once it is established that a patient has hypertension, several strategies are available for use before drug therapy is begun. Because the majority of patients have "essential" hypertension, a history, a physical examination, and only a limited laboratory examination should be necessary. In chapter 60A, clues are discussed that should suggest possible secondary and curable forms of hypertension. These clues include severe hypertension, sweating spells, decreased femoral pulses, and renal bruits. Various historical, physical, and laboratory findings make a significant difference in therapeutic choices, however, even among patients with essential hypertension.

From the history (Table 60B-3) we try to learn whether the patient is likely to follow our therapy: that is, whether there had been previous treatment and, if so, why the patient no longer was on it. Were there side effects from the drugs? Was it inconvenient to come to the physician's office for rechecks? Perhaps having the patient take his or her own pressure or having it taken at the place of work would be better. In particular, the current medical program should be assessed, especially regarding the use of birth control pills, nasal decongestants, antidepressant medications, and nonsteroidal anti-arthritic medications, because all these can interfere with therapy.

Choice of therapy often will also depend on the nature of other problems encountered in the patient's medical history. If the patient has a history of depression, a number of antihypertensive agents such as methyldopa, reserpine, and certain β-adrenergic blockers should be avoided. Historical clues to other disease states such as migraine headaches, strokes or transient ischemic attacks, asthma, coronary artery disease, liver or ulcer disease, diabetes, gout, Raynaud's disease, and intermittent claudication should be sought. The presence of one of these problems may make it necessary to choose one drug program rather than another.

The physical examination (Table 60B-4) may offer clues to secondary causes of hypertension, but it also can reveal conditions that will affect the choice of medical therapy. There may be retinopathy, suggesting the need for more urgent and aggressive therapy. Carotid bruits would suggest the avoidance of drugs causing a postural decrease in the blood pressure. Signs of heart failure should be noted so that use of β-blocking drug therapy can be avoided. Absent or decreased pulses suggest that a β-blocking drug be used with caution to prevent worsening of intermittent claudication.

Table 60B-3 History in the hypertensive patient

Family history of hypertension
Previous history of hypertension
Previous therapy of hypertension
Previous side effects of antihypertensive agents
Previous stroke, heart disease, renal disease, liver disease, "spells," diabetes, gout, asthma, intermittent claudication, Raynaud's phenomenon, depression
Current use of alcohol and tobacco
Use of other drugs, especially birth control pills, nasal vasoconstrictors, antidepressants, nonsteroidal anti-inflammatory agents

Table 60B-4 Physical examination in the hypertensive patient

Serial blood pressure determinations
Blood pressure in both arms
Funduscopic examination
Palpation of thyroid
Auscultation
Lungs for wheezing and rales
Cardiac
Abdominal and cervical
Palpation of pulses, especially femoral

Table 60B-5 Laboratory testing in the hypertensive patient

Blood hemoglobin
Serum creatinine
Serum potassium
Blood uric acid
Blood glucose
Urinalysis
Electrocardiogram
Chest radiograph
Serum cholesterol
Serum triglycerides
Echocardiogram(?)
Plasma renin activity(?)

Table 60B-6 Aids to increase patient compliance

Educate the patient about hypertension
Use simplest program possible
Make follow-up convenient
Make prescription size fit follow-up visits
Consider home or workplace blood pressure determinations
Make follow-up visits valuable for further education

Table 60B-7 Education of the patient

Explain what high blood pressure is
Explain complications and effects of hypertension
Explain that drug therapy is not a cure for hypertension
Emphasize importance of follow-up visits and laboratory testing
Discuss possible side effects of therapy
Discuss other risk factors and their importance

Appropriate laboratory testing is essential before any drug therapy is begun. The extent of this testing will depend on clues derived from the history and physical examination. For instance, a prolonged carotid bruit suggests the need for duplex ultrasound scanning of the carotid artery; rales in the lung bases indicate the need for a chest radiograph. A number of laboratory tests should be done in most patients with newly diagnosed hypertension before therapy is begun (Table 60B-5). Results of these baseline tests will help in choosing therapy and in detecting future abnormalities during the drug program.

COMPLIANCE

With modern drug therapy it is possible, given the opportunity, to achieve a normal blood pressure in almost all patients. The usual cause of failure to control the pressure is lack of patient compliance—either failure to take the medicine as prescribed or simply dropping out of the treatment program completely.

Various strategies have been used to increase compliance (Table 60B-6). The two most important seem to be patient education and convenience of recheck examination. Patients expect and demand answers; they want to know the reason for taking each medicine and are concerned about the possible side effects of the drugs. Either directly or through paramedical personnel or by use of written material, movies, or videotapes, the treating physician should impart this information to the patient (Table 60B-7).

For the busy homemaker or income earner, convenience of recheck is paramount. It has been shown that compliance is better with treatment programs at the workplace than in a clinic or physician's office.[4] Teaching the patient to measure blood pressure at home also has a number of advantages: more convenient, more readings, cheaper, and the patient shares the responsibility and develops an interest in the success of the program. In the "self-measurement" program, the patient mails or brings the records to the treatment center or physician's office periodically. One should allot time under this method for intermittent office visits, because the patient usually has other medical concerns to discuss and therefore feels that these visits are of double benefit. If the office visit is to a paramedical therapist, a physician should be available to discuss these other medical concerns when they arise in addition to consulting regarding changes needed in the program.

NONPHARMACOLOGIC THERAPY AND LIFESTYLE MODIFICATION

In patients with significant hypertension, it seems most reasonable to begin with drug therapy, with the gradual addition of nonpharmacologic measures later. If successful, the drug therapy can be gradually reduced. Conversely, in patients with mild or borderline hypertension who are well motivated, nonpharmacologic therapy may be considered as the initial treatment. Under these circumstances, however, the patients must be convinced that they have hypertension, that they need to undergo close follow-up, and that they may need the addition of drugs if the initial program fails to normalize pressure.

Nonpharmacologic treatment consists of behavior modification, weight reduction, exercise, and reduced salt intake. Other factors that appear to play some part in blood pressure elevation or are associated with increasing risk of cardiovascular disease include excessive alcohol intake,[5] smoking, and elevated cholesterol and lipid values. Caffeine seems to elevate blood pressure only in subjects who are not regular users of coffee or caffeine-containing soft drinks, and thus there does not seem to be a reason to restrict the use of these beverages in reasonable amounts.

Exercise

One possible benefit of exercise is a reduction in weight, thus resulting in a lowering of the blood pressure. Clearly, patients who can be stimulated to begin an exercise program, whether it consists of a simple walking program or is a more vigorous program (e.g., jogging/running, bicycling, swimming), benefit in that they have an increased health consciousness. They are more likely to stop smoking, to lose weight, and to restrict their cholesterol intake.

The direct effect of an exercise program on the blood pressure appears to be related to weight reduction.[6,7] Currently, the best strategy is to include exercise as part of a weight reduction program in the therapy of the hypertensive patient.[8,9]

Salt restriction

Advice to avoid adding salt to one's food at the table, in addition to avoiding high-sodium foods such as bacon, ham, and salted peanuts, should be part of the early discussion with the patient. After the first few weeks, most patients find that their tolerance for these restrictions rises. More formal salt restriction can be maintained by instructions from a dietitian or from one of the many manuals available through voluntary health agencies, such as the American Heart Association.

The goal in most moderate sodium restriction diets is an intake of approximately 90 mEq of sodium per day. This level of intake usually can be approached by avoiding obviously salty foods and by not adding salt at the table. The new federal regulations that require labeling of processed foods to indicate sodium content plus the new, highly advertised "low-salt soups" also make it easier for the well-motivated patient to follow a salt-restricted diet. If there is doubt that a patient is indeed following a low-salt program, 24-hour urine sodium content can be determined. If sodium content is high, more formal dietary instructions might be indicated in addition to further encouragement to the patient. "Salt substitutes" sometimes can be used by those patients who cannot tolerate sodium restriction, but this is seldom needed.

Because the goal of treating hypertension is not just obtaining normal blood pressure but is the prevention of the cardiovascular and renal complications that arise in these patients, part of the advice we give these patients should include dietary instructions for those patients with increased lipid or cholesterol values. Few would not know that cigarette smoking should be stopped, but this should be emphasized because the patient may be more receptive to such advice at the time that the antihypertensive therapy is begun.

Alcohol intake of 2 oz/day or less need not be restricted. Both epidemiologic and clinical studies have confirmed that excessive alcohol consumption is directly related to higher blood pressures. Fortunately, this increase in blood pressure is totally reversible in this group of heavy drinkers.

A diet high in potassium may protect against development of hypertension. A normal plasma potassium value should be maintained. Hypokalemia that occurs during diuretic therapy may require potassium supplements or the use of a potassium-sparing diuretic agent. This type of drug must be used with caution in patients receiving angiotensin-converting enzyme inhibitors or those susceptible to hyperkalemia. Higher calcium and magnesium intakes have been associated with lower blood pressure, but as yet there is no convincing evidence to justify recommending increases in dietary supplements in the treatment or prevention of hypertension.[1]

APPROACH TO THERAPY–GENERAL GUIDELINES

For most adult hypertensive patients, once it has been established that the patient requires drug treatment, the goal is a pressure of 140/90 mm Hg or below. This should be an average pressure obtained in the sitting position. Periodic casual readings may be higher, and the measurement should be repeated over several hours or days before it is assumed that the pressure is high and that additional drug therapy is needed (just as the original diagnosis of hypertension requires multiple readings). In patients who are nervous about their blood pressure, it is best to use home readings by having them purchase their own equipment and learn how to measure the blood pressure themselves. In addition to the advantage of convenience, more frequent readings are easily obtained.

Obtaining a normal blood pressure is rarely an urgent problem, and therefore each change of drug therapy can be instituted after several days or weeks of observation, depending on convenience to the patient, the age of the patient, and the rate of drug effectiveness. A cautious approach is also indicated to give time to assess the extent of minor or major side effects after each increase in dosage of a given drug or addition of a drug. Finally, time will be available to note the effect of nonpharmacologic measures such as salt restriction, exercise, and weight reduction. Often, 6 weeks to 3 months or more are required before satisfactory blood pressures are obtained.

Once normotension is attained, periodic visits are needed to check the pressures, reinforce the importance of continued therapy, adjust dosage, and answer questions. Periodic laboratory tests are also needed, depending on which drugs the patient is using. Those patients who are normotensive and taking their blood pressures at home require fewer office visits but still require periodic laboratory testing.

The goal in treating hypertension is overall improvement of cardiovascular health, and the initial antihypertensive therapy should achieve and maintain diastolic blood pressure below 90 mm Hg without compromising renal, cerebral, or myocardial function or producing symptoms that might unfavorably affect quality of life. Hence, the effects of different antihypertensive drug therapies on morbidity and mortality from cardiovascular disease have been, and continue to be, extensively studied. Side effects are a major factor in determining whether a patient will comply with a prescribed treatment regimen. For example, 20% to 40% of patients stop taking antihypertensive medications because of treatment-related side effects. Thus, it is important to educate patients about the disease as well as the known side effects of available antihypertensive agents.

Initiation of drug therapy for uncomplicated mild or moderate hypertension should be with a single drug. Because diuretics and β-blockers have been shown in controlled clinical trials to reduce cardiovascular mortality, the Joint National Committee[1] considers these the "preferred" drugs for initial therapy. Treatment in black patients, however, may be an exception, as it has been shown that they respond less well to β-blockers.

Alternative drugs—calcium antagonists, angiotensin-converting enzyme inhibitors, α_1-receptor blockers, and α- and β-blockers—have been shown to adequately control pressure but have as yet not been used in long-term trials to demonstrate a reduction in cardiovascular events.

Direct vasodilation, the α_2-agonists, and the peripherally acting adrenergic neuron antagonists are thus not recommended by the Joint National Committee for initial monotherapy.[1]

The choice of drug depends greatly on concomitant diseases. For example, β-blockers are avoided in insulin-dependent diabetic patients or patients with asthma, whereas a β-blocker may be the preferred drug in a patient with angina or migraine headaches.

Drug choice is more complex in the current era of cost containment. Although low at initiation, the cost of the use of a diuretic should include the expense of needed

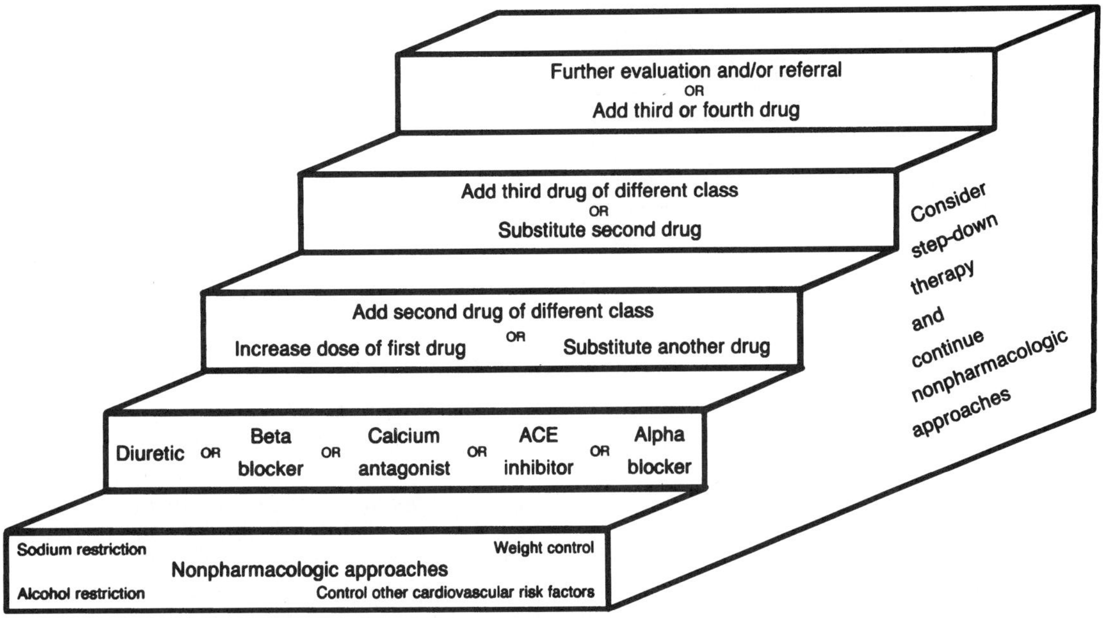

Fig 60B-1 Individualized step-care therapy for hypertension. ACE, angiotensin-converting enzyme. (Modified from 1988 Joint National Committee: The 1988 Report of the Joint National Committee on Detection, Evaluation, and Treatment of High Blood Pressure. *Arch Intern Med* 148:1023-1038, 1988.)

monitoring and laboratory tests, such as potassium, glucose, uric acid, and lipid determinations; in contrast, these expenses are unnecessary with the use of a calcium blocking agent. The increasing use of formulas of approved drugs by payers also restricts the prescribing physician in the choice of drugs and at the very least reduces the choices in a specific group to less expensive drugs.

If the initiation of a single drug does not control the pressure, increasing the dosage, switching to another drug, and adding additional drugs are alternatives (Fig 60B-1).

DRUG THERAPY

Diuretics

Diuretics administered alone or in combination with other agents form the basis of therapy for the majority of hypertensive patients. Even after 35 years of their use, the exact mechanism of their antihypertensive action is not known. Diuretics increase the urine volume. They all inhibit tubular reabsorption of sodium and chloride. At the beginning of daily administration, there is a urinary loss of salt and water that decreases plasma and extracellular volume. Venous filling pressures and cardiac output fall. Blood pressure falls, although peripheral resistance does not and may even increase at this initial stage. Plasma and extracellular fluid volume return nearly to normal and, as a result, cardiac output returns to normal. However, the blood pressure remains low because peripheral resistance decreases during this period. Why this occurs is not known, but one reason may be a decrease in intracellular sodium and water in blood vessel walls.

Diuretics used in hypertension therapy are listed in Table 60B-8. They are prescribed for most patients with hypertension for four reasons.

1. They are effective without additional drugs in a large number of hypertensive patients with mild to moderate blood pressure elevation. Generally, a lowering of pressure by 15/10 mm Hg can be expected with few or no side effects.
2. In patients who require multiple drug therapy, they enhance or augment the hypertensive action of most drugs.
3. They reduce the salt- and water-retaining effects of a number of other antihypertensive agents—particularly β-blockers, calcium blockers, and minoxidil.
4. They produce diuresis in patients who have heart failure complicating hypertension.

Thiazide diuretics. A thiazide or related drug is often used as initial therapy in mild to moderate hypertension, and several weeks are required before the effect is noted. There is no benefit from exceeding the maximum thera-

Table 60B-8 Diuretic agents

Type of drug	Usual dosage range, total mg/day	Frequency	Common or important side effects
Thiazides and related agents			
Bendroflumethiazide	2.5-5	Daily	Hypokalemia, hyperuricemia, hypomagnesemia, hyperglycemia, hypercalcemia, hyponatremia, pancreatitis, rash, increased low-density cholesterol and triglycerides (may be transient), impotence
Benzthiazide	12.5-50	Daily	
Chlorothiazide	125-500	Twice daily	
Chlorthalidone	12.5-50	Daily	
Cyclothiazide	1-2	Daily	
Hydrochlorothiazide	12.5-50	Daily	
Hydroflumethiazide	12.5-50	Daily	
Indapamide	2.5-5	Daily	
Methylclothiazide	2.5-5	Daily	
Metolazone	0.5-5	Daily	
Polythiazide	1-4	Daily	
Quinethazone	25-100	Daily	
Trichlormethiazide	1-4	Daily	
Loop diuretics			
Bumetanide	0.5-5	Twice daily	Hypokalemia, hyperuricemia, hypocalcemia, hyperglycemia, dehydration, hypomagnesemia, blood dyscrasias, rashes, lipid changes, ototoxicity
Ethacrynic acid	25-100	Twice daily	
Furosemide	20-320	Twice daily	
Potassium-sparing diuretics			
Amiloride	5-10	Once or twice	Hyperkalemia, rash, gastrointestinal disturbance
Spironolactone	25-100	Twice or thrice	Hyperkalemia, gynecomastia, menstrual abnormalities, rash
Triamterene	50-150	Once or twice	Hyperkalemia, nephrolithiasis, gastrointestinal disturbances

peutic dose because there is no increase in effect on the blood pressure with increased dosage and adverse effects may be increased. Thiazide diuretics are much more effective with moderate sodium restriction. All these drugs are similar except metolazone and indapamide, which may be effective in patients with renal insufficiency when thiazides are not.

Loop diuretics. Loop diuretics are potent diuretics but as antihypertensive agents are no more potent than the thiazides. They act over a shorter period of time, producing an intense polyuria for about 6 hours after administration. They are particularly useful in patients with renal insufficiency or heart failure. Thiazide drugs are rarely effective in patients with creatinine levels above 2.5 mg/dL, whereas the loop diuretics at increased dosage retain their ability to produce diuresis.

Potassium-sparing diuretics. These diuretics are rarely used alone because they are weak as diuretic and antihypertensive agents. The exception is spironolactone, an aldosterone antagonist, which may be effective alone in treatment of primary or secondary hyperaldosteronism. In addition to spironolactone, triamterene and amiloride are most frequently used in combination with thiazide drugs, mainly for their potassium-sparing action. These drugs, in addition, can be used with loop diuretics in order to avoid the need for potassium supplements, which are quite unpalatable to many patients.

Side effects. A number of points in relation to the side effects (see Table 60B-8) should be made for the use of diuretics in hypertension. By using a thiazide or related drug, marked electrolyte and volume depletion with resulting hypotension can be avoided in most hypertensive patients. When it is necessary to avoid use of thiazide diuretics because of the development of an idiosyncratic reaction such as a skin rash, a related nonthiazide diuretic or a nondiuretic drug can be used.

Pretreatment blood levels of potassium, uric acid, and fasting sugar should be determined (if the potassium value is low, further study to eliminate secondary causes of hypertension such as hyperaldosteronism should be considered). If the potassium value becomes low (less than 3.2 mEq/L) after therapy is started, a potassium-sparing diuretic can be added to the program, or a drug from a nondiuretic group can be used. To decrease the possibility of hypokalemia, and thus avoid the use of oral potassium agents, diuretic therapy is begun with a combination of a thiazide and a potassium-sparing drug, such as hydrochlorothiazide/triamterene or hydrochlorothiazide/amiloride. The potassium-sparing drugs may cause hyperkalemia and, if they are used, potassium supplements should not be given without close monitoring, and they should not be used concurrently with the beginning of therapy with a potassium-sparing agent.

A similar approach can be used with an increased uric acid level. If the pretreatment value of uric acid is high or there is a history of gout, use of diuretics should be avoided. There is little evidence that uric acid values up to 10.0 mg/dL produce renal damage, and up to this blood level no treatment is indicated. If clinical gout develops, either a nondiuretic antihypertensive program can be used or allopurinol or probenecid can be added to the program. When allopurinol is added, we usually also give colchicine for several months to prevent attacks of gout, which sometimes are initiated by allopurinol therapy.

Thiazides sometimes increase the blood sugar level. In some patients, overt diabetes develops, and thus it is reasonable to check the blood sugar level periodically. Recent recommendations favor reduced dosage of thiazides. At doses of hydrochlorothiazide between 12.5 mg and 50 mg, significant changes in glucose or cholesterol values are infrequent. In patients with diet-controlled diabetes, it seems wise to choose nondiuretic antihypertensive therapy. With insulin-dependent diabetes there is little reason to avoid diuretics, because the insulin dosage can be adjusted upward a few units if necessary to control the increase in hyperglycemia.

In clinical practice, one of the common side effects with the use of diuretics is the development of a fine petechial rash over the anterior tibial areas. Changing to a related nonthiazide diuretic usually resolves this problem.

Potassium supplements. Diuretics decrease the serum potassium concentration. Our practice is to use prevention by restricting sodium intake, urging the patient to eat fruit at least twice daily, and prescribing a thiazide with a potassium-sparing agent when beginning antihypertensive therapy. A salt substitute containing KCl also can be used if indicated. If the potassium value remains above 3.2 mEq/L, we rarely add oral potassium supplements, unless the patient complains of muscle weakness or muscle cramps.

Potassium supplements can be given in liquid form, as wax-matrix KCl, or in a microencapsulated form of KCl. We find that the liquid forms often are not tolerated over a long time by most patients because of taste and gastrointestinal effects such as nausea and diarrhea. Some studies suggest that the wax-matrix forms of KCl may produce more gastric erosion than previously believed, but this is not completely proved.[10]

Adrenergic inhibitors

β-blockers. Atenolol, betaxolol, bisoprolol, metoprolol, nadolol, propranolol, and timolol are drugs available in the United States that block the β-adrenergic receptors of the sympathetic nervous system (Table 60B-9). Acebutolol, carteolol, penbutolol, or pindolol added to β-adrenergic receptor blockage has intrinsic sympathomimetic activity that reduces the bradycardiac effect of the β-blockade. In addition, these drugs produce fewer metabolic effects. Labetalol, in addition to β-blockage, has α_1-blockade effects. This drug, which decreases blood pressure more promptly than the other β-blockers, is used intravenously to treat hypertensive emergencies. Finally, atenolol, betaxolol, metoprolol, and acebutolol are cardioselective; that is, in lower doses, they are less likely to inhibit β_2 receptors in the pulmonary vessels.

These drugs decrease blood pressure primarily by blockade of the β-adrenergic receptors of the heart, leading to decreased myocardial contractility. β-Blockade results in a decreased resting heart rate, decreased myocardial oxygen consumption, decreased atrioventricular (AV) conduction, and decreased cardiac output.

Table 60B-9 Adrenergic inhibitors

Type of drug	Usual dosage range, total mg/day	Frequency	Adverse affects
β-Blockers			
Atenolol	25-100	Daily	Fatigue, depression, bradycardia, congestive heart failure, increased airway resistance, Raynaud's phenomenon, aggravation, peripheral vascular disease, increased triglycerides, decreased high-density lipoprotein cholesterol, masking of insulin-induced hypoglycemia
Betaxolol	5-40	Daily	
Bisoprolol	5-20	Daily	
Metoprolol	50-200	Once or twice	
Nadolol	20-240	Once or twice	
Propranolol	40-240	Twice daily	
Timolol	20-40	Twice daily	
β-Blockers with ISA			
Acebutolol	200-1,200	Twice daily	Same as β-blockers with perhaps less bradycardia
Carteolol	2.5-10	Daily	
Penbutolol	20-80	Once	
Pindolol	10-60	Twice	
α- and β-Blocker			
Labetalol	200-1,200	Twice	Same as β-blockers
α_1-Receptor blockers			
Doxazosin	1-16	Once	Orthostatic hypotension, syncope, palpitation, headache, weakness
Prazosin	1-20	Twice or thrice	
Terazosin	1-20	Once	

ISA, intrinsic sympathomimetic activity.

Because β_2-blockade also occurs in the blood vessels, there may be coronary vasoconstriction along with peripheral vasoconstriction. Further effects of β_2-blockade may include bronchoconstriction and decreased glycogenolysis and delay of response to hypoglycemia.

The β-blockers also decrease renin levels. However, studies suggest that this is not an important part of the antihypertensive effect of the drugs.[11] Patients with high renin levels either before therapy or secondary to diuretic therapy may respond impressively to β-blockers. Because most patients without increased renin levels respond to β-blockade, a trial of these drugs when indicated seems more reasonable than performing renin level measurements in the majority of hypertensive patients.

There are differences among the drugs, although they all lower the blood pressure in a similar manner and to a similar extent. For instance, propranolol has greater lipid solubility and crosses the blood-brain barrier to a greater extent than does metoprolol or nadolol; thus, propranolol may have greater central nervous system effects. Metoprolol and atenolol are β_1-blockers (cardiac), and thus in low doses have less effect on the bronchoconstriction produced by nonselective drugs. In higher doses, β_1-blockers also block β_2-receptors, but in some patients with mild asthma a trial with a β_1-blocker might be indicated.

The β-blockers often are used as a second-step drug along with a diuretic in moderate to severe hypertension. They can be used in single-drug therapy in mild to moderate hypertension. If needed, a third drug can be added, usually a vasodilator, such as hydralazine, or a calcium entry blocker, such as nifedipine.

Side effects of the β-blockers include fatigue and depression. Utilizing β-blockers such as metroprolol and atenolol can often decrease this side effect. Patients with asthma or chronic obstructive pulmonary disease are often made more symptomatic when a β-blocker is used, and it is well to avoid this group of drugs if possible in these patients. When this cannot be done, the addition of a β_2-stimulating drug such as terbutaline may be tried. Patients with Raynaud's phenomenon or peripheral vascular disease with claudication are often made more symptomatic with β-blocking drugs, but, again, symptoms can be decreased or avoided by giving small to moderate doses of β_1-selective drugs. Use of a β-blocker may lead to heart failure and AV block; therefore, these drugs must be avoided or used cautiously in patients with these problems. Combining β-blockers with verapamil, the calcium channel antagonist with the most significant effects on AV conduction, occasionally produces advance AV block. This combination should be used with caution.

In the treatment of patients with hypertension and coexisting angina pectoris, β-blockers are especially advantageous. Sudden withdrawal of β-blocking drugs should be avoided because rebound hypertension may develop or angina pectoris may worsen.

Labetalol has especially attractive properties for the treatment of hypertension because in addition to β_1- and

Table 60B-10 Calcium antagonists

Type of drug	Usual dosage range, total mg/day	Frequency	Side effects
Diltiazem	90-360	Thrice	Bradycardia, AV tachycardia, constipation (verapamil), peripheral edema, headache, dizziness, possible aggravation of congestive heart failure, gingival hyperplasia
Verapamil	80-480	Twice	
Dihydropyridines			
Amlodipine	2.5-10	Once	Headache, dizziness, tachycardia, peripheral edema, gingival hyperplasia, possible aggravation of angina
Felodipine	5-20	Once	
Isradipine	2.5-10	Twice	
Nicardipine	60-120	Thrice	
Nifedipine	30-120	Thrice	

β_2-blocking effects, it has α-adrenergic receptor blocking effects. This latter effect results in a decrease in peripheral resistance and a marked fall in blood pressure.[12] A rare side effect is itching of the scalp.

α_1-Receptor blockers. Doxazosin, prazosin, and terazosin all block peripheral α_1-receptors (see Table 60B-9). They cause little or no increase in heart rate. The reason is that only α_1-adrenergic receptors are blocked on the vascular smooth muscle cell, allowing α_2-receptors located on the nerve ending to continue uptake of norepinephrine; thus, no increase in circulating norepinephrine results.[13] These drugs can be used alone to treat mild to moderate hypertension, but fluid retention often occurs, so that addition of a diuretic is often necessary.

The major side effect of these drugs is postural hypotension, particularly with the first dose, so that titration should be based on standing blood pressure. It can be prevented by initiating therapy with a low dose, having the patient take the first dose at bedtime, and withholding diuretic for the 24 hours before the start of therapy. The α_1-receptor blockers have the advantage of producing no adverse metabolic or lipid effects, and occasionally they relieve mild degrees of urinary outflow symptoms in men with prostatic hypertrophy.

Calcium antagonists

Calcium entry blockers decrease calcium entry into vascular smooth muscle cells and thereby reduce vascular tone and contractility (Table 60B-10). Many investigators believe that excessive intracellular calcium maintains the hypertensive state. Thus, calcium entry blockers act at the site of hemodynamic abnormality of hypertension by decreasing total peripheral resistance both at rest and during exercise.

Seven calcium antagonists or blockers are now available in the United States: diltiazem, verapamil, amlodipine, felodipine, isradipine, nicardipine, and nifedipine. Diltiazem, verapamil, and nifedipine are available as long-acting preparations for once-daily dosing.

Verapamil and, to a lesser extent, diltiazem slow heart rate and decrease myocardial contractility; thus, if a calcium antagonist is to be used in combination with a β-adrenergic blocker, one of the other calcium antagonists should be used, such as nifedipine. These other drugs, classified as dihydropyridines (see Table 60B-10), are more potent vasodilators than diltiazem and verapamil and thus cause more dizziness, edema, flushing, headache, and tachycardia. Verapamil often produces troubling constipation in some patients.

Calcium entry blockers show promise as the therapeutic agents of choice for hypertensive patients who are either elderly or black or have low renin profiles—those traditionally treated with diuretics. Hypertensive patients with angina pectoris, left ventricular diastolic dysfunction, diabetes mellitus, chronic obstructive lung disease, Raynaud's phenomenon, or severe occlusive peripheral vascular disease are logical candidates for treatment with a calcium entry blocker.

Angiotensin-converting enzyme inhibitors

The angiotensin-converting enzyme (ACE) inhibitors exert their effects by blocking the conversion of angiotensin I to angiotensin II and thereby inhibiting the vasoconstrictive effects of angiotensin II and decreasing total peripheral resistance.[14] ACE is also responsible for inactivating bradykinin, a vasodilator substance. In addition to inducing vasodilation directly, bradykinin releases vasoactive prostaglandins from various organs. However, the major hypotensive action of ACE inhibitors is considered to be reduction of generation of angiotensin II. ACE inhibition decreases total peripheral resistance with little change in cardiac output or heart rate. In patients with congestive heart failure, these agents may increase cardiac output, and the drug often is used for this purpose and has been shown to prolong life in patients with cardiomyopathy and after myocardial infarction. As a result of the decrease in angiotensin II levels, plasma renin activity increases and aldosterone production decreases. The antihypertensive effectiveness of ACE inhibitors is enhanced when they are used in combination with a diuretic. Effectiveness of ACE inhibitors is quite similar in white and black hypertensive patients who are also receiving a diuretic. In addition, ACE inhibitors blunt diuretic-induced hypokalemia.

At present, 10 ACE inhibitors are available: benazepril, captopril, cilazapril, enalapril, fosinopril, lisinopril, per-

Table 60B-11 Angiotensin-converting enzyme inhibitors

Type of drug	Usual dosage range, total mg/day	Frequency	Adverse effects
Benazepril	10-40	Once or twice	Cough, rash, angioneurotic edema, hypercalcemia, dysgeusia, renal failure in patients with bilateral renal artery stenosis, occasional hypotension in patients receiving diuretics, neutropenia, proteinuria
Captopril	12.5-150	Twice	
Cilazapril	2.5-50	Once or twice	
Enalapril	2.5-40	Once or twice	
Fosinopril	10-40	Once or twice	
Lisinopril	5-40	Once or twice	
Perindopril	1-16	Once or twice	
Quinapril	5-80	Once or twice	
Ramipril	1.25-20	Once or twice	
Spirapril	12.5-50	Once or twice	

indopril, quinapril, ramipril, and spirapril (Table 60B-11). Food reduces the absorption of captopril. Once-daily dosing is possible with all except captopril.

Class-specific side effects of ACE inhibitors include hypotension, cough,[15] hyperkalemia, acute renal failure, and angioedema. Hypotension is more common in patients who are in a high renin state, usually as the result of associated diuretic use. Cough may be the most common side effect of the ACE inhibitors. Although earlier studies suggested an incidence of 1% to 3%, newer studies suggest a much higher incidence, in the range of 13% to 24%.[16] The cough tends to be nocturnal and nonproductive. Rash, angioneurotic edema, and taste disturbances are other side effects, but they are less commonly noted with this class of drugs. ACE inhibitors can cause reversible acute renal failure in patients with severe bilateral renal artery stenosis (or in patients with a solitary kidney and unilateral stenosis).[17] Hyperkalemia can occur in persons with renal insufficiency or hyporeninemic hypoaldosteronism.

ACE inhibitors do not seem to produce glucose intolerance or any significant changes in lipid metabolism. The role of ACE inhibitors in decreasing proteinuria and the rate of progression of chronic renal failure is gaining interest, especially in diabetic patients. An important feature of ACE inhibitors is the reduction of efferent arteriolar tone in the kidney. These agents thereby reduce transcapillary glomerular pressures and reduce proteinuria, particularly in diabetes. Whether this effect slows progression of renal failure is currently under study. However, the potential for ACE inhibitors to produce hyperkalemia should be recognized when these agents are considered for use in an azotemic patient.

Overall, the ACE inhibitors are extremely well tolerated and have a low incidence of side effects, attributes that may improve long-term adherence to therapy. Although these agents are expensive, their relative lack of side effects and their antihypertensive effectiveness in patients with a variety of disease states make them of interest for use.

Central agonists

Drugs of this group—methyldopa, clonidine, guanabenz, and guanfacine (Table 60B-12)—are currently believed to lower arterial pressure by stimulation of central inhibitory α-adrenergic receptors. The blood pressure falls due to a decrease in peripheral resistance. These drugs act centrally to reduce sympathetic activity, and they all tend to have similar side effects, including sedation and dry mouth. Before β-blocking drugs became available, methyldopa was the most common second-step drug. Guanabenz can be used alone as well as with other drugs.

Methyldopa. This is most often used with a diuretic but may be used alone.[18] It does not affect cardiac function, but there may be some slowing of the heart rate due to the decrease in sympathetic outflow. Renal function does not decrease, and thus the drug frequently is used in patients with renal impairment. Renin levels may decrease.

There are three major side effects: drug fever, hepatic disease, and Coombs-positive hemolytic anemia. The drug fever presents early in the course of therapy as a flulike illness and abates quickly with discontinuation of the drug. Liver abnormalities occur later with elevated transaminase value, fever, and jaundice. Hepatic necrosis with fatality is rare. Patients who have active hepatic disease should not be given methyldopa. With prolonged therapy (usually 6 to 12 months), 10% to 20% of patients have a positive Coombs test. Rarely is this associated with a hemolytic anemia. Although it cannot be predicted in which patients the hemolytic anemia will develop, usually a positive Coombs test does not necessitate discontinuation of the drug, only close monitoring.

The usual starting dose of methyldopa is 250 mg two to four times daily. Sedation is the most frequent side effect. Fortunately, this abates somewhat with prolonged therapy, and most patients tolerate the drug well.

Clonidine. This drug stimulates central α-adrenoceptors in the pons and medulla, causing a decrease in arterial pressure and heart rate.[19] Clonidine can be used as single-drug therapy[20] or in combinations in patients with mild to moderate hypertension. This drug does not have the potentially serious side effects of methyldopa,

Table 60B-12 Adrenergic agonists, rauwolfia alkaloids, and vasodilators

Type of drug	Usual dosage range, total mg/day	Frequency	Adverse effects
Centrally activating α-agonists			
Clonidine	0.1-1.2	Twice	Sedation, dry mouth, fatigue, dizziness, rebound hypertension with abrupt discontinuance
Clonidine-TTS (patch)	0.1-0.3	Once weekly	
Guanabenz	4-64	Twice	
Guanfacine	1-3	Once	
Methyldopa	250-2,000	Twice daily	
Peripherally acting adrenergic antagonists			
Guanadrel	10-75	Twice	Diarrhea, exercise and orthostatic hypotension
Guanethidine	10-100	Once	
Rauwolfia alkaloids			
Rauwolfia root	50-200	Once	Lethargy, nasal congestion, depression
Reserpine	0.05-0.25	Once	
Direct vasodilators			
Hydralazine	50-300	Twice or four times	Tachycardia, lupus erythematosus syndrome, aggravation of angina, fluid retention
Minoxidil	2.5-80	Once or twice	Tachycardia, hypertrichosis, aggravation of angina, fluid retention

but sedation and dry mouth are frequent problems. These effects also seem to decrease somewhat with continued therapy. One serious problem that occurs with clonidine (and also may occur with β-blockers, methyldopa, and guanabenz) is the "acute withdrawal syndrome." This is the development of exacerbation of the hypertension on abrupt withdrawal of the drug.[21] Although this response is uncommon, patients should be warned (as are patients with coronary artery disease taking β-blockers) about the advisability of not discontinuing the drug abruptly. When this complication does arise, reinitiation of clonidine therapy or the intravenous administration of phentolamine will decrease the blood pressure.

Clonidine is usually given as 0.1 mg twice daily with gradual increases to 0.8 mg a day if needed. A transdermal patch is available to be applied only once weekly in doses of 0.1 to 0.3 mg.

Guanabenz. The mechanism of action of this drug is similar to that of the two drugs above. The major advantage of it is that sodium retention, leading to edema formation, is less frequent and thus there is less need for concomitant diuretic therapy than with methyldopa or clonidine. Drowsiness and dry mouth still occur, however, but also are reported to abate with prolonged therapy. The "acute withdrawal syndrome" occurs with this drug as with the other two drugs in this group.

Guanabenz can be used as a single drug in mild to moderate hypertension.[22] The usual starting dose is 4 mg twice daily.

Guanfacine. This central-acting α_2-adrenoceptor agonist is used in patients with mild to moderate hypertension who have not had an adequate response to a thiazide-type diuretic. Sedation or drowsiness is the major side effect. Patients should be cautioned not to stop taking the drug abruptly, because rebound can occur, manifested by increases in blood pressure, nervousness, or anxiety. The usual dose is 1 mg (given in the evening to minimize somnolence) along with thiazide diuretic therapy.

Peripherally acting adrenergic antagonists and rauwolfia alkaloids

These drugs—reserpine, rauwolfia root, guanethidine, and guanadrel (see Table 60B-12)—are peripherally acting adrenergic blocking agents: they act by interfering with the release of norepinephrine at the sympathetic nerve terminal. Reserpine acts by inhibiting norepinephrine uptake into storage vesicles, thereby depleting norepinephrine in the postganglionic neurons.[23] Guanethidine also acts in the postganglionic neurons but by displacing norepinephrine in the storage vesicles; thus, less norepinephrine is available for release from the nerve ending.[24] Guanadrel inhibits norepinephrine release from storage sites and causes depletion of norepinephrine from nerve endings.[25]

Reserpine is used less than it once was because of the availability of more potent antihypertensive drugs with more tolerable side effects. Reserpine is most effective when combined with a diuretic and is most often used with the "fixed-combination" type of antihypertensive. These combinations add convenience to a drug program but are not recommended for initial therapy, because the physician cannot adjust the dosage to establish an ideal medical program. Reserpine is one of a number of the rauwolfia alkaloids and derivative drugs used. All of these, such as rauwolfia serpentina and deserpidine, have similar actions.

The major side effects that cause reserpine to be less than an ideal drug are nasal congestion, drowsiness, sedation, and depression. Often, patients with these side effects will not recognize them as caused by the drug until the drug is discontinued; then, their sense of well-being is improved.

Reserpine is usually given in a dosage of 0.1 to 0.25 mg/day in a single dose. Up to 1.0 mg/day can be used but with increasing side effects.

Guanethidine is used in the management of more severe hypertension. Unlike reserpine, it does not enter the brain, and thus two major side effects, fatigue and depression, do not occur. The use of this drug also is declining because of more effective therapy with newer drugs. However, guanethidine is an extremely potent agent, and because its dose-response curve is steep, increasing dosage markedly increases the hypotensive effect in the upright position. The drug has little effect on the supine blood pressure. Thus, the major side effect is postural hypotension, particularly upon arising.

Guanethidine is usually used in combination with a diuretic drug or a diuretic plus another agent such as α-methyldopa. Most often, therapy with this drug is reserved for the patient in whom other drugs have failed or cannot be used. From 10 mg up to several hundred milligrams can be administered, but most often the range is 10 to 50 mg before intolerable side effects occur. For patients with postural hypotensive side effects, we recommend that they arise slowly (especially in the morning), elevate the head of their bed at night, and wear elastic stockings. Another common side effect of the drug is loose stools or diarrhea, most often occurring in the morning. Often this can be tolerated by the addition of an antidiarrhea agent such as diphenoxylate when it is necessary to add guanethidine.

Guanadrel does not cross the blood-brain barrier and thus central nervous system side effects are said not to occur. However, the major side effects do include fatigue and drowsiness. It is approved for use in patients not responding to diuretic therapy, and its effectiveness is enhanced with a thiazide diuretic. The drug reduces both systolic and diastolic pressures, heart rate, and total peripheral resistance. The usual starting dose is 5 mg twice daily.

Vasodilators

Vasodilator drugs—hydralazine[26] and minoxidil[27] (see Table 60B-12)—act directly on the blood vessel wall to produce vasodilation.

Hydralazine. The mechanism of action is complex and may involve chelation of certain metallic ions.[28] The drug acts by producing relaxation of the smooth muscle of the vessel wall, predominantly in arterioles and small arteries rather than in veins. This vasodilation results in a decrease in blood pressure, which induces a reflex tachycardia, and this is a major side effect of the drug. The tachycardia is controlled by the use of β-blocking drugs. The increase in plasma renin level that would result from the vasodilation is prevented by the β-blocker.

The lupus-like syndrome that is a complication of hydralazine therapy is infrequent with dosages of 200 mg/day or less. Most patients who have had this complication were taking 400 mg or more a day.[29] When hydralazine is added to a diuretic-plus-β-blocker program, the usual starting dose is 10 to 25 mg four times daily.

Minoxidil. This is a potent antihypertensive drug that acts directly on vascular smooth muscle.[27] Its use generally is reserved for patients with severe hypertension or with renal insufficiency. It is a potent vasodilator, and fluid retention is a problem; the use of a diuretic is needed. It can cause not only severe fluid retention but also occasionally pericardial effusion and even tamponade. Minoxidil can be used with a β-blocker as part of a "triple-therapy" program.

An unusual side effect of the drug is the production of increased hair growth over the face and extremities. This effect is reversible.

The recommended initial dose is 5 mg once daily; the dose can be increased to 50 mg/day as needed.

Individualized therapy

Although the agents currently available are effective, with relatively few side effects, additional considerations may favor one agent over another. Safety and efficacy should be considered in selecting antihypertensive therapy. Safety considerations must include both objective manifestations of toxic effects and subjective experiences that may affect patient acceptance.

The demographics of hypertension have assumed a more important role in therapeutic decisions. Specifically, it is becoming increasingly apparent that factors such as age and race of a patient, levels of hormonal indices, such as plasma renin activity, and coexisting disease may dictate the choice of one agent rather than another. In older hypertensive patients, in whom low-renin status is common, calcium entry blockers and diuretics have increased efficacy. In younger hypertensive patients, in whom renin-dependent mechanisms are usually important, β-adrenergic blockers and ACE inhibitors are more effective. However, this strategy is not absolute.

It has become increasingly clear that antihypertensive therapy will be successful only if it is effective in reducing arterial pressure and is well tolerated by the patient. To accomplish this, one must consider patient-related factors such as age, race, and duration of increased blood pressure. The hemodynamic characteristics of hypertension vary with age and other factors. In addition, different antihypertensive agents produce different hemodynamic effects. The most appropriate therapeutic strategy matches the needs of the individual patient with the actions of the drug.

In stage 1 or stage 2 hypertension, single-drug therapy, usually with a diuretic or β-blocker, often is adequate. Stage 3 or stage 4 hypertension often does not respond to single-drug therapy and may require double- or triple-drug therapy. The choice of drugs often depends on concomitant disease or conditions. Hypertension should be considered resistant if blood pressure cannot be controlled with maximum triple therapy. Reassessment of causes of hypertension should be considered in addition to reviewing whether the patient is indeed taking the medication as prescribed.

Isolated systolic hypertension often occurs in older patients and is characterized by loss of arterial compliance due to aging. Lifestyle modifications should be attempted, but if the systolic pressure remains above 160 mm Hg, drug therapy should be strongly considered. Alternatively, lowering the diastolic pressure excessively in older patients may increase the risks in those with coronary artery disease ("J-curve" hypothesis).[30,31] Cautious attempts to lower the systolic pressure below 160 mm Hg and the diastolic below 90 mm Hg are supported by evidence, even in the elderly.[32]

As many as 60% of patients with hypertension have concomitant disease and may be unable to tolerate certain classes of drugs. A list of preferred drugs for those with concomitant disease is outlined in Table 60B-13.

Table 60B-13 Concomitant diseases and recommended monotherapy

Disease	Recommended drug	Relative contraindication
Angina	β-blocker, Ca entry blocker	Direct vasodilators
Congestive heart failure		
Systolic	Diuretic, ACE inhibitor	Ca entry blocker,* β-blocker*
Diastolic	Ca entry blocker, β-blocker	
Peripheral vascular disease	Ca entry blocker, ACE inhibitor	β-blocker, diuretic
Diabetes	ACE inhibitor, Ca entry blocker	β-blocker, diuretic
Chronic obstructive pulmonary disease	Ca entry blocker, ACE inhibitor, diuretic	β-blocker
Hyperlipidemia	ACE inhibitor, Ca entry blocker	β-blocker, diuretic
Arrhythmia	β-blocker, Ca entry blocker	Diuretic
Gout		Diuretic

ACE, angiotensin-converting enzyme; Ca, calcium.
*May be useful in some circumstances.

HYPERTENSIVE URGENCIES AND EMERGENCIES

A list of drugs useful in the treatment of hypertensive urgencies and emergencies is in Tables 60B-14 and 60B-15. The term "hypertensive urgency" refers to severe systolic or diastolic hypertension, the systolic exceeding 200 mm Hg and the diastolic, 120 mm Hg. Patients presenting in this hypertensive state rarely have target-organ damage, and the pressure should be reduced over hours to days. Oral therapy may be adequate. A hypertensive emergency is severe elevation causing functional disturbance in the central nervous system, heart, or kidneys and requires rapid reduction of the pressure to prevent worsening of the underlying clinical conditions. Hypertensive emergencies cannot be defined by a specific systolic or diastolic pressure. Parenteral therapy is usually indicated.

A diastolic pressure of 120 mm Hg is severe hypertension but may not require rapid or even early treatment. Alcoholic patients or very apprehensive persons sometimes present with blood pressure in this range. However, such blood pressure values may indicate the presence of severe sustained, so-called urgent, hypertension, malignant hypertension, or hypertensive encephalopathy. Usually, a brief history and physical examination will aid in deciding whether an emergency exists. Patients who have a history of marked variations in blood pressure, are mentally clear, and have negative results on neurologic examination and normal funduscopic findings are unlikely to require emergency treatment. On the other hand, a patient with severe headache, confusion, funduscopic hemorrhages, cotton-wool exudates, and papilledema needs immediate hospitalization and therapy.

Because more patients with mild or moderate essential hypertension are receiving successful drug therapy, malignant hypertension occurs less often. Currently, many patients who present with severe or malignant hypertension have recognizable underlying causes. There are a number of conditions in which the outstanding physical finding at presentation is severe elevation of the blood pressure; these include cerebral hemorrhage, reactions to lysergic acid diethylamide or phencyclidine ("angel dust"), pulmonary edema, and dissecting aortic aneurysm. Whatever the cause, severely elevated blood pressure with cerebral and funduscopic abnormalities requires therapy.

Patients with hypertensive encephalopathy have headache, neurologic abnormalities, nausea, and vomiting. They may have convulsions and progress to coma. Treatment is a true medical emergency.

Malignant hypertension (presence of papilledema is mandatory by definition) most often is a change from previous mild or moderate hypertension with "acceleration." A necrotizing arteriolitis is the underlying pathologic state. Renal failure, congestive heart failure, cerebral hemorrhage, microangiopathic hemolytic anemia, and hypertensive encephalopathy may be part of the clinical picture. Urgent treatment is clearly necessary.

Today, a large number of useful drugs are available for therapy. With control of the acute hypertension, the most frequent problem is renal insufficiency of varying degree. With prolonged and successful antihypertensive therapy there may be some improvement in renal function, but if

Table 60B-14 Orally administered drugs for hypertension urgencies and emergencies

Type of drug	Dosage, mg	Frequency	Onset of action, minutes	Adverse effects
Captopril	25	Repeat as needed	15-30	Hypotension, renal failure in bilateral renal artery stenosis
Clonidine	0.1-0.2	Every hour as required	30-60	Hypotension, dry mouth, heart block
Labetalol	100	Repeat in 1-2 hr	30-120	Heart block, bronchoconstriction
Minoxidil	2.5-5	Repeat after 2-3 hr	30-120	Hypotension, tachycardia
Nifedipine	10	Repeat as needed	15-30	Hypotension

Table 60B-15 Parenterally administered drugs for hypertension urgencies and emergencies

Type of drug	Dosage	Onset, minutes	Adverse effects
Vasodilators			
Nitroprusside	0.25-10 μg/kg/min IV infusion	Instantaneous	Nausea, vomiting, muscle twitching, methemoglobinemia, thiocyanate intoxication
Nitroglycerin	5-100 μg/min IV infusion	2-5	Headache, tachycardia, vomiting, flushing, methemoglobinemia
Diazoxide	50-150 mg IV bolus IV infusion	1-2	Hypotension, increase in angina, nausea, vomiting, hyperglycemia
Hydralazine	10-40 mg IV bolus 10-40 mg IM/10 min	20-30	Tachycardia, headache, vomiting, increase in angina
Enalaprilat	0.625-1.25 mg IV every 6 hr	15	Hypotension, renal failure in patients with bilateral renal artery stenosis
Nicardipine	5-10 mg/hr IV	10	Tachycardia, headache, flushing, local phlebitis
Adrenergic inhibitors			
Phentolamine	5-15 mg IV bolus	1-2	Tachycardia, flushing
Trimethaphan	1-4 mg/min IV infusion	1-5	Paresis of bowel and bladder, orthostatic hypotension, dry mouth, blurred vision
Esmolol	500 μg/kg/min for 4 min 50-300 μg/kg/min IV	1-2	Hypotension
Labetalol	20-80 mg IV bolus every 10 min	5-10	Bronchoconstriction, heart block, orthostatic hypotension
Methyldopa	250-500 mg IV infusion every 6 hr	30-60	Drowsiness

severe impairment is present, normal function cannot be expected to return.

A drug often used for immediate treatment is sodium nitroprusside;[33] it has a direct action on the smooth muscle of arteries and veins. All types of hypertension are responsive to this drug. It must be given intravenously, and it has an immediate effect. By titrating the dose carefully, one can establish nearly any desired blood pressure level. In patients with congestive heart failure, afterload reduction is an added benefit. Another advantage of the drug is the almost immediate disappearance of its effects when its administration is stopped. The major toxic effect is due to its metabolic product, thiocyanate, which is excreted by the kidneys and may accumulate rapidly in the presence of renal failure. Symptoms of thiocyanate toxicity include nausea, anorexia, and confusion. Blood levels of thiocyanate may be determined if a question of toxicity arises, but because the drug usually is required for only 24 to 48 hours, this measurement is rarely needed if other antihypertensive therapy is begun. Cyanide toxicity is a potential but rare problem and occurs in individuals with a deficiency of a specific enzyme.

Several of the newer drugs may have a place in the urgent therapy of hypertension. These include captopril,[34] clonidine,[35] nifedipine,[36] prazosin,[13] minoxidil,[27] and labetalol.[37] They have been used by "oral loading" in a limited number of patients.

Nifedipine has been particularly useful in the treatment of "urgent" hypertension (severe hypertension without end-organ damage). A chewed capsule of 10 or 20 mg of nifedipine can be expected to result in a 20- to 30-mm decrease in diastolic pressure in 45 minutes in most but not all patients.[38] Labetalol or esmolol given intravenously by bolus and by infusion results in a significant decrease in diastolic pressure. Esmolol is effective in 1 to 2 minutes, labetalol in 5 to 10 minutes.

THERAPY OF SECONDARY HYPERTENSION

Although the majority of hypertensive patients have essential hypertension, a small number of patients have a known cause for their increased blood pressure. These causes include conditions such as acute or chronic glomerulonephritis, scleroderma with renal disease, and periarteritis nodosa. These diseases require specific medical therapy and dietary restrictions in addition to antihypertensive drug therapy. The most common problem in these diseases with secondary hypertension is the presence of renal insufficiency. Loop diuretics, β-adrenergic blockers, calcium blocking drugs, clonidine, methyldopa, hydralazine, and minoxidil are particularly useful for chronic therapy of these types of problems. Captopril is also useful in reduced dosage (because it is excreted mainly by the kidney).

Patients with mineralocorticoid excess may require surgical therapy, depending upon the underlying adrenal lesion. In some patients who produce aldosterone excess, spironolactone and amiloride can be used successfully as antihypertensive therapy. In others, drugs such as clonidine, methyldopa, or prazosin may be needed.

In patients with pheochromocytoma, surgical removal after preoperative preparation is the appropriate treatment. Preoperative preparation by blocking α-adrenergic receptors with phenoxybenzamine followed by β-blockade usually will normalize the blood pressure. β-Blockade should not be used until α-blockade is achieved; otherwise, severe hypertension can result. Prazosin, an α-receptor blocker, has also been used in a limited number of patients. Finally, in patients with inoperable malignant pheochromocytoma, L-methyltyrosine can be used to block catecholamine synthesis. Phentolamine or nitroprusside given intravenously can be used to control the pressure on an emergency basis or during operation.

Many patients with renal artery disease will be treated medically in the same manner as patients with essential hypertension because of the presence of other serious medical conditions, age, or the mildness of the blood pressure elevation. Percutaneous transluminal renal angioplasty can now be offered to many patients in place of surgical repair. The advantage of this method is that it can be used in many patients who would be considered inoperable by any other approach.

SUMMARY

The following points discussed in this chapter regarding therapy are likely to remain as basic principles.

1. Establish the presence of hypertension by appropriate examination.
2. By means of the history, physical examination, and selected laboratory tests, ensure that the patient is unlikely to have a secondary form of hypertension.
3. By means of the history, physical examination, and selected laboratory tests, be sure that associated conditions that may affect the choice of therapy are identified.
4. Educate the patient about his or her disease.
5. Use nonpharmacologic therapy in selected patients.
6. Begin drug therapy with the simplest program possible.
7. Add to or change the drug program slowly.
8. Establish a pattern of periodic blood pressure checks along with selected laboratory tests.

REFERENCES

1. The Fifth Report of the Joint National Committee on the Detection, Evaluation, and Treatment of High Blood Pressure (JNCV). NIH Publication, 1992

2. Blood Pressure Study, 1979. Chicago, Society of Actuaries and Association of Life Insurance Medical Directors of America, 1980

3. The National High Blood Pressure Education Program Coordinating Committee: National High Blood Pressure Education Program Working Group report on ambulatory blood pressure monitoring. *Arch Intern Med* 150:2270-2280, 1990

4. Foote A, Erfurt JC: Hypertension control at the work site: comparison of screening and referral alone, referral and follow-up, and on-site treatment. *N Engl J Med* 308:809-813, 1983

5. Arkwright PD, Beilin LJ, Rouse I, et al: Effects of alcohol use and other aspects of lifestyle on blood pressure levels and prevalence of hypertension in a working population. *Circulation* 66:60-66, 1982

6. Sannerstedt R: Hemodynamic response to exercise in patients with arterial hypertension. *Acta Med Scand* [*Suppl*] 458:1-83, 1966

7. Román O, Camuzzi AL, Villalón E, et al: Physical training program in arterial rehabilitation: a long-term prospective follow-up. *Cardiology* 67:230-243, 1981

8. Physical exercise in the management of hypertension: a consensus statement by the World Hypertension League. *J Hypertens* 9:283-287, 1991

9. Arroll B, Beaglehole R: Does physical activity lower blood pressure: a critical review of the clinical trials. *J Clin Epidemiol* 45:439-447, 1992

10. McMahon FG, Ryan JR, Akdamar K, et al: Upper gastrointestinal lesions after potassium chloride supplements: a controlled trial. *Lancet* 2:1059-1061, 1982

11. Alhenc-Gelas F, Plouin P-F, Ducrocq M-B, et al: Comparison of the antihypertensive and hormonal effects of a cardioselective beta-blocker, acebutolol, and diuretics in essential hypertension. *Am J Med* 64:1005-1012, 1978

12. Fagard R, Amery A, Reybrouck T, et al: Response of the systemic and pulmonary circulation to alpha- and beta-receptor blockade (labetalol) at rest and during exercise in hypertensive patients. *Circulation* 60:1214-1219, 1979

13. Colucci WS: Alpha-adrenergic receptor blockade with prazosin: consideration of hypertension, heart failure, and potential new applications. *Ann Intern Med* 97:67-77, 1982

14. Vidt DG, Bravo EL, Fouad FM: Captopril. *N Engl J Med* 306:214-219, 1982

15. Williams GH: Converting-enzyme inhibitors in the treatment of hypertension. *N Engl J Med* 319:1517-1525, 1988

16. Goldszer RC, Lilly LS, Solomon HS: Prevalence of cough during angiotensin-converting enzyme inhibitor therapy. *Am J Med* 85:887, 1988

17. Hricik DE, Browning PJ, Kopelman R, et al: Captopril-induced functional renal insufficiency in patients with bilateral renal-artery stenoses or renal-artery stenosis in a solitary kidney. *N Engl J Med* 308:373-376, 1983

18. Frohlich ED: Methyldopa: mechanisms and treatment 25 years later. *Arch Intern Med* 140:954-959, 1980

19. Van Zwieten PA, Timmermans PB: Basic pharmacology of centrally acting antihypertensive drugs. *Cardiovasc Rev Rep* 3:1079-1093, 1982

20. Thananopavarn C, Golub MS, Eggena P, et al: Clonidine, a centrally acting sympathetic inhibitor, as monotherapy for mild to moderate hypertension. *Am J Cardiol* 49:153-158, 1982

21. Lilja M, Jounela AJ, Juustila HJ, et al: Abrupt and gradual change from clonidine to beta blockers in hypertension. *Acta Med Scand* 211:375-380, 1982

22. McMahon FG, Ryan JR, Jain AK, et al: Guanabenz in essential hypertension. *Clin Pharmacol Ther* 21:272-277, 1977

23. Koelle GB: Neuromuscular blocking agents. In *The Pharmacological Basis of Therapeutics.* Fifth edition. Edited by LS Goodman, A Gilman. New York, Macmillan Publishing Co, 1975, pp 575-588

24. Woosley RL, Nies AS: Guanethidine. *N Engl J Med* 295:1053-1057, 1976

25. Nugent CA, Palmer JD, Ursprung JJ: Guanadrel sulfate compared with methyldopa for mild and moderate hypertension. *Pharmacotherapy* 2:378-383, 1982

26. Freis ED, Rose JC, Higgins TF, et al: The hemodynamic effects of hypotensive drugs in man. IV. 1-Hydrazinophthalazine. *Circulation* 8:199-204, 1953

27. Pettinger WA: Minoxidil and the treatment of severe hypertension. *N Engl J Med* 303:922-926, 1980

28. Merrill DH, Kenyon K: 1-Hydrazinophthalazine (Apresoline) in the treatment of hypertensive disease: a clinical trial with a control group. *Am J Med Sci* 226:623-631, 1953

29. Alarcón-Segovia D, Wakim KG, Worthington JW, et al: Clinical and experimental studies on the hydralazine syndrome and its relationship to systemic lupus erythematosus. *Medicine (Baltimore)* 46:1-33, 1967

30. Farnett L, Mulrow CD, Linn WD, et al: The J-curve phenomenon and the treatment of hypertension. Is there a point beyond which pressure reduction is dangerous? *JAMA* 265:489-495, 1991

31. Fletcher AE, Bulpitt CJ: How far should blood pressure be lowered? *N Engl J Med* 326:251-254, 1992

32. SHEP Cooperative Research Group: Prevention of stroke by antihypertensive drug treatment in older persons with isolated systolic hypertension. Final results of the Systolic Hypertension in the Elderly Program (SHEP). *JAMA* 265:3255-3264, 1991

33. Ahearn DJ, Grim CE: Treatment of malignant hypertension with sodium nitroprusside. *Arch Intern Med* 133:187-191, 1974

34. Case DB, Atlas SA, Sullivan PA, et al: Acute and chronic treatment of severe and malignant hypertension with the oral angiotensin-converting enzyme inhibitor captopril. *Circulation* 64:765-771, 1981

35. Anderson RJ, Hart GR, Crumpler CP, et al: Oral clonidine loading in hypertensive urgencies. *JAMA* 246:848-850, 1981

36. Guazzi MD, Fiorentini C, Olivari MT, et al: Short- and long-term efficacy of a calcium-antagonistic agent (nifedipine) combined with methyldopa in the treatment of severe hypertension. *Circulation* 61:913-919, 1980

37. Cosentino F, Vidt DG, Orlowski JP, et al: The safety of cumulative doses of labetalol in perioperative hypertension. *Cleve Clin J Med* 56:371-376, 1989

38. Jaker M, Atkin S, Soto M, et al: Oral nifedipine vs oral clonidine in the treatment of urgent hypertension. *Arch Intern Med* 149:260-265, 1989

CHAPTER

61

Pulmonary hypertension

Michael D. McGoon, M.D., Valentin Fuster, M.D., William K. Freeman, M.D., William D. Edwards, M.D., and John P. Scott, M.D.

DEFINITION

The term "pulmonary hypertension" does not refer to a disease in itself but is a description of the hemodynamic consequence of various conditions that lead to a chronic increase in the pulmonary arterial pressure. Pulmonary arterial pressure consistently in excess of 35 mm Hg systolic, 15 mm Hg diastolic, and 25 mm Hg mean may be regarded as indicative of pulmonary hypertension. Pulmonary arterial pressure (PA) is related to the pulmonary venous pressure (PV), pulmonary arterial blood flow (Qp), and pulmonary vascular or arteriolar resistance (R):

$$\text{Qp (L/min/m}^2\text{)} = \frac{\text{PA} - \text{PV (mm Hg)}}{\text{R (U} \cdot \text{m}^2\text{)}}$$

The pathophysiology, pathology, clinical and diagnostic features, and treatment are determined by the underlying cause (Table 61-1) as well as by the degree of pulmonary hypertension per se.

PATHOPHYSIOLOGY

The stimulus for development of pulmonary hypertension may occur at any point in the pulmonary circuit, from the left-sided vascular region and cardiac chambers to the right-sided cardiac chambers. Pulmonary arterial hypertension may be produced by four different pathophysiologic mechanisms (Fig 61-1).

1. *High pulmonary venous pressure* leads to a passive increase in the pulmonary artery pressure and, often, to superimposed arteriolar constriction. The increase in pulmonary vascular resistance may further increase the pulmonary arterial pressure.

2. In *pulmonary parenchymal disease,* hypoxia-related constriction and anatomic destruction of the microvascular bed lead to an increase in the pulmonary vascular resistance, and so to pulmonary arterial hypertension.

3. In *primary vascular obstructive disorders* of the lungs, there is a predominant increase in the pulmonary vascular resistance which leads to pulmonary arterial hypertension.

4. In *congenital left-to-right shunts,* as in atrial septal defect, over a period of many years the large pulmonary flow can produce a reactive hyperplasia in the arteriolar wall and anatomic reduction of the vascular bed. This increase in pulmonary vascular resistance occasionally may lead to progressive pulmonary arterial hypertension, reversal of the shunt, and appearance of cyanosis (Eisenmenger's syndrome).

In other anomalies, such as large ventricular septal defect, the combination, from birth, of a large pulmonary flow and high pulmonary pressure (due to the open communication between the systemic and pulmonary circulations) with pulmonary venous hypertension (due to the left ventricular volume overload causing failure) contributes to the development of Eisenmenger's syndrome. This process may take up to 2 decades. In addition, when cyanosis with polycythemia supervenes, the increased blood viscosity further impedes blood flow.

PATHOLOGY

Normal pulmonary vasculature

The pulmonary arteries, both elastic and muscular, normally are thin walled (Fig 61-2). In the systemic arteries, the ratio of the medial thickness to the external arterial diameter is normally 20% to 25%, but in pulmonary arteries the ratio is less than 10% and usually averages about 5% (Table 61-2). Elastic arteries function as compliant conduits and generally are larger than 1 mm in diameter, whereas the muscular pulmonary arteries, which primarily control vascular resistance, tend to be smaller than 1 mm in diameter (Table 61-3).

Because pulmonary arterioles lie within the alveolar walls and normally contain little or no medial smooth muscle (see Fig 61-2), they contribute little to pulmonary vascular resistance. Hence, the clinical term "pulmonary arteriolar resistance" is anatomically inaccurate.

Pulmonary capillaries and lymphatics form the microcirculation. Normally, most capillary beds in the lungs are only partially open. However, if pulmonary blood flow increases (with exercise, for example), capillary beds open to accommodate the increased blood volume. In this manner, pulmonary blood flow may increase without an appreciable increase in pulmonary vascular resistance.

The pulmonary veins and venules are normally thin walled (see Fig 61-2); the medial thickness averages 3% to

Table 61-1 Pathophysiologic and etiologic classification of pulmonary hypertension

1. Pulmonary venous hypertension
   - Thoracic aorta
     - Coarctation of the aorta
     - Supravalvular aortic stenosis
   - Left ventricle
     - Aortic stenosis or insufficiency
     - Congenital subaortic stenosis
     - Hypertrophic cardiomyopathy
     - Constrictive pericarditis
     - Myocardial disease of various etiologies
     - Mitral stenosis or incompetence
   - Left atrium
     - Ball-valve thrombus
     - Myxoma
     - Cor triatriatum
   - Pulmonary veins
     - Congenital pulmonary vein stenosis
     - Mediastinitis or mediastinal fibrosis
     - Mediastinal neoplasm
2. Chronic hypoxia
   - Residence at high altitude
   - Inadequate respiratory excursion
     - Extreme obesity (Pickwickian syndrome)
     - Severe kyphoscoliosis
     - Neuromuscular disorders
     - Extreme pleural fibrosis or lung resection
   - Chronic upper airway obstruction
     - Congenital webs
     - Enlarged tonsils
   - Chronic lower airway obstruction
     - Chronic bronchitis
     - Asthmatic bronchitis
     - Bronchiectasis
   - Cystic fibrosis
     - Emphysema
   - Chronic diffuse pulmonary parenchymal disease
     - Interstitial fibrosis (idiopathic, chronic pneumonitic, toxic, etc.)
     - Pneumoconioses (silicosis, asbestosis, etc.)
     - Granulomatous diseases (sarcoidosis, tuberculosis, etc.)
     - Alveolar filling disorders (alveolar proteinosis, etc.)
     - Connective tissue disorders (rheumatoid lung, systemic sclerosis, etc.)
3. Vascular disorders of the lung
   - Primary vascular disease
     - Plexogenic pulmonary arteriopathy
     - Connective tissue disorders (lupus, systemic sclerosis)
   - Thrombotic disease
     - Sickle cell disease
     - Pulmonary veno-occlusive disease
   - Embolic disease
     - Persistent large pulmonary emboli
     - Recurrent pulmonary emboli
     - Tumor emboli (e.g., breast carcinoma)
     - Schistosomiasis
4. Left-to-right shunts
   - Extracardiac shunts
     - Patent ductus arteriosus
     - Aortopulmonary window
     - Rupture of aortic sinus
   - Intracardiac shunts
     - Ventricular septal defect
     - Atrial septal defect

Table 61-2 Comparison of pulmonary and systemic circulations

	Circulation	
Feature	**Pulmonary**	**Systemic**
Arterial pressure, mm Hg	22/10 (mean, 13)	120/80 (mean, 90)
Capillary pressure, mm Hg	6-9 (7)	10-30 (17)
Venous pressure, mm Hg	1-4 (2)	0-10 (6)
Arterial M:D ratio, %	3-8 (5)	15-25 (20)
Venous M:D ratio, %	2-5 (3)	3-6 (4)
Vascular resistance, U · m^2	1-4 (3)	10-25 (15)
Blood flow, L/min	5	5

M:D ratio is the ratio of thickness of media to external diameter of the vessel.

Table 61-3 Diameters of histologic types of pulmonary arteries

Histologic type	Diameter, μm	Adjacent airways
Elastic	>1,000 (1 mm)	Lobar, segmental, and subsegmental bronchi
Musculoelastic	500-1,500	Subsegmental bronchus
Muscular	50-1,000	Subsegmental bronchus, terminal bronchiole
Arteriole	15-150	Respiratory bronchiole, alveolar duct, and alveolar wall

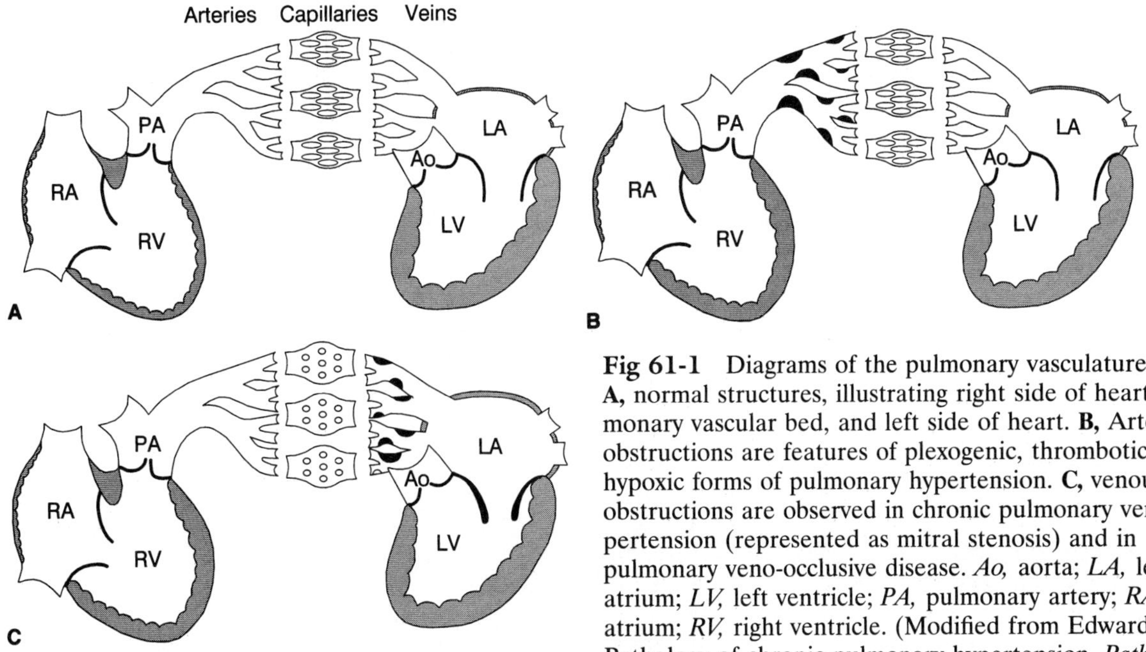

Fig 61-1 Diagrams of the pulmonary vasculature. **A,** normal structures, illustrating right side of heart, pulmonary vascular bed, and left side of heart. **B,** Arterial obstructions are features of plexogenic, thrombotic, and hypoxic forms of pulmonary hypertension. **C,** venous obstructions are observed in chronic pulmonary venous hypertension (represented as mitral stenosis) and in pulmonary veno-occlusive disease. *Ao,* aorta; *LA,* left atrium; *LV,* left ventricle; *PA,* pulmonary artery; *RA,* right atrium; *RV,* right ventricle. (Modified from Edwards JE: Pathology of chronic pulmonary hypertension. *Pathol Annu* 9:1-25, 1974.)

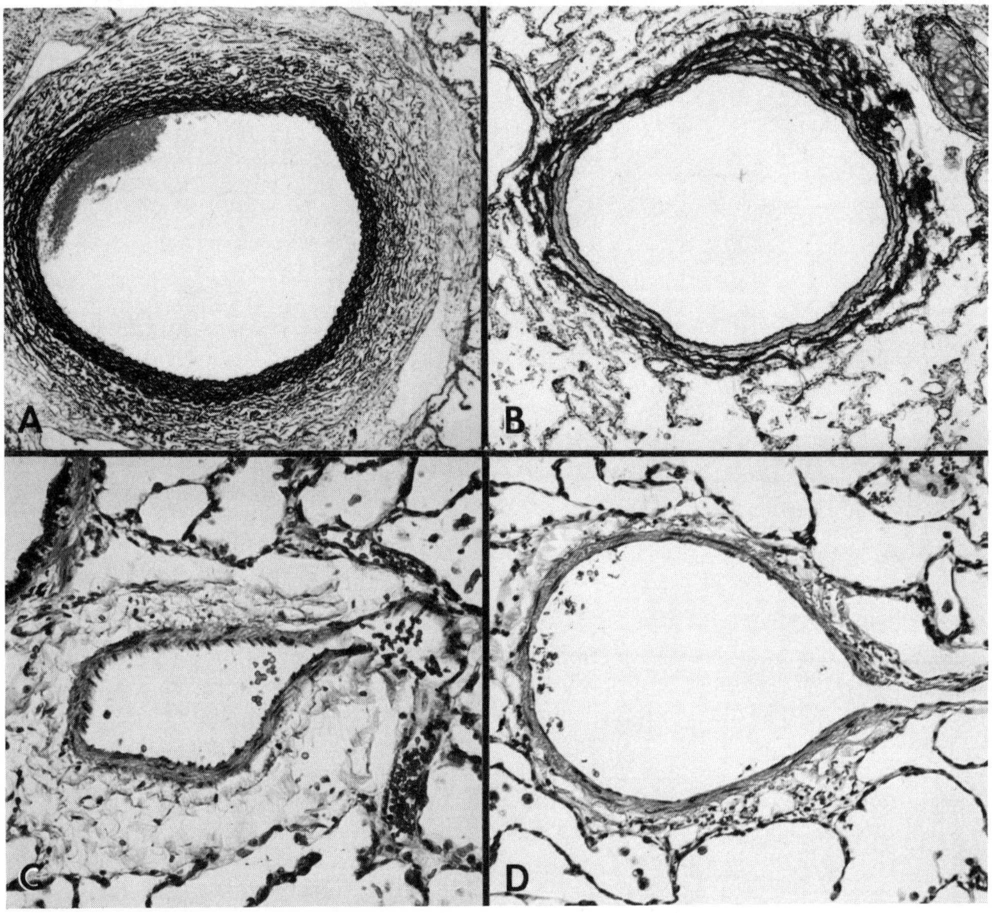

Fig 61-2 Normal pulmonary vasculature. **A,** elastic pulmonary artery. **B,** muscular pulmonary artery. **C,** small muscular pulmonary artery and nonmuscular arteriolar branch. **D,** pulmonary vein. (Elastic van Gieson; **A,** ×27, **B,** ×70; hematoxylin and eosin; **C,** ×140, **D,** ×140.)

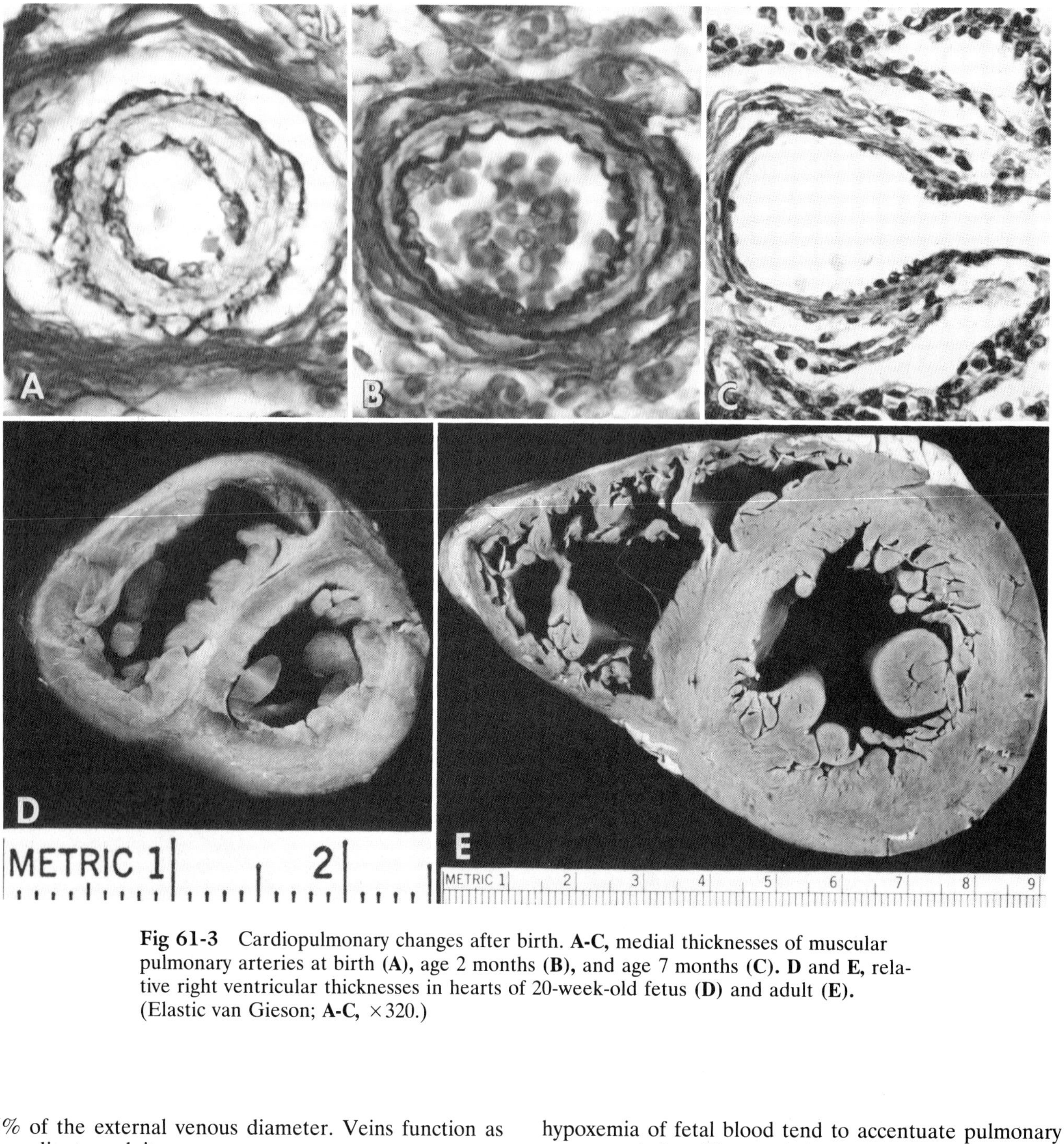

Fig 61-3 Cardiopulmonary changes after birth. **A-C,** medial thicknesses of muscular pulmonary arteries at birth **(A),** age 2 months **(B),** and age 7 months **(C). D** and **E,** relative right ventricular thicknesses in hearts of 20-week-old fetus **(D)** and adult **(E).** (Elastic van Gieson; **A-C,** ×320.)

5% of the external venous diameter. Veins function as compliant conduits.

In human lungs, arteries travel with their respective bronchi and bronchioles (and are similar in size), and veins travel within the interlobular septa. Lymphatics course through the interlobular septa and within the pleura. The bronchial arteries and veins travel along or within the bronchial walls and tend to be small.

Physiologic fetal pulmonary hypertension

During fetal life, the ductus arteriosus allows free communication between the systemic and pulmonary arteries. The collapsed state of the lungs and the relative hypoxemia of fetal blood tend to accentuate pulmonary vasoconstriction. The result is a relatively high-pressure, high-resistance pulmonary circulation with medial hypertrophy of elastic and muscular pulmonary arteries and with right ventricular hypertrophy.

At birth, changes occur that transform the pulmonary circulation into a low-pressure, low-resistance vascular bed, relative to the systemic circulation. The ductus arteriosus closes functionally during the first day of life and anatomically during the first 2 to 3 months. Furthermore, after birth, pulmonary vasoconstriction abates as the lungs expand and as arterial oxygen saturation increases. Consequently, within 4 to 6 months after birth, the anatomic hallmarks of physiologic fetal pulmonary

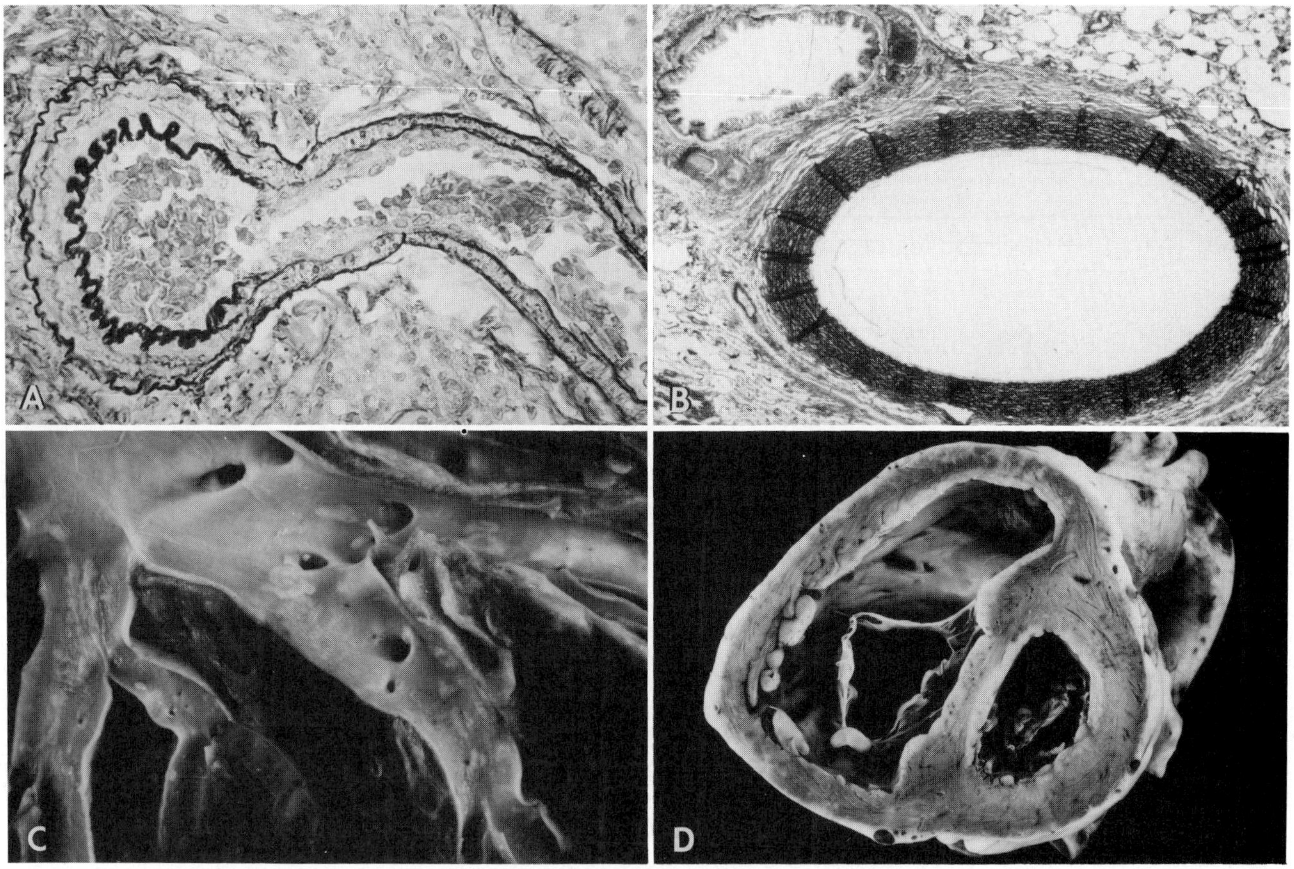

Fig 61-4 General features of chronic pulmonary hypertension. **A,** medial hypertrophy of muscular pulmonary artery, with muscular extension into arteriole. **B,** medial hypertrophy and dilatation of elastic pulmonary artery; diameter of normal artery should be similar to that of adjacent bronchus *(left upper corner).* **C,** shallow atheromas of large elastic pulmonary arteries. **D,** right ventricular hypertrophy and dilatation, with straightening of ventricular septum. (Elastic van Gieson; **A,** ×245, **B,** ×25.) (**D,** from Edwards WD, Tajik AJ, Seward JB: Standardized nomenclature and anatomic basis for regional tomographic analysis of the heart. *Mayo Clin Proc* 56:479-497, 1981. By permission, Mayo Foundation.)

hypertension have regressed: the pulmonary arteries have become thin walled, and the right ventricle is no longer hypertrophied (Fig 61-3).

General features of pulmonary hypertension

All forms of chronic pulmonary hypertension share certain features in common (Fig 61-4). The specific pathologic features of the different types of pulmonary hypertension are summarized in Table 61-4.

Secondary pulmonary hypertension. *Pulmonary venous hypertension* (Fig 61-5), the most common form of pulmonary hypertension, results from obstruction downstream from the small pulmonary veins. The vascular lesions are reversible if the cause of the obstruction can be removed, but several months to several years may be required for the vessels to return to a relatively normal functional and structural state.

Chronic alveolar hypoxia may cause pulmonary hypertension by its potent vasoconstrictor effects and eventually may result in right heart failure (cor pulmonale). The histopathologic features are summarized in Table 61-4. In cases associated with pulmonary fibrosis, the small pulmonary arteries may contain organized thrombus or may be occluded by retracted fibroelastic plugs (Fig 61-6). The nonfibrotic lesions may regress if the chronic alveolar hypoxia is reversed.

Chronic thromboembolic pulmonary hypertension (Table 61-4 and Fig 61-7) may result from recurrent or persistent pulmonary thromboembolism (usually from the deep leg veins or pelvic venous plexus). In situ thrombosis may occur with pulmonary hypertension from other causes or as a component of primary pulmonary hypertension.

Clinical primary pulmonary hypertension. Among patients with pulmonary hypertension for which no cause can be identified, three major histopathologic types have

Table 61-4 Pathologic features of pulmonary hypertension

Type of pulmonary hypertension	Right ventricle	Pulmonary arteries
Pulmonary venous hypertension (chronic)	Hypertrophy with or without dilatation	• Medial hypertrophy • Eccentric intimal proliferation or fibrosis • Dilatation and shallow intimal atheromas of elastic arteries
Chronic hypoxia	Hypertrophy with or without dilatation	• Medial hypertrophy • Eccentric intimal proliferation or fibrosis • Longitudinal smooth muscle bundles within intima, media, or adventitia of muscular arteries • Organized thrombus or retracted fibroelastic plugs may be present • Dilatation and shallow intimal atheromas of elastic arteries
Chronic major vessel thromboembolism	Hypertrophy with or without dilatation	• Organized, recanalized, endothelialized thrombi in main, lobar, or segmental elastic arteries • Fibrous webs in elastic arteries • Dilatation and shallow intimal atheromas of elastic arteries
Plexogenic pulmonary hypertension (primary or associated with left-to-right shunt)	Hypertrophy with or without dilatation	• Medial hypertrophy • Extension of smooth muscle into arterioles • Concentric intimal proliferation • Concentric laminar intimal fibrosis • Fibrinoid degeneration • Necrotizing arteritis • Dilatation lesions • Plexiform lesions • Dilatation and shallow intimal atheromas of elastic arteries
Thrombotic primary pulmonary hypertension	Hypertrophy with or without dilatation	• Medial hypertrophy less severe than in other forms • Dilatation and shallow intimal atheromas of elastic arteries • Recent thrombi in muscular arteries • Organized thrombi in muscular arteries appearing as recanalized channels, luminal webs, or fibrocalcific pads
Pulmonary veno-occlusive disease	Hypertrophy with or without dilatation	• Medial hypertrophy • Dilatation and shallow intimal atheromas of elastic arteries • Arteries may be dilated • Eccentric and concentric nonlaminar intimal fibrosis
Pulmonary capillary hemangiomatosis	Hypertrophy with or without dilatation	• Medial hypertrophy • Dilatation and shallow intimal atheromas of elastic arteries

Pulmonary capillaries	Pulmonary veins	Other
Engorged with blood	• Engorged with blood • Medial hypertrophy of veins and venules ("arterialization") • Eccentric intimal fibrosis	• Edema of pleura and interlobular septa • Dilatation of pleural and septal lymphatics • Alveolar edema • Focal microhemorrhages and hemosiderosis Parenchymal abnormalities of chronic obstructive pulmonary disease
		May be associated with evidence of prior deep vein thrombosis
		Possible intracardiac right-to-left shunt
Congestion	• Organized and recanalized thrombi in veins and venules • Medial hypertrophy	• Edema of pleura and interlobular septa • Dilatation of pleural and septal lymphatics • Alveolar edema • Focal microhemorrhages and hemosiderosis
Proliferation of thin-walled microvessels, which infiltrate the lung parenchyma, pleura, and walls of pulmonary vessels and bronchi	Microvessel infiltration and fibrous luminal obstruction	Alveolar hemosiderin-laden macrophages

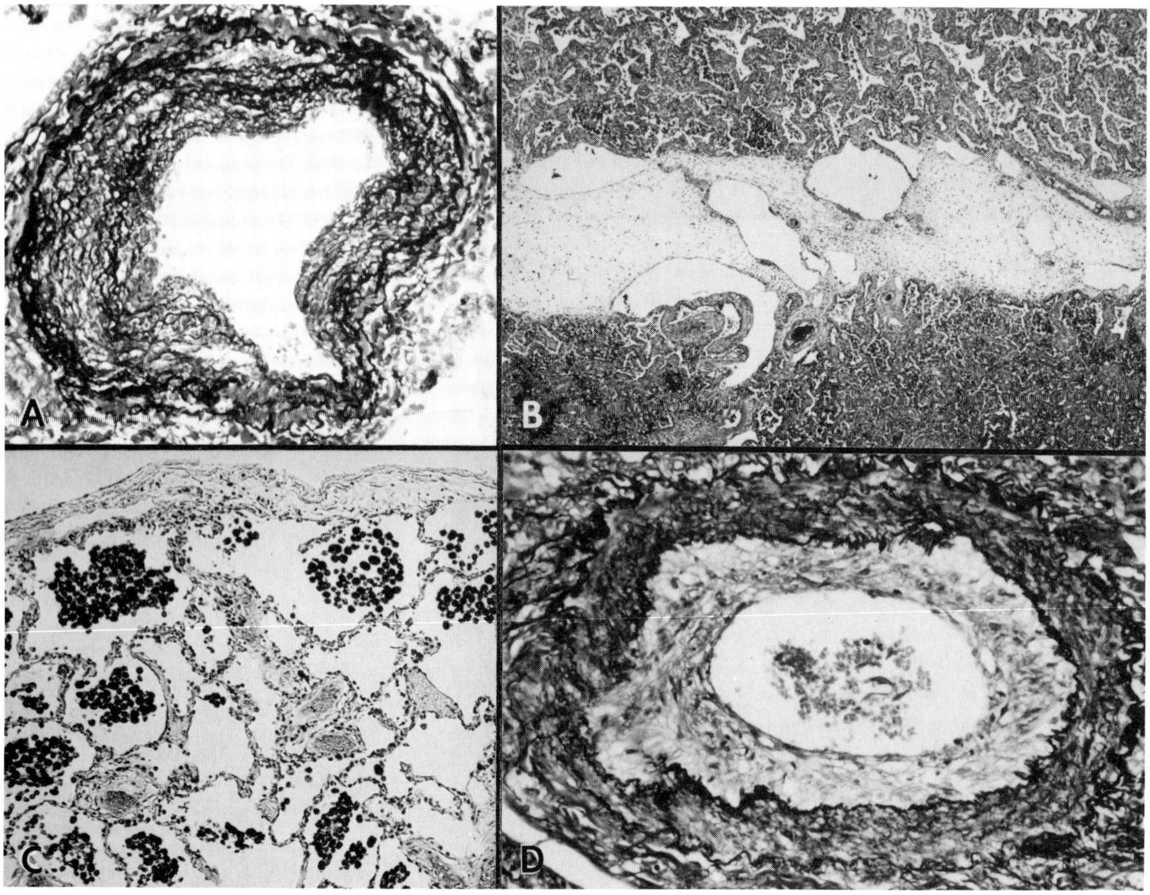

Fig 61-5 Chronic pulmonary venous hypertension. **A,** medial hypertrophy and eccentric intimal fibrosis of pulmonary vein. **B,** septal edema and dilated lymphatics. **C,** alveolar hemosiderin-laden macrophages. **D,** medial hypertrophy and intimal fibrosis of muscular pulmonary artery. (Elastic van Gieson; **A** and **D,** ×140; hematoxylin and eosin; **B,** ×27, **C,** ×70.)

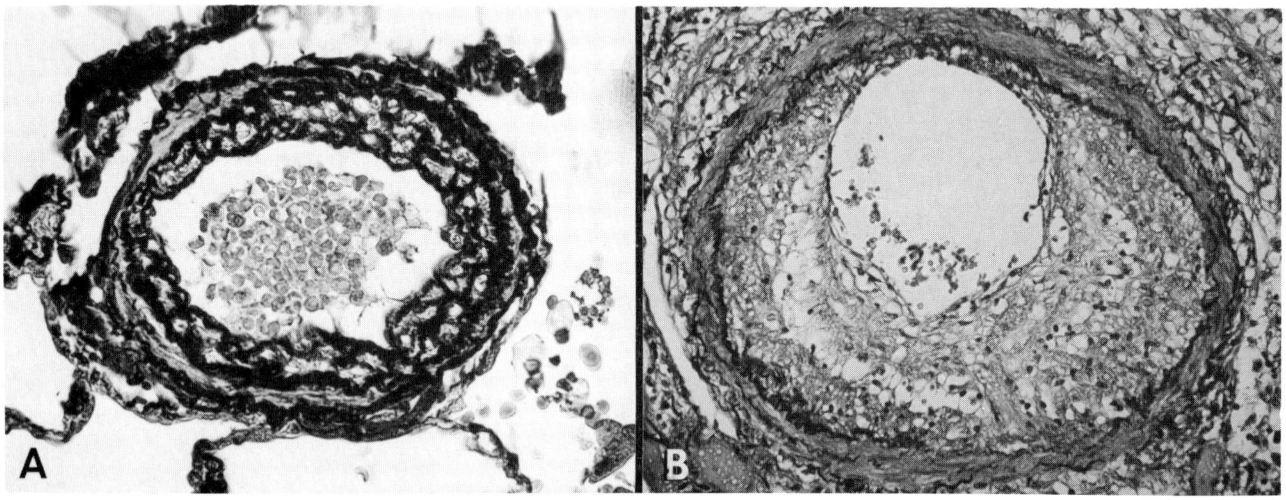

Fig 61-6 Hypoxic pulmonary hypertension. **A,** longitudinal bundles of intimal smooth muscle cells in pulmonary artery, in pulmonary emphysema. **B,** eccentric intimal fibrosis in pulmonary artery, in polymyositis with interstitial pulmonary fibrosis. (Elastic van Gieson; **A,** ×330, **B,** ×160.)

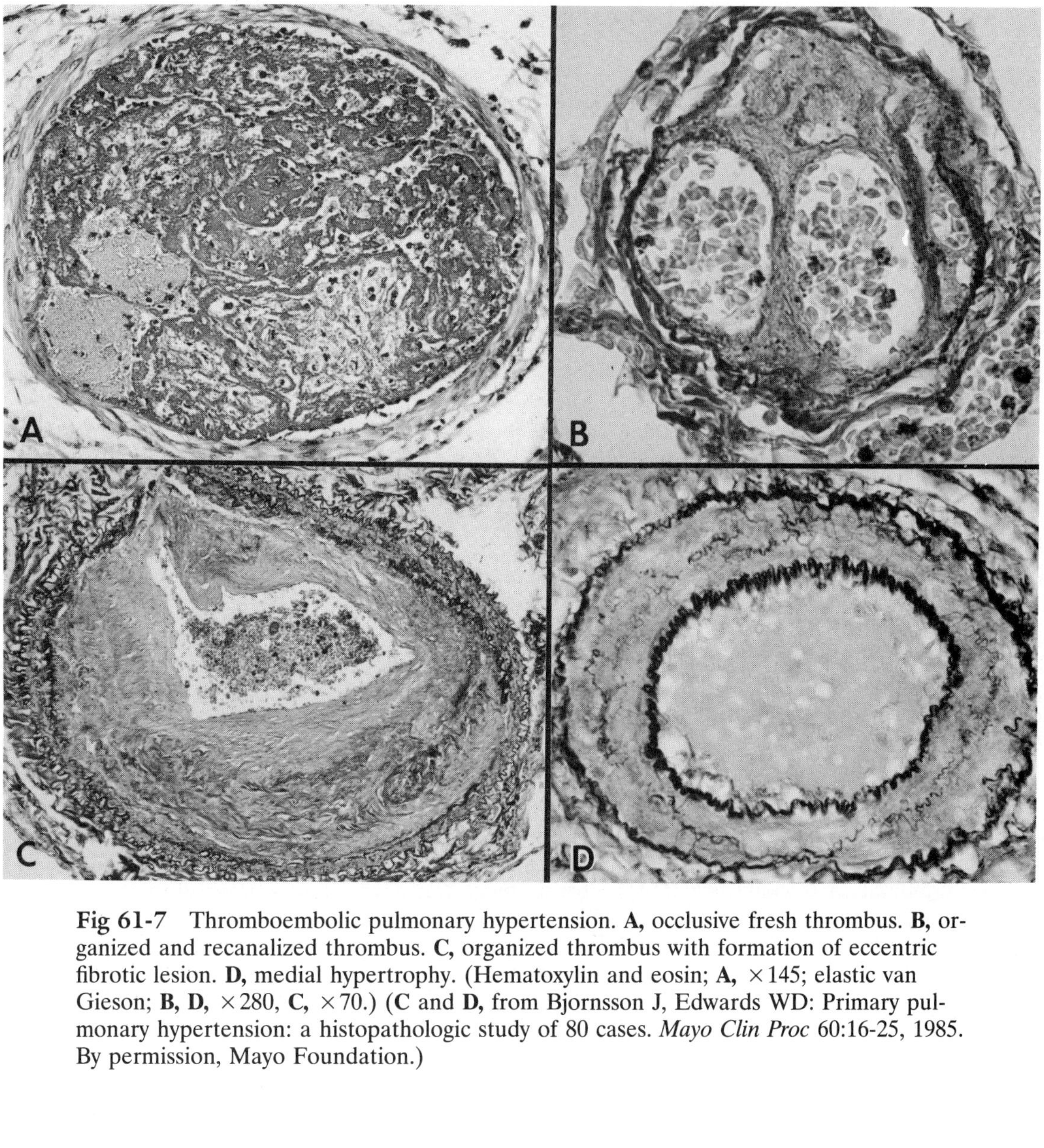

Fig 61-7 Thromboembolic pulmonary hypertension. **A,** occlusive fresh thrombus. **B,** organized and recanalized thrombus. **C,** organized thrombus with formation of eccentric fibrotic lesion. **D,** medial hypertrophy. (Hematoxylin and eosin; **A,** ×145; elastic van Gieson; **B, D,** ×280, **C,** ×70.) (**C** and **D,** from Bjornsson J, Edwards WD: Primary pulmonary hypertension: a histopathologic study of 80 cases. *Mayo Clin Proc* 60:16-25, 1985. By permission, Mayo Foundation.)

been recognized:[1-5] (1) primary plexogenic pulmonary arteriopathy, (2) pulmonary veno-occlusive disease, and (3) pulmonary capillary hemangiomatosis. Rarely, idiopathic pulmonary hypertension may be characterized by arterial medial hypertrophy only or by isolated pulmonary arteritis.[6]

Thromboembolic findings are common in primary pulmonary hypertension and may be considered a histopathologic subtype.[3,5,7,8] Obstructing thrombi may not be embolic but are likely to have developed in situ secondary to endothelial damage. Platelets associated with the obstructive plexiform and thrombotic lesions may contribute to the progression of primary pulmonary hypertension, either by luminal obstruction or by release of platelet-derived smooth muscle growth factor.

Plexogenic pulmonary arteriopathy (see Table 61-4) may be primary or associated with congenital left-to-right shunts (e.g., ventricular septal defect or patent ductus arteriosus).[3-5] In primary pulmonary arteriopathy, all grades of lesions may be observed in different vessels (Fig 61-8). This may reflect the advanced state of the disease at the time of histopathologic diagnosis in most instances.

Pulmonary veno-occlusive disease (see Table 61-4) is associated mainly with thrombotic obstruction of the small pulmonary veins and secondary pulmonary congestion and edema[3-5] (Fig 61-9), although eccentric and concentric nonlaminar intimal fibrosis of muscular pulmonary arteries may also be observed.[1]

Pulmonary capillary hemangiomatosis is a rare entity in which thin-walled microvessels infiltrate peribronchial-perivascular interstitium, lung parenchyma, and pleura. Microvascular infiltration of pulmonary vein walls results in destruction of medial elastic fibers and in fibrous luminal obstruction.[1,6]

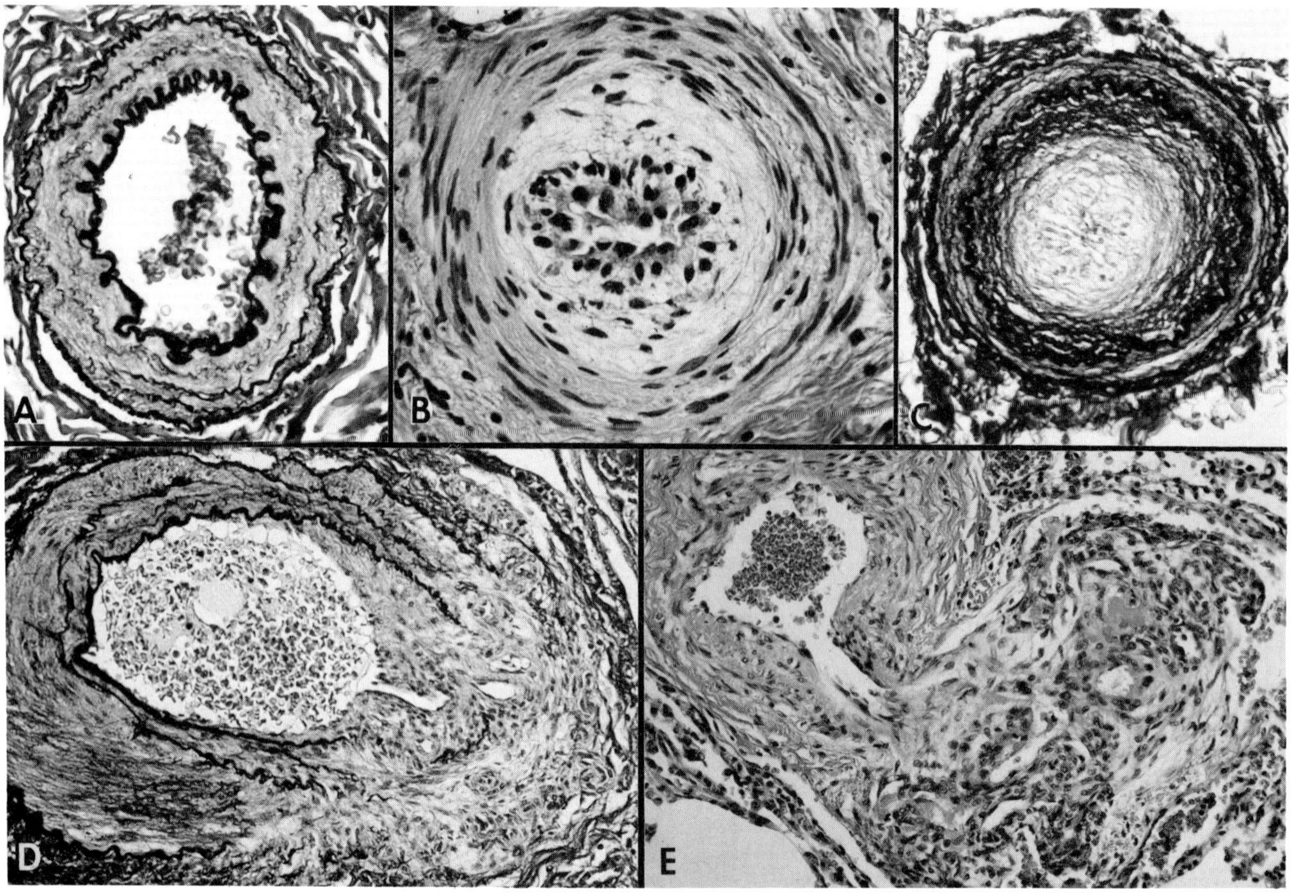

Fig 61-8 Plexogenic pulmonary arteriopathy. **A,** medial hypertrophy. **B,** intimal cellular proliferation. **C,** concentric intimal fibroelastosis. **D,** healing arteritis. **E,** plexiform lesion. (Elastic van Gieson; **A,** ×270, **C, D,** ×140; hematoxylin and eosin; **B,** ×270, **E,** ×140.) (**D,** from Bjornsson J, Edwards WD: Primary pulmonary hypertension: a histopathologic study of 80 cases. *Mayo Clin Proc* 60:16-25, 1985. By permission, Mayo Foundation.)

CLINICAL FEATURES

The clinical features of pulmonary hypertension depend in large part on the nature of the underlying lesion. They are summarized in Table 61-5.

PHYSICAL EXAMINATION

The physical examination provides valuable clues about the presence, severity, and underlying cause of pulmonary hypertension. Its critical role as both a screening tool and a diagnostic procedure should not be overlooked. The important components of the physical examination in relation to pulmonary hypertension are shown in Tables 61-6, 61-7, and 61-8.

LABORATORY EVALUATION

Chest radiograph

Radiographic examination of the chest discloses that in patients with significant pulmonary hypertension, the pulmonary trunk and main branches are dilated (Fig 61-10). As a consequence of constriction of the smaller arteries, the vascular markings in the peripheral lung fields are diminished, leading to a typical "pruned" appearance of the pulmonary vascular tree. Although pulmonary venous congestion may be present early in the course of syndromes that cause obstruction to pulmonary venous outflow, the constriction of the smaller arteries and occurrence of significant pulmonary arterial hypertension are associated with decrease in the prominence of pulmonary venous congestion.

Patients with pulmonary venous hypertension associated with right cardiac failure or systemic venous hypertension tend to have pleural effusions.

Right ventricular enlargement may be visible, as suggested by anterior enlargement of the heart shadow and enlargement of the right heart border.

Electrocardiography

The electrocardiographic changes in pulmonary hypertension reflect right ventricular and right atrial enlarge-

Table 61-5 Chronic secondary pulmonary hypertension

Category	Pathophysiology	Clinical profile	Treatment
Pulmonary venous hypertension (early)	Passive increase in pulmonary arterial pressure due to elevated pulmonary vein, left heart, or systemic arterial resistance	• Dyspnea • Pulmonary edema • Hemoptysis	Remove underlying cause if possible
Pulmonary venous hypertension (late)	Reactive pulmonary arteriolar vasoconstriction, medial hypertrophy, and intimal proliferation	• Dyspnea • Fatigue • Cough • Right ventricular failure • Tricuspid regurgitation • Hepatomegaly • Peripheral edema	Remove underlying cause if possible
Chronic obstructive lung disease, parenchymal lung disease	• Alveolar hypoxia causing vasoconstriction • Ventilation-perfusion mismatch • Secondary erythrocytosis[9] • Structural loss of vascular bed contributory (emphysema)	Bronchitis > emphysema[10,11]	• Oxygen • Lung transplant • Vasodilator • Consider phlebotomy • Consider anticoagulation • Consider diuretic
Obesity, obstructive sleep apnea,[12] hypoventilation	• Nocturnal upper airway obstruction • Reduced respiratory drive • Alveolar hypoventilation • Hypoxia • Vasoconstriction	• Disordered sleep • Somnolence • Dyspnea	• Positive airway pressure (CPAP, BiPAP) • Respiratory stimulants (medroxyprogesterone) • Weight reduction
Restrictive lung disease • Skeletal • Fibrotic • Neuromuscular	• Alveolar hypoventilation • Hypoxia • Vasoconstriction	• Stigmata of underlying disease • Dyspnea	• Oxygen • BiPAP • Vasodilators • Anticoagulation • Lung transplant (fibrotic) • Consider phrenic nerve stimulation (neuromuscular)
High altitude	• Hypoxia • Vasoconstriction	• Dyspnea • Right heart failure	• Oxygen • Lower altitude
Vascular	• Persistence of large vessel thromboemboli • Anatomic vascular obstruction • Continuing platelet activation • Vasoconstriction	May mimic primary pulmonary hypertension • Dyspnea • Chest pain or angina • Syncope	• Thromboendarterectomy • Inferior vena cava filter • Anticoagulation • Vasodilators • Oxygen
Intracardiac shunt	• Left-to-right shunt • High pulmonary blood flow • Increased pulmonary vascular impedance • Reversal of shunt (Eisenmenger's complex)	• Dyspnea • Cyanosis • Clubbing • Hemoptysis	• Lung transplant with repair of intracardiac defect • Heart-lung transplant

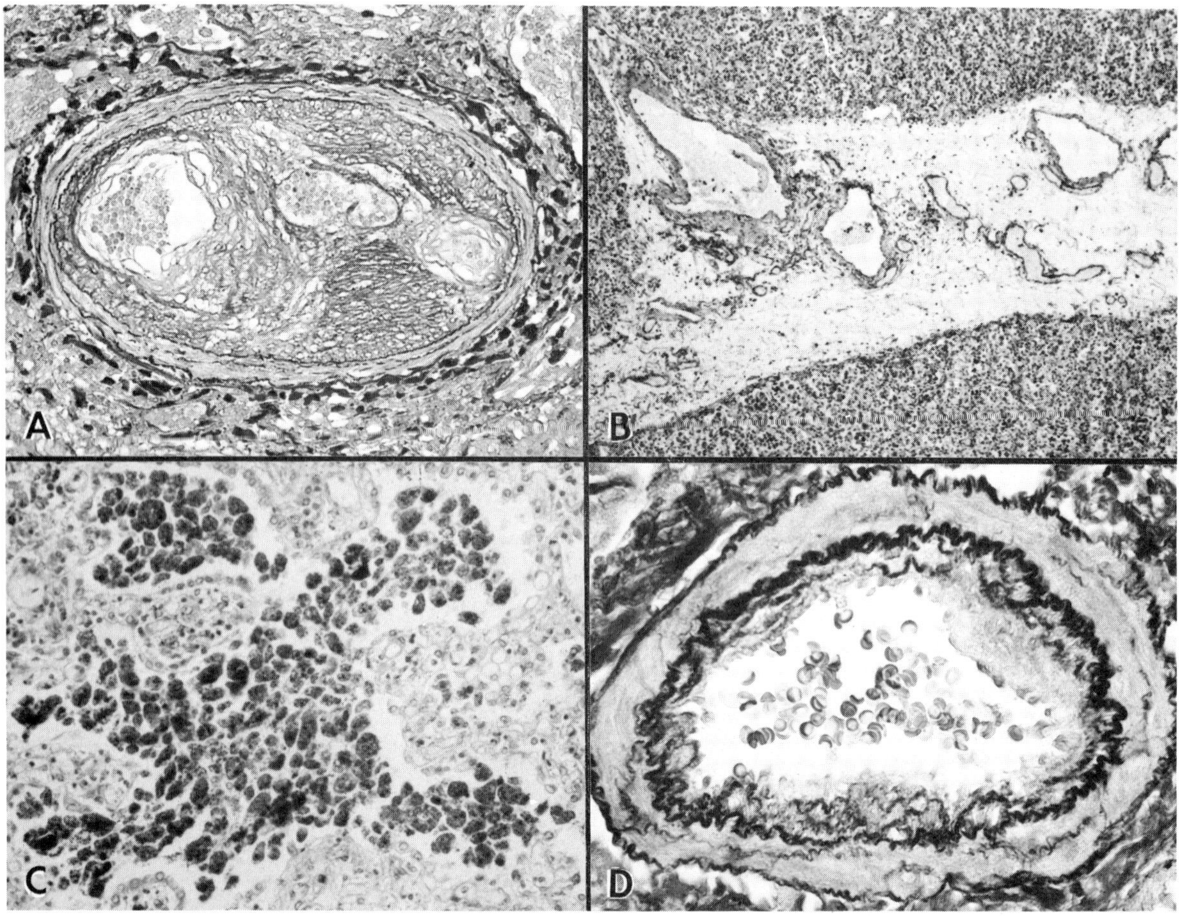

Fig 61-9 Pulmonary veno-occlusive disease. **A,** organized and recanalized thrombus in "arterialized" vein. **B,** septal edema and dilated lymphatics. **C,** alveolar hemosiderin-laden macrophages. **D,** medial hypertrophy of muscular pulmonary artery. (Elastic van Gieson; **A,** ×145, **D,** ×280; hematoxylin and eosin; **B,** ×35, **C,** ×145.) (**A, B,** and **D,** from Bjornsson J, Edwards WD: Primary pulmonary hypertension: a histopathologic study of 80 cases. *Mayo Clin Proc* 60:16-25, 1985. By permission, Mayo Foundation.)

Table 61-6 Physical signs that reveal pulmonary hypertension

Signs	Implication	Diagnostic utility
Accentuated pulmonary component of S_2 (audible at apex)	High pulmonary pressure increases force of pulmonary valve closure	Suspect pulmonary hypertension
Early systolic click	Sudden opening of pulmonary valve into high-pressure artery	
Midsystolic ejection murmur	Turbulent transvalvular pulmonary outflow	
Left parasternal lift	High right ventricular pressure and hypertrophy present	
Increased jugular "a" waves	High right ventricular filling pressure	

Table 61-7 Physical signs that indicate severity of pulmonary hypertension

Signs	Implication	Diagnostic utility
Diastolic murmur	Pulmonary regurgitation	Moderate to severe pulmonary hypertension
Holosystolic murmur that increases with inspiration	Tricuspid regurgitation	
Increased jugular v waves	Tricuspid regurgitation	
Hepatojugular reflux	Tricuspid regurgitation	
Pulsatile liver	Tricuspid regurgitation	
Right ventricular S_3	Right ventricular dysfunction	Advanced pulmonary hypertension with right ventricular failure
Marked distention of jugular veins	Right ventricular dysfunction or tricuspid regurgitation or both	
Hepatomegaly	Right ventricular dysfunction or tricuspid regurgitation or both	
Peripheral edema	Right ventricular dysfunction or tricuspid regurgitation or both	
Ascites	Right ventricular dysfunction or tricuspid regurgitation or both	
Low blood pressure, diminished pulse pressure, cool extremities	Reduced cardiac output, peripheral vasoconstriction	

Table 61-8 Physical signs that indicate possible underlying cause or associations of pulmonary hypertension

Signs	Implication	Diagnostic utility
Central cyanosis	Hypoxemia, right-to-left shunt	Severe pulmonary hypertension or congenital heart disease, Eisenmenger physiology
Clubbing	Congenital heart disease	Eisenmenger physiology
Cardiac auscultatory findings, including systolic murmurs, diastolic murmurs, opening snap, and gallop	Congenital or acquired heart or valvular disease	Eisenmenger physiology, high left-sided pressures with secondary pulmonary hypertension
Rales, dullness, or decreased breath sounds	Pulmonary congestion or effusion or both	High left-sided pressures with secondary pulmonary hypertension
Fine rales, accessory muscle use, wheezing, protracted expiration, or productive cough	Pulmonary parenchymal disease	Pulmonary hypertension secondary to parenchymal or hypoxic lung disease
Obesity, kyphoscoliosis, or enlarged tonsils	Possible substrate for disordered ventilation	Hypoxic pulmonary hypertension
Sclerodactyly, arthritis, or rash	Connective tissue disorder	Pulmonary hypertension associated with vasculitis
Peripheral venous insufficiency or obstruction	Possible venous thrombosis	Chronic thromboembolic pulmonary hypertension

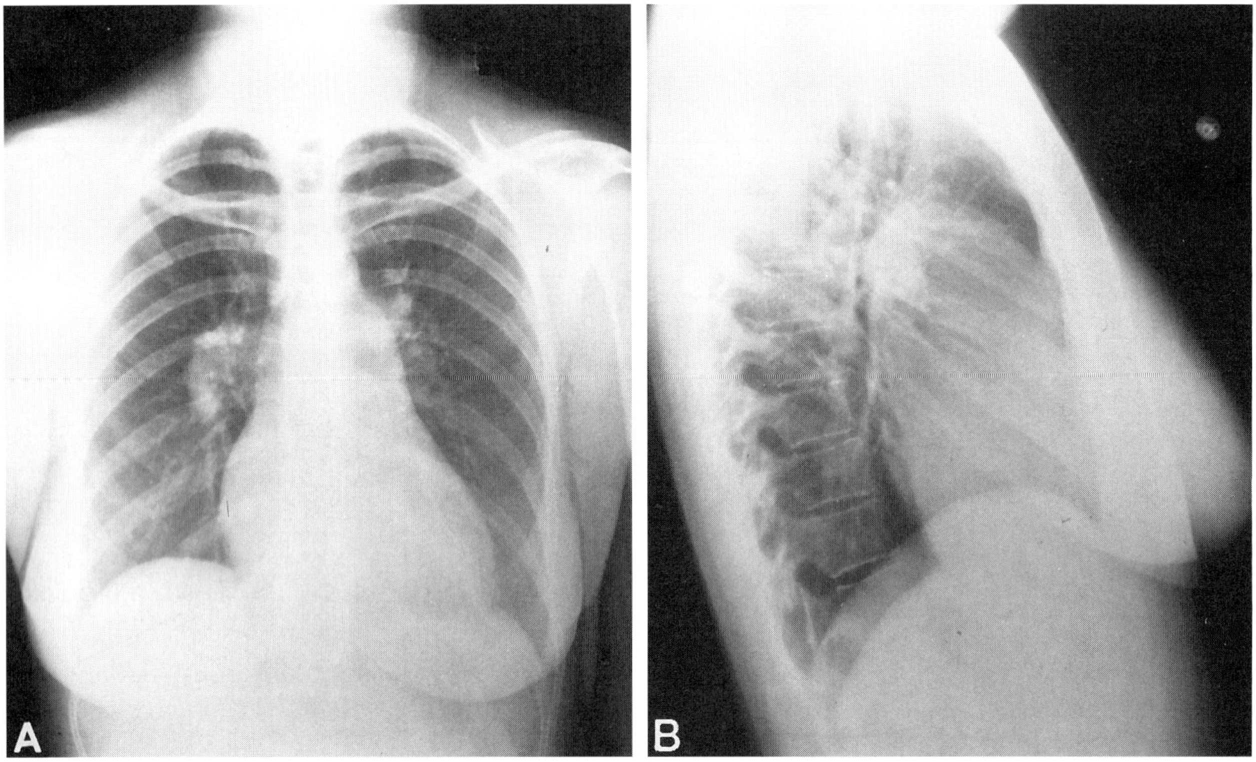

Fig 61-10 Posteroanterior (**A**) and lateral (**B**) chest radiographs demonstrate hilar pulmonary artery prominence, decreased peripheral vascular markings, and right ventricular enlargement.

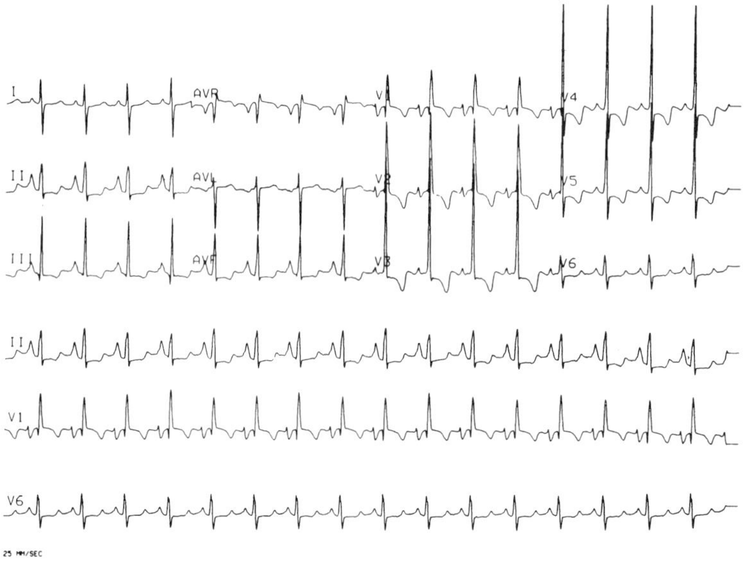

Fig 61-11 Electrocardiogram of young female patient with primary pulmonary hypertension shows evidence of right ventricular hypertrophy, right-axis deviation, and right atrial enlargement.

ment (Fig 61-11). Criteria of right ventricular hypertrophy include abnormal right-axis deviation, a tall R wave and small S wave with R/S ratio >1 in lead V_1, a qR complex in V_1, a large S wave and small R wave with R/S ratio <1 in lead V_5 or V_6, an rSR′ pattern in lead V_1, or an S_1, S_2, S_3 pattern. ST-segment depression and T-wave inversions are frequently present in the right precordial leads. Right atrial abnormalities may be manifested as a tall P wave (height >2.5 mm) in leads II, III, and aVF and P-wave frontal axis ≥ 75°. The presence of concurrent left atrial enlargement, as in mitral stenosis, may produce a notched P wave of duration >120 msec and a P terminal force in lead V_1 more negative than −0.04 mm · sec.

Echocardiography

Multiple causes of secondary pulmonary hypertension can be delineated by echocardiography, including hemodynamically significant stenosis or regurgitation of the aortic or mitral valves, cardiomyopathic states, ischemic left ventricular dysfunction, left ventricular inflow obstruction (e.g., left atrial myxoma or cor triatriatum), and intracardiac or extracardiac left-to-right shunts.

Various degrees of concentric right ventricular hypertrophy, enlargement, and global dysfunction are seen. The right atrium and main pulmonary arteries are often also enlarged. Flattening of the interventricular septum with D-shaped deformation of the left ventricle in later systole and throughout diastole is an important finding of right ventricular pressure overload.[13]

In the absence of right ventricular outflow tract obstruction or pulmonary valvular stenosis, systolic pulmonary arterial pressure can be determined by obtaining the maximal tricuspid regurgitant velocity by continuous-wave Doppler echocardiography. By use of the modified Bernoulli equation[14] $\Delta P = 4V^2$, in which V = the maximal Doppler velocity, the maximal systolic pressure gradient (ΔP) across the tricuspid valve can be estimated. If estimated right atrial pressure (RAP) is added, the right ventricular systolic pressure (RVSP) and, hence, systolic pulmonary artery pressure can be calculated: $RVSP = \Delta P + RAP$. Right atrial pressure can be estimated by jugular venous pressure (JVP) examination, but even closer correlation has been found by regression equations derived from simultaneous catheterization and Doppler study: $RVSP = \Delta P + 14$ (if JVP <20 cm H_2O) or $RVSP = 1.1\ \Delta P + 20$ (if JVP ≥ 20 cm H_2O).[15] Approximately 60% of patients with normal and 80% of patients with increased pulmonary artery pressures have analyzable tricuspid regurgitant Doppler spectra for determination of right ventricular systolic pressure.[15,16]

Pulsed-wave Doppler analysis of central laminar flow in the distal right ventricular outflow tract[17] or proximal main pulmonary artery[18] can also determine mean pulmonary artery pressure. Normally, the peak velocity of right ventricular outflow occurs in midsystole. In pulmonary hypertension, decreasing pulmonary vascular compliance increases impedance to right ventricular ejection and causes maximal acceleration of blood to occur earlier in systole. This shortens the pulmonary acceleration time, the time from onset of right ventricular ejection to the peak Doppler flow velocity. The pulmonary acceleration time (PAT) is obtainable in 88% to 98% of patients.[16-19] On the basis of correlative catheterization studies, the mean pulmonary artery pressure (MPAP) can be accurately estimated from linear regression equations using the PAT obtained at the distal right ventricular outflow tract[17] ($\log_{10} MPAP = -0.0068 \times PAT + 2.1$) or proximal main pulmonary artery[18] ($MPAP = 90 - 0.62 \times PAT$).

The end-diastolic pulmonary regurgitant velocity (V_{PR}) can be determined by continuous-wave Doppler examination, reflecting the pressure gradient between the pulmonary artery and the right ventricle at end-diastole. In the absence of tricuspid inflow stenosis, right ventricular end-diastolic pressure approximates right atrial pressure (RAP, estimated by jugular venous pressure examination), and the pulmonary artery diastolic pressure (PAP_D) can be estimated by the following relationship:[14] $PAP_D = 4V^2{}_{PR} + RAP$.

Radionuclide studies

Ventilation-perfusion scanning is useful primarily for determining whether pulmonary embolism is likely to be a cause of pulmonary hypertension. The presence of a perfusion defect in a segmental distribution without corresponding ventilation abnormalities indicates high probability of pulmonary embolism. Matched perfusion-ventilation defects may reflect parenchymal lung disease, heart failure, or atelectasis. In cases of primary pulmonary hypertension, perfusion lung scans may be normal, may demonstrate small subsegmental abnormalities, or may have a diffuse granular appearance.

Pulmonary artery imaging

A segmental (or greater) perfusion defect on ventilation-perfusion lung scan warrants further investigation to assess the possibility of thromboembolic pulmonary hypertension, since significant remediable chronic thromboembolism may be present despite a minimally abnormal scan.[20] Pulmonary angiography has been regarded as the definitive examination of pulmonary intraluminal anatomy and remains an essential part of the evaluation. However, in thromboembolic pulmonary hypertension, chronic thrombi may have organized and become an integral component of the vascular wall. Consequently, the angiogram may underestimate the degree of vascular obstruction by proximal clots.

Alternative imaging modalities that have shown promise in enhancing the diagnosis of pulmonary thromboembolic disease are magnetic resonance imaging, angioscopy, intravascular ultrasonography, and electron-beam computed tomography[1,21-23] (Fig 61-12).

Hemodynamic studies

Direct hemodynamic assessment with invasive studies may be required for confirmation and quantification of pulmonary hypertension. In addition, these investigations may be necessary to evaluate underlying cardiac disease

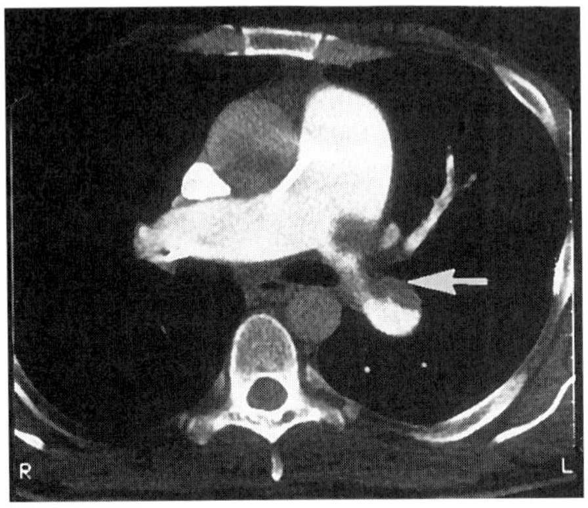

Fig 61-12 Electron-beam computerized tomogram shows chronic thromboembolic material in the descending trunk of the left pulmonary artery *(arrow)*.

Table 61-9 Hemodynamic results of pulmonary thromboendarterectomy in 131 patients

Measurement	Preoperative	Postoperative
Cardiac output, L/min	3.8 ± 1.2	5.6 ± 1.5
Systolic pulmonary artery pressure, mm Hg	78.8 ± 22.3	47.0 ± 16.9
Mean pulmonary artery pressure, mm Hg	48.5 ± 13.7	18.9 ± 10.8
Pulmonary vascular resistance, dyn · sec/cm^{-5}	936.9 ± 44.5	299.4 ± 16.0

Modified from Jamieson SW, Auger WR, Fedullo PF, et al: Experience and results with 150 pulmonary thromboendarterectomy operations over a 29-month period. *J Thorac Cardiovasc Surg* 106:116-126, 1993.

and to provide information regarding the short-term response to pharmacologic intervention.[24] Right atrial pressure may be increased, and direct evaluation of tricuspid regurgitation may be accomplished from the increased systolic v wave on right atrial pressure tracings. Measurement of pulmonary blood flow provides the necessary data for calculation of pulmonary vascular resistance. Capillary wedge pressure measurements, which may be difficult to obtain reliably, will distinguish between precapillary pulmonary hypertension, in which case the wedge pressure is not significantly abnormal, and postcapillary hypertension, in which case the wedge pressure is increased.

TREATMENT

Treatment of pulmonary hypertension (see Table 61-5) is most effective when instituted early. When an underlying cause is identified, it should be corrected whenever possible. This includes repair of cardiac defects that produce a left-to-right shunt or pulmonary venous hypertension as well as the avoidance of smoking by patients with chronic obstructive disease. In pulmonary parenchymal disease, some disorders, such as the pneumoconioses and the fibrotic stage of inflammatory disease, are virtually unresponsive to therapy whereas others, such as the inflammatory stage of the chronic interstitial pneumonias and alveolar proteinosis, may be managed effectively with specific therapy such as corticosteroids or bronchoalveolar lavage.[25,26] For this reason, lung biopsy may establish a specific diagnosis.

When the diagnosis of pulmonary hypertension is established, in most patients the disease is relatively late in its course, and correction of underlying causes may no longer be feasible or possible. In these cases, the success of any therapeutic intervention is limited, and treatment is generally directed toward palliation of symptoms (see Table 61-5).

One form of pulmonary hypertension that is now recognized as virtually curable by treatment is chronic major vessel thromboembolic pulmonary hypertension, which is thought to occur in approximately 0.1% to 0.2% (or 540 to 1,080) of the 540,000 survivors of acute pulmonary embolism per year.[27] Since this entity can present clinically as primary pulmonary hypertension, its recognition (by ventilation-perfusion scanning, pulmonary angiography, and computed tomography [see Fig 61-12] or other imaging modalities) and treatment are vital.

Cumulative experience indicates that thromboendarterectomy can be performed with a high rate of success and acceptable mortality for this otherwise debilitating and untreatable disease. Bilateral thromboendarterectomy in which operative techniques such as median sternotomy, cardiopulmonary bypass, and deep hypothermia are used has yielded a surgical mortality as low as 9% and substantial hemodynamic improvement[27] (Table 61-9).

PRIMARY PULMONARY HYPERTENSION

Primary pulmonary hypertension, defined as "pulmonary arterial hypertension of unknown cause,"[2] is a rare entity, with an incidence among all patients at the Mayo Clinic of approximately 2 cases per 10,000 patients. The incidence of clinically apparent disease in the general population is likely even smaller. Despite the infrequency of its occurrence, it constitutes a significant clinical problem because of its devastating impact and the absence of reliable palliative or curative therapy.

Epidemiology

Primary pulmonary hypertension has been regarded generally as a disease of young, predominantly female, adults. The age range reported in five large series[7,28-31] comprising 459 patients extends from 1 to 81 years, with a normal distribution and mean age of 35 years. The female-to-male ratio in these studies was 2.4:1. A familial clustering of the disease has been noted in 2% to 14% of cases. Racial distribution appears to reflect the popula-

Table 61-10 Possible causes of primary pulmonary hypertension

Proposed etiologic mechanism	Evidence
Occult thromboembolism or thrombosis in situ	Pathologic studies[5] Response to anticoagulation[7]
Genetic factors	Family clusters[32,33]
Connective tissue disorder	High incidence of ANA[34] Occasional Raynaud's phenomenon Similarities with PSS-related pulmonary hypertension[35]
Exogenous toxins	Examples: aminorex fumarate,[36] toxic rapeseed oil,[37] *Crotalaria,* and L-tryptophan
Inadequate hepatic detoxification mechanisms	Occasional association with cirrhosis and portal hypertension[38-42]
Hormonal factors	Female preponderance Possible oral contraceptive role[43]
Vasospasm, chronic or recurrent	Occasional Raynaud's phenomenon Occasional vasodilator benefit

ANA, antinuclear antibody; PSS, progressive systemic sclerosis.

Table 61-11 Hemodynamic features of primary pulmonary hypertension at diagnosis ($n = 120$)

Measurement	Mean	Range
Pulmonary artery pressure, mm Hg		
Peak	98	53-208
Mean	64	36-120
Pulmonary flow index, L/min/m^2	2.2	0.7-5.0
Total pulmonary resistance, units · m^2	33	11-95
Right ventricular end-diastolic pressure, mm Hg	13	2-30
Right ventricular work index, kg/min/m^2	1.6	0.4-5.8
Systemic arterial oxygen saturation, %	91	42-99
Pulmonary arterial oxygen saturation, %	60	20-80

From Fuster V, Steele PM, Edwards WD, et al: Primary pulmonary hypertension: natural history and the importance of thrombosis. *Circulation* 70:580-587, 1984. By permission of American Heart Association.

tion at large, although female preponderance may be more apparent in the black population (4.3:1).[28]

Etiology

Although causal mechanisms are, by definition, not known in primary pulmonary hypertension, a number of possible mechanisms have been suggested on the basis of limited evidence (Table 61-10). Very likely, primary pulmonary hypertension is a clinical manifestation common to a variety of unrecognized etiologic mechanisms.

Clinical features

Symptoms. The most frequent symptoms at presentation and throughout the course of primary pulmonary hypertension are dyspnea on exertion and fatigue. Syncope, dizziness, and anginal chest pain are less common at presentation but not infrequently occur during the course of the disease. Sudden death also may be an initial manifestation of primary pulmonary hypertension.[44]

The mechanism of syncope is probably multifactorial. Systemic vasodilation, regardless of mechanism, can result in profound sudden hypotension because of the inability to increase cardiac output through the high-resistance pulmonary vasculature. Commonly occurring arrhythmias that are normally benign, such as accelerated junctional rhythms, have been associated with syncope, perhaps because of loss of a critically important atrial systolic contribution to cardiac output. It is of interest that patients with atrial fibrillation are seldom, if ever, identified,[28] a suggestion that this arrhythmia, in combination with significant primary pulmonary hypertension, may not be compatible with life.

Angina most likely is related to right ventricular ischemia secondary to high myocardial oxygen demand provoked by increased ventricular wall tension and increased right ventricular mass. Unlike the left ventricle, the right ventricle receives much of its coronary blood flow during systole because of the high gradient between the aortic and the right ventricular systolic pressures. The reduction of this gradient resulting from high right ventricular systolic pressure contributes to right ventricular ischemia.

Physical examination and laboratory studies. The features of the physical examination are those seen secondary to pulmonary hypertension of any cause (see Tables 61-6 and 61-7), as are the findings on the chest radiograph and electrocardiogram (see above).

Hemodynamic and angiographic features

Hemodynamic evaluation at the time of diagnosis characteristically reveals markedly increased pulmonary artery pressures and resistances and diminished cardiac output (Table 61-11).

Although originally thought to be prohibitively risky, pulmonary angiography can be performed safely in patients with significant pulmonary hypertension.[28,45,46] This procedure is advisable if there is a suspicion of pulmonary embolism on the basis of the clinical history, examination, or ventilation-perfusion radionuclide scan, since confirmation of the diagnosis has important therapeutic significance. Documentation of thromboembolic pulmonary hypertension mandates use of anticoagulants, if possible, and prompt consideration of thromboendarterectomy.[45] Indeed, since ventilation-perfusion scans

Table 61-12 Primary pulmonary hypertension: predictors of survival

Category	Observation
Pulmonary vascular resistance and pulmonary arterial mean pressure (PA_m)	PA_m < 55 mm Hg: medial survival, 48 mo $PA_m \geq$ 85 mm Hg: median survival, 12 mo[47]
Response to vasodilator therapy	1. Patients in whom pulmonary arteriolar resistance decreases with short-term administration of vasodilators tend to survive longer, and this benefit may be independent of subsequent treatment status.[48] 2. Treatment with vasodilators may also enhance survival.[49,50]
New York Heart Association (NYHA) functional classification	NYHA I-II: median survival, 58.6 mo NYHA III: median survival, 31.5 mo NYHA IV: median survival, 6 mo[47]
Right atrial pressure (RAP)	RAP > 20 mm Hg: median survival, 1 mo RAP < 10 mm Hg: median survival, 46 mo[47]
Cardiac index (CI)	CI < 2.0 L · m^2/min: median survival, 17 mo CI ≥ 4.0 L · m^2/min: median survival, 43 mo[47]
Pulmonary arterial (mixed venous) oxygen saturation (SvO_2)	SvO_2 < 63%: mean 3-year survival, 17% $SvO_2 \geq$ 63%: mean 3-year survival, 55%[7]

Table 61-13 Vasodilators used to treat primary pulmonary hypertension

α-Adrenoceptor antagonists
Tolazoline
Phentolamine
Phenoxybenzamine
Prazosin
β-Adrenoceptor agonists
Isoproterenol
Terbutaline
Direct-acting vasodilators
Diazoxide
Hydralazine
Nitroprusside
Isosorbide dinitrate
Calcium entry blockers
Nifedipine
Verapamil
Diltiazem
Angiotensin-converting enzyme inhibitor
Captopril
Prostaglandins and cyclo-oxygenase inhibitors
Prostaglandin E_1
Prostaglandin I_2 (prostacyclin)
Indomethacin
Anticholinergic agent
Acetylcholine
Serotonergic blockers
Ketanserin
Oxygen

may underestimate the severity of embolic pulmonary vascular obstruction,[20] angiography should be advised to assess the potential for therapy with thromboendarterectomy when scans show any segmental defects.

Patients with primary pulmonary hypertension who undergo pulmonary angiography typically have dilatation of the central pulmonary arteries and their lobar and segmental branches, with abrupt narrowing of more distal branches but no discrete occlusion, producing a so-called pruned tree appearance.[7] Pulmonary transit time frequently is very slow.[7]

Clinical course

The clinical course of primary pulmonary hypertension is generally one of inexorable progression toward death. Among patients who do not undergo heart-lung transplantation, actuarial survival at 1 year is 68% to 77%, 2 years 52% to 58%, 3 years 40% to 56%, 4 years 30% to 43%, and 5 years 22% to 38%.[7,31,47] The usual causes of death are right ventricular failure (63%), pneumonia (7%), and sudden death (7%).[7]

A variety of indicators appear to have predictive value for survival (Table 61-12).

An individual patient's chances of survival can be predicted by the formula[47]

$$P(t) = [H(t)]^{A(x,y,z)}$$
$$H(t) = [0.88 - 0.14t + 0.01t^2]$$
$$A(x,y,z) = e^{(0.007325x + 0.0526y - 0.3275z)}$$

in which P(t) is a patient's chances of survival at t years, t equals 1, 2, or 3 years, x is mean pulmonary arterial pressure, y is mean right atrial pressure, and z is cardiac index.

Graphs based on this equation (Fig 61-13) provide a useful means of estimating survival so that one can determine whether treatment modalities such as lung transplantation should be considered.

Therapy

Vasodilators. Since the underlying hemodynamic abnormality of primary pulmonary hypertension is

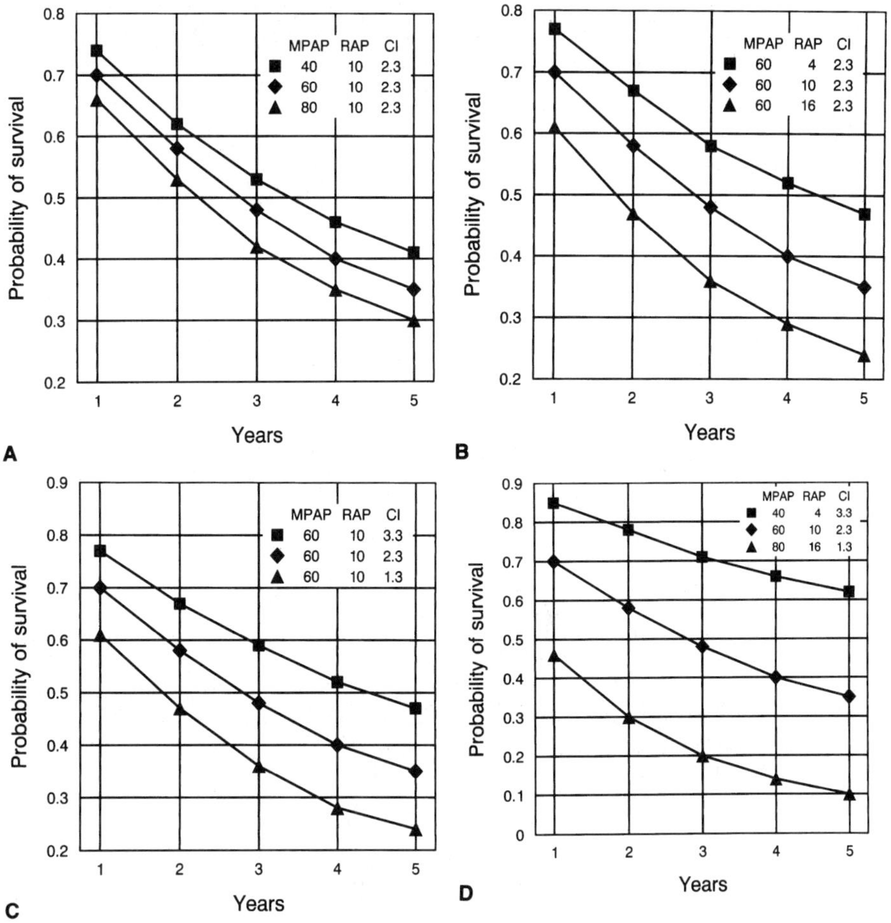

Fig 61-13 Probability of survival for medically treated patients with primary pulmonary hypertension. Differences in survival probability are depicted according to variation of baseline mean pulmonary artery pressure (*MPAP,* mm Hg) **(A),** mean right atrial pressure (*RAP,* mm Hg) **(B),** cardiac index (*CI,* L/min/m^2) **(C),** and combinations of all three variables **(D).** (**A-C,** from Rubin LJ: Primary pulmonary hypertension. *Chest* 104:236-250, 1993. By permission of American College of Chest Physicians; **D,** data from D'Alonzo GE, Barst RJ, Ayres SM, et al: Survival in patients with primary pulmonary hypertension. Results from a national prospective registry. *Ann Intern Med* 115:343-349, 1991.)

augmented pulmonary vascular resistance, continuing attempts have been made to afford hemodynamic and symptomatic improvement with vasodilators (Table 61-13). Although optimistic reports have appeared for most of the vasodilators tried, it has become clear that regardless of which medication is used, the number of patients responding is limited, the degree of response in terms of pulmonary hemodynamics or symptoms is minimal, and the duration of response is uncertain. Nevertheless, evidence is accumulating that some patients do have a salutary response to vasodilators.[49,51] Symptomatic and survival benefits appear to be conferred by long-term use of prostacyclin[50,52] (Fig 61-14) and by the use of high doses of calcium entry blockers in patients who demonstrate an initial beneficial hemodynamic response[53] (Fig 61-15).

Administration of vasodilators should be begun during careful monitoring of pulmonary artery pressure, cardiac output, and systemic blood pressure.[24] Therapy with these drugs should never begin in the outpatient setting. Monitoring is done both to document efficacy and to rapidly identify adverse outcomes, including hypotension and exacerbation of pulmonary hypertension. Increasing venous return to the right side of the heart as a consequence of systemic vasodilation may exacerbate right ventricular pressure overload and failure. Although the effect of any vasodilator can be determined by systematic monitoring during careful titration, the highest level of success with conventional vasodilators seems to be achieved with nifedipine or diltiazem, often in high doses.[54]

Potent very short-acting vasodilators, such as adenosine

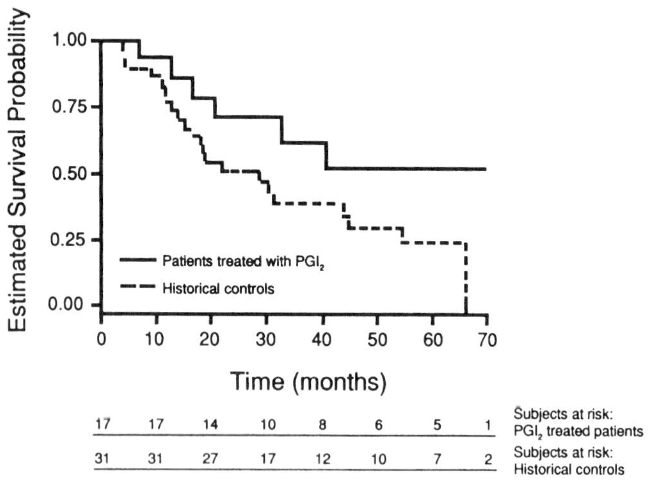

Fig 61-14 Probability of survival for patients with symptomatic primary pulmonary hypertension treated with prostacyclin[50] ($n = 17$) compared with that for patients in the Patient Registry for the Characterization of Primary Pulmonary Hypertension receiving standard therapy ($n = 31$).[47] Survival was significantly better in the prostacyclin-treated group ($P < 0.05$). (From Barst RJ, Rubin LJ, McGoon MD, et al: Survival in primary pulmonary hypertension with long-term continuous intravenous prostacyclin. *Ann Intern Med* 121:409-415, 1994. By permission of American College of Physicians.)

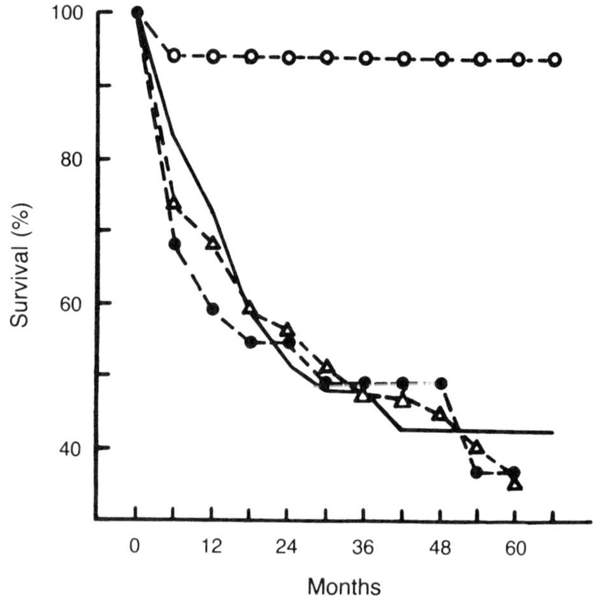

Fig 61-15 Probability of survival for patients with primary pulmonary hypertension who had a response to treatment with high doses of calcium blockers *(open circles)* compared with probability for those who did not have a response *(solid line)*, patients in the Patient Registry for the Characterization of Primary Pulmonary Hypertension (PRCPPH) at the same institution *(solid circles)*, and the entire PRCPPH cohort *(triangles)*. The difference between the responders and the other groups was highly significant ($P = 0.003$). (From Rich S, Kaufmann E, Levy PS: The effect of high doses of calcium-channel blockers on survival in primary pulmonary hypertension. *N Engl J Med* 327:76-81, 1992. By permission of the journal.)

and prostacyclin, can be used to determine whether a patient has any vasodilatory capabilities.[55-57] Absence of a response to these agents suggests a very low likelihood of benefit from longer acting agents and may obviate further low-yield testing. However, a beneficial response to a potent intravenous agent may not accurately predict a beneficial effect from a longer acting medication, so that testing with these conventional agents is still required in the individual patient.

Anticoagulation. The recommendation for anticoagulation in patients with clinical primary pulmonary hypertension is based on several factors. First, the thromboembolic form of primary pulmonary hypertension accounts for more than half the cases;[5] whether this is due to emboli or thrombosis in situ, or both, the interruption of an ongoing thrombotic process is of theoretical importance even if clinically apparent clotting is not observed. Second, patients treated with anticoagulants appear to have a better long-term survival than untreated patients (Fig 61-16).[7] Third, right ventricular failure may predispose a patient to deep venous or intracardiac thrombus formation, thereby potentially exacerbating the situation. Thus, if there is no contraindication, therapeutic long-term anticoagulation with warfarin is warranted.

Diuretics. When right ventricular failure intervenes, edema develops and may become a predominant symptom. Complete alleviation with diuretics may be impossible, especially if systemic or postural hypotension supervenes. Some relief can usually be afforded by cautious incremental use of diuretics.

Digitalis glycosides. Inotropic augmentation should be attempted for treatment of right-sided heart failure, although the benefit is likely to be relatively minimal in cor pulmonale and the likelihood of toxicity is increased.

Oxygen. Oxygen is a pulmonary vasodilator and may provide some advantage on that basis. More directly, it will help overcome decreased diffusing capacity and thereby promote symptomatic benefit and improved arterial saturation.

Cardiopulmonary transplantation. Primary pulmonary hypertension constitutes one of the most common indicators for heart-lung transplantation despite its infrequency in the general population. This therapeutic option (see chapter 18) should be considered for appropriate candidates, although it should be recognized that the procedure is still investigational, the potential recipients outnumber the available donors, and the waiting period may exceed the life span of the patient. Nevertheless, transplantation has been of benefit to properly selected patients. Single-lung and double-lung transplantation have been used in the treatment of pulmonary vascular disease. Early survival rates were relatively low (60% to 70% at 1 year), but survival is improving as experience accrues.[58,59]

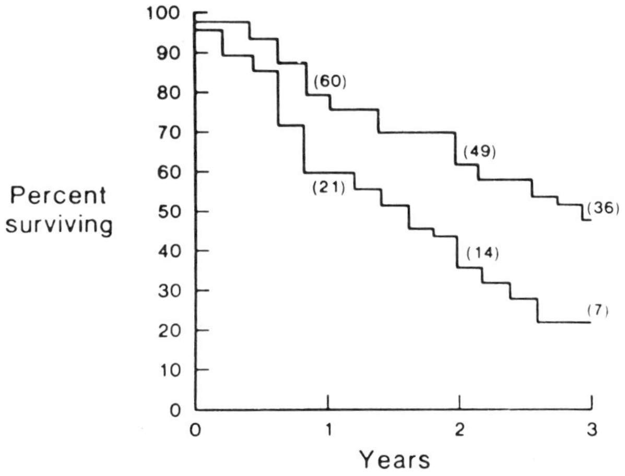

Fig 61-16 Observed survival with *(upper line)* and without *(lower line)* anticoagulant treatment in primary pulmonary hypertension (patients who survived diagnostic catheterization) ($P = 0.02$, log-rank test). Parentheses enclose numbers of patients living and under observation at end of each year. (From Fuster V, Steele PM, Edwards WD, et al: Primary pulmonary hypertension: natural history and the importance of thrombosis. *Circulation* 70:580-587, 1984. By permission of American Heart Association.)

REFERENCES

1. Rubin LJ: Primary pulmonary hypertension. *Chest* 104:236-250, 1993
2. Hatano S, Strasser T (eds): *WHO Meeting on Primary Pulmonary Hypertension.* Geneva, World Health Organization, 1975, pp 7-43
3. Edwards WD, Edwards JE: Clinical primary pulmonary hypertension: three pathologic types. *Circulation* 56:884-888, 1977
4. Wagenvoort CA, Wagenvoort N: Primary pulmonary hypertension: a pathologic study of the lung vessel in 156 clinically diagnosed cases. *Circulation* 42:1163-1184, 1970
5. Bjornsson J, Edwards WD: Primary pulmonary hypertension: a histopathologic study of 80 cases. *Mayo Clin Proc* 60:16-25, 1985
6. Edwards WD: Pathology of pulmonary hypertension. *Cardiovasc Clin* 18 no 2:321-359, 1988
7. Fuster V, Steele PM, Edwards WD, et al: Primary pulmonary hypertension: natural history and the importance of thrombosis. *Circulation* 70:580-587, 1984
8. Pietra GG, Edwards WD, Kay JM, et al: Histopathology of primary pulmonary hypertension: a qualitative and quantitative study of pulmonary blood vessels from 58 patients in the National Heart, Lung and Blood Institute Primary Pulmonary Hypertension Registry. *Circulation* 80:1198-1206, 1989
9. Dayton LM, McCullough RE, Scheinhorn DJ, et al: Symptomatic and pulmonary response to acute phlebotomy in secondary polycythemia. *Chest* 68:785-790, 1975
10. Edelman NH: Cor pulmonale. In *Clinical Medicine.* Vol. 6, Chap 22. Edited by JA Spittell Jr. Philadelphia, Harper & Row, Publishers, 1981, pp 1-13
11. Thurlbeck WM, Henderson JA, Fraser RG, et al: Chronic obstructive lung disease: a comparison between clinical, roentgenologic, functional and morphologic criteria in chronic bronchitis, emphysema, asthma and bronchiectasis. *Medicine (Baltimore)* 49:81-145, 1970
12. Weitzenblum E, Krieger J, Apprill M, et al: Daytime pulmonary hypertension in patients with obstructive sleep apnea syndrome. *Am Rev Respir Dis* 138:345-349, 1988
13. Ryan T, Petrovic O, Dillon JC, et al: An echocardiographic index for separation of right ventricular volume and pressure overload. *J Am Coll Cardiol* 5:918-924, 1985
14. Hatle L, Angelsen B: *Doppler Ultrasound in Cardiology: Physical Principles and Clinical Applications.* Second edition. Philadelphia, Lea & Febiger, 1985
15. Currie PJ, Seward JB, Chan K-L, et al: Continuous wave Doppler determination of right ventricular pressure: a simultaneous Doppler-catheterization study in 127 patients. *J Am Coll Cardiol* 6:750-756, 1985
16. Chan K-L, Currie PJ, Seward JB, et al: Comparison of three Doppler ultrasound methods in the prediction of pulmonary artery pressure. *J Am Coll Cardiol* 9:549-554, 1987
17. Kitabatake A, Inoue M, Asao M, et al: Noninvasive evaluation of pulmonary hypertension by a pulsed Doppler technique. *Circulation* 68:302-309, 1983
18. Dabestani A, Mahan G, Gardin JM, et al: Evaluation of pulmonary artery pressure and resistance by pulsed Doppler echocardiography. *Am J Cardiol* 59:661-668, 1987
19. Stevenson JG: Comparison of several noninvasive methods for estimation of pulmonary artery pressure. *J Am Soc Echo* 2:157-171, 1989
20. Ryan KL, Fedullo PF, Davis GB, et al: Perfusion scan findings understate the severity of angiographic and hemodynamic compromise in chronic thromboembolic pulmonary hypertension. *Chest* 93:1180-1185, 1988
21. Shah HR, Buckner CB, Purnell GL, et al: Computed tomography and magnetic resonance imaging in the diagnosis of pulmonary thromboembolic disease. *J Thorac Imaging* 4:58-61, 1989
22. Teigen CL, Maus TP, Sheedy PF II, et al: Pulmonary embolism: diagnosis with electron-beam CT. *Radiology* 188:839-845, 1993
23. Ricou F, Nicod PH, Moser KM, et al: Catheter-based intravascular ultrasound imaging of chronic thromboembolic pulmonary disease. *Am J Cardiol* 67:749-752, 1991
24. McGoon MD: The role of catheterization in the treatment of pulmonary hypertension. In *Interventional Cardiology.* Edited by DR Holmes Jr, RE Vlietstra. Philadelphia, FA Davis Company, 1989, pp 197-209
25. Bergofsky EH, Turino GM, Fishman AP: Cardiorespiratory failure in kyphoscoliosis. *Medicine (Baltimore)* 38:263-317, 1959
26. Hunninghake GW, Kawanami O, Ferrans VJ, et al: Characterization of the inflammatory and immune effector cells in the lung parenchyma of patients with interstitial lung disease. *Am Rev Respir Dis* 123:407-412, 1981
27. Jamieson SW, Auger WR, Fedullo PF, et al: Experience and results with 150 pulmonary thromboendarterectomy operations over a 29-month period. *J Thorac Cardiovasc Surg* 106:116-126, 1993
28. Rich S, Dantzker DR, Ayres SM, et al: Primary pulmonary hypertension: a national prospective study. *Ann Intern Med* 107:216-223, 1987
29. Rozkovec A, Montanes P, Oakley CM: Factors that influence the outcome of primary pulmonary hypertension. *Br Heart J* 55:449-458, 1986
30. Hughes JD, Rubin LJ: Primary pulmonary hypertension: an analysis of 28 cases and a review of the literature. *Medicine (Baltimore)* 65:56-72, 1986
31. Glanville AR, Burke CM, Theodore J, et al: Primary pulmonary hypertension: length of survival in patients referred for heart-lung transplantation. *Chest* 91:675-681, 1987
32. Loyd JE, Atkinson JB, Pietra GG, et al: Heterogeneity of pathologic lesions in familial primary pulmonary hypertension. *Am Rev Respir Dis* 138:952-957, 1988
33. Melmon KL, Braunwald E: Familial pulmonary hypertension. *N Engl J Med* 269:770-775, 1963
34. Rich S, Kieras K, Hart K, et al: Antinuclear antibodies in primary pulmonary hypertension. *J Am Coll Cardiol* 8:1307-1311, 1986
35. Trell E, Lindström C: Pulmonary hypertension in systemic sclerosis. *Ann Rheum Dis* 30:390-400, 1971
36. Gurtner HP: Pulmonary hypertension, "plexogenic pulmonary arteriopathy" and the appetite depressant drug aminorex: post or propter? *Bull Eur Physiopathol Respir* 15:897-923, 1979
37. Gomez-Sanchez MA, Saenz de la Calzada C, Gomez-Pajuelo C, et al: Clinical and pathologic manifestations of pulmonary vascular disease in the toxic oil syndrome. *J Am Coll Cardiol* 18:1539-1545, 1991
38. Edwards BS, Weir EK, Edwards WD, et al: Coexistent pulmonary and portal hypertension: morphologic and clinical features. *J Am Coll Cardiol* 10:1233-1238, 1987
39. Lebrec D, Capron J-P, Dhumeaux D, et al: Pulmonary hypertension complicating portal hypertension. *Am Rev Respir Dis* 120:849-856, 1979
40. McDonnell PJ, Toye PA, Hutchins GM: Primary pulmonary

hypertension and cirrhosis: are they related? *Am Rev Respir Dis* 127:437-441, 1983

41. Hadengue A, Benhayoun MK, Lebrec D, et al: Pulmonary hypertension complicating portal hypertension: prevalence and relation to splanchnic hemodynamics. *Gastroenterology* 100:520-528, 1991

42. Robalino BD, Moodie DS: Association between primary pulmonary hypertension and portal hypertension: analysis of its pathophysiology and clinical, laboratory and hemodynamic manifestations. *J Am Coll Cardiol* 17:492-498, 1991

43. Kleiger RE, Boxer M, Ingham RE, et al: Pulmonary hypertension in patients using oral contraceptives: a report of six cases. *Chest* 69:143-147, 1976

44. Ackermann DM, Edwards WD: Sudden death as the initial manifestation of primary pulmonary hypertension: report of four cases. *Am J Forensic Med Pathol* 8:97-102, 1987

45. Moser KM, Auger WR, Fedullo PF: Chronic major-vessel thromboembolic pulmonary hypertension. *Circulation* 81:1735 1743, 1990

46. Nicod P, Peterson K, Levine M, et al: Pulmonary angiography in severe chronic pulmonary hypertension. *Ann Intern Med* 107:565-568, 1987

47. D'Alonzo GE, Barst RJ, Ayres SM, et al: Survival in patients with primary pulmonary hypertension. Results from a national prospective registry. *Ann Intern Med* 115:343-349, 1991

48. Rich S, Brundage BH, Levy PS: The effect of vasodilator therapy on the clinical outcome of patients with primary pulmonary hypertension. *Circulation* 71:1191-1196, 1985

49. Rubin LJ, Mendozo J, Hood M, et al: Treatment of primary pulmonary hypertension with continuous intravenous prostacyclin (epoprostenol): results of a randomized trial. *Ann Intern Med* 112:485-491, 1990

50. Barst RJ, Rubin LJ, McGoon MD, et al: Survival in primary pulmonary hypertension with long-term continuous intravenous prostacyclin. *Ann Intern Med* 121:409-415, 1994

51. Reeves JT, Groves BM, Turkevich D: The case for treatment of selected patients with primary pulmonary hypertension. *Am Rev Respir Dis* 134:342-346, 1986

52. Higenbottam TW, Spiegelhalter D, Scott JP, et al: Prostacyclin (epoprostenol) and heart-lung transplantation as treatments for severe pulmonary hypertension. *Br Heart J* 70:366-370, 1993

53. Rich S, Kaufmann E, Levy PS: The effect of high doses of calcium-channel blockers on survival in primary pulmonary hypertension. *N Engl J Med* 327:76-81, 1992

54. Rich S, Brundage BH: High-dose calcium channel-blocking therapy for primary pulmonary hypertension: evidence for long-term reduction in pulmonary arterial pressure and regression of right ventricular hypertrophy. *Circulation* 76:135-141, 1987

55. Rubin LJ, Groves BM, Reeves JT, et al: Prostacyclin-induced acute pulmonary vasodilation in primary pulmonary hypertension. *Circulation* 66:334-338, 1982

56. Schrader BJ, Inbar S, Kaufmann L, et al: Comparison of the effects of adenosine and nifedipine in pulmonary hypertension. *J Am Coll Cardiol* 19:1060-1064, 1992

57. Rozkovec A, Stradling JR, Shepherd G, et al: Prediction of favourable responses to long term vasodilator treatment of pulmonary hypertension by short term administration of epoprostenol (prostacyclin) or nifedipine. *Br Heart J* 59:696-705, 1988

58. Levine SM, Gibbons WJ, Bryan CL, et al: Single lung transplantation for primary pulmonary hypertension. *Chest* 98:1107-1115, 1990

59. Girard C, Mornex JF, Gamondes JP, et al: Single lung transplantation for primary pulmonary hypertension without cardiopulmonary bypass. *Chest* 102:967-968, 1992

CHAPTER

62

Venous thromboembolism

Jay H. Ryu, M.D., Thom W. Rooke, M.D., and Edward C. Rosenow III, M.D., M.S.

Venous thromboembolism is common, has a potentially serious, even fatal, outcome, and cannot be diagnosed without a high degree of acuity and suspicion and the performance of expensive procedures. Table 62-1 highlights some of the facts relevant to the diagnosis of venous thromboembolism.

The true incidence of venous thromboembolism is unknown; accurate statistics are extremely difficult to obtain. The most widely quoted numbers are those of Dalen and Alpert[1] (Fig 62-1). They estimated that more than half a million people suffered acute pulmonary embolism per year in the United States, and approximately 10% died within 1 hour of the event. If the preliminary deep venous thrombosis, or even the initial embolic episode, could have been recognized, perhaps many of these deaths—estimated to be more than 60,000/year in the United States—could have been prevented. A large number of these patients are terminally ill with metastatic cancer, infirmities of age, intractable congestive heart failure, etc., but many are not. They are recovering from elective surgery, orthopedic procedures, or uncomplicated myocardial infarction, only to die from the consequences of pulmonary embolism.

Table 62-1 Points to be remembered in diagnosis of pulmonary embolism

It is one of the most underdiagnosed and overdiagnosed conditions. There are no reliably characteristic or typical historical, physical, laboratory, or roentgenographic abnormalities.
Fewer than 50% of patients in whom venous thromboembolism is clinically suspected turn out to have it.
Normal perfusion scan results rule it out.
An abnormal ventilation-perfusion lung scan does not mean pulmonary embolism; for this diagnosis, the result must be in the "high-probability" range with a compatible clinical picture.
If there is any diagnostic doubt, a pulmonary arteriogram or venogram, or both, should be obtained.
An impedance plethysmogram or duplex ultrasound examination is nearly as accurate as a venogram for diagnosis of deep venous thrombosis of the thigh and pelvic veins.

The overdiagnosis of pulmonary embolism is a major problem. This error occurs because of the relative nonspecificity of the usual diagnostic measures, particularly the misconception that any abnormality of the ventilation-perfusion lung scan means the presence of pulmonary embolism.[2,3] Only the interpretation "high probability" by a nuclear medicine expert reading a ventilation-perfusion lung scan correlates well with pulmonary embolism demonstrated by pulmonary angiography. Overreading of a lung scan occurs most commonly in young women on oral contraceptives or the postoperative patient with chest pain and dyspnea whose abnormal lung scan may well be on the basis of atelectasis, pneumonia, congestive heart failure, or aspiration pneumonitis. These conditions plus asthma, emphysema, myocardial infarction, and pleuritic chest pain from many causes mimic pulmonary embolism. On the other hand, pulmonary embolism mimics many of these conditions, which further emphasizes the point that the clinician must be aggressive and pursue the diagnosis to a satisfactory conclusion.

Of those patients initially considered as possibly having pulmonary embolism on the basis of clinical grounds, fewer than 30% to 40% actually do.[4-9] In the Prospecive Investigation of Pulmonary Embolism Diagnosis (PIOPED) study[9] of 933 patients referred with the tentative diagnosis of pulmonary embolism, 251 (33%) of the 755 patients in whom pulmonary angiography was completed had thromboemboli. The clinicians in this study rated the prior probability for pulmonary embolism high (80% to 100% likelihood), intermediate (20% to 79% likelihood), or low (0 to 19% likelihood) on the basis of clinical presentation. Pulmonary embolism was confirmed in 68% of those with high, 30% of those with intermediate, and 9% of those with low likelihood. The majority (64%) of referred patients were rated as having an intermediate likelihood. This points out the nonspecificity and inaccuracy of clinical findings in the diagnosis of venous thromboembolism. The opposite is also true—many cases are never diagnosed or even suspected until found at autopsy.

Adding to the confusion are the statistics coming from autopsy series, with wide variation in incidence from 6%

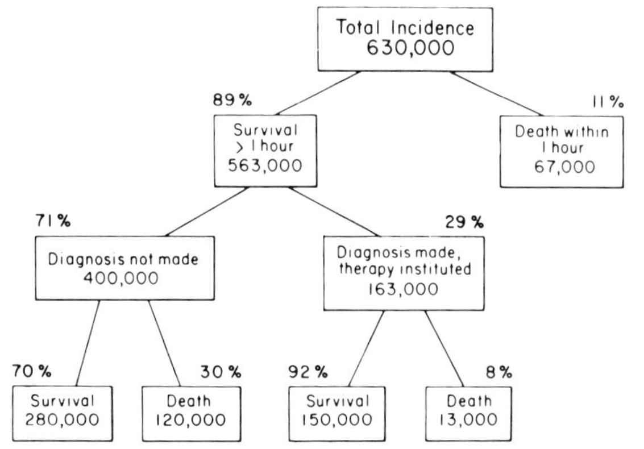

Fig 62-1 Incidence of pulmonary embolism per year in the United States. (From Dalen JE, Alpert JS: Natural history of pulmonary embolism. *Prog Cardiovasc Dis* 17:259-270, 1975. By permission of Grune & Stratton.)

to 64% of autopsies! This discrepancy generally is related to the thoroughness of the pathologist. More recent studies have shown major pulmonary embolism to be the cause of death or a major contributing factor in 3% to 9% of patients dying in general hospitals.[10-12]

Over 95% of pulmonary emboli are thrombi that originate in thigh and pelvic veins. Other possible sources of embolic material are air, fat, amniotic fluid, and tumor. Embolisms from these sources usually occur under readily identifiable circumstances, with the exception of tumor emboli, which tend to present insidiously in a recurrent fashion rather than acutely as the others do. Deep venous thrombi of the upper extremities can embolize to the lungs but not nearly as commonly as those from the lower extremities or pelvis, possibly because of an increase in the intrinsic fibrinolytic system in the veins of the upper extremities. However, this potential source of pulmonary embolism as well as the right side of the heart and the inferior vena cava should be considered in patients who have no evidence of thrombosis in the lower extremities.[13,14]

DIAGNOSIS OF DEEP VENOUS THROMBOSIS

Approximately half of the patients with clinical signs compatible with venous thrombosis have normal venograms.[15,16] Conversely, many venous thrombi detected by leg scanning with isotope-labeled fibrinogen were not detected clinically.[17] Although many of these silent vein thrombi are small and in the calf veins, a substantial portion are in the thigh veins.[18]

Patients particularly prone to the development of deep venous thrombosis are those who are seriously ill and have been at bed rest for prolonged periods. Some of the patients who are at highest risk are those who have congestive heart failure or recent myocardial infarction, advanced malignant disease, or a shock syndrome. Postoperative deep venous thrombosis occurs with increased frequency after pelvic, abdominal, or thoracic surgery and in those patients who have had orthopedic procedures. Post-traumatic deep venous thrombosis is also a major clinical problem, particularly with prolonged immobilization.

Other medical conditions predisposing to deep venous thrombosis are antithrombin III deficiency, protein C or S deficiency, obesity, polycythemia vera, dysproteinemias, sickle cell anemia, pregnancy, and estrogen therapy. Persons more than 60 years old have an increased incidence of deep venous thrombosis, as do patients with varicose veins and a history of prior venous thromboembolic disease.

Three mechanisms for the development of venous thrombosis were postulated by Virchow more than a century ago: (1) venous stasis, (2) abnormality of the blood which produces a hypercoagulable state, and (3) abnormality of the vein itself. Venous stasis appears to be the major factor in most cases. Most venous thrombi are thought to begin in the sinuses of the venous valves.[19] The thrombotic process then propagates into the adjacent vein. The process may become apparent clinically as it produces major venous obstruction or if an inflammatory process develops in the involved or contiguous vein.

Approximately 50% of deep thrombi in the iliofemoral venous system will embolize if untreated, although the factors determining which patients will experience embolization and which will not are not well known. Rarely, if ever, is there embolization of thrombi that are localized to the superficial venous system. Calf vein thrombosis also rarely embolizes to cause clinically significant pulmonary embolism.[20,21] However, in 5% to 20% of patients with calf vein thrombosis, there is propagation to the deep veins of the thigh, which do constitute a source for pulmonary emboli.

The signs and symptoms of deep venous thrombosis involving the lower extremities vary with the location and the extent of the disease. When there is extensive involvement of the iliofemoral venous system, abrupt onset of swelling of one lower extremity with tenderness to palpation over the involved veins is typical. Often there will be newly prominent superficial veins, skin suffusion, and increased skin temperature in the involved extremity. When there is less extensive iliofemoral venous thrombosis, the signs may be more subtle or even absent.

Venous thrombosis involving only the veins of the calf typically presents with calf pain and tenderness. The calf may be swollen, with increased turgor of the musculature. If there is edema of the ankle, it is usually mild. A great many conditions may simulate calf vein thrombosis and must be included in the differential diagnosis. These include plantaris tendon rupture, acute muscle strain or tear, popliteal cysts, and popliteal aneurysms.

Because the clinical diagnosis of deep venous thrombosis is highly inaccurate, particularly when the findings are subtle or when only calf vein thrombosis is present,[22] it is essential to corroborate the clinical impression with objective tests (Table 62-2).

Table 62-2 Procedures for diagnosis of deep venous thrombosis involving lower extremities

Procedure	Accuracy, by site			Advantages and disadvantages			
	Calf vein	Thigh vein	Inferior vena cava, iliac vein	Availability	Cost	Potential complications	Repeatability
Physical examination	±	++	++	++++	+	0	++++
Doppler ultrasound blood flow detector	+	+++	++	++++	+	0	++++
Impedance plethysmography	+	+++	+++	++	++	0	+++
Contrast venography	+++	++++	++++	+++	+++	+	+
Isotope venography	+	++++	++++	++	++	0	+
Duplex scanning*	++	++++	+	+++	++	0	++++

*Doppler ultrasound blood flow detection plus two-dimensional real-time ultrasound imaging.

Doppler examination

The continuous-wave venous Doppler examination is satisfactorily accurate in the diagnosis of deep venous thrombosis involving the thigh but is unsatisfactory in the diagnosis of venous thrombosis below the knee.[23,24] It is inexpensive, readily available, repeatable, and useful in the detection of deep venous valvular incompetence.

It is customary to examine the common femoral veins, superficial femoral veins, popliteal veins, and posterior tibial veins. The findings from one limb should be compared to those from the other. For each vein examined, observations are made and recorded pertaining to the patency of the vein in question along with a notation as to whether the venous signal is heard spontaneously or only with augmentation. The venous signal is augmented by compressing the limb distal to the examining site or releasing limb compression proximal to the examining site or releasing the Valsalva maneuver (the last, particularly when the common femoral veins are examined). There may be varying degrees of abnormality in reduced augmentation when deep venous thrombosis is present, depending on the severity of the venous obstruction. The venous Doppler signal normally is phasic with respiration, and this characteristic may be altered in the presence of venous obstruction to varying degrees. Venous Doppler signals obtained from collateral veins usually do not have normal respiratory phasicity. The incompetence or absence of valves in the deep veins is deduced from venous Doppler examination by demonstrating retrograde venous flow with a Valsalva maneuver at the common femoral veins or by inducing retrograde flow by compressing the extremity proximal to the examination site.[24]

Plethysmography

This noninvasive method for detecting venous occlusive disease is based on measuring blood volume changes in the extremity. Several different methods have been used, including electrical impedance,[25] strain gauge,[26] and pneumatic cuff.[27] Of the techniques reported, electrical impedance has been the most carefully studied in comparisons with venography and isotope-labeled fibrinogen leg scanning. The electrical impedance method, as originally performed, relied on changes in calf blood volume produced by maximum respiratory effort, and there were major problems in the performance and interpretation of the test.[28,29] The technique was subsequently modified to determine changes in electrical impedance of the calf in response to blood volume changes produced by inflating a pneumatic thigh cuff to pressures in excess of venous pressure and then rapidly deflating it.[25] The increase in blood volume with cuff occlusion has been termed "venous capacitance." The second measurement, the decrease in blood volume during the first 3 seconds after cuff deflation, reflects the maximum rate of venous outflow. The test results customarily are plotted on a graph with the vertical axis indicating venous outflow and the horizontal axis, the venous capacitance (Fig 62-2). The results can be interpreted as normal or abnormal; of course, some results are equivocal.

Impedance plethysmography has been compared with venography in a study of 346 consecutive patients with suspected venous thromboembolic disease.[30] It achieved a specificity of 97% and a sensitivity of 93% in detecting occlusive proximal venous thrombi.[30] The sensitivity for detection of nonocclusive proximal venous thrombi in this

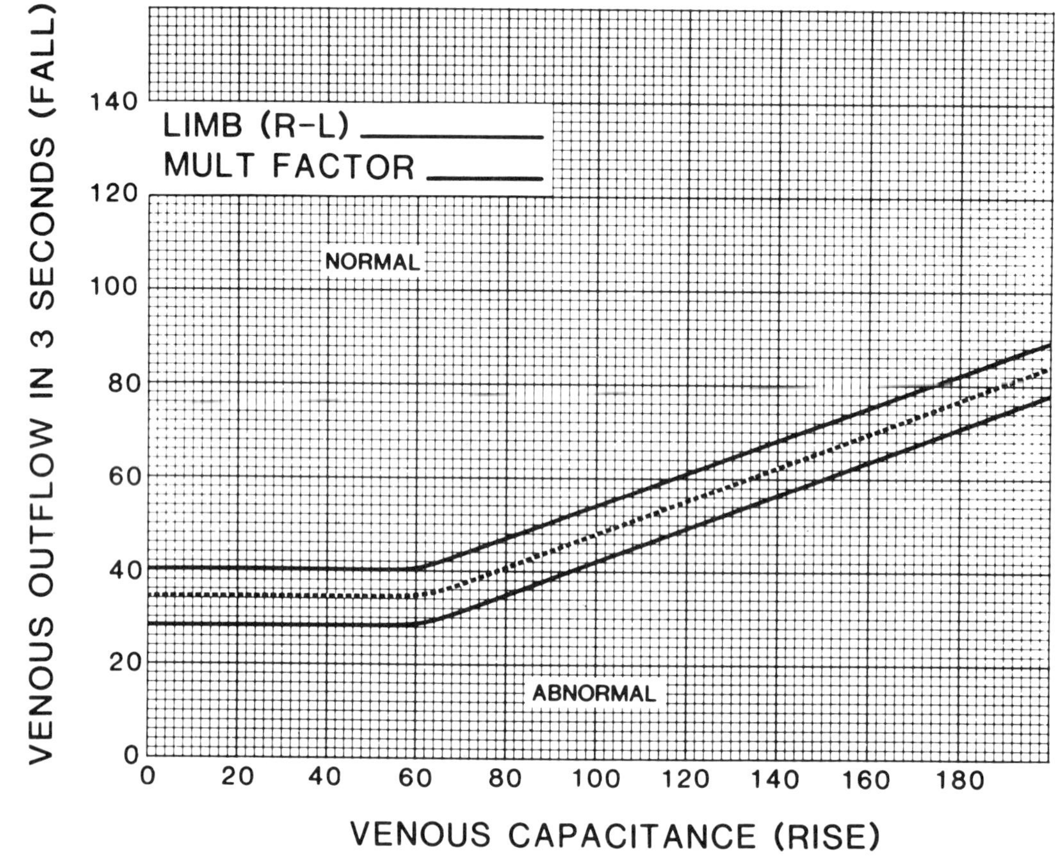

Fig 62-2 Form for plotting results of impedance plethysmography.

study was 78%. The major limitation of impedance plethysmography is its insensitivity to thrombi in the calf vein. Also, the test requires a certain amount of cooperation from the patient in regard to proper limb position. The test can be invalidated by the coexistence of severe arterial insufficiency or congestive heart failure.

Venography (phlebography)

Contrast venography has become the reference standard for the diagnosis of deep venous thrombosis. When the clinical situation calls for the most definitive diagnostic test, venography is indicated. Different methods have been employed, some using tourniquets to enhance filling of the deep veins and others using a dependent position of the lower extremities. The objective is to achieve as complete filling of the deep venous system as possible. Unequivocal evidence for deep venous thrombosis is a definite filling defect in an opacified vein or a partially occluding defect surrounded by a rim of contrast medium (Table 62-3). Venographic patterns that suggest deep venous thrombosis but are not definitive are altered venous flow and the presence of collaterals.[31,32] Special techniques must be used to assess competence of valves in the deep veins.

Disadvantages of venography are the invasive nature of the test, the potential for extravasation of contrast medium outside the vein, the possibility of a sensitivity reaction to the contrast medium, and the possibility of producing or worsening phlebitis in a small percentage of patients.

Radionuclide venography

Isotope venography provides an alternative method of imaging the deep venous system.[33] Isotope-labeled human

Table 62-3 Peripheral venography (phlebography) for diagnosis of deep venous thrombosis

Unequivocal
- Definite filling defect in a well-opacified vein
- Partially occluding defect surrounded by contrast medium

Suggestive but not definitive
- Lack of filling of vein(s) when adjacent veins are well opacified
- Extensive venous collateral circulation

albumin microspheres are injected into the dorsal veins of the feet, and radioactivity is subsequently measured in the more proximal veins up to and including the inferior vena cava. This method is reliable for the diagnosis of thrombosis in the inferior vena cava, iliac veins, and femoral veins but is inaccurate in the detection of deep venous thrombosis in the veins below the knee. Its use in diagnosis is limited, but it is a method to consider if the patient has a history of sensitivity reactions to radiographic contrast medium or if one wishes to combine a perfusion lung scan with an imaging study to search for thrombosis in the inferior vena cava or iliac or femoral veins.

Duplex scanning

Duplex scanning combines real-time two-dimensional ultrasound imaging with Doppler ultrasound (continuous- or pulsed-wave) blood flow analysis to evaluate the venous system.[34] Thrombosed veins can be identified by their failure to compress or collapse when pressure (provided by pushing the transducer against the skin) is applied over them. The accuracy of this technique for diagnosing femoral or popliteal deep venous thrombosis approaches 100%;[35] the ability to detect calf vein thrombosis is not as good but is still substantial. Old thrombus can often be differentiated from fresh thrombus by the presence of increasing echogenicity within the clot. The Doppler component of the duplex scanner can be used to assess flow augmentation, changes in flow with respiration, and valvular incompetence, as previously described for Doppler studies. Duplex scanning has the advantage of being able to diagnose hematomas, popliteal cysts, and many other nonvenous causes of leg pain and swelling. Because of its accuracy and versatility, duplex scanning is rapidly becoming the method of choice for assessing proximal deep venous thrombosis, and it may become increasingly useful in studying calf thrombosis as well.

Combinations of studies

The diagnosis of deep venous thrombosis has achieved greater accuracy when two noninvasive tests have been combined. The combination of impedance plethysmography and isotope-labeled fibrinogen leg scanning has been reported to be a satisfactory alternative to venography in selected patients with clinically suspected deep venous thrombosis.[36,37] The combination of impedance plethysmography and venous Doppler examination has also achieved greater accuracy than either test individually and is a frequently used combination for the detection of deep venous thrombosis.[38] Nevertheless, when the clinical situation calls for the most definitive test, venography is indicated.

CLINICAL PRESENTATIONS OF PULMONARY EMBOLISM

There are no characteristic clinical cardiopulmonary signs or symptoms, chest radiograph abnormalities, or arterial or venous blood test results that clearly define pulmonary embolism. Not many years ago, the triad of acute onset of chest pain, dyspnea, and hemoptysis was thought to be characteristic of pulmonary embolism, but it is now recognized that this occurs in fewer than 15% of patients with proved pulmonary embolism and can also occur in nonembolic disorders.

Table 62-4 Possible presentations of pulmonary embolism

Acute onset of symptoms with normal chest radiograph
Acute onset of symptoms with abnormal chest radiograph
Acute cor pulmonale with dyspnea, anginoid type of chest pain, and abnormal chest radiograph (may be read as normal in 10% to 15%)
Insidious onset of dyspnea over months; chest radiograph may be normal

There appear to be four different types of presentation of pulmonary embolism – three acute and one chronic and insidious (Table 62-4). Of the three acute varieties of presentation, that of acute onset of dyspnea, with or without chest pain, and an abnormal chest radiograph is the most common. Acute onset of the same symptoms with a normal chest radiograph occurs in about 15% to 20% of cases. In the presentation with acute cor pulmonale, severe dyspnea, and chest pain similar to that of angina pectoris, the chest radiograph may be normal or, in retrospect, only subtly abnormal. This presentation occurs more commonly in massive embolism – i.e., more than 40% of the vascular system occluded. The electrocardiogram is more likely to show changes of acute right ventricular strain in this setting. It is not uncommon for a patient to have two or all three of these presentations sequentially with the occurrence of subsequent embolisms over a period of hours or days.

The fourth presentation of pulmonary embolism is the occurrence of repeated small emboli over a period of weeks and months until enough vascular occlusion has occurred that pulmonary hypertension develops.[39] It is uncommon for this type to be preceded by one or more of the acute varieties. In addition, chronic pulmonary hypertension almost never occurs as a result of acute pulmonary embolism that has been treated appropriately.

A substantial number of patients with pulmonary embolism may have subtle presentations and are never recognized by physicians. This, in part, may explain why autopsy studies show that in only 20% to 30% of patients dying of pulmonary embolism is the disorder suspected or diagnosed ante mortem.[11,12] In addition, a study of 101 consecutive patients with deep venous thrombosis but without symptoms of pulmonary embolism showed a 51% occurrence of high-probability lung scan.[40] Thus, asymptomatic pulmonary embolism appears to occur frequently, at least in patients with symptomatic deep venous thrombosis.

A thromboembolus is a thrombus that has migrated downstream to a new location; a mesh of fibrin, erythrocytes, and platelets coats the surface of the thrombus. The sequelae of pulmonary emboli are related to both the degree of mechanical obstruction and the degranulation of platelets on the surface of the thrombi, with the release of a number of vasoactive and bronchoactive substances, such as catecholamines, prostaglandins, serotonin, histamine, and thromboxanes. All this occurs within seconds of the time the thrombus reaches the pulmonary artery and can be prevented by use of heparin (see below). The reactions to these mediators account for many of the nonspecific signs and symptoms of pulmonary embolism. It is hoped that in the future, the measurement of one or more of these substances in the blood will be a sensitive and specific test for the noninvasive diagnosis of pulmonary embolism.

Three factors tend to predict the cardiovascular response to a pulmonary embolus: (1) the extent of the mechanical obstruction, (2) the degree of smooth muscle constriction of the pulmonary arteries and arterioles, and (3) the presence or absence of underlying cardiopulmonary disease.[41-43] At the time of the embolization, it is not always evident whether underlying cardiopulmonary disease is present; however, if the episode is adequately treated and cardiac catheterization studies performed a few months later give abnormal results, it is likely that underlying cardiopulmonary disease is present. If the right heart hemodynamic data return to normal, it can be assumed that no underlying cardiopulmonary disease was present at the time of the pulmonary embolism.[42] In "normals" it is not possible for the mean pulmonary artery pressure to exceed 40 mm Hg, because the normal right ventricle cannot generate pressures greater than this, even if a massive embolism had recently occurred (Fig 62-3).

The increase in the pulmonary artery pressure generally correlates with the percentage of vascular obstruction in the normal person. Pulmonary hypertension usually does not occur in the normal patient, unless there is at least 30% obstruction of the pulmonary vascular system as noted on angiography. In patients with preexisting cardiopulmonary disease, however, the hemodynamic response does not correlate as closely with the extent of vascular obstruction. Again, it can be assumed that if the pulmonary artery pressure is above 40 mm Hg at the time of embolization, preexisting cardiopulmonary disease was present.

Pulmonary embolism causes pulmonary hypertension by three different mechanisms, and all probably play a role: (1) mechanical obstruction of the pulmonary arteries, (2) vasoconstriction from substances such as serotonin, and (3) vasoconstriction produced by hypoxemia.[42] Chronic pulmonary hypertension probably does not occur as the result of a single episode of pulmonary embolism. It appears that multiple, relatively small emboli must occur over at least several months before irreversible changes occur. It would seem that, in this setting of untreated (and unsuspected) recurrent small pulmonary emboli, the intrinsic fibrinolytic system never really catches up.

Cardiovascular collapse rarely occurs with less than 40% obstruction (submassive) unless there is underlying cardiopulmonary disease or another process is going on.

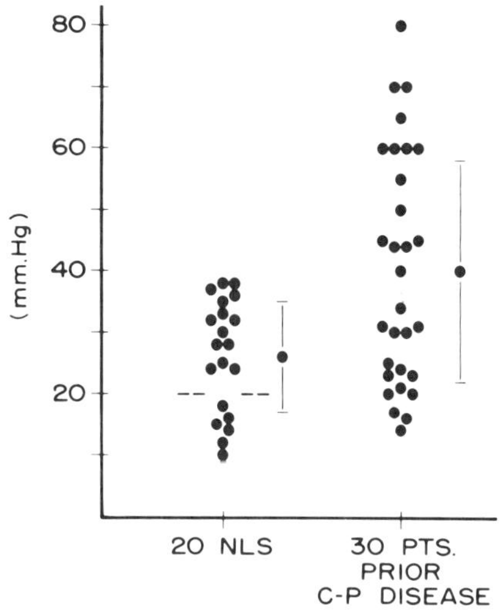

Fig 62-3 Postembolic pulmonary artery mean pressure (in mm Hg) for 20 patients with no prior cardiopulmonary disease *(NLS)* and for 30 patients with prior cardiopulmonary *(C-P)* disease. (From McIntyre KM, Sasahara AA: Determinants of cardiovascular responses to pulmonary embolism. In *Pulmonary Thromboembolism.* Edited by KM Moser, M Stein. Chicago, Year Book Medical Publishers, 1973, pp 144-159. By permission.)

Systemic hypotension occurs in fewer than 20% of patients with acute pulmonary embolism; if in this setting there is uncertainty as to whether or not pulmonary embolism has occurred, a normal or low central venous pressure rules it out.

Bronchoconstriction occurs in most patients with pulmonary embolism, but it is limited to the small peripheral airways that are perfused only by the pulmonary artery that is occluded by the embolus. This includes the terminal bronchioles and the alveolar ducts; everything proximal to these is perfused by a bronchial artery. These small peripheral airways contribute very little to the total airway resistance, and, therefore, features resembling asthma do not occur. However, this peripheral airway constriction contributes to an appreciable loss of lung volume (pneumoconstriction), producing one of the more common findings on the chest radiograph in pulmonary embolism—an elevated hemidiaphragm. Previously, it was thought that the elevated hemidiaphragm was caused by a "splinting" reaction of the chest wall to the pleuritic pain. Untreated, this peripheral airway bronchoconstriction persists 24 to 48 hours, but it can be blocked or quickly reversed with heparin.

The mediators released by the degranulating platelets in the pulmonary vessels act on three different lung receptors: (1) lung irritant receptors in the airways, which possibly are responsible for reflex bronchoconstriction, (2) receptors in the alveolar wall, and (3) pulmonary stretch receptors in smooth muscle in the airway (Hering-Breuer inflation reflex).[41] These receptors are mediated vagally and are blocked by vagotomy on the side of the embolus in the experimental animal. The first two receptors are thought to contribute to the dyspnea and tachypnea found in almost all patients with pulmonary embolism.

The assessment of the arterial oxygen partial pressure (Pa_{O_2}) is of little value in the diagnosis of pulmonary embolism; there are too many other nonembolic pulmonary conditions that will also lower this value, and a normal value (80 mm Hg or greater at sea level) is found in up to 26% of patients with pulmonary embolism.[2,3,8,44,45] A widened alveolar-arterial gradient (determined by using the alveolar gas equation and subtracting the Pa_{CO_2} value from the PA_{O_2} value) is more sensitive than the Pa_{O_2} alone.[46] This is because the reflex tachypnea and hyperventilation falsely elevate the Pa_{O_2}, possibly up to normal values. The Pa_{O_2} frequently is low because of the hyperventilation but is not diagnostic. The exact mechanism of pulmonary embolism-induced hypoxemia is not understood; it appears to involve ventilation-perfusion imbalance and decreased mixed venous P_{O_2}.[44,47,48]

Pulmonary infarction—the necrosis of lung tissue from lack of blood supply—occurs in only 10% of patients with pulmonary embolism. Contrary to what might be imagined, infarction is more likely to occur with smaller, subsegmentally located emboli than with larger, more proximal ones. Occlusion of a main pulmonary artery by massive emboli is not usually associated with infarction. This is not well understood, but the collateral bronchial circulation does not supply the lung periphery beyond the segmental level. However, there likely are other reasons, because subsegmental level emboli do not necessarily cause infarction. Underlying cardiopulmonary disease probably predisposes the patient to infarction, but it is not a consistent finding. A pulmonary infiltrate consisting of hemorrhage or edema or both occurs in about half of the patients with pulmonary embolism in the absence of infarction; in some this goes on to infarction, but in the majority it resolves spontaneously or with treatment.

Dyspnea and chest pain, frequently pleuritic, are the most common symptoms of acute pulmonary embolism[1,8,45,49-51] (Table 62-5). The sensation of dyspnea is thought to be primarily a manifestation of the vagally mediated reflex as a result of mediators from degranulating platelets stimulating the lung receptors as well as of acute hypoxemia, if present. Pleuritic chest pain is present in 70%, with a pleural friction rub heard in 5% to 20%. Pleuritic chest pain does not mean pulmonary embolism, even in the high-risk patient, and is not an indication to initiate anticoagulant therapy until more definitive studies have been done.

Hemoptysis is present in 15% to 30% of patients and is not necessarily related to the occurrence of infarction. It may begin as bright red and gradually, over several days, become darker; but this is not pathognomonic for pulmonary embolism. Surprisingly, cough is a relatively uncommon complaint (present in 40% to 50%), in spite of mediator stimulation of lung receptors and in spite of the presence of blood in the airways.[8]

A relative increase in the respiratory rate (tachypnea) occurs in almost all patients with pulmonary embolism, probably as a result of mediator stimulation of lung

Table 62-5 Incidence of symptoms and signs in 327 patients with pulmonary embolism

Symptoms	Incidence, %	Signs	Incidence, %
Chest pain	88	Respirations > 16/min	92
Pleuritic	74	Rales	58
Nonpleuritic	14	↑ S_2P	53
Dyspnea	84	Pulse > 100/min	44
Apprehension	59	Fever, > 37.8°C	43
Cough	53	Phlebitis	32
Hemoptysis	30	Gallop	34
Sweats	27	Diaphoresis	36
Syncope	13	Edema	24
		Murmur	23
		Cyanosis	19

Data from Bell WR, Simon TL, DeMets DL.[10]

receptors. Again, this is a nonspecific sign, because it occurs in many conditions with pleuritic pain, fever, or acute onset of hypoxemia. However, if the patient is acutely dyspneic in the absence of chest pain or fever and the tachypnea is enough to produce hypocarbia, pulmonary embolism should be suspected. Crackles are heard in 50% to 60% of patients. Fever is present in at least half of the patients and may go as high as 40°C. Chills are uncommon. An increase in the intensity of the pulmonic component of the second sound occurs not uncommonly, depending on the pulmonary artery pressure, but it is a very subjective finding and of little relative value. A right ventricular S_3 gallop is heard in most patients with acute cor pulmonale.

The electrocardiogram is abnormal in up to 85% of patients with acute pulmonary embolism, but in the majority the changes are nonspecific and generally transient.[45,52] The classic S_1,Q_3,T_3 is present in about 10%. The two most common abnormalities are QRS changes and ST- and T-wave changes, each occurring in about half of the patients. Except for sinus tachycardia, which is usually present, arrhythmias are relatively uncommon and, when present, usually are atrial in origin. Pulmonary embolism should always be suspected in any patient with electromechanical dissociation.

The chest radiograph is read as normal in 15% to 30% of patients with pulmonary embolism but, once the diagnosis is confirmed, it is not difficult in retrospect to see changes that are thought by some to be typical of pulmonary embolism, particularly when they occur acutely.[45,50,51,53,54] However, the usual abnormalities are generally so nonspecific that they rarely lead to the suggestion of the correct diagnosis (Table 62-6).

The chest radiograph of a patient with suspected pulmonary embolism should be compared with a recent radiograph made before the embolism. One of the more

Table 62-6 Chest radiograph in acute pulmonary embolism

Finding	Incidence, %
Normal	15-30
Abnormal	
High hemidiaphragm	25-60
Infiltrate	
Infarction	10
Hemorrhage	50
Pleural effusion	40-50
Enlarged pulmonary arteries	15-20
Atelectasis	20
Focal oligemia	15-50

common abnormalities is an elevated hemidiaphragm, occurring in up to half of the cases. Platelike atelectasis may occur above this elevated hemidiaphragm or in the absence of this elevation.

A parenchymal infiltrate is found in nearly half of the cases but represents true infarction in only about 20%; the rest have been referred to as "pseudo-infarction," which is a temporary transudation of fluid or blood.[55] This pseudo-infarct usually clears in less than 1 week, whereas a true infarct takes weeks or longer to resolve. A pulmonary infarct will occasionally resolve in the form of a melting ice cube—that is, it shrinks uniformly on all sides. An infarction in the form of a pyramidal-shaped infiltrate with the peak directed toward the hilus (Hampton's hump) is very uncommon. Otherwise, the appearance of an infarct is nonspecific.

Pleural effusion is found in nearly one-third of the patients, and probably the percentage would be higher if decubitus views had been done on all patients with proved pulmonary embolism.[56] It is bilateral in less than 10% and only rarely is massive. It is bloody in the majority of cases when it is associated with infarction and less commonly so when there is no infarction. Rarely, a cytologic study gives a false-positive result in an effusion associated with infarction. The fluid is an exudate. Beware of pulmonary embolism in the patient in congestive heart failure with a bloody effusion that is an exudate.

Enlargement of the pulmonary artery may occur as a result of an embolism. Acute cor pulmonale with enlargement of the right ventricle, as noted on the posteroanterior and lateral chest radiographs, may be an important observation in massive pulmonary embolism (i.e., occlusion of more than 40% of the vascular bed). An increased radiolucency due to decreased vascular filling, referred to as oligemia or Westermark's sign, is a common finding but often is a retrospective observation.

No studies of the venous blood are of diagnostic value either to suggest or to rule out a pulmonary embolus.[57] The Wacker triad of elevated lactate dehydrogenase and bilirubin values with a normal liver transaminase value occurs in about 15% of cases but is not of the diagnostic value once given it. Most patients with pulmonary embolism have increased levels of circulating cross-linked fibrin degradation products (D-dimers).[58-60] However, this finding is nonspecific, and normal results do not exclude the possibility of pulmonary embolism.

In patients presenting with dyspnea, echocardiography may provide the first clues that eventually lead to the diagnosis of pulmonary embolism. Echocardiographic findings have included dilated right ventricle, reduced left ventricular cavity dimension, decreased ejection fraction slope of the mitral valve, dilatation of the right pulmonary artery, abnormal motion of the interventricular septum, and right-sided thrombi (including thrombi in the pulmonary artery, right ventricle, right atrium, superior vena cava, and innominate vein).[61]

LUNG SCANS

A normal six- or eight-view perfusion scan virtually rules out the possibility of pulmonary embolism, provided that it has been done within 48 to 72 hours of the event. A normal perfusion scan is not difficult to interpret. It is more than 99% accurate in eliminating the diagnosis of acute pulmonary embolism.[9,62] However, it does not eliminate the possibility of deep venous thrombosis.[4] If the results of a test do not fit the clinical situation, further studies may be needed. If a lung scan is not normal, it is described as high-, intermediate-, or low-probability for pulmonary embolism.

The principle of perfusion lung scanning is based on the trapping of radioactively tagged particulate matter in the pulmonary capillary bed. Macroaggregates of albumin or albumin microspheres in the size range 10 to 40 μm are used; the radionuclide label is ^{99m}Tc. This particulate material is injected into a peripheral vein and imaged immediately with a gamma camera to demonstrate the functional pulmonary blood flow. The standard perfusion lung scan consists of six views.

There are several ways of performing ventilation-perfusion scans. In some institutions the perfusion scan is done first, and if it is normal, no further studies are done. If it is abnormal, a ventilation scan is performed immediately. However, other nuclear medicine specialists prefer to begin with the ventilation scan, because there is background radioactivity if the ^{99m}Tc-tagged albumin has been injected. In doing a ventilation scan, a radioactive inert gas such as ^{133}Xe is used. The procedure is performed by having the patient take an initial breath followed by rebreathing to equilibrium through a closed system; then, the washout of the radioactive material from the lungs is monitored for 3 to 5 minutes.

A normal ventilation scan will show a uniform distribution of radioactive gas in the first-breath and equilibrium views and a uniform washout from the lung fields. Abnormal areas of ventilation can be seen in any or all of the phases of washin, equilibrium, and washout; the most common cause of abnormal ventilation is chronic obstructive pulmonary disease (COPD). This is particularly true when there is a delay in the washout of radioactive tracer from the lung fields. This uneven washout in COPD would explain (1) the subsegmental perfusion defects that also are likely to be seen in this patient and (2) the frequent misinterpretation of abnormal perfusion scans as being consistent with pulmonary embolism.

As with so many features already discussed in regard to the diagnosis of pulmonary embolism, the major limiting factor in use of ventilation-perfusion lung scans is the nonspecificity of the findings. To compound the problem even further, in nearly one-third of the cases in the Urokinase-Streptokinase Pulmonary Embolism Trial, three experts could not agree on the interpretation of the extent of perfusion defects.[63] This was less of a problem in the PIOPED study.[9]

Many clinical conditions other than pulmonary embolism—such as pulmonary infiltrates of any kind, obstructive lung disease, and centrally located lung tumors—will cause perfusion abnormalities. When an asthmatic patient presents with chest pain and dyspnea and an abnormal lung scan is found, an erroneous diagnosis of pulmonary embolism frequently is made, and inappropriate treatment is initiated without further investigative studies. This happens not infrequently, especially in women taking an oral contraceptive.[2,3]

The nuclear medicine specialist looks for perfusion defects at the segmental or lobar level, where the scan shows normal ventilation. However, the lung fields must be clear on the chest radiograph where the perfusion defects are seen; otherwise, the scan is not easily interpreted and may be called "indeterminate." A perfusion defect with normal ventilation is a mismatch ($\dot{V}/\dot{Q}$ mismatch), and two or more segmental defects represent a high probability for pulmonary embolism.

Why it is that not all cases of pulmonary embolism show high probability is not known. The sensitivity of high-probability lung scan in the diagnosis of pulmonary embolism was 41% in the PIOPED study.[9] The finding of a high-probability lung scan is usually sufficient for a diagnosis of acute pulmonary embolism, provided that the clinical situation fits. If the area or areas of perfusion defect did not ventilate well or there was delayed washout, as would be expected in COPD, this is a ventilation-perfusion match and a low probability for pulmonary embolism. Between high and low probability is intermediate probability or indeterminate scan, which is not acceptable to support or to rule out the disorder; at this point more studies are necessary. The results in different series vary, mostly depending on the expertise and interest of the nuclear medicine specialist, but approximately 40% of all ventilation-perfusion studies done for the evaluation of possible pulmonary embolism fall in the intermediate-probability classification.[9]

Several interpretation schemes define the criteria for lung scan categories of high, intermediate (indeterminate), and low probability.[4,9,64-66] Although they share some similarities, many differences exist. Prevalence of pulmonary embolism found in two large prospective studies on the diagnosis of pulmonary embolism[4,9] is listed for each lung scan category in Table 62-7. High-probability lung scans provide an adequate basis for the diagnosis of pulmonary embolism in appropriate clinical situations. However, patients at high risk for serious bleeding complications from anticoagulant therapy should have pulmonary angiography for an unequivocal diagnosis. In addition, the positive predictive value of a high-probability lung scan is reduced to 75% in patients with a history of pulmonary embolism.[9] Further diagnostic evaluation may also be required if the high-probability lung scan is at odds with the clinical impression, i.e., low clinical suspicion for pulmonary embolism.

Intermediate probability or indeterminate lung scans are not helpful, and further diagnostic steps are necessary in these patients. Low-probability scans are also generally not helpful. However, patients with low clinical suspicion and low-probability lung scan have a very low prevalence (4%) of pulmonary embolism, and follow-up may be done without further tests.[9,67]

The clinician's assessment of the likelihood ("prior probability") of pulmonary embolism has a place in the diagnostic use of lung scan results. The prevalence of pulmonary embolism according to clinical assessment in each lung scan category, as derived from the PIOPED data,[9] is shown in Table 62-8. Clinical assessment has

Table 62-7 Probability of pulmonary embolism (PE) by lung scan categories

Lung scan category	Prevalence of PE, % PIOPED[9]	Hull et al.[4]
High probability	88	86
Intermediate probability (indeterminate)	33	21
Low probability	16	15-46

PIOPED, Prospective Investigation of Pulmonary Embolism Diagnosis.

Table 62-8 Probability of pulmonary embolism (PE) by clinical likelihood assessment

Clinical likelihood	Prevalence of PE, % All patients	Lung scan categories High	Intermediate	Low
High suspicion	68	96	66	40
Intermediate suspicion	30	88	28	16
Low suspicion	9	56	16	4

Modified from The PIOPED Investigators: Value of the ventilation/perfusion scan in acute pulmonary embolism: results of the Prospective Investigation of Pulmonary Embolism Diagnosis (PIOPED). *JAMA* 263:2753-2759, 1990.

substantial influence on the positive predictive value of lung scan results. It is apparent that in patients with discordance between clinical assessment and lung scan results, e.g., low clinical suspicion with high-probability lung scan or high clinical suspicion with low-probability scan, further diagnostic evaluation is necessary beyond the lung scan. Overall, lung scanning is useful in 30% to 40% of patients with suspected pulmonary embolism undergoing this procedure.

Lung scans should be performed as soon as possible in the course of the workup of a patient thought to have pulmonary embolism—preferably within 48 hours—because the intrinsic fibrinolytic system will decrease the size of the thrombus. As the thrombus shrinks, the perfusion defects will get smaller with time, and a high-probability scan will quickly become intermediate-probability. Even when pulmonary angiography is contemplated, a properly performed perfusion scan can be used to guide the angiographer to the specific areas of abnormality.

PULMONARY ARTERIOGRAPHY

Pulmonary arteriography is the definitive study. As with lung scans, it should be done within 24 to 48 hours after the embolism is suspected. Otherwise, resolution of the thrombus may make interpretation of the arteriogram difficult. A pulmonary arteriogram that is positive for embolism shows either intraluminal filling defects or cutoffs of pulmonary arteries or both. In the series by Hull et al.,[4] 94% of the positive angiograms showed intraluminal defects. Asymmetry of blood flow and oligemia are suggestive but not diagnostic findings, because these changes can occur with other conditions. If the results of the arteriogram are indeterminate, as they are in 5% to 15% of cases, the angiographer might do selective magnification arteriography to clarify the abnormalities. On the other hand, a normal pulmonary arteriogram virtually eliminates the possibility of pulmonary embolism.[68]

The mortality with the procedure is less than 0.2% and the morbidity is about 4%. Risk and expense are associated with arteriography, but they are less than those associated with anticoagulation therapy for 3 to 6 months. Computed tomography, digital subtraction angiography, and magnetic resonance imaging do not give the resolution necessary for detecting pulmonary emboli, with the exception of large proximal thrombi. However, encouraging results have recently been reported on the use of contrast-enhanced electron-beam computed tomography.[69]

A pulmonary arteriogram should be considered in the following situations: (1) when there is discrepancy between the level of clinical suspicion and the results of ventilation-perfusion lung scan; (2) when the results of ventilation-perfusion lung scan yield indeterminate or intermediate probability; (3) when pulmonary embolism is suspected in the presence of pulmonary parenchymal lung disease, significant COPD, or congestive heart failure; (4) when consideration is being given to inferior vena cava ligation, plication, or umbrella placement; (5) when there is probable pulmonary embolism but a high risk with use of anticoagulants and thus a "need to know"; (6) when there is a history of unconfirmed "recurrent pulmonary emboli," usually with episodes of dyspnea and chest pain and a low- or intermediate-probability lung scan, especially if the events occur during treatment with anticoagulants; and (7) when the situation is massive pulmonary embolism with hemodynamic instability, and the use of expensive and potentially hazardous fibrinolytic therapy or pulmonary embolectomy is contemplated. In summary, if there is any uncertainty about whether or not pulmonary embolism has occurred in the last 72 hours, pulmonary arteriography should be performed.

DIAGNOSIS OF PULMONARY EMBOLISM

When pulmonary embolism is suspected, several diagnostic pathways are available. In hemodynamically unstable patients, pulmonary angiography may be the best option to reach an unequivocal diagnosis rapidly. For stable patients, either noninvasive evaluation of the lower extremity veins or lung scan may serve as the initial diagnostic step. Positive findings by impedance plethysmography (in the absence of conditions causing false-positive results) or duplex ultrasonography provide an end point to treat and the diagnosis of venous thromboembolism. If the results are equivocal, a venogram may be necessary. High-probability lung scan results in patients highly likely to have primary embolism also provide a secure diagnosis. Normal lung scan results or low-probability lung scan in a patient with low clinical suspicion adequately excludes pulmonary embolism. If neither the lung scan nor the lower extremity venous evaluation has satisfactorily resolved the diagnostic problem, pulmonary angiography most likely is needed.

TREATMENT OF VENOUS THROMBOEMBOLISM

The treatment of venous thromboembolism can be divided into preventive and definitive measures. Preventive measures include the use of anticoagulants and venous interruption; anticoagulation can be further subclassified into whether or not the venous thromboembolism has already occurred. Definitive measures include the use of thrombolytic therapy and embolectomy.

Table 62-9 shows the various ways venous thromboembolism is prevented.[70-75] Even though pulmonary embolism or deep venous thrombosis has occurred, anticoagulants and venous interruption are used to prevent further formation of thrombi and embolization; they have no effect on preexisting thrombi or emboli (except for the heparin effect on platelets, which will be discussed later). It is easy to say that the most effective way to treat deep venous thrombosis and subsequent pulmonary embolism is to prevent it, but this means that virtually every patient at risk would need some form of preventive therapy. What is needed is some method of identifying, with a blood test, the patient at risk—e.g., on the basis of antithrombin III deficiency or protein C or S deficiency.[76] Until such a

Table 62-9 Prevention of venous thromboembolism (VTE)

Risk category	Examples	Risk of VTE, % DVT	Risk of VTE, % Fatal PE	Prophylaxis
Low	Patients <40 yr undergoing minor surgery	<10	<0.01	Early ambulation
Moderate	Patients with MI or CHF; medical ICU patients; patients >40 yr undergoing major abdominal surgery	10-40	0.1-0.7	Low-dose heparin or intermittent leg compression
High	Patients undergoing total hip replacement; major abdominal surgery in patients >40 yr with history of recent VTE; patients with hip fractures	40-80	1-5	Warfarin, low-molecular-weight heparin, or adjusted-dose heparin

Data from Salzman EW: Progress in preventing venous thromboembolism (editorial). *N Engl J Med* 309:980-982, 1983, Hirsh J (guest editor): Venous thromboembolism: prevention, diagnosis and treatment. *Chest* 89 Suppl:S369-S437, 1986, and Clagett GP, Anderson FA Jr, Levine MN, et al: Prevention of venous thromboembolism. *Chest* 102 Suppl 4:391-407, 1992.

CHF, congestive heart failure; DVT, deep venous thrombosis; ICU, intensive care unit; MI, myocardial infarction; PE, pulmonary embolism.

group of tests is available, we have to rely on clinical judgment to select who should receive prophylactic or preventive drug therapy. It is extremely important to remember that the low doses of drugs used to prevent the formation of venous thrombi must be given *before* the initiation of the thrombus, which in many cases is on the operating table or in the emergency room while the patient is waiting to be evaluated for a fractured hip.

Several investigators[77-81] popularized the use of low doses of heparin, averaging 10,000 to 15,000 units/day divided into two or three doses given subcutaneously, beginning before operation; this regimen produced a two-thirds reduction in the incidence of deep venous thrombosis and, in turn, of pulmonary embolism. It is continued until the patient is fully ambulatory.

Although low-dose heparin is an effective form of deep venous thrombosis prophylaxis, it is not applicable to all patients at risk for venous thromboembolism. In choosing the optimal mode of prophylaxis for a patient, the physician must first assess the likelihood of venous thromboembolism by considering the number and nature of risk factors (see Table 62-9). The likelihood of serious bleeding complications from the use of anticoagulants also needs to be addressed. For example, a patient with hip fracture is at high risk (43%) for deep venous thrombosis. Low doses of heparin with or without dihydroergotamine reduce this risk only slightly. Oral anticoagulants provide effective prophylaxis for this group of patients by almost halving the risk of deep venous thrombosis. Combining different modes of prophylaxis, such as addition of intermittent leg compression to oral anticoagulation, may prove to be even better prophylaxis in high-risk groups. Patients at risk for venous thromboembolism who may suffer serious bleeding complications from the use of anticoagulants are candidates for physical methods of prophylaxis. For example, in most patients undergoing elective intracranial neurosurgery, intermittent leg compression with or without elastic stockings is appropriate. Prophylaxis of deep venous thrombosis is an active area of continuing investigation. Current recommendations are described in detail in a recent consensus conference on antithrombotic therapy.[82]

Larger doses of heparin are required to treat acute deep venous thrombosis with pulmonary embolism than to prevent it.[83] Also, the half-life of heparin is shorter in patients with pulmonary embolism than it is in patients with only deep venous thrombosis. If there is any question of whether or not pulmonary embolism has occurred, heparin treatment should be initiated immediately and then appropriate studies done. The urgency is not quite as great with deep venous thrombosis if one can be certain that embolization has not occurred.

In current guidelines for anticoagulant treatment of acute venous thromboembolism, therapy begins with heparin, 5,000 U intravenously in a bolus, when the disorder is suspected.[84] When imaging studies have confirmed venous thromboembolism, another bolus of heparin, 5,000 to 10,000 U given intravenously, is followed by maintenance intravenous infusion of 1,300 U/L. After several hours of infusion, activated partial thromboplastin time is checked and the heparin infusion rate is adjusted to keep the time between 1.5 and 2.5 times the control value. The optimal route of heparin administration cannot be determined from currently available studies. Intermittent intravenous injection and subcutaneous injection are other options for heparin administration. Heparin requirements are usually greater during the first several days after an acute episode of venous thromboembolism. The platelet count should be checked daily. Heparin-induced thrombocytopenia may occur during the first day of heparin therapy, although it is more common between 3 and 18 days after heparin therapy is begun. It is more common with bovine than with porcine heparin.

The incidence of bleeding complications from heparin therapy in venous thromboembolism is 4% to 5% in contemporary studies.[85,86] Other complications include osteoporosis, anaphylactic reactions, skin necrosis, local urticaria, and hypoaldosteronism.

Heparin is not without its side effects, which are estimated to occur in 3% to 8% of patients, mostly in the form of excessive bleeding.[5,51,86] Death from exsanguination can occur.[5,86] Mild to severe thrombocytopenia occurs in up to one-fourth of the patients receiving heparin.[84-86] Large amounts of citrate-dextrose-converted blood have anticoagulant activity that is aggravated by heparin and oral anticoagulants. Protamine sulfate stoichiometrically neutralizes heparin and may be administered if overdosage of heparin or bleeding occurs.

When it is possible that an acute embolization has occurred, heparin therapy should be initiated immediately. It is uncommon for bleeding complications from heparin to occur before 48 hours. There is no contraindication to angiography or venography while the patient is receiving heparin. The problem of active bleeding, such as from a peptic ulcer or cerebral hemorrhage, prior to initiation of heparin therapy must be dealt with accordingly and may be a contraindication to anticoagulation. In this case, vena cava interruption will be needed, but this should be done only after pulmonary embolism has been proven. If hypotension or significant hypoxemia is present, oxygen should be given and a vasopressor started. Persistent hypotension is an indication for use of thrombolytic agents or possibly embolectomy. If cardiopulmonary arrest has occurred, closed-chest massage may fragment the thrombus and cause it to be pushed more peripherally, reducing the amount of major vessel obstruction. One should suspect a massive pulmonary embolus if electromechanical dissociation occurs.

A more delayed method of anticoagulation is the use of the coumarin derivatives (dicumarol, sodium warfarin [Coumadin, Panwarfin]). These drugs require 4 to 7 days to become effective. Warfarin is the compound most widely used in North America.

Heparin and oral anticoagulant therapy are usually begun together at the time of venous thromboembolism diagnosis. Heparin therapy may be discontinued after 4 to 5 days of combined administration if the prothrombin time has reached the therapeutic range.[84,85] The average duration of anticoagulation for pulmonary embolism is about 3 months, but this varies according to the circumstances. After 3 months, recurrence is rare in patients having their first episode of venous thrombosis, unless there is a persistent underlying risk factor.[75] In patients with recurrent venous thrombosis, discontinuation of therapy after 3 months is associated with a 20% incidence of recurrence within the next year. In this setting, anticoagulation should be continued for at least a year. In patients with an irreversible risk factor such as antithrombin III or protein C or S deficiency, anticoagulant therapy should be continued indefinitely.

TREATMENT OF PULMONARY EMBOLISM OTHER THAN WITH ANTICOAGULANTS

There are three intrinsic mechanisms that prevent the natural tendency of blood to clot (30 mL of blood contains enough of the clotting factors to clot nearly all the blood in the body): antithrombin III, the protein C and protein S system, and an intrinsic fibrinolytic system of which plasminogen (fibrinolysin) is a part. Through this delicate balance of clotting vs. inhibition of clotting and fibrinolysis of clots, overcoagulation and excessive bleeding are normally prevented.[87] The fibrinolytic system is not affected by anticoagulants, but it is responsible for bringing about the resolution of a thrombus once the basic disorder that caused its formation either is controlled with anticoagulants or spontaneously reverses, as it must in thousands of people each year.

Plasminogen is directly or indirectly stimulated by the plasminogen activators streptokinase (SK), urokinase (UK), and tissue plasminogen activator.[88-90] These activators convert the inactive enzyme precursor plasminogen to the active fibrinolytic enzyme plasmin (fibrinolysin). The Urokinase-Streptokinase Pulmonary Embolism Trial showed that these enzymes definitely improved lung reperfusion and hemodynamic status during the first 24 hours compared to heparin alone.[91-93] Goldhaber et al.[94] showed that treatment with recombinant tissue plasminogen activator caused more rapid lysis of clot than UK at currently recommended doses in patients with pulmonary embolism. Appropriate use of thrombolytic agents in the treatment of venous thromboembolism needs to be defined further. The optimal dosing regimen of currently available thrombolytic agents is being investigated.[95] Thrombolytic therapy should be considered for patients with clinically serious or massive pulmonary embolism or with extensive proximal deep venous thrombosis in the absence of serious contraindications.[75,84]

The clinician using these drugs should become familiar with the indications and method of administering them, because there may not be enough time to start this educational preparation with the presentation of an acutely ill, hemodynamically unstable patient. Angiographic or other definitive confirmation of pulmonary embolism must be obtained first. If angiographic facilities are not available, a high-probability lung scan in conjunction with invasive or noninvasive confirmation of deep venous thrombosis of the thigh or pelvic vessels is an alternative approach.

There are two absolute contraindications to using these drugs: current bleeding problems and recent cerebrovascular hemorrhage. Relative contraindications include recent (within 7 to 10 days) surgery, recent intra-arterial investigative procedures, renal or hepatic biopsy within 14 days, pregnancy, intracranial malignancy, gastrointestinal ulcerative disease, severe hypertension, and recent trauma. Specimens for blood gas analysis should be obtained only with a small needle in the radial artery, and pressure should be applied for 30 minutes or more afterward.

Heparin therapy is not used during thrombolytic therapy and cannot be resumed until the thrombin time or activated partial thromboplastin time is less than twice the upper limit of normal after the therapy is given. However, heparin therapy almost always needs to be resumed.

Generally, SK is given for 24 hours and UK for 12 hours for pulmonary embolism and longer for deep venous thrombosis. After 24 hours, these agents have little advantage over heparin for the treatment of pulmonary embolism. Tissue plasminogen activator is given for 2 hours. Shorter dosing regimens may be equally effective, with fewer bleeding complications.[95]

It is estimated that interruption of the inferior vena cava is performed in about 2% of all proved cases of pulmonary emboli. It is a preventive and adjuvant form of therapy and is indicated (1) when anticoagulant therapy fails, (2) when anticoagulant therapy is contraindicated or leads to complications, (3) for certain high-risk situations, such as free-floating inferior vena cava clots, massive pulmonary embolism, and recurrent episodes of venous thromboembolism, and (4) after pulmonary embolectomy or thromboendarterectomy. Inferior vena cava interruption includes surgical ligation or plication or the passage of an intraluminal umbrella or filter type of device through the internal jugular vein or femoral vein under fluoroscopic guidance. Because the surgical procedures are done using general anesthesia and because these patients are acutely ill, the risk is such that many inferior vena cava interruptions are now in the form of the percutaneous insertion of an umbrella or balloon. Surgical ligation is preferred over plication and use of filter devices, however, for septic and small recurrent emboli.

The Greenfield filter and Mobin-Uddin umbrella (Fig 62-4) are two of the several devices currently in use. Each has its own type of complications and none is totally effective in preventing embolization[96-101] (Table 62-10), because there is an incidence of recurrence of emboli of up to 5%. Anticoagulants should be continued for at least a few months after insertion of the umbrella if not contraindicated. Umbrellas and balloons are inserted under local anesthesia by a surgeon or radiologist with the aid of fluoroscopy. Perforation of the vena cava and migration of the filter are the most common complications. Others include technical difficulties during placement, insertion-site deep venous thrombosis, and inferior vena cava obstruction.

Pulmonary embolectomy for acute embolism is not nearly as popular now as it once was, because of the high mortality associated with it[102] and because intensive heparin and fibrinolytic therapy have replaced it. The mortality varies from 30% to 70%.[103] Transvenous pulmonary embolectomy by a catheter device has been used

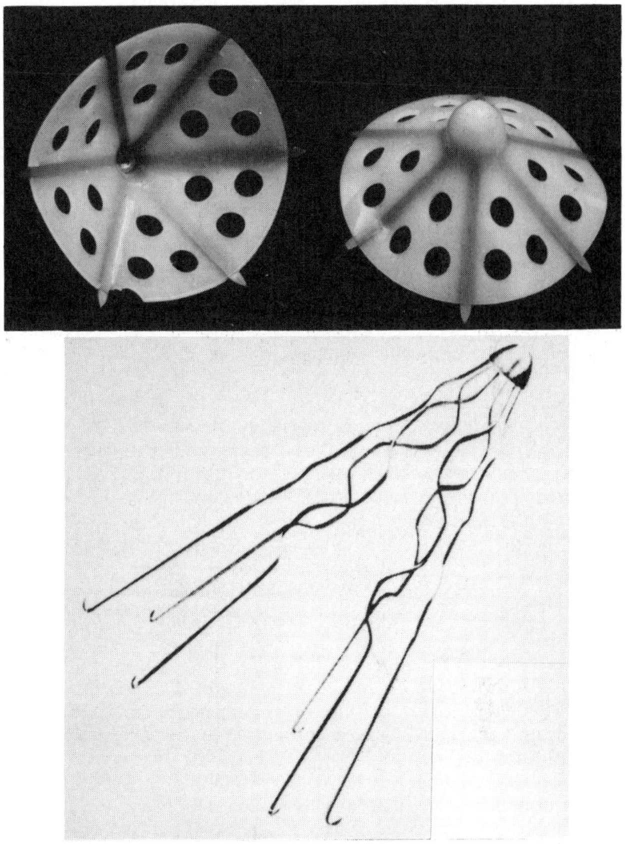

Fig 62-4 Intraluminal devices for interruption of the inferior vena cava. **Upper,** Mobin-Uddin umbrella. **Lower,** Greenfield filter.

Table 62-10 Cumulative results of transvenous methods

Operative method	Patients, no.	Operative mortality, %	Recurrent PE, %	New or worsened venous sequelae, %	IVC patency, %
Mobin-Uddin umbrella	2,966	0.6	3.4	9	40
Greenfield filter	141	3.5	2	15	96
Hunter balloon	60	0	1	24	–
Total	3,167	0.7	3.3	–	–

IVC, inferior vena cava; PE, pulmonary embolism.
From Bomalaski JS, Martin GJ, Hughes RL, et al: Inferior vena cava interruption in the management of pulmonary embolism. *Chest* 82:767-774, 1982. By permission of American College of Chest Physicians.

in recent years, with more favorable results.[104] Thromboendarterectomy has been performed in patients with thromboembolic hypertension resulting from unresolved central pulmonary artery thromboemboli.[105,106] Postoperative mortality was 16.6%, although the survivors had substantial hemodynamic and symptomatic improvement.[105]

REFERENCES

1. Dalen JE, Alpert JS: Natural history of pulmonary embolism. *Prog Cardiovasc Dis* 17:259-270, 1975
2. Robin ED: Overdiagnosis and overtreatment of pulmonary embolism: the emperor may have no clothes. *Ann Intern Med* 87:775-781, 1977
3. Letters to the Editor: Pulmonary embolism. *Ann Intern Med* 88:711-715, 1978
4. Hull RD, Hirsh J, Carter CJ, et al. Diagnostic value of ventilation-perfusion lung scanning in patients with suspected pulmonary embolism. *Chest* 88:819-828, 1985
5. Cheely R, McCartney WH, Perry JR, et al: The role of noninvasive tests versus pulmonary angiography in the diagnosis of pulmonary embolism. *Am J Med* 70:17-22, 1981
6. Stein PD, Willis PW III: Diagnosis, prophylaxis, and treatment of acute pulmonary embolism. *Arch Intern Med* 143:991-994, 1983
7. McNeil BJ: Ventilation-perfusion studies and the diagnosis of pulmonary embolism: concise communication. *J Nucl Med* 21:319-323, 1980
8. Bell WR, Simon TL, DeMets DL: The clinical features of submassive and massive pulmonary emboli. *Am J Med* 62:355-360, 1977
9. The PIOPED Investigators: Value of the ventilation/perfusion scan in acute pulmonary embolism: results of the Prospective Investigation of Pulmonary Embolism Diagnosis (PIOPED). *JAMA* 263:2753-2759, 1990
10. Dismuke SE, Wagner EH: Pulmonary embolism as a cause of death: the changing mortality in hospitalized patients. *JAMA* 255:2039-2042, 1986
11. Rubinstein I, Murray D, Hoffstein V: Fatal pulmonary emboli in hospitalized patients. An autopsy study. *Arch Intern Med* 148:1425-1426, 1988
12. Karwinski B, Svendsen E: Comparison of clinical and postmortem diagnosis of pulmonary embolism. *J Clin Pathol* 42:135-139, 1989
13. Monreal M, Lafoz E, Ruiz J, et al: Upper-extremity deep venous thrombosis and pulmonary embolism. A prospective study. *Chest* 99:280-283, 1991
14. Becker DM, Philbrick JT, Walker FB IV: Axillary and subclavian venous thrombosis. Prognosis and treatment. *Arch Intern Med* 151:1934-1943, 1991
15. Johnson WC: Evaluation of newer techniques for the diagnosis of venous thrombosis. *J Surg Res* 16:473-481, 1974
16. Sigel B, Felix R Jr, Popky GL, et al: Diagnosis of lower limb venous thrombosis by Doppler ultrasound technique. *Arch Surg* 104:174-179, 1972
17. Palko PD, Nanson EM, Fedoruk SO: The early detection of deep venous thrombosis using I^{131}-tagged human fibrinogen. *Can J Surg* 7:215-226, 1964
18. Mavor GE, Galloway JMD: Iliofemoral venous thrombosis: pathological considerations and surgical management. *Br J Surg* 56:45-59, 1969
19. Hirsh J, Hull RD, Raskob GE: Epidemiology and pathogenesis of venous thrombosis. *J Am Coll Cardiol* 8 Suppl B:104-113, 1986
20. Kakkar VV, Howe CT, Flanc C, et al: Natural history of postoperative deep-vein thrombosis. *Lancet* 2:230-233, 1969
21. Moser KM, LeMoine JR: Is embolic risk conditioned by location of deep venous thrombosis? *Ann Intern Med* 94:439-444, 1981
22. Hirsh J, Hull RD, Raskob GE: Clinical features and diagnosis of venous thrombosis. *J Am Coll Cardiol* 8 Suppl B:114-127, 1986
23. Strandness DE Jr, Sumner DS: Ultrasonic velocity detector in the diagnosis of thrombophlebitis. *Arch Surg* 104:180-183, 1972
24. Barnes RW: Doppler ultrasonic diagnosis of venous disease. In *Noninvasive Diagnostic Techniques in Vascular Disease.* Second edition. Edited by EF Bernstein. St Louis, CV Mosby Company, 1982, pp 452-458
25. Wheeler HB, Pearson D, O'Connell D, et al: Impedance phlebography: technique, interpretation, and results. *Arch Surg* 104:164-169, 1972
26. Barnes RW, Collicott PE, Mozersky DJ, et al: Noninvasive quantitation of maximum venous outflow in acute thrombophlebitis. *Surgery* 72:971-978, 1972
27. Nicholas GG, Miller FJ Jr, Demuth WE Jr, et al: Clinical vascular laboratory diagnosis of deep venous thrombosis. *Ann Surg* 186:213-215, 1977
28. Dmochowski JR, Adams DF, Couch NP: Impedance measurement in the diagnosis of deep venous thrombosis. *Arch Surg* 104:170-173, 1972
29. Harris WH, Sara SM, Salzman EW, et al: Impedance phlebography: a correlation with lower limb venography in the diagnosis of deep vein thrombosis. *Surgery* 74:385-389, 1973
30. Hull R, van Aken WG, Hirsh J, et al: Impedance plethysmography using the occlusive cuff technique in the diagnosis of venous thrombosis. *Circulation* 53:696-700, 1976
31. Rabinov K, Paulin S: Roentgen diagnosis of venous thrombosis in the leg. *Arch Surg* 104:134-144, 1972
32. Thomas ML: Phlebography. *Arch Surg* 104:145-151, 1972
33. Yao JST, Bergan JJ, Dean RH: Radionuclide venography and simultaneous lung scanning. In *Noninvasive Diagnostic Techniques in Vascular Disease.* Second edition. Edited by EF Bernstein. St Louis, CV Mosby Company, 1982, pp 502-507
34. Rooke TW, Martin RP: Lower extremity venous imaging for the echocardiologist. *J Am Soc Echocardiogr* 3:158-169, 1990
35. Lensing AWA, Prandoni P, Brandjes D, et al: Detection of deep-vein thrombosis by real-time B-mode ultrasonography. *N Engl J Med* 320:342-345, 1989
36. Hull R, Hirsh J, Sackett DL, et al: Combined use of leg scanning and impedance plethysmography in suspected venous thrombosis: an alternative to venography. *N Engl J Med* 296:1497-1500, 1977
37. Hull R, Hirsh J, Sackett DL, et al: Replacement of venography in suspected venous thrombosis by impedance plethysmography and ^{125}I-fibrinogen leg scanning. *Ann Intern Med* 94:12-15, 1981
38. Lepore TJ, Savran J, Van De Water J, et al: Screening for lower extremity deep venous thrombosis: an improved plethysmographic and Doppler approach. *Am J Surg* 135:529-534, 1978
39. Moser KM, Spragg RG, Utley J, et al: Chronic thrombotic obstruction of major pulmonary arteries: results of thromboendarterectomy in 15 patients. *Ann Intern Med* 99:299-305, 1983
40. Huisman MV, Buller HR, ten Cate JW, et al: Unexpected high prevalence of silent pulmonary embolism in patients with deep venous thrombosis. *Chest* 95:498-502, 1989
41. Widdicombe JG: Reflex mechanisms in pulmonary thromboembolism. In *Pulmonary Thromboembolism.* Edited by KM Moser, M Stein. Chicago, Year Book Medical Publishers, 1973, pp 178-186
42. McIntyre KM, Sasahara AA: Determinants of cardiovascular responses to pulmonary embolism. In *Pulmonary Thromboembolism.* Edited by KM Moser, M Stein. Chicago, Year Book Medical Publishers, 1973, pp 144-159
43. Elliott CG: Pulmonary physiology during pulmonary embolism. *Chest* 101 Suppl 4:162-171, 1992
44. Dantzker DR, Bower JS: Alterations in gas exchange following pulmonary thromboembolism. *Chest* 81:495-501, 1982
45. Stein PD, Terrin ML, Hales CA, et al: Clinical, laboratory, roentgenographic, and electrocardiographic findings in patients with acute pulmonary embolism and no pre-existing cardiac or pulmonary disease. *Chest* 100:598-603, 1991
46. Cvitanic O, Marino PL: Improved use of arterial blood gas analysis in suspected pulmonary embolism. *Chest* 95:48-51, 1989
47. D'Alonzo GE, Bower JS, DeHart P, et al: The mechanisms of abnormal gas exchange in acute massive pulmonary embolism. *Am Rev Respir Dis* 128:170-172, 1983
48. Manier G, Castaing Y, Guenard H: Determinants of hypoxemia during the acute phase of pulmonary embolism in humans. *Am Rev Respir Dis* 132:332-338, 1985
49. Moser KM: Venous thromboembolism. *Am Rev Resp Dis* 141:235-249, 1990
50. Wenger NK, Stein PD, Willis PW III: Massive acute pulmonary embolism: the deceivingly nonspecific manifestations. *JAMA* 220:843-844, 1972
51. American Heart Association (Monograph No 9): The urokinase

pulmonary embolism trial: a national cooperative study. *Circulation* 47 Suppl 2:1-108, 1973
52. Stein PD, Dalen JE, McIntyre KM, et al: The electrocardiogram in acute pulmonary embolism. *Prog Cardiovasc Dis* 17:247-257, 1975
53. Simon M: Plain film and angiographic aspects of pulmonary embolism. In *Pulmonary Thromboembolism*. Edited by KM Moser, M Stein. Chicago, Year Book Medical Publishers, 1973, pp 197-215
54. Talbot S, Worthington BS, Roebuck EJ: Radiographic signs of pulmonary embolism and pulmonary infarction. *Thorax* 28:198-203, 1973
55. Dalen JE, Haffajee CI, Alpert JS, et al: Pulmonary embolism, pulmonary hemorrhage and pulmonary infarction. *N Engl J Med* 296:1431-1435, 1977
56. Bynum LJ, Wilson JE III: Radiographic features of pleural effusions in pulmonary embolism. *Am Rev Respir Dis* 117:829-834, 1978
57. Szucs MM Jr, Brooks HL, Grossman W, et al: Diagnostic sensitivity of laboratory findings in acute pulmonary embolism. *Ann Intern Med* 74:161-166, 1971
58. Rowbotham BJ, Egerton-Vernon J, Whitaker AN, et al: Plasma cross linked fibrin degradation products in pulmonary embolism. *Thorax* 45:684-687, 1990
59. Bounameaux H, Cirafici P, de Moerloose P, et al: Measurement of D-dimer in plasma as diagnostic aid in suspected pulmonary embolism. *Lancet* 337:196-200, 1991
60. Leitha T, Speiser W, Dudczak R: Pulmonary embolism. Efficacy of D-dimer and thrombin-antithrombin III complex determinations as screening tests before lung scanning. *Chest* 100:1536-1541, 1991
61. Kasper W, Meinertz T, Henkel B, et al: Echocardiographic findings in patients with proved pulmonary embolism. *Am Heart J* 112:1284-1290, 1986
62. Kipper MS, Moser KM, Kortman KE, et al: Longterm follow-up of patients with suspected pulmonary embolism and a normal lung scan: perfusion scans in embolic suspects. *Chest* 82:411-415, 1982
63. Novelline RA, Baltarowich OH, Athanasoulis CA, et al: The clinical course of patients with suspected pulmonary embolism and a negative pulmonary arteriogram. *Radiology* 126:561-567, 1978
64. Biello DR, Mattar AG, McKnight RC, et al: Ventilation-perfusion studies in suspected pulmonary embolism. *AJR* 133:1033-1037, 1979
65. McNeil BJ: A diagnostic strategy using ventilation-perfusion studies in patients suspect for pulmonary embolism. *J Nucl Med* 17:613-616, 1976
66. Webber MM, Gomes AS, Roe D, et al: Comparison of Biello, McNeil, and PIOPED criteria for the diagnosis of pulmonary emboli on lung scans. *AJR* 154:975-981, 1990
67. Kelley MA, Carson JL, Palevsky HI, et al: Diagnosing pulmonary embolism: new facts and strategies. *Ann Intern Med* 114:300-306, 1991
68. Bell WR, Simon TL: A comparative analysis of pulmonary perfusion scans with pulmonary angiograms. *Am Heart J* 92:700-706, 1976
69. Tiegen CL, Maus TP, Sheedy PF II, et al: Pulmonary embolism: diagnosis with contrast-enhanced electron-beam CT and comparison with pulmonary angiography. *Radiology* 194:313-319, 1995
70. Francis CW, Marder VJ, Evarts CM, et al: Two-step warfarin therapy: prevention of postoperative venous thrombosis without excessive bleeding. *JAMA* 249:374-378, 1983
71. Leyvraz PF, Richard J, Bachmann F, et al: Adjusted versus fixed-dose subcutaneous heparin in the prevention of deep-vein thrombosis after total hip replacement. *N Engl J Med* 309:954-958, 1983
72. Sautter RD, Koch EL, Myers WO, et al: Aspirin-sulfinpyrazone in prophylaxis of deep venous thrombosis in total hip replacement. *JAMA* 250:2649-2654, 1983
73. Hirsh J: Oral anticoagulant drugs. *N Engl J Med* 324:1865-1875, 1991
74. Hirsh J, Dalen JE, Deykin D, et al: Oral anticoagulants. Mechanism of action, clinical effectiveness, and optimal therapeutic range. *Chest* 102 Suppl 4:312-326, 1992
75. Hirsh J, Hull RD: Treatment of venous thromboembolism. *Chest* 89 Suppl:S426-S433, 1986
76. Schafer AI: The hypercoagulable states. *Ann Intern Med* 102:814-828, 1985
77. An International Multicentre Trial: Prevention of fatal postoperative pulmonary embolism by low doses of heparin. *Lancet* 2:45-51, 1975
78. Kiil J, Kiil J, Axelsen F, et al: Prophylaxis against postoperative pulmonary embolism and deep-vein thrombosis by low-dose heparin. *Lancet* 1:1115-1116, 1978
79. Hirsh J, Genton E: Low-dose heparin prophylaxis for venous thromboembolism. In *Prophylactic Therapy of Deep Vein Thrombosis and Pulmonary Embolism* (DHEW Publication No [NIH] 76-866). Edited by J Fratantoni, S Wessler. Washington, DC, Government Printing Office, 1975, pp 183-206
80. The Multicenter Trial Committee: Dihydroergotamine-heparin prophylaxis of postoperative deep vein thrombosis: a multicenter trial. *JAMA* 251:2960-2966, 1984
81. Salzman EW: Progress in preventing venous thromboembolism (editorial). *N Engl J Med* 309:980-982, 1983
82. Dalen JE, Hirsh J (eds): Third ACCP consensus conference on antithrombotic therapy. *Chest* 102 Suppl:303-549, 1992
83. Hirsh J (guest editor): Venous thromboembolism: prevention, diagnosis and treatment. *Chest* 89 Suppl:S369-S437, 1986
84. Hyers TM, Hull RD, Weg JG: Antithrombotic therapy for venous thromboembolic disease. *Chest* 102 Suppl 4:408-425, 1992
85. Hirsh J: Heparin. *N Engl J Med* 324:1565-1574, 1991
86. Levine MN, Hirsh J, Landefeld S, et al: Hemorrhagic complications of anticoagulant treatment. *Chest* 102 Suppl 4:352-363, 1992
87. Verstraete M, Collen D: Thrombolytic therapy in the eighties. *Blood* 67:1529-1541, 1986
88. Volgesang GB, Bell WR: Treatment of pulmonary embolism and deep vein thrombosis with thrombolytic therapy. *Clin Chest Med* 5:487-494, September 1984
89. Marder VJ, Sherry S: Thrombolytic therapy: current status. *N Engl J Med* 318:1512-1520 (part I); 1585-1595 (part II), 1988
90. Goldhaber SZ: Tissue plasminogen activator in acute pulmonary embolism. *Chest* 95 Suppl:S282-S289, 1989
91. Urokinase Pulmonary Embolism Trial Study Group: Urokinase-Streptokinase Embolism Trial: phase 2 results; a cooperative study. *JAMA* 229:1606-1613, 1974
92. Urokinase Pulmonary Embolism Trial Study Group: Urokinase Pulmonary Embolism Trial: phase 1 results; a cooperative study. *JAMA* 214:2163-2172, 1970
93. Tow DE, Simon AL: Comparison of lung scanning and pulmonary angiography in the detection and follow-up of pulmonary embolism: the urokinase-pulmonary embolism trial experience. *Prog Cardiovasc Dis* 17:239-245, 1975
94. Goldhaber SZ, Kessler CM, Heit J, et al: Randomised controlled trial of recombinant tissue plasminogen activator versus urokinase in the treatment of acute pulmonary embolism. *Lancet* 2:293-298, 1988
95. Goldhaber SZ: Evolving concepts in thrombolytic therapy for pulmonary embolism. *Chest* 101 Suppl 4:183-185, 1992
96. Wingerd M, Bernhard VM, Maddison F, et al: Comparison of caval filters in the management of venous thromboembolism. *Arch Surg* 113:1264-1269, 1978
97. Greenfield LJ, Cho KJ, Proctor M, et al: Results of a multicenter study of the modified hook-titanium Greenfield filter. *J Vasc Surg* 14:253-257, 1991
98. Becker DM, Philbrick JT, Selby JB: Inferior vena cava filters. Indications, safety, effectiveness. *Arch Intern Med* 152:1985-1994, 1992
99. Goldhaber SZ, Buring JE, Lipnick RJ, et al: Interruption of the inferior vena cava by clip or filter. *Am J Med* 76:512-516, 1984
100. Greenfield LJ, Wakefield TW: Prevention of venous thrombosis and pulmonary embolism. *Adv Surg* 22:301-323, 1989
101. Welch TJ, Stanson AW, Sheedy PF II, et al: Percutaneous placement of the Greenfield vena caval filter. *Mayo Clin Proc* 63:343-347, 1988
102. Hirsh J: Diagnosis of venous thrombosis and pulmonary embolism. *Am J Cardiol* 65:45C-49C, 1990
103. Gray HH, Miller GAH, Paneth M: Pulmonary embolectomy: its place in the management of pulmonary embolism. *Lancet* 1:1441-1445, 1988
104. Timsit JF, Reynaud P, Meyer G, et al: Pulmonary embolectomy by catheter device in massive pulmonary embolism. *Chest* 100:655-658, 1991
105. Moser KM, Daily PO, Peterson K, et al: Thromboendarterectomy for chronic, major-vessel thromboembolic pulmonary hypertension: immediate and long-term results in 42 patients. *Ann Intern Med* 107:560-565, 1987
106. Rich S, Levitsky S, Brundage BH: Pulmonary hypertension from chronic pulmonary thromboembolism. *Ann Intern Med* 108:425-434, 1988

CHAPTER

63

Endocrines and the heart

Charles F. Abboud, M.D., and Emilio R. Giuliani, M.D.

THE THYROID GLAND AND THE HEART

Hyperthyroidism

The causes, diagnosis, and management of hyperthyroidism are summarized in Table 63-1.

Cardiovascular abnormalities are common features of the hyperthyroid state and, in some patients, may be its predominant clinical manifestation.[1-5]

The cardiovascular effects of hyperthyroidism result from the increased metabolic demands of the body tissues (due to hypermetabolism, increased peripheral oxygen requirements, and increased need to dissipate the excess heat produced) and from the direct chronotropic and inotropic effects of excess thyroid hormone on the heart. The circulatory changes include increases in heart rate, stroke volume, and cardiac output. Myocardial work is increased, coronary vascular resistance is decreased, and coronary blood flow, along with blood flow for all of the body tissues except the liver, is increased. Peripheral resistance is decreased, and the pulse pressure is widened. The systemic venous pressure is normal. There is a disproportionate increase in cardiac output during exercise.

The hemodynamic changes of hyperthyroidism strongly resemble those of increased catecholamine effects. Total catecholamine production in hyperthyroidism, however, is decreased (levels of dopamine β-hydroxylase and total catecholamines are low).[6-8] It has been demonstrated that there is no increased sensitivity to catecholamines in thyrotoxicosis[9,10] despite a demonstrable increase in β-catecholamine receptors in some tissues.[11] It appears that the effects of thyroid hormones and catecholamines on the cardiovascular system are additive. Both act via the intracellular adenylate cyclase system, although through activation of different cellular receptors.[12] Studies indicate that a direct action of thyroid hormone on the myocardium is responsible for the enhanced inotropic and chronotropic effects.[9,13] Adrenergic blockade therapy, although it does not abolish the increased myocardial contractility and rhythmicity, ameliorates many of the features of the hyperthyroid, hyperdynamic cardiovascular status.[9,14] It is possible that the sympathomimetic manifestations of hyperthyroidism are related to reduced catecholamine uptake by intravascular nervous tissue from the intersynaptic space,[8] or thyroxine (T_4) may serve as a substrate for tyrosine hydroxylase, a rate-limiting enzyme in catecholamine biosynthesis, and thus increase the intracellular production and action of catecholamines.[8]

Clinically, the hyperthyroid patient typically complains of palpitations, tachycardia, and exertional dyspnea. The pulse is rapid, full, and bounding, and the apical impulse is forceful and diffuse. The heart sounds are loud and ringing. Systolic ejection murmurs are common. In many patients a scratchy systolic sound is heard along the left sternal border, resembling a pericardial friction rub—the Means-Lerman crunch. The sound is believed to be due to apposition of the pericardial and pleural surfaces brought about because of the hyperdynamic heart and the dilated pulmonary artery; it is best heard at the second intercostal space to the left of the sternum and at the end of expiration. A jugular venous hum is often heard. There are no distinctive electrocardiographic (ECG) features of hyperthyroidism. The ECG in uncomplicated cases shows sinus tachycardia, increased voltage in precordial leads, and nonspecific ST-segment changes and T-wave abnormalities.[15,16] One study revealed that the left ventricular ejection fraction is high at rest in hyperthyroid patients and paradoxically decreases during exercise. This abnormal left ventricular function is restored to normal with management of the hyperthyroid state.[17]

Cardiac arrhythmias are common and are almost invariably supraventricular in type, primarily premature beats or atrial fibrillation. Atrial fibrillation is estimated to occur in about 10% to 20% of patients with thyrotoxicosis, in approximately half of whom there is no evidence of antecedent heart disease. About 10% of patients with otherwise unexplained atrial fibrillation prove to be thyrotoxic.[18] Arterial embolization in patients with thyrotoxicosis and atrial fibrillation is rare.[19] Paroxysmal supraventricular tachycardia and flutter are rare. Both intra-atrial and intraventricular conduction disturbances occur,[20,21] manifested by prolongation or notching of the P wave, prolongation of the P-R interval, and right bundle-branch block. Complete heart block and the Wolff-Parkinson-White syndrome are rarely present.[22-24]

Preexisting cardiac disease is markedly aggravated by the increased demands of the thyrotoxic state. Angina pectoris is worsened. The frequency of coronary heart disease in thyrotoxicosis is uncertain, but myocardial

Table 63-1 Etiology, diagnosis, and treatment of hyperthyroidism

Etiology

- Graves' disease
- Toxic nodular goiter (single or multinodular)
- Thyroiditis
  - Subacute thyroiditis
  - Painless lymphocytic thyroiditis
  - Radiation thyroiditis
- Exogenous
  - Iatrogenic
  - Factitial
  - Iodide-induced
- Rare causes
  - Ectopic tumor (struma ovarii)
  - Metastatic thyroid follicular carcinoma
  - Thyrotropin excess—pituitary and trophoblastic tumors

Diagnosis

- Is hyperthyroidism present?
  - Measure total and free serum T_4 or free-T_4 index:
    - If hormone levels are normal, check serum T_3
    - Obtain serum-sensitive TSH
- What is the cause of the hyperthyroidism?
  - Clinical
    - Drug history: iodides, thyroid hormones
    - Ophthalmopathy: Graves' disease
    - Goiter: Diffuse—Graves' disease or painless thyroiditis
      - Nodular—nodular toxic goiter
      - Painful—subacute thyroiditis
    - No palpable thyroid: exogenous or factitial; struma ovarii
- Radioiodide uptake: differential diagnosis, Graves' disease vs. thyroiditis

Treatment

- Remove cause if possible
- Ablate the gland
  - Radioiodine
  - Surgery
- Block hormone formation or release
  - Thionamides
  - Iodides
  - Lithium
- Inhibit peripheral conversion of T_4 to T_3
  - Propylthiouracil
  - Glucocorticoids
  - Propranolol
- Ameliorate thyroid hormone tissue effects with β-blockers

infarction is distinctively rare. Some reports have documented the development of angina and myocardial infarction in young thyrotoxic patients who had arteriographically normal coronary arteries.[25-28]

In most thyrotoxic patients without underlying heart disease, cardiac compensation is maintained. The cardiovascular effects of thyrotoxicosis, however, can produce congestive heart failure in patients with underlying nonthyrotoxic cardiac disease who are otherwise well compensated, and the presence of such heart disease often cannot be determined until the thyrotoxic state has been relieved.[29,30] Rarely, high-output cardiac failure may develop in thyrotoxic patients who have no evidence of other forms of heart disease.[31,32] Infants with neonatal thyrotoxicosis and without underlying cardiac disease have cardiomegaly and congestive heart failure, which respond to the usual regimen of digitalis, diuretics, and antithyroid therapy and usually resolve spontaneously within a few weeks.[33]

Mitral valve prolapse is twice as frequent in patients with Graves' disease as in euthyroid persons.[34] In one study,[35] about 50% of the thyrotoxic subjects had clinical and echocardiographic findings of mitral valve prolapse. Rarely, the thyrotoxic patient may have hemodynamically severe mitral or tricuspid regurgitation, which is attributed to papillary muscle dysfunction and which disappears with adequate antithyroid therapy.[36,37]

The clinician should be aware that the symptoms and signs of hypermetabolism may not be dramatic in the elderly thyrotoxic patient. The dominant manifestations of thyrotoxicosis in these patients frequently are congestive heart failure, most often with atrial fibrillation, significant weight loss, small goiter, proximal myopathy, lethargy, and blepharoptosis—the so-called apathetic hyperthyroid state.[38] This presentation is of clinical importance because of the relative ease with which the diagnosis can be overlooked and because of the potentially reversible nature of the condition. The presence of atrial fibrillation or congestive heart failure of "obscure" etiology, of "resistance" to digitalis therapy, and of the failure of cardiac decompensation to respond to a therapeutic regimen that is usually adequate should always suggest the possibility of thyrotoxicosis.

Cardiovascular drugs and the thyroid. Normally, thyroid triiodothyronine production accounts for only about 20% of the circulating triiodothyronine (T_3) levels, the remainder being produced in the peripheral tissues, primarily liver and kidney, by monodeiodination of T_4 by 5'-deiodinase. Some drugs commonly used in cardiovascular therapeutics are known to influence the metabolism of thyroid hormones and can, therefore, induce alterations in serum concentrations. Propranolol[39] and amiodarone[40,41] inhibit 5'-deiodinase and thus the conversion of T_4 to T_3 in the peripheral tissues. The decrease of T_3 in the pituitary thyrotrope leads to a mild, transient increase in serum thyroid-stimulating hormone (TSH), an increase in T_4 production, and a new equilibrium in which T_4 levels are slightly increased, T_3 levels are normal, and the patient remains euthyroid. In addition, amiodarone has been reported to induce T-cell abnormalities and lead to an autoimmune state.[42]

It is important to remember that amiodarone also serves as a source of exogenous iodides, providing 75 mg of iodine per 200-mg tablet. In normals, intrathyroidal regulatory mechanisms maintain a euthyroid state in the face of this iodine overload induced by amiodarone administration. In patients with intrinsic thyroid disease, however, such adaptation does not take place. Iodide-induced thyrotoxicosis or hypothyroidism can occur.[43-46] Iodide-induced thyroid dysfunction can be found in patients with or without identifiable underlying thyroid disease. Thyrotoxicosis occurs more commonly in geographic areas of marginal or deficient iodide intake, and hypothyroidism occurs in patients with Hashimoto's thyroiditis, Graves' disease treated with radioactive iodine, or cystic fibrosis. In the fetus and neonate, the thyroid gland is particularly prone to development of iodide-induced thyroid dysfunction. Amiodarone is stored in fat and muscle and requires about 3 months for excretion. Its clinical and biochemical abnormalities may persist for months after administration is discontinued.

Diagnosis. In the approach to diagnosis, the clinician has to document the presence of hyperthyroidism and define its cause.[47-49] In the usual case of hyperthyroidism, the thyroid gland produces supraphysiologic quantities of both T_4 and T_3. The measurement of serum total and free T_4 or their equivalent (for example, free-T_4 index) should suffice for the diagnosis of the hyperthyroid state. However, in 10% to 20% of patients, only T_3 is produced in excess, the so-called T_3 toxicosis. Therefore, in a patient with suspected hyperthyroidism, if the total and free serum T_4 are found to be normal or low, measurement of serum T_3 is in order. In the usual case of hyperthyroidism, TSH production by the anterior pituitary gland is suppressed and TSH is undetectable in the serum. The conventional radioimmunoassays for serum TSH are generally insensitive to low levels of circulating hormone, and serum TSH will be undetectable in some normal individuals. When these assays are used, the fact that TSH is undetectable cannot differentiate normal from hyperthyroid individuals. Sensitive TSH assays are available that can detect levels of TSH of 0.05 μU/mL or less. These assays can differentiate normal TSH concentrations from the suppressed concentrations seen in hyperthyroid patients. Clinically hyperthyroid patients generally have undetectable values for sensitive TSH. A normal sensitive TSH level excludes hyperthyroidism, except in the rare case of TSH-producing pituitary hyperplasia or tumor. Sensitive TSH measurements have made thyrotropin-releasing hormone testing unnecessary.[50]

In determining the cause of hyperthyroidism, a drug history is important. The clinician should specifically ask about iodide or thyroid hormone administration. Two physical findings are important in the etiologic diagnosis of hyperthyroidism: the presence of ophthalmopathy/dermopathy and the presence of goiter. If ophthalmopathy or dermopathy is present, the diagnosis is obviously Graves' disease. A diffuse goiter usually indicates Graves' disease or painless thyroiditis, a nodular goiter indicates single or multinodular toxic goiter, and a painful goiter indicates subacute thyroiditis. If the clinician cannot discern palpable thyroid tissue in the neck in a patient with hyperthyroidism, exogenous or factitial hyperthyroidism is probable. A radioiodine scan will delineate ovarian mass in those patients with struma ovarii. Radioactive iodine uptake is an essential study in the differential diagnosis of a patient who presents with hyperthyroidism and diffuse goiter but without ophthalmopathy or dermopathy; an appropriately high uptake of radioactive iodine is diagnostic of Graves' disease, whereas a suppressed radioactive iodine uptake in hyperthyroid patients without recent previous exposure to iodides is compatible with the diagnosis of thyroiditis.

Other laboratory values occasionally may prove helpful in the differential diagnosis of the hyperthyroid state. The erythrocyte sedimentation rate is typically elevated and the radioiodine uptake is suppressed in subacute thyroiditis. Assays for thyroid-stimulating immunoglobulins are positive in 90% of patients with Graves' disease.

Treatment. For a patient with thyrotoxic heart disease, therapy has two goals: an immediate one of reducing demands on the heart by reducing the hyperdynamic state and the levels of circulating thyroid hormone as rapidly as possible, and an ultimate one of treating the hyperthyroid state definitively.[51,52]

The hyperdynamic state and supraventricular arrhythmias respond well to the use of β-adrenergic blocking drugs with appropriate caution concerning contraindications to their use and side effects.[14] The patient should be maintained on an effective dosage of the β-blocker until the euthyroid state has been achieved by the necessary means.

β-Adrenergic blockade ameliorates many of the clinical manifestations of thyrotoxicosis but does not alter the intrinsic thyroid abnormality. Such blockade may decrease the high cardiac output and relieve the tachycardia, arrhythmia, heat intolerance, tremor, restlessness, myopathy, and other neurologic manifestations. However, it has little effect on increased oxygen consumption or weight loss. Therefore, β-blockers are used as adjunctive therapy to achieve rapid control of thyrotoxicosis symptoms. They are not recommended as first-line therapy. Propranolol is the agent of choice; it is given orally at 40 to 200 mg/day in divided doses. In emergency situations, it may be given intravenously in much smaller doses with continuous ECG monitoring. In addition to β-adrenergic blockade, propranolol inhibits the peripheral conversion of T_4 to T_3. The effects of selective β-adrenergic blockers in thyrotoxicosis have been less well studied than those of propranolol.

The most expedient and safest avenue for control of the hyperthyroid state in a patient with significant thyrotoxic cardiac disease is the use of an antithyroid agent. Propylthiouracil, in the usual dosage of 300 to 600 mg/day in divided doses given every 8 hours, is the agent of choice because, in addition to blocking thyroid hormone synthesis, it decreases the peripheral conversion of T_4 to T_3. It takes more than 3 to 6 weeks for antithyroid agents to produce euthyroidism. Concomitant β-adrenergic blocking therapy will help tide the patient through this latent period. After the euthyroid state has been reached, antithyroid drug therapy is continued for a few more months to allow depletion of thyroid hormone in the gland before a decision is made regarding definitive treatment of the thyrotoxic state. Such an approach will prevent the postsurgical or postradioactive iodine release of large amounts of thyroid hormone into the circulation.

We regard radioactive iodine as the definitive therapy for most adults with Graves' disease. Surgery is reserved for the thyrotoxic child and the pregnant woman after preoperative medical management has controlled the thyrotoxic state and its cardiac manifestations.

With restoration of euthyroidism, the manifestations of the hyperdynamic cardiovascular state abate; atrial fibrillation, if present, reverts to normal sinus rhythm in about 60% of patients.[53] Systemic anticoagulation is indicated in the presence of atrial fibrillation; it should be continued until sinus rhythm has been restored for at least 3 to 6 months. Attempts to convert atrial fibrillation or other supraventricular tachyarrhythmias to sinus rhythm by specific means are usually of no avail until the thyrotoxic state has been controlled. About half the patients with concurrent onset of hyperthyroidism and angina experience complete remission of angina after the control of their hyperthyroidism.[54]

The therapeutic considerations in thyrotoxic patients with congestive heart failure and atrial fibrillation are the same as those for euthyroid patients with these disorders. However, the clinician should be aware that hyperthyroid patients with congestive heart failure are particularly resistant to therapy; that digitalis requirements are often greater, possibly because of increased clearance of the drug, increased tissue distribution, and decreased cardiac sensitivity; that digitalis blood levels may be misleading, possibly as a result of altered distribution of the drug; and that great caution needs to be exercised in determining the therapeutic vs. the toxic dosage of digitalis.[55]

Hypothyroidism

The causes, diagnosis, and treatment of hypothyroidism are summarized in Table 63-2.

The cardiovascular effects of hypothyroidism result from the decrease in metabolic rate of body tissues, and thus the circulatory demands, and from the direct effect on the myocardium of lack of thyroid hormone.

The heart rate is slowed, and there is a decrease in myocardial contractility and stroke volume, a decrease in blood and plasma volume,[56] and an increase in peripheral resistance with a decrease in blood flow to the skin, kidneys, and brain. Peripheral oxygen requirements are decreased, and circulation time is prolonged. With exercise, there is an appropriate increase in stroke volume, heart rate, and cardiac output, and a decrease in peripheral resistance.

Clinically, the heart is often enlarged in primary hypothyroidism, and the heart sounds are distant but distinct. A small heart in the presence of hypothyroidism should raise the possibility of secondary or tertiary hypothyroidism. The ECG changes include bradycardia, low voltage, and nonspecific T-wave changes. The chest radiograph often shows an enlarged cardiac silhouette with a globular appearance and without evidence of pulmonary congestion.

The cardiac enlargement is related both to intrinsic myocardial disease and to pericardial effusion. Pathologically, the heart in significant or long-standing hypothyroidism is pale, flabby, and grossly dilated with interstitial edema, swelling and degeneration of the myocardial fibers, and interstitial fibrosis. The rate and force of cardiac muscle contractility are reduced, and systolic time intervals are prolonged.[57,58] These myocardial, pathologic, and functional changes are believed to be related to a direct effect of hypothyroidism on the heart, and they resolve spontaneously with thyroid hormone replacement. Echocardiographic changes of hypertrophic cardiomyopathy have been reported in patients with primary hypothyroidism; they resolve with adequate thyroid hormone replacement therapy. There is an increased incidence of atrioventricular and intraventricular conduction disturbances in patients with hypothyroidism.[59] Ventricular arrhythmias are rare.[60,61] These conduction disturbances resolve with thyroid hormone replacement.

Pericardial effusion is estimated to occur in about one-third of all patients with hypothyroidism[62] and may be the presenting feature of the syndrome.[63] It is probably due to increased capillary permeability and protein extravasation and to relatively slow lymphatic drainage.

Table 63-2 Etiology, diagnosis, and treatment of hypothyroidism

Etiology

Primary thyroprival
- Without goiter
  - Postablative: postsurgical, postradioiodine
  - Primary atrophy
  - Congenital developmental defects
- With goiter
  - Chronic autoimmune thyroiditis (Hashimoto's)
  - Defective biosynthesis
    - Drugs: lithium, iodides, antithyroid
    - Iodide deficiency
    - Genetic biosynthetic defects

Secondary (pituitary) or tertiary (hypothalamic) – diseases of hypothalamus-pituitary area

Peripheral resistance to thyroid hormones

Diagnosis

Is hypothyroidism present?
- Measure serum total and free T_4 or free-T_4 index
- Serum T_3 is unreliable in the diagnosis of hypothyroidism

What is the cause of the hypothyroidism?
- Search for goiter:
  - If goiter is present, primary hypothyroidism is the diagnosis
  - If no goiter is present, determine serum TSH
    - If TSH is increased, the diagnosis is primary hypothyroidism
    - If TSH is low or normal, the diagnosis is secondary or tertiary hypothyroidism
  - If secondary or tertiary hypothyroidism is present, evaluate the hypothalamus-pituitary axis

Treatment

Treat or remove a reversible cause if possible

Administer thyroid hormone replacement

Cholesterol crystals may accumulate in the fluid and give it an appearance of "gold paint." Fifty percent of patients with pericardial effusion have associated pleural effusion, and some have ascites as well. The pericardial fluid accumulates slowly in most patients, and cardiac tamponade is extremely rare.[64] The usual ECG and radiologic changes are not reliable indicators of the presence of pericardial effusion. Echocardiography is the most useful procedure for establishing the diagnosis.[62,65] Thyroid hormone treatment leads to spontaneous resolution of the pericardial fluid. Pericardial effusion is rare in congenital hypothyroidism.

The above findings, together with decreased exercise tolerance and ankle swelling, which are all common manifestations of hypothyroidism, often lead to a suspicion that congestive heart failure is present. Heart failure is, in fact, a rare occurrence in hypothyroidism in the absence of associated cardiac disease.[66,67] In left heart failure, cardiac output fails to increase normally, and pulmonary artery pressure is elevated during exercise. The opposite occurs in hypothyroidism.[68,69]

There is controversy over the incidence of hypertension in patients with hypothyroidism. Some studies show that diastolic hypertension is present in about one-third of older patients with hypothyroidism, and in the majority of patients, it is corrected or significantly relieved with adequate thyroid hormone therapy.[70-72] It has been suggested that increased production of norepinephrine and dominance of the α-adrenergic system contribute to the development of hypertension in the elderly patient with hypothyroidism.[73] In one study, however, the incidence of hypertension in hypothyroidism was similar to that in an age-matched euthyroid group.[74]

Coronary atherosclerosis was found to occur twice as often in patients with myxedema as in age- and sex-matched controls.[75] The pathogenesis is unknown. Lipid abnormalities are common in hypothyroidism. Although almost all types of lipoprotein abnormalities have been reported to occur in hypothyroidism, types IIa and IIb are the most commonly encountered. The degree of lipidemia correlates directly with the severity of the hypothyroidism. The contribution of hyperlipidemia to the development of coronary atherosclerosis has not been clearly established. For a comprehensive discussion of the relationship between hypothyroidism and atherosclerotic heart disease, the reader is referred to the review by Becker.[76]

Clinical angina pectoris and myocardial infarction are relatively uncommon occurrences in hypothyroidism. In a patient with known coronary heart disease, angina may improve as hypothyroidism develops and worsen with thyroid hormone replacement therapy. However, in some hypothyroid patients with angina, treatment with thyroid hormone may lead to amelioration of the angina.[77]

Serum concentrations of enzymes such as aspartate transaminase, lactic dehydrogenase, and creatine kinase are usually elevated in patients with hypothyroidism,[78] but the specific myocardial isoenzymes are normal. The mechanism of these enzyme changes is uncertain but may be related to mild skeletal and cardiac muscle damage with release of enzymes and to reduced clearance of enzymes. The enzyme abnormalities are reversed in days to a few weeks after thyroid hormone therapy.

Patients who have normal serum thyroid hormone levels and elevated serum TSH are believed to be in a state of decreased thyroid reserve and subclinical hypothyroidism. Such patients may have subtle impairment of left ventricular function which is corrected by thyroid hormone therapy.[79]

Diagnosis. In the diagnostic approach, the physician seeks to establish whether hypothyroidism is present or not and, if it is present, its cause. For documentation of the presence of hypothyroidism, reliance is placed on measurement of serum total and free T_4 (or their equivalent). Since 80% of serum T_3 is formed by peripheral tissues from the deiodination of serum T_4, and since serum T_3 can be low in nonthyroidal disease, determination of serum T_3 is unreliable in the diagnosis of hypothyroidism.[80,81]

In the physical examination, the clinician looks for evidence of hypothalamic pituitary disease and signs of a goiter. If a goiter is present in a hypothyroid patient, the diagnosis of primary hypothyroidism is almost certain. If a goiter is not present, the disorder may be primary atrophic thyroid failure or secondary (pituitary) or tertiary (hypothalamic) hypothyroidism. Determining the cause of hypothyroidism in this case would depend on measurement of serum TSH. If the level of TSH is increased, the diagnosis of primary hypothyroidism is made. Serum TSH is inappropriately normal or low in patients who have secondary or tertiary hypothyroidism. A thyrotropin-releasing hormone determination can differentiate pituitary (no TSH response) from hypothalamic (normal but delayed TSH response) causes of hypothyroidism.

A wide variety of abnormalities of pituitary thyroid function, serum hormone binding, and extrathyroidal metabolism of thyroid hormones occur in patients with nonthyroidal acute or chronic illnesses and revert to normal with recovery. These include decreased serum T_3 concentrations (decreased T_4, 5′-deiodinase activity), decreased serum T_4 levels (decreased binding proteins and presence of inhibitors of T_4 binding), decreased serum T_3 and T_4 levels and decreased serum TSH concentration (decreased TSH secretion), and increased serum T_4 concentrations (decreased T_4 clearance).[82,83] Therefore, care must be taken in the diagnosis of thyroid dysfunction in patients who have nonthyroidal illness.

Treatment. The objective of treatment in hypothyroidism is to restore and to maintain a euthyroid state. This necessitates administration of thyroid hormones in physiologic doses on a lifelong replacement basis.

Although rapid restoration of normal metabolic activity is usually without hazard in the young, such rapid replacement may precipitate angina pectoris, cardiac arrhythmias, congestive heart failure, and even sudden death in older patients who have latent or overt cardiac disease. Therefore, in older patients with hypothyroidism of indeterminate or long-standing duration, the clinician should start with a low dosage of a given thyroid hormone and increase the dosage gradually and only after the full effects of the previous dosage have been obtained (4 to 6 weeks for levo-T_4 and 2 to 3 weeks for T_3) until euthyroidism has been achieved.

We prefer to use levo-T_4 for replacement purposes. With such therapy, the increase in serum levels of T_4 and T_3 is gradual and physiologic replacement dosages normalize serum T_4 and T_3 levels; also, with a single daily dose of levo-T_4, there is no fluctuation in serum levels of T_4, T_3, and TSH. In contrast, in therapy with T_3 or levo-T_4 and T_3 in combination, serum levels of T_3 fluctuate widely after a single daily dose and may reach two to four times the normal levels a few hours after the administration of the drug or drugs, and the physician cannot rely on serum T_3 (fluctuates widely) or serum T_4 (low or low normal in T_3-treated patients) values for an assessment of the adequacy of therapy.

Levo-T_4 is started in a dosage of 0.025 to 0.05 mg/day, and increments of the same amount can be given every 4 to 6 weeks or longer until the optimal metabolic state for the patient has been achieved.

With such replacement therapy, the pulse rate increases and diuresis sets in within 1 to 2 weeks; most symptoms are diminished or disappear in 1 to 2 months.

If frank congestive heart failure is present, it demands an intensive search for other underlying cardiac disease. Treatment of heart failure may be more difficult in the presence of hypothyroidism. Responsiveness to digitalis appears to be decreased; serum levels of digitalis tend to be elevated (as a result of a decrease in volume of distribution), and therefore digitalis intoxication occurs more readily.[55] Such treatment may be further complicated by the effects of administered thyroid hormone on the ailing heart.

Patients with severe angina pectoris and untreated hypothyroidism pose a difficult therapeutic problem. The usual medical management of angina with β-blocking drugs may induce severe bradycardia. Angina may be exacerbated by thyroid hormone therapy. Thyroid hormone replacement therapy should be administered with very small doses, and increases in dosage should be made in small increments over a longer time; often the physician and the patient have to accept a suboptimal metabolic state. It is important to remember that coronary revascularization, if deemed appropriate, can be performed with minimal thyroid replacement. After successful revascularization, optimal thyroid hormone replacement can then be achieved gradually and safely without recurrence of angina.[84-86] In a patient with known or strongly suspected secondary or tertiary hypothyroidism, thyroid replacement should not be instituted until treatment with cortisol has been started, since thyroid hormone treatment in the adrenocortical-insufficient patient may cause acute adrenocortical insufficiency.

THE PARATHYROID GLANDS AND THE HEART

Hyperparathyroidism

The causes, diagnosis, and treatment of primary hyperparathyroidism are summarized in Table 63-3.

Table 63-3 Etiology, diagnosis, and treatment of primary hyperparathyroidism

Etiology	
Parathyroid adenoma	85%
Hyperplasia	12%
Carcinoma	3%
Diagnosis	
Hypercalcemia—with "normal" or increased serum parathyroid hormone	
Exclusion of other causes of hypercalcemia	
Treatment	
Elective: surgical excision of abnormal parathyroid tissue	
Hypercalcemic crisis	
Supportive therapy	
Hydration	
Saline diuresis	
Furosemide	
Other antihypercalcemic agents, if needed	
Elective parathyroid surgery	

The cardiovascular effects of hyperparathyroidism are due primarily to hypercalcemia and they include hypertension and cardiac dysfunction.

Hypertension. The incidence of hypertension is increased in hypercalcemic states.[87,88] Hypertension is estimated to occur in about 50% to 70% of patients with primary hyperparathyroidism and in up to about 35% of patients with hypercalcemia of other disorders.[89] In primary hyperparathyroidism, the occurrence of hypertension is related to the level of hypercalcemia and to the presence of renal dysfunction. The pathogenesis may be multifactorial, but the disorder is mainly caused by an increase in peripheral vascular resistance, which is thought to be related to a direct effect of calcium on the vascular smooth muscle cells.[90] Increased myocardial contractility and altered release of or sensitivity to angiotensin or catecholamines have also been suggested.

The course of hypertension after successful parathyroid surgery for primary hyperparathyroidism is variable. Although normalization of blood pressure may ensue in a significant proportion of patients, hypertension may persist and even progress despite achievement of normocalcemia, especially in patients with renal impairment.[91,92]

Cardiac dysfunction. In the usual patient with hyperparathyroidism, parathyroid hormone excess or hypercalcemia appears to have no direct adverse effect on cardiac function despite the occasional calcium deposition in the heart and blood vessels.[93] Chronic hypercalcemia, however, may be a risk factor for accelerated atherosclerosis.[94] Extreme hypercalcemia (serum calcium levels more than 16 mg/dL) as seen in hypercalcemic crisis may cause arrhythmias or even cardiac arrest. The major ECG change in hypercalcemia is shortening of the Q-T interval. Less frequent are disorders of intraventricular conduction, shortened P-R interval, and, rarely, complete heart block. Parathyroid hormone has direct positive inotropic and chronotropic myocardial effects[95] that probably are mediated by increased entry of calcium into the myocardial cell and by increased release of myocardial norepinephrine. This may be responsible for cardiac calcification in uremia.[96] One report described left ventricular hypertrophy as an almost invariable accompaniment of primary hyperparathyroidism.[97]

Patients with hypercalcemia may be more predisposed to the complications of digitalis intoxication.

Thiazide-induced hypercalcemia. It should be mentioned here that thiazides and related diuretics (such as chlorthalidone) can alter calcium homeostasis. They decrease clearance of urinary calcium (by a decrease in glomerular filtration and a direct renal tubular absorption effect)[98] and increase the release of calcium from bones (especially when bone turnover is already elevated) and absorption of calcium from the intestines. These agents may therefore cause hypercalcemia, which is usually mild and intermittent in persons with otherwise normal calcium metabolism but may be sustained in the presence of underlying disorders of calcium homeostasis.

On the basis of these considerations, we recommend that serum calcium be determined in all hypertensive patients before antihypertensive treatment is instituted and that the calcium status be checked periodically in patients who are being treated with thiazides. If hypercalcemia develops in a thiazide-treated person, use of the drug should be stopped and serum calcium should be rechecked in 2 to 3 months. If the level is still elevated, a search for other causes of hypercalcemia is in order.

Diagnosis. The hypercalcemia may be mild and intermittent, especially in early primary hyperparathyroidism. The differential diagnosis includes familial benign hypocalciuric hypercalcemia, hypercalcemia of malignancy, sarcoidosis and other granulomatous diseases, multiple myeloma, vitamin A and vitamin D intoxication, milk-alkali syndrome, thyrotoxicosis, adrenal insufficiency, and idiopathic hypercalcemia of infancy. Exclusion of these secondary causes of hypercalcemia and the finding of "normal" or elevated serum immunoreactive parathyroid hormone in the face of hypercalcemia are diagnostic of primary hyperparathyroidism (see Table 63-3).

Treatment. Definitive treatment consists of surgical excision of the hyperfunctioning parathyroid tissue. Surgery by an experienced parathyroid surgeon is usually indicated in patients with significant hypercalcemia (a level 1.0 to 1.6 mg/dL above normal); a history of episodes of life-threatening hypercalcemia; significant hypercalciuria, kidney stones, or renal failure; reduced bone mass; or age less than 50 years. Surveillance may be justified in patients with minimal calcium elevation when renal function and bone mass are normal and remain so.

Table 63-4 Etiology, diagnosis, and treatment of hypoparathyroidism

Etiology

Parathyroid disease
- Congenital
- Acquired
  - Idiopathic autoimmune
  - Postsurgical
  - Magnesium depletion

Parathyroid hormone resistance: pseudohypoparathyroidism

Diagnosis

Hypocalcemia
Hyperphosphatemia
Normal renal function
Inappropriately low parathyroid hormone level in parathyroid disease and elevated parathyroid hormone level in pseudohypoparathyroidism

Treatment

Calcium and vitamin D therapy
Ancillary: thiazides

Hypoparathyroidism

The causes, diagnosis, and treatment of hypoparathyroidism are outlined in Table 63-4.

The cardiovascular manifestations in most hypoparathyroid patients are clinically insignificant. The ECG changes are those of hypocalcemia – prolongation of the Q-T interval, which results from a lengthened ST segment. In hypoparathyroid patients with coexisting heart disease and congestive heart failure, restoration of eucalcemia may lead to improvement in cardiac function. Hypoparathyroidism may cause a cardiomyopathy that probably is related to the effects of hypocalcemia, hypomagnesemia, and lack of parathyroid hormone.[99-101]

An acute decrease in blood pressure and even shock may be associated with acutely induced hypocalcemia as occurs with rapid intravenous infusion of phosphate in the treatment of hypercalcemic crisis.[102] These circulatory changes probably result from acute reduction in peripheral vascular tone and in cardiac contractility.

THE PANCREAS AND THE HEART
Diabetes mellitus

The vascular disease associated with diabetes mellitus is of two types: (1) the nonspecific atherosclerosis and arteriosclerosis that primarily involve the large vessels, especially of the lower extremities, brain, and heart, and that affect the older patient – such disease is more severe and extensive in the diabetic than the nondiabetic patient[103] – and (2) the specific diabetic microangiopathy that produces a characteristic thickening of the basement membrane of capillaries of the retina, glomerulus, and myocardium, among other tissues, and that may be associated, in some patients, with proliferation of endothelial cells leading to occlusion of small arteries. This microangiopathy may be seen in diabetic patients of all ages.

Coronary heart disease. Coronary atherosclerosis in diabetic patients is characterized by its increased incidence, its prematurity and frequent occurrence in younger age groups, its severity, and its increased prevalence among female patients.[104-108] The atherosclerotic lesions are almost invariably present in patients who have had diabetes for 5 to 10 years or longer, and they increase both with the age of the patient and with the duration of the diabetes. Such disease and fatal myocardial infarction are known to occur at least twice as often in diabetic men and three times as often in diabetic women as in the nondiabetic population.[109] The risk of atherosclerotic coronary artery disease is also substantially increased in patients with asymptomatic hyperglycemia.[110,111]

The lesions tend to develop 10 to 12 years earlier in diabetic than in nondiabetic persons. There is an unusually high incidence of subclinical diabetes among patients with premature coronary atherosclerosis.[105]

Diabetes accelerates coronary atherosclerosis more significantly in women than in men. There is a striking increase in coronary heart disease in diabetic women, including those who are premenopausal, normolipemic, and normotensive. The incidence of angina and fatal ischemic heart disease is equal in both sexes in patients more than 40 years old.[104]

The atherosclerotic lesion in the diabetic person has the same pathologic features as in the nondiabetic. The pathogenesis is still incompletely understood. There is an increased prevalence of hypertension among diabetic patients, and hyperlipidemia is common. Epidemiologic studies suggest that the risk factors of hypertension and hyperlipidemia, although more prevalent among diabetics, do not satisfactorily account for the increased risk of coronary heart disease.[111] Roles for insulin, the sorbitol (polyol) pathway, and enhanced platelet adhesiveness have been suggested.

Myocardial infarction in the diabetic patient is noted for its high mortality, frequent recurrence, and poor long-term prognosis in survivors.[112-123] Studies show that, despite the significant development of coronary care units and newer pharmacologic modalities of treatment, myocardial infarction in the diabetic patient continues to carry a high risk.[124,125] Diabetic patients have a higher incidence of cardiogenic shock, congestive heart failure, and ventricular rupture. Mortality is adversely affected by poor diabetes control. After infarction, persistently abnormal ^{99m}Tc pyrophosphate myocardial scintigrams have been found, and these have correlated with poor prognosis.[126] Patients with myocardial infarction and poor control of diabetes before hospital admission have a significantly higher mortality than those with good control, but there appears to be no significant difference in mortality between well-controlled diabetic and nondiabetic patients.[125]

It is important to stress that both angina and myocardial infarction occurring in the diabetic patient are often manifested by atypical symptoms. These unusual symptoms may delay the diagnosis and contribute to excess mortality. The pain pattern is more variable and there is an unusually high incidence of painless infarction in diabetic patients.[127] Abrupt onset of congestive heart failure, nausea or vomiting, or abrupt decompensation in diabetic control may be the presenting manifestations of infarction. Recent reports have indicated that silent ischemia occurs commonly in diabetic individuals with coronary artery disease and not necessarily in those with autonomic neuropathy.[128-134]

The occurrence of myocardial infarction has a distinctly adverse effect on intermediate carbohydrate and lipid metabolism.[135,136] Stimulation of the sympathetic nervous system and the consequent increase in catecholamine production, an increase in the production of growth hormone, cortisol, and glucagon, and an associated decrease in the release of insulin lead to increased production of glucose by the liver and to insulin resistance. Carbohydrate intolerance is common after myocardial infarction even in "nondiabetics." Such hyperglycemia in the "nondiabetic" patient may be transient but is often a reflection of latent diabetes. The hormonal changes also lead to increased lipolysis, and the high concentration of free fatty acids may increase the propensity for the development of ventricular arrhythmias.

Hypertension. There is an increased incidence of hypertension in diabetic patients. Most studies report that it affects 40% to 80% of the diabetic population,[89, 137-140] the incidence being directly related to the age of the patient and the duration of the diabetes. The onset of diabetic nephropathy is almost invariably accompanied by hypertension.

There is an additive effect of hypertension and diabetes on the severity, extent, and rate of progression of atherosclerosis. In addition, hypertension increases the severity and accelerates the course of diabetic microangiography, and control of the hypertensive state retards the progress of this complication of diabetes.[89,137,141]

The cause of hypertension in diabetes mellitus is most likely multifactorial. Alterations in the renin-angiotensin-aldosterone system, the sympathetic nervous system, and the blood volume and sodium regulatory mechanisms have been reported.[89]

A strong association between type II diabetes and a cluster of disorders that includes obesity, atherosclerosis, hyperlipidemia, and hypertension has been known for years. Insulin resistance and the consequent hyperinsulinism may be the underlying pathogenetic mechanism, the so-called syndrome X proposed by Reaven. Hyperinsulinemia promotes renal tubular absorption of sodium, is associated with increased sympathetic activity and increased hepatic production of very-low-density lipoproteins, and is atherogenic.[142-144]

Cardiomyopathy. There is experimental and clinical evidence of the association of diabetes with a form of cardiomyopathy unrelated to coronary or other recognizable forms of heart disease.[145-148] Diabetic mice have been shown to have a primary myocardial disease.[149] Patients with idiopathic cardiomyopathy have a significant increase in the frequency of diabetes.[150,151] Epidemiologic evidence from the Framingham Study has suggested that the frequency of congestive heart failure in diabetic patients is greater than that predicted from atherosclerotic risk factors.[114,152] Other studies have suggested that heart failure may be due to coronary small vessel disease similar to that seen in the retina and kidney, with relatively normal coronary arteries on angiography[153] and at autopsy.[150] Histologic studies of the diabetic heart have revealed abnormalities of the small vessels, with intimal proliferation and thickened walls, interstitial and perivascular fibrosis, and deposition of glycoproteins and lipids.[153-155] Thickening of capillary basement membrane[156] and capillary microaneurysms[157] have been found in the myocardium. Diabetes can be associated with abnormalities of the myocardial membrane and enzyme systems (Ca^{2+}-ATPase and Na^+, K^+-ATPase).[158,159]

Studies have also shown that left ventricular function, as assessed by noninvasive methods, is often impaired in the absence of clinical coronary heart disease.[160,161] Such impairment has been documented in young asymptomatic diabetic persons,[162] in persons with maturity-onset diabetes,[163] and in those with clinical microangiopathy,[164] in whom the degree of dysfunction appears to parallel the extent of the microangiopathy.[165] The left ventricular functional impairment is predominantly diastolic, with delayed opening of the mitral valve and prolongation of isovolumetric relaxation time. Systolic functional impairment, with reduced ejection and abnormal systolic time intervals, is probably a late occurrence.[163-166] The cause of the left ventricular dysfunction in diabetic patients is probably multifactorial; in addition to large and small coronary vessel disease, diabetic persons have platelet and coagulation abnormalities,[167] increased blood viscosity,[168] and abnormal erythrocyte mechanics,[169] all of which may add to the decrease in tissue perfusion.

A transient form of hypertrophic cardiomyopathy with cardiomegaly, septal hypertrophy with features of outflow obstruction, and hypertrophy of the right ventricular free wall is seen in some infants of diabetic mothers. Its exact mechanism is unclear. Usually, it resolves by the end of the first 6 months of life.[170-172]

Autonomic neuropathy and the heart. Some diabetic patients with autonomic neuropathy or retinopathy have a defect in the autonomic control of the heart.[173-179] This may be expressed by parasympathetic denervation (tachycardia, decreased rate changes with respiration) or sympathetic denervation (decreased rise in heart rate with standing).[180] Parasympathetic denervation is more frequent and occurs earlier in the course of diabetes. Data indicate that it may be associated with diminished survival and increased risk of ventricular arrhythmias and sudden death, which may reflect the high incidence of Q-T prolongation at rest or after exercise.[181,182] Symptomatic postural hypotension occurs in diabetics with autonomic neuropathy, especially with the use of diuretics or other antihypertensives or after bed rest. As a consequence of neuropathy, the anginal threshold may be increased.[183]

Management of heart disease in the diabetic patient. Diet and insulin or oral antidiabetic agents form the mainstay of treatment of the diabetic state. Evidence is accumulating that tight metabolic control of diabetes may be important in reducing the incidence and severity of the long-term complications of diabetes.

The objectives and avenues of treatment of cardiovascular disease in the diabetic are similar to those in the nondiabetic population. However, several points have to be emphasized in the management of ischemic heart disease in the diabetic patient:

1. A conscientious, sustained effort is needed to control the other coronary risk factors: hypertension, hyperlipidemia, and cigarette smoking.
2. Nitrate-induced hypotension is of concern, because cardiovascular responses may be impaired by diabetic autonomic neuropathy. Such an effect may result in orthostatic hypotension, syncope, or aggravation of symptomatic coronary or cerebrovascular ischemic disease.
3. Hypoglycemia is of particular concern in the insulin-dependent diabetic patient treated with β-blockers. Such therapy may potentiate hypoglycemia and at the same time impair the recognition of its hyperepinephrinic cardiovascular premonitory manifestations, such as changes in pulse rate and blood pressure, although sweating and hunger sensations remain intact. Propranolol-treated hypoglycemic patients may also show a significant hypertensive response, presumably because of unopposed α-adrenergic stimulation. Therefore, β-blockers should probably not be given to hypertensive patients who are prone to the development of hypoglycemic attacks. Caution is also required in the institution and maintenance of β-blocking therapy because of the potential risk of aggravating conduction abnormalities and its propensity to decrease myocardial reserve.
4. Significant proliferative diabetic retinopathy may be a contraindication to the use of anticoagulants when such therapy is contemplated for prophylaxis and management of thromboembolism.
5. In general, coronary angiography is well tolerated by the diabetic patient. Because of the known hazards of iodinated contrast agents in the presence of renal failure, the volume of contrast material given should be limited and attention must be paid to the maintenance of hydration, blood pressure, and urinary output.

In the evaluation of patients for possible coronary artery bypass surgery, the same considerations apply to the diabetic as to the nondiabetic patient. The perioperative management of diabetes is the same as for any other major surgical procedure. Although the risk during coronary artery bypass grafting may be slightly higher in the diabetic than in the nondiabetic patient, surgery can be performed safely in most cases. Hypotension or a decreasing cardiac output, which may occur during cardiopulmonary bypass, is of particular concern in the diabetic patient who has nephropathy or cerebrovascular or peripheral vascular disease. The significant amelioration of angina by coronary artery bypass is the same for diabetic and nondiabetic patients.

The management of acute myocardial infarction in the diabetic is similar to that in the nondiabetic population.

Patients in whom the diabetes had been adequately controlled by diet, with or without oral agents, may require insulin during the initial part of hospitalization. The blood sugar is maintained at 150 to 200 mg/dL, if possible. Hypoglycemia is to be avoided because of the known hazard of the effect of release of catecholamines.

Hypertension, because of its effects on atherosclerosis and microvascular disease, markedly affects morbidity and mortality in diabetic patients. Early and vigorous antihypertensive therapy is essential.[184,185] Caution is needed in the use of potassium-wasting diuretics because potassium depletion can cause further impairment in glucose tolerance. Diabetic patients may be particularly susceptible to orthostatic hypotension, and blood pressure in supine and upright positions should be monitored closely if antihypertensive agents that are capable of causing orthostatism are used. β-Blockers can significantly reduce peripheral blood flow and aggravate symptomatic peripheral vascular disease. Special consideration needs to be given to the potential effects of antihypertensive medication on glycemic control and lipid profile, insulin action, and plasma levels of insulin. Angiotensin-converting enzyme inhibitors, calcium channel blockers, and α-adrenergic blockers have a more favorable metabolic profile than diuretics and β-blockers and should be used for initial drug therapy.

Hyperinsulinism

Hyperinsulinism, whether fasting or postprandial, spontaneous or induced, has no direct effects on cardiovascular function. Its cardiovascular effects are mediated by the resulting acute hypoglycemia, the attendant catecholamine secretion, and the transient hypokalemia due to the movement of potassium from the extracellular to the intracellular fluid compartment. Slowly developing or chronic low-grade hypoglycemia is not usually accompanied by cardiovascular manifestations.

In patients with underlying heart disease, such as coronary atherosclerosis, the well-known catecholamine-induced cardiovascular effects of acute or severe hypoglycemia may produce arrhythmias, angina, or myocardial infarction. The ECG changes of acute hypoglycemia include a depressed ST-T segment, prolonged Q-T interval, and flattening of the T waves. These changes mimic those of hypokalemia and can be corrected somewhat by the administration of potassium chloride. They are believed to be due to β-adrenergic stimulation and can be prevented or abolished by β-blockade.

THE ADRENAL GLANDS AND THE HEART

Adrenocortical insufficiency

Adrenocortical insufficiency results from decreased production of glucocorticoids or mineralocorticoids by the adrenal cortex. Its causes are outlined in Table 63-5.

Table 63-5 Etiology of adrenocortical failure

Primary
Acquired
Idiopathic (presumed autoimmune)
Tuberculosis
Miscellaneous vascular: hemorrhage, infarction
Fungal infections
Infiltration: hemochromatosis, amyloidosis
Malignancy: metastasis, lymphoma
Congenital
Hypoplasia
Steroidogenic enzyme deficiency
Secondary
ACTH deficiency
Hypothalamic pituitary disease
Exogenous glucocorticoid therapy
Angiotensin deficiency: hyporeninemic hypoaldosteronism

Adrenocortical insufficiency is important to the cardiologist because (1) it may present with clinical features that mimic primary cardiovascular disease, (2) it may occur as a consequence of primary cardiovascular disease or its management (adrenal hemorrhage in severe congestive heart failure or anticoagulant therapy), and (3) it may occur in association with cardiovascular disease in certain infiltrative diseases, such as hemochromatosis and amyloidosis.

The most common cardiovascular finding in adrenocortical insufficiency is arterial hypotension (more than 90% of cases), which is often associated with complaints of orthostatic dizziness and occasionally syncope.[186,187] The heart is small, and peripheral pulses are decreased. ECG abnormalities appear in most patients[16] and consist of sinus bradycardia, low or inverted T waves, prolonged Q-T interval, and low voltage. Conduction defects may occur. These changes resolve with glucocorticoid therapy. Hyperkalemic ECG changes are not common and resolve with mineralocorticoid therapy.

Acute adrenal crisis develops in the addisonian patient who is exposed to stress in the form of infection, injury, surgery, or dehydration. Significant hypotension or shock is an almost universal finding. Other symptoms include weakness, apathy, confusion, nausea, vomiting, anorexia, dehydration, abdominal pains, hyperthermia, and hypoglycemia. The possibility of adrenal insufficiency must be considered in any patient with unexplained shock. Hyperpigmentation, hyponatremia, hyperkalemia, lymphocytosis, and eosinophilia should suggest the diagnosis. Without appropriate therapy, death ensues rapidly.

Adrenal hemorrhage[188,189] may cause rapid and total adrenal destruction and acute loss of steroid secretion. In adults, one-third of the cases result from anticoagulant therapy (the most common cause). Among other causes are overwhelming infection with sepsis and severe life-threatening major medical illnesses such as congestive heart failure, pulmonary embolism, acute renal failure, and malignancy.

The usual presenting symptoms in adrenal hemorrhage are abdominal, flank, or back pain and tenderness;

Table 63-6 Diagnosis of adrenocortical failure

1. Rapid exogenous ACTH (Cortrosyn) test
   - ↙ Normal response
     - ↓ Excludes primary failure, but patient could have secondary failure
     - ↓ 2. Metyrapone or insulin hypoglycemia test
       - ↙ Normal response ↓ Excludes secondary failure
       - ↘ Impaired response ↓ Secondary adrenocortical failure
   - ↘ Impaired response
     - ↓ Adrenocortical failure. Is it primary or secondary?
     - ↓ 2. Serum ACTH
       - ↙ High ↓ Primary adrenocortical failure
       - ↘ Inappropriately low ↓ Secondary adrenocortical failure

hypotension or shock; dehydration; nausea and vomiting; and fever and confusion progressing to coma and death. The classic clinical features of Addison's disease, such as hyperpigmentation and weight loss, are absent. The diagnosis should be considered in the patient whose condition is deteriorating and who has abdominal or flank pain, shock, hyperpyrexia, or hypoglycemia. Steroid therapy may enhance survival, and adrenal damage may not be permanent.

Diagnosis. An approach to the diagnosis of adrenocortical failure is outlined in Table 63-6. Faced with a patient who is suspected of having adrenocortical insufficiency, the clinician has to take steps to confirm the diagnosis and to establish whether the failure is due to disease that is primary in the adrenal cortex or to disease of the hypothalamus-pituitary axis. The third phase of the diagnostic process is aimed at finding the basic disease that has caused the endocrinopathy.

Treatment. It is important to remember that adrenocortical failure may be a life-threatening disease and, therefore, that treatment (Table 63-7) should not be delayed, especially in acutely ill patients, until the results of the laboratory tests have been obtained. Treatment should be started promptly after appropriate blood samples have been obtained for diagnosis. When laboratory results are received, treatment can be appropriately modified.[190]

Table 63-7 Treatment of adrenocortical failure

Acute

Hydrocortisone, 100 mg IV every 6 hr for 24 hr; decrease to 50 mg every 6 hr, then taper to oral maintenance therapy by day 4 or 5
Saline and glucose infusion to correct hypovolemia and electrolyte and glucose abnormalities
General supportive measures
Steps to correct precipitating or coexisting disorders

Chronic

Primary failure
- Glucocorticoid: hydrocortisone, 20 mg A.M., 10 mg P.M., every day or other glucocorticoid in equivalent dosage
- Mineralocorticoid: 9α-fluorocortisol, 0.05 to 0.1 mg every day
- Steroid stress precautions

Secondary failure
- Glucocorticoid therapy as in primary failure
- Steroid stress precautions

Hyporeninemic hypoaldosteronism

The hallmarks of hyporeninemic hypoaldosteronism[191,192] are hyperkalemia, hyperchloremic acidosis, decreased renin and aldosterone secretion that is unresponsive to salt depletion and upright posture, and associated renal disease, mainly interstitial nephritis and diabetic nephropathy. Treatment consists of the use of mineralocorticoids or, if the patient is hypertensive, loop diuretics. Administration of fludrocortisone at 100 to 300 μg/day generally results in a prompt increase in renal excretion of potassium and hydrogen ion and amelioration of hyperkalemia and metabolic acidosis. Furosemide in doses of 40 to 120 mg/day has the same effects. β-Blockers and calcium channel blockers can exacerbate this condition by further impairing aldosterone production.[193]

Cushing's syndrome

The major causes of Cushing's syndrome are outlined in Table 63-8.

Hypertension. Hypertension[194,195] is present in about 80% to 90% of patients with spontaneous Cushing's syndrome in contrast to fewer than 20% of those with the

Table 63-8 Etiology of Cushing's syndrome

Endogenous
- ACTH-dependent
  - Cushing's disease
  - Ectopic ACTH syndrome
- ACTH-independent – adrenal tumors (adenoma, carcinoma)

Exogenous – glucocorticoid therapy

Table 63-9 Diagnosis of Cushing's syndrome

Does the patient have Cushing's syndrome?

Document increased cortisol production
- Best test: 24-hr urinary free cortisol excretion

Document abnormal cortisol suppressibility
- Overnight dexamethasone (1 mg) test, or standard dexamethasone (2 mg) test, or both

What is the cause of the syndrome?

Serum ACTH
High-dose (8 mg) dexamethasone suppression test
Metyrapone test
Radiologic tumor localization

exogenous iatrogenic type. The cause of this discrepancy is not known but may be related to the fact that most exogenous glucocorticoids are analogues of cortisol and have a negligible mineralocorticoid effect. The hypertension may be quite severe, lead to chronic and severe hypertensive sequelae, and contribute greatly to the mortality and morbidity in spontaneous Cushing's syndrome. In one series, 40% of those dying with the syndrome did so directly as a result of hypertension or atherosclerosis.[196] Cure or improvement of the hypertension usually follows successful treatment of the syndrome.

The mechanism of the hypertension in spontaneous Cushing's syndrome is not clear, and several factors may be operative:[194,197-199] (1) mineralocorticoid effects of excess cortisol or other mineralocorticoid excess; (2) induction of excess renin substrate by hypercortisolism and, therefore, increased angiotensin production (saralasin, the angiotensin II antagonist, can lower the blood pressure in Cushing's syndrome); (3) increased sensitivity to β-adrenergic agonists because of cortisol and thus increased vascular reactivity; and (4) production of other steroids by the adrenal glands, which can cause hypertension.

Recently, severe disproportionate hypertrophy of the interventricular septum was reported in patients with Cushing's syndrome who were hypertensive. Such hypertrophy regressed after successful treatment of the hypercortisol state. The frequency of left ventricular hypertrophy and asymmetric septal hypertrophy appears to be much greater in Cushing's syndrome than in essential hypertension or other forms of secondary hypertension; it appears that excess cortisol may be a direct significant etiologic factor.[200,201]

Coronary atherosclerosis. Coronary atherosclerosis is believed to be accelerated in patients who have Cushing's syndrome of long duration. Hypertension, diabetes mellitus, and hyperlipidemia are undoubtedly contributing factors. Hypercholesterolemia and hypertriglyceridemia have long been known to accompany Cushing's syndrome;[202] the extent of increase in cholesterol exceeds that in triglycerides. Both very-low-density and low-density lipoproteins are increased, and if steroidogenic diabetes sets in, mixed hyperlipidemia may occur.

Cardiomegaly and heart failure due to hypertensive coronary cardiovascular disease are often present in patients with untreated Cushing's syndrome of long duration.

Cushing's syndrome due to primary adrenocortical nodular disease has recently been reported to occur in a rare familial syndrome, Carney's complex,[203] that also may include cardiac myxomas, pigmentation, mammary fibroadenomas, testicular tumors, and gigantism/acromegaly.[204,205]

Diagnosis. The diagnosis of Cushing's syndrome is outlined in Table 63-9.[206,207]

In the differential diagnosis of Cushing's syndrome, reliance is placed on the anatomic localization of the tumor, the level of serum ACTH, and the behavior of the hypothalamus-pituitary-adrenal axis in the face of provocative suppression or stimulation tests. In Cushing's disease, the axis is suppressible with high doses of dexamethasone and is responsive to metyrapone stimulation, and serum ACTH is normal or increased. In ectopic Cushing's syndrome, the overproduction of cortisol is unresponsive to high-dose dexamethasone suppression, and metyrapone stimulation and serum ACTH are usually markedly increased. In adrenal tumors, the cortisol overproduction is also unresponsive to high doses of dexamethasone and metyrapone, but serum ACTH is undetectable. In selected cases, bilateral inferior petrosal sinus sampling for ACTH gradient may be resorted to for diagnostic etiologic clarification.

Treatment. The definitive treatment of Cushing's syndrome is outlined in Table 63-10.

Primary aldosteronism

The causes of hyperaldosteronism are listed in Table 63-11.

The cardiovascular effects of primary aldosteronism are related to those of hypertension and hypokalemia. Excessive production of aldosterone causes sodium retention, increased total body sodium and extracellular fluid volume, and suppression of the renin-angiotensin system. Despite the increased extracellular fluid volume, overt edema does not occur, because of cardiohormonal and renal adjustments that enable the kidneys to compensate for and come into equilibrium with the sodium intake. Hyperaldosteronism, in addition, causes increased renal

Table 63-10 Treatment of Cushing's syndrome

Cushing's disease

Transsphenoidal adenectomy
or
Pituitary irradiation
If not successful, bilateral adrenalectomy

Ectopic ACTH syndrome

If feasible, resection of primary tumor
If not, bilateral adrenalectomy or adrenolytic drug therapy with mitotane (*o,p'*-DDD)
or
Adrenocortical blocking drugs: aminoglutethimide, metyrapone, and ketoconazole

Adrenal tumor

Unilateral adrenalectomy
If surgically incurable, adrenolytic drug therapy with mitotane (*o,p'*-DDD)

Table 63-11 Etiology of aldosteronism

Primary aldosteronism	
Adrenocortical adenoma	80%
Hyperplasia	<20%
Carcinoma	<1%
Dexamethasone suppressible	
Secondary aldosteronism	
Without hypertension	
Extracellular fluid depletion—e.g., diuretics, gastrointestinal fluid losses	
Extracellular fluid redistribution—e.g., nephrosis, cirrhosis, congestive heart failure	
Bartter's syndrome	
With hypertension	
Renal artery stenosis	
Malignant hypertension	
Estrogen therapy	
Reninoma	

tubular loss of potassium and hydrogen, depletion of total body potassium, hypokalemia, and metabolic alkalosis.

Systemic hypertension[195] is one cardinal manifestation of the disease. The incidence of primary aldosteronism in the hypertensive population is 0.5% to 2%. The cause of hypertension in primary aldosteronism is probably multifactorial[208] and is related to increased plasma volume, increased sodium concentration in the arteriolar wall, and increased vasoconstriction, possibly because of the effect of increased body sodium in decreasing the uptake of norepinephrine by the neuronal endings in the circulatory system.

Table 63-12 Diagnosis of primary aldosteronism

Document unprovoked hypokalemia
- Serum potassium
- Exclude other causes of hypokalemia, especially gastrointestinal and nonaldosterone-dependent renal losses

Document inappropriate kaliuresis in face of hypokalemia
- Urine potassium

Document aldosterone overproduction
- Serum or urinary aldosterone
- Glucocorticoid parameters

Document the cause of the hyperaldosteronism (Is it primary or secondary?)
- Plasma renin activity under provoked state

Document the cause of primary aldosteronism (Is it adrenal tumor or hyperplasia?)
- Anatomic
  - CT scan of adrenal glands
  - Isotope scanning
  - Adrenal venography
  - Selective adrenal vein sampling
- Functional: serum aldosterone response to upright posture

The hypertension in primary aldosteronism is usually mild to moderate in severity. Malignant hypertension is rare. In time, the usual features of hypertensive vascular disease may make their appearance. Hypertensive retinopathy is usually mild; nephropathy is very infrequent. Cardiomegaly is present in some patients, but congestive heart failure is rarely seen.

Hypokalemia is the other cardinal manifestation of primary aldosteronism. It may express itself as muscle weakness (rarely periodic paralysis), areflexia, orthostatism due to the impairment of vascular reflexes, and paresthesias and tetany from increased neuromuscular irritability due to the hypokalemic alkalosis and the associated magnesium depletion. Polyuria and polydipsia may be caused by the development of diabetes mellitus or more commonly by nephrogenic diabetes insipidus due to the kaliopenic nephropathy. Hypokalemia may also cause electrophysiologic alterations in the myocardium and disturbances in cardiac conduction or rhythm.

Diagnosis. The diagnostic approach is outlined in Table 63-12.[209,210] The first step in the evaluation of a patient with suspected aldosteronism is the demonstration of unprovoked hypokalemia. It is important, in taking the history, to exclude use of drugs such as diuretics and steroids, ingestion of licorice, and gastrointestinal losses of fluid. Since excretion of potassium by the distal nephron is, in part, a function of the quantity of sodium reaching that part of the nephron, a low-sodium intake may mask the hypokalemia. Therefore, a normal serum concentration of potassium in a patient who is suspected of having primary aldosteronism should not exclude the diagnosis. If feasible, such a patient should be salt loaded to unmask the kaliuretic effect of hyperaldosteronism. A normal serum level of potassium after about 3 to 4 days of salt loading excludes the presence of primary aldosteronism.

The next step is to determine whether inappropriate urinary loss of potassium is present in the face of hypokalemia. Urinary excretion of potassium of more than 30 mEq/24 hours in the presence of hypokalemia indicates a renal potassium-losing state. The next diagnostic step is to determine whether the hypokalemia and the inappropriate kaliuresis are due to increased aldosterone production or to other causes. Hypokalemia must be corrected and a period of adequate salt intake must be ensured before aldosterone measurements are made. A demonstrable increase in serum or urinary level of aldosterone, after correction of the electrolyte abnormalities, is diagnostic of aldosteronism. The renin status after salt depletion (use of diuretic) and in the upright posture is then assessed. Suppressed renin activity that fails to increase normally with physiologic stimuli of upright posture, salt restriction, and diuretic therapy in a patient with hypokalemia, inappropriate kaliuresis, and increased aldosterone production is diagnostic of primary aldosteronism.[211]

All antihypertensive drugs have some effect on the renin-angiotensin-aldosterone axis. Plasma renin activity is increased by diuretics, direct vasodilators, and angiotensin-converting enzyme inhibitors and is decreased by β-blockers,[211] calcium channel blockers, and centrally active agents. If at all possible, antihypertensive medications should be discontinued prior to the diagnostic evaluation. If the blood pressure increases to unacceptably high levels, methyldopa or hydralazine can be administered because they have the least effect on renin activity.

Since the modality of therapy in primary aldosteronism depends on the underlying pathology, diagnostic steps are then taken to ascertain whether the cause of the disease is an adrenal tumor or bilateral adrenal hyperplasia.[212] Anatomic localization of the lesion is most commonly accomplished by a computed tomography scan of the adrenals[213] or by selective sampling of both adrenal veins for aldosterone. Reliance is also placed on the response of aldosterone secretion to upright posture. An increased aldosterone response to upright posture favors hyperplasia (renin sensitive), whereas absence of a response or an actual decrease in serum aldosterone after upright posture favors adrenal adenoma (diurnal ACTH effect).[214]

Treatment. Adenomas are best treated surgically, and excellent results are usually obtained in restoration of normotension and reversal of biochemical effects.[215] Because bilateral adrenalectomy can reverse hypertension in only one-third of patients with idiopathic hyperaldosteronism, medical treatment is usually advised for this condition. Drug therapy with spironolactone, an aldosterone antagonist, is the modality of choice in the treatment of the patient with idiopathic hyperaldosteronism, the treatment of the patient with adenoma who refuses or is ineligible for surgery, and the preoperative preparation of the patient with adenoma. The hypertension and hypokalemia are usually controlled by 25 to 100 mg of spironolactone every 8 hours. Such long-term therapy in men is usually limited by the common occurrence of decreased libido, impaired potency, and gynecomastia. When spironolactone is not tolerated, amelioride, a potassium-sparing diuretic, in 10 to 40 mg/day is usually successful. Alternatives such as trilostane, a 3β-hydroxysteroid inhibitor, and calcium channel blockers have been studied.[216] For bilateral hyperplasia, surgery is indicated only when significant symptomatic hypokalemia cannot be controlled by medical therapy.

If congestive heart failure is present, caution must be exercised during treatment with cardiac glycosides because of the hypokalemia.

Pheochromocytoma

This catecholamine-producing tumor arises from the adrenal medulla (90%) or from extra-adrenal, abdominal, or extra-abdominal paraganglion tissue (10%), can be either benign (90%) or malignant (10%), and in the adrenal can be either unilateral (90%) or bilateral (10%). The vast majority of pheochromocytomas occur sporadically, but in approximately 5% to 10% of cases they are inherited as an autosomal trait and occur in association with a pluriglandular neoplastic syndrome. The syndrome of multiple endocrine neoplasia type II (MEN II) is characterized by medullary carcinoma of the thyroid gland, pheochromocytoma, and hyperparathyroidism, whereas the MEN III syndrome consists of multiple mucosal neuromas, medullary carcinoma of the thyroid gland, and pheochromocytoma and is often associated with a marfanoid habitus. In this familial form of pheochromocytoma, nearly half of the patients have bilateral adrenal tumors.

The clinical manifestations of pheochromocytoma are expressions of the pharmacologic effects of catecholamines and depend on whether the secretion of these catecholamines by the tumor is persistent or intermittent and whether the predominant catecholamine secreted is norepinephrine or epinephrine.[217-219]

Hypertension is one cardinal manifestation of pheochromocytoma. In some patients, the secretion of catecholamines is episodic, and the resulting symptoms and hypertension are paroxysmal. Episodic symptoms include prominent severe headache, sweating, palpitations, tremor, nervousness, apprehension, a sense of impending doom, pallor, paresthesias (occasionally frank tetany), abdominal pain (infrequently associated with nausea, vomiting, or diarrhea), and angina. Occasionally, the episode is heralded by a cerebrovascular accident. These paroxysms of pheochromocytoma may be precipitated by an emotional event, physical upset, or straining at stool and, if the tumor is in the bladder, by micturition. They may last from a few minutes to several days. The patient may be normotensive and symptom-free during the interval between the paroxysms.

An increase in blood pressure may be sustained with or without accompanying spells. A small number of subjects have paroxysmal hypertension, but nonetheless almost all have increased circulating and urinary catecholamines and metabolites all of the time.[217] Probably fewer than

0.1% of all hypertensive patients have pheochromocytomas. The presence of pheochromocytoma in such patients should be suspected if there is a history of classic symptoms of sudden headache, excessive perspiration, and palpitations; if there is an otherwise unexplained tendency to have cardiac arrhythmias; if a significant increase in the blood pressure occurs during abdominal palpation or induction of anesthesia; and if orthostatic hypotension is present. Orthostatic hypotension is common in pheochromocytoma and is believed to be due to impairment of the sympathetic postural reflexes and, to a lesser extent, to hypovolemia. Pheochromocytoma should be suspected also if the hypertensive patient has manifestations of hypermetabolism such as loss of weight or diabetes. The degree of weight loss in the diabetic patient with pheochromocytoma is usually out of proportion to the degree of carbohydrate intolerance. Typical features of malignant hypertension will occur in some patients with untreated disease of long duration.

The majority of patients with pheochromocytoma secrete large amounts of norepinephrine. Predominantly epinephrine- or dopamine-secreting pheochromocytomas do occur, although rarely. Such patients may present with hypotension and shock[220] or with cardiomyopathy.[221]

Cardiac dysfunction often occurs in patients with pheochromocytoma. In addition to the cardiac effects of the hypertensive process, direct catecholamine-induced structural and biochemical abnormalities in myocardial tissue often occur—so-called catecholamine myocarditis.[222] The structural changes include focal degeneration and necrosis of the myocardial fibers, infiltration with inflammatory cells, fibrosis, and internal medial thickening of the small and medium-sized coronary arteries. The biochemical changes include defective storage of endogenous amines and increased concentration of free fatty acids in cardiac tissue. Autopsy series of patients who died from pheochromocytoma revealed that about half had active myocarditis, usually associated with left ventricular failure and pulmonary edema.[223]

ECG abnormalities occur in the majority of patients and include T-wave inversion, left ventricular hypertrophy, sinus tachycardia or bradycardia, and other disturbances in rhythm such as supraventricular premature beats and paroxysmal supraventricular tachycardia. These cardiac arrhythmias, which resemble those of thyrotoxicosis, are believed to result from the direct cardiac chronotropic effects of catecholamines, from reflex bradycardia mediated by baroreceptor stimulation, from sudden increases in blood pressure, and from catecholamine-induced myocarditis. When the blood pressure is increased suddenly and markedly, ECG changes may occur that suggest myocardial damage, such as transient elevation of ST segments, inversion of T waves, and depression of ST segments. These changes are transient, however, and are reversible with control of the hypertensive state.[224] The echocardiogram is usually normal in patients with pheochromocytoma who have no clinical evidence of heart disease.[225]

Diagnosis. The diagnostic approach is outlined in Table 63-13.

Table 63-13 Diagnosis of pheochromocytoma

Document reproducible increase in catecholamine production
Plasma and urinary catecholamines
Urinary catecholamine metabolites
Perform pheochromocytoma provocative tests, if needed
Clonidine suppression test
Rarely, histamine, tyramine, and glucagon tests
Localize the tumor
Oblique chest radiograph
Abdominal CT scan
Radioisotope scanning
Arteriography (rarely used)

The most reliable screening test for pheochromocytoma is determination of 24-hour urinary excretion of metanephrines.[226] Urinary levels of free catecholamines and vanillylmandelic acid are slightly less reliable. Another reliable screening test is measurement of metanephrines and creatinine in a single-voided urine specimen; more than 1 μg of metanephrines per milligram of creatinine is suggestive of pheochromocytoma.[227] Measurement of plasma catecholamines is also a sensitive indicator and is widely used at present.[228] The diagnostic yield from all these tests is increased if blood or urinary samples are obtained during a hypertensive attack. It is important to know the methods for and accuracy of measurements of catecholamines and metabolites in the laboratory as well as the influence of various drugs on these measurements.

Measurements of circulating and urinary catecholamines and their metabolites have replaced provocative tests such as with histamine, glucagon, and tyramine. These provocative tests can be hazardous and therefore are warranted only in unusual circumstances. If suspicion of pheochromocytoma is high and these tests are deemed necessary, the patient should be pretreated with phenoxybenzamine; plasma catecholamine levels are used as end points for assessment of the patient's response to the provocative tests.

The clonidine suppression test[229] is used in conjunction with plasma catecholamine determination. In patients with pheochromocytoma, the plasma catecholamine levels are unaffected by the administration of clonidine, whereas in those with hypertension of other causes, catecholamine levels are suppressed.

Computed tomography is the most accurate means of localizing the tumor, provided that it is larger than 0.5 cm in diameter. In unusual cases, radioisotopic scanning or angiography after appropriate medical preparation may be necessary. A radioisotope, *m*-iodobenzylguanidine (MIBG), is useful in visualizing catecholamine-containing tissues, including ectopic and metastatic pheochromocytoma. Magnetic resonance imaging of the chest, neck, and abdomen is the procedure currently used for the identification of extra-adrenal and perivertebral pheochromocytomas.[218]

Treatment. Surgery is the only definitive treatment. Preoperative stabilization with medical treatment is essential to reduce the risk of the operation.[229] This includes prior treatment with α-blockade (phenoxybenzamine) to control the hypertension, followed by β-blockade (propranolol) to prevent or treat sinus tachycardia or other catecholamine-induced arrhythmias. β-Adrenergic-mediated vasodilatation must not be inhibited before adequate α-blockade has been achieved. Phenoxybenzamine is started at a dosage of 10 mg two times a day, and the dose is gradually increased every 2 days until the blood pressure becomes normal. A single 120-mg dose of long-acting propranolol is added. Side effects of phenoxybenzamine include postural hypotension and, occasionally, the emergence of cardiac arrhythmias. The relatively selective α_1-adrenergic antagonist prazosin (Minipress) can be used as an alternative to phenoxybenzamine, with an initial dose of 0.5 mg.

Careful monitoring during surgery is essential. The anesthesiologist-surgeon team must be prepared to treat fluctuations in blood pressure and pulse rate in the perioperative period which are related to the induction of anesthesia or manipulation and removal of the tumor.

Long-term blockade of catecholamines with phenoxybenzamine and propranolol and therapy with α-methyl-*p*-tyrosine (a competitive inhibitor of tyrosine hydroxylase) are used in the management of inoperable tumors.

ACROMEGALY AND THE HEART

Chronic hypersecretion of growth hormone results in gigantism in children and acromegaly in adults. It is caused in almost all patients by a growth hormone-producing pituitary tumor. Rarely, the syndrome can be caused by an ectopic tumor, a bronchial or pancreatic carcinoid that elaborates a growth hormone-releasing hormone that causes pituitary somatotropic hyperplasia and consequent hypersecretion of growth hormone, or by an ectopic growth hormone-producing tumor. The clinical presentations of gigantism and acromegaly are related to the effects of excess growth hormone on the tissues, largely mediated by the increased production of insulin-like growth factor I (IGF-I or somatomedin C) by the liver and other peripheral tissues, and to the anatomic effects of the pituitary or extrapituitary causative tumor.

Hypertension is the most common cardiovascular manifestation of the syndrome, occurring in 20% to 70% of patients.[230-232] It has significant positive correlation with the serum concentration of growth hormone, the age of the patient, and the duration of the disease. It is usually mild, uncomplicated, and readily responsive to antihypertensive drugs.[230] Its pathogenesis is uncertain. In acromegaly there is an increase in total body sodium, extracellular fluid and plasma volumes, renal blood flow, and glomerular filtration rate.[233] The renin-angiotensin-aldosterone system is usually suppressed,[234,235] although aldosterone levels may rarely be increased and are sometimes related to associated primary aldosteronism.[236] Increased vasomotor responsiveness to angiotensin II is frequently present in both normotensive and hypertensive acromegalic patients.[237]

The acromegalic state is believed to be associated with an increased incidence of premature coronary atherosclerosis. This may be due in part to the associated hypertension and diabetes mellitus. Impaired glucose tolerance occurs in more than 50% of patients, with acromegaly and frank diabetes mellitus in about 10%. Blood lipids tend to be normal except in patients with clinical diabetes mellitus.

Cardiomegaly of a magnitude greater than would be expected from the generalized organomegaly is present in the great majority of patients.[238-242] Most patients, including those who are normotensive, have echocardiographic changes of left ventricular hypertrophy.[243,244] These patients have significantly higher serum levels of growth hormone than do those without evidence of left ventricular hypertrophy.[243] In addition, most acromegalic patients without clinical hypertension and coronary atherosclerosis have evidence of cardiac dysfunction, with shortening of left ventricular ejection time and prolongation of the preejection period.[245] More than half of all acromegalic patients have ECG abnormalities, most commonly ST depression and T-wave abnormalities, and often changes of left ventricular hypertrophy and intraventricular conduction disturbances, usually right bundle-branch block. Cardiac arrhythmias are present in about 25% of patients and most commonly occur as ventricular premature beats or atrial fibrillation and flutter.[16,246] Congestive heart failure occurs in 10% to 20% of patients, and in about 25% of these patients there is no known predisposing cause. Sudden death has been reported and has been found to be associated with inflammatory degenerative changes in the sinoatrial and atrioventricular nodal tissue.[247]

The frequent occurrence of cardiac dysfunction in acromegaly could be due to a specific cardiomyopathy. Histologically, myocardial hypertrophy, interstitial fibrosis, and myofibrillar degeneration with lymphomononuclear cell infiltrate and small-vessel disease of the myocardium have been reported.[248] Acromegaly has been reported to occur in a rare familial syndrome, Carney's complex, that may include among its various manifestations cardiac myxomas, cutaneous spotty pigmentation, mammary fibroadenomas, testicular tumors, and Cushing's syndrome due to adrenocortical nodular disease.[204]

The diagnostic steps are outlined in Table 63-14.[249,250] It is important to remember that in the hypertensive patient with acromegaly, steps have to be taken to exclude associated pheochromocytoma or primary aldosteronism. In those with cardiac arrhythmias, coexisting hyperthyroidism has to be ruled out.

Once the diagnosis of acromegaly has been made, active treatment is essential[251,252] (see Table 63-14), because untreated patients with acromegaly have a shortened life span, mainly because of the cardiovascular complications.[232,239,253] Hypertension, arrhythmias, and heart failure are treated by conventional means. Patients with hypertension can be particularly responsive to volume-depleting maneuvers, and those with congestive heart failure can be particularly resistant to therapy. Bromocriptine,[254] an investigational agent, can normalize secretion of growth hormone in 20% to 25% of patients

Table 63-14 Diagnosis and treatment of acromegaly

Diagnosis

High or normal serum levels of growth hormone unsuppressible with glucose loading
Elevated serum somatomedin-C level (IGF-I)5
Anatomic evidence of pituitary tumor (great majority) or ectopic tumor (rare)

Treatment

Surgical – adenectomy:
- Transsphenoidal (majority)
- Transfrontal (rare)

Radiotherapeutic
- External
- Internal

Pharmacologic – dopaminergic agonists (bromocriptine [investigational]) and somatostatin analogue (Sandostatin [investigational])

and cause a reduction in secretion of growth hormone in an additional 50% of patients. Subjective improvement in features of the acromegalic syndrome occurs in most treated patients. Bromocriptine can be considered as an interim medical therapy in patients who are poor risks for definitive surgical or radiotherapeutic treatment and for those in whom ablative treatment has failed. A long-acting somatostatin analogue (Sandostatin)[255] is available for investigational use in the treatment of acromegaly. It can be given by intermittent injections or by continuous infusion subcutaneously. Normalization of serum concentrations of growth hormone and IGF-I in 60% to 75% of patients and shrinkage of the growth hormone-producing tumor in <50% of patients can be expected with only minor and transient side effects. Pharmacologic treatment, whether by bromocriptine or somatostatin analogue, is only temporizing, since discontinuation of therapy results in resurgence of active acromegaly.[256] It is not clear whether active treatment of acromegaly leads to improvement in the associated cardiac disease.[257-259]

ORAL CONTRACEPTIVES AND THE HEART

Of all types of contraception known, the oral contraceptive (OC) is the most popular and effective form. It is estimated that, worldwide, OCs are currently used by more than 50 million women. This extensive use for the past 2 decades has been associated with an increasing incidence of cardiovascular disease in young women. Thromboembolic disease, hypertension, coronary atherosclerotic heart disease, diabetes, and cerebrovascular disease occur with greater frequency in users of "the pill."[260-265] Only venous thromboembolic disease, hypertension, and myocardial infarction will be discussed here.

Venous thromboembolism

It has been estimated from a variety of studies that the relative risk of venous thromboembolism in OC users varies from 4.2- to 11-fold.[266,267] This risk is limited to current users of the pill, the risk being the same in ex-users as in never-users, and it is unrelated to age or duration of pill use. The major identifiable risk factor for venous thromboembolism in OC users is a history of venous thromboembolism.[268] The presence of varicose veins in OC users increases the risk of superficial thrombophlebitis and only slightly the risk of deep venous thrombosis.[269] The risk appears to be increased after surgery.[270] Smoking does not increase the risk.

The mechanism of thromboembolism in OC users is still debatable. The weight of evidence to date indicates that the increased incidence is due to estrogen-induced hypercoagulability, which is thought to be related to increased platelet aggregation,[271] to increased levels of several clotting factors (most strikingly, factor XII), to decreased antithrombin III,[272] or to other factors. The incidence of thromboembolic complications in OC users has been shown to be related to the dose of estrogen:[273] the relative risk of venous thromboembolism with 100 μg of ethinyl estradiol was 2.5 times greater than that with 50 μg. The estrogen content of the pill therefore has been progressively reduced to the minimum level (30 μg) necessary for suppression of ovulation without allowing breakthrough bleeding. As a result, there has been a significant decrease in the incidence of venous thromboembolism in OC users.

Oral contraceptives therefore should not be prescribed for women who have other identifiable risk factors for venous thromboembolism, such as history of venous thromboembolism, heart disease, significant obesity, chronic disease leading to immobility, and malignancy. Use of the OC should be discontinued 1 month before elective surgery or in the event of significant leg trauma. The lowest effective dose of estrogen should be prescribed.

Hypertension

Elevation of both systolic and diastolic blood pressure occurs in almost all patients who use OCs. Systolic readings average 4.5 mm Hg higher and diastolic readings average 1.5 mm Hg higher in users than in nonusers.[260] It has been estimated that 5% of patients become overtly hypertensive.[274,275] The hypertension could take months or years to develop after the use of OCs has been started. It is usually reversible after discontinuation of the drug, although it may take months to subside; however, a significant minority of patients remain hypertensive. In some patients who have had OC-associated hypertension and have had normalization of their blood pressure after discontinuation of the pill, spontaneous hypertension may develop later.[276]

The OC-related hypertension is usually mild to moderate but can be severe. Malignant hypertension can occur; it may be reversible with discontinuation of use of the pill[277] or lead to irreversible renal failure.[278]

The factors that predispose a person to the development of hypertension during use of OCs include older age, family history or history of hypertension, and chronic renal disease.[279]

The pathogenesis of hypertension caused by OCs is still not clear. Both estrogen and progestin have been implicated as being causative. The effect may be mediated through the renin-angiotensin system. With OC use, there is an increase in the concentration of plasma renin substrate, a consequent increase of plasma renin activity and plasma angiotensin II concentration, an increase of aldosterone secretory rate and plasma aldosterone, and a lowering of plasma renin concentration.[280] However, no significant differences have been found in these changes during therapy with OCs between women who are normotensive and those who are hypertensive. Angiotensin may still be implicated in the pathogenesis, since administration of saralasin, an angiotensin-blocking agent, has been shown to lower the blood pressure in patients with hypertension due to OCs.[281]

A patient should be started on OC therapy only after a careful history has been obtained to exclude factors predisposing her to hypertension. Continued blood pressure monitoring for the duration of therapy is indicated. An increase in blood pressure of 15/10 mm Hg or more or the development of overt hypertension should lead to the cessation of OC therapy.

Myocardial infarction

Women who use OCs are at increased risk for fatal or nonfatal myocardial infarction;[282-287] the relative risk is on the order of 4.0. Since myocardial infarction is rare in premenopausal women, the actual risk of infarction is small in OC users. The risk does not apply to all users equally. It increases with age and is greatest in women who have other risk factors for premature coronary atherosclerosis. Cigarette smoking,[285] hypertension,[286] diabetes mellitus,[288] and hyperlipidemia[288] have a definite synergistic adverse effect. The increased risk is limited to current OC users and is not seen in ex-users. It is not related to the duration of OC use.

The mechanism of myocardial infarction in OC users is still not clear. OCs may contribute to the progression of coronary atherosclerosis[289] by their impact on serum lipids, glucose tolerance, and blood pressure. Other factors must be operative, because the increased risk is limited to current OC users and is not seen in ex-users. OCs do predispose users to arterial thrombosis[290] and may predispose them to coronary artery spasm.

The OCs should not be used by women who are at increased risk for premature coronary atherosclerosis. Women with diabetes, hypertension, or hyperlipidemia or those who are over the age of 35 years, are cigarette smokers, or have a family history of premature coronary artery disease should not use OCs. Such a limitation on the use of OCs can nearly eliminate the excess risk of myocardial infarction in OC users.

REFERENCES

1. Forfar JC, Caldwell GC: Hyperthyroid heart disease. *Clin Endocrinol Metab* 14:491-508, 1985
2. Skelton CL: The heart and hyperthyroidism. *N Engl J Med* 307:1206-1208, 1982
3. Vlase H, Lungu G, Vlase L: Cardiac disturbances in thyrotoxicosis: diagnosis, incidence, clinical features and management. *Endocrinologie* 29:155-160, 1991
4. Popovici D, Hertoghe J: Cardiothyreosis. *Endocrinologie* 29:119-136, 1991
5. Woeber KA: Thyrotoxicosis and the heart. *N Engl J Med* 327:94-98, 1992
6. Stoffer SS, Jiang N-S, Gorman CA, et al: Plasma catecholamines in hypothyroidism and hyperthyroidism. *J Clin Endocrinol Metab* 36:587-589, 1973
7. Nishizawa Y, Hamada N, Fujii S, et al: Serum dopamine-β-hydroxylase activity in thyroid disorders. *J Clin Endocrinol Metab* 39:599-602, 1974
8. Spaulding SW, Noth RH: Thyroid-catecholamine interactions. *Med Clin North Am* 59:1123-1131, September 1975
9. Levey GS: The heart and hyperthyroidism: use of beta-adrenergic blocking drugs. *Med Clin North Am* 59:1193-1201, September 1975
10. Aoki VS, Wilson WR, Theilen EO: Studies of the reputed augmentation of the cardiovascular effects of catecholamines in patients with spontaneous hyperthyroidism. *J Pharmacol Exp Ther* 181:362-368, 1972
11. Williams LT, Lefkowitz RJ, Watanabe AM, et al: Thyroid hormone regulation of β-adrenergic receptor number. *J Biol Chem* 252:2787-2789, 1977
12. Levey GS, Epstein SE: Myocardial adenyl cyclase: activation by thyroid hormones and evidence for two adenyl cyclase systems. *J Clin Invest* 48:1663-1669, 1969
13. Morkin E, Flink IL, Goldman S: Biochemical and physiologic effects of thyroid hormone on cardiac performance. *Prog Cardiovasc Dis* 25:435-464, 1983
14. Ingbar SH: The role of antiadrenergic agents in the management of thyrotoxicosis. *Cardiovasc Rev Rep* 2:683, 1981
15. Hoffman I, Lowrey RD: The electrocardiogram in thyrotoxicosis. *Am J Cardiol* 6:893-904, 1960
16. Surawicz B, Mangiardi ML: Electrocardiogram in endocrine and metabolic disorders. *Cardiovasc Clin* 8 No 3:243-266, 1977
17. Forfar JC, Muir AL, Sawers SA, et al: Abnormal left ventricular function in hyperthyroidism: evidence for a possible reversible cardiomyopathy. *N Engl J Med* 307:1165-1170, 1982
18. Ciaccheri M, Cecchi F, Arcangeli C, et al: Occult thyrotoxicosis in patients with chronic and paroxysmal isolated atrial fibrillation. *Clin Cardiol* 7:413-416, 1984
19. Staffurth JS, Gibberd MC, Ng Tang Fui S: Arterial embolism in thyrotoxicosis with atrial fibrillation. *Br Med J* 2:688-690, 1977
20. Kramer MR, Shilo S, Hershko C: Atrioventricular and sinoatrial block in thyrotoxic crisis. *Br Heart J* 54:600-602, 1985
21. Nakagawa S, Higa A, Kondoh H, et al: Cyclic sinus node dysfunction in a patient with hyperthyroidism. *Arch Intern Med* 145: 2126-2127, 1985
22. Sanghvi LM, Banerjee K: Wolff-Parkinson-White syndrome associated with thyrotoxicosis. *Am J Cardiol* 8:431-437, 1961
23. Campus S, Rappelli A, Malavasi A, et al: Heart block and hyperthyroidism: report of two cases. *Arch Intern Med* 135:1091-1095, 1975
24. Muggia AL, Stjernholm M, Houle T: Complete heart block with thyrotoxic myocarditis: report of a case. *N Engl J Med* 283:1099-1100, 1970
25. Proskey AJ, Saksena F, Towne WD: Myocardial infarction associated with thyrotoxicosis. *Chest* 72:109-111, 1977
26. Featherstone HJ, Stewart DK: Angina in thyrotoxicosis: thyroid-related coronary artery spasm. *Arch Intern Med* 143:554-555, 1983
27. Carey D, Hurst JW Jr, Silverman ME: Coronary spasm and cardiac arrest after coronary arteriography in unsuspected thyrotoxicosis. *Am J Cardiol* 70:833-834, 1992
28. Moliterno D, DeBold CR, Robertson RM: Case report: coronary vasospasm – relation to the hyperthyroid state. *Am J Med Sci* 304:38-42, 1992

29. Ikram H: The nature and prognosis of thyrotoxic heart disease. *Q J Med* 54:19-28, 1985

30. Bauerlein EJ, Chakko CS, Kessler KM: Reversible dilated cardiomyopathy due to thyrotoxicosis. *Am J Cardiol* 70:132, 1992

31. Graettinger JS, Muenster JJ, Selverstone LA, et al: A correlation of clinical and hemodynamic studies in patients with hyperthyroidism with and without congestive heart failure. *J Clin Invest* 38:1316-1327, 1959

32. Cavallo A, Joseph CJ, Casta A: Cardiac complications in juvenile hyperthyroidism. *Am J Dis Child* 138:479-482, 1984

33. Shapiro S, Steier M, Dimich I: Congestive heart failure in neonatal thyrotoxicosis: a curable cause of heart failure in the newborn. *Clin Pediatr (Phila)* 14:1155-1156, 1975

34. Brauman A, Algom M, Gilboa Y, et al: Mitral valve prolapse in hyperthyroidism of two different origins. *Br Heart J* 53:374-377, 1985

35. Channick BJ, Adlin EV, Marks AD, et al: Hyperthyroidism and mitral-valve prolapse. *N Engl J Med* 305:497-506, 1981

36. Reynolds JL, Woody HB: Thyrotoxic mitral regurgitation. *Am J Dis Child* 122:544-548, 1971

37. Dougherty MJ, Craige E: Apathetic hyperthyroidism presenting as tricuspid regurgitation. *Chest* 63:767-772, 1973

38. Davis PJ, Davis FB: Hyperthyroidism in patients over the age of 60 years: clinical features in 85 patients. *Medicine (Baltimore)* 53:161-181, 1974

39. Cooper DS, Daniels GH, Ladenson PW, et al: Hyperthyroxinemia in patients with high-dose propranolol. *Am J Med* 73:867-871, 1982

40. Burger A, Dinichert D, Nicod P, et al: Effect of amiodarone on serum triiodothyronine, reverse triiodothyronine, thyroxine, and thyrotropin: a drug influencing peripheral metabolism of thyroid hormones. *J Clin Invest* 58:255-259, 1976

41. Gammage MD, Franklyn JA: Amiodarone and the thyroid. *Q J Med* 62:83-86, 1987

42. Rabinowe SL, Larsen PR, Antman EM, et al: Amiodarone therapy and autoimmune thyroid disease: increase in a new monoclonal antibody-defined T cell subset. *Am J Med* 81:53-57, 1986

43. Martino E, Safran M, Aghini-Lombardi F, et al: Environmental iodine intake and thyroid dysfunction during chronic amiodarone therapy. *Ann Intern Med* 101:28-34, 1984

44. Brennan MD, van Heerden JA, Carney JA: Amiodarone-associated thyrotoxicosis (AAT): experience with surgical management. *Surgery* 102:1062-1067, 1987

45. Fradkin JE, Wolff J: Iodide-induced thyrotoxicosis. *Medicine* 62:1-20, 1983

46. Georges JL, Normand JP, Lenormand ME, et al: Life-threatening thyrotoxicosis induced by amiodarone in patients with benign heart disease. *Eur Heart J* 13:129-132, 1992

47. Ross DS: Subclinical thyrotoxicosis. *Adv Endocrinol Metab* 2:89-105, 1991

48. Hay ID, Klee GG: Thyroid dysfunction. *Endocrinol Metab Clin North Am* 17:473-509, 1988

49. Bayer MF: Effective laboratory evaluation of thyroid status. *Med Clin North Am* 75:1-26, 1991

50. Klee GG, Hay ID: Assessment of sensitive thyrotropin assays for an expanded role in thyroid function testing: proposed criteria for analytic performance and clinical utility. *J Clin Endocrinol Metab* 64:461-471, 1987

51. Orgiazzi J: Management of Graves' hyperthyroidism. *Endocrinol Metab Clin North Am* 16:365-389, 1987

52. Solomon B, Glinoer D, Lagasse R, et al: Current trends in the management of Graves' disease. *J Clin Endocrinol Metab* 70:1518-1524, 1990

53. Nakazawa HK, Sakurai K, Hamada N, et al: Management of atrial fibrillation in the post-thyrotoxic state. *Am J Med* 72:903-906, 1982

54. Sandler G, Wilson GM: The nature and prognosis of heart disease in thyrotoxicosis: a review of 150 patients treated with ^{131}I. *Q J Med* 28:347-370, 1959

55. Doherty JE, Perkins WH: Digoxin metabolism in hypo- and hyperthyroidism: studies with tritiated digoxin in thyroid disease. *Ann Intern Med* 64:489-507, 1966

56. Graettinger JS, Muenster JJ, Checchia CS, et al: A correlation of clinical and hemodynamic studies in patients with hypothyroidism. *J Clin Invest* 37:502-510, 1958

57. Hillis WS, Bremner WF, Lawrie TDV, et al: Systolic time intervals in thyroid disease. *Clin Endocrinol (Oxf)* 4:617-624, 1975

58. Vora J, O'Malley BP, Petersen S, et al: Reversible abnormalities of myocardial relaxation in hypothyroidism. *J Clin Endocrinol Metab* 61:269-272, 1985

59. Vanhaelst L, Neve P, Chailly P, et al: Coronary-artery disease in hypothyroidism: observations in clinical myxoedema. *Lancet* 2:800-802, 1967

60. Hansen JE: Paroxysmal ventricular tachycardia associated with myxedema: a case report. *Am Heart J* 61:692-697, 1961

61. Pechter RA, Osborn LA: Polymorphic ventricular tachycardia secondary to hypothyroidism. *Am J Cardiol* 57:882-884, 1986

62. Kerber RE, Sherman B: Echocardiographic evaluation of pericardial effusion in myxedema: incidence and biochemical and clinical correlations. *Circulation* 52:823-827, 1975

63. Zimmerman J, Yahalom J, Bar-On H: Clinical spectrum of pericardial effusion as the presenting feature of hypothyroidism. *Am Heart J* 106:770-771, 1983

64. Smolar EN, Rubin JE, Avramides A, et al: Cardiac tamponade in primary myxedema and review of the literature. *Am J Med Sci* 272:345-352, 1976

65. Khaleeli AA, Memon N: Factors affecting resolution of pericardial effusions in primary hypothyroidism: a clinical, biochemical and echocardiographic study. *Postgrad Med J* 58:473-476, 1982

66. Aber CP, Thompson GS: The heart in hypothyroidism. *Am Heart J* 68:428-430, 1964

67. Shenoy MM, Goldman JM: Hypothyroid cardiomyopathy: echocardiographic documentation of reversibility. *Am J Med Sci* 249:1-9, 1987

68. McBrien DJ, Hindle W: Myxoedema and heart-failure. *Lancet* 1:1066-1068, 1963

69. Wieshammer S, Keck FS, Waitzinger J, et al: Left ventricular function at rest and during exercise in acute hypothyroidism. *Br Heart J* 60:204-211, 1988

70. Dratman MB: Thyroid function and high blood pressure. *Cardiovasc Med* 1:319-331, 1976

71. Saito I, Ito K, Saruta T: Hypothyroidism as a cause of hypertension. *Hypertension* 5:112-115, 1983

72. Streeten DH, Anderson GH Jr, Howland T, et al: Effects of thyroid function on blood pressure: recognition of hypothyroid hypertension. *Hypertension* 11:78-83, 1988

73. Christensen NJ: Increased levels of plasma noradrenaline in hypothyroidism. *J Clin Endocrinol Metab* 35:359-363, 1972

74. Endo T, Komiya I, Tsukui T, et al: Re-evaluation of a possible high incidence of hypertension in hypothyroid patients. *Am Heart J* 98:684-688, 1979

75. Steinberg AD: Myxedema and coronary artery disease: a comparative autopsy study. *Ann Intern Med* 68:338-344, 1968

76. Becker C: Hypothyroidism and atherosclerotic heart disease: pathogenesis, medical management, and the role of coronary artery bypass surgery. *Endocr Rev* 6:432-440, 1985

77. DeGroot LJ: Thyroid and the heart. *Mayo Clin Proc* 47:864-871, 1972

78. Griffiths PD: Serum enzymes in diseases of the thyroid gland. *J Clin Pathol* 18:660-663, 1965

79. Forfar JC, Wathen CG, Todd WTA, et al: Left ventricular performance in subclinical hypothyroidism. *Q J Med* 57:857-865, 1985

80. Cooper DS: Subclinical hypothyroidism. *Adv Endocrinol Metab* 2:77, 1991

81. Robuschi G, Safran M, Braverman LE, et al: Hypothyroidism in the elderly. *Endocrinol Rev* 8:142-153, 1987

82. Gooch BR, Isley WL, Utiger RD: Abnormalities in thyroid function tests in patients admitted to a medical service. *Arch Intern Med* 142:1801-1805, 1982

83. Kaplan MM, Larsen PR, Crantz FR, et al: Prevalence of abnormal thyroid function test results in patients with acute medical illnesses. *Am J Med* 72:9-16, 1982

84. Paine TD, Rogers WJ, Baxley WA, et al: Coronary arterial surgery in patients with incapacitating angina pectoris and myxedema. *Am J Cardiol* 40:226-231, 1977

85. Drucker DJ, Burrow GN: Cardiovascular surgery in the hypothyroid patient. *Arch Intern Med* 145:1585-1587, 1985

86. Weinberg AD, Brennan MD, Gorman CA, et al: Outcome of anesthesia and surgery in hypothyroid patients. *Arch Intern Med* 143:893-897, 1983

87. Kleerekoper M, Rao DS, Frame B: Hypercalcemia, hyperparathyroidism, and hypertension. *Cardiovasc Med* 3:1283-1295, 1978

88. Christensson T, Hellström K, Wengle B: Blood pressure in subjects with hypercalcaemia and primary hyperparathyroidism detected in a health screening programme. *Eur J Clin Invest* 7:109-113, 1977

89. Sowers JR, Tuck ML: Hypertension associated with diabetes mellitus, hypercalcaemic disorders, acromegaly and thyroid disease. *Clin Endocrinol Metab* 10:631-650, November 1981

90. Weidmann P, Massry SG, Coburn JW, et al: Blood pressure effects of acute hypercalcemia: studies in patients with chronic renal failure. *Ann Intern Med* 76:741-745, 1972

91. Hellström J, Birke G, Edvall CA: Hypertension in hyperparathyroidism. *Br J Urol* 30:13-24, 1958

92. Resnick LM: Calcium, parathyroid disease, and hypertension. *Cardiovasc Rev Rep* 3:1341, 1982

93. Roberts WC, Waller BF: Effect of chronic hypercalcemia on the heart: an analysis of 18 necropsy patients. *Am J Med* 71:371-384, 1981

94. Roberts WC, Walker BF: Chronic hypercalcemia as a risk factor for coronary atherosclerosis. *Cardiovasc Rev Rep* 4:1275, 1983

95. Bogin E, Massry SG, Harary I: Effect of parathyroid hormone on rat heart cells. *J Clin Invest* 67:1215-1227, 1981

96. Palmieri GMA, Nutting DF, Bhattacharya SK, et al: Parathyroid ablation in dystrophic hamsters: effects of Ca content and histology of heart, diaphragm, and rectus femoris. *J Clin Invest* 68:646-654, 1981

97. Symons C, Fortune F, Greenbaum RA, et al: Cardiac hypertrophy, hypertrophic cardiomyopathy, and hyperparathyroidism—an association. *Br Heart J* 54:539-542, 1985

98. Jørgensen FS: Effect of thiazide diuretics upon calcium metabolism. *Dan Med Bull* 23:223-230, 1976

99. Giles TD, Iteld BJ, Rives KL: The cardiomyopathy of hypoparathyroidism: another reversible form of heart muscle disease. *Chest* 79:225-229, 1981

100. Csanady M, Forster T, Julesz J: Reversible impairment of myocardial function in hypoparathyroidism causing hypocalcaemia. *Br Heart J* 63:58-60, 1990

101. Mano T, Kamiya H, Kawakita S, et al: A case of primary hypoparathyroidism complicated by heart failure. *Jpn J Med* 30:464-467, 1991

102. Shackney S, Hasson J: Precipitous fall in serum calcium, hypotension, and acute renal failure after intravenous phosphate therapy for hypercalcemia: report of two cases. *Ann Intern Med* 66:906-916, 1967

103. Waller BF, Palumbo PJ, Lie JT, et al: Status of the coronary arteries at necropsy in diabetes mellitus with onset after age 30 years: analysis of 229 diabetic patients with and without clinical evidence of coronary heart disease and comparison to 183 control subjects. *Am J Med* 69:498-506, 1980

104. Bradley RF, Partamian JO: Coronary heart disease in the diabetic patient. *Med Clin North Am* 49:1093-1104, July 1965

105. West KM: *Epidemiology of Diabetes and Its Vascular Lesions.* New York, Elsevier, 1978

106. Boucher CA, Fallon JT, Johnson RA, et al: Cardiomyopathic syndrome caused by coronary artery disease. III. Prospective clinicopathological study of its prevalence among patients with clinically unexplained chronic heart failure. *Br Heart J* 41:613-620, 1979

107. Dash H, Johnson RA, Dinsmore RE, et al: Cardiomyopathic syndrome due to coronary artery disease. II. Increased prevalence in patients with diabetes mellitus: a matched pair analysis. *Br Heart J* 39:740-747, 1977

108. Jarrett RJ: Risk factors for coronary heart disease in diabetes mellitus. *Diabetes* 41 Suppl 2:1-3, 1992

109. Manson JE, Colditz GA, Stampfer MJ, et al: A prospective study of maturity-onset diabetes mellitus and risk of coronary heart disease and stroke in women. *Arch Intern Med* 151:1141-1147, 1991

110. Herman MV, Gorlin R: Premature coronary artery disease and the preclinical diabetic state (editorial). *Am J Med* 38:481-483, 1965

111. Stamler R, Stamler J: Asymptomatic hyperglycemia and coronary heart disease: a series of papers by the International Collaborative Group, based on studies in fifteen populations; introduction. *J Chronic Dis* 32:683-691, 1979

112. Butler WJ, Ostrander LD Jr, Carman WJ, et al: Mortality from coronary heart disease in the Tecumseh study. Long-term effect of diabetes mellitus, glucose tolerance and other risk factors. *Am J Epidemiol* 121:541-547, 1985

113. Pan W-H, Cedres LB, Liu K, et al: Relationship of clinical diabetes and asymptomatic hyperglycemia to risk of coronary heart disease mortality in men and women. *Am J Epidemiol* 123:504-516, 1986

114. Kannel WB, McGee DL: Diabetes and cardiovascular disease: the Framingham Study. *JAMA* 241:2035-2038, 1979

115. Partamian JO, Bradley RF: Acute myocardial infarction in 258 cases of diabetes: immediate mortality and five-year survival. *N Engl J Med* 273:455-461, 1965

116. Kereiakes DJ: Myocardial infarction in the diabetic patient. *Clin Cardiol* 8:446-450, 1985

117. Ulvenstam G, Aberg A, Bergstrand R, et al: Long-term prognosis after myocardial infarction in men with diabetes. *Diabetes* 34:787-792, 1985

118. Jacoby RM, Nesto RW: Acute myocardial infarction in the diabetic patient: pathophysiology, clinical course and prognosis. *J Am Coll Cardiol* 20:736-744, 1992

119. Savage MP, Krolewski AS, Kenien GG, et al: Acute myocardial infarction in diabetes mellitus and significance of congestive heart failure as a prognostic factor. *Am J Cardiol* 62:665-669, 1988

120. Abbott RD, Donahue RP, Kannel WB, et al: The impact of diabetes on survival following myocardial infarction in men vs women. The Framingham study. *JAMA* 260:3456-3460, 1988

121. Stone PH, Muller JE, Hartwell T, et al: The effects of diabetes mellitus on prognosis and serial left ventricular function after acute myocardial infarction: contribution of both coronary disease and diastolic left ventricular dysfunction to the adverse prognosis: the MILIS Study Group. *J Am Coll Cardiol* 16:49-57, 1989

122. Herlitz J, Malmberg K, Karlson BW, et al: Mortality and morbidity during a five-year follow-up of diabetics with myocardial infarction. *Acta Med Scand* 224:31-38, 1988

123. Woods KL, Samanta A, Burden AC: Diabetes mellitus as a risk factor for acute myocardial infarction in Asians and Europeans. *Br Heart J* 62:118-122, 1989

124. Soler NG, Bennett MA, Pentecost BL, et al: Myocardial infarction in diabetics. *Q J Med* 44:125-132, 1975

125. Harrower ADB, Clarke BF: Experience of coronary care in diabetics. *Br Med J* 1:126-128, 1976

126. Nicod P, Lewis SE, Corbett JC, et al: Increased incidence and clinical correlation of persistently abnormal technetium pyrophosphate myocardial scintigrams following acute myocardial infarction in patients with diabetes mellitus. *Am Heart J* 103:822-829, 1982

127. Margolis JR, Kannel WB, Feinleib M, et al: Clinical features of unrecognized myocardial infarction—silent and symptomatic: eighteen year follow-up; the Framingham Study. *Am J Cardiol* 32:1-7, 1973

128. Chipkin SR, Frid D, Alpert JS, et al: Frequency of painless myocardial ischemia during exercise tolerance testing in patients with and without diabetes mellitus. *Am J Cardiol* 59:61-65, 1987

129. Hume L, Oakley GD, Boulton AJM, et al: Asymptomatic myocardial ischemia in diabetes and its relationship to diabetic neuropathy: an exercise electrocardiography study in middle-aged diabetic men. *Diabetes Care* 9:384-388, 1986

130. Felsher J, Meissner MD, Hakki A-H, et al: Exercise thallium imaging in patients with diabetes mellitus: prognostic implications. *Arch Intern Med* 147:313-317, 1987

131. Naka M, Hiramatsu K, Aizawa T: Silent myocardial ischemia in patients with non-insulin-dependent diabetes mellitus as judged by treadmill exercise testing and coronary angiography. *Am Heart J* 123:46-53, 1992

132. O'Sullivan JJ, Convoy RM, MacDonald K, et al: Silent ischaemia in diabetic men with autonomic neuropathy. *Br Heart J* 66:313-315, 1991

133. Weiner DA, Ryan TJ, Parsons L, et al: Significance of silent myocardial ischemia during exercise testing in patients with diabetes mellitus: a report from the Coronary Artery Surgery Study (CASS) Registry. *Am J Cardiol* 68:729-734, 1991

134. Langer A, Freeman MR, Josse RG, et al: Detection of silent myocardial ischemia in diabetes mellitus. *Am J Cardiol* 67:1073-1078, 1991

135. Oliver MF: Metabolic response during impending myocardial infarction. II. Clinical implications. *Circulation* 45:491-500, 1972

136. Ceremuzynski L: Hormonal and metabolic reactions evoked by acute myocardial infarction. *Circ Res* 48:767-776, 1981

137. Mogensen CE: Diabetes and hypertension (letter to the editor). *Lancet* 1:388-389, 1979

138. Statement on hypertension in diabetes. *Diabetes Care* 10:764-776, 1987

139. Feher MD: Hypertension in noninsulin dependent diabetes mellitus and its management. *Postgrad Med J* 67:938-946, 1991

140. Simonson DC: Etiology and prevalence of hypertension in diabetic patients. *Diabetes Care* 11:821-827, 1988
141. Mogensen CE: Renal function changes in diabetes. *Diabetes* 25 Suppl 2:872-879, 1976
142. Reaven GM: Insulin resistance and compensatory hyperinsulinemia: role in hypertension, dyslipidemia, and coronary heart disease. *Am Heart J* 121:1283-1288, 1991
143. Karam JH: Type II diabetes and syndrome X: pathogenesis and glycemic management. *Endocrinol Metab Clin North Am* 21:329-350, 1992
144. Reaven GM: Role of insulin resistance in human disease (syndrome X): an expanded definition. *Annu Rev Med* 44:121-131, 1993
145. Fein FS, Sonnenblick EH: Diabetic cardiomyopathy. *Prog Cardiovasc Dis* 27:255-270, 1985
146. Regan TJ, Weisse AB: Diabetic cardiomyopathy (editorial). *J Am Coll Cardiol* 19:1165-1166, 1992
147. Galderisi M, Anderson KM, Wilson PW, et al: Echocardiographic evidence for the existence of a distinct diabetic cardiomyopathy (the Framingham Heart Study). *Am J Cardiol* 68:85-89, 1991
148. van Hoeven KH, Factor SM: The diabetic heart: clinical, experimental and pathological features. *Acta Cardiol* 46:329-339, 1991
149. Giacomelli F, Wiener J: Primary myocardial disease in the diabetic mouse: an ultrastructural study. *Lab Invest* 40:460-473, 1979
150. Hamby RI, Zoneraich S, Sherman L: Diabetic cardiomyopathy. *JAMA* 229:1749-1754, 1974
151. Zoneraich S (ed): *Diabetes and the Heart.* Springfield, Illinois, Charles C Thomas, Publisher, 1978
152. Kannel WB, Hjortland M, Castelli WP: Role of diabetes in congestive heart failure: the Framingham Study. *Am J Cardiol* 34:29-34, 1974
153. Pearce MB, Bulloch RT, Kizziar J-C: Myocardial small vessel disease in patients with diabetes mellitus (abstract). *Circulation* 48 Suppl 4:6, 1973
154. Regan TJ, Lyons MM, Ahmed SS, et al: Evidence for cardiomyopathy in familial diabetes mellitus. *J Clin Invest* 60:885-899, 1977
155. Ledet T: Diabetic cardiopathy: quantitative histological studies of the heart from young juvenile diabetics. *Acta Pathol Microbiol Scand [A]* 84:421-428, 1976
156. Fischer VW, Barner HB, Leskiw ML: Capillary basal laminar thickness in diabetic human myocardium. *Diabetes* 28:713-719, 1979
157. Factor SM, Okun EM, Minase T: Capillary microaneurysms in the human diabetic heart. *N Engl J Med* 302:384-388, 1980
158. Tahiliani AG, McNeill JH: Diabetes-induced abnormalities in the myocardium. *Life Sci* 38:959-974, 1986
159. Dhalla NS, Pierce GN, Innes IR, et al: Pathogenesis of cardiac dysfunction in diabetes. *Can J Cardiol* 1:263-281, 1985
160. Shapiro LM: Echocardiographic features of impaired ventricular function in diabetes mellitus. *Br Heart J* 47:439-444, 1982
161. Rynkiewicz A, Semetkowska-Jurkiewicz E, Wyrzykowski B: Systolic and diastolic time intervals in young diabetics. *Br Heart J* 44:280-283, 1980
162. Ahmed SS, Jaferi GA, Narang RM, et al: Preclinical abnormality of left ventricular function in diabetes mellitus. *Am Heart J* 89:153-158, 1975
163. Shapiro LM, Leatherdale BA, Coyne ME, et al: Prospective study of heart disease in untreated maturity onset diabetics. *Br Heart J* 44:342-348, 1980
164. Seneviratne BIB: Diabetic cardiomyopathy: the preclinical phase. *Br Med J* 1:1444-1446, 1977
165. Shapiro LM, Leatherdale BA, Mackinnon J, et al: Left ventricular function in diabetes mellitus. II. Relation between clinical features and left ventricular function. *Br Heart J* 45:129-132, 1981
166. Shapiro LM, Howat AP, Calter MM: Left ventricular function in diabetes mellitus. I. Methodology, and prevalence and spectrum of abnormalities. *Br Heart J* 45:122-128, 1981
167. Fuller JH, Keen H, Jarrett RJ, et al: Haemostatic variables associated with diabetes and its complications. *Br Med J* 2:964-966, 1979
168. Barnes AJ, Locke P, Scudder PR, et al: Is hyperviscosity a treatable component of diabetic microcirculatory disease? *Lancet* 2:789-791, 1977
169. McMillan DE, Utterback NG, La Puma J: Reduced erythrocyte deformability in diabetics. *Diabetes* 27:895-901, 1978
170. Wolfe RR, Way GL: Cardiomyopathies in infants of diabetic mothers. *Johns Hopkins Med J* 140:177-180, 1977
171. Gutgesell HP, Speer ME, Rosenberg HS: Characterization of the cardiomyopathy in infants of diabetic mothers. *Circulation* 61:441-450, 1980
172. Mace S, Hirschfeld SS, Riggs T, et al: Echocardiographic abnormalities in infants of diabetic mothers. *J Pediatr* 95:1013-1019, 1979
173. Lloyd-Mostyn RH, Watkins PJ: Total cardiac denervation in diabetic autonomic neuropathy. *Diabetes* 25:748-751, 1976
174. Lloyd-Mostyn RH, Watkins PJ: Defective innervation of heart in diabetic autonomic neuropathy. *Br Med J* 3:15-17, 1975
175. Smith SE, Smith SA, Brown PM: Cardiac autonomic dysfunction in patients with diabetic retinopathy. *Diabetologia* 21:525-528, 1981
176. Watkins PJ, Mackay JD: Cardiac denervation in diabetic neuropathy. *Ann Intern Med* 92:304-307, 1980
177. Fisher BM, Gillen G, Lindop GBM, et al: Cardiac function and coronary arteriography in asymptomatic Type 1 (insulin-dependent) diabetic patients: evidence for a specific diabetic heart disease. *Diabetologia* 29:706-712, 1986
178. Vered Z, Battler A, Segal P, et al: Exercise-induced left ventricular dysfunction in young men with asymptomatic diabetes mellitus (diabetic cardiomyopathy). *Am J Cardiol* 54:633-637, 1984
179. Roy TM, Peterson HR, Snider HL, et al: Autonomic influence on cardiovascular performance in diabetic subjects. *Am J Med* 87:382-388, 1989
180. Oikawa N, Umetsu M, Sakurada M, et al: Discrimination between cardiac para- and sympathetic damage in diabetics. *Diabetes Res Clin Pract* 1:203-209, 1985
181. Ewing DJ, Campbell IW, Clarke BF: The natural history of diabetic autonomic neuropathy. *Q J Med* 49:95-108, 1980
182. Kahn JK, Sisson JC, Vinik AI: QT interval prolongation and sudden cardiac death in diabetic autonomic neuropathy. *J Clin Endocrinol Metab* 64:751-754, 1987
183. Ambepityia G, Kopelman PG, Ingram D, et al: Exertional myocardial ischemia in diabetes: a quantitative analysis of anginal perceptual threshold and the influence of autonomic function. *J Am Coll Cardiol* 15:72-77, 1990
184. Chriestlieb AR: Treatment selection considerations for the hypertensive diabetic patient. *Arch Intern Med* 150:1167-1174, 1990
185. Arauz-Pacheco C, Raskin P: Management of hypertension in diabetes. *Endocrinol Metab Clin North Am* 21:371-394, 1992
186. Dunlop D: Eighty-six cases of Addison's disease. *Br Med J* 2:887-891, 1963
187. Irvine WJ, Barnes EW: Adrenocortical insufficiency. *Clin Endocrinol Metab* 1:549-594, July 1972
188. Xarli VP, Steele AA, Davis PJ, et al: Adrenal hemorrhage in the adult. *Medicine (Baltimore)* 57:211-221, 1978
189. Rao RH, Vagnucci AH: The clinical profile and management of bilateral massive adrenal hemorrhage. *Adv Endocrinol Metab* 3:213-236, 1992
190. Werbel SS, Ober KP: Acute adrenocortical insufficiency. *Endocrinol Metab Clin North Am* 22:303-328, 1993
191. Schambelan M, Sebastian A: Hyporeninemic hypoaldosteronism: review. *Adv Intern Med* 24:385-405, 1979
192. Schambelan M, Sebastian A, Biglieri EG: Prevalence, pathogenesis, and functional significance of aldosterone deficiency in hyperkalemic patients with chronic renal insufficiency. *Kidney Int* 17:89-101, 1980
193. Lee TH, Salomon DR, Rayment CM, et al: Hypotension and sinus arrest with exercise-induced hyperkalemia and combined verapamil/propranolol therapy. *Am J Med* 80:1203-1204, 1986
194. Taylor AA, Bartter FC: Hypertension in licorice intoxication, acromegaly, and Cushing's syndrome. In *Hypertension: Physiopathology and Treatment.* Edited by J Genest, E Koiw, O Kuchel. New York, McGraw-Hill Book Company, 1977, pp 755-767
195. Kaplan NN: Adrenal causes of hypertension. *Arch Intern Med* 133:1001-1006, 1974
196. Plotz CM, Knowlton AI, Ragan C: The natural history of Cushing's syndrome. *Am J Med* 13:597-614, 1952
197. Ross EJ, Marshall-Jones P, Friedman M: Cushing's syndrome: diagnostic criteria. *Q J Med* 35:149-192, 1966
198. Krakoff L, Nicolis G, Amsel B: Pathogenesis of hypertension in Cushing's syndrome. *Am J Med* 58:216-220, 1975
199. Dalakos TG, Elias AN, Anderson GH Jr, et al: Evidence for an angiotensinogenic mechanism of the hypertension of Cushing's syndrome. *J Clin Endocrinol Metab* 46:114-118, 1978

200. Sugihara N, Shimizu M, Shimizu K, et al: Disproportionate hypertrophy of the interventricular septum and its regression in Cushing's syndrome: report of three cases. *Intern Med* 31:407-413, 1992

201. Sugihara N, Shimizu M, Kita Y, et al: Cardiac characteristics and postoperative courses in Cushing's syndrome. *Am J Cardiol* 69:1475-1480, 1992

202. Soffer LJ, Iannaecone A, Gabrilove JL: Cushing's syndrome: a study of fifty patients. *Am J Med* 30:129-146, 1961

203. Young WF Jr, Carney JA: Cushing's syndrome: primary pigmented nodular adrenal disease. *Adv Endocrinol Metab* 3:179-197, 1992

204. Carney JA, Gordon H, Carpenter PC, et al: The complex of myxomas, spotty pigmentation, and endocrine overactivity. *Medicine (Balt)* 64:270-283, 1985

205. Danoff A, Jormark S, Lorber D, et al: Adrenocortical micronodular dysplasia, cardiac myxomas, lentigines, and spindle cell tumors: report of a kindred. *Arch Intern Med* 147:443-448, 1987

206. Carpenter PC: Diagnostic evaluation of Cushing's syndrome. *Endocrinol Metab Clin North Am* 17:445-472, 1988

207. Loriaux DL, Nieman L: Cushing's syndrome: advances in diagnosis and treatment. *Adv Endocrinol Metab* 1:23, 1990

208. Tarazi RC, Ibrahim MM, Bravo EL, et al: Hemodynamic characteristics of primary aldosteronism. *N Engl J Med* 289:1330-1335, 1973

209. Melby JC: Diagnosis of hyperaldosteronism. *Endocrinol Metab Clin North Am* 20:247-255, 1991

210. Young WF Jr, Hogan MJ, Klee GG, et al: Primary aldosteronism: diagnosis and treatment. *Mayo Clin Proc* 65:96-110, 1990

211. Conn JW, Cohen EL, Rovner DR: Suppression of plasma renin activity in primary aldosteronism: distinguishing primary from secondary aldosteronism in hypertensive disease. *JAMA* 190:213-221, 1964

212. Melby JC: Solving the adrenal lesion(s) of primary aldosteronism (editorial). *N Engl J Med* 294:441-442, 1976

213. White EA, Schambelan M, Rost CR, et al: Use of computed tomography in diagnosing the cause of primary aldosteronism. *N Engl J Med* 303:1503-1507, 1980

214. Schambelan M, Brust NL, Chang BCF, et al: Circadian rhythm and effect of posture on plasma aldosterone concentration in primary aldosteronism. *J Clin Endocrinol Metab* 43:115-131, 1976

215. Ferriss JB, Brown JJ, Fraser R, et al: Results of adrenal surgery in patients with hypertension, aldosterone excess, and low plasma renin concentration. *Br Med J* 1:135-138, 1975

216. Kremer D, Boddy K, Brown JJ, et al: Amiloride in the treatment of primary hyperaldosteronism and essential hypertension. *Clin Endocrinol* 7:151-157, 1977

217. Sheps SG, Jiang N-S, Klee GG, et al: Recent developments in the diagnosis and treatment of pheochromocytoma. *Mayo Clin Proc* 65:88-95, 1990

218. Sheps SG, Jiang N-S, Klee GG: Diagnostic evaluation of pheochromocytoma. *Endocrinol Metab Clin North Am* 17:397-414, 1988

219. Bravo EL, Gifford RW: Pheochromocytoma. *Endocrinol Metab Clin North Am* 22:329-341, 1993

220. Page LB, Raker JW, Berberich FR: Pheochromocytoma with predominant epinephrine secretion. *Am J Med* 47:648-652, 1969

221. Baker G, Zeller NH, Weitzner S, et al: Pheochromocytoma without hypertension presenting as cardiomyopathy. *Am Heart J* 83:688-693, 1972

222. Van Vliet PD, Burchell HB, Titus JL: Focal myocarditis associated with pheochromocytoma. *N Engl J Med* 274:1102-1108, 1966

223. Sjoerdsma A, Engelman K, Waldmann TA, et al: Pheochromocytoma: current concepts of diagnosis and treatment; combined clinical staff conference at the National Institutes of Health. *Ann Intern Med* 65:1302-1326, 1966

224. Cheng TO, Bashour TT: Striking electrocardiographic changes associated with pheochromocytoma: masquerading as ischemic heart disease. *Chest* 70:397-399, 1976

225. Shub C, Cueto-Garcia L, Sheps SG, et al: Echocardiographic findings in pheochromocytoma. *Am J Cardiol* 57:971-975, 1986

226. Gitlow SE, Mendlowitz M, Bertani LM: The biochemical techniques for detecting and establishing the presence of a pheochromocytoma: a review of ten years' experience. *Am J Cardiol* 26:270-279, 1970

227. Kaplan NM, Kramer NJ, Holland OB, et al: Single-voided urine metanephrine assays in screening for pheochromocytoma. *Arch Intern Med* 137:190-193, 1977

228. Bravo EL, Tarazi RC, Gifford RW, et al: Circulating and urinary catecholamines in pheochromocytoma: diagnostic and pathophysiologic implications. *N Engl J Med* 301:682-686, 1979

229. Boutros AR, Bravo EL, Zanettin G, et al: Perioperative management of 63 patients with pheochromocytoma. *Cleve Clin J Med* 57:613-617, 1990

230. McGuffin WL Jr, Sherman BM, Roth J, et al: Acromegaly and cardiovascular disorders: a prospective study. *Ann Intern Med* 81:11-18, 1974

231. Gordon DA, Hill FM, Ezrin C: Acromegaly: a review of 100 cases. *Can Med Assoc J* 87:1106-1109, 1962

232. Nabarro JDN: Acromegaly. *Clin Endocrinol* 26:481-511, 1987

233. Strauch G, Lego A, Therain F, et al: Reversible plasma and red blood cells volumes increases in acromegaly. *Acta Endocrinol (Copenh)* 85:465-478, 1977

234. Cain JP, Williams GH, Dluhy RG: Plasma renin activity and aldosterone secretion in patients with acromegaly. *J Clin Endocrinol Metab* 34:73-81, 1972

235. Strauch G, Vallotton MB, Touitou Y, et al: The renin angiotensin system in normotensive and hypertensive patients with acromegaly. *N Engl J Med* 287:795-799, 1972

236. Dluhy RG, Williams GH: Primary aldosteronism in a hypertensive acromegalic patient. *J Clin Endocrinol Metab* 29:1319-1324, 1969

237. Moore TJ, Thein-Wai W, Dluhy RG, et al: Abnormal adrenal and vascular responses to angiotensin II and an angiotensin antagonist in acromegaly. *J Clin Endocrinol Metab* 51:215-222, 1980

238. Mather HM, Boyd MJ, Jenkins JS: Heart size and function in acromegaly. *Br Heart J* 41:697-701, 1979

239. Csanady M, Gaspar L, Hogye M, et al: The heart in acromegaly: an echocardiographic study. *Acta Cardiol* 42:1, 1987

240. Erbas T, Erbas B, Usman A, et al: Assessment of left ventricular dysfunction in acromegalic patients using radionuclide ventriculography parameters. *Cardiology* 80:172-179, 1992

241. Kahaly G, Stover C, Beyer J, et al: Relation of endocrine and cardiac findings in acromegalics. *J Endocrinol Invest* 15:13-18, 1992

242. Morvan D, Komajda M, Grimaldi A, et al: Cardiac hypertrophy and function in asymptomatic acromegaly. *Eur Heart J* 12:666-672, 1991

243. Smallridge RC, Rajfer S, Davia J, et al: Acromegaly and the heart: an echocardiographic study. *Am J Med* 66:22-27, 1979

244. Savage DD, Henry WL, Eastman RC, et al: Echocardiographic assessment of cardiac anatomy and function in acromegalic patients. *Am J Med* 67:823-829, 1979

245. Jonas EA, Aloia JF, Lane FJ: Evidence of subclinical heart muscle dysfunction in acromegaly. *Chest* 67:190-194, 1975

246. Kahaly G, Olshausen KV, Mohr-Kahaly S, et al: Arrhythmia profile in acromegaly. *Eur Heart J* 13:51-56, 1992

247. Rossi L, Thiene G, Caregaro L, et al: Dysrhythmias and sudden death in acromegalic heart disease: a clinicopathologic study. *Chest* 72:495-498, 1977

248. Lie JT, Grossman SJ: Pathology of the heart in acromegaly: anatomic findings in 27 autopsied patients. *Am Heart J* 100:41-52, 1980

249. Abboud CF, Laws ER Jr: Diagnosis of pituitary tumors. *Endocrinol Metab Clin North Am* 17:241-280, 1988

250. Chang-De Moranville BM, Jackson IM: Diagnosis and endocrine testing in acromegaly. *Endocrinol Metab Clin North Am* 21:649-668, 1992

251. Fahlbusch R, Honegger J, Buchfelder M: Surgical management of acromegaly. *Endocrinol Metab Clin North Am* 21:669-692, 1992

252. Eastman RC, Gorden P, Glatstein E, et al: Radiation therapy of acromegaly. *Endocrinol Metab Clin North Am* 21:693-712, 1992

253. Wright AD, Hill DM, Lowy C, et al: Mortality in acromegaly. *Q J Med* 39:1-16, 1970

254. Jaffe CA, Barkan AL: Treatment of acromegaly with dopamine agonists. *Endocrinol Metab Clin North Am* 21:713-735, 1992

255. Lamberts SWJ, Reubi JC, Krenning EP: Somatostatin analogs in the treatment of acromegaly. *Endocrinol Metab Clin North Am* 21:737-752, 1992

256. Barkan AL: Acromegaly: diagnosis and therapy. *Endocrinol Metab Clin North Am* 18:277-310, 1989

257. Hayward RP, Emanuel RW, Nabarro JDN: Acromegalic heart disease: influence of treatment of the acromegaly on the heart. *Q J Med* 62:41-58, 1987

258. Editorial: Acromegalic heart disease. *Lancet* 2:254-255, 1987

259. Pereira JL, Rodriguez-Puras MJ, Leal-Cerro A, et al: Acromegalic cardiopathy improves after treatment with increasing doses of octreotide. *J Endocrinol Invest* 14:17-23, 1991

260. Kaplan NM: Hypertension with pregnancy and the pill. In *Clinical Hypertension.* Fifth edition. Edited by NM Kaplan. Baltimore, Williams & Wilkins, 1990, pp 325-349

261. Dalen JE, Hickler RB: Oral contraceptives and cardiovascular disease. *Am Heart J* 101:626-639, 1981

262. Stadel BV: Oral contraceptives and cardiovascular disease. *N Engl J Med* 305:612-618; 672-677, 1981

263. Stampfer MJ, Willett WC, Colditz GA, et al: A prospective study of past use of oral contraceptive agents and risk of cardiovascular disease. *N Engl J Med* 319:1313-1317, 1988

264. Castelli WP: Cardiovascular disease in women. *Am J Obstet Gynecol* 158:1553-1560, 1988

265. Knopp RH: Cardiovascular effects of endogenous and exogenous sex hormones over a woman's lifetime. *Am J Obstet Gynecol* 158:1630-1643, 1988

266. Vessey M, Mant D, Smith A, et al: Oral contraceptives and venous thromboembolism: findings in a large prospective study. *Br Med J* 292:526, 1986

267. Meade TW: Risks and mechanisms of cardiovascular events in users of oral contraceptives. *Am J Obstet Gynecol* 158:1646-1652, 1988

268. Vessey MP, Doll R: Investigation of relation between use of oral contraceptives and thromboembolic disease. *Br Med J* 2:199-205, 1968

269. Royal College of General Practitioners' Oral Contraception Study: Oral contraceptives, venous thrombosis, and varicose veins. *J R Coll Gen Pract* 28:393-399, 1978

270. Sagar S, Stamatakis JD, Thomas DP, et al: Oral contraceptives, antithrombin-III activity, and postoperative deep-vein thrombosis. *Lancet* 1:509-511, 1976

271. Montanari CMD, Vittoria A, Rossi U, et al: Human platelet aggregation curve and oral contraception. *Acta Haematol (Basel)* 61:230-232, 1979

272. Howie PW, Mallinson AC, Prentice CRM, et al: Effect of combined oestrogen-progestogen oral contraceptives, oestrogen, and progestogen on antiplasmin and antithrombin activity. *Lancet* 2:1329-1332, 1970

273. Inman WHW, Vessey MP, Westerholm B, et al: Thromboembolic disease and the steroidal content of oral contraceptives: a report to the committee on safety of drugs. *Br Med J* 2:203-209, 1970

274. Royal College of General Practitioners: *Oral Contraceptive Study: Oral Contraceptives and Health; An Interim Report.* New York, Pitman Publishing Co, 1974, pp 37-42

275. Woods JW: Oral contraceptives and hypertension. *Hypertension* 11 Suppl 2:11, 1988

276. Woods JW, Algary WA, Stier FM: Oral contraceptives and hypertension (abstract). *Circulation* 46 Suppl 2:82, 1972

277. Harris PWR: Malignant hypertension associated with oral contraceptives. *Lancet* 2:466-467, 1969

278. Zacherle BJ, Richardson JA: Irreversible renal failure secondary to hypertension induced by oral contraceptives. *Ann Intern Med* 77:83-85, 1972

279. Woods JW: Oral contraceptives and hypertension. *Lancet* 2:653-654, 1967

280. Weir RJ, Fraser R, McElwee G, et al: The effect of estrogen-progestogen oral contraceptives on blood pressure and on the renin-angiotensin-aldosterone system. In *Oral Contraceptives and High Blood Pressure.* Edited by MJ Fregly, MS Fregly. Gainesville, Florida, Dolphin Press, 1974, pp 68-78

281. Streeten DHP, Anderson GH Jr, Dalakos TG: Angiotensin blockade: its clinical significance. *Am J Med* 60:817-824, 1976

282. Jick H, Dinan B, Herman R, et al: Myocardial infarction and other vascular diseases in young women: role of estrogens and other factors. *JAMA* 240:2548-2552, 1978

283. Mann JI, Inman WHW: Oral contraceptives and death from myocardial infarction. *Br Med J* 2:245-248, 1975

284. Mann JI, Inman WHW, Thorogood M: Oral contraceptive use in older women and fatal myocardial infarction. *Br Med J* 2:445-447, 1976

285. Shapiro S, Slone D, Rosenberg L, et al: Oral-contraceptive use in relation to myocardial infarction. *Lancet* 1:743-747, 1979

286. Rosenberg L, Hennekens CH, Rosner B, et al: Oral contraceptive use in relation to nonfatal myocardial infarction. *Am J Epidemiol* 111:59-66, 1980

287. Krueger DE, Ellenberg SS, Blood S, et al: Fatal myocardial infarction and the role of oral contraceptives. *Am J Epidemiol* 111:655-674, 1980

288. Mann JI, Doll R, Thorogood M, et al: Risk factors for myocardial infarction in young women. *Br J Prev Soc Med* 30:94-100, 1976

289. Kannel WB: Possible hazards of oral contraceptive use (editorial). *Circulation* 60:490-491, 1979

290. Ratnoff OD, Kaufman R: Arterial thrombosis in oral contraceptive users (editorial). *Arch Intern Med* 142:447-448, 1982

CHAPTER

64

Heart disease in the elderly

Eric G. Tangalos, M.D., and Bernard J. Gersh, M.B.,Ch.B., D.Phil

THE aging of America is the most important demographic development in our nation's 20th century history. The texture of society has changed greatly since the 1960s, and we will not realize its full implications until the postwar baby boomers officially join the ranks of the retired, beginning in 2010. The experience will be that of a sexagenarian explosion as this segment increases by 1 million persons per year for the next 20 years (a 59% change). In actual numbers, approximately 34 million elderly currently accounting for 12.5% of the population will become 67 million elderly composing almost 22% of the U.S. population in the year 2040.[1]

In caring for the elderly patient, the physician must remember that the aging process is far more random, unorganized, and unpredictable than normal human growth and development. We are now only beginning to establish norms and expectations for the population over age 85. With advancing age, the incidence of chronic disease increases and the complexity of patient care becomes more challenging (Fig 64-1). Many of the cardiovascular problems encountered by the elderly are not unique to them and are covered in other chapters of this text. The purpose of this chapter is not to duplicate other information but instead to consider studies that have been purposely designed with the elderly population in mind, particularly the clinical outcome of these studies.

Several clinical studies have reported a high prevalence (nearly 50%) of heart disease in those aged over 65 years. Heart disease is the largest single cause of death in these persons and accounts for a major portion of the health-care costs in this age group.[2,3] Between 80% and 85% of cardiac disease deaths are attributed to ischemic heart disease, and deaths from hypertensive and rheumatic valvular disease add 5% to the rate. Congestive heart failure accounts for about 6% in the group aged 65 to 69 but rises to approximately 15% in the 85 and older group.[2,3]

In 1980, there were about 2 million persons in the United States aged 65 and over with diagnosed coronary heart disease. Ischemic heart disease, defined by angina pectoris, previous myocardial infarction, abnormal Q waves on the electrocardiogram, or a combination thereof, has a reported prevalence of about 20% in men and 12% in women over 65.[3] As of 1986, 3.6 million people over age 65 had symptomatic coronary artery disease, and of all patients hospitalized with an acute myocardial infarction, approximately 60% were over age 65. Hypertensive heart disease, defined by blood pressures greater than 180/100 mm Hg and probable left ventricular hypertrophy on the electrocardiogram, has a prevalence of about 10% in older men and 14% in older women. Combined ischemic and hypertensive heart disease, valvular heart disease, and pulmonary heart disease are the other major kinds of heart disease in elderly persons. Unfortunately, the notable decline in heart disease rates in the 1970s was much less in those over age 65 than in those under age 65.[4,5]

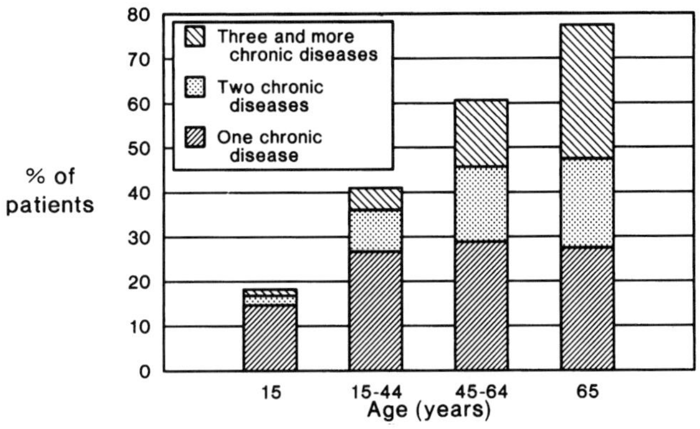

Fig 64-1 Incidence of chronic disease with advancing age. (From Lamby PP: Modifying drug dosage in elderly patients. In Covington TR, Walker JI [eds]: *Current Geriatric Therapy.* Philadelphia, WB Saunders Company, 1984. pp 35-72. By permission.)

PHYSIOLOGY OF THE CARDIOVASCULAR SYSTEM WITH AGING

Normal aging of the cardiovascular system produces important changes in hemodynamics, especially diminished cardiac reserve. Aging of collagen and other structural elements leads to a loss of elasticity in the arterial system and an increase in peripheral resistance. The significance of hypertension in the elderly has been greatly debated, but most researchers now agree that an elderly person is at increased risk for end-organ damage from increased blood pressure.[5,6]

From an epidemiologic perspective, the relationship between aging and cardiovascular disease has long been appreciated. The extended Framingham Study has shown that the overall mortality due to cardiovascular disease is higher among hypertensive elderly than their normotensive counterparts.[5] The strength of this association is evident regardless of which disease variables are studied—hospital admission rates, myocardial infarctions, mortality, or even economic costs.

The effects of aging alter the normal myocardial response during relaxation and impede diastolic function. Sinoatrial node activity slows, as does ventricular contraction. Frequently, the aged heart has difficulty maintaining output against a high afterload in the face of impaired contractility and a blunted chronotropic response (Fig 64-2). End-diastolic volumes increase to maintain stroke output (as ejection fraction decreases), but this increases left ventricular wall tension and myocardial oxygen demand. Often, the elderly heart fails, because increased left ventricular end-diastolic pressures dilate an already weak myocardium.

Slight increases in blood pressure in many elderly patients may be regarded as part of the normal loss of capacitance. However, systolic pressures over 200 mm Hg and diastolic pressures over 95 mm Hg are always abnormal, no matter what the age. Arteriosclerosis should be considered a disease entity no matter what the patient's age. Serum cholesterol plays an important role in determining the extent of atherosclerosis. Cigarette smoking and tobacco abuse certainly exacerbate this process.[7]

Other factors that influence cardiovascular fitness are kidney performance to clear salt and water and adrenal gland production of catecholamines and corticosteroids. The autonomic nervous system also loses functional performance during aging, a loss contributing to the elderly patient's inability to respond quickly to postural and positional changes. Several studies have documented

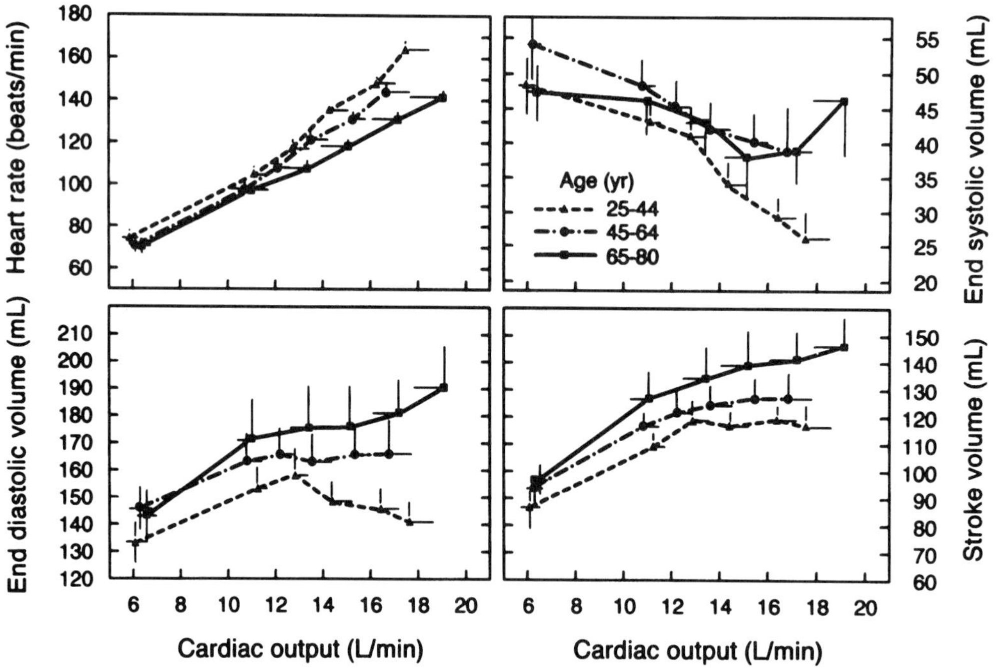

Fig 64-2 Cardiac performance measured by radionuclide ventriculography during upright cycle ergometry in normal subjects carefully screened to exclude coronary artery disease. The population has been divided into three age groups. In older subjects, a given cardiac output during exercise is achieved with a lower heart rate *(upper left)* and higher left ventricular end-diastolic *(lower left)*, end-diastolic *(upper right)*, and stroke *(lower right)* volumes. (Modified from Rodeheffer RJ, Gerstenblith G, Becker LC, et al: Exercise cardiac output is maintained with advancing age in healthy human subjects: cardiac dilatation and increased stroke volume compensate for a diminished heart rate. *Circulation* 69:203-213, 1984. By permission of American Heart Association.)

higher plasma catecholamine levels in older than in younger subjects during exercise.[8] The most likely interpretation of these findings suggests a functional β-adrenergic blockade with age.

In summary, a wide variety of variables determine cardiovascular performance in the elderly. They allow for multiple interventions and opportunities for the clinician to affect outcome. Many medications can be used to act on preload or afterload conditions, and other drugs can be used to modify heart rate and contractility.[9,10] Training programs using aerobic exercises make the heart a more efficient pump, and being at or near ideal weight reduces cardiovascular demand. Hypertension in the elderly should not be left untreated, and preventive strategies include stopping smoking and reducing salt intake. Invasive therapies have also taken their place in the management of this population.

CORONARY ARTERY DISEASE

Angina pectoris

Symptoms of ischemic heart disease do not differ significantly in the elderly. Dyspnea, the exception, may be a common presenting symptom of ischemic heart disease.[7] In persons aged 65 and older, atherosclerotic coronary disease accounts for about 85% of all deaths due to heart disease.[8] The prevalence of coronary artery disease exceeds 20% in the population aged 65 and over, and ischemic myocardial disease (old or recent, or both) is found at autopsy in 10% of hearts of all persons older than 65 years.[11,12] Significant coronary atherosclerosis, that is, fibrous plaques and calcium deposition in the vascular intima and luminal narrowing of more than 50%, has been demonstrated at autopsy in more than half the hearts from persons aged 55 to 64 years.[13] An extensive autopsy study of Olmsted County, Minnesota, residents showed that since 1970, more than 60% of persons aged 60 years or older had occlusion of 75% to 100% in at least one major coronary artery.[14] Thus, occult significant coronary artery disease is present during life in most elderly persons.[13,14]

The pharmacologic opportunities available for the treatment of coronary artery disease should be available to all patients without age limitation. However, the clinician should have a better understanding of the alteration in body composition and metabolism in this age group, because differences in the host significantly alter drug effect (see chapter 66).

The frequency of adverse drug reactions is twofold to threefold greater in the elderly than in young adults. Adverse reactions in young patients are easily recognized, whereas the same reaction in an older patient may mimic a disease state and therefore be mistaken.[15] The clinician must be particularly watchful, since decreased total body water and lean body mass with increased body fat affects drug distribution. Serum protein levels also affect drug distribution, and chronic diseases that may lower protein levels increase the free fraction of protein-bound drugs, leading to an exaggeration of their chemical effects.[16]

Several factors contribute to poor compliance in the elderly and require expectant management by the treating physician. Adverse side effects increase with the use of multiple drugs, particularly in cognitively impaired patients.[17] In the care of the elderly, one might sacrifice an elegant dosing schedule for a simple one that the patient can understand. Newer and more expensive once-a-day drugs may also be more appropriate for these patients, despite the cost. With repeat hospitalizations come changes in drug therapy, and patients are often displeased when large quantities of medication from an old regimen are discarded. However, discarding discontinued drugs may indeed be better than stockpiling at home. The latter practice may promote self-treatment with outdated and inappropriate medications.

The elderly are now regularly considered for special therapies and invasive procedures. Age as an independent risk factor is minimal in well-selected surgical case studies. In fact, most of the growth in invasive cardiology has occurred in the population over age 65. The number of patients over age 65 undergoing bypass grafting in the United States increased fivefold from 1975 to 1980; and by 1985, more than one-third of coronary artery bypass grafting procedures were in patients older than 65.[4] At the Mayo Clinic and at other major centers in the United States, the median age for bypass grafting is now 65 to 67 years, reflecting the steady increase over the past 2 decades, even though most elderly patients have "high-risk" or severe coronary artery disease.[18]

The number of patients over age 65 undergoing percutaneous transluminal coronary angioplasty also is rapidly increasing, but controlled comparisons with medical therapy are lacking. The National Heart, Lung, and Blood Institute percutaneous transluminal coronary angioplasty registry initially reported that in-hospital mortality associated with angioplasty was increased and that the success rate was lower in patients older than 65.[19] Later studies reported a lower mortality (0.8%), one not different from that in younger patients.[20]

Recent technical advances appear to have improved the primary success rate of dilatation in the elderly. Hartzler et al.[21] reported on 750 multiple-lesion percutaneous transluminal coronary angioplasty procedures performed in patients older than 70. The initial success rate in these patients (93%) was quite similar to that in patients younger than 70 (91%), and the development of myocardial infarction (2%) and the need for emergency coronary artery bypass grafting (1%) were quite low. At Mayo, the primary success rate of angioplasty in the elderly exceeds 90% and is similar among different age groups within the context of the elderly.[22] The complication rate and overall mortality, however, were greater in patients over age 75 who had angina and a higher incidence of congestive heart failure and multiple-vessel disease.

Early mortality in elderly patients who undergo bypass surgery is 5% to 6%.[23] This is higher than the rate for younger patients but is still very low and should not prevent either the patient or the physician from considering this option. In the Coronary Artery Surgery Study (CASS) registry, isolated coronary artery bypass in 1,087 patients 65 years old or older was compared with the same procedure in 7,827 patients younger than 65.[23] The older patients had more symptoms and a greater frequency of unstable angina and congestive heart failure. Other medical conditions, such as diabetes, hypertension, obstructive lung disease, cerebrovascular disease, and peripheral vascular disease, may have contributed to increased associated risk. At angiography, the elderly had a higher incidence of triple-vessel disease, left main disease, and decreased left ventricular function.[23] Similar profiles obtained by other investigators point to the elderly as a sicker population with a greater burden of disease.[24,25]

In the CASS registry study of patients entered from 1975 to 1979, perioperative mortality was 5.2% in patients older than 65 and only 1.9% in patients younger than 65.[23] Predictors of perioperative mortality were (1) left main coronary stenosis greater than 70% in association with left dominant circulation, (2) increased left ventricular end-diastolic pressure, (3) current cigarette smoking, (4) pulmonary rales on auscultation, and (5) number of associated medical diseases. Predictors of five-year mortality in the same study (in perioperative survivors) were (1) number of associated medical diseases, (2) functional impairment due to congestive heart failure, (3) severity of abnormal left ventricular wall motion (determined angiographically), and (4) increased left ventricular end-diastolic pressure.[26]

Acute myocardial infarction

The diagnosis of acute myocardial infarction is more difficult in the elderly. Dyspnea is a far more common complaint than chest pain, with a classic chest pain syndrome occurring in only about one-third of patients older than 85. Acute pulmonary edema and arterial embolism also are frequent presenting manifestations.[27] Myocardial infarction in elderly patients is characterized by a marked increase in morbidity and mortality.[28,29] Given the greater burden of disease, a history of myocardial infarction in the Bronx Aging Study[30] predicted a threefold greater risk of recurrent unrecognized myocardial infarction. Although myocardial infarction occurs with equal frequency in men and women older than 70, the prognosis is worse for women. In many elderly patients hospitalized for classic chest pain syndromes, myocardial infarction or unstable angina is never confirmed.[31] Laboratory proof is also vexing in this population. The high frequency of non-Q-wave myocardial infarction and baseline electrocardiographic abnormalities secondary to left ventricular hypertrophy and conduction abnormalities obscures the recognition of myocardial infarction. Diagnostic elevations of creatine kinase-MB levels may occur with stable total creatine kinase values.[32]

Patients 65 years of age and older compose over 60% of those dismissed from the hospital with a diagnosis of acute myocardial infarction.[33] Elderly patients more frequently have heart failure, cardiogenic shock, atrial arrhythmia, and cardiac rupture. A tenfold increase in hospital mortality in elderly patients (17.8% at 75 years or older compared with 2% below 55 years) was described in the Myocardial Infarction Triage and Intervention study.[34] In a multivariate analysis of outcome in older patients (more than 65 years), adverse events were related to both history of heart failure (odds ratio, 3:9) and increasing age (odds ratio, 1.4 for each decade of age). Outcomes were not improved by treatment with thrombolytic drugs, but these agents were prescribed for only 12% of patients older than 65, and thereby the power for detecting such an effect was reduced.

Thrombolytic therapy (intracoronary and intravenous) is being increasingly used to treat a greater number of elderly patients examined within the first few hours after an acute myocardial infarction.[23,35,36] Although no data from a prospective study are available for comparison of results between elderly and younger patients, overall successful reperfusion seems to be somewhat lower in the elderly than in younger patients.[37] Several randomized studies assessing the effectiveness of early thrombolysis on survival and preservation of left ventricular function in patients with known and suspected infarction reported analyses of patient subsets of different ages.[38,39] These studies indicated a striking severalfold increase in mortality in the older patient subsets in the placebo groups. The benefit of thrombolysis appears to increase with age up to 75 years. Beyond age 75, the benefit decreases and the risk of cerebral hemorrhage increases.[40] This is a study area of rapid evolution, and assessing the benefit-risk ratio and deciding whether to use thrombolytic therapy will become more obvious within the next few years. Benefit will most likely vary with the size of the infarct, that is, older patients with large anterior infarcts will probably receive the most benefit, whereas the contraindications of severe hypertension and previous cerebrovascular accidents will work against the decision to use thrombolytic therapy.

CONGESTIVE HEART FAILURE

Congestive heart failure is a very common problem in clinical geriatrics. Its prevalence rises dramatically with increasing age, beginning in the fifth decade.[3,41,42] The incidence of heart failure increases so greatly with age that approximately 75% of all ambulatory patients with heart failure are 60 years of age or older.[41,42] Congestive heart failure may result from a compromise of either systolic or diastolic function or of both, resulting in increased ventricular end-diastolic pressures. The average annual incidence of congestive heart failure according to age and sex based on 16-year follow-up results of the Framingham Heart Study[41] is shown in Figure 64-3.

Several studies have documented the high prevalence of diastolic dysfunction with preserved systolic function in elderly patients with congestive heart failure.[43,44] Between 50% and 60% of older persons with congestive heart failure have normal or slightly reduced ejection fractions.[43,45] Elderly patients with impaired diastolic function are often erroneously treated for systolic heart failure with medications such as diuretics and vasodilators, which may exacerbate rather than relieve their cardiac disease. Postmortem studies of elderly patients with heart failure reveal that the underlying pathologic conditions are similar to those found in middle-aged persons.[46]

Coexisting pathologic processes, each of which in itself would not otherwise cause heart failure, occasionally may be responsible for heart failure in the elderly.[46] Although

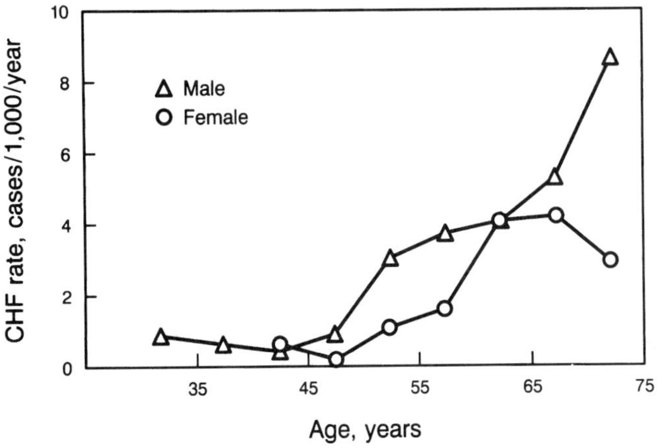

Fig 64-3 Average annual incidence of congestive heart failure (CHF) by sex and age. (Data from McKee PA, Costelli WP, McNamara PM, et al: The natural history of congestive heart failure: The Framingham study. *N Engl J Med* 285:1441-1446, 1971.)

amyloid deposition is frequently found in the senescent heart and occurs primarily in the atria, in the vast majority of cases it is not significant enough to contribute to heart failure. The responsiveness to β-adrenergic stimulation decreases with age, and there is greater dependence in elderly persons on the Frank-Starling mechanism.[9,47,48] Data in animals suggest that the hypertrophic response of the myocardium to a given increase in afterload may be decreased in old age.[49] The age-related prolongation of ventricular relaxation time together with increased myocardial stiffness of the aged heart results in increases in left ventricular end-diastolic pressures at rest or during exercise, so that pulmonary and systemic venous congestion may occur to produce heart failure despite preserved systolic function. Clinically apparent disease occurs when the heart is unable to adapt to increased workloads through a combination of the following three functions: (1) increased sympathetic nervous system stimulation, (2) myocardial hypertrophy, and (3) the Frank-Starling mechanism.[11,45]

Two factors have changed the approach to elderly patients with heart failure. The first is the recognition of ventricular diastolic dysfunction as an important pathophysiologic mechanism among elderly patients;[50] it occurs in as many as half of all very elderly patients with heart failure. The identification of persons with diastolic dysfunction can result in a far more favorable prognosis with a correctly designed treatment regimen.[51] The second factor is that elderly women, who constitute most of this population, tend to have a less favorable prognosis, which may be related to the characteristics of their underlying disease.

Vasodilator therapy reduces afterload and thereby enhances myocardial shortening and increasing stroke volume.[52] The most frequently used vasodilators are the nitrates. Alone or in combination with hydralazine, nitrates may be effective in reducing filling pressure, increasing cardiac output, increasing renal blood flow, and improving exercise tolerance.[52,53] Clinical trials that included some elderly patients showed that vasodilator drugs improve symptomatic status, functional capacity, and survival in patients with heart failure and ventricular systolic dysfunction. Improvement has occurred with combinations of isosorbide dinitrate and hydralazine[53] and with several angiotensin-converting enzyme inhibitor drugs.[54,55]

The administration of long-term digitalis therapy to elderly patients has again come under scrutiny.[45,56] Digitalis is useful in managing acute and severe congestive heart failure in patients with either sinus rhythm or atrial fibrillation.[45,56] The inotropic response to cardiac glycosides may be diminished in senescent mammalian cardiac muscle, but the toxic effects of digitalis may not be decreased in old age.[57] Higher steady-state levels and prolonged plasma half-lives of digoxin in the elderly are due partly to the age-related decline in renal excretory capacity.[58] Decreased renal clearance and wide variability in extrarenal clearance further reduce the predictability of serum digoxin levels in the elderly. Because of these age-related changes, including a possible decrease in inotropic response, the indication for digitalis should be considered in the context of its known toxicity.

If angiotensin-converting enzyme inhibitor therapy has been initiated, a long-acting agent such as lisinopril is much easier on the patient and caregiver to use. In all instances of providing therapy to the elderly, a simple program requiring fewer or longer acting medications is usually worth the expense of these newer agents.

ARRHYTHMIAS

Age-associated histologic changes occur throughout most of the cardiac impulse and conduction system.[12] Idiopathic bundle-branch fibrosis is the most common cause of chronic atrioventricular block in patients over age 65. Lev[59] described a type of fibrosis that occurs predominantly in the proximal portions of the bundles, and Lenegre[60] described a diffuse process involving the entire bundle branch. The intrinsic sinus node rate and parasympathetic and sympathetic tone decrease with age, as does the respiratory variation in sinus rate.[61] Maximum heart rate decreases with age.[9,62] In nonselected populations and in patients free of cardiovascular disease, the prevalence of ectopy increases with age.[63,64]

Atrial and ventricular arrhythmias are common in the elderly, including those without clinically apparent heart disease. The incidence of frequent or complex arrhythmias is related to the presence and extent of underlying heart disease and reportedly is between 20% and 75%, with ventricular arrhythmias accounting for two-thirds and supraventricular arrhythmias for one-third of the cases.[2,64,65] The clinical significance of supraventricular arrhythmias varies from trivial to life-threatening, and proper management depends on accurate diagnosis of the rhythm disturbance and knowledge of the clinical setting.[2,64,65] Both benign and potentially malignant ventricular arrhythmias are common in asymptomatic and otherwise healthy elderly individuals. Although minor ventricular arrhythmias also occur frequently in the elderly with symptoms, serious episodic arrhythmias are less common and often occur in relation to the onset of systemic dysfunction. Prognosis of chronic arrhythmias is related to the severity of underlying heart disease.

The Cardiac Arrhythmia Suppression Trial (CAST) tested the hypothesis that pharmacologic suppression of ventricular premature depolarizations or asymptomatic or mildly symptomatic nonsustained ventricular tachycardia in patients after myocardial infarction would reduce deaths caused by arrhythmias.[66] Patients aged 66 to 79 had more previous myocardial infarctions, congestive heart failure, hypertension, nonsustained ventricular tachycardia repolarization abnormalities, digitalis use, and diuretic therapy.[67] The observation that this age group did less well with encainide, flecainide, and moricizine than their younger counterparts suggests that the elderly are even more susceptible to the adverse effects of these antiarrhythmic agents than the general population.[68]

Many antiarrhythmic drugs given to suppress ventricular arrhythmias are potentially proarrhythmic.[69] Cardiac failure may be precipitated or exacerbated by some agents, such as disopyramide, with prominent negative inotropic properties, and the sick sinus syndrome is exacerbated by many of these antiarrhythmic drugs. Decreased dosage of most antiarrhythmic agents is required to avert drug toxicity,[70] because impaired hepatic metabolism, decreased rate of renal excretion, and drug interactions predispose to excessive drug levels.

Treatment of symptomatic supraventricular arrhythmias is similar for all age groups. Atrial fibrillation may be treated with drugs, cardioversion, or pacing. The experience with pacemaker therapy has been good in the elderly, and long-term survival in elderly patients with pacemakers is identical to that of an age-matched population without pacemakers.[71] For those with sick sinus syndrome, a permanent pacemaker is indicated only when the patient has symptoms, since pacemaker implantation does not alter life expectancy.[72,73]

SUMMARY

As the population over age 65 continues to increase rapidly, care of the elderly will consume an ever-greater proportion of each physician's practice. Cardiovascular disease will remain the leading cause of death and disability in this population, and cardiovascular risk will continue to increase with age for the foreseeable future. The differences in physiologic age and chronologic age must be understood by the practitioner and adjustments made accordingly. Optimal management of these persons requires a general understanding of the effects of aging on the entire human organism and a specific understanding of the new treatments for cardiovascular disease in this population. Advanced age should never preclude appropriate therapy. Aggressive medical and surgical approaches should be considered for select individuals. The population over age 85 will provide the most opportunities for further research, and its rapid expansion creates challenges for clinical practice.

REFERENCES

1. United States population estimates by age, sex and race: 1980 to 1987. In *Current Population Reports,* SER p-25, No 1022. Washington, DC, US Bureau of the Census, Government Printing Office, 1988
2. Wei JY: Heart disease in the elderly. *Cardiovasc Med* 9:971-982, 1984
3. Caird FI, Kennedy RD: Epidemiology of heart disease in old age. In *Cardiology in Old Age.* Edited by FI Caird, JLC Dall, RD Kennedy. New York, Plenum Press, 1976, pp 1-10
4. Wenger NK, Marcus FI, O'Rourke RA: Cardiovascular disease in the elderly. *J Am Coll Cardiol* 10 Suppl A:80-87, 1987
5. Kannel WB, Dawber TR, McGee DL: Perspectives on systolic hypertension. The Framingham study. *Circulation* 61:1179-1182, 1980
6. Hypertension Detection and Follow-up Program Cooperative Group: Five-year findings of the Hypertension Detection and Follow-up Program. II. Mortality by race-sex and age. *JAMA* 242:2572-2577, 1979
7. Pathy MS: Clinical features of ischemic heart disease. In *Cardiology in Old Age.* Edited by FI Caird, JLC Dall, RD Kennedy. New York, Plenum Press, 1976, pp 193-208
8. Milch RA: Matrix properties of the aging arterial wall. *Monogr Surg Sci* 2:261-341, 1965
9. Rodeheffer RJ, Gerstenblith G, Becker LC, et al: Exercise cardiac output is maintained with advancing age in healthy human subjects: cardiac dilatation and increased stroke volume compensate for a diminished heart rate. *Circulation* 69:203-213, 1984
10. Hossack KF, Bruce RA: Prognostic value of exercise testing: the Seattle Heart Watch experience. *J Card Rehabil* 5:9-19, 1985
11. Wei JY: Cardiovascular anatomic and physiology changes with age. *Top Geriatr Rehabil* 2:10-16, 1986
12. Davies MJ: Pathology of the conduction system. In *Cardiology in Old Age.* Edited by FI Caird, JLC Dall, RD Kennedy. New York, Plenum Press, 1976, pp 57-59
13. Tejada C, Strong JP, Montenegro MR, et al: Distribution of coronary and aortic atherosclerosis by geographic location, race, and sex. *Lab Invest* 18:509-526, 1968
14. Elveback L, Lie JT: Continued high incidence of coronary artery disease at autopsy in Olmsted County, Minnesota, 1950 to 1979. *Circulation* 70:345-349, 1984
15. Herd JA, Wood AJ, Blumenthal J, et al: Medical therapy in the elderly. *J Am Coll Cardiol* 10 Suppl A:29-34, 1987
16. Vestal RE: Drug use in the elderly? A review of problems and special considerations. *Drugs* 16:358-382, 1978
17. Larson EB, Kukull WA, Buchner D, et al: Adverse drug reactions associated with global cognitive impairment in elderly persons. *Ann Intern Med* 107:169-173, 1987
18. Backes RJ, Gersh BJ: The treatment of coronary artery disease in the elderly. *Cardiovasc Drugs Ther* 5:449-455, 1991
19. Mock MB, Holmes DR Jr, Vlietstra RE, et al: Percutaneous transluminal coronary angioplasty (PTCA) in the elderly patient: experience in the National Heart, Lung, and Blood Institute PTCA Registry. *Am J Cardiol* 53:89C-91C, 1984
20. Raizner AE, Hust RG, Lewis JM, et al: Transluminal coronary angioplasty in the elderly. *Am J Cardiol* 57:29-32, 1986
21. Hartzler GO, Rutherford BD, McConahay DR, et al: Late results of multiple lesion coronary angiography in an aged population (abstract). *J Am Coll Cardiol* 7 Suppl A:21, 1986
22. Thompson RC, Holmes DR Jr, Gersh BJ, et al: Percutaneous transluminal coronary angioplasty in the elderly: early and long-term results. *J Am Coll Cardiol* 17:1245-1250, 1991
23. Gersh BJ, Kronmal RA, Frye RL, et al: Coronary arteriography and coronary artery bypass surgery: morbidity and mortality in patients ages 65 years or older. A report from the Coronary Artery Surgery Study. *Circulation* 67:483-491, 1983
24. Ennabli K, Pelletier LC: Morbidity and mortality of coronary artery surgery after the age of 70 years. *Ann Thorac Surg* 42:197-200, 1986
25. Mullany CJ, Darling GE, Pluth JR, et al: Early and late results after isolated coronary artery bypass surgery in 159 patients aged 80 years and older. *Circulation* 82 Suppl 5:229-236, 1990
26. Gersh BJ, Kronmal RA, Schaff HV, et al: Comparison of coronary artery bypass surgery and medical therapy in patients 65 years of age or older. A nonrandomized study from the Coronary Artery Surgery Study (CASS) registry. *N Engl J Med* 313:217-224, 1985

27. O'Rourke RA, Chatterjee K, Wei JY: Cardiovascular disease in the elderly. Coronary heart disease. *J Am Coll Cardiol* 10 Suppl A:52-56, 1987

28. Tofler GH, Muller JE, Stone PH, et al: Factors leading to shorter survival after acute myocardial infarction in patients ages 65 to 75 years compared with younger patients. *Am J Cardiol* 62:860-867, 1988

29. Marcus FI, Friday K, McCans J, et al: Age-related prognosis after acute myocardial infarction (the Multicenter Diltiazem Postinfarction Trial). *Am J Cardiol* 65:559-566, 1990

30. Nadelmann J, Frishman WH, Ooi WL, et al: Prevalence, incidence and prognosis of recognized and unrecognized myocardial infarction in persons aged 75 years or older: The Bronx Aging Study. *Am J Cardiol* 66:533-537, 1990

31. Solomon CG, Lee TH, Cook EF, et al: Comparison of clinical presentation of acute myocardial infarction in patients older than 65 years of age to younger patients: the Multicenter Chest Pain Study experience. *Am J Cardiol* 63:772-776, 1989

32. Hong RA, Licht JD, Wei JY, et al: Elevated CK-MB with normal total creatine kinase in suspected myocardial infarction: associated clinical findings and early prognosis. *Am Heart J* 111:1041-1047, 1986

33. Graves EJ: Detailed diagnoses and procedures, National Hospital Discharge Survey, 1989. *Vital Health Stat* Series 13, No. 108, 1991, pp 1-236

34. Weaver WD, Litwin PE, Martin JS, et al: Effect of age on use of thrombolytic therapy and mortality in acute myocardial infarction. The MITI Project Group. *J Am Coll Cardiol* 18:657-662, 1991

35. Gersh BJ: Clinical manifestations of coronary heart disease in the elderly. In *Working Conference on Recognition and Management of Coronary Heart Disease in the Elderly* (in press)

36. O'Rourke RA, Chatterjee K, Wei JY: Atherosclerotic coronary heart disease in the elderly. *J Am Coll Cardiol* (in press)

37. Fuentes F, Smalling RW, Hicks CH, et al: Thrombolytic therapy in myocardial infarction in the elderly patient. In *Geriatric Heart Disease.* Edited by EL Coodley. Littleton, Massachusetts, PSG Publishing Company, 1985, pp 404-410

38. Gruppo Italiano per lo Studio della Streptochinasi nell'Infarto Miocardico (GISSI): Effectiveness of intravenous thrombolytic treatment in acute myocardial infarction. *Lancet* 1:397-402, 1986

39. ISIS-2 (Second International Study of Infarct Survival) Collaborative Group: Randomised trial of intravenous streptokinase, oral aspirin, both, or neither among 17,187 cases of suspected acute myocardial infarction: ISIS-2. *Lancet* 2:349-360, 1988

40. Lew AS, Hod H, Cercek B, et al: Mortality and morbidity rates of patients older and younger than 75 years with acute myocardial infarction treated with intravenous streptokinase. *Am J Cardiol* 59:1-5, 1987

41. McKee PA, Castelli WP, McNamara PM, et al: The natural history of congestive heart failure: the Framingham study. *N Engl J Med* 285:1441-1446, 1971

42. Klainer LM, Gibson TC, White KL: The epidemiology of cardiac failure. *J Chronic Dis* 18:797-814, 1965

43. Dougherty AH, Naccarelli GV, Gray EL, et al: Congestive heart failure with normal systolic function. *Am J Cardiol* 54:778-782, 1984

44. Echeverria HH, Bilsker MS, Myerburg RJ, et al: Congestive heart failure: echocardiographic insights. *Am J Med* 75:750-755, 1983

45. Luchi RJ, Ware T: Congestive heart failure. In *Recent Advances in Geriatric Medicine.* Edited by B Isacs. New York, Churchill Livingstone, 1985, pp 19-36

46. Pomerance A: Pathology of the myocardium and valves. In *Cardiology in Old Age.* Edited by FI Caird, JLC Dall, RD Kennedy. New York, Plenum Press, 1976, pp 11-55

47. Vestal RE, Wood AJ, Shand DG: Reduced beta-adrenoceptor sensitivity in the elderly. *Clin Pharmacol Ther* 26:181-186, 1979

48. Feldman RD, Limbird LE, Nadeau J, et al: Alterations in leukocyte beta-receptor affinity with aging. A potential explanation for altered beta-adrenergic sensitivity in the elderly. *N Engl J Med* 310:815-819, 1984

49. Isoyama S, Wei JY, Fort P, et al: Does the capacity for left ventricular hypertrophy diminish with age? (Abstract.) *Circulation* 74 Suppl 2:174, 1986

50. Wong WF, Gold S, Fukuyama O, et al: Diastolic dysfunction in elderly patients with congestive heart failure. *Am J Cardiol* 63:1526-1528, 1989

51. Soufer R, Wohlgelernter D, Vita NA, et al: Intact systolic left ventricular function in clinical congestive heart failure. *Am J Cardiol* 55:1032-1036, 1985

52. Chatterjee K, Parmley WW: Vasodilator therapy for acute myocardial infarction and chronic congestive heart failure. *J Am Coll Cardiol* 1:133-153, 1983

53. Cohn JN, Archibald DG, Ziesche S, et al: Effect of vasodilator therapy on mortality in chronic congestive heart failure. Results of a Veterans Administration Cooperative Study. *N Engl J Med* 314:1547-1552, 1986

54. The CONSENSUS Trial Study Group: Effects of enalapril on mortality in severe congestive heart failure. Results of the Cooperative North Scandinavian Enalapril Survival Study (CONSENSUS). *N Engl J Med* 316:1429-1435, 1987

55. Furberg CD, Yusuf S, Thom TJ: Potential for altering the natural history of congestive heart failure: need for large clinical trials. *Am J Cardiol* 55:45A-47A, 1985

56. Lee DC, Johnson RA, Bingham JB, et al: Heart failure in outpatients: a randomized trial of digoxin versus placebo. *N Engl J Med* 306:699-705, 1982

57. Gerstenblith G, Spurgeon HA, Froehlich JP, et al: Diminished inotropic responsiveness to ouabain in aged rat myocardium. *Circ Res* 44:517-523, 1979

58. Greenblatt DJ, Sellers EM, Shader RI: Drug therapy: drug disposition in old age. *N Engl J Med* 306:1081-1088, 1982

59. Lev M: The pathology of complete atrioventricular block. *Prog Cardiovasc Dis* 6:317-326, 1964

60. Lenegre J: Etiology and pathology of bilateral bundle branch block in relation to complete heart block. *Prog Cardiovasc Dis* 6:409-444, 1964

61. Jose AD: Effect of combined sympathetic and parasympathetic blockade on heart rate and cardiac function in man. *Am J Cardiol* 18:476-478, 1966

62. Julius S, Amery A, Whitlock LS, et al: Influence of age on the hemodynamic response to exercise. *Circulation* 36:222-230, 1967

63. Chiang BN, Perlman LV, Ostrander LD Jr, et al: Relationship of premature systoles to coronary heart disease and sudden death in the Tecumseh epidemiologic study. *Ann Intern Med* 70:1159-1166, 1969

64. Fleg JL, Lakatta EG: Prevalence and prognosis of exercise-induced nonsustained ventricular tachycardia in apparently healthy volunteers. *Am J Cardiol* 54:762-764, 1984

65. Dreifus LS: Cardiac arrhythmias in the elderly: clinical aspects. *Cardiol Clin* 4:273-283, 1986

66. The Cardiac Arrhythmia Suppression Trial (CAST) Investigators: Preliminary report: effect of encainide and flecainide on mortality in a randomized trial of arrhythmia suppression after myocardial infarction. *N Engl J Med* 321:406-412, 1989

67. Smith SC Jr, Gilpin E, Ahnve S, et al: Outlook after acute myocardial infarction in the very elderly compared with that in patients aged 65 to 75 years. *J Am Coll Cardiol* 16:784-792, 1990

68. Akiyama T, Pawitan Y, Campbell WB, et al: Effects of advancing age on the efficacy and side effects of antiarrhythmic drugs in post-myocardial infarction patients with ventricular arrhythmias. The CAST Investigators. *J Am Geriatr Soc* 40:666-672, 1992

69. Dunbar DN: Ventricular arrhythmias in elderly patients. Evaluation and management. *Postgrad Med* 81:281-288, 1987

70. Podrid PJ, Levine PA, Klein MP: Effect of age on antiarrhythmic drug efficacy and toxicity. *Am J Cardiol* 63:735-739, 1989

71. Siddons H: Deaths in long-term paced patients. *Br Heart J* 36:1201-1209, 1974

72. McAnulty JH, Rahimtoola SH, Murphy E, et al: Natural history of "high-risk" bundle-branch block: final report of a prospective study. *N Engl J Med* 307: 137-143, 1982

73. Ginks W, Leatham A, Siddons H: Prognosis of patients paced for chronic atrioventricular block. *Br Heart J* 41:633-636, 1979

CHAPTER

65

Heart disease in women

Pamela B. Morris, M.D.

The impact of cardiovascular disease (CVD) on the health and well-being of women is a subject of growing concern. CVD, including coronary heart disease (CHD) and stroke, is the leading killer of women. Nearly 500,000 women die each year from CVD, and these deaths exceed those due to all other major causes combined[1] (Fig 65-1). Cardiovascular deaths in women are a greater threat than the combined risk of breast, uterine, ovarian, and cervical cancers and the risk of death due to childbirth[2] (Fig 65-2).

CVD is not a disease primarily of middle-aged men. More women than men die annually from CVD[1] (Fig 65-3). CHD accounts for 24% of all deaths and 52% of all CVD deaths in women.[3] Although the prevalence of CVD is higher at all ages in men than in women, after age 65 the prevalence is higher in women. Although women represent only 24% of persons younger than age 65 who die of acute myocardial infarction, they constitute 64% of elderly persons who die of myocardial infarction.[4] Because women outlive men by 7.5 years on average (Fig 65-4) and women predominate in the growing elderly population in the United States, CVD emerges as a major cause of morbidity and mortality for women and as a serious national public health problem.

Deaths due to CVD have declined among women by 43% since the mid-1960s.[3] However, data from 1965 to 1982 showed an alarming 28% increase in the incidence of myocardial infarction, sudden unexpected death, and angina in women, compared with a 21% reduction in men.[5] An increasing incidence of nonfatal CHD among women was also reported in data from the National Health Interview Survey, which evaluated trends in prevalence and incidence of coronary disease from 1980 to 1989[6] (Fig 65-5). During the observed decade, the incidence nearly doubled among white women, with much of the increase noted among elderly women (Fig 65-6). Even if the observed trends represent better diagnosis and increasing awareness, these data only further emphasize the burden of CVD among women. Declining mortality rates despite an increasing incidence of CHD in women may in part be due to a decrease in the case fatality rate for myocardial infarction and improvement in survival in

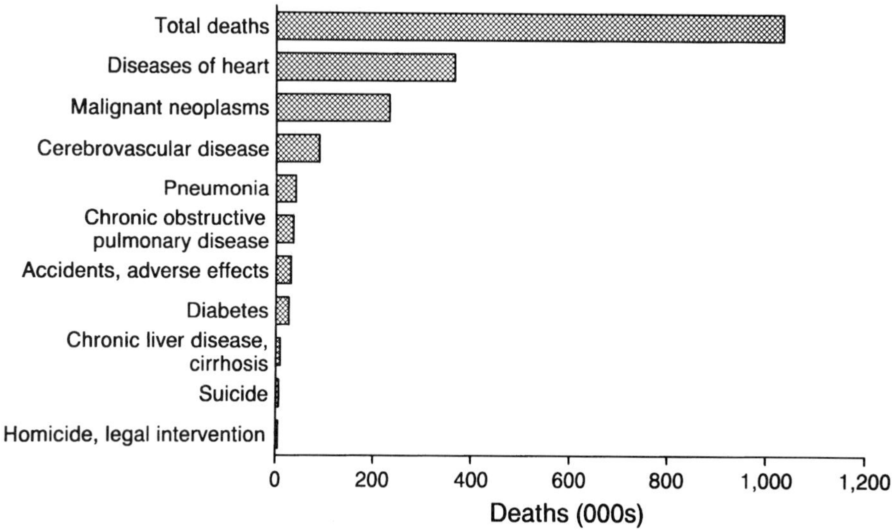

Fig 65-1 Leading causes of death among women, 1989. (Data from US Bureau of the Census, Statistical Abstract of the United States: 1992 [112th edition]. Washington, DC, 1992.)

women with angina pectoris. However, early and late morbidity and mortality rates remain higher in women than in men with heart disease.[7] These sex-specific trends in CHD are striking and further highlight the magnitude of the problem of CVD in women.

CVD is a leading cause of disability in women in the United States. In 1989, women accounted for 46% of hospital dismissals for management of heart disease. Rates of hospitalized days of care for heart disease are nearly equal in men and women. In recent years, the number of medical procedures performed on women for the diagnosis of CVD has increased dramatically. In 1989, 37% of cardiac catheterizations were performed on women. From 1985 to 1989, the number of cardiac catheterizations performed increased 48% in women and 37% in men. The number of cardiovascular surgical

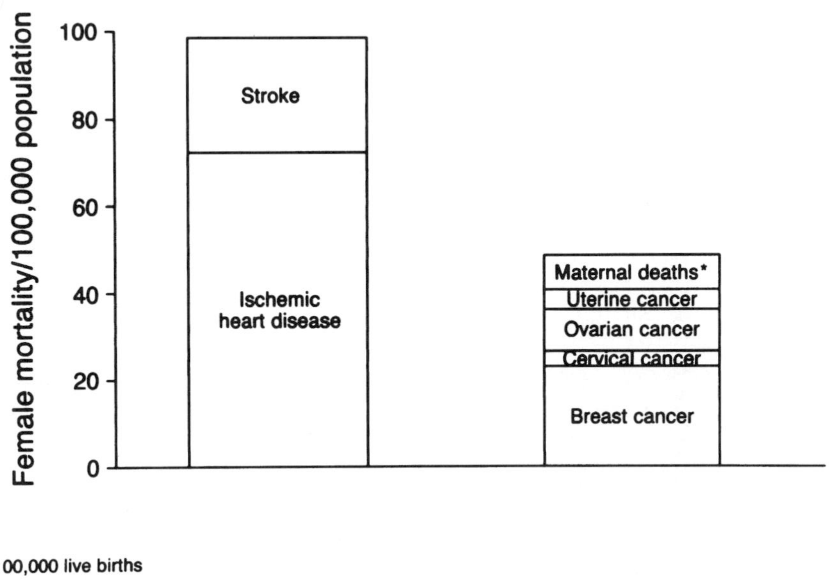

Fig 65-2 According to final 1989 data, deaths from coronary heart disease and stroke among women increased to a combined annual rate of 98.6 per 100,000 population. The cardiovascular death rate in women was thus more than double the cumulative toll of maternal mortality and that of breast, uterine, ovarian, and cervical cancers (48.6 per 100,000). (From Wenger NK: Coronary heart disease in women: a 'new' problem. *Hosp Pract* 27:59-74, November 15, 1992. By permission of HP Publishing Company.)

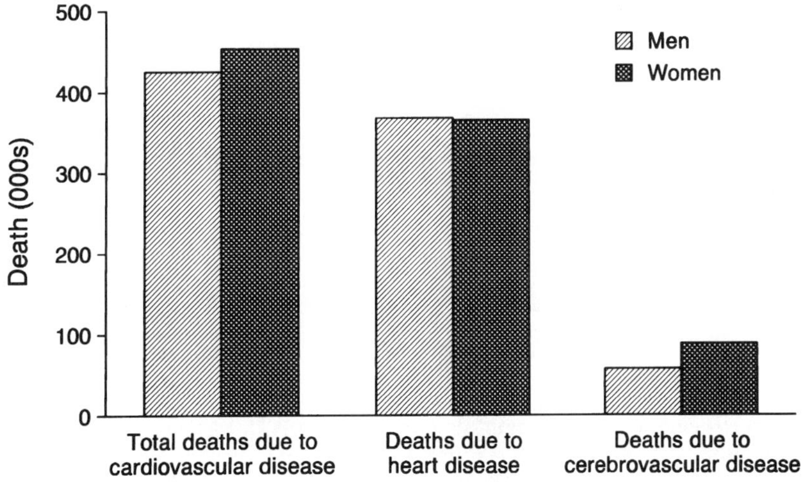

Fig 65-3 Cardiovascular death rates among women and men. (Data from US Bureau of the Census, Statistical Abstract of the United States: 1992 [112th edition]. Washington, DC, 1992.)

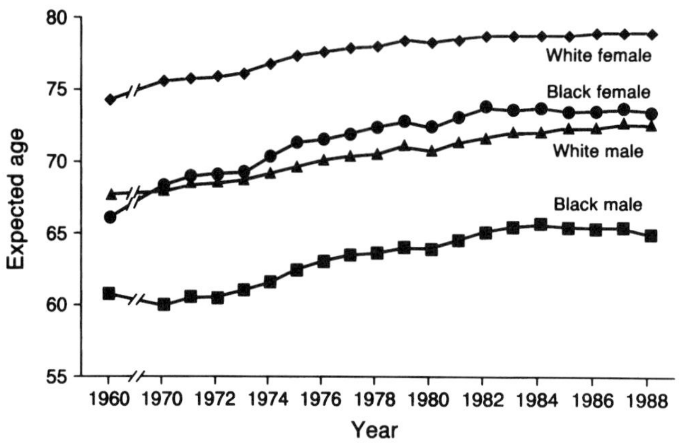

Fig 65-4 Life expectancy at birth, according to sex and race: United States, 1960 and 1970-1988. (From National Center for Health Statistics. Health, United States, 1990. Hyattsville, Maryland, Public Health Service, 1991.)

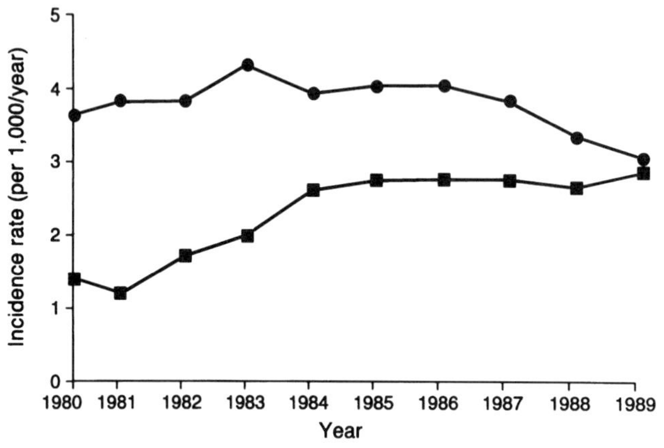

Fig 65-5 Incidence rates of nonfatal coronary heart disease among white men *(circles)* and women *(squares)* in the United States from 1980 through 1989. (From DeStefano F, Merritt RK, Anda RF, et al: Trends in nonfatal coronary heart disease in the United States, 1980 through 1989. *Arch Intern Med* 153:2489-2494, 1993. By permission of American Medical Association.)

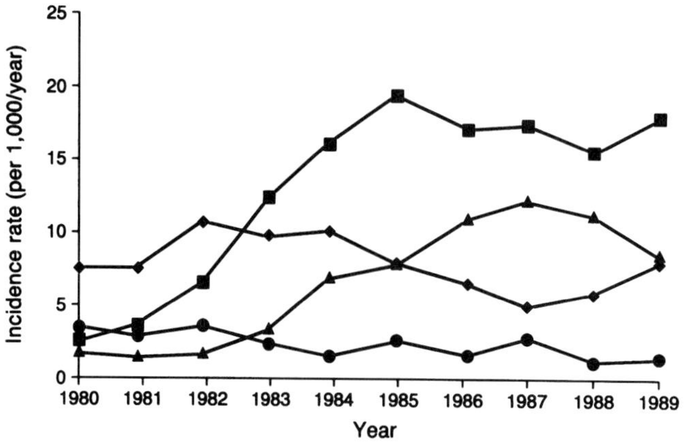

Fig 65-6 Incidence rates of nonfatal coronary heart disease among women by age in the United States from 1980 through 1989. *Circles* indicate age 45 to 54 years; *triangles,* 55 to 64 years; *diamonds,* 65 to 74 years; and *squares,* 75 to 84 years. (From DeStefano F, Merritt RK, Anda RF, et al: Trends in nonfatal coronary heart disease in the United States, 1980 through 1989. *Arch Intern Med* 153:2489-2494, 1993. By permission of American Medical Association.)

procedures performed has increased as well, with nearly 25% of all coronary artery bypass procedures taking place in women.[8]

The magnitude of the health-care costs incurred by CVD in women is substantial. Although CVD mortality is less common in women, 58% of the personal health-care expenditure for CVD is in women,[8] at an annual cost of more than $9 billion.[9] More than half of women who die of heart disease rely on Medicare as the major source of health payments, creating a significant national health-care burden.[10]

Despite clear evidence of the impact of CVD on the health of women, few clinical trials have had sufficient numbers of female participants to effectively evaluate therapy for prevention and treatment of CVD in women. Although it is not clear to what extent available data from middle-aged men can be extrapolated to women, particularly elderly women, therapy for CVD still tends to be based on the male model. Recently, increasing awareness of the gap in our knowledge of descriptors of CVD in women led to additional research efforts and funding to elucidate the gender-related differences in the biology and pathogenesis of atherosclerosis and the clinical course of CVD and its management.[11]

Table 65-1 Framingham Study: 10-year incidence of coronary heart disease excluding angina pectoris in men and women aged 50 to 59 years*

Variable	Coefficient	RR†	P
Systolic blood pressure	0.02	1.37	<0.001
Relative weight	0.00		NS
Serum cholesterol	0.01	1.35	<0.001
Cigarette smoking	0.61	1.84	<0.001
Glucose intolerance	0.56	1.75	<0.001
Gender	−1.33	3.78	<0.001

NS, not significant.
*3,562 men and women, 267 cases; multiple logistic regression analysis
†Relative risks for the differences: systolic blood pressure, 20 mm Hg; Metropolitan relative weight, 20%; serum cholesterol, 50 mg/100 mL; cigarette smoking, smoker or nonsmoker; glucose intolerance, yes or no.
From Havlik RJ, Liu BM, Kovar MG, et al: Health statistics on older persons, United States, 1986. *Vital Health Stat [3]* No 25, 1987.

CORONARY RISK FACTORS IN WOMEN

Coronary risk factors may be considered as those that influence CVD risk similarly in men and women (age, race, family history, smoking, hypertension, plasma lipoprotein concentrations, obesity, diabetes, and physical activity) and those unique to women (menopause, oral contraceptive use, and postmenopausal hormone use). With the exception of diabetes, the absolute risk for CVD is lower in women for each of the traditional coronary risk factors.[12]

Differences in the prevalence of coronary risk factors in men and women do not fully explain gender differences in CHD risk and morbidity[8,13] (Table 65-1). Even after traditional coronary risk factors are controlled for, men have a relative risk of CVD of 3.78 compared with women. Gender differences in CVD risk remain incompletely explained.

Nonmodifiable risk factors

Age. Age is the most powerful predictor of CVD incidence and mortality in men and women. Cardiovascular death rates increase by approximately 50% in each succeeding 5-year age group for both men and women, and the shapes of the mortality curves are similar[14] (Fig 65-7). However, whereas men experience a sharp increase in CVD incidence and mortality during the fifth decade of life, CVD rates in women lag 7 or 8 years behind those in men. The reasons for the delay in onset of CVD as an important cause of death and disability in women are not completely understood.

Race. Black women are particularly at risk of death due to CVD, with mortality rates nearly twice those in white women before the age of 75.[3,14] Death rates from myocardial infarction are 35% higher in black women, and death due to stroke is three times as likely.[14] Black women with symptomatic CHD have greater morbidity and mortality than do white women and men. Black women with myocardial infarction have the highest in-hospital mortality, highest 4-year mortality, and higher morbidity with complications, including more postinfarction angina and congestive heart failure.[7]

Family history. Parental history of death due to CHD is an independent risk factor for the occurrence of heart disease in both men and women.[15] Women with a positive family history of death of either parent due to CHD are at increased risk of CHD, but the relative risk is greatest in women with mothers who died of CHD. Women with either parent dying of CVD at an age less than 65 years are at the greatest risk (relative risk, 1.6).

The predictive power of a family history of CVD is strongest for young women. Among women older than 50 years, the association of a family history of CVD with CVD death remains unclear and is at best perhaps modestly predictive.[16,17]

Modifiable risk factors

Cigarette smoking. Cigarette smoking is a strong independent predictor of CVD among women and is as strong a risk factor as it is in men. Cigarette smoking accounts for at least 30% to 40% of deaths due to CHD in addition to being responsible for a significant portion of cardiovascular mortality from stroke, peripheral vascular disease, and other complications of atherosclerosis.[18]

Despite these well-defined risks associated with smoking, the rate of cigarette use among women has declined only slightly in recent years.[3] From 1983 to 1988, reduction in cigarette smoking in white and black women older than 18 was only 13%. The introduction in 1967 of tobacco

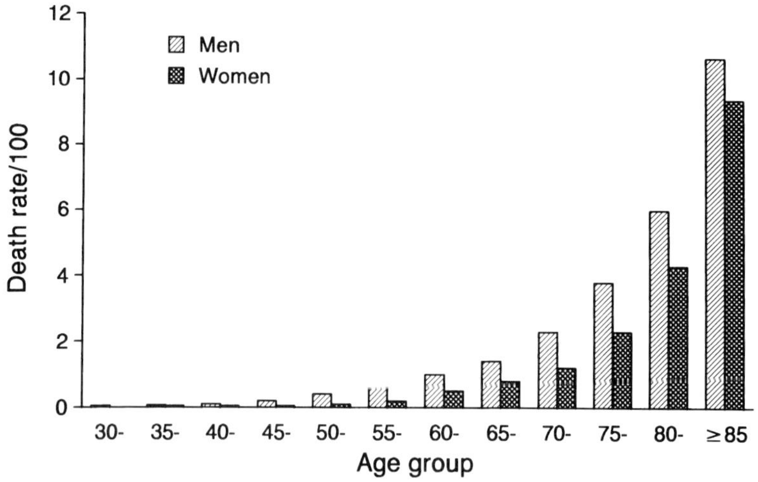

Fig 65-7 Cardiovascular disease death rates (per 100) in women and men by 5-year age groups, United States, 1984. (Data from National Center for Health Statistics: Vital statistics of the United States 1984. Vol. II. Mortality, Part B. Public Health Service, Washington, DC: United States Government Printing Office, DHHS Publication #87-1114, 1987.)

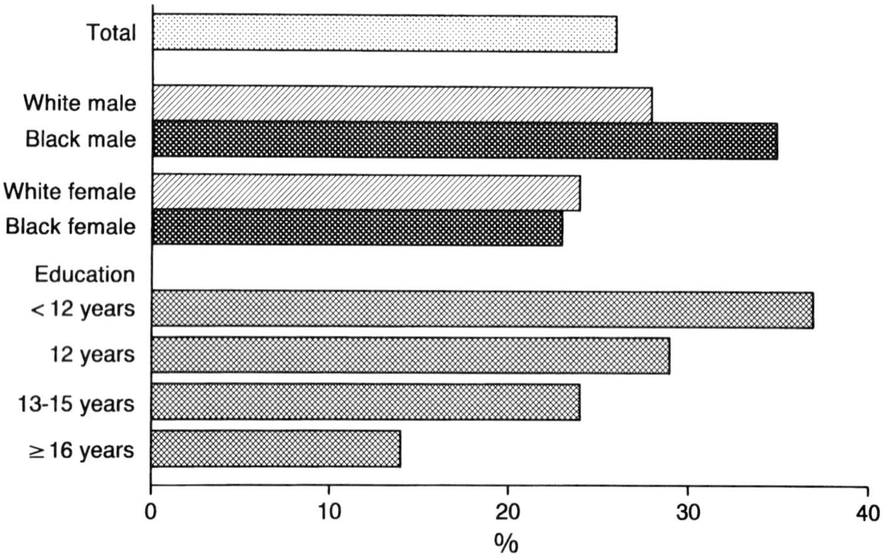

Fig 65-8 Current cigarette smokers among persons 25 years of age and older, according to selected characteristics, United States, 1990. (From National Center for Health Statistics. Health, United States, 1990. Hyattsville, Maryland, Public Health Service, 1991.)

advertising campaigns aimed at women was associated with a major increase in smoking initiation in women under age 18.[19] The rate of tobacco use is closely related to educational factors, because rates of smoking are from 25% to 50% lower in women with 1 or more years of education beyond high school than in women who complete a high school education or have less education[3] (Fig 65-8).

The risk of CVD death associated with smoking in women is dose-dependent, similar to that in men.[16,20,21] CVD mortality is increased in women with even modest tobacco use. Women who smoke as few as 10 cigarettes a day have a 50% greater risk of cardiovascular death than nonsmokers. This risk is more than doubled in women who smoke a pack or more a day. The risk of myocardial infarction for current smokers of more than 35 cigarettes a day is 10 times that of women who never smoked (Table 65-2). In one study of myocardial infarction in women younger than 50, a population generally at low CHD risk, an estimated 65% of heart attacks were attributable to cigarette smoking.[16] Smoking is also strongly associated with coronary vasospasm in young women with normal coronary angiograms.[22]

Passive exposure to cigarette smoke increases the risk

Table 65-2 Cigarette smoking among patients with myocardial infarction and controls

Cigarettes per day	Cases No.	Cases %	Controls No.	Controls %	Relative risk estimate*	95% confidence interval
Never smoked	24	9	250	31	1.0†	...
Ex-smoker‡	18	7	126	16	1.4	0.7-2.6
1-14	8	3	89	11	0.9	0.4-2.2
15-24	66	26	172	22	4.3	2.6-7.0
25-34	54	21	73	9	8.3	5.0-14
≥35	85	33	86	11	10	6.5-16

*Allowance made for age.
†Reference category.
‡Last smoked at least 1 year before admission.
From Rosenberg L, Miller DR, Kaufman DW, et al: Myocardial infarction in women under 50 years of age. *JAMA* 250:2801-2806, 1983. By permission of American Medical Association.

of CVD among nonsmoking women. Women whose husbands are current or former smokers have an increased risk of CVD death and are significantly more likely to suffer a myocardial infarction than are wives of men who have never smoked.[23]

Although there is a powerful causal association between smoking and myocardial infarction in young women, whether smoking remains a determinant of CVD in older women is controversial. In a recent prospective study of older persons, current smoking among women older than 65 was shown to be associated with a 70% increase in risk of cardiovascular mortality over that in nonsmokers.[24]

The CVD risk among women who quit cigarette smoking is reduced. Women who are former smokers appear to have similar rates of CHD and nonfatal myocardial infarction as women who have never smoked.[20] Furthermore, survival in women who suffer a myocardial infarction is improved if they discontinue smoking. In a study of smoking cessation in women with myocardial infarction, the 5-year survival rate was 85% in those who quit but only 73% among those who continued to smoke.[25] In 12 years of follow-up in the Nurses' Health Study, risk of stroke among women who smoke declined within 2 to 4 years of cessation.[26] Benefits were evident regardless of smoking history, age at cessation, and other risk factors for stroke. Additional evidence indicates that smoking cessation after the age of 65 can reduce the risk of CVD mortality among women as well as reduce the risk of myocardial infarction and death among older smokers with existing coronary disease.[24,27] A recent radiographic study of progression of atherosclerosis in women suggested that the rate of atherosclerotic change may be reduced by cessation of smoking, but a significant excess risk persisted 5 to 10 years after quitting.[28]

Because of the health hazards of smoking for women, counseling in smoking cessation is a critical aspect of preventive health care. Although success rates are low and recidivism is high, this preventive medical practice in women is cost-effective and has health benefits equal to other preventive health measures, such as management of hypercholesterolemia or hypertension and prescription for nicotine gum.[29]

Hypertension. Approximately 20% of adult white women and 40% of adult black women are hypertensive.[30] The overall prevalence of hypertension (controlled and uncontrolled) is nearly equal in white men and women and is slightly higher in black women than in black men[31] (Table 65-3). After age 50, the prevalence of hypertension is higher in women regardless of race.[3] Because women outnumber men in the growing elderly United States population, more women than men have hypertension.

Increased blood pressure, either systolic or diastolic, whether fixed or labile, is predictive of increased CVD risk in women of all ages.[32,33] In the Framingham cohort, hypertension was the most significant and consistent predictor of the development of all forms of CVD in women aged 35 to 64 years. For every 10 mm Hg increase in systolic blood pressure, the risk of CVD or CVD death increases 20% to 40%.[34-36]

Table 65-3 Percentage of persons screened who had controlled and uncontrolled hypertension

Study	Women, % Black	Women, % White	Men, % Black	Men, % White
NHEFS (follow-up)	48.4	30.0	49.9*	30.0
NHANES II	39.8	20.0	28.3†	21.2
CHEC	26.0	21.4	22.0†	20.1
HDFP	38.0	18.0	36.0†	19.0

NHEFS, National Health and Nutrition Examination Survey I Epidemiologic Follow-up Study; NHANES II, National Health and Nutrition Examination Survey II; CHEC, Community Hypertension Evaluation Clinic Study; HDFP, Hypertension Detection and Follow-up Program.
**P* not significant (prevalence difference between black men and black women).
†$P < 0.001$ (prevalence difference between black men and black women).
From Anastos K, Charney P, Charon RA, et al: Hypertension in women: What is really known? The Women's Caucus, Working Group on Women's Health of the Society of General Internal Medicine. *Ann Intern Med* 115:287-293, 1991. By permission of American College of Physicians.

Table 65-4 Hypertension intervention studies from 1967 to 1985

Study	Number of subjects	Percentage of women	Analysis by gender
Hypertension Detection and Follow-Up Program[37]	10,940	46	Decreased mortality in black women and in all men Possible increased mortality in white women
The Australian Therapeutic Trial[38]	3,427	37	36% decrease in adverse outcome in women (P is not significant) 26% decrease in adverse outcome in men ($P < 0.05$)
Medical Research Council[39]	17,354	48	26% increased mortality in women 15% decreased mortality in men
European Working Party on Hypertension in the Elderly[40]	840	70	18% reduction in cardiovascular mortality in women 47% reduction in cardiovascular mortality in men
Multiple Risk Factor Intervention Trial[41]	12,866	0	Not applicable
The Oslo Study[42]	785	0	Not applicable
Veterans Administration Cooperative Study[43,44]			Not applicable
Severe	143	0	
Moderate	380	0	

From Anastos K, Charney P, Charon RA, et al: Hypertension in women: What is really known? The Women's Caucus, Working Group on Women's Health of the Society of General Internal Medicine. *Ann Intern Med* 115:287-293, 1991. By permission of American College of Physicians.

Hypertensive women have lower cardiovascular morbidity and mortality at all ages than hypertensive men.[12] When men and women with similar blood pressure levels are compared, the risks of stroke, CHD, congestive heart failure, and sudden death are significantly lower among women. However, the attributable risk percentage (the proportion of cardiovascular end points that could be eliminated by removal of hypertension as a risk factor) in persons with hypertension is higher for women than for men. Because the number of hypertensive complications is somewhat greater in elderly women than in men older than 65, control of hypertension in women has important public health implications.[31]

The number of women receiving antihypertensive therapy and the number of women with medication-controlled hypertension have nearly doubled over recent decades.[8] The current guidelines for management of hypertension do not distinguish between men and women. The evidence that treatment of hypertension reduces cerebrovascular and possibly cardiovascular mortality is conclusive only in men[31] (Table 65-4). Of the seven hypertension intervention studies considered, three did not include women, and in three studies the clinical interpretation must be limited because of the small numbers of women.[37-39,41-44] Clinical trials suggest a benet of therapy in black hypertensive women but no clear benefit in white women. The most recent data indicate that treatment of hypertension reduces CVD risk in women, but the benefit is significantly less than that in men.[40]

The potential adverse effects of antihypertensive agents are poorly characterized in women. An increase in total cholesterol has been reported in women treated with bendroflumethiazide, propranolol, and methyldopa.[39] Chlorthalidone has been noted to cause menopause-dependent increases in total and low-density lipoprotein (LDL) cholesterol.[45] Information on other side effects of antihypertensive agents in women, such as sexual dysfunction, metabolic abnormalities, and cardiovascular complications, is limited. Amlodipine, chlorthalidone, acebutolol, enalapril, and doxazosin are equally well tolerated and effective in women and men.[46]

The practice of instituting antihypertensive therapy in women according to guidelines defined for men is under question. Evidence supports aggressive treatment in black women with hypertension. Recommendations for treatment in white women are unclear, because treatment may actually be harmful.

Lipids and lipoproteins. There is a strong, consistent association between total cholesterol concentration and CHD in women younger than 65.[47] In middle-aged women, the association is as strong as it is in men. For older women, the strength and consistency of the relationship are somewhat diminished.

Important preanalytical variables in laboratory measurement of lipids are unique to the female population[48] (Table 65-5). Variations in lipoprotein levels occur during the menstrual cycle, apparently from hemodilutory effects. These fluctuations can be limited by correcting for

Table 65-5 Preanalytic variables for lipid determination in women

Fasting: 12 to 14 hours overnight, water only
Stable weight, diet, and activity over past 3 to 6 weeks
No recent illness, surgery, or injury; at least 12 weeks since myocardial infarction or coronary artery bypass surgery
Not currently pregnant and at least 12 weeks postpartum
Stable (4 to 8 weeks) after menopause or after oral contraceptive therapy
Stable doses of medications or no other medications known to affect lipid and lipoproteins, e.g., corticosteroids, androgenic steroids, thyroid hormone, thiazide and other loop diuretics, nonselective β-blockers, carbamazepine
Menstrual cycle
Phlebotomy position, e.g., sitting rather than recumbent
Prolonged venous occlusion
Sample handling before serum or plasma isolation
Biologic variation

From Stein EA: Use of the clinical laboratory for lipid evaluation. In *Lipids and Women's Health.* Edited by GP Redmond. New York, Springer-Verlag, 1991, pp 39-47. By permission.

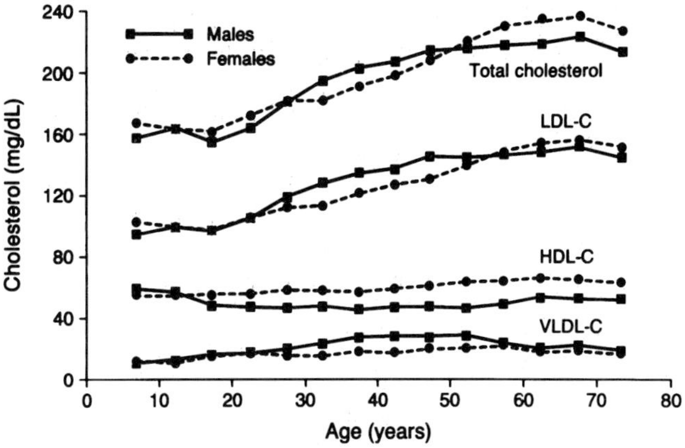

Fig 65-9 Mean plasma total, LDL, HDL, and VLDL cholesterol values by 10-year age groups for 3,581 males and 3,426 females, Lipid Research Clinics Prevalence Study, visit 2, random sample. (From Rifkind BM, Tamir I, Heiss G, et al: Distribution of high density and other lipoproteins in selected LRC prevalence study populations: a brief survey. *Lipids* 14:105-112, 1979. By permission of AOCS Press.)

total protein levels. Hormone therapy, including use of oral contraceptives and postmenopausal administration of estrogens and progestins, alters lipid levels; stabilization of the lipid profile generally occurs after 1 to 2 months of therapy. LDL levels increase significantly with pregnancy, returning to their baseline state within 8 to 12 weeks unless breastfeeding is continued.

There are important gender differences in age-related changes in lipid levels throughout adult life[49] (Fig 65-9). Until age 20, total cholesterol levels in men and women are similar. After the second decade of life, however, men experience a sharp increase in total cholesterol to an average level of 235 mg/dL by about age 45 years[8] (Fig 65-10). The average total cholesterol level in women younger than 45 is 200 to 215 mg/dL. There is a gradual increase until midlife, and then a steeper increase occurs. Between the ages of 45 and 55 years, the mean cholesterol value in women increases to 240 to 260 mg/dL, remaining higher than average levels in men. Very-low-density lipoprotein (VLDL) cholesterol levels increase with advancing age but remain consistently lower in women than in men.[49] In both sexes, high-density lipoprotein (HDL) cholesterol shows little variation with age, but levels are consistently higher in men. Various subpopulations of HDL cholesterol are characterized by particles of different sizes and composition.[50] Little information is available on sex- and age-related changes in these HDL subfractions.

From 1960 to 1991, serum total cholesterol levels declined continuously and substantially among U.S. adults, according to data from the National Health and Nutrition Examination Surveys (NHANES)[51] (Fig 65-11). This decline was evident in all age and sex categories, with the greatest decreases in middle-aged and elderly women

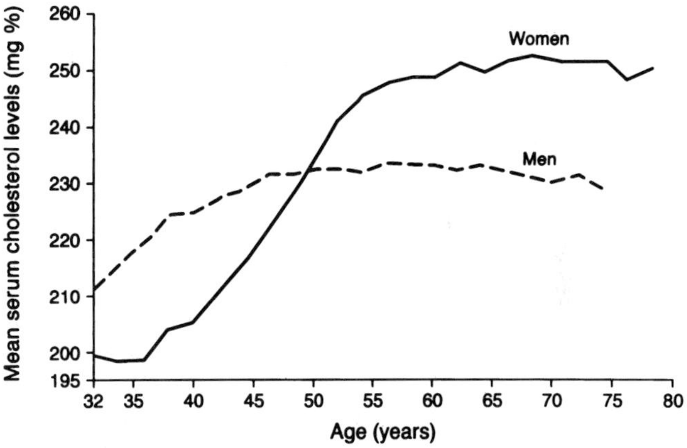

Fig 65-10 Average age trends in serum cholesterol levels for cohort data, Framingham study, examinations 1 to 10. (From Havlik RJ, Liu BM, Kovar MG, et al: Health statistics on older persons, United States, 1986. *Vital Health Stat* [3] No 25, 1987.)

and elderly men. From 1960 to 1991, the mean total cholesterol concentration among women aged 20 to 74 decreased from 222 to 205 mg/dL. The percentage of women with increased total cholesterol levels (>240 mg/dL) also decreased from 1976 to 1991 (28% to 20%).[52]

Numerous factors are known to influence the concentrations of blood lipids in women.[53] Abnormalities in genetic determinants of total cholesterol, LDL, and HDL concentrations are not sex-linked and contribute similarly to lipid regulation in men and women. However, genetic influences have a minor place in lipid disorders in women,

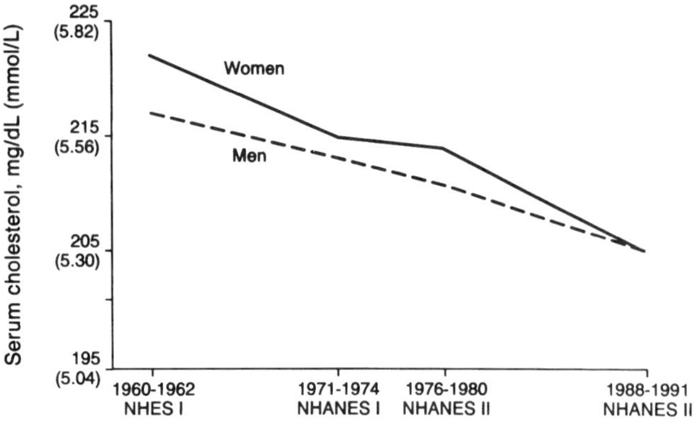

Fig 65-11 Trends in age-adjusted mean serum total cholesterol levels. NHES, National Health Examination Survey; NHANES, National Health and Nutrition Examination Survey. (Data from Sempos CT, Cleeman JI, Carroll MD, et al: Prevalence of high blood cholesterol among US adults: the National Health and Nutrition Examination surveys. *JAMA* 269:3009-3014, 1993.)

as less than 2% of hypercholesterolemia is due to genetic factors.

Dietary factors are less influential on blood lipid levels in women than in men.[14] Although diets low in cholesterol or with a high ratio of polyunsaturated fat to saturated fat consistently result in reductions in total and LDL cholesterol concentrations in women, the magnitude of the decreases is somewhat less than that in men. Lowering of HDL levels in women receiving low-cholesterol diets may also be less, but information is equivocal.[54] Obesity has similar detrimental effects on lipid levels in men and women, and the effects are independent of other risk factors, such as smoking, estrogen use, and alcohol use. Obesity is associated with increased total and LDL cholesterol levels[55] and reduced HDL cholesterol.[56]

Exercise has beneficial effects on blood lipid levels in women, although conclusions are limited by small sample sizes and few clinical trials including women.[53] Exercise in combination with weight loss may increase HDL levels by as much as 10% to 20% in women; however, exceedingly high volumes of exercise accompanied by body fat reduction are required to increase HDL levels in premenopausal women.[50,57] In older women, even intense exercise training has not been shown to raise HDL cholesterol levels. Exercise training may attenuate the age-related increase in total cholesterol concentration in older women. The decrease in HDL resulting from low-fat, low-cholesterol diets can be attenuated or prevented by regular aerobic exercise in women as well as in men.[54,57]

Alcohol consumption is strongly associated with increased levels of HDL cholesterol in women,[58,59] and the magnitude of the effect does not differ between the sexes. Information on changes in HDL subfractions associated with alcohol use in women is limited. In one study, HDL_3 cholesterol levels were significantly greater in women who consumed alcohol, whereas HDL_2 cholesterol levels were only modestly higher.[59] Moderate alcohol consumption may protect against CHD in women as well as in men,[60] possibly because of beneficial alterations in HDL. The reduction in risk has been estimated at approximately 20% for women reporting any use of alcohol and is greatest for women who consume one-half to two drinks per day.[61] This protective effect is modest, however, and because of the potentially harmful effects of alcohol does not justify recommendations for more widespread use of alcohol among women.

Smoking is strongly associated with reduced levels of HDL cholesterol in men and women, and the effect is more pronounced in women.[62,63] Reductions in HDL levels vary from 8% to 14% in women, depending on the number of cigarettes smoked. Passive cigarette smoke exposure also reduces HDL cholesterol.[50] Smoking cessation results in an increase in HDL cholesterol levels in women, with levels returning to normal within as few as 30 days.[64] Cigarette smoking is also associated with increased levels of total and LDL cholesterol, although the effect is modest and less consistent than changes in HDL cholesterol.[65]

Use of exogenous hormones is associated with significant alterations in the concentrations of blood lipids.[66,67] Most formulations of oral contraceptives increase LDL, with the magnitude of the increase depending on the relative estrogen and progestin content. Only the newer preparations containing desogestrel have a neutral or LDL-lowering effect. Triglyceride levels are consistently increased by all contraceptive formulations. Alterations in HDL cholesterol levels induced by oral contraceptives are inversely related to the androgenicity of the formulation. The most androgenic progestins can reduce HDL levels by as much as 10% to 15%. The newer gonane, desogestrel, is less androgenic and has a positive effect on HDL. When used in combination with estrogen, desogestrel has the most favorable effect on lipoproteins of all the oral contraceptive agents.

Postmenopausal hormone therapy can significantly influence lipid and lipoprotein levels in women, and alterations depend on whether unopposed estrogen or combined estrogen-progestin replacement is used. The lipid and lipoprotein effects of estrogen and progestins are summarized in Table 65-6. Estrogen effects on the lipid profile tend to be antiatherogenic, whereas the progestin effects could potentially increase the risk of CHD. The magnitude of estrogen- and progestin-induced changes in lipoproteins is great enough to have a significant effect on CVD risk.[53] Estrogen therapy may increase HDL levels by 9% to 13% and decrease LDL levels by 4% to 10%. Progestin effects vary with androgenicity, but HDL levels may be decreased by 25% to 31% and LDL levels increased by 6% to 13%. Because progestins prevent estrogen-induced endometrial hyperplasia, they are a necessary part of postmenopausal hormone therapy in women with an intact uterus. The optimal combined estrogen-progestin preparation to both protect the endometrium and have acceptable effects on lipid levels and cardiovascular risk is uncertain.

The Postmenopausal Estrogen/Progestin Interventions trial, a 3-year, multicenter, randomized, placebo-controlled study of unopposed estrogen and combination hormone replacement therapy, confirmed that unopposed estrogen has a more favorable effect on HDL cholesterol

Table 65-6 Effects of estrogens and synthetic progestins on lipids and lipoproteins

Lipid	Estrogen effect	Progestin effect*
HDL-C	Increased	Decreased
HDL_2	Increased	Decreased
HDL_3	Increased	Decreased
Apo A-I	Increased	Decreased
Apo A-II	Increased	Variable
LDL-C	Decreased	Increased
Apo B	Decreased	Increased
VLDL-C	Increased	Decreased
Triglycerides	Increased	Decreased

*Newer gonanes do not follow this progestin pattern of effect.
From Miller VT, La Rosa JC: Sex steroids and lipoproteins. In *Lipids and Women's Health.* Edited by GP Redmond. New York, Springer-Verlag, 1991, pp 48-65. By permission.

than estrogen with a continuous or cyclic progestin. The combination regimen of estrogen and cyclic micronized progesterone had a more pronounced effect on HDL than estrogen and cyclic or continuous medroxyprogesterone acetate. Both progestins were equally effective in prevention of endometrial hyperplasia.[68]

Lipids and cardiovascular risk in women. Total cholesterol levels are strongly predictive of fatal CHD in women. The pooled relative risk of fatal CHD associated with cholesterol levels greater than 240 mg/dL is 2.44 compared with cholesterol levels of less than 200 mg/dL in middle-aged (under 65 years) and older (over 65 years) women.[47] Thus, women with cholesterol levels of 240 mg/dL or higher have a 144% increased risk of CHD. The strength of the association between cholesterol and fatal CHD is stronger in middle-aged women than in men. There is a positive relationship between total cholesterol concentration and fatal CHD in women older than 65, but the association is not as strong or consistent, with a pooled relative risk of 1.12.[47,69]

The risk of coronary events, including myocardial infarction, increases with increasing levels of total cholesterol in women.[70,71] Nonfatal CHD events are not increased at total cholesterol levels of less than 264 mg/dL. However, women with cholesterol levels greater than 265 mg/dL have a twofold to threefold increased risk over that in women with levels of less than 200 to 204 mg/dL. In the Framingham Study, 61% of CHD events in middle-aged women were attributable to cholesterol values of 240 mg/dL or greater.[72]

Total cholesterol value is a risk factor for CHD recurrence in women with symptomatic CHD. Among women who have recovered from myocardial infarction, high total cholesterol levels are associated with increased risk for reinfarction, CHD death, and all-causes mortality.[73]

LDL cholesterol levels predict CHD in middle-aged women only, although the association is less consistent and strong. The association of increased triglyceride levels and cardiovascular risk remains controversial. In the Framingham population, triglyceride levels were strongly and consistently associated with fatal CHD in older women, and a positive but not significant relationship was noted in middle-aged women. In the Lipid Research Clinics Follow-up Study, triglyceride levels were not independently associated with coronary mortality in men or women after adjustment for the plasma glucose level.[74]

The strongest lipid determinant of cardiovascular risk in women is HDL cholesterol.[12,34,36,70,75-78] HDL is a strong negative, independent predictor of CHD in women. An increase in HDL of 10 mg/dL is associated with a 40% to 50% reduction in CHD risk. There is also evidence that high concentrations of HDL in women neutralize the risk associated with increased concentrations of total cholesterol.[70,79]

Controversy exists about modification of blood lipid levels in women. Although high cholesterol level and nonfatal CHD are strongly associated in women, there is no association with overall cardiovascular deaths.[80] The reason is that cholesterol levels and the risk of hemorrhagic stroke deaths are not associated in women. No studies have directly addressed whether altering lipid and lipoprotein concentrations in women influences CVD risk. There is evidence that estrogen-induced increases in HDL cholesterol lower the risk of fatal CVD in women.[77]

In women with CHD, the average total and LDL cholesterol values are only slightly above the values recommended for diet and drug therapy.[81] Current guidelines would require aggressive lipid therapy in a large proportion of the female population, because 20% of adult women have total cholesterol values greater than 240 mg/dL.[52] Until more information is available, a more conservative approach to drug therapy has been suggested to be appropriate in low-risk premenopausal women.[82] However, high-risk women with multiple cardiovascular risk factors and those with manifest CHD should be treated for high cholesterol concentrations in the blood.

Diabetes. In women, diabetes is strongly associated with CVD, including CHD and ischemic stroke, and with cardiovascular mortality.[83,84] In the largest prospective study, the Nurses' Health Study cohort, diabetic women had a greater than sixfold increase in risk for both nonfatal myocardial infarction and fatal CHD (relative risk, 6.7).[83] Risks of nonfatal and fatal stroke among diabetic women were increased fourfold (RR, 4.1). Total cardiovascular mortality was increased in diabetic women (RR, 6.3), and a smaller but highly significant increase in all-causes mortality was noted (RR, 3.0). In this study population, 13.8% of coronary events and 12.1% of ischemic strokes were attributable to diabetes. Of all cardiovascular deaths, 14.8% were attributable to diabetes.

Even in women with newly diagnosed diabetes, the risk of nonfatal myocardial infarction and fatal CHD is greater than in nondiabetic women. There appears to be a cumulative deleterious effect, however, with a near-doubling of risk when the duration of diabetes exceeds 15 years.

Diabetes is an independent predictor of CVD events, and the association cannot be entirely explained by known coronary risk factors often present in patients with diabetes. Diabetic women still have a threefold increase in

CVD risk after hypertension, cholesterol, obesity, and other variables are controlled for in multivariate analyses. The impact of diabetes on CVD risk is increased by other coronary risk factors. Thus, in addition to regulation of diabetes in women, loss of weight and control of traditional coronary risk factors are critical to reduce CVD risk.

At every level of other cardiovascular risk factors, women have lower CVD rates than men with comparable levels. However, diabetes reduces the favored status of women and is associated with similar CVD disease rates in men and women.[85] This greater relative hazard in women may largely be due to the superior survival of women over men in the nondiabetic population.[86]

Obesity. Obesity associated with other coronary risk factors, including hypertension, hypercholesterolemia, reduced HDL cholesterol levels, and hyperglycemia, is causally related to CVD risk.[14] Some limited data show an independent effect of obesity alone after other risk factors are controlled for.[87] Because more than 27% of adult white women and 46% of adult black women are overweight (defined as body mass index greater than or equal to 27.3 kg/m^2), the relationship between obesity and CVD has major public health implications.[3]

Regional patterns of obesity, or the distribution of body fat, may be more important than the overall degree of obesity.[88] In the Framingham study, after adjustment for all other cardiovascular risk factors, the subscapular-to-triceps skinfold ratio independently predicted CHD, cardiovascular, and all-causes mortality in women.[89] Another measure of body fat distribution, the waist-hip circumference ratio, has been strongly and positively associated with cardiovascular mortality in women aged 55 to 69 years.[90]

Despite controversy about the independent effect of obesity on CVD risk and the appropriate measure of body fat distribution, excess body weight remains an important modifiable risk factor in women. Obesity is likely to be causally related to potent cardiovascular risk factors, such as hypertension, hyperlipidemia, and hyperglycemia, and should be targeted for aggressive intervention in women.

Risk factors unique to women

Changes in endogenous hormone levels throughout a woman's life and exposure to exogenous hormone therapy have an important effect on CVD risk.

Endogenous hormones

PARITY. Data from the Framingham Heart Study and the NHANES Follow-up Study have suggested that having six or more pregnancies is associated with a small but consistent increase in the risk of CHD and CVD.[91] Other evaluations of parity and CVD risk in women have not shown a consistent relationship.[92-95] Although there may be biologically plausible mechanisms, such as pregnancy-related increases in LDL cholesterol, for an association between an increased number of pregnancies and CVD risk, evidence remains unclear.

MENOPAUSE. Because CVD risk does not pose a major health threat in women until the age of about 55, it has been suggested that the premenopausal hormonal status confers relative gender protection and that menopause is responsible for the increased risk of CVD. Vital statistics do not entirely support this hypothesis. Some studies do not show an acceleration in the rate of increase of CVD after menopause and thus suggest that menopause may not have a direct effect on CVD risk.[96,97] The rate of increase in CVD mortality between ages 30 and 49 is nearly identical to that between ages 50 and 69, so that age, not menopause, appears to account for the increase in CVD risk[14] (see Fig 65-7). However, Framingham data showed that age-adjusted rates of CHD increase after menopause.[98] At this time, it remains unclear whether natural menopause increases a woman's risk of CVD.

There is evidence that early surgical menopause is associated with an increased risk of CVD.[99] The risk of CVD increases as the age of surgically induced menopause decreases.[100] In one study, women older than 45 years who underwent hysterectomy with bilateral oophorectomy had a 30% increased risk of CHD over that in age-matched premenopausal women. Women who underwent hysterectomy with bilateral oophorectomy before age 35 had nearly an eightfold increase in CHD risk. If one or both ovaries were retained, no relationship between CHD risk and age of surgical menopause was noted. Oophorectomy does not result in an increase in CVD risk in women who received estrogen replacement therapy.[101]

Exogenous hormone use. Confusion about the potential cardiovascular risks and benefits associated with use of exogenous hormones in women has resulted from a failure to consider important differences between hormone therapy used for contraceptive purposes and that intended to treat postmenopausal symptoms. Estrogens used for menopausal symptoms are primarily the natural steroidal agents, with conjugated equine estrogens (Premarin) accounting for more than 75% of all prescriptions.[66] Formulations for contraceptive purposes contain only the more potent synthetic estrogens. The synthetic estrogens appear to have a greater effect on coronary risk factors, including blood pressure, lipids and lipoproteins, glucose tolerance, and clotting variables.[102]

In the United States, more than 90% of women receive medroxyprogesterone acetate (Provera) for combination postmenopausal hormone replacement. This agent is less androgenic than the *19-nor* agents used in combination-contraceptive therapy. The more androgenic progestins are known to most adversely affect blood lipid and lipoprotein levels. Newer, less androgenic progestational agents have been developed for use in combination-contraceptive therapy and may demonstrate a beneficial effect on lipoproteins.[66]

Estrogen and progestin doses in current oral contraceptive formulations have been significantly reduced. The early preparations contained up to 5 times the current dose of estrogen and 10 times the dose of progestin.[103]

ORAL CONTRACEPTIVES. Limited data are available on the effect of newer oral contraceptive formulations on coronary risk factors, CVD risk, and safety of use in older women. Because the increased risk of CVD associated with oral contraceptive use has been attributed to the thromboembolic effect of high doses of estrogen, the risk of current formulations may be less. However, even some of the newer formulations may have a negative effect on blood lipids and lipoproteins and blood pressure.[104] A reduction in the dose of progestin and change in the type of progestin can significantly reduce the lipid abnormalities associated with use of the low-dose oral contraceptives.[105,106]

In most early studies, current use of oral contraceptives is associated with increased risk of CHD, particularly in older premenopausal women.[99] The risk is greatest in older women who smoke, with a more than 20-fold increased risk of myocardial infarction alone.[94] There is no increase in risk of CHD in women who are past users of oral contraceptives, and duration of past oral contraceptive use is not related to risk of CHD.

As a result of decreased hormone doses and aggressive screening for coronary risk factors, the Food and Drug Administration recommended in 1989 that no upper age limit be imposed on nonsmoking women who have no other risk factors.[103]

POSTMENOPAUSAL HORMONE REPLACEMENT. Information on noncontraceptive hormone use and CVD risk is based on the use of unopposed oral conjugated equine estrogen, which was the usual practice from the 1960s until 1975. At that time, evidence became available to show that unopposed estrogen therapy increased the risk of endometrial cancer and that the addition of a progestational agent reduced this risk.[107,108] Combination hormone therapy is now considered necessary in women with an intact uterus, but limited data are available on the effect of combined estrogen and progestin therapy on CVD risk. The cardiovascular arm of the Women's Health Initiative will provide definitive data on the effect of unopposed estrogen and combination hormone therapy on cardiovascular disease events. However, results will not be available until 2006.

Observational studies indicate a significant reduction in CHD risk among women using unopposed estrogen therapy.[99,109-111] Cardiovascular end points in studies of estrogen use and reduced CHD risk have included angiographically defined CHD, nonfatal myocardial infarction, all CVD, and sudden death. These studies indicate that current estrogen use is associated with a 50% reduction in risk of CHD from that in nonusers. This reduction in risk persists after other coronary risk factors are controlled for. Estrogen use has also been found to be associated with lower levels of subclinical CVD as measured by electrocardiogram (ECG), left ventricular mass, carotid intimal-medial thickness, carotid stenosis grade, and Doppler mitral peak flow velocities.[112]

The relationship between postmenopausal hormone use and stroke remains unclear, as available studies show conflicting results.[113] In the NHANES study, postmenopausal estrogen therapy was associated with a 63% reduction in stroke mortality and a 31% reduction in the incidence of stroke, with benefits persisting after other CVD risk factors were controlled for.[114] Similar results suggesting a protective effect have been found in other studies,[110,115,116] whereas the Framingham study found an increase in risk of stroke associated with estrogen use.[117]

Potential mechanisms for an estrogen effect on reduction of CHD include beneficial lipid and lipoprotein effects,[53,118] improved carbohydrate metabolism,[118-120] and lower blood pressure.[121] The cardioprotective effects of estrogen may also be mediated in part by a direct effect on the arterial wall, perhaps due to changes in arterial tone or alterations in lipoprotein metabolism.[122-124] Few data support a significant effect on clotting mechanisms. In the Postmenopausal Estrogen/Progestin Interventions trial, both unopposed estrogen and combination hormone therapy resulted in reductions in fibrinogen levels in postmenopausal women.[68] In two analyses of estrogen use and CHD risk, between 25% and 50% of the reduction in CHD risk in estrogen users could be attributed to beneficial changes in HDL and LDL cholesterol.[77,99,125] The nonlipid mechanisms responsible for the remaining 50% to 75% reduction in risk require further study.

CARDIOVASCULAR DIAGNOSTIC TESTING IN WOMEN

The accuracy of noninvasive diagnostic testing for the detection of CHD in women has been disappointing. A number of explanations for observed gender differences in the response to exercise stress testing have been considered. Most importantly, the prevalence of CHD is lower among women than among men except in the elderly population. Because the predictive accuracy of a diagnostic test is greatest in populations with a high prevalence of disease, the diagnostic value of noninvasive tests for CHD is less for women. Single-vessel disease is more common in women (42%) than in men (22%) with CHD, a phenomenon that contributes to the difficulty of detection of disease.[126] In addition, conditions associated with false-positive responses to stress testing, including mitral valve prolapse and coronary vasospasm without atherosclerosis, are more prevalent among women.[127,128] Some progress in noninvasive detection of CHD in women has been made with computer analysis of exercise data, multivariate statistical techniques, new radionuclides for imaging with fewer artifactual results, and exercise echocardiography.

Exercise stress testing

The stress ECG is the least expensive and least invasive of techniques to evaluate coronary perfusion and ventricular function. It has moderate sensitivity and specificity for the detection of CHD in women.[129-140] The magnitude, time course, and configuration of ST segment changes are not as reliable for detection of CHD in women as in men. Nearly half of all abnormal test results in women may be false-positive, particularly in those with nonspecific chest pain.[133]

The specificity of exercise stress testing is comparable in men (78% to 83%) and women (74% to 86%).[133,141] There are significant gender differences in specificity when men and women with resting ST-T wave changes are considered. The specificity of the stress ECG is only 54% in men and 36% in women with abnormal resting ECGs. Thus, in men and women with abnormal resting ST-T waves, the exercise stress test may have little utility.

The predictive value of exercise ECG depends on the population of women being studied.[142] In asymptomatic women without known CHD, abnormal stress ECG events have not been shown to be associated with an increase in

CHD events.[143] In this population, the criteria for interpretation of the stress ECG are different in men than in women, because ST-segment depression and evaluation of R-wave amplitude do not predict an increased incidence of CHD. Most predictive of CHD among women free of symptoms is poor exercise tolerance.

The predictive value of a positive stress ECG has also been shown to be lower among women than among men with atypical or nonspecific chest pain. In long-term follow-up, CHD develops in only about 5% of women with such pain but in almost 20% of men.[136] The angiographic prevalence of significant CHD in such patients is generally low, with estimates ranging from 4% to 20% among men[144] and 2% to 8% among women.[132,137,144] Given this low disease prevalence among women with atypical chest pain, the stress ECG is likely to be of low diagnostic yield and most abnormal results are false-positive.[133,144]

Even in women with typical angina, the diagnostic value of the stress ECG is less than that in men. When typical chest pain is associated with an abnormal stress ECG, CHD is highly probable in men (98%) but is present in only 75% of women.[132] The false-positive rates are lower in women with typical angina (18% to 25%), but rates remain considerably higher than false-positive rates in men (<5%).[133]

There is a gender difference in the sensitivity of the exercise ECG. Even after adjustment for other factors, including disease severity and maximal exercise heart rate, the sensitivity of the stress ECG is significantly lower in women (57%) than in men (72%). The explanation for the sex difference in test sensitivity is not certain.[141]

A true gender difference in the response to exercise has been shown in populations of men and women with a similar prevalence of CHD.[134] In a study of patients with chest pain who had angiography, disease prevalence did not differ significantly between men and women (36% and 33%, respectively). Although a negative stress ECG accurately ruled out disease in both men and women (predictive values of 81% and 78%, respectively), a positive test result did not necessarily predict disease in women. Only 47% of women with a positive test result had CHD compared with 77% of men with abnormal stress ECGs.

The problems associated with use of ST-segment depression for detection of CHD in women have prompted study of other diagnostic criteria to improve the accuracy of the stress ECG. Additional diagnostic information in women has been derived from the R-wave response to exercise;[143,145] logistic discriminant analysis of exercise variables, including workload, heart rate (HR), and ST depression in lead X;[146] heart rate adjustment of ST depression by the simple ST-segment/HR (ST/HR) index;[147,148] and the ST/HR slope and HR-recovery loop.[149] These more computationally complex criteria can improve the sensitivity and specificity of the stress ECG in women. However, clinical application of these methods has been limited, probably because of their complexity.

Exercise thallium-201 scintigraphy

Exercise thallium-201 scintigraphy, a reliable diagnostic method to detect CHD, is superior to exercise ECG, but most studies have been conducted in men. In three clinical studies that included women (245 subjects), the sensitivity of thallium scintigraphy in women was 71% to 75% (82% in men) and the specificity 91% to 97% (91% in men).[129,131,150] The combination of thallium scintigraphy with exercise ECG significantly improves the specificity of the stress ECG, whereas the sensitivity is comparable to stress ECG alone. The effect of gender on the sensitivity and specificity of thallium-201 scintigraphy has not been rigorously studied.

The major problem with interpretation of thallium scintigrams in women is attenuation of signals in the high anteroseptal and anterolateral segments of the heart due to interposition of breast tissue. A fixed perfusion defect in these anatomic regions may represent breast artifact rather than flow-limiting CHD. There is a widely held opinion that breast artifact is more readily recognized with technetium-99m sestamibi images, but this is as yet unproven.

Dipyridamole thallium-201 scintigraphy

When used in conjunction with thallium-201, dipyridamole, a coronary vasodilator given intravenously, is useful for detecting myocardial perfusion abnormalities caused by flow-limiting coronary atherosclerosis. Overall sensitivity for detection of CHD in women is 87%, specificity is 58%, and results are comparable between the sexes.[151]

Radionuclide angiography

Exercise radionuclide angiography is of limited value in the detection of CHD in women because of gender differences in the response to exercise. In men, significant disease is suggested by failure of the resting left ventricular ejection fraction to increase by 5%.[152] In healthy women, however, stroke volume increases with exercise through an increase in end-diastolic volume without an increase in ejection fraction from rest to maximal exercise.[153] By this criterion, radionuclide angiography has a low specificity in women. Whether use of other measurements, such as peak ejection fraction, will improve the diagnostic value of radionuclide angiography in women remains to be shown.

Exercise echocardiography

A normal exercise echocardiogram in women with good exercise capacity has been shown to be predictive of a low rate of CHD events, even in those with abnormal stress ECGs.[154] The only study to specifically examine the effectiveness of this procedure in women demonstrated a sensitivity of 86% and a specificity of 86%.[155] However, the women in this study had a high prevalence of disease and frequency of typical angina, so that the sample may have been somewhat nonrepresentative. A study of 228 patients, including 75 women, showed that exercise echocardiography was more sensitive (97%) and specific (64%) than stress ECG (51% and 62%, respectively) and had better positive and negative predictive values.[156] However, gender differences in diagnostic accuracy were not reported.

Clinical applications of noninvasive tests in women

Noninvasive diagnostic testing can provide important information on the likelihood of CHD, the severity of disease, and the prognosis in women with known CHD. Until it is clear whether gender-specific criteria are necessary to improve their diagnostic accuracy, these techniques must be used critically. The exercise ECG provides the most reliable information in women with a normal resting ECG and typical angina. The utility of the stress ECG in women with atypical symptoms and resting ST-T wave changes is questionable. Exercise thallium-201 scintigraphy, exercise echocardiography, and dipyridamole thallium-201 scintigraphy have improved sensitivity and specificity in some groups of patients, such as women with resting ST-T wave changes and women unable to exercise to adequate intensity levels.

CLINICAL SYNDROMES OF CORONARY HEART DISEASE IN WOMEN

There are established gender differences in the clinical presentation and course of CHD and in the response to methods of revascularization.

Angina pectoris

The predominant clinical expression of CHD in women is angina pectoris, occurring in 56% of women (compared with 39% of men.)[12] Angina in women is less likely to be complicated by myocardial infarction, which occurs in only about 15% of women with angina. Twenty-five percent of men are likely to sustain a myocardial infarction within 5 years. Women with angina pectoris have longer survival and lower risk of myocardial infarction and cardiac death than do men.[157]

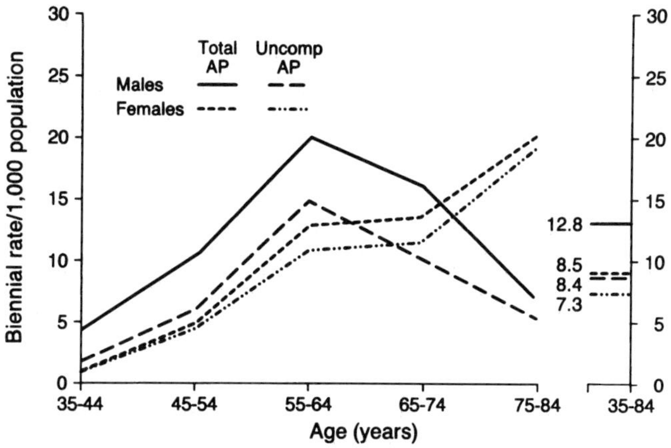

Fig 65-12 Sex- and age-specific incidence of uncomplicated angina pectoris (AP) and total angina pectoris in subjects aged 35 to 84 years, Framingham study, 26-year follow-up. (From Lerner DJ, Kannel WB: Patterns of coronary heart disease morbidity and mortality in the sexes: a 26-year follow-up of the Framingham population. *Am Heart J* 111:383-390, 1986. By permission of Mosby–Year Book.)

The age trend in the incidence of angina pectoris is unique in women. In men, the incidence of angina increases sharply, reaches a peak between ages 55 and 65 years, and then declines in old age. In women, the incidence of angina continues to increase with advancing age, so that after age 75, angina is predominantly a disease of women[12] (Fig 65-12).

In women, the description of typical or probable angina is a less reliable indicator of CHD than in men. Only 72% of women with typical angina pectoris have significant coronary obstruction at angiography, whereas 93% of men with typical angina have obstruction[144] (Table 65-7). The gender differences in angiographically confirmed CHD are even more striking when angina is probable or atypical.

Acute myocardial infarction

Approximately one-third of women with CHD present initially with acute myocardial infarction, compared with nearly half of men. When women do present with myocardial infarction, they are more likely to experience silent or unrecognized myocardial infarction (women, 34%; men, 27%).[12,158] There is a trend toward an increase in non-Q-wave myocardial infarction in women.[7,158] Women are at greater risk of reinfarction (relative risk, 4.9, or 25% of women) than are men (relative risk, 2.2, or 22% of men) when comparisons are made to age-matched controls in the general population.[158]

The clinical presentation of myocardial infarction is similar in women and men.[159,160] Gender-related differences in presentation of myocardial infarction in women are attributable to the older age of women at occurrence of infarction.[160] Both male and female elderly patients tend to have more atypical signs and symptoms of CHD.

Location and size of acute myocardial infarctions do not appear to be significantly different between men and women.[7,161,162] Assessment of infarct size by myocardial enzyme determination yields similar results in men and women when creatine kinase values are adjusted for body surface area.[161]

Although the incidence of some complications appears to be increased in women, when data are age-adjusted to account for the typically older age of women presenting with myocardial infarction, some gender differences are not significant.[163] Cardiac rupture may occur more frequently in women, although the increased incidence

Table 65-7 Radiographic prevalence of coronary artery disease

	Men, %	Women, %
Typical angina	93	72
Probable angina	66	36
Nonspecific chest pain	14	6

Data from Chaitman BR, Bourassa MG, Davis K, et al: Angiographic prevalence of high-risk coronary artery disease in patient subsets (CASS). *Circulation* 64:360-367, 1981.

may be due to a higher prevalence of postinfarction hypertension[7,164,165] as well as to older age at presentation. Ventricular arrhythmias,[162] supraventricular arrhythmias (including atrial fibrillation and supraventricular tachycardia), and electrical complications (including bundle-branch block and atrioventricular block) are not increased in women when data are age-adjusted.[7,161]

Women have a higher postinfarction ejection fraction than men with comparable infarct size and location.[7] Despite preserved left ventricular function, morbidity is not less in women than in men. The risks of stroke in the postinfarction period[158] and infarct extension[166] may be increased in women. Limited data do not suggest gender differences in the incidence of mitral regurgitation or right ventricular infarction.[162,167,168]

It is unclear whether immediate, short-term, and long-term prognoses in women after myocardial infarction are worse than in men[7,12,169] or whether gender differences in prognosis are attributable to the older age of women and other known risk factors for mortality (hypertension, diabetes, impaired left ventricular function, and clinical heart failure).[170] Available data on gender differences in prognosis after myocardial infarction were obtained before the thrombolytic era, so that mortality information for current standards of care is limited. The major trials of thrombolysis support gender differences in mortality associated with myocardial infarction, even when modern regimens are used.[171]

Although historically there have been gender biases in the management of myocardial infarction, current patterns in pharmacologic treatment of men and women are similar. There are no statistically significant gender-related differences in the use of anticoagulants, β-blockers, calcium channel blockers, digoxin, nitrates, and thrombolytic agents.[172] Women are more likely than men to receive diuretics and less likely to receive antiplatelet agents, lidocaine, and other antiarrhythmic agents. Previous results had shown that only 55% of eligible women received thrombolytic agents in comparison with 78% of eligible men.[173] However, an approximate sixfold increase in the use of thrombolytic therapy occurred between 1986 and 1990, and in 1990 rates of use in men and women were comparable.[172]

Thrombolytic therapy

There are no significant gender differences in the systemic response to thrombolytic therapy.[174] Minor differences noted reflect an effect of higher dose of the lytic agent per unit of body weight in women. Coronary artery patency rates and rates of reperfusion after thrombolytic therapy are similar in men and women. Successful coronary reperfusion is established in 64% to 100% of men and 72% to 100% of women.[174] No data have yet compared reocclusion rates and lysis time in women with those in men. Further study is needed on weight-, age-, and gender-based dosage modifications of thrombolytic agents.

Gender analyses of the effect of thrombolytic therapy on left ventricular function and recurrent cardiac events have not been performed. Subgroup analyses from the large clinical trials provide information on gender differences in mortality after thrombolytic therapy.[171,174]

Table 65-8 reviews trials that examined mortality data by gender.[175-178] Mortality rates after myocardial infarction were higher among women, both in the thrombolysis group and in the control group. In the control group, mortality rates ranged from 8.6% to 26.2% for men and 10.9% to 31.3% for women. Thrombolytic therapy in acute myocardial infarction reduced mortality rates in both men (6.7% to 18.1%) and women (2.9% to 28.3%). Absolute reductions in mortality were similar in men and women.[171] Because of their high baseline mortality rates with myocardial infarction, women had somewhat lower relative reductions in mortality with thrombolysis. A recent report suggested that after adjustment for gender differences in baseline clinical variables (age, history of prior infarction, antecedent angina, hypertension, diabetes, anginal class, and time to therapy), women and men had similar mortality rates after administration of tissue plasminogen activator.[182] In both men and women, thrombolysis now offers the greatest potential pharmaco-

Table 65-8 Thromboloytic therapy in women: mortality by gender in thrombolysis trials

		Mortality rate, %				Reduction in mortality, %			
		Thrombolysis group		Control group		Relative		Absolute	
Study	Treatment	Women	Men	Women	Men	Women	Men	Women	Men
ISIS-2[175]	SK/ASA	12.2	6.7	17.5	12.0	31	45	53	53
GISSI-1[176]	SK	18.5	8.8	22.6	10.6	19	17	41	18
GISSI-1 (FU)[177]	SK	28.3	14.5	31.3	16.0	10	10	30	15
ASSET[178]	TPA/H	8.6	6.8	10.9	9.4	21	28	23	26
EWP[179]	SK	20.3	18.1	26.6	26.2	24	31	63	81
WWT (12 mo)[180]	IC-SK	13.3	7.5	21.0	13.4	37	44	77	59
WWT[181]	SK	2.9	7.0	16.0	8.6	82	19	131	16

ASA, aspirin; H, heparin; IC, intracoronary; SK, streptokinase; TPA, tissue plasminogen activator.
Modified from Eysmann SB, Douglas PS: Reperfusion and revascularization strategies for coronary artery disease in women. *JAMA* 268:1903-1907, 1992.

logic reduction in mortality during acute myocardial infarction. Appropriate patient selection for thrombolytic therapy will include sizable numbers of women who derive substantial benefit from treatment.

Data on gender differences in complications associated with thrombolytic therapy are limited. An increased incidence of hemorrhagic events, including intracranial hemorrhage, cardiac tamponade, hemoglobin decrease of more than 5.0 g/L, death due to exsanguination, and minor hemorrhagic complications, has been reported in women.[183] A higher incidence of hemorrhagic stroke has been noted in women (5.9%) than in men (3.8%).[182,184] It remains unclear whether this increase in hemorrhagic events in women is due to a true gender difference in response to thrombolysis or due to the older age and smaller body size of women with acute myocardial infarction.

Gender differences in response to combined thrombolytic therapy and interventional strategies compared with conservative strategies have not been reported.

Congestive heart failure

Few studies examine gender differences in the incidence and survival rates of congestive heart failure. Some data suggest that women have an increased incidence of congestive heart failure after myocardial infarction but that the increase is due to the older age of women presenting with infarction.[159,161] Other studies have shown an increased risk of congestive heart failure after infarction that can be attributed to female gender even after age adjustment.[7,158,185,186] Although women are more likely than men to have unrecognized or silent myocardial infarctions, men are at greater risk of congestive heart failure in this situation.[158]

Gender differences in survival after postinfarction congestive heart failure have not been established, but results indicate that women have a better prognosis, with longer median survival and better 1- and 5-year survival rates.[187,188] Median survival after the diagnosis of congestive heart failure is 1.7 years in men and 3.2 years in women. The 1-year and 5-year survival rates are 64% and 38% in women compared with 57% and 25% in men. Congestive heart failure is most lethal in elderly patients of both sexes.

Although the large randomized trials of vasodilator therapy for treatment and prevention of congestive heart failure and for improvement of survival after myocardial infarction have included women, detailed gender analysis of results has not been performed in most studies.[189-192] The Cooperative North Scandinavian Enalapril Survival Study (CONSENSUS) II did analyze results by gender but did not show any benefit of early therapy with enalapril in men and women with acute myocardial infarction.[191] Treatment begun within 24 hours of the onset of myocardial infarction did not improve 6-month survival.

In the Survival and Ventricular Enlargement (SAVE) trial, the benefits of long-term therapy with captopril were examined in men and women with myocardial infarction and asymptomatic left ventricular dysfunction.[190] The number of women eligible for inclusion in the trial was small, and an excess of women were excluded because of lack of data from cardiac catheterization.[193] In the entire study population, long-term administration of captopril resulted in an improvement in survival and reduced cardiovascular morbidity and mortality. Data in women, however, showed only a 2% reduction in risk of death from all causes, whereas men had a 22% reduction. Treatment with captopril reduced the risk of cardiovascular morbidity and death by 28% in men but by only 4% in women. At this point, it appears to be premature to draw conclusions on gender differences in the use of angiotensin-converting enzyme inhibitors in women after myocardial infarction.

Studies of congestive heart failure from multiple causes, including ischemic cardiomyopathy, have also included women. An unpublished analysis of CONSENSUS I showed no improvement in long-term survival in women with congestive heart failure of multiple causes treated with the angiotensin-converting enzyme inhibitor enalapril.[185] The Studies of Left Ventricular Dysfunction (SOLVD) investigators found that in patients (20.5% women) with chronic congestive heart failure, enalapril reduced mortality and hospitalizations for congestive heart failure in men and women, although the effect was greater in men.[192] Overall mortality for congestive heart failure remained high. The reduction in rate of myocardial infarction was greater in women. Women in this trial were older and had a high mortality not due to older age or other factors.[193]

Limited data are currently available to guide the use of vasodilator therapy in women with asymptomatic left ventricular dysfunction and postinfarction congestive heart failure. Recommendations await analyses of gender-specific risks and benefits of therapy.

PERCUTANEOUS TRANSLUMINAL CORONARY ANGIOPLASTY IN WOMEN

There are important gender differences in baseline clinical variables and acute and long-term outcomes in patients referred for percutaneous transluminal coronary angioplasty (PTCA). Women referred for PTCA are older than men by approximately 4.5 to 5 years.[194-200] Cardiovascular risk factors, including hypertension, diabetes, and hypercholesteremia, are more common in women. Tobacco use among women is not significantly different than that among men undergoing PTCA.[194,196,200] Only one series has tried to characterize the relation between body size and gender differences in PTCA outcomes. In the National Heart, Lung, and Blood Institute (NHLBI) PTCA Registry cohorts, height, weight, and body surface area were all less in women.[194] However, body mass index was similar in men and women. Other severe noncardiac medical illnesses are also more common in women.

Women undergoing PTCA are more likely to have angina, and their symptoms are more severe. They have more class III and IV angina, more unstable angina, more new-onset angina or angina with a changing clinical pattern, and more angina refractory to medical therapy.[194-196,198,200] A history of congestive heart failure is more common in women, but overall, women have better left ventricular function as measured by ejection fraction.[194,196,198]

The angiographic severity of disease is similar in men and women, with multivessel disease in 49% to 69% of patients.[194,196] In the NHLBI PTCA Registry cohorts, women were more often judged to have inoperable disease or to be high-risk surgical candidates. In women undergoing PTCA, the likelihood of a history of myocardial infarction is similar to, or perhaps less than, that in men and the likelihood of previous surgical revascularization is less than that in men.[194-197,200] In the Cleveland Clinic series, men and women had a similar prevalence of repeat PTCA procedures.[200]

Technologic advances and accumulated experience with the technique of PTCA have resulted in changes in the patient population referred for this procedure. Patients are now older, with a greater prevalence of multivessel disease, congestive heart failure, reduced ventricular function, acute myocardial infarction, and history of surgical revascularization.[196,201] The increase in congestive heart failure, previous bypass surgery, and multivessel disease is greater among women than among men. There has been a significant increase in hypertension, diabetes, and hypercholesterolemia among both men and women undergoing PTCA. Cigarette smoking is less common in more recent series. Overall, patients are now older and have more acute and advanced disease and more concomitant medical illnesses, and these changes are more prominent among women.[196,201]

Although early data suggested a lower angiographic success rate for women (60%) than for men (66%),[197] more recent series have shown that PTCA is an equally effective form of revascularization for men and women.[194-196,198,200,202] Reported angiographic success rates vary from 84% to 95% in women and 80% to 95% in men.

Acute complications of PTCA

The relation between female gender and acute nonfatal complications of PTCA has been variable in reported clinical series. Women in the NHLBI PTCA Registry cohorts from 1979 to 1983 and 1985 to 1986 were more likely to have coronary dissection and major entry site complications.[194,197] In the Emory PTCA database, female gender was a strong independent predictor of acute coronary closure after PTCA.[203] However, women in the series from the Cleveland Clinic, Beth Israel Hospital, and Mid-America Heart Institute did not have a significant increase in acute closure, coronary dissection, or other nonfatal complications,[195,198,200] except perhaps those older than 70.[198] There is no increase in myocardial infarction or emergency surgical revascularization after PTCA in women.[194-198,200] A gender difference was noted, however, in the mortality associated with emergency surgery in the early NHLBI PTCA Registry cohort.[197] The mortality with emergency CABG was more than five times higher in women than in men (17.4% versus 3.2%). Complications of PTCA for total coronary artery occlusions may be increased in women.[204]

Reports of gender differences in procedural or in-hospital mortality associated with PTCA differ. Women in the Cleveland Clinic and Beth Israel series did not have an increase in early mortality after PTCA,[198,200] although the Cleveland Clinic series reported only deaths occurring in the cardiac catheterization laboratory, not total in-hospital deaths.[196] The Mayo Clinic, NHLBI PTCA Registry, Mid-America Heart Institute, and extended follow-up data from the Cleveland Clinic, however, have clearly shown a higher procedural mortality in women (women, 1.4% to 2.9%; men, 0.3% to 1.4%).[194-196,205-207] The gender difference in mortality is in part due to the increased age of women and an increased prevalence of diabetes, congestive heart failure, multivessel disease, and more advanced symptoms. After adjustment for these factors, an independent effect of gender on mortality remains, with an odds ratio of 2.21 to 4.53.[194,196]

Periprocedural mortality has remained unchanged in men in recent years, even though patients undergoing PTCA are generally "sicker" and have more advanced coronary disease.[196] However, mortality reported from 1979 to 1990 has significantly increased in women. The higher in-hospital mortality in women and the increase in mortality reported over recent years are explained in part by the significant increase (nearly 50%) in the proportion of high-risk women undergoing PTCA right after infarction.

Long-term outcome of PTCA

Although female gender is a predictor of early mortality after PTCA, the long-term outcome for women who survive the initial procedure is said to be similar to that for men. The relation between gender and restenosis rates after PTCA is uncertain. In the NHLBI-1 cohort, women had a lower acute success rate and more early complications but had lower restenosis and repeat PTCA rates, lesser likelihood of late coronary artery bypass grafting, and a lower late mortality than men.[197] A higher risk of restenosis among men has been observed in a number of other studies. In a recent meta-analysis, men had a highly significant but small increased risk of restenosis over that in women (36% and 28%).[208,209] Other analyses have not confirmed gender differences in restenosis rates.[210]In several recent series with follow-up ranging from 20 to 48 months, need for repeat PTCA, long-term survival rates, incidence of myocardial infarction, and need for late bypass grafting were similar in men and women.[194,198,200,211,212]

Gender differences in reduction of anginal symptoms are unclear. Women in the NHLBI cohort reported symptomatic improvement similar to that in men, even though they reported more angina and were more likely to require cardiac medications.[194] In the Cleveland Clinic series, reported remission in angina was similar in men and women, but women were more likely to be hospitalized for chest pain.[200]

Gender differences in complications during new procedures for percutaneous coronary revascularization, such as directional atherectomy and intracoronary stenting, are not defined. In one study of atherectomy, female gender was associated with an independent risk of major complications.[213] Female gender did not predict restenosis after intracoronary stenting in a series of 250 patients, including 70 women, from Beth Israel Hospital.[214]

Techniques for PTCA are important management strategies for women with manifest coronary artery disease. Although early in-hospital and procedural mortality are increased, the long-term outcome for women is excellent and comparable to that in men.

CORONARY ARTERY BYPASS SURGERY

Gender differences in the baseline clinical characteristics of patients undergoing coronary artery bypass surgery have been observed.[126,215-219] Women tend to be slightly older than men at the time of surgery and are more likely to have associated cardiac risk factors, including diabetes, hypertension, hyperlipidemia, morbid obesity, sedentary lifestyle, and tobacco use. Women are more likely to have concomitant medical illnesses, such as peripheral vascular disease, valvular heart diseases, pulmonary and renal disease, thrombophlebitis, and neoplasm.[219]

Women undergoing surgical revascularization have more anginal symptoms and more severe and unstable angina than men.[216,220-222] A higher proportion of women have been treated with prescription cardiac medications before surgery, including antihypertensive drugs, antianginals, digitalis, diuretics, and hypoglycemic agents.[219] Reported gender differences in the history of previous myocardial infarction are inconsistent.[126,215-219] Women tend to have better left ventricular function at the time of surgery but an increased likelihood of a history of congestive heart failure. The frequency of left main coronary artery disease is similar in men and women, but women have less three-vessel disease and more single-vessel disease.[126,216,219]

Outcome after coronary artery bypass surgery

Accurate assessment of gender differences in outcome after surgical revascularization has been difficult for several reasons. Advances in the technique of cardiac surgery have improved outcomes for cardiac patients over the period of observation and follow-up for many reported surgical series. Improvements in cardioprotection during surgery and the routine use of antiplatelet agents have contributed to noted differences in survival and short- and long-term rates of graft patency.[223] Many of the reported surgical series antedate the routine use of internal mammary artery grafts. Compared with saphenous vein grafts, internal mammary artery grafts have increased rates of patency in men and women.[224] A trend toward improvement in survival has also been observed in women receiving internal mammary artery grafts.[225] Use of the internal mammary graft accelerated throughout the 1970s and 1980s, so that assessment of gender influences on outcomes from earlier studies is less meaningful in today's clinical practice. In addition, body or coronary artery size may be more important than gender in determining outcome after surgical revascularization.[126,220,221,226,227] In many reported series, this information is unavailable.

Operative mortality

Most early surgical series observed that operative mortality after coronary bypass surgery is nearly twice as likely overall in women as in men.[126,217,218,228-232] (Table 65-9). More recent surgical series have confirmed these findings. Gender differences in mortality were noted in 12,448 patients in 1989 (women, 3.08%; men, 5.43%), with a relative risk of in-hospital death of 1.52 in women compared with men.[215] Elderly women and women with left main coronary artery disease and increased end-diastolic pressure have the greatest risk of perioperative death.[231,233-235]

Gender differences in operative mortality may be the result of clinical factors. In one series, adjustment for gender differences in baseline clinical variables (age, anginal classification, extent of coronary disease) resulted in a similar operative mortality rate of 2% in

Table 65-9 Operative mortality for men and women after coronary artery bypass graft surgery

Author and affiliation	Study period	Operative mortality, % Men (*n*)	Operative mortality, % Women (*n*)	Relative risk
Bolooki et al. (U of Miami)[228]	1969-1973	2.0 (51)	8.8 (34)	4.84
Tyras et al. (St. Louis U)[217]	1970-1977	2.4 (1,300)	3.7 (241)	1.58
Kennedy et al. (CASS)[231]	1975-1978	1.9 (5,569)	4.5 (1,061)	2.44
Douglas et al. (Emory U)[218]	1973-1979	1.0 (2,663)	2.2 (492)	2.15
Killen et al. (Mid-America Heart Inst)[229]	1970-1976	0.9 (2,243)	1.3 (385)	1.46
Loop et al. (Cleveland Clinic)[225]	1967-1981	1.3 (18,079)	2.9 (2,445)	2.20
Hall et al. (Texas Heart Inst)[232]	1970-1981	2.6 (19,175)	5.3 (3,109)	2.10
Laird-Meeter et al. (Rotterdam)[230]	1971-1980	1.0 (915)	2.4 (126)	2.46
Gardner et al. (Johns Hopkins)[227]	1974-1983	3.0 (2,640)	7.4 (639)	2.57

The relative risk is the ratio of the mortality rate for women and the mortality rate for men.
n, number of patients; CASS, Coronary Artery Surgery Study.
From Davis KB: Coronary artery bypass graft surgery in women. In *Coronary Artery Disease in Women.* Edited by ED Eaker, B Packard, NK Wenger, et al. New York, Haymarket-Doyma, 1987, p 249.

men and women.[218] Several studies have found that after adjustment for body surface area, female gender is not a risk factor for operative mortality.[126,220,221]

Surgical revascularization may be less complete in women than in men. Men have been noted to receive more grafts at the time of bypass surgery than women and to be more likely to receive a graft to each coronary artery with a proximal stenosis.[218] Internal mammary artery grafting is less often performed in women than in men, and the absence of internal mammary artery grafting is also associated with increased risk of death from heart failure in both sexes.[221]

An overall improvement in surgical survival has been reported in women in recent surgical study periods.[227,236] Observed gender differences in operative mortality in patients undergoing coronary artery bypass surgery are most likely the result of patient, disease, and treatment factors. Older age, greater coexisting medical illness, advanced symptoms, smaller body surface area and coronary artery luminal size, and lack of internal mammary artery grafting all contribute to excessive mortality among women.[221]

Long-term outcome after coronary artery bypass surgery

Long-term clinical follow-up confirms that surgical revascularization may be technically less satisfactory in women. Women have less efficacy of coronary artery bypass grafting for relief of anginal symptoms than do men.[126,218,228,237,238] However, in no series has adjustment for the preoperative gender differences in anginal classification and frequency been performed. Long-term rates of graft patency have also been consistently lower in women.[126,217,218,228,239]

There are no gender differences in long-term survival after successful coronary artery bypass surgery. In follow-up periods ranging from 42 months to 10 years, there are no statistically significant differences in survival between men and women.[126,217-219] The reported 5-year survival rate is more than 90% and the 10-year survival rate more than 75% for both sexes.[240] Although the baseline clinical variables noted more frequently in women predict an increased risk of early operative mortality, the favorable long-term results of coronary artery bypass surgery support its importance as an excellent therapeutic management option in women.

GENDER BIAS IN MANAGEMENT OF CORONARY HEART DISEASE

Decisions to use cardiovascular diagnostic and therapeutic procedures may be influenced by patient gender. Several studies indicate that women are less likely to be referred for invasive cardiovascular diagnostic and therapeutic procedures.[241-243] In one study of patients with abnormal radionuclide scans (exercise-gated blood-pool scans and exercise thallium scans), only 4% of women but 40% of men were referred for coronary arteriography.[241] This sex difference in referral persisted after adjustment for age, previous myocardial infarction, and nature of symptoms (typical or atypical angina). Women are less likely to undergo coronary arteriography, PTCA, or coronary artery bypass surgery during hospitalization for myocardial infarction, unstable angina, or chest pain of chronic ischemic heart disease.[242] Women enrolled in the SAVE trial after myocardial infarction were also less likely to undergo invasive cardiac procedures.[243] However, after coronary angiography, there was no gender difference in referral for coronary artery bypass surgery. Women tend to be referred late in their clinical course and have advanced symptoms of CVD, including more unstable angina, postmyocardial infarction angina, congestive heart failure, and class IV angina.[222]

A recent series studied referral for invasive cardiac procedures among men and women with confirmed acute myocardial infarction.[244] No gender difference was noted in referral for coronary angiography when results were age-adjusted. Women had a significantly lower rate of severe coronary artery stenosis (left main stenosis >50%, three-vessel disease, or two-vessel disease with a proximal left anterior descending stenosis of >70%). Women and men were equally likely to be referred for angioplasty. When adjusted for age and severity of disease, gender differences in referral for surgical revascularization were of only borderline significance.

Gender differences in referral for diagnostic and therapeutic management of cardiac disease may represent more appropriate treatment referral for women than for men.[216] In a study of patients who underwent cardiac catheterization between 1969 and 1984, no gender difference was noted in patients referred for surgical revascularization. There was no statistical difference in duration of symptoms before referral for coronary angiography. The effect of referral bias on patient outcome was evaluated by estimating the baseline risk of cardiac death and the potential survival benefit of coronary artery bypass graft surgery relative to medical therapy. Gender differences in referral pattern were noted when higher risk patients were compared with lower risk patients. Low-risk men with little to gain from revascularization were more often referred for surgery than similarly low-risk women, who were more often treated medically. Among high-risk men and women in whom surgery offered the greatest survival benefit, men and women were equally likely to be referred for surgery. This pattern of referral may have resulted in more appropriate treatment strategies among women.

PREVENTION OF CORONARY HEART DISEASE IN WOMEN

Primary prevention

Definitive clinical trials of management of hyperlipidemia, hypertension, and diabetes for primary prevention of heart disease in women are not available. The benefits of tobacco cessation are documented and likely to be evident even in elderly women. Available information supports the recent recommendation by the Scientific Advisory Committee of the American Heart Association to improve cardiovascular health in women: "The three most important health-related behaviors for women are to avoid smoking, eat a balanced, low-saturated-fat diet to control blood lipid levels, and maintain a moderate level of physical activity to help control body weight."[245]

The recent revision of the National Cholesterol Education Program (NCEP) Expert Panel guidelines for management of high blood cholesterol levels in adults has incorporated new principles for treatment of women.[82] Because of the relatively low risk of CVD in premenopausal women without other cardiac risk factors, drug therapy should generally be delayed. Only dietary therapy, weight reduction, and increased physical activity are indicated in such women. Lipid-lowering drug therapy should be considered in premenopausal women without other cardiac risk factors if nonpharmacologic measures are unsuccessful in lowering LDL cholesterol values below the range of 190 to 220 mg/dL. Premenopausal women with multiple cardiac risk factors should be considered for nonpharmacologic and drug therapy according to guidelines established for men. In postmenopausal women with increased LDL cholesterol levels, estrogen therapy should be considered to potentially obviate lipid-lowering drug therapy. The established goals of therapy for hyperlipemia to prevent primary CVD are similar in men and women: total cholesterol <200 mg/dL, LDL <130 mg/dL, and HDL >35 mg/dL.

The role of exercise in cardiac disease prevention is uncertain, because clinical trials have not been conducted in women. In an overview of available observational studies, only 5 of 43 studies of exercise included women.[246] Four of these studies indicated that low levels of physical activity were associated with an increased risk of cardiac end points. Statistical considerations in these papers suggest that the beneficial effects may actually have been underestimated, but at this time strong evidence for a causal relation between physical activity and coronary artery disease in women is lacking. Exercise has been documented to have beneficial effects on cardiac risk factors. Blood pressure, body weight, glucose tolerance, and blood lipid status are all affected positively in physically active women.[247]

Aspirin in low doses may have a beneficial role in the primary prevention of CHD in women. The Nurses' Health Study, an observational study of 87,678 women aged 34 to 65 years, concluded that use of one to six aspirin tablets a week was associated with a 25% reduction in risk of first myocardial infarction in women older than 50 years.[248] No beneficial effect was noted in women younger than 50 or with use of seven or more aspirin per week.

The use of β-blockade in the primary prevention of CHD in hypertensive men has been associated with a reduction in cardiac events.[249] Data are lacking in women in these preventive trials because of the low incidence of cardiac events in middle-aged white women.

Secondary prevention

Women with established CHD should be managed as aggressively as men for prevention of recurrent cardiac events. Counseling for tobacco cessation is critical in the treatment program for women with known cardiac disease. Tobacco cessation is associated with improved prognosis in women with acute myocardial infarction.[25] There is also a suggestion that tobacco cessation in women can delay progression of atherosclerosis, as detected and followed radiographically.[28]

No clinical trials of lipid-lowering therapy for secondary prevention of cardiac events have been performed in women to date. Two angiographic studies of regression of coronary atherosclerosis with aggressive lipid lowering have included women.[250,251] The number of women in these trials was small, but both studies suggested that women may have a greater ability than men to undergo coronary atherosclerotic regression. The goals of therapy for lipid lowering in women with known CHD are total cholesterol <180 mg/dL, LDL <100 mg/dL, and HDL >35 mg/dL.[82]

Data on the value of exercise in the secondary prevention of CHD in women are lacking. Women represented only 3% of patients (143 women, 4,411 men) in 22 trials included in two reviews.[252,253] Information is limited to guide the exercise rehabilitation of women with manifest CHD.

The effectiveness of aspirin in secondary prevention of CHD is uncertain because men predominate in available trials. Overall, studies evaluating the effect of aspirin on platelet function have shown no significant gender differences.[254] Most studies reporting no beneficial effect of aspirin or a reduction in cardiac events with aspirin use are compromised by lack of separate analysis of data for women.

In women and men, β-blockade after myocardial infarction has resulted in equivalent reduction in nonfatal reinfarctions and overall mortality.[255-257] Use of propranolol or timolol reduced mortality by 39% to 41% and reinfarction by 28% to 48% in women.

Hormone therapy for prevention of cardiovascular disease in women

Because of the extensive evidence that unopposed estrogen therapy decreases the risk of CHD, all women should consider preventive hormone therapy. The overall effect of treatment with combined estrogen and progestin is difficult to assess for CHD, stroke, and breast cancer. Combination therapy reduces the risk of endometrial cancer and does not attenuate the beneficial effects of estrogen for prevention of hip fracture.

The American College of Physicians recently reviewed the risks and benefits of hormone therapy for postmenopausal women and published guidelines for counseling patients and instituting treatment.[258,259] The decision to use preventive hormone therapy, whether unopposed estrogen or estrogen and progesterone combined, should be based on estimation of the expected beneficial effects and the potential risks associated with treatment (Table 65-10). Each woman, after counseling on her risk for disease and likely changes in life expectancy, potential side effects, and necessary monitoring, must participate in the decision to use preventive hormone therapy. The American College of Physicians has provided tables for estimation of relative risks of CHD, stroke, hip fracture, and breast and endometrial cancer (Table 65-11). This infor-

Table 65-10 Management strategy for hormone therapy in postmenopausal women

Assessment of hysterectomy status and risk for coronary heart disease, breast cancer, and osteoporotic fractures
Estimation of the benefits and risks of hormone therapy based on risk group
Patient information and education
Management decision based on estimated effect of hormone therapy on life expectancy, lifetime probability of disease developing, side effects, bleeding, and need for endometrial monitoring
Surveillance

Data from American College of Physicians: Guidelines for counseling postmenopausal women about preventive hormone therapy. *Ann Intern Med* 117:1038-1041, 1992.

Table 65-11 Relative risk of selected conditions for a 50-year-old white woman treated with long-term hormone replacement

	Relative risk, %*	
Condition	Estrogen therapy	Estrogen plus progestin
Coronary heart disease	0.65	0.65 to 0.80
Stroke	0.96	0.96
Hip fracture	0.75	0.75
Breast cancer	1.25	1.25 to 2.00
Endometrial cancer	8.22	1.00

*Best estimates of the relative risk for each condition developing in long-term hormone users compared with nonusers. The same relative risk estimate was used for dying of each condition in long-term users compared with nonusers except for endometrial cancer, in which a relative risk of 3.0 was used.
From Grady D, Rubin SM, Petitti DB, et al: Hormone therapy to prevent disease and prolong life in postmenopausal women. *Ann Intern Med* 117:1016-1037, 1992. By permission of American College of Physicians.

information is useful for predicting the likelihood of benefit from hormone therapy.

Women who have undergone a hysterectomy are likely to benefit from unopposed estrogen therapy for both primary and secondary prevention of CVD. No progestin or additional monitoring is necessary other than the routine breast cancer surveillance recommended for all women.

Women with manifest CHD or with multiple cardiac risk factors are likely to benefit from preventive hormone therapy. The cardioprotective benefits of estrogen may be even greater in women who have known heart disease than in healthy women (relative risk of recurrent disease, 0.16; i.e., risk reduction of 84%). Combined therapy with estrogen and a progestin should be used if such women have a uterus, unless cautious endometrial monitoring is performed.

Preventive hormone therapy is not recommended in women at increased risk of breast cancer, unless in the judgment of physician and patient the potential reduction in CVD morbidity and mortality outweighs the risk of breast cancer.

For administration of unopposed estrogen to prevent CVD, the oral route is preferred because estrogen delivered orally increases levels of HDL cholesterol.[77,99,125] This increase is responsible for 30% to 40% of the reduction in cardiovascular risk associated with estrogen therapy. The estrogen patch, which bypasses the systemic "first-pass" effect of metabolism in the liver, is most useful in treatment of menopausal symptoms or prevention of osteoporosis in women at low risk of CVD. Estrogen should be prescribed as conjugated estrogen, 0.625 mg or the equivalent, taken daily without interruption. The benefits of therapy are more likely to be achieved with long-term use (10 to 20 years), because CHD is a chronic, progressive disease. However, the potential risk of endometrial and breast cancers increases with duration of estrogen use as well.

Combination preventive hormone therapy should consist of estrogen and cyclic progestin (medroxyprogesterone acetate), 5 to 10 mg orally per day, or micronized progesterone, 200 mg orally per day, for 10 to 14 days a month. Alternatively, medroxyprogesterone acetate may be prescribed on a continuous basis at a dose of 2.5 mg orally per day or the equivalent.

There is currently no upper age limit to initiation of preventive hormone therapy. The recommendations of the American College of Physicians suggest that because CHD and osteoporosis are diseases of later life in women, beginning treatment in older women may be beneficial.

REFERENCES

1. US Bureau of the Census, Statistical Abstract of the United States: 1992 (112th edition). Washington, DC, 1992
2. Wenger NK: Coronary heart disease in women: a 'new' problem. *Hosp Pract* 27:59-74, November 15, 1992
3. National Center for Health Statistics. Health, United States, 1990. Hyattsville, Maryland, Public Health Service, 1991
4. Kapantais G, Powell-Griner E: Characteristics of persons dying of disease of heart: preliminary data from the 1986 National Mortality Followback Survey. Hyattsville, Maryland. National Center for Health Statistics; 1989. Advance data from Vital and Health Statistics No. 172
5. Elveback LR, Connolly DC, Melton LJ III: Coronary heart disease in residents of Rochester, Minnesota. VII. Incidence, 1950 through 1982. *Mayo Clin Proc* 61:896-900, 1986
6. DeStefano F, Merritt RK, Anda RF, et al: Trends in nonfatal coronary heart disease in the United States, 1980 through 1989. *Arch Intern Med* 153:2489-2494, 1993
7. Tofler GH, Stone PH, Muller JE, et al: Effects of gender and race on prognosis after myocardial infarction: adverse prognosis for women, particularly black women. *J Am Coll Cardiol* 9:473-482, 1987
8. Eaker ED, Packard B, Thom TJ: Epidemiology and risk factors for coronary heart disease in women. *Cardiovasc Clin* 19:129-145, 1989
9. Havlik RJ, Liu BM, Kovar MG, et al: Health statistics on older persons, United States, 1986. *Vital Health Stat* [3] No 25, 1987
10. National Mortality Followback Survey: Characteristics of persons who died from diseases of the heart—United States, 1986. *JAMA* 262:1587-1591, 1989

11. Rossouw JE, Finnegan LP, Harlan WR, et al: The evolution of the Women's Health Initiative: perspectives from the NIH. *J Am Med Wom Assoc* 50:50-55, 1995

12. Lerner DJ, Kannel WB: Patterns of coronary heart disease morbidity and mortality in the sexes: a 26-year follow-up of the Framingham population. *Am Heart J* 111:383-390, 1986

13. McGill HC Jr, Stern MP: Sex and atherosclerosis. *Atherosclerosis Rev* 4:157-242, 1979

14. Bush TL: Epidemiology of cardiovascular disease in women. In *Lipids and Women's Health.* Edited by GP Redmond. New York, Springer-Verlag, 1991, pp 6-20

15. Schildkraut JM, Myers RH, Cupples LA, et al: Coronary risk associated with age and sex of parental heart disease in the Framingham Study. *Am J Cardiol* 64:555-559, 1989

16. Rosenberg L, Miller DR, Kaufman DW, et al: Myocardial infarction in women under 50 years of age. *JAMA* 250:2801-2806, 1983

17. Barrett-Connor E, Khaw KT, Wingard DL: A ten-year prospective study of coronary heart disease mortality among Rancho Bernardo women. In *Coronary Heart Disease in Women.* Edited by E Eaker, B Packard, N Wenger, et al. New York, Haymarket Doyma, 1987, pp 117-121

18. Department of Health and Human Services: The health consequences of smoking: cardiovascular disease. A report of the Surgeon General. Rockville, Maryland, 1983

19. Pierce JP, Lee L, Gilpin EA: Smoking initiation by adolescent girls, 1944 through 1988: an association with targeted advertising. *JAMA* 271:608-611, 1994

20. Willett WC, Green A, Stampfer MJ, et al: Relative and absolute excess risks of coronary heart disease among women who smoke cigarettes. *N Engl J Med* 317:1303-1309, 1987

21. Bush TL, Comstock GW: Smoking and cardiovascular mortality in women. *Am J Epidemiol* 118:480-488, 1983

22. Caralis DG, Deligonul U, Kern MJ, et al: Smoking is a risk factor for coronary spasm in young women. *Circulation* 85:905-909, 1992

23. Garland C, Barrett-Connor E, Suarez L, et al: Effects of passive smoking on ischemic heart disease mortality of nonsmokers. A prospective study. *Am J Epidemiol* 121:645-650, 1985

24. LaCroix AZ, Lang J, Scherr P, et al: Smoking and mortality among older men and women in three communities. *N Engl J Med* 324:1619-1625, 1991

25. Johansson S, Bergstrand R, Pennert K, et al: Cessation of smoking after myocardial infarction in women. Effects on mortality and reinfarctions. *Am J Epidemiol* 121:823-831, 1985

26. Kawachi I, Colditz GA, Stampfer MJ, et al: Smoking cessation and decreased risk of stroke in women. *JAMA* 269:232-236, 1993

27. Hermanson B, Omenn GS, Kronmal RA, et al: Beneficial six-year outcome of smoking cessation in older men and women with coronary artery disease: results from the CASS registry. *N Engl J Med* 319:1365-1369, 1988

28. Witteman JC, Grobbee DE, Valkenburg HA, et al: Cigarette smoking and the development and progression of aortic atherosclerosis. A 9-year population-based follow-up study in women. *Circulation* 88:2156-2162, 1993

29. Cummings SR, Rubin SM, Oster G: The cost-effectiveness of counseling smokers to quit. *JAMA* 261:75-79, 1989

30. Rowland M, Roberts J: Blood pressure levels and hypertension in persons aged 6-74 years: United States, 1976-80. Advancedata No 84, October 8, 1982

31. Anastos K, Charney P, Charon RA, et al: Hypertension in women: What is really known? The Women's Caucus, Working Group on Women's Health of the Society of General Internal Medicine. *Ann Intern Med* 115:287-293, 1991

32. Kannel WB: Status of risk factors and their consideration in antihypertensive therapy. *Am J Cardiol* 59:80A-90A, 1987

33. Stamler J, Stamler R, Neaton JD: Blood pressure, systolic and diastolic, and cardiovascular risks. US population data. *Arch Intern Med* 153:598-615, 1993

34. Bush TL, Criqui MH, Cowan LD, et al: Cardiovascular disease mortality in women: results from the Lipid Research Clinics follow-up study. In *Coronary Heart Disease in Women.* Edited by E Eaker, B Packard, N Wenger, et al. New York, Haymarket Doyma, 1987, pp 106-111

35. Keil JE, Gazes PC, Loadbolt CB, et al: Coronary heart disease mortality and its predictors among women in Charleston, South Carolina. In *Coronary Heart Disease in Women.* Edited by E Eaker, B Packard, N Wenger, et al. New York, Haymarket Doyma, 1987, pp 90-98

36. Eaker ED, Castelli WP: Coronary heart disease and its risk factors among women in the Framingham Study. In *Coronary Heart Disease in Women.* Edited by ED Eaker, B Packard, N Wenger, et al. New York, Haymarket Doyma, 1987, pp 122-130

37. Hypertension Detection and Follow-up Program Cooperative Group: Five-year findings of the Hypertension Detection and Follow-up Program. II. Mortality by race-sex and age. *JAMA* 242:2572-2577, 1979

38. The Australian Therapeutic Trial in Mild Hypertension. Report by the Management Committee. *Lancet* 1:1261-1267, 1980

39. Medical Research Council Working Party: MRC trial of treatment of mild hypertension: principal results. *Br Med J* 291:97-104, 1985

40. Amery A, Birkenhager W, Brixko P, et al: Mortality and morbidity results from the European Working Party on High Blood Pressure in the Elderly trial. *Lancet* 1:1349-1354, 1985

41. Multiple Risk Factor Intervention Trial: Risk factor changes and mortality results. *JAMA* 248:1465-1477, 1982

42. Helgeland A: Treatment of mild hypertension: a five year controlled drug trial. The Oslo study. *Am J Med* 69:725-732, 1980

43. Veterans Administration Cooperative Study Group on Antihypertensive Agents: Effects of treatment on morbidity in hypertension. Results in patients with diastolic blood pressure averaging 115 through 129 mm Hg. *JAMA* 202:1028-1034, 1967

44. Veterans Administration Cooperative Study Group on Antihypertensive Agents: Effects of treatment on morbidity in hypertension. II. Results in patients with diastolic blood pressure averaging 90 through 114 mm Hg. *JAMA* 213:1143-1152, 1970

45. Boehringer K, Weidmann P, Mordasini R, et al: Menopause-dependent plasma lipoprotein alterations in diuretic-treated women. *Ann Intern Med* 97:206-209, 1982

46. Neaton JD, Grimm RH Jr, Prineas RJ, et al: Treatment of Mild Hypertension Study: final results. *JAMA* 270:713-724, 1993

47. Manolio TA, Pearson TA, Wenger NK, et al: Cholesterol and heart disease in older persons and women. Review of an NHLBI workshop. *Ann Epidemiol* 2:161-176, 1992

48. Stein EA: Use of the clinical laboratory for lipid evaluation. In *Lipids and Women's Health.* Edited by GP Redmond. New York, Springer-Verlag, 1991, pp 39-47

49. Rifkind BM, Tamir I, Heiss G, et al: Distribution of high density and other lipoproteins in selected LRC prevalence study populations: a brief survey. *Lipids* 14:105-112, 1979

50. NIH Consensus Development Panel on Triglyceride, High-Density Lipoprotein, and Coronary Heart Disease: Triglyceride, high-density lipoprotein, and coronary heart disease. *JAMA* 269:505-510, 1993

51. Johnson CL, Rifkind MB, Sempos CT, et al: Declining serum total cholesterol levels among US adults. *JAMA* 269:3002-3008, 1993

52. Sempos CT, Cleeman JI, Carroll MD, et al: Prevalence of high blood cholesterol among US adults: the National Health and Nutrition Examination surveys. *JAMA* 269:3009-3014, 1993

53. Bush TL, Fried LP, Barrett-Connor E: Cholesterol, lipoproteins, and coronary heart disease in women. *Clin Chem* 34(8B):B60-B70, 1988

54. Wood PD, Stefanick ML, Williams PT, et al: The effects on plasma lipoproteins of a prudent weight-reducing diet, with or without exercise, in overweight men and women. *N Engl J Med* 325:461-466, 1991

55. National Center for Health Statistics, Harlan WR, Hill AL, Schmouder RP, et al: Dietary intake and cardiovascular risk factors, part II. Serum urate, serum cholesterol, and correlates: United States, 1971-75. *Vital Health Stat [11]* No 227, 1983

56. Glueck CJ, Taylor HL, Jacobs D, et al: Plasma high-density lipoprotein cholesterol: association with measurements of body mass. The Lipid Research Clinics Program Prevalence Study. *Circulation* 62 Suppl 4:62-69, 1980

57. Taylor PA, Ward A: Women, high-density lipoprotein cholesterol, and exercise. *Arch Intern Med* 153:1178-1184, 1993

58. Ernst N, Fisher M, Smith W, et al: The association of plasma high-density lipoprotein cholesterol with dietary intake and alcohol consumption. The Lipid Research Clinics Prevalence Study. *Circulation* 62 Suppl 4:41-52, 1980

59. Meilahn EN, Kuller LH, Matthews KA, et al: Potential for increasing high-density lipoprotein cholesterol, subfractions HDL2-C and HDL3-C, and apoprotein AI among middle-age women. *Prev Med* 20:462-473, 1991

60. Criqui MH, Cowan LD, Tyroler HA, et al: Lipoproteins as

mediators for the effects of alcohol consumption and cigarette smoking on cardiovascular mortality: results from the Lipid Research Clinics Follow-Up Study. *Am J Epidemiol* 126:629-637, 1987

61. Garg R, Wagener DK, Madans JH: Alcohol consumption and risk of ischemic heart disease in women. *Arch Intern Med* 153:1211-1216, 1993

62. Taylor KG, Carter TJ, Valente AJ, et al: Sex differences in the relationships between obesity, alcohol consumption and cigarette smoking and serum lipid and apolipoprotein concentrations in a normal population. *Atherosclerosis* 38:11-18, 1981

63. Criqui MH, Wallace RB, Heiss G, et al: Cigarette smoking and plasma high-density lipoprotein cholesterol. The Lipid Research Clinics Program Prevalence Study. *Circulation* 62 Suppl 4:70-76, 1980

64. Moffatt RJ: Effects of cessation of smoking on serum lipids and high density lipoprotein-cholesterol. *Atherosclerosis* 74:85-89, 1988

65. Muscat JE, Harris RE, Haley NJ, et al: Cigarette smoking and plasma cholesterol. *Am Heart J* 121:141-147, 1991

66. Miller VT, La Rosa JC: Sex steroids and lipoproteins. In *Lipids and Women's Health.* Edited by GP Redmond. New York, Springer-Verlag, 1991, pp 48-65

67. Vaziri SM, Evans JC, Larson MG, et al: The impact of female hormone usage on the lipid profile: the Framingham Offspring Study. *Arch Intern Med* 153:2200-2206, 1993

68. The Writing Group for the PEPI Trial: Effects of estrogen/progestin regimens on heart disease risk factors in postmenopausal women. The Postmenopausal Estrogen/Progestin Interventions (PEPI) Trial. *JAMA* 273:199-208, 1995

69. Kronmal RA, Cain KC, Ye Z, et al: Total serum cholesterol levels and mortality risk as a function of age: a report based on the Framingham data. *Arch Intern Med* 153:1065-1073, 1993

70. Brunner D, Weisbort J, Meshulam N, et al: Relation of serum total cholesterol and high-density lipoprotein cholesterol percentage to the incidence of definite coronary events: twenty-year follow-up of the Donolo-Tel Aviv Prospective Coronary Artery Disease Study. *Am J Cardiol* 59:1271-1276, 1987

71. Kannel WB, Gordon T (eds): The Framingham Study: an epidemiological investigation of cardiovascular disease. Section 30: Some characteristics related to the incidence of cardiovascular disease and death: Framingham Study, 18-year follow-up. DHEW publication NIH 74-599. Washington, DC, US Government Printing Office, February 1974

72. Kannel WB, Wilson PW: Efficacy of lipid profiles in prediction of coronary disease. *Am Heart J* 124:768-774, 1992

73. Wong ND, Wilson PW, Kannel WB: Serum cholesterol as a prognostic factor after myocardial infarction: the Framingham Study. *Ann Intern Med* 115:687-693, 1991

74. Criqui MH, Heiss G, Cohn R, et al: Plasma triglyceride level and mortality from coronary heart disease. *N Engl J Med* 328:1220-1225, 1993

75. Gordon T, Castelli WP, Hjortland MC, et al: High density lipoprotein as a protective factor against coronary heart disease. The Framingham Study. *Am J Med* 62:707-714, 1977

76. Kannel WB: Metabolic risk factors for coronary heart disease in women: perspective from the Framingham Study. *Am Heart J* 114:413-419, 1987

77. Bush TL, Barrett-Connor E, Cowan LD, et al: Cardiovascular mortality and noncontraceptive use of estrogen in women: results from the Lipid Research Clinics Program Follow-up Study. *Circulation* 75:1102-1109, 1987

78. Jacobs DR, Mebane IL, Bangdiwala SI, et al: High density lipoprotein cholesterol as a predictor of cardiovascular disease mortality in men and women: the follow-up study of the Lipid Research Clinics Prevalence Study. *Am J Epidemiol* 131:32-47, 1990

79. Castelli WP, Garrison RJ, Wilson PW, et al: Incidence of coronary heart disease and lipoprotein cholesterol levels. The Framingham Study. *JAMA* 256:2835-2838, 1986

80. Jacobs D, Blackburn H, Higgins M, et al: Report of the Conference on Low Blood Cholesterol: mortality associations. *Circulation* 86:1046-1060, 1992

81. Kannel WB: Low high-density lipoprotein cholesterol and what to do about it (editorial). *Am J Cardiol* 70:810-814, 1992

82. Summary of the second report of the National Cholesterol Education Program (NCEP) Expert Panel on Detection, Evaluation, and Treatment of High Blood Cholesterol in Adults (Adult Treatment Panel II). *JAMA* 269:3015-3023, 1993

83. Manson JE, Colditz GA, Stampfer MJ, et al: A prospective study of maturity-onset diabetes mellitus and risk of coronary heart disease and stroke in women. *Arch Intern Med* 151:1141-1147, 1991

84. Palumbo PJ, Elveback LR, Connolly DC: Coronary heart disease and congestive heart failure in the diabetic: epidemiologic aspects. The Rochester Diabetes Project. In *Clinical Cardiology and Diabetes.* Vol. 1. Edited by RC Scott. Mount Kisco, New York, Futura Publishing Company, 1981, pp 13-27

85. Barrett-Connor E, Orchard T: Diabetes and heart disease. In *Diabetes in America.* NIH Publication 85-1468. Edited by the National Diabetes Data Group. Bethesda, Maryland, National Institutes of Health, 1985, pp XVI-1-41

86. Barrett-Connor EL, Cohn BA, Wingard DL, et al: Why is diabetes mellitus a stronger risk factor for fatal ischemic heart disease in women than in men? The Rancho Bernardo Study. *JAMA* 265:627-631, 1991

87. Manson JE, Colditz GA, Stampfer MJ, et al: A prospective study of obesity and risk of coronary heart disease in women. *N Engl J Med* 322:882-889, 1990

88. Lapidus L, Bengtsson C, Larsson B, et al: Distribution of adipose tissue and risk of cardiovascular disease and death: a 12 year follow up of participants in the population study of women in Gothenburg, Sweden. *Br Med J* 289:1257-1261, 1984

89. Kannel WB, Cupples LA, Ramaswami R, et al: Regional obesity and risk of cardiovascular disease: the Framingham Study. *J Clin Epidemiol* 44:183-190, 1991

90. Folsom AR, Kaye SA, Sellers TA, et al: Body fat distribution and 5-year risk of death in older women. *JAMA* 269:483-487, 1993

91. Ness RB, Harris T, Cobb J, et al: Number of pregnancies and the subsequent risk of cardiovascular disease. *N Engl J Med* 328:1528-1533, 1993

92. Beard CM, Griffin MR, Offord KP, et al: Risk factors for sudden unexpected cardiac death in young women in Rochester, Minnesota, 1960 through 1974. *Mayo Clin Proc* 61:186-191, 1986

93. Colditz GA, Willett WC, Stampfer MJ, et al: A prospective study of age at menarche, parity, age at first birth, and coronary heart disease in women. *Am J Epidemiol* 126:861-870, 1987

94. Croft P, Hannaford PC: Risk factors for acute myocardial infarction in women: evidence from the Royal College of General Practitioners' Oral Contraception Study. *BMJ* 298:165-168, 1989

95. Talbott EO, Kuller LH, Detre K, et al: Reproductive history of women dying of sudden cardiac death: a case-control study. *Int J Epidemiol* 18:589-594, 1989

96. Tracy RE: Sex difference in coronary disease: two opposing views. *J Chronic Dis* 19:1245-1251, 1966

97. Heller RF, Jacobs HS: Coronary heart disease in relation to age, sex, and the menopause. *Br Med J* 1:472-474, 1978

98. Gordon T, Kannel WB, Hjortland MC, et al: Menopause and coronary heart disease. The Framingham Study. *Ann Intern Med* 89:157-161, 1978

99. Barrett-Connor E, Bush TL: Estrogen and coronary heart disease in women. *JAMA* 265:1861-1867, 1991

100. Rosenberg L, Hennekens CH, Rosner B, et al: Early menopause and the risk of myocardial infarction. *Am J Obstet Gynecol* 139:47-51, 1981

101. Colditz GA, Willett WC, Stampfer MJ, et al: Menopause and the risk of coronary heart disease in women. *N Engl J Med* 316:1105-1110, 1987

102. Barrett-Connor E, Bush TL: Estrogen replacement and coronary heart disease. *Cardiovasc Clin* 19:159-172, 1989

103. Mishell DR Jr: Oral contraceptives for women over the age of 35. *Int J Fertil* 36 Suppl 2:55-64, 1991

104. Leaf DA, Bland D, Schaad D, et al: Oral contraceptive use and coronary risk factors in women. *Am J Med Sci* 301:365-368, 1991

105. Godsland IF, Crook D, Simpson R, et al: The effects of different formulations of oral contraceptive agents on lipid and carbohydrate metabolism. *N Engl J Med* 323:1375-1381, 1990

106. Godsland IF, Crook D, Wynn V: Coronary heart disease risk markers in users of low-dose oral contraceptives. *J Reprod Med* 36 Suppl 3:226-237, 1991

107. Smith DC, Prentice R, Thompson DJ, et al: Association of exogenous estrogen and endometrial carcinoma. *N Engl J Med* 293:1164-1167, 1975

108. Ziel HK, Finkle WD: Increased risk of endometrial carcinoma among users of conjugated estrogens. *N Engl J Med* 293:1167-1170, 1975

109. Hong MK, Romm PA, Reagan K, et al: Effects of estrogen replacement therapy on serum lipid values and angiographically defined coronary artery disease in postmenopausal women. *Am J Cardiol* 69:176-178, 1992

110. Stampfer MJ, Colditz GA, Willett WC, et al: Postmenopausal estrogen therapy and cardiovascular disease. Ten-year follow-up from the Nurses' Health Study. *N Engl J Med* 325:756-762, 1991

111. Wolf PH, Madans JH, Finucane FF, et al: Reduction of cardiovascular disease-related mortality among postmenopausal women who use hormones: evidence from a national cohort. *Am J Obstet Gynecol* 164:489-494, 1991

112. Manolio TA, Furberg CD, Shemanski L, et al: Associations of postmenopausal estrogen use with cardiovascular disease and its risk factors in older women: the CHS Collaborative Research Group. *Circulation* 88:2163-2171, 1993

113. Psaty BM, Heckbert SR, Atkins D, et al: A review of the association of estrogens and progestins with cardiovascular disease in postmenopausal women. *Arch Intern Med* 153:1421-1427, 1993

114. Finucane FF, Madans JH, Bush TL, et al: Decreased risk of stroke among postmenopausal hormone users: results from a national cohort. *Arch Intern Med* 153:73-79, 1993

115. Henderson BE, Paganini-Hill A, Ross RK: Decreased mortality in users of estrogen replacement therapy. *Arch Intern Med* 151:75-78, 1991

116. Falkeborn M, Persson I, Terent A, et al: Hormone replacement therapy and the risk of stroke: follow-up of a population-based cohort in Sweden. *Arch Intern Med* 153:1201-1209, 1993

117. Wilson PW, Garrison RJ, Castelli WP: Postmenopausal estrogen use, cigarette smoking, and cardiovascular morbidity in women over 50: the Framingham Study. *N Engl J Med* 313:1038-1043, 1985

118. Nabulsi AA, Folsom AR, White A, et al: Association of hormone-replacement therapy with various cardiovascular risk factors in postmenopausal women: the Atherosclerosis Risk in Communities Study Investigators. *N Engl J Med* 328:1069-1075, 1993

119. Bush TL, Miller VT: Effects of pharmacologic agents used during menopause: impact on lipids and lipoproteins. In *Menopause: Physiology and Pharmacology*. Edited by DR Mishell Jr. Chicago, Year Book Medical Publishers, 1987, pp 187-208

120. Barrett-Connor E, Laakso M: Ischemic heart disease risk in postmenopausal women. Effects of estrogen use on glucose and insulin levels. *Arteriosclerosis* 10:531-534, 1990

121. Bush TL, Barrett-Connor E: Noncontraceptive estrogen use and cardiovascular disease. *Epidemiol Rev* 7:80-104, 1985

122. Lobo RA: Hormones, hormone replacement therapy, and heart disease. In *Cardiovascular Health and Disease in Women.* Edited by PS Douglas. Philadelphia, WB Saunders Company, 1993, pp 153-173

123. Gilligan DM, Quyyumi AA, Cannon RO III: Effects of physiological levels of estrogen on coronary vasomotor function in postmenopausal women. *Circulation* 89:2545-2551, 1994

124. Reis SE, Gloth ST, Blumenthal RS, et al: Ethinyl estradiol acutely attenuates abnormal coronary vasomotor responses to acetylcholine in postmenopausal women. *Circulation* 89:52-60, 1994

125. Gruchow HW, Anderson AJ, Barboriak JJ, et al: Postmenopausal use of estrogen and occlusion of coronary arteries. *Am Heart J* 115:954-963, 1988

126. Loop FD, Golding LR, MacMillan JP, et al: Coronary artery surgery in women compared with men: analyses of risks and long-term results. *J Am Coll Cardiol* 1:383-390, 1983

127. Selzer A, Langston M, Ruggeroli C, et al: Clinical syndrome of variant angina with normal coronary arteriogram. *N Engl J Med* 295:1343-1347, 1976

128. Pasternak RC, Hutter AM Jr, DeSanctis RW, et al: Variant angina: clinical spectrum and results of medical and surgical therapy. *J Thorac Cardiovasc Surg* 78:614-622, 1979

129. Hung J, Chaitman BR, Lam J, et al: Noninvasive diagnostic test choices for the evaluation of coronary artery disease in women: a multivariate comparison of cardiac fluoroscopy, exercise electrocardiography and exercise thallium myocardial perfusion scintigraphy. *J Am Coll Cardiol* 4:8-16, 1984

130. Sketch MH, Mohiuddin SM, Lynch JD, et al: Significant sex differences in the correlation of electrocardiographic exercise testing and coronary arteriograms. *Am J Cardiol* 36:169-173, 1975

131. Melin JA, Wijns W, Vanbutsele RJ, et al: Alternative diagnostic strategies for coronary artery disease in women: demonstration of the usefulness and efficiency of probability analysis. *Circulation* 71:535-542, 1985

132. Detry JM, Kapita BM, Cosyns J, et al: Diagnostic value of history and maximal exercise electrocardiography in men and women suspected of coronary heart disease. *Circulation* 56:756-761, 1977

133. Weiner DA, Ryan TJ, McCabe CH, et al: Exercise stress testing. Correlations among history of angina, ST-segment response and prevalence of coronary-artery disease in the Coronary Artery Surgery Study (CASS). *N Engl J Med* 301:230-235, 1979

134. Barolsky SM, Gilbert CA, Faruqui A, et al: Differences in electrocardiographic response to exercise of women and men: a non-Bayesian factor. *Circulation* 60:1021-1027, 1979

135. Åstrand I: Exercise electrocardiograms recorded twice with an 8-year interval in a group of 204 women and men 48-63 years old. *Acta Med Scand* 178:27-39, 1965

136. Manca C, Dei Cas L, Albertini D, et al: Different prognostic value of exercise electrocardiogram in men and women. *Cardiology* 63:312-319, 1978

137. Guiteras P, Chaitman BR, Waters DD, et al: Diagnostic accuracy of exercise ECG lead systems in clinical subsets of women. *Circulation* 65:1465-1474, 1982

138. Linhart JW, Laws JG, Satinsky JD: Maximum treadmill exercise electrocardiography in female patients. *Circulation* 50:1173-1178, 1974

139. Cumming GR, Dufresne C, Kich L, et al: Exercise electrocardiogram patterns in normal women. *Br Heart J* 35:1055-1061, 1973

140. Profant GR, Early RG, Nilson KL, et al: Responses to maximal exercise in healthy middle-aged women. *J Appl Physiol* 33:595-599, 1972

141. Hlatky MA, Pryor DB, Harrell FE Jr, et al: Factors affecting sensitivity and specificity of exercise electrocardiography: multivariate analysis. *Am J Med* 77:64-71, 1984

142. Osbakken MD: Exercise stress testing in women: diagnostic dilemma. *Cardiovasc Clin* 19:187-203, 1989

143. Allen WH, Aronow WS, Goodman P, et al: Five-year follow-up of maximal treadmill stress test in asymptomatic men and women. *Circulation* 62:522-527, 1980

144. Chaitman BR, Bourassa MG, Davis K, et al: Angiographic prevalence of high-risk coronary artery disease in patient subsets (CASS). *Circulation* 64:360-367, 1981

145. Ilsley C, Canepa-Anson R, Westgate C, et al: Influence of R wave analysis upon diagnostic accuracy of exercise testing in women. *Br Heart J* 48:161-168, 1982

146. Robert AR, Melin JA, Detry JM: Logistic discriminant analysis improves diagnostic accuracy of exercise testing for coronary artery disease in women. *Circulation* 83:1202-1209, 1991

147. Deckers JW, Rensing BJ, Simoons ML, et al: Diagnostic merits of exercise testing in females. *Eur Heart J* 10:543-550, 1989

148. Deckers JW, Rensing BJ, Tijssen JG, et al: A comparison of methods of analysing exercise tests for diagnosis of coronary artery disease. *Br Heart J* 62:438-444, 1989

149. Okin PM, Kligfield P: Identifying coronary artery disease in women by heart rate adjustment of ST-segment depression and improved performance of linear regression over simple averaging method with comparison to standard criteria. *Am J Cardiol* 69:297-302, 1992

150. Friedman TD, Greene AC, Iskandrian AS, et al: Exercise thallium-201 myocardial scintigraphy in women: correlation with coronary arteriography. *Am J Cardiol* 49:1632-1637, 1982

151. Kong BA, Shaw L, Miller D, et al: Comparison of accuracy for detecting coronary artery disease and side-effect profile of dipyridamole thallium-201 myocardial perfusion imaging in women versus men. *Am J Cardiol* 70:168-173, 1992

152. Okada RD, Boucher CA, Strauss HW, et al: Exercise radionuclide imaging approaches to coronary artery disease. *Am J Cardiol* 46:1188-1204, 1980

153. Higginbotham MB, Morris KG, Coleman RE, et al: Sex-related differences in the normal cardiac response to upright exercise. *Circulation* 70:357-366, 1984

154. Sawada SG, Ryan T, Fineberg NS, et al: Exercise echocardiographic detection of coronary artery disease in women. *J Am Coll Cardiol* 14:1440-1447, 1989

155. Sawada SG, Ryan T, Conley MJ, et al: Prognostic value of a normal exercise echocardiogram. *Am Heart J* 120:49-55, 1990

156. Crouse LJ, Harbrecht JJ, Vacek JL, et al: Exercise echocardiography as a screening test for coronary artery disease and correlation with coronary arteriography. *Am J Cardiol* 67:1213-1218, 1991

157. Orencia A, Bailey K, Yawn BP, et al: Effect of gender on long-term outcome of angina pectoris and myocardial infarction/sudden unexpected death. *JAMA* 269:2392-2397, 1993

158. Johansson S, Bergstrand R, Schlossman D, et al: Sex differences

in cardioangiographic findings after myocardial infarction. *Eur Heart J* 5:374-381, 1984

159. Henning R, Lundman T: Swedish Co-operative CCU Study. A study of 2008 patients with acute myocardial infarction from 12 Swedish hospitals with coronary care unit. Part I. A description of the early stage. *Acta Med Scand Suppl* 586:1-64, 1975

160. Solomon CJ, Lee TH, Crook EF, et al: Comparison of clinical presentation of acute myocardial infarction in patients older than 65 years of age to younger patients. The Multicenter Chest Pain Study experience. *Am J Cardiol* 63:772-776, 1989

161. Robinson K, Conroy RM, Mulcahy R, et al: Risk factors and in-hospital course of first episode of myocardial infarction or acute coronary insufficiency in women. *J Am Coll Cardiol* 11:932-936, 1988

162. Puletti M, Sunseri L, Curione M, et al: Acute myocardial infarction: sex-related differences in prognosis. *Am Heart J* 108:63-66, 1984

163. Hendel RC: Myocardial infarction in women. *Cardiology* 77 Suppl 2:41-57, 1990

164. Dellberg M, Held P, Swedberg K, et al: Rupture of the myocardium: occurrence and risk factors. *Br Heart J* 54:11-16, 1985

165. Pohjola-Sintonen S, Muller JE, Stone PH, et al: Ventricular septal and free wall rupture complicating acute myocardial infarction: experience in the Multicenter Investigation of Limitation of Infarct Size. *Am Heart J* 117:809-818, 1989

166. Muller JE, Rude RE, Braunwald E, et al: Myocardial infarct extension: occurrence, outcome and risk factors in the Multicenter Investigation of Limitation of Infarct Size. *Ann Intern Med* 108:1-6, 1988

167. Murdaugh CL, O'Rourke RA: Coronary heart disease in women: special considerations. *Curr Probl Cardiol* 13:79-156, 1988

168. Moro AG, Cohen LS, Roberts WC, et al: Severe mitral regurgitation following acute myocardial infarction and ruptured papillary muscle: hemodynamic findings and results of operative treatment in four patients. *Circulation* 37 Suppl 2:124-132, 1968

169. Greenland P, Reicher-Reiss H, Goldbourt U, et al: In-hospital and 1-year mortality in 1,524 women after myocardial infarction. Comparison with 4,315 men. *Circulation* 83:484-491, 1991

170. Fiebach NH, Viscoli CM, Horwitz RI: Differences between women and men in survival after myocardial infarction. Biology or methodology? *JAMA* 263:1092-1096, 1990

171. Eysmann SB, Douglas PS: Reperfusion and revascularization strategies for coronary artery disease in women. *JAMA* 268:1903-1907, 1992

172. Pagley PR, Yarzebski J, Goldberg R, et al: Gender differences in the treatment of patients with acute myocardial infarction: a multihospital, community-based perspective. *Arch Intern Med* 153:625-629, 1993

173. Maynard C, Althouse R, Cerqueira M, et al: Underutilization of thrombolytic therapy in eligible women with acute myocardial infarction. *Am J Cardiol* 68:529-530, 1991

174. Becker RC: Coronary thrombolysis in women. *Cardiology* 77 Suppl 2:110-123, 1990

175. ISIS-2 (Second International Study of Infarct Survival) Collaborative Group: Randomised trial of intravenous streptokinase, oral aspirin, both, or neither among 17,187 cases of suspected acute myocardial infarction: ISIS-2. *Lancet* 2:349-360, 1988

176. Gruppo Italiano per lo Studio della Streptochinasi nell'Infarto Miocardico (GISSI): Effectiveness of intravenous thrombolytic treatment in acute myocardial infarction. *Lancet* 1:397-402, 1986

177. Gruppo Italiano per lo Studio della Streptochinasi nell'Infarto Miocardico (GISSI): Long-term effects of intravenous thrombolysis in acute myocardial infarction: final report of the GISSI study. *Lancet* 2:871-874, 1987

178. Wilcox RG, von der Lippe G, Olsson CG, et al: Trial of tissue plasminogen activator for mortality reduction in acute myocardial infarction. Anglo-Scandinavian Study of Early Thrombolysis (ASSET). *Lancet* 2:525-530, 1988

179. European Working Party: Streptokinase in recent myocardial infarction: a controlled multicentre trial. *Br Med J* 3:325-331, 1971

180. Kennedy JW, Ritchie JL, Davis KB, et al: The Western Washington Randomized Trial of Intracoronary Streptokinase in Acute Myocardial Infarction. A 12-month follow-up report. *N Engl J Med* 312:1073-1078, 1985

181. Kennedy JW, Martin GV, David KB, et al: The Western Washington Intravenous Streptokinase in Acute Myocardial Infarction Randomized Trial. *Circulation* 77:345-352, 1988

182. White HD, Barbash GI, Modan M, et al: After correcting for worse baseline characteristics, women treated with thrombolytic therapy for acute myocardial infarction have the same mortality and morbidity as men except for a higher incidence of hemorrhagic stroke: the Investigators of the International Tissue Plasminogen Activator/Streptokinase Mortality Study. *Circulation* 88:2097-2103, 1993

183. Bovill EG, Terrin ML, Stump DC, et al: Hemorrhagic events during therapy with recombinant tissue-type plasminogen activator, heparin, and aspirin for acute myocardial infarction. Results of the Thrombolysis in Myocardial Infarction (TIMI), Phase II Trial. *Ann Intern Med* 115:256-265, 1991

184. Maggioni AP, Franzosi MG, Santoro E, et al: The risk of stroke in patients with acute myocardial infarction after thrombolytic and antithrombotic treatment. Gruppo Italiano per lo Studio della Sopravvivenza nell'Infarto Miocardico II (GISSI-2), and the International Study Group. *N Engl J Med* 327:1-6, 1992

185. Kimmelstiel C, Goldberg RJ: Congestive heart failure in women: focus on heart failure due to coronary artery disease and diabetes. *Cardiology* 77 Suppl 2:71-79, 1990

186. Kannel WB, Savage D, Castelli WP: Cardiac failure in the Framingham Study: twenty-year follow-up. In *Congestive Heart Failure: Current Research and Clinical Applications.* Edited by E Braunwald, MB Mock, JT Watson. New York, Grune & Stratton, 1982, pp 15-30

187. McKee PA, Castelli WP, McNamara PM, et al: The natural history of congestive heart failure: The Framingham Study. *N Engl J Med* 285:1441-1446, 1971

188. Ho KKL, Anderson KM, Kannel WB, et al: Survival after the onset of congestive heart failure in Framingham Heart Study subjects. *Circulation* 88:107-115, 1993

189. The CONSENSUS Trial Study Group: Effects of enalapril on mortality in severe congestive heart failure: results of the Cooperative North Scandinavian Enalapril Survival Study (CONSENSUS). *N Engl J Med* 316:1429-1435, 1987

190. Pfeffer MA, Braunwald E, Moye LA, et al: Effect of captopril on mortality and morbidity in patients with left ventricular dysfunction after myocardial infarction. Results of the Survival and Ventricular Enlargement trial. *N Engl J Med* 327:669-677, 1992

191. Swedberg K, Held P, Kjekshus J, et al: Effects of the early administration of enalapril on mortality in patients with acute myocardial infarction. Results of the Cooperative New Scandinavian Enalapril Survival Study II (CONSENSUS II). *N Engl J Med* 327:678-684, 1992

192. The SOLVD Investigators: Effect of enalapril on mortality and the development of heart failure in asymptomatic patients with reduced left ventricular ejection fractions. *N Engl J Med* 327:685-691, 1992

193. Wenger NK, Speroff L, Packard B: Cardiovascular health and disease in women. *N Engl J Med* 329:247-256, 1993

194. Kelsey SF, James M, Holubkov AL, et al: Results of percutaneous transluminal coronary angioplasty in women. 1985-1986 National Heart, Lung, and Blood Institute's Coronary Angioplasty Registry. *Circulation* 87:720-727, 1993

195. Kahn JK, Rutherford BD, McConahay DR, et al: Comparison of procedural results and risks of coronary angioplasty in men and women for conditions other than acute myocardial infarction. *Am J Cardiol* 69:1241-1242, 1992

196. Bell MR, Holmes DR Jr, Berger PB, et al: The changing in-hospital mortality of women undergoing percutaneous transluminal coronary angioplasty. *JAMA* 269:2091-2095, 1993

197. Cowley MJ, Mullin SM, Kelsey SF, et al: Sex differences in early and long-term results of coronary angioplasty in the NHLBI PTCA Registry. *Circulation* 71:90-97, 1985

198. Lorell BH, McCabe CH, Sipperly ME, et al: Women and PTCA: no feminine mystique (abstract). *Circulation* 76 Suppl 4:400, 1987

199. Detre KM, Myler RK, Kelsey SF, et al: Baseline characteristics of patients in the National Heart, Lung, and Blood Institute Percutaneous Transluminal Coronary Angioplasty Registry. *Am J Cardiol* 53:7C-11C, 1984

200. McEniery PT, Hollman J, Knezinek V, et al: Comparative safety and efficacy of percutaneous transluminal coronary angioplasty in men and women. *Cathet Cardiovasc Diagn* 13:364-371, 1987

201. Detre K, Holubkov R, Kelsey S, et al: Percutaneous transluminal coronary angioplasty in 1985-1986 and 1977-1981. The National Heart, Lung, and Blood Institute Registry. *N Engl J Med* 318:265-270, 1988

202. Savage MP, Goldberg S, Hirshfeld JW, et al: Clinical and angiographic determinants of primary coronary angioplasty success. M-HEART investigators. *J Am Coll Cardiol* 17:22-28, 1991

203. Ellis SG, Roubin GS, King SB III, et al: In-hospital cardiac mortality after acute closure after coronary angioplasty: analysis of risk factors from 8,207 procedures. *J Am Coll Cardiol* 11:211-216, 1988

204. Stone GW, Rutherford BD, McConahay DR, et al: Procedural outcome of angioplasty for total coronary artery occlusion: an analysis of 971 lesions in 905 patients. *J Am Coll Cardiol* 15:849-856, 1990

205. Ellis SG, Roubin GS, King SB III, et al: Angiographic and clinical predictors of acute closure after native vessel coronary angioplasty. *Circulation* 77:372-379, 1988

206. Holmes DR Jr, Holubkov R, Vlietstra RE, et al: Comparison of complications during percutaneous transluminal coronary angioplasty from 1977 to 1981 and from 1985 to 1986: the National Heart, Lung, and Blood Institute Percutaneous Transluminal Coronary Angioplasty Registry. *J Am Coll Cardiol* 12:1149-1155, 1988

207. Simpfendorfer C, Dorosti K, Franco I, et al: Risk factors for in-hospital mortality associated with coronary angioplasty. *Cleve Clin J Med* 58:25-27, 1991

208. Califf RM, Ohman EM, Frid DJ, et al: Restenosis: The clinical issues. In *Textbook of Interventional Cardiology.* Edited by EJ Topol. Philadelphia, WB Saunders Company, 1990, pp 363-394

209. Califf RM, Fortin DF, Frid DJ, et al: Restenosis after coronary angioplasty: an overview. *J Am Coll Cardiol* 17 Suppl B:2-13, 1991

210. Bobbio M, Detrano R, Colombo A, et al: Restenosis rate after percutaneous transluminal coronary angioplasty: a literature overview. *J Invasive Cardiol* 3:214-224, 1991

211. Weintraub WS, Ghazzal ZMB, Douglas JS Jr, et al: Long-term clinical follow-up in patients with angiographic restudy after successful angioplasty. *Circulation* 87:831-840, 1993

212. Hollman J, Badhwar K, Beck CJ, et al: Risk factors for recurrent stenosis following successful coronary angioplasty. *Cleve Clin J Med* 56:517-523, 1989

213. Casale PN, Whitlow PL, Franco I, et al: Women have a higher major complication rate with new devices for percutaneous coronary revascularization (abstract). *J Am Coll Cardiol* 19 Suppl A:94, 1992

214. Carrozza JP Jr, Kuntz RE, Levine MJ, et al: Angiographic and clinical outcome of intracoronary stenting: immediate and long-term results from a large single-center experience. *J Am Coll Cardiol* 20:328-337, 1992

215. Hannan EL, Bernard HR, Kilburn HC Jr, et al: Gender differences in mortality rates for coronary artery bypass surgery. *Am Heart J* 123:866-872, 1992

216. Bickell NA, Pieper KS, Lee KL, et al: Referral patterns for coronary artery disease treatment: gender bias or good clinical judgment? *Ann Intern Med* 116:791-797, 1992

217. Tyras DH, Barner HB, Kaiser GC, et al: Myocardial revascularization in women. *Ann Thorac Surg* 25:449-453, 1978

218. Douglas JS Jr, King SB III, Jones EL, et al: Reduced efficacy of coronary bypass surgery in women. *Circulation* 64 Suppl 2:11-16, 1981

219. Eaker ED, Kronmal R, Kennedy JW, et al: Comparison of the long-term, postsurgical survival of women and men in the Coronary Artery Surgery Study (CASS). *Am Heart J* 117:71-81, 1989

220. Fisher LD, Kennedy JW, Davis KB, et al: Association of sex, physical size, and operative mortality after coronary artery bypass in the Coronary Artery Surgery Study (CASS). *J Thorac Cardiovasc Surg* 84:334-341, 1982

221. O'Connor GT, Morton JR, Diehl MJ, et al: Differences between men and women in hospital mortality associated with coronary artery bypass graft surgery. *Circulation* 88:2104-2110, 1993

222. Khan SS, Nessim S, Gray R, et al: Increased mortality of women in coronary artery bypass surgery: evidence for referral bias. *Ann Intern Med* 112:561-567, 1990

223. Chesebro JH, Clements IP, Fuster V, et al: A platelet-inhibitor-drug trial in coronary-artery bypass operations. Benefit of perioperative dipyridamole and aspirin therapy on early postoperative vein-graft patency. *N Engl J Med* 307:73-78, 1982

224. Loop FD, Irarrazaval MJ, Bredee JJ, et al: Internal mammary artery graft for ischemic heart disease. Effect of revascularization on clinical status and survival. *Am J Cardiol* 39:516-522, 1977

225. Loop FD, Lytle BW, Cosgrove DM, et al: Influence of the internal-mammary-artery graft on 10-year survival and other cardiac events. *N Engl J Med* 314:1-6, 1986

226. Myers WO, Davis K, Foster ED, et al: Surgical survival in the Coronary Artery Surgery Study (CASS) Registry. Presented at the 31st annual meeting of the Southern Thoracic Surgical Association, Hilton Head Island, South Carolina, November 1 to 3, 1984

227. Gardner TJ, Horneffer PJ, Gott VL, et al: Coronary artery bypass grafting in women. A ten-year perspective. Presented at the 96th annual meeting of the Southern Surgical Association, Palm Beach, Florida, December 3 to 5, 1984

228. Bolooki H, Vargas A, Green R, et al: Results of direct coronary artery surgery in women. *J Thorac Cardiovasc Surg* 69:271-277, 1975

229. Killen DA, Reed WA, Arnold M, et al: Coronary artery bypass in women: long-term survival. *Ann Thorac Surg* 34:559-563, 1982

230. Laird-Meeter K, Penn OC, Haalebos MM, et al: Survival in 1041 patients with consecutive aorto-coronary bypass operations. *Eur Heart J* 5:35-42, 1984

231. Kennedy JW, Kaiser GC, Fisher LD, et al: Multivariate discriminant analysis of the clinical and angiographic predictors of operative mortality from the Collaborative Study in Coronary Artery Surgery (CASS). *J Thorac Cardiovasc Surg* 80:876-887, 1980

232. Hall RJ, Elayda MA, Gray A, et al: Coronary artery bypass: long-term follow-up of 22,284 consecutive patients. *Circulation* 68 Suppl 2:20-25, 1983

233. Loop FD, Lytle BW, Cosgrove DM, et al: Coronary artery bypass graft surgery in the elderly. Indications and outcome. *Cleve Clin J Med* 55:23-34, 1988

234. Gersh BJ, Kronmal RA, Schaff HV, et al: Long-term (5-year) results of coronary bypass surgery in patients 65 years old or older: a report from the Coronary Artery Surgery Study. *Circulation* 68 Suppl 2:190-199, 1983

235. Jeffery DL, Vijayanagar RR, Bognolo DA, et al: Results of coronary bypass surgery in elderly women. *Ann Thorac Surg* 42:550-553, 1986

236. Miller DC, Stinson EB, Oyer PE, et al: Discriminant analysis of the changing risks of coronary artery operations: 1971-1979. *J Thorac Cardiovasc Surg* 85:197-213, 1983

237. Johnson WD, Kayser KL, Pedraza PM: Angina pectoris and coronary bypass surgery: patterns of prevalence and recurrence in 3105 consecutive patients followed up to 11 years. *Am Heart J* 108:1190-1197, 1984

238. Richardson JV, Cyrus RJ: Reduced efficacy of coronary artery bypass grafting in women. *Ann Thorac Surg* 42 Suppl 6:16-21, 1986

239. Golding LR, Groves LK: Results of coronary artery surgery in women. *Cleve Clin Q* 43:113-115, 1976

240. Eysmann SB, Douglas PS: Coronary heart disease: therapeutic principles. In *Cardiovascular Health and Disease in Women.* Edited by PS Douglas. Philadelphia, WB Saunders Company, 1993, pp 43-61

241. Tobin JN, Wassertheil-Smoller S, Wexler JP, et al: Sex bias in considering coronary bypass surgery. *Ann Intern Med* 107:19-25, 1987

242. Ayanian JZ, Epstein AM: Differences in the use of procedures between women and men hospitalized for coronary artery disease. *N Engl J Med* 325:221-225, 1991

243. Steingart RM, Packer M, Hamm P, et al: Sex differences in the management of coronary artery disease. *N Engl J Med* 325:226-230, 1991

244. Krumholz HM, Douglas PS, Lauer MS, et al: Selection of patients for coronary angiography and coronary revascularization early after myocardial infarction: Is there evidence for a gender bias? *Ann Intern Med* 116:785-790, 1992

245. Eaker ED, Chesebro JH, Sacks FM, et al: Cardiovascular disease in women. *Circulation* 88:1999-2009, 1993

246. Douglas PS, Clarkson TB, Flowers NC, et al: Exercise and atherosclerotic heart disease in women. *Med Sci Sports Exerc* 24 Suppl:266-276, 1992

247. O'Toole ML: Exercise and physical activity. In *Cardiovascular Health and Disease in Women.* Edited by PS Douglas. Philadelphia, WB Saunders Company, 1993, pp 253-267

248. Manson JE, Stampfer MJ, Colditz GA, et al: A prospective study of aspirin use and primary prevention of cardiovascular disease in women. *JAMA* 266:521-527, 1991

249. Wikstrand J, Berglund G, Tuomilehto J: β-blockade in the primary prevention of coronary heart disease in hypertensive patients. Review of present evidence. *Circulation* 84 Suppl 6:93-100, 1991

250. Kane JP, Malloy MJ, Ports TA, et al: Regression of coronary atherosclerosis during treatment of familial hypercholesterolemia with combined drug regimens. *JAMA* 264:3007-3012, 1990

251. Ornish D, Brown SE, Scherwitz LW, et al: Can lifestyle changes reverse coronary heart disease? The Lifestyle Heart Trial. *Lancet* 336:129-133, 1990

252. May GS, Eberlein KA, Furberg CD, et al: Secondary prevention after myocardial infarction: a review of long-term trials. *Prog Cardiovasc Dis* 24:331-352, 1982

253. O'Connor GT, Buring JE, Yusuf S, et al: An overview of randomized trials of rehabilitation with exercise after myocardial infarction. *Circulation* 80:234-244, 1989

254. Weksler BB: Hemostasis and thrombosis. In *Cardiovascular Health and Disease in Women.* Edited by PS Douglas. Philadelphia, WB Saunders Company, 1993, pp 231-251

255. β-Blocker Heart Trial Research Group: A randomized trial of propranolol in patients with acute myocardial infarction. I. Mortality results. *JAMA* 247:1707-1714, 1982

256. β-Blocker Heart Trial Research Group: A randomized trial of propranolol in patients with acute myocardial infarction. II. Morbidity results. *JAMA* 250:2814-2819, 1983

257. Furberg CD, Friedman LM, MacMahon SW: Women as participants in trial of the primary and secondary prevention of cardiovascular disease: Part II. Secondary prevention: the beta-blocker heart attack trial and the aspirin myocardial infarction study. In *Coronary Artery Disease in Women.* Edited by ED Eaker, B Packard, NK Wenger, et al. New York, Haymarket-Doyma, 1987, pp 241-246

258. Grady D, Rubin SM, Petitti DB, et al: Hormone therapy to prevent disease and prolong life in postmenopausal women. *Ann Intern Med* 117:1016-1037, 1992

259. American College of Physicians: Guidelines for counseling postmenopausal women about preventive hormone therapy. *Ann Intern Med* 117:1038-1041, 1992

CHAPTER

66

Pharmacologic considerations in the use of cardiovascular drugs

Craig N. Mattson, R.Ph., M.S., M.B.A., and Michael D. McGoon, M.D.

RATIONAL drug therapy is guided by the principles of pharmacokinetics and pharmacodynamics. Optimization of drug therapy is accomplished by minimizing the probability of toxicity without compromising efficacy or by maximizing the probability of efficacy without unacceptable toxicity.

Pharmacokinetics has been described as "what the body does to the drug."[1] Pharmacodynamics is "what the drug does to the body" (Fig 66-1).

The pharmacologic effect of a drug results from an interaction of the drug and its physiologic receptor. Drug receptor sites are for the most part impossible to measure or monitor clinically. However, drug concentrations can be measured in the blood or plasma, urine, saliva, and other easily sampled body fluids. For many drugs, there is frequently a constant dynamic equilibrium between receptor site concentration and serum concentration, resulting in a strong correlation (often linear) between the plasma drug concentration and the pharmacologic effect.

Pharmacokinetic calculations are not necessary for all drugs, especially those with significant differences between therapeutic and toxic serum concentrations. In practice, these drugs can be given in sufficient doses to ensure "therapeutic concentrations" without undue concern about potential toxicities. Measuring serum levels of these types of drugs might be useful if there is a question of noncompliance or malabsorption.

Drugs that may be toxic at dosages or serum concentrations near those required to achieve the optimal therapeutic effect are commonly monitored (Table 66-1). These drugs, best characterized as having a narrow "therapeutic range," require relatively precise dosage scheduling. The therapeutic range is defined as the range of drug concentrations within which the probability of the desired clinical response is relatively high and the probability of unacceptable toxicity is relatively low (Fig 66-2). For drugs with a narrow therapeutic range, pharmacokinetic principles can improve the quality of an individual dosage prediction.

PHARMACOKINETIC MODELS

Most pharmacokinetic drug calculations use the one-compartment model, in which body tissues and fluids are

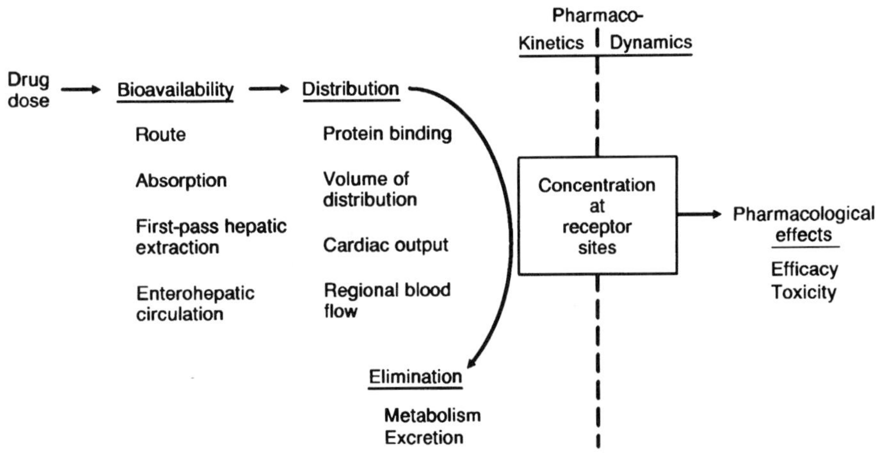

Fig 66-1 Interrelationship of pharmacokinetic and pharmacodynamic considerations.

Table 66-1 Usefulness of monitoring drug concentration

Therapeutic drug monitoring is useful when
1. A good correlation exists between the pharmacologic response (i.e., therapeutic or toxic) and the plasma concentration.
2. Wide intersubject variation in drug plasma levels results from a given dose, i.e., for individualizing therapy.
3. The drug has a narrow therapeutic range.
4. The potential exists for drug-drug or drug-food interactions.
5. Compliance is uncertain.

Therapeutic drug monitoring is limited when
1. There is no well-defined therapeutic plasma concentration (e.g., propranolol).
2. The parent compound is metabolized to pharmacologically active metabolites (e.g, propafenone).
3. Toxic effects may occur at unexpectedly low drug concentrations as well as at high concentrations.
4. Therapeutic response is best measured by a clinical variable rather than the serum level of the drug, e.g., blood pressure response to a calcium channel blocker.

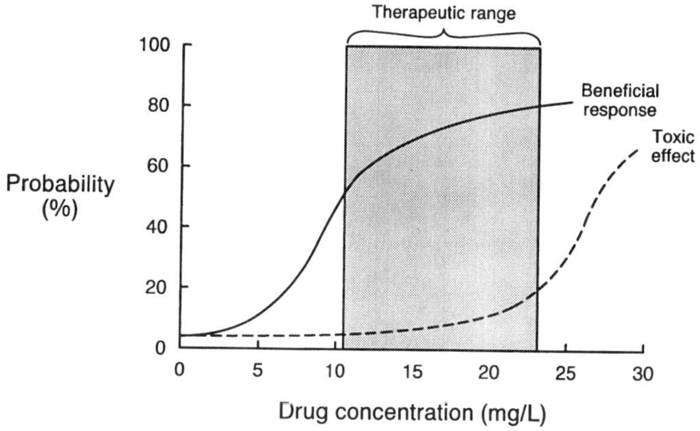

Fig 66-2 The probability of the desired therapeutic effect is very low when the drug concentration is low. The probability of toxicity is also very low. As the drug concentration increases between 5 and 20 mg/L, the probability of a therapeutic response increases from less than 10% to about 80% and then plateaus. Over this concentration range, the probability of toxicity increases more slowly (≤5% to only about 10%). The probability of toxicity increases more rapidly as the concentration exceeds 20 mg/L. The "therapeutic range" would be 10 to 20 mg/L, with up to 50% of patients having a response at a drug concentration of 10 mg/L. Increasing the drug concentration to 20 mg/L would increase the probability of response to 80% while increasing the probability of toxicity to only 10%.

considered to be a single compartment. The assumption is made that when a dose of a drug is administered, it is distributed instantaneously to all parts of the body.

The pharmacokinetic behavior of some drugs, e.g., digoxin and lidocaine, does not fit this model and is more accurately described by a two-compartment model. In a two-compartment model, the drug is rapidly distributed to the central compartment and then more slowly distributed to the peripheral compartment. The half-time for the distribution phase is the alpha (α) half-life, and the time for drug elimination from the body is the beta (β) half-life (Fig 66-3). The drug is distributed between the two compartments to maintain equilibrium (Fig 66-4).

The volume of distribution is an indicator of the extent of drug distribution into body fluids and tissues. It is an important factor in determining proper drug dosing regimens. The size of the volume of distribution dictates the size of the dose necessary to achieve the target concentration. A large volume of distribution usually indicates that a large portion of the administered drug permeates the peripheral compartment (e.g., amiodarone).

When a drug has extensive tissue distribution, the volume of distribution calculated from plasma concentrations is much higher than any conceivable volume in the body. Since the volume of distribution for digoxin is large (at approximately 7 L/kg in an adult), it can be concluded that digoxin is extensively bound outside the plasma, especially in muscle tissue. For other drugs, tissue concentrations may not be as great as the plasma concentration, so that it may appear that these drugs are distributed in a relatively small volume.

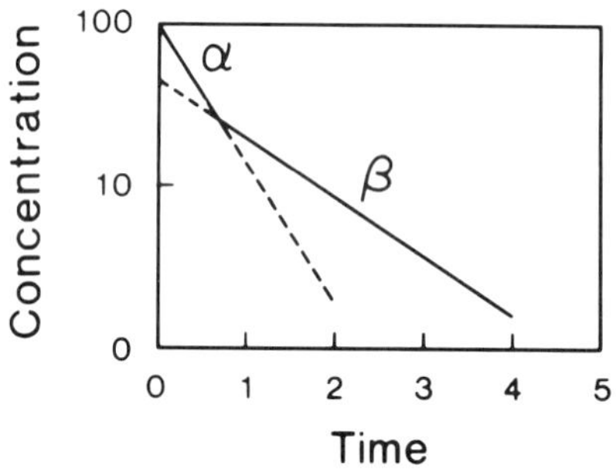

Fig 66-3 Decreasing plasma concentration reflects drug distribution during the alpha (α) phase and drug elimination during the beta (β) phase.

Knowing the volume of distribution (Vd) of a specific drug and what plasma drug concentration (Cp) is correlated with the therapeutic range, one can calculate the loading dose that results in the desired Cp by the following formula.

$$\text{Loading dose} = \frac{(\text{Vd})(\text{Cp})}{\text{F}}$$

in which F is the fraction of the administered dose that reaches the systemic circulation.

For calculation of the loading dose of digoxin required to produce a plasma concentration of 1.5 μg/L in a 70-kg patient, the following information is used. The Vd of

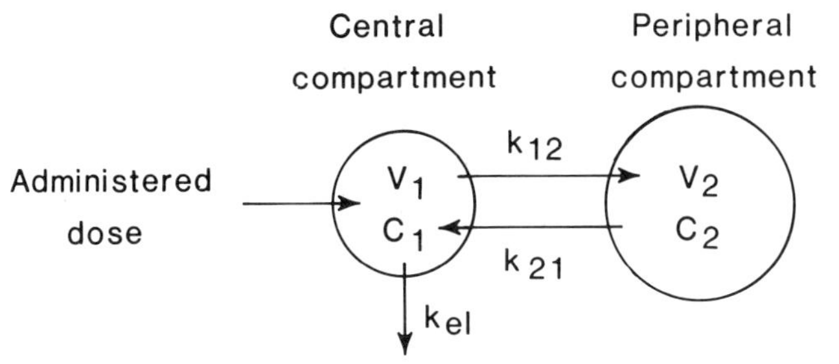

Fig 66-4 Two-compartment model. The drug enters and is eliminated from the central compartment, and it is distributed to and from the peripheral compartment. V_1 and V_2 represent the apparent volumes of, and C_1 and C_2 the drug concentrations in, the central and peripheral compartments; k_{12} and k_{21} are the first-order rate constants for transfer of drug between the two compartments; and k_{el} is the rate constant for elimination. (From Bresnahan JF, Vlietstra RE: Series on pharmacology in practice. 3. Digitalis glycosides. *Mayo Clin Proc* 54:675-684, 1979. By permission, Mayo Foundation.)

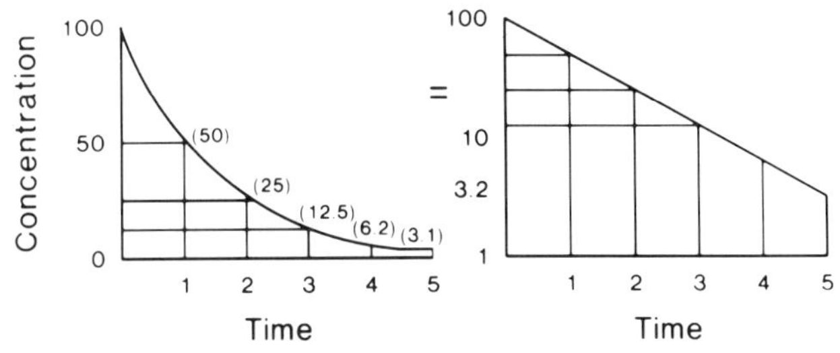

Fig 66-5 First-order elimination kinetics. The concentration of drug decreases logarithmically with time because a constant fraction of drug is eliminated per unit of time. The concentration-time curve is linear when plotted semilogarithmically (*right side*).

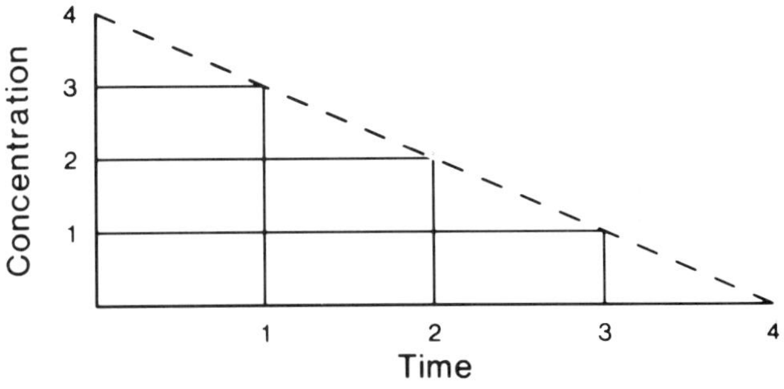

Fig 66-6 Zero-order elimination kinetics. The concentration of drug decreases linearly with time because a constant amount of drug is eliminated per unit of time. This situation applies when a metabolic mechanism is saturated.

digoxin is approximately 7 L/kg, or 490 L for a 70-kg person (7 L/kg × 70 kg = 490 L). The F for digoxin tablets is 0.7. The calculated loading dose is as follows:

$$\text{Loading dose} = \frac{(\text{Vd})(\text{Cp})}{\text{F}} = \frac{(490\text{L})(1.5\ \mu\text{g/L})}{\text{F}} = 1{,}050\ \mu\text{g}$$

This formula can be modified to calculate a loading dose that will produce a different concentration (Cp desired) for a patient already receiving digoxin with a known steady-state concentration (Cp observed).

$$\text{Loading dose} = \frac{(\text{Vd})(\text{Cp desired - Cp observed})}{\text{F}}$$

For example, if the trough steady-state digoxin value is 1.0 μg/L and a 1.5-μg/L level is desired, the additional loading dose is as follows:

$$\text{Loading dose} = \frac{(490)(1.5\ \mu\text{g/L} - 1\ \mu\text{g/L})}{0.7} = 350\ \mu\text{g}$$

DRUG KINETICS

Movement of most drugs into, between, and out of compartments proceeds at rates proportional to the concentration of the drug. This behavior is said to follow first-order kinetics; that is, the rate of drug movement out of a compartment is a function of the first power of the concentration of the drug in the compartment. With first-order kinetics, the fraction of the drug removed from the compartment per unit of time is constant (Fig 66-5). In zero-order kinetics, elimination of the drug from the compartment is a function of concentration to the zero power; the amount of drug removed per unit of time is constant (Fig 66-6). Zero-order kinetics describes the elimination of some drugs (e.g., phenytoin) that undergo biotransformation by mechanisms that easily become saturated.

Another factor that influences the distribution of drugs is binding to proteins, primarily albumin, α_1-acid glycoprotein (AAG), and lipoproteins. Most anionic drugs and weak acids are bound to albumin. Many cationic drugs, e.g., lidocaine, and neutral drugs bind principally to AAG in addition to albumin.

Although only the unbound portion of drug exerts a pharmacologic effect, most drug assays measure total drug concentration--both bound and unbound. Therefore, changes in the binding characteristics of a drug could affect the pharmacologic response to the drug. AAG is an acute phase reactant and may increase as many as four or five times during stress or trauma, e.g., myocardial infarction. As a result, drugs highly bound to AAG (such as quinidine, disopyramide, propranolol, and lidocaine) may have a significant decrease in their unbound fraction.

Only in the case of highly bound drugs, i.e., 80% to 90%, is the change in binding of therapeutic importance. Warfarin, salicylates, and phenytoin are highly bound drugs in which changes in proteins or the binding characteristics of the drugs may have clinical significance.

ELIMINATION

Drug biotransformation generally involves conversion in the liver of the parent compound into water-soluble metabolites that are ionized at physiologic pH and are excreted, usually by the kidneys. The liver may remove a drug from the systemic circulation or from the splanchnic circulation on the first passage of the drug through the liver before it reaches the systemic circulation.

Hepatic disease may adversely affect the elimination of drugs metabolized primarily by the liver. Drugs may also adversely affect metabolizing enzymes. For example, cimetidine reversibly inhibits cytochrome P-450, and rifampin induces hepatic metabolism.

An initial dosing guideline in patients with cirrhosis or chronic active hepatitis may be to start with one-half the usual dose of an oxidatively metabolized drug. First-pass metabolism may not occur in patients with cirrhosis or a portacaval shunt.

Regional clearance (by the liver or kidney) is a function of perfusion of the organ, proportion of free drug to bound drug in the blood, and intrinsic capability of the organ to clear unbound drug. For the kidney, creatinine clearance is a reasonable index of drug elimination; digoxin renal clearance, for example, is linearly related to creatinine clearance. Creatinine clearance can be determined directly:

$$Cl_{cr} = \frac{U_{cr}V}{C_{cr}}$$

in which Cl_{cr} is creatinine clearance, U_{cr} and C_{cr} are the urinary and plasma concentrations of creatinine, respectively, and V is the volume of urine per unit of time.

Creatinine clearance can be estimated as follows:[2]

$$Cl_{cr}\ (\text{mL/min})\ \text{for males} = \frac{(140 - \text{age})W}{72\ Cl_{cr}}$$

$$Cl_{cr}\ (\text{mL/min})\ \text{for females} = Cl_{cr}\ \text{for males} \times 0.85$$

in which W is patient weight in kilograms and age is in years.

Total body clearance refers to the removal of drug from plasma and correlates with the rate at which the drug is administered and eliminated to the resulting plasma concentrations. Clearance (Cl) and volume of distribution (Vd) of the drug determine the rate of drug removal (Kd) from the body. This can be expressed as

$$Kd = \frac{Cl}{Vd}$$

The elimination rate constant (Kd) represents the fraction of drug removed per unit of time and is expressed in units of reciprocal time (e.g., minute^{-1} or hour^{-1}). For example, Kd = 0.25/hr means that the body is removing 25% of the drug every hour. The total clearance of a drug from the body is a composite of clearance by mechanisms such as biotransformation, renal excretion, and biliary excretion.

When the clearance of a drug is known, the maintenance dose required to sustain an average steady-state plasma concentration can be calculated as follows:

$$\text{Maintenance dose} = \frac{(Cl)(Cpss)(\tau)}{F}$$

in which Cpss is the desired average plasma concentration at steady state, τ (tau) is the dosing interval, and F is the fraction of the dose that reaches the systemic circulation.

The half-life is the time necessary for the concentration of drug in the plasma to decrease by one-half after a first-order elimination process. A drug's half-life is important in determining when a drug will be at steady state on a constant dosage regimen. In most clinical situations, steady-state conditions can be assumed after four half-lives. Drug elimination can also be described by half-life ($T_{1/2}$), which is related to the calculation of clearance by

$$T_{1/2} = \frac{0.693\ Vd}{Cl}\ \text{or}\ \frac{0.693}{Kd}$$

BIOAVAILABILITY

The term "bioavailability" refers to the fraction (F) of the drug dose that reaches the systemic circulation. This concept is important, because only the portion of the drug that gains access to the systemic circulation (a component of the central compartment) has an opportunity to reach the receptor sites and exert a pharmacologic effect. Bioavailability depends on several variables: route of administration, completeness of absorption, and extent of extraction or metabolism between the site of absorption and the systemic circulation (Table 66-2).

Because intravenous injection of a drug places the entire dose directly into the systemic circulation, bioavailability is considered to be 100%; hence, F = 1. The

Table 66-2 Determinants of bioavailability

Route of administration
Intravenous
Buccal
Transdermal
Swallowed
Gastric
Intestinal
Rectal
Absorption
Drug formulation
Solubility
Stability
Metabolism in gastrointestinal tract
Destruction by intestinal organism
Surface area of absorbing mucosa
Binding within gastrointestinal tract
Competitive presence of food
Rate of stomach emptying
Intestinal blood flow
Extraction
First-pass hepatic elimination
"Enterohepatic circulation"

Table 66-3 Selected cardiac drug interactions*

Drug	Interacting drug	Outcome and recommendations
Warfarin	Anabolic steroids	Increased anticoagulant response, usually in first week.
	Bile acid sequestrants	Reduced anticoagulant response due to binding in gastrointestinal tract. Optimal dosage separation by at least 6 hours.
	Enzyme inducers (barbiturates, phenytoin, primidone, rifampin, etc.)	Reduced anticoagulant response over 1 to 2 weeks. Important to reduce warfarin dosage if enzyme inducer is discontinued.
	Enzyme inhibitors (allopurinol, amiodarone, cimetidine, ciprofloxacin, fluconazole, trimethoprim-sulfamethoxazole, etc.)	Increased anticoagulant response, usually in first week. Generally, decrease warfarin dosage and follow prothrombin time more closely.
	Gemfibrozil	Increased anticoagulant response in first few days. Increase may continue for 2 weeks. Interindividual variation. Unknown mechanism.
	NSAIDs	Increased anticoagulant response, usually after 1 to 2 days.
	Salicylates (aspirin, choline magnesium trisalicylate, etc.)	May increase risk of bleeding because of platelet function inhibition. Large doses may increase anticoagulant response.
	Thyroid hormones	Gradual increase in anticoagulant response over 2 to 3 weeks.
Calcium channel blockers: nefedipine, verapamil	Rifampin	Reduction in blood levels over 3 to 5 days. May need to increase dose of calcium channel blocker.
Clonidine	Tricyclic antidepressants	Inhibition of antihypertensive response, usually after 1 week. May increase rebound hypertension after withdrawal of clonidine.
Cyclosporine	Enzyme inducers (barbiturates, phenytoin, rifampin, etc.)	Marked decrease in cyclosporine levels over several days. Increase cyclosporine dose by 50% or more.
	Enzyme inhibitors (anabolic steroids, diltiazem, erythromycin, ketoconazole, nicardipine, verapamil, etc.)	Marked increase in cyclosporine levels over 3 to 5 days. Decrease cyclosporine dose by 50% or more.
Digoxin	Calcium channel blockers (bepridil, diltiazem, verapamil)	Increase in digoxin levels of 50% to 70%. Maximal effect in 5 to 7 days. May require digoxin dose reduction of 25% to 50%.
	Quinidine	Increase in digoxin levels of 50%. Maximal effect in 5 to 7 days may require digoxin dose reduction of 25% to 50%.
	Amiodarone	Increase in digoxin levels of up to 200%. Maximal effect may be over weeks. Digoxin dose reduction of 25% to 50% or more.
Potassium-sparing diuretics: amiloride, spironolactone, triamterene	ACE inhibitors (captopril, enalapril, lisinopril, etc.)	Additive potassium-retaining effects may result in hyperkalemia in predisposed patients.
	Potassium	Increased potassium levels over several days. Decrease potassium supplementation.
Quinidine	Enzyme inducers (phenobarbital, phenytoin, rifampin, etc.)	Quinidine levels gradually decrease over a week or more. May need to increase quinidine dose. If enzyme inducer is discontinued, may need to decrease quinidine.

*Not including interactions of drugs with alcohol, food, or smoking.

bioavailability of drugs given by other routes is defined as the ratio of the amount that gains access to the systemic circulation to the amount that gains access when the same dose is administered intravenously.

PHARMACODYNAMICS

Pharmacodynamics is the study of the body's response to a drug. The relationship between the drug concentration and the pharmacologic response depends on the mechanism by which the drug exerts its effect. Some drugs exert their effects by binding directly to a specific receptor, for example, α- and β-adrenergic blockers. For other drugs, the effect is indirect. For example, warfarin blocks the synthesis of vitamin K-dependent clotting factors but has no effect on the degradation of these clotting factors, which ultimately determines the onset of warfarin's activity. Although most pharmacologic effects are reversible, some effects of drugs on cells are irreversible, such as those of bactericidal antibiotics and antineoplastic agents.

A decrease in cardiac output affects drug absorption, distribution, and elimination. In cardiac failure and shock, regional perfusion is shifted to favor cerebral and cardiac flow at the expense of muscle, splanchnic, and renal flow. Decreased mesenteric flow and the presence of intestinal mucosal edema decrease the rate of absorption of orally administered drugs. Perfusion redistribution may significantly limit the rate and extent of drug distribution into the peripheral compartment (such as skeletal muscle), thereby decreasing the volume of distribution. Conversely, organs in which perfusion is selectively maintained (such as the heart and brain) may be susceptible to high or even toxic local drug concentrations for any given plasma concentration in contrast to that in patients with normal cardiac function. Decreased hepatic blood flow decreases clearance of drugs whose intrinsic hepatic clearance is high. Similarly, decreased renal blood flow may lead to decreased glomerular filtration rate and lower renal clearance of certain drugs. Both of these effects produce a longer elimination half-life than would otherwise be expected. Coadministration of cardioactive drugs, such as quinidine or verapamil with digoxin, may lead to decreased volume of distribution or reduced clearance, or both, and thus to higher plasma levels of digoxin than occur during single-drug therapy (Table 66-3). All these factors must be considered in tailoring drug therapy or monitoring potential adverse effects in cardiac patients.

Age can affect the response to drugs. This factor is not always taken into consideration, as evidenced by the higher incidence of adverse reactions in the elderly population. Some of the known physiologic changes that occur with age may have clinically significant effects on the pharmacokinetic aspects of drug therapy in the elderly. These potential relationships are shown in Table 66-4.

Despite known gastric changes, the absorption of many cardiac drugs is unaffected by age. However, some cardiac drugs with first-pass metabolism, e.g., propranolol, may have increased bioavailability because of reduced first-pass hepatic extraction. The bioavailability of sustained-release products that depend on pH for their dissolution is unknown.

Table 66-4 Physiologic determinants of drug disposition in the elderly

Pharmacokinetic process	Physiologic change with aging
Absorption	↑ Gastric pH
	↑ Gastric emptying time
	↓ Gastrointestinal blood flow
Distribution	↓ Total body water
	↓ Lean body mass
	↑ Body fat
	↓ Serum albumin
Metabolism	↓ Liver blood flow
	↓ Liver size
	↓ Enzymatic activity
Excretion	↓ Glomerular filtration rate
	↓ Renal blood flow
	↓ Tubular function

As a result of changes in body composition, larger doses of lipophilic drugs and smaller doses of hydrophilic drugs may be needed to achieve the same serum level in the elderly as in the young. This is clinically true with digoxin; the volume of distribution decreases with age, and lower doses should be used to avoid high serum levels in the elderly.

Renal and hepatic function decrease with age. Hepatic metabolism of drugs, such as nitrates, lidocaine, propranolol, and benzodiazepines, is reduced with age. The age-associated decreases in renal function are probably responsible for the single largest pharmacokinetic change in the elderly. Between the ages of 25 and 65 years, renal perfusion decreases by 40% to 50%. Therefore, drugs that are renally eliminated have decreased clearance in the elderly and a resultant increase in half-life.

Age-related pharmacodynamic changes have not been widely studied. The elderly have an attenuated reduction in heart rate in response to β-blockers; attenuation may be due to alterations in receptor affinity or in the postreceptor response rather than to a change in β-adrenergic receptor density.[3] Elderly patients may also have an exaggerated response to warfarin because of a reduction in circulating clotting factors. Reduced activation of the renin-angiotensin-aldosterone system may also occur in the elderly. Decreased activation may result in a more pronounced blood pressure reduction by angiotensin-converting enzyme inhibitors. Postural hypotension can also be a problem in the elderly and may be exacerbated by a number of cardiovascular drugs.

When drug levels are requested, there are a few points to remember. The first is the timing of the sample blood draw. If the drug has not achieved steady state, the sampled blood level must be interpreted from the perspective that the final steady-state level will be higher. It is also important to know when in the dosing interval the blood sample was drawn. The most easily interpreted sampling time is a trough level. Peak levels are difficult to determine, because the absorption characteristics of an orally administered drug in an individual patient often are not known. Peak drug levels are rarely necessary in clinical cardiology unless there is a question of toxicity. Generally, it is more relevant to know that a certain minimum drug concentration is always present, and this is ascertained by a trough blood level.

REFERENCES

1. Benet LZ, Massoud W: Pharmacokinetics. In *Pharmacokinetic Basis for Drug Treatment*. Edited by LZ Benet, N Massoud, JG Gambertoglio. New York, Raven Press, 1984, pp 1-28

2. Cockcroft DW, Gault MH: Prediction of creatinine clearance from serum creatinine. *Nephron* 16:31-41, 1976

3. Feldman RD, Limbird LE, Nadeau J, et al: Alterations in leukocyte beta-receptor affinity with aging. A potential explanation for altered beta-adrenergic sensitivity in the elderly. *N Engl J Med* 310:815-819, 1984

CHAPTER

67

Anesthesia and noncardiac surgery in patients with heart disease

Martin D. Abel, M.D., and J. Christopher Sill, M.B.,B.S.

RISK OF ANESTHESIA AND SURGERY

Risk in patients with coronary artery disease

The prevalence of coronary artery disease in the American population is so great that someone with this disease is on the surgical list in nearly every hospital every day. Of the 20 million patients undergoing surgery annually in the United States, approximately 15%, or 3 million, have or are at risk for coronary artery disease.[1] The risk of noncardiac surgery in patients with coronary artery disease is due primarily to the unmasking of clinically silent or apparently stable disease by the stress of surgery.[2] The preoperative evaluation of the patient with ischemic heart disease must therefore consider the risk factors relevant to each patient. Often, a simple clinical assessment is all that is needed. When there is uncertainty or the patient is considered to be at high risk, further investigations may be required.

Retrospective studies indicate that the risk of myocardial infarction during the 7-day period after anesthesia and noncardiac surgery in patients who have never had a myocardial infarction is approximately 0.15%[3] (Table 67-1). In sharp contrast, in patients who undergo anesthesia and surgery after one or more previous episodes of myocardial infarction, the risk of postoperative reinfarction in the 7-day period after anesthesia and surgery is approximately 5% to 6%. In patients with a recent myocardial infarction—that is, within 3 months—the risk of reinfarction may be as much as 30%. For patients who had a myocardial infarction 3 to 6 months ago, the risk of reinfarction after anesthesia and surgery is 15%; thereafter, it levels off to 5% to 6%. There appears to be little difference in the risk of perioperative reinfarction if the previous infarction was subendocardial (non-Q-wave) or transmural (Q-wave).[4] The peak incidence of perioperative infarction is within 72 hours of surgery.[5-9]

In 1983, Rao et al.[5] reported a dramatic reduction in the risk of reinfarction (see Table 67-1). In this study, 733 patients (group 2) were compared with a historical control group of 364 patients (group 1). The overall incidence of reinfarction was 1.9% in group 2 compared with 7.7% in group 1. If the interval between myocardial infarction and anesthesia was less than 3 months, the incidence was reduced from 36% in group 1 to 5.8% in group 2. If the interval between myocardial infarction and anesthesia and surgery was between 4 and 6 months, the incidence was reduced to 2.3% in group 2 from 26% in group 1. The decrease in reinfarction rate was attributed to intensive perioperative hemodynamic monitoring. In this way, more nearly complete treatment of the hyperdynamic circulatory state that frequently accompanies recovery from surgery was possible. Major criticisms of this study are the use of historical controls and the identification of factors responsible for the reduction in mortality by statistical testing of multiple subgroups.[10] Because of these deficiencies and lack of corroboration of the findings, we believe that insufficient data exist to alter our approach to patients with a history of recent myocardial infarction. We still recommend that elective surgery, other than myocardial revascularization, be postponed for at least 6 months after a subendocardial or transmural myocardial infarction.

If the patient has not had a myocardial infarction, the next step in evaluation is to search for factors associated with an increased incidence of life-threatening cardiac events in the perioperative period. A number of important

Table 67-1 Risk of perioperative myocardial infarction (MI) within 7 days of anesthesia and surgery*

History	Risk, % Literature[3-15]	Rao et al.[5]
No prior MI	0.15	...
Prior MI	6	1.9
Prior MI within 3 months	30	5.8
Prior MI 4-6 months earlier	15	2.3
Mortality from perioperative MI	15-70	36

*See text for explanation of results obtained in this series.

risk factors have been identified by a multifactorial approach to the estimation of cardiac risk for noncardiac surgical procedures. In addition to a previous myocardial infarction, significant risk factors include coronary artery disease, left ventricular dysfunction, aortic stenosis, dysrhythmias, advanced age (more than 70 years), associated medical conditions, site of surgery, and the urgency of the surgical procedure (Table 67-2). Poorly controlled hypertension before the operation doubles the risk of perioperative reinfarction.[4] The belief that control of perioperative hypertension significantly lowers the risk of reinfarction is supported by the absence of hypertension as a risk factor in many of the multivariate analyses of risk factors that have been published.[11-14]

In an analysis of patients entered into the Coronary Artery Surgery Study (CASS) who underwent noncardiac surgical procedures, only left ventricular dysfunction was independently predictive of cardiac-related morbidity and mortality.[14] A preoperative history of myocardial infarction was not an independent predictor of cardiac outcome; thus, the degree of left ventricular dysfunction, not simply a history of myocardial infarction, may be the most important determinant of cardiac risk.[14] Symptoms of left ventricular function that were important determinants of poor outcome were dyspnea on exertion and left ventricular wall motion abnormalities determined by angiography. If one excludes the operative mortality associated with myocardial revascularization itself (2.3% overall for CASS registry patients), patients who had undergone prior coronary artery bypass operation and those without severe coronary artery disease evident on angiography had similar operative mortality in association with noncardiac surgery. Thus, for purposes of preoperative evaluation, patients who have successfully undergone bypass grafting are at low risk in subsequent noncardiac procedures.[15,16] It is uncertain how long this benefit continues after myocardial revascularization. The high rate of reocclusion in vein bypass grafts suggests that the benefit conferred by myocardial revascularization is not lifelong. The Veterans Affairs Cooperative Study of Coronary Artery Bypass Surgery concluded that the benefits of coronary artery bypass surgery on survival, symptoms, and postinfarction mortality were transient and lasted fewer than 11 years. The benefits began to diminish after 5 years, when graft closure accelerated.[17] Coronary angioplasty probably also affords protection against perioperative myocardial infarction, although data to demonstrate such a beneficial effect are scant.[18]

Table 67-2 Factors that increase the risk of perioperative infarction

Ischemic heart disease
Previous myocardial infarction
Angina
Silent ischemia
Multivessel disease
Left coronary artery stenosis
Left ventricular dysfunction
Congestive heart failure
Left ventricular aneurysm
Multiple left ventricular regional wall motion abnormalities
Elevated left ventricular end-diastolic pressure
Ventricular dysrhythmias
Aortic stenosis
Older age
Associated medical conditions
Operative site
Great vessels
Thoracic noncardiac
Upper abdomen
Emergency surgery
Uncontrolled hypertension

The type of surgery, the magnitude and duration of the procedure, and the development of untoward intraoperative events all influence the outcome of noncardiac surgery. Ophthalmologic surgery, even in patients with a history of myocardial infarction, carries a very low risk of cardiac complications.[19,20] Operations on the great vessels, noncardiac intrathoracic surgery, and upper abdominal procedures, including "open" cholecystectomy, are associated with greater risks of myocardial infarction than other types of operations.[4] When these operations exceed 3 hours in duration, even higher infarction rates may result.[4] Other operations are not linked in this way with duration of anesthesia.

Attempts have been made to quantitate the factors mentioned above and to construct a "point scale" that might be of use in predicting perioperative cardiac morbidity. In a 1977 study of 1,001 patients, Goldman et al.[11] weighted the various factors obtained from a multivariate analysis of risk to construct a multifactorial risk index in which points were assigned to the various risk factors for stratification of patients to various risk categories. The results of various studies undertaken to validate the Goldman risk index prospectively have been conflicting. Zeldin[12] found a clear difference in risk of perioperative cardiac events among patients categorized to different risk classes. Jeffrey et al.,[6] on the other hand, found that the cardiac risk index was unable to discriminate between patients at low risk for life-threatening events and those at high risk.[21] Detsky et al.[13] modified the Goldman index by incorporating angina pectoris, a factor noticeably absent from the original index, and claimed improved predictive accuracy. Mangano et al.[9] prospectively studied 474 men undergoing elective noncardiac surgery. All patients either had or were at high risk for coronary artery disease. Using a multivariate analysis, they found that the only preoperative variables associated with adverse cardiac outcome were dysrhythmia, congestive heart failure requiring digoxin, and vascular surgery (Table 67-3). The increased cardiac risk in patients undergoing vascular surgery is related, in part, to the high prevalence of coronary artery disease in patients who have peripheral vascular disease. Nearly one-fourth of patients without a history of cardiac disease who underwent routine coronary angiography before vascular surgery had

Table 67-3 Prospective evaluation of preoperative predictors of adverse cardiac outcome[9]*

Univariate model	Multivariate model
History of dysrhythmia	History of dysrhythmia
Congestive heart failure	Congestive heart failure (on digoxin)
Vascular surgery	Vascular surgery
Claudication	
Diabetes mellitus (on medication)	
Digoxin or nitrates	
Creatinine >2 mg/dL	
Coronary artery disease	
Previous myocardial infarction	

*See text for explanation of results obtained in this series.

Table 67-4 Factors influencing cardiac morbidity in patients with valvular heart disease

Type of valvular lesion
Severity of valvular lesion
Left ventricular function
Clinical presentation

severe, diffuse coronary artery disease.[22] Not surprisingly, the early mortality after abdominal aortic operations is cardiac-related in 70% of cases,[23] and late mortality is attributable to cardiac causes in 38% of cases.[21] In data obtained from CASS, Rihal et al.[24] found that coronary revascularization improved long-term survival in patients with three-vessel coronary artery disease and peripheral vascular disease.

In assessing the overall risk, the physician must take into account not only patient-related factors but also the magnitude, site, and duration of the proposed surgical procedure and the local experience related to outcome in comparable patients undergoing similar surgical procedures.

Risk in patients with valvular heart disease

Unlike patients with coronary artery disease, patients with valvular heart disease undergoing noncardiac surgery have been the subject of few clinical outcome studies. Patients with valvular heart disease usually experience a gradual decline in cardiac performance without discrete events on which to base numerical risk studies. Nonetheless, considerable evidence has accumulated to show that patients with moderate to severe degrees of congestive heart failure are at major risk for anesthesia and surgery. In patients with valvular heart disease, the risk of noncardiac surgery is influenced by the type and severity of the valvular lesion, the adequacy of left ventricular function, and the patient's clinical presentation (Table 67-4).

Aortic stenosis. Severe symptomatic aortic stenosis poses the highest risk for noncardiac surgery.[11] Because of this risk, patients with severe aortic stenosis are generally advised to undergo surgical correction of the aortic stenosis before an elective noncardiac operation. However, increasing numbers of patients are seen for noncardiac surgery in whom aortic valve operation is precluded because of advanced age or coexisting serious medical problems. O'Keefe et al.,[25] in a retrospective review, reported on 48 patients with severe aortic stenosis who underwent noncardiac procedures between 1985 and 1987. Fifty percent of these patients had congestive heart failure, 40% had angina, and 15% had syncope. Doppler echocardiography, performed in all 48 patients, revealed a mean transvalvular gradient of 76 mm Hg and a calculated aortic valve area (in 22 patients) of 0.6 cm^2. Seven patients had significant perioperative events, including intraoperative hypotension in five. However, none had major sequelae and there were no intraoperative deaths. It was concluded that even patients with severe aortic stenosis can undergo noncardiac surgery with low risk, a result that was attributed to modern-day anesthesia care. It should be noted, however, that because most patients in this study had normal left ventricular systolic function, this conclusion should not be extended to patients with severe aortic stenosis and significant left ventricular systolic dysfunction.[25]

In aortic stenosis, in addition to abnormalities of systolic and diastolic function, coronary vascular reserve is decreased and myocardial ischemia can occur, even in the absence of coronary artery disease.[26] Patients with severe aortic stenosis are at increased risk from the stresses of surgery despite the most meticulous anesthetic management. The patients at highest risk, we believe, are those who have critical aortic stenosis (valve area <0.7 cm^2), patients with secondary left ventricular dysfunction, and patients who have symptoms of heart failure or angina secondary to aortic stenosis (Table 67-5). These patients require relief of stenosis before surgery.

Mitral stenosis. The major risk of mitral stenosis is elevation of left atrial pressure secondary to tachycardia, resulting in pulmonary venous hypertension and subsequent pulmonary edema. Increased pressure usually occurs only in patients who have a moderate to severe degree of mitral stenosis (valve area <1.5 cm^2). Patients with symptoms usually have a significant increase in left atrial pressure at rest. Pulmonary hypertension secondary to long-standing mitral stenosis poses an increased risk for right heart failure.

Aortic and mitral regurgitation. Patients with aortic or mitral valve regurgitant lesions are probably at less risk for noncardiac surgery than those with stenotic lesions. In this group of patients, the risk of surgery depends more on coexistent left ventricular dysfunction than on the valvular lesion itself. Patients with significant symptoms due to left

Table 67-5 Factors that increase the risk of noncardiac surgery in patients with aortic stenosis

Critical aortic stenosis (valve area <0.7 cm^2)
Left ventricular dysfunction
Congestive heart failure
Angina

ventricular dysfunction before noncardiac surgery have a much higher risk than patients without congestive heart failure.[11,27] Symptoms of congestive failure are not always caused by impairment of systolic pumping function but instead may be related to impaired diastolic relaxation.[28,29] However, whatever the cause of pulmonary congestion, drug therapy with vasodilators or even the vasodilating effects of anesthesia itself can frequently reduce increased intracardiac and pulmonary arterial pressures.

Risk in patients with myocardial disease (cardiomyopathies)

There are no clinical outcome studies in patients with cardiomyopathies undergoing noncardiac surgery. Although grouped here under a common heading, cardiomyopathies may differ significantly from one another, both in the natural history of the underlying disease process and in the pathophysiologic processes. The evaluation and treatment of the two most common cardiomyopathies, dilated cardiomyopathy and hypertrophic cardiomyopathy, should be considered separately.

Dilated cardiomyopathy. In dilated cardiomyopathy, there is a primary abnormality of systolic function with diminished myocardial contractility and left ventricular dilatation.[30] Symptoms are related to increased venous pressure and low cardiac output. Dilated cardiomyopathy is often idiopathic but may be secondary to ischemic heart disease, alcohol abuse, parturition, or viral myocarditis. The risk of noncardiac surgery in patients with dilated cardiomyopathy is related to congestive heart failure or dysrhythmias. For example, in the patient with increased jugular venous pressure or a loud third heart sound, or in the patient with ventricular dysrhythmias, the risk of noncardiac surgery is increased. In patients with dilated cardiomyopathy who do not have any signs or symptoms of heart failure and few dysrhythmias, the risk of noncardiac surgery is comparatively lower.

Hypertrophic cardiomyopathy. Hypertrophic cardiomyopathy is a disease in which hypertrophy of the myocardium is associated with an impairment of normal muscular relaxation that, in turn, may be secondary to abnormal handling of Ca^{2+} by the cell.[31] Ventricular hypertrophy results in diastolic dysfunction, increased cardiac filling pressures, and symptoms of dyspnea. Hypertrophy also reduces coronary vascular reserve, and the result is susceptibility to myocardial ischemia and angina. Some patients also have an associated dynamic left ventricular outflow obstruction due to systolic anterior motion of the mitral valve. Patients who have a nonobstructive form of hypertrophic cardiomyopathy run a slightly increased risk of pulmonary congestion from fluid overload. However, in patients with the obstructive form of hypertrophic cardiomyopathy, hemodynamic changes, such as decreased peripheral vascular resistance secondary to anesthetics or adrenergic stimulation resulting from surgery, may increase the outflow gradient and exacerbate coexistent mitral regurgitation, effects that may lead to marked hemodynamic deterioration.[32]

Risk in patients with congenital heart disease

It is not possible to quantify risk in patients with congenital heart disease because anatomy and pathophysiology can vary significantly among patients who superficially carry identical diagnoses and because these diseases are progressive rather than associated with discrete events as in patients with coronary artery disease.[33] In patients with an atrial septal defect, uncomplicated ventricular septal defect, or other relatively well-tolerated congenital cardiac defects, risks of anesthesia for noncardiac surgery are low. Risk is higher in patients with such complex congenital cardiac lesions as pulmonary atresia, tricuspid atresia, double-outlet right ventricle, and single ventricle. In patients with complex congenital heart disease, hypoxemia, polycythemia, and pulmonary vascular obstructive disease increase the risk of any operative procedure.

PREOPERATIVE EVALUATION AND PREPARATION

Patients with coronary artery disease

Patients scheduled for elective surgery who have coronary artery disease and who die in the perioperative period nearly always die of complications related to the coronary artery disease, regardless of the operation or the severity of the other disease or diseases. The cardiac risk associated with noncardiac surgery is due primarily to clinically silent or apparently stable coronary artery disease that is unmasked by the stress of surgery.[2] Therefore, patients thought to have coronary disease should undergo cardiovascular system assessment before elective surgery. A thorough clinical history can usually provide most of the information necessary to determine the patient's cardiovascular functional status. Risk stratification based primarily on a clinical assessment of the patient (see Tables 67-1 through 67-5) allows the physician to determine which patients may benefit from special preoperative testing (Table 67-6). Obviously, patients without angina or a history of a previous myocardial infarction or who have few risk factors for coronary artery disease are at least risk. Those at increased risk include older men, patients with known coronary artery disease, and patients with symptoms of left ventricular dysfunction. Patients in the intermediate-risk category may appear clinically stable, and therefore the severity of their

Table 67-6 Risk stratification to identify the need for further cardiovascular testing

Low risk (no special tests required)	Intermediate risk (individualize testing)	High risk (additional testing indicated)
No history of ischemic heart disease; few risk factors for ischemic heart disease, e.g., related to age, gender, smoking, hypertension, lipids, family history	Stable ischemic heart disease • Myocardial infarction >6 months ago • Angina, class I or II (NYHA) Risk factors for ischemic heart disease	Unstable ischemic pattern • Recent myocardial infarction • Angina, changing pattern or accelerating or class III or IV (NYHA) • Postinfarction angina
No history of dysrhythmias	History of supraventricular dysrhythmias requiring digoxin	History of ventricular dysrhythmias, especially "sudden death"
Unlimited physical activity	Mild-to-moderate limitation of physical activity	Congestive heart failure Pulmonary edema
Normal valvular function	Moderate aortic stenosis	Severe symptomatic aortic stenosis
No associated medical conditions	Diabetes mellitus	Insulin-dependent diabetes mellitus
Low-risk surgery, e.g., surgery of short duration outside abdominal or thoracic cavities	Upper abdominal or thoracic surgery Surgery of longer duration	Vascular surgery Prolonged thoracic or upper abdominal procedures

NYHA, New York Heart Association.

underlying coronary artery disease cannot be readily determined at the bedside. Patients in a very-high-risk category are those with compensated heart failure, particularly pulmonary edema, those who have recently sustained a myocardial infarction, and those with manifestations of ischemic instability, for example, changing pattern of angina, accelerating angina, postinfarction angina, and New York Heart Association class III or IV angina.[1,2,34,35]

In the assessment of the stability of ischemia, changing or new symptoms of angina, escalation of medical therapy, and curtailment of activity are important guides to ischemic instability. Patients with unusual chest pain syndromes or atypical angina also merit further investigation. Clues that have important implications for the clinician taking care of these patients may be obtained from unusual symptoms of ischemia. For example, dyspnea suggests left ventricular dysfunction with an increase in left ventricular end-diastolic pressure. Palpitations suggest ischemia-induced dysrhythmias. Dizziness or syncope may be the result of a reduction in cardiac output.[36]

Baseline tests. Baseline testing in patients with known or suspected coronary artery disease should include a 12-lead electrocardiogram (ECG), the hemoglobin or hematocrit value, an electrolyte panel, and a chest radiograph (Table 67-7). The initial ECG provides a basis for later comparison. A knowledge of the hemoglobin is particularly important in patients scheduled to undergo noncardiac surgery in which large blood losses are anticipated, for example, vascular surgery. In addition, significant reductions in the hemoglobin or hematocrit value result in a compensatory increase in cardiac output that may place an increased demand on a myocardium already ischemic. The measurement of electrolytes, including an estimate of renal function with use of blood urea nitrogen or creatinine, is important, particularly in patients with a history of congestive heart failure who may be taking diuretics or digitalis and who may require intravenous (IV) administration of contrast agents for radiologic imaging procedures. The chest radiograph provides important information about cardiac size and pulmonary edema. A decision to proceed with further laboratory testing should be made only after a full clinical history has been taken, as described above. As suggested, when the risks are thought to be very low, it is probably unnecessary to proceed further. If preoperative screening

Table 67-7 Baseline tests indicated in all patients with a history of cardiac disease who are to have noncardiac surgery

Test	Rationale
ECG	• Baseline record for later comparison • Abnormal ST-T pattern suggests the need for alternative intraoperative monitors for ischemia
Hemoglobin	• Anemia produces a compensatory increase in cardiac work to maintain oxygen delivery • Operations associated with increased blood loss
Electrolyte panel	• Assessment of renal function, particularly if radiologic contrast agents will be used • Use of diuretics may alter electrolytes and increase risk of dysrhythmias in patients receiving digoxin
Chest radiograph	• Cardiac size • Pulmonary edema

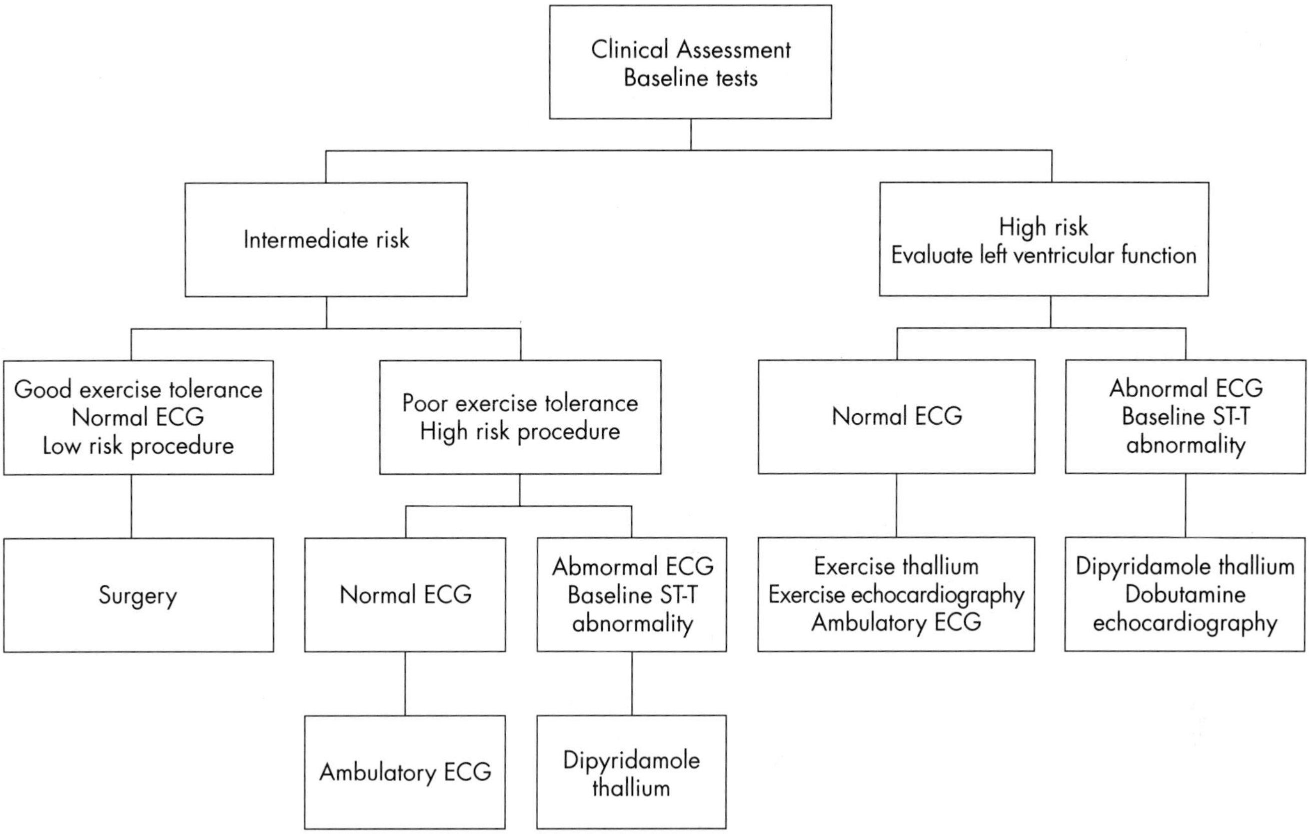

Fig 67-1 Algorithm used to evaluate patients at risk for perioperative cardiac morbidity. A positive test result may warrant coronary angiography if coronary revascularization or angioplasty is an option. Negative test results should permit noncardiac surgery to be undertaken at relatively low risk.

by history suggests moderate to high risk or if adequate stress testing cannot be performed because of factors such as claudication, further testing should be undertaken.

Risk stratification*[35] *(Fig 67-1)

EXERCISE STRESS TEST. In patients who have normal ST-T segments on their preoperative ECG and can exercise, which usually excludes patients with peripheral vascular disease, an exercise stress test performed with ECG monitoring can provide useful information. If the exercise ECG is positive at a low heart rate, elective surgery should be postponed until a coronary angiographic examination can be performed. If the exercise ECG is not positive until after an adequate workload has been reached, there is little increased risk for elective noncardiac surgery. The anesthesiologist also gains useful information from the results of the exercise stress test. Helpful data include the limits of the rate-pressure product (double product) at which ischemia occurred and the occurrence of dysrhythmias in association with ischemia. Hypotension provoked by exercise stress testing is an ominous finding and suggests left main coronary artery stenosis.

AMBULATORY ECG MONITORING. Patients with peripheral vascular disease are often unable to exercise. When able to undergo exercise stress testing, they often perform with an inadequate workload, so that the test results cannot be usefully interpreted. Raby et al.[8] found that 48-hour preoperative ambulatory ECG monitoring used to detect episodes of myocardial ischemia in everyday life was a useful method for assessing cardiac risk in patients who subsequently underwent elective vascular surgery. However, the low predictive accuracy of the test precludes its value in clinical practice.

THALLIUM SCINTIGRAPHY AND STRESS ECHOCARDIOGRAPHY. An alternative approach to better define risk in moderate-to-high-risk patients with ST-T abnormalities and ischemic heart disease undergoing noncardiac surgery is the use of exercise, dipyridamole, or adenosine thallium scintigraphy[2,37-39] or exercise or dobutamine stress echocardiography.[36,40] A reversible defect on thallium scintigraphy (thallium redistribution) or a new regional wall motion abnormality with echocardiography is associated with a significantly higher cardiac risk for patients undergoing high-risk surgical procedures. These tests, used in conjunction with either exercise or pharmacologic stress, often can identify the distribution and severity of coronary artery disease. Pharmacologic stress testing is reserved for patients with coronary artery disease who are unable to exercise optimally. Because of low predictive accuracy, these tests are most useful in the population with a moderate pretest probability of postoperative complications.

CORONARY ANGIOGRAPHY. Despite the high prevalence of coronary artery disease in patients undergoing peripheral vascular surgery (95% for aortic aneurysm surgery and 64% for aortoiliac surgery), routine coronary angiography in this category of patients cannot be recommended[22] because of the considerable cost and risk. If, however, a patient has a highly positive exercise stress test result, multiple areas of redistribution on dipyridamole thallium scintigraphy, or multiple new regional wall motion abnormalities on stress echocardiography, coronary angiography may be an appropriate next step. Coronary angiography should be performed only if angioplasty or myocardial revascularization is a suitable treatment option for the patient before noncardiac surgery.

RADIONUCLIDE ANGIOGRAPHY. If the clinical history suggests that the patient has reduced left ventricular function, additional tests may be required to determine the severity of left ventricular compromise. If cardiac catheterization data are lacking, radionuclide angiography or two-dimensional echocardiography can provide useful information. Patients with an abnormal ejection fraction and patients with increased left ventricular end-diastolic pressure are at increased risk for surgery and anesthesia; therefore, an accurate estimate of the degree of left ventricular dysfunction before anesthesia may influence the conduct of anesthesia and surgery. For example, vasodilator therapy may be instituted during surgery for patients with impaired ventricular function. In contrast, patients with normal ventricular function may tolerate more liberal use of depressant volatile anesthetics, such as halothane and isoflurane.

SUMMARY. Once all the information has been gathered, patients with cardiac disease can be managed before surgery in a number of ways, ranging from myocardial revascularization to review and adjustment of medical therapy. A final option is cancellation of the noncardiac surgical procedure itself. However, recent data suggest that even patients at high risk can be successfully guided through noncardiac surgery and recovery with low mortality.[5,8,41]

Patients with valvular heart disease

Aortic stenosis. Of all patients with valve lesions, those with aortic stenosis pose the highest risk for noncardiac surgery,[11,13] although one report suggests that recent improvements in anesthesia care have reduced this risk.[25] Before noncardiac surgery, it is essential not only to determine the severity of the aortic stenosis but also to evaluate coexistent left ventricular function. Although symptoms such as angina, dyspnea, and syncope offer insight into the degree of dysfunction, special testing is also needed. Echocardiography is particularly useful and can determine both valvular severity and left ventricular function. A Doppler echocardiographic evaluation of the aortic valve gradient and valve area should be obtained, and left ventricular function can be assessed by two-dimensional echocardiography.

In the patient who has mild-to-moderate aortic stenosis (valve area >1 cm^2) without symptoms, noncardiac surgery is associated with low risk. The only preoperative management necessary is infective endocarditis prophylaxis. In the patient who has severe aortic stenosis (valve area <1 cm^2) with symptoms, noncardiac surgery carries a high risk. If the surgery is elective, it is recommended that the patient undergo aortic valve replacement before noncardiac surgery.

In the patient who urgently needs a noncardiac operation or in a patient who is at high risk for aortic valve surgery because of associated medical conditions or advanced age, percutaneous aortic balloon valvuloplasty can stabilize the patient's condition and improve multiorgan function.[42,43] However, because long-term survival is poor, aortic valvuloplasty should be viewed as a temporizing measure in selected patients with critical aortic stenosis and multiple organ failure.[44]

In a patient who has moderately severe aortic stenosis without symptoms, there is still disagreement about the best approach. One study suggests that most patients can be managed safely during noncardiac surgery.[25] However, if the patient has coexistent left ventricular dysfunction, either the operation should be canceled or a lesser procedure under local anesthesia should be considered if aortic valve replacement or aortic balloon valvuloplasty is not feasible.[25]

Mitral stenosis. Patients with mitral stenosis may not have symptoms or have only mild symptoms for long periods after the initial diagnosis. The cardinal symptom of dyspnea reflects increased left atrial pressure and lung water. Subsequently, orthopnea and paroxysmal nocturnal dyspnea become prominent features. Acute pulmonary edema can occur suddenly and is usually precipitated by an external event like pulmonary infection, thyrotoxicosis, pregnancy, or the onset of atrial fibrillation. Tachycardia is common to all the precipitating events and leads to a reduction in cardiac output by shortening diastolic filling time. Long-standing mitral stenosis may result in pulmonary hypertension, right ventricular hypertrophy, and dilatation with secondary tricuspid regurgitation. As with aortic stenosis, echocardiography permits assessment of the severity of mitral stenosis, the size of the cardiac chambers, and the pulmonary artery pressure. In patients who have severe symptoms (New York Heart Association class III or IV) and have severe mitral stenosis (valve area <1 cm^2), mitral valve replacement or percutaneous mitral balloon valvuloplasty is indicated before noncardiac surgery.[45,46] The patient with mild mitral stenosis without symptoms probably can undergo noncardiac surgery safely if care is taken to control the heart rate and the rate of fluid administration. When there is a discrepancy between Doppler echocardiographic findings and the patient's symptoms—usually in a patient without symptoms who appears to have severe mitral stenosis on echocardiographic examination—exercise stress testing before noncardiac surgery should be considered. In these patients, the long-standing valvular abnormality may have led to a sedentary lifestyle, so that the patient may be unaware of his or her physical limitations. If the patient's functional aerobic capacity is limited to less than 50% of predicted on a treadmill exertion test, some type of intervention should be considered before noncardiac surgery.

Valvular regurgitation. Patients with chronic aortic and mitral regurgitation may be without symptoms for long periods. Mild-to-moderate aortic and mitral regurgitation that is not progressive is extremely well tolerated. Documentation of signs and symptoms of ventricular function before noncardiac surgery is important. Patients with significant symptoms of congestive heart failure from regurgitant lesions should undergo diuresis and afterload reduction to optimize their medical condition before noncardiac surgery. However, if the patient has minimal symptoms, even with significant regurgitation, noncardiac surgery is usually well tolerated. Patients with acute aortic regurgitation or mitral regurgitation may have rapid decompensation and usually require cardiac surgery.

Anticoagulation. The approach to anticoagulation therapy in patients with valvular prostheses is variable. Patients with bioprostheses usually do not require long-term anticoagulation. Primarily, patients with mechanical valvular prostheses are at risk for thromboembolism. Discontinuation of oral anticoagulant administration several days before anesthesia and surgery to allow the prothrombin time to return toward normal has been shown to be safe, even without low-dose heparin therapy.[47] Oral anticoagulant therapy can be reinstituted after noncardiac surgery between the second and the fifth postoperative days, depending on the type of surgical procedure and any surgical bleeding problems that may be present.[47] Some patients are at a higher risk of thromboembolism, such as those with mechanical mitral prostheses, left atrial enlargement, left ventricular dysfunction, atrial fibrillation, or a history of embolic phenomena. In these patients, continuous infusion heparin therapy should be considered after oral anticoagulant therapy has been stopped. It is used until the time of surgery and restarted as soon as possible postoperatively.

Endocarditis prophylaxis. Guidelines for prophylaxis against bacterial endocarditis in patients with valvular heart disease should follow the recommendations of the American Heart Association.[48]

Patients with myocardial disease

An objective assessment of left ventricular function should be obtained in patients with dilated cardiomyopathy. This can be done with either echocardiography or radionuclide angiography. However, the major determinant of the preoperative management of these patients still depends on the patient's clinical symptoms. The patient with significant symptoms of shortness of breath (New York Heart Association class III or IV) is at high risk for noncardiac surgery. Especially thorough treatment of heart failure should be done before noncardiac surgery, including afterload reduction and diuresis. Frequently, this kind of therapy can be guided by use of a pulmonary artery catheter and is best done in an intensive care unit before surgery. If the patient claims to have no symptoms but on clinical examination has evidence of congestive heart failure—for example, increased jugular venous pressure or a loud third heart sound—similar precautions and treatment should be instituted. The end points of treatment in patients with dilated cardiomyopathy are return of the venous pressure to normal and disappearance of the third heart sound. If invasive hemodynamic monitoring has been instituted, reduction in the pulmonary artery occlusion pressure to less than 18 mm Hg is ideal. In patients with dilated cardiomyopathy, even if there is objective evidence of a significant reduction in left ventricular function by echocardiography or radionuclide angiography, absence of symptoms and signs of heart failure usually implies a relatively low risk for noncardiac surgery. In this situation, however, a knowledge of the patient's cardiac disease may guide the anesthesiologist in the judicious use of fluid therapy and myocardial depressant anesthetics in the operative period.

Patients with nonobstructive hypertrophic cardiomyopathy have a relatively low risk with noncardiac surgery. In patients with the obstructive variety, however, hemodynamic deterioration can occur rapidly. In these patients, it is essential to document the severity of the left ventricular outflow obstruction. Doppler echocardiography can quantitate the pressure gradient across the left ventricular outflow tract. Provocative tests, such as amyl nitrate inhalation or exercise during the Doppler echocardiographic examination, may be used to ascertain the dynamic nature and severity of a labile obstruction. If there is a resting or labile left ventricular outflow tract obstruction, β-blockade should be instituted before noncardiac surgery and continued until the time of surgery. It is probably best to continue calcium antagonist therapy until the time of surgery. However, because both calcium antagonists and anesthetics are vasodilators, together their effect on peripheral vascular tone may be surprisingly marked. In addition, because hypovolemia exacerbates the left ventricular outflow tract gradient, hydration on the night before surgery is prudent, particularly if the planned noncardiac surgery is scheduled for late the following day.

Patients with congenital heart disease

The adult patient with congenital heart disease scheduled for noncardiac surgery is likely to have undergone previous corrective surgery. In the assessment of the patient with corrected or uncorrected congenital heart disease, the following questions should be answered. Is congestive heart failure present? Has pulmonary hypertension occurred, and is there any residual valvular or subvalvular obstruction? If there are any residual intracardiac or extracardiac shunts, how would they respond to alterations in pulmonary or systemic vascular resistance? And, finally, is the patient polycythemic consequent to cyanotic congenital heart disease? Cyanotic patients who are polycythemic are predisposed to thrombotic complications, particularly if dehydration is allowed to occur in the preoperative period. Therefore, consideration should be given to the placement of an IV catheter for preoperative hydration. These patients also have an abnormality in platelet function and abnormal blood clotting, and they are at risk for intraoperative coagulopathy.

Depending on the type of surgery planned and the anticipated blood loss during surgery, precautions can be taken in regard to the hemostatic abnormality. These precautions might include preoperative hemodilution, further testing of the coagulation system, and crossmatching for the appropriate blood products. Patients with congestive heart failure should undergo maximum medical management, which might include optimization of digitalis therapy, diuresis, and afterload reduction, if appropriate. A right-to-left shunt alerts the anesthesiologist to the possibility of paradoxical air embolism occurring intraoperatively. In addition, patients with a right-to-left shunt and those with reduced pulmonary blood flow may be compromised by systemic vasodilatation secondary to anesthetic agents. (Systemic vasodilatation may exacerbate right-to-left shunting and may also decrease perfusion pressure, further reducing blood flow to the lungs.) An increased degree of right-to-left shunting under anesthesia may exacerbate arterial hypoxemia.

Finally, a detailed knowledge of the surgical history of the patient with congenital heart disease is important. A shunting procedure such as the Blalock-Taussig operation, having obliterated the peripheral pulse in the upper extremity, makes it difficult to obtain a blood pressure recording in that extremity. In the evaluation of patients with congenital heart disease presenting for noncardiac surgery, all the considerations above may affect the decision on whether proposed elective noncardiac surgery should be postponed until corrective cardiac surgery can be performed. Antibiotic prophylaxis for patients with congenital heart disease should follow the guidelines of the American Heart Association.[48]

Table 67-8 Perioperative use of common cardiac medications

Medication	Perioperative use
β-Blockers	• Continue throughout the perioperative period • Administer <4 hours before surgery to ensure adequate blood levels
Calcium channel blockers	• Continue preoperatively • Perioperative use dictated by angina control
Nitrates	• Continue preoperatively • Not indicated prophylactically • Useful for perioperative hypertension control
Diuretics	• Exclude hypokalemia • Consider reduced dose preoperatively to avoid volume contraction
Antihypertensives	• Continue preoperatively • Avoid abrupt withdrawal of clonidine
Digitalis	• Continue perioperatively if used for heart rate control • Not indicated prophylactically except possibly for pneumonectomy

Medications (Table 67-8)

β-Blockers. The patient's preoperative drug therapy is of concern, not only because of the need to provide optimal conditions for the operation but also because of the many potential drug interactions. Patients with coronary artery disease taking a β-adrenergic blocking agent should continue to take this medication until the morning of surgery.[49,50] Among 440 patients about to have coronary artery bypass surgery, ischemia was significantly less frequent in those receiving β-adrenergic blocking drugs than in those receiving either calcium channel antagonists alone or no medication.[50] Perioperative ischemia, usually caused by tachycardia, is closely related to perioperative myocardial infarction.[51] These findings support the continued use of β-adrenergic blockade, not only in the preoperative period but also after surgery.

The duration of action of β-adrenergic blocking drugs such as propranolol and metoprolol is determined by the dose administered and by the plasma half-life. Sill et al.[52] demonstrated that in patients receiving β-blocker therapy, the commonly prescribed dose schedules of propranolol and metoprolol did not consistently result in plasma levels within the therapeutic range at the time of anesthesia and surgery. Furthermore, therapeutic levels at the time of anesthesia and surgery were achieved only if the final β-blocker dose had been administered within a few hours of departure for the operating room. They concluded that low-dose propranolol therapy (40 to 80 mg/day) was ineffective in producing therapeutic plasma levels and that if therapeutic levels were desired at the time of anesthesia and surgery, the dosage should be increased. Medium doses of propranolol (160 mg/day) and metoprolol (100 mg/day) were more likely to result in therapeutic levels, but such levels would become subtherapeutic unless oral therapy was maintained until the time of departure for the operating room.[52]

Calcium channel blockers. Recommendations for patients taking calcium channel blocking drugs are less certain. The calcium channel blocking agents have various degrees of direct negative inotropic effects. They relieve vasospastic ischemia by decreasing the overall myocardial oxygen demand (negative inotropy) and by direct coronary and peripheral vasodilatation. They may actually improve myocardial performance by improving the oxygen supply and demand balance. Although calcium antagonists and anesthetics have additive vasodilator and negative inotropic effects, patients taking even high doses of calcium antagonists can be anesthetized safely, and patients undoubtedly benefit from their continuance until the time of surgery. Calcium antagonist drugs have not yet been shown to provide the dramatic protective effect against intraoperative myocardial ischemia observed with β-blocking drugs. However, their antianginal effects in the conscious patient are beyond dispute.

In two studies, patients treated with calcium channel blocking drugs alone had a significantly higher incidence of perioperative ischemic ECG changes than did patients receiving β-adrenergic blocking drugs alone or in combination with calcium channel blocking drugs.[50,53] In a review, Packer[54] concluded that controlled clinical trials "did not support the concept that combined therapy with a β-blocker and a calcium entry blocker produces additive or synergistic clinical benefits in most patients with coronary artery disease." In fact, "combined treatment is likely to be accompanied by more adverse effects than is the use of a single antianginal drug." Notwithstanding these reports, we believe that calcium entry blockers, even when used in conjunction with β-blockers, should be continued until the time of surgery.

Nitrates. Patients with coronary artery disease taking nitroglycerin or longer acting nitrates should be permitted to use the drug ad libitum preoperatively. The prophylactic use of nitroglycerin in patients with coronary artery disease is less certain. Two studies did not demonstrate that IV administration of nitroglycerin helped prevent intraoperative myocardial ischemia in patients undergoing coronary artery bypass grafting.[55,56] There is some evidence, however, that hypertensive episodes can be diminished by the use of nitroglycerin in the perioperative period.[56]

Antihypertensives. Antihypertensive medications should be continued up until the time of surgery because uncontrolled hypertension per se increases the risk of perioperative cardiac morbidity. Most patients on an antihypertensive regimen are receiving potassium-losing diuretics that may lead indirectly to dysrhythmias and problems of digitalis toxicity. In this situation, preoperative hypokalemia indicates a large total deficit of potassium, and correction should be begun early and achieved over the course of a few days rather than overnight before surgery. The abrupt withdrawal of the centrally acting β-adrenergic agonist clonidine may result in severe rebound hypertension in the perioperative period in patients accustomed to high doses of clonidine.[57] Consideration should be given to altering the patient's antihypertensive regimen preoperatively if the patient is taking clonidine or, alternatively, ensuring that no abrupt cessation of clonidine therapy occurs in the perioperative period. The latter course can be accomplished by converting from oral clonidine to the transdermal preparation 2 to 3 weeks before surgery. However, rebound hypertension responds to conventional treatment with drugs such as labetalol. The newer antihypertensive agents, such as the angiotensin-converting enzyme inhibitors (e.g., captopril), direct vasodilators (e.g., minoxidil), α-adrenergic receptor antagonists (e.g., prazosin), are not known to pose particular problems with anesthesia. Good control of blood pressure preoperatively in hypertensive patients, that is, a diastolic pressure of less than 100 mm Hg, ensures that the patient's blood volume will be normalized. This may minimize the marked swings in blood pressure to which hypertensive patients are prone.

Digitalis. Digitalis is used in patients with congestive heart failure and to control supraventricular tachydysrhythmias. In the evaluation of the patient receiving digitalis who also is taking potassium-losing diuretics, particular care should be taken to ensure that a normal plasma level of potassium is present preoperatively. If digitalis is being used for rate control in patients with atrial fibrillation, administration should be continued at the same dosage before anesthesia. The respiratory alkalosis that often occurs with controlled ventilation during general anesthesia results in a lowered level of extracellular potassium, with the potential for digitalis-induced dysrhythmias. The large fluid and electrolyte shifts that are possible during major surgery may also result in hypokalemia. Digitalis, catecholamines released during sympathetic stimulation, and volatile anesthetics (especially halothane) may interact and lead to symptoms that are indistinguishable from those of digitalis toxicity. The concept that some patients, especially the elderly, should be prophylactically digitalized preoperatively is no longer tenable. Digitalis should be used preoperatively to control heart rate or to treat congestive heart failure. An exception to the avoidance of prophylactic use of digitalis can be made for patients undergoing pneumonectomy in whom the incidence of tachydysrhythmias is high and is associated with a significant mortality.[58]

Pacemakers

Temporary pacemaker insertion is indicated only if grounds exist for the placement of a permanent cardiac pacemaker.[59] In patients with asymptomatic conduction system disease, such as bundle-branch block, bifascicular block, or even trifascicular block, the long-term risk of complete heart block is increased, but the probability of intraoperative complete heart block is so low ($<1\%$) that prophylactic pacemaker insertion is virtually unnecessary.[60] Patients who have symptoms with bradyarrhythmias, on the other hand, are usually candidates for a permanent pacemaker, and in this situation, prophylactic temporary pacemaker insertion should be considered before urgent noncardiac surgery. In patients who have had a transvenous pacemaker placed within the preceding 2 weeks, the possibility exists that the transvenous pacing wire could be dislodged with the introduction of a pulmonary artery balloon flotation catheter. If invasive hemodynamic monitoring is indicated in this subset of patients, we believe that the pulmonary artery catheter is best placed under fluoroscopic guidance in the cardiac catheterization laboratory. In patients in whom the transvenous pacing wire has been present for more than 2 weeks and has had enough time to imbed itself into the right ventricular wall, problems do not usually occur in the placement of a pulmonary artery catheter.

INTRAOPERATIVE MANAGEMENT

Monitoring

Blood pressure. Close monitoring of blood pressure is essential, because patients who experience periods of hypotension during anesthesia (arbitrarily defined as a decrease of 30% from control preoperative blood pressures for 10 minutes or more at one time or more) have approximately double the perioperative infarction rate of those who do not have hypotension.[4] Noninvasive measurements of blood pressure are commonly obtained with semiautomated oscillometric or ultrasonic equipment. Blood pressure monitoring with an intra-arterial catheter is indicated if large or abrupt changes in arterial pressure are anticipated, there is a risk of major bleeding, sudden changes in afterload are likely (e.g., with aortic cross-clamping), or the patient's cardiac status is such that compensation for hemodynamic changes induced by anesthesia or surgery is impaired. Use of an intra-arterial catheter is also desirable if frequent sampling of arterial blood will be necessary during anesthesia and surgery. Occasionally, noninvasive and invasive blood pressure measurements are discordant. In this situation, a search should be made for factors that may produce false readings, such as inappropriate size of a blood pressure cuff for noninvasive measurements and an air bubble between the transducer and the arterial catheter. In the absence of confounding factors, clinical judgment should direct therapy toward the more appropriate measurement. In general, direct arterial pressure measurements are more accurate at low blood pressures and indirect measurements are better when the blood pressure is high.

Electrocardiography. Intraoperative myocardial ischemia is an independent predictor of perioperative cardiac morbidity, and every effort should be made to detect and treat ischemia intraoperatively.[51] If more sophisticated methods of ischemia detection are not available, the ECG remains the only meaningful way to do this, because most ischemic episodes are silent and not associated with any hemodynamic aberration.[51,61] The ECG is a simple, noninvasive monitor. An ideal intraoperative ECG monitoring system allows observation of the 12 standard ECG leads. In the operating room, however, leads II and V_5 are usually monitored and usually reveal the vast majority of intraoperative ischemic episodes. A knowledge of the results of preoperative exercise stress testing and the lead system that detected the ischemic episode is most helpful in determining intraoperative lead placement. Although the ECG is neither the earliest nor the most sensitive marker of myocardial ischemia, it remains the simplest, safest, and most widely available method for detection of ischemia. Newer directions in intraoperative ECG monitoring include the use of computer-assisted methods for analysis of ST segments and arrhythmias. One major drawback of ECG monitoring for ischemia is its inability to detect ischemia in patients with left bundle-branch block, patients with left ventricular hypertrophy and a strain pattern, and patients who have a digitalis effect on the ECG. In these circumstances, alternative methods of ischemia detection, such as transesophageal echocardiography, may be used if the clinical situation warrants it.

Pulmonary artery catheterization. Practice guidelines for the perioperative use of pulmonary artery catheterization have recently been developed by the American Society of Anesthesiologists[62] (Table 67-9). In patients with cardiopulmonary disease or even in the elderly surgical patient, right heart pressures are unreliable determinants of left ventricular filling pressures. The pulmonary artery catheter allows measurements of intracardiac pressures, cardiac output, and oxygen content or saturation of mixed venous blood. From these data, further information can be derived about pulmonary vascular and systemic vascular resistance, stroke volume, and oxygen consumption. Although a wide variety of complications have resulted from pulmonary arterial catheterization, these complications are relatively infrequent.[62,63] Pulmonary artery and, in particular, pulmonary artery occlusion pressures provide a useful guide to intraoperative fluid replacement and, together with measurement of cardiac output, allow inotropic and vasodilator therapy to be optimized. It is important to remember that, particularly in patients with valve disease, discrepancies among pulmonary artery diastolic pressure, pulmonary artery occlusion pressure, and left ventricular end-diastolic pressure are common. For example, in patients with mitral stenosis, left atrial pressure exceeds left ventricular end-diastolic pressure, and similarly in patients with mitral regurgitation, a large v wave can lead to an erroneous estimation of the left ventricular end-diastolic pressure.

Transesophageal echocardiography. Transesophageal echocardiography (TEE) has been used increasingly in anesthetic practice to monitor high-risk patients having surgery. After induction of general anesthesia, TEE may be used during the operation to monitor global and regional left ventricular function.[64] The fractional area change of the left ventricle may be used as a guide to changes in contractility, and regional left ventricular wall motion abnormalities may be used to monitor patients for myocardial ischemia. TEE may be a more sensitive and

Table 67-9 Guidelines for the perioperative use of the pulmonary artery catheter[62]*

Patient	Procedure	Practice setting
Cardiovascular disease Pulmonary dysfunction Renal insufficiency Multiorgan dysfunction Hemodynamic instability, e.g., • Sepsis • Trauma • Burns • Advanced age • Endocrine disorders	Surgery associated wth an increased risk of complications from hemodynamic changes, e.g., • Cardiac surgery • Vascular surgery • Severe preeclampsia • Neurosurgery	Physician skills Duration of procedure Technical support Postoperative factors, e.g., • Nursing training and experience • Ancillary and technical support • Specialists and equipment available to manage complications of catheterization

*In general, at least two of the three listed indicators (patient's health, procedure, and practice setting) should be present to warrant catheterization.

specific monitor of myocardial ischemia that can detect changes earlier than ECG monitoring.[65] In patients having cardiac surgery, TEE was helpful in predicting postoperative cardiac morbidity.[66] However, in patients undergoing noncardiac procedures, primarily vascular surgery, TEE was not as helpful.[67] Whether TEE monitoring for myocardial ischemia can be safely used in real-time in the operating room is yet to be determined. On the other hand, TEE estimates of left ventricular end-diastolic area provide a better assessment of preload than pulmonary capillary wedge pressure in patients with cardiac disease.[68]

Practice guidelines for the intraoperative use of TEE are being developed by the American Society of Anesthesiologists. In general, these guidelines should follow the example developed for the use of the pulmonary artery catheter and require that the patient's health, proposed surgical procedure, and practice setting are taken into account in determining the appropriateness of using TEE.

Anesthetic management

The choice of anesthetic technique and intraoperative monitoring takes into consideration the patient's clinical status, the results of any special investigations, the patient's wishes, and the impact of anesthesia and surgery on the patient's condition. As each case has its own unique problems, the overall management of the patient, including the choice of anesthetic, needs to be individualized.

Regional anesthesia. Major regional anesthesia, especially subarachnoid block (spinal), although of enormous potential benefit because of isolating the cardiovascular system from reflex stimulation resulting from the stress of surgery, can be associated with major hemodynamic perturbations. In addition to a blockade of motor and sensory nerves, spinal anesthesia blocks sympathetic fibers. The higher the level of the block, the greater the sympathetic blockade. Because of the greater sensitivity of sympathetic nerves, the autonomic blockade is usually two or three dermatome levels higher than the sensory level. With a T-4 dermatome sensory level, there is at least a T-2 and possibly a total (including cardiac) sympathetic block (C-8 to L-2). Sympathetic blockade results in peripheral vasodilatation and hypotension. Autonomic blockade of the cardiac sympathetic outflow exacerbates hypotension. With a spinal or subarachnoid block, the onset of motor, sensory, and sympathetic nerve blockade is rapid, and severe hypotension and bradycardia may ensue. To prevent these untoward effects, 1 to 2 L of crystalloid solution is usually given immediately before administration of the spinal anesthetic. In patients with a history of congestive heart failure or in patients with increased left ventricular end-diastolic pressure or left atrial pressure (mitral stenosis), appropriate fluid therapy becomes more difficult to manage. In patients with a low fixed cardiac output, such as those with severe aortic stenosis, compensatory mechanisms may be inadequate to restore the blood pressure to normal, and a vicious cycle of hypotension, myocardial ischemia, and further hypotension may ensue.

With epidural blockade, the rapid hemodynamic changes seen with subarachnoid block are less likely, primarily because induction of the block is slower. Fluid loading before onset of the block can therefore be accomplished in a more paced manner, thereby perhaps reducing the risk of precipitating acute pulmonary edema. Eventually, the degree of sympathetic blockade for a given sensory block is about the same with an epidural block as with a spinal block.

Upper extremity blocks, for example, axillary blocks, and other specific nerve blocks constitute a less major regional form of anesthesia that does not usually produce such major hemodynamic changes. Other approaches include local anesthetic infiltration to the surgical site combined with sedation of the patient with narcotics (e.g., fentanyl), minor tranquilizers (e.g., midazolam), or anesthetics (e.g., propofol). Sedation increases the risk of respiratory depression and hypoventilation with ensuing hypoxemia; thus, oxygen therapy and pulse oximetry are essential parts of this technique. In general, if the patient's preoperative cardiac status warrants a high level of noninvasive or invasive monitoring, it should be undertaken irrespective of the type of anesthetic used.

General anesthesia

INDUCTION. General anesthesia is invariably required for surgery in the thorax or upper abdomen. General anesthesia is conveniently divided into three phases: the induction period, the maintenance period, and the emergence period. The induction and emergence periods perhaps carry the highest risk for the patient with cardiac disease. During the induction of anesthesia, the patient is taken from a conscious state to a level of unconsciousness deep enough to allow surgery to take place. Most commonly, induction of anesthesia is achieved by the use of ultrashort, rapidly acting, IV administered anesthetic agents. These drugs include sodium thiopental (first introduced into clinical practice by Lundy[69] at the Mayo Clinic in 1935), methohexital, etomidate, ketamine, and, most recently, propofol. Not only do these drugs have markedly different chemical structures but also they differ in many other respects. Sodium thiopental, for example, the best known of the IV anesthetic agents, produces direct myocardial depression and peripheral vasodilatation, so that caution needs to be exercised in its administration to patients with severe left ventricular dysfunction or fixed cardiac output, for example, aortic stenoses.[70] Methohexital has an action similar to that of thiopental but is slightly shorter acting. Etomidate, conversely, maintains hemodynamic stability through preservation of both sympathetic outflow and autonomic reflexes.[71] Propofol, introduced into clinical practice in the United States in 1989, is the shortest acting of these IV anesthetic agents and is recommended for use in outpatient or ambulatory surgery because it produces little hangover effect and is associated with a lower incidence of postanesthetic nausea and vomiting.[72,73] However, propofol may cause significant decreases in blood pressure mediated by an inhibition of the sympathetic nervous system and impairment of baroreflex regulatory mechanisms,[71] and it therefore has a limited role as an induction agent in patients with diminished cardiovascular reserve.

ENDOTRACHEAL INTUBATION. Laryngoscopy and endotracheal intubation, frequently performed soon after induction of anesthesia, constitute a significant stress to the patient. Most importantly, dysrhythmias, hypertension, and tachycardia may be associated with laryngoscopy and intubation. To avoid these untoward side effects in patients at risk, anesthesiologists commonly administer a relatively large dose of a short-acting narcotic, for example, fentanyl, sufentanil, or alfentanil, to attenuate the response to laryngoscopy. Choosing the right dose of medication and the speed of administration to avoid extreme swings of blood pressure and heart rate cannot be scientifically predetermined and must be guided by the anesthesiologist's experience and judgment. Small doses of esmolol, a short-acting β-adrenergic blocking drug, can also be very effectively used to attenuate the adverse cardiovascular responses to endotracheal intubation.[74]

MAINTENANCE. Anesthesia is usually maintained with an inhalational anesthetic agent, for example, halothane, enflurane, or isoflurane, or a continuous infusion of an intravenous agent, for example, propofol. The potent inhalational agents are usually supplemented during the maintenance of anesthesia with either nitrous oxide, which has analgesic and weak anesthetic activity, or the potent narcotics, for example, morphine, fentanyl, sufentanil, and alfentanil. The synthetic narcotics like fentanyl are particularly useful for patients in whom tachycardia may be disadvantageous, for example, patients with coronary artery disease and those with mitral and aortic stenosis. These drugs have a potent vagotonic effect and may induce quite profound levels of bradycardia. The inhalational agents are volatile liquids that are so potent that concentrations of less than 2% by volume are usually adequate to produce anesthesia. Each of the volatile anesthetic agents is a direct negative inotropic agent as well as a direct peripheral vasodilator, acting on both the arteriolar and the capacitance vessels (Table 67-10). If peripheral vasodilatation predominates, afterload and preload decrease. In the absence of narcotics or β-adrenergic blockade, isoflurane may cause an increase in heart rate. Halothane and, to a lesser extent, enflurane depress the sinoatrial node and thus minimize the tendency to tachycardia. These properties of the inhalational agents are often useful, especially in patients with relatively normal ventricular contractility. The blood levels of inhalational agents can be rapidly adjusted and easily monitored, both by hemodynamic response and by the analysis of end-tidal gas composition. The inhalational anesthetics are of proven value and are extremely safe drugs, even in patients with ventricular dysfunction. In patients with more marked cardiac deterioration, the volatile anesthetics are best used as a supplement to some form of IV narcotic anesthesia.

None of these anesthetic techniques has been shown to be superior to any other, at least in patients undergoing coronary artery bypass surgery.[75] A prospective, randomized clinical trial of enflurane, fentanyl, halothane, and isoflurane involving 17,201 patients (>90% American Society of Anesthesiologists physical status 1 or 2) found that the anesthetic-related mortality was 0.04%.[76] The rates of death, myocardial infarction, and stroke were too low (<0.15%) to discern differences among these anesthetics. However, the rates of 16 minor adverse events were significantly different among the four study agents. Significant ventricular arrhythmias were more common with halothane, whereas severe tachycardia was associated with isoflurane. Hypertension and bronchospasm were more common with fentanyl.[76]

Table 67-10 Characteristics of inhalational anesthetic agents at equipotent anesthetic doses

Effect	Halothane	Enflurane	Isoflurane
Myocardial depression	++	++	+
Peripheral vasodilatation	+	+	++
Heart rate	↓	↓	↑

+, slight effect; ++, moderate effect; ↑, increase; ↓, decrease.

NEUROMUSCULAR BLOCKADE. Muscle relaxation is usually required in surgical procedures involving the abdomen and, to a lesser extent, the thorax. In addition, muscle relaxants are used to facilitate endotracheal intubation. Muscle relaxants may be classified into two broad groups: depolarizing, for example, succinylcholine, and nondepolarizing (competitive antagonists), for example, tubocurarine, pancuronium, vecuronium, and atracurium (Table 67-11). Side effects associated with the use of muscle relaxants differ among the various agents. For example, pancuronium is vagolytic and may be associated with significant increases in heart rate. Tubocurarine is no longer commonly used in clinical practice, having been replaced by pancuronium and metocurine. Newer agents, like vecuronium and atracurium, are short-acting muscle relaxants relatively free of side effects.

EMERGENCE. The final period of anesthesia that needs to be considered is the emergence from a state of unconsciousness. Patients awakening with an endotracheal tube in place may become sufficiently agitated by its presence, particularly during a light state of anesthesia, that they become tachycardiac and hypertensive. General anesthesia and particularly the use of narcotics, which may stimulate the chemoemetic trigger zone in the medulla, may provoke retching and its associated autonomic side effects. In addition, because it is often difficult to balance adequate pain control with a minimum amount of respiratory depression, patients often emerge with some degree of discomfort, and this may, in turn, produce autonomic side effects. Thus, as much skill is required in reversing anesthesia as in inducing and maintaining it. For this reason, modern-day anesthesia care does not end with the emergence of the patient from anesthesia but continues into a postanesthesia recovery period during which the patient is closely monitored for any untoward side effects related to either the surgical procedure or the administration of anesthesia.

Table 67-11 Autonomic effects of muscle relaxants

Drug	Histamine release	Cardiac	Autonomic ganglia	Duration of action
Succinylcholine	+	↓ heart rate	Stimulation	Ultrashort
Tubocurarine	+ +	↔	Blockade	Long
Pancuronium	↔	↑ heart rate	↔	Long
Atracurium	+	↔	↔	Intermediate
Vecuronium	↔	↔	↔	Intermediate

↔, no effect; ↑, increase; ↓, decrease; +, slight effect; + +, moderate effect.

Cardiovascular adjuvants

VASOCONSTRICTORS. Many adjuvant drugs are used during anesthesia and surgery to reverse the adverse effects of anesthetic drugs, to control autonomic system reflexes, and to support the failing heart and circulation. Vasoconstrictors are used to restore arterial perfusion pressure and to reverse the decrease in peripheral vascular resistance that may accompany either regional[77] or general[78] anesthesia. Pure α-adrenergic agonists like phenylephrine and methoxamine exhibit no cardiac sympathomimetic activity. It is therefore not surprising that phenylephrine given as an IV bolus to anesthetized patients with coronary artery disease causes an increase in systemic blood pressure, albeit at the expense of a transient impairment in left ventricular global function.[77,78] In patients with valvular aortic stenosis, however, bolus administration of phenylephrine is well tolerated. If, on the other hand, both peripheral vasoconstriction and some inotropic or chronotropic effect is desirable, ephedrine, an α- and β-adrenergic agonist, may be a better choice.[79]

VASODILATORS. Vasodilator therapy is often required in patients with a history of hypertension, particularly to control adverse responses to anesthesia and surgery, such as intubation and laryngoscopy, or responses consequent to surgical intervention, such as aortic cross-clamping. In addition, vasodilators can be used in specific cardiac conditions either to treat myocardial ischemia or to reduce preload or afterload, as may be necessary in patients with valvular heart disease. In some surgical settings, induced hypotension may be a prerequisite to a successful surgical outcome, for example, in some neurosurgical and craniofacial procedures. Nitroglycerin is the first-choice vasodilator in managing patients with ischemic heart disease, because it not only has peripheral vasodilator effects but also has a pronounced and beneficial vasodilator effect on epicardial coronary arteries. Alternatively, in patients requiring more marked reduction in peripheral vascular resistance, nitroprusside can be infused. Sublingual administration of nifedipine is occasionally useful in reducing arterial pressure, although this method does not permit ready titration of effect. Labetalol is a versatile drug that can be used to control both heart rate and blood pressure responses to surgical stimulation.[80]

INOTROPES. Inotropic support is occasionally required in patients with cardiac disease undergoing noncardiac surgery, especially vascular surgery. If the use of a bolus of calcium chloride or ephedrine is too short-lasting or fails to support the circulation in these patients, consideration must be given to the use of a continuous infusion of an inotrope, for example, dopamine. The use of epinephrine in combination with potent inhalational anesthetics, particularly halothane, may predispose the patient to an increased risk of dysrhythmias.[76,81] Isoflurane and, to a greater extent, enflurane carry a much lower risk for this interaction.[81] Inotropes are often used in conjunction with vasodilator therapy because of their synergistic effects that result in augmentation of myocardial contractility and a reduction in left ventricular afterload.

β-BLOCKERS. β-Blockers are commonly used during anesthesia and surgery in patients with cardiac disease, primarily ischemic heart disease. β-Blockade can potentiate the myocardial depressant action of many anesthetic agents and, therefore, needs to be used with caution during anesthesia and surgery. Until the recent introduction of esmolol, the choice of β-blockers was limited to agents with a relatively long duration of action. Esmolol is a relatively cardioselective β-blocker that because of rapid metabolism to inactive products has a very short duration of action.[82] The clinical effects of esmolol closely parallel the plasma levels of the drug. Its elimination half-life is between 8 and 12 minutes, and by 20 to 30 minutes its effect is essentially gone. Esmolol may be administered by bolus dose with or without continuous infusion until an appropriate reduction in the heart rate is achieved. Esmolol has been demonstrated to be useful in a number of perioperative clinical situations. Examples include acute β-blockade in patients with chronic obstructive pulmonary disease and cardiac disease with little risk of bronchospasm,[83] attenuation of the hypertension and tachycardia response to laryngoscopy and endotracheal intubation,[74,84] treatment of perioperative hypertension,[85] and treatment of intraoperative myocardial ischemia.[86] Another drug that has achieved some popularity in the treatment of perioperative hypertension is labetalol,[80,87] which has a mixed α- and β-blocking action (ratio of α:β blocking potency, 1:7). All β-blockers carry the potential risk of producing bronchospasm, and caution needs to be exercised in their use in patients with bronchospastic disease.

ANTIDYSRHYTHMIC AGENTS. Dysrhythmias are common in the perioperative period, particularly in patients with cardiac disease.[88] Of some concern is the predisposition to ventricular dysrhythmias caused by use of high concentrations of the potent inhalational anesthetic agents, particularly in conjunction with sympathetic stimulation or the administration of a sympathomimetic agent.[81,88] The management of ventricular ectopy in the perioperative period follows the same guidelines as those used in any cardiology practice. It is customary for anesthesiologists to choose lidocaine as the first agent in the treatment of patients with ventricular ectopy. If there is no response to a repeat dose of lidocaine, an alternative agent may be chosen, for example, procainamide or bretylium. Occasionally, atropine is required to treat sinus bradycardia resulting from excessive vagal stimulation, as may occur with traction on the extraocular eye muscles or from the use of high IV doses of narcotics, for example, fentanyl. IV administration of verapamil is occasionally required in the treatment of paroxysmal supraventricular tachyarrhythmias, although extreme caution needs to be exercised in its use during the intraoperative period because it can cause myocardial depression, peripheral vasodilatation, and a profound decrease in arterial blood pressure.

The role of hypokalemia in the development of ventricular ectopy during general anesthesia is uncertain.[89] The common practice of replacing potassium overnight probably carries more risk than benefits; alternatively, there is little evidence to support cancellation of surgery because of hypokalemia.[89] The management of preoperative hypokalemia should focus on the precipitating causes for the electrolyte imbalance, the duration and severity of the potassium deficit, potential interactions with medications, and the presence of associated electrolyte disturbances.[89]

Patients with a pacemaker. In emergencies, a temporary transvenous pacemaker can be placed, when indicated.[59,60] A pacing pulmonary artery catheter can be used as a temporary pacemaker or in the uncommon situation of a drug-induced bradycardia or a cardiac event producing severe bradycardia. In patients with a permanent pacemaker, the possibility of intraoperative failure should be considered. Failure is usually related to electrocautery interference but may be due to electrolyte abnormalities (primarily potassium), myopotentials, or myocardial ischemia and infarction. Programmable pacemakers may be reprogrammed during electrocautery or after a magnet has been placed over the generator. This may result in ventricular fibrillation due to an R-on-T electrical impulse. For this reason, a pacemaker programmer should be available to reprogram a pacemaker that has been affected by the intraoperative use of electrocautery. In patients with pacemakers, electrocautery should be used in short bursts and the electrocautery ground plate should be located as far as possible from the generator.[90] Pulse oximetry monitoring is a useful method of ensuring that an arterial pulse is present during the use of electrocautery, because ECG monitoring is invalidated by the degradation of the ECG signal by electrocautery.

Patients with an implantable cardioverter-defibrillator. The implantable cardioverter-defibrillator (ICD) may be temporarily or permanently inhibited by electromagnetic interference from electrocautery. The manufacturer recommends deactivating the generator before using electrocautery in patients with an ICD. In addition, magnets should be kept away from the ICD generator. Repeated induction of ventricular fibrillation and subsequent defibrillation to determine the defibrillation threshold during ICD placement may lead to a significant reduction in myocardial performance, particularly in patients with preexisting left ventricular function.[91]

POSTOPERATIVE MANAGEMENT

In addition to the usual problems associated with any surgical procedure, patients with cardiac disease may experience problems in the perioperative period specific to their underlying cardiac status. Surgical repair, either curative or palliative, is undertaken because it offers less risk of death and greater quality of life than medical management.[92] However, for almost all patients with cardiac disease undergoing cardiac and noncardiac surgery, the intraoperative and immediate postoperative periods are times of high risk for cardiac dysrhythmia, organ system failure, and sudden death. Care for these patients often requires complex cardiopulmonary supportive measures and invasive monitoring. The low mortality currently achieved is due, in part, to improved surgical technique and improved intraoperative and postoperative monitoring and support of failing organ systems.[5,8,21,92]

The general philosophy for postoperative care of the patient with cardiac disease takes into account the possible complications attendant upon the surgical procedure itself, the underlying cardiac lesion, secondary subsystem abnormalities engendered by the cardiac disease, age, drug therapy, and other factors that alter the general condition of the patient. Taking all these factors into account, one can estimate the risks for organ dysfunction during the perioperative period and can design the monitoring technique, using either continuous or intermittent repetitive measurement, that will provide information about organ function.[92] Changes in organ function trigger appropriate actions, as directed by specific guidelines for discrete events. These guidelines should be provided to the medical and paramedical staff who will be caring for the patient. A concept of progressive patient care is important for the efficient use of resources. The patient proceeds from the operating room to the postanesthesia recovery room, to a period in an intensive care unit, or "step-down" unit, where ECG monitoring may be available, to rehabilitation on an open floor area, and finally to recuperation at home.[92]

Cardiac complications occur much more frequently during the postoperative period than during the intraoperative period. The peak incidence of myocardial infarction is within the first few days after surgery.[3-16] One can speculate on the reasons for this. In the operating room, there is close supervision of the patient by the anesthesiologist. In the postoperative period, a combination of poor pain control, hypothermia,[93] anemia, hypovolemia or hypervolemia, hypoxemia, fever, and electrolyte abnormalities may occur and be less closely managed

Table 67-12 Factors that influence myocardial oxygen balance in the postoperative period

Decrease myocardial oxygen supply	Increase myocardial oxygen demand ($M\dot{V}O_2$)
Respiratory depression → hypoventilation → ↑ $PaCO_2$ and ↓ PaO_2 Respiratory complications, e.g., atelectasis → ↓ PaO_2 Fluid overload → ↑ LVEDP → ↑ subendocardial ischemia → further ↑ LVEDP → pulmonary edema → ↓ PaO_2 Anemia Hypercoagulable state?	Hypothermia → shivering → ↑ $M\dot{V}O_2$ Pain → sympathetic stimulation → ↑ $M\dot{V}O_2$ Hypoventilation → ↑ $PaCO_2$ → sympathetic stimulation → ↑ $M\dot{V}O_2$ Hypertension → ↑ $M\dot{V}O_2$ Tachycardia → ↑ $M\dot{V}O_2$

LVEDP, left ventricular end-diastolic pressure.

(Table 67-12). Arrhythmias, thromboembolic disease, and respiratory complications are more common in patients with cardiac disease. Close monitoring should therefore be continued in the postoperative period. Almost half of 230 male patients with known coronary artery disease or at high risk of coronary artery disease undergoing major noncardiac surgical procedures had frequent or major ventricular arrhythmias perioperatively.[94] Specific attention should be paid to the control of postoperative tachycardia in patients with ischemic heart disease.[95]

Patients taking β-blockers are subject to withdrawal supersensitivity. Administration of these medications should be resumed as soon as possible postoperatively, provided that there is no clinical contraindication. Calcium channel blockers should also be administered again as soon as possible after surgery. For patients who are unable to take medications orally, transdermal administration of nitroglycerin can be used as an alternative method. The resumption of digoxin therapy should be predicated on the basis of the patient's clinical status and whether postoperative dysrhythmias or electrolyte abnormalities are present. Administration of antihypertensive medications should also be resumed as soon as possible after noncardiac surgery. The problem of clonidine withdrawal is significant and can possibly be managed by transdermal administration of the drug.

The high incidence of postoperative ischemia and myocardial infarction in patients with coronary artery disease and also the high prevalence of silent ischemia[61] suggest that these patients should have ECG monitoring, serial 12-lead ECG studies, and creatine kinase analysis, at least for the first few days after major noncardiac surgery. Many patients with coronary artery disease or a history of hypertension become hypertensive in the postoperative period, especially if they have undergone major surgery, such as aortic aneurysm resection. Hypertension may be related to untreated pain, anxiety, depression over an unfavorable diagnosis, hypoxemia, and the failure to reinstitute antihypertensive medication in the immediate postoperative period. Postoperative hypertension can usually be managed with β-blockers and vasodilator therapy. Esmolol, as previously mentioned, is a useful short-acting, intravenously administered β-blocker that can prevent reflex tachycardia, which often accompanies the lowering of arterial pressure with vasodilators. Nitroglycerin can be a particularly beneficial vasodilator for patients with coronary artery disease. At times, however, the effect of this drug on peripheral vascular resistance may be insufficiently potent to effectively reduce increased arterial pressure. Nitroprusside is an alternative, although in rare instances, a coronary steal syndrome may be induced in a subset of patients.

SUMMARY AND CONCLUSIONS

The past decade has seen major strides in the diagnosis and management of patients with cardiac disease. Improvements in anesthetic management, both intraoperatively and postoperatively, and in surgical results have kept pace with these improvements. These improvements have come at the expense of escalating costs of medical care and, consequently, government intrusion into the practice of medicine. It is increasingly likely that external pressures will force changes in eligibility for medical services, dictate where these services will be provided (outpatient or inpatient facilities), and even cause rationing of services. There will be an increasing demand for outcome studies to determine the efficacy of diagnostic procedures and of therapeutic techniques. The challenge to medicine in the 1990s is to respond to these factors proactively. Medical societies should develop clinical practice guidelines based on a review of the relevant scientific evidence and expert opinion about effectiveness.[62,96]

REFERENCES

1. Mangano DT: Perioperative cardiac morbidity. *Anesthesiology* 72:153-184, 1990
2. Eagle KA, Boucher CA: Cardiac risk of noncardiac surgery (editorial). *N Engl J Med* 321:1330-1332, 1989
3. Tarhan S, Moffitt EA, Taylor WF, et al: Myocardial infarction after general anesthesia. *JAMA* 220:1451-1454, 1972
4. Steen PA, Tinker JH, Tarhan S: Myocardial reinfarction after anesthesia and surgery. *JAMA* 239:2566-2570, 1978
5. Rao TL, Jacobs KH, El-Etr AA: Reinfarction following anesthesia in patients with myocardial infarction. *Anesthesiology* 59:499-505, 1983
6. Jeffrey CC, Kunsman J, Cullen DJ, et al: A prospective evaluation of cardiac risk index. *Anesthesiology* 58:462-464, 1983

7. Charlson ME, Ales KL, Simon R, et al: Why predictive indexes perform less well in validation studies. Is it magic or methods? *Arch Intern Med* 147:2155-2161, 1987

8. Raby KE, Goldman L, Creager MA, et al: Correlation between preoperative ischemia and major cardiac events after peripheral vascular surgery. *N Engl J Med* 321:1296-1300, 1989

9. Mangano DT, Browner WS, Hollenberg M, et al: Association of perioperative myocardial ischemia with cardiac morbidity and mortality in men undergoing noncardiac surgery. The Study of Perioperative Ischemia Research Group. *N Engl J Med* 323:1781-1788, 1990

10. Lowenstein E, Yusuf S, Teplick RS: Perioperative myocardial reinfarction: a glimmer of hope – a note of caution (editorial). *Anesthesiology* 59:493-494, 1983

11. Goldman L, Caldera DL, Nussbaum SR, et al: Multifactorial index of cardiac risk in noncardiac surgical procedures. *N Engl J Med* 297:845-850, 1977

12. Zeldin RA: Assessing cardiac risk in patients who undergo noncardiac surgical procedures. *Can J Surg* 27:402-404, 1984

13. Detsky AS, Abrams HB, McLaughlin JR, et al: Predicting cardiac complications in patients undergoing non-cardiac surgery. *J Gen Intern Med* 1:211-219, 1986

14. Foster ED, Davis KB, Carpenter JA, et al: Risk of noncardiac operation in patients with defined coronary disease: the Coronary Artery Surgery Study (CASS) registry experience. *Ann Thorac Surg* 41:42-50, 1986

15. Mahar LJ, Steen PA, Tinker JH, et al: Perioperative myocardial infarction in patients with coronary artery disease with and without aorta-coronary artery bypass grafts. *J Thorac Cardiovasc Surg* 76:533-537, 1978

16. Nielsen JL, Page CP, Mann C, et al: Risk of major elective operation after myocardial revascularization. *Am J Surg* 164:423-426, 1992

17. The VA Coronary Artery Bypass Surgery Cooperative Study Group: Eighteen-year follow-up in the Veterans Affairs Cooperative Study of Coronary Artery Bypass Surgery for stable angina. *Circulation* 86:121-130, 1992

18. Gagnon RM, Dumont G, Sestier F, et al: The role of coronary angioplasty in patients with associated noncardiac medical and surgical conditions. *Can J Cardiol* 6:287-292, 1990

19. Backer CL, Tinker JH, Robertson DM, et al: Myocardial reinfarction following local anesthesia for ophthalmic surgery. *Anesth Analg* 59:257-262, 1980

20. Spirito P, Chiarella F, Carratino L, et al: Clinical course and prognosis of hypertrophic cardiomyopathy in an outpatient population. *N Engl J Med* 320:749-755, 1989

21. Hollier LH, Plate G, O'Brien PC, et al: Late survival after abdominal aortic aneurysm repair: influence of coronary artery disease. *J Vasc Surg* 1:290-299, 1984

22. Hertzer NR, Young JR, Kramer JR, et al: Routine coronary angiography prior to elective aortic reconstruction: results of selective myocardial revascularization in patients with peripheral vascular disease. *Arch Surg* 114:1336-1344, 1979

23. Brown OW, Hollier LH, Pairolero PC, et al: Abdominal aortic aneurysm and coronary artery disease. *Arch Surg* 116:1484-1488, 1981

24. Rihal CS, Eagle KA, Mickel MC, et al: Surgical therapy for coronary artery disease among patients with combined coronary artery and peripheral vascular disease. *Circulation* 91:46-53, 1995

25. O'Keefe JH Jr, Vlietstra RE, Bailey KR, et al: Natural history of candidates for balloon aortic valvuloplasty. *Mayo Clin Proc* 62:986-991, 1987

26. Marcus ML, Doty DB, Hiratzka LF, et al: Decreased coronary reserve: a mechanism for angina pectoris in patients with aortic stenosis and normal coronary arteries. *N Engl J Med* 307:1362-1366, 1982

27. Tinker JH, Noback CR, Vlietstra RE, et al: Management of patients with heart disease for noncardiac surgery. *JAMA* 246:1348-1350, 1981

28. Labovitz AJ, Pearson AC: Evaluation of left ventricular diastolic function: clinical relevance and recent Doppler echocardiographic insights. *Am Heart J* 114:836-851, 1987

29. Nishimura RA, Housmans PR, Hatle LK, et al: Assessment of diastolic function of the heart: background and current applications of Doppler echocardiography. Part I. Physiologic and pathophysiologic features. *Mayo Clin Proc* 64:71-81, 1989

30. Kopecky SL, Gersh BJ: Dilated cardiomyopathy and myocarditis: natural history, etiology, clinical manifestations, and management. *Curr Probl Cardiol* 12:569-647, 1987

31. Wagner JA, Sax FL, Weisman HF, et al: Calcium-antagonist receptors in the atrial tissue of patients with hypertrophic cardiomyopathy. *N Engl J Med* 320:755-761, 1989

32. Maron BJ, Bonow RO, Cannon RO III, et al: Hypertrophic cardiomyopathy. Interrelations of clinical manifestations, pathophysiology, and therapy. Parts 1 and 2. *N Engl J Med* 316:780-789; 844-852, 1987

33. Baum VC, Perloff JK: Anesthetic implications of adults with congenital heart disease. *Anesth Analg* 76:1342-1358, 1993

34. Freeman WK, Gibbons RJ, Shub C: Preoperative assessment of cardiac patients undergoing noncardiac surgical procedures. *Mayo Clin Proc* 64:1105-1117, 1989

35. Fleisher LA, Barash PG: Preoperative cardiac evaluation for noncardiac surgery: a functional approach. *Anesth Analg* 74:586-598, 1992

36. Bach DS, Armstrong WF: Dobutamine stress echocardiography. *Am J Cardiol* 69:90H-96H, 1992

37. Boucher CA, Brewster DC, Darling RC, et al: Determination of cardiac risk by dipyridamole-thallium imaging before peripheral vascular surgery. *N Engl J Med* 312:389-394, 1985

38. Leppo J, Plaja J, Gionet M, et al: Noninvasive evaluation of cardiac risk before elective vascular surgery. *J Am Coll Cardiol* 9:269-276, 1987

39. Eagle KA, Singer DE, Brewster DC, et al: Dipyridamole-thallium scanning in patients undergoing vascular surgery. Optimizing preoperative evaluation of cardiac risk. *JAMA* 257:2185-2189, 1987

40. Ryan T, Feigenbaum H: Exercise echocardiography. *Am J Cardiol* 69:82H-89H, 1992

41. Eagle KA, Coley CM, Newell JB, et al: Combining clinical and thallium data optimizes preoperative assessment of cardiac risk before major vascular surgery. *Ann Intern Med* 110:859-866, 1989

42. Roth RB, Palacios IF, Block PC: Percutaneous aortic balloon valvuloplasty: its role in the management of patients with aortic stenosis requiring major noncardiac surgery. *J Am Coll Cardiol* 13:1039-1041, 1989

43. Smedira NG, Ports TA, Merrick SH, et al: Balloon aortic valvuloplasty as a bridge to aortic valve replacement in critically ill patients. *Ann Thorac Surg* 55:914-916, 1993

44. Otto CM, Mickel MC, Kennedy JW, et al: Three-year outcome after balloon aortic valvuloplasty. Insights into prognosis of valvular aortic stenosis. *Circulation* 89:642-650, 1994

45. Nishimura RA, Holmes DR Jr, Reeder GS: Percutaneous balloon valvuloplasty. *Mayo Clin Proc* 65:198-220, 1990

46. Cohen DJ, Kuntz RE, Gordon SP, et al: Predictors of long-term outcome after percutaneous balloon mitral valvuloplasty. *N Engl J Med* 327:1329-1335, 1992

47. Tinker JH, Tarhan S: Discontinuing anticoagulant therapy in surgical patients with cardiac valve prostheses. Observations in 180 operations. *JAMA* 239:738-739, 1978

48. Dajani AS, Bisno AL, Chung KJ, et al: Prevention of bacterial endocarditis. Recommendations by the American Heart Association. *JAMA* 264:2919-2922, 1990

49. Romagnoli A, Keats AS: Plasma and atrial propranolol after preoperative withdrawal. *Circulation* 52:1123-1127, 1975

50. Slogoff S, Keats AS: Does chronic treatment with calcium entry blocking drugs reduce perioperative myocardial ischemia? *Anesthesiology* 68:676-680, 1988

51. Slogoff S, Keats AS: Does perioperative myocardial ischemia lead to postoperative myocardial infarction? *Anesthesiology* 62:107-114, 1985

52. Sill JC, Nugent M, Moyer TP, et al: Plasma levels of beta-blocking drugs prior to coronary artery bypass surgery. *Anesthesiology* 62:67-70, 1985

53. Chung F, Houston PL, Cheng DC, et al: Calcium channel blockade does not offer adequate protection from perioperative myocardial ischemia. *Anesthesiology* 69:343-347, 1988

54. Packer M: Drug therapy. Combined beta-adrenergic and calcium-entry blockade in angina pectoris. *N Engl J Med* 320:709-718, 1989

55. Thomson IR, Mutch WA, Culligan JD: Failure of intravenous nitroglycerin to prevent intraoperative myocardial ischemia during fentanyl-pancuronium anesthesia. *Anesthesiology* 61:385-393, 1984

56. Gallagher JD, Moore RA, Jose AB, et al: Prophylactic nitroglycerin infusions during coronary artery bypass surgery. *Anesthesiology* 64:785-789, 1986

57. Bruce DL, Croley TF, Lee JS: Preoperative clonidine withdrawal syndrome. *Anesthesiology* 51:90-92, 1979

58. Krowka MJ, Pairolero PC, Trastek VF, et al: Cardiac dysrhythmia following pneumonectomy. Clinical correlates and prognostic significance. *Chest* 91:490-495, 1987

59. Frye RL, Collins JJ, DeSanctis RW, et al: Guidelines for permanent cardiac pacemaker implantation, May 1984. A report of the Joint American College of Cardiology/American Heart Association Task Force on Assessment of Cardiovascular Procedures (Subcommittee on Pacemaker Implantation). *Circulation* 70:331A-339A, 1984

60. Pastore JO, Yurchak PM, Janis KM, et al: The risk of advanced heart block in surgical patients with right bundle branch block and left axis deviation. *Circulation* 57:677-680, 1978

61. Knight AA, Hollenberg M, London MJ, et al: Perioperative myocardial ischemia: importance of the preoperative ischemic pattern. *Anesthesiology* 68:681-688, 1988

62. Anonymous: Practice guidelines for pulmonary artery catheterization. A report by the American Society of Anesthesiologists Task Force on Pulmonary Artery Catheterization. *Anesthesiology* 78:380-394, 1993

63. Shah KB, Rao TL, Laughlin S, et al: A review of pulmonary artery catheterization in 6,245 patients. *Anesthesiology* 61:271-275, 1984

64. Abel MD, Nishimura RA, Callahan MJ, et al: Evaluation of intraoperative transesophageal two-dimensional echocardiography. *Anesthesiology* 66:64-68, 1987

65. Smith JS, Cahalan MK, Benefiel DJ, et al: Intraoperative detection of myocardial ischemia in high-risk patients: electrocardiography versus two-dimensional transesophageal echocardiography. *Circulation* 72:1015-1021, 1985

66. Leung JM, O'Kelly B, Browner WS, et al: Prognostic importance of postbypass regional wall-motion abnormalities in patients undergoing coronary artery bypass graft surgery. SPI Research Group. *Anesthesiology* 71:16-25, 1989

67. London MJ, Tubau JF, Wong MG, et al: The "natural history" of segmental wall motion abnormalities in patients undergoing noncardiac surgery. S.P.I. Research Group. *Anesthesiology* 73:644-655, 1990

68. Thys DM, Hillel Z, Goldman ME, et al: A comparison of hemodynamic indices derived by invasive monitoring and two-dimensional echocardiography. *Anesthesiology* 67:630-634, 1987

69. Lundy JS: Intravenous anesthesia: preliminary report of the use of two new thiobarbiturates. *Proc Staff Meet Mayo Clin* 10:536-543, 1935

70. Conway CM, Ellis DB: The haemodynamic effects of short-acting barbiturates. *Br J Anaesth* 41:534-542, 1969

71. Ebert TJ, Muzi M, Berens R, et al: Sympathetic responses to induction of anesthesia in humans with propofol or etomidate. *Anesthesiology* 76:725-733, 1992

72. McLeskey CH, Walawander CA, Nahrwold ML, et al: Adverse events in a multicenter phase IV study of propofol: evaluation by anesthesiologists and postanesthesia care unit nurses. *Anesth Analg* 77 Suppl 4:3-9, 1993

73. Borgeat A, Wilder-Smith OH, Saiah M, et al: Subhypnotic doses of propofol possess direct antiemetic properties. *Anesth Analg* 74:539-541, 1992

74. Cucchiara RF, Benefiel DJ, Matteo RS, et al: Evaluation of esmolol in controlling increases in heart rate and blood pressure during endotracheal intubation in patients undergoing carotid endarterectomy. *Anesthesiology* 65:528-531, 1986

75. Slogoff S, Keats AS: Randomized trial of primary anesthetic agents on outcome of coronary artery bypass operations. *Anesthesiology* 70:179-188, 1989

76. Forrest JB, Cahalan MK, Rehder K, et al: Multicenter study of general anesthesia. II. Results. *Anesthesiology* 72:262-268, 1990

77. Goertz AW, Seeling W, Heinrich H, et al: Effect of phenylephrine bolus administration on left ventricular function during high thoracic and lumbar epidural anesthesia combined with general anesthesia. *Anesth Analg* 76:541-545, 1993

78. Goertz AW, Lindner KH, Seefelder C, et al: Effect of phenylephrine bolus administration on global left ventricular function in patients with coronary artery disease and patients with valvular aortic stenosis. *Anesthesiology* 78:834-841, 1993

79. Goertz AW, Hubner C, Seefelder C, et al: The effect of ephedrine bolus administration on left ventricular loading and systolic performance during high thoracic epidural anesthesia combined with general anesthesia. *Anesth Analg* 78:101-105, 1994

80. Goa KL, Benfield P, Sorkin EM: Labetalol. A reappraisal of its pharmacology, pharmacokinetics and therapeutic use in hypertension and ischaemic heart disease. *Drugs* 37:583-627, 1989

81. Johnston RR, Eger EI II, Wilson C: A comparative interaction of epinephrine with enflurane, isoflurane, and halothane in man. *Anesth Analg* 55:709-712, 1976

82. Blanski L, Lutz J, Laddu A: Esmolol, the first ultra-short-acting intravenous beta blocker for use in critically ill patients. *Heart Lung* 17:80-89, 1988

83. Gold MR, Dec GW, Cocca-Spofford D, et al: Esmolol and ventilatory function in cardiac patients with COPD. *Chest* 100:1215-1218, 1991

84. Helfman SM, Gold MI, DeLisser EA, et al: Which drug prevents tachycardia and hypertension associated with tracheal intubation: lidocaine, fentanyl, or esmolol? *Anesth Analg* 72:482-486, 1991

85. Gibson BE, Black S, Maass L, et al: Esmolol for the control of hypertension after neurologic surgery. *Clin Pharmacol Ther* 44:650-653, 1988

86. Harrison L, Ralley FE, Wynands JE, et al: The role of an ultra short-acting adrenergic blocker (esmolol) in patients undergoing coronary artery bypass surgery. *Anesthesiology* 66:413-418, 1987

87. Muzzi DA, Black S, Losasso TJ, et al: Labetalol and esmolol in the control of hypertension after intracranial surgery. *Anesth Analg* 70:68-71, 1990

88. Atlee JL III, Bosnjak ZJ: Mechanisms for cardiac dysrhythmias during anesthesia. *Anesthesiology* 72:347-374, 1990

89. Wong KC, Schafer PG, Schultz JR: Hypokalemia and anesthetic implications. *Anesth Analg* 77:1238-1260, 1993

90. Simon AB: Perioperative management of the pacemaker patient. *Anesthesiology* 46:127-131, 1977

91. Keyl C, Tassani P, Kemkes B, et al: Hemodynamic changes due to intraoperative testing of the automatic implantable cardioverter defibrillator: implications for anesthesia management. *J Cardiothorac Vasc Anesth* 7:442-447, 1993

92. Marsh HM, Abel MD: Postoperative management of adult cardiac surgical patients. In *Cardiovascular Anesthesia and Postoperative Care.* Second edition. Edited by S Tarhan. Chicago, Year Book Medical Publishers, 1989, pp 609-630

93. Frank SM, Beattie C, Christopherson R, et al: Unintentional hypothermia is associated with postoperative myocardial ischemia. The Perioperative Ischemia Randomized Anesthesia Trial Study Group. *Anesthesiology* 78:468-476, 1993

94. O'Kelly B, Browner WS, Massie B, et al: Ventricular arrhythmias in patients undergoing noncardiac surgery. The Study of Perioperative Ischemia Research Group. *JAMA* 268:217-221, 1992

95. Mangano DT, Wong MG, London MJ, et al: Perioperative myocardial ischemia in patients undergoing noncardiac surgery—II: incidence and severity during the 1st week after surgery. The Study of Perioperative Ischemia (SPI) Research Group. *J Am Coll Cardiol* 17:851-857, 1991

96. Woolf SH: Practice guidelines: a new reality in medicine. III. Impact on patient care. *Arch Intern Med* 153:2646-2655, 1993

CHAPTER

68

Genetics of heart disease

Virginia V. Michels, M.D., and David J. Driscoll, M.D.

GENETIC factors play a role in the development of many types of heart disease, including most congenital heart defects, some cardiomyopathies, and heart diseases as components of some systemic disorders. The genetic determinants may be single gene defects, mitochondrial mutations, chromosomal abnormalities, or multifactorial. A glossary of terms appears at the end of this chapter.

CHROMOSOMAL ABNORMALITIES

Approximately 5% of all congenital heart defects are due to chromosomal abnormalities. Chromosomal abnormalities occur in approximately 1 per 180 live births. One-third of these abnormalities involve an abnormal number (aneuploidy) of non-sex chromosomes (autosomes). The only factors known to result in a higher-than-average risk for having a child with autosomal aneuploidy are maternal age of 35 years or older and having previously had an affected child. Pregnant women at increased risk can be offered prenatal diagnosis by karyotype of fetal cells obtained by amniocentesis or chorionic villus sampling.

The most common autosomal aneuploidy syndrome in term infants is the Down syndrome, with an incidence of 1 per 880. Forty percent of patients with the Down syndrome have a congenital heart defect, most frequently ventricular septal defect or atrioventricular (AV) canal defect, although other congenital heart defects may occur. Most patients with the Down syndrome have trisomy 21 (Fig 68-1) as a result of a new mutation nondysjunctional event; in these cases, the risk to the parents of having another affected child is 1% to 2% or higher, depending on maternal age. In 3% of patients with the Down syndrome, a translocation chromosomal abnormality is present (Fig 68-2). These translocation chromosomes may be inherited in an unbalanced form from a parent carrying a balanced form of the translocation; these parents have a 5% to 15% risk of having another affected child. To identify these high-risk families, chromosome analysis should be performed on all patients with the Down syndrome. Even if the parents have completed their childbearing, the karyotype of the affected child should be determined so that other relatives may be counseled appropriately. The same principles are presumed to be true for other autosomal aneuploidy syndromes.

Approximately 35% of the chromosomal abnormalities in live-born infants involve sex chromosome aneuploidy. These patients may have an additional X or Y chromosome or be lacking one. Patients with 47,XXX, 47,XYY, or 47,XXY karyotype do not have an increased risk for congenital heart defects. However, patients with Turner's syndrome (45,X karyotype) or its variants (with one structurally abnormal X or Y) have a risk of approximately 30% for a congenital heart defect. Bicuspid aortic valve with or without coarctation of the aorta is particularly common. Ordinarily, parents of patients with sex chromosome aneuploidy are not at increased risk for having another affected child, and these parents do not routinely need chromosome analyses.

Thirty-four percent of chromosomal abnormalities involve structural changes such as deletions (Fig 68-3), duplications (Fig 68-4), inversions, or translocations. The translocations may be balanced (no net loss or gain of genetic material) or unbalanced. People with balanced translocations usually are phenotypically normal and healthy, but they may be at increased risk for miscarriages or their children may have birth defects. Patients with net loss or gain of genetic material by any of the mechanisms listed above have phenotypic abnormalities that usually include mental retardation and frequently include congenital heart defects. The parents of all patients with a structural chromosomal abnormality should have a chromosome analysis to determine if they are carriers of a balanced translocation.

PATTERNS OF INHERITANCE

Autosomal dominant

Autosomal dominant inheritance implies that the responsible gene is located on one of the autosomes and that the gene overrides or dominates its homologue in terms of clinical effect. Therefore, one copy of the gene is sufficient for the trait to be expressed or for the disease to be present. For diseases inherited in this way, heterozygotes (persons carrying one normal gene and one abnormal gene) have the disease. There is a 50% chance that any child born to an affected person will inherit the abnormal gene.

The severity of the disease caused by the abnormal gene may be quite uniform for some conditions, such as

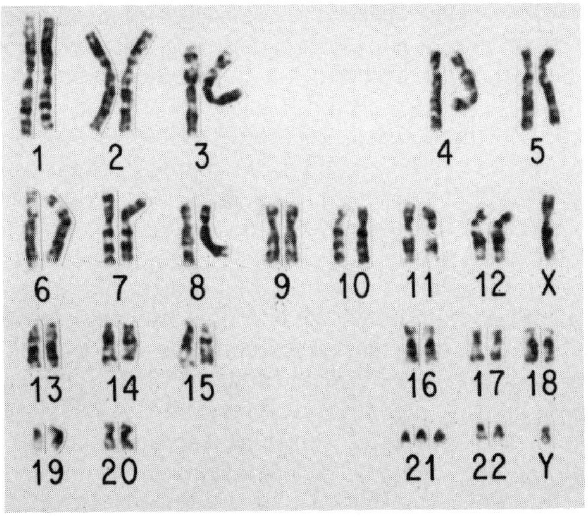

Fig 68-1 Karyotype of a patient with the Down syndrome due to trisomy 21; 47,XY, +21. (Courtesy of Gordon Dewald, Ph.D.)

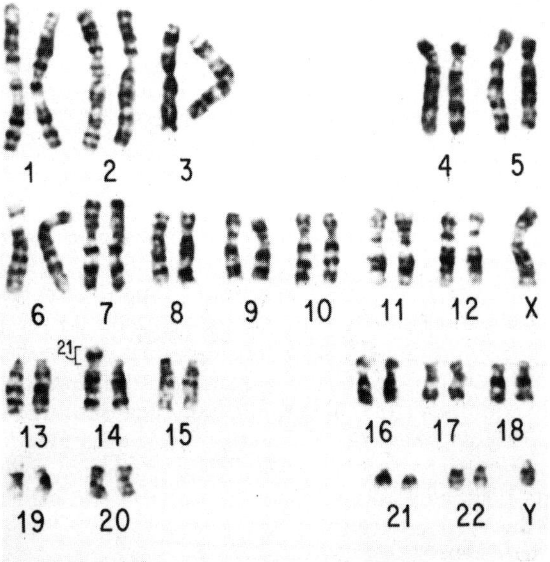

Fig 68-2 Karyotype of a patient with the Down syndrome due to an unbalanced translocation—46,XY,der(21), t(14;21) (q11;p11)pat—inherited from the father, who carried a balanced form of the translocation. (Courtesy of Gordon Dewald, Ph.D.)

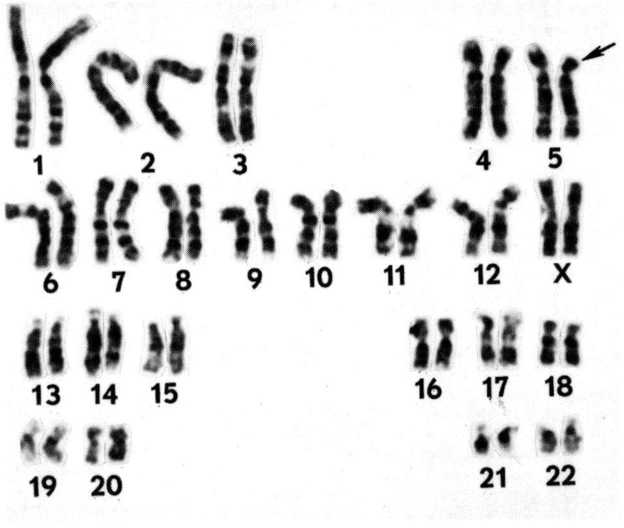

Fig 68-3 Karyotype of a patient with deletion of part of the short arm of one chromosome 5, resulting in cri du chat syndrome; 46,XX,del(5)(p15). (Courtesy of Gordon Dewald, Ph.D.)

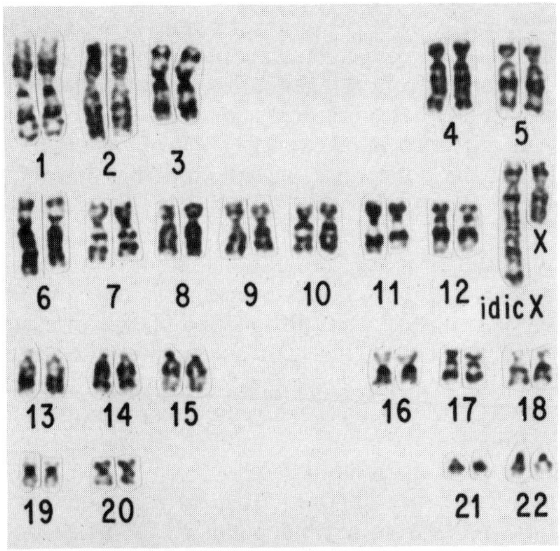

Fig 68-4 Karyotype of a patient with duplication of the short arm and most of the long arm of chromosome X, resulting in primary amenorrhea; 46,X,idic(X)(q28). (Courtesy of Gordon Dewald, Ph.D.)

achondroplasia, but for other conditions, such as neurofibromatosis and Marfan syndrome, the severity may be variable. This difference of severity is referred to as "variable expression." In contrast, the term "incomplete penetrance" means that some persons who have inherited the gene show no signs of it. Obviously, the clinical decision regarding whether or not a person has signs of the gene defect depends on the thoroughness of the examination and the sensitivity of the investigative techniques—for example, many families with hypertrophic cardiomyopathy were thought to include instances of incomplete penetrance until asymptomatic patients were examined by echocardiography. Although transmission of a disease through members of either sex through multiple generations of a family is strongly suggestive of autosomal dominant inheritance, it is equally important to remember that autosomal dominant diseases can occur without a positive family history. This can occur because of incomplete penetrance, incorrect assignment of paternity, new mutation, or somatic mosaicism. New mutation events represent changes that occur in the genetic material of the individual egg or sperm that gives rise to the fetus. Although the risk for siblings of a person whose disease arose by new mutation is not increased over that in the general population, the risk for the offspring still is 50%. Somatic mosaicism refers to the possibility that one of the parents may have the gene defect in only some cells, including the reproductive cells (germinal mosaicism), so that the person has no or few signs of the disease but potentially can transmit the disease to one or more children.

Autosomal recessive

Autosomal recessive diseases also occur because of abnormal genes that are located on the autosomes. However, one copy of the abnormal gene is not sufficient to cause disease, and heterozygotes (carriers) clinically are no different from the general population. When two persons who are heterozygotes for a given gene defect mate, the children are at a 25% risk of inheriting the abnormal gene from both parents and thus having the disease.

Because the heterozygous state may be transmitted silently through many generations before the chance mating of two heterozygotes occurs, it is not surprising that there rarely is a family history of the disease in previous generations. The occurrence of multiple affected siblings within a family suggests autosomal recessive inheritance; however, because of the small average family size in this country, many autosomal recessive diseases appear to occur as isolated cases.

The risk for the children of a person who has an autosomal recessive disease depends on the frequency of the abnormal gene in the population. The risk is usually quite small, provided that this person does not marry a relative or a person who has a family history of the same disease.

Many diseases that are caused by an identified metabolic defect, such as homocystinuria, are autosomal recessive diseases due to an enzyme deficiency. When the enzymatic defect is established, carrier testing and prenatal diagnosis sometimes are possible.

X-linked recessive

X-linked recessive diseases are caused by abnormal genes located on the X chromosome. Female heterozygotes, who have one abnormal gene on one chromosome and one normal gene on the other X chromosome, usually are clinically normal. Exceptions may occur because of the phenomenon of lyonization, in which one X chromosome is inactivated at random early in fetal life; if the normal gene is inactivated in a critical number of cells, the woman may have symptoms or clinical signs of the disease. However, the disease usually is less severe than in males. The likelihood of clinical signs of the disease developing in a female is quite variable for different diseases. For example, it is rare for female carriers of hemophilia A to have significant bleeding problems, but it is relatively common for carriers of ornithine carbamoyltransferase (ornithine transcarbamylase) deficiency to have intermittent symptoms.

Males who inherit the abnormal gene have no corresponding genetic loci on the Y chromosome and therefore are referred to as "hemizygotes." Any male child born to a heterozygous female is at 50% risk for having the disease; female children are at 50% risk for inheriting the gene and being carriers. All the daughters of affected males are carriers, and all the sons are unaffected—i.e., male-to-male transmission cannot occur.

X-linked recessive diseases also may arise by new mutation affecting either the mother or the afflicted son. Genetic counseling is difficult in these situations because if the mother represents the new mutation, the risk for her future male children is 50%. However, if the child represents the new mutation, there is no significant risk for siblings of that child. For carrier detection for some diseases, advances in methodology for DNA-based diagnosis have resulted in new opportunities that circumvent problems created by lyonization.

X-linked dominant

X-linked dominant inheritance is uncommon. Heterozygous females have the disease in a less severe form than do hemizygous males. Some X-linked dominant disorders are lethal in males. Both male and female children born to an affected mother have a 50% risk of being affected. Affected fathers have all affected daughters but no affected sons.

Y-linked

No human disease has been proved to be transmitted as a Y-linked trait. Clearly, the Y chromosome encodes important genetic information related to maleness and reproduction. However, mutations in genes on the Y chromosome often result in infertility, so that heritable transmission of the mutation cannot occur.

Mitochondrial

Mitochondria contain several circular copies of their own genetic material, mitochondrial DNA. This mitochondrial DNA, approximately 16,000 base pairs in length, encodes for transfer RNA and several proteins involved in the mitochondrial respiratory chain. Many mitochondrial enzymes, including some others of the respiratory chain complex, are encoded by nuclear DNA and transported into the mitochondria. Mitochondrial DNA mutations recently were found to cause Leber's optic atrophy and the multisystem syndromes of multiple episodes of lactic acidosis and stroke (MELAS) and myoclonic epilepsy with ragged red fibers (MERRF). Many cases of Kearns-Sayre syndrome of cardiomyopathy and ophthalmologic disorders have been shown to be due to mitochondrial mutations.[1] Mitochondrial disorders can arise as new mutations or be maternally inherited; only the egg, not the sperm, contributes mitochondria to the zygote. The mitochondrial mutations may be homoplasmic (present in all mitochondrial DNA) or heteroplasmic (present in only some of the mitochondrial DNA). It has been suggested that accumulation of acquired mutations may contribute to aging,[2] and there is evidence that mitochondrial mutations have a role in the pathogenesis of ischemic heart disease.[3]

MULTIFACTORIAL CAUSATION

This means that the disease or trait is determined by the interaction of environmental influences and a polygenic predisposition. Human conditions that may be due to multifactorial causation include many common birth defects—such as congenital heart defects, cleft lip and palate, and neural tube defects—and many common diseases—such as diabetes mellitus, asthma, hypertension, and atherosclerotic coronary artery disease.

The multifactorial model predicts that there will be a tendency for familial aggregation of the condition but without a strict mendelian pattern of inheritance.[4] Familial aggregation also can be due to common environmental factors, so familial aggregation by itself is not sufficient to prove multifactorial causation. Adoption studies and twin studies, especially when the study subjects are reared apart from their biologic relatives from an early age, are helpful in this regard.

Because familial aggregation exists for multifactorial disorders, it is implicit that the occurrence risk will be increased for members of an affected family over that of the general population. As expected, the risk is highest for first-degree relatives (parents, siblings, children), who have half of their genes in common. The risk is less for second-degree relatives (grandparents, aunts, uncles, grandchildren, nephews, nieces), who share one-quarter of their genes. The risk decreases exponentially thereafter; third-degree relatives (great-grandparents, cousins, great-grandchildren) share only one-eighth of their genes. Empiric (observed) risk figures for some well-studied multifactorial disorders fit well with the predicted risks.[5]

The genetic liability in multifactorial causation is due to the cumulative effect of many genes, each having a small effect, rather than to the effect of one major gene. These genes create a liability that presumably is continuously distributed within the population. If the genetic liability is strong enough, under an unfortunate set of environmental circumstances, the disorder will occur.[6]

For many, but not all, multifactorial conditions, there is a difference in predilection between males and females that could result directly from genetic differences or from different internal (e.g., hormonal) or external environmental factors. Furthermore, if a member of the less commonly affected sex has the condition, his or her genetic liability was probably greater and therefore the risk for his or her relatives is greater. Similarly, if a person has a more severe form of the disease, the risk for relatives is higher. In those disorders in which disease frequency increases with age, earlier onset sometimes implies a greater risk for relatives. Finally, the greater the number of affected individuals within the family, the higher the risk for other relatives.

There also are ethnic differences in frequency for many disorders of multifactorial causation, and in some cases these differences persist after the family members migrate to another geographical area. When the ethnic differences persist for several generations after migration, the evidence for genetic predisposition is strengthened.

When attempting to determine the inheritance pattern of any disease, the possibility of genetic heterogeneity always must be taken into account. For example, there are both autosomal dominant and multifactorial causes of atrial septal defect that may be indistinguishable clinically. Failure to recognize that different genetic diseases can cause the same or similar clinical entities can result in confusion when determining risks.

CONGENITAL HEART DISEASE

General considerations

Congenital cardiac defects occur in 1 per 125 total births (stillbirths and live births).[7] Approximately 90% of congenital cardiac defects had been considered to be due to multifactorial causation, 8% to chromosomal or single gene defects, and 2% to primarily environmental factors.[8] However, another subgroup of patients with submicroscopic chromosomal deletions has recently been defined, and they may account for another 5% or less of patients with heart defects.

Risks of recurrence for a congenital heart defect of multifactorial cause in a sibling of an affected patient are well established and tend to range between 2% and 4%.[8] Before counseling is given, it should be determined that the congenital heart defect in the proband is not due to a chromosomal or single gene defect. Although the recurrence risk is low, it is increased over the general population risk of approximately 0.8%. Some parents may wish to have ultrasound monitoring of subsequent pregnancies; such monitoring should be performed by an ultrasonographer with expertise in the prenatal diagnosis of birth defects. If the fetus is found to have a congenital heart defect, and depending on its severity and the gestational age at which it is detected, the parents may opt

Table 68-1 Recurrence of congenital heart defects in children born to affected parents

	VSD	ASD	AS
Nora and Nora, 1987*[14]			
No. of fathers	99	157	36
Total children	201	296	71
Affected children	5 (2.5%)	4 (1.4%)	2 (2.8%)
No. of mothers	152	405	50
Total children	275	721	93
Affected children	32 (11.6%)	37 (5.1%)	15 (16%)
Driscoll et al., 1989[16]			
No. of fathers	151	ND	123
Total children	318		227
Affected children	10 (3.1%)		3 (1.3%)
No. of mothers	190	ND	35
Total children	382		66
Affected children	11 (2.9%)		0 (0%)
Zellers et al., 1990[17]			
No. of fathers	ND	ND	ND
Total children			
Affected children			
No. of mothers	ND	ND	ND
Total children			
Affected children			
Ferencz, 1986[15]			
No. of fathers	5	1	6
Total children	8	1	6
Affected children	0 (0%)	0 (0%)	0 (0%)
(No women studied)			
Rose et al., 1985[12]			
No. of fathers	ND	32	37
Total children		56	61
Affected children		4 (7.1%)	?† (17%)
No. of mothers	ND	72	26
Total children		138	35
Affected children		19 (13.7%)	?† (8.2%)
Total			
No. of fathers	255	190	165
Total children	527	353	304
Affected children	15 (2.8%)	8 (2.2%)	5 (1.6%)
No. of mothers	342	477	85
Total children	657	859	159
Affected children	43 (6.5%)	56 (6.5%)	15 (0.9%)

AS, aortic stenosis; ASD, atrial septal defect; AV, atrioventricular canal; Coarc, coarctation of aorta; ND, no data; PDA, patent ductus arteriosus; PS, pulmonary stenosis; ToF, tetralogy of Fallot; VSD, ventricular septal defect.

*Adapted from Nora JJ, Nora AH: Maternal transmission of congenital heart diseases: new recurrence risk figures and the questions of cytoplasmic inheritance and vulnerability to teratogens. *Am J Cardiol* 59:459-463, 1987, which includes the data of Whittemore R, Hobbins JC, Engle MA: Pregnancy and its outcome in women with and without surgical treatment of congenital heart disease. *Am J Cardiol* 50:641-651, 1982.

†Because percentage of affected offspring given in report does not match number of affected children stated in report, this number is excluded from calculation of totals.

Parental cardiac defect				
Coarc	**PS**	**PDA**	**ToF**	**AV**
112 193 4 (2.0%)	71 147 3 (2.0%)	95 176 5 (2.8%)	46 45 1 (2.2%)	16 16 0 (0%)
63 135 5 (3.7%)	98 188 13 (6.9%)	332 614 31 (5.0%)	43 41 2 (4.8%)	36 36 5 (13.9%)
ND	92 169 3 (1.8%)	ND	ND	ND
ND	106 204 8 (3.9%)	ND	ND	ND
ND	ND	ND	66 130 2 (1.5%)	ND
ND	ND	ND	63 126 1 (0.8%)	ND
5 7 0 (0%)	3 9 0 (0%)	3 6 0 (0%)	1 1 0 (0%)	1 1 0 (0%)
30 59 2 (3.4%)	ND	ND	ND	ND
19 31 2 (6.5%)	ND	ND	ND	ND
147 259 6 (2.3%)	166 325 6 (1.8%)	98 182 5 (2.7%)	113 176 3 (1.7%)	17 17 0 (0%)
82 166 7 (4.2%)	204 392 21 (5.3%)	332 614 31 (5.0%)	106 167 3 (1.8%)	36 36 5 (13.9%)

for termination of the pregnancy. Alternatively, the parents may prepare for the birth of the affected child, and delivery of the infant in a tertiary medical center with immediate availability of a pediatric cardiologist or surgeon may be indicated. If ultrasonographic imaging of the heart does not reveal a congenital heart defect, the parents should realize that some heart malformations may not be detected in utero.[9,10]

It must be emphasized that recurrence risks are for congenital cardiac defects in general and are not for a specific defect, although there is a tendency for recurrence of defects with similar embryologic origins, such as septal defects and conotruncal abnormalities. Thus, when counseling families in regard to congenital cardiac defects, it should be stressed that the risk for future offspring is for a congenital cardiac defect that could be similar to, less severe than, or more severe than that of the proband.

There is debate regarding the risk for congenital heart defects in children born to affected parents. In 1983, Nora,[8] in a summary of risks derived from studies published up to that time, found the range to be 2% to 4% for children born to parents with several types of congenital heart defects. Subsequently, Whittemore et al.[11] published results of a prospective study that showed a much higher overall recurrence risk of 14.2% for children born to mothers with congenital heart defects. Depending on the type of defect in the mother, the risk ranged from 11% for atrial septal defect and patent ductus arteriosus to 26% for left ventricular outflow obstruction. A retrospective study reported by Rose et al.[12] showed a 7% recurrence risk for children born to affected fathers and a 13% risk for children born to affected mothers. Whittemore,[13] in another study of children born to affected fathers, found that 9% of children had a congenital heart defect. Nora and Nora[14] summarized the results of several studies available before 1987; the overall recurrence risk was 2.5% for children born to fathers with a congenital heart defect and 7.6% for children born to affected mothers. In contrast, Ferencz[15] found no instance of congenital heart defect in 52 children born to fathers with a defect. Copel et al.[9] found no instance of congenital heart defect in 49 fetuses examined in utero by ultrasound in mothers with a defect, and Allan et al.[10] found no affected fetuses in a similar study of 30 women with a defect. Most recently, in the single largest study reported thus far, the risk for a clinically significant congenital heart defect in children born to a parent with ventricular septal defect was 3%, with aortic stenosis was 1%, and with pulmonary stenosis was 3%.[16] In another recent study, the risk to parents with tetralogy of Fallot for having a child with a defect was 1.2%.[17] These results are similar to those of early studies and suggest lower risk figures than those published in Whittemore et al.[11] and Rose et al.[12] Data on risks to children from studies in which the sex and type of congenital heart defect in the parent are specified are summarized in Table 68-1.

The reason for the discrepancies among various studies for risks for children born to affected parents is not clear. Possible explanations include random variation based on relatively small sample sizes, the intense follow-up evaluation in the children in the study of Whittemore et al.,[11] and bias of ascertainment. For example, in the prospective study of Whittemore et al.,[11] women who already had one or more healthy children may have declined participation. In addition, children with defects, such as ventricular septal defect, that may have subsequently closed may not have been detected in the retrospective studies. In the retrospective study of Rose et al.,[12] many of the adult patients could not be located to be invited to participate; those with children with a congenital heart defect would be more likely to be in contact with the medical center and to have a current address on file. Although additional studies will be needed to further clarify these risks, available data suggest that the risks for significant heart disease in children born to affected parents are relatively low and generally fall in the range of 2% to 6%. If one includes risks for minor or hemodynamically insignificant heart defects, the risk may be slightly higher.

Patent ductus arteriosus

Persistent patency of the ductus arteriosus occurs in 1 of 1,600 live births and constitutes approximately 12% of all congenital heart defects.[18] Incidence is higher in infants born prematurely than in those born at full term and in infants born at high altitudes than in those born at sea level.

In the majority of instances, the cause is multifactorial with an empiric risk of 3% for individuals with one affected sibling.[8] There have been rare reports of families in which autosomal dominant genetic transmission seems likely.[19-21] Some of these families may have Char syndrome, with unusual facial features, such as long philtrum, downslanting palpebral fissures, and thick lips.[22]

Persistent patency of the ductus arteriosus occurs commonly in the congenital rubella syndrome. Histologically, there is a paucity of elastic tissue in the ductus arteriosus in patients with congenital rubella.[23] However, the cardiac malformations observed in the rubella syndrome are not limited to patent ductus arteriosus and include generalized vascular abnormalities, peripheral pulmonary artery stenosis, transposition of the great arteries, tetralogy of Fallot, atrial septal defect, and valvular stenoses.

Patent ductus arteriosus also may be associated with fetal hydantoin syndrome and chromosome abnormalities, including 4p-, 5p- (cri du chat), 9p-, trisomy 13, trisomy 18, trisomy 21, XXXXY, and XXXXX syndromes. Occasionally it may occur with single gene defects, including the Carpenter, Conradi, Seckel, Smith-Lemli-Opitz, Weill-Marchesani, Hay-Wells, Meckel-Gruber, and Treacher Collins syndromes and camptomelic dysplasia. Patent ductus arteriosus also occurs in the CHARGE association, DiGeorge sequence, Rubinstein-Taybi syndrome, facioauriculovertebral syndrome, and thanatophoric dysplasia.[24]

Ventricular septal defect

This is the most common form of congenital cardiac defect (perhaps with the exception of mitral valve prolapse and bicuspid aortic valve), occurring in 1 of 420 to 770 live births[25,26] and constituting 20% of congenital heart defects. Because the ventricular septum is formed from three embryologic components (the muscular septum, the conotruncus, and the endocardial cushions), the genetic determinants of ventricular septal defect may differ depending upon the mechanism of malformation of the ventricular septum.

For isolated ventricular septal defect, the risk is 3%, assuming one affected sibling.[8] Genetic counseling for ventricular septal defect associated with other conotruncal malformations (tetralogy of Fallot, transposition of the great arteries, truncus arteriosus, interrupted aortic arch, etc.) should be based on risks for conotruncal abnormalities.

Ventricular septal defects can be associated with many chromosome abnormalities, including trisomy 21, trisomy 13, trisomy 18, triploidy, trisomy 20p, and 9p- syndromes. Genetic defects that may be associated with ventricular septal defect are the Holt-Oram, Shprintzen, thrombocytopenia-absent radius, Meckel-Gruber, Waardenburg, Carpenter, Coffin-Siris, and Hay-Wells syndromes. The defect also may be seen in association with the Aase, Rubinstein-Taybi, Williams, Cornelia de Lange, facioauriculovertebral, and linear sebaceous nevus syndromes and the CHARGE and VATER associations. Maternal phenylketonuria, congenital rubella, infection, and hydantoin or trimethadione ingestion during pregnancy also have been associated with ventricular septal defect in some offspring.[24]

Atrial septal defect

Secundum atrial septal defect occurs in 1 per 1,667 live births and constitutes 7% of congenital cardiac malformations. The female-to-male ratio is 2:1.[27,28] The suggested risk is 2.5% for individuals with one affected sibling and 7.5% for individuals with two affected siblings.[8] Although multifactorial causation seems likely in the majority of cases, there are numerous reports of recurrence of atrial septal defect in three and four generations of a family, suggesting autosomal dominant inheritance. Incomplete penetrance has been observed in some of these families.[29-38]

In 1966, Kahler et al.[39] described two families with atrial septal defect and AV conduction abnormalities, including first-degree or complete AV block. Bizarro et al.[40] and Pease et al.[41] also observed families that had atrial septal defect and AV conduction abnormalities in three generations. Some family members had only AV conduction abnormalities, some had atrial septal defect, and some had both. These data suggest an autosomal dominant form of inheritance.

The Holt-Oram syndrome is characterized by congenital heart disease and malformations of an upper extremity.[42] The upper extremity malformations can range from minor thumb abnormalities (triphalangeal, absent, hypoplastic, bifid, etc.) to phocomelia (Fig 68-5). Although atrial septal defect is the most common form of congenital heart disease associated with the Holt-Oram syndrome, most forms of congenital heart disease can be associated with upper extremity malformations. Ventricular septal defect is the second most common defect associated with Holt-Oram syndrome. It is important to examine family members for evidence of upper extremity malformations or heart disease. The Holt-Oram syndrome is inherited in an autosomal dominant fashion. Some cases represent a new mutation. The gene defect that causes Holt-Oram syndrome has been mapped to chromosome 12q2.[43]

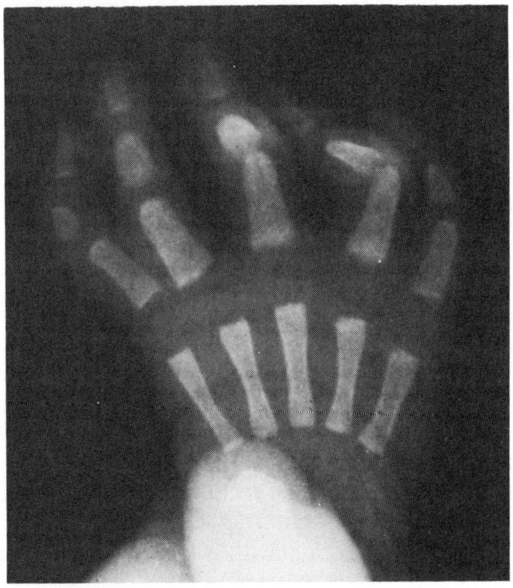

Fig 68-5 Hand radiograph demonstrating triphalangeal thumb of a patient with Holt-Oram syndrome.

Atrial septal defect also may be associated with the Down, cri du chat, trisomy 13, trisomy 18, triploidy, Turner, XXXXY, Ellis-van Creveld, Williams, Robinow, facioauriculovertebral, Treacher Collins, fetal alcohol, congenital cytomegalovirus, and rubella syndromes, thanatophoric dysplasia, maternal thalidomide embryopathy, maternal phenylketonuria, and the CHARGE association.[24]

Endocardial cushion defects

These defects include ostium primum atrial septal defect, complete AV canal, common atrium, and isolated cleft of the mitral valve. AV septal defects account for approximately 4.3% of congenital heart defects, with an incidence in live-born infants of approximately 1 per 500.[44] Assuming multifactorial inheritance, the risk is 2% to 4% with one affected sibling.[8] Recurrence of endocardial cushion defect in more than two generations is unusual but has been reported as an autosomal dominant condition in some families.[45,46] There is an association between endocardial cushion defect and secundum atrial septal defect. Also, there is a strong association between complete AV canal and the Down syndrome; in most series, AV canal defects are the most common cardiac defect associated with the Down syndrome, accounting for approximately 40% of heart defects in these patients.

Endocardial cushion defects also can occur with other chromosome anomalies, autosomal dominant Holt-Oram syndrome and Alagille arteriohepatic dysplasia, and autosomal recessive Ellis-van Creveld, hydrolethalus, hydrometrocolpos-polysyndactyly, and Smith-Lemli-Opitz syndromes. The teratogenic effects of alcohol and maternal diabetes also have resulted in endocardial cushion defects.[47]

Coarctation of the aorta

Coarctation of the aorta occurs in 1 of 4,000 children between birth and 15 years of age[48] and constitutes approximately 6% of congenital cardiac malformations. There is a male preponderance (male-to-female ratio, 1.7:1.0).[49] Abnormalities of the aortic valve (usually a bicuspid aortic valve) occur in up to 85% of patients with isolated coarctation of the aorta.

In almost all instances (excluding Turner's syndrome) the cause of coarctation of the aorta is multifactorial; the risk is 2% for individuals with one affected sibling.[8] Hall et al.[50] reported a pair of male first cousins with coarctation of the aorta whose mothers had been exposed to an insect repellant. However, this may have been a coincidental rather than a teratogenic event.

Turner's syndrome[24] (45,X karyotype) is characterized by a female phenotype, short stature, streak gonads, low hairline, webbing of the neck, highly arched palate, lymphedema of the hands and feet in infancy, renal abnormalities, cubitus valgus, short fourth metacarpals, failure of development of secondary sexual characteristics, and sterility. Approximately 14% of patients with Turner's syndrome have coarctation of the aorta, and this defect is relatively more common in those with webbed neck. There is a suggestion that the aorta of patients with Turner's syndrome is more friable than normal and that these patients may be at an increased risk for bleeding after repair of coarctation of the aorta.[51] Some patients have had progressive aortic dilatation, so that periodic echocardiograms are recommended. Aortic atresia, aortic valve stenosis, and bicuspid aortic valve also have been described in patients with Turner's syndrome. Turner's syndrome occurs in approximately 1 per 5,000 newborn infants. It usually is a sporadic event unrelated to maternal or paternal age, and the chance of a second affected offspring seems to be no greater than that for the general population. All patients suspected of having Turner's syndrome must have a chromosome analysis. In some patients, a 46,XY cell line also is present, which results in an increased risk for gonadal malignancy; prophylactic removal of the nonfunctioning gonads is indicated in these patients.

Coarctation of the abdominal aorta may occur with multiple renal stenoses in neurofibromatosis type 1. Coarctation of the aorta also can occur in association with autosomal chromosome abnormalities, with autosomal dominant Alagille arteriohepatic dysplasia, and with autosomal recessive Meckel-Gruber and Smith-Lemli-Opitz syndromes. Coarctation of the aorta occasionally occurs in babies born to mothers who had rubella during pregnancy or who have phenylketonuria or diabetes mellitus. It also has been associated with intrauterine exposure to hydantoin, isotretinoin, or lithium. It has been observed in patients with the following disorders: the Beckwith-Wiedemann, Cornelia de Lange, facioauriculovertebral, Kabuki make-up, linear sebaceous nevus, Robinow, and Rubinstein-Taybi syndromes, the Pierre Robin sequence, and the VATER association.[47]

Conotruncal abnormalities

Abnormalities of conotruncal development result in a spectrum of congenital cardiac diseases, including semilunar valve malformation, transposition of the great arteries, tetralogy of Fallot, truncus arteriosus, pulmonary artery atresia or stenosis, and some forms of ventricular septal defect. Assuming multifactorial inheritance, when there is one affected sibling, the generally quoted risks are: ventricular septal defect, 3%; tetralogy of Fallot, 2.5%; pulmonary valve stenosis, 2%; aortic valve stenosis, 2%; transposition of the great arteries, 2%; truncus arteriosus, 1%; and pulmonary artery atresia, 1%.[8] However, a recent study suggested recurrence risks for siblings of patients with simple and complex truncus arteriosus of 6.6% and 13%, respectively.[52]

There have been other purported hereditary patterns in patients with conotruncal abnormalities.[53] Pitt[54] reported six cases of tetralogy of Fallot among 275 descendants of one man. This was interpreted as autosomal dominant inheritance with incomplete penetrance. Miller and Smith[55] described a family in which at least two and possibly three generations had conotruncal abnormalities, including tetralogy of Fallot and pulmonary valve stenosis. However, these observations also are consistent with multifactorial etiology. Some familial cases may represent instances of syndromes associated with a submicroscopic deletion of chromosome 22, as described below.

There is an important association between conotruncal abnormalities and the DiGeorge sequence.[24,56] The DiGeorge sequence consists of absence or hypoplasia of the thymus and parathyroid glands, which results in deficits of cellular immunity and in hypocalcemia. It may or may not be associated with ocular hypertelorism, a short philtrum, down-slanting palpebral fissures, and ear anomalies. The absence of these facial features does not preclude the presence of the DiGeorge or partial DiGeorge sequence. The DiGeorge sequence is associated with a spectrum of conotruncal abnormalities, particularly interrupted aortic arch but also tetralogy of Fallot and right-sided aortic arch. It is important to recognize the presence of the DiGeorge or partial DiGeorge sequence in patients with congenital heart disease who may require blood transfusion, because administration of leukocytes to a patient with deficient cellular immunity can result in a graft-vs.-host reaction. Usually, the occurrence of the DiGeorge sequence is sporadic, but cases of affected siblings or affected parent and child have been reported. Also, the DiGeorge sequence has been associated with 22q- syndrome and other chromosome abnormalities. In particular, DiGeorge sequence can be associated with microdeletions of chromosome 22q11. A microdeletion refers to a chromosomal deletion that is too small to be seen by routine microscopic karyotype analysis. The deletion can be detected only by the use of a DNA probe combined with fluorescent in situ hybridization (FISH) analysis. The phenotype in these patients may overlap with those of the Shprintzen velocardiofacial syndrome, and sometimes this complex phenotype is referred to as CATCH 22. Shprintzen syndrome is characterized by a characteristic facies, with long prominent nose, square nasal bridge, narrow alar base, long face, and malar hypoplasia in association with variable combinations of cleft of the secondary palate, ear abnormalities, carious teeth, and long tapering fingers. Conotruncal anomalies are common, often in association with severe abnormalities of the arborization of the pulmonary arterial tree.[57]

Goldenhar's syndrome[24,58] (oculoauriculovertebral dysplasia) consists of unilateral facial hypoplasia, epibulbar dermoids or lipodermoids, preauricular tags, antetragal fistulas, and vertebral anomalies. In 14% to 53% of patients with Goldenhar's syndrome, congenital heart disease is present, and approximately half of those with congenital heart disease have tetralogy of Fallot. Other cardiac anomalies include ventricular septal defect, coarctation of the aorta, corrected transposition of the great arteries, and atrial septal defect. Goldenhar's syndrome has been reported in multiple family members, but it is usually a sporadic disorder. The empiric risk of recurrence is approximately 2%.

Tetralogy of Fallot has been seen in the CHARGE association, autosomal recessive thrombocytopenia-absent radius syndrome, fetal trimethadione syndrome, and trisomy 20p. Limb reduction ichthyosis syndrome may be associated with truncus arteriosus.

Pulmonary valve stenosis was observed to affect three generations of one family.[59] A combination of pulmonary valve stenosis and atrial septal defect has been reported in multiple family members.[60] However, in most cases, pulmonary valve stenosis is probably multifactorial with a risk of 2.7% when one sibling is affected.[8] Beagle dogs have an unusually high incidence of pulmonary valve stenosis. It has been postulated that genes at more than one locus account for this phenomenon, which is compatible with the observations in humans.[61] Pulmonary valve stenosis also has been associated with chromosome abnormalities and the Alagille arteriohepatic dysplasia, asplenia, polysplenia, Rubinstein-Taybi, Williams, Holt-Oram, LEOPARD, McDonough, Meckel-Gruber, Carpenter, and Noonan syndromes[47] (see "Noonan's Syndrome" and "Hypertrophic Cardiomyopathy"). Occasionally, pulmonary stenosis is present in infants whose mothers had collagen vascular disease, diabetes mellitus, or rubella infection during pregnancy or in infants who had intrauterine exposure to hydantoin, retinoic acid, or alcohol. Carpenter's syndrome also has been associated with transposition of the great arteries. Pulmonary valve stenosis has been seen with Williams syndrome, fetal hydantoin syndrome, congenital cytomegalovirus infection, and chromosome abnormality 9p-.[24]

Aortic valve stenosis may be an isolated birth defect or may be present in patients with chromosome abnormalities, autosomal dominant LEOPARD and Williams syndromes, autosomal recessive geleophysic dwarfism and Smith-Lemli-Opitz syndromes, and intrauterine exposure to hydantoin or rubella virus.[47]

Supravalvular aortic stenosis

Supravalvular aortic stenosis is much less common than aortic valve stenosis but occurs in two important conditions, Williams syndrome and autosomal dominant forms of supravalvular aortic stenosis.[39,62]

Williams syndrome[24] (formerly known as idiopathic hypercalcemic syndrome) is characterized by microcephaly, mental retardation, a friendly personality, short palpebral fissures, depressed nasal bridge, epicanthal folds, anteverted nares, long philtrum, prominent lower lip, partial anodontia, enamel hypoplasia, and cardiovascular abnormalities. The cardiovascular abnormalities may include supravalvular aortic stenosis, peripheral pulmonary branch stenosis, ventricular septal defect, atrial septal defect, stenoses of the renal, carotid, and brachiocephalic arteries, and hypertension. Mitral valve abnormalities have been reported rarely.[63] Some of these patients have unexplained hypercalcemia in infancy. Some of the cardiovascular abnormalities can be produced in rabbits exposed to high doses of vitamin D in utero.[62] Williams syndrome usually is sporadic with a low risk for siblings, although there have been a few reported cases of affected siblings, cousins, or parents and children. Williams syndrome is a contiguous gene syndrome that involves deletion of the elastin gene on chromosome 7q and deletion of one or more genes adjacent to the elastin locus. Although standard chromosome analysis is generally normal, this microdeletion can be detected with an elastin DNA probe with FISH. Sporadic cases are due to a new mutation, and recurrence risk for affected persons' children is 50%.

Isolated supravalvular aortic stenosis can be a sporadic event, but autosomal dominant forms with variable expression exist.[39] In many cases, autosomal dominant supravalvular aortic stenosis is due to elastin gene abnormalities, and the mutations are too subtle to be detected even by the elastin DNA-FISH technique.[64] Occasionally, supravalvular aortic stenosis can be associated with peripheral pulmonary artery stenosis.

Hypoplastic left heart syndrome

Aortic or mitral atresia without ventricular septal defect (the hypoplastic left heart syndrome) occurs in less than 1 per 3,300 total births. Recurrence risk for siblings is approximately 2%.[65,66] Although there have been reports of siblings with hypoplastic left heart syndrome, the number of cases is not sufficient to prove autosomal recessive inheritance.[66,67] Hypoplastic left heart syndrome can be diagnosed in utero by utilizing two-dimensional echocardiography.[68] This syndrome has been associated with chromosome abnormalities, so any infant with dysmorphic facial features or additional birth defects should have a chromosome analysis. Hypoplastic left heart also can occur in infants with syndromes such as Apert's, Holt-Oram, Ellis-van Creveld, Smith-Lemli-Opitz, asplenia, polysplenia, and Beckwith-Wiedemann and with Saldino-Noonan chondrodysplasia, DiGeorge sequence, and VATER association. It has been reported in infants of diabetic mothers and those with intrauterine exposure to retinoic acid, trimethadione, and increased phenylalanine levels because of maternal phenylketonuria.[47]

Mitral valve prolapse

Mitral valve prolapse frequently is familial.[69,70] Weiss et al.[71] found it in 47% of first-degree relatives of probands; 56% of female children and 36% of male children had it. This and other studies have led many geneticists to consider mitral valve prolapse to be an autosomal dominantly inherited condition in at least some families.

Mitral valve prolapse frequently is present in patients with connective tissue defects such as Marfan syndrome and the Ehlers-Danlos syndromes.

Asplenia (Ivemark's syndrome) and polysplenia

Ivemark's syndrome consists of asplenia and complex congenital heart disease, including transposition of the great arteries, pulmonary stenosis or atresia, total anomalous pulmonary venous return, complete AV canal, common ventricle, dextrocardia, bilateral superior venae cavae, and absence of the coronary sinus.[72] Twenty percent of patients with Ivemark's syndrome have genitourinary abnormalities, and 5% to 10% have bronchopulmonary and skeletal abnormalities.[73] There is a male preponderance of asplenia (male-to-female ratio, 1.7:1). There have been at least eight reports of Ivemark's syndrome in siblings, and consanguinity has been identified in four families, supporting autosomal recessive inheritance patterns in some cases.[74-80] However, most cases have appeared to be sporadic, and the recurrence risk was estimated at approximately 5% if parental consanguinity is not present.[81k]

The cardiac anomalies associated with polysplenia include anomalous pulmonary venous connection to the right-sided atrium, absence of the hepatic segment of the inferior vena cava, atrial septal defect, bilaterally bilobed lungs, bilaterally left-sided atria, pulmonary valve stenosis, and double-outlet right ventricle. In contrast to asplenia, transposition of the great arteries and common ventricle are uncommon.[72]

Mutations in the connexon 43 gap junction gene have recently been reported in six children with visceroatrial heterotopic syndromes with complex cardiac malformations and asplenia or polysplenia. The mutation studies in these children support autosomal recessive inheritance, but genetic heterogeneity may exist. Thus, a risk to siblings of 25% may exist in some cases.[74]

Patients suspected of having Ivemark's syndrome should have abdominal ultrasound examination in an attempt to visualize the spleen. Erythrocyte pitting and the presence of Howell-Jolly bodies are evidence of functional hyposplenia.

Kartagener's syndrome

This syndrome consists of situs inversus totalis, bronchiectasis, sinusitis, and immotile cilia and sperm.[82-85] It occurs in 1 per 68,000 persons and affects males and females equally.[82] The inheritance pattern is autosomal recessive. It has been suggested that situs may be controlled by a single gene and that absence of the gene results in random situs.[86] The immotility of the cilia and sperm is related to abnormal formation or function of the dynein arms that form cross-bridges between the microtubules of the axonemal structures that comprise cilia and sperm or of the protein that binds the dynein arms to the microtubules. Intermittent attachments of the dynein arm forming cross-bridges to adjacent microtubules are vital to the sliding relationship of the microtubules that produces ciliary or sperm motion.

Primary pulmonary hypertension

Primary pulmonary hypertension (idiopathic pulmonary vascular obstructive disease) results from intimal proliferation and obstruction of the pulmonary arterioles. The cause is obscure. It was identified in 29 of 22,000 cases of heart disease in children at the Hospital for Sick Children (Toronto, Ontario).[87] Characteristically, it is a disease of young women (female-to-male ratio, 2.5:1) but occurs at all ages and in either sex. The principal clinical features are dyspnea, fatigue, syncope, and increased intensity of the pulmonary component of the second heart sound. Most cases of primary pulmonary hypertension are sporadic, but several instances of multiple family members being affected have supported autosomal dominant inheritance with female preponderance in some instances and autosomal recessive inheritance in others.[81h]

Arterial calcification of infancy

Idiopathic arterial calcification of infancy is a rare (approximately 80 cases have been reported), usually fatal condition of unknown cause.[81j,88,89] It is characterized by deposition of calcium salt in the interna lamina of arteries, particularly the pulmonary arteries (Fig 68-6). Death usually occurs in the first year of life as a result of myocardial ischemia and congestive heart failure. There is no apparent sex predilection. In four families, two siblings were affected. In one of the four families, the parents of the siblings were first cousins, supporting an autosomal recessive mode of inheritance.[90-93]

Arrhythmias

Cardiac arrhythmias can be of multifactorial causation or can be due to single gene defects, chromosomal abnormalities, or environmental factors. Møller and Heiberg[94] studied members of families of women with either a long or a short P-R interval and found a significantly longer P-R interval in relatives of those with long intervals than in relatives of those with short intervals. They concluded that length of the P-R interval was an inherited characteristic possibly influenced by major genes. Since Morquio's[95] first report of five of eight siblings with syncope and bradycardia, there have been numerous reports of familial congenital complete AV block.[96-100] Lynch and Engle[97] described two siblings with complete AV block in a family with multiple members who had polydactyly. Wagner and Hall[92] reported congen-

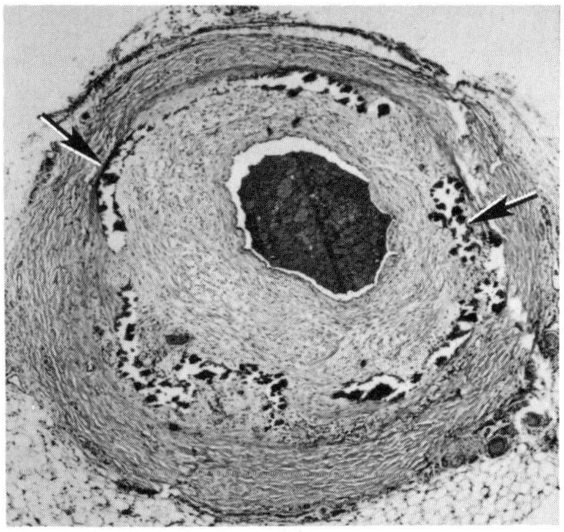

Fig 68-6 Right coronary artery from 14-month-old boy with idiopathic arterial calcification of infancy. The internal elastic membrane is calcified *(arrows),* and secondary internal proliferation has produced marked luminal narrowing. The small residual lumen is filled with barium sulfate from postmortem coronary arteriography. (Hematoxylin and eosin; ×27.) (Courtesy of William D. Edwards, M.D.)

ital complete AV block in three siblings whose mother had atrial fibrillation. Crittenden et al.[100] reported congenital complete AV block in four of eight siblings. One form of autosomal dominant progressive heart block involving the bundle-branch conduction system has been mapped to chromosome 19q13.[101] Also, there is an association between atrial septal defect and conduction abnormalities (see under "Atrial Septal Defect" above).

Wolff-Parkinson-White syndrome has occurred in multiple family members. Massumi[102] described it in a mother and her two children, and Schneider[103] noted it in a mother and a daughter. Gillette et al.[104] reported Wolff-Parkinson-White syndrome in three generations of one family and suggested autosomal dominant inheritance in the family. Familial forms of Wolff-Parkinson-White syndrome may be more common than is appreciated because family members may be asymptomatic and the presence of AV accessory pathways may not be apparent on the surface ECG. Wolff-Parkinson-White syndrome also has been observed in a patient with a chromosome abnormality (8p-), in two members of a family with dilated cardiomyopathy[105] and in patients with mitochondrial DNA abnormalities.

Atrial fibrillation was reported in multiple members of a family in four generations by Gould.[106] Phair[107] described a woman and her two sons with atrial fibrillation.

Brodsky et al.[108] reported the familial occurrence of Lown-Ganong-Levine syndrome. In this family it appeared to be an autosomal dominant trait.

The Jervell and Lange-Nielsen syndrome and the Romano-Ward syndrome are genetically determined disorders associated with prolongation of the Q-T interval and a propensity toward ventricular fibrillation and sudden death.[109-113] The Jervell and Lange-Nielsen syndrome is associated with congenital deafness and is an autosomal recessively inherited disorder. The Romano-Ward syndrome is not associated with congenital deafness and is inherited as an autosomal dominant trait. The autosomal dominant form of prolonged Q-T interval recently has been mapped to chromosome 11p15.5 on the basis of linkage analyses in affected families.[114] However, heterogeneity is present, with other families showing linkage to 3p21-24 or 7q35-36. The mutations causing long Q-T interval on chromosome 7 are in the HERG potassium channel gene.[115]

McRae et al.[116] described four siblings with familial paroxysmal ventricular fibrillation, short P-R interval, and prominent U waves. The relationship of this disorder to other disorders with short P-R interval (Wolff-Parkinson-White syndrome and Lown-Ganong-Levine syndrome) or to familial prolongation of the Q-T interval is unclear.

A number of investigators have reported an association between maternal collagen disease (systemic lupus erythematosus) and congenital complete heart block in offspring.[117,118] This may be due to transplacental passage of maternal SS-A/Ro antibodies.[119]

METABOLIC DISEASES ASSOCIATED WITH ARRHYTHMIAS

Refsum's disease

Refsum's disease is an autosomal recessive neurodegenerative disease characterized by cerebellar ataxia, hypertrophic polyneuropathy, and retinitis pigmentosa. Deafness, ichthyosis, and cardiac conduction defects are frequently present. Onset of the disorder may be in infancy or in middle age, and the course is progressive. Cerebrospinal fluid protein concentration is increased, and phytanic acid accumulates in serum and organs. Hypertrophic interstitial neuritis and degenerative changes of nuclei and fiber tracts are observed histologically in the brain stem. The ECG is characterized by a prolonged P-Q interval and ST-segment and T-wave changes. Impaired AV conduction, bundle-branch block, and sudden death from cardiac arrhythmia may occur. Myocardial fibrosis has been reported.[120]

Phytanic acid is a fatty acid present in dairy products and fat from grazing animals. Patients with Refsum's disease are deficient in the catabolic enzyme phytanic acid α-hydroxylase, which results in accumulation of ingested phytanic acid in fatty deposits in the involved organ systems. The enzyme deficiency is expressed in cultured skin fibroblasts, and prenatal diagnosis is possible.

Dietary restriction of phytanic acid results in clinical improvement[121] and stabilization of the disease. ECG changes have resolved in some patients after treatment. Plasmapheresis removes phytanic acid from the body and may allow liberalization of the diet; it can be extremely valuable in the management of acutely ill patients.[122]

Fabry's disease

Fabry's disease is a lysosomal storage disease due to deficiency of α-galactosidase A.[123] The inheritance pattern is X-linked recessive, although females may have less severe signs of the disease than males. Glycosphingolipids accumulate in the endothelium, perithelium, and smooth muscle of blood vessels. There is a lesser degree of accumulation in ganglion cells, myocardial cells, reticuloendothelial cells, and connective tissue cells.

The first signs of the disease may be telangiectatic angiokeratomas of the skin and mucous membranes. Acroparesthesias and episodes of severe burning pain in the palms and soles with proximal radiation also may occur in childhood and adolescence. Whorl-shaped corneal opacities and cataracts develop. In adulthood, cardiovascular and renal disease are the major causes of morbidity and mortality. Cardiac problems, including ischemia, infarction, congestive failure, mitral insufficiency, and aortic stenosis, may result from progressive glycosphingolipid infiltration. Systemic hypertension secondary to infiltration of renal parenchymal vessels may aggravate the cardiac disease. The ECG may show signs of left ventricular hypertrophy, ST-segment changes, and T-wave inversion. Occasionally, patients have arrhythmias and a short P-R interval.

The interventricular septum and posterior left ventricular wall may be thickened. Cardiomegaly, especially involving the left atrium and ventricle, is observed. The right atrium and ventricle may be dilated. Myocardial cells show extensive glycosphingolipid deposited around the nucleus and between myofibrils. Endothelial cells and smooth muscle cells are hypertrophied. The mitral valve frequently is thickened, with normal or thick papillary muscles; the tricuspid valve may be involved but the aortic and pulmonary valves usually are normal. Lipid-filled cells can be seen within the fibrous tissue of the involved valves.

Neurologic signs result from small vessel involvement in the brain. The most frequent cause of death is renal failure.

Dilantin and carbamazepine are useful for treating the pain. Renal transplantation can prolong life. The gene has been cloned, and presymptomatic and prenatal diagnoses are possible.[120]

CARDIOMYOPATHY

Hypertrophic cardiomyopathy

It is well documented that isolated hypertrophic cardiomyopathy frequently is inherited as an autosomal dominant disorder.[81i] In two series of 30 patients[81b] and 14 patients,[124] 93% were found to have an affected parent or child or both when studied by echocardiography. Investigation of first-degree relatives is necessary. Even if parents are normal by echocardiography, the possibility of new mutation cannot be excluded,[125] and children born to an affected parent must be considered to be at risk and should be evaluated. The possibility of an autosomal dominant disorder can never be excluded on the basis of a negative family history.

As with any autosomal dominant disorder, the risk of passing on the abnormal gene to each offspring is 50%. Although there is a high degree of penetrance, the degree of penetrance ranges from 65% to 95%, depending on the specific genetic defect. The course of the disease may be variable, even within a family; therefore, the age at onset cannot be predicted precisely. It is not rare to study a child who presents with symptoms and to discover, after family investigations, that an asymptomatic parent is affected. Clinical manifestations usually occur in the second or third decade of life but have been described in infants and children.[126]

Hypertrophic cardiomyopathy with or without outflow obstruction has been observed within single families. This is compelling evidence that they are different manifestations of the same disease.

Some families with hypertrophic cardiomyopathy have a defect in the β cardiac myosin heavy chain gene on chromosome 14q.[127] Approximately 30 different mutations in the myosin gene have been discovered thus far. However, other families with hypertrophic cardiomyopathy have genetic defects in cardiac troponin T on chromosome 1 or α-tropomyosin on chromosome 15.[128]

It has been suggested that some patients with hypertrophic cardiomyopathy may have structural or functional abnormalities of skeletal muscle that usually are asymptomatic.[129] Several other genetic disorders have been reported in association with hypertrophic cardiomyopathy; however, these diseases can be distinguished easily on the basis of additional clinical and pathologic signs and symptoms.

Friedreich's ataxia

This is an autosomal recessive disorder associated with ECG or echocardiographic evidence of cardiomyopathy in most cases.[121] The first sign of the disease is an ataxic gait; the mean age at onset is approximately 12 years. Dysarthria, hypotonic muscle weakness, loss of vibration and position senses, and loss of deep tendon reflexes develop subsequently. In some patients, diabetes mellitus, nystagmus, optic atrophy, dementia, respiratory dysfunction due to kyphoscoliosis, and decreased sensory nerve conduction velocities also develop.

In one series,[130] 60 of 82 patients had clinical evidence of cardiac dysfunction 4 months to 4 years prior to death, and 56% died of heart failure. The mean age at death was 36.6 years. Cardiac arrhythmias, particularly atrial fibrillation, were common and occurred in 50% of fatal cases. At autopsy, in the majority of cases there was marked thickening of the left ventricle with extensive interstitial fibrosis and focal degeneration of muscle fibers. Muscle fibers were hypertrophied and many had large nuclei.[131] The cardiomyopathy may be of the hypertrophic type with subaortic stenosis.[132-134]

The risk for a sibling being affected is 25%. The basic biochemical defect remains unknown. However, the gene has been localized to chromosome 9q12-21.1 by genetic linkage studies of affected families. This potentially allows for prenatal or presymptomatic diagnosis of cases when one affected child already has been found.[135]

Multiple lentigines syndrome

The multiple lentigines syndrome (LEOPARD syndrome) is another hereditary disorder that has been associated with hypertrophic cardiomyopathy.[136] Histologic examination of the heart in some cases showed classic features of hypertrophic cardiomyopathy with large but variable-sized fibers and large nuclei.[137] The syndrome is characterized by lentigines, mild growth deficiency, ocular hypertelorism, prominent ears, mild to moderate sensorineural deafness, and sometimes hypogonadism and mental deficiency. It is autosomal dominant in inheritance with a wide range of expression.[24]

Noonan's syndrome

Hypertrophic cardiomyopathy has been detected in up to 25% of patients with Noonan's syndrome with or without pulmonary valve stenosis.[138] One patient with Noonan's syndrome and nonobstructive hypertrophic cardiomyopathy who died at age 14 years had a thickened right ventricle. She had no associated cardiac lesions. Histologically, the ventricular myocardium showed a mixture of normal-sized and hypertrophied fibers with scattered foci of myocytolysis, proliferation of myocardial histiocytes, and crisscrossing fiber disarray.[139] Other cardiac lesions, including pulmonary valvular or infundibular stenosis, peripheral pulmonary artery stenosis, patent ductus arteriosus, atrial septal defect, and tetralogy of Fallot, have been described in 35% to 55% of patients.[140] The Noonan syndrome is perhaps a heterogeneous group of clinically similar disorders, and this has resulted in confusion about the hereditary aspects of the disorder. Autosomal dominant inheritance seems likely in some families, but in many other cases the disease is sporadic, possibly because of new mutations. The prominent clinical features are short stature, webbed neck, low-set ears or folded auricular helices, ocular hypertelorism, ptosis of the eyelids, downward-slanting palpebral fissures, highly arched palate, cubitus valgus, proximal pectus carinatum with distal pectus excavatum, cryptorchidism in males, and mental retardation in 50%.

Although hypertrophic cardiomyopathy rarely has been reported in association with other genetic diseases such as tuberous sclerosis and neurofibromatosis,[27,141] it is unclear if these cases represented coincidental occurrences or rare manifestations of these relatively common diseases.

Cardiomyopathy associated with metabolic diseases

The cardiomyopathies of some metabolic diseases can resemble idiopathic hypertrophic cardiomyopathy clinically, but they often are distinct histologically.

Glycogen storage diseases. Glycogen storage disease type II (Pompe's disease) is an autosomal recessive disorder due to deficiency of the lysosomal enzyme α-1,4-glucosidase (acid maltase). The infantile form is characterized by hypotonia, macroglossia, and progressive cardiomyopathy resulting in death within the first year of life. The ECG is characterized by high-voltage QRS complexes in all leads and a short P-R interval. Cardiac catheterization frequently reveals biventricular hypertrophy with left outflow tract obstruction.[142] The myocardium is different histologically from the myocardium in isolated hypertrophic cardiomyopathy. There is evidence of glycogen storage with vacuolation of heart muscle. Histologic examination of tissues such as liver and kidney may reveal engorged lysosomes, but in muscle the lysosomes may have ruptured and cytoplasmic glycogen is seen. Myofibrils are displaced and destroyed.[143] The diagnosis can be confirmed by determination of α-1,4-glucosidase activity in skeletal muscle or leukocytes. Prenatal diagnosis through enzyme analysis of amniotic fluid cells is available.[142]

Juvenile and adult forms of glycogen storage disease type II also exist. The presenting characteristic is skeletal muscle weakness, and cardiac involvement usually is absent or minimal.[144,145] At least one patient had a cardiac arrhythmia that required implantation of a ventricular pacemaker, but her echocardiogram showed no cardiomegaly.[146]

Glycogen storage disease type III is due to an autosomal recessively inherited deficiency of amylo-1,6-glucosidase (debrancher) activity. The enzyme is deficient in liver and, in some patients, also is deficient in skeletal muscle, cultured skin fibroblasts, and leukocytes. Clinically, the disorder is characterized by hepatomegaly and growth retardation, which resolves at puberty. There may be hypoglycemia and hyperlipidemia. Skeletal muscle weakness may develop in adult life.[147] Clinical evidence of cardiomyopathy is rare but, when present, may be life-threatening and mimic hypertrophic cardiomyopathy. Histologic evaluation of cardiac tissue reveals increased intracellular glycogen with no disarray of myofibers or myofibrils (Fig 68-7). Deficiency of the enzyme has been documented in cardiac muscle from one patient.[148]

Other storage diseases. Other rare metabolic storage diseases may be associated with cardiomyopathy. Ethanolaminosis resembles Pompe's disease clinically.[149] The cardiomyopathy sometimes associated with the lysosomal storage diseases, such as Sandhoff's disease[150] and the mucopolysaccharidoses,[151,152] only rarely comes to medical attention because of cardiac problems.[153] Cardiac valvular disease is more likely to be a presenting feature in the milder variants of the mucopolysaccharidoses, with survival into adulthood.

Dilated cardiomyopathy. Idiopathic dilated cardiomyopathy usually had not been considered familial in the United States or Western Europe, and frequently it is omitted from discussion of genetic cardiomyopathies.[154] However, the disease is familial in more cases than previously recognized. In Japan, several groups of patients with dilated cardiomyopathy were studied and a high proportion of familial cases was found. In one series, 52% of cases were familial, and it was stated that there seemed to be an equal number of autosomal dominant and autosomal recessive cases, although details about how the inheritance patterns were determined were not provided in the paper.[155] In another Japanese study, 64% of patients had consanguineous parents, which is very suggestive of autosomal recessive inheritance.[156] It is possible that autosomal recessive inheritance of dilated cardiomyopathy is relatively common in Japan, but this does not seem to be the case in Western Europe or the United States.

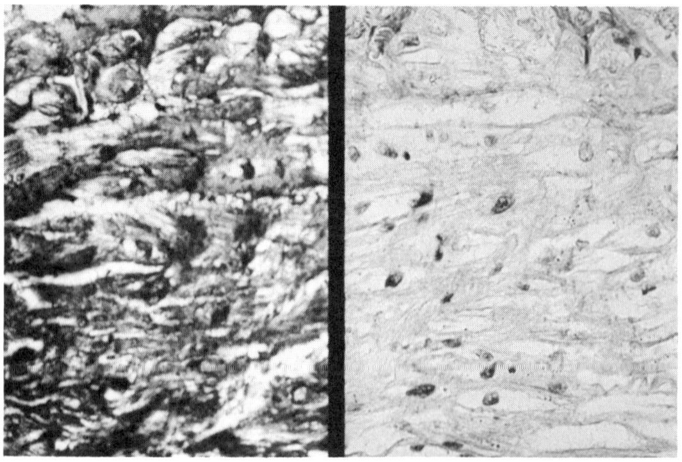

Fig 68-7 Endomyocardial biopsy in patient with glycogen storage disease type III. **Left,** before digestion with diastase, showing glycogen within myocardial cells. **Right,** after digestion with diastase, glycogen is absent. (Periodic acid-Schiff stain; ×275.) (From Olson LJ, Reeder GS, Noller KL, et al: Cardiac involvement in glycogen storage disease type III: morphologic and biochemical characterization with endomyocardial biopsy. *Am J Cardiol* 52:980-981, 1984. By permission of Technical Publishing Company.)

The incidence of dilated cardiomyopathy is higher in South Africa and some other countries where certain segments of the population are undernourished. Selenium deficiency is known to be responsible for cardiomyopathy in some parts of China (Keshan disease), but the role of nutritional deficiency in the pathogenesis of cardiomyopathy in other countries is unclear. Whether or not the causes of cardiomyopathy in other countries are similar to those in Western countries is unknown.[157]

The proportion of cases of dilated idiopathic cardiomyopathy that are familial is underestimated when this diagnosis is based only on a family history. In a retrospective study specifically performed for the purpose of determining the proportion of familial cases, a positive family history was obtained in 6.4% of patients.[158] In several families the onset of cardiomyopathy in different family members spanned many years and several generations, so that a common viral exposure would not be likely to account for the familial aggregation.

In a series of patients with idiopathic dilated cardiomyopathy who underwent cardiac transplantation, 16 of 84 (8.7%) had familial disease on the basis of review of family histories.[159] In a prospective series of 95 patients with idiopathic dilated cardiomyopathy, 457 first-degree relatives had physical examinations, electrocardiograms, and M-mode and two-dimensional echocardiograms. Twelve (24%) index patients were shown to have familial disease, and in most, the familial nature of the cardiomyopathy had not been suspected by review of the family history. Some relatives had dilated cardiomyopathy, and had considered themselves healthy. In addition, a significant number of healthy relatives of index patients with idiopathic dilated cardiomyopathy had slight enlargement of the left ventricle. These relatives with ventricular enlargement had a lower mean left ventricular ejection fraction than did relatives with a normal-sized ventricle. Whether ventricular enlargement reflects a genetic marker or a predisposition for idiopathic dilated cardiomyopathy to develop is unknown.[160] It is likely that idiopathic and familial dilated cardiomyopathies are a heterogeneous group of nongenetic and genetic diseases. In familial cases, the pattern of affected members varies from one family to another and is consistent with autosomal recessive, X-linked recessive, mitochondrial, or, most frequently, autosomal dominant inheritance.[160]

Although familial aggregation does not necessarily mean that the disease is genetic, a better understanding of the role of genetic factors in the development of cardiomyopathy may lead to a better understanding of the disease in all patients.

Endocardial fibroelastosis of infancy is probably a common pathologic end point that can result from several different diseases. Endocardial fibroelastosis without associated congenital heart disease seems to be an autosomal recessive condition in some families, although there have been rare reports in which the family pattern was compatible with X-linked recessive inheritance.[161] In other families the disease appears to be sporadic and nongenetic. Empiric risks of 4% to 17% have been reported.[162,163]

Carnitine deficiency. Carnitine deficiency is an important cause of cardiomyopathy. The diagnosis is made on the basis of low levels of carnitine in plasma and tissues. Carnitine facilitates transfer of long-chain fatty acids into the mitochondria, where they undergo oxidation. Deficiency of carnitine results in lipid accumulation in the cytoplasm. Although the incidence of carnitine deficiency is unknown, it causes one of the few forms of cardiomyopathy that are amenable to specific treatment. In the first reported family[164] that presented with cardiomyopathy without clinical evidence of hypoglycemia or skeletal muscle disease, there was biventricular hypertrophy and endocardial fibroelastosis. Light microscopy revealed extensive lipid vacuolization of the myocardial fibers. Aggregates of bizarrely shaped mitochondria with disrupted cristae and electron-dense inclusions were evident by electron microscopy. One surviving patient in this family improved after oral administration of L-carnitine, as has a second patient from another family.[165] The primary defect resulting in carnitine deficiency in some patients remains unknown, whereas other patients have been shown to have specific carnitine transport defects.[166]

Cardiac enlargement with congestive heart failure also has been reported with the myopathic form of skeletal carnitine deficiency.[167,168]

Cardiomyopathies have occurred in many patients with secondary carnitine deficiency due to long-chain fatty acyl CoA dehydrogenase deficiency as well as in organic acidemias, such as β-ketothiolase deficiency,[169] and isovaleric, methylmalonic, and propionic acidemias.[170,171] In these disorders, secondary carnitine deficiency may develop because of urinary excretion of accumulated intermediate metabolites as carnitine esters.

Hereditary hemochromatosis. The cardiomyopathy associated with familial hemochromatosis probably is due to tissue damage by iron overload, although the extent of iron overload in an organ does not always correspond exactly to the severity of tissue damage. Other clinical features of the disease are gray-brown skin pigmentation, hepatomegaly with fibrosis or cirrhosis, diabetes mellitus, hypogonadism, and bone demineralization. Biochemical abnormalities include increased serum iron and ferritin levels, increased transferrin saturation, and increased urinary iron excretion, especially in response to deferoxamine administration. The hemochromatosis gene is linked to the HLA complex on chromosome 6, and this linkage association was instrumental in proving the autosomal recessive inheritance pattern.

The risk for siblings of an affected patient is 25%, and therefore all should be screened for biochemical evidence of the disease. Patients with iron overload should have phlebotomy until the excess iron is removed, regardless of whether or not clinical signs of the disease are present. The risk for offspring of affected individuals is relatively low (approximately 1/36) but is not negligible because of the relatively high gene frequency in the general population. Therefore, offspring should be screened to determine if they are at risk for having the disease.[172]

Heart disease is seen in 15% to 20% of patients with clinically evident hemochromatosis, and the earliest signs may be ECG changes characterized by decreased QRS amplitude and T-wave flattening or inversion. Later, congestive heart failure and arrhythmias may occur. Resolution of the heart condition sometimes occurs after phlebotomy treatments.[173]

Cardiomyopathy associated with neuromuscular diseases

Cardiomyopathy can be associated with many forms of neuromuscular diseases, including Duchenne's and Becker's muscular dystrophies,[174] myotonic dystrophy, limb-girdle and facioscapulohumeral muscular dystrophies, ocular myopathies,[175] mitochondrial cytopathies,[176] centronuclear myopathy,[177] and scapuloperoneal[178] and humeroperoneal[179] neuromuscular diseases. Although skeletal muscle involvement dominates the clinical symptoms in these disorders, the possibility of skeletal muscle involvement in patients presenting with cardiomyopathy always should be considered. There have been several families in which patients presented with cardiomyopathy and no or minimal skeletal muscle symptoms but were found to have electromyographic or histologic evidence of skeletal muscle disease.[180,181]

Duchenne's muscular dystrophy is one of the most common types of muscular dystrophy; its incidence is approximately 1 per 3,500 newborn males. It is an X-linked recessive disease, and approximately one-third of the cases arise by new mutation. Progressive skeletal weakness beginning at 2 to 5 years of age, with death in the late teens or 20s, is characteristic. The diagnosis is made on the basis of clinical findings plus markedly increased creatine kinase levels. The muscle biopsy findings are relatively nonspecific.

The genetic defect that results in both Duchenne's and Becker's muscular dystrophies involves the dystrophin gene located on chromosome X at band p21. Approximately two-thirds of patients have a submicroscopic partial gene deletion, and the rest have undetected deletions, duplications, or other abnormalities. The dystrophin gene is very large, consisting of at least 60 exons and 1,800 kilobases. The entire gene has been cloned. The protein product of this gene, dystrophin, is a rod-shaped cytoskeletal protein that is predominantly localized to the surface membrane of striated muscle cells.[182] Identification of the molecular defect has resulted in improved ability to determine carrier status in female relatives by DNA analysis. This represents a significant improvement over carrier testing by measurement of creatine kinase levels, since increased levels are found in only 70% of obligate carriers.[183] DNA analysis also can be used for prenatal diagnosis. All mothers and sisters of patients with Duchenne's or Becker's muscular dystrophy should have genetic counseling.

The heart disease in patients with Duchenne's muscular dystrophy is characterized by significant changes in systolic time intervals suggestive of compromised left ventricular function. There are histologic changes characterized by multifocal dystrophic areas with fibrosis and loss of myofilaments. These changes are most marked in the posterobasal segment and contiguous lateral and inferior walls of the left ventricle.[184]

Myotonic dystrophy, the most common form of muscular dystrophy in adults, occurs with an incidence of approximately 1 per 20,000 to 30,000. The inheritance pattern is autosomal dominant with extremely variable expression. Although average age at onset is in the second to third decade of life, the disease may be evident at birth or first be noticed in the seventh decade. The disease is characterized by myotonia, muscle atrophy and weakness, ptosis of the eyelids, and expressionless facies resulting from particularly severe involvement of the facial and temporal muscles. Rate of progression of the disease is variable, but disability is usually severe within 15 to 20 years after onset. Associated abnormalities include premature frontal baldness, testicular atrophy or menstrual irregularities, gastrointestinal symptoms related to smooth muscle involvement, and cardiac disease. Distinctive refractile posterior subcapsular cataracts often are evident by slit-lamp examination; this finding is helpful in making the diagnosis, but the cataracts rarely interfere with vision. Although glucose intolerance is common, overt diabetes mellitus occurs in only about 6% of patients.

The diagnosis is based on clinical findings and a typical electromyographic pattern characterized by prolonged rhythmic discharges. The risk for children born to an affected parent is 50%. However, affected females also need to be aware of the additional risk of having an affected infant with severe, sometimes fatal, hypotonia and mental deficiency. These infants may not have myotonia, and this infantile form of the disease does not occur when the father is the affected parent.[185]

The gene for myotonic dystrophy is located on chromosome 19 at band q13, and genetic counseling is warranted for the patient and family members. The molecular basis of myotonic dystrophy recently has been shown to be an expansion of a CTG trinucleotide repeat sequence in a gene encoding a protein kinase.[186] Thus, direct DNA-based diagnosis of the disease is possible and can be used presymptomatically and prenatally.

Cardiac disease is present in approximately two-thirds of patients with myotonic dystrophy, and sudden death is not uncommon. There is prolongation of the P-R or QRS interval and changes in the T wave or ST segment. Intra-atrial and His-Purkinje conduction may be prolonged, and heart block may require implantation of a pacemaker. There seems to be degeneration of the conducting tissue before other cardiac muscle is involved.[187] If general anesthesia is required, caution must be taken, because many of these patients have central and alveolar hypoventilation, and there is a serious risk of postanesthetic respiratory depression,[188] which can occur several hours after the patient seems to be alert and stable.

Amyloidosis

There are at least 13 forms of inherited amyloidosis. All are autosomal dominant with the exception of autosomal recessive familial Mediterranean fever and X-linked recessive cutaneous amyloidosis. Autosomal recessive inheritance of three types of localized amyloidoses (gingival, corneal, and bullous cutaneous) has been suggested but not proved.

Cardiac involvement is most prominent in amyloidosis type III, also referred to as cardiac amyloidosis and Denmark type amyloidosis. The patients present with bradycardia, syncope, or heart failure in the third to fifth decade of life. The underlying cause of Denmark cardiac amyloidosis is a mutation in the prealbumin (transthyretin) gene that results in substitution of methionine for leucine at amino acid 111. A substitution of isoleucine for leucine at amino acid 122 has been found in several black Americans with cardiac amyloidosis, but other forms of "senile" amyloidosis are not yet understood biochemically and may be unrelated to the prealbumin gene.[189]

Cardiac amyloid infiltration also may be seen in some of the other forms of genetic amyloidosis, including amyloidosis types I and II (Portuguese or Andrade type and Rukavina or Indiana type, respectively). Neuropathy is the initial abnormality in these types.[81a] Type I is usually more severe and onset is earlier, in the fourth to fifth decade. Development of symmetric sensory polyneuropathy is followed by autonomic nerve involvement that results in constipation, diarrhea, hypohidrosis, and postural hypotension. In one series of 22 patients, 15 had cardiac conduction disturbances after 4 years of illness.[190] Cranial neuropathy and corneal lattice dystrophy are most prominent in amyloidosis V (Finland or Meretoja type), although some degree of cardiac involvement can occur.[191]

At least six forms of autosomal dominant amyloidosis, including types I and II, Danish, Jewish, Appalachian, and Illinois/German amyloidoses, are due to different point mutations in the prealbumin (transthyretin) gene. These findings make presymptomatic or prenatal diagnoses possible in some families.[192]

CONNECTIVE TISSUE DISORDERS

Marfan syndrome

The Marfan syndrome is the prototype of the connective tissue disorders and is relatively common, with an incidence of 1 per 20,000. It is an autosomal dominant disorder with extremely variable expression, and approximately 20% of cases arise by new mutation. There are no well-documented instances of nonpenetrance.

The disease involves the musculoskeletal, cardiovascular, and ocular systems. Skeletal abnormalities include tall stature, a low upper/lower segment ratio because limbs are relatively long compared to the trunk, scoliosis or kyphosis, and pectus deformities. These features result from overgrowth of the tubular bones. Increased joint laxity and hyperextensibility are common, but occasionally patients have limited extension of fingers and elbows. The face may be long and thin, and the palate may be narrow and highly arched. This "marfanoid habitus" may be present in patients with other disorders, such as other connective tissue dysplasias, mucosal neuroma syndrome (multiple endocrine neoplasia, type IIB) Stickler syndrome, and homocystinuria. The characteristic body habitus is never sufficient evidence for making the diagnosis of Marfan syndrome in the absence of other characteristic features or a well-documented family history of Marfan syndrome.

The ocular abnormalities associated with Marfan syndrome include subluxation of the lenses, myopia, and retinal detachment. As the most specific ocular feature, dislocation of the lenses is very helpful in making the diagnosis of Marfan syndrome, although ectopia lentis also can be seen in other disorders, such as homocystinuria and Weill-Marchesani syndrome. Dislocations occur in 50% to 80% of patients; the lens frequently is displaced upward, but this is not always the case. Gross dislocations may be evident without the aid of special equipment, but lesser degrees of dislocation may be evident only by slit-lamp examination. Therefore, all patients suspected of having Marfan syndrome must have a complete ophthalmologic evaluation, including slit-lamp examination. Patients with Marfan syndrome should have frequent ophthalmologic examinations to permit early detection of complications such as retinal detachment or glaucoma.

The life expectancy of patients with Marfan syndrome is shortened because of cardiovascular disease. The most common manifestation is mitral valve prolapse with or without mitral regurgitation. Dilation of the ascending aorta is the next most common cardiovascular disorder; it may lead to aortic regurgitation, aortic rupture, or dissecting aneurysm.[193] Although fewer than 70% of patients have evidence of cardiovascular disease by physical examination, more than 80% have abnormalities detected by echocardiography.

Mitral valve prolapse in patients with Marfan syndrome initially may involve only the posterior leaflet; it may be late systolic or pansystolic and often is progressive. The prevalence of mitral valve prolapse is similar in males and females.[194] In one retrospective series of 166 patients who had had at least one echocardiogram before age 22 years, 8 patients died as a result of mitral valve dysfunction or required valve replacement; severe mitral regurgitation developed in an additional 15 patients.[195] Mitral insufficiency may be present in young infants with Marfan syndrome.[196] Acute onset of severe mitral regurgitation due to rupture of chordae tendineae may occur even in childhood.[197] The finding of mitral valve prolapse in a patient with a "marfanoid" body habitus is not a sufficient basis for the diagnosis of Marfan syndrome in the absence of a positive family history of Marfan syndrome or other characteristic findings. Patients with some forms of Ehlers-Danlos syndrome and nonspecific connective tissue dysplasias can have a similar body habitus, joint laxity, and mitral valve prolapse.

Aortic abnormalities were found in 60% to 94% in two series of patients.[193,198] The prevalence of aortic root enlargement is greater in males than in females.[194] In children and adults, the diameter of the aortic root usually is abnormal in proportion to body surface area. Aortic dilation is progressive, with symmetric involvement in the region of the sinus of Valsalva and sinotubular ridge.

The risk of cardiovascular complications during pregnancy poses a special problem for women with Marfan syndrome. Acute aortic dissection may occur before, during, or after labor. A retrospective review[199] of one series of patients suggested that the risk of maternal death was "low in patients with minimal pre-existing vascular disease," but the risk may be significant in those with moderate degrees of aortic root dilation. Therefore, the aortic root diameter must be taken into account in counseling women who are considering childbearing. It is recommended by some that if aortic root dilation is present, pregnancy should not be undertaken.[200] Those who decide to become pregnant should receive care appropriate for "high-risk" obstetric patients.[199] Patients with Marfan syndrome also are prone to traumatic aortic rupture, and contact sports should be avoided.

Additional features sometimes associated with Marfan syndrome include decreased amounts of subcutaneous tissue, skin striae, inguinal hernias, pneumothorax, and degenerative joint disease.

In addition to physical examination, the diagnostic evaluation of patients suspected of having Marfan syndrome should include chest radiograph, ophthalmologic examination (including slit-lamp evaluation of the lenses), and echocardiography. A thorough family history should be obtained. For patients with a well-documented family history of Marfan syndrome, characteristic involvement of any one of the three organ systems may be sufficient for the diagnosis to be made. However, in patients without a positive family history, the patient must have the characteristic body habitus plus either aortic root dilation or ectopia lentis. In those with ectopia lentis, homocystinuria must be excluded. In patients with the characteristic body habitus plus mitral valve prolapse but without aortic root dilation, the diagnosis cannot be made definitely. If skin hyperextensibility, poor skin and wound healing, or atrophic skin scarring is present, the patient probably has a form of Ehlers-Danlos syndrome. If no other abnormality is present, it may be impossible to exclude the diagnosis of Marfan syndrome, and subsequent evaluations are warranted.

Investigation of first-degree relatives should be undertaken even if they have no obvious stigmas of the Marfan syndrome. Families have been observed in which a child may present with obvious phenotypic features of Marfan syndrome, but a parent was found to be affected only after echocardiography revealed aortic root dilation or slit-lamp examination revealed ectopia lentis.

The basic cause of Marfan syndrome has been found to be a defect in fibrillin; the gene encoding fibrillin is on chromosome 15q15-21.[201] This discovery potentially makes presymptomatic and prenatal diagnosis possible in families known to have the disease, and in the near future it also may allow for diagnostic testing in patients with equivocal signs of the disease.

Ehlers-Danlos syndrome

There may be up to 15 forms of Ehlers-Danlos syndrome. Type I, or gravis type, was the first described and serves as a prototype for discussion of this group of genetically heterogeneous disorders.[81b] The syndrome is inherited as an autosomal dominant condition, and the basic defect in type I disease has not been defined. The disorder is characterized by velvety-textured, hyperextensible, fragile skin that splits easily and heals poorly, resulting in wide, thin scars. Many tissues are friable, which is an important consideration when surgical procedures are considered. Even the fetal membranes are affected and frequently rupture before term, resulting in premature birth. "Molluscoid pseudotumors" are areas of sagging, wrinkled, redundant skin that may develop over the knee and elbow joints (Fig 68-8). Small fat- or mucin-containing spherules may be present in the subcutaneous tissue and may become calcified. The joints are hyperextensible and

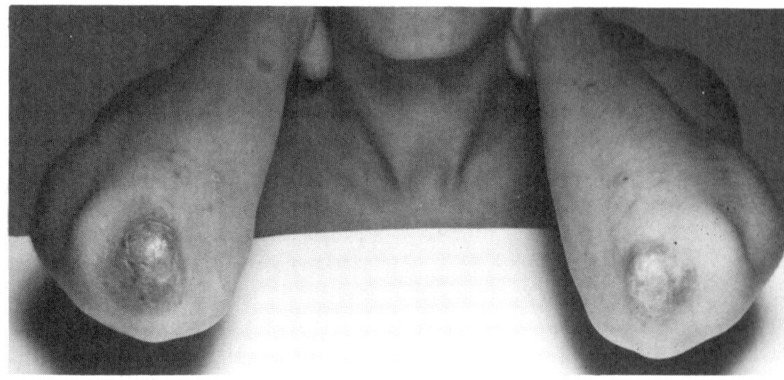

Fig 68-8 Molluscoid pseudotumors on the elbows of a patient with Ehlers-Danlos syndrome type I.

prone to dislocations. Pes planus, scoliosis, degenerative arthritis, visceral diverticulosis, and spontaneous pneumothorax may occur.[24]

Involvement of small blood vessels results in easy bruisability. Mitral valve prolapse may occur in 50% of the patients.[202] Dilation of the aortic root or pulmonary artery and prolapse of the tricuspid valve may occur. Vascular rupture is relatively rare. Structural congenital heart defects, including atrial septal defect, ventricular septal defect, tetralogy of Fallot, bicuspid tricuspid valve, and dextrocardia, have been reported in a few patients.[203]

Ehlers-Danlos syndrome type II, or mitis type, is similar to type I but milder; it also is inherited as an autosomal dominant disorder. A significant number of patients have mitral valve prolapse. It is uncertain if this disorder results from a mutation at the same locus as for type I or at a different one.[81c]

The joint hypermobility of Ehlers-Danlos type III, or benign familial hypermobility syndrome, is similar to that in type I and may result in joint dislocations. However, skin hyperextensibility and scarring are minimal or absent. There is a wide range of expression both within and between families. Families with the mildest manifestations merge with the general population in terms of normal variation in joint mobility. It is an autosomal dominant disorder.[81d]

Type IV, or vascular Ehlers-Danlos syndrome, is genetically heterogeneous with both autosomal dominant and autosomal recessive forms. It is usually due to deficiency of type III collagen synthesis or secretion in skin, aorta, uterus, and intestine. This is the most severe form of Ehlers-Danlos syndrome and is characterized by rupture of large arteries, the colon, or the gravid uterus. Angiography and other invasive procedures may precipitate vascular or organ rupture and should be done only after careful consideration of the risk-to-benefit ratio. Mitral valve prolapse frequently is present.[204] In some patients the skin is extremely thin, allowing visualization of the underlying venous network. In spite of this, there is a tendency to form keloid scars and contractures. In contrast to patients with other forms of Ehlers-Danlos syndrome, in these patients the skin and connective tissues may not be hyperextensible. Occasional complications include spontaneous pneumothorax and severe periodontal disease. This defect is expressed in cultured skin fibroblasts, so prenatal diagnosis theoretically is possible.[205] It has been suggested that type III collagen also is deficient in some patients with congenital cerebral aneurysms who do not have Ehlers-Danlos syndrome.[81e,206]

Ehlers-Danlos type V is an X-linked recessive disease that may be secondarily associated with lysyl oxidase deficiency, although this has not been a universal finding. Skin hyperextensibility is severe, but joint hypermobility is mild to moderate. Mitral and tricuspid valve prolapse or insufficiency may be present, and at least one patient had an atrial septal defect.[81n,207]

Ehlers-Danlos type VI is called the ocular type because blindness from retinal detachment or ocular rupture is a serious complication. In some cases the disease is due to an autosomal recessively inherited deficiency of procollagen lysyl hydroxylase. Severe scoliosis, recurrent joint dislocations, aortic rupture, and gastrointestinal hemorrhage also can occur.[81l,208] Prenatal diagnosis is possible in families with a documented biochemical defect.

Ehlers-Danlos type VII, or arthrochalasis multiplex congenita, is characterized by extreme joint laxity and dislocations. Some patients have defective conversion of procollagen to collagen, which is an autosomal recessive defect. However, others have structural abnormalities of half their $\alpha 2$ chains of type I collagen that interfere with the enzymatic conversion of procollagen to collagen. The latter is an autosomal dominant condition.[81f]

Ehlers-Danlos type VIII is similar to types I and II but includes particularly severe periodontal disease. It is an autosomal dominant disorder, and the basic defect is unknown.[81m]

It is apparent that there is marked genetic heterogeneity in all the Ehlers-Danlos syndromes that have been chemically defined, and it is probable that an equal degree of heterogeneity will be found in the more common types I, II, and III.

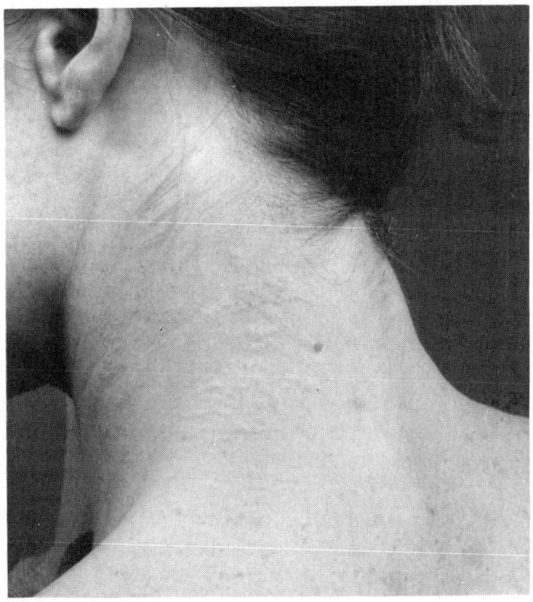

Fig 68-9 Yellow skin papules on neck of patient with pseudoxanthoma elasticum.

Pseudoxanthoma elasticum

There are two hereditary forms of pseudoxanthoma elasticum, autosomal dominant and autosomal recessive. Both forms are characterized by yellowish skin papules, especially on the neck and flexural areas (Fig 68-9), angioid streaks and choroiditis of the retina, and vascular complications including angina pectoris, claudication, calcification of peripheral arteries, and renal vascular hypertension. In one series of patients, 19% had angina pectoris, 14% had calcification of peripheral arteries, and 18% had intermittent claudication. The age at onset of these complications is variable, and they may occur in early adolescence.[209] Endocardial thickening may result in deformity of the valves, and the conduction system also may be involved, resulting in arrhythmias.[210] Histologically, the arteries show fragmented elastic fibers with granular deposits in place of amorphous elastin.[211] The basic defect is not known but seems to be either an intrinsic abnormality of elastin or secondary destruction of elastin.

Osteogenesis imperfecta

There are several types of autosomal dominant osteogenesis imperfecta. Mitral valve prolapse is increased in frequency but infrequently progresses to significant regurgitation. The mean aortic root diameter is said to be slightly but significantly increased, and aortic regurgitation occurs in 1% to 2% of the patients.[81g]

The disease is characterized by multiple bone fractures, and some patients have opalescent teeth, blue sclerae, and child- or adult-onset hearing loss. The clinical expression is extremely variable between and within families. Multiple different defects in the genes encoding the α1 and α2 chains of type I collagen have been reported, so that the disease is extremely heterogeneous at the DNA level.

Homocystinuria

The classic form of homocystinuria is due to autosomal recessively inherited deficiency of cystathionine β-synthase. The gene is expressed in skin fibroblasts and amniocytes, so prenatal diagnosis by determination of enzyme activity in amniocytes is feasible.

The incidence of the disease is approximately 1 per 200,000. Clinically it is characterized by tall stature with a low upper segment/lower segment ratio, pectus deformities, scoliosis, genu valgum, pes planus, and a highly arched palate. Lens dislocation is progressive, and the direction of displacement is usually, but not always, downward. Myopia, retinal detachment, secondary glaucoma, fair hair and skin, cutaneous flushing, and hernias may be present. Approximately 50% of patients are mentally retarded, but this is variable even within a sibship. The electroencephalogram may be abnormal, and some patients have seizures, focal neurologic signs, and hemiatrophy of the brain. Acute episodes of "nervousness" or schizophrenic behavior may occur. Osteoporosis with a tendency to fractures and "codfish"-shaped, collapsed vertebrae may be evident radiographically. It is important to realize that none of the features is present consistently in all patients, and some affected individuals appear normal.

Cardiovascular abnormalities include arterial or venous thrombosis, angina pectoris, coronary occlusions at a young age, renal artery narrowing resulting in hypertension and renal atrophy, cerebrovascular accidents, thrombophlebitis, and pulmonary emboli. Dilation of the pulmonary artery and left atrial endocardial fibroelastosis have been reported. Thrombi are particularly likely to occur after surgical procedures,[212] venipuncture, or catheterization.

Histologic examination of the arteries reveals marked fibrous thickening of the intima. Aortic intimal fibrosis may be severe enough to mimic coarctation. Medial changes consist of thrombosis and dilation with widely spaced, frayed muscle fibers. The elastic fibers of the large arteries may be fragmented, and dilation of the ascending aorta has been observed.[213] No consistent platelet defect has been observed.[214]

The disease sometimes may be diagnosed by a positive urinary nitroprusside test with confirmation by the more sensitive method of elevated urinary homocystine excretion by amino acid chromatography. Levels of plasma homocystine and its precursor, methionine, are increased. The goal of treatment is to lower plasma homocystine, which seems to result in slower progression and fewer symptoms of the disease; 50% of patients respond to pyridoxine therapy (25 to 1,000 mg/day). Supplemental folate also should be given because patients who are potentially capable of responding to pyridoxine may not do so in the presence of folate deficiency. A low-protein, low-methionine diet can be useful, but adult patients may find it difficult to comply with this diet. For infants, a low-methionine formula is available. Betaine[215] and penicillamine[216] also have been reported to be of benefit in decreasing plasma homocystine levels.

There is a rare form of homocystinuria that is due to *N*-methyltetrahydrofolate-homocysteine methyltransferase deficiency.[217] These patients have additional neurologic symptoms, and the plasma methionine levels may be normal. Patients with homocystinuria due to abnormal cobalamin metabolism also have normal plasma methionine levels and may have methylmalonic acidemia and megaloblastic anemia as well.[218] There is increasing evidence that mild hyperhomocystinemia is associated with arterial vascular disease. The cause of the elevation may be related to carrier status for one of the classic homocystinurias, vitamin deficiency, or other unknown genetic or environmental mechanisms.

CONCLUSION

In summary, there are many forms of heart disease that are genetically determined to some extent. The clinical geneticist can assist the cardiologist in the evaluation of some of these patients in various ways.

Parents of children with congenital heart defects should be informed of the risk of occurrence in future children. In most cases the cardiologist will take the family history as part of the routine medical evaluation and can relate the appropriate risk figures. However, in families with multiple affected members, the geneticist may be of assistance in obtaining a more detailed family history, sending for medical records, or arranging for medical investigations of family members in an attempt to determine the inheritance pattern and provide accurate estimates of risks. The geneticist can be of particular assistance in the evaluation of children with multiple congenital anomalies who have an underlying chromosomal abnormality or other recognizable syndrome. Methods of prenatal diagnosis can be discussed with the family when appropriate. Patients with congenital heart disease who enter their reproductive years also can benefit from this type of counseling.

Patients with heart disease as a component of an inherited disease such as Marfan syndrome frequently benefit from a genetic evaluation. Investigation of family members is often warranted. The patient can be counseled about general prognosis, and appropriate evaluation of other involved organ systems can be arranged. Many geneticists are skilled in the treatment of rare metabolic disorders, such as phenylketonuria and glycogen storage disease. Risk of occurrence for siblings or children and options for prenatal diagnosis can be discussed.

GLOSSARY

Autosome: Chromosome other than sex chromosome.

Chromosome: Long strands of double-stranded deoxyribonucleic acid (DNA) that encode genes and that are associated with a protein framework. The normal human has 46 chromosomes per cell.

Deletion: Structural abnormality in which part of a chromosome is missing.

Duplication: Structural abnormality in which an extra copy of part of a chromosome is present.

Gene: A portion of a deoxyribonucleic acid (DNA) molecule that codes for a specific RNA or protein product.

Hemizygote: A person who has a gene form on one chromosome but no homologous chromosome with a corresponding gene site. The term usually refers to males because they have only one X chromosome.

Heterozygote: A person who has different gene forms at a given site on two homologous chromosomes.

Homozygote: A person who has the same gene forms at a given site on two homologous chromosomes.

Inversion: Structural abnormality characterized by reversal of a segment within the chromosome.

Karyotype: The chromosome complement of an individual person.

Linkage (genetic linkage): Close physical proximity of two gene loci on the same chromosome such that segregation is nonrandom.

Phenotype: The observable biochemical or physical characteristics of an individual as determined by genetic material and environment.

Proband: The index patient.

Recurrence: Occurrence of another case of a specific condition in the same family.

Translocation: Structural abnormality characterized by transfer of a piece of one chromosome to another chromosome.

REFERENCES

1. Goto Y, Nonaka I, Horai S: A mutation in the tRNA (Leu) (UUR) gene associated with the MELAS subgroup of mitochondrial encephalomyopathies. *Nature* 348:651-653, 1990

2. Linnane AW, Marzuki S, Ozawa T, et al: Mitochondrial DNA mutations as an important contributor to ageing and degenerative diseases. *Lancet* 1:642-645, 1989

3. Corral-Debrinski M, Stepien G, Shoffner JM, et al: Hypoxemia is associated with mitochondrial DNA damage and gene induction. Implications for cardiac disease. *JAMA* 266:1812-1816, 1991

4. Edwards JH: Familial predisposition in man. *Br Med Bull* 25:58-64, 1969

5. Smith C: Recurrence risks for multifactorial inheritance. *Am J Hum Genet* 23:578-588, 1971

6. Falconer DS: The inheritance of liability of certain diseases, estimated from the incidence among relatives. *Ann Hum Genet* 29:51-76, 1965

7. Mitchell SC, Korones SB, Berendes HW: Congenital heart disease in 56,109 births: incidence and natural history. *Circulation* 43:323-332, 1971

8. Nora JJ: Etiologic aspects of heart diseases. In *Moss' Heart Disease in Infants, Children, and Adolescents.* Third edition. Edited by FH Adams, GC Emmanouilides. Baltimore, Williams & Wilkins Company, 1983, pp 2-10

9. Copel JA, Pilu G, Green J, et al: Fetal echocardiographic screening for congenital heart disease: the importance of the four-chamber view. *Am J Obstet Gynecol* 157:648-655, 1987

10. Allan LD, Crawford DC, Chita SK, et al: Familial recurrence of congenital heart disease in a prospective series of mothers referred for fetal echocardiography. *Am J Cardiol* 58:334-337, 1986

11. Whittemore R, Hobbins JC, Engle MA: Pregnancy and its outcome in women with and without surgical treatment of congenital heart disease. *Am J Cardiol* 50:641-651, 1982

12. Rose V, Gold RJM, Lindsay G, et al: A possible increase in the incidence of congenital heart defects among the offspring of affected parents. *J Am Coll Cardiol* 6:376-382, 1985

13. Whittemore R: Maternal transmission of congenital heart disease (letter to the editor). *Am J Cardiol* 61:499-500, 1988

14. Nora JJ, Nora AH: Maternal transmission of congenital heart diseases: new recurrence risk figures and the questions of cytoplasmic inheritance and vulnerability to teratogens. *Am J Cardiol* 59:459-463, 1987

15. Ferencz C: Offspring of fathers with cardiovascular malformations (letter to the editor). *Am Heart J* 111:1212-1213, 1986

16. Driscoll DJ, Michels VV, Gersony WM, et al: Occurrence risk for congenital heart defects in relatives of patients with aortic stenosis, pulmonary stenosis, or ventricular septal defect. *Circulation* 87 Suppl 2:114-120, 1993

17. Zellers TM, Driscoll DJ, Michels VV: Prevalence of significant congenital heart defects in children of parents with Fallot's tetralogy. *Am J Cardiol* 65:523-526, 1990

18. Rowe RD: Patent ductus arteriosus. In *Heart Disease in Infancy and Childhood.* Third edition. Edited by JD Keith, RD Rowe, P Vlad. New York, Macmillan Publishing Co, 1978, pp 418-451

19. Lynch HT, Grissom RL, Magnuson CR, et al: Patent ductus arteriosus: study of two families. *JAMA* 194:135-138, 1965

20. Taussig HB: *Congenital Malformations of the Heart.* Vol 1. Second edition. Cambridge, Massachusetts, Harvard University Press, 1960

21. Burman D: Familial patent ductus arteriosus. *Br Heart J* 23:603-604, 1961

22. Pierpont ME, Sletten LJ: Char syndrome: a cause of familial patent ductus arteriosus (abstract). *Am J Hum Genet* 55 Suppl:89, 1994

23. Rowe RD: Cardiovascular disease in the rubella syndrome. In *Heart Disease in Infancy and Childhood.* Third edition. Edited by JD Keith, RD Rowe, P Vlad. New York, Macmillan Publishing Co, 1978, pp 958-966

24. Smith DW: Recognizable patterns of human malformation: genetic, embryologic and clinical aspects. *Major Probl Clin Pediatr* 7:1-653, 1982

25. Hoffman JIE, Rudolph A: The natural history of ventricular septal defects in infancy. *Am J Cardiol* 16:634-653, 1965

26. Yerushalmy J: The California Child Health and Development Studies: study design and some illustrative findings on congenital heart disease. *Excerpta Medica International Congress Series* No 204, 1969, pp 299-306

27. Keith JD: Atrial septal defect: ostium secundum, ostium primum, and atrioventricularis communis (common AV canal). In *Heart Disease in Infancy and Childhood.* Third edition. Edited by JD Keith, RD Rowe, P Vlad. New York, Macmillan Publishing Co, 1978, pp 380-404

28. Feldt RH, Edwards WD, Puga FJ, et al: Atrial septal defects and atrioventricular canal. In *Moss' Heart Disease in Infants, Children, and Adolescents.* Third edition. Edited by FH Adams, GC Emmanouilides. Baltimore, Williams & Wilkins Company, 1983, pp 118-134

29. Sánchez Cascos A: Genetics of atrial septal defect. *Arch Dis Child* 47:581-588, 1972

30. Richer TJ, Gallen WJ, Friedberg DZ: Familial atrial septal defect in a single generation. *Br Heart J* 34:198-200, 1972

31. Howitt G: Atrial septal defect in three generations. *Br Heart J* 23:494-496, 1961

32. Campbell M, Polani PE: Factors in the aetiology of atrial septal defect. *Br Heart J* 23:477-493, 1961

33. Zetterqvist P: Multiple occurrence of atrial septal defect in a family. *Acta Paediatr* 49:741-747, 1960

34. Lynch HT, Bachenberg K, Harris RE, et al: Hereditary atrial septal defect: update of a large kindred. *Am J Dis Child* 132:600-604, 1978

35. Zuckerman HS, Zuckerman GH, Mammen RE, et al: Atrial septal defect: familial occurrence in four generations of one family. *Am J Cardiol* 9:515-520, 1962

36. Nora JJ, McNamara DG, Fraser FC: Hereditary factors in atrial septal defect. *Circulation* 35:448-456, 1967

37. Johansson BW, Sievers J: Inheritance of atrial septal defect (letter to the editor). *Lancet* 1:1224-1225, 1967

38. Williamson EM: A family study of atrial septal defect. *J Med Genet* 6:255-261, 1969

39. Kahler RL, Braunwald E, Plauth WH Jr, et al: Familial congenital heart disease: familial occurrence of atrial septal defect with A-V conduction abnormalities; supravalvular aortic and pulmonic stenosis; and ventricular septal defect. *Am J Med* 40:384-399, 1966

40. Bizarro RO, Callahan JA, Feldt RH, et al: Familial atrial septal defect with prolonged atrioventricular conduction: a syndrome showing the autosomal dominant pattern of inheritance. *Circulation* 41:677-683, 1970

41. Pease WE, Nordenberg A, Ladda RL: Familial atrial septal defect with prolonged atrioventricular conduction. *Circulation* 53:759-762, 1976

42. Smith AT, Sack GH Jr, Taylor GJ: Holt-Oram syndrome. *J Pediatr* 95:538-543, 1979

43. Basson CT, Cowley GS, Solomon SD, et al: The clinical and genetic spectrum of the Holt-Oram syndrome (heart-hand syndrome). *N Engl J Med* 330:885-891, 1994

44. Samanek M: Prevalence at birth, "natural" risk and survival with atrioventricular septal defect. *Cardiol Young* 1:285-289, 1991

45. Emanuel R, Nichols J, Anders JM, et al: Atrioventricular defects: a study of 92 families. *Br Heart J* 30:645-653, 1968

46. Yao J, Thompson MW, Trusler GA, et al: Familial atrial septal defect of the primum type: a report of four cases in one sibship. *Can Med Assoc J* 98:218-219, 1968

47. Michels VV, Riccardi VM: Congenital heart defects. In *Principles and Practice of Medical Genetics.* Vol. 2. Second edition. Edited by AEH Emery, DL Rimoin. Edinburgh, Churchill Livingstone, 1990, pp 1207-1237

48. Keith JD: Coarctation of the aorta. In *Heart Disease in Infancy and Childhood.* Third edition. Edited by JD Keith, RD Rowe, P Vlad. New York, Macmillan Publishing Co, 1978, pp 736-760

49. Gersony WM: Coarctation of the aorta. In *Moss' Heart Disease in Infants, Children, and Adolescents.* Third edition. Edited by FH Adams, GC Emmanouilides. Baltimore, Williams & Wilkins Company, 1983, pp 188-199

50. Hall JG, McLaughlin JF, Stamm S: Coarctation of the aorta in male cousins with similar maternal environmental exposure to insect repellent and insecticides. *Pediatrics* 55:425-427, 1975

51. Ravelo HR, Stephenson LW, Friedman S, et al: Coarctation resection in children with Turner's syndrome: a note of caution. *J Thorac Cardiovasc Surg* 80:427-430, 1980

52. Pierpont ME, Gobel JW, Moller JH, et al: Cardiac malformations in relatives of children with truncus arteriosus or interruption of the aortic arch. *Am J Cardiol* 61:423-427, 1988

53. Boon AR, Farmer MB, Roberts DF: A family study of Fallot's tetralogy. *J Med Genet* 9:179-192, 1972

54. Pitt DB: A family study of Fallot's tetrad. *Aust Ann Med* 11:179-183, 1962

55. Miller ME, Smith DW: Conotruncal malformation complex: examples of possible monogenic inheritance. *Pediatrics* 63:890-892, 1979

56. Raatikka M, Rapola J, Tuuteri L, et al: Familial third and fourth pharyngeal pouch syndrome with truncus arteriosus: DiGeorge syndrome. *Pediatrics* 67:173-175, 1981

57. Jedele KB, Michels VV, Puga FJ, et al: Velo-cardio-facial syndrome associated with ventricular septal defect, pulmonary atresia, and hypoplastic pulmonary arteries. *Pediatrics* 89:915-919, 1992

58. Greenwood RD, Rosenthal A, Sommer A, et al: Cardiovascular malformations in oculoauriculovertebral dysplasia (Goldenhar syndrome). *J Pediatr* 85:816-821, 1974

59. David TJ: A family with congenital pulmonary valve stenosis. *Humangenetik* 21:287-288, 1974

60. Weil MH, Allenstein BJ: A report of congenital heart disease in five members of one family. *N Engl J Med* 265:661-667, 1961

61. Patterson DF, Haskins ME, Schnarr WR: Hereditary dysplasia of the pulmonary valve in beagle dogs: pathologic and genetic studies. *Am J Cardiol* 47:631-641, 1981

62. Friedman WF, Benson LN: Aortic stenosis. In *Moss' Heart Disease in Infants, Children, and Adolescents.* Third edition. Edited by FH Adams, GC Emmanouilides. Baltimore, Williams & Wilkins Company, 1983, pp 171-188

63. Driscoll DJ, Friedberg DZ, Gallen WJ: Idiopathic hypercalcemic syndrome with mitral stenosis. *Wis Med J* 73:S115-S116, September 1974

64. Anonymous: A 30kb deletion within the elastin gene results in familial supravalvular aortic stenosis. *Hum Mol Genet* (in press)

65. Child AH, Dennis NR: The genetics of congenital heart disease. *Birth Defects* 13 No 3A:85-91, 1977

66. Brownell LG, Shokeir MHK: Inheritance of hypoplastic left heart syndrome (HLHS): further observations. *Clin Genet* 9:245-249, 1976

67. Rao SS, Gootman N, Platt N: Familial aortic atresia: report of a case of aortic atresia in siblings. *Am J Dis Child* 118:919-922, 1969

68. Silverman NH, Enderlein MA, Golbus MS: Ultrasonic recognition of aortic valve atresia in utero. *Am J Cardiol* 53:391-392, 1984

69. Fortuin NJ, Strahan NV, Come PC, et al: Inheritance of the mitral valve prolapse syndrome (abstract). *Clin Res* 25:470A, 1977

70. Devereux RB, Brown WT: Genetics of mitral valve prolapse. *Prog Med Genet* 5:139-161, 1983

71. Weiss AN, Mimbs JW, Ludbrook PA, et al: Echocardiographic detection of mitral valve prolapse: exclusion of false positive diagnosis and determination of inheritance. *Circulation* 52:1091-1096, 1975

72. Ruttenberg HD: Corrected transposition (L-transposition) of the great arteries and splenic syndromes. In *Moss' Heart Disease in Infants, Children, and Adolescents.* Third edition. Edited by FH Adams, GC Emmanouilides. Baltimore, Williams & Wilkins Company, 1983, pp 333-350

73. Freedom RM: The asplenia syndrome: a review of significant extracardiac structural abnormalities in 29 necropsied patients. *J Pediatr* 81:1130-1133, 1972

74. Britz-Cunningham SH, Shah MM, Zuppan CW, et al: Mutations of the Connexin43 gap-junction gene in patients with heart malformations and defects of laterality. *N Engl J Med* 332:1323-1329, 1995

75. Chen S-C, Monteleone PL: Familial splenic anomaly syndrome (letter to the editor). *J Pediatr* 91:160-161, 1977

76. Simpson J, Zellweger H: Familial occurrence of Ivemark syndrome with splenic hypoplasia and asplenia in sibs. *J Med Genet* 10:303-304, 1973

77. Ursell PC, Wigger HJ: Asplenia syndrome in conjoined twins: a case report. *Teratology* 27:301-304, 1983

78. Hurwitz RC, Caskey CT: Ivemark syndrome in siblings. *Clin Genet* 22:7-11, 1982

79. Schidlow DV, Katz SM, Turtz MG, et al: Polysplenia and Kartagener syndromes in a sibship: association with abnormal respiratory cilia. *J Pediatr* 100:401-403, 1982

80. Rose V, Izukawa T, Moës CAF: Syndromes of asplenia and polysplenia: a review of cardiac and non-cardiac malformations in 60 cases with special reference to diagnosis and prognosis. *Br Heart J* 37:840-852, 1975

81. McKusick VA: *Mendelian Inheritance in Man: Catalogs of Autosomal Dominant, Autosomal Recessive, and X-Linked Phenotypes.* Eighth edition. Baltimore: Johns Hopkins University Press, 1988, pp *a,* 44-51; *b,* 217-218; *c,* 218; *d,* 218; *e,* 218-219, 917-918; *f,* 219; *g,* 551-553; *h,* 647; *i,* 755-756; *j,* 821; *k,* 826-827; *l,* 918; *m,* 918-919; *n,* 1276

82. Goldstein JL, Brown MS: Genetics and cardiovascular disease. In *Heart Disease: A Textbook of Cardiovascular Medicine.* Vol. 2. Edited by E Braunwald. Philadelphia, WB Saunders Company, 1980, pp 1683-1722

83. Afzelius BA: A human syndrome caused by immotile cilia. *Science* 193:317-319, 1976

84. Holmes LB, Blennerhassett JB, Austen KF: A reappraisal of Kartagener's syndrome. *Am J Med Sci* 255:13-28, 1968

85. Resouly A: Kartagener's syndrome: a case report and review of the literature. *J Laryngol Otol* 86:1237-1240, 1972

86. Layton WM Jr: Random determination of a developmental process: reversal of normal visceral asymmetry in the mouse. *J Hered* 67:336-338, 1976

87. Rowe RD, Godman MJ: Cor pulmonale. In *Heart Disease in Infancy and Childhood.* Third edition. Edited by JD Keith, RD Rowe, P Vlad. New York, Macmillan Publishing Co, 1978, pp 262-274

88. Bird T: Idiopathic arterial calcification in infancy. *Arch Dis Child* 49:82-89, 1974

89. Witzleben CL: Idiopathic infantile arterial calcification—a misnomer? *Am J Cardiol* 26:305-309, 1970

90. Menten ML, Fetterman GH: Coronary sclerosis in infancy: report of three autopsied cases, two in siblings. *Am J Clin Pathol* 18:805-810, 1948

91. Meradji M, de Villeneuve VH, Huber J, et al: Idiopathic infantile arterial calcification in siblings: radiologic diagnosis and successful treatment. *J Pediatr* 92:401-405, 1978

92. Moran JJ, Becker SM: Idiopathic arterial calcification of infancy: report of 2 cases occurring in siblings, and review of the literature. *Am J Clin Pathol* 31:517-529, 1959

93. Hunt AC, Leys DG: Generalized arterial calcification of infancy. *Br Med J* 1:385-386, 1957

94. Møller P, Heiberg A: Atrioventricular conduction time—a heritable trait? II. Family studies. *Clin Genet* 18:454-455, 1980

95. Morquio L: Sur une maladie infantile et familiale: caractérisée par des modifications permanentes du pouls, des attaques syncopales et épileptidormes et la mort subite. *Arch Med Enfants* 4:467-475, 1901

96. Fuhrman BP, Bass JL, Lawrence C, et al: Progressive cardiac conduction defect and cardiomyopathy in siblings with syncope. *Pediatr Cardiol* 2:57-62, 1982

97. Lynch RJ, Engle MA: Familial congenital complete heart block: its occurrence in 2 children with another genetically determined anomaly. *Am J Dis Child* 102:210-217, 1961

98. Wagner CW Jr, Hall RJ: Congenital familial atrioventricular dissociation: report of three siblings. *Am J Cardiol* 19:593-596, 1967

99. James TN, McKone RC, Hudspeth AS: De subitaneis mortibus. X. Familial congenital heart block. *Circulation* 51:379-388, 1975

100. Crittenden IH, Latta H, Ticinovich DA: Familial congenital heart block. *Am J Dis Child* 108:104-108, 1964

101. Brink PA, Ferreira A, Moolman JC, et al: Gene for progressive familial heart block type I maps to chromosome 19q13. *Circulation* 91:1633-1640, 1995

102. Massumi RA: Familial Wolff-Parkinson-White syndrome with cardiomyopathy. *Am J Med* 43:951-955, 1967

103. Schneider RG: Familial occurrence of Wolff-Parkinson-White syndrome. *Am Heart J* 78:34-36, 1969

104. Gillette PC, Freed D, McNamara DG: A proposed autosomal dominant method of inheritance of the Wolff-Parkinson-White syndrome and supraventricular tachycardia. *J Pediatr* 93:257-258, 1978

105. Schmidt MA, Michels VV, Edwards WD, et al: Familial dilated cardiomyopathy. *Am J Med Genet* 31:135-143, 1988

106. Gould WL: Auricular fibrillation: report on a study of a familial tendency, 1920-1956. *Arch Intern Med* 100:916-926, 1957

107. Phair WB: Familial atrial fibrillation. *Can Med Assoc J* 89:1274-1276, 1963

108. Brodsky M, Wu D, Denes P, et al: Familial atrial tachyarrhythmia with short PR interval. *Arch Intern Med* 137:165-169, 1977

109. Ward OC: A new familial cardiac syndrome in children. *J Ir Med Assoc* 54:103-106, 1964

110. Karhunen P, Luomanmäki K, Heikkilä J, et al: Syncope and Q-T prolongation without deafness: the Romano-Ward syndrome. *Am Heart J* 80:820-823, 1970

111. Garza LA, Vick RL, Nora JJ, et al: Heritable Q-T prolongation without deafness. *Circulation* 41:39-48, 1970

112. Jervell A, Lange-Nielsen F: Congenital deaf-mutism, functional heart disease with prolongation of the Q-T interval, and sudden death. *Am Heart J* 54:59-68, 1957

113. Hashiba K: Hereditary QT prolongation syndrome in Japan: genetic analysis and pathological findings of the conducting system. *Jpn Circ J* 42:1133-1150, 1978

114. Keating M, Atkinson D, Dunn C, et al: Linkage of a cardiac arrhythmia, the long QT syndrome, and the Harvey ras-1 gene. *Science* 252:704-706, 1991

115. Curran ME, Splawski I, Timothy KW, et al: A molecular basis for cardiac arrhythmia: HERG mutations cause long QT syndrome. *Cell* 80:795-803, 1995

116. McRae JR, Wagner GS, Rogers MC, et al: Paroxysmal familial ventricular fibrillation. *J Pediatr* 84:515-518, 1974

117. Chameides L, Truex RC, Vetter V, et al: Association of maternal systemic lupus erythematosus with congenital complete heart block. *N Engl J Med* 297:1204-1207, 1977

118. McCue CM, Mantakas ME, Tingelstad JB, et al: Congenital heart block in newborns of mothers with connective tissue disease. *Circulation* 56:82-90, 1977

119. Reed BR, Lee LA, Harmon C, et al: Autoantibodies to SS-A/Ro in infants with congenital heart block. *J Pediatr* 103:889-891, 1983

120. Steinberg D: Phytanic acid storage disease (Refsum's disease). In *The Metabolic Basis of Inherited Disease.* Fifth edition. Edited by JB Stanbury, JB Wyngaarden, DS Fredrickson, et al. New York, McGraw-Hill Book Company, 1983, pp 732-734

121. Skre H: Spinocerebellar disorders. In *Principles and Practice of Medical Genetics.* Vol 1. Edited by AEH Emery, DL Rimoin. Edinburgh, Churchill Livingstone, 1983, pp 267-283

122. Moser HW, Braine H, Pyeritz RE, et al: Therapeutic trial of plasmapheresis in Refsum disease and in Fabry disease. *Birth Defects* 16 No 1:491-497, 1980

123. Desnick RJ, Sweeley CC: Fabry's disease: α-galactosidase A deficiency. In *The Metabolic Basis of Inherited Disease.* Fifth edition. Edited by JB Stanbury, JB Wyngaarden, DS Fredrickson, et al. New York, McGraw-Hill Book Company, 1983, pp 906-944

124. Van Dorp WG, ten Cate FJ, Vletter WB, et al: Familial prevalence of asymmetric septal hypertrophy. *Eur J Cardiol* 4:349-357, 1976

125. Jörgensen G: Genetische Untersuchungen bei funktionellobstruktiver subvalvulärer Aortenstenose (irregulär hypertrophischer Kardiomyopathie). *Humangenetik* 6:13-28, 1968

126. Bingle GJ, Dillon J, Hurwitz R: Asymmetric septal hypertrophy in a large Amish kindred. *Clin Genet* 7:255-261, 1975
127. Smith ER, Heffernan LP, Sangalang VE, et al: Voluntary muscle involvement in hypertrophic cardiomyopathy: a study of eleven patients. *Ann Intern Med* 85:566-572, 1976
128. Watkins H, McKenna WJ, Thierfelder L, et al: Mutations in the genes for cardiac troponin T and alpha-tropomyosin in hypertrophic cardiomyopathy. *N Engl J Med* 332:1058-1064, 1995
129. Geisterfer-Lawrence AAT, Kass S, Tanigawa G, et al: A molecular basis for familial hypertrophic cardiomyopathy: A β cardiac myosin heavy chain gene missense mutation. *Cell* 62:999-1006, 1990
130. Hewer RL: Study of fatal cases of Friedreich's ataxia. *Br Heart J* 3:649-652, 1968
131. Hewer RL: The heart in Friedreich's ataxia. *Br Heart J* 31:5-14, 1969
132. Boehm TM, Dickerson RB, Glasser SP: Hypertrophic subaortic stenosis occurring in a patient with Friedreich's ataxia. *Am J Med Sci* 260:279-284, 1970
133. Glasser SP: Friedreich's ataxia and myocardiopathies (letter to the editor). *Am Heart J* 84:843, 1972
134. Elias G: Muscular subaortic stenosis and Friedreich's ataxia (letter to the editor). *Am Heart J* 84:843, 1972
135. Pandolfo M, Sirugo G, Antonelli A, et al: Friedreich ataxia in Italian families: genetic homogeneity and linkage disequilibrium with the marker loci D9S5 and D9S15. *Am J Hum Genet* 47:228-235, 1990
136. Polani PE, Moynahan EJ: Progressive cardiomyopathic lentiginosis. *Q J Med* 41:205-225, 1972
137. Somerville J, Bonham-Carter RE: The heart in lentiginosis. *Br Heart J* 34:58-66, 1972
138. Nora JJ, Lortscher RH, Spangler RD: Echocardiographic studies of left ventricular disease in Ullrich-Noonan syndrome. *Am J Dis Child* 129:1417-1420, 1975
139. Battiste CE, Feldt RH, Lie JT: Congestive cardiomyopathy in Noonan's syndrome. *Mayo Clin Proc* 52:661-664, 1977
140. Summitt RL: Noonan syndrome. In *Birth Defects Compendium.* Second edition. Edited by D Bergsma. New York, Alan R Liss, 1979, pp 778-779
141. Elliott CM, Tajik AJ, Giuliani ER, et al: Idiopathic hypertrophic subaortic stenosis associated with cutaneous neurofibromatosis: report of a case. *Am Heart J* 92:368-372, 1976
142. Howell RR, Williams JC: The glycogen storage diseases. In *The Metabolic Basis of Inherited Disease.* Fifth edition. Edited by JB Stanbury, JB Wyngaarden, DS Fredrickson, et al. New York, McGraw-Hill Book Company, 1983, pp 152-154
143. McAdams AJ, Hug G, Bove KE: Glycogen storage disease, types I to X: criteria for morphologic diagnosis. *Hum Pathol* 5:463-487, 1974
144. Askanas V, Engel WK, DiMauro S, et al: Adult-onset acid maltase deficiency: morphologic and biochemical abnormalities reproduced in cultured muscle. *N Engl J Med* 294:573-578, 1976
145. Matsuishi T, Yoshino M, Terasawa K, et al: Childhood acid maltase deficiency: a clinical, biochemical, and morphologic study of three patients. *Arch Neurol* 41:47-52, 1984
146. Francesconi M, Auff E: Cardiac arrhythmias and the adult form of type II glycogenosis (letter to the editor). *N Engl J Med* 306:937-938, 1982
147. Brunberg JA, McCormick WF, Schochet SS Jr: Type III glycogenosis: an adult with diffuse weakness and muscle wasting. *Arch Neurol* 25:171-178, 1971
148. Olson LJ, Reeder GS, Noller KL, et al: Cardiac involvement in glycogen storage disease III: morphologic and biochemical characterization with endomyocardial biopsy. *Am J Cardiol* 53:980-981, 1984
149. Vietor KW, Havsteen B, Harms D, et al: Ethanolaminosis: a newly recognized, generalized storage disease with cardiomegaly, cerebral dysfunction and early death. *Eur J Pediatr* 126:61-75, 1977
150. Blieden LC, Desnick RJ, Carter JB, et al: Cardiac involvement in Sandhoff's disease: inborn error of glycosphingolipid metabolism. *Am J Cardiol* 34:83-88, 1974
151. Young ID, Harper PS: Long-term complications in Hunter's syndrome. *Clin Genet* 16:125-132, 1979
152. Stevenson RE, Howell RR, McKusick VA, et al: The iduronidase-deficient mucopolysaccharidoses: clinical and roentgenographic features. *Pediatrics* 57:111-122, 1976
153. Beaudet AL, DiFerrante NM, Ferry GD, et al: Variation in the phenotypic expression of β-glucuronidase deficiency. *J Pediatr* 86:388-394, 1975
154. Emanuel R, Withers R: The cardiomyopathies. In *Principles and Practice of Medical Genetics.* Vol. 2. Edited by AEH Emery, DL Rimoin. Edinburgh, Churchill Livingstone, 1983, pp 979-986
155. Ando M: The mode of inheritance of idiopathic cardiomyopathy: preliminary report. *Jpn Circ J* 42:1193-1195, 1978
156. Yamaguchi M, Toshima H, Yanase T: Genetic heterogeneity of idiopathic cardiomyopathies. *Jpn Circ J* 42:1131-1132, 1978
157. Johnson RA, Palacios I: Dilated cardiomyopathies of the adult. *N Engl J Med* 307:1051-1058, 1982
158. Michels VV, Driscoll DJ, Miller FA Jr: Familial aggregation of idiopathic dilated cardiomyopathy. *Am J Cardiol* 55:1232-1233, 1985
159. Valantine HA, Hunt SA, Fowler MB, et al: Frequency of familial nature of dilated cardiomyopathy and usefulness of cardiac transplantation in this subset. *Am J Cardiol* 63:959-963, 1989
160. Michels VV, Moll PP, Miller FA, et al: The frequency of familial dilated cardiomyopathy in a series of patients with idiopathic dilated cardiomyopathy. *N Engl J Med* 326:77-82, 1992
161. Westwood M, Harris R, Burn L, et al: Heredity in primary endocardial fibroelastosis. *Br Heart J* 37:1077-1084, 1975
162. Rose V: Endocardial fibroelastosis: family studies with special reference to assessment of recurrence risk. *Birth Defects* 8 No 5:27-29, 1972
163. Katcher ML, Segar WE, Wolfson JJ, et al: Clinicopathologic conference: a six-month-old infant with sudden onset of metabolic acidosis and shock. *Am J Med Genet* 11:77-96, 1982
164. Tripp ME, Katcher ML, Peters HA, et al: Systemic carnitine deficiency presenting as familial endocardial fibroelastosis: a treatable cardiomyopathy. *N Engl J Med* 305:385-390, 1981
165. Waber LJ, Valle D, Neill C, et al: Carnitine deficiency presenting as familial cardiomyopathy: a treatable defect in carnitine transport. *J Pediatr* 101:700-705, 1982
166. Eriksson BO, Gustafson B, Lindstedt S, et al: Transport of carnitine into cells in hereditary carnitine deficiency. *J Inherit Metab Dis* 12:108-111, 1989
167. Hart ZH, Chang C-H, DiMauro S, et al: Muscle carnitine deficiency and fatal cardiomyopathy. *Neurology (Minneap)* 28:147-151, 1978
168. VanDyke DH, Griggs RC, Markesbery W, et al: Hereditary carnitine deficiency of muscle. *Neurology (Minneap)* 25:154-159, 1975
169. Henry CG, Strauss AW, Keating JP, et al: Congestive cardiomyopathy associated with β-ketothiolase deficiency. *J Pediatr* 99:754-757, 1981
170. Stanley CA, Hale DE, Whiteman DEH, et al: Systemic carnitine (carn) deficiency in isovaleric acidemia (IVA) (abstract). *Pediatr Res* 17:296A, 1983
171. Benke PJ, Foradada J: Carnitine is low in well patients with vitamin unresponsive organic acidurias (OA) (abstract). *Am J Hum Genet* 35:37A, 1983
172. Cartwright GE, Edwards CQ, Kravitz K, et al: Hereditary hemochromatosis: phenotypic expression of the disease. *N Engl J Med* 301:175-179, 1979
173. Simon M: Disorders of iron metabolism: idiopathic haemochromatosis and atransferrinaemia. In *Principles and Practice of Medical Genetics.* Vol 2. Edited by AEH Emery, DL Rimoin. Edinburgh, Churchill Livingstone, 1983, pp 1329-1338
174. Katiyar BC, Misra S, Somani PN, et al: Congestive cardiomyopathy in a family of Becker's X-linked muscular dystrophy. *Postgrad Med J* 53:12-15, 1977
175. Tanaka H, Uemura N, Toyama Y, et al: Cardiac involvement in the Kugelberg-Welander syndrome. *Am J Cardiol* 38:528-532, 1976
176. Egger J, Lake BD, Wilson J: Mitochondrial cytopathy: a multisystem disorder with ragged red fibres on muscle biopsy. *Arch Dis Child* 56:741-752, 1981
177. Verhiest W, Brucher JM, Goddeeris P, et al: Familial centronuclear myopathy associated with "cardiomyopathy." *Br Heart J* 38:504-509, 1976
178. Chakrabarti A, Pearce JMS: Scapuloperoneal syndrome with cardiomyopathy: report of a family with autosomal dominant inheritance and unusual features. *J Neurol Neurosurg Psychiatry* 44:1146-1152, 1981
179. Waters DD, Nutter DO, Hopkins LC, et al: Cardiac features of an unusual X-linked humeroperoneal neuromuscular disease. *N Engl J Med* 293:1017-1022, 1975
180. Sengers RCA, Stadhouders AM, Jaspar HHJ, et al: Cardiomyopathy and short stature associated with mitochondrial and/or lipid storage myopathy of skeletal muscle. *Neuropaediatrie* 7:196-208, 1976

181. Lochner A, Hewlett RH, O'Kennedy A, et al: A study of a family with inherited disease of cardiac and skeletal muscle. II. Skeletal muscle morphology and mitochondrial oxidative phosphorylation. *S Afr Med J* 59:453-461, 1981

182. Lindlöf M, Kiuru A, Kääriäinen H, et al: Gene deletions in X-linked muscular dystrophy. *Am J Hum Genet* 44:496-503, 1989

183. Caskey CT, Nussbaum RL, Cohan LC, et al: Sporadic occurrence of Duchenne muscular dystrophy: evidence for new mutation. *Clin Genet* 18:329-341, 1980

184. Sanyal SK, Tierney RC, Rao PS, et al: Systolic time interval characteristics in children with Duchenne's progressive muscular dystrophy. *Pediatrics* 70:958-964, 1982

185. Grimm T, Harper PS: Genetic aspects of congenital myotonic dystrophy (abstract). *Clin Genet* 23:212, 1983

186. Brook JD, McCurrach ME, Harley HG, et al: Molecular basis of myotonic dystrophy: expansion of a trinucleotide (CTG) repeat at the 3′ end of a transcript encoding a protein kinase family member. *Cell* 68:799-808, 1992

187. Griggs RC, Davis RJ, Anderson DC, et al: Cardiac conduction in myotonic dystrophy. *Am J Med* 59:37-42, 1975

188. Harper PS: Myotonic dystrophy and related disorders. In *Principles and Practice of Medical Genetics.* Vol 1. Edited by AEH Emery, DL Rimoin. Edinburgh, Churchill Livingstone, 1983, pp 426-441

189. Jacobson DR, Buxbaum JN: Genetic aspects of amyloidosis. *Adv Hum Genet* 20:69-123, 1991

190. Suzuki T, Tsuge I, Higa S, et al: Catecholamine metabolism in familial amyloid polyneuropathy. *Clin Genet* 16:117-124, 1979

191. Meretoja J: Genetic aspects of familial amyloidosis with corneal lattice dystrophy and cranial neuropathy. *Clin Genet* 4:173-185, 1973

192. Wallace MR, Conneally PM, Benson MD: A DNA test for Indiana/Swiss hereditary amyloidosis (FAP II). *Am J Hum Genet* 43:182-187, 1988

193. Brown OR, DeMots H, Kloster FE, et al: Aortic root dilatation and mitral valve prolapse in Marfan's syndrome: an echocardiographic study. *Circulation* 52:651-657, 1975

194. Come PC, Fortuin NJ, White RI Jr, et al: Echocardiographic assessment of cardiovascular abnormalities in the Marfan syndrome: comparison with clinical findings and with roentgenographic estimation of aortic root size. *Am J Med* 74:465-474, 1983

195. Pyeritz RE, Wappel MA: Mitral valve dysfunction in the Marfan syndrome: clinical and echocardiographic study of prevalence and natural history. *Am J Med* 74:797-807, 1983

196. Hohn AR, Webb HM: Cardiac studies of infant twins with Marfan's syndrome. *Am J Dis Child* 122:526-528, 1971

197. Simpson JW, Nora JJ, McNamara DG: Marfan's syndrome and mitral valve disease: acute surgical emergencies. *Am Heart J* 77:96-99, 1969

198. Pyeritz RE: Marfan syndrome. In *Principles and Practice of Medical Genetics.* Vol. 2. Edited by AEH Emery, DL Rimoin. Edinburgh, Churchill Livingstone, 1983, pp 820-835

199. Pyeritz RE: Results and maternal risks of pregnancy in the Marfan syndrome (abstract). *Am J Hum Genet* 32:124A, 1980

200. Ferguson JE, Ueland K, Stinson EB, et al: Marfan's syndrome: acute aortic dissection during labor, resulting in fetal distress and cesarean section, followed by successful surgical repair. *Am J Obstet Gynecol* 147:759-762, 1983

201. Dietz HC, Cutting GR, Pyeritz RE, et al: Marfan syndrome caused by a recurrent de novo missense mutation in the fibrillin gene. *Nature* 352:337-339, 1991

202. Byers PH, Holbrook KA, Barsh GS: Ehlers-Danlos syndrome. In *Principles and Practice of Medical Genetics.* Vol 2. Edited by AEH Emery, DL Rimoin, Edinburgh, Churchill Livingstone, 1983, pp 836-850

203. Leier CV, Call TD, Fulkerson PK, et al: The spectrum of cardiac defects in the Ehlers-Danlos syndrome, types I and III. *Ann Intern Med* 92:171-178, 1980

204. Jaffe AS, Geltman EM, Rodey GE, et al: Mitral valve prolapse: a consistent manifestation of type IV Ehlers-Danlos syndrome; the pathogenetic role of the abnormal production of type III collagen. *Circulation* 64:121-125, 1981

205. Pope FM, Martin GR, Lichtenstein JR, et al: Patients with Ehlers-Danlos syndrome type IV lack type III collagen. *Proc Natl Acad Sci USA* 72:1314-1316, 1975

206. Pope FM, Nicholls AC, Narcisi P, et al: Some patients with cerebral aneurysms are deficient in type III collagen. *Lancet* 1:973-975, 1981

207. DiFerrante N, Leachman RD, Angelini P, et al: Lysyl oxidase deficiency in Ehlers-Danlos syndrome type V. *Connect Tissue Res* 3:49-53, 1975

208. Dembure P, Priest J, Snoddy S, et al: Prenatal assessment of lysyl hydroxylase deficiency (abstract). *Am J Hum Genet* 35:41A, 1983

209. Schachner L, Young D: Pseudoxanthoma elasticum with severe cardiovascular disease in a child. *Am J Dis Child* 127:571-575, 1974

210. Goodman RM: Pseudoxanthoma elasticum and related disorders. In *Principles and Practice of Medical Genetics.* Vol 2. Edited by AEH Emery, DL Rimoin. Edinburgh, Churchill Livingstone, 1983, pp 851-862

211. Sandberg LB, Soskel NT, Leslie JG: Elastin structure, biosynthesis, and relation to disease states. *N Engl J Med* 304:566-579, 1981

212. Mudd SH, Levy HL: Disorders of transsulfuration. In *The Metabolic Basis of Inherited Disease.* Fifth edition. Edited by JB Stanbury, JB Wyngaarden, DS Fredrickson, et al. New York, McGraw-Hill Book Company, 1983, p 536

213. Schimke RN, McKusick VA, Huang T, et al: Homocystinuria: studies of 20 families with 38 affected members. *JAMA* 193:711-719, 1965

214. Uhlemann ER, TenPas JH, Lucky AW, et al: Platelet survival and morphology in homocystinuria due to cystathionine synthase deficiency. *N Engl J Med* 295:1283-1286, 1976

215. Smolin LA, Benevenga NJ, Berlow S: The use of betaine for the treatment of homocystinuria. *J Pediatr* 99:467-472, 1981

216. Kang DS, Wong PWK, Curley K: Effect of D-penicillamine on plasma homocystine in homocystinurics (abstract). *Am J Hum Genet* 32:44A, 1980

217. Wong PWK, Justice P, Hruby M, et al: Folic acid nonresponsive homocystinuria due to methylenetetrahydrofolate reductase deficiency. *Pediatrics* 59:749-756, 1977

218. Matalon R, Michals K: Methylmalonic acidemia with homocystinuria: lack of clinical improvement to treatment with hydroxycobalamin and choline despite biochemical improvement (abstract). *Pediatr Res* 17:293A, 1983

Index

B

D

M

W

X

Y